MW00843354

# Rudolph's
# PEDIATRICS

## 23rd EDITION

## VOLUME ONE

# Rudolph's PEDIATRICS

## 23rd EDITION

## VOLUME ONE

### EDITOR-IN-CHIEF

**Mark W. Kline, MD**
Physician-in-Chief, Texas Children's Hospital
J.S. Abercrombie Professor and Chairman
Ralph D. Feigin Chair
Department of Pediatrics
Baylor College of Medicine
Houston, Texas

### EDITORS

**Susan M. Blaney, MD**
Professor and Executive Vice-Chair
Department of Pediatrics, Baylor College of Medicine
Director, Texas Children's Cancer Center, Texas Children's Hospital
Houston, Texas

**Angelo P. Giardino, MD, PhD**
Senior Vice President/Chief Quality Officer
Texas Children's Hospital
Professor and Chief, Academic General Pediatrics
Baylor College of Medicine
Houston, Texas

**Jordan S. Orange, MD, PhD**
Chief, Immunology, Allergy and Rheumatology
Director, Center for Human Immunobiology
Louis and Marybeth Pawleek Endowed Chair
Texas Children's Hospital
Professor of Pediatrics, Pathology, and Immunology
Vice Chair for Research, Department of Pediatrics
Baylor College of Medicine
Houston, Texas

**Daniel J. Penny, MD, PhD**
Professor of Pediatrics, Baylor College of Medicine
Chief of Cardiology, Texas Children's Hospital
Houston, Texas

**Gordon E. Schutze, MD**
Professor of Pediatrics
Executive Vice Chairman
Martin I. Lorin MD Endowed Chair in Medical Education
Department of Pediatrics, Baylor College of Medicine
Texas Children's Hospital
Houston, Texas

**Lara S. Shekerdemian, MD, MHA**
Professor and Chief, Critical Care
Vice Chair for Clinical Affairs, Department of Pediatrics
Baylor College of Medicine, Texas Children's Hospital
Houston, Texas

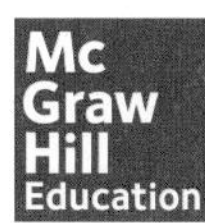


New York Chicago San Francisco Athens London Madrid Mexico City
Milan New Delhi Singapore Sydney Toronto

**Rudolph's Pediatrics, Twenty-Third Edition.**



1 2 3 4 5 6 7 8 9 LWI 23 22 21 20 19 18

Set ISBN 978-1-259-58859-4; MHID 1-259-58859-9
Volume One ISBN 978-1-260-01140-1; MHID 1-260-01140-2
Volume Two ISBN 978-1-260-01141-8; MHID 1-260-01141-0

The book was set in Minion Pro by Cenveo® Publisher Services.
The editors were Andrew Moyer and Christie Naglieri.
The production manager was Richard Ruzycka.
Project management was provided by Tania Andrabi, Cenveo Publisher Services.
The text designer was Alan Barnett.
The cover designer was Owen Sears, Assistant Director, Creative Services/Marketing, Texas Children's Hospital.
Cover photography was provided by Smiley N. Pool.

This book is printed on acid-free paper.

**Library of Congress Cataloging-in-Publication Data**

Names: Kline, Mark, editor.
Title: Rudolph's pediatrics / editor-in-chief, Mark W. Kline ; associate editors, Susan Blaney [and 5 others].
Other titles: Pediatrics
Description: 23rd edition. | New York : McGraw-Hill Education, [2018] | Includes bibliographical references and index.
Identifiers: LCCN 2017017351 | ISBN 9781259588594 (hardcover : alk. paper) | ISBN 1259588599 (hardcover : alk. paper)
Subjects: | MESH: Pediatrics
Classification: LCC RJ45 | NLM WS 200 | DDC 618.92—dc23

To health professionals everywhere for their dedication to improving the health and well-being of children and families;

To mothers, fathers, and families across the globe who drive, ride, fly, and walk across cities, states, jungles, and deserts every day in search of answers and cures for their ill children;

To our teachers for their patience, faith, and inspiration during the formative stages of our careers; and

To our families for the love, support, and sacrifices that have made us who we are today.

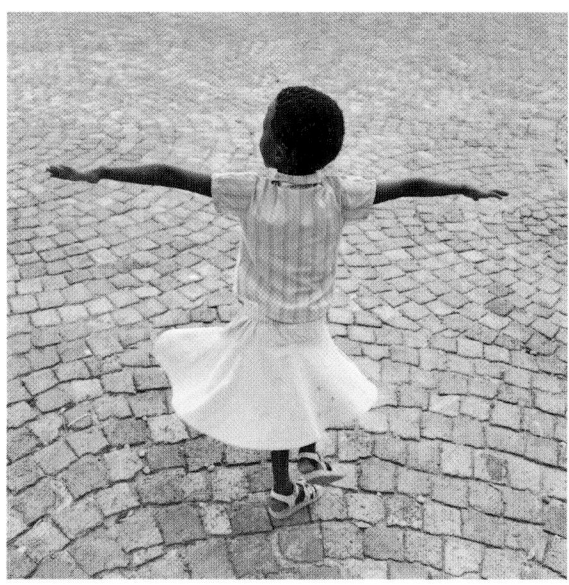

# CONTENTS

# SECTION 4 Newborn

*Section Editors: Gautham K. Suresh and Haresh Kirpalani*

## PART 1 CARE OF THE NEWBORN



## PART 2 INFANTS AT RISK



## PART 3 NONSPECIFIC NEONATAL CONDITIONS



## PART 4 DISORDERS SPECIFICALLY RELATED TO PRETERM BIRTH



# SECTION 5 Principles of Adolescent Care

*Section Editors: Albert C. Hergenroeder and Mariam R. Chacko*

## PART 1 GROWTH AND DEVELOPMENT



## PART 2 HEALTH PROBLEMS OF ADOLESCENTS



## PART 3 MENTAL HEALTH DISORDERS IN THE ADOLESCENT



## PART 4 REPRODUCTIVE HEALTH PROBLEMS

# SECTION 6 Developmental and Behavioral Pediatrics

*Section Editor: Robert G. Voigt*



# SECTION 7 Pediatric Mental Health

*Section Editor: Efrain Bleiberg*



# SECTION 8 Acute and Critical Illness

*Section Editors: Lara S. Shekerdemian and Desmond Bohn*

## PART 1 THE PATHOPHYSIOLOGY OF ACUTE AND CRITICAL ILLNESS



## PART 2 STABILIZATION AND MANAGEMENT OF THE ACUTELY ILL INFANT AND CHILD



## PART 3 INJURIES AND UNTOWARD EVENTS



# SECTION 9 Children with Medical Complexity

*Section Editors: Carl D. Tapia and Christopher J. Stille*

# SECTION 10 Palliative Care

*Section Editor: Tammy I. Kang*



# SECTION 11 Inherited Disorders of Metabolism

*Section Editor: William J. Craigen*

## PART 1 INTRODUCTION



## PART 2 AMINO ACIDS



## PART 3 VITAMINS



## PART 4 CARBOHYDRATES



## PART 5 DISORDERS OF OXIDATIVE PHOSPHORYLATION AND PYRUVATE OXIDATION



## PART 6 ORGANELLE DISORDERS



## PART 7 CHOLESTEROL AND BILE ACID DISORDERS



## PART 8 NUCLEIC ACID, HEME, AND METALS DISORDERS

## SECTION 12 Clinical Genetics and Dysmorphology

*Section Editor: James R. Lupski*



## SECTION 13 Immunological Disorders

*Section Editors: William T. Shearer and Jordan S. Orange*



## SECTION 14 Allergic Disorders

*Section Editor: Carla M. Davis*



## SECTION 15 Rheumatology

*Section Editor: Robert P. Sundel*



## SECTION 16 The Musculoskeletal System

*Section Editor: John P. Dormans*

## SECTION 17 Infectious Diseases

*Section Editors: Laurence B. Givner, Mobeen H. Rathore, Gordon E. Schutze, Bernhard L. Wiedermann*

### PART 1 PRINCIPLES OF INFECTIOUS DISEASE



### PART 2 INFECTIONS OF ORGAN SYSTEMS



### PART 3 INFECTIONS OF THE RESPIRATORY SYSTEM



### PART 4 TREATMENT AND PREVENTION OF INFECTIOUS DISEASES



### PART 5 BACTERIAL INFECTIONS

## PART 6 FUNGAL INFECTIONS



## PART 7 VIRAL INFECTIONS



## PART 8 PARASITIC INFECTIONS—NEMATODES

# VOLUME TWO

## SECTION 18 Disorders of the Skin

*Section Editor: Carrie L. Kovarik*



## SECTION 19 Disorders of the Ear, Nose, and Throat

*Section Editor: Ellis M. Arjmand*



## SECTION 20 Disorders of the Oral Cavity

*Section Editors: Howard L. Needleman and Stephen Shusterman*

## SECTION 21 Disorders of the Gastrointestinal System

*Section Editor: Mitchell B. Cohen*



## SECTION 22 Disorders of the Liver and Biliary Tract

*Section Editor: Benjamin L. Shneider*



CONTENTS

## SECTION 23 Disorders of the Blood

*Section Editor: Amber M. Yates*



## SECTION 24 Neoplastic Disorders

*Section Editors: Susan M. Blaney and Peter C. Adamson*

## SECTION 25 Disorders of the Kidney and Urinary Tract

*Section Editor: Michael C. Braun*

### PART 1 PRINCIPLES OF NEPHROLOGY



### PART 2 ABNORMALITIES OF THE KIDNEY AND URINARY TRACT



### PART 3 CHRONIC KIDNEY DISEASE



## SECTION 26 Disorders of the Cardiovascular System

*Section Editors: Daniel J. Penny and Robert E. Shaddy*

### PART 1 PRINCIPLES OF CARDIOLOGY



### PART 2 APPROACH TO THE PATIENT WITH CARDIOVASCULAR DISEASE



### PART 3 ACQUIRED CARDIOVASCULAR DISEASE



### PART 4 DIAGNOSTIC TOOLS IN HEART DISEASE



### PART 5 MANAGEMENT OF PATIENTS WITH CARDIOVASCULAR DISEASE



## SECTION 27 Disorders of the Respiratory System

*Section Editor: Andrew Bush*

### PART 1 PRINCIPLES OF PULMONOLOGY

# CONSULTING AND SECTION EDITORS



## CONSULTING EDITORS

Abraham M. Rudolph, MD
Colin D. Rudolph, MD, PhD

## SECTION EDITORS

### Section 1: Foundations in Pediatric Practice and Child Care

**Jean L. Raphael, MD,** Baylor College of Medicine, Texas Children's Hospital
**Angelo P. Giardino, MD, PhD,** Baylor College of Medicine, Texas Children's Hospital

### Section 2: Nutrition

**Dennis Bier, MD,** Baylor College of Medicine, Texas Children's Hospital

### Section 3: Social-Environmental Factors

**Christopher S. Greeley, MD, MS,** Baylor College of Medicine, Texas Children's Hospital
**Andrea G. Asnes, MD, MSW,** Yale College of Medicine, Yale-New Haven Hospital

### Section 4: Newborn

**Gautham K. Suresh, MD, DM, MS, FAAP,** Baylor College of Medicine, Texas Children's Hospital
**Haresh Kirpalani, MD,** Perelman School of Medicine, University of Pennsylvania, Children's Hospital of Philadelphia

### Section 5: Principles of Adolescent Care

**Albert C. Hergenroeder, MD,** Baylor College of Medicine, Texas Children's Hospital
**Mariam R. Chacko, MD,** Baylor College of Medicine, Texas Children's Hospital

### Section 6: Developmental and Behavioral Pediatrics

**Robert G. Voigt, MD, FAAP,** Baylor College of Medicine, Texas Children's Hospital

### Section 7: Pediatric Mental Health

**Efrain Bleiberg, MD,** Baylor College of Medicine, Texas Children's Hospital

### Section 8: Acute and Critical Illness

**Lara S. Shekerdemian, MD,** Baylor College of Medicine, Texas Children's Hospital
**Desmond Bohn, MB, FRCPC,** University of Toronto, The Hospital for Sick Children

### Section 9: Children with Medical Complexity

**Carl D. Tapia, MD, MPH,** Baylor College of Medicine, Texas Children's Hospital
**Christopher J. Stille, MD, MPH,** University of Colorado School of Medicine, Children's Hospital Colorado

### Section 10: Palliative Care

**Tammy I. Kang, MD, MSCE,** Baylor College of Medicine, Texas Children's Hospital

### Section 11: Inherited Disorders of Metabolism

**William J. Craigen, MD, PhD,** Baylor College of Medicine

### Section 12: Clinical Genetics and Dysmorphology

**James R. Lupski, MD, PhD, DSc (Hon),** Baylor College of Medicine

### Section 13: Immunological Disorders

**William T. Shearer, MD, PhD,** Baylor College of Medicine, Texas Children's Hospital
**Jordan S. Orange, MD, PhD,** Baylor College of Medicine, Texas Children's Hospital

### Section 14: Allergic Disorders

**Carla M. Davis, MD,** Baylor College of Medicine, Texas Children's Hospital

### Section 15: Rheumatology

**Robert P. Sundel, MD,** Harvard Medical School, Boston Children's Hospital

### Section 16: The Musculoskeletal System

**John P. Dormans, MD, FACS,** Baylor College of Medicine, Texas Children's Hospital

### Section 17: Infectious Diseases

**Laurence B. Givner, MD,** Wake Forest School of Medicine, Wake Forest Baptist Health Medical Center
**Mobeen H. Rathore, MD, FAAP,** University of Florida School of Medicine, Wolfson Children's Hospital
**Gordon E. Schutze, MD,** Baylor College of Medicine, Texas Children's Hospital
**Bernhard L. Wiedermann, MD, MA,** George Washington University School of Medicine, Children's National Health System

### Section 18: Disorders of the Skin

**Carrie L. Kovarik, MD,** Perelman School of Medicine, University of Pennsylvania

### Section 19: Disorders of the Ear, Nose, and Throat

**Ellis M. Arjmand, MD, PhD,** Baylor College of Medicine, Texas Children's Hospital

### Section 20: Disorders of the Oral Cavity

**Howard L. Needleman, DMD,** Harvard Medical School, Boston Children's Hospital
**Stephen Shusterman, DMD,** Harvard Medical School, Boston Children's Hospital

### Section 21: Disorders of the Gastrointestinal System

**Mitchell B. Cohen, MD,** University of Alabama at Birmingham, Children's of Alabama

### Section 22: Disorders of the Liver and Biliary Tract

**Benjamin L. Shneider, MD,** Baylor College of Medicine, Texas Children's Hospital

### Section 23: Disorders of the Blood

**Amber M. Yates, MD,** Baylor College of Medicine, Texas Children's Hospital

### Section 24: Neoplastic Disorders

**Susan M. Blaney, MD,** Baylor College of Medicine, Texas Children's Hospital
**Peter C. Adamson, MD,** Perelman School of Medicine, University of Pennsylvania, Children's Hospital of Philadelphia

### Section 25: Disorders of the Kidney and Urinary Tract

**Michael C. Braun, MD,** Baylor College of Medicine, Texas Children's Hospital

### Section 26: Disorders of the Cardiovascular System

**Daniel J. Penny, MD, PhD,** Baylor College of Medicine, Texas Children's Hospital
**Robert E. Shaddy, MD,** Keck School of Medicine, The University of Southern California, Children's Hospital of Los Angeles

### Section 27: Disorders of the Respiratory System

**Andrew Bush, MD,** Imperial College London, Royal Brompton and Harefield NHS Foundation Trust

### Section 28: Disorders of the Endocrine System

**Jake Kushner, MD,** Baylor College of Medicine, Texas Children's Hospital
**Lefkothea P. Karaviti, MD, PhD,** Baylor College of Medicine, Texas Children's Hospital

### Section 29: Disorders of the Nervous System

**Gary D. Clark, MD,** Baylor College of Medicine, Texas Children's Hospital
**Timothy E. Lotze, MD,** Baylor College of Medicine, Texas Children's Hospital

### Section 30: Disorders of the Eye

**Amit Bhatt, MD,** Baylor College of Medicine, Texas Children's Hospital
**David K. Coats, MD,** Baylor College of Medicine, Texas Children's Hospital

**Kjersti M. Aagaard, MD, PhD, FACOG**
Henry and Susan E. Meyer Chair in Obstetrics and Gynecology; Professor and Vice Chair of Research, Baylor College of Medicine, Department of Obstetrics & Gynecology, Division of Maternal-Fetal Medicine, Texas Children's Hospital, Houston, Texas

**Nahed Abdel-Haq, MD**
Professor of Pediatrics, Wayne State University School of Medicine, Division of Infectious Diseases, Children's Hospital of Michigan, Detroit, Michigan

**Sakena Abedin, MD**
Assistant Professor of Pediatrics, Yale School of Medicine, New Haven, Connecticut

**Farida Abid, MD, FAAP**
Assistant Professor of Pediatrics, Baylor College of Medicine, Texas Children's Hospital, Houston, Texas

**Andrew Abreo, MD**
Allergy and Immunology Fellow, Division of Allergy, Pulmonary, and Critical Care Medicine, Vanderbilt University Medical Center, Nashville, Tennessee

**Maisam Abu-El-Haija, MD**
Associate Professor, University of Cincinnati Department of Pediatrics, Division of Gastroenterology, Hepatology, and Nutrition, Cincinnati Children's Hospital Medical Center, Cincinnati, Ohio

**Karen P. Acker, MD**
Pediatric Infectious Disease Fellow, Department of Pediatrics, Columbia University Medical Center and New York-Presbyterian Hospital, New York, New York

**Amy Acosta, PhD**
Assistant Professor of Pediatrics, Baylor College of Medicine; Attending Psychologist, Texas Children's Hospital, Houston, Texas

**Elisha Acosta, MD**
Assistant Professor of Internal Medicine and Pediatrics, Baylor College of Medicine, Texas Children's Hospital, Houston, Texas

**Denise M. Adams, MD**
Associate Professor of Pediatrics, Harvard Medical School; Co-Director of the Vascular Anomalies Center (VAC); Boston Children's Hospital, Boston, Massachusetts

**Peter C. Adamson, MD**
Professor of Pediatrics, Perelman School of Medicine, University of Pennsylvania; Chair, Children's Oncology Group, Children's Hospital of Philadelphia, Philadelphia, Pennsylvania

**Anne Ades, MD**
Associate Professor of Clinical Pediatrics, Perelman School of Medicine, University of Pennsylvania; Attending Neonatologist, Children's Hospital of Philadelphia; Fetal Consultant, Center for Fetal Diagnosis and Treatment, Philadelphia, Pennsylvania

**N. Scott Adzick, MD, MM, FACS, FAAP**
Professor of Pediatrics, Obstetrics and Gynecology, Perelman School of Medicine, University of Pennsylvania; Surgeon-in-Chief, Department of Surgery; Chief, General, Thoracic and Fetal Surgery; C. Everett Koop Endowed Chair, Pediatric Surgery; Director, Center for Fetal Diagnosis and Treatment, Children's Hospital of Philadelphia, Philadelphia, Pennsylvania

**Hitesh Agrawal, MD**
Fellow in Cardiology, Department of Pediatrics, Baylor College of Medicine, Houston, Texas

**Iram Ahmad, MD, MME**
Fellow, Pediatric Otolaryngology, University of Iowa Health Care/Carver College of Medicine, Department of Otolaryngology—Head and Neck Surgery, Iowa City, Iowa

**Amina Ahmed, MD, FAAP**
Division of Pediatric Infectious Disease, Department of Pediatrics, Levine Children's Hospital at Carolinas Medical Center, Charlotte, North Carolina

**Lemuel O. Aigbivbalu, MD**
Associate Professor, Department of Pediatrics, Division of Infectious Disease, University of Texas Medical Branch, Galveston, Texas

**Nicole Akar-Ghibril, MD**
General Pediatrician, University of Miami Health System, Miami, Florida

**Andrés E. Alarcón, MD**
Assistant Professor, Division of Infectious Diseases, Department of Pediatrics, Children's Hospital of New Orleans/The Louisiana State University Health Sciences Center, School of Medicine, New Orleans, Louisiana

**Adam C. Alder, MD, MSCS, FACS, FAAP**
Assistant Professor of Surgery, University of Texas Southwestern; Chief, Division of Pediatric Surgery, Children's Medical Center, Plano, Texas

**Carl Allen, MD, PhD**
Associate Professor of Pediatrics, Baylor College of Medicine; Co-Director Fayez Sarofim Lymphoma Program; Co-Director TXCH Histiocytosis Program; Texas Children's Cancer and Hematology Centers, Houston, Texas

**Mohammed Almannai, MD**
Medical Biochemical Genetics Fellow, Molecular and Human Genetics department, Baylor College of Medicine, Texas Children's Hospital, Houston, Texas

**Sharonda Alston-Taylor, MD**
Assistant Professor, Department of Pediatrics, Section of Adolescent Medicine and Sports Medicine, Baylor College of Medicine, Houston, Texas

**Muhammad A. Altaf, MD**
Interim Chief, Division of Pediatric Gastroenterology, University of Oklahoma Health Sciences Center, Oklahoma City, Oklahoma

**Martha Isabel Alvarez-Olmos, MD, MPH**
Chief, Section of Pediatric Infectious Diseases, Fundación Cardioinfantil IC University Hospital; Director, Pediatric Infectious Diseases Fellowship Program, Universidad El Bosque, Bogotá, District of Columbia

**Chad Andersen, MBBS, FRACP**
Neonatologist, Robinson Research Institute, Adelaide Medical School, University of Adelaide; Medical Unit Head, Department of Neonatal Medicine, Women's and Children's Health Network, North Adelaide, South Australia

**Diane M. Anderson, PhD, RD**
Associate Professor of Pediatrics, Baylor College of Medicine, Texas Children's Hospital, Department of Pediatrics, Section of Neonatology, Houston, Texas

**Scott A. Anderson, MD**
Associate Professor, Division of Pediatric Surgery, University of Alabama at Birmingham, Children's Hospital of Alabama, Birmingham, Alabama

**Dean B. Andropoulos, MD, MHCM**
Professor of Anesthesiology and Pediatrics, Baylor College of Medicine; Anesthesiologist-in-Chief, Texas Children's Hospital, Houston, Texas

**Joseph Angelo, MD**
Assistant Professor of Pediatrics, Renal Section, Baylor College of Medicine, Texas Children's Hospital, Houston, Texas

**Sara Anvari, MD**
Assistant Professor, Baylor College of Medicine, Allergy and Immunology Service, Texas Children's Hospital, Houston, Texas

**Peter D. Aplan, MD**
Senior Investigator, Genetics Branch, Head, Leukemia Biology Section, Center for Cancer Research, National Cancer Institute, Bethesda, Maryland

**Charles J. Aprahamian, MD**
Assistant Clinical Professor of Surgery and Pediatrics, University of Illinois College of Medicine, Children's Hospital of Illinois at OSF Medical Center, Peoria, Illinois

**Monica I. Ardura, DO, MSCS**
Associate Professor of Pediatrics, The Ohio State University, Nationwide Children's Hospital, Pediatric Infectious Diseases and Immunology, Columbus, Ohio

**Ayse Akcan Arikan, MD**
Assistant Professor, Department of Pediatrics, Baylor of College of Medicine, Sections of Critical Care Medicine and Renal; Medical Director, Critical Care Nephrology, Texas Children's Hospital, Houston, Texas

**Ellis M. Arjmand, MD, MMM, PhD**
Bobby Alford Endowed Chair in Pediatric Otolaryngology; Professor of Otolaryngology and Pediatrics, Baylor College of Medicine; Chief, Otolaryngology, Texas Children's Hospital, Houston, Texas

**Lisa M. Arkin, MD**
Assistant Professor of Dermatology and Pediatrics, University of Wisconsin School of Medicine and Public Health, American Family Children's Hospital, Madison, Wisconsin

**Saro Armenian, DO, MPH**
Associate Professor of Pediatrics, Director, Division of Outcomes Research, City of Hope Comprehensive Cancer Center, Duarte, California

**Sandra R. Arnold, MD, MSc**
Professor of Pediatrics; Chief, Division of Infectious Diseases, University of Tennessee Health Science Center, Le Bonheur Children's Hospital, Memphis, Tennessee

**Jennifer Arnold, MD, MSc**
Assistant Professor of Pediatrics, Medical Director of Simulation, Johns Hopkins All Children's Hospital, Tampa, Florida

**Amy S. Arrington, MD, PhD**
Assistant Professor of Pediatrics, Section Chief, Global Biologic Preparedness, Baylor College of Medicine; Medical Director, Pediatric Special Isolation Unit, Texas Children's Hospital, Houston, Texas

**Basim I. Asmar, MD**
Professor of Pediatrics, Wayne State University School of Medicine; Director, Division of Infectious Diseases, Children's Hospital of Michigan, Detroit, Michigan

**Andrea G. Asnes, MD, MSW**
Associate Professor of Pediatrics, Yale School of Medicine, New Haven, Connecticut

**Elizabeth V. Asztalos, MD, MSc, FRCPC**
Associate Professor of Pediatrics, University of Toronto; Neonatologist, Department of Newborn & Developmental Pediatrics, Women and Babies Program, Sunnybrook Health Sciences Centre, Toronto, Ontario, Canada

**Ioanna Athanassaki, MD**
Assistant Professor of Pediatrics, Section of Diabetes and Endocrinology, Baylor College of Medicine, Texas Children's Hospital, Houston, Texas

**Shean J. Aujla, MD**
Associate Professor of Pediatrics, Division of Pediatric Pulmonology, MUSC Children's Health, Medical University of South Carolina, Charleston, South Carolina

**Jeffery J. Auletta, MD**
Associate Professor of Clinical Pediatrics, Department of Pediatrics, The Ohio State University College of Medicine; Director, Host Defense Program; Director, Blood and Marrow Transplant Program, Hematology/Oncology/BMT and Infectious Diseases, Nationwide Children's Hospital, Columbus, Ohio

**Fida Bacha, MD**
Associate Professor of Pediatrics, Baylor College of Medicine, Pediatric Endocrinology and Diabetes, Texas Children's Hospital, Houston, Texas

**Carlos A. Bacino, MD**
Professor, Department of Molecular and Human Genetics, Baylor College of Medicine; Chief, Clinical Genetics Division, Texas Children's Hospital, Houston, Texas

**Carl H. Backes, MD**
Assistant Professor of Pediatrics, Center for Perinatal Research, Nationwide Children's Hospital, The Heart Center, Nationwide Children's Hospital, Department of Obstetrics/Gynecology, The Ohio State University Wexner Medical Center, Columbus, Ohio

**Razan Bader, MBBS, MPH**
Advanced Pediatric Transplant Hepatology Fellow, Center for Childhood Liver Disease, Division of Gastroenterology, Hepatology and Nutrition, Boston Children's Hospital, Boston, Massachusetts

**Rochelle Bagatell, MD**
Associate Professor of Pediatrics, Division of Oncology, Perelman School of Medicine, University of Pennsylvania, The Children's Hospital of Philadelphia, Philadelphia, Pennsylvania

**K. Scott Baker, MD, MS**
Professor of Pediatrics, University of Washington School of Medicine; Director, Pediatric Blood and Marrow Transplantation and Survivorship Programs, Fred Hutchinson Cancer Research Center, Seattle, Washington

**M. Douglas Baker, MD**
Professor, Department of Pediatrics, Johns Hopkins University School of Medicine, Baltimore, Maryland

**Cristina Baldassari, MD, FAAP, FACS**
Associate Professor, Eastern Virginia Medical School, Children's Hospital of the King's Daughters, Norfolk, Virginia

**Robert S. Baltimore, MD**
Attending Physician, Yale-New Haven Children's Hospital; Associate Director, Infection Prevention, Quality Improvement Support Services, Yale-New Haven Hospital; Professor of Pediatrics and Epidemiology, Yale School of Medicine, New Haven, Connecticut

**Manisha Balwani, MD**
Associate Professor, Department of Genetics and Genomic Sciences, Icahn School of Medicine at Mount Sinai, New York, New York

**Anuja Bandyopadhyay, MBBS**
Fellow, Division of Pediatric Pulmonology, Allergy, and Sleep Medicine, Indiana University School of Medicine, Indianapolis, Indiana

**Ritu Banerjee, MD, PhD**
Associate Professor, Pediatric Infectious Diseases, Vanderbilt University, Nashville, Tennessee

**Chantay Banikarim, MD, MPH**
Physician, Adolescent Medicine, Dignity Health, St. Joseph's Hospital and Medical Center, Phoenix, Arizona

**Nidhi Bansal, MD, MPH**
Clinical Assistant Professor, Department of Pediatrics, Section of Endocrinology, University of Iowa, Iowa City, Iowa

**Victoria R. Barrio, MD**
Associate Clinical Professor of Dermatology and Pediatrics, University of California, San Diego, California

**Karyl S. Barron, MD**
Deputy Director, Division of Intramural Research, National Institute of Allergy and Infectious Diseases, National Institutes of Health, Bethesda, Maryland

**Lee M. Bass, MD**
Associate Professor of Pediatrics, Northwestern University Feinberg School of Medicine; Clinical Practice Director and Director of Endoscopy, Gastroenterology, Hepatology and Nutrition, Ann & Robert H. Lurie Children's Hospital of Chicago, Chicago, Illinois

**Patricia Bastero, MD**
Assistant Professor of Pediatrics, Baylor College of Medicine, Texas Children's Hospital, Houston, Texas

**J. Bronwyn Bateman, MD**
Clinical Professor of Ophthalmology, David Geffen School of Medicine, University of California, Los Angeles, Los Angeles, California

**Surabhi Batra, MD**
Clinical Assistant Professor, Department of Pediatrics, Pediatric Hematology Oncology, University of Illinois College of Medicine at Peoria, St. Jude Affiliate Clinic, Peoria, Illinois

**Michel Baum, MD**
Professor of Pediatrics and Internal Medicine; Sara M. and Charles E. Seay Chair in Pediatric Research, University of Texas Southwestern Medical Center, Dallas, Texas

**Laurie J. Bauman, PhD**
Professor of Pediatrics; Director, Preventive Intervention Research Center, Albert Einstein College of Medicine, Jack and Pearl Resnick Campus, Bronx, New York

**John Beca, MB ChB, FCICM**
Director of Pediatric Intensive Care, Starship Children's Hospital, Auckland, New Zealand

**Elizabeth A. Beierle, MD**
Charles D. McCrary Chair in Pediatric Surgery; Professor, Division of Pediatric Surgery, University of Alabama at Birmingham, Children's Hospital of Alabama, Birmingham, Alabama

**Bryce Bell, MD, BS**
Assistant Professor, Baylor College of Medicine, Hand and Upper Extremity Surgery, Texas Children's Hospital, Houston, Texas

**Lionel Bercovitch, MD**
Professor of Dermatology, Department of Dermatology, Warren Alpert Medical School of Brown University, Providence, Rhode Island

**Robert A. Berg, MD, FAAP, FCCM, FAHA**
Professor of Anesthesiology and Critical Care Medicine, and Pediatrics, The University of Pennsylvania; Division Chief, Critical Care Medicine and Russell Raphaely Endowed Chair, The Children's Hospital of Philadelphia, Philadelphia, Pennsylvania

**Brad D. Berman, MD**
Clinical Professor of Pediatrics, UCSF Benioff Children's Hospital, Progressions: Developmental and Behavioral Pediatrics, Walnut Creek, California

**William Bernal, MD**
Assistant Professor of Pediatrics, University of California, San Francisco, San Francisco, California

**Marcia Berretta, LCSW**
Instructor of Pediatrics, Baylor College of Medicine, Meyer Center for Developmental Pediatrics, Texas Children's Hospital, Houston, Texas

**Leslie R. Berry, BSc (Hons)**
Assistant Professor of Pediatrics, McMaster University, Hamilton, Ontario, Canada

**Vidit Bhargava, MBBS**
Pediatric Resident, Department of Pediatrics, University of Texas Medical Branch, Galveston, Texas

**Amit Bhatt, MD**
Assistant Professor of Ophthalmology, Baylor College of Medicine, Houston, Texas

**Dennis Bier, MD**
Professor, Baylor College of Medicine, Children's Nutritional Center, Texas Children's Hospital, Houston, Texas

**John G. Birch, MD**
Assistant Chief of Staff Emeritus, Texas Scottish Rite Hospital for Children; Professor, University of Texas, Southwestern Medical Center, Dallas, Texas

**Steven Black, MD**
Professor of Pediatrics, Division of Infectious Disease, Cincinnati Children's Hospital, Cincinnati, Ohio

**Susan M. Blaney, MD**
Professor and Executive Vice-Chair, Department of Pediatrics, Baylor College of Medicine; Director, Texas Children's Cancer Center, Texas Children's Hospital, Houston, Texas

**Efrain Bleiberg, MD**
Professor of Psychiatry and Pediatrics and Vice Chair, Menninger Department of Psychiatry and Behavioral Sciences; Director, Child and Adolescent Psychiatry, Baylor College of Medicine, Houston, Texas

**Joseph R. Block, MD**
Assistant Professor, Department of Pediatrics (Cardiology), Medical College of Wisconsin, Milwaukee, Wisconsin

**Desmond Bohn, MB, FRCPC**
Department of Critical Care Medicine, The Hospital for Sick Children, Toronto; Professor, Anesthesia and Pediatrics, University of Toronto, Toronto, Canada

**Christopher F. Bolling, MD**
General Pediatrician, Pediatric Associates, PSC, Crestview Hills, Kentucky; Volunteer Associate Professor of Pediatrics, Division of General and Community Pediatrics, University of Cincinnati College of Medicine, Cincinnati, Ohio

**William Borkowsky, MD**
Professor of Pediatrics, Division of Pediatric Infectious Diseases, New York University School of Medicine, New York, New York

**Bret L. Bostwick, MD**
Assistant Professor, Department of Molecular and Human Genetics, Baylor College of Medicine, Texas Children's Hospital, Houston, Texas

**Scarlett Boulos, MD**
Fellow, Pediatric Dermatology, Children's Hospital of Philadelphia, University of Pennsylvania, Philadelphia, Pennsylvania

**Annemarie Boyan, JD**
Associate General Counsel, The Children's Hospital of Philadelphia, Philadelphia, Pennsylvania

**Brendan M. Boyle, MD, MPH**
Assistant Professor of Pediatrics, Division of Pediatric Gastroenterology, Hepatology, and Nutrition, The Ohio State University College of Medicine, Nationwide Children's Hospital, Columbus, Ohio

**Renée Boynton-Jarrett, MD, ScD**
Associate Professor of Pediatrics, Boston University School of Medicine, Boston Medical Center, Boston, Massachusetts

**Jennifer M. Brady, MD**
Assistant Professor of Pediatrics, Cincinnati Children's Hospital Medical Center, University of Cincinnati College of Medicine, Cincinnati, Ohio

**Ken Brady, MD**
Associate Professor of Pediatrics and Anesthesia, Baylor College of Medicine, Texas Children's Hospital, Houston, Texas

**Rebecca C. Brady, MD**
Associate Professor of Clinical Pediatrics, Cincinnati Children's Hospital Medical Center, Division of Infectious Diseases, Cincinnati, Ohio

**Denise Bratcher, DO**
Professor of Pediatrics, Pediatric Infectious Diseases; Associate Dean, Pediatrics, University of Missouri—Kansas City School of Medicine; Chair, Graduate Medical Education, Children's Mercy Hospital—Kansas City, Kansas City, Missouri

**Dylan Braun, BS**
Research Coordinator, Columbia University Medical Center, New York, New York

**Michael C. Braun, MD, FASN**
Professor of Pediatrics, Renal Section, Baylor College of Medicine; Chief of Renal Services, Texas Children's Hospital, Houston, Texas

**Nancy Braverman, MD**
Associate Professor, Department of Pediatrics, Faculty of Medicine, Research Institute of the McGill University Health Center, Montreal, Canada

**Joe Brierley, MB ChB, FRCPCH, MA**
Consultant in Intensive Care and Bioethics, Great Ormond Street Hospital for Children, London, United Kingdom

**Mark Brittan, MD, MPH**
Assistant Professor of Pediatrics, University of Colorado School of Medicine, Children's Hospital Colorado, Aurora, Colorado

**Justin Brockbank, MD**
Assistant Professor of Pediatrics, Children's Hospital of Richmond at Virginia Commonwealth University, Richmond, Virginia

**Ronald A. Bronicki, MD, FCCM, FACC**
Professor of Pediatrics, Baylor College of Medicine, Texas Children's Hospital, Houston, Texas

**Jason Brophy, MD, MSc, DTM, FRCPC**
Assistant Professor of Pediatrics, University of Ottawa, Division of Infectious Diseases, Department of Pediatrics, Children's Hospital of Eastern Ontario, Ontario, Canada

**Richard Bruun, DDS**
Assistant Professor of Developmental Biology, Harvard School of Dental Medicine; Senior Associate in Dentistry, Boston Children's Hospital, Boston, Massachusetts

**Sara M. Buckelew, MD, MPH**
Associate Clinical Professor of Pediatrics, Medical Director, Eating Disorders Program, Division of Adolescent and Young Adult Medicine, Department of Pediatrics, UCSF Benioff Children's Hospital, University of California, San Francisco, San Francisco, California

**Fernando J. Bula-Rudas, MD**
Fellow, Pediatric Infectious Diseases and Immunology, University of Florida College of Medicine, Jacksonville, Florida

**Anthony Ernest Burgos, MD**
Kaiser Permanente Medical Group, Oakland, California

**Lindsay C. Burrage, MD, PhD**
Assistant Professor, Department of Molecular and Human Genetics, Baylor College of Medicine, Texas Children's Hospital, Houston, Texas

**Andrew Bush, MD**
Professor of Pediatrics and Head of Section (Pediatrics), Imperial College; Professor of Pediatric Respirology, National Heart and Lung Institute; Consultant Pediatric Chest Physician, Royal Brompton and Harefield NHS Foundation Trust, London, United Kingdom

**Tina L. Butera, MD, FAAO, AAPOS, FAAP**
Pediatric Ophthalmologist, The Eye Center, Pediatric Ophthalmology and Strabismus, Alexandria, Virginia

**Warwick Butt, MBBS, FRACP, FCICM**
Associate Professor of Pediatrics, University of Melbourne; Director of Intensive Care, The Royal Children's Hospital, Melbourne, Australia

**Miguel M. Cabada, MD, MSc**
Assistant Professor, Division of Infectious Diseases, Department of Internal Medicine, University of Texas Medical Branch, Galveston, Texas; Director, Tropical Medicine Institute—Cusco Branch, Universidad Peruana Cayetano Heredia, Cusco, Peru

**David A. Cabral, MD**
Clinical Professor, University of British Columbia, Division of Rheumatology, BC Children's Hospital, Vancouver, British Columbia, Canada

**Antonio G. Cabrera, MD**
Assistant Professor and Pediatric Cardiology Fellowship Program Director, Baylor College of Medicine; Attending Cardiologist, Texas Children's Hospital, Houston, Texas

**Cary Cain, MPH, BSN, RN**
Research Associate, Department of Pediatrics, Baylor College of Medicine, Houston, Texas

**Nicholas CaJacob, MD**
Assistant Professor of Pediatrics, Division of Pediatric Gastroenterology, Hepatology, and Nutrition, University of Alabama at Birmingham, Birmingham, Alabama

**Chadi Calarge, MD**
Thomas S. Trammell Research Professor in Child Psychiatry, Baylor College of Medicine, Texas Children's Hospital, Child and Adolescent Psychiatry, Houston, Texas

**Casey M. Calkins, MD**
Professor, Division of Pediatric Surgery, The Medical College of Wisconsin, Children's Hospital of Wisconsin, Milwaukee, Wisconsin

**Scott R. Callahan, MD**
Medical Director, PCMH Learning Collaborative, Cincinnati Children's Hospital, Cincinnati, Ohio

**Judith R. Campbell, MD**
Professor of Pediatrics, Section of Infectious Diseases, Baylor College of Medicine; Medical Director, Infection Control and Prevention, Texas Children's Hospital, Houston, Texas

**Alexandra Canetti, MD**
Assistant Professor of Psychiatry, Columbia University Medical Center, New York, New York

**Joseph A. Carcillo, MD**
Professor of Critical Care Medicine and Pediatrics, Department of Critical Care Medicine, University of Pittsburgh School of Medicine, Pittsburgh, Pennsylvania

**Aaron L. Cardon, MD, MSc**
Clinical Instructor, Department of Neurology, Division of Child Neurology, Stanford University School of Medicine, Palo Alto, California

**David P. Carlton, MD**
Marcus Professor of Pediatrics, Chief of Neonatal-Perinatal Medicine, Emory University School of Medicine, Atlanta, Georgia

**Beth A. Carter, MD**
Associate Professor, Department of Pediatrics, Baylor College of Medicine, Texas Children's Hospital, Houston, Texas

**Heidi Castillo, MD**
Assistant Professor of Pediatrics, Baylor College of Medicine, Meyer Center for Developmental Pediatrics, Texas Children's Hospital, Houston, Texas

**Jonathan Castillo, MD, MPH**
Assistant Professor of Pediatrics, Baylor College of Medicine, Meyer Center for Developmental Pediatrics, Texas Children's Hospital, Houston, Texas

**Melissa Del Castillo, MD**
Fellow, Pediatric Infectious Disease, Children's National Medical Center, Washington, District of Columbia

**Mariam R. Chacko, MD**
Professor, Pediatrics/Adolescent Medicine, Baylor College of Medicine, Texas Children's Hospital, Houston, Texas

**Rana Chakraborty, MD, MSc, FRCPCH, DPhil**
Professor of Pediatrics, Emory University School of Medicine, Atlanta, Georgia

**Anthony K. C. Chan, MBBS, FRCPC, FRCPCH, FRCPI, FRCP (Glas), FRCPath**
Professor of Pediatrics, Thrombosis and Atherosclerosis Research Institute (TaARI), McMaster University, McMaster Children's Hospital, Hamilton, Ontario, Canada

**Isabelle I. Chase, DDS, FRCD(C)**
Assistant Professor of Developmental Biology (Pediatric Dentistry); Director, Postdoctoral Pediatric Dentistry, Harvard School of Dental Medicine; Associate in Dentistry, Boston Children's Hospital, Boston, Massachusetts

**Talal A. Chatila, MD, MSc**
Professor of Pediatrics, Harvard Medical School, Boston, Massachusetts

**Ira Cheifetz, MD**
Professor of Pediatrics, Chief, Division of Pediatric Critical Care Medicine, Duke University School of Medicine, Durham, North Carolina

**Daniel C. Chelius, MD**
Assistant Professor of Otolaryngology—Head and Neck Surgery, Baylor College of Medicine; Director, Pediatric Head and Neck Tumor Program, Texas Children's Hospital, Houston, Texas

**Yuan-Tsong Chen, MD, PhD**
Professor of Pediatrics, Duke University; Distinguished Research Fellow, Institute of Biomedical Sciences, Academia Sinica, Taipei, Taiwan

**Mike K. Chen, MD**
Joseph M. Farley Chair in Pediatric Surgery; Professor and Director, Division of Pediatric Surgery, University of Alabama at Birmingham; Surgeon-in-Chief, Children's Hospital of Alabama, Birmingham, Alabama

**Min-Jye Chen, MD**
Assistant Professor, Section of Diabetes and Endocrinology, Department of Pediatrics, Baylor College of Medicine, Texas Children's Hospital, Houston, Texas

**Karen A. Chernoff, MD**
Assistant Professor of Dermatology and Pediatrics, Weill Cornell Medical College, New York, New York

**Erica Chin, PhD**
Assistant Clinical Professor of Medical Psychology, Columbia University Medical Center; Director of Psychology, New York Presbyterian Hospital, New York, New York

**Javier Chinen, MD, PhD**
Associate Professor of Pediatrics, Baylor College of Medicine; Chief, Immunology Allergy and Rheumatology Service, Texas Children's Hospital The Woodlands, The Woodlands, Texas

**Ivan K. Chinn, MD**
Assistant Professor of Pediatrics, Baylor College of Medicine, Section of Immunology, Allergy, Rheumatology, and Retrovirology, Texas Children's Hospital, Houston, Texas

**Murali Chintagumpala, MD**
Professor of Pediatrics, Baylor College of Medicine; Director, Solid Tumor Program; Co-Director, Neuro-Oncology Program, Texas Children's Cancer Center, Houston, Texas

**Brett Chiquet, DDS, PhD**
Assistant Professor of Pediatric Dentistry, University of Texas Health Science Center at Houston School of Dentistry, Houston, Texas

**Tasnee Chonmaitree, MD**
Professor, Department of Pediatrics, Division of Infectious Diseases, University of Texas Medical Branch, Galveston, Texas

**Eric J. Chow, MD, MPH**
Associate Professor of Pediatrics, University of Washington School of Medicine; Medical Director, Cancer Survivor Program, Seattle Children's Hospital, Seattle, Washington

**Robin B. Churchill, MD**
Attending Physician, Pediatric Infectious Diseases, Golisano Children's Hospital, Fort Myers, Florida

**Thomas M. Ciecierega, MD**
Assistant Professor of Pediatrics, Weill Cornell Medical College, New York, New York

**Gary D. Clark, MD**
Blue Bird Circle Endowed Chair of Neurology and Developmental Neuroscience; Professor of Pediatrics, Baylor College of Medicine; Chief of the Neurology Service, Texas Children's Hospital, Houston, Texas

**David K. Coats, MD**
Professor of Ophthalmology, Chief of Pediatric Ophthalmology, Baylor College of Medicine, Texas Children's Hospital, Houston, Texas

**Mitchell B. Cohen, MD**
Katharine Reynolds Ireland Chair of Pediatrics, University of Alabama at Birmingham; Physician in Chief, Children's of Alabama, Birmingham, Alabama

**Kenneth J. Cohen, MD, MBA**
Professor of Oncology, Johns Hopkins University School of Medicine; Clinical Director of Pediatric Oncology, The Sidney Kimmel Comprehensive Cancer Center at Johns Hopkins, Baltimore, Maryland

**Peter D. Cole, MD**
Associate Professor of Pediatrics, Albert Einstein College of Medicine, The Children's Hospital at Montefiore, Bronx, New York

**Talia Collier, MD**
Assistant Professor of Pediatrics, Baylor College of Medicine, Texas Children's Hospital, Houston, Texas

**Beverly L. Connelly, MD**
Emeritus Professor of Pediatrics, Division of Infectious Diseases, Cincinnati Children's Hospital Medical Center, University of Cincinnati College of Medicine, Cincinnati, Ohio

**Despina Contopoulos-Ioannidis, MD**
Clinical Associate Professor, Pediatrics—Infectious Diseases, Stanford University, Palo Alto, California

**M. Brett Cooper, MD**
Fellow, Pediatrics/Adolescent Medicine, Baylor College of Medicine, Texas Children's Hospital, Houston, Texas

**Rohini Coorg, MD**
Assistant Professor of Pediatrics, Baylor College of Medicine, Texas Children's Hospital, Houston, Texas

**Lawson A. B. Copley, MD**
Staff Orthopedist, Texas Scottish Rite Hospital for Children, Children's Medical Center of Dallas; Associate Professor of Orthopedic Surgery, University of Texas Southwestern, Dallas, Texas

**Michael J. Corwin, MD**
Associate Professor of Pediatrics and Epidemiology, Boston University Schools of Medicine and Public Health; Senior Epidemiologist, Slone Epidemiology Center, Boston University, Boston, Massachusetts

**C. Michael Cotten, MD**
Professor of Pediatrics, Duke University School of Medicine, Durham, North Carolina

**William J. Craigen, MD, PhD**
Professor, Department of Molecular and Human Genetics, Baylor College of Medicine, Houston, Texas

**Shelley E. Crary, MD, MS**
Associate Professor of Pediatrics, University of Arkansas for Medical Sciences, Arkansas Children's Hospital, Little Rock, Arkansas

**Haidee Custodio, MD**
Assistant Professor, Division of Pediatric Infectious Diseases, University of South Alabama College of Medicine, Mobile, Alabama

**Cori L. Daines, MD**
Professor of Pediatrics, University of Arizona, Tucson, Arizona

**Basil T. Darras, MD**
Professor of Neurology, Harvard Medical School; Associate Neurologist-in-Chief; Director, Neuromuscular Center and Spinal Muscular Atrophy Program, Boston Children's Hospital, Boston, Massachusetts

**Carla M. Davis, MD**
Associate Professor, Baylor College of Medicine, Allergy and Immunology Service, Texas Children's Hospital, Houston, Texas

**Bouke C. de Jong, MD, PhD**
Mycobacteriology Unit, Department of Biomedical Sciences, Institute of Tropical Medicine, Antwerp, Belgium

**C. G. de Waal, MD, PhD**
Neonatologist, Department of Neonatology, Emma Children's Hospital, Academic Medical Center, Amsterdam, The Netherlands

**Walter Dehority, MD, MSc**
Pediatric Infectious Disease Physician, Department of Pediatrics, University of New Mexico, Albuquerque, New Mexico

**Monte A. Del Monte, MD, FAAP**
Division Chief, Pediatric Ophthalmology and Adult Strabismus; Skillman Professor of Pediatric Ophthalmology, Professor of Ophthalmology and Visual Sciences, Professor of Pediatrics and Communicable Diseases, Kellogg Eye Center, Mott Children's Hospital, University of Michigan, Ann Arbor, Michigan

**Sara B. DeMauro, MD, MSCE**
Assistant Professor of Pediatrics, Perelman School of Medicine, University of Pennsylvania, Children's Hospital of Philadelphia, Philadelphia, Pennsylvania

**Craig S. Derkay, MD, FACS, FAAP**
Professor Otolaryngology and Pediatrics, Eastern Virginia Medical School; Director, Pediatric Otolaryngology, Children's Hospital of the King's Daughters, Norfolk, Virginia

**Moreshwar Desai, MD**
Assistant Professor of Pediatrics, Section of Critical Care Medicine, Department of Pediatric Intensive Care, Baylor College of Medicine, Texas Children's Hospital, Houston, Texas

**Daniel DeSalvo, MD**
Assistant Professor, Section of Diabetes and Endocrinology, Baylor College of Medicine, Texas Children's Hospital, Houston, Texas

**Robert J. Desnick, MD, PhD**
Dean, Genetics and Genomic Medicine; Professor and Chair Emeritus, Genetics and Genomic Sciences, Icahn School of Medicine at Mount Sinai, New York, New York

**Jenny M. Despotovic, DO**
Associate Professor of Pediatrics, Baylor College of Medicine; Director, Immune Hematology Program, Texas Children's Hospital, Houston, Texas

**Prasad Devarajan, MD**
Louise M. Williams Endowed Chair; Professor of Pediatrics and Developmental Biology; Director of Nephrology and Hypertension, Cincinnati Children's Hospital Medical Center, University of Cincinnati College of Medicine, Cincinnati, Ohio

**Thomas G. DeWitt, MD**
Professor and Director, Division of General and Community Pediatrics, Cincinnati Children's Hospital Medical Center, Cincinnati, Ohio

**Shweta U. Dhar, MD, MS, FACMG**
Associate Professor, Department of Molecular and Human Genetics, Baylor College of Medicine; Chief, Section of Genetic Medicine, Michael E. DeBakey Veterans Affairs Medical Center, Houston, Texas

**Lucia Z. Diaz, MD**
Assistant Professor of Pediatrics, Dell Medical School, University of Texas at Austin, Austin, Texas

**Rosa Diaz, MD**
Assistant Professor of Pediatrics, Baylor College of Medicine, Texas Children's Hospital, Houston, Texas

**Shannon DiCarlo, MD**
Assistant Professor of Pediatrics, Baylor College of Medicine, Texas Children's Hospital, Houston, Texas

**Salvatore DiMaur, MD**
Lucy G. Moses Professor of Neurology, Department of Neurology, Columbia University, New York

**Linda A. DiMeglio, MD, MPH**
Professor of Pediatrics, Department of Pediatrics, Section of Pediatric Endocrinology/Diabetology, Indiana University School of Medicine, Indianapolis, Indiana

**Reed A. Dimmitt, MD**
David E. Dixon Endowed Chair in Pediatric Gastroenterology; Professor of Pediatrics, Division of Pediatric Gastroenterology, Hepatology, and Nutrition, University of Alabama at Birmingham, Birmingham, Alabama

**Jeffrey S. Dome, MD, PhD**
Professor of Pediatrics, George Washington University School of Medicine and Health Sciences; Vice President, Center for Cancer and Blood Disorders, Children's National Medical Center, Washington, DC

**John P. Dormans, MD, FACS**
Chief of Pediatric Orthopedic and Scoliosis Surgery; Professor of Orthopedic and Scoliosis Surgery, Baylor College of Medicine, LE Simmons Chair in Orthopedic Surgery, Texas Children's Hospital, Houston, Texas

**Cicely Dowdell-Smith, MD**
Assistant Professor of Pediatrics, Baylor College of Medicine, Texas Children's Hospital, Houston, Texas

**Irina F. Dragan, DDS, MS**
Assistant Professor of Periodontology, Tufts University School Dental Medicine, Boston, Massachusetts

**Steven G. DuBois, MD, MS**
Director, Experimental Therapeutics, Dana-Farber/Boston Children's Cancer and Blood Disorders Center, Harvard Medical School, Boston, Massachusetts

**Howard Dubowitz, MD, MS**
Professor, Department of Pediatrics; Head, Division of Child Protection, University of Maryland School of Medicine, Baltimore, Maryland

**Gueorgui Dubrocq, MD**
Pediatric Infectious Disease Specialist, Baylor Scott and White McLane Children's Medical Center; Assistant Clinical Professor of Pediatrics, Texas A&M Health Science Center College of Medicine, Temple, Texas

**Holly Dudley-Harrell, MD**
Assistant Professor of Pediatrics, Baylor College of Medicine, Texas Children's Hospital, Houston, Texas

**Trevor Duke, MD, FRACP, FCICM**
Professor of Pediatrics, University of Melbourne; Director, Centre for International Child Health, University of Melbourne, The Royal Children's Hospital, Melbourne, Australia; Adjunct Professor of Child Health, School of Medicine, University of Papua New Guinea, Port Moresby, Papua New Guinea

**Daniel E. Dulek, MD**
Assistant Professor, Pediatric Infectious Diseases, Vanderbilt University Medical Center, Monroe Carell Jr. Children's Hospital at Vanderbilt, Nashville, Tennessee

**James J. Dunn, PhD, D(ABMM)**
Director of Medical Microbiology and Virology, Department of Pathology, Texas Children's Hospital; Associate Professor, Department of Pathology and Immunology, Baylor College of Medicine, Houston, Texas

**Teresa Duryea, MD**
Associate Professor of Pediatrics, Baylor College of Medicine; Clinic Chief, Primary Care Practice at Palm Center; Co-Program Director, Primary Care LEAD Residency; Associate Section Head for Clinical Affairs, Academic General Pediatrics, Texas Children's Hospital, Houston, Texas

**Christopher C. Dvorak, MD**
Associate Professor of Clinical Pediatrics, University of California San Francisco School of Medicine; Chief, Division of Pediatric Allergy/Immunology/Bone Marrow Transplant, Benioff Children's Hospital, San Francisco, California

**R. Blaine Easley, MD**
Professor of Anesthesiology and Pediatrics, Baylor College of Medicine; Medical Director, Surgical Intensive Care Unit, Texas Children's Hospital, Houston, Texas

**Tanya N. Eble, MS, CGC**
Assistant Professor, Department of Molecular and Human Genetics, Baylor College of Medicine, Houston, Texas

**Darius Ebrahimi-Fakhari, MD, Dr med**
Resident, Department of Neurology, Harvard Medical School and Boston Children's Hospital, Boston, Massachusetts

**Olive Eckstein, MD**
Assistant Professor of Pediatrics, Baylor College of Medicine, Texas Children's Hospital, Houston, Texas

**Allison A. Eddy, MD**
Chair, Department of Pediatrics, University of British Columbia; Chief of Pediatric Medicine, British Columbia Children's Hospital, Vancouver, British Columbia, Canada

**Tracy R. Ediger, MD, PhD**
Assistant Professor of Pediatrics, The Ohio State University College of Medicine, Nationwide Children's Hospital, Columbus, Ohio

**Jennifer C. Edman, MD, MPH**
Staff Physician, Health and Counseling Center, Reed College, Portland, Oregon

**Morven S. Edwards, MD**
Professor of Pediatrics, Section of Pediatric Infectious Diseases, Baylor College of Medicine and Texas Children's Hospital, Houston, Texas

**Lawrence F. Eichenfield, MD**
Chief, Pediatric and Adolescent Dermatology, San Diego School of Medicine and Rady Children's Hospital; Professor of Dermatology and Pediatrics, University of California, San Diego, California

**Despina Eleftheriou, MBBS, MRCPCH, PhD**
Clinical Senior Lecturer, UCL Great Ormond Street Institute of Child Health, and Arthritis Research UK Centre for Adolescent Rheumatology, University College London, London, United Kingdom

**M. Tarek Elghetany, MD**
Professor of Pathology and Immunology, Baylor College of Medicine, Texas Children's Hospital, Houston, Texas

**Ayman W. El-Hattab, MD**
Consultant and Chief, Division of Genetic and Metabolic Disorders, Department of Pediatrics, Tawam Hospital, Al Ain, United Arab Emirates

**Lisa T. Emrick, MD**
Assistant Professor of Pediatrics, Baylor College of Medicine, Texas Children's Hospital, Houston, Texas

**Moshe Ephros (Efrat), MD**
Associate Clinical Professor of Pediatrics, Faculty of Medicine, Technion—Israel Institute of Technology; Director, Pediatric Infectious Disease Unit, Carmel Medical Center, Haifa, Israel

**Howard R. Epps, MD**
Associate Professor of Orthopedic Surgery, Baylor College of Medicine; Medical Director, Pediatric Orthopedics and Scoliosis, Texas Children's Hospital, Houston, Texas

**Guliz Erdem, MD**
Professor, Department of Pediatrics, Nationwide Children's Hospital, The Ohio State University, Section of Infectious Diseases, Columbus, Ohio

**Steven H. Erdman, MD**
Professor of Pediatrics, Director, Gastroenterology Fellowship Training Program, The Ohio State University College of Medicine, Nationwide Children's Hospital, Columbus, Ohio

**Rebecca K. Erenrich, MPH**
Staff Research Associate, Division of Adolescent and Young Adult Medicine, Department of Pediatrics, University of California, San Francisco, San Francisco, California

**Ruth A. Etzel, MD, PhD**
Professor of Epidemiology, Joseph J. Zilber School of Public Health, University of Wisconsin, Milwaukee, Wisconsin

**Nicholas Evans, DM, MRCPCH, CCPU (Neonatal)**
Clinical Associate Professor, Department of Neonatal Medicine, University of Sydney, Royal Prince Alfred Hospital, Sydney, Australia

**Marybeth Ezaki, MD**
Professor, University of Texas-Southwestern Medical School; Texas Scottish Rite Hospital for Children; The Charles E. Seay, Jr. Hand Center, Dallas, Texas

**Cicely W. Fadel, MD, PhD**
Neonatology Fellow, Harvard Neonatal-Perinatal Training Program, Boston Children's Hospital, Boston, Massachusetts

**Christine B. Falkensammer, MD**
Attending Cardiologist, Division of Cardiology, Department of Pediatrics, University of Pennsylvania Perelman School of Medicine; Attending Cardiologist, The Children's Hospital of Philadelphia, Philadelphia, Pennsylvania

**Leland L. Fan, MD**
Professor of Pediatrics, The Breathing Institute at Children's Hospital Colorado, The University of Colorado, Aurora, Colorado

**Avroy A. Fanaroff, MD**
Emeritus Professor, Department of Pediatrics; Emeritus Eliza Henry Barnes Professor of Neonatology, Case Western Reserve University School of Medicine, Rainbow Babies and Children's Hospital, Cleveland, Ohio

**Bethany J. Farr, MD**
Resident, Department of Surgery, LSU Health Science Center, New Orleans, Louisiana

**James A. Feinstein, MD, MPH**
Assistant Professor of Pediatrics, University of Colorado School of Medicine, Children's Hospital Colorado, Aurora, Colorado

**Amy G. Feldman, MD**
Assistant Professor of Pediatrics, Children's Hospital Colorado, Digestive Health Institute, University of Colorado Denver School of Medicine, Section of Gastroenterology, Hepatology and Nutrition, Aurora, Colorado

**Sing-Yi Feng, MD**
Associate Professor of Pediatrics; Medical Toxicologist, University of Texas Southwestern Medical Center Dallas, Division of Emergency Medicine, Dallas, Texas

**Ada M. Fenick, MD**
Associate Professor of Pediatrics, Yale University School of Medicine, New Haven, Connecticut

**Chris Feudtner, MD, PhD, MPH**
Director, Department of Medical Ethics, Children's Hospital of Philadelphia; Professor, Pediatrics and Medical Ethics and Health Policy, Perelman School of Medicine of the University of Pennsylvania, Philadelphia, Pennsylvania

**Zameera Fida, DMD**
Instructor of Developmental Biology (Pediatric Dentistry), Harvard School of Dental Medicine; Assistant in Dentistry, Boston Children's Hospital, Boston, Massachusetts

**Lauren Fiechtner, MD, MPH**
Instructor of Pediatrics, Harvard Medical School; Director of Nutrition, MassGeneral Hospital for Children, Boston, Massachusetts

**Jonathan D. Finder, MD**
Professor of Pediatrics, University of Pittsburgh School of Medicine; Pediatric Pulmonologist Children's Hospital of Pittsburgh, Pittsburgh, Pennsylvania

**Douglas S. Fishman, MD**
Associate Professor of Pediatrics, Baylor College of Medicine, Director, Gastrointestinal Endoscopy and Therapeutic Endoscopy, Texas Children's Hospital, Houston, Texas

**Linda S. Flannery, BSN, RN**
Diagnostic Nurse Manager—Central Access Team, Children's Hospital of Wisconsin, Milwaukee, Wisconsin

**Tim Flerlage, MD**
Specialist, Pediatric Critical Care Medicine, St. Jude Children's Research Hospital, Memphis, Tennessee

**John Flibotte, MD**
Assistant Professor of Clinical Pediatrics, Perelman School of Medicine, University of Pennsylvania; Attending Neonatologist, Children's Hospital of Philadelphia, Philadelphia, Pennsylvania

**Patricia M. Flynn, MD**
Member, Department of Infectious Diseases, St. Jude Children's Research Hospital, Memphis, Tennessee

**Joseph T. Flynn, MD, MS**
Professor of Pediatrics, Dr. Robert O. Hickman Endowed Chair in Pediatric Nephrology, Division of Nephrology, Seattle Children's Hospital, Seattle, Washington

**Marc Foca, MD**
Associate Professor of Pediatrics, Columbia University Medical Center, Division of Pediatric Infectious Diseases, New York, New York

**Mark A. Fogel, MD**
Professor of Pediatrics and Radiology, Perelman School of Medicine at the University of Pennsylvania; Director of Magnetic Resonance Imaging, Children's Hospital of Philadelphia, Philadelphia, Pennsylvania

**Elizabeth E. Foglia, MD**
Assistant Professor, Department of Pediatrics, Division of Neonatology, Perelman School of Medicine, University of Pennsylvania; Attending Neonatologist, Children's Hospital of Philadelphia, Philadelphia, Pennsylvania

**Robert P. Foglia, MD**
Helen J. and Robert S. Strauss Professor and Chief of Pediatric Surgery, University of Texas, Southwestern Medical Center; Surgeon-In-Chief, Children's Medical Center at Dallas, Texas

**Lisa Forbes, MD**
Assistant Professor of Pediatrics, Baylor College of Medicine; Medical Director Center for Human Immunobiology, Texas Children's Hospital, Houston, Texas

**John W. Foreman, MD**
Consulting Professor, Department of Pediatrics, Duke University Health System, Durham, North Carolina

**Elizabeth Fox, MD**
Associate Professor of Pediatrics, Perelman School of Medicine, University of Pennsylvania; Head, Developmental Therapeutics, Division of Oncology, Children's Hospital of Philadelphia, Philadelphia, Pennsylvania

**María Victoria Fraga, MD**
Assistant Professor of Clinical Pediatrics, Perelman School of Medicine, University of Pennsylvania; Attending Neonatologist, Children's Hospital of Philadelphia, Philadelphia, Pennsylvania

**A. Lindsay Frazier, MD, ScM**
Associate Professor of Pediatrics, Harvard Medical School; Associate Professor of Epidemiology, Harvard T.H. Chan School of Public Health, Boston Children's Hospital and Dana Farber Cancer Institute, Boston, Massachusetts

**Heather M. French, MD, MSEd**
Associate Professor of Clinical Pediatrics, Perelman School of Medicine, University of Pennsylvania; Attending Neonatologist, Children's Hospital of Philadelphia, Philadelphia, Pennsylvania

**Juanita Neira Fresneda, MD**
Assistant Professor, Emory University School of Medicine, Atlanta, Georgia

**Ilona J. Frieden, MD**
Professor of Dermatology and Pediatrics, University of California, San Francisco, California

**Glenn T. Furuta, MD**
Professor of Pediatrics; Director, Digestive Health Institute, Gastrointestinal Eosinophilic Diseases Program, Children's Hospital Colorado, University of Colorado School of Medicine, Aurora, Colorado

**Marta Grisel Galarza, MD, FAAP**
Assistant Professor of Clinical Pediatrics, Division of Neonatology, University of Miami Miller School of Medicine; Medical Director, Newborn Nursery and Intermediate Care NICU, Miami, Florida

**David P. Galloway, MD**
Assistant Professor of Pediatrics, Division of Pediatric Gastroenterology, Hepatology and Nutrition, Birmingham, Alabama

**Zoe W. Gao, MBBS (Hon), FRANZCO, BMedsc, MPhil (Ophth)**
Consultant Ophthalmologist, Precision Eye Clinic, Hobart, Australia; Honorary Consultant, Royal Victorian Eye and Ear Hospital, Melbourne, Australia

**Christopher Gappy, MD**
Clinical Assistant Professor, Kellogg Eye Center, Mott Children's Hospital, University of Michigan, Ann Arbor, Michigan

**Andrea K. Garber, PhD, RD**
Associate Professor of Pediatrics, Division of Adolescent and Young Adult Medicine, UCSF Benioff Children's Hospital, University of California, San Francisco, San Francisco, California

**Héctor H. Garcia, MD, PhD**
Director, Center for Global Health, Universidad Peruana Cayetano Heredia, Tumbes, Peru; Professor, Department of Microbiology, Universidad Peruana Cayetano Heredia; Head, Cysticercosis Unit, Instituto Nacional de Ciencias Neurologicas, Lima, Peru

**Angela Garcia Cazorla, MD, PhD**
Associate Professor of Pediatrics; Head of the Neurometabolic Unit and the Synaptic Metabolism Laboratory, Hospital Sant Joan de Déu, Barcelona, Spain

**Maria Garcia Lloret, MD**
Assistant Clinical Professor, Pediatric Allergy, Immunology and Rheumatology, University of California Los Angeles, Los Angeles, California

**Beth H. Garland, PhD**
Assistant Professor, Department of Pediatrics, Adolescent Medicine and Sports Medicine Section, Baylor College of Medicine, Texas Children's Hospital, Houston, Texas

**Evan F. Garner, MD**
Resident, Department of Surgery, University of Alabama at Birmingham, Birmingham, Alabama

**Andrea Garrod, MD**
Assistant Professor of Pediatrics, University of Virginia, Charlottesville, Virginia

**Aditya H. Gaur, MD**
Member, St. Jude Faculty; Medical Director, Occupational Health; Director, Translational Trials Unit; Director, Clinical Research, Infectious Diseases, St. Jude Children's Research Hospital, Memphis, Tennessee

**Charles T. Gay, MD**
Associate Professor of Pediatrics, Baylor College of Medicine, Texas Children's Hospital, Houston, Texas

**Alex George, MD, PhD**
Assistant Professor of Pediatrics, Baylor College of Medicine; Co-Director, Texas Children's Sickle Cell Center, Texas Children's Hospital, Houston, Texas

**Angelo P. Giardino, MD, PhD**
Senior Vice President/Chief Quality Officer, Texas Children's Hospital; Professor and Chief, Academic General Pediatrics, Baylor College of Medicine, Houston, Texas

**Francis Gigliotti, MD**
Professor of Pediatrics; Chief, Pediatric Infectious Diseases, Microbiology, and Immunology; Lindsey Distinguished Professorship for Pediatric Research, University of Rochester Medical Center, School of Medicine and Dentistry, Rochester, New York

**Michael Giladi, MD, MSc**
Associate Professor of Medicine, Sackler Faculty of Medicine, Tel Aviv University; The Infectious Disease Unit and the Bernard Pridan Laboratory for Molecular Biology of Infectious Diseases, Sourasky Medical Center, Tel Aviv, Israel

**Laurence B. Givner, MD**
Professor, Department of Pediatrics, Wake Forest School of Medicine; Associate Chief Medical Officer, Wake Forest Baptist Health Medical Center Blvd, WinstonSalem, North Carolina

**Aharon Z. Gladstein, MD**
Assistant Professor of Orthopedics, Baylor College of Medicine, Pediatric Orthopedics and Sports Medicine, Texas Children's Hospital, Houston Texas

**Carol Glaser, MD, DVM, MPVM**
Kaiser Permanente, Pediatric Infectious Diseases, Oakland, California; Associate Clinical Professor of Pediatrics, Infectious Disease, Department of Pediatrics, University of California, San Francisco, California

**Daniel G. Glaze, MD, FAASM**
Professor of Pediatrics, Baylor College of Medicine; Medical Director, The Children's Sleep Center; Medical Director, The Blue Bird Circle Rett Center, Texas Children's Hospital, Houston, Texas

**Praveen S. Goday, MBBS, CNSC**
Professor of Pediatrics, Medical College of Wisconsin; Director, Clinical Nutrition, Children's Hospital of Wisconsin, Milwaukee, Wisconsin

**Dinah L. Godwin, LCSW**
Instructor of Pediatrics, Baylor College of Medicine, Meyer Center for Developmental Pediatrics, Texas Children's Hospital, Houston, Texas

**Vi Lier Goh, MD**
Instructor, Boston University, Boston Medical Center, Boston, Massachusetts

**Ganga Gokulakrishnan, MD**
Assistant Professor of Pediatrics, Baylor College of Medicine and Texas Children's Hospital, Houston, Texas

**David B. K. Golden, MD**
Associate Professor of Medicine, Johns Hopkins University, Baltimore, Maryland

**Blanca E. Gonzalez, MD**
Assistant Professor of Pediatrics, Cleveland Clinic Lerner College of Medicine of Case Western Reserve, Center for Pediatric Infectious Diseases, Cleveland Clinic Children's, Cleveland, Ohio

**Regino P. González-Peralta, MD**
Professor, Department of Pediatrics, Assistant Dean for Diversity and Health Equity, University of Florida College of Medicine, Jacksonville, Florida

**Richard Gorlick, MD**
Professor and Mosbacher Pediatrics Chair; Division Head and Department Chair, Division of Pediatrics, The University of Texas MD Anderson Cancer Center, Houston, Texas

**Mark P. Gorman, MD**
Assistant Professor of Neurology, Harvard Medical School; Director, Pediatric Neuroimmunology, Boston Children's Hospital, Boston, Massachusetts

**Collin S. Goto, MD**
Professor of Pediatrics; Medical Toxicologist, University of Texas Southwestern Medical Center at Dallas, Division of Emergency Medicine, Dallas, Texas

**Manjula Gowrishankar, MD, FRCPC**
Professor, Department of Pediatrics, Division of Pediatric Nephrology, University of Alberta, Edmonton, Alberta

**David Gozal, MD, MBA**
Herbert T. Abelson Professor of Pediatrics, Neuroscience, and Neurobiology, The University of Chicago, Chicago, Illinois

**Brett H. Graham, MD, PhD**
Associate Professor, Department of Molecular and Human Genetics, Baylor College of Medicine, Houston, Texas

**Christopher S. Greeley, MD, MS**
Chief, Section of Public Health Pediatrics, Texas Children's Hospital; Professor of Pediatrics, Baylor College of Medicine, Houston, Texas

**John H. Greinwald, Jr., MD, FAAP**
Professor, Division of Otolaryngology Head and Neck Surgery, Cincinnati Children's Hospital, Cincinnati, Ohio

**Adda Grimberg, MD**
Associate Professor of Pediatrics, Perelman School of Medicine, University of Pennsylvania; Scientific Director, Diagnostic and Research Growth Center, The Children's Hospital of Philadelphia, Philadelphia, Pennsylvania

**Markus Grompe, MD**
Professor of Pediatrics, Ray Hickey Chair of the Pape' Family Pediatric Research Institute Oregon Health and Science University, Portland, Oregon

**Thomas G. Gross, MD**
Deputy Director of Science, NCI-Center of Global Health, National Cancer Institute, Rockville, Maryland

**Melvin M. Grumbach, MD**
Edward B. Shaw Professor of Pediatrics, Emeritus Chairman of Department of Pediatrics, University of California, San Francisco, California

**Ruth Grychtol, MD**
Clinical Respiratory Fellow, Respiratory Unit, Great Ormond Street Hospital for Children, London, United Kingdom

**Anne-Marie Guerguerian, MD, PhD**
Senior Scientist, Neuroscience and Mental Health Program Research Institute, University of Toronto; Staff Physician, Pediatric Intensive Care Unit, The Hospital for Sick Children, Toronto, Canada

**Anna C. Gunz, MD, FRCPC, FAAP**
Assistant Professor, Department of Pediatrics, Children's Hospital, London Health Sciences Centre, Ontario, Canada

**Deepti Gupta, MD**
Assistant Professor, University of Washington School of Medicine, Seattle Children's Hospital, Seattle, Washington

**Howard P. Gutgesell, MD**
Professor, Department of Pediatrics, University of Virginia Health System, Charlottesville, Virginia

**Marietta M. de Guzman, MD**
Associate Professor of Pediatrics, Baylor College of Medicine; Clinic Chief, Pediatric Rheumatology, Texas Children's Hospital, Houston, Texas

**Fareeda Haamid, DO**
Assistant Professor of Clinical Pediatrics, Division of Adolescent Medicine, Nationwide Children's Hospital, Columbus, Ohio

**Ellen S. Haddock, AB, MBA**
Resident Physician, School of Medicine, University of California, San Diego, California

**Anita N. Haggstrom, MD**
Associate Professor of Dermatology, Indiana University and Riley Children's Hospital, Indianapolis, Indiana

**Amy B. Hair, MD**
Assistant Professor of Pediatrics, Baylor College of Medicine; Program Director of Neonatal Nutrition, Section of Neonatology, Texas Children's Hospital, Houston, Texas

**Neal Halfon, MD, MPH**
Professor of Pediatrics, Public Health and Public Policy; Director, UCLA Center for Healthier Children, Families & Communities, Los Angeles, California

**Stuart R. Hall, MD**
Assistant Professor of Anesthesiology and Pediatrics, Baylor College of Medicine, Texas Children's Hospital, Houston, Texas

**Gail Halliday, MBBS, MRCPCH, MClinRes**
Department of Pediatric Oncology, Great North Children's Hospital, Newcastle upon Tyne, United Kingdom

**Eric B. Hamill, MD**
Medical Resident in Ophthalmology, Cullen Eye Institute, Baylor College of Medicine, Houston, Texas

**Jin-Young Han, MD, PhD**
Assistant Professor of Clinical Pediatrics, Division of Infectious Diseases, Department of Pediatrics, Weill Cornell Medicine, New York, New York

**Benjamin Hanisch, MD**
Attending in Infectious Diseases and Assistant Professor of Pediatrics, Children's National Health System and George Washington University School of Medicine and Health Sciences, Washington, District of Columbia

**Tamar Harel, PhD, MD**
Senior Clinical Geneticist, Hadassah-Hebrew University Medical Center, Department for Genetics and Metabolic Diseases, Hadassah Ein Kerem, Jerusalem, Israel

**Nada Harik, MD**
Attending Physician, Division of Infectious Diseases, Children's National Health System, Washington, District of Columbia

**Dorothy Y. Harris, MD**
Assistant Professor of Orthopedic Surgery, Baylor College of Medicine, Orthopedic Surgery, Texas Children's Hospital, Houston, Texas

**Lee S. Haruno, BS**
Medical Student, Baylor College of Medicine, Texas Children's Hospital Division of Orthopedic Surgery, Houston, Texas

**Philip J. Hashkes, MD, MSc**
Associate Professor of Pediatrics, Hebrew University School of Medicine; Head, Pediatric Rheumatology Unit, Shaare Zedek Medical Center, Jerusalem, Israel

**Julie Hauer, MD**
Medical Director, Seven Hills Pediatric Center, Division of General Pediatrics, Boston Children's Hospital; Assistant Professor of Pediatrics, Harvard Medical School, Groton, Massachusetts

**Douglas S. Hawkins, MD**
Professor of Pediatrics, University of Washington School of Medicine; Associate Division Chief, Hematology/Oncology, Seattle Children's Hospital, Seattle, Washington

**William W. Hay, Jr., MD**
Professor, University of Colorado School of Medicine, Anschutz Medical Campus, Perinatal Research Center, Aurora, Colorado

**Mary Fran Hazinski, RN, MSN**
Professor, Division of Trauma and Surgical Critical Care, Vanderbilt University School of Nursing, Nashville, Tennessee

**Patrick J. Healey, MD**
Chief, Division of Transplantation, Seattle Children's Hospital; Associate Professor, Department of Surgery, University of Washington School of Medicine, Seattle Children's Hospital, Seattle, Washington

**C. Mary Healy, MD**
Associate Professor of Pediatrics, Infectious Diseases Section, Baylor College of Medicine; Director, Vaccinology and Maternal Immunization, Center for Vaccine Awareness and Research, Texas Children's Hospital, Houston, Texas

**Matthew M. Heeney, MD**
Assistant Professor of Pediatrics, Harvard Medical School; Associate Chief, Hematology, Dana-Farber/Boston Children's Cancer and Blood Disorders Center, Boston, Massachusetts

**Desmond B. Henry, MD**
Professor of Anesthesiology and Pediatrics; Vice Chair, Department of Anesthesiology and Pain Management, University of Texas Southwestern Medical Center; Anesthesiologist-in-Chief, Dallas Children's Hospital, Dallas, Texas

**Honey H. Herce, MD**
Assistant Professor, Departments of Ophthalmology and Pediatrics, Baylor College of Medicine, Texas Children's Hospital, Houston, Texas

**Albert C. Hergenroeder, MD**
Professor, Chief of Section of Adolescent Medicine and Sports Medicine, Department of Pediatrics, Baylor College of Medicine, Houston, Texas

**John A. Herring, MD**
Chief of Staff, Texas Scottish Rite Hospital; Professor, Orthopedic Surgery, UT Southwestern Medical School, Dallas, Texas

**Gurjit K. Khurana Hershey, MD, PhD**
Endowed Professor of Pediatrics; Kindervelt Endowed Chair in Asthma Research; Director, Division of Asthma Research; Attending Physician, Allergy and Immunology, Cincinnati Children's Hospital Medical Center, Cincinnati, Ohio

**Heather Y. Highsmith, MD, MSc**
Assistant Professor of Pediatrics, University of Arkansas for Medical Sciences, Arkansas Children's Hospital, Little Rock, Arkansas

**Friedhelm Hildebrandt, MD**
Professor of Pediatrics, Harvard Medical School; Chief, Division of Nephrology, Boston Children's Hospital, Boston, Massachusetts

**Jaclyn F. Hill, MD**
Assistant Professor of Orthopedic Surgery, Baylor College of Medicine, Orthopedic Surgery, Texas Children's Hospital, Houston, Texas

**Ivor D. Hill, MD**
Professor of Pediatrics, Division of Pediatric Gastroenterology, Hepatology, and Nutrition, The Ohio State University College of Medicine, Nationwide Children's Hospital, Columbus, Ohio

**Christine E. Hill-Kayser, MD**
Assistant Professor of Radiation Oncology, Perelman School of Medicine at the University of Pennsylvania and the Hospital of the University of Pennsylvania, Philadelphia, Pennsylvania

**Ryan Himes, MD**
Clinic Chief, Ambulatory Gastroenterology Clinics, Texas Children's Hospital; Assistant Professor of Pediatrics, Baylor College of Medicine, Houston, Texas

**Linda Tayeko Hiraki, MD, FRCPC, MS, ScD**
Staff Rheumatologist, Hospital for Sick Children, Toronto, Canada

**Nicolette A. Hodyl, PhD, BSc (Hons)**
MS McLeod Research Fellow, Robinson Research Institute, Adelaide Medical School, University of Adelaide, Women's and Children's Health Network, North Adelaide, South Australia

**Mary Ellen Hoehn, MD**
Associate Professor, Departments of Ophthalmology and Pediatrics, Hamilton Eye Institute, University of Tennessee Health Science Center, Memphis, Tennessee

**Edward J. Hoffenberg, MD**
Professor of Pediatrics, University of Colorado School of Medicine; Director, Inflammatory Bowel Diseases Program, Children's Hospital of Colorado, Aurora, Colorado

**Julien I. E. Hoffman, MD, MB BCh**
Professor Emeritus, Department of Pediatrics and Senior Member, Cardiovascular Research Institute, University of California, San Francisco, California

**Michelle A. Hoffman, MD**
Pediatric Infectious Diseases Specialist, Golisano Children's Hospital of Southwest Florida, Pediatric Infectious Diseases, Fort Myers, Florida

**J. Lloyd Holder, Jr., MD**
Assistant Professor of Pediatrics, Baylor College of Medicine, Texas Children's Hospital, Houston, Texas

**Michelle Holick, MD**
Assistant Professor of Pediatrics, Baylor College of Medicine, Texas Children's Hospital, Houston, Texas

**Kristen E. Holland, MD**
Medical Director, Dermatology, Children's Hospital of Wisconsin; Associate Professor, The Medical College of Wisconsin; Children's Hospital of Wisconsin-Milwaukee Campus, Milwaukee, Wisconsin

**Eboni Smith Hollier, MD**
Assistant Professor of Pediatrics, Baylor College of Medicine, Meyer Center for Developmental Pediatrics, Texas Children's Hospital, Houston, Texas

**Jonathan Honegger, MD**
Assistant Professor, Department of Pediatrics, Nationwide Children's Hospital, The Ohio State University, Section of Infectious Diseases, Columbus, Ohio

**Rachel K. Hopper, MD**
Assistant Professor, Department of Pediatrics, Perelman School of Medicine at the University of Pennsylvania; Associate Director, Pulmonary Hypertension Program, Division of Cardiology, Children's Hospital of Philadelphia, Philadelphia, Pennsylvania

**Lisa K. Hornberger, MD**
Professor of Pediatrics and Obstetrics & Gynecology, Pediatric Cardiology, University of Alberta; Section Head, Pediatric Echocardiography; Director, Fetal & Neonatal Cardiology Program, Stollery Children's Hospital, Edmonton, Alberta, Canada

**Peter J. Hotez, MD, PhD**
Dean, National School of Tropical Medicine, Baylor College of Medicine, Houston, Texas

**Gene O. Huang, MD**
Pediatric Urology Fellow, Texas Children's Hospital, Baylor College of Medicine, Houston, Texas

**Walter T. Hughes, MD**
Emeritus, St Jude Faculty, Department of Infectious Diseases, St. Jude Research Hospital, Memphis, Tennessee

**Lisa Humphrey, MD**
Director, Palliative and Hospice Medicine, Nationwide Children's Hospital; Assistant Professor of Pediatrics, The Ohio State University School of Medicine, Columbus, Ohio

**W. Garrett Hunt, MD**
Associate Professor, Department of Pediatrics, Nationwide Children's Hospital, The Ohio State University, Section of Infectious Diseases, Columbus, Ohio

**Raegan Hunt, MD, PhD**
Assistant Professor of Pediatrics and Dermatology, Baylor College of Medicine, Texas Children's Hospital, Houston, Texas

**Thy N. Huynh, MD**
Research Fellow, Department of Pediatric Dermatology, Northwestern University, Feinberg School of Medicine, Chicago, Illinois

**Loris Y. Hwang, MD**
Associate Professor of Pediatrics, Division of Adolescent and Young Adult Medicine, Department of Pediatrics, University of California San Francisco, San Francisco, California

**Sindhu Idicula, MD**
Assistant Professor of Psychiatry and Pediatrics, Menninger Department of Psychiatry, Baylor College of Medicine; Attending Psychiatrist, Texas Children's Hospital, Houston, Texas

**Terrie E. Inder, MB ChB, MD**
Chair, Department of Pediatric Newborn Medicine, Brigham and Women's Hospital; Mary Ellen Avery Professor of Pediatrics in the Field of Newborn Medicine, Harvard Medical School, Boston, Massachusetts

**Charles E. Irwin, Jr., MD**
Distinguished Professor of Pediatrics; Director, Division of Adolescent & Young Adult Medicine; Director, Health Policy, Department of Pediatrics; Director, Adolescent and Young Adult Health National Resource Center, University of California, San Francisco, San Francisco, California

**Reena Isaac, MD**
Assistant Professor of Pediatrics, Section of Public Health Pediatrics, Baylor College of Medicine, Houston, Texas

**Sherwin J. Isenberg, MD**
Lorraine and David Gerber Professor of Ophthalmology, Stein Eye Institute, Department of Ophthalmology, UCLA School of Medicine, Los Angeles, California

**Jaak Jaeken, MD, PhD**
Emeritus Professor of Pediatrics, University Hospital Gasthuisberg, Leuven, Belgium

**Adam Jaffe, MBBS, MD, FRCPCH, FRCP, FRACP, FThorSoc**
John Beveridge Professor of Pediatrics; Faculty of Medicine, University of New South Wales; Head of Discipline of Pediatrics, School of Women's and Children's Health, Sydney, Australia

**Julie Jaffray, MD**
Assistant Professor of Clinical Pediatrics, Keck School of Medicine of University of Southern California, Children's Hospital Los Angeles, Los Angeles, California

**Mahim Jain, MD, PhD**
Assistant Professor, Johns Hopkins School of Medicine, Osteogenesis Imperfecta Clinic, Kennedy Krieger Institute, Baltimore, Maryland

**Katherine A. Janeway, MD, MMSc**
Assistant Professor of Pediatrics, Harvard Medical School; Director, Solid Tumor Service, Dana-Farber/Boston Children's Cancer and Blood Disorders Center, Boston, Massachusetts

**Barbara A. Jantausch, MD**
Professor of Pediatrics, Division of Infectious Diseases, Department of Pediatrics, Children's National Health System/George Washington University School of Medicine, Washington, District of Columbia

**Imad T. Jarjour, MD, FAAN, FAAP**
Associate Professor of Pediatrics, Baylor College of Medicine; Director of Clinic for Autonomic Dysfunction, Texas Children's Hospital, Houston, Texas

**Jill Ann Jarrell, MD, MPH**
Assistant Professor, Section of Palliative Care and Section of Academic General Pediatrics, Baylor College of Medicine, Texas Children's Hospital, Houston, Texas

**Aamir Jeewa, MD**
Assistant Professor, Department of Cardiology, The University of Toronto; Section Head, Cardiomyopathy and Heart Function Program, Hospital for Sick Children, Toronto, Canada

**George S. Jeha, MD**
Assistant Professor, Section of Diabetes and Endocrinology, Baylor College of Medicine, Texas Children's Hospital, Houston, Texas

**Michael Jellinek, MD**
CEO, Lahey Health Community Network; Executive Vice-President, Lahey Health; Professor Emeritus of Psychiatry and of Pediatrics, Harvard Medical School, Boston, Massachusetts

**Erik A. Jensen, MD, MSCE**
Instructor of Pediatrics, Perelman School of Medicine, University of Pennsylvania; Attending Neonatologist, Children's Hospital of Philadelphia, Philadelphia, Pennsylvania

**Traci Jester, MD, RD**
Assistant Professor of Pediatrics, Division of Pediatric Gastroenterology, Hepatology, and Nutrition, University of Alabama at Birmingham, Birmingham, Alabama

**Chandy C. John, MD, MS**
Ryan White Professor of Pediatrics; Professor of Medicine, Microbiology and Immunology, Indiana University School of Medicine; Director, Ryan White Center for Pediatric Infectious Disease and Global Health, Riley Hospital for Children at IU Health, Indianapolis, Indiana

**Candace Johnson, MD**
Postdoctoral Clinical Fellow; Associate Professor of Pediatrics, Division of Pediatric Infectious Diseases, Columbia University Medical Center, New York, New York

**Charles E. Johnston, MD**
Associate Chief of Staff, Texas Scottish Rite Hospital; Professor, Orthopedic Surgery, UT Southwestern Medical School, Dallas, Texas

**Christopher D. Jolley, MD**
Professor, Department of Pediatrics; Chief, Division of Gastroenterology, Hepatology, and Nutrition, University of Florida College of Medicine, Jacksonville, Florida

**Maureen M. Jonas, MD**
Professor of Pediatrics, Harvard Medical School, Center for Childhood Liver Disease, Division of Gastroenterology, Hepatology, and Nutrition, Boston Children's Hospital, Boston, Massachusetts

**Barbara L. Jones, PhD, MSW**
Associate Dean for Health Affairs and Professor, Co-Director, Institute for Collaborative Health Research and Practice, The University of Texas at Austin School of Social Work, Austin, Texas

**Cassandra D. Josephson, MD**
Professor of Pathology and Pediatrics; Director of Clinical Research, Center for Transfusion and Cellular Therapies, Emory University School of Medicine; Medical Director of Tissue Transfusion and Apheresis, Children's Healthcare of Atlanta, Atlanta, Georgia

**Henri Justino, MD**
Associate Professor, Department of Pediatrics, Section of Cardiology, Baylor College of Medicine, Texas Children's Hospital, Houston, Texas

**Stephen G. Kaler, MD**
Senior Investigator, Section on Translational Neuroscience; Molecular Medicine Branch Eunice Kennedy Shriver National Institute of Child Health and Human Development, Bethesda, Maryland

**Sameer Kamath, MD**
Associate Professor, Department of Pediatrics, Division of Critical Care, Duke Children's Hospital, Duke University Medical Center, Durham, North Carolina

**Akinobu Kamei, MD**
Research Associate, Department of Infectious Diseases, St. Jude Children's Research Hospital, Memphis, Tennessee

**Peter B. Kang, MD**
Chief, Division of Pediatric Neurology, Department of Pediatrics, University of Florida College of Medicine, Gainesville, Florida

**Tammy I. Kang, MD, MSCE**
Chief, Palliative Care; Associate Vice Chair, Clinical Affairs, Department of Pediatrics, Baylor College of Medicine, Texas Children's Hospital, Houston, Texas

**Shibani Kanungo, MD, MPH**
Associate Professor, Department of Pediatric and Adolescent Medicine, Western Michigan University Homer Stryker MD School of Medicine, Kalamazoo, Michigan

**Lina Boujaoude Karam, MD**
Assistant Professor, Section of Gastroenterology, Hepatology and Nutrition, Department of Pediatrics, Baylor College of Medicine, Texas Children's Hospital, Houston, Texas

**Lefkothea P. Karaviti, MD, PhD**
Professor, Section of Diabetes and Endocrinology, Department of Pediatrics, Baylor College of Medicine, Texas Children's Hospital, Houston, Texas

**Nadeem Y. Karimbux, DMD, MMSc**
Professor of Periodontology; Associate Dean of Academic Affairs, Tufts University School of Dental Medicine, Boston, Massachusetts

**Lori A. Karol, MD**
Professor of Orthopedic Surgery, University of Texas-Southwestern; Assistant Chief of Staff, Texas Scottish Rite Hospital for Children, Dallas, Texas

**Daniel J. Karr, MD, FAAO, FAAP**
Elks of Oregon Pediatric Ophthalmology Professor, Professor of Ophthalmology and Pediatrics; Director, Elks Children's Eye Clinic, Casey Eye Institute, Oregon Health and Science University, Portland, Oregon

**Clifford E. Kashtan, MD**
Professor of Pediatrics, University of Minnesota Medical School, Minneapolis, Minnesota

**Bhushan Katira, MD**
Fellow in Critical Care Medicine, Hospital for Sick Children, University of Toronto, Toronto, Canada

**Howard M. Katzenstein, MD**
Professor of Pediatrics, Scott and Tracie Hamilton Chair in Cancer Survivorship, Vanderbilt University; Medical Director, Pediatric Hematology-Oncology, Ingram Cancer Center, Nashville, Tennessee

**Beth D. Kaufman, MD**
Clinical Associate Professor of Cardiology, Stanford University, School of Medicine, Lucille-Packard Children's Hospital, Palo Alto, California

**Rajniderpal Kaur, MD**
Child and Adolescent Psychiatry Fellow, Baylor College of Medicine, Houston, Texas

**Brian Kavanagh, MB, FRCPC, FFARCSI (Hon.)**
Professor of Anesthesia, Medicine, and Physiology, University of Toronto; Dr Geoffrey Barker Chair in Critical Care Medicine, Hospital for Sick Children, Toronto, Canada

**Simon Kayyal, MD**
Assistant Professor of Pediatrics, Baylor College of Medicine, Texas Children's Hospital, Houston, Texas

**Amy Keir, MBBS, MPH, FRACP**
Clinical Senior Lecturer, Robinson Research Institute, Adelaide Medical School, University of Adelaide; Consultant Neonatologist, Women's and Children's Health Network, North Adelaide, South Australia

**Andrea Kelly, MD**
Associate Professor of Pediatrics, Department of Pediatrics, University of Pennsylvania Perelman School of Medicine, The Children's Hospital of Philadelphia, Philadelphia, Pennsylvania

**Kara M. Kelly, MD**
Professor of Pediatrics, University at Buffalo Jacobs School of Medicine and Biomedical Sciences; Chair, Pediatric Oncology, Roswell Park Cancer Institute, Buffalo, New York

**Michael E. Kelly, MD, PhD**
Director, Pediatric Cancer Program, Children's Hospital of Wisconsin; Associate Professor of Pediatrics, Medical College of Wisconsin, Milwaukee, Wisconsin

**John M. Kelso, MD**
Division of Allergy, Asthma and Immunology, Scripps Clinic; Clinical Professor of Pediatrics, University of California San Diego School of Medicine, San Diego, California

**Leila Kheirandish-Gozal, MD, MSc**
Professor of Pediatrics, The University of Chicago, Chicago, Illinois

**Monica R. Khitri, MD**
Clinical Instructor, UCLA Doheny Eye Center, Pasadena, California

**David M. Kim, DDMs, DMSc**
Associate Professor of Oral Medicine, Infection, and Immunity; Director of the Postgraduate Program in Periodontology and the Continuing Education, Harvard School of Dental Medicine; Clinical Associate in Dentistry, Oral and Maxillofacial Surgery, Massachusetts General Hospital, Boston, Massachusetts

**Jeffrey J. Kim, MD**
Director, Electrophysiology and Pacing, Section of Pediatric Cardiology, Department of Pediatrics, Baylor College of Medicine, Texas Children's Hospital, Houston, Texas

**David W. Kimberlin, MD**
Professor and Vice Chair for Clinical and Translational Research, Department of Pediatrics; Sergio Stagno Endowed Chair in Pediatric Infectious Diseases, The University of Alabama at Birmingham, Birmingham, Alabama

**Yukiko Kimura, MD**
Chief, Pediatric Rheumatology Joseph M. Sanzari Children's Hospital, Hackensack University Medical Center, Hackensack, New Jersey

**Kristi King, MPH, RDN, LD, CNSC**
Instructor, Baylor College of Medicine, Section of Gastroenterology, Hepatology, and Nutrition, Texas Children's Hospital, Houston, Texas

**Haresh Kirpalani, MD**
Professor of Pediatrics, Perelman School of Medicine, University of Pennsylvania, Children's Hospital of Philadelphia, Philadelphia, Pennsylvania

**Priya S. Kishnani, MD**
C.L. and Su Chen Professor of Pediatrics; Medical Director, YT and Alice Chen Pediatrics Genetics and Genomics Center; Division Chief, Medical Genetics, Duke University Medical Center, Durham, North Carolina

**Niranjan Kissoon, MD, FRCP(C), FAAP, MCCM, FACPE**
Professor, BCCH and UBC Global Child Health, Department of Pediatrics and Emergency Medicine, University of British Columbia; Vice President, Medical Affairs, BC Children's Hospital and Sunny Hill Health Centre; Clinical Investigator, Child and Family Research Institute, Vancouver, British Columbia, Canada

**Ronald Kleinman, MD**
Charles Wilder Professor of Pediatrics, Harvard Medical School; Physician in Chief, MassGeneral Hospital for Children, Boston, Massachusetts

**Katherine M. Knapp, MD**
Staff Physician, Infectious Diseases, St. Jude Children's Research Hospital, Memphis, Tennessee

**Richard Ko, MD, MS**
Assistant Professor of Clinical Pediatrics, Keck School of Medicine of University of Southern California; Medical Director, Clinical Coagulation Laboratory, Children's Hospital Los Angeles, Los Angeles, California

**David M. Koeller, MD**
Professor of Molecular and Medical Genetics, Oregon Health and Science University, Portland, Oregon

**Chester J. Koh, MD, FACS, FAAP**
Associate Professor of Urology (Pediatric), Pediatrics, and Obstetrics and Gynecology, Texas Children's Hospital, Baylor College of Medicine, Houston, Texas

**E. Anders Kolb, MD**
Associate Professor and Vice Chairman for Research, Department of Pediatrics, Sidney Kimmel Medical College at Thomas Jefferson University; Director, Nemours Center for Cancer and Blood Disorders, Nemours/Alfred I. duPont Hospital for Children, Wilmington, Delaware

**Katja Kovacic, MD**
Assistant Professor, Center for Pediatric Neurogastroenterology, Motility, and Autonomic Disorders, Division of Gastroenterology, Hepatology and Nutrition, Department of Pediatrics, Medical College of Wisconsin, Milwaukee, Wisconsin

**Claire Kovalchin, BS**
Center for Perinatal Research, Nationwide Children's Hospital, Columbus, Ohio

**Carrie L. Kovarik, MD**
Associate Professor, Dermatology, Dermatopathology, and Infectious Diseases, University of Pennsylvania, Philadelphia, Pennsylvania

**Eva Morava Kozicz, MD, PhD**
Professor of Pediatrics, Hayward Genetics Center, Tulane University Medical School, New Orleans, Louisiana

**Peter J. Krause, MD**
Senior Research Scientist, Yale School of Public Health and Yale School of Medicine, New Haven, Connecticut

**Jacqueline Kreutzer, MD**
Professor of Pediatrics, University of Pittsburgh School of Medicine; Chief of Cardiology, Children's Hospital of Pittsburgh, Pittsburgh, Pennsylvania

**Subra Kugathasan, MD**
Professor of Pediatrics, Division of Pediatric Gastroenterology, Hepatology, and Nutrition, Emory University School of Medicine, Atlanta, Georgia

**Manisha Kulkarni, PhD**
Assistant Professor, School of Epidemiology, Public Health and Preventive Medicine, University of Ottawa, Ontario, Canada

**Madan Kumar, DO**
Pediatric Infectious Diseases Fellow, Children's National Health System, Washington, DC

**Annie F. Kuo, MD**
Assistant Professor of Ophthalmology, Casey Eye Institute, Oregon Health and Science University, Portland, Oregon

**Geoffrey Kurland, MD**
Professor of Pediatrics, University of Pittsburgh School of Medicine, Pittsburgh, Pennsylvania

**Indranil Kushare, MD**
Assistant Professor of Orthopedic Surgery, Baylor College of Medicine; Pediatric Orthopedic Surgeon, Texas Children's Hospital, Houston, Texas

**Jake Kushner, MD**
Associate Professor, Departments of Pediatrics, Baylor College of Medicine, Houston, Texas

**Satyan Lakshminrusimha, MD**
Professor and Vice-Chair of Pediatrics, State University of New York at Buffalo; Chief, Division of Neonatology, Women and Children's Hospital of Buffalo, Buffalo, New York

**Seema R. Lalani, MD**
Associate Professor, Molecular and Human Genetics Department, Baylor College of Medicine/Texas Children's Hospital; Assistant Laboratory Director, Cytogenetics Laboratory, Baylor Genetics, Houston, Texas

**Fong Lam, MD, FAAP**
Assistant Professor of Pediatrics, Baylor College of Medicine, Texas Children's Hospital, Houston, Texas

**Elton M. Lambert, MD**
Assistant Professor, Baylor College of Medicine, Department of Otolaryngology, Texas Children's Hospital, Houston, Texas

**Wendy Gwirtzman Lane, MD, MPH**
Associate Professor, Department of Epidemiology and Public Health, Department of Pediatrics, University of Maryland School of Medicine, Baltimore, Maryland

**Valerie Langlois, MD, FRC**
Staff Nephrologist, Division of Nephrology, The Hospital for Sick Children; Assistant Professor, University of Toronto, Toronto, Ontario, Canada

**Charles Larson, MDCM, FRCPC**
Intensivist, Pediatric Intensive Care Unit, The Royal Children's Hospital, Melbourne, Australia

**Catherine Larson-Nath, MD**
Assistant Professor, Department of Pediatrics, University of Minnesota; Pediatric Gastroenterology, Hepatology, and Nutrition, University of Minnesota Masonic Children's Hospital, Minneapolis, Minnesota

**Javier J. Lasa, MD, FAAP**
Assistant Professor of Pediatrics, Baylor College of Medicine, Texas Children's Hospital, Houston, Texas

**Kathleen M. Leack, MS, RN, CNS**
Clinical Nurse Specialist—Pediatric General Surgery, Children's Hospital of Wisconsin, Milwaukee, Wisconsin

**Ann-Marie Leahey, MD**
Clinical Professor of Pediatrics, Perelman School of Medicine of the University of Pennsylvania, Children's Hospital of Philadelphia, Philadelphia, Pennsylvania

**Brendan Lee, MD, PhD**
Professor, Department of Molecular and Human Genetics, Baylor College of Medicine, Texas Children's Hospital, Houston, Texas

**Henry C. Lee, MD**
Associate Professor of Pediatrics, Stanford University Division of Neonatal and Developmental Medicine, Lucile Packard Children's Hospital, Palo Alto, California

**Deborah Lehman, MD**
Clinical Professor, Pediatrics Infectious Diseases, David Geffen School of Medicine at UCLA, Los Angeles, California

**Daniel Spencer Lemke, MD**
Assistant Professor of Pediatrics, Baylor College of Medicine, Texas Children's Hospital, Houston, Texas

**David S. Leslie, MD**
Attending Physician, Franciscan Hospital for Children, Brighton, Massachusetts

**Ariadne Letra, DDS, MS, PhD**
Associate Professor of Diagnostic and Biomedical Sciences, University of Texas Health Science Center at Houston School of Dentistry, Craniofacial Research Center, Houston, Texas

**Daniel Leung, MD, MSc**
Assistant Professor of Medicine, Division of Infectious Diseases, University of Utah School of Medicine, Salt Lake City, Utah

**John M. Leventhal, MD**
Professor of Pediatrics, Yale School of Medicine, New Haven, Connecticut

**Alex V. Levin, MD, MHSc, FRCSC**
Chief, Pediatric Ophthalmology and Ocular Genetics; Robison D. Harley, MD Endowed Chair in Pediatric Ophthalmology and Ocular Genetics, Wills Eye Hospital; Professor, Departments of Ophthalmology and Pediatrics, Sidney Kimmel Medical College at Thomas Jefferson University, Philadelphia, Pennsylvania

**John E. Levine, MD, MS**
Professor of Pediatrics and Internal Medicine, Icahn School of Medicine at Mount Sinai; Director of BMT Clinical Research, Tisch Cancer Institute, New York, New York

**Saul Levine, MD**
Professor Emeritus of Psychiatry, University of California, San Diego, San Diego, California

**Moise L. Levy, MD**
Physician-in-Chief, Dell Children's Medical Center; Professor of Pediatrics Dell Medical School, University of Texas at Austin; Pediatric/Adolescent Dermatology, Austin, Texas

**Shih-Ning Liaw, MD**
Site Director, Boston Children's Hospital; Harvard Interprofessional Palliative Care Fellowship, Division of Pediatric Palliative Care, Department of Psychosocial Oncology and Palliative Care, Dana-Farber Cancer Institute; Instructor in Pediatrics, Harvard Medical School, Boston, Massachusetts

**Bryan Liming, MD, MAJ(USA)**
Fellow, Pediatric Otolaryngology, University of Iowa Health Care/Carver College of Medicine, Department of Otolaryngology—Head and Neck Surgery, Iowa City, Iowa

**Tom K. Lin, MD**
Associate Professor, University of Cincinnati Department of Pediatrics, Division of Gastroenterology, Hepatology and Nutrition, Cincinnati Children's Hospital Medical Center, Cincinnati, Ohio

**Yuezhen Lin, MD**
Assistant Professor of Pediatrics, Section of Diabetes and Endocrinology, Baylor College of Medicine, Texas Children's Hospital, Houston, Texas

**Pengfei Liu, PhD, FACMGG**
Assistant Professor of Molecular and Human Genetics; Assistant Laboratory Director of Baylor Genetics, Baylor College of Medicine, Houston, Texas

**Yi-Chun Liu, MD**
Assistant Professor, Baylor College of Medicine, Otolaryngology, Texas Children's Hospital, Houston, Texas

**Maya B. Lodish, MD, MHSc**
Staff Clinician, Section on Endocrinology and Genetics, Eunice Kennedy Shriver National Institute of Child Health and Human Development, National Institutes of Health, Bethesda, Maryland

**Lindsey Loomba-Albrecht, MD**
Assistant Clinical Professor, Department of Pediatrics, UC Davis, Sacramento, California

**Kimberly Kay Lopez, DrPH, MPH**
Assistant Professor, Public Health Pediatrics, Baylor College of Medicine, Houston, Texas

**Michael A. Lopez, MD, PhD**
Child Neurology Resident, Section of Pediatric Neurology and Developmental Neuroscience, Baylor College of Medicine, Texas Children's Hospital, Houston, Texas

**Michelle Lopez, MD**
Assistant Professor of Pediatrics, Baylor College of Medicine, Texas Children's Hospital, Houston, Texas

**Timothy E. Lotze, MD**
Associate Professor of Pediatrics, Baylor College of Medicine, Texas Children's Hospital, Houston, Texas

**James R. Lupski, MD, PhD, DSc (Hon)**
Professor of Pediatrics, Integrative, Molecular, Biomedical Sciences and Translational Biology, Molecular and Human Genetics, Baylor College of Medicine, Houston, Texas

**Keren Machol, MD, PhD**
Assistant Professor, Department of Molecular and Human Genetics, Baylor College of Medicine, Houston, Texas

**Charles G. Macias, MD, MPH**
Associate Professor of Pediatrics, Department of Pediatrics, Baylor College of Medicine; Chief Clinical Systems Integration Officer, Texas Children's Hospital, Houston, Texas

**Jeanine Maclin, MD, MPH**
Associate Professor of Pediatrics, Division of Pediatric Gastroenterology, Hepatology and Nutrition, University of Alabama at Birmingham, Birmingham, Alabama

**Pilar L. Magoulas, MS, CGC**
Assistant Professor, Department of Molecular and Human Genetics, Baylor College of Medicine; Chief, Division of Genetic Counseling, Texas Children's Hospital, Houston, Texas

**Sheilagh M. Maguiness, MD**
Assistant Professor, Dermatology and Pediatrics, Department of Dermatology, University of Minnesota, Minneapolis, Minnesota

**Ilan Maizlin, MD**
Research Fellow, Division of Pediatric Surgery, University of Alabama at Birmingham, Children's Hospital of Alabama, Birmingham, Alabama

**Joseph A. Majzoub, MD**
Chief, Division of Endocrinology, Professor of Pediatrics and Medicine Harvard Medical School, Boston Children's Hospital, Boston, Massachusetts

**Yvonne (Bonnie) A. Maldonado, MD**
Senior Associate Dean for Faculty Development and Diversity; Professor of Pediatrics and Health Research and Policy; Director, Global Child Health; Chief, Division of Pediatric Infectious Diseases, Stanford University School of Medicine; Berger-Raynolds Distinguished Fellow and Attending Physician, Lucile Packard Children's Hospital, Stanford, California

**George B. Mallory, MD**
Professor of Pediatrics, Baylor College of Medicine; Medical Director, Lung Transplant Program; Texas Children's Hospital, Houston, Texas

**Mark J. Manary, MD**
Helene Roberson Professor of Pediatrics, Washington University School of Medicine, St. Louis, Missouri

**Pedro Mancias, MD**
Professor, Department of Pediatrics, McGovern Medical School at The University of Texas Health Science Center, Houston, Texas

**George Thomas Mandy, MD**
Associate Professor of Pediatrics, Baylor College of Medicine, Texas Children's Hospital, Houston, Texas

**Mona E. Mansour, MD**
Professor of Pediatrics, Cincinnati Children's Hospital, Cincinnati, Ohio

**Nizar F. Maraqa, MD, FAAP, FPIDS**
Associate Professor, Pediatric Infectious Diseases and Immunology, University of Florida College of Medicine, University of Florida Center for HIV/AIDS, Research, Education & Service (UF CARES); CMS HIV Program Director, Jacksonville, Florida

**Monica L. Marcus, DO**
Assistant Professor of Pediatrics, Baylor College of Medicine, Texas Children's Hospital, Houston, Texas

**Peter Margolis, MD, PhD**
Professor of Pediatrics, University of Cincinnati College of Medicine, Cincinnati Children's Hospital, Cincinnati, Ohio

**Ketzela J. Marsh, MD, MS**
Fellow, Infectious Diseases, University of Minnesota, Minneapolis, Minnesota

**Colin A. Martin, MD**
Associate Professor, Division of Pediatric Surgery, University of Alabama at Birmingham, Children's Hospital of Alabama, Birmingham, Alabama

**Bernadette Martineau, MS**
Clinical Nutritionist, Inflammatory Bowel Disease Program, Emory University School of Medicine, Division of Pediatric Gastroenterology, Hepatology, and Nutrition, Department of Pediatrics, Atlanta, Georgia

**Ahmed I. Marwan, MD**
Assistant Professor of Surgery and Pediatrics, Colorado Fetal Care Center, Children's Hospital Colorado, University of Colorado School of Medicine, Aurora, Colorado

**Douglas P. Marx, MD**
Assistant Professor of Ophthalmology, Cullen Eye Institute, Baylor College of Medicine, Houston, Texas

**Roshni Mathew, MD**
Clinical Assistant Professor, Department of Pediatrics, Division of Infectious Diseases, Stanford University, Stanford, California

**Sravan Reddy Matta, MBBS**
Assistant Professor of Pediatrics, George Washington University; Attending Physician, Pediatric Gastroenterology, Children's National Medical Center, Washington, District of Columbia

**Thomas Wm. Mayo, JD**
Associate Professor, Southern Methodist University, Dedman School of Law; Adjunct Associate Professor, Internal Medicine, University of Texas Southwestern Medical School, Dallas, Texas

**Bonnie McCann-Crosby, MD**
Assistant Professor, Division of Pediatric Endocrinology, Baylor College of Medicine, Texas Children's Hospital, Houston, Texas

**Kenneth McClain, MD, PhD**
Professor, Department of Pediatrics, Baylor College of Medicine; Co-Director TXCH Histiocytosis Program, Texas Children's Cancer and Hematology Centers, Houston, Texas

**George McDaniel, MD**
Assistant Professor, Department of Pediatrics, University of Virginia Health System, Charlottesville, Virginia

**Scott D. McKay, MD**
Assistant Professor, Baylor College of Medicine, Orthopedic Surgery, Texas Children's Hospital, Houston, Texas

**Siripoom McKay, MD**
Assistant Professor, Section of Diabetes and Endocrinology, Baylor College of Medicine, Texas Children's Hospital, Houston, Texas

**Holly Meany, MD**
Associate Professor of Pediatrics, George Washington University School of Medicine and Health Sciences, Children's National Medical Center, Washington, District of Columbia

**Jennifer Mehl, MD**
Resident, Department of Pediatrics, Baylor College of Medicine, Houston, Texas

**Deepak K. Mehta, MD, FRCS**
Associate Professor of Otolaryngology, Baylor College of Medicine; Director, Pediatric Aerodigestive Center, Texas Children's Hospital, Houston, Texas

**H. Cody Meissner, MD**
Professor of Pediatrics, Tufts University School of Medicine; Director, Pediatric Infectious Disease Division, Tufts Medical Center, Boston, Massachusetts

**Asuncion Mejias, MD, PhD, MsCS**
Associate Professor of Pediatrics, Nationwide Children's Hospital—The Ohio State University, Columbus, Ohio

**Meenal Mendiratta, MD**
Pediatric Endocrinologist, Valley Children's Healthcare, Madera, California

**Noel Mensah-Bonsu, MD**
Developmental-Behavioral Pediatrics Fellow, Baylor College of Medicine, Meyer Center for Developmental Pediatrics, Texas Children's Hospital, Houston, Texas

**Nadia Merchant, MD**
Clinical Postdoctoral Fellow, Section of Diabetes and Endocrinology, Baylor College of Medicine, Texas Children's Hospital, Houston, Texas

**Soheil Meshinchi, MD, PhD**
Professor of Pediatrics, University of Washington School of Medicine; Full Member, Fred Hutchinson Cancer Research Center; Attending Physician, Seattle Children's Hospital, Seattle, Washington

**Mindl M. Messinger, PharmD**
Instructor in Pediatrics, Baylor College of Medicine; Clinical Pharmacy Specialist, Texas Children's Hospital, Houston, Texas

**Jose Mestre, MD**
Professor of Pediatrics, Division of Pediatric Gastroenterology, Hepatology, and Nutrition, University of Alabama at Birmingham, Birmingham, Alabama

**Janel A. Meyer, BSN, RN**
Gastrostomy Resource Nurse Clinician, Children's Hospital of Wisconsin, Milwaukee, Wisconsin

**Wayne M. Meyers, MD, PhD**
Department of Environmental and Infectious Disease Sciences, Armed Forces Institute of Pathology, Washington, District of Columbia

**Mohammad Mhaissen, MD**
Clinical Instructor (Affiliated), Stanford University School of Medicine, Valley Children's Hospital, Madera, California

**Walter L. Miller, MD**
Distinguished Professor of Pediatrics, Emeritus, University of California, San Francisco, San Francisco, California

**Tamir Miloh, MD**
Associate Professor, Section of Pediatric Gastroenterology, Hepatology, and Nutrition, Texas Children's Hospital and Baylor College of Medicine, Houston, Texas

**Adnan Mir, MD, PhD**
Assistant Professor, Pediatric Dermatology and Dermatopathology, University of Texas Southwestern Medical Center, Dallas, Texas

**Adrian Miranda, MD**
Associate Professor, Center for Pediatric Neurogastroenterology, Motility, and Autonomic Disorders, Division of Gastroenterology, Hepatology and Nutrition, Department of Pediatrics, Medical College of Wisconsin, Milwaukee, Wisconsin

**Ayesha Mirza, MD, FAAP**
Associate Professor, Department of Pediatrics, Division of Pediatric Infectious Diseases and Immunology, University of Florida; Program Director, Pediatric Residency Program, University of Florida, Jacksonville, Florida

**Sanghamitra M. Misra, MD, FAAP, ABIHM**
Assistant Professor of Pediatrics, Section of Academic General Pediatrics, Baylor College of Medicine/Texas Children's Hospital, Houston, Texas

**Sunita N. Misra, MD, PhD**
Instructor in Pediatrics, Baylor College of Medicine, Texas Children's Hospital, Houston, Texas

**Joseph P. Mizgerd, ScD**
Professor of Medicine, Microbiology, and Biochemistry, Pulmonary Center, Boston University School of Medicine, Boston, Massachusetts

**Brady S. Moffett, PharmD, MPH**
Assistant Professor of Pediatrics, Baylor College of Medicine; Clinical Pharmacy Specialist, Texas Children's Hospital, Houston, Texas

**Silvana Molossi, MD, PhD**
Medical Director, Community and Program Development, Cardiology, Baylor College of Medicine, Texas Children's Hospital, Houston, Texas

**Erica B. Monasterio, MN, FNP-BC**
Nursing Faculty, Division of Adolescent and Young Adult Medicine, University of California, San Francisco, San Francisco, California

**Sonia Monteiro, MD**
Assistant Professor of Pediatrics, Baylor College of Medicine, Meyer Center for Developmental Pediatrics, Texas Children's Hospital, Houston, Texas

**Nicole Montgomery, MD**
Assistant Professor, Baylor College of Medicine, Orthopedic Surgery, Texas Children's Hospital, Houston, Texas

**Heather Moore, MD**
Assistant Professor of Pediatrics, Baylor College of Medicine, Texas Children's Hospital, Houston, Texas

**Lee E. Morris, MD, MSPH, DTM&H**
Associate Professor, Pediatric Infectious Disease and Immunology, Levine Children's Hospital, Department of Pediatrics, Carolinas HealthCare System, Charlotte, North Carolina

**Wynne Morrison, MD, MBE**
Director, Pediatric Advanced Care Team, The Children's Hospital of Philadelphia; Associate Professor, Department of Anesthesiology and Critical Care, Perelman School of Medicine at the University of Pennsylvania, Philadelphia, Pennsylvania

**Vincent E. Mortellaro, MD**
Assistant Professor, Division of Pediatric Surgery, University of Alabama at Birmingham, Children's Hospital of Alabama, Birmingham, Alabama

**Anna-Barbara Moscicki, MD**
Professor of Pediatrics; Chief, Division of Adolescent and Young Adult Medicine, Department of Pediatrics, David Geffen School of Medicine, University of California, Los Angeles, California

**Salina Mostajabian, MD**
Clinical Postdoctoral Fellow, Department of Pediatrics, Section of Adolescent Medicine and Sports Medicine, Baylor College of Medicine, Houston, Texas

**Kathleen J. Motil, MD, PhD**
Professor, Pediatric-Gastroenterology, Hepatology and Nutrition, Baylor College of Medicine, Texas Children's Hospital, Houston, Texas

**Dennis L. Murray, MD, FAAP, FIDSA**
Clinical Professor, Department of Pediatrics, Augusta University, Augusta, Georgia

**Thomas S. Murray, MD, PhD**
Attending Physician, Infectious Disease, Connecticut Children's Medical Center, Hartford, Connecticut; Associate Professor Frank H Netter MD School of Medicine, Quinnipiac University, Hamden, Connecticut

**Eyal Musca, MD**
Associate Professor of Pediatrics, Baylor College of Medicine, Texas Children's Hospital, Houston, Texas

**Mary Frances Musso, DO, BA**
Assistant Professor, Ear, Nose and Throat Service, Baylor College of Medicine, Texas Children's Hospital, Houston, Texas

**Michael. J. Muszynski, MD, FAAP**
Regional Campus Dean, Associate Dean for Clinical Research, Professor of Clinical Sciences and Pediatric Infectious Disease, Florida State University College of Medicine, Orlando, Florida

**Sandesh C. S. Nagamani, MBBS, MD**
Assistant Professor; Director, Clinical Research Division, Department of Molecular and Human Genetics, Baylor College of Medicine, Texas Children's Hospital, Houston, Texas

**Suresh Nagappan, MD, MSPH**
Pediatric Teaching Program, Cone Health, Greensboro, North Carolina

**Kirsti Näntö-Salonen, MD, PhD**
Pediatric Endocrinologist, Department of Pediatrics, Turku University Hospital, Turku, Finland

**Anupama Narla, MD**
Assistant Professor of Pediatrics, Stanford University School of Medicine, Lucile Salter Packard Children's Hospital, Stanford, California

**Girija Natarajan, MD**
Associate Professor, Department of Pediatrics, Wayne State University; Children's Hospital of Michigan and Hutzel Women's Hospital, Detroit, Michigan

**Pamela G. Nathanson, MBE**
Program Manager, Department of Medical Ethics, The Children's Hospital of Philadelphia, Philadelphia, Pennsylvania

**Heather E. Needham, MD, MPH**
Assistant Professor of Pediatrics, Division of Adolescent Medicine and Sports Medicine, Department of Pediatrics, Baylor College of Medicine, Texas Children's Hospital, Houston, Texas

**Howard L. Needleman, DMD**
Professor of Developmental Biology (Pediatric Dentistry), Harvard School of Dental Medicine; Senior Associate in Dentistry, Boston Children's Hospital, Boston, Massachusetts

**Mark S. Needles, MD**
Medical Officer, Center for Drug Evaluation and Research, US Food and Drug Administration, White Oak, Maryland

**Linda P. Nelson, DMD, MScD**
Lecturer, Developmental Biology (Pediatric Dentistry), Harvard School of Dental Medicine; Senior Associate in Dentistry, Boston Children's Hospital, Boston, Massachusetts

**Marie V. Nelson, MD**
Assistant Professor of Pediatrics, George Washington University School of Medicine and Health Sciences; Attending Physician, Division of Oncology, Children's National Health System, Washington, District of Columbia

**Josef Neu, MD**
Professor of Pediatrics, University of Florida, Jacksonville, Florida

**Jane W. Newburger, MD, MPH**
Commonwealth Professor of Pediatrics, Harvard Medical School; Associate Chief for Academic Affairs, Department of Cardiology, Boston Children's Hospital, Boston, Massachusetts

**Beverley Newman, BSc, MB BCh, FACR**
Professor of Radiology, Stanford University; Associate Chief of Pediatric Radiology, Lucile Packard Children's Hospital, Stanford, California

**Man Wai Ng, DDS, MPH**
Associate Professor of Developmental Biology (Pediatric Dentistry), Harvard School of Dental Medicine; Dentist-In-Chief, DentaQuest Endowed Chair in Pediatric Oral Health and Dentistry, Boston Children's Hospital, Boston, Massachusetts

**Vicky Lee Ng, MD**
Professor of Pediatrics, Hospital for Sick Children, University of Toronto, Toronto, Canada

**Thuy L. Ngo, DO, MEd**
Assistant Professor, Department of Pediatrics, Johns Hopkins University School of Medicine, Baltimore, Maryland

**Nathalie Nguyen, MD**
Assistant Professor of Pediatrics, Digestive Health Institute, Gastrointestinal Eosinophilic Diseases Program, Children's Hospital Colorado, University of Colorado School of Medicine, Aurora, Colorado

**Trung C. Nguyen, MD**
Associate Professor of Pediatrics, Baylor College of Medicine, Texas Children's Hospital, Houston, Texas

**Christian Niedzwecki, DO**
Assistant Professor of Pediatrics, Baylor College of Medicine, Texas Children's Hospital, Houston, Texas

**Peter A. Nigrovic, MD**
Associate Professor of Medicine, Harvard Medical School; Staff Rheumatologist, Boston Children's Hospital; Director, Center for Adults with Pediatric Rheumatic Illness (CAPRI), Brigham and Women's Hospital, Boston, Massachusetts

**Harri Niinikoski, MD, PhD**
Professor, Department of Pediatrics, Turku University Hospital, Turku, Finland

**Richard J. Noel, MD, PhD**
Assistant Professor; Section Chief, Division of Pediatric Gastroenterology, Hepatology, and Nutrition, Duke University Medical Center, Durham, North Carolina

**Cory V. Noel, MD**
Pediatric Cardiologist, Department of Pediatrics, Baylor College of Medicine; Medical Director of MRI (Cardiology), Texas Children's Hospital, Houston, Texas

**Damien Noone, MB BCh, BAO, MSc**
Assistant Professor, University of Toronto; Staff Nephrologist, Division of Nephrology, The Hospital for Sick Children, Toronto, Ontario, Canada

**Luigi D. Notarangelo, MD**
Chief, Laboratory of Clinical Immunology and Microbiology, National Institute of Allergy and Infectious Diseases, National Institute of Health, Bethesda, Maryland

**Aura M. Obando, MD**
Family Team Medical Director, Boston Health Care for the Homeless Program, Massachusetts General Hospital/Harvard Medical School, Boston, Massachusetts

**Matthew J. O'Connor, MD**
Assistant Professor of Clinical Pediatrics, Division of Cardiology, Department of Pediatrics, University of Pennsylvania Perelman School of Medicine; Attending Cardiologist, The Children's Hospital of Philadelphia, Philadelphia, Pennsylvania

**Teresia O'Connor, MD, MPH**
Associate Professor of Pediatrics, Baylor College of Medicine, USDA/ARS Children's Nutrition Research Center, Academic General Pediatrics, Houston, Texas

**Scott Oishi, MD**
Professor, University of Texas Southwestern Medical School; Director, Hand Services, Texas Scottish Rite Hospital for Children, The Charles E. Seay, Jr. Hand Center, Dallas, Texas

**Chee Y. Ooi, MBBS, Dip Paeds, FRACP, PhD**
Senior Lecturer and Consultant in Pediatric Gastroenterology, School of Women's and Children's Health, UNSW Medicine, UNSW, Sydney, Australia

**Jordan S. Orange, MD, PhD**
Chief, Immunology, Allergy and Rheumatology; Director, Center for Human Immunobiology; Louis and Marybeth Pawleek Endowed Chair, Texas Children's Hospital; Professor of Pediatrics, Pathology, and Immunology; Vice Chair for Research, Department of Pediatrics, Baylor College of Medicine, Houston, Texas

**Kathryn K. Ostermaier, MD**
Associate Professor of Pediatrics, Baylor College of Medicine, Meyer Center for Developmental Pediatrics, Texas Children's Hospital, Houston, Texas

**Gary D. Overturf, MD**
Professor of Pathology; Professor Emeritus Pediatric Infectious Diseases, The University of New Mexico Health Sciences Center, Department of Pediatrics, University of New Mexico, Albuquerque, New Mexico

**Elizabeth M. Ozer, PhD**
Professor, Division of Adolescent and Young Adult Medicine, Department of Pediatrics, UCSF Benioff Children's Hospital; Director of Research, UCSF Office of Diversity and Outreach, University of California, San Francisco, San Francisco, California

**Bonnie L. Padwa, MD, DMD**
Associate Professor, Department of Plastic and Oral Surgery, Harvard School of Dental Medicine; Oral Surgeon-in-Chief, Boston Children's Hospital, Boston, Massachusetts

**Elizabeth L. Palavecino, MD**
Professor of Pathology; Director of Clinical Microbiology Laboratory, Wake Forest School of Medicine, Medical Center Boulevard, Winston Salem, North Carolina

**Debra L. Palazzi, MD, MEd**
Associate Professor of Pediatrics, Infectious Diseases Section, Baylor College of Medicine; Chief, Infectious Diseases Clinic, Texas Children's Hospital, Houston, Texas

**Joseph J. Palermo, MD, PhD**
Associate Professor, University of Cincinnati Department of Pediatrics, Division of Gastroenterology, Hepatology, and Nutrition, Cincinnati Children's Hospital Medical Center, Cincinnati, Ohio

**Judith S. Palfrey, MD, FAAP**
T. Berry Brazelton Professor of Pediatrics, Professor of Global Health and Social Medicine, Harvard Medical School, Boston Children's Hospital, Boston, Massachusetts

**Sirish K. Palle, MD**
Assistant Professor of Pediatrics, Division of Pediatric Gastroenterology, Department of Pediatrics, Oklahoma University Health Sciences Center, Oklahoma City, Oklahoma

**Amy S. Paller, MS, MD**
Chair, Department of Dermatology; Director, Northwestern University Skin Disease Research Center (SDRC); Walter J. Hamlin Professor of Dermatology, Lurie Children's Hospital of Chicago, Chicago, Illinois

**Mohan Pammi, MD, PhD, MRCPCH**
Associate Professor of Pediatrics, Baylor College of Medicine; Medical Director, NICU at Pavilion for Women, Texas Children's Hospital, Houston, Texas

**Charalampia Papadopoulou, MD**
Clinical Research Fellow in Pediatric Rheumatology, UCL Great Ormond Street Institute of Child Health, London, United Kingdom

**Nethnapha Paredes, BSc (Hons)**
Department of Pediatrics, McMaster University, Hamilton, Ontario, Canada

**Mered Parnes, MD**
Assistant Professor of Pediatrics, Baylor College of Medicine; Director, Pediatric Movement Disorders Clinic, Texas Children's Hospital, Houston, Texas

**Juan M. Pascual, MD, PhD**
Associate Professor, The University of Texas Southwestern Medical Center, Neurology and Neurotherapeutics, UT Southwestern Medical Center, Dallas, Texas

**Ravi Mangal Patel, MD, MSc**
Assistant Professor of Pediatrics, Emory University School of Medicine and Children's Healthcare of Atlanta, Atlanta, Georgia

**Maria Jevitz Patterson, MD, PhD**
Professor Emerita, Departments of Microbiology/Molecular Genetics and Pediatrics, Michigan State University, Flint, Michigan

**Andrew T. Pavia, MD**
George and Esther Gross Presidential Professor of Pediatrics and Medicine; Chief, Division of Pediatric Infectious Disease, University of Utah, Salt Lake City, Utah

**Cynthia Peacock, MD**
Associate Professor of Internal Medicine and Pediatrics, Baylor College of Medicine, Texas Children's Hospital, Houston, Texas

**Davut Pehlivan, MD**
Clinical Fellow at Division of Pediatric Neurology, Baylor College of Medicine, Houston, Texas

**Stephen I. Pelton, MD**
Professor of Pediatrics and Epidemiology, Boston University Schools of Medicine and Public Health; Chief, Section of Pediatric Infectious Diseases, Boston Medical Center, Boston, Massachusetts

**Daniel J. Penny, MD, PhD**
Professor of Pediatrics, Baylor College of Medicine; Chief of Cardiology, Texas Children's Hospital, Houston, Texas

**Lena Perger, MD**
Assistant Professor of Surgery and Pediatrics, Texas A&M College of Medicine, Baylor Scott and White Healthcare, McLane's Children's Hospital, Temple, Texas

**Mark J. Peters, MB ChB, MRCP, FRCPCH, PhD**
Professor of Pediatric Intensive Care, University College of London; Consultant Intensivist, Great Ormond Street Hospital, London, UK

**Sarah M. Phillips, RD, LD**
Instructor, Nutrition Services, Baylor College of Medicine, Texas Children's Hospital, Houston, Texas

**William A. Phillips, MD**
Professor, Orthopedics and Pediatrics, Pediatric Orthopedics and Scoliosis, Baylor College of Medicine, Texas Children's Hospital, Houston, Texas

**Sharon E. Plon, MD, PhD**
Professor, Departments of Pediatrics and Molecular and Human Genetics; Member, Human Genome Sequencing Center, Baylor College of Medicine; Chief, Cancer Genetics Clinic, Texas Children's Hospital, Houston, Texas

**David A. Podeszwa, MD**
Associate Professor, University of Texas Southwestern Medical Center; Attending Surgeon, Texas Scottish Rite Hospital for Children, Dallas, Texas

**Henry Pollack, MD**
Associate Professor of Pediatrics, Division of Pediatric Infectious Diseases, New York University School of Medicine, New York, New York

**Ian F. Pollack, MD, FACS, FAAP, FAANS**
Professor of Neurological Surgery, University of Pittsburgh School of Medicine; Chief, Department of Neurosurgery, Children's Hospital of Pittsburgh, Pittsburgh, Pennsylvania

**Claudette L. Poole, MD**
Fellow of Pediatric Infectious Disease, Department of Pediatrics, University of Alabama at Birmingham, Birmingham, Alabama

**Françoise Portaels, PhD**
Head, Mycobacteriology Unit, Department of Microbiology, Institute of Tropical Medicine, Antwerp, Belgium

**Jennifer E. Posey, MD, PhD**
Assistant Professor, Department of Molecular and Human Genetics, Baylor College of Medicine, Houston, Texas

**Lorraine Potocki, MD, FACMG**
Professor and Vice Chair for Education, Department of Molecular and Human Genetics, Baylor College of Medicine, Texas Children's Hospital, Houston, Texas

**Jacquelyn M. Powers, MD, MS**
Assistant Professor of Pediatrics, Baylor College of Medicine, Texas Children's Hospital, Houston, Texas

**Krista Preisberga, MD**
Assistant Professor of Pediatrics; Director of Pediatric Sedation Course, Baylor College of Medicine, Houston, Texas

**Julie Prendiville, MB BCh, BAO, MRCPI, DCH, FRCPC**
Clinical Professor of Pediatrics, University of British Columbia; Head, Division of Pediatric Dermatology, British Columbia's Children's Hospital, Vancouver, British Columbia, Canada

**Christopher Prestel, MD**
Fellow, Pediatric Infectious Diseases, Emory University School of Medicine, Atlanta, Georgia

**Jack Price, MD**
Associate Professor of Pediatrics, Baylor College of Medicine, Texas Children's Hospital. Houston, Texas

**Jason Primus, MD**
Resident, Department of Surgery, Mayo Clinic, Scottsdale, Arizona

**Monica Proud, MD, MS**
Assistant Professor of Pediatrics, Baylor College of Medicine, Texas Children's Hospital, Houston, Texas

**Anthony C. Puliafico, PhD**
Assistant Professor of Medical Psychology, Columbia University Medical Center, Tarrytown, New York

**Jyotinder Nain Punia, MD**
Assistant Professor of Pathology and Immunology, Baylor College of Medicine, Texas Children's Hospital, Houston, Texas

**Amol Purandare, MD**
Fellow, Pediatric Infectious Diseases, Children's National Health System, Washington, District of Columbia

**Michael M. Quach, MD**
Assistant Professor of Pediatrics, Baylor College of Medicine, Texas Children's Hospital, Houston, Texas

**Anthony G. Quinn, MB ChB, DCH, FRANZCO**
Consultant Ophthalmologist, West of England Eye Unit, Royal Devon and Exeter NHS Foundation Trust, University of Exeter School of Medicine, Exeter, Devon, United Kingdom

**Athar M. Qureshi, MD, FSCAI, FAAP**
Associate Director, CE Mullins Cardiac Catheterization Laboratories, The Lillie Frank Abercrombie Section of Cardiology, Texas Children's Hospital; Associate Professor of Pediatrics, Baylor College of Medicine; Attending Physician, Internal Medicine/Cardiology, Baylor St. Luke's Medical Center, Houston, Texas

**Elizabeth A. Raetz, MD**
Professor, Department of Pediatrics, University of Utah School of Medicine; Medical Director, High Risk Leukemia and Lymphoma Program, Primary Children's Hospital, Salt Lake City, Utah

**Jennifer A. Rama, MD, MEd**
Assistant Professor, Section of Pediatric Pulmonology, Baylor College of Medicine, Texas Children's Hospital, Houston, Texas

**Tara M. Randis, MD, MS**
Assistant Professor of Pediatrics and Microbiology, Division of Neonatology, New York University School of Medicine, New York, New York

**Jean L. Raphael, MD, MPH**
Associate Professor of Pediatrics, Baylor College of Medicine; Director, Center for Child Health Policy and Advocacy; Associate Vice Chair for Community Health, Texas Children's Hospital, Houston, Texas

**Karl E. Rathjen, MD**
Professor of Orthopedic Surgery, University of Texas Southwestern Medical Center; Orthopedic Staff, Texas Scottish Rite Hospital for Children; Chief of Clinical Service, Department of Orthopedic Surgery, Children's Medical Center, Dallas, Texas

**Mobeen H. Rathore, MD, FAAP, CPE, FPIDS, FIDSA, FSHEA, FACPE**
Professor and Associate Chairman, Department of Pediatrics, University of Florida, Jacksonville; Chief, Pediatric Infectious Diseases and Immunology, Wolfson Children's Hospital; Director, University of Florida Center for HIV/AIDS Research, Education and Service (UF CARES); Co-Director, Community Engagement Research Program, University of Florida Clinical and Translational Science Institute, Jacksonville, Florida

**Adam J. Ratner, MD, MPH**
Associate Professor of Pediatrics; Chief, Division of Pediatric Infectious Diseases, New York University School of Medicine, New York, New York

**Chitra Ravishankar, MD**
Attending Cardiologist, Heart Failure/Transplant Program, The Children's Hospital of Philadelphia; Associate Professor Pediatrics, The Perelman School of Medicine at the University of Pennsylvania, Philadelphia, Pennsylvania

**Gregory H. Reaman, MD**
Professor of Pediatrics, George Washington University School of Medicine and Health Sciences, Children's National Health System, Washington, DC; Associate Director for Oncology Sciences, Office of Hematology and Oncology Products, Office of New Drugs, Center for Drug Evaluation and Research, US Food and Drug Administration, Silver Spring, Maryland

**Carol A. Redel, MNS, MD**
Assistant Professor of Pediatrics, Pediatric Gastroenterology, Hepatology, and Nutrition, Baylor College of Medicine, Texas Children's Hospital, Houston, Texas

**Surya Rednam, MD**
Assistant Professor of Pediatrics, Pediatric Hematology-Oncology, Baylor College of Medicine, Texas Children's Hospital, Houston, Texas

**Maria J. Redondo, MD, PhD, MPH**
Associate Professor, Section of Diabetes and Endocrinology, Baylor College of Medicine, Texas Children's Hospital, Houston, Texas

**Perry Ann Reed, MBA**
Director, Ethics and Palliative Care, Texas Children's Hospital, Houston, Texas

**Travis D. Reeves, MD**
Assistant Professor, Pediatric Otolaryngology-Head and Neck Surgery, Eastern Virginia Medical School and the Children's Hospital of the King's Daughters, Norfolk, Virginia

**Sophie Remoue-Gonzales, MD**
Adolescent Medicine Fellow, Baylor College of Medicine, Texas Children's Hospital, Department of Pediatrics, Adolescent Medicine and Sports Medicine Section, Houston, Texas

**Clement L. Ren, MD, MBA**
Professor of Clinical Pediatrics; Associate Chief, Division of Pediatric Pulmonology, Allergy, and Sleep Medicine, Indiana University School of Medicine; Cystic Fibrosis Center Director, Riley Hospital for Children, Indianapolis, Indiana

**Cory M. Resnick, MD, DMD**
Assistant Professor of Oral and Maxillofacial Surgery, Harvard School of Dental Medicine; Oral and Maxillofacial Surgeon, Boston Children's Hospital, Boston, Massachusetts

**Elizabeth A. Rider, MSW, MD**
Director of Academic Programs, Institute for Professionalism and Ethical Practice; Director, Faculty Education Fellowship in Medical Humanism and Professionalism, Division of General Pediatrics, Department of Medicine, Boston Children's Hospital; Assistant Professor of Pediatrics, Harvard Medical School; Chair, Medicine Academy, and Carlton Horbelt Senior Fellow, National Academies of Practice; Founding Member, International Research Centre for Communication in Healthcare; Boston, Massachusetts

**Lisa G. Rider, MD**
Deputy Chief, Environmental Autoimmunity Group, National Institute of Environmental Health Sciences, National Institutes of Health, Bethesda, Maryland

**Marc A. Riedl, MD, MS**
Professor of Medicine, Clinical Director—US HAEA Angioedema Center, Division of Rheumatology, Allergy, and Immunology, University of California, San Diego, La Jolla, California

**Natalie Rintoul, MD**
Associate Professor of Clinical Pediatrics, Perelman School of Medicine, University of Pennsylvania; Attending Neonatologist, Children's Hospital of Philadelphia; Fetal Consultant, Center for Fetal Diagnosis and Treatment, Philadelphia, Pennsylvania

**Sarah Risen, MD**
Assistant Professor of Pediatrics, Baylor College of Medicine, Meyer Center for Developmental Pediatrics, Texas Children's Hospital, Houston, Texas

**Brian K. Rivera, MS**
Research Associate, Center for Perinatal Research, Nationwide Children's Hospital, Columbus, Ohio

**William B. Rizzo, MD**
Professor, Division of Inherited Metabolic Diseases, Department of Pediatrics, University of Nebraska Medical Center, Omaha, Nebraska

**Laurie A. Robak, MD, PhD**
Instructor, Department of Molecular and Human Genetics, Baylor College of Medicine, Texas Children's Hospital Neurological Research Institute, Houston, Texas

**Kenneth B. Roberts, MD**
Pediatric Teaching Program, Cone Health, Greensboro, North Carolina

**Alyssa Robinson, BS**
Clinical Research Coordinator at Massachusetts General Hospital, Tufts University School of Medicine, Boston, Massachusetts

**Renee S. Rodrigues-D'Souza, MD**
Assistant Professor of Pediatrics, Baylor College of Medicine, Meyer Center for Developmental Pediatrics, Texas Children's Hospital, Houston, Texas

**Margo R. Rollins, MD**
Assistant Professor of Pathology, Emory University School of Medicine; Assistant Medical Director of Tissue Transfusion and Apheresis, Children's Healthcare of Atlanta, Atlanta, Georgia

**José R. Romero, MD, FAAP, FIDSA, FPIDS**
Professor of Pediatrics; Horace C. Cabe Endowed Chair in Infectious Diseases; Director, Pediatric Infectious Diseases Section, University of Arkansas for Medical Sciences and Arkansas Children's Hospital, Arkansas Children's Hospital, Little Rock, Arkansas

**Chokechai Rongkavilit, MD**
Medical Director, Pediatric Infectious Diseases, Valley Children's Hospital, Madera, California; Clinical Professor (affiliated), Department of Pediatrics, Stanford University School of Medicine, Stanford, California

**Allan Root, MD**
Pediatric Endocrinologist, Johns Hopkins All Children's Hospital, St. Petersburg, Florida

**Rachel Rosen, MD, MPH**
Director, Aerodigestive Center, Boston Children's Hospital; Associate Professor of Pediatrics, Harvard Medical School, Boston, Massachusetts

**Tara L. Rosenberg, MD**
Assistant Professor, Baylor College of Medicine; Surgical Director, Vascular Anomalies Center, Texas Children's Hospital, Houston, Texas

**Norman D. Rosenblum, MD**
Department of Pediatrics, Physiology, Laboratory Medicine, and Pathology, The University of Toronto; Canada Research Chair, Department of Nephrology, The Hospital for Sick Children, Toronto, Canada

**Scott B. Rosenfeld, MD**
Associate Professor of Orthopedic Surgery, Baylor College of Medicine; Director, Hip Preservation Program, Texas Children's Hospital, Houston, Texas

**Alexander Rotenberg, MD, PhD**
Associate Professor of Neurology, Harvard Medical School; Director, Neuromodulation Program; Division of Epilepsy and Clinical Neurophysiology, Boston Children's Hospital, Boston, Massachusetts

**Tracey A. Rouault, MD**
Senior Investigator, Section on Human Iron Metabolism; Molecular Medicine Branch, Eunice Kennedy Shriver National Institute of Child Health and Human Development, Bethesda, Maryland

**Paul J. Rozance, MD**
The Frederick C. Battaglia Chair in Neonatology Research; Associate Professor, Department of Pediatrics, Children's Hospital Colorado and University of Colorado School of Medicine, Aurora, Colorado

**Rodrigo Ruano, MD, PhD**
Associate Professor, Department of Obstetrics and Gynecology, Mayo Clinic, Rochester, Minnesota

**Daniel M. Rubalcava, MD**
Assistant Professor of Pediatrics, Baylor College of Medicine, Texas Children's Hospital, Houston, Texas

**Lorry G. Rubin, MD**
Director, Pediatric Infectious Diseases, Steven and Alexandra Cohen Children's Medical Center of New York of Northwell Health, New Hyde Park, New York; Professor of Pediatrics, Hofstra Northwell School of Medicine, Hempstead, New York

**Fadel E. Ruiz, MD**
Assistant Professor, Department of Pediatrics, Baylor College of Medicine; Director of The Cystic Fibrosis Center, Section of Pulmonology, Texas Children's Hospital, Houston, Texas

**Robert Russell, MD, MPH**
Associate Professor, Division of Pediatric Surgery, University of Alabama at Birmingham, Children's Hospital of Alabama, Birmingham, Alabama

**Melissa Russo, MD**
Assistant Professor of Obstetrics and Gynecology, Brown University; Maternal-Fetal Medicine and Clinical Genetics, Women and Infants Hospital, Providence, Rhode Island

**Moira Rynn, MD**
Director, Division of Child and Adolescent Psychiatry, Columbia University Medical Center, New York, New York

**Camille Sabella, MD**
Director, Center for Pediatric Infectious Diseases, Cleveland Clinic Children's Hospital; Associate Professor of Pediatrics, Cleveland Clinic Lerner College of Medicine of Case Western Reserve University, Cleveland, Ohio

**Vishal Saddi, MBBS, DCH**
Department of Pediatric Respiratory Medicine, Monash Medical Centre, Melbourne, Australia

**Sejal Saglani, MRCPCH, MD**
Professor of Respiratory Pediatrics, National Heart and Lung Institute, Imperial College London and The Royal Brompton Hospital, London, United Kingdom

**Mustafa Sahin, MD, PhD**
Professor of Neurology, Department of Neurology, Boston Children's Hospital, Harvard Medical School, Boston, Massachusetts

**Lisa Saiman, MD**
Professor of Pediatrics, Department of Pediatrics, Columbia University Medical Center and Department of Infection Prevention and Control, New York-Presbyterian Hospital, New York, New York

**Joshua Samuels, MD, MPH**
Professor of Pediatrics and Internal Medicine, Division of Pediatric Nephrology and Hypertension, University of Texas Health Science Center Houston, Houston, Texas

**John T. Sandlund, MD**
Member, St. Jude Children's Research Hospital; Medical Director, Leukemia/Lymphoma Clinic; Medial Director, Russia Program, St. Jude Global, Memphis, Tennessee

**René Santer, MD**
Professor, Department of Pediatrics, University Medical Center Hamburg-Eppendorf, Germany

**Sarah E. Sartain, MD**
Assistant Professor of Pediatrics, Baylor College of Medicine, Texas Children's Hospital, Houston, Texas

**Jean-Marie Saudubray, MD**
Honorary Professor of Pediatrics, Metabolic Consultant at Neurometabolic Unit, Hopital Pitié Salpétriére, Paris, France

**Hemant Sawnani, MD**
Associate Professor of Pediatrics, Cincinnati Children's Hospital Medical Center, University of Cincinnati, Cincinnati, Ohio

**Anju Sawni, MD, FAAP, FSAHM**
Director of Adolescent Medicine, Hurley Children's Hospital/Hurley Medical Center; Assistant Professor, Department of Pediatrics and Human Medicine, Michigan State University College of Human Medicine, Flint, Michigan

**Kirti Saxena, MD**
Associate Professor of Psychiatry, Department of Psychiatry, Baylor College of Medicine, Texas Children's Hospital, Houston, Texas

**Fernando Scaglia, MD, FACMG**
Professor of Genetics, Department of Molecular and Human Genetics, Baylor College of Medicine; Attending Physician, Genetics and Metabolic Service, Texas Children's Hospital, Houston, Texas

**Christian P. Schaaf, MD, PhD**
Assistant Professor of Molecular and Human Genetics, Baylor College of Medicine; The Joan and Stanford Alexander Endowed Chair for Neuropsychiatric Genetics, Texas Children's Hospital, Houston, Texas

**Julie V. Schaffer, MD**
Pediatric Dermatology Fellowship Director, Division of Pediatric Dermatology, Hackensack University Medical Center, Hackensack, New Jersey

**Joshua K. Schaffzin, MD, PhD**
Assistant Professor of Pediatrics, University of Cincinnati College of Medicine; Director, Infection Prevention & Control Program, Division of Infectious Diseases, Cincinnati Children's Hospital Medical Center, Cincinnati, Ohio

**Theodore E. Schall, MSW**
Research Assistant, Department of Medical Ethics, The Children's Hospital of Philadelphia, Philadelphia, Pennsylvania

**Michael E. Scheurer, PhD, MPH**
Associate Professor, Department of Pediatrics, Baylor College of Medicine, Texas Children's Cancer Center, Houston, Texas

**Manuel Schiff, MD, PhD**
Head of Metabolic Unit, Reference Center for Inborn Errors of Metabolism, Robert-Debré University Hospital, Paris, France

**Elizabeth P. Schlaudecker, MD, MPH**
Assistant Professor of Pediatrics, Division of Infectious Diseases, Global Health Center, Cincinnati Children's Hospital Medical Center, Cincinnati, Ohio

**Mark R. Schleiss, MD**
Professor, Division of Pediatric Infectious Diseases and Immunology; Co-Director, Center for Infectious Diseases and Microbiology Translational Research; American Legion and Auxiliary Endowed Research Foundation Chair, University of Minnesota Medical School, Minneapolis, Minnesota

**Fernanda Bellodi Schmidt, MD**
Assistant Professor, Departments of Pediatrics and Dermatology, University of Cincinnati College of Medicine; Attending Physician, Division of Pediatric Dermatology, Cincinnati Children's Hospital Medical Center, Cincinnati, Ohio

**David J. Schonfeld, MD, FAAP**
Professor of the Practice in the School of Social Work and Pediatrics, University of Southern California and Children's Hospital Los Angeles; Director, National Center for School Crisis and Bereavement, Los Angeles, California

**Herbert Schreier, MD**
Associate Psychiatrist, Department of Psychiatry, UCSF Benioff Children's Hospital, Oakland, California

**Rebecca J. Schultz, PhD, RN, CPNP-PC**
Assistant Professor of Pediatrics, Baylor College of Medicine, Comprehensive Epilepsy Program and Blue Bird Circle Rett Center, Texas Children's Hospital, Houston, Texas

**Gordon E. Schutze, MD**
Professor of Pediatrics; Executive Vice Chairman, Martin I. Lorin MD Endowed Chair in Medical Education, Department of Pediatrics, Baylor College of Medicine, Texas Children's Hospital, Houston, Texas

**Aloysia Schwabe, MD**
Associate Professor of Pediatrics, Baylor College of Medicine; Chief of Physical Medicine and Rehabilitation, Texas Children's Hospital, Houston, Texas

**Bernd Christian Schwahn, MD, FRCPCH**
Consultant in Pediatric Metabolic Medicine, Willink Biochemical Genetics Unit, Manchester Centre for Genomic Medicine, Central Manchester University Hospitals NHS Foundation Trust, Saint Mary's Hospital, Manchester, United Kingdom

**Heidi Schwarzwald, MD, MPH**
Associate Professor and Vice Chair for Community Pediatrics, Department of Pediatrics, Baylor College of Medicine; Chief Medical Officer, Texas Children's Health Plan, Houston, Texas

**Meghna R. Sebastian, MD**
Assistant Professor, Section of Adolescent Medicine and Sports Medicine, Department of Pediatrics, Baylor College of Medicine, Houston, Texas

**Robert Sege, MD, PhD, FAAP**
Chief Medical Officer, Health Resources in Action, Boston, Massachusetts; Senior Fellow, Center for the Study of Social Policy, Washington, District of Columbia

**Elaine S. Seto, MD, PhD**
Assistant Professor of Pediatrics, Baylor College of Medicine, Texas Children's Hospital, Houston, Texas

**Robert E. Shaddy, MD**
Chair, The Department of Pediatrics, Keck School of Medicine, The University of Southern California; Pediatrician-in-Chief, Children's Hospital of Los Angeles, Los Angeles, California

**Ajay Shah, MD**
Child and Adolescent Psychiatry Fellow, Baylor College of Medicine, Houston, Texas

**Ankoor Y. Shah, MD, MPH**
Assistant Professor of Pediatrics, George Washington University School of Medicine and Health Sciences, Division of General and Community Pediatrics, Children's National Health System, Washington, District of Columbia

**Kara N. Shah, MD, PhD**
Associate Professor, Departments of Pediatrics and Dermatology, University of Cincinnati College of Medicine; Attending Physician, Division of Pediatric Dermatology, Cincinnati Children's Hospital Medical Center, Cincinnati, Ohio

**Shweta Shah, MD**
Assistant Professor, Renal Section, Baylor College of Medicine, Texas Children's Hospital, Houston, Texas

**Veeral S. Shah, MD, PhD**
Assistant Professor of Ophthalmology, Pediatric Neuro-Ophthalmology, Adult Neuro-Ophthalmology, Texas Children's Hospital/Baylor College of Medicine, University of Texas MD Anderson Cancer Center, Houston, Texas

**Furqan Shaikh, MD, MSc**
Assistant Professor of Pediatrics, University of Toronto, Division of Hematology/Oncology, The Hospital for Sick Children, Toronto, Canada

**Seetha Shankaran, MD**
Professor of Pediatrics, Wayne State University School of Medicine, Children's Hospital of Michigan and Hutzel Women's Hospital, Detroit, Michigan

**Eugene D. Shapiro, MD**
Professor of Pediatrics, of Epidemiology and of Investigative Medicine, Yale University Schools of Medicine, and of Public Health and Graduate School of Arts and Sciences; Attending Pediatrician, Children's Hospital at Yale-New Haven, New Haven, Connecticut

**Mary C. Shapiro, MD**
Assistant Professor of Pediatrics, Baylor College of Medicine, Texas Children's Hospital, Houston, Texas

**Judith S. Shaw, EdD, MPH, RN, FAAP**
Professor of Pediatrics and Nursing, Executive Director, Vermont Child Health Improvement Program (VCHIP) and National Improvement Partnership Network (NIPN), University of Vermont Larner College of Medicine, Burlington, Vermont

**Oleg A. Shchelochkov, MD**
Senior Investigator, Medical Genomics and Metabolic Genetics Branch, National Human Genome Research Institute, National Institutes of Health, Bethesda, Maryland

**William T. Shearer, MD, PhD**
Professor of Pediatrics and Pathology and Immunology; Distinguished Service Professor, Baylor College of Medicine, Allergy and Immunology Service, Texas Children's Hospital, Houston, Texas

**Lara S. Shekerdemian, MD, MHA**
Professor and Chief, Critical Care; Vice Chair for Clinical Affairs, Department of Pediatrics, Baylor College of Medicine, Texas Children's Hospital, Houston, Texas

**Vinitha Shenava, MD**
Assistant Professor, Department of Orthopedic Surgery, Baylor College of Medicine, Texas Children's Hospital, Houston, Texas

**Rohit P. Shenoi, MD**
Associate Professor of Pediatrics, Baylor College of Medicine, Texas Children's Hospital, Houston, Texas

**Avinash K. Shetty, MD**
Professor, Pediatrics, Wake Forest School of Medicine, Winston-Salem, North Carolina

**Jeffrey S. Shilt, MD**
Associate Professor of Orthopedics and Scoliosis Surgery, Baylor College of Medicine; Chief Surgical Officer, The Woodlands, Texas Children's Hospital, Houston, Texas

**Benjamin L. Shneider, MD**
George Peterkin Endowed Chair; Professor of Pediatrics and Head of Section, Pediatric Gastroenterology, Hepatology, and Nutrition, Baylor College of Medicine; Chief of Service, Pediatric Gastroenterology, Hepatology, and Nutrition, Texas Children's Hospital, Houston, Texas

**Robert J. Shulman, MD**
Professor of Pediatrics, Children's Nutrition Research Center, Baylor College of Medicine, Texas Children's Hospital, Houston, Texas

**Stephen Shusterman, DMD**
Associate Professor of Developmental Biology (Pediatric Dentistry), Harvard School of Dental Medicine; Dentist-in-Chief, Emeritus, Boston Children's Hospital, Boston, Massachusetts

**Jennifer N. Avari Silva, MD**
Director, Pediatric Electrophysiology; Assistant Professor, Pediatrics, Washington University School of Medicine, St. Louis Children's Hospital, St. Louis, Montana

**Earl Dean Silverman, MD**
Professor, University of Toronto, Rheumatology Service, The Hospital for Sick Children, Toronto, Ontario, Canada

**Narong Simakajornboon, MD**
Professor and Director, Sleep Center; Director, Sleep Medicine Fellowship Training Program; Cincinnati Children's Hospital Medical Center, Cincinnati, Ohio

**Jeffrey M. Simmons, MD**
Associate Professor of Pediatrics, Cincinnati Children's Hospital Medical Center, Cincinnati, Ohio

**Rebecca A. Simmons, MD**
Professor of Pediatrics, Perelman School of Medicine, University of Pennsylvania; Attending Neonatologist, Children's Hospital of Philadelphia, Philadelphia, Pennsylvania

**Stephanie Sisley, MD**
Assistant Professor of Pediatrics, Divisions of Nutrition and Pediatric Endocrinology, Baylor College of Medicine, Texas Children's Hospital, Houston, Texas

**V. Ben Sivarajan, MD, MS, FRCPC**
Associate Professor of Pediatrics, University of Alberta; Pediatric Cardiac Intensivist, Stollery Children's and University of Alberta Hospitals, Alberta, Canada

**Gwenn Skar, MD**
Instructor, Division of Pediatric Infectious Diseases, University of Nebraska Medical Center, Omaha, Nebraska

**Peter D. Sly, MBBS, MD, DSc, FRACP**
Director, Children's Lung, Environment, and Asthma Research, Child Health Research Centre, The University of Queensland, Brisbane, Australia

**Richard J. H. Smith, MD**
Professor of Otolaryngology, Pediatrics, Internal Medicine, Molecular Physiology, and Biophysics, Carver College of Medicine, Department of Molecular Physiology and Biophysics, University of Iowa Health Care, Iowa City, Iowa

**Malcolm A. Smith, MD, PhD**
Associate Branch Chief, Pediatrics, Cancer Therapy Evaluation Program, National Cancer Institute, Bethesda, Maryland

**Charles V. Smith, PhD**
Professor, Center for Developmental Therapeutics, Seattle Children's Research Institute, University of Washington School of Medicine, Seattle, Washington

**Jessica Snowden, MD**
Associate Professor, Division of Pediatric Infectious Diseases, University of Nebraska Medical Center, Nebraska Medical Center, Omaha, Nebraska

**Michael J. G. Somers, MD**
Director, Clinical Services, Division of Nephrology, Boston Children's Hospital, Boston, Massachusetts

**Mary Beth F. Son, MD**
Assistant Professor, Harvard Medical School, Division of Immunology, Boston Children's Hospital, Boston, Massachusetts

**Andrew L. Sonis, DMD**
Professor of Developmental Biology (Pediatric Dentistry), Harvard School of Dental Medicine; Senior Associate in Dentistry, Boston Children's Hospital, Boston, Massachusetts

**Manu R. Sood, FRCPCH, MD**
Professor of Pediatrics; Director, Division of Pediatric Gastroenterology, Hepatology and Nutrition, The Medical College of Wisconsin, Children's Hospital of Wisconsin, Milwaukee, Wisconsin

**Ilene R. Sosenko, MD**
Professor of Pediatrics, Division of Neonatology, University of Miami; Associate Director of Clinical Development and Outreach; Medical Director, Newborn Services Jackson North Hospital, Miami, Florida

**Katherine A. Sota**
Medicine Student, Universidad Peruana Cayetano Heredia; Assistant Investigator, Cysticercosis Unit, Instituto Nacional de Ciencias Neurologicas, Lima, Peru

**Carmen L. Soto-Rivera, MD**
Pediatric Endocrinologist, Division of Endocrinology, Department of Pediatrics and Medicine Harvard Medical School, Boston Children's Hospital, Boston, Massachusetts

**Logan G. Spector, PhD**
Professor of Pediatrics, University of Minnesota Medical School; Director, Division of Epidemiology/Clinical Research, Minneapolis, Minneapolis

**Adiaha I. A. Spinks-Franklin, MD, MPH, FAAP**
Assistant Professor of Pediatrics, Baylor College of Medicine, Meyer Center for Developmental Pediatrics, Texas Children's Hospital, Houston, Texas

**Joseph A. Spinner, MD, BA**
Fellow, Pediatric Cardiology, Baylor College of Medicine, Houston, Texas

**Sheri L. Spunt, MD, MBA**
Endowed Professor of Pediatric Cancer, Stanford University School of Medicine, Stanford, California

**James E. Squires, MD, MS**
Assistant Professor of Pediatrics, Division of Gastroenterology, Hepatology, and Nutrition, Pittsburgh Liver Research Center, Pittsburgh, Pennsylvania

**Robert H. Squires, MD**
Professor of Pediatrics, Division of Gastroenterology, Hepatology, and Nutrition, Children's Hospital of Pittsburgh, Pittsburgh, Pennsylvania

**Deepak Srivastava, MD**
Director, Gladstone Institute of Cardiovascular Disease; Professor, Departments of Pediatrics and Biochemistry and Biophysics, University of California, San Francisco, San Francisco, California

**Poyyapakkam Srivaths, MD**
Associate Professor of Pediatrics, Department of Pediatrics, Baylor College of Medicine and Renal Section, Texas Children's Hospital, Houston, Texas

**Laura L. Stafman, MD**
Resident, Department of Surgery, University of Alabama at Birmingham, Birmingham, Alabama

**Charles A. Stanley, MD**
Professor Emeritus of Pediatrics at the University of Pennsylvania, Perelman School of Medicine, Congenital Hyperinsulinism Center at the Children's Hospital of Philadelphia, Philadelphia, Pennsylvania

**Michael Stark, BSc(Hons), MB ChB, MRCP, FRACP, PhD**
Assistant Professor, Robinson Research Institute, Adelaide Medical School, University of Adelaide, Women's and Children's Health Network, North Adelaide, South Australia

**Jeffrey R. Starke, MD**
Professor of Pediatrics, Baylor College of Medicine, Texas Children's Hospital, Houston, Texas

**Russell W. Steele, MD**
Professor of Pediatrics; Division Head, Pediatric Infectious Diseases, Ochsner Children's Health Center, University of Queensland School of Medicine, Ochsner Clinical School; Clinical Professor, Department of Pediatrics, Tulane University School of Medicine, New Orleans, Louisiana

**Ruth E. K. Stein, MD**
Professor of Pediatrics, Albert Einstein College of Medicine, Bronx, New York

**Robert D. Steiner, MD**
Chief Medical Officer, Acer Therapeutics, Departments of Pediatrics and Genetics, University of Wisconsin School of Medicine and Public Health, Madison, Wisconsin

**Robin H. Steinhorn, MD**
Professor of Pediatrics; Senior Vice President, Center for Hospital Based Specialties, Children's National Health System, Washington, District of Columbia

**Richards B. Stephens, MD**
Professor of Orthopedic Surgery, University of Texas Southwestern Medical Center, Chief Medical Officer, Texas Scottish Rite Hospital for Children, Dallas, Texas

**Christopher J. Stille, MD, MPH**
Professor of Pediatrics, University of Colorado School of Medicine, Children's Hospital Colorado, Aurora, Colorado

**Sylvia Stockler-Ipsiroglu, MD, PhD**
Professor and Head, Division of Biochemical Diseases, Department of Pediatrics, University of British Columbia, Canada

**Stephanie H. Stovall, MD**
Pediatric Infectious Diseases Specialist, Golisano Children's Hospital of Southwest Florida, Fort Myers, Florida

**Constantine A. Stratakis, MD, D(Med)Sc**
Senior Investigator, Section on Endocrinology and Genetics, Eunice Kennedy Shriver National Institute of Child Health and Human Development, National Institutes of Health, Bethesda, Maryland

**Haley Streff, MS, CGC**
Certified Genetic Counselor, Baylor College of Medicine, Houston, Texas

**Dennis M. Styne, MD**
Professor of Pediatric Medicine, Department of Pediatrics, UC Davis, Sacramento, California

**Ruthie R. Su, MD**
Assistant Professor, Department of Urology, Division of Pediatric Urology, University of Wisconsin School of Medicine and Public Health, American Family Children's Hospital, Madison, Wisconsin

**Daniel J. Sucato, MD, MS**
Professor of Orthopedic Surgery, University of Texas-Southwestern, Chief of Staff, Texas Scottish Rite Hospital for Children, Dallas, Texas

**Frederick J. Suchy, MD**
Chief Research Officer; Director, Research Institute; Professor of Pediatrics, Children's Hospital Colorado; Associate Dean for Child Health Research, Denver School of Medicine, University of Colorado, Aurora, Colorado

**Kathleen E. Sullivan, MD, PhD**
Professor of Pediatrics, Perelman School of Medicine, University of Pennsylvania; Chief, Allergy Immunology, The Children's Hospital of Philadelphia, Philadelphia, Pennsylvania

**Cecille G. Sulman, MD**
Associate Professor of Pediatric Otolaryngology, Medical College of Wisconsin; Chief, Pediatric Otolaryngology Division, Children's Hospital of Wisconsin, Milwaukee, Wisconsin

**Rosalyn M. Sulyanto, DMD, MS**
Instructor of Developmental Biology (Pediatric Dentistry), Harvard School of Dental Medicine; Associate in Dentistry, Boston Children's Hospital, Boston, Massachusetts

**Robert P. Sundel, MD**
Associate Professor of Pediatrics, Harvard Medical School; Fred S. Rosen Chair in Pediatric Rheumatology, Boston Children's Hospital, Boston, Massachusetts

**Gautham K. Suresh, MD, DM, MS, FAAP**
Professor of Pediatrics, Baylor College of Medicine; Section Head and Service Chief of Neonatology, Texas Children's Hospital, Houston, Texas

**Melissa A. Suter, PhD**
Assistant Professor, Department of Obstetrics and Gynecology, Baylor College of Medicine, Houston, Texas

**Bernhard Suter, MD**
Assistant Professor of Pediatrics, Baylor College of Medicine; Associate Medical Director of the MECP2 Duplication Clinic; The Blue Bird Circle Rett Center, Texas Children's Hospital, Houston, Texas

**V. Reid Sutton, MD**
Professor, Department of Molecular and Human Genetics, Baylor College of Medicine; Chief, Inborn Errors of Metabolism Service, Texas Children's Hospital, Houston, Texas

**Sarah J. Swartz, MD**
Associate Professor of Pediatrics, Renal Section, Baylor College of Medicine, Texas Children's Hospital, Houston, Texas

**Sylvia Szentpeterry, MD**
Assistant Professor of Pediatrics, Division of Pediatric Pulmonary and Sleep Medicine, Medical University of South Carolina, Charleston, South Carolina

**Theresa A. Tacy, MD**
Associate Professor, Department of Pediatrics, Stanford University, School of Medicine, Lucile Packard Children's Hospital, Palo Alto, California

**Carl D. Tapia, MD, MPH**
Assistant Professor of Pediatrics, Baylor College of Medicine, Texas Children's Hospital, Houston, Texas

**Sarah K. Tasian, MD**
Assistant Professor of Pediatrics, Perelman School of Medicine at the University of Pennsylvania, Children's Hospital of Philadelphia, Philadelphia, Pennsylvania

**David F. Teitel, MD**
Professor of Pediatrics, Division of Pediatric Cardiology, University of California, San Francisco, San Francisco, California

**Jonathan E. Teitelbaum, MD, FAAP, AGAF**
Director, Pediatric Gastroenterology and Hepatology, The Unterberg Children's Hospital at Monmouth Medical Center; Associate Professor of Pediatrics, Drexel University School of Medicine; Director, Pediatric Gastroenterology and Hepatology, The Unterberg Children's Hospital at Monmouth Medical Center; Associate Professor of Pediatrics, Drexel University School of Medicine, Philadelphia, Pennsylvania

**Grzegorz Telega, MD**
Associate Professor, Medical College of Wisconsin; Program Director, Liver Transplant Hepatology, Children's Hospital of Wisconsin, Milwaukee, Wisconsin

**Jeff R. Temple, PhD**
Professor and Licensed Psychologist Director, Behavioral Health and Research, Department of Obstetrics and Gynecology, The University of Texas Medical Branch at Galveston, Galveston, Texas

**Andreas A. Theodorou, MD, FCCM, FAAP**
Professor and Vice Chair, Department of Pediatrics, University of Arizona College of Medicine; Regional Chief Medical Officer, Banner Health Tucson, Arizona

**Matthew J. Thomas, ScM, CGC**
Genetic Counselor, Department of Pediatrics, University of Virginia Health System, Charlottesville, Virginia

**James A. Thomas, MD**
Professor of Pediatrics, Section of Critical Care Medicine, Baylor College of Medicine; Medical Director of ECMO, Texas Children's Hospital, Houston, Texas

**James Tibballs, B Med Sc (Hon), MBBS, MEd, MBA, MD, MHlth&MedLaw, PGDipArts(Fr), DALF, FANZCA, FCICM, FACLM**
Principal Fellow, Australian Venom Research Unit, Department of Pharmacology and Therapeutics and Department of Pediatrics, the University of Melbourne; Senior Physician, Pediatric Intensive Care Unit The Royal Children's Hospital, Melbourne, Australia

**Neelesh A. Tipnis, MD**
Professor of Pediatrics, Division of Pediatric Gastroenterology, Hepatology, and Nutrition, University of Alabama at Birmingham, Birmingham, Alabama

**Gail E. Tomlinson, MD, PhD**
Professor of Pediatrics; Division Director, Pediatric Hematology-Oncology, University of Texas Health Science Center at San Antonio, San Antonio, Texas

**Leidy Tovar Padua, MD**
Clinical Assistant Professor, University of California San Diego Rady, Children's Hospital of San Diego, San Diego, California

**Jeffrey A. Towbin, MD**
Co-Director, Heart Institute; St. Jude Chair, Pediatric Cardiology; Vice Chair, Strategic Advancement Le Bonheur Children's Hospital; Chief, Cardiology, St. Jude Children's Research Hospital; Chief, Pediatric Cardiology, The University of Tennessee Health Science Center, Memphis, Tennessee

**Christopher Towe, MD**
Assistant Professor of Pediatrics and Medicine, Departments of Pediatrics, University of Cincinnati College of Medicine, Cincinnati Children's Hospital Medical Center, Cincinnati, Ohio

**Bruce C. Trapnell, MD**
Professor of Translational Pulmonary Medicine, Departments of Medicine and Pediatrics, University of Cincinnati College of Medicine, Cincinnati Children's Hospital Medical Center, Cincinnati, Ohio

**James R. Treat, MD**
Associate Professor of Clinical Pediatrics, Perelman School of Medicine at the University of Pennsylvania; Associate Professor of Dermatology, Perelman School of Medicine at the University of Pennsylvania, Philadelphia, Pennsylvania

**Indi Trehan, MD, MPH, DTM&H**
Associate Professor, Emergency Medicine; Associate Professor, Infectious Diseases, Washington University School of Medicine, St. Louis, Missouri

**Nicole Triggs, MSN, APRN, CPNP-PC, CPN**
Pediatric Nurse Practitioner, Pediatric Gastroenterology, Hepatology, and Nutrition, Texas Children's Hospital, Houston, Texas

**Amy Trowbridge, MD**
Assistant Professor, Division of Hospital Medicine and Pediatric Advanced Care Team, Seattle Children's Hospital, Seattle, Washington

**Lori B. Tucker, MD, FRCPC**
Professor of Pediatrics, University of British Columbia, Division of Pediatric Rheumatology, BC Children's Hospital, Vancouver, British Columbia, Canada

**David Tunkel, MD**
Director of Pediatric Otolaryngology; Professor of Otolaryngology—Head and Neck Surgery, Johns Hopkins University School of Medicine, Baltimore, Maryland

**Marie Turcich, LPC, LMFT, LSSP**
Instructor of Pediatrics, Baylor College of Medicine, Meyer Center for Developmental Pediatrics, Texas Children's Hospital, Houston, Texas

**Jeremy Udkoff, MA**
Pediatric and Adolescent Dermatology, University of California, San Diego School of Medicine and Rady Children's Hospital, San Diego, California

**Luis A. Umana, MD**
Assistant Professor, Department of Genetics, University of Texas Southwestern Medical Center, Dallas, Texas

**Joyee Goswami Vachani, MD, MEd**
Assistant Professor of Pediatrics; Director of Pediatric Hospital Medicine Fellowship; Director of Quality and Safety, Section of Pediatric Hospital Medicine; Director of Education, Clinical Systems Integration, Baylor College of Medicine/Texas Children's Hospital, Houston, Texas

**Aldo Vagge, MD**
International Pediatric Ophthalmology Fellow, Pediatric Ophthalmology and Ocular Genetics, Wills Eye Hospital, Philadelphia, Pennsylvania

**George F. Van Hare, MD**
Louis Larrick Ward Professor of Pediatrics, Washington University School of Medicine; Director, Division of Pediatric Cardiology, St. Louis Children's Hospital, St. Louis, Montana

**Johan L. K. Van Hove, MD, PhD**
Professor of Pediatrics, Section of Clinical Genetics and Metabolism, University of Colorado School of Medicine, Aurora, Colorado

**A. H. van Kaam, MD, PhD**
Professor, Department of Neonatology, Emma Children's Hospital, Academic Medical Center, Amsterdam, the Netherlands

**Kristof Van Schelvergem, MD, FEBO**
Ocular Genetics Fellow, Wills Eye Hospital, Pediatric Ophthalmology and Ocular Genetics, Philadelphia, Pennsylvania

**Sivabalan Vasudavan, BDSc, MDSc, MPH, M Orth RCS, MRACDS, FDS RCS**
Senior Research Fellow, University of Western Australia, Perth, Australia

**Charles P. Venditti, MD, PhD**
Senior Investigator, Medical Genomics and Metabolic Genetics Branch, National Human Genome Research Institute, National Institutes of Health, Bethesda, Maryland

**Claudia P. Vicetti Miguel, MD**
Fellow, Pediatric Infectious Diseases, Nationwide Children's Hospital—The Ohio State University, Columbus, Ohio

**Vini Vijayan, MD**
Assistant Professor of Pediatrics, University of Arkansas for Medical Sciences, Arkansas Children's Hospital, Little Rock, Arkansas

**Tibisay Villalobos-Fry, MD, FAAP**
Assistant Clinical Professor of Pediatrics, Pediatric Infectious Diseases, USF Morsani College of Medicine-Lehigh Valley; Director Pediatric Antibiotic Stewardship, Children's Specialty Center, Children's Hospital of Lehigh Valley, Allentown, Pennsylvania

**Sherry Sellers Vinson, MD, MEd**
Assistant Professor of Pediatrics, Baylor College of Medicine, Meyer Center for Developmental Pediatrics, Texas Children's Hospital, Houston, Texas

**Jerry Vockley, MD, PhD**
Professor of Pediatrics and Human Genetics, University of Pittsburgh School of Medicine; Chief of Medical Genetics, Children's Hospital of Pittsburgh, Pittsburgh, Pennsylvania

**Robert G. Voigt, MD, FAAP**
Professor of Pediatrics, Head, Section of Developmental Pediatrics, Baylor College of Medicine; Director, Autism Center and Meyer Center for Developmental Pediatrics, Texas Children's Hospital, Houston, Texas

**Amy Vyas, MD**
Child and Adolescent Psychiatry Chief Resident, Menninger Department of Psychiatry and Behavioral Sciences, Baylor College of Medicine, Houston, Texas

**Ellen R. Wald, MD**
Chair, Department of Pediatrics, University of Wisconsin School of Medicine and Public Health, American Family Children's Hospital, Madison, Wisconsin

**Carol A. Wallace, MD**
Professor, Rheumatology Service, University of Washington School of Medicine, Seattle Children's Hospital, Seattle, Washington

**Colin Wallis, MD, FRCP, FRCPCH, DCH, FCP(SA)**
Consultant Pediatrician and Senior Lecturer, Respiratory Unit, Great Ormond Street Hospital for Children, London, United Kingdom

**Douglas S. Walsh, MD, MS**
Chief, Dermatology Service; Associate Chief of Staff for Research, Veterans Affairs Medical Center, Syracuse, New York

**Brian H. Walsh, MB BCh, BAO, PhD**
Instructor, Department of Pediatrics, Harvard Medical School; Neonatologist, Department of Pediatric Newborn Medicine, Brigham and Women's Hospital, Boston, Massachusetts

**David S. Walton, MD**
Clinical Professor of Ophthalmology and Pediatrician, Department of Ophthalmology, Massachusetts Eye and Ear Infirmary and Department of Pediatrics, Massachusetts General Hospital, Harvard Medical School, Boston, Massachusetts

**Michael Wangler, MD, MS, BS**
Assistant Professor, Department of Molecular and Human Genetics, Baylor College of Medicine, Texas Children's Hospital Neurological Research Institute, Houston, Texas

**Stephanie Ware, MD, PhD**
Professor of Pediatrics and Medical and Molecular Genetics, Indiana University School of Medicine; Vice Chair of Clinical Affairs, Medical and Molecular Genetics, Indiana University Health, Indianapolis, Indiana

**Matthew C. Washam, MD, MPH**
Assistant Professor, Division of Pediatric Infectious Disease, Cincinnati Children's Hospital Medical Center, Cincinnati, Ohio

**Alicia M. Waters, MD**
Resident, Department of Surgery, University of Alabama at Birmingham, Birmingham, Alabama

**Joshua R. Watson, MD**
Assistant Professor, Department of Pediatrics, Nationwide Children's Hospital, The Ohio State University, Section of Infectious Diseases, Columbus, Ohio

**Howard L. Weiner, MD**
Professor and Vice Chairman of Neurosurgery, Baylor College of Medicine; Chief of Neurosurgery, Texas Children's Hospital, Houston, Texas

**Michael Weiss, MD**
Associate Professor of Pediatrics, Division of Neonatology, University of Florida, Gainesville, Florida

**Carol Cohen Weitzman, MD**
Professor of Pediatrics and Child Study Center; Director, Developmental-Behavioral Pediatrics, Yale School of Medicine, New Haven, Connecticut

**Scott E. Wenderfer, MD, PhD**
Department of Pediatrics, Baylor College of Medicine and Renal Section, Texas Children's Hospital, Houston, Texas

**Kristen A. Wendorf, MD, MS**
Public Health Medical Officer, Infectious Diseases, California Department of Public Health, San Francisco, California

**William E. Whitehead, MD**
Associate Professor, Department of Neurosurgery, Baylor College of Medicine, Texas Children's Hospital, Houston, Texas

**Bernhard L. Wiedermann, MD, MA**
Professor of Pediatrics/Director, Pediatric Infectious Diseases Fellowship Program, Division of Infectious Diseases, Department of Pediatrics, Children's National Health System/George Washington University School of Medicine, Washington, District of Columbia

**Constance M. Wiemann, PhD**
Associate Professor and Director of Research, Department of Pediatrics, Adolescent Medicine and Sports Medicine Section, Baylor College of Medicine, Texas Children's Hospital, Houston, Texas

**Eric Williams, MD**
Associate Professor of Pediatrics, Baylor College of Medicine, Texas Children's Hospital, Houston, Texas

**Laurel Williams, DO**
Interim Chief of Psychiatry, Texas Children's Hospital; Director of Residency Training, Child & Adolescent Psychiatry; Director of the Baylor Child & Adolescent Psychiatry Clinic; Associate Professor, Menninger Department of Psychiatry & Behavioral Sciences, Baylor College of Medicine, Houston, Texas

**Rodney E. Willoughby, MD**
Professor, Department of Pediatrics (Infectious Diseases), Medical College of Wisconsin, Milwaukee, Wisconsin

**Erin Wilmer, MD**
Resident, Department of Dermatology, Warren Alpert Medical School of Brown University, and Hasbro Children's Hospital, Providence, Rhode Island

**Philip Wilson, MD**
Assistant Professor of Orthopedic, University of Texas Southwestern Medical Center, Pediatric Orthopedic Staff Surgeon, Texas Scottish Rite Hospital for Children, Children's Medical Center Dallas, Dallas, Texas

**Kenneth D. Winkel, B Med Sc, MBBS, PhD, FACTM**
Senior Research Fellow, Australian Venom Research Unit, Department of Pharmacology and Therapeutics, The University of Melbourne, Melbourne, Australia

**Joshua Wolf, MBBS, FRACP**
Assistant Member, Infectious Diseases Department, St Jude's Research Hospital, Memphis, Tennessee

**Rachel Wolfe, PhD**
Assistant Professor of Pediatrics, Baylor College of Medicine; Attending Psychologist, Texas Children's Hospital, Houston, Texas

**Suzanne L. Woodbury, MD**
Assistant Professor of Pediatrics, Baylor College of Medicine, Texas Children's Hospital, Houston, Texas

**Charles R. Woods, MD, MS**
Chairman, Department of Pediatrics; Billy F. Andrews Endowed Chair in Pediatrics; Professor, Pediatric Infectious Diseases, University of Louisville School of Medicine; Chief of Staff, Norton Children's Hospital, Louisville, Kentucky

**Lisa Nassif Wright, MD**
Assistant Professor of Pediatrics, Baylor College of Medicine, Texas Children's Hospital, Houston, Texas

**Clyde J. Wright, MD**
Assistant Professor of Pediatrics, Section of Neonatology, University of Colorado School of Medicine and Children's Hospital Colorado, Aurora, Colorado

**Myra H. Wyckoff, MD**
Professor of Pediatrics, Division of Neonatal-Perinatal Medicine, The University of Texas Southwestern Medical Center, Dallas, Texas

**Paula Yanes-Lukin, PhD**
Assistant Professor of Clinical Psychology; Director of Psychology, Pediatric Anxiety and Mood Research Clinic and Children's Day Unit, Columbia University Medical Center, New York, New York

**Amber M. Yates, MD**
Assistant Professor of Pediatrics, Baylor College of Medicine; Assistant Director, Clinical Division (Outpatient), Texas Children's Hospital, Houston, Texas

**Donald L. Yee, MD**
Associate Professor of Pediatrics, Baylor College of Medicine; Director, Texas Children's Hemophilia and Thrombosis Center, Texas Children's Hospital, Houston, Texas

**Helen H. Yeung, MD**
Instructor, Department of Ophthalmology, Yale School of Medicine, New Haven, Connecticut

**Guy Young, MD**
Professor of Pediatrics, University of Southern California Keck School of Medicine; Director, Hemostasis and Thrombosis Center, Children's Hospital Los Angeles, Los Angeles, California

**David C. Yu, MD**
Assistant Professor of Clinical Surgery, LSU Health Science Center, Children's Hospital New Orleans, Section of Pediatric Surgery, New Orleans, Louisiana

**Jason T. Yustein, MD, PhD**
Assistant Professor of Pediatrics, Baylor College of Medicine; Director, Faris D. Virani Ewing Sarcoma Center, Texas Children's Hospital, Houston, Texas

**Andrea L. Zaenglein, MD**
Professor of Dermatology and Pediatrics, Penn State College of Medicine/Hershey Medical Center, Hershey, Pennsylvania

**Jessica A. Zagory, MD**
Resident, Department of Surgery, LSU Health Science Center, New Orleans, Louisiana

**Heather J. Zar, MB BCh, FRCP, PhD**
Professor and Chair, Department of Pediatrics and Child Health, Red Cross War Memorial Children's Hospital; Director, MRC Unit on Child and Adolescent Health, University of Cape Town, Cape Town, South Africa

**Jose J. Zayas, DO**
Assistant Professor of Pediatrics; Director, Pediatric Residency Program, University of Florida, Jacksonville, Florida

**Huayan Zhang, MD**
Associate Professor of Clinical Pediatrics, Perelman School of Medicine, University of Pennsylvania; Attending Neonatologist and Medical Director, Newborn and Infant Chronic Lung Disease Program, Children's Hospital of Philadelphia, Philadelphia, Pennsylvania

**Barry S. Zuckerman, MD**
Professor, Department of Pediatrics, Boston Medical Center/Boston University School of Medicine, Boston, Massachusetts

**Francesco Zulian, MD**
Associate Professor of Pediatrics, University of Padua; Chief, Pediatric Rheumatology Unit, Department of Woman and Child Health, Padua, Italy

# PREFACE



We are honored and privileged to have assumed editorial responsibilities for the 23rd edition of this iconic, 120-year-old textbook of pediatrics, originated as *Diseases of Infancy and Childhood* by Dr. Luther Emmett Holt in 1896. The book was published through 11 editions into the 1940s by Dr. Holt and subsequently by his son, Dr. Luther Emmett Holt, Jr., and eventually through another 7 editions by Dr. Abraham Rudolph, who turned *Rudolph's Pediatrics* into one of the world's most widely recognized and read medical textbooks. This 23rd edition represents the first complete transition of editorial responsibilities in more than 40 years. It comes as pediatric practice advances at a dizzying pace. Each new month brings reports in the medical literature of new diagnostic tools and therapeutic strategies. Revolutionary advances in human genomics are illuminating the etiologies and pathogenesis of many of the most vexing medical conditions pediatricians have faced over the course of decades and generations. Fields as diverse as oncology, immunology, and neurology are being transformed by these advances. At the same time, pediatricians are being asked to do more with less, to be more efficient, to provide better patient access, and to become better stewards of the limited resources entrusted to us. We treat children, and families, not diseases, and our patients depend on us to be as straightforward and pragmatic as possible. Change is inherently challenging, but big challenges invariably represent big opportunities. There has never been a better time to be a pediatrician or a more hopeful time to be the parent of a seriously ill child. The years ahead will bring better treatments and more cures for a multitude of medical conditions afflicting children. Our fondest hope is that in the pages of this textbook the reader will find not only relevant facts and information but also the inspiration to do more for the children and families we serve.

Mark W. Kline

Susan M. Blaney

Angelo P. Giardino

Jordan S. Orange

Daniel J. Penny

Gordon E. Schutze

Lara S. Shekerdemian

# ACKNOWLEDGMENTS

The 23rd edition of *Rudolph's Pediatrics* was made possible by the creative input and hard work of an outstanding team of co-editors from the Department of Pediatrics at Texas Children's Hospital and Baylor College of Medicine, including Susan Blaney, Angelo Giardino, Jordan Orange, Dan Penny, Gordon Schutze, and Lara Shekerdemian. Abraham Rudolph and Colin Rudolph provided invaluable perspective and input during the planning phase of textbook production. All of us are indebted to the 44 section editors and 845 authors who contributed to this 2950-page textbook. We also are indebted to Julie O'Brien, Mark Meyer, and Lee Ligon at the Texas Children's Hospital and Baylor College of Medicine for administrative support and editorial assistance, and to Andrew Moyer, Tania Andrabi, and the entire editorial staff at McGraw-Hill for their partnership, support, and guidance. I want to thank my longtime friend Smiley Pool for the stunning cover photography. Finally, special thanks to Sandra Queen for allowing us to use the photograph of her darling and much loved late daughter Janie in the swimming pool.

Mark W. Kline

# 1 Evolution of Pediatric Practice

Thomas G. DeWitt and Neal Halfon

## INTRODUCTION

As pediatrics and the delivery of children's health care enter the third decade of the 21st century, the role of the pediatrician continues to evolve and change. Guided by the knowledge, skills, and tools that the profession has accumulated over many decades, pediatricians must strategically respond to changing conditions, health determinants, and the epidemiology of childhood, as well as to shifting social and cultural norms of what constitutes healthy child development. Our knowledge of the pathophysiology of many diseases has evolved from simple causal models based on germ theory to more complex multilevel and developmentally informed models of gene–environment interactions. As pediatric care has triumphed over many infectious diseases and made significant strides in the management of chronic disease, newer morbidities continue to emerge as the social conditions of children and families evolve and inequality and adversity become more prevalent. The growing prevalence of developmental, behavioral, and mental health conditions is indicative of these changes. To impact child health, forward-looking pediatricians must provide care with an expanded concept of healthy child development and must acquire skills to effectively practice in collaboration with other individuals and entities involved in promoting and supporting that development.

Societal expectations for healthy child development are a reflection of our collective hopes for what our children should achieve and what challenges they must successfully face in their transition to adulthood. These expectations are being transformed by an expanded understanding of what constitutes a healthy child as well as by a globalized economy that places a higher value on cognitive and emotional performance in rapidly evolving work environments.

The 2004 Institute of Medicine's landmark report, *Children's Health, The Nation's Wealth*, presents a new definition of child health and three associated, measurable domains:

> *Children's health should be defined as the extent to which individual children or groups of children are able or enabled to (a) develop and realize their potential, (b) satisfy their needs, and (c) develop the capacities to allow them to interact successfully with their biological, physical, and social environments.*

The domains include *health conditions*, capturing the traditional notions of health measured by disorders or illnesses of body systems; *functioning*, assessing how health affects an individual's daily life; and *health potential*, identifying the assets and positive aspects of health, such as competence, capacity, and developmental potential.

The new definition and domains help establish the goals of child health care, which go beyond diagnosing and treating disease and preventing and managing chronic health conditions. They include promoting the health capacities of each child and optimizing the health potential of all children. Underlying this definition and these goals is a new and more dynamic conceptual model of how health develops; the model can be represented by a health trajectory that is influenced by a range of biopsychosocial and environmental risks, as well as by protective and promoting factors (Fig. 1-1).

Pediatricians play an important, collaborative role in influencing factors that can optimize the child health trajectory. For one, the role and professional responsibility of the pediatrician are greatly expanded by ever-increasing medical knowledge and new, more powerful and expensive technologies. In addition, evolving performance guidelines of healthcare systems redefine expectations and attributes of the well-trained pediatrician. These expectations include the areas of professionalism, systems-based practice, patient care, interpersonal and communication skills, medical knowledge, and practice-based learning and improvement. As such, pediatricians of the 21st century, in striving to improve child health, whether at the individual or population level, must master a new, important array of knowledge, skills, and attitudes (Table 1-1).

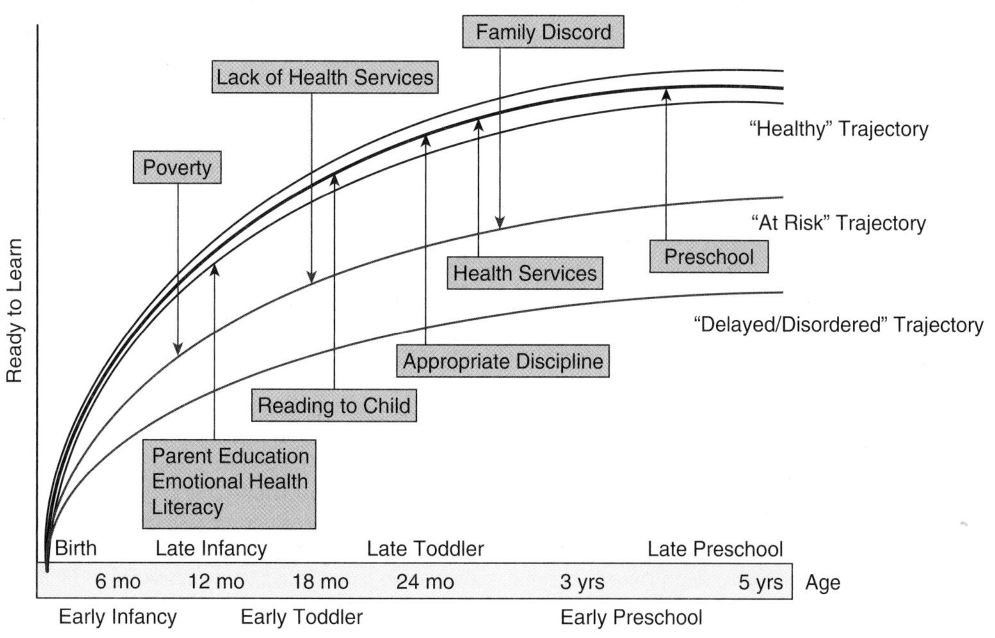


**FIGURE 1-1** Strategies to improve health development trajectories.

**TABLE 1-1 CHANGE IN ROLE AND PRACTICE ENVIRONMENT BETWEEN 20TH AND 21ST CENTURIES**

| | 20th-Century Pediatrician | 21st-Century Pediatrician |
|---|---|---|
| **Focus of clinical knowledge** | Infections and syndromes, empiric behavior and development | Genomics, environment, neuroscience-based behavior and development |
| **Access to and application of knowledge** | Delayed (months/years) | Immediate and ongoing |
| **Who controls care** | Physician | Patient/family |
| **Consistency of care** | Highly variable: individual provider based | Highly reliable: system based and evidence based |
| **Settings of care** | Inpatient and outpatient | Inpatient, outpatient, or community |
| **Role in child health** | Insular, focused on biological and developmental health | Collaborative, integrates biologic and developmental aspects of health with broader domains |

This evolution includes a shift in focus from dealing with the symptoms and empiric treatment of diseases, as well as with syndromic identification, to a greater understanding of underlying mechanisms of health and disease development. This leads to multilevel interventions that target factors that span from the genetic and cellular mechanisms to the social and family factors that are increasingly appreciated as important causal influences. In many situations, this evolution has moved medical care from a more limited focus on symptomatic treatments and palliative care to a healthcare model utilizing more sophisticated diagnostics and therapeutics, spanning from gene manipulation to modifying social influences.

The ability to deal with the inherent complexity of 21st-century medical care is facilitated by information systems, including the Internet and electronic health records. These systems also create immediacy with regard to new knowledge that is available not only to pediatricians but also to patients and families, with an expectation of more timely application of that knowledge.

As patients and families have gained increased access to medical information, a corresponding emphasis on more patient-centered and family-centered medical care has developed. Decision-making is shifting from a traditional physician-focused process to one determined by informed patient and family preferences. Widespread access to evidence-based guidelines and benchmarked systems transparent about patient outcomes have created an expectation that pediatric health care will be highly reliable with systems in place to assure safety, consistency, and high quality. It also has underscored the need for medical homes that not only provide continuous care but can translate the barrage of information. Further, family-centered models of care require that pediatricians are skilled at collaborative service delivery efforts that include the variety of settings and professionals that serve children within the context of their families. All these dimensions of care have been particularly driven this century by the Institute of Medicine's 2001 report, *Crossing the Quality Chasm*, which stipulates that health care should be safe, effective, patient centered, timely, efficient, and equitable.

Many influences are now making it difficult for an individual practitioner to care for children in multiple settings: inpatient, outpatient, or community health facilities. This is particularly true for generalists and not as true for pediatricians in more rural settings or for subspecialists. As a result, there is an increasing focus on providing care in one setting, whether inpatient or outpatient, with a few practitioners focusing on community health. This trend underscores the importance of collaboration across sectors (eg, education, family support, child welfare) to effectively influence and promote optimal child health.

Even with all these changes in pediatric health care, child health from a whole population perspective has only slightly improved. While all-cause mortality in childhood continues to decline, the proportion of children with chronic health conditions and disabilities has continued to rise. For specific disease entities, such as cancer, congenital heart disease, cystic fibrosis, and type 1 diabetes, important new treatment modalities have achieved cures and extended life. However, persistently disparate and high infant mortality rates; increasing incidence of some diseases, such as autism and attention deficit hyperactivity disorder; and an epidemic of obesity that is leading to chronic medical diseases such as type 2 diabetes in younger populations underscore the continued challenge of improving child health. Our advances in understanding the determinants and meaning of child health, as reflected in the Institute of Medicine's new developmentally focused definition, is evidence of the complementary nature of technical knowledge and collaborative strategies.

In this new era of child health, pediatricians and pediatric care need to continue to focus on care at the level of the individual child but also need to incorporate a population and community health perspective. Solutions to ongoing child health issues will be found within the context of the pediatrician's medical practice and also within the larger environmental context that now also includes the physician. In this context, the pediatrician can serve as the interpreter and synthesizer of clinical, public health, and social factors, moving beyond the confines of individual-focused care models to one that also captures and incorporates a population and community health perspective. Pediatricians skilled in these arenas can and should play a significant role in impacting the health of children in an increasingly complex world that presents many challenges to healthy development.

## SUGGESTED READINGS


Committee of Evaluation of Child Health, National Research Council and Institute of Medicine. *Children's Health, The Nation's Wealth: Assessing and Improving Child Health*. Washington, DC: National Academies Press; 2004.

Committee on Quality of Health Care in America, Institute of Medicine. *Crossing the Quality Chasm: A New Health System for the 21st Century*. Washington, DC: National Academies Press; 2001.

Halfon N, Houtrow A, Larson K, Newacheck PW. The changing landscape of disability in childhood. *Future Child*. 2012;22(1):13-42.

Halfon N, Larson K, Lu M, Tullis E, Russ S. Lifecourse health development: past, present and future. *Matern Child Health J*. 2014;18(2):344-365.


# 2 Decision-Making in Pediatrics: Use of Evidence-Based Medicine

Suresh Nagappan and Kenneth B. Roberts

## INTRODUCTION

Making thoughtful decisions about patient care is at the core of a physician's responsibilities. Multiple factors feed into clinical decision-making for a given patient with a given problem: a physician's experience, the values and preferences of the patient and patient's family, socioeconomic factors, available resources, and the best evidence that exists at the time. Physicians may have an understandable tendency to be influenced by a past missed diagnosis or an emotional case or to ignore information that conflicts with preconceived theories. Evidence-based practice can help mitigate some of these biases. Despite the trend toward peer-reviewed evidence, however, a management plan based solely on evidence from the literature may fail if not adapted to individual patient circumstances or accepted by the family. Peer-reviewed evidence is therefore a necessary but insufficient basis for clinical decision-making.

Satisfying the need for evidence typically comes in three forms: keeping up to date, building expertise in a specific field, and answering questions related to the care of specific patients. Patient-centered evidence, the focus of this chapter, demands a streamlined approach. For most clinicians, it is not feasible to spend hours reading dozens of studies to answer every clinical question that arises. The clinician must prioritize the most important patient-centered questions. A useful approach is as follows, using the mnemonic PARCA:

1. ***P***rioritize the most important patient-centered questions.
2. ***A***ssemble the four elements of an answerable question (PICO, described shortly).
3. ***R***etrieve the evidence.
4. ***C***ritically appraise the evidence.
5. ***A***pply the evidence to the particular patient.

The following vignette demonstrates the application of this process:

*The parents of a term 4-month-old are worried about their infant's frequent emesis after feedings. They tried positioning her upright after feedings, but she has continued to vomit, and her weight gain has been inadequate. Would a trial of a thickened formula help?*

## PRIORITIZING THE QUESTIONS

The physician must first decide whether it is important enough to warrant the time and effort of a literature review. If the question pertains to the mechanism of action of medications or the pathophysiology or signs and symptoms of a disease (a background question), the answers are likely found in textbooks or review articles. If the question aims to ascertain which therapy is most effective or whether a diagnostic test is useful (a foreground question), the answer is likely found in systematic reviews or original journal articles. For some foreground questions, clinical guidelines or predigested evidence may be sufficient. For other questions, clinicians may decide that they are an important enough part of their practice that it is worth looking at the evidence in more detail by following the steps below.

## ASSEMBLING THE QUESTION

The preliminary question (*Will thickened formula help?*) must be converted into a more complete, answerable format. One method, from Sackett, is summarized by *PICO: patient or problem, intervention, comparison, outcome.* The time invested in framing clinical questions in such a way is rewarded in efficiency by weeding out inapplicable evidence, irrelevant comparisons, and clinically unimportant outcomes. The focus should be on patient-centered outcomes (eg, hospitalization rate, length of stay, decrease in pain). Studies with disease-oriented outcomes (eg, improvement in laboratory values) can be a guide to future investigation but have limited application to patient care. Reframing the preliminary question in PICO format might lead to the following: *In children with gastroesophageal reflux and poor weight gain* (P), *does thickened formula* (I), *compared with positioning alone* (C), *result in improved weight gain* (O)?

## RETRIEVING THE EVIDENCE

Once the question is clearly stated, the search strategy begins by seeking current systematic reviews, such as in the Cochrane Library. In addition to saving time, well-done systematic reviews can find statistical significance in the aggregate that was not reached in any individual study because they pool the results of multiple studies. A search can then be conducted for original studies published since the review was completed. A convenient method of doing this is by using the National Library of Medicine PubMed Web site portal (https://pubmedhh.nlm.nih.gov/nlmd/pico/piconew.php) that permits clinicians to directly enter each part of the PICO question. Specifying a 4-month-old infant with reflux as the patient and problem and "thickened formula" as the intervention yields more than 2 dozen articles. To efficiently and effectively determine which articles are worth reading, clinicians can survey the article titles (and occasionally the abstracts) and compare them to the PICO question. Among the retrieved titles are the following:

1. *A thickened formula does not reduce apneas related to gastroesophageal reflux in preterm infants*
2. *Effect of cereal-thickened formula and upright positioning on regurgitation, gastric emptying, and weight gain in infants with regurgitation*
3. *Efficacy of a pre-thickened infant formula: a multicenter, double-blind, randomized, placebo-controlled parallel group trial in 104 infants with symptomatic gastroesophageal reflux*
4. *Effects of thickened feeding on gastroesophageal reflux in infants: a placebo-controlled crossover study using intraluminal impedance*

Since the patient population of interest is term infants and the issue is weight gain, not apneas, article 1 can be skipped. The desired outcome measure is weight gain, so studies that use disease-oriented outcomes, such as article 4 (intraluminal impedance), can also be skipped. Using this strategy, the number of studies to be appraised is reduced to a manageable number.

### Study Types

The "best" study type depends on the question. Systematic reviews and randomized control trials best address questions about therapy. To determine the efficacy of a diagnostic test, a prospective, blinded comparison trial is most useful. Questions about prognosis are best addressed in cohort studies, followed, in order of value, by case-control studies and case series; randomized control trials about prognosis or harm can be difficult to conduct, may have ethical problems, or may not even be feasible if the harm event is rare.

In *cohort studies* (Fig. 2-1A), investigators start by finding a group of children with a particular exposure and a group without such exposure.

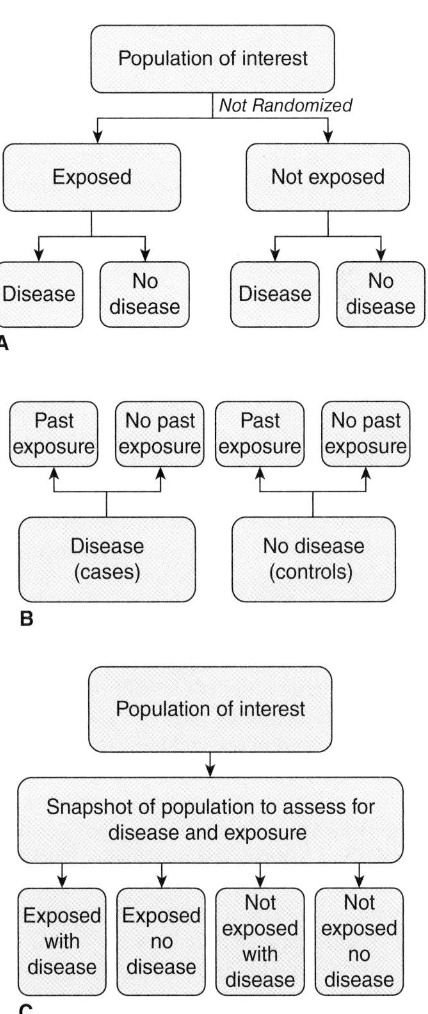


**FIGURE 2-1** What is the best type of study to answer a clinical question: (**A**) cohort study, (**B**) case-control study, or (**C**) cross-sectional study?

The groups are then followed to see whether disease develops. If a greater proportion of exposed than unexposed children develops disease, an *association* between the exposure and disease exists. Because the individuals in the groups are not randomly assigned, cohort trials are not as useful as randomized controlled trials for determining *causation*. The strength of associations in cohort trials is limited by the possibility of confounders or extraneous variables that may influence the association being studied.

In *case-control studies* (Fig. 2-1B), investigators begin with a group of children with a disease (the cases) and then match them as closely as possible to individuals who do not have the disease (the controls). The proportion of each group with the exposure of interest is determined. If there is a significant difference (eg, if 90% of the case group were exposed but only 20% of the control group were exposed), then there may be an association between the exposure and the disease. Case-control studies are practical for rare diseases. (Imagine the size of a cohort study needed for a disease with an incidence of 1 per 1 million.) The disadvantage of case-control studies is the problem of recall bias (control cases might not remember past exposures) and the inability to calculate incidence or prevalence of disease.

A third type of observational study is the *cross-sectional study* (Fig. 2-1C). A population is surveyed at one moment in time for both the presence of disease and the presence of exposure. The prevalence of disease in exposed children is then compared with that of non-exposed children. Cross-sectional studies are easier to perform than cohort or case-control studies. While they cannot establish causation, they can give useful information about prevalence and can suggest associations that can then be studied in depth using a randomized control trial or stronger observational study.

## CRITICAL APPRAISAL OF THE EVIDENCE

The fundamental determination is whether a study is valid (ie, what is claimed as true is actually true). Seven questions aid in determining the validity of a study:

1. *Were the patients randomized and was the randomization concealed?* Randomization is the only way to equalize study groups for known and unknown confounding factors. A cohort study with carefully matched groups might achieve the former but not the latter.
2. *Were treatment and control patients similar at the start of the study (ie, did randomization work)?* Most studies provide a table of demographic data and other potentially relevant characteristics of the individuals in the study groups. Comparability of the groups is necessary to assure that randomization was effective.
3. *Were patients analyzed in the groups to which they were randomized (intent to treat)?* What should be done with participants who do not follow the assigned protocol? If 10% of children who were supposed to get thickened formula received regular formula instead, should they be counted in the treatment group? In the control group? Dropped from the study? The problem with the third option is that, in real practice, nonadherence is common. The clinically important result is how a potential treatment performs in real-world use. Moving nonadherent participants into a different group might reduce the benefit of randomization, since a factor relevant to the study's outcome also might affect compliance with the intervention (eg, children with the worst reflux may have given up on the thickened formula and tried something else). Ideally, a study will analyze nonadherent patients in the original randomized category (intent-to-treat analysis) and do a separate analysis based on patients who actually follow the protocol (per-protocol analysis).
4. *Were clinicians, patients, and study personnel blinded to the group assignment?* If clinicians or patients know which intervention is being received, they might introduce bias into treatment plans or assessments and either exaggerate or minimize the true treatment effect.
5. *How many patients were lost to follow-up? Was the length of follow-up reasonable?* If a large number of patients drop out of a study, it is difficult to assess the outcome in each group fairly (especially if, for instance, the patients dropped out because the new therapy was not working or had intolerable side effects). Some loss to follow-up is unavoidable. One way of assessing whether the loss is acceptable is by using a worst-case scenario analysis. The authors could assume the worst case, that all of the children lost to follow-up did poorly, and recalculate the results using that assumption. If the results still indicate a benefit, the conclusion is strengthened. As a rule of thumb, loss to follow-up of more than 20% significantly reduces the validity of the study.
6. *Is it possible that the results could have been due to chance ($P > .05$)?* Another threat to the validity of a study is that the difference between groups is not real but is simply due to chance (a type I error). The probability of this error is expressed as *P*. By convention, up to a 5% likelihood of the results occurring by chance ($P \leq .05$) is accepted. The confidence interval is the range of values that the authors are 95% certain contains the actual value.
7. *Is it possible that results could have been skewed by a small sample size? (When does* n *matter?)* In a "positive" study (ie, a difference is demonstrated between intervention and control groups), statistical significance ($P < .05$) assures that the sample size ($n$) was adequate. In a "negative" study (ie, no statistically significant difference between groups), it is possible that a real difference between the study groups was missed (a type II error, or β). In these studies, in order to decide if the sample size was large enough to avoid this error, the clinician must examine the methods section of the study for an explanation of how the sample size was determined. The authors should specify their sample size calculation based on the difference in response they want to detect, the estimated success rate in the control group, and the minimum acceptable probability of correctly finding a clinically meaningful difference ($1 - \beta$, also known as power and generally set at 80% by convention). The importance of clinically meaningful differences is discussed later in the chapter. Using these assumptions, the authors should have calculated—and should state—the sample size needed to demonstrate a difference.

Additional measures are often useful beyond statistical significance: relative risk, odds ratio, absolute risk reduction, and the number needed to treat (the inverse of absolute risk reduction). Many published studies apply a statistic incorrectly (eg, relative risk is given in a study in which it is not valid to calculate), so it is important that clinicians aspiring to practice evidence-based medicine understand which statistics can be calculated from which types of studies and how to interpret those statistics (Table 2-1).

The *relative risk* helps clinicians decide the degree to which a new treatment shows benefit (or harm). It is a comparison of the risk of disease in the experimental group (or, in a cohort trial, the exposed children) with the risk in the control group (or the non-exposed children). Consider a fictitious randomized control trial of a new vaccine for the prevention of malaria in sub-Saharan Africa (Table 2-2).

The risk of malaria in the experimental group is 400/1220 = 33%. The risk in the control group is 800/1160 = 69%. The relative risk is thus 33%/69% = 0.48. If the relative risk is less than 1, the new treatment is beneficial; if it is greater than 1, the new treatment causes harm. A relative risk of 1 indicates that the treatment makes no difference. If the example had been a cohort study instead of a randomized control trial, "exposed" and "non-exposed" would be substituted for "treatment group" and "control group"; the relative risk would indicate whether exposure increased the risk of disease.

**TABLE 2-1 APPROPRIATE MEASURES IN CLINICAL TRIALS**

| Randomized Control Trial | Cohort Study | Case-Control Study | Cross-Sectional (Prevalence) Study |
|---|---|---|---|
| Absolute risk reduction | Relative risk | Odds ratio | Prevalence |
| Number needed to treat | Odds ratio | | |
| Relative risk | | | |

**TABLE 2-2 FICTITIOUS EXAMPLE OF RANDOMIZED CONTROLLED TRIAL OF NEW VACCINE FOR PREVENTING MALARIA IN SUB-SAHARAN AFRICA**

| | Contracted Malaria | No Malaria | Total |
|---|---|---|---|
| Vaccine (experimental group) | 400 | 820 | 1220 |
| Placebo (control group) | 800 | 360 | 1160 |

**TABLE 2-4 FICTITIOUS EXAMPLE OF SAME MALARIA VACCINE TRIAL DONE IN A MUCH LOWER PREVALENCE POPULATION**

| | Contracted Malaria | No Malaria | Total |
|---|---|---|---|
| Vaccine (experimental group) | 4 | 1216 | 1220 |
| Placebo (control group) | 8 | 1152 | 1160 |

Relative risk should not be used for case control or cross-sectional (prevalence) studies because it requires knowing the number of new cases (incidence) in each of the two groups. In our example, the children in the malaria study started disease free and were followed to determine how many contracted malaria. In a case-control study, however, the starting point would be a group that already has the disease and another that does not; because children enter the study already having the disease, the rate of *new* cases cannot be determined. To approximate relative risk in case-control trials, the **odds ratio** is used. Consider the malaria study done as a case-control study, starting with a group of children with malaria and a matched group that is malaria free (Table 2-3).

The proportion of each group that received the vaccine is measured. We must then convert from probability to odds.

The odds that a child with malaria (a case) received the vaccine is:

$$\begin{aligned} \textit{Odds that case got vaccine} &= \textit{Proportion who got vaccine/} \\ &\quad \textit{proportion who did not} \\ &= P/(1 - P) \text{ where } P \text{ is } 400/1200 \\ &= (400/1200)/[1 - (400/1200)] \\ &= 0.33/0.67 = 0.5. \end{aligned}$$

The odds that a malaria-free child (a control) received the vaccine are:

$$\begin{aligned} \textit{Odds that control got vaccine} &= \textit{Proportion who got vaccine/} \\ &\quad \textit{proportion who did not} \\ &= P/(1 - P) \text{ where } P \text{ is } 820/1180 \\ &= (820/1180)/[1 - (820/1180)] \\ &= 0.7/0.3 = 2.3. \end{aligned}$$

The odds ratio is the ratio of the above two numbers:

$$\begin{aligned} \textit{Odds ratio} &= \textit{Odds that a case got vaccine/} \\ &\quad \textit{Odds that a control got vaccine} \\ &= 0.5/2.3 = 0.22. \end{aligned}$$

Note that the relative risk (0.48) and the odds ratio (0.22) are quite different. The odds ratio is a good estimate of the relative risk only when the disease is a rare one. The high prevalence of malaria in the example explains the divergence between the two statistics and is a reminder to interpret odds ratio with caution.

There are instances in which the relative risk can also be misleading. Here, **absolute risk reduction** and **number needed to treat** become valuable. Consider the malaria study done in a much lower prevalence population (say, South America) (Table 2-4).

The relative risk is (4/1220)/(8/1160) = 0.48, identical to our African study. The study authors could still make the claim that the vaccine reduces the risk of malaria by 52%. It is clear, however, that the decision about whether to vaccinate is very different for South American doctors than for their African counterparts. The absolute risk reduction and the number needed to treat highlight this difference. The absolute risk reduction is the risk of disease in the control group minus the risk in the treatment group.

In the South American study, the absolute risk reduction is 8/1160 – 4/1220 = 0.69% – 0.33% = 0.36%.

The number needed to treat (NNT) is the reciprocal (inverse) of the absolute risk reduction, which is 1/0.36% = 278. The number needed to treat indicates that 278 children would need to be vaccinated to prevent one case of malaria.

In the African study, the absolute risk reduction is 800/1160 – 400/ 1160 = 69% – 33% = 36%. The number needed to treat (NNT) is 1/ 36% = 2.78. While the relative risk is the same, the number of children who would have to be vaccinated to prevent 1 case of malaria is 100-fold higher in South America, so a consideration of risks and costs is very different. Thus, unless the side-effect profile is intolerable, the malaria vaccine makes sense in Africa, but the decision is not as clear in South America. Reliance solely on relative risk would have masked this clinically important distinction.

**TABLE 2-3 FICTITIOUS EXAMPLE OF SAME MALARIA VACCINE TRIAL DONE AS A CASE-CONTROL STUDY**

| | Have Malaria (Cases) | No Malaria (Controls) |
|---|---|---|
| History of vaccine | 400 | 820 |
| No history of vaccine | 800 | 360 |
| **Total** | **1200** | **1180** |

## APPLYING THE EVIDENCE

If we decide the study results are valid, we must decide whether the results are applicable to our patient. Even if the outcome is relevant and statistically significant, it may still not be clinically meaningful. If, for example, a 1-oz weight gain can be demonstrated to be statistically significant in a very large study of infants with reflux treated with thickened formula, the clinician and family must decide whether such a modest gain is meaningful and whether it is worth the costs and risks of the intervention. Also, a valid study may have a patient population that does not match that of your own patients. In such cases, the study may be of little use in your clinical practice.

## CARING FOR THE PATIENT

Proceeding through the PARCA steps to determine the quality and applicability of the evidence is not the end of the process. The physician must return to the decision-making philosophy discussed at the beginning of this chapter. The evidence is only as good as the clinical acumen of the physician: In this particular case, how certain is the physician that reflux is the cause of this infant's poor weight gain? How concerning are the symptoms to the family? What is the family's preference and willingness to thicken the formula? Current best evidence provides one piece of the ultimate management plan for the patient. Clinical experience and judgment remain essential.

## SUGGESTED READINGS

Gordis L. *Epidemiology*. 5th ed. Philadelphia, PA: Saunders; 2014.

Straus S, Glasziou P, Richardson WS, Haynes EB. *Evidence-Based Medicine*. 4th ed. Edinburgh, UK: Elsevier; 2011.

Walsh M, Perkovic V, Manns B, et al. Therapy (randomized trials). In: Guyatt G, Rennie D, Meade MO, Cook DJ, eds. *Users' Guides to the Medical Literature: A Manual for Evidence-Based Clinical Practice*. 3rd ed. New York, NY: McGraw-Hill Professional; 2015.

# 3 Communication with Children and Families

Elizabeth A. Rider

## INTRODUCTION

*The practice of medicine is an art, not a trade; a calling, not a business; a calling in which your heart will be exercised equally with your head.*
—Sir William Osler

Despite the extraordinary scientific and technological advances in modern medicine, the core skills and sine qua non for the delivery of quality pediatric health care remain those of skillful communication and building and maintaining therapeutic and caring relationships with children, adolescents, and their families. The quality of the relationship with the child and family affects all aspects of patient care—the diagnostic process, treatment decisions, adherence with recommendations, and both patient and physician satisfaction.

Evidence-based studies show a direct association between the physician's competency with communication and relationship building and healthcare quality and outcomes. Good communication between physicians and their patients improves the physician's diagnostic acumen and promotes more efficient, accurate, and supportive interviews. Most physicians agree that good communication with their patients is a desirable goal.

In this chapter, we briefly consider the evidence for enhancing physician-patient communication, the concepts of patient-centered and relationship-centered care, interpersonal and communication skills, a framework for enhancing attention to values in healthcare interactions, and several evidence-based models for communication and relational skills. We examine specific strategies and techniques for communicating and building relationships with children and families throughout the pediatric interview. The overlay of children's understanding of illness and the related developmental stages of childhood are presented.

### Why Learn Communication Skills?

In one of the earliest research studies on physician-patient communication, pediatrician Barbara Korsch described communication lapses in the care of children in an emergency department. The central tenet of her groundbreaking paper, that communication is an essential factor in quality of care, is supported by numerous evidence-based studies, including the Institute of Medicine's 2001 report *Crossing the Quality Chasm*. Studies show that good communication between physician and patient correlates directly with symptom improvement; better management of chronic conditions; improved efficiency of care, including a significant reduction in diagnostic testing and referrals; increased patient satisfaction and adherence; greater physician satisfaction; and fewer medication errors and malpractice claims. The majority of malpractice claims arise from communication errors.

In pediatrics, effective physician-parent communication is associated with parental satisfaction with care, adherence to treatment recommendations, and enhanced discussion of psychosocial issues. Parents highly value physicians who attend to both their own and their child's feelings and concerns and who seek to understand their perspective. Greater parent satisfaction with care is positively associated with more active communication between physician and child, adequate attention to parental concerns regarding the child's illness, and parents' perceptions of the physicians' interpersonal sensitivity, partnership building, and ability to provide information.

Kahn and colleagues found that psychosocial issues motivate 65% of primary care pediatric visits, and 85% of mothers with young children indicate they would welcome or not mind being asked about emotional and psychosocial stressors. Studies show that parents are more likely to disclose psychosocial issues when the pediatrician directly questions, shows interest and attention while listening, and shows interest in managing parenting and behavioral concerns.

In 2008, the Committee on Bioethics of the American Academy of Pediatrics published a technical report that reviewed evidence for effective communication in various pediatric situations, provided additional practical suggestions, and, like previous authors, called for greater emphasis on communication with patients and families in pediatric education, practice, and research. Rider, Volkan, and Hafler studied pediatric residents' attitudes about communication skills and their perceptions of the importance of learning, and confidence in, 15 specific pediatric communication skills. Most residents reported confidence in core communication skills (interviewing, listening, building rapport, and demonstrating caring and empathy), yet half or fewer felt confident about their skills in 7 more advanced communication competencies (ability to discuss end-of-life issues, speaking with children about serious illness, giving bad news, dealing with the "difficult" patient/parent, cultural awareness/sensitivity, understanding psychosocial aspects, and understanding patients' perspectives).

International guidelines, consensus statements such as the Kalamazoo Consensus Statement, and certification standards reflect the increasing emphasis on interpersonal and communication skills at all levels of medical training. The Liaison Committee on Medical Education (LCME) and the Accreditation Council for Graduate Medical Education (ACGME) in the United States, and accreditation organizations internationally, require medical schools and residency programs to teach and assess interpersonal and communication competencies. Licensing and medical specialty boards also require competency in these areas.

Interpersonal and communication competencies in pediatric education continue to evolve. Rider and Keefer provide further definitions of effective communication with diverse patients and families, understanding and responding to emotions, interprofessional communication and working effectively as a leader or member of healthcare teams, and acting as a consultant to other physicians and healthcare professionals.

### Patient-Centered and Relationship-Centered Care

Patient-centered care places a focus on the patient's disease and illness experience. Each patient is acknowledged as a unique individual, and the patient's and family's perspectives, culture, personalities, and related factors are relevant to the process of health care. As noted in the Pew-Fetzer Task Force's document, *Health Professions Education and Relationship-Centered Care*, "The phrase 'relationship-centered care' captures the importance of the interaction among people as the foundation of any therapeutic or healing activity" (p. 11).

With its focus on how physicians and patients relate to each other, relationship-centered care is a natural next step for conceptualizing health care. Beach and colleagues note that the focus on the patient expands to include ways in which both physician and patient relate together and also includes additional relationships around the patient and doctor.

Relationship-centered care in the clinician-patient relationship includes the following concepts: relationships are the medium of care; relationships are therapeutic; both patients and physicians are active participants; and partnership and respect for patients' participation in decision-making are valued. In addition, the physician's capacity for self-awareness and self-reflection is an important component of relationship-centered care and includes an awareness of ideas, feelings, and values that influence the relationship, being "present" for self and others, and paying attention to one's own behavior. The relationship-centered clinician understands that the way in which they participate in an interaction with patients essentially shapes the course and outcome of care.

### Interpersonal and Communication Skills

*The treatment of a disease may be entirely impersonal; the care of a patient must be completely personal. The significance of the intimate personal relationship between physician and patient cannot be too strongly emphasized, for in an extraordinarily large number of cases both diagnosis and treatment are directly dependent on it, and the failure of the young physician to establish this relationship accounts for much of his ineffectiveness in the care of patients.*
—Francis W. Peabody (1927)

Medicine has traditionally defined interpersonal and communication skills as a set of specific behaviors or tasks. Dyche, Duffy and colleagues, and Rider describe how interpersonal and communication skills are distinct, even though they are considered components of the same competency for all physicians to master. Communication skills are behavioral and task-oriented (eg, making eye contact, greeting each person in the room). Alone, these behaviors can neither build nor maintain a therapeutic relationship. Rider notes that the ability to form a deeper level of relationship and connection with patients and families goes beyond developing a set of communication behaviors with which to carry out the interview.

Interpersonal skills are relationship and process oriented and include a focus on humanistic qualities and the effects of communication on others. Examples of interpersonal skills include empathy, with an accurate understanding of patients' and families' emotions, caring, and emotional responsiveness; and as Rider and Keefer note, the capacity to provide a sustainable relationship that includes authenticity and honesty and allows repair when mistakes are made.

#### Values as the Foundation of Care

Browning notes that all healthcare interactions between patients and healthcare professionals, and among healthcare teams and colleagues, occur within a broader moral universe of human standards that include personal integrity, professionalism, and the everyday ethics of practice. Attention to core values and skilled communication are vital to the practice of high-quality, safe, compassionate healthcare. Excellent relationships and communication, grounded by attention to values and patient engagement, improve health outcomes, patient safety, and patient and clinician satisfaction. The International Charter for Human Values in Healthcare delineates core values fundamental to all healthcare interactions, and provides a framework of values that is used to inform clinical practice, training, research, and organizational change efforts.

Rider, Kurtz, Slade, and colleagues describe the development of the Charter and the identification of 5 categories of core values—Compassion, Respect for Persons, Commitment to Integrity and Ethical Practice, Commitment to Excellence, and Justice in Healthcare—that are central to every healthcare interaction. Attention to values along with skilled communication not only inform everyday practice, but can help guide and support physicians' and other clinicians' approaches to unexpected, difficult situations such as conversations about end-of-life decisions.

The late pediatrician Steven Z. Miller, a long-time advocate of compassionate clinical care, developed with Hilary Schmidt a conceptual framework to encourage the infusion of humanism into every patient encounter and into the medical culture as a whole. Their "habit of humanism" includes the following:

1. Identifying the multiple perspectives in each encounter (ie, that of the patient, family member or other support person, and physician).
2. Reflecting on possible conflicts that could help or hinder forming a relationship with the patient.
3. Choosing to act altruistically (ie, supporting the patient's perspective above all, even if it conflicts with the physician's agenda or personal interest).

### FRAMEWORKS FOR INTERPERSONAL AND COMMUNICATION SKILLS AND RELATIONSHIP ABILITIES

The pediatric encounter is unique in medicine. Communicating with children and their families is complex, routinely involves the physician-parent-child triad and other family members, and is influenced by the developmental and cognitive stage of the child. The interaction dynamics of physician-parent-child communication are particularly challenging when the child and the parent have different needs.

In addition to covering medical issues, anticipatory guidance, and parent education, the pediatric interview often includes psychosocial and developmental concerns. Increasingly, more children are seen for behavioral, developmental, and psychosocial problems, especially in primary care. The varied needs and perspectives of both children and family members and the complexity of issues require physician flexibility and the ability to adjust interview and physical examination techniques as needed.

A variety of communication models or frameworks exist and can be learned and/or adapted for pediatric care. These frameworks are evidence based and include specific communication competencies associated with improved health outcomes. The conceptual frameworks for interpersonal and communication skills presented here can be used or adapted for clinical practice, teaching, and assessment.

#### Expanded Definitions of Interpersonal and Communication Skills Competencies

Rider and Keefer used an expert consensus group model with an international group of medical education leaders to further define and expand the original ACGME interpersonal and communication skills competencies. The international expert consensus group's expanded competencies that address the physician-patient relationship are presented in Table 3-1.

#### The Four Habits Model

The Four Habits Model, described by Frankel and Stein, organizes communication tasks into 4 interrelated groups of skills and provides techniques for performing these "habits" as well as the benefits of each (Tables 3-2 and 3-3). The Four Habits Model was originally created for use within Kaiser Permanente and was derived from a blend of clinical experience and empirical literature.

#### Kalamazoo Consensus Statement

The Kalamazoo Consensus Statement, developed by a group of 21 medical education leaders and communication experts from the United States and Canada, identifies 7 evidence-based "essential elements" of effective physician-patient communication and provides tasks for each element. The essential elements are (1) build a relationship, (2) open the discussion, (3) gather information, (4) understand the patient's perspective, (5) share information, (6) reach agreement, and (7) provide closure. The framework considers building a relationship an ongoing task throughout each encounter (see Table 3-3).

Similarly, the Academic Pediatric Association, with help from 300 pediatric experts, developed guidelines for education in pediatric residencies. These guidelines include core communication skills that were developed, in part, from the Kalamazoo Consensus Statement framework.

### COMMUNICATION SKILLS AND RELATIONSHIP STRATEGIES IN THE PEDIATRIC ENCOUNTER

The models for communication and relationship skills presented in the previous section can be used or adapted for clinical practice with children and their families. The combined components of the Four Habits Model and the Kalamazoo Consensus Statement framework are presented in Table 3-3. The components of these frameworks overlap significantly because they stem from the same literature. We can use these frameworks as a guide to examining techniques and strategies for working with children and their family members.

#### Building Relationships with Children and Families

Building and sustaining relationships and building a therapeutic alliance with children and their family members remain ongoing tasks within all clinical encounters. Components that underlie an effective physician-parent-child relationship include getting to know the patient and parent as individuals, expressing interest in the child as a person, giving attention to the child's and family's values, and understanding the way each family member experiences the child's illness. Other important components of effective relationships include listening skills, nonverbal communication, and understanding the role of play and children's different developmental stages. As noted by Rider, Kurtz, Slade, and colleagues, awareness of and attention to core values such as compassion, respect, integrity, excellence, and justice remain essential in healthcare interactions.

**The Child's Participation** Children understand more about concepts of health and illness than previously thought and can provide unique and valuable information about themselves. When appropriate, children should be involved in decisions about their own health care. Studies show that direct communication between physician and child contributes to

**TABLE 3-1 INTERPERSONAL AND COMMUNICATION SKILLS COMPETENCIES: EXPANDED DEFINITIONS**

| Expanded Competencies and Subcompetencies |
|---|
| **1. Create and sustain a relationship that is therapeutic for patients and supportive of their families.** |
| (a) Be "present," paying attention to the patient, caring for the patient, and working collaboratively and from strengths. |
| (b) Accept and explore the patient's feelings, including negative feelings. |
| (c) Provide a sustainable relationship that allows for repair when mistakes are made, and includes authenticity, honesty, and admission of and sorrow for mistakes. |
| (d) Communicate with the patient's family honestly and supportively. In some cases (eg, pediatrics and geriatrics), the doctor-patient relationship is imbedded in and extends to the family; in other circumstances, the doctor's relationship with the family may be separate from that with the patient. |
| **2. Use effective listening skills to facilitate relationship. Elicit and provide information using effective nonverbal, explanatory, questioning, and writing skills. Respond promptly to patients' queries and requests.** |
| (a) Demonstrate effective listening by hearing and understanding in a way that the patient feels heard and understood. Use nonverbal cues such as nodding, pausing, and maintaining eye contact, and verbal skills including back-tracking, reflecting, and mirroring. |
| (b) Recognize the patient's preferred (or current) mode of communication and selectively choose the most effective mode of communication for the situation. Assess patient's understanding of problem and desire for more information; explain using words that are easy for the patient to understand. |
| (c) Understand the patient's perspective, including the patient's individual concerns, beliefs, and expectations; respect the patient's cultural and ethnic beliefs, practices, and language. |
| (d) Create an atmosphere of mutuality and respect through patient participation and involvement in decision-making. |
| 1. Include patient in choices and decisions to the extent he or she desires. |
| 2. Collaboratively set agenda for encounters. |
| 3. Negotiate mutually acceptable plans in partnership with patient. |
| **3. Work effectively with others as a member or leader of the healthcare team or other professional group. In all areas of communication and interaction, show respect and empathy toward colleagues and learners.** |
| (a) Demonstrate excellent collaboration and cooperation with other members of the healthcare team involved in the patient's care |
| 1. Be specific with questions asked of, and answers given to, colleagues; ensure that the communication is clearly understood. |
| 2. Include adequate and complete information in all documentation and written communication about a patient's care. |
| 3. Resolve conflict and give constructive feedback on mistakes. |
| (b) Communicate clearly in the role of teacher. |
| 1. Assess the educational needs of learners. |
| 2. Collaboratively set realistic learning expectations with learners. |
| 3. Identify and eliminate barriers in team teaching; maintain an appropriate balance between patient care and teaching. |
| 4. Offer, seek, and accept honest, constructive, and timely feedback. |

Reproduced with permission from Rider EA, Keefer CH: Communication skills competencies: definitions and a teaching toolbox, *Med Educ.* 2006 Jul;40(7):624-629.

improved relationships, treatment adherence, satisfaction with care, and better health outcomes.

Physicians can collaborate with parents to help children have a voice in medical encounters. Differing communication needs of the child and parents sometimes present a challenge to relationship-centered care in pediatrics. Physicians can facilitate the child's participation and at the same time address parents' needs and call on parents' expertise and knowledge of their child.

Strategies that enhance the child's participation in the pediatric encounter include addressing the child by name, inviting the child to state the problem, and encouraging the child to participate in the conversation both verbally, by directing questions to the child, and nonverbally, by using eye contact, nodding, and smiling. Physicians should give advice and explain treatment plans to the child in words he or she can understand. Utilizing these and similar strategies allows physicans to model for parents the direct inclusion of the child.

### Listening Skills

*I suspect that the most basic and powerful way to connect to another person is to listen. Just listen. Perhaps the most important thing we ever give each other is our attention. And especially if it's given from the heart.... We connect through listening.*

—Rachel Remen, MD

Effective listening skills facilitate relationships and promote collaboration between physician and patient. Listening inattentively or without mindfulness may lead to suboptimal diagnostic and treatment decisions.

Active listening enables the physician to hear and address the concerns of children and their families. Listening includes being "present" and attending fully. Physicians demonstrate effective listening by reflecting, summarizing, and checking whatever seems unusual in the context of the patient's story so that the patient can correct or add information that completes the picture. Patients appreciate the physician's attempts to understand.

**Nonverbal Communication** Effective use of nonverbal communication helps to promote an environment of trust and support. Nonverbal communication includes body language as well as tone, pace, and pitch of speaking. To focus the interview on the patient as well as the illness, the physician must demonstrate, nonverbally, that what the patient and parents have to say is important. Use of nonverbal cues such as nodding, pausing, maintaining eye contact, and posture show attentiveness and concern. Congruence between words, tone, and body language is important for effective communication. Strategies for nonverbal communication that promote relationship building are presented in Table 3-4.

### Invest in the Beginning

The Four Habits Model identifies 3 tasks to accomplish at the beginning of the interview: create rapport quickly, elicit the patient's concerns, and plan the visit with the patient. The Kalamazoo Consensus Statement identifies similar tasks in its first 3 essential elements for communication in medical encounters: build a relationship, open the discussion, and gather information (see Table 3-3).

**Opening the Interview** Rapport begins from the opening moments of the interview and includes mutual interest and respect among the physician, child, and parents. The pediatric visit often includes a variety of individuals (eg, siblings, 1 or both parents, or other caregivers). Open the interview with an inclusive greeting and introduction, acknowledge everyone in the room, use their names, and find out how they are related to the patient. Greet and welcome the child. Even with infants, the physician can smile and interact with the infant for several seconds. This also gives the physician a moment to assess the child.

Address and acknowledge siblings in the room: "I see your baby brother came today. Does he make lots of noise?" "Sometimes babies do funny things!" Siblings can be disruptive if they feel displaced by a new baby or another sibling, so your early interaction with a patient's sibling may have an important calming effect on the entire visit. Your role modeling also engages and assists the parents.

**Elicit Concerns and Plan the Visit** Important components of investing in the beginning of the interview include planning the visit and setting an agenda with the parents and patient. Dyche and Swiderski's study showed that physicians who solicited an agenda from their patients and allowed them to complete a statement of concerns were able to report their patients' problems more accurately, while failure to ask the patients' agenda correlated with a 24% reduction in physician understanding.

**TABLE 3-2 THE FOUR HABITS MODEL**

| Habit | Skills | Techniques and Examples | Benefits |
|---|---|---|---|
| Invest in the Beginning | Create rapport quickly | • Introduce self to everyone in the room.<br>• Refer to the patient by last name and title (eg, Mr. or Ms.) until a relationship has been established.<br>• Acknowledge wait.<br>• Make a social comment or ask a nonmedical question to put the patient at ease.<br>• Convey familiarity by commenting on prior visit or problem.<br>• Consider the patient's cultural background and use appropriate gestures, eye contact, and body language. | • Establishes a welcoming atmosphere<br>• Allows faster access to real reason for visit<br>• Increases diagnostic accuracy<br>• Requires less work<br>• Minimizes "Oh by the way ..." at the end of the visit.<br>• Facilitates negotiating an agenda<br>• Decreases potential for conflict |
| | Elicit the patient's concerns | • Start with open-ended questions:<br>"What would you like help with today?"<br>"I understand that you're here for.... Could you tell me more about that?"<br>• Speak directly with the patient when using an interpretor. | |
| | Plan the visit with the patient | • Repeat concerns back to check understanding.<br>• Let the patient know what to expect: "How about if we start with talking more about ___, then I'll do an exam, and then we'll go over possible ways to treat this? Sound OK?"<br>• Prioritize when necessary: "Let's make sure we talk about ___ and ___. It sounds like you also want to make sure we cover ___. If we can't get to the other concerns, let's ..." | |
| Elicit the Patient's Perspective | Ask for the patient's ideas | • Assess the patient's point of view:<br>"What do you think might be causing your symptoms?"<br>"What concerns you most about this problem?"<br>"What have you done to treat your illness so far?"<br>• Ask about ideas from loved ones or from community.<br>• Express respect toward alternative healing practices. | • Respects diversity<br>• Allows the patient to provide important diagnostic clues<br>• Uncovers hidden concerns<br>• Reveals use of alternative treatments or requests for tests<br>• Improves diagnosis of depression and anxiety |
| | Elicit specific requests | • Determine the patient's goal in seeking care: "How were you hoping I could help?" | |
| | Explore the impact on the patient's life | • Check context: "How have your symptoms affected your daily activities/work/family?" | |
| Demonstrate Empathy | Be open to the patient's emotions | • Respond in a culturally appropriate manner to changes in body language and voice tone. | • Adds depth and meaning to the visit<br>• Builds trust, leading to better diagnostic information, adherence, and outcomes<br>• Makes limit-setting or saying "no" easier |
| | Make an empathetic statement | • Look for opportunities to use brief empathetic comments: "You seem really worried."<br>• Compliment the patient on efforts to address problem. | |
| | Convey empathy nonverbally | • Use a pause, touch, or facial expression. | |
| Invest in the End | Deliver diagnostic information | • Frame the diagnosis in terms of the patient's original concerns. | • Increases potential for collaboration<br>• Influences health outcomes<br>• Improves adherence<br>• Reduces return calls and visits<br>• Encourages self-care<br>• Enhances confidence and trust |
| | Provide education | • Explain rationale for tests and treatments in plain language<br>• Review possible side effects and expected course of recovery.<br>• Discuss options that are consistent with the patient's lifestyle, cultural values, and beliefs.<br>• Provide written materials in the patient's preferred language when possible. | |
| | Involve the patient in making decisions | • Discuss treatment goals to ensure mutual understanding and agreement.<br>• Assess the patient's ability and motivation to carry out plan.<br>• Explore barriers: "What do you think would help overcome any problems you might have with the treatment plan?" | |
| | Complete the visit | • Summarize visit and review next steps.<br>• Verify comprehension by asking the patient to repeat instructions.<br>• Ask: "What questions do you have about what we discussed today?"<br>• Give the patient a written summary of the visit, including relevant Web sites.<br>• Close the visit in a positive way: "It's been nice seeing you. Thanks for coming in." | |

**TABLE 3-3 A COMPARISON OF THE COMMUNICATION AND RELATIONSHIP COMPETENCIES OF THE FOUR HABITS MODEL AND THE KALAMAZOO CONSENSUS STATEMENT FRAMEWORK**

| The Four Habits Model | Kalamazoo Consensus Statement Framework |
|---|---|
| **Habit 1. Invest in the Beginning** | **1. Build a relationship (throughout interview)** |
| • Create rapport quickly | • Greet and show interest in patient as a person |
| • Elicit the patient's concerns | • Use words that show care and concern throughout the interview |
| • Plan the visit with the patient | • Use tone, pace, eye contact, and posture that show care and concern |
| | **2. Open the discussion** |
| | **3. Gather information** |
| **Habit 2. Elicit the Patient's Perspective** | **4. Understand the patient's perspective** |
| • Ask for the patient's ideas | • Ask about life events, circumstances, other people that might affect health |
| • Elicit specific request | • Elicit patient's beliefs, concerns, and expectations about illness and treatment |
| • Explore impact on the patient's life | • Respond explicitly to patient statements about ideas, feelings, and values |
| **Habit 3. Demonstrate Empathy** | Incorporated in |
| • Be open to the patient's emotions | 1. Build a relationship |
| • Make an empathic statement | 4. Understand the patient's perspective |
| • Convey empathy nonverbally | |
| **Habit 4. Invest in the End** | **5. Share information** |
| • Deliver diagnostic information | **6. Reach agreement** |
| • Provide education | **7. Provide closure** |
| • Involve patient in making decisions | |
| • Complete the visit | |

Data from Frankel RM, Stein T. Getting the most out of the clinical encounter: the Four Habits Model. *Permanente J.* 1999;3:79-88; Bayer-Fetzer Conference on Physician-Patient Communication in Medical Education. Essential elements of communication in medical encounters: the Kalamazoo consensus statement. *Acad Med.* 2001;76:390-393; and Rider EA. Interpersonal and Communication Skills. In: Rider EA, Nawotniak RH, eds. *A Practical Guide to Teaching and Assessing the ACGME Core Competencies.* 2nd ed. Marblehead, MA: HCPro, Inc; 2010:1-137.

In today's healthcare environments, the short time allowed for many office visits and time a parent needs to discuss issues may prove incompatible. Prioritizing concerns, both parents' and physician's, and being explicit about the time allowed for a visit, conveys respect to the patient and saves time. The physician can invite the child and parent to return for subsequent visits if concerns remain.

The words physicians use are important. For example, a parent will experience the words "I wish we had time to talk about your concerns about your child's sleep today. Let's make a follow-up appointment to talk further" differently from the words "I don't have time to deal with all these problems now." The following questions may help to plan the visit.

1. *Agenda-setting questions:* "What is concerning you today?" "Anything else?" "I see you have a list; is there anything else you would like us to talk about today?" "Your child was scheduled for a 10-minute visit. I want to make sure I've heard all of your concerns, and then we can decide together what we can accomplish today."
2. *Prioritizing questions:* "What is most important for us to address today?" "What is at the top of your list?" The physician may need to take the lead in efficiently negotiating and prioritizing both the physician's agenda and the parents. "Let's make sure we discuss A and B; if we don't get to C, we can talk by phone or set up another visit."

**TABLE 3-4 STRATEGIES FOR NONVERBAL COMMUNICATION THAT PROMOTE RELATIONSHIP BUILDING**

| Nonverbal Communication Strategies |
|---|
| • Acknowledge and briefly interact with the child at the beginning of the visit. |
| • Establish eye contact with the infant and child from across the room. Talk with the parent and acknowledge and smile at the child, while the child becomes more comfortable with your presence. This strategy brings the child into the interaction nonverbally. |
| • Adapt your own pace, tone, and posture in response to the child and parent. Tone and pace of speech sometimes communicate feelings more effectively than the words themselves. |
| • Be present, appear unhurried, and convey interest and caring. |
| • During the physical examination, respect the child's personal distance. If your face is too close to an infant's face, she may look away and cry. Toddlers often avoid unfamiliar people in their personal space. A good strategy is to look away when you are close (eg, listening to heart and lungs). Approach school-aged children calmly and respectfully. |
| • Adults appear large to small children. Make yourself appear less threatening by sitting at the child's eye level while the child remains in the parent's lap, or having the child sit on the examination table with the parent nearby. |
| • Avoid interruptions of patient visits. This includes interruptions from phone calls and beepers, reading the chart, or using the computer while listening to or talking with the child and family. |

Adapted with permission from Rider EA. Communication and relationships with children and parents. In: Novack DH, Clark W, Saizow R, Daetwyler C, eds. *DocCom: an interactive learning resource for healthcare communication.* 2006. Available at: http://webcampus.drexelmed.edu/doccom/user/. Accessed October 10, 2016.

### Understand the Patient's and Family's Perspective

Effective communication requires an understanding of the patient in his or her world context. Understanding the patient's and family's perspectives includes understanding their individual concerns, beliefs, values, and expectations about diagnosis and treatment, and also depends on the child's developmental stage. Inherent is respect for the patient's and family's cultural and ethnic beliefs.

The Four Habits Model identifies 3 skills to elicit the patient's perspective: assessing patient attribution, identifying the patient's requests for care, and exploring the impact of the patient's symptoms on his or her life and well-being. The Kalamazoo Consensus Statement adds asking about life events, circumstances, and other people that might affect health, and responding explicitly to the patient's statements about ideas, feelings, and values (see Table 3-3).

Listen to the patient's or family's story, identify their major concerns, and ask about their understanding of the causes of illness and possible treatment. "What concerns you the most about your child's illness?" "What do you think has caused the problem?"

Elicit expectations about illness and treatment. Find out what the patient and family want: "How were you hoping I might help?" Explore the impact of the illness on the patient and family, considering their physical, emotional, and social well-being. How do they experience the child's illness? Respond explicitly to the patient's and parents' expressed thoughts and feelings: "You seem worried about…."

As noted by Rider (2002), even young children reveal clues about their concerns and perspectives through their questions and comments:

*After a 3-year-old well-child visit, Sarah's mother shares that Sarah has seemed anxious and worried since the 9/11 terrorist attacks. We talk further. I kneel down to Sarah's eye level and tell her, "Your mommy is safe, your daddy is safe, and you are safe." She looks at me with big, attentive eyes and I know I have connected. With solemn seriousness, she slowly pulls her lollipop out of her mouth and says, with great emphasis, "And my kitty cat." "Yes, your kitty cat is safe too."*

#### Demonstrate Empathy and Compassion

Demonstrating empathy and compassion help the child and family to feel validated and understood. Evidence-based studies support the positive value of empathy in health care and suggest an association between the physician's caring and empathy and the effectiveness and appropriateness of care. Conveying empathy increases diagnostic accuracy and patient adherence, yet remains time efficient. Empathy also has been shown to increase both patient and physician satisfaction.

Conveying empathy requires the physician to perceive the patient's emotions and experience and then respond to them in ways that the patient and family feel understood. Much of empathic communication is subtle and subject to cultural differences, particularly in its nonverbal components. Because of this subtlety, empathy may be lost if the physician is preoccupied with the cognitive work of organizing complex data about diagnosis and treatment, and the patient is preoccupied with confusion, worry, or perceived social rules for medical visits. The ability to convey empathy and compassion in countless diverse and complex medical interview situations requires a mindful approach to interactions, listening to feedback, and continuing practice.

The words we use with patients help us to recognize patient clues and to elicit and respond to the patient's emotions. What we say may promote empathic discussion, or miss it, or actually end it. By exercising basic empathic skills, physicians can attend to connectedness and relationship and remain empathic in spite of obstacles. Possessing a toolbox of strategies to promote empathic communication promotes the physician's efficiency and enhances satisfaction. Strategies and words to use to convey empathy and to handle emotions are presented in Table 3-5.

**TABLE 3-5 STRATEGIES THAT CONVEY EMPATHY AND FACILITATE HANDLING EMOTIONS**

| Strategy | Content and Words to Use |
|---|---|
| Elicit emotions | • Recognize when the child or parent has emotions that are present but not directly expressed in words. The child may hide behind the examination table or cling to a parent. A parent may appear distracted or skeptical.<br>• Invite exploration of unexpressed feelings.<br>  • With the child we can ask, "Are you worried?" "How are you doing right now?" "Anything else?"<br>  • With the parent, we can ask, "What are you most concerned about?" "What has this been like for you?" "Can you tell me more?" or note, "You look skeptical."<br>• Explicitly acknowledge and accept feelings: "You seem worried by this; you've been through a lot."<br>• Accept children's expressions of upset or grief. Crying usually brings relief and can be helpful to the child. Avoid overreacting to tears or trying to distract children from their feelings. Ignore temper tantrums. |
| Respond to the child's and parent's emotions | • "I can see that this is bothering you."<br>• "That sounds really hard."<br>• "It seems like that might feel ..."<br>• "You must feel proud about that. That's great!"<br>• "You were really brave. Good for you!"<br>• "It's okay to cry. No one likes to have a shot."<br>• "I am here to help you in any way I can."<br>• "Most people feel overwhelmed when this happens."<br>• "You must have been up all night too (with your child). I imagine you are tired." |
| Reflect content and check in with child and parent | • "It sounds like you think ... Did I leave anything out?"<br>• "What I am hearing is ... Do I have it right?"<br>• "I want to make sure I understand what you have shared with me."<br>• "Are you worried about having a shot?"<br>• "You sound sad (or unhappy, skeptical, etc)." |

Adapted with permission from Rider EA. Communication and relationships with children and parents. In: Novack DH, Clark W, Saizow R, Daetwyler C, eds. *DocCom: an interactive learning resource for healthcare communication.* 2006. Available at: http://webcampus.drexelmed.edu/doccom/user/. Accessed October 10, 2016; and Coulehan JL, Platt FW, Egener B, et al. "Let me see if I have this right ...": words to help build empathy. *Ann Intern Med.* 2001;135:221-227.

#### Invest in the End of the Visit

Investing in the end of the visit includes sharing information and providing education, partnering with the child and family members, and including them in choices and decisions to the extent they desire. The physician also works with the child and parents to reach agreement on plans and to complete the visit by summarizing, clarifying follow-up plans, and providing closure.

**Share Information and Provide Education** Determine the patient's and family's understanding of the issues and their desire for additional information: "Is there a particular issue you would like information on now?" "What is your understanding of why your child is receiving this medication?" Consider the child's developmental and cognitive perspective, and use this knowledge when sharing information. Provide education for both child and parents, including the rationale for diagnostic tests and treatment options, expectations, and resources.

The impact of the physician's words is often powerful, and patients and worried parents may be easily frightened by careless word choices, especially about prognosis. Share diagnostic and treatment information gently, and use words that are easy for the child and family to understand. Intersperse the telling of information with asking about understanding and impact. Patients value these demonstrations of respect and consideration.

**Establish a Partnership with the Child and Family** Tuckett and colleagues describe the clinical encounter as a "meeting between experts." The patient is an expert in describing his or her problems, experience of disease, and preferences. The physician is an expert in disease identification and management and in sorting the patient's issues into a format that provides therapeutic direction.

Studies show that involving the patient and parents in making decisions corresponds with improved outcomes. Invite active child and family collaboration throughout the encounter, with attention to involving them in decision making to the extent they wish. Most patients prefer information and discussion, and some prefer mutual or joint decisions. Strategies for partnering with patients include inviting the child and parents to help establish the agenda for the visit, checking for mutual understanding of information about diagnosis and treatment, exploring barriers, and collaborating in negotiation about mutually acceptable diagnostic and treatment plans.

**Provide Closure for the Visit** Ask if the patient has additional questions or concerns, summarize what was discussed, and clarify any follow-up plans. Complete the visit by acknowledging the patient and reassuring the patient of ongoing care.

## COMMUNICATING WITH CHILDREN AT DIFFERENT DEVELOPMENTAL STAGES

#### Children's Concepts of Illness

Children's understanding of illness and their cognitive, social, and emotional abilities vary by developmental stage. Understanding children's perspectives at different ages helps the pediatrician to communicate more effectively and accurately. During the pediatric visit, the physician can educate parents about child development and

**TABLE 3-6 CHILDREN'S COGNITIVE DEVELOPMENT AND CONCEPTS OF ILLNESS AT DIFFERENT AGES**

| | Preschool Children (3–5 Years) | School-Aged Children (6–12 Years) | Adolescents (≥ 13 Years) |
|---|---|---|---|
| **Cognitive development** | Magical thinking; circular reasoning | Begins to think relationally and to generalize | Capable of cognitive problem solving and decision making |
| | Sees 1 or 2 aspects at a time; may ignore the whole of the situation | Emergence of clear differentiation between self and others | Can think abstractly and hypothetically |
| | Does not differentiate well between self and outside world; lives in the immediate environment | Begins to integrate variables in causal relationships | Uses generalization to fill in gaps in knowledge |
| **Child's concept of the cause of illness** | Does not spontaneously conceptualize the internal parts of the body | Can distinguish what is internal and external to self | Integrates multiple factors/causes in understanding illness; imagines alternative possibilities |
| | Illness results from wrongdoing; medical procedures are seen as a punishment | Cause of illness is a person, object, or action outside of the child: "You get a cold from not wearing a hat;" "You breathe too much air in your nose." | Cause of illness lies in internal physiologic organ or process; may have additional psychological cause |
| | Illness is caused by external concrete phenomenon: contagion, magic, "from the sun," "from outside" | Cause of illness is the presence of "germs" | Understands illness as internal systems that dysfunction and cause external symptoms: "A virus gets into the bloodstream and causes a cold." |

Adapted with permission from Rider EA. Communication and relationships with children and parents. In: Novack DH, Clark W, Saizow R, Daetwyler C, eds. *DocCom: an interactive learning resource for healthcare communication.* 2006. Available at: http://webcampus.drexelmed.edu/doccom/user/. Accessed October 10, 2016.

support good parenting. Table 3-6 presents information about children's cognitive development and their concepts of illness at different developmental stages.

### Approaches to Children at Different Stages

Both child and family members have different needs based on the child's developmental stage. Each developmental stage requires different interviewing, examination, and counseling approaches. Placement of the child in the room, relationship-building strategies, play and interaction techniques, and history taking are important variables to consider (Table 3-7).

### Children and Play

The use of play is a particularly effective strategy for communicating with young children. Children use play to gain understanding of themselves and others, to learn about the world, and to explore their abilities to cope with its complexities. As you observe young children at play, you will see family-related themes and action plans for helping and healing and for avoiding fears. Children's play becomes increasingly complex and varied as they grow older. Creating a playful atmosphere helps the physician to complete necessary tasks and enhances enjoyment for both the child and the physician (Table 3-8).

## CONCLUSION

*Expertise in interviewing is the key to the pediatrician's psychotherapeutic effectiveness.... Skill in interviewing involves more than asking the right questions; it also requires an ability to empathize, to observe, and to listen carefully.*

—Morris Green, MD

Skillful communication and relationship abilities are essential to the practice of high-quality pediatric care. Effective communication among child, family, and physician consists of a 2-way,

**TABLE 3-7 APPROACHES TO THE PEDIATRIC INTERVIEW WITH CHILDREN AT DIFFERENT DEVELOPMENTAL STAGES**

| | Infants (0–15 Months) | Toddlers (15 Months–2 Years) | Preschool Children (3–5 Years) | School-Aged Children (6–12 Years) | Adolescents (≥ 13 Years) |
|---|---|---|---|---|---|
| **Location of child during interview** | Parent's lap or arms | Parent's lap or arms | Freely moving about room | Exam table | Exam table |
| | Exam table | Freely moving about room | Exam table | Chair | Chair |
| **Relationship-building strategies** | Talk with child | Talk with child | Talk with child | Talk with child | Talk with adolescent |
| | Play | Play | Playful interaction | Playful interaction | Ask about school, relationships with peers, family, feelings, activities |
| | Make sounds | Share books, toys | Share books, toys | Share books, toys | |
| | Share board books, toys | | | | |
| **Play and interaction strategies** | Respond to baby's sounds, smile | Pretend-play, guessing games | Engage in discussion | Engage in discussion | Engage in discussion by using nonintrusive questions, listening, reflecting back |
| | Play peek-a boo, pat-a-cake, hiding games | Tell stories | Make-believe games, hide-and-seek, counting and number games, mimic animals, hand puppets, read | Make-believe games, improvise, jokes and riddles, magic tricks, guessing games, talk about hobbies, sports | |
| | Name objects as you give them to baby | Hide and find things | | | |
| **Can obtain some history from child** | No | Minimal; ask older toddler, "Can you put your finger on where it hurts?" | Yes | Yes | Yes |

Data from Rider EA. Communication and relationships with children and parents. In: Novack DH, Clark W, Saizow R, Daetwyler C, eds. *DocCom: an interactive learning resource for healthcare communication.* 2006. Available at: http://webcampus.drexelmed.edu/doccom/user/. Accessed October 10, 2016; and Mendelsohn JS, Quinn MT, McNabb WL. Interview strategies commonly used by pediatricians. *Arch Pediatr Adolesc Med.* 1999;153:154-157.

**TABLE 3-8 USING DEVELOPMENTALLY BASED COMMUNICATION DURING THE 2-YEAR-OLD WELL-CHILD VISIT**

**The Examination**

*Using the language of play and metaphor builds relationships and enables physicians to examine young children in ways that create positive experiences.*

"No doctor! No doctor!" exclaims my next patient, his small hands pressed tightly over his ears, a determined scowl on his face. Ryan is 2 years old. I smile at him and say, "Hi." "No doctor!" he replies. After talking with his mother and letting him get used to me, I approach him slowly. He looks at me with big blue eyes beneath his brown, spiking crew cut.

"Would you like to see a pink finger?" I ask as I put my finger on the otoscope light and it lights up pink. I note, playfully, how silly that is. A skeptical smile forms on his face. We play peek-a-boo with the light and I examine his eyes. "Show me the biggest mouth in the world!" I exclaim. Ryan opens his mouth wide. His hands remain tightly clamped over his ears.

"Where is your heart? Is it here?" I ask, pointing to Ryan's head. He looks at me and points to his chest. "We'd better check," I note calmly and then exclaim, "I hear it right there!" "Do you have Elmo back here?" I ask as I listen for various Sesame Street characters on his back.

"Do you have birthday cake in your tummy?" I inquire. "Let's check!" Ryan remains skeptical but allows his mother to lay him on his back on the examination table. I listen to his heart, then quickly search for birthday cake in his abdomen. "Do you have pizza in there? Milk? Goldfish?" He smiles and removes his hands from his ears.

When Ryan sits up again, I pull out the reflex hammer. "Would you like to see my hammer?" I say as I lightly tap it on my nose. "It's very soft. Let's check your knees!" Curiosity has the best of him, and he smiles as I check his reflexes.

"Do you have bunny rabbits in your ears?" I ask. "Which ear should we check first?" He points to his right ear. After I look for bunny rabbits in one ear, he turns his head so I can check the other. He's now relaxed and more comfortable with me. "You're perfect," I tell him as we finish the examination.

Ryan's mother and I talk, and she helps Ryan put on his coat. When he realizes our time is up, he lags, pulling on his mother's arm so he can remain in the examination room. "More doctor! More doctor!" he exclaims.

*Elizabeth A. Rider, MSW, MD*



relationship-centered process involving flexibility in interaction and relationships rather than simply information exchange.

Numerous studies support the importance of enhancing physician-patient communication and confirm the value of relationship-centered care. Building and sustaining relationships with children and their family members is an ongoing responsibility and is enhanced by the physician's development of communication and relationship abilities. The physician's skill in these areas improves with knowledge, reflection, and practice.

## ACKNOWLEDGMENTS

Parts of this chapter were adapted from Rider EA. Interpersonal and communication skills. In: Rider EA, Nawotniak RH, eds. *A Practical Guide to Teaching and Assessing the ACGME Core Competencies*. 2nd ed. Marblehead, MA: HCPro, Inc; 2010:1-137; and from Rider EA. Communication and relationships with children and parents. In: Novack DH, Clark W, Saizow R, Daetwyler C, eds. *DocCom: an interactive learning resource for healthcare communication*. 2006. Available at: http://webcampus.drexelmed.edu/doccom/user/. Accessed October 10, 2016.

## SUGGESTED READINGS

Bayer-Fetzer Conference on Physician-Patient Communication in Medical Education. Essential elements of communication in medical encounters: the Kalamazoo consensus statement. *Acad Med.* 2001;76(4):390-393.

Beach MC, Inui T; Relationship-Centered Care Research Network. Relationship-centered care. A constructive reframing. *J Gen Intern Med.* 2006;21(suppl 1):S3-S8.

Browning DM. Microethical and relational insights from pediatric palliative care. *Virtual Mentor.* 2010;12(7):540-547.

Duffy FD, Gordon GH, Whelan G, et al; participants in the American Academy on Physician and Patient's Conference on Education and Evaluation of Competence in Communication and Interpersonal Skills. Assessing competence in communication and interpersonal skills: the Kalamazoo II report. *Acad Med.* 2004;79(6):495-507.

Dyche L. Interpersonal skill in medicine: the essential partner of verbal communication. *J Gen Intern Med.* 2007;22(7):1035–1039.

Dyche L, Swiderski D. The effect of physician solicitation approaches on ability to identify patient concerns. *J Gen Intern Med.* 2005:20(3):267-270.

Frankel RM, Stein T. Getting the most out of the clinical encounter: the Four Habits Model. *Permanente J.* 1999;3:79-88. http://www.swselfmanagement.ca/uploads/ResourceTools/Getting%20the%20most%20out%20of%20the%20clinical%20encounter.pdf. Accessed November 21, 2016.

Miller SZ, Schmidt HJ. The habit of humanism: a framework for making humanistic care a reflexive clinical skill. *Acad Med.* 1999;74(7):800-803.

Rider EA. Advanced communication strategies for relationship-centered care. *Pediatr Ann.* 2011;40(9):447-453.

Rider EA. Interpersonal and communication skills. In: Rider EA, Nawotniak RH, eds. *A Practical Guide to Teaching and Assessing the ACGME Core Competencies*. 2nd ed. Marblehead, MA: HCPro, Inc; 2010:1-137.

Rider EA. It's because they didn't know our names. *Arch Pediatr Adolesc Med.* 2002;156(6):531.

Rider EA, Keefer CH. Communication skills competencies: definitions and a teaching toolbox. *Med Educ.* 2006;40(7):624-629.

Rider EA, Kurtz S, Slade D, et al. The International Charter for Human Values in Healthcare: an interprofessional global collaboration to enhance values and communication in healthcare. *Patient Educ Counseling.* 2014;96(3):273-280.

Rider EA, Volkan K, Hafler JP. Pediatric residents' perceptions of communication competencies: implications for teaching. *Med Teach.* 2008;30(7):e208-e217.

# 4 Interviewing Techniques

Christopher F. Bolling

## INTRODUCTION

The medical history represents the single most important opportunity to obtain individualized medical information. Since it is an opportunity and not a guaranteed source of information, the caregiver or patient during the interview may unknowingly miss critical data. Language proficiency, patient and caregiver cognitive abilities, readiness to change behavior, interest in seeking health care, and personal comfort with the practitioner are only a few factors that may influence the ability to obtain vital information. The information in this chapter can enhance the clinician's ability to obtain patient information and to delve more deeply into patient motivation and understanding than the classically structured patient history. It assumes that it is a caregiver of a patient that is being interviewed, but the principles described apply to interviewing patients when developmentally appropriate.

## THE CLASSIC HISTORY

Table 4-1 describes the traditional patient history. The typical history focuses on gathering a variety of specific information in a brief period of time. The very important information recorded in the traditional

**TABLE 4-1 COMPONENTS OF THE CLASSIC PATIENT HISTORY**

| | Content |
|---|---|
| Chief complaint (CC) | The patient- or primary caregiver–stated reason for being present at the visit |
| History of the present illness (HPI) | A detailed synopsis of factors most pertinent to the chief complaint; focuses on timing, duration, severity, and symptoms associated with the chief complaint |
| Past medical history (PMH) | A listing of medications, allergies, surgeries, hospitalizations, chronic illnesses, and other significant medical occurrences |
| Review of systems (ROS) | An organ system–based evaluation of complaints and previous diagnoses not otherwise covered in the past medical history |
| Family history (FH) | A summary of illnesses present in the patient's family history, recorded in relation to the patient |
| Social history (SH) | A synopsis of psychosocial and other factors affecting care; at a minimum, social history should include living situation, school/work history, and support system |

history is an organized synopsis and a necessary summary of medications, surgeries, and major medical events. The degree of detail present in the various components is highly variable and should be tailored in response to the purpose and duration of the visit. The traditional history provides early valuable insight into factors influencing a patient's motivation for seeking care.

The challenge of the medical history is to not lose sight of the patient and caregiver's often unstated goals. A significant hazard of the traditional medical history is losing valuable information that may not present itself if the patient feels the clinician is not listening to them. A clinician may unwittingly prevent a patient or caregiver from expressing concerns and from identifying barriers to care. Often, large parts of the medical history can be obtained from patients and caregivers in the form of surveys or questionnaires completed either independently or with the assistance of trained staff. Additionally, the first two components of the history, the chief complaint and history of the present illness, may be adequately addressed in some of the less directive techniques discussed in this chapter. Questions that necessarily lend themselves to simple answers can be sandwiched between more evocative and collaborative questions. In the context of a busy office visit, a question that elicits a one-word answer is often preferable. For example, a question like "Have you had an appendectomy?" seeks a simple answer and is most efficiently asked in a direct or closed fashion.

## WHY IS A COLLABORATIVE ARRANGEMENT BENEFICIAL?

Interviewing techniques represent far more than an information-gathering technique. Talking with caregivers lays the groundwork for later therapeutic intervention. Considering that the health status of adults in the United States is determined by behavior 50% of the time, and that the leading attributable causes of death are dominated by conditions modified by behaviors, such as diet, smoking, and safety, the clinician's ability to assist productive behaviors for health maintenance are highly desirable.

The hierarchical nature of the doctor–patient relationship is long standing and established in a variety of disciplines. Rogers, in response to a culture of therapist-directed counseling, in the 1940s and 1950s described how therapists may be more effective in helping patients by forming a more collaborative relationship. In the 1970s, Prochaska and DiClemente introduced the transtheoretical model as a construct emphasizing the importance of patient readiness to accept prescribed treatment. They described a linear progression of patient readiness to change from a precontemplative state to contemplative, preparative, action, and ultimately maintenance stages regarding specific behaviors. Miller and Rollnick further posited in the 1980s that physicians, counselors, dietitians, and other clinicians in advice-giving professions may actually be harming their ability to modify patient behavior in a positive fashion.

Motivational interviewing, developed by Miller and Rollnick, provides a useful framework to improve the depth of data collected by the clinician and can provide deeper insight into patient behavior. Motivational interviewing follows the patient centeredness of Rogerian theory, but unlike stricter interpretations of Rogerian practice, motivational interviewing is a directive technique. Clinicians may have identified harmful behaviors, but they hypothesized that consistent and repeated advice giving may actually promote patients to continue detrimental behaviors. Current research by Resnicow goes further in describing the role of the clinician as that of a facilitator who helps set the stage for behavior change. The clinician can increase the likelihood of behavior change by various actions and statements, but ultimate responsibility lies with patient and caregiver. Motivational interviewing suggests that the path to behavior adoption is not linear, as proposed by Prochaska and DiClemente, but rather is chaotic, progresses forward and back in readiness, and is fraught with expected relapses, failures, and false starts.

## USING MOTIVATIONAL INTERVIEWING

In a collaborative environment, health counseling involves a partnership that honors patient and caregiver expertise and perspectives. The atmosphere is conducive rather than coercive. Miller and Rollnick describe the four processes of motivational interviewing: engagement, guiding (or focus), evocation, and planning. When talking with patients, *engagement* refers to taking time to establish a relationship between clinician and patient. *Guiding* refers to setting a shared goal that is set by the patient but can be endorsed and supported by the clinician. *Evocation* is the development of motivation for changing behavior by activating the patient's internal values and priorities. Only after establishing a respectful relationship, creating a shared focus for action, and evoking internal motivation, should the clinician start the *planning* phase. Even at that point, the plan devised should mostly come from the patient.

These processes are used to resolve the central dilemma of behavior change—ambivalence—a natural response to proposed change and the patient's thoughtful consideration and balancing of changing versus sustaining current behavior. Tools for resolving ambivalence include increased use of open-ended questions, affirmations, reflections, summarizations, readiness rulers, and a technique known as elicit-provide-elicit. Examples of these tools are given in Table 4-2.

**Open-ended questions** are questions that do not allow one-word, simple, or yes/no answers. Furthermore, they are not leading or suggestive on the part of the clinician. When discussing behavior, experts recommend 4 open-ended questions to every 1 closed-ended question. Open-ended questions are structured to require an engagement with the clinician. They encourage caregivers to discuss their thoughts and to reflect on their own impression. They also indicate the clinician's desire to know more about the caregivers' experiences.

**Affirmations** are often simple acknowledgments of the caregiver's struggles. Clinicians may enhance the collaborative environment by acknowledging the caregiver's struggles without judging. Focusing on positive progress or simply seeking assistance can augment confidence, leading to an improved therapeutic relationship and a greater willingness to discuss sensitive topics. Therefore, affirmations are a critical piece of the engagement process of motivational interviewing.

The central skill in motivational interviewing is the ability to make **reflections**, which may reflect the content of what was just said, the underlying feelings the caregiver is expressing, or the conjectured meaning of the patient's statement. Clinicians may be reluctant to attempt reflecting the meaning or feeling of a statement for fear of conjecturing incorrectly. Motivational interviewing encourages this attempt knowing that it will result either in affirmation that the clinician understands the caregiver or an opportunity for the caregiver to clarify the feeling or meaning. Reflections should be phrased in such a way as not to imply a desired answer. Skilled motivational

**TABLE 4-2 TYPICAL MOTIVATIONAL INTERVIEWING TOOLS FOR USE IN BRIEF CLINICAL ENCOUNTERS**

| Tool | Example in Practice |
|---|---|
| Open-ended questions | Instead of asking "Have you been taking your asthma medication?" ask "Tell me about your asthma medication schedule." |
| Affirmations | "I know it must be difficult to talk about your diabetes. I am very glad that you decided to keep your appointment today." |
| Reflections | Instead of asking a question reflexively, respond with either the content or feeling of the patient/caregiver statement. In response to "Despite what everyone says, my child is not overweight in my opinion," the clinician may reflect:<br>*Content:* "I understand that you feel your child is not overweight."<br>*Feeling:* "It sounds like you are frustrated by everyone's opinion about your child's weight."<br>*Meaning:* "Your experience seems to indicate that your child's current weight status is not a problem." |
| Summarizations | Recap the visit in a series of nonjudgmental statements, often in the patient/caregiver's own words. Joint creation of a change plan may also be undertaken. |
| Readiness rulers | *Responding to importance and confidence:* "On a scale of 1 (not at all confident [or important]) to 10 (very confident [or important]), how confident are you (or how important is it to you) that you will be able to convince your boyfriend to use a condom?"<br>After patient responds, the clinician may ask, "Why not lower?" to identify strengths and "Why not higher?" to identify barriers. |
| Elicit-provide-elicit | *Elicit:* "What are your current thoughts on making your toddler take his anticonvulsant medication?"<br>Patient response.<br>*Provide:* "May I give some information on how some other parents have had success in giving this medication?"<br>Wait for parent permission.<br>*Elicit:* "What do you think about that approach?"<br>Patient response. |

interviewing clinicians do not exhibit an "upward" concluding tone to declarative statements that will often elicit a confirmatory "yes" response. The desired intonation is a "downward" declarative tone that stimulates a conversational response. As clinicians become more skilled with reflections, they become comfortable with action reflections. Rather than advice giving, *action reflections* are statements made by the clinician that restate a patient's stated plan to change behavior. Another complex form of reflection is reframing. In *reframing*, a negative statement can be reworked by the clinician into a statement for change. For example, a statement like "I smoke because I don't want my husband to be alone or ostracized" could be reframed into "It is important for you to spend quality time with him." Motivational interviewing also acknowledges that periods of silence sometimes follow in the normal course of conversation. Not "filling the vacuum" will often lead to the stating of important information or insights.

**Summarizations** are commonly used by clinicians and caregivers in collaborative relationships. They are effective as a tool to affirm the clinician's understanding and to clarify agreed-upon goals. Summarization provides an opportunity to formulate a collaborative care plan and incorporate other patient-tracking tools. In these ways, summarization can help keep a clinician-caregiver-patient interaction moving in a positive direction.

**Readiness rulers** or scales can help clinicians to assess the importance a caregiver attributes to a particular behavior and to assess a caregiver's confidence in his or her ability to carry out that behavior. Caregivers may be asked to rate a behavior on a scale of 1 (low importance or confidence) to 10 (high importance or confidence). The clinician can then help the caregiver identify strengths that will help carry out a behavior by asking why the score was not lower and can identify barriers by asking why the score was not higher.

**Elicit-provide-elicit** is a summative strategy guiding a clinician through a motivational interviewing–based sequence that seeks the caregiver's thoughts (elicit), allows the exchange of information (provide), and follows the exchange with a further exposition of the caregiver's thoughts (elicit). Central to elicit-provide-elicit are safeguards to avoid returning to unsolicited advice giving. Knowledge is often not the central deficit when detrimental behaviors are being followed. In the interest of providing a collaborative environment that respects the caregiver's autonomy, permission must be granted by the caregiver before the clinician supplies factual knowledge or expert opinion. Bracketing this specific information with reflections and open-ended questions promotes evocation powered by the caregiver's inherent values, perceptions, and goals.

In motivational interviewing, patient responses can be characterized as either *change talk* or *sustain talk*. Change talk is language the patient uses to suggest a change in behavior is desired. On the other hand, sustain talk is language that the patient uses to defend current behavior or the status quo. The role of the clinician is to identify and accentuate change talk to help patients effectively argue for positive behavior. The clinician's role is similarly to identify sustain talk and, without being dismissive of it, avoid emphasizing it, but help patients identify and overcome barriers they describe.

## THE CHALLENGE OF AGE

A particularly vexing problem in pediatrics is deciding when a behavior is in the domain of an adult caregiver and when that behavior is in the domain of the pediatric patient. The preverbal 1-year-old is clearly primarily influenced by the decisions of his caregiver. Conversely, the 18-year-old adolescent is making the transition to adulthood and is often not heavily influenced by parents on daily decisions. No comprehensive studies have been performed to definitively say when these collaborative techniques should be transitioned from caregiver to patient in pediatric settings. Clinicians should consider patient cognition, family dynamics, school situation, and age in making this transition. For most children reaching typical developmental milestones, 8 years of age generally represents a transition point from primary parental control to patient decision making. Clinicians are well-served by engaging both parties from 6 years of age on.

## GOING FORWARD

Collaborative interviewing techniques such as motivational interviewing show great promise and are currently incorporated into a variety of clinical settings. Motivational interviewing has been identified as a preferred method for clinicians to discuss behavior change with their patients in a variety of clinical recommendations. A growing body of evidence has reinforced the efficacy of motivational interviewing in brief clinical encounters. As such, motivational interviewing can be viewed as the "why" of behavior change. Other strategies based on cognitive behavioral theory, behavioral economics, and self-management can be valuable adjuncts to motivational interviewing. Motivational interviewing has been said to answer the question "Why should I change?" These other strategies can answer the questions "What should I change" and "How can I do it? Clinicians interested in these techniques are encouraged to participate in ongoing evaluation of training validity and fidelity and to evaluate for clinical effectiveness. Further information on these techniques and training opportunities are available at http://www.motivationalinterviewing.org.

## SUGGESTED READING

Miller WR, Rollnick S. *Motivational Interviewing: Helping People Change*. 3rd ed. New York, NY: Guilford Press; 2013.

# 5 Law, Ethics, and Clinical Judgment

Thomas Wm. Mayo, Perry Ann Reed, and Angelo P. Giardino

In pediatrics, it is the child—not the parent—who is the patient, and the pediatrician's professional, ethical, and legal obligations are owed to the child. While parents in our society have been given wide latitude to raise children as they see fit, there are matters with respect to which the state can appropriately intervene: Parents may spank their children, but child abuse is not permitted. Parents may choose a variety of educational settings and resources for their children, but the state does demand that children achieve some level of literacy. Pediatricians, therefore, care for children and work with their parents in a social context that requires their intervention in ways that may range from working with parents to make decisions of great medical complexity (see Chapter 123) to notifying the state of suspected neglect or abuse (see Chapter 36).

This chapter focuses on three areas in which the law, ethics, and clinical judgment intertwine: (1) Who makes decisions when it comes to caring for children and adolescents? (2) Who is able to refuse treatment—the child and/or the parent for the child? (3) When is confidentiality an issue for an older child or adolescent?

## CONSENT TO TREATMENT: WHO DECIDES?

*Informed consent* is a legal notion of relatively recent vintage. At its core, it requires physicians to provide truthful, relevant information to patients/surrogates in the process of obtaining their consent to treatment. Although the concept began to appear in legal opinions in the late 19th and early 20th centuries, it wasn't until the 1950s that courts undertook in earnest the hard work of delineating its contours and requirements. The applicability of informed-consent principles to pediatric decision-making was confirmed by the American Academy of Pediatrics (AAP) in its 1976 statement on the subject and has since been reaffirmed by the AAP in statements published in 1995 and 2016.

At the same time that informed consent was being worked out in the courts, the moral and legal status of children was undergoing a vast upheaval. Before the 20th century, children (until recently, all those under 21 years, and now almost universally those under 18) were considered a form of chattel with no recognizable legal rights. Since that time, courts have increasingly recognized that children and adolescents have rights separate from those of their parents. While parents, of course, have the right (and duty) to make decisions about their children's health care, the "children's rights" movement over the last 50 years has recognized the rights of adolescents to participate in making decisions about their health care, just as they do in a variety of other socio-legal contexts. However, minors do not have the legal authority to consent to medical treatment (subject to certain exceptions discussed below). *Assent* is the legal and ethical term that connotes the minor patient's right to participate in the decision-making process. The combination of parental decision-making authority, the traditional role of the pediatrician, and the somewhat uncertain scope of patient assent predictably sets the stage for multiple layers of conflicts among the decision-makers.

Parents may vary greatly in their subjective values, tolerance for prognostic uncertainty, and many other factors that typically influence medical decision-making for children. This variance requires that pediatricians bring a comparable degree of sensitivity to treatment decisions subject to a broad array of parental expectations and perspectives. In addition, the United States has become a nation of diverse cultures; thus, sensitivity toward and understanding of child-raising practices from other parts of the world are increasingly important. While some practices may seem abusive in the context of American cultural values, it is important to realize that the intent behind the practices is almost always benevolent and not abusive. In addition, the decision-making process itself can vary across cultures, which in turn may determine who speaks for the patient, who within the family is entitled to receive information about the patient's diagnosis and prognosis, and the identity of the ultimate decision-maker. When societal, cultural, familial, and personal values clash, sometimes explanations and education, not legal interventions, may help to resolve disagreements.

The ethical concept of *respect for persons* does not have a minimum age. While demonstrating respect for a 16-year-old will be quite different from demonstrating respect for a 6-year-old, which is different from the respect due an infant, the principle is the same at any age. Both informed consent and the right to assent reflect this bedrock principle.

Elements of informed consent to medical treatment include a description of the proposed procedure, the risks and the benefits of the proposed therapy, and what alternatives are available. In many cases, an alternative is to do nothing, and, if applicable, the consequences of doing nothing should be explained to the parents and, as appropriate, to the patient. Whether a particular risk must be disclosed, as well as the degree of detail that must be disclosed, varies from state to state. A majority of states rely on a professional or objective standard to address these questions (ie, what a reasonable practitioner would disclose to a patient under similar circumstances). A substantial minority, however, employ a subjective or patient-oriented standard to determine what risks must be disclosed and to what degree of detail.

The doctrine of assent requires a similar level of transparency and truthfulness. The process of obtaining a patient's assent is based on respect for the patient—and for the patient's autonomy—even if the law does not allow the minor patient under most circumstances to consent to treatment. Beginning as early as a patient is capable of understanding what she is being told, the process of assent involves the patient in discussions about her medical condition and treatment choices. Disclosures to minors need to be age-appropriate and calibrated to the patient's developmental stage. It is somewhat risky to generalize based solely upon the patient's chronological age. Because children mature at different rates, their ability at the same chronological age to process information may differ, as well. One rule of thumb is to be guided by the patient's own questions, on the assumption that patients—including minors—typically do not ask questions unless and until they are developmentally capable of processing the answers.

The physician–patient interaction described above reflects the notion that informed consent is a process, not simply a piece of paper to be signed by the patient's surrogate decision-maker. Understood in this light, both informed consent and assent bring patients and parents into a relationship with their physician over time that promotes understanding, trust, and cooperation, as well as an understanding of the patient as an autonomous being entitled to respect in her own right.

### Young Children

Parents are almost always asked to consent to treatment of a small child except in case of an emergency when parental consent cannot immediately be obtained. As a general rule, if parents or guardians cannot be found in a timely manner, consent to treatment of an emergency medical condition will be presumed. Emergencies are broadly construed by courts and include situations in which a child is in pain, not just cases of life-threatening illness or injury. For example, if a child in day care falls and cuts her head and is brought to the emergency department by a teacher, if the parents are not immediately available, the child's cut will be sutured on the basis of presumed consent. On the other hand, if a child has a nonemergent medical condition that allows for discussion of treatment options without the need for speed, the child should not be treated without discussion with and permission from his parents.

Even when children are too young to be able to assent to medical care, it is respectful to them and is likely to increase their cooperation if the procedure is explained to them and they are allowed to make some choices, even if it is what color Band-Aid they get after their immunization. To the extent the child seems to understand, explaining what is wrong with him or her, why the problem needs to be treated, and what the options are is respectful of the child's personhood and is likely to produce increased understanding and thus cooperation.

#### The Adolescent Patient

Early in the 1960s, there was an epidemic of sexually transmitted infections among teenagers. Because they did not want their parents to find out that they had been sexually active, they forewent treatment rather than ask for parental consent to therapy, thus spreading the infections. State legislatures enacted statutes allowing minors of any age to receive treatment for sexually transmitted infections without parental involvement, and in subsequent years, almost all state legislatures extended the same exemption from parental knowledge to treatment for alcohol or drug problems. In many states, statutes specifically provide that parents may not be billed for these services without the consent of the patient, since the parents would discover the problem from the bill they received. Because this is a topic governed almost entirely by state law, and states may vary in their approach to disclosures to parents, pediatricians should be familiar with the laws of the state in which they practice.

As the concept of minors' rights began to expand in the second half of the 20th century, some state legislatures recognized the right of minors of a given age (ranging from 14 to 17) or status (high-school graduate) to consent to some or all medical or surgical treatments without parental involvement. Even in those states without consent statutes, some courts began to carve out what is known as the mature minor doctrine. If the patient is over 13 (or 14 in some recent cases) and the physician feels that she understands the reasons for the recommended therapy and what its risks and benefits are, she is a mature minor capable of giving legal consent to medical treatment. At present, 14 states permit mature minors to consent to some or all medical and surgical treatments. Three states recognize the same right regardless of the minor's age or maturity, and 34 states have no legal rule on the subject. Thus, in a considerable majority of jurisdictions, the general rule requiring the consent of a lawful surrogate decision-maker applies.

Mature-minor rules may be subject to exceptions requiring parental consent to specific interventions (eg, all surgeries) or procedures. An example of the latter is abortion. Currently, 3 states and the District of Columbia permit minors to consent to abortion services, while 39 states require either the consent or the notification of at least one parent or both notification and consent. Federal courts have generally upheld notification/consent statutes as long as the laws also provided for a meaningful judicial bypass process for minors who could demonstrate sufficient maturity, in cases of a medical emergency, or when there is evidence of abuse or neglect.

Emancipated minors have the legal authority to make their own decisions about all aspects of their lives, not just about medical care. State laws vary, but emancipated minors typically include those who are married, those who are in the military, and, in most states, those who are self-supporting and living away from their families. In some states, parents and a child of 16 or older may go to court and ask for a declaration of emancipation, meaning that the parents have no further responsibility, financial or otherwise, for their child. College students living away from home are almost always considered emancipated, even if their parents are paying their college expenses. Many of the medical interventions needed by runaways will fall under one of the exceptions discussed above, and some runaways may be able to establish their independent living (including finances).

Most states authorize minors to consent to medical treatment for their own children even when the teenaged parent does not meet the requirements for mature-minor status or emancipation. Depending upon the applicable statutory language, the right to make medical decisions may extend to prenatal treatment decisions. The state laws tend not to be clear as to whether treatment decisions during pregnancy include decisions about the pregnant minor's own medical treatments. In cases of doubt, legal counsel may be helpful.





#### Insistence on Unorthodox "Therapy" or Treatments the Physician Thinks Are Wrong

Almost always, children and their parents agree with the pediatrician on the need for medical care, the physician finds their choices of therapy reasonable, and treatment proceeds. However, this is not always the case. What is the physician's ethical responsibility when an adolescent, parents, or both ask the pediatrician to provide a treatment that the physician thinks is either unwise or wrong?

Suppose, for example, a 14-year-old with cancer and his parents insist that the physician treat his disease with an alternative therapy such as laetrile. The assessment of the situation should include the following considerations:

1. Is the alternative dangerous? Can the physician even determine whether it might be harmful? If a parent presents a bottle of laetrile and demands that it be given to his child with cancer, the physician has no way of knowing what contaminants may be in the liquid, aside from the potential danger of the laetrile itself.
2. If the alternative is not dangerous and the parents and the patient are willing to accept conventional therapy as long as the alternative is added, the physician might reasonably decide to go along with their request, although she is perfectly within her legal and ethical rights to decline.
3. If the parents insist on the alternative as the only method of therapy and the alternative would not be dangerous, the child's condition should be the first decision point. If the child is likely to recover or at least gain a long-term remission with conventional therapy, there is always the option of obtaining a court order to treat the patient.
4. If the child is dying and conventional therapy may prolong the process but will not affect the outcome, the alternative is not harmful, and the parents are desperate in their beliefs that it may help, the physician has to make a very difficult judgment call. To refuse their request and thus close the door between physician and parents, however, means that as the child is dying, she or he may have no access to the physician because the parents are too angry to call for help. (For further discussion of this topic, see Chapter 128.)

Where there is serious disagreement between the adolescent and his parents, the pediatrician must be sure that the decision is made in the best interests of the patient, not the best interests of the parents. Suppose, for example, a 16-year-old Jehovah's Witness accepts a needed blood transfusion to which his parents object. Of course, the patient would be transfused (pursuant to a court order, if time permits), but in the process, the medical team should consider the effects of this conflict on the family unit and attempt to provide support as necessary. For example, the parents might consider refusing to let the "sinful" child come home after discharge from the hospital. How can the physician help the family unit recover?

### REFUSAL OF TREATMENT: WHO DECIDES?

If a minor (of any age) has an illness or injury for which medical care can produce a cure or at least a recovery with minimal disability, courts will almost always override the parents' refusal. For example, if a child is hit by a car and requires surgery, but the parents refuse to allow a necessary blood transfusion because their religion does not permit it, most courts will order the transfusion to be given. In practical terms, however, a court order may also require that physical custody of the child must be secured during the treatment period. A blood transfusion during surgery is one thing, but court-ordered chemotherapy, occurring over months, might require placing the child in foster care so his parents will not respond to the order by taking him out of the country. That trauma to the parent–child relationship must be factored into the initial decision to go to court, and the physicians must be quite sure that the intervention is reasonably predicted to succeed. (Parental refusal of treatment when the child's prognosis is not good is discussed in Chapter 128.)

Adolescents may object to treatment their parents wish them to have. Short of physical restraint during the treatment, it is often best to negotiate a course acceptable to the adolescent patient if at all possible. A simple refusal may not be the real agenda, and the physician should make efforts to find out what the real problem is. A teenager who is responding well to chemotherapy and suddenly refuses to continue may want to go to her prom with hair—and helping her find and pay for a wig may resolve the treatment issue. The younger child's or adolescent's feelings of helplessness in the face of serious medical problems should be understood and taken very seriously. Dealing honestly with those feelings may lessen the possibility of outright refusal.

Adolescents in most circumstances may refuse any treatment to which they can consent. If the proposed therapy is elective, the patient may certainly refuse. Decisions about life-sustaining therapies are more controversial. As explained by the American Academy of Pediatrics in a 2016 report, "Many bioethicists support limiting a child's or adolescent's short-term autonomy by overriding a treatment refusal to preserve long-term autonomous choice and an open future." The AAP report concludes that, in general, adolescents should not be allowed to refuse life-saving therapy even if the patient's parents agree.

## CONFIDENTIALITY

### Disclosures to Parents

Pediatricians who have long-time relationships with their patients—perhaps from hospital nursery to college entrance—must make decisions about the age and stage of maturity at which patients may legitimately demand that information be received in confidence and, in particular, not be disclosed to the patient's parents. A promise of confidentiality from the physician to an adolescent patient may be the only way to obtain honest information necessary to make a correct diagnosis. In general, if a minor is legally capable of consent or refusal of treatment, that treatment may be given in confidence. State laws largely dominate this subject and, of course, vary from highly protective of confidentiality to not protective at all.

Younger children probably do not understand, much less expect, confidentiality. In most cases, younger children assume that their parents know everything about them, and in the context of medical care, the parent is usually present.

Many pediatricians have developed an explicit policy in their practices about confidentiality, when it will be maintained and when parents will be notified, and patients and their parents are informed of this at an appropriate age or when an adolescent is accepted as a new patient. If the parents are not willing for their child's confidences to be respected by a physician, this conversation in advance of any conflict would put them on notice to seek another source of regular medical care. The patient also should understand that, while there is a general adherence to confidentiality at his age, there are times—for example, when the teenager might be dangerous to himself or others—when the parents' need to know will override the adolescent's desire for confidentiality. To promise, either explicitly or implicitly, that a conversation will be confidential and then to inform the parent without the adolescent's knowledge is a clear violation of the ethical principles underlying the physician–patient relationship. It is also likely to cause mistrust of all physicians for years to come. In some families, as well, disclosure of information the adolescent wanted for good reasons to be kept confidential may lead to abuse, rejection, or having the parent expel the child from the home.

### Disclosures to State Agencies

In some cases, such as child abuse or neglect, reports to state agencies are required. The ages for reporting vary among the states, but most age out of the requirement by 16, if not earlier. In determining abuse stemming from sexual activity among adolescents, the context determines whether abuse has occurred. If a 15-year-old girl is having a sexual relationship with her 16-year-old boyfriend and the physician becomes involved when she asks for contraceptives, confidentiality is almost certainly required. If, however, the girl is 11, clearly abuse should be presumed. If the 15-year-old is having a sexual relationship with her mother's 38-year-old boyfriend, this is almost certainly statutory rape as well as child abuse under the criminal laws in most states. In that instance, of course, the mother will be informed of the situation by the police if not by the pediatrician.

Infectious diseases, particularly sexually transmitted diseases, are also reportable to the state public health authorities or to designated local health authorities, even though the adolescent patient has the right of confidentiality with regard to his or her parents.

### Disclosures to Schools

Reports to schools may very well not be confidential. Even if the report is made to a school nurse, in some schools, principals take the position that they have the right to all information, including medical information and family information, about all the students in the school. Once the information leaves the control of the school nurse, there is nothing to prevent its dissemination to the faculty. Parents and physicians should understand that informing a school nurse about a child's medical condition is by no means the same thing as sharing the same medical information with other physicians or clinics. In the early days of human immunodeficiency virus (HIV), this lack of privacy, coupled with demonstrated invasions of the children's and their families' privacy and unfair treatment and abuse in schools, caused many pediatricians to refuse to notify a school that a patient was HIV positive. Those caring for these children instead hoped that teachers understood that universal precautions were necessary in dealing with all the children.

In all circumstances, parents and adolescents should be told exactly what information is being sent to the school, and in most cases, they have the right to decline to allow the disclosure.


## ACKNOWLEDGMENT

We appreciate the contributions of the author of this chapter in the 22nd edition, Angela Roddey Holder, LLB, LLM (1938–2009).


## SUGGESTED READINGS


Berlinger N, Jennings B, Wolf SM. Guidelines concerning neonates, infants, children, and adolescents. In: *The Hastings Center Guidelines for Decisions on Life-Sustaining Treatment and Care Near the End of Life* (revised and expanded). 2nd ed. New York, NY: Oxford University Press; 2013:67–87.

Coleman DL, Rosoff PM. The legal authority of mature minors to consent to general medical treatment. *Pediatrics.* 2013;131(4):786-793.

Committee on Bioethics, American Academy of Pediatrics. Informed consent in decision-making in pediatric practice. *Pediatrics.* 2016;138(2):1-7.

Diekema DS, Mercurio MR, Adam MB, eds. *Clinical Ethics in Pediatrics: A Case-Based Textbook.* Cambridge, UK: Cambridge University Press; 2011.

Maguire AL, Bruce CR. Keeping children's secrets: confidentiality in the physician-patient relationship. *Houston J Health Law Policy.* 2008;8(2):315-333.

# 6 US Healthcare System

Jean L. Raphael and Angelo P. Giardino

## INTRODUCTION

In order to provide high-quality care to children in an evolving healthcare landscape, it is becoming increasingly imperative that pediatricians become familiar with the fundamental components of the US healthcare system. Over the past decade, healthcare providers have experienced reforms across a diverse set of areas—frameworks of health and health care, reimbursement, performance measurement and performance-based incentives, healthcare coverage, quality improvement, and information technology. All of these reforms critically impact the environment in which pediatricians practice, the types of functions to which they are accountable, and how they can best advocate for the needs of children. As pediatricians attempt to adapt and thrive in the new environment of health care, they do so with the understanding that many reforms are based on adult models of care that do not reflect the unique characteristics and experiences of children within the healthcare system. According to a model first conceptualized by Forrest et al in 1997, and later modified by Stille et al in 2010, children differ from adults in the 5 Ds:

- Demographics
- Differential epidemiology
- Development over time
- Dependency on adults
- Dollars

Understanding the changing demographics of US children is critical to informing both health and healthcare policy. The number of children and how they use health care influence the demands for access to care, insurance provision, and models of care. Children currently make up approximately 23% of the US population with increasing racial/ethnic diversity. Racial/ethnic minority children account for over half of US children. The population of the US is projected to grow even more diverse in the coming decade. In terms of epidemiology, an increasing percentage of children experience chronic conditions or medical complexity. This may impact the composition of practices and how pediatricians allocate resources and time. The prevalence of chronic conditions among the pediatric population is estimated to be 15% to 20%. Also important to the health care of children is that their needs and engagement in health care evolve over time as they progress through the stages of infancy, early childhood, school age, adolescence, and adulthood. Therefore, children's engagement in their health care will change over time. Children rely heavily on adults for their health care. Consequently, the health of the entire family is an important consideration in care. Lastly, children have greater reliance on public insurance relative to adults. Roughly 40% of US children are publicly insured through Medicaid or the Children's Health Insurance Program (CHIP). Despite the importance of the unique attributes of children, these factors are not routinely incorporated into current reforms. Therefore, knowledge of the US healthcare system is paramount for both aspiring pediatricians and those well established in their practices as a first step in understanding their practice environment and ensuring that children receive the best health care possible according to their unique needs.

## INSURANCE COVERAGE FOR CHILDREN

While many children receive health insurance coverage through private insurance, a significant proportion of low-income children rely on public insurance for coverage (Fig. 6-1). Public insurance plays a critical role in providing adequate healthcare coverage for these children and their families. At its inception in 1965, Medicaid provided coverage to children in low-income families. CHIP was created in 1997 to address insurance coverage gaps for children who were not eligible for Medicaid but whose families could not afford private insurance. More recently, under the Patient Protection and Affordable Care Act, parents of low-income children have gained coverage through Medicaid expansion and subsidies available for marketplace coverage. Public health insurance has demonstrated a number of benefits to low-income children and their families. The availability of Medicaid and CHIP has reduced the number of children without health insurance coverage. Furthermore, it has increased access to and utilization of healthcare services. Public insurance has reduced families' financial strain attributable to medical care. Lastly, it has improved material well-being for families.

## EFFORTS TO ADDRESS COSTS AND QUALITY OF CARE

Health care accounts for a substantial proportion of the US economy, with an estimated $3 trillion spent on health care annually. The US spends approximately 18% of its gross domestic product on health care. Expenditures attributable to health care grow faster than many other sectors of the US economy, including education, transportation, and agriculture. Such costs may have significant impact on families, making insurance less affordable and, consequently, resulting in children not receiving the healthcare services they need. Although children account

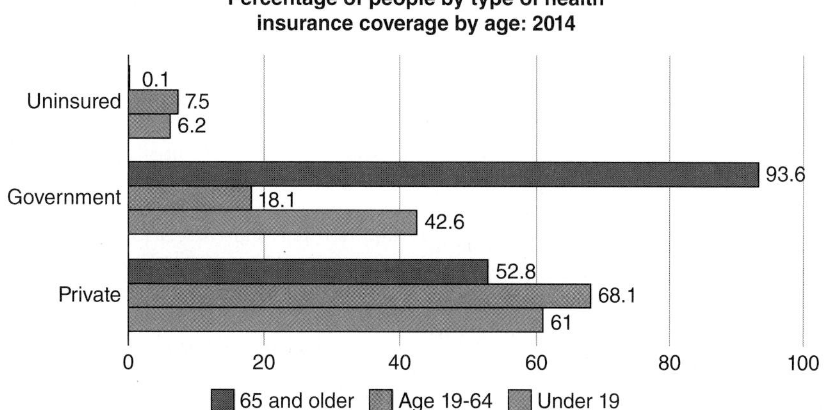


**FIGURE 6-1** Percentage of people by type of health insurance coverage by age: 2014. (Data from Smith JC, Medalia C: *Health Insurance Coverage in the United States: 2014*. US Census Bureau, Current Population Reports, P60-253. https://www.census.gov/content/dam/Census/library/publications/2015/demo/p60-253.pdf. Published September 2015.)

for approximately 23% of the US population, they only account for roughly 13% of healthcare spending. In contrast, individuals ages 65 and older account for approximately 35% of US healthcare spending, although they comprise only 13% of the population. Since children are generally healthy and the cost of covering them relative to other populations is low, they may take less priority in efforts to address healthcare quality and spending. Given the significant costs attributable to older adults, efforts and strategies to improve quality and reduce healthcare expenditures predominantly focus on adult models, with assumptions that such approaches should apply to children.

A number of strategies have been proposed to address quality and escalating medical expenditures. Value-based purchasing (VBP) refers to a broad set of performance-based payment strategies that couple financial incentives to a physician's provision of high-quality care and performance on a set of defined measures. Such strategies have been implemented by both public and private payers to drive improvements and curb spending. Despite modest results in improving performance, VBP models continue to be used by payers. Current VBP programs assess performance on measures of quality (eg, structure, process, outcomes, access, and patient experience) and resource use. Three broad models of VBP currently are in use. *Pay-for-performance* refers to a payment program in which providers are rewarded (bonuses) or penalized (payment reductions) based on achieving benchmarks for measures of quality and/or efficiency. *Accountable care organizations* (ACO) refers to health organizations comprised of physicians, hospitals, and other clinical providers who agree to work together to provide coordinated care and be held accountable for overall costs and quality of care for an assigned population of patients. Provider reimbursements are coupled to performance on quality measures and reductions in cost of care. In an ACO model, providers accept financial risk and are eligible for shared savings achieved through improved care. *Bundle payments* are a strategy in which payments to providers are based on the anticipated costs for a clinically defined episode of related health services. The agreement includes quality and financial performance accountability for the episode of care.

Fundamental to a VBP approach is the development and articulation of established quality measures. While many quality measures exist for adults, few exist for children. Most measures have focused on preventive aspects of primary care, including vaccine administration, developmental screening, and preventive counseling. Recent federal initiatives have accelerated efforts toward identifying performance measures for pediatrics. The Children's Health Insurance Program Reauthorization Act (CHIPRA) in 2009 funded a number of pediatric quality measurement projects and launched the Core Set of Children's Health Care Quality Measures for Medicaid and CHIP. The American Recovery and Reinvestment Act set forth a roadmap for universal adoption of health information technology in order to better assess and monitor quality. The Patient Protection and Affordable Care Act of 2010 called for a comprehensive national approach to healthcare quality. Measures of quality fall into 4 categories: structure, process, outcome, and patient experience. Structural measures assess the infrastructure of the healthcare setting and policies related to healthcare delivery. Process measures evaluate whether services align with care guidelines. Outcome measures assess whether services lead to changes in health or behavior. Patient experience measures provide feedback from the patient on their experiences with their medical care. Surveys such as the Consumer Assessment of Healthcare Providers and Systems (CAHPS) serve as tools for documenting patient experience.

The field of quality improvement (QI) is increasingly used as a core strategy for improving healthcare quality. QI encompasses systematic activities that are organized and implemented by an organization to monitor, assess, and improve its quality of health care. QI focuses on testing different strategies on a small scale to ascertain if they achieve their intended results before large-scale implementation occurs across a practice or system. Techniques specific to QI include standardized clinical pathways, benchmarking, performance incentives, public reporting, provider reminder systems, and decision aids. The Model for Improvement with the readily recognized Plan-Do-Study-Act (PDSA) cycle serves as the conceptual framework for most QI initiatives (Fig. 6-2). Strategies with promising results can be spread and adopted on a wide-scale basis. Fundamental to the PDSA model is that QI must be a continuous, iterative activity that incorporates emerging evidence-based guidelines and innovations in healthcare delivery. QI is now an integral part of the American Board of Pediatrics' (ABP's) Maintenance of Certification (MOC) Program. The rationale is that focusing on performance at the practice level and supporting improvement across practices addresses gaps in quality and has the potential to improve care for diverse pediatric populations. The ABP requires that pediatricians demonstrate with data that they can determine the quality of care their team delivers. Furthermore, it asks that pediatricians learn to systematically apply QI methods to improve care in order to receive Part 4 MOC credit. The ABP has developed standards for what constitutes meaningful pediatrician involvement in QI endeavors to qualify for Part 4 credits.

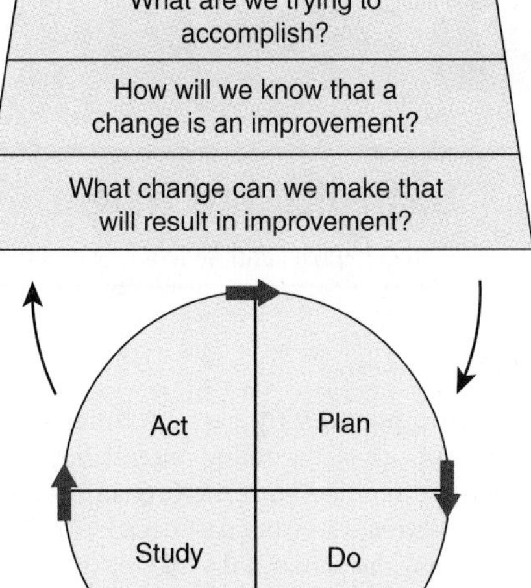


**FIGURE 6-2** The Plan-Do-Study-Act cycle. (Reproduced with permission from Langley GJ, Moen RD, Nolan KM, et al: *The Improvement Guide: A Practical Approach to Enhancing Organizational Performance*, 2nd ed. San Francisco, CA: Jossey-Bass; 2009.)

Efforts to fully invest in the promise of health information technology are also being employed to improve care and reduce costs. They increasingly impact how pediatricians practice across medical settings. The American Recovery and Reinvestment Act (ARRA) set forth guidelines for universal adoption of health information technology for the purposes of electronic health records (EHR) and health information exchanges. The Health Information Technology for Economic and Clinical Health (HITECH) Act authorized incentives payments through Medicare and Medicaid to clinicians and hospitals when they utilize EHRs privately and securely to reach specified improvements in care delivery. In addition to adoption, the HITECH Act also aimed to achieve "meaningful use" of EHRs, such that their use by providers achieves substantial improvements in health care. To be considered meaningful users, providers and hospitals must meet a set of core objectives that serve as a baseline expectation for meaningful use of EHRs. Core objectives include entry of basic data (eg, demographics, active medications, drug allergies, up-to-date problem lists, and current and active diagnoses), implementation of clinical decision support tools, and use of computer order entry. Additionally, providers and hospitals must select for implementation from a separate menu of additional important activities. This gives providers the ability to choose their own path toward full EHR adoption and meaningful use. The HITECH Act lastly requires that meaningful use include electronic reporting of data on the quality of care.

## TRIPLE AIM

Historically, care improvement efforts have centered on fulfilling all 6 dimensions identified by the Institute of Medicine: safety, effectiveness, patient-centeredness, timeliness, efficiency, and equity.

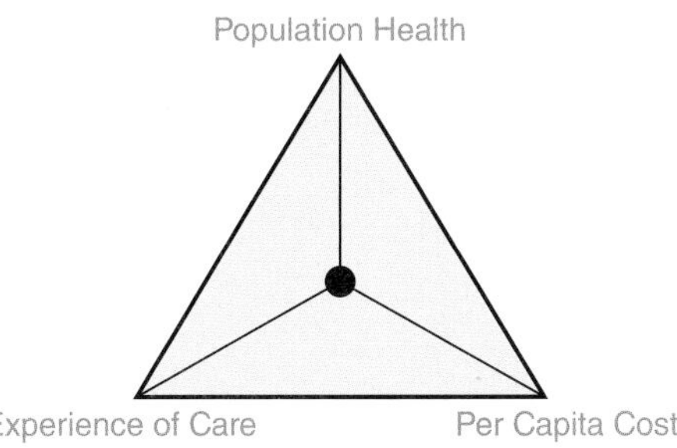


**FIGURE 6-3** The Triple Aim. (The IHI Triple Aim framework was developed by the Institute for Healthcare Improvement in Massachusetts, USA [ihi.org].)

As policy makers have endeavored to address quality and costs through the efforts described above, the Triple Aim has emerged as a roadmap of linked goals to guide efforts (Fig. 6-3). Created by the Institute for Healthcare Improvement, the Triple Aim promotes the pursuit of 3 aims: improving the experience of care, improving the health of populations, and reducing per capita costs of health care. These components function interdependently. Pursuing any 1 aim can impact the other 2. These effects may be positive or negative. Improving the health of populations may lead to improved patient experience. Alternatively, improving care for individuals may result in increased healthcare costs depending on the types of therapies and technologies used. Consequently, pursuit of the Triple Aim must be balanced across its aims. Furthermore, achieving the Triple Aim requires several shifts in approaches to health care. First, patients and families must be educated on the benefits and limitations of individual healthcare practices and procedures. This requires an emphasis on shared decision-making and efforts to change the perception that more care equates to better care. Second, primary care services and structures must be redesigned to expand the functions of a healthcare team. Expanded functions through a patient-centered medical home may include creating shared plans of care, coordinating care, providing enhanced access to care, connecting families to community resources, and collaborating with schools. Third, more efforts must increasingly focus on the health of populations in addition to individuals. This will facilitate more efficient and equitable deployment of resources.

As the US healthcare system continues to evolve in response to the aspirations of the Triple Aim, the practice of pediatrics must change accordingly, particularly with respect to implementation of reforms that may be more tailored to the needs of adults rather than children. As a first step, pediatricians must familiarize themselves with concepts such as value-based purchasing, quality improvement, meaningful use, and the Triple Aim. Subsequently, pediatricians must determine how to best practice in the evolving healthcare landscape while effectively advocating strategies that work for children and their families.

## SUGGESTED READINGS

Berwick DM, Nolan TW, Whittington J. The Triple Aim: care, health, and cost. *Health Aff.* 2008;27(3):759-769.

Blumenthal D, Tavenner M. The "meaningful use" regulation for electronic health records. *N Engl J Med.* 2010;363(6):501-504.

Brooks T. *Measuring and Improving Health Care Quality for Children in Medicaid and CHIP: A Primer for Child Health Stakeholders.* Washington, DC: Georgetown University Health Policy Institute, Center for Children and Families; 2016. http://ccf.georgetown.edu/wp-content/uploads/2016/03/Measuring_Health_Quality_Medicaid_CHIP_Primer.pdf. Accessed November 14, 2016.

Damberg CL, Sorbero ME, Lovejoy SL, Martsolf G, Raaen L, Mandel D. *Measuring Success in Health Care Value-Based Purchasing Programs: Findings from an Environmental Scan, Literature Review, and Expert Panel Discussions*; 2014. Rand Corporation Research Report. http://www.rand.org/content/dam/rand/pubs/research_reports/RR300/RR306/RAND_RR306.pdf. Accessed November 14, 2016.

Forrest CB, Simpson L, Clancy C. Child health services research: challenges and opportunities. *JAMA.* 1997;277(22):1787-1793.

Kaiser Family Foundation. *Health Care Costs: A Primer*; 2012. https://kaiserfamilyfoundation.files.wordpress.com/2013/01/7670-03.pdf. Accessed November 14, 2016.

Lassman D, Hartman M, Washington B, Andrews K, Catlin A. US health spending trends by age and gender: selected years 2002–10. *Health Aff.* 2014;33(5):815-822.

Stille C, Turchi RM, Antonelli R, et al; Academic Pediatric Association Task Force on the Family-Centered Medical Home. The family-centered medical home: specific considerations for child health research and policy. *Acad Pediatr.* 2010;10(4):211-217.

Wherry LR, Kenney GM, Sommers BD. The role of public health insurance in reducing child poverty. *Acad Pediatr.* 2016;16(3 suppl):S98-S104.

# 7 Population Health Management and Pediatrics

Heidi Schwarzwald and Charles G. Macias

## BACKGROUND

Population health is a term that reflects the health of patients across continuums of care with a goal of improving health outcomes. Its definition reflects the users' relationship to that continuum: public health, advocacy and policy, research, or clinical care delivery. Public health has traditionally been focused on the safety and health of families and communities by preventing and treating diseases and injuries where children and their families live, learn, work, and play. Population health differs from public health in two main ways. First, it is dictated less by governmental health departments, and second, it is more inclusive of the healthcare delivery system. The focus of population health may span geography (eg, a region), a condition (eg, children with a chronic condition such as asthma), a payer (eg, patients in an accountable care organization or within a health plan), or any characteristic that would link accountability for outcomes for that group of patients. This gives rise to the concept of population management, where a common condition or other linking element may drive the practitioner to create and implement prevention or care strategies and promote health for groups of patients.

Population health is defined as the art and science of preventing disease, prolonging life, and promoting health through recognized efforts and informed choices of society, organizations, public and private communities, and individuals. It encompasses a number of critical components for ensuring improved outcomes of care. Most importantly, it expands the reach (and the obligation) of the clinician from bedside care alone to a goal of ensuring the health of the patient, including helping the patient and family overcome barriers to access and coordinating care. Clinicians must also identify and mitigate the effects of social determinants of health and engage the patient and family in their own health management and disease and injury prevention. Social determinants may include education, economic stability, social and community context, and neighborhood and physical environments. The concepts of prevention and health promotion are not foreign to the pediatrician; however, population health introduces a great challenge for the provider to engage a great number of factors that influence health outcomes but are not within the locus of control of the clinician unless actively attempting to work in concert with other aspects of the healthcare system. Childhood obesity, asthma, and dental caries are not only prevalent in the US child population, but they have a reciprocal interaction with family dysfunction and school

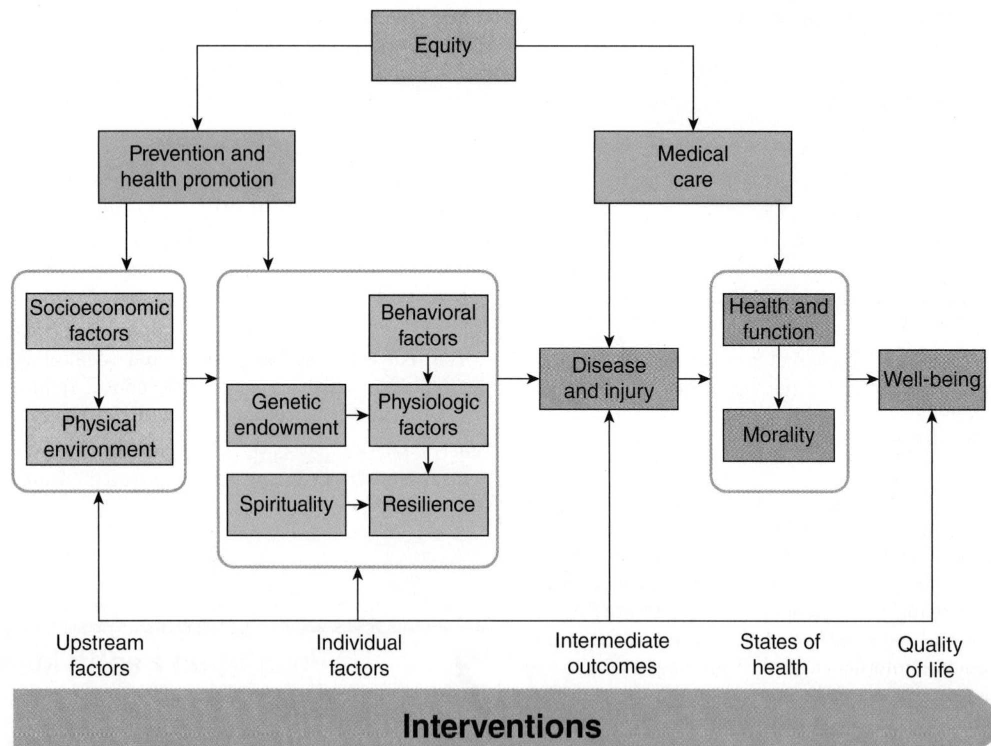


**FIGURE 7-1** The Institute for Healthcare Improvement population health composite model. (Reprinted from www.ihi.org with permission of the Institute for Healthcare Improvement (IHI), Copyright © 2011.)

stress, necessitating that a provider address these social determinants in order to achieve improved outcomes of care. The Institute for Healthcare Improvement has described a composite model that best explains the interventions necessary to improve outcomes and thus quality of life. Prevention and health promotion include upstream factors in the patient and families' environment (eg, physical or socioeconomic factors) that are further influenced by individual factors (eg, behavioral, spiritual, genetic factors). The practitioner must consider a broader array of determinants of health than is typical in bedside disease management. Moreover, measurement of population health may include any array of metrics spanning from upstream factors to quality of life, thus expanding beyond simple health outcomes (Fig. 7-1).

## OPERATIONALIZING POPULATION HEALTH AS A PROVIDER

As healthcare systems and governments move to value-based payment models (models that reward high-quality outcomes rather than provide a fee for service), providers are faced with external pressures to engage in population management to meet the demands of payers. The impact to the provider may be thought of in four domains of healthcare transformation within population health: business models, clinical integration, technology, and payment models.

The first domain encompasses changes in business models, where expansion of facilities and services by healthcare systems are aligned to provide a more comprehensive menu of services and better access to those services, for example, an expanded number of clinics, urgent care settings, freestanding ERs, or other innovative settings in which a patient may access care and for which a provider must consider in attempting to establish a medical home and a continuum of care for that patient.

The second domain, clinical integration, involves the ability to provide care and services across a continuum. Specifically, the American Medical Association has described clinical integration as the means to facilitate the coordination of patient care across conditions, providers, settings, and time in order to achieve care that is safe, timely, effective, efficient, equitable, and patient-focused. Rather than care focused on episodes or strategies created in silos, care must be integrated in a patient-centric model. In other words, hospital-based care must be synchronized and transitioned within its own departments and across to the primary care provider and the engaged patient and family. For the provider, care coordination becomes a critical element of care delivery.

In the third domain, technology empowers the creation and transfer of information, in retrospect, real time, or near time. Information may be utilized, transmitted, or transformed into meaningful analytics, and shared across a system or systems. Electronic medical records and the systems of hardware and analytics that support them become critical vehicles for the exchange of clinical data and data regarding the outcomes of a population of children for ensuring the right outcomes are achieved. Mechanisms for improving utilization and efficiency of the electronic health record (EHR) have been endorsed and incentivized through federally funded programs such as Meaningful Use.

The fourth and final domain is a change in payment models. More and more systems are engaged in shared savings models, where improvement in outcomes, including reductions in cost of care, is paid back in part to the providers as an incentive. An improvement aim for the broader healthcare systems has been described as *the triple aim*; improvement initiatives are focused on three dimensions: improved patient experience, improved health of the population determined by improved health outcomes, and reduced per capita cost of care. Primary care providers engaged in population management may be engaged as members linked further through *clinically integrated networks* (CINs). CINs are legal arrangements in which employed or affiliated physicians negotiate with payers and work toward measuring and improving practice in an ongoing and cooperative fashion to control costs and improve quality.

In addition to these external forces shaping care delivery, the provider must also be cognizant of how these infrastructure forces require a more holistic view of the patient: understanding the community and environment in which the patient lives and the family works, recognizing the patient's access to preventive medical care and helping reduce potential barriers to that access, understanding measurement of quality of life, and assessing data that addresses disease burden in a providers' practice and/or system. This demands that the practitioner's office, partnership, or system maintain collaborations with public health departments, local agencies, and community organizations to understand local population health needs and to jointly address them if patient outcomes are to be improved. Only a relatively small proportion of a population's health outcomes is the result of the medical care system, while over half of outcomes are related to individual behaviors. Strategies that will effectively change health-related behaviors must reach beyond the clinical setting, incorporate community and public health systems, and engage the patients and their families.

Quality improvement (QI) remains at the core of better outcomes through population health. An attention to outcomes means an increasing attention to measurement. Efforts to enhance QI applications to the healthcare industry are pervasive, and payment reform is only a part of it. Academically, the American Board of Medical Specialties and its member boards have changed certification principles to lifelong learning strategies with the inclusion of requirements for demonstration of QI applications to patient panels and the populations they serve (eg, Maintenance of Certification Part 4).

## LEGISLATION THAT AFFECTS POPULATION HEALTH

### The Affordable Care Act

The Affordable Care Act (ACA) was passed in 2010 and upheld by the Supreme Court in 2012. The ACA's intent was to "put consumers back in charge of their healthcare." The provisions of the bill were designed to remove barriers to care by increasing access to health insurance, removing preexisting condition exemptions, and making preventive care available without copays. It created or strengthened organizations such as the Patient-Centered Outcomes Research Institute (PCORI) and the Agency for Healthcare Research and Quality (AHRQ). These organizations focus on quality of care and encourage the creation of systems that provide care to specific populations, such as accountable care organizations (ACO).

### Community Needs Assessments: IRS Rule Change

Another provision of the ACA changed the methodology by which nonprofit hospitals qualify for tax exemptions. In order to achieve nonprofit status, hospitals must conduct a community health needs assessment (CHNA) at least every 3 years. Prior to this, in order to achieve tax-exempt status, a hospital had to show it was charitable by serving "a public rather than a private interest." Most hospitals met this obligation through charity care programs. With the implementation of the ACA and a change to the tax code, however, this was no longer adequate to maintain tax-exempt status. Hospital systems are now obligated to partner with community and governmental organizations to take an approach to care delivery integrated with public health strategies.

Community health needs assessments and implementation create an important opportunity to improve the health of communities. They ensure that hospitals have the information they need to provide community-centered benefits. They also provide an opportunity to improve coordination of hospital community benefits with other efforts to improve community health. By statute, the CHNAs must take into account input from "persons who represent the broad interests of the community served by the hospital facility, including those with special knowledge of or expertise in public health."

## SUCCESSFUL STRATEGIES IN POPULATION HEALTH

The following case studies illustrate the implementation of population health strategies.

### Obesity

The most recent statistics from the Centers for Disease Control state that 17% of children ages 2 to 19 years are obese. Obesity rates are different based on race, ethnicity, household income, and whether the household has one or two primary caregivers. If a family is at or below the poverty level, the children in that household have a 14.5% prevalence of obesity as compared to a prevalence of 11.8% in households where the income is between 151% and 185% of the federal poverty level. Prevalence among 2 to 4 year olds who receive supplemental food from the Women, Infants, and Children (WIC) program also varies by state with Utah being the lowest (8.7%) and Alaska the highest (20.6%). Poverty and geography are examples of social determinants of health. Reducing obesity requires a population health approach.

While many community-based programs are successful at targeting obesity, the pediatric patient-centered medical home has a significant role to play in any program. When compared to schools or other community resources, the longitudinal nature of the relationship between a family and its medical home is unique because it often ranges from birth to age 20. Understanding and addressing the societal and community drivers of obesity particular to the community while in the office is one approach to population health. The patient-centered medical home can also take a broader population health approach within the practice.

The practice can begin by defining the population to be addressed, for example: all pediatric patients at a particular clinic with a body mass index (BMI) greater than the 85th percentile, all children who attend a particular school system, or all obese children covered by Medicaid in a particular city.

Using Figure 7.1, the upstream factors for obesity would include poverty level; availability of fresh, healthy food in the community; and safe spaces for physical activity. Individual factors may include race/ethnicity; eating behaviors, such as use of food as a reward, knowledge of caregivers about food preparation, time to prepare food vs. buying food; and willingness to alter habits or current practices.

Cultural differences in the psychological effects of obesity are also present. Obese white adolescent females are more likely than obese black adolescent females to have mental health disorders tied to feelings of worthlessness. This may reflect differences in societal norms in black communities that do not tie personal worth as tightly to weight as in white communities.

Disease burden may become more obvious in older children and adolescents as they develop prediabetes or elevated cholesterol. The longer-term health outcomes can include diabetes, heart disease, and poor quality of life. As a pediatric provider, addressing these medical outcomes is one part of addressing the health issue. The most successful programs, however, have combined medical and community approaches.

One successful population health approach to obesity comes from Mississippi where the target population is defined as elementary students in the state. In 2015, Mississippi reported a decrease in combined overweight and obesity among elementary school–aged children from 43% to 38%, over the years 2005 to 2013 ($P$ = .0002). Decreases in weight were more significant in white than in black students. The success in Mississippi is based on many factors, such as new legislative efforts changing the foods available in schools, changes in school practices for physical education, and public/private initiatives to increase grocery availability in food deserts. Funding for other activities came from insurance companies and other businesses.

In Wisconsin, the local medical society worked with the school district to obtain a federal grant to increase areas for physical activity. Other studies have looked at interventions focused on the primary care office. Measurements and structured anticipatory guidance has been shown to alter some behaviors (eg, television time). However, the most successful interventions are those in which the medical community partners with local organizations and governments to reduce weight in populations. An example is the use of the Mind, Exercise, Nutrition, Do It! (MEND) program in which local pediatricians make referrals to a community-based health center where the program has been implemented. The pediatric office then reinforces the program in the office. The American Academy of Pediatrics Institute for Childhood Obesity (www.ihcw.org) has many tools to assist the pediatric provider in optimizing health care through motivational interviewing, engaging families, and catalyzing communities.

### Behavioral/Mental Health

Behavioral and mental health issues in a pediatric population can also be approached from a population health perspective. As an example, a pediatric provider may keep a registry of all the patients within the clinic who have been diagnosed with attention-deficit/hyperactivity disorder (ADHD). This allows staff within the practice to track medication refills, completion of standardized questionnaires, and most recent appointments. The utilization of a registry can also allow a practice to manage a group of patients with a similar diagnosis.

The practice may be motivated to take this approach for different reasons. They may be utilizing registries as part of a strategy for seeking recognition for providing a patient-centered medical home. Larger payers may be offering incentives to practices in their area that can demonstrate improved quality metrics.

Many insurance companies, particularly those that provide Medicaid through Medicaid managed care contracts, are required to track and report a set of quality metrics called the Healthcare Effectiveness Data and Information Set (HEDIS). Several of these metrics relate to care for ADHD. One example is ensuring that any patient starting medication for ADHD is seen within 30 days of initiation by the provider who prescribed the medication. The payer develops this list based on members who have chosen that provider or been assigned to that provider. The provider may only develop the list from the patients actually seen in the practice. In this case, the populations may not align exactly. Population health theory would include patients/members who have and have not been seen in clinic.

Insurance companies offer additional payments ("pay for performance") to providers who improve on this metric in the shared savings model previously described. This type of arrangement has no risk for the provider, but it does allow the provider the possibility of earning additional monies to offset the cost of additional staff required to maintain and manage a registry of patients. This approach to population health has been shown to improve quality metrics. In this case, the provider and payer's incentives are aligned. The payer might even supply the provider with a list of assigned patients with the diagnosis of ADHD. This type of population health initiative focuses on the medical aspect of Fig. 7-1.

Additional stakeholders would include the schools. If a pediatric provider had many patients with a particular school or school district, another aspect of population health would be to develop streamlined communication tools and workflow with the school personnel to ensure timely communication of medication changes and return of standardized questionnaires to determine progress. Further, the participation of pediatric providers in the school accommodation process could be eased.

#### Asthma

Another population health approach can be hospital centric. In this example, the population is defined as the 70,000 asthmatics who have been seen in a particular healthcare system in Houston, Texas. This system includes two hospitals, over 50 primary care clinics, specialty clinics, and an insurance company. The system uses a unified EHR, allowing for improved data sharing. The first step in creating a unified approach to asthma care is defining the population. The most basic approach to defining the population is using diagnoses from health record encounters. However, this proved to be a process with low sensitivity or specificity.

Collaborative teams were developed to determine the best definition of the asthma population. The current definition utilized combined patient characteristics (eg, age), medication prescriptions and use, encounter diagnosis, and other criteria. This rigorous process of correctly defining the population is a crucial first step to any population health or quality project. Without the correct denominator, it is difficult to correctly assess the progress or effect of various interventions.

Starting with medical management (Fig. 7-1, right side), the system developed a common asthma action plan so that patient instructions across the enterprise are universal. Next, universal order sets were developed. Initial data revealed that nearly 60% of patients with an asthma exacerbation underwent a chest radiograph, an unnecessary procedure for most children with asthma. Furthermore, only 54% of patients with asthma received an asthma action plan (AAP) upon discharge, which is a metric of quality asthma care according to the National Asthma Education and Prevention Program.

A multidisciplinary team began their improvement efforts by building clinical decision support into the EHR through an evidence-based order set. This guided providers toward a predetermined course of action and decreased variation. Run charts showing results of interventions were made easily available to providers on the inpatient wards and in the emergency rooms. Chest radiograph rates currently remain below target—under 30%—and 97% of children currently receive an AAP at discharge. The decrease in unwanted variation in practice and decrease in waste have allowed for a decrease in length of stay from 3.4 days at baseline to 1.7 days. Furthermore, survey samplings of families of children with asthma have demonstrated greater confidence in self-management and a better understanding of care delivery. The subsequent reduction in cost of care has driven care delivery from an average loss per inpatient asthma visit, to a positive average margin contribution (profitability), while providing a better patient experience and better outcomes of care, thus achieving the triple aim with this population.

The system has concurrently increased community involvement, including schools, nonprofit organizations, environmental/pollution monitoring groups, and other key stakeholders. Asthma prevention has included active antismoking campaigns/education for parents and others and improvement in housing through city government–health department partnerships to decrease exposure to molds, cockroaches, and other environmental triggers.

## ENABLERS AND BARRIERS TO POPULATION HEALTH

#### EHR

Electronic health records are one of the primary enablers to population health. The ability to collect data in discrete predetermined fields allows for unprecedented analyses. Reminders and order sets (ie, clinical decision support) can assist with quicker dissemination of best practices and evidence-based care.

Despite their benefits, many find EHRs as obstructions to care. Acknowledging that they can be difficult at times in a daily workflow, they can also assist with decision-making. Best practice alerts remind providers of health maintenance needs for individual patients during an encounter. Medication alerts can reduce re-work when prescriptions are not covered on a particular formulary. The EHR also is the platform where a provider can begin collecting data that can inform healthcare changes at a population level that ultimately will be translated into analytics to drive improved health at an individual level.

#### Analytics/Benchmarking

Population health today differs from public health campaigns of the past primarily because of data and data analytics. The analytics industry has suggested that healthcare data will double in a 5-year period within 2010–2020 decade. Most large institutions today have some way to collect and analyze the data being generated within the health system. Generally, the data is abstracted from various sources: pharmacy distribution and payment data, clinical data, and payer or claims information. When this data is aggregated, a more complete picture of healthcare utilization can be developed and used to drive quality improvement and cost containment. By agreeing on the measures to be tracked and changed, providers, healthcare systems, and payers also can come to an agreement on value-based payments, which align the patient, provider, and payer incentives toward better health as defined by the individual patient. This is only possible with analytics and benchmarking. As in the example of asthma, analytics and benchmarking allow for the rapid detection of variants and the improvement of care. Electronic data warehouses abstract data from claims as well as health records to create a more complete picture of a population. Linking that data to a provider's panel allows the provider to execute mass orders and communication to his or her patients.

#### Disparate Measures

As enabling as analytics and benchmarking are, the proliferation of process measures and relatively few outcome measures can also be a hindrance to better health. In the recently published white paper "Vital Signs," it is noted that over 16 different metrics for obesity exist within the U.S. Department of Health and Human Services. Another study found that hospitals report on over 120 quality measures to various payers or regulators. One percent of patient revenue is utilized in the cost of measure collection and analysis. Recently the National Committee for Quality Assurance (NCQA) has proposed new measures for quality, particularly for patient-centered medical home recognitions. These measures acknowledge a reduced emphasis on process and a greater emphasis on outcomes. For instance, sections focused on care coordination no longer ask for policies on care coordination, but instead ask for outcomes of populations managed within a clinic (NCQA proposed 2017 revision). "Vital Signs" calls for a complete simplification of measures to the 15 core elements of health. Some examples are life expectancy, well-being, patient safety, and preventative services.

#### Data Integration

Although great strides have been made in data integration, barriers remain. Some cities are far advanced in the ability to utilize integrated data to improve care and reduce duplication. Both San Antonio, Texas, and Cincinnati, Ohio, have integrated health records via a city-wide health connection. These platforms are cloud based, using common data fields across multiple hospitals, systems, and EHRs to allow providers to know when patients receive care in another hospital or in the emergency room. This allows for improvement in care transitions and continuity. Diagnostic examinations are less likely to be repeated when data can be easily shared. Patient consent and privacy should be protected in such systems, and allowing individuals to opt out of the system is important. One small study found that 88% of the 62 persons interviewed felt comfortable sharing their health information via health exchanges once educated on the intent. The concept behind Meaningful Use measures and the ACA were to allow for waste reduction via data integration. This remains a work in progress.

### SUMMARY

The one-on-one clinician–patient dyad will always be important but alone cannot accommodate the demands of the healthcare system to improve outcomes for the entire population. Increasing attention to the integration of population health competencies into professional training is giving rise to new demands on continuing education, for example, managing chronic disease in a patient panel or practice, engaging in interprofessional teams, or collaborating with others on health promotion. Thus, many academic institutions have developed public health and/or population health departments while many healthcare systems and/or hospitals have developed population health strategies. Competencies for population health have been described by educators within the domains of public health and community engagement. These include (but are not limited to) defining the role of communities in health, addressing the role of social determinants of health, leveraging community assets and resources to improve health, participating in population-based prevention strategies, engaging essential functionality of public health systems, and supporting principles of accountability at the community or public health agency level. Additional competencies address community engagement in academic partnerships, critical thinking and application to evidence-based practice, data and analytics, health literacy, quality improvement tenets, program evaluation, interprofessional team skills, communication, and navigation of complex healthcare organizations.

### SUGGESTED READINGS


Blumenthal D, Malphrus E, McGinnis JM, eds; Committee on Core Metrics for Better Health at Lower Cost; Institute of Medicine. *Vital Signs: Core Metrics for Health and Health Care Progress.* Washington DC: National Academies Press; 2015.

Kaprielian VS, Silberberg M, McDonald MA, et al. Teaching population health: a competency map approach to education. *Acad Med.* 2013;88(5):626-637.

Macias, CG, Bartley KA, Rodkey TL, Russell HV. Creating a clinical systems integration strategy to drive improvement. *Curr Treat Options Pediatr.* 2015;1(4):334-346. doi: 10.1007/s40746-015-0031-7.

Social determinants of health. Office of Disease Prevention and Health Promotion Web site. http://www.academyhealth.org/publications/2013-02/population-health-affordable-care-act-era. Accessed September 2, 2016.

Stiefel M, Nolan K. A guide to measuring the triple aim: population health, experience of care, and per capita cost. IHI Innovation Series white paper. Cambridge, MA: Institute for Healthcare Improvement; 2012. http://www.ihi.org/resources/pages/ihiwhitepapers/aguidetomeasuringtripleaim.aspx. Accessed September 2, 2016.

Stoto MA. Population health in the Affordable Care Act era. 2013. *Academy Health.* http://www.academyhealth.org/files/AH2013pophealth.pdf. Accessed September 2, 2016.

Taveras EM, Gortmaker SL, Hohman KH, et al. Randomized controlled trial to improve primary care to prevent and manage childhood obesity: The High Five for Kids Study. *Arch Pediatr Adolesc Med.* 2011;165(8):714-722. doi:10.1001/archpediatrics.2011.44.

Whaley AL, Smith M, Hancock A. Ethnic/racial differences in the self-reported physical and mental health correlates of adolescent obesity. *J Health Psychol.* 2011;16(7):1048-1057.

Zhang L, Kolbo JR, Kirkup M, et al. Prevalence and trends in overweight and obesity among Mississippi public school students, 2005-2013. *J Miss State Med Assoc.* 2014;55(3):80-87.


# 8 Patient and Family–Centered Care and the Patient-Centered Medical Home

Scott R. Callahan, Mona E. Mansour, and Jeffrey M. Simmons

### DEFINITION OF PATIENT AND FAMILY–CENTERED CARE

The philosophy of patient and family–centered care is founded on the belief that health outcomes are improved by partnering among healthcare providers, patients, and their families. This belief permeates the healthcare system and does not represent a specific therapy that is applied as part of a treatment plan. In the literature, there is no uniform definition of patient and family–centered care. Therefore, it is best described by its fundamental principles: *respect and dignity, information control, participation, collaboration,* and *flexibility.*

#### Respect and Dignity

Although individual healthcare providers typically are respectful in their interaction with patients, the healthcare system was not designed to afford dignity and respect to patients. The system often values providers' needs and time over that of patients. Many of the routine policies and practices that seemingly disregard patients' comfort and dignity are now changing. Treating patients and families with honor, addressing them as they wish to be addressed, and learning about their strengths and human history in addition to their medical history exemplifies this core principle of respect and dignity.

#### Information Control

Implementing the patient and family–centered care philosophy involves transfer of control of information from the healthcare system to the patient and family. As we become a predominantly electronic healthcare system, designers of electronic health records are faced with the decision of who "owns" the information. Patient portals now give patients and families facile access to their health information. Access also includes information regarding the performance of the healthcare system, such as comparative outcome data and patient safety issues.

**Participation**

Perhaps this principle can best be summed up by the phrase "nothing about me, without me." Families and patients have the fundamental right to make decisions regarding their care. Therefore, families need to be presented with choices. Shared decision-making is gaining attention as an important aspect of caring for children with chronic and serious conditions. Increasing emphasis is placed on presenting information in a clear manner and allowing patients to make choices when they desire with evidence indicating improved engagement and compliance.

**Collaboration**

Many healthcare organizations have found families are a great resource of energy and expertise that often goes underutilized. Most pediatric health systems have developed family advisory councils; some also have advisory councils composed of patients. Families are more frequently becoming members of governing boards and serving on quality improvement teams and facility design teams. In addition, there is support from the literature that parent-to-parent support may be crucial for families whose child has a chronic or serious condition.

**Flexibility**

It is important to recognize that illness places a significant burden on families. To truly partner with patients and families, systems must be flexible and address families' and patients' unique circumstances and needs. Offering expanded and flexible hours for office visits, tests, and even surgery may be necessary. Phone visits, e-mail advice, text messaging, telemedicine, and alternative sites of care (eg, school-based health centers) all allow for flexibility. In hospital settings, flexibility that allows increased control of daily schedules by the patient can both assure that appropriate care is provided in a timely manner and empower patients to become more engaged in their care.

## PARADIGM SHIFT

As entire organizations, healthcare clinics, hospital units (microsystems), and individual providers work toward the principles of patient and family–centered care, a paradigm shift takes place. Table 8-1 summarizes some key distinctions of patient and family–centered care in comparison to the more provider-centric care that is waning in influence.

## EVOLUTION OF THE PATIENT-CENTERED MEDICAL HOME

The first reference of a medical home is made in an American Academy of Pediatrics text entitled *Standards of Child Health Care.* Published by the AAP Counsel of Pediatric Practice in 1967, a key emphasis is placed on the importance of having the medical records of a child centralized, particularly when providing care for children with special healthcare needs. As the benefits and necessity of establishing a patient-centric clinical method to healthcare delivery have subsequently developed, the medical home model has evolved, but always with the theme of a partnership between a primary care provider and a parent and/or patient.

The definition of a patient-centered medical home (PCMH) is exceedingly varied, but there are a number of generally recognized requirements. In 2007, the American Academy of Family Practice, the American Academy of Pediatrics, the American College of Physicians, and the American Osteopathic Association issued a joint statement describing 7 principles that PCMHs should be expected to demonstrate: patients having a personal physician, physician-directed practice, whole person orientation, care integration, quality and safety, enhanced access, and payment recognizing the value added with the PCMH model. Current descriptions of the model articulate the need for continuity of care, accessibility, comprehensiveness, coordination, compassion, and culturally competent care with a focus not only on individual patient care but population management. There is a push for practices to participate in voluntary recognition by a nongovernmental entity of services consistent with the medical home model. This process, which can be burdensome to the practice from an administrative standpoint, allows the patient and payers to engage in healthcare decision-making and reimbursement strategies with practices that have demonstrated the ability to meet various measures that align with goals of improved patient experience, population health management, and increased value for services provided. Table 8-2 summarizes some key distinctions of the PCMH in comparison to a more traditional practice model, representing another paradigm shift.

The future of the PCMH will involve expanding the scope of impact on patient and family health by aligning community resources with patient need. The patient-centered medical home is uniquely positioned to screen for toxic stress generators and social determinants of health such as maternal depression, food insecurity, interpersonal violence, substance abuse, and harsh discipline techniques, and then align preidentified geographical relevant agencies to assist in mitigation. As payment reform continues to drive toward better management of population health, decreased total expenditures, and improved patient satisfaction with care delivered, the PCMH model will be more fully embraced. Implementing PCMH has potential to improve not only patient satisfaction, but provider satisfaction with care; however, attention will need to be paid to how PCMH can potentially shift workloads for the primary care provider.

**TABLE 8-1 CARE DELIVERY PARADIGM SHIFT**

| Provider-Centered Model: Deficit Based | Patient/Family-Centered Model: Strength Based |
|---|---|
| Control | Collaboration |
| Expert model | Partnership model |
| Information gate keeping | Information sharing |
| No systematic support | Support built into the system |
| Rigidity | Flexibility |
| Dependence | Empowerment |

Data from Brinkman WB, Geraghty SR, Lanphear BP, Khoury JC, Gonzalez del Rey JA, Dewitt TG, Britto MT; Effect of multisource feedback on resident communication skills and professionalism: a randomized controlled trial. *Archives of Pediatrics and Adolescent Medicine.* January 2007; 161(1):44-49

## IMPLEMENTATION OF PATIENT AND FAMILY–CENTERED CARE

Because each practice, clinic, and other healthcare facility has its unique norms and culture, the approach to implement the philosophy of patient and family–centered care must be customized to the environment: there is no one-size-fits-all approach. To ensure sustainability of your patient and family–centered care strategies, a 3-pronged approach is recommended. Strategies must be aimed at the strategic or organizational level, the microsystem or point-of-care level (eg, on the unit, in the clinic), and the individual practitioner level. Short-term gains may be achieved if a specific clinical setting is targeted, but families can become frustrated by variation in care approaches across an organization. Thus, full implementation of a patient and family–centered care approach requires organizational change. Ideas for establishing a culture of patient and family–centered care are presented in Table 8-3.

**Strategic or Organizational Level**

On an organizational level, support from senior leadership is a key component of success. Executive champions should promote a culture change that is solidly built on the principles of patient and family–centered care. This group of leaders sets the tone for the organization by weaving the core concepts of patient and family–centered care throughout the vision and mission statements and strategic plans.

Collaboration is recommended for any point at which families interact with the healthcare system. Such collaboration might mean family involvement in areas as diverse as policy and procedure development, human resources practices, and facilities renovation and design. Standing committees benefit from the perspective that family members bring, and there are many examples where families have helped drive quality improvement initiatives. When working with patients and families in an advisory capacity, consider allocating resources for stipends for family involvement to cover their travel

**TABLE 8-2 MEDICAL HOME PARADIGM SHIFT**

| | Traditional Office/Hospital Practice | Patient-Centered Medical Home (PCMH) |
|---|---|---|
| **Personal Provider/Team** | Visits directed and based on practice preference and schedule accessibility, rather than alignment with patient preferences | An ongoing relationship with a single personal provider and associated team, which is recorded and known to the practice and patient |
| **Comprehensive Care** | Care limited to office, emergent, or hospital events and provided without surveillance for chronic or preventive services, or coordination of end-of-life needs | Addressing the whole person and all the patient's acute, preventive, chronic, and end-of-life healthcare needs |
| **Patient Centered** | Treatment is provider prescribed, with plans and goals provided to the patient without assessment of personal preference or barriers | Treatment plans include items such as language and spiritual preferences, barriers, and patient directed goals |
| **Coordinated Care** | Fractured care with various providers; no single responsible physician leading a team and coordinating care, resulting in redundancy and gaps in care | Care coordinated across the healthcare spectrum to include behavioral health and community resources in the neighborhood |
| **Accessible** | Provider centered with daily schedules kept full for productivity and only access during routine business hours; communication pathways limited and not interconnected | Open access, same-day scheduling, shorter waiting times, afterhour care, alternative communication methods that are often technologically enhanced and integrated |
| **Quality and Safety** | Improvement and safety work occur without time restraints or transparency; usually driven by provider and practice interests | Continuous and sustained work on improvement and safety; patient and family identify and participate in QI priority setting and projects |
| **Payment** | Payment aligned with fees for services provided; little incentive for disease prevention or whole person care | Payment model that moves toward shared savings and value-based reimbursement; aligned with and incentivizes population health measures and disease prevention |

| | Traditional Office/Hospital Practice | Patient-Centered Medical Home (PCMH) |
|---|---|---|
| **Personal Provider/Team** | Visits directed and based on practice preference and schedule accessibility, rather than alignment with patient preferences | An ongoing relationship with a single personal provider and associated team, which is recorded and known to the practice and patient |
| **Comprehensive Care** | Care limited to office, emergent, or hospital events and provided without surveillance for chronic or preventive services, or coordination of end-of-life needs | Addressing the whole person and all the patient's acute, preventive, chronic, and end-of-life healthcare needs |

and childcare costs, which demonstrates respect for their time and commitment.

#### Microsystem or Point-of-Care Level

Strategic patient and family-centered care expectations are operationalized at the microsystem level, whether on a nursing unit or in a clinic. Leaders of the microsystem must embrace the patient and family-centered care philosophy to create a culture where patient and family–centered care can flourish. Unit leaders and staff should partner with families on microsystem-specific initiatives. Systems must be put in place to support staff both during the transition to patient and family–centered care and in coping with challenges as they arise.

Consider inviting family members to staff meetings to tell their stories, highlight an actual family experience demonstrating exemplary patient and family–centered care at monthly staff meetings, and conduct physician and nursing grand rounds. Education must be ongoing because of staff turnover and the need to reinforce positive behaviors.

Measure progress over time from both quantitative and qualitative perspectives. Consider overall measures of patient and family satisfaction with their involvement in care (eg, "Did the staff listen to your concerns about your child?") and specific measures of unit strategies (eg, "Was the adolescent involved in the daily plan of care discussions at the bedside?"). Staff satisfaction should also be considered, as joy in work for staff is increasingly recognized as a critical factor in realizing patient satisfaction. Informal discussions about challenging situations help the staff to understand family behaviors and coping mechanisms during stressful times.

To maintain enthusiasm for patient and family–centered care, celebration of both small and large gains is important. When individual practitioners are observed demonstrating top-notch patient and family–centered care, consider a written award highlighting their practice. Especially meaningful for staff is when family advisors arrive on the unit and distribute a small token of appreciation to them.

#### Individual Practitioner Level

Providers, not the family, are the true "visitors" in the child's life. In general, the healthcare experience is imposed upon families by healthcare providers and their systems, and to a great extent, the family role is regulated by the staff. To change the role of the family, individual practitioners must first change their own approach and role.

Staff must support the family/parental role at the point of care. Parents bring to the care experience their intimate knowledge of the child's responses, cues, and patterns of behavior. Staff must recognize this strength, capitalize on the family's knowledge, and partner with the family in the care of the child. Parental choices for involvement in the child's care need to be explored, supported, and communicated to all caregivers. Parental involvement might range from administering a medication to being present during resuscitation in the emergency department or intensive care unit. On an ongoing basis, families need to have opportunities to share their insights, observations, and questions.

At the individual practitioner level, information that families need and want must be provided or recommended. With a wealth of information at the public's fingertips through the Internet, discussions about value-added information are more important than ever. Individual practitioners must develop a new appreciation of the effort involved when a family hands them a stack of computer printouts on the information they have researched and the plan of care they are proposing. Practitioners should recognize this as the new way of doing business and view it as an opportunity to learn and collaborate, not as a threat to their "authority."

#### Health Provider Education

An important challenge in implementing patient and family–centered care in many healthcare environments is how to train new providers—medical students, residents, nursing students, and other allied health trainees—to deliver care that is patient and family–centered. Part of

**TABLE 8-3 ESTABLISHING A CULTURE OF PATIENT AND FAMILY–CENTERED CARE**

| |
|---|
| **Hospital-wide policies and procedures** |
| Involve families in emergency situations |
| Eliminate the word *visitor* when referring to families |
| Welcome families 24 hours a day to care for and be with their child |
| **Human resources interviewing/job standards** |
| Incorporate behavioral interviewing with a patient and family–centered care focus on human resources and on clinical units |
| Structure position descriptions to reflect staff behaviors surrounding core concepts |
| Evaluate employee performance based on the core concepts of patient and family–centered care |
| **Facilities planning/signage** |
| Provide families with access to resource library |
| Ensure that all written materials express belief that families are partners |
| Present information in correct language and format, including attention to literacy level |
| Provide funds for training family members |
| Invite family and youth involvement in design of programs and facilities |
| **Support for staff** |
| Acknowledge the difficulties/challenges staff may face with increased family engagement in care |
| Share care, then discuss how to move forward |
| **Roles of family leaders** |
| Parent coordinators |
| Hospital ambassadors |
| Committees: patient safety, medication reconciliation, cultural competence, bioethics |
| Signage |
| Billing initiatives |
| Focus groups |
| Interview leadership and staff hires |
| Unit/department-specific initiatives |
| Renovations |
| Strategic plan subgroups |
| New employee orientation |
| Liaison to other families |
| **Families on committees** |
| Get families involved from the beginning |
| Communicate, check in with, and follow up on their ideas |
| Identify common attitudes staff and families have toward making change |
| Imagine what you can learn from each other |

the challenge is in introducing new personnel to the patient and family–centered care philosophy, which may differ from their previous training, while another part is the frequent turnover of new trainees. Many health education credentialing bodies now mandate direct observation and feedback about professionalism and communication skills, and patient and family–centered care skills should be included in these mandates.

The old paradigm in medical education—"see one, do one, teach one"—applies, in part, to learning the principles of patient and family-centered care. Trainees need to observe the approaches used by skilled practitioners in this care setting, be given the chance to demonstrate their evolving skills, and, perhaps most importantly, be given concrete feedback about their skills and performance. In this tradition, Dr. Steven Miller developed a theoretical framework for medical education to make humanism more of a "habit" for trainees. His approach is delineated in Chapter 3, and it applies equally well to teaching principles of patient and family–centered care. To extend the humanism framework to education in patient and family–centered care, trainees must be placed in situations in which they can identify—concretely—a patient's and family's perspective. Teaching is therefore best done at the bedside, where a more experienced provider can demonstrate how to identify the family's perspective. Then, trainees must be asked to reflect on and identify potential conflicts between their own and the patient's or the family's perspectives. Trainees need to be regularly engaged in this conversation using concrete examples from their daily work. Finally, education within an environment focused on patient and family–centered care requires a universal expectation that all staff and trainees act in accordance with these principles of care. Behaviors that are patient and family centered become normative, and both informal and formal evaluation and feedback take these behaviors into account.

Multiple practical methods of teaching principles of patient and family–centered care have been described. Family, faculty, parents, and caregivers of children with chronic medical needs can be utilized in a variety of instructional methods: as lecturers, small group discussion leaders, participants in role plays, and hosts of home visits. Their participation in multidisciplinary bedside hospital rounds (often called family-centered rounds) also facilitates learning of patient and family–centered care principles, as do bedside nursing change-of-shift handoffs. Both techniques blend previously separated functions of teaching and working to create a care environment in which the patient and family are the center of and are included in conversations about both care and teaching.

A curriculum to introduce learners to the core principles of patient and family–centered care is a worthy undertaking. A powerful adjunct to, and perhaps replacement of, typical lectures or question-and-answer sessions is the use of anecdotes to illustrate patient and family–centered principles. Ideally, these stories come from day-to-day experiences within the care environment and are shared during the course of regularly scheduled educational sessions to allow for interaction between audience and storyteller.

Finally, patients and families should be included in the learner evaluation process. Incorporating patient and family evaluations into formal evaluation and feedback processes provides perspective beyond that gained by direct observation by instructors and can lead to improved overall skill and performance.

## SUGGESTED READINGS


About Us. Patient-Centered Primary Care Collaborative. https://www.pcpcc.org/about. Accessed September 7, 2016.

Brinkman WB, Geraghty SR, Lanphear BP, et al. Effect of multisource feedback on resident communication skills and professionalism: a randomized controlled trial. *Arch Pediatr Adolesc Med.* 2007;161(1):44-49.

Clarke R, Bharmal N, Di Capua P, et al. Innovative approach to patient-centered care coordination in primary care practices. *Am J Manag Care.* 2015;21(9):623-630.

Coller RJ, Kiltzner TS, Saenz AA, Lerner CF, Nelson BB, Chung PJ. The medical home and hospital readmissions. *Pediatrics.* 2015;136(6):e1550-e1560.

Institute for Patient- and Family-Centered Care. http://www.ipfcc.org/. Accessed September 7, 2016.

Jackson GL, Powers BJ, Chatterjee R, et al. Improvingpatient care: the patient centered medical home:asystematic review. *Ann Intern Med.* 2013;158(3):169-178.

Johnson AM, Yoder J, Richardson-Nassif K. Using families as faculty in teaching medical students family-centered care: What are students learning? *Teach Learn Med.* 2006;18(3):222-225.

Miller SZ, Schmidt HJ. The habit of humanism: a framework for making humanistic care a reflexive clinical skill. *Acad Med.* 1999;74(7):800-803.

Muething SE, Kotagal UR, Schoettker PJ, Gonzalez del Rey J, DeWitt TG. Family-centered bedside rounds: a new approach to patient care and teaching. *Pediatrics.* 2007;119(4):829-832.

National Committee for Quality Assurance. http://www.ncqa.org/HomePage.aspx. Accessed September 7, 2016.

Rosenthal MB, Sinaiko AD, Eastman D, et al. Impact of the Rochester Medical Home Initiative on primary care practices, quality, utilization, and costs. *Med Care.* 2015;53(11):967-973.

Stewart M, Brown JB, Weston WW, McWhinney IR, McWilliam CL, Freeman TR. *Patient-Centered Medicine: Transforming the Clinical Method.* 3rd ed. London, UK: Radcliffe Publishing Ltd; 2014.

# 9 Systems of Practice and Office Management

Peter Margolis and Eric Williams

## SYSTEMS-BASED PRACTICE AND QUALITY OF CARE

Better design and organization of healthcare service is a priority for healthcare systems because of ongoing gaps in the outcomes of care, changes in the nature of morbidity, rapid changes in technology and new payment models, and the explosive growth of new knowledge. Ongoing redesign of systems of care delivery will be required to keep pace with these changes. The Institute of Medicine (IOM) proposed a set of 6 expectations that high-performing health care should achieve—safety, effectiveness, patient-centeredness, timeliness, efficiency, and equity—and described steps to promote more evidence-based practice. More recently, the IOM proposed a vision for Learning Health Systems in which patients and clinicians base decisions on evidence and discovery is a natural outgrowth of care.

Pediatricians want to provide the best care they can for their patients. Extensive research indicates that much of the quality of care achieved is determined by the specific *processes* or *systems* of care delivery in place in the practice. For example, addressing psychosocial morbidities, managing the growing prevalence of children with chronic illness, the complexity of immunization schedules, and using electronic medical record systems effectively requires ongoing efforts to adopt new approaches, tools, and linkages to accomplish many of the things that cannot be done in the office. Thus, processes for care delivery cannot remain static. They must evolve over time as patients' needs and patterns of illness change and new discoveries emerge.

Multiple studies have documented the long interval between healthcare innovation and use in practice. Traditional methods of translating research findings into practice, such as peer-reviewed publications and continuing medical education, are passive and slow, and the passive provision of information is rarely effective in helping busy clinicians adapt new knowledge to practice. However, change is possible. Sinsky et al reported on the changes made by 23 primary care practices to become high-functioning teams with improved professional satisfaction.

All healthcare domains have systems and processes to organize the work of caring for patients. Practice systems often develop on a somewhat ad hoc basis to address specific issues or problems. More contemporary approaches create practice-based systems that are linked directly to improving the IOM's 6 dimensions of quality. A partnership between the IOM and the National Academy of Engineering highlighted underutilized methodologies from systems engineering that could be applied to optimizing delivery of health care. A practical approach for organizing care is to institute processes to manage the most common types of conditions encountered. This chapter highlights major practice systems for four key areas of care (prevention, acute care, chronic care, and access and efficiency). The evidence-based resources cited can be adapted to support efforts in all types of care delivery settings to optimize patients' health outcomes.

### What Is a System?

A system is a "set of interrelated processes carried out by multiple individuals to achieve a purpose." A primary practice, a specialty clinic, or a unit in a hospital can be thought of as a small, organized group of clinicians and staff working together with a shared clinical purpose to provide care for a defined set of patients. Many practices are part of a larger organization and are embedded in a legal, financial, social, and regulatory environment. Note that the term *system* does not necessarily involve an elaborate operational structure. Well-engineered systems often outline how specific tasks are accomplished and who is responsible to ensure that the necessary tools and training are available to support responsible individuals. Healthcare engineering has recently been suggested to not only encompass design in healthcare interventions and treatments, but more importantly, to provide design for the delivery of health care, including logistics, information systems, and networks.



## OFFICE SYSTEMS TO SUPPORT CLINICAL CARE

### Prevention

Preventive care is the most frequent reason for pediatric office visits, accounting for 29% of visits by all children and young adults 21 years of age and younger, and 52% of all visits by infants. The scope of well-child care is very broad, and the number of potential topics to be covered during preventive care visits far exceeds the average 20 minutes that are typically available. Therefore, effective delivery of preventive care depends on tailoring the visit to closely meet families' needs. Evidence shows that the use of structured tools to elicit parents' concerns, the identification of psychosocial risk factors, anticipatory guidance about developmental concerns, and problem-focused counseling about behavior and development are efficacious in tailoring care to families' needs. There is accumulating evidence that implementing these approaches through specific practice-based systems that support preventive care make it possible to meet parents' needs and improve the quality of care.

Table 9-1 lists specific processes that can be implemented to achieve the goals of providing needed anticipatory guidance; addressing parents' concerns about their child's learning, development, and behavior; identifying children at risk; providing a strong and streamlined link to community resources for families who need or want them; and promoting optimal parent-child relationships. These changes emphasize several key points. First, establishing officewide guidelines or standards about the timing and content of preventive care enables practices to adopt tools, such as preventive services summaries and structured developmental assessment instruments, which can be implemented by staff other than the physician. Second, previsit planning reduces total visit time and helps to focus the content of the visit on identified risks and concerns. Third, the content and duration of preventive care visits should be based on the unique needs of the child and family. Higher-risk/higher-need families should receive more targeted screening and a substantially greater amount of information in anticipation of normal developmental transitions and in response to identified risks and problems. Such families are likely to need more services from other service providers in the community, which will require more clinician and office staff time to integrate and coordinate care. In summary, these changes promote tiered or risk-based care that is more individualized, more appropriate, and more effective. Additional resources for improving preventive care are provided at the following Web sites: http://www.commonwealthfund.org/, http://www.ahrq.gov/professionals/prevention-chronic-care/resources/index.html, and http://www.ihi.org/resources/Pages/Tools/ResourcesforPublicHealth.aspx.

### Chronic Illness Care

Wagner's chronic illness care model (Fig. 9-1) provides a useful, evidence-based framework for organizing changes to the system of chronic illness care that result in improved outcomes for patients. The model includes clinical information systems, delivery-system design, decision support, and patient and family self-management support. The *clinical information system* enables caregivers to access data and use registries for care and to provide regular feedback; this information technology also facilitates scheduling and patient tracking. The *delivery-system design* component comprises the use of planned

**TABLE 9-1 OFFICE SYSTEMS TO SUPPORT PREVENTIVE SERVICES DELIVERY**

| |
|---|
| **Use Officewide Care Protocols and Visit-Planning Tools and Processes** |
| Develop practicewide guidelines for the provision and documentation of preventive services and anticipatory guidance and parent education (AGPE) |
| Utilize standardized, structured tools to encourage parents to consider their informational needs prior to the visit (eg, Parental Evaluation of Developmental Status, and Ages and Stages questionnaire) to screen for developmental delay and/or to elicit parent concerns |
| Use structured tools to conduct psychosocial screening for maternal depression, substance abuse, and domestic violence to identify children at risk |
| Configure the electronic health record to identify what preventive services and age-appropriate anticipatory guidance has been offered, and provide decision alerts |
| Organize, make accessible, and provide patient education materials that are consistent with practice guidelines |
| Review and update guidelines for the provision and documentation of preventive services and AGPE annually |
| **Provide Team-Based Care** |
| Train office staff to use the preventive services summary to identify and prompt clinicians about needed preventive services |
| Prioritize family needs before the visit |
| Use medical record screening and prompting tools at well-child *and* non–well-child visits |
| **Develop Relationships with Community Resources to Meet the Needs of Young Children** |
| Organize and make accessible a list of the most commonly used community resources |
| Identify and train a staff person to regularly update the community resources list |
| Identify and utilize (if available) a community clearinghouse (eg, resource and referral line) for needed community referrals |
| Establish a relationship with personnel at organizations serving your practice population |
| Create or adapt standardized referral forms within your practice for sending information to and requesting information from community agencies |
| **Use a Reminder/Recall System and Immunization Registry, and Measure Performance Regularly** |
| Use an immunization registry to assess immunization status at every visit and measure coverage monthly |
| Utilize a recall system to identify children who have missed well-child appointments, and follow up on referrals to community agencies |
| Use the registry and/or parent surveys to measure provision and delivery of preventive services and AGPE regularly |

encounters, clarity in the roles and responsibilities of team members, appropriate training of team members, and the use of regular meetings of the care team to review performance. *Decision support* means access to evidence-based information and the use of care protocols that are integrated into the practice systems. Family and patient *self-management support* refers to the methods used by the clinical practice to increase families' confidence and skills to effectively manage chronic illness at home on a daily basis.

The specific changes practices can make to promote better chronic illness care are in many respects similar to those described for preventive care. A registry is a powerful tool that enables staff other than the physician to identify patients with chronic illnesses and implement needed care. Registries can also serve as a tool for implementing a recall system by enabling the practice to identify which patients have not returned at appropriate intervals. Implementation of a population registry requires adoption of practicewide guidelines and standards. Agreement about which services to provide and when to provide them enables staff to take responsibility for core elements of care delivery. Care protocols also minimize the risk that patient needs are overlooked. Once a practice decides on a guideline for care, protocols can be developed to identify the role of the care team in distributing the work of undertaking chronic care. Agreement on guidelines also supports the concept of stratifying care on the basis of severity of illness so that resources for care management can be more effectively deployed. Once these basic changes have been accomplished, practices can concentrate more effort on selecting appropriate educational materials and promoting patients' and families' ability to manage their own disease (eg, through motivational interviewing). More detailed information about tools and strategies to support chronic illness care are available at the following Web sites: http://www.improvingchroniccare.org, http://www.acponline.org/clinical_information/guidelines, http://www.aafp.org/online/en/home.html, https://www.aap.org/en-us/professional-resources/practice-support/Pages/Chronic-Condition-Management-Resources.aspx, http://shop.aap.org/Caring-for-Children-with-ADHD-A-Resource-Toolkit-for-Clinicians, and https://eqipp.aap.org/.

### Acute Care

The core processes for supporting acute care are in many ways similar to those required to achieve effective preventive and chronic care. Developing processes for the management of the most common acute problems, such as otitis media, pharyngitis, fever, gastroenteritis, and asthma, enables practices to provide more consistent and reliable care.

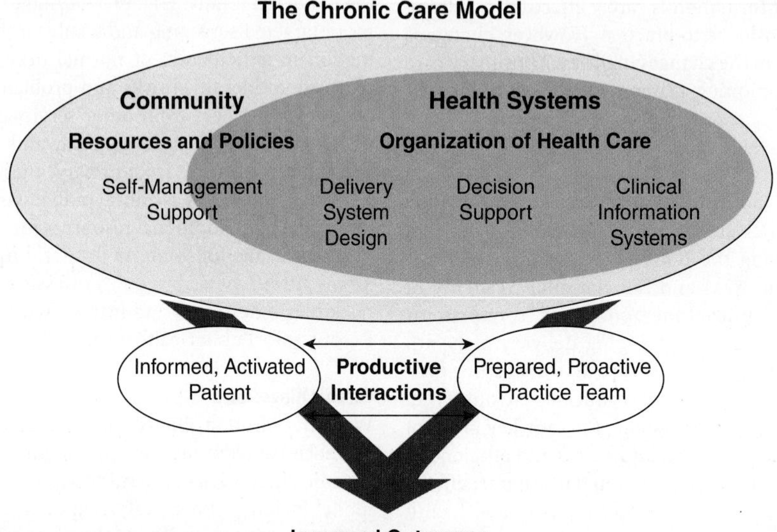


**FIGURE 9-1** The chronic care model. (Adapted with permission from Wagner EH: Chronic Disease Management: What Will It Take to Improve Care for Chronic Illness? *Effective Clinical Practice* 1998; Aug-Sep;1(1):2-4.)

Clinical practice guidelines are now readily accessible for many of these conditions. Guidelines can provide a much-needed interface between evidence and practice. By distilling relevant clinical research and making it readily available, guidelines can point the way to higher-quality, evidence-based, and more cost-effective care. Many guideline recommendations are embedded in companion documents and processes to promote easy access to the best evidence at the point of care. These tools may include a clinical pathway, standing order sets, a parent edition of the guideline, an education record, and discharge goals and instructions for patients.

#### Access and Efficiency

Managing the flow of operations remains the mainstay of applied industrial engineering principles, and the need in health care is to change the delivery system from provider centric to patient centric. Modern approaches to scheduling and management of office flow make it possible to create processes that provide patients the opportunity to see their own physician when they choose. To improve office flow, a practice must manage its total resources (supply) to provide care. When the resources are managed well, openness or space in the clinic (capacity) is created. In an optimal system, a practice provides enough capacity for health services to meet the demands of its patient population *at the time* the demand occurs. This is a fundamental shift from the complex scheduling systems and wide variety of appointment types and lengths that resulted in long waits to see clinicians.

Systems known as *open* or *advanced* access take advantage of practices' ability to predict demand and respond to it effectively. Although many pediatric practices allow same-day appointments for acute care visits, these newer approaches expand same-day access to include routine and preventive care. This model is based on the principle that when supply and demand are in balance (or equilibrium), there is no need for waits in the system. Evidence is emerging that such systems result in higher continuity of patients with their own physician, resulting in improvements in outcomes of preventive and chronic illness care.

Strategies for creating a system for advanced access involve 3 main principles: (1) reducing the amount of demand, making it easier for the system to absorb current or future levels of demand by maximizing activity at appointments and increasing the interval between appointments; (2) redesigning the system to increase supply by making the clinic more efficient; and (3) matching supply with demand through effective use of appointment data. A more detailed list of changes is given in Table 9-2. In addition, the Institute of Industrial and Systems Engineers provides resources for healthcare entities to better understand the impact of ergonomics, information systems, and operations research on work in a socio-technical system. See http://www.iienet2.org.

#### Leadership, Planning, and Practice Infrastructure

Managing the types of changes required to provide effective clinical operations depends on effective leadership and support systems to create an ongoing emphasis on the continual improvement of the practice system. Many resources are available through the American Academy of Pediatrics and other practice management organizations to enable practices to develop and implement approaches to financial management, human resources management, and information systems. As a general principle of system development and continual improvement, it is advisable to introduce changes in a single area of the clinical setting to gain experience and achieve improved results before implementing changes to the next area. This incremental approach minimizes the risk of disrupting the practice and promotes confidence that change can be made without compromising care delivery during transition. It is also important to remember that health care is not a product manufactured by the healthcare system, but a service that is co-created by patients and health professionals.

**TABLE 9-2 PRINCIPLES OF ADVANCED ACCESS**

| Principle | Examples |
|---|---|
| Balance appointment supply with patient demand | Predict appointment supply by accounting for holidays, vacations, and nonclinical work |
| | Predict patient demand for appointments by collecting appointment data |
| Work down the backlog (waiting list) | Distinguish between "good" (planned care) and "bad" (delayed care) backlog |
| | Measure the extent of the backlog and make a plan for reducing it, including a start and end date |
| Reduce appointment types | Reduce number of appointment types (new preventive, established brief, acute, etc) |
| | Standardize appointment lengths (eg, consider 20-minute appointments for all visits) |
| Plan for contingencies | Increase capacity at peak times |
| | Plan for predictable seasonal increases in appointment demand |
| Reduce future patient demand | Maximize activity at appointments to reduce future demand |
| | Extend intervals for return appointments |
| Manage the bottlenecks | Identify bottlenecks in clinic flow |
| | Drive unnecessary work away from the bottlenecks |
| Synchronize patient, provider, and information | First morning and afternoon appointments start on time |
| | Patient registration done by phone if confirming patient appointment |
| Predict and anticipate patient needs at the time of the appointment | Use regular "huddles" to anticipate and plan for contingencies in schedule |
| | Use notepads, whiteboards, flag systems, and so on, to communicate during the day |
| Optimize rooms and equipment | Use "open rooming" to maximize flexibility |
| | Standardize supplies in all rooms, and keep stocked at all times |
| Use continuous flow strategies | Do this moment's work now (eg, dictate immediately after visits) |
| | Use scheduled pauses to apply continuous flow approach to nonappointment activities (eg, returning phone calls) |

## SUGGESTED READINGS


Balas E, Boren S. *Managing Clinical Knowledge for Health Care Improvement*. Stuttgart, Germany: Schattauer Verlagsgesellschaft; 2000.

Batalden M, Batalden P, Margolis P, et al. Coproduction of healthcare service. *BMJ Qual Saf*. 2016;25(7):509-517.

Bero L, Grilli R, Grimshaw J, Harvey E, Oxman A, Thompson M. Closing the gap between research and practice: an overview of systematic reviews of intervention to promote the implementation of research findings. The Cochrane Effective Practice and Organization of Care Review Group. *BMJ*. 1998;317(7156):465-468.

Bloom B. Effects of continuing medical education on improving physician clinical care and patient health: a review of systematic reviews. *Int J Technol Assess Health Care*. 2005;21(3):380-385.

Cabana M, Rand C, Powe N, et al. Why don't physicians follow clinical practice guidelines? A framework for improvement. *JAMA*. 1999;282(15):1458-1465.

Grol R, Grimshaw J. From best evidence to best practice: effective implementation of change in patients' care. *Lancet*. 2003;362: 1225-1230.

Haines A, Jones R. Implementing findings of research. *BMJ*. 1994;308: 1488-1492.

Healthy Steps for Young Children. http://healthysteps.org/. Accessed June 8, 2016.

National Center for Medical Legal Partnership. http://medical-legalpartnership.org/. Accessed June 8, 2016.

Reach Out and Read. http://www.reachoutandread.org/. Accessed June 8, 2016.

Rogers E. *Diffusion of Innovations*. 4th ed. New York, NY: Free Press; 1995.



# 10 Environmental Pediatrics

Ruth A. Etzel

## INTRODUCTION

It is only in the last 50 years that diseases linked to environmental contamination have been recognized in pediatrics. Most environmental exposures now understood to be harmful to children were initially identified as a result of acute epidemics of illness affecting groups of people. For example, polluted outdoor air was not well understood to be unhealthy until the Great Smog of 1952 in London. An estimated 4000 people died from exposures to the very heavy air pollution; deaths were unusually high among the very young and the elderly. This led to the development of the first laws to regulate air pollution. Mercury was not understood to be harmful until an epidemic of cerebral palsy occurred among infants living near Minamata Bay, Japan, in the 1950s (called Minamata disease). Between 1959 and 1972 in Iraq, seed grain treated with a mercury fungicide was accidentally eaten by humans instead of being planted in the fields, and thousands of Iraqi people developed mercury poisoning.

The harmful effects of polychlorinated biphenyls (PCBs) came to light in 1968 when an epidemic of acne occurred among people in Japan; the disease was traced to the use of cooking oil inadvertently mixed with PCBs. About 2000 Japanese people exposed to the oil were diagnosed with *Yusho* (oil disease). Dioxin's health effects were not well known until 1975 when a chemical plant explosion in Seveso, Italy, released large amounts of dioxin, and children in the area near the explosion developed chloracne, especially on areas of the body unprotected by clothing. Drinking water contamination became well recognized in 1986 when a cluster of childhood leukemia was uncovered in Woburn, Massachusetts, and was epidemiologically linked to drinking water supplied from 2 municipal wells contaminated with seepage of the animal carcinogens trichloroethylene, tetrachloroethylene, and chloroform from area chemical disposal pits that had been in use for several decades. Natural toxins began being recognized as potentially important indoor contaminants when, in 1994, a cluster of cases of acute pulmonary hemorrhage among infants was linked to inhalation exposures to natural toxins produced by molds that grow in chronically water-damaged environments.

One of the most important themes that emerged from these acute epidemics of environmental diseases was that, unlike some other specialty areas of pediatrics, in environmental pediatrics, treatment of the individual patient is not sufficient; it is critical to identify and eliminate the sources of exposure so that disease does not recur in the known patients and so that additional cases do not occur.

### Diagnosing Environment-Related Illness

Most signs and symptoms of illnesses linked to environmental contaminants are nonspecific and may occur only in association with fairly high-level exposures. The signs and symptoms of high-level, acute poisoning are relatively well characterized for most chemicals. In contrast, the effects of low-level, chronic, and mixed exposures are poorly studied, particularly in infants and children. Establishing the environmental cause of a given illness is further complicated by the similarity of pollutant effects to those of other diseases. For example, a respiratory illness from an environmental pollutant may closely resemble an allergy or a respiratory infection. Diagnosis of an environmental disease requires a high index of suspicion and a thorough environmental history. Although clinicians cannot assess the causal association between pollutant exposures and health effects, they should consider environmental causes of disease when children's illnesses do not follow usual expected patterns.

A comprehensive intake of a new patient and ongoing anticipatory guidance should include an assessment of possible environmental risks to the child in the home environment. This includes discussion of the age and condition of the residence, source of drinking water, and potential access or exposure to toxins in the home environment or parental workplace. Anticipatory guidance differs by the age of the child because environmental risks differ by age. When the baby is 2 months old, the clinician should ask about nitrate in drinking water, smoking, and water damage and mold growth in the home. At 6 months, clinicians should ask about lead in the home. When the child reaches school age, the pediatrician should ask questions about radon, mercury, carbon monoxide, ultraviolet light, and pesticides. Families should be advised to prevent excessive exposure to contaminants and their possible adverse effects.

Commonly-encountered environmental toxins and pollutants are described individually in this chapter. Discussions of specific toxins and management of exposures are also found in Chapter 114.

## CARBON MONOXIDE

Carbon monoxide (CO) is an odorless gas produced by incomplete combustion of carbon-containing material. Common sources of exposure include house fires, automobile exhaust, and improperly ventilated water heaters, stoves, furnaces, fireplaces, and space heaters. Inhalation of CO is the leading cause of poisoning death in the United States. The diagnosis of CO poisoning is readily suspected in the patient found unconscious in a house fire or running automobile. However, the diagnosis is difficult when the patient presents with nonspecific symptoms after an unrecognized exposure. Mild to moderate exposures present with malaise, nausea, vomiting, dyspnea, headache, dizziness, and confusion. Such patients are often misdiagnosed with influenza or gastroenteritis. Severe poisoning is characterized by syncope, seizures, coma, cardiorespiratory depression, and death. Diagnosis and treatment of CO exposure is discussed in detail in Chapter 114.

## LEAD

The major source of lead exposure among children in the United States is ingestion of lead-containing paint chips or lead-contaminated dust or dirt by hand-to-mouth activity. Although lead-based paint was banned in 1978 for use in homes, as many as three quarters of dwellings built before 1980 have lead-containing paint on their interior surfaces. Lead paint on interior and exterior window components becomes abraded into dust by repetitive opening and closing of the window. Lead poisoning also may result from use of certain herbal remedies, traditional cosmetics, imported spices, and ceramic cooking utensils. Lead poisoning has been caused by drinking water contaminated from lead pipes used in some older municipalities, and solder in home plumbing. Inhalation of lead-containing air may occur in children living in the vicinity of lead smelting and automobile battery plants and from clothing brought into the home by family members working in lead-related industries. Fishing weights, stained glass, or ceramics may also lead to exposure. Gasoline containing tetraethyl lead, used to prevent engine "knocking," was extensively used in the United States until the early 1980s and contributed to an increased concentration of lead in the soil.

Lead serves no physiologic function. Ingested material containing lead is solubilized by gastric hydrochloric acid and then absorbed primarily in the upper gastrointestinal tract. Although adults absorb about 10% of ingested lead, children absorb as much as 50%. Absorption may be increased further by deficiencies of iron and other trace metals, malnutrition, and increased fat in the diet. About 70% to 90% of absorbed lead is deposited in the bones and about

5% is present in the red blood cells and their precursors in the bone marrow. Lead is very slowly excreted from the body, primarily in the urine, and its biological half-life has been estimated to be more than 15 years. The toxic effects of lead are primarily related to its binding to sulfhydryl ligands, leading to inhibition of a large number of enzymes. Lead toxicity is a function of the level of lead in the blood and tissues as well as the duration of exposure. In the red blood cell precursors, lead interferes with several steps in the heme synthetic pathway, which leads to an increased level of heme precursors, free erythrocyte protoporphyrin, and zinc protoporphyrin in the mature red blood cells. At higher levels, lead reduces iron utilization, resulting in anemia.

In the immature, developing brain, even moderate elevations of lead are associated with neurobehavioral abnormalities and decreased intelligence quotients, which appear to be permanent. Lead can cause neuronal demyelinization, decreased numbers of neurons, decreased neuronal growth, interference with neuronal transmission, and sensorineural hearing loss that may result in significant delays in the acquisition of language and difficulty in auditory processing. At very high levels, lead can cause encephalopathy and cerebral edema, resulting in death or severe neurologic damage in survivors. Peripheral neuropathy and nephropathy that occur in lead-poisoned adults are unusual in children.

The magnitude of body lead is indicated by the blood lead level (BLL), and laboratory assessment is based primarily on blood levels determined by atomic absorption analysis. Blood lead concentrations can be measured in capillary blood, but abnormal findings should be confirmed using venous blood because finger-stick capillary blood can be contaminated by trace amounts of lead-containing dust on the skin.

The Centers for Disease Control and Prevention uses a reference level of 5 μg/dL to identify children with BLLs that indicate an elevated source of exposure in the child's environment. This is based on the 97.5th percentile of blood lead distribution in US children aged 1 to 5 years old in the National Health and Nutrition Examination Survey. This level does not, however, define a threshold for the harmful effects of lead. The development of a child's nervous system can be affected at BLLs of less than 5 μg/dL.

Symptoms that may be associated with lead poisoning are relatively nonspecific and include gastrointestinal complaints such as anorexia, constipation, abdominal pain, and vomiting. Signs and symptoms suggestive of central nervous system involvement include irritability, lethargy, changes in sleep pattern, and alterations in behavior and coordination. Seizures, hypertension, coma, and signs of increased cranial pressure are indicative of lead encephalopathy, which is usually associated with blood levels higher than 70 μg/dL.

In all exposed children, a health department inspection should be conducted to ascertain possible sources of lead in the home. Until this is possible, the child should be relocated to a known lead-free environment. If home therapy is being considered, a health department inspection should be done prior to starting treatment. A randomized controlled trial indicated that chelation therapy for children with BLLs between 25 and 45 μg/dL did not have a beneficial effect on chronic neuropsychological abnormalities; therefore, chelation therapy is usually reserved for children with a BLL higher than 45 μg/dL. However, medical evaluation, repeated testing, nutritional intervention to increase iron and calcium intake and decrease fat consumption, treatment of iron deficiency anemia, and investigation of the source of lead exposure are indicated.

## MERCURY

Mercury has been used for more than 3000 years in medicine and industry. Mercury occurs in three forms: the metallic element (quicksilver or elemental mercury), inorganic salts (mercurous or mercuric salts), and organic compounds (methylmercury, ethylmercury, and phenylmercury). Solubility, reactivity, biological effects, and toxicity vary among these forms.

Elemental mercury has been used in thermometers, sphygmomanometers, and thermostat switches. Dental amalgams contain mercury, silver, and other metals. Fluorescent light bulbs (usually 2- to 4-foot tubes) and disk ("button") batteries also contain mercury. Elemental mercury also is used in some folk remedies.

Elemental mercury is a liquid at room temperature and readily volatilizes to a colorless and odorless vapor. When inhaled, it easily passes through pulmonary alveolar membranes and distributes into red blood cells and the central nervous system. Less than 0.1% is absorbed after ingestion, and only minimal absorption occurs through the skin.

Inhalation of high concentrations of mercury vapor can cause a fatal acute necrotizing bronchitis and pneumonitis. Fatalities have resulted from heating elemental mercury in inadequately ventilated areas.

Children may present with rash, vomiting, muscle pain, and tachycardia. Clinicians may miss the diagnosis unless they ask the child about mercury exposures.

Long-term exposure to mercury vapor primarily affects the central nervous system. Early signs include insomnia, forgetfulness, loss of appetite, and mild tremor. These symptoms may be misdiagnosed as a psychiatric illness. Continued exposure results in progressive tremor and erethism, characterized by red palms, emotional lability, and memory impairment. Salivation, excessive sweating, and hemoconcentration may follow.

Although dental amalgams are a source of mercury exposure and are associated with slightly higher urinary mercury excretion, amalgams should not be replaced merely to reduce mercury exposure. Increased mercury vapor concentrations can be measured in exhaled air from persons with dental amalgams, but the biological significance is uncertain. Also unclear is the significance of the slight increase in urinary mercury excretion detected after dental amalgams are placed.

### Inorganic Mercury

Acrodynia, or childhood mercury poisoning, was frequently reported in the 1940s among infants exposed to calomel teething powders containing mercurous chloride. Acrodynia has developed in infants exposed to phenylmercury used as a fungicidal diaper rinse and in children exposed to phenylmercuric acetate from interior latex paint.

Inorganic mercury exposure is measured by urinary mercury determination, preferably using a 24-hour urine collection. Results greater than 10 to 20 μg/L are evidence of excessive exposure, and neurologic signs may be present at values greater than 100 μg/L. However, the urinary mercury concentration does not necessarily correlate with chronicity or severity of toxic effects, especially if the mercury exposure has been intermittent or variable in intensity. Whole blood mercury can be measured acutely, but values tend to return to normal (< 0.5–1.0 μg/dL) within 1 to 2 days after the end of the exposure to metallic mercury vapor. In a representative sample of the US population, the geometric mean blood mercury levels were 0.3 μg/L for children 1 to 5 years old and 1.2 μg/L for women 16 to 49 years old.

Mercury accumulates in blood and in central nervous system and renal tissues and is very slowly eliminated. Chelating agents have been used to enhance mercury elimination, but it is not known whether chelation reduces toxic effects or speeds recovery in persons who have been poisoned. Mercury poisoning should be treated in consultation with a physician experienced in managing children with mercury poisoning.

### Organic Mercury

Unlike inorganic mercury, organic mercury compounds are lipid soluble and essentially 100% absorbed after ingestion. Ethylmercury is found in thimerosal, an antiseptic and preservative for vaccines and other drug therapies. Thimerosal contains 49.6% mercury by weight. Before the fall of 1999, there was 12.5 to 25 μg of mercury in each dose of most diphtheria and tetanus toxoids, hepatitis B, acellular pertussis, *Haemophilus influenzae* type B, influenza, meningococcal, pneumococcal, and rabies vaccines. In 1999, recognizing the potential for excessive exposure, the American Academy of Pediatrics, along with the American Academy of Family Physicians, the Advisory Committee on Immunization Practices, and the US Public Health Service, issued a joint recommendation that thimerosal be removed from vaccines as quickly as possible. Currently, all routinely recommended vaccines manufactured for administration to infants in the United States are available in thimerosal-free formulation.

Organic mercury toxicity affects the central nervous system. Signs progress from paresthesia to ataxia, followed by generalized weakness, visual and hearing impairment, tremor and muscle spasticity, and then coma and death. Organic mercury also is teratogenic, causing disruption of the normal patterns of neuronal migration and nerve cell histology in the developing brain. In the Minamata Bay disaster and the Iraq epidemic, mothers who were asymptomatic or showed mild toxic effects gave birth to severely affected infants. The infants seemed normal at birth, but psychomotor retardation, blindness, deafness, and seizures developed over time.

A reference dose is a dosage of a chemical that has been determined to be safe on the basis of available toxicity information, which is used to provide a basis for establishing safety standards and guidelines. The National Academy of Sciences, after reviewing methylmercury toxicity, determined that the reference dose for mercury, based on the development of neurobehavioral toxicity, should be established at 0.1 μg/kg/d.

Ethylmercury has been less well studied than methylmercury. Very high exposures to thimerosal-containing products have resulted in toxicity.

The effects of low-dose exposure are not known. There has been recent concern that organic mercury exposure from thimerosal-containing vaccines and other sources has played a role in the increased incidence of autism. The National Academy of Sciences reviewed this issue and determined that there is insufficient scientific evidence for a causal relationship.

Organic mercury compounds concentrate in red blood cells, so whole blood may be used to diagnose excessive exposure. Blood mercury levels rarely exceed more than 1.5 μg/dL in the unexposed population, and a blood concentration of 5 μg/dL or greater is considered the threshold for symptoms of toxicity. Methylmercury also distributes into growing hair, thus providing a noninvasive means to estimate body burden and blood concentration over time. In the general population, the mercury level in hair is usually 1 ppm or less. There is no chelation agent approved by the US Food and Drug Administration (FDA) that is effective for methylmercury poisoning, although succimer has been used for the treatment of severe organic mercury poisoning.

Children who have had mercury poisoning should undergo periodic follow-up neurologic examinations by a pediatrician.

The Environmental Protection Agency has established a guideline for maximum exposure to mercury at 0.1 μg/kg/d. The FDA and most states advise that pregnant women, young children, and women of childbearing age should not eat fish with mercury levels greater than 0.5 ppm. Most state health agencies advise limiting intake of freshwater fish having greater than 0.2 ppm of mercury, and the FDA advises that people at higher risk eat no more than 12 oz of fish a week, on average. Other states simply recommend that women and children not eat any large predator fish that tend to concentrate mercury. The levels of mercury in commercial fish and shellfish are reported at http://www.fda.gov/food/foodborneillnesscontaminants/metals/ucm115644.htm.

In the United States, state specific recommendations for consumption of sport fish are available on the Environmental Protection Agency Web site noted above. The level of mercury in canned tuna differs by the type of tuna. Albacore tuna contains about 3 times more mercury than light tuna.

Although the levels of mercury in commercial fish are regulated by the FDA, the federal government does not regulate the levels of mercury in fish caught for sport. Because of the potential for mercury contamination, many states have issued advisories recommending that the public limit or avoid consumption of certain fish caught for sport from specific bodies of water. In some areas of the United States, certain freshwater species (eg, walleye, pike, muskie, and bass) have levels of mercury that, if consumed, would result in substantial mercury intakes. Most state health agencies advise limiting intake of freshwater sport fish having mercury concentrations of more than 0.2 to 1 ppm. Current state fish consumption advisories can be found on the Environmental Protection Agency Web site (http://www.epa.gov/OST/fish/).

## NITRATES AND NITRITES IN WATER

High nitrate levels in water can have adverse health effects. Nitrate and other nutrients have been linked to blue-green algal blooms, which can produce toxic bacteria. Methemoglobinemia in infants may be caused by ingestion of water contaminated with nitrate that is converted to nitrite by intestinal bacteria, which then oxidizes fetal hemoglobin to methemoglobin. Infants younger than 4 months of age who are fed formula reconstituted with nitrate-containing well water are at the greatest risk.

Evaluation and treatment of methemoglobinemia is discussed in Chapter 114. It is critical to identify and eliminate the exposure source prior to discharge. Reconstitution of formula with well water is generally not recommended and, if used, well water should be tested.

*N*-nitroso compounds are some of the strongest known carcinogens and induce cancer in a variety of organs in more than 40 animal species, including higher primates. Exposures to nitrate in drinking water may be associated with increased risks of non-Hodgkin lymphoma, gastric cancer, bladder cancer, hyperthyroidism, and insulin dependent diabetes.

## PESTICIDES

Pesticides are widely available consumer products. Many aerosol products marketed for use in the home, sometimes called "over-the-counter bug bombs," contain insecticides. Insecticides for garden and agricultural uses have a higher potential for toxicity because they are intrinsically more toxic and more concentrated. Acute organophosphate and carbamate toxicity diagnosis and management are discussed in Chapter 114.

Long-term effects of low-level exposures to pesticides have been documented. Organophosphate exposure has been linked to neurodevelopmental delays. Epidemiologic studies demonstrate associations between pesticide exposures and certain childhood cancers, including leukemia, all brain cancers, and non-Hodgkin lymphoma. A comprehensive review of studies showing an association between pesticides and childhood leukemia revealed higher risks among children whose parents were exposed to pesticides at work or who used pesticides in the home or garden. Several studies have linked home use of pesticides with childhood brain tumors. Using sprays or foggers to dispense flea or tick treatments, flea collars, home pesticide bombs, fumigation for termites, and pest strips were associated with brain tumors in children. Studies in agricultural workers linked chronic exposures to chlorophenoxy herbicides with non-Hodgkin lymphoma. Pediatricians should ask questions about exposures to pesticides at home and suggest adoption of integrated pest management programs.

## POLYCHLORINATED BIPHENYLS, DIBENZOFURANS, AND DIBENZODIOXINS

PCBs are clear, nonvolatile, hydrophobic oils that resist metabolism and persist in the environment. They were used primarily in the electrical industry as insulators until the late 1970s, when they were banned in the United States and northern Europe. There are still detectable levels of PCBs in human tissue and human milk. Polychlorinated dibenzofurans (PCDFs) are partially oxidated PCBs.

The source of exposure for most people to all of these compounds is contaminated food. Because the chemicals are not well metabolized or excreted, even very small daily doses accumulate to measurable amounts over years. The most concentrated source is sport fish from contaminated waters because the residues bioconcentrate, and fish is the food that is usually at the highest trophic level consumed by humans. Alaska Native people who consume the blubber of sea mammals and fishermen who eat their own catch from contaminated waters may have high exposures. The major dietary source for young children is human milk. Some children may be exposed in schools that still have old fluorescent light ballasts.

Chronic exposure to commonly encountered levels of PCBs is associated with lower developmental and intelligence test scores, including lower psychomotor scores, defects in short-term memory, and lowered intelligence quotients. Acute exposure has been documented twice in Asia, and affected children are found to have persistent behavioral abnormalities and cognitive impairment.

Although many laboratories can measure PCBs, there are no agreed-on methods or quality assurance programs that would enable such measurements to be used in diagnosis or therapy. No regimen is known to lower body burden of these compounds.

Fish advisories for Lake Michigan recommend that individuals not eat more than 1 meal per month of salmon (with an average of 0.7 ppm PCBs), for a maximum of 12 meals per year. Women and children are advised to wait 1 month before eating another meal of Lake Michigan salmon to prevent PCBs from building up in the body.

PCB exposures from fish can be reduced by cleaning (eg, fat removal) and cooking methods. Old fluorescent light ballasts should be replaced.

## IONIZING RADIATION

Types of radiation are shown in Figure 10-1. On average, the annual effective dose equivalent of ionizing radiation on a person in the United States is 0.006 Sv (0.6 rem), 37% of which is from radon, 13% from other natural sources, 24% from computerized tomography, 12% from nuclear medicine, 7% from interventional fluoroscopy, 5% from medical x-rays, and 2% from other man-made sources (see Fig. 10-2).

Radiation exposure may be instantaneous (atomic bomb), chronic (uranium miners), fractionated (radiotherapy), or partial-body. For a given dose, whole-body exposure is more harmful than partial-body exposure. Radioisotopes decay with time into stable elements and have physical half-lives of various lengths, from fractions of a second to millions of years. They also have biological half-lives related to the rate at which they are excreted from the body.

Acute effects of overexposure include acute radiation sickness (nausea, vomiting, diarrhea, declining white blood cell count, and thrombocytopenia), epilation (loss of hair), and death. Delayed effects largely are due to mutagenesis, teratogenesis, and carcinogenesis.

Ionizing radiation causes chromosome breaks in somatic cells (eg, lymphocytes and skin fibroblasts) that are detectable decades after exposure and presumably account for the increased rates of cancer observed after exposure in childhood or adulthood.

Intrauterine exposure to ionizing radiation may cause small head size, alone or with severe mental retardation. Susceptibility to severe mental retardation is greatest at 8 to 15 weeks of gestational age, with some occurring during the 16th to 25th week. The lowest dose that caused severe mental retardation from atomic bomb exposure was 0.6 Sv, far above diagnostic exposures in medical radiology. The lowest dose that caused small head size without mental retardation was 0.10 to 0.19 Sv among conceptuses exposed at 4 to 17 weeks of gestational age.

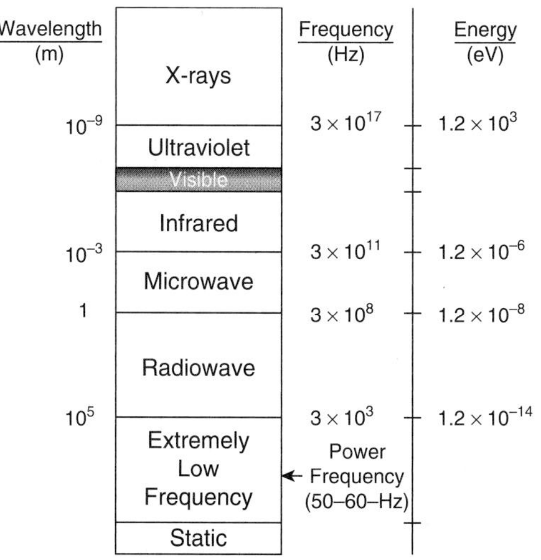


**FIGURE 10-1** Approximate range of wavelength, frequency, and energy for different types of electromagnetic radiation or fields. Adapted with permission of the National Council on Radiation Protection and Measurements, http://ncrponline.org/.

### Cancers after Radiation Exposure

An excess of thyroid cancer occurred in Japanese children exposed to the atomic bomb beginning at 11 years of age. An excess of breast cancer after childhood exposure to the atomic bomb was found when the cohort reached 30 years old. Thyroid ablation in 2 infants and thyroid neoplasia in Marshall Islanders were due to fallout from nuclear weapons tests.

Accidental release of radiation from nuclear reactors can cause thyroid cancer. In 1986, a partial meltdown at a nuclear reactor in Chernobyl, Ukraine, occurred, and substantial amounts of radioactive isotopes were released into the atmosphere. Fallout occurred primarily in the Ukraine and Belarus, in neighboring countries, and, to a lesser extent, throughout the world. Twenty-five thousand people who lived 3 to 15 km from the plant were estimated to have received 350 to 550 mSv (35–55 rem) from external irradiation. This amount is 7 to 11 times the annual dose limit for radiation workers. Additional exposures occurred from the ingestion of radioisotopes (fallout) that contaminated food and water. Thyroid cancer developed in nearly 5000 children.

### Radon

The US population is constantly exposed to radon, which accounts for 74% of background radiation (see Fig. 10-2). Radon gas comes from radioactive decay of radium, a product of uranium deposits in rocks and soil. Radon enters homes through cracks in the foundation, porous cinderblocks, and granite walls. Thus, radiation exposures in basements may be higher than those on the first-floor level.

When inhaled, radon decay products (also known as radon daughters or radon progeny) caused an increase in rates of lung cancer in uranium miners. There also is an increased risk of lung cancer after lifelong residential radon exposure. A meta-analysis of 8 epidemiologic studies indicated a linear dose-response relationship with lung cancer detectable down to 4 pCi/L, the level at which home remediation is recommended. Although most of the dose of radon and radon decay products is delivered to the lungs, increasing the risk of lung cancer, some goes to the bone marrow. An ecological study in France showed an association between indoor radon concentration and acute myeloid leukemia in children under 10 years old.

The Environmental Protection Agency recommends that homes be tested for radon. Radon exposure can be reduced by increasing ventilation and by reducing the influx of radon in the home. Several methods of reducing exposure include sealing cracks in the foundation, creating negative pressure under the basement floor, and prohibiting the use of building materials containing excessive radium. When levels of radon higher than 4 pCi/L are found, repairs should be made to reduce the radon level.

## SOLAR RADIATION

Skin cancers may be induced by ultraviolet (UV) light. Because of the long latent period, skin cancers rarely occur in childhood except when there is markedly heightened sensitivity, as in xeroderma pigmentosum or in albinism. The incidence of melanoma has increased more rapidly than that of most cancers, and children who experience repeated sunburns are at risk.

## AIR POLLUTION

In children, acute health effects associated with outdoor air pollution include increased respiratory symptoms, such as wheezing and cough, serious lower respiratory tract infections, and exacerbation of asthma. Increases in the number of hospital emergency department admissions have been observed when air pollution levels are elevated, which commonly occurs in major urban areas. Historically, episodes of very heavy air pollution (such as the Great Smog of 1952 in London) have been linked with increased death rates among adults and children. Most of the short-term respiratory effects of outdoor air pollution, such as symptoms of cough or shortness of breath, are thought to be reversible. The effects of repeated or long-term exposures to outdoor air pollution on the developing lungs of children are not as well understood.

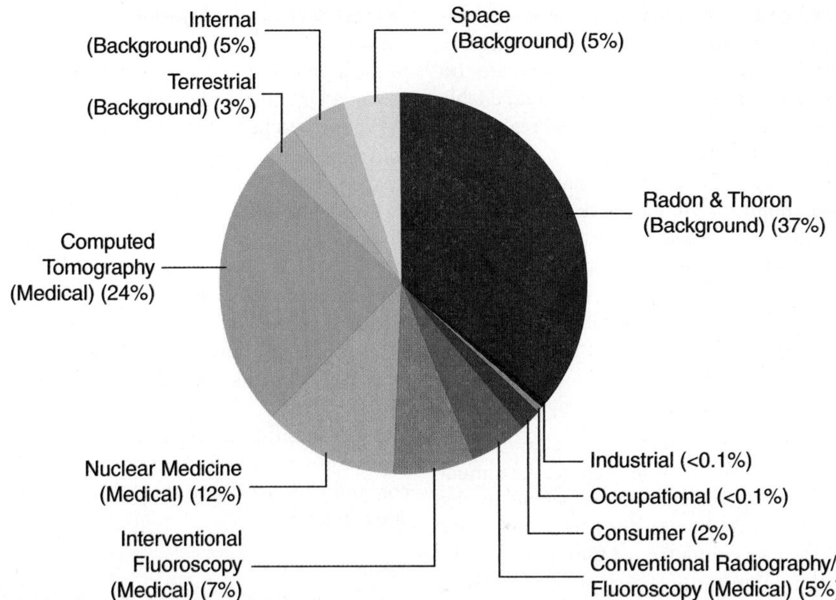


**FIGURE 10-2** Population exposure to ionizing radiation in the United States (average annual). (Adapted with permission of the National Council on Radiation Protection and Measurements, http://NCRPonline.org.)

Individual air pollutants typically exist as part of a complex mixture of multiple pollutants. Only a few air pollutants, however, are regularly monitored by the US government to assess outdoor (ambient) air quality. Those that are monitored regularly are respirable particulate matter, sulfur compounds, CO, lead, nitrogen oxides, and ozone.

#### Particulate Matter

*Particulate matter* is a generic term for a variety of materials with many different characteristics. Both solid particles and liquid droplets are included, and the particle or droplet size can range from slightly above the molecular level (invisible to the naked eye) to large dust particles several hundred microns in diameter. Solid particulate matter, including soot and smoke, is generated by the incomplete combustion of organic matter. Particulate matter also can include dusts that come from the mechanical breakdown of solid matter (such as rocks, soil, and dust). Fine and ultrafine particulate matter is emitted by diesel engines, can be found in the smoke of forest fires, and is emitted by power plants in which the coarse particle fraction is filtered out.

Particle size is the major determinant of where the particles will be deposited in the respiratory system. Although particles larger than 10 μm in diameter are filtered out when air passes through the nose, smaller particles reach the lower airways. Children, however, frequently breathe through their mouths, thus bypassing the nasal filtration mechanism. Particles smaller than 2.5 μm can penetrate deeply into the lungs. The particles that reach the alveoli stay there permanently. The concentration of particulate matter smaller than 10 μm in air is called $PM_{10}$. The concentration of particulate matter smaller than 2.5 μm in air is called $PM_{2.5}$. The fine particles often contain the most toxic compounds.

Diesel automotive exhaust generates particles smaller than 1 μm that remain suspended in the atmosphere for longer periods of time and are more likely to be inhaled.

Several studies have noted an association between particulate air pollution and mortality among persons of all ages, as well as low birth weight and other outcomes such as intrauterine growth retardation and postneonatal infant death.

#### Sulfur Compounds

Sulfur-containing compounds include sulfur dioxide ($SO_2$), sulfuric acid ($H_2SO_4$) aerosol, sulfate particles, and hydrogen sulfide ($H_2S$). The primary source of $SO_2$ is from burning coal; thus, major emitters of $SO_2$ include coal-fired power plants, smelters, and pulp and paper mills. $H_2SO_4$ aerosol is formed in the atmosphere from the oxidation of $SO_2$ in the presence of moisture. Facilities that either manufacture or use acids also can emit $H_2SO_4$ aerosol. $H_2S$ is emitted from a variety of industrial processes, including oil refining, wood pulp production, and waste water treatment, as well as from the operation of geothermal plants and landfills. $H_2S$ which has an odor similar to that of rotten eggs, can be detected at $H_2S$ levels that are far below those associated with physiological effects.

#### Carbon Monoxide and Lead

Large amounts of CO may enter the outdoor air primarily through the incomplete combustion of motor vehicle fuels. CO poisoning is discussed in Chapter 114. Leaded gasoline was once an important source of lead exposure for children in the United States until it was discontinued. Lead exposure from this source continues to occur in emerging nations. Treatment of lead exposure is discussed earlier in this chapter. Newer automobiles produce far less CO than do older vehicles. (See "Carbon Monoxide," above.)

#### Nitrogen Oxides

Although motor vehicle emissions contribute to outdoor levels of nitrogen oxides, emissions of nitrogen oxides from natural sources far outweigh those generated by human activity. Natural sources include intrusion of stratospheric nitrogen oxides, bacterial and volcanic action, and lightning. Most atmospheric nitrogen dioxide is emitted as nitric oxide, which is rapidly oxidized by ozone to nitrogen dioxide.

The levels of nitrogen oxides outdoors are generally lower than those found indoors. Infants living in homes with a nitrogen dioxide concentration exceeding 17.4 ppb had more days with wheeze, persistent cough, and shortness of breath than infants in homes with nitrogen dioxide concentrations lower than 5.1 ppb.

#### Ozone

Ozone ($O_3$) is a pervasive outdoor air pollutant. Outdoor $O_3$ and other photochemical oxidants are secondary pollutants formed in the atmosphere from a chemical reaction between volatile organic compounds and nitrogen oxides in the presence of sunlight. The primary sources of these precursor compounds include motor vehicle exhaust, chemical factories, and refineries. $O_3$ is the principal component of urban summer smog. Levels of $O_3$ are generally highest on hot summer days and increase to maximum levels in the late afternoon. It is common for air pollutants to occur together; for example, on days when $O_3$ levels are high, outdoor air levels of fine particles and acid aerosols may also be high.

Long-term exposure to $O_3$ is linked to chronic respiratory symptoms and small deficits in pulmonary function tests. Chronic exposure to ozone pollution has been associated with de novo development of chronic lung disease, with mild pulmonary fibrosis, and with modest increases in small airway obstruction. $O_3$ also may increase allergic response, possibly directing the immune response toward a Th2 pattern under certain conditions.

Dietary antioxidant supplementation (400 IU vitamin E and 500 mg vitamin C) may affect $O_3$-induced bronchial hyperresponsiveness in persons with asthma. In several, but not all, studies of adults, dietary supplementation was associated with higher lung function values during periods of $O_3$ pollution. It is not yet known whether dietary antioxidant supplementation is helpful for children exposed to $O_3$.

#### Mycotoxins

Emerging evidence points to the importance of considering novel sources of indoor air pollution when an infant presents with recurrent respiratory illnesses. In immunocompetent children, indoor exposure to water damage and fungi has been clearly linked to asthma and allergic diseases. Some children who are exposed to fungi have persistent upper respiratory tract symptoms such as rhinitis, sinusitis, sneezing, and eye irritation, as well as lower respiratory tract symptoms such as coughing and wheezing. Less well recognized is disease linked to toxins from molds. Cases of acute pulmonary hemorrhage have occurred among infants living in homes with severe water damage and fungal growth. Clinicians should recognize and manage health effects related to mold exposure and moisture indoors.

## WATER POLLUTANTS

More than 15,000 chemicals are produced at a rate of more than 10,000 pounds per year in the United States, and thousands of new chemicals are introduced into use each year. Few of these chemicals have been tested. Even among the 2800 chemicals used at more than a million pounds per year, more than half have not been tested for toxic effects on humans.

Common chemical contaminants in water are listed in Table 10-1. Children drink more water per kilogram of body weight than adults do, putting them at increased risk for health effects from contaminated water. Household water supplies can result in inhalation exposures as well. If volatile substances (eg, organic solvents) or gases (eg, radon gas) are present, these will enter the home during showering, bathing, and other activities.

Acute exposures to high levels of pollutants in water (and in foods) may result in acute gastrointestinal symptoms. There are numerous chemical exposures that can result in vomiting in children (see Table 10-2). Although less common than bacterial or viral causes of vomiting, toxins causing vomiting should be included in the differential diagnosis of vomiting in children, especially those with very rapid onset of gastrointestinal symptoms after eating or drinking.

**TABLE 10-1 WATER POLLUTANTS, COMMON SOURCES, AND SYSTEMS AFFECTED**

| Pollutant Category (Specific Examples) | Common Sources | Systems Affected/Health Effects |
|---|---|---|
| **Inorganic Chemicals** | | |
| Arsenic | Ores, smelting, pesticides | Lung, kidney, and skin cancer; cardiovascular; neurodevelopmental |
| Chromium | Ores, steel and pulp mills | Cancer (chromium VI) |
| Lead | Pipes, solder, soil | Neurologic, hematologic |
| Mercury (inorganic) | Waste incineration, burning coal, mercury use, volcanoes | Kidney damage, neurologic |
| Nitrates | Nitrogen fertilizer, leaching from septic tanks, sewage, erosion of natural deposits | Methemoglobinemia in infants |
| **Organic Chemicals** | | |
| Benzene, other organic chemicals | Leaking gasoline storage tanks | Leukemia, aplastic anemia |
| Pesticides | Agricultural use, urban runoff | Multiple |
| Polychlorinated biphenyls | Transformers, industry | Multiple |
| Trichloroethylene | Degreasing, dry cleaning | Cancer |
| **Disinfectants and Disinfection By-products** | | |
| Chloramines | Water chlorination | Eye/nose irritation, upper and lower airway irritation, stomach discomfort, anemia |
| Chlorine | Water chlorination | Eye/nose irritation, stomach discomfort |
| Chlorine dioxide | Water chlorination | Anemia, nervous system effects |
| Haloacetic acid | Byproduct of drinking water disinfection | Increased risk of cancer |
| Trihalomethanes | Byproduct of drinking water disinfection | Increased risk of cancer |
| **Radionuclides** | | |
| Radon | Natural uranium | Lung cancer |
| **Natural Toxins** | | |
| Microcystins | Cyanobacteria | Gastrointestinal tract, neurologic |
| *Pfiesteria* toxins | *Pfiesteria piscicida* | Neurologic, dermatologic |

Adapted with permission from Etzel RA: *Pediatric Environmental Health*, 3rd ed. Elk Grove Village, IL: American Academy of Pediatrics; 2012.

#### Nonorganic Chemicals in Water

Arsenic is ubiquitous in the environment. Human activities, such as smelting, coal burning, wood preservation, pesticide distribution, and other industrial processes, produce at least 3 times more arsenic than natural processes. The toxicity of arsenic to humans depends on the form, with organic being less toxic than inorganic and pentavalent being less toxic than trivalent. Except in electronics, industrial uses of arsenicals are decreasing. Drinking water and food represent the major sources of arsenic for humans. Arsenic is a known human carcinogen that naturally occurs in drinking water in many parts of the United States.

Chromium in drinking water is regulated to protect against exposure to one of the valence states of chromium, chromium VI, which is a carcinogen.

Drinking water also represents a potential route of exposure to lead.

Combustion sources that release mercury into the air, such as coal-fired power plants used for generating electrical energy and municipal waste incinerators that burn garbage are sources of atmospheric mercury that are deposited into lakes and rivers by rain and snow. Risks of mercury ingestion are discussed earlier in this chapter. Mercury is converted by sediment bacteria in the water into methylmercury, which becomes concentrated in fish by biomagnification up the food chain. Mercury is a drinking water contaminant; however, the most important route of exposure is through consumption of methylmercury-contaminated fish.

#### Organic Chemicals in Water

**Components of Gasoline** Gasoline is stored in underground tanks that can develop leakages over time, causing toxic chemicals to rapidly move into groundwater and eventually into drinking water supplies. The most toxic component of gasoline is benzene. It enters the water when gasoline is spilled or when gasoline tanks leak into the ground. Benzene is known to cause leukemia in humans, and aplastic anemia at high doses.

Nitrates and pesticides enter the water supply from urban and agricultural runoff of nitrogen fertilizers. Their effects are discussed earlier in this chapter. Pesticides may not be removed by conventional water treatment, and private wells may become contaminated with agricultural pesticides.

In 1986, an association was found between childhood leukemia and drinking water supplied from 2 municipal wells in Woburn,

**TABLE 10-2 TOXINS CAUSING VOMITING IN CHILDREN**

| Etiology | Incubation Period | Signs and Symptoms of Illness | Duration | Associated Items |
|---|---|---|---|---|
| Nuclear accident fallout | 3–16 hr | Nausea, vomiting, and diarrhea usually < 2 days after exposure | < 2 days | Acute radiation syndrome |
| Aflatoxins | ~8 hr | Vomiting, fever, abdominal pain, hematemesis, dizziness, diarrhea, seizures | Several weeks | Peanuts, maize, soybeans, cassava |
| Antimony | 5 min to 8 hr, usually <1 hr | Vomiting, metallic taste | Usually self-limited | Metallic container |
| Arsenic | Few hours | Vomiting, colic, diarrhea | Several days | Contaminated food |
| Cadmium | 5 min to 8 hr, usually <1 hr | Nausea, vomiting, myalgia, increase in salivation, stomach pain | Usually self-limited | Seafood, oysters, clams, lobster, grains, peanuts |
| Carbon monoxide | Varies | Nighttime vomiting, headache, lethargy, nausea, drowsiness, dizziness, weakness | Several hours | Combustion of carbon-based fuels |
| Copper | 5 min to 8 hr, usually <1 hr | Nausea, vomiting, blue or green vomitus | Usually self-limited | Metallic container |
| Fumonisins | Unknown | Nausea, vomiting | Unknown | Foods made from corn |
| Lead | Varies | Headache, abdominal pain, vomiting, loss of appetite, constipation | Several weeks | Lead dust, paint chips |
| Nitrite | 1–2 hr | Nausea, vomiting, cyanosis, dizziness, weakness, loss of consciousness, chocolate-brown–colored blood | Usually self-limited | Cured meats, any contaminated foods, spinach exposed to excessive nitrification |
| Patulin | Unknown | Nausea, vomiting | Unknown | Apple juice, other nonfermented apple products |
| Pesticides | Few minutes to few hours | Nausea, vomiting, abdominal cramps, diarrhea, headache, nervousness, blurred vision, twitching, convulsions, salivation and meiosis | Usually self-limited | Any contaminated food, home fumigation |
| Sodium fluoride | Few minutes to 2 hr | Salty or soapy taste, numbness of mouth, vomiting, diarrhea, dilated pupils, spasms, pallor, shock, collapse | Usually self-limited | Dry foods (such as dry milk, flour, baking powder, cake mixes) contaminated with sodium fluoride–containing insecticides and rodenticides |
| T-2 | 5 min to1 hr | Nausea, vomiting, abdominal pain, bloody diarrhea, dizziness, "burning" in mouth | 3–9 days | Food made with wheat, rice, corn or millet |
| Thallium | Few hours | Nausea, vomiting, diarrhea, painful paresthesias, motor polyneuropathy, hair loss | Several days | Contaminated food |
| Tin | 5 min to 8 hr, usually <1 hr | Nausea, vomiting, diarrhea | Usually self-limited | Metallic container |
| Vomitoxin | Few minutes to 3 hrs | Nausea, headache, abdominal pain, vomiting | Usually self-limited | Grains such as wheat, corn, barley |
| Zinc | Few hours | Stomach cramps, nausea, vomiting, diarrhea, myalgia | Usually self-limited | Metallic container |

Massachusetts. The two wells were contaminated with trichloroethylene, tetrachloroethylene, and chloroform. Childhood leukemia rates in Woburn reported between 1964 and 1983 were twice the national rates.

In the 1970s, chlorination of waters having high natural organic content was found to cause the formation of chloroform and other chlorinated compounds called trihalomethanes. Residual levels of the disinfectants chlorine and chlorine dioxide are now found in some tap water. Epidemiologic studies show a correlation between trihalomethane-containing drinking water and increases in the rates of rectal and bladder cancer.

#### Natural Toxins

Natural toxins may produce either acute or chronic illnesses and a variety of clinical syndromes. Water from ponds and lakes may contain Cyanobacteria (blue-green algae), including *Microcystis aeruginosa.* These bacteria produce cyanotoxins such as microcystins, some of which are hepatotoxic and neurotoxic compounds.

Water from the rivers flowing into the Chesapeake Bay on the Atlantic coast of the United States has been contaminated with *Pfiesteria piscicida* and dinoflagellates that can produce neurotoxins. Chronic exposure to toxin-producing *Pfiesteria* dinoflagellates has been associated with learning and memory difficulties.

## CLIMATE CHANGE

Children may be especially vulnerable to the effects of climate change because they often play outdoors and may become dehydrated during periods when temperatures are higher. They have a higher risk than their parents of becoming ill or dying from extreme heat.

## SUGGESTED READINGS

American Academy of Pediatrics Council on Environmental Health; Etzel RA, ed. *Pediatric Environmental Health.* 3rd ed. Elk Grove Village, IL: American Academy of Pediatrics; 2012.

American Academy of Pediatrics Council on Environmental Health. Global climate change and children's health. *Pediatrics.* 2015;136(5):992-997. doi: 10.1542/peds.2015-3232.

American Academy of Pediatrics Council on Environmental Health. Prevention of childhood lead toxicity. *Pediatrics.* 2016;138(1). pii: e20161493. doi: 10.1542/peds.2016-1493.

Etzel RA. What the primary care pediatrician should know about syndromes associated with exposures to mycotoxins. *Curr Probl Pediatr Adolesc Health Care.* 2006;36(8):282-305.

Landrigan PL, Etzel RA, eds. *Textbook of Children's Environmental Health.* New York, NY: Oxford University Press; 2014.

United Nations Scientific Committee on the Effects of Atomic Radiation. Sources, effects and risks of ionizing radiation. UNSCEAR 2013: Report to the General Assembly with Scientific Annexes. Vol. II, Scientific Annex B. Effects of radiation exposure of children. Available at: http://www.unscear.org/docs/publications/2013/UNSCEAR_2013_Annex-B.pdf. Accessed September 15, 2016.

# 11 Well-Child Care

Judith S. Shaw and Judith S. Palfrey

## INTRODUCTION

Health supervision visits, the cornerstone of primary care pediatrics, provide healthcare professionals the opportunity to promote the optimal health and well-being of children and their families in the communities in which they live. The value of contributing to and influencing the developmental trajectory of a child cannot be overstated. Through promoting children's health, nurturing their growth, anticipating their needs, and guiding their families, child healthcare professionals support and contribute to the healthy and positive development of children and youth.

Children have many "homes" where they receive care, but it is the medical home that looks after their health. Health supervision entails a variety of interrelated activities, including health promotion, prevention, surveillance, and management, and the coordination of care for children and youth with special healthcare needs. Going beyond diagnosis, management, and treatment of health-related problems, the medical home is foremost a place for promoting health and development and building on the recognized strengths of the child and family.

Although most children remain healthy, there is an increasing population of children living with chronic illness, disability, mental health problems, and other special needs. Child healthcare professionals are in a unique position to coordinate the often complex care, advocate for appropriate services, and facilitate optimum communication among the various individuals involved. In addition, societal and community forces, such as poverty, racism, and stigma, limit the life chances of far too many children. By getting at the root causes of these issues and working in tandem with families, schools, community agencies (such as public health and mayors' offices), child healthcare professionals can greatly improve the life situations and long-term health and development of all children and youth.

Caring for children's health provides many rewards and challenges for child healthcare providers. The interplay between environmental influence and factors intrinsic to the child becomes evident in many aspects of pediatric health and development. Continuity care is based on a developmental framework that recognizes the constancy of growth and change throughout childhood. Appreciating the impact of physical and psychosocial health not only on the child but also on the people in the child's life, child healthcare professionals have responsibilities beyond the traditional medical model that include health promotional activities, such as consideration for emotional, spiritual, and environmental health, and for community and societal health as well as their influences on the child's future development.

Most children are generally healthy and grow along a predictable trajectory. The first task of well-child care is to determine that the child is following a normal course, to document the growth and development parameters, and to celebrate and reinforce with the family their accomplishments in raising a healthy child. However, when a deviation in growth and/or development occurs, it is the role of child healthcare providers to detect the problem early and to provide the child and family with prompt, appropriate treatment. It is also important for child healthcare professionals to work with the family on crafting a plan for preventing future sequelae or problems.

Continuity of care and relationship building are essential elements of well-child care. Through the regular health supervision visits from birth to late adolescence, children and families often develop a special bond with their healthcare professional team. Well-child care is most successful when it is based on a partnership between the family and the healthcare team. Effective health promotion involves a bidirectional relationship of receptivity that values the agenda and needs of the family while recognizing the importance of providing services essential to the health and well-being of the child and family.

This chapter provides an overview of health supervision of infants, children, and adolescents; covers specific aspects of the visits and other important areas pertaining to health supervision; and discusses considerations in the office practice to support excellence in health supervision.

## HEALTH SUPERVISION GUIDELINES

### Introduction

The goal of primary care pediatrics is to facilitate optimal health, well-being, and development of children and their families. This is accomplished through a variety of interrelated activities, including monitoring of health and growth, anticipatory guidance and prevention, screening, early identification and intervention for problems, health maintenance and health promotion, coordination of care for children with special needs, and advocacy for improvement of community and societal situations that impact on children and youth.

Well-child care is a proactive venture. The traditional focus on problem diagnosis and management has been broadened to include screening for disease and its precursors in an asymptomatic population. Pediatric providers have long recognized the value of preventive programs such as mass immunization and continue to lead the way in this area through an emphasis on regular health surveillance, anticipatory guidance, and involvement in community-based prevention strategies. Emphasis is placed on the related concept of health promotion, whereby optimal health and well-being are positively encouraged. These areas form the foundation for current recommendations for health supervision guidelines.

At each visit, the age and developmental level of the child dictate the approach to the patient and much of the visit's content. In pediatrics, the therapeutic alliance includes both the child and the family; the importance of establishing a trusting longitudinal relationship cannot be overemphasized.

The American Academy of Pediatrics' *Bright Futures: Guidelines for Health Supervision of Infants, Children, and Adolescents* is a consolidation of the many health supervision guidelines into a single set of guidelines for healthcare professionals. These guidelines, based on the latest evidence and expert opinion on standards of care, offer a roadmap for the healthcare professional to follow and provide a structure for health supervision in primary care.

### What Is New in *Bright Futures*

Experienced healthcare professionals see the well-child visit as an opportunity to improve the health and well-being of children and their families. However, most report feeling tension as they seek to provide care that includes a personal assessment of the child's health and the family's ability to promote continued health in the limited time available during office encounters.

Resolving this tension is important to the success of the visit and is key to family and healthcare professional satisfaction. *Bright Futures* proposes solutions to improve the organization of clinical processes and well-child care. Using the *Bright Futures* materials, a healthcare professional working with office staff can create effective encounters that meet their goals of disease detection, disease prevention, and health promotion.

The third edition of *Bright Futures* was published in 2007 following a careful examination of the evidence supporting each recommendation, and with a goal of improving the structure and format for delivery of primary care. Ten years later, in 2017, the 4th edition will be published and contains new updates to the health supervision guidelines, including new recommendations for medical screening. Some of the changes include screening for newborn bilirubin, maternal depression, adolescent depression, dyslipidemia, and human immunodeficiency virus (HIV). Anticipatory guidance changes include new priorities focusing on the social determinants of health (both the risks and the strengths and protective factors), and new areas that focus on social media including screen time for young children. The *Bright Futures Guidelines* are aligned with the AAP's periodicity schedule, which is the standard for child preventive services that are covered without cost-sharing according to the Affordable Care Act (ACA). The 4th edition guidelines and associated periodicity schedule can be found at http://brightfutures.aap.org.

### Overview of the *Bright Futures* Visit

*Bright Futures* outlines the health supervision visit using four areas of importance: context, priorities, health supervision, and anticipatory guidance. The 4th edition has added review of symptoms (Table 11-1).

The "Context" section in *Bright Futures* recommendations provides a brief overview of the child at different age levels, including the developmental tasks and milestones to be achieved, thereby setting the context for the visit. It points out the unique attributes, strengths, and assets of the child and special considerations for ensuring healthy growth and development.

For the "Priorities for the Visit" section, the *Bright Futures* Expert Panel identified 5 priority topics to be discussed during visits once the concerns of the child and family have been elicited and addressed.

"Health Supervision" includes 7 subsections: "History" offers questions relevant to the child and family to assess interval and past medical history. "Surveillance of Development" suggests questions for assessing developmental milestones and tasks at those visits when a structured developmental screening tool is not used. "Review of Systems" suggests questions and recommends a complete review of systems as a part of every health visit. "Observation" provides ideas for observing the child and family as a starting point for the visit. "Physical Examination" emphasizes that a complete physical examination "is included as part of every health supervision visit" and describes aspects of the examination that are important for children of specific ages. "Screening" provides tables for universal (done for all children) and selective (based on risk assessment) screening. The tables list the method of screening and the action to take if the risk assessment is positive. "Immunizations" refers readers to the appropriate Web sites for the most current recommendations.

The "Anticipatory Guidance" section describes in more detail each of the 5 priorities identified by the expert panel, including sample questions and guidance in the exact words that the clinician could use.

**TABLE 11-1 *BRIGHT FUTURES* VISIT OUTLINE, USING A STRENGTH-BASED APPROACH**

A. Context (brief overview of developmental tasks and milestones usually achieved at specific age levels)

B. Priorities for the Visit
- The first priority is to attend to the concerns of the parents.
- The Bright Futures Expert Panel has given priority to 5 topics for discussion in each visit.

C. Health Supervision
- C1. History
- C2. Surveillance of Development
- C3. Review of Systems
- C4. Observation of Parent-Child Interaction
- C5. Physical Examination
  - Assessment of Growth
    - Younger than 2 years: weight, length, head circumference, and weight-for-length
    - Older than 2 years: weight, height, and BMI
  - Listing of particular components of the examination that are important for the child at each age visit
- C6. Screening
  - Universal screening, including action if screen is positive
  - Selective screening, including risk assessment and action if risk assessment is positive
- C7. Immunizations

D. Anticipatory Guidance
- Information for the healthcare professional
- Health promotion questions for the 5 priorities for the visit
- Anticipatory guidance for the parent and child

Reproduced with permission from Hagan JF, Shaw JS, Duncan PM, eds. *Bright Futures: Guidelines for Health Supervision of Infants, Children, and Adolescents.* 4th ed. Elk Grove Village, IL: American Academy of Pediatrics; 2017.

## CONDUCTING A HEALTH SUPERVISION VISIT

### Priorities

Primary care pediatrics is changing as healthcare professionals are challenged to provide more service in less time and with shrinking reimbursement. The luxury of extended face-to-face time between the patient and clinician is disappearing. Healthcare administrators approach health supervision visits as a business, limiting nonreimbursed activities, seeking greater efficiencies, and measuring return on investment and relative-value units. Insurers often tie performance to payment, through such initiatives as pay-for-performance and value-based payments. Recognizing that the long list of anticipatory guidance topics that could and should be discussed at each visit was unrealistic, and in response to a plea from healthcare professionals to help focus the topics, the *Bright Futures* authors were challenged with how to design a comprehensive visit, yet acknowledging the limited time available during the visit, to hone in on those areas most important to a child at each age level. The first priority is to attend to the concerns of the child and parents. Beyond that, the *Bright Futures* Expert Panel developed 5 priorities through an exhaustive process considering and reviewing the available evidence, expert opinions, and numerous discussions with experts in preventive services. The 4th edition kept the same commitment to having only 5 priorities and the priorities were updated based on new evidence (eg, newborns and infants sleeping in parents' room until at least 6 months of age) and new morbidities (eg, impact of social media).

In addition to 5 priorities for each visit, *Bright Futures* provides detailed information about each priority along with sample questions, dialog, and anticipatory guidance. The numerous individuals who contributed to the writing of *Bright Futures* recognized that it was important to explain not only what should be done but also how to do it and how to say it. For example, rather than just recommending "screen for domestic violence," *Bright Futures* offers the clinician sample questions such as "Because violence is so common in many people's lives, I've begun to ask about it. I don't know if this is a problem for you, but many children I see have parents who have been hurt by someone else. Some are too afraid or uncomfortable to bring it up, so I've started asking about it routinely. Do you always feel safe in your home? Are you scared that your partners or someone else may try to hurt you or your child?" It offers anticipatory guidance such as "One way that I and other healthcare professionals can help you if your partner is hitting or threatening you is to support you and provide information about local resources that can help you."

### History Taking

For a more detailed discussion of interview techniques, see Chapter 4.

**Taking a History: Process** As with any health encounter, the history is the central element of the health supervision visit. How the history is taken sets the tone for the entire visit. The information gleaned sets the agenda for the visit and for subsequent visits. In most cases, the information that healthcare providers learn through the history affirms that the child is doing well on all health and developmental parameters. Families' input into the history and their voicing of current concerns and questions are key components of the history process. As with all well-child care, the more that the history process can be a "joint venture" the more successful it will be. Through a careful history taking, the child health clinician and parent can identify those areas that require further discussion or action. Occasionally during the history taking, a serious unmet health, developmental, or social need is uncovered. When this occurs, the clinician and family can readjust the content of the visit and establish a plan of consultations and further visits to meet the child's and family's needs.

Health supervision visits are best accomplished when parents and providers see the enterprise as a shared task or partnership. It is helpful for the child healthcare provider to make this partnership explicit by using words like *we* and *us* when taking a history. The history helps align the expectations of the parent with those of the provider.

The health supervision visit should be conducted in private, and the family should feel confident that the information they provide will be handled professionally and shared only with those who need to know the information for the benefit of the patient. With the advent of electronic recordkeeping, some parents may be wary about discussing information they consider personal. The child health clinician should take the time to explain how the records system works and that there are layers of security and privacy protection.

The parents, children/adolescents, and clinician should be seated during history taking to emphasize the importance of the activity and show that the clinician is eager to listen to the families' answers and concerns. The clinician should record the information at the time of history taking (ideally in an electronic form). The clinician should also review with the family the prescreening questionnaire that may have been completed. While the computer is a valuable tool for recording and monitoring information, the child health clinician should make it a point to face the family during the history taking and establish eye contact whenever possible. The history should be taken in the family's preferred language whenever feasible. If the child healthcare provider does not speak the family's language, a well-trained interpreter (not a family member) should be used. It should be recognized, however, that even the best interpreters often miscommunicate key questions and answers. While conducting a child supervision history through an interpreter, the clinician should not hesitate to ask the interpreter to rephrase a question or answer if the information seems unclear. (See Chapter 14 for further discussion of culturally competent care.) The healthcare provider should have the opportunity to speak with adolescents alone to ask a number of personal questions regarding their health behaviors (smoking, drug and alcohol use, exposure to violence, sexual experience, etc).

**Taking a History: Content** As with any health encounter, the child health clinician should first ask the parents (or older child) whether they are concerned about any pressing issues. If the child is sick on the day of the well-child visit, or if a destabilizing event has occurred in the household, such as a death or the loss of a job, these issues may take precedence over the more routine questions. If there are no pressing issues, the well-child care clinician should ask an open-ended question about the parents' concerns and elicit what they hope to accomplish through this visit. The answers to these questions help assure that the visit is appropriately addressing the issues that are on the family's agenda.

At a family's first well-child–care health supervision visit, important baseline information about the family and child is gathered. At subsequent visits, the child healthcare professionals ask if there have been any changes in this baseline information since the last visit. Table 11-2 provides suggestions for history taking at the first and subsequent visits.

### Observation

The astute clinician utilizes all aspects of the visit to glean information about the child and family. Information is gained not only through physical examination and by asking questions but also by observing interactions between the child and family. Observation, while generally not formally taught, can provide important information about the child and family that may not be elicited through questions. *Bright Futures* provides a list of questions to ask at each visit to guide the clinician in observing the child and family. For example, at the 12-month visit, the clinician is prompted to observe the family interaction when the child is given a book as part of a Reach Out and Read program. Observing what the child does with the book and how the parents respond can provide important information about their interaction.

### Conducting a Physical Examination





**Physical Examination Process** The physical assessment begins with obtaining and recording the child's height, weight, head circumference (for infants and toddlers), and vital signs. This information is often collected by a nurse or clinical assistant and plotted on the age-appropriate growth chart. For infants and children ages 0 to 2 years of age, the World Health Organization growth chart should be used. For children age 2 years and older, the Centers for Disease Control and Prevention growth chart should be used. These charts can be found at: http://www.cdc.gov/growthcharts. These charts indicate the child's growth percentile. The clinic should have an alert system for children whose measurements are above or below clinically specified cutoffs or whose percentiles are shifting up or down. Body mass index should also be recorded and monitored to detect children who are at risk for undernutrition or overweight status. For further discussion of nutritional evaluation, see Chapter 20. The approach to the child with poor weight gain is discussed in Chapter 22, and growth impairment is discussed in Chapter 515. The management of overweight or obesity is discussed in Chapter 24.

Ideally, vision and hearing screenings take place at selected health supervision visits along with other medical screenings, such as for anemia, lead poisoning, developmental problems, and signs of autism, according to the AAP's periodicity schedule found at http://brightfutures.aap.org.

An anxious child is difficult to examine. Using calming techniques can help put the child at ease, allowing for a stress-free, more accurate examination. Table 11-3 provides suggestions for calming prior to and during the examination. The physical examination should be conducted with the child wearing minimal clothing so the clinician can conduct the examination with fewer time lags. The clinician determines how comprehensive an examination to conduct depending on (1) the history, (2) the age of the child, and (3) how recently a comprehensive examination was recorded in the child's record. *Bright Futures* describes the age-appropriate components of the physical examination that are important for each visit.

The child and family should be assured of privacy during the physical examination. Parents should always be present when children are examined. Teenagers should be given the choice of having their parent present. Teenagers should ideally be examined by a healthcare professional of the same gender or have someone (a chaperone, usually a healthcare professional) of the same gender as the patient also present if the person doing the full examination is of the opposite gender. In some cases, it may also be appropriate to have a chaperone even if the clinician and adolescent are of the same gender. The AAP policy on the use of chaperones is a useful guide for establishing office routines. The examination room should afford privacy for the child or adolescent, and the door should be kept closed while they are undressing or dressing and during the physical examination. Please refer to the *Bright Futures* Web site for age-specific physical exam recommendations.

**Closing the Visit** Health supervision visits are greatly enhanced when the clinician takes a minute or 2 at the end of the visit to review the high-priority areas that were emphasized in the visit. This is a great time for the clinician to reinforce the health promotion messages by handing out materials or referring the parent or child to a content-appropriate Web site. At this time, it may be appropriate to ask the parent or child where they obtain health information and to talk about the pros and cons of information that is widely available through social media. The *Bright Futures* Tool and Resource Kit contains single-page visit-summary sheets for parents, 1 for each visit, with the priorities listed and the anticipatory guidance for each priority written for the parent and/or child. The brochures and summary sheets can be distributed before the visit to allow the clinician to point out the information or after the visit to reinforce what was discussed.

The end of the visit is also a good time for the clinician to model positive reinforcement techniques by praising the child for maintaining good health habits. A wonderful way to end the visit is by rewarding the child for his or her participation by giving an age-appropriate book from a program such as Reach Out and Read.

**TABLE 11-2 HISTORY TAKING AT FIRST AND SUBSEQUENT VISITS TO THE PRACTICE**

**Initial History at First Visit**

Pregnancy information
- Age and health of the mother, parity, other pregnancy losses
- Use of drugs and/or alcohol during pregnancy
- Prenatal care (number of visits, health or social concerns)

Birth history
- Length of gestation
- Birth weight
- Delivery complications
- Infections, jaundice, or other cause for hospitalization
- More extensive questioning for premature and low–birth-weight babies

Health history
- Has the child been diagnosed with any health condition?
- Is the child taking any medications prescribed by a healthcare provider?
- Is the child taking any home remedies or complementary therapies?
- Does the child use any durable medical equipment, specialized diet, or other medical intervention?
- Has the child been hospitalized at any time? What for? For how long?
- Is the child allergic to medicines, foods, other?

Social history
- Who lives at home with the child?
- What type of living arrangement is it: house, apartment, etc.?
- If the family is homeless, are they on the street, in a shelter, or doubled up with other families?
- Was the housing stock built before 1957? If so, has it been deleaded?
- Does the family have current financial problems?
- Does the family have enough food?
- Employment of parents
- Daycare arrangements
- Other concerns or stresses on the family (a family member who is ill, in jail, or unemployed; domestic violence; community violence; exposure to racism or other stigma; uncertain citizenship status)

**History at Subsequent Visits**

Interim health events
- Has the child had any health events since the last visit?
- If so, is the child on any new medicines or health regimes?

Interim social events
- Have there been any major changes at home (eg, new baby, move, new job or loss of a job, separation or divorce, death in the family, domestic violence event, community violence event)?

Feeding/sleep/elimination patterns (infants)
- Does infant have own crib (eg, not co-sleeping) and is sleeping on back?
- Is the child being breastfed? How often? Any concerns?
- If on formula, which one? How often? Any concerns?
- Is the child receiving solid food? Tolerating well?
- Does the child receive vitamin and iron supplements?
- How much water does the child drink? Is the water fluoridated?
- What is the child's sleep pattern? Any concerns?
- What is the child's elimination pattern? Any concerns?

Eating/sleeping/elimination patterns (toddlers/preschoolers)
- Questions about the solid foods in the child's diet and weaning from breast or bottle
- Questions about transition from crib to bed
- How is toilet training going? Any concerns?

Eating/sleeping/elimination patterns (older children and adolescents)
- Questions about the amount and type of food the children and adolescents are eating: Too much? Too little?
- Unusual eating behaviors?
- Questions about sleep patterns with an emphasis on an optimum sleep routine
- Questions about daytime and nighttime wetting and/or soiling
- Questions about sleep patterns with an emphasis on an optimum sleep routine
- Questions about daytime and nighttime wetting and/or soiling

Activity (a formal developmental screen can substitute for the milestone questions)
- For infants and toddlers, questions about milestone development
- For older children and adolescents, questions about routine exercise and sports activities

(Continued)

**TABLE 11-2 HISTORY TAKING AT FIRST AND SUBSEQUENT VISITS TO THE PRACTICE (CONTINUED)**

Screen time (starting during toddler years)
- How much television does the child watch? With an adult present?
- What types of video games does the child play, and how much time is spent playing?
- For adolescents, are they involved in excessive online interactions?

Language, literacy, and numeracy (a formal developmental screen can substitute for this)
- How often does the family read to the child?
- Is the family concerned about the child's language development?
- For older children, what reading level has the child attained?
- Are the parents concerned about the child's progress in reading or in math?

School functioning (starting in preschool)
- What are the teachers reporting about the child?
- Has the family been attending regular parent-teacher meetings at the school?
- What are the child's interests and strengths?
- If there are concerns, have they been adequately addressed?

Safety
- Does the family have any safety concerns?
- Is there a gun in the house? Is there a lock on the gun?
- Have smoke detectors been installed in the home?
- Local safety questions (pool guards, window guards, safe storage of farm equipment, etc.)
- Is use of car seats and bicycle helmets reinforced?

Confidential questions with adolescents and young adults (questions vary with age)
- School performance and aspirations
- Life and career goals
- Smoking, vaping, marijuana use
- Alcohol and/or drug use or dependency
- Gender identification
- Sexual intimacy; sexual intercourse; birth control, pregnancies, and/or abortions
- Interpersonal violence, gun possession
- Sleep
- Social media, video games, and other Internet use

### Other Important Areas

**Privacy and Confidentiality** Issues of privacy and confidentiality may arise during any health supervision visit and for children of any age. They should be addressed as they arise. They must, however, be addressed during the adolescent years. Clinicians and practices are encouraged to establish rules of privacy and confidentiality and to share them with the children and families. Beginning in the early adolescent years (ages 11–14 years, according to *Bright Futures*), part of the visit may be conducted with the child alone. This is especially important for young adolescents who many not share certain information when a parent is present. Establishing a trusting relationship between the adolescent and clinician is extremely important at this stage of the young person's development to assure the discussion of information that will help the clinician to support the adolescent's health and development. Sharing is bidirectional as the clinician seeks to learn about the adolescent while sharing information to promote health, assessing for strengths and assets, and promoting a supportive and open environment for discussing issues that might transpire during the often tumultuous period of adolescence.

During the visit, the physical examination may invoke embarrassment for young adolescents, and they may be uncomfortable responding to seemingly private, personal questions. Privacy during the physical examination is essential; many clinicians ask for a chaperone when conducting the physical examination of both girls and boys. Confidentiality is addressed with the assurance that information is not disclosed or shared with parents or anyone else unless the information indicates that someone is in immediate danger.

## HEALTH SUPERVISION IN THE OFFICE PRACTICE

### How Do I Look at My Practice?

In the United States, it is reported that 38.3% of children received the recommended well-child care, according to a report on the quality of ambulatory care. Delivering high-quality primary care is an active process shared by all personnel in the primary care office.

The health supervision visit entails more than just the face-to-face time between the clinician and the child and parent. Other actions take place, such as completion of paperwork and questionnaires; psychosocial and developmental screening; interactions with nursing that may include history taking and immunization administration; and conducting, documenting, and plotting various anthropomorphic measures. These activities can consume considerable time, and when combined with a clinical encounter that is estimated to be 15 to 18 minutes, the actual time spent in the primary care practice can be substantial.

Given the significant amount of time the child and family spend on the entire visit, it is not surprising that increased attention is being paid to examining the effectiveness and efficiency of how care is delivered in the primary care setting. For further discussion of approaches to improving systems of care, refer to Chapter 9. Practice managers seek to make the encounter a valuable experience for the patient while limiting inefficiencies in the system of care. Time spent gathering information from the child and family prior to the clinical encounter can contribute to increased face-to-face time between the clinician and family. Examining the practice for ways to improve the system of care, streamline processes, and maximize the use of resources will help to create an environment that delivers high-quality primary care. Table 11-4 provides a comprehensive list of tips and strategies for practice improvement.

### *Bright Futures* Tools and Resources

Healthcare professionals have the opportunity to reflect on their current system of providing well-child care and consider new approaches to improving how that care is delivered. Owning a *Bright Futures* book and having knowledge of the recommendations does not translate into

**TABLE 11-3 CALMING TECHNIQUES TO IMPROVE EXAMINATION ACCURACY IN CHILDREN AGES 1 TO 4 YEARS**

**Preparation:** Read stories about health check-ups or health visits before the appointment.

**Parent contact:** The child sits or lies in the parent's lap or is held chest-to-chest by the parent.

**Establishing alliance with the child:** The examiner "aligns" with the parent first so that the child knows the parent approves of the exam and will be "with" the child throughout.

**Establishing friendly relationship with the child:** Examiner gets down to child's level, notes something about the child's shirt or shoes, jokes about something in the room—nice if both child and parent join in the joke

**Distraction:**

- **Auditory:** Gentle, relaxed, reassuring constant banter from the examiner or parent; singing or music; or nonsense buzzing noises or whispering.
- **Manual:** The child holds a tongue blade in each hand or feels the stethoscope head, holds jingling keys, or brings dolls or toys to the appointment.
- **Visual:** The otoscope is shown to the child while lighting the examiner's palm, then the child's, before the ear examination; or the examiner puts the otoscope into his or her own ear declaring, "See! It's okay! Just a flash-light. Do you have a flashlight at home?"

**Demonstration:** A doll or stuffed animal is examined before the patient, or the child's shoe is "listened" to with the stethoscope before listening to the patient.

**Recruitment:** Request the child's help in holding the stethoscope head or tongue blade; "blowing out" the otoscope light; or while listening to the chest, ask the child to blow on a piece of tissue held in front of the mouth to encourage deep breathing.

**Comfort measures:**

- **Avoidance of fear-inducing actions:** Avoid direct looks into the eyes of a young toddler until the eyes are examined; delay invasive portions of the examination (eg, otoscopy) until last; or examine toes or fingers first.
- **Pleasant office surroundings:** Books, toys, and pictures or drawings on the walls.

Reproduced with permission from Hagan JF, Shaw JS, Duncan PM, eds. *Bright Futures: Guidelines for Health Supervision of Infants, Children, and Adolescents.* 4th ed. Elk Grove Village, IL: American Academy of Pediatrics; 2017.

**TABLE 11-4 TIPS AND STRATEGIES FOR PRACTICE IMPROVEMENT**

| **Tips** |
|---|
| View guidelines as an opportunity |
| Re-examine how things are done |
| Educate staff in quality-improvement methods |
| Reward innovation |
| Involve all members of the staff |
| Start small |
| Turn frustration into ideas for change |
| Post your progress in a visible place so all can share in the success |
| Seek out partnerships and leverage others' expertise (eg, state or local chapter of the AAP, quality-improvement organizations, improvement partnerships, managed care organizations) |
| Celebrate your successes no matter how small they are |
| Think outside the box, be creative, and be willing to try new ideas; change is not easy! |
| **Strategies** |
| Small, sequential steps are better than one large step: You will learn more along the way and be more likely to achieve success |
| Begin simply: one area, one visit, one screening |
| Measure: you change what you measure and monitor (pull charts, review billing data, review managed care organization data, review state data such as immunization audits) |
| Designate a lead person or "owner" of the process |
| Identify possible strategies and ideas; brainstorm creatively so everyone contributes |
| Pick one idea to test, or encourage a few simultaneous ideas |
| Stay open to change: Change is not often viewed as a good thing and is not easy; minimize resistance |
| Recognize all improvements that result from change |
| Explore how this effort might benefit others (eg, State Title V program's National Performance Measures, managed care organizations, Department of Health, Medicaid) |
| Share and learn in community, region, and state |
| Seek free labor: undergraduates and graduate students; groom the next generation. |
| Involve parents and youth in identifying areas for improvement and solutions |

Reproduced with permission from Shaw JS: Practice Improvement: Child Healthcare Quality and Bright Futures, Pediatric Annals Mar;37(3):159-164, 2008.

improved care. Making the guidelines "come to life" in the practice involves a proactive, systematic approach to guideline implementation. Assuring adherence to guidelines and high-quality care is typically accomplished with the support of tools, materials, and strategies. The *Bright Futures* Tool and Resource Kit provides a comprehensive set of tools and materials matched to the recommendations at each visit. *Bright Futures* anticipatory guidance handouts and summary sheets for parents and children are available for each visit, covering the 5 priorities and other visit interventions. Parent and child previsit questionnaires cover screening questions to ascertain risks of each of the universal and selective screening topics. Questionnaires used prior to the visit can assess the parents' and child's concerns and needs and help to focus priorities for the visit. Clinical documentation forms align with the clinical recommendations at each visit.

The tools that accompany the *Bright Futures* guidelines are a resource for the practices that want to implement the guidelines. Despite this resource, each practice must decide what to implement, and how and when to do so, in order to best meet the practice's unique needs. Knowing the most efficient and effective way to replace previous tools and methods and to phase in a new approach will challenge all practices faced with implementation. Those with electronic medical records systems must review their existing systems and match them to the *Bright Futures* recommendations and guidelines. Many companies are working to align their electronic medical records templates and child health sections with the *Bright Futures* guidelines, so for some practices, a software upgrade may smooth the transition. There is no one "correct" way to implement new guidelines; there are many.

Systems improvement through quality improvement is one approach to implementing new or changes to guidelines. Attention to quality improvement, prompted by the recognition of medical errors and the increasing evidence of poor healthcare quality, has prompted clinicians to reexamine their own practices and how care is delivered. Many practices now participate in quality improvement activities and share methods and strategies for implementation as they learn from one another. Physician licensure recertification in many specialties, including pediatrics, requires competence in quality improvement as demonstrated by participating in or carrying out practice-based quality improvement. A common approach is using the principles of quality improvement, such as the model for improvement, which involves choosing an area for improvement, typically based on data, and then completing the Plan-Do-Study-Act (PDSA) cycle of improvement (Table 11-5). For example, a practice wants to improve its rates of lead screening at the 12-month visit. The data may come from a recent audit by the insurer or public health authorities, or it may have been researched by a curious clinician. Once the area for improvement is identified, the PDSA approach is applied, making small, sequential, and incremental changes, often referred to as *tests of change*, toward the ultimate goal. The *plan*, for example, is to implement a system to prompt all clinicians that the lead screening is due. They will *do* the prompting for 1 week and will *study* by examining 5 to 8 charts of 12-month-olds seen during that time to see if the lead screening was done. Once the data has been collected, the practice will *act* on the results by determining if their approach achieved the desired result of increasing lead screening. If the prompting system does not achieve the desired results

**TABLE 11-5 PDSA WORKSHEET FOR TESTING CHANGE**

| *Aim (overall goal): Every goal will require multiple smaller tests of change* | | | |
|---|---|---|---|
| Describe your first (or next) test of change | Person responsible | When to be done | Where to be done |
| *Plan* | | | |
| List the tasks needed to set up this test of change | Person responsible | When to be done | Where to be done |
| Predict what will happen when the test is carried out | Measures to determine if prediction succeeds | | |
| *Do:* Describe what actually happened when you ran the test | | | |
| *Study:* Describe the measured results and how they compared to the predictions | | | |
| *Act:* Describe what modifications to the plan will be made for the next cycle from what you learned | | | |



or is deemed cumbersome or inappropriate for the practice, then a new test is implemented with a new PDSA cycle. While the approach is simple in concept, applying PDSA can be a challenge, starting with choosing an area for improvement. In our example, the practice may choose to improve lead screening rates, but this goal requires further clarification: Does the practice want to improve the ordering of lead screening tests or improve the documentation of the screening values in the charts? Each option requires a different approach and consequently a different PDSA cycle. Further information on these methods can be obtained from the Improvement Guide or online resources such as the Institute for Healthcare Improvement (http://www.ihi.org). Using quality improvement principles help practices to systematically examine how they deliver care and what aspects of that care might be amenable to change.

## SUGGESTED READINGS

Hagan J, Shaw J, Duncan P, eds. *Bright Futures: Health Supervision Guidelines for Infants, Children, and Adolescents*. 4th ed. Elk Grove Village, IL: American Academy of Pediatrics; 2017 (*In press*).

Langley GJ, Moen RD, Nolan KM, Nolan TW, Norman CL, Provost LP. *The Improvement Guide: A Practical Approach to Enhancing Organizational Performance*. 2nd ed. San Francisco, CA: Jossey-Bass; 2009.

Mangione-Smith R, DeCristofaro AH, Setodji CM, et al. The quality of ambulatory care delivered to children in the United States [see comment]. *N Engl J Med*. 2007;357(15):1515-1523.

# 12 Oral Health Supervision

Ada M. Fenick and Rosalyn M. Sulyanto

## INTRODUCTION

The condition of children's teeth and the associated tissues are critical to their well-being. A child with poor dentition may be experiencing chronic pain and thus may have difficulties achieving proper nutrition. He or she may also be at risk of malocclusion and life-threatening infection. Further, dental problems such as early childhood caries can affect the secondary dentition if not addressed, with consequences extending through the life span. Caries are the most common dental problem encountered; the National Health and Nutrition Examination Survey of 2011-2012 showed that 37% of children from ages 2 to 8 have some evidence of caries in their primary teeth, and 21% of children from ages 6 to 11 have evidence of caries in their secondary dentition. Unfortunately, a large proportion of these children have untreated caries. At higher risk of caries are children living in low-income and moderate-income households, children of color, and children with special healthcare needs. However, caries can and do occur in children of all backgrounds. As the health professional most likely to encounter new mothers and their infants at a young age, the pediatric clinician has a unique opportunity to provide anticipatory guidance that may help to prevent or slow the development of caries. Therefore, it behooves the provider to evaluate a child's current dental status from an early age, to advise the child and the primary caregiver about positive and negative practices that may bear on future dentition, and to assist the family in establishing a dental home.

## EVALUATION OF CURRENT DENTITION

The evaluation of a child's current dental status begins with age-appropriate history gathering regarding the child's current practices. Data should be accumulated to assess risk for caries (Table 12-1). Fixed events such as known decay, special healthcare needs, low socioeconomic status, and familial history of caries raise the child's overall assessed risk for developing decay and should be noted in early life. However, mutable practices such as the use of a dental home, exposure to fluoride, exposure to simple sugars, and frequency of brushing are potentially modifiable by behavioral intervention and are critical to assess with every health supervision visit. In addition, sucking habits, including bottle, pacifier, and thumb, should be addressed to evaluate for the risk of malocclusion.

Once historical risk factors for poor dentition have been assessed, the pediatric provider should perform a physical screening as part of the general physical examination. The oral screening is different from a formal dental examination: The former is meant to assess for risk factors; the latter provides specific diagnoses. The screening should be conducted with the child feeling comfortable and safe, preferably on the lap of the primary caregiver at younger ages and with the primary caregiver close by for older children. Projection of a calm demeanor and use of distraction techniques will help to smooth the examination. With a gloved hand, the provider should palpate the outside of the mouth and then lift the lips away from the surface of the teeth to examine the teeth and gum line and to palpate the gum line. Using a tongue depressor, or a mirror if available, the provider can encourage the child to open his or her mouth in order to examine the facing surfaces of the molars, if any, and the inner surfaces of the teeth.

Teeth form, erupt, and exfoliate predictably (Fig. 12-1), and the provider should assess this timing. In addition, the provider should be alert for signs of caries, including both overt cavities and the demineralized (chalky white) areas that may form initially. The provider should be on alert for discolored, abnormally shaped, or traumatized teeth; plaque formation; and signs of current infection (such as dental abscess).

As the enamel is forming, during late pregnancy and early infancy, it is very sensitive to systemic changes in the child, such as temperature changes or nutritional changes. Like the rings of a tree, the enamel records these changes that then become hypoplastic defects or hypocalcified areas within the enamel (Fig. 12-2). Enamel hypoplasia, a defect in the maturation process that results in voids in the enamel structure and predisposes the tooth to dental caries, is common in children with low birth weight or systemic illness in the neonatal period. There is considerable presumptive evidence that malnutrition or undernutrition during this period causes hypoplasia. A consistent association exists between clinical hypoplasia and early childhood caries.

**TABLE 12-1 AAPD CARIES-RISK ASSESSMENT TOOL (CAT)**

| | Risk Indicators | | |
|---|---|---|---|
| **Risk Factors to Consider** | ***High*** | ***Moderate*** | ***Low*** |
| (For each item below, circle the most accurate response found to the right under "Risk Indicators") | | | |
| **Part 1. History (Determined by Interviewing the Parent/Primary Caregiver)** | | | |
| Child has special health care needs, especially any that impact motor coordination or cooperation[a] | Yes | | No |
| Child has condition that impairs saliva (dry mouth)[b] | Yes | | No |
| Child's use of dental home (frequency of routine dental visits) | None | Irregular | Regular |
| Child has decay | Yes | | No |
| Time lapsed since child's last cavity | < 12 mo | 12–24 mo | > 24 mo |
| Child wears braces or orthodontic/oral appliances[c] | Yes | | No |
| Child's parent and/or sibling(s) have decay | Yes | | No |
| Socioeconomic status of child's parent[d] | Low | Midlevel | High |
| Daily between-meal exposures to sugars/cavity-producing foods (includes on-demand use of bottle/sippy cup containing liquid other than water; consumption of juice, carbonated beverages, or sports drinks; use of sweetened medications)[e] | > 3 | 1–2 | Mealtime only |
| Child's exposure to fluoride[f,g] | Does not use fluoridated toothpaste; drinking water is not fluoridated and is not taking fluoride supplements | Uses fluoridated toothpaste; usually does not drink fluoridated water and does not take fluoride supplements | Uses fluoridated toothpaste; drinks fluoridated water or takes fluoride supplements |
| Times per day that child's teeth/gums are brushed | < 1 | 1 | 2–3 |
| **Part 2. Clinical Evaluation (Determined By Examining the Child's Mouth)** | | | |
| Visible plaque (white, sticky buildup) | Present | | Absent |
| Gingivitis (red, puffy gums)[h] | Present | | Absent |
| Areas of enamel demineralization (chalky white spots on teeth) | More than 1 | 1 | None |
| Enamel defects, deep pits/fissures[i] | Present | | Absent |
| **Part 3. Supplemental Professional Assessment (Optional)[j]** | | | |
| Radiographic enamel caries | Present | | Absent |
| Levels of *S. mutans* or *Lactobacillus* | High | Moderate | Low |
| *Each child's overall assessed risk for developing decay is based on the highest level of risk indicator circled above (ie, a single risk indicator in any area of the "high risk" category classifies a child as being high risk).* | | | |

[a]Children with special healthcare needs are those who have a physical, developmental, mental, sensory, behavioral, cognitive, or emotional impairment or limiting condition that requires medical management, healthcare intervention, and/or use of specialized services. The condition may be developmental or acquired and may cause limitations in performing daily self-maintenance activities or substantial limitations in a major life activity. Health care for special needs patients is beyond that considered routine and requires specialized knowledge, increased awareness and attention, and accommodation.

[b]Alteration in salivary flow can be the result of congenital or acquired conditions, surgery, radiation, medication, or age-related changes in salivary function. Any condition, treatment, or process known or reported to alter saliva flow should be considered an indication of risk unless proven otherwise.

[c]Orthodontic appliances include both fixed and removable appliances, space maintainers, and other devices that remain in the mouth continuously or for prolonged time intervals and which may trap food and plaque, prevent oral hygiene, compromise access of tooth surfaces to fluoride, or otherwise create an environment supporting caries initiation.

[d]National surveys have demonstrated that children in low-income and moderate-income households are more likely to have caries and more decayed or filled primary teeth than children from more affluent households. Also, within income levels, minority children are more likely to have caries. Thus, socioeconomic status should be viewed as an initial indicator of risk that may be offset by the absence of other risk indicators.

[e]Examples of sources of simple sugars include carbonated beverages, cookies, cake, candy, cereal, potato chips, french fries, corn chips, pretzels, breads, juices, and fruits. Clinicians using caries-risk assessment should investigate individual exposures to sugars known to be involved in caries initiation.

[f]Optimal systemic and topical fluoride exposure is based on use of a fluoride dentifrice and American Dental Association/American Academy of Pediatrics (AAP) guidelines for exposure to fluoride drinking water and/or supplementation.

[g]Unsupervised use of toothpaste and at-home topical fluoride products is not recommended for children unable to expectorate predictably.

[h]Although microbes responsible for gingivitis may be different from those primarily implicated in caries, the presence of gingivitis is an indicator of poor or infrequent oral hygiene practices and has been associated with caries progression.

[i]Tooth anatomy and hypoplastic defects (eg, poorly formed enamel, developmental pits) may predispose a child to develop caries.

[j]Advanced technologies such as radiographic assessment and microbiologic testing are not essential for using this tool.

Reproduced with permission from American Academy on Pediatric Dentistry Council on Clinical Affairs: Policy on use of a caries-risk assessment tool (CAT) for infants, children, and adolescents, *Pediatr Dent.* 2008-2009;30(7 Suppl):29-33.

## ANTICIPATORY GUIDANCE

The provision of oral health anticipatory guidance is a partnership between the pediatrician, the dentist, and the family. The success of this partnership can be measured by good oral hygiene, fluoride exposure, sealants, and the resulting absence of dental caries, as well as trauma prevention in the use of a mouthguard during sports.

### The Infant

Every child should begin to receive oral health risk assessments by 6 months of age from a pediatrician or a qualified healthcare professional. Infants identified as having significant risk of caries or assessed to be in one of the high-risk groups (children with special healthcare needs; children of mothers with high caries rate; children with demonstrable caries, plaque, demineralization, and/or staining; children who sleep with a bottle or breastfeed throughout the night; late-order offspring; children in families of low socioeconomic status) should be entered into an aggressive anticipatory guidance and intervention program provided by a dentist between 6 and 12 months.

Infancy is perhaps the most important time to discuss risk factors that can be altered by behavior change, such as the vertical and horizontal transmission of *Streptococcus mutans.* Horizontal transmission is the transmission of bacteria among members of a group, such as among children at day care or between siblings. Vertical transmission,

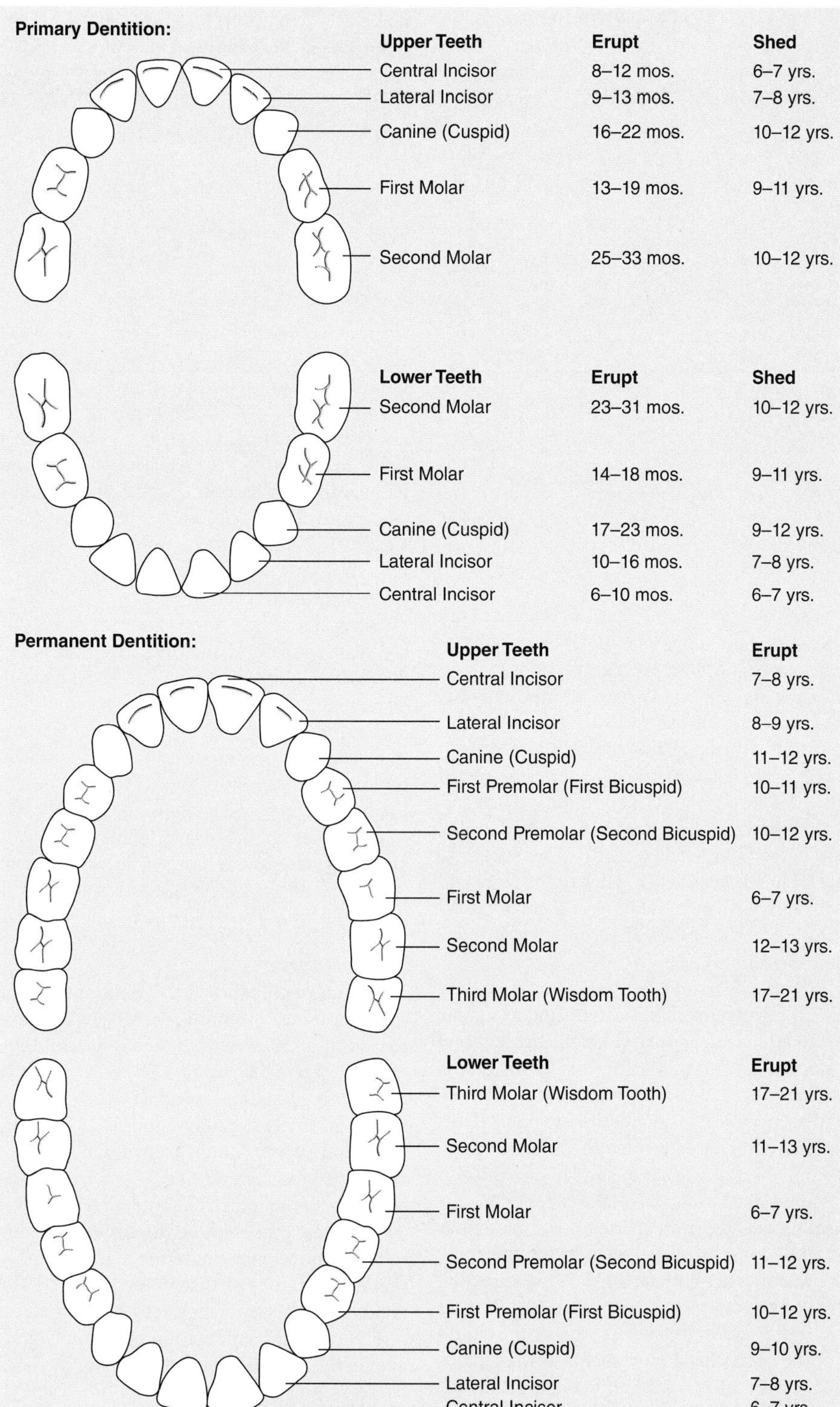


**FIGURE 12-1** Tooth eruption chart. Primary Teeth: (Reproduced with permission from ADA Division of Communications; Journal of the American Dental Association; ADA Council on Scientific Affairs: For the dental patient. Tooth eruption: The primary teeth, J Am Dent Assoc. 2005 Nov;136(11):1619. Permanent Teeth: Reproduced with permission from ADA Division of Communications; Journal of the American Dental Association; ADA Council on Scientific Affairs: For the dental patient. Tooth eruption: the permanent teeth, J Am Dent Assoc. 2006 Jan;137(1):127.)

the transfer of bacteria via the saliva from the primary caregiver to the child, occurs when a mother tests the temperature of the bottle with their own mouth, tastes the food on a spoon and then feeds the child with the same utensil, or cleans the pacifier or bottle nipple with her mouth. The mother's saliva has been shown to be the main reservoir from which infants acquire *S. mutans.* A mother with a high level of these bacteria continually recolonizes her infant when she employs such practices.

The timing of bacterial transmission is important, because acquisition of *S. mutans* before age 2 is a significant risk factor for development of early childhood caries and future dental caries. During infancy, or better still, during late pregnancy, the mother and other intimate caregivers should be counseled to reduce their *S. mutans* count by having all their own dental caries restored and by setting up a routine to brush their own teeth twice a day with fluoridated toothpaste and to floss daily. To reduce the *S. mutans* inoculum, they

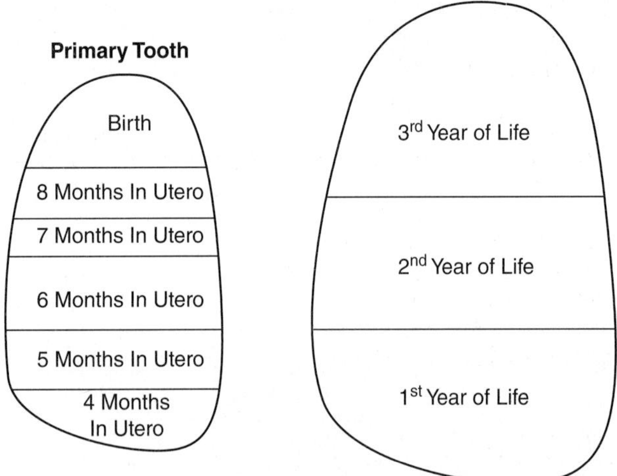


**FIGURE 12-2** Timing of enamel insult to maxillary central incisor. (Used with permission from Linda P. Nelson, DMD, MScD.)

may wish to rinse every night with an alcohol-free over-the-counter fluoride mouth rinse if they have more than 4 relatively recent fillings in their mouth or if they live in a non-fluoridated community.

Infancy is the optimal time for the family to examine their diet and eating practices. The family should eat foods containing sugar at mealtimes only, as limiting the frequency of consumption of fruit juices, candy, cookies, and cakes to mealtimes will decrease the risk of dental caries. Additionally, the family should be mindful of "sticky" foods that adhere to the teeth and thereby increase the risk of caries, such as dried fruit, rolled dry fruits, and sticky candy. If the carbohydrate sticks to the fingers and hand, it is likely to stick to the teeth and increase the risk of caries. Parents also should wean themselves off carbonated beverages. The pH of most of the soda products sold today is 3; below pH 5, *S. mutans* thrives.

Predentate children can harbor *S. mutans* in the mouth at as early as 3 months old. The primary caregiver should clean the infant's gums with a clean, damp cloth after each feeding to develop the habit of oral care and reduce the *S. mutans* levels. When the first tooth erupts (Fig. 12-1), the caregiver can move on to a soft-bristled toothbrush with a very small head and a smear of fluoride toothpaste. For infants at high risk, the plain water may be replaced with a tiny smear of fluoridated toothpaste. As the child grows, either a standard toothbrush or an electric one may be used; the latter may make it easier for the child to accept dental cleaning due to prior experience with vibratory sensations. The caregiver should not brush the teeth facing the child, but rather turn the child so that they are both facing the same direction with the child either sitting on the caregiver's lap or standing in front of the caregiver, so that the adult will have a better view of the child's teeth and better control of the child's head movements. If the child is particularly squirmy, the caregiver can place the child on his or her lap so that the child is facing up with the top of the head against the adult's stomach. The caregiver should brush the teeth from the gum line to the top of the tooth, including the backside of the tooth, while rotating the brush in small circles, not horizontally. To see the gum line, the caregiver must lift the child's lip. While brushing, the caregiver should inspect the teeth for any changes, such as staining, white demineralized areas (white spot lesions), or frank caries, which often look yellow or brown and cavitated.

Infants 6 months of age and older should receive fluoride supplements based on the risk for dental caries and known level of fluoride in the infant's drinking water (Table 12-2). For families that prefer to drink bottled water, drinking a brand that adds fluoride should be considered after the child is 6 months of age. Formula should not be reconstituted with fluoridated water in infants due to a risk of receiving too much fluoride, causing fluorosis.

During this developmental period, teething is a major concern for many parents. Sore gums from teething can be reduced by giving the

**TABLE 12-2 DAILY RECOMMENDED DIETARY FLUORIDE SUPPLEMENTATION DEPENDING ON DRINKING WATER CONTENT**

| Age | <0.3 ppm | 0.3–0.6 ppm | >0.6 ppm |
|---|---|---|---|
| Birth to 6 mo | 0 | 0 | 0 |
| 6 mo to 3 y | 0.25 mg | 0 | 0 |
| 3–6 y | 0.50 mg | 0.25 mg | 0 |
| 6 y up to at least 16 y | 1.00 mg | 0.50 mg | 0 |

Reproduced with permission from American Academy of Pediatrirc Dentistry Guideline on Flouride Therapy. Reference Manual/Clinical Guidelines, 37(6):176-179, 2014 (revised).

infant a wet wash cloth to suck on, a chilled teething ring, or using a clean finger to massage the child's gum (being careful to not get bitten). Benzocaine gels are not recommended for infants.

Once the primary teeth begin to erupt, it is important to discuss not putting the infant to bed with a bottle or sippy cup with anything other than water. Also, ad libitum nocturnal breast-feeding should be avoided at this point. In addition, frequent or prolonged bottle feedings or sippy cup usage with beverages with high sugar content, such as fruit juices, soda, milk, or formula, during the day should be discouraged. These sugary fluids pool around the teeth and increase the risk for dental caries.

Nonnutritive sucking is sucking that extends beyond that needed for nourishment. It provides emotional security and is thought to be a self-calming behavior. Pacifier use is preferable to digital habits because it can be more easily disrupted. Be sure that the pacifier is not tied around the child's neck and that it is kept clean and not dipped in a sugary substance such as honey to encourage sucking. Again, to discourage colonization of *S. mutans,* the caregiver should not clean the pacifier by placing it in his or her own mouth.

Anticipatory guidance in infancy also includes placing the dentist's emergency telephone contact information in a highly visible place. As infants become mobile, tooth trauma is a common result of falls. Avulsed primary teeth should not be reimplanted.

### The Preschooler

Anticipatory guidance at this developmental age includes all the relevant recommendations for infancy if they have not been reviewed with the family at prior visits. By age 3, the child should be using a pea-sized amount of fluoridated toothpaste when brushing. Monitoring the use of fluoride-containing products, including toothpaste, may help prevent ingestion of excessive amounts of fluoride that cause fluorosis. The child's teeth should be brushed twice a day, after breakfast and before bed, because *S. mutans* can recolonize every 24 hours. Infants and preschool children should have their teeth brushed by an adult. Young preschool children do not have the fine motor skills necessary to brush, nor do they have the object permanence to brush back teeth that they cannot visualize in the mirror. The rule of thumb is that if a child can tie his own shoelaces, he can independently brush his teeth.

Fluoride supplementation based on risk of developing tooth decay and on the known level of fluoride in the child's drinking water should be reexamined during this period (Table 12-2). The family's diet should be reviewed again for frequency of juice and soda consumption as well as for frequent consumption of foods high in sugar, especially candy, cookies, cake, and sticky carbohydrates, such as dried fruits and rolled dried fruits. The child should be encouraged to drink from a cup at this age.

Injury prevention should be reviewed with parents of preschoolers. They should be aware that injuries to the face and mouth are common at this age. Because of the risk of harm to the permanent tooth, they should never reimplant a primary tooth.

### The School-Aged Child

At this age, anticipatory guidance for oral health includes discussion with the child. The child should be well entrenched in a dental home by now and should be seeing the dentist twice a year or more frequently depending on the risk factors for dental caries. At this age, the child may experience the discomfort of tooth eruption as the permanent teeth erupt and primary (baby) teeth begin to exfoliate.

The dentist will begin to place sealants on the permanent molars as they erupt into the mouth.

The child should be brushing his or her own teeth twice a day, after breakfast and before bed, with a pea-sized amount of fluoridated toothpaste. If the child cannot tie shoelaces at this age, the parent should continue to brush the child's teeth until those fine motor skills have developed. The child may be placed on a supplemental fluoride rinse if they are found to be at high risk for dental caries. Oral fluoride supplementation still depends on the fluoride content of the water that the child drinks, whether it is from a community water source or from bottled water (Table 12-2).

The dietary recommendations from infancy and preschool development are still important, but school vending machines become an important discussion point. The child should be encouraged to choose water or milk rather than sweetened fruit drink or soda. If the child enjoys chewing gum, xylitol (sugar substitute) gum has been shown with varying results to reduce dental caries by lowering the plaque index scores.

Most children will have discontinued nonnutritive sucking on their own by this age. The eruption of the anterior permanent teeth makes nonnutritive sucking less enjoyable. If the child has not stopped nonnutritive sucking by the time the permanent anterior teeth are erupting, discussions about helping the child discontinue the habit should begin. If the child wants help to stop the habit, a positive reinforcement system can be used, such as stars on a calendar for every night the child does not suck his or her thumb before bed. On the first night, the child gets a star for 1 minute of not sucking his or her thumb; every 3 nights, the duration is increased by 1 minute. The reward for a week of consecutive stars should be something motivating to the child. Usually, by the time the child has reached 5 minutes of non–thumb sucking, he or she will have stopped the habit if the parent has been consistent in the criteria for awarding the star. If a reward system does not work and the child and family wish additional help, an orthodontic appliance can be fabricated. In severe and very prolonged cases of nonnutritive sucking, a psychological consult may be necessary.

Discussions about preventive orthodontics may be introduced as a form of injury prevention. Very protrusive maxillary incisors place the child at great risk for dental trauma. Interceptive or phase I orthodontics may be indicated to reduce the protrusion, known as overjet. The parent should know how to handle oral injuries. At this age, fractured anterior teeth are very common. The use of mouthguards when participating in all contact sports and physical activities that could result in trauma to the mouth must have occurred by this age. A boil and bite–type of mouthguard can be used, or the dentist can fabricate a custom-made mouthguard for the child. The annual cost of sports-related injuries sustained by school-aged children has been estimated to be $1.8 billion.

Infants and children exposed to environmental tobacco smoke have higher rates of caries in the primary dentition. Thus, the dangers of cigarette smoking and chewing tobacco should be discussed with the child and parents.

#### The Adolescent

At this age, the discussion may involve only the adolescent or may include the parents. All of the previously mentioned anticipatory guidance issues still should be discussed as necessary, but the use of mouthguards should be reinforced at this age for contact sports or for any physical activity that could result in trauma to the mouth. The frequent intake of soda and/or sports drinks throughout the day is seen frequently in this age group and accounts for a spike in dental caries formation. Early adolescence is also the time when many children engage in active orthodontic treatment, increasing their risk for developing caries. Good oral hygiene during this period is of utmost importance. Supplemental fluoride is often prescribed during active orthodontic treatment as a preventive modality. The adolescent can also benefit from continuing oral fluoride supplementation throughout the teenage years and into early adulthood as part of the framework of positive youth development.

The adolescent should be counseled on the dangers of oral piercings, which can damage the tongue and gums. It is not unusual to see lingual gingival recession in an adolescent with tongue piercing when the adolescent rolls the pierced object against the lower front teeth. Thus, tongue piercing may predispose the adolescent to future localized gingival disease on the lingual aspects of the mandibular incisors. Additionally, oral piercings of the tongue, lips, cheeks, and uvula have been associated with pathological conditions of pain, infection, scar formation, tooth fractures, metal hypersensitivity reactions, speech impediment, and nerve damage.

Through news stories and advertisements, adolescents are becoming more aware of the advances in cosmetic dentistry and may request information on whitening or dental bleaching of the teeth. Dental whitening may be achieved by using either professional or at-home (gels, whitening strips, or brush-on agents) bleaching modalities. Most of the research on bleaching has been performed on adult patients; very little data has been accumulated using child or adolescent patients. The more common side effects associated with bleaching vital (non–root-canal treated) teeth are tooth sensitivity and tissue irritation. Sensitivity affects 8% to 66% of patients and often occurs during early stages of treatment. Both sensitivity and tissue irritation are temporary and cease with the discontinuation of treatment. If tooth whitening is initiated too early, when the teeth are still erupting, the result may be mismatched coloration. The adolescent should consult with the dentist before using any bleaching product to determine the right product and timing of dental whitening.

Smoking and smokeless tobacco use almost always are initiated during adolescence. Oral consequences of smoking and using smokeless tobacco include oral cancer, periodontal disease, and poor wound healing. Avoidance or cessation of all forms of tobacco use, including cigarettes, pipes, cigars, smokeless tobacco, and alternative nicotine delivery systems (ANDS) such as nicotine lozenges, nicotine water, nicotine lollipops, or "heated tobacco" cigarette substitutes, should be discussed with adolescents.

If the adolescent has been seeing a pediatric dentist, discussions about transitioning to an adult or family dentist should begin during late adolescence. This transition can be difficult for both the provider and the patient after a multiyear relationship. This is especially true for children with special healthcare needs, when there may be few providers who feel comfortable dealing with persons with special healthcare needs and a dearth of providers willing to accept state-funded dental insurance.

## TREATMENT AND REFERRAL

In-office treatment by pediatric providers is limited. If the child is between 6 months and 16 years of age and is not regularly exposed to fluoridated water, then fluoride supplementation should be prescribed using published guidelines. Pediatric providers in some areas have been trained to administer 5% sodium fluoride varnish to infants and children at moderate or high risk for caries. Administration of fluoride varnish by a pediatric provider is not, however, a substitute for referral to a dentist for establishment of a dental home.

Every infant, child, adolescent, and child with special healthcare needs should have a dental home. The American Academy of Pediatric Dentistry has adopted the concept of a dental home, derived from the AAP's definition of a medical home. A dental home is a comprehensive, individualized preventive dental health program based on risk assessment, established by 12 months of age, that provides periodic supervision, anticipatory guidance, plans for acute dental trauma, and referrals to dental specialists when care cannot be provided within the dental home. Strong clinical evidence exists for the efficacy of early professional dental care complemented with caries-risk assessment, anticipatory guidance, and periodic supervision. Children should be referred to a dental home as early as 6 months of age, 6 months after the eruption of the first tooth, and no later than 1 year of age. Although trained dentists generally see children in their offices, many defer the first visit until 3 years of age. In contrast, a pediatric dentist has undergone a minimum of 2 years of specialty training in an accredited program with a standardized curriculum and will see children of any age. Care frequency will be at the discretion of the dentist, will depend on the caries risk assessment and need for treatment, and will be no less than twice per year.

## SUGGESTED READINGS


Adirim T, Cheng T. Overview of injuries in the young athlete. *Sports Med.* 2003;33(1):75-81.

American Academy of Pediatric Dentistry. Policy on dental bleaching for child and adolescent patients. *Pediatr Dent.* 2007;29(suppl): 59-61.

American Academy of Pediatric Dentistry. Policy on early childhood caries (ECC): classification, consequences, and preventive strategies. *Pediatr Dent.* 2007;29(suppl):39-41.

American Academy of Pediatric Dentistry. Policy on intraoral and perioral piercing. *Pediatr Dent.* 2007;29(suppl):54-55.

American Academy of Pediatric Dentistry. Policy on tobacco use. *Pediatr Dent.* 2007;29(suppl):51-53.

American Academy of Pediatric Dentistry. Policy on use of a caries-risk assessment tool (CAT) for infants, children, and adolescents. *Pediatr Dent.* 2007;29(suppl):29-33.

American Academy of Pediatric Dentistry. Policy on use of fluoride. *Pediatr Dent.* 2007;29(suppl):34-35.

Berkowitz RJ. Mutans streptococci: acquisition and transmission. *Pediatr Dent.* 2006;28:106-109.

Dye BA, Tan S, Smith V, et al. Trends in oral health status: United States, 1988–1994 and 1999–2004. National Center for Health Statistics. *Vital Health Stat.* 2007;11(248).

Hagan JF, Shaw JS, Duncan PM, eds. *Bright Futures: Guidelines for Health Supervision of Infants, Children, and Adolescents.* 3rd ed. Elk Grove Village, IL: American Academy of Pediatrics; 2008.

Section on Pediatric Dentistry. American Academy of Pediatrics Policy Statement. Oral health risk assessment timing and establishment of the dental home. *Pediatrics.* 2003;111(5):1113-1116.

Seow WK, Humphrys C, Tudehope DI. Increased prevalence of developmental defects in low-birthweight children: a controlled study. *Pediatr Dent.* 1987;9:221-225.


# 13 Complementary and Integrative Pediatrics

Anju Sawni and Sanghamitra M. Misra

## INTRODUCTION

Integrative medicine (IM) is a newly emerging field of comprehensive healthcare that emphasizes wellness and healing of the whole person with a focus on mental and spiritual health. It is the integration into mainstream medicine of complementary therapies for which there is evidence of safety and effectiveness. Integrative physicians strengthen the physician–patient relationship and empower the patient. The Academic Consortium for Integrative Medicine and Health, which consists of 56 academic medical centers, defines IM as "the practice of medicine that reaffirms the importance of the relationship between practitioner and patient, focuses on the whole person, is informed by evidence, and makes use of all appropriate therapeutic approaches, healthcare professionals and disciplines to achieve optimal health and healing." This concept is illustrated in Figure 13-1.

The knowledge and use of complementary and alternative medicine (CAM) is an important aspect of IM. CAM refers to a large range of therapies outside the domain of mainstream conventional/Western medicine that are used for the purpose of medical intervention, health promotion, and disease prevention. CAM includes therapies such

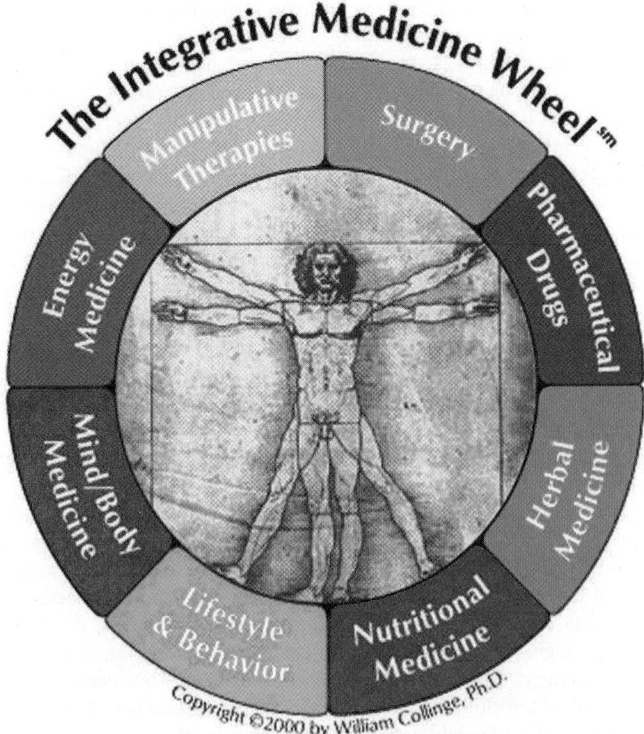


**FIGURE 13-1** The integrative medicine wheel. (Used with permission from William Collinge, PhD.)

as alternative/whole medical systems (homeopathy, naturopathy, Ayurveda, and traditional Chinese medicine), mind-body interventions (meditation, prayer for healing, biofeedback, yoga, and art and music therapy), biologically based therapies (megavitamins, nutritional supplements, and herbs), manipulative and body-based methods (chiropractic manipulations, osteopathy, and massage), and energy therapies (Reiki and Therapeutic Touch).

With increasing interest in the integration of CAM therapies into conventional pediatrics, a more appropriate term of pediatric integrative medicine (PIM) has emerged. Interestingly, the growing trend in conventional medicine toward the patient and family–centered medical home, with a focus on prevention and health promotions of the whole child, is the core of PIM.

The pediatric medical landscape has evolved over the last 20 years primarily due to increasing prevalence of complex and chronic conditions such as diabetes, autism, attention-deficit disorder, asthma, obesity, cancer, chronic pain, and depression/anxiety. Many pediatricians are developing interest in learning new skills and embracing new therapies to better care for these complex patients. The current conventional biomedical model of treating illness is not very effective in preventing the development of disease or in altering the course of chronic physical illness. In fact, the current model does not adequately address the mental, emotional, and spiritual needs of an individual. As pediatricians are becoming more aware of the need for holistic care, a trend toward the integration of CAM therapies within the practice of conventional medicine is occurring. Children's hospitals are commonly offering CAM therapies, health insurances are covering such therapies, and a growing number of physicians are using CAM therapies in their practices. IM centers and clinics are being established, many with close ties to medical schools and teaching hospitals.

As a result of increasing interest in CAM and the realization of our limited understanding of these modalities, the National Center for Complementary and Integrative Health (NCCIH), a sub-office of the National Institutes of Health (NIH), was established by a mandate in 1998 to facilitate and conduct research and education on complementary and integrative health approaches. The NCCIH generally uses the term "complementary health approaches" to discuss practices and products of nonmainstream origin and uses "integrative health" when incorporating complementary health approaches into mainstream medicine.

The use of complementary health approaches is common among children and adolescents in the United States. The 2007 and 2012 National Health Interview Surveys (NHIS), conducted by the Centers for Disease Control and Prevention's (CDC) National Center for Health Statistics (NCHS), of parents of 17,300 children ages 4–17 years, found that approximately 12% of children used some form of complementary health approaches. The most commonly used complementary health approach in children were natural products (dietary supplements other than vitamins and minerals), and pain was the most common condition for which children used complementary health approaches.

Studies of CAM use in primary care and in healthy children show a prevalence of 12% to 21%. However, CAM use among children from special populations or with chronic, recurrent conditions such as cystic fibrosis, cancer, asthma, ADHD, and cerebral palsy is even higher, ranging from 11% to 80%. CAM use among parents is the number one predictor of CAM use among children. Most patients use CAM in conjunction with conventional medical care. Parents and patients generally do not use CAM because they are dissatisfied with conventional medicine. They simply consider CAM therapies to be more congruent with their own culture, values, beliefs, and philosophical orientation toward health and life. Parents may seek CAM therapies for their children because of fear of drug side effects or because they are seeking a "cure" for a chronic medical problem. Some parents hear about complementary therapies by word of mouth or get referrals from family members. Most commonly, parents desire more personal care and attention.

CAM also appears to be slowly gaining acceptance among pediatricians. Two studies performed in 2001 and 2004 of American Academy of Pediatrics' fellows found that over 80% of pediatricians had been asked about CAM by their patients. Most believed CAM therapies could enhance recovery or relieve symptoms and would consider referring for CAM. However, less than half of the pediatricians asked about CAM use it as part of routine pediatric history and over 80% wanted education on CAM so that they could counsel families appropriately.

In response to this need for more CAM education and training for pediatricians, the American Academy of Pediatrics (AAP) formed the Section on Complementary and Integrative Medicine (SOCIM) in 2005, and the section received full AAP Section status in 2009. In 2011, the section was renamed the Section on Integrative Medicine (SOIM) reflective of more appropriate nomenclature. Pediatric educators are also cognizant that training and education in PIM need to start in pediatric residency. A national survey of academic pediatric institutions in 2012 identified integrative pediatric programs at only 16 of 143 academic pediatric programs. This led to the development of a pilot curriculum embedded into conventional residency training: the Pediatric Integrative Medicine in Residency (PIMR) program, a 100-hour online curriculum created by the University of Arizona Center for Integrative Medicine.

The growing interest in PIM for pediatricians as well as the public may reflect increasing trends in the use of CAM by adults and children, growing acceptance of CAM among conventionally trained pediatricians, and an increase in the amount of information on this subject (continuing medical education courses, medical journals, research, the media, and the Internet). Pediatricians are reacting by becoming more aware of CAM therapies and by having open discussions about complementary health approaches with their patients/families. Patients are increasingly seeking pediatricians who are knowledgeable about both conventional medicine and CAM. Pediatricians recognize this and are requesting more education in PIM from leaders in the field. Pediatricians need not be experts on every CAM therapy and product or seek specialized training, nor should they reject their conventional biomedical training. However, pediatricians need to be knowledgeable and comfortable in communicating about PIM. Many medical schools and postgraduate medical training centers are developing new competencies regarding CAM that include inquiring about CAM use, counseling on CAM from an evidence-based approach, and referring to and partnering with CAM practitioners. IM is now recognized as a medical specialty with board certification through the American Board of Integrative Medicine.

This next section describes CAM modalities, provides some evidence-based approaches to CAM, and suggests how to counsel about and refer for CAM.

## MIND-BODY MEDICINE

Mind-body medicine is a philosophy and a system of health practices based on the concept that the mind and the body work together for healing. Mind-body medicine includes modalities such as meditation and relaxation training, guided imagery, self-hypnosis, yoga, art and music therapy, biofeedback, prayer, and tai chi. Children suffering from chronic medical problems can benefit from mind-body therapies to help with symptoms like pain and anxiety. In addition, children experiencing emotional stress who complain of chronic physical symptoms often respond poorly to medications. Evidence suggests that higher cognitive centers and limbic emotional centers are capable of regulating virtually all aspects of the immune system and therefore have a profound effect on health and illness. The autonomic nervous system and the hormonal system can generate a wide variety of messages that can modulate the immune system. Mind-body approaches can improve quality of life by reducing stress and symptom burden, and also may improve self-monitoring and coping skills. The physical and emotional risk of using these techniques is minimal, cost is low, and many techniques can be taught by paraprofessionals. Most can easily be applied along with conventional medical care. Mind-body therapies have been shown to be safe and effective for many pediatric conditions, including headaches, asthma, enuresis, sleep disorders, pain, and stress-related conditions.

### Meditation and Yoga

Meditation is a self-directed practice for relaxing the body and stilling the mind. It is a form of concentration that nurtures the development of focused attention and personal awareness. Nearly all religions include some form of meditative practice. Examples of meditations include transcendental meditation, Tibetan meditation, mindfulness meditation (being in the moment), and walking meditation. Teaching children approaches that calm the mind has shown to be helpful in a variety of conditions such as attention-deficit/hyperactivity disorder (ADHD) and mood disorders.

Yoga is an ancient practice from India that aims to unify body and mind with universal spirit, thereby encouraging physical and mental well-being. Yoga seeks to alter the body's physiology through breathing techniques, postures, and meditation, which activate the parasympathetic autonomic system and decrease the sympathetic system. An increase in parasympathetic activity leads to a decrease in blood pressure, heart rate, and respiratory rate and an increase in galvanic skin resistance, as well as providing psychological benefits such as improved concentration, mood, memory, self-actualization, and cognitive functions. Research studies have shown yoga's benefit in improving cognitive functions, heart rate, and mental focus in children specifically with chronic conditions such as ADHD, asthma, and sickle cell disease. Evidence also shows that school curricula incorporating yoga along with stress management programs improve academic performance, self-esteem, classroom behaviors, concentration, and emotional balance. The central nervous system effects, as well as yoga's perceived benefits in stress reduction and improved concentration, provide the rationale for yoga as a treatment modality. Meditation and yoga classes are now readily available for children in schools, summer camps, after-school programs, and yoga studios. Yoga Alliance, a national credentialing organization for yoga teachers, ensures a set of educational standards for yoga schools. A minimum of 200 hours of training is needed for beginner teacher certification and many experienced yoga teachers have over 500 hours of training.

### Hypnosis

Self-hypnosis is an altered state of consciousness within a relaxed physical state of intense, focused concentration aimed at improving mental or physical health. It is an internal, imaginative process (using the imagination to see, hear, touch, smell, and taste things) to focus attention and become absorbed so that a hypnotic state is entered. In this altered state, perceptions and sensations can be enhanced, modified, or changed to decrease anxiety, stress, or discomfort and to increase self-esteem. All hypnosis is self-hypnosis. When taught by a trained facilitator, clinical hypnosis has 6 stages: introduction, induction, intensification, therapeutic suggestion, re-alerting, and debriefing. School-aged children and adolescents enter into the hypnotic trance far more easily and rapidly than adults. Hypnotherapy allows a child to gain a sense of control, increase self-esteem and competence, and reduce stress. Children usually readily accept therapeutic suggestions, and hypnosis bridges the child's inner world of imagination and therapeutic change. Self-hypnosis is a teachable coping skill that most children are able to learn with minor effort. Hypnosis can be useful in treating pain (chronic pain related to diseases such as malignancy, sickle cell disease, chronic headaches, abdominal pain, or acute pain associated with procedures such as lumbar puncture, needle sticks, suturing, and injuries), behavioral problems (tics, habit problems, enuresis, encopresis, smoking, weight control, nightmares, ADHD), anxiety associated with procedures or illness, performance anxiety (tests, athletes), and nausea and vomiting. Hypnosis is considered safe when implemented by a skilled practitioner. There are two organizations that teach clinical hypnosis in children: the American Society of Clinical Hypnosis (ASCH) and the National Pediatric Hypnosis Training Institute (NPHTI). Both have a certification program of training for licensed healthcare workers.

Hypnotherapy's benefits can be enhanced by the use of biofeedback to induce physiological changes. Biofeedback is a mind-body therapy that uses visual and auditory stimuli to give the participant information about autonomic nervous system functions (heart rate, blood pressure, skin temperature, muscle contraction) using a computerized feedback system. Children's ready acceptance of suggestion and the ease of mobilizing physiologic responses into a computerized feedback system make these modalities appealing, and this positive feedback helps them improve more rapidly. The Biofeedback Certification International Alliance (BCIA) is the certification body for the clinical practice of biofeedback and regionally accredited institutions in the United States have adopted the BCIA blueprints of knowledge for standardization. There are 13 accredited schools of biofeedback in the United States. Some insurance companies now cover biofeedback.

By using mind-body techniques such as self-hypnosis, relaxation, meditation, and yoga, children and adolescents can be taught to self-manage anxiety, boost self-esteem, and increase their capacity to focus.

#### Spirituality

Spirituality is considered to be a person's sense of connection to a higher being. It may or may not involve formal religion. The discussion of spirituality and religiosity in pediatrics often focuses on parents' beliefs and not on the beliefs of the child or adolescent. Children often have strong beliefs about a religion, God, and spirituality. However, extent of belief and regularity of practices such as prayer vary widely among pediatric patients. Prayer is a way to communicate directly with a spiritual energy or higher being. Children with chronic conditions are often strongly connected with God or a higher being. Prayer can help pediatric patients find an inner sense of meaning, and it may strengthen their belief in a higher being. Strong spiritual connections may be associated with better coping, faster recovery, and better quality of life. Interestingly, most pediatricians believe that spirituality impacts illness but few ask their patients about it.

#### Creative Arts Therapy

Creative arts therapies include therapies such as art therapy, dance and movement therapy, drama therapy, music therapy, poetry therapy, and psychodrama. These therapies use art modalities in therapeutic, rehabilitative, community, hospital, and educational settings to foster health, communication, and expression. These therapies strengthen the mind-body connection and improve relaxation by promoting the integration of physical, cognitive, and social functioning as well as emotional self-awareness. Music therapy is an example of a creative arts intervention that can be integrated into daily or weekly activities, and that may be beneficial for children, who naturally respond to music and rhythm. Music therapy has been studied extensively and has been shown to be beneficial in premature infants. Music therapy is utilized in pediatric patients with conditions such as cancer, autism spectrum disorders, pain, and ADHD; it is also used for preoperative and postoperative anxiety.

### MANIPULATIVE AND BODY-BASED PRACTICES

Manipulative and body-based practices such as chiropractic, osteopathy, massage, and reflexology incorporate physical touch and focus on the structures and systems of the body, including the bones, joints, soft tissues, and circulatory and lymphatic systems. These practices are based on the principle that the human body is self-regulating and has the ability to heal itself and that all parts of the human body are interdependent.

#### Massage

Massage therapy (the laying on of hands for health purposes) is used all over the world and dates back thousands of years. Massage involves manipulation, compression, and stretching of the skin, muscle, and joints, and activates a variety of mechanisms that lead to enhanced blood flow to the muscles and soft tissues and also enhanced lymphatic flow to create a sense of well-being. There are various forms of massage techniques including Swedish massage, deep-tissue massage, trigger-point massage, and shiatsu massage. It can also include many different techniques such as Rolfing, movement integration (Feldenkrais method, Alexander Technique), pressure-point techniques (acupressure), cranial sacral therapy, reflexology, and many others.

Massage is used to promote relaxation and to reduce stress. Clinical studies of selected physiological parameters suggest that massage can alter various neurochemical, hormonal, and immune markers. Several studies in infants and children have shown benefits of massage therapies for various conditions such as ADHD, cystic fibrosis, and asthma. Massage therapy has also been shown to improve weight gain in premature infants, decrease pain and anxiety, and enhance mood.

The massage experience is sometimes enhanced through the use of clinical aromatherapy, which is the therapeutic application of oils distilled from plants. Topical oils that enhance blood flow and engender a sense of warmth (called rubefacients) are also often used. Massage may be provided by parents or other family members as well as by professional massage therapists. Massage therapists are regulated in most states in the form of a license, registration, or certification. Cities, counties, or other local governments also may regulate massage therapists. Massage therapists are licensed in 40 states. The largest professional national organization of body workers and massage therapists is the American Massage Therapy Association (AMTA), and therapists may choose to become board certified in massage therapy. Membership in AMTA requires a minimum of 500 hours of supervised, in-class massage therapy training including anatomy and physiology from an accredited school. Most massage therapy visits last approximately one hour and are rarely covered by insurance, although some massage therapies are incorporated into physical rehabilitation medicine.

#### Osteopathy and Chiropractic

Doctors of osteopathy (DOs) are mainstream physicians and are fully licensed in all 50 states to practice medicine (prescribe drugs, perform surgery) but are also trained in musculoskeletal manipulation. Osteopathic philosophy is holistic; focuses on the mind, body, and spirit; and emphasizes the promotion of health and illness prevention. On a musculoskeletal level, osteopaths are primarily concerned with barriers to normal physiologic motion. The American Association of Colleges of Osteopathic Medicine represents the 33 accredited colleges of osteopathic medicine teaching at 48 locations in 31 states in the United States.

Doctors of chiropractic (DCs) are trained only in chiropractic spinal manipulation and do not prescribe drugs or do surgery.

Chiropractic is based on the belief that spinal problems are the cause of health problems and that spinal manipulations ("adjustments") can restore and maintain health. According to chiropractic concepts, the nervous system coordinates all of the body's functions, and disease results from a lack of normal nerve function due to displacement (subluxation) of a spinal vertebral body. This subluxation, misalignment, and nerve pressure can cause problems not only in the local area but also at some distance from it.

Chiropractors are the most commonly utilized CAM practitioners in the United States. According to the 2007 NHIS, more than 18 million adults and more than 2 million children had chiropractic or osteopathic manipulation in the past 12 months. Considerable numbers of children and adolescents receive chiropractic care for musculoskeletal conditions as well as for chronic illness such as asthma, allergies, infant colic, otitis media, and enuresis. However, there is an absence of randomized controlled clinical trials suggesting that chiropractic is a significantly helpful or cost-effective therapy for any major pediatric disease. Chiropractors tend to take few radiographs of children and use lighter force when making adjustments. Some adult studies suggest that chiropractic manipulation may be beneficial for acute back pain. Although serious adverse events (AEs) are rare, and much less common than medication-related adverse events, mild to moderate AEs that are self-limited have been associated with spinal manipulation in children. Further studies are necessary to determine the safety and benefits of chiropractic care in children.

The United States, Canada, and many European countries have accredited postgraduate degrees to obtain a DC. The profession is regulated and chiropractors are licensed in all 50 states. The Council on Chiropractic Education (CCE) sets minimum guidelines for the 18 chiropractic colleges in the United States.

## ENERGY HEALING THERAPIES

Energy healing therapies are based on the concept that human beings are infused with a subtle form of biophysical energy. These include therapies such as Healing Touch, Therapeutic Touch, reiki, qigong, and acupressure/acupuncture. This vital energy or life force is known by different names in different cultures such as *qi* (chi) in Chinese medicine, *ki* in the Japanese Kampo system, *doshas/prana* in Ayurvedic medicine, etheric energy, and energy or life force. Therapists believe that they can work with this subtle energy, see it with their own eyes, and use it to effect changes and influence health in the physical body. Practitioners of energy medicine theorize that illness results from disturbances of the biofield, which is an energy field that is proposed to surround and flow throughout the human body. Biofields have not been measured by conventional instruments. Healing or Therapeutic Touch, reiki, and qigong are examples of therapies that involve movement of the practitioner's hands over the patient's body to become attuned to the condition of the patient, with the idea that by so doing, the practitioner can strengthen and reorient the patient's energies. Even though energy therapies are among the most controversial of CAM practices, because neither the external energy fields nor their therapeutic effects have been demonstrated convincingly by any biophysical means, they are gaining popularity in the United States. Acupuncture, which could be considered a variant of energy therapy, is discussed later in this chapter.

Therapeutic Touch was developed in the 1970s by Dolores Krieger, a nurse, and Dora Kunz, a lay healer. It is taught in nursing schools and in many hospitals, including children's hospitals, in the United States. Therapeutic Touch has shown potential efficacy for wound healing, osteoarthritis, migraine headaches, and anxiety in burn patients.

Reiki, an energy practice similar to Therapeutic Touch, comes from a Japanese tradition based on a belief that an invisible energy may be transmitted from healer to patient through intention; the energy is focused by placing the hands on particular parts of the patient's body or even from distant healing through intention. Practitioners are trained by a reiki master through apprenticeship and spiritual/energetic initiation. Neither Therapeutic Touch nor reiki have national certifying examinations or state licensure. Therapeutic Touch is taught in more than 70 US nursing schools and medical schools in almost 100 countries. Credentialing for Therapeutic Touch is provided through Therapeutic Touch International Association. Reiki practitioners are trained by a reiki master and are apprenticed. While there are no good studies evaluating the effectiveness of these energy therapies, there are no reported side effects from such treatments.

## WHOLE MEDICAL SYSTEMS

Whole medical systems, as defined by the NCCIH, are complete systems of theory and practice that have evolved independently from or parallel to allopathic (conventional) medicine. Many are traditional systems of medicine that are practiced by individual cultures throughout the world. Major Eastern whole medical systems include traditional Chinese medicine (TCM) and Ayurvedic medicine (a whole medical system that originated in India). Major Western whole medical systems include homeopathy and naturopathy (both originated in Europe). Other systems have been developed by Native American, African, Middle Eastern, Tibetan, and Central and South American cultures.

### Homeopathy

Homeopathy is a whole medical system that was founded by a German physician, Samuel Christian Hahnemann (1755–1843), in the late 18th and early 19th centuries. Homeopathy is based on 2 principles: (1) the Law of Similars or "like cures like" and (2) the Law of Dilutions. The Law of Similars states that a remedy that would cause a symptom in a healthy person is used to treat the same symptom in a sick person: "like cures like." Hahnemann proceeded to give repeated doses of many common remedies to healthy volunteers and carefully recorded the symptoms they produced. This procedure is called a "proving" or, in modern homeopathy, a "human pathogenic trial." As a result of this experience, Hahnemann developed his treatments for sick patients by matching the symptoms produced by a drug to symptoms in sick patients. For example, a treatment (remedy) made from an onion skin (*Allium cepa*) might be used to treat a child with rhinorrhea and watery eyes from either allergies or a cold.

Homeopathic remedies are made from plant, animal, and mineral substances that are diluted to extremely small doses such that only the "medicinal energy," and not the actual substance, remains in the end product. This is based on the second principle, the Law of Dilutions, which states that the more a remedy is diluted, the more powerful it becomes. This is counter-intuitive to conventional medications, where the larger the dose, the more powerful the effects. In homeopathy, the most powerful remedies are ones that have been diluted hundreds, thousands, or even millions of times. Homeopathic potencies are labeled with a combination of a number and a letter. Dilutions of 1:10 are designated by the Roman numeral X (decimal method) (1X = 1/10; 3X = 1/1000; 6X = 1/1,000,000). Dilutions of 1:100 are designated by the Roman numeral C (centesimal) (1C = 1/100; 3C = 1/1,000,000; and so on). Dilutions beyond 12X or 24C do not contain any of the original molecules. Most remedies range from 6X to 30X, but some are as dilute as 200C. Serious side effects from homeopathic treatment are very rare, far less common than side effects from standard over-the-counter and prescription medications. Generally, homeopathy is considered to be safe in children. True homeopathic treatment is individualized to the unique characteristics of each patient's experience and symptoms. Homeopaths also believe that illness results from disrupted "vital energies" and these very dilute solutions contain an energy, or information, that is used by the patient to heal his or her symptoms. The appropriate remedy may cause an initial aggravation of symptoms briefly but this is regarded favorably and subsides over time. The concept of homeopathy is hard for mainstream physicians to understand and many believe that the remedies are nothing more than placebos that trigger the patient's psychoneuroimmunological healing systems.

Homeopathic remedies are available over the counter, through mail-order catalogs, and over the Internet without a prescription. Common over-the-counter remedies include combination products for colds, teething, colic, allergies, injuries, and bedwetting.

The 2012 NHIS estimated that 5 million adults and 1 million children used homeopathy in the previous year, and that although about 1.8% of children used homeopathy, only 0.2% of children visited a homeopathic practitioner. Practitioners of homeopathy are licensed in fewer than 10 states and can be lay practitioners, chiropractors, physicians, naturopaths, nurses, or other healthcare professionals. Certification is offered through the Council for Homeopathic Certification and the National Board of Homeopathic Examiners. Children and adolescents comprise between 20% and 30% of the patient load of the typical homeopathic practitioner.

**Naturopathic Medicine**

Naturopathy is a whole medical system that has its roots in Germany. The word *naturopathy* comes from Greek and Latin and literally translates as "nature disease." A central belief in naturopathy is that nature has a healing power (a principle known as *vis medicatrix naturae*). Another belief is that living organisms (including the human body) have the power to maintain (or return to) a state of balance and health and to heal themselves. Naturopathic physicians are educated and trained in a 4-year, graduate-level program in the same basic sciences as an MD, but also focus on holistic, nontoxic natural therapies and approaches to health with an emphasis on wellness and disease prevention. Graduates receive the degree of ND (Doctor of Naturopathic Medicine). Naturopathic doctors (NDs) prefer to use treatment approaches that they consider to be the most natural and least invasive, instead of using drugs and more invasive procedures. The core modalities supporting these principles include diet modification and nutritional supplements, herbal medicine, acupuncture and TCM, hydrotherapy, massage and joint manipulation, and lifestyle counseling. Naturopathy is not a complete substitute for conventional medical care. Some therapies used in naturopathy have the potential to be harmful if not used properly or under the direction of a trained practitioner. For example, herbs can cause side effects on their own and interact with prescription or over-the-counter medicines. Restrictive or other unconventional diets can be unsafe for some people. Some practitioners of naturopathy do not recommend using all or some of the childhood vaccinations that are standard practice in conventional medicine. A few studies of naturopathic remedies in children have been published with mixed results.

There are 7 accredited naturopathic medical programs and 8 campus locations in North America, and naturopathic physicians have to pass an extensive postdoctoral board examination (NPLEX) in order to receive a license. Currently, the American Association of Naturopathic Physicians lists 17 states, the District of Columbia, the US territories of Puerto Rico and the US Virgin Islands, and 5 Canadian provinces as have licensing or regulation laws for naturopathic doctors. Licensed naturopathic physicians must fulfill state-mandated continuing education requirements annually, and many states have licensing laws for naturopathic physicians with a specific scope of practice. There is no insurance coverage for naturopathic doctors; visits are paid out of pocket by families and are typically 60 to 90 minutes for an initial visit and 30 to 45 minutes for follow-up. Some families choose NDs as the only source of primary care. Children and adolescents account for 20 to 30 percent of NDs' patient loads.

**Ayurveda**

Ayurveda, which literally means "the science of life," is a natural healing system developed in India. It is a comprehensive system of medicine that places equal emphasis on the body, mind, and spirit, and strives to restore the innate harmony of the individual. Some of the primary Ayurvedic treatments include diet, exercise, yoga, meditation, herbs, massage, exposure to sunlight, and controlled breathing. Ayurveda also has some basic beliefs about the body's constitution. *Constitution* refers to a person's general health, how likely he or she is to become out of balance, and his or her ability to resist and recover from disease or other health problems. The constitution is called the *prakriti*. Three qualities called *doshas* form important characteristics of the constitution and control the activities of the body. Practitioners of Ayurveda call the *doshas* by their original Sanskrit names: *vata*, *pitta*, and *kapha*. It is also believed that each *dosha* is made up of one or two of the 5 basic elements: space, air, fire, water, and earth. Each *dosha* has a particular relationship to body functions and can become upset for different reasons. *Doshas* are constantly being formed and reformed by food, activity, and bodily processes. It is believed that a person's chances of developing certain types of diseases are related to the way *doshas* are balanced. There is very little research done on Aryuvedic medicine and its benefits in children. There are a few schools that offer 400–800 hours of training over 9–15 months, but there is no licensing body for Ayurvedic practitioners in the United States.

**Traditional Chinese Medicine**

TCM is a complete system of healing that dates back to 200 B.C. in written form. Korea, Japan, and Vietnam have all developed their own unique versions of traditional medicine based on practices originating in China. In the TCM view, the body is a delicate balance of two opposing and inseparable forces: *yin* and *yang*. *Yin* represents cold, slow, or passive aspects of the person, while *yang* represents hot, excited, or active aspects. Health is achieved through balancing *yin* and *yang*, and disease is caused by an imbalance leading to a blockage of the flow of *Qi*, which is the vital energy or life force proposed to regulate a person's spiritual, emotional, mental, and physical health and to be influenced by the opposing forces of *yin* and *yang* and of blood along pathways known as meridians. TCM practitioners typically use herbs, massage, and acupuncture to help unblock *Qi* and restore normal blood flow in patients in an attempt to bring the body back into harmony and wellness. Acupuncture is the most common form of TCM that is practiced in the United States. There are more than 50 master's programs in Oriental medicine and acupuncture in the United States. The National Certification Commission for Acupuncture and Oriental Medicine (NCCAOM) offers board certification in TCM.

**Acupuncture**

Acupuncture, a component of TCM, originated over 2000 years ago as a therapeutic treatment. Acupuncture is the stimulation of specific points on the body along the energy meridians by a variety of techniques. In the traditional Chinese system of medicine, acupuncture is intended to remove blockages in the flow of *Qi*. Disease occurs when the flow of vital energy is disrupted or blocked. Health returns when the flow is restored, balanced, and harmonized by acupuncture. It is believed that there are 12 main meridians and 8 secondary meridians, and over 2000 acupuncture points on the human body that connect these meridians. Acupuncture techniques used to stimulate these points include insertion of thin metal needles that are manipulated by the hand or by electrical stimulation, heat (moxibustion), laser, or vigorous massage (shiatsu). In the Western system of medicine, it is proposed that acupuncture produces its effects by the conduction of electromagnetic signals at a greater-than-normal rate, thus aiding the activity of pain-killing biochemicals such as endorphins and immune system cells at specific sites in the body. In addition, studies have shown that acupuncture may alter the release of neurotransmitters and neurohormones affecting the parts of the central nervous system related to sensation and involuntary body functions. This can positively affect immune reactions and processes thus regulating a person's blood pressure, blood flow, and body temperature.

Data from the 2007 NHIS found that an estimated 3.1 million US adults and 150,000 children had used acupuncture in the previous year. The NIH consensus development conference in 1997 concluded that acupuncture was effective for treating pain such as postoperative pain, chemo-related nausea, and vomiting and dental pain in adults. There is promising evidence that the use of acupuncture as an alternative or in conjunction with conventional medical care is beneficial in headaches, back pain, dysmenorrhea, fibromyalgia, myofacial pain, tennis elbow, carpal tunnel syndrome, and tendonitis. Acupuncture is used in pediatric patients as well. Nearly one-third of the major teaching hospitals with a pediatric pain service offer acupuncture to treat chronic pain in children. Most children are open and receptive to acupuncture, despite the perception that children fear needles. Many acupuncturists who treat children use special techniques, including non-needle methods (eg, heat, magnets, lasers, and vigorous massage or tapping) to stimulate points along the energy meridians.

Studies show that acupuncture has potential benefits for recurrent headaches, nausea, pain (acute and chronic), and allergy. Large systematic reviews have concluded that AEs associated with pediatric needle acupuncture are generally mild in severity. Many AEs might have been caused by substandard practice, therefore supporting that acupuncture is safe for children when performed by appropriately trained practitioners who follow detailed protocols.

In the United States, there are approximately 50 accredited acupuncture schools. The National Certification Commission for Acupuncture and Oriental Medicine (NCCAOM) is the governing body for certification. Acupuncturists are licensed in more than 43 states and the District of Columbia. Approximately 80% of licensed acupuncturists also recommend dietary changes, herbs and other supplements, and changes in lifestyle, exercise, rest, and relationships to enhance health. Acupuncture visits increasingly are covered by insurance. Thus, pediatricians are likely to see increased availability of affordable acupuncture services for their patients. Initial visit length is approximately 90 minutes and follow-up visits last approximately 30–60 minutes. Acupuncture has been demonstrated to be a reasonably safe therapy in the hands of experienced and qualified practitioners as evidenced by several large prospective studies.

## NUTRITIONAL/DIETARY SUPPLEMENTS

Herbs, vitamins, minerals, and other dietary supplements are among the most commonly used CAM therapies with use increasing over the past 20 years. According to the 2012 NHIS, natural products (nonvitamin, nonmineral dietary supplements) represented the complementary health approach most frequently used by almost 18% of adults and 5% of children with fish oils, probiotics, melatonin, and Echinacea as the most common dietary supplements used by children. Some studies indicate that 20% to 40% of children and adolescents have used dietary supplements and use is even higher in sub-populations of children, like those with chronic medical problems. Table 13-1 lists common herbs used by children and adolescents.

Integrative pediatricians and even many conventional pediatricians recommend nutritional and herbal supplements. Many neurologists recommend feverfew, butterbur, and vitamin $B_2$ to prevent migraine headaches. Neonatologists routinely use probiotics to reduce the risk of necrotizing enterocolitis (NEC). Gastroenterologists may recommend probiotics for irritable bowel syndrome, antibiotic-induced diarrhea, and inflammatory bowel disease (IBS). Research now supports that the addition of probiotics to conventional treatment may be helpful in NEC, IBS, antibiotic-induced diarrhea, constipation, and possibly asthma and eczema.

It is important that pediatricians are cognizant of the reasons families and patients use herbs (ie, part of their culture, parental beliefs about health, preventing disease, and treating chronic or acute illness). Also, with the explosion of the Internet, mass media, and multilevel marketing companies for herbs and dietary supplements, parents are inundated with information and proposed claims of herbal supplements for various medical conditions. Nutritional supplements such as vitamin C, zinc, omega-3 fatty acids (fish oils/flaxseed oil), melatonin, and probiotics are being used with increasing frequency. Multivitamins and minerals are promoted as therapies for children who have developmental disabilities, autism spectrum disorder, and Down syndrome. Fish oils, antioxidants, and herbs are marketed for children with ADHD. Adolescents commonly spend money on dietary supplements to lose weight, build strength, enhance mood, and treat acne.

Many patients take herbs, believing they are safe because they are natural. The safety and efficacy of herbal remedies remains largely unknown and many herbal remedies have been associated with adverse effects and herb-drug interactions. Some herbal remedies have been found to contain heavy metals such as lead and arsenic as well as drugs such as steroids and benzodiazepines. The Dietary Supplement Health and Education Act (DSHEA) of 1994 defined herbal medicines and supplements as neither food nor drugs. These substances are regulated by the Food and Drug Administration (FDA) but with less stringent requirements than drugs. They are not tested according to the same safety and efficacy regulations as are prescription and over-the-counter drugs. Under DSHEA, herbal supplements can be sold claiming to "stimulate, maintain, support, regulate, and promote health" rather than to treat disease. For example, an herbal supplement company can claim on a supplement bottle that the product supports bone health but not that it treats osteopenia. Supplements can only be removed from the market if the FDA can prove them unsafe under ordinary conditions of use. In 2003, the FDA proposed Good Manufacturing Practices (GMPs) for the dietary supplement industry. The proposed GMPs require that herbal medicines be properly labeled, free of adulterants, and manufactured according to specified standards for personnel and equipment. Despite this effort, there is substantial variation in the quality of herbal products in the United States and abroad and this impacts a product's efficacy and safety. The clinical usefulness of an herbal supplement for a particular patient or condition depends on its evidence for quality, efficacy, and safety. Another concern is that families do not always disclose their use of herbal/nutritional supplements to their pediatrician because they do not consider them to be medications. Therefore, it is critical that pediatricians ask specifically about herb use as part of the routine pediatric history.

Modification of a child's diet is also used commonly by families who pursue CAM approaches. Parents may have their children follow vegetarian, vegan, macrobiotic, or other special diets for religious, ethical, or health reasons. Parents may not be aware that some restrictive diets have a potential for nutritional deficiencies. Families often seek advice regarding diet from other healthcare professionals like nutritionists, naturopathic doctors, chiropractors, and licensed acupuncturists instead of their pediatrician. Although diet is discussed by pediatricians as part of routine health supervision visits, most pediatricians do not inquire specifically about special diets. This is a lost opportunity to address potential nutritional deficiencies from special diets.

## TALKING TO FAMILIES ABOUT CAM

With increasing interest and use of integrative CAM therapies, it is important that pediatricians obtain a complete CAM history from every family/patient as part of the routine pediatric history. This is best done in a culturally sensitive, open-minded, and nonjudgmental manner. Table 13-2 provides examples of how to talk to families about CAM.

CAM is typically used as an adjunct rather than an alternative to conventional/mainstream medical care, but families/patients do not always discuss their use of CAM with their pediatrician or primary healthcare provider. There are multiple reasons why families may not disclose CAM use to their pediatrician; for example, pediatricians may not ask about CAM use, or families may be fearful that the pediatrician may disapprove or abandon care, especially if they perceive the pediatrician to be judgmental or antagonistic. Despite this, studies have shown that families/patients want and appreciate their pediatrician's input, guidance, and professional recommendations regarding CAM. Therefore, to provide optimal care, pediatricians should ask all patients about all the therapies they use to treat their illness or promote health. Families often see CAM therapists who offer personal attention, hope, time, and therapies as consistent with their own health beliefs, culture, and values.

CAM providers may not communicate with pediatricians regarding the care they are providing to patients. This lack of coordination is of particular concern when care is provided by CAM providers such as acupuncturists and naturopathic physicians who prescribe herbs that can interact with medications. Pediatricians can facilitate open conversation by inquiring, "Which other healthcare professionals has your child visited?" When medical information is not obtained completely, the doctor–patient relationship is attenuated and medical care can be compromised. When communication is open and comprehensive, especially about CAM, it almost always strengthens the doctor–patient relationship and bridges potential gaps in beliefs about health and illness. In the best interest of children, it is important to provide balanced advice about therapeutic options, to guard against bias, and to establish and maintain a trusting relationship

**TABLE 13-1 COMMON HERBS USED IN CHILDREN AND ADOLESCENTS**

| Herb | Typical Uses | Side Effects and Drug Interactions |
|---|---|---|
| Aloe vera | *External use*: Applied topically to treat minor burns, abrasions, insect bites, acne, poison ivy, sunburn, skin irritations, frostbite, and canker sores | *Side effect* of leaf lining taken internally: Contact dermatitis, gastric cramping, or diarrhea.[a] |
| | | *Pregnancy and lactation*[b] |
| | *Internal use*: Gel taken as a peptic ulcer remedy and treatment for digestive disorders | *Drug interactions* for leaf lining: May potentiate digitalis and cardiac glycosides because of increased potassium loss; may enhance potassium loss with corticosteroids and thiazide diuretics |
| | Leaf lining used as a laxative | *Other*: Reduced absorption of drugs due to decreased bowel transit time |
| Astragalus (*Astragalus membranaceus*) | To strengthen and regulate the immune system | *Side effects*: Few side effects but very high doses might cause immunosuppression |
| | To increase production of blood cells, especially in patients with cancer | *Pregnancy and lactation*[b] |
| | Has antibacterial, antiviral, and anti-inflammatory properties | *Drug interactions*: Might interfere with immunosuppressive therapy such as cyclophosphamide |
| Calendula (*Calendula officinalis*) | *External use*: Skin irritations, rashes, cold sores, eczema, and conjunctivitis | *Side effects*[a] |
| | | *Pregnancy and lactation*[b] |
| | | *Drug interactions*: None known |
| Cascara (*Ramnus purshiana*) | As a laxative for constipation | *Side effects*: Orally, mild gastric cramping, colic; long-term use can lead to potassium depletion |
| | Bitter tonic for liver ailments, gallstones | *Pregnancy and lactation*[b] |
| | | *Drug interactions*: May enhance potassium loss with corticosteroids and thiazide diuretics; may potentiate digitalis and cardiac glycosides because of increased potassium loss |
| Catnip (*Nepeta cataria*) | Low-grade fever, upper respiratory tract infection, colic, headache, nervousness, sleep disorders, indigestion | *Side effects*: One case report of central nervous system depression in toddler[a] |
| | | *Pregnancy and lactation*[b] |
| | | *Drug interactions*: None known |
| Chamomile (*Anthemis nobilis*) | *External use*: Skin irritation, prevention and treatment of cracked nipples | *Side effects*[a] |
| | | *Pregnancy and lactation*: No known adverse effects in pregnancy, lactation, and childhood |
| | *Internal use*: Colic, peptic ulcer disease, teething pain, sleep problems, anxiety | *Drug interactions*: None known |
| Clove oil (*Syzygium aromaticum*) | Topically for toothaches, mouth and throat inflammation | *Side effects*: Inhalation of clove can cause respiratory distress; topically can cause oral mucosal irritation |
| | Orally for gastrointestinal upset | *Pregnancy and lactation*: Possibly safe |
| | | *Drug interactions*: Theoretically, may potentiate the effects of anticoagulant/antiplatelet drugs |
| Dandelion (*Taraxacum officinale*) | Mild diuretic, liver tonic | *Side effects*: Orally can cause gastric hyperacidity, topically can cause dermatitis[a] |
| | | *Pregnancy and lactation*: Possibly safe |
| | | *Drug interactions*: Dandelion contains large amounts of potassium and therefore should not be used with potassium-sparing drugs |
| | | Theoretically, since it increases gastric acid, should not be used with antacids, $H_2$ blockers, proton pump inhibitors |
| Dill (*Anethum graveolens*) | Antispasmodic, colic, decreases flatulence | *Side effects*[a] |
| | | *Pregnancy and lactation:* Safe if used in amounts same as found in foods[b] |
| | | *Drug interactions*: None known |
| Echinacea (*Echinacea angustifolia, E purpurea, or E pallida*) | *External use*: Boils, ulcerations, burns, herpes simplex | *Side effects*: Dermatitis[a] |
| | *Internal use*: Immune stimulation, anti-inflammatory | *Pregnancy and lactation*[b] |
| | Prevention and supportive therapy for upper respiratory infection, yeast infection, and some bacterial infections | *Drug interactions*: Possible unknown interactions with other immunomodulators |
| Fennel (*Foeniculum vulgare*) | Colic, dyspnea, bloating, fullness, flatulence, and diarrhea in infants | *Side effects*[a] |
| | | *Pregnancy and lactation*[b] |
| | Cough, bronchitis, upper respiratory tract infection, conjunctivitis | *Drug interactions*: None known |
| Feverfew (*Tanacetum parthenium*) | Migraine headache, nausea and vomiting, arthritis, fever | *Side effects*: Rebound headache, oral ulcers, and gastric disturbances[a] |
| | | *Pregnancy and lactation*[b] |
| | | *Drug interactions*: May potentiate effects of anticoagulants and aspirin |

(*Continued*)

**TABLE 13-1 COMMON HERBS USED IN CHILDREN AND ADOLESCENTS (CONTINUED)**

| Herb | Typical Uses | Side Effects and Drug Interactions |
|---|---|---|
| Garlic (*Allium sativum*) | Ear infections, upper respiratory tract infections, cough/bronchitis, atherosclerosis, high cholesterol, hypertension, gastrointestinal disorders, menstrual disorders, diabetes mellitus | *Side effects*: Flatulence, heartburn, gastric disturbances[a]<br>*Pregnancy and lactation*: Reported emmenagogue in large amounts[b]<br>*Drug interactions*: Inhibits platelet aggregation, prolongs bleeding and clotting times, and has fibrinolytic activity; use large doses with caution for patients taking anticoagulants and anti-inflammatory drugs |
| Ginger (*Zingiber officinale*) | Colic, anorexia, indigestion; prevention of vomiting and nausea in motion sickness, morning sickness, and postoperative nausea; upper respiratory tract infection, cough, and bronchitis | *Side effects*: Heartburn[a]<br>*Contraindications*: Patients with gallstones due to cholagogue effect<br>*Pregnancy and lactation*[b]<br>*Drug interactions*: May potentiate anticoagulants |
| Ginseng (*Panax* species) | Adaptogen: general tonic for improving well-being; stimulant: enhances endurance and performance, improves immune function and cognitive function | *Side effects*: Generally safe when used for less than 3 months; can cause insomnia<br>*Pregnancy and lactation*: Avoid in pregnancy and lactation; not recommended for infants<br>*Drug interactions*: Might decrease platelet aggregation; might have additive hypoglycemic effects; might potentiate stimulant drug effects |
| Goldenseal (*Hydrastis canadensis*) | *External use*: Conjunctivitis, boils, inflammation of gums, hemorrhoids, fungal infections<br>*Internal use*: Diarrhea and other digestive disorders, upper respiratory tract infection, postpartum bleeding | *Side effects*: For large doses, nausea, vomiting, diarrhea, mucocutaneous irritation; increased cardiac and uterine contractility, vasoconstriction, central nervous system stimulation, and neonatal jaundice<br>*Pregnancy and lactation*: Avoid in pregnancy and lactation; not recommended for infants; berberine displaces bilirubin from albumin<br>*Drug interactions*: None known |
| Hops (*Humulus lupulus*) | Nervousness, irritability, insomnia, indigestion | *Side effects*: Skin irritation[a]<br>*Pregnancy and lactation*[b]<br>*Drug interactions*: Sedative activity increases the sleeping time induced by phenobarbital |
| Lavender (*Lavandula* species) | Sedative, headaches, gastrointestinal upset, insect repellent | *Side effects*: Generally recognized as safe[a]<br>*Pregnancy and lactation*[b]<br>*Drug interactions*: Theoretically, can potentiate the effects of central nervous system depressants |
| Lemon balm (*Melissa officinalis*) | Oral and genital herpes, insomnia, anxiety, depression | *Side effects*[a]<br>*Pregnancy and lactation*[b]<br>*Drug interactions*: None known |
| Licorice (*Glycyrrhiza glabra*) | Asthma, cough, sore throat, upper respiratory tract infection, bronchitis, stomach ulcers and digestive disturbances, constipation, colic, cholestatic liver disorders and liver disease, adrenocorticoid insufficiency, hypokalemia, hypertonia, arthritis | *Side effects*: Long-term use may lead to a mineralocorticoid effect, hypertension, potassium wasting, and arrhythmias[a]<br>*Pregnancy and lactation*[b]<br>*Contraindications*: Patients who have hypertension, diabetes, hypokalemia, liver disorders, or kidney disease<br>*Drug interactions*: May potentiate digitalis and cardiac glycosides because of increased potassium loss; may increase potassium loss in patients taking corticosteroids and thiazide diuretics |
| Milk thistle (*Silybum marianum*) | Hepatoprotection, cirrhosis, hepatitis | *Side effects*: Possibly safe; mild laxative[a]<br>*Pregnancy and lactation*[b]<br>*Drug interactions*: Might inhibit cytochrome P450 (2C9 and 3A4) |
| Oats (*Avena byzantina*) | Skin inflammation, eczema, antipruritic, hypercholesterolemia, constipation | *Side effects*: Generally recognized as safe[a]<br>*Pregnancy and lactation*[b]<br>*Drug interactions*: None known |
| Rhubarb root (*Rheum officinale*) | Constipation, dyspepsia<br>Topically used for cold sores | *Side effects*: Generally recognized as safe[a]<br>Spasmodic gastrointestinal discomfort, diarrhea, uterine contractions; chronic use can cause potassium loss<br>*Pregnancy and lactation*: Avoid in pregnancy and lactation; not recommended for infants/children under 12 years<br>*Drug interactions*: Overuse with corticosteroids and diuretics might cause potassium loss; increase digoxin toxicity due to potassium loss |
| Peppermint (*Mentha piperita*) | *External use*: Muscle aches, neuralgia, headache<br>*Internal use*: Indigestion, nausea, diarrhea, flatulent, colic, anorexia, inflammatory bowel disease, spastic complaints of the gastrointestinal tract as well as gall bladder and bile ducts, upper respiratory tract infection, cough, tension headache | *Side effects*: Abdominal pain, heartburn, and perianal burning or hypersensitivity reactions[a]<br>*Contraindications*: Biliary duct occlusion, gallbladder inflammation, liver disease, and gastroesophageal reflux disease; patients who have gallstone could develop colic due to peppermint's cholagogic effect<br>*Pregnancy and lactation*[b]<br>*Drug interactions:* None known |

(*Continued*)

**TABLE 13-1 COMMON HERBS USED IN CHILDREN AND ADOLESCENTS (CONTINUED)**

| Herb | Typical Uses | Side Effects and Drug Interactions |
|---|---|---|
| Skullcap (*Scutellaria lateriflora*) | Sedative; dermatitis, inflammation | *Side effects*: Large amounts can cause stupor, confusion, seizures<br>*Pregnancy and lactation*[b]<br>*Drug interactions*: None known |
| Slippery elm bark (*Ulmus fulva*) | *External use*: Minor skin irritations, cold sores, ulcers, abscesses, and boils<br>*Internal use*: Diarrhea, colic, inflammation or ulcerations of stomach or duodenum, urinary tract infections, sore throats, upper respiratory tract infections, abortifacient | *Side effects*: Dermatitis[a]<br>*Pregnancy and lactation*:[b] The whole bark has been used to induce abortions; there are no reported problems with the use of powdered slippery elm<br>*Drug interactions*: None known |
| St John's wort (*Hypericum perforatum*) | *External use*: Wounds, burns, neuralgia, contusions<br>*Internal use*: Depression, nervousness, anxiety | *Side effects*: Gastrointestinal symptoms, sedation, dizziness, and confusion; photosensitivity is rare but can be severe[a]<br>*Pregnancy and lactation*[b]<br>*Drug interactions*: None known |
| Tea Tree Oil | *External use*: Antimicrobial; acne; minor skin infections, including fungal and yeast infections | *Side effects*: Safe for most people when put on the skin, but it can cause skin irritation and swelling; in people with acne, it can sometimes cause skin dryness, itching, stinging, burning, and redness<br>*Pregnancy*: Safe when applied to the skin; however, it is likely unsafe if taken by mouth; ingestion of tea tree oil can be toxic<br>*Drug Interactions*: None known |
| Thyme (*Thymus vulgaris*) | *Internal use*: antimicrobial; colds, sore throats; cough; expectorant | *Side effects*: Generally safe with few side effects but it can cause digestive system upset<br>*Drug Interactions*: None known |
| Valerian (*Valeriana officinalis*) | Insomnia, restlessness, menstrual cramps, rheumatic pain | *Side effects*: Headache, insomnia[a]<br>*Pregnancy and lactation*[b]<br>*Drug interactions*: Sedative activity increases the sleeping time induced by pentobarbital |
| Witch hazel (*Hamamelis virginia L*) | Internally used for diarrhea, mucus colitis, colds, fevers<br>Topically used for skin inflammation/irritation, antiseptic, hemorrhoids | *Side effects*: Dermatitis; orally in high doses can cause gastrointestinal problems, kidney and liver damage[a]<br>*Pregnancy and lactation*[b]<br>*Drug interactions*: None known |

[a]Allergic reactions are possible with any natural product.

[b]Insufficient clinical data on safety during pregnancy and lactation.

Adapted with permission from Gardiner P, Kemper KJ. Herbs in pediatric and adolescent medicine, *Pediatr Rev*. 2000 Feb;21(2):44-57.

**TABLE 13-2 HOW TO TALK WITH CAREGIVERS/PATIENTS ABOUT THERAPEUTIC OPTIONS FOR CHILDREN AND ADOLESCENTS**

**Do** talk about the different kinds of therapies families may have tried to help their child.

Do **not** wait for families to bring it up.

Ask in an open-minded, nonjudgmental fashion. Avoid using potentially pejorative terms such as "unproven," "unconventional," or "alternative."

Elicit further information with questions about specific therapies:

- Have you tried any **herbal** therapies, such as Echinacea or ginkgo?
- Have you tried any **dietary** therapies, like avoiding wheat or milk?
- Have you sought care from any **other healthcare professionals**, such as acupuncturists or chiropractors?

Elicit the values, beliefs, and influences that led parents to these therapies:

- Suggested by family members?
- Consistent with their religious, spiritual, or cultural beliefs?
- Value of natural or organic approaches?
- Fear of side effects of mainstream treatments?

Whenever possible, join with the parents and support their decision to pursue avenues that may help their child; be an ally rather than a tyrant.

Ask how well the family thinks the therapies worked or didn't work **before** offering your opinion.

Offer to talk with other therapists involved in the child's care to better maintain coordinated, comprehensive care.

Offer to learn more to help answer the family's questions.

Offer families additional information and resources to address their questions about alternative and complementary therapies.

Reproduced with permission from Kemper KJ. Complementary and alternative medicine in pediatrics. In: UpToDate, Post TW (Ed), UpToDate, Waltham, MA. (June 7, 2017) Copyright © 2017 UpToDate, Inc. For more information visit www.uptodate.com.

with families. In 2001, the AAP came out with the policy statement "Counseling Families Who Choose CAM for their Children." This statement recommends that pediatricians "seek information," evaluate the scientific merits of specific therapeutic approaches, and "identify risks or potential harmful effects." These recommendations are summarized in Table 13-3.

## MEDICOLEGAL AND ETHICAL CONSIDERATIONS

Legal issues about CAM center on individual liability and integration of care. Pediatricians have an ethical responsibility to guard the welfare of children by ensuring that any treatment they endorse is in accordance with science and proven evidence and experience. There is also a duty not only to avoid harm but also to do good—that is, to act in the patient's best interests. This duty of beneficence takes precedence over any self-interest. Cohen and Kemper have summarized the ethical issues of CAM by acknowledging the dilemmas: lack of pediatrician knowledge about the safety and effectiveness of many CAM therapies, scope of practice, licensing requirements, credentialing of CAM practitioners, concerns about safety and legal liability, and how to translate principles of medical ethics into CAM. They have suggested a framework for assessing the medicolegal risks regarding CAM therapies (Table 13-4).

Following a standard approach can help guide pediatricians toward clinical conduct that is responsible, ethically appropriate, and legally defensible. Pediatricians recommend, tolerate, and in some cases, actively prescribe CAM therapies to patients, but this occurs on the basis of an individualized risk–benefit assessment.

The Federation of State Medical Boards recommends that, in addition to the standard documentation of the history, physical examination, diagnostic test results, and reports from consultants,

**TABLE 13-3 AMERICAN ACADEMY OF PEDIATRICS RECOMMENDATIONS FOR PEDIATRICIANS WHO DISCUSS COMPLEMENTARY AND ALTERNATIVE THERAPIES WITH THEIR FAMILIES**

1. Seek information for yourself and be prepared to share it with families.

   Families are likely to be appreciative of information you have obtained through literature searches. Reviews of CAM discuss currently popular alternative approaches and their attendant risks.

2. Evaluate the scientific merits of specific therapeutic approaches.

   Critical evaluation of claims of effectiveness requires training in the scientific method and an understanding of processes of disease. This training is equally important for evaluating conventional biomedical treatments and alternative therapies. Many CAM approaches are based on inconsistent or implausible biomedical explanations, and claims of effectiveness rest on anecdotal information and testimonials. The pediatrician can be uniquely helpful to parents seeking an assessment of the merits of specific therapies by evaluating such therapies and providing guidance.

3. Identify risks or potential harmful effects.

   Alternative therapies may be directly harmful by causing direct toxic effects, compromising adequate nutrition, interrupting beneficial medications or therapies, or postponing biomedical therapies of proven effectiveness. Indirect harm may be caused by the financial burden of the alternative therapy, other unanticipated costs (eg, the time investment required to administer the therapy), and feelings of guilt associated with inability to adhere to rigorous treatment demands. If a child receiving alternative therapy is at direct or indirect risk of harm, the pediatrician should advise against the therapy. In some circumstances, it may be necessary for the pediatrician to seek an ethics consultation or to refer to child welfare agencies. If there is no risk of direct or indirect harm, a pediatrician should be neutral.

4. Provide families with information on a range of treatment options (avoid therapeutic nihilism).

   Although effective treatments to cure the underlying condition or restore function may be lacking, there may be adjunctive treatments to improve quality of life, address specific concerns of the child or family, or modify environmental conditions that may be causing additional problems. Consultation with pediatric specialists may suggest therapeutic options. Discussion of a range of treatment options may avert feelings of frustration and powerlessness that drive families to alternative sources of care.

5. Educate families to evaluate information about all treatment approaches.

   Families should be informed about placebo effects and the need for controlled studies. The pediatrician should explain that anecdotal and testimonial evidence is very weak. Families also should be advised to be vigilant for exaggerated claims of cure, especially if such claims are for treatments requiring intense commitment of time, energy, and money on the part of the family.

6. Avoid dismissal of CAM in ways that communicate a lack of sensitivity or concern for the family's perspective.

   Some alternative therapies considered by families may warrant independent review and evaluation of scientific merit by the pediatrician. Respectful family-centered care rests on the pediatrician's willingness to listen carefully and to acknowledge the family's concerns, priorities, and fears, including social and cultural factors that may affect their choice of therapies. If CAM is chosen against the advice of the pediatrician, he or she should continue to offer care to the child.

7. Recognize feeling threatened and guard against becoming defensive.

   Families may express their opinions in ways that challenge the professional expertise of the pediatrician. They may bring to the discussion of CAM a number of biased assumptions that contribute to an atmosphere of distrust and an adversarial relationship. It may be helpful for the pediatrician to make empathic statements that acknowledge the families' deep concerns, thereby avoiding angry or defensive reactions.

8. If the CAM approach is endorsed, offer to assist in monitoring and evaluating the response.

   The pediatrician can help to establish clinical outcomes and target behaviors or symptoms that can be observed and measured. Sometimes, the pediatrician and family can agree on a time-limited trial of the proposed approach.

9. Actively listen to the family and the child with chronic illness.

   The pediatrician should be aware of their concerns, their understanding of the condition, and their needs for support. Support groups and community networks can greatly enhance family comfort with the management of the chronic illness or disability.

Data from American Academy of Pediatrics. Counseling families who choose complementary and alternative medicine for their child with chronic illness or disability. Committee on Children with Disabilities, *Pediatrics*. 2001 Mar;107(3):598-601.

**TABLE 13-4 MEDICOLEGAL CONSIDERATIONS IN THE USE OF COMPLEMENTARY THERAPIES IN CHILDREN**

**Do parents elect to abandon effective care when the child's condition is serious or life threatening?**

Courts are likely to respect parental choices that are supported by some medical authority and that present reasonable alternatives as long as the child's life is not in danger and conventional care is not imminently necessary. The child's condition should be monitored so that conventional interventions can be used if necessary.

**Will the use of CAM therapy otherwise divert the child from imminently necessary conventional treatment?**

If not, a "time-limited" trial of the proposed approach may be appropriate provided that the child can be monitored conventionally and conventional therapy can be continued as appropriate.

**Are the CAM therapies that have been selected known to be unsafe or ineffective?**

The medical evidence can be categorized as follows, with increasing risk of liability

1) Medical evidence supports efficacy and safety—the therapy can be **recommended**; efficacy should be monitored.

2) Medical evidence supports safety, but evidence regarding efficacy is inconclusive—the therapy can be **tolerated**; efficacy should be monitored.

3) Medical evidence supports efficacy, but evidence regarding safety is inconclusive—the therapy should be **monitored closely or discouraged**.

4) Medical evidence indicates serious risk and inefficacy—the therapy should be **avoided and actively discouraged**.

The clinician caring for the patient should continue to monitor the patient and the literature for new information that would change the category.

**Have the proper parties consented to the use of the CAM therapy?**

Informed consent is particularly important when informing the patient about CAM therapies may affect the patient's choice of treatment.

**Is the risk–benefit ratio of the proposed CAM therapy acceptable to a reasonable, similarly situated clinician, and does the therapy have at least minority acceptance or support in the medical literature?**

Data from Cohen MH, Kemper KJ: Complementary therapies in pediatrics: a legal perspective, *Pediatrics*. 2005 Mar;115(3):774-780.

**TABLE 13-5 FEDERATION OF STATE MEDICAL BOARDS MODEL GUIDELINES FOR MEDICAL RECORD DOCUMENTATION REGARDING COMPLEMENTARY/ALTERNATIVE THERAPIES**

| |
|---|
| The conventional medical therapies that have been discussed, offered, tried, or refused |
| Discussion of the risks and benefits of the recommended CAM treatment |
| That the physician has determined the extent to which the CAM therapy could interfere with any other recommended or ongoing treatment |
| Appropriate informed consent |
| Treatments and medications (including date, type, dose, and quantity prescribed) |
| Instructions and agreements |
| Periodic reviews |

Data from Model Guidelines for the Use of Complementary and Alternative Therapies in Medical Practice. Federation of State Medical Boards. Policy, April 2002.

the documentation in the medical record should include information about CAM (Table 13-5).

The weighing of risks and benefits is at times complicated by variables such as a family's personal beliefs, cultural values, practices, therapeutic goals, and the type and severity of illness. Additionally, the efficacy and safety of a particular treatment may not be well studied in certain populations such as children. While scientific evidence exists regarding some CAM therapies, for most, there are key questions yet to be answered through well-designed scientific studies, including whether particular therapies are safe and effective for certain diseases or medical conditions in children. Although the same principles and standards of evidence of treatment effectiveness should apply to all treatments, certain characteristics of many CAM therapies make it difficult or impossible to conduct standard randomized controlled trials. For these therapies, innovative methods of evaluation are needed. Pediatricians should be aware of relevant professional guidelines and the 4 basic principles of biomedical ethics: autonomy, nonmaleficence, beneficence, and justice.

## CONCLUSION

CAM therapies are used frequently in the pediatric population and pediatricians are in an ideal position to inquire about CAM use, have open communication about CAM use, work with families regarding safe and effective remedies, and be culturally sensitive, open minded, educated, supportive, and candid with their families regarding integration of CAM therapies within conventional medicine. In addition, pediatricians should seek high-quality information regarding CAM therapies, evaluate the scientific merits of specific therapeutic approaches, and identify risks or potential harmful effects of CAM therapies. Scientific evidence of safety and efficacy supporting use of certain CAM therapies for many pediatric conditions is increasing. Multidisciplinary care in pediatrics, especially in children with chronic illnesses, often includes opportunities for pediatricians to collaborate with CAM providers such as chiropractors, acupuncturists, massage therapists, and naturopathic doctors. Continued research of well-designed, well-conducted clinical trials to determine the safety and efficacy of CAM therapies as adjuncts to standard treatments or as primary treatments for children is warranted. By asking about CAM use and by considering CAM as part of an overall treatment plan in families who are interested, pediatricians can enhance improved communication and strengthen the patient–physician relationship.

## SUGGESTED READINGS


Cohen M, Kemper KJ. Complementary therapies in pediatrics: a legal perspective. *Pediatrics*. 2005;115(3):774-780.

Culbert T, Olness K. *Integrative Pediatrics*. 1st ed. Weil Integrative Medicine Library. New York, NY: Oxford University Press; 2009.

Kemper KJ. *The Holistic Pediatrician: A Pediatrician's Comprehensive Guide to Safe and Effective Therapies for the 27 Most Common Ailments of Infants, Children, and Adolescents*. 3rd ed. New York, NY: Harper Paperbacks; 2016.

Kemper KJ, Vohra S, Walls R; Task Force on Complementary and Alternative Medicine; Provisional Section on Complementary, Holistic, and Integrative Medicine; American Academy of Pediatrics. The use of complementary and alternative medicine in pediatrics. *Pediatrics*. 2008;122(6):1374-1386.

Longwood Herbal Task Force Web site. http://www.longwoodherbal.org/. Accessed September 6, 2016.

Loo M. *Integrative Medicine for Children*. St. Louis, MO: Saunders Elsevier; 2008.

McClafferty H, ed. Pediatric integrative medicine: an emerging field of pediatrics. *Children*. 2015 (special issue). Basel, Switzerland: MDPI. Available at: http://www.mdpi.com/journal/children/special_issues/pediatric_integrative_medicine. Accessed September 6, 2016.

Misra S, Verissimo AM. *A Guide to Integrative Pediatrics for the Healthcare Professional*. Basel, Switzerland: Springer International Publishing; 2014.

National Center for Complementary and Integrative Health. National Institutes of Health Web site. https://nccih.nih.gov/. Accessed September 6, 2016.

PedCAM: Pediatric Complementary and Alternative Medicine Research and Education Network. www.pedcam.ca. Accessed September 6, 2016.

Rakel D. *Integrative Medicine*. 3rd ed. Toronto, Canada: Saunders; 2012.

Section on Integrative Medicine.American Academy of Pediatrics Web site. http://www2.aap.org/sections/chim/default.cfm. Accessed September 6, 2016.


# 14 Health Disparities in Practice

Sakena Abedin and Michelle Lopez

## INTRODUCTION

Health disparities are the result of population differences that lead to preventable and unfair or unjust barriers to health equity. Health disparities research has demonstrated significant racial gaps in health outcomes. For example, in the United States, infants born to black mothers are more than twice as likely to die before their first birthday as infants born to white mothers. However, health disparities go beyond race and ethnicity as other vulnerable populations can also experience obstacles to health, based on religion, socioeconomic status, gender, age, mental health, disability, sexual orientation or gender identity, geographic location, or other characteristics linked to discrimination or exclusion. For example, children in poor families are twice as likely not to receive preventive medical and dental care as children in families earning 400% or more of the federal poverty level. There is a complex interaction of biological, behavioral, social, and physical environmental factors contributing to health disparities and addressing these gaps requires interventions at the patient, provider, and system level. This chapter will enhance the clinicians' ability to care for diverse patient populations.

## APPROACHING HEALTH DISPARITIES

Medicine has traditionally emphasized the role of individual behavior on health. While personal responsibility is important to health, the picture is more complicated when we are trying to examine health disparities. Race, ethnicity, and culture are part of social context, which contributes to an individual's social position and stratification. Based on this stratification, individuals or groups are differentially exposed to health-damaging conditions and experience differential vulnerability based on the availability of and access to resources. Children's health deserves special attention because of children's dependency on adults, demographic differences, epidemiology, and separate system of healthcare financing. Additionally, developmentally, the circumstances a child is born into, including biological, social, and environmental factors, have ongoing and long-lasting effects on their health outcomes. Through circumstances beyond their control, certain disadvantaged children and adults are more vulnerable to poor health outcomes and health inequities than more advantaged groups.

The life course model emphasizes the cumulative effects of these early-life adversities on adult health. In the Adverse Childhood Experiences (ACE) Study, a graded relationship was observed between ACE scores (based on self-reported abuse and household dysfunction in childhood) and adverse health outcomes measured by depression, anxiety, substance abuse, and sexual risk behaviors in adulthood. ACEs were also associated with increased risk of chronic conditions and premature death. The ACE risk factors are hypothesized to produce a toxic stress response, the result of significant, repetitive or prolonged activation of the body's stress response systems and stress hormones without the buffering protection of a supportive relationship. This response may cause a cumulative stress-induced burden called allostatic load on overall brain and body functioning that results in physical and mental illnesses.

Toxic stress is one of the mechanisms postulated to lead to persistent racial disparities in health. There is a long-standing and persistent difference with increased infant mortality, higher low–birth weight births, and preterm deliveries among black infants compared to non-Hispanic white infants. While sociodemographic, environmental, and behavioral risk factors contribute to these differences in outcomes, studies have demonstrated persistent racial gaps in outcomes independent of maternal education and prenatal care in black mothers. The allostatic stress response related to childhood experiences and the effects of various forms of racism may contribute to some of the persistent disparities.

It is essential that we work toward a better understanding of the issues surrounding health disparities and factors contributing to adverse outcomes in historically disadvantaged groups. Building the knowledge base and skill set needed to care for diverse patient populations enhances our ability to positively influence health outcomes for all of our patients.

The remainder of this chapter borrows from the humanities and social sciences and covers two different kinds of competencies that we think physicians need to develop to address health disparities in medical practice. The first we are calling interactional competence, and it addresses the role of social, cultural, gender, and other forms of difference on the interaction between doctor and patient. The second approach, structural competence, takes a larger view, and examines the role of physicians in addressing the social structures that create health disparities.

## INTERACTIONAL COMPETENCE

Interactional competence, as we are defining it, relates to the interaction between doctor and patient, and the ways in which physicians can improve the outcomes of these conversations. Our promotion of interactional competence is based on the idea that health disparities may arise, in part, from deficiencies in communication between doctor and patient. We take the approach of emphasizing the importance of understanding difference—racial, socioeconomic, cultural, gender, and other forms of difference—between doctor and patient, and how that difference between doctor and patient shapes their interaction.

Narrative medicine, in the work of physician Rita Charon, is based on the idea that medical practice is a series of narrative situations, interactions between doctors and patients, where each is engaged in trying to interpret and understand the narratives produced by the other. Thinking about the interaction between doctor and patient as a process of interpretation explicitly acknowledges the role of the physician as a listener in this process. According to Charon:

> *As the physician listens to the patient, he or she follows the narrative thread of the story, imagines the situation of the teller (the biological, familial, cultural, and existential situation), recognizes the multiple and often contradictory meanings of the words used and events described, and in some way enters into and is moved by the narrative world of the patient.*

In making meaning of a patient's story, a physician calls upon his or her own previous experiences and cultural understanding, as well as the culture of medicine. By naming this process, instead of taking it for granted, we can pay attention to how it works in clinical practice, and the particular role that racial, gender, and socioeconomic difference can play in a physician's interpretation of a patient's story. For physicians to elicit, receive, and interpret their patient's stories effectively requires a mindset that promotes listening and suspends judgment, while acknowledging the potential effects of a physician's own personal biases.

Narrative medicine is based in the premise that *both* doctors and patients are engaged in constructing narratives, which are shaped by their point of view. The distinction between illness and disease, as described by medical anthropologist and physician Arthur Kleinman and his colleagues, draws attention to the differences in these viewpoints. Diseases, abnormalities in the structure and function of body organs and systems, are what physicians are trained to diagnose and treat. The culture of medicine, with its optimistic belief in medical science and technology and its focus on the individual, shapes understandings of disease. Illnesses, on the other hand, are what patients experience, and the experience of illness is shaped by culture and previous experiences, as well as by social factors. An explanatory model is the sum of ideas about a particular sickness; given the differences between illness and disease, we can see how the explanatory models held by physicians and patients would differ.

Kleinman and colleagues offer a guide to eliciting patients' explanatory models through direct questions. These questions help the physician obtain a better understanding of how a patient views the physiologic disease processes affecting him or her. Explanatory models are relevant "to a greater or lesser degree in *all* clinical transactions." Kleinman recounts the story of a 38-year-old university professor who was diagnosed with angina but refused to accept the diagnosis and demanded instead the diagnosis of pulmonary embolus. Eventually, the treating team discovered that the professor felt that a diagnosis of angina signified the end of an active lifestyle; uncovering this misconception allowed his cardiologist to address the patient's concerns in a way that eventually allowed the patient to accept his diagnosis.

In primary care pediatrics, disease and illness are not always the issue, especially when dealing with problems or concerns relating to sleep, feeding, and development. With some modification, the explanatory model questions can be used by a pediatrician interacting with the family of a patient to address the kinds of issues that arise during well visits (Table 14-1). The questions can be used to understand a parent's anxieties, assess the parent's understanding of or particular interpretation of a child's problem, or to understand a parent's expectations regarding intervention. Finally, taken as a whole, the questions help to reveal the meaning that the problem has taken on for the family of the patient. Listening carefully to patients' illness narratives and asking questions that encourage patients to speak their minds create opportunities to improve communication and have the potential to reduce disparities in health.

**TABLE 14-1 ELICITING EXPLANATORY MODELS**

| |
|---|
| Question 1. What do you think caused your child's problem? |
| Question 2. Why do you think it started when it did? |
| Question 3. What do you think your child's problem does to him or her? How does it work? |
| Question 4. How severe is your child's problem? Do you think it will have a short or a long course? |
| Question 5. What kind of treatment do you think that your child requires? |
| Question 6. What are the most important results that you hope to obtain for your child through treatment? |
| Question 7. What are the chief problems that your child's problem has caused for him or her? |
| Question 8. What do you fear most about your child's problem? |

Data from Kleinman A, Eisenberg L, Good B. Culture, illness, and care: clinical lessons from anthropologic and cross-cultural research, *Ann Intern Med.* 1978 Feb;88(2):251-258.

**TABLE 14-2 USING AN INTERPRETER**

| |
|---|
| According to the 2010 US Census, approximately 25 million people, or 8.6 percent of the US population, have limited English proficiency (LEP), meaning that they speak English less than very well. This represents a greater than 50% increase in people with LEP from 1990. For physicians, this means an increased likelihood of seeing LEP patients and needing to use an interpreter. Not using an interpreter with an LEP patient can lead to misunderstandings that affect patient care and lead to poor outcomes. |
| Unless a physician is thoroughly fluent in a patient's language, he or she should use a trained interpreter. Problems with accuracy and confidentiality can occur with the use of untrained interpreters and family members. In-person interpretation by a trained interpreter, where available, is preferable. If an interpreter phone is being used, a speaker phone can be used to maintain some of the normal conversational flow of the encounter. |
| At the beginning of the encounter, the physician should allow a moment for introductions between patient, physician, and interpreter. The physician should also explain the purpose of the visit briefly to the interpreter (eg, follow-up, acute, or routine visit). If an in-person interpreter is present during the encounter, the physician should position himself or herself so that he or she can see both the interpreter and the patient. Having the patient, interpreter, and physician positioned as the points of an equilateral triangle is one way to accomplish this. The physician should make an effort to speak slowly and clearly, avoiding slang and jargon. It is better to speak in sentences, then pause for translation, than to speak in paragraphs. |
| If, during the course of the encounter, concerns arise about the quality or consistency of the interpretation, the physician should repeat or return to concerning points later in the conversation. Use of handwritten visual aids and repetition through back translation can aid in both solidifying and assessing patients' understanding. The physician should involve the interpreter in the creation of patient instructions, and, if possible, the interpreter should accompany the patient to make any necessary follow-up appointments. |

Doctors need to pay attention to how they speak as well as to how they listen to or interpret stories. In cases where doctor and patient speak different languages, the use of an interpreter is extremely important, and the failure to provide appropriate interpreter services can be considered discrimination based on national origin, which is prohibited by Title VI of the Civil Rights Act of 1964. Table 14-2 provides helpful information about using an interpreter to ensure accurate communication with patients and families who are not proficient in the English language.

## STRUCTURAL COMPETENCE

Interactional competence, by definition, functions at the level of the individual provider and patient. Health disparities may be the product of these interactions, but they are clearly also a product of the social and economic factors that influence the health of patients. Physicians need to be aware of and willing to address the structural factors that influence overall disparities in health; we are calling this structural competence.

In the context of their interactions with patients, physicians need to understand the effect of the material reality of socioeconomic status on children's and families' access to health care. This includes issues such as health insurance, transportation, and health literacy. The first step in addressing these issues as they arise in practice is to be aware of their existence. One approach is to divide social concerns into 4 major domains: (1) social stress and support networks, (2) change in environment (particularly relevant for recent immigrants or refugees), (3) life control, and (4) literacy. A list of questions, modified for pediatrics, can be found in Table 14-3.

Structural competence, as defined by physician-historian Jonathan Metzl and physician-anthropologist Helena Hanson, goes beyond even these individual level questions about the impact of socioeconomic status. At its core is the idea that physicians need to understand the economic and political conditions that produce inequalities in health, and to pay attention to the organization of institutions, policies, neighborhoods, and cities, not just patients' beliefs or attitudes. Race, class, gender, and ethnicity shape interactions between doctor and patient, but this effect is magnified by a larger structural context; as Metzl and Hanson point out, stigma is not produced in the clinical encounter, but it is enacted there. In addition to recognizing the structures that shape clinical interactions, Metzl and Hanson discuss 4 core structural competencies for physicians, as well as suggestions for how to attain them (see Suggested Readings).

**TABLE 14-3 ENGAGING SOCIAL CONTEXT: SAMPLE QUESTIONS**

| |
|---|
| What is causing the most stress in your child's life? What is causing the most stress in your family? How do you, your child, and your family deal with this stress? |
| Do you have friends or relatives whom you can call on for help? |
| How long have you and your child lived in this country and city? |
| How do you feel that your child is adjusting to life in this country and city? |
| What was your child's medical care like in your home country compared with here? |
| Do you ever feel that you are not able to afford food, medications, or medical expenses for your child? |
| Do you have any difficulties with transportation to and from the clinic? |
| Do you have trouble reading medication bottles, instructions, or other patient information? |

Data from Green AR, Betancourt JR, Carrillo JE. Integrating social factors into cross-cultural medical education, *Acad Med.* 2002 Mar;77(3):193-197.

Medical education, with its focus on the individual, effectively renders structure invisible. Physician and anthropologist Paul Farmer's work on structural violence is an example of what it might look like to make structure visible. Farmer defines structural violence as

> *one way of describing social arrangements that put individuals in harms' way. The arrangements are* structural *because they are embedded in the political and economic organization of our social world; they are* violent *because they cause injury to people.*

He also provides examples of the kinds of medical interventions that address structure. He relates the story of researchers and clinicians at an HIV clinic in Baltimore who wanted to alleviate the effect of race and insurance status on mortality from HIV among their patients. They were able to do this by making care more convenient, community based, and acceptable for patients. This work is just one example of the ways in which structural competence among physicians can impact disparities in health.

## SUGGESTED READINGS

### Health Disparities


Braveman P, Barclay C. Health disparities beginning in childhood: a life-course perspective. *Pediatrics.* 2009;124(5)(suppl 3):S163-S175.

Felitti VJ, Anda RF, Nordenberg D, et al. Relationship of childhood abuse and household dysfunction to many of the leading causes of death in adults: the Adverse Childhood Experiences (ACE) Study. *Am J Prev Med.* 1998;14(4):245-258.

Institute of Medicine. *Children's Health, the Nation's Wealth: Assessing and Improving Child Health.* Washington, DC: National Academies Press; 2004. Available at: http://www.ncbi.nlm.nih.gov/books/NBK92206/. Accessed September 6, 2016.doi: 10.17226/10886

Shonkoff JP, Garner AS; Committee on Psychosocial Aspects of Child and Family Health; Committee on Early Childhood, Adoption, and Dependent Care; and Section on Developmental and Behavioral Pediatrics. American Academy of Pediatrics technical report. The lifelong effects of early childhood adversity and toxic stress. *Pediatrics.* 2012;129:e232-e246.

Smedley BD, Stith AY, Nelson AR, eds; Committee on Understanding and Eliminating Racial and Ethnic Disparities in Health Care, Board on Health Sciences Policy, Institute of Medicine. Unequal treatment: confronting racial and ethnic disparities in health care. Washington, DC: National Academies Press; 2003.

World Health Organization. Commission on Social Determinants of Health. A conceptual framework for action on the social determinants of health. April 2007. Available at: http://www.who.int/social_determinants/resources/csdh_framework_action_05_07.pdf. Accessed September 6, 2016.

**Interactional and Structural Competence**

Charon R. Narrative and medicine. *N Engl JMed.* 2004;350(9): 862-864.

DelVecchio Good MJ, Willen SS, Hannah SD, Vickery K, Park LT, eds. *Shattering Culture: American Medicine Responds to Cultural Diversity.* New York, NY: Russell Sage Foundation; 2011.

Farmer PE, Nizeye B, Stulac S, Keshavjee S. Structural violence and clinical medicine. *PLOS Med.* 2006;3(10): e449.

Kleinman A, Eisenberg L, Good B. Culture, illness, and care: clinical lessons from anthropologic and cross-cultural research. *Ann Intern Med.* 1978; 88(2):251-258.

Metzl JM, Hansen H. Structural competency: theorizing a new medical engagement with stigma and inequality. *SocSci Med.* 2014;103:126-133.

# 15 Normal Nutritional Requirements

Catherine Larson-Nath and Praveen S. Goday

## INTRODUCTION

Every infant or child has a genetic potential for physical, mental, and emotional growth. Providing nutrition that fulfills all aspects of that growth potential represents *optimal nutrition.* When nutrition either limits growth or results in excessive body mass, because of either inadequate quality or inappropriate quantity, an individual is suffering from malnutrition (ie, undernutrition or obesity).

All published dietary requirements are guidelines designed to assure that most individuals will be well nourished. They are not meant to be rigidly followed by any specific individual. Also, precise adherence to these guidelines by any one person does not guarantee that an individual will be well nourished.

## DIETARY GUIDELINES AND THE BASIC FOOD GROUPS

In 1988, the first *Surgeon General's Report on Nutrition and Health* concluded that overconsumption of certain dietary components now is a major concern for Americans. The disproportionate consumption of foods that are high in fats, often at the expense of foods that are high in complex carbohydrates and fiber (eg, vegetables, fruits, and whole-grain products), increased the risk of diet-related diseases. The report reiterated the dietary guidelines issued jointly by the US Department of Agriculture (USDA) and the US Department of Health and Human Services. The recommendations of the Dietary Guidelines for Americans were revised in 2015 to focus on healthy eating patterns instead of specific food groups, as people do not eat foods in isolation. These guidelines are summarized here:

- Follow a healthy eating pattern across the lifespan.
- Focus on variety, nutrient density, and amount.
- Limit calories from added sugars and saturated fats and reduce sodium intake.
- Switch to healthier food and beverage choices.
- Support healthy eating patterns for all.

The USDA has defined a system of 6 basic food groups that, when combined appropriately, should provide the average American with his or her nutritional needs. These 6 groups are vegetables, fruits, grains (eg, breads, cereals, pastas), dairy products, proteins (eg, meat, poultry, fish eggs, nuts, legumes), and oils. Saturated fats, trans fats, added sugars, and sodium are separated, and it is recommended that their consumption be limited.

## DIETARY REFERENCE INTAKES

The Food and Nutrition Board (FNB) of the Institute of Medicine, National Academy of Science, has collaborated since 1992 to revise the recommended dietary allowances (RDAs). Following an explosion of nutrition-related scientific data, the FNB decided to replace the RDAs with *dietary reference intakes* (DRIs), which broadened the focus of the FNB as well as provided guidelines for the United States and Canada. The DRIs were established to meet a variety of uses, those focused on the intake and adequacy of populations as well as individuals. The FNB investigated the connection between nutrient intake and the risk reduction for chronic disease. In addition, upper limits (ULs) for nutrients were established, specifically addressing therapeutics and toxicities. The following are 4 categories that comprise the general heading of DRIs:

- *Estimated average requirement (EAR)*: an estimated nutrient intake value that meets the requirement of half the healthy individuals in a group or population according to accepted scientific research. This level is set at the mean of the standard deviation curve. Proposed usage is to assess the adequacy of intakes of population groups. These values are utilized to establish the RDAs.
- *Recommended dietary allowance (RDA)*: the averaged daily dietary intake level that is sufficient to meet the nutrient requirements of virtually all (97–98%) healthy individuals in a group or population. These levels were developed based on the average requirements of a population with an adjusted factor to account for variability among individuals. An RDA can be set only if the EAR is known.
- *Adequate intake (AI)*: a recommended daily intake based on scientific observation or approximations of nutrient intakes of healthy group(s). If the EAR is not known because of inadequate data, the RDAs cannot be set. In that case, an AI is estimated. AIs are levels at which deficiency has not been observed. They are to be applied to individual intake as well as to groups.
- *Tolerable upper limit (UL)*: the highest level of daily nutrient intake found to pose no risks of adverse effects in individuals of a healthy population. The risk of adverse effects and toxicities increases with an increase in consumption above these limits. The tolerable UL is used to guide and limit intake as well as to examine the possibility of overconsumption for the individual.

The safe range of intake is the area between the RDA and the tolerable UL. This is the area where deficiency and toxicity for the individual are most likely not to occur. The recommended intakes for macronutrients and the DRIs of calcium, vitamin D, phosphorus, magnesium, fluoride, folate, vitamin $B_{12}$, and other B vitamins and choline, along with a variety of minerals, have been published by the US National Academy of Sciences. Recommended pediatric intakes will be discussed in this chapter and summarized in the corresponding tables (Tables 15-1, 15-2, and 15-3).

An important distinction between AIs and RDAs should be noted. The AIs do not provide the same margin of safety that the RDAs do for other nutrients. Therefore, these levels are only an approximation of daily dietary intake observed for healthy individuals. For example, despite the limited understanding of the relationship between

**TABLE 15-1 ESTIMATED DAILY MAINTENANCE FLUID REQUIREMENTS**

| Body Weight | Fluid Requirements |
|---|---|
| 1–10 kg | 100 mL/kg |
| 11–20 kg | 1000 mL plus an additional 50 mL for each kg over 10 |
| ≥ 21 kg | 1500 mL plus an additional 20 mL for each kg over 20 |

**TABLE 15-2 ESTIMATED ENERGY REQUIREMENTS**

| Age | Estimated Energy Requirements Equations |
|---|---|
| 0–3 mo | (89 × weight [kg] −100) + 175 kcal |
| 4–6 mo | (89 × weight [kg] −100) + 56 kcal |
| 7–12 mo | (89 × weight [kg] −100) + 22 kcal |
| 13–36 mo | (89 × weight [kg] −100) + 20 kcal |
| Boys, 3–8 y | 88.5 (61.9 × age [y]) + PA × (26.7 × weight [kg] + 903 × height [m]) + 20 kcal |
| Girls, 3–8 y | 135.3 (30.8 × age [y]) + PA × (10.0 × weight [kg] + 934 × height [m]) + 20 kcal |
| Boys, 9–18 y | 88.5 (61.9 × age [y]) + PA × (26.7 × weight [kg] + 903 × height [m]) + 25 kcal |
| Girls, 9–18 y | 135.3 (30.8 × age [y]) + PA × (10.0 × weight [kg] + 934 × height [m]) + 25 kcal |

Where PA is the physical activity coefficient:
PA = 1.00 if physical activity level (PAL) is estimated to be sedentary
PA = 1.16 if PAL is estimated to be low active
PA = 1.31 if PAL is estimated to be active
PA = 1.56 if PAL is estimated to be very active

**TABLE 15-3 DIETARY REFERENCE INTAKES (DRIs): RECOMMENDED INTAKES FOR INDIVIDUALS; MACRONUTRIENTS**

| | Carbohydrate (g/d) | Total Fiber (g/d) | Fat (g/d) | Linoleic Acid (g/d) | α-Linolenic Acid (g/d) | Protein (g/d) |
|---|---|---|---|---|---|---|
| **Infants** | | | | | | |
| 0–6 mo | 60 | ND | 31 | 4.4 | 0.5 | 9.1 |
| 7–12 mo | 95 | ND | 30 | 4.6 | 0.5 | **11** |
| **Children** | | | | | | |
| 1–3 y | **130** | 19 | ND | 7 | 0.7 | **13** |
| 4–8 y | **130** | 25 | ND | 10 | 0.9 | **19** |
| **Males** | | | | | | |
| 9–13 y | **130** | 31 | ND | 12 | 1.2 | **34** |
| 14–18 y | **130** | 38 | ND | 16 | 1.6 | **52** |
| **Females** | | | | | | |
| 9–13 y | **130** | 26 | ND | 10 | 1.0 | **34** |
| 14–18 y | **130** | 26 | ND | 11 | 1.1 | **46** |
| **Pregnancy** | | | | | | |
| 14–18 y | **175** | 28 | ND | 13 | 1.4 | **71** |
| **Lactation** | | | | | | |
| 14–18 y | **210** | 29 | ND | 13 | 1.3 | **71** |

**Acceptable Macronutrient Distribution Ranges**

| **Macronutrient** | Range (percent of energy) | |
|---|---|---|
| | **Children, 1–3 y** | **Children, 4–18 y** |
| **Fat** | 30–40 | 25–35 |
| n-6 polyunsaturated fatty acids (linoleic acid)[a] | 5–10 | 5–10 |
| n-3 polyunsaturated fatty acids (α-linolenic acid)[a] | 0.6–1.2 | 0.6–1.2 |
| **Carbohydrate** | 45–65 | 45–65 |
| **Protein** | 5–20 | 10–30 |

[a]Approximately 10% of the total can come from longer-chain n-3 or n-6 fatty acids.

This table presents RDAs in bold type and AIs in ordinary type. Additional macronutrient recommendations suggest that consumption of saturated cholesterol, *trans*-fatty acids, and saturated fat be kept as low as possible while consuming a nutritionally adequate diet and that added sugars be limited to no more than 25% of total energy. ND, not determined.

adequate calcium intake and the risk of osteoporosis, an AI for calcium has been established. It can be inferred that inadequate scientific data exist to provide recommended daily intakes for calcium that would meet 97% of the needs of the healthy population. Furthermore, the guidelines for infants for many nutrients are AIs as well. These values are based on observations of breastfed babies. For this population, because of limitations of reliable experimental data, the healthy breastfed baby serves as the paradigm for adequate nutrient intake to support normal growth and development.

In addition to the nutrients found naturally in foods, the FNB took into consideration nutrients obtained from other sources, including fortification and supplementation. This is particularly true for folic acid because the bioavailability of folic acid derived from supplementation is greater than that from fortification, which is greater than that of folate ingested in folate-containing foods. Therefore, a separate measure of dietary folate equivalent (DFE) has been developed.

These dietary guidelines are meant for healthy groups and individuals. They cannot be applied to individuals with acute or chronic disease without significant adjustment. For the ill patient, the required amounts of nutrients vary among individuals as a result of malabsorption, increased use, or a need to replenish decreased stores.

## SPECIFIC NUTRITIONAL REQUIREMENTS

It is useful to partition nutrients into 8 major categories: (1) water, (2) energy, (3) proteins, (4) carbohydrates, (5) fats, (6) vitamins, (7) major minerals, and (8) trace elements. Each category is discussed in the context of the requirements in healthy children and considerations regarding changing requirements during illness.

### Water

Water comprises approximately 50% to 60% of body weight in young adults and 70% to 75% of body weight in infants. Total body water, expressed as a percentage of body weight, is a function of age, sex, and body composition. Total body water decreases with age and changes in body fat content. Water and electrolyte balance are exquisitely controlled, as discussed in greater detail in Chapter 462.

Providing adequate amounts of nutrients without adequate amounts of fluid will result in dehydration, excessive renal solute load, and inefficient use and wasting of calories. An individual's requirement for water is determined by total water losses, which reflect sensible and insensible losses, renal concentrating ability, and total nutrient and water intake. Infants are especially susceptible to dehydration; their requirement for water is much greater because of insensible losses from their large surface area. They also have a higher percentage of body water, their kidneys have a limited capacity for handling solute load, they have an impaired capacity to concentrate their urine, and they are unable to consistently communicate their thirst.

An individual's water requirement is highly variable and quite complex. An AI for water has been established; from a clinical perspective, Table 15-1 provides a useful method for estimating maintenance fluid requirements. Additional water must be provided when losses occur because of diarrhea, renal disease, cardiopulmonary compromise, fever, or catabolic stress.

For infants, breast milk or infant formula provides the majority of fluid requirements. Human milk and commercial formulas of standard energy density (ie, 20 kcal/oz or 0.66 kcal/mL) consist of approximately 89% water. Additional water that is produced from the oxidation of the ingested milk results in approximately 95% of the volume consumed being available as free water. The concentration of solutes that require excretion by the kidney must be considered during the design and manufacture of infant formula. This renal solute load includes primarily urea formed from protein catabolism and electrolytes. The potential renal solute load (PRSL) in infancy is calculated as

$$\text{PRSL} = \text{N}/28 + \text{Na} + \text{Cl} + \text{K} + \text{P}_a$$

where the units are in millimoles (or milliosmoles) except for N, which is total nitrogen in milligrams, and the term N/28 represents nitrogenous solutes. Na is sodium, Cl is chloride, K is potassium, and

$P_a$ is available phosphorus (which is assumed to be total phosphorus of milk-based formulas and two-thirds of the phosphorus of soy-based formula). To convert milligrams to millimoles, divide Na by 23, Cl by 35, K by 39, and P by 31.

The PRSL of commercially available milk-based formulas is about 135 mOsm/L (20 mOsm/100 kcal), and of soy protein–based formulas is about 160 mOsm/L (24 mOsm/100 kcal). In contrast, whole cow's milk is 308 mOsm/L (46 mOsm/100 kcal), and skim milk is 326 mOsm/L (93 mOsm/100 kcal). The use of formula with a high PRSL places the infant at increased risk for hypertonic dehydration, whereas formulas providing 20 to 26 mOsm/100 kcal offer a margin of safety with respect to water balance and are therefore recommended. Maintaining an appropriate PRSL is achieved by not exceeding a protein content of 3.2 g/100 kcal and a phosphorus concentration of less than 93 mg/100 kcal. Maximum PRSL will then be 221 mOsm/l (33 mOsm/100 kcal). Concentrated formulas are often indicated for infants who require fluid restrictions for cardiac, pulmonary, or renal indications as well as those who have insufficient volume intake resulting in inadequate caloric intake. Formula can often be safely concentrated to 24 kcal/oz by adding more powder/concentrate and less water, but careful attention must be paid to fluid status and hydration of the infant, particularly during an illness associated with decreased fluid intake or increased fluid losses. If higher–caloric-density formula is desired, carbohydrate or fat supplementation without additional protein or electrolyte being added to the formula is desirable.

## Energy

Energy is required to carry out the biochemical processes of life and to perform physical work. The energy provided by foods is chemical energy obtained after digestion. The unit of measure for energy is either the joule or the calorie (1 joule = 4200 cal). The kilocalorie is equal to 1000 calories, or the amount of heat energy that is required to raise 1 kg of water by 1 °C. Energy from foods that are consumed in a child's diet derives from carbohydrate (4 kcal/g), fat (9 kcal/g), and protein (4 kcal/g). In adults (and some adolescents), calories from ethanol (7 kcal/g) also may be a contributing source of energy.

The World Health Organization defines the energy requirements of an individual as the level of energy intake from food that will balance energy expenditure when the individual has a body size and composition and level of physical activity consistent with long-term good health and that will allow for the maintenance of economically necessary and socially desirable physical activity. In children and pregnant or lactating women, the energy requirement also includes the energy needs associated with the deposition of tissues or secretion of milk.

Energy requirements are highly individualized and vary widely among healthy persons. In states of disease and activity, energy requirements must be further adjusted to account for additional stresses. In most clinical situations, energy requirements for children are estimated from age, with the assumption of a similarity regarding body size, physical activity, and rate of growth. Provided one recognizes that recommendations for energy requirements are based on assumptions of size and activity, the energy needs of the healthy individual may be estimated from the estimated energy requirement (EER) equations that allow for growth and levels of physical activity.

The equations used to obtain EERs are shown in Table 15-2. Over 3 years of age, the recommended energy needs of boys and girls differ because of evolving activity patterns and later, because of the onset of puberty. Variability in the timing and intensity of the pubertal growth spurt as well as activity lead to substantial variation in the energy requirements of individual adolescents.

For the well-nourished, growing child, calculation of the EERs may be sufficient to evaluate caloric adequacy. However, these calculations are not an adequate tool for determining the energy needs of sick or malnourished children. In these instances, more precise, individualized calculations are necessary to assess a child's energy needs. The most reliable indicators of caloric adequacy in the sick child, however, are measurements of appropriate weight gain or loss, height, or skinfold thickness over time. Continual monitoring of growth parameters provides the only truly reliable method for determining the adequacy of energy intake. If growth is normal, it is reasonable to assume that the energy intake is adequate.

A number of methods are used to estimate the energy needs of ill children. These include indirect calorimetry, pediatric basal metabolic rate tables with appropriate activity, and growth and stress factors, as well as nitrogen balance studies. These studies are useful in the clinical setting to a certain extent. They should not be perceived as absolute values because all have a margin of error. The calculations that are products of these methods can only be utilized as a rough guideline by which to provide adequate energy to the acutely or chronically ill child. However, as stated previously, it is the growth and development of these patients that remain the gold standard of adequate energy intake or administration.

## Protein

Protein intake is required to supply nitrogen and amino acids for the synthesis of constituent proteins and other nitrogen-containing compounds such as polypeptide hormones. Nitrogen cannot be synthesized from fat or carbohydrate. Growth and regeneration of body components requires the constant replenishment of protein stores because of nitrogen losses from skin, hair, feces, and urine.

*Protein quality* refers to the distribution and the proportion of amino acids that the body is not capable of synthesizing from a particular protein source. A protein of high quality contains a large proportion of all essential amino acids. The required intake of protein varies inversely with the quality of the protein ingested; with intake of the higher-quality proteins, requirements will decrease. When low-quality proteins are ingested, excessive nonessential amino acids must be ingested to provide all of the essential amino acid requirements. These nonessential amino acids are either metabolized and excreted or can be deaminated and utilized as energy via gluconeogenesis. This process is not an efficient route of energy metabolism; it is both nutrient and energy consuming. Therefore, ingestion of higher-quality proteins is desirable.

Protein needs range from 2.0 to 2.4 $g{\cdot}kg^{-1}{\cdot}d^{-1}$ during the first month after birth and gradually fall to approximately 1.5 $g{\cdot}kg^{-1}{\cdot}d^{-1}$ by 6 months of age, where it remains throughout the infant's first year. DRIs for protein have been established but are tabulated in grams/day rather than the more useful $g{\cdot}kg^{-1}{\cdot}d^{-1}$ (Table 15-3).

During the second year of life, as table foods replace milk, the dietary requirement of protein increases from 1.5 $g{\cdot}kg^{-1}{\cdot}d^{-1}$ to approximately 2 $g{\cdot}kg^{-1}{\cdot}d^{-1}$ because the quality of mixed dietary protein is about 75% that of milk protein. Dietary protein requirements beyond infancy are met relatively easily by most Western diets. There is a surprising lack of appreciation of how much (or, more accurately, how little) protein actually is necessary in the diet to meet individual needs. The RDA for a 15-year-old boy is approximately 60 g of dietary protein. A 5-oz hamburger will meet over 50% of this protein need.

Of some concern is the current popularity of so-called high-protein body-building diets, which are aggressively marketed to male adolescents. There is no proof that ingestion of these high-protein diets is of any greater benefit than intake of a normal, well-balanced diet combined with vigorous training for the acquisition of muscle mass. Furthermore, those diets that truly are high in protein pose a potential though unproven risk of nephrotoxicity.

## Carbohydrate

Dietary carbohydrate may be either digestible or nondigestible. Digestible carbohydrates provide an important source of energy for metabolism. Glucose, stored as glycogen in the liver, is the preferred energy substrate for the brain. Carbohydrates also are structural elements in glycoproteins. If adequate dietary energy is not provided, additional energy must be expended to convert protein to glucose. The converted protein loses its value as a synthetic building block, with the nitrogen being lost in urine. An alternative means of deriving energy is via fatty acid oxidation. When carbohydrate is unavailable, fatty acids undergo β-oxidation, which results in acetyl-CoA, an intermediate of the citric acid cycle. This results in energy production. However, as in the case of gluconeogenesis, this alternative means of energy production requires energy itself. Therefore, inadequate provision of carbohydrate, which is an important source of calories, results in a net loss of body protein and fat stores, which may progress to protein-calorie malnutrition. Furthermore, inadequate energy intake from all sources can result in starvation, in which the body derives energy from ketone bodies. Carbohydrates are the predominant macronutrient in the promoted healthy diet.

Human milk provides approximately 40% of its calories as lactose, which is hydrolyzed to glucose and galactose. Fruits and vegetables contain simple sugars, including glucose and fructose; sucrose (table sugar) is a combination of glucose and fructose. In the child and adult, the majority of dietary carbohydrate is consumed in the form of polysaccharides, especially plant starches. Dietary carbohydrates provide from 35% to 60% of the average American diet. Complex carbohydrates should be promoted, and simple and refined starches should be minimized. This will help limit the overconsumption of "empty calories" and fructose, which are often found in foods with high concentrations of refined sugars (eg, soda, sweets, candy, and various "fruit" drinks).



Nondigestible carbohydrates, or dietary fiber, derive from plants and consist of a number of polysaccharides and lignins that are present in the cell walls of all plants. There are 2 forms of dietary fiber: soluble and insoluble. Soluble fiber includes pectins, gums, mucilages, and some hemicelluloses. Pectins are found primarily in fruits and vegetables. Oat bran, barley, and legumes are examples of dietary sources of soluble fiber. Insoluble fiber consisting of predominantly cellulose and hemicellulose provides structure to plant cells. The major source of insoluble fiber is the bran layer of whole grains.

A number of potential benefits are reported to result from the ingestion of high-fiber diets. Dietary increases in fiber are proven to be useful for the treatment of constipation and irritable bowel syndrome. Increasing fecal bulk by combining both soluble and insoluble fiber increases the nondigestible particles as well as the water-holding capacity in the colon. Furthermore, dietary fiber reduces intestinal transit time. Decreased transit time and increased volume of colonic fluids are potential mechanisms for the suggested (but unproven) beneficial effects of dietary fiber. In addition, the addition of soluble fiber to a low-fat diet has been found to lower total cholesterol and low density lipoprotein (LDL) cholesterol.

Short-chain fatty acids are metabolic by-products of fermented undigested carbohydrate, including fiber and lactose. Acetate, propionate, and butyrate comprise 95% of the short-chain fatty acids in the colon, which are absorbed by the normal colon and stimulate fluid and electrolyte absorption (especially sodium transport). They are also the preferred source of energy for the epithelial lining of the colon. Short-chain fatty acids stimulate intestinal mucosal cell turnover and blood flow. Although experimental data suggest that short-chain fatty acids can act as a trophic factor for the colon, adverse effects of excessive fiber and short-chain fatty acids include gastrointestinal obstruction (especially with motility disturbances), diarrhea, bloating, gas, and a metabolic acid load.

The importance of dietary fiber for infant nutrition is unknown. Its role in the appropriate nutrition of the toddler, child, and adolescent is inferred from studies on adults. It is important that an excessive emphasis on high-fiber intakes does not compromise the caloric intake of children.

### Fat

Fat (or lipid) provides an important, concentrated source of energy and plays a key role in the formation of the lipid bilayer membrane structure. In addition, the essential fatty acid arachidonic acid provides substrate for the formation of prostaglandins, leukotrienes, and thromboxanes. There are 3 major categories of lipids in Western diets: (1) triglycerides, (2) phospholipids, and (3) sterols. Triglycerides are the main dietary lipid. Each triglyceride consists of 3 esterified fatty acids that are bound to a molecule of glycerol. Triglycerides are characterized on the basis of the chain length of the bound fatty acids as short-chain fatty acids (fewer than 8 carbons), medium-chain fatty acids (8–12 carbons), and long-chain fatty acids (greater than 12 carbons). There are 3 predominant forms of phospholipid in the diet: (1) phosphatidylcholine (lecithin), (2) phosphatidylserine, and (3) phosphatidylethanolamine. These are structurally similar except for the bases (choline, serine, ethanolamine). The main dietary sterol is cholesterol, which is not present in foods of plant origin.

The main dietary lipid in North America is the long-chain fatty acid (each fatty acid contains 14, 16, 18, or 20 carbon units). The long-chain fatty acids are further classified according to their degree of saturation; that is, *saturated* (contain the maximum number of hydrogens bound to the chain), *monounsaturated* (1 double bond), and *polyunsaturated* (two or more double bonds). Typical American diets contain approximately 40% each of monounsaturated and saturated fatty acids. Polyunsaturated fatty acids and glycerol account for approximately 10% each. The proportion of unsaturated to saturated fatty acids in the diet is referred to as the P/S ratio (after the contribution of monounsaturated fatty acids has been excluded). In general, animal fats are highly saturated and have a lower P/S ratio than do vegetable fats. These distinctions are important because there is compelling evidence that links the ingestion of diets that are high in saturated fat to the development of atherosclerosis.

*Trans*-fatty acids are formed when manufacturers add hydrogen to liquid oils to create semisolid and more stable fats. This process results in the formation of a *trans* configuration (the *cis* configuration exists naturally in unsaturated fats). Recent studies have shown that consuming *trans*-fatty acids at levels similar to those in the average American diet (3% of kilocalories) will raise LDL cholesterol and increase the risk of coronary heart disease and that increased *trans*-fatty acid intake may have adverse effects on infant neurodevelopment. *Trans*-fatty acids are found in stick margarine, commercial frying fats, and high-fat baked goods. Natural sources of *trans*-fatty acids include butter, beef, and milk fats.

Humans are able to synthesize most fatty acids de novo by elongation and saturation of shorter unsaturated fatty acids. However, linoleic acid (an 18-carbon fatty acid with 2 unsaturated bonds) and longer polyunsaturates cannot be synthesized and therefore must be provided in the diet. Linoleic acid can be lengthened to form arachidonic acid (a 20-carbon fatty acid with 4 unsaturated bonds), which is therefore not essential if there is adequate linoleic acid in the diet. Linolenic acid (an 18-carbon fatty acid with 3 double bonds) generally also is considered to be an essential fatty acid, although dietary deficiency is rare. The benefits of supplementation of infants and lactating mothers with docosahexaenoic acid, an ω-3 polyunsaturated fatty acid, and arachidonic acid, an ω-6 polyunsaturated acid, on infant neurodevelopmental outcomes are unclear.

Essential fatty acid deficiency occurs when levels of linoleic acid are too low to maintain normal fatty acid metabolism. Clinically, symptoms that are most likely to be recognized are those of a scaly dermatitis, hair loss, diarrhea, and poor wound healing. Those children who are most at risk to develop essential fatty acid deficiency include premature infants who receive inadequate linoleic acid, children with fat malabsorption from hepatobiliary or pancreatic disease, and children receiving long-term parenteral nutrition without intravenous lipid. Although the exact requirement for linoleic acid is unclear, there is general agreement that 2% to 10% of calories should be ingested as linoleic acid. The diagnosis of essential fatty acid deficiency is established by demonstrating abnormally low plasma linoleic acid levels based on analysis of either total lipid extracts or isolated phospholipids. In addition, classically there is a decrease in arachidonic acid levels and a rise in 5,8,11-eicosatrienoic acid, which reflects a high rate of conversion of oleic acid to an abnormal triene. This generally is thought to occur as a compensatory mechanism with production of more longer-chain polyunsaturated fatty acids. The increased triene and decreased arachidonic acid (tetraene levels) result in a triene: tetraene ratio above 0.2, which is diagnostic of essential fatty acid deficiency.

Human milk contains 3% to 7% of calories from linoleic acid and significant amounts of linolenic acid. The actual fatty acid content varies depending on the mother's diet. Most commercial formulas derive over 10% of their calories from linoleic acid, and all contain at least some linolenic acid. Cow's milk has only approximately 1% linoleic acid, which is less than one half of the recommended level (2.4% of calories from linoleic acid), but essential fatty acid deficiency has not been observed in healthy babies who have been fed cow's milk.

Medium-chain fatty acids comprise approximately 10% of the fatty acids in milk from the mother of a full-term infant and approximately 17% in that of the mother of a premature infant. Medium-chain triglycerides do not require bile acids to achieve solubilization and absorption. Additionally, they are absorbed directly into the portal system rather than via the lymphatic circulation. Thus, medium-chain triglycerides are better absorbed by premature infants compared with long-chain triglycerides, since bile acid secretion and pancreatic enzyme excretion is relatively deficient in the infant. Excessive use of medium-chain triglycerides (> 60% of total fat intake) as a replacement for long-chain triglycerides decreases the intake of essential fatty acids, thus increasing the risk of essential fatty acid deficiency.

Concerns regarding excessive caloric and cholesterol intake have led to the recommendation that overall fat intake should be limited, because elevated cholesterol levels early in life are linked to the later development of atherosclerosis in adulthood. Therefore, in all healthy children and adolescents over the age of 2 years, nutritional adequacy should be achieved by eating a wide variety of foods, with total fat providing no more than 30% of total calories and saturated fatty acids less than 10% of total calories. Intake of dietary cholesterol should not exceed 300 mg/d. Each of these recommendations refers to an average nutrient intake over a period of several days. The hope is that children will adopt these healthy eating habits and guidelines early in life, thereby fostering healthy eating patterns throughout life. Children who are younger than 2 years of age are specifically excluded from these recommendations because fat provides an important dietary source of energy. Therefore, emphasis on limiting fat intake can lead to inadequate caloric intake.

### Vitamins

Vitamins serve as cofactors in a wide range of vital metabolic reactions. Their biochemical actions, effects of deficiency, toxicities, and dietary sources are enumerated in Table 15-4; acceptable ranges of vitamin intake are listed in Table 15-5. Vitamins are widely used as dietary supplements. These supplements are of no demonstrated value for the healthy infant, child, adolescent, or adult who is consuming an adequate and varied diet. Although there is no demonstrated adverse effect to the use of a daily multivitamin supplement containing the RDA for vitamins, supplementation is expensive and unnecessary. For the otherwise well patient, use of a vitamin supplement may undermine the concept that adequate nutrition is provided through the intake of a mixed, varied diet.

### Major Minerals

Approximately 98% of the body's mineral content consists of calcium, phosphorus, and magnesium, with bone containing 99% of the calcium, 80% of the phosphorus, and 60% of the magnesium. Table 15-6 outlines the principal biochemical actions, effects of deficiency, toxicity, and dietary sources of these 3 major minerals. Acceptable intakes are listed in Table 15-7. Total body calcium rapidly increases during the last 2 months of gestation and during adolescence. Bone mineralization continues through the third decade, when peak bone density is achieved. The height of this peak appears to influence the development of osteoporosis later in life, reinforcing the importance of early nutrition on later health.

Milk or infant formula supplies these minerals to the infant and young child. Therefore, children with decreased intake of milk, for whatever reason, are at increased risk of dietary calcium deficiency. The ratio of calcium to phosphorus (Ca:P ratio) strongly affects net mineral absorption and varies widely in different foods. Green vegetables have a Ca:P ratio of 2.8:1, human milk of 2:1, cow's milk of 1.2:1, and meat of 0.6:1. Foods that are high in phosphates (eg, cola drinks) may predispose to bone loss. The favorable Ca:P in human milk is particularly important to assure adequate bone mineralization in infancy. Specially formulated premature and low–birth-weight formulas contain Ca:P ratios of approximately 2:1 to assure adequate bone mineralization for this high-risk population. The control of calcium metabolism is discussed in detail in Chapter 535.

Calcium absorption is inhibited by dietary phosphate, oxalate, fiber, alkali, and malabsorbed fat. Calcium absorption is enhanced by lactose-containing formulas and the activated form of vitamin D [1,25-$(OH)_2D_3$]. Phosphorus absorption is decreased by dietary calcium and aluminum-containing or magnesium-containing antacids.

### Trace Elements, Iron, and Zinc

Trace elements constitute less than 0.0001 of the total body weight, yet many are considered to be essential for life, health, and reproduction. Table 15-8 summarizes the biochemical actions, effects of deficiency, toxicity, and dietary sources of the trace elements. Trace elements serve as cofactors in enzyme reactions, components of body fluids, sites for binding oxygen, and structural components for nonenzymatic macromolecules. Except for deficiencies of iron and iodine, which have been well known, deficiencies of other trace elements are only beginning to be recognized as health-related problems. For example, fluoride deficiency has been linked to an increased risk of dental caries, zinc deficiency to growth failure, chromium deficiency to glucose intolerance, copper deficiency to hypercholesterolemia, and selenium deficiency to cardiomyopathy. Adequate iron intake is a concern throughout childhood. This is especially significant in periods of rapid growth. The exclusively breast-fed infant receives adequate iron and zinc from breast milk for the first 4 to 6 months of life. It has been shown that iron from breast milk is better absorbed than iron from formula. However, both breastfed and formula-fed infants should receive additional sources of iron by age 6 months. This includes iron-fortified cereals and meats.

## SUGGESTED READINGS

Delgado-Noguera MF, Calvache JA, BonfillCosp X, Kotanidou EP, Galli-Tsinopoulou A. Supplementation with long chain polyunsaturated fatty acids (LCPUFA) to breastfeeding mothers for improving child growth and development. *Cochrane Database Syst Rev.* 2015 Jul 14;(7):CD007901.

Dietary Guidelines for Americans 2015–2020. US Department of Health & Human Services Web site. Available at: http://health.gov/dietaryguidelines/2015/resources/2015-2020_Dietary_Guidelines.pdf. Accessed July 11, 2016.

Dietary Reference Intakes. Institute of Medicine of the National Academies Web site. Available at: http://www.nationalacademies.org/hmd/Activities/Nutrition/SummaryDRIs/DRI-Tables.aspx. Accessed July 11, 2016.

Sun H, Como PG, Downey LC, Murphy D, Ariagno RL, Rodriguez W. Infant formula and neurocognitive outcomes: impact of study endpoint selection. *J Perinatol.* 2015 Oct;35(10):867-74. doi10.1038/jp.2015.87.

**TABLE 15-4 SUMMARY OF CLINICALLY RELEVANT INFORMATION ON FAT-SOLUBLE AND WATER-SOLUBLE VITAMINS**

| | Biochemical Action | Effects of Deficiency | Effects of Toxicity | Dietary Sources |
|---|---|---|---|---|
| | ***Fat-Soluble Vitamins*** | | | |
| **Vitamin A** | Component of retinal pigments and rhodopsin for vision in dim light, bone and tooth development; preserves integrity of epithelial cells; promotes wound healing and growth | Night blindness, xerophthalmia, photophobia, conjunctivitis, Bitot spots, keratomalacia, hyperkeratosis of the skin and mucous membranes, poor growth, impaired resistance to infection | Carotenemia with xanthosis cutis, night sweats, dry and cracking skin, vertigo, hepatomegaly, vomiting, alopecia, increased cerebrospinal fluid pressure | Liver, fish-liver oils, milk fat, egg yolk, butter, green and deep yellow vegetables |
| **Vitamin D** | Regulates absorption and deposition of calcium and phosphorus, formation of calcium transport protein in duodenal mucosa, synthesis of calcium-binding protein in epithelial cells | *In infants and children:* rickets.<br>*In adults:* osteomalacia | *In infants and children:* hypercalcemia, anorexia, poor growth<br>*In adults:* nausea, vomiting, polydipsia, polyuria, calcification of soft tissue including heart, renal tubules, and bronchi | Fortified milk, egg yolk, liver, salmon, butter, sardines, mackerel |
| **Vitamin E** | Antioxidant, role in red blood cell fragility, stabilizes cell membranes, prevents peroxidation of unsaturated fatty acids | Hemolytic anemia in premature infants, loss of neural integrity, muscle lesions, ceroid pigment deposition | Unknown | Vegetable oils, beef liver, seed oils, peanuts, soybeans, milk fat, turnip greens, eggs, butter, leafy vegetables |
| **Vitamin K** | Catalyzes prothrombin synthesis; coagulation factors II, VII, IX, X; proteins C, S, Z | Hemorrhagic manifestations | Kernicterus (water-soluble analogs only) | Vegetable oils, liver, pork, green leafy vegetables (also synthesized by normal intestinal flora) |
| | ***Water-Soluble Vitamins*** | | | |
| | **Biochemical Action** | **Effects of Deficiency** | **Effects of Toxicity** | **Dietary Sources** |
| **Thiamin** | Combines with phosphorus to form thiamin pyrophosphate, which acts in various oxidative decarboxylations, including pyruvic acid | *Wet beriberi:* congestive heart failure, tachycardia, peripheral edema<br>*Dry beriberi:* neuritis, paresthesia, irritability, anorexia | Unknown | Liver, meat, milk, pork, whole grains, legumes, nuts |
| **Riboflavin** | Part of the flavin coenzymes, FAD and FMN, necessary for tissue oxidation and respiration and synthesis of FMN and FAD essential for growth, retinal pigment for light adaptation | Photophobia, loss of visual acuity, burning and itching of eyes, corneal vascularization, glossitis, seborrheic dermatitis, poor growth, cheilosis | Unknown | Milk, cheese, eggs, organ meats, fish, green leafy vegetables, whole and enriched grains |
| **Niacin** | Component of coenzymes I and II (NAD, NADP), cofactors in a number of dehydrogenase systems, necessary for synthesis of glycogen and breakdown of fatty acids | *Pellagra:* dermatitis, apathy, anorexia, peripheral neuropathy, encephalopathy with some degree of dementia, diarrhea secondary to atrophy of mucosa | Nicotinic acid has transient vasodilating effects, skin flushing, tingling, itching, dizziness, nausea; may induce liver abnormalities | Lean meats, poultry, peanuts, organ meats, brewer's yeast, green vegetables, enriched cereals and grains |
| **Folate** | Tetrahydrofolic acid is the active form; essential in the biosynthesis of purines, pyrimidines, and nucleoproteins; methylation reactions; 1-carbon acceptor | Megaloblastic anemia (should also suspect concurrent vitamin $B_{12}$ deficiency), impaired cellular immunity, poor growth, glossitis, gastrointestinal disturbances | Unknown | Liver, green leafy vegetables, legumes, asparagus, broccoli, nuts, cheese |
| **Vitamin $B_6$ (Pyridoxine)** | Constituent of many coenzymes for decarboxylation, transamination, transsulfuration, role in hemoglobin synthesis and fatty acid metabolism | Dermatitis, cheilosis, stomatitis, peripheral neuritis (in patients on isoniazid), microcytic, hypochromic anemia, irritability, convulsions | Sensory neuropathy with progressive ataxia, altered sense of touch, pain, fever | Liver, meat, whole grains, yeast, potatoes, corn, soybeans, bananas, peanuts |
| **Vitamin $B_{12}$ (Cobalamin)** | Essential for red blood cell maturation in bone marrow, coenzyme for methylmalonyl CoA mutase, transfer of 1-carbon units in purine metabolism, affects central nervous system metabolism | Pernicious anemia, neurologic deterioration because of demyelination of large nerve fibers of the spinal cord, methylmalonic aciduria, homocystinuria | Unknown | Liver, organ meats, meat, eggs, cheese, fish |
| **Biotin** | Coenzyme of all carboxylases and of carbon dioxide | Leiner dermatitis, anorexia, glossitis, alopecia, nausea, anorexia, muscle pain, insomnia | Unknown | Liver, kidney, milk, egg yolk, yeast, mushrooms, banana, watermelon, strawberries, grapefruit |
| **Pantothenic acid** | Component of CoA; necessary for fat, protein, and CHO metabolism; fatty acid biosynthesis | Observed with use of antagonists, can cause depression, hypotension, muscle weakness, nausea, sleep disturbances, abdominal pain, loss of antibody production | Unknown | Most foods |
| **Vitamin C** | Integrity maintenance of all intercellular materials, collagen biosynthesis, iron absorption and transport, metabolism of tyrosine, synthesis of corticosteroids | *Scurvy:* diffuse tissue bleeding, pinpoint peripheral hemorrhages, easy bone fracture, poor wound healing, friable bleeding gums with loose teeth | Nausea, diarrhea, cramps; massive doses may predispose to kidney stones | Citrus fruits, tomatoes, berries, green vegetables, cabbage, human milk |

CHO, carbohydrate; CoA, coenzyme A; FAD, flavin adenine dinucleotide; FMN, flavin mononucleotide; NAD, nicotinamide adenine dinucleotide; NADP, nicotinamide adenine dinucleotide phosphate.

**TABLE 15-5 ACCEPTABLE INTAKES FOR VITAMINS**

| | Vitamin A (mg/d) | Vitamin C (mg/d) | Vitamin D (μg/d)[b] | Vitamin E (mg/d)[c] | Vitamin K (μg/d) | Thiamin (mg/d) | Riboflavin (mg/d) | Niacin (mg/d) | Vitamin $B_6$ (mg/d) | Folate (mg/d)[d] | Vitamin $B_{12}$ (μg/d) | Pantothenic Acid | Biotin (mg/d) | Choline (mg/d) |
|---|---|---|---|---|---|---|---|---|---|---|---|---|---|---|
| **Infants** | | | | | | | | | | | | | | |
| 0–6 mo | **400[a]**–600 | **40[a]** | **10[a]**–25 | **4[a]** | **2.0[a]** | **0.2[a]** | **0.3[a]** | **2[a]** | **0.1[a]** | **65[a]** | **0.4[a]** | **1.7[a]** | **5[a]** | **125[a]** |
| 7–12 mo | **500[a]**–600 | **50[a]** | **10[a]**–38 | **5[a]** | **2.5[a]** | **0.3[a]** | **0.4[a]** | **4[a]** | **0.3[a]** | **80[a]** | **0.5[a]** | **1.8[a]** | **6[a]** | **150[a]** |
| **Children** | | | | | | | | | | | | | | |
| 1–3 y | 300–600 | 15–400 | 15–63 | 6–200 | **30[a]** | 0.5 | 0.5 | 6–10 | 0.5–30 | 150–300 | 0.9 | **2[a]** | **8[a]** | **200[a]**–1000 |
| 4–8 y | 400–900 | 25–650 | 15–75 | 7–300 | **55[a]** | 0.6 | 0.6 | 8–15 | 0.6–40 | 200–400 | 1.2 | **3[a]** | **12[a]** | **250[a]**–1000 |
| **Males** | | | | | | | | | | | | | | |
| 9–13 y | 600–1700 | 45–1200 | 15–100 | 11–600 | **60[a]** | 0.9 | 0.9 | 12–20 | 1–60 | 300–600 | 1.8 | **4[a]** | **20[a]** | **375[a]**–2000 |
| 14–18 y | 900–2800 | 75–1800 | 15–100 | 15–800 | **75[a]** | 1.2 | 1.3 | 16–30 | 1.3–80 | 400–800 | 2.4 | **5[a]** | **25[a]** | **550[a]**–3000 |
| **Females** | | | | | | | | | | | | | | |
| 9–13 y | 600–1700 | 45–1200 | 15–100 | 11–600 | **60[a]** | 0.9 | 0.9 | 12–20 | 1–60 | 300–600 | 1.8 | **4[a]** | **20[a]** | **375[a]**–2000 |
| 14–18 y | 700–2800 | 65–1800 | 15–100 | 15–800 | **75[a]** | 1 | 1 | 14–30 | 1.2–80 | 400–800 | 2.4 | **5[a]** | **25[a]** | **400[a]**–3000 |
| **Pregnancy** | | | | | | | | | | | | | | |
| 14–18 y | 750–2800 | 80–1800 | 15–100 | 15–800 | **75[a]** | 1.4 | 1.4 | 18–30 | 1.9–80 | 600–800 | 2.6 | **6[a]** | **30[a]** | **450[a]**–3000 |
| **Lactation** | | | | | | | | | | | | | | |
| 14–18 y | 1200–2800 | 115–1800 | 15–100 | 19–800 | **75[a]** | 1.4 | 1.6 | 17–30 | 2–80 | 500–800 | 2.8 | **7[a]** | **35[a]** | **550[a]**–3000 |

[a]Where the RDA is unavailable, AIs are shown in bold and marked with an asterisk; in some instances, where tolerable ULs are unavailable, only the AIs are shown.

[b]As cholecalciferol; 1 μg cholecalciferol = 40 IU vitamin D.

[c]As α-tocopherol.

[d]As dietary folate equivalents (DFE); 1 DFE = 1 μg food folate = 0.6 μg of folic acid from fortified food or as a supplement consumed with food.

These ranges reflect the RDAs as the lower limit and the tolerable upper intake levels as the UL. For thiamin, riboflavin, and niacin beyond the age of 1 year, only RDAs without the ULs are available.

**TABLE 15-6 SUMMARY OF CLINICALLY RELEVANT INFORMATION ON MINERALS**

| | Biochemical Action | Effects of Deficiency | Effects of Toxicity | Dietary Sources |
|---|---|---|---|---|
| **Calcium** | Structure of bone and teeth; activates smooth, skeletal, cardiac muscle contraction and neural transmitter release, blood coagulation | Poor mineralization of bone and teeth, osteomalacia, osteoporosis, rickets, tetany, growth impairment, possibly hypertension | *Dietary:* excessive calcification of bone, calcification of soft tissue<br>*Parenteral:* heart block and renal stones | Cheese, milk, turnip and mustard greens, collards, kale, broccoli, canned salmon and sardines with bones, clams, oysters |
| **Magnesium** | Cofactor for many enzyme systems, including ATP formation, protein synthesis, nerve impulse transmission, phosphate transfer systems, muscle contraction, principal cation of soft tissue structure of bone and teeth | Muscle tremors, convulsions, irritability, tetany, hyperreflexia or hyporeflexia | Rare dietary toxicity, toxicity more common with intravenous infusions | Whole grains, nuts, dried beans, peas, meat, milk |
| **Phosphorus** | Constituent of bones and teeth; structure of cytoplasm and nucleic acids; phospholipids; coenzyme for CHO, fat, and protein metabolism | Rickets may develop in low-birth-weight babies; neuromuscular, renal, and skeletal abnormalities | High-phosphorus infant formulas (Ca:P ratio 1:1) may contribute to hypocalcemia, tetany in early infancy | Milk, cheese, dairy products, egg yolk, meat, legumes, nuts, poultry, fish |

ATP, adenosine 5′-diphosphate; CHO, carbohydrate; Ca:P, Calcium:Phosphorus.

**TABLE 15-7 ACCEPTABLE INTAKES FOR MINERALS**

| | Calcium (mg/d) | Chromium (μg/d) | Copper (μg/d) | Fluoride (mg/d) | Iodine (μg/d) | Iron (mg/d) | Magnesium (mg/d)[b] | Manganese (mg/d) | Molybdenum (μg/d) | Phosphorus (mg/d) | Selenium (μg/d) | Zinc (mg/d) | Potassium (g/d) | Sodium (g/d) | Chloride (g/d) |
|---|---|---|---|---|---|---|---|---|---|---|---|---|---|---|---|
| **Infants** | | | | | | | | | | | | | | | |
| 0–6 mo | **200[a]**–1000 | **0.2[a]** | **200[a]** | **0.01[a]**–0.7 | **110[a]** | **0.27[a]**–40 | **30[a]** | **0.003[a]** | **2[a]** | **100[a]** | **15[a]**–45 | **2[a]**–4 | **0.4[a]** | **0.12[a]** | **0.18[a]** |
| 7–12 mo | **260[a]**–1500 | **5.5[a]** | **220[a]** | **0.5[a]**–0.9 | **130[a]** | 11–40 | **75[a]** | **0.6[a]** | **3[a]** | **275[a]** | **20[a]**–60 | 3–5 | **0.7[a]** | **0.37[a]** | **0.57[a]** |
| **Children** | | | | | | | | | | | | | | | |
| 1–3 y | 700–2500 | **11[a]** | 340–1000 | **0.7[a]**–1.3 | 90–200 | 8–40 | 80 | **1.2[a]**–2 | 17–300 | 460–3000 | 20–90 | 3–7 | **3.0[a]** | **1.0[a]**–1.5 | **1.5[a]**–2.3 |
| 4–8 y | 1000–2500 | **15[a]** | 440–3000 | **1[a]**–2.2 | 90–300 | 10–40 | 130 | **1.5[a]**–3 | 22–600 | 500–3000 | 30–150 | 5–12 | **3.8[a]** | **1.2[a]**–1.9 | **1.9[a]**–2.9 |
| **Males** | | | | | | | | | | | | | | | |
| 9–13 y | 1300–3000 | **25[a]** | 700–5000 | **2[a]**–10 | 120–600 | 8–40 | 240 | **1.9[a]**–6 | 34–1100 | 1250–4000 | 40–280 | 8–23 | **4.5[a]** | **1.5[a]**–2.2 | **2.3[a]**–3.4 |
| 14–18 y | 1300–3000 | **35[a]** | 890–8000 | **3[a]**–10 | 150–900 | 11–45 | 410 | **2.2[a]**–9 | 43–1700 | 1250–4000 | 55–400 | 11–34 | **4.7[a]** | **1.5[a]**–2.3 | **2.3[a]**–3.6 |
| **Females** | | | | | | | | | | | | | | | |
| 9–13 y | 1300–3000 | **21[a]** | 700–5000 | **2[a]**–10 | 120–600 | 8–40 | 240 | **1.6[a]**–6 | 34–1100 | 1250–4000 | 40–280 | 8–23 | **4.5[a]** | **1.5[a]**–2.2 | **2.3[a]**–3.4 |
| 14–18 y | 1300–3000 | **24[a]** | 890–8000 | **3[a]**–10 | 150–900 | 15–45 | 360 | **1.6[a]**–9 | 43–1700 | 1250–4000 | 55–400 | 9–34 | **4.7[a]** | **1.5[a]**–2.3 | **2.3[a]**–3.6 |
| **Pregnancy** | | | | | | | | | | | | | | | |
| 14–18 y | 1300–3000 | **29[a]** | 1000–8000 | **3[a]**–10 | 220–900 | 27–45 | 400 | **2.0[a]**–9 | 50–1700 | 1250–3500 | 60–400 | 12–34 | **4.7[a]** | **1.5[a]**–2.3 | **2.3[a]**–3.6 |
| **Lactation** | | | | | | | | | | | | | | | |
| 14–18 y | 1300–3000 | **44[a]** | 1300–8000 | **3[a]**–10 | 290–900 | 10–45 | 360 | **2.6[a]**–9 | 50–1700 | 1250–4000 | 70–400 | 13–34 | **5.1[a]** | **1.5[a]**–2.3 | **2.3[a]**–3.6 |

[a]Where the RDA is unavailable, AIs are shown in bold and marked with an asterisk; in some instances, where tolerable ULs are unavailable, only the AIs are shown.

[b]The tolerable ULs for magnesium are based on intake from pharmaceutical agents only and are not shown.

These ranges reflect the RDAs as the lower limit and the tolerable upper intake levels as the UL.

**TABLE 15-8 SUMMARY OF CLINICALLY RELEVANT INFORMATION ON TRACE ELEMENTS**

| | Biochemical Action | Effects of Deficiency | Effects of Toxicity | Dietary Sources |
|---|---|---|---|---|
| **Chromium** | Required for normal glucose metabolism, potentiates the action of insulin | Glucose intolerance, impaired growth, peripheral neuropathy, negative nitrogen balance, decreased respiratory quotient | Unknown | Meat, cheese, brewer's yeast |
| **Copper** | Necessary for red blood cell and hemoglobin formation, constituent of ceruloplasmin, component of key metalloenzymes, role in connective tissue biosynthesis, iron absorption | Sideroblastic anemia, neutropenia, leukopenia, depigmentation, ataxia, erythropoiesis dysfunction, anorexia, bone demineralization, increased serum cholesterol | Wilson disease, copper deposition in the cornea and liver (leading to cirrhosis), deterioration of neurologic status | Liver, oysters, kidney, shellfish, legumes, raisins, chocolate, meat, fish, nuts |
| **Fluoride** | Helps protect against tooth decay, may minimize bone loss | Increased tendency to dental caries | Fluorosis: mottled and discolored teeth, calcified muscle insertions, and exostosis | Drinking water, seafood, plant and animal foods (dependent on content in water and soil) |
| **Iodine** | Component of thyroid hormones thyroxine and triiodothyronine | Hypothyroidism, simple goiter, endemic cretinism | Thyrotoxicosis, medicinally induced goiter | Iodized salt, seafood, seaweed |
| **Iron** | Structure of hemoglobin and myoglobin for $O_2$ and $CO_2$ transport, oxidative enzymes, cytochrome c, and catalase | Hypochromic, microcytic anemia, growth failure | Hemochromatosis | Liver, lean meat, egg, poultry, oysters, legumes, fortified cereals, grains, dark molasses |
| **Manganese** | Cofactor for pyruvate and acetyl-CoA carboxylases, mitochondrial superoxide dismutase, and other enzymes | Weight loss, transient dermatitis, nausea and vomiting, slow hair growth, change in hair color | Neurologic changes like those of Parkinson or Wilson disease | Widely distributed, deficiency reported only with experimental diets |
| **Molybdenum** | Cofactor for xanthine, aldehyde, and sulfite oxidases | Severe brain damage, tachycardia, headache | Gout-like syndrome | Widely distributed, deficiency reported only with parenteral nutrition and genetic syndromes |
| **Selenium** | Growth factor and cofactor for glutathione peroxidase and other enzyme systems | Cardiomyopathy, muscle pain, macrocytosis | Hair loss, polyneuritis, metallic taste | Widely distributed, deficiency reported in some areas of China (Keshan) and rarely with parenteral nutrition |
| **Zinc** | Cofactor of more than 90 enzymes, including erythrocyte carbonic anhydrase and superoxide dismutase | Growth failure, hypogonadism, hypogeusia, diarrhea, dermatoses | Vomiting and diarrhea, dermatoses, copper deficiency | Widely distributed, deficiency in chronic diarrhea and parenteral nutrition |



# 16 Breastfeeding

Lauren Fiechtner, Alyssa Robinson, and Ronald Kleinman

## BACKGROUND

All major national and international organizations focused on nutrition and infant and child health support breastfeeding to provide optimal nutrition for healthy full-term infants. The recommended period of exclusive breastfeeding during which the infant receives "no other food or drink, not even water, except breast milk (including milk expressed or from a wet nurse)"—although the infant can receive oral rehydration solution, drops, and syrups (vitamins, minerals, and medicines)—has been the subject of much discussion and varies from 3 to 4 months to 6 months. The American Academy of Pediatrics (AAP) recommends that children be exclusively breastfed for approximately the first 6 months of life, followed by continued breastfeeding as complementary foods are introduced for 1 year or longer as mutually desired by the mother and infant. The World Health Organization's (WHO) growth standards reflect the growth of breastfed infants and are now commonly used to plot the growth of infants and young children.

Benefits of breastfeeding are numerous. In addition to providing nutrition to the infant and supporting early development, breastfeeding may impart additional health benefits to both child and mother. Cost analyses suggest significant economic benefits of breastfeeding.

## COMPOSITION

Breast milk is a complex biologic fluid with nutrients that support the growth and development of infants as well as the health of the mother. It contains all the nutrients necessary for infant survival during the first 4 to 6 months of life, including fat, protein, carbohydrates, vitamins (with the exception of vitamin K in the postpartum period and then vitamin D), minerals, and water. The level of nutrients in human milk varies within a single lactation, during the period of lactation and also between mothers, with maternal diet playing a role in the levels of selected nutrients. Generally, about one half of the energy content of breast milk comes from fats, including long-chain polyunsaturated fatty acids (LCPUFA) that are not found in other milks/infant formulas, although the formulas are now routinely fortified with selected LCPUFA. The protein in breast milk is well suited to infant development in both quantity and quality, relative to other animal milks. With the exception of vitamin D, breast milk of a healthy mother contains all the vitamins and minerals that an infant needs in sufficient quantities, although the concentrations of zinc and iron decline substantially beginning at 4 months of age. Breast milk also contains a number of non-nutrient, biologically active substances, including hormones, immunoglobulins, growth factors (both human and microbial), digestive enzymes, cytokines, pheromones, and its own microbiota (Table 16-1 and Table 16-2).

### Physiology of Lactation

As early as 16 weeks of gestation, the breast is prepared for lactation. Lactation is regulated by the interaction of various hormones, nerves, and glands. Sensory nerves at the nipple are stimulated when a baby suckles at the breast, stimulating the "let-down reflex" and ultimately the release of prolactin from the anterior pituitary and oxytocin from the posterior pituitary. Increased prolactin levels in the blood stimulate milk production by the alveoli. Suckling also suppresses ovulation and menstruation following childbirth through its effects on levels of other pituitary hormones, including gonadotropin releasing hormone, luteinizing hormone, and follicle stimulating hormone.

**TABLE 16-1 NUTRIENT COMPOSITION OF BREAST MILK**

| | Preterm | | Postpartum | | |
|---|---|---|---|---|---|
| | Early | Late | Colostrum | Transitional | Mature |
| Fat (%) | — | 2 | 2 | 2.9 | 3.6 |
| Fat (g) | — | — | 2.9 | 3.6 | 3.8 |
| Lipid (g/dL) | 1.15 | 1.28 | 3.16 | 3.49 | 4.14 |
| Phospholipid (mg/dL) | 37 | 40 | 35 | 31 | 27 |
| Percentage of total lipid | 3.2 | 3.1 | 1.1 | 0.9 | 0.6 |
| Cholesterol (mg/dL) | — | — | 29 | 20 | 13.5 |
| Protein (g/L) | 54 | | — | — | 10.5 |
| Lactose | 79.78 mM | | — | — | 72.0 (g/L) |

Adapted with permission from Lawrence RA: Biochemistry of Human Milk. *Breastfeeding: A Guide for the Medical Professional,* 8th edition. Philadelphia: Elsevier; 2016.



Oxytocin release leads to contraction of the myoepithelial cells surrounding the alveoli, pushing milk out of the alveoli and into the ducts. The let-down reflex may also become activated when a mother sees, hears, smells, or thinks about her baby and can be inhibited if a mother is experiencing extreme stress or pain.

A complex feedback system exists to ensure a proper balance between the amount of breast milk the baby needs and the amount of milk produced. Milk production in each individual breast is controlled independently and depends on the release of milk either through suckling by the infant or expression by the mother.

## EPIDEMIOLOGY

The Centers for Disease Control and Prevention (CDC) has estimated that the overall rate of initiation of breastfeeding for the US population is 81%, with 44% and 22% of mothers reporting "exclusive breastfeeding" at 3 and 6 months, respectively; reports of "any breastfeeding" at 6 months and 1 year remain below Healthy People 2020 targets, although they continue to increase steadily. The rates of initiation of breastfeeding as well as duration of exclusive or any breastfeeding vary significantly by age, race/ethnicity, income level, and employment status of the mother (and these factors contribute to the uncertainty associated with observational studies that have examined and ascribed certain positive health outcomes associated with breastfeeding, as discussed below).

In general, women who breastfeed have higher education levels are more likely to be white, have a higher level of income/employment rate and are older. For example, 80.6% of Hispanic women initiate breastfeeding as compared to 58.1% of non-Hispanic Black women. Among low-income mothers participating in the special supplemental nutrition program for Women, Infants, and Children (WIC), breastfeeding initiation rate was 67.5%, but in those with a higher income it was 84.6%. Women who are 20 years and younger have a lower initiation rate of 59.7% compared to 79.3% of women 30 years and older.

**TABLE 16-2 NON-NUTRITIVE CONTENTS OF BREAST MILK**

| | |
|---|---|
| Immunoglobulins | IgG, IgA |
| Nonimmunoglobulins | Mucins, sialic acid-containing glycoproteins |
| Polyamines | Putrescine, spermidine, spermine |
| Nonprotein nitrogen | Peptide hormone/growth factors, epidermal growth factor, amino sugars of oligosaccharides, free amino acids, amino alcohols of phospholipids, nucleotides and carnitine, lactoferrin |
| Minerals | Potassium, sodium, chloride, magnesium |
| Trace elements | Iron, zinc, fluorine, iodide |
| Carotenoids | Lutein |
| Vitamins | Vitamin A, vitamin $B_1$, vitamin $B_2$, niacin, vitamin $B_6$, pantothenic acid, folic acid, vitamin $B_{12}$ |
| Enzymes | Amylases, lipases, glucose-6-phosphate dehydrogenase, lactic and malic acid dehydrogenases, lactose synthase, lysozymes, phosphatases proteases and antiproteases, xanthine oxidase |
| Hormones | T4, T3, reverse T3, cortisol, progesterone, pregnanediol, estrogens, erythropoietin, EGF, insulin, IGF-1, nerve growth factor, TGF-α, gastrin, gastric inhibitory peptide, gastric regulatory peptide, neurotensin, peptide histidine methionine, peptide YY |
| Prostaglandins | PGE, PGF |
| Bile Salts | Cholate and chenodeoxycholate |

Data from Lawrence RA: Biochemistry of Human Milk. *Breastfeeding: A Guide for the Medical Professional,* 8th edition. Philadelphia: Elsevier; 2016.

## NUTRITIONAL RECOMMENDATIONS

Nutritional supplementation for breastfed infants should include a vitamin K injection within 6 hours of life, which can be given after the first breastfeeding. Children who are breastfed should also be started on 400 IUs daily of vitamin D beginning at hospital discharge. Finally, because breast milk is low in iron and zinc, complementary foods rich in these micronutrients should be introduced at about 6 months of age. There are no routine recommendations for maternal diet while breastfeeding, but many women continue use of prenatal vitamin supplements. The USDA's dietary guidelines for 2015–2020 recommend that women who are breastfeeding consume at least 8 ounces of cooked seafood per week, from choices that are higher in eicosapentaenoic acid (EPA) and docosahexaenoic acid (DHA) and lower in methylmercury, including salmon, anchovies, herring, shad, sardines, Pacific oysters, trout, and Atlantic and Pacific mackerel

## BREASTFEEDING SUPPORT AND GUIDANCE

Mothers' breastfeeding practices are influenced significantly by the healthcare providers that they interact with during both the prenatal and postpartum periods. However, studies have shown that breastfeeding promotion and support is inadequate in both hospital and outpatient pediatric settings. The Ten Steps to Successful Breastfeeding program designed by the WHO and the United Nations Children's Fund (UNICEF) outlines strategies that have been shown to improve breastfeeding practices and has been endorsed by the AAP. Nationally, the percentage of hospitals implementing more than half of the Ten Steps has increased substantially over the past decade to more than 50%, and successful efforts have been made to expand these recommendations to outpatient practices.

Greater support from healthcare professionals is needed not only to optimize rates of initiation of breastfeeding, but also to ensure that mothers feel that they have adequate support and resources to deal with potential barriers to continuation of breastfeeding for the recommended duration. Although mothers are often aware of the benefits of breastfeeding and may intend to breastfeed, the challenges and discomfort sometimes associated with breastfeeding often lead to premature termination. More than half of mothers who terminate breastfeeding do so earlier than desired. Mothers are more likely to terminate early if they are concerned about lactation difficulties, infant nutrition and weight, their own health or need for medication, and the effort required to pump milk if they work outside the home. Healthcare professionals are well positioned to work with mothers to address these challenges and alleviate concerns. Adequate training in breastfeeding management is critical for health profession trainees.

Healthcare professionals should encourage mothers to begin breastfeeding within the first hour after birth whenever possible. Subsequent feeding schedules should be based on the infant's cues, although frequent feeding (at least 8 to 12 feeds daily) is recommended. Guidance on latching techniques, including video tutorials, can be found at http://med.stanford.edu/newborns/professional-education/breastfeeding.html, http://www.womenshealth.gov/breastfeeding/index.html, and http://www.llli.org/llleaderweb/LV/LVAugSep00p63.html. Safe sleep practices during breastfeeding are particularly important and should be reviewed and emphasized during the period of initiation of breastfeeding.

Some of the most common problems a mother may experience during breastfeeding are nipple discomfort (soreness, cracks, bleeding), plugged duct, engorgement, mastitis, and candida infection. For additional information regarding management of specific breastfeeding issues, refer to the Academy of Breastfeeding Medicine Web site at http://www.bfmed.org.

## HEALTH OUTCOMES

It has been widely reported that breast milk may confer advantages for cardiovascular health and cognitive development, contribute to the development of a diverse and biologically appropriate infant microbiome, and reduce the risk of necrotizing enterocolitis in preterm infants. However, various methodological issues limit the extent to which current research findings on these health outcomes can be applied to the overall population.

It is generally not possible to conduct randomized trials of feeding practices, due to both practical and ethical considerations. Thus, most research on breastfeeding health outcomes has relied on observational study designs, preventing inference of a causal relationship between breastfeeding and the outcome measured. Other study limitations include underestimation of random error, small sample sizes, selection bias, recall error and bias, differences in the definition of breastfeeding (duration, exclusivity, volume), and inadequate adjustment for genetic, behavioral, and social confounders.

### Promotion of Breastfeeding Intervention Trial

The Promotion of Breastfeeding Intervention Trial (PROBIT) was a multicenter cluster-randomized controlled trial in the Republic of Belarus. The intervention sites were modeled on the WHO Baby-Friendly Hospital Initiative list. Over 17,000 mother–infant pairs were recruited and the researchers followed 81% up until the age of 11.5 years. Infants in the intervention sites were more likely to be breastfed to any degree at 12 months and exclusively breastfed at 3 and 6 months. However, long-term, secondary outcomes were less robust. There was no association with body mass index (BMI) and blood pressure at 6.5 and 11.5 years, and no difference in the risk of respiratory infections or atopic eczema.

### Respiratory and Gastrointestinal Diseases

Studies have shown a decrease in the risk of hospitalization for lower respiratory tract infections for those exclusively breastfed for 4 months, a decrease in pneumonia for those infants exclusively breastfed for more than 6 months, and a decrease in severity of respiratory syncytial virus associated bronchiolitis for those exclusively breastfed for 4 months. Receiving any breast milk compared with infant formula was associated with a 23% reduction in otitis media, and exclusive breastfeeding for greater than 3 months decreased the risk of otitis media by 50%. However, multiple other studies have demonstrated a null relationship between breastfeeding and episodes of otitis media. In a prospective cohort, children who were exclusively breastfed until 4 months and then partially after had a 59% reduction in gastrointestinal infections (adjusted odds ratio [aOR]: 0.41; confidence interval [CI]: 0.26, 0.64). In a different study of over 500,000 children adjusting for confounders, children who were fed a mix of formula and breast milk as well as exclusively formula at 6 to 8 weeks of life had a higher risk of hospitalization for gastrointestinal infections from birth to 27 months. Finally a meta-analysis of 4 randomized clinical trials that evaluated the use of human milk and the incidence of necrotizing enterocolitis, there was a 58% reduction in the incidence among those receiving human milk.

### Sudden Infant Death Syndrome and Infant Mortality

A meta-analysis of 18 case–control studies found a protective association of any breastfeeding with sudden infant death syndrome (SIDS). However, many of the studies included in the analysis did not adjust for confounders, and it is unclear if the authors of the meta-analysis adjusted their results for confounders. Because many epidemiological studies have shown differing results and after adjustment for confounders the results are often null, the AAP task force on SIDS believes there is insufficient evidence that breastfeeding reduces SIDS. Sleep practices appear to provide the strongest risk prediction, along with smoking and use of alcohol and other mood altering drugs by mothers, on the risk of SIDS.

In a cost analysis examining all pediatric diseases for which the Agency for Healthcare Research and Quality reported favorable risk ratios, it was estimated that if 90% of mothers breastfed exclusively for 6 months there would be a savings of $13 billion per year and it would prevent 911 deaths. However, this assumes that there would be a reduction in multiple long-term health disorders, for which evidence remains to be substantiated (see below). In the developing world, it is estimated that more than 1 million infant deaths could be prevented if infants were exclusively breastfed for 6 months and weaned after 1 year.

### Allergic, Celiac, and Inflammatory Bowel Disease

The literature on allergic diseases including asthma and atopic diseases remains controversial. There are multiple studies that do not demonstrate an association with breastfeeding and long-term prevention of atopy and asthma. IgE-mediated food allergy is considered separately in light of new data regarding early introduction of certain proteins to promote tolerance is compelling (see Chapter 191). With regard to celiac disease, previous research suggested that there was a protective effect of breastfeeding during the introduction of gluten-containing foods. However, two recent randomized trials tested early versus late introduction of gluten-containing foods and found no difference in the incidence of celiac disease. They also found no association with breastfeeding. In a meta-analysis of 7 studies, breastfeeding was associated with a reduced odds of developing early-onset inflammatory bowel disease (IBD), but there was a null relationship between breastfeeding and ulcerative colitis and Crohn disease.

### Neurodevelopment

Although differences in neurodevelopmental outcomes between breastfed and formula-fed infants have been reported, these findings have frequently been confounded by several genetic, social, and environmental factors. For example, data from the PROBIT study group suggested some adjusted outcomes of intelligence and teacher ratings are greater in breastfed infants at 6.5 years of age, although this was a secondary outcome so the study could not control for many of the most important confounding variables that influence these outcomes. In a Cochrane Review on exclusive breastfeeding, the authors found that "Exclusive breastfeeding for six months does not seem to confer any long-term (at least to early school age) ... benefits in cognitive ability or behaviour, compared with exclusive breastfeeding for three to four months with continued partial breastfeeding to six months."[1]

#### Obesity

As with cognitive and developmental outcomes, obesity is a complex condition with genetic background, socioeconomic status, and environment all playing a role in its development. Previous research has shown that there is a 15% to 30% reduction in teen and adult obesity rates if any breastfeeding occurred. However, much of the obesity and breastfeeding literature is limited because of residual confounding and the complex causes of obesity. Also, it is unclear what the biological mechanism for the observed effects might be. It has been suggested that breast milk itself and perhaps its effect on the microbiome may be responsible for observed long-term benefits with regard to body fat accretion; others have proposed improved self-regulation of energy intake compared to bottle feeding.

Given the data and considering the potential bias and confounding that was not accounted for in published studies, it has been concluded that there is not sufficient evidence that breastfeeding does or does not cause (1) a reduction in the risk of obesity in early childhood or (2) a reduction in the risk of obesity that persists into adulthood.



## CONTRAINDICATIONS TO BREASTFEEDING

### Maternal Medical Contraindications

There are very few medications that are contraindicated or lack substitutions during breastfeeding. However, in general, breastfeeding is not recommended when mothers are receiving amphetamines, chemotherapy, ergotamines, or statins. A list of up-to-date information on the safety of medications can be found online at LactMed, which is published by the National Library of Medicine and the National Institutes of Health at https://toxnet.nlm.nih.gov/newtoxnet/lactmed.htm.

**Transmission of Infectious Agents** Group B *Streptococcus* and *Staphylococcus aureus* could theoretically be transmitted during breastfeeding from the mother's skin to the infant, although it seldom causes illness in the infant. Thus, in cases of mastitis, breastfeeding on the affected side is generally recommended. For women with a breast abscess or cellulitis, it is recommended to temporarily discontinue breastfeeding on the affected side for 24 to 48 hours until surgical drainage and appropriate antimicrobial therapy are initiated.

Breastfeeding is not contraindicated for women with tuberculosis who have been treated appropriately for 2 or more weeks and who are not contagious (negative sputum). However, those who are thought to be contagious should refrain from breastfeeding and avoid close contact with the infant to prevent spreading the infection.

Viruses that may cause issues include but are not limited to hepatitis B and C, human immunodeficiency virus (HIV), human T-lymphotropic virus 1 (HTLV-1), and herpes simplex virus (HSV). Hepatitis B surface antigen (HbSAg) has been detected in the milk of HbSAg-positive women; however, studies have indicated that breastfeeding does not increase the risk of infection. Children in the United States born to HbSAg-positive mothers should receive the vaccine and immunoglobulin within 12 hours of birth to avoid any risk of transmission through breastfeeding.

Transmission of hepatitis C via breastfeeding has not been documented for those who are HIV negative. Mothers should be counseled to consider not breastfeeding with cracked or bleeding nipples because transmission is possible from breastfeeding alone but has not been documented.

HIV can be transmitted through human milk. The risk is highest for women who acquire HIV during lactation as opposed to those with preexisting infection. Based on a meta-analysis, the risk of HIV infection through breast milk is estimated to be 22%. In the United States, where safe alternatives exist, it is recommended that HIV-positive women not breastfeed. In regions where infectious diseases and malnutrition are frequent causes of infant mortality and no safe alternatives are available, it is recommended the mother breastfeed exclusively for the first 6 months of life.

In the United States, women who are HTLV-1 seropositive should be advised not to breastfeed or donate milk. Data is unknown about HTLV type 2, so the current recommendation is for mothers with HTLV type 2 to refrain from breastfeeding as well.

Women with HSV lesions on the breasts or nipples should not breastfeed from an affected breast until lesions have resolved. As long as the affected breast is covered completely, women can breastfeed from the unaffected breast. A more extensive and complete discussion of the infectious contraindications to breastfeeding can be found in the AAP's *Red Book: 2015 Report of the Committee on Infectious Diseases*, 30th Edition.

**Severe Combined Immunodeficiency** Almost all states in the United States screen newborns for severe combined immunodeficiency (SCID) via T-cell receptor excision circle testing. An abnormal screen indicates a risk for SCID and prompts rapid evaluation (see Chapter 184). Infants with SCID are treated with bone marrow transplantation. Infants suspected to have SCID should not be breastfed if their mothers have been previously infected with cytomegalovirus (CMV) owing to a risk of transmission to the severely immunocompromised baby.

**Maternal Substance Use Disorder** Maternal substance use disorder is not an absolute contraindication to breastfeeding. If a narcotic-dependent mother is well nourished, is enrolled in a methadone maintenance program, and is HIV negative, she can breastfeed. Conversely, phencyclidine (PCP), cocaine, and cannabis can be found in human milk and may have long-term neurobehavioral development effects and thus are contraindicated. Alcohol can blunt prolactin response to suckling and negatively affect infant motor development. Alcohol intake while breastfeeding should be limited to 0.5 g alcohol per kg maternal body weight and nursing should take place at least 2 hours after intake. Smoking is not an absolute contraindication, but efforts should be made to help the mother quit given increased incidence of infant respiratory allergy and SIDS; smoking is also a risk factor for low milk supply and poor weight gain.

## CONCLUSION

In conclusion, breast milk and breastfeeding provide optimal nutrition for healthy full-term infants. Although the validity of most of the proposed long-term health outcomes that have been associated with breastfeeding share significant methodological challenges and thus require confirmation, there is no challenge to the importance of supporting breastfeeding for all healthy infants. The racial/ethnic and socioeconomic disparities in the rates of initiation of breastfeeding in the United States speak to the ongoing challenges to achieve the goals outlined in Healthy People 2020 and to the need for all involved with maternal child health to provide support for mothers to surmount these disparities.

## SUGGESTED READINGS


Breastfeeding and the use of human milk. *Pediatrics* 2012, 129(3).

CDC Progress in increasing breastfeeding and reducing racial/ethnic differences—United States, 2000–2008 births. *MMWR Morb Mortal Wkly Rep* 2013, 62(5):77-80.

Cope MB, Allison DB. Critical review of the World Health Organization's (WHO) 2007 report on 'evidence of the long-term effects of breastfeeding: systematic reviews and meta-analysis' with respect to obesity. *Obes Rev* 2008, 9(6):594-605.

Ip S, Chung M, Raman G, Trikalinos TA, Lau J. A summary of the Agency for Healthcare Research and Quality's evidence report on breastfeeding in developed countries. *Breastfeed Med* 2009, 4 Suppl 1:S17-30.

Kramer MS, Kakuma R. Optimal duration of exclusive breastfeeding. *Cochrane Database Syst Rev* 2012(8):CD003517.


[1] Kramer MS, Kakuma R. Optimal duration of exclusive breastfeeding. Cochrane Database Syst Rev 2012(8):CD003517.

Martin RM, Patel R, Kramer MS, et al. Effects of promoting longer-term and exclusive breastfeeding on adiposity and insulin-like growth factor-I at age 11.5 years: a randomized trial. *JAMA* 2013, 309(10):1005-1013.

Patel R, Oken E, Bogdanovich N, et al. Cohort profile: the Promotion of Breastfeeding Intervention Trial (PROBIT). *Int J Epidemiol* 2014, 43(3):679-690.

The World Health Organization's infant feeding recommendation. WHO website. http://www.who.int/nutrition/topics/infantfeeding_recommendation/en/. Accessed.

U.S. Department of Health and Human Services and U.S. Department of Agriculture. 2015–2020 Dietary Guidelines for Americans, 8th ed. December 2015. http://health.gov/dietaryguidelines/2015/guidelines/.

# 17 Infant Formula and Complementary Foods

Sarah M. Phillips and Robert J. Shulman

## INFANT FORMULA

For the first 6 months after birth, breast milk or infant formula is the primary source of nutrients for optimal growth. Despite successful efforts to increase breastfeeding to levels that exceed 90% in developing countries and 50% to 90% in industrialized countries following birth, fewer than half of infants in many countries are exclusively breastfed by 3 to 4 months postpartum. Thus, infant formulas provide a significant portion of the nutrient intake for many infants. Infant formulas are designed to be an acceptable substitute for human milk. Their use is indicated for (1) infants whose mothers choose not to breastfeed; (2) infants for whom human milk is contraindicated; (3) infants who require a supplement to human milk because of slow growth; and (4) infants whose mothers choose to discontinue breastfeeding before the infant is 1 year old. All infant formulas are nutritionally complete and have concentrations of macronutrients (protein, fat, and carbohydrate) that are similar to breast milk. Infant formulas are the only acceptable alternative nutrient source for infants who are unable to take breast milk.

Guidelines for specific nutrient intakes for infants are detailed in Chapter 15. Infant formulas are regulated by the US Food and Drug Administration (FDA) and the European Food Safety Authority to ensure that they provide adequate nutrients at optimum bioavailability for complete nutrition for the first 4 to 6 months after birth. Regulatory requirements include (1) nutrient content and quantity requirements, with minimum levels for 29 nutrients and maximum levels for 9 nutrients; (2) quality control procedures ensuring bioavailability of nutrients, adequate content throughout the shelf life of the product, and avoidance of contamination; (3) record keeping on testing; (4) recall procedures for removal of unsafe formulas; and (5) labeling requirements.

Infant formulas commonly available in the United States are detailed in Table 17-1. They generally are available in ready-to-feed, powder, and liquid concentrate forms. Nutrient composition is nearly identical among the various formulations within any specific formula brand, although there may be small differences due to technological requirements in production. The *Pediatric Nutrition Handbook* from the American Academy of Pediatrics (AAP) reports the caloric density of human milk as ~19.2–20.7 kcal/fl oz with an osmolarity of 280 to 300 mOsm/kg. Some standard infant formulas contain 19 kcals/oz and others 20 kcal/oz; refer to Table 17-1 for specific formula compositions. Infant formulas can be categorized as either standard term infant formulas or specialized formulas. Standard term infant formulas are further categorized according to their protein type and composition: cow-milk based, soy based, hydrolyzed, or elemental or amino-acid based. Specialized formulas have altered macronutrient or electrolyte content specific for management of a medical condition.

The AAP recommends cow-milk-based, iron-fortified formula as the feeding of choice during the first year of life for infants who are not breastfed. Unmodified cow milk is not recommended for infants in the first year of life because of the poor digestibility of the fat; inadequate amounts of vitamin C, iron, zinc, and essential fatty acids; and the high amount of protein, sodium, chloride, and phosphorus that increase the potential renal solute load (see Chapter 15). Mature human milk provides a protein content of approximately 0.9 g/100 mL as 60% whey and 40% casein compared with 3.3 g/100 mL protein in cow milk with 18% whey and 82% casein.

## COW-MILK INFANT FORMULAS

Cow-milk infant formulas are derived from cow milk, with the components being reformulated or replaced to better simulate the protein, fat, carbohydrate, and mineral content of human milk. The protein content is reduced to decrease the renal solute load to the developing kidney. The protein quality is improved by adding taurine, which is in much higher concentration in human-milk protein than in cow-milk protein. The ratio of casein and whey milk proteins is altered to simulate the ratio in human milk. The fat content of mature human milk varies during feeding from about 3 g (foremilk) to 5 g/100 mL (hind milk), whereas that of infant cow-milk formula is 3.3 g/100 mL. Formulas are usually composed of a mixture of vegetable fats, and occasionally animal fats, to improve digestibility and absorption, increase essential fatty acid content, and provide a balance of polyunsaturated, saturated, and monounsaturated fatty acids that more closely resembles that of human milk. Standard vegetable oils used include coconut oil, providing saturated, short-chain, and medium-chain fatty acids; palm oil, providing saturated long-chain fatty acids; and soy, corn, and safflower oils, providing polyunsaturated fatty acids. Although human milk contains cholesterol, there is little or no cholesterol in cow-milk-based formulas, and there is no currently known value of adding cholesterol to formulas. (See "New Additives in Infant Formula" in this section for further discussion of fatty acid composition.) The carbohydrate content of human milk is 7.3 g/100 mL compared with 4.7 g/100 mL in cow milk. The primary carbohydrate source in both milks is lactose, so additional lactose is added to cow milk to achieve a macronutrient balance similar to that of human milk.

## SOY FORMULAS

Soy formulas are not recommended by the AAP Committee on Nutrition except for infants whose parents have a preference for a vegetarian diet; infants with hereditary lactase deficiency (which is exceedingly rare); or infants with galactosemia. The AAP specifically recommends against the use of soy formulas in preterm infants, for prevention or management of colic or allergy, for infants with cow-milk-protein-induced enterocolitis or enteropathy, or for prevention of atopic disease in infants. Soy provides a low biological value protein and, therefore, protein is provided in higher amounts than in cow-milk formula, with additional supplementation of methionine and taurine. The fat content of soy formula contains a blend of vegetable oils and is similar to that of cow-milk-based formula, with additional carnitine. Lactose is avoided in soy formulas primarily because it lacks milk protein. It is replaced with sucrose, cornstarch hydrolysates, or a mixture of both. Due to interference of soy phytates with adequate mineral absorption, most soy formulas contain increased amounts of calcium, phosphorus, zinc, and iron. Although there has been some previous unease that soy phytoestrogens affect human development, reproduction, or endocrine function, these concerns have not been substantiated.

## SPECIALIZED FORMULAS

**Protein Hydrolysate Formula** Protein hydrolysate formula is useful in infants with cow- and soy-protein intolerance and for infants with malabsorption due to gastrointestinal or hepatobiliary disease.

**TABLE 17-1 COMMON INFANT FORMULAS AVAILABLE IN THE UNITED STATES**

| Formula Name | Protein Source | CHO Source | % CHO | Fat Source | % Fat | Miscellaneous Information |
|---|---|---|---|---|---|---|
| **Cow Milk-Based Formulas** | | | | | | |
| Similac Advance/Similac (Ross) | Nonfat milk | Lactose | 100 | High-oleic safflower oil | 40 | Available with and without DHA/ARA |
| | Whey protein | | | Soy oil | 30 | |
| | | | | Coconut oil | 29 | |
| Enfamil Lipil (Mead Johnson) | Nonfat milk | Lactose | 100 | Palm olein | 44 | 60:40 whey-to-casein ratio |
| | Whey | | | Soy oil | 19.5 | |
| | | | | Coconut oil | 19.5 | |
| | | | | High-oleic sunflower oil | 14.5 | |
| | | | | DHA/ARA oil blend | 2.5 | |
| Good Start Supreme/ Supreme DHA & ARA (Nestlé) | Whey protein, partially hydrolyzed | Lactose | 70 | Palm olein | 46 | |
| | | Corn maltodextrin | 30 | Soy oil | 26 | |
| | | | | Coconut oil | 20 | |
| | | | | High-oleic safflower oil | 6 | |
| | | | | DHA/ARA oil blend | 1 | |
| Ultra Bright Beginnings Milk (Bright Beginnings, PBM Products) | Casein | Lactose | 100 | Palm olein | 41 | |
| | Whey protein | | | Soy oil | 20 | |
| | | | | Coconut oil | 20 | |
| | | | | High-oleic sunflower oil | 15 | |
| | | | | Soy lecithin | 2.5 | |
| Similac Organic (Ross) | Nonfat milk | Corn maltodextrin | 46 | High-oleic sunflower oil | 40 | Organic protein, carbohydrate, and fat sources |
| | | Lactose | 27 | Soy oil | 29 | |
| | | Sucrose | 27 | Coconut oil | 29 | Contains DHA/ARA |
| Ultra Bright Beginnings Organic (Bright Beginnings, PBM Products) | Casein | Lactose | 100 | Palm olein | 35 | Organic protein, carbohydrate, and fat sources |
| | Whey protein | | | High-oleic safflower oil | 21 | |
| | | | | Coconut oil | 21 | May contain sunflower oil instead of safflower oil |
| | | | | Soy oil | 21 | |
| | | | | DHA/ARA oil blend | | |
| Similac Sensitive (Ross) | Milk protein isolate | Corn maltodextrin | 55 | High-oleic safflower oil | 40 | |
| | | Sucrose | 45 | Soy oil | 30 | |
| | | | | Coconut oil | 29 | |
| Similac Sensitive R.S. (Ross) | Milk protein isolate | Corn syrup solids | 50 | High-oleic safflower oil | 40 | Thickened for term infant with frequent spit-ups |
| | | Rice starch | 30 | Soy oil | 30 | |
| | | Sucrose | 20 | Coconut oil | 29 | Lactose-free with rice starch added |
| | | | | | | Contains DHA/ARA |
| Enfamil Gentlease Lipil (Mead Johnson) | Nonfat milk, partially hydrolyzed | Corn syrup solids | | Palm olein | 44 | Contains ~1/5 the lactose of regular formula |
| | | Lactose | | Soy oil | 19.5 | |
| | Whey protein, partially hydrolyzed | | | Coconut oil | 19.5 | |
| | | | | High-oleic sunflower oil | 14.5 | |
| | | | | DHA/ARA oil blend | 2.5 | |
| Ultra Bright Beginnings Gentle (Bright Beginnings, PBM Products) | Casein | Corn syrup solids | 75 | Palm olein | 41 | Lactose 1/4 of standard, milk-based formula |

(Continued)

**TABLE 17-1 COMMON INFANT FORMULAS AVAILABLE IN THE UNITED STATES (CONTINUED)**

| Formula Name | Protein Source | CHO Source | % CHO | Fat Source | % Fat | Miscellaneous Information |
|---|---|---|---|---|---|---|
| | Whey protein, partially hydrolyzed | Lactose | 25 | Coconut oil | 20 | |
| | | | | Soy oil | 20 | |
| | | | | High-oleic safflower oil | 15 | |
| | | | | DHA/ARA oil blend | | |
| Enfamil A.R. Lipil (Ready-to-Feed) (Mead Johnson) | Nonfat milk | Lactose | 66 | Palm olein | 43.5 | Thickened for term infant with frequent spit-ups |
| | | Rice starch | 20 | Soy oil | 19.5 | |
| | | Maltodextrin | 14 | Coconut oil | 19.5 | |
| | | | | High-oleic sunflower oil | 14.5 | |
| | | | | DHA/ARA oil blend | 3 | |
| Enfamil A.R. Lipil (Powder) (Mead Johnson) | Nonfat milk | Lactose | 59 | Palm olein | 43.5 | Thickened for term infant with frequent episodes of regurgitation or spitting up |
| | | Rice starch | 29 | Soy oil | 19.5 | |
| | | Maltodextrin | 12 | Coconut oil | 19.5 | |
| | | | | High-oleic sunflower oil | 14.5 | |
| | | | | DHA/ARA oil blend | 3 | |
| Similac Go & Grow Milk-Based (Ross) | Nonfat milk | Lactose | 100 | High-oleic safflower oil | 40 | Milk-based formula for 9–24 month old |
| | Whey protein | | | Soy oil | 30 | Higher calcium, phosphorus, iron, vitamin C, vitamin E |
| | | | | Coconut oil | 29 | |
| | | | | | | Contains DHA/ARA |
| Enfamil Next Step Lipil (Mead Johnson) | Nonfat milk | Lactose | 55 | Palm olein | 44 | Milk-based formula for 9–24 month old |
| | | Corn syrup solids | 45 | Soy oil | 19.5 | Higher calcium, phosphorus, iron |
| | | | | Coconut oil | 19.5 | |
| | | | | High-oleic sunflower oil | 14.5 | |
| | | | | DHA/ARA oil blend | 2.5 | |
| Good Start Supreme 2 DHA & ARA (Nestlé) | Whey protein, partially hydrolyzed | Lactose | 70 | Palm olein | 46 | Milk-based formula for infants eating solid foods |
| | | Corn maltodextrin | 30 | Soy oil | 26 | |
| | | | | Coconut oil | 20 | Higher calcium, phosphorus, vitamin C, iron |
| | | | | High-oleic safflower oil | 6 | |
| | | | | DHA/ARA oil blend | 1 | |
| Ultra Bright Beginnings 2 (Follow On) (Bright Beginnings, PBM Products) | Casein | Lactose | 71 | Palm olein | 36 | For infants 4 months and older started on foods |
| | Whey protein | Corn syrup solids | 29 | Coconut oil | 21 | |
| | | | | High-oleic safflower oil | 21 | Higher vitamin and mineral content |
| | | | | Soy oil | 21 | May contain sunflower oil instead of safflower oil |
| | | | | DHA/ARA oil blend | | |
| Good Start Natural Cultures (Nestlé) | Whey protein, partially hydrolyzed | Lactose | 70 | Palm olein | 46 | Contains probiotic *Bifidobacterium lactis* |
| | | Corn maltodextrin | 30 | Soy oil | 26 | |
| | | | | Coconut oil | 20 | |
| | | | | High-oleic safflower oil | 6 | |
| | | | | DHA/ARA oil blend | 1 | |

*(Continued)*

**TABLE 17-1 COMMON INFANT FORMULAS AVAILABLE IN THE UNITED STATES (CONTINUED)**

| Formula Name | Protein Source | CHO Source | % CHO | Fat Source | % Fat | Miscellaneous Information |
|---|---|---|---|---|---|---|
| **Soy-Based Formulas** | | | | | | |
| Similac Isomil Advance/ Similac Isomil (Ross) | Soy protein isolate | Corn syrup solids | 80 | High-oleic safflower oil | 41 | Milk and lactose free |
| | L-methionine | Sucrose | 20 | Soy oil | 30 | Available with and without DHA/ARA |
| | | | | Coconut oil | 29 | |
| Enfamil ProSobee Lipil (Mead Johnson) | Soy protein isolate | Corn syrup solids | 100 | Palm olein | 44 | Milk, sucrose, and lactose free |
| | L-methionine | | | Soy oil | 19.5 | |
| | | | | Coconut oil | 19.5 | |
| | | | | High-oleic sunflower oil | 14.5 | |
| | | | | DHA/ARA oil blend | 2.5 | |
| Ultra Bright Beginnings Soy (Bright Beginnings, PBM Products) | Soy protein isolate | Corn syrup solids | 75 | Palm olein | 36 | Milk and lactose free |
| | L-methionine | Sucrose | 25 | High-oleic safflower oil | 21 | |
| | | | | Coconut oil | 21 | |
| | | | | Soy oil | 21 | |
| | | | | DHA/ARA oil blend | | |
| Good Start Supreme Soy DHA & ARA (Nestlé) | Soy, partially hydrolyzed | Corn maltodextrin | 79 | Palm olein | 46 | Milk and lactose free |
| | | Sucrose | 21 | Soy oil | 26 | May contain sunflower oil instead of safflower oil |
| | | | | Coconut oil | 20 | |
| | | | | High-oleic safflower oil | 6 | |
| | | | | DHA/ARA oil blend | 1 | |
| Similac Go & Grow Soy-Based (Ross) | Soy protein isolate | Corn syrup solids | 80 | High-oleic safflower oil | 41 | Soy-based formula for 9–24 month old with DHA/ARA |
| | L-methionine | Sucrose | 20 | Soy oil | 30 | |
| | | | | Coconut oil | 29 | Milk and lactose free |
| | | | | | | Higher calcium, phosphorus, iron, vitamin C |
| Enfamil ProSobee Next Step Lipil (Mead Johnson) | Soy protein isolate | Corn syrup solids | 100 | Palm olein | 44 | Soy-based formula for 9–24 month old |
| | L-methionine | | | Soy oil | 19 | Milk, sucrose, and lactose free |
| | | | | Coconut oil | 19 | |
| | | | | High-oleic sunflower oil | 15 | |
| | | | | DHA/ARA oil blend | 3 | |
| Good Start 2 Supreme Soy DHA & ARA (Nestlé) | Soy, partially hydrolyzed | Corn maltodextrin | 79 | Palm olein | 46 | Soy-based formula for infants eating solid foods |
| | | Sucrose | 21 | Soy oil | 26 | |
| | | | | Coconut oil | 20 | Milk and lactose free |
| | | | | High-oleic safflower oil | 6 | Higher calcium, phosphorus, iron, manganese |
| | | | | DHA/ARA oil blend | 1 | |
| **Protein Hydrolysate Formulas** | | | | | | |
| Nutramigen Lipil (Mead Johnson) | Casein hydrolysate | Corn syrup solids | 86 | Palm olein | 44 | Hypoallergenic |
| | | Modified corn starch | 14 | Soy oil | 19.5 | Lactose and sucrose free |
| | | | | Coconut oil | 19.5 | |
| | | | | High-oleic sunflower oil | 14.5 | |
| | | | | DHA/ARA oil blend | 2.5 | |
| Pregestimil Lipil (Powder) (Mead Johnson) | Casein hydrolysate | Corn syrup solids | 65 | Medium-chain triglyceride oil | 55 | Hypoallergenic |
| | | Dextrose | 20 | | | Lactose and sucrose free |
| | | Modified corn starch | 15 | Soy oil | 25 | |

(Continued)

**TABLE 17-1 COMMON INFANT FORMULAS AVAILABLE IN THE UNITED STATES (CONTINUED)**

| Formula Name | Protein Source | CHO Source | % CHO | Fat Source | % Fat | Miscellaneous Information |
|---|---|---|---|---|---|---|
| | | | | Corn oil | 10 | |
| | | | | High-oleic vegetable oil | 7.5 | |
| | | | | DHA/ARA oil blend | 2.5 | |
| Pregestimil Lipil (Ready-to-Feed) (Mead Johnson) | Casein hydrolysate | Corn syrup solids | 75 | Medium-chain triglyceride oil | 55 | Hypoallergenic |
| | | Modified corn starch | 25 | | | Lactose and sucrose free |
| | | | | Soy oil | 35 | |
| | | | | High-oleic vegetable oil | 7.5 | |
| | | | | DHA/ARA oil blend | 2.5 | |
| Alimentum (Powder) (Ross) | Casein hydrolysate | Corn maltodextrin | | Safflower oil | 38 | Hypoallergenic and lactose -free |
| | | Sucrose | | Medium-chain triglyceride oil | 33 | Contains DHA/ARA |
| | | Soy oil | | 28 | | |
| Alimentum (Ready-to-Feed) (Ross) | Casein hydrolysate | Sucrose | 70 | Safflower oil | 38 | Hypoallergenic with DHA/ARA |
| | | Modified tapioca starch | 30 | Medium-chain triglyceride oil | 33 | Corn and lactose free |
| | | | | Soy oil | 28 | |
| **Elemental Formulas** | | | | | | |
| Neocate Infant DHA & ARA/Neocate Infant (Nutricia) | Free L-amino acids | Corn syrup solids | 100 | Soy oil | | Indicated for intolerance of intact or hydrolyzed protein |
| | | | | Coconut oil | | |
| | | | | High-oleic sunflower oil | | |
| | | | | DHA/ARA oil blend | | |
| Elecare (Ross) | Free L-amino acids | Corn syrup solids | 100 | High-oleic safflower oil | 39 | Indicated for intolerance of intact or hydrolyzed protein |
| | | | | Medium-chain triglyceride oil | 33 | Can be made to 20 or 30 calories/oz |
| | | | | Soy oil | 28 | |
| **Other Specialized Formulas** | | | | | | |
| Enfamil LactoFree Lipil (Mead Johnson) | Milk protein isolate | Corn syrup solids | 100 | Palm olein | 44 | Milk based |
| | | | | Soy oil | 19.5 | Lactose and sucrose free |
| | | | | Coconut oil | 19.5 | |
| | | | | High-oleic sunflower oil | 14.5 | |
| | | | | DHA/ARA oil blend | 2.5 | |
| Similac Isomil DF (Ross) | Soy protein isolate | Corn syrup solids | 60 | Soy oil | 60 | Added soy fiber for diarrhea management |
| | L-methionine | Sucrose | 40 | Coconut oil | 40 | For infants > 6 months |
| Similac PM 60/40 (Ross) | Whey protein | Lactose | 100 | High-oleic safflower oil | 41 | Lower mineral content |
| | Casein | | | Soy oil | 30 | Impaired renal function and calcium disorders |
| | | | | Coconut oil | 29 | Additional iron should be supplied from other sources |
| | | | | | | Additional electrolytes may be needed |
| | | | | | | Infants with birth weight < 1500 g may need additional Ca, P, and Na |
| Ross Carbohydrate Free (RCF) (Ross) | Soy protein isolate | Customize | | High-oleic safflower oil | | Used for carbohydrate intolerance |
| | L-methionine | | | Coconut oil | | Requires added carbohydrate |
| | | | | Soy oil | | |

(*Continued*)

**TABLE 17-1 COMMON INFANT FORMULAS AVAILABLE IN THE UNITED STATES (CONTINUED)**

| Formula Name | Protein Source | CHO Source | % CHO | Fat Source | % Fat | Miscellaneous Information |
|---|---|---|---|---|---|---|
| Portagen (Mead Johnson) | Casein | Corn syrup solids | 75 | Medium-chain triglyceride oil | 87 | Not nutritionally complete; not intended for long-term use |
| | | Sucrose | 25 | | | |
| | | | | Corn oil | 13 | Indicated for defects in fat digestion, absorption |
| | | | | | | Add essential fatty acids/minerals if long term |
| 3232A (Mead Johnson) | Casein hydrolysate | Modified tapioca starch | 30 | Medium-chain triglyceride oil | 85 | Not nutritionally complete; not intended for long-term use |
| | L-Cystine | | | | | |
| | L-Tyrosine | Customize | 70 | Corn oil | 15 | Used for carbohydrate intolerance |
| | L-Tryptophan | | | | | Requires added carbohydrate |
| | | | | | | Add essential fatty acids if long term |

Used with permission from Elaine Danner, RD, CNSD, and Margaret Kirby, MS, RD, CSP, Department of Clinical Nutrition, Children's Hospital of Wisconsin, Milwaukee.



Cow-milk protein is heat-treated and enzymatically hydrolyzed to yield a combination of free amino acids and peptides of varying lengths, which are then supplemented with additional amino acids to replace those lost in manufacturing. Most of these formulas are also lactose-free, with tapioca starch, corn syrup solids, sucrose, or cornstarch as the carbohydrate sources. Fat blends also vary among products, used with some providing medium-chain fats to aid in absorption in the face of gastrointestinal and/or liver disease.

**Amino-Acid-Based Formulas** Amino-acid formulas are useful in infants with extreme protein allergies because they utilize only free amino acids as the protein source. Fat and carbohydrate sources vary but are similar to the protein hydrolysate formulas. Although the protein hydrolysate and elemental formulas are useful in specific clinical situations, they should not be used indiscriminately because they do have disadvantages, including higher cost, poor taste, and often, higher osmolality.

**Other Specialized Formulas** Other specialized formulas and medical foods are designed to manage specific conditions. They include protein-altered formulas to treat inborn errors of metabolism, protein-altered and electrolyte-altered formulas for management of renal disease, calcium/vitamin D-altered formula for William's syndrome, and carbohydrate-modified formulas for certain gastrointestinal disorders in which specific carbohydrates are poorly digested or absorbed. In addition, specific formulas are designed for use in preterm infants and for these infants following discharge. Recently, formulas have been marketed for the treatment of transient conditions of infancy, such as lactose-free, cow-milk-based formulas for postviral diarrhea, modified carbohydrate formulas (carbohydrates that thicken upon exposure to gastric acid) to limit gastroesophageal reflux, and transitional formulas with higher protein and mineral content for older infants and toddlers. The nutritional advantage of transitional formulas is uncertain.

## NEW ADDITIVES

Continuing research on the optimal composition of infant formulas as a substitute for human milk recently has focused on alterations in fatty acid composition and the addition of nucleotides, selenium, prebiotics, and probiotics.

Infant formulas have traditionally have contained the essential fatty acids linoleic and α-linolenic acid as the precursors to arachidonic acid and docosahexaenoic acid (DHA), which are the predominant long-chain polyunsaturated fats found in the central nervous system. Some studies demonstrated improved neurodevelopmental outcomes in infants fed human milk, which contains higher concentrations of DHA than cow-milk formulas, leading many formula companies to add arachidonic acid and DHA to formulas. This modification is not yet required by most regulatory bodies, but recommendations to assure DHA levels between 0.2% and 0.5% of fatty acids with arachidonic acid levels at least equal to the DHA level were endorsed by several international bodies. In addition to arachidonic acid and DHA palm oil and palm olein are now added to many formulas to provide a fatty acid composition that is similar to the higher palmitic acid content of human milk. However, concerns have been raised regarding the potential for lower bone-mineral density of infants fed these formulas due to decreases in calcium and fat absorption.

Nucleotides are nitrogen-containing compounds that function as metabolic regulators, constituents of coenzymes, and sources of energy. Nucleotides also play a role in the development of the gastrointestinal tract and the immune system. Nucleotides represent 2% to 5% of the nonprotein nitrogen in human milk and are virtually absent from cow milk, which has led several manufacturers to add nucleotides to infant formulas, but the benefit for immunologic function or intestinal mucosal development has not been established in humans. Currently, there is no minimum recommendation for nucleotide content of formulas, but there is a maximum permitted level.

Selenium is an essential micronutrient and a component of glutathione peroxidase, which is needed to prevent oxidative damage in cell membranes. The selenium concentration in human milk is much higher than that in unsupplemented cow-milk-based formula, leading to the addition of selenium to some commercial formulas. This addition may have clinical relevance for preterm infants who have lower plasma concentrations at birth and are at higher risk of oxidative stress, although a clear benefit has yet to be demonstrated.

Prebiotics are nutrients that support the proliferation of nonpathogenic organisms, whereas probiotics are living bacteria that when ingested provide a health benefit. Human milk contains oligosaccharides that appear to promote the establishment of the intestinal microbiota (the microbiome) and, therefore, may have positive consequences for subsequent overall health. Various probiotics are being added to infant formulas with increasing frequency. The value of probiotics should not be generalized; each individual probiotic strain should be considered as a separate "drug." Data regarding probiotics also should be interpreted with caution because there are no clearly established regulatory guidelines to ensure the safety and quality of commercially available probiotic preparations.

Several studies have suggested that the addition of certain oligosaccharides to infant formula can reduce the development of atopy and decrease the rate of infections during the first 2 years of life. Preterm infants with birth weight <1500 g may benefit from probiotics through a lower incidence of necrotizing enterocolitis. Thus, emerging data suggest that there may be benefits for addition of prebiotics and probiotics to infant formula. The specific composition of the prebiotics and probiotics that may be beneficial at certain ages (eg, the preterm infant) or for specific disorders is the subject of intense investigation.

Plant-based milks and drinks such as rice, almond, coconut, and hemp and other "milk beverages" should be avoided during the first year of life. These beverages are not regulated by the FDA and are poor

**TABLE 17-2 GUIDE FOR INFANT FEEDING IN THE FIRST 2 YEARS OF LIFE**

| Age of Child | Introduction of New Foods | Reason for Introduction | Developmental Skills |
|---|---|---|---|
| 0–4 mo | 8–12 feedings of 2–6 oz per feed (16–34 oz/day) breast milk or iron-fortified formula (until 1 year of age). | Meets all of the infant's needs for the first 4–6 months | Develops a suck-swallow-breathe pattern during breast or bottle feeding<br>Tongue moves forward and back to suck |
| 4–6 mo | 4–6 feedings of breast milk or iron-fortified formula (22–28 oz/day).<br>Iron-fortified infant cereal mixed with breast milk or formula; typically start with rice cereal, then oatmeal and barley; in the breastfed infant, consider meats | Provides a dietary source of iron when the body stores from birth are depleting; meat provides a source of zinc for the breastfed infant | Sits with support<br>Holds head steady<br>Reaches for objects and can grab them<br>On tummy, pushes up on arms with straight elbows |
| 6–8 mo | 3–5 feedings of breast milk or iron-fortified formula<br>Strained fruits and vegetables<br>Sips of 100% fortified juice from a cup; limit juice to 4–6 oz per day | Provides dietary sources of vitamins, minerals, and calories<br>Introduces new food flavors | Sits without support<br>Holds small objects in hand<br>Eats with up-and-down munching movement<br>Leans toward food or spoon<br>Learns to keep thick purees in mouth<br>Pulls head downward and presses upper lip to draw food from spoon |
| 8–10 mo | 3–4 feedings breast milk or iron-fortified formula<br>Wheat cereal, strained chicken and other meats, mashed cooked beans; finger foods such as crackers, small pieces of meat, and cheese sticks | Provides additional protein, vitamins, and iron for rapid growth; encourages chewing when teeth erupt | Can bite into foods<br>Uses finger and thumb to grab pieces of food<br>Can feed self finger foods<br>Can drink from a cup with help |
| 10–12 mo | 3–4 feedings breast milk or iron-fortified formula<br>Mashed table food, plain yogurt, cottage cheese, and cooked scrambled eggs<br>Pasteurized whole milk can be added at age 1 year | Encourages the development of hand-to-mouth coordination and proper chewing; infant gains more experience with self-feeding; can drink from a cup and should be weaned from bottle | Is able to coordinate hand-eye movements<br>Can hold and use a spoon<br>Can drink with a straw |
| 12–24 mo | 3–4 feedings breast milk or iron-fortified formula<br>Mixed table food diet<br>Avoid foods that may pose choking hazard (grapes, nuts, hot dogs, raisins, raw vegetables, peanut butter) | Foods of high nutrient value should be offered, because intake declines with decreased rate of growth | Names food, expresses preferences, and may go on food jags |

Data from Butte N, Cobb K, Dwyer J, et al: The Start Healthy Feeding Guidelines for Infants and Toddlers, *J Am Diet Assoc.* 2004 Mar;104(3):442-454.



sources of protein, calcium, vitamin D, and many other vitamins and minerals when unfortified (see Table 17-2). Soy milks or drinks are not equivalent to infant soy formulas. Many soy drinks are not fortified and are poor sources of calcium. The use of these foods in patients with allergies or other food intolerances requires close, frequent nutritional monitoring.

## COMPLEMENTARY FOODS

Complementary feeding (or *beikost*) refers to the introduction of non-breast milk, non-formula foods, and liquids into the infant diet. Between 4 and 6 months of age, these foods supplement the energy, vitamins, trace minerals, and iron needed for optimal growth as well as assist in the acquisition of oral motor development and eating behaviors. At 1 year of age, most infants will consume about one half of their energy needs from these foods. There continue to be major differences in the timing and types of introduced complementary foods across cultures and over time, prompting ongoing research attempts to identify the nutritional, growth, and health consequences of various complementary feeding patterns. The World Health Organization (WHO), the AAP, and the United Nations Children's Fund (UNICEF) have recommended exclusive breast feeding for 4 to 6 months, but there is controversy regarding the exact timing of the introduction of complementary foods. The European Society for Pediatric Gastroenterology, Hepatology, and Nutrition (ESPGHAN) recommendations are to delay the introduction of complementary foods until 17 weeks of age but not beyond 26 weeks. The AAP recommends that, particularly in developing countries, where the use of potentially contaminated and/or low-nutrient-dense foods puts infants at risk for diarrhea and undernutrition, infants should be exclusively breastfed for 6 months. When these risks are lessened in developed countries, complementary foods may be introduced when the infant is between 4 and 6 months of age. In infants fed an iron-fortified formula, no complementary solid foods are required before approximately 6 months of age to assure attainment of adequate nutrient intakes.

For most infants, age in general is an indication of readiness to eat solid food. Between 4 and 6 months of age, infants have doubled their birth weight, and the volume of breast milk or formula becomes insufficient to meet all the infant's nutritional needs. However, infants should be developmentally ready for *beikost* feeding as demonstrated by the ability to sit up and to hold the head without support, by the disappearance of the extrusion reflex (pushing food out of the mouth with the tongue), and by increasing exploratory feeding behaviors. Solid foods often change the proportion of ingested types of macronutrients, vitamins, and minerals.

The general guidelines for introducing complementary foods are to (1) provide a safe, non-contaminated food; (2) select food for nutritional advantage; (3) use single-ingredient foods; (4) introduce 1 new food for 1 week, monitoring for allergy or intolerance as suggested by rash, wheezing, vomiting, or diarrhea; (5) initially provide as a thin puree, and advance texture as developmentally appropriate, minimizing risk of aspiration; (6) avoid juice until after 6 months of age, and then limit to a maximum of 4 to 6 ounces per day; (7) avoid cow milk until 1 year of age (see Table 17-2).

The types of food that are presented to infants are influenced by culture, tradition, and parental preference. The following recommendations are some of those of the AAP and ESPGHAN committees on nutrition:

1. Introduce single ingredient foods first. Single-grain cereals supply energy and iron. Rice cereal traditionally has been offered first, but many parents are concerned because of potential contamination with arsenic. Recent studies in infants support the introduction of meat as a first food for the exclusively breastfed infant, demonstrating improved zinc levels and increased head circumference

compared to infants who received iron-fortified cereal as their first food.

2. Single strained or pureed vegetables and fruits may be added next.
3. Fat and cholesterol are not restricted in infants.
4. Avoid adding sugar and salt.
5. In infants older than 6 months of age, fruit juice may be offered. Fruit juice should be pasteurized, offered only from a cup, and not exceed 4 to 6 ounces per day.

## OTHER RECOMMENDED NUTRIENT SUPPLEMENTS

Recommendations for vitamin and mineral supplements for infants include vitamin K injection at birth, vitamin D supplementation for exclusively breastfed infants by 2 months of age, a supplemental iron source for exclusively breastfed infants by 4 to 6 months of age, and supplemental fluoride source for all infants older than 6 months of age. Ready-to-feed infant formulas are produced with water that does not contain fluoride. Fluoride supplementation is warranted for infants who are fed ready-to-feed formulas and for exclusively breastfed infants. Vitamin $B_{12}$ supplementation is recommended for breastfed infants of vegan mothers.

## SUGGESTED READINGS


Agostoni C, Decsi T, Fewtrell M, et al.; and ESPGHAN Committee on Nutrition. Complementary feeding: a commentary by the ESPGHAN Committee on Nutrition. *J Pediatr Gastroenterol Nutr.* 2008;46(1):99.

Arslanoglu S, Moro GE, Schmitt J, et al. Early dietary intervention with a mixture of prebiotic oligosaccharides reduces the incidence of allergic manifestations and infections during the first two years of life. *J Nutr.* 2008;138:1091-1095.18492839.

American Academy of Pediatrics Committee on Nutrition. The use and misuse of fruit juice in pediatrics. *Pediatrics.* 2001;107(5):1210-3.

American Academy of Pediatrics Committee on Nutrition. Water-soluble vitamins. In: Kleinman RE, Greer FR, eds. *Pediatric Nutrition*, 7th ed, . Elk Grove Village, IL: American Academy of Pediatrics; 2014:517.

Beer SS, Bunting KD, Canada N, Rich S, Spoede E, Turybury K, eds. Texas Children's Hospital Pediatric Nutrition Reference Guide 2016. 11th ed. Published by Texas Children's Hospital, Houston, Texas. https://www.texaschildrens.org/sites/default/files/TCH%20PNRG%2011th%20ed%20Order%20Form.pdf

Bhatia J, Greer F; and Committee on Nutrition. Use of soy protein-based formulas in infant feeding. *Pediatrics.* 2008;121:1062-1067. 18450914.

Chen A, Rogan WJ. Isoflavones in soy infant formula: a review of evidence for endocrine and other activity in infants. *Annu Rev Nutr.* 2004;24: 33-5415189112.

Heird WC. Progress in promoting breast-feeding, combating malnutrition, and composition and use of infant formula, 1981-2006. *J. Nutr.* 2007;137:499S-502S.

Karagas MR, Punshon T, Sayarath V, Jackson BP, Folt CL, Cottingham KL. Association of rice and rice-product consumption with arsenic exposure early in life. *JAMA Pediatr.* 2016;170(6):609.

Koletzko B, Lien E, Agostoni C, et al. The roles of long-chain polyunsaturated fatty acids in pregnancy, lactation and infancy: review of current knowledge and consensus recommendations. *J Perinat Med.* 2008;36:5-14.18184094.

Krebs NF, Westcott JE, Butler N, Robinson C, Bell M, Hambidge KM. Meat as a first complementary food for breastfed infants: feasibility and impact on zinc intake and status. *J Pediatr Gastroenterol Nutr.* 2006;42:207-214.16456417.

Lin HC, Hsu CH, Chen HL, et al. Oral probiotics prevent necrotizing enterocolitis in very low birth weight preterm infants: a multicenter, randomized, controlled trial. *Pediatrics.* 2008;122: 693-700.18829790.


# 18 Postdischarge Nutrition for the Premature Infant

Amy B. Hair and Diane M. Anderson

## INTRODUCTION

Nutrition for the premature infant following discharge from the neonatal intensive care unit (NICU) varies based on risk factors such as gestational age, birth weight (BW), occurrence of postnatal complications that affect nutrition (such as bowel resection for necrotizing enterocolitis), and the need for specialized nutritional supplementation caused by an inability to take adequate calories resulting from either volume limitation or inability to feed by mouth. Feeding issues are discussed in Chapter 23, and specialized nutritional support is discussed in Chapter 25. This chapter discusses the special postdischarge nutritional needs of infants born <37 weeks gestation.

## THE PREMATURE INFANT IN THE NEONATAL INTENSIVE CARE UNIT

The growth of premature infants in the NICU should be similar to in utero growth rates; however, this growth is difficult to achieve due to inability to provide adequate nutrition in the NICU. Premature infants are at high risk of nutrient deficiencies because they do not receive the in utero transfer of nutrients such as protein, iron, and minerals. Over the years, we have learned that early nutrition is important to maintain in utero accretion rates, especially of protein. In addition, premature infants, especially infants <1000 g (extremely low birth weight [ELBW]), are at significant risk for failure to maintain postnatal growth and growth percentiles. Dusick et al (2003) found that although 16% of ELBW infants were born with a birth weight below the 10th percentile, 89% of these infants had weights at 36 weeks that had fallen below the 10th percentile, leading to postnatal growth failure. As in-hospital growth has been linked to improved neurodevelopmental outcomes, it is essential that premature infants receive appropriate nutrition not only in the NICU but postdischarge to assure optimal catch-up growth in the first year of life.

## THE PREMATURE INFANT AFTER DISCHARGE

During the NICU course, cumulative energy and protein deficits frequently accrue in infants born at 31 weeks' gestation or earlier. These deficits tend to worsen when infants are fed a formula designed for healthy full-term infants or if they are fed with unsupplemented breast milk at discharge. Bone mineral content usually is decreased in premature infants after discharge from the hospital, so attention to intake of calcium, phosphorus, and vitamin D is also critical to catch-up bone-mass accretion. The postdischarge options for feeding premature infants depend on the infant's hospital course and medical history and may include breast milk with or without supplementation with formula or fortification of breast milk. Formula determination is based on gestational age, birth weight, and clinical history but may include postdischarge transitional formula, term infant formula, and more recently available bovine human milk fortifier and premature infant formula. Other factors to be considered include maternal preference, prenatal history, and growth of the infant.

## POSTDISCHARGE FEEDING STRATEGIES

### Human Milk

Breast milk is recognized by the American Academy of Pediatrics (AAP) Section on Breastfeeding as the optimal nutrition for infants. Breast milk has many significant benefits and is rich in immune factors. Although breast milk is optimal, due to the increased nutritional needs of premature infants, especially infants <1800 g, breast milk may not provide adequate calories, protein, calcium, phosphorus, and vitamins to these infants. Therefore, these infants often require supplementation of breast milk with these nutrients, either as bovine fortifier or supplemental formula feeds. Table 18-1 compares macronutrient

**TABLE 18-1 MILK AND INFANT FORMULA NUTRIENT COMPARISON BASED ON INTAKE OF 160 ML/KG**

| Nutrient (160 mL/kg) | HM | BF × 6 + PDF × 2[a] | HM + PDF = 22 kcal/oz[b] | PDF[c] | BF × 4 + HM with HMF × 4[d] | BF × 7 + 30 kcal/oz PT × 1[e] | PT 24 kcal/oz[f] | Term Formula[g] |
|---|---|---|---|---|---|---|---|---|
| Energy (kcal) | 109 | 111, 112 | 118 | 120 | 118 | 116 | 129 | 109 |
| Protein (g) | 1.4 | 1.9 | 1.7 | 3.3, 3.4 | 3.1 | 1.9 | 4.3, 4.7 | 2.2, 2.4 |
| Carbohydrate (g) | 12.8 | 12.6, 12.7 | 13.7 | 12.1, 12.5 | 14 | 12.8, 13.4 | 12.9, 13.6 | 12.2, 12.5 |
| Fat (g) | 5.6 | 5.8 | 6.1 | 6.4, 6.6 | 5.8 | 6, 6.2 | 6.5, 7.0 | 5.6, 5.8. 5.9 |
| Calcium (mg) | 37 | 59, 64 | 48, 50 | 125, 144 | 127 | 66, 69 | 213, 232 | 72, 85 |
| Phosphorus (mg) | 21 | 34, 35 | 27, 28 | 74, 79 | 73 | 37, 38 | 116, 129 | 42, 45, 46 |
| Iron (mg) | 0.1 | 0.6 | 0.29 | 2.2 | 0.37 | 0.45 | 2.3 | 1.6, 1.9 |

[a]Breastfeeding (BF) 6 times + 2 feedings of 22 kcal/oz postdischarge infant formula (PDF; Enfamil Enfacare or Similac Neosure)

[b]Human milk (HM) + Enfamil Enfacare or Similac Neosure = 22 kcal/oz

[c]PDF = Enfamil Enfacare or Similac Neosure, 22 kcal/oz

[d]BF 4 times + 4 feedings of HM + Similac Human Milk Fortifier (HMF), powdered (24 kcal/oz)

[e]BF 7 times + 1 feeding of 30 kcal/oz premature infant formula (PT) Enfamil Premature or Similac Special Care

[f]Premature infant formula: 24 kcal/oz Enfamil Premature High Protein or Similac Special Care High Protein

[g]Term formula = Enfamil Infant, Similac Advance, and Gerber Good Start Gentle 20 kcal/oz, all feeds



and minerals among different postdischarge nutrition regimens fed at 160 mL/kg.

Former premature infants should be fed on demand with a minimum of 160 mL/kg/day of formula volume, unless fluid is restricted, or with direct breastfeeding. Common strategies for premature infants <1800 g BW who are receiving breast milk or who are breastfeeding is to provide 2 to 3 supplemental feedings a day of transitional formula (see Table 18-1). The supplemental formula feeding strategy promotes the breastfeeding dyad with relatively less interruption of breastfeeding. Other strategies may include fortification of breast milk with a transitional formula; however, this strategy does not allow for as many direct breastfeeds.

Liquid formula is sterile, so there are no concerns about possible bacterial contamination, as opposed to powdered formula. In addition, the United States Food and Drug Administration does not recommend the use of powdered formula for premature or immunocompromised infants due to sterility concerns and risk of bacterial infection.

If discharged infants are receiving any breast milk, then they should also receive 1 mL of a multivitamin with iron daily. The vitamin/mineral supplement will provide the 400 IU of vitamin D per day that is recommended for premature infants. The 10 mg of iron contained in this supplement will meet the suggested 2 to 3 mg iron/kg intake. If a mother has a low milk supply, the premature infant should be discharged on liquid transition formula (see Table 18-1). If infants are discharged receiving transitional formula, then they should receive 0.5 mL of a multivitamin with iron. At this dose, 200 IU vitamin D will be provided in the supplement, which is in addition to the vitamin D content of the infant formula. When the infant consumes greater than 800 mL (26.5 oz) of the discharge formula, the goal of 400 IU vitamin D per day will be met and vitamin supplementation will not be indicated. The infant formula label or the formula company Web site will provide current formula vitamin D concentrations.

### Iron

The premature infant, compared to the term infant, has an increased need for iron due to decreased iron stores at birth, limited iron intake, frequent blood sampling, and rapid growth. Iron needs to be provided sooner and at a higher dose for the premature infant. Iron can be started at 2 weeks of age and at the recommended dose of 2 to 3 mg/kg. The iron dose of 2 mg/kg continues through the first year of life, and some infants may require 3 mg/kg. Iron intake can be met with a multivitamin with iron, iron supplements, iron-fortified formula, and iron-containing complementary foods (iron-fortified cereals and meats). Complementary foods should be introduced when the infant is 6 months corrected gestational age (CGA).

### Infant Formulas

Specialized premature formulas are designed for the hospitalized premature infant to assure adequate protein and essential nutrient intake provided the infant receives full enteral feedings. In comparison to standard term infant formula, preterm formulas contain more protein, sodium, calcium, phosphorus, and vitamins (Table 18-1). Despite data documenting that infants fed preterm formulas have better growth, these formulas are not recommended following discharge because of concerns that infants may ingest a dangerous level of certain nutrients if they are fed a high volume of the preterm formula. This concern has led to the development and marketing of separate transitional formulas or preterm, postdischarge formulas designed to promote catch-up growth while minimizing the possibility of nutritional toxicities. The nutrient levels of these formula are at the upper end of the nutrient level range for healthy term infants; they contain a higher protein and energy content than that of term formula (but not in sufficient amounts to promote excess fat deposition); additional calcium and phosphorus to promote bone mineralization; and additional zinc, vitamins, and trace elements to support growth (Table 18-1).

Unless medically necessary, premature infants should not receive any specialty formulas because they are not designed to meet the nutrient needs of premature infants. For example, soy formulas are not recommended due to decreased bioavailability of calcium and phosphorus. Specialty formulas are usually low in calcium and phosphorus, which are important for bone formation.

The most common question from pediatricians and parents is how long a premature infant requires this postdischarge feeding strategy. The AAP recommends continuing transitional formula or supplementary formula feeds until weight for length is maintained above the 25th percentile or the infant reaches 6 months CGA. It is helpful to include length and head circumference above the 25th percentile in addition to weight. In clinical practice, infants receive this diet until at least 48 weeks postmenstrual age (PMA) if their growth is adequate because this is the most critical time for brain growth and bone mineralization. Growth should be monitored closely, with attention given to head circumference and length as well as weight. Another guideline is to continue the diet until 9 months CGA (which is close to the first year of life chronologically in very premature infants) for infants not gaining excessive weight.

## MONITORING

To ensure consistent growth past discharge, early medical follow-up in the pediatrician's office is essential and follow-up weight/feeding assessments should be scheduled as needed. The late premature infant is also at risk for jaundice, feeding difficulties, dehydration, and sepsis, which can lead to readmission to the hospital. Postdischarge lactation support needs to be continued. Referrals to the Special Supplemental Nutrition Program for Women, Infants, and Children (WIC) should be made.

Monitoring of growth parameters (weight, length, head circumference) is critical so that nutritional deficiencies are recognized. Growth charts have been developed by Fenton and Kim (2013) and provide large set of combined data of premature infants that includes gender-based growth curves. The Fenton growth curves are for premature infants but transition to the World Health Organization (WHO) growth curves at 50 weeks PMA. Former premature infants are corrected for gestational age (CGA = chronological age – weeks of prematurity) and plotted using this CGA until 2 years of age.

Routine laboratory follow-up in the otherwise healthy premature infant who is receiving appropriate nutrient and supplement intake is not recommended. Exclusively breastfed infants will need close follow-up for growth parameters, anemia, and bone disease (low serum phosphorus and an elevated alkaline phosphatase). Much of the data available on optimal postdischarge nutrition is based on growth data of former premature infants at 1 to 2 years of age. Long-term data on the impact of various nutritional management approaches on neurodevelopmental outcomes and on the risk for other disorders, such as obesity and metabolic syndrome, are lacking.



## SUGGESTED READINGS


Adamkin DM. Postdischarge nutritional therapy. *J Perinatol.* 2006; 26:S27-S30.

American Academy of Pediatrics Committee on Nutrition; Kleinman RE, Greer FR, eds. *Pediatric Nutrition.* 7th ed. Elk Grove Village, IL: American Academy of Pediatrics. 2014.

American Academy of Pediatrics Section on Breastfeeding. Breastfeeding and the use of human milk. *Pediatrics.* 2012;129:e827-84.

Bhatia J. Post-discharge nutrition of preterm infants. *J Perinatol.* 2005;25:S15-S16.

Denne SC, Poindexter BB. Evidence supporting early nutritional support with parenteral amino acid infusion. *Semin Perinatol.* 2007;31:56-60.

Domellof M, Georgieff MK. Postdischarge iron requirements of the preterm infant. *J Pediatr.* 2015;167:S31-S35.

Dusick AM, Poindexter BB, Ehrenkranz RA, Lemons JA. Growth failure in the preterm infant: can we catch up? *Semin Perinatol.* 2003;27:302-310.

Ehrenkranz RA, Dusick AM, Vohr BR, Wright LL, Wrage LA, Poole KW. Growth in the neonatal intensive care unit influences neurodevelopmental and growth outcomes of extremely low birth weight infants. *Pediatrics.* 2006;117:1253-1261.

Fenton TR, Kim JH. A systematic review and meta-analysis to revise the Fenton growth chart for preterm infants. *BMC Pediatrics.* 2013;13:59.

Kleinman RE. Expert recommendations on iron fortification in infants. *J Pediatr.* 2015;167:S48-S49.

Koletzko B, Poindexter B, Uauy R, eds. *Nutritional Care of Preterm Infant:s Scientific Basis and Practical Guidelines.* Basel, Germany: Karger AG. 2014. World Review of Nutrition and Dietetics 110.


# 19 Nutritional Issues: Toddler to Adolescent

Sravan Reddy Matta and Praveen S. Goday

## CHANGING REQUIREMENTS DURING DEVELOPMENT

Nutritional requirements change substantially in early childhood. The rate of physical growth in toddlers is lower than in infancy. This requirement goes up again during the pubertal growth spurt. Nutrient needs vary substantially according to the age, gender, and health status. Dietary reference intakes (DRIs) for various age ranges are outlined in Chapter 15.

Protein requirements are based on age and weight, with the requirement decreasing with age relative to weight but the total requirement increases with age. Additional factors, such as growth rate and state of health or illness, impact protein needs. It is important to recognize that recommended protein intakes assume high-quality protein providing amino acids essential to humans, such as eggs, milk, meat, poultry, and fish. If protein is primarily derived from lower-quality plant protein sources, the total requirement is increased. North American childhood diets generally contain more than adequate amounts of protein, but certain groups, including vegetarians, children with severe food allergies, those with limited access to foods, and children with severe food selectivity, are at risk for inadequate protein intake.

Fat requirements decrease from infancy through early childhood. Fat provides 40% to 50% of total calorie intake for infants. Restriction of fat intake in children under 2 years old is not advised because it may compromise growth. However, fat intake should gradually be decreased to approximately 30% by age 5 years and through adolescence. This decrease occurs as children transition from breast milk or infant formula during the first year, to whole milk during the second year, and then to lower fat milk after age 2. Low fat milk (2%) is recommended for children aged 1 to 2 years who are at risk of obesity or have a family history of lipid disorders, obesity, or cardiovascular disease. Intake of fruits, vegetables, and whole grains products should gradually increase.

Children from age 5 years to early adolescence grow slowly but steadily. During this age, they learn to eat by themselves and expand the spectrum of food groups they consume. It is widely noted that appetite drops and they become pickier. It is recommended that the diet include a variety of nutrient-dense foods and beverages from the basic food groups and the intake of saturated and *trans* fats, cholesterol, added sugars, and salt should be limited. In this age group, dietary intakes of iron, calcium, zinc, and vitamins $B_6$, A, D, and C are less than recommended, but deficiencies are unlikely in most children in the United States because of easy access to fortified foods. Required quantities of vitamins and minerals are usually obtained from whole grain cereals, fruits, and vegetables.

Nutritional requirements for the preadolescent and adolescent age groups rapidly increase. Also, individual teenagers differ greatly depending upon their growth rate more than upon their chronological age. Needless to say, adolescence is very challenging because teens make decisions independently to assert their authority among family members and peers. An increase in appetite is noted around the age of 10 in girls and 12 in boys. Energy demands also surge during this period to meet metabolic needs. Girls require an average of 2200 calories per day, and boys require around 2400 calories per day.

Adolescents are at increased risk of deficiencies in 2 important minerals: iron and calcium. Typically during mid- and late adolescence, girls consume 25% fewer calories than boys, making them susceptible to mineral and vitamin deficiencies. In adolescent girls, blood loss due to menstruation puts them at a greater risk of iron deficiency. The DRIs for iron for 14- to 18-year-olds are 11 mg/day in boys and 15 mg/day in girls. Teenagers should be encouraged to eat more iron-rich foods from animal sources (lean meats and fish) and from plant sources (beans, dark green vegetables, nuts, and iron-fortified cereals). Iron from animal foods (heme iron) is much better absorbed than iron from nonanimal sources (non-heme iron).

The DRIs provide guidelines for vitamin and mineral intake throughout development and this intake is best achieved by encouraging ingestion of food choices from all major food groups, including dairy, protein sources, fruits, vegetables, and whole grains. Clinical signs of specific nutrient deficiencies are rare in the United States. The Feeding Infant and Toddler Study (2008) found that intakes of usual nutrients were adequate for the majority of toddlers and preschoolers, except for a subset of older infants at risk for inadequate iron and zinc intakes; macronutrient distributions were within acceptable ranges, except for dietary fat distribution in some toddlers and preschool children; and dietary fiber intake was low in the vast majority of toddlers and preschoolers, while saturated fat intake exceeded recommendations for the majority of preschoolers.

| TABLE 19-1 DIETARY SUBGROUPS AT RISK FOR NUTRIENT DEFICIENCIES | | |
|---|---|---|
| **Dietary Subgroup** | **Nutrient at Risk** | **Intervention** |
| High milk intake | Iron | Recommend milk intake of 16–24 oz/day<br>Encourage increased intake of meat, fish, and poultry as iron-rich foods<br>Encourage foods high in vitamin C to improve iron absorption |
| Excess juice intake | Calories, protein, calcium, vitamin D | Avoid juice before 6 months of age<br>Limit juice to 4–6 oz for children 1–6 years old and 8–12 oz for children 7–12 years old |
| Children allergic to or avoiding milk | Calcium, vitamin D | Appropriate milk substitute (eg, soy milk enriched with calcium/vitamin D) |
| Children allergic to wheat or other grain, or children following gluten-free diet | B vitamins | Use enriched grain substitutes |
| Children with moderate-to-severe food selectivity | Multiple vitamins and minerals | Begin children's chewable complete vitamin mineral supplement, crushed if necessary to prevent choking |
| Vegetarian diets | Iron, zinc | Encourage increased intake of non-heme sources of iron with foods high in Vitamin C |
| Vegan diets | Vitamin $B_{12}$, vitamin D, calcium, iron, zinc | Foods enriched with vitamin $B_{12}$<br>Appropriate supplements |

## COMMON CAUSES OF NUTRITIONAL INADEQUACY

Table 19-1 lists subgroups of otherwise healthy young children whose feeding patterns place them at risk for specific nutrient deficiencies. Obtaining information from parents regarding their young child's intake can be an important tool for screening for nutrient inadequacy. Children with chronic disorders that cause malabsorption of nutrients (see Chapter 403) or increased nutrient requirements due to excessive energy needs (eg, chronic infection, cardiac disorders, cerebral palsy, endocrine or metabolic disorders) may require substantial increases in caloric intake. Those with substantial protein loss from the skin, urine, or gastrointestinal tract may require increased protein intake. Micronutrient and vitamin requirements may be increased with specific disorders.

## CHANGES IN DIET DURING DEVELOPMENT

Family members provide the primary influence on the attitudes and behaviors of children with regard to food. Foods offered early in a child's life shape the child's future food preferences. Parents can also guide their children by modeling healthy food choices and portion sizes. Regular family mealtimes also encourage healthy eating habits. Regular consumption of meals and healthy snacks are essential for a child's nutritional health. All children and adolescents should eat a diet containing whole-grain foods, fruits, and vegetables. Iron-containing foods should be encouraged, along with a diet rich in calcium and vitamin D. Breakfast is perhaps the most important meal but is the most often overlooked. Regular physical activity will help prevent obesity and osteoporosis. Snacks and fast foods are problematic when they are high in sugar or fats, and availability of these should be limited in quantity and frequency.

The diet changes from 100% liquid to a combination of liquids and solids as children advance from infancy through childhood. Texture advances parallel the development of oral-motor and swallowing skills (see Table 17-2). These transitions occur over the first several years of life and support the gradual development of independence in feeding, appropriate selection of foods, and independent acquisition of appropriate healthy foods.



### Food Selectivity

The development of feeding independence includes learning to express food preferences. A child's food choices are strongly influenced by culture, family food preferences, food access, and regulation of food intake. This learning process can be associated with difficulties when children become overly picky and selective in their food choices. Approximately 20% of parents view their toddler as having feeding problems. For most children, these problems consist of typical "picky eating" behavior and reflect a normal developmental process characterized by erratic appetite, easy distractibility at mealtimes, variable food intake, food jags, preference for sweets, and limited acceptance of vegetables and meats. Overly picky eating can usually be avoided if caregivers recognize these behaviors as part of normal development. Providing a supportive feeding environment that includes regular mealtime and snack schedules, limiting grazing behavior between meals, and offering a variety of nutritious foods in appropriate portion sizes generally prevents major problems from developing. Repeated exposures of nonpreferred foods facilitates acceptance of a healthy, culturally appropriate diet.

Some children become highly selective such that it may limit growth, impinge on normal social interactions, or have health consequences due to either macronutrient or micronutrient deficiencies. This may occur in otherwise healthy children (eg, refusal of solids due to a choking phobia following an episode of choking), but it is more frequent in children with autism spectrum disorder or developmental delays. In these instances, consultation with a pediatric dietitian to obtain a complete nutrient analysis and assure adequate nutrient intake is warranted. Behavioral therapy can be effective in promoting expansion of the diet.



### Risk of Choking with Diet Advancement

Choking due to provision of inappropriate food textures and bite sizes is problematic during the initial introduction of solids and remains a concern up to the age of 4 years. Adequate skills for chewing and swallowing develop steadily through the first 3 years of life. Simple precautions recommended to prevent choking include the following: (1) Food textures should be gradually advanced from smooth to mashed or ground, and then to soft, chewable table foods to support development of chewing skills. (2) Certain high-risk choking foods should be avoided in children younger than 3 years, including nuts, hard pieces of fruits and vegetables, popcorn, peanut butter, hot dogs, and round or hard, sticky candy. (3) Children should not be allowed to eat while running or playing or while in the car, and they should be monitored at all times during meals and snacks. (4) Children should be monitored when playing with older children because the older child can provide dangerous toys or food to a younger child. A study from a nationwide representative sample in the Unted States reported that improving surveillance, labeling foods, and social awareness could reduce the risk of children choking on food.

## DIET EFFECTS ON HEALTH

Childhood dietary intake has myriad potential effects on long-term health, including potential impact on the later development of atherosclerosis, bone health, and metabolic syndrome. The World Health Organization (WHO; 2002) recommended ranges for nutrient intakes *in adults* that are intended to reduce the long-term risk of chronic disorders such as atherosclerosis, diabetes, and osteoporosis. These include recommendations for total fat intake of 15% to 20% of total energy intake with less than 10% total as saturated fatty acids, and less than 1% as *trans* fatty acids; total carbohydrate intakes of 55% to 75% of total energy intake with less than 10% as added sugars to foods or as sugars from honey, syrups, or fruit juices; and 10% to 15% of energy from protein. Adult recommendations suggest cholesterol intakes of less than 300 mg/day and suggest limiting sodium to under 2 g/day. This maximum level of sodium intake should be adjusted downward based on the energy requirements of children relative to those of adults. Be aware that lowering dietary fat and cholesterol intakes in adults to those recommended more than a decade ago by the WHO are no longer recommended today by other authoritative bodies since newer data question their clinical efficacy in reducing cardiovascular disease. Likewise, current data suggest that severe sodium restriction may have adverse consequences in elderly adults. In childhood, there are no systematic data to support recommending very low fat diets, cholesterol restricted diets, or severe restriction of dietary sodium intakes. These should not be considered without prior consultation with a dietitian. Diet selections may affect specific health issues, such as defecation patterns, oral health, and bone health, in early childhood and adolescence.



### Constipation

Dietary selections may contribute to problems of constipation, and constipation may impair appetite. While formula selection may alter stool consistency in infants, iron-containing formulas do not contribute to constipation despite a widely held belief that they do so. Cow's milk protein allergy should be considered in infants and children with constipation. Recent evidence suggests that fiber supplementation, excess fluid intake, and pre- or probiotic usage is effective for treatment of functional constipation in children. However, excess fiber intake can impair absorption of micronutrients. This can occur with high intake of phytate-containing foods, impairing absorption of calcium, iron, copper, magnesium, and zinc. The recommended goal for fiber intake is calculated as the child's age plus 5 to 10 g/day. For example, in a 3-year-old child, this would be equivalent to a recommended 8 to 13 g/day. This is lower than the recommended DRI adequate intake of 19 grams/day for a 1- to 3-year-old, but there is no strong evidence to support the health benefits of this higher intake of fiber in young children.

### Oral Health

Adequate intake of protein; calories; vitamins A, C, and D; calcium; and fluoride affect the timing of tooth eruption, tooth size, or tooth mineralization. Poor oral health can impair a child's intake, particularly of chewable foods. Dietary intake and feeding practices that negatively impact oral health include sleeping with or grazing on a bottle of milk, juice, or liquid other than water (promoting "milk caries"); use of a pacifier dipped in sugar or other sweetened substances; and frequent grazing during the day, especially with sucrose-containing or other sweetened foods. Intake of excessive soda beverages is associated with poor oral health. Good oral hygiene and healthful dietary practices are positively associated with oral health.

### Bone Health

Peak bone mass is achieved during adolescence. Bone mass acquisition during adolescence is vital to reduce the risk of later osteoporosis. During peak adolescent growth, calcium retention is, on average, about 200 mg/day in girls and 300 mg/day in boys. Because the efficiency of calcium absorption is only around 30%, the diet needs to supply adequate calcium to improve peak bone mass. The recommended Dietary Allowance (RDA) for calcium in adolescents is 1300 mg/day. Eight ounces of milk provides 275 to 305 mg of calcium and a similar serving of yogurt provides 345 to 452 mg of calcium. Nondairy products like sardines, spinach, and beans are good sources of calcium. Dietary sources of calcium should be encouraged over calcium supplementation because of good bioavailability and to promote healthy dietary habits.

RDA for vitamin D is 400 ID/day for infants younger than 1 year and 600 IU/day for children 1 year and older. Children who are obese or on certain medications (antifungals, antiretrovirals, corticosteroids, and antiepileptic medications) may require higher intakes than normal children to achieve acceptable serum 25(OH)D levels. Fortified milk, yogurt, juices, and breakfast cereal are good sources of vitamin D. Salmon, sardines, tuna, and shitake mushrooms are good, natural nonlactose sources of vitamin D. In addition to calcium and vitamin D, phosphorus is necessary for optimum bone health. The other crucial element is physical activity with weight-bearing exercise.

## VEGETARIAN DIETS

Vegetarianism is becoming increasingly popular in the United States. About 4% (approximately 2 million) of American youth aged 8 to 18 years follow a vegetarian diet and consume no fish, seafood, meat, or poultry. The American Dietetic Association acknowledges that properly planned, balanced vegetarianism (including veganism) is healthy, nutritionally adequate, and useful in prevention and treatment of certain diseases.

Vegetarians typically are classified according to the types of protein they are willing to consume. *Pollovegetarians* will eat poultry but no red meat; *pescovegetarians* will eat only fish and other seafood; and *lactoovovegetarians* consume milk, dairy products, and eggs but no seafood or meat. The total or strict vegetarian, or vegan, will not eat any animal products, and he or she eats exclusively foods of plant origin. The risks of malnutrition are greatest in the vegan. For children on vegan diets, the greatest problem is attaining adequate caloric intakes because they consume foods with a low caloric density. Pregnant and lactating women, infants, and children are at most risk from these diets because they have increased nutritional demands from anabolism. Adolescents are also at particular risk. Although dietary experimentation is part of the normal developmental process, when vegetarianism occurs at the time of the pubertal growth spurt and there is lack of knowledge among adolescents and parents regarding ingestion of a safe vegetarian diet, the risks are compounded. The risks associated with vegetarianism increase in relation to the restrictiveness of the diet and/or lack of adequate planning. Children consuming a partial or semi-vegetarian diet are at little risk and are actually more likely to be complying with dietary recommendations for the prevention of chronic illness than are children on a typical Western diet.

Vegetarian diets that contain a complete source of protein containing the essential amino acids required by humans, such as eggs, milk, fish, or poultry, can easily be planned for nutritional adequacy. Diets that contain only plant proteins, which are incomplete (they do not contain a full complement of essential amino acids) require much more detailed planning. Typically, nuts, seeds, and grains (foods containing methionine) are combined with legumes (containing lysine) at the same meal so that adequate amounts of all essential amino acids are available for protein synthesis. This process, known as mutual supplementation, assures that there are no unduly limiting amino acids and that there is adequate dietary protein for protein synthesis. Recent research suggests that complementary proteins need not be consumed at the same meal. The consumption of essential amino acids over the course of the day should ensure adequate nitrogen retention and usage in healthy individuals. On the introduction of protein-rich foods into the infant's diet, pureed tofu or legumes are recommended.

Intake of adequate minerals, especially iron, calcium, and zinc, is also difficult without consumption of animal products. Plant foods contain only non-heme iron, which is more susceptible to inhibitors of iron absorption than is heme iron (derived from meat, chicken, and fish). Therefore, even when a vegetarian diet consists of a higher total iron content than the standard Western diet, poor absorption of iron from plant sources can result in decreased body iron stores. Ingestion of high vitamin C-containing foods aids in non-heme iron absorption.

Adequate calcium intake is of particular concern for children who consume a vegan diet. Foods rich in calcium, such as calcium-fortified soy milk and juices, should be encouraged. Vegan diets also tend to be deficient in vitamin D, and it is therefore recommended that children be exposed to sunlight and provided with vitamin D-fortified foods to meet their needs. Infants and young children receiving a vegetarian diet should receive a sufficient amount (~1000 mL) of milk (breast milk or formula) and dairy products to meet their vitamin D needs.

The bioavailability of zinc from plant sources is low. As a result, vegetarians show a lower intake of zinc than do non-vegetarians. It is recommended that vegetarians strive to exceed the RDA for zinc. Supplementation of vitamins and minerals may be necessary to prevent deficiency.

Vitamin $B_{12}$ is found only in products of animal origin, and this poses an important and serious risk to those vegetarians who do not consume animal products. Vegans must obtain vitamin $B_{12}$ by using supplements or by eating vitamin $B_{12}$-fortified foods, including soy milk, yeast, and cereals. Although adults may take several years to develop vitamin $B_{12}$ deficiency, infants who are breastfed by mothers who are marginally deficient themselves are likely to be at risk of vitamin $B_{12}$ deficiency. Vegan mothers should be supplemented with vitamin $B_{12}$ throughout pregnancy and lactation. Breastfed vegan infants of mothers without adequate vitamin $B_{12}$ intake need supplementation. Vegan infants are also at risk of deficiencies in energy, protein, vitamin D, riboflavin, calcium, iron, and zinc. A combination of these deficiencies can lead to poor growth and psychomotor retardation. It is recommended that infants and young children not receive a vegan diet.

Dietary counseling is important to aid vegetarians in selection of appropriate food combinations to maintain good health. The more restrictive the diet and the younger the child, the greater is the need for professional nutritional advice.

## VITAMIN AND MINERAL SUPPLEMENTATION

The use of vitamin and mineral supplements is fairly common among children and adolescents in the United States. Healthy children who eat adequate amounts of a variety of foods probably do not need supplements. The requirement for a supplement depends on a child's nutrient intake, age, stage of growth, and medical status. If caregivers choose to give their child a supplement, a standard pediatric vitamin and mineral supplement with nutrients no higher than the DRI should be used, and mega doses avoided. The components of typical multivitamin supplements are listed in Table 19-2. Megavitamin and mega mineral therapies are often advocated as "natural therapies" by various healers, but there is little evidence to support these contentions, and there are associated risks of such therapy.

Subgroups of young children who may be at nutritional risk and may benefit from an appropriate supplement prescription are (1) children with anorexia and poor growth, (2) children with chronic illness such as cystic fibrosis, (3) children with multiple food allergies, (4) children receiving a vegetarian diet, and (5) children with severe food selectivity who avoid 1 or more basic food groups. Evaluation of the dietary intake of these children provides a guideline for appropriate supplement recommendation.

## FOOD FADDISM AND NUTRITION QUACKERY

Food faddism and nutrition quackery involve unusual patterns of food behavior that are often enthusiastically promoted and/or adopted by their adherents. Typically, nutrition faddists and quacks claim that a particular food or nutrient has a specific therapeutic value, can cure disease, or has only positive effects. They downplay or totally ignore any negative or side effects. They may claim that dietary supplements such as vitamins or special nutrients are routinely needed to achieve a healthy balanced diet or that amino acid supplements have special values unto themselves and that supplements will enhance stamina, endurance, and muscle growth. A particular regimen often is claimed to achieve particular benefits (eg, to cure obesity). Frequently, the proposed beneficial product can be purchased through only 1 particular company or source, and proponents discredit "conventional" sources of information as not being credible, while providing testimonials or a celebrity endorsement as their evidence of efficacy.

Food faddism and quackery cause harm in many ways. They cost the economy billions of dollars a year in useless expense. Sometimes, patients are harmed indirectly through delays in seeking useful treatment or advice. Direct harm ensues when a so-called alternative treatment causes death, serious injury, or unnecessary suffering. Psychological harm is inevitable when vulnerable and sometimes



**TABLE 19-2 CHILDREN'S CHEWABLE VITAMIN MINERAL SUPPLEMENTS**

| Nutrients | Centrum Kids[a] | Flintstones Complete[b] | One-A-Day Trolls Complete Multivitamin Gummies[c] | Walgreens Multivitamin Children's Gummies[d] |
|---|---|---|---|---|
| Vitamin A, IU | 1500 | 3000 | 2000 | 2000 |
| Vitamin C, mg | 60 | 60 | 30 | 30 |
| Vitamin D, IU | 400 | 600 | 600 | 600 |
| Vitamin E, IU | 30 | 30 | 18 | 18 |
| Vitamin K, mcg | 10 | 55 | — | — |
| Thiamin, mg | 1.5 | 1.5 | — | — |
| Riboflavin, mg | 1.7 | 1.7 | — | — |
| Niacin, mg | 20 | 15 | — | — |
| Vitamin $B_6$, mg | 2 | 2 | 1 | 1 |
| Folic Acid, mcg | 400 | 400 | 200 | — |
| Vitamin $B_{12}$, mcg | 6 | 6 | 3 | 3 |
| Biotin, mcg | 45 | 40 | 75 | 150 |
| Pantothenic acid, mg | 10 | 10 | 5 | 200 |
| Calcium, mg | 108 | 100 | — | — |
| Iron, mg | 8 | 18 | — | — |
| Phosphorus, mg | 50 | — | — | — |
| Iodine, mcg | 150 | 150 | 30 | 30 |
| Magnesium, mg | 40 | — | — | — |
| Zinc, mg | 15 | 12 | 2.5 | 2.5 |
| Copper, mg | 2 | 2 | — | — |
| Manganese, mg | 1 | — | — | — |
| Chromium, mcg | 20 | — | — | — |
| Molybdenum, mcg | 20 | — | — | — |
| Sodium, mg | — | 10 | 10 | — |

[a]Values listed are for 1 tablet; recommended serving size: 1 tablet for children 4 years and older

[b]Values listed are for 1 tablet; recommended serving size: 1 tablet for adults and children 4 years of age and older

[c]Values listed are for 2 gummies; recommended serving size: 2 gummies for adults and children 4 years of age and older

[d]Values listed are for 2 gummies; recommended serving size: 2 gummies

desperate individuals blame themselves for ineffective therapy. Surprisingly, this may result in making them even more susceptible to future deception. Finally, there is an incalculable harm to our society when the general public uses erroneous and unfounded beliefs as a foundation for unrealistic expectations about nutrition and health. These unrealistic expectations often seriously undermine confidence in the scientific approach to problems in general and to legitimate providers of health care in particular.

## SUGGESTED READINGS


Aggett PJ. Iron. In: Erdman JW, Macdonald IA, Zeisel SH, eds. *Present Knowledge in Nutrition*. 10th ed. Washington, DC: Wiley-Blackwell; 2012:506-20.

Craig WJ, Mangels AR; American Dietetic Association. Position of the American Dietetic Association: Vegetarian Diets. *J Am Diet Assoc.* 2009;109: 1266-1282.

Golden NH, Abrams SA. Optimizing Bone Health in Children and Adolescents. *Pediatrics*. 2014; 134: e1229.

Holt K, Wooldridge N, Story M, Sofka D. *Bright Futures: Nutrition*, 3rd ed. Elk Grove, IL: American Academy of Pediatrics; 2011.

Shelov SP, Altmann TR. *Caring for Your Baby and Young Child: Birth to Age 5*, 6th ed. Elk Grove, IL: American Academy of Pediatrics; 2014.

World Health Organization, Food and Agriculture Organization. Joint WHO/FAO Expert Consultation on Diet, Nutrition and the Prevention of Chronic Diseases. Geneva, Switzerland; 2002. WHO Technical Report Series. Available at: http://www.fao.org/docrep/005/ac911e/ac911e01.htm. Accessed October 29, 2016.

Wright CM, Parkinson KN, Shipton D, et al. How do toddler eating problems relate to their eating behavior, food preferences, and growth? *Pediatrics*. 2007;120:e1069-e1075.




# 20 Assessment of Nutritional Adequacy

Vi Lier Goh and Praveen S. Goday

## INTRODUCTION

A complete nutritional assessment integrates a combination of subjective medical evaluations and objective evaluation of the medical and nutritional history, including past and present dietary intake; physical examination, including anthropometric measurements and growth assessment; biochemical and metabolic parameters; and anticipation of the future medical course (including likely complications) and effects of therapy.

## ROUTINE NUTRITIONAL ASSESSMENT

Nutritional assessment of an otherwise well child at a health maintenance examination differs from that of an infant or child with a chronic illness. A routine history should include a nutritional history with questions regarding family attitudes toward health foods, junk foods, dieting, fad diets, nutritional supplements, herbal remedies, and general nutrition. A healthy child on a routine visit to the doctor requires only a measurement of height, weight, and, for infants, head circumference (plotted on either the World Health Organization [WHO] growth standards or the Centers for Disease Control and Prevention [CDC] charts), along with a routine history and physical examination. It is important that either a weight for length (for ≤ 2 years) or body mass index (for > 2 years) be assessed as part of growth assessment. If growth is normal and there are no unusual dietary habits, further assessment is not required.

Both the CDC and WHO growth charts provide meaningful data, especially when tracked over time. However, assessment of normal height and weight percentiles vary slightly when applying the 5th to 95th percentile ranges to the same children. The WHO charts are more likely to suggest shortness and overweight and are less likely to suggest underweight when compared to the CDC charts when 5th and 95th percentile cutoffs for normalcy are utilized. However, when the WHO-recommended cutoff values of z-scores of −2 and +2 are applied to the WHO charts, these differences are lessened for shortness and overweight. The WHO charts consistently classify fewer children as underweight in early childhood years than do the CDC charts. The CDC growth charts are available at http://www.cdc.gov/growthcharts, and the WHO growth charts are available at http://www.who.int/childgrowth/standards/chart_catalogue/en/index.html. Computer software to facilitate calculations of anthropomorphic data using the WHO charts is available at http://www.who.int/childgrowth/software/en. The current recommendations are that the WHO growth standards be used for children younger than 2 years of age and the CDC 2000 growth reference charts be used for children older than 2 years of age. With the gradual acceptance of electronic medical records, z-score values for all anthropometric data (as opposed to percentiles) should be used.

The patient with poor growth or weight gain requires a more careful nutritional assessment. Any child with a history of poor growth or a chronic disorder placing him or her at risk for malnutrition should have periodic nutritional assessment.

## MEDICAL AND NUTRITIONAL HISTORY

It is challenging to obtain an accurate nutritional history. A 24-hour recall is the most commonly used method to obtain information about a child's intake and is useful as a screening tool. Parents and other caregivers are asked to describe the types and amounts of food eaten by the child in the previous 24-hour period. This may not represent a typical day's intake, so the recall may not accurately describe a child's nutrient intake, and foods consumed between meals often are not recorded. Accuracy is improved by the use of food models for estimating portion sizes or newer technology such as applications on smartphones, but errors are still common. The 24-hour recall is helpful during clinic follow-up to measure adherence to dietary recommendations. A 3-day or 7-day food record provides a more accurate assessment of dietary intake than the 24-hour food recall. The type and quantity of intake are recorded prospectively. Analysis of these records by a pediatric dietitian provides valuable information on caloric intake and intake of specific nutrients.

The medical history may suggest inadequate intake or malabsorption. Factors that increase energy expenditure, such as fever, tachypnea, and tachycardia, should be recognized. Chronic disorders, including cardiac, endocrine, and neurologic disorders, may increase caloric utilization. Malabsorption interferes with nutrient absorption (see Chapter 403). Increased protein losses may occur through the gastrointestinal tract, skin, or kidneys.

## NUTRITIONAL MONITORING

The most useful measure of nutritional status in the healthy child or in one with chronic disease is the longitudinal assessment of height and weight and correlation with normative values for age. Slowing of growth will occur before specific indicators of malnutrition are apparent; however, the physical examination can identify signs of overt nutritional deficiency, including angular stomatitis, cheilosis, glossitis, wasting, and edema. Pubertal development is affected by nutritional status, and the Tanner stage of sexual development should be recorded. Measurements of temperature, heart rate, and blood pressure are important in the assessment of a child with severe malnutrition because hypothermia and bradycardia are grave prognostic signs.

Accurate measurement of the child is essential for interpretation of serial values. Infants and children should be weighed unclothed on the same scale each visit. Length should be measured on an infantometer or recumbent measurement board for children until the age of 2 years. After age 2, a stadiometer should be used for height measurement. Head size is obtained by measuring the greatest occipitofrontal circumference using a tape measure. Plotting the child's weight, height, and head circumference on standardized growth charts allows the physician to compare the individual child to others of the same sex and age and is an indicator of chronic malnutrition (growth stunting). Weight-for-length assesses the appropriateness of an individual's weight compared to his length, even in those patients with chronic malnutrition. Body mass index replaces the weight-for-height calculation in children older than 2 years. Ideal body weight is the weight at the 50th percentile on the weight-for-height growth chart and can be calculated from the 50th percentile of body mass index-for-age using the child's height.

Measurement of triceps skinfold thickness and mid-arm circumference provide a useful estimate of adipose tissue and lean body mass respectively (see http://www.who.int/childgrowth/standards/en). These measurements are reliable, however, only when performed by an experienced individual such as a pediatric dietitian, and they are most useful when measured serially, being subject to intraobserver and interobserver variability. Training guides on methods of anthropometry for nutritional assessment are available at http://www.who.int/childgrowth/training/en.

Subjective global nutritional assessment (SGNA), a method of nutritional assessment based on clinical judgment has also been shown to be a useful tool for assessing nutritional status in children and identifying those at higher risk of nutrition-associated complications and prolonged hospitalizations. Clinical assessment is done based on information gathered from questionnaires regarding child's change in height, weight, caloric intake, gastrointestinal symptoms, functional capacity, and lastly, a nutritional-related physical examination.

## BIOCHEMICAL ASSESSMENT OF NUTRITIONAL STATUS

Several laboratory tests may reflect nutritional status, but none alone may be considered a useful parameter of nutritional assessment. Only in the correct clinical context do any biochemical measures become useful. Hemoglobin concentration, iron, total serum proteins, albumin, transferrin, cholesterol, triglyceride, and blood levels of some vitamins may be helpful in specific disease states. Measurement of visceral proteins allows some assessment of overall nutritional adequacy. Serum albumin values vary with acute infection, trauma, or stress, and they may be abnormal because of liver or renal disease. In addition to albumin, other more rapidly metabolized proteins that may be useful to monitor nutritional status include transferrin, prealbumin, fibronectin, and retinol-binding protein.

## SUGGESTED READINGS

Grummer-Strawn LM, Reinold C, Krebs NF; Centers for Disease Control and Prevention (CDC). Use of the World Health Organization and CDC growth charts for children aged 0–59 months in the United States. *MMWR Recomm Rep*. 2010;59:1-15.

Mehta NM, Corkins MR, Lyman B, et al. Defining pediatric malnutrition: a paradigm shift toward etiology-related definitions. *JPEN J Parenter Enteral Nutr*. 2013;37:460-81.

# 21 Childhood Undernutrition in Resource-Limited Settings

Indi Trehan and Mark J. Manary

## INTRODUCTION

### Scope of the Problem

Childhood malnutrition—both the timeless scourge of the various forms of *under*nutrition as well as the exploding epidemic of obesity that is the hallmark of *over*nutrition—is arguably the most important disease cluster in pediatrics, given our discipline's all-encompassing emphasis on the optimal growth and development of children and the essential role of nutrition in the optimal functioning of all other organ systems. Childhood malnutrition, in all its forms, contributes to the deaths of no less than 45% of all children younger than 5 years of age worldwide (under-5 mortality). Decreasing maternal, prenatal, infant, and childhood malnutrition remain among the highest priorities for improving child health worldwide, an effort that obligates pediatricians to look beyond the individual patient and to work toward the greater health of entire societies and communities. The vast majority of the world's undernourished children live in low- and middle-income countries, predominantly in sub-Saharan Africa and South Asia, emphasizing the pervasive link between poverty and malnutrition.

### Undernutrition, Infection, and the Gut

Most profoundly, undernutrition and acute infectious diseases both exacerbate each other, leading to a vicious cycle of impaired growth, high rates of infection-related morbidity, and unacceptably high rates of early mortality. When considering the global mortality attributed to undernutrition and infectious diseases, aggregate estimates of deaths are far larger than the actual observed deaths worldwide. That is because 2 coincident conditions, such as a nutrient deficiency and a microbial infection, may lead to death; however, when these conditions occur in isolation, death does not occur. Thus, a child's death may be attributed to both the nutrient deficiency and the microbe, and counted as 2 deaths. Rather than see this as "double-counting" or overestimating mortality, it is better to consider this as 2 opportunities to save the child's life.

At the center of this balance lies the gut, which acts not only as the agent of nutrient absorption, but also as the symbiotic host of the enteric microbiome and the most intimate interface between the immune system and the environment. In order to ensure adequate absorption and bioavailability of all the essential nutrients in the diet, the gut must properly balance inflammation such that acute infections are controlled but that a chronic catabolic state is avoided.

## STUNTING

### Risk Factors and Mechanism

The pathway to undernutrition begins in the prenatal period with undernourished mothers, with gestations often marked by relative food insecurity, poor micronutrient intake, and intermittent infections such as malaria, leading to growth retardation. Affected infants are thus more likely to be born premature, underweight, and short for gestational age, and have small head circumferences for their gestational age. This physical stunting often continues through the rest of the critical 1000-day window encompassing pregnancy through the first 2 years of life. During this time, the road to stunting is often irreversibly paved and significant deficits are often difficult or impossible to ameliorate after this time.

During these first 2 years of life, a number of additional insults may occur that perpetuate and worsen stunting. Among these are the premature cessation of exclusive breastfeeding prior to 6 months of age; poor complementary feeding practices; poor water, sanitation, and hygiene (WASH) practices resulting in frequent bouts of diarrhea; recurrent acute infections; exposure to a range of environmental mycotoxins and byproducts of biomass combustion; and poor infant stimulation and nurturing, which may be due to maternal depression. The net sum of these events contributes further to physical and cognitive stunting throughout low- and middle-income countries (LMICs) worldwide.

### Diagnosis and Prevalence

To diagnose stunting, an individual child's height or recumbent length is compared to the World Health Organization (WHO) growth standards. Stunted children are defined as those who are at least 2 standard deviations below the international median of height-for-age standards; severely stunted are those at least 3 below. Other causes of stunted height should be considered in the differential diagnosis, including hypothyroidism, growth hormone deficiency, selected micronutrient deficiencies, and familial short stature, but any of these is relatively rare relative to chronic undernutrition in vulnerable populations.

Stunting rates worldwide have decreased significantly over the past 25 years, from approximately 40% of all children to approximately 25%, yet remain far behind the consensus international aims set out in the United Nations Millennium Development Goals and the newer Sustainable Development Goals. An estimated 15% of total under-5 mortality worldwide can be attributed to stunting. The most impressive progress in decreasing the prevalence of stunting has been made in South Asia, with rates declining nearly in half. While the proportion of children with stunting has decreased in Africa as well, the population of children continues to grow, and thus the total number of stunted children continues to increase on the continent.



## INTERVENTIONS FOR STUNTING

A number of large multicenter longitudinal randomized controlled trials have been conducted that test individual interventions to decrease childhood stunting. Interventions that have been studied include micronutrient supplementation, low-dose macronutrient supplementation of pregnant women and infants, antimicrobial prophylaxis, and community-wide WASH improvements, among others, but the observed decreases in stunting have generally been negligible. The inability of individual interventions to decrease stunting emphasizes the multifactorial, synergistic, and longitudinal nature of the factors leading to this chronic growth faltering. On the whole, increasing dietary diversity to ensure a full complement of all essential nutrients, dietary quantity to ensure adequate energy intake, and dietary quality, especially of complete protein sources, will likely contribute greatly to rectifying this problem.

### Consequences of Stunting

The consequences of stunting are pervasive and lifelong. Short stature is merely the most easily recognized physical marker of a wide range of pathologies, most significantly reduced neurocognitive development, reduced effectiveness of vaccines, greater susceptibility to acute and chronic infections, increased risk of developing MAM and SAM, short stature in adulthood, diminished earning capacity, and an increased risk of chronic disease in adulthood. When a large proportion of a society's children suffers from stunting, the entire community suffers diminished economic productivity and limitations in overall development. More recently, there is increasing evidence for links between stunting and chronic adult diseases such as diabetes, hypertension, obesity, and hyperlipidemia; this "double burden" of malnutrition in developing societies is yet another way that prenatal and early childhood malnutrition hinders optimal individual and societal achievement.

## ENVIRONMENTAL ENTERIC DYSFUNCTION

### Pathophysiology

Environmental enteric dysfunction (EED, previously known as *environmental enteropathy* and earlier as *tropical enteropathy*) is a nefarious, poorly understood inflammatory condition of the small bowel that is strongly linked to poor growth and development of children worldwide. The etiology of EED has not been elucidated clearly, but in vulnerable children there are clear epidemiologic links to poor early sanitation and hygiene (including close contact with domesticated farm animals), inadequate nutritional intake (both premature cessation of exclusive breastfeeding as well as poor complementary feeding), and repeated—almost incessant—exposure to a variety of enteric pathogens.

EED is in many ways histologically similar to tropical sprue or celiac disease: Its most prominent features include disrupted architecture and flattening of intestinal villi, increased crypt depth between the villi, and a marked lymphocytic infiltration into the lamina propria. Children with EED suffer from diminished absorption of ingested nutrients, bacterial pathogen and toxin translocation across the gut, decreased effectiveness of enteric vaccines, and a chronic catabolic state that leads to the futile consumption of calories and nutrients. All of these pathophysiological changes lie on a continuum, and there is no specific diagnostic threshold for EED. When investigated closely, significant metabolic alterations involving serum phosphatidylcholines, sphingomyelins, and several amino acids have been identified in children with EED.

### Clinical Presentation

Despite these relatively profound histologic, immunologic, and metabolic perturbations, children with EED are clinically asymptomatic without any overt signs of acute illness. Instead, they suffer from marked growth and developmental stunting, relative immunocompromise, and greater susceptibility to acute infections, particularly diarrhea. It is this recognition of a synergistic cycle of early life growth faltering and infections leading to stunting and EED, which then lead to further undernutrition and illness, that has led to the appreciation of the EED-afflicted gut at the center of childhood malnutrition.

### Diagnosis

Diagnosing and measuring EED are not yet possible in a real-time basis that would alter clinical management; nevertheless, it can be safely assumed that in many impoverished communities, nearly all children will suffer some degree of EED. No specific biomarker for EED has been universally accepted as a replacement for invasive endoscopic intestinal biopsy, but the dual-sugar absorption test remains the most widespread and accepted method at this time in research settings.

### Interventions

A number of interventions have been attempted to ameliorate EED in individual children and on a population-wide basis. These have included probiotics, non-absorbable enteric antibiotics, micronutrient supplementation, deworming therapy, and others; none has proven markedly successful in either decreasing EED or stunting. A recent trial in Kenya among severely malnourished children demonstrated some benefit of the anti-inflammatory agent mesalazine. Ongoing and upcoming work using specific nutritional and environmental (WASH) interventions may yet prove beneficial, although given the multifactorial nature of EED, a combined package of interventions may ultimately be necessary to improve EED in children in order to ultimately improve their growth and development.

## MICRONUTRIENT DEFICIENCIES

### Overview

There are 32 micronutrients, small organic molecules or minerals required in the diet for healthy function of the human body. Rather than micronutrient sufficiency being a dichotomous state, micronutrient deficiency has a graded effect on human physiology: the more severe the deficiency, the more detrimental the physiologic dysfunction. Thus, large swaths of the world's population, particularly populations living in resource-constrained circumstances, may have seemingly subclinical deficiency. Minerals are absorbed from the gastrointestinal tract to a lesser extent than organic molecules, for example, 10% to 30% for zinc and iron absorption would be typical, compared to over 90% for organic molecules. Table 21-1 summarizes the extent and impact of a few of the most important and prevalent micronutrient deficiencies. The 3 most significant deficiencies are briefly reviewed here; see individually referenced chapters elsewhere in this text for further details about the clinical deficiency states associated with these micronutrients. Daily home fortification with multiple micronutrient powders, either on their own or as part of small-quantity lipid-based nutrient supplements that also contain essential fatty acids and macronutrients, have shown significant promise in helping reduce the burden of morbidity and mortality in many vulnerable populations.

### Vitamin A

Vitamin A deficiency is the best understood micronutrient deficiency because of its obvious ocular manifestations. Population estimates of night blindness have been used in a variety of settings to identify deficiency for many decades. The synergy between infection and malnutrition was recognized between measles and vitamin A more than a century ago. Like all micronutrients, vitamin A is needed in all cells, and thus deficiency creates pathology in multiple organ systems. A growing appreciation of this in the 1980s and 1990s led to large clinical trials that demonstrated significant

**TABLE 21-1 SELECTED MICRONUTRIENT DEFICIENCIES**

| Micronutrient | Epidemiology of Deficiency | Global Significance | Prevention Strategies |
|---|---|---|---|
| Vitamin A | Found worldwide in significant numbers, but concentrated in South Asia and sub-Saharan Africa | 33.3% prevalence worldwide; 2.3% of all deaths | Supplementation every 6 months in high risk countries; fortification of vegetable oil and sugar |
| Calcium | 90% of deficiency occurs in South Asia and sub-Saharan Africa | 3.5 million at high risk for deficiency | Supplementation for at-risk pregnant women to prevent eclampsia |
| Vitamin D | Both calcium and vitamin D intakes contribute to clinical manifestations of deficiency; severe deficiency manifesting in central Asia | 10% with subclinical deficiency in LMICs; 0.3% of children in LMICs have rickets | Supplementation through the health system to all individuals; coverage achieved using this strategy is dependent on access to health care and economic resources; food fortification used in Scandinavia |
| Folic Acid | Of clinical significance in least developed countries and among populations averse to processed foods | Unknown, but approaches 30% in screening programs in middle-income countries | 63 of the most developed countries mandate food fortification; supplementation during pregnancies routine in LMICs |
| Iodine | Found in the least developed locations worldwide where salt is not fortified; consider this in populations averse to processed food products | 29% of world's population affected although most children not severely affected; accounts for 0.5% of childhood DALYs | Commercial salt fortified with iodine in all countries; 71% of all households use this salt, thereby eliminating deficiency |
| Iron | Distributed equally in all geographic regions | 18.1% prevalence; accounts for 2% of childhood DALYs | Supplementation in pregnancy is routine worldwide; food fortification highly effective where processed foods such as milk or wheat are consumed |
| Niacin | Primarily in populations that consume corn as staple crop, eg, sub-Saharan Africa, Latin America | True burden unknown; present in 33% of women consuming corn as staple crop | Corn flour can be fortified with niacin for use in populations where pellagra is seen; peanuts are a rich source of niacin |
| Selenium | Amount in diet directly related to selenium content of rocks and soil from which food was produced; China and Europe with lowest levels | Of clinical significance only in central China and in children consuming specialized diets due to chronic illness | No fortification programs implemented since therapeutic range is relatively narrow, with only a 10-fold difference between deficiency and toxicity |
| Zinc | Highest in southern and western Africa, India, Indonesia | 17% prevalence; accounts for 1.7% of all deaths | Daily supplementation with or without other micronutrients is offered widely by UNICEF throughout LMICs; extra supplementation in children with diarrhea |

DALYs, disability-adjusted life-years; LMICs, low- and middle-income countries; UNICEF, United Nations Children's Fund.

survival benefits to populations of children in LMICs receiving vitamin A, even outside the context of measles and night blindness. Successful public health interventions to boost vitamin A status include fortification of oil, sugar, and other foods, and community-wide administration of high-dose vitamin A supplementation to pregnant and lactating women and to children every 6 months from 6 to 60 months of age. Neonatal vitamin A supplementation provided during the first month of life has not shown consistent mortality benefits, and may even lead to increased mortality in certain populations, and thus should be reserved for select populations only.

#### Iron

Iron deficiency is the most common nutrient deficiency worldwide, affecting one-third of the world's population. In addition to causing chronic anemia, iron deficiency significantly stunts neurocognitive development. Although young children with rapidly developing brains are at risk, adolescent girls are an especially vulnerable population and the consequences of their anemia is carried on to the next generation via adverse pregnancy outcomes, such as lower birth weight and higher rates of premature delivery. Management of iron deficiency is best achieved by increased consumption of flesh foods, rather than iron salts, which are much less bioavailable. Consumption of iron salts also has been shown to adversely affect gut health due to alterations of the intestinal microbiota.

#### Zinc

Zinc deficiency is primarily due to its low bioavailability from plant-based foods, rather than the absence of zinc in the diet. The primary consequences of zinc deficiency are manifested as growth faltering, impaired gastrointestinal integrity, and higher morbidity and mortality with routine infections, such as pneumonia, diarrhea, and malaria. Community-wide zinc supplementation in vulnerable populations reduces overall mortality by 9%. Targeted supplementation to children with diarrhea has also been found to reduce the duration and severity of dehydration associated with the acute illness and is recommended as part of the care of all children with dehydrating diarrhea in LMICs.

## ACUTE MALNUTRITION

### Definition

Acute malnutrition is primarily a macronutrient deficiency that can range in the spectrum from mild acute malnutrition, or mild wasting, to moderate acute malnutrition (MAM), or moderate wasting, to 1 of several manifestations of severe acute malnutrition (SAM). SAM includes (1) all children with edematous malnutrition, generally referred to as kwashiorkor, regardless of their weight or other anthropometric criteria; (2) children with severe wasting of lean body mass, also known as marasmus, as measured by either severely diminished weight-for-height or mid-upper-arm circumference (MUAC); or (3) marasmic kwashiorkor, when children suffer from both severe wasting and the development of edematous malnutrition simultaneously. Children with SAM have almost 10 times the mortality rate as those without acute malnutrition; children with MAM have more than double the mortality rate.

## EPIDEMIOLOGY

Given the transient nature of acute malnutrition, population prevalence surveys tend to underestimate the number of children per year who develop acute malnutrition. Prevalence surveys estimate that some 8% of children suffer from marasmus and the number who suffer from kwashiorkor remains unknown due to few attempts at high-quality surveillance. It is not unusual for therapeutic feeding programs in the region with the greatest burden of kwashiorkor, southern Africa, to report more than 50% of their cases of SAM as being 1 of the edematous forms. An estimated 12% of worldwide under-5 mortality is due to wasting.

### Severe Acute Malnutrition

**Wasting (Marasmus)** Wasted children are weak and emaciated, having suffered rapid weight loss over a short time frame. Often described as looking like an old man, wasting is usually visible first in the groin or axilla, eventually progressing to the buttocks, thighs, abdomen, arms, and face (Fig. 21-1). Many of these children are remarkably irritable and difficult to console.

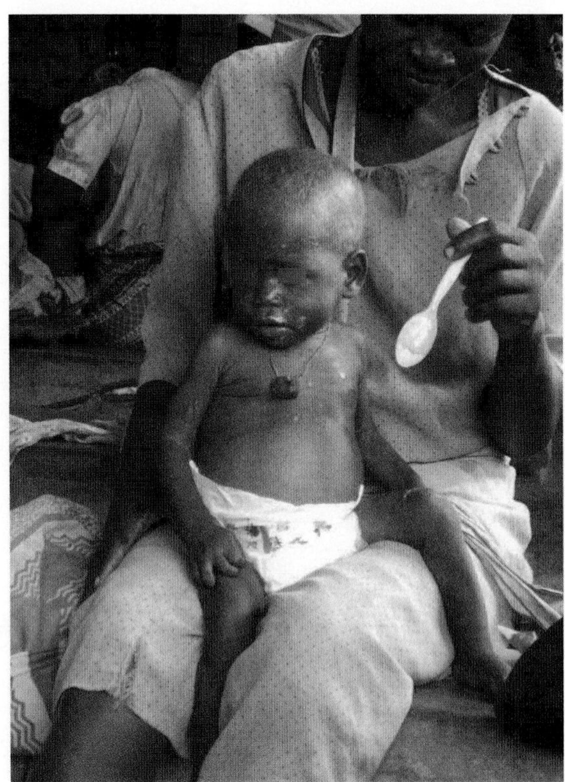

**FIGURE 21-1** Child with severe wasting (marasmus). Note the loss of muscle and lean tissue in the arms and groin. In this image, the child is being treated with RUTF.

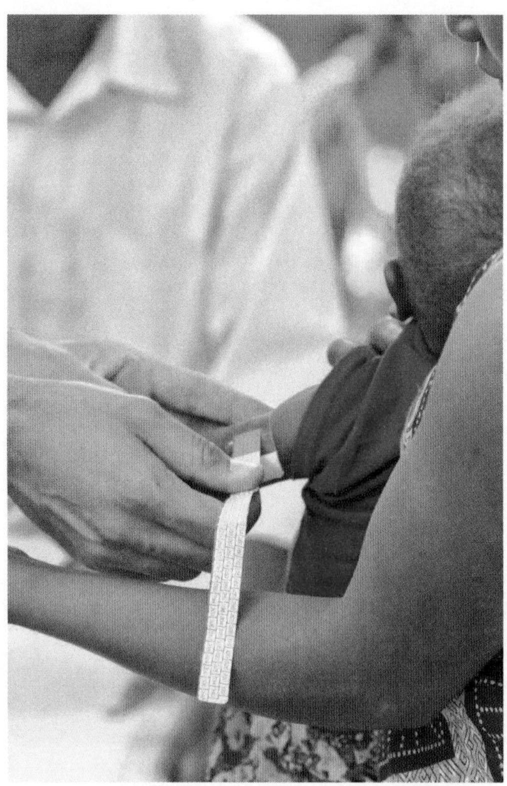

**FIGURE 21-2** Measuring MUAC to quantify wasting. Color-coded bands are often used in the field in order to quickly diagnose children with moderate (115–125 mm) or severe wasting (less than 115 mm).

The traditional way of quantifying the degree of wasting is to compare a child's weight and height with international growth standards developed by longitudinal and cross-sectional surveys of large numbers of children drawn from multiple diverse populations. Anthropometric measurements must be collected carefully and precisely, with length measurements obtained using flat, rigid boards precise to at least to the nearest 0.5 cm and scales with weight precise to at least 100 grams. Children who are 3 or more standard deviations below the median (ie, weight-for-height z-score [WHZ] < –3) are diagnosed as having SAM.

Even more useful in diagnosing MAM or SAM is the measurement of the child's MUAC, by convention in the left upper arm and ideally to at least the nearest 2 mm (Fig. 21-2). Children aged 6 to 59 months without acute malnutrition should generally have a MUAC above 125 mm; children with a MUAC of less than 115 mm have SAM.

Screening children by MUAC or weight-for-height measurements mostly will identify the same population of acutely malnourished children, but there will be a significant population that will only be diagnosed by 1 criterion or the other. Generally, the population diagnosed by MUAC will be younger and have a higher mortality rate than those diagnosed by weight-for-height criteria, and thus MUAC is preferable if resources are only available for 1 form of anthropometric screening for wasting. Simply using criteria such as "visible severe wasting" is no longer considered appropriate, as it lacks sufficient sensitivity and specificity.

Other than acute malnutrition, children may become wasted due to a wide variety of other illnesses, including severe dehydrating diarrhea, malabsorption due to intestinal infections, tuberculosis, HIV/AIDS, and congenital heart disease. Nevertheless, a child who meets the anthropometric criteria for wasting should receive nutritional therapies while the initiating insult is concomitantly evaluated and treated.

**Edematous Malnutrition (Kwashiorkor)** All children in vulnerable populations should be evaluated for evidence of edematous malnutrition in addition to routine anthropometry. This is performed by depressing firmly down to the 3rd to 4th tarsal bones with the pad of the examiner's thumb on the dorsal aspect of the child's foot for 3 to 5 seconds and then observing for pitting edema for 2 to 3 seconds. The presence of symmetric bilateral pedal pitting edema in a vulnerable child in a high-risk population, regardless of other anthropometric values, necessarily places kwashiorkor at the top of the differential diagnosis. The more pronounced the disease is, either as a function of greater severity or of longer duration, the more likely the edema is to be observed more proximally up the child's body. Edema may be graded as 1+ if limited to the feet and lower legs (Fig. 21-3A), 2+ if present in the arms (Fig. 21-3B), and 3+ if found on the face (Fig. 21-3C), although this classification scheme is of relatively limited direct clinical utility. Despite this, these children generally do not have frank ascites, although studies have demonstrated fatty infiltration of the liver, and some degree of hypoalbuminemia. Upon examination, the skin may demonstrate "flaky pain" dermatitis, with denuded areas that make the child susceptible to infection or sepsis from bacterial contamination across the skin. It has also long been noted that children with kwashiorkor often have dry, brittle, yellow-brown hair, but this is a relatively nonspecific finding and seen often in chronically malnourished children even in the absence of kwashiorkor.

First described in the published literature in 1935, the prototypical child with kwashiorkor is one who was previously doing well but then is rapidly weaned from breast milk after a younger sibling is born. The child then consumes a predominantly protein-poor and micronutrient-deficient diet consisting mostly of staple carbohydrate-heavy crops with little dietary diversity. The differential diagnosis includes the typical cardiac, hepatic, and renal causes of edema seen in resource-rich settings. In LMICs, the differential diagnosis also must be expanded to include congenital or rheumatic heart disease, tuberculosis, postinfectious glomerulonephritis, and severe anemia. On most occasions, however, kwashiorkor will remain the most likely diagnosis of a child presenting with peripheral edema in this epidemiologic context.

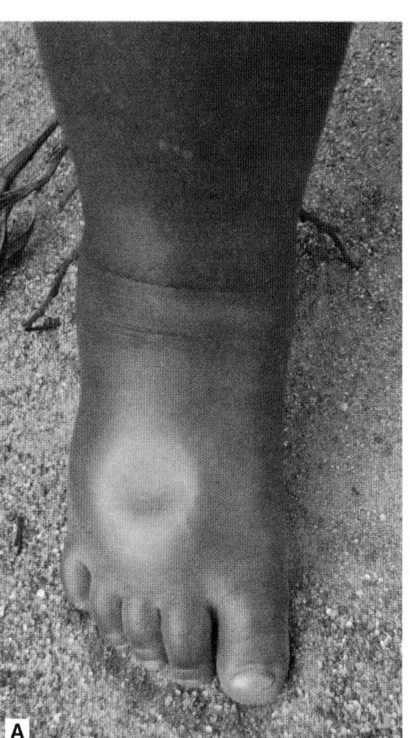


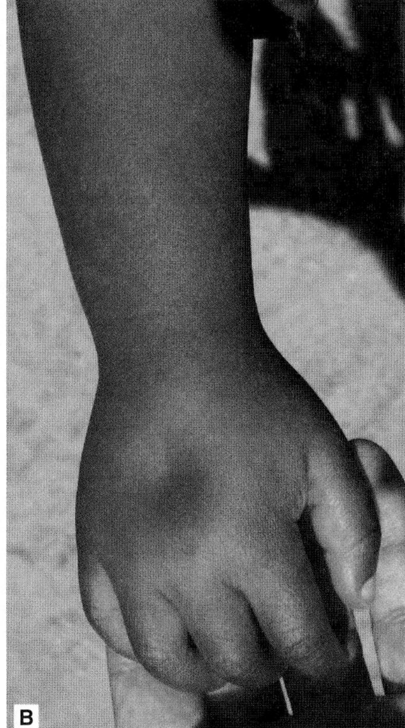


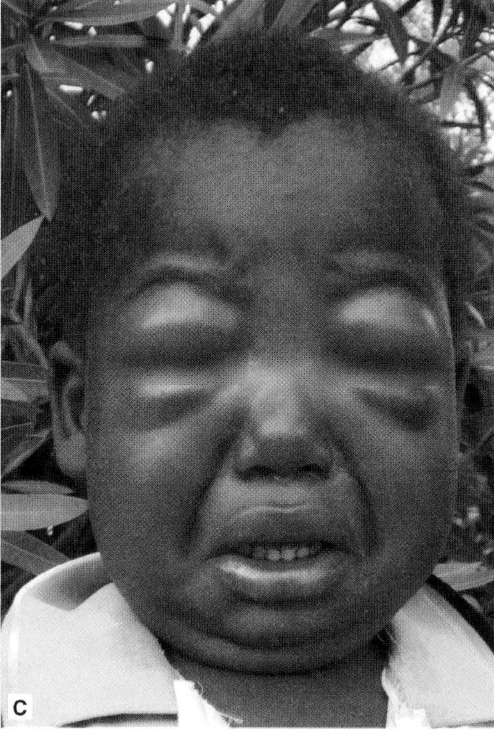


**FIGURE 21-3** Child with edematous malnutrition (kwashiorkor). This child has uncomplicated kwashiorkor marked by nutritional edema in the **A:** feet, **B:** hands, and **C:** face.



One of the major mysteries of malnutrition is why children who live in close proximity of each other, harking from the same genetic background, exposed to the same environmental pathogens and toxins, and eating essentially the quantity and quality of foods, manifest these different forms of SAM. Some have theorized that this may be due to a poor adaptive response to acute or subacute caloric and protein deprivation; other hypotheses include a recent loss of diversity in the commensal intestinal microbiome, significant exposure to aflatoxins or other environmental triggers, increased oxidative stress, and disruption of sulfated glycosaminoglycans. Unfortunately, none of these hypotheses has proven sufficiently complete to explain the pathophysiology of nutritional edema, thus hampering our ability to optimally prevent disease and treat cases.

A small percentage of children will manifest both the severe wasting of marasmus as well as the nutritional edema of kwashiorkor, giving them an overlap syndrome known as marasmic kwashiorkor. These children have a significantly worse prognosis than those with either marasmus or kwashiorkor alone, with higher rates of mortality, opportunistic infections, and failure to respond to therapy.

**Inpatient Management** For decades, the care of severely malnourished children has taken place in inpatient settings where patients would ideally be provided with round-the-clock nutritional rehabilitation. The key element in this care is the provision of highly fortified and balanced milk-based formulas. In the initial *stabilization phase*, frequent small feedings (every 2–3 hours) of F-75 formula (so named because it provides 75 kcal per 100 mL). Initially, the goal is to provide children with approximately 100 kcal/kg/d of energy for the first several days while their physiology stabilizes, but many children will tolerate these feedings quite well and will actually be hungry for more. In contrast, consideration can be given to using a nasogastric tube to schedule feedings for those with severe anorexia or vomiting.

Following the stabilization phase, children should proceed to the *rehabilitation phase* within 1 to 7 days, depending on how quickly the child gains weight and/or progresses in the resolution of the edema, how well he or she tolerates feedings without vomiting or diarrhea, and how well the overall clinical status improves. There is no specific recommendation to guide the timing of this transition, and it often involves some trial and error as children who are moved too quickly into the rehabilitation phase may have to take a step back in their feeding regimen. The therapeutic food administered in rehabilitation phase itself has traditionally been another fortified milk formula, F-100 (providing 100 kcal per 100mL), delivered in sufficient quantities over the course of a day to provide 150 to 220 kcal/kg/d and 4 to 6 grams of protein per kg.

The more recent development and greater availability of ready-to-use therapeutic food (RUTF) has made this a preferable option for most children in the rehabilitation phase. RUTF allows for more frequent round-the-clock feedings by the child's mother or other caretaker at the bedside without the significant work required to prepare F-100. Another advantage is that if a child is found to be clinically improving with RUTF, they can then also be more quickly discharged to complete their therapy as outpatients with RUTF at home.

Other components of inpatient care include careful attention to hydration status, electrolyte balance, the provision of empiric antimicrobial medications, and psychosocial support of children and their caregivers. This approach has been codified for some time by the WHO and other bodies (Fig. 21-4), but remains largely grounded in mechanistic studies and expert opinion, rather than truly rigorous clinical trials. Nevertheless, rigorous implementation of this protocol has led to marked improvements in morbidity and mortality among severely malnourished children.

**Outpatient Management** The vast majority of children with SAM do not require inpatient care; instead, it is preferable that they be managed as outpatients using the community-based management of acute malnutrition model of care, which has several significant advantages including lower resource needs, greater acceptability for caretakers, and ultimately higher success rates. Outpatient care, both as the initial form of care for children with uncomplicated SAM and for the continued care of children who have improved significantly following hospitalization, relies upon a steady supply of RUTF that can be provided in quantities sufficient to feed the child at home for 1 to 2 weeks at a time.

If, at the time of screening and diagnosis, a child has a normal mental status and clinically demonstrates an appropriate appetite, strong consideration should be given to pursuing outpatient care. Significant complications such as severe dehydration, respiratory distress, severe

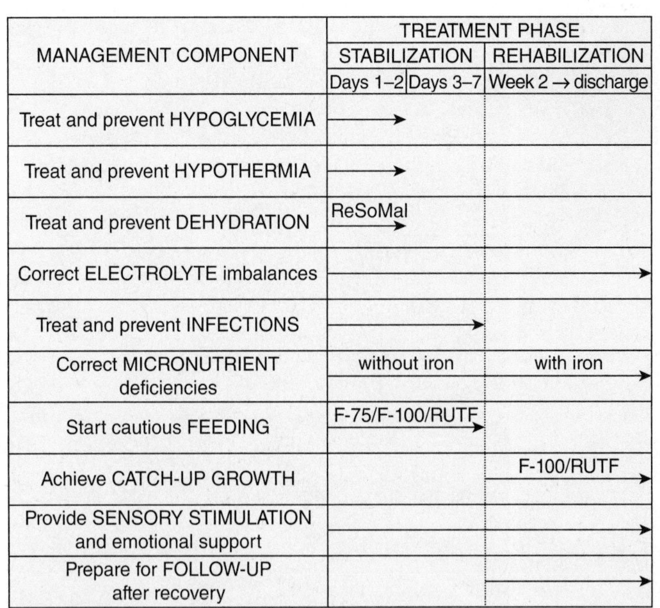


**FIGURE 21-4** Components of comprehensive inpatient management of SAM. (Adapted with permission from World Health Organization guidelines.)

anemia, high fevers, or other evidence of significant toxicity should be ruled out prior to performing an appetite test, wherein a test feeding of 20 to 30 grams of RUTF is provided. Severely malnourished children who successfully complete this test feeding under direct observation by a trained health worker can be discharged home with sufficient RUTF to provide 150 to 200 kcal/kg/d, with clear instructions to the caretaker that the RUTF should be not be shared with other members of the household and that the child should have no other intake other than breast milk or clean water during this time (Fig. 21-5).

An empiric 1-week course of a broad-spectrum oral antibiotic such as amoxicillin or cefdinir should also be provided to all children at the outset of therapy due to the risk of overwhelming bacterial sepsis, even in the clinically well-appearing child; this has been shown to reduce mortality, improve nutritional recovery, and decrease the need for hospitalization. If resources are available for other appropriate health interventions, such as linkage to HIV care for the child and mother, WASH interventions, deworming therapy, catch-up of any missing routine immunizations, and general health and nutritional counseling, these would be expected to lead to even better outcomes.

Clinical reassessment and anthropometry should be repeated every 1 to 2 weeks. This will allow for more intensive therapy for children who are not recovering appropriately, ranging from further directed counseling of the caretakers, to an assessment of social or home factors making it difficult for the child to receive all of the RUTF intended, to an evaluation for infection or other comorbidities, to possibly having

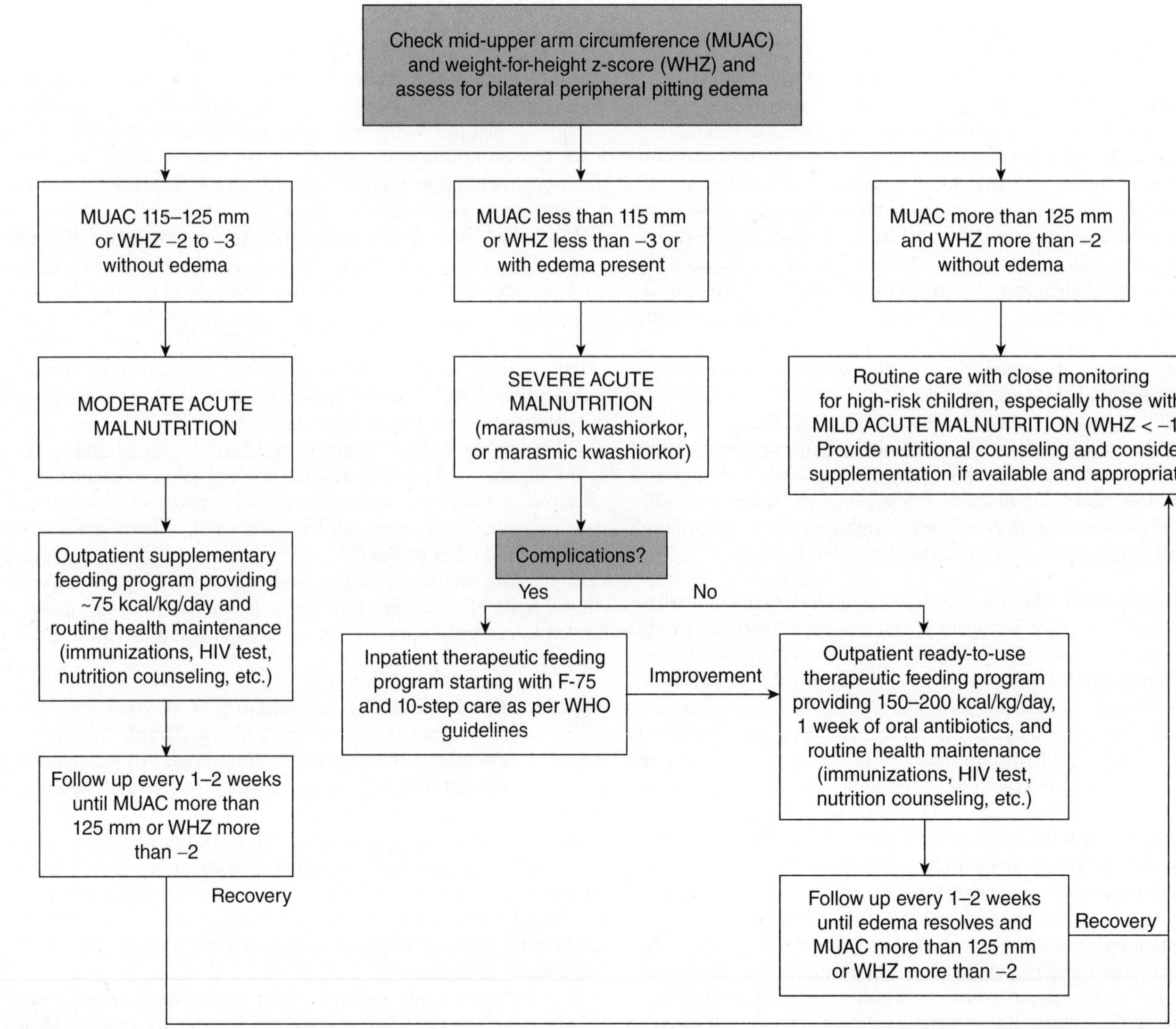

Check mid-upper arm circumference (MUAC) and weight-for-height z-score (WHZ) and assess for bilateral peripheral pitting edema

MUAC 115–125 mm or WHZ –2 to –3 without edema

MUAC less than 115 mm or WHZ less than –3 or with edema present

MUAC more than 125 mm and WHZ more than –2 without edema

MODERATE ACUTE MALNUTRITION

SEVERE ACUTE MALNUTRITION (marasmus, kwashiorkor, or marasmic kwashiorkor)

Routine care with close monitoring for high-risk children, especially those with MILD ACUTE MALNUTRITION (WHZ < –1). Provide nutritional counseling and consider supplementation if available and appropriate.

Outpatient supplementary feeding program providing ~75 kcal/kg/day and routine health maintenance (immunizations, HIV test, nutrition counseling, etc.)

Complications?

Yes

No

Inpatient therapeutic feeding program starting with F-75 and 10-step care as per WHO guidelines

Improvement

Outpatient ready-to-use therapeutic feeding program providing 150–200 kcal/kg/day, 1 week of oral antibiotics, and routine health maintenance (immunizations, HIV test, nutrition counseling, etc.)

Follow up every 1–2 weeks until MUAC more than 125 mm or WHZ more than –2

Recovery

Follow up every 1–2 weeks until edema resolves and MUAC more than 125 mm or WHZ more than –2

Recovery

**FIGURE 21-5** Decision tree for diagnosis and treatment of acute malnutrition. (Adapted with permission from World Health Organization guidelines.)

to refer the child for inpatient care. For the vast majority of children who will improve on this regimen (at least 80–90%), therapeutic feeding can be discontinued when the child's edema has resolved, WHZ is no more than 2 standard deviations below the median, and MUAC is at least 125 mm, depending on which SAM criteria led to the initial enrollment. Most children can be expected to recover within 12 weeks of therapy; any child who does not recover in this time should have a careful assessment for comorbidities or insufficient administration of RUTF, and may need to be referred for inpatient care.

#### Moderate Acute Malnutrition

Children without the bilateral pitting edema of kwashiorkor, but who are 2 to 3 standard deviations below the median of WHO growth standards and/or have an MUAC of 115 to 125 mm are diagnosed as having MAM. Roughly 10% of children under 5 years of age in LMICs suffer from MAM at any given time. These children are at high risk for progression to SAM, with the consequent physical and cognitive stunting, morbidity, and mortality associated with SAM. Even though far more children worldwide suffer from MAM than from SAM, the optimal management of this disease is less clear. A number of different interventions for MAM have been tested with varying degrees of efficacy, including intensive nutritional counseling and education, targeted supplementary feeding with either ready-to-use supplementary foods or fortified blended flours, blanket supplementary feeding to all vulnerable children and families in food insecure situations, and direct cash transfers to families of malnourished children.

Given the lack of consensus on the optimal management of MAM, the large variety of contexts in which children with MAM will be encountered, the varied causes of MAM, and the wide range of resources that might be available in any given context, only general principles of nutritional management can be offered. There is little controversy that each child with MAM should receive sufficient nutrition to achieve normal growth and development and that essential nutrition actions such as optimal breastfeeding practices be included. Children with MAM undoubtedly benefit from the inclusion of nutrient-dense foods to aid their nutritional recovery and achieve appropriate catch-up growth.

Despite these principles, the optimal choice of supplementary foods for children with MAM remains unclear. Lipid-nutrient spreads (LNS), for example reformulations of peanut-based RUTF, have shown fairly good results with regard to nutritional recovery and mortality. These spreads may or may not need to contain animal-source proteins such as milk powder or whey protein, and in head-to-head comparisons, replacing milk powder with extruded soy flour have led to very similar recovery rates. Given the resources required to manufacture LNS, a fortified blended flour called Super Cereal Plus is offered by the World Food Programme for the targeted treatment of children with MAM. This is a corn-soy blend fortified with an advanced micronutrient mixture, milk powder, and oil, and has been shown to lead to similar recovery rates as LNS.

Except for the rare child with severe infectious or other complications, children with MAM should be treated in the community as children with SAM are (except for the empiric use of antibiotics), with supplies of supplementary foods administered every 1 to 2 weeks and repeat clinical assessments on this schedule. Children should be treated at least until their WHZ exceeds −2 and their MUAC exceeds 125 mm, although emerging evidence suggests that treating to higher thresholds will lead to lower rates of relapse in the months following completion of treatment.

#### Mild Acute Malnutrition

There is no consensus definition for what constitutes mild acute malnutrition, but WHZ between 1 and 2 standard deviations below the median is often used in research contexts. Unfortunately, resources are generally not available to provide specific therapies for the very large number of children with mild acute malnutrition. The primary reason for identifying children with mild acute malnutrition is because this helps identify a high-risk patient population that is at risk for progressing to MAM or SAM and is more likely to be a cohort of children with chronic forms of malnutrition such as stunting, underweight, and EED. It is also useful to identify these children for the purpose of risk-stratifying those children seeking medical attention for acute infections or other illnesses, as they are relatively less likely to recover successfully from their presenting illness.

Given the lack of specific clinical management for mild acute malnutrition (on those rare occasions that this illness is even specifically diagnosed), appropriate dietary, hygiene, and primary health counseling, particularly the maintenance of exclusive breastfeeding during the first 6 months of life and continued breastfeeding for at least the first 2 years of life, is to be encouraged. Ensuring the child is kept up to date with other routinely recommended preventive therapies appropriate for the local context, such as vaccinations, periodic deworming, and vitamin A; the use of intermittent preventive therapy for malaria; and the use of insecticide-treated mosquito nets will also help the child's nutritional status. Communities with high rates of global acute malnutrition will likely benefit from agricultural and WASH interventions in addition to community-wide micro- and macronutrient supplementation when possible.

### SUGGESTED READINGS

Annan RA, Webb P, Brown R. *Management of Moderate Acute Malnutrition (MAM): Current Knowledge and Practice*. Oxford: CMAM Forum; 2014.

Black RE, Victora CG, Walker SP, et al. Maternal and child undernutrition and overweight in low-income and middle-income countries. *Lancet*. 2013;382(9890):427-51.

Crane RJ, Jones KD, Berkley JA. Environmental enteric dysfunction: an overview. *Food Nutr Bull*. 2015;36(1 Suppl):S76-87.

de Onis M, Branca F. Childhood stunting: a global perspective. *Matern Child Nutr*. 2016;12(Suppl 1):12-26.

Guerrant RL, DeBoer MD, Moore SR, Scharf RJ, Lima AA. The impoverished gut—a triple burden of diarrhoea, stunting and chronic disease. *Nat Rev Gastroenterol Hepatol*. 2013;10(4):220-9.

Kennedy E, Branca F, Webb P, Bhutta Z, Brown R. Setting the scene: an overview of issues related to policies and programs for moderate and severe acute malnutrition. *Food Nutr Bull*. 2015;36(1 Suppl):S9-14.

Prendergast AJ, Humphrey JH. The stunting syndrome in developing countries. *Paediatr Int Child Health*. 2014;34(4):250-65.

Semba RD, Shardell M, Trehan I, et al. Metabolic alterations in children with environmental enteric dysfunction. *Sci Rep*. 2016;6:28009.

Tickell KD, Denno DM. Inpatient management of children with severe acute malnutrition: a review of WHO guidelines. *Bull World Health Organ*. 2016;94(9):642-51.

Tickell KD, Walson JL. Nutritional enteric failure: neglected tropical diseases and childhood stunting. *PLoS Negl Trop Dis*. 2016;10(4):e0004523.

Trehan I, Banerjee S, Murray E, et al. Extending supplementary feeding for children younger than 5 years with moderate acute malnutrition leads to lower relapse rates. *J Pediatr Gastroenterol Nutr*. 2015;60(4):544-9.

Trehan I, Manary MJ. Management of severe acute malnutrition in low-income and middle-income countries. *Arch Dis Child*. 2015;100(3):283-287.

WHO. Management of severe malnutrition: a manual for physicians and other senior health workers. (World Health Organization, Geneva, 1999).

WHO. Updates on the management of severe acute malnutrition in infants and children. (World Health Organization, Geneva, 2013).

WHO, UNICEF. WHO child growth standards and the identification of severe acute malnutrition in infants and children. (World Health Organization, United Nations Children's Fund, Geneva, 2009).

WHO, WFP, UNSCN, UNICEF. Community-based management of severe acute malnutrition. (World Health Organization, World Food Programme, United Nations System Standing Committee on Nutrition, United Nations Children's Fund, Geneva, 2007).

# 22 Poor Weight Gain

Teresa Duryea and Kathleen J. Motil



## INTRODUCTION

Poor weight gain is the finding of weight loss or a deceleration in the rate of weight gain. Failure to thrive describes the condition of infants and toddlers under age 2 years who have an abnormally low weight relative to their stature for their age and sex. With prolonged and/or severe malnutrition, linear growth and head circumference can be secondarily affected. The term *failure to thrive* is not a singular disorder; rather, poor growth is a sign of an underlying problem that leads to insufficient usable nutrition. A wide variety of medical and psychosocial factors can contribute to poor weight gain.

The prevalence of failure to thrive is reported to be 5% to 10% in primary care settings. Community studies indicate that up to 50% of children with failure to thrive are not identified. Recurrent failure to thrive is reported in 5% of children due to diarrhea, respiratory infections, urinary tract infections, discontinuation of breastfeeding, teething, and age of initiating complementary feeding. Regardless of specific etiology, failure to thrive may have profound effects on the growing child, including persistent short stature, decreased resistance to infection, and developmental impairment and/or disabilities.

## DEFINITION

Failure to thrive is characterized by insufficient growth recognized by the observation of growth over time using standard growth curves for age and gender. This condition is also called *weight faltering* or *growth failure*. There is a lack of consensus regarding the specific anthropometric criteria required to classify failure to thrive. Thus, many "definitions" for failure to thrive are commonly used in children under 2 years of age. These include weight less than 3rd percentile for corrected gestational age, weight-for-length less than 5th percentile, or downward crossing of 2 or more major percentiles on the growth chart. Other definitions include weight less than 80th percentile of ideal weight-for-age, triceps skinfold thickness of 5 mm or less, or a depressed rate of weight gain compared to that expected for age and gender. The interpretation of failure to thrive based on the pattern of height and weight from growth charts may be misleading because 25% of children demonstrate normal growth rate shifts during infancy and early childhood. Hence, a fall in growth velocity that persists is key and accuracy in obtaining and plotting growth measurements is implicit to the diagnosis. Special growth charts for prematurity and selected genetic syndromes should be used when indicated.

## PATHOGENESIS

Three basic mechanisms underlie poor weight gain: (1) inadequate nutrient intake, (2) insufficient utilization or impaired absorption of consumed nutrition, and (3) increased metabolic requirements. There are numerous specific etiologies for failure to thrive (see Table 22-1). However, most commonly, it results from insufficient intake of dietary energy and nutrients due to lack of food offered, chewing and swallowing dysfunction, and/or behavioral problems that limit a young child's intake. In many cases, a specific organic etiology for a child's failure to thrive is never identified, and when one is, it rarely presents with growth failure in isolation. Gestational age, birth weight, and age at first visit are lower in children with organic failure to thrive. Preceding infection and persecutory feeding have been reported as the most common triggering factors of inorganic failure to thrive. Behavioral and psychosocial feeding problems are common and should not be considered diagnoses of exclusion.

Prematurity and low birth weight are likely risk factors for the development of feeding problems. Many other factors potentially contribute to inadequate weight gain in infants or children and may lead to failure to thrive. These can be categorized as (1) medical problems of the infant/child, or (2) psychosocial issues related to the family or parent–child relationship (Table 22-2). Poverty is the single largest risk factor for undernutrition or failure to thrive.

Often, the underlying medical problems (organic disease) and psychosocial or environmental factors (inorganic causes) related to failure to thrive are intertwined. For instance, difficulty in establishing breastfeeding or bottle-feeding in infancy can be due to underlying medical problems, and this can lead to dysfunctional maternal–child bonding. Resultant disruption of the mutually rewarding parent–child relationship then may negatively affect the child's mealtime behavior and consequently the child's food intake. Weaning is a prime time for the emergence of problems with weight gain. It is at this time that a child's oral motor skills have developed to allow the consumption of more solid foods. For some children, refusal of new textures and/or flavors presented as these solid foods are introduced into the diet leads

**TABLE 22-1 MAJOR ETIOLOGIES OF FAILURE TO THRIVE**

| Inadequate Nutrient Intake | Insufficient Utilization/Impaired Absorption of Consumed Nutrition or Excessive Energy Losses | Increased Metabolic Requirements |
|---|---|---|
| Error in formula preparation | Cystic fibrosis | Hyperthyroidism |
| Poor diet (eg, excessive juice intake, fad foods) | Inflammatory bowel disease | Chronic hypoxemia |
| Grazing feeding behavior | Celiac disease | Chronic lung disease |
| Behavioral problems affecting food consumption (eg, feeding refusal, oral aversion) | Liver disease | Acquired or congenital heart disease |
| Anorexic states (eg, inflammatory bowel disease) | Short-gut syndrome | Renal disease |
| Mechanical feeding difficulties (eg, oromotor abnormalities, neurological disorders, congenital abnormalities affecting oronasalpharyngeal and/or upper gastrointestinal tract) | Chromosomal abnormalities/syndromes (eg, trisomies 13, 18, and 21) | Chronic/recurrent infection(s) |
| Inadequate food supply/poverty | Genetic diseases | Trauma |
| Poor child–parent relationship | Congenital infection | Burns |
| Neglect | Metabolic disorders/inborn errors of metabolism | Malignancy |
| | Persistent vomiting | Spasticity |
| | Gastroesophageal reflux | Hyperactivity |
| | Pancreatic insufficiency | |
| | Enzyme deficiency (eg, disaccharidase deficiency) | |
| | Microvillus inclusion disease | |
| | Protein-losing enteropathy | |
| | Chronic immunodeficiency | |
| | Allergic gastroenteropathy | |
| | Chronic enteric infections/parasite infestation | |
| | Diabetes mellitus | |

**TABLE 22-2 POTENTIAL RISK FACTORS FOR POOR WEIGHT GAIN**

| Medical (Infant/Child-Related Factors) | Psychosocial (Family-Related Factors) |
|---|---|
| Prematurity | Single parent |
| Intrauterine growth retardation | Young parental age |
| Perinatal infection | Lower educational level |
| Exposure to teratogens | Lack of social support |
| Anemia | Poverty |
| Lead poisoning | Breastfeeding problems |
| Acute illness | Disordered feeding techniques |
| Chronic disease | Underfeeding |
| Malabsorption states | Postpartum depression |
| Food intolerance/allergies | Family dysfunction |
| Neurologic disease | Substance abuse |
| Oromotor dysfunction | Mental illness |
| Anatomic abnormalities | Aberrant health/nutrition beliefs |
| Developmental delay | Poor parent–child attachment |
| Chromosomal/genetic disease | Abuse/neglect |
| Temperament | |
| Sensory-based feeding issues | |
| Victim of abuse/neglect | |

to inadequate energy consumption. Oral motor dysfunction, especially when accompanied by developmental delay and dysmorphic features may have a genetic basis for "failure to feed." Family-related factors may directly contribute to the child's failure to thrive. Likewise, the child's acute or chronic medical problems, including developmental and behavioral issues that may lead to poor weight gain, can heighten psychosocial concerns in the family.

## EVALUATION

### Medical History

A thorough medical history, including review of past and present growth data, and physical examination are the first steps in the evaluation of poor weight gain. Often, the history will yield clues that may either direct further evaluation or eliminate the need for extensive testing. The physician's role is to determine whether the child's failure to thrive primarily is due to insufficient nutritional intake, energy wasting, increased metabolic requirements, or altered growth potential. Important historical details include age of onset, perinatal history, dietary intake and feeding practices, review of systems focusing on associated gastrointestinal complaints, past medical history, family history, and social history (Table 22-3).

### Diet History

Detailed information regarding nutritional intake and feeding practices should be obtained. Parental report via a 24-hour dietary recall is often a good initial assessment of dietary intake. Completion of a 3-day food diary and observation of feeding may be important in cases of moderate to severe failure to thrive. The impact of psychosocial factors, such as poverty and food insecurity, parenting skills and nutrition knowledge, family disruption, and lack of access to resources, should always be considered when evaluating the diet history.

### Physical Examination

The goals of the physical examination are to assess the nutritional state and identify signs or symptoms of any underlying medical or genetic disorders that may be contributory to the inadequate growth. Accurate measurement and interpretation of the child's growth parameters (weight, length or height, and head circumference) are essential to establishing the diagnosis of failure to thrive. The appropriate tools and techniques for measurement must be used; plus, standardized growth curves for gender, age, and specific genetic disorders must be applied. It is recommended that the growth parameters of former premature infants be corrected for gestational age; however, there is no consensus regarding how long to continue this correction.

Obtaining accurate serial measurements provides key information, because the growth trajectory, the timing of the change in slope, and the proportionality of the growth parameters often provide clues to the etiology of the diminished weight. For instance, decreased weight in proportion to length often reflects inadequate usable energy or

**TABLE 22-3 HISTORICAL INFORMATION THAT AIDS IN DIAGNOSING FAILURE TO THRIVE**

| |
|---|
| **Perinatal History** |
| Birth weight |
| Intrauterine growth retardation |
| Prematurity |
| Postnatal complications |
| Maternal illness/infections |
| Exposure to drugs |
| **Dietary Intake and Feeding Practices** |
| Breast milk or formula fed |
| Established milk supply and schedule |
| Formula preparation |
| Introduction of solids |
| Duration of mealtimes |
| Number of meals/snacks daily |
| Location of meals (family table, on-the-go) |
| Parent–child feeding behaviors |
| Variety and types of foods/beverages offered |
| Amount of foods/beverages offered |
| Consumption of foods/beverages |
| Problems with chewing and/or swallowing |
| Special diets/formulas |
| Supplements |
| Unusual feeding behaviors |
| **Associated Gastrointestinal Symptoms** |
| Persistent vomiting: Consider congenital abnormalities (malrotation, strictures, webs), pyloric stenosis, gastroesophageal reflux, gastroparesis, food allergies/allergic gastropathy, eosinophilic esophagitis |
| Dysphagia: Consider eosinophilic esophagitis, oromotor abnormalities, neurologic disorders, congenital abnormalities affecting the oropharyngeal tract or esophagus |
| Persistent diarrhea: Consider malabsorption syndromes, pancreatic insufficiency, disaccharidase deficiency, microvillus inclusion disease, allergic gastroenteropathy, celiac disease, chronic enteric infections/parasite infestations, enteropathy, inflammatory bowel disease, excessive fructose or sorbitol intake |
| Food preferences: Consider child avoidance of certain textures or symptoms of intolerance, autism spectrum; parent imposed dietary restrictions |
| **Other** |
| Age of onset |
| Review of growth parameters from previous medical encounters |
| Presence of other systemic signs and symptoms |
| Underlying medical problems or genetic syndromes |
| Child's development, behavior, and temperament |
| Tone of child–caregiver interactions |
| Mid-parental height |
| Growth patterns in family members |
| Family history of chronic medical conditions |
| Family history of mental illness or substance abuse |
| Household composition |
| Number of caregivers |
| Employment status and financial state of family |
| Food insecurity/accessibility |
| History of neglect or abuse |

nutrient intake or increased losses. When weight and length are decreased proportionately, longstanding nutritional deficiency may be a cause, yet other etiologies such as endocrine, genetic, or familial conditions should be considered. When head growth is impaired more than weight or length, the variety of conditions that can lead to microcephaly (eg, intrauterine infection, exposure to teratogens, congenital syndromes) should be contemplated.

Clinical signs of protein-energy malnutrition that may be present on physical examination include loss of skin turgor, decreased subcutaneous fat and muscle mass, lack of activity (apathy), sparse or lusterless hair, poor nail growth, pigmentation changes of the skin, rash, and edema. The astute physician should perform a thorough and careful examination to look for signs of an underlying medical condition, anatomic abnormality, genetic syndrome, nutrient deficiency, delayed development, neurologic problems, and abuse or neglect. Observation of the parent–child interactions during encounters is also an important part of the evaluation.



### Diagnostic Studies

When needed, investigations should be selected on the basis of patient history and physical examination rather than ordered as a matter of routine. Tests that are not suggested by the patient history and physical examination are rarely helpful. A stepwise approach should be used in planning the evaluation. Baseline laboratory tests that are obtained often include complete blood count, lead level, C-reactive protein, erythrocyte sedimentation rate, urinalysis, and urine culture. These tests may identify the consequences of malnutrition (eg, anemia) or screen for general medical conditions that may contribute to poor weight gain (eg, chronic infection, inflammation, malignancy, lead poisoning, renal disease). If the history and/or physical examination are suggestive of particular conditions, additional tests or imaging studies may be necessary in the initial evaluation. Other more specialized or advanced testing may be warranted if specific conditions are suspected or when a patient is not responding to dietary modification and no etiology has been found (Table 22-4).

**TABLE 22-4 STEPWISE EVALUATION OF FAILURE TO THRIVE**

| **Baseline Laboratory** |
|---|
| Complete blood count |
| Lead level |
| Inflammatory markers (erythrocyte sedimentation rate, C-reactive protein) |
| Urinalysis and urine culture |
| **Additional Tests** |
| Chemistry panel: |
| Electrolytes, BUN, creatinine, glucose, calcium, phosphorus, magnesium, albumin, total protein, liver enzymes, amylase, lipase |
| Stool studies: |
| Guaiac, culture for enteric pathogens, smear for ova and parasites, giardia antigen |
| Stool for *Helicobacter pylori* antigen |
| Stool reducing substances, $\alpha_1$-antitrypsin, calprotectin, elastase |
| **Advanced or Specialized Tests** |
| Human immunodeficiency virus antibody |
| Sweat chloride test |
| Tuberculin skin testing |
| Celiac screen (total immunoglobulin A, anti-tissue transglutaminase immunoglobulin A [anti-tTG IgA]) |
| Quantitative immunoglobulins |
| Newborn screen or metabolic workup: serum amino acids, urine organic acids, urine reducing substances, acylcarnitine profile, plasma lactate |
| Genetic testing |
| Growth hormone levels |
| Thyroid studies (thyroid-stimulating hormones, free $T_4$) |
| Inflammatory bowel disease panel for anti-*Saccharomyces cerevisiae* antibodies (ASCA), perinuclear antineutrophil cytoplasmic antibodies (p-ANCA), and anti-ompC antibodies |
| Serum IgE, radioallergosorbent tests (RAST), and skin tests to selected food antigens |
| Serum antinuclear antibodies (ANA), anti-endomysial antibodies, and anti-LKM antibodies |
| Hepatitis panel |
| Cytomegalovirus (CMV) and Epstein-Barr virus (EBV); immunoglobulin M (IgM) and immunoglobulin G (IgG) |
| Chest x-ray |
| Electrocardiogram |
| Upper gastrointestinal series with small bowel follow through |
| Swallowing function study |
| Abdominal ultrasound |
| Endoscopic studies with biopsies |
| Bone age |
| Skeletal survey |
| Magnetic resonance imagery (MRI) of brain or abdomen |

## MANAGEMENT

The role of the physician in the management of failure to thrive is multifaceted: He or she must be an astute diagnostician, clinician, and advocate for the patient. Frequent follow-up visits with growth monitoring are essential. Hospitalization is indicated if the child is severely malnourished, when a serious organic cause is probable, and any time there is concern for neglect or abuse. Hospitalization also may be necessary to verify reported feeding patterns when the history seems discordant with growth values.

The first steps in management are nutritional counseling and dietary interventions. Assisting parents in the care of their child with failure to thrive must be accomplished in a sensitive, nonjudgmental manner. Management involves the following: (1) increasing nutritional intake, (2) evoking catch-up growth, (3) resolving feeding difficulties if possible, and (4) strengthening positive feeding interactions between parent and child.

Failure to thrive is largely managed by dietary intervention; the ultimate goal is to increase the energy intake of the child to enable catch-up growth, which is weight gain at a rate more rapid than the basal requirement for age, such that the weight deficit is overcome. Energy needs for catch-up growth can be calculated: estimated energy requirement for age (kcal/kg) multiplied by ideal weight-for-height (kg) divided by actual weight (kg), where ideal weight-for-height is the median weight for the patient's height (as determined from the weight-for-height curves). One method for initiating catch-up growth is increasing the energy intake by 50%. In practice, recommendations include a focus on intake of high-energy foods, addition of extra energy to foods, limited consumption of low-energy foods (especially juice), and structured mealtimes and snacks.

Incorporating high-energy foods into a young child's diet may be challenging because of patient and family food preferences. Strategies for increasing energy consumption in toddlers and children include frequent child-sized meals, energy-dense foods, and the addition of extra energy via high-fat condiments such as oils, butter, and cheese. Children should be offered 3 meals and 2 to 3 snacks daily, or 5 to 6 small meals daily. Portion size should be individualized to fit the size of the child; portions that are too large often are overwhelming. Energy-dense foods include cheese, eggs, peanut butter, whole milk, avocado, and meats. Energy can be boosted by adding margarine, honey, gravy, creamy dips or sauces, powdered milk, or ice cream. The addition of supplemental vitamins and minerals may be offered.

Mealtime behavior should be structured. Meals for the toddler should be offered in a high chair at the table, and distractions should be minimized. The child should be allowed to experiment with the food, and forceful feeding should be avoided. The "2-spoon method" is a commonly employed strategy in which the child is allowed to play with 1 spoon while the parent feeds with the other. Parents should be instructed to keep relaxed and calm at mealtime and offer praise for the child when he or she eats well. The child should be allowed to determine when he or she is finished eating and should not be forced to finish portions of food. Grazing behavior in between meals/snacks and drinking juice should be minimized. Beverages should be limited at mealtime because drinking too much can make a child feel full and preclude the intake of solids. The consumption of milk should be tailored to patient age but, in general, should be between 16 and 24 ounces daily. The use of high-calorie drinkable supplements, shakes, and puddings may be helpful.

Close follow-up of the patient recovering from malnutrition is essential. In the early refeeding phase, the child with substantial malnourishment may be at risk for refeeding syndrome. Additionally, some children with malnutrition experience nutritional recovery syndrome. This is characterized by hepatomegaly (secondary to increased glycogen deposition in the liver), sweatiness, mild irritability or hyperactivity, and widening of the cranial sutures in infants with open sutures (as brain growth is more rapid than skull growth). If weight gain has not occurred after 4 to 6 weeks, further investigation may be pursued and referrals to specialists may be warranted. Depending upon the degree of failure to thrive, hospitalization for evaluation and initiation of supplemental feeding with a nasogastric tube may be considered. In children requiring prolonged supplemental nasogastric feeding, placement of a gastrostomy tube may be indicated. Feeding assessment by a speech pathologist or occupational therapist may allow for the development of strategies to improve sucking and swallowing, chewing, and oral aversion. A multidisciplinary team approach involving the primary care physician, pediatric specialists, psychologist, and dietitian, in addition to the occupational therapist and/or speech pathologist, may be helpful for improving oral intake in the most difficult cases of failure to thrive.

## OUTCOMES

Adequate nutrition is especially important in the first 3 years of a child's life, the period when exponential development of the brain and cognitive processes takes place. Malnutrition in this period may carry the risk of a negative impact on cognitive development. The prognosis with respect to stature and weight is good for children with failure to thrive; however, up to 60% of infants with failure to thrive remain below the 20th percentile for height and weight. Approximately 50% of children with failure to thrive have below-normal cognitive function. Additionally, behavioral problems and learning difficulties are identified in a significant portion of this population. Of note, cognitive recovery in children with failure to thrive appears to mirror their nutritional recovery; this finding emphasizes the need for quick nutritional interventions for these children.

## SUGGESTED READINGS


Barron MA, Makhija M, Hagen LE, Peencharz P, Grunebaum E, Roifman CM. Increased resting energy expenditure is associated with failure to thrive in infants with severe combined immunodeficiency. *J Pediatr.* 2011;159(4):628-32.

Black MM, Dubowitz H, Krishnakumar A, Starr RH Jr. Early intervention and recovery among children with failure to thrive: follow-up at age 8. *Pediatrics.* 2007;120(1):59-69.

Cole SZ, Lanham JS. Failure to thrive: an update. *Am Fam Physician.* 2011;83(7):829-34.

Jaffe AC. Failure to thrive: current clinical concepts. *Pediatr Rev.* 2011;32(3):100-7.

Larson-Nath C, Blank VF. Clinical review of failure to thrive in pediatric patients. *Pediatr Ann.* 2016;45(2):e46-9.

Larson-Nath CM, Goday PS. Failure to thrive: a prospective study in a pediatric gastroenterology clinic. *J Pediatr Gastroenterol Nutr.* 2016;62(6):907-13.

Perrin EC, Cole, CH, Frank DA, et. al. Criteria for determining disability in infants and children: failure to thrive: summary. *Evid Rep Technol Assess (Summ).* 2003;(72):1-5.

Rabago J, Marra K, Allmendinger N, Shur N. The clinical geneticist and the evaluation of failure to thrive versus failure to feed. *Am J Med Genet C Semin Med Genet.* 2015;169(4):337-48.

Saki Malehi A, Hajideh E, Ahmadi K, Kholdi N. Modeling the recurrent failure to thrive in less than two-year children: recurrent events survival analysis. *J Res Health Sci.* 2014;14(1):96-9.

ud Din Z, Emmett P, Steer C, Emond A. Growth outcomes of weight faltering in infancy in ALSPAC. *Pediatrics.* 2013;131(3);e843.

Walker SP, Grantham-McGregor SM, Powell CA, Chang SM. Effects of growth restriction in early childhood on growth, IQ, and cognition at age 11 to 12 and benefits of nutritional supplementation and psychosocial stimulation. *J Pediatr.* 2000;137(1):36-41.

Yoo SD, Hwang EH, Lee YJ, Park JH. Clinical characteristics of failure to thrive in infant and toddler: organic vs. nonorganic. *Pediatr Gastroenterol Hepatol Nutr.* 2013;16(4):261-8.




# 23 Feeding Difficulties in Infants and Children

Carol A. Redel

## INTRODUCTION

From the time of birth, acquisition of nutrients essential for growth and development of the infant is determined by a complex interplay of hunger, feeding and swallowing skills, and the social environment meeting those nutrient needs. Appropriate interplay results in a mutually satisfying feeding and mealtime experience for both infant and caregiver, reinforcing bonding. A deficit in any of these areas is termed feeding difficulties, or feeding disorder.

Functionally feeding and swallowing are complex processes divided into 4 phases, as shown in Figures 23-1 and 23-2. The first phase is the *preoral phase*, which is dependent upon the infant/child's sensation and communication of hunger. The second phase, the *oral phase*, is the oral cavity–food processing phase where food or liquid is formed into a bolus, enabling safe passage through the pharynx. The next steps in the swallow process are reflexive, and therefore, involuntary. In the ensuing *pharyngeal phase*, the bolus contacts the tonsillar pillars and pharyngeal wall, resulting in elevation of the larynx, closure of the vocal cords, and relaxation of the esophageal sphincter. Then, contraction of the pharynx deposits the food bolus in the esophagus. During the passage of the food bolus through the pharynx, coordination between breathing and swallowing is essential to prevent aspiration. The final phase, *the esophageal phase*, moves the food bolus into the stomach and then small intestine, where the processes of digestion and nutrient absorption occur. Any developmental change in the phases of swallowing occurring from infancy through adulthood will impact the ability to feed successfully.

Feeding difficulties in infancy and childhood can present in a number of ways, including total feeding refusal, frequent emesis, poor weight gain, recurrent pneumonia, and chronic lung disease. The

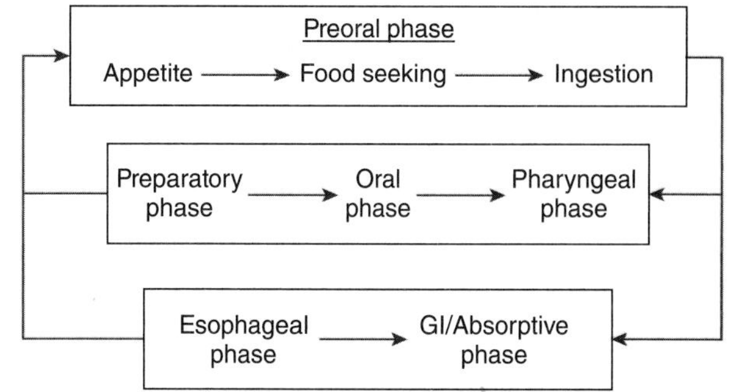


**FIGURE 23-1** Model of normal phases of swallowing in infants and children. The complexity of interactions between phases often complicates determination of the primary cause of feeding difficulty.

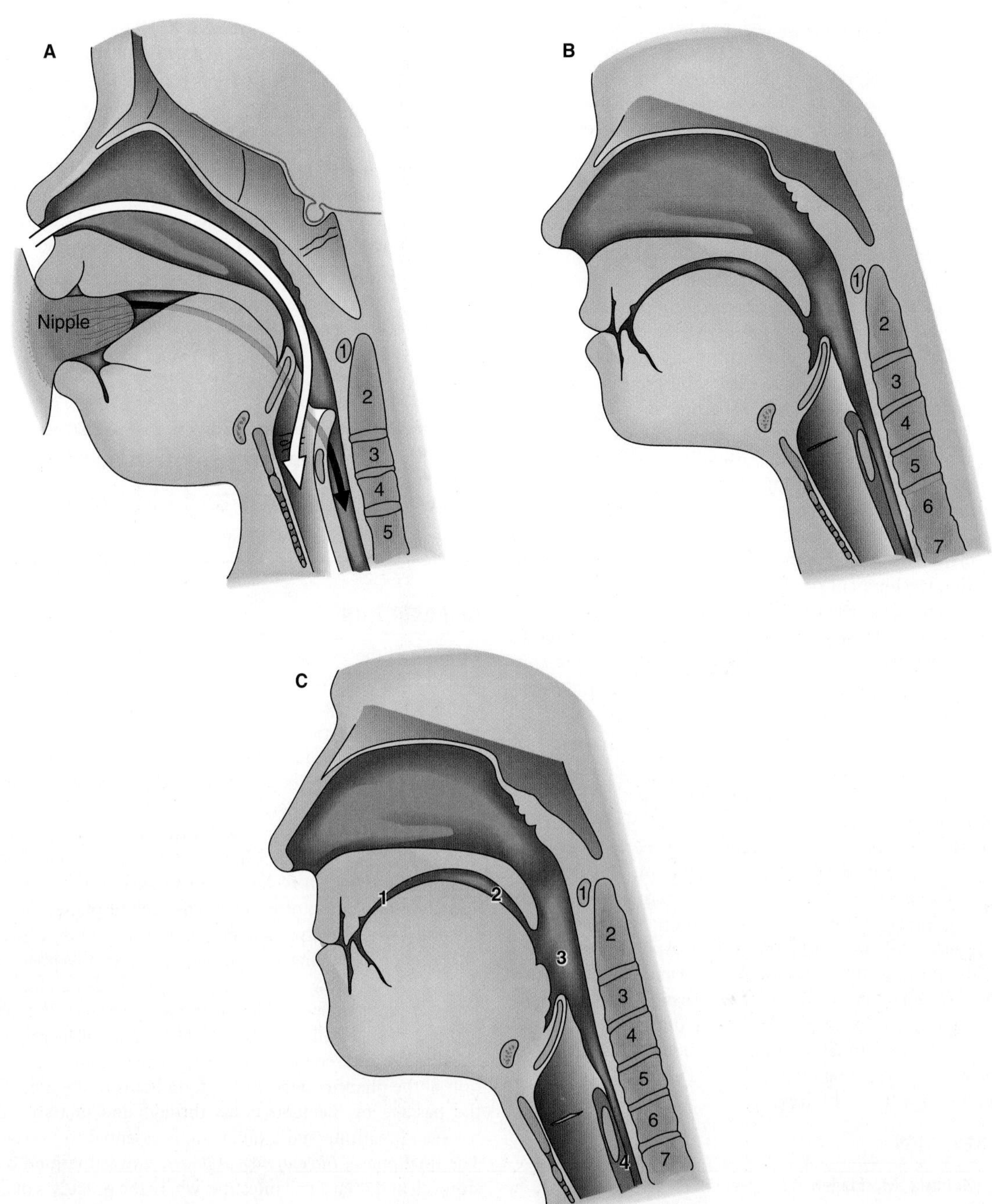


**FIGURE 23-2** **A:** The infant oropharynx has anatomical differences from the mature oropharynx. The larynx is elevated with the contact between the epiglottis and soft palate, so that there is a functional separation between air passages (white arrow) and food passages (black/gray arrow) in the pharynx. Food moves around the epiglottis into the pharyngeal recess, and then finally into the esophagus. **B:** The toddler (aged 2–3 years old) oropharynx. **C:** The adult oropharynx: (1) oral preparatory phase, (2) oral phase, (3) pharyngeal phase, (4) esophageal phase. The infant oral cavity is much smaller than the toddler or adult oral cavity, thus providing little space for manipulation of the food bolus. The larynx is elevated so that the epiglottis nearly touches the soft palate, and the larynx is at the level of the first to third cervical vertebrae. The tongue is entirely in the oral cavity, with no oral region of the pharynx. In the toddler, the larynx has descended to the fifth cervical vertebra, and by adulthood, to the sixth to seventh cervical vertebrae.

etiologies for these swallowing and feeding difficulties a can be multifactorial, and are included in Table 23-1. Feeding and swallowing difficulties may present at any point in the acquisition of oral motor skills during infancy and the toddler years. Since organic and nonorganic etiologies can occur alone and in combination, their evaluation and treatment can be challenging. The first step in the process is the determination of physical causes of the feeding difficulty. With this approach, any correctable cause can be dealt with. Nonorganic causes are more appropriately evaluated once organic processes are ruled out. In many cases, by the time of diagnosis, feeding difficulties may have both organic and nonorganic contributors. Success in treatment is improved if the child and caregiver behaviors surrounding feeding are identified and addressed, thus resulting in a more mutually enjoyable feeding relationship between caregiver and child.

## PREORAL PHASE

### Hunger and Appetite

Hunger, or the recognition of the physiological need to ingest food, is somewhat distinct from appetite, which represents desire to consume.

**TABLE 23-1 PARTIAL LIST OF MEDICAL ETIOLOGIES OF FEEDING DIFFICULTIES IN CHILDREN**

| | |
|---|---|
| Disorders affecting appetite, food seeking behavior, and consumption | Congenital esophageal stenosis due to tracheobronchial remnants |
| Anorexia nervosa | Esophageal web, stricture, or ring |
| Deprivation | Esophageal tumor/mass |
| Depression | Foreign body |
| Central nervous system disorders | Aberrant right subclavian artery |
| Metabolic diseases | Disorders affecting suck/swallow coordination with breathing |
| Sensory defects | Choanal atresia |
| Neuromuscular disorders | Chronic lung disease/bronchopulmonary dysplasia |
| Oral hypersensitivity or aversion secondary to lack of feeding experience during critical time periods | Cardiac disease |
| Conditioned dysphagia | Any disorder causing tachypnea |
| Aspiration | Disorders affecting neuromuscular coordination of swallowing |
| Oral inflammation | Infantile botulism |
| Gastroesophageal reflux disease (GERD) | Cerebral palsy |
| Eosinophilic esophagitis | Bulbar or brain stem glioma |
| Gastroparesis | Arnold–Chiari malformation |
| Dumping syndrome or gas bloat | Familial dysautonomia |
| Fatigue secondary to cardiac or pulmonary disease | Myelomeningocele |
| Poverty | Diphtheria or poliomyelitis postinfectious paralysis |
| Caregiver psychopathology, including eating disorders | Moebius syndrome |
| Anatomical abnormalities of the oropharynx | Myasthenia gravis |
| Cleft lip and/or palate | Tardive dyskinesia |
| Ankyloglossia/macroglossia | Muscular dystrophies |
| Pierre Robin sequence/Stickler syndrome | Congenital myotonic dystrophy |
| Velopharyngeal insufficiency (VPI) | Dermatomyositis, polymyositis |
| Retropharyngeal abscess or mass | Rheumatoid arthritis |
| Tonsillar hypertrophy | Disorders of esophageal peristalsis |
| Dental abscess or caries | Achalasia |
| Anatomical abnormalities of larynx and trachea | Chagas disease |
| Laryngeal clefts or cysts | Systemic lupus erythematosus |
| Laryngomalacia/tracheomalacia | Scleroderma |
| Subglottic stenosis | Mixed connective tissue disorders |
| Tracheoesophageal cleft | Diffuse esophageal spam |
| Vascular ring/sling causing tracheoesophageal compression | Pseudo-obstruction |
| Infectious and inflammatory disorders causing difficulty swallowing (dysphagia) | Miscellaneous disorders affecting feeding and swallowing |
| Adenotonsillitis | Hypothyroidism |
| Epiglottitis | Neonatal hyperparathyroidism |
| Deep neck space infections | Syndromic chromosomal abnormalities (trisomies, deletions) |
| Laryngopharyngeal reflux secondary to GERD | Prader-Willi syndrome (during infancy) |
| Caustic ingestion | Allergies and atopic disorders |
| Viral esophagitis due to cytomegalovirus (CMV) or herpes simplex virus (HSV) | Lipid/lipoprotein metabolic defects |
| Candidal esophagitis or pharyngitis | Russell-Silver syndrome |
| Crohn disease | Coffin-Siris syndrome |
| Behçet disease | Williams syndrome |
| Chronic graft-versus-host disease (GVHD) | Coloboma, heart defect, atresia choanae, retarded growth and development, genital abnormality, and ear abnormality (CHARGE) syndrome |
| Anatomical abnormalities of the esophagus | Congenital disorders of glycosylation |
| Esophageal atresia/tracheoesophageal fistula | Epidermolysis bullosa dystrophica |
| | Globus hystericus |

The hypothalamic center for hunger receives signals from a variety of source: the gastrointestinal (GI) tract, blood nutrient levels, hormones, and psychological factors. This complex interaction appears to be functional even in newborns. Unfortunately, this relationship, and subsequently appetite, can be impacted negatively by early events such as social deprivation and any illness associated with negative eating experiences. For example, infants and children whose hunger has not been satisfied by a caregiver may have both reduced hunger and reduced appetite. Disorders associated with negative eating experiences result in decreased appetite; some examples include food allergies, metabolic disorders and gastroesophageal reflux disease (GERD)-associated emesis, and prolonged ventilation and tube feeding. These infants and children may progress to the point of oral defensiveness, or the unwillingness to have anything near the mouth. Although these children may feel hunger, they appear to not associate eating with satisfying that hunger.

**Food Seeking and Consumption**

Preverbal infants and children may cry, lip smack, or extend the tongue to indicate hunger; these cues must be identified and satisfied by the caregiver. Neurotypical toddlers are able to communicate hunger, and they are able to secure available food themselves. Gross and fine motor developmental skills ensure the child's ability to self-nourish using utensils to self-feed. Disorders interfering with the acquisition of these skills will necessitate caregiver training in feeding techniques appropriate for the child's needs. Failure to recognize the need for alteration in feeding techniques has the potential to disrupt the caregiver–child relationship.

## SWALLOWING

### Oral Phase

In the oral cavity, food is formed into a bolus, readying it for movement toward the pharynx. The development of the oral phase requires normal anatomy, sensation, muscle development, and coordination. Any difficulty swallowing foods or liquids is termed dysphagia, regardless of the defect. In utero development of mouthing and sucking is seen at 15 weeks gestation. An uncoordinated pattern of suck followed by pause emerges by 32 weeks gestation, with rhythmicity of suck and swallow attained by 34 to 36 weeks gestation. Once the infant is born, swallowing occurs with a certain liquid volume in the mouth. Tongue motion and coordination are both necessary for this oral phase.

During early infancy, changes occur in the oral cavity that coincide with development of motor skills necessary for safe liquid feeding (see Fig. 23-2). The brain stem regulates sucking, which is the process of extension/retraction movements of the tongue. The size of the tongue is large relative to the size of the oral cavity, and the presence of large buccal fat pads assists in sucking upon a nipple. By coordination of the mouth seal around a nipple and then the tongue seal up against the palate, suction pressure to express a bolus of approximately 0.2 mL liquid per suck is achieved. More rapid flow has potential to overwhelm the initiation of the swallow, resulting in gagging, choking, and/or aspiration.

By 3 to 6 months of age, though, the anatomy of the oral cavity and pharynx changes, resulting in a more mature suck pattern. As the buccal fat pads regress, there is more space in the oral cavity; an accompanying developmental drop in the jaw also contributes to this increased space. These changes allow for development of an up/down tongue motion, eventual bolus formation, and an overall more mature suck pattern. Up/down and lateral tongue movements enable oral motor processing of both semisolid and liquid food sources. Then, during the time period from 6 to 12 months of age, chewing motions begin, allowing the oral processing of increasing textures of foods, especially assisted by appearance of deciduous teeth. At approximately 1 year of age, the infantile suck pattern disappears, enabling cup drinking. Maturation of chewing skills from mashing to rotary jaw movements allows transition to foods of varied textures, and an adult feeding pattern.

For infants and children unable to progress through the above steps in oral motor development during infancy and the toddler years, lengthy periods of therapy may be necessary to garner these skills. Some children may not progress beyond a certain point in these developmental processes, requiring lifelong alterations in food consistency or feeding appliance for delivery of nutrition.

### Pharyngeal Phase of Feeding

Anatomical and developmental changes in the involuntary pharyngeal phase of swallowing occur during early life. Bolus contact with the pharyngeal wall initiates the involuntary swallow; at that point the nasal cavity is sealed off by closure of the upper pharynx and soft palate. During pharyngeal contraction, the larynx elevates, the vocal cords close, and breathing stops in order to prevent aspiration into the lower airway. The upper esophageal sphincter relaxes, allowing pharyngeal peristalsis to move the bolus past the closed, elevated larynx, and into the upper esophagus. Anatomical relationships during infancy allow for swallowing without aspiration into the airway; recall that the larynx is at the level of the first to third cervical vertebrae, allowing the velum, tongue, and epiglottis to meet, thus separating the airway from the GI tract. Therefore, most babies are able to coordinate breathing and sucking. Reduced minute ventilation and mild hypoxemia may occur in healthy infants with vigorous sucking and swallowing; this hypoxemia is worsened in cardiac or pulmonary disorders.

The anatomical change occurring early in the toddler years is the downward movement of the larynx to the fifth cervical vertebra. This in effect decreases the distance between the swallowing process and the GI tract. Hence, developed oral motor skills as well as laryngeal function are necessary to prevent aspiration. This anatomical change should be considered when evaluating the toddler suspected of aspiration, even in the absence of aspiration during infancy.

Multiple disorders may interfere with swallowing coordination. GERD and neurological disorders affecting laryngeal function increase the risk of aspiration. Other anatomical problems of the larynx, including clefts, cysts, or laryngomalacia, can place a child at risk for aspiration. Central nervous system disorders, tumors, foreign bodies, myopathies, inflammatory processes involving the larynx and surrounding structures, and esophageal motility disorders can additionally place a child at risk for aspiration. The process of coordination of swallowing and breathing may additionally be disrupted by cardiac disorders or any disorder causing tachypnea.

### Esophageal and GI Phases

Abnormal GI motility, esophageal inflammatory disorders such as GERD and eosinophilic esophagitis, allergy, infection, and mechanical obstruction of the upper GI tract may all result in feeding difficulties. In fact, any disorder causing odynophagia or postprandial discomfort from any pathology can result in feeding difficulties.

## EVALUATION OF THE CHILD WITH FEEDING DIFFICULTIES

The evaluation of a child with issues such as poor weight gain, refusal to eat or drink, texture aversion, recurrent pneumonia, and chronic lung disease of uncertain etiology is best accomplished by a multidisciplinary team of pediatric specialists trained in the management of feeding disorders. The team may include pediatric subspecialists in gastroenterology, otolaryngology and pulmonary medicine, radiology, neurology, and physical medicine and rehabilitation medicine; dentists; behavioral psychologists; nurses; speech and language pathologists; occupational therapists; and dietitians. The multidisciplinary approach evaluates both organic and nonorganic factors contributing to a feeding difficulty.

The first goal of this group of professionals is determination of the safest feeding route for the infant or child. Hence, a complete medical, feeding, and developmental history, coupled with physical exam, is essential. In this way, identification of anatomical, functional, developmental, psychosocial, and behavioral factors contributing to current feeding difficulties is made. Specific details of current feeding, including child position; feeding frequency and child's ability to self-feed; current diet; and texture modifications already in use are pertinent. Medical comorbidities affecting intake, as well as history of stridor or upper airway congestion with feeding should be evaluated. A history of recurrent pneumonia may suggest aspiration. Additionally, any history of airway or GI surgeries is included.

A nutritional evaluation will include growth and weight gain for age and medical status and adequacy of kilocalories and nutrients for age in the current diet, regardless of mode of delivery. From a behavior standpoint, evaluation by a psychologist will assess current behaviors of the child and caregivers impacting meal and snack time intake.

A feeding therapist with a background in either speech and language pathology or occupational therapy will conduct both non-nutritive and nutritive oral motor evaluation. Prior to the actual feeding, the therapist looks at posture, neuromuscular tone, and position for feeding. Some children may have incomplete lip closure, resulting in food and liquid loss while eating or drinking. Oral structures are evaluated by the therapist: tonsillar hypertrophy may negatively impact both desire to eat and oral motor skill in initiating the swallow, while loss of gag reflex is suggestive of cranial nerve IX or X involvement. The feeding observation itself will include lip closure and handling of secretions, sucking or bolus formation, pace of feeding, gagging, choking, coughing or emesis, and airway sounds. Involvement of the behavioral psychologist while the caregiver is feeding the infant or child provides information about positive and negative aspects of the caregiver–child interaction at mealtime.

Vocal evaluation enables consideration of velopharyngeal insufficiency (VPI), which typically presents with hypernasal speech. VPI is the consequence of anatomically or neurologically based failure to close the velopharynx, resulting in nasal regurgitation and poor pharyngeal movement of the orally formed bolus.

Based on oral-motor and feeding assessments, the team will make recommendations regarding safety maneuvers to prevent aspiration, optimal food consistency, and nutritional intake. There may be some sense that behavior problems are contributing, but anatomical and physiological disorders must be excluded prior to behavioral intervention.

## DIAGNOSTIC TESTS

Since the clinical oral motor evaluation will miss silent aspiration, that is, aspiration without cough or gag, radiological testing is often indicated to assess oral, pharyngeal, and laryngeal anatomy and function. Many centers use imaging studies, although direct visualization and manometry may provide complementary information.

Contrast radiological studies are used to evaluate for the presence of anatomical and structural abnormalities including fistulas, strictures, or mass effect. The videoflouroscopic swallow study is recommended for the functional assessment of any infant and child with feeding difficulties. This test utilizes the expertise of the speech pathologist to orally feed the infant or child, while real-time radiological evaluation of anatomy and function occurs. In this study, velopharyngeal closure, pharyngeal function, laryngeal penetration and pooling in the laryngopharynx, aspiration, and early stage of esophageal motility can be evaluated. Frank aspiration is concerning. Laryngeal pooling as a risk factor for aspiration is currently thought not to be a risk for aspiration. It is center specific how much esophageal detail is obtained, so that typically this study does not substitute for an esophagram. Food consistencies provided during the swallow study are determined by the clinical feeding evaluation. Infants may be nipple fed barium or spoon fed a barium-coated pureed food. Toddlers with age-appropriate development may be evaluated with up to 3 textures: liquid, pureed, or solids. Additionally, when there is concern for aspiration of thin liquids, therapeutic modifications such as nectar-thick and honey-thick liquids may be tested, as well as accommodations in position or feeding devices.

Unfortunately, there are limitations of the video swallow study. First, the study requires cooperation of the infant or child to drink or eat sufficient barium to complete the exam; this need for cooperation precludes study of totally aversive children. Repeated exams to check for progress in the development of oral motor skills are limited due to the amount of radiation exposure inherent in the study. The risk versus benefit of additional radiation exposure warrants consideration when ordering follow-up studies.

Other imaging studies may be indicated as based on the medical evaluation. In cases of suspected aspiration pneumonia, an esophagram is indicated for the possible diagnosis of H-type tracheoesophageal stricture.

MRI of the chest may be helpful in cases of dysphagia or feeding-associated stridor, to determine the possibility of vascular ring or sling. If any study is suspicious for cranial nerve IX or X involvement, an MRI of the brain may elucidate lesions responsible for swallowing difficulties: Chiari malformations with tonsillar herniation, hydromyelia with myelomeningocele, and cervicomedullary junction compression.

If there is suspicion for laryngeal cleft, rigid laryngoscopy is indicated.

Some centers are currently using flexible endoscopic evaluation of swallowing (FEES) for real-time feeding evaluation. A flexible laryngoscope is passed by an otolaryngologist through the nose to directly see the larynx and pharynx; a speech pathologist then feeds the child multiple consistencies under direct observation. For children who are orally aversive, green food coloring can be mixed with oral secretions, and the child's management of secretions via swallowing can be evaluated. With the primary advantage of no radiation exposure, this study clearly defines anatomy and can evaluate velopharyngeal closure, pharyngeal function, laryngeal penetration, secretion management, and aspiration.

In cases of suspected upper gastrointestinal pathology, upper GI endoscopy may assist with diagnosis of inflammatory processes contributing to aversion: reflux esophagitis, eosinophilic esophagitis, and candidal esophagitis, to name a few. Finally, an upper GI manometry study can be used to study pharyngeal and esophageal motility and lower esophageal sphincter function via pressure readings at multiple sites. These studies are typically conducted in specialized centers for pediatric manometry given difficulty performing them.

## TREATMENT OF FEEDING DIFFICULTIES

Multidisciplinary evaluation of infant or child with feeding difficulties allows for the assessment of anatomical, functional, and behavior-based difficulties upon which to base recommendations for oral motor therapy. Children may benefit from oral motor therapy, plus or minus behavioral therapy, or alternative methods to provide or supplement nutrition. Although medical practitioners typically see these difficulties and their management as intrinsic to the child, caregivers are more likely to view these difficulties and management in the context of family life. Hence, family involvement is essential for understanding the evaluation and proposed treatment. It will be the responsibility of the caregivers and family in the future to implement these changes within the home.

Safety of oral feeding is of paramount importance, and it necessitates balancing the risks of aspiration pneumonia and chronic lung disease with the social and emotional rewards of eating. When aspiration has been observed clinically or on swallow study, recommendations may include thickness or texture changes, as well as feeding position modifications, to allow safe feeding. At this time, there is lack of evidence on restricting water in children with aspiration of thin liquids. In other cases of aspiration involving all thicknesses, tube feeding may be indicated to supply all nutrient needs.

Another consideration includes ability to consume nutrition safely within a reasonable time; lengthy times are typically related to poor oral motor skills or fatigue. Families often spend excessive time—1 to 2 hours for a feeding—to achieve or maintain oral feeding. These lengthy feedings result in frustration in both caregiver and child, compromising the quality of family life. Partial or complete nutrition by tube feeding should not be perceived as a caregiver failure, especially in syndromes or significant neurological comorbidities where children are unlikely to make significant progress with feeing therapy.

Oral motor therapy, otherwise known as feeding therapy, involves a 1-on-1 relationship between the infant/child and an occupational therapist or speech and language pathologist skilled in feeding techniques. Based on prior studies, the therapist determines (1) method of food/liquid delivery: mesh bag, bottles, cups, utensils—including adaptive forms of each; (2) upgrading or downgrading thickness or texture; (3) alterations in bolus flow rate; and (4) pacing for bites, chews, and swallows. Positioning during feeding is equally important, as changes in head and body position may compensate for difficulty moving food through the oropharynx, thus avoiding aspiration in the at-risk child.

For many children, behavioral therapy is indicated for acquisition of normal eating behaviors. The behavioral therapist typically works with the feeding therapist and caregiver to overcome aversive eating behaviors. These behaviors may include refusing to sit for meals, turning away from food, gagging at the sight of food, refusal to accept progressively upgraded textures, severely restricting foods accepted, gagging instead of swallowing, and expelling food from the mouth. Young children may respond to behavioral methods, including positive reinforcement, ignoring negative behaviors, and shaping behaviors. The active involvement of a caregiver with a healthy relationship with eating is essential for success of behavior therapy, given the need to sustain the techniques at home.

In many instances, the severity of feeding difficulties may necessitate intensive outpatient or even inpatient treatment. Such intensive programs provide multiple therapeutic feeding sessions daily, caregiver instruction and observation of caregiver implementation of therapeutic techniques, and psychosocial support to enable transition to home mealtime experiences. The goal of intensive feeding programs is consumption of nutrients appropriate for age in the least restrictive form tolerated by the child.

Adil E, Al Shemari H, Kacprowicz A, et al. Evaluation and management of chronic aspiration in children with normal upper airway anatomy. *JAMA Otolaryngol Head Neck Surg.* 2015;141(11):1006-1011.

Estrem HH, Pados BF, Thoyre S, Knafl K, McComish C, Park J. Concept of pediatric feeding problems from the parents' perspective. *MCN Am J Matern Child Nurs.* 2016;41(4):212-220.

Kemps G, Sewictch M, Birnbaum H, Daniel SJ. Contrast pooling in videoflouroscopic swallowing study as a risk factor for pneumonia in children with dysphagia. *Int J Pediatr Otorhinolaryngeal.* 2015;79(8):1306-1309.

Link DT, Willging JP, Miller CK, Cotton RT, Rudolph CD. Pediatric laryngopharyngeal sensory testing during flexible endoscopic evaluation of swallowing: feasible and correlative. *Ann Otol Rhino Laryngol.* 2000;109(10 Pt 1):899-905.

O'Donoghue S, Bagnall A. Videoflouroscopic evaluation in the assessment of swallowing disorders in pediatric and adult populations. *Folia Phoniatr Logop.* 1999;51(4-5):158-171.

Rudolph CD, Link DT. Feeding disorders in infants and children. *Pediatr Clin North Am.* 2002;49(1):97-112.

Weir K, McMahon S, Chang AB. Restriction of oral intake of water for aspiration lung disease in children. *Cochrane Database Syst Rev.* 2012;(9):CD005303.



# 24 The Overweight or Obese Child

Teresia O'Connor, Stephanie Sisley, and Fida Bacha

## INTRODUCTION

### Epidemiology of Obesity Among Children in the United States

Childhood obesity has been identified as a critical medical and public health problem due to both an increase in prevalence of overweight and obesity among children and the increased risk for obesity-associated diseases and conditions in these children. Reports from the National Health and Nutrition Examination Survey (NHANES) by the Centers for Disease Control and Prevention (CDC) estimate that 31.8% of the US pediatric population, 2 to 19 years old, were overweight in 2011–12, and 16.9% were obese. The incidence of overweight and obesity has tripled in the United States over the past 3 decades, leading to the prediction that the current generation of children will have a shorter life expectancy than that of their parents. Also alarming is the increasing prevalence of extreme obesity among children, with 6% of youth aged 2 to 19 years old meeting that criteria in 2013–14. Children who have extreme obesity are at particularly high risk for developing obesity-associated comorbidities and diseases, including some that were previously considered only of adult onset, such as type 2 diabetes.

The incidence of both overweight and obesity increases as children get older. Many physicians recommend greater efforts to prevent the development of obesity starting in early childhood to reverse this troubling trend. Ethnic minority children in the United States, specifically Hispanic and non-Hispanic black children, are at greatest risk for overweight and obesity. Health disparities due to differences in access to healthy environments, resources, and health care may be contributing to this difference in prevalence. A child's weight status is influenced by a combination of genetic, behavioral, environmental, and psychosocial variables. Interventions that attempt to prevent or treat obesity among children need to consider the complex interactions of these variables and ensure that the underlying factors for the current health disparities in obesity rates are addressed.

### Pathophysiology of Weight Regulation

Weight gain typically is considered as being related simply to the imbalance between energy intake and energy expenditure. However, this simple energy balance equation is heavily influenced by very complex mechanisms. Most people are aware that physical activity is important in increasing energy expenditure and, not unexpectedly, the weight gain of the Western world has paralleled a decrease in overall activity levels. New research has shown that small increments of exercise throughout the day are equivalent to larger sessions. Nutritional choices influencing energy intake are also important. Previously, high-fat diets were thought to be a culprit of the obesity epidemic. Current research is mixed on the role of total fat and fat subtypes in mediating excessive weight gain and, more importantly, shows a probable role of refined carbohydrates in accelerating weight gain. Additionally, sleep has an important role in maintaining a healthy weight through the establishment of normal circadian rhythms.

The brain is also vitally important in maintaining an individual's weight and can match intake and expenditure with less than a 1.25% error. This is due in large part due to regulation by the nucleus accumbens to control hedonic responses to food and by the hypothalamus to control food intake. In brief, the hypothalamus contains 2 important sets of neurons: anorexigenic (appetite suppressing) proopiomelanocortin (POMC) neurons and orexigenic (appetite promoting) neuropeptide Y (NPY) neurons. Hormones that are direct measures of the energy status of an individual (ie, fasting or fed) can directly activate or suppress these neurons to bring the individual back to equilibrium. Insulin, glucose, leptin, lipids, and the gut-derived peptides cholecystokinin, amylin, peptide YY (PYY), glucagon-like peptide-1 (GLP-1), ghrelin, and gastric inhibitory peptide (GIP) all have actions within the brain to control food intake. For instance, after a meal, glucose levels rise along with insulin levels. Insulin can activate POMC neurons and inhibit NPY neurons, which promotes satiety and the cessation of eating. However, in an obese state, the anorexigenic pathway is not activated appropriately by signaling molecules. There is also evidence that the body will defend a higher body weight through decreased energy expenditure and/or increased hunger after weight loss. These pathways are highly complex and contribute to the difficulty in losing weight and maintaining weight loss in the obese individual.

## ASSESSMENT OF WEIGHT STATUS

Obesity refers to excess body fat or adiposity. However, accurate direct measurement of adiposity often is impractical in the clinical setting, and various surrogate indices have been used to assess adiposity indirectly. The most common method for clinically identifying a child as being overweight or obese relies on the CDC definition for children using the body mass index (BMI), an approach that has been endorsed by multiple other agencies including the American Academy of Pediatrics. BMI percentile is used and recommended most frequently because it is easy and inexpensive to obtain. This index is a reflection of weight for height. As a child grows, normal BMI values vary with age and sex, thus, a single absolute cutoff of BMI as a measure of obesity is not available in youth. Rather, BMI is converted into a percentile or a z-score relative to distribution of BMI for age and sex in a reference population, most often based on the 2000 CDC growth charts (http://www.cdc.gov/growthcharts). The CDC also provides BMI calculators for clinicians and families to use to identify a child's weight status. Overweight for children is defined as a BMI at or above the 85th percentile but below the 95th percentile for the child's age and gender. Obesity is defined as BMI at or above the 95th percentile for the child's age and gender. Severe or extreme levels of pediatric obesity have also been defined using several different criteria. Extreme obesity has been reported as BMI at the 97th and 99th percentiles; at the 120th percentile above the 95th percentile; or as excess overweight calculated as 100 × (BMI / 50th percentile BMI for child age and gender). These additional assessments can be helpful in evaluating weight and change in weight status in severely obese children.

Nonetheless, the BMI measure is an imperfect measure of body fat because it does not distinguish between fat and muscle mass contributions to body weight, which may result in misclassification of obesity status. The BMI percentile or z-score is likely to correlate with body fatness, but a specific BMI percentile may not reflect the same percentage of body fatness at different ages, in different children, in different genders, among different racial or ethnic groups, or among children with different athletic builds. However, in heavier children, the relationship of BMI to body fat percentage is much stronger. BMI for age at ≥ 95th CDC percentile has moderately high (70–80%) sensitivity and adequate specificity to identify children with excess body fatness. Although there are no risk-based cutoffs for obesity in childhood, children with a high BMI have been shown to have higher prevalence of cardiometabolic disease risk factors, such as insulin resistance, dyslipidemia, and increased blood pressure, and are at higher risk of developing prediabetes and type 2 diabetes. They are also at higher risk of becoming obese adults. Clinicians also must exercise caution when diagnosing a child as overweight or obese based on the CDC-defined BMI percentile. An athletic build with greater musculature, especially in adolescent athletes, can result in an elevated BMI percentile even when the adolescent does not have excess adiposity.

In addition to total body fat, ectopic fat deposition such as intra-abdominal (visceral) or in the liver (hepatic) confers added metabolic risk. These fat deposits also vary with age, sex, and ethnicity and are not completely reflected by the BMI. Other clinical measures of adiposity include skinfold thicknesses, neck circumference, and waist and hip circumference. They are useful to further identify children with moderately elevated levels of BMI who may have greater adiposity and may be at higher risk for the complications of childhood obesity. However, some methodological issues may impede the clinical application of such assessments, and some studies suggest that they may only slightly improve the estimation of body fatness among obese children beyond that obtained using the BMI. Additional methods to more accurately determine body composition include bioelectric impedance, air displacement plethysmography (BodPod), total body potassium content, and dual-energy x-ray absorptiometry. Computer tomography (CT) and magnetic resonance imaging (MRI) scans allow more detailed assessment of body fat topography and the distribution of abdominal fat. The clinical applicability of these methods is limited and cost prohibitive on a population level.

## CLINICAL EVALUATION

The evaluation of obesity has 3 main purposes: (1) to exclude underlying pathology, (2) to evaluate potential comorbidities of obesity, and (3) to identify underlying behavioral and environmental variables that can be targeted to improve the child's weight status. Given that most parents are concerned their child's obesity is secondary to a hormonal cause, understanding when to evaluate/refer for a possible secondary cause is an important aspects of care.

### Evaluation of Underlying Pathology

Possible identifiable causes of obesity include iatrogenic, endocrine, or genetic conditions. Iatrogenic causes include glucocorticoids, appetite stimulants, certain antidepressants, antipsychotics, oral hypoglycemic agents, or surgical injury to the hypothalamus. Endocrine causes, such as hypothyroidism or Cushing syndrome, are almost always accompanied by decreased linear growth. Very early-onset obesity, developmental delays, and/or impaired learning may be signs of a genetic disorder. Melanocortin-4 receptor mutations are the most common genetic form of obesity and are associated with early-onset obesity and a strong family history of severe obesity. Prader-Willi syndrome (loss of imprinted genes on 15q11-q13) is the most common syndromic form of obesity. Given the rarity of genetic syndromes in causing obesity in the general population, further discussion is outside the scope of this chapter. A good history and physical exam are often sufficient to identify whether there is any concern for an underlying genetic or hormonal etiology of obesity.

### Evaluation for Comorbidities

The second purpose in the evaluation of obesity is to evaluate for comorbidities. The comorbidities of overweight and obesity are summarized by organ systems in Figure 24-1. The history should obtain

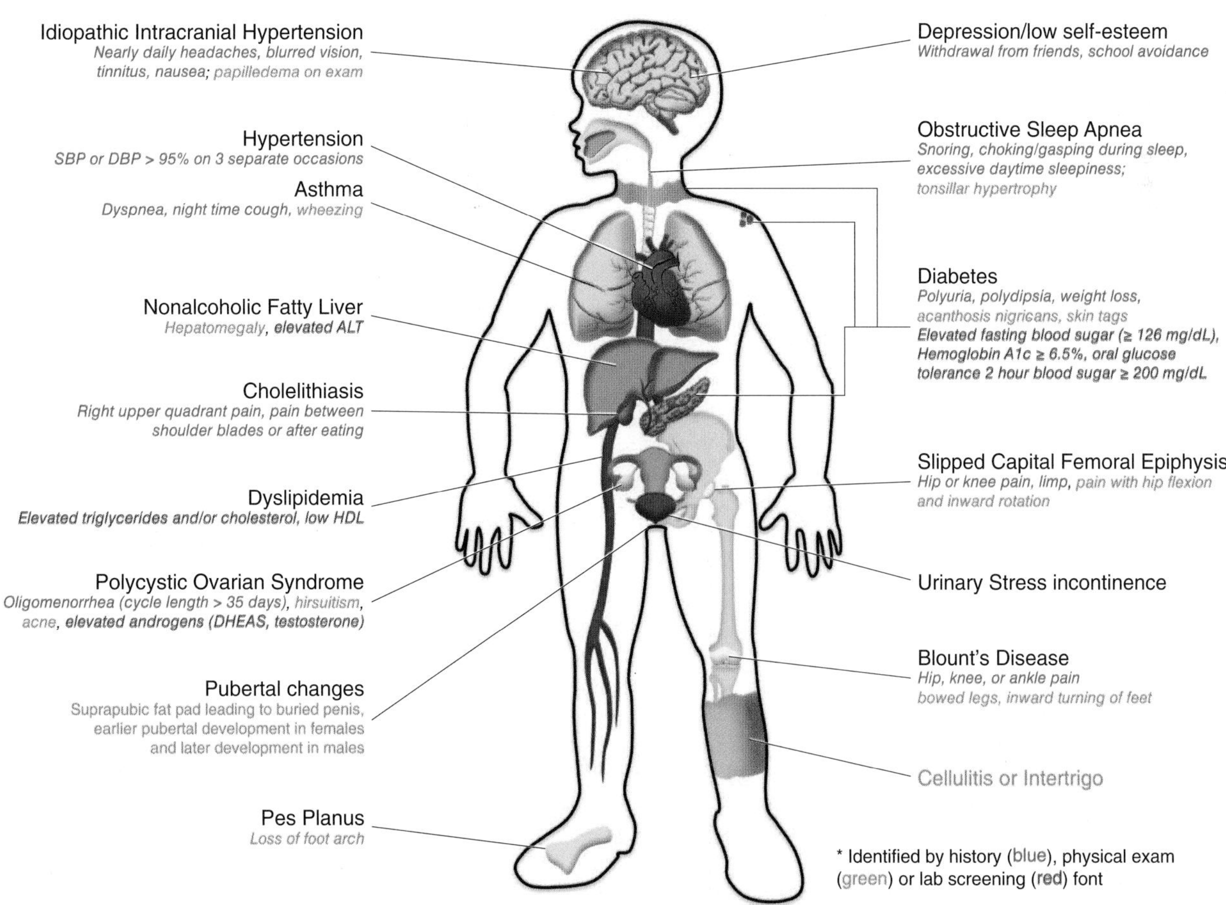


**FIGURE 24-1** Possible comorbidities of obesity among children and adolescents. The symptoms of each condition that should be identified by history and review of symptoms are in blue. The findings found on physical exam are in green. The findings found on laboratory screening are in red.

information on the timing of weight gain, especially in the infant/toddler years, and any triggers for sudden weight gain. The review of systems should include the presence of headache, tinnitus, blurred vision, abdominal pain, abnormal menstrual cycles, joint/foot pain, depression, snoring, excessive daytime sleepiness, asthma symptoms, polyuria, polydipsia, unintentional weight loss, incontinence, or skin rashes or infections. Family history should include presence of genetic disorders, severe obesity, hypertension, cardiovascular disease, diabetes, fatty liver disease, or dyslipidemia.



#### Assessment of Lifestyle Behaviors

Thirdly, a history of the child's obesity-related behaviors will help identify areas in which the family can work to help improve the child's weight status. Assessment of children's typical behaviors can be challenging due to potential biases introduced by self- or parent-report and social desirability. Some clinicians use screening forms to help them identify potential behavioral or environmental targets. Others have found patient-centered communication techniques for obtaining a behavioral history helpful because it also incorporates behavioral counseling. An example is motivational interviewing, which tries to elicit the patient's or parent's intrinsic motivation to engage in and explore their ambivalence toward behavior change. A detailed description is beyond the scope of this chapter (see Chapter 4). However, a behavioral assessment that includes the child's typical dietary intake, physical activity, screen media use, and other sedentary behaviors, as well as sleep habits, is critical to help the family develop a management plan. The dietary history should include information about the number of meals and snacks consumed per day, with a focus on intake of foods and beverages with added sugar, consumption of foods from different food groups, and the portion sizes consumed by the child. The assessment of physical activity should include the frequency and duration of moderate to vigorous physical activity that the child is engaged in, and use of screen media should differentiate the time spent using screens for academic versus entertainment purposes. Lastly, the child's typical bed time and sleep duration should be assessed.

#### Physical Exam

The physical exam should include assessment of the child's growth pattern over time and the child's vital signs, particularly blood pressure. The exam should include assessing the skin for acanthosis, skin tags, violaceous striae, hirsutism, severe acne, or cellulitis; the eyes for papilledema; the mouth for tonsillar hypertrophy; the lungs for wheezing; the abdomen for hepatomegaly; the joints for pain with hip flexion/internal rotation, bowing of legs, and flat feet; and genitourinary exam for pubertal progression. Initial lab screening tests may include fasting blood sugar and/or hemoglobin A1c, alanine aminotransferase (ALT), aspartate aminotransferase (AST), and a fasting lipid panel, to assess for metabolic dysfunction. Further lab evaluation for polycystic ovary syndrome or hypertension should be performed as needed. Unless the history and physical exam suggest concern for other conditions, such as hypothyroidism, additional lab screening is not necessary. Although the initial screening (eg, thyroid-stimulating hormone [TSH]) tests for the evaluation of obesity are consistent across guidelines, there is no clear consensus on when subsequent screening should be performed. The American Diabetes Association recommends diabetes screening should be done every other year; however, many tertiary care centers obtain screening for most comorbidities on an annual basis.

## PREVENTION OF OBESITY

Preventing children from becoming overweight or obese should be at the forefront of the primary care efforts for combating the obesity epidemic. Promoting healthy lifestyle behaviors is the mainstay for prevention of obesity and should be done at the family, school, and community levels. Key recommendations are to increase physical activity to at least 60 minutes daily, reduce or stop consumption of sugar-sweetened beverages, eat 5 servings of fruits and vegetables daily, have 2 hours or less of screen time daily, decrease total sugar intake to less than 25 grams per day (World Health Organization guideline), and achieve normal sleep times and patterns. Many public health promotional campaigns are available to be implemented in healthcare clinics, such as those found at the National Institute of Children's Health Quality Web site. Another good healthy eating resource for clinicians and families is the USDA MyPlate Web site (http://www.choosemyplate.gov).

Families should be encouraged to create health-promoting environments at home, by removing sugar-sweetened drinks and reducing access to snacks with added sugar or high fat content, and to make fruit and vegetable snacks accessible for children. Children are more active when outdoors, particularly in parks and playgrounds. Therefore, promoting daily outdoor active play for children in safe and fun environments should be encouraged when possible. Setting rules and monitoring children's screen use can also reduce the amount of time children spend on screens. Efforts are most likely to be successful when the whole family is targeted for change, and parents are encouraged to use proactive parenting to support their child toward healthy lifestyles, rather than use reactive parenting. This approach includes making known family expectations regarding eating, physical activity, and screen use; creating a healthy home environment; role modeling healthy eating and activity; engaging the child to help with healthy food selection and preparation (eg, vegetables); allowing the child choice from healthy food options and activities; and actively playing with the child. Such parenting practices help support children in healthy lifestyle behaviors, but often take planning in advance. Parenting practices that are coercive or overly controlling, such as threatening to take away privileges, bribing the child, or using psychological threats or punishment, are reactive and should be discouraged. Instead, physicians should help families provide autonomy and support for the child to learn healthy lifestyle behaviors over time.

## MANAGEMENT OF OBESITY IN YOUTH

#### Weight Management in Primary Care

To prevent long-term consequences of childhood obesity, aggressive intervention is needed early in childhood. Obesity interventions at an early age appear to be more effective than in adolescence. In growing children, relatively small weight losses or even weight maintenance can bring an obese child to a healthy weight range. Several strategies can be employed. Randomized controlled trials and meta-analyses have demonstrated the superiority of multicomponent behavioral interventions (including nutrition counseling, physical activity counseling, and behavioral management techniques) over education only or usual care for treating childhood obesity. The US Preventive Services Task Force (USPSTF) has reported the greatest evidence exists for programs that can provide 26 to 75 hours of therapy over at least 6 months. This intervention often requires referral to a community-based program or tertiary care treatment center, which may not be possible for all children or in all regions, due to lack of access or availability of such programs. Becoming familiar with the programs in your area is important to best help the families under your care. Importantly, family-based interventions demonstrate greater effectiveness than those focusing on the child alone.

The key nutritional and physical activity targets remain the same for weight management as those listed above for obesity prevention. However, some children and adolescents will require a more restrictive diet or structured exercise program. In such cases, it is advised to work with a registered dietitian or physical therapist to ensure the child still obtains adequate nutrients and/or appropriate exercises for healthy development. Several behavioral management techniques, such as motivational interviewing or strategies from social cognitive theory can be employed to help families. Examples of helpful strategies include goal setting, implementation plans, behavior monitoring, and changing the environment. Addressing 1 or 2 behavioral goals at a time with frequent follow-up is important to help keep the child and family motivated and accountable, address any problems that arise, and help them move toward additional behavior changes. Regardless of the behavioral management approach used, it is imperative for the clinician to be empathetic and nonjudgmental during the discussions and to consider the cultural differences in children's and families' behaviors when treating a child to improve his or her weight status. Using themed office visits, such as those through the Healthy Active Living for Families (American Association of Pediatrics; infant through preschool), is 1 way to systematically address the myriad of factors that need to be addressed in developing a healthy weight.

#### Who to Refer for Weight Management

Community and tertiary care weight management programs are available for children and adolescents in some areas of the United States. Deciding who may benefit from a referral to such programs can be difficult. It is best to refer only to programs that are evidence-based and have the expertise and training for weight management among children and adolescents. In referring patients, their motivation to engage in a program should be carefully considered. Youth with comorbidities may require referral to both weight management and subspecialty clinics to help manage the comorbidity.

Immersion treatment is an intensive therapy program designed to remove the child from the obesogenic environment into a therapeutic environment that reinforces healthy weight loss behaviors and includes a restricted diet and at least 6 days per week of physical activity. The most effective programs include a cognitive behavioral therapy component. In a recent meta-analysis of 22 studies of immersion programs, participants decreased their percent overweight by 23.9% during treatment and by 20.6% at follow-up. In comparison, outpatient programs targeting lifestyle changes resulted in 8.2% reductions in percent overweight during treatment and 8.9% at follow-up. For severely obese youth, prolonged inpatient programs are successful in the short term, but long-term weight maintenance has not been demonstrated.

#### Pharmacotherapy

Given the difficulty of achieving adequate, sustained weight management with lifestyle intervention methods, safe and effective pharmacotherapeutic agents are desirable, particularly in severely obese youth. Currently, such agents are not available. Two medications (orlistat, sibutramine) have been tested in randomized control trials. Orlistat is a gastrointestinal lipase inhibitor, and sibutramine is a serotonin and norepinephrine reuptake inhibitor. Combined with behavioral interventions, these 2 drugs resulted in small to moderate short-term weight loss in obese adolescents (BMI reduction of 2.6 kg/m$^2$ more for sibutramine, 0.85 kg/m$^2$ more for orlistat compared to placebo). Potential side effects include increase in heart rate and blood pressure with sibutramine and gastrointestinal side effects with orlistat that can be prohibitive for continued use. There have also been reports of liver injury, cholelithiasis, and pancreatitis with orlistat. Data on weight maintenance after interruption of therapy are not available. Only orlistat is FDA (US Food and Drug Administration) approved for use in children and adolescents 12 years and older. Sibutramine was voluntarily withdrawn in 2010 because of an association with increased incidence of cardiovascular events among adults at high risk for cardiovascular disease. Metformin, an insulin sensitizer, is approved for the treatment of type 2 diabetes in children 10 years of age and older. It can result in modest weight loss among children with type 2 diabetes. Glucagon-like peptide-1 receptor analogs are approved by the FDA for the treatment of both obesity and type 2 diabetes in adults. One such agent showed modest efficacy in 2 small trials of extremely obese youth. In adults, lorcaserin (a selective 5-HT2C receptor agonist; increases satiety) and combination therapies of agents such as phentermine/topiramate or bupropion/naltrexone appear to be useful adjuncts to lifestyle therapy in the treatment of obesity, with variable efficacy and safety profiles. Pharmacotherapy may need to be considered in patients with weight-related complications that can be ameliorated by weight loss. However, to use pharmacotherapy in pediatrics, randomized controlled studies in children are urgently needed to assess efficacy, tolerability, adverse events, and long-term safety profiles of agents currently approved for treatment of adult obesity.

#### Bariatric Surgery

Bariatric surgery is a consideration in the setting of severe obesity in adolescents, particularly if associated with comorbidities. However, experts recommend that adolescents should be considered for bariatric surgery only if they are severely obese (BMI $\geq$ 40 kg/m$^2$) and have serious medical comorbidities associated with their obesity, have reached Tanner stage of 4 or greater to ensure skeletal maturity, have a demonstrated commitment to lifestyle change, have failed at least 6 months of a structured weight loss program, and have a stable psychosocial environment. It may also be appropriate with BMI $\geq$ 35 kg/m$^2$ if associated with severe comorbidities such as type 2 diabetes mellitus, moderate to severe sleep apnea, or pseudotumor cerebri. These factors are best assessed in a pediatric tertiary care center in the context of a multidisciplinary program.

Different surgical modalities, including restrictive or malabsorptive procedures, or a combination, can be employed. They include the Roux-en-Y gastric bypass (RYGB), biliopancreatic diversion, adjustable gastric banding (AGB), and the vertical sleeve gastrectomy (VSG). Bariatric surgery can lead to massive reductions in body weight, BMI, and fat mass, with reports of 50% to 60% of excess weight loss in the first year, with absolute BMI reduction of about 30%. This reduction is associated with marked improvement or resolution of obesity-related comorbidities and improvement in mental health and quality of life. Significant beneficial metabolic changes include changes in hormones that regulate glucose homeostasis (insulin, incretin hormones), energy homeostasis (leptin, adiponectin, thyroid), and satiety and hunger (incretins, PYY, and ghrelin). Side effects include potential serious surgical complications, including pneumonia, deep venous thrombosis, pulmonary embolus, gastrointestinal hemorrhage, anastomotic obstruction, wound infections, risk for cholelithiasis, and even death. Postoperatively, nutritional status should be closely monitored and supplementation provided to avoid macronutrient (mostly protein) and micronutrient (fat-soluble vitamins, iron, and calcium) deficiencies, which are particularly concerning in the growing adolescent. Bariatric surgery and continued management of adolescents should be done only by a multidisciplinary team with pediatric expertise.

### SUMMARY

Obesity remains a common pediatric medical condition that most clinicians will have to address among their patients due to the impact that obesity has on many disease processes and conditions. In pediatric primary care, overweight and obesity should be screened for and, depending on the weight status of the child, either obesity prevention or weight management should be addressed during well-child and/or follow-up visits. Clinicians should help advocate for children both in their clinical practice and in their community for healthy eating and physical activity behaviors, along with health-promoting environments for children.

### SUGGESTED READINGS

AAP Council of School Health, Committee on Nutrition. Snacks, sweetened beverages, added sugars, and schools. *Pediatrics.* 2015;135(3):D1-D4.

ADA Position Statement. Standards of medical care in diabetes—2016. *Diabetes Care.* 2016;39(supp 1):S86-S93.

Barlow SE. Expert Committee recommendations regarding the prevention, assessment, and treatment of child and adolescent overweight and obesity: summary report. *Pediatrics.* 2007;120(Suppl 4): S164-S192.

Daniels SR. Hassink, SG; Committee on Nutrition. The role of the pediatrician in primary prevention of obesity. *Pediatrics.* 2015;136(1):e275-e292.

Danielsson P, Kowalski J, Ekblom Ö, Marcus C. Response of severely obese children and adolescents to behavioral treatment. *Arch Pediatr Adolesc Med.* 2012;166(12):1103-1108.

Goldschmidt AB, Wilfley DE, Paluch RA, Roemmich JN, Epstein JH. Indicated prevention of adult obesity: how much weight change is necessary for normalization of weight status in children? *JAMA Pediatr.* 2013;167(1):21-26

Inge T, Courcoulas AP, Jenkins TM. et al; Teen-LABS Consortium. Weight loss and health status 3 years after bariatric surgery in adolescents. *N Engl J Med.* 2016;374(2):113-23.

National Heart, Lung, and Blood Institute. Expert Panel on integrated guidelines for cardiovascular health and risk reduction in children and adolescents: summary report. *Pediatrics.* 2011;128(Suppl 5): S213-S256.

Ogden CL, Carroll MD, Kit BK, Flegal K. Prevalence of childhood and adult obesity in the United States, 2011–2012. *JAMA.* 2014;311(8):806-814.

Ogden CL, Carroll MD, Lawman HG, et al. Trends in obesity prevalence among children and adolescents in the United States, 1988–1994 through 2013–2014. *JAMA.* 2016;315(21):2292-2299.

Sherafat-Kazemzadeh R, Yanovski S, Yanovski J. Pharmacotherapy for childhood obesity: present and future prospects. *Int J Obes (Lond).* 2013;37(1):1-15.

US Preventive Services Task Force; Barton M. Screening for obesity in children and adolescents: US Preventive Services Task Force recommendation statement. *Pediatrics.* 2010;125(2):361-367.

Whitlock EP, O'Connor EA, Williams SB, Beil TL, Lutz KW. Effectiveness of weight management interventions in children: a targeted systematic review for the USPSTF. *Pediatrics.* 2010;125(2):e396-e418.



# 25 Specialized Nutrition Support

Kristi King and Robert J. Shulman

## GENERAL PRINCIPLES

Specialized nutrition support is required to provide either total or partial nutrient supplementation for patients with general undernutrition or other specific nutritional deficiencies. Nutrition support can be provided enterally, intravenously (parenteral nutrition), or by a combination of both routes.

The decision to provide specialized nutrition support starts with nutrition screening to identify patients who are malnourished, or those with risk factors that place the patient at risk for nutrition-related problems. The nutrition screen may determine the need for a more careful nutrition assessment. The assessment should consist of a detailed history, physical examination (including anthropometric measurements), and biochemical parameters in order to assess the presence of malnutrition as discussed in Chapter 20. Thus, the assessment should lead to nutrition risk stratification and specific nutrition therapy recommendations, including energy, protein, and micronutrient requirements; route of administration; and treatment goals and monitoring parameters.

The goal of appropriate nutrition therapy is to improve the outcome of a patient's primary illness, although data supporting this goal are typically lacking. An individual's requirements for nutrients are initially estimated and cannot be accurately predicted. Therefore, careful evaluation of nutritional status, including evaluation of growth and developmental parameters, diet history, physical examination, anthropometric measurements, and laboratory determinations, is required at regular intervals in all patients receiving specialized nutritional support. Teams that provide pediatric nutrition support services typically include physicians, nurse specialists, dietitians, pharmacologists, social workers, and feeding therapists. Such teams are now available at major medical centers to provide guidance and to monitor nutrition support for pediatric patients.

## ENTERAL SUPPLEMENTATION

Enteral alimentation provides nutrition via a functioning gastrointestinal tract. It is preferable to intravenous feeding because it is significantly less costly and is associated with far fewer and less serious complications. Nevertheless, proper caution must be exercised to avoid deleterious effects from enteral feeding.

Nutrients can be introduced into the gastrointestinal tract orally or by orogastric, nasogastric, nasoduodenal, esophagostomy, gastrostomy, jejunostomy, or gastrojejunostomy feeding tubes. The route selected depends on patient tolerance and the underlying medical condition necessitating nutritional support. The orogastric route, most commonly employed in preterm infants with immature suck and swallow mechanisms, is useful to provide access for bolus feedings directly into the stomach. In older infants and children, nasogastric intubation permits more prolonged feedings because the tube can be secured and left in position for up to several weeks. Gastrostomy feedings are implemented when the oral and nasal routes cannot be used, when patients have severe neuromuscular problems with dysphagia, or if enteral tube feeding is warranted for more than 2 to 3 months. Nasoduodenal or jejunostomy tubes are used in patients who may have abnormal gastric emptying or gastroesophageal reflux and aspiration. Additionally, with specially designed tubes and the assistance of a gastroenterologist or radiologist, a gastrostomy tube can be converted into a gastrojejunostomy tube. Potential indications and contraindications for tube feedings are listed in Table 25-1. Tube choice and route selection are 2 of the most important components in the delivery of enteral nutrition (see Chapter 26).

Once a decision is made to start a patient on tube feedings, careful consideration must be taken to select the proper formula. The strength, rate of infusion, and route of administration should be determined and an appropriate feeding tube selected. An appropriate formula must be carefully chosen with the patient's age, underlying disease process, and gastrointestinal function all in mind. Commonly available formulas in the United States for use in infants are listed in Table 17-1, and those for toddlers and older children are listed in Table 25-2. Human breast milk or special formulas for premature infants can be administered either by bolus or continuous infusion.

Lactose-free, low-residue, isotonic formulas may be useful in patients with chronic diarrhea. If these are not tolerated, or a patient has deficient digestive and absorptive function, a semi-elemental (ie, chemically defined) formula that is specifically designed to meet the nutritional needs of infants (eg, Pregestimil [Mead Johnson], Nutramigen [Mead Johnson], or Alimentum [Abbott Nutrition]] or older children (eg, Peptamen [Nestlé Nutrition] or PediaSure Peptide Abbott Nutrition]) can be instituted. Under certain circumstances, such as in patients with severe malabsorption or exquisite protein intolerance, elemental formulas may be required. Most elemental formulas provide protein as free amino acids, adequate long-chain fatty acids to meet essential fatty acid requirements, glucose and glucose polymers, minerals, vitamins, and trace elements. Neocate (Nutricia), EleCare (Abbott Nutrition), and Alfamino (Nestlé Nutrition) are designed to meet the nutritional needs of infants. For toddlers and older children, EleCare Jr (Abbott Nutrition), Neocate Junior (Nutricia), E028 Splash (Nutricia), and Alfamino Junior (Nestlé Nutrition) are elemental formulas that can be used to meet their specific nutritional requirements. In the event that formulas are used that have been formulated to meet adult requirements, such as Tolerex or Vivonex Plus (Nestlé Nutrition), an assessment of nutrient needs should be completed to ensure no additional vitamin or mineral supplements are needed.

Modular solutions that are nutritionally complete offer the opportunity to cater the regimen to meet specific needs. As examples, fat (Microlipid [Nestlé Nutrition]), protein (Beneprotein [Nestlé Nutrition]), and carbohydrate (SolCarb [Solace Nutrition]) can be added to a formula to modify its composition and meet the specific needs of selected patients. Considerations in choosing an enteral formula include the underlying diagnosis; nutritional status; gastrointestinal function; formula osmolality; protein source and quantity; lipid content and composition; mineral, vitamin, and trace element content; feeding route; fiber content; and cost.

Enteral feedings should be initiated slowly in patients with significant gastrointestinal dysfunction. Because hypotonic and hypertonic solutions may adversely affect gastric emptying and using a dilute formula plus any additional parenteral alimentation may compromise

| TABLE 25-1 INDICATIONS AND CONTRAINDICATIONS FOR ENTERAL TUBE FEEDING |
|---|
| **Potential Indications** |
| Inadequate intake |
| Inability to coordinate swallowing |
| Prematurity |
| Oropharyngeal disease |
| Craniofacial trauma, especially fractured jaw |
| Esophageal disorders, especially obstructive |
| Central nervous system disorders |
| Coma |
| Severe cerebral palsy |
| Cerebral trauma |
| Encephalopathy |
| Degenerative neurologic disorders |
| Myopathies |
| Anorexia |
| Psychiatric disorders |
| Anorexia nervosa |
| Severe depression |
| Inflammatory disorders (eg, collagen vascular disease, AIDS) |
| Surgery |
| Neoplasms |
| Significant failure to thrive |
| Transition from parenteral to enteral nutrition |
| Inflammatory bowel disease |
| Inherited metabolic disorders (eg, glycogen storage disease) |
| Gastrointestinal disease |
| Crohn disease |
| Short bowel syndrome |
| Chronic diarrhea with malabsorption |
| Severe gastroesophageal reflux[a] |
| Pancreatitis |
| Distal small intestinal fistulas |
| Cystic fibrosis |
| Trauma |
| Sepsis |
| Burns |
| Severe cardiac anomalies |
| Severe respiratory failure |
| **Potential Contraindications** |
| Intestinal obstruction |
| Persistent emesis |
| Severe respiratory distress |
| Prolonged upper gastrointestinal bleeding |
| Necrotizing enterocolitis |
| Intestinal ischemia |

[a]Placement of a tube distal to the pylorus may be preferable.

fluid status, a full-strength isotonic formula can be started at a slow, continuous rate (1–2 mL/kg/h). As the infusion rate is increased, the parenteral infusion rate can be decreased, keeping in mind that parenteral solutions usually are more energy dense than formulas. Tolerance is continuously assessed by monitoring clinical changes, such as abdominal distension, intake and output (including diarrhea and vomiting), and stool reducing substances and pH.

Monitoring patients who receive enteral nutrition is important to ensure the patient is free from complications and that the nutrition regimen is meeting the patient's nutrition goals. Common complications include aspiration, diarrhea, nausea, vomiting, dehydration, abdominal distention, abdominal cramps, constipation, bacterial contamination of the formula or the upper intestinal tract, nasal or skin ulcers, obstruction or infection of nasal passages, and electrolyte or mineral imbalances. Severe complications such as perforation of the posterior pharynx, esophagus, or cribriform fossa (resulting in intracranial placement of the feeding tube) are rare and generally avoidable by use of proper precautions and techniques. Additionally, complications can be avoided by reinforcing to healthcare providers and families proper preparation and administration of nutrients as well as assessing metabolic imbalances before they become clinically evident.





## PARENTERAL NUTRITION

Parenteral nutrition support should be used for patients who are unable to maintain adequate nutrition status orally or by tube feedings via the gastrointestinal tract. Supplemental parenteral nutrition is useful when the intestinal tract can assimilate some but not all of the nutrients necessary for normal maintenance and growth. Enteral nutrients stimulate gut hormones and other secretions that may be trophic factors to the intestinal tract and thus may be beneficial where gut regeneration is necessary. Because prolonged use of parenteral nutrition is associated with significant complications as well as expense, careful selection of patients and judicious use of available enteral and parenteral solutions are particularly important.

As in enteral support, patient selection begins with nutrition assessment. This process includes determining the gastrointestinal tract's ability to absorb sufficient nutrients; if it cannot, then parenteral nutrition may be required. Potential indications for parenteral nutrition support are listed in Table 25-3. This list is not meant to be definitive or exhaustive; rather, it provides examples of conditions for which parenteral nutrition has been used with some success. Improved technology, newer formulations, and a better understanding of safe approaches to enteral nutritional support have allowed the replacement of total parenteral nutrition with either complete or partial enteral support for many of the disorders listed. Each patient should be evaluated individually regarding needs and possible benefits and risks of parenteral versus enteral therapy.

Parenteral nutrition may be infused via peripheral veins in patients with good venous access who require short-term (ie, < 2 weeks) support and no fluid restriction. The maximum recommended concentration through a peripheral vein is 12.5% dextrose; this reduces the risk of thrombophlebitis, which occurs when the osmolality of the solution exceeds 900 mOsm/kg. Patients in whom caloric needs cannot be met by the peripheral venous route, or those who may require parenteral nutrition for > 2 weeks' duration will require a central venous catheter. The dextrose concentration then can be raised to 20% to 30% (ie, 2000–3000 mOsm/kg) or greater when infused through a central line placed appropriately, usually by an experienced pediatric surgeon or pediatric interventional radiologist. Percutaneous intravenous central catheters (PICC lines) also are utilized for medium duration venous access including parenteral nutrition.

After placement of a central line, the physician must always document the correct location of the catheter tip by radiography before initiating the parenteral nutrition infusion. The catheter tip should be located just proximal to the junction of the superior vena cava and right atrium. Infusion of the solution through an improperly placed catheter can be dangerous. Complications associated with catheter insertion include pneumothorax, hemothorax, hydrothorax, arterial puncture, myocardial perforation, catheter embolism, air embolism, cardiac arrhythmias, cardiac tamponade, and thrombosis of the jugular or vertebral vein, and catheter malposition can result in placement in the central nervous system.

## PARENTERAL NUTRITION SOLUTIONS

The goal of parenteral nutrition is to provide the necessary fluid and nutrients, either alone or in combination with enteral nutrition, for maintenance or replenishment of normal nutrition status. In children, "normal" nutrition support includes nutrients for growth. Calculations therefore must be made to infuse adequate fluid, energy, fat, protein, electrolytes, minerals, vitamins, and trace elements to meet each patient's requirements. Estimates of nutrient needs are based on oral intakes, balance studies, and accepted standards. Fluid and

**TABLE 25-2 ENTERAL FEEDING PRODUCTS AVAILABLE IN THE UNITED STATES[a]**

| Formula | Manufacturer | kcal/oz | Prot. g/L | mOsm/kg | Protein Source | Carbohydrate Source | Fat Source | Comments |
|---|---|---|---|---|---|---|---|---|
| ***Formulas for Children (1–10 years old)[a]*** | | | | | | | | |
| Compleat Pediatric | Nestlé Nutrition | 30 | 38 | 380 | Chicken<br>Sodium caseinate | Vegetable<br>Fruit<br>Corn syrup | MCT oil<br>Vegetable oil | Unflavored<br>Commercial blenderized formula<br>Contains fiber from fruit and vegetable sources (4.4 g/L) |
| Nutren Junior (also with fiber) | Nestlé Nutrition | 30 | 30 | 350 | Milk protein concentrate<br>Whey protein concentrate | Maltodextrin<br>Sugar | Soybean oil<br>MCT oil<br>Canola oil | Vanilla flavored<br>Also available with fiber (6 g/L) |
| PediaSure Enteral (also with fiber) | Abbott Nutrition | 30 | 30 | 335<br>350 (w/fiber) | Milk protein concentrate | Corn maltodextrin<br>Sugar | MCT oil<br>High-oleic safflower oil<br>Soy oil | Available in vanilla, strawberry, banana, chocolate, and vanilla flavors<br>Also available with fiber (5 g/L) |
| Boost Kid Essentials (vanilla) | Nestlé Nutrition | 30 | 29 | 550–600 | Sodium and calcium caseinate<br>Whey protein concentrate | Sucrose<br>Maltodextrin | High-oleic sunflower oil<br>Soybean oil<br>MCT oil | Available in vanilla, chocolate, and strawberry |
| **Special Formulas for Children (1–10 years old)** | | | | | | | | |
| EleCare Jr (powder) | Abbott Nutrition | 30 | 31 | 590 | Free amino acids | Corn syrup solids | High-oleic safflower oil<br>MCT oil<br>Soy oil | Also available in vanilla<br>Hypoallergenic |
| Neocate Junior (powder) | Nutricia | 30 | 33 | 550–650 | Free amino acids | Corn syrup solids | Refined vegetable oil | Available in unflavored, vanilla, strawberry, chocolate<br>Hypoallergenic |
| Peptamen Junior<br>Unflavored | Nestlé Nutrition | 30 | 30 | 260 | Hydrolyzed whey | Maltodextrin<br>Sugar<br>Corn starch | MCT oil<br>Canola oil<br>Soy oil | Also available in vanilla, chocolate, strawberry<br>Note flavor does increase mOsm (365–400) |
| PediaSure Peptide<br>Unflavored | Abbott Nutrition | 30 | 30 | 250 | Hydrolyzed whey and caseinate | Corn maltodextrin<br>scFOS | Structured lipid | Available in vanilla and strawberry<br>Note flavors increase to 390 mOsm |
| Vivonex Pediatric (unflavored) | Nestlé Nutrition | 24 | 24 | 360 | Free amino acids | Maltodextrin<br>Modified corn starch | MCT oil<br>Soy oil | Available as a powder<br>Low in fat |
| Tolerex | Novartis | 30 | 21 | 550 | Free amino acids | Corn maltodextrin<br>Modified corn starch | Safflower oil | Available as a powder<br>1% of kcal as fat<br>Calcium, phosphorus, and vitamin D inadequate for children |
| **Other Milks[b,c]** | | | | | | | | |
| Evaporated whole milk | Assorted | 42 | 70.7 | N/A | Casein<br>Whey | Lactose | Butterfat | Inadequate vitamin A and D unless fortified; inadequate vitamin C, iron, zinc, and essential fatty acids |
| Goat's milk | Assorted | 30 | 36 | N/A | Casein<br>Whey | Lactose | Butterfat | Inadequate vitamin D, $B_6$, folate, iron, and essential fatty acids |

***Adult Formulas and Supplements***

| Formula | Manufacturer | Contents | Comments |
|---|---|---|---|
| **Whole-Protein Supplements** | | | |
| Carnation Instant Breakfast (powder) | Nestlé Nutrition | Casein, egg white, whey, lactose, sucrose | Nutritionally incomplete |
| Compleat-B | Nestlé Nutrition | Meat- and nonfat-milk-based blenderized tube feeding | |
| Ensure | Abbott Nutrition | Lactose-free, casein, and soy proteins; 1 kcal/mL; flavored for oral use | |
| Boost | Nestlé Nutrition | Lactose-free, casein and soy proteins; 1 kcal/mL; flavored for oral use | |

(Continued)

**TABLE 25-2 ENTERAL FEEDING PRODUCTS AVAILABLE IN THE UNITED STATES[a] (CONTINUED)**

| | | |
|---|---|---|
| **High-calorie or Protein-Dense Supplements** | | |
| Ensure Plus | Abbott Nutrition | Lactose-free, casein and soy proteins; 1.5 kcal/mL; flavored for oral use |
| Isosource HN | Nestlé Nutrition | High-nitrogen feeding for volume-restricted patients |
| Nutren 2.0 | Nestlé Nutrition | Lactose-free, casein; 2.0 kcal/mL; flavored for oral use |
| Promote | Abbott Nutrition | Lactose-free, high-protein (casein and soy) tube feeding |
| Scandishake | Scandipharm | Nonfat milk, high-calorie oral feeding supplement (2 kcal/mL) |
| TwoCal HN | Abbott Nutrition | High-calorie and nitrogen (casein) for volume-restricted patients |
| **Elemental or Protein Hydrolysate** | | |
| Peptamen | Nestlé Nutrition | Whey hydrolysate, 70% MCT |
| Vital HN | Abbott Nutrition | Partially hydrolyzed whey, meat, and soy, with low fat |
| Vivonex TEN | Nestlé Nutrition | Free amino acids, higher nitrogen, minimal fat |
| **Specialized Formulas** | | |
| Glucerna | Abbott Nutrition | High-fiber, low-carbohydrate, high-fat |
| Glytrol | Nestlé Nutrition | Higher fiber, support glycemic control |
| Impact | Nestlé Nutrition | Increased RNA, arginine |
| Pulmocare | Abbott Nutrition | Lactose-free, high-fat, low-carbohydrate formula |
| Suplena | Abbott Nutrition | High-calorie (1.8 kcal/mL), low-protein, low renal solute load |

**Modular Additives**

| Formula | Manufacturer | kcal | Fat Source | Protein Source | Carbohydrate Source |
|---|---|---|---|---|---|
| Benefiber | Novartis | 22 per tbsp | — | — | Wheat dextrin |
| Beneprotein | Nestlé Nutrition | 17 per tbsp | Soy lecithin | Whey | — |
| MCT Oil | Nestlé Nutrition | 7.7 per mL | Coconut and/or palm | — | — |
| Microlipid | Nestlé Nutrition | 4.5 per mL | Safflower | — | — |
| Duocal | Nutricia | 40 per tbsp | Corn, coconut, palm | — | Hydrolyzed corn starch |
| SolCarb | Solace Nutrition | 23 per tbsp | — | — | Maltodextrin |

[a]All of these formulas are ready-to-feed.

[b]Not recommended for infants because of increased renal solute load and poorly digestible fat.

[c]Increased risk of contamination and improper dilution.

COPD, chronic obstructive pulmonary diseases; MCT, medium-chain triglyceride; scFOS, short-chain fructooligosaccharides.

**TABLE 25-3 CLINICAL SITUATIONS THAT MAY BENEFIT FROM PARENTERAL NUTRITION SUPPORT**

**Medical**

- Prematurity/low birth weight
- Inflammatory bowel disease
- Sepsis with ileus
- Severe malabsorption syndromes
- Severe respiratory distress (cystic fibrosis, ECMO)
- Short-bowel syndrome
- Necrotizing enterocolitis
- Malignancies
  - Radiation therapy
  - Chemotherapy-induced gastrointestinal injury
- Bone marrow transplantation
- Pseudoobstruction syndrome

**Surgical**

- Major trauma
- Severe burns
- Preoperative and postoperative support
- Gastroschisis/omphalocele
- Enterocutaneous fistula

ECMO, extracorporeal-membrane oxygenation.

energy requirements are calculated for weight and age. Specific considerations for each component utilized in parenteral solutions are discussed in the following sections.

### Glucose

Glucose, in the form of dextrose monohydrate, provides 3.4 kcal/g of dextrose and can be infused safely through a central line in concentrations up to 35 g/dL or a 35% dextrose solution. The usual starting dose of dextrose to maintain a normal blood glucose concentration is 5 mg/kg/min. The dose can be increased as tolerated to 10 to 15 mg/kg/min under normal circumstances; tolerance is judged by the absence of glycosuria and hyperglycemia. As noted earlier, the maximum recommended dextrose concentration administered via a peripheral vein is 12.5%. Premature infants often are unable to metabolize glucose at even relatively low doses and may require lower amounts and slower increases of dextrose infusions. If glucose intolerance appears in a previously stable patient, infection and sepsis must be considered; insulin may be required in selected patients to control glucose intolerance. The initial dose of insulin (usually 0.5–1.0 unit per 10 g of dextrose in solution) may be difficult to predict accurately because the insulin binds variably to the bottle and tubing. The goal should be to have no glucose or only trace amounts in the urine, although the serum glucose concentrations may still be as high as 150 mg/dL. It may be beneficial to avoid prolonged hyperglycemia in critically ill children, but this needs to be balanced with the avoidance of hypoglycemia.

Parenteral nutrient infusions containing a large concentration of dextrose cannot be discontinued abruptly unless another source of glucose (enteral or intravenous) is assured. High plasma insulin levels persist for 15 to 30 minutes after cessation of the glucose infusion and can lead to hypoglycemia. Problems with hypoglycemia on cessation of parenteral glucose infusions are routinely prevented by gradual tapering of the infusion rate.

#### Lipid

Lipid emulsions in a 10% solution (1.1 kcal/mL; generally not recommended because of the high concentration of phospholipids predisposing to hyperlipidemia) or a 20% solution (2 kcal/mL) are composed of triglycerides stabilized with egg phospholipids and are isotonically balanced with glycerol. They provide a concentrated calorie source with relatively low osmolality. At least 0.25 g/kg/d of linoleic acid should be given to preterm infants (0.1 g/kg/d to older infants and children) to prevent essential fatty acid deficiency. The maximum recommended amount of intravenous lipid administered daily is 2.5 to 3.0 g/kg/d in adults and up to 4 g/kg/d in neonates, infants, and children. Usually, 25% to 40% of the infused calories are provided by lipids. Tolerance should be assessed by occasionally monitoring serum triglyceride concentration 4 hours after initiating the lipid infusion or with changes in the infusion rate. If the serum triglyceride level is greater than 250 mg/dL in infants and 400 mg/dL in older children, the lipid infusion rate should be reduced. Side effects of lipid emulsion include allergic reactions (particularly in persons allergic to eggs), metallic taste, hepatomegaly, splenomegaly, transiently elevated serum transaminase (alanine aminotransferase, aspartate aminotransferase) concentrations, and hyperlipidemia. The fat overload syndrome, which is characterized by jaundice, fever, leukocytosis, bleeding secondary to a coagulopathy, focal seizures, and possibly shock, occurs with extreme hyperlipidemia and has been reported in infants receiving lipid dosages of 4 g/kg/d or greater. Stable infants on a lipid infusion regimen may develop the fat overload syndrome consequent to an acquired viral or bacterial infection. Recently, it has been suggested that the lipid dose be limited to 1 g/kg/d to decrease the risk of developing parenteral nutrition–associated cholestasis and to treat parenteral nutrition–associated cholestasis. Evidence suggests that this strategy is effective although concern has been raised regarding the potential for an associated increased risk of essential fatty acid deficiency.

Newer lipid solutions composed of fish oils (Omegaven [Fresenius Kabi]), which contain omega-3 fatty acids, may reduce inflammatory responses (such as tumor necrosis factor-α) to a variety of stimuli compared to traditional vegetable oil–based lipid emulsions. These solutions are not available for general use in the United States where they are currently under investigation. In Europe, fish oil–derived lipid emulsion for intravenous administration is available commercially. In some clinical scenarios, these lipid emulsions may reduce morbidity and mortality. Promising data suggest that they may be particularly beneficial for reversal or prevention of parenteral nutrition–associated liver disease in infants and children. Recently, SMOF lipid (soy oil, medium chain triglycerides, olive oil, and fish oil) has been approved for use in adults in the United States. However, experience with these emulsions in children is limited.

#### Protein (as Amino Acids)

Protein requirements are estimated from studies of fetal nitrogen accumulation (mean nitrogen retention of 320 mg/kg/d or of 2 g/kg/d protein) or by analysis of breastfed infant data. Current guidelines suggest giving premature and term infants a minimum of 1.5 g/kg/d of protein to prevent a negative nitrogen balance, with a maximum of 4 g/kg/day in preterm infants and 3.5 g/kg/day in term infants. Increasing the nonprotein calories above a minimum of 50 to 60 kcal/kg/d appears to enhance the efficiency of protein accretion in a growing infant. The amount of protein necessary to attain positive nitrogen balance declines with age, so by adulthood, the amount of protein required is 0.6 to 0.8 g/kg/d.

Most currently available amino acid solutions are not made specifically for infants and children. Formulations such as TrophAmine (B. Braun Medical) and Aminosyn PF (Abbott Laboratories) yield a plasma amino acid pattern resembling that seen in breastfed infants. Addition of cysteine and other amino acids that may be essential for neonates is being considered, although evidence to support their routine use is not conclusive. Addition of cysteine is useful to lower the pH of the parenteral nutrition solution and thereby enhance the solubility of calcium and phosphorus.

**TABLE 25-4 RECOMMENDED ELECTROLYTE AND MINERAL REQUIREMENTS[a]**

| Nutrient | Infant and Child mEq/kg | Adolescent (mEq/kg) |
|---|---|---|
| Sodium | 2–4 | 1–2 |
| Potassium | 2–4 | 1–2 |
| Calcium | 0.5–4 | 10–20/day |
| Magnesium | 0.3–0.5 | 10–30/day |
| Phosphorous (mmol) | 0.5–2 | 10–40/day |
| Chloride | To balance, adjust as indicated | To balance, adjust as indicated |
| Acetate | To balance, adjust as indicated | To balance, adjust as indicated |

[a]A pharmacist should be consulted to determine solution compatibility to avoid calcium phosphate precipitation. To meet recommendations for premature infants, a solution containing calcium (50–60 mg/dL), magnesium (5–7 mg/dL), and phosphate (40–45 mg/dL) should be used; this solution is applicable for central parenteral infusions where the fluid intake is 120 to 150 mL/kg/d and includes 2.5 g of amino acids per deciliter.

Data from Mirtallo J, Canada T, Johnson D, et al; Task Force for the Revision of Safe Practices for Parenteral Nutrition. Safe practices for parenteral nutrition. *JPEN J Parenter Enteral Nutr.* 2004 Nov-Dec;28(6):S39-S70.

#### Electrolytes and Minerals

Electrolyte and mineral requirements can be met by using the guidelines listed in Table 25-4 and adjusting them as indicated for losses from vomiting, diarrhea, and also from nasogastric suction, gastrostomy, ileostomy, colostomy, or fistula outputs. Potassium, magnesium, and particularly phosphorus should be monitored especially carefully when parenteral nutrition is given to a severely undernourished patient because as the patient becomes anabolic, there is a flux of these minerals into cells, resulting in what is known as refeeding syndrome—a preventable condition. Symptoms of hypophosphatemia, hypokalemia, and hypomagnesemia can be severe and life threatening in these patients (see Chapter 21). Acetate can be added to the parenteral nutrition in the form of sodium acetate or potassium acetate. The acetate is metabolized to bicarbonate and can be adjusted as desired to achieve acid–base equilibrium.

Precipitation of calcium phosphate in solution presents a problem in the supply of calcium and phosphorus to premature and term neonates, infants, and young children. Current solutions often do not contain adequate amounts to meet the patient's metabolic requirements for both minerals, so infants who are on long-term parenteral nutrition have a high prevalence of bone demineralization, rickets, and fractures. Studies suggest that the ratio of calcium to phosphorus should be approximately 1.3:1 to 1.7:1. A higher ratio of calcium to phosphorus can lead to precipitation in the parenteral nutrition bag. Ratios can be checked using the calcium phosphate solubility curves. High concentrations of calcium and phosphorus should not be infused by peripheral vein because of the risk of the potentially caustic solution infiltrating into the soft tissues. Oral supplementation may be beneficial for selected patients.

#### Vitamins and Trace Elements

All 13 vitamins are available in a single solution to meet the guidelines established for intravenous vitamin infusions (Table 25-5). The multivitamin preparation solution is available in a 5-mL vial. The dose for children weighing more than 3 kg is 5 mL/day. Additional vitamin D (25,000 IU intramuscularly per month) may be necessary to prevent rickets in infants receiving long-term total parenteral nutrition. In the past, extra water-soluble vitamins have been available as an additive for intravenous solutions, and these may be necessary for patients with excess losses, such as those undergoing hemodialysis or peritoneal dialysis.

**TABLE 25-5 GUIDELINES FOR VITAMINS IN PEDIATRIC PARENTERAL NUTRITION SOLUTION**

| Vitamin | RDD | MVI-Pediatric[a] | RDD/kg Premature Infants |
|---|---|---|---|
| A (mg)[b] | 0.7 | 0.7 | > 0.2 |
| D (µg)[b] | 10 | 10 | 4 |
| E (mg)[b] | 7 | 7 | 2.8 |
| $K_1$ (µg) | 200 | 200 | 100 |
| Ascorbic acid (mg) | 80 | 80 | 32 |
| Thiamine (mg) | 1.2 | 1.2 | 0.48 |
| Riboflavin (mg) | 1.4 | 1.4 | 0.15 |
| Niacin (mg) | 17 | 17 | 6.8 |
| Pyridoxine (mg) | 1 | 1 | 0.18 |
| Folic acid (mcg) | 140 | 140 | 56 |
| $B_{12}$ (µg) | 1.0 | 1 | 0.4 |
| Biotin (µg) | — | 20 | 8 |
| Pantothenic acid (mg) | — | 5 | 2 |
| Total recommended dose | — | 5 mL/d (1 vial) | 2.0 mL/kg (max 5.0 mL) |

[a]Multivitamin infusion for pediatrics (Hospira, Inc).

[b]Vitamin A: 1 µg = 1 retinol equivalent (RE) = 3.33 IU; vitamin D: 10 µg = 400 IU; vitamin E: 1 mg tocopherol = 1 IU.

RDD, recommended daily dose.

Several trace elements have been associated with documented deficiency states in humans. Four are routinely provided in parenteral nutrition solutions: (1) zinc, (2) copper, (3) chromium, and (4) manganese (Table 25-6). Normal excretion routes for trace elements must be considered in assessing a patient's requirements. Extra zinc may be needed in diarrheal or high ostomy output states. Conversely, manganese should be limited or totally withheld when cholestasis is present because it is excreted mainly in bile. Copper levels should be monitored frequently in the presence of cholestasis and titrated to maintain normal serum levels. Selenium supplementation also may be necessary for patients on prolonged (ie, > 6 weeks) total parenteral nutrition with no enteral intake, but excess selenium should be avoided because it also can cause significant toxicity. Selenium, chromium, and molybdenum should not be administered to patients with renal failure. Iron is provided enterally if possible or by intravenous bolus infusion of iron dextran or sucrose solutions as indicated. Intramuscular injections of iron should be avoided because of complications of pain, pigmented staining of skin, and difficulties in managing allergic reactions. The addition of iron to routine parenteral nutrition solutions is controversial because it may lead to sensitization and allergic reactions, and it is incompatible with lipid preparations. Additionally, prolonged intravenous iron administration may predispose patients to iron overload, gram-negative septicemia, or oxidant injury, especially in premature infants. Additional molybdenum and iodide may be useful to prevent deficiency states in patients receiving prolonged total parenteral nutrition, although adequate iodide appears to be provided by topical agents that are used routinely for catheter and wound care. Fluoride may be important in children with developing teeth who take no oral fluid containing fluoride, even though no data support this recommendation.

**TABLE 25-6 GUIDELINES FOR DAILY AMOUNT OF TRACE ELEMENTS IN PARENTERAL NUTRITION INFUSIONS[a]**

| Nutrient | Premature and Low-Birth-Weight Infants (µg/kg/d) | Infants and Children (µg/kg/d) | Adults |
|---|---|---|---|
| Copper | 20 | 20 | 0.3–0.5 mg/d |
| Zinc | 450–500 | 250 (< 3 mo)<br>50 (> 3 mo)<br>50 (child) | 2.5–5 mg/d |
| Chromium | 0.2 | 0.2 | 10–15 µg |
| Manganese | 1.0 | 1 | 0.6–1 mg/d |
| Selenium | 2–3 | 1–3 | 20–60 mg/d |
| Molybdenum | 1 | 0.25 | |
| Iodide[b] | 1 | 1 | |
| Iron[c] | | | |
| Fluoride[d] | | | |

[a]Trace elements usually are provided as Pediatric Multiple Trace Element Solution, which contains copper, 0.1 mg/mL; zinc, 0.5 mg/mL; chromium, 1 µg/mL; and manganese, 30 µg/mL. No selenium, molybdenum, iodide, iron, or fluoride is supplied in the commercially available trace element solution.

[b]Most patients appear to absorb adequate iodide through the skin from topical application.

[c]The safest approach for iron supplementation appears to be bolus infusion if oral intake is not possible.

[d]Fluoride supplementation may help dental development and have a role in bone mineral homeostasis, although no data currently support its routine use in intravenous solutions. Oral drops may be an effective alternative.

Data from Vanek VW, Borum P, Buchman A, et al. A.S.P.E.N. position paper: recommendations for changes in commercially available parenteral multivitamin and multi-trace element products. *Nutr Clin Pract.* 2012 Aug;27(4):440-491.

### Other Additives

A variety of medications can be added safely to parenteral nutrition regimens. The compatibility of each drug with a specific solution should be confirmed before it is added to the solution. Common additives include heparin, $H_2$-receptor antagonists (famotidine, ranitidine), additional albumin, and insulin. Antibiotics that are compatible with the solution can be infused in "piggyback" fashion so that the parenteral nutrient infusion does not have to be discontinued. Many pharmacologic agents precipitate in parenteral nutrient solutions and therefore cannot be infused into the same venous line as the total parenteral nutrition solution.

## CARE AND MONITORING

Careful clinical observation, laboratory assessment, and catheter care technique can prevent complications that are associated with parenteral nutrition regimens. A pediatric nutrition support team, including a parenteral nutrition nurse specialist designated specifically for catheter care, has been shown to improve outcome and minimize complication rates. Complications are divided into 3 main categories: (1) infectious, (2) metabolic, and (3) mechanical (Table 25-7). The most common and potentially serious complications are sepsis (1–5% of patients), usually with *Staphylococcus*, *Streptococcus*, gram-negative organisms, and *Candida* species; catheter thrombosis; and metabolic problems because of deficiencies (eg, refeeding syndrome), excesses, or imbalance of nutrients. This increased risk of sepsis requires that febrile patients with a central line be treated presumptively for infection.

Long-term parenteral nutrition may lead to hepatobiliary disorders, including cholestasis or fibrosis, and skeletal demineralization. Early initiation of enteral supplementation may help to prevent the development or progression of these problems. Use of a fish oil–based lipid emulsion may be beneficial in children with cholestasis on chronic total parenteral nutrition. Chronic use of loop diuretics and acid–base abnormalities especially predispose those infants receiving total parenteral nutrition to cholelithiasis and bone mineral loss. Increased experience with prolonged parenteral nutritional support may reveal other unrecognized nutrient deficiencies or parenteral nutrition–associated toxicities such as aluminum accumulation. Diminished renal function in patients on total parenteral nutrition for 4 years or longer also has been reported; further studies are pending to determine the significance of this observation. Another often overlooked problem with both enteral and parenteral nutritional support in infants and children is poor acquisition of oral feeding skills. Infants and toddlers acquire these skills at specific ages, so if the child has oral feeding entirely withheld, later acquisition of feeding skills is very challenging. Allowing a child to swallow even small amounts of water, breast milk, and/or formula several times a day or to eat and chew

**TABLE 25-7 COMPLICATIONS ASSOCIATED WITH PARENTERAL NUTRITION**

| |
|---|
| **Infectious** |
| Sepsis, bacteremia, fungemia |
| Catheter site infection |
| **Metabolic** |
| Fluid overload, dehydration |
| Hyperglycemia, hypoglycemia |
| Hypernatremia, hyponatremia |
| Hyperkalemia, hypokalemia |
| Hyperchloremia, hypochloremia |
| Hyperphosphatemia, hypophosphatemia |
| Hypercalcemia, hypocalcemia |
| Hypermagnesemia, hypomagnesemia |
| Vitamin or trace element deficiency |
| Essential fatty acid deficiency |
| Hyperlipidemia |
| Fat overload syndrome |
| Amino acid imbalance |
| Hyperammonemia |
| Acidosis |
| **Mechanical** |
| Venous thrombosis |
| Superior vena cava syndrome |
| Catheter occlusion because of Ca-P crystals |
| Embolism |
| Air embolism |
| Hydrocephalus |
| Extravasation of solution |
| Cardiac arrhythmia |
| Deep vein or myocardial perforation |
| Pneumothorax |
| Hydrothorax |
| Hemothorax |
| Catheter dislodgment |
| **Other** |
| Bone demineralization |
| Osteoporosis, rickets |
| Hepatobiliary dysfunction |
| Cholestasis, cholelithiasis |
| Hepatic abnormalities |
| Steatosis, fibrosis |
| Renal abnormalities (decreased GFR?) |
| Psychological (depression) |
| Feeding problems (aversion) |

GFR, glomerular filtration rate.

minimal amounts of food at developmentally appropriate times may either minimize or avoid problems with later acquisition of feeding skills.

Careful observation and reassessment are paramount to the successful implementation of parenteral nutrition regimens. Proper monitoring is necessary to detect or prevent complications and to assess the efficacy and appropriateness of the solution being infused. Clinical monitoring will determine whether mechanical or infectious problems are likely to occur. Biochemical abnormalities can be uncovered by appropriate laboratory assessment before they become clinically significant. Suggested guidelines are listed in Table 25-8. The frequency of monitoring will depend on the clinical status of each patient. Close monitoring of all patients on parenteral nutrition regimens is essential to assure optimal nutritional support and minimize complications.

**TABLE 25-8 GUIDELINES FOR MONITORING INFANTS AND CHILDREN RECEIVING PARENTERAL NUTRITION**

| Parameter | Recommended Frequency[a] | |
|---|---|---|
| **Clinical Status** | | |
| Strict intakes and output records | Daily | |
| Total intake: calories, protein, lipids, fluid, other | Daily | |
| Total output: urine, stool, other | Daily | |
| Vital signs (temperature) | Daily, and as indicated[a] | |
| Physical findings | As indicated | |
| **Growth Measurements (Anthropometrics)** | | |
| Weight | Daily | |
| Length | Weekly | |
| Head circumference (infants < 2y) | Weekly | |
| Triceps skinfold | Biweekly | |
| Mid-arm circumference | Biweekly | |
| **Laboratory** | **Initial** | **Steady State[a]** |
| Glucose | Every 4–6 hours[a] | As indicated |
| Serum electrolytes (including bicarbonate) | Daily | Weekly |
| Blood urea nitrogen | 3 times weekly | Weekly |
| Calcium, magnesium, phosphate | 3 times weekly | Weekly |
| Albumin | 2 times weekly | Biweekly |
| γ-Glutamyl trans peptidase | Weekly | Biweekly |
| AST (SGOT) | Weekly | Biweekly |
| Bilirubin (total) | Weekly, or as indicated | Biweekly |
| Complete blood count with differential | 2 times weekly, or as indicated | Biweekly |
| Platelet count | Weekly | Biweekly |
| Serum triglycerides | 2–3 times weekly[a] | Biweekly |
| Urine glucose | Each void | As indicated |
| Zinc | Baseline | Bimonthly, or as indicated |
| Iron/total iron-binding capacity/ferritin | | Bimonthly, or as indicated |
| Copper, selenium, manganese, molybdenum | | As indicated |

[a]These recommendations apply to infants and children during the initiation of parenteral nutrition, or when physiologic status is potentially changing. Some parameters need less frequent monitoring in stable infants and children receiving long-term parenteral nutrition. The frequency of monitoring *premature* and *low-birth-weight infants,* as well as *critically ill* older infants and children, will be guided by the clinical situation. Glucose tolerance should be monitored more frequently in these patients. Every urine voided should be tested for glucosuria, and blood levels should be obtained when the urine tests positive. Lipid tolerance in such patients also should be monitored more closely, with daily triglyceride levels obtained until the patient is on a fixed regimen and clinically stable. Premature infants require close monitoring of bilirubin levels, both conjugated and unconjugated, during parenteral nutrition infusions to assess for potential lipid interactions and hepatoxicity. Calcium and phosphorus levels also should be checked 1 to 3 times weekly, even in stable premature infants on parenteral nutrition regimens. Ammonia levels are useful in premature infants and metabolically imbalanced patients.

AST, aspartate aminotransferase; SGOT, serum glutamic oxaloacetic transaminase.

## SUGGESTED READINGS

American Society for Parenteral and Enteral Nutrition Board of Directors and the Clinical Guidelines Task Force. Guidelines for the use of parenteral and enteral nutrition in adult and pediatric patients. *JPEN J Parenter Enteral Nutr*. 2002;26(1 Suppl):1SA-138SA.

Koletzko B, Goulet O, Hunt J, Krohn K, Shamir R; Parenteral Nutrition Guidelines Working Group; European Society for Clinical Nutrition and Metabolism; European Society of Paediatric Gastroenterology, Hepatology and Nutrition (ESPGHAN); European Society of Paediatric Research. Guidelines on paediatric parenteral nutrition of the European Society of Paediatric Gastroenterology, Hepatology and Nutrition (ESPGHAN) and the European Society for Clinical Nutrition and Metabolism (ESPEN). *J Pediatr Gastroenterol Nutr.* 2005;41(Suppl 2):S1-S87.

Mayer K, Seeger W. Fish oil in critical illness. *Curr Opin Clin Nutr Metab Care.* 2008;11(2):121-127.

Gura KM, Duggan CP, Collier SB, et al. Reversal of parenteral nutrition–associated liver disease in two infants with short bowel syndrome using parenteral fish oil: implications for future management. *Pediatrics.* 2006;118(1):e197-e201.

# 26 Nutritional Access Devices

Kathleen M. Leack, Janel A. Meyer, and Linda S. Flannery

## INTRODUCTION

A variety of nutritional access devices are available to provide enteral supplementation and parenteral nutrition (PN) safely and effectively to children.

## PARENTERAL ACCESS DEVICES

Peripheral intravenous access is usually insufficient to provide adequate nutrition to patients as the nutrient concentrations need to be limited to prevent thrombophlebitis. Central venous line access is essential to patients requiring long- and short-term intravenous nutrition. A central venous access device (CVAD) is a line with a catheter tip that lies in the subclavian vein, superior/inferior vena cava, or right atrium. The type of CVAD is determined by the medical diagnosis and length of therapy. Insertion sites may include jugular, subclavian, femoral, antecubital, and umbilical veins. These lines may be tunneled or non-tunneled and may have 1 or more lumens. Line placement can be done in surgery, in interventional radiology, or at the bedside.

Tunneled central lines (Broviac/Hickman, Cook, Groshong) are placed through a subcutaneous tunnel away from the vein insertion site. These lines have a Dacron cuff to provide stability to the line and function as an antimicrobial barrier. Both placement and removal of tunneled central lines are done by a surgeon or radiologist. Children requiring prolonged PN need a tunneled central venous line.

Non-tunneled central venous catheters are generally placed directly into a jugular, subclavian, or femoral vein. These lines are typically placed in the hospital setting at the bedside for use while the patient is in the hospital. Since they do not have a Dacron cuff, they are sutured into place. They can also be removed at the bedside.

Peripherally inserted central catheters (PICC lines) are chosen for short-term intravenous therapies lasting weeks or months. Generally, they are placed in an arm or a leg and threaded to a central vein or right atrium. These lines can be placed at the bedside or in interventional radiology.

Implanted medication ports are tunneled lines implanted beneath the skin that contain a single or double reservoir pocketed between the subcutaneous layers and sutured in place. Placement is done in surgery or interventional radiology. Access to the reservoir is obtained with a non-coring needle. These ports are ideal for patients needing repeated but intermittent therapies, such as chemotherapy. They only need special care when accessed.



## CARE AND MANAGEMENT OF CVADs

Presence of a CVAD increases a child's risk for central line–associated bloodstream infection (CLABSI). It is of utmost importance that CVADs are managed using a "bundle" of care activities that include using sterile technique when accessing the line; scrubbing the access points with appropriate products; and keeping the dressing dry, intact, and occlusive. Many national initiatives have focused on CLABSI prevention, as CLABSI is a known source of morbidity and mortality. All levels of care providers/caregivers should be well versed in CLABSI prevention.

A torn or broken catheter puts the patient at risk for CLABSI. Repair kits, available for each of the long-term silastic catheters, allow for repair of the external portion of the CVAD. However, if the catheter breaks beneath the surface of the skin or has been repaired multiple times, it will need to be removed and a new catheter placed. Other CVAD problems and their management are shown in Table 26-1.

In patients with CVADs, fever or other signs or symptoms of suspected CLABSI demands immediate evaluation. Hospitalization may be indicated to observe and treat a patient for presumed sepsis if no obvious source for the fever is found. Apart from a full physical examination, laboratory tests, including complete blood counts and blood cultures (both through the line and by peripheral vein), are mandatory. In most cases, and in all infants and young children, antibiotics are started until the culture results are available. Depending on the clinical setting, antibiotics may be discontinued if cultures are negative after 48 to 72 hours. Repeat blood cultures often are drawn through the catheter until the cultures are negative.

Children with CVADs are encouraged to continue with age- and developmentally appropriate activities. Exercise, including swimming, is allowable with these catheters. Active children, especially toddlers, may need additional securement techniques and devices, to prevent accidental line dislodgement.

Caregivers need to be trained on all aspects of CVAD care. To avoid complications that are associated with infusions, appropriate preparation and infusion of the nutrient solution is critical. The patient and caregiver also need to be trained on pumps and other home equipment. They must be able to troubleshoot problems that arise in the home setting.

Close partnership between the patient, family, and care team is essential. Monitoring for CVAD and therapy-related complications is indicated. This may be done through clinic appointments or home-nursing visits. It is important to train families to notify the physician or a member of the nutrition support team whenever unusual or abnormal symptoms or signs occur. This will help to decrease potential morbidity and mortality that are associated with these therapies.

## ENTERAL ACCESS DEVICES

Nasogastric (NG) tubes and nasojejunal (NJ) tubes are used as initial or temporary feeding tubes. NG tubes can usually be placed at the bedside while NJ tubes are placed under fluoroscopy. Generally, the smallest size enteral tube should be chosen and the tube should be replaced only when necessary. If long-term feedings are anticipated, tubes should be polyurethane or silicone to reduce the frequency of tube replacement and minimize trauma. Use of weighted tubes should be avoided to decrease the risk of bowel perforation. These tubes can be used for a maximum of 2 to 3 months before considering durable enteral feeding tube placement.

For patients requiring long-term enteral feeding access, gastrostomy (G) tubes, transgastric-jejunal (GJ) tubes, and jejunal (J) tubes are used. Durable enteral feeding tubes can be placed using endoscopic, surgical, or interventional radiologic techniques when

**TABLE 26-1 TROUBLESHOOTING CENTRAL VENOUS ACCESS DEVICE PROBLEMS**

| Problem | Possible Causes | Recommendations |
|---|---|---|
| Occlusion | Line clamped or kinked | Assess line; open all clamps and straighten catheter and tubing |
| | Medication precipitation | Consult with pharmacist on possible medication precipitate; use pharmacist recommendations |
| | Thrombosis | CVL contrast study to determine presence of thrombosis; use t-PA (Activase, Alteplase) |
| Redness and/or rash at exit site | Sensitivity to cleansing agent, type of dressing, and/or adhesive used | Assess and use alternative products |
| | Site is moist | Assess and maintain a clean, dry, and occlusive dressing at all times |
| | Infection | Use antimicrobial ointment with dressing changes; if redness persists, obtain site culture |
| Fever | Central line–associated blood stream infection (CLABSI) | CLABSIs can be prevented or minimized by (1) good handwashing technique prior to handling CVAD and equipment; (2) good sterility techniques; (3) proper disinfection of all injection ports of CVAD prior to connections and accessing; (4) prevention of contamination of IV tubing ends and tips of needles; and (5) assessing dressings routinely and changing when needed (*Note:* Dressings need to be clean, dry, and occlusive at all times.); obtain blood culture and treat with intravenous antibiotics until cultures are negative |
| Bleeding at exit site | Line is accidentally tugged | Stabilize and secure line at all times |
| | Hole in line | Assess for puncture in line (refer to breakage or puncture guideline solutions) |
| Drainage at the site | Line is accidentally tugged | Stabilize and secure line at all times |
| | Infection | Obtain site culture (*Note:* If fever present then blood culture may be obtained.); assess site and change dressing as needed; maintain a clean, dry, and occlusive dressing at all times |
| Breakage or puncture in line | Line is accidentally cut | Clamp between the patient and the break; repair or replace the line |
| | Forceful flushing of line | If resistance is met when flushing line, determine line patency (refer to occlusion guideline solutions) |
| | Needle puncture | Clamp between patient and puncture site; repair or replace the line |
| | PICC line is severed | Assess exit site and if PICC line is not visible then immediately apply a tourniquet to the patient's extremity; keep child sedentary; have extremity evaluated by radiologist; retrieval of catheter may be necessary under fluoroscopy |
| Accidental removal | Line is pulled out | Apply pressure and occlusive dressing to exit site; keep child sedentary; may need surgical intervention if there is significant bleeding or shock |

CVL, central venous line; CVAD, central venous access device; IV, intravenous; PICC line, peripherally inserted central catheter.

**TABLE 26-2 ENTERAL FEEDING DEVICES**

| Route | Indications | Tube Selection |
|---|---|---|
| Nasogastric | For children with a functional gastrointestinal tract requiring 2 months or less of enteral feeding | Available in 5–18 French (Fr) |
| | | Choose the smallest tube through which formula will flow, usually 6–10 Fr |
| | | Use 5 Fr for preterm infants |
| | | Polyurethane and silicone are softer and longer lasting |
| | | Tube and tip are radiopaque |
| Nasoduodenal or Nasojejunal | For children with a functional gastrointestinal tract requiring 2 months or less of enteral feeding; may be used postoperatively following gastric surgery | Available in a variety of sizes but longer than nasogastric tubes |
| | | Usually 8 Fr, 120 cm used |
| | | Some are weighted |
| | | Radiopaque |
| Gastrostomy | For children requiring intragastric feeding for longer than 2 months | Usual pediatric sizes are 12–24 Fr |
| | | Available with or without external fixation device |
| | | Tubes have an external fixation device and an internal mushroom or balloon to secure placement |
| | | Balloon sizes are 2.5–14 mL |
| | | Low-profile devices are available and are recommended for children when possible |
| | | Radiopaque |
| Gastrojejunostomy | For children requiring jejunal feedings due to intolerance of gastrostomy feeds (eg, risk of aspiration or poor gastric emptying) | Designed for placement through a gastrostomy site |
| | | Some have poor gastric venting abilities |
| | | Radiopaque |
| Jejunostomy | For children who have had a GJ tube for 3–6 months, and cannot tolerate G tube feeds. | Surgically placed sizes range from 12–24 Fr |
| | | Many gastrostomy tubes can be used as jejunostomy tubes |
| | | Radiopaque |

long-term feeding access is indicated. When caring for a patient with any enteral tube, it is important to know the location, purpose, and type of tube in place. The commonly used enteral feeding devices are summarized in Table 26-2.

Gastrostomy tubes are placed to avoid complications and trauma associated with repeated replacement of the nasogastric tube. This is particularly important with infants and young children who may develop a severe feeding aversion that is exacerbated by irritation of the nasal passages and oropharynx by the nasogastric tube. Placement of a gastrostomy tube may facilitate progression of oromotor development in some of these children even though they still depend on tube feedings for a portion of their nutrition.

Gastrostomy tubes are frequently placed by percutaneous endoscopic gastrostomy (PEG) procedure which is typically done under general anesthesia in children. The principal contraindications to placement of a PEG are overlying organs (eg, liver, colon), ascites, a coagulopathy, failure to transilluminate the stomach, or a history of esophageal stricture or other esophageal surgery. PEG tubes have been successfully placed in patients who have undergone prior abdominal surgical procedures, including those with indwelling ventriculoperitoneal (VP) shunts, intestinal malrotation, or severe scoliosis.

Complications of PEG tube placement include pneumoperitoneum, transient fever, pain, bleeding, gastric ulceration from direct erosion of the gastric mucosa by the internal portion of the gastrostomy tube, ileus, gastric separation, gastric fistula, gastrocolic fistula, "buried bumper syndrome," and tube extrusion. Surgical site infection is decreased by use of prophylactic antibiotics. Site-related complications include persistent gastric leakage, hypergranulation tissue, cellulitis, abscess, and unplanned tube removal.

Exchange of the primary PEG device for replacement with a standard gastrostomy tube is usually not performed for 3 months after placement to allow for complete healing and maturation of the gastrostomy tract. Several tubes are available for use in a gastrostomy, ranging from skin-level, low-profile "buttons" to standard long gastrostomy tubes. Both types of tubes offer water balloon or mushroom-type internal bumpers. The choice of tube depends on the patient's and caretaker's needs and tolerance. Following tube exchange, parents can generally be instructed on the tube replacement procedure.

Transgastric-jejunal tubes are used when a patient cannot tolerate gastric feedings. GJ tubes, which are placed in interventional radiology, have both a gastric and jejunal port and lumen. Feedings are delivered via the jejunal lumen. The clinician must determine the appropriate route for medication administration. Some children are unable to tolerate their gastric secretions, resulting in the need for continuous gastric drainage. Fluid losses and replacement need to be considered in this situation.

Jejunal feeding tubes are placed when a patient has demonstrated inability to return to gastric feeding. Many children retain their gastrostomy tube even after a jejunostomy tube is placed.

## CARE AND MANAGEMENT OF ENTERAL FEEDING TUBES

### Nasogastric Tubes

Ensuring the gastric location of an NG tube is of utmost importance. Parents may be taught to check the pH of aspirated gastric contents. Secure with a clamping device or tape. Assess the nose for pressure or breakdown, the nose being most vulnerable. Assess the skin on the face for tape-related breakdown.

### Nasojejunal Tubes

Nasojejunal tubes are placed via fluoroscopy. They are secured in the same manner as NG tubes and pressure and breakdown should be assessed accordingly.

### Skin Site Care

Assess the peristomal site daily for overall health of the site as well as for site complications. A small amount of erythema and serosanguineous drainage is normally present for the first 2 weeks post placement. The site should be cleansed daily and as needed with soap and water, rinsed, and thoroughly dried. Dressings may be placed if indicated.

### Stabilization of the Tube

The durable enteral feeding tube is stabilized by holding the balloon/mushroom up against the stomach wall. The tube should exit the site at a 90-degree angle to prevent pressure along the edges of the tract, which could lead to skin breakdown or pressure necrosis. If an external fixation device (bar, disc, elbow) is present, ensure that the stabilizer is not too tight. If the fixation device is absent, tape or another dressing method should be used to prevent migration or excessive movement of the tube. The ultimate goals of tube stabilization are to (1) protect tube and site; (2) prevent excess movement of the tube; and/or (3) prevent the tube from being pulled out.

### Flushing the Tube

After all feeding and medication administration, the tube should be briskly flushed with water to clear the tube. This is necessary to prevent clogging and to ensure that all formula and medication are cleared from the tube. With continuous drip feeding, the feeding needs to be interrupted every 8 hours in order to flush the tube with water to minimize the risk of clogging.

### Medication Administration

When possible, administer liquid medication through enteral tubes. If only pill form is available, crush all medication to a fine powder and mix with water until dissolved. Flush well with water after each medication.

### Care of Feeding Equipment

With proper care and cleaning, feeding equipment can be reused many times. This step is important in preventing the growth of bacteria. Wash the feeding equipment in liquid dish detergent and warm water to prevent the growth of bacteria. Rinse well and air dry between feedings. If the feeding equipment becomes "cloudy," a 3:1 water: vinegar solution, followed by thorough water rinsing, can be used.

### Management of Complications

Management approaches for the most common complications of enteral tube feeding and enteral feeding devices are summarized in Table 26-3. These include inadvertent removal of the tube, movement of the tube (eg, causing pyloric obstruction), leakage around the tube, development of granulation tissue, local infections, and clogging of the tube.

### Caregiver Education and Support

Caregivers must be educated on the rationale for and method of tube placement, feeding and medication administration, site cares, and troubleshooting. Psychosocial support in the form of alternate caregivers and respite care is necessary. Patients will be reintegrated into daily activities such as day care, school, and other social activities. All of this will require frequent reinforcement from all care team members. Pediatricians should be aware of the tubes, equipment, and resources (eg, nursing, nutritional, pharmaceutical, and home care companies) that are available in the local area. With the current emphasis on shorter hospital stays, more patients will be discharged quickly on enteral feeding regimens and require follow-up care from their primary physicians.

**TABLE 26-3 COMPLICATIONS OF ENTERAL FEEDINGS AND ENTERAL FEEDING DEVICES**

| Problem | Possible Cause | Solution |
|---|---|---|
| **Mechanical Tube-Related Problems** | | |
| Impairment of child development (all tubes) | Enteral feeding and tube interfere with feeding skill development and normal activity | Develop feeding schedule so that child learns association between oral activity and satiety. Establish a non-nutritive program. If possible, offer small amounts of food from spoon and fluids from a cup. These offerings should be before enteral feedings. |
| | | Instruct family to secure tube and place child on abdomen to promote upper body development and encourage crawling. |
| | | Encourage normal clothing. |
| | | Consider skin-level device as early as possible. |
| | | If oral food refusal results, consult an occupational therapist and/or speech pathologist. |
| Leaking of gastric/jejunal contents onto the abdomen (G tube, GJ tube, J tube) | Balloon or mushroom of tube has slipped away from the stomach wall | Check marking on tube and gently pull back on to assure that balloon/mushroom is snug against stomach wall. |
| | Balloon has deflated | Add water to the balloon or change tube.[a] |
| | Child has increased pressure in stomach from air, delayed gastric emptying, or coughing, causing formula to leak | Vent tube before or after feeding. |
| | | Protect skin with barrier creams and skin protectants. Use absorptive dressing. |
| | Tube is too small for size of stoma | Placing a larger tube is usually not recommended. Take tube out to allow stoma to shrink. Check stoma diameter every half hour. |
| | Frequent positioning of child onto the left side | Limit the time spent on the left side after feeding. |
| | Frequent pulling at tube | Use 1-piece T-shirts, extra clothing, or "belly band" devices as needed. |
| | Antireflux valve of skin-level device is defective | Change tube.[a] |
| Redness or drainage around tube/stoma (G tube, GJ tube, J tube) | Some redness and drainage are normal | Assess area more frequently. |
| | Skin irritation results from dampness and/or leaking around tube | Keep skin dry. Protect skin with barrier creams and skin protectants. |
| | | Utilize dressing methods that promote absorption and stability. |
| | | Consult stoma resource nurse/wound nurse. |
| | | Antacid therapy may increase pH of enteric leakage, which will be less caustic to peristomal skin. |
| | Ineffective cleaning | Clean area with mild soap and water. |
| | | Avoid routine use of hydrogen peroxide. |
| | | Address patient discomfort or anxiety with site cares as needed. |
| | | Reinforce parental teaching. |
| | Tube has not been rotated | Rotate tube once a day. |
| | External fixation device (bar, disc, elbow) is too tight | Loosen fixation device and assess daily for ability to move slightly. (Space between the abdomen and fixation device should be about the depth of a dime.) |
| | Peristomal wound infection | Enteral antibiotics, antibiotic ointments, or antifungals should be used only with signs of infection. |
| | Ill child | It is not uncommon that a patient's tube site will become irritated when ill (due to coughing, distension, etc). Address site concerns. They may not resolve until primary illness does. |
| Clogged tube or inability to irrigate tube (all tubes) | Lack of routine flushing | Flush tube after feedings. Use warm water with a syringe and slight pulsating pressure twice daily. |
| | Medication–formula interaction | Flush tube in between and after medications. |
| | Aspirating gastric contents frequently | Flush tube before and after residual checks. |
| Feedings will not flow or increased formula in reflux bag | Inadequately crushed medications through the tube | Assess medication–formula compatibility. |
| | | Crush medications finely. |
| | | Use liquid when possible. |
| | Gastric reflux | Consider intestinal feedings. |
| | Formula too viscous | Use formula designed for tube diameter. Change formula to one with a lower viscosity. |
| | | Consider milking the tube to alleviate the obstruction. |
| Nasal/pharyngeal/esophageal irritation and erosion (NG tube, NJ tube) | Prolonged intubation with nasogastric/nasojejunal tube | Use the softest/smallest-caliber feeding tube when possible. |
| | | Perform regular assessment of nares. Moisten and clean nares every 8 hours. Lubricate lips. |
| | | Secure tube properly. Assess securement device/method. Avoid pressure on nare. Adjust device as needed. |
| | | Consider gastrostomy or jejunostomy tubes for long-term feeding (> 2 months). |

*(Continued)*

**TABLE 26-3 COMPLICATIONS OF ENTERAL FEEDINGS AND ENTERAL FEEDING DEVICES (CONTINUED)**

| Problem | Possible Cause | Solution |
|---|---|---|
| Granulation tissue build-up around gastrostomy tube | Small amount of epithelial tissue is normal and not painful | Skin care prevents irritation. |
| | | Avoid hydrogen peroxide. |
| | Tissue may increase with increased movement | Secure tube to minimize movement. |
| | Some children are more prone than others | Apply silver nitrate or triamcinolone cream to the tissue. |
| Bleeding (G tube, GJ tube, J tube) | May occur with tube change | Lubricate the new tube well before insertion. |
| | Excessive tension on the tube | Allow slight movement in tube between gastric and abdominal walls. |
| | Movement of tube against mucosa | Secure tube. |
| | Gastric ulcers or pressure necrosis from internal bumper | Acid inhibition, endoscopy. |
| | | Tube change may be indicated.[a] |
| Migration of tube (all tubes) | Movement or migration of tube | Stop feeding if tube position is unknown. |
| Stomach into esophagus (retching, vomiting, coughing) | | May need to verify tube position with x-ray. |
| Stomach into intestines (increase in stools) | | Reposition tube. |
| Jejunal extension into stomach (retching, vomiting, coughing, formula in gastric aspirate) | | Secure tube and monitor length of external tube. |
| Tube into the tract (G tube, GJ tube, J tube) | Movement or migration of tube | Reposition tube. |
| | | Tract may need to be remeasured. |
| | | May need to verify tube position with x-ray. |
| | | Reevaluate tube securement technique. |
| Perforation (esophageal, gastric, intestinal) | Esophageal perforation with NG tube insertion | Surgical consultation. |
| | Gastric disruption with G tube replacement | Surgical consultation. |
| | Jejunal perforation with NJ/GJ tube placement | Surgical consultation. |
| | | Use of guidelines for GJ tube placement. |
| Accidental removal of tube (G tube, GJ tube, J tube) | Tube out[a] | Cover the area with a small dressing and cover with tape. |
| | | Replacement should occur within 1 hour. |
| | | Determine if bedside replacement is safe or if fluoroscopic guided replacement is indicated. |
| | Balloon deflated[a] | Reinflate balloon. |
| | | If balloon is defective, tube should be replaced. |
| | Child pulls on tube | Secure tube. |
| | Caregiver pulls on tube | Secure tube. |
| | | Reinforce tube location awareness prior to repositioning/transfer. |
| **Gastrointestinal Problems** | | |
| Aspiration (all tubes) | Seek to determine cause | Stop feeding immediately if aspiration is suspected. |
| | Tube malposition | Check placement of tube. |
| | Gastroesophageal reflux | Consider antireflux medication. |
| | Delayed gastric emptying/gastroparesis | Never feed if child feels full or is vomiting. |
| | | Consider jejunal feeding. |
| Vomiting (all tubes) | Position during feeding | Never feed child flat. Place on right side, sit up, or raise head of bed 30°–45°. |
| | Rapid formula administration | Offer smaller and more frequent feedings. |
| | | For bolus feedings, increase length of time for feedings. |
| | | Consider pump feeding rather than gravity. |
| | | Consider continuous feeding rather than bolus. |
| | | For continuous feedings, reduce rate of administration. |
| | Gastroparesis | Consider jejunal feeding. |
| | | Place gastric port of GJ tube to gravity drainage. |
| | High osmolality | Select isotonic formula. |
| | Gastric retention | Avoid adding other food to formula (eg, strained or dehydrated baby food). |
| | | Consider prokinetic agent to promote gastric emptying, continuous feedings, or postpyloric feedings. |
| | Air in stomach | Vent tube during feedings or allow for short breaks. |
| | | Elevate child's head during feeding and for 30 minutes after meals. |
| | | Decompress routinely. |

*(Continued)*

**TABLE 26-3 COMPLICATIONS OF ENTERAL FEEDINGS AND ENTERAL FEEDING DEVICES (CONTINUED)**

| Problem | Possible Cause | Solution |
|---|---|---|
| | Tube migration from stomach to small intestine | Stop feeding and reposition tube against stomach wall. |
| | | May need to verify the tube position with x-ray. |
| | Medications given with feeding | Change times of medication, if possible. Check contents of medications. |
| | Obstruction (bilious vomiting) | Stop feedings. |
| | | Obtain imaging studies and surgical consult as warranted. |
| Diarrhea (all tubes) | Rapid formula administration | Reduce rate of administration or initiate feedings at low rate. |
| | Hyperosmolar or low-residue formulas | Rule out formula-related causes. Select isotonic or fiber-supplemented formula. Consider diluting formula concentration and gradually increase the strength. |
| | Intolerance of formula (allergy/lactose intolerance) | Use formula lacking intolerant component. |
| | Malabsorption | Consider use of elemental or semielemental formula, medium-chain triglyceride. |
| | | If diarrhea persists, measure stool electrolytes and osmolality. Consider holding feedings for 24 hours and monitor effect on stool output. |
| | | If osmotic diarrhea persists or if secretory diarrhea is diagnosed, begin parenteral nutrition. |
| | Hypoalbuminemia | If absorptive capacity of the small intestine is compromised, consider use of hydrolyzed, peptide-based formulas or parenteral nutrition. |
| | Bacterial contamination | Use commercially prepared sterile formulas. |
| | | Use aseptic techniques in handling and administering feedings. |
| | | Avoid hanging feedings over a prolonged time. |
| | | Do not use a delivery set for over 24 hours. |
| | | Throw away any opened formula refrigerated over 48 hours |
| | Rapid gastrointestinal transit time | Select formula with fiber supplement. |
| | Prolonged antibiotic therapy or other medications | Send stool for *C. difficile* toxin and culture. |
| | | Monitor medications (eg, sorbitol content) and eliminate causative medication if possible. |
| | | Check time medications are given. |
| Cramping, gas, abdominal distention (all tubes) | Rapid administration of formula | Reduce rate of formula administration and deliver according to patient tolerance. |
| | Administration of cold formula | Administer formula at room temperature. |
| | Malabsorption of formula | Select hydrolyzed formula. |
| Constipation (all tubes) | Inadequate fluid | Monitor and increase fluids. |
| | Inadequate fiber | Consider formula with fiber or add fiber supplement. Try prune juice. |
| | Inadequate activity | Encourage activity. |
| | Fecal impaction | Disimpact and add stool softeners. |
| | Obstruction | Stop feedings. |
| | | Obtain imaging studies and surgical consult as warranted. |

[a]Tube change/replacement: It is important for the provider to know the age of the gastrostomy tract. Patients that have not had a primary tube change are at risk for gastric disruption with early tube replacement/manipulation. Following primary tube change, bedside replacement is a safe intervention assuming the individual has had training in the technique. Fluoroscopic tube change/replacement is indicated when integrity of the tract is a concern.

G, gastrostomy; GJ, transgastric-jejunal; J, jejunal; NG, nasogastric; NJ, nasojejunal.

## SELECTED READINGS


Baskin JL, Pui C-H, Reiss U, et al. Management of occlusion and thrombosis associated with long-term indwelling central venous catheters. *Lancet*. 2009;374(9684):159-169.

Doellman D, Pettit J, Catudal JP, et al. Best practice guidelines in the care and maintenance of pediatric central venous catheters. *Pedivan, Association of Vascular Access Practice Guidelines*. 2010.

Egnell C, Eksborg S, Grahnquist L. Jejunostomy enteral feeding in children: outcome and safety. *JPEN J Parenter Enteral Nutr*. 2014;38(5):631-636.

Farber LD. Care and management of patients with tubes and drains. In: Browne N, Flanigan L, McComiskey C, Pieper P, eds. *Nursing Care of the Pediatric Surgical Patient*. 3rd ed. Burlington, MA: Jones & Bartlett Learning; 2013: 95-120.

O'Grady NP, Alexander M, Burns LA, et al; the Healthcare Infection Control Practices Advisory Committee (HICPAC). Guidelines for the prevention of intravascular catheter-related infections, 2011. Centers for Disease Control Web site. https://www.cdc.gov/hicpac/pdf/guidelines/bsi-guidelines-2011.pdf. Accessed April 6, 2017.

Soscia J, Friedman J. A guide to the management of common gastrostomy and gastrojejunostomy tube problems. *Paediatr Child Health*. 2011;16(5):281-287.

# 27 Families in the 21st Century: An Introduction to Families

Laurie J. Bauman and Ruth E. K. Stein

## INTRODUCTION

Pediatricians provide care for children who live in a variety of family situations. Children may live with 2 working parents, unmarried parents, grandparents, or other nonparental caregiver; or they may live in single-parent families where the mother or father may be divorced or never married; or they may live with lesbian, gay, bisexual, or transgendered (LGBT) parents; in foster homes; or in blended families. The traditional nuclear family, consisting of a mother and a father who are married and living with their biological children, is becoming rare; in fact, only 25% of households fit this description. Although it was the norm decades ago, today only one-half of American households include a married couple, and only one-half of those have children. Only 14% of children are raised in a 2-parent home with a working father and a mother who stays home full time. Given the diversity of family forms, it is important to identify the ideas central to the definition of *family*.

The notion of family is universal in all cultures and societies, but the definition is changing and is often vague. At a broad, conceptual level, the family is a system of social relationships that are shaped by expectations and values and that are based on distinctions of age and gender. Each member occupies a particular position or status that governs behavior toward other family members. On a more practical level, the US Bureau of the Census defines a *family* as 2 or more persons who live together and are related by blood, marriage, or adoption.

## CHARACTERISTICS OF FAMILIES

Given the difficulty in defining *family*, it may be useful to conceptualize the characteristics and functions of family units. First, many families share biology, including temperament, personality, talent, and disease vulnerability. Second, families typically have a power hierarchy that is determined in part by age, generation, culture, personality characteristics, and gender. Third, families tend to have their own "culture," which includes a family-specific set of values, goals, and expectations. Although they are unique to each family, these "microcultures" reflect the larger societal and ethnic cultures. Fourth, every family has an "invisible boundary" that defines who is a member and who is not.

Another set of family characteristics is developmental and arises from a family's common history and future. Family history may be completely unknown or extend back for generations, reflecting both ethnic and religious beliefs and the dramatic life-altering events that have affected the family. A family's future course usually follows a pattern of successive developmental phases that depend in part on both biology and social norms. The *phase of expansion* includes the initial parental union and continues until the youngest child becomes an adult. This period spans fertility and the physical and emotional maturation of children. The *phase of dispersion* occurs when the first child achieves adulthood and leaves home. The *phase of independence* begins when all the children have left and the parents are alone. The *phase of replacement* covers the period of retirement to death.

## SOCIETAL FUNCTIONS OF THE FAMILY

Historically, the family as a social institution has served several functions. Its primary purpose has been the care, rearing, and socialization of children and the legitimization of sexual union. Families have had the major role in child rearing and in regulating sexual relationships. Marriage has been the social institution used to legitimize sexual union; however, over time, sexual liaisons outside of marriage have become more common, and childbirth frequently occurs outside of the marital tie. In 1950, only 4% of US children were born out of wedlock; today, almost half (48%) of first births are to unmarried mothers. This is accepted in many cultures. In addition, the family is expected to meet the subsistence needs of its members, but 11% of US families with children have no working members. Another role of the family is to provide love and emotional intimacy. This is more characteristic of Western than of Eastern societies, but American notions include the expectation that partners will provide affection and emotional support to each other and their children. Depending on the cultural background of the family, there may be differences in the role of children, their degree of autonomy, and the authority of parents. For non-native-born families, this may put stress on children who are negotiating 2 worlds.

## TYPES OF FAMILIES

There are many ways to classify families, but family types are most often described by their structure. For children in the United States today, changes in family type are the norm rather than the exception, and it is no longer uncommon for a family to undergo multiple changes in composition during a child's lifetime.

In its simplest form, a family consists of the husband, wife, and nonadult children, and it is called the *nuclear, conjugal, elementary, immediate,* or *simple family.* This family structure consists of 2 generations, parents and children. In industrial societies, nuclear families tend to live in a separate household that often is far removed from relatives.

In *extended families,* several generations live together, and grandparents often have some responsibility for child rearing. As a result of parent incapacity, abandonment, or death, 7% of US children live with a grandparent and no parent, 3 million have a grandparent as their main caregiver, and 5.4 million live in households headed by a grandparent. In this configuration, the children may have experienced the loss of a parent and may have had to move, leaving behind home, friends, and school. Sometimes, custody is a matter of legal question or family controversy.

Most children develop loving, caring relationships with new caregivers, but some relationships between children and custodians are ambivalent or antagonistic, and on occasion, custodians may be antagonistic to the living biological parent(s). If the parent has died, all may be grieving. Little is known about the custodial arrangements of many of these vulnerable children. Regardless of the reason for the transfer of custody, many grandparents find it difficult to parent again.

*Single-parent families* are increasingly common, and most are headed by women. Almost 30% of all children under 18 years of age live in single-parent families, and more than one-half of black children in the United States live in single-parent families. Single-parent families also include never-married mothers, some of whom choose to parent alone, and parents who are divorced, some of whom share the custody of their children. Fathers are 16% of single parents.

Single parents face special challenges. Most importantly, they tend to have far fewer economic resources and a much lower standard of living. If the parent is working outside the home, they must make childcare arrangements, which can be complex, costly, and difficult to find. Divorced parents and their children find the first year to be very painful, but research suggests that children who have a supportive, understanding, and affectionate parent tend to do well. Although divorced fathers are sometimes uninvolved with their children, many children remain emotionally connected to both parents, even when contact with the noncustodial parent is limited. It is becoming somewhat more common for fathers to share custody or to become the custodial parent. Seven out of 10 single mothers are working or looking for work, and adequate sources of childcare are difficult to find. Older siblings may be given significant responsibility, and some may experience school and peer problems. Despite the many issues that single parents face, there is strong evidence that most single families raise healthy, secure children. Resources facilitating a positive outcome include parental organizational skills, adequate support networks, and closer proximity to extended family.

Blended families are becoming increasingly more common and sometimes more than 1 parent is in a blended family situation. Three-quarters of divorced people remarry, usually within 3 years. Remarriage often eases the financial problems of single parenthood, but complex new family relationships result. In some instances, 1 partner lives with children who are from the other partner's previous relationship. Moreover, there may be significant friction between the child and the stepparent as the child struggles for the biological parent's attention and tries to negotiate new roles. These relationships may be more complicated when both of the child's biological parents are involved with new partners. In addition, new siblings may be introduced from the stepparent's family or as a product of the parent's new relationship. It may be difficult for the child to maintain these multiple new relationships and live by the rules and standards of his or her different families, especially if they have different cultural values.

About 7% of children live with *unmarried parents* who have made a commitment to stay together. Although this arrangement may be a transitional step toward planned marriage, this cannot be assumed. The lack of permanence can be difficult for all family members; there may be conflict between partners about where the relationship is going. The instability of the relationship may draw attention away from the children, but if the parental figure and the child have a strong bond, this family form can work well.

*LGBT families* are becoming more common and accepted as a family form. Sometimes a parent realizes after having children that he or she is gay or transsexual. Divorce may result, and the child may live with or visit an LGBT parent. Both the family separation and the need for the child to adjust to a new adult in the home may be stressful. Furthermore, the child may experience rejection from the larger community or from the other parent. To avoid the many possible problems, some parents choose secrecy. In other instances, an LGBT couple forms a primary relationship and actively chooses to parent a child. Some of these may require surrogate parent arrangements or adoption. Research on the children of homosexual parents has found that children can be nurtured effectively in this family form.

Few adolescents are prepared for the demands of *teenaged parenthood*. Married teenagers with children are more likely than married teenagers without children to have marital problems, to have additional children at an accelerated pace, and to leave school earlier. Inherent in "children parenting children" is the tension between the developmental needs of the adolescent and those of the child. Some teenaged mothers set up an independent household, either as a single parent or with the infant's father. However, most adolescent parents live at home with their parents, which creates an extended family system. There may be conflict between the adolescent and her mother over caregiving responsibilities for the infant and the adolescent's own independence and autonomy.

About 2 million US men are stay-at-home dads. Although this family arrangement is increasingly common, fathers may not find full acceptance by their peers, even when this is a choice rather than an economic necessity. Working mothers may welcome or regret being the family breadwinner, and be conflicted about their children's stronger attachment to their father. Studies are few on the consequences for children of this family form, but children may benefit from the full engagement of both parents and in most cases both parents play an important role in child development.

## EFFECTS OF SOCIAL TRENDS ON FAMILIES

Several social changes in the United States are affecting families of many types. One that affects an increasing number of families is the deinstitutionalization of elderly, disabled, and mentally ill persons. Mothers of young and adolescent children may confront the additional demands of caring for an ill or elderly parent, spouse, or child. Social, economic, and psychological supports for these women are often inadequate, which may adversely impact child rearing and the responsibilities of older children in the family unit.

Another societal evolution that will continue to affect families is changing gender roles. More married mothers are in the workforce, and more men are sharing or taking primary responsibility for child rearing. Recent economic trends have forced many families to rely on 2 incomes. In 66% of nuclear households with children under 18, both parents work, 70% of mothers with children under 18 work, and 60% of mothers with children under 3 years work. Families with 2 working parents tend to be smaller, younger, and more educated and have a higher income. Child rearing in families with 2 working parents can be stressful, and it requires effective and flexible external sources of childcare. However, lack of stable childcare arrangements may be difficult—for the parents and the children—and is especially problematic when there are significant ongoing health conditions. When both parents work, there may be special concerns; these families are likely to have latchkey children—children who are left alone after school until the parents come home from work. It is especially important to provide guidance concerning when this is developmentally appropriate and to provide guidelines for accident prevention.

## CLINICAL IMPLICATIONS OF THE CHANGING FAMILY

The variability of family forms, and the different values and norms that go along with them, pose challenges to clinicians. Families often behave in ways that are counter to the healthcare provider's own beliefs or to traditional health advice. Doctors, nurse practitioners, or social workers may find that their own values and standards differ from those of the patients. At times, these differences may create problems in communication or may lead to inappropriate attempts to enforce family conformity.

The clinician must be aware of the potential for encountering a wide range of different family types and must recognize them during interactions with families. There are many ways that family structure and values influence child development and behavior. The degree to which understanding of the family affects practice depends on the nature of the encounter and the type of information and interaction that are required to meet the child's needs and to care for the child's condition. Sensitivity to differences in family structure is important during all care provider interactions with families. Because family structure may not be stable, the clinician should inquire periodically and without judgment about changes in caregiving, living arrangements, and responsibility for the child.

Issues of family organization and management often are relevant in the care of children with acute intercurrent illness. When a child is on a short course of antibiotics, for example, it may be desirable to know whether the person who brings in the child for care can depend on other caregivers to adhere to the medication schedule and whether the babysitter or day care provider will cooperate. It also may be important to obtain history about the onset of symptoms from the person who was actually with the child when the problem first presented. These issues become even more critical in the presence of an ongoing or chronic health condition. When there are marked differences in health beliefs, other family frictions, or conflicting agendas, such as in custody disputes, cooperation may be impaired and the acute or ongoing care of the child jeopardized. The clinician may need to address such issues if they interfere with the delivery of effective pediatric care and can often help by taking a proactive role in inviting participation by other caregivers in subsequent appointments so that 1 caregiver is not in the position of having to tell others what care is needed.

All pediatricians take family histories focused on special medical risks that run in the family and that may affect the child's health. However, it is equally important to take social histories and to inquire about who is in the family and household, both at baseline and subsequently, and to inquire about whether there have been any changes at home when seeing a family periodically. It is not uncommon to find that different members of the family group may have differing views of the roles and relationships. It can be critical to understand the ways the members of the living unit interact and relate to one another and to the child. When there are serious health problems, it is important to consider the way family health and social issues affect the child's psychological and social development. All these factors play central roles in the child's development and well-being, so pediatricians should include social histories routinely in their interactions with their patients and parents.

The majority of children who are reared in any given family type will grow and thrive. During the course of normal child development, the stability of caregiving arrangements and provision of supportive and affectionate nurturance of the child are central issues, and the availability of multiple adults who are related to the child may offer some advantage to the child's emotional development. The clinician who has a trusting and respectful relationship with a child and family can play a critical role in helping them through a wide range of adaptive challenges.

## SUGGESTED READINGS


American Academy of Pediatrics Committee on Hospital Care and Institute for Patient- and Family-Centered Care. Patient- and family-centered care and the pediatrician's role. *Pediatrics.* 2012;129(2):394-404.

Chambers D. *A Sociology of Family Life: Change and Diversity in Intimate Relations.* Cambridge, UK: Polity Press; 2012.

Fadiman A. *The Spirit Catches You and You Fall Down: A Hmong Child, Her American Doctors, and the Collision of Two Cultures.* New York, NY: Farrar, Straus and Giroux; 1997.

Kotlowitz A. *There Are No Children Here: The Story of Two Boys Growing Up in the Other America.* New York, NY: Anchor Books; 1991.

LeBlanc AN. *Random Family: Love, Drugs, Trouble, and Coming of Age in the Bronx.* New York, NY: Schribner; 2003.


# 28 Childhood Adversity and Toxic Stress

Andrea G. Asnes and Christopher S. Greeley

## INTRODUCTION

While some degree of trauma and exposure to adversity in childhood is both commonplace and may even be an asset to healthy development, sustained exposure to trauma or severe trauma can result in long-term negative health consequences. This trauma may be physical, but it is often the more insidious emotional, psychological, or social forms of trauma. Early traumatic experiences can affect the way the genome is read, the development of the hypothalamic–pituitary–adrenal (HPA) axis, and the way the developing brain is wired. Because a child's brain continues to grow long after birth, environmental exposures, both positive and negative, can profoundly impact the developing child. The first 3 years of life are a particularly vulnerable period, given the plasticity of the brain in infancy and early childhood. Traumatic exposures (often collectively referred to as *adversities*) can influence learning, behavior, and health in children as well as result in adult risky behaviors, serious health problems, and early death. An understanding of the ways in which adversity affects the growing child can help the pediatric provider both to mitigate the influence of traumatic exposures in children and to shore up community resources that promote resiliency and protect against some of the negative lifelong consequences of childhood trauma.

## ETIOLOGY AND PATHOGENESIS

Pediatricians began to appreciate the importance of developmental, social, and behavioral problems in children in the 1970s. These problems were dubbed the "new morbidities," as they represented new threats to the well-being of children. This shift in focus on aspects of child health beyond infectious diseases, nutritional deficiencies, high infant mortality, and epidemics to include emotional disorders, educational needs, and family dysfunction paved the way for the consideration of other important realms of child health and functioning. These include child abuse and neglect, community violence, parental mental health, food insecurity, poverty, and socioeconomic disparity and social inequality.

**TABLE 28-1 ADVERSE CHILDHOOD EXPERIENCES**

| |
|---|
| Abuse |
| • Physical |
| • Emotional |
| • Sexual |
| Neglect |
| • Physical |
| • Emotional |
| Household Dysfunction |
| • Substance abuse |
| • Mental illness |
| • Violence against mother |
| • Parental separation/divorce |
| • Incarcerated household member |
| • Criminal behavior |

The lifelong impact of childhood adversity was most clearly reported in the landmark Adverse Childhood Experiences (ACE) Study in the late 1990s. This study linked childhood exposure to trauma and adversity, particularly the cumulative exposure, to multiple negative downstream health outcomes in adults. This study, which enrolled over 17,000 members of an employment-based health insurance plan, queried participants about their exposure to a list of ACEs including abuse, neglect, and household dysfunction such as parental substance abuse and having a family member become incarcerated. See Table 28-1 for a list of the original ACEs.

There were 2 main findings of the original ACE Study that transformed our appreciation and understanding of the importance of childhood adversity. First, the study found an extremely high prevalence of ACEs in its participants. Over 28% of subjects reported they had been physically abused in childhood, over 20% reported sexual abuse, and over 26% reported having lived with a substance-abusing adult as a child. Many subjects reported multiple ACEs, and a striking 12.5% reported 4 or more ACEs. The study linked the number of ACEs a person reported (the ACE score) to multiple negative health behaviors and morbidities in adulthood, such as depression, ischemic heart disease, obesity, intravenous drug use, and smoking.

The second important finding of the ACE Study was the dose-response relationship between childhood adversity and adult medical and psychosocial outcomes. The greater the adversity was, the worse the adult outcomes were. This gradient is a well-described phenomenon in public health. A graded and dose-related response to the degree of exposure to childhood trauma was found for all the negative health outcomes tracked in the ACE Study, and it has continued to be identified for over 40 negative health outcomes in adults exposed to childhood adversity. ACEs also are linked to limited academic attainment and poor graduation rates, as well to missed time at work. Importantly, ACEs are connected in a graded and dose-dependent fashion to early death. The gradient between childhood adversity and adult outcomes provides some insights into possible mechanisms of effect. The Center for Disease Control and Prevention (CDC) has constructed an ACE pyramid that illustrates this mechanism (Fig. 28-1). The risky behaviors manifested by those subjects with multiple ACEs can be understood in the context of untreated symptoms of trauma exposure. Nicotine, for example, is a powerful anxiolytic. Overeating and substance use can be employed to numb painful emotions. The more ACEs an adult reported having, the more likely that adult was to exhibit a risky behavior or have a medical problem in adulthood.

While the ACE Study was performed 2 decades ago, data published in 2016 demonstrated that a large national sample of children of all age ranges reported that they currently were experiencing similar levels and types of ACEs. This has prompted professional child-serving

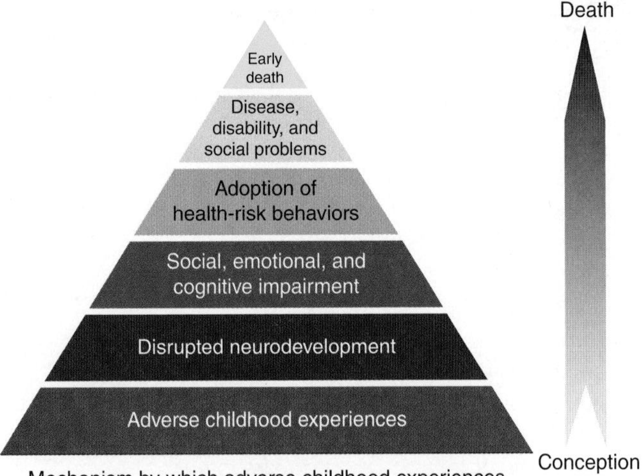


**FIGURE 28-1** Mechanism by which adverse childhood experiences influence health and well-being throughout the lifespan. (Reproduced with permission from Centers for Disease Control and Prevention. Adverse childhood experiences (ACEs). https://www.cdc.gov/violenceprevention/acestudy/index.html. Accessed September 30, 2016.)



agencies to begin to focus effort on childhood adversities. The American Academy of Pediatrics (AAP) endorses the ecobiodevelopmental framework for pediatricians to better understand the role of childhood adversity (Fig. 28-2). The cornerstone of the ecobiodevelopmental framework is *stress*. The dynamic construct of *toxic stress* provides insight into the mechanism by which exposure to adversity in childhood leads to adult health problems and dysfunction. Stress is a part of life for all children and all people, but stress can be categorized into 3 types. The first, *positive stress*, occurs when a child faces challenges that build resilience. Positive stress results in mild and transient activation of a child's hormonal response to stressors that are relatively easily overcome, such as that experienced by a child on the first day of preschool. Positive stress results from difficult but ultimately managed situations that teach a child that she or he can and will manage later stressors, which leads to resiliency. The presence of secure social

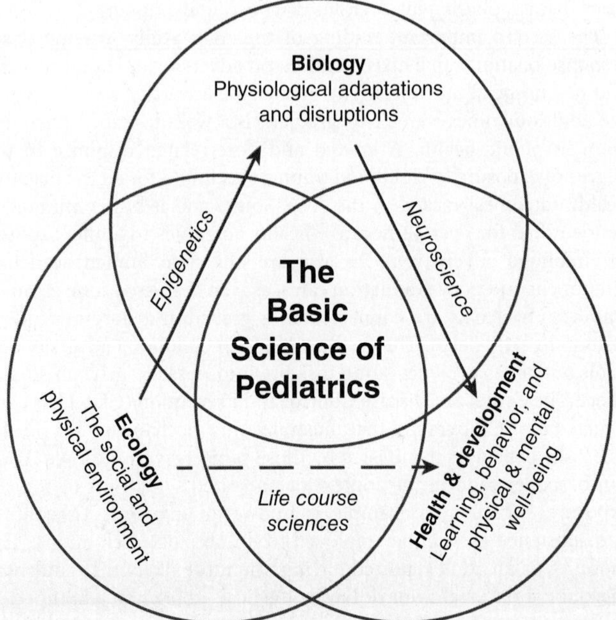


**FIGURE 28-2** The ecobiodevelopmental framework. (Reproduced with permission from Shonkoff JP et al. The lifelong effects of early childhood adversity and toxic stress, *Pediatrics*. 2012 Jan;129(1):e232-e246.)

and emotional buffering in the form of supportive adults adds to the likelihood that a given stressor may result in positive stress. *Tolerable stress* occurs when a child is exposed to a degree of adversity that is not overwhelming, in the setting of adequate social and emotional buffering. With tolerable stress, such as would occur with the death of a family member or during a natural disaster, the child's physical response to stress is stronger than with positive stress, but because it occurs in the context of adequate support, it does not have a long-lasting physical impact on the child. *Toxic stress* occurs when a child is exposed to severe or unremitting stress in the absence of adequate sources of buffering and support from adults. In toxic stress, the child's physical response to stress is overactivated, which leads to potentially permanent alterations in the way the child's genome is read (epigenetic changes), the way the HPA axis functions, and the child's brain structure.

Children may have both vulnerabilities and strengths that either protect them from toxic stress or predispose them to it. Children with medical complexities or disabilities, for example, as well as children with challenging temperaments, are even more vulnerable to toxic stress than are children without these challenges. Similarly, children with innate strengths and learned positive social and emotional behaviors (often referred to as *resilience* or *hardiness*) may be protected from toxic stress, often the result of increased adult support. The overall life well-being trajectory is determined by a continuous tension between adversities and resilience. Like children, families also have innate strengths and vulnerabilities. Families living in poverty or with a mentally ill or substance-abusing parent are inherently more vulnerable to toxic stress when exposed, for example, to the adversity of a natural disaster than would be a family not faced with these challenges. In this way, adverse events may generate either toxic or tolerable stress, depending on the strengths and vulnerabilities of a particular child or family. The toxic stress model advances what was previously understood about ACEs in that exposure to adversity alone does not determine the health and behavioral outcomes of that exposure for a child. Rather, these outcomes depend on the context in which the exposure occurs. (For further discussion of resilience, see Chapter 29.)

Severe and sustained adversity in the absence of adequate, protective adult support leads to toxic stress in children as a result of the plasticity of the growing brain (often attributed to the chronic effects of cortisol on the growing brain and body). The term *allostatic load* has been used to describe the body's degree of exposure to stress-activating events and the subsequent return to homeostasis when the stress-activating event has ceased. When activation is high and chronic and stress hormones are persistently elevated in the developing child, this can lead to permanent dysregulation in the body's stress response mechanisms. Overactivation of the stress response in children also can result in permanent alterations in epigenetic mechanisms, and to indelible changes in the architecture of the brain—specifically in the amygdala, the hippocampus, and the prefrontal cortex—leading to a lifelong impact on learning and resiliency.

## CLINICAL MANIFESTATIONS

Children exposed to trauma can exhibit a multitude of symptoms that affect their daily functioning. These symptoms are often behavioral, developmental, or social, and may range from subtle to obvious. Sleep may be impaired, with children experiencing difficulty falling and staying asleep as well as nightmares. Traumatized children may display dysfunctional eating behaviors, including food hoarding, rapid eating, loss of appetite, and lack of satiety. Abnormal toileting behaviors can include regression of previously obtained toileting skills, enuresis, constipation, and encopresis. Traumatized children may dissociate or become aggressive, be hypervigilant and anxious, or demonstrate an exaggerated response to even minor stress. Children may develop post-traumatic stress disorder (PTSD) and experience distressing memories of or flashbacks to traumatic events, emotional numbness, avoidant behavior, and difficulty concentrating. Traumatic exposure in the absence of adequate buffering also can lead to negative impact on a child's working memory, inhibitory control, and cognitive flexibility. Dysfunction in these arenas can limit a child's ability to learn, function in social settings, display self-control, and stay focused.

## DIAGNOSIS

Children exhibiting symptoms of trauma exposure may be misdiagnosed as having other developmental, psychological, or even psychiatric problems. For example, children who dissociate may be misdiagnosed as depressed, as having the inattentive form of attention-deficit disorder, or even to be developmentally delayed. Hypervigilant and aggressive children may be diagnosed with attention-deficit/hyperactivity disorder, conduct disorder, or oppositional defiant disorder, or as having anger management problems. Identifying victims of trauma is crucial in order for appropriate treatment to be provided to these children. Clinicians should have a low threshold to explore the possibility of trauma exposure in children exhibiting behavior dysfunction.

Traumatized children who exhibit behavior disturbance are best understood once the trauma exposure is identified because their dysfunctional behavior may be adaptive in another sphere. For example, a child exposed to intimate partner violence in his home may display hypervigilance and overarousal that, at home, may in fact be protective. That same behavior at preschool, however, is maladaptive and may be misdiagnosed.

## PREVENTION AND TREATMENT

Recognition of childhood adversity and an understanding of the potent health consequences of this adversity are important first steps for the pediatric provider to take. As noted earlier, the AAP has promoted the ecobiodevelopmental model of human health and disease (Fig. 28-2). This model and its policies direct the focus of health care toward positive community-based strategies for children in need. This model also combines the important roles of early experiences and exposures in a child's life (the ecology) with a given child's genetic makeup (the biology) in leading to the development of behaviors and health in adulthood that may be healthy or unhealthy and adaptive or maladaptive. The ecobiodevelopmental model also directs pediatric providers to move beyond simply recognizing morbidities in children and to identify and work to ameliorate sources of significant adversity in children's lives. Furthermore, the pediatric provider is in a potent position to shore up and strengthen parents and other adult caregivers in a child's life, thereby bolstering protection against the development of toxic stress in children exposed to adversity. Efforts to prevent domestic violence, or to teach positive parenting, may lead to more nurturing and safe environments for children, which can buffer against future adverse event exposures.

As there has been increased attention to the social determinants of health, there is more interest in screening tools that can be utilized within the healthcare setting to identify these "nonmedical" factors affecting patients' lives. Screening for adversity is a key responsibility of pediatric providers. Asking families, for example, about food insecurity can allow the pediatric provider to link needy families to local food banks. An example of 1 such tool is the Safe Environment for Every Kid (SEEK) program at the University of Maryland. This screening tool is a parent questionnaire for use in pediatric primary care clinics. The instrument screens for substance abuse, domestic violence, maternal depression, and parental stress, and then providers link parents to a social worker to help with these problems or directly to community services.

Once childhood adversity is identified, pediatric providers need resources with which to address specific problems and threats to health. Medical–legal partnerships (MLPs) are another example of how pediatric primary care can effectively link to community resources and embrace the ecobiodevelopmental model. MLPs embed lawyers and paralegals within health systems in order to address health-harming social problems. MLP staff may prevent homelessness by assisting families facing illegal eviction, help families to avoid having utilities such as heat shut off, and effectively address community health risks such as unsafe levels of lead in drinking water. MLPs also build capacity among providers both to recognize health-harming social problems early and to act to address such problems.

Many children will present to pediatric care with trauma-related symptoms or PTSD. After they are recognized by the pediatric practitioner, traumatized children may be referred to 1 of several evidence-based treatment modalities for PTSD. The most studied of these is trauma-focused cognitive behavioral therapy (TF-CBT), which has been shown to be effective in abused children, those exposed to domestic violence, those who have experienced grief, and victims of natural disasters and terrorist attacks. In this treatment model, traumatized children undergo gradual exposure to memories of the traumatic event(s) that they have experienced. A primary focus is the understanding of the ways in which the trauma can affect how a child feels and acts. TF-CBT helps both the child and the child's family to manage memories and feelings related to the trauma and teaches strategies to stay safe. Another key component of this treatment modality is the recounting of the child's trauma narrative, which may be accomplished by writing, drawing, or acting out what happened. TF-CBT has been shown to lessen PTSD symptoms, decrease fears, and improve social competence. The model also has demonstrated improvement in symptoms in the parents of traumatized children.

## SUMMARY

The world has changed dramatically for children and families since the times of the first American pediatrician, Dr. Abraham Jacobi, at the turn of the 20th century. While the diseases of yesteryear, such as diphtheria, tetanus, scurvy, and tuberculosis ("consumption") are, for the most part, in the rearview mirror, newly recognized threats and challenges to the well-being of children must be addressed and overcome. Although these adversities can be subtle and insidious, the *new morbidities* can have immediate and lifelong negative effects on the developing child. The crippling stress of living in poverty, with household or community violence, without adequate food, with familial mental illness, or with the effects of racism can embed in the makeup of children, and requires both careful surveillance and, once recognized, a meaningful, comprehensive response.

## SUGGESTED READINGS


American Academy of Pediatrics; Dave Thomas Foundation for Adoption. *Helping Foster and Adoptive Families Cope With Trauma.* 2015. https://www.aap.org/en-us/advocacy-and-policy/aap-health-initiatives/healthy-foster-care-america/documents/guide.pdf. Accessed September 30, 2016.

Centers for Disease Control and Prevention. Adverse childhood experiences (ACEs). https://www.cdc.gov/violenceprevention/acestudy/index.html. Accessed September 30, 2016.

Cohen JA, Mannarino AP, Deblinger E. *Treating Trauma and Traumatic Grief in Children and Adolescents.* New York, NY: Guilford Press; 2006.

Dubowitz H, Lane WG, Semiatin JN, Magder LS, Venepally M, Jans M. The safe environment for every kid model: impact on pediatric primary care professionals. *Pediatrics.* 2011;127(4):e962-e970.

Felitti VJ, Anda RF, Nordenberg D, et al. Relationship of childhood abuse and household dysfunction to many of the leading causes of death in adults: the Adverse Childhood Experiences (ACE) Study. *Am J Prev Med.* 1998;14(4):245-258.

Garner AS, Shonkoff JP; American Academy of Pediatrics Committee on Psychosocial Aspects of Child and Family Health; Committee on Early Childhood, Adoption, and Dependent Care; Section on Developmental and Behavioral Pediatrics. Early childhood adversity, toxic stress, and the role of the pediatrician: translating developmental science into lifelong health. *Pediatrics.* 2012;129(1):e224-e231.

Harvard University Center on the Developing Child. Toxic stress. http://developingchild.harvard.edu/science/key-concepts/toxic-stress/. Accessed September 30, 2016.

National Center for Medical Legal Partnership Web site. http://medical-legalpartnership.org/. Accessed September 30, 2016.

128 Shonkoff JP, Garner AS; American Academy of Pediatrics Committee on Psychosocial Aspects of Child and Family Health; Committee on Early Childhood, Adoption, and Dependent Care; Section on Developmental and Behavioral Pediatrics. The lifelong effects of early childhood adversity and toxic stress. *Pediatrics.* 2012;129(1):e232-e246.

# 29 Resiliency in Children and Adolescents

Cary Cain, Kimberly Kay Lopez, and Saul Levine

## INTRODUCTION

Resiliency is the ability to rebound from real, experienced adversity. It refers to an individual's use of inner strengths and outer resources to overcome seriously adverse, even traumatic, circumstances and still continue to pursue and succeed in one's endeavors. Resiliency varies according to personal hardiness and social supports, as well as the nature and degree of the imposed hardship or impediment. Refer to Chapter 28 for a discussion on adversity.

Research studies over the last three decades have shown that, even without therapeutic interventions, most at-risk children do remarkably well over the course of their lives. Contrary to absolutist opinions, a proportion of children who suffer early oppressive circumstances grow up to be productive, law-abiding, fulfilled, and generative adults. In a large population of children followed over 4 decades, it has been discovered that one-third of the most at-risk children, defined by having at least 4 early risk factors, such as poverty, family conflict, perinatal stress, and abuse, developed well personally, socially, and educationally. In another longitudinal study of 300 mother–infant dyads in which the mother was exposed to partner violence, it was found that the intergenerational impact of violence on the child's functioning was lessened by maternal self-efficacy and social support. Additional studies support the findings that children can overcome the lasting effects of adversity.

This chapter reviews the factors that impact the individual's makeup and determine his or her inherent resilience in relation to external and societal influences.

## POSITIVE ATTRIBUTES FOR RESILIENCE

Prospective studies indicate that there are consistent enhancing personal characteristics that contribute to resiliency. These include individual, familial, and community attributes and factors such as secure early attachments, physical health, interpersonal skills, self-awareness, supportive relationships, and access to services, as detailed in Table 29-1. These are cumulative in nature and positively enhance each other; the result is a strengthening of the individual's inner resolve. They are also bidirectional, in that a severe trauma or deficit can cause a decrease in the positive attributes. Although these positive attributes are correlated with personal resilience, none of the attributes by itself is uniquely sufficient to determine success.

## RISK FACTORS

The most salient finding demonstrated in many studies is that we can all meet our Waterloo—even the most resilient person can be downtrodden, degraded, and ultimately defeated if there is a sufficient confluence of risk factors and a concomitant absence of personally enhancing factors. Potential risk factors for psychosocial problems include poor pre- and perinatal care for the mother and child; abject poverty; abuse, neglect, and molestation; family discord; parental psychopathology; poor schools; lack of nurturing adults; absence of mentors; community violence; and occurrence of war or natural disasters during childhood, as detailed in Table 29-2. In addition, early

**TABLE 29-1 ATTRIBUTES THAT ARE POSITIVE FOR RESILIENCE**

| Individual Attributes and Factors | Description |
|---|---|
| Secure early attachments | Early attachment relationships provide a model for trust and are an important source of resilience and foster the ability for one to manage stress. |
| Temperament | A temperamental style that is fluid and easy acts as a facilitator of social involvement, adaptability, coping, belonging, and resilience. |
| Intelligence | A basic modicum of intellectual/cognitive skills is paramount to adequate comprehension and functioning. (Brilliance, however, does not guarantee exceptional resiliency skills.) |
| Health | Both physical health and emotional stability are correlated with coping skills and resilience. |
| Social attractiveness and social skills | Individuals with a positive interpersonal manner, who can interact with facility and warmth, who can read their companion's mood and receptivity, who have empathy for others' situations, who inspire confidence and trust, and who are engaging and communicative are much more likely to have help and opportunities proffered to them. |
| Self-awareness | Like empathy for others, the capacity to understand oneself, to recognize strengths and weaknesses, and to have some insight into one's own moods and relationships is of salient importance in dealing with adversity. |
| Optimism | Believing "the glass is half full" goes a long way toward enabling one to cope. |
| Sense of humor | To be able to laugh, to be amused by one's own foibles and frailties and by the vagaries of life, is a wonderfully enhancing attribute. |
| Purpose and planning (organization) | The most resilient individuals are seemingly more purposeful and committed to an organized, analytical approach and to a sequential plan of dealing with difficulties or challenges and resolving problems. |
| Productivity | Resilient people tend to be dedicated workers and task-oriented, with an eye on successful fulfillment and completion of duties and responsibilities. |
| Compartmentalization | This attribute enables individuals to cope with the inevitable vicissitudes of life by temporarily walling off or circumscribing worries about other significant problems in their lives so that they do not become debilitated. |
| Recreation | This refers to the ability to play, relax, and enjoy one's leisure time, and appreciate the time and space afforded by lack of time- and task-inspired duties and demands. |
| Approachability | While this is related to the social-skills characteristic, it more specifically refers to the ability to respond to another's offer of help during a particularly tough time. |
| **Familial Attributes and Factors** | **Description** |
| Supportive relationships | Positive child–caregiver relationships |
| Networks | Relationships with extended family members and peers |
| Stability | Stable living environment |
| Health | Healthy caregivers |
| **Community Attributes and Factors** | **Description** |
| Access to services | Basic needs, advocacy, and health services |
| Schools | Positive school climate, social supports, and fosters educational attainment |
| Neighborhood cohesion | Safe and connected neighborhood communities, positive organizations, and emergency services |

**TABLE 29-2 NEGATIVE ENVIRONMENTAL FACTORS FOR RESILIENCE: RISK FACTORS FOR PSYCHOSOCIAL PROBLEMS**

| Factor | Impact |
|---|---|
| Poor pre-, peri-, and postnatal care of mother and child | Highly implicated in cognitive, behavioral, or emotional dysfunction |
| Abject poverty | Adds deprivation and stress on families, making coping more difficult and diminishing opportunities for personal growth |
| Abuse, neglect, and molestation | Remarkably associated with difficult development and later manifestation of symptoms |
| Family discord | Imposes an environment of chaos and instability on children, who benefit most from stability, predictability, and nurturance |
| Parental psychopathology | If not treated or managed, affects offspring either by genetic vulnerability or by adding to the chaos and turmoil |
| Inadequate/poor schools | Underperforming schools do not provide the child the educational foundation for academic or career success. |
| Lack of significant nurturing adults | Perhaps the most salient, crucial loss of all the necessary ingredients in the life of a child |
| Absence of mentors and models | Related to the above but is often adjunctive or can even serve as a surrogate or replacement, especially for older youth |
| War/culture of violence and chaos | Impacts the prevalence of mental health disorders, especially post-traumatic stress disorder |
| Natural disasters | Can destroy families, inflict brutalizing injuries and losses, and remove any semblance of stability |

risk factors can potentiate each other, allowing cumulative risk to be magnified, and the chances of symptomatology or dysfunction are in turn significantly increased. However, none of these risks individually is predictive of inevitable problems. Many of the external stressors and burdens in Table 29-2 coexist and interact in a cumulative manner. Conversely, most of these risk factors can be significantly ameliorated or even overcome with the presence of protective factors.

## POSITIVE EMOTIONAL FACTORS FOR RESILIENCE

In studies of youth and young adults in a variety of settings, and in research interviews with the elderly population, 4 psychosocial determinants were found when individuals evaluated self-perceived satisfaction and worth of one's life (Table 29-3).

**TABLE 29-3 THE TETRAD OF Bs**

| Determinant | Description |
|---|---|
| Being (personal) | One's self-image and accommodation to one's sense of identity: It includes an appreciation of strengths and an awareness of limitations, and it reflects a perception of being "grounded," or comfortable in one's skin. |
| Belonging (social) | A sense of being an integral, accepted, appreciated part of a community: It is more than merely being with like-minded people; support and nurturance are necessary. It encompasses the sharing of noteworthy personal (pain and pleasure) experiences, mutual empathy, common goals, and a sense of being affiliated and "connected" in a basic, meaningful way. |
| Believing (ideological) | The sense of having a personal overriding system of values and principles of life, beyond the everyday mundane aspects of living: This is especially so beyond unbridled competition, materialism, and acquisitiveness. It refers to a higher order raison d'être, a moral compass, and even a spiritual guide (although it need not be religious in nature). |
| Benevolence (altruism) | The degree to which an individual is authentically generous and generative: It is related to being, belonging, and believing and depends on the existence of others. This is the ultimate criterion in the personal evaluation of one's self-image—the extent of self-initiated mentoring and magnanimity; caring for and charity to others; being nurturing and supportive; giving of one's self for the benefit of family, friends, the less fortunate, and so on. This is particularly meaningful in the healing process following deprivation, where a battered individual is still committed to sharing, giving, and mentoring. |

In children and adolescents who have risk factors that are potentially detrimental to development, a variety of factors appear to foster the development of a sense of personal satisfaction and fulfillment that improves their later coping skills. These include the following:

- *A primary attachment.* The single most important factor in an infant's life is the bond formed with a primary caretaker. This is the foundation of an awareness that needs can be met, comfort can be provided, pain can be alleviated, and self-regulation can be achieved.
- *Love.* Love in childhood represents affection, appreciation, nurturance, commitment, dedicated time, interest, and caring—all constant reminders of being regarded as a vital presence.
- *Limits.* Rules, laws, and consequences define expectations and, by implication, the boundaries of safety and social interaction in every community.
- *Stimulation.* Without stimulation of the senses through visual, auditory, olfactory, and tactile explorations and cognitive stimulation, the child lacks opportunities to learn, inquire, and discover.
- *Relationships with peers.* Contacts with family, friends, and companions help a child to answer questions like "Where do I fit in?" "What am I all about?" and "Who am I?"
- *Models and mentors.* Older peers or trustworthy adults can guide, counsel, and inspire a child or youth.
- *Space.* Children need both physical and emotional privacy, and they need physical space for exploration. Space to be alone, to experiment, to fantasize, and to make mistakes is necessary, within limits of safety, for their self-regulated social and emotional development.
- *Respect.* By modeling civility in everyday discourse and empathy for others, respect is evident in words and deeds and can be "transferred" to future generations.
- *Consistency.* Children need a sense of predictability, stability, routine, and ritual. They need to know that those who care for them are reliable, dependable, and stable and are there in good times and in bad.
- *Responsibilities.* Holding children responsible for certain obligations invites them to share in the adult's reality, teaches mutual dependence, and dispels the notion of a perpetual free ride.
- *Safety and subsistence.* Freedom from fear and want is a prerequisite of freedom for growth, exploration, and opportunity.
- *Opportunities.* All children should have access to quality medical care, education, recreational activities, and vocational choice.
- *Traditions.* Ritual and repetitive family, cultural, or religious events enhance the present, enrich the future, and endow the past with a sense of continuity and community.
- *Altruism.* To receive or bestow a kindness can be a moving experience for anyone, at any age. Children model their parents' generosity and altruism.
- *Values.* Young people need to be inspired and to believe in a reason for being. Idealism can more readily be kindled in youth than at any other time in life.

## FOSTERING RESILIENCE

This leads us to the most crucial and salient question on the concept of resiliency. Given that (1) individuals can recover from adversity and go on to lead meaningful productive lives; (2) there are social risk factors associated with the appearance of personal difficulties, symptoms, and maladaptive or destructive behaviors; and (3) there are equally well-documented personal characteristics that are shared by those who demonstrate resiliency in their personal trajectories, are there active preventive and interventional programs that can help foster

**TABLE 29-4 APPROACHES USED BY SUCCESSFUL PREVENTION AND INTERVENTION PROGRAMS**

| Approach | Description |
| --- | --- |
| Family-centered programs | Utilizing parent support, parental training and education, babysitting, respite care, recreational activities, hotlines, case management, parent groups, child support, advocacy, and welfare |
| School-centered programs | Using good teaching (teachers, space, materials), tutoring, special education classes, counseling programs, health centers, after-school programs, and parental involvement |
| Neighborhood-centered programs | Removal of firearms; use of safety committees, block parents (crime prevention), community-based institutions (church, school, recreation centers), police patrol, mentorship programs, and parental involvement |
| Private sector | Use of apprentice programs, paid/part-time and summer jobs, educational equivalency credits, at-school presentations, tours and visits, mentorships, and parental involvement |
| Police, corrections | Use of visits to schools, "cop-on-the-beat" programs, friendship emphasis (as opposed to purely punitive), tours of facilities, community officers, and recreational programs |
| Effective therapeutic interventions | For children with serious disorders and high-risk circumstances, a child-centered aggregation of parents, case managers, physicians, nurses, social workers, teachers, librarians, neighbors, police, recreation supervisors, and employers; any or all of those listed above in this table, as dictated by the individual child's needs |

resiliencies? Such programs will need to prospectively demonstrate efficacy by significantly reducing social risk factors, ameliorating personal distress and debilitating behaviors, significantly improving the resiliency potential of individuals at risk, and dramatically improving the outcomes of children. A key component in interventional programs designed to improve resiliency in children, adolescents, and adults is the presence of at least one supportive relationship that allows for capacity building of coping skills.

Fortunately, such programs do exist. Numerous prospective studies confirm the positive effects of early interventions in children and adolescents (eg, Carolina Abecedarian Project, National Scientific Council on the Developing Child, HighScope Educational Research Foundation, Center on the Developing Child). These programs have shown that early childhood education from infancy through age 5 years results in improved long-term outcomes for at-risk children.

However, implementing these protective interventions requires a *societal commitment* due to their expense. All these programs involve similar approaches (Table 29-4).

## PROTECTIVE FACTORS FRAMEWORK

Pediatricians have ongoing access to children and their parents; therefore, they have the opportunity to promote resilience. The AAP recommends that pediatricians identify and increase protective factors to reduce risk and create optimal outcomes for all children, adolescents, and families. These protective factors include:

- Parental resilience
  - Assess parents' mental health, including postpartum depression, and encourage positive coping strategies for stress reduction.
- Social connections
  - Offer parenting groups or support parents to form positive connections with others.
- Knowledge of parenting and child development
  - Provide anticipatory guidance and share knowledge on realistic expectations of the child based on his or her developmental stage.
- Concrete support in times of need
  - Assist parents in navigating available resources in the community, such as family resource centers, parent education programs, home visiting programs, food pantries, and support groups.
- Social and emotional competence of children
  - Help parents understand the importance of attachment and social and emotional development with their child and provide resources to assist them in nurturing that development.

## LESSONS LEARNED REGARDING RESILIENCE

From many studies of resilience and interviews with resilient individuals, the following salient and instructive lessons have been learned:

- Early trauma and destitution do not inevitably lead to permanent scarring and debilitation.
- Early devastating trauma can take many forms: severe, acute, or chronic illness; abject poverty; brutality; abuse; natural disasters (earthquakes, floods, fire, landslides, drought, hurricanes); persecution; omnipresent danger and fear. The nature and severity of the trauma, the presence or absence of internal and external resources, and the immediate and subsequent mobilization of these resources determine the quality of the coping process and the resiliency of the individual.
- Nobody is invulnerable. All children and adults have their limitations and breaking points. Given an existing stress or, more often, a confluence of different stressors with sufficient severity, any individual can succumb to these oppressive forces and become debilitated.
- Few are helpless. Almost all children, adolescents, and adults have some resources (biopsychosocial fortifications) that can be strengthened and built upon to enhance their resiliency potential.
- Nobody does it alone. In cases of resilience, it has been found that there is at least one crucial individual who took an interest and served as a nurturer or mentor to help recalibrate a corrective trajectory.
- Individuals have different levels of personal resources and levels of tolerance for stress.
- The resilient individual utilizes social skills, trust, initiative, and motivation to grasp the extended arm.
- Even those resilient people who have thrived after calamitous losses will have suffered some ill effects down the road.
- The presence of a personally committed, consistent, nurturing caregiver in the first year of life is a vital advantage to any child.
- As risk factors increase in a population, so, too, does the appearance of deleterious problems in children and adolescents.
- As resources (preventive or interventional) develop in a community, at-risk children and adults manifest increased evidence of coping skills and resilience.
- It does, indeed, take a village to raise a child (Zulu proverb).

In this era of seemingly omnipresent conflicts, turmoil, and wars, humanity does have the capacity to take a quantum leap forward in assuring the health-promoting growth and development of children. This can be done by enhancing children's innate resources and, in turn, by capturing their resiliency, fostering their maturation into adults who can maximize their potential and contribute significantly to society and to themselves.

## SUGGESTED READINGS


American Academy of Pediatrics Committee on Psychosocial Aspects of Child and Family Health. The new morbidity revisited: a renewed commitment to the psychosocial aspects of pediatric care. *Pediatrics.* 2001;108(5):1227-1230.

American Academy of Pediatrics Committee on Psychosocial Aspects of Child and Family Health; Committee on Early Childhood, Adoption, and Dependent Care; Section on Developmental and Behavioral Pediatrics. Early childhood adversity, toxic stress, and the role of the pediatrician: translating developmental science into lifelong health. *Pediatrics.* 2012;129(1):e224-e231.

Dubowitz H, Thompson R, Proctor L, et al. Adversity, maltreatment, and resilience in young children. *Acad Pediatr*. 2016;16(3):233-239.

Felitti V, Anda R. Relationship of childhood abuse and household dysfunction to many of the leading causes of death in adults: the Adverse Childhood Experiences (ACE) Study. *Am J Prev Med*. 1998;14(4):245-258.

Garmezy N. Resilience in children's adaptation to negative life events and stressed environments. *Pediatr Ann*. 1991;20(9):459-466.

Levine S. *Against Terrible Odds: Lessons in Resilience from Our Children*. Palo Alto, CA: Bull Publishing Co; 2002.

Masten AS. Promoting resilience in development: a general framework for systems of care. In: Flynn RJ, Dudding PM, Barber JG, eds. *Promoting Resilience in Child Welfare*. Ottawa, Canada: University of Ottawa Press; 2006:3-17.

National Scientific Council on the Developing Child. Supportive relationships and active skill-building strengthen the foundations of resilience: Working Paper No. 13; 2015. http://developingchild.harvard.edu/resources/supportive-relationships-and-active-skill-building-strengthen-the-foundations-of-resilience/. Accessed October 10, 2017.

Shonkoff JP. Building a new biodevelopmental framework to guide the future of early childhood policy. *Child Dev*. 2010;81(1):357-367.

Werner E. Vulnerable but invincible: high-risk children from birth to adulthood. *Acta Paediatr*. 1997;86(S422):103-105.

# 30 Poverty, Homelessness, and Social Disorganization

Barry S. Zuckerman and Aura M. Obando

## POVERTY AND CHILD DEVELOPMENT

Children who live in poor families face profound challenges to their health, development, and educational achievement. These challenges lead to increased rates of illness, developmental delays, behavioral problems, school failure, and social dysfunction. Poverty, adverse exposures, and unmet basic needs amplify the impact of biological vulnerabilities on the child. However, as with other threats to health and development, the effects of poverty can be offset by individual, family, community, and professional buffering factors that offer both protection and support. Pediatricians are in a prime position to screen for poverty-related complications and offer support through appropriate community referrals in order to mitigate the long-term detrimental consequences of poverty

## THE EPIDEMIOLOGY OF POVERTY

The federal poverty level (FPL) is derived from the estimated cost of food multiplied by 3; this is based on the assumption that food accounts for one-third of a family's income after taxes, which for a family of four with two children in 2015 was $24,036 or less. The level was adjusted for size of household but not for regional variations in cost of living or actual expenditures and income. The 2014 Census data reported that 15.5 million children under the age of 18, or 21.1% of all US children, were considered to reside in "poor" households (ie, those with incomes below 100% of the FPL). Children living in "deep poverty" (50% of the FPL) numbered 6.8 million, or 9.3% of children in the United States. Even families whose incomes are twice the federal poverty level have trouble making ends meet. Thirty-one million children live in such "low-income" families. Poverty disproportionally affects children of color: 33% of all black children (3.6 million), 27% of all Latino children (4 million), and 40% of American Indian children (200,000) live in poverty, as compared to 10% of white children (4.2 million). Poverty may be cyclical for families, a brief experience, or a prolonged state, and as a result, about 37% of US children will experience poverty at some point during their childhood.



## THE DIMENSIONS OF POVERTY

The concept of "poverty" encompasses insufficient income and the range of conditions that poor families endure. Poverty's impact varies, depending on whether it is normative within a given society; urban or rural; brief, intermittent, or chronic; relative; or at a level that compromises physical survival. Income inequality is now thought to be a more sensitive indicator of health problems than mean income is. This may be mediated through social marginalization, or the end product of the experience of social inequalities such as poor schools, poor health services, and poor homes. Some US families may have members who are disabled by mental illness, substance use disorders, or other chronic conditions, and local economic stagnation or systemic racism may limit their access to educational opportunities, quality healthcare, and better jobs, leading to multigenerational poverty.

Families in such variable settings experience different social environments and have different expectations for themselves and for their children. For example, families who fall under the poverty level for shorter periods because of transient unemployment may have more economic and psychological reserves with which to endure poverty's effects than families who have been in poverty for several generations. Families living in urban poverty have increased exposure to lead, violence, household allergens, and airborne pollutants, while rural families typically have less access to the array of supportive agencies that may be available in cities. As the demographics of poverty shift, resources must be adapted in order to meet new needs.

## RISKS AND PROTECTIVE FACTORS IN POVERTY

The biomedical risks of poverty affect children starting prenatally and are compounded by the ongoing social environment of poverty. The stress of poverty can lead to poor maternal mental health, reducing maternal responsiveness and subsequently reducing social and verbal interactions between mother and child. Witnessing violence in the home is a significant source of potentially toxic stress, which leads to prolonged activation of the hypothalamic–pituitary–adrenal (HPA) axis and can result in chronic trauma symptoms. Substance use disorders arise as maladaptive coping mechanisms to poverty, and not only perpetuate poverty but often lead to dangerous or neglectful child-rearing situations. These risk factors, which can be cumulative, impair the child's brain development, behavior, learning, and resiliency, and are associated with worse health outcomes for both parents and children. Take for example a child who is born prematurely to a depressed mother, is exposed to second-hand smoke, suffers from inadequate nutrition due to insufficient household income, and is subjected to conflict and violence due to parental stress. This child is at high risk for early language delay, poor self-regulation, subsequent learning problems, and school failure, along with health problems such as iron deficiency anemia and asthma. Such a child is less likely to succeed in school or at work unless these risks are either prevented or recognized, and treatment, including early intervention, and appropriate community support are provided.

Although families living in poverty face many obstacles, they can also develop protective factors that serve as buffers when faced with adversity. Pediatricians should approach families from a strengths-based perspective, helping them identify assets on which they can draw during times of economic and social hardship, such as spiritual beliefs, individual resilience, resourcefulness, or special skills. Poor families can also mitigate the stressors associated with poverty by developing strong and flexible networks among extended family and friends, and among community resources such as churches and neighborhood associations. These networks can provide assistance with childcare, a sense of belonging, and help with practical needs such as food and shelter. The ability to form such relationships (social capital) is critical to the survival of families in poverty.

## THE IMPACT OF POVERTY ON CHILDREN AND FAMILIES

Prolonged poverty fosters a number of coping styles that are maladaptive in other settings. For example, children who are raised in poorer families may be socialized for early independence and toughness, traits that are adaptive to their neighborhood, if not for school. Poor children of school age are less likely to participate in extracurricular activities, and missing these activities is associated with antisocial behavior and lower scores on standardized tests. Furthermore, living amid a culture that has much higher material expectations, chronically poor families endure a sense of persistent helplessness and hopelessness, which can grow into a depression and anxiety that can be as debilitating as the lack of access to goods or services.

Without the buffer of loving, positive relationships, living in poverty can lead to toxic stress: a disruption of neuronal connections in the brain, maladaptive coping strategies, and fragmented social supports, all leading to poor health (diabetes and cardiovascular disease, substance use disorders) and poor socioeconomic outcomes (school failure, financial difficulties). Pediatricians can advocate for interventions that reduce the effect of toxic stress, such as referrals to mental health services for parents as well as children, particularly at school age or adolescence. Providing trauma-informed, compassionate care to patients also promotes trusting relationships that buffer stress, and facilitates the identification of the source of the stressors.

The effects of poverty also influence parents' behavior and create many pathways for poor child health. Parents in poor families may read less to their young children, which contributes to lack of school readiness. Low-income or poverty status can also lead to parents having to make budget trade-offs, such as deciding whether to pay for food or for heating their house. Research shows increased hunger and malnutrition in the winter compared to the summer, a phenomenon called "heat or eat." Also, children from families that are on waiting lists for housing subsidies are more likely to have nutrition problems as compared to children who received such subsidies.

The persistently high levels of stress that are associated with poverty undermine parents' physical and mental health as well, leading to high rates of stress-related medical conditions (such as hypertension and asthma) and psychological problems (such as depression, anxiety, troubled relationships, and substance use disorders). Parental stress may interfere with daily interactions that are needed to establish trust, safety, a sense of cause and effect, and the ability to express curiosity, and contributes to abuse and neglect. The ability to climb out of poverty can be limited by joblessness, particularly of fathers, which is linked to domestic violence and child abuse. In addition, many institutions that are intended to serve poor families (eg, welfare and public housing agencies) impose further stress through demeaning and time-consuming hurdles. These stressors can impact the parental ability to provide a sensitive and nurturant environment that optimizes brain development, and this may have a lifelong impact as discussed in Chapter 28.

## FOOD INSECURITY

Poor families often struggle with food insecurity, due to their tenuous financial state, making it difficult at times to purchase nutritious meals. Food insecurity has been associated with poor overall child health, more hospitalizations, lower bone density, lower cognitive indicators, dysregulated behavior, and developmental problems. The health impacts of early childhood food insecurity can persist into adulthood, with associations between childhood malnutrition and adult diabetes, hyperlipidemia, and cardiovascular disease. There are multiple programs in place on both state and national levels to mitigate the effects of food insecurity, including the Women, Infants, and Children (WIC) program, the Supplemental Nutritional Assistace Program (SNAP), and the National School Lunch Program. The American Academy of Pediatrics currently recommends that pediatricians screen all patients for food insecurity, familiarize themselves with local resources in case a problem is identified, and advocate for improved access to nutritious food at the local and national policy levels.

## HOMELESS CHILDREN AND FAMILIES

Stable, safe housing is necessary for children's health and development. It has been estimated that there are currently 2.5 million children in the United States who are experiencing homelessness, representing 1 in every 30 children in the United States. Homelessness and housing instability are associated with several negative biomedical and psychosocial outcomes, including injuries, lead poisoning, higher rates of asthma and respiratory illnesses, stunted growth, higher rates of developmental delays and learning disabilities, early onset of mental health problems, and higher rates of exposure to physical and sexual abuse.

Homeless children cannot count on a quiet place to sleep or a safe place to play and learn. They do not have the security of regular routines, and their parents are often stressed and preoccupied by the struggle to survive and obtain housing. They may spend their days on the streets and their nights in cars or doorways, or they may live in homeless shelters or motels. Such shelters can be noisy and dangerous, often infested and unclean, leaving children tired and hypervigilant when and if they reach school. Shelters and motels often restrict families' abilities to prepare meals by limiting cooking implements to microwaves and mini-refrigerators, making conditions such as obesity, insulin resistance, and hypertension nearly impossible to manage. Because shelter placement tends to prioritize availability over location of origin, children and families are often distanced from their medical homes. As such, access to medical care becomes further impaired given limited income to use toward transportation expenses. Homeless children also experience disruptions in schooling due to frequent moves in the setting of housing instability and within the shelter system, leading to poor educational outcomes. Given that homeless families are able to provide an address where they are being sheltered, and due to shame around overtly reporting homeless status, these children often go unrecognized as homeless. As such, it is imperative to conduct screening around housing instability/homelessness at medical visits in order to mobilize the appropriate resources to support these incredibly vulnerable children.

## THE ROLE OF HEALTHCARE PROVIDERS FOR POOR CHILDREN

Although adequate health care can buffer children from some of the adverse consequences of poverty, broad-based social policies that can provide for basic needs such as food, affordable housing, and income support have the greatest potential to attenuate these consequences. Gaps in the implementation of available programs and policies are well documented. In addition to providing preventive and acute medical care and supportive relationships, healthcare providers can screen and advocate for unmet basic needs. Programs such as Health Leads and We Care, implemented in primary care settings, connect families to community-based resources that address key unmet needs. It is also important for child healthcare providers to identify and refer problems of maternal mental health (depression and trauma), poor health behaviors (cigarette smoking and substance use disorders), and unmet family planning needs.

The American Academy of Pediatrics has put forth policy statements with recommendations around the care of children in poverty, homeless families, food insecurity, and early childhood adversity. Table 30-1 provides an outline of social history screening questions that focus on basic needs and on factors that influence health and are amenable to direct intervention. While social workers, case managers, or other members of the healthcare team help families with these unmet basic needs, attorneys have been added to the pediatric healthcare team in a growing number of health settings. Legal professionals have the knowledge and skills to address many of the social determinants of poor health associated with poverty; in fact, poor people have been shown to have three to four unmet legal needs. Disenfranchised families facing multiple crises generally have difficulties convincing community agencies, landlords, or government agencies of their eligibility. Medical–legal partnerships, healthcare providers partnering with lawyers, can be particularly effective voices for such families and their children, whether through individual advocacy or through policy-related research.

**TABLE 30-1 EXAMPLES OF POTENTIAL SOCIAL HISTORY QUESTIONS: "I HELLP" TO ADDRESS BASIC NEEDS**

| Domain | Areas | Examples of Questions |
|---|---|---|
| Income | General | Do you ever have trouble making ends meet? |
| | Food income | Is there ever a time when you don't have enough food? |
| | | Do you have WIC? Food stamps? |
| Housing | Housing | Is your housing ever a problem for you? |
| | Utilities | Do you ever have trouble paying your electric/heat/phone bill? |
| Education | Appropriate school placement | How is your child doing in school? |
| | | Is he/she getting the help to learn what he/she needs? |
| | Early childhood program | Is your child in Head Start or preschool or other early childhood enrichment? |
| Legal status | Immigration | Do you have questions about your immigration status? |
| | | Do you need help accessing benefits or services for your family? |
| Literacy | Child literacy | Do you read to your child every night? |
| | Parent literacy | How happy are you with how you read? |
| Personal safety | Domestic violence | Have you ever taken out a restraining order? |
| | | Do you feel safe in your relationship? |
| | General safety | Do you feel safe in your home? Neighborhood? |

Reproduced with permission from Kenyon C, Sandel M, Silverstein M, Shakir A, Zuckerman B. Revisiting social history for children, *Pediatrics.* 2007 Sep;120(3):e734-e738.

## SUGGESTED READINGS

American Academy of Pediatrics Council on Community Pediatrics. Poverty and child health in the United States. *Pediatrics.* 2016:137(4):e20160339.

American Academy of Pediatrics Council on Community Pediatrics. Providing care for children and adolescents facing homelessness and housing insecurity. *Pediatrics.* 2013;131(6):1206-1210.

American Academy of Pediatrics Council on Community Pediatrics, Committee on Nutrition. Promoting food security for all children. *Pediatrics.* 2015:136(5):e1431-e1438.

Garner AS, Shonkoff JP; Committee on Psychosocial Aspects of Child and Family Health; Committee on Early Childhood, Adoption, and Dependent Care; Section on Developmental and Behavioral Pediatrics. Early childhood adversity, toxic stress, and the role of the pediatrician: translating developmental science into lifelong health. *Pediatrics.* 2012;129(1):e224-e231.

Hair NL, Hanson JL, Wolfe BL, Pollack SD. Association of child poverty, brain development, and academic achievement. *JAMA Pediatrics.* 2015;169(9):822-829.

Halfon N, Wise PH, Forrest CB. The changing nature of children's health development: new challenges require major policy solutions. *Health Aff.* 2014;33(12):2116-2124.

# 31 Family Discord and Divorce

Michael Jellinek

## INTRODUCTION

Chronic parental discord and divorce can have profound, long-lasting effects on children. A child's need to be loved, to be cared for, and to be a central priority of both parents is often shattered by seeing parents frequently sad, clinically depressed, unavailable (emotionally and/or physically), and preoccupied by their personal anger. If the tension leads to divorce, and especially if the discord continues after divorce, children may feel insecure, suffer diminished self-esteem, and not trust that love and attachment to others is reliable. The severity of long-term consequences may be considerably ameliorated if parents can focus on their love of the child in the midst of their own discord and loss. It is critical to remember that marriages can end, but parenting is forever.

Family discord and divorce are common in pediatric practice, with many divorces occurring in the first 5 to 10 years of marriage. The divorce rate per thousand marriages is at the highest during child-bearing years.

Divorce is the loss of the family unit, and its impact can be divided into 3 broad areas. One area is the child's psychological development. Divorce makes a strong statement that relationships once thought to represent the definition of stability may be unreliable and that the expectation of a permanent family unit can be lost. The second impact relates to parental functioning. Fathers and mothers in the midst of discord and divorce often suffer depression and anger, are preoccupied for many months or years with the divorce process, and are no longer spontaneously available in the same home. The third area is financial. The same family resources are now spread over 2 households, and additional, often major, expenses accrue in lawyer fees and other unanticipated costs. Most families cannot sustain a major increase in monthly expense, and over time, mothers often suffer the more serious financial harm.

Pediatricians should screen family functioning ("On a scale of 1 to 10, with 10 being most satisfied, rate your overall satisfaction in your marriage?" Or, "Are there ongoing tensions or arguments within your marriage or family?") as part of every annual physical. This question will help pediatricians be aware of discord, pending divorces, changes in living circumstances and custody, and remarriages. Knowing the impact of divorce and related life changes offers opportunities to assess the risks for the child and parent and then give anticipatory guidance or, if there is intense discord, referral for mental health services.

## EXPECTED PSYCHOLOGICAL REACTIONS

Parents may ask whether it is better to stay married for the sake of the children than to put them through a divorce. The answer depends on the intensity of the marital discord and the quality of relationships after the divorce is finalized. The tensions in discordant marriages may result in verbal or physical confrontations, compound other psychological problems such as depression or substance use, and create a bitter emotional tone in the home. Children who live with chronic family discord, tension, and unhappiness become vigilant as to how their parents are feeling and assume responsibility for trying to relieve tension and unhappiness. Many children wonder if they are causing the problems, why one or both parents are so unhappy, and experience the impact of the marital tension on their relationship with each parent. Over time, these children often harbor intense anger at their parents and grow up distrustful of, yet longing for, intimacy. Thus, as young adults, they may feel unable to tolerate intimacy, or they may begin their own marriages dominated by the ghosts related to their parents' discord. If the divorce ends chronic discord, abuse, neglect, and domestic violence (sadly, this is not always the outcome), and the quality of the child's relationship to one or both parents is positive, then the child or adolescent may actually be relieved and benefit from the divorce.

For parents, divorce represents a loss of initial marital hopes, the initial dream for an adult life, and the family unit. Dashed hopes, selfish behavior, scorn, substance use, or infidelity may fuel one spouse's intense anger and disappointment about the other. As a consequence of this rage, some parents prioritize hurting their spouse and fail to see the needs of the children. Such parents may become preoccupied with divorce issues embedded in rage and may become clinically depressed. The consequences are a deteriorating relationship with their children, poor judgement, use of substances, and great risk of "accidents" due to lack of parental oversight.

The anger between parents can spill into the pediatrician's office during a visit or through requests by one parent to protect the child from the other, which may or may not be valid (eg, true risk of danger from parental abuse, neglect, or substance use versus using the pediatrician as a tool to express anger or in a shortsighted, legal strategy). During the divorce, and often for a year or more thereafter, both parents will undergo a difficult period of grieving often characterized by depression, anger, and preoccupation that can impact their relationship with their children.

For the child, divorce is a loss that is re-experienced with varying intensity throughout childhood, adolescence, and adulthood in their own relationships and parenting. Some children recall feelings of loss when they see well-functioning two-parent families and during events such as birthdays, holidays, graduation, or college visits. Some will carry into their own relationships what they saw and felt in their parents' marriage, including longings, self-esteem, expectations, and how they treat others they care about. While many children experience difficulty adjusting, commonly evidenced by lowered school performance in the first year of divorce, those exposed to ongoing discord generally experience sustained emotional difficulties and dysfunction through adolescence and young adulthood and commonly require mental health services.

The causes of the divorce and the child's perspective of each parent are questioned, reframed, and grieved again at major development transitions, such as when the young adolescent starts high school, achieves varsity status on a team, begins to date, considers moving away from home for college or work, falls in love as a young adult, marries, and becomes a parent.

The specific impact of the divorce on children depends in part on their developmental level. Infants and toddlers are heavily influenced by the emotional state of the caregivers; thus, these children suffer most overtly when their custodial parent (most commonly their mother) is preoccupied, overwhelmed, or clinically depressed. Children under 3 years old require special consideration in terms of visitation, because they have less tolerance for long absences, especially if one parent is the predominant caregiver.

Children 4 and 5 years old, although more verbal, have important cognitive limitations on their ability to understand concepts, longer time frames, and thus the implications of a divorce. These children have a rich fantasy life, and their limited understanding of causality facilitates their taking responsibility for most of what happens, including parental discord. Children in this age group may feel guilty about having caused the divorce and parental tension, which is reinforced by any overheard arguments.

School-aged children can begin to understand more realistically and in concrete terms the issues causing and related to the divorce. These children often feel caught in loyalty conflicts, wishing their parents would reunite and wondering about whether the parents would have divorced if they (ie, the children) had been "better." School-aged children often are moody and preoccupied by the divorce, and boys, for example, are commonly more aggressive, especially toward their mother. The sources of this increased aggression may be the inherent propensity for boys to be more aggressive, a mother's depression or vulnerability, the son possibly eliciting some of the mother's unresolved anger toward her husband, longings for the father, or a father's conscious or unconscious encouragement of anger toward the mother.

Older school-aged children and adolescents may react less directly, such as with increasing complaints of psychosomatic disorders, which may be an emotional solution to avoiding angry feelings directed at the parents or reflecting their helplessness during the divorce. A secondary result of both psychosomatic symptoms and oppositional behavior might be to gain the attention of both parents, sometimes jointly, such as during medical visits when worry about a potential illness temporarily replaces parental tensions or when meeting with a school principal focuses the parents' attention on the child's behavior.

Although adolescents have the cognitive capacity to understand the divorce process, they are at a particularly vulnerable point in the process of developing their own sense of autonomy, identity, and capacity for intimacy. This process of separation and identity formation starts in early adolescence and lasts into young adulthood. A virulent divorce calls into question the adolescent's basic assumptions about the meaning of sustained trust and intimacy. Faced with the rapid, real loss of what was their home, adolescents may flee into young adult behavior, such as premature sexual activity or substance abuse, or give up their own developmental path to take care of other family members, whether a parent or siblings. Given the stress, achievement in school may suffer during this period of adjustment or in a world of ongoing discord.

Remarriage adds complexity and new opportunities. Accepting the reality that remarriage ends any hope of reuniting the family, the child or adolescent must negotiate a new relationship with a stepparent and possibly additional siblings. Sometimes remarriage adds to the conflict as angry emotions are rekindled; alternatively, remarriage offers new happiness to the parent and new perspectives that give the child options for supportive relationships with stepparents and step-siblings.

## PRACTICE ISSUES

Divorce has a major impact on the child's life outside the home. Joint custody by mutually cooperative parents is overwhelmingly positive. However, even under a well-intentioned understanding, many activities become complicated by visitation schedules, a decrease in disposable income, or any parental disagreement. Everyday experiences, such as planning a sleepover, team practice, music lessons, and summer camp, now might have to be approved by 2 often independent households. In addition to scheduling problems, the costs of summer camp or school tuition may be beyond the family's means or may rekindle tense negotiations through lawyers or the courts. Divorce is a major financial event and a major factor in pulling families below the poverty line. If the family's home is a major asset, it may have to be sold, with the consequence that the child will have to change communities, thereby threatening the social fabric of school, friends, and recreational activities.

Pediatricians should be wary of requests for letters or recommendations that draw them into custody battles. Pediatricians may be biased by having seen one parent more than the other. Unless the pediatrician has a clear, full view of the issues or knows of risks to the child on a first-hand basis, he or she should be wary of submitting anything to a court. Whenever possible, medical instructions and reports should be given to both parents. If the child has a serious acute or chronic disease, routine scheduling of meetings with both parents should be a high priority.

The goal of custody and visitation decisions should be the child's long-term optimal development, including having the necessary warm and unencumbered relationship with each parent as needed at each developmental stage. Although mothers, unless deemed incompetent (eg, because of substance abuse), commonly retain physical custody, especially of young children, agreements for joint parenting are often more effective in supporting the benefits of a strong relationship with the father and the father's ongoing involvement. Increasingly, courts and legislative statutes encourage parents to negotiate the details of joint physical and legal custody. Joint physical custody implies a close to equal time-sharing arrangement; legal custody relates to shared authority in decision making, which is relevant to such issues as obtaining consent for medical care. If joint physical or legal custody is used to expedite contentious cases, implementation of joint custody often becomes the basis for ongoing discord. Under such circumstances, every hour, activity, vacation, and option in the child's life is a potential vehicle to express anger and initiate another round of poor-faith negotiations. In a positive context, joint custody offers an opportunity for both parents to remain highly involved in their child's daily life and facilitates appropriate changes in schedule and even physical custody as the child grows older. However, such arrangements require cooperative, flexible parents who are able to focus on the child's needs and who are willing to live in reasonable proximity (ideally reasonably close to the child's school) of each other for many years.

A parent may come to the pediatrician because the child refuses to spend time with the other parent. The issue may result from the child's inability to cope, the parent's behavior caring for the child during visitation, or the custodial parent attempting to control or alienate. Pediatricians should consider possible abuse, neglect, or substance use, as well any other safety risks to the child. Often a mental health referral will be needed to assess and treat children limiting time or refusing to see a parent.

With the increase in same-sex marriages, pediatricians will provide anticipatory guidance for discord in these marriages. These circumstances do not alter the core principles of advising for the child's best interest or attempting discord.

When either parent begins to date, a common concern is how to introduce the new individual into the child's life. Children often react negatively as they see the new adult as further confirmation that their parents are not reuniting and as a usurper of their priority in the family. It is often wise to limit these introductions to as few as possible and only when the relationship is serious and very likely to be long lasting. Asking the child to relate to too many, too brief relationships could ultimately distance the child from both the biological parent and future stepparent.

## MANAGEMENT

As the pediatrician becomes aware of a pending divorce, anticipatory guidance should include recommending a long-term view of what is in the best interest of the child in terms of parental relationships, discussing the very serious impact of ongoing discord, and alerting parents to the risks of depression and preoccupation (eg, "accidental" injury to the child as a pool gate is left open, a seat belt not buckled, or a gun not safely stored). An approach to management of a family with discord is shown in Figure 31-1. Pediatricians should use questionnaires or ask standardized questions that facilitate recognition of family discord, domestic violence, and psychosocial dysfunction. Larger group practices are likely to have so many families in various stages of divorce that facilitating educational sessions, Web-based resources, or self-help groups, in conjunction with a mental health professional, can be a highly valued clinical service to try to prevent either the divorce itself or the harm of ongoing discord.

Any evidence of significant marital discord, separation, or intention to divorce should initiate a multiyear protocol that assesses the child's acute reaction, the level of parental interpersonal anger, the capacity of the parents to understand the child's needs distinct from their own feelings of anger and loss, and the screening for symptoms of impaired functioning in any member of the family. Specifically, pediatricians should ask about depression; use of substances, especially alcohol; and intensity of preoccupation. The best time to initiate help is early in the divorce process when parents usually prioritize their child's well-being. Recommending a mediator to decrease hostility and potential costs of an extended legal process might help to focus attention on the child's needs. Psychiatric referral for treatment of depression or substance use is a critical priority. Focusing on the needs of the child, the pediatrician can recommend mental health evaluation and counseling for the child or parent as indicated. Evidence of ongoing discord after the separation and divorce is a poor prognostic sign. The pediatrician should recommend that the

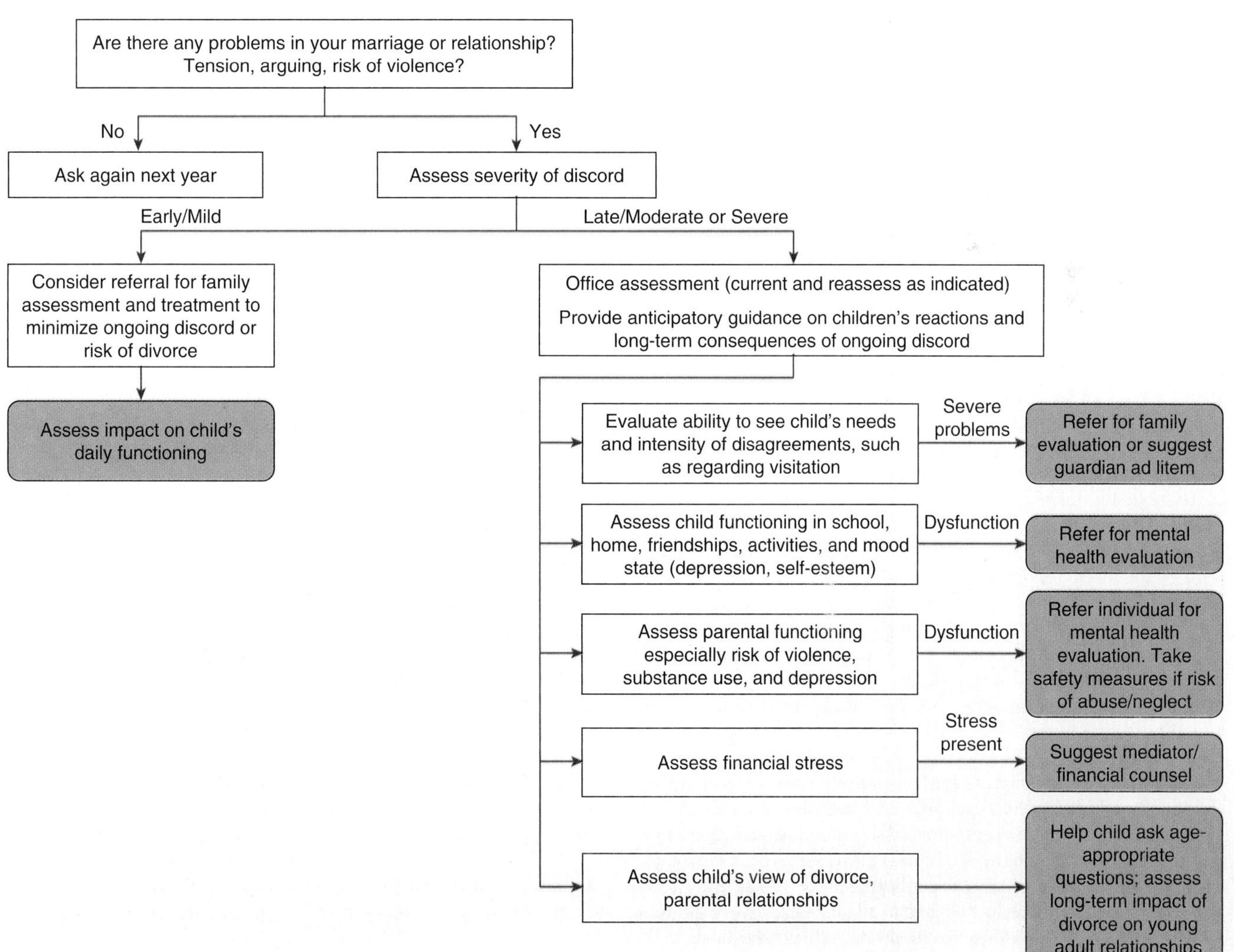


**FIGURE 31-1** Approach to assessment and management of a family with discord.

parents urgently address the tension and, if necessary, consider a court-appointed mediator or a guardian ad litem, generally a lawyer or mental health specialist with investigatory and arbitration authority to serve on behalf of the child's best interest.

After divorce, pediatric guidance and review should span through adolescence into early young adulthood. A trusted pediatrician may ask at each major developmental stage whether the child's view of the divorce has changed, whether he or she might want any information or have new questions, and what he or she senses are any ongoing effects of the divorce. Providing an opportunity for children to discuss, question, and reframe these feelings over time and helping them develop a better understanding of the divorce is an invaluable and professionally rewarding opportunity.

## SUGGESTED READINGS


Hetherington ME. The adjustment of children with divorced parents: a risk and resiliency perspective. *J Child Psychol Psychiatry.* 1999;40(1):129-140.

Jellinek M, Patel BP, Froehle MC, eds. *Bright Futures in Practice: Mental Health.* Vol 1, *Practice Guide.* Arlington, VA: National Center for Education in Maternal and Child Health; 2001.

Kleinsorge C, Covitz LM. Impact of divorce on children: developmental considerations. *Pediatr Rev.* 2012;33(4):147-154.

Wallerstein JS, Lewis JM. The unexpected legacy of divorce: report of a 25-year study. *Psychoanal Psychol.* 2004;21(3):353-370.




# 32 Family and Community Violence

Renée Boynton-Jarrett and Robert Sege

## INTRODUCTION

Violence is among the leading causes of death and disability for American children and adolescents. The epidemic of murder took the lives of approximately 2000 young people annually between 1980 and 2002. During this period, approximately 1 out of every 4 youth homicides was committed by juveniles. Overall, homicide was the third leading cause of death for youth aged 13 to 21 and *the* leading cause of death for African American young men in this age category. Altogether, violence claimed the lives of 6849 Americans under 22 years old in 2014 (7.5 per 100,000); homicide and suicide were among the top three causes of death in the pediatric population. Despite a recent national decline in the homicide rate, the United States continues to have one of the highest homicide rates in the world.

While homicide is the most extreme form of community violence, many more young people are injured: In 2009, over 7000 children were hospitalized for firearms injuries alone; black children were hospitalized far more often than white children, and boys were hospitalized more often than girls. When surveyed in 2013, over one-third of high school students reported having been in a physical fight in the past 12 months (40% of males and 25% of females); in fact, the rate of injuries due to fighting has remained steady for decades. One in 6 youths reported carrying weapons in the past month, and 1 in 14 reported having avoided school due to fear of violence.

The quality of the family and community environment during childhood and adolescence has profound and lasting effects, which persist into adulthood. Recent studies have demonstrated that exposure to violence is among the earliest and most pervasive adverse experiences. Childhood adversities have been linked to future physical, mental, and developmental health and to all major causes of morbidity and mortality in adulthood. While recent data are not available, in the 1990s, 1 out of every 10 children attending a Boston, Massachusetts, city hospital pediatric primary care clinic witnessed a shooting or stabbing in their homes or communities before the age of 6. This high prevalence of exposure to violence underscores the importance of violence as a public health problem.

Pediatricians play a crucial role in preventing, identifying, and intervening in such situations. Contrary to the perception that violence consists of random acts in society, violence is most likely to be perpetrated by individuals known to the victim. Hospital readmission for subsequent assaults and homicide are high. Moreover, violence is associated with known risk and resilience factors that may be routinely assessed during the course of medical care.

Well-established risk factors for violence-related injury include access to firearms, history of fighting or injury, violent discipline, alcohol and drug use, exposure to familial violence, media violence, and gang involvement. As this list of risk factors makes evident, distinct forms of violence rarely occur in isolation. In addition to these individual risk factors, violence also tends to be highly correlated with other social adversities, particularly poverty, substance abuse, housing insecurity, parental mental health challenges, and neighborhood disadvantage.

The accumulation of violence exposure and other social risks may overwhelm a young person's ability to cope with adversities effectively. Indeed, the adverse effects of exposure to violence on mental, physical, and developmental health are often cumulative.

This chapter reviews the epidemiology, health, and developmental impact of familial, dating, and community violence and exposure to violence. The intent is to provide an overview of the pattern of exposure to violence among youth in the United States and useful approaches to prevention, identification, and intervention for pediatricians in the clinical setting.

## FAMILY VIOLENCE

Family violence refers to acts of violence between family members. While all forms of family violence may have grave consequences, this section highlights intimate partner and sibling violence. Intimate partner violence (IPV) includes the actual or threatened emotional, physical, psychological, or sexual abuse between 2 individuals in a close (ie, current or former dating/marital) relationship. Although IPV is present in relationships across class, culture, race/ethnicity, and sexual orientation, this phenomenon is characterized by a gender disparity; in 2001, the US Bureau of Justice Statistics reported that 85% of victims of IPV are women. Between 3 and 10 million children are exposed to IPV annually. The risk of child maltreatment increases as the level of violence in the household increases: Children exposed to IPV are 6 to 15 times more likely to be abused. Children who witness IPV in their homes are at an increased risk of violence in future intimate relationships. Parental history of abuse in childhood, substance abuse, and poor mental health increases the likelihood of family violence. Although IPV spans the socioeconomic gradient, poorer children may be at higher risk of exposure.

The impact of intimate partner violence on child health, behavior, cognitive development, and academic performance may vary by age and developmental stage (Table 32-1). An expansive body of research has documented an association between toxic family environments and mental health problems, including externalizing symptoms such as aggression, conduct disorder, and antisocial behavior, and internalizing symptoms such as anxiety disorders, depression, and suicidal behavior. Moreover, the association between childhood adversities, such as IPV exposure and household dysfunction, with subsequent poor physical health is well-established. Youth residing in environments characterized by aggression, conflict, and neglect are more likely to exhibit health-threatening behaviors (eg, smoking, alcohol and drug abuse, and risky sexual practices). Violence exposure may impact development of strategies to process emotions and coping responses and ultimately lead to higher emotional reactivity. Social competence—social skills, cognition, and prosocial behaviors—may be impacted by deficits in the ability to temper emotions and by lack of role modeling and socialization in the home. Not surprisingly, adaptation to school, academic performance, and peer relations may be subsequently influenced.

**TABLE 32-1 POTENTIAL EFFECTS OF WITNESSING FAMILY VIOLENCE, BY AGE AND DEVELOPMENTAL STAGE**

| Age | Physical Functioning | Cognitive | Emotional and Mental Health | Behavioral |
|---|---|---|---|---|
| Infant | FTT/nutrition | Poor socialization skills | Impaired attachment | Eating problems |
| | Irritability | | Distress | Disordered sleeping |
| | Injury/abuse | | Fear of isolation | Excessive crying |
| Preschool | Insomnia | Developmental delays | Perceived lack of safety | Separation anxiety |
| | Enuresis | Stuttering | Hypervigilance | Regression |
| | Nightmares | | | |
| School-aged | Somatic complaints | Lower verbal and quantitative skills | Self-blame | Regression |
| | PTSD | Violence for conflict resolution | Shame | Aggression |
| | Injury | Immaturity | Guilt | School refusal |
| | | | Powerlessness | Externalized and internalized behaviors |
| | | | Anxiety/fear | Truancy |
| Adolescent | STIs | | Low self-esteem | Recidivism |
| | | | Distrust | Delinquency |
| | | | Depression | Substance abuse |
| | | | Suicidal ideation and attempt | Early sexual initiation |

FTT, failure to thrive; PTSD, posttraumatic stress disorder; STI, sexually transmitted infection.

When the family environment is a source of both threat and protection, the parental role can be severely compromised. Parent–child relationships may be strained by caregiver depression, emotional unavailability, feelings of helplessness to protect the child, and social stress associated with battering. Therefore, the parental response to violence may compound the child's vulnerability in the context of violence exposure. Witnessing a life-threatening act against a caregiver is ranked among the most traumatic experiences a child can face and may lead to post-traumatic stress disorder or associated symptoms.

## SIBLING VIOLENCE

Sibling violence is commonly discounted as more benign and less harmful than other forms of peer violence. Approximately 35% to 50% of children report being hit or attacked by a sibling annually. Overall, sibling violence tends to result in fewer serious injuries than peer violence and involves the use of fewer potentially injurious weapons; however, sibling violence is more likely to be chronic and therefore may hold greater potential for trauma symptoms. Sibling violence may vary depending on the age of the perpetrator; for example, impulsivity and inability to foresee consequences may imbue child aggressors with the greatest potential to cause harm.

## CLINICAL RECOMMENDATIONS

The American Academy of Pediatrics and the American Medical Association recommend incorporating screening for parental IPV into routine health care of children. Screening should take place during new patient visits, annual well-child visits, if a new intimate relationship is disclosed, or if concerning symptoms arise. Symptoms of emotional distress, including somatic complaints and behavioral and emotional problems, or an obvious physical injury should prompt screening for family violence. Among younger children, regression from established milestones for language, communication, and bowel and bladder control should raise concern for the possibility of family violence. Details on whom, when, and how to screen are summarized in Table 32-2.

An approach to management following disclosure of IPV is provided in Figure 32-1. Safety planning may be complex and time consuming; many physicians refer affected caregivers to a social worker or advocate. Clinicians can establish a clinical protocol for IPV screening, assessment, anticipatory guidance, and response if familial violence is identified. Establishment of a multidisciplinary team or collaboration with community agencies may enhance clinical training and resources available for patient care.

Children may benefit from referral to comprehensive mental health services or to specific programs that provide trauma-informed care and allow parent and child to communicate about violent episodes safely. Referrals are particularly warranted in the setting of behavioral change, symptoms persisting longer than 3 months, witnessing severe violence, or an emotionally unavailable caregiver. In those cases in which a report to the state child protective services is warranted, the report should include information regarding the presence of IPV, and the response of child protective services should be designed in a way to promote safety for both adult and child victims.

The acceptability of screening for IPV in the pediatric setting is high and is associated with improved parental satisfaction. Many abused parents will not seek medical care for themselves but will seek care for their children, and disclose the IPV in the context of their children's health, further supporting the inclusion of IPV screening in routine care.

Parents and youth should be screened routinely regarding the nature and pattern of sibling disagreements. Screening provides a valuable opportunity for prevention and early identification. The introduction of alternative forms of conflict resolution is important. Sibling violence resulting in injuries or trauma symptoms should be referred to mental health specialists, family counselors, or family crisis intervention. Serious intentional injuries or threats and repeat injuries should be referred or reported to appropriate services.

## DATING VIOLENCE

Teen dating violence may represent a bridge between exposure to family violence in childhood and violent adult intimate relationships. Patterns of intimacy are established during adolescence. Unfortunately, approximately 6% of high school boys and 14% of high school girls reported experiencing physical and/or sexual dating violence in 2014.

Dating violence includes physical, sexual, verbal, and emotional violence. Although both young men and young women inflict and receive physical abuse, females are more likely to experience severe physical and sexual violence; they are at least twice as likely to experience dating violence.

There is consistent evidence that both the perpetrators and victims of youth dating violence are at an elevated risk of serious health concerns, including suicidal ideation, lower health-related quality of life, risky sexual behaviors, illicit drug use, antisocial behaviors, disordered eating, and unhealthy weight control behaviors. Greater awareness of the multiple health risks associated with dating violence may elevate the index of suspicion and lead to more timely identification and intervention.

Further discussion of teen dating violence, including clinical implications, may be found in Chapter 33.

TABLE 32-2 INTIMATE PARTNER VIOLENCE SCREENING TIPS

| When to Screen | How to Screen[a] | Goals of Screening and Tips |
|---|---|---|
| **Routine screening** | **Introduction** | **Goals** |
| New patient visit<br>Routine healthcare maintenance | "Because violence is so common, I have begun to ask all parents in my practice about it routinely." | Establish the importance of healthy relationships for child health.<br>Send a message to caregivers that IPV is important and they can receive help in the clinical setting.<br>Set foundation for possible future discussion or disclosure. |
| **Opportunities to screen** | **Indirect questions** | **Empathize** |
| Disclosure of new intimate relationship<br>Symptoms of emotional distress (somatic complaints, behavioral or emotional problems, regression of milestones)<br>Physical injury<br>Concern for physical abuse or sexual abuse | "What happens when there is a disagreement with other adults in your home?"<br>"Do you feel safe at home?" | Express concern for safety of caregiver and child.<br>Empathize with complexity of situation. |
| | **Direct questions** | **Documentation** |
| | "Are you in a relationship with a person who physically hurts or threatens to hurt you?"<br>"Do you ever feel afraid of your partner?"<br>"Has your child witnessed a violent event in your home?"<br>"Has your child been hurt during an argument between you and your partner?" | Document findings in a sensitive area of the chart.<br>Use nonjudgmental language. |
| | **Assess safety** | **Quality improvement** |
| | "Do you feel safe in your home?"<br>"Have there been threats to harm you or your children?"<br>"Do you need access to a shelter?"<br>"Do you want police intervention?" | Establish a clinical protocol for screening and staff responsibilities.<br>Consider system of chart prompts for screening.<br>Audit medical records to review compliance. |

[a]Screen caregiver and adolescent.

## COMMUNITY VIOLENCE

American youth are at heightened risk of being victims of, witnessing, and hearing about violence or knowing a relative or peer who died violently. In comparison to suburban youth, youth residing in urban areas report higher rates of witnessing severe violence—stabbings and shootings—while youth in rural areas report high rates of witnessing threats, psychological abuse, and beatings by peers.

Fortunately, death rates due to homicide in the pediatric population (birth to age 21 years) have been declining since the turn of the century. As shown in Figure 32-2, overall homicide rates in this age group have fallen over 27%, from 5.1 to 3.7 per 100,000. Large declines were also noted during the 1990s; Douglas and Bell offer evidence that suggests that these declines may have resulted from effective violence programs that reduce risk factors and help build positive ones. Despite this progress, homicide remains the third leading cause of death, trailing only unintentional injuries and suicide.

Minority youth are at particularly high risk of exposure to community violence. Racial/ethnic disparities in the homicide rates have actually grown; the death rate for young blacks in the United States is now 6.8 times the rate for whites. In 1999, the same ratio was 5.3. In addition, all children, regardless of race, are at high risk of violence-related injury. The risk of being killed at home increases dramatically whenever there is a handgun in the home. Alcohol and drug use are associated with violent events and injury.

Witnessing violence has been associated with psychological, social, academic, cognitive, and physical challenges as well as with propensity to engage in violent acts in the future. Young persons in violent communities have a higher likelihood of weapon-carrying and aggression. Although exposure to firearm violence has been associated with a heightened risk for perpetration of serious violence, the majority of youth exposed to violence do not perpetrate abuse or engage in criminal behavior. Moreover, youth are less likely to carry concealed firearms if they reside in neighborhoods that are safe, have greater social and physical order, and have higher collective efficacy, that is, social cohesion and informal social control.

Exposure to community violence influences perceptions of safety and security, which may undermine development of trust and autonomy and thereby hinder efforts to obtain mastery of the social environment. Somatic symptoms, anxiety, depressive symptoms, irritability, sleep disturbances, and post-traumatic stress disorder and associated symptoms result from acute or chronic exposure to community violence. Approximately one-third of urban youth exposed to community violence meet criteria for post-traumatic stress disorder, and nearly two-thirds of adolescent girls exposed to community violence have the symptomatology.

Exposure to violence impacts global developmental and social morbidity for children and adolescents. Peer relations may suffer from violence exposure; these youth appear to be more antisocial and socially isolated and may have difficulty building healthy relationships with peers. Academically, violence exposure is linked to difficulties with memory and concentration and poorer school performance. Finally, witnessing violence is linked to substance abuse and dependency.

## CLINICAL IMPLICATIONS

Although a majority of parents believe that pediatricians should discuss community violence during routine office visits, only 10% of parents reported that their pediatricians did so. The American Academy of Pediatrics and other professional societies have developed violence prevention training programs, such as Connected Kids, to provide resources for practitioners and families. These programs provide training and resources that support child healthcare providers in clinical, community, and social advocacy and policy settings. Specific approaches to prevention and intervention around community violence exposure are discussed in "Assessment of Risk" and "Prevention and Intervention," below.

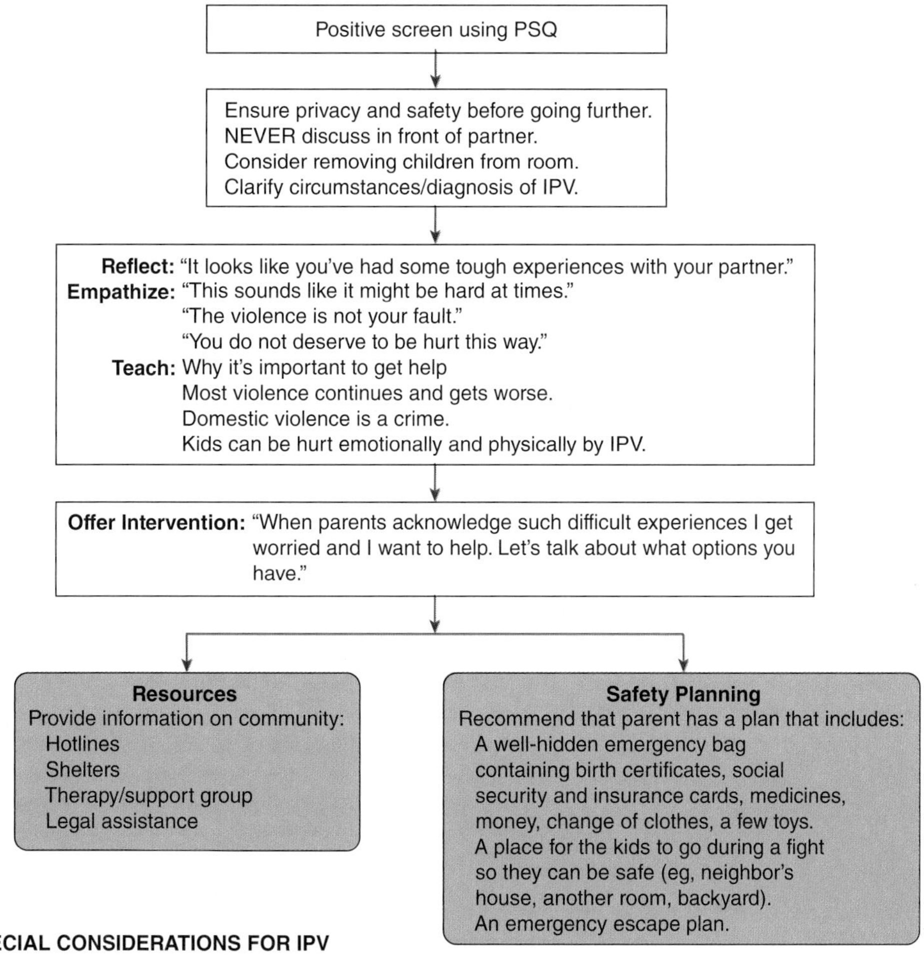

Positive screen using PSQ

↓

Ensure privacy and safety before going further.
NEVER discuss in front of partner.
Consider removing children from room.
Clarify circumstances/diagnosis of IPV.

↓

**Reflect:** "It looks like you've had some tough experiences with your partner."
**Empathize:** "This sounds like it might be hard at times."
"The violence is not your fault."
"You do not deserve to be hurt this way."
**Teach:** Why it's important to get help
Most violence continues and gets worse.
Domestic violence is a crime.
Kids can be hurt emotionally and physically by IPV.

↓

**Offer Intervention:** "When parents acknowledge such difficult experiences I get worried and I want to help. Let's talk about what options you have."

↓

**Resources**
Provide information on community:
Hotlines
Shelters
Therapy/support group
Legal assistance

**Safety Planning**
Recommend that parent has a plan that includes:
A well-hidden emergency bag containing birth certificates, social security and insurance cards, medicines, money, change of clothes, a few toys.
A place for the kids to go during a fight so they can be safe (eg, neighbor's house, another room, backyard).
An emergency escape plan.

**SPECIAL CONSIDERATIONS FOR IPV**

*(I) In some states (eg, Connecticut), a child's exposure to IPV can be considered maltreatment. Pediatricians practicing in these states are required to report this maltreatment to CPS.*

*(II) Parent declines referrals,* ***no*** *immediate safety concerns:*
Encourage meeting with a social worker or a community resource.
Encourage developing a safety plan.
Offer a private clinic phone to call a hotline.
Follow-up at next visit, sooner than regular appointment.

*(III) Parent declines referral, child(ren) is clearly affected:*
Inform parent that most children know when IPV occurs, even when adults try to hide it from them.
Tell parent that IPV can really harm children (eg, learning problems, psychosomatic complaints, behavior problems, high anxiety, depression, sleep and eating disturbance).
Clearly state how the child's presenting problem(s) may be due to the IPV, and that counseling should help.
If the child exhibits suicidal ideation/gestures or self-injurious behavior, inform parent of the limits of confidentiality (eg, "This is serious. We need to make sure that _____ gets help so he/she doesn't hurt him/herself. This information cannot be kept private. We have to make a referral so that ______ gets the help he/she needs."). Refer child for an immediate mental health evaluation (eg, local emergency department).

*(IV) Child maltreatment is a significant concern:*
Refer to a social worker or other resource for further assessment and services.
Refer to Child Protective Services if child abuse or neglect is suspected (eg, "I'm worried about you, and your child. I think your child may be harmed by this situation. So, I need to call Child Protective Services. They will assess the situation and help make sure your child is safe.")
Plan a follow-up visit and reassess.

*(V) If the parent is afraid to return home:*
Refer to a social worker or a hotline before leaving the office to consider options including emergency shelter.
Discuss a safety plan for parent and child(ren).

**FIGURE 32-1** Assessment and management of intimate partner violence. (Used with permission from Wendy Gwirtzman Lane, MD, MPH, and Howard Dubowitz, MB, ChB.)



Children who have been exposed to violence, whether in the home or in the community, may suffer from a variety of behavioral and somatic complaints. The evaluation of behavioral problems, in particular, should include a careful and sympathetic examination of any past exposure to violence, including experiences as a victim or perpetrator. Enuresis, insomnia, and sudden emergence of problems at school (including inattention) may be particularly likely to result from violence exposure. Similarly, when patients or family members discuss a history of violence exposure, clinicians may assess for symptoms and/or refer for mental health treatment. Depending on the

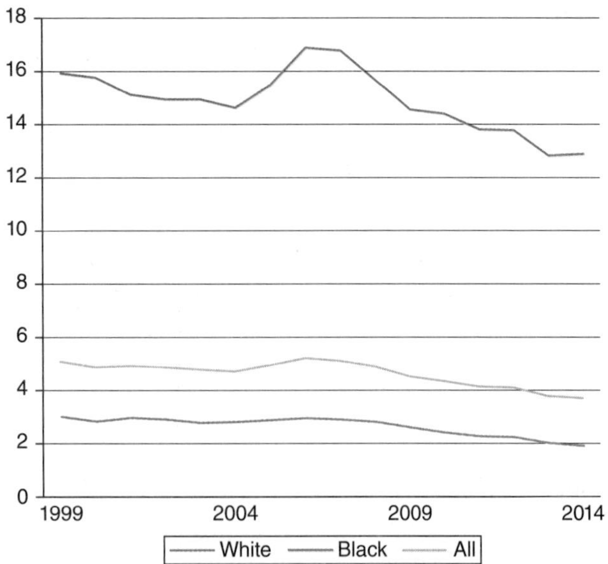


**FIGURE 32-2** Homicide rates in the United States, 1999–2014. Rates are reported in deaths per 100,000. (Data from the US Centers for Disease Control and Prevention, Web-based Injury Statistics Query and Reporting System [WISQARS™].)



child's age, severity of exposure, and symptomatology, any of a number of evidence-based treatment options have been shown to mitigate the behavioral and emotional sequelae to violence.

## SPECIAL RISKS AND GROUPS AT RISK FOR VIOLENCE

### Bullying

Bullying, a worldwide phenomenon of middle childhood, occurs when a bully (usually larger and stronger than the victim) repeatedly acts and behaves negatively toward a specific victim, often at school or on the way to or from school. Nearly 10% of students in 6th through 12th grade report having been bullied at school, during school-related activities, or en route to or from school. Bullying not only causes injury to the victim but may engender resentment and lead to retaliatory violence. Bullied youth are at greater risk of low self-esteem, disordered eating, anxiety, depression, somatic symptoms, and school absence.

Bullies themselves have the greatest risk of long-term adverse outcomes and are more likely to come from disordered homes. Unchecked, bullying behavior becomes destructive and ineffective for the bully in the middle school and high school years. Male bullies, in particular, are unlikely to complete their schooling and are at elevated risk of unemployment, incarceration, and living in poverty as adults. They are also less likely to have stable adult relationships.

An effective anti-bullying strategy for use in schools has been adapted from a Scandinavian model by the US Maternal and Child Health Bureau. This evidence-based approach can reduce bullying in the school by 90%. For the individual parent who brings the child who is the victim of bullying to the physician's office, it is most important to acknowledge the difficulty that the victim faces and suggest that the caregiver talk with the principal and school counselor at the school in order to ensure a safe environment for the child. At the same time, introduction of the child to an alternative social environment may help insulate him or her from the negative effects of bullying. For example, many parents enroll their child in a martial arts program, scouting, or a youth program sponsored by faith-based organizations. In each of these settings, the youngster may experience social success and ameliorate the negative consequences of bullying. Efforts to prevent bullying provide an opportunity for the healthcare practitioner to engage with the school administrators and identify important research-backed approaches.

### GLBTQ Youth and Violence

Gay, lesbian, bisexual, transgender, and questioning (GLBTQ) youth are at an increased risk of violent victimization. GLBTQ youth are more likely to be harassed, attacked, and/or threatened at school. Approximately 17% of anti-GLBTQ incidents of violence reported in a national study in 2002 occurred among individuals 22 years old and younger. Hate crimes, or incidents of violence fueled by discrimination, can be unusually humiliating, cruel, and brutal acts. GLBTQ youth are also at increased risk of depression, hopelessness, alcohol abuse, and suicidal ideation and attempts.

Youth in same-sex relationships are at a particularly elevated risk of violence in intimate relationships. Among young men, the number of same-sex male partners correlated with higher frequency of dating violence. Vulnerability to violence may be linked to social isolation; moreover, concerns for social acceptance may increase challenges to seeking care.

Only a minority of GLBTQ youth discuss their sexual orientation with their healthcare providers, although most report that they would be open to such a discussion. Relieving concerns about confidentiality and creating an atmosphere that is open to discussion of sexual orientation and avoids the assumption of heterosexuality can enable discussion of violence prevention and facilitate care for physical and mental health concerns.

### Youth in the Juvenile Justice System

Despite a decline in crimes committed by juveniles over the past decade, 3% of youth ages 10 to 17 years were arrested in 2014. The rate at which boys were arrested for violent crimes in 2014 (252/100,000) was less than half of the rate in 1980 (519/100,000); however, the arrest rate for girls (59 vs 62 per 100,000) was virtually unchanged. Approximately 14% of those involved in juvenile crimes are placed in correctional facilities, where young men in racial/ethnic minority groups are significantly overrepresented. Over the past decade, the number of adolescent girls involved in juvenile arrests and incarceration has increased dramatically; girls now account for 19% of all juvenile arrests for violent crime.

The mental health profile of juvenile offenders differs by sex. Girls and young women offenders have a higher prevalence of reported traumatic exposures and psychiatric disorders. Nearly two-thirds of male and three-fourths of female detainees meet criteria for at least 1 psychiatric disorder. Among this population, approximately 93% have experienced at least 1 traumatic incident (often child abuse), and 11% meet criteria for post-traumatic stress disorder. Nearly half have substance use disorders, and a large percentage have disruptive behavior disorders. Youth who have been involved in the juvenile justice system have higher rates of suicide attempts and tend to use more lethal means. Youth in juvenile detention are also at an elevated risk of intentional injuries, including physical and sexual abuse perpetrated by other detainees or staff. Not surprisingly, many develop physical and mental health problems during incarceration, and access to health services is often limited.

Recently, increased attention has been paid to the death of adolescents, particularly young black men, at the hands of law enforcement. Although the overall rate of death is low in the pediatric age group (45 deaths = 0.05 per 100,000 in 2014), 41 of the 45 (90%) of those deaths were male. Black boys and youths died from legal intervention at three times the rate of whites. Clinicians may want to consider the increased vulnerability of minority children and youths, particularly boys and young men, when discussing violence and self-protection.

### Firearms in the Home

The safest home for a child is a home without guns. Firearms are the third leading cause of death among children 10 to 14 years old and the second leading cause of death among those 15 to 19 years old. Approximately 43% of homes in the United States have firearms. The presence of firearms in the home is associated with a fivefold increase in the risk of adolescent suicide. More than 50% of adolescent suicides involve the use of firearms; moreover, greater than 90% of suicide attempts involving the use of firearms are lethal.

Firearms in the home present a unique risk factor for adolescents, both for interpersonal violence and for suicide attempts. Providers should routinely screen parents and youth for the presence of guns in the home, their storage, and the ability to access a fatal weapon.

Developmentally, adolescents are inclined to make more spontaneous decisions, a characteristic that poses an even greater risk for the impulsive use of firearms. Public health data suggest that access to firearms increases the rate of completed suicide. Families should be counseled regarding the dangers of in-home firearms and advised to remove guns from the home for the sake of those who are at high risk, including adolescents with a history of depression, drug abuse, or affective disorders.

## MEDIA VIOLENCE

Television viewing is the most time-consuming activity for youth aside from sleep. Increasing numbers of violent incidents are aired on television. Presently, nearly two-thirds of television shows contain violence. By the end of grade school, children will witness an estimated 8000 murders and 100,000 acts of violence on television. Not only is violence often glamorized on television, it often exists to the exclusion of other means of resolving conflicts, and televised perpetrators do not suffer consequences for their actions, thus endorsing violent behavior as socially acceptable.

Younger children tend to have difficulty distinguishing fantasy from reality on television and appear to be more affected by television violence. Media violence has been associated with an increased state of arousal for youth, identification with the aggressor, and justification of the acts of violence. Television viewing has been associated with aggressive behavior, desensitization to witnessed violent acts, increased feelings of threat and danger, and fear of victimization. Reduction in television viewing has been associated with reduced fighting-related behaviors.

Although total screen time, beyond television, is less well-studied, a recent report suggests that total screen time, not television per se, is associated with physical violence. The American Academy of Pediatrics recommends that parents monitor and provide guidance for television viewing, limit television viewing to less than 2 hours daily, remove televisions from bedrooms or potentially unmonitored locations, discuss the content of television shows, and supervise DVDs and video games. At the community level, pediatricians can support campaigns to increase media literacy among children and their parents and support community-based programs that encourage alternative forms of entertainment for youth.

## RESILIENCE

Resilience factors help children overcome adversities; in particular, they may buffer stressors by promoting recovery, facilitating adaptation during exposure, or protecting an individual from exposure to a stressor. The interplay of the type of exposure, developmental stage, and specific vulnerability determines the ability for resilience factors to help buffer stressors. Individual traits associated with resiliency include social competence, self-esteem, problem-solving skills, autonomy, and sense of purpose. Establishment of a secure attachment between child and primary caregiver in early life also contributes to resiliency. Parents also model resilient behaviors and attitudes for their children. Supportive family relationships, parental monitoring, clearly established rules, high expectations for prosocial behavior, and participation of children in family activities can help improve resiliency in children exposed to violence in the community. Finally, meaningful connections to the larger community promote resiliency in youth.

Positive youth development programs provide settings for adolescent development that view young people as important contributors to their communities. After-school arts programs, music programs, volunteer opportunities, and athletic programs have all been adopted as a method of reducing youth risk behavior. There is strong evidence to support the effectiveness of these programs. From a clinical perspective, helping young people engage with these programs is one key to successful modification of risk factors and is likely to be more effective than brief in-office behavioral counseling. Neighborhood characteristics, such as collective efficacy—related to social cohesion and informal social control—and the availability of institutional resources in the community have been linked to increased resilience of youth exposed to violence.

**TABLE 32-3 FISTS: FIGHTING, INJURIES, SEX, THREATS, SELF-DEFENSE**

| | |
|---|---|
| **Fighting** | How many fights have you been in during the past year? |
| | When was your last fight? |
| **Injuries** | Have you ever been injured in a fight? |
| | Have you ever injured someone else in a fight? |
| **Sex** | Are you scared of disagreeing with your partner? |
| | Does your partner criticize or humiliate you in front of others? |
| | Are you scared by your partner's violent or threatening behavior? |
| | Has your partner ever forced you to do something sexual you didn't want to do? |
| | Every family argues. What are fights like in your family or with people you're dating? Do they ever become physical? |
| | Do you think that couples can stay in love when one partner makes the other one afraid? |
| **Threats** | Has someone carrying a weapon ever threatened you? |
| | What happened? |
| | Has anything changed since then to make you feel safer? |
| **Self-defense** | What do you do if someone tries to pick a fight with you? |
| | Have you ever carried a weapon in self-defense? |

Data from Spivak H, Sege R, Flanigan E, Licenziato V, eds. *Connected Kids: Safe, Strong, Secure Clinical Guide*. Elk Grove Village, IL: American Academy of Pediatrics; 2006.

## ASSESSMENT OF RISK

Several risk-based screening instruments are published for use in identifying adolescents at risk for interpersonal violence. The American Medical Association's Guidelines for Adolescent Preventive Services (GAPS) provides the most widely used general adolescent primary care protocols. GAPS includes the recommendation that healthcare providers "counsel (patients) to resolve interpersonal conflicts without violence and to avoid the use of weapons and/or promote weapon safety." The American Academy of Pediatrics' Connected Kids program, discussed in the next section, recommends the fighting, injuries, sex, threats, self-defense (FISTS) screener, which probes specific risk factors associated with subsequent violence (Table 32-3). Youth at moderate risk for violence exposure report fighting once or twice in the past 12 months or occasional drug or alcohol use. High-risk individuals are truant from school or have dropped out, report 2 or more fights in the past year, or use illicit drugs. Counseling and referral may be needed for moderate to high-risk individuals.

## PREVENTION AND INTERVENTION

Universal strategies to prevent violence include efforts to reach all children and families. Resources and Web sites for families, schools, children, and medical professionals are listed in Table 32-4. From a clinical standpoint, these strategies can be directed at promoting resilience and risk reduction. Effective strategies are developmentally appropriate and comprehensive—intervening at individual, family, school, and community levels—and begin with infants and toddlers. This comprehensive developmental philosophy forms the basis for the American Academy of Pediatrics' Connected Kids: Safe, Strong, Secure program for prevention of violence in the primary care setting. Preschool anticipatory guidance focuses on development of family support and highlights parent understanding of child behavior and the use of alternatives to corporal punishment. Violence prevention for school-age children focuses specifically on the issue of bullying and more generally on helping children acquire adequate communication and conflict resolution skills.

*Universal* prevention for adolescents centers on identifying engaging, prosocial activities for adolescents that allow them to develop and grow and meet their developing need for independence, mastery, and belonging. Health care providers may serve as resources for information about after-school and community-based programs for teenagers and young adults. Comprehensive violence prevention programs that

**TABLE 32-4 RESOURCES AND WEB SITES**

| URL | Web Site | Description |
|---|---|---|
| **Web Resources for Families and Schools** | | |
| http://www.stopbullying.gov | US Department of Health and Human Services stopbullying.gov | Provides information and technical support for school-based bullying prevention; features webisodes, brief video scenarios to support better understanding of bullying and bullying prevention |
| http://vetoviolence.cdc.gov/apps/stryve/ | US Centers for Disease Control and Prevention STRYVE Program | Provides support for youth violence prevention at the community level |
| http://www.girlsinc.org | Girls Incorporated National Resource Center | A national youth organization dedicated to inspiring girls |
| **Web Resources for Health Professionals** | | |
| http://www.nctsn.org/ | National Child Traumatic Stress Network (NCTSN) | Has extensive resources for the diagnosis and treatment of stress-related disorders in children |
| http://www.aap.org/connectedkids | American Academy of Pediatrics' youth violence prevention program Connected Kids: Safe, Strong, Secure | Provides clinical information and parent/patient handouts to support resilience-based anticipatory guidance |
| http://vetoviolence.cdc.gov/links | US Centers for Disease Control and Prevention's comprehensive violence prevention resources | A rich, searchable database of resources, training, and technical support materials |
| http://www.cdc.gov/injury/wisqars/fatal.htm | US Centers for Disease Control and Prevention Web-based injury statistics query and reporting system | Allows exploration of injury rates, including violence-related injuries, by demography, geography, mechanism, and intent |
| http://www.endabuse.org | The Family Violence Prevention Fund (FVPF) | Provides resources and materials for healthcare settings and professionals focusing on domestic violence education, prevention, and policy reform |



focus on the promotion of resilience and the reduction of risk factors appear to have contributed to the decline in violence in the past decade. In some communities, information may need to be gathered and maintained by the personnel at the clinical site. In many others, however, city, school, or community organizations may collect and disseminate this type of information; clinicians may be able to access centralized resources.

Providers also have an opportunity to engage in community and social policy efforts to prevent exposure to community violence and intervene in a systematic and efficacious manner. Clinicians may lead efforts to reduce violence in society by coordinating educational campaigns to raise awareness of the impact of violence on child health, community-based prevention efforts and interventions, and support for socially responsible gun laws.

*Selective* prevention interventions are focused on youth identified as high-risk on the basis of risk behavior profiles or because of exposure to violence. Selective interventions directly address the social networks and resources for adolescents and their families, particularly by establishing adult mentors, supporting supervised enrichment activities, providing intensive psychotherapy for individuals and families exposed to violence, and providing meaningful career pathways.

*Indicated* interventions are activated once adolescents have been injured or become involved in the juvenile justice system. These include facilitating appropriate physical and mental health services for youth, recommending comprehensive programs to help reform criminal behavior, addressing the root causes of antisocial and/or violent behavior, and providing options to gang involvement.

## SUGGESTED READINGS


Committee on Psychosocial Aspects of Child and Family Health; Committee on Early Childhood, Adoption, and Dependent Care; Section on Developmental and Behavioral Pediatrics; Shonkoff JP, Siegel BS, Dobbins MI, et al. Early childhood adversity, toxic stress, and the role of the pediatrician: translating developmental science into lifelong health. *Pediatrics*. 2012;129(1):e224-e231.

Douglas K, Bell CC. Youth homicide prevention. *Psychiatr Clin North Am*. 2011;34(1):205-216.

Dubowitz H, Prescott L, Feigelman S, Lane W, Kim J. Screening for intimate partner violence in a pediatric primary care clinic. *Pediatrics*. 2008;121(1):e85-e91.

Felitti VJ, Anda RF, Nordenberg D, et al. Relationship of childhood abuse and household dysfunction to many of the leading causes of death in adults: the Adverse Childhood Experiences (ACE) study. *Am J Prev Med*. 1998;14(4):245-258.

Finkelhor D, Ormrod R, Turner H, Hanby SL. The victimization of children and youth: a comprehensive national survey. *Child Maltreat*. 2005;10(1):5-25.

Grinshteyn E, Hemenway D. Violent death rates: the US compared with other OECD countries, 2010. *Am J Med*. 2016;129(3):263-271.

Janssen I, Boyce WF, Pickett W. Screen time and physical violence in 10- to 16-year-old Canadian youth. *Int J Public Health*. 2012;57(2):325-331.

Leventhal JM, Gaither JR, Sege R. Hospitalizations due to firearm injuries in children and adolescents. *Pediatrics*. 2014;133(2):219-225.

Olweus D. *Bullying at School*. Oxford, England: Blackwell Publishers; 1993.

Repetti RL, Taylor SE, Seeman TE. Risky families: family social environments and the mental and physical health of offspring. *Psychol Bull*. 2002;128:330-366.

Sege RD, Dowd M. Firearm-related injuries affecting the pediatric population. *Pediatrics*. 2012;130(5):e1416-e1423.


# 33 Teen Dating Violence

Jeff R. Temple and Constance M. Wiemann

Teen dating violence (TDV), which includes physical violence, sexual aggression, and psychological abuse, is a major public health concern in the United States. New forms of sexual harassment and avenues for TDV are emerging through the use of blogs, chat rooms, texting, sexting, and social networking sites, placing an increasing number of teens at risk of becoming victims of TDV. This chapter provides an overview of different forms of abuse, including terminology and prevalence, as well as screening for TDV and anticipatory guidance, risk and protective factors, consequences, prevention, and treatment.

## TERMINOLOGY

While our attention to and understanding of TDV have increased rapidly over the previous 2 decades, how researchers, advocates, and practitioners label and define this form of abuse is far from settled. The debate over labels is not merely academic; what something is called can impact policy, funding, measurement, and programming. For example, the term we use for this chapter—TDV—could be considered limited to a specific age group (ie, teens) and to a specific form of abuse (ie, physical violence). Others have suggested that a more inclusive term, such as *adolescent relationship abuse*, incorporates a wider age range and multiple forms of abusive behavior (eg, physical violence, psychological abuse, sexual aggression, stalking, cyber abuse). Paralleling the differences in how TDV is labeled, there is a general lack of consistency in the timeframe used (eg, lifetime, past year, past month) and how it is measured (eg, current vs. recent partner), resulting in varying estimates of prevalence. Rates of reported victimization are generally higher than rates of perpetration. Moreover, context is rarely included in TDV measurement, resulting in potentially misleading findings related to rates by gender (see "Gender, Sexual Orientation, and Ethnicity," below). Complicating matters, and specific to TDV, is the transient nature of adolescent relationships and the fact that what teens consider, label, and define as "dating" varies by context, time, and region (see "Screening for TDV and Discussing TDV with Adolescent Patients," below).

## TYPES AND PREVALENCE OF TDV

### Physical Abuse

Physical TDV is any form of abuse that is physical in nature, including acts such as biting, hair-pulling, slapping, strangling, punching, kicking, pushing, or use of a weapon. Threatening these behaviors could also fit within the definition of physical violence (note that, depending on the situation, threats may also be considered a form of psychological abuse). The Centers for Disease Control and Prevention's biannual Youth Risk Behavior Survey (YRBS) consistently finds that approximately 10% of teens report past-year physical TDV, with even higher rates in more recent YRBS surveys when only teens who have a history of dating are included. Research among high-risk youth—for instance, teens who misuse substances or those who are victims of or witnesses to family or community violence—often finds rates of physical TDV over 50%.

### Sexual Abuse

Sexual TDV can vary from sexual coercion (eg, psychological manipulation) to unwanted or nonconsensual kissing and touching to forced sexual intercourse. As is common with estimating risky behaviors, the prevalence of sexual TDV varies by methodology. When defined as forced sexual intercourse or rape (also commonly referred to as *date rape*), the prevalence ranges between 4% and 10%, with substantially higher rates (~50%) when the definition includes more broadly defined forced sexual acts. Reproductive coercion, which involves attempts to sabotage use of birth control, can also be considered a form of sexual aggression. While research is in its infancy, it has been reported that approximately 5% to 15% of teen and young adult women experience reproductive coercion.

### Psychological Abuse

Psychological TDV includes a range of behaviors intending to exert control over one's partner, and can include subtle (eg, controlling activities) and overt (eg, ridiculing, excessively yelling, threatening suicide) forms of abuse. Withholding money or providing a conditional allowance (ie, economic abuse), threatening or abusing a pet, and constant surveillance also fit under the umbrella of psychological abuse. Because most relationships, even healthy ones, involve some acts that could be considered psychologically abusive, its prevalence in the literature varies considerably: from a low of 20% to a high of over 90%. From a clinical perspective, psychological abuse should be considered problematic when it is severe or excessive in nature, includes multiple acts, or is paired with physical or sexual abuse. Most importantly, if psychological abuse is causing distress, then regardless of the above qualifiers, it should be taken seriously. Indeed, psychological abuse has repeatedly been shown to be at least as harmful to mental health as physical violence. Psychological abuse is present in nearly all physically violent relationships, and in fact may be a precursor to physical violence. Stalking, or harassing, intrusive, and unwanted behaviors that elicit fear in a partner or ex-partner, may be considered a severe form of psychological abuse and is often predictive of severe physical violence.

### Cyber or Electronic Abuse

Cyber or electronic abuse may not be a distinct form of TDV, but rather a method used to threaten, stalk, and perpetrate psychological abuse. The small but accumulating research on cyber dating abuse indicates a prevalence rate similar to other forms of TDV, especially psychological abuse.

## SCREENING FOR TDV AND DISCUSSING TDV WITH ADOLESCENT PATIENTS

Providers often want to use measures of adult partner violence to evaluate TDV in adolescent patients. However, developmental differences suggest this downward extension may be inappropriate and not accurately reflect violence in teen intimate relationships. Adolescents are generally less mature, have underdeveloped sexual identity and experiences, are new to romantic relationships, and are just beginning to experience mixed-gender peer groups. Moreover, behaviors interpreted as problematic in adulthood (eg, impulsivity, a sense of invulnerability) are common and developmentally normal in adolescence. Near daily conflict with family members, peers, and dating partners is also common among adolescents. To complicate screening for TDV, teens may view jealousy and partners' controlling behaviors as evidence of love, and they may not label coerced sexual contact at the hands of a dating partner as sexual assault. Overall, compared to young adult relationships, adolescent dating relationships are more superficial and of shorter duration; less sexually intimate and committed; more likely to be between partners of similar status; and have different strategies for conflict resolution. These differences between teens and adult relationships suggest we need to ask adolescents about all perpetration and victimization in a specific time period and follow up with assessment of context.

### Anticipatory Guidance

While reliable and valid research measures of TDV have been normed and repeatedly used on adolescents (eg, Conflict in Adolescent Relationship Inventory), their length and complexity make them difficult to use in a clinical setting. Instead, tween and teen healthcare professionals should directly ask patients about their dating relationships in general and about TDV specifically. Anticipatory guidance about healthy dating should be provided to both males and females. Conversations about TDV should be interactive and occur at each visit. It is important to avoid lectures to present the facts while listening to patient reactions and concerns. Although adolescents may be reluctant to disclose TDV to adults, including healthcare professionals, routinely and universally asking about TDV will let teens know that (1) these behaviors are not normal or healthy, (2) the practitioner considers TDV a health problem, and (3) the practitioner is someone they can talk with should they choose to disclose. For these reasons, teen-serving pediatric, family, and obstetrics/gynecology clinics should have visible posters about TDV and pamphlets on healthy relationships, and should make the TDV hotline number (866-331-9474) available. Items assessing TDV could also be included in screening paperwork as teens may be more willing to disclose TDV when answering written questions as opposed to providing verbal responses when interviewed. An example of a brief measure that could be included with other health-related items is the 4-item and easily interpreted Hurt, Insulted, Threatened with Harm, and Screamed (HITS) tool (ie, How often does your partner "physically hurt you," "insult or talk down to you," "threaten you with harm," and "scream at you"?). This, or any measure, should be augmented with a question on cyber dating abuse or by asking, "Did any of these behaviors occur via text or social media?"

### Risk and Protective Factors

While universal screening is recommended, careful attention should be directed to teen patients who (1) have been exposed to relationship, family, or community violence; (2) report a history of any TDV victimization or perpetration; (3) associate with delinquent or violent peers; (4) have been exposed to adverse childhood experiences; (5) have a history of risky behaviors, including alcohol and other substance use/misuse and early or risky sexual behavior; (6) are pregnant; (7) evidence symptoms of depression or anxiety; (8) display attitudes dismissive or accepting of violence; or (9) have irregular medical care histories. In addition, teens with partners who are jealous and possessive, who embarrass or demean the teen in front of others, make all relationship decisions, and have a history of losing their temper are at particularly high risk of being in a violent relationship.

## GENDER, SEXUAL ORIENTATION, AND ETHNICITY

Accumulating research on adolescent and adult samples indicates that females are at least as likely as males to perpetrate TDV and that violent relationships are generally characterized by mutual violence, in which both male and female partners engage in aggressive behavior. However, much of this research lacks context and simply asks about acts of violence, which may be misleading. Take the case of professional football player Ray Rice, who was captured on a surveillance video punching and knocking his then-fiancée unconscious. Prior to Mr. Rice punching his fiancée, it appears that she pushed him. Despite the clear distinction in strength and resulting harm, many partner violence measures would count these acts equally (ie, he pushed, shoved, punched, or kicked her; she pushed, shoved, punched, or kicked him). While females are substantially more likely to be injured (or killed), sustain sexual aggression, and be otherwise harmed, the reality of mutual violence indicates that prevention and intervention programs must consider both genders/partners in addressing dating violence. Indeed, even acts that are often (erroneously) considered exclusively male-to-female violence, such as sexual assault, can be initiated and perpetrated by females. Moreover, when surveyed, many high-school teens report responding to TDV victimization with the perpetration of physical violence or verbal abuse. Similarly, a recent longitudinal study found that men's and women's perpetration of dating violence tended to be a response to their partners' aggression. Mutual violent relationships have also been shown to be more severe and injurious, compared with relationships in which only one partner was violent.

The limited existing studies on gay, lesbian, bisexual, transgender, and questioning (GLBTQ) teens suggest that sexual minority youth—especially transgender and bisexual teens—may be at higher risk for all forms of TDV victimization and perpetration, relative to their heterosexual peers. Preliminary research suggests that TDV may be more stable in GLBTQ couples and that traditional risk factors often observed in heterosexual couples may not apply to sexual minority youth. From a clinical standpoint, healthcare professionals should be aware of this potentially higher risk, but screening and discussing TDV with GLBTQ patients should follow the same nonjudgmental structure as screening for TDV with heterosexual patients.

Accumulating evidence suggests that TDV perpetration and victimization may be higher among African American and Hispanic teens, relative to their white counterparts. However, this is not consistently found and may be due to a third variable, such as low socioeconomic status. The recent YRBS, of nearly 10,000 adolescents, found the following rates of TDV among white, African American, and Hispanic teens, respectively: 14.5%, 15.5%, and 17.2%.

## CONSEQUENCES OF TEEN DATING VIOLENCE

Compared with adolescents without a history of TDV, those with a history exhibit higher rates of depression, anxiety, suicidal ideation, substance use, posttraumatic stress disorder, risky sexual behavior, sexually transmitted infections, teen pregnancy, and eating disorders. They are also more likely to perform poorly in school and to experience difficulties in future relationships. Indeed, studies indicate that violence in adolescence predicts violence in adulthood, with one study finding that youth who were victims of TDV as high school students were three times more likely than nonvictims to experience TDV in college. A longitudinal study of adverse health outcomes found that TDV victimization predicted adult partner violence victimization (males and females), as well as heavy episodic drinking (females), depression (females), suicidality (males and females), smoking (females), marijuana use (males), and antisocial behaviors (males). Perhaps most relevant for clinicians is recent research showing that approximately 17% of female teens and 13% of male teens treated at a suburban emergency room had a positive history of TDV. Even higher rates (40%) were found in a study of female teens seeking care (for any reason) at urban primary care clinics. Importantly, presenting problems will often not be directly associated or identified with patient experiences of TDV (bruises, broken bones). Instead, patients experiencing TDV may present with depressed mood, stress, anxiety, or idiopathic head and stomach aches.

## PREVENTION AND TREATMENT

TDV can be prevented, and early intervention is now recognized as a crucial step in preparing youth for sustained healthy relationships in later life. Several individual, relationship, family, and school/community factors appear to protect teens against the occurrence or progression of TDV. Individual factors include knowledge of healthy relationships and available resources, good communication and decision-making skills, and self-efficacy for engaging in nonviolent behavior. In addition, empathic youth, those with prosocial attributes (ie, the tendency to help others), and those with adaptive coping and conflict resolution skills are less likely to engage in TDV. Parental factors inversely related to TDV include parental monitoring, warmth, and closeness, as well as awareness, recognition, and open communication regarding violent relationships. Finally, youth who feel connected to their school and community and who have prosocial models are less likely to engage in TDV, relative to less connected teens.

Most existing TDV prevention programs are school based, which makes sense given the resources that are available in schools and the fact that youth spend a third of their lives in these institutions. Empirically evaluated programs have demonstrated some potential in eliciting change. For example, several studies have shown that adolescents who undergo a school-based prevention program exhibit increased knowledge of, reduced intentions for, and more appropriate attitudes about dating violence. However, prevention programs (eg, Safe Dates, Shifting Boundaries, Ending Violence, Coaching Boys into Men, Stepping Stones, and Fourth R) have only recently been evaluated using rigorous research methods with long-term measures of actual behaviors. The Safe Dates prevention program was evaluated in 8th and 9th grade students in 14 schools randomized to receive either a dating violence prevention curriculum or the control condition. This school-based program includes a theatrical production, community-based activities, and ten 45-minute sessions targeting mediating variables (ie, dating violence norms, gender-role norms, and conflict management skills) in an attempt to prevent the onset (primary prevention) or stop the continuation (secondary prevention) of dating aggression. In general, the program has been found to be effective in reducing physical, severe physical, and sexual dating violence victimization and perpetration. Notably, these effects were observed 4 years post-treatment.

Shifting Boundaries is a 6-session classroom and school-based curriculum designed to prevent sexual dating violence and harassment in middle school students. The focus is on (1) presenting consequences for perpetrating sexual dating violence and harassment, (2) setting and communicating personal space boundaries in interpersonal relationships, (3) identifying unsafe areas on the school campus (ie, "hotspots"), and (4) a building-based component involving restraining orders and placement of violence awareness posters. The building-only intervention and combined classroom/building intervention were found to be effective in reducing sexual violence victimization.

One of the more promising programs, Fourth R, integrates the promotion of healthy relationship skills and the prevention of dating violence into existing health and physical education courses. The program includes a school-level component in which teachers receive specialized training on healthy relationships and teen dating violence, and students form "safe school committees." A cluster randomized trial of Fourth R revealed that Canadian adolescents in the treatment group evidenced reduced physical dating violence 2.5 years post-treatment, relative to adolescents in the control group.

## SUMMARY AND RECOMMENDATIONS

Physical, sexual, and psychological TDV are prevalent and widespread, with consequences ranging from mild distress to suicide and homicide. While TDV may occur in any relationship, adolescents with a history of TDV who have experienced or been exposed to any form of violence and who participate in risky behaviors (eg, substance use, risky sexual behavior) are especially vulnerable to victimization and perpetration. Pediatric healthcare professionals should familiarize themselves with local and national TDV resources, advocate for evidence-based school- and community-based prevention programs, discuss and promote healthy relationships with all patients and their parents, and routinely screen for TDV. All staff should be trained in recognizing and responding to TDV, and clinics should be equipped with practical resources (relevant phone numbers and Web sites) and informational pamphlets and posters describing characteristics of healthy and unhealthy relationships.

## SUGGESTED READINGS


Break the Cycle Web site. www.breakthecycle.org. Accessed February 2, 2017.

Cutter-Wilson E, Richmond T. Understanding teen dating violence: practical screening and intervention strategies for pediatric and adolescent healthcare providers. *Curr Opin Pediatr.* 2011;23:379-383.

Exner-Cortens D, Eckenrode J, Rothman E. Longitudinal associations between teen dating violence victimization and adverse health outcomes. *Pediatrics.* 2013;131:71-78.

Mulford C, Giordano PC. Teen dating violence: A closer look at adolescent romantic relationships. *Natl Inst Justice J.* 2008; 261:34-40.

National Domestic Violence Hotline and Break the Cycle. Loveisrespect Web site. www.loveisrespect.org. Accessed February 2, 2017.

Nemours. Teens Health. https://kidshealth.org/en/teens/. Accessed May 6, 2017.

Teen dating violence. Centers for Disease Control and Prevention Web site. www.cdc.gov/violenceprevention/intimatepartnerviolence/teen_dating_violence.html. Accessed February 2, 2017.

Temple JR, Le VD, Muir A, Goforth L, McElhany AL. The need for school-based teen dating violence prevention. *J Appl Res Child.* 2013;4(1).

That's Not Cool Web site. www.thatsnotcool.com. Accessed February 2, 2017.


# 34 Child Trafficking


Reena Isaac and Salina Mostajabian


## INTRODUCTION

It is perplexing to consider that, in the modern era of vast accomplishments of the human condition, the concept of slavery continues to thrive. Trafficking in persons (TIP) is a form of slavery that sits at the junction of human rights, immigration, criminal justice, global public health, and politics. Most troubling is the discovery of children becoming ensnared and exploited by others for commercial profit. From the child beggars on the streets of Calcutta, to the young girls of the Far East whose nimble fingers weave intricate products for the carpet industry, to the child soldiers of Uganda who are abducted from their homes and trained to kill within their homeland, to the wayward teenaged runaway selling sex on the streets of Houston, the umbrella of child trafficking shades many different faces and industries. The trauma that child victims are subjected to and endure includes physical, psychological, sexual, and mental abuse. Such multilayered and chronic suffering can have significant medical and psychological manifestations long after a victim has left the life as a captive, and change a community for generations.



## DEFINITION

While the exploitation of persons for profit has been a stain on human history since the beginning of time, the last few decades have revealed greater recognitions of, and responses to, increased numbers of marginalized and displaced individuals who become entrapped in various industries for ill-gained profit. The end of the Cold War, dissolving of national borders, increased economic disparities, and the effects of globalization have been cited as some of the causes from the global vantage. In an effort to unite various definitions to combat trafficking, the United Nations (UN) put forth the Protocol to Prevent, Suppress and Punish Trafficking in Persons, Especially Women and Children, also known as the Palermo protocol, where human trafficking is defined in Article 3 as the recruitment, transportation, transfer, harboring or receipt of persons, by means of threat or use of force or other forms of coercion, of abduction, of fraud, of deception, of abuse of power or of a position of vulnerability or of the giving or receiving of payments or benefits to achieve the consent of a person having control over another person, for the purpose of exploitation. Exploitation shall include, at a minimum, the exploitation of the prostitution of others or other forms of sexual exploitation, forced labor or services, slavery or practices similar to slavery, servitude or the removal of organs.

### Scope of the Problem

Given the elusive and criminal nature of the entity, research of victims, traffickers, and clients is difficult and the statistics are highly speculative. Victim identification is difficult due to the fluidity of trafficking and its clandestine nature. Consistent, uniform collection of data by regions is not occurring, and no central database currently exists. Many of the statistics offered have been provided without clear constructs of methodologies, and terms and definitions used in different studies may vary to include different populations. The majority of data collected emerges from the post-trafficking assistance organizations such as non-governmental organizations (NGO) or homeless shelters to detention centers and law enforcement both at the local and national levels. Those victims providing permission for study may not completely reflect the greater body of victims still unrealized; thus, such data may have limited generalizability depending on the sample population. With this understanding, while the true incidence and prevalence of trafficking is unknown, it has been estimated that more than 21 million victims are being trafficked worldwide each year. There is a paucity of data on male victims and children especially in non–sex-related trafficking; however, the available global data does indicate that women and children are particularly vulnerable. Of the estimated total $150 billion generated as annual illegal profit, two-thirds, or $99 billion, is derived from commercial sexual exploitation, while another $51 billion results from forced economic exploitation, including domestic work, agriculture, and other economic activities.

## CLASSIFICATION OF TRAFFICKING

### Labor Trafficking

Labor trafficking is defined as the use of force, fraud, or coercion for the purpose of subjection to involuntary service, peonage, debt bondage, or slavery. Given the many vulnerabilities of children and adolescents, the inclusion of "force, fraud, or coercion" is not required to meet the definition of child trafficking. Trafficking can include, but does not require, movement of persons to perform their expected duties. At the heart of the issue is the traffickers' goal of exploitation and entrapment of victims for profit. There are limited data and studies on the issue of child labor trafficking, though the phenomenon is pervasive throughout the globe. Labor trafficking can include work in agricultural, food, hospitality, construction, or domestic servitude industries, to name a few. Poor or dangerous work conditions, long work hours, unsanitary living and working environments, exposure to toxic chemicals, and limits to social and family contacts are some of the situations that child victims in various industries (eg, gold mines of Africa, tobacco industry of Bangladesh, peddling industry in the

United States) may be subjected to. Elements of trafficking have been used as tactics in armed conflicts in regions around the world as a means of intimidating populations through the use of violence, fear, and oppression. Children can be abducted and trained as child soldiers in regional conflicts, and/or used as cooks, servants, and brides for extreme militant or political groups.

### Sex Trafficking

Sex trafficking of a minor (STM) refers to trafficking of a person under the age of 18 in commercial sex, where the inclusion of force, fraud, or coercion is not required. Commercial sexual exploitation of children (CSEC) is closely tied with sex trafficking and can be expanded to any sexual practice involving children for economic benefit. Commercial exchanges for sexual activities or performances include exchanges of money, drugs, food, clothing, or shelter or basic survival. Commercial sex industries include prostitution, pornography production, strip performances at shows, and mail-order brides. Survival sex or trade sex practiced by many homeless youths in exchange for basic necessities (eg, food, shelter, or money) is classified under CSEC by some sources. Shared Hope International has suggested that the term "child prostitution" be replaced with the term "domestic minor sex trafficking" in order to clarify the child's status as a victim. Although women and children are the majority of sex trafficking victims, a growing body of evidence shows previously unidentified male victims of sexual exploitation.

### International Victims

International or transnational trafficking requires movement of victims away from their native country to a destination or host nation for the purpose of exploitation. The majority of foreign victims identified in the United States originate from Mexico and the Philippines, but many others, including Guatemalan, Thai, Honduran, and Indonesian nationals, have also been identified. As violence and economical and political instability erupt in many countries in various parts of the world, they create waves of human displacement, including an increasing number of unaccompanied minors, crossing international borders. Such minors are extremely vulnerable to exploitation.

### Domestic Victims

Domestic victims are US citizens or legal permanent residents. Most domestic victims are children being exploited for the commercial sex industry. Those vulnerable to domestic sex trafficking include children with past sexual/physical abuse, children with low self-esteem, kidnapped children, and children with disabilities and mental illness. Sexual minorities and marginalized youth such as runaways, homeless, and throwaway youth, and those with unstable housing, with disproportionate numbers of LGBTQ youth, are especially at risk.

## ENTRY INTO THE WORLD OF SHADOWS

### Push and Pull Factors

An analysis of the *push-pull factors* of human migration, when viewed through the lens of personal finance and aspiration, may illuminate the causes for entry by often unwitting pawns into the world of trafficking. Push factors produce the migration of persons from one land to another with the hope and promise of financial gain or safety, and pull factors attract persons to regions of economic and individual hope; these factors include but are not limited to those listed in Table 34-1.

**TABLE 34-1 PUSH AND PULL FACTORS OF MIGRATION**

| Push Factors of Migration | Pull Factors of Migration |
|---|---|
| War, calamity, political unrest, regional conflicts | Demand for workers and low-wage labor |
| Paucity of employment opportunity | Possibility of improved opportunity |
| Disintegration of the family: substance abuse, homelessness, parental illness, death, abandonment | Hope and dreams of a better life (false promises) |
| Economic disparities | |
| Corruption within political and authoritarian factions | |
| Poor border control | |
| Gender and ethnic discrimination | |
| Prior victimization (sexual abuse, physical abuse, neglect) | |
| Poverty | |

### Supply and Demand

The economic concepts of supply and demand further contribute to the multifaceted exploitations of vulnerable and marginalized populations seeking financial opportunities from trafficking profiteers who barter services to an increasingly demanding clientele. Children and adolescents form a sizeable portion of trafficking victims and are particularly vulnerable, as they are still developing cognitively, socially, and physically, and due to their concrete thinking and lack of life experience to discern harm and deception, are easy targets for predators. One study estimates that 1 out of every 3 teens on the street will be lured into prostitution within 48 hours of leaving home. It is due to this susceptibility that the involvement of fraud, force, or coercion is nullified in definitions of trafficking as they relate to minors. Recruitment of victims often occurs in early adolescents as young as 12, from common places such as schools, shopping areas, and movie theaters. Internet-based platforms (eg, social media networks, chatrooms, microblogs) are being used to facilitate commercial sex, thereby extending the criminal reach beyond the metropolitan cities into the rural communities. Digital currency, such as Bitcoin, enhances online escort sites by further allowing secretive financial exchanges and anonymity of all parties involved.

Adolescent girls make up a significant portion of trafficking victims, especially in sex trafficking. Younger age acts as a risk factor when it is combined with negative emotions within the victim, which increases her vulnerability to psychological games. Predatory tactics can involve the emotional manipulation of children and adolescents such as validating feelings of love and attention and promise of financial security through appealing jobs or gifts.

### The Socio-Ecological Model

**Risk Factors** Although victimization can occur to any youth, the available literature overwhelmingly places children with a history of family violence, sexual or physical abuse, or neglect at higher risk. The factors putting an individual at risk of becoming a trafficking victim are manifold and can be analyzed from a multilevel standpoint including individual, local, and larger societal factors that have been known to have adverse health effects. On an individual level, vulnerability to recruitment plays a fundamental role in the cascade of trafficking. Factors that are taken into consideration include individual health, financial crisis, psychological state, and risk behaviors.

**Individual Level** Childhood abuse can impact cognition, behavior, and affect in exposed children with negative effects lasting into adulthood, especially in the absence of social support. Studies in the United States have shown a high rate of 30% to 40% of childhood sexual abuse, which is reflected in surveys of women in post-trafficking service centers, showing a rate of 59% experiencing abuse prior to their involvement in trafficking. A study from 2010 by Wilson and Widom indicated that victims of abuse were more than twice as likely as nonabused children to become involved in prostitution later in life. The experience of trafficking becomes another abusive situation endured by the victim with adverse psychological consequences added to previous trauma, which puts victims at risk of re-trafficking.

**Relationship Level** Family dysfunction, such as a history of domestic abuse, plays a critical role in victimization risk. Parental mental illness, especially depression and substance abuse, as well as system involvement such as child protective custody or juvenile detention make for tenuous social support systems for children. Chronic stress from a singular or recurring event such as abuse can lead to anxiety, depression, and other adverse psychological as well as physical sequelae.

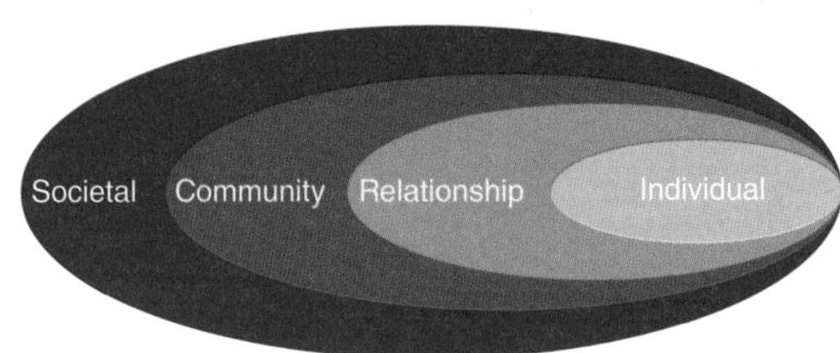


**FIGURE 34-1** The social-ecological model. (Reproduced with permission from The Social-Ecological Model: A Framework for Prevention. Centers for Disease Control and Prevention. http://www.cdc.gov/violenceprevention/overview/social-ecologicalmodel.html. Published 2015.)

**Community Level** At the community level, there are also multiple elements contributing to the expanding human trafficking levels. Factors for involvement into human trafficking both as victim or perpetrator include exposure to violence, abuse, and poor economic opportunities at the local level. There is an increasing level of gang involvement and organized crime entities, which have influenced the patterns of business conduct and use of violence. A study analyzing survey responses from victims to prosecutors in eight US cities shows a correlation between the drug trade and human trafficking, specifically underground sex trafficking, and the overlapping of these economies. This is congruent with evidence that there is increased risk of trafficking for youth living in areas with high crime rates. Other local/geographic factors such as military bases, truck stops, or large athletic venues serve as destinations for large transient male populations that could increase demand for sexual services and thus increase the risk for exploitation of potential trafficking victims.

**Societal Level** On the larger societal level, political instability, armed conflict, and corruption contribute to the problem of human trafficking. Corruption within the law enforcement sector in many cities or countries can precipitate escalating levels of community violence. Such disturbances in turn can lead to increased recruitment risk, facilitating movement of victims through transit routes, and to inadequate enforcement of existing anti-trafficking laws.

From the socio-ecological model vantage, the interplay of the risk factors involved in the telescoping social levels of the individual, family, community, and society showcases how the cumulative nature of each risk factor within each rubric can create the environment for which violence and abuse may fester, and how individuals, families, and communities may fall prey (Figure 34-1).

Understanding and addressing the various risk factors and how they each contribute to the possibility of a state of violence and exploitation that leaves children at risk may provide avenues for both intervention and prevention programs that seek to thwart the perpetuating cycle.

## HEALTHCARE SIGNIFICANCE

The health consequences in a trafficked victim are legion. Many victims suffer physical, mental, and/or sexual abuse during their time of entrapment. Access to healthcare among trafficking victims is variable. While some may have access to regular and preventive care, including contraceptive and sexually transmitted infection (STI) screening/treatment needs, others only interact with the healthcare system during life-threatening situations or acute exacerbation of chronic problems. It is noteworthy, therefore, that victims and survivors reported that they had interfaced at some point with the healthcare industry during their captivity, with a range of 28% to 88% reporting such contact. One study reported that 46% of CSEC victims had been to a medical provider within the past 2 months. These statistics underscore the need for enhanced screening and identification of potential victims by healthcare professionals.

Many of the health problems experienced by trafficking victims can be nonspecific, such as headaches, back pain, weight loss, and sexual health concerns, while others may be more specific to the type of exploitation, including reproductive health care, infections, overdose, or physical injury. They may present to different settings, such as emergency departments, urgent care clinics, reproductive clinics, school clinics, private clinics, or correctional facility clinics. Pediatricians are in a unique position in that they may encounter a teen who is trafficked as well as possibly the child's parent, who may actually be the victim.

### Mental Health

Trafficked victims repeatedly experience physical, sexual, and emotional abuse, all of which are used as means of manipulation and control by those who seek to exploit them. Economic as well as social isolation further perpetuates the feelings of helplessness and fear. Children who are exposed to multiple traumatic events or complex trauma at a young age can sustain serious impairment in all domains of their development and functioning. The seven domains of impairment of children exposed to complex trauma are:

- Attachment: How victims view and relate to personal relationships with others (eg, seeking out abusive partners, poor reader of people, antisocial behaviors)
- Biology: How the physical body reacts or is perceived to react to trauma (eg, somatization, increase in medical problems, may span multiple organ systems, elevated hypertension)
- Affect or emotional regulation: How victims regard and emote social cues (eg, flat affect, difficulty voicing desires, diminished empathy)
- Dissociation: How victims may have alternate states of consciousness (eg, amnesia, impaired memory of events, depersonalization).
- Behavioral control: How victims react in common life situations (eg, self-destructive behaviors, tantrums, threats to others, aggressiveness)
- Cognition: How victims think, and how they may appear to be slower (eg, difficulty processing new information, poor school performance, inability to do simple math or balance a home budget)
- Self-concept: How victims view themselves (eg, low self-esteem, distorted body image, self-blame, guilt).

The persistent toxic stress that a trafficked victim endures during a time filled with unknown dangers, constant threats, and limited freedoms (whether realized or not) changes the emotional and physical makeup of the individual, resulting in adaptive measures to cope with an environment for survival. This fight-or-flight state continues long after rescue and reintegration are attempted.

One study of US victims of sexual exploitation and trafficking found that 69% suffered from post-traumatic stress disorder (PTSD). Suicidal ideations, low self-esteem, and high-risk behaviors are often associated and confronted. The effect of these adversities can lead to depressive and anxiety disorders with some evidence suggesting direct correlation with the duration of exploitation. Symptoms often persist for years after the trafficking experience, especially if there is preexisting trauma, which is common to many victims. Substance abuse may begin during the period of exploitation when a trafficker may dispense drugs to victims to make them compliant; alternatively drugs and alcohol may be consumed by victims as a means of escape and a coping tool continuing far after the time of containment.

### Sexual Health

Sex trafficking victims are at high risk for sexually STIs, pregnancy, and complications from unsafe abortions. The majority of studies show that trafficked minors and women who were trafficked as minors are at risk of contracting HIV and hepatitis. In various samples, an average of one-third have been identified as HIV positive with increased risk for those who were trafficked at a younger age. Violent sexual assaults, gang rapes, and other forms of sexual violence may also occur. Gynecologic issues, such as pain during intercourse, abnormal vaginal discharge and odor, ectopic pregnancies, and pelvic inflammatory disease, may also be signs and sequelae of the life.

### Physical Health

Exposure to violence is common among trafficking victims in various settings. Extreme exhaustion and body aches from intense labor without adequate rest, nutrition, and hydration are observed. Physical violence from inflicted trauma, such as beatings, may result in limited function of a part of the body. Tattoos, burns, or other branding measures serve to mark a victim as a product of commerce and may further diminish or depersonalize the victim by its psychological effect. Trafficked women in the sex industry continue to suffer more physical and sexual violence compared to other sex workers. Headaches are one of the most common physical problems reported by trafficked victims in addition to fatigue, dizziness, back pain, abdominal and pelvic pain, and skin conditions. When evaluating pain in this population, somatoform disorders also need to be considered. Certain medical conditions (eg, diabetes, asthma) that existed prior to captivity may be exacerbated by inadequate or infrequent medical access and availability. Unsanitary and unhealthy work and living conditions may result in respiratory and other infections. Those trafficked into the labor force may suffer from work-related injuries related to inadequate protective gear, training, or rest.

**The Medical Evaluation**

Suspicious factors could emerge from a clinical history, physical finding, or social history, or a combination of the three. It is critical to be able to obtain accurate information from the patient independently and to build rapport. Interviewing can be difficult in these situations. Taking the time to build rapport may yield a more relaxed and productive exchange. The first steps to a positive interaction can include separating the patient, if the victim is accompanied by another person. If language is a barrier, locating an interpreter is important. Traumatic bonding may steep the victim in the reluctance to reveal information of the trafficker and "family" and denial of current exploitation. Clinicians must be familiar with the laws regarding mandated reporting where they practice, and the limitations of confidentiality should be discussed with patients prior to asking sensitive questions. In addition, youth should be reassured that they can choose to answer questions based on their comfort level to minimize re-traumatization.

The physical evaluation serves to

1. determine and treat acute complaints and conditions.
2. document physical injuries, including potential branding sites (eg, tattoos).
3. document and treat chronic conditions.
4. document general physical health and nutritional status.
5. potentially obtain a sexual assault evidence kit, if determined.
6. document anogenital injuries.
7. test and treat for STIs.
8. test for pregnancy and offer emergency contraception.
9. assess and test for alcohol and drugs.
10. assess mental health, imminent harm, and self-injurious injuries.

**Safety and Consent** The clinician should be familiar with state laws relating to conducting a physical exam and sexual assault evidence collection kit on a minor without the permission of a guardian. Most states allow clinicians to evaluate and assess minors without guardian consent when the clinician suspects child maltreatment. Patient assent for the exam, testing, and treatment are essential in these cases. Allowing the patient to dictate what occurs to his or her body is critical in returning control and enhancing trust. If a patient consistently refuses all or part of the examination, and it is safe to defer examination or treatment, the patient's wishes should be respected. The forensic evidence collection kit is not medically necessary, but if permitted to be obtained by the patient, it may be completed when appropriate. Some counties and jurisdictions have specially trained clinicians at specific sites, such as emergency centers and child advocacy centers, who conduct acute sexual assault examinations and completion of the forensic evidence collection kit. The medical evaluation and its purpose should be clearly and carefully discussed with the patient. The patient should be asked if he or she prefers to have a friend or caregiver in the room during the examination for comfort and support; however, care must be made that a suspected exploiter is not present during the evaluation. Separation is crucial in these circumstances. It is prudent for the clinician to have a staff chaperone present during the examination. If the suspected victim patient declines further evaluation, attempt to arrange a follow-up visit a few days following the initial encounter, as this may allow time for further reflection and possible compliance by the patient.

**TABLE 34-2 POTENTIAL INDICATORS OF TRAFFICKED VICTIMS IN A CLINICAL SETTING**

| |
|---|
| Poor or inconsistent history |
| Hesitation to answer basic questions such as living or work situations |
| Avoiding eye contact and exhibiting fear and anxiety |
| A companion who stays with the patient at all times or patient's refusal to be interviewed alone |
| Hostile behavior, disorientation, or hypervigilance |
| Not having access to identification and other documents and money |
| Physical injuries with a repetitive pattern or involving readily visible areas of the body; external injuries should prompt further evaluation, including diagnostic imaging or potential internal injuries |
| Tattoos or branding that could be subtle or explicit with only male names or various symbols indicating sale or property |
| Sexual history indicating trade sex in minors or high number of sexual partners |
| Repeated STI or pregnancy |
| Poor oral health |
| Repeated somatic complaints |

**Potential Indicators in the Clinical Setting** Clinical clues can come from rising discomfort during certain examination routines. Clinicians should approach such situations with respect for the patient's wishes while walking the patient through the examination process. Red flags, or potential indicators, of trafficked victims that may prompt concern during an evaluation include but are not limited to those in Table 34-2.

**Screening Tools** The ability of healthcare providers to recognize adolescents at high risk of CSEC/sex trafficking is critical to offering victims needed services. As many victims may not self-identify as victims, maintaining a very narrow definition of trafficking may cause clinicians to overlook those hiding in plain sight. To date, a validated screening tool is not currently available; however, one study created a short, data-driven screening tool, a six-item questionnaire, specifically designed for youth in a healthcare setting:

- Is there a previous history of drug and/or alcohol use?
- Has the youth ever run away from home?
- Has the youth ever been involved with law enforcement?
- Has the youth ever broken a bone, had traumatic loss of consciousness, or sustained a significant wound?
- Has the youth ever had a STI?
- Does the youth have a history of sexual activity with more than 5 partners?

With the constructed 6-item screen, a cutoff score of 2 positive answers had a sensitivity of 92%, specificity of 73%, positive predictive value of 51%, and negative predictive value of 97%. An intervention prompted by a positive screen would result in additional questions about high-risk sexual activity and commercial sexual exploitation using a trauma-informed approach. Such inquiries are performed in a nonjudgmental, open-minded manner, being sensitive and observant of any undue stress in the patient.

**Treatment and Resources** The elements of trust and safety must be evaluated for effective treatments. Applying a trauma-informed outlook into those in the medical workforce who will most likely interface with young, potentially exploited victims would set the stage for establishing a safe harbor for treatment and recovery.

The National Human Trafficking Hotline (1-888-373-7888) can assist in finding local resources for the victim and developing a safety plan that is amenable to the patient. The accompanying Web site (http://nhtrc.polarisproject.org) also provides additional resources. Transnational victims may also benefit from additional resources such as the U.S. Immigration and Customs Enforcement (ICE) Victim Assistance Program (1-866-872-4973). If the victim is a minor, the healthcare professional is under legal obligation to contact Child Protective Services for any suspicion of child maltreatment, including exploitation.

The needs for many victims caught in the complicated web of trafficking are vast. Medical and mental health assessment and therapy, housing, legal representation, schooling and training, and financial resources are a few of the most common and important needs in the immediate and expected futures of victims. Painting broad strokes that implement programs and establish resources in larger cities may not effectively and efficiently serve more rural communities, given the differences in resources, trafficked victims, accommodations, and transportation. The concept of "think globally, act locally" addresses the scope and scale of the problem, while delivering the practical allotment of known resources within an affected community.

## CONCLUSION

Child trafficking is multifaceted problem and global public health issue that requires a robust multidisciplinary response. The adverse health outcomes are considerable for victims, and the medical community is a major stakeholder in the areas for early intervention, prevention, identification, and rehabilitation of victims and children at risk.

## SUGGESTED READINGS


Fong R, Cardoso JB. Child human trafficking victims: challenges for the child welfare system. *Eval Program Plann.* 2010;33(3):311-316. doi:10.1016/j.evalprogplan.2009.06.0

Greenbaum J, Crawford-Jakubiak JE. Child sex trafficking and commercial sexual exploitation: health care needs of victims. *Pediatrics.* 2015;135(3):566-574. doi:10.1542/peds.2014-4138

Isaac R, Solak J, Giardino AP. Health care providers' training needs related to human trafficking: maximizing the opportunity to effectively screen and intervene. *J Appl Res Child.* 2011;2(1). http://digitalcommons.library.tmc.edu/childrenatrisk/vol2/iss1/8. Accessed February 3, 2017.

National Human Trafficking Hotline. National Human Trafficking Resource Center Web site. https://traffickingresourcecenter.org/. Accessed February 3, 2017.

Office on Trafficking in Persons Administration for Children and Families Web site. http://www.acf.hhs.gov/programs/endtrafficking. Accessed February 3, 2017.

Polaris Web site. http://polarisproject.org/. Accessed February 3, 2017.

Reid JA. Exploratory review of route-specific, gendered, and age-graded dynamics of exploitation: applying life course theory to victimization in sex trafficking in North America. *Aggress Violent Beh.* 2012;17(3):257-271. doi:10.1016/j.avb.2012.02.005.

U.S. Department of State. Trafficking in persons report, July 2015. Available at http://www.state.gov/j/tip/rls/tiprpt/2015/index.htm. Accessed February 3, 2017.


# 35 Infant Colic

Krista Preisberga and Joyee Goswami Vachani

## INTRODUCTION

Crying in infants is considered a normal developmental behavior with great variability between individuals in the amount of crying. There has been no clear singular definition of what constitutes normal versus excessive crying, known as colic. Observational studies in various settings have shown certain patterns that could constitute normal crying patterns in infants:

1. Crying increases progressively from birth and peaks at about 6 weeks of life and subsequently decreases. One meta-analysis showed an average duration of crying to be 110 to 118 min per day in the first 6 weeks and then decreasing to 70 minutes per day by week 12.
2. There appears to be a diurnal rhythm, with peak crying clustering during the evening hours, and this is most apparent during the peak crying time at 2 months.
3. Considerable variability exists in the amount of crying not only between different individuals but also day-to-day differences in the same infant.

## DIAGNOSIS

Colic is a descriptive term for the amount and quality of crying that appears to be outside the expected or "normal" crying behavior observed in otherwise well infants. As a descriptive term, it does not imply any pathology and is generally believed to be a benign process that self-resolves with time.

The pattern of crying observed in infants with colic is the same as that observed in normal infants in terms of peak at 6 weeks and then a steady decline in frequency, and duration of crying, but the episodes of crying are longer and more high-pitched and fail to improve with the normal soothing behaviors such as carrying or rocking. Additionally, family dynamics, psychosocial factors, and expectations affect the parent perception of what constitutes excessive crying. Infants perceived to be crying excessively by their parents cause a considerable amount of distress in the caretakers and are at higher risk for harm such as shaken baby syndrome. One study found that 5.6% of parents had admitted to having shaken, slapped, or smothered the baby to stop the crying.

There are several clinical definitions for qualifying what constitutes excessive crying for diagnostic purposes:

- The most recognized in clinical practice and research is Wessel's "rule of threes." It requires that in an otherwise well and fed infant the crying episodes last 3 or more hours per day, occur on 3 or more days per week, and persist for at least 3 weeks.
- The Rome IV criteria is another classification system that requires confirmation of total crying time by a parental diary to be 3 or more hours per day, in addition to lack of failure to thrive or evidence of other systemic illness. The episodes of crying have to start and stop without obvious precipitating factors.
- Another term used to describe colic is a period of PURPLE crying. This acronym describes the timing as well as the morphology of crying, taking into account the facial grimacing and stiffening of the extremities and the environmental factors.

  **P**eak: There is increase in crying that peaks at about 6 to 8 weeks. There is a subsequent decrease to resolution by 4 months of age.
  **U**nexpected: Cry starts and stops seemingly without a cause.
  **R**esists soothing.
  **P**ain-like grimacing.
  **L**ong-lasting: Crying can last for several hours a day.
  **E**vening: Clustering of crying in late afternoon and evening.

The occurrence rate of colic has been reported anywhere from 8% to 33%; however, the data is based on varied definitions and relies on self-reporting and recall by parents. Data collection methods have ranged from audio recordings and parental diaries to varied questionnaires and interviews. There is no racial, socioeconomic, or gender prevalence for colic, and it occurs equally in breastfed and formula-fed infants.

## ETIOLOGY

While there is no single mechanism that has been identified as a clear cause for colic, many different possibilities have been proposed in past years. There are several interesting associations that have been drawn; however, the cause-and-effect relationship has not been reliably demonstrated with any single source.

The thought that colic represents pain or discomfort originating in the gastrointestinal tract was based on observations of borborygmus, passage of flatus or stool at the end of the crying episode, drawing up of the legs, and tensing of the abdomen. This belief has not been substantiated by evidence but has geared many investigations to seek the source of pain in the abdomen. Other investigative paths have focused on the neurologic and developmental aspects with possible interplay between the intestinal and central nervous system (CNS) communication.

The ever-changing environment of the gastrointestinal tract is influenced by the complex network between the CNS, the autonomic nervous system, the intestinal microbiota, and the very plastic enteric nervous system. This bidirectional communication between the gut and the brain is commonly referred to as the brain-gut-microbiota axis. The microbiota supports normal digestion, modulates motility, maintains barrier function, prevents colonization by pathogens, and shapes immunologic responses. Perturbations in this fine balance can lead to functional intestinal disorders, and colic could be classified in this category.

#### Gastrointestinal Etiologies

Visceral hypersensitivity is suggested as a possible mechanism for perception of pain in the absence of identifiable pathology in functional gastrointestinal disorders. Stress-induced inflammation mediated by mast cells can stimulate the enteric nerve endings and lead to an increase in density and altered function of the enteric neurons. Even after resolution of initial insult and inflammation, the altered enteric signaling persists. A recent study found that even minor stress of gastric suction in infants at birth appears to lead to visceral hypersensitivity and an increase in functional intestinal disorders in later life.

Altered microbiome has been shown to present in infants with colic with a more restrictive pattern of organisms detected. There is evidence from recent studies that showed increased presence of *Klebsiella* spp and *Escherichia coli* as well as Proteobacteria in infants with colic, whereas *Bifidobacterium* spp and *Lactobacillus* spp were increased in control infants. One study demonstrated an increase in fecal calprotectin, indicating a possible underlying inflammation. It is not yet clear if the inflammation is the cause of the altered microbiome or vice versa. There is emerging evidence of the benefits of *Lactobacillus reuteri* supplementation in colic with decrease in crying severity.

Abnormal intestinal motility has been proposed to lead to perception of pain in the presence of hyperperistalsis. While there is no direct evidence available that there is alteration in motor activity in colic, two hormones that play a key role in intestinal contractions—motilin and ghrelin—are elevated in infants with colic. There is evidence of motility and hypersensitivity being linked closely to the altered microbiome, and likely all three mechanisms are highly interdependent. In breastfed infants, the lipid content of the milk is increased toward the end of a feed, which stimulates cholecystokinin release to produce satiety and decrease gut transit time. One study demonstrated that infants with colic had lower plasma cholecystokinin concentrations.

Gastroesophageal reflux (GER) and gastroesophageal reflux disease (GERD) have been implicated in colic. GER, however, is not a disease process, and regurgitation occurs in up to 50% of all infants. GERD develops when frequent reflux leads to esophagitis, aspiration pneumonia, failure to thrive, and hematemesis, which are pathologic symptoms that should not be present in infants with colic. Also, there is no evidence that increased use of acid suppressive medications has resulted in remittance of colic symptoms.

Cow's milk protein allergy (CMA) is the most common food allergy in infants. The presence of dysmotility, visceral hypersensitivity, and an altered microbiome in children with food allergies is similar to that postulated in colic. The diagnosis of CMA is generally made by elimination diet in the mother or use of hydrolyzed formulas in the absence of a confirmatory diagnostic test. The results of these dietary interventions, however, have been equivocal with regard to length of crying in infants with colic, except in a small subset that likely have allergy to whey or casein.

Functional lactose overload occurs when increased levels of lactose are delivered to the colon due to malabsorption. The fermentation of lactose by bacteria leads to formation of hydrogen gas that can be readily measured as exhaled gas. Several studies have found an increased concentration of exhaled hydrogen gas in infants with colic compared to controls. This theory links in with the abnormal motility causing rapid delivery of carbohydrates to the colon. The presence of more hydrogen producing bacteria in an altered microbiome leads to increase in gas production and colonic dissension. In individuals with gut hypersensitivity, this cascade of events leads to perception of pain and discomfort.

#### Neurodevelopmental Etiologies

Developmental immaturity of the motor functions could contribute to feeding difficulties, such as underfeeding, overfeeding, swallowing excessive amounts of air, and difficult coordination of the suck–swallow–breath mechanism. There appears to be an association between breastfeeding difficulty and excessive crying. Problems of attachment and positioning, ankyloglossia, and sensory processing problems can put susceptible infants at risk for persistent aversive feeding behaviors.

Circadian rhythm immaturity is another mechanism that can contribute to the pattern and explain the timing of the crying. The organization of sleep and wake cycles matures in the first 3 months of life, coinciding with a decrease in length of the crying episodes. Melatonin and serotonin secretions are increased in the evenings and follow a circadian pattern. One of the actions of melatonin is to relax intestinal smooth muscle while serotonin increases the contractions. Increased levels of serotonin metabolite have been found in infants with colic, while it is believed that melatonin secretion does not become fully functional until 3 months of age, leaving serotonin action unopposed. Cortisol, another hormone with a circadian pattern, is involved in regulation of the early-morning awakening. A recent study found that infants with colic lacked the circadian variation in cortisol levels when compared with controls.

An association between colic and migraine onset later in life has been shown in a few retrospective studies, and a recent prospective study found a 2.7 relative risk increase in developing migraine without aura by 18 years of age in infants with colic. While some have postulated that colic could be a variant of abdominal migraine versus true headache in the infant, the mechanism behind this in unknown at this time.

Family stress, maternal anxiety, and depression during pregnancy are also associated with colic. The psychosocial factors bear a large significance in how the caregivers cope and perceive the crying infant and their perceptions of their own parenting skills. The transference of tension from the caregiver to the child is a possible contributing theory. Additionally, the parents' temperament and expectations can affect their perceptions of what constitutes excessive crying and their decision to seek medical evaluation. The hypothesis that colic is an early manifestation of a difficult temperament has not been supported by a prospective longitudinal study in which the authors found no differences in temperament between infants with colic and the control group.

### EVALUATION

The presentation of the crying infant can pose a diagnostic dilemma to the provider and is one of the most common complaints by parents. In general, a thorough history and physical examination is sufficient to establish the diagnosis without the use of specific laboratory tests or imaging. A review of the evidence has shown that no more than 5% to 10% of infants presenting to clinicians because of prolonged crying have an identifiable underlying pathology.

A thorough history should include the pattern of crying; inciting events; feeding and sleeping disturbances; associated symptoms, such as emesis and stool and urine output changes; maternal drug use to evaluate for abstinence syndrome; social history to evaluate support structure; and infant–mother bonding. The importance of a complete and thorough physical examination cannot be overstated. Table 35-1 highlights important aspects of the exam and findings that should prompt further evaluation for an underlying pathology.

A recent study of infants presenting to the emergency room for excessive crying found that only 5% had significant pathology and a quarter of those were infants with urinary tract infections. Other sources were clavicle fracture, acute lymphoblastic leukemia, acute cholecystitis, epidural hematoma, intussusception, spinal muscular atrophy I, and dislocated elbow. It is not currently indicated to

**TABLE 35-1 PHYSICAL EXAM FINDINGS IMPLYING PATHOLOGIC CAUSES OF CRYING**

| Exam | Concerning Findings for Underlying Pathology |
|---|---|
| **Anthropomorphic parameters and vital signs** | **Failure to thrive** (broad differential) |
| | **Macrocephaly or microcephaly** (hydrocephalus, number of underlying genetic syndromes) |
| | **Fever, tachycardia** (sepsis, UTI, congestive heart failure) |
| **General appearance** | **Decreased activity** (sepsis, abusive head trauma, metabolic derangements) |
| | **High-pitched cry, excess sweating** (neonatal abstinence syndrome) |
| **HEENT** | **Photophobia, conjunctival erythema** (corneal abrasion) |
| | **Mouth breathing** (choanal stenosis, nasal mass) |
| | **Sneezing and congestion** (URI, neonatal abstinence) |
| | **Oral ulcers** (herpangina) |
| | **Bulging tympanic membrane** (acute otitis media) |
| | **Decreased neck range of motion** (retropharyngeal abscess) |
| **Cardiac** | **Irregular rate** (SVT) |
| | **Gallop** (congestive heart failure, myocarditis) |
| **Respiratory** | **Asymmetric breath sounds** (foreign body aspiration) |
| | **Wheezing, crackles** (bronchiolitis) |
| | **Stridor** (croup or foreign body) |
| **Neurologic** | **Full fontanelle** (hydrocephalus, meningitis, encephalitis) |
| | **Delayed motor skills or altered tone** (neurologic disease) |
| **GI** | **Distended abdomen** (malrotation, obstruction) |
| | **Tender to palpation** (appendicitis, volvulus, gastroenteritis) |
| | **Presence of mass** (pyloric stenosis, malignancy) |
| | **Rectal tone increased** (Hirschsprung's disease) |
| | **Inguinal hernia** (incarcerated hernia) |
| **Musculoskeletal** | **Full range of motion of joints** (septic joint, dislocation) |
| | **Deformity or palpable mass on long bones** (fracture, malignancy) |
| | **Crying elicited by palpation of extremities** (osteomyelitis) |
| | **Mucous or bloody stool in diaper** (CMA, intussusception) |
| **Skin** | **Pallor** (anemia, malignancy) |
| | **Jaundice** (hyperbilirubinemia, sepsis, UTI) |
| | **Bruises or burn marks** (abuse) |
| | **Eczema** (food allergy) |
| | **Hair tourniquet** |
| **GU** | **Testicular mass or swelling** (torsion) |

perform urinary culture and analysis in all afebrile, well-appearing children, but should be considered in infants younger than 1 month.

## MANAGEMENT

Infantile colic is often a challenging illness to diagnose and treat. Management algorithms in the literature suggest first stratifying treatment plans based on red flags related to potential organic disease (eg, reflux, atopy, failure to thrive) or parental coping (eg, parental anxiety or depression, child maltreatment). If red flags are identified, appropriate steps should be taken and referrals should be made. Assessment of the family dynamic—including postpartum depression screening and intervention, and discussion of coping strategies—is necessary to support families affected by infantile colic. If there are no red flags and there is no improvement with patient and family support, CMA can be considered and treated with a cow's milk–free diet for breastfeeding mothers or hydrolysate formula for formula-fed infants. If the patient does not improve, next steps to consider include hospitalization for observation or referral to a gastroenterologist.

Although numerous therapies have been suggested for infantile colic, a recent systematic review found little evidence to support the use of several commonly used medications (simethicone, dicyclomine hydrochloride, cimetropium bromide, lactase), fiber, or behavioral interventions. There is some evidence to support the use of casein hydrolysate formula for formula-fed infants and a low-allergen maternal diet for breastfed infants, although further research is necessary.

Several recent studies support the use of the probiotic *Lactobacillus reuteri* DSM 17938 for infantile colic in bottle-fed and breastfed infants, citing benefits that include decreases in crying time, functional gastrointestinal disorders, and maternal depression. Additional research regarding the mechanism of action and long-term consequences is needed.

## NATURAL PROGRESSION AND PROGNOSIS

There is no evidence to suggest that children who cry excessively until 4 months of age are at increased risk of problems associated with growth or development; however, parental perception of their children as more temperamental is increased. Any child who has excessive crying at over 4 to 5 months of age should be further evaluated.

## SUGGESTED READINGS


Akhnikh S, Engelberts AC, van Sleuwen BE, L'Hoir MP, Benninga MA. The excessively crying infant: etiology and treatment. *Pediatr Ann.* 2014;43(4):e69-e75.

Barr RG, Paterson J, Macmartin L, Lehtonen L, Young S. Prolonged and unsoothable crying bouts in infants with and without colic. *J Dev Behav Pediatr.* 2005;26:14-23.

Batchelor N, Kelly J, Choi H, Geary B. Towards evidence-based emergency medicine: best BETs from the Manchester Royal Infirmary. BET 2: Probiotics and crying time in babies with infantile colic. *Emerg Med J.* 2015;32(7):575-576.

Douglas P, Hill P. Managing infants who cry excessively in the first few months of life. *BMJ.* 2011;343:d7772.

Freedman SB, Al-Harthy N, Thull-Freedman J. The crying infant: diagnostic testing and frequency of serious underlying disease. *Pediatrics.* 2009;123:841-848.

Gelfand A. Infant colic. *Semin Pediatr Neurol.* 2016; 23:79-82.

Hall, B, Chesters J, Robinson A. Infantile colic: a systematic review of medical and conventional therapies. *J Paediatr Child Health.* 2012;48(2):128-137.

Nocerino R, Pezzella V,Cosenza L, et al. The controversial role of food allergy in infantile colic: evidence and clinical management. *Nutrients.* 2015;7(3):2015-2025.

Rhoads, M. Altered fecal microflora and increased fecal calprotectin in infants with colic. *J Pediatr.* 2009;155:823.

Shamir R, St James-Roberts I, Di Lorenzo C, et al. Infant crying, colic, and gastrointestinal discomfort in early childhood: review of the evidence and plausible mechanisms. *J Pediatr Gastroenterol Nutr.* 2013;57(suppl 1):S1-S45.

Vandeplas Y, Gutierrez-Castrellon P, Velasco-Benitez C, et al. Practical algorithms for managing common gastrointestinal symptoms in infants. *Nutrition.* 2013;29(1):184-194.

Wolke D, Samara M, Alvarez Wolke M. Meta-analysis of fuss/cry durations and colic prevalence across countries. Presented at: 11th Internationational Infant Cry Research Workshop; June 8–10, 2011; the Netherlands.

Xu M, Wang J, Wang N, Sun F, Wang L, Liu XH. The efficacy and safety of the probiotic bacterium *Lactobacillus reuteri* DSM 17938 for infantile colic: a meta-analysis of randomized controlled trials. *PLoS One.* 2015;10(10):e0141445.

# 36 Child Maltreatment: Neglect to Abuse

Andrea G. Asnes and John M. Leventhal

## INTRODUCTION

The spectrum of parental feelings and behaviors toward children can extend from those that are positive and nurturing to those that are negative, harmful, and culturally unacceptable. At the negative extreme are behaviors that result in child maltreatment, including physical abuse, neglect, and sexual abuse. While most children are not abused or neglected, "normal" parents may have feelings and behaviors that may extend to those considered to be maltreatment. Thus, a parent's anger at the child and use of physical punishment may border on physical abuse, ignoring the child and providing inadequate nurturance or supervision may border on neglect, and close bodily contact and sensual feelings toward the child may border on sexual abuse.

## DEFINITIONS

Maltreatment of children includes physical abuse, neglect, sexual abuse, exploitation, and emotional maltreatment. Physical abuse is an act of commission toward the child by a parent or other caregiver that results in harm or intends harm to the child. It can include bruises from a beating, broken bones, or even death. Violence toward children may not result in a serious injury but is still a form of abuse. The World Health Organization defines *physical abuse* as "the intentional use of physical force against a child that results in—or has a high likelihood of resulting in—harm for the child's health, survival, development, or dignity."

Neglect is an act of omission, such as failure to provide adequate nutrition, shelter, clothing, or supervision; abandonment; or failure to ensure that the child receives adequate health care, dental care, or education. Physical abuse and neglect must be distinguished from *unintentional* or *"accidental" injuries*, and *health neglect* must be distinguished from less serious lapses in attending to a child's medical care, such as poor adherence to medical recommendations or missing a few appointments for health care.

Sexual abuse is the involvement of children or adolescents in sexual activities that they do not fully understand, to which they cannot give informed consent because of their developmental understanding, and that break societal or family taboos. It includes behaviors such as sexual intercourse, genital fondling, and exposing children to pornography. Exploitation is the use of a child in work or other activities for the benefit of others, such as child labor or sex trafficking.

Emotional maltreatment, which is the most difficult form of maltreatment to define, includes repeated verbal denigration, belittling, or scapegoating so that the child develops a sense of worthlessness and low self-esteem. Because emotional maltreatment often coexists with other forms of maltreatment, it is difficult to identify and enumerate as a separate type, and thus is substantially underreported. A degree of emotional maltreatment is a component of every form of child maltreatment.

## EPIDEMIOLOGY

Although abuse of children and infanticide have occurred over the centuries, pediatric recognition of and concern about the *battered child syndrome* did not begin formally until the 1960s. By the 1970s, each state had passed laws requiring the reporting of suspected maltreatment to the state's child protection agency.

Since 1990, the United States Department of Health and Human Services has maintained a voluntary national reporting system, the National Child Abuse and Neglect Data System (NCANDS), which publishes a yearly report, *Child Maltreatment*, after collection and analysis of data from participating states. The results of the 2014 *Child Maltreatment* report identified approximately 3.6 million referrals, including 6.6 million children under 18 years of age and 1580 deaths due to abuse or neglect. Of the children who died, 70.7% were younger than 3 years of age, highlighting the importance of young age related to lethal and serious injuries. The types of maltreatment substantiated were neglect (75%), physical abuse (17%), sexual abuse (8%), psychological maltreatment (6%), medical neglect (2%), and other (7%), with some children being victims of more than 1 type of maltreatment. Reports were approximately equal for males and females.

Of the reported cases, 19.2% were substantiated, meaning that the protective service agency found enough evidence to believe that maltreatment occurred. Thus, 702,000 children were substantiated victims of maltreatment at a rate of 9.4 victims per s1000 children annually. An unsubstantiated report does not necessarily mean that maltreatment did not occur; rather, it means that there was insufficient evidence to meet the state's definition of maltreatment. In a study of investigated cases that were closed without substantiation, more than one-third of closed cases were reported within 2 to 3 years of the original report. Low socioeconomic status was found to be a key predictor of which closed cases were likely to be rereferred.

Because states have different requirements for reporting, use different criteria to decide whether a report is a substantiated case of maltreatment, and use different approaches to classification and to counting multiple reports on the same child, it is difficult to compare rates from 1 state to another. Since yearly national statistics were first collected by NCANDS in 1990, reports of maltreatment have tended to increase annually. One explanation for this increase is that changes in society have made it more difficult for parents to care for their children; an alternative explanation, however, is that professionals caring for children have broadened their definition of maltreatment and both parents and professionals have become more aware of the problem and are more likely to recognize less serious forms of maltreatment.

In spite of these consistent increases in the overall number of reports annually, there has been a 55% decrease in cases of substantiated physical abuse and a 64% decrease in cases of sexual abuse based on NCANDS data from 1990 to 2013. The authors of this study speculate that possible explanations for these marked decreases include improvements in the economy, increased rates of incarceration of criminals, increased availability and dissemination of effective psychiatric medication, and a possible generational shift in behavior and attitudes. Rates of neglect, on the other hand, have remained fairly stable, with a decline of only 13%. Whether this decrease reflects a lack of change in actual rates of neglect or a shift in what defines neglect is not known.

Most maltreatment occurs in the child's home. In 2014, 78% of perpetrators of child maltreatment were parents, and 54% of perpetrators were women. In a study of child deaths due to inflicted injuries, over 70% of known perpetrators were male. Perpetrators of sexual abuse are almost all males, and between 20% and 25% of them are juveniles, 16 years old or younger. The child who has been sexually abused most often knows the perpetrator, who may be the father, stepfather, another male relative, or a family friend. The small proportion of sexually abused children who do not know the perpetrator are usually older children or adolescents who are victims of forceful sexual assault or rape.

Reported cases of maltreatment are those that are recognized by clinicians and therefore may substantially underestimate the true rate of maltreatment that occurs in society. For example, it is thought that sexual abuse of boys is common but likely to be both under-recognized and under-reported. Two additional epidemiologic approaches have been used to determine the true prevalence of the problem. First, parents have been interviewed to determine both their behaviors toward their children and their knowledge of their children's victimization by others. A telephone survey of mothers in North Carolina and South Carolina found dramatically higher reported rates of physical abuse and sexual victimization than were reflected in local child protective services data. The incidence of physical abuse as determined by maternal survey was 40 times higher than that of official child protective services reports, and the reported incidence of sexual abuse was 15 times greater. Interviewing parents is a method that has also been used internationally to determine incidence when child protective services data are scarce or absent. In a cross-national collaborative study, investigators in Chile, Egypt, India, and the Philippines queried mothers between 1997 and 2003 about discipline practices. During the 6 months prior to the start of the study, 36% to 45% of mothers reported that they used an object to hit a child not on the buttocks. In Egypt, 25% of mothers reported beating a child within the last 6 months, while in rural India, 10% of mothers reported kicking a child.

A second epidemiologic approach surveyed adults about how they were treated as children. In a random survey of 2869 young adults in the United Kingdom conducted in 1998 and 1999, 16% of the respondents reported that they had experienced some form of child maltreatment. Seven percent of respondents reported experiencing physical abuse, 6% reported emotional abuse, 6% reported absence of care, 5% reported absence of supervision, and 11% reported sexual abuse involving contact. With respect to serious physical abuse, it is to be noted that most serious physical abuse occurs in children 3 years old and younger. Therefore, it is possible that adults recalling their own childhoods may be likely to underestimate their abuse histories.

Rates of reported past sexual abuse vary based on the population sampled, the type and number of questions asked of adults, and the operational definitions used. A review of 19 studies of adults in the United States or Canada found that the rates of sexual abuse reported by men were 3% to 16% and those reported by women were 3% to 62%. The review determined that a reasonable estimate of the rate of sexual abuse of girls under age 18 years is 20% and that of boys under 18 years is 5% to 10%.

## ETIOLOGY

The causes of child maltreatment are complex, and no single factor can be identified as certain to lead to child maltreatment. Belsky wrote that "there is no one pathway to disturbances in parenting; rather, maltreatment seems to arise when stressors outweigh supports and risks are greater than protective factors." A helpful framework for understanding what may place a child at risk of maltreatment involves the construction of an ecological model consisting of child, parent, family, and societal factors. The factors associated with the occurrence of abuse and neglect are listed in Table 36-1.

Child factors include the age of the child because younger children, those under 3 years of age, are significantly more likely than older children to die from physical abuse or neglect. Younger children are also most dependent upon caretakers for meeting basic human needs and are thus most vulnerable to neglect. Children born of unwanted pregnancies, disabled children, multiple births (eg, twins), and premature infants are at an increased risk of child maltreatment.

Parent factors that can lead to abuse or neglect include young parental age and abuse of alcohol or drugs. Some parents have limitations that can seriously interfere with parenting, as in the case of a parent with intellectual disability who may lack the basic skills necessary to provide appropriate food or stimulation to a child, or a depressed mother who may lack the energy and vigilance to supervise the child adequately. It is not likely that any single parent factor will lead to abuse. For example, although there is a strong association between a history of abuse as a child and abusing one's own child (the "intergenerational transmission of abuse"), the majority of parents who were abused as children do not abuse their own children.

Family factors associated with abuse and neglect include single-parent families, socially isolated families, families in which the household composition is frequently in flux, and families in which there are many children under the age of 5 years. The presence of an unrelated male in the household, such as a boyfriend of the mother, increases the risk of physical abuse, especially in households with young children. Intrafamilial violence, such as intimate partner violence, is an independent risk factor for subsequent child maltreatment.

Societal factors that contribute to child maltreatment are poverty and poor community resources and infrastructure, such as lack of adequate jobs and poor education. Because reported cases of maltreatment come from all social classes, the fact that abuse and neglect are reported more commonly in families who are poor and less educated suggests that these factors contribute heavily to the ability (or failure) of a parent to form an adequate and protective relationship with a child. Other neighborhood-level factors found to have an association with maltreatment include male unemployment rates, residential turnover, and median residential property value.

Reporting bias can play a worrisome role in the setting of suspected abuse and can lead to both over- and under-reporting of abuse. For example, in a study of young children (ages 1 and 2 years old) evaluated for long-bone or skull fractures, minority children who had accidental injuries were evaluated and reported for suspected abuse at higher rates than were nonminority children. Similarly, in a study of cases of abusive head trauma that were initially missed by medical providers, cases in white children and those living with both parents were significantly more likely to be missed than were cases in minority children.

**TABLE 36-1 BUILDING AN ECOLOGICAL MODEL: FACTORS ASSOCIATED WITH ABUSE OR NEGLECT**

| |
|---|
| **Child** |
| Unwanted |
| Disabled (including cognitive or emotional problems) |
| Twin |
| Premature |
| **Parent** |
| Younger than 19 years of age at child's birth |
| Substance abuse |
| Intellectual disability |
| Serious psychiatric illness |
| Maltreated as child |
| **Family** |
| Single parent |
| Isolated family |
| Inadequate supports |
| Family violence |
| Many children under 5 years of age |
| **Social Setting** |
| Poverty |
| Unemployment |
| High level of violence |

## PATHOGENESIS

Within the ecological framework, clinicians have focused on the nature of the relationship between a parent and a child. Two interrelated ways of understanding this relationship are an examination of a parent's attitudes and feelings about a child and the quality of the attachment between a parent and a child.

Bavolek has framed 4 types of attitudes and behaviors that are seen in abusive or neglecting parents. The first is an inappropriate parental expectation of the child, such as expecting a newborn to sleep through the night or an 8-month-old to be toilet trained. The second is a failure of empathy between parent and child, or an inability of the parent to understand and participate in the child's emotional experience and ideas. This failure may stem from a low self-worth on the part of the abusive parent, as the degree of self-worth is a predictor of how a person will treat and respond to others. The third is a placement of inherent value on the use of physical punishment. Fourth, abusive or neglecting parents may reverse the parent-child roles and see children as the source for family comfort and happiness. When faced with the persistent neediness and dependence of children, parents who expect their children to care for them can experience profound disappointment, which can lead to further abuse or neglect.

An assessment of the quality of the relationship between the parent and the child also is helpful in understanding the factors that lead to abuse and neglect. Secure attachment between a parent and a child is a protection against abuse or neglect, and a poor or failed attachment is a risk factor. Sensitive and responsive parents help ensure attachment, while parents who are insensitive, rejecting, or inconsistent threaten a successful attachment. Parents may be unable to be sensitive, accepting, and consistent for a host of reasons, including their own parents' failure to provide a secure, nurturing environment to them or other traumatic experiences that led to mental health problems, such as depression or substance abuse.

It is likely that a constellation of factors, such as a combination of ecological risk factors, a parent's negative feelings about a child, and a poor parent-child attachment, must exist for maltreatment to occur.

It is important to recognize that risk factors for child maltreatment tend to vary with the type of maltreatment. Physical abuse, for example, typically occurs when a parent loses control and injures a child. In cases of both abusive head trauma and abusive fractures, males are significantly more likely than females to be the perpetrators. Parents who use and value physical discipline at baseline are more likely to experience such a loss of control, and use of physical punishment is a known risk factor for more serious physical abuse. Similarly, predictably challenging periods in a child's development are frequently linked with physical abuse. For example, normal infant crying that peaks within the first months of life is associated as a prime trigger for abusive head trauma. Another trigger for physical abuse is toilet training and the inevitable demands that this period can bring. An important factor to consider is parental drug or alcohol abuse, which can have profound negative influences on parents' abilities to care for their children. Substance abuse is also an important precursor to neglect. National spikes in drug use, such as the epidemic of crack cocaine in the 1980s and 1990s, result in a marked increase in the incidence of neglect.

The sexual abuse of children is more difficult for most clinicians to understand than is the occurrence of physical abuse or neglect. The 2 prerequisites for this form of maltreatment include sexual arousal to children and the willingness to act upon this arousal. Factors that may contribute to this willingness include alcohol or drug abuse, poor impulse control, and a belief that the sexual behaviors are acceptable and not harmful to the child. The past history of the perpetrator (eg, having been sexually abused during childhood), the particular vulnerability of the child (eg, a developmental delay), and a circumstance that enables the perpetrator to have increased contact with the child (eg, a mother who is hospitalized) all contribute to the likelihood that sexual abuse may occur. Recent work suggests that while identified perpetrators of child sexual abuse may have levels of generalized empathy comparable to nonperpetrators, perpetrators are likely to lack empathy specifically for their child victim. This finding suggests that even in an adult capable of empathy, a failure or suspension of understanding and regard for a child victim is an important component of sexual abuse.

## CLINICAL MANIFESTATIONS

Like other forms of family violence, the maltreatment of children usually occurs in the privacy of a home and is seldom witnessed by another person. Because the child is often too young or too frightened to explain what happened and the correct history often is not known or not provided by the parents, clinicians should be aware of suspicious histories and recognize the typical behaviors and physical findings of maltreated children. Children may be victims of multiple types of maltreatment.

### Physical Abuse

Five types of histories should raise the suspicion of abuse: (1) a child with a serious injury, such as a fracture, but no history of preceding trauma (eg, "I noted that his arm was limp"); (2) a history that is inconsistent with the severity, mechanism, or timing of the injury; (3) a delay in seeking medical care for a significant injury; (4) a history that changes during the course of the evaluation; and (5) a history of recurrent injuries, especially those that are poorly explained.

Children who have been abused display a variety of behaviors. They may be excessively fussy, frightened, or depressed due to recurrent pain, maltreatment, and the impact of living in a threatening and unpredictable environment. Older children may demonstrate role reversal in their interactions with their parents: Instead of the parent caring for the child's needs, the children learn to be particularly sensitive to the parents' needs and, in part, to avoid being hurt, may provide care for the parents. Such children may attempt to be well behaved around adults in order to avoid offending them and being punished. Some children who have been abused repeatedly do not cry during medical procedures, such as blood drawing, because crying at home may have resulted in additional punishment.

The spectrum of physical abuse extends from a single episode, such as a slap on the face, to recurrent and more serious injuries. Children who sustain injuries from abuse that are mistakenly diagnosed as unintentional injuries are at substantial risk of being more seriously hurt or even of dying from abuse. Abusive injuries may be medically mild (such as a small bruise on an infant unable to move around under her own power), but forensically significant in that they represent physical abuse. Such medically mild abusive injuries are known as "sentinel injuries" as they indicate abusive caregiver behavior and are "sentinel" because they may precede and therefore predict the occurrence of more serious abusive injuries. It is crucial for pediatric providers to recognize these injuries for what they are in order to prevent more serious physical abuse. In a study of abused infants who were hospitalized, more than one-quarter had a history of a sentinel injury noted by caregivers and medical providers before abuse was recognized.

Soft tissue injuries are the most common clinical manifestation of physical abuse. These include hand marks from slapping; bruises from punches; linear and curved marks from belts, cords, or switches; and bite marks. In evaluating injuries to the skin, it is important to consider the child's developmental level. For example, 1-year-olds who are learning to walk often fall forward and bruise their faces, and it is not uncommon for preschool children to bruise their shins. Studies of bruises in young children have demonstrated that it is unusual to see bruises in children who are not cruising. In children under 4 years of age, bruising on the torso, ear, and neck are worrisome for physical abuse. Pierce has put forth a useful mnemonic to help clinicians recall the locations of bruises that suggest physical abuse: TEN-4. Bruising on the **t**orso, **e**ar, and **n**eck of any child under the age of 4 years and any bruising at all in an infant under 4 months of age should prompt clear concern. Bruising occurs after bleeding into the skin or subcutaneous tissues. Fresh bruises are usually tender and swollen, with maximum swelling in 1 or 2 days. Bruises may change color from deep purple/red to green to yellow/brown. The rate of these changes depends on the depth of the bruise, the amount of bleeding, the location of the injury, possible drugs the child has taken, or the inherent clotting ability of the child. Because of the many factors involved in bruise progression, dating an injury based on the appearance of a bruise is inexact.

Burns are another common type of abusive injury. These can include scald burns from hot liquids or burns from hot objects, such as irons, stoves, or cigarettes. Although burns that are due to abuse are often difficult to distinguish from unintentional injuries or those due to neglect, the location and pattern can be helpful. Children who have been immersed in hot water may have bilateral burns of the upper or lower extremities or burns of the buttocks or back. These inflicted burns often have a sharp demarcation between the injured and noninjured skin. A child who has been held in hot water in a tub may have a spared area of the buttocks, as a result of the area having been pressed against the tub. In contrast, nonabusive scalds tend to be asymmetric from 1 extremity to the other, have less sharply demarcated borders, and reveal splash marks that indicate the child tried to avoid the injury. Other commonly occurring unintentional scald burns occur when young children spill containers of hot liquid on themselves.

Cigarette burns are another type of suspicious injury. An isolated, unintentional cigarette burn, which tends to be superficial, can occur when a young child comes in contact with a cigarette held by an adult. In contrast, inflicted cigarette burns tend to be deeper, are located on areas to which accidental contact would be unlikely, and may be multiple.

Head injuries are the most common serious abusive injury, with an incidence of 30 to 40 per 100,000 children between 0 and 12 months of age, and they are the leading cause of death from abuse. Abusive head trauma can occur from shaking alone, blunt impact to the head, or a combination of both mechanisms. An analysis of perpetrator confessions of abusive head trauma indicates that shaking is the most common mechanism of abusive head trauma. Because in most cases the actual mechanism of injury is not observed, the use of a general term such as *abusive head trauma* is preferable to a specific term like *shaken baby syndrome*, which implies a single mechanism of injury. An important secondary mechanism involved in abusive head trauma is hypoxic-ischemic injury that occurs as a result of the initial trauma. These injuries, best detected on diffusion weighted imaging (DWI) sequences on magnetic resonance imaging (MRI), can have important prognostic implications for the brain-injured child. Abusive head trauma can result in intracranial bleeding due to repeated accelerations and decelerations of the brain that produce shearing of the bridging veins (resulting in subdural or subarachnoid hemorrhages) and retinal hemorrhages, which often can be extensive, involve different layers of the retina, and extend to the periphery (see Chapter 577).

Children with abusive head injuries may present with seizures, signs of increased intracranial pressure, coma, or apnea and cardiac arrest. Often, there are other signs of physical abuse, such as bruises or healing fractures. Rib fractures can be seen in conjunction with abusive head trauma; these fractures occur when the infant is held around the thorax, and the abuser squeezes the chest, causing anteroposterior compression and posterior rotation. Because rib fractures are usually not visible on chest radiographs until callus formation has begun to occur 10 to 14 days after an injury, the presence of an acute head injury and healing rib fractures indicates that the child has been injured on at least 2 occasions.

In head injuries due to abuse, there usually is no clear history of severe head trauma to direct the clinician toward the right diagnosis. In contrast, when children sustain serious unintentional intracranial injuries, such as those due to major falls or automobile accidents, there is a clear history to explain the injury, and retinal hemorrhages occur much less commonly. Most minor falls from heights of less than 36 inches do not result in serious head injuries, although skull fractures, with and without small, transient, and localized areas of subdural bleeding near the fractures, as well as epidural bleeding, can occur. Scalp hematomas are more common in children who sustain accidental falls than in children with abusive head injuries.

Fractures of bones are another common type of abusive injury in young children. In a series of 215 children under 3 years of age with fractures, 24% of the fractures were believed to be due to abuse. The highest occurrence of abusive fractures is in children under 1 year of age. Skull fractures that are depressed, branching, or diastatic have been associated with physical abuse; the most common type of skull fracture, however, found as a result of abuse (as well as with unintentional injuries) is a linear fracture of the parietal bone. Fractures of the humerus (especially the midshaft or the proximal end) and fractures of the femur (especially in children under 1 year of age) should be considered suspicious of abuse. In contrast, a 2- or 3-year-old child may have a supracondylar fracture of the humerus from a fall on an outstretched arm or a spiral fracture of the femur or tibia from falling and twisting. Whether the fracture is spiral or transverse is not by itself diagnostic of abuse. Rather, a careful consideration of the nature and severity of the injury, the proposed mechanism of injury, and the developmental abilities of the child should be undertaken. Two types of fractures more specific for abuse are classic metaphyseal, or bucket handle, fractures and rib fractures, particularly those that are posterior and adjacent to the spine. Several studies have indicated that rib fractures are unlikely to occur during cardiopulmonary resuscitation in young children.

Other types of injuries that should raise the suspicion of abuse are intentional poisonings and abdominal injuries (including lacerations of the liver, spleen, or intestines). Children with abdominal injuries are at particular risk of hypovolemic shock and even death when the internal injury is unrecognized and the history of blunt trauma is not provided by the caregiver. Multiple abdominal injuries, a high severity of injury, and a delay in seeking care should prompt particular concern for abuse.

An additional form of abuse that is often difficult to recognize is medical child abuse, or caregiver-fabricated illness in a child. In this form of abuse, the caregiver (usually the mother) fabricates symptoms of an illness in the child, resulting in an extensive medical evaluation, or causes the child to be ill by poisoning or some other means (eg, injecting contaminated fluid into an intravenous line) in order to assume the sick role by proxy (see Chapter 37).

### Neglect

Neglected children are recognizable by the chronic failure of their parents to provide adequate physical care or ensure appropriate medical care or education, or when the child is brought for medical attention because of an injury or ingestion due to failure of adequate supervision. While neglect may be chronic, even 1 instance of supervisory neglect may be severe, as in the case of a small child left at home alone. Worrisome histories include evidence of inadequate provision for the child's basic needs, inadequate supervision, or a delay in seeking medical care. It should be noted, however, that neglect in its less obvious forms can be quite difficult to define.

In infants and young children, a common manifestation of neglect is poor growth and developmental delay due to decreased nutritional intake and understimulation. Such children, who are labeled as having nonorganic failure to thrive, often are recognized first because of poor weight gain or because they fall off the growth curve. Initially, the child's length and head circumference may be relatively spared, but if the nutritional deprivation continues, these parameters also are affected. The general pattern of growth for decreased nutritional intake, regardless of the cause, is for weight to be most affected and head circumference least affected; this pattern can be ascertained by plotting each of the growth parameters on the 50th percentile curve and determining the child's age at the respective points (eg, the child's "weight age"). In many children whose failure to thrive is due to neglect, there also is a developmental delay, particularly affecting the child's language and social interactions. Such children may appear listless, have a flat affect, and demonstrate indiscriminate attachment behaviors. Older children who are neglected often appear as emotionally needy. They may be depressed or adult like in their behaviors as a result of having to learn to care for themselves. Acute problems, such as ingestions, burns, or injuries from falls, are common presentations in neglected children and should be distinguished from abuse or unintentional injuries.

### Sexual Abuse

Children who have been sexually abused generally come to the attention of clinicians because the child has told an adult about an uncomfortable experience (eg, "My uncle touches me down there, and I don't like it"), the parent becomes concerned about the child's behaviors (eg, sexualized acting out), or, much more rarely, symptoms (eg, vaginal discharge), a genital or anal abnormality noted on physical examination, or a positive culture.

Although the child's statement is one of the clearest indications that the child has been sexually abused, a very young child may have difficulty explaining what happened, and an older child may retract a relatively clear statement after the child begins to understand how upsetting the disclosure is to the family. In certain circumstances, such as disputes about custody or visitation, it may be particularly difficult to determine the truthfulness of the child's statements because of the complexities of the relationships in the family.

Children who have been sexually abused may demonstrate a variety of behaviors and symptoms. Many are nonspecific and are seen in response to other childhood stresses as well, such as poor school performance, generalized anxiety, encopresis, or suicidal gestures. Others are more suggestive, but not specific, such as excessive masturbation, sexualized behaviors, vaginal discharge or bleeding, or rectal bleeding. Even a symptom such as vaginal discharge, however, has a low likelihood of being due to sexual abuse. In several studies of premenarcheal girls with the complaint of vaginal discharge, the most frequent diagnosis was poor hygiene, and sexual abuse was found in less than 5% of cases.

Although all children suspected of being sexually abused should have a complete physical examination, most are likely to have normal findings on examination. In a study of 2384 children referred for possible sexual abuse to a tertiary referral center, the investigators found that only 4% of the children had an abnormal genital or anal examination at the time of evaluation. A normal examination does not rule out sexual abuse, as there may have been no injury to the genital area or, if there was an injury, it might have healed without leaving any signs. In cases in which there has been a conviction of a perpetrator, it is unusual for victims to have an abnormal physical finding. In a series of 236 children whose perpetrators were convicted, 23% of genital examinations of girls and 7% of anal examinations of all children were considered abnormal or suspicious. In a study of 36 adolescent girls who became pregnant as a result of suspected sexual abuse, only 2 of the 36 girls had definitive genital findings of penetration.

Considerable research has been conducted to define normal and abnormal genital and anal anatomy in prepubertal children. The appearance of the hymen is often thickened in early childhood because of the effects of maternal estrogen in utero; in preschool and school-age girls, the hymenal tissue becomes thinner until the effects of estrogen during puberty result in a thickening of the tissue and the development of redundant folds. Studies of normal prepubertal girls have described the shapes of the hymen as crescentic, annular, and fimbriated (or redundant) and have noted the frequency of normal variations, including hymenal mounds, intravaginal ridges, and adhesions of the labia minora.

Bruising, petechiae, or abrasions on the hymen, acute laceration of the hymen, vaginal laceration, and perianal laceration with exposure of tissues below the dermis are physical signs that indicate acute trauma. A healed hymenal transection or complete hymen cleft, noted as a defect in the hymen between 4 o'clock and 8 o'clock that extends to the base of the hymen, with no hymenal tissue discernible at that location, and a defect in the posterior (inferior) half of the hymen wider than a transection with an absence of hymenal tissue extending to the base of the hymen are signs suggestive of healed genital trauma.

Anal findings, such as acute fissures, also can be seen in sexually abused children. Normal findings in the prone, knee-chest position include skin tags in the midline, fan-shaped areas in the midline superiorly, perianal erythema, venous congestion, and anal dilation up to 2 cm. Children who sustain anal trauma as a result of sexual abuse may not have abnormalities on examination if the event is not acute. In a study of children with documented anal injuries followed from acute injury to healing, 29 of 31 children healed completely, with scar formation in only the 2 cases requiring acute surgical repair.

Infections known to be transmitted sexually and, therefore, of significant concern for sexual abuse in children include genital, rectal, or pharyngeal *Neisseria gonorrhoeae* infection; syphilis; genital or rectal *Chlamydia trachomatis* infection; *Trichomonas vaginalis* infection; and HIV, if transmission by blood transfusion or perinatally has been ruled out. Human papillomavirus (HPV) presents a special case in the evaluation for possible sexual abuse. Although previously believed to be the result of perinatal transmission, HPV is either rarely or never vertically transmitted. Young children may acquire HPV from nonsexual horizontal transmission, either by autoinoculation if a child has common skin warts or horizontally from nonabusive contact by a person who has common warts, and the likelihood of sexual abuse as a possible cause increases with age. History and full medical evaluation are of particular importance in ascertaining the possibility of sexual abuse in a child with HPV. Similarly, genital herpes in a child can and should raise a concern of sexual abuse (unless there is a clear history of autoinoculation). The likelihood of sexual transmission of herpes is unknown. In children over 5 years of age with isolated genital lesions and where herpes simplex virus type 2 (HSV2) is isolated, sexual transmission is more likely but not a certainty. HSV, even HSV2, is not diagnostic of sexual abuse.

Physical findings that are diagnostic of sexual contact in children include pregnancy and semen identified in forensic specimens taken directly from a child's body.

## ASSESSMENT AND DIAGNOSIS

When evaluating a child for suspected maltreatment, the clinician must decide whether an alternative explanation, such as an unintentional injury, a medical problem, or an acceptable parental behavior, can help explain the child's problem. The evaluation should include a complete history, careful physical examination, appropriate imaging studies and laboratory tests, and full documentation of the findings. In many settings, these tasks are divided among professionals so that a physician might obtain a medical history and conduct the examination while a social worker obtains a psychosocial history. When available, community-based or hospital-based child-protection teams can guide clinicians in their assessments and offer specialized evaluations or treatment services.

A careful history concerning the events leading to the child's condition, the child's health status and development, and the family's strengths and weaknesses can help determine what happened to the child and the important contributory factors (Table 36-2). Data should be collected from the parents, from the professionals who know the child and family, and from the child directly.

It is not uncommon for caregivers who were not actually present when the child was injured to report about the events causing the injury as if they were present. Careful questioning can help distinguish eyewitness accounts from secondhand information. It is important to note inconsistencies in reports (either from different caregivers or, over time, from the same caregiver) about how an injury occurred or how an injury/behavior evolved. Sometimes, however, inconsistencies may reflect different styles of history taking or variable documentation rather than inconsistencies because of intentionally confusing and misleading information. When maltreatment is being considered, supportive interviews of the parents alone and together may result in an admission of an abusive episode, a chronic pattern of neglect, or failure to nurture the child adequately.

When failure to thrive due to neglect is suspected, a careful feeding history should be obtained to estimate the child's caloric intake and to determine how the formula (or food) is prepared, what is offered to the child and how the child responds, whether feeding problems have occurred in the past, and what the parental concerns and fears are. Information also should be obtained about the child's developmental milestones, temperament, affect, and interactions with parents and others.

**TABLE 36-2 HISTORY TO EVALUATE SUSPECTED MALTREATMENT**

| Event(s) "Causing" Injury |
|---|
| What happened to child |
| Who was present |
| How the child responded |
| How the adults responded |
| Who cares for the child |
| **Child** |
| Previous injuries or concerns |
| Past medical history, including immunizations and missed appointments |
| Developmental history |
| Parents' descriptions of child |
| Parents' feelings toward child |
| **Family** |
| Care of other children |
| Parents' own nurturing |
| Parents' physical and mental health |
| Family violence |
| Previous involvement with child protective services or police |
| Substance abuse |
| Resources and supports |
| Recent stresses |

When sexual abuse is suspected, the parents must be asked explicitly about what the child said as well as about the child's symptoms, such as vaginal discharge or bleeding, rectal bleeding, constipation, encopresis, sexualized behaviors, or unusual or recurrent fears. If possible, information should be gathered from sources other than the child in order both to minimize additional trauma to the child and to prevent contamination of information necessary to the investigation and possible prosecution of a crime. Important additional data to be obtained about the family include whether the parents are separated or divorced and, if so, what kind of visitation schedule exists, and whether there is a dispute about custody or visitation.

After a referral to child protective services is made, developmentally appropriate children suspected of being sexually abused are likely to be interviewed directly about what may have happened to them by a trained forensic interviewer. This interview should be done with the child alone, and the interviewer should be skilled at such assessments and careful to avoid leading questions. An evidence-based protocol for forensic interviews has been developed and is in widespread use. Interviews are usually conducted behind a 1-way mirror with representatives of child protective services and law enforcement observing, and in many jurisdictions, these interviews are video recorded. To help young children describe what may have happened to them, interviewers have used stimulus props, such as anatomic drawings, for clarification of a child's initial statements.

The physical examination should focus on the child's growth, development, affect, and interactions with parents and health professionals as well as on the state of hygiene, signs of new and old injuries, and signs of sexual abuse. A careful skin examination is of particular importance with attention paid to the identification of any sentinel injuries. Physical findings such as extensive dental caries and severe diaper dermatitis may be indicative of neglect. Tattoos may be a sign of sex trafficking (see Chapter 34).

The examination of children suspected of having been sexually abused should include a careful inspection of the genitals and anus. The clinician should remain alert to signs that might point to an alternative diagnosis. In girls, the genital examination is best performed in the supine position; when abnormalities of the hymen are noted, the child also should be examined in the prone, knee-chest position to determine whether the abnormality persists. The physical examination is best approached as a healing step for abused children. A carefully performed examination can reassure an abused child that his or her body is healthy and normal.

To visualize the hymen, the examiner can use 2 maneuvers: labial separation—separating the labia majora and pulling down at an angle of 45 degrees—and labial traction—gently pinching the labia majora and pulling out and toward the examiner. Girls with suspicious findings should be examined by an expert examiner who uses a videocolposcope or photocolposcope, which provides magnification and the ability to document the findings. During the examination, careful attention must be paid to avoid any additional trauma to the child who may have been sexually abused. A clear explanation of the nature and purpose of the examination, as well as the presence of a supportive adult, will help to assure the child's comfort in this setting.

In some cases, more extensive diagnostic studies are indicated. For children with serious head injuries, an ophthalmologic examination should be performed to determine whether retinal hemorrhages are present. This examination is best performed on dilated pupils by a pediatric ophthalmologist or an ophthalmologist with pediatric experience, and photographs of the findings can be very helpful. The location and extent of retinal hemorrhages have been found to be very helpful in differentiating accidental from inflicted head trauma. A child's course can be followed clinically, and magnetic resonance scans can be helpful in delineating the injuries and location of intracranial bleeds. Where there is a suspicion of abuse or neglect in a child under 2 years of age, a skeletal survey can reveal unsuspected recent or old fractures as well as provide information about an underlying medical problem, such as osteogenesis imperfecta. In children in whom abuse is highly suspected, a follow-up skeletal survey 2 weeks after the first is also indicated. The rate of detection of unsuspected fractures depends on the sample investigated; in a study of children up to 36 months of age who had a skeletal survey for suspected abuse, the survey identified a previously undetected fracture in 18%.

In children with bruises or bleeding, a complete blood count, a platelet count, prothrombin time, partial thromboplastin time, von Willebrand factor (vWF) antigen and activity (Ristocetin cofactor), and factor VIII and IX levels should be obtained as an initial screen. When suspected clinically or when initial screening tests are abnormal, more detailed tests for bleeding disorders should be ordered. Children with liver transaminases greater than 80 IU/L should be evaluated for possible occult abdominal trauma.

In children with failure to thrive, a careful history, physical examination, feeding observation, and home visit are significantly more likely than laboratory testing to reveal the cause of poor or failed growth. Any additional tests to search for an underlying disease should be directed by concerns noted in the history or abnormalities noted on the physical examination.

When a pubescent child is evaluated within 72 hours of an episode of suspected sexual abuse, forensic evidence collection, including body swabs, clothing and linen collection, and hair samples are indicated. In prepubertal children, the recommended window for DNA collection is 24 hours. Tests for sexually transmitted diseases, including gonorrhea, chlamydia, syphilis, trichomonas, hepatitis C, and HIV infection, should be obtained in children when the abuse might have resulted in transmission of such a disease. In adolescents, a pregnancy test may be necessary. Emergency contraception as well as postexposure prophylaxis for sexually transmitted infection (including HIV) should be provided as indicated.

Detailed documentation of the data collected, with direct quotations of the parents' or child's statements, and a clear description of the child's injuries both in writing and with sketches are important. Many states have a specific form for recording information from an examination to determine whether sexual abuse has occurred. Photographs of the child's injuries, labeled with the date and the child's name and record number, can be very helpful.

### Differential Diagnosis

The most common distinction that must be made in a case of suspected maltreatment is between abuse or neglect and an unintentional injury or inadequate nurturance. In addition, a variety of alternative explanations should be considered in the differential diagnosis. Bruises must be distinguished from birthmarks (eg, congenital dermal melanocytosis), coagulation abnormalities (eg, idiopathic thrombocytopenic purpura), dermatitis (eg, phytophotodermatitis), or the result of folk medicine practices (eg, coin rubbing). Burns due to maltreatment can be confused with skin diseases that develop bullae, unintentional scalds, or unusual burns, such as laxative-induced dermatitis of the buttocks due to ingestion of senna. Cigarette burns may be confused with impetigo. When evaluating a young child with a fracture, the clinician must consider the possibility of an underlying disease such as osteogenesis imperfecta, rickets, or congenital syphilis. In such cases, there usually are other clinical signs or radiographic features to help make the correct diagnosis.

When evaluating concerns of sexual abuse, the clinician should consider the possibility of a false allegation in the differential diagnosis. In young children, particular attention should be paid to using open-ended questions and to avoiding the overinterpretation of vague statements, such as "He touched me." Also, clinicians should consider the possibility of a false allegation if the child has a serious mental health problem; if the child is caught in a bitter dispute, such as a custody battle, between parents; or if the child's statements about what happened have important inconsistencies or are vague and lack details.

In cases of suspected sexual abuse, the examiner must identify abnormalities that are secondary to trauma due to sexual abuse from normal variations of anatomy. Physical conditions also can be mistaken for sexual abuse. Common examples are lichen sclerosis, which can cause thinning of the skin and subepidermal hemorrhages of the vulva and perianal area, and prolapsed urethra, which can mimic acute trauma.

Straddle injuries, which usually have a clear history of a fall and are associated with external injuries of the female genitalia, also must be distinguished from sexual abuse. A foreign body, such as toilet paper in the vagina, can present with foul smelling, serosanguinous fluid and can be confused with sexual abuse.

Children with failure to thrive due to neglect must be distinguished from children who are not growing well because of an underlying disease (eg, cystic fibrosis or a congenital infection) or whose poor nutritional intake is due to an interactional problem between the primary caregiver (usually the mother) and the child. For example, if an infant is fussy and spitting during feeding, a vulnerable mother may not enjoy feeding her child, lose patience, and thus provide inadequate calories.

## MANAGEMENT AND TREATMENT

There are 6 important steps in the management of suspected child maltreatment. First, there must be appropriate communication with the family about the child's condition and the physician's concerns. The physician must communicate clearly that there are questions about how the child got hurt and there is worry that the child may have been abused. The family should be informed that the physician is a mandated reporter who must notify the state's child protection agency about suspected maltreatment and not just cases of confirmed abuse. The second step is appropriate medical care for the child; third is ensuring the child's safety. Although some abused and neglected children are admitted to the hospital for protection and further evaluation, it is not uncommon for children who are not seriously injured to be placed in foster care or with relatives by the child protection agency. Fourth, the physician must assess the child's medical, developmental, emotional, and educational needs so that appropriate services can be provided. Fifth, the parents' and family's needs also must be evaluated so that adequate parenting can be ensured. And sixth, siblings should be assessed carefully to determine whether they have been maltreated.

These steps, which usually are carried out over time by professionals from several disciplines, including primary care clinicians, pediatric experts in child abuse, child protective services workers, police, and mental health clinicians, help determine the kinds of interventions needed. Services for the child might include ensuring appropriate medical care, participation in an early intervention program or a crisis nursery, or mental health counseling for an older child. For families, services might include concrete assistance (eg, ensuring adequate housing or transportation for the child's medical care), treatment programs for the parents' own problems (eg, drug treatment, mental health counseling, or counseling for domestic violence), or treatment programs that focus on parenting (eg, parent-child programs).

If the suspected maltreatment is substantiated, child protective services can help the family obtain the necessary services and monitor the child's safety. Unfortunately, most state protective service agencies are understaffed because of budgetary constraints and often have difficulty providing the necessary supervision of families whom they are mandated to serve. Pediatricians can help monitor families by providing follow-up care that focuses on the child's needs. This includes rereporting the child to protective services if new injuries occur or if the child continues to be at substantial risk of maltreatment.

Maltreated children whose safety cannot be ensured in the home usually are placed in foster care or with relatives.

Physically and sexually abused children and those children separated from parents for any reason, including neglect, will benefit from trauma-focused care. Evidence-based models of trauma-focused mental health care such as trauma-focused cognitive behavioral therapy (TF-CBT) can diminish posttraumatic symptoms and may mitigate the downstream effects of child maltreatment.

## NATURAL HISTORY AND PROGNOSIS

Maltreatment can have long-lasting and devastating effects on the development of children, adolescents, and adults. Although a child can be physically harmed from maltreatment, and brain injuries can have serious, long-term consequences, it is likely that the major consequences of maltreatment are related to its emotional impact. Also, studies have shown that childhood stressors such as physical and sexual abuse can affect brain development and disrupt the hypothalamic–pituitary–adrenal axis. In addition, studies have documented that the long-term effects of abuse can be determined by an interaction between genetic predisposition (or protection) and an abused child's environment. Many other factors also can affect the development of a maltreated child, such as malnutrition, placement in multiple foster homes, or exposure to family violence. Thus, the link between child maltreatment and subsequent outcomes is not straightforward.

Studies of abused and neglected children indicate that they have a higher rate of delayed intellectual development, poor school performance, aggressive behaviors, and social and relationship deficits compared to nonmaltreated children. There also is an increased occurrence of emotional difficulties, including depression, suicide attempts, and self-mutilation. Children who were maltreated are likely to have difficulty in forming trusting relationships with adults and in viewing adults as helpful people in their lives. Children who were neglected may be indiscriminate in seeking adult relationships.

There is clear evidence that children who have been maltreated have substantial problems with social interactions with peers. Children who were physically abused, in particular, have been noted to be physically aggressive and antisocial. Both abused and neglected children are at an increased risk of juvenile delinquency, substance abuse, and self-destructive behaviors during adolescence.

Adults who were abused or neglected as children often have difficulty forming intimate relationships and often choose partners with similar problems. Parents who were abused as children are at increased risk of abusing their own children (intergenerational transmission of abuse), but the link between experiencing childhood abuse and abusing one's own child is not a simple linear association. Although some investigators have estimated that 30% of abused parents will abuse their own children, further research is needed to define this risk more clearly. Adult survivors of childhood abuse suffer at significantly higher rates than others from depression, anxiety disorders, eating disorders, posttraumatic stress disorder, and chronic pain syndromes. Furthermore, adults maltreated as children are more likely than nonabused adults to be obese or physically inactive; to engage in smoking, substance use, and unsafe sex; to attempt suicide; and to have an unintended pregnancy.

Sexual abuse also has a major adverse impact on development. Children who have been victims of sexual abuse may develop low self-esteem and feelings of guilt and shame and may learn to use sexual behaviors inappropriately in their interactions with peers and adults. Teenage girls and adult women are at increased risk of promiscuity, have difficulties forming intimate relationships, and may be revictimized. They also are at increased risk of having mental health problems, such as depression, suicide, eating disorders, multiple personality disorder, and posttraumatic stress disorder. Males who were sexually abused as children are at increased risk of having mental health problems, abusing substances, or becoming perpetrators.

Little data exist about the long-term effects of specific treatments of maltreated children. The expectation is that early recognition and appropriate treatment for the child and family will minimize adverse outcomes. The presence of a supportive adult who is able to respond to the emotional needs of the child seems to minimize the short-term psychological effects of maltreatment, but less is known about its importance regarding long-term sequelae.

## SUGGESTED READINGS

Adams JA, Kellogg ND, Farst KJ, et al. Updated guidelines for the medical assessment and care of children who may have been sexually abused. *J Pediatr Adolesc Gynecol.* 2016;29(2):81-87.

Anderst JD, Carpenter SL, Abshire TC; Section on Hematology/Oncology and Committee on Child Abuse and Neglect of the American Academy of Pediatrics. Evaluation for bleeding disorders in suspected child abuse. *Pediatrics.* 2013;131(4):e1314-e1322.

Bavolek S. The nurturing parenting programs. In: US Department of Justice, ed. *Juvenile Justice Bulletin.* Family Strengthening Series. Rockville, MD: Juvenile Justice Clearinghouse; 2000. https://www.ncjrs.gov/pdffiles1/ojjdp/172848.pdf. Accessed September 7, 2016.

Bechtel K, Stoessel K, Leventhal JM, et al. Characteristics that distinguish accidental from abusive injury in hospitalized young children with head trauma. *Pediatrics.* 2004;114(1):165-168.

Christian CW; Committee on Child Abuse and Neglect, American Academy of Pediatrics. The evaluation of suspected child physical abuse. *Pediatrics.* 2015;135(5):e1337-e1354.

Cohen JA, Deblinger E, Mannarino AP. Trauma-focused cognitive behavioral therapy for children and families. *Psychother Res.* 2016;22:1-11.

Kleinman P. *Diagnostic Imaging of Child Abuse.* 3rd ed. Cambridge, UK: Cambridge University Press; 2015.

Kempe CH, Silverman FN, Steele BF, Droegemueller W, Silver HK. The battered-child syndrome. *JAMA.* 1962;181:17-24.

Krug EG, Dahlberg LL, Mercy JA, Zwi AB, Lozano R, eds. *World Report on Violence and Health.* Geneva, Switzerland: World Health Organization; 2002. http://apps.who.int/iris/bitstream/10665/42495/1/9241545615_eng.pdf. Accessed September 7, 2016.

Pierce MC, Kaczor K, Aldridge S, O'Flynn J, Lorenz DJ. Bruising characteristics discriminating physical child abuse from accidental trauma. *Pediatrics.* 2010;125(1):67-74.

Sheets LK, Leach ME, Koszewski IJ, Lessmeier AM, Nugent M, Simpson P. Sentinel injuries in infants evaluated for child physical abuse. *Pediatrics.* 2013;131(4):701-707.

Starling SP, Patel S, Burke BL, Sirotnak AP, Stronks S, Rosquist P. Analysis of perpetrator admissions to inflicted traumatic brain injury in children. *Arch Pediatr Adolesc Med.* 2004;158(5):454-458.

Sugar NF, Taylor JA, Feldman KW. Bruises in infants and toddlers: those who don't cruise rarely bruise. Puget Sound Pediatric Research Network. *Arch Pediatr Adolesc Med.* 1999;153(4):399-403.

# 37 Factitious Disorder by Proxy

Herbert Schreier

## INTRODUCTION

Factitious disorder by proxy, previously known as Munchausen by proxy, occurs when a caretaker (usually a mother) directly causes her child to be, or to appear to be, ill or impaired and obtains medical and/or psychiatric interventions. A child may be hospitalized unnecessarily or may receive inappropriate procedures and treatments that may have devastating effects on the child as well as the physician.

## CLINICAL DEFINITIONS AND PREVALENCE

The American Professional Society on the Abuse of Children (APSAC) proposed *pediatric condition falsification* (PCF) as a diagnostic description for abuse through illness fabrication. Conditions may be exaggerated, falsified, or induced. *Factitious disorder by proxy* (FDP) refers to a form of PCF in which a caretaker abuses a child for personal psychological motivations. The *Diagnostic Statistical Manual of Mental Disorders*, 5th edition, recognizes this condition as *factitious disorder imposed on another.* Some pediatricians use the term *medical child abuse*, but this term refers only to the child's maltreatment, not the psychopathology of the perpetrator. Although often difficult to discern, the motivation in FDP is important to know, because this form of abuse often has a guarded prognosis and may need interventions different from those for other forms of child abuse. PCF is child abuse regardless of the motivation. The historical term Munchausen by proxy continues to be used by some pediatricians, psychologists, and other child advocacy specialists.



Approximately 140 new cases of the most serious forms of FDP (eg, suffocation, poisoning) can be expected annually in the United States; less dramatic forms are often undetected or not reported.

## ETIOLOGY

The self-serving psychological needs in FDP vary. Some individuals appear to need or thrive on the attention that results from their own perception as the devoted parent of a sick child; others appear to be motivated by the need to covertly control or deceive clinicians and/or other authority figures. These mothers appear to have the ability to convince others of their essential goodness and caring. External incentives such as monetary rewards or wresting a child from a spouse may be present but are not the paramount motivation. Self-aggrandizement through the use of social media is now commonly found.

The abuse in FDP frequently involves the physician as an unsuspecting agent in harming the child. Qualities that we value in doctors, such as empathic caring and an interest in and need to solve complicated medical problems, may make some clinicians more susceptible to these manipulations. This is often the case when a perpetuator is a colleague or someone with impressive medical knowledge.

Despite signs and symptoms that are not consistent or that are ambiguous, or despite surgical procedures and medications that do not change the reported symptoms, the pediatrician is so often taken in that he or she disregards these results and the suspicions of others and prolongs the child's suffering. Unfortunately, it is common to find a principal physician who resists the diagnosis even when strongly approached by colleagues and refuses to report. Physicians who have failed to file mandated reports for suspected illness falsification have been sued and are open to criminal charges in at least two states. Death rates in reported cases are between 6% and 15%. When a new case occurs, other siblings who died mysteriously may be discovered. In a study with covert video surveillance of 38 women and 1 father suspected of suffocating their children, 33 were observed abusing their child on camera, and 3 others later admitted abuse. Eventually, 38 out of 39 parents were found to have abused their children. Among the 42 siblings of these children, 12 died previously from suspicious causes, 11 were classified as sudden infant death syndrome, and 4 parents admitted to killing 8 siblings of the index children. An additional 15 were abused. Typically, the abuse in FDP persists for an average of 14 to 22 months before a diagnosis is established. In another study, 17% of FDP victims had been treated through central venous catheters. Sepsis occurred in 56%, and the mean time until diagnosis was 82 months.

## CLINICAL PRESENTATIONS

Over 100 clinical presentations of FDP have been described, including failure to thrive, vomiting, acute life-threatening events, over- and undertreated asthma, mitochondrial illness, and dermatologic conditions. FDP can also present as a psychiatric condition and school-related disabilities.

Clinical profiles can be useful to suspect FDP in a child who is abused by a parent (Table 37-1). However, the parent profiles overlap substantially with behaviors commonly seen in mothers of truly ill children, anxious mothers, parents who are strong advocates for their genuinely ill children, and difficult parents. Careful chart review can often help distinguish these.

## DIAGNOSTIC PROCESS

A careful review of all relevant medical records is important in order to uncover FDP and factitious conditions. When FDP is suspected, action should be taken immediately to protect the child and confirm the diagnosis. Separating the parent from the child may be useful but only if carried out with the utmost of rigor and concern for the child and parent. Establishing the diagnosis of condition falsification is the first priority. Discovering the motivation for falsification is the next step.

Professionals from other disciplines who have experience with this disorder should be enlisted in the diagnostic process and in assessing

**TABLE 37-1 CLINICAL PROFILES SUSPICIOUS FOR FACTITIOUS DISORDER BY PROXY**

| |
|---|
| **Child Presentations** |
| A child who presents with medical problems that do not respond to treatment or that follow an unusual course |
| Signs and symptoms of a child's illness fail to occur in the parent's absence |
| **Parent Presentations** |
| A parent who is medically knowledgeable and/or fascinated with medical details and hospital gossip |
| A parent who appears unusually calm or even giddy in the face of serious difficulties in the course of her child's illness and may at the same time be very supportive of the physician; some parents may become demanding and angry when further investigations and procedures are resisted by staff |
| Discrepancies in the medical history or presentation as reported by the parent |
| A parent who makes self-serving efforts at public acknowledgment |



a potential underlying motivation of the perpetrator. There are no specific psychological tests to diagnose FDP.

The psychological assessment to discern a mother's mental health condition should only be performed by a professional who is familiar with the disorder, as inexperienced evaluators are often taken in by the mother's dissimulating abilities. In some cases of FDP, a mother may appear emotionally healthy on psychological tests. There are other situations of child abuse in which illness fabrication takes place for reasons other than that described in FDP (Table 37-2).

Guides for clinicians who are faced with the challenge of differentiating suffocation from sudden infant death syndrome in an infant (Table 37-3) and falsification of bowel symptoms from chronic intestinal pseudo-obstruction in toddlers are useful. Algorithms for differentiating FDP from failure to thrive have been described and include the red flags of involvement of more than five organs and more than five allergies. In such cases, one should be suspicious of the need for multiple parenteral feeding tube replacements.

## MANAGEMENT AND TREATMENT

The most difficult aspect of this disorder is ascertaining if symptoms are falsified. It is in the nature of this process that the clinician closest to the case is often least able to recognize that a child is being abused in this way. It is incumbent on the child's clinician to protect the child. Consultation with a professional child abuse expert is the first step. Care must be taken to avoid false accusations and to balance the parents' rights against those of the child, often one who is preverbal.

## PROGNOSIS

The prognosis in FDP is grim. Recidivism rates are high, and abuse has often recurred even on supervised visits. Mothers rarely concede their behavior, and as they continue their denial, they may extend the process of manipulation to social service and the court personnel. Treating someone with great dissimulating skills is difficult, clinicians with experience are essential, and it is tough to be confident in honest progress.

**TABLE 37-2 FABRICATION OF SYMPTOMS BY A PARENT IN SITUATIONS OTHER THAN FACTITIOUS DISORDER BY PROXY**

| |
|---|
| "Masquerade syndrome": Amplification or falsification of an illness to keep a child with mother at home |
| Delusion: A belief that the child is ill as part of a psychotic process in the mother (resolves with treatment of mother's condition) |
| Help seeker: Trying to obtain help for herself by presenting the baby as in need; usually, harm is minimal to child |
| Doctor-shopping and overly anxious parent: Belief that the child is not being diagnosed or treated appropriately; this is not FDP unless it is with the motivations described above |
| Hypochondria: Overreacting to normal conditions and exaggerating their seriousness |
| Obsessive-compulsive disorder: Focus on child being sick and obtaining unnecessary treatment |
| Malingering motivation is secondary gain such as monetary reward |

**TABLE 37-3 SUFFOCATION VS. SUDDEN INFANT DEATH SYNDROME—WHEN TO SUSPECT SUFFOCATION**

| |
|---|
| Multiple episodes of reported apnea |
| A child older than 6 months |
| A sibling with a major illness |
| A sibling who has died |
| Index child or sibling on the child abuse list |
| Blood in the nose and mouth in a child with an apparent life-threatening event (ALTE) |
| ALTE only by mother's report or only happens when she is present |

## SUGGESTED READINGS


Ayoub C. Munchausen by proxy. In: Plante TG. *Mental Disorders of the New Millennium: Biology and Function.* Wesport, CT: Praeger Press; 2006;3:173-193.

Ayoub C, Schreier HA, Alexander R. Guest editors' introduction: Munchausen by proxy. *Child Maltreat.* 2002;7(2):103-165.

Feldman KW, Hickman RO. The central venous catheter as a source of medical chaos in Munchausen syndrome by proxy. *J Pediatr Surg.* 1998;33:623-637.

Hyman P, Bursch B, Beck D, et al. Discriminating pediatric condition falsification from chronic intestinal pseudo-obstruction in toddlers. *Child Maltreat.* 2002;7:132-137.

McClure R, Davis P, Meadow SR, et al. Epidemiology of Munchausen by proxy in non-accidental suffocation and non-accidental poisoning. *Arch Dis Child.* 1996;75:57-61.

Schreier HA. Munchasuen by proxy. *Curr Probl Pediatr Adolesc Health Care.* 2004;34:121-148.

Schreier HA, Libow J. *Hurting for Love: Munchausen by Proxy Syndrome.* New York, NY: Guilford Press; 1993.

Sanders MJ, Bursch B. Forensic assessment of illness falsification, Munchausen by proxy, and factitious disorder NOS. *Child Maltreat.* 2002;7:112-124.


# 38 Foster Care and Adoption

Brad D. Berman and Carol Cohen Weitzman

## INTRODUCTION

Raising a child outside the child's biological family of origin, as in foster care or adoption, presents a unique set of psychosocial challenges involving an interplay between transition and adaptation. The child must contend with separation from and possible reunification with the birth parent, adjustments to 1 or more families, and changes in physical environment, social support, and care providers. The foster or adoptive parents are challenged with helping the child integrate into a new family, taking into account the child's previous experiences, and facing the possibility of further transitions in the future. The child's and family's success in adapting to these changes in care are influenced by a complex interaction between innate, individual capabilities and external resources. Nowhere is the traditional role of the pediatric provider more important in providing continuity of care, family guidance, and support for the physical, neurodevelopmental, and emotional needs of the child and family.

## EPIDEMIOLOGY AND DEFINITIONS

### Foster Care

The primary purpose of a child entering foster care is to provide a "temporary haven" for those who have been neglected and/or abused and cannot remain safely with their birth parents or family. The goals then are to provide for child and adolescent well-being, safety, health, and permanence of care. Approximately 415,000 children were in foster care on any given day in 2014 with about 653,000 children being served by the foster care system in a year. To characterize this population further, 108,000 children were awaiting adoption in 2014 and just over 50,000 were actually adopted out of foster care. After a peak number of 800,000 children in 2006, the overall number of children in the foster care system has slowly declined due to an increased emphasis on permanency planning. The overall number of children in foster care has remained relatively stable for the past 4 years. Of those children living in foster care in 2014, 49% were living in a *nonrelative* foster home, 29% in a *relative or kinship care* foster home, and the remainder in various care arrangements including group homes, other institutions, and pre-adoptive homes.

The Adoption and Foster Care Analysis and Reporting System (AFCARS) estimates that the median age for entering foster care is just over 6 years old, with a trend toward younger age of entry into the system for the past decade. Fifty-two percent of the foster care population is male. This report further describes the ethnic/racial distribution as 42% white, 24% African American, 22% Hispanic, and the remainder multiracial or undetermined. The median length of stay for a child in foster care in 2014 was 13.3 months with 26% remaining in this system for longer than 2 years. Of youth in foster care, 50% experienced at least more than one foster care placement with 25% experiencing three or more.

In contrast to the early years of foster care when foster placement often resulted because of illness or death of parents or extreme poverty, approximately 70% of children today are placed because of parental abuse and/or neglect. Often there is neglect of basic health care, safety, and educational needs for the child. Children enter foster care for a variety of reasons, including the negative impact of acute and chronic family stressors that include parental substance abuse, domestic violence, parental mental health problems and homelessness, living in poverty, abandonment, and increasingly, child neglect and/or physical and sexual abuse. Foster care is intended to be a temporary legal arrangement in which the child is protected and nurtured while supportive services are provided to the biological parent(s) to achieve family reunification.

Adolescents in foster care represent a unique group who may enter this system directly from the juvenile justice system, placed by their parents due to unmanageable behavioral or care challenges, or because they have grown up in long-term foster care. Adolescents often have the greatest placement instability. They have often had repeated exposures to maltreatment and sexual abuse with an accumulative impact on neurodevelopment and mental health. Adolescents in foster care are at risk of sexually transmitted infections (STIs) and unwanted pregnancy, negative self-concept, and lower self-esteem.

### Adoption

As of 2007, an estimated 1.8 million children under 17 years of age lived with an adoptive parent(s), representing 2% of the US child population. Approximately 130,000 children are adopted in the United States each year. The majority are domestic adoptions, with just over 5600 children of intercountry origin. The percentage of all adoptions by type is represented in Figure 38-1. Adoption trends have stabilized in the past few years, with the majority occurring via public agency/foster care and nonrelative sources. There has been a significant decline in intercountry adoptions in the past few years due to increasing expenses related to the adoption process, efforts to encourage domestic adoptions, political unrest, exploitation of children and families, and difficulties implementing the Hague Adoption Convention—an international agreement enacted in 2008 to ensure that adoptions occur in the best interest of the child. Approximately 10% of all adoptions are voluntarily relinquished infant adoptions. Increasing numbers of children are being adopted by transracial, transcultural, single-parent, and same-sex couples. Slightly more girls than boys are adopted, all of broad racial and ethnic groups. Thirty-nine percent of adopted children had reported special healthcare needs with higher than background rates of attention-deficit/hyperactivity disorder (ADHD) and behavioral challenges.

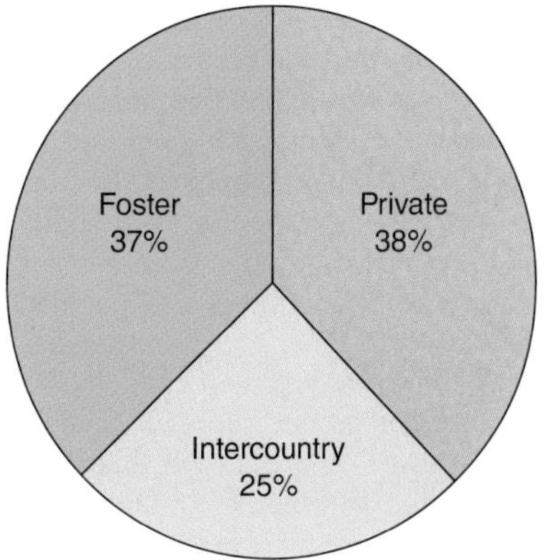


**FIGURE 38-1** Percent of all adoptions in the United States by type, as of 2013 (N = 1,782,000). (Data from Adoption USA: National Survey of Adoptive Parents, U.S. Department of Health and Human Services. 2016 Statistic Brain Research Institute.)

The typology of adoption has expanded from the traditional *closed* adoption, in which there is little ongoing communication between the birth parents and adoptive parents, to include *open* adoption, in which there is a greater sharing of information. In an open adoption, which is seen more commonly in domestic infant adoptions, the birth parents may meet the adoptive parents and agree on future communication and contacts between them and the child.

## FOSTER CARE: CHARACTERISTICS OF CHILDREN PLACED IN OUT-OF-HOME CARE

Children in foster care suffer from high rates of medical, developmental, and mental health problems (Table 38-1) that have often been identified prior to placement. Young children experiencing

**TABLE 38-1 COMMON MEDICAL AND MENTAL HEALTH OR DEVELOPMENTAL PROBLEMS SEEN IN CHILDREN IN FOSTER CARE**

| Medical Problems |
|---|
| Growth failure and failure to thrive |
| Consequences of prematurity |
| Microcephaly |
| Recurrent otitis media |
| Asthma |
| Anemia |
| Lead poisoning |
| Dental caries and poor dentition |
| Eczema |
| Sickle cell anemia |
| Sexually transmitted infections |
| Occult fractures |
| **Mental Health or Developmental Problems** |
| Developmental delay |
| Learning disability |
| Borderline intelligence/cognitive impairment |
| Attention-deficit/hyperactivity disorder |
| Depression or bipolar disorder |
| Conduct disorder |
| Anxiety disorder |
| Oppositional defiant disorder or other disruptive behavior disorder |
| Post-traumatic stress disorder |
| Fetal alcohol spectrum disorder |

early, extreme, and chronic adversity and trauma are at high risk of deleterious neurobiologic effects on behavior, cognition, and learning. Estimates are that at least 40% of children in foster care are believed to have a chronic medical condition; children under 2 have the highest prevalence. At least 60% of preschool children in foster care have some type of neurodevelopmental delay or disability. Up to 70% of children entering foster care have a significant mental health problem as compared with 16% to 22% in the general population. Children in foster care are also 10 to 15 times more likely to have been exposed to alcohol prenatally, but nearly 90% of children in care with a fetal alcohol spectrum disorder go undiagnosed. Fetal alcohol spectrum disorder is a nondiagnostic umbrella term that includes the specific diagnoses of fetal alcohol syndrome (FAS), partial fetal alcohol syndrome (pFAS), and neurobehavioral disorder associated with prenatal alcohol exposure (ND-PAE).

Neuromaturational lags, mild to moderate developmental delays, and speech or language disorders are frequent. As a group, children in foster care often function in the low-average range of cognitive abilities, and they are overrepresented in grade retention, school failure, and need for special education services. Findings from the National Survey of Child and Adolescent Well-Being indicated that approximately 50% of children in foster care engaged in at least one high-risk behavior, including pregnancy and sexual intercourse, alcohol and substance use, and carrying a weapon. A total of 40% met criteria for at least one mental health problem, including depression and suicidality, substance abuse, ADHD, or anxiety. There is a significant need in this population for both inpatient and outpatient mental health services. A 2012 report by the Administration of Children and Families indicated that 18% of children in foster care were taking a psychotropic medication and yet 30% were still awaiting mental health services. In a review of Ohio Medicaid data, 5.4% of children in foster care received 4 or more psychotropic medications. Further, the use of prescription psychotropic medications was 2 to 3 times greater for children in foster care than for a comparison group of children living in family care. However, some children show improvement in school attendance and academic growth when they are placed in a supportive foster home environment.



#### Challenges to Adjustment to Foster Care

**Children** Transition to care can often exacerbate underlying problems for children due to the abrupt and traumatic separation from their biological families. Young children may blame themselves for these events and may resist developing a relationship with their foster parents out of a sense of loyalty to their biological parent. Older children may experience more feelings of anger and have maladaptive coping strategies. It is not unusual for children to experience a honeymoon period during the initial months in foster care, after which more significant problems emerge. Children who have experienced abuse and neglect are less likely to have a secure attachment with their biological parents and are less likely to view caregivers as consistently available and nurturing. Because of this attachment insecurity, foster children respond to foster parents with dysfunctional behavior patterns, causing the foster parent to withdraw at times from the relationship or even inflict further abuse and maltreatment. Between 12% and 25% of children are maltreated in their foster homes. Further compounding the challenges for these youth is the potential separation from siblings, relatives, and friends, as well as familiar environments such as neighborhoods and schools. The McKinney–Vento Homeless Assistance Act passed in 2002 requires school districts to allow children placed in foster care the option of staying in their district of origin until the end of the academic school year, even if the district must provide transportation. There are also the transitional realities of being accepted by, and blending with, the new foster family (or families). Common behaviors seen in children placed in foster care are listed in Table 38-2.

**Biological Parents** Biological parents experience a traumatic separation and loss after the child's placement even when it occurs as a result of abuse or neglect. Removal often occurs in the acute setting of an abusive event and the co-occurrence of substance use and violence, which heightens the emotional tension and chaos surrounding the removal. Biological parents often face many socioeconomic and legal stressors, and they can experience complex feelings of grief, remorse, inadequacy, powerlessness, guilt, and resentment. Many of these families distrust and fear authority figures such as health professionals and child protective workers, and these feelings may interfere with taking appropriate steps to regain custody of their children. The removal of the child from the home may motivate some families to alter current parenting practices and to obtain help. About half of all children in foster care are returned to their biological families within the first 6 months after their initial removal. For some families, however, their longstanding dysfunctional patterns are entrenched and may interfere with compliance with visitation and permanency planning.

| TABLE 38-2 COMMON BEHAVIORS SEEN AFTER PLACEMENT |
|---|
| Sleep disturbances |
| Difficulty falling asleep |
| Frequent awakenings |
| Nightmares |
| Reluctance to sleep alone |
| Eating disturbances |
| Overeating |
| Poor appetite regulation |
| Hoarding of food |
| Poor appetite |
| Food refusal |
| Developmental regression |
| Loss of toileting skills |
| Regression in language, attention, and adaptive skills |
| Mood lability or instability |
| Temper tantrums |
| Irritability |
| Impulsivity |
| Apathy and withdrawal |
| Hypervigilance and exaggerated fear response |
| Indiscriminate sociability |
| Self-stimulating behaviors |
| Excessive masturbation |
| Rocking |
| Repetitive movements |
| Aggression |

**Foster Parents** In recent years, there has been a greater emphasis on placing children with extended family members or in kinship care, with a more than 300% increase in children placed in this setting. This type of care is believed to be more culturally appropriate and to maintain stronger ties to family members in an effort to minimize the trauma of separation for the child. Kinship care providers tend to be older and poorer than nonrelative foster placements and often they receive less financial assistance as well as less oversight and supervision than nonrelative foster care providers. There is great variability in caregivers who provide nonrelative care, but these families tend to be married, middle or lower income, and religiously observant. Approximately 50% of foster parents, however, have been shown to have a high school diploma or less education. Only a very small number of foster families receive specialized training, and even well-educated families often have limited knowledge of child behavior and development, particularly for traumatized or abused children. Foster parents often receive limited information about the child who is placed in their care. They may feel unsupported and ill equipped to care for highly challenging and vulnerable children.

#### Outcomes

Approximately 10% of children in foster care remain in the child welfare system for a number of years, while approximately 50% of children return to their biological families within 6 months of placement. In 2014, 21% of children in foster care were adopted and another 9% were emancipated. The median length of stay for those exiting foster care has shifted over the years to just over 13 months; however, 26% of children were in foster care for longer than 24 months with 13% for greater than 3 years. While there are efforts to develop permanency plans quickly, to use kinship care more frequently, and to enhance efforts to promote family reunification, the amount of time spent in foster care has actually increased for those children who do not exit the system after 1 month. The greatest predictors of length of stay in foster care are the biological families' cooperation with reunification plans, with minority and older children remaining in care longer. Children experiencing at least 1 placement change tend to be adolescents and those children with behavior problems, specifically defiant and externalizing behaviors. These children can be expected to experience multiple placements, with about 50% experiencing more than 1 and 25% having 3 or more placements. These multiple shifts exacerbate children's feelings of rejection, poor self-esteem, and uncertainty for their future and often can cause children to relive the initial trauma of separation. Those adolescents who age-out of foster care experience significantly higher rates of chronic medical and mental health problems, homelessness, uncompleted education and underemployment, and life in poverty. Laws that are designed to help transition children who age-out of foster care include the John H. Chafee Foster Care Independence Program, which provides states with federal funds for independent living services and extends Medicaid coverage until age 21.

Despite the significantly higher rates of mental health, medical, and developmental problems for children in foster care, it has been shown that children in foster care show improvements in their levels of conduct disorder behaviors, hyperactivity, and emotional stability, and better school attendance and performance. Children who displayed long-term healthy social adjustment and well-being after placement in foster care reported (1) the presence of a lasting and important relationship with at least one parental figure, (2) the ability to maintain contact with the biological families, (3) that the foster families were accepting and engaged in a collaborative relationship with the biological families, and (4) that they were made to feel like part of the family.

Pediatricians and primary healthcare providers therefore occupy a unique and vital role to provide a medical home in supporting children, adolescents, and caregivers; identifying potential problems with health, behavior, and neurodevelopment; and coordinating referrals as appropriate.

#### Common Issues

Two important issues that need to be negotiated for children and foster and biological families are visitation and permanency planning. Visitation can be a difficult aspect of foster care for all involved. Biological parents may not appear for visits due to poor organizational abilities; barriers such as transportation, guilt, ambivalence, fear of criminal punishment, and anger; and resistance toward supervision by a child welfare worker. Ambivalence toward their child, their role as a parent, and the child welfare system may cause biological families to act in inconsistent and unpredictable ways.

When biological parents do not appear for visits, children may experience feelings of rejection, unworthiness, and further abandonment, and they may relive earlier traumas. Visitations themselves may stimulate feelings of fear and anxiety in children that may compete with their feelings of grief, loss, and love for their biological parents. Children's responses to these stressors are often misdirected toward the foster parents, who also may be struggling with their feelings of anger and ambivalence toward the biological parents. Foster parents also report feeling excluded from important decisions surrounding visitation and permanency planning. This triad of the child, foster parents, and biological parents can become entangled in shifting alliances and conflicting loyalties and may threaten the ability of each party to maintain the best interest of the child.



### ADOPTION

Adoptive families represent a unique group. The prospective adoptive parents must go through the effort and expense of working with an adoption agency to fulfill the legal requirements of both the United States and the child's country of origin in the case of an international adoption and of traveling to that country to receive the child, commonly with only scant or inaccurate information about the child, the child's family history, and the child's health.

The core participants in the adoption process—the child, birth parents, and adoptive parents—are called the *adoption triad*. Each member of the adoption triad must adjust to the transition of the child moving from the care of one family to the care of another. The birth mother may experience a sense of loss and unresolved grief long after the adoption process ends. The adopted child must blend life experiences and feelings toward the adoptive family with the reality of a birth mother who resides outside the family. Confusion over identity, fantasies about the birth parents and their reasons for relinquishing the child, and feelings of rejection all may arise and influence the child's sense of belonging and self-esteem. An open and accepting family attitude toward adoption has been shown to be predictive of a child's positive adjustment to these psychological issues.



#### Adoptive Parents

The decision to adopt a child may often be the culmination of a history of failed pregnancies, infertility, and loss of the imagined child. Adoptive parents may be reluctant to express the complex feelings associated with the decision to adopt because of feelings of guilt, inadequacy, and uncertainty. Adoptive families frequently get mixed messages from places such as schools, early intervention programs, and healthcare providers that may over-pathologize the behaviors and attitudes of the child or may fail to recognize the needs of the child. Single parent, same-sex parents, and mixed-racial adoptions may further add to these mixed and often judgmental messages. Pediatricians, too, sometimes underreact or overreact to the child's possible developmental delays and behavior problems. They may either intervene and become alarmed prematurely or, conversely, wait too long to refer children for services with the belief that they simply need more time to catch up.

#### Internationally Adopted Children

Parents of international adoptees tend to be white, married, well educated, and economically stable. Some of these characteristics, such as age and marital status, may be requirements by the foreign country, and the high cost of international adoption accounts for the higher socioeconomic status among this population. According to a 2013 report by the US Department of State, adoption service providers charge up to $64,000 for all adoption services with a median of $28,000. While the internationally adopted child shares many similarities with the child in foster care, there are a few important distinctions. Often, the child's history prior to adoption is not well known or is ambiguous or incorrect. Similar to children in foster care, many international adoptees have experienced early instability in their caregiving environment; multiple transitions, losses, and traumas; and early adversity and deprivation prior to adoption. More than 50% of adoptees have spent a portion of their lives in institutional care. The quality of care in these settings is highly variable: Child ratio, nutrition, and health care may be inadequate, and children are exposed to a high turnover of caregivers who often have limited training in child development. Some international adoptees have experienced abuse and neglect in the homes of their biological family, although this is rarely reported on the records that adoptive parents receive.

Internationally adopted children also may have sustained some neurobiological insult as a result of poor prenatal care and nutrition and prenatal substance and alcohol abuse. The country of origin may influence some of these variables. For example, there are high rates of maternal alcohol consumption in Eastern Europe and Russia with up to 30% of women of childbearing age reported to regularly consume alcohol. Acute and chronic medical problems are common and include infections, such as HIV, syphilis, hepatitis, and tuberculosis; inadequate immunizations; developmental delays; fetal alcohol spectrum disorders; speech and language disorders; and disrupted emotional development and behavior, including abnormal stress responses and attachment disorders. These risk factors place these children, similar to children in foster care, at higher risk for medical, behavioral, developmental, and mental health issues. International adoptees also face a loss of culture and their family of origin, and they must deal with complex issues of acculturation to a strange country, home, and language.

#### Rules and Regulations

The Department of Homeland Security and the US Department of State have outlined steps to be taken by prospective adoptive parents. A home study must be completed prior to adoption approval.

Safeguarding the rights of children has been an important aspect of international adoption, and controversy exists as to whether international adoption is beneficial to children. The United Nations Convention on the Rights of the Child (UNCRC) emphasized "the right of the child to preserve his or her identity including nationality, name and family relations." The UNCRC stressed that international adoption should be viewed as the last option except institutional care after all efforts to place a child with existing family members or within their community have been exhausted. The Hague Convention on Protection of Children and Cooperation in Respect of Intercountry Adoption, on the other hand, was drafted in 1993 to recognize the legitimacy of international adoption and establish a set of minimum requirements and procedures to ensure that children are not exploited, trafficked, abducted, or sold.

#### Outcomes

The Bucharest Early Intervention Project (BEIP), a longitudinal study that began in 2000 looking at children placed in institutions at or shortly after birth, provides much data about our understanding of the long-term consequences of early institutional care. The BEIP showed that removing young children from institutions and placing them in foster care resulted in improved attachment patterns, reduced signs of emotionally withdrawn/inhibited attachment, improved measures of positive affect, and reduced prevalence of internalizing disorders. Overall, adopted children show somewhat higher rates of neurodevelopmental and psychological morbidity, especially early in childhood. Adopted children are overrepresented among those with learning disabilities, with an estimated prevalence of school problems 3 to 4 times national norms. These children represent 5% of children seen in outpatient mental health settings and 10% to 15% of children in inpatient mental health facilities. Externalizing behaviors such as oppositional defiant and conduct disorders, reactive attachment disorders, disinhibited social engagement disorder, executive functioning deficits, and ADHD occur more frequently, as does substance abuse. Prolonged exposure to adversity is believed to negatively affect the circuitry in the prefrontal cortex. However, most adopted individuals perceive their experiences positively and mature as healthy, normal children with successes and failures similar to those of their nonadopted peers. Reports suggest that adoptees have self-esteem similar to that of their nonadopted peers. The longer children have lived in their adoptive homes, the fewer behavioral problems are reported. Age at adoption, which is often a proxy for length of institutional care, is the best predictor of mental health and developmental and learning problems.

Most adoptions are final. The rates, however, of adoption disruption (terminating an adoption before it is legally finalized) and dissolution (terminating an adoption after it is legally finalized) may be as high as 10%. Older children and children with a history of multiple placements, longer duration of time spent in foster care, and significant behavioral and mental health needs are at greater risk for disruption and dissolution.

#### Common Issues

As greater numbers of children are living in adoptive homes, adoptive families have become increasingly open and interested in discussing adoption and adapting some of their child's original cultural practices into their home. Parents sometimes feel unsure about when and how to discuss adoption with their children. Discussing adoption with children can begin from the moment they enter their adoptive home and particularly when children become curious and ask questions about themselves and their background. However, it is not until children are ages 5 to 7 that they can begin to understand cognitively the difference between an adoptive parent and a birth parent. Feelings of adoption-related loss may certainly emerge by this time. From 8 to 11 years, questions regarding their permanence within the adoptive family may arise, possibly mixed with fantasies of being reclaimed by a birth parent. During early to mid-adolescence, young teens struggle to consolidate different notions of self with beginning interest about information on the birth family and heritable traits. By mid- to late adolescence, there is a clearer understanding of the emotional and legal permanence of the adoption. At this time, adopted children also may begin to seek contact with their birth mother or other members of the birth family. Recommended approaches for adoptive parents about discussing themes of adoption with their child include early and periodic discussion, ongoing emotional availability, and to begin the "adoption story" with the child's birth and family diversity. Validation of feelings, including those of the adoptive parent(s) and a nonjudgmental attitude toward the child's biologic family of origin can be supportive. There are many books and resources available to aid parents in discussing adoption with their children, and it is important that parents respond with answers that are appropriate to a child's developmental understanding of adoption and identity formation.

## HEALTHCARE PROVIDER'S ROLE

The pediatric provider occupies an ideal position to assist in the foster or adoptive child's adaptation to a new family by (1) providing thorough health supervision through the medical home model, (2) assisting families in coordination of services and providing professional advocacy, and (3) serving as a counselor to the child and family (Table 38-3.)

The health professional also is in a unique position to provide a global view of the child's strengths and needs within the context of the family, thus helping to facilitate planning for individual or family interventions when necessary. The pediatric provider is also a key resource for families in advocating for appropriate educational interventions. Such a role requires a working familiarity with special education laws and the rights of families, and local educational, social, legal, and mental health resources for children. Often children in foster care or adoptees require complex care that includes care coordination that links children and families with needed and appropriate services.

Physicians may find themselves in the role of counseling the adoptive or foster family, the child, and the biological parents. Feelings of guilt, confusion, and frustration require an empathic ear. An understanding, open, and *neutral* health professional can be a valuable resource for children as questions of self-identity arise in the middle-school years. Clinicians also may serve as a sounding board to prospective parents about decisions regarding foster or adoptive care. Families often need guidance as they try to understand their child's development and behavior within the context of foster care and adoption. At times, appropriate referral to a mental health professional will be necessary. The pediatric healthcare provider and the medical home model thus occupy a central role in monitoring the well-being of the child and family and of supporting their adaptation to the sequence of transitions experienced in foster care and adoption.

**TABLE 38-3 SUPPORTIVE ROLE OF THE PEDIATRICIAN IN THE CARE OF THE FOSTER OR ADOPTIVE CHILD**

| |
|---|
| **Prior to Adoption** |
| Preview information on the child (eg, medical records, prenatal information, family history, videotape of child) |
| Advise on supplies to take to pick up the child (eg, medicines, formula) |
| Advise on vaccines, medicines for parents traveling to a foreign country |
| Plan for evaluation of the child upon return |
| Refer family to support group for domestic or international adoption |
| Provide anticipatory guidance for new parents |
| Perform medical evaluation |
| **Immediate Visit (First Week)** |
| Obtain available records, including prenatal and birth history with particular attention to prenatal alcohol exposure, growth curves, immunization records, hospitalizations, results of health screening (eg, lead, anemia), and medications |
| Evaluate/treat acute illnesses |
| Measure baseline growth; check nutritional status of the child |
| For the foster child, become familiar with key personnel, including caseworkers and attorneys |
| Address any immediate concerns of the family |
| Assess immediate family coping and adjustment |
| **Comprehensive Examination (4–6 Weeks)** |
| Perform complete physical examination: check for congenital anomalies, chronic conditions, nutritional disorders |
| Screen vision, hearing, dental |
| Update immunizations |
| Recheck newborn screening if child is under 3 months old |
| Perform screening medical tests when appropriate to include complete blood count, lead, iron (look for hemoglobinopathies), urinalysis, tuberculosis (purified protein derivative), stool ova and parasites, hepatitis B and C, human immunodeficiency virus, syphilis, malaria (if appropriate) |
| Perform developmental evaluation: gross and fine motor, communication, adaptive and cognitive skills, initial behavior, and coping responses |
| Developmental screen for language, autistic spectrum disorders, fetal alcohol spectrum disorders, learning and attentional difficulties |
| Provide anticipatory guidance: refer to support groups, appropriate literature |
| **Periodic Surveillance** |
| Examine children in sensitive and compassionate settings (eg, it may be stressful to child if both biological and foster parents are present at a visit) |
| Perform well-child care; complete and update immunization schedules |
| Monitor own emotional responses to biological and foster parents and child; avoid being pulled into adversarial relationships or taking sides |
| Monitor growth, nutrition |
| Check for late signs of infection |
| Provide close developmental and behavioral surveillance (at any age) |
| Perform episodic developmental screening using standardized instruments to detect developmental and/or behavioral problems |
| Counsel or refer for developmental or behavioral problems |
| Monitor events related to visitation and permanency planning for the child in foster care and communicate episodically with caseworkers |
| Advocate for the rights and needs for adoptive and foster children in the educational and legal sectors |

## SUGGESTED READINGS


American Academy of Pediatrics. Healthy Foster Care America. American Academy of Pediatrics Web site. www.aap.org/fostercare. Accessed February 6, 2017.

Bos K, Zeanah C, Fox N, Drury S, McLaughlin K, Nelson C. Psychiatric outcomes in young children with a history of institutionalization. *Harv Rev Psychiatry.* 2011;19(1):15-24.

Brodzinsky DM. Children's understanding of adoption: developmental and clinical implications. *Prof Psychol Res Pr.* 2011:42(2):200-207.

Jones VF; American Academy of Pediatrics Committee on Early Childhood, Adoption, and Dependent Care; High PC, Donoghue E, Fussell JJ, et al. Comprehensive health evaluation of the newly adopted child. *Pediatrics.* 2012;129(1):e214-e223.

Jones VF, Schulte EE; American Academy of Pediatrics Committee on Early Childhood; Council on Foster Care, Adoption, and Kinship Care. The pediatrician's role in supporting adoptive families. *Pediatrics.* 2012;130(4):e1040-e1049.

Kerker BD, Dore MM. Mental health needs and treatment of foster youth: barriers and opportunities. *Am J Orthopsychiatry.* 2006:76(1):138-147.

Mason P, Johnson D, Prock L. *Adoption Medicine: Caring for Children and Families.* Elk Grove Village, IL: American Academy of Pediatrics; 2014.

Szilagyi M, Rosen D, Rubin D, Zlotnik S; American Academy of Pediatrics Council on Foster Care, Adoption, and Kinship Care; Committee on Adolescence; Council on Early Childhood. Health care issues for children and adolescents in foster care and kinship care. *Pediatrics.* 2015;136(4):e1142-e1166.

Weitzman C, Albers L. Long-term developmental, behavioral, and attachment outcomes after international adoption. *Pediatr Clin North Am.* 2005;52(5):1395-1419.




# 39 Preventing Child Abuse and Neglect: What Pediatricians Can Do

Wendy Gwirtzman Lane and Howard Dubowitz

## THE IMPORTANCE OF PREVENTION

Preventing child abuse and neglect (ie, maltreatment) fits well with the goals and scope of pediatrics, as expressed by the commitment of the American Academy of Pediatrics (AAP) to "prevention, early detection, and management of behavioral, developmental, and social problems as a focus in pediatric practice." The prevention of child maltreatment has benefits at the level of the individual child, the family, the community, and society at large. Sparing a child from the physical, cognitive, behavioral, emotional, and social problems associated with maltreatment is intuitively and morally preferable to intervening after the fact.

Beyond the individual child, the prevention of child maltreatment has at its heart the goal of supporting parents, strengthening families, and enhancing childrearing. Effective interventions may achieve much more than the narrow goal of preventing maltreatment. Additional outcomes may include enhancing children's cognitive, emotional, social, and behavioral development; improving maternal health and communication with the children; decreasing use of public assistance; and decreasing involvement in the criminal justice system. Child maltreatment has significant costs, human and economic, that need to be weighed against the cost of prevention. Though more research is needed, several studies have demonstrated the cost-effectiveness of specific child maltreatment preventive strategies.

## ROLES OF PEDIATRIC HEALTHCARE PROVIDERS

Pediatric practice has focused primarily on the important issues of identifying abuse and neglect, providing medical care, reporting to the public agencies, and facilitating referrals for assessment and treatment. In order to fulfill their responsibility to promote children's health and well-being, pediatricians should also focus on preventing maltreatment. Pediatricians can do so by identifying and helping to manage child and family risk and protective factors, referring families to effective community-based services, and advocating for the development of policies and programs that promote family well-being. As primary care pediatricians generally enjoy excellent relationships with children and families, they may play a role that other professionals cannot. Pediatricians are usually perceived as credible, supportive, and caring, without the stigma often attached to social work and mental health. This rapport can facilitate a remarkable entrée into families' lives, with sharing of sensitive information.

## RISK FACTORS FOR MALTREATMENT

The ecological framework of child maltreatment posits that physically abusive and/or neglectful behavior derives from the complex set of interactions between the child, parent, community, and society. Child characteristics, such as difficult temperament or chronic physical or mental health problems, may challenge parents, heighten parental stress, and increase the risk of maltreatment. Specific patterns of behavior observed within the parent–child dyad can serve as important indicators of possible physical abuse or neglect. The relationship between parent and child in maltreating families may involve harsh, inattentive, and inconsistent parenting. Maltreating parents, particularly physically abusive ones, have often reported feeling "out of control" as parents.

Research has identified strong associations between parental problems and child maltreatment. For example, maternal depression has been linked to child maltreatment, and a study demonstrated that treating depressed mothers improved child outcomes. Maltreating parents have higher rates of substance abuse than their nonabusive counterparts, and children of substance-abusing parents have higher rates of maltreatment. Intimate partner violence (IPV) frequently co-occurs with child abuse; studies have estimated that 33% to 77% of children living in homes with IPV are physically abused. Given the strong association between these problems and maltreatment, the identification and amelioration of these risk factors could help prevent child abuse and neglect.

Family and community contexts, although less immediately observable to pediatricians, nonetheless also contribute to maltreatment. Studies across age groups have documented that family stressors such as poverty, unemployment, negative life events, or geographic moves heighten the risk of maltreatment.

One of the central stressors identified in maltreatment risk is that of family poverty. Families reported to Child Protective Services (CPS) are more likely to have single mothers, have unemployed fathers, receive public assistance, and/or live in poor neighborhoods. It is not difficult to understand how the burdens associated with poverty may compromise a family. At the same time, it is important to highlight that most impoverished families are never identified as maltreating. And, maltreatment certainly does occur in middle-class and wealthy families.

Another contributor to child maltreatment is the quality of social support available to families. Compared with non-maltreating families, maltreating families have smaller social networks with which they have less contact and fewer reciprocal exchanges. Pediatricians assist families with poor social support by conveying that they care and by referring families to community-based programs such as parent support groups.

Cultural influences are also an important consideration in child maltreatment. Wide variation has been noted across cultural contexts regarding, for example, the extent of child supervision, the belief in corporal punishment, and acceptance or resistance to mental health care. Finally, societal influences such as the availability and affordability of child care and health care may contribute to maltreatment.

While the factors described above may increase the risk of maltreatment, families usually also have protective factors that lower their risk. These may be internal characteristics (eg, parental caring for the child) or external (eg, social support). There is longstanding support for the protective effect of a strong social network. Good social support is associated with lower rates of physical neglect and increased use of nonphysical disciplinary methods. Healthy family functioning appears to be another critical protective factor in preventing child maltreatment. Consideration of a family's strengths and ability to cope with adversity is important to the prevention of child maltreatment, as well as to the promotion of children's health and safety. Research has shown that even maltreated children can have positive outcomes in the presence of protective family functioning (eg, a nurturing caregiver).

## IDENTIFICATION OF FAMILIES AT RISK

High-risk families often lack insight into their problems and may not know where help is available. They thus underutilize both formal and informal helping systems but may be more likely to seek medical care for their children. Healthcare services provide a critical, near-universal access point for identifying and addressing psychosocial problems, such as parental depression, facing many families. Primary care, therefore, provides a logical starting point for efforts to prevent maltreatment.

Many risk factors are unlikely to be detected unless specific screening efforts are made. For example, parental depression is often well masked and is not recognized by pediatricians. IPV is usually a well-kept, dark family secret. For these reasons, the AAP has specifically recommended that pediatricians screen for IPV, parental substance abuse, and other family risk factors. An approach to identify these possible problems is to screen *all* families at certain pediatric visits (eg, initially, and then periodically) with a brief questionnaire, which can be completed before selected checkups or be incorporated into the interview during the visit. Relying on clinical judgment as to who, for example, appears "high" will result in many problems remaining hidden.

A number of screening questionnaires have been developed to identify parental problems such as depression, substance abuse, and IPV. Given the range of issues to be covered in a pediatric primary care visit and the limited time available, brief tools are critical. Introducing questions in a sensitive manner may make parents comfortable in disclosing information. For example: "Being a parent is not always easy. We want to help families have a safe environment for kids, so we're asking everyone these questions. They are about problems that affect many families. If there's a problem, we'll try to help. This is voluntary. You don't have to answer any question you prefer not to." It is useful to begin with some well-accepted safety issues such as bike helmets and smoke alarms. Building on pediatricians' longstanding interest in children's safety, this is a logical transition to areas such as corporal punishment, parental depression, substance abuse, domestic violence, and other environmental hazards. An example of a 1-page screening questionnaire is the evidence-based Parent Questionnaire developed for the Safe Environment for Every Kid (SEEK) model of pediatric primary care (Fig. 39-1), in which pediatricians are trained to screen, briefly assess, and initially address child maltreatment–related risk factors.

In addition to questions directed to parents, valuable information can be obtained directly from children and teenagers, and pediatricians have an interest in children's perceptions and history. It is now customary to spend some time alone with adolescents and to obtain a history independently; this practice can be extended to younger children as well. It is important first to establish rapport, by asking general open-ended questions such as "What are you doing this summer? What's school like? What kind of things do you like to do?" and "Who lives with you?" One can then ask how family members get along and what kinds of things the child likes to do with each of them. More sensitive issues can then be raised, such as "All kids sometimes behave badly. What happens when you behave badly?" "Is there anyone at home who gives you a hard time?" and "Whom do you tell when you have a problem?" It is generally a good principle to talk to children alone if possible. If problems are uncovered, it is important to tell the child of the concern and the need to involve the parent(s).

### Confidentiality

Screening raises issues pertaining to confidentiality. If information is gathered on sensitive problems, particularly IPV, it is prudent to assess the problem privately, without the child or partner present. Women may be understandably reluctant to disclose violence in the presence of others, and there is the risk of aggravating the situation. Children may be later coerced to report on what was said during the visit. A child who

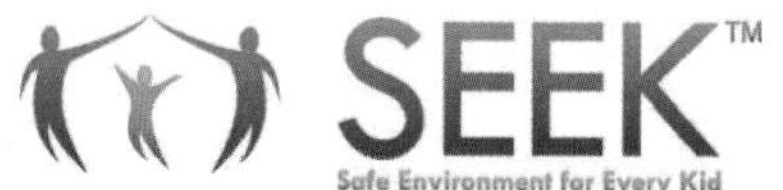


**Parent Questionnaire (PQ)**

**Dear Parent or Caregiver:** Being a parent is not always easy. We want to help families have a safe environment for kids. So, we're asking everyone these questions. They are about problems that affect many families. If there's a problem, we'll try to help.

Please answer the questions about your child being seen today for a checkup. If there's more than one child, please answer "yes" if it applies to any one of them. This is voluntary. You don't have to answer any question you prefer not to.

Today's Date: __/__/___ Child's Name: ________________

Child's Date of Birth: __/__/___ Relationship to Child: ________________

**PLEASE CHECK**

- ☐ Yes ☐ No Do you need the phone number for Poison Control?
- ☐ Yes ☐ No Do you need a smoke detector for your home?
- ☐ Yes ☐ No Does anyone smoke tobacco at home?
- ☐ Yes ☐ No In the last year, did you worry that your food would run out before you got money or Food Stamps to buy more?
- ☐ Yes ☐ No In the last year, did the food you bought just not last and you didn't have money to get more?
- ☐ Yes ☐ No Do you often feel your child is difficult to take care of?
- ☐ Yes ☐ No Do you sometimes find you need to hit/spank your child?
- ☐ Yes ☐ No Do you wish you had more help with your child?
- ☐ Yes ☐ No Do you often feel under extreme stress?
- ☐ Yes ☐ No In the past month, have you often felt down, depressed, or hopeless?
- ☐ Yes ☐ No In the past month, have you felt very little interest or pleasure in things you used to enjoy?
- ☐ Yes ☐ No In the past year, have you been afraid of your partner?
- ☐ Yes ☐ No In the past year, have you had a problem with drugs or alcohol?
- ☐ Yes ☐ No In the past year, have you felt the need to cut back on drinking or drug use?
- ☐ Yes ☐ No Are there any other problems you'd like help with today?

**Please give this form to the doctor or nurse you're seeing today. Thank you!**



**FIGURE 39-1** Parent Questionnaire. (©2012, University of Maryland School of Medicine.)

is present when a parent denies ongoing violence may learn to keep all maltreatment secret. There is also an issue of documentation, given that the partner may have access to the child's medical record. One approach is to place sensitive information in a separate section of the chart or to use code terms, such as "family conflict discussed."

### Assessment

If screening identifies possible risk factors, there is a need for further brief assessment, which can be done by pediatricians or by behavioral health professionals when available (examples are Fig. 39-2 and Fig. 39-3). If the screen identifies a parent with depressive symptoms, a brief assessment (Fig. 39-3) should focus on prioritized concerns such as how the parent thinks the problem is affecting the family, whether the parent is receiving treatment, and whether the parent is interested in obtaining help. Incorporating principles of motivational interviewing helps understand the parent's perception of the problem and how to address it. By jointly developing a plan that is based on the parent's ideas and that the parent "owns," there's a greater likelihood of the recommendations being implemented.

Some families have more than 1 problem, increasing their risk of child abuse or neglect. Ideally, a comprehensive assessment is done by a behavioral health professional to understand the family's needs and strengths. This more comprehensive understanding is key to intervening appropriately. It is also important to know what interventions have been tried and with what results.

## PREVENTIVE INTERVENTIONS

A critical criterion for screening is that the person benefits from having a problem recognized. Following screening and a brief assessment, there may be a need for further evaluation and intervention. In some instances, pediatricians can provide education and guidance, such as helping a parent manage the child's challenging behaviors or supporting a parent suffering a loss. Alternatively, a behavioral health professional may play this role. In other instances, such as IPV or substance abuse, pediatricians serve primarily as "gate keepers," facilitating referrals—a potentially pivotal role that, with knowledge and skill, may take only a few strategic minutes.

To provide a child adequate or excellent health care and to prevent maltreatment, pediatricians need to be familiar with the family's structure, child rearing practices, stresses and strengths, and barriers to care. Rooted in a trusting relationship, this understanding builds over time, and it is a dynamic process as circumstances change. While it is often difficult to change others' behavior, the approach used in the SEEK model, including empathy, support, and motivation, conveys an important message that the pediatrician cares about the parent; this may facilitate a later disclosure of a problem and willingness to engage in help.

The following are general principles concerning preventive efforts:

- The needs of parents, children, and families should be considered, following the vision of Bright Futures. Effective interventions focus

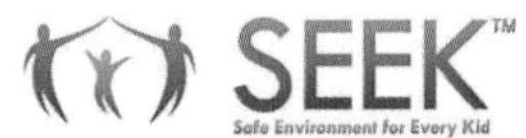

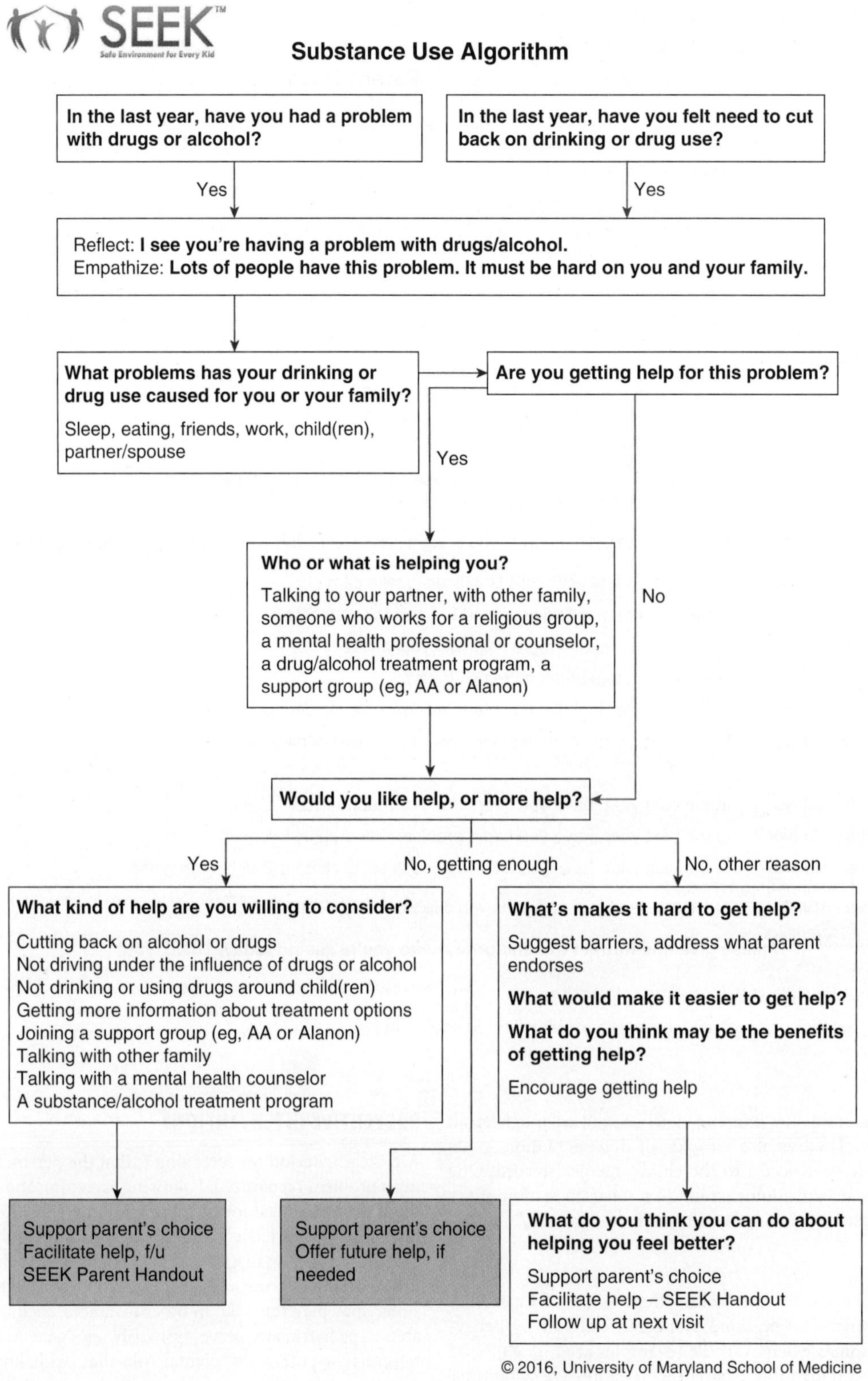

**Substance Use Algorithm**

**In the last year, have you had a problem with drugs or alcohol?** → Yes

**In the last year, have you felt need to cut back on drinking or drug use?** → Yes

Reflect: **I see you're having a problem with drugs/alcohol.**
Empathize: **Lots of people have this problem. It must be hard on you and your family.**

**What problems has your drinking or drug use caused for you or your family?**
Sleep, eating, friends, work, child(ren), partner/spouse

**Are you getting help for this problem?**

Yes → **Who or what is helping you?**
Talking to your partner, with other family, someone who works for a religious group, a mental health professional or counselor, a drug/alcohol treatment program, a support group (eg, AA or Alanon)

No → **Would you like help, or more help?**

Yes → **What kind of help are you willing to consider?**
Cutting back on alcohol or drugs
Not driving under the influence of drugs or alcohol
Not drinking or using drugs around child(ren)
Getting more information about treatment options
Joining a support group (eg, AA or Alanon)
Talking with other family
Talking with a mental health counselor
A substance/alcohol treatment program

→ Support parent's choice
Facilitate help, f/u
SEEK Parent Handout

No, getting enough → Support parent's choice
Offer future help, if needed

No, other reason → **What's makes it hard to get help?**
Suggest barriers, address what parent endorses
**What would make it easier to get help?**
**What do you think may be the benefits of getting help?**
Encourage getting help

→ **What do you think you can do about helping you feel better?**
Support parent's choice
Facilitate help – SEEK Handout
Follow up at next visit



**FIGURE 39-2** Substance Use Algorithm. (©2016, University of Maryland School of Medicine.)

on basic problem-solving skills and concrete family needs, provide behavior management strategies, *and* help address environmental factors. Parents often require attention to their own needs in order to nurture their children.

- Identification of a family's strengths and resources is key to comprehending the situation and to intervening. Strengths may include coping abilities, intelligence, determination, and/or religious faith. Resources may include informal supports (eg, family, friends), as well as formal community resources. Informal support may be especially useful for families who are resistant to interventions from public agencies or behavioral health professionals. Formal support through a religious affiliation may be valuable, and professionals too often overlook this important source of support and guidance. However, some fundamentalist religious groups may encourage corporal punishment, exacerbating the risk for physical abuse. It is, therefore, important to have a sense of the nature of support that is likely from such resources before simply recommending them. Incorporating strengths into one's approach helps address problems more constructively (eg, "I can see how much you love your child. How can we make sure she stays healthy?"). By conveying caring, pediatricians become valuable resources to parents needing support.

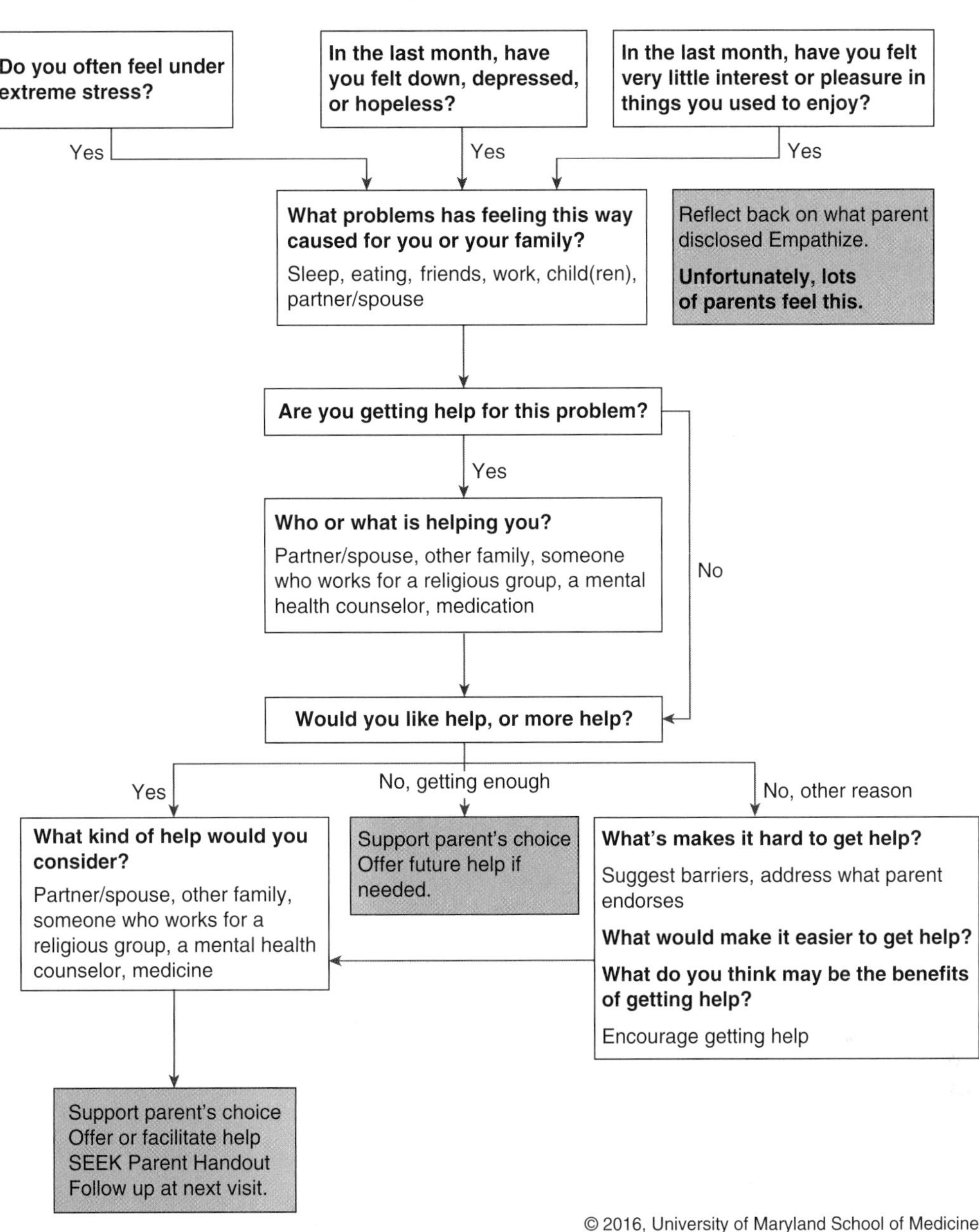


**FIGURE 39-3** Stress/Depression Algorithm. (©2016, University of Maryland School of Medicine.)

- Risk factors for maltreatment need to be identified and addressed. Figures 39-2 and 39-3 offer approaches to assessing and addressing 2 of these risk factors: depression and substance abuse.
- Be knowledgeable about community resources, and facilitate referrals. Pediatricians serve as an important conduit to community services and are in a good position to encourage reluctant or ambivalent families to accept or try services. Alternatively, this role may be played by a behavioral health colleague. Office staff can also help with referrals, the way they do for many issues.

## COMMUNITY-BASED PREVENTION PROGRAMS

Pediatricians need to consider community resources as they aim to address risk factors for abuse and neglect. Therefore, pediatricians should be aware of local resources and should periodically update their information. Community resource information may be available from the local or state health department, United Way agency, and/or through an Internet search, supplemented by phone calls and requests for brochures and information. Families in need of services may be more willing to engage when their pediatrician is familiar with staff and services.

Pediatricians should also be knowledgeable about the quality and effectiveness of the available programs; some may have had little or no formal program evaluation. Several online resources provide information about the quality of community-based prevention programs. These include the Home Visiting Evidence of Effectiveness (http://homvee.acf.hhs.gov/), the California Evidence-Based Clearinghouse for Child Welfare (http://www.cebc4cw.org/), the Centers for Disease Control and Prevention's Child Abuse and Neglect: Prevention Strategies (www.cdc.gov/violenceprevention/childmaltreatment/prevention.html), and the Community Guide (www.thecommunityguide.org/violence/index/html).

### Home Visiting

Home visitation services assign a professional (often a nurse or social worker) or layperson to deliver parent education, case management, and sometimes role-modeling, emotional support, and other parent assistance in the home. Whether a professional or layperson, home visitors are trained, receive intense supervision, and follow a structured curriculum. Often beginning during prenatal care or shortly after birth and continuing over several years, home visitation programs should include close partnerships with healthcare providers, helping parents to learn when to seek medical care, assuring medical follow-up, and providing careful monitoring. Home visitors may also assist families by connecting them to services for public assistance, Medicaid, mental health, substance abuse, or IPV, or to other community supports.

The 2010 federal Patient Protection and Affordable Care Act included funding for evidence-based home visiting through the Maternal, Infant, and Early Childhood Home Visiting Program (MIECHV). At least 75% of MIECHV community funding must be spent on evidence-based home visiting programs. Twelve programs have been designated by the US Department of Health and Human Services (DHHS) as evidence-based (http://homvee.acf.hhs.gov). It is important to note that while all DHHS-designated programs have shown positive outcomes for children, not all have demonstrated effectiveness in preventing child abuse and neglect.

### Parent Support Programs

Parent support programs typically aim to improve parents' comfort and competence with parenting. Examples include Triple P, Sure Start, Family Connections, Parents as Teachers, and Together for Kids. There is variability in services among these programs, several of which involve home-based interventions. Program components may include psychoeducation regarding child development, responsiveness, promoting sensitivity and nurturing toward the child, positive interactions, emotional communication, and disciplinary approaches. Some programs have shown improvements in parents' self-esteem and attitudes toward child rearing. One of the most effective programs is Triple P, the Positive Parenting Program. Triple P focuses on addressing children's behavioral, emotional, and developmental problems, enhancing family protective factors, and reducing family risk factors for maltreatment. Five tiers of Triple P services are available, and the services are tailored to family need. An evaluation of Triple P implementation in South Carolina demonstrated lower rates of substantiated maltreatment, fewer out-of-home placements, and fewer maltreatment injuries in counties that implemented the model compared to counties providing usual care.

Several meta-analyses of parent training programs have identified characteristics that may increase program effectiveness. For example, programs that include multiple modalities, such as office-based and home visitation services or group and individual services, may have better outcomes than more limited programs. This information may be helpful for pediatricians fortunate enough to have more than 1 available program, or for those who are advocating for the development of new programs.

### Prevention of Abusive Head Trauma

Approximately 30 of every 100,000 infants suffer from abusive head trauma (AHT), which is the leading cause of child abuse–related death. The observation, and later demonstration, of a temporal association between peak frequency of infant crying and peak incidence of AHT have led to an interest in educating parents of infants about ways to cope with infant crying and to refrain from shaking their babies. One program that has had some success focused on educating parents of newborns during their postpartum hospital stay, using a brochure and video. Parents were also asked to sign a commitment statement stating that they had received the AHT information and they understood that shaking is harmful. An evaluation of the intervention showed a decrease in the rate of AHT, while AHT rates in a neighboring state without the intervention were unchanged. While these preliminary findings were encouraging, more recent evaluations of similar programs, including the National Center for Shaken Baby's Period of PURPLE Crying program, have not demonstrated significant prevention of AHT.

### Prevention of Child Sexual Abuse

Most existing sexual abuse prevention programs are specifically directed at children, teaching them about personal safety, body safety, saying "no," and telling a trusted adult. Critics of these child-focused educational programs have argued that they unreasonably burden children with the responsibility for preventing sexual abuse, rather than targeting those who may abuse children. Parents have also expressed concern that it may be harmful to tell children that someone close to them could possibly abuse them, though program evaluations have identified few negative consequences. A recent meta-analysis of school-based prevention programs demonstrated improvements in children's protective behaviors in hypothetical situations, in knowledge—sustained up to 6 months later—and in reporting previous or current sexual abuse.

Assessing the direct effect of a program on the rate of sexual abuse is methodologically difficult and, therefore, has generally not been done. One study that did demonstrate effectiveness was a retrospective study in which college students were asked about their participation in school-based sexual abuse programs and their possible history of sexual abuse. Rates of abuse were significantly higher in the group that did not participate in prevention programs. This study, several program evaluations, and documentation of a decline in the incidence of sexual abuse over the past 20 years have led 1 expert to support the continuation of high-quality prevention-education programs.

Several public health media campaigns have been conducted in recent years. Stop It Now! (http://www.stopitnow.org) is a program first introduced in Vermont that incorporated public service announcements on television and radio, newspaper articles, bus advertising, and an interactive Web site. Evaluation demonstrated greater awareness about sexual abuse and an increased number of helpline calls. Darkness to Light (http://www.d2l.org) educates parents and child-serving organizations about methods to keep children safe, including the avoidance of 1 adult–1 child situations. A media campaign evaluation found that the program led to increased knowledge of sexual abuse, and improvements in protective behavior regarding hypothetical situations. Unfortunately, these effects did not persist 9 months post-intervention. The Enough Abuse Campaign (http://www.enoughabuse.org) takes a multipronged approach, incorporating education of adults and children and advocacy to ensure policies and regulations are focused on child safety.

Little or no data are available regarding effective primary care–based interventions to prevent child sexual abuse. However, pediatricians can provide children and parents with basic information about sexual safety. Some examples of safety messages follow:

- During the genital exam, the pediatrician can point out to the child that only their doctor and specific adult caregivers should be allowed to see their "private parts." Parents can be engaged in this conversation by asking to clarify which caregivers are permitted to do so.
- Pediatricians can counsel parents on how to maintain open channels of communication with their children, including a child informing the parent if anyone makes them feel bad. At the same time, the pediatrician can encourage children to talk with their parents when something is troubling them.
- Parents can be given information on how to minimize the opportunity for perpetrators to access children (eg, limiting 1 adult-1 child situations), how to discuss issues of sexual abuse with children, and how to recognize potential behavioral and medical signs of sexual abuse. The Stewards of Children program, developed by Darkness to Light, has developed educational materials to address these issues (http://www.d2l.org).

## ADVOCACY

Pediatricians can be advocates for the prevention of child maltreatment on different levels, including that of the individual child, parent, family, community, and society. Helping parents meet their children's needs is advocacy on behalf of children unable to express or meet their own needs. Acknowledging the stress a parent may feel and facilitating help is also a form of advocacy. While most pediatricians do not have direct involvement in community-based prevention programs, they can advocate individually or through their state's AAP chapter for policies and programs at the local, state, and federal level that help children and families. Enhancing access to health care represents advocacy at the broadest societal level. These examples illustrate the various ways that pediatricians' advocacy can be valuable in helping promote children's health, development, and safety, and in preventing child abuse and neglect.

## CHALLENGES

Addressing risk factors for child maltreatment within primary care may be novel to many pediatricians. Some pediatricians may raise concerns about the feasibility of implementing systematic screening, assessment, and referral for psychosocial problems in the family. Below are responses to commonly cited concerns.

1. **"There's not enough time to delve into psychosocial problems, such as a mother who is depressed."** It may add time, but there are ways to briefly assess and address these problems, playing a valuable gatekeeper role. It is also a matter of setting priorities. If there are serious and prevalent problems affecting children, they deserve attention; other issues may be given less time (eg, listening to the lungs in an asymptomatic child). Knowledge, practice, and skills enhance efficiency in addressing these problems. Having parents complete a questionnaire while waiting saves time, obviating the need to ask these questions during the visit.
2. **"What will this cost me?"** When efficiently incorporated into practice, the financial costs should be minimal, given the above. Access to behavioral health is helpful, and costs are reduced when families function better and child abuse and neglect are prevented.
3. **"I'm not sure how to handle problems like IPV."** It is clear that most pediatricians have had little training is some of these problems. There is a need to obtain some training and to identify local resources for consultation and referral. There is also online training that is readily available (eg, http://www.seekwellbeing.com). As with a worrisome peripheral blood smear, it may amount to knowing whom to call. Someone on the office staff should be able to readily identify a few key local resources.
4. **"These problems are very sensitive. I don't feel comfortable raising them."** The issues are sensitive, but important. If framed carefully (eg, "Lots of families have these problems, so I'm asking everyone. . . ."), most families will not be offended, and some will be grateful. Discomfort is also related to not knowing what to do; knowledge and skill help. As an analogy, asking adults about sexual practices was awkward for many, but the prevalence of HIV disease warranted overcoming that discomfort.
5. **"What if the screen is incorrect? There's the problem of false-positives and false-negatives."** First, it is important to recognize that a screen is just a screen. A brief assessment should clarify whether the problem exists. Screening questionnaires will miss some at-risk parents. These false-negatives may occur when a parent is in denial about a problem or is not ready to acknowledge the problem to others or begin to address it. An ongoing, supportive relationship with families and periodic repetition of screening may increase a parent's comfort in disclosing sensitive information and in engaging in help. It is also important to remember that while screening misses some at-risk parents, many others will be identified who would have otherwise gone undetected.
6. **"Appropriate services are often not available to address the family's needs."** This issue naturally varies in different regions. However, a little scouting on the Internet often identifies local resources. Even when these are less than ideal, they may still provide valuable assistance to families.
7. **"We don't really know that these approaches work."** There is mounting evidence supporting preventive strategies. For example, the US Preventive Services Task Force recommended screening for IPV in their most recent policy update. Evaluations of the SEEK model in 2 randomized controlled trials yielded promising findings. Motivational interviewing has increased the effectiveness in engaging those with a substance abuse problem in seeking treatment. There is also considerable clinical experience suggesting that pediatricians can successfully facilitate referrals for mental health and social services. Their positive relationships with families enable them to be trusted confidants and to offer valuable support and guidance.

## SUGGESTED READINGS


Avellar S, Paulsell D, Sama-Miller E, Del Grosso P. Home visiting evidence of effectiveness review: executive summary. Washington, DC: Office of Planning, Research and Evaluation, Administration for Children and Families, US Department of Health and Human Services; 2014. http://homvee.acf.hhs.gov/HomVEE_Executive_Summary_2013.pdf. Accessed October 17, 2016.

Avellar SA, Supplee LH. Effectiveness of home visiting in improving child health and reducing child maltreatment. *Pediatrics.* 2013:132:S90-S99.

Dias MS, Smith K, deGuehery K, et al. Preventing abusive head trauma in infants and young children: a hospital-based, parent education program. *Pediatrics.* 2005;115:e470-e477.

Dubowitz H, Feigelman S, Lane W. Pediatric primary care to help prevent child maltreatment: the Safe Environment for Every Kid (SEEK) model. *Pediatrics.* 2009;123:858-864.

Dubowitz H, Lane WG, Semiatin JN, Magder LS. The SEEK model of pediatric primary care: can child maltreatment be prevented in a low-risk population? *Acad Pediatr.* 2012;12(4):259-268.

Flaherty EG, Stirling J Jr; American Academy of Pediatrics Committee on Child Abuse and Neglect. Clinical report: the pediatrician's role in child maltreatment prevention. *Pediatrics.* 2010;126(4):833-841.

Mikton C, Butchart A. Child maltreatment prevention: a systematic review of reviews. *Bull World Health Organ.* 2009;87:1-9.

Prinz RJ, Sanders MR, Shapiro CJ, Whitaker DJ, Lutzker JR. Population-based prevention of child maltreatment: the U.S. Triple P System population trial. *Prev Sci.* 2009;10:1-12. doi: 10.1007/s11121-00900123-3.

Walsh K, Zwi K, Woolfenden S, Shlonsky A. School-based educational programmes for the prevention of child sexual abuse: a systematic review. *Campbell Systematic Rev.* 2015;11(10). doi: 10.4073/csr.2015/10. http://www.campbellcollaboration.org/lib/project/28/. Accessed October 17, 2016.

Zolotor AJ, Runyan DK, Shanahan M, et al. Effectiveness of a statewide abusive head trauma prevention program in North Carolina. *JAMA Pediatr.* 2015;169(12):1126-1131. doi: 10.1001/jamapediatrics.2015.2690.

# PART 1 CARE OF THE NEWBORN

# 40 Historical Perspectives

Haresh Kirpalani and Gautham K. Suresh

*"Any society, any nation, is judged on the basis of how it treats its weakest members—the last, the least, the littlest."*

—Cardinal Roger Mahony

Modern, well-resourced societies in the 21st century expect most newborn infants to survive, especially when they are full term or near term. But in the past, newborn infants frequently died at birth or soon thereafter. As recently as in the 18th century, Queen Anne of England died childless in 1714, despite bearing 17 children. Over the last several hundred years, and especially in the last 50 years, advances in the care of healthy and sick neonates have led to dramatic improvements in their survival and outcomes. These remarkable improvements are the result of changing societal attitudes toward the care of neonates, advances in technology that led to the modern neonatal intensive care unit (NICU), regionalization of neonatal care, and incorporation over time of scientific advances and the principles of evidence-based medicine into neonatal practice. In parallel, improved obstetric care of pregnant women during pregnancy and delivery has also improved neonatal survival and outcomes.

## SOCIETY'S VIEW OF THE NEWBORN AND CHANGES OVER TIME

From a teleological and evolutionary standpoint, individual adults are primed to react to a baby with tender emotions. However, attitudes of societies to the baby have varied through history. An underlying theme is that as society got more complex and richer, it could afford a more caring approach to the infant. In addition, by the 1800s, society generally viewed that a healthy individual contributed to the economic and social wellbeing of the nation.

Silverman noted that "infanticide is the oldest method of human family planning." This was exemplified in the Greek Spartan approach. But this was gradually superseded by strictures against infanticide. By 52 BC, Roman law passed by the Consul Pompeius warned against any murder of any relative, but was still often flouted. In the Justinian Code of AD 529, "foundlings" were not to be made slaves, but at the same time, fathers had rights to destroy "deformed" children and had absolute power over the life of the child. By the 1500s, court records in Nuremberg, Germany, show that women convicted of infanticide were buried alive, yet the practice remained rife. In England, unwanted infants were placed into "baby farms" staffed by "killer nurses" plying "Godfrey's cordial" (a mixture of opium, treacle, and sassafras). In the 1860s the British press carried "frequent reports of dead infants found under bridges, in parks, in culverts and ditches, and in cesspools." An outcry led to the first Infant Life Protection Act, in 1872. Yet, at the same time, the Industrial Revolution placed no value on children's lives, nor on the expectant mothers, as records of medical commissions reported.

Following the Franco-Prussian War in 1870, French society realized that a strong, healthy conscripted army was needed for society, which led to efforts to improve the health of "feeble" infants. The Boer War was another example of war as a societal driver of healthcare reforms because of the need for a healthy population from which the army can recruit.

The French example inspired other countries. Ballantyne, an obstetrician in Scotland, pointed out the economic benefits of improving the outcomes of the premature infant, given the falling birth rate in England and Wales:

> The problem of the premature infant is . . . a very real and a very pressing one. The steady fall in the birth-rate in the British Isles as well as in some foreign countries and in our own colonies, has, so to say, caused an appreciation in the value, economic as well as sentimental, of the premature infant. When it is borne in mind that in England and Wales in 1871 the birth-rate was nearly 35 per 1000 (34.7 was the exact figure), that it had fallen to 29.3 in 1899, to 28.9 in 1900, and that it was as low as 28.5 in 1901, it is evident that there is a pressing need to conserve the lives of the infants that are actually born, even although they are prematurely born. It may not be possible exactly to define their value to the State and the community, but manifestly it is greater now than it was when the birth rate was 35 per 1000. The problem of the premature infant is urgent.

Such wider considerations guided the first enacted healthcare welfare acts. Chancellor Bismarck introduced the first comprehensive old age, pension, and healthcare insurance scheme, in Germany in 1883. His inspiration was revealed in an 1849 address: "The social insecurity of the worker is the real cause of their being a peril to the state."

In summary, throughout history, society's view of the newborn reflected the socioeconomic and political fault lines. Ballantyne's is an explicit example of the survival of the preterm being viewed as a contribution to the economic well-being of a society.

In the era of high neonatal mortality, it was expected that prematurely born neonates and those with birth defects would not survive. Some pioneers started to care for premature babies and others tried to save those with birth defects (including congenital cardiac anomalies) by operating upon them. Around 1900, preterm babies were displayed in fairs and public exhibitions as curiosities. Gradually, attitudes shifted toward the acceptance of these babies as survivors. This shift in attitudes was helped by a recognition that surviving neonates would eventually contribute to the economic well-being of society. Over time, the gestational threshold at which neonatologists attempted to provide intensive care to babies shifted lower and lower. Nowadays, it is not uncommon for neonatologists to offer resuscitation and a trial of intensive care to neonates with a gestation as low as 22 weeks at birth. In addition, many congenital abnormalities which were previously considered lethal, are now amenable to surgical repair. These factors have dramatically impacted the prognosis of vast numbers of newborns with complex disease.

## STEADY ADVANCEMENT OF TECHNOLOGY

This trend toward saving more neonates, including the higher-risk and more fragile ones, was helped by technology. Figure 40-1 shows the birth weight at which an approximate 50% survival rate is seen in infants, over the period from the 1930s to the end of the 20th century. This trend has been accompanied by an overall increase in survival. Depicted along the curve are also some selected key technological advances in the care of newborns, as seen by 1 if the pioneers of the field—M. E. Avery.

Starting in the 1950s, devices to improve the survival and outcomes of sick neonates began to be introduced, and they continue to evolve. These included devices to maintain infants at the optimal temperature (incubators, radiant warmers), devices to provide respiratory support (mechanical ventilators, continuous positive airway pressure devices), vital signs monitors, and infusion pumps. In addition, the ability to perform laboratory test on very small volumes of blood, and

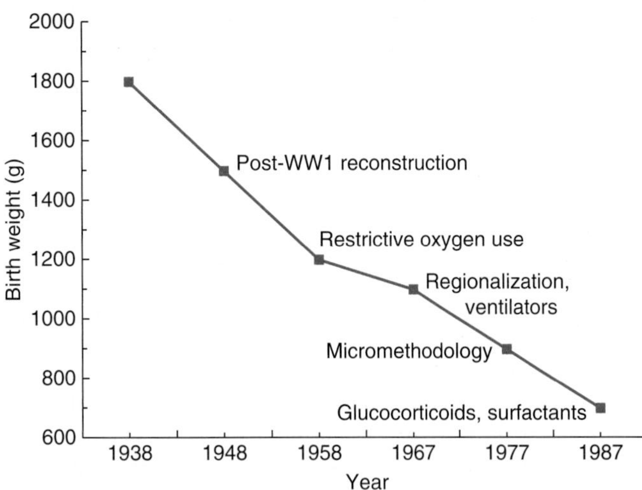


**FIGURE 40-1** Birth weight and survival in the 20th century. Birth weights at which approximately 50% of infants survived up to 28 postnatal days between 1938 and 1987, with some of the significant perinatal advances of this period. WWI, World War I.

refinements in radiological imaging, improved the ability to perform diagnostic tests in these fragile infants. Many of these devices and techniques represented adaptations of similar technology evolving for adult and pediatric critical care units. However, others, such as incubators, radiant warmers, and transcutaneous oxygen monitors, were developed exclusively for use in NICUs.

Only some of these advances have been adopted with the support of randomized evidence. In some situations, in which a huge death rate is reduced immediately by a new technology, no randomized controlled trial (RCT) is needed. Such was the case with the introduction of penicillin and, indeed, with the widespread uptake of neonatal ventilation in respiratory distress syndrome.



## EVOLVING PARADIGMS AND PHILOSOPHY OF MEDICINE AND EVIDENCE-BASED MEDICINE

As enthusiasm for saving infants using technology burgeoned, the focus moved from mere survival to ensuring that surviving neonates were free of medical morbidity and neurodevelopmental impairment. There was also increasing recognition of the amount of preventable iatrogenic harm that NICU patients were suffering. This recognition of iatrogenic harm became particularly dramatic when neonatologists identified an epidemic of retrolental fibroplasia (subsequently termed *retinopathy of prematurity*) and linked it to liberal use of supplemental oxygen in preterm infants with immature retinal development. This led to a realization of the need to study therapeutic interventions rigorously and assess both benefits and harms before implementing them. Thus, neonatology became 1 of the earliest specialties to adopt the principles of evidence-based medicine. But this adoption of a modern paradigm of evidence-based medicine was the most recent of 4 shifts in the prevailing medical paradigm driven by developments in science.

The first paradigm of medicine was a purely descriptive and experience-based philosophy of care, and can be termed a "magical theory" of medicine. While early "physicians" were shamans or magic men, they carefully observed nature, in an attempt to control it. Even in the Stone Age, magnificent cave paintings displayed a mastery of external anatomy. Such intense observation of nature allowed later physicians to lay a basis for medical care, which shifted to the second paradigm in medicine: careful observation coupled with an abstracted theorization. This approach is exemplified by Hippocrates (c. 460–c. 370 BC) who said, in *On Forecasting Diseases*:

> First of all the doctor should look at the patient's face. If he looks his usual self, this is a good sign. If not, however, the following are bad signs—sharp nose, hollow eyes, cold ears, dry skin on the forehead, strange face colour such as green, black, red or lead coloured. If the face is like this at the beginning of the illness, the doctor must ask the patient if he has lost sleep, or had diarrhoea, or not eaten.

Unsurprisingly, such a focus fostered a very realist and material approach, that denied any "mystery" or "magic":

> It seems to me that the disease called sacred is no more divine than any other. It has a natural cause, just as other diseases have. Men think it is divine because they do not understand it. . . . [I]n Nature all things are alike in this, that they can all be traced to preceding causes.

Yet its reliance upon an abstract theory usually devoid of experimental proof was a major source of dogmatism and ineffectiveness.

The teachings of the Greeks were largely lost in the chaos of the so-called Dark Ages. Waves of invaders buried the teachings in the rubble of battles to take over the Greek and Romans empires. Their writings were only preserved in far corners of the world. Ironically, given the vituperation they were to later receive in the 20th century, the Arabs transmitted the corpus of ancient Greek philosophy, medicine, and science down through the ages. They added and reinvigorated this, as evidenced by great physicians such as Avicenna. By the 10th to 12th centuries, Salerno, Italy, had become a European modernizing spearhead on the basis of the Arab-transmitted texts. But this received wisdom itself became transformed by the new scientific discoveries.

As towns and cities grew, enveloping the countryside, interest grew in physics and mechanics and in biomechanics. Now, physiological and anatomical experimentation could be incorporated into medicine. This led to the third medical paradigm: a physiology-based medicine. The rapid rise of capability in this era led to a certain authoritarianism in medicine.

However, due to its incomplete understanding, this physiological-era medicine was often reductionist. It did fuel intense research that, with time, was to become applicable to patient care. Moreover, this investigation was combined with the print revolution, to result in magnificent books such as *De Humanis Corporis Fabrica*, by Andreas Vesalius (1514–1564). His anatomical dissections laid bare the reality of the human anatomy and was a brave challenge to church dogma and prohibition on science.

Increasingly, it became commonplace to conceive of humans as a machine, and thereby comprehensible by natural physical laws. This formed the Renaissance ideology espoused by Rene Descartes (1596–1650) and others. It was accompanied by an explosion of observational science. This was the era of the discovery of transmissible agents. One such example, cholera, had been investigated by John Snow (1813–1858), who mapped an outbreak in London by observing those using a single water pump. Increasingly, it was understood that data was crucial. Sir William Petty (1620–1687) first built an economic database in England, which inspired the physician William Farr (1807–1883) to set up the routine recording of causes of death in the United Kingdom in 1838. This was the first national health registry.

After a long interval, this led to the observations and brilliant interventions of Pierre Budin (1846–1907). Budin observed an enormous death rate in the Paris Foundlings Hospital, and correlated it to the temperature of the infant. He then instituted warmth (and feeding) to newborns from birth, and restored the survival rate dramatically (Fig. 40-2).

This was a major therapeutic intervention instituted on the basis of an observational study. However, we now appreciate that in evaluating therapies, the observational study has pitfalls, in comparison to the RCT study. Above all, it was William Silverman (1917–2004) who pointed this out to neonatologists. Figure 40-3 depicts the difference between association and causation involved in the new epidemic of retinopathy of prematurity.

The inherent bias of observational studies prompted a recognition of the need for tighter scientific methods. The word *bias* here refers to a systematic deviation from the truth. In reality, the RCT was born in ignorance of the play of bias. A quasi RCT was actually first performed by James Lind (1716–1794), who divided 12 sailors suffering from scurvy into groups who consumed cider, sulfuric acid, vinegar,

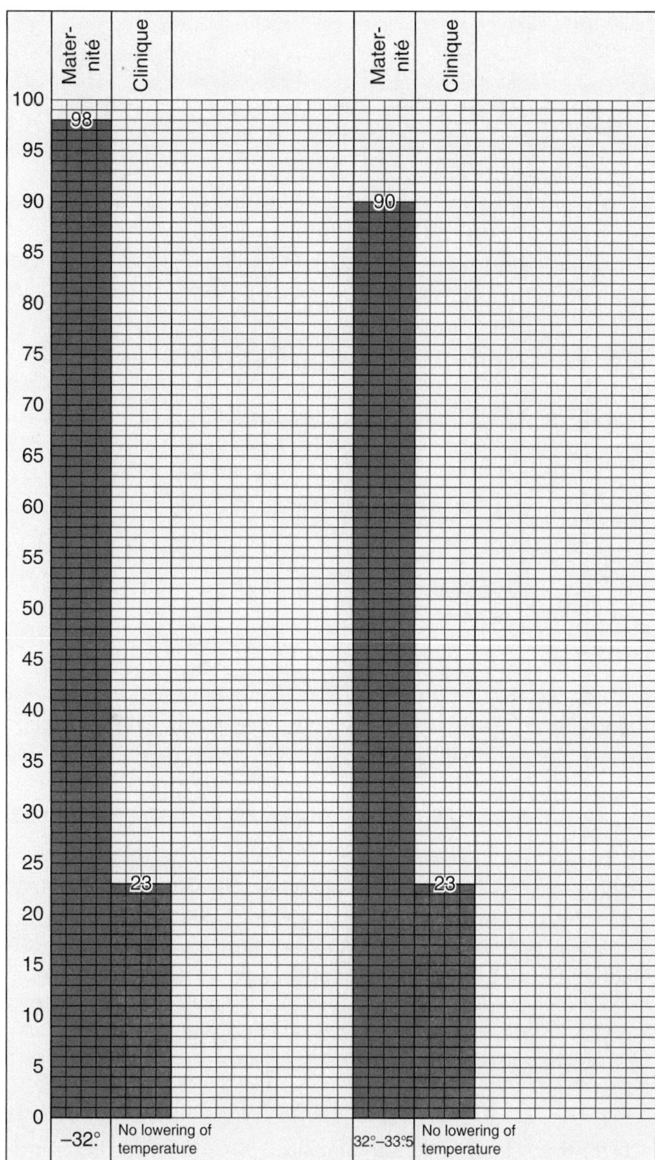


**FIGURE 40-2** Body temperature and neonatal death. Pierre Budin's charts showing the percentage of neonates who died in Paris at the maternity hospital, when temperatures were either at the 32–33.5°C range or lower, as compared to his experimental clinics, where there was no hypothermia. The *y*-axis shows mortality in percent. (From http://www.neonatology.org/pinups/default.html.)

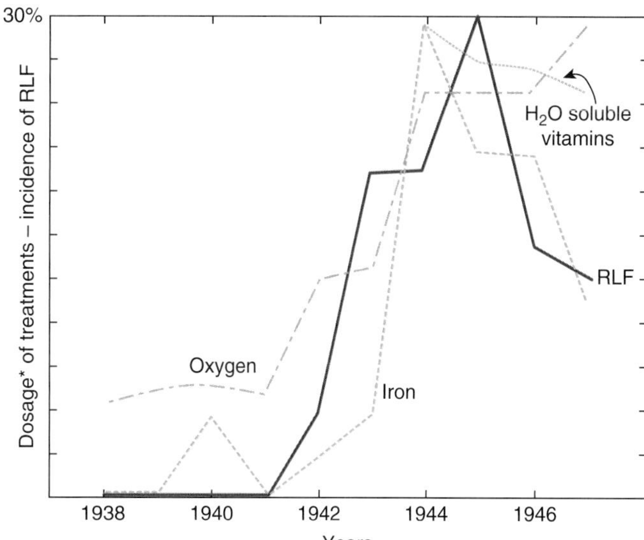


**FIGURE 40-3** Incidence of retrolental fibroplasia. This graph shows the incidence of retrolental fibroplasia (RLF) now known as retinopathy of prematurity (ROP), during the years 1938 to 1946. The solid black line shows that rates of RLF rapidly rose until 1945. This rise was paralleled by the rise in use of 3 therapies: oxygen, iron, and vitamins. For many years, the medical profession mistakenly blamed vitamins and iron as the etiological agent for RLF. This association delayed the understanding of oxygen as the main etiological agent. This is a classic case of confusion of association rather than causation. *Days in oxygen, drops of water-miscible vitamins, and drams of ferrous sulfate. (Reproduced with permission from Silverman, WA: *Retrolental Fibroplasia: A Modern Parable*. Philadelphia: Grune & Stratton; 1980.)

seawater, barley water, or oranges and lemons. Without having a correct theory for it or even knowing the active ingredient of vitamin C, he abolished scurvy in the latter group. However, the advance of this method stagnated for many centuries.

By the 20th century, many pioneers incorporated statistical techniques allowing large trials to be performed on a scientific basis. These large scientific trials, coupled with an increased awareness of the limitations of authoritarian medicine, led to the current and fourth paradigm: evidence-based medicine.

An important development occurred when Archibald Cochrane (1909–1988) in Scotland strongly advocated the use of randomized control trials. After his death, the Cochrane Library, a database of systematic reviews, was established in his name at Oxford and became the international Cochrane Collaboration. Coincident with these developments was the development of the school of medicine at McMaster University in Hamilton, Ontario, Canada, which pioneered evidence-based medicine as an explicit teaching and clinical strategy. Led by David Sackett, Gordon Guyatt, Mike Gent, and Brian Haynes, they championed evidence-based medicine. A wide awareness of their view of a hierarchy of evidence, commonly depicted as a pyramid, became common (Fig. 40-4). The terminology *evidence-based medicine*, as coined by Guyatt, provoked intense dissent from the more physiologically established clinical schools. However, it became accepted as the norm around 2000.

Neonatologists, facing both scientific and moral-ethical dilemmas, were in the thick of debates about evidence. The ferment was led by William Silverman (1917–2004), his mentee Jack Sinclair (1933–2014) in the United States and Canada, and Edmund Hey (1934–2009) in the United Kingdom. Sinclair and Michael Bracken went on to develop the first set of neonatal and obstetric systematic reviews together with

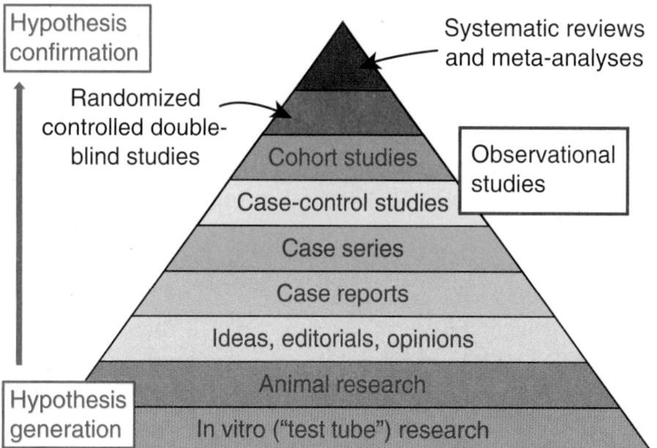


**FIGURE 40-4** Study hierarchy for human therapies. For human therapy, the lower part of the pyramid is a good source for hypothesis generation. However, for definitive evaluation (hypothesis confirmation) of the risk, the benefit ratio, the randomized controlled study, and the pooling of these results into a meta-analysis or systematic review are the highest level of evidence.

Iain Chalmers, Murray Enkin, and Marc J. N. C. Keirse, in 1989. This effort turned into the Neonatal Review Group of the Cochrane Collaboration, edited by Roger Soll, which contains a host of evidence that is easy and free to access.

One of the first large maternal-neonatal databases, the UK's Northern Region Perinatal Mortality Survey, was pioneered by Edmund Hey. It showed the potential of large databases, but it was more fully harnessed by the Vermont Oxford Network in Burlington, Vermont, led by Jerry Lucey, Jeff Horbar, and Roger Soll. It was soon followed by worldwide networks. The tension between observational and randomized data was ongoing. The observation of differences between their findings led to much discussion about the methods to avoid bias. John Ioannides did a pivotal study that, overall, appeared to show no difference between observational and randomized studies on effects of a therapy. However, worryingly, when they did differ, results of observational therapies appeared to show a greater treatment effect overall.

Since not all potential therapies can be subject to RCT evaluation, and since resources are limited and trials are expensive, the tension certainly reflected an objective reality. McMaster University in fact defused the tension by moving toward a synthesis that emphasized the interconnectedness of several types of evidence, from clinical "gut" sense and anecdotal experience, to formal RCT evaluation, with observational studies in between. This synthesis has had a natural outgrowth into the current era of grading evidence developed by the Grading of Recommendations, Assessment, Development, and Evaluations (GRADE) Working Group, in which recommendations for therapy and practice are based on a range of considerations, performed by unbiased panels. A major challenge in neonatology today is that although there is widespread awareness of the need to practice evidence-based medicine, there is paucity of randomized trials for many of the medications and therapies available. In fact, most drugs in the NICU are used off-label and many useless medications are used.



## LONG TERM OUTCOMES FOR HIGH RISK NEONATES

The astonishing improvements in outcome of the modern era of neonatology are evident. Figure 40-5 shows the fall in neonatal mortality rates from the year 1910 on, in the United States, as 1 example. It shows a remarkable fall in overall infant and neonatal mortality from 1915 to 1985. However, the neonatal mortality proportion of infant mortality rose from 44% to 75% of the total. These data demonstrate that the riskiest period of childhood life is the neonatal period. It also highlights that more needs to be done here, which brings up the role of technology.

That we have grown more sophisticated and able to ensure survival is beyond debate. However, improved survival rates have come with an increasing burden of more chronic illness (eg, bronchopulmonary dysplasia). The earlier the infant is born, the less mature the lungs are, and injury to the lungs at the canalicular stage of development may impact long-term lung function. This has implications for how the development of neonatal care fares in the 21st century. The identification of the limitations of short-term outcomes of randomized trials caused the development of an awareness of the importance of incorporating long-term outcomes into trials, such as in the Caffeine for Apnea of Prematurity Trial, which has reported a series of outcomes up to 11 years of age.

Multidisciplinary care providers of newborn intensive care should feel proud about these achievements. However, the turn from the mere survival of extremely preterm infants to their ultimate function and well-being in society inspires some humility. Initial small selected studies suggested that increased survival was associated with an inferior long-term health-related quality of life. However, this observation has been challenged by the findings reported from large, comprehensive datasets, including those from a Finnish cohort. In a large cohort of infants born between 1967 and 1988, as well as higher childhood (ie, post-neonatal) mortality rates for survivors of preterm NICU care (22–27 weeks), boys had a relative risk of death that ranged from 5.3% in early childhood to 9.7% in late childhood. Girls had corresponding rates of 1.71% and 9.7%, respectively. The data for these children were accompanied by considerably lower rates of childbearing in adult life.

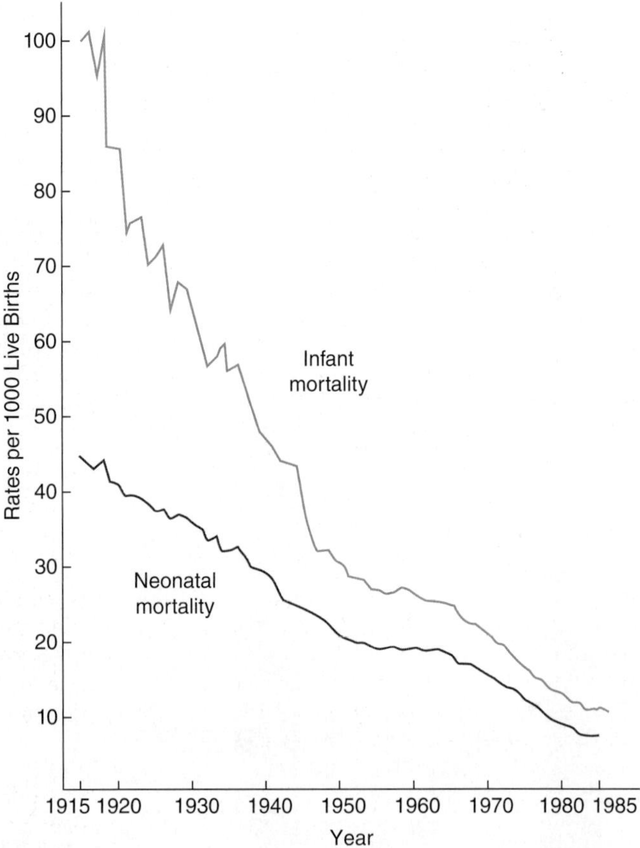


**FIGURE 40-5** Infant and neonatal mortality rates in the United States, 1916–1985. The greatest decline in mortality was between 1935 and 1949. From Desmond MM. A review of newborn medicine in America: European past and guiding ideology. (Reproduced with permission from Desmond MM: A review of newborn medicine in America: European past and guiding ideology, *Am J Perinatol.* 1991 Sep;8(5):308-322.)

These underlying issues have sparked both ethical and economical discussions. The ethical issues have tended largely to be resolved by providing parents with comprehensive information and supporting data regarding the risks associated with preterm delivery. To do this well is not a trivial matter and decision aids or information aids can help to standardize and anticipate key parental concerns. Economic concerns about the cost of NICU care and the ongoing cost for survivors with sequelae reflect societal issues. However, such concerns are alleviated by the realization that NICU care is actually remarkably cost effective, as compared to aspects of adult care. For example, the cost per quality-adjusted life year (QALY) gained for NICU care (birth weight of 500–999 g) in Victoria, Australia, was A$8630 compared to the cost of A$7290 per QALY gained over a similar time period for coronary artery bypass of the left main coronary artery (in adults), or A$33,170 for treatment of mild hypertension (diastolic pressure of 95–104 mm Hg for males aged 40).

## OTHER RECENT DEVELOPMENTS IN NEONATOLOGY AND ONGOING CHALLENGES

### Increased Focus on Measuring and Improving the Quality of Care

In the 1990s, monitoring of neonatal clinical outcomes and process measures to assess the quality of care became increasingly common. In North America, multicenter databases such as those from the Vermont Oxford Network, the Pediatrix Medical Group, the Neonatal Research Network, and the Canadian Neonatal Network were developed. Similar databases evolved in other countries as well. These databases demonstrated large variations from NICU to NICU in clinical practices and in outcomes even after statistical risk adjustment, raising the possibility that the quality of care in some NICUs was worse than in others. This led to the introduction of intentional, methodical attempts to improve neonatal care and clinical outcomes using quality improvement, both within single institutions as well as within multicenter quality improvement projects (ie, collaboratives).

#### Family-Centered Care and Social and Economic Determinants of Health

In the past 2 decades, there has been increasing recognition of the need to involve the infant's family in the ongoing medical care of the infant, to support their psychosocial needs, and to have them participate in making decisions about their infant's care. Such participation is enhanced by the use of decision aids—visual displays of quantitative information about risks and benefits of potential interventions in easily comprehensible formats. There is also increasing recognition that health professionals should identify and address high-risk social and economic factors (such as parental smoking, quality of housing, and health literacy) related to the family that affect the health of neonates after discharge from the intensive care unit.

#### Evolving Ethical Challenges

As neonatal care has advanced over the past several decades, so too have the ethical dilemmas in the field. Currently, health professionals and families struggle with dilemmas about initiating and withdrawing intensive care after birth for preterm infants born at the threshold of viability, and those with severe chromosomal anomalies and other disorders previously considered lethal for which intensive care was not offered. There are also emerging dilemmas about whether or not fetal surgical interventions should be used to treat prenatally diagnosed conditions such as twin–twin transfusion syndrome and congenital diaphragmatic hernia.

#### Neonatal Care in Low- and Middle-Income Countries

Much of the description above involves neonatal care in high-income countries. Neonatal mortality rates in low- and middle-income countries (LMICs) are still high, and comprise an increasing proportion of mortality in children under 5 years of age, as mortality in older children descreases. In such countries, high-risk pregnant mothers and sick neonates have poor access to medical care and experience delays in receiving care. The health facilities in which they receive care often have inadequate resources and inferior quality of care, even if the care is provided in a NICU. This often leads to poor outcomes, with higher mortality and increased morbidity, including a high rate of ROP and blindness secondary to poorly controlled oxygen delivery. Addressing some of the more basic gaps in care delivery, coupled with appropriate education, would undoubtedly result in significantly improved outcomes in LMIC settings.

### SUGGESTED READINGS

Avery ME. Changes in care of the newborn: personal reflections over forty years. *Neonatal Netw.* 1994;13(6):13-14.

Desmond MM. A review of newborn medicine in America: European past and guiding ideology. *Am J Perinatol.* 1991;8(5):308-322.

Doyle LW. Cost evaluation of intensive care for extremely tiny babies. *Semin Neonatol.* 1996;1(4):289-296.

Dukhovny D, Pursley DM, Kirpalani HM, Horbar JH, Zupancic JA. Evidence, quality, and waste: solving the value equation in neonatology. *Pediatrics.* 2016;137(3):e20150312.

Dunn PM. Professor Pierre Budin (1846-1907) of Paris, and modern perinatal care. *Arch Dis Child Fetal Neonatal Ed.* 1995;73(3); F193-F195.

Guillén Ú, Suh S, Munson D, et al. Development and pretesting of a decision-aid to use when counseling parents facing imminent extreme premature delivery. *J Pediatr.* 2012;160(3):382-387.

Guyatt G, Sackett DL, Cook DJ; Evidence-Based Medicine Working Group. Users guides to the medical literature. II. How to use an article about therapy or prevention. A. Are the results of the study valid? *JAMA.* 1993;270(21):2598-2601.

Haynes RB, Sackett DL, Gray JM, Cook DJ, Guyatt GH. Transferring evidence from research into practice: 1. The role of clinical care research evidence in clinical decisions. *ACP J Club.* 1996;125(3): A14-A16.

Ho T, Dukhovny D, Zupancic JA, Goldmann DA, Horbar JD, Pursley DM. Choosing wisely in newborn medicine: five opportunities to increase value. *Pediatrics.* 2015;136(2):e482-e489.

Ioanndis JP. Comparison of evidence of treatment effects in randomized and nonrandomized studies. *JAMA.* 2011;286(7);821-830.

Lussky RC, Cifuentes RF, Siddappa AM. A history of neonatal medicine—past accomplishments, lessons learned, and future challenges. Part 1—the first century. *J Pediatr Pharmacol Ther.* 2005;10(2):76-89.

Schmidt B, Roberts RS, Davis P, Caffeine for Apnea of Prematurity Trial Group. Long-term effects of caffeine therapy for apnea of prematurity. *N Engl J Med.* 2007;357(19):1893-1902.

Sigerist HE. From Bismarck to Beveridge: developments and trends in Social Security legislation. *J Public Health Policy.* 1999;20(4):474-496.

Silverman WA. Mismatched attitudes about neonatal death. *Hastings C Rep.* 1981;11(6):12-16.

Swamy GK, Ostbye T, Skjaerven R. Association of preterm birth with long-term survival, reproduction, and next-generation preterm birth. *JAMA.* 2008;299(12):1429-1436.

# 41 Care of the Fetus

Rodrigo Ruano



The care of the child begins with the care of the fetus. Accurate prenatal diagnosis and optimal perinatal management strongly affect the outcomes of the future infant, not just in childhood but throughout life. Careful planning of perinatal care for high risk pregnancies improves neonatal outcomes. Optimal maternal and fetal care with high-risk pregnancies improves neonatal outcomes and also decreases mortality and morbidity of mothers. Over the last 3 decades, fetal medicine has evolved into a distinct discipline that primarily focuses on the fetus as a patient. Many hospitals now have fetal medicine programs with coordinated and integrated care provided by subspecialists and support staff from maternal-fetal medicine and pediatric subspecialties such as neonatology, surgery, neurosurgery, urology, cardiology, genetics, palliative care, and ethics. This chapter will provide a brief overview of assessment of fetal well-being, prenatal screening and diagnostic tests, common problems that affect the fetus (including disorders of fetal growth, fetal anomalies, prematurity, and multiple pregnancies), and fetal therapy.

## FETAL GESTATION AND GROWTH

The accurate assessment of gestational age and fetal growth are essential for care of the fetus. The assignment of gestational age is more accurate in early gestation and decreases with advancing gestation. The standard method to assign fetal gestation uses the last menstrual period (LMP), often with confirmation using ultrasonographic measurement of the crown–rump length in the first trimester or biparietal diameter, head circumference, abdominal circumference, and femur length in the second trimester. Serial biometric measurements can be used in combination to evaluate fetal growth.

Although fetal biometric measurement is the gold standard method of estimating fetal gestational age and assessing fetal growth, there can be some differences when assessing fetal patients with different ethnic backgrounds. According to studies conducted at the National Institutes of Health, current ultrasonographic standards for evaluating fetal growth may result in up to 15% of fetuses to be misclassified as small for gestational age (SGA). Prenatal growth charts were first derived from ultrasound measurements of 139 predominantly middle-class white pregnant women during the 1980s. Currently, many population-based studies are being conducted to develop more accurate ultrasonographic fetal growth standards. Of these, the most prominent one is the Intergrowth-21st project.

Fetal growth assessment detects abnormalities of growth that are associated with fetal and neonatal morbidity and mortality. As in children, fetal growth is assessed by the percentile of the estimated fetal weight (EFW) at a particular gestational age. Fetuses whose weight is on percentile curves below the tenth percentile are considered SGA, and those above the 90th percentile are considered large for gestational age (LGA). The cutoff at the tenth percentile is arbitrary, and some fetuses who are SGA do not have any identifiable disease. They may simply be constitutionally small, with their small size attributable to factors such as maternal ethnicity, parity, and body mass. However, some fetuses may have pathologic conditions leading to attenuation of growth, and are said to have intrauterine growth restriction (IUGR). The terms *SGA* and *IUGR* are related but not synonymous.

The causes of IUGR can be fetal, placental, and maternal; the most common fetal causes include chromosomal abnormalities, structural malformations, fetal infections, and multiple gestation. IUGR caused by placental insufficiency (a common cause of which is pregnancy-induced hypertension) may present with different degrees of severity, which is reflected by the presence of abnormal placental-fetal hemodynamics. Pregnancies complicated by IUGR due to severe placental insufficiency may have abnormal Doppler studies including absent or reversed end-diastolic blood flow in the umbilical artery, elevated blood flow in the middle cerebral artery, and abnormal blood flow in the ductus venosus. There are 2 patterns of IUGR: asymmetric and symmetric. Of all fetuses with IUGR, 70% to 80% have asymmetric growth (preservation of head size with decrease in body weight and length), usually due to placental insufficiency. Symmetric IUGR (decrease in head size, body weight. and length), may be the result of chromosomal anomalies, congenital malformations, or intrauterine infections, but can also be caused by placental insufficiency during early gestation.



## FETAL ANOMALIES

The timely detection of anatomic fetal anomalies and physiologic derangements that can cause mortality or morbidity is a major goal of fetal care. This is accomplished primarily by prenatal diagnosis and screening. Current diagnostic and screening methods are able to identify various problems such as neural tube defects, genetic syndromes, and lower urinary tract obstruction. Common screening tests include noninvasive maternal serum testing for a variety of analytes, and ultrasonography, while invasive tests include chorionic villus sampling and amniocentesis.

Maternal serum screening has been available since the late 1980s as a screening test for Down syndrome and neural tube defects. Abnormal levels of 3 main biomarkers in the maternal blood were originally used during the second trimester of pregnancy to identify fetal abnormalities. These were maternal serum α-fetoprotein, human chorionic gonadotropin, and unconjugated estradiol. Inhibin A was later added to this list, and this quad screen improved the sensitivity and specificity. These biomarkers are normally found in the fetal blood, brain, spinal fluid, and amniotic fluid. Together, these quad screen markers are widely used today for prenatal identification of fetal anomalies such as Down syndrome and neural tube defects. Over the last decade, screening has moved into the first trimester using ultrasound measurement of a clear space behind the back of the neck called the nuchal translucency and a combination of serum analytes. More recently, cell-free DNA in the maternal serum has become an alternative method to screen for aneuploidy.

Another useful tool to identify fetal anomalies is prenatal ultrasonography, which can identify a range of structural anatomic fetal abnormalities. Findings such as increased nuchal translucency signals an increased risk for chromosomal abnormalities and polyhydramnios signals possible anatomic defects. Ultrasound can also help identify the sex of the fetus (which is important when an X-linked genetic disorder is suspected). Doppler ultrasound screening can detect functional abnormalities in the fetus, and doppler velocimetry allows the assessment of the fetal circulation.

## PREMATURITY

In women at risk of delivering preterm (ie, at less than 37 weeks' gestation), fetal assessment should include confirmation of the assigned gestational age for prenatal records when available, estimation of the exact gestation, assessment of fetal well-being, and the risks to the fetus from maternal conditions such as preterm prolonged rupture of membranes, placental abruption, or pregnancy-induced hypertension. Neonatal respiratory distress syndrome is the leading cause of mortality and morbidity associated with prematurity. The incidence is inversely related to the gestational age. Fetal lung maturity (FLM) can be determined by the presence of pulmonary surfactant components in the amniotic fluid. Although these tests were widely employed in the past, several recent studies have shown that demonstration of a mature fetal lung index by antenatal testing does not improve neonatal outcomes. Instead, decreased respiratory and nonrespiratory morbidities are most highly correlated with gestational age of the fetus. In addition, the amniocentesis needed to obtain amniotic fluid for this test increases risks. For these reasons, these tests are rarely used today.

Whenever there is a disorder of pregnancy or an abnormal fetal condition, the risks to the baby and mother from delaying delivery have to be balanced against the risks of prematurity and possible operative delivery if the baby is delivered immediately. This balance of risks should be repeatedly reassessed if the pregnancy is continued. When a pregnant woman is at risk of delivering a preterm infant prior to 34 weeks' gestation, glucocorticoids are given to accelerate FLM and decrease neonatal morbidity and mortality. Attempts can also be made to prevent preterm birth. In most cases, tocolytics are used to allow time for antenatal corticosteroids to be administered to the mother.

## MULTIPLE GESTATION

Multiple gestation is associated with increased risk of prematurity, neurodevelopmental delay and perinatal death. The number of fetuses and the characteristics of the placentas are the main factors related to those complications. Triplet pregnancies have higher risks of obstetrical and perinatal complications than twin gestations. With ultrasonography a determination can be made about whether the placentation is monochorionic or dichorionic and whether it is monoamniotic or diamniotic. Monochorionic pregnancies have also more complications than dichorionic gestations. Monochorionic pregnancies are at risk of severe complications, including twin-to-twin transfusion syndrome, selective intrauterine fetal growth restriction, and twin anemia-polycythemia sequence. In these conditions, perinatal mortality and morbidity are extremely high, and care is often provided by maternal-fetal medicine specialists. Sometimes, prenatal interventions including selective cord occlusion or fetoscopic laser ablation of placental anastomoses may be necessary.

## INVASIVE AND NONINVASIVE PRENATAL DIAGNOSTIC TESTS

*Chorionic villus sampling, amniocentesis, and cordocentesis* (also known as percutaneous umbilical blood sampling, or PUBS) are invasive prenatal tests that are used to diagnose chromosomal/genetic diseases and congenital infection as well as to investigate fetal metabolic disorders. These invasive tests increase the risk of premature rupture of the membranes and preterm birth, and rarely may cause pregnancy loss. Fetal biochemistry can be used to determine fetal renal function, pulmonary maturity, fetal anemia, and fetal hormonal status, such as hyper- or hypothyroidism. Fetal renal function is sometimes determined by vesicocentesis or tapping the fetal bladder. In current practice, these invasive tests are gradually being displaced by less invasive tests, such as maternal blood testing for fetal cells to identify chromosomal disorders (ie, noninvasive prenatal testing [NIPT]), Doppler of the fetal middle cerebral artery (used to screen for fetal anemia), and fetal anatomy scan. Invasive prenatal tests are still indicated when a specific condition such as thalassemia or congenital adrenal hyperplasia is suspected, or when a noninvasive screening test is positive.

## FETAL THERAPY

Current fetal therapies and interventions are aimed at reducing morbidity and mortality in fetuses with conditions that were previously considered lethal. The scope of fetal interventions includes medical therapies aimed at managing fetal conditions, ultrasound-guided percutaneous in utero interventions, fetoscopic or open fetal surgery, and ex utero intrapartum treatment (EXIT) procedures. These are discussed in detail in Chapter 42.

## CONCLUSION

Many disorders that cause fetal or neonatal death or morbidity can now be identified and treated before birth. Care of mothers and fetuses with complex, high-risk conditions is best provided at specialized treatment centers by an integrated team of specialists from different disciplines. All diagnostic and therapeutic decisions should involve careful balancing of benefits and risks both to the unborn fetus and to the mother.

## SUGGESTED READINGS


Aditya I, Tat V, Sawana A, Mohamed A, Tuffner R, Mondal T. Use of Doppler velocimetry in diagnosis and prognosis of intrauterine growth restriction (IUGR): a review. *J Neonatal Perinatal Med.* 2016;9(2):117-26.

Altman DG, Chitty LS. Charts of fetal size: 1. methodology. *Br J Obstet Gynaecol.* 1994;101(1):29-34.

Altman DG, Chitty LS. New charts for ultrasound dating of pregnancy. *Ultrasound Obstet Gynecol.* 1997;10(3):174-191.

Benson CB, Doubilet PM. Sonographic prediction of gestational age: accuracy of second- and third-trimester fetal measurements. *AJR Am J Roentgenol.* 1991;157(6)1275-1277.

Besnard AE, Wirjosoekarto SA, Broeze KA, Opmeer BC, Mol BW. Lecithin/sphingomyelin ratio and lamellar body count for fetal lung maturity: a meta-analysis. *Eur J Obstet Gynecol Reprod Biol.* 2013;169(2):177-183.

Das UG, Sysyn GD. Abnormal fetal growth: intrauterine growth retardation, small for gestational age, large for gestational age. *Pediatr Clin North Am.* 2004;51(3):639-654.

Gee RE, Dickey RP, Xiong X, Clark LS, Pridjian G. Impact of monozygotic twinning on multiple births resulting from in vitro fertilization in the United States, 2006-2010. *Am J Obstet Gynecol.* 2014;210(5):468.e1-e6.

Gnanendran L, Bajuk B, Oei J, Lui K, Abdel-Latif ME; NICUS Network. Neurodevelopmental outcomes of preterm singletons, twins and higher-order gestations: a population-based cohort study. *Arch Dis Child Fetal Neonatal Ed.* 2015;100(2):F106-F114.

Huerta-Enochian G, Katz V, Erfurth S. The association of abnormal alpha-fetoprotein and adverse pregnancy outcome: does increased fetal surveillance affect pregnancy outcome? *Am J Obstet Gynecol.* 2001;184(7):1549-1553; discussion 1553-1545.

Lepage N, Chitayat D, Kingdom J, Huang T. Association between second-trimester isolated high maternal serum maternal serum human chorionic gonadotropin levels and obstetric complications in singleton and twin pregnancies. *Am J Obstet Gynecol.* 2003;188(5):1354-1359.

Lin CC, Santolaya-Forgas J. Current concepts of fetal growth restriction: part I. Causes, classification, and pathophysiology. *Obstet Gynecol.* 1998;92(6)1044-1055.

Papageorghiou AT, Kennedy SH, Salomon LJ, et al. International standards for early fetal size and pregnancy dating based on ultrasound measurement of crown-rump length in the first trimester of pregnancy. *Ultrasound Obstet Gynecol.* 2014;44(6):641-648.

Papageorghiou AT, Ohuma EO, Altman DG, et al; International Fetal and Newborn Growth Consortium for the 21st Century (INTERGROWTH-21st). International standards for fetal growth based on serial ultrasound measurements: the Fetal Growth Longitudinal Study of the INTERGROWTH-21st Project. *Lancet.* 2014;384(9946):869-879.


# 42 Fetal Therapy

Natalie Rintoul, Anne Ades, and N. Scott Adzick

## INTRODUCTION

One in 28 babies is born with a structural birth defect. Advances in prenatal diagnosis have provided a window into the womb to accurately elucidate the precise details of anatomic defects and assess their impact on development (Table 42-1). These allow new possibilities for targeted innovation in prenatal therapy. Further, fetal therapy offers the ability to alter the natural history of some fetal disorders, converting a previously lethal diagnosis to a nonlethal diagnosis. In some cases, the progress of a disorder can be halted prior to irreversible damage. The scope for fetal therapy includes both medical interventions and surgical interventions, fetoscopic and open.

Embarking on fetal interventions requires a dedicated multidisciplinary team. The team should be comprised of a specialized group of individuals with expertise in fetal disease. At a minimum, the team should include maternal fetal medicine specialists, obstetricians, radiologists, pediatric surgeons, cardiologists, ultrasonographers, anesthesiologists, nurses, geneticists, neonatologists, social workers, and other pediatric subspecialists as needed. State-of-the art fetal imaging techniques such as high resolution 3-dimensional (D) and 4-D ultrasound, computed tomography (CT), magnetic resonance imaging (MRI), and echocardiography are paramount to the success of the fetal enterprise for accurate fetal diagnosis and detailed anatomy. Recent advances in techniques such as 3-D printing are increasingly used in treatment planning. In addition, advances in molecular diagnosis allows for the diagnosis of many genetic diseases in utero.

Deciding whether a mother and fetus are candidates for fetal therapy is very complex. Maternal factors such as overall health, cervical length, uterine abnormalities, and placental positioning are all determinants of candidacy. Fetal considerations for candidacy for fetal therapy include evaluation for genetic disorders or other associated congenital anomalies. Gestational age and severity at diagnosis are other key factors as the success of many of these interventions are dependent on being done in a time-sensitive critical window. In

**TABLE 42-1 DEFECTS AFFECTING THE FETUS AND THEIR SEQUELAE**

| Anatomic Defect | Effect on Development |
|---|---|
| Cystic adenomatoid malformation (CCAM) | Pulmonary hypoplasia<br>Hydrops |
| Sacrococcygeal teratoma (SCT) | High output failure |
| Laryngeal atresia | Congenital high airway obstruction syndrome (CHAOS)<br>Hydrops |
| Twin-twin transfusion syndrome (TTTS) and twin-reversed arterial perfusion (TRAP) syndrome | Vascular steal<br>Hydrops |
| Myelomeningocele (MMC) | Paraplegia<br>Hydrocephalus |
| Urethral obstruction | Pulmonary hypoplasia<br>Renal dysplasia |
| Congenital diaphragmatic hernia (CDH) | Pulmonary hypoplasia |
| Aortic stenosis | Hypoplastic left heart syndrome |

addition, in some cases, delivery of the fetus early for postnatal therapy rather than fetal therapy may be indicated.

In the past, fetal intervention was limited to conditions in singleton pregnancies in which the life of the fetus was threatened. In recent years, the indications for fetal intervention have been extended to non–life-threatening but potentially devastating conditions, such as myelomeningocele, and to multiple gestations for twin-twin transfusion syndrome (TTTS).

The evolution of fetal intervention holds tremendous promise for altering the prenatal natural history of a disorder in ways not possible after delivery. However the decision to pursue fetal intervention must always be balanced with the risk for prematurity and maternal morbidity. This requires very careful parental counseling and sensitive and transparent information giving.

## MEDICAL FETAL THERAPY

Medical fetal therapy refers to the administration of medications to the mother with the goal of transplacental transfer to achieve therapeutic dosages in the fetal circulation. Less commonly, direct medication administration to the fetus occurs through cordocentesis, accessing the fetal circulation. There is a growing list of conditions in which such approaches are used. Some of these are now well established, but some are still at an early developmental stage.

### Fetal Arrhythmia

Medical fetal therapy has been widely used to treat fetal cardiac conditions such as tachyarrhythmias and complete heart block seen with maternal autoimmune disorders. The most common fetal arrhythmia is supraventricular tachycardia (SVT), which can be treated successfully in utero through maternal administration of antiarrhythmic drugs. Medications that have been used to treat fetal SVT include digoxin, sotalol, amiodarone, and flecainide. Digoxin is the first-line drug of choice unless hydrops is present. Hydrops limits the transplacental transfer of digoxin. Thus, in cases of fetal SVT with hydrops, sotalol or flecainide may be used as first-line treatment to ensure adequate transplacental transfer. Another common fetal arrhythmia that may need intervention is atrial flutter. As with any attempt to treat a fetus with maternal administration of a medication, the mother needs careful monitoring. For instance, signs of maternal adverse effects when cardiac medications are used include maternal arrhythmias and prolonged QT.

Fetal complete heart block can cause significant bradycardia and potential development of hydrops and subsequent death. Fetal complete heart block is usually seen in the setting of a structurally normal heart, with the transplacental passage of anti-Ro/SSA maternal antibodies, which cross-react with antigens expressed in the conduction system of the fetal heart. Maternal steroids in fetal complete heart block can improve the degree of atrioventricular (AV) block and treat any associated myocarditis. In addition, maternal administration of β-mimetics, including salbutamol and terbutaline, has been reported to increase the ventricular rate when coadministered with steroids.

### Congential Cystic Adenomatoid Malformation

*Congenital cystic adenomatoid malformations* (CCAMs) grow in utero up to about 28 weeks of gestation. Most remain small and do not cause any adverse fetal effects. However, in some fetuses, the CCAM grows quite large. In this case, it can interfere with normal lung growth with resultant pulmonary hypoplasia, and it can create mediastinal shift with compression of the heart and great vessels and consequent hydrops (Fig. 42-1). The presence of hydrops carries a poor prognosis with a high likelihood of mortality. Maternal administration of steroids (eg, betamethasone) has been shown in many patients to arrest the growth of the solid component of the CCAM and prevent the development of hydrops, and allow the fetus to grow. Prenatal steroids are typically reserved for large lesions that are microcystic and do not have dominant cysts amenable to in utero decompression. In addition, reversal of hydrops has been documented after maternal betamethasone administration. Some fetuses who have not responded adequately to a first course of steroids may respond to repeat courses. However, the response is variable and some fetuses will still require surgical intervention either in the fetal or immediate postnatal period. The risks and benefits of repeated maternal administration of betamethasone need to be closely weighed and discussed with the family by an experienced team given the known adverse effects on growth and potentially on brain development.

### Congenital Adrenal Hyperplasia

In the most common form of *congenital adrenal hyperplasia* (CAH), 21-hydroxylase deficiency, 17-hydroprogesterone accumulates and can be detected in the amniotic fluid. Maternal steroid administration prior to 9 weeks' gestation may prevent virilization in genotypic female fetuses. However, there is significant risk treating the early gestation fetus at risk for CAH with dexamethasone, including decreased birth weight, orofacial clefts, and adverse neurocognitive outcomes. Thus, accurate prenatal diagnosis of CAH is necessary before this fetal therapy can be recommended outside of trials.

### Stem Cell and Gene Therapy

Intense work is currently underway to develop fetal treatments with stem cell or gene therapy to prevent postnatal diseases. This includes prenatal stem cell therapy to target sickle cell disease with the premise that stem cells injected into the preimmune fetus would engraft and treat the underlying deficiency. While experimental, there is potential to target hemophilias, muscular dystrophy, and central nervous system disorders with gene therapies.

In summary, medical fetal therapy has seen some successes anecdotally, but there have not been any randomized controlled trials performed to truly demonstrate benefit. However, given the rarity of these disorders, embarking on such trials would be very challenging. Thus, it remains key that a multidisciplinary care team review each case and develop an intervention plan with the parents that accounts for the potential benefits as well as the known risks.

If a fetus fails medical therapy, or if the underlying condition is not amenable to medical therapy, more invasive approaches can be considered. These range from moderately invasive to fully invasive interventions, which may involve ultrasound guidance or open fetal surgeries.

## PERCUTANEOUS ULTRASOUND-GUIDED INTERVENTIONS

### Thoracoamniotic Shunt

Prenatal lung lesions, such as large pleural effusions or CCAMs with a large dominant cyst, may cause mediastinal shift and compress the heart and lungs. Fetuses with such lesions are at risk for the development of hydrops and pulmonary hypoplasia. In general, initial therapies are targeted at decompressing the thorax with needle thoracentesis alone. If the lesions recur, then thoracoamniotic shunt placement can be considered. Placement of these shunts has been effective at decreasing the relative and absolute size of the CCAMs, and result in complete drainage of effusions in up to 25% of patients. In addition, hydrops has been reported to resolve in up to 90% of patients with CCAMs and 70% of patients with pleural effusions after shunt placement (Fig. 42-1). Chest wall deformities have been seen in babies following fetal shunt placement. In one series, early shunt placement at less than 21 weeks' gestation, resulted in chest wall deformities (eg, concavity, rib thinning) in 77% of newborns (Fig. 42-2).

### Vesicoamniotic Shunt

Fetuses with obstructive uropathies are at risk for the development of renal dysplasia as well as oligo-/anhydramnios with subsequent development of pulmonary hypoplasia. Potentially by decompressing the obstructed bladder and improving amniotic fluid volume, these complications can be ameliorated by ultrasound-guided fetal intervention. Most commonly, the patients eligible for vesicoamniotic shunt placement are male fetuses with posterior urethral valves or urethral atresia, prior to the development of presumed irreversible renal disease based on fetal urinary laboratory values and sonographic renal assessment. There is suggestive evidence of an improvement in mortality with vesicoamniotic shunt placement in male fetuses but there is still high

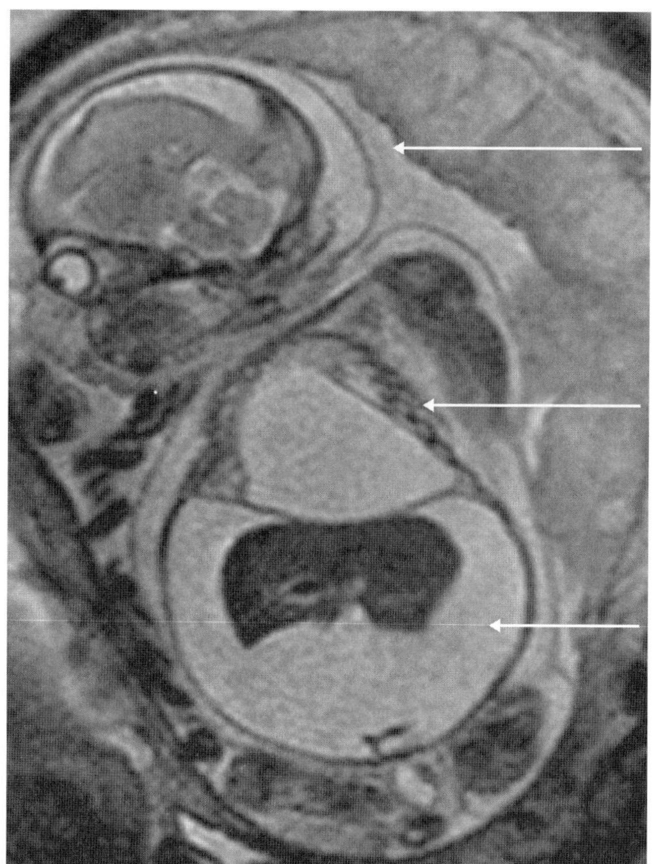


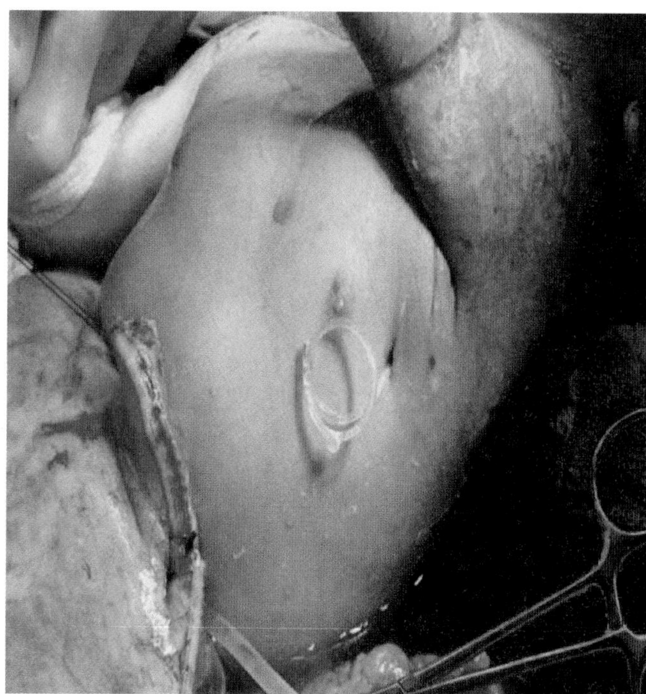


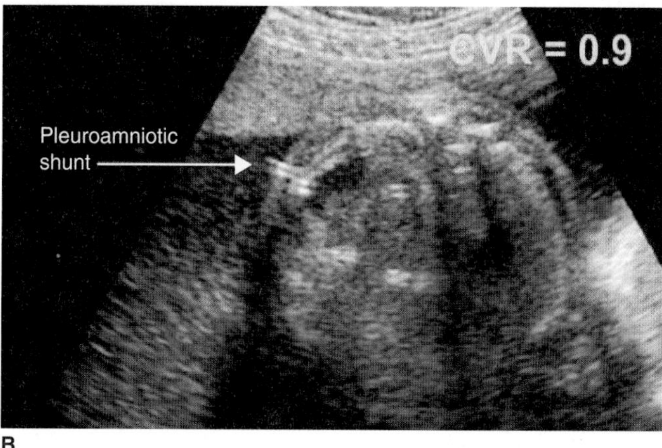




**FIGURE 42-1** Congenital cystic adenomatous malformation (CCAM). **A:** A 24-week fetus with a macrocystic CCAM and hydrops. *Upper arrow* shows scalp edema, *middle arrow* shows the CCAM, and *lower arrow* shows ascites. **B:** Resolution of hydrops following thoracoamniotic shunt insertion. **C:** Appearance of thoracoamniotic shunt at delivery.

renal postnatal morbidity. Work is underway to examine if restoration of amniotic fluid volume can lead to improved pulmonary outcomes.

### Cardiac Interventions

A small number of high-risk fetal centers now perform fetal cardiac percutaneous interventions to reverse the progression and improve the fetal-to-neonatal transition in fetuses with congenital heart disease. The 3 most common cardiac conditions for which fetal interventions are performed are severe aortic valve stenosis with concern for evolving hypoplastic left heart syndrome (HLHS), HLHS with intact or very restrictive atrial septum, and pulmonary atresia with intact ventricular septum.

In severe aortic stenosis, a transuterine fetal percutaneous balloon valvotomy can be performed. The goal of this procedure is to dilate the stenotic aortic valve and enhance left ventricular volume before irreversible left ventricle hypoplasia has occurred. Fetuses with HLHS with a severely restrictive or intact atrial septum can develop significant pulmonary venous hypertension due to the high left atrial pressures. When left untreated, high left atrial pressure results in postnatal hypoxemia and acidosis, and is associated with a high mortality. Fetal treatment for HLHS with intact atrial septum involves relieving the atrial-level obstruction with an in utero septostomy with dilation, with or without subsequent stent placement. In severe cases of pulmonary atresia with intact ventricular septum, fetal pulmonary valvotomy has been attempted in order to increase the chance of achieving a biventricular circulation.

## FETOSCOPIC SURGERY

### Twin-Twin Transfusion Syndrome

The most common fetoscopic procedure performed is selective laser photocoagulation for TTTS. TTTS occurs exclusively in monochorionic gestations, affects 10% to 15% of monochorionic twin pregnancies, and accounts for 17% of all prenatal mortality in twins. While the cause of TTTS is not known, chorioangiopagus, the vascular connections between twins that normally occurs in monochorionic

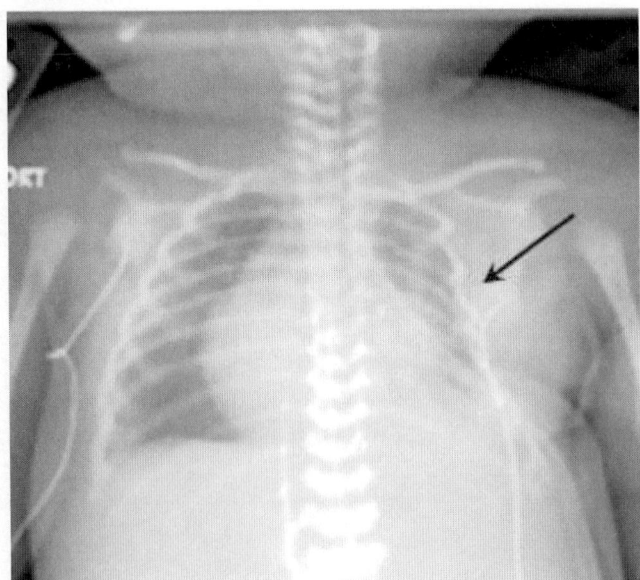

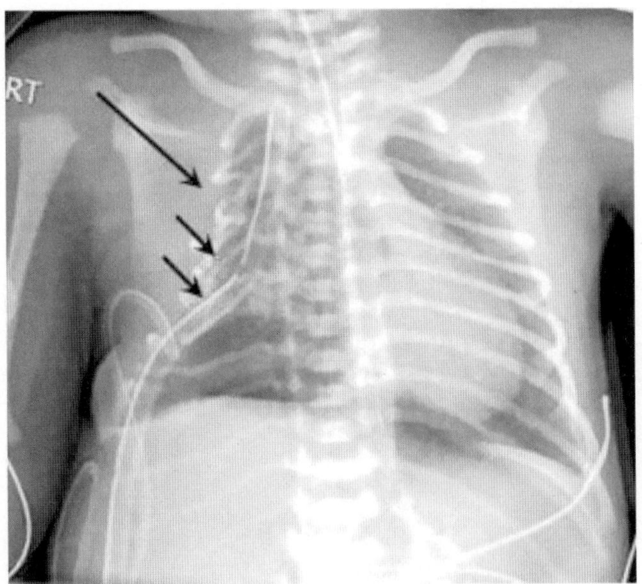


**FIGURE 42-2** Chest wall deformity after shunt placement. Chest radiographs in 2 newborns after shunt placement for congenital cystic adenomatous malformation. There is rib thinning, concavity, and fractures (*arrows*). Findings are more severe the earlier in gestation the shunt is placed, and with rapid decompression of massive cysts.



pregnancies, is a necessary prerequisite for this disease. In TTTS, polyhydramnios develops in the "recipient" twin (the twin receiving blood) and severe oligohydramnios in the "donor" twin. In addition, the recipient twin is at risk for developing a hypertrophic cardiomyopathy (Fig. 42-3).

Historically, amnioreduction was the primary treatment of choice for TTTS, but this has been superceded by selective fetoscopic laser photocoagulation. Amnioreduction is still used in cases to manage polyhydramnios in the recipient twin. Selective fetoscopic laser photocoagulation of vascular connections can arrest the progression of TTTS and, as a result, has become the primary therapeutic modality. Untreated, TTTS is almost uniformly fatal. With selective fetoscopic laser photocoagulation, survival rates of 70% to 77% have been reported, with up to 64% of pregnancies having both twins survive and 92% of pregnancies having 1 or both fetuses survive. Cerebral injury occurs in TTTS-affected pregnancies in utero. One study reported an incidence of cerebral injury of 8.6% in TTTS, half of which were acquired antenatally. Ultrasound-guided radiofrequency umbilical cord ablation may be indicated as salvage therapy to protect 1 twin from the death of the co-twin.

Twin-reversed arterial perfusion sequence is another highly lethal anomaly in which vascular connections between a "pump" twin and an acardiac acephalic twin result in polyhydramnios, preterm labor, heart failure, and death in the pump twin. Intrafetal radiofrequency

**Recipient** Plethoric, hypervolemic, macrosomic

→ Hypertensive, polyuric (elevated atrial natriuretic peptide)

→ Hypertrophic cardiomyopathy, **polyhydramnios**

→ Hydrops -> fetal death, **PROM/PTL**

**Donor** Anemic, hypovolemic, growth restricted

→ Hypotension, oliguric (elevated ADH and renin)

→ Hypoxia, anhydramnios (stuck twin)

**FIGURE 42-3** Fetal pathophysiology of twin-twin transfusion syndrome. ADH, antidiuretic hormone; PROM, premature rupture of membranes; PTL; preterm labor.

ablation of the umbilical cord of the acardiac fetus results in 95% survival of the pump twin in cases in which adverse pregnancy outcome is anticipated.

### Congenital Diaphragmatic Hernia

Congenital diaphragmatic hernia (CDH) is a congenital anomaly in which pulmonary hypoplasia and pulmonary hypertension can be life limiting. Midgestation fetal lung development is characterized by an increase in lung liquid volume and secretion rate and, as a result, lung growth. However, in patients with CDH, this lung growth is compromised due the mass effect of the abdominal organs herniated into the thorax. Experimental tracheal occlusion (TO) has been found to accelerate fetal lung growth by blocking egress of tracheal fluid. This results in increased intratracheal pressure and accelerated lung growth. Fetoscopic endoluminal tracheal occlusion (FETO) was first applied clinically in 2004 in fetuses with severe, isolated left-sided CDH in order to increase lung growth. Investigators in Leuven, Belgium, reported their nonrandomized observational results of FETO showing an improved survival (49%) as compared to standard postnatal management (24%) in 175 patients with isolated, severe left CDH from 24% to 49%. The Tracheal Occlusion to Accelerate Lung (TOTAL) growth trial is an international randomized trial to further investigate the role of fetal therapy for severe and moderate pulmonary hypoplasia.

### Amniotic Band Syndrome

Fetoscopic surgery has been successfully used to treat amniotic band syndrome. Amniotic bands may form as a result of amniocentesis, or they may spontaneously encircle a limb and result in a tourniquet-like effect with diminished blood flow distally and subsequent limb amputation. Death may occur if the band involves the umbilical cord. Fetoscopic laser release of amniotic bands has prevented not only limb amputation, but death from cord accidents. The limbs affected by amniotic bands may have abnormalities from amniotic bands, even if released, that include a secondary form of lymphedema or failure of the distal limb to grow.

### Congenital High Airway Obstruction Syndromes

Congenital high airway obstruction syndrome results from complete airway obstruction due to tracheal or laryngeal atresia. Up to one-third of fetuses with congenital high airway obstruction syndrome will spontaneously perforate through the atresia into the larynx or esophagus with resolution of hydrops. Several patients have now undergone fetoscopic laser perforation of laryngeal or tracheal atresia to allow hydrops to resolve. An EXIT (ex utero intrapartum treatment) procedure (discussed later in this chapter) is necessary for delivery of these infants, but the resolution of hydrops can result in much healthier newborns.

## OPEN FETAL SURGERY

The indications for open fetal surgery remain relatively few. The maternal risks with open fetal surgery are higher than with fetoscopic intervention because of the large laparotomy incision, the hysterotomy, and the aggressive tocolytic regimen required for management. With the notable exception of myelomeningocele, open fetal surgery is usually indicated for cases in which the life of the fetus is in jeopardy.

In open fetal surgery for CCAM, a thoracoabdominal incision is used for exposure, and care is taken to preserve the remaining hypoplastic lobe(s), as CCAM is usually lobar. The fetal survival rate following an open fetal surgery for hydropic CCAM is 60%. However, fetal demise is common when patients are referred late in the course of the disease with end-stage nonimmune hydrops. Those fetuses that are followed closely and show progression to hydrops despite steroid administration are better risk candidates if the surgery is performed earlier in the course of the disease.

### Sacrococcygeal Teratoma

Sacrococcygeal teratoma (SCT) is a rare condition that occurs in 1 in 25,000 live births. It can grow rapidly, causing high-output cardiac failure, polyhydramnios, preterm labor and/or delivery, or death in utero from nonimmune hydrops, and in the longer term can undergo malignant transformation. Almost uniformly fatal in the setting of hydrops, successful resections in utero have been reported. The key to successful cases has been intervention early in the development of hydrops. The goal of fetal surgery in SCT is to debulk the tumor and interrupt the large vascular connections responsible for nonimmune hydrops. Care is taken to preserve the anorectal sphincter complex, and a complete resection of the SCT is not attempted. The resection of the pelvic component of the fetal SCT and the coccyx is performed postnatally. These infants must be followed for at least 3 years with serial α-fetoprotein levels, serial MRIs, and physical examinations as surveillance for recurrent SCT or malignant transformation.

Open fetal surgery has also been employed to treat other life-threatening conditions for which no other therapy exists or conventional approaches have failed. An example of this being a case of a resection of a pericardial teratoma.

### Myelomeningocele

Perhaps the most significant change in the field of fetal surgery has been the application of open fetal surgery to non–life-threatening conditions such as myelomeningocele (Fig. 42-4). Although folic acid supplementation has reduced the incidence of myelomeningocele, it still occurs in up to 1 in 2000 births.

Early reports suggested that in utero surgery to repair fetal myelomeningocele (fMMC) might reverse the hindbrain herniation of the associated Chiari II malformation, thus slowing the rate of enlargement of the ventriculomegaly, and perhaps decrease the need for postnatal ventriculoperitoneal shunting. The Management of Myelomeningocele Study (MOMS) Trial was a National Institutes of Health–sponsored prospective randomized clinical trial to test this. The trial compared fetal repair to standard neonatal repair. The trial demonstrated that fMMC repair led to decreased rate of ventricular shunting for hydrocephalus at 12 months of age, reversal of hindbrain herniation, and improved outcomes, including the ability to walk at 30 months of age. Since the trial concluded, fMMC repair has become a standard of care option for prenatally diagnosed spina bifida in appropriately selected fetal surgery candidates at specialty sites. Experience with fMMC repair in 1 center after the trial has shown similar results. Deliveries are by scheduled cesarean section near term. In the event of premature rupture of membranes, deliveries are performed at 34 weeks. The average gestational age at delivery is 34.3 weeks.

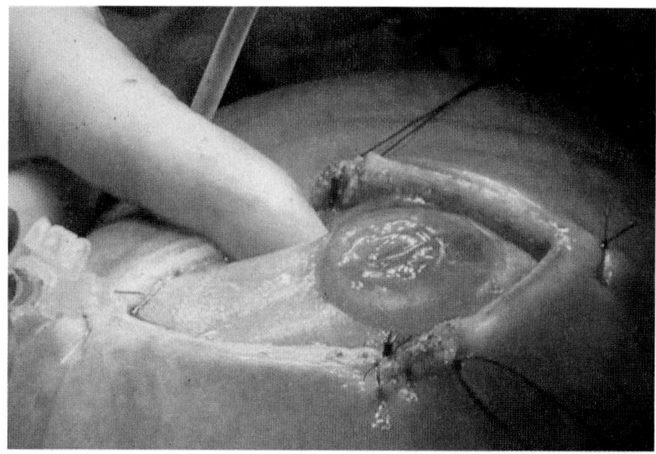
A

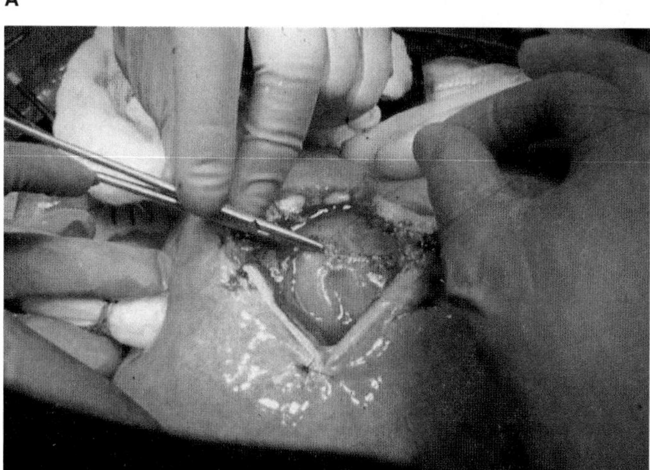
B

**FIGURE 42-4** Fetal myelomeningocele. **A:** Surgical exposure of fetal myelomingocele. **B:** Surgical closure of fetal myelomeningocele.

Approximately 10% deliver before 30 weeks. Of note, these infants are at risk of postnatal apnea. Some infants require caffeine and apnea monitoring at discharge. This is distinct from the apnea that is seen in infants who have undergone postnatal repair, as this may be a Chiari symptom and requires shunting or posterior fossa decompression.

The development of minimally invasive (fetoscopic) surgical techniques for MMC closure are currently underway, though to date the early results are inferior to those seen with open fetal repair.

## EX UTERO INTRAPARTUM TREATMENT

Prenatal diagnosis has implications for the optimal timing and mode of delivery. In highly select circumstances, delivery via an ex utero intrapartum therapy procedure is necessary for safe postnatal transition. Ex utero intrapartum therapy (EXIT) procedures were initially developed to secure the airway before delivery in fetuses that had undergone in utero tracheal occlusion for CDH. The procedure uses fetal surgical techniques. For 60 to 80 minutes, the fetus is partially delivered and while on placental support, care is taken to secure an airway and, if needed, to resect a mass. During this time, uteroplacental gas exchange and hemodynamic stability are maintained.

Delivery via an EXIT procedure is indicated in cases of anticipated life-threatening neonatal airway compromise or cardiovascular instability. Examples include large neck masses such as cervical teratoma (Fig. 42-5) and lymphangioma causing airway obstruction, large oropharyngeal masses, severe micrognathia, congenital high airway obstruction syndrome, large lung lesions, and large mediastinal lesions with airway compression. In select cases, an EXIT-to-ECMO (extracorporeal membrane oxygenation) procedure has been performed for fetuses with severe CDH, but has shown no survival benefit.

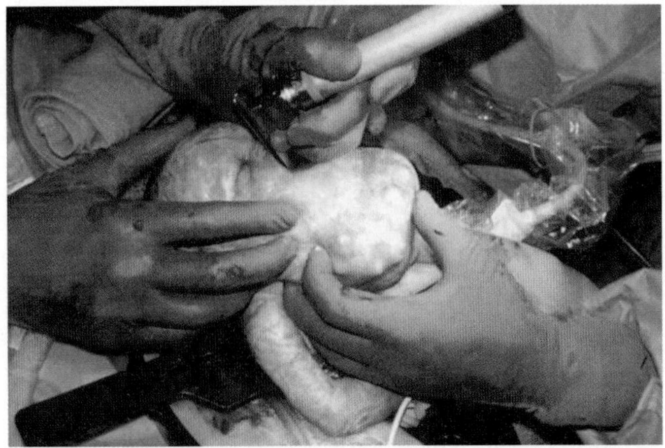

**FIGURE 42-5** Ex utero intrapartum treatment procedure for fetus with cervical teratoma. Laryngoscopy after fetal head delivered prior to cord clamping.

## SUGGESTED READINGS


Adzick NS. Open fetal surgery for life-threatening fetal anomalies. *Semin Fetal Neonatal Med.* 2010;15(1):1-8.

Adzick NS, Thom EA, Spong CY, et al; MOMS Investigators. A randomized trial of prenatal versus postnatal repair of myelomeningocele. *N Engl J Med.* 2011;364(11):993-1004.

Deprest J, Brady P, Nicolaides K, et al. Prenatal management of the fetus with isolated congenital diaphragmatic hernia in the era of the TOTAL trial. *Semin Fetal Neonatal Med.* 2014;19(6): 338-348.

Hedrick HL, Flake AW, Crombleholme TM, et al. Sacrococcygeal teratoma: prenatal assessment, fetal intervention, and outcome. *J Pediatr Surg.* 2004;39(3):430-438; discussion 430-438.

Lim FY, Crombleholme TM, Hedrick HL, et al. Congenital high airway obstruction syndrome: natural history and management. *J Pediatr Surg.* 2003;38(6):940-945.

Maeno Y, Hirose A, Kanbe T, et al. Fetal arrhythmia: prenatal diagnosis and perinatal management. *J Obstet Gynecol Res.* 2009;35(4): 623-629.

Mann S, Johnson M, Wilson R. Fetal thoracic and bladder shunts. *Semin Fetal Neonatal Med.* 2010;15(1):28-33.

Mathis J, Raio L, Baud D. Fetal laser therapy: applications in the management of fetal pathologies. *Prenat Diagn.* 2015;35(7):623-636.

Moldenhauer JS. Ex utero intrapartum therapy. *Semin Pediatr Surg.* 2013;22(1):44-49.

Pearson EG, Flake AW. Stem cell and genetic therapies for the fetus. *Semin Pediatr Surg.* 2013;22(1):56-61.

Peranteau W, Adzick S, Boelig M, et al. Thoracoamniotic shunts for the management of fetal lung lesions and pleural effusions: a single institution review and predictors of outcome in 75 cases. *J Pediatr Surg.* 2015;50(2):301-305.

Peranteau WH, Boelig M, Khalek N, et al. Effect of single and multiple courses of maternal betamethasone on prenatal congenital lung lesion growth and fetal survival. *J Pediatr Surg.* 2016;51(1): 28-32.

Ryan G, Somme S, Crombleholme TM. Airway compromise in the fetus and neonate: prenatal assessment and perinatal management. *Semin Fetal Neonatal Med.* 2016;21(4):230-239.

Schidlow D, Tworetzky W, Wilkins-Haug L. Percutaneous fetal cardiac intervention for structural heart disease. *Am J Perinatol.* 2014;31(7):629-636.




# 43 Neonatal Mortality and Morbidity

Avroy A. Fanaroff

## INTRODUCTION

The accurate definition and reporting of perinatal deaths (ie, fetal and neonatal deaths) is a critical first step in understanding the magnitude and causes of these important events, and in ultimately reducing mortality and morbidity. Infant mortality is an important outcome measure of the health services of a population. In the United States, where there are approximately 4 million births each year, the infant mortality is around 6 per 1000 live births. The highest risk period for infant death is within 24 hours of birth, but mortality and morbidity rates remain high during the neonatal period, until the 28th day of life. The fetus and newborn are most vulnerable during labor, delivery, and the neonatal period because central nervous system injury may result in lifelong morbidity and neurodevelopmental impairment. The perinatal period, from 28 weeks of gestation to the 28th day of life, is the period of greatest mortality. In the modern era, with survival of extremely-low-birth-weight (ELBW) infants, postneonatal mortality also contributes significantly to the infant mortality rate (IMR).

## TERMINOLOGY AND DEFINITIONS

The reduction in maternal and infant mortality and the improved health of mothers and infants in the United States are high priorities. Statistical comparisons among countries, states, regions, and individual centers have been hampered by differences in definitions. In order to compare outcomes and plan interventions, it is imperative that standard definitions be utilized.

1. *Gestational age*: The number of weeks that have elapsed between the first day of the last normal menstrual period (LMP) (not the presumed time of conception) and the date of delivery, irrespective of whether the gestation results in a live birth or a fetal death. Beginning with the 2014 data year, the National Center for Health Statistics is transitioning to a new standard for estimating the gestational age of a newborn. The new measure, the obstetric estimate of gestation at delivery (OE), replaces the measure based on the date of the LMP. This transition is being made because of increasing evidence of the greater validity of the OE compared with the LMP-based measure.
2. *Appropriate for gestational age (AGA)*: An infant with a birth weight between the 10th and 90th percentiles for that gestational age. Those below the 10th percentile are regarded as small for gestational age (SGA), or growth restricted, whereas those above the 90th percentile are considered large for gestational age (LGA).
3. *Birth weight*: The weight of a neonate determined immediately after delivery or as soon thereafter as feasible, expressed to the nearest gram.
4. *Fetal death*: Death before the complete expulsion or extraction from the mother of a product of human conception, fetus and placenta, irrespective of the duration of pregnancy; the death is indicated by the fact that after such expulsion or extraction, the fetus does not breathe or show any other evidence of life, such as beating of the heart, pulsation of the umbilical cord, or definite movement of voluntary muscles. Heartbeats are to be distinguished from transient cardiac contractions; respirations are to be distinguished from fleeting respiratory efforts or gasps. This definition excludes induced termination of pregnancy.
5. *Infant death*: Any death at any time from birth up to, but not including, 1 year of age.
6. *Live birth*: The complete expulsion or extraction from the mother of a product of human conception, irrespective of the duration of pregnancy, which, after such expulsion or extraction, breathes or shows any other evidence of life, such as beating of the heart, pulsation of the umbilical cord, or definite movement of voluntary muscles, whether or not the umbilical cord has been cut or the

placenta is attached. Heartbeats are to be distinguished from transient cardiac contractions; respirations are to be distinguished from fleeting respiratory efforts or gasps.

7. *Low birth weight*: Any neonate, regardless of gestational age, whose weight at birth is less than 2500 g.
8. *Neonatal death*: Death of a live-born neonate before the neonate becomes 28 days old.
9. *Perinatal death*: Indices of perinatal mortality combine fetal deaths and live births with only brief survival (up to a few days or weeks) on the assumption that similar factors are associated with these losses. Three definitions of perinatal deaths are in use: (1) Infant deaths that occur at less than 7 days of age and fetal deaths with a stated or presumed period of gestation of 28 weeks or more; (2) infant deaths that occur at less than 28 days of age and fetal deaths with a stated or presumed period of gestation of 20 weeks or more; (3) infant deaths that occur at less than 7 days of age and fetal deaths with a stated or presumed gestation of 20 weeks or more.
10. *Post-term*: Any neonate whose birth occurs from the beginning of the first day of the 43rd week (295th day) following the onset of the LMP.
11. *Preterm*: Any neonate whose birth occurs through the end of the last day of the 37th week (259th day) following the onset of the LMP.
12. *Term*: Any neonate whose birth occurs from the beginning of the first day of the 38th week (260th day) through the end of the last day of the 42nd week (294th day) following the onset of the LMP.

## MORTALITY AND MORBIDITY: CAUSES AND STATISTICS

### Infant Mortality

Congenital anomalies, infection, asphyxia, disorders relating to short gestation and low birth weight (LBW), and sudden infant death syndrome globally accounted for more than half of all infant deaths in 2015. However, while prematurity remains an important cause of infant mortality, advances in neonatal and perinatal care including antenatal corticosteroids, surfactant therapy, continuous positive airway pressure (CPAP), and mechanical ventilation have reduced the IMR due to respiratory distress syndrome.

The US IMR—the ratio of infant deaths to live births in a given year—is generally regarded as a good indicator of the overall health of a population. The IMR, expressed as the number of infant deaths per 1000 live births, was 5.9 in 2015. The 10 leading causes of infant death in 2015 accounted for 68.6% of all infant deaths in the United States. The leading causes remained the same as in 2014. These rates are similar to the rates in 2013 (5.96) and 2012 (5.98). For multiple births, the IMR was 25.84, 5 times the rate of 5.25 for singleton births. In 2013, 36% of infant deaths were due to preterm-related causes of death, and an additional 15% were due to causes grouped into the sudden unexpected infant death category. Fetal deaths are greatest in pregnancies in teenagers, in mothers over age 35, and with multiple fetuses. Race played a major role, and persistent racial discrepancies are noted with IMRs among non-Hispanic black women, non-Hispanic white women, and Hispanics.

In 2011, 15 per 1000 term newborns in the United States were coded as SGA, a 30% increase since 2002. Compared with other term newborns, SGA term newborns were significantly more likely to be female, receive public insurance, and reside in lower income zip codes. Comorbidities, including perinatal complications, metabolic disorders, central nervous system diseases, infection, and neonatal abstinence syndrome were more common among SGA-coded term newborns. These newborns also had higher odds of in-hospital death, longer mean length of stay, and higher mean hospital charges.

### Causes of Perinatal and Neonatal Mortality and Morbidity

Leading causes of death in the neonatal period include respiratory distress syndrome, newborn complications of pregnancy, newborn complications related to placental disorders, cord accidents, membrane disorders, neonatal infections, intrauterine hypoxia, and birth asphyxia. Patel reported that from 2000 through 2011, overall mortality declined among extremely premature infants. Deaths related to pulmonary causes, immaturity, infection, and central nervous system injury decreased, while necrotizing enterocolitis–related deaths increased

Infant and neonatal mortality rates for the United States from the Centers for Disease Control and Prevention are presented in Figure 43-1. Advances in perinatal care have improved the chances for survival of infants with major congenital anomalies in addition to those with cardiorespiratory disorders and other major organ system failures. Approximately 0.5% of all births occur before the third trimester of pregnancy, and these very early deliveries result in the majority of neonatal deaths and more than 40% of infant morbidity. An increasing number of ELBW neonates now survive with proactive care. Many factors influence neonatal mortality. In addition to race,



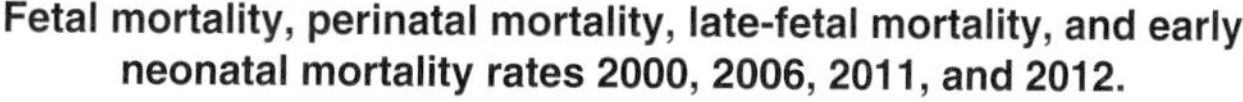


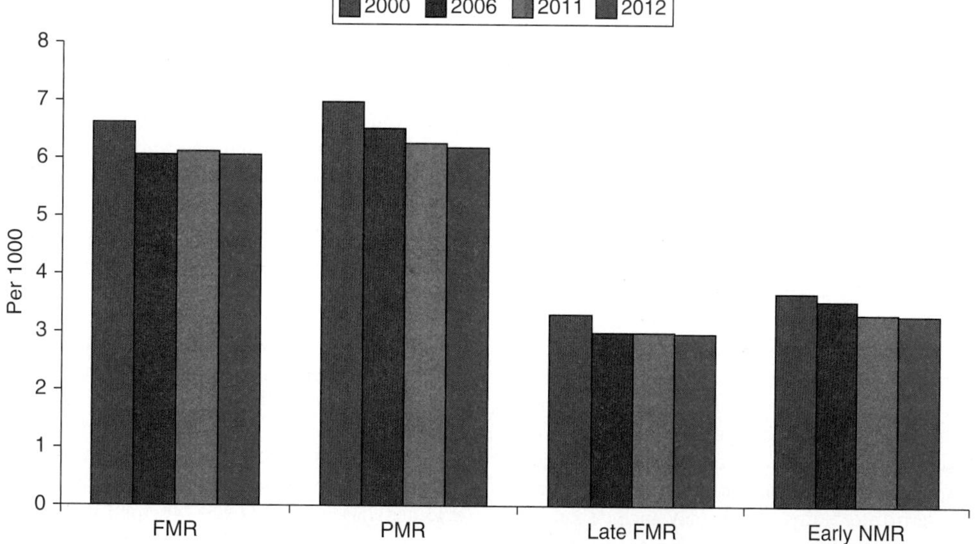


**FIGURE 43-1** Fetal (F), perinatal (P), late-fetal, and early neonatal (N) mortality rates (MR). (Reproduced with permission from Centers for Disease Control and Prevention/NCHS, National Vital Statistics System.)

birth weight, gestational age, gender, place of delivery, and intrauterine growth, there are wide variations in population descriptions, in the criteria used for starting or withdrawing treatment, in the reported duration of survival, and in care. The perinatal mortality rate in the United States has consistently declined with an overall decrease of 10% from 1990 to 2003.

In 2002 to 2003, the perinatal mortality rate reached its nadir of 6.74 deaths per 1000 live births and fetal deaths. The decline is attributable to a drop in late fetal deaths. In the United States in 2013, the fetal mortality rate for gestations of at least 20 weeks (5.96 fetal deaths per 1000 live births and fetal deaths) was similar to the IMR. Depending on the definition used, fetal mortality contributes to approximately 40% to 60% of perinatal mortality.

Stoll reported on trends in morbidity and mortality among extremely preterm infants born at US academic centers over the last 20 years. Changes in maternal and infant care practices and modest reductions in several morbidities were observed, although bronchopulmonary dysplasia increased. Use of antenatal corticosteroids increased from 1993 to 2012 (24–87%), as did cesarean delivery (44–64%). Delivery room intubation decreased from 80% in 1993 to 65% in 2012. Although most infants were ventilated, CPAP without ventilation increased from 7% in 2002 to 11% in 2012. Despite lack of improvement from 1993 to 2004, rates of late-onset sepsis declined between 2005 and 2012 for infants of each gestational age. Survival increased most markedly for infants born at 23 and 24 weeks' gestation and survival without major morbidity increased for infants aged 25 to 28 weeks.

### Factors Affecting Infant and Neonatal Morbidity and Mortality

Although IMRs continue to decrease, specific factors—including prematurity, lack of or inadequate prenatal care, inadequate weight gain in pregnancy, and African American ethnicity—increase mortality rates several-fold.

**Race** American women have many more preterm and very early preterm births, which, in part, explain the doubling of their fetal and IMRs. In general, however, the racial discrepancies in preterm birth and other pregnancy outcomes remain unexplained. Although there has been a noticeable decline in the perinatal mortality rates for the past few decades, the prematurity rate has remained fairly constant, and African American infants continue to have a higher mortality rate than their white counterparts. The relative differences in perinatal and neonatal mortality between different racial/ethnic populations have not substantially changed. Non-Hispanic black newborns are twice as likely as non-Hispanic white and Hispanic black infants to die within the first year of life. Although for the total birth cohort, blacks have a higher mortality risk than whites, the reverse is noted at the lower weight group/gestational age distributions.

In summary, neonatal mortality rates are higher in infants who are non-Hispanic black, preterm, or a product of a multifetal pregnancy.

**Maternal Factors** IMRs are higher for pregnancies in which prenatal care is initiated after the first trimester of pregnancy and in infants born to teenagers or to women 40 years of age or older who did not complete high school, were unmarried, or smoked during pregnancy. Infant mortality is also higher for male infants, multiple births, and infants born preterm or at LBW. In many instances, the precipitating cause of preterm delivery remains undetected, but risk factors for premature birth include uterine abnormalities, placental bleeding including abruptio placentae associated with cocaine use, maternal chronic illnesses, multifetal gestation, premature rupture of the membranes, chorioamnionitis, and bacterial vaginosis. Bacterial vaginosis, a short cervix, and the presence of fetal fibronectin in the vaginal tract are predictors of preterm delivery, but treatment of the bacterial vaginosis has been ineffective in preventing prematurity. Premature delivery complicates over 10% of births but contributes disproportionately to at least two-thirds of infant deaths and to a significant amount of neonatal and long-term morbidity, which may include cerebral palsy, mental restriction, physical handicap, blindness, and deafness in addition to major and minor school adaptive and learning problems. Although there has been a substantial decline in the number of medically preventable deaths and deaths from respiratory distress syndrome, the number of deaths from extremely LBW has increased relative to other causes; asphyxia, birth trauma, early-onset sepsis, and meconium aspiration syndrome have been reduced to a minimum. Nonetheless, congenital malformation is the leading cause of infant death in the United States and accounts for a much greater proportion of infant mortality than does premature birth. To further reduce neonatal mortality, the incidence of lethal congenital malformations and very-low-birth-weight infants must be addressed; congenital anomalies cause approximately 23% of infant mortality, and short gestation and LBW cause about 15%.

**Multiple Gestation** Perinatal morbidity and mortality are significantly increased in multiple gestation, and the incidence of severe handicap is increased in survivors of multiple gestation, predominantly because of preterm delivery. In the United States, the number and rate of multiple births have risen dramatically. An ever-increasing number of multiple births is related to infertility treatments: The rates of triplet and higher-order multiple births jumped 16% between 1996 and 1997, and in 2012, the incidence of higher order multiple gestations was 0.12 per 1000 live births. Multiple gestation accounts for 26% of deliveries with birth weight below 1500 g. In addition to multiple gestation, aggressive interventions for fetal compromise identified in extremely immature infants contribute to the continuing toll of preterm birth.

**Preterm Birth** In the United States in the last 2 decades, despite increasing availability of prenatal care, nutrition supplementation programs, drugs to stop preterm contractions, and an overall decline over recent years, the preterm birth rate remains higher than in many other developed countries.

The preterm birth rate in the United States declined for the seventh straight year in 2013 to 11.39%; the LBW rate was essentially unchanged at 8.02%. The IMR was 5.96 infant deaths per 1000 live births in 2013, down 13% from 6.86 in 2005. The LBW rate rose slightly to 9.63% from 2014 to 2015. Part of this increase is due to multiple births associated with infertility treatments, but many preterm births occur spontaneously. Multiple births accounted for 3.3% of all births in 2003 but account for at least 25% of births below 1.5 kilograms. The triplet and higher-order birth rate declined 41% from 1998 to 2014, or from about 1 in every 515 births in 1998 to 1 in every 880 births in 2014. Triplet and higher-order birth rates fell by about 50% or more for women aged 25 and over.

The medical or public health strategies used to reduce preterm birth have overall not succeeded. However, for women with a previous history of preterm birth, progesterone therapy has reduced the rate of prematurity. Because of their high risk of mortality and serious morbidity, most studies on prematurity (defined as birth at less than 37 weeks) have focused on very preterm infants (birth at < 32 weeks). However, the all-cause risk of mortality among singletons born at 32 through 33 gestational weeks were increased over 6-fold in the United States and 15-fold in Canada, whereas among singletons born at 34 through 36 gestational weeks, the relative risks were increased at least 3-fold. Late preterm births are more numerous than ELBW infants and are responsible for an important fraction of infant deaths. Intense focus has been placed on this population because much of their morbidity and mortality may be prevented.

Neonatal mortality increases with decreasing gestational age and birth weight (Fig. 43-2A). Survival at 22 weeks of gestation ranges from 5% to 40%; at 23 weeks from 13% to 60%, at 24 weeks from 35% to 80%, and at 35 weeks from 56% to 85%. Survival varies by nation with the best results reported from Japan (Fig. 43-2B). A number of European countries do not provide active care before 25 weeks' gestation.

Whereas there has been little to no success at reducing the incidence of preterm birth, intrauterine growth restriction, and congenital malformations over the past 20 years, the survival of ELBW infants (< 1500 g) has increased from 74% to 85%. Although the validity of the Apgar scoring system continues to be challenged, a 5-minute Apgar score below 4 remains a better predictor of mortality than does severe metabolic acidosis (pH < 7.0) measured from the cord blood. Male sex,

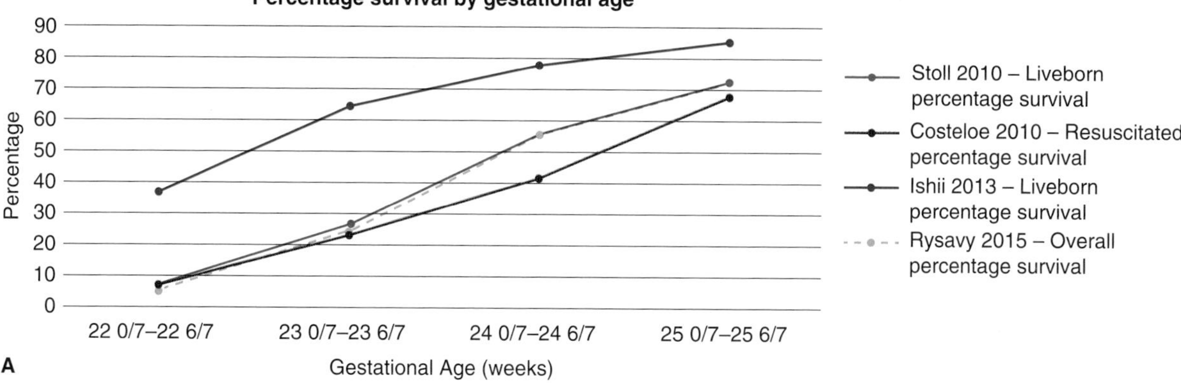


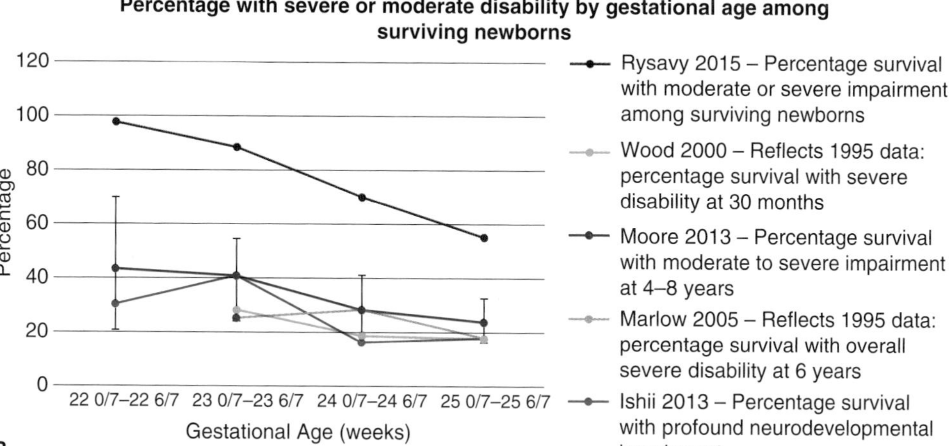


**FIGURE 43-2** **A:** Overall survival according to gestational age. **B:** Disability amongst surviving newborns according to gestational age. Survival rates from Japan as reported by Ishi are superior to the United States and the United Kingdom for these periviable infants. **A** demonstrates the difference in outcomes when only the live births (Stoll) or all births (Rysavy) are considered. The morbidity data (**B**) shows similar trends. We should be encouraged by the finding that in addition to having a high survival rate, Ishii's cohort has lower morbidity than the USA multicenter Neonatal Research Network data. (Reproduced with permission from American College of Obstetricians and Gynecologists; Society for Maternal-Fetal Medicine: Obstetric Care consensus No. 6: Periviable Birth, *Obstet Gynecol.* 2017 Oct;130(4):e187-e199.)

failure to receive antenatal steroids, persistent bradycardia at 5 minutes, hypothermia, and poor intrauterine growth all independently increase the risk for death.

**Fetal Growth Restriction** The most common causes of inadequate fetal growth relate to maternal hypertension, malnutrition, and smoking. These disorders may be associated with intrauterine fetal demise, neonatal adaptive problems including severe hypoglycemia, or long-term abnormalities of growth and neurodevelopment. Cigarette smoking remains a major cause of intrauterine growth restriction, preterm birth, fetal and neonatal deaths, and sudden infant death syndrome. Alcohol and drug use may also affect pregnancy outcome. Prenatal alcohol exposure is an important cause of fetal growth restriction, including microcephaly, which results in long-term growth failure in addition to substantial neurodevelopmental delay and mental restriction. Mortality and morbidity are increased among infants born at term whose birth weights are at or below the third percentile for their gestational age. The incidence of intubation at birth, seizures during the first day of life, and sepsis also were significantly increased among term infants with birth weights at or below the third percentile.

**Gender** The sex of the newborn infant is a major determinant of survival, with the female advantage most noticeable at the youngest gestational ages. For example, the mortality rate of a girl who weighs 700 g at 24 weeks of gestation is 30% to 40%, whereas a boy of equal weight and gestational age has a mortality risk of 50%. In addition to a higher mortality than girls, boys are more likely to need cardiopulmonary resuscitation at delivery and are at greater risk for most adverse neonatal outcomes, including chronic lung disease, intracranial hemorrhage, and nosocomial infections.

Figure 43-3 illustrates well the widespread distribution of mortality risk for a given gestation, and shows that the larger infants at each gestational age have a greater chance of surviving. Similarly, there is variability in the morbidity at each gestational age, and babies in the bottom percentiles for weight are more likely to be acidotic, require

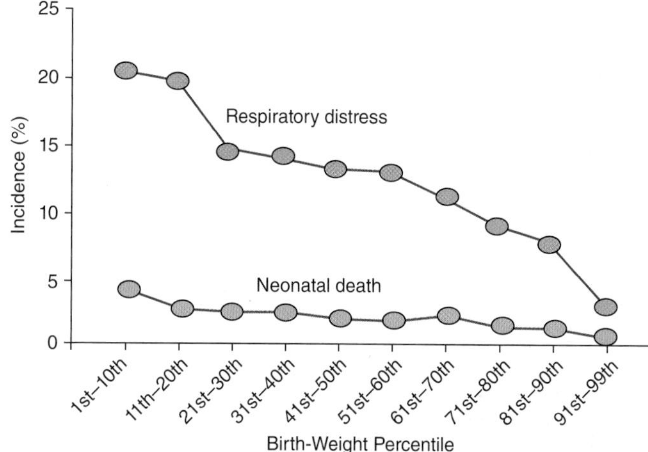


**FIGURE 43-3** Incidence of respiratory distress and neonatal death in infants born at 24 to 36 weeks of gestation. (Reproduced with permission from American College of Obstetricians and Gynecologists; Society for Maternal-Fetal Medicine: Obstetric Care consensus No. 6: Periviable Birth, *Obstet Gynecol.* 2017 Oct;130(4):e187-e199.)

admission to the intensive care unit, develop major morbidities including respiratory failure, or die.

#### Factors Contributing to Mortality and Morbidity Trends

During the 1990s, 2 significant factors contributed to the improved outcome after preterm birth. These are the introduction of surfactant therapy for respiratory distress syndrome in 1990 and the widespread use of antenatal steroids that followed the National Institutes of Health consensus conference in 1994.

Some reports indicate that the survival chances for infants between 501 and 1500 g at birth improved in the 1990s, but concerns about morbidity and the high rates of chronic lung disease persist. For those born at 23 weeks of gestation, chronic lung disease affects 57% to 86% of survivors; at 24 weeks, it affects 33% to 89%; and at 25 weeks, it affects 16% to 71% of survivors. Additional significant morbidities—necrotizing enterocolitis (7%), severe (grade III or IV) intraventricular hemorrhage (11%), and retinopathy of prematurity (6%)—have fluctuated only slightly between 1991 and 2012.

**Regionalization of Perinatal Care** Regionalization of perinatal care to various levels (see Table 43-1), first introduced in the 1970s, is cost effective and has reduced morbidity and mortality. Market forces and economics disrupted regionalization in the 1990s. Nonetheless, the evidence continues to demonstrate that the best outcomes for LBW infants are achieved when they are delivered at the larger subspecialty centers (formerly known as level III), with an average neonatal intensive care unit (NICU) daily census in excess of 15. There has been a large increase in both the number of NICUs in community hospitals and the complexity of the cases treated in these units. The mortality among very-low-birth-weight infants was lowest for deliveries that occurred in hospitals with NICUs that had both a high level of care and a high volume of such patients, implying that increased use of such facilities might reduce mortality among very-low-birth-weight infants. Risk-adjusted neonatal mortality for infants born in smaller level III NICUs and in level II+ and level II NICUs (specialty), regardless of size, was not significantly different from that in hospitals without a NICU and was significantly higher than in hospitals with large subspecialty NICUs.

Despite the differences in outcomes, hospital costs for the birth of infants born at hospitals with large subspecialty NICUs were not more than those for infants born at other hospitals with NICUs. The centralization of high-risk subspecialty NICU care has the potential to decrease neonatal mortality without increasing costs. The concept of specialized LBW units has been introduced with a reduction in both mortality and number of invasive and noninvasive tests. It is the commitment by an experienced team to both provide evidenced-based care and continued learning rather than the structural facility that is most important.

#### Neurodevelopmental Outcomes

Advances in perinatal care have led to increased survival of children born at the lower limits of viability. Children with birth weights of 1000 g or lower have poorer outcomes relative to normal-birth-weight term-born controls in their neurologic and health status, cognitive-neuropsychological skills, school performance, academic achievement, and behavior. Outcomes are highly variable but are related largely to medical complications of prematurity and social risk factors.

Factors associated with risk of impaired neurodevelopmental outcome include LBW, male gender, the presence of cerebral ultrasound abnormalities including periventricular leukomalacia and persistent ventriculomegaly, bronchopulmonary dysplasia, and growth failure. In addition to gross neurologic deficits including cerebral palsy,

**TABLE 43-1 LEVELS OF IN-HOSPITAL PERINATAL CARE**

| Maternal | Neonate |
|---|---|
| **Basic Care** | |
| • Monitoring and care for low-risk patients<br>• Identification of high risk for transfer<br>• Detection and care of unanticipated labor/delivery problems<br>• Emergency cesarean delivery within 30 minutes<br>• Blood bank, anesthesia, radiology, ultrasound<br>• Care of postpartum problems<br>• Involvement of obstetrician, certified nurse midwife, anesthesiologist | • Examination and care of healthy neonate<br>• Resuscitation and stabilization<br>• Consultation and transfer protocols<br>• Nursery care<br>• Parent/sibling visitation<br>• Involvement of general pediatrician staff (capable of neonatal resuscitation) and laboratory support |
| **Special Care** | |
| *Basic services plus:*<br>• Involvement of obstetrician with experience in maternal-fetal medicine<br>• Care of high-risk pregnancies<br>• Triage, transfer of high-risk pregnancies (< 32 weeks, IUGR, pre-eclampsia, severe anomalies, chorioamnionitis, severe maternal medical illnesses) | *Basic services plus:*<br>• Involvement of physicians, specialized nurses, respiratory therapies, radiology technicians, laboratory technicians, and equipment<br>• Care of high-risk neonate with short-term problems<br>• Stabilization before transfer (< 1500 g, < 32 weeks, critically ill)<br>• Accepting of convalescing back (reverse) transfers |
| **Subspecialty Care** | |
| *Basic plus specialty care plus:*<br>• Involvement of experienced perinatologist (24-hour coverage)<br>• Evaluation of high-risk therapies<br>• Care for severe maternal medical or obstetric illnesses<br>• High-risk fetal care (Rh disease, nonimmune hydrops, life-threatening anomalies) and surgical capabilities<br>• Research<br>• Community education<br>• Anesthesiologist with maternal-fetal medicine experience | *Basic plus specialty care plus:*<br>• Care of < 1000 g, < 28 weeks, capable of providing advanced respiratory support and ECMO<br>• Involvement of experienced neonatologist (24-hour coverage)<br>• Inborn plus transferred patients<br>• Evaluation of high-risk therapies<br>• All pediatric medical, radiologic, and surgical subspecialties<br>• NICU with operating room capabilities<br>• High-risk follow-up<br>• Outcomes research<br>• Community education |

ECMO, extracorporeal membrane oxygenation; IUGR, intrauterine growth restriction; NICU, neonatal intensive care unit.

Data from American Academy of Pediatrics; American College of Obstetricians and Gynecologists; March of Dimes Birth Defects Foundation. *Guidelines for Perinatal Care*. 6th ed., Elk Grove Village, IL: American Academy of Pediatrics; 2007.

hydrocephalus, and hemiplegia, these infants are susceptible to growth failure, deafness, and blindness.

The rates of severe abnormalities on cerebral ultrasound range from 10% to 83% at 23 weeks of gestation, 9% to 64% at 24 weeks, and 7% to 22% at 25 weeks. Of 77 survivors at 23 weeks of gestation, 26 (34%) were reported to have severe disability (defined as subnormal cognitive function, cerebral palsy, blindness, and/or deafness). At 24 weeks of gestation, the rates of severe neurodevelopmental disability range from 22% to 45%, and at 25 weeks of gestation, they range from 12% to 35%. The continuing toll of major neonatal morbidity and neurodevelopmental handicap is of serious concern. Neurodevelopmental impairment of ELBW infants increased in the 1990s.

Vohr, on the basis of evaluation of a multicenter cohort at 18 to 22 months corrected age, noted ELBW infants (< 1 kg) to be at significant risk of neurologic abnormalities, developmental delays, and functional delays. Twenty-five percent of the children had an abnormal neurologic examination; 37% had a Bayley Scales of Infant Development (BSID) II Mental Developmental Index (referenced to a population mean of 100) below 70; 29% had a Psychomotor Developmental Index below 70; 9% had vision impairment; and 11% had hearing impairment. Neurologic, developmental, neurosensory, and functional morbidities increased with decreasing birth weight. Factors significantly associated with increased neurodevelopmental morbidity include bronchopulmonary dysplasia, grades III or IV intraventricular hemorrhage/periventricular leukomalacia, the use of steroids for bronchopulmonary dysplasia, necrotizing enterocolitis, and male gender. Factors significantly associated with decreased morbidity include increased birth weight, female gender, higher maternal education, antenatal corticosteroids, and white race.

Since 2000, neurodevelopmental impairment has decreased among ELBW infants in the Cleveland cohort. This improvement has been attributed to a number of perinatal and neonatal factors, including increased antenatal steroid use and cesarean section delivery as well as decreased rates of sepsis, decreased rates of severe cranial ultrasound abnormalities, and reduced postnatal steroid use. The initial Epicure study group from a national cohort in 1995 at a median age of 30 months had mean BSID Mental and Psychomotor Developmental Indices of 84 ± 12 and 87 ± 13, respectively. Nineteen percent had severely delayed development (with scores more than 3 standard deviations [SD] below the mean), and 11% had scores from 2 SD to 3 SD below the mean. Twenty-eight children (10%) had severe neuromotor disability, 7 (2%) were blind or perceived light only, and 8 (3%) had hearing loss that was uncorrectable or required aids. This cohort included 49% of survivors with no disability. At age 6 years, many in this cohort demonstrated impairment of motor, visuospatial, and sensorimotor function, including planning, self-regulation, inhibition, and motor persistence, contributing to excess cognitive impairment in extremely preterm children compared to term infants. These factors contribute independently to poor classroom performance at 6 years of age. Global problems with executive function persists with age so that preterm infants perform worse in the classroom, are more likely to repeat grades, and are less likely to attain college degrees.

Survival and impairment in early childhood are both closely related to gestational age for infants born at less than 27 weeks' gestation. Extremely preterm children are at high risk for comorbid intellectual and learning disabilities. Educational professionals should be aware of the complex nature of these children's difficulties and the need for multidomain assessments to guide intervention. Extremely preterm children are also at increased risk for attention-deficit/hyperactivity disorder (ADHD) symptoms, predominantly inattention, for which the antecedents differ by symptom domain. Attention deficits after extremely preterm birth were associated with poor brain growth and neurological function. Furthermore, LBW babies are up to 5 times more likely to be later diagnosed with autism than children born at a normal weight. Joseph and colleagues reported that low gestational age is associated with increased risk for autism spectrum disorder irrespective of intellectual ability, whereas severe fetal growth restriction is strongly associated with autism spectrum disorder without intellectual disability.

#### Global Neonatal Mortality



Globally, 2.9 million infants die in the first month of life, and an additional 2.6 million are stillborn. Four out of 5 newborn deaths result from 1 or more of 3 preventable or treatable conditions: complications from prematurity and LBW, complications during childbirth (including birth asphyxia), or infection. Proven low-cost interventions, health commodities, and medicines can prevent more than two-thirds of newborn deaths.

## SUMMARY

There have been marked improvements in the perinatal outcomes so that in the United States in 2016, the expectation of life at birth is 79 years for all gender and race groups combined. However, US perinatal mortality rates still lag behind those of other industrialized countries, and in spite of advances in neonatal intensive care, the infant mortality in the United States for black infants persistently remains higher than for whites. Globally, neonatal mortality—often from easily preventable causes—continues to remain high and comprises an increasing proportion of childhood deaths, and much work remains to be done in this arena.

## SUGGESTED READINGS


Bhutta ZA, Das JK, Bahl R, et al; Lancet Newborn Interventions Review Group; The Lancet Every Newborn Study Group. Can available interventions end preventable deaths in mothers, newborn babies, and stillbirths, and at what cost? *Lancet*. 2014;384(9940):347-370.

Centers for Disease Control and Prevention National Center for Health Statistics. 2003 revisions of the U.S. standard certificates of live birth and death and the fetal death report. http://www.cdc.gov/nchs/nvss/vital_certificate_revisions.htm. Accessed August 8, 2016.

Costeloe KL, Hennessy EM, Haider S, Stacey F, Marlow N, Draper ES. Short term outcomes after extreme preterm birth in England: comparison of two birth cohorts in 1995 and 2006 (the EPICure studies). *BMJ*. 2012;345:e7976.

Dickson KE, Simen-Kapeu A, Kinney MV, et al; Lancet Every Newborn Study Group. Every Newborn: health-systems bottlenecks and strategies to accelerate scale-up in countries. *Lancet*. 2014;384(9941):438-454.

Ishii N, Kono Y, Yonemoto N, Kusuda S, Fujimura M; Neonatal Research Network, Japan. Outcomes of infants born at 22 and 23 weeks' gestation. *Pediatrics*. 2013;132(1):62-71.

Joseph RM, Korzeniewski SJ, Allred EN et al; ELGAN Study Investigators. Extremely low gestational age and very low birthweight for gestational age are risk factors for autism spectrum disorder in a large cohort study of 10-year-old children born at 23-27 weeks' gestation. *Am J Obstet Gynecol*. 2017;216(3):304.e1-304.e14.

Linsell L, Malouf R, Morris J, Kurinczuk JJ, Marlow N. Prognostic factors for cerebral palsy and motor impairment in children born very preterm or very low birthweight: a systematic review. *Dev Med Child Neurol*. 2016;58(6):554-569.

MacDorman MF, Gregory ECW. Fetal and perinatal mortality: United States, 2013. *Natl Vital Stat Rep*. 2015;64(8):1-24.

Marlow N, Bennett C, Draper ES, Hennessy EM, Morgan AS, Costeloe KL. Perinatal outcomes for extremely preterm babies in relation to place of birth in England: the EPICure 2 study. *Arch Dis Child Fetal Neonatal Ed*. 2014;99(3):F181-F188.

Marlow N, Wolke D, Bracewell MA, Samara M; EPICure Study Group. Neurologic and developmental disability at six years of age after extremely preterm birth. *N Engl J Med*. 2005;352(1):9-19.

Martin JA, Hamilton BE, Osterman MJK, Curtin SC, Matthews TJ. Births: final data for 2013. *Natl Vital Stat Rep*. 2015;64(1):1-65.

Moore GP, Lemyre B, Barrowman N, Daboval T. Neurodevelopmental outcomes at 4 to 8 years of children born at 22 to 25 weeks' gestational age: a meta-analysis. *JAMA Pediatr*. 2013;167(10):967-974.

Obstetric Care Consensus No. 4: periviable birth. *Obstet Gynecol.* 2016; 127(6):e157-e169.

Osterman M, Kochanek K, MacDorman M, Strobino D, Guyer B. Annual summary of vital statistics: 2012-2013. *Pediatrics.* 2015; 135(6):1115-1125.

Patel RM, Kandefer S, Walsh MC, et al; Eunice Kennedy Shriver National Institute of Child Health and Human Development Neonatal Research Network. Causes and timing of death in extremely premature infants from 2000 through 2011. *N Engl J Med.* 2015;372(4):331-340.

Rysavy MA, Li L, Bell EF, et al; Eunice Kennedy Shriver National Institute of Child Health and Human Development Neonatal Research Network. Between-hospital variation in treatment and outcomes in extremely preterm infants. *N Engl J Med.* 2015;372(19):1801-1811.

Stoll BJ, Hansen NI, Bell EF, et al; Eunice Kennedy Shriver National Institute of Child Health and Human Development Neonatal Research Network. Neonatal outcomes of extremely preterm infants from the NICHD Neonatal Research Network. *Pediatrics.* 2010;126(3):443-456.

Stoll BJ, Hansen NI, Bell EF, et al; Eunice Kennedy Shriver National Institute of Child Health and Human Development Neonatal Research Network. Trends in care practices, morbidity, and mortality of extremely preterm neonates, 1993-2012. *JAMA.* 2015;314(10):1039-1051.

Wood NS, Marlow N, Costeloe K, Gibson AT, Wilkinson AR. Neurologic and developmental disability after extremely preterm birth. EPICure Study Group. *N Engl J Med.* 2000;343(6):378-384.



# 44 Delivery Room Resuscitation of the Newborn Infant

Elizabeth E. Foglia and Myra H. Wyckoff

## THE IMPACT OF NEWBORN RESUSCITATION

The vast majority of newborn infants have a successful transition from intrauterine to extrauterine life without need of assistance; however, approximately 10% require some degree of resuscitative support in the delivery room. The presence of certain antepartum, intrapartum, or postpartum risk factors predicts many but certainly not all infants who require help in the delivery room (Table 44-1). Premature infants, when compared to term infants, are at particular risk for a difficult transition following birth. The most common contributing factor for infants in need of resuscitation is asphyxia. Asphyxia results in concomitant hypoxia and hypercapnia and causes a mixed metabolic and respiratory acidosis. The asphyxia can result from either failure of placental gas exchange before birth or deficient pulmonary gas exchange once the newborn is delivered.

Prompt, effective reversal of asphyxia (with a major focus on *effective ventilation*) can potentially prevent or minimize multiorgan failure, death, and disability. Nearly 1 million newborns worldwide die from birth asphyxia. As a result, development of competence in effective newborn resuscitation could make a profound global impact on the health of children.

## ANTICIPATION AND PREPARATION

Anticipation and planning for both expected and unexpected neonatal emergencies is essential for success. If a fetus is at high risk for needing resuscitation in the delivery room, antepartum triage to a center with expertise in high-risk stabilization should be attempted if it is safe to do so. Regardless, every birth should have at least 1 person immediately available to focus solely on the newborn to assess the need for and to perform resuscitation, if required. That person should be able to call for additional immediate assistance if necessary. If a high-risk delivery is anticipated, a team of at least 2 or more people with comprehensive resuscitation skills should be present and prepared. Ideally, 1 person should be the resuscitation leader who assigns tasks among the available team members before the delivery, and helps coordinate the entire resuscitation while limiting his or her own active involvement in the individual tasks. Additional personnel must stabilize the airway by maintaining an open airway with good positioning of the head. This person may need to intubate and stabilize the endotracheal tube and/or provide assisted ventilation. Other team members should be assigned to monitor the infant's condition by auscultation, pulse oximetry, or cardiac monitoring and keep an accurate written record; to perform cardiac compressions when needed; to establish vascular access and administer epinephrine or volume; and to perform other emergency procedures as indicated by the infant's condition. A dedicated, well-trained resuscitation team is ideal to coordinate all these tasks.

Obtaining a clear history from the obstetrical team as to why resuscitation providers were called is a critical first step in preparation. At a bare minimum, the resuscitation provider must know how many babies are delivering, the estimated gestational age, whether meconium is present in the amniotic fluid, and if there are any additional risk factors (Table 44-2). If there is time, discussion to plan timing of cord clamping with the obstetrical team is helpful. All equipment for a complete resuscitation, including personal protection gear for the resuscitation providers, must be present, in working order, and ready for use at every delivery (Table 44-3). Appropriate equipment should be immediately checked for presence and function with particular attention to provision of a warm resuscitation environment. Hypothermia of the newborn is associated with hypoglycemia, metabolic acidosis, and increased mortality (particularly for preterm infants). The International Liaison Committee on Resuscitation (ILCOR) recommends that in order to minimize heat loss for the newborn,

**TABLE 44-1 ANTEPARTUM, INTRAPARTUM, AND POSTPARTUM FACTORS ASSOCIATED WITH NEED FOR NEWBORN RESUSCITATION**

| Antepartum Factors | Intrapartum Factors | Postpartum Factors |
|---|---|---|
| Maternal diabetes | Breech or other abnormal presentation | Drug-induced respiratory depression |
| Maternal hypertension | Placental abruption | Central nervous system anomalies or injury |
| Preeclampsia or eclampsia | Placenta previa | Lung immaturity |
| Fetal anemia | Cord compression or prolapse | Spinal cord injury |
| Previous fetal death | Precipitous labor | Airway obstruction |
| Previous neonatal death | Prolonged labor (> 24 hours) | Immaturity |
| Bleeding in 2nd or 3rd trimester | Shoulder dystocia | Severe lung disease |
| Maternal infection | Narcotics given to the mother < 4 hours before delivery | Sepsis, infection |
| Polyhydramnios | Maternal magnesium therapy | Diaphragmatic hernia |
| Oligohydramnios | Chorioamnionitis | Pneumothorax |
| Premature rupture of membranes | Meconium-stained amniotic fluid | Deformities |
| Fetal hydrops | Emergency cesarean section | Abdominal anomalies |
| Gestational age ≥ 41 0/7 weeks | Category 2 or 3 fetal heart rate pattern | Heart anomalies |
| Gestational age ≤ 36 0/7 weeks | Forceps or vacuum-assisted delivery | |
| Multiple gestation | Preterm labor | |
| Fetal macrosomia | Ruptured membranes > 24 hours | |
| Intrauterine growth restriction | Maternal general anesthesia | |
| Maternal drug abuse | Intrapartum bleeding | |
| No prenatal care | | |
| Fetal malformations | | |

Data from Weiner GM: *Textbook of Neonatal Resuscitation*, 7th ed. Elk Grove Village, IL: American Academy of Pediatrics and American Heart Association; 2016.

**TABLE 44-2 HISTORY TO GATHER PRIOR TO DELIVERY**

| |
|---|
| **Essential Prebirth Questions** |
| Singleton or multiple pregnancy |
| Obstetrical EGA |
| Presence or absence of meconium-stained amniotic fluid |
| Additional risk factors? |
| **Potential Risk Factors** |
| Quality of maternal prenatal care (accuracy of dating criteria?) |
| Social risk factors (smoking, alcohol, drug use during pregnancy) |
| Maternal complications during pregnancy |
| Maternal medications |
| Maternal screenings |
| Infection screens |
| Maternal serum α-fetoprotein screen |
| Diabetes screen |
| Maternal blood type |
| Antenatal sonogram results |
| When labor began and when membrane ruptured |
| Labor complications |
| Gestational hypertension |
| Chorioamnionitis |
| Type of maternal anesthesia |
| Fetal heart rate tracing patterns |
| Tachycardia |
| Variability |
| Decelerations (What kind? How low? How long? Recovering?) |
| Position of the fetus |
| Other maternal medications during labor |
| Illicit substance screen during labor |

EGA, estimated gestational age.

the delivery area temperature should be maintained at 74°F to 77°F (23–25°C). Additional heat loss–prevention strategies include maximally powered radiant warmers, warm blankets for drying, heated, humidified resuscitation gases, and warming aids such as hats, plastic occlusive wrap, and thermal mattresses for preterm infants.

The following equipment should always be immediately available: functional positive pressure ventilation device capable of delivering oxygen, suction devices (bulb syringe as well as wall suction and suction catheters), a functional laryngoscope with appropriate-sized blades, and appropriate endotracheal tubes and end-tidal $CO_2$ detectors. Pulse oximetry monitoring should be available for every delivery. Cardiac monitoring may help to monitor infants receiving positive pressure ventilation and is recommended if cardiac compressions are initiated. In certain potentially dire circumstances, an umbilical venous line should be prepared and resuscitation medications drawn up and labeled for potential use.

## INDICATIONS FOR NEED FOR RESUSCITATION

Most term newborns respond to birth with good respiratory effort, a rising or stable heart rate greater than 100 beats per minute (bpm), and movement of the arms and legs with good tone. Preductal oxygen saturations will improve steadily over the first 5 to 10 minutes, although clinical judgment of pink color is notoriously unreliable. Term babies who respond vigorously to birth with adequate respiratory effort and good heart rate need only routine care, such as providing warmth (drying) and opening of the airway, can often remain with the mother. Infants with poor, gasping, or absent respiratory effort; with inadequate heart rate below 100 bpm; or who are born preterm should be taken to the radiant warmer for further assessment and possible resuscitation interventions (Fig. 44-1). Heart rate may initially be assessed by listening to the precordium with a stethoscope but cardiac monitoring can be used at any time as well. Palpation of the base of the

**TABLE 44-3 NEONATAL RESUSCITATION SUPPLIES AND EQUIPMENT**

| |
|---|
| **Suction Equipment** |
| Bulb syringe |
| Mechanical suction and tubing |
| Suction catheters: 5F or 6F, 8F, 10F, 12F, or 14F |
| 8F feeding tube and 20-mL syringe |
| Meconium aspirator |
| **Positive-Pressure Ventilation Equipment** |
| Device for delivering positive-pressure ventilation |
| Face masks, newborn and premature sizes (cushioned-rim masks preferred) |
| Oxygen source with flowmeter (flow rate up to 10 L/min) and tubing |
| Compressed air source |
| Oxygen blender to mix oxygen and compressed air with flow meter (flow rate set to 10L/min) and tubing |
| Pulse oximeter with sensor and cover |
| Target oxygen saturation table |
| **Intubation Equipment** |
| Laryngoscope with straight blades, size 0 (preterm) and size 1 (term) |
| Extra bulbs and batteries for laryngoscope |
| Endotracheal tubes, 2.5-, 3.0-, and 3.5-mm internal diameter |
| Stylet (optional) |
| Measuring tape |
| Endotracheal tube insertion depth table |
| Scissors |
| Waterproof tape or tube-securing device |
| Alcohol pads |
| $CO_2$ detector or capnograph |
| Laryngeal mask (or similar supraglottic device) and 5-mL syringe |
| 5F or 6F orogastric tube if insertion port present on laryngeal mask |
| **Medications** |
| Epinephrine 1:10,000 (0.1 mg/mL), 3-mL or 10-mL ampules |
| Normal saline for volume expansion: 100 or 250 mL |
| Dextrose 10%, 250 mL (optional) |
| Normal saline for flushes |
| Syringes (1-mL, 3-mL, or 5-mL, 20- to 60-mL) |
| **Umbilical Vessel Catheterization Supplies** |
| Sterile gloves |
| Scalpel or scissors |
| Antiseptic prep solution |
| Umbilical tape |
| Small clamp (hemostat) |
| Forceps (optional) |
| Umbilical catheters (single lumen), 3.5F, 5F |
| 3-way stopcock |
| Syringes (3- to 5-mL) |
| Needles (25-, 21-, 18-gauge) or puncture device for needleless system |
| Normal saline for flushes |
| Clear adhesive dressing to temporarily secure umbilical venous catheter to abdomen (optional) |
| **Miscellaneous** |
| Gloves and appropriate personal protection |
| Radiant warmer or other heat source |
| Temperature sensor with sensor cover for radiant warmer (for use during prolonged resuscitation) or thermometer |
| Firm, padded resuscitation surface |
| Timer/clock with second hand |
| Warmed linens |
| Infant hat |
| Stethoscope (neonatal head preferred) |
| Tape, $^1/_2$- or $^3/_4$-inch |
| Cardiac monitor and electrodes |
| Resuscitation record forms |
| **For Very Preterm Babies** |
| Food-grade plastic bag (1-gallon size) or plastic wrap |
| Chemically activated warming pad |
| Transport incubator to maintain baby's temperature during move to the nursery |

Reproduced with permission from Weiner GM: *Textbook of Neonatal Resuscitation*, 7th ed. Elk Grove Village, IL: American Academy of Pediatrics and American Heart Association; 2016.

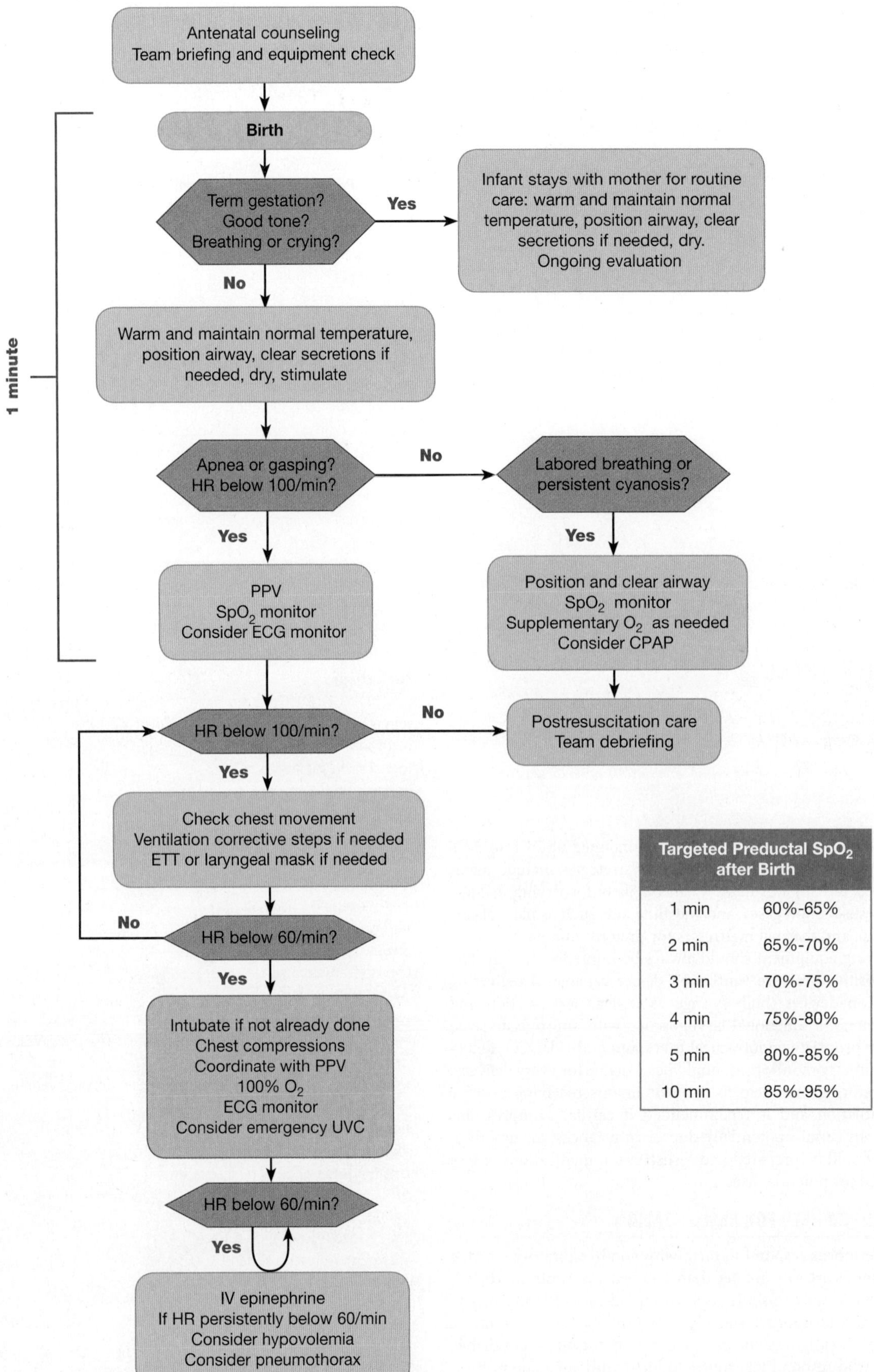


| Targeted Preductal $SpO_2$ after Birth | |
|---|---|
| 1 min | 60%-65% |
| 2 min | 65%-70% |
| 3 min | 70%-75% |
| 4 min | 75%-80% |
| 5 min | 80%-85% |
| 10 min | 85%-95% |

**FIGURE 44-1** American Academy of Pediatrics/American Heart Association Neonatal Resuscitation Program Algorithm. CPAP, continuous positive airway pressure; ECG, electrocardiogram; ETT, endotracheal tube; HR, heart rate; IV, intravenous; PPV, positive pressure ventilation; $SpO_2$, oxygen saturation level; UVC, umbilical venous catheter. (Reproduced with permission from Wyckoff MH, Aziz K, Escobedo MB, et al: Part 13: Neonatal Resuscitation: 2015 American Heart Association Guidelines Update for Cardiopulmonary Resuscitation and Emergency Cardiovascular Care, *Circulation*. 2015 Nov 3;132(18 Suppl 2):S543-S560.)

cord should not be performed as this is not accurate. Gasping, apnea, and a heart rate below 100 bpm are signs that indicate the need to clear the airway and provide positive pressure ventilation.

## UMBILICAL CORD MANAGEMENT

*Delayed cord clamping* (DCC) after birth provides transfusion of placental blood to the newly born infant. In full-term infants, the placental blood volume at birth is approximately 35 mL/kg of birth weight. If the infant is held at the level of the introitus after birth, 40% of this blood volume will be transferred to the infant within 1 minute after birth. In full-term infants, DCC improves hemoglobin levels at birth and iron stores throughout infancy. Improved neurodevelopment at 4 years of age has been reported. The only known negative outcome of DCC is hyperbilirubinemia, leading to increased need for phototherapy. In preterm infants, DCC improves short-term outcomes. For example, it reduces the need for blood transfusion and reduces intraventricular hemorrhage (all grades) and necrotizing enterocolitis. Based on the available data, DCC should be performed in preterm and term infants who do not require resuscitation at birth. Other investigations to examine the risks and benefits of cord milking compared to DCC are underway. Until more data are known, infants who require resuscitation after birth should have immediate cord clamping to enable initiation of resuscitative steps.

## INITIAL STEPS OF NEWBORN RESUSCITATION

All babies should have an immediate assessment and initial steps of resuscitation (provision of warmth, airway opened, and drying and stimulation) provided. If the infant is term estimated gestational age and vigorous at birth with good respiratory effort, heart rate, and tone, these steps can be done on the mother's abdomen or chest. If the infant is preterm, nonvigorous, or has anomalies, then he or she should be taken to the prepared radiant warmer for further action, using the following steps:

1. *Provide warmth:* The infant should be wrapped in warm blankets and placed under a preheated radiant warmer. The initial wet blanket must be removed and the infant dried with particular attention to the head. Consider a wool or plastic hat. If the infant is preterm, place the infant on a portable, chemically activated heating pad under a layer of warm blankets. If the baby is less than 32 weeks' estimated gestational age, place the trunk and extremities into a food-grade resealable polyethylene bag or plastic wrap. It is useful to measure the infant's temperature while in the delivery room to guide further intervention, in addition to preventing iatrogenic hyperthermia, which is detrimental as well. Additional measures to prevent heat loss in preterm infants include use of warm, humidified resuscitation gases and increased environmental temperature of the delivery room.
2. *Open the airway:* The infant should be placed with the neck in mild extension so that the airway is maximally patent. Sometimes a shoulder roll helps to maintain correct position of the head. If the airway is obstructed or positive pressure ventilation is required, secretions should be gently suctioned from the mouth and then nose with a bulb syringe or suction catheter. Take care to avoid vigorous or deep suction because it can cause vagal stimulation with apnea and bradycardia (the very state you are trying to avoid!).
3. *Stimulate:* Once the airway is clear, the infant should be dried thoroughly and briefly stimulated by rubbing the back. An infant in primary apnea will respond to almost any form of stimulation. If, however, the baby remains apneic, gasping, or with an inadequate heart rate, the infant is in secondary apnea, and effective positive pressure ventilation must be initiated without delay.

## MECONIUM-STAINED AMNIOTIC FLUID

Depressed infants born through meconium-stained amniotic fluid are at risk for aspiration of the meconium into the lungs, increasing the risk of severe respiratory failure. Until recently, nonvigorous infants born through meconium stained amniotic fluid were immediately intubated for tracheal suctioning with the aim to prevent meconium aspiration syndrome. However, this historical practice was never evidence based, and the available limited evidence does not support tracheal suctioning.

Thus, initial steps of resuscitation for infants born through meconium-stained amniotic fluid should be the same as infants born through clear fluid. Nonvigorous infants born through meconium-stained fluid should be brought to the radiant warmer, and initial management steps should include providing warmth, opening the airway, and stimulating the neonate. Intubation for tracheal suction should be reserved only for those infants with evidence of airway obstruction. After the initial steps, positive pressure ventilation should be initiated for infants who are apneic, gasping, or have a heart rate below 100 bpm.

## EFFECTIVE POSITIVE PRESSURE VENTILATION

Effective ventilation of the lungs is the most critical step in stabilization of the newborn infant who is not transitioning well at birth. Three different devices (self-inflating bag, flow-inflating bag, and T-piece resuscitator (Table 44-4) are currently available for ventilation of the newborn in the delivery room, each with its particular positive and negative features. Ventilation can be provided via an appropriately sized face mask, laryngeal mask, or endotracheal tube. In order to provide effective ventilation via face mask, the first step is to make sure the infant is maintained in the open airway position. The mask must be appropriately sized to achieve a good seal. It should fit snugly around the mouth, supported by the chin and bridge of nose. The

**TABLE 44-4 TYPES OF POSITIVE-PRESSURE VENTILATION DEVICES FOR THE NEWBORN**

| Characteristic | Self-Inflating Bag | Flow-Inflating Bag | T-Piece Resuscitator |
|---|---|---|---|
| Appropriate-sized masks | Available | Available | Available |
| Oxygen concentration | | | |
| 90–100% capability | Only with reservoir | Yes | Yes |
| Variable concentration | Only with blender plus reservoir<br>~ 40% $O_2$ delivered with no reservoir attached | Only with blender | Only with blender |
| Peak inspiratory pressure | Amount of squeeze measured by pressure gauge | Amount of squeeze measured by pressure gauge | Peak inspiratory pressure determined by adjustable mechanical setting |
| PEEP | No direct control (unless optional PEEP valve attached) | Flow-control valve adjustment | PEEP control |
| Inspiratory time | Duration of squeeze | Duration of squeeze | Duration that PEEP cap is occluded |
| Appropriate-sized bag | Available | Available | Available |
| Safety features | Pop-off valve<br>Optional pressure gauge | Pressure gauge | Maximum pressure relief valve<br>Pressure gauge |

PEEP, positive end-expiratory pressure.

Data from Weiner GM: *Textbook of Neonatal Resuscitation*, 7th ed. Elk Grove Village, IL: American Academy of Pediatrics and American Heart Association; 2016.

**TABLE 44-5 STRATEGIES TO ACHIEVE CHEST RISE DURING BAG MASK VENTILATION**

| | | |
|---|---|---|
| M | Mask adjustment | Check the seal of the mask and reapply if needed. |
| R | Reposition airway | Make sure the infant is truly in the open airway (mild extension) position. |
| S | Suction mouth and nose | Remove obstructing secretions. |
| O | Open the mouth | Sometimes in an effort to get a good seal, the mouth is accidentally closed. The higher resistance of the nasal passages will limit effective ventilation. |
| P | Pressure increase | Try increasing the inflation pressure if possible. |
| A | Advanced airway | If all previous steps have failed to achieve chest rise, it is time to intubate or place a laryngeal mask! |

Reproduced with permission from Weiner GM: *Textbook of Neonatal Resuscitation*, 7th ed. Elk Grove Village, IL: American Academy of Pediatrics and American Heart Association; 2016.

**TABLE 44-6 LARYNGOSCOPE BLADE SIZE, ENDOTRACHEAL TUBE SIZE, AND DEPTH OF INSERTION FOR BABIES OF VARIOUS ESTIMATED GESTATIONAL AGES**

| Blade Size | ETT Size (mm) | EGA (wks) | Depth of Insertion (cm) |
|---|---|---|---|
| No. 0 or No. 00 | 2.5 | 23–24 | ~ 5.5 |
| No. 0 or No. 00 | 2.5 | 25–26 | ~ 6.0 |
| No. 0 | 2.5–3.0 | 27–29 | ~ 6.5 |
| No. 0 | 3.0 | 30–34 | ~ 7.0–7.5 |
| No. 1 | 3.5 | 34–38 | ~ 8.0–8.5 |
| No. 1 | 3.5–4.0 | > 38 | ~ 9.0–10.0 |

EGA, estimated gestational age; ETT, endotracheal tube.

Data from Weiner GM: *Textbook of Neonatal Resuscitation*, 7th ed. Elk Grove Village, IL: American Academy of Pediatrics and American Heart Association; 2016.

mask should not rest on the eyes because adequate pressure to achieve an adequate seal often elicits an adverse vagal reflex. Lack of appropriate airway position and poor seal are common causes of inadequate ventilation and resultant poor response to positive pressure ventilation in the delivery room. The best sign that effective ventilation is underway is a rapid rise in heart rate, followed by improvement in oxygen saturation and tone. If there is not rapid improvement, then look for the presence of chest rise with each ventilation and listen for breath sounds. If no chest rise is noted with positive pressure breaths, then attempt a series of specific measures to achieve chest rise, summarized by the acronym MR SOPA and listed in Table 44-5. Ventilation rates of 40 to 60 breaths per minute are recommended. It is easy for an inexperienced provider to deliver much higher rates than are beneficial, so counting out loud to maintain a steady rhythm of 1 breath per second can be helpful. Initial inflation pressures may be high to inflate the lungs, but having done so, adjust the inspiratory pressure to maintain a heart rate greater than 100 bpm avoiding overdistending the lungs. The optimum inspiratory pressure, inflation time, and flow rate required to maintain effective ventilation varies. If the heart rate (> 100 bpm), oxygen saturations, and tone improve, and the baby begins to breathe spontaneously, then the bagging rate can be gradually reduced. The stomach should be decompressed to prevent gas distention and aspiration of stomach contents (which can further impede effective ventilation) via placement of an orogastric tube if prolonged bagging is needed. If there is not full improvement, then the infant may need to have the trachea intubated or laryngeal mask placed for continued support. If the heart rate remains less than 60 bpm despite apparent effective ventilation with chest rise, then external cardiac compressions are indicated.

## CONTINUOUS POSITIVE AIRWAY PRESSURE

Continuous positive airway pressure (CPAP) should be used after birth in spontaneously breathing preterm infants with labored breathing. Compared with empiric intubation for surfactant and mechanical ventilation, early application of CPAP has been shown to reduce the risk of chronic lung disease among preterm infants. While CPAP may help establish and maintain a functional residual capacity in stiff, noncompliant lungs, thus improving respiratory distress, it should never be used in place of positive pressure ventilation when respiratory effort is poor or absent.

## INTUBATION

Intubation may be performed for a variety of indications during resuscitation. These include suctioning an obstructed airway, inadequate response and/or poor chest rise during bag-mask ventilation, need for positive pressure ventilation beyond a few minutes, need for external chest compressions, endotracheal delivery of epinephrine if the intravenous route is inaccessible, surfactant administration, and suspected diaphragmatic hernia. For endotracheal tube size, laryngoscope blade size, and depth of insertion, see Table 44-6. Use of a stylet is an option as long as care is taken that the tip does not protrude beyond the tube and it is secured so that accidental trauma does not occur. Intubation is a skill that takes practice (Fig. 44-2). An increasing heart rate and end-tidal carbon dioxide detection after several breaths are the primary methods of confirming ventilation. Once the tube is inserted, the intubator confirms that the tip-to-lip measurement seems reasonable. For infants greater than 1000 g birth weight, the distance (in cm) of 6 + the weight in kilograms measured at the lip is a practical starting point. For infants 30 weeks' gestation or less, this rule frequently results in right main-stem tube placement. Thus for very immature infants, 2 other estimates of depth of insertion are useful. Either measure the distance from the septum of the nose to the tragus of the ear and add 1 cm for tube insertion depth, or use the gestational age–based depth of insertion table (Table 44-6). Secondary confirmation includes seeing chest rise after beginning positive pressure breaths through the tube, listening for equal breath sounds, and seeing condensation within the tube. Subsequent radiographic confirmation of proper placement is needed. Prolonged or repetitive intubation attempts should be interrupted for reapplication of bag mask ventilation to avoid exacerbation of hypoxia and hypoventilation.

## OXYGEN USE

In utero, the oxygen tension of the fetus is relatively low compared to adult levels. Healthy term newborns take 5 to 10 minutes for preductal oxygen saturations to reach 90% without intervention. Although 100% oxygen was widely used to resuscitate infants for years, evidence from randomized trials demonstrated that initiating resuscitation with ambient air for full-term infants reduces mortality and oxidative injury. Thus, in term infants, resuscitation should be initiated with 21% fraction of inspired oxygen ($FiO_2$) and the oxygen subsequently adjusted to meet normal oxygen saturation goals per minute of life for healthy term infants.

Oxygen use during resuscitation of preterm infants remains controversial. Preterm infants are often hypoxemic due to lung immaturity and impaired gas exchange. However, they are also deficient in antioxidant protection and thus face potential adverse effects from exposing developing organs to high concentrations of inspired oxygen or high blood oxygen tension. In pooled analysis of the available trials comparing low versus high oxygen concentration to resuscitate preterm infants, there is no clear benefit for either strategy to prevent mortality or major neonatal morbidities. Larger trials of initial oxygen concentration for resuscitation of preterm infants are ongoing. Until results of these trials are available, resuscitation of preterm infants should be initiated with a low concentration of blended oxygen (≤ 30% $FiO_2$) and subsequently titrated to limit excessive oxygen exposure.

For all infants who require respiratory support or supplemental oxygen during resuscitation, pulse oximetry should target oxygen saturations based on published nomograms of preductal oxygen saturations during the first 10 minutes of life.

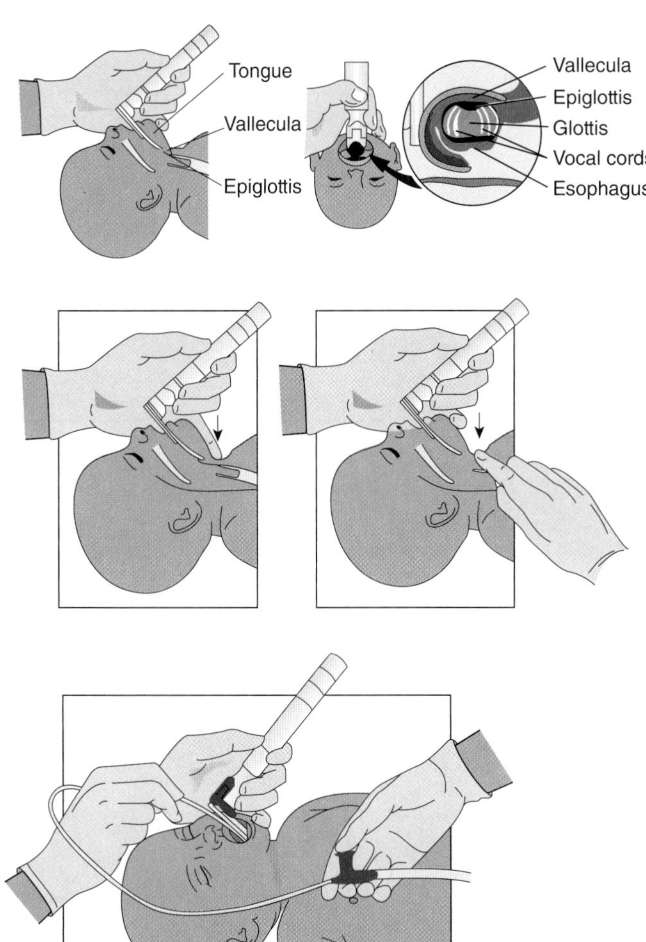


**FIGURE 44-2** Critical anatomic structures for neonatal intubation. The infant is placed in the open airway position. Holding the laryngoscope in the left hand, the intubator opens the newborn's mouth and inserts the blade gently and gradually into the vallecula (the space between the base of the tongue and epiglottis). Gently lifting upward in a 45-degree angle (no rocking, which can put pressure on the alveolar ridge and cause damage) exposes the glottic structures. The cords of a newborn are pink and shaped as an upside-down V. Using the right hand, the intubator inserts the endotracheal tube from the right side, using care to maintain visualization of the vocal cords. The tube is inserted to the level of the vocal cord guide printed on the tube. If the cords are closed, the intubator must wait for them to open because touching the cords themselves with the tube can cause spasm.

## EXTERNAL CARDIAC COMPRESSIONS

Effective ventilation is typically all that is required for stabilization of most newborns in the delivery room, and cardiac compressions are rarely needed in the delivery room. Current resuscitation guidelines recommend cardiac compressions for a newborn infant with a heart rate below 60 bpm despite adequate ventilation with supplementary oxygen for 30 seconds. Because ventilation is the most effective action in newborn resuscitation and because chest compressions are likely to interfere with effective ventilation, resuscitation providers are strongly encouraged to optimize assisted ventilation via endotracheal tube before initiating chest compressions. Once compressions are initiated, the oxygen concentration should be increased to 100%. Compressions should be delivered to the lower third of the sternum to a depth of approximately one-third the anteroposterior diameter of the chest, which should be adequate to produce a palpable pulse. The 2-thumb method, in which the hands encircle the newborn chest while the thumbs compress the sternum, provides the best reliability in achieving the desired depth of compression over time with less fatigue, higher generated blood pressures, and less concerning drift of hand placement that could cause traumatic injury. Once the airway is secured, cardiac compressions using the 2-thumb method can be done from the head of the bed which allows open access to the baby from the side for a provider to obtain intravenous access via an umbilical venous catheter (Fig. 44-3). A compression-to-ventilation ratio of 3:1, such that 90 compressions and 30 breaths are achieved per minute, is currently recommended in order to optimize ventilation. Although vital signs should be checked, the less interruption there is of the cardiac compressions, the easier it is to maintain perfusion pressure. Use of cardiac monitoring during chest compressions is recommended to limit the time it takes to assess for return of heart rate. Coordinated chest compressions and ventilations should continue until the spontaneous heart rate is 60 bpm or greater.

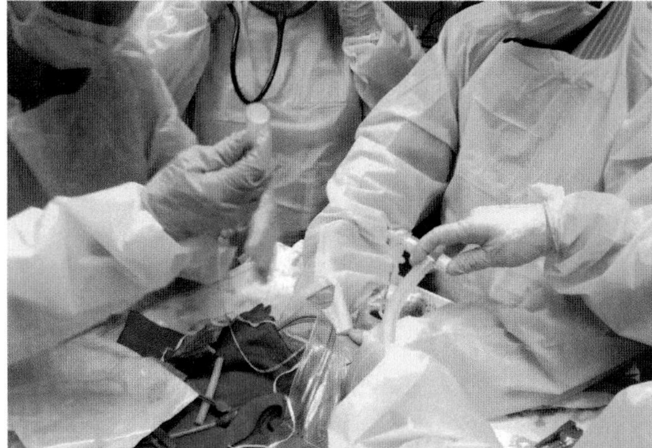

**FIGURE 44-3** Two-thumb method of neonatal cardiac compressions. Note that providing compressions from the head of the bed allows another provider easy access to the umbilical cord for umbilical catheter placement.

The goal of cardiac compressions is to perfuse the heart and the brain. If severe asphyxia results in asystole or agonal bradycardia, the newborn myocardium is depleted of energy substrate. Adequate coronary perfusion must be reestablished with oxygenated blood in order to regenerate sufficient adenosine 5′-triphosphate required for effective myocardial function and return of spontaneous circulation. Coronary perfusion pressure is the difference between the aortic diastolic blood pressure and the right atrial end-diastolic blood pressure. Thus, cardiac compressions and adequate systemic vascular resistance are needed to generate an adequate diastolic blood pressure in order to achieve return of spontaneous circulation. Given the profound vasodilation that typically results from the significant acidemia induced by asphyxia, a vasopressor agent such as epinephrine will frequently be required to achieve an adequate aortic diastolic pressure for sufficient coronary perfusion.

## MEDICATION USE FOR AGONAL BRADYCARDIA/ASYSTOLE

### Epinephrine

Although based primarily on adult and animal studies, epinephrine has long been the preferred vasopressor agent for treatment of ventilation-resistant neonatal cardiac arrest. As mentioned in the previous section, during cardiopulmonary resuscitation, the most important action of epinephrine is to stimulate α-adrenergic receptor–mediated vasoconstriction in order to elevate the diastolic blood pressure and thus the coronary perfusion pressure. Consequently, during neonatal cardiac arrest, if effective ventilation and cardiac compressions have failed to reestablish perfusion, epinephrine should be given rapidly. Current guidelines recommend that if agonal bradycardia (heart rate < 60 bpm) or asystole persists despite 30 seconds of effective positive pressure ventilation, followed by 30 seconds of coordinated cardiac compressions and ventilation, then 0.1 to 0.3 mL/kg of 1:10,000 epinephrine solution should be given rapidly via the intravenous route

**TABLE 44-7 APGAR SCORE**

| Sign | 0 | 1 | 2 | 1 min | 5 min | 10 min | 15 min | 20 min |
|---|---|---|---|---|---|---|---|---|
| **Color** | Blue or pale | Acrocyanotic | Completely pink | | | | | |
| **Heart rate** | Absent | < 100/min | > 100/min | | | | | |
| **Reflex irritability** | No response | Grimace | Cry or active withdrawal | | | | | |
| **Muscle tone** | Limp | Some flexion | Active motion | | | | | |
| **Respiration** | Absent | Weak cry; hypoventilation | Good, crying | | | | | |
| **Comments:** | | | **RESUSCITATION** | | | | | |
| | | | **Minutes** | 1 | 5 | 10 | 15 | 20 |
| | | | **Oxygen** | | | | | |
| | | | **PPV/CPAP** | | | | | |
| | | | **ETT** | | | | | |
| | | | **Chest Compressions** | | | | | |
| | | | **Epinephrine** | | | | | |

ETT, endotracheal tube; PPV/CPAP, positive pressure ventilation/continuous positive airway pressure.

Modified with permission from American Academy of Pediatrics Committee on Fetus and Newborn, American College of Obstetricians and Gynecologists Committee on Obstetric Practice. The Apgar Score. *Pediatrics.* 2015 Oct;136(4):819-822.

followed by 0.5 to 1.0 mL of normal saline flush. The emphasis on intravenous delivery of epinephrine rather than the previously acceptable endotracheal route mandates that delivery room resuscitation providers be well trained in rapid placement of umbilical venous catheters. The endotracheal route is not efficacious or reliable, but if it must be used due to persistent lack of intravenous access, a higher dose (0.5–1.0 mL/kg) of epinephrine should be used in hopes of improving efficacy. The higher endotracheal dose should always be drawn up in a larger 3- to 5-mL syringe to help alert the resuscitation team of the route for which the dose is intended, because high doses of epinephrine should not be given intravenously.

#### Volume Infusion

Volume infusion should be given only if there is a high suspicion for blood loss as a cause of shock given the clinical circumstances surrounding the delivery (cord avulsion, velamentous insertion of the cord, traumatic abruption, etc); or if the baby appears to be in shock and unresponsive to apparently adequate resuscitation. If there is a suspicion of significant blood loss, then the best replacement fluid is emergency supply O-negative blood, but normal saline is acceptable until blood is available. It should be given in 10-mL/kg aliquots slowly over 5 to 10 minutes with assessment for response. It is important to remember, though, that the majority of severely depressed infants have suffered an asphyxial injury and are not hypovolemic. In an asphyxia-induced hypotension and bradycardia model (without hypovolemia), volume infusion during resuscitation increased pulmonary edema, decreased pulmonary dynamic compliance, and did not improve blood pressure either during or after the resuscitation. Thus, volume infusions during delivery room resuscitation may be detrimental and exacerbate poor cardiac output when hypovolemia is not present.

#### Sodium Bicarbonate

There is no evidence to support use of sodium bicarbonate during resuscitation of the newborn. Its use in the newborn should be moved to postresuscitation care that can be guided by assessment of acid-base balance. Bicarbonate should never be given unless the lungs are being adequately ventilated. Otherwise, acidemia will be increased due to increased respiratory acidosis.

## ASSIGNMENT OF APGAR SCORES

Virginia Apgar, an obstetrical anesthesiologist, devised a rapid standardized scoring system to assess the clinical status of the infant at birth. She sought to focus the attention of medical providers on the newborn during the critical window of transition from intrauterine to extrauterine life so that they could offer assistance as needed. The Apgar score consists of 5 components: heart rate, respiratory effort, muscle tone, reflex irritability, and color (Table 44-7). Each component is given a score from 0 to 2 for a total composite score ranging from 0 to 10. Scores are assigned at 1 and 5 minutes for every delivery. If the 5-minute score is lower than 7, it is suggested to keep assigning scores every 5 minutes until the score is 7 or higher or until resuscitation efforts are withdrawn. A change between the 1- and 5-minute Apgar score is a useful index of the newborn's response to resuscitation. However, Apgar scores are poor predictors of outcome and should not be used as sole criteria to diagnose asphyxia or hypoxic-ischemic encephalopathy.

## OTHER CONSIDERATIONS

There are a variety of other conditions that may lead to severe respiratory depression or distress at birth and that require early resuscitation. Many of these conditions are fetal anomalies or abnormal fluid collections that interfere with effective ventilation and oxygenation and therefore may require specific interventions, such as insertion of an oral airway, fluid removal from the chest or abdomen, or specific surgical intervention. Special planning is indicated for possible ex utero intrapartum treatment (EXIT) procedures for fetuses with possible severe airway obstructions. With specialized surgical teams, it is possible to partially deliver the infant and obtain a surgical airway while the infant is sustained on placental bypass.

If an infant has not responded and remains asystolic after more than 10 minutes of complete and adequate resuscitative measures, it may be reasonable to discontinue assisted ventilation and compressions. At this point in resuscitation efforts, there are few survivors and those few who do survive often bear a heavy burden of disability. However, the decision to continue or stop must be individualized. Variables such as whether the prior resuscitation was optimal, the availability of advanced neonatal care such as therapeutic hypothermia, special circumstances prior to delivery (such as a known timing of insult), and wishes of the family should be taken into consideration.

## SUGGESTED READINGS

American Academy of Pediatrics Committee on Fetus and Newborn; American College of Obstetricians and Gynecologists Committee on Obstetric Practice. The Apgar score. *Pediatrics.* 2015;136(4):819-822.

Chettri S, Adhisivam B, Bhat BV. Endotracheal suction for nonvigorous neonates born through meconium stained amniotic fluid: a randomized controlled trial. *J Pediatr.* 2015;166(5):1208-1213.e1.

Dawson JA, Kamlin CO, Vento M, et al. Defining the reference range for oxygen saturation for infants after birth. *Pediatrics.* 2010;125(6):e1340-e1347.

Harrington DJ, Redman CW, Moulden M, Greenwood CE. The long-term outcome in surviving infants with Apgar zero at 10 minutes: a systematic review of the literature and hospital-based cohort. *Am J Obstet Gynecol.* 2007;196(5):463.e1-e5.

Kapadia V, Wyckoff MH. Chest compressions for bradycardia or asystole in neonates. *Clin Perinatol.* 2012;39(4):833-842.

McDonald SJ, Middleton P, Dowswell T, Morris PS. Effect of timing of umbilical cord clamping of term infants on maternal and neonatal outcomes. *Cochrane Database Syst Rev.* 2013;(7):CD004074.

Nangia S, Sunder S, Biswas R, Saili A. Endotracheal suction in term non vigorous meconium stained neonates—a pilot study. *Resuscitation.* 2016;105:79-84.

Oei JL, Vento M, Rabi Y, et al. Higher or lower oxygen for delivery room resuscitation of preterm infants below 28 completed weeks gestation: a meta-analysis. *Arch Dis Child Fetal Neonatal Ed.* 2017;102(1):F24-F30.

Perlman J, Kjaer K. Neonatal and maternal temperature regulation during and after delivery. *Anesth Analg.* 2016;123(1):168-172.

Perlman JM, Wyllie J, Kattwinkel J, et al; Neonatal Resuscitation Chapter Collaborators. Part 7: neonatal resuscitation: 2015 international consensus on cardiopulmonary resuscitation and emergency cardiovascular care science with treatment recommendations. *Circulation.* 2015;132(16 Suppl 1):S204-S241.

Rabe H, Diaz-Rossello JL, Duley L, Dowswell T. Effect of timing of umbilical cord clamping and other strategies to influence placental transfusion at preterm birth on maternal and infant outcomes. *Cochrane Database Syst Rev.* 2012;(8):CD003248.

Saugstad OD, Aune D, Aguar M, Kapadia V, Finer N, Vento M. Systematic review and meta-analysis of optimal initial fraction of oxygen levels in the delivery room at ≤32 weeks. *Acta Paediatr.* 2014;103(7):744-751.

Saugstad OD, Ramji S, Soll RF, Vento M. Resuscitation of newborn infants with 21% or 100% oxygen: an updated systematic review and meta-analysis. *Neonatology.* 2008;94(3):176-182.

Subramaniam P, Ho JJ, Davis PG. Prophylactic nasal continuous positive airway pressure for preventing morbidity and mortality in very preterm infants. *Cochrane Database Syst Rev.* 2016;(6):CD001243.

Weiner GM. *Textbook of Neonatal Resuscitation*, 7th ed. Elk Grove Village, IL: American Academy of Pediatrics and American Heart Association; 2016.

# 45 Transitional Changes in the Newborn

Satyan Lakshminrusimha and David P. Carlton

## INTRODUCTION

Birth involves changes in numerous organ systems in the infant, but only a few of these are required to undergo relatively rapid postnatal adjustment. The most important of these birth-related changes involve transitional function in the respiratory, cardiovascular, gastrointestinal, renal, thermoregulatory, and metabolic systems. Common factors that influence transition at birth include delivery by cesarean section, prematurity, and delayed cord clamping.

## THE RESPIRATORY SYSTEM

Within minutes after birth, regular breathing efforts are sustained, lung compliance improves, airway resistance diminishes, and a functional residual capacity is established. With these changes, the tensions of both oxygen and carbon dioxide in the blood gradually approach those expected in the mature postnatal infant. The physiological triggers for establishing regular breathing efforts are probably the loss of the umbilical circulation and the increase in systemic oxygen content.

### Surfactant Production

A critical element necessary for pulmonary adaptation after birth is surfactant (Fig. 45-1). Surfactant facilitates respiratory and gas exchange by lowering the surface tension of the alveolar lining layer, which is the shallow pool of liquid that overlies the cells of the distal airspaces. Without a very low surface tension at end-expiration, the airspaces become atelectatic with exhalation. Surfactant deficiency underlies the respiratory distress syndrome (RDS) observed after premature birth.

Surfactant is synthesized in the type II cells that line the distal airspaces. It is composed primarily of lipids, including the desaturated phospholipids, which are responsible for its biophysical properties. Associated with these lipids are a small but critical collection of proteins, the surfactant-associated proteins A, B, C, and D. Proteins B and C are water-insoluble, hydrophobic proteins that are closely associated with the lipid component of surfactant. The pivotal role of these latter 2 proteins is exemplified by RDSs that result from their genetic alteration. Specifically, the absence of surfactant protein B results in severe neonatal respiratory failure unresponsive to routine supportive care.

During the latter stages of intrauterine development, the enzymes important in surfactant production increase and this results in an increase in intracellular surfactant content. Surfactant release into the alveolar space is stimulated by lung inflation and the increase in circulating catecholamine concentration that accompanies birth. The lungs of premature infants release less surfactant into the airspace at the time of birth than do those of a term infant.

In addition to an adequate concentration of surfactant, postnatal lung adaptation also depends on the clearance of fluid from the lumen of the lung. Before birth, the potential airspaces are filled with liquid, and failure to remove this liquid after birth results in respiratory difficulty and hypoxemia. Fetal lung liquid is produced by a process that is dependent on the secretion of chloride ($Cl^-$) ions across the respiratory epithelium into the lung lumen. The importance of fetal lung liquid derives from its ability to act as a dynamic template around which the lung develops in utero. If the fetal airspaces are inadequately distended with liquid, lung growth is stunted and lung cell differentiation is disturbed.

Clearance of fetal lung liquid at the time of birth does not occur primarily by egress of fluid from the lungs by way of the trachea. Rather, the liquid contained within the fetal airspaces at the time of birth is reabsorbed across the respiratory epithelium, a process that is driven by transcellular movement of sodium ($Na^+$) ions from the lung liquid into the interstitium through channels on the apical surface of the distal lung cells (Fig. 45-1). The complete characterization of events that initiate and maintain $Na^+$ and liquid reabsorption from the lung is not clear but likely involves changes in oxygen tension and circulating catecholamines associated with delivery.

## THE CIRCULATION

Profound changes in central circulatory patterns occur after birth and are necessary for the successful transition to extrauterine life. The extent to which this transition fails to take place influences not only the clinical condition of patients who have structural heart disease but also infants whose primary illness may appear to have little, if any, relationship to the circulation.

### The Fetal Circulation

The blood flow pattern of the fetus can be considered to be composed of 2 parallel circuits, as contrasted with the circulation of the adult, which involves 2 circuits linked in series (Fig. 45-2). That is, in the mature adult circulation, venous blood enters the right atrium and is ejected from the right ventricle into the pulmonary circulation. This same blood then drains from the pulmonary venous system into the left atrium and is ejected from the left ventricle into the systemic circulation. The right and left ventricular outputs are essentially equivalent

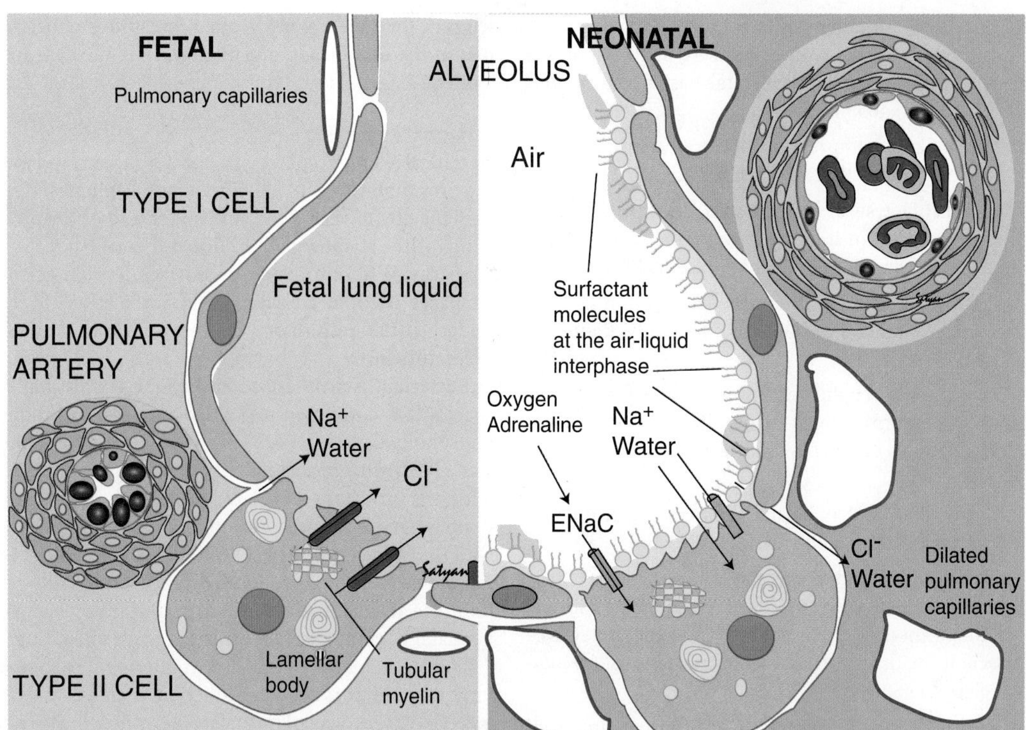


**FIGURE 45-1** Respiratory transition at birth. During fetal life, the alveoli are filled with chloride ($Cl^-$)-rich fluid secreted by the alveolar epithelium. In a term fetus, the type II cells have lamellar bodies and tubular myelin. The pulmonary vascular resistance is high secondary to pulmonary vasoconstriction. Following birth, air enters the alveoli and lung liquid is absorbed secondary to sodium ($Na^+$) transport via the epithelial sodium channels (ENaC). Pulmonary vasodilation and surfactant release lead to the formation of a layer of surfactant at the air-fluid interphase, which leads to establishment of lungs as the site of gas exchange. (Used with permission from Satyan Lakshminrusimha.)



and either accurately represents cardiac output. However, in the fetus, the output from the right and left ventricles each contribute, in parallel, to systemic blood flow because a portion of the right ventricular output traverses the ductus arteriosus and contributes to blood flow to the descending aorta. Because cardiac output to regional vascular beds in the fetus has to be considered with this arrangement in mind, both right and left ventricular outputs are important when considering fetal cardiac function.

In contrast to the mature circulation in which all of the right ventricular output perfuses the pulmonary circulation, in the fetus, most of the blood exiting the right ventricle perfuses the systemic circulation by way of the ductus arteriosus, which is an important right-to-left shunt in the fetus. Thus, as a result of the elevated pulmonary vascular resistance (PVR), only 10% to 15% of the right ventricular output perfuses the pulmonary circulation during fetal life. Just as in the adult circulation, all of the blood leaving the fetal left ventricle perfuses the systemic circulation, although the fractional distribution to regional vascular beds differs from that observed in the mature circulation.

In the fetus, the placenta is the organ of gas exchange, a function that is assumed by the lungs after birth. Unlike the mature postnatal circulation in which all of the cardiac output perfuses the pulmonary circulation and participates in gas exchange, in the fetal circulation, only about one-half of the combined ventricular output perfuses the placenta and participates in gas exchange. The placental vascular resistance is low during fetal life, contributing to low systemic blood pressure. About one-half of this oxygenated blood from the placenta returns directly to the right atrium by way of the ductus venosus and inferior vena cava, the balance entering the portal circulation in the liver. As a result of intraluminal streaming in the inferior vena cava, the oxygenated blood returning to the fetal heart preferentially flows from the right atrium, through the foramen ovale, and into the left atrium, resulting in different oxygen saturations in the right and left ventricles. Blood exiting the left ventricle and preferentially perfusing the coronary and cerebral circulations has an oxygen tension of approximately 25 mm Hg, whereas blood exiting the right ventricle and perfusing the lower body and placenta has a lower oxygen tension of about 20 mm Hg.

### Circulatory Changes after Birth

After delivery, PVR and pulmonary arterial pressure decrease and pulmonary blood flow increases. Under normal postnatal circumstances, both the mechanical stimulus of lung inflation and the increase in alveolar oxygen concentration contribute to the increase in pulmonary blood flow after birth. There are likely a number of mediators involved in the regulation of pulmonary vascular tone around the time of birth, including arachidonic acid metabolites, endothelin, and nitric oxide. The increase in pulmonary blood flow allows for complete oxygen saturation of the entire cardiac output and helps to meet the demand of the doubling of oxygen consumption that occurs after delivery.

Although the reduction in PVR is the most important immediate event that occurs in the central circulation after birth, there are also other changes. Clamping the umbilical cord and removing the placental circulation increases systemic vascular resistance, decreases blood flow through the ductus venosus, and decreases blood return to the right atrium by way of the inferior vena cava. The decrease in right atrial blood return results in a decrease in right atrial pressure. When this decrease in right atrial pressure is coupled with the expected increase in pulmonary venous return and left atrial pressure, the interatrial shunt diminishes and leads to at least functional closure of the foramen ovale.

**The Ductus Arteriosus** Functional closure of the ductus arteriosus occurs within 3 days after birth in healthy term infants but may be delayed in some preterm infants. Permanent anatomic closure occurs in the weeks that follow. Prostaglandins, specifically prostaglandin $E_2$, are an important class of compounds that maintain ductal patency in utero and in small premature infants after birth. As opposed to factors that control ductal patency, the modulators of ductal closure are less well studied, but oxygen is 1 of the important physiologic triggers for ductal constriction. Blocking prostaglandin formation

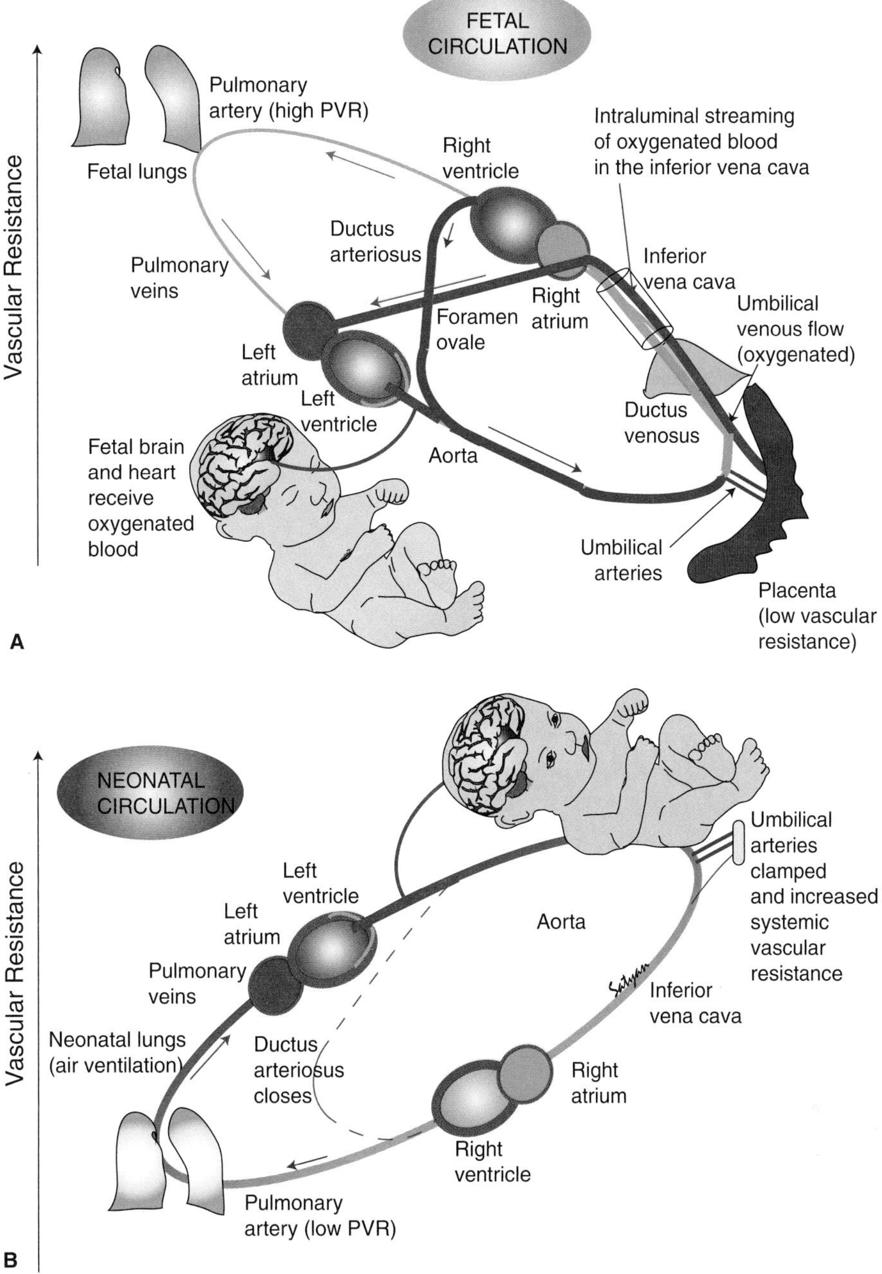


**FIGURE 45-2** Cardiovascular transition at birth. (**A**) Fetal circulation and (**B**) neonatal circulation are shown demonstrating flow from areas of high resistance to low resistance. During fetal life, pulmonary vascular resistance (PVR) is high and placental vascular resistance is low. Therefore, right ventricular output flows away from the lungs through the ductus arteriosus and perfuses the placenta to pick up oxygen from the maternal blood. Oxygenated blood flows through the umbilical vein and ductus venosus and streams along the inferior vena cava and enters the left atrium through the foramen ovale to perfuse the heart and brain. Following birth, the onset of ventilation and clamping of the umbilical cord lead to a decrease in pulmonary vascular resistance and an increase in systemic vascular resistance, respectively. Right ventricular output perfuses the lung, and the left ventricle pumps blood to the systemic circulation. Increased oxygenation leads to closure of the ductus arteriosus. (Used with permission from Satyan Lakshminrusimha.)

by cyclooxygenase inhibition results in ductal constriction, probably because the dilating effect of prostaglandin $E_2$ is eliminated.

Newborn infants with structural heart disease characterized by cyanosis or inadequate systemic perfusion are often deemed to have heart lesions that are "ductal dependent" (see also Chapter 51). Maintenance of blood flow through the ductus arteriosus with prostaglandin $E_1$ in patients with these types of lesions can temporarily provide sufficient blood flow to the pulmonary or systemic circulations to prevent otherwise life-threatening consequences.

Patency of the ductus arteriosus associated with an otherwise structurally normal heart can be undesirable, particularly in the premature infant who has respiratory distress after birth. Within several days after delivery, PVR is often low enough to result in a significant left-to-right shunt through the ductus arteriosus and accompanying overperfusion of the pulmonary circulation. In these infants, cyclooxygenase inhibition with indomethacin or ibuprofen is often used to decrease endogenous prostaglandins and allow ductal closure.

In some infants after birth, PVR fails to decrease as expected. In patients with the most severe form of this condition, called *persistent pulmonary hypertension of the newborn* or *persistent fetal circulation*, blood destined for the pulmonary circulation is diverted right to left into the descending aorta through a patent ductus arteriosus. The severe right-to-left shunting seen in this condition may result in life-threatening hypoxemia. Reducing PVR, for instance, by inhalation of nitric oxide, can play an important role in the early management of this condition.

### Fetal Thermoregulation

In utero, the fetus consumes oxygen to maintain normal cellular respiration and produce energy (Fig. 45-3A). Heat is generated as an expected by-product of these reactions. When values are normalized to body weight, the fetus generates about twice as much heat as an adult of the same species. Most of the heat generated by the fetus is dissipated in the placenta as fetal blood is cooled by the maternal circulation. The balance, perhaps 10% to 20% of the total fetal heat production, is dissipated through the fetal skin, amniotic fluid, and uterine wall. Under conditions in which the efficiency of heat transfer in the placental circulation is diminished, the fetal skin and amniotic fluid can assume a greater role in heat removal. The uterus and placenta are metabolically active, but most of the heat generated in the uterus is a result of fetal metabolism.

At equilibrium, the sum of fetal heat generation and dissipation results in a fetal temperature that is about 0.5°C greater than maternal temperature. An increase in maternal temperature will result in an increase in fetal temperature, and this observation highlights the disadvantage the fetus has to overcome in regulating body temperature. This disadvantage extends to hypothermic situations as well, although this condition is encountered much less frequently than maternal fever.

Unlike the newborn, the fetus has a limited capacity for thermogenesis. The biological basis for this limitation is unclear but is likely the result of substances from the placenta that circulate in the fetus and diminish after birth with removal of the umbilical circulation. Replicating in utero those events that occur after birth, including inflating the lungs, exposure to oxygen, body cooling, and thyroid hormone infusion, do not induce a substantial thermogenic response, whereas cord occlusion does.

### Thermoregulation after Birth

After delivery, the relatively low ambient environmental temperature and evaporation of the residual amniotic fluid from the skin combine to increase heat loss from the newborn infant (Fig. 45-3B). In addition to these environmental challenges, the newborn is intrinsically disadvantaged compared to the adult by virtue of the increased surface area of the newborn relative to body weight. Thus, heat production, relative to body weight, must be greater in the newborn to maintain a normal body temperature. Measurements of perinatal thermal balance suggest that heat production increases by about 2-fold shortly after birth to overcome the relative disadvantage of a greater surface area.

Heat production postnatally is the result of shivering and nonshivering thermogenesis. In adults, heat production from shivering thermogenesis contributes significantly to maintenance of body temperature under conditions of cold stress. An increase in metabolic rate and heat production occurs as a result of shivering thermogenesis, which is characterized by involuntary muscle contractions that may be initially undetectable except with electromyography. The increase in heat production from shivering is substantial but limited in its long-term ability to maintain heat production.

The proportion of heat generated from shivering and nonshivering thermogenesis after birth depends on the species studied. In general, nonshivering thermogenesis is thought to be more important than shivering thermogenesis in the newborn, but there are species in which shivering thermogenesis supplies most, if not all of the heat production even within hours after delivery. Interestingly, in some species that rely entirely on nonshivering thermogenesis after birth, shivering thermogenesis can be induced if nonshivering thermogenesis is inhibited. This observation suggests that although under usual circumstances nonshivering thermogenesis may be the primary means by which heat is generated in the newborn, at least some capacity for shivering may exist.

The immediate control of thermogenesis, both shivering and nonshivering, is by way of the central nervous system. Cutaneous receptors responsive to thermal stimuli are present on the skin, and such receptors respond independently to cold and warm stimuli. Nearly all skin surfaces have receptors for both cold and warm stimuli, but receptors responsive to cold are more abundant than are receptors responsive to heat. The thermoreceptive afferent signals are ultimately processed in several areas of the brain, including the midbrain and hypothalamus. Efferent signaling responsible for initiating shivering thermogenesis is by way of the motor neurons. Nonshivering thermogenesis is also mediated by efferents from the central nervous system.

An important intracellular source of energy for thermogenesis is the generation of free fatty acids from triglycerides. The glycerol

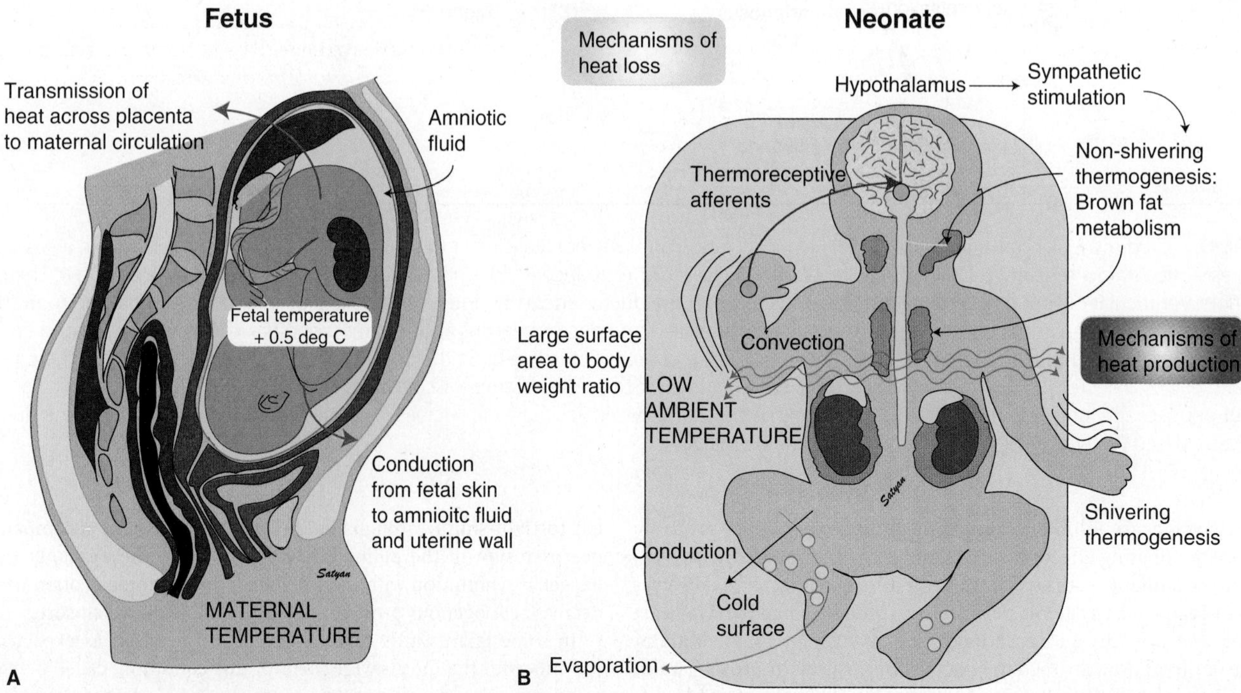


**FIGURE 45-3** Temperature regulation during (**A**) fetal life and (**B**) after birth. Heat produced by the fetus is conducted from the fetal skin to the amniotic fluid and uterine wall by conduction and to the maternal circulation through the placenta. After birth, heat loss by conduction (to a cold surface or blanket), convection (cold air currents), or evaporation of amniotic fluid from the skin can lead to rapid decrease in body temperature. Such heat loss is more profound in preterm infants due to large ratio of surface area to body weight. Afferents from the skin activate the thermoregulatory center in the hypothalamus and induce shivering and nonshivering (through brown fat) thermogenesis. (Used with permission from Satyan Lakshminrusimha.)

produced as part of this reaction is released into the circulation and is 1 of the means by which thermogenesis is measured indirectly in experimental studies. Lipoprotein lipase is developmentally regulated, and its activity is increased after birth. Free fatty acids generated by lipoprotein lipase may contribute to intracellular sources of energy for heat production. Circulating free fatty acids probably do not serve as an acute source of energy during periods of cold stress but rather replenish depleted intracellular fat stores.

**Brown Adipose Tissue** *Brown adipose tissue (BAT)* is responsible for the generation of heat associated with nonshivering thermogenesis. Although BAT can be found in a variety of locations within the body, the upper back and neck, mediastinum, and perinephric areas are major sites of brown fat storage in the newborn. While BAT is relatively more abundant in the newborn than in the adult, BAT increases in abundance postnatally, at least for some period of time. The degree to which it supplies significant amounts of heat in the premature infant is less clear than it is in the term newborn.

The thermogenic response attributed to BAT is the result of both neurogenic and biochemical responses. Sites within the hypothalamus coordinate input from thermoreceptive afferents and also regulate sympathetic output to the brown fat stores in the body. Sympathetic stimulation of nerves in the BAT results in the release of norepinephrine. Subsequent binding of norepinephrine to β-adrenergic receptors on the fat cell triggers an increase in cyclic adenosine monophosphate through the action of adenylate cyclase. An intracellular lipase then liberates fatty acids from cytoplasmic stores of triglycerides, making them available for mitochondrial processing, oxidation, and heat generation.

An important finding in the study of thermogenesis was the discovery of uncoupling protein 1 (UCP1). UCP1 represents a critical factor in the mechanism of heat generation in nonshivering thermogenesis, exemplified by the observation that genetically altered mice that lack UCP1 are unable to produce heat efficiently when exposed to cold and therefore become hypothermic. During mitochondrial respiration, protons are generated outside the inner mitochondrial membrane and contribute to the electrochemical gradient for protons across this barrier. Under conditions in which adenosine 5′-diphosphate is plentiful, the adenosine 5′-triphosphate (ATP) synthase present on the inner mitochondrial membrane uses protons as the driving force for ATP synthesis. In the absence of this pathway for proton entry, mitochondrial respiration slows. UCP1 acts as an ion transport protein, allowing the entry of protons so that respiration can continue, albeit generating heat instead of ATP, a process called *uncoupling*. It is activated by free fatty acids and inhibited by purine nucleotides. The long-term regulation of UCP1 has not been well characterized.

### Ambient Temperature and Metabolic Rate

There exists an ambient temperature range in which the newborn infant's body temperature is normal and its metabolic rate at a minimum. The ambient temperature around this point is designated the *neutral thermal environment*. In this temperature range, there is no requirement for there to be extra metabolic energy expenditure for heat production, the infant does not need to dissipate any extra heat. If heat loss occurs (commonly by exposure to a lower ambient temperature or by evaporative heat loss), then the infant must use thermogenesis to maintain body temperature. This results in an increase in energy consumption and oxygen demand.

As heat loss continues, body temperature will begin to decrease if the increase in metabolic rate cannot keep up with heat loss. Although the newborn infant has the capacity to respond to a cold stress by increasing heat production, the absolute extent to which a newborn can sustain a cold stress and maintain a normal temperature is limited when compared to an adult. In a term infant with little or no clothing, the ambient temperature threshold is approximately 25°C as contrasted with adults under similar conditions in whom 5°C might represent an equivalent stress. The length of time that such a stress may be tolerated without becoming hypothermic is short. Thermal insulation with clothing can lower these temperatures, as will maneuvers that reduce radiative, conductive, and convective heat losses.

As the ambient temperature increases above the neutral thermal environment, body temperature will increase unless heat loss can be enhanced by sweating or changes in the environment. Vasomotor responses will have already been recruited maximally by the time an increase in ambient temperature causes the infant's body temperature to increase. Thus, if sweating is limited, neutral thermal environment is likely near that ambient temperature at which the infant's body temperature begins to increase.

Increased heat loss in the delivery room is associated with morbidity in preterm infants. Strategies to prevent heat loss in preterm infants include (1) increasing delivery room temperature, (2) placing an infant in a plastic bag to minimize convective and evaporative losses, (3) using a radiant warmer, (4) using a thermal mattress, and (5) placing a cap on the infant's head (Fig. 45-4). In contrast, in term

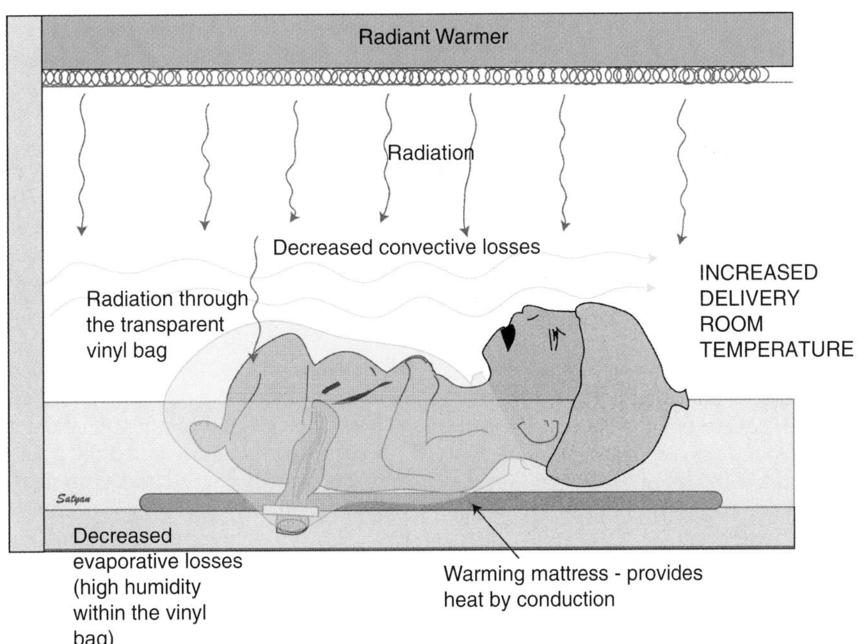


**FIGURE 45-4** In preterm infants, heat loss can be prevented by increasing the delivery room temperature (convection), placing the infant on a heated mattress (conduction) and in a plastic bag (limit evaporation), or using a cap to cover the head under a preheated radiant warmer (radiation). (Used with permission from Satyan Lakshminrusimha.)

infants with perinatal asphyxia and hypoxic ischemic encephalopathy, whole-body or selective head cooling is associated with improved neurodevelopmental outcomes.

## ENDOCRINOLOGIC TRANSITION

The endocrinologic regulation of the fetus is determined to a great extent by the fetus itself, although placental and maternal hormones are important. The capacity for self-regulation occurs early in development. The fetal hypothalamus has demonstrable concentrations of releasing hormones by the late first or early second trimester, and hormone appearance in the pituitary occurs during a similar time frame. Placentally derived hormones include estrogens, progesterone, human chorionic gonadotropin, and human placental lactogen, but the importance to the fetus of many of the placental hormones is uncertain. Although the placenta restricts the movement of many maternal hormones into the fetus, important maternal hormones that cross the placenta directly or do so after modification in the placenta include steroid hormones and thyrotropin-releasing hormone. Cortisol and thyroid hormone are both involved indirectly in postnatal adaptation.

### The Adrenal Gland and Cortisol Production

The fetal adrenal gland develops early in the first trimester and contains the full spectrum of enzymes important in steroidogenesis in the mature adrenal gland. Corticotropin-releasing factor is present in the fetal hypothalamus during early development, and adrenocorticotropin is present at the same time in the pituitary. Adrenocorticotropin has the dual effect of not only increasing steroid synthesis but also promoting growth and maturation of the adrenal gland. Most of the circulating fetal cortisol derives from the fetal adrenal gland with the remainder being transplacental. The synthetic capability of the fetal adrenal gland, at least for cortisol, is at least as great as that in the adult.

Circulating cortisol concentrations increase through development, beginning near the end of the first trimester and increasing more rapidly during the final weeks of gestation. The increase in cortisol during the third trimester appears to have at least a permissive effect on the development of several major organ systems, including the lung, in which the molecular processes important in surfactant homeostasis and in lung water removal are induced circulating cortisol. Although the fetal adrenal gland provides the cortisol needed by the fetus for normal development, under conditions in which sufficient fetal cortisol is unavailable, placental or maternal steroids appear adequate for normal development. At the time of birth, both adrenocorticotropin and cortisol concentrations are increased, at least as compared to their values several days after delivery.

### The Thyroid Axis

Similar to cortisol, thyroid hormone also plays a permissive role in postnatal adaptation. In utero, thyroid hormone concentrations begin to increase near midgestation, increasing more rapidly during the last few weeks before birth and then decreasing during the days to weeks after delivery. At the time of birth, there is an increase in thyroid-stimulating hormone and a several-fold increase in circulating thyroid hormone concentration. The increase in thyroid-stimulating hormone at birth appears to be a result of the thermal stress associated with delivery.

Transplacental passage of maternal thyrotropin-releasing hormone occurs readily, but maternal thyroid-stimulating hormone and thyroid hormone transfer less well. Despite this inefficiency, adequate maternal thyroid hormone is now known to be important for optimal childhood neurologic development. This observation provides an important impetus for treatment of maternal hypothyroidism during pregnancy.

Thyroid hormone appears to play a role in regulating nonshivering thermogenesis and postnatal cardiovascular function, but the role of thyroid hormone in the successful extrauterine transition of the newborn infant is unclear. Patients who are diagnosed with congenital hypothyroidism rarely have clinical abnormalities that bring them to medical attention immediately after birth. This empiric observation highlights the importance of newborn screening programs.

### Glucose Balance

Glucose concentration in the fetal blood during the third trimester of pregnancy is approximately 80% that of the maternal concentration. In the fetus, glucose is supplied transplacentally, and most of this glucose is metabolized by the fetus for energy. There is little, if any, glucose synthesized by the fetus under normal conditions. The small portion of transplacental glucose that is not used immediately as energy is stored as glycogen in the fetal liver, but little glycogen is stored prior to the third trimester. Energy sources other than glucose are available to the fetus, including lactate, free fatty acids, ketones, and amino acids, but glucose is the major metabolic fuel during intrauterine development.

Disturbances of glucose homeostasis are common during the neonatal period (see also Chapter 53). At the time of birth, the maternal glucose delivery to the fetus ceases with clamping of the umbilical cord. Circulating glucose concentrations in the infant must then be maintained by a combination of glycogenolysis and gluconeogenesis until enteral or intravenous glucose is supplied. During the initial 1 to 2 hours after birth, glucose concentration in the newborn decreases substantially and then increases over the next several hours to days to a value of 70 mg/dL. The production of glucose in the newborn averages 4 to 6 mg/kg body weight per minute and exceeds by 2- to 3-fold the basal synthetic rate in adults. The brain consumes a significant amount of the circulating glucose in the newborn because of the disproportionate size of the brain in relation to body weight compared to the adult. The usual postnatal increase in circulating catecholamine and glucagon concentrations, and the simultaneous decrease in insulin concentration, are important factors in the modulation of glucose concentrations in the newborn shortly after birth.

Hepatic glycogen content begins to decrease after delivery and is nearly exhausted by 12 hours after birth in the absence of exogenous glucose. After this time, gluconeogenesis and enteral or intravenous sources of glucose are necessary to assure glucose concentrations remain in an acceptable range. Glycogen stores in the liver release glucose in response to increases in glucagon and circulating catecholamines, changes that are associated with the mechanical event of cord clamping. The normal decrease in insulin concentration after birth also participates in the maintenance of normal circulating concentrations of glucose, although the decline in insulin concentration is not a result of the decrease in glucose concentrations after delivery. The relative contribution of epinephrine, norepinephrine, and glucagon in the regulation of hepatic glycogenolysis postnatally in human infants is incompletely understood because the circulating concentrations of each of these are interdependent. Receptor-mediated stimulation of glycogenolysis occurs with both glucagon and catecholamines. Because hepatic glycogen stores increase significantly only during the latter part of gestation, premature birth increases the risk for hypoglycemia because of the relatively limited supply of glucose from glycogenolysis.

One of the enzymes important in liberating glucose from glycogen is glycogen phosphorylase, an enzyme regulated in part by catecholamines, glucagon, and thermal stress. As a result of the action of this enzyme, glucose-1-phosphate is generated and is itself converted to glucose-6-phosphate. Tissues containing glucose-6-phosphatase can then use it to synthesize glucose and subsequently release it into the circulation. There are, however, a number of tissues that lack glucose-6-phosphatase, and in these tissues, glucose cannot be produced, necessitating that glucose-6-phosphate be metabolized intracellularly.

Because glycogen stores are limited, gluconeogenesis plays a critical role in regulating glucose concentration in the newborn. In animal studies, inhibition of gluconeogenesis after birth results in a profound decrease in circulating glucose concentrations. Lactate, pyruvate, and selected amino acids are substrates from which glucose can be synthesized. The enzymes responsible for the conversion of these compounds include glucose-6-phosphatase, fructose-1,6-diphosphatase, pyruvate carboxylase, and phosphoenolpyruvate carboxykinase. The cytosolic form of phosphoenolpyruvate carboxykinase is the rate-limiting enzyme in gluconeogenesis during development. It increases in concentration rapidly after birth as a result of an increase in transcription.

Events associated with birth are considered the physiologic trigger for the increase in cytosolic activity of phosphoenolpyruvate carboxykinase, but the specific downstream effector molecules associated with birth that increase enzyme activity are unknown.

Although gluconeogenic precursors are essential to hepatic glucose production postnatally, fatty acid oxidation also influences gluconeogenesis. Energy stored as fat exceeds the energy stored as glycogen by 5 to 10 times in the term infant at birth. Medium-chain triglycerides increase gluconeogenesis and circulating glucose concentrations even in the absence of exogenous gluconeogenic precursors. Conversely, inhibition of long-chain fatty acid oxidation results in a significant decrease in circulating glucose concentration.

## GASTROINTESTINAL TRANSITION

The small intestine increases its length (125 cm at 20 weeks' gestation to 275 cm at term and 380 cm at 1 year) and absorptive surface area during the fetal and neonatal periods. Suck-swallow coordination develops at approximately around 34 weeks' gestation. The near-term fetus swallows approximately 50% of the amniotic fluid daily. Amniotic fluid is rich in growth factors that promote intestinal development, and a wide spectrum of proteins, which can be transferred to the fetus through absorption.

Most newborn mammals can absorb intact proteins during the early postnatal period, which allows them to acquire passive immunity by absorbing immunoglobulins in colostrum and breast milk. The ability of the gastrointestinal tract to exclude intact antigenic food proteins increases with gestational age. In both preterm and term infants, intestinal permeability is higher in the first 2 days after birth (a period when colostrum is rich in immunoglobulins) than it is 3 to 6 days after birth.

During fetal life, the gastrointestinal tract receives approximately 5% of the combined ventricular output or 12% of left ventricular output (this has been shown to be 25–30 mL/kg body weight/min in fetal lambs). Intestinal oxygen uptake and blood flow increase dramatically after birth to sustain rapid growth and demands of enteral nutrition. Postnatally, the splanchnic circulation accounts for 20% of cardiac output at baseline (60–70 mL/kg body weight/min). However, splanchnic blood flow increases 30% to 130% after feeds (postprandial hyperemia). The increase in intestinal blood flow in neonates is mediated by components of enteral feeds and other luminal contents: Glucose and solubilized long-chain fatty acids increase jejunal blood flow; bile and bile salts increase ileal flow; and volatile fatty acids from fermentation of undigested carbohydrates increase colonic blood flow. In preterm infants, dietary mixed nucleotides increase superior mesenteric blood flow. The increase in intestinal blood flow after birth following enteral feeding enables the switch from placenta to intestinal tract as the main source of nutrition.

## RENAL TRANSITION

During fetal life, the placenta "excretes" waste products into the maternal circulation. The kidney is involved in the production of hypotonic urine (100–250 mOsm/kg $H_2O$) and is the primary contributor to amniotic fluid during later gestation. Systemic blood pressure (~40–60 mm Hg) is low and the fetal kidney receives only 3% of cardiac output. The renin-angiotensin system is upregulated and renal vascular resistance is high in the fetus. Formation of urine begins by 12 weeks of gestation. The urinary flow increases 10-fold from 6 mL/h at 20 weeks to 60 mL/h at 40 weeks of gestational age (~15 mL/kg/h).

In term newborns, nephrogenesis is complete at birth. As mentioned previously, the transition from the fetal circulation to extrauterine life is characterized by a rapid increase in systemic blood pressure. Renal blood flow is low and increases markedly in the first 24 hours after birth. At birth, the glomerular filtration rate (GFR) is low compared to adult values: 20 mL/min/1.73 $m^2$ in term newborns and less than 15 mL/min/1.73 $m^2$ in preterm newborns. Renal blood flow increases from 6% of cardiac output to 10% after the first postnatal week and GFR increases 2.5- to 3-fold during the first month of postnatal life.

## WATER BALANCE

During fetal development, the proportion of body weight composed of water decreases from 80% to 85% at 24 weeks' gestation to 75% to 80% at term. In term infants at birth, intracellular water accounts for two-thirds of total body water, and extracellular water accounts for the remaining one-third. During the first week after birth, body weight decreases, an effect that is the result of water loss. The changes in water balance associated with birth appear to begin shortly before delivery. The biological basis of these changes is not completely understood but likely arises from perinatal changes in circulating hormone concentrations, which result in a loss of fluid from the circulation into the interstitial space and a simultaneous increase in hematocrit. Longer-term changes in body water balance occur after birth as well. During the first week after delivery, infants born at term tend to lose about 5% of their birth weight as a result of a decrease in both intracellular and interstitial fluid.

### Postnatal Weight Loss

In the preterm infant, body weight decreases after birth in a fashion similar to that seen in term infants, but in an exaggerated fashion. Infants born modestly preterm may lose 5% to 10% of their birth weight, whereas the youngest of premature infants may lose 15% to 20% of their birth weight with no apparent ill effects. This weight loss results from salt and water loss during the first week of life, and the fluid is lost primarily from the interstitial space. Whether this weight loss is "normal" is a matter of definition. The spontaneous feeding and apparent health of term newborns lends itself well to describing the observed weight loss in term infants as normal. However, because fluid intake in small premature infants is often determined by rates of intravenous fluid infusions, these smallest of preterm infants cannot be considered to regulate fluid intake in the same manner as term infants. Thus, the range of "normal" for variables such as weight loss in this population is somewhat arbitrary and probably should be abandoned in favor of what is most desirable for optimal health. In this regard, the interpretation of epidemiological and prospective intervention studies suggests that there is a direct relationship between morbidity and the abundance of salt and water intake, at least in the early newborn period. Thus, the most prudent extrapolation of this information would lead to a strategy in which fluid intake is adjusted to allow a gradual loss of body weight over the first postnatal week, with restriction of sodium intake until near the time when the target weight loss has occurred. Frequent measurement of body weight, urine output, and serum concentrations of electrolytes help to assure this gradual transition.

## OTHER FACTORS INFLUENCING THE TRANSITION TO NEWBORN LIFE

The changes at birth described above typically refer to term infants delivered by spontaneous vaginal delivery. Infants delivered by elective or emergent cesarean section experience a delay in resorption of fetal lung liquid and decrease in PVR after birth and are at higher risk for respiratory problems such as transient tachypnea of newborn (TTN) and persistent pulmonary hypertension of the newborn (PPHN). Preterm infants have a lower surfactant pool and are at risk for RDS. Preterm infants are also at risk for electrolyte imbalance due to renal immaturity, hypoglycemia due to impaired glucose homeostasis, and hypothermia. "Delayed" cord clamping refers to avoiding clamping the umbilical cord soon after birth and allowing transfusion of fetal blood from the placenta to the neonate. This practice increases the blood volume of the newborn and has been found to be beneficial in reducing intraventricular hemorrhage in preterm infants and increasing iron load in term infants.

## SUGGESTED READINGS

Downs CA, Kriener LH, Yu L, Eaton DC, Jain L, Helms MN. β-Adrenergic agonists differentially regulate highly selective and nonselective epithelial sodium channels to promote alveolar fluid clearance in vivo. *Am Journal Physiol Lung Cell Mol Physiol.* 2012;302(11):L1167-L1178.

Fawcett K. Preventing admission hypothermia in very low birth weight neonates. *Neonatal Netw*. 2014;33(3):143-149.

Guemes M, Rahman SA, Hussain K. What is a normal blood glucose? *Arch Dis Child*. 2016;101(6):569-574.

Hooper SB, Te Pas AB, Kitchen MJ. Respiratory transition in the newborn: a three-phase process. *Arch Dis Child Fetal Neonatal Ed*. 2016;101(3):F266-F271.

Jain L. Alveolar fluid clearance in developing lungs and its role in neonatal transition. *Clin Perinatol*. 1999;26(3):585-599.

Kiserud T. Physiology of the fetal circulation. *Semin Fetal Neonatal Med*. 2005;10(6):493-503.

Kota S, Gayatri K, Jammula S, et al. Fetal endocrinology. *Indian J Endocrinol Metab*. 2013;17(4):568-579.

Lakshminrusimha S, Saugstad OD. The fetal circulation, pathophysiology of hypoxemic respiratory failure and pulmonary hypertension in neonates, and the role of oxygen therapy. *J Perinatol*. 2016;36 Suppl 2:S3-S11.

Laptook AR, Watkinson M. Temperature management in the delivery room. *Semin Fetal Neonatal Med*. 2008;13(6):383-391.

Polin RA, Abman SH, Rowitch D, Benitz WE, Fox WW, eds. *Fetal and Neonatal Physiology*. 5th ed. Philadelphia, PA: Elsevier Health Sciences; 2016.

Prsa M, Sun L, van Amerom J, et al. Reference ranges of blood flow in the major vessels of the normal human fetal circulation at term by phase-contrast magnetic resonance imaging. *Circ Cardiovasc Imaging*. 2014;7(4):663-670.

Saint-Faust M, Boubred F, Simeoni U. Renal development and neonatal adaptation. *Am Journal Perinatol*. 2014;31(9):773-780.

Steinhorn RH. Advances in neonatal pulmonary hypertension. *Neonatology*. 2016;109(4):334-344.

Whitsett JA, Wert SE, Weaver TE. Diseases of pulmonary surfactant homeostasis. *Annu Rev Pathol*. 2015;10:371-393.

Wood CE. Development and programming of the hypothalamus-pituitary-adrenal axis. *Clin Obstet Gynecol*. 2013;56(3):610-621.



# 46 Examination of the Newborn Infant

John Flibotte and Ganga Gokulakrishnan

## GENERAL PRINCIPLES

The newborn examination is largely seen as a screening examination for congenital anomalies or for problems that are expected to present soon after birth. The recommendations as to the optimal timing of the examination vary, and while a thorough examination can be carried out in the delivery room, recent years have seen a renewed emphasis on the importance of this time for families to bond with their newborn, for the establishment of successful breastfeeding, and for limiting medicalization. Moreover, while some major anomalies should be apparent at birth, other conditions are less apparent and may evolve over time, making later examination of higher value. For these reasons, and following from the United Nations Children's Fund (UNICEF)/World Health Organization (WHO) Baby Friendly Initiatives, many hospitals now seek to limit initial examination of newborns immediately after birth to a health screen with a more thorough examination taking place later on but prior to hospital discharge (Table 46-1).

The neonatal examination is best performed in an appropriately equipped, well lit, warm, draft-free room, with the parents present. Examining the infant under a servo-controlled radiant warmer is an alternative. Thorough hand-washing before and after handling each infant is essential to prevent the spread of pathogenic organisms, and if the infant has not had a first bath, gloves should be worn.

Parental presence is important so that one can address their specific concerns. Observation of the undisturbed infant's appearance, posture, and state of consciousness should precede the formal aspects of palpation and auscultation. Isolated minor congenital anomalies are quite common, with some studies reporting these in as many as 15% of the newborn population, but the presence of 3 or more increases the risk of the infant having a syndrome. Evidence of trauma in 1 part of the baby should lead to a search for trauma in other areas, particularly in large infants and in infants who underwent difficult deliveries such as breech or forceps delivery. It is also important to be able to distinguish malformations from deformations as the etiology and managements differ.

A thorough history that includes the maternal medical, antenatal, and obstetric history is crucial as this will allow the clinician to focus on aspects of the newborn physical examination that are pertinent to the history. For example, polyhydramnios may signal bowel obstruction and oligohydramnios may signal renal anomalies and pulmonary insufficiency. Small-for-gestational-age and postmature infants are at increased risk for hypoglycemia and polycythemia. Prolonged rupture of the membranes, maternal fever, and fetal tachycardia may signal neonatal sepsis. The neonatal consequences of intrauterine growth restriction, prematurity, multiple births, maternal diabetes, and meconium-stained amniotic fluid are discussed in detail elsewhere.

## PHYSICAL EXAMINATION

### Gestational Age and Size

The infant's gestational age should be estimated and body size compared with appropriate normal standards. There are several ways to estimate gestational age, including reliable maternal history, prenatal ultrasound scan performed before 20 weeks of gestation, and physical examination of the infant's skin, external genitalia, ears, breasts, and neuromuscular behavior (Fig. 46-1). Infants are classified as *preterm* (born at less than 37 completed weeks of gestation), *early term* (37–38 weeks), *term* (39 to 41 weeks), and *postterm* (> 42 weeks).

Birth weight, head circumference, and length should be measured. Length is measured from vertex to heel with the infant's legs fully extended. These measurements are then compared for gestational age against standard population-based growth charts. An infant is considered to be appropriate for gestational age (AGA) if the birth weight for gestational age falls between the 10th and 90th percentile. Twenty percent of infants with serious congenital malformations are small for gestational age (see Chapter 49).

In the following sections, elements of the physical examination of the newborn are reviewed by organ system with a focus on how to perform the exam and normal or expected findings. Table 46-2 summarizes common abnormal findings and provides brief descriptions of each as well as diagnoses that should be considered.

### General Inspection

Most babies born at term cry at birth, quickly establish regular breathing, and may remain awake and active for 30 minutes or more, during which their eyes are open; they make sucking, chewing, and swallowing movements; and they may have bursts of flexion and extension of extremities with facial grimaces. Term infants spend approximately 80% of the time in active or quiet sleep. The remaining 20% of the time is spent awake in varying states of activity with or without crying.

Initially, infants often adopt a position similar to that assumed in utero. Placing a crying infant into this posture often calms the infant. About 2% of infants have significant deformities caused by mechanical forces that are often the result of oligohydramnios, uterine malformations, or multiple gestation.

### Temperature

The normal infant is pink and well-perfused and feels warm to the touch, but exposure to even a moderately cold environment leads to the hands and feet quickly becoming cool and slightly cyanotic. The *normal*

**TABLE 46-1 DIAGNOSTIC PERFORMANCE OF THE NEONATAL PHYSICAL EXAM FOR DETECTING TARGET CONDITIONS**

| Target Condition | Sens | Spec | PPV | NPV | LR+ |
|---|---|---|---|---|---|
| Cardiac disease[a] | 63% | 98% | 1.35 | 99.98 | 32.4 |
| Developmental hip dysplasia[b] | 74–99% | 98–99% | NR | NR | 37–99 |
| Congenital cataract[c] | 85 | 94.3 | 18.7–42[d] | 99.96 | 14.9 |
| Neurologic abnormality[e] | 91 | 79 | 76 | 92 | 4.3 |

[a]de-Wahl Granelli, Wennergren, Sandberg, et al, 2009.

[b]Witt, 2003.

[c]Ruttum, Nelson, Wamser, Bailliff, 1987.

[d]Eventov-Friedman, Leiba, Flidel-Rimon, Juster-Reicher, Shinwell, 2010.

[e]Wusthoff, 2013.

LR, likelihood ratio; NPV, negative predictive value; NR, not reported; PPV, positive predictive value; Sens, sensitivity; Spec, specificity.

*axillary temperature* is between 36.5°C and 37.4°C. The most common reasons for a low or high temperature are exposure to a cool environment and overheating.

### Skin

**Gestational Changes** Fine, soft, *lanugo hair* covers the entire body in very preterm infants and disappears from the face and lower back between 32 and 37 weeks. The term infant has lanugo hair on the upper back and dorsal aspects of the limbs. *Vernix caseosa*, a thick, white material with the consistency of soft cheese, covers the skin of the entire body until 35 to 37 weeks. By term, the amount of vernix is limited mainly to the flexor creases. The subcutaneous tissue is relatively thick, and the fingernails and toenails are fully formed and extend slightly beyond the ends of the digits. If fetal stress occurs at term, *meconium* may be passed into the amniotic fluid. If meconium has been in the amniotic fluid for several hours, it will also stain the skin, fingernails, toenails, and umbilical cord with a greenish hue. Fetuses at less than 34 weeks of gestation rarely pass meconium. The postmature infant (beyond 42 weeks) may have a somewhat wasted appearance with dry, peeling skin, a decreased amount of subcutaneous tissue, long fingernails, and an alert appearance.

**Skin Abnormalities** Neonates often have skin rashes, some of which indicate a serious systemic issue. These are summarized in Table 46-2. Much more common than these serious rashes are many benign skin lesions that are important to recognize and explain to parents. Disorders of the skin are also described in detail in Section 18.

**Color** Abnormalities of skin color that exist after completing the transition from birth are important and may suggest serious underlying pathology, examples of which are summarized in Table 46-2. There may be cyanosis of the hands and feet (*acrocyanosis*), which is normal immediately after birth or if the infant has been exposed to a cold environment. *Harlequin skin* describes a transient change in the skin color of no known pathologic significance: 1 side of the body turns pale while the other side remains pink with a sharp line of demarcation in the midline.

*Ecchymoses* or localized *petechiae* generally result from birth trauma and are often present over the head after vertex delivery or on



| Physical Findings | | Gestation (week) 20 21 22 23 24 25 26 27 28 29 30 31 32 33 34 35 36 37 38 39 40 41 42 43 44 45 46 47 48 | | | | | |
|---|---|---|---|---|---|---|---|
| Vernix | | Appears | Covers body, thick layer | On back, scalp, in the creases | Scant, in the creases | No vernix | |
| Breast Tissue and Areola | | Areola and nipple barely visible No palpable breast tissue | Areola raised | 1–2 mm nodule | 3–5 mm | 5–6 mm | 7–10 mm |
| Ear | Form | Flat, shapeless | Beginning incurving superior | Incurving upper 2/3 pinnae | Well-defined incurving to lobe | | |
| | Cartilage | Pinna soft, stays folded | Cartilage scant, returns slowly from folding | Thin cartilage, springs back from folding | Pinna firm, remains erect from head | | |
| Sole Creases | | Smooth soles without creases | 1–2 anterior creases | 2–3 anterior creases | Creases anterior 2/3 sole | Creases involving heel | Deeper creases over entire sole |
| Skin | Thickness and Appearance | Thin, translucent skin, piethoric, venules over abdomen, edema | Smooth, thicker, no edema | Pink | Few vessels | Some desquamation, pale pink | Thick, pale, desquamation over entire body |
| | Nail Plates | Appear | | Nails to finger tips | Nails extend well beyond finger tips | | |
| Hair | | Appear on head | Eyebrows and lashes | Fine, wooly; bunches out from head | Silky, single strands, lays flat | Receding hairline or loss of baby hair, short/fine underneath | |
| Lanugo | | Appears | Covers entire body | Vanishes from face | Present on shoulders | No lanugo | |
| Genitalia | Testes | | Testes palpable in inguinal canal | In upper scrotum | In lower scrotum | | |
| | Scrotum | | Few rugae | Rugae, anterior portion | Rugae cover | Pendulous | |
| | Labia and Clitoris | | Prominent clitoris; labia majora small, widely separated | Labia majora larger, nearly covers clitoris | Labia minora and clitoris covered | | |
| Skull Firmness | | Bones are soft | Soft to 1 in from anterior fontanelle | Spongy at edges of fontanelle, center firm | Bones hard, sutures easily displaced | Bones hard, cannot be displaced | |

**FIGURE 46-1** Examination: first hours of life. (Adapted with permission from Kempe C, Silver H, O'Brien D: *Current Pediatric Diagnosis and Treatment*, 3rd ed. Los Altos: Lange; 1974.)

TABLE 46-2 **PHYSICAL EXAMINATION AND SUGGESTED DIAGNOSES BY SYSTEM**

| System | Finding | Description | Conditions Associated with the Finding |
|---|---|---|---|
| General inspection | Abnormal cry | Weak/whimpering | General illness, hypotonia, other |
| | | High-pitched/shrieking | Neurologic issue, drug withdrawal, mild hypoxic ischemic encephalopathy |
| | | Hoarse cry | Vocal cord paralysis, hypothyroidism, trauma to the hypopharynx |
| Temperature | Hypothermia | < 36.5°C | Sepsis, hypoglycemia, hypoxia, hypothyroidism |
| | Hyperthermia | ≥ 38°C | Drug withdrawal, intracranial hemorrhage, adrenal hemorrhage |
| Skin | Thrombocytopenia purpura | Red or purple nonblanching spots | Impaired platelet production or function, infection, sites of pressure, nuchal cord (if limited to face) |
| | Blueberry muffin rash | Macular or slightly raised purple lesions | Congenital rubella or congenital leukemia |
| | Maculopapular rash | Red, flat rash with merging spots | Toxoplasmosis |
| | | Pink, later turning brown and/or hemorrhagic | Syphilis, especially if on palms and soles |
| | Vesicles on a red base | Thin, fluid-filled blister | Herpes simplex |
| | Pustules and/or generalized erythema | | Staphyloccoal infection, including scalded skin syndrome, toxic epidermal necrolysis, or Ritter disease |
| | Purple military granulomas | | Listeria monocytogenes |
| | Macerated red skin, especially in diaper area | | Cutaneous moniliasis |
| | Abnormal color | Pallor | Poor perfusion (if also delayed capillary refill), anemia (if involving mucous membranes) |
| | | Gray | Metabolic acidosis |
| | | Mottling | Sepsis, hypothermia |
| | | Plethora | Polycythemia (infant of diabetic mother) |
| | | Cyanosis | Hypoxemia, methemoglobinemia |
| Scalp | Caput succedaneum | Edema of the scalp, crosses suture lines | Local pressure/trauma during labor |
| | Subgaleal hemorrhage | Blood collection under the galea aponeurotica, palpable fluid wave, tensely distended scalp with potential displacement of ears forward and laterally | Trauma; can evolve into shock |
| | Cephalohematomas | Subperiosteal hemorrhages that are confined to suture lines, firm fluctuant masses typically on occipital or parietal bones | Trauma during labor |
| Eyes | Congenital lid ptosis | Drooping lid | Horner syndrome (if with miosis and enophthalmos) |
| | Failure to close eyes fully | | Facial paralysis |
| | Congenital microphthalmia | Small eyes | Genetic syndromes |
| | Proptosis | Bulging eyes | Mass lesions, retrobulbar hemorrhage |
| | Conjunctivitis | Red injection of the sclera | *Staphylococcus aureus*, streptococci, coliform bacteria, gonococcal infections, *Chlamydia trachomatis* (especially if toward end of first week) |
| | Eye drainage | Yellowish discharge from 1 or both eyes in absence of conjunctivitis | Lacrimal duct obstruction (dacryostenosis) |
| Ears/nose/throat | Ear abnormalities | Preauricular pits/skin tags | Normal variant and inherited in autosomal dominant fashion, may warrant hearing testing |
| | | Malformed auricles | Result from in utero positioning, may also be seen in genetic syndromes |
| | | Low-set ears (below lateral epicanthus) | Suggestive of genetic syndrome |
| | Nasal obstruction | May manifest as respiratory distress except when crying | Choanal atresia, encephalocele |
| Chest/lungs | Tachypnea | > 60 breaths per minute | Acidosis, respiratory distress syndrome, pneumonia, meconium aspiration, cardiac disease |
| | Asymmetric chest movement | | Phrenic nerve palsy, intrathoracic mass/congenital diaphragmatic hernia |
| Heart and vasculature | Bradycardia | < 80 beats per minute | Birth asphyxia, increased intracranial pressure, hypothyroidism, heart block |
| | Tachycardia | > 160 beats per minute | Hypovolemia, fever, pain, drug withdrawal, poor perfusion, tachyarrhythmias, anemia, hyperthyroidism |

(Continued)

**TABLE 46-2 PHYSICAL EXAMINATION AND SUGGESTED DIAGNOSES BY SYSTEM (CONTINUED)**

| System | Finding | Description | Conditions Associated with the Finding |
|---|---|---|---|
| Abdomen | Scaphoid abdomen | Hollow/scooped out | Congenital diaphragmatic hernia |
| | Distended abdomen | Large, firm, visible superficial veins | Bowel obstruction, volvulus, intra-abdominal mass |
| | Prune belly | Absent abdominal musculature, shriveled skin | Urinary tract abnormalities and obstruction |
| | Abdominal wall defects | Visible intestinal structures outside the abdominal wall | Omphalocele and gastroschisis (**Chapters 63** and **391**) |
| | Umbilical cord drainage | | Vitelline duct remnants, persistent urachus |
| | Abdominal mass | | Usually renal in origin (> 50%), also consider neuroblastoma, anterior meningomyelocele |
| | Red abdominal wall | | Omphalitis |
| Genitalia | Hydrometrocolpos | Collection of blood in the uterus | Imperforate hymen, vaginal atresia |
| | Micropenis | Penile length < 2.5 cm | Suggests potential endocrinopathy |
| | Hypospadias | Ventral defect of varying length along the penis | Can require surgical intervention |
| | Chordee | Ventral bend in penis | |
| | Epispadias | Dorsal defect on the penis | Variant of bladder exstrophy |
| | Hydroceles | Fluid collections in remnants of the processus vaginalis | Common variants |
| | Testicular enlargement/ discoloration | | Testicular torsion (can be present at birth) |
| Limbs | Hemihypertrophy/ hemiatrophy | Limbs on each side of body are different in size but normally proportioned | Genetic syndromes |
| | Phocomelia | Underdevelopment and abnormal shape of limbs to a variable degree | In utero toxic exposures, genetic syndromes |
| | Arthrogryposis multiplex congenita | Severe contractions of multiple joints that cannot correct with manual pressure | Neurologic injury, genetic syndromes |
| | Syndactyly | Fusion of digits | Genetic syndromes |
| | Polydactyly | Extra digits | Genetic syndromes; often can be an inherited normal variant in families (postaxial polydactyly) |

the feet, lower limbs, and buttocks following breech delivery. More generalized petechiae suggest thrombocytopenia. *Subcutaneous fat necrosis* appears as red lesions where the subcutaneous tissue is hard and sharply demarcated, and is usually seen over the cheeks, buttocks, limbs, or back.

Neonatal *jaundice* is caused by an elevation in indirect-reacting bilirubin, resulting in a yellow-to-green discoloration of skin. It is assessed by briefly pressing on the infant's skin with a finger and observing the color in the blanched area. One must be cautious in interpreting the intensity of jaundice based on physical exam as visual assessment of jaundice has been shown to be unreliable. Mild physiologic jaundice usually develops 2 to 4 days after birth. However, jaundice in the first day warrants prompt investigation; it is usually from sepsis or hemolytic anemia (see Chapter 56).

### The Head

The *head shape* is influenced by their presentation in utero. After vertex presentation and vaginal delivery, infants demonstrate pronounced vertical elongation of the head referred to as molding. Breech infants often have occipital-frontal head elongation, with a prominent occipital shelf.

The cranial sutures should be palpably open and may be separated by up to several millimeters at birth. Temporary overlap of bones, due to molding, should be distinguished from *craniosynostosis* (premature closure of a suture). If a suture closes in utero, it prevents growth of the skull perpendicular to the fused suture line, resulting in a sustained, abnormal skull configuration. In contrast, after molding occurs, the bones return to their normal positions in a few days, sometimes with a small concomitant decrease in head circumference.

Normally, the *anterior fontanelle* is open, soft, and flat, and the mean diameter is less than 3.5 cm. The *posterior fontanelle* is often fingertip size or just palpably open. A *bulging* or *tense fontanelle*, with separation of the bony sutures, indicates increased intracranial pressure. A *circular hematoma* may be seen at the site of application of a vacuum extractor. Other typical findings are summarized in Table 46-2.

### Face

The newborn's face may indicate the presence of a dysmorphic syndrome. There may be obvious malformations, such as cleft lip or a small mandible (micrognathia). Intrauterine position may cause asymmetry of the face. Pressure over the stylomastoid foramen during labor may cause a peripheral *facial paralysis*, which is obvious during crying. The paralysis usually resolves and should be distinguished from congenital absence of the depressor anguli oris muscle, which also results in an *asymmetric crying facies*. *Fracture* of the zygomatic arch can occur and is detectable by palpation. *Forceps* often leave bruises on the face, usually in the shape of the forceps blade.

### Eyes

Newborns generally open their eyes when they are awake, held upright, and shaded from bright light. An infant who is quiet and alert will fix on the examiner's face and follow it.

Birth trauma may cause *subconjunctival hemorrhages* or hemorrhages in the *anterior chamber*, *vitreous*, and *retina*. Forceps deliveries can result in *lacerations* of the lid or globe. A rupture of the Descemet membrane in the cornea may result in corneal clouding.

Ophthalmoscopic examination should be performed in newborn infants prior to their discharge. One holds the ophthalmoscope close to the examiner's eye with the lens power set at 0. In a dark room, light is allowed to project simultaneously in both eyes and then individually from 18 inches away. It should begin by focusing on the anterior portion of the eye and then progressing back to the retina. This allows detection of anterior lesions, such as cataracts and *colobomas* of the iris. In fair babies, a *red reflex* is transmitted back through the lens, whereas in darker skinned infants a *paler orange-tan* color may be seen. It should be symmetrical in color and intensity. Visualizing retinal vessels verifies focusing on the retina. A diminished or absent red reflex suggests a cataract or other opacities. A *white pupillary reflex* is abnormal and may occur with a large retinoblastoma or developmental abnormalities such as retinal coloboma, retinopathy of prematurity, and persistent hypoplastic primary vitreous.

### Ears

At term, the ears are well formed and contain sufficient cartilage to retain a normal shape and resist deformation. Gently pulling the pinna back and down aids examination of the *ear canal* and *tympanic membrane*. An alert, normal newborn will turn toward human speech and startle to a loud noise, which is a considered a crude estimate of hearing.

### Nose

Most newborn infants are nose breathers. Occasional sneezing is the normal mechanism infants use to clear the nose. Nasal patency can be verified by checking each naris for a good airstream with a thin strip of tissue or cotton and if in doubt confirmed with passage of a thin catheter. *Nasal stuffiness* can occur as a result of retained mucus or trauma but could also suggest drug withdrawal.

### Mouth

Examination of the mouth includes inspection and palpation. A *cleft palate* may not be seen but may be detectable by palpation; a *cleft uvula* should raise suspicion of a palatal defect. Small, shiny white masses on the gums (*epithelial pearls*) are common. White *Epstein pearls* are found in the midline on the roof of the mouth, at the junction of the hard and soft palate. A *ranula* is a small benign mass (ie, mucocele) that arises from the floor of the mouth. A *high-arched* or *narrow palate* is found in many dysmorphic syndromes.

The tongue may be attached to a short central *frenulum* (ie, *ankyloglossia*). An enlarged or *protruding tongue* can be seen with hemangiomas, isolated macroglossia, hypothyroidism, or in Down and Beckwith syndromes. The normal, awake newborn will usually suck vigorously on a finger placed in the mouth. *Natal teeth*, if present, usually erupt in the lower incisor position. These can either be supernumerary teeth or true, deciduous "milk" teeth. If very loose or the cause of painful breast feeding, they may be removed.

### Neck

The neck of the newborn should have a full range of motion; limitation may indicate an abnormality of the cervical spine. Cervical masses, such as a *goiter*, *cavernous hemangioma*, or *cystic hygroma*, may compress the trachea and cause inspiratory obstruction. *Brachial cleft anomalies* include cysts or sinuses along the anterior edge of the sternocleidomastoid muscle. *Thyroglossal duct cysts* usually occur in the ventral midline. *Torticollis* is seen with a tightened sternocleidomastoid muscle on 1 side and an atretic sternocleidomastoid muscle on the side toward which the head is turned; facial asymmetry is a common accompaniment.

Lateral traction during delivery may damage the upper root of the brachial plexus (C5 or C6 vertebra), resulting in paralysis of the shoulder and arm. The arm is held alongside the body in internal rotation (ie, Duchenne-Erb paralysis). The lower root of the brachial plexus (C8 or T1 vertebra) may be damaged, particularly during breech delivery. When this occurs, the small muscles of the hand are paralyzed, resulting in the absence of grasp reflex (ie, Klumpke paralysis). When there is neck trauma, the cervical sympathetic nerves may be damaged (ie, Horner syndrome), and the phrenic nerve may be injured, causing diaphragmatic paralysis.

### Chest

The chest of the normal newborn is barrel-shaped, with the xiphoid often prominent. The most frequent birth injury to the thoracic region is *fracture of the clavicles*, identified by crepitation upon clavicle palpation. *Supernumerary nipples* are a common minor anomaly; *wide spacing* of nipples is seen in Turner syndrome. *Breast engorgement* may occur in boys or girls and increases over the first few days.

### Lungs

The *normal respiratory rate* is 35 to 60 breaths per minute. Excursion of the abdomen is quite prominent, as infants breathe principally with their diaphragms. With normal breathing, the chest and abdomen move together. When the airway is obstructed or the lungs are stiff, the abdomen appears to enlarge and the chest cage appears to get smaller with inspiration (ie, *thoracoabdominal asynchrony*). *Intercostal retractions* are normal during the first few minutes after birth. Thereafter, they are usually a sign of increased inspiratory effort from noncompliant lungs or airway obstruction. Mild *expiratory grunting*, *nasal flaring*, and *tachypnea* occur during the first few minutes after birth. Scattered crackles caused by residual retained intra-alveolar lung fluid often clears rapidly. Persistence or worsening of respiratory symptoms may indicate more serious problems (see Table 46-2).

### Heart and Vasculature

The point of *maximal cardiac impulse* is at the fourth to fifth intercostal space and medial to the midclavicular line on the left side of the chest. This may be displaced if there is a pneumothorax or space-occupying lesion.

The heart rate may be 160 to 180 beats per minute (bpm) during the first few hours after birth. Thereafter, the normal *awake heart rate* averages 120 to 130 bpm. Occasionally, a normal newborn infant may have a heart rate of 80 bpm, which may fall transiently to 60 bpm for short periods. Heart rates outside these ranges should be investigated (see Table 46-2).

Despite the rapid heart rate, *heart sounds* can be clearly distinguished. The pulmonic component of $S_2$ may be prominent on the first day. Splitting of the second sound is audible along the left upper and midsternum. While postnatal circulatory adjustments are occurring, transient benign *murmurs* can be heard over the pulmonic area or cardiac apex. Murmurs, other physical signs such as cyanosis, poor perfusion, tachypnea, difficulty in palpating pulses or brachiofemoral delay require further evaluation (see Chapters 51, 478, and 479).

### Abdomen

Infants often have abdomens that are bulging at the sides but they should be soft. History of maternal polyhydramnios should raise concern for possible intestinal obstruction. A gap between the abdominal rectus muscles in the midline (ie, *diastasis recti*), most noticeable with crying, is quite common. There is also often a small defect in the periumbilical musculature of the anterior abdominal wall, which may allow an *umbilical hernia*; this usually closes as the muscles develop toward the end of the first year.

The *umbilical cord* normally contains 2 arteries and 1 vein, with the vein being larger than the arteries. Approximately 1% of newborns have a *single umbilical artery*, and 15% of these have 1 or more congenital anomalies, usually involving the nervous, gastrointestinal, genitourinary, pulmonary, or cardiovascular system.

Palpation of the abdomen should be gentle and not be done immediately after a feed. The edge of the *liver* is normally felt 1 to 2 cm below the right costal margin. The *spleen* tip may be palpable but usually is no more than 1 cm below the rib margin. In some pathologic conditions, the liver and spleen may be so massively enlarged that their edges are in the pelvis and not initially identified. Renal examination is easiest on the first day, before the bowel is filled with gas. The lower portion of each *kidney* is normally palpable on each side; the lateral and lower edges can be felt above the level of the umbilicus and lateral to the midclavicular line. The right kidney is situated slightly lower than the left kidney, and the palpable portion of the kidney normally feels about 2 cm wide.

The *umbilical cord* usually falls off between 10 and 14 days, releasing a small amount of opaque, yellowish discharge. Delayed separation of the cord, past 3 weeks, often occurs in infants with defective phagocyte function. A small, raw-appearing granuloma at the site of cord separation is termed an *umbilical polyp*. During the first week, a small amount of erythema at the rim of the umbilical stump is common and of no consequence, but more extensive erythema or edema may indicate the onset of *omphalitis*.

### External Genitalia

In preterm female infants, separation of the labia majora may give the illusion that the *clitoris* is enlarged. In term female infants, the labia majora meet in the midline, covering the rest of the genitalia. It is important to identify the *urethra*, which is just below the clitoris, and the vagina as distinct orifices; a single orifice or urogenital sinus is abnormal. Normally, the vagina has white secretions secondary to fetal stimulation by maternal hormones; the secretions persist for a week and occasionally become blood tinged.

The term male newborn has a *penis* approximately 3 to 4 cm long and a *scrotum* that is pigmented and has extensive rugae. The *testes* are usually in the scrotum but, if not fully descended, are often palpable in the upper scrotum or inguinal canal. Specific abnormalities of both female and male genitalia are summarized in Table 46-2.

*Ambiguous genitalia* is a term that encompasses a wide range of findings such as enlargement of the clitoris and varying degrees of labial fusion in females or micropenis, hypospadias with bifid scrotum, and cryptorchidism in males. As the distinction between a male and female can often be difficult, the assistance of a pediatric endocrinologist is warranted. In such situations, it may be prudent to avoid assigning a sex until further investigation (see Chapter 532).

#### Anus

A thorough examination is required to confirm anal patency, as an imperforate anus is not always obvious on inspection. A normal appearing anal dimple can exist with no opening. A fistula that opens onto the perineum, ventral to the normal anus, may also accompany the imperforate anus. However, this fistula will not have the radiating skin creases of a normal anus. Presence of meconium on the perineum and perianal area does not rule out imperforate anus; meconium in the anal area may have been passed by way of the skin fistula or, in a girl, a fistula from the rectum to the vagina.

#### Spine

The spine of the newborn is quite flexible in both the dorsoventral and lateral axes; restricted movement suggests vertebral anomalies. The entire length of the spine, including the sacrum, should be palpated for bony defects and asymmetries. A *midline abnormality* of the skin over the spine, such as a small dimple, tufts of hair, or a pilonidal sinus, may indicate an occult spina bifida or a *diastematomyelia* (ie, a division of the spinal cord into 2 parts, which may become tethered as the child grows). Neural tube defects (ie, *meningocele* and *myelomeningocele)* and tumors of the spine (ie, teratomas) also may be present at birth (see Chapter 542).

#### Limbs

Traumatic injuries to the limbs can occur as a consequence of intrauterine positioning and delivery. These include fractures in the shaft of the femur, humerus, or clavicles and injury to the brachial plexus, causing paralysis of the hand and arm.

It is important to be able to distinguish normal variations in joint positions from joints that are deformed. As a rule, if simple manual pressure will correct a deformed joint back to its neutral position, then corrective positioning or simple exercise and stretching will correct the deformity. If the deformity cannot be corrected by gentle pressure, orthopedic evaluation is needed.

With the hips flexed to 90 degrees, the legs normally can be abducted until the knees touch the table the infant is lying on. If this cannot be done, there may be *developmental dysplasia of the hip.* Female infants constrained in a breech position in utero are at a higher risk. In this condition, the head of the femur is displaced posteriorly, out of the acetabular fossa. The affected leg may appear shorter. The examiner will feel a click when abducting and adducting the hips in about 10% of all infants. However, only 10% of infants with hip clicks have developmental dysplasia of the hip. The Ortolani and the Barlow maneuvers can test for a dislocatable hip (see Chapter 212).

Malformations of the limbs are often obvious and are the subject of other chapters. However, terms associated and used to describe abnormalities are summarized in Table 46-2. Often, limb abnormalities are indicators of underlying genetic syndromes. The notable exceptions are those associated with traumatic amputation from amniotic band syndrome. These intrauterine constriction bands may amputate the digits or cause localized edema by obstructing lymphatic drainage.

## THE NEUROLOGIC EXAMINATION

Interpretation of neurologic signs in a newborn infant requires knowledge of normal development because maturational changes parallel increase in level and complexity of neurologic function. It is useful to retain the basic approach in evaluating neurologic function, including



**TABLE 46-3 CRANIAL NERVE EXAMINATION**

| Observation | Cranial Nerve Assessed |
|---|---|
| Pupillary light reflex (> 28 weeks) | II, III |
| Blinking (> 28 weeks) | II, VII |
| Fixing on objects and tracking (> 34 weeks) | II-IV, VI |
| Corneal reflex | V |
| Withdrawal to pinprick to face | V |
| Ptosis and asymmetric facies while crying | VII |
| Blinking to a loud noise | VIII |
| Sucking | V, VII, VIII |
| Swallowing | IX, X |
| Atrophy/fasciculation of tongue | XI |
| Atrophy/contracture of sternocleidomastoid | XII |

a systematic assessment of mental status (ie, level of alertness), cranial nerve function, the motor and sensory systems, and the evoked reflexes.

#### Mental Status

Mental status examination consists of observing spontaneous eye opening and movements of the eyes, face, and extremities, as well as the response to stimulation. A preterm infant born before 32 weeks of gestation spends much of the time sleeping but can be aroused by gentle stimulation. After 32 weeks of gestation, there are periods of spontaneous eye opening with roving eye movements and movements of the face and extremities. The irritable and agitated infant cries spontaneously with minimal stimulation and cannot be calmed. Delayed or poorly maintained response to stimulation suggests lethargy. In coma, arousal is impossible.

#### Cranial Nerve Examination

The cranial nerves are assessed by a series of observations of the neonate and are listed in Table 46-3.

#### Motor Examination

The motor examination assesses spontaneous movements and muscle tone. Posture and resistance of muscles to passive movement evaluate passive tone. Evoked changes in extremity tone and evoked postures of the head, trunk, and extremities assess active tone.

During the last trimester of gestation, changes occur in tone and primitive reflexes. Flexor tone increases in the lower extremities and progresses cephalad between 28 and 40 weeks of gestation. After 40 weeks of gestation, maturation of tone and coordination begins rostrally and progresses caudally. For example, the infant at 28 weeks of gestation lies with both upper and lower extremities fully extended with little or no resistance to passive movement of the extremities. As the infant matures, by 34 weeks, the lower extremities are flexed, and by 36 weeks, the upper extremities are flexed. Term infants demonstrate flexion in both upper and lower extremities. At term, both neck flexors and extensors can maintain the head in the axis of the trunk for more than a few seconds. Figure 46-2 demonstrates the transitional stage of motor function seen in the term newborn infant, based on the timing and direction of motor pathway myelination.

#### Involuntary Movements

The frequency and symmetry of spontaneous movements vary with the infant's level of arousal; normal spontaneous movements of the extremities in the term infant are organized and smooth. The ability to abduct the thumb is particularly meaningful, as persistent adduction suggests a corticospinal tract lesion. Jitteriness and seizures are involuntary movements that require further evaluation (see Chapter 54). Jitteriness consists of tremor-like movements of extremities that are very sensitive to stimuli and can be stopped with gentle passive flexion. Jitteriness may be found in hypoglycemia,

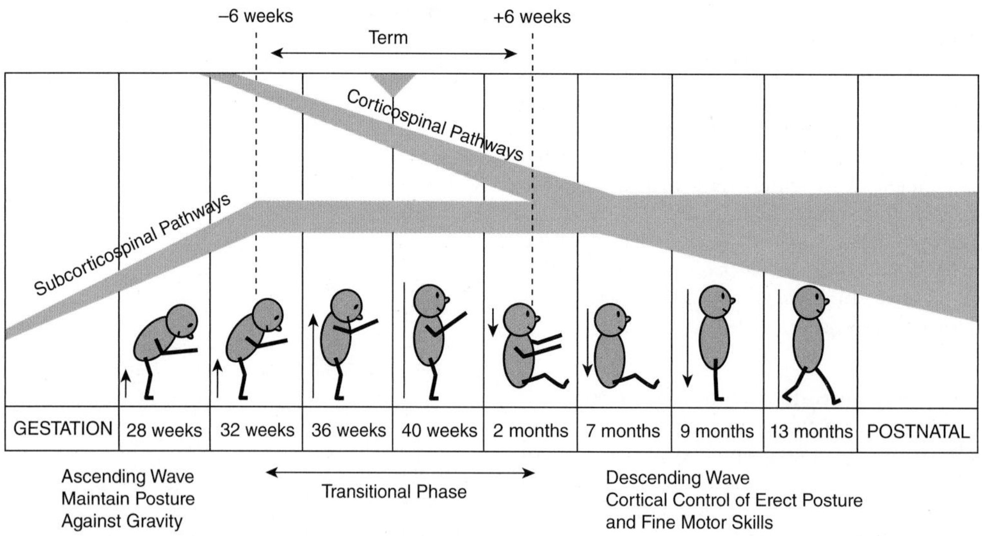


**FIGURE 46-2** Maturation in motor control from fetal life through infancy. The *subcorticospinal pathways* derive from the brainstem with myelination taking place between 24 and 32 weeks of gestation and proceeding upward, starting in the spinal cord. Their essential role is to maintain posture against gravity. The *corticospinal pathways* originate in the motor and the premotor cortex; 80% of the descending fibers cross the midline in the medulla (pyramidal tract). Their myelination starts around 32 weeks of gestation, proceeds downward from the pons to the spinal cord very slowly, reaching completion at about 12 years of age. They are responsible for control of erect posture and for movements of the extremities, including fine motor skills. From term onward, corticospinal control takes over, allowing development of mature head control, sitting, and walking.



hypocalcemia, and hypoxic ischemic encephalopathy, but often no specific cause is identified. Seizures are difficult to diagnose clinically and suspicion requires confirmation with electroencephalography. Many infants demonstrate myoclonic jerks during the onset of sleep that are mistaken for seizures.

### Posture and Passive Tone

The symmetry and maturity of passive tone are evaluated by observing the resting posture of the infant and by moving the extremities while the infant is awake and quiet. The degree of resistance to slow, gentle movement of the extremities and extremity angles ascertain passive tone. The infant's head must be in the midline position during the motor examination to avoid eliciting asymmetries in tone provoked by the asymmetric tonic neck reflex. Six maneuvers of posture and passive tone are summarized in Table 46-4. Maturational changes in tone and reflexes of these and other maneuvers are shown in Figure 46-3. In a normal baby, *flexion always exceeds extension.*

### Active Tone and Primitive Reflexes

Active tone refers to the infant's tone during active movement in reaction to certain situations. Active tone and evoked reflexes are evaluated by observing changes in the infant's posture in response to changes in position with respect to gravity or by observing the infant's responses to other stimuli, such as touch and pressure (Table 46-5). Of the many primitive reflexes described in neonates, only a few, including the 'righting reaction' and 'raise-to-sit' maneuver (see Figs. 46-4 and 46-5), are routinely assessed (Table 46-6). These are normally present in term and preterm infants and do not disappear until the infant reaches several months of age. Absence of primitive reflexes in the newborn infant indicates central nervous system depression.

### Maturational Changes in Tone and Reflexes

Maternal menstrual history or early fetal sonography provide the best possible dating before 32 weeks of gestation; from 32 weeks on, it appears reasonable to confirm gestational age by physical criteria and central nervous system function of the infant according to the normal steps of development (Fig. 46-3). In this assessment, structured evaluation of passive tone, active tone, and primary reflexes are used to determine gestational age within 2-week periods. A definite conclusion on neurologic maturation is reached only if 7 of the 10 responses correspond to the same 2-week gestation period. When more than 3 responses are out of line, no firm conclusion can be made. Such a result also raises the probability of a neurologic abnormality.

### Sensory Examination

The sensory examination usually is limited to the evaluation by touch. A positive response is identified by a change in facial expression or in level of alertness. The response to stimulation of individual dermatomes, including the sacral area (anal wink), may be necessary to localize the level of a spinal lesion.

### Tendon Reflexes

In the term infant, biceps, knee, and ankle jerks can be elicited readily, and ankle clonus is also common. Asymmetry or absence of reflexes may indicate a significant central or peripheral nervous system abnormality. Eliciting a plantar response is of limited value.

**TABLE 46-4 MANEUVERS OF POSTURE AND PASSIVE TONE**

| Maneuver | Description |
|---|---|
| Popliteal angle | Flex the infant's thighs laterally beside the abdomen, and then extend the knee to its limit. Measure the angle formed at the knee, which is the popliteal angle. |
| Foot dorsiflexion angle | With the knee extended, dorsiflex the ankle by applying pressure with a finger on the sole of the foot. Measure the angle between the dorsum of the foot and the anterior aspect of the leg. Foot dorsiflexion angle is a physical criterion of gestational age because the result depends on the progressive restriction of space in utero up to term. |
| Scarf sign | With 1 hand, support the infant in a semireclining supine position, keeping the head straight. Pull 1 of the infant's hands across the chest toward the opposite shoulder and note the position of the elbow. |
| Forearm recoil | This reflex can be elicited only when the infant is in a spontaneously flexed position. Extend the arm passively at the elbow by pulling on the hand. Then immediately release the hand and observe the speed of recoil of the forearm to its former position. If the forearm recoils normally, the test can be repeated after the forearm has been held in extension for 20–30 seconds. |
| Ventral flexion in the axis | With the child supine, grasp the lower limbs and push both legs and pelvis toward the head in order to achieve the maximum curvature of the spine. Some passive flexion of the trunk is normally present. |
| Dorsal extension in the axis | With the infant lying on his or her side, place the flat of the palm of 1 hand on the lumbar region and pull both legs backward with the other hand. Extension is normally minimal or absent. |

| | Weeks Gestation | Below 32 | 32–33 | 34–35 | 36–37 | 38–39 | 40–41 |
|---|---|---|---|---|---|---|---|
| PASSIVE TONE | Popliteal angle | 130° or more | 120°–110° | 110°–100° | 100°–90° | 90° | 90° or less |
| PASSIVE TONE | Scarf-sign | No resistance | Very weak resistance | Largely passes midline | Slightly passes midline | Does not reach midline | Very tight |
| PASSIVE TONE | Return to flexion of forearms | Posture in extension most of the time | | Weak or absent | Present, less than 4 times | 4 Times or more brisk but inhibited | 4 Times or more very strong & not inhibited |
| PASSIVE TONE | Foot-dorsiflexion angle | ≥50° | 40°–30° | | 20°–10° | | Null |
| ACTIVE TONE | Righting reaction lower limbs and trunk | No support | Brief support lower limbs only | Begins to maintain trunk | Trunk more firm | Begins to raise head | Complete righting for a few seconds |
| ACTIVE TONE | Raise-to-sit (neck flexor muscles) | No movement of the head forward | | Face View<br>Head rolls on the shoulder | Passes briskly in the axis | More powerful | Perfect, minimal lag |
| ACTIVE TONE | | | | Better Backward | Progressive Equalization | | Symmetrical |
| ACTIVE TONE | Back-to-lying (neck extensor muscles) | No movement of the head backward | Head begins to lift but cannot pass backward | Passes briskly in the axis | Powerful movement backward | | Perfect, minimal lag |
| PRIMARY REFLEX | Finger grasp and response to traction | Absent | | Very weak or absent | Able to lift part of the body weight | Able to lift all body weight for 1 second | Maintains 2 to 3 second with head passing forward |
| PRIMARY REFLEX | Crossed extension | | Good extension but no adduction | | Tendency to adduction | Reaches the simulated foot | Crosses immediately |
| PRIMARY REFLEX | Sucking | Sucks/burst<br>Rate of sucks<br>Negative pressure<br>interburst time | 3 or less<br>1/second<br>Weak or none<br>15–20 second | 4–7<br>1.5/second<br>intermediate<br>5–10 second | 8 or more<br>2/second<br>high<br>5–10 second | Idem | Idem |

**FIGURE 46-3** Neurologic criteria described at 2-week intervals, from 32 to 40 weeks' gestation. Periods of rapid modifications are enclosed by heavy borders, indicating the most discriminative period for each observation. Idem = refers to same response as 36–37 weeks; null = no flexion. (Adapted with permission from Levene MI, Bennett MJ, Puni J: *Fetal and Neonatal Neurology and Neurosurgery*, 2nd ed. London: Churchill Livingstone; 1995.)

**TABLE 46-5 MANEUVERS TO ASSESS ACTIVE TONE**

| Maneuver | Description |
|---|---|
| Righting reaction | Placement of the infant in the standing position with the feet on a horizontal surface while supporting the trunk evokes extension of the legs and trunk so that the infant supports his or her own weight |
| Neck flexor tone tested by the raise-to-sit maneuver | The infant demonstrates active contraction of the neck flexor muscles in an attempt to raise the head to a vertical position when pulled from the lying to the sitting position |
| Neck extensor tone tested by the back-to-lying maneuver | The infant contracts the head extensor muscles, tending to lift the head before the trunk when the infant, held in the sitting position and the head hanging forward on the chest, is gently moved backward |

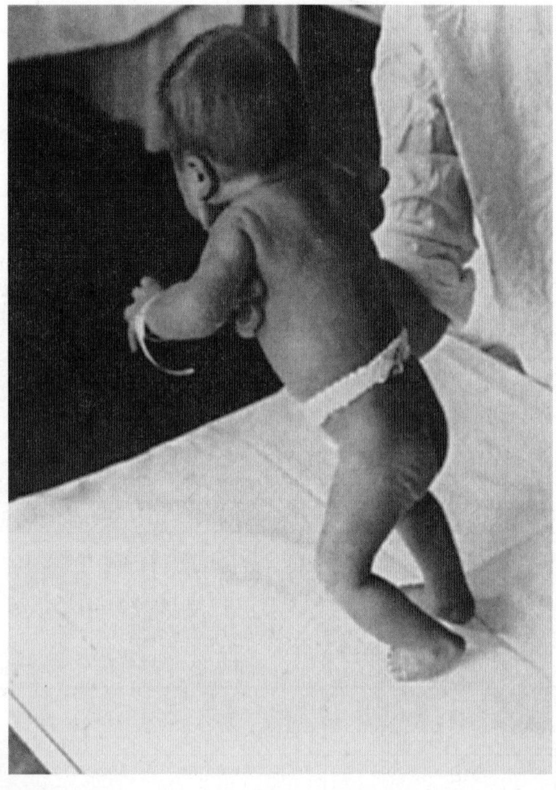

**FIGURE 46-4** Righting reaction.

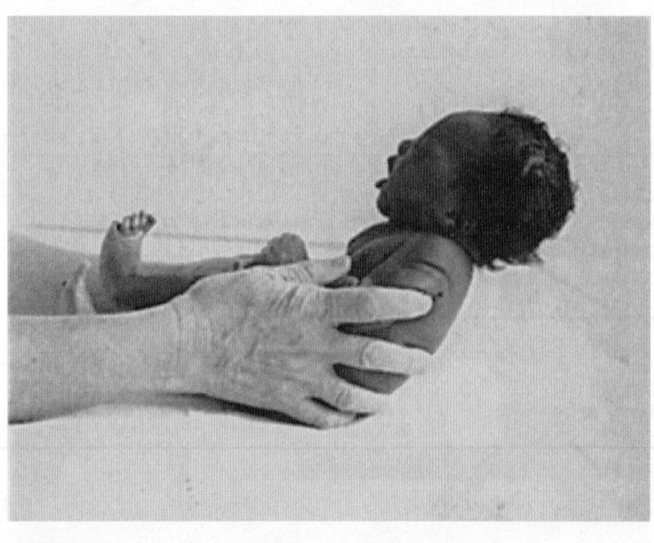

**FIGURE 46-5** Raise-to-sit maneuver.

**TABLE 46-6 PRIMITIVE REFLEXES ROUTINELY ASSESSED**

| Reflex | Description |
|---|---|
| Moro reflex | The Moro reflex is a rapid abduction and extension of the arms, followed by complete opening of the hands, which presents after holding both hands of the infant in abduction, lifting the infant's shoulders a few inches off the bed, and then releasing the hands briskly. |
| Finger grasp and response to traction | Placement of adult index fingers into a supine infant's hands results in flexion of the infant's fingers, amounting to a palmar grasp that is sufficiently strong to take the infant's weight when lifted by the adult. This "response to traction" provides a very good estimate of the strength of active tone. |
| Automatic walking | Tilting the infant while holding the infant upright with the feet on a table in a standing position results in the infant making a step forward. |
| Crossed extension | Holding 1 leg in extension and gently stroking the plantar surface of the foot produces a sequence of 3 movements of the opposite leg: (1) a rapid movement of withdrawal followed by extension of the leg, (2) fanning of the toes, and (3) adduction of the leg toward the stimulated side. The third component shows a distinct maturational change, first appearing at 26 weeks and becoming fully developed at 40 weeks. |
| Suck-swallow reflex | Placing a clean finger in the infant's mouth allows evaluation of sucking strength and rhythm, and synchrony with swallowing, as well as estimation of the number of movements in a burst, the rate, the negative pressure perceived, and the interburst time. |

## SUGGESTED READINGS


Benitz WE; Committee on Fetus and Newborn, American Academy of Pediatrics. Hospital stay for healthy term newborn infants. *Pediatrics.* 2015;135(5):948-953.

de-Wahl Granelli A, Wennergren M, Sandberg K, et al. Impact of pulse oximetry screening on the detection of duct dependent congenital heart disease: a Swedish prospective screening study in 39,821 newborns. *BMJ.* 2009;338:a3037.

Engel M, Kochilas L. Pulse oximetry screening: a review of diagnosing critical congenital heart disease in newborns. *Med Devices (Auckl).* 2016;9:199-203.

Eventov-Friedman S, Leiba H, Flidel-Rimon O, Juster-Reicher A, Shinwell ES. The red reflex examination in neonates: an efficient tool for early diagnosis of congenital ocular diseases. *Isr Med Assoc J.* 2010;12(5):259-261.

Green K, Oddie S. The value of the postnatal examination in improving child health. *Arch Dis Child Fetal Neonatal Ed.* 2008;93(5): F389-F393.

The newborn examination: clinical rotations for students. Stanford University School of Medicine website. http://med.stanford.edu/newborns/clinical-rotations/students/students-newborn-exam.html. Accessed October 10, 2016.

Ruttum MS, Nelson DB, Wamser MJ, Balliff M. Detection of congenital cataracts and other ocular media opacities. *Pediatrics.* 1987;79(5):814-817.

Volpe JJ. *Neurology of the Newborn.* 5th ed. Philadelphia, PA: Saunders; 2008.

WHO, United Nations Population Fund, UNICEF. *Pregnancy, Childbirth, Postpartum and Newborn Care: A Guide for Essential Practice.* 3rd ed. Geneva, Switzerland: WHO Press; 2015.

Witt C. Detecting developmental dysplasia of the hip. *Adv Neonatal Care.* 2003;3(2):65-75.

Wusthoff CJ. How to use: the neonatal neurological examination. *Arch Dis Child Educ Pract Ed.* 2013;98(4):148-153.

# 47 Postnatal Care and Observation of Low-Risk Newborns

George Thomas Mandy and Anthony Ernest Burgos

## GENERAL CONSIDERATIONS

This chapter will describe the care of hospital-born low-risk newborn infants between birth and discharge home. Routine care usually begins with an initial assessment of the infant in the newborn nursery.

The goals of postnatal neonatal care for low-risk newborns are to

1. ensure transition to extra-uterine life,
2. prevent or treat neonatal conditions arising from maternal or infant medical and social risk factors, and
3. ensure a successful transition to home care.

## PHYSICAL ASSESSMENT

The infant should be examined by the primary provider within the first 24 hours after birth. Generally, immediately after birth, healthy infants will remain with their mothers for a period of transition, skin-to-skin contact, breastfeeding, and bonding. This time together helps maintain the infant's body temperature and facilitates successful breastfeeding. Guidelines suggest that the newborn's condition should be evaluated after birth every 30 minutes until it has been stable for 2 hours. Thereafter, observations can be less frequent if the infant appears well. Nursing staff, medical staff, or a midwife in the postpartum area should perform a full assessment of the infant to identify potential problems.

### Body Temperature

In the first few hours after birth, the infant's body temperature should be measured on a regular basis. Skin temperature is usually lower than central body or core temperature, but it is still a reliable indicator of optimal temperature. Rectal temperature is a good indicator of core temperature, but insertion of a rectal temperature probe carries with it a risk of large bowel perforation. Measurement of axillary temperature is the preferred and safe alternative, and the normal range is 36.5°C to 37.4°C.

At delivery, the skin is wet and covered with amniotic fluid; the infant is usually exposed to low ambient temperature in the delivery room and frequently is kept unclothed to allow adequate initial observation. Therefore, heat is lost by evaporation, radiation, and convection. If measures are not taken to prevent heat loss in the newborn, body temperature can fall precipitously. Drying the infant immediately after birth, wrapping the infant in a warm, dry towel, and placing a knit cap on the head all help to reduce heat loss. Delivery room assessments and resuscitation should be performed under a radiant warmer, ideally with a servo-controlled feedback device that attaches to the infant's skin. Infants may also be placed in an incubator for observation in a neutral thermal environment of 31°C to 34°C at 50% humidity. In this range of ambient temperature and humidity, heat loss, metabolic demands, and oxygen consumption are lowest.

The nursery should be free of drafts at a temperature of 24°C to 26°C to assure a proper thermal environment for the healthy term infant. An infant who is hypothermic soon after birth should be warmed in an incubator or beneath a radiant warmer at a moderate rate to avoid the adverse consequences of cold stress and of excessive application of external heat. When an infant is in an incubator, both the infant's temperature and the ambient temperature inside the incubator should be monitored and recorded. When an infant achieves a stable normal temperature, care can be provided in an open crib with adequate clothing and a blanket to prevent cooling. Temperature instability may be an important indicator of illness and, in particular, of infection.

### Cardiopulmonary Function

The majority of life-threatening cardiopulmonary conditions appear during the first 6 hours after birth. The newborn's heart rate, blood pressure, respiratory rate, quality of respirations, oxygenation, and color of skin and mucous membranes should be monitored and recorded frequently during this time.

In the first 10 minutes after birth, the average heart rate is 160 beats per minute (bpm) but may vary from 120 to 180 bpm. Thereafter, the average is 120 to 130 bpm (range 90–175 bpm). A consistently low or high heart rate suggests a pathologic condition. Tachycardia may be a sign of low intravascular volume, cardiovascular or respiratory disease, drug withdrawal, pain, or hyperthyroidism. Rates greater than 200 bpm should prompt consideration of tachydysrhythmias such as supraventricular tachycardia. Bradycardia is often seen after perinatal asphyxia and also may be an ominous sign in association with apnea, airway obstruction, or infection. An irregular rhythm is occasionally encountered during auscultations, most frequently due to premature atrial contractions. These are typically benign and resolve within 48 hours. More than 6 ectopic beats per minute should be evaluated with a 12-lead electrocardiogram and referral to a cardiologist if a conductive defect is suspected.

Normal newborns breathe approximately 40 times per minute. This rate is variable between 30 and 60 breaths per minute. Breathing may not be regular. Periodic breathing, characterized by brief respiratory pauses, is considered to be normal. These are usually 5 seconds or less in duration but occasionally last as long as 10 to 15 seconds. A prolonged respiratory pause of longer than 20 seconds is abnormal and is considered to be apnea, especially if it results in bradycardia. These episodes require investigation. It is a nonspecific sign; it may be caused by such diverse conditions as infection, cardiac disease, hypoglycemia, polycythemia, and intracranial hemorrhage.

Tachypnea (respiratory rate > 60 breaths/min) in the newborn is also a nonspecific sign. Tachypnea is very common during the first few hours of transition, and in the first 24 hours. Tachypnea is most often due to retained fetal lung fluid (transient tachypnea of the newborn). In addition to the causes noted above for apnea, tachypnea may also be caused by disorders such as respiratory distress syndrome, meconium aspiration, pneumonia, and pneumothorax.

The normal range of blood pressure measured with a properly fitting limb cuff in term infants within 12 hours after birth is 65 to 95 mm Hg systolic and 30 to 60 mm Hg diastolic, with a mean blood pressure ranging from 40 to 55 mm Hg. An abnormal gradient of upper extremity to lower extremity blood pressures and absent or weak femoral pulses may be signs of coarctation of the aorta.

Oxygenation is best assessed with a pulse oximeter. After 10 minutes of life, the oxygen saturation should be in the 90s. Pulse oximeter probes should be attached to the right hand to assess preductal oxygenation. Oxygen saturation measured on other extremities may be affected by right-to-left shunting across the ductus arteriosus in the newborn.

### Gastrointestinal Function

Feeding can be initiated once the infant has been initially assessed and vital signs are stable. If the mother has chosen to breastfeed, this should occur in the first hour after delivery. Careful observation during the first 1 or 2 feeds may yield valuable information regarding coordination of suck and swallow, possible presence of gastrointestinal obstruction, and the potential for aspiration of gastric contents.

Choanal and esophageal atresia should be excluded if the infant experiences difficulty breathing during feeding or if the infant regurgitates during or after each feeding. A soft catheter can be passed orally into the stomach to assure patency of the esophagus; however, an H-type tracheoesophageal fistula will not be recognized this way and needs to be ruled out by other methods. Inability to pass a catheter nasally can reveal choanal atresia.

Newborns commonly regurgitate a small amount of milk with some feedings. Recurrent vomiting, or larger amounts or bile-stained emesis, may reflect intestinal obstruction that requires immediate diagnostic evaluation. During the first day, infants who have large amounts of mucus or swallowed blood in the stomach may repeatedly regurgitate small amounts of material or have difficulty in feeding. If vomiting persists, further assessment, including abdominal radiography, should be pursued.

All mothers should be encouraged to breastfeed, unless there are clear contraindications. Exclusive breastfeeding for 3 to 6 months may help prevent allergic conditions from occurring in infancy and early childhood. In infants who are breastfed, feeding behavior, frequency of feeding, stool characteristics, and initiation of maternal milk production should be noted and recorded. If there are any concerns regarding nutritional intake, the change in weight before and after breastfeeding can be measured. In babies who are fed milk formula, nutritional intake can be judged by the volume of formula ingested.

Approximately 70% of normal newborn infants excrete meconium during the first hours, and 95% of infants pass at least 1 stool within 24 hours. An infant who does not pass meconium in the first 24 hours should be evaluated. Passage of meconium may be delayed in infants with distal intestinal obstruction, as in meconium plug syndrome, or in infants with aganglionic colon (Hirschsprung disease). Other causes of abnormal gastrointestinal motility and delayed stool excretion are premature birth, sepsis, hypothyroidism, and various drugs, including narcotics.

Infants with high gastrointestinal obstruction usually present with vomiting but may not have abdominal distension or abnormal stool frequency during the first 24 hours after birth. Infants with lower intestinal obstruction are less likely to exhibit vomiting early but often exhibit abdominal distension and absent stools. Plain films of the abdomen are simple and effective in the initial evaluation of abdominal distention.

The color and consistency of stools change from green-black and viscous on the first day to green-yellow and paste-like by the third or fourth postnatal day. Normal stools are not watery, but those of breastfed infants are often softer and less formed than are the stools of formula-fed infants. During the first week, the normal frequency of stool output varies from 1 to 10 per day, usually averaging 3 to 5 stools daily. Delayed or infrequent stool passage increases the risk of hyperbilirubinemia during the first week.

Stools that are dark red and tarlike in consistency are indicative of old blood, usually maternal in origin, which was swallowed at the time of delivery. This can be distinguished from the infant's blood by a test that differentiates between adult and fetal hemoglobin (the Apt test for alkali resistance of fetal hemoglobin). Small streaks of bright red blood in the stools often reflect the presence of a rectal fissure. If no fissure is found, or if there are large quantities of blood in the stools, further evaluation is indicated. Diarrhea is a common sign of systemic or gastrointestinal infection, feeding intolerance, or drug withdrawal.

#### Urinary Function

Newborn babies very frequently urinate shortly after birth in the labor and delivery setting and virtually all normal infants have voided at least once within 24 hours. An absence of urine output may be of prerenal origin (severe hypovolemia and hypotension, myocardial failure, dehydration); or it may reflect renal anomalies, such as absent kidneys, acute tubular necrosis from ischemia, or renal vein thrombosis; or it may signal obstruction to urinary outflow, possibly from posterior urethral valves or from a blocked urethra.

An infant who does not pass urine in the first 24 hours should be examined for genital abnormalities and for a distended bladder. The prenatal records should be reviewed for the presence or absence of oligohydramnios. The delivery summary should be reviewed for documentation of possible void at the time of delivery. The infant may also be challenged with a supplemental feeding. If no urine is excreted, a straight catheter may be passed to detect presence of urine in the bladder. If the bladder remains dry, initial work up would include blood urea nitrogen, creatinine, and renal and bladder ultrasound.

Neonatal urine is normally yellow or light brown. Urate crystals, which vary from brick red to tan in color, are a common source of diaper stain in the newborn period and are often misinterpreted as blood. True hematuria is pathologic and requires urgent evaluation. During the first week of life, female infants may experience estrogen withdrawal and have vaginal bleeding which may complicate the clinical picture. Such bleeding should be brief (1 day) and occurs in tiny amounts.

#### Size and Weight

The newborn infant should be weighed in the hospital at birth, and daily thereafter, upon discharge from hospital. At postnatal follow-up examinations, hospital staff should determine whether the infant is small, appropriate, or large for gestational age. A maturational assessment such as the Ballard score may be useful for preterm infants. Infants who are small or large for gestational age may be at risk for postnatal complications, such as hypoglycemia or polycythemia.

The normal newborn loses approximately 5% to 10% of the birth weight during the first few days after birth and usually begins to regain weight by the second half of the first week. Weight loss beyond 7% should prompt an evaluation of feeding effectiveness. Weight loss of more than 10% in a term infant is considered abnormal.

Infant length is best measured with the infant supine, using a calibrated length board. In practice, a less accurate method using a measuring tape is common. It should be secured at the top of the head. The infant's knees should be held together and pressed gently to straighten the legs. Then the measuring tape is used to calculate the distance from the top of the infant's head to the infant's heels. Body length does not change measurably during this newborn period.

Occipital-frontal head circumference should be measured by placing a measuring tape above the eyebrows and the ears and wrapping it around the largest part of the occiput. The circumference may decrease by up to 1 cm as tissue edema abates during the week after birth. In some infants, head circumference may increase by up to 1 cm as the cranial molding that occurred during labor resolves. Rapid expansion of the head size in the first week may be a sign of ventricular enlargement and merits evaluation by cranial imaging studies. Infants who were delivered with instrumentation (vacuum or forceps) may be at increased risk for cephalohematoma, subgaleal hemorrhage, and intracranial hemorrhage and should have serial examinations and serial measurement of occipital-frontal head circumference.

## PROPHYLAXIS

#### Prevention of Neonatal Ophthalmia

Ophthalmia neonatorum is defined as conjunctivitis occurring in the first month of life. Several organisms can infect the eyes of the newborn, including *Chlamydia trachomatis*, *Neisseria gonorrhoeae*, herpes simplex virus, or other bacterial microbes like skin, respiratory, vaginal, and gastrointestinal tract pathogens. *Neisseria gonorrhoeae* infects the eyes in 1% of the cases but can penetrate the intact corneal epithelium and cause microbial keratitis, ulceration, and perforation. To prevent gonococcal ophthalmia, all newborn infants should have 2 drops of a solution of 1% silver nitrate or a 1- to 2-cm ribbon of ophthalmic antimicrobial ointment, containing either 1% tetracycline or 0.5% erythromycin, placed in each eye within 1 hour after birth. The solution or ointment should reach all parts of the conjunctival sac and should be dispensed from a single-use container. The eyes should not be rinsed after treatment because doing so decreases effectiveness.

It is important to note that neither silver nitrate nor erythromycin ointment is effective treatment for an already established case of gonococcal ophthalmia and systemic antimicrobial therapy is required. Typical side effects of eye prophylaxis include chemical conjunctivitis, especially with silver nitrate prophylaxis.

#### Prevention of Hemorrhagic Disease of the Newborn: Vitamin K

Hemorrhagic disease of the newborn has become a rare entity because of vitamin K prophylaxis. Vitamin K is necessary for synthesis of factors II (prothrombin), VII, IX, and X, and yet vitamin K is undetectable in cord blood. *Lactobacillus*, the primary gut flora in breastfed babies, does not synthesize vitamin K, and breast milk contains only small amounts of vitamin K (1–9 mcg/L versus 53–66 mcg/L in formula).

All newborns should receive a single dose of vitamin K (1 mg, intramuscularly) during the first few hours after birth to prevent the development of hemorrhagic disease of the newborn. Classically, vitamin K deficiency can cause gastrointestinal, intracranial, or generalized bleeding between 2 and 7 days after birth (0.25–1.7% incidence).

However, the early form of the disease may present in the first 24 hours, and the late form may present anywhere between 2 weeks and 6 months of age. The late form of hemorrhagic disease occurs mainly in babies who are exclusively breastfed but may also be associated with cystic fibrosis, celiac disease, chronic diarrhea, $\alpha_1$ antitrypsin deficiency, or hepatitis.

For infants of parents who refuse the intramuscular injection, a 2-mg oral dose of vitamin K maintains normal coagulation status in the first few days, but the effect may be transient and the dose should be repeated. The recommended timing of additional dosing varies. Some recommend an additional dose of 2 mg at 6 to 8 weeks of age, while others recommend weekly dosing while breastfeeding. The intramuscular form of vitamin K can be given safely orally.

### Hepatitis B Vaccine

It is now public policy in the United States to immunize all infants against hepatitis B infection. In infants born to mothers who are negative for hepatitis B surface antigen, the first dose of recombinant vaccine should be administered before 2 months of age. Infants who receive the first dose in the delivery hospital are more likely to complete the 3-dose series. Delivery hospital protocols that encourage vaccination in the first 12 hours of life also protect the infant against maternal hepatitis B surface antigen conversion that may have occurred during the pregnancy. If the vaccine is given prior to discharge in the nursery, an immunization record should be filled out and given to the parents. Due to the effective vaccination policy, the incidence of acute hepatitis B virus infection among US children younger than 19 years decreased by 98% between 1990 and 2010.

Infants born to mothers who are positive for hepatitis B surface antigen or to mothers of unknown hepatitis status need special management. Proper prophylaxis can prevent transmission in approximately 95% of exposed newborns that complete the 3-dose vaccine series. If the mother is positive for hepatitis B surface antigen, the infant should be bathed soon after birth to remove infectious bloody material, and the skin should be swabbed carefully with disinfectant before any drug injection or blood drawing. In addition, the infant should receive hepatitis B immune globulin (0.5 mL) intramuscularly at 1 site and recombinant hepatitis vaccine concurrently in another site within the first 12 hours after birth. Infants whose mothers are positive for hepatitis B surface antigen should be immunized on an accelerated schedule, with the second dose at 1 month and the third at 6 months after birth.

If the mother is of unknown hepatitis B status at the time of delivery, her blood should be sent for immediate testing, and the infant should receive the vaccine within 12 hours as described above for the infant whose mother is positive for hepatitis B surface antigen. If the mother is proven to be positive for hepatitis B surface antigen, the infant should then receive hepatitis B immune globulin as soon as possible and no later than 7 days postnatally. If the mother is hepatitis B surface antigen negative, the regular schedule of immunizations should be followed.

### Umbilical Cord Care

Umbilical cords tend to dry quickly, naturally, and without any additional care. This simple observation has called into question the various methods of care previously thought necessary to prevent infection. Cord care is best accomplished by leaving the umbilicus exposed to air and keeping it clean and dry. Topical application of antiseptic agents such as triple dye, chlorhexidine, or alcohol to the cord has no advantage over dry umbilical cord care. Regardless, parental education regarding the signs and symptoms of omphalitis is imperative.

## SCREENING

### Hypoglycemia

Routine monitoring of blood glucose concentration is only recommended for symptomatic infants and infants at risk for hypoglycemia. At-risk infants should be fed by 1 hour of age and have a screening blood glucose test 30 minutes after feeding. In at-risk or symptomatic newborns, blood sugar should be measured with a rapid bedside screening method within 2 to 3 hours of life, before breastfeeding, and whenever clinical signs of hypoglycemia are noted. Hospital protocols specifying serial glucose measurements, early feedings, and transfer criteria should be developed for infants at risk for hypoglycemia.

Risk factors for neonatal hypoglycemia include being infants of diabetic mothers (IDM); small or large for gestational age (SGA or LGA) infants; preterm or postmature infants; or intrapartum asphyxia, polycythemia, hypothermia, or stress related to clinical conditions such as infection. Clinical signs of hypoglycemia include changes in level of consciousness, apnea or cyanosis, poor feeding, hypothermia, hypotonia, tremor, and seizures. Blood glucose measurement of below 40 mg/dL by the screening technique should be evaluated using a specific assay for serum or plasma glucose, and treatment for hypoglycemia should be initiated while the result is pending. Hypoglycemia may also occur in a variety of neonatal conditions.

Hypoglycemia is defined as a blood glucose concentration low enough to cause signs and symptoms of impaired brain function. Most healthy term infants have a serum or plasma glucose concentration higher than 40 mg/dL on the first day of life and over 45 to 50 mg/dL thereafter. However, there is a physiologic dip in blood glucose concentrations during the first 2 hours of life, and at this time, blood glucose levels as low as 30 mg/dL may be tolerated in an otherwise healthy term infant who is able to feed appropriately. A steady state rate of glucose production has been measured in normal infants by 3 to 4 hours of life. It is important to note that individual infants exposed to high glucose levels in utero may become symptomatic at "normal" glucose concentrations above 40 mg/dL.

Hospital nurseries should define operational thresholds, or levels at which nurses and physicians should consider intervention, and have clear protocols for treatment of hypoglycemia, using guidelines from the American Academy of Pediatrics and the Pediatric Endocrine Society for detection and treatment of neonatal hypoglycemia.

### Screening for Critical Congenital Heart Disease

Critical congenital heart disease (CCHD) is a group of heart conditions that are present at birth, and can be cyanotic or acyanotic. In the United States, the frequency of these lesions is 18 per 10,000 deliveries. The most common lesions presenting in the early neonatal period are coarctation of the aorta, double outlet right ventricle, d-transposition of the great arteries, Ebstein anomaly, hypoplastic left heart syndrome, interrupted aortic arch, total anomalous venous return, tetralogy of Fallot, tricuspid atresia, and truncus arteriosus. Many of these conditions are life threatening and generally require intervention soon after birth. CCHD commonly presents within hours or a few days of life. Clinical signs and symptoms can include a heart murmur, reduced pulses, tachypnea, hypotension, hypoxemia, or cyanosis. If untreated, CCHD can lead to shock, coma, and death. CCHD affects the flow of blood into, out of, or through the heart. Sometimes the defect is in the heart itself, while other times it affects the valves that regulate the blood flow within the heart. Newborn screening for CCHD includes a thorough physical examination including auscultation of the heart and palpation of peripheral pulses, and includes pre and post ductal oxygen saturation screening. This should be done after 24 hours of life or just prior to discharge from hospital if within 24 hours of birth.

### Polycythemia and Anemia

In infants at risk, hematocrit/hemoglobin can be measured to exclude possible anemia or polycythemia. Anemia may result from hemolysis or blood loss, or other conditions such as suspected subgaleal hemorrhage that may require measurement of serial hematocrits. Suspected fetomaternal hemorrhage can be detected by performing a Kleihauer-Betke acid elution test on maternal blood. Polycythemia is more common than anemia and is often associated with delayed cord clamping at birth, when the infant is held below the level of the uterus or placenta for a prolonged time (more than 1 minute) (placental-to-infant transfusion), postmaturity, severe intrauterine growth restriction, large size for gestational age, monozygotic twins, or infants born to diabetic or hypertensive mothers.

### Isoimmunization and Hyperbilirubinemia

It is the standard of care to obtain a mother's blood type and Rh during pregnancy in order to avoid Rh sensitization and isoimmune hemolytic disease. Some centers obtain the mother's blood type and Rh upon admission to labor and delivery in order to avoid transcription errors of prenatal laboratory results. If a mother's Rh status is negative, her infant's blood type and Rh should be determined and a direct Coombs test should be performed. Blood type and direct Coombs test also should be performed if the mother has a positive antibody titer.

Risk factors for hyperbilirubinemia include predischarge total serum bilirubin (TSB) or transcutaneous bilirubin (TcB) in the high-risk or high intermediate risk zone, lower gestational age (late preterm gestation 34 0/7 to 36 6/7 weeks), exclusive breastfeeding, especially if nursing is not going well and weight loss is excessive, jaundice observed in the first 24 hours of life, isoimmune or other hemolytic disease (eg, G6PD deficiency), history of a sibling who was jaundiced or required phototherapy in the newborn period, East Asian race, polycythemia, cephalohematoma, or bruising.

Guidelines from the American Academy of Pediatrics recommend predischarge bilirubin measurement and/or assessment of clinical risk factors to evaluate the risk of subsequent severe hyperbilirubinemia. Some hospitals have implemented the guideline by obtaining a predischarge total serum or transcutaneous bilirubin and determining risk based on an hour-specific nomogram. The American Academy of Pediatrics and the Centers for Disease Control and Prevention have developed toolkits to assist birthing centers in following the guidelines for management of hyperbilirubinemia. (See Chapter 55 for further information.)



### Metabolic Diseases and Hemoglobinopathies

Inborn errors of metabolism are rare but potentially serious, even lethal if untreated. Advances in laboratory technology such as tandem mass spectrometry (MS/MS) have increased the number of genetic conditions that can be diagnosed at birth through neonatal screening programs. Newborn screening policies and availability of tests greatly vary around the world. In the United States, in 2005, the American Academy of Pediatrics endorsed the report from the American College of Medical Genetics, which recommended that all states should screen newborn infants for a core panel of 29 treatable conditions and an additional 25 conditions that may be detected by screening. Newborn screening blood specimens are collected on a test paper between 24 and 48 hours after birth. If the initial testing is obtained before 24 hours of life, in most states it is recommended that a second sample should be obtained. Some states also mandate or recommend that an additional newborn screening blood specimen be collected on all infants at 10 to 14 days of age.

Newborn nurseries should have protocols in place to ensure that initial testing is performed on all infants at the proper time, that conditions affecting results are noted (eg, blood transfusion), that results are followed up in a timely manner, and that infants with positive results are referred for diagnostic testing and treatment. Hospitals should perform regular audits of live births as well as outborn transfers, and certify that each infant was tested or retested at the appropriate time, review all abnormal test results, and document referral for appropriate evaluation and treatment.

### Hearing Screening

Screening newborn infants for deafness and auditory abnormalities is recommended by the American Academy of Pediatrics so that infants with sensorineural or conductive hearing loss can be diagnosed by 3 months of age and early intervention initiated by 6 months of age. Hearing screening should be completed prior to discharge from the hospital, and hospital programs must ensure that tracking, follow-up, identification, intervention, and evaluation can be carried out when necessary. According to the recommendations of the American Academy of Pediatrics Task Force on Improving the Effectiveness of Newborn Hearing Screening, Diagnosis, and Intervention, and the Joint Committee on Infant Hearing, all infants should be screened by 1 month of age.

Currently, there are 2 methods of automated testing: the auditory brain stem response and the otoacoustic emissions test. Both of these tests can be performed by nursery personnel trained in their use. Infants who fail these screening tests in 1 or both ears should be referred, not later than 3 months of age, for formal diagnostic studies at an audiology center that is capable of testing young infants. The prevalence of newborn hearing loss is 1 to 2 per 1000 live births, and the incidence in normal newborns is 1 per 1000. The referral rate for diagnostic testing after failed hearing screening should be less than 4%.

### Exposure to Toxic Substances

Infants who have been exposed in utero to drugs of abuse should be identified in the neonatal period so that they can be monitored carefully for signs of neonatal abstinence syndrome. Every nursery should have a protocol that defines specific criteria based on maternal risk factors and on infant symptoms to determine those patients for whom a urine or meconium sample should be sent for detection of illicit drugs. Common maternal risk factors include history of drug use; limited prenatal care; history of hepatitis B, HIV, syphilis, gonorrhea, or prostitution; and unexplained placental abruption. Clinical suspicion is increased when these risk factors are accompanied by preterm labor.

Infant risk factors include unexplained neurologic complications, unexplained intrauterine growth retardation, and evidence of drug signs of withdrawal. The signs and symptoms of neonatal abstinence syndrome include neuroexcitability or central nervous system dysfunction; metabolic, vasomotor, and respiratory disturbances; and gastrointestinal dysfunction. The onset of symptoms depends on the drug, the time and extent of the last exposure, as well as the metabolism and excretion of the drug and its metabolites. Abstinence scores should be obtained regularly in exposed infants and may be used to guide therapy, which may be with morphine, methadone, or phenobarbital. Abstinence scores may also be elevated in infants who have been exposed to stimulants, as these infants may have higher levels of excitability and may appear to be irritable or hungry. This usually represents drug effect rather than withdrawal.

Toxicology testing may be performed on the infant's urine, meconium, or umbilical cord. Urine testing is the most readily available, although collection with a urine bag can be difficult. The first void contains the highest concentration of drug or metabolites, but generally detects drug use in only the prior 72 hours. As such, negative urine toxicology results are common even with known drug use. Chronic use of certain drugs (marijuana, barbiturates, or phencyclidine) may allow detection up to 30 days after last use. Meconium screening may allow detection of drugs used a month or more before birth when collected in the first 2 days of life. Meconium is easier to collect than urine, but delayed passage of stool will also delay drug detection. Regardless of method used, positive results should ideally be confirmed by a second test. Umbilical cord testing for substances of abuse is increasingly being used in many hospitals. Its main advantage is that it obviates the need to wait to collect urine or meconium and thus every eligible baby can have a sample sent to the lab with a more rapid turnaround.

A physician or other allied health professional should order the screening, document the indication, and inform the infant's mother. Mothers with a history of drug use should also receive a social services evaluation, the focus of which should be the health and well-being of the mother, infant, and family. Such infants are not candidates for early discharge, and arrangements should be made for appropriate care and follow-up evaluation. Issues for long-term follow-up include increased risk of sudden infant death syndrome, high-risk social situations, and abnormal cognitive and behavioral development.

### Renal Pelviectasis and Hydronephrosis

Approximately 1% of infants will have urinary dilatation detected in utero by ultrasound. Most children with this diagnosis will have a benign course, but some will suffer renal deterioration due to infection or obstruction. Of all cases with dilatation, the order of significant uropathy is approximately 20%. Currently, there is no consensus regarding subsequent evaluation once mild antenatal renal pelviectasis is noted. Most agree that a newborn infant with mild unilateral pelviectasis or hydronephrosis (< 7 mm of dilatation) does not require further evaluation. Those with greater than 7 mm of dilatation should have a renal ultrasound. The use of prophylactic antibiotics during this period is controversial but still widely practiced. Infants with a positive ultrasound should be placed on prophylactic antibiotics and a repeat renal ultrasound obtained at 1 month of age. A negative study at this time would warrant no further workup, while persistent findings should trigger referral to a specialist. Whether or not to perform a voiding cystourethrogram if the first renal ultrasound is negative is also controversial. Approximately 25% of infants with vesicoureteral reflux on complete evaluation (ultrasound plus voiding cystourethrogram) have a negative ultrasound. Grades 1, 2, and 3 vesicoureteral reflux also often have normal ultrasounds, as the findings of hydronephrosis with vesicoureteral reflux are often transient.

Newborns with more serious prenatal diagnoses, such as fetally diagnosed severe bilateral hydronephrosis, bilateral hydroureteronephrosis, multicystic dysplastic kidney, or male fetal hydronephrosis with prenatal history of oligohydramnios, should be evaluated with a consult from a pediatric urologist, a same-day renal/bladder ultrasound, a chemistry panel at 12 hours of life, and a voiding cystourethrogram based on the recommendations of the consulting specialist. These infants also require antibiotic prophylaxis.

#### Developmental Dysplasia of the Hip

Hip instability occurs in approximately 1% of newborns, while the incidence of dislocation is only 1 to 1.5 per 1000. All newborns should be screened for developmental dysplasia of the hip (DDH) through physical examination (the Ortolani and Barlow maneuvers) and review of risk factors. Developmental dysplasia of the hip is more common in girls and with breech presentation and in those with a positive family history, and more commonly involves the left hip. Infants with a positive Ortolani or Barlow sign at the time of newborn examination should receive a consultation by a pediatric orthopedist, and those with equivocal examinations at birth should have a follow-up hip examination at 2 weeks of age, followed by a referral to a pediatric orthopedist if the examination remains positive.

Routine radiologic screening is not recommended for newborn infants with negative examinations. However, infants with 1 risk factor present should be reexamined at 2 weeks of age and then according to the periodicity schedule. Radiologic screening (ultrasound at 6 weeks *or* plain radiographs at 4 months) is recommended for female infants who were carried in the breech position, as these represent the 2 greatest risk factors for DDH.

#### Infection

Acute infections acquired during the perinatal period are common. Sepsis and pneumonia commonly coexist, and spread of the infection to the central nervous system can lead to long-term disability or death. Prolonged rupture of membranes (> 18 hours), fetal tachycardia, maternal fever, premature delivery, maternal chorioamnionitis, and birth depression are major risk factors in the perinatal period.

Signs and symptoms of neonatal sepsis include abnormal body temperature, poor feeding, abdominal distension, lethargy, hypoglycemia or glucose intolerance, hypotension, cyanosis, respiratory distress, petechiae, apnea, and irritability or seizures. Sepsis is often associated with poor peripheral perfusion, pallor or cyanosis, and mottled skin. Umbilical erythema, sometimes accompanied by a generalized rash, is indicative of serious infection and merits prompt evaluation and treatment with antibiotics. Jaundice in the first 24 hours after birth also may indicate the presence of infection.

Serious neonatal infections may present with either low or high white blood cell counts (< 5000/mm$^3$ or > 30,000/mm$^3$ of blood) with a high percentage of immature cells (bands, myelocytes, metamyelocytes). However, healthy newborns often have high white blood cell and absolute band counts because of the demargination that occurs during the stress of delivery. C-reactive protein has a good negative predictive value for sepsis when at least 2 values are obtained 24 hours apart and are both negative (< 1 mg/dL). Conversely, C-reactive protein has positive predictive value for sepsis only when elevated above 6 mg/dL.

The subtleties of presentation and potential gravity of neonatal sepsis are cause for a high index of suspicion and low threshold for conducting a careful diagnostic evaluation. The presence of multiple risk factors should prompt diagnostic tests for infection and immediate antibiotic treatment. Conditions associated with a modest risk of sepsis (eg, prolonged rupture of membranes) may warrant screening laboratory studies, including a white blood cell count and C-reactive protein, and careful clinical observation. Blood culture should also be considered during this period of observation.

Any infant with signs or symptoms of sepsis, regardless of laboratory values, should undergo a complete sepsis evaluation, including white blood cell count, blood culture, and cerebrospinal fluid culture, and should be started on empiric antibiotics immediately.

#### Group B Streptococcal Infection

Intrapartum antibiotic prophylaxis is recommended for group B *Streptococcus*–positive mothers in order to minimize the risk of infection to the newborn. One dose of antibiotics (penicillin, ampicillin, or cefazolin) received 4 hours prior to delivery is considered adequate to achieve effective antibacterial levels in the fetus and amniotic fluid.

Infants of group B *Streptococcus*–positive mothers who have received adequate intrapartum antibiotic prophylaxis can simply be observed for 48 hours. Gestational age at birth of less than 37 weeks or prolonged rupture of membranes (greater than 18 hours) warrant diagnostic evaluation, as well as 48 hours' observation. Infants born to mothers whose group B streptococcal status is unknown should be observed and evaluated for sepsis according the general principles discussed here. The Centers for Disease Control and Prevention recommends that infants born to mothers with chorioamnionitis, infants with premature prolonged rupture of membranes, and infants with a sibling who had group B streptococcal sepsis should receive a full diagnostic evaluation and empiric antibiotic therapy. Above all, clinical signs and symptoms of systemic illness warrant prompt evaluation and treatment.

### PROCEDURES

#### Circumcision

Circumcision, or removal of the penile foreskin to near the coronal sulcus, is frequently performed to prevent late inflammatory diseases of the penis (eg, balanoposthitis) and stenotic or constrictual foreskin problems (phimosis and paraphimosis). Many times circumcision is done for personal, religious, or cultural reasons.

Evaluation of current evidence indicates that the health benefits of newborn male circumcision outweigh the risks of the procedure and benefits justify access to this procedure for families who choose it, though the policy statement of the American Academy of Pediatrics states that the potential medical benefits are not sufficient to warrant its recommendation as a routine procedure. Circumcision is associated with decreased risk of penile cancer, urinary tract infection, and sexually transmitted diseases, including human papillomavirus, syphilis, gonorrhea, and human immunodeficiency virus (HIV). The complication rate of circumcision is less than 1%, and complications typically involve bleeding and infection at the surgical site.

Circumcision is contraindicated in infants with a family history of bleeding disorder (hemophilia) and infants with structural abnormalities of the penis, including hypospadias, epispadias, chordee, or ambiguous genitalia. Other relative contraindications include prematurity, small or concealed penis, curvature or penile torsion, large hydroceles, and clinical instability or illness.

Circumcision is performed by either a surgical clamp technique (eg, Gomco or Mogen) or use of a PlastiBell circumcision device. With the former procedures, the diaper adhesion to the surgical site is prevented postoperatively by petrolatum gauze dressing or petrolatum applied to the diaper or penis. With the PlastiBell device, the underlying tissue is normally healed by the time the ring falls off. Circumcision should be performed using local anesthesia, most commonly with local dorsal penile nerve block or penile ring block. Use of topical anesthetic cream (mixture of lidocaine and prilocaine) is recommended if local injection of anesthetic is not available.

Parents of infants who remain uncircumcised should receive instruction soon after delivery and at subsequent physician office visits regarding proper hygiene. Parents should be discouraged from forcibly retracting the foreskin of the uncircumcised penis, until such time as the foreskin becomes naturally softened and detached from adhesions.

### Sublingual Frenulotomy

Ankyloglossia, or tongue-tie, is a condition in which the sublingual frenulum extends out toward the tip of the tongue. Ankyloglossia occurs in rates ranging from 0.1% to 10.7%, but definitive incidence and prevalence is unknown due to an absence of standard diagnostic criteria. When ankyloglossia is present, 25% to 80% incidence of breastfeeding difficulties is reported, including failure to thrive, maternal nipple damage, maternal breast pain, poor milk supply, maternal breast engorgement, and refusing the breast. Ineffective latch is hypothesized to underlie these problems. A small body of evidence suggests that frenulotomy may be associated with improvements in breastfeeding as reported by mothers, and potentially in nipple pain. However, the strength of evidence is low to insufficient.

Complications of frenulotomy are rare but include bleeding, infection, and salivary gland injury.

## BREASTFEEDING AND LACTATION SUPPORT

Neonatal nutrition is ideally provided through breastfeeding. Initiation of breastfeeding should start shortly after birth and effectiveness should be continuously monitored until discharge home. There are very few contraindications of breastfeeding. The numerous benefits of breastfeeding and management approaches to encourage and facilitate breastfeeding are discussed elsewhere.

Successful breastfeeding depends on early initiation and support. Newborn infants should breastfeed within the first hour of life unless medically contraindicated. Hospital staff should be trained to recognize breastfeeding difficulties and to help mothers achieve proper position and latch. Regular nursing assessments should include documentation of breastfeeding efficacy using a lactation scoring system. Mothers identified with greater needs should be referred for additional consultation with a lactation specialist.

Hospitals should also consider developing preventive management guidelines for infants at risk for feeding difficulties, which may exacerbate weight loss and hyperbilirubinemia. Mothers of premature infants, late preterm infants, and multiples often require additional lactation consultation, care planning, and close, frequent follow-up. Although use of formula and pacifiers may negatively affect breastfeeding duration, early supplementation (with pumped milk or formula) may be appropriate for certain at-risk groups and in certain clinical situations.

Breastfeeding is contraindicated in maternal conditions that may result in transmission of infection to the infant, such as active pulmonary tuberculosis (until treatment is started and the mother is considered to be noncontagious), herpetic breast lesions, or infection with HIV. Possible effects on the infant of maternal medications and chemical exposures also should be considered, as many drugs and other chemicals can pass from mother to infant in breast milk.

## BIRTH PLANS AND REFUSAL OF ROUTINE CARE

Birth plans play an important role in the relationships parents have with their newborn children and with their care providers. Preferences regarding childbirth, feeding, and routine care (such as location; length of stay; administration of prophylactic erythromycin, vitamin K, and hepatitis B vaccine; or circumcision) should be discussed prenatally with the obstetrician or midwife.

Care providers should make every effort to discuss the birth plan by presenting the family evidence- based standard of care guidelines, and to address contingency plans in case of emergency (neonatal resuscitation, transfers to higher level of care, transports). Hospitals should ensure that policies are in place to obtain waivers of liability from parents when required by law.

## LATE-PRETERM AND EARLY-TERM DELIVERIES

Newborn nurseries frequently have admissions of infants whose gestational age falls in the category of late-preterm (34 0/7 to 36 6/7 weeks of gestation) or early term (37 0/7 to 38 6/7 weeks of gestation). Currently, in the United States, 6.8% of all deliveries occur in the late preterm period, and 24.8% occur in the early term period. Delivery can be indicated medically at such an early gestational age due to placental/uterine, fetal, maternal, or obstetric issues.

Mortality and morbidity are higher in these infants than in term newborns and there should be a low threshold for transfer to the neonatal intensive care unit. These preterm infants require increased observation, particularly with respect to symptoms of respiratory distress, dysregulation of body temperature and blood sugar control, inconsistencies in feeding ability/performance, hyperbilirubinemia, or meeting criteria for discharge from hospital. Administration of antenatal betamethasone for women at risk for late preterm delivery significantly reduces the rate of neonatal respiratory complications, although this intervention is associated with a higher risk of neonatal hypoglycemia.

Timing of discharge for late preterm infants depends on the infant's competency in thermoregulation and feeding, stable weight, absence of medical illness and social risk factors, and the readiness of the family to provide a safe environment post discharge. Early medical follow up should be scheduled for 24 to 48 hours post discharge.

## PREPARATION FOR DISCHARGE

The time that a newborn infant spends in the hospital nursery provides an important opportunity for maternal education as well as for critical infant evaluation. Although in the United States, legislation has guaranteed a 48-hour stay for vaginal deliveries and a 72-hour stay for delivery via Cesarean section, the needs of each mother–infant dyad dictate the amount of preparation deemed to be sufficient. Before the infant is discharged from the hospital, the mother should receive sufficient practical instruction to ensure appropriate home management of feeding, bathing, and general care of the infant, including recognition of well-being and illness.

The adequacy of the home situation should be evaluated, as well as the presence of particular stresses, such as domestic violence, isolation, depression, and homelessness. Social services and public health nurse referrals may be very helpful in ensuring a safe and nurturing environment for the baby after discharge. Additional anticipatory counseling should be done to promote infant safety and to prevent exposure to potential infections and toxins.

The discharge examination of the infant should be done, if possible, in the parents' presence to allow ample opportunity to express their concerns and ask questions about the findings they may think are abnormal. Plans for subsequent well-baby care of the infant should be established and instructions given for communicating concerns to the appropriate medical provider.

Term, healthy infants who are discharged within 48 hours after birth should be seen again in 2 to 3 days. Infants with risk factors such as prematurity, weight loss, poor feeding, or early jaundice may require earlier and more frequent follow-up visits. The hospital staff should document the location and date of the infant's anticipated follow-up, ensure parental understanding of the time interval and any significant clinical conditions, and facilitate the transfer of information to the provider who will assume care of the infant.

### Car Seat Selection and Testing

Every hospital should have policies to ensure that each newborn is transported home properly restrained safely in a car seat. The policies should ensure that parents are informed about the importance and proper use of car seats, that hospital staff are trained to assess infant car seat needs, that all infants less than 37 weeks' gestation have a period of observation in a car seat prior discharge from hospital, that all printed materials are reviewed periodically for accuracy, and that provisions are made for parents to obtain free or low-cost seats when needed.

## SUGGESTED READINGS


Adamkin DH; Committee on Fetus and Newborn. Postnatal glucose homeostasis in late-preterm and term infants. *Pediatrics.* 2011;127(3): 575-579.

American Academy of Pediatrics. Newborn screening for CCHD. American Academy of Pediatrics Web site. https://www.aap.org/en-us/advocacy-and-policy/aap-health-initiatives/PEHDIC/Pages/Newborn-Screening-for-CCHD.aspx. Accessed January 25, 2017.

American Academy of Pediatrics and the American College of Obstetricians and Gynecologists. *Guidelines for Perinatal Care.* 7th ed. Elk Grove Village, IL: American Academy of Pediatrics; 2012.

American Academy of Pediatrics Subcommittee on Hyperbilirubinemia. Management of hyperbilirubinemia in the newborn infant 35 or more weeks of gestation. *Pediatrics.* 2004;114(1):297-331.

American Academy of Pediatrics Task Force on Circumcision. Circumcision policy statement. *Pediatrics.* 2012;130(3):585-586.

American College of Medical Genetics. Newborn screening: toward a uniform screening panel and system. *Genet Med.* 2006; 8 (Suppl 1): 1S-252S.

Committee on Infectious Diseases; American Academy of Pediatrics; Kimberlin DW, Brady MT, Jackson MA, Long SS. *Red Book 2015.* 30th ed. Elk Grove Village, IL: American Academy of Pediatrics; 2015: 400-423.

Harlor AD Jr, Bower C; Committee on Practice and Ambulatory Medicine; Section on Otolaryngology—Head and Neck Surgery. Hearing assessment in infants and children: recommendations beyond neonatal screening. *Pediatrics.* 2009;124(4):1252-1263.

Jegatheesan P, Song D, Angell C, Devarajan K, Govindaswami B. Oxygen saturation nomogram in newborns screened for critical congenital heart disease. *Pediatrics.* 2013;131(6):e1803-e1810.

Sachs HC; Committee on Drugs. The transfer of drugs and therapeutics into human breast milk: an update on selected topics. *Pediatrics.* 2013;132(3):e796-e809.

Section on Breastfeeding. Breastfeeding and the use of human milk. *Pediatrics.* 2012;129(3):e827-e841.

Thornton PS, Stanley CA, De Leon DD, et al.; Pediatric Endocrine Society. Recommendations from the Pediatric Endocrine Society for evaluation and management of persistent hypoglycemia in neonates, infants, and children. *J Pediatr.* 2015;167(2):238-245.


# PART 2 INFANTS AT RISK



# 48 Multiple Births

Elizabeth V. Asztalos

## INTRODUCTION

Since antiquity, multiple births have fascinated humanity. Twins, triplets, and higher order births attract public attention and bemusement that often belies appreciation of specific management challenges not associated with singleton pregnancies. In addition, certain complications of pregnancy, such as preterm birth, occur more frequently with higher order gestations. Optimal management requires knowledge of issues associated with multifetal gestation during pregnancy, at delivery, and into the neonatal period.

The incidence of multiple births in developed countries has risen significantly. The increase in twin and higher order multiple births has occurred in conjunction with increases in maternal age and the use of assisted reproductive technologies (ART), ovulation-inducing agents, and artificial insemination. At least a quarter of successful ART procedures result in multiple pregnancies which, in turn, account for 2% to 3% of all live births. Multiple pregnancies are associated with higher risks for both the mothers and the infants. Preterm birth occurs in 50% of twin pregnancies, with 10% taking place before 32 weeks' gestation. Multiple pregnancies in general, but also as a result of ART, are associated with high direct costs for the medical system of any country as well as for the families. Consequently, many colleges of obstetrics and gynecology and professional bodies associated with ART have endorsed the implementation of a mandatory 2-embryo transfer policy with further consideration of a selective single embryo transfer policy.

The increase in the number of multiple births is recognized as a significant public health concern because of the associated mortality and morbidity risks that will be discussed in this chapter.

## THE ASSESSMENT OF MULTIPLE PREGNANCY

Because multiple pregnancies are at higher risk of morbidity and mortality for the infants compared to singleton pregnancies, early assessment is crucial so that appropriate care for these pregnancies can be provided which, in turn, will optimize outcomes. Early ultrasound assessment is crucial for (1) determination of chorionicity, (2) appropriate pregnancy dating, and (3) proper labeling of the fetuses.

Multifetal gestations are classified on the basis of zygosity and chorionicity. *Dizygotic twins* arise from independent fertilization of separate ova. *Monozygotic twins* develop from a single fertilized ovum that subsequently divides at or before the blastocyst stage of embryogenesis. The factors promoting fission of the conceptus are poorly understood. The timing of embryonic division determines whether the monozygotic twins will be separated by amnion and chorion (dichorionic, diamniotic), amnion only (monochorionic, diamniotic), or not separated (monoamniotic, monochorionic). Dizygotic twins account for approximately two-thirds of spontaneous twin births and are almost always dichorionic, diamniotic. Monochorionic twins share a single placenta with a shared circulation. Higher order multiples can be a combination of monozygotic and dizygotic gestations. Monozygotic triplets arising from a single fertilized ovum are extremely rare. Monochorionic pregnancies experience more complications and loss compared to dichorionic pregnancies. Determination of chorionicity is critical to determine which pregnancies are at risk and require careful monitoring. Ultrasound determination of chorionicity is best achieved in the first trimester of the pregnancy.

Accurate dating of the pregnancy is needed to provide optimal antenatal care and prevent unnecessary complications and poorly timed delivery. Multiple pregnancies are scanned by ultrasound frequently because of their increased risk of having congenital anomalies, chromosomal abnormalities, and growth discrepancies. This risk necessitates accurate labeling of the fetuses to ensure that the same fetus is being assessed consistently over time. Correct labeling according to orientation in relation to the mother as lateral (maternal left and maternal right), or vertical (upper and lower), is better than assigning a fetus number alone. In addition, in utero labeling does not predict the order at birth.

## COMPLICATIONS OF MULTIPLE PREGNANCIES

**Chromosomal and Structural Abnormalities** There is a higher risk of Down syndrome and other aneuploidies in multiple pregnancies.

First trimester screening is encouraged with all multiple pregnancies; however, screening is fraught with concerns: (1) the detection rate is lower as compared to singleton pregnancies; (2) the false-positive rate is high; (3) this higher rate leads to a higher rate of invasive diagnostic screening such as amniocentesis; and (4) the options, in the event of a true positive, are complex and pose risks to the surviving normal fetus/fetuses. For twins, in particular, combining screening methods is best.

Structural abnormalities are common in multiple pregnancies. They are due, in part, to the higher incidence of abnormalities in monozygotic twins. The management of pregnancies in which a structural abnormality is present is complex and should involve specialists from genetics and pediatrics to appropriately plan postnatal care.

**Growth Retardation** Fetuses of multiple pregnancies are at increased risk of being small for gestational age (because the uterus is less able to address the needs of more than 1 fetus) or growth restricted (if there is placental dysfunction). More information is available regarding the management of growth in twins as compared to higher multi-fetal gestations. The growth of twins is similar to that of singletons until 32 weeks' gestation, at which time overall growth velocity slows down. Regular ultrasound scanning is crucial after pregnancy dating and chorionicity have been established. Poor growth can occur in 1 or both twins.

Monochorionic twins are more commonly small for gestational age than are their dichorionic counterparts, suggesting that sharing a single placenta is a disadvantage for the twins. In discordant growth, 1 twin, usually the larger twin, grows appropriately and the smaller 1 becomes more growth-restricted. The average growth discordance in monochorionic as well as in dichorionic twin pregnancies is 10%. The threshold for clinically relevant discordant growth is set at a difference in estimated fetal weight of more than 25%, which affects approximately 10% of twin pregnancies, and is as common in monochorionic as in dichorionic twins. Despite the equal incidence of discordant growth in monochorionic and dichorionic twins, the risk of any adverse perinatal outcome is higher for monochorionic than for dichorionic twins at every level of discordance, again suggesting that sharing a single placenta is a disadvantage to the fetuses. Further, growth discordance in monochorionic twins must be distinguished from twin–twin transfusion syndrome.

Dichorionic twins can be viewed as 2 singleton pregnancies sharing a single uterus at the same time. The pattern for growth restriction in these twins follows a pattern similar to that of a singleton pregnancy. Worsening of flow within the fetoplacental unit may lead to a derangement of the biophysical profile, which in turn often becomes the trigger for elective preterm births for the fetuses. Any clinical decision to deliver early (ie, an iatrogenic preterm birth) to prevent fetal demise has to be balanced against risk. Here, the risks of demise and handicap for each fetus are determined by both gestational age and the weight of each fetus.

**Twin–Twin Transfusion Syndrome** Monochorionic twin pregnancies are at risk for complications related to the unique angio-architecture of the monochorionic placenta. Monochorionic twins share a single placenta with vascular anastomoses that connect the fetal circulations, thereby allowing intertwin transfusion of blood. When the flow is balanced, it is considered a physiologic phenomenon and no pathology ensues. However, an unbalanced intertwin flow leads to a variety of abnormalities. Of these, the best-known syndrome is twin–twin transfusion syndrome (TTTS), which can affect as many as 9% of monochorionic twins.

TTTS is diagnosed prenatally by ultrasound and typically presents in the second trimester of pregnancy. Diagnosis is based on the presence of twin oligo-polyhydramnios sequence (TOPS). The severity of TOPS is based on a classification system presented by Quintero et al. Higher stages are associated with more severe forms of TTTS and, in turn, with a poorer prognosis. Early diagnosis is essential to optimize the outcome (see also Chapter 42).

**Demise of a Twin** The rate of a single intrauterine fetal demise after 20 weeks' gestation is estimated to be as high as 6.2% of all twin pregnancies. Chorionicity is a key variable influencing the outcome of this complication. Monochorionic twins are at higher risk because of the placental angio-architecture, with rates being highest among monochorionic, monoamniotic pregnancies. Numerous reasons for the demise of a twin are present, with the more common ones outlined in Table 48-1. The etiology of the fetal demise plays a significant role in management of the pregnancy and the viability of the surviving twin. Preterm delivery is a common outcome of a pregnancy with a fetal demise occurring in the second or third trimester. The preterm birth can lead to complications of prematurity, which can include neonatal death, pulmonary hypoplasia, and enterocolitis.

**TABLE 48-1 CAUSES OF FETAL DEMISE IN MULTIPLE PREGNANCY**

| | |
|---|---|
| Fetal | Infection |
| | Chromosomal anomaly |
| | Structural anomaly |
| | Cord anomaly (eg, entanglement and velamentous cord insertion) |
| | Placental (eg, twin–twin transfusion syndrome, twin anemic polycythemia sequence, and selective intrauterine growth retardation) |
| Maternal | Hypertensive disorders (eg, preeclampsia) |
| | Thrombophilia, abruption |
| Iatrogenic | Selective feticide |
| | Complication after laser therapy for twin–twin transfusion syndrome |

Reproduced with pemission from Shek NW, Hillman SC, Kilby MD: Single-twin demise: pregnancy outcome, *Best Pract Res Clin Obstet Gynaecol.* 2014 Feb;28(2):249-263.

The management of a pregnancy compromised by a demise is determined by the gestation of the pregnancy and the chorionicity. A conservative approach is recommended with a previable pregnancy. Upon reaching viability, risks of the surviving twin are based on chorionicity. In dichorionic pregnancies, a goal is to prevent preterm delivery unless there is another obstetric indication. Regular growth assessment and maternal surveillance are initiated. In monochorionic pregnancies, the risks for the surviving twin are more problematic and include preterm delivery, intrauterine death, or ischemic brain damage.

**Preterm Birth** Multiple pregnancies account for 2% to 3% of all pregnancies but contribute to at least 10% of preterm births. Prevention of preterm delivery is ultimately a goal for all multiple pregnancies. Several modalities of care have been studied to varying degrees in managing pregnancies deemed at high risk for preterm birth. Cervical length measurements done at 20 to 24 weeks' gestation can identify those pregnancies at high risk of preterm delivery; a cervical length less than 25 mm has been identified as being a critical cut-off measurement for increased surveillance. Other modalities in care, such as progesterone, cervical cerclage, and cervical pessary, are still being studied to determine how they may help reduce preterm delivery in multiple pregnancies, in this case, twins.

## DELIVERY OF MULTIPLE PREGNANCY

Multiple pregnancies are associated with an increased risk of stillbirth near term compared to singleton pregnancies, even in low-risk twin pregnancies. The stillbirth rate of singletons at 42 weeks is equivalent to that of twins at 38 weeks, suggesting that twins should be delivered around 38 weeks. Chorionicity again plays a role in the risk of stillbirth. Because the risk of stillbirth does not change from 28 to 38 weeks, the consensus is that expectant management can be in place until 38 weeks. The risk for monochorionic twins is higher than for dichorionic twins but does not change significantly between 32 and 37 weeks, indicating that elective delivery should be considered at 37 weeks.

Determining the method of delivering a twin pregnancy is a challenge for most obstetricians. It is generally accepted that an elective cesarean delivery should be done with all monoamniotic twins, conjoined twins, and twin pregnancies in which the leading twin, A, is in a nonvertex position. For twin pregnancies in which the leading twin is in a vertex position, an elective vaginal delivery is acceptable. A nonvertex twin B can be delivered by a vaginal approach as long as the obstetrician is comfortable and skilled in a breech delivery.

## OUTCOMES OF MULTIPLE PREGNANCY

In general, multiple pregnancies have a higher incidence of preterm birth compared to singleton pregnancies, due, in part, to twin pregnancies' increased probability of preterm birth. Complications for infants born preterm include respiratory disorders, sepsis, patent ductus arteriosus, varying degrees of intraventricular hemorrhages and their sequelae, necrotizing enterocolitis, and retinopathy of prematurity. The key variables that affect these outcomes are related to the degree of prematurity; the earlier the birth occurs, the higher the chances are for many of these outcomes to occur. In general, the incidence of these specific outcomes is not different from that of singletons at their comparable gestations. Infants born preterm are predisposed to long-term sequelae in cognition, language, and motor outcomes, and poor achievement in school.

A single fetal demise, particularly in monochorionic pregnancies, predisposes the surviving twin to a high rate of cerebral lesions as demonstrated on magnetic resonance imaging (fetal and/or neonatal). Absence of any lesion was associated with a normal neurodevelopmental outcome.

Growth discordance in general is associated with an increased probability of adverse outcomes both in the neonatal period and in the long term. In dichorionic twins, these presentations may be similar to what is seen in singleton pregnancies associated with growth restriction. In monochorionic pregnancies, adverse perinatal outcomes are higher because of the disadvantage of sharing a single placenta.

The method of delivery does not affect the incidence of morbidities, both in the neonatal period and in 2-year neurodevelopmental outcomes, as evidenced by the largest trial to date involving twins and the approach to planned deliveries.

## SUGGESTED READINGS


Asztalos EV, Hannah ME, Hutton EK, et al. Twin Birth Study: 2-year neurodevelopmental follow-up of the randomized trial of planned cesarean or planned vaginal delivery for twin pregnancy. *Am J Obstet Gynecol.* 2016;214(3):371.e1-371.e19.

Barrett JF. Twin delivery: method, timing, and conduct. *Best Pract Res Clin Obstet Gynaecol.* 2014;28(2):327-338.

Bricker L. Optimal antenatal care for twin and triplet pregnancy: the evidence base. *Best Pract Res Clin Obstet Gynaecol.* 2014;28(2):305-317.

Denbow ML, Cox P, Taylor M, Hammal DM, Fisk NM. Placental angioarchitecture in monochorionic twin pregnancies: relationship to fetal growth, fetofetal transfusion syndrome, and pregnancy outcome. *Am J Obstet Gynecol.* 2000;182:417-26.

Dias T, Arcangeli T, Bhide A, Napolitano R, Mahsud-Dornan S, Thilaganathan B. First-trimester ultrasound determination of chorionicity in twin pregnancy. *Ultrasound Obstet Gynecol.* 2011;38(5):530-532.

Dias T, Contro E, Thilaganathan B, et al. Pregnancy outcome of monochorionic twins: does amnionicity matter? *Twin Res Hum Genet.* 2011;14(6):586-592.

Dias T, Patel D, Bhide A, et al; Southwest Thames Obstetric Research Collaborative (STORK). Prospective risk of late stillbirth in monochorionic twins: a regional cohort study. *Ultrasound Obstet Gynecol.* 2012;39(5):500-504.

Goldenberg RL, Culhane JF, Iams JD, Romero R. Epidemiology and causes of preterm birth. *Lancet.* 2008;371(9606):75-84.

Hack KE, Derks JB, Elias SG, et al. Increased perinatal mortality and morbidity in monochorionic versus dichorionic twin pregnancies: clinical implications of a large Dutch cohort study. *BJOG.* 2008;115(1):58-67.

Hillman SC, Morris RK, Kilby MD. Co-twin prognosis after single intrauterine fetal death: a systematic review and meta-analysis. *Obstet Gynecol.* 2011;118(4):928-940.

Jatzko B, Rittenschober-Böhm J, Mailath-Pokorny M, et al. Cerebral lesions at fetal magnetic resonance imaging and neurologic outcome after single fetal death in monochorionic twins. *Twin Res Hum Genet.* 2015;18(5):606-612.

Lewi L, Gucciardo L, Huber A, et al. Clinical outcome and placental characteristics of monochorionic diamniotic twin pairs with early- and late-onset discordant growth. *Am J Obstet Gynecol.* 2008;199(5):511.e1-7.

Martin JA, Hamilton BE, Osterman MJ, Curtin SC, Matthews TJ. Births: final data for 2013. *Natl Vital Stat Rep.* 2015;64(1):1-65.

Mouzon de J, Goossens V, Bhattacharya S, et al.; European IVF-Monitoring (EIM) Consortium for the European Society on Human Reproduction and Embryology (EHSRE). Assisted reproductive technology in Europe, 2007: results generated from European registers by ESHRE. *Hum Reprod.* 2012;27(4):954-966.

Quintero RA, Morales WJ, Allen MH, Bornick PW, Johnson PK, Kruger M. Staging of twin-twin transfusion syndrome. *J Perinatol.* 1999;19(8 Pt 1):550-555.

Sperling L, Kiil C, Larsen LU, et al. Detection of chromosomal abnormalities, congenital abnormalities and transfusion syndrome in twins. *Ultrasound Obstet Gynecol.* 2007;29(5):517-526.

Zádori J, Kozinszky Z, Orvos H, Katona M, Kaáli SG, Pál A. Birth weight discordance in spontaneous versus induced twins: impact on perinatal outcome. *J Assist Reprod Genet.* 2004;21(3):85-88.


# 49 The Small-for-Gestational-Age Infant

William W. Hay, Jr.

## INTRODUCTION

Newborn infants are classified according to birth weight as small, average, or large for gestational age (Table 49-1).

### Small-for-Gestational-Age

Small-for-gestational-age (SGA) infants are a heterogeneous group of infants who are smaller than normal at birth due to genetic or constitutional conditions, diseases such as congenital infections, or growth restriction from a smaller or poorly functioning placenta that reduces oxygen and nutrient supplies to the fetus. SGA infants are commonly defined as having a birth weight less than the 10th percentile of a population-specific birth weight versus gestational age relationship. They also can simply be thinner than normal, in which case their weight-to-length ratio (or the ponderal index = [weight, g]/[length, cm]$^3$) is less than normal. Being thinner as an SGA infant most commonly is the result of late gestation nutritional deficiency

**TABLE 49-1 CLASSIFICATION OF FETAL GROWTH[a]**

| | | |
|---|---|---|
| SGA | Small for gestational age | Birth weight < 10th percentile for gestational age |
| AGA | Average for gestational age | Birth weight between 10th and 90th percentile for gestational age |
| LGA | Large for gestational age | Birth weight > 90th percentile for gestational age |
| IUGR | Intrauterine growth restriction | Slower than normal rate of fetal growth |
| LBW | Low birth weight | Less than 2500 g |
| VLBW | Very low birth weight | Less than 1500 g |
| ELBW | Extremely low birth weight | Less than 1000 g |

[a]Normal birth weight is > 2500 g at term gestation.

due to placental insufficiency. It is important that all anthropometric measurements (weight, length, head circumference, ponderal index), not just weight, are used to define fetal growth as deviations in each of these can represent unique causes and specific adverse outcomes.

#### Intrauterine Growth Restriction

Intrauterine growth restriction (IUGR) is defined as a rate of fetal growth that is less than normal for the population and for the growth potential of a specific infant. Infants with IUGR, therefore, can be SGA or simply smaller than they could have been. The latter point is important because adverse outcomes of growth restriction are due to the processes that produce slower growth and the fetal adaptations to them, not just whether the infant is less than the 10th percentile in anthropometric measurements. Infants with moderate or severe IUGR tend to have asymmetric growth restriction (ie, growth restriction of muscle, fat, and organs is greater than that of the brain and the long bones). Importantly, however, such infants do have growth restriction of the brain, which can include fewer neurons, shorter axons, fewer dendrites, and less dendritic arborization and synapse formation. These adverse conditions can lead to limited cognitive capacity and behavioral problems later in life. Particularly at risk for developmental complications are very preterm infants who already are growth-restricted at birth. Constitutionally small infants (from normal but small mothers who have small uteruses) tend to have more symmetrical brain and body growth, but even when asymmetrically grown, their head circumference and brain size and development tend to be in the normal range without evidence of later life cognitive deficiencies.

#### Low Birth Weight

Most infants with low birth weights are the result of a shorter than normal gestation (ie, they are born preterm). Also, a large fraction of preterm infants are already growth-restricted at birth; indeed, many causes of growth restriction also lead to preterm delivery.



## FETAL GROWTH

### REGULATION OF FETAL GROWTH

Fetal growth is regulated by maternal, placental, and fetal factors, representing a mix of genetic mechanisms and environmental influences through which fetal genetic growth potential is expressed and modulated. Maternal genotype is more important than is fetal genotype in the overall regulation of fetal growth. However, the paternal genotype is essential for trophoblast development, which secondarily regulates fetal growth by the provision of nutrients. The major maternal factors that regulate fetal growth include maternal size (height and prepregnancy weight) and maternal weight gain during pregnancy.

Normal variations in maternal nutrition have relatively little impact on fetal growth because changes in maternal nutrition, unless extreme and prolonged, do not markedly alter maternal plasma concentrations of nutrient substrates or the rate of uterine blood flow. They are the principal determinants of maternal nutrient substrate delivery to the placenta and transport to the fetus by the placenta. The placental trophoblast surface area is the primary regulator of fetal growth via its nutrient transport capacity (glucose, amino acids, lipids, oxygen) and its interaction with maternal (uterine) and fetal (umbilical) circulations. The placenta also integrates maternal and fetal nutritional and endocrine signals to balance fetal nutrient needs with the ability of the mother to support pregnancy by regulating maternal physiology, placental growth, and placental nutrient transport. At more advanced stages of placental development, placental production of growth factors and growth regulating hormones (human placental lactogen [hPL] and placental growth hormone [PGH]) leads to significant autocrine regulation of placental growth and placental regulation of fetal growth processes.

In the fetus, oxygen and nutrient supplies are the primary regulators of fetal growth. Oxygen is necessary for production of energy to maintain metabolism and allow protein synthesis. Nutritional regulation of fetal growth depends primarily on amino acids for protein synthesis and secondarily on energy from glucose oxidation in fetal tissues. Mineral supply (calcium and phosphorous) is essential to promote bone structure. In addition, nutrient-stimulated secretion of insulin and IGFs promote fetal growth via their signal transduction effects on protein synthesis and energy storage in glycogen and lipid.

### ETIOLOGY OF GROWTH RESTRICTION

Intrinsic abnormalities that limit fetal growth usually begin early in fetal life, whereas the onset of extrinsic adverse factors, such as under nutrition or hypoxia from placental insufficiency, develop at variable times during later gestation (Table 49-2). Abnormalities that limit the growth of both the fetal brain and body include chromosomal anomalies (particularly trisomy conditions), congenital infections (eg, toxoplasmosis, rubella, and cytomegalovirus), dwarf syndromes, some inborn errors of metabolism, and some drugs (eg, maternal smoking and excessive alcohol consumption). Most other cases of fetal growth restriction are the result of a small or poorly functioning placenta.

The most common cause of late-gestation fetal growth restriction is placental insufficiency, which limits oxygen and nutrient transport to the fetus. Relative hypoxia diminishes the production of fetal insulin by limiting fetal pancreatic beta cell replication and promotes catecholamine secretion, principally noradrenaline, which suppresses insulin secretion. These changes in anabolic hormone production lead to diminished fetal tissue amino acid uptake, protein synthesis, and protein accretion (net positive protein balance). Hypoxia, catecholamine secretion, and reduced insulin secretion also lead to increased production of hepatic glucose, which reduces glucose uptake from the placenta. Such mechanisms appropriately reduce fetal growth and the corresponding need for nutrient uptake from the poorly or insufficiently functioning placenta.

### GROWTH CURVES

#### Neonatal Growth Curves

Cross-sectional growth curves from anthropometric measurements in populations of newborn infants born at different gestational ages demonstrate whether an infant's birth weight is within the normal range for a given gestational age and thus whether that infant's in utero growth was greater or less than normal. Estimating gestational age has considerable error, derived from variability in dating the time of conception, the physical features of maturation in the infant, and interobserver assessments of an infant's developmental stage.

#### Fetal Growth Curves

Fetal growth curves have been developed from serial ultrasound measurements of fetuses that subsequently were born at term in healthy condition and with normal anthropometric measurements, providing longitudinal indices of fetal growth. Serial ultrasound measurements of fetal growth more accurately determine how environmental factors

| TABLE 49-2 MATERNAL CONDITIONS ASSOCIATED WITH INTRAUTERINE GROWTH RESTRICTION |
|---|
| Both very young and advanced maternal age |
| Maternal prepregnancy short stature and thinness |
| Poor maternal weight gain during the third trimester of pregnancy |
| Maternal illness during pregnancy |
| Failure to obtain normal medical care during pregnancy |
| Lower socioeconomic status |
| Black race (in the United States) |
| Multiple gestation |
| Uterine and placental anomalies |
| Polyhydramnios |
| Preeclampsia |
| Hypertension, both chronic and pregnancy-induced |
| Chronic, severe diabetes |
| Intrauterine infections |
| Cigarette smoking, cocaine use, and other substance abuse |

(eg, severe maternal illness and undernutrition) inhibit fetal growth and how maternal overnutrition and gestational diabetes enhance fetal growth, particularly of adipose tissue. They are much more useful than anthropometric indices at birth as measures of fetal growth rate and deviations from normal growth patterns. Regardless of the growth curve, however, normal average fractional human fetal growth during most of the second half of gestation is relatively constant at approximately 17 g/kg/day.

## CLINICAL EVALUATION AND TREATMENT OF THE SGA INFANT

### General Evaluation and Treatment in the Delivery Room

SGA infants lose heat rapidly because of their large surface area relative to body mass and their scant subcutaneous insulation. They should be dried quickly and completely at birth, placed under a radiant warmer, and protected from drafts with warmed blankets. Severely undergrown SGA infants often experience marked oxygen and substrate deprivation in utero, which can lead to cardiopulmonary failure at birth.

**Physical Examination** Markedly SGA infants who have had severe IUGR usually have disproportionately large heads relative to their undergrown trunks and extremities. Their abdomen can appear shrunken or scaphoid. Their extremities often appear scrawny, with thin skin folds, decreased subcutaneous tissue, loose skin that often is rough and dry, long fingernails, and hands and feet that appear large for the size of the body. The anterior fontanel often is larger than expected, representing diminished membranous bone formation. The umbilical cord often is thinner than usual. SGA infants also have an increased incidence of severe malformations and chromosomal abnormalities accompanied by dysmorphic features and congenital anomalies, abnormal hands and feet, and the presence of palmar creases.

**Gestational Age Assessment** Gestational age assessed using physical criteria often is erroneous in SGA infants. Specific organ maturity often continues at normal developmental rates despite diminished somatic growth. Cerebral cortical convolutions, renal glomerular development, and alveolar maturation correlate better with gestational age than with body size.

**Neurological and Behavioral Examination** SGA infants often appear to have advanced neurological maturity, although this observation is derived primarily from comparisons with infants of similar birth weight rather than with similar gestational age. They can be hyperexcitable but show mixed aberrations in tone, from hypertonia to hypotonia. Abnormalities in tone occur more frequently among infants with severe IUGR in whom neurological abnormalities usually reflect brain injury during fetal development.

### Early Clinical Problems of the SGA Neonate

#### IUGR/SGA Status vs Preterm Birth and Effects on Mortality and Morbidity

Among preterm SGA infants, problems associated with preterm birth have a much greater impact on outcome than whether infants are SGA or average for gestational age (AGA). In contrast, more mature infants may suffer more from the impact of growth restriction. Perinatal mortality rates of markedly SGA infants with severe IUGR can be 5 to 20 times those of AGA infants of the same gestational age, related primarily to hypoxic-ischemic conditions and lethal congenital anomalies.

**Perinatal Depression** Severely SGA fetuses with marked IUGR frequently show signs of distress (eg, fetal bradycardic arrhythmias and decreased movement) from hypoxia-ischemia and often do not tolerate labor and vaginal delivery when exposed to the added stress of diminished blood flow during uterine contractions.

**Hypoglycemia** Hypoglycemia is common in SGA infants, increasing with the severity of IUGR. Early hypoglycemia usually results from increased brain glucose utilization relative to a reduced capacity to mobilize hepatic and skeletal muscle glycogen stores. Less commonly, it reflects transient hyperinsulinemia and increased peripheral sensitivity to insulin and glucose. Transient hyperinsulinemia appears to develop from increased insulin secretion capacity in fetal pancreatic β cells following reduced β cell replication. Usually, this potential for increased insulin secretion is suppressed in the fetus by hypoxia-induced catecholamine secretion. After birth, reductions in catecholamines allow increased insulin secretion to develop quite quickly, leading to hypoglycemia from increased insulin-mediated glucose uptake by peripheral tissues. The liver has a relatively lower insulin resistance to promote hepatic glucose production, but peripheral tissues have increased insulin and glucose sensitivity, in part because of maintained or up-regulated expression and activity of glucose transporters.

All SGA infants should have early and frequent measurements of plasma glucose concentrations, which should be kept greater than 45 mg/dL in the first 48 hours after birth and greater than 60 mg/dL thereafter. Plasma or serum glucose concentrations are preferable to whole blood measurements, as SGA infants and especially infants with IUGR often have relative polycythemia. It reduces whole blood glucose concentration values relative to plasma and tends to reduce plasma glucose delivery to tissues. Early enteral feeding, particularly with milk, usually can limit the development of hypoglycemia. The lactose in milk is hydrolyzed in the gut to glucose and galactose; the reduced amount of glucose limits excessive glucose absorption and increased plasma concentrations while the galactose promotes glycogen formation. In less mature infants or those with other clinical problems, intravenous glucose should be started at 6 to 8 mg/min/kg body weight as soon after birth as possible and adjusted frequently to maintain plasma glucose concentrations in the normal range. A slightly higher dextrose infusion rate compensates for the greater brain-to-body weight ratio and the increased peripheral glucose and insulin sensitivity that tend to increase glucose utilization and lead to hypoglycemia.

**Hyperglycemia** SGA preterm infants often have low insulin secretion rates and plasma insulin concentrations from hypoxia-induced catecholamine secretion in utero, as well as persistent hepatic glucose production due to hepatic insulin resistance. These problems add to the common problem of hyperglycemia that is principally caused by excessive rates of glucose infusion (usually greater than 11 mg/min/kg). Higher concentrations of stress-induced hormones, such as norepinephrine and epinephrine, glucagon, and cortisol, contribute to hyperglycemia. Insulin treatment in these infants usually decreases glucose concentrations promptly, indicating that they have appropriate or even increased insulin sensitivity. If an insulin infusion is used to reduce very high rates of glucose concentration, it is imperative that a simultaneous glucose infusion be maintained and glucose concentrations be measured frequently to prevent hypoglycemia. Enteral feeding also helps reduce hyperglycemia by promoting secretion of incretins, which are gut-derived endocrine factors that promote insulin secretion.

**Lipid Metabolism** SGA infants tend to have low concentrations of plasma free fatty acid, as a result of reduced stores of body fat. Fasting glucose concentrations in SGA infants indirectly correlate with plasma concentrations of free fatty acids and ketoacids. When fed intravenously, however, SGA infants often have deficient cellular uptake and metabolism of plasma triglycerides, which produce relatively higher plasma concentrations of fatty acids and triglycerides but reduced concentrations of ketoacids.

**Energy Expenditure** SGA infants have higher oxygen consumption and total energy expenditure rates than do infants with normal growth at the same gestational age, primarily because their resting energy expenditure rate also is higher. This rate reflects an increase in cell number relative to body mass, greater heat production in response to increased heat loss due to their larger body surface area relative to tissue mass, and their higher brain-to-body weight ratio (the brain has the highest metabolic rate of all organs).

**Protein Metabolism** Because SGA infants are particularly deficient in muscle mass, providing adequate nutrition for accretion of skeletal muscle and total body protein is a priority in these infants. There is conflicting information, however, about how well SGA infants tolerate higher rates of amino acid and protein nutrition, as they may have adapted metabolically to limit their capacity for protein synthesis in response to both amino acid supply and insulin action. Also, infants with IUGR have reduced capacity for insulin production due to having fewer pancreatic β cells and islets, further limiting anabolic capacity. Gestational age–specific rates of protein intake in both enteral and parenteral feedings should be used, but very high rates of protein intake, greater than 3.5 to 4.0 g/kg/day, should be used cautiously, particularly during the parenteral nutrition phase right after birth.

**Polycythemia-Hyperviscosity Syndrome** SGA infants have an increased incidence of polycythemia, probably because of chronic intrauterine hypoxia, which induces increased erythropoiesis. Some SGA infants can have a central hematocrit greater than 60% to 65%; only 5% of term AGA infants have a central hematocrit greater than 65%.

#### Longer Term Problems

**Immune Function and Infectious Diseases** Immunologic function of SGA infants can be impaired at birth and even in childhood. SGA infants often have deficiencies in lymphocyte numbers and function, low immunoglobulin levels during infancy, and attenuated antibody responses to vaccines.

**Neurodevelopmental Outcome** Neurological disorders occur 5 to 10 times more often in SGA than in AGA infants. Such disorders include hyperactivity, short attention span, learning disabilities associated with substandard school performance, and subtle neurological and behavioral problems, including fine motor incoordination, hyperreflexia, speech problems, and diffuse electroencephalographic abnormalities. Relative microcephaly at birth that resulted from growth restriction or congenital infections is especially associated with poor developmental outcomes in severely SGA infants.



**Somatic Growth** SGA infants with severe IUGR continue to have short stature, and males particularly may remain relatively underweight as they age. The short stature persists into adulthood, indicating permanence of the growth deficits. SGA infants who have had mild to moderate IUGR that developed in later gestation tend to have accelerated growth velocity during the first 6 months, and some achieve a growth rate and body size similar to those of AGA infants. Overfeeding such infants, however, can promote obesity, indicating that such approaches to nutrition and feeding of SGA infants carry significant risks.

**Impact on Adult Health Status** Recent epidemiologic evidence indicates that insulin resistance, glucose intolerance, obesity, diabetes, and cardiovascular disease are more common among adults who were SGA secondary to IUGR compared to those who were AGA at birth. Adaptive mechanisms that develop in the fetus in response to nutrient deprivation, such as increased glucose and insulin sensitivity, may underlie or contribute to these disorders by enhancing the formation of fat in adipose tissue in response to increased caloric intake, as is common in modern Western diets.

## SUGGESTED READINGS


Committee on Fetus and Newborn, Adamkin DH. Postnatal glucose homeostasis in late-preterm and term infants. *Pediatrics.* 2011; 127(3):575-579.

Dearden L, Ozanne SE. The road between early growth and obesity: new twists and turns. *Am J Clin Nutr.* 2014;100(1):6-7.

Dimasuay KG, Boeuf P, Powell TL, Jansson T. Placental responses to changes in the maternal environment determine fetal growth. *Front Physiol.* 2016;7:12.

Fowden AL, Sibley C, Reik W, Constancia M. Imprinted genes, placental development and fetal growth. *Horm Res.* 2006;65(Suppl 3): 50-58.

Gluckman PD, Hanson MA, Cooper C, Thornburg KL. Effect of in utero and early life conditions on adult health and disease. *N Engl J Med.* 2008;359(1):61-73.

Green AS, Rozance PJ, Limesand SW. Consequences of a compromised intrauterine environment on islet function. *J Endocrinol.* 2010;205(3): 211-224.

Guellec I, Lappillonne A, Renolleau S, et al; EPIPAGE Study Group. Neurologic outcomes at school age in very preterm infants born with severe or mild growth restriction. *Pediatrics.* 2011;127(4): e883-e891.

Hack M. Effects of intrauterine growth retardation on mental performance and behavior outcomes during adolescence and adulthood. *Eur J Clin Nutr.* 1998;52(Suppl. 1):S65-S70.

Hack M, Breslau N, Weissman B, Aram D, Klein N, Borawski E. Effect of very low birth weight and subnormal head size on cognitive abilities at school age. *N Engl J Med.* 1991;325(4):231-237.

Peeling AN, Smart JL. Review of literature showing that undernutrition affects the growth rate of all processes in the brain to the same extent. *Metab Brain Dis.* 1994;9(1):33-42.

Regnault TRH, Limesand SW, Hay WW Jr. Aspects of fetoplacental nutrition in intrauterine growth restriction and macrosomia. In: Thureen PJ, Hay WW Jr., eds. *Neonatal Nutrition and Metabolism.* 2nd ed. Cambridge: Cambridge University Press; 2006:32-46.

Rozance PJ, Brown LD, Thorn SR, Anderson, MS, Hay WW Jr. Intrauterine growth restriction and the small-for-gestational-age infant. In: MacDonald MG, Seshia MMK, eds. *Avery's Neonatology: Pathophysiology and Management of the Newborn.* 7th ed. Philadelphia, PA: Lippincott Williams & Wilkins; 2015:357-376.

Smart JL. Undernutrition, learning and memory: review of experimental studies. In: Taylor TG, Jenkins NK, eds. *Proceedings of XII International Congress of Nutrition.* London, UK: John Libbey; 1986:74.

Smart JL. Vulnerability of developing brain to undernutrition. *Ups J Med Sci Suppl.* 1990;48:21-41.

van Wassenaer A. Neurodevelopmental consequences of being born SGA. *Pediatr Endocrinol Rev.* 2005;2(3):373-377.


# 50 Infant of a Diabetic Mother

Heather M. French and Rebecca A. Simmons

## INTRODUCTION

The true prevalence of diabetes in pregnancy (including gestational diabetes and pregestational diabetes) is unknown, but most studies report rates as high as 10% in the United States. Whereas 90% of cases encountered during pregnancy are caused by gestational diabetes mellitus (GDM), the incidence of pregestational diabetes mellitus is rapidly increasing, in large part due to the increased incidence of obesity-related type 2 diabetes. Unfortunately, the prevalence of type 2 diabetes has been increasing in every age group and ethnicity in the United States for the past 10 years. The epidemic of childhood obesity in the United States causing a sharp increase in childhood and adolescent diabetes will have a profound impact on obstetric and pediatric practices for the next generation.

## COMPLICATIONS IN THE INFANT

The infant of a diabetic mother (IDM) is at increased risk for development of periconceptional, fetal, neonatal, and long-term morbidities. Most, if not all, of the complications are related to maternal glycemic control, both before and during pregnancy. Before insulin was available to the pregnant mother, perinatal mortality rates were as high as 75%. With the addition of insulin therapy and good prenatal care, perinatal mortality rates now approach those seen in the nondiabetic population.

However, even with strict glycemic control, fetal and infant complications persist. Congenital anomalies are 3 to 4 times greater in the diabetic versus nondiabetic pregnancies. Macrosomia and related birth injuries occur 10 times more frequently in diabetic pregnancies. Hypoglycemia, electrolyte abnormalities, and hyperviscosity syndrome can render management in the neonatal period challenging for pediatricians. Commonly encountered complications in the perinatal and neonatal period include the following:

- Intrauterine fetal demise
- Macrosomia or intrauterine growth restriction
- Birth trauma
- Perinatal depression
- Congenital anomalies
- Respiratory distress syndrome
- Neonatal hypoglycemia
- Electrolyte abnormalities such as hypocalcemia and hypomagnesemia
- Polycythemia and hyperviscosity syndrome
- Hyperbilirubinemia
- Cardiomyopathy

No single pathogenic mechanism has been identified to explain the diversity of problems encountered in the IDM. Nonetheless, most researchers agree that many of the effects can be attributed to maternal metabolic control. In 1977, the hypothesis of "hyperinsulinism" in the IDM was proposed by Jorgen Pedersen. The hypothesis recognized that maternal hyperglycemia causes fetal hyperglycemia, which results in fetal islet cell hypertrophy and β cell hyperplasia due to chronic fetal pancreas stimulation. Insulin, an anabolic hormone, and the hyperinsulinemic state lead to visceromegaly and macrosomia. At delivery, with the sudden loss of maternal glucose supplies, hypoglycemia quickly ensues. However, this hypothesis does not tell the whole story, as birth weight is not always correlated with mean maternal plasma glucose concentration. Further, the large Hyperglycemia and Adverse Pregnancy Outcome (HAPO) study found a significant association between infant adverse outcomes and higher levels of maternal glucose within what is currently considered a nondiabetic range. It is likely that control of fetal growth and fetal glucose homeostasis is multifactorial.

### Congenital Anomalies

Major congenital anomalies are the leading causes of perinatal mortality in pregnancies complicated by pregestational diabetes, occurring in 6% to 12% of IDMs, compared to a 2% to 3% incidence in the general population. Most studies support that the risk of major malformations is related to the degree of maternal glycemic control during organogenesis in the first trimester. Unfortunately, the critical window for glycemic control may occur before pregnancy or very early in pregnancy, before there is even recognition that a pregnancy has occurred. Elevated glycosylated hemoglobin levels (Hb $A_{1C}$) directly correlate with the frequency of anomalies, but as noted above, even with a Hb $A_{1C}$ in the normal range, the rate of congenital anomalies is increased in diabetic women. A level of Hb $A_{1C}$ of 7% to 8.5% is associated with a 5% to 6% risk of congenital anomaly, and a level of Hb $A_{1C}$ greater than 10% is associated with an anomaly rate of 20% to 25%.

What precisely leads to congenital malformations in IDMs remains unknown. Attempts to answer this question definitely in animal models and human studies have been unsuccessful. Hypoglycemia, hyperglycemia, insulin, ketone bodies, tumor necrosis factor-α, free oxygen radicals, and disordered metabolism of arachidonic acid and prostaglandin all have been proposed as candidate teratogens, but each lacks solid scientific support to be declared the sole responsible teratogen.

Congenital heart defects are anomalies frequently reported in IDMs. Ventral septal defects are the most prevalent congenital heart defect, but more severe defects, such as atrial septal defects, transposition of the great arteries, and left-sided obstructive lesions, also are reported. Neural tube defects, including myelomeningocele, encephalocele, anencephaly, and hydrocephalus, have an increased incidence in IDMs compared to the general population. Gastrointestinal atresia, gastroschisis, intestinal malrotation, renal and urinary tract malformations, and skeletal malformations also are reported. Spinal agenesis associated with caudal regression syndrome is a congenital anomaly that is found exclusively in IDMs. Additionally, small left colon syndrome is a rare but well described anomaly associated with IDM. Presenting symptoms of gastrointestinal obstruction are caused by a transient but decreased diameter of the descending and sigmoid colon and rectum. This syndrome mimics Hirschsprung disease, but colonic innerviation and, ultimately, function are normal.

### Body Size and Macrosomia

Insulin is the major anabolic hormone and glucose is the major anabolic fuel for fetal growth. In the setting of excess glucose and cellular uptake, glycogen and fat synthesis increase, especially during the third trimester after 32 weeks. Macrosomia, which is defined as a birthweight above the 90th percentile for gestational age or greater than 4000 grams, is the result of excess fuel deposition, causing increased body fat, increased muscle mass, and organomegaly, especially of the heart and liver. Skeletal growth is largely unaffected. Therefore, IDMs have higher weight than length and head circumference percentiles. This disproportionate head/body size explains the increased incidence of shoulder dystocia. Macrosomia occurs in 15% to 45% of cases, which is 3 times higher than in the general population.

Most of the excess fat in IDMs is deposited centrally in the abdomen and intrascapular areas, placing the infant at risk for shoulder dystocia and delivery by cesarean section. Although linear relationships between insulin levels and birthweight have been shown, other metabolic fuels may contribute to macrosomia in the IDM as well. Positive correlations have been demonstrated between maternal triglyceride levels, amino acids, and free fatty acids with birth weight. Thus, macrosomia likely is multifactorial in nature.

The rate of delivery by cesarean section in diabetic women is 3 times higher than that of the general population, but the difference is not entirely attributable to macrosomia. Given the concerns over shoulder dystocia and perinatal depression, caregivers are more prone to perform cesarean deliveries because of the concerns for a poor outcome and the imperfect clinical ability to predict which infants are at the highest risk. Macrosomia can lead to a difficult vaginal delivery due to shoulder dystocia, with resultant birth injury or perinatal depression. Birth injuries, which include cephalohematoma, subdural or ocular hemorrhage, facial palsy, brachial plexus injuries, clavicular fractures, and abdominal organ injury, are 2 to 4 times more common among IDMs, with macrosomic infants having the highest risk.

Not all IDMs are macrosomic. Mothers with advanced pregestational diabetes are at risk for giving birth to a small-for-gestational-age infant. Advanced maternal vascular disease, seen in pregnant women with diabetes-associated retinal or renal vasculopathies and/or chronic hypertension, leads to placental insufficiency and can cause fetal growth restriction and a deficiency of nutrients and oxygen.

### Neonatal Hypoglycemia

At delivery, the maternal supply of glucose is abruptly terminated, and hypoglycemia, defined as a blood glucose less than 40 mg/dL, can occur in all infants. It is particularly likely to occur in IDMs, especially if they are macrosomic, for several reasons. Most IDMs have elevated C-peptide or insulin levels at baseline, which quickly leads to clearance of available serum glucose. Hypoglycemia normally leads to cathecholamine and glucagon release, in turn resulting in glycogen breakdown and gluconeogenesis. In the IDM, this response to hypoglycemia may be blunted. Additionally, if perinatal stress was experienced, catecholamine release and glycogen depletion may have occurred. Therefore, the IDM has increased glucose clearance from serum as well as decreased glucose production.

Hypoglycemia usually develops within the first 24 hours of life. Infants can be asymptomatic or present with nonspecific symptoms, such as jitteriness, irritability, tachypnea, apnea, lethargy, hypotonia, poor feeding, or frank seizure activity. Hypoglycemia, even if asymptomatic, can cause brain injury and lead to long-term neurodevelopmental complications.

Hypocalcemia occurs in 20% to 50% of IDMs during the neonatal period. Unlike hypoglycemia, hypocalcemia usually arises later—between 48 and 72 hours of life. Serum calcium levels lower than 7 mg/dL are frequently observed. Clinical signs of hypocalcemia include tremors, twitching, sweating, irritability, arrhythmia seizures, and, occasionally, decreased myocardial contractility. A prolonged QT interval is associated with hypocalcemia but is not often observed in IDMs.

During fetal life, calcium is transferred by active transport across the placenta. The fetus, especially during the third trimester, has low parathyroid hormone (PTH) due to the relatively high serum calcium levels. At birth, with the abrupt end of maternal calcium transfer, infant PTH levels rise to compensate for decreasing serum calcium. In the IDM, PTH levels and end-organ sensitivity to PTH are lower than those in age-matched controls during the first 4 days after birth. Additionally, PTH secretion may be hampered by hypomagnesemia via limited magnesium-dependent adenylate cyclase action, seen more commonly in infants born to mothers with diabetes who have renal insufficiency. Hypocalcemia can be magnified if the IDM is born prematurely or suffers from acidosis or perinatal depression. Persistently high levels of calcitonin and alterations in vitamin D metabolism also may play roles.

Hypomagnesemia (< 1.5 mg/dL) occurs in as many as one-third of IDMs but rarely is of clinical significance. Neonatal magnesium levels correspond to the mother's levels as well as with maternal insulin requirements. Mothers with advanced diabetes and renal insufficiency may have significant renal losses of magnesium, which contribute to low placental transfer of this electrolyte. Magnesium treatment should be considered for the infant with documented clinical signs of hypocalcemia and low plasma calcium and magnesium concentrations.

Total and ionized serum calcium should be measured at least daily during the first 72 to 96 hours of life. Daily calcium requirements are 100 to 200 mg/kg, and IDMs may require up to 3 times that amount. Although treatment rarely is necessary, symptomatic infants should be treated with 10% calcium gluconate given intravenously under careful monitoring because of the risk of arrhythmias and intravenous (IV) infiltrates. Daily maintenance therapy (50–60 mg/kg/day) can be considered based on feeding status and laboratory value trends. It should be noted that if a hypocalcemic infant is also hypomagnesemic, calcium therapy is futile unless magnesium levels are replete.



### Hyperbilirubinemia and Polycythemia

Hyperbilirubinemia occurs more frequently in the IDM than in the general population. The pathogenesis remains uncertain as red blood cell lifespan, osmotic fragility, and deformability are not different between the 2 groups. Some research points to increased hemoglobin turnover. However, other information points to delayed clearance of bilirubin by the liver. Other risk factors for hyperbilirubinemia are macrosomia, which increases the risk for birth trauma, bruising and cephalohematoma, and polycythemia. Because of an increased hemoglobin load, bilirubin levels rise more rapidly and peak later in IDMs than in neonates of nondiabetic women. Serum bilirubin levels should be measured earlier and more frequently in IDMs compared to age-matched controls and may need to be monitored for up to 5 to 7 days. Hyperbilirubinemia is exacerbated in the preterm IDM population given delayed enteral feedings and decreased bilirubin excretion.

Chronic fetal hyperglycemia and hyperinsulinemia increase the fetal metabolic rate and increase oxygen consumption. Given that the fetus develops in a relatively hypoxic environment and oxygen extraction from maternal blood is at a maximal rate, the fetus increases its oxygen-carrying capacity by increasing erythropoiesis. Additionally, increased insulin and insulin-like growth factors also can increase production of red blood cells, putting the infant at risk for development of polycythemia (hematocrit > 65), which can occur at the expense of other bone marrow cell lines, producing transient leukopenia and/or thrombocytopenia. As many as 20% of IDMs have polycythemia. The associated hyperviscosity and vascular sludging that occur puts this group of infants at risk for development of persistent hypoglycemia, respiratory distress due to vascular congestion, heart failure, stroke, seizures, necrotizing enterocolitis, renal vein or sinus venous thrombosis, and persistent pulmonary hypertension of the newborn. Symptomatic polycythemic infants should be treated with a partial exchange transfusion to decrease the central hematocrit to less than 55%.

Thrombosis occurs more frequently in IDMs caused by both polycythemia with hyperviscosity, and low blood concentrations of anticoagulant proteins, protein C, protein S, and antithrombin, the result of the hyperinsulinemic state. Elevated insulin levels also increase the production of procoagulant proteins. Intravenous or low molecular-weight heparin treatment should be considered when significant deep vessel thrombosis is documented by Doppler flow ultrasound.

### Respiratory Disorders

Respiratory distress syndrome (RDS) requiring admission to a NICU occurs almost 6 times as frequently in IDMs compared to infants of nondiabetic mothers. Infants of diabetic mothers are at increased risk for development of RDS for several reasons. Surfactant deficiency due to delayed maturation of type II alveolar cells and their subsequent decreased synthesis and secretion of surfactant phospholipids and surfactant proteins has been observed, but it is unclear whether this state is caused by hyperglycemia, hyperinsulinemia, or both.

Glycogen levels in the lung normally decline with increasing gestational age. This decrease corresponds with increased surfactant production. Insulin inhibits glycogen breakdown, decreasing available substrate for the synthesis of phosphatidylglycerol (PG), an important component of surfactant. The presence of PG in the amniotic fluid is an indicator of lung maturity. There are several reports in the literature of delayed appearance of PG in diabetic pregnancies. Even when amniotic fluid analysis documents maturation of the surfactant production system, there is still a 10% incidence of RDS in IDMs. Other causes of respiratory distress in the IDM include increased rates of premature birth, congenital heart disease, diaphragmatic paralysis from a brachial plexus injury (due to large size and difficulty of delivery), and persistent pulmonary hypertension of the newborn caused by hyperviscosity from polycythemia or chronic fetal hypoxia.

### Cardiomyopathy

Reversible cardiomyopathy with intraventricular hypertrophy and outflow tract obstruction can occur in as many as 30% of IDMs. Cardiomyopathy may be caused by congestive failure due to a poorly functioning myocardium or hypertrophy of the intraventricular septum and 1 or both ventricular walls. Occasionally, the outflow tract obstruction becomes so profound as to require extracorporeal membrane oxygenation (ECMO) while awaiting regression of the obstruction. With supportive care, most symptoms related to septal hypertrophy resolve spontaneously within 2 weeks, with the hypertrophy itself resolving by 4 months.

The mechanism by which hypertrophic cardiomyopathy occurs is not completely understood. The human heart has been shown to be rich in insulin receptors. It is postulated that the fetus of the diabetic mother in whom hyperinsulinism develops will have increased myocardial receptor sites and increased affinity for insulin. These increases could lead to increased protein, glycogen, and fat synthesis in the myocardium and subsequent hyperplasia and hypertrophy of the myocardium. Postnatally, as serum insulin levels and the number of insulin receptors decrease, the septal hypertrophy should decrease as well. Although this hypothesis is consistent with the natural history of this disease process, other yet unidentified factors may be important as well. Other research has shown that fetuses of diabetic mothers who were thought to be in good diabetic control, as compared with normal controls, had evidence of cardiac hypertrophy at the level of the intraventricular septum and at the right and left ventricular free wall by late gestation. More sensitive markers of maternal metabolic control may be needed to better define the in utero environment that promotes this type of cardiac growth.

## OUTCOMES FOR INFANTS OF DIABETIC MOTHERS

Complications of the IDM occurring in the neonatal period are of great concern to the pediatrician. However, equal concern should be given to the long-term outcomes on growth and development, psychosocial intellectual capabilities, and the subsequent risk of developing diabetes and obesity later in life. Research suggests that the IDM is more vulnerable to intellectual impairment, which can be exacerbated by iron deficiency in the newborn and during infancy. Several studies have shown problems with memory formation, verbal conceptualization ability, acquired knowledge, spatial ability, and sequencing ability in IDMs. How much of this intellectual impairment is due to birth trauma, perinatal depression, hypoglycemia in the neonatal period, or other neonatal morbidities remains unknown. Vigilant obstetric care of the mother to maintain euglycemia during pregnancy and medical care of the infant to manage associated symptoms can greatly reduce the risk of complications developing in the neonatal period and childhood.

Even if the infant does not suffer from any early complications of maternal disease, the risk of developing obesity and diabetes later in life appears to be increased. However, unanswered questions remain regarding the size effect of the maternal intrauterine environment exposure compared to inherited genetic traits. Additional influences include the child's postnatal environment and lifestyle. Macrosomic infants of diabetic or obese mothers are at significant risk of developing metabolic syndrome (obesity, hypertension, dyslipidemia, glucose intolerance) in childhood. Oxidative stress and epigenetic alterations have been proposed as possible mechanisms for this increased risk. Given the relationship of obesity and gestational diabetes, it is likely that gestational diabetes will continue to increase in future generations.

## SUGGESTED READINGS


HAPO Study Cooperative Research Group; Metzger BE, Lowe LP, Dyer AR, et al. Hyperglycemia and adverse pregnancy outcomes. *N Engl J Med*. 2008;358(9):1991-2002.

Hay WW Jr. Care of the infant of the diabetic mother. *Curr Diab Rep*. 2012;12(1):4-15.

Mitanchez D, Yzydorczyk C, Siddeek B, Boubred F, Benahmed M, Simeoni U. The offspring of the diabetic mother: short- and long-term implications. *Best Pract Res Clin Obstet Gynaecol*. 2015;29(2):256-269.

VanHaltren K, Malhotra A. Characteristics of infants at risk of hypoglycaemia secondary to being "infant of a diabetic mother." *J Pediatr Endocrinol Metab*. 2013;26(9-10):861-865.


# PART 3 NONSPECIFIC NEONATAL CONDITIONS



# 51 Approach to the Cyanotic Infant

Satyan Lakshminrusimha and Robin H. Steinhorn

## INTRODUCTION

Cyanosis, or bluish discoloration of the skin, is derived from the Greek word *kuaneos*, meaning "dark blue." Cyanosis is caused by the presence of deoxygenated hemoglobin in the blood vessels that is most visible on the surface of the skin and mucosa. The mechanisms of cyanosis are outlined in Table 51-1 and Figure 51-1. In general, cyanosis occurs because (1) the binding of oxygen to hemoglobin is abnormal, so that blood does not carry much oxygen despite having a normal partial pressure of oxygen, or $PO_2$ (eg, methemoglobin or carboxyhemoglobin); (2) the perfusion of the skin is poor, such that the venous and capillary blood are very deoxygenated even though the arterial blood may be well oxygenated (eg, cold environment or circulatory shock); or (3) the arterial, and therefore the capillary and venous blood, is poorly oxygenated (eg, a right-to-left shunt with congenital cardiac disease, parenchymal pulmonary disease, or hypoventilation).

Cyanosis typically becomes apparent when there is about 3 to 5 g/dL of deoxygenated hemoglobin, but detection varies widely depending on lighting, observer differences, and pigmentation of the skin, among other factors. The oxygen binding capacity of the fetal hemoglobin in the newborn also alters the degree of desaturation at a given $PaO_2$. For example, at a $PaO_2$ 45 mmHg, the saturation of adult hemoglobin would fall below 80%, typically creating a cyanotic appearance, but fetal hemoglobin saturation would remain in the mid 80s, which may not be associated with overt cyanosis. There is urgency to determine the cause of cyanosis because of the high risk of tissue injury or death posed by poor oxygenation and in order to guide important interventions to improve tissue oxygenation. Although a specific diagnosis may not necessarily be determined at the bedside without special investigations, the underlying nature of the disturbance usually can be derived with common clinical tools and the physical examination.

## ASSESSMENT OF CYANOSIS

### Pulse Oximetry

Arterial $O_2$ saturation using pulse oximetry should immediately be measured in any cyanotic newborn infant. Visual perception of cyanosis in a newborn is very subjective and cannot reliably detect or rule out hypoxemia. New guidelines for resuscitation and screening rely on pulse oximetry. The neonatal resuscitation program recommends application of a pulse oximeter (with the sensor attached to right hand or wrist) if resuscitation is anticipated at birth. Simultaneous preductal and postductal oxygen saturations by pulse oximetry ($SpO_2$) are recommended as a screen for critical congenital heart disease (CCHD) for all newborn infants. Functional saturation ($HbO_2$/[Hb+$HbO_2$]) is measured by traditional pulse oximeters and can display normal values in the presence of carboxyhemoglobin (COHb) and fixed saturation in the mid to high 80s with methemogloblin (MetHb). The newer pulse oximeters can measure fractional saturation of hemoglobin and detect methemoglobinemia and carboxyhemoglobinemia. It is particularly important to measure the oxygen saturation of tissue that is likely perfused from the aorta proximal to the ductus arteriosus—generally, the right hand or, if possible, an ear lobe—and from a lower extremity. Although there is some imprecision in oximeters, especially if perfusion is poor, this approach will help establish whether the hypoxemia is a valid finding. Furthermore, right-to-left shunting across the ductus arteriosus may be detected when the upper and lower body saturations differ consistently by more than 3% to 5%. If there is indeed hypoxemia, measurement of arterial blood gas tensions and pH is also important to help determine whether there is an acidemia of respiratory (from hypoventilation or fatigue) or metabolic (from tissue hypoxia) origin.

### Physical Examination

A rapid assessment of the circulatory and respiratory systems can establish a few important issues. By evaluating central and peripheral pulses, capillary refill, and extremity warmth, it should be apparent whether poor perfusion with peripheral vasoconstriction is contributing to the cyanotic appearance. The clinician should simultaneously assess the breathing pattern to determine whether the child has signs of respiratory distress or quiet and unlabored respiration. Pulmonary

**TABLE 51-1 PATHOGENESIS OF CYANOSIS IN THE NEWBORN INFANT**

| Mechanism for Cyanosis | Key Findings | Examples |
|---|---|---|
| Abnormal hemoglobin, normal arterial $PO_2$ (rare) | Normal perfusion, normal respiratory pattern | COHb (usually $SpO_2$ normal); MetHb ($SpO_2$ 85%), |
| High hemoglobin concentration, slightly decreased arterial $PO_2$ and arterial $SpO_2$, normal venous and capillary $PO_2$ | Cyanotic extremities, normal central pulses, normal respiratory pattern, or tachypnea | Polycythemia |
| Normal or slightly decreased arterial $PO_2$, very decreased venous and capillary $PO_2$ | Cyanotic extremities, normal central pulses, normal respiratory pattern | Acrocyanosis, cold environment |
| | Cyanotic or pale extremities, poor pulses, prolonged capillary refill, tachycardia; respiratory distress; consistent with circulatory shock | Aortic atresia, coarctation; myocardial dysfunction<br>Note: if pulses greater in upper vs lower extremities, consider coarctation or interrupted aortic arch; if $SpO_2$ greater in upper vs lower extremities, consider pulmonary hypertension or coarctation with R-L ductus shunt; if $SpO_2$ greater in lower vs upper extremities, consider transposition with aortic arch obstruction |
| Decreased arterial $PO_2$ | Normal respiratory pattern, decreased pulmonary blood flow, normal perfusion with or without murmurs → intracardiac R-L shunt | Tetralogy of Fallot, tricuspid atresia, pulmonary stenosis or atresia |
| | Normal respiratory pattern, normal or increased pulmonary blood flow, normal perfusion → intracardiac R-L shunt | Transposition |
| | Respiratory distress and pulmonary edema with poor systemic perfusion | Left heart inlet or outlet obstruction |
| | Severe respiratory distress, consolidation, collapse, airway obstruction | Pulmonary parenchymal disease or airway obstruction |
| Decreased arterial $PO_2$ with increased arterial $PCO_2$ | Diminished respiratory effort | Hypoventilation |

COHb, carboxyhemoglobin; MetHb, methemoglobin; $PCO_2$, partial pressure of carbon dioxide; $PO_2$, partial pressure of oxygen; R-L, right-to-left; $SpO_2$, oxygen saturation measured by pulse oximetry.



edema, alveolar consolidation, or collapse sufficient to cause cyanosis is invariably accompanied by an increase in inspiratory work, including tachypnea, retractions, grunting, accessory muscle use, or nasal flaring. In contrast, the child with normal pulmonary mechanical function would be expected to breathe somewhat more quickly and more deeply than normal in the presence of hypoxemia but would not have signs of markedly increased work. Finally, if an infant has slow and shallow respirations and appears to have depressed responses, this might be caused by respiratory depression, in which case the hypoxemia is caused by hypoventilation.

Based on the initial oximetry and blood gas data and the physical examination, a few preliminary conclusions might be derived regarding the potential underlying disease (Fig. 51-2).

## CARDIOPULMONARY ADAPTATION AT BIRTH

At birth, profound changes in the cardiovascular and respiratory systems occur to allow the infant to adapt to air breathing (see Chapter 45). An understanding of these normal transitional changes is important in evaluating a cyanotic infant, as their disruption is likely to lead to cyanosis. The fetus has a unique circulatory pattern because the placenta, not the lung, serves as the organ of gas exchange. Approximately 10% to 20% of the combined ventricular cardiac output is circulated through the pulmonary vascular bed, and the placenta receives nearly half of the cardiac output. Pulmonary blood flow remains low due to elevated pulmonary vascular resistance; pulmonary pressure is equivalent to systemic pressure due to active vasoconstriction. Fetal circulation shunts blood from the right to left atrium across the foramen ovale and from the pulmonary artery to the descending aorta through the ductus arteriosus, providing direct blood flow to the placenta.

The fetal lungs produce fluid that fills the alveoli, bronchi, and trachea. At birth, catecholamines and other hormones that increase during labor cause a rapid switch from net secretion to net absorption of liquid in alveolar spaces. As the lungs fill with air, lung fluid is removed via the trachea and via absorption by the pulmonary capillaries and lymphatics. Pulmonary vascular resistance drops dramatically and permits an 8-fold to 10-fold rise in pulmonary blood flow. Simultaneously, the low vascular resistance bed of the placenta is removed and systemic vascular resistance increases. As pulmonary pressure falls to less than systemic pressure, pulmonary blood flow increases and blood flow through the patent ductus arteriosus reverses direction. Functional closure of the ductus usually occurs over the first several hours of life, largely in response to the increased oxygen tension. Left atrial pressure also increases, leading to closure of the foramen ovale. These events therefore eliminate the fetal right-to-left shunts and establish the normal postnatal circulatory pattern of pulmonary and systemic circulations. Within 24 hours after birth, pulmonary artery pressure typically decreases to approximately 50% of mean systemic arterial pressure and continues to drop over the next 2 to 6 weeks.

The initiation of air breathing and a drop in pulmonary vascular resistance allow arterial oxygen tension to rise after birth. $SpO_2$ measured by pulse oximetry rises slowly after birth and does not usually reach 90% until after the first 5 minutes of life. Further, the postductal $SpO_2$ level may be lower than the preductal level for as long as 15 minutes, because right-to-left ductal shunting across the ductus arteriosus frequently occurs during early transition.

## DIFFERENTIAL DIAGNOSIS OF CYANOSIS IN INFANTS

Utilizing an ABC (airway, breathing, circulation) algorithm of evaluation permits a rapid and systematic consideration of the most common causes of cyanosis in the newborn period (Table 51-2 and Fig. 51-3). It is important to recognize that cyanosis is more difficult to recognize at lower hemoglobin values due to the altered concentration of deoxygenated hemoglobin (Table 51-3).

### Upper and Lower Airway Disease

**Upper Airway Obstruction** Abnormalities of the airway will generally present shortly after birth. Choanal atresia occurs in about 1 in 5000 infants, with unilateral disease being more common. Choanal atresia should be suspected when an infant's distress is more obvious in a quiet state and improves during crying. It can be confirmed by the inability to pass a suction catheter through the nares into the oropharynx, as well as by computer tomography scanning. Placement

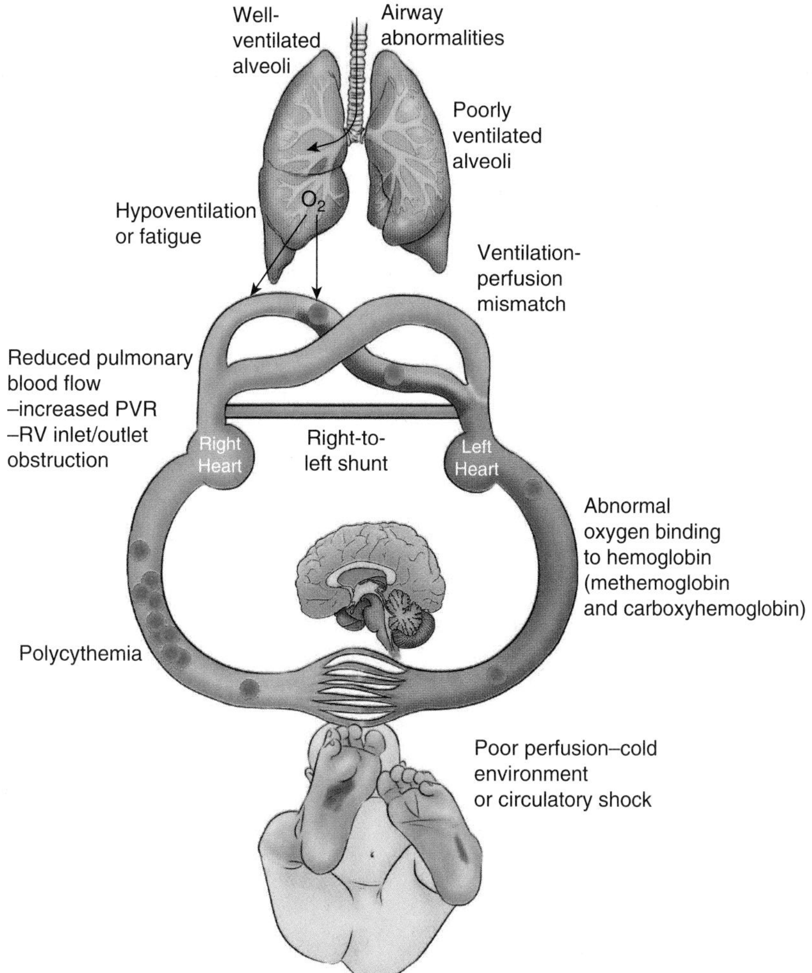


**FIGURE 51-1** Mechanisms of cyanosis in newborn infants. Decreased inspired oxygen concentration, airway abnormalities, lung disease (by ventilation-perfusion mismatch), abnormalities of hemoglobin, poor perfusion, polycythemia, heart disease (reduced pulmonary blood flow or right-to-left shunting or poor perfusion), and hypoventilation and fatigue can result in cyanosis. PVR, pulmonary vascular resistance; RV, right ventricle. (Used with permission from Satyan Lakshminrusimha and Robin Steinhorn.)

of an oral airway should provide immediate improvement. Other associated anomalies are very common; in particular, the CHARGE sequence (coloboma, heart disease, atresia of choana, retarded growth and development, genitourinary anomalies, ear/hearing anomalies) should be considered.

Micrognathia, retrognathia, or the Pierre Robin sequence generally presents early in life and will be obvious on physical examination. The airway obstruction from the posterior tongue is more pronounced in the supine position. When present, a cleft palate does not cause respiratory distress unless feeding difficulties are severe. These infants may require tracheostomy for several years until the mandible grows enough to maintain the tongue in a more anterior position. A tongue-lip adhesion procedure and mandibular distraction osteogenesis (MDO) to slowly lengthen the lower jaw may be effective in relieving airway obstruction.

Laryngomalacia is a congenital abnormality of the larynx and is the most common cause of inspiratory stridor in infants. While it may be noted immediately after birth, it commonly presents at several weeks of age. Airway symptoms typically worsen with crying, feeding, and respiratory infections. Gastroesophageal reflux is a common association. Subglottic stenosis may occur as a congenital malformation or be acquired after prior airway manipulation. Infants present with stridor, respiratory distress, or obstructive apnea.

Vocal cord paralysis may occur in association with birth or surgical trauma and is another common cause of stridor in the newborn. It is typically unilateral, causing a hoarse cry and minimal respiratory symptoms. In contrast, bilateral vocal cord paralysis can cause severe respiratory distress, and a tracheostomy may be required. In these cases, central nervous system anomalies such as the Arnold-Chiari malformation should be considered.

**Tracheal Stenosis or Compression** Other conditions may cause intrinsic or extrinsic compression of the trachea. Tracheal stenosis is characterized by inspiratory and expiratory stridor, respiratory distress, wheezing, and persistent cough. Symptoms typically worsen after an upper airway infection. The diagnosis is confirmed by direct bronchoscopic visualization. Tracheal stenosis is often associated with complete tracheal rings, which may require extensive surgical repair in the case of multiple rings or long-segment stenosis. A number of conditions may produce extrinsic airway compression. Abnormal development of the great vessels (eg, vascular ring) can compress or deviate the trachea, causing airway obstruction. An anomalous distal origin of the innominate artery from the aortic arch is the most common cause of extrinsic vascular compression, but other anomalies include double aortic arch or an aberrant right subclavian artery. Specialized cardiac computerized tomography or magnetic resonance imaging studies are helpful in accurately defining the anatomy. Neck or mediastinal masses, such as teratomas and cystic hygromas, represent large lesions that can cause extrinsic compression of the trachea; these typically are associated with visible neck masses. Subglottic hemangiomas should be considered in infants who have skin hemangiomas. Because hemangiomas typically increase in size over the first 6 to 12 months of life, symptoms often

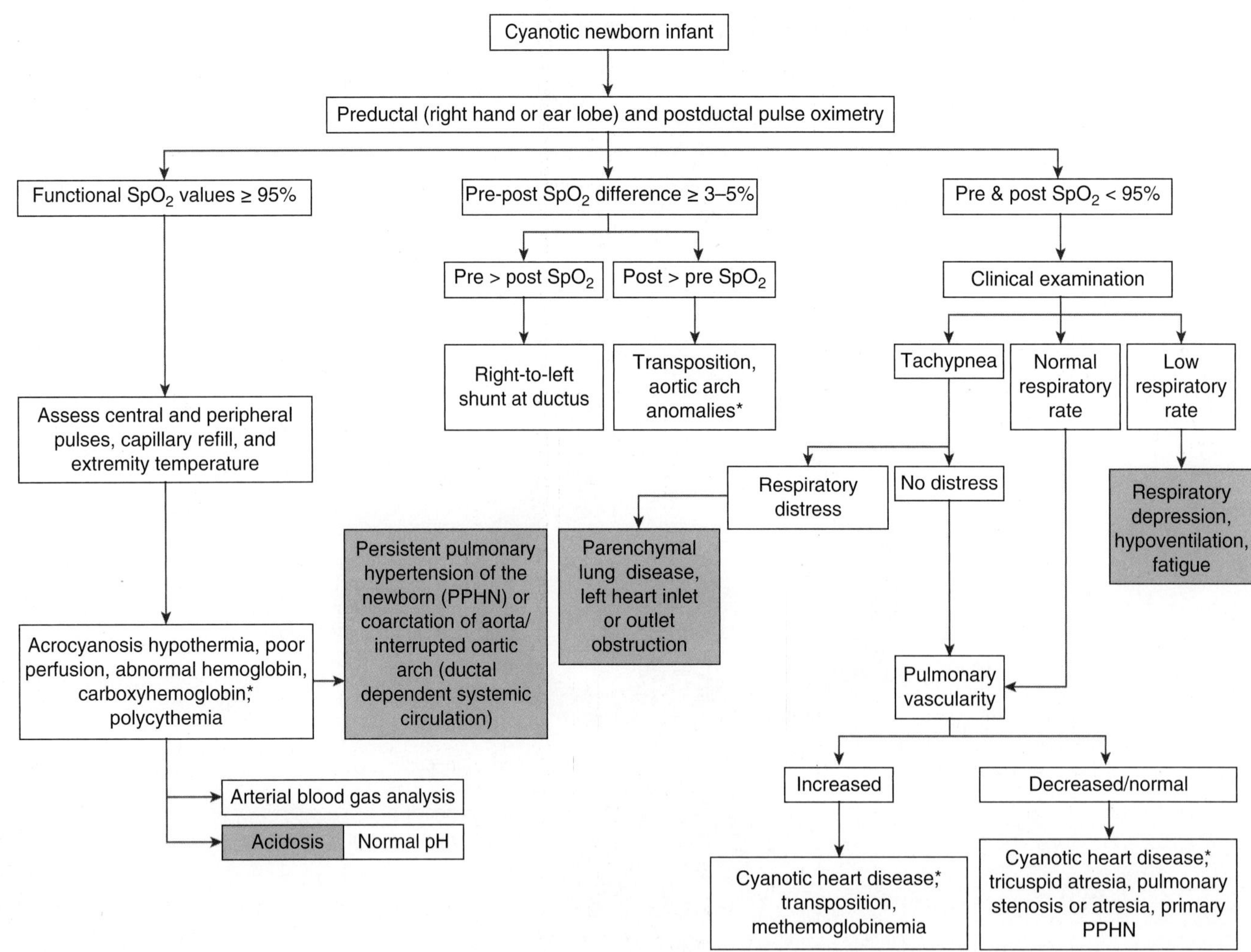


**FIGURE 51-2** Approach to a newborn infant with cyanosis. Obtaining preductal and postductal oxygen saturation by pulse oximetry ($SpO_2$) is the first step in evaluation. Final diagnosis in black boxes represents conditions most likely to be associated with acidosis on an arterial blood gas analysis. Conditions that may be associated with normal pH (at least in the initial phases) are shown in white boxes. It is important to remember that prolonged hypoxemia will eventually result in acidosis. *May present with acidosis following hypoxemia and/or hypoperfusion.



emerge after an initially benign history. The trachea can also be compressed by masses such as teratomas, cystic hygromas, or hemangiomas.

### Lung Disease

**Respiratory Distress Syndrome** Respiratory distress syndrome (RDS; see also Chapter 57) occurs almost exclusively in premature infants. The cause of RDS is surfactant deficiency, which results in decreased lung compliance and functional residual capacity and increased dead space. While the incidence and severity of RDS decreases in more mature infants, it is important to remember that a significant percentage of late preterm infants (defined as 34 0/7 to 36 6/7 weeks' gestation) will develop RDS. Infants will present visible respiratory distress (tachypnea, grunting, nasal flaring, subcostal and intercostal retractions) associated with their cyanosis. A chest radiograph will show poor lung expansion association with a homogenous "ground-glass" appearance and air bronchograms (which are produced by air-filled bronchi superimposed on collapsed alveoli).

**Neonatal Pneumonia** Neonatal pneumonia is most commonly acquired at the time of birth and usually causes diffuse rather than lobar infiltrates. The initial chest radiograph may be indistinguishable from the ground-glass appearance of RDS, although pleural effusions are more characteristic of pneumonia. Bacterial pneumonia is most common, and frequent pathogens include group B β-hemolytic streptococci (GBS) and Gram-negative enteric bacilli (*Escherichia coli, Klebsiella, Enterobacter*). Important elements of the maternal history will include colonization with group B β-hemolytic streptococci with or without adequate intrapartum prophylaxis (more than 2 doses of penicillin prior to delivery) as well as a history of prolonged rupture of membranes (> 18 hours) or a history of maternal fever or chorioamnionitis. Herpes simplex and cytomegalovirus are viral causes of neonatal pneumonia but typically present as components of disseminated infections. Congenital chlamydia infections can cause pneumonia that presents between 2 and 8 weeks of age, typically with upper respiratory symptoms associated with a cough and apnea.

**Meconium Aspiration Syndrome** Approximately 13% of all live births are associated with meconium-stained fluid, although only 5% of these infants develop meconium aspiration syndrome. The traditional belief was that aspiration occurs with the first breath after birth, leading to the practice of aggressive suctioning protocols. More recent data suggest that in utero aspiration may be responsible for the most severely affected infants and the neonatal resuscitation program no longer recommends routine tracheal suctioning for infants born through meconium-stained amniotic fluid. Meconium aspiration can injure the lungs through multiple mechanisms, including mechanical obstruction of the airways, chemical pneumonitis, inactivation of surfactant, and vasoconstriction of pulmonary vessels, all of which prevent adequate ventilation and oxygenation in the immediate postnatal period. Air trapping substantially increases the risk of pneumothorax. Infants tend to present shortly after birth with a variable degree of respiratory distress and hypoxemia; the latter is often in proportion to the severity of pulmonary hypertension. The chest radiograph typically reveals coarse, patchy infiltrates with hyperinflation of the lung fields, although the severity of radiographic findings does not correlate well with the clinical disease.

**TABLE 51-2 COMMON CAUSES OF CYANOSIS**

| A: Airway | B: Breathing | C: Circulation |
|---|---|---|
| Choanal atresia | Respiratory distress syndrome | Oxygen carrying capacity |
| Micrognathia | Pneumonia | Polycythemia |
| Pierre Robin sequence | Meconium aspiration syndrome | Anemia |
| Laryngomalacia | Congenital diaphragmatic hernia | Methemoglobinemia |
| Vocal cord paralysis | Congenital cystic adenomatoid malformation | Congenital heart disease |
| Tracheal stenosis | Pulmonary sequestration | Decreased pulmonary blood flow |
| Vascular slings/rings | Congenital lobar emphysema | Tricuspid atresia |
| Cystic hygroma | Pulmonary hypoplasia | Pulmonary atresia |
| Hemangioma | Phrenic nerve palsy | Pulmonary stenosis |
| Other neck masses | Hypoventilation | Tetralogy of Fallot |
| | | Ebstein anomaly |
| | | Inadequate mixing |
| | | Transposition of the great arteries |
| | | Persistent pulmonary hypertension |

**Congenital Lung Abnormalities** Congenital lung abnormalities are rare but important causes of respiratory distress in the newborn. In many cases, infants are initially asymptomatic, with respiratory distress developing over time. Careful review of the chest x-ray should reveal most of these lesions. Congenital diaphragmatic hernia is a relatively common birth defect, occurring in approximately 1 per 3000 births. Due to its frequent association with significant pulmonary hypoplasia and pulmonary hypertension, infants with congenital diaphragmatic hernia typically present shortly after birth with respiratory distress. Congenital cystic adenomatoid malformations (CCAM) are extremely rare lung abnormalities composed of cystic lung tissue with communication to the bronchial tree. In some cases, medical imaging is needed to differentiate this lesion from a congenital diaphragmatic hernia. Pulmonary sequestration is a rare condition characterized by nonfunctioning primitive lung tissue that does not communicate with the tracheobronchial tree and receives vascular supply from the systemic circulation (thoracic or abdominal aorta). Sequestrations may occasionally present in the neonatal period with signs of congestive heart failure due to the "runoff" circulation but more commonly present later in life with recurrent infections. Congenital lobar emphysema

**TABLE 51-3 EFFECT OF HEMOGLOBIN CONCENTRATION ON THE RECOGNITION OF CYANOSIS**

| Hb (g) | Reduced Hb (g) | $SaO_2$ | Total Hb–Reduced Hb/Total Hb |
|---|---|---|---|
| 20 | 3 | 85 | (20–3)/20 |
| 8 | 3 | 62 | (8–3)/20 |

These data show the expected levels of saturation for 2 hypothetical babies: 1 with a normal hemoglobin (20 g/dL) and 1 with a low hemoglobin (8 g/dL). Both babies have a fixed reduced hemoglobin level of 3 grams. The infant with the hemoglobin of 20 will have a saturation of 85% and may appear cyanotic. However, the severely anemic infant may not appear cyanotic until the saturation is critically low.

Hb, hemoglobin; $SaO_2$, arterial oxygen saturation.

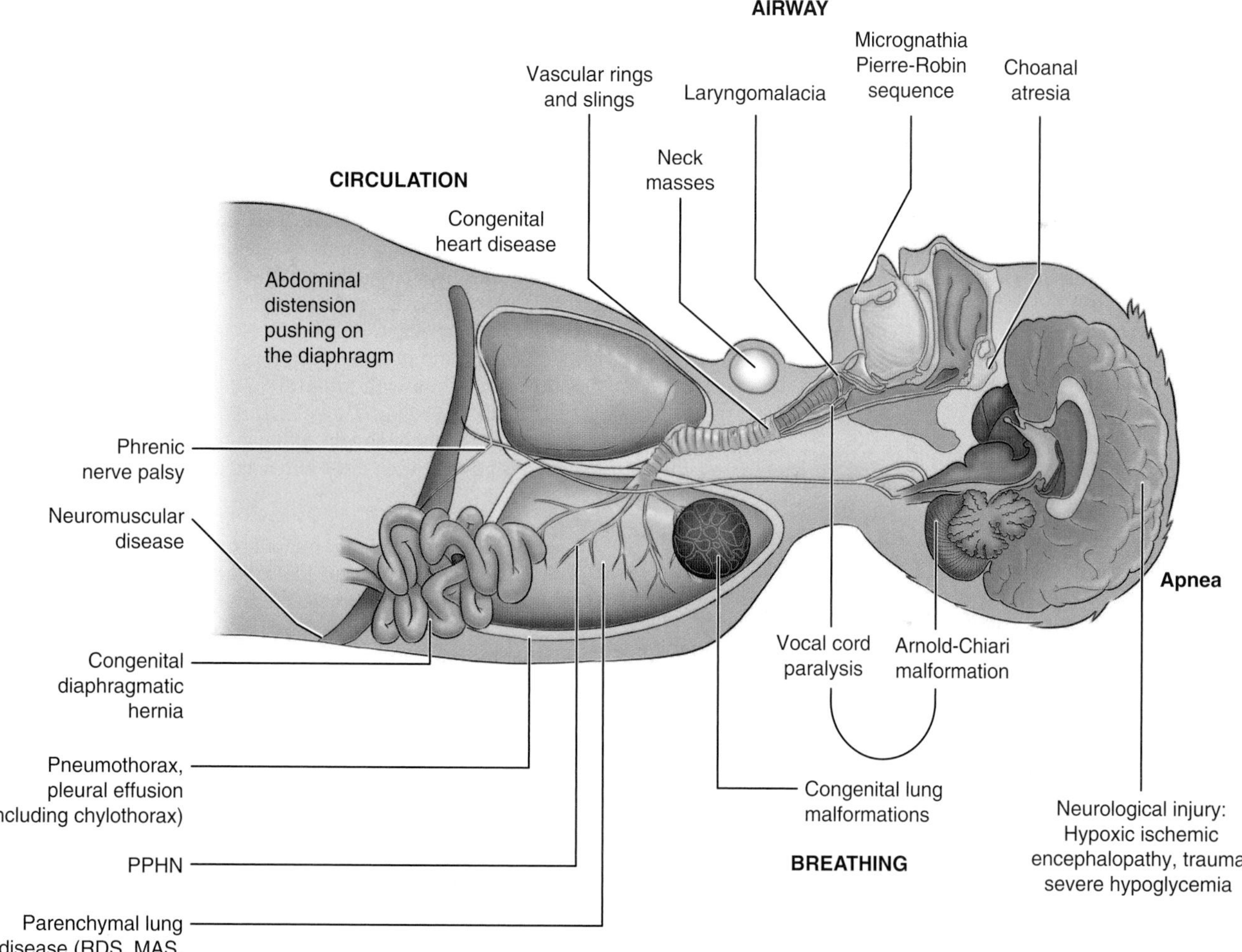


**FIGURE 51-3** Causes of cyanosis in newborn infants. MAS, meconium aspiration syndrome; PPHN, persistent pulmonary hypertension of the newborn; RDS, respiratory distress syndrome. (Used with permission from Satyan Lakshminrusimha and Robin Steinhorn.)

(CLE) is an overinflated, hyperplastic area of the lung surrounded by otherwise normal lung tissue. These are most common in the upper lobes. Symptoms are progressive but are occasionally evident at birth. Surgical excision is usually curative, although overinflation of remaining lung areas can occur.

**Central Nervous System Disease and Hypoventilation** It is important to remember that respiratory failure and cyanosis may occur secondary to neurological or other organ dysfunction. For instance, birth injury associated with neurological depression or hypoxic-ischemic encephalopathy is commonly associated with hypoventilation. Phrenic nerve injury may cause diaphragmatic paresis. In addition, excessive oral secretions and inadequate swallowing may obstruct the airway and cause respiratory distress. Hypoglycemia may cause central nervous system depression and secondary respiratory distress; this is most commonly seen in small-for-gestational-age infants, large-for-gestational-age infants, infants of diabetic mothers, and infants with birth asphyxia, or in rare cases, due to primary hyperinsulinism (eg, nesidioblastosis or Beckwith-Wiedemann syndrome).

**Other Respiratory Causes** Abdominal distension may compress the thorax and interfere with normal respiration. This may be seen as a result of gastrointestinal pathology (eg, obstruction) or large intra-abdominal mass effect (eg, renal/genitourinary masses, severe ascites). Finally, later preterm or even term infants may present with apneic episodes as a cause of cyanosis.

### Cardiovascular Disease

Severe cyanosis is a prominent feature of congenital heart disease associated with separate circulations and poor mixing (eg, transposition of the great arteries), obstruction to pulmonary blood flow (eg, critical pulmonary stenosis, pulmonary atresia, tetralogy of Fallot), or obstruction to systemic flow with ductal-dependent systemic circulation (eg, hypoplastic left heart syndrome and its variants). In these circulations, arterial oxygen saturation is a function of the relative amounts of pulmonary and systemic blood flow and the relative oxygenation in the pulmonary and systemic venous return. Hence, hypoxemia can result from markedly diminished pulmonary blood flow, but can also occur in the presence of excessive pulmonary blood flow with poor systemic blood flow, which reduces the oxygenation of systemic venous return. Thus, cardiac disease associated with complete mixing may be associated with a variable degree of cyanosis. In conditions in which pulmonary blood flow is dependent on blood directed to the lungs through a patent ductus arteriosus, cyanosis can worsen at the time of ductus closure and tends to improve rapidly after the ductus is reopened following initiation of an infusion of prostaglandin $E_1$ ($PGE_1$).

**Transposition of the Great Arteries** The systemic and pulmonary circulations are normally in series with each other, but in *complete transposition*, the circulations are in parallel. Therefore, deoxygenated systemic venous blood returns to the right atrium, enters the right ventricle, and exits through the aorta. Infants with transposition of the great arteries are dependent on communication between the pulmonary and systemic circuits for mixing. If the ventricular septum is intact, life-threatening cyanosis will develop when the foramen ovale and ductus arteriosus become restrictive or in the hours or days after birth. While a patent ductus arteriosus will improve atrial mixing to a variable degree, an interatrial communication is needed for adequate mixing and oxygenation. Infants with a large ventricular septal defect may be less symptomatic early on, but may present after the first few days of life with cyanosis and signs of pulmonary overcirculation.

**Persistent Pulmonary Hypertension of the Newborn** Persistent pulmonary hypertension of the newborn (PPHN) describes the failure of the normal circulatory transition that occurs after birth and is characterized by marked pulmonary hypertension that causes hypoxemia and right-to-left extrapulmonary shunting of blood through fetal channels (ie, the foramen ovale and ductus arteriosus). The combination of inadequate pulmonary perfusion and extrapulmonary shunting leads to severe, refractory hypoxemia. PPHN often complicates parenchymal lung diseases such as meconium aspiration syndrome in newborn infants, because pulmonary vessels readily constrict in response to alveolar hypoxia. However, PPHN can also occur as an idiopathic condition in the absence of underlying parenchymal disease. In these cases, the syndrome is believed to be the result of an abnormally remodeled vasculature that develops in utero in response to prolonged fetal stress, hypoxia, and/or pulmonary hypertension. Lung hypoplasia, as seen in congenital diaphragmatic hernia is commonly associated with PPHN.

### Hematologic Causes

**Polycythemia** Polycythemia can cause pulmonary hypertension due to increased viscosity of the blood interfering with pulmonary perfusion. This may be seen in infants of diabetic mothers, chronic fetal hypoxia (eg, placental insufficiency, preeclampsia), recipient twins of twin–twin transfusion syndrome, and conditions such as trisomy 21.

**Hemoglobinopathies** Abnormalities of the hemoglobin molecule itself may interfere with the normal chemical combination of hemoglobin with oxygen, but these are very rare in neonates. The most common cause is methemoglobinemia, which results from the oxidation of hemoglobin molecules from the normal ferrous to ferric state. Infants are more susceptible to methemoglobinemia because fetal hemoglobin is more easily oxidized than is adult hemoglobin and because levels of methemoglobin reductase are relatively low in infants. Methemoglobinemia may result from exposure to oxidants (eg, nitrites, sulfonamides, prilocaine, metoclopramide) or, rarely, from a congenital deficiency of methemoglobin reductase. The characteristic clinical scenario is a blue-gray–appearing infant without respiratory distress who has decreased oxygen saturation but normal arterial oxygen tension.

## INITIAL DIAGNOSTIC EVALUATION OF THE CYANOTIC INFANT

### Perinatal History

The evaluation should systematically assess the infant for airway, pulmonary, and circulatory causes as described previously. The history should include an assessment of the pregnancy, labor, and newborn risk factors. A history of maternal diabetes increases the risk of RDS and congenital heart disease, as well as polycythemia and hypoglycemia, which may be associated with lethargy and hypoventilation. The presence of oligohydramnios may suggest renal abnormalities associated with hypoplastic lungs, whereas polyhydramnios may suggest airway, esophageal, or neurological abnormalities. A history of a difficult delivery may result in intracranial hemorrhage or phrenic nerve paralysis, and prolonged rupture of membranes or a history of cervical colonization with group B *Streptococcus* may suggest bacterial infection. Screening results for cervical colonization of group B *Streptococcus* should be sought, although it is important to realize that infection is possible even if the antenatal culture was negative.

### Physical Examination

A detailed physical examination should be performed when the infant has been appropriately warmed and quieted. The growth characteristics should be noted on physical examination, because infants who are small or large for gestational age are more prone to polycythemia. The initial focus is on determining the degree of respiratory distress and systemic perfusion. Because neurological conditions are potential causes of cyanosis due to hypoventilation and may be associated with slow or irregular respirations, it is also important to evaluate the infant's tone and activity and to assess for periodic breathing and/or apneic spells.

The cardiac examination is described in Chapter 478. Although auscultation of heart murmurs is often not helpful, attention to the second heart sound, which will be loud and single (or narrowly split) in pulmonary hypertension, as well as transposition and pulmonary atresia, can be helpful.

A chest radiograph is an integral part of the initial assessment of the cyanotic newborn. The locations of stomach, liver, and heart should be determined to rule out dextrocardia and situs inversus. Examining the lung fields may reveal parenchymal lung disease or lung abnormalities such as cystic adenomatoid malformation. Elevation of either hemidiaphragm by more than 2 intercostal spaces relative to the opposite side suggests diaphragmatic paralysis due to phrenic nerve injury. Hyperinflated lung fields are seen occasionally in lobar emphysema or cystic lesions of lungs. Decreased pulmonary vascular markings are characteristic of pulmonary stenosis or pulmonary atresia with inadequate ductal shunting and may be seen in infants with idiopathic persistent pulmonary hypertension of the newborn. The size and shape of the heart may yield some clues to the diagnosis, for example, the so-called "wall-to-wall" cardiomegaly characteristic of Ebstein anomaly.

An electrocardiogram can occasionally be useful to determine the absence of ventricular forces, which suggests a cardiac anomaly (eg, an infant with left axis deviation and reduced right ventricular forces, which suggests tricuspid atresia). Normal newborns have a predominance of right-sided forces, and moderate right ventricular hypertrophy is a common finding with many types of respiratory and cardiac disease. Therefore, the electrocardiogram can also be completely normal even in infants with serious disease such as transposition.

Some clinicians advocate for the hyperoxia test as a clinical tool to differentiate between pulmonary and cardiac disease in cyanotic infants. The test is based on the principle that in the absence of fixed cardiac shunts, 100% oxygen will increase the alveolar partial pressure of oxygen ($PO_2$), leading to an increase in pulmonary venous and systemic arterial $PO_2$. In cyanotic congenital heart disease (eg, decreased pulmonary blood flow or transposition of the great arteries), little or no rise in the arterial partial pressure of oxygen ($PaO_2$) would be expected after breathing 100% oxygen. However, there can be limited increase in $PaO_2$ with parenchymal lung disease or persistent pulmonary hypertension. Given the current wide availability of echocardiography, the hyperoxia test may still be used as an adjunct to the clinical evaluation, but cannot reliably rule out (or confirm) congenital heart disease.

## INITIAL TREATMENT

### Basic Supportive Measures

Severe cyanosis requires urgent supportive therapy while a diagnosis is established. Supportive therapy includes intravenous fluids and withholding of enteral feedings. The infant should be maintained in a thermoneutral environment using a radiant warmer. Hypoglycemia is common in critically ill infants; therefore, glucose levels should be monitored and glucose infusions provided to maintain a blood glucose greater than 55 mg/dL. An airway and assisted ventilation should be considered for infants with respiratory distress but should be deferred for the infant breathing comfortably. If the infant is less than 10 days old and the umbilical stump is still attached, umbilical venous and arterial lines can be rapidly placed by experienced practitioners for rapid central access. Hypocalcemia is often associated with cardiac disease and critical illness and should be corrected on the basis of the ionized calcium.

### Oxygen

Oxygen should be provided once cyanosis is documented. The Neonatal Resuscitation Program guidelines recommend initiating positive pressure ventilation with 21% oxygen for the infant requiring acute resuscitative measures, and increasing inspired oxygen based on preductal $SpO_2$. Escalation to 100% oxygen is recommended if circulatory support is required in the form of chest compressions. The potential risks of excessive oxygen exposure to a newborn infant with immature antioxidant defense should be kept in mind during therapy. Even brief (30-minute) exposures to extreme hyperoxia are increasingly recognized to increase oxidative stress. These events potentially damage lung parenchymal and vascular function, even in term infants, and have been suggested to have long-term effects, including an increase in childhood cancer. Therefore, except in the scenario of acute resuscitation including circulatory support, the use of 100% oxygen should generally be avoided at the outset. Initiating oxygen therapy with 40% to 60% oxygen will allow the caregiver to provide support, assess for improvement, and seek advice from a cardiologist. It is important to remember that high inspired oxygen levels can promote closure of the ductus arteriosus, and may increase pulmonary blood flow and decrease systemic blood flow.

In the infant who does not require assisted ventilation, oxygen may be delivered via a head hood or nasal cannula. A head hood is the only method that allows the fraction of inspired oxygen to be determined precisely. The oxygen concentration should be measured by an oxygen analyzer placed near the baby's mouth. Relatively high flows are needed to achieve adequate concentrations of oxygen and avoid carbon dioxide accumulation, although humidification is generally not necessary. While head-hood oxygen is generally well tolerated, this method limits the infant's mobility, and oxygen concentrations fall quickly when the hood is lifted to provide care to the infant. Therefore, this method is typically not used when prolonged oxygen treatment is required.

Oxygen is frequently delivered by a nasal cannula. The disadvantage of this method is that the infant entrains variable amounts of room air around the nasal cannula. Therefore, it cannot provide 100% oxygen, and the oxygen concentration in the hypopharynx (a good proxy for the tracheal concentration) will be much lower than the concentration of oxygen at the cannula inlet. Both the oxygen concentration and the cannula flow rate are the major factors that determine the fraction of oxygen actually delivered. Therefore, it is generally better to titrate delivery to achieve the desired oxygen saturation levels, generally 90% to 95% by pulse oximetry. High-flow, humidified oxygen through a nasal cannula is commonly used to supplement oxygen and provide positive pressure. However, the amount of pressure provided is variable and offers no distinct advantages over traditional nasal continuous positive airway pressure (CPAP).

### Prostaglandin $E_1$

If congenital heart disease is suspected, then there is rarely, if ever, a contraindication to starting $PGE_1$ to maintain ductal patency. $PGE_1$ can maintain pulmonary blood flow (eg, congenital heart disease with pulmonary stenosis or pulmonary atresia), systemic blood flow (eg, hypoplastic left heart syndrome), or sufficient mixing (eg, transposition of the great arteries). It is given by constant intravenous infusion, with typical doses starting at approximately 0.01 mcg/kg/min. Apnea is a common side effect after initiation of $PGE_1$, and a period of observation is recommended prior to transporting nonintubated infants on prostaglandin. Other common side effects include flushing, irritability, fever, and diarrhea. There are no absolute contraindications to beginning an infusion of prostaglandin, although it may worsen the pulmonary edema associated with obstructed total anomalous pulmonary venous return.

### Indications for Transfer

Infants with intractable cyanosis and hypoxemia who do not respond to the above measures, and all infants with suspected CCHD, require urgent evaluation at a tertiary center that can provide immediate diagnostic work-up and appropriate medical and surgical interventions, including ECMO, as necessary.

## SUGGESTED READINGS

Frey B, Shann F. Oxygen administration in infants. *Arch Dis Child Fetal Neonatal Ed.* 2003;88(2):F84-F88.

Iyer NP, Mhanna MJ. Association between high-flow nasal cannula and end-expiratory esophageal pressures in premature infants. *Respir care.* 2016;61(3):285-290.

Kemper AR, Mahle WT, Martin GR, et al. Strategies for implementing screening for critical congenital heart disease. *Pediatrics.* 2011;128(5):e1259-e1267.

Lakshminrusimha S, Russell JA, Steinhorn RH, et al. Pulmonary arterial contractility in neonatal lambs increases with 100% oxygen resuscitation. *Pediatr Res.* 2006;59(1):137-141.

Lakshminrusimha S, Steinhorn RH. Pulmonary vascular biology during neonatal transition. *Clin Perinatol.* 1999;26(3):601-619.

Lees MH. Cyanosis of the newborn infant. Recognition and clinical evaluation. *J Pediatr.* 1970;77(3):484-498.

Manley BJ, Owen LS. High-flow nasal cannula: Mechanisms, evidence and recommendations. *Semin Fetal Neonatal Med.* 2016;21(3): 139-145.

Saugstad OD, Ramji S, Vento M. Oxygen for newborn resuscitation: how much is enough? *Pediatrics.* 2006;118(2):789-792.

Sasidharan P. An approach to diagnosis and management of cyanosis and tachypnea in term infants. *Pediatr Clin North Am.* 2004;51(4): 999-1021, ix.

Spector LG, Klebanoff MA, Feusner JH, Georgieff MK, Ross JA. Childhood cancer following neonatal oxygen supplementation. *J Pediatr.* 2005;147(1):27-31.

Steinhorn RH. Advances in neonatal pulmonary hypertension. *Neonatology.* 2016;109(4):334-344.

Wyckoff MH, Aziz K, Escobedo MB, et al. Part 13: neonatal resuscitation: 2015 American Heart Association guidelines update for cardiopulmonary resuscitation and emergency cardiovascular care. *Circulation.* 2015;132(18 Suppl 2):S543-S560.

# 52 Lung Abnormalities in the Newborn

Marta Grisel Galarza and Ilene R. Sosenko



## INTRODUCTION

Respiratory distress, the most common indication for neonatal intensive care, manifests with 1 or more of the following: tachypnea, grunting, nasal flaring, and chest retractions. In addition, the infant may also have cyanosis, gasping, apnea, stridor, or choking. Conditions that cause respiratory distress in the newborn are listed in Table 52-1.

## TRANSIENT TACHYPNEA OF THE NEWBORN

Transient tachypnea of the newborn (TTN) is a self-limiting, usually benign disease, affecting term or late preterm infants soon after birth. It occurs in approximately 11 infants per 1000 live births and is more common in males. It is associated with cesarean section delivery, the use of analgesia or anesthesia during labor, gestational diabetes, and perinatal asphyxia.

### PATHOGENESIS

TTN results from inadequate or delayed absorption of fetal lung fluid leading to a persistent postnatal pulmonary edema.

### CLINICAL FEATURES AND DIAGNOSIS

Infants with TTN present shortly after birth with mild to moderate respiratory distress. They have mild cyanosis and often require oxygen therapy but rarely need mechanical ventilation. On physical examination, diffuse crackles and rhonchi during the first few hours after birth result from residual fluid within the air spaces of the lungs. Blood gas analysis may be normal or may reveal mild alkalosis and hypoxemia. The characteristic radiographic findings are prominent pulmonary vascular markings, especially around the hila; diffuse parenchymal infiltrates; widened interlobar fissures; and some degree of hyperinflation with flattening of the diaphragm. Pleural effusions may also be present and the cardiac silhouette may appear enlarged on the chest radiograph (Fig. 52-1).

A diagnosis of TTN in a newborn infant with respiratory distress can only be made once other lung and cardiac diseases have been excluded.

**TABLE 52-1 CAUSES OF RESPIRATORY DISTRESS IN THE NEWBORN**

| |
|---|
| **Respiratory Diseases** |
| *1. Obstructive* |
| Stenosis/atresia |
| Nasal |
| Choanal |
| Laryngeal, tracheobronchial |
| Anatomical abnormalities |
| Vocal cord paralysis |
| Vascular rings |
| Hemangioma |
| *2. Chest wall abnormalities/diaphragmatic hernia* |
| *3. Malformations of the mediastinum and lung parenchyma* |
| Congenital cystic adenomatoid malformation (CCAM) |
| Congenital lobar emphysema |
| Congenital pulmonary cyst |
| Pulmonary arteriovenous malformations |
| Bronchopulmonary sequestrations |
| Tumors/masses |
| *4. Lung parenchymal and vascular diseases* |
| Transient tachypnea of the newborn |
| Hyaline membrane disease |
| Pneumonia |
| Meconium aspiration syndrome |
| Bronchopulmonary dysplasia |
| Pulmonary edema/hemorrhage |
| Persistent pulmonary hypertension |
| Congenital alveolar proteinosis or genetic abnormalities of surfactant system |
| **Cardiac** |
| *1. Cyanotic* |
| Tetralogy of Fallot |
| Transposition of the great vessels |
| Tricuspid atresia |
| Total anomalous pulmonary venous return |
| Pulmonic stenosis |
| Ebstein anomaly |
| *2. Acyanotic* |
| Patent ductus arteriosus |
| Interrupted aortic arch |
| Hypoplastic left heart syndrome |
| Coarctation of the aorta |
| Severe congestive heart failure |
| **Other Disease Processes** |
| *1. Neurological* |
| Trauma |
| Intraventricular hemorrhage |
| Hypoxic ischemic encephalopathy |
| Seizure disorder |
| Meningitis |
| *2. Sepsis* |
| *3. Polycythemia* |

### MANAGEMENT AND OUTCOME

Most infants with uncomplicated TTN only require supportive care and supplemental oxygen. Infants with moderate disease may require nasal continuous positive airways pressure (CPAP) to increase the functional residual capacity and help clear lung fluid. Mechanical ventilation is rarely required and the need for this may indicate another lung process. Most infants with TTN are also evaluated for

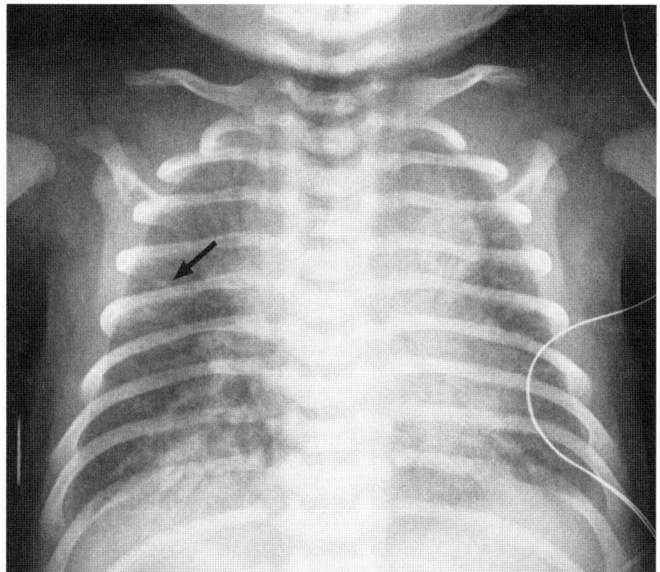

FIGURE 52-1 Transient tachypnea of the newborn. An anteroposterior radiograph of a term newborn on day 1 with transient tachypnea shows bilateral linear opacities (*arrow*) extending from the lung hila to peripheral lung fields.

sepsis, and empiric antibiotic therapy is given for 48 to 72 hours while awaiting blood culture results, clinical improvement, and radiographic evolution. Diuretics do not change the clinical course and may cause electrolyte problems. For infants with uncomplicated disease, clinical improvement within 2 to 4 days is typical, and prognosis is good without long-term pulmonary sequelae.

## CONGENITAL PNEUMONIA

### ETIOLOGY

Infectious organisms causing pneumonia can enter the fetal lungs by the hematogenous route from a maternal bloodstream infection; by ascent through the birth canal, after which it spreads to the fetal membranes; or by aspiration in utero caused by fetal gasping after an asphyxial event and aspiration of infected amniotic fluid. Ascending transmission of organisms may be increased by amniocentesis, repeated pelvic examinations, or placement of intrauterine catheters, and it may occur with or without rupture of amniotic membranes. Early-onset pneumonia may also occur secondary to intrapartum acquisition of infectious organisms during the passage of the newborn through the birth canal. Many pathogens may lead to neonatal pneumonia, but the most common are those that cause early-onset neonatal sepsis—group B *Streptococcus* (GBS), *Escherichia coli*, *Listeria*, and rarely *Candida albicans* or herpes simplex virus. The incidence of congenital pneumonia has fallen to less than 1% in full-term infants and to approximately 10% in ill preterm and low–birth-weight infants, due to universal screening of all pregnant women for GBS and the recently instituted guidelines for maternal intrapartum antibiotic treatment.

### CLINICAL FEATURES AND DIAGNOSIS

Congenital pneumonia is diagnosed by a combination of historical, physical, and radiographic findings (Fig. 52-2). Prenatal risk factors are the same as those associated with neonatal sepsis: maternal fever and uterine tenderness, rupture of membranes for longer than 18 hours, foul-smelling amniotic fluid, maternal history of recurrent or recent untreated urinary tract infection, and a previous infant with neonatal infection. Peripartum signs associated with congenital pneumonia include fetal tachycardia, loss of beat-to-beat variability, meconium-stained amniotic fluid, and unexplained premature labor.

Congenital pneumonia should be suspected in any newborn presenting with respiratory distress at or soon after birth. The clinical

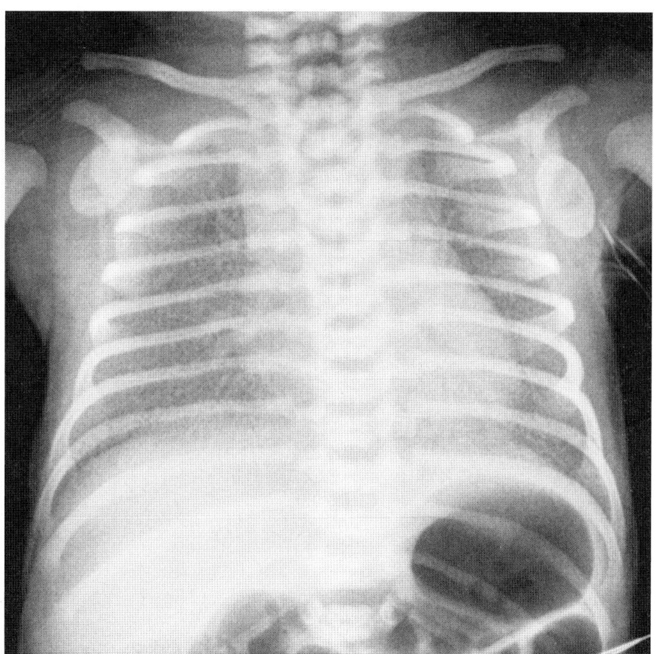

FIGURE 52-2 Congenital pneumonia. An anteroposterior radiograph of term infant with diffuse, relatively homogeneous infiltrates with a "ground-glass" appearance similar to hyaline membrane disease. Pleural effusions (not present here) if present support an infectious process.

presentation of congenital pneumonia may resemble neonatal sepsis, and may include temperature instability, hypoglycemia, hyperglycemia, lethargy, abdominal distention, and poor feeding. Some infants may progress to develop septic shock, disseminated intravascular coagulation, pulmonary hemorrhage, air leaks, effusions, or pulmonary hypertension.

Radiographic and laboratory data for congenital pneumonia are also nonspecific and share findings not only with neonatal sepsis but also with noninfectious processes, such as TTN, hyaline membrane disease, and meconium aspiration syndrome (MAS). Blood cultures usually do not yield a pathogen (especially if maternal antimicrobial treatment was given during labor) but should be obtained. The yield of a pathogen from cerebrospinal fluid examination is very low (< 1%). Culture and gram stain of tracheal aspirate from a newly placed (within 8 hours of delivery) endotracheal tube may provide an early and specific diagnosis in some infants with congenital pulmonary infection. The use of inflammatory markers to support a diagnosis of infection, including pneumonia, is controversial.

### THERAPY AND PROGNOSIS

Supportive care should be provided, along with antibiotic treatment with a broad-spectrum penicillin and an aminoglycoside until cultures are reported. Antibiotics are continued for 7 to 10 days if a clinical diagnosis of congenital pneumonia is likely, even if blood cultures remain negative.

Prognosis is good for term infants with mild to moderate disease who have prompt treatment and no complications. Those infants with severe symptomatology also may have pulmonary hypertension and additional treatment options may include inhaled nitric oxide therapy or even extracorporeal membrane oxygenation (ECMO). Those who develop complications may have an increased risk of chronic lung disease, reactive airway disease, and childhood otitis media.

## PULMONARY HEMORRHAGE

Massive pulmonary hemorrhage in the newborn infant is a catastrophic event that usually occurs in the first 4 days of life in 1 to 12 per 1000 live births. It occurs most commonly in preterm infants, and is usually associated with a patent ductus arteriosus. Rarer associations are preeclampsia, erythroblastosis fetalis, breech delivery, maternal cocaine use, coagulopathies, infection, asphyxia, hypothermia, congenital heart disease, and aspiration.

### PATHOGENESIS

Pulmonary hemorrhage is, in most cases, a hemorrhagic pulmonary edema due to high pulmonary capillary pressures, increased filtration of fluid into the lung, and disruptions in the endothelial–epithelial barrier that cause hemorrhagic fluid to enter the air spaces. Underlying conditions may be acute left ventricular failure from hypoxia and severe acidosis or a patent ductus arteriosus. Surfactant therapy has also been associated with pulmonary hemorrhage, perhaps related to the rapid increase in pulmonary blood flow that occurs with the improvement in lung function after surfactant administration. Sepsis may be a contributory factor in some cases.

### CLINICAL FEATURES AND DIAGNOSIS

Increased respiratory distress, apnea, pallor, peripheral vasoconstriction, and bradycardia minutes before the onset of hemorrhage are common. Severe metabolic acidosis may precede the onset of hemorrhage. With massive hemorrhage, blood may flow out from the nose and mouth or from an endotracheal tube. The fluid may have a normal to low hematocrit. Chest radiographic findings are varied and nonspecific and may range from patchy infiltrates to complete opacification of the lung fields.



### MANAGEMENT

A large pulmonary hemorrhage is a life-threatening event that requires immediate support and resuscitative measures that include clearing the airway and providing supportive mechanical ventilation. Underlying conditions such as sepsis, asphyxia, coagulopathy, or a patent ductus arteriosus should be treated promptly. Interventions commonly used without high-quality evidence to support them include a high positive end expiratory pressure (PEEP) to control the bleeding, endotracheal administration of epinephrine to cause constriction of the pulmonary vessels, activated recombinant factor VII, and exogenous surfactant therapy. In a massive pulmonary hemorrhage, transfusion with packed red blood cells may be necessary to maintain adequate perfusion and blood volume. However, caution should be used with excessive transfusion volumes, which can increase in left atrial pressure and pulmonary edema.

### OUTCOMES

Mortality rates following pulmonary hemorrhage are high, and range from 30% to 60% in premature infants. Approximately 60% of the survivors develop chronic lung disease. Mortality in term infants with pulmonary hemorrhage is related to the underlying precipitating disease process, as well as the consequences of the shock-like state that may complicate this.

## MECONIUM ASPIRATION SYNDROME

### INCIDENCE

Meconium staining of amniotic fluid occurs in approximately 10% to 15% of all live births, with 4% to 5% of these infants developing MAS. Passage of meconium in utero is rare prior to 32 weeks of gestation. Advanced gestation of 42 weeks or more increases the risk of fetal meconium passage (30–50% of post-term infants), putting these infants at higher risk of MAS, compared to term infants (7–22%) and preterm infants (< 2%).

### PATHOGENESIS

Aspiration of meconium may occur in utero if there is fetal distress secondary to hypoxia, acidosis, or infection, as well as when there are conditions that cause intestinal peristalsis and relaxation of the anal sphincter. Oligohydramnios with meconium passage results from compression of the umbilical cord or fetal head, promoting a fetal vagal response. Fetal gasping movements then cause entry of meconium-stained amniotic fluid into the lungs. Abnormal fetal heart tracings and low Apgar scores are associated with meconium-stained fluid and MAS. Aspiration of meconium may also occur during and soon after delivery. The timing of aspiration is unclear in most infants.

Respiratory failure typically is associated with the aspiration of thick or particulate meconium, but also may occur with thin meconium-stained fluid, and in newborns with no meconium recovered from below the vocal cords. Aspirated meconium may partially obstruct the airways, leading to air trapping (ball-valve effect), overdistension of the lungs, and air leaks. It also may completely obstruct the airways (stop-valve effect) leading to atelectasis. The aspiration of meconium induces an inflammatory response and chemical pneumonitis, and also inactivates surfactant. These mechanisms may result in decreased lung compliance, increased airway resistance, ventilation-perfusion mismatching, hypoxia, hypercapnia, acidosis, and inflammation. MAS often is associated with persistent pulmonary hypertension (PPHN) of the newborn.

### PULMONARY FUNCTION

Reduced lung compliance and increased airway resistance in infants with MAS, together lead to an increased work of breathing and result in alveolar hypoventilation and $CO_2$ retention. If there is complete small airway obstruction (a stop-valve effect), distal alveolar gas is absorbed, resulting in collapse of the alveoli, which can then increase intrapulmonary shunting and lead to more severe arterial hypoxemia. The later stages of MAS are characterized by pulmonary inflammation, which causes microvascular endothelial damage, further increasing intrapulmonary shunt and alveolar collapse. Infants with severe MAS have a marked reduction in dynamic lung compliance, which may be secondary to the inflammation as well as inactivation of surfactant by meconium.

### CLINICAL FEATURES

MAS is a disorder affecting near-term, term, and post-term infants. There may be fetal distress, and at delivery the infant with MAS may have low Apgar scores and may require resuscitation, and may demonstrate other signs of asphyxia. The skin, nails, and umbilical cord may be stained with meconium. Meconium may be found in the mouth and pharynx or may be suctioned from the trachea. Signs of respiratory distress include tachypnea, retractions, and cyanosis. Signs of air-trapping include a barrel-shaped chest and coarse bronchial sounds, with prolonged expiration. Occasionally, infants with MAS may have minimal symptomatology or even be asymptomatic.

The radiographic findings of MAS do not always correlate with the severity of the clinical disease. With severe aspiration, the chest radiograph may reveal areas of patchy infiltrates with regions of atelectasis and overinflation with a flattened diaphragm (Fig. 52-3). Pneumomediastinum and pneumothorax occur in as many as 10% to 15% of infants with MAS. Early in the clinical course of MAS, hypoxemia and some degree of metabolic acidosis may represent perinatal asphyxia. Later in the course of the disease, the partial pressure of carbon dioxide ($CO_2$) in arterial blood ($PaCO_2$) may increase and the hypoxia may worsen.

### PREVENTION

#### Antenatal Prevention

A policy of labor induction at 41 completed weeks is associated with a reduction in MAS. The incidence of MAS is not reduced by fetal monitoring during labor, elective cesarean delivery when there is meconium-stained amniotic fluid, and amnioinfusion (injection of hypotonic fluid into the amniotic cavity with the intent of diluting the meconium).

#### Postnatal Prevention

The historical practice of suctioning of the oropharynx and nasopharynx after delivery of the head but before delivery of the shoulders, and routine endotracheal intubation at birth and suction to clear the

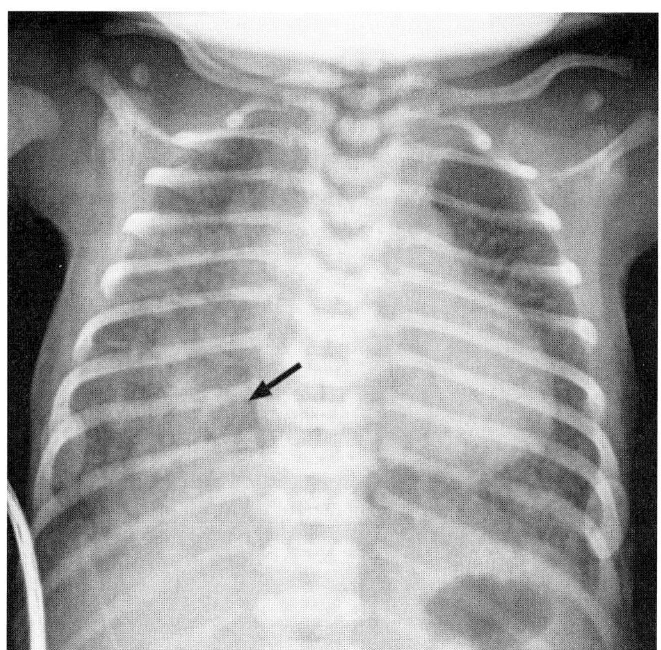

**FIGURE 52-3** Meconium aspiration syndrome. An anteroposterior radiograph of a term newborn showing lung opacities (*arrow*), predominantly involving the right lung fields.

trachea of meconium have been shown to be of no benefit in randomized controlled trials. Thus, current neonatal resuscitation guidelines from the American Heart Association do not recommend routine endotracheal suction at birth for vigorous and nonvigorous infants born through meconium-stained amniotic fluid, although gentle bulb suction of the oropharynx is suggested. The incidence of MAS has decreased in recent years, and this is most likely due to improved fetal surveillance and aggressive intervention for fetal distress as well as the avoidance of postmaturity.

### MANAGEMENT

The infant with MAS should have continuous pulse oximetry to monitor oxygenation, as well as careful monitoring of blood gases and radiographic evaluation. Supplemental oxygen should be provided to maintain partial pressure of arterial oxygen ($PaO_2$) above 70 to 80 mm Hg or preductal oxygen saturation in the low-to-mid 90s. Metabolic acidosis should be addressed to decrease the risk of pulmonary vasoconstriction and pulmonary hypertension. As the disease progresses, mechanical ventilation may be required. High-peak inspiratory pressures may be necessary to overcome reduced lung compliance and increased airway resistance associated with meconium plugging or injured lungs, which may increase the risk of air leak and further lung injury. The use of high-frequency ventilation in MAS may be necessary to avoid excessive peak inspiratory pressures or if pulmonary hypertension complicates the clinical course of MAS. However, hyperventilation should be avoided because of the associations with lung and brain injury. Sedation may be necessary during the first 24 to 48 hours since agitation may worsen pulmonary hypertension, and may interfere with ventilator synchrony and gas exchange.

MAS may inactivate endogenous surfactant. Small trials have demonstrated improved outcome and a reduced rate of ECMO when exogenous surfactant is used early in the course of the disease. Clinical trials have reported better outcomes in infants with MAS treated with surfactant therapy and high-frequency ventilation. Meta-analysis suggests lavage of the MAS lung with surfactant may improve the clinical outcome, specifically preventing death or the need for ECMO in infants with MAS.

MAS may cause chemical pneumonitis and inflammation and increase the risk of bacterial invasion and infection. Clinical infection in the setting of MAS cannot be distinguished from MAS alone. In addition, maternal infection may be the trigger for fetal distress, leading to meconium passage in utero and subsequent MAS. Therefore, infants with MAS born to mothers with chorioamnionitis, fever during labor, or history of untreated urinary tract or other infection should have a sepsis evaluation and antibiotic therapy.

Inhaled nitric oxide (iNO) is an effective treatment of pulmonary hypertension in term newborns. The use of iNO in MAS complicated by pulmonary hypertension may improve oxygenation and prevent the need for ECMO.

## PULMONARY AIR LEAKS

Air leaks may present as extrapulmonary gas collections in the pleural space or other locations, and can cause significant morbidity and even mortality. Prompt diagnosis and intervention are essential with significant air leaks.

### INCIDENCE

*Spontaneous pneumothorax* occurs in approximately 1% of infants born vaginally at term and in approximately 2% of those born via cesarean section. Small air leaks in asymptomatic infants may go undetected and resolve spontaneously. Air leaks are more common in infants with lung disease, and are significantly higher in infants who require respiratory interventions at birth. However, the use of antenatal steroids, gentler ventilation strategies and surfactant therapy in the preterm infant have led to a decline in the incidence of air leaks in newborn infants.

### PATHOGENESIS

Air leaks often manifest with pulmonary interstitial emphysema. Air that has leaked from the alveoli may track through the perivascular and peribronchial cuffs to the hilum of the lung and rupture into the mediastinum (to produce a pneumomediastinum) or into the pleural space (to produce a pneumothorax). More rarely, air may track from the mediastinum to the pericardial space (producing a pneumopericardium) or to the peritoneal cavity (producing a pneumoperitoneum).

### CLINICAL FEATURES AND DIAGNOSIS

Distinguishing the various types of air-leak requires radiography (Fig. 52-4). Clinical signs and symptoms of air leaks depend on the location and size of the accumulated air. A small pneumothorax or the presence of a small degree of pulmonary interstitial emphysema may be asymptomatic and resolve spontaneously. However, an infant with a large air leak, either into the interstitium or the pleural space, may present with respiratory distress or a sudden deterioration in clinical status. Tachypnea is a universal finding and may be accompanied by grunting, pallor, or cyanosis. When a pneumothorax is present, chest asymmetry and/or abdominal distention may be present. Breath sounds may be decreased on the affected side, and heart sounds may be displaced or muffled by the air. With a large air leak, particularly involving the pericardial sac, compression of the great veins can decrease stroke volume, cardiac output, and systemic blood pressure. Pneumomediastinum alone is often asymptomatic, but air can dissect into the soft tissues of the neck, producing subcutaneous emphysema, or can rupture into the intrapleural space. A pneumoperitoneum, if large, may cause respiratory or cardiorespiratory compromise and require drainage. To differentiate this from a gastric or bowel perforation, ultrasound, and eventually needle aspiration may be necessary. If needle aspiration reveals green or brown peritoneal fluid, then a primary bowel perforation is more likely.

Pulmonary interstitial emphysema most often occurs in a preterm infant with significant lung disease requiring ventilatory support and presents with respiratory deterioration, requiring increased ventilator settings. A small pneumothorax or the presence of pulmonary interstitial emphysema may be an incidental finding on chest radiograph of a newborn with mild distress.

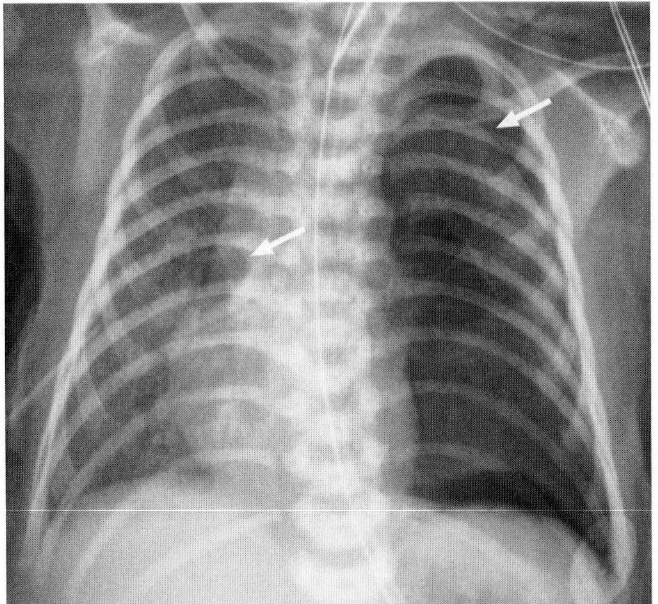

**FIGURE 52-4** Air leak syndrome. An anteroposterior radiograph demonstrating a moderate left-sided pneumothorax. The *arrow* on the left outlines the partially collapsed left lung. Cardiac silhouette and mediastinal structures are shifted to the right. A small anterior pneumothorax is also visualized on the right side as a round lucency (*arrow on the right*).

In an emergency, if there is a sudden worsening of clinical status, translumination of the chest may be a very useful technique to diagnose a large pneumothorax at the bedside. The technique is best performed using a fiber optic light probe placed on the infant's chest wall in a darkened room. The hemithorax on the affected side will light up when a large pneumothorax is present. The contralateral side will have diminished transillumination secondary to lung compression. Immediate decompression is necessary and need not await radiographic confirmation if the infant is unstable. If transillumination is questionable and the infant is stable, radiographic confirmation is appropriate. A chest radiograph allows for better localization and quantification of the pneumothorax and differentiation from pulmonary interstitial emphysema, pneumomediastinum, or a pneumopericardium.

A large pneumothorax is easily identified on a chest radiograph. Air in the pleural cavity separates the parietal and visceral pleura of the lung. The ipsilateral lobes will be collapsed, the mediastinum may be displaced to the contralateral side, and the diaphragm may be displaced downward (Fig. 52-4). If there are bilateral tension pneumothoraces, the heart will appear small on radiograph. The chest radiograph of an isolated pneumomediastinum may demonstrate a hyperlucent area lateral to the heart borders, elevating the thymus away from the pericardium in the characteristic "spinnaker-sail" sign. The classic radiographic finding in a pneumopericardium is that of air completely surrounding the heart on all borders.

### MANAGEMENT

A small pneumothorax in an asymptomatic infant may not require any intervention. Close monitoring of vital signs is essential, and repeat chest radiographs may be necessary to follow the evolution of the air leak. The use of 100% oxygen to help accelerate resorption of the pneumothorax is not recommended in the newborn as the high oxygen tension in arterial blood may cause retinopathy of prematurity, and high concentrations of inspired oxygen may cause lung damage and generalized oxidative stress.

Infants with pulmonary interstitial emphysema require close clinical and radiographic monitoring as well as ventilation with low peak pressures. High-frequency oscillatory ventilation may be preferable to conventional mechanical ventilation in the presence of this and other air leaks. The definitive treatment for an air leak is insertion of a chest tube (thoracostomy).

## PERSISTENT PULMONARY HYPERTENSION OF THE NEWBORN

*Persistent pulmonary hypertension of the newborn* (PPHN) is a condition in which increased pulmonary vascular resistance and decreased perfusion of the lungs lead to hypoxia. MAS is the most common cause, with PPHN occurring in 40% to 75% of cases of severe MAS. Other conditions associated with PPHN are parenchymal lung diseases (including pneumonia, sepsis, or surfactant deficiency), abnormalities of the structure of the pulmonary vasculature as in congenital diaphragmatic hernia (CDH), and certain congenital heart anomalies. PPHN occurs in 1 to 2 infants per 1000 live births, most commonly in near-term or term infants. Perinatal conditions associated with an increased risk for PPHN are maternal asthma, diabetes, and obesity; maternal exposure to nonsteroidal anti-inflammatory drugs (NSAIDs) and selective serotonin reuptake inhibitors; fetal distress (including meconium-stained amniotic fluid); malpresentation at delivery; perinatal asphyxia; cesarean delivery; postmaturity; neonatal infection; pneumonia; and polycythemia and hyperviscosity. These conditions lead to acidosis, hypoxia, hypercarbia, and inflammation, which decrease the production and release of endogenous vasodilators (nitric oxide, cyclic guanosine monophosphate, prostacyclin) and increase endogenous vasoconstrictors (endothelin 1 and thromboxane), resulting in pulmonary vascular constriction.

Some infants may develop PPHN without parenchymal lung disease, termed *idiopathic* PPHN. In this condition, there is significant remodeling of the pulmonary vasculature that is already present at birth, possibly secondary to in utero asphyxia. At autopsy, the pulmonary vessel walls are thickened with extension of muscle into nonmuscular pulmonary arteries. As a result, infants are not able to dilate or relax the pulmonary vasculature adequately at birth and have severe hypoxemia and acidosis. The chest radiograph typically has clear, hyperlucent, underperfused lung fields ("black lung fields"). Disruptions of the endogenous nitric oxide–cyclic guanosine monophosphate, prostacyclin–cyclic adenosine monophosphate, and endothelin pathways may also contribute to idiopathic PPHN (see Chapter 45). Constriction of the ductus arteriosus in utero from maternal use of NSAIDs during the last trimester of pregnancy is an additional risk factor for PPHN.

PPHN frequently is present in infants with CDH and other causes of lung hypoplasia. Because the pulmonary vasculature develops in parallel with the conducting airways, hypoplasia of the pulmonary vascular bed accompanies lung hypoplasia. There is reduced total cross-sectional area of the pulmonary vascular bed and increased muscularization of the intra-acinar pulmonary arteries that decrease pulmonary blood flow.

### CLINICAL FEATURES AND DIAGNOSIS

The infant with PPHN may be normal at birth and then progress to show signs of respiratory distress within hours after birth, or may present with cyanosis and distress at birth. Physical examination may reveal a systolic murmur from tricuspid insufficiency and a loud second heart sound as a result of a more forceful pulmonic valve closure. Differential cyanosis may be observed, with greater preductal (right upper extremity) than postductal oxygen saturation due to a large right-to-left shunt at the level of the ductus arteriosus. Arterial blood gas analysis usually shows severe arterial $O_2$ desaturation with relatively normal $CO_2$ tension, and marked acidosis reflecting poor tissue perfusion. Chest radiographs may reflect the underlying lung disease process in infants with PPHN associated with MAS, CDH, and pneumonia. The infant with idiopathic PPHN has clear, hyperlucent, or undervascularized lung fields and an enlarged cardiac silhouette.

Definitive diagnosis of PPHN requires echocardiography with Doppler flow. This is used to exclude cyanotic congenital heart disease, to diagnose right-to-left shunts across the foramen ovale and ductus arteriosus, and to measure the peak velocity of the tricuspid regurgitant jet, which in turn provides an estimate of right ventricular systolic pressure. The persistently elevated pulmonary vascular resistance also increases right ventricular afterload and oxygen demand and impairs oxygen delivery to the right ventricle, the posterior wall of the left ventricle, and the subendocardial regions of the right ventricle. The ischemia can cause right and left ventricular failure, papillary muscle necrosis, and tricuspid insufficiency. The increased right ventricular afterload causes displacement of the septum into the left ventricle, impairs left ventricular filling, and reduces cardiac output.

### MANAGEMENT

Clinical goals for the management of infants with PPHN include lowering pulmonary vascular resistance, reversing right to left shunting, improving oxygenation and tissue perfusion, and maintaining systemic perfusion while reducing oxygen demand. Metabolic derangements such as hypoglycemia, hypocalcemia, cold stress, and acidosis should be corrected promptly. Cardiac evaluation should urgently exclude congenital heart disease. Cardiac function and systemic arterial pressure should be optimized with pressors such as dopamine and/or dobutamine and with careful use of volume expansion. If the central hematocrit is greater than 60% to 65%, a partial exchange transfusion may be performed to lower the hematocrit and reduce the effects of hyperviscosity on pulmonary artery pressure. Intravenous antibiotics should be started immediately if infection is suspected.

If the infant is breathing spontaneously and maintaining a normal or low $PaCO_2$, supplemental oxygen by nasal cannula or hood should be provided to maintain adequate $PaO_2$. Oxygen at high concentrations can be lifesaving, but it is also toxic to the developing lung with formation of reactive oxygen species that can react with arachidonic acid to form potent vasoconstrictors. Superoxide also inactivates endogenous nitric oxide, and the resulting peroxynitrite can cause vasoconstriction, cytotoxicity, and damage to surfactant proteins and lipids.

If supplemental oxygen fails to maintain adequate oxygenation, then mechanical ventilation is required, with the goal of achieving optimal lung volumes that allow for alveolar recruitment while minimizing lung injury. Infants with parenchymal lung disease and hypoplastic lungs may have a better response to high-frequency oscillatory ventilation, which allows adequate gas exchange with smaller tidal volumes and lower airway pressures with effective recruitment of the lung. Caution is essential during mechanical ventilation because excessive pressures and hyperventilation can exacerbate lung injury, inflammation, and pulmonary edema, and decrease lung compliance. Overexpansion of the lung may also produce pulmonary air leaks and the resulting overdistended alveoli can compress the small arterioles and capillaries diminishing flow further. Pharmacological alkalinization in the treatment of PPHN has been shown not to reduce mortality and is associated with an increased risk for the use of ECMO and prolonged oxygen dependency. Hyperventilation strategies and hypocarbia are associated with worse outcomes in PPHN. Gentle ventilation strategies that allow for normal $PaCO_2$ or even permissive hypercarbia are effective and potentially less damaging to the lung. Infants with PPHN may be very sensitive to stimulation; therefore, a quiet environment and sedation as needed should be provided. Hands-on activities such as bathing and weighing should be avoided. Paralytic agents should be avoided if possible, as they are associated with an increased risk for mortality. Surfactant therapy may improve ventilation and oxygenation, and reduce the need for ECMO in infants with MAS and with sepsis associated with PPHN.

Inhaled NO, a potent vasodilator that can be delivered directly to the lungs with minimal systemic effects, decreases the need for ECMO in infants with severe PPHN but not in infants with PPHN secondary to CDH. Low-dose iNO reduces pulmonary vascular resistance, improves pulmonary blood flow, and improves ventilation-perfusion mismatch in the treatment of severe parenchymal lung diseases. Sildenafil, a potent and highly specific systemic phosphodiesterase type 5 inhibitor, is presently used for the treatment of pulmonary hypertension in adults. It may improve oxygenation in infants with PPHN when iNO is not readily available, and also attenuates rebound pulmonary hypertension after withdrawal of iNO. Kinsella and colleagues found that therapy with combined iNO and high-frequency ventilation was more successful than either individual therapy in severe PPHN. Some infants may not respond to iNO therapy and require ECMO. Several newer therapies for PPHN are also being investigated.



### OUTCOMES

PPHN is fatal in less than 10% of cases treated at tertiary care centers. Survivors are at increased risk for serious, long-term sequelae as a result of the hypoxemia associated with this condition and the aggressive therapies used for treatment.

## CONGENITAL DIAPHRAGMATIC HERNIA

*Congenital diaphragmatic hernia occurs* once in every 2000 to 3000 live births and accounts for 8% of all major congenital anomalies. It is more common in male infants and occurs mostly on the left side (85%). It can be associated with chromosomal disorders, such as trisomy 13, 18, and 21; tetraploidy; Pallister-Killian syndrome; Turner syndrome; and single gene disorders, such as Fryns syndrome. However, most cases of CDH occur as isolated events in nonsyndromic infants. The rate of recurrence in future siblings is approximately 2% and familial CDH is rare (< 2% of all cases).

### TYPES OF DIAPHRAGMATIC HERNIA

The most common type of CDH, a Bochdalek hernia, occurs through a posterior defect in the diaphragm. Defects in the central and lateral portions of the diaphragm result in a less common anterior retrosternal hernia, a Morgagni hernia. Often, the stomach, spleen, and most of the intestines herniate into the thorax. In rare instances, the liver and kidneys may also be in the thoracic cavity. Herniation of the abdominal contents interferes with lung development and growth, and the resulting lung compression results in pulmonary hypoplasia that is most severe on the ipsilateral side, although both lungs may be affected. There is a marked reduction in the number of bronchi and alveoli associated with a decrease in cross-sectional area of the pulmonary vasculature. In addition to parenchymal maldevelopment, the intra-acinar pulmonary arteries have increased muscularization. Pulmonary capillary blood flow is decreased because of the small cross-sectional area of the pulmonary vascular bed, and flow may be further decreased by abnormal pulmonary vasoconstriction. Surfactant production may also be affected by pulmonary hypoplasia in infants with CDH.



### PRENATAL DIAGNOSIS

Diaphragmatic hernia is often diagnosed by fetal ultrasound, which can reveal abdominal organs and fluid-filled bowel with peristalsis in the thorax, and a shift of the heart and mediastinum away from the side of the hernia. Polyhydramnios, pleural effusions, and ascites often are present. The differential diagnosis of these sonographic findings includes congenital cystic adenomatoid malformation, bronchogenic cysts, cystic teratoma, and neurogenic tumors. If CDH is suspected, fetal echocardiography and karyotype should be performed for potential prenatal diagnosis of common associated malformations. The patient should be referred to a quaternary treatment center for prenatal counseling and delivery. Fetal surgical procedures for CDH have failed to improve survival or decrease morbidity and are not routinely recommended at present (see also Chapter 42). Minimally invasive fetal endoscopic tracheal occlusion (FETO) has been studied in fetuses diagnosed with CDH and a large randomized controlled trial is underway.

### CLINICAL FEATURES

Clinical presentation of CDH depends on the type and size of the hernia. Infants with a large left-sided hernia may present with a scaphoid abdomen and significant respiratory symptoms in the delivery room.

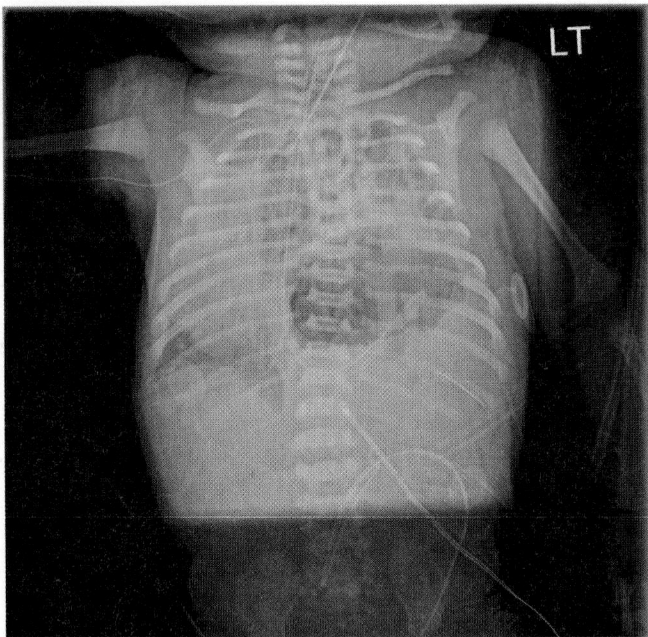


**FIGURE 52-5** Left-sided congenital diaphragmatic hernia. An anteroposterior radiograph of a near-term infant with known left diaphragmatic hernia, intubated in delivery room. Note the bowel in the left chest, with displacement of the heart to the right. Incidental finding on the radiograph was the orogastric tube noted high in the esophagus. This patient also had esophageal atresia.



On examination, breath sounds may not be heard on either side of the chest, bowel sounds may be audible in the chest, and the heart sounds may be better heard on the right side. The infant's respiratory status may worsen as air is swallowed and fills the bowel in the chest, compressing the lungs. The diagnosis can be made with chest and abdominal radiographs, after an orogastric tube is placed. These will reveal the abdominal organs and feeding tube in the thoracic cavity and displacement of the heart and mediastinum to the contralateral side (Fig. 52-5). The infant with a right-sided hernia may be asymptomatic at birth, and the diagnosis may be incidental if not made prenatally. With right-side hernias, the liver and some intestine may occupy the right hemithorax, but little or no displacement of the heart may occur (Fig. 52-6). These infants have a better prognosis because they generally have less lung hypoplasia. Further evaluation of the infant with CDH should include heart echocardiography, chromosomal analysis, and renal ultrasonography secondary to the high incidence of associated malformations.

Approximately 40% of infants with CDH have associated anomalies, most with minimal effect on survival, and others that significantly affect survival, including chromosomal and complex cardiac defects. During fetal life, the left ventricle is often small (probably as a result of increased intrathoracic pressure) and left ventricular output is reduced. Postnatally, the left ventricular size and output may improve with correction of the hernia.

## MANAGEMENT

If CDH has been diagnosed prenatally, or as soon as the diagnosis is suspected, a double-lumen orogastric tube should be placed into the infant's stomach in the delivery room to reduce air in the bowel and decrease compression of the lung. If assisted ventilation is required, it should be performed via an endotracheal tube, using the lowest peak pressure ($\leq$ 25 cm $H_2O$) possible to prevent air leaks and lung injury. Bag and mask ventilation should be avoided. Close monitoring of oxygenation and radiological evaluation should be promptly initiated, and umbilical catheters should be placed for medications and for blood gas monitoring. Sedation may be needed to avoid the need for higher pressures and occurrence of pneumothorax.

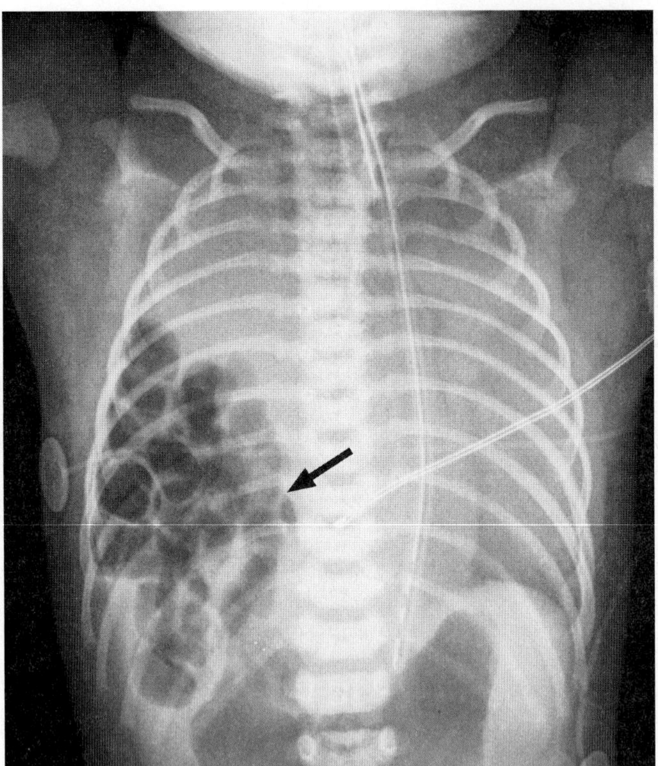

**FIGURE 52-6** Right-sided congenital diaphragmatic hernia. An anteroposterior chest radiograph reveals gas-distended bowel loops (*arrow*) projecting over the liver shadow as well as right lower lung fields. There is opacification of the bilateral lung fields and little or no displacement of the heart.

## POSTNATAL CARE

Postnatal care should be directed toward lung function and pulmonary hypertension. Surgical intervention is delayed where possible, until the infant is hemodynamically stable and pulmonary hypertension is controlled. Mechanical ventilation is currently based on principles of "gentle ventilation." These medical and surgical strategies have resulted in better outcomes at tertiary care institutions that can provide ECMO and surgical repair.

## MEDICAL INTERVENTIONS

### Surfactant

Studies have not shown a primary surfactant deficiency in patients with CDH compared to age-matched control infants. Surfactant therapy in CDH has no reported benefits, and may cause clinical deterioration and increased mortality.

### Ventilation Strategy

Pulmonary hypoplasia and pulmonary hypertension are significant contributors to mortality in CDH. Pulmonary hypertension has a reactive component, due to the changing resistance of the pulmonary arterioles, and a fixed component due to the diminished cross-sectional area of the pulmonary vascular bed. Mechanical ventilation should aim to maintain appropriate lung volumes and adequate oxygenation while minimizing lung injury. The previous use of hyperventilation and alkalosis in CDH has been replaced by a gentler ventilation strategy, which allows for higher $PaCO_2$ and lower preductal oxygen saturation as long as blood pressure and tissue perfusion are maintained. Many centers prefer to use high-frequency ventilation, especially high-frequency oscillatory ventilation, before and after surgery.

### Nitric Oxide

Although iNO is an effective treatment for infants with PPHN in general, it has not had the same success for infants with CDH, and may actually increase the death rate. Nonetheless, it is still widely used in the management of CDH.

#### Extracorporeal Membrane Oxygenation

ECMO is often used as rescue therapy for CDH, although its efficacy is uncertain and its use is declining. The criteria for initiation of ECMO vary widely across centers. With the onset of delayed surgical repair, ECMO is now used more frequently during preoperative stabilization.

### SURGICAL REPAIR

Surgical repair of the diaphragmatic defect should be performed during the neonatal period. The exact timing of surgery depends on a number of variables, but over the past 2 decades practice has changed. In the past, surgical intervention was considered emergent, and as a consequence, postoperative management was characterized by severe pulmonary hypertension and tension pneumothoraces, resulting in poor outcomes. Currently, the preferred management strategy for CDH is medical stabilization with appropriate cardiorespiratory support, including high-frequency oscillatory ventilation, iNO, or ECMO for several days to allow for physiologic stabilization and improvement in pulmonary hypertension. The surgical approach is through a subcostal opening with primary repair if enough diaphragm tissue is available. For those with a more significant defect, closure with a patch may be required. The use of chest drains or tubes postoperatively has also decreased in the past few years, but a consensus on their use has not been reached.

### OUTCOMES

Several antenatal and postnatal prognostic tools have been evaluated in CDH. The most widespread currently in use is the antenatal determination of position of the liver and the lung area–to–head circumference ratio (LHR) via ultrasound. Postnatally, the McGoon index is also used, which is the sum of the diameters of the immediately prebranching left and right pulmonary arteries to the descending aorta just above level of the diaphragm, as measured by echocardiography.

The overall survival rate for CHD is between 60% and 85% for infants with a gestational age of more than 34 weeks, those with no associated chromosomal or severe cardiac defects, and those delivered at a tertiary center with adequate experience in medical and surgical management of CDH. Survivors are at risk for chronic lung disease, feeding difficulties, gastroesophageal reflux, scoliosis, pectus excavatum, hearing loss, neurodevelopmental delay, brain injury, and recurrence of the diaphragmatic hernia. Overall survival of patients with CDH and significant cardiac defects is lower than those without heart abnormalities.

### SUGGESTED READINGS


Abman SH. Recent advances in the pathogenesis and treatment of persistent pulmonary hypertension of the newborn. *Neonatology*. 2007;91(4):283-290.

Aziz A, Ohlsson A. Surfactant for pulmonary haemorrhage in neonates. *Cochrane Database Syst Rev*. 2012;(7):CD005254.

Berger TM, Allred EN, Van Marter LJ. Antecedents of clinically significant pulmonary hemorrhage among newborn infants. *J Perinatol*. 2000;20(5):295-300.

Centers for Disease Control and Prevention. Prevention of perinatal group B streptococcal disease. Revised guidelines from CDC, 2010. MMWR. 2010;59(RR-10):1-32.

Choi HJ, Hahn S, Lee J, et al. Surfactant lavage therapy for meconium aspiration syndrome: a systematic review and meta-analysis. *Neonatology*. 2012;101(3):183-191.

Dargaville PA, Copnell B; Australian and New Zealand Neonatal Network. The epidemiology of meconium aspiration syndrome: incidence, risk factors therapies, and outcome. *Pediatrics*. 2006;117(5):1712-1721.

Elias N, O'Brodovich H. Clearance of fluid from airspaces of newborns and infants. *Neoreviews*. 2006;7(2):88-93.

Graziano JN; Congenital Diaphragmatic Hernia Study Group. Cardiac anomalies in patients with congenital diaphragmatic hernia and their prognosis: a report from the Congenital Diaphragmatic Hernia Study Group. *J Pediatr Surg*. 2005;40(6):1045-1050.

Hernández-Diaz S, Van Marter LJ, Werler MM, Louik C, Mitchell AA. Risk factors for persistent pulmonary hypertension. *Pediatrics*. 2007;120(2):e272-e282.

Kluckow M, Evans N. Ductal shunting, high pulmonary blood flow, and pulmonary hemorrhage. *J Pediatr*. 2000;137(1):68-72.

Kuhns LR, Bednarek FJ, Wyman ML, Roloff DW, Borer RC. Diagnosis of pneumothorax or pneumomediastinum in the neonate by transillumination. *Pediatrics*. 1975;56(3):355-360.

Lally KP, Lally PA, Van Meurs KP; Congenital Diaphragmatic Hernia Study Group. Treatment evolution in high-risk congenital diaphragmatic hernia: ten years' experience with diaphragmatic agenesis. *Ann Surg*. 2006;244(4):505-513.

Nissen MD. Congenital and neonatal pneumonia. *Paediatr Respir Rev*. 2007;8(3):195-203.

Ogata E, Gregory GA, Kitterman JA, Phibbs RH, Tooley WH. Pneumothorax in respiratory distress syndrome: incidence and effect on vital signs, blood gases and pH. *Pediatrics*. 1976;58(2):177-183.

Olver RE, Walters DV, Wilson SM. Developmental regulation of lung liquid transport. *Annu Rev Physiol*. 2004;66:77-101.

Tiruvoipati R, Vinogradova Y, Faulkner G, Sosnowski AW, Firmin RK, Peek GJ. Predictors of outcome in patients with congenital diaphragmatic hernia requiring extracorporeal membrane oxygenation. *J Pediatr Surg*. 2007;42(8):1345-1350.

Weiner GM, ed. *Textbook of Neonatal Resuscitation*, 7th ed. Elk Grove Village, IL: American Academy of Pediatrics; 2016.


# 53 Disorders of Glucose, Electrolytes, and Acid–Base Balance

Paul J. Rozance, William W. Hay, Jr, and Clyde J. Wright

## DISORDERS OF GLUCOSE METABOLISM

Normal postnatal glucose homeostasis is established by increased glucose production and utilization. Factors that promote glucose production include catecholamines and glucagon, which activate glycogenolysis. A high glucagon-to-insulin ratio, which induces synthesis and activity of the enzymes, is required for there to be gluconeogenesis. Once normal feedings are established, glycerol and amino acids continue to fuel gluconeogenesis while dietary fatty acids activate the enzymes responsible for gluconeogenesis. Additionally, galactose derived from the hydrolysis of milk sugar (lactose) in the gut increases hepatic glycogen production for sustained between-feeding hepatic glucose release from glycogen breakdown. Feeding also induces production of intestinal peptides, or incretins, that promote insulin secretion. Insulin decreases hepatic glucose production and increases glucose utilization for energy production and storage as glycogen. These opposing conditions of glucose production and utilization continue in response to normal feed-fast cycles, regulating normal plasma glucose concentrations.

## HYPOGLYCEMIA

Glucose is the major source of energy for organ function. All organs use glucose, and glucose deficiency leads to impaired cardiac performance, cerebral energy failure, hepatic glycogen depletion, and muscle weakness. Cerebral glucose metabolism accounts for as much as 90%

of total glucose consumption in the newborn. Thus, maintenance of glucose delivery to all organs, particularly the brain, is an essential physiological function. Although alternate fuels can substitute for glucose metabolism, concentrations of these substances often are low in newborn infants, especially preterm infants. Newborns, therefore, are especially susceptible to hypoglycemia when they are exposed to conditions that impair glucose homeostasis during the transition from intrauterine to extrauterine life.

## DEFINITION

Ideally, hypoglycemia should be defined as a glucose concentration below the lower limit of the normal range of blood or plasma/serum glucose concentrations. This concentration, however, is uncertain, controversial, and is variably defined. Early statistical evaluations in term infants historically defined hypoglycemia as a blood glucose concentration below 35 mg/dL, or a plasma glucose value below 40 mg/dL; and even lower concentrations were applied in preterm infants. Such statistical definitions, however, have limited biological or clinical significance. This is because physiological hypoglycemia is present when the concentration of glucose in the plasma yields glucose delivery rates that are inadequate to meet essential requirements for glucose utilization, which vary considerably. Definitions of normal and hypoglycemic glucose concentrations vary according to postnatal feeding practices and timing of the measurement. Postnatally, the blood glucose concentration normally decreases to its lowest value between 1 and 3 hours after birth, followed by a progressive increase to greater than 50 to 60 mg/dL by 12 to 24 hours (Fig. 53-1).

The absolute glucose concentration below which short- or long-term organ dysfunction occurs remains undefined, although animal studies suggest that concentrations below 20 mg/dL sustained over several hours can result in brain injury. Conditions that should be present before relating long-term neurological impairment to neonatal hypoglycemia are given in Table 53-1. Unfortunately, there are no sufficiently large, randomized controlled trials to establish the efficacy of any diagnostic and/or treatment approach, or any set of guidelines for the management of hypoglycemia (however defined). Thus, the key to preventing complications from glucose deficiency, is to focus less on numerical values of glucose concentration. Management should be directed toward identification of infants at risk, promotion of early and frequent feedings, normalization of glucose homeostasis, measurement of glucose concentrations early and frequently in infants at risk, and prompt treatment when glucose deficiency is marked and symptomatic.

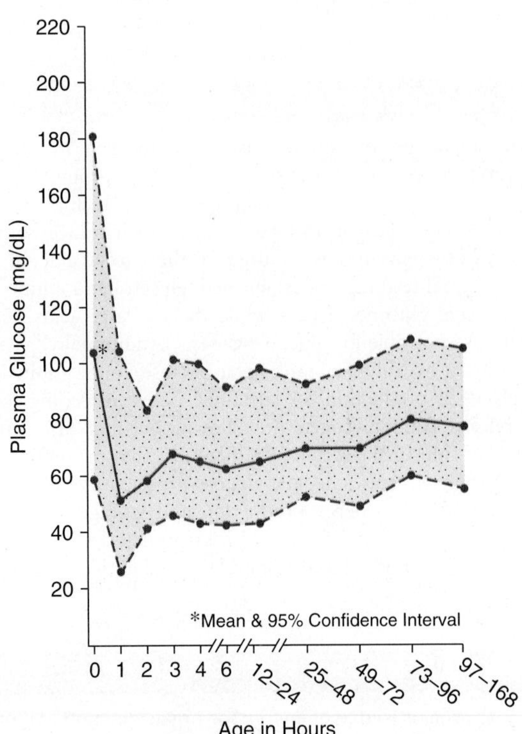


**FIGURE 53-1** Plasma glucose concentrations during the first week of life in healthy, appropriate-for-gestational-age term infants.

| **TABLE 53-1** NECESSARY CONDITIONS FOR ATTRIBUTING LONG-TERM NEUROLOGICAL IMPAIRMENT TO NEONATAL HYPOGLYCEMIA |
|---|
| Blood or plasma glucose concentrations below 18 mg/dL. Such values definitely are abnormal, although if transient, there is no study in the literature confirming that they lead to permanent neurological injury. |
| Persistence of such severely low glucose concentrations for prolonged periods (hours, probably > 2–3 hr, rather than minutes, although there is no study in human neonates that defines this period). |
| Early mild to moderate clinical signs (primarily those of increased adrenalin [epinephrine] activity), such as alternating central nervous system signs of jitteriness/tremulousness versus stupor/lethargy or even a brief convulsion, that diminish or disappear with effective treatment that promptly restores the glucose concentration to the statistically normal range (> 45 mg/dL). |
| More serious clinical signs that are prolonged (many hours or longer), including coma, seizures, respiratory depression and/or apnea with cyanosis, hypotonia or limpness, high-pitched cry, hypothermia, and poor feeding after initially feeding well. These are more refractory to short-term treatment. |
| Concurrence of associated conditions, particularly persistent excessive insulin secretion and hyperinsulinemia with repeated episodes of acute, severe hypoglycemia with seizures and/or coma (although subclinical, often severe, hypoglycemic episodes occur in these conditions and might be just as injurious). |

Most clinicians today use higher values than previously accepted to define hypoglycemia. Several recent studies support this practice. Repeated blood glucose concentrations below 48 mg/dL in preterm infants were associated with adverse neurodevelopmental outcomes. Among a group of normal term infants, most achieved a serum glucose concentration greater than 50 mg/dL by 12 to 24 hours after birth. Human fetuses have a blood glucose concentration greater than 50 mg/dL during normal development. In clinical practice, blood glucose concentrations of 45 to 50 mg/dL (50–60 mg/dL plasma or serum) commonly represent the acceptable lower limit for neonatal glucose concentrations.

## DIAGNOSIS

The gold standard for measuring blood or plasma/serum glucose concentration is the hexokinase method used by most diagnostic laboratories. Colorimetric reagent strip methods are commonly used at the bedside to screen for hypoglycemia, but they are often inaccurate and must be confirmed by a standard laboratory method as soon as possible.

## INCIDENCE

The incidence of neonatal hypoglycemia, defined by a blood glucose of less than 45 mg/dL, is estimated at being between 1 and 5 per 1000 live births. The reported incidence varies depending on the definition, the time after birth when the concentration of glucose is measured, and the method used to measure the blood, plasma, or serum glucose concentration. In a group of at-risk newborns whose glucose was measured frequently throughout the first 48 hours of life, approximately half were found to have a blood glucose less than 47 mg/dL.

## CLINICAL PRESENTATION

Hypoglycemia is classified as *symptomatic* or *asymptomatic*, to indicate the presence or absence of physical signs that accompany a low glucose concentration. The most common and least specific signs include tremulousness and irritability (often alternating with mild hypotonia), diminished arousal (often noted as stupor or lethargy as manifestations of mild changes in level of consciousness), and failure to eat after first eating well.

These signs occur, however, with other common, similarly transient neonatal disorders, including hypocalcemia, subarachnoid hemorrhage, and in the early stages of sepsis. If due to hypoglycemia, signs usually correct quickly upon restoration of normal glucose concentrations. More severe and prolonged hypoglycemia may be associated with abnormal respiratory patterns, such as respiratory depression or apnea leading to cyanosis; cardiovascular signs, such as tachycardia or bradycardia; and neurological signs, such as temperature instability, loss of consciousness or coma, limpness and hypotonia, and seizures. Hypoglycemia should be excluded in any infant who exhibits any of these serious signs, since, if left untreated, severe, prolonged, or repeated, hypoglycemia can impair the function of many organs, especially the brain. In those infants known to be at risk for hypoglycemia, careful observation and screening is required since intermittent, asymptomatic injury that can lead to neurologic injury may occur.

## RISK FACTORS

Risk factors for hypoglycemia, such as maternal diabetes or abnormal glucose tolerance, maternal administration of drugs associated with neonatal hypoglycemia, ultrasound evidence of intrauterine growth restriction, or preterm birth, should be identified (Table 53-2). Growth parameters should be plotted on a growth chart to establish whether the infant is small or large for gestational age. Sepsis should be suspected if the infant has no apparent risk factors for hypoglycemia. If hypoglycemia persists for more than 1 week, hyperinsulinism, other endocrine disorders, and inborn errors of metabolism should be investigated, especially if the hypoglycemia is refractory to standard treatment.

## ETIOLOGY

The most common cause of neonatal hypoglycemia is an imbalance of reduced glucose production and increased glucose utilization (Table 53-3). Decreased substrate availability is common among preterm and small-for-gestational-age infants with intrauterine growth restriction (see Chapter 49). Hepatic glycogen stores are diminished in all preterm infants and many small-for-gestational-age infants. These 2 groups of infants also have a relatively increased brain-to-body weight ratio. This will increase glucose demand relative to the capacity for glucose production. Infants with stressful conditions (including asphyxia, hypothermia, or respiratory distress) can break down their glycogen stores more rapidly in response to increased secretion of catecholamines and glucagon. Even normal body stores of glycogen, however, may be inadequate to meet the increased rates of glucose utilization imposed by such conditions. Gluconeogenic and ketogenic enzymes also can be low in preterm and small-for-gestational-age infants, further preventing normal rates of new glucose production, or producing alternative fuel substrates from fatty acids. Infants of diabetic mothers are predisposed to hypoglycemia, due to persistent hyperinsulinemia following the excessive intrauterine glucose stimulation of their pancreas by maternal hyperglycemia. This leads to a persistently high insulin-to-glucagon ratio after birth, when placental glucose supply is abruptly discontinued. The high insulin-to-glucagon ratio inhibits enzymes regulating glycogenolysis (ie, glycogen phosphorylase), gluconeogenesis (ie, phosphoenolpyruvate carboxykinase), and hepatic glucose release (ie, glucose-6-phosphatase). Insulin also increases peripheral glucose utilization in insulin-sensitive tissues such as skeletal muscle, myocardium, and adipose tissue. Infants with erythroblastosis fetalis have increased levels of insulin and an increase in the number of pancreatic β cells. β-Adrenergic drugs, such as terbutaline, which are used to inhibit preterm uterine contractions and labor, also are associated with hyperinsulinemia and reduced glycogen stores.

Hypoglycemia that persists for more than 5 to 7 days most often results from 1 of several types of congenital hyperinsulinism. Although uncommon, these are serious metabolic disorders and are associated with a markedly increased risk of neurologic complications. Several of these disorders are genetic, including those that cause diffuse β-cell/islet hyperplasia or, less commonly, focal β-cell/islet adenomas. Many of these forms of congenital hyperinsulinism have been linked to defects in the sulfonylurea receptor or $K^+$-ATP channel. These genetic defects can be autosomal dominant or recessive. A syndrome of congenital hyperinsulinemia and asymptomatic hyperammonemia associated with mutations in the glutamate dehydrogenase gene also has been described. *Beckwith-Wiedemann syndrome* is associated with hyperplasia of multiple organs, including the pancreas, with increased insulin secretion.

**TABLE 53-2 RISK FACTORS FOR NEONATAL HYPOGLYCEMIA**

| **Maternal Conditions** |
|---|
| Presence of diabetes or abnormal result from glucose tolerance test |
| Preeclampsia and pregnancy-induced or essential hypertension |
| Previous macrosomic infants |
| Substance abuse |
| Treatment with β-agonist tocolytics |
| Treatment with oral hypoglycemic agents |
| Late antepartum to intrapartum administration of intravenous glucose |
| **Neonatal Conditions** |
| Preterm birth |
| Intrauterine growth restriction |
| Perinatal hypoxia-ischemia |
| Sepsis |
| Hypothermia |
| Polycythemia-hyperviscosity |
| Erythroblastosis fetalis |
| Iatrogenic administration of insulin |
| Congenital cardiac malformations |
| Persistent hyperinsulinemia |
| Endocrine disorders |
| Inborn errors of metabolism |
| Late antepartum to intrapartum administration of intravenous glucose |
| Poor feeding, especially new onset after previously feeding well |

Reproduced with permission from Gardner SL, Carter BS, Enzman Hines M, et al: *Merenstein G & Gardner's Handbook of Neonatal Intensive Care*. 8th ed, St. Louis: Elsevier; 2016.

**TABLE 53-3 NEONATAL HYPOGLYCEMIA: ETIOLOGIES AND TIME COURSE**

| Clinical Mechanism | Setting | Expected Duration |
|---|---|---|
| Decreased substrate availability | Intrauterine growth restriction | Transient |
| | Prematurity | Transient |
| | Glycogen storage disease | Prolonged |
| | Inborn errors (eg, fructose intolerance) | Prolonged |
| Increased utilization | Perinatal asphyxia | Transient |
| | Hypothermia | Transient |
| **Endocrine Disturbances** | | |
| Hyperinsulinemia | Infant of diabetic mother | Transient |
| | Beckwith-Wiedemann syndrome | Prolonged |
| | Congenital hyperinsulinism | Prolonged |
| | Erythroblastosis fetalis | Transient |
| | Exchange transfusion | Transient |
| | Islet cell dysplasias | Transient |
| | Maternal β-agonist tocolytics | Prolonged |
| | Improperly placed umbilical artery catheter | Transient |
| Other endocrine disorders | Hypopituitarism | Prolonged |
| | Hypothyroidism | Prolonged |
| | Adrenal insufficiency | Prolonged |
| Miscellaneous/multiple mechanisms | Sepsis | Transient |
| | Congenital heart disease | Transient |
| | Central nervous system abnormalities | Prolonged |

Reproduced with permission from Gardner SL, Carter BS, Enzman Hines M, et al: *Merenstein G & Gardner's Handbook of Neonatal Intensive Care*. 8th ed, St. Louis: Elsevier; 2016.

Inborn errors of metabolism can limit availability of gluconeogenic precursors or the function of the enzymes required for hepatic glucose production. Metabolic defects that present with hypoglycemia include some forms of glycogen storage disease, galactosemia, fatty acid oxidation defects, carnitine deficiency, several of the amino acidemias, hereditary fructose intolerance (fructose-1,6-diphosphatase deficiency), and defects of other gluconeogenic enzymes. Rare endocrine disorders, such as hypopituitarism and adrenal failure, also lead to hypoglycemia because of inadequate hormonal responses, including inadequate growth hormone and adrenal corticosteroid secretion.

## HYPOGLYCEMIA AND THE BRAIN

Severe hypoglycemia in the newborn is associated with selective neuronal necrosis in multiple brain regions, including the superficial cortex, dentate gyrus, hippocampus, and caudate-putamen. Energy failure leads to decreased cerebral electrical activity followed by neuronal cell membrane breakdown. Energy failure also prevents postsynaptic uptake of the principal neurotransmitter glutamate. Excess glutamate concentrations then activate NMDA (*N*-methyl D-aspartate) receptors in the neuronal membranes, which increases cellular entry and cytoplasmic concentrations of sodium and calcium, causing osmotic swelling and acute neuronal necrosis. The high calcium concentrations also activate cellular phospholipases and proteases and prevent normal mitochondrial metabolism, which leads to increased toxic free radical formation. These processes disrupt synaptic transmission and eventually lead to delayed neuronal necrosis. Hypoglycemia also can exacerbate pre-existing cerebral hypoxic brain injury.

## MANAGEMENT

Symptomatic neonatal hypoglycemia must be corrected rapidly, and further episodes of hypoglycemia must be prevented by providing adequate substrate until normal glucose homeostasis is established (Fig. 53-2). Early enteral feeding is usually successful in treating mild hypoglycemia in asymptomatic infants. Human milk or standard infant formulas provide carbohydrate in the form of lactose without excessively stimulating insulin secretion, and also include protein and fat, which provide a sustained supply of substrates for gluconeogenesis and alternative fuels. Fat intake also decreases cellular glucose uptake. Blood glucose concentrations should increase by 20 to 30 mg/dL within the first hour after a feeding of 30 to 60 mL of milk or formula.

Intravenous glucose infusion should be used when infants are symptomatic or are unable to tolerate enteral feedings and when hypoglycemia does not respond to enteral feeding. Intravenous glucose also should be used early after birth in those high-risk infants who are likely to experience severe and prolonged disturbances in glucose homeostasis, such as preterm infants, small-for-gestational-age infants with intrauterine growth restriction, infants of diabetic mothers, and infants who have underlying etiologies for hypoglycemia, such as sepsis, known or suspected inborn errors of metabolism, endocrine defects, or erythroblastosis.

In symptomatic newborns, an initial rapid intravenous infusion of 200 mg/kg (2 mL/kg) of 10% dextrose solution should be followed by continuous infusion of 5 to 8 mg/kg/min of glucose—that is, the glucose utilization rate of a healthy term infant (Fig. 53-3). The blood glucose concentration should be measured approximately 30 minutes after the initial rapid infusion and then every 1 to 2 hours until it is stable within the normal range. If the glucose level subsequently falls into the hypoglycemic range, then the rapid infusion should be repeated, and the infusion rate increased by 10% to 15%. In asymptomatic hypoglycemic newborns it may be appropriate to start a continuous infusion of 5 to 8 mg/kg/min of glucose without an initial rapid infusion, and then to follow the glucose response closely, and adjust the infusion rate to obtain a glucose in the normal range.

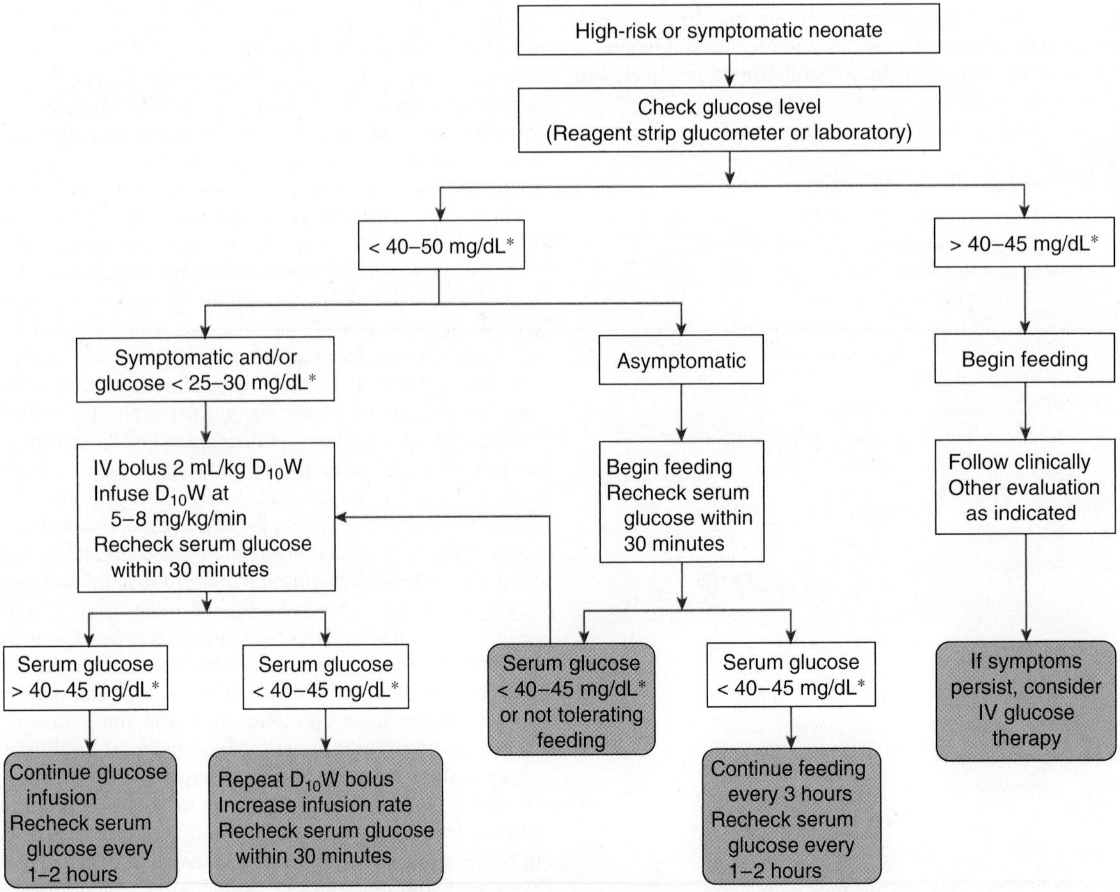


**FIGURE 53-2** Algorithm for management of the neonate with hypoglycemia. $D_{10}W$, 10% dextrose; IV, intravenous.

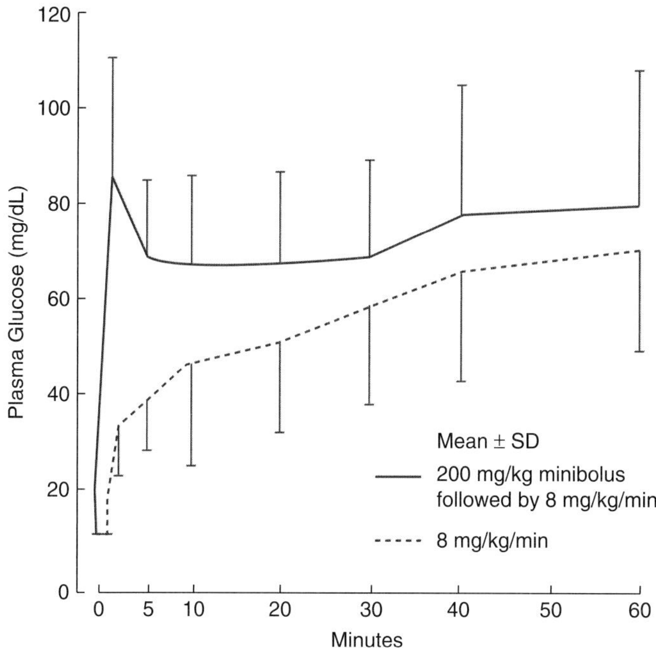


**FIGURE 53-3** Plasma glucose response to glucose "minibolus" followed by continuous glucose infusion of 8 mg/min/kg as therapy for severe neonatal hypoglycemia.

Infants with hyperinsulinemia often require as much as 12 to 15 mg/kg/min of intravenous glucose to maintain normoglycemia. At these rates, it is safest to use a central venous catheter to allow infusion of dextrose concentrations greater than 12.5%. Infants requiring intravenous therapy for hypoglycemia should continue feedings as long as there is no evidence of feeding intolerance. An alternate feeding strategy is to provide some carbohydrate as galactose, 1 of the sugars that compose lactose. This can be useful for infants of diabetic mothers and other infants with hyperinsulinism, because the pancreatic production of insulin in response to galactose is less than its response to an equivalent amount of glucose. When a normal blood glucose concentration has been established, and the requirement for intravenous glucose has been stable for 12 to 24 hours, the infant can be weaned. The safest method is to measure preprandial blood glucose concentrations and decrease the infusion rate by 10% to 20% each time the blood glucose is greater than 50 to 60 mg/dL. Failure to tolerate weaning from intravenous glucose may indicate the presence of a pervasive disorder, such as a metabolic defect or idiopathic hyperinsulinemia and warrants further diagnostic investigation, and may require adjunctive therapies (Table 53-4).

**TABLE 53-4 ADJUNCT THERAPIES FOR PERSISTENT NEONATAL HYPOGLYCEMIA**

| Therapy | Effect | Dose |
|---|---|---|
| Corticosteroids | Decreases peripheral glucose utilization | Hydrocortisone 5–15 mg/kg/d or prednisone 2 mg/kg/d |
| Glucagon | Stimulates glycogenolysis | 30 μg/kg with normal insulin |
| | | 300 μg/kg with hyperinsulinemia |
| Diazoxide | Inhibits insulin secretion | 15 μg/kg/d |
| Somatostatin (long-acting: octreotide acetate) | Inhibits insulin and growth hormone release | 5–10 μg/kg every 6–8 h |
| Pancreatectomy | Decreases insulin secretion | |
| | Causes diabetes and pancreatic insufficiency | |



## OUTCOME

The long-term effects of severe neonatal hypoglycemia remain controversial. Repeated episodes of symptomatic hypoglycemia, particularly in infants with persistent hyperinsulinism, have been associated with selective neuronal necrosis and impaired cognitive and motor function. There is little evidence of long-term sequelae in late preterm and term infants who have experienced relatively few, brief episodes of hypoglycemia, especially if asymptomatic. In preterm infants, however, the evidence with respect to long-term outcomes following repeated daily glucose concentrations below 46 mg/dL is mixed. Thus, mild to moderate hypoglycemia might affect the outcome in high-risk infants, particularly those who cannot respond adequately to hypoglycemia, although such infants have many other confounding problems that independently or in combination lead to abnormal neurodevelopment.

# HYPERGLYCEMIA

Hyperglycemia is relatively common in infants who are born extremely preterm (< 26 weeks of gestation). It is most often caused by excessive rates of intravenous glucose infusion in the presence of physiological and biochemical mechanisms that lead to excess glucose production, insulin resistance, and glucose intolerance.

## DEFINITION

Hyperglycemia refers to a blood glucose concentration greater than 120 to 125 mg/dL (plasma concentration > 145–150 mg/dL), regardless of gestational age, weight, or postnatal age.

## EPIDEMIOLOGY

Hyperglycemia is most common in neonates that are extremely preterm (< 26 weeks of gestation) and of extremely low birth weight (< 1000 g). The incidence of hyperglycemia is inversely related to birth weight in the preterm infant, ranging from about 2% in infants who weigh more than 2000 g to about 45% in those who weigh less than 1000 g, and up to 80% in infants weighing less than 750 g.

## ETIOLOGY

Hyperglycemia affects around half of all preterm infants receiving continuous intravenous dextrose infusions at glucose rates greater than 10 to 11 mg/kg/min, and almost all infants at rates greater than 14 mg/kg/min. Even after dextrose infusion rates are decreased to treat hyperglycemia, infusion rates as low as 3 to 4 mg/kg/min can result in persistent hyperglycemia, especially during prolonged periods of stress. Previously stable glucose values becoming hyperglycemic on a stable glucose input may herald new sepsis. Hyperglycemia is associated with the severity of clinical problems in neonates, as estimated by low Apgar scores, high fractional concentrations of inspired oxygen, and respiratory distress. Intravenous lipid infusion also increases the incidence and degree of hyperglycemia, as increased plasma concentrations of free fatty acids decrease peripheral glucose utilization by competing with glucose for oxidation and by stimulating the activity of enzymes that specifically promote fatty acid oxidation.

Stress, as measured by increased plasma cortisol concentrations, is an important risk factor for hyperglycemia, most frequently among infants receiving catecholamine infusions, or undergoing painful procedures such as surgery, venipuncture, vascular cutdowns, and endotracheal tube insertion without adequate analgesia or anesthesia. Narcotic treatment during and after surgery lowers the incidence of hyperglycemia. Recent observations indicate that postsurgical hyperglycemia is likely caused by increased cortisol secretion during surgery, whereas hyperglycemia immediately after the induction of anesthesia more likely is related to increased catecholamine secretion. Thus, narcotic treatment with fentanyl or morphine during and after surgery has been associated with lower circulating concentrations of catecholamines, glucocorticoids, and glucagon as well as a lower incidence of hyperglycemia.

Catecholamines reduce insulin secretion and interfere with peripheral insulin action. Glucagon promotes glycogenolysis and release of hepatic glucose. Glucocorticoids promote gluconeogenesis by increasing protein breakdown and the supply of amino acids. Glucocorticoids also enhance hepatic enzyme activity in the gluconeogenic pathway, particularly phosphoenolpyruvate carboxykinase, the rate-limiting enzyme for gluconeogenesis, and glucose-6-phosphatase, which releases glucose into the circulation. Hyperglycemia also occurs more commonly among preterm and small-for-gestational-age infants, who have increased plasma concentrations of counter-regulatory (anti-insulin) hormones. Other, more common causes of neonatal hyperglycemia include the use of medications such as theophylline and dexamethasone. It has also been associated with prostaglandin $E_1$ infusions.

*Insulin-dependent diabetes mellitus*, either transient or permanent, is an unusual but important cause of hyperglycemia in newborn infants. Neonatal diabetes mellitus usually presents early in postnatal life with weight loss, polyuria, dehydration, glycosuria, and hyperglycemia. It usually does not resolve for several weeks or even months and sometimes is permanent, and it may be associated with chromosomal abnormalities or pancreatic agenesis.

#### PATHOPHYSIOLOGY

The principal mechanism responsible for hyperglycemia in preterm infants is intravenous infusion of dextrose at rates that exceed the capacity for glucose utilization. Glucose utilization is limited by relatively inadequate insulin secretion rates as well as by decreased peripheral insulin sensitivity (primarily in skeletal muscle) in infants who experience stress and relatively increased secretion rates of catecholamines, glucocorticoids, and glucagon. Some preterm infants also appear to maintain glucose production during insulin, glucose, and lipid infusions, indicating central (hepatic) insulin resistance. Excessive or inappropriate (according to insulin secretion rates and plasma insulin concentrations) glucose production rates also can promote or prolong hyperglycemia. Even extremely low-birth-weight preterm infants can have high rates of glucose production (4–8 mg/min/kg), primarily from gluconeogenesis, relatively soon after birth.

#### COMPLICATIONS

Hyperglycemia in newborn infants is seldom if ever so severe as to cause osmotic injury to tissues, particularly in the brain, unlike the well-known brain damage caused by salt poisoning. Another potential effect of aggressive glucose administration is steatosis, with associated impaired secretion of hepatic triglycerides. Steatosis rarely causes clinical signs in the neonate, but it can be detected by modest elevations of liver transaminases. Another complication of hyperglycemia is electrolyte imbalance in neonates who have glycosuria and increased sodium excretion. Hyperglycemia in older, more mature infants may jeopardize respiratory function by increasing lipogenesis, producing increased amounts of carbon dioxide. This requires an increase in minute ventilation that, theoretically, might compromise infants who already have significant respiratory distress.

#### MANAGEMENT

Treatment of hyperglycemia must include the simultaneous treatment of underlying conditions. With modest hyperglycemia (plasma glucose concentration < 300 mg/dL), reducing the exogenous glucose (dextrose) infusion rate to as low as 3 to 4 mg/kg/min usually is sufficient to ameliorate or resolve the hyperglycemia. The rate of infusion should be decreased gradually by 1 to 2 mg/kg/min every 2 to 4 hours, with frequent measurement of glucose concentrations until normoglycemia is achieved. Early intravenous amino acid infusions should be considered to prevent or treat hyperglycemia. The rationale for this approach is that certain amino acids are known insulin secretagogues and are important for normal growth and development of the pancreas and the pancreatic islets and β cells. Limiting intravenous lipid infusions also should be considered, as they promote gluconeogenesis and inhibit glucose utilization. Even a minimal enteral feeding regimen may be beneficial unless the infant is very ill or there are clear signs of feeding intolerance, as enteral feeds promote the secretion of insulin by inducing gut production of *enteroinsular hormones*, also known as *incretins*. These hormones increase insulin secretion by direct actions on the pancreatic cells.

Intravenous infusion of short-acting, regular insulin should be reserved for infants who have severe hyperglycemia (> 300 mg/dL) that persists despite reducing the glucose infusion rate to less than 3 to 4 mg/kg/min. These infants also may have a metabolic acidosis, lactic acidosis, hyperkalemia, and osmotic diuresis. Infusion rates should be started at 0.02 to 0.05 U/kg/h. Hypokalemia can be prevented by addition of potassium to intravenous fluids. Blood glucose concentrations should be measured frequently, every 1 to 2 hours, or whenever signs of possible hypoglycemia develop.

## DISORDERS OF CALCIUM REGULATION

### HYPOCALCEMIA

#### DEFINITION

Neonatal hypocalcemia is generally defined as a serum total calcium concentration of less than 2 mmol/L (< 8 mg/dL) in term infants and less than 1.75 mmol/L (< 7 mg/dL) in preterm infants or an ionized calcium concentration of less than 0.75 to 1.1 mmol/L (< 3.0–4.4 mg/dL). Early-onset neonatal hypocalcemia typically is transient and occurs during the first 24 to 48 hours after birth; later-onset hypocalcemia usually occurs after the first week of life and commonly involves lasting pathology.

#### ETIOLOGY

Early-onset hypocalcemia is most commonly associated with preterm birth, perinatal depression (from hypoxic-ischemic conditions), maternal insulin-dependent diabetes, gestational exposure to anticonvulsants, and maternal hyperparathyroidism. Previous experience was that transient hypocalcemia often occurred in approximately 30% of all preterm infants (up to 90% in those born extremely preterm), approximately 30% of infants who have an Apgar score below 5 at 1 minute of age, and approximately 10% to 20% of infants of insulin-dependent diabetic mothers. However, much lower rates are currently reported, with earlier postnatal administration of intravenous solutions that contain calcium and earlier onset of enteral feeding. Subcutaneous fat necrosis (SCFN) is a rare form of panniculitis in infants that generally occurs following birth trauma, meconium aspiration, or therapeutic cooling. Severe hypercalcemia occurs in a subset of these patients. In addition to the local signs, fever is common, and there is a high incidence of persistent nephrocalcinosis without evidence of adverse renal outcomes.

Later-onset hypocalcemia is much less frequent and is most commonly associated with relatively high phosphate-containing diets, disturbed maternal vitamin D metabolism, intestinal malabsorption of calcium, hypomagnesemia, and hypoparathyroidism.

#### PATHOPHYSIOLOGY

A normal physiological neonatal calcium nadir occurs at about 48 hours after birth in normal term infants. Early neonatal hypocalcemia generally represents a transient failure of calciotropic hormone secretion in response to the loss of placental calcium supply at birth. Preterm infants often do not appropriately increase parathyroid hormone secretion. This can be aggravated by restricted intravenous and oral calcium intake, end-organ resistance to 1,25-dihydroxyvitamin D [$1,25(OH)_2D$], and increased serum calcitonin. Other contributing factors in infants exposed to hypoxia-ischemia, include an increased endogenous phosphate load, low neonatal glomerular filtration rate that limits phosphorous excretion, bicarbonate therapy, and an increased serum calcitonin concentration. Hypocalcemia in infants of insulin-dependent diabetic mothers appears related to magnesium insufficiency from renal losses and impaired fetal parathormone secretion. Formulas usually contain more phosphorus than human milk, and formula-fed infants often have lower serum ionized calcium and higher serum phosphorus concentrations in the first week of life compared to breastfed infants.

Congenital hypoparathyroidism is the most significant cause of late-onset hypocalcemia that has to be treated early in life. Congenital hypoparathyroidism also occurs as part of the 22q11.2 deletion syndrome (also called DiGeorge syndrome or DiGeorge sequence). Insufficiency of vitamin D arises from maternal vitamin D deficiency, lack of exposure to sunlight coupled with insufficient dietary vitamin D intake, reduced production of vitamin D or its active metabolites caused by liver or renal disease, congenital deficiency of renal 1α-hydroxylase, and $1,25(OH)_2D$ resistance. Deficiency of vitamin D or its metabolites causes decreased intestinal calcium absorption and renal calcium reabsorption. Most infant vitamin D disturbances are not apparent until several months of age.

Magnesium concentrations should be measured in all infants with hypocalcemia because magnesium is necessary for parathyroid secretion and end-organ action.

### CLINICAL PRESENTATION

Most cases of neonatal hypocalcemia are asymptomatic. When severe, the main clinical signs are jitteriness, irritability, tremors, twitching movements, and generalized or focal convulsions. Other nonspecific features include lethargy, poor feeding, vomiting, and abdominal distension. Arrhythmias may occur, but the characteristic prolongation of the electrocardiogram QT interval is not consistently found. Frank convulsions are seen more commonly with late neonatal hypocalcemia (usually calcium < 6 mg/dL). The classical signs of peripheral hyperexcitability of motor nerves (carpopedal spasm and laryngospasm) are uncommon in newborn infants.

### DIAGNOSIS

The diagnosis of hypocalcemia is based on the determination of serum total and ionized calcium as well as serum phosphorus, magnesium, and glucose concentrations and blood pH. Prolongation of the corrected QT interval on the electrocardiogram should always raise the suspicion of hypocalcemia, and this can may be useful in monitoring the response to calcium therapy.

Symptomatic hypocalcemia that is refractory to therapy may be secondary to less common causes such as primary hypoparathyroidism, malabsorption, and disorders of vitamin D metabolism. Elevated serum phosphorus concentration (> 8 mg/dL) indicates phosphorus loading (a clue to high dietary phosphorus intake), renal insufficiency, or hypoparathyroidism. Absence of a thymic shadow on chest radiograph suggests DiGeorge syndrome. Hypercalciuria associated with hypocalcemia indicates deficient parathyroid hormone. Low serum 25-hydroxyvitamin D concentration (< 11 ng/mL) indicates vitamin D deficiency.

### MANAGEMENT

Asymptomatic hypocalcemia is treated by providing intravenous calcium salts followed by formula or milk feeding that provides 75 mg/kg/d of calcium. After normocalcemia is achieved, a stepwise reduction of intravenous calcium may prevent rebound hypocalcemia: 75 mg/kg/d for the first day, half the dose the next day, half again, and discontinue. Infants of diabetic mothers often require as much as 100 to 200 mg/kg daily, and some require 2 to 3 times that amount. If infants can tolerate oral fluids, calcium gluconate can be given enterally at the same total daily dose (divided into 4 to 6 doses) after initial correction. Use of the intravenous form of calcium for enteral administration may cause less gut stimulation than syrup-based (high osmolar) preparations.

Symptomatic hypocalcemia usually responds rapidly to intravenous calcium therapy, and this also helps to confirm the diagnosis. In mildly symptomatic cases, attempts to correct hypocalcemia with rapid bolus infusions are less successful than slower infusions or repeated low dose bolus injections; this approach also helps prevent cardiac dysrhythmias. If hypocalcemia is associated with seizures, calcium can be replaced rapidly with 1 to 2 mL of 10% calcium gluconate per kg (9–18 mg elemental calcium/kg) given intravenously over 5 to 10 minutes; heart rate should be measured continuously during the infusion because of bradycardia, for which the infusion should be stopped temporarily. Additional calcium should be given intravenously as 100 to 200 mg/kg/dose every 4 to 6 hours if symptoms persist. A central venous catheter is preferable for acute intravenous calcium administration, particularly in severely symptomatic cases (eg, with seizures). If a peripheral catheter is used, its patency and the skin around the catheter's skin entry site should be checked for signs of extravasation before every dose of calcium, as calcium can cause considerable tissue injury with extravasation from the vein. This is more common with calcium chloride, which should only be used in extreme emergencies using a central venous catheter. Vitamin D metabolites are not recommended for treatment of early hypocalcemia because of their variable responses and potential side effects.

Most cases of neonatal hypocalcemia require only 2 to 3 days of treatment, but such treatment is important to prevent adverse cardiovascular and central nervous system (CNS) complications of low serum calcium concentrations. Calcium supplementation usually is required for long periods in cases of hypocalcemia caused by malabsorption or hypoparathyroidism. If hypocalcemia is associated with hypomagnesemia (serum magnesium concentration below 0.6 mmol/L or 1.5 mg/dL), magnesium sulfate 50% solution (500 mg or 4 mEq/mL), 0.1 to 0.2 mL/kg intravenously or intramuscularly, providing 50 to 100 mg/kg, should be given and repeated after 12 to 24 hours. Serum magnesium should be obtained before each dose.

Late hypocalcemia is usually symptomatic and requires treatment. The goals of therapy are to reduce the phosphorus load and to increase calcium absorption by using feedings with a calcium/phosphorus ratio greater than or equal to 4:1. This can be accomplished by the use of low-phosphorus feedings, such as human milk or low-phosphorus formula, in conjunction with an oral calcium supplement. Phosphate binders generally are not necessary. Hypoparathyroidism requires therapy with vitamin D or preferably one of its metabolites: $1,25(OH)_2D$ (or 1α-hydroxyvitamin $D_3$, a synthetic analog) and lifelong calcium supplementation.

### PREVENTION

Early neonatal hypocalcemia can be prevented by oral or intravenous calcium supplementation (80 mg elemental calcium gluconate/kg/d [100 mg/kg/d of calcium gluconate = 9.3 mg of elemental calcium]). Use of continuous calcium infusion by central catheter to maintain a total calcium higher than 8.0 mg/dL and an ionized calcium level higher than 1.0 mmol/L (4.0 mg/dL), may prevent hypocalcemia in sick newborns with cardiovascular compromise requiring cardiotonic drugs or pressor support. Maintenance of normal maternal vitamin D status with exogenous vitamin D supplements may help to maintain adequate amounts of fetal vitamin D; which, in turn, may prevent late hypocalcemia. In addition, the judicious use of bicarbonate administration and avoidance of respiratory alkalosis reduce the risk of developing symptomatic hypocalcemia in ill infants.

## HYPERCALCEMIA

### DEFINITION

Neonatal hypercalcemia is defined as a serum total calcium concentration greater than 2.75 mmol/L (11 mg/dL) or an ionized calcium concentration greater than 1.4 mmol/L (5.6 mg/dL). Pathological hypercalcemia includes increased ionized and total calcium, although increased total calcium may occur without increased ionized calcium.

### ETIOLOGY

Hypercalcemia is uncommon but more frequent in preterm infants. It is usually iatrogenic in the setting of excessive vitamin D and/or calcium supplementation, or following the use of parenteral nutrition with insufficient phosphate administration (with or without excessive calcium). Hypercalcemia of the mother and the neonate may result from chronic maternal exposure to excess vitamin D or its metabolites during treatment of maternal hypocalcemia or by maternal self-medication. Chronic maternal diuretic therapy with thiazides during pregnancy also can cause lead to neonatal hypercalcemia.

Much rarer causes of hypercalcemia in the newborn have a metabolic or familial basis, such as primary hyperparathyroidism, familial hypocalciuric hypercalcemia, hypercalcemia associated with subcutaneous fat necrosis, idiopathic infantile hypercalcemia (part of Williams syndrome), severe infantile hypophosphatasia, and Bartter syndrome variant.

### PATHOPHYSIOLOGY

Normally, an increase in serum calcium inhibits parathyroid hormone and $1,25(OH)_2D$ synthesis and thereby prevents or reduces hypercalcemia by decreasing calcium mobilization from bone, absorption from intestine, and reabsorption from kidney. A sustained elevation in serum calcium concentration implies an inappropriately increased calcium efflux from 1 of these pools into the extracellular fluid.

Hypophosphatemia can cause elevated circulating $1,25(OH)_2D$ with increased intestinal absorption of calcium and increased bone resorption; calcium cannot be deposited in bone in the absence of phosphate and thereby contributes to hypercalcemia. Pathological conditions associated with parathyroid hormone or vitamin D overactivity that lead to hypercalcemia include increased bone turnover, intestinal calcium absorption, and renal calcium absorption.

### CLINICAL PRESENTATION

Hypercalcemia may be asymptomatic. Mild clinical signs include lethargy, irritability, feeding difficulties, emesis, constipation, polyuria, dehydration, and poor growth. More serious signs include seizures, hypertension, respiratory distress (from hypotonia, demineralization, and deformation of the rib cage), and nephrocalcinosis. Long-standing hypercalcemia can lead to metastatic calcifications such as nephrocalcinosis.

### DIAGNOSIS

An increased serum calcium concentration confirms the diagnosis. A maternal dietary and drug history (eg, excessive vitamin A or D, thiazides) or history of possible calcium-phosphorus imbalance or polyhydramnios during pregnancy, or a family history of disturbed calcium metabolism, should prompt further evaluation. Very elevated serum calcium level (> 15 mg/dL) usually indicates primary hyperparathyroidism or, in very low–birth-weight infants, phosphate depletion. Further evaluation should include serum phosphorus concentration, percentage of renal tubular phosphorus reabsorption, serum parathyroid hormone concentration, urinary calcium–urinary creatinine ratio, serum alkaline phosphatase concentration, and serum 25-hydroxyvitamin D concentration. Bone x-ray films will identify demineralization and/or osteolytic lesions or osteosclerotic lesions consistent with the etiology of the hypercalcemia.

### MANAGEMENT

The treatment of neonatal hypercalcemia consists of correcting specific underlying causes and removing iatrogenic or external causes. This includes the surgical removal of parathyroid glands, stopping of excessive vitamin D intake, and reducing or temporarily stopping calcium supplementation of human milk (mother's or donor) given to preterm infants. In mild cases in which patients are asymptomatic, maintenance of hydration may suffice. In the first 2 to 3 days after birth, adjustments in the intravenous calcium–phosphorous ratio usually prevent further hypercalcemia. For a moderately to severely hypercalcemic infant, prompt investigation and therapy must be instituted with the following goals: correction of dehydration, enhancement of renal excretion of calcium, inhibition of intestinal absorption or bone resorption (eg, with hydrocortisone treatment), restriction of dietary calcium intake, oral phosphorous supplementation if hypophosphatemia is present, and treatment of the underlying disorder.

For the short-term treatment of acute symptomatic hypercalcemia (or serum calcium > 14 mg/dL), expansion of the extracellular fluid compartment with 10 to 20 mL/kg of 0.9% sodium chloride intravenously, followed by an intravenous injection of a potent loop diuretic such as 1 mg/kg of furosemide every 6 to 8 hours, may increase urinary calcium excretion. In patients with low serum phosphorus concentrations, oral phosphate supplements of 0.5 to 1.0 mmol (16–31 mg) of elemental phosphorus per kilogram per day in divided doses mixed with feeds may normalize the serum phosphorus concentration and lower serum calcium concentration. Parenteral phosphate, however, should be avoided in severely hypercalcemic patients (serum total calcium > 12 mg/dL) unless hypophosphatemia is severe (< 1.5 mg/dL), because extraskeletal calcification may occur. Calcitonin, glucocorticoids and bisphosphonate also have been used for severe hypercalcemia. For severe and unremitting hypercalcemia, either hemodialysis if the infant is hemodynamically stable or peritoneal dialysis may be helpful. Virtually all cases of primary hyperparathyroidism require subtotal or total parathyroidectomy, because the hypercalcemia may be life threatening and does not respond to medical management. The need for treatment should be reassessed at regular intervals because some instances of neonatal hypercalcemia may resolve spontaneously.

# DISORDERS OF SODIUM BALANCE

## HYPERNATREMIA

### DEFINITION

Hypernatremia is defined as a serum sodium concentration of greater than 150 mEq/L.

### INCIDENCE AND EPIDEMIOLOGY

Hypernatremia is common in preterm infants, particularly in those born before 28 weeks' gestation and in those of extremely low birth weight (< 1000 g). The frequency of severe hypernatremia has diminished in recent years with improved fluid and electrolyte management.

### ETIOLOGY AND PATHOPHYSIOLOGY

The most common cause of neonatal hypernatremia is dehydration from free water deficiency. In the preterm neonate, multiple factors contribute to free water loss. Excessive evaporative water loss in the first 24 hours especially, across the very underdeveloped skin of extremely premature infants contributes to dehydration and hypernatremia. Evaporation is aggravated by radiant warmers, high environmental temperatures, increased body temperatures, low ambient or inspired humidity, congenital skin defects (eg, omphalocele), and phototherapy. Other contributing factors include the poor concentrating capacity of the underdeveloped renal medulla with high urinary water loss.

Hypernatremia in preterm infants can be exacerbated by injudicious use of sodium-containing solutions, including normal saline boluses and sodium bicarbonate. Sodium-containing medications often are overlooked as contributors to hypernatremia. Rarely, congenital or acquired reduction in antidiuretic hormone (diabetes insipidus) can lead to excessive, relatively sodium-free urinary water loss. In the term neonate, dehydration secondary to breast feeding failure is often complicated by various degrees of hypernatremia.

Sodium is the principal cation of extracellular fluid, including the plasma. Hypernatremia from dehydration will deplete intracellular fluid, in any organ and tissue in the body, but most worryingly in the brain. This must be taken into consideration, as rapid correction of hypernatremia can cause complications from cerebral edema.

### CLINICAL PRESENTATION

Mild to moderate hypernatremia usually is well tolerated in both the preterm and term neonate. More severe hypernatremia (> 175 mEq/L) can manifest with symptoms referred to the CNS. Hypernatremia leads to osmotic shifts in capillaries and cells in the

CNS, which can rupture and produce neuronal cell necrosis and intracerebral hemorrhage. Late-occurring seizures can occur with very severe hypernatremia, with or without venous thrombosis or intracranial hemorrhage. Dehydrated term infants can present with lethargy, irritability, hypotonia and with seizures if hypernatremia is severe.

### PREVENTION AND MANAGEMENT

For the preterm neonate, interventions to prevent the development of hypernatremia include the use of polyethylene occlusive wrapping or plastic bags to minimize evaporative water loss during resuscitation, and the use of humidified isolettes in the NICU. Fluid administration should be guided by frequent measurements of weight and urinary flow rate to adjust fluid intake to prevent dehydration, and judicious use of sodium-containing infusions.

Treatment is directed toward correcting the cause, either free water deficit or total body sodium overload. Serum sodium should be reduced slowly to prevent osmotic swelling in cells, particularly in the CNS. It is appropriate to aim to correct no more than 10 to 12 mEq/L of serum sodium concentration over 24 to 36 hours. Extremely severe hypernatremia, particularly if the infant has CNS signs such as seizures and intracerebral hemorrhage, can be treated with whole blood exchange transfusion.

### OUTCOME

Multiple studies have correlated hypernatremia with an increased risk of long-term neurologic complications in both the preterm and term neonate. However, given that the clinical course of the neonate with hypernatremia often complicated, it is difficult to link causality between hypernatremia and neurologic injury.

## HYPONATREMIA

### DEFINITION

Hyponatremia is defined as a serum sodium concentration of less than 130 mEq/L.

### INCIDENCE AND EPIDEMIOLOGY

Hyponatremia is common in extremely small preterm infants. It is not uncommon for these infants to be treated in the first 2 to 3 days of life with high intravenous fluid infusion rates to prevent dehydration. However, during this time, glomerular filtration rates and urinary flow rates are low, especially when associated with pulmonary disorders. The imbalance between fluid administration and fluid loss results in hyponatremia. Late hyponatremia also is common in preterm infants, and usually occurs as a result of diuretic use. Hyponatremia in the term infant is rare. When it does occur, it is often the result of excessive fluid administration in the critically ill neonate.

### ETIOLOGY AND PATHOPHYSIOLOGY

Hyponatremia in preterm infants is most commonly iatrogenic. This can occur at birth if the mother has received high intravenous infusion rates during labor or cesarean section; water diffuses across the placenta more rapidly than do solutes. Decreased effective blood volume prevents the suppression of antidiuretic hormone (vasopressin) secretion, common with perinatal depression secondary to hypoxic-ischemic conditions, intracranial hemorrhage, sepsis, respiratory distress, intrathoracic air leak syndromes, and medications such as morphine, barbiturates, or carbamazepine. Low glomerular filtration rates at early gestational ages also limit high urine flow rates in response to fluid boluses, particularly in the first 2 to 3 days of life. Further dilution of serum sodium often is augmented by coincident hyperglycemia, which osmotically pulls water from intracellular and extravascular extracellular fluid spaces. Later hyponatremia occurs frequently as a result of renal loss of sodium from diuretic therapy, particularly the potent loop diuretics such as furosemide. The syndrome of inappropriate antidiuretic hormone secretion also can produce hyponatremia. This should be suspected clinically when decreased serum sodium concentrations and urine output occur simultaneously, usually in response to a sudden, often catastrophic change in CNS and cardiovascular status, such as with acute, severe intracranial hemorrhage. Suboptimal sodium intake at any stage contributes to hyponatremia, as does urinary sodium loss once the very preterm infant enters its natural diuretic phase after the first 2 to 3 days of life. Late hyponatremia has been noted with exclusive breast milk feedings without supplements of milk fortifiers that include salts and protein and with certain low-sodium formulas.



### CLINICAL PRESENTATION

Hyponatremia often is asymptomatic because of chronic rather than acute development of sodium imbalance, but a late clinical sign is the onset of seizures. Infants fed unsupplemented breast milk or low-sodium formulas often develop peripheral edema with hyponatremia that sometimes is aggravated by hypoproteinemia from low protein in the diet.

Severe and persistent hyponatremia can lead to pathologic conditions in the CNS (eg, seizures), lung (eg, patent ductus arteriosus, pulmonary edema), and acid–base balance (eg, hypochloremic alkalosis from diuretic therapy, often worsened by bicarbonate generation from retained carbon dioxide in infants with chronic lung disease), as well as poor growth that often is accompanied by peripheral edema.

### DIAGNOSIS AND MANAGEMENT

Diagnostic criteria include (1) low serum sodium, (2) continued urine sodium loss, (3) urine osmolality greater than plasma, and (4) normal adrenal and renal function. The usual management is with water restriction until diuresis follows and is directed toward the etiology. Diuretics to reduce pulmonary edema, particularly in infants with chronic lung disease, will typically aggravate the hyponatremia and promote hypochloremic alkalosis.

### OUTCOME

Infants with hyponatremia may grow more slowly, although this probably is related to associated nutritional and acid–base disturbances, and they more commonly develop cerebral palsy, although this has not been demonstrated to be an independent risk factor separate from associated pathologies (eg, intracranial hemorrhage) and preterm birth itself.

## DISORDERS OF POTASSIUM REGULATION

## HYPERKALEMIA

### DEFINITION

Hyperkalemia is defined as a serum potassium concentration greater than 7 mEq/L, but the rate of rise is more important than the exact concentration.

### INCIDENCE AND EPIDEMIOLOGY

Hyperkalemia occurs frequently in very preterm infants, usually in the first few days of life in association with other serious conditions and aggressive forms of treatment. It is important to note that most neonates do not need supplemental potassium in the first 2 to 4 days of life, when normal glomerular filtration rates and urinary flow are being established.

### ETIOLOGY AND PATHOPHYSIOLOGY

Causes of hyperkalemia include (1) acidosis with or without tissue destruction; (2) renal failure, particularly with continued potassium treatment; and (3) adrenal insufficiency, which is relatively uncommon. Hyperkalemia often occurs with hyperglycemia in very preterm infants receiving high dextrose infusion rates, and some even refer to this problem as the *hyperglycemia–hyperkalemia syndrome*.

Potassium is the main cation of intracellular space and contributes to polarization of the cell membrane. High extracellular fluid potassium concentrations, therefore, tend to depolarize the cell membrane and contribute to reduced action potentials in nerves and conductive cells in skeletal, cardiac, and smooth (eg, gut) myocytes.

### CLINICAL PRESENTATION

Clinical signs of hyperkalemia include muscle weakness (hypotonia), ileus, and a variety of cardiac dysrhythmias. Electrocardiographic changes include prolonged PR interval, peaked T waves, widened QRS duration, and subsequently a sine-wave pattern of the QRS-T waves and ventricular arrhythmias.

When severe, hyperkalemia can produce life-threatening cardiac dysrhythmias, including ventricular fibrillation and asystole. Ileus can contribute to feeding intolerance. Muscle weakness in the diaphragm and thoracic muscles can aggravate other causes of respiratory failure.

### DIAGNOSIS AND MANAGEMENT

Hyperkalemia is determined by serum electrolyte concentrations; its severity, along with clinical and electrocardiographic signs, determines the need for and urgency of treatment. Serum electrolytes should be measured frequently. Management is directed toward the causes and nonspecific treatment, depending on the severity of the hyperkalemia. Non–potassium-containing volume expanders can acutely lower high serum potassium concentrations.

When hyperkalemia is severe, the following actions are urgent:

- Stop all potassium administration.
- Infuse calcium gluconate (100 to 200 mg/kg intravenously [IV]) to lower the cell membrane threshold. This is transient but may be lifesaving.
- Infuse sodium bicarbonate (1 to 2 mEq/kg IV, over at least 30 minutes). This transient therapy enhances intracellular sodium and hydrogen exchange for potassium and is particularly useful when the hyperkalemia is associated with acidosis. If hyperkalemia is associated with acute renal failure, the volume of fluid necessary to deliver the sodium bicarbonate may be excessive.
- Administer cation exchange resin (sodium polystyrene-sulfonate [Kayexalate], 1 g/kg) as an oral or rectal solution. Little experience has been reported in neonates, and technical problems of retention can be substantial. Furthermore, this may not be an option if the infant is restricted to nothing by mouth or has an injured gastrointestinal tract. When this resin is used, sodium from the resin is exchanged for serum potassium, which may result in hypernatremia, requiring frequent serial electrolyte measurements and increased fluid administration, often with diuretics. This therapy should be used with caution in newborns, and is contraindicated in premature neonates, as it has been associated with the development of necrotizing enterocolitis.
- An insulin infusion (0.1 U/kg/hr IV), given simultaneously with a dextrose infusion, can help shift potassium intracellularly. Complications of insulin infusion can occur with this treatment for severe hyperkalemia, and frequent monitoring of blood glucose levels is required.
- Administer inhaled albuterol (0.15 mg/kg every 20 minutes for 3 doses then 0.15–0.3 mg/kg) to shift potassium intracellularly. While this is transient, it can be lifesaving.
- Administer furosemide (orally [PO]: 1–4 mg/kg/dose 1–2 times/day; IV: 1–2 mg/kg/dose given every 12–24 hours) to increase the urinary excretion of potassium.
- Perform renal replacement therapy. This takes time to set up and may be technically impractical in very preterm infants.

## HYPOKALEMIA

### DEFINITION

Hypokalemia is defined by a serum potassium concentration less than 3.5 mEq/L.

### INCIDENCE AND EPIDEMIOLOGY

Hypokalemia is most common in very preterm infants during diuretic therapy.

### ETIOLOGY AND PATHOPHYSIOLOGY

The most common causes of hypokalemia are (1) increased gastrointestinal losses from an ostomy or drainage from a nasogastric tube when there is lower intestinal obstruction, and (2) renal losses, common in diuretic therapy. Hypokalemia also can occur when insulin and glucose infusions are used to treat severe hyperglycemia.

About 90% of total potassium is intracellular. Loss of intracellular potassium depolarizes cells, leading to cellular dehydration and diminished action potentials in nerves, cardiomyocytes (particularly those involved in contractile conduction), and gut myocytes (leading to ileus).

### CLINICAL PRESENTATION AND COMPLICATIONS

Clinical signs of hypokalemia are related to muscle weakness (eg, generalized hypotonia and reduced respiratory effort), cardiac dysrhythmias (eg, abnormal conductions, but most seriously, asystole and cardiac arrest), and diminished gut peristalsis (producing ileus and feeding intolerance).

### DIAGNOSIS AND MANAGEMENT

Serum electrolyte concentrations should be measured frequently to document the disorder. Early electrocardiographic changes include decreased T-wave amplitude and ST-segment depression.

Management is directed toward the causes, such as correction of metabolic acidosis and ostomy and renal losses. Low serum potassium always implies significant intracellular depletion, but intracellular potassium can be low with normal serum potassium. When intravenous treatment is used, the correction dose should be low (0.5 mEq/kg), and usually should not contain more than 40 mEq/L of potassium, and the treatment should be over hours, not by bolus (except for life-threatening cardiac dysrhythmias) *and only in the setting of normal renal function.* Diuretic-induced hypokalemia can be minimized by using a potassium-sparing diuretic such as spironolactone and increasing potassium salt supplements of milk or formula.

## DISORDERS OF ACID-BASE BALANCE

## METABOLIC ACIDOSIS

### DEFINITION

Metabolic acidosis is a decrease in pH due to increased acid ($H^+$ [hydrogen ion or proton]) production greater than any coincident increase in bicarbonate ($HCO_3^-$) or decrease in the partial pressure of carbon dioxide ($PCO_2$) or a loss of bicarbonate greater than any coincident decrease in $PCO_2$ or decrease in acid production. Metabolic acidosis can be further divided into those with an elevated anion gap and those with a normal anion gap. The anion gap reflects the balance between certain unaccounted cations and acidic anions in the extracellular fluid. The unmeasured anions normally include the serum proteins, phosphates, sulfates, organic acids, and lactate, whereas the unaccounted cations are the serum potassium, calcium, and magnesium. Thus, the anion gap is estimated using the formula

$$\text{Anion gap} = [Na^+]_{serum} - ([CL^-]_{serum} + [HCO_3^-]_{serum})$$

The normal serum anion gap in newborns is 8 to 16 mEq/L, and can be slightly higher in very premature newborns. Accumulation of strong acids because of increased intake, increased production, or decreased excretion results in an increased anion gap acidosis, whereas loss of bicarbonate ($HCO_3^-$) or accumulation of $H^+$ results in a normal anion gap acidosis.

## INCIDENCE AND EPIDEMIOLOGY

The most common cause of anion gap metabolic acidosis in preterm infants is hypoxia-ischemia with lactic acidosis. The most common cause of normal anion gap metabolic acidosis in the preterm newborn is a mild, developmentally regulated, proximal renal tubular acidosis with renal $HCO_3^-$ wasting. Other causes include as well as bicarbonate loss in the urine or plasma dilution by rapid fluid expansion of the blood volume and extracellular fluid.

## ETIOLOGY AND PATHOPHYSIOLOGY

Increased anion gap acidosis occurs with additional acid to the blood and extracellular fluid, such as with lactic acidosis, renal failure, and metabolic disorders. The serum chloride concentration is normal in these disorders. Normal anion gap acidosis occurs with bicarbonate loss in the urine (proximal renal tubular acidosis), ostomy drainage, the inability to excrete acid due to defects in distal nephron function (distal renal tubular acidosis), or administration of Cl-containing compounds (eg, arginine HCl, HCl, $CaCl_2$, $MgCl_2$, $NH_4Cl$ hyperalimentation, high-protein formula). The serum chloride is increased in these disorders. Mild to moderate chronic metabolic acidosis occurs in infants fed too much protein (> 4–5 g/kg/d) and may contribute to growth failure. Acute and relatively severe metabolic acidosis has been associated with decreased cardiac contractile performance and increased pulmonary vascular tone (pulmonary hypertension), although the degree that such conditions are only due to increased acid in the blood is controversial and probably not as marked as previously assumed.

## CLINICAL PRESENTATION

Acute metabolic acidosis usually is associated with clinical conditions that produce it. Chronic metabolic acidosis often is accompanied by growth failure. Complications of metabolic acidosis usually are those of underlying causes or inappropriate treatments.

## DIAGNOSIS AND MANAGEMENT

Metabolic acidosis is measured by blood gas analysis. It is expected with acute abnormalities that include hypoxia, ischemia, hypovolemia, hypotension, and aggressive intravenous fluid treatment. It should be anticipated and looked for in more chronic conditions with high urinary flow rates, excessive ostomy or gastric drainage, and poor growth.

Acid production should be diminished by correcting the underlying pathophysiology. Acute intravenous sodium bicarbonate bolus infusion has been commonly used to treat severe and persistent metabolic acidosis, but this treatment generally is unproven and risky. Bicarbonate infusions in small infants can produce volume overload, intracranial hemorrhage, hypernatremia, respiratory acidosis, decreased capillary oxygen exchange from increased hemoglobin-oxygen affinity, and a paradoxical intracellular acidosis as carbon dioxide, produced when the bicarbonate reacts with water via carbonic anhydrase, diffuses into cells. This treatment should be reserved for severely unstable and acidotic infants when other measures fail. Infants should be intubated and ventilated or spontaneously breathing well enough to lower their $PCO_2$ easily. Infants with dilutional acidosis should have their fluid balance corrected. Chronic metabolic acidosis from bicarbonate loss responds well to daily addition of bicarbonate to feedings.

## OUTCOME

Chronic metabolic acidosis produces reversible growth failure. Outcomes from acute, severe metabolic acidosis are usually due to its underlying causes or overly aggressive treatment with sodium bicarbonate bolus infusions.

# METABOLIC ALKALOSIS

## DEFINITION

Metabolic alkalosis is an increase in pH due to loss of acid or gain of bicarbonate without sufficient increase in $PCO_2$.

## INCIDENCE AND EPIDEMIOLOGY

Metabolic alkalosis occurs frequently in newborns but is common to only a few specific conditions.

## ETIOLOGY AND PATHOPHYSIOLOGY

Three basic mechanisms contribute to metabolic alkalosis: loss of acid, such as hydrochloric acid from vomiting, or intestinal obstruction and drainage; excessive treatment with, or ingestion of a base, such as alkali bolus infusions during resuscitations; and contraction of the extracellular fluid from dehydration (contraction alkalosis) or loss of fluids containing more chloride than bicarbonate (as occurs with chronic diuretic treatment). Common causes of metabolic alkalosis in neonates include acid loss from vomiting with pyloric stenosis, duodenal stenosis/atresia, or other high intestinal obstructions, or gastric drainage following intestinal surgery or with persistent ileus. Potassium depletion promotes metabolic alkalosis by stimulating renal ammonia genesis and inhibiting movement of hydrogen ions out of cells. Chloride depletion or chronic respiratory acidosis also maintains a metabolic alkalosis.

Bicarbonate is normally excreted by the kidney, except with dehydration and reduced glomerular filtration rate that diminishes urine flow rate and distal tubule chloride-bicarbonate exchange. This condition also promotes proximal bicarbonate resorption that occurs readily with sodium resorption promoted by aldosterone secreted in response to low glomerulus filtration rate or blood volume, as well as hyponatremia.

## CLINICAL PRESENTATION

Metabolic alkalosis is usually asymptomatic but should be suspected in infants with high urine flow rates, ostomy, and gastric drainage, and those treated with alkali and/or hyperventilation. Complications of metabolic alkalosis usually are those of associated conditions.

## DIAGNOSIS AND MANAGEMENT

Metabolic alkalosis is diagnosed by blood gas measurements. The underlying pathophysiology must be corrected. Chronic and marked contraction alkalosis can occur with intracellular potassium deficiency that often is more severe than indicated by the serum potassium concentration.

## OUTCOME

Chronic alkalosis has been associated with sensorineural hearing loss that is distinct from commonly associated loop diuretic ototoxicity. Neurodevelopmental outcomes appear to be worse with acute, severe alkalosis produced by hyperventilation (respiratory alkalosis) and alkali treatment, though the pathophysiology causing this adverse outcome is not clearly defined.

## SUGGESTED READINGS

Aschner JL, Poland RL. Sodium bicarbonate: basically useless therapy. *Pediatrics.* 2008;122(4):831-835.

Bhatia J. Fluid and electrolyte management in the very low birth weight neonate. *J Perinatol.* 2006;26(suppl 1):S19-S21.

Bockenhauer D, Zieg J. Electrolyte disorders. *Clin Perinatol.* 2014;41(3):575-590.

Cowett RM, Farrag HM. Selected principles of perinatal-neonatal glucose metabolism. *Semin Neonatol.* 2004;9(1):37-47.

Jain A, Agarwal R, Sankar MJ, Deorari A, Paul VK. Hypocalcemia in the newborn. *Indian J Pediatr.* 2010;77(10):1123-1128.

Kelly A, Levine MA. Hypocalcemia in the critically ill patient. *J Intensive Care Med.* 2013;28(3):166-177.

Lavagno C, Camozzi P, Renzi S, et al. Breastfeeding-associated hypernatremia: a systematic review of the literature. *J Hum Lact.* 2016;32(1):67-74.

Levy-Shraga Y, Dallalzadeh K, Stern K, Paret G, Pinhas-Hamiel O. The many etiologies of neonatal hypocalcemic seizures. *Pediatr Emerg Care*. 2015;31:197-201.

McKinlay CJ, Alsweiler JM, Ansell JM, et al; CHYLD Study Group. Neonatal glycemia and neurodevelopmental outcomes at 2 years. *NEJM*. 2015;373(16):1507-1518.

McNeilly JD, Boal R, Shaikh MG, Ahmed SF. Frequency and aetiology of hypercalcaemia. *Arch Dis Child*. 2016;101(4):344-347.

Nyp M, Brunkhorst JL, Reavey D, Pollotto EK. Fluid and electrolyte management. In: Gardner SL, Carter BS, Hines ME, Hernandez JA. eds. *Merenstein & Gardner's Handbook of Neonatal Intensive Care*. 8th ed. St. Louis, MO: Elsevier; 2016: 315-336.

Quigley R, Baum M. Neonatal acid base balance and disturbances. *Semin Perinatol*. 2004;28(2):97-102.

Rodd C, Goodyer P. Hypercalcemia of the newborn: etiology, evaluation, and management. *Pediatr Nephrol*. 1999;13(6):542-547.

Rozance PJ, Hay WW Jr. Hypoglycemia in newborn infants: features associated with adverse outcomes. *Biol Neonate*. 2006;90(2): 74-86.

Rozance PJ, Hay WW Jr. New approaches to management of neonatal hypoglycemia. *Matern Health Neonatol Perinatol*. 2016;2:3.

Rozance PJ, Hay WW Jr. Neonatal hyperglycemia. *Neoreviews*. 2010;11(11):e632-e639.

Rozance PJ, McGowan JE, Price-Douglas W, Hay WW Jr. Glucose homeostasis. In: Gardner SL, Carter BS, Enzman-Hines ME, Hernandez JA, eds. *Merenstein & Gardner's Handbook of Neonatal Intensive Care*. 8th ed. St. Louis, MO: Elsevier; 2016: 337-359.

Stanley CA, Rozance PJ, Thornton PS, et al. Re-evaluating "transitional neonatal hypoglycemia": mechanism and implications for management. *J Pediatr*. 2015;166(6):1520-1525.

Thornton PS, Stanley CA, De Leon DD, et al; Pediatric Endocrine Society. Recommendations from the Pediatric Endocrine Society for evaluation and management of persistent hypoglycemia in neonates, infants, and children. *J Pediatr*. 2015;167(2):238-245.

Thomas TC, Smith JM, White PC, Adhikari S. Transient neonatal hypocalcemia: presentation and outcomes. *Pediatrics*. 2012;129(6): e1461-e1467.

# 54 Neonatal Encephalopathy

Girija Natarajan, Michael Weiss, C. Michael Cotten, and Seetha Shankaran

## INTRODUCTION

Neonatal encephalopathy is a clinically defined syndrome of disturbed neurological function in the early postnatal days of life in the term infant. It is manifested by a combination of signs, including altered consciousness, abnormal muscle tone or reflexes, altered autonomic function, or seizures. Etiologies of neonatal encephalopathy include the following: (1) a combination of intrapartum or antepartum hypoxia and ischemia (hypoxic-ischemic encephalopathy [HIE]), which may be accompanied by prenatal signs of fetal distress, and vascular pathologies, including intracranial bleeding and stroke; (2) injuries secondary to birth trauma; (3) infections; (4) genetic disorders; (5) metabolic disorders; and (6) congenital brain abnormalities. This chapter focuses on neonatal encephalopathy in term newborn infants, with particular emphasis on infants who present with biochemical and clinical evidence of HIE, and the current diagnostic and treatment approaches to such injury. Other etiologies associated with central nervous system damage including vascular malformations and birth trauma are briefly discussed as well.

## EPIDEMIOLOGY OF ENCEPHALOPATHY

Neonatal encephalopathy occurs in 1 to 6 per 1000 live full-term births, with a recent population-based estimate of 1.9 to 3.8 per 1000 live births. Mortality ranges from 7% to 26%, and an additional 25% of infants will have long-term disabilities. In a few recent studies, neonates with mild encephalopathy have been noted to have an increased risk of motor, cognitive, or behavioral deficits on long term follow-up. Neonates with severe encephalopathy have an increased risk (> 60%) of death or of cerebral palsy and mental retardation. Infants with severe HIE related to an intrapartum event develop either spastic quadriplegia or a dyskinetic type of cerebral palsy. Neonates with moderate encephalopathy also are at risk of death or deficits, such as cognitive impairment, visual motor or visual perceptive dysfunction, hyperactivity, and delayed school readiness, although the risk is approximately half that of those with severe encephalopathy.

The cause and timing of such injuries leading to encephalopathy is usually unknown. Since neonatal encephalopathy has multiple causes, the American College of Obstetrics and Gynecology–American Academy of Pediatrics Executive Summary delineates certain criteria that may suggest a hypoxic-ischemic insult secondary to an acute intrapartum event. These include metabolic acidosis with a cord pH below 7 or a base deficit of 12 mmol/L or greater, Apgar scores less than 5 at 5 and 10 minutes, multisystem organ involvement apparent within 72 hours of birth and neuroimaging consistent with hypoxia-ischemia, along with early-onset of encephalopathy, and exclusion of other etiologies such as trauma, coagulation disorders, and genetic and metabolic causes. Signs consistent with an acute peripartum or intrapartum event are a sentinel event occurring immediately before or during labor; a sudden sustained fetal bradycardia; or absence of fetal heart rate variability in the presence of persistent, late, or variable decelerations, usually after a sentinel event before which the fetal heart rate pattern was normal.

The vast majority of infants with encephalopathy do not have an identifiable intrapartum event such as cord prolapse or uterine rupture. Neuroimaging studies identifying injury to the basal ganglia and parasagittal white matter suggest an injury that occurred to tissues susceptible to hypoxic-ischemic injury in the perinatal period rather than long-standing antenatal compromise or an acute vascular event. Although the neuroimaging results may identify presence and severity of perinatal injury, precise timing of perinatal injury based on imaging alone is not possible.

## PATHOPHYSIOLOGY OF HYPOXIC-ISCHEMIC BRAIN INJURY

The pathophysiology of brain injury secondary to hypoxia-ischemia has 2 phases that culminate in sustained brain injury. These phases are termed primary and secondary energy failure based on the temporal sequence that has been observed in studies in newborn animals. *Primary energy failure* is characterized by reductions in cerebral blood flow and delivery of oxygen and substrates to brain tissue. High-energy phosphorylated compounds such as adenosine triphosphate and phosphocreatine are reduced, and tissue acidosis is prominent. This phase is a prerequisite for all deleterious events that follow. Primary energy failure is associated with acute intracellular derangements, such as loss of membrane ionic homeostasis, excessive release or blocked reuptake of excitatory neurotransmitters, defective osmoregulation, and inhibition of protein synthesis. Excessive stimulation of neurotransmitter receptors and loss of ionic homeostasis mediate an increase in intracellular calcium and osmotic dysregulation. Elevation in intracellular calcium triggers a number of destructive pathways by activating lipases, proteases, and endonucleases.

Resolution of hypoxia-ischemia reverses the fall in high-energy phosphorylated metabolites and intracellular pH and promotes recycling of neurotransmitters. There is a potential time window, within which there may be successful recovery of cerebral energy state in hypoxia-ischemia. This window is influenced by maturation, preconditioning events, substrate availability, body temperature, and coexisting disease processes. A second interval of energy failure may then occur at a later time. *Secondary energy failure* differs from primary energy failure in that declines in phosphocreatine and adenosine triphosphate are not accompanied by brain acidosis. The presence and severity of secondary energy failure depends on the degree of primary energy failure. The pathogenesis of secondary energy failure is not as well understood as that of primary energy failure. It likely involves multiple processes, including accumulation of excitatory neurotransmitters, oxidative injury, apoptosis, inflammation, and altered growth factors and protein synthesis. Much later injury is secondary to the process of apoptosis, or programmed cell death. Apoptosis occurs in normal brain development and is useful for refining cell connections and pathways. The cellular signals after hypoxic-ischemic injury accelerate this process in normal brain tissue, contributing to the later evolving injury noted in infants with HIE.

The interval between primary and secondary energy failure is the latent phase that corresponds to a potential therapeutic window. However, clinicians usually do not know the precise time of primary energy failure. Initiation of therapies during this latent phase in perinatal animals has been successful in reducing brain damage, substantiating the concept of a therapeutic window. The duration of the therapeutic window is approximately 6 hours in near-term fetal sheep based on the neuroprotection associated with brain cooling initiated within this timeframe following brain ischemia.

## DIAGNOSIS AND INVESTIGATION OF ENCEPHALOPATHY

Neonatal encephalopathy is characterized by the presence of an abnormal neurologic examination in the first postnatal days, including decreased activity or lethargy, hypotonia, hypertonia, or a normal appearance with the sudden occurrence of apnea or seizures. The seizures can be subclinical or clinically evident and can be focal or generalized. Many infants may also present with myoclonus, which may appear to be seizures. In extreme cases, an otherwise apparently well grown, healthy term neonate may present with coma after extremely low Apgar scores and severe metabolic acidosis on cord blood gases.

The first step in diagnosis of neonatal encephalopathy is to obtain a detailed history of the pregnancy and intrapartum period. Any event likely to compromise blood or oxygen supply to the fetus, such as placental abruption, uterine rupture, amniotic fluid embolism, tight nuchal cord, cord prolapse or avulsion, maternal hemorrhage, trauma or cardiorespiratory arrest, severe and sustained fetal bradycardia, or prolonged labor, may be causative. Most infants with encephalopathy do not have an obvious cause for the encephalopathy. A history of maternal elevation of temperature increases the risk of neonatal encephalopathy and cerebral palsy. A history of fetal tachycardia and maternal tachycardia may also raise suspicions of chorioamnionitis. The placenta should be examined to determine if there was placental infection or noninfectious etiologies for HIE.

All neonates with encephalopathy should have detailed neurologic examinations repeatedly during the first postnatal days to evaluate the presence of mild (stage 1), moderate (stage 2), or severe encephalopathy (stage 3) based on the Sarnat classification (Table 54-1). The physical examination, acid–base data, intrapartum history and Apgar scores provide useful indicators of status. Ongoing encephalopathy through the first postnatal week, and continuing burst suppression on electroencephalograph, are poor prognostic signs.

Clinicians caring for neonates with HIE rely on the neurologic exam, magnetic resonance imaging (MRI), and the full or amplitude-integrated electroencephalogram (EEG) to monitor a neonate's response to medical therapy and to predict the neonate's long-term prognosis. Protein biomarkers of brain injury have also been used, largely in the research setting, as indicators of severity and prognosis.

### Neuroimaging of Encephalopathic Term Infants

*Magnetic resonance imaging* findings in near-term and term infants with HIE differ depending upon the severity of hypotension or ischemia in the perinatal/neonatal period. In mild to moderate hypotension, the typical MRI features are characterized by parasagittal lesions involving the vascular boundary zones, whereas profound hypotension involves primarily the lateral thalami, posterior putamina, the hippocampi, and the corticospinal tract including the perirolandic area but mainly sparing the remaining cortex. *Positron emission tomography* has demonstrated that lesions in the basal ganglia, perirolandic area, and hippocampi are related to impairment of energy substrates in areas with higher metabolic requirements. The major patterns of brain injury detectable by conventional MRI in near-term and term newborns with encephalopathy include the watershed-predominant pattern involving the white matter, particularly in the vascular watershed extending to the cortical gray matter when severe, and a basal nuclei–predominant pattern involving the deep gray nuclei and perirolandic cortex extending to the whole cortex when severe ischemia occurs. Involvement of specific structures at the posterior limb of the internal capsule is also noted with acute perinatal asphyxia. Clinicians should note that the neuroimaging picture, even on specialized MRI scans, is quite dynamic even in the first 2 postnatal weeks following hypoxic-ischemic injury. Areas that appear abnormal on initial examination may appear normal later, and tissue that initially appeared normal may worsen.

There is an association between the neonatal MRI findings and outcome in childhood. Abnormal signal intensity with the posterior limb of the internal capsule in the neonatal MRI predicts abnormal outcome in term infants with HIE. Basal ganglia and thalamic (BGT) lesions give rise to motor impairment in cerebral palsy. Approximately 50% of neonates with these lesions have extensive concurrent white matter abnormalities. White matter involvement is often associated with cognitive deficits. Severe BGT injury may be associated with spastic quadriplegia, cognitive impairment, feeding difficulties, and poor head growth. Moderate BGT injury may be associated

**TABLE 54-1 STAGES OF ENCEPHALOPATHY ACCORDING TO THE SARNAT CLASSIFICATION**

| Variable | Stage 1 | Stage 2 | Stage 3 |
|---|---|---|---|
| Level of consciousness | Hyper-alert, apparent awareness, responses to minimal stimuli | Lethargic | Stupor, coma |
| Spontaneous activity | Normal or decreased | Decreased | No activity |
| Posture | Mild flexion of distal joints (fingers, wrist usually) | Strong distal flexion, complete extension | Intermittent decerebration |
| Tone | Normal | Hypotonia, hypertonia | Flaccid, rigid |
| Reflexes | | | |
| Suck | Weak | Weak or absent bites | Absent |
| Moro | Intact, low threshold to illicit | Incomplete | Absent |
| Autonomic | | | |
| Pupils | Mydriasis | Miosis | Variable, often unequal, disconjugate eye movement, nonreactive |
| Heart rate | Tachycardia | Bradycardia (< 100 bpm) | Variable heart rate |
| Respirations | Regular respirations | Periodic breathing | Apnea, on ventilator |
| Seizures | None | Yes/No | Yes/No |

with athetoid or dyskinetic cerebral palsy with normal cognition and normal head growth. Purely dyskinetic cerebral palsy has been noted with a mild pattern of brain injury in the BGT region, purely spastic cerebral is seen with severe BGT pattern, and dyskinetic or spastic cerebral palsy is seen with either moderate or severe BGT or white matter injury pattern.

No relationship between antenatal and perinatal conditions and the pattern of predominant brain injury has been shown. Antenatal conditions such as maternal substance use, gestational diabetes, premature rupture of the membranes, preeclampsia, and intrauterine growth restriction do not differ across MRI patterns. The BGT pattern has been associated with the most severe neonatal events, including more intensive resuscitation at birth, severe encephalopathy, and seizures. Among infants born following a sentinel event such as placenta abruption, BGT lesions are likely to be isolated. BGT and white matter lesions may coexist in a large proportion of neonates presenting without an apparent precipitating event.

It can be logistically challenging to obtain brain MRI scans for neonates being treated with hypothermia, as the maintenance of hypothermia during transport and scanning is difficult. As a result, MRIs are usually not performed until the fourth day of life or after rewarming is completed and the neonate is clinically stable. In addition, hypothermia therapy may limit the early predictive value of the amplitude-integrated EEG (aEEG) and the neurologic exam. Biomarkers may potentially aid the clinician by stratifying neonates with HIE within the first 24 hours of life as follows: (1) responders to hypothermia alone with good neurodevelopmental prognosis, (2) nonresponders to hypothermia who survive but are at high risk for neurological injury and/or neurodevelopmental deficits and subsequently may be candidates for other clinical interventions. Early stratification of neonates into these groups allows the clinician to make decisions related to neuroprotective interventions and systemic supportive care.

Randomized controlled trials of hypothermia for neonatal HIE include data on MRI as biomarkers of outcome in the hypothermia era. The CoolCap trial documented that brain injury was decreased following hypothermia for neonatal HIE. In the Neonatal Research Network (NRN) hypothermia randomized controlled trial (RCT), 136 infants had neonatal MRI scans and outcome data at 18 months of age. A pattern of brain injury was described with each level reflecting a greater involvement of brain injury: 0, normal; 1A, minimal cerebral lesions with no involvement of basal ganglia or thalamus (BGT) or anterior or posterior limb of the internal capsule (ALIC, PLIC) and no watershed infarction; 1B, extensive cerebral lesions only; 2A, any BGT, ALIC, PLIC, or watershed involvement only; 2B, 2A and additional cerebral lesions; and 3, cerebral hemispheric devastation. Normal MRI scans were noted among 38 of 73 infants (52%) in the hypothermia group and 22 of 63 (35%) in the control group. Infants in the hypothermia group had significantly fewer areas of infarction (12%) compared to control infants (22%). Fifty-one of 136 participants had death or moderate/severe disability at 18 months. The brain injury pattern described correlated with outcome of death or disability, and with disability among survivors. Each point increase in the severity of the pattern of brain injury was independently associated with a 2-fold increase of death or disability. Another study confirmed that abnormal MRI findings are prognostic of moderate/severe HIE at 2 years of age.

Recently, the NRN hypothermia RCT data was used to examine the ability of neonatal MRI imaging to predict death or an IQ of less than 70 at 6 to 7 years of age. This composite outcome occurred in 4 of 50 (8%) children with pattern 0, 1 of 6 (17%) with 1A, 1 of 4 (25%) with 1B, 3 of 8 (38%) with 2A, 32 of 49 (65%) with 2B, and 7 of 7 (100%) with 3 ($P < 0.001$). A similar association was seen within hypothermia and control subgroups. The IQ was 90±13 among the 46 children with a normal MRI and 69±25 among the 50 children with an abnormal MRI. In childhood, for a normal outcome, a normal neonatal MRI had a sensitivity of 61%, a specificity of 92%, a positive predictive value (PPV) of 92% and a negative predictive value (NPV) of 59%; for death or IQ less than 70, the 2B and 3 pattern combined had a sensitivity of 81%, a specificity of 78%, a PPV of 70%, and an NPV of 87%. Thus, the National Institute of Child Health and Human Development (NICHD) NRN MRI pattern of neonatal brain injury is considered to be predictive of outcome at 6 to 7 years of age.

#### Physiologic (Vital Signs) Monitoring

Physiologic monitoring may also be utilized as a real-time biomarker. The intervals between beats of the heart or heart periods are constantly changing. This beat-to-beat variability is regulated by neural inputs from the sympathetic and parasympathetic branches of the autonomic nervous system. Twenty neonates undergoing hypothermia were evaluated for heart rate variability. At 24 hours of age, the low-frequency relative power (ie, sympathetic and parasympathetic activity) was higher in neonates with good outcomes at 15 months of age. The high-frequency relative power (ie, parasympathetic activity) was higher in neonates with poor outcomes at 15 months of age. A clinical scoring system based on examination and history has also been developed, with a correct classification rate of 78% for death/disability and 71% for death.

#### Cerebral Function Monitoring

A bedside tool that is currently used for cerebral function monitoring in term and near-term infants is the aEEG, which correlates well with conventional EEG. The aEEG records a sing-le-channel EEG from biparietal electrodes; the signal is then filtered, rectified, and smoothed, and its amplitude is integrated. The aEEG interpretation is based on pattern recognition. It appears to be predictive of neurodevelopmental outcome in term infants with HIE, and coupled with an early neurologic examination, the aEEG correlates well with persistent encephalopathy. It has been suggested that aEEG should become part of the initial evaluation of late preterm and term infants with HIE. It can be combined with measures of regional cerebral oxygen saturation and fractional cerebral tissue oxygen extraction (FTOE) measured by near-infrared spectroscopy. Early work suggests the aEEG plus the FTOE may predict outcome. Coupling regional saturation and FTOE may identify the period of secondary injury and energy failure that may be our best target for therapeutic intervention. The aEEG should not be used for the detection and treatment of neonatal seizures because it does not reliably detect subclinical seizures.

#### Protein Biomarkers

Biomarkers can measure a biological state or condition. An ideal biomarker is obtained with minimal invasion, is specific to the target organ of interest, and provides results that are obtained rapidly. Sources of biomarkers include serum, plasma, saliva, urine, cerebrospinal fluid (CSF) and umbilical cord blood. Several pilot studies have identified promising protein biomarkers that are indicative of brain injury. These include ubiquitin C-terminal hydrolase L1 (UCH-L1), glial fibrillary acidic protein (GFAP), phosphorylated heavy-chain neurofilament (pNF-H), S100B, neuron specific enolase (NSE), inflammatory cytokines, creatine kinase-brain (CK-BB), and myelin basic protein (MBP). Table 54-2 summarizes the protein biomarker characteristics.

**UCHL-1 and GFAP** A highly abundant neuronal protein, UCHL-1 is thought to play a critical role in cellular protein degradation during both normal and pathological conditions. GFAP is a type III intermediate filament that forms part of the cytoskeleton of mature astrocytes and other glial cells but is not found outside the central nervous system. Injury to the central nervous system and subsequent gliosis upregulate GFAP, which makes it an attractive candidate biomarker for brain injury screening. Concentrations of UCHL-1 also were higher in neonates with more severe brain injury as measured at 0 to 6 hours of age by MRI and developmental follow-up. In addition, the concentrations of UCHL-1 in umbilical cord samples have been shown to correlate with the severity of HIE. In neonates undergoing hypothermia, GFAP concentrations were increased in neonates with severe injury as measured by MRI at 24 hours. These GFAP concentrations predicted poor neurodevelopmental outcomes when increased at 6 to 24 hours of age. Concentrations of GFAP were increased during the first week of life in neonates with abnormal MRIs compared to those

**TABLE 54-2 SUMMARY OF PROTEIN BIOMARKER CHARACTERISTICS**

| Biomarker | Description | Cell Specificity | Pathophysiology of High Plasma Concentrations |
|---|---|---|---|
| UCHL-1 | Plays a critical role in cellular protein degradation during both normal and pathological conditions | Neuronal cell body | Released following neuronal cell body injury |
| S100β | A protein that binds calcium and is a major component of the cytosol in various cell types | Astroglial cells have a high concentration of S100β; other cells can release S100β | Released predominantly after astrocyte death but can be released from other tissue damage |
| GFAP | A cytoskeletal intermediate filament protein found in the astrocytes | Specific marker of differentiated astrocytes | Released after astrocyte death |
| Neuron specific enolase (NSE) or enolase 2 | Glycolytic isoenzyme (γγ) | High concentrations of NSE found in mature central and peripheral neurons; trace amounts of similar isoenzyme (ag) in platelets | Released after neuronal death |
| pNF-H | A cytoskeletal intermediate filament protein found in the astrocytes | Specific marker of differentiated astrocytes | Released after astrocyte death |

with normal MRIs. Studies have not found GFAP to be elevated in the umbilical cord blood of neonates with HIE compared to controls. These data suggest that UCHL-1 may be an early marker of injury, while GFAP becomes detectable later after injury. The bedside clinician may be able to identify a responder to hypothermia when a rapid decrease in the concentration of UCHL-1 by 24 hours of treatment is combined with the absence of an increase in GFAP.

**pNF-H** Phosphorylated heavy-chain neurofilament is 1 of the major subunits of neurofilaments, the main components of the axonal cytoskeleton, and if found, represents injury to the subcortical white matter. In neonates not undergoing hypothermia, pNF-H concentrations were higher in those with HIE compared to controls. Concentrations of pNF-H were higher in neonates with abnormal MRIs compared to those with normal MRIs.

**S100B** S100B is a calcium binding protein and is a major component of the cytosol in glial cells. S100B concentrations in both the cord blood, and in the first urine passed after birth, were significantly higher in infants with HIE compared with healthy controls. A S100B concentration in cord blood of greater than 2.02 μg/L has been shown to have a sensitivity of 86.7% and a specificity of 88.0% for predicting moderate or severe HIE. A recent meta-analysis of thirteen S100B studies concluded that levels are increased in neonates with HIE compared with controls, and that they are proportional to the severity of HIE.

**NSE** Neuron specific enolase is an enzyme involved in the glycolytic pathway and is found primarily in neurons. In 43 babies with birth asphyxia, serum NSE above 40 mcg/L obtained between 4 and 48 hours of life distinguished infants with no or mild HIE from infants with moderate or severe HIE. Additionally, serum NSE concentrations above 45.4 mcg/L distinguished infants with poor outcomes from infants with normal outcomes at 1 year of age.

**Inflammatory Cytokines** Researchers also have examined inflammatory cytokine profiles. In neonates undergoing hypothermia, serum concentrations of interleukin 6 (IL-6), IL-1, IL-8, and vascular endothelial growth factor (VEGF) obtained at 6 to 24 hours of age predicted long-term outcomes observed at 20 ± 5 months of age. Similarly, elevated IL-6 and monocyte chemotactic protein-1 obtained within 9 hours after birth, and low macrophage inflammatory protein 1a obtained at 60 to 70 hours of age were associated with death or severely abnormal neurodevelopment at 12 months of age. Metabolomics and microRNA are additional potential biomarkers being investigated.

## THERAPIES FOR NEONATAL HYPOXIC-ISCHEMIC ENCEPHALOPATHY

The management of neonatal HIE has traditionally consisted of supportive intensive care. This includes correction of hemodynamic and pulmonary disturbances (hypotension and hypoventilation), correction of metabolic disturbances (related to glucose, calcium, magnesium, and electrolytes), treatment of seizures, and monitoring for other organ system dysfunction, especially hepatic, renal, and coagulation status. Avoiding hyperthermia may also be beneficial, as is monitoring of urine output to guide fluid maintenance and drug dosing. This management approach is directed at avoiding injury from secondary events associated with hypoxia-ischemia.

### Therapeutic Hypothermia

Therapeutic hypothermia to attenuate the cascade of events triggered by hypoxia and ischemia is of proven benefit in reducing death and disability in multiple clinical trials. This is summarized in the Cochrane meta-analysis of the randomized controlled trials. There are 2 modalities of cooling. The NICHD trial (n = 208) tested whole-body hypothermia to an esophageal temperature of 33.5°C for 72 hours for neonatal HIE. The CoolCap trial (n = 234) tested head cooling with mild systemic cooling (34–35°C for 72 hours) for infants with moderate or severe HIE and an abnormal aEEG. Head cooling for infants with the most severe aEEG changes was not protective; however, head cooling for infants with less severe aEEG changes (n = 172) was protective (odds ratio, 0.42 [0.22–0.80]; $P = 0.009$). The rates of death or disability based on currently available evidence are summarized in Tables 54-3 and 54-4.

Therapeutic hypothermia is also safe. In a smaller randomized, controlled pilot study performed at 7 centers with 65 infants, moderate systemic whole-body hypothermia to 33°C for 48 hours was compared to normothermia maintained at 37°C. Infants in the hypothermia group had more significant bradycardia, longer dependence on pressor medications, higher prothrombin times, more seizures, and need for more plasma and platelets transfusions. In the larger trials, growth parameters were similar between survivors, while rehospitalization rates were 27% in the hypothermia and 42% in the control group.

All of the major RCTs targeting hypothermia as a neuroprotective strategy have targeted death or disability at 18 months of age as their primary outcome. This is the earliest age at which major disability can be ruled out with a high level of confidence. Since hypothermia may influence not only major motor and cognitive deficits detected at 18 months but also more subtle effects of brain injury in childhood, longer term outcomes are relevant. These include behavior, learning, fine motor development, executive function, attention, and psychosocial

**TABLE 54-3 HYPOTHERMIA RANDOMIZED CONTROLLED TRIALS: DEATH OR DISABILITY AT 18 MONTHS**

| Study Name | Hypothermia | Control | OR (95% CI) |
|---|---|---|---|
| CoolCap | 55% | 66% | 0.61 (034–1.09) |
| NICHD | 44% | 62% | 0.72 (0.54–0.95) |
| TOBY | 45% | 53% | 0.86 (0.68–1.07) |
| Neo.nEURO | 51% | 83% | 0.21 (0.09–0.54) |
| China | 31% | 49% | 0.47 (0.26–0.84) |
| ICE | 51% | 66% | 0.77 (0.62–0.98) |

CI, confidence interval; ICE, Infant Cooling Evaluation; NICHD, National Institute of Child Health and Human Development; OR, odds ratio; TOBY, Total Body Hypothermia for Neonatal Encephalopathy.

**TABLE 54-4 HYPOTHERMIA RANDOMIZED CONTROLLED TRIALS: RATES OF CEREBRAL PALSY AT 18 MONTHS**

| Study Name | Hypothermia | Control | OR (95% CI) |
|---|---|---|---|
| CoolCap | 32% | 43% | 0.75 (0.48–1.16) |
| NICHD | 19% | 30% | 0.68 (0.38–1.22) |
| TOBY | 28% | 41% | 0.67 (0.47–0.96) |
| Neo.nEURO | 12% | 48% | 0.15 (0.04–0.60) |
| China | 14% | 28% | 0.40 (0.17–0.92) |
| ICE | 27% | 29% | 0.92 (0.54–1.59) |

CI, confidence interval; ICE, Infant Cooling Evaluation; NICHD, National Institute of Child Health and Human Development; OR, odds ratio; TOBY, Total Body Hypothermia for Neonatal Encephalopathy.

outcome. The NICHD and Total Body Hypothermia for Neonatal Encephalopathy (TOBY) trials have also evaluated cognitive and neurological outcomes at 6 to 7 years of age (Table 54-5).

Multiple published systemic reviews of this data and statements from pediatric societies conclude that therapeutic hypothermia (1) significantly reduces both death and disability after perinatal encephalopathy, (2) is safe, and (3) results in homogeneous outcomes both within and between trials.

#### Treatment of Seizures

Because neonatal seizures may have adverse effects, their prevention and treatment with prophylactic administration of anticonvulsants has been considered. However, the consequences of subclinical or electroencephalogram-detected neonatal seizures on neurodevelopmental outcome has not been adequately evaluated. No data demonstrates that treatment with anticonvulsants or barbiturates reduces cerebral palsy or developmental disability in infants with encephalopathy. The existing studies are small and there is concern that treatment may have adverse effects on the central nervous system. Therefore, larger scale clinical trials of anticonvulsant and barbiturate therapy are needed before these agents are routinely prescribed.

#### Emerging Therapies

In animal models, higher than physiologic doses of erythropoietin after hypoxic-ischemic injury as well as neonatal strokes have been associated with clinical benefits. Human clinical trials of erythropoietin and stem cell therapy in HIE are currently in the early phases of investigation.

### ENCEPHALOPATHY CAUSED BY BIRTH TRAUMA AND VASCULAR INJURIES

Encephalopathy secondary to birth trauma and vascular events often presents with seizures in the first postnatal days without other preceding neurologic signs. Since these early seizures may be due to other causes, including metabolic disorders, infection, hypoglycemia, hypocalcemia, hyponatremia, acidosis, and hyperbilirubinemia, it is important to consider these diagnoses in assessing for possible vascular injury with neuroimaging.

Perinatal stroke is estimated to occur in approximately 1 out of 4000 births, while the overall incidence of birth trauma–related brain injury that may influence neurologic outcome is much smaller in developed countries. There is an increased risk for major trauma, including depressed skull fracture, intracranial hemorrhage, or brachial plexus palsy in vaginal deliveries assisted with instrumentation, either forceps or vacuum. There does not appear to be a difference in mortality risk for infants born via vacuum versus forceps assist, but vacuum may be associated with a higher risk of cephalohematomas than forceps delivery. When both modalities are used sequentially, risk of any injury is greatly increased. Infants with these injuries often present with seizures in the first postpartum hours to days. Appropriate diagnostic testing includes the evaluation of coagulation factors, platelet counts, and hemoglobin and hematocrit to assess the degree of blood loss and need for replacement.

#### Perinatal Stroke

Perinatal arterial stroke as a cause of cerebral palsy in term and near-term infants occurs in approximately 17 per 100,000 live births. It is important to note that perinatal stroke may present after the immediate neonatal period. Peripartum risk factors for perinatal stroke include maternal preeclamptic toxemia and intrauterine growth restriction. Approximately two-thirds of all neonatal strokes are arterial in origin, while the remainder are secondary to sinovenous thrombosis.

Arterial stroke usually causes wedge-shaped infarcts, often in the distribution of the middle cerebral artery. Antenatal infarcts can occur in cases of monozygotic twins with demise of 1 twin, with passage of thromboplastin-rich blood to the survivor. Significant fetomaternal hemorrhage can also result in hypoperfusion and infarction in watershed areas of the brain. Birth trauma may be contributory to ischemic stroke, with increased pressure from subdural bleeding putting pressure on internal vascular structures. Postnatal arterial strokes may be related to congenital heart lesions. Clearly delineated diagnostic and risk factor analyses, as well as mechanism-based rapid intervention treatment approaches, similar to the "brain attack" approach in adults, are still in development.

Venous infarction is less common than arterial infarction. It has been related to problems with blood flow, such as hypovolemia, polycythemia, and poor flow related to preeclampsia. Thrombosis has also been associated with infection. Neuroimaging with MRI, with added magnetic resonance venography, may reveal the occluded venous structure, but development of collateral circulation or recanalization of the vessel often has occurred between injury and imaging. The diagnostic workup for venous thrombosis should include, in addition to consideration of systemic illness, activity assays for antithrombin, protein C, protein S, and the lupus anticoagulant; immunologic assays for anticardiolipin antibody; and molecular assays for the presence of factor V Leiden. In addition, the *G20210A* mutation in the prothrombin gene, and the methylenetetrahydrofolate reductase (MTHFR) mutations *C677T* and *A1298C*. Recent work, however, casts doubt on the importance of these and other polymorphisms for the pathogenesis of neonatal stroke. To date, there are no large randomized trials of anticoagulant therapies for venous stroke in neonates. The American College of Chest Physicians recently published evidence-based clinical practice guidelines for antithrombotic therapy in neonates and children. The guidelines include dose and duration recommendations for antithrombotic therapies and thrombolytic therapies, as well as diagnostic and therapeutic guidance. Further information for clinicians, in the absence of informative definitive clinical trials, is currently available from 1-800-NOCLOTS, the toll-free pediatric stroke telephone consultation service initiated in the United States in 1994. This program has 3 goals: first, to provide free telephone consultation to physicians requesting advice on the management of children with stroke on the basis of best available evidence; second, to document the patient characteristics and most urgent questions facing these physicians; and third, to make these data available for planning future clinical trials in pediatric stroke.

**TABLE 54-5 SUMMARY OF CHILDHOOD OUTCOMES OF THERAPEUTIC HYPOTHERMIA AS REPORTED IN RANDOMIZED CONTROLLED TRIALS**

| Trial Follow-Up | Outcome Measures | Results |
|---|---|---|
| NICHD | Death or IQ < 70 | 47% in hypothermia vs. 62% in controls, $P = 0.06$ |
| | Death or severe disability | 41% vs. 60%, $P = 0.03$ |
| | Moderate/severe disability | 35% vs. 38%, $P = 0.87$ |
| | Death | 28% vs. 44%, $P = 0.04$ |
| CoolCap study | WeeFIM ratings | Disability status at 18 m strongly associated with WeeFIM ratings, $P < 0.001$ |
| TOBY trial | IQ ≥ 85 | 52% in hypothermia vs. 39% in controls; RR, 1.31; $P = 0.04$ |

IQ, intelligence quotient; NICHD, Neonatal Research Network; RR, relative risk; TOBY, Total Body Hypothermia for Neonatal Encephalopathy; WeeFIM, Functional Independence Measure for Children.

## SUGGESTED READINGS


Azzopardi D, Strohm B, Marlow N, et al; TOBY Study Group. Effects of hypothermia for perinatal asphyxia on childhood outcomes. *N Engl J Med.* 2014;10(371):140-149.

Badawi N, Kurinczuk JJ, Hall D, Field D, Pemberton PJ, Stanley FJ. Newborn encephalopathy in term infants: three approaches to population-based investigation. *Semin Neonatol.* 1997;2(3):181-188.

Committee on Fetus and Newborn; Papile LA, Baley JE, Benitz W, et al. Hypothermia and neonatal encephalopathy. *Pediatrics.* 2014;133(6):1146-1150.

Douglas-Escobar MV, Heaton SC, Bennett J, et al. UCH-L1 and GFAP serum levels in neonates with hypoxic-ischemic encephalopathy: a single center pilot study. *Front Neurol.* 2014;5:273.

Douglas-Escobar M, Weiss MD. Biomarkers of hypoxic-ischemic encephalopathy in newborns. *Front Neurol.* 2012;3:144.

Executive summary: Neonatal encephalopathy and neurologic outcome, second edition. Report of the American College of Obstetricians and Gynecologists' Task Force on Neonatal Encephalopathy. *Obstet Gynecol.* 2014;123(4):896-901.

Ferriero DM. Neonatal brain injury. *N Engl J Med.* 2004;351(19):1985-1995.

Jacobs SE, Berg M, Hunt R, Tarnow-Mordi WO, Inder TE, Davis PG. Cooling for newborns with hypoxic ischemic encephalopathy. *Cochrane Database Syst Rev.* 2013;(1):CD003311.

Lynch JK, Hirtz DG, DeVeber G, Nelson KB. Report of the National Institute of Neurological Disorders and Stroke workshop on perinatal and childhood stroke. *Pediatrics.* 2002;109(1):116-123.

Monagle P, Chalmers E, Chan A, et al. Antithrombotic therapy in neonates and children: American College of Chest Physicians evidence-based clinical practice guidelines (8th edition). *Chest.* 2008;133(suppl 6):887S-968S.

Rutherford M, Ramenghi LA, Edwards AD, et al. Assessment of brain tissue injury after moderate hypothermia in neonates with hypoxic-ischemic encephalopathy: a nested substudy of a randomized controlled trial. *Lancet Neurology.* 2010;9(1):39-45.

Sarnat HB, Sarnat MS. Neonatal encephalopathy following fetal distress. A clinical and electroencephalographic study. *Arch Neurol.* 1976;33(10):696-705.

Shankaran S, Barnes PD, Hintz SR, et al; Eunice Kennedy Shriver National Institute of Child Health and Human Development Neonatal Research Network. Brain injury following trial of hypothermia for neonatal hypoxic-ischemic encephalopathy. *Arch Dis Child Fetal Neonatal Ed.* 2012;97(6):F398-F404.

Shankaran S, Laptook AR, Pappas A, et al; Eunice Kennedy Shriver National Institute of Child Health and Human Development Neonatal Research Network. Effect of depth and duration of cooling on deaths in the NICU among neonates with hypoxic ischemic encephalopathy: a randomized clinical trial. *JAMA.* 2014;312(24):2629-2639.

Shankaran S, Pappas A, Laptook AR, et al; NICHD Neonatal Research Network. Outcomes of safety and effectiveness in a multicenter randomized, controlled trial of whole-body hypothermia for neonatal hypoxic-ischemic encephalopathy. *Pediatrics.* 2008;122(4):e791-e798.

Shankaran S, Pappas A, McDonald SA, et al; Eunice Kennedy Shriver National Institute of Child Health and Human Development Neonatal Research Network. Childhood outcomes after hypothermia for neonatal encephalopathy. *N Engl J Med.* 2012;366(22):2085-2092.

van Handel M, Swaab H, de Vries LS, Jongmans MJ. Behavioral outcome in children with a history of neonatal encephalopathy following perinatal asphyxia. *J Pediatr Psychol.* 2010;35(3):286-295.


# 55 Hematologic Abnormalities in the Newborn

Chad Andersen, Amy Keir, Nicolette A. Hodyl, and Michael Stark

## RED CELL DISORDERS

## NUCLEATED RED BLOOD CELLS

Circulating erythrocyte precursors (nucleated red blood cells or normoblasts) are frequently found in the peripheral blood of newborns. In the normal term neonate, nucleated red blood cells (nRBCs) are rapidly cleared from the bloodstream after birth. However, in the preterm neonate, low numbers of nRBCs may persist throughout the first week of life. Absolute numbers of nRBCs may be reported in relation to the number of white blood cells (nRBCs/100 white blood cells) or expressed as an absolute number per unit volume (nRBCs/$mm^3$). The upper limit of the normal range for nRBCs in the term infant is 1000 nRBCs/$mm^3$, with preterm newborns typically having greater numbers of nRBCs in the immediate postnatal period compared to term neonates.

Elevated nRBC numbers or their persistence in the peripheral circulation may result from either increased erythropoiesis and/or stress-related release of normoblasts from the bone marrow. Increased erythropoiesis can occur as a result of pathological events, such as fetal hypoxia secondary to placental insufficiency and/or preeclampsia, or can be secondary to blood loss, including hemolysis. In infants of diabetic mothers, elevated nRBC concentrations are also observed, driven by an increase in erythropoiesis secondary to elevated erythropoietin concentrations and a direct hematopoietic action of hyperinsulinemia. Maternal smoking during pregnancy can also increase nRBCs.

Hypoxia does not need to be chronic to result in increased nRBCs in the immediate newborn period. Nucleated RBCs have been shown to be raised in infants following acute perinatal asphyxia. This is thought to result from an increase in interleukin-6 immediately following the hypoxic insult. A prolonged elevation in nRBCs then continues, secondary to erythropoietin stimulation. Previously, nRBCs were thought to represent a useful biomarker for the degree of perinatal asphyxia. While they may discriminate mild from moderate/severe encephalopathy in normothermic infants, this association is lost in infants receiving therapeutic hypothermia.

## ANEMIA

Hemoglobin, located in the red cell, is a heme-containing metalloprotein comprising 4 globin chains. These chains undergo conformational change in the context of oxygen binding, with each gram capable of carrying 1.34 mL of oxygen. The globin chains change from fetal life to infancy with adult globin chain predominating by 6 months of age. The mean hemoglobin concentration in the term newborn ranges from 14 to 20 g per 100 mL. The thalassemia syndromes (α and β) occur from abnormalities in globin chain synthesis (see Chapter 430).

### CAUSES OF ANEMIA

*Erythropoietin* (EPO) is a glycoprotein produced by the kidney in the setting of hypoxia. Stimulation of EPO release in the context of relative hypoxia in utero, results in a surge of RBC production leading to high red cell population at birth. After birth, EPO is subsequently down-regulated as a result of the transition to the relatively oxygen-rich extra-uterine environment thus leading to a fall in hemoglobin (Hb), termed *physiologic anemia*, with a nadir at around 6 to 8 weeks of age. Preterm newborns have an exaggerated relative anemia, termed *anemia of prematurity*, as a result of phlebotomy losses and relatively poor bone marrow response to EPO.

Blood loss resulting in physiological anemia may occur before, during, or after birth. Fetal to maternal hemorrhage can be detected by the observation of fetal red blood cells in the maternal blood using the Betke-Kleihauer test. Twin–twin transfusion can occur in monozygotic twins with monochorionic placentae. Placental disorders such as abruption (acute, chronic, or acute on chronic) and previa, including vasa previa, can all result in significant anemia with risk of morbidity and mortality.

Closed hemorrhage into body spaces may also result in anemia in the newborn period. Cephalohematomas are generally self-limiting and resolve spontaneously, often with significant hyperbilirubinemia. Subgaleal hematomas, often associated with vacuum extraction, may lead to rapid anemic shock and thus require careful observation following delivery. Other areas of hidden bleeding include abdominal viscera and the retroperitoneum.

### BLOOD TRANSFUSION

Transfusion thresholds based on Hb levels in the context of relative anemia in the preterm newborn remain imprecise. There are very few studies to guide transfusion practice in the newborn. Mostly, transfusion is based on Hb or hematocrit (Hct) levels alone. It is clear, however, that the newborn with hypovolemic anemia requires urgent transfusion often with group-O rhesus-negative blood whereas the newborn with normovolemic anemia can tolerate a much lower Hb level without suffering from hypoxic ischemia. However, the precise clinical cutoffs remain unclear.

## ERYTHROBLASTOSIS FETALIS

*Erythroblastosis fetalis* or hemolytic disease of the fetus and newborn (HDFN) was first described in 1932 as a distinct condition comprising anemia, universal edema of the fetus (hydrops fetalis), and neonatal jaundice. It is caused by maternal red cell alloantibodies that are actively transported across the placenta and destroy fetal erythroid cells carrying the involved red blood cell antigen. Typically, this is the rhesus (Rh) antigen, though hemolysis may occur with sensitization to any number of other red blood cell antigens. The most important of the Rh membrane antigens is the D antigen, with mothers lacking this designated as Rh-negative. Despite the introduction of anti–D immunoglobulin prophylaxis, between 1 and 3 in 1000 D-negative women will develop anti-D. Further, an additional 1 in 500 pregnancies will be complicated by HDFN secondary to red cell antibodies other than anti-D.

Maternal alloimmunization is generally the result of fetomaternal hemorrhage and rarely occurs during a first pregnancy. The majority of pregnant women are typed for ABO and D early in pregnancy and screened for the presence of red cell antibodies. In addition, in many Western countries, additional screening is performed later in the second and/or third trimesters in an attempt to detect all clinically relevant alloimmunizations. Antenatal assessment of high-risk cases is now predominantly by Doppler ultra-sonographic measurement of the peak systolic velocity of the middle cerebral artery, which demonstrates high sensitivity and specificity for the detection of fetal anemia. In severe fetal anemia, the use of intrauterine transfusion prevents the development of hydrops fetalis and fetal death and has resulted in a reduction in overall perinatal mortality in severe HDFN to less than 10%, with normal long-term neurodevelopmental outcome reported in more than 95% of cases.

### FETAL MANIFESTATIONS

Hemolysis and fetal anemia, secondary to alloantibody mediated red blood cell destruction, leads to compensatory increases in fetal cardiac output, a hyperdynamic circulation, and ultimately, hydrops fetalis. If the presence of red cell alloantibodies is not detected during pregnancy, initial presentation may be nonspecific, for instance with reduced fetal movements, or sudden intrauterine death my occur. While hemolysis of fetal red cells results in significant production of bilirubin, jaundice may be absent immediately following delivery due to the placenta's capacity to clear lipid-soluble unconjugated bilirubin. However, hemolysis continues following birth with jaundice becoming evident over the first 24 hours of life. This early hyperbilirubinemia has the potential to rapidly reach extremely high levels carrying the risk of bilirubin encephalopathy and kernicterus.

### MANAGEMENT

The mainstay of the management of hyperbilirubinemia is intensive phototherapy, which has significantly reduced the requirement for exchange transfusion. However, in severe disease, exchange transfusion may be required. Exchange transfusion removes both maternal alloantibodies and bilirubin, and corrects anemia but carries a significant risk of associated complication in up to 24% of infants. Administration of intravenous immunoglobulin has been postulated to reduce the severity of hemolysis with HDFN. A recent systematic review reported a significant reduction in the requirement for exchange transfusion following intravenous immunoglobulin, but this review included a number of earlier trials of low quality. When confined to those studies with an overall low risk of bias, no beneficial effect of intravenous immunoglobulin was observed. Therefore, the efficacy of intravenous immunoglobulin treatment has not conclusively been proven.

## POLYCYTHEMIA

*Neonatal polycythemia* is usually defined as a central venous hematocrit of greater than 65%, although this does not discriminate between symptomatic and asymptomatic infants or define those at risk of complications. Polycythemia occurs as a result of increased red cell mass, regardless of plasma volume. Hematocrit generally peaks 4 to 6 hours after delivery then declines to cord blood levels by 12 to 18 hours of life, after which it remains stable.

### INCIDENCE AND ETIOLOGY

The prevalence of polycythemia and its associated hyperviscosity syndrome varies between 1% and 5% of newborns, dependent upon the altitude of the population studied. Exposure to acute or chronic hypoxia in utero (eg, placental insufficiency, maternal hypertension, maternal smoking) is associated with an increased incidence of polycythemia, while it is less common in the preterm compared to term infant due to a lower red cell mass. The practice of deferred umbilical cord clamping has also resulted in an increased incidence of polycythemia.

### POSTNATAL CONSEQUENCES

Polycythemia can affect multiple organ systems; therefore, the affected neonate may present with a wide range of clinical symptoms. The most common clinical features include lethargy, tachypnea, irritability, and poor feeding in a neonate who appears ruddy (rubeosis) with poor peripheral perfusion and slow capillary return. Hypoglycemia affects 12% to 40% of infants, with hyperbilirubinemia common due to the breakdown of the increased red blood cell mass.

### MANAGEMENT

With plasma volume likely to be normal in neonatal polycythemia, isovolemic partial exchange transfusion has been recommended for treatment of the symptomatic infant. The volume to be exchanged is calculated using the following formula:

$$\text{Volume (mL)} = \text{Circulating blood volume} \times \frac{\text{Hct current} - \text{Hct desired}}{\text{Hct current}}$$

where circulating blood volume can be estimated as 90 mL/kg for term infants and 100 mL/kg for preterm infants and crystalloid solutions used instead of plasma or albumin. In neonates in a stable condition or with few symptoms, there is no clinical data supporting either a short-term or long-term benefit of partial exchange transfusion. Indeed, partial exchange transfusion may increase the risk of necrotizing enterocolitis in these infants. Further, studies evaluating the long-term outcome of neonates with symptomatic polycythemia undergoing partial exchange transfusion have found no clear benefit with regard to neurocognitive development.

## WHITE BLOOD CELL DISORDERS

## NEUTROPENIA

*Neutropenia* is often seen in the newborn period and may be due to decreased production or increased destruction of white cells. While classically defined as a blood neutrophil concentration below 2 standard deviations of the appropriate mean, the definition in the newborn is more arbitrary, including less than the fifth percentile and less than 1500 per μL. Neutropenia generally occurs in the first postnatal week and is transient. Up to 8% of all neonatal intensive care patients will be neutropenic during their hospital stay.

Neutropenia is more common in small-for-gestational-age infants, affecting up to 50% of infants with a birth weight of less than 1500 g. In preterm infants, neutropenia is associated with sepsis, maternal hypertension, and severe asphyxia, and may be associated with increased risk of early-onset sepsis and nosocomial infection. The neutropenia seen in neonatal sepsis syndromes is a result of accelerated neutrophil use and depleted bone marrow neutrophil storage pools. There is usually a left shift and other morphologic characteristics, such as toxic granulation and vacuolization.

### INVESTIGATION OF NEUTROPENIA

If neutropenia persists for longer than 5 days, additional diagnostic measures are recommended. *Congenital neutropenia* (Kostmann syndrome) presents with profound neutropenia, often with an absolute neutrophil count of less than 200/μL. This condition is characterized by maturational arrest at the promyelocyte stage in the bone marrow. Although originally described in a family with autosomal recessive inheritance, the majority of reported cases are sporadic mutations with an autosomal dominant inheritance pattern. *Alloimmune neonatal neutropenia* is caused by maternal sensitization to a paternal granulocyte antigen present on the fetal neutrophils. Symptomatic infants may present with delayed separation of the umbilical cord, skin infections, or pneumonia in the first 2 weeks of life, and although most infections are mild, mortality may reach 5%. Alloimmune neonatal neutropenia is a self-limiting condition, however, with resolution seen over a period of weeks to months, as transplacentally acquired maternal antibodies diminish.

### MANAGEMENT

Various treatments have been proposed to enhance neutrophil production and function, including intravenous immunoglobulin and granulocyte colony stimulating factor. Although their use in infants with severe chronic neutropenia may be associated with benefit, there is little evidence to support their use in other varieties of neonatal neutropenia. For further discussion of granulocyte disorders see Chapter 437.

## LEUKEMIAS

Neonatal or congenital leukemia has an estimated incidence of 1 to 5 cases per million live births. Neonatal leukemia differs from leukemia in later childhood and poses significant clinical challenges due to the requirement for aggressive treatment, generally very poor prognosis, and concerns about longer-term morbidity.

### PRESENTATION AND DIFFERENTIAL DIAGNOSIS

*Leukemia* may present in utero with hydrops, polyhydramnios, and ultimately, stillbirth. Presentation in the neonatal period is commonly associated with a tumoral syndrome characterized by hepatosplenomegaly in up to 80% of cases and nodular cutaneous infiltrates or "blueberry muffin spots" in up to 60% of cases. Hyperleukocytosis is a common finding, with the cells exhibiting atypical morphology. It is important to differentiate leukemia in neonates from leukemoid reactions secondary to other pathological conditions such as infection, hypoxia, and hemolytic disease of the newborn.

A transient clonal myeloproliferation, also termed *transient myelopoiesis,* is observed in up to 10% of neonates with trisomy 21. More than 80% of patients have spontaneous regression; however, some present with severe disease, with increased risk of death secondary to sepsis, hepatic fibrosis, and/or cardiopulmonary failure. Further, 16% to 30% of cases are complicated by the development of myeloid leukemia of Down syndrome (ML-DS) within the first 4 years of life.



## PLATELET DISORDERS

## THROMBOCYTOPENIA

Estimates of the prevalence of neonatal thrombocytopenia range between 1% and 5% of all neonates. Prevalence is higher, approximately 25%, when only neonates admitted to the intensive care unit are included. The incidence of neonatal thrombocytopenia increases with lower gestational age and lower birth weight.

### ETIOLOGY

Causes of thrombocytopenia can be related to its timing of onset. Thrombocytopenia occurring within 72 hours of delivery is most often due to antenatal and peripartum factors (eg, placental insufficiency, perinatal hypoxia, and antenatal/perinatal infection) with reduced megakaryopoiesis. Less common causes of neonatal thrombocytopenia at 72 hours or less include thrombosis (eg, renal vein, aortic), congenital/inherited (eg, thrombocytopenia absent radius syndrome), congenital infection (eg, cytomegalovirus, toxoplasmosis, rubella), and inborn errors of metabolism (eg, propionic and methylmalonic acidaemia). Severe thrombocytopenia occurring beyond 72 hours of age is most likely due to postnatally acquired infection or necrotizing enterocolitis. If these more common etiologies have been ruled out, then congenital infections, Kasaback-Merritt syndrome, drug-induced thrombocytopenia, and Fanconi anaemia should be considered. Algorithms are widely available to assist in the diagnosis of neonatal thrombocytopenia. The pathophysiology involves both the suppression of platelet production due to cytokine release and increased consumption. In term neonates with thrombocytopenia who are otherwise well and with no history of maternal idiopathic thrombocytopenic purpura, neonatal alloimmune thrombocytopenia (NAIT) should be considered. See also Chapter 435.

### PLATELET TRANSFUSION

Use of platelet transfusions in neonatal intensive care units is highly variable with studies reporting that up to 45% of neonates with a birth weight of 1000 g or less are transfused with platelets, and approximately 10% receive platelets when all birth weights and gestational ages are included. The vast majority of neonates that receive prophylactic platelet transfusions do so in the absence of significant bleeding, despite the fact that no data exist to demonstrate the benefit in maintaining high platelet counts in preterm neonates for prevention of major haemorrhage.

At this time, there is no evidence base with which to inform safe and effective practice for prophylactic platelet transfusions in neonates. Suggested thresholds for stable neonates range from 20 to 50 × 100 per L. When prescribing platelet transfusion, both risks and benefits should be considered.

## COAGULATION DISORDERS

Several coagulation factors in neonates have values outside the normal adult range. Neonates have increased levels of thrombomodulin, tissue plasminogen activator (tPA), and plasminogen activator-1 compared to adults, and decreased levels of factors II, VII, IX, XI, and XII, predisposing neonates to bleeding. This is balanced by lower levels of antithrombin, protein C and protein S, and larger and more abundant von Willebrand Factor. The net result is prolongation of prothrombin time and activated partial thromboplastin time, resulting in a shortened bleeding time.

## VITAMIN K DEFICIENCY

The most common acquired causes of bleeding in the neonate are *vitamin K deficiency, disseminated intravascular coagulation,* and *liver disease.* These conditions typically present as petechiae, purpura, or internal hemorrhage. Vitamin K deficiency results in impaired carboxylation of vitamin-K dependent clotting factors, which renders them functionally inactive. The classical form of vitamin K deficiency presents on days 2 to 7 of life in breastfed healthy full-term neonates. This is due to poor placental transfer of vitamin K and marginal vitamin K content in breast milk. As commercial formulae are supplemented with vitamin K, vitamin K deficiency is rarely observed in formula-fed infants. It is important to note that bleeding secondary to vitamin K deficiency is not confined to the immediate newborn period and may occur beyond the first month of life.

### DIAGNOSIS

Laboratory findings of vitamin K deficiency classically include prolonged prothrombin time and activated partial thromboplastin time in neonates with a normal fibrinogen and platelet count. The diagnosis is confirmed by demonstration of reduced vitamin K–dependent factors (factors II, VII, IX, and X).

### MANAGEMENT

Vitamin K deficiency is treated by administration of intravenous vitamin K. If major bleeding is the initial presentation, consideration should be given to factor replacement therapy with fresh frozen plasma, prothrombin complex concentrate (factor II, factor IX, and factor X), or a 4-factor concentrate containing all the vitamin-K dependent factors. Routine newborn prophylaxis with intramuscular vitamin K is optimal to prevent vitamin K deficiency.

## INHERITED BLEEDING DISORDERS

Inherited conditions also can present with significant bleeding, with *hemophilia A and B* the most common of the inherited bleeding disorders. Over 50% of affected infants are diagnosed during the neonatal period, with approximately 15% presenting with clinically significant bleeding. Unlike the presentation of these conditions in later life, continued oozing of excessive hematoma formation following venipuncture, heel stab blood collection, or administration of intramuscular vitamin K are the most common patterns of bleeding seen in neonates with hemophilia. Both hemophilia A and B typically result in an isolated prolongation of the activated partial thromboplastin time, but definitive diagnosis requires measurement of factor VIII and IX, respectively. It is important to note that factor IX levels are reduced in normal newborns; therefore, confirmation by molecular analysis may be required for mildly affected cases. Von Willebrand disease generally does not present in the neonatal period due to the physiologic increased in von Willebrand factor at birth. See also Chapter 432.

## THROMBOTIC DISORDERS

Whilst thromboembolic events in the perinatal period are rare, the incidence of both neonatal venous and arterial thrombosis is increasing with venous and arterial thrombosis each accounting for approximately 50% of cases. Catheter-related thrombosis accounts for a significant proportion of thrombotic events during the neonatal period. The commonest cause of non–catheter-related neonatal thrombosis is renal vein thrombosis. This condition is more common in preterm neonates and classically presents with hematuria, a flank mass, and thrombocytopenia. Whilst it may be a spontaneous occurrence, a significant proportion of affected neonates will subsequently be found to have an underlying thrombophilic disorder.

Thromboembolic events may also be related to the presence of underlying prothrombotic states such as factor V Leiden and mutations in the 5,10-methylenetetrahydrofolate reductase (*MTHFR*) gene. In these situations, clinical presentation may be a perinatal stroke. A number of maternal factors may also increase the risk of thromboembolic events including preeclampsia, diabetes, systemic lupus erythematosus, and antiphospholipid syndrome, as well as intrapartum events such as asphyxia and traumatic delivery.

### PRESENTATION

Clinical presentations of thrombophilic disorders are variable. Ischemic skin lesions or unprovoked extensive thrombosis suggest homozygous or biheterozygous protein C or protein S deficiency. Perinatal stroke may present with focal seizures. Outcomes are related to the presence of underlying prothrombotic risk factors, particularly factor V Leiden, with significantly higher rates of hemiplegia and global developmental delay observed in infants diagnosed with a thrombophilic disorder.

### INVESTIGATION

Laboratory testing for the evaluation of thrombophilia includes quantification of factor V Leiden, demonstration of antithrombin deficiency, proteins C and S deficiencies, and genetic testing for the prothrombin and *MTHFR* gene mutations. Similar to the diagnosis of the hemophilia, confirmation of mild deficiency states can be difficult, as many of these factors are normally lower than adult levels during the neonatal period.

### MANAGEMENT

There continues to be uncertainty regarding the most appropriate anticoagulant and thrombolytic therapy in neonates. The American College of Chest Physicians has recently updated its guidance on the management of thrombosis in neonates and children. Management of neonatal thrombosis centers on 3 treatment options: anticoagulation with unfractionated or low–molecular-weight heparin, thrombolysis with recombinant tPA, or vascular microsurgery. Although unfractionated heparin has the benefit of a relatively short half-life, it is necessary to monitor its effect by frequent measurement of activated partial thromboplastin time. Low–molecular-weight heparin is becoming the preferred treatment option due to its ability to be administered subcutaneously, its predictable pharmacokinetics, and therefore, the reduced requirement of monitoring. Both unfractionated and low–molecular-weight heparin require higher doses in neonates than in adults to achieve therapeutic effects. The main side effect of both is bleeding, although this risk is probably lower for low–molecular-weight heparin. As all potential treatments carry the risk of major bleeding, supportive care and close observation are optimal. Detection of thrombus at any site should result in the immediate assessment of any potential reversible contributory factors, such as polycythemia, dehydration, hypoxia, and sepsis. Catheter removal is critically important in the management of catheter-related thrombosis, but where lines must remain, therapeutic anticoagulation should be continued for 6 to 12 weeks, followed by heparin prophylaxis until lines can be removed.

*Tissue plasminogen activator* is indicated in neonates with extensive thrombosis or thrombosis that places life, organ function, or a limb in danger. It is most often administered systemically but can be locally infused directly into the affected blood vessel. Because neonates have low levels of plasminogen, supplementation by infusion of fresh frozen plasma may be considered prior to the use of tissue plasminogen activator. While there is no simple laboratory test available to monitor its effect, effective fibrinolysis can be inferred by a postinfusion elevation in d-dimers. Oral anticoagulation with warfarin is challenging in neonates, as warfarin is a vitamin K antagonist and vitamin K–dependent factors are already low. Overall, warfarin is not generally recommended as first line therapy for neonatal thrombolysis.

## SUGGESTED READINGS


Chalmers EA. Neonatal coagulation problems. *Arch Dis Child Fetal Neonatal Ed*. 2004;89(6):F475-F478.

de Haas M, Thurik FF, Koelewijn JM, van der Schoot CE. Haemolytic disease of the fetus and newborn. *Vox Sang*. 2015;109(2):99-113.

Del Vecchio A, Christensen RD. Neonatal neutropenia: what diagnostic evaluation is needed and when is treatment recommended? *Early Hum Dev*. 2012;88(Suppl 2):S19-S24.

Hermansen MC. Nucleated red blood cells in the fetus and newborn. *Arch Dis Child Fetal Neonatal Ed*. 2001;84(3):F211-F215.

Isaacs H, Jr. Fetal and neonatal leukemia. *J Pediatr Hematol Oncol*. 2003;25(5):348-361.

Mimouni FB, Merlob P, Dollberg S, Mandel D; Israeli Neonatal Association. Neonatal polycythaemia: critical review and a consensus statement of the Israeli Neonatology Association. *Acta Paediatr*. 2011;100(10):1290-1296.

Monagle P, Chan AK, Goldenberg NA, et al. Antithrombotic therapy in neonates and children: antithrombotic therapy and prevention of thrombosis, 9th ed: American College of Chest Physicians evidence-based clinical practice guidelines. *Chest*. 2012;141(2 Suppl): e737S-e801S.

Monagle P, Massicotte P. Developmental haemostasis: secondary haemostasis. *Semin Fetal Neonat Med*. 2011;16(6):294-300.

National Blood Authority (NBA). *Patient Blood Management Guidelines: Module 6—Neonatal and Paediatrics*. Canberra, Australia; NBA; 2016.

Stanworth SJ. Thrombocytopenia, bleeding, and use of platelet transfusions in sick neonates. *Hematology Am Soc Hematol Educ Program*. 2012;2012:512-516.

Whyte R, Kirpalani H. Low versus high haemoglobin concentration threshold for blood transfusion for preventing morbidity and mortality in very low birth weight infants. *Cochrane Database Syst Rev*. 2011;(11):CD000512.

Williams MD. Thrombolysis in children. *Br J Haematol*. 2010;148(1): 26-36.


# 56 Neonatal Jaundice

Mohan Pammi, Henry C. Lee, and Gautham K. Suresh

## INTRODUCTION

*Jaundice*, a yellow discoloration of the skin and sclerae resulting from bilirubin deposition in tissues arises when the rate of bilirubin production exceeds the rate of its elimination. Newborn infants have a rate of bilirubin formation that is 2 to 3 times higher than that of adults due to the higher hematocrit and the shorter lifespan of the red blood cells. The decrease in bilirubin elimination results from the limited ability of the newborn liver to conjugate bilirubin and the increased enterohepatic circulation. Although jaundice can result from an increase in either unconjugated (indirect) or conjugated (direct) bilirubin, a rise in the indirect fraction is the most common cause of newborn jaundice and is the focus of this chapter.

## BILIRUBIN METABOLISM

*Bilirubin* is derived from the catabolism of heme. Approximately 75% of bilirubin is derived from the breakdown of hemoglobin from senescent red blood cells and the rest from ineffective erythropoiesis and breakdown of hemoproteins, such as cytochromes, myoglobin, nitric oxide synthase, glutathione peroxidase, and catalase (Fig. 56-1).

Heme is degraded in a 2-step process by the enzyme heme oxygenase resulting in formation of biliverdin and carbon monoxide in equimolar amounts. Carbon monoxide, which diffuses from the cell, binds to hemoglobin in circulating red blood cells to form carboxyhemoglobin (COHb) and is eventually excreted during exhalation (measurable as end-tidal carbon monoxide). Bilirubin is produced from biliverdin by the action of biliverdin reductase, and on entering the circulation, bilirubin binds to albumin and is transported to the liver. Fat-soluble, nonpolar bilirubin crosses the plasma membrane of the hepatocyte and binds to cytoplasmic ligandin, for transport to the endoplasmic reticulum. Conjugation with glucuronic acid in a reaction catalyzed by uridine diphosphate glucuronosyltransferase (UGT) transforms bilirubin into a water-soluble form, bilirubin glucuronide, which is easily excretable. Distribution of bilirubin into tissues depends on its binding to albumin and the serum pH. The greater the binding to albumin is and the more alkaline the pH is, the more likely it is that bilirubin will remain in circulation until it enters the liver. Conjugated bilirubin is excreted into the intestine via the bile, where it is either deconjugated by the enzyme μ-glucuronidase and reabsorbed into the circulation (enterohepatic circulation), or converted by bacteria to nonabsorbable breakdown products. Because the newborn infant has few intestinal bacteria, the enterohepatic circulation of bilirubin is active in the newborn and contributes to the increased propensity for jaundice.

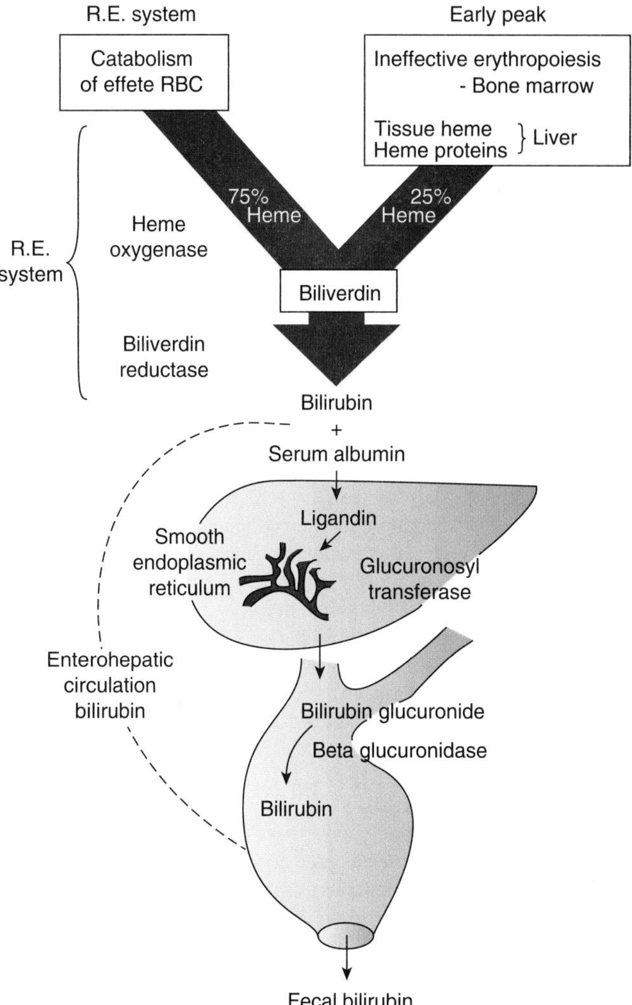


FIGURE 56-1 Bile pigment metabolism in the newborn. RBC, red blood cells; R.E. system, reticulo-endothelial system. (Adapted with permission from MacDonald MG, Mullett MD, Seshia M: *Avery's Neonatology: Pathophysiology and Management of the Newborn*, 6th ed. Philadelphia: Lippincot Williams & Wilkins; 2005.)

Although not all full-term infants become visibly jaundiced, nearly all have a higher total serum bilirubin (TSB) concentration (hyperbilirubinemia > 1 mg/dL) compared to adults. The range of normal TSB levels in a population depends on race, ethnicity, genetic factors, and rates of breastfeeding. In term, healthy infants, jaundice resolves by 2 weeks of age but may take longer in late preterm infants (35 to 37 weeks of gestation).

## PATHOLOGIC HYPERBILIRUBINEMIA

Delayed physiologic processes or pathologic conditions can result in severe hyperbilirubinemia requiring treatment. Jaundice occurring in the first 24 hours of life or persisting beyond 2 weeks of age in a term infant, a rapid rate of rise of bilirubin greater than 0.2 mg/dL/h, a serum bilirubin level greater than the 95th percentile for age in hours, or a direct bilirubin level greater than 1 mg/dL are all suggestive of pathologic jaundice.

Pathologic jaundice is due to an imbalance between bilirubin production and elimination. Increased production can result from hemolysis arising from blood group incompatibilities, erythrocyte enzyme deficiencies, or structural defects of the erythrocytes. Increased bilirubin production is also seen in premature infants because of the shortened red cell lifespan; in infants of diabetic mothers due to polycythemia or ineffective erythropoiesis; in infants with closed-space bleeding, such as bruising or hemorrhage into internal organs due to the breakdown of extruded blood; in infants with polycythemia; and in infants with sepsis. Decreased elimination of bilirubin can result from either a genetic defect in hepatic uptake, as seen in newborn infants with a polymorphic variant of the *organic anion transporter protein (OATP-2) gene*, or impaired conjugation of bilirubin from inherited defects in UGT as seen in *Gilbert syndrome* and *Crigler-Najjar syndrome* types I (severe deficiency) and II (less severe form). In Gilbert syndrome, the mildly decreased UGT activity is related to an increased number of the thymine-adenine repeats in the promoter region of the *UG1TA* gene, the principal gene encoding for this enzyme. Similar polymorphisms may contribute to the variations in conjugating capacity observed in infants, independent of their maturity. In Asian infants, a DNA sequence variant (Gly71Arg), resulting in an amino acid change in the UGT protein, has been associated with neonatal hyperbilirubinemia.

Increased enterohepatic circulation of bilirubin (and decreased elimination) occurs if there is a failure to establish breastfeeding or with conditions that result in decreased intestinal motility such as ileus, pyloric stenosis, or intestinal obstruction. In breastfeeding failure characterized by a decreased feeding frequency, weight loss, and dehydration, there is not only increased enterohepatic circulation but also caloric deprivation. True breast milk jaundice syndrome develops more gradually, presents typically in the second week of life, and requires the exclusion of other causes of unconjugated hyperbilirubinemia and generally resolves between 1 and 3 months of age. The etiology of breast milk jaundice is unclear but probably multifactorial. Exaggerated enterohepatic circulation, variations in the β-glucuronidase gene, and variations in the breast milk microbiome have been implicated as factors contributing to the development of breast milk jaundice.

### BILIRUBIN TOXICITY AND KERNICTERUS

Prevention and treatment of indirect hyperbilirubinemia is directed at preventing neurological injury and long-term neurodevelopmental impairment. Acute bilirubin encephalopathy in the infant presents with a poor suck, lethargy, hypotonia in the first 2 days of age followed by hypertonia of extensor muscles, opisthotonus, retrocollis, and fever in the middle of the first week and hypertonia after the first week. Surviving infants may have exaggerated deep tendon reflexes, obligatory tonic neck reflexes, delayed motor skills, and after the first year, movement disorder (choreoathetosis, ballismus, tremor), upward gaze, paralytic palsies, intellectual deficits, and sensorineural hearing loss. *Kernicterus* is characterized pathologically by staining and necrosis of neurons in the basal ganglia, hippocampus, and subthalamic nuclei of the brain. Magnetic resonance imaging of infants with kernicterus has shown abnormalities in these regions. Bilirubin may also cause changes in brain-stem–evoked responses and abnormal infant cry in the acute phase, and sensorineural hearing loss long term. No clear association can be made between a specific serum bilirubin level or the duration of exposure to high bilirubin levels and the risk of neurotoxicity, although the risk is higher with a serum bilirubin level of greater than 25 mg/dL. Low serum albumin levels and the use of agents that displace bilirubin from albumin such as sulfisoxazole, benzyl alcohol, or ceftriaxone, can increase the risk of bilirubin encephalopathy. A decrease in blood pH may render unbound (free) bilirubin lipophilic, thereby enhancing tissue uptake. Premature infants are particularly at risk of encephalopathy because of low serum albumin concentrations and frequency of acidosis. Albumin-bound bilirubin and conjugated bilirubin do not cross the blood-brain barrier but when the barrier is disrupted, as in prematurity, asphyxia, meningitis, sepsis, and intracranial hemorrhage, bilirubin may access vulnerable areas of the developing brain.

### EVALUATION AND TREATMENT OF INDIRECT HYPERBILIRUBINEMIA

#### Evaluation

Evaluation of a jaundiced infant should try to identify the type of hyperbilirubinemia (indirect or direct), its severity, the risks of bilirubin encephalopathy, and the cause of the hyperbilirubinemia.

A review of the maternal, family, and infant history should aim to identify blood group incompatibilities, congenital infections, maternal diabetes, maternal drugs, birth trauma, closed space bleeding in the newborn, familial causes such as hereditary spherocytosis, glucose-6-phosphate dehydrogenase (G6PD) deficiency, family history of liver disease, and siblings with jaundice (which may suggest blood group incompatibilities, breast milk jaundice, or Lucey-Driscoll syndrome). The newborn should be assessed for poor feeding, decreased stooling or urination, excessive weight loss, and poor breastfeeding or poor milk intake.

Physical examination of the infant should try to identify whether the infant is preterm, small for gestational age, or large for gestational age. The infant should be assessed for ruddiness (suggestive of polycythemia), pallor, presence of extravasated blood (eg, cephalohematoma), petechiae, hepatosplenomegaly, chorioretinitis, omphalitis, evidence of sepsis, and features of congenital hypothyroidism. Finally, careful examination and documentation should be made of features of bilirubin encephalopathy.

Visual inspection of the degree of yellow discoloration of the skin is unreliable, and a total serum bilirubin level should be obtained. Other common laboratory tests to identify the presence of hemolysis and its etiology and severity may be indicated. These include a maternal and infant ABO and Rh blood types, indirect and direct antiglobulin test, complete blood count, reticulocyte count, peripheral blood smear, a G6PD level, and if necessary, specific tests such as an osmotic fragility test. Finally, assessment of serum albumin, and if the infant appears ill, the blood pH may be helpful to assess the risk of bilirubin encephalopathy. Evaluation for infection may be warranted depending on the history and physical examination. ABO hemolytic disease is the most common form of hemolysis diagnosed in the newborn. Only half of those infants with a positive direct antibody (Coombs) test are likely to have significant hemolysis. On the other hand, some infants with a negative direct Coombs test have increased rates of hemolysis. Reticulocytosis and the presence of microspherocytes on a peripheral blood smear may help confirm the diagnosis but are not pathognomonic. Routine testing for G6PD deficiency is indicated when family history or ethnic or geographic origin suggests the likelihood of G6PD deficiency. However, not all infants with G6PD deficiency have hemolysis, and G6PD levels can be high in the presence of hemolysis. Also, such testing is not available currently in all institutions and, when done, the results are usually not timely enough for immediate decision making. Careful follow-up is required for all discharged newborn infants who have hemolysis.

Transcutaneous bilirubinometry has been investigated as a substitute for serum bilirubin assessment. Noninvasive transcutaneous bilirubin (TcB) measurements have been shown to underestimate TSB measurements, especially with advancing chronological age and in African-American infants but may be a reasonable surrogate in certain situations. End-tidal carbon monoxide concentration, an index of hemolysis and bilirubin production, may be useful, but there is insufficient data to make a recommendation for clinical practice.

If an infant is significantly jaundiced clinically, it is prudent to immediately institute phototherapy while waiting for the laboratory test results. If the serum bilirubin exceeds thresholds described in published guidelines, then phototherapy should be continued and periodic serum bilirubin assessments performed until the bilirubin drops below the phototherapy threshold.

### Phototherapy

Phototherapy and exchange transfusion are the main modalities used to treat hyperbilirubinemia (the American Academy of Pediatrics' Practice Guidelines for infants of more than 35 weeks' gestation are shown in Fig. 56-2). Consensus-based guidelines for the management of jaundice in preterm infants less than 35 weeks based on gestational age and birth weight have been published.

Bilirubin absorbs blue light mainly at the wavelength of 450 nm and is converted to lumirubin, a water-soluble isomer of bilirubin, which is excreted in the urine. The efficacy of phototherapy is determined by the dose (irradiance) and the amount of body surface area exposed. The irradiance is determined by the type of light source and the distance of the light from the infant. Intensive phototherapy is recommended for infants with high TSB, rapidly rising TSB, or hemolysis. It requires irradiance in the range of 30 ÂµW/cm$^2$/nm at the effective wavelength range (430–490 nm) to the largest body surface area of the infant. A bank of special blue fluorescent lights is placed approximately 10 to 12 cm above the infant along with either a fiber-optic blanket or special blue fluorescent lights under the infant to increase the exposed surface area. Newer devices using high-intensity gallium nitride light-emitting diodes (LEDs) can generate high irradiance and have greater efficacy than conventional phototherapy. When phototherapy is administered, temperature and hydration status must be monitored and the infant's eyes must be shielded. Unless the TSB is approaching exchange transfusion levels, phototherapy can be interrupted for breastfeeding or for other brief periods of time to attend to the infant without compromising its effectiveness.

Total serum bilirubin levels should be repeated within 2 to 4 hours after initiation and followed to ensure that the levels are decreasing. Phototherapy can be discontinued once the TSB concentration has dropped significantly below threshold levels for age. Except in the context of hemolytic disease, rebound hyperbilirubinemia after discontinuation of phototherapy is unusual. Infants with direct hyperbilirubinemia should have a focused diagnostic workup. In infants with hepatic dysfunction, phototherapy can result in significant discoloration of the skin, referred to as *bronze baby syndrome*, which may last for weeks to months.

Filtered sunlight has been proposed as an alternative to conventional phototherapy in resource limited settings such as countries in Africa. A randomized trial found that filtered sunlight therapy was noninferior to conventional phototherapy for the treatment of hyperbilirubinemia in African neonates. Prophylactic phototherapy in preterm or low–birth-weight infants decreases peak TSB levels and the rate of exchange transfusion and should be considered in high-risk infants.

**Exchange Transfusion** Exchange transfusion was the first therapy available to treat jaundice of the newborn. It removes not only bilirubin but also circulating antibodies that can target the erythrocytes and antibody-coated erythrocytes, which might hemolyze later. A complete exchange transfusion involves removing and replacing twice the infant's blood volume (~160 mL/kg). The complications associated with exchange transfusion include hypocalcemia, thrombocytopenia, portal vein thrombosis, necrotizing enterocolitis, electrolyte imbalance, and infection. Mortality after exchange transfusion is usually less than 1%. Anticipatory management of hyperbilirubinemia and intense phototherapy can avoid the need for exchange transfusion in most cases. The American Academy of Pediatrics' Practice Guidelines outline criteria for exchange transfusion. The role of intravenous immune globulin therapy to avoid exchange transfusion in Rh or ABO hemolytic disease is not clear but may be helpful in infants with excessive hemolysis. Tin mesoporphyrin, an inhibitor of heme oxygenase, may decrease bilirubin concentrations in newborns in the short term but its role in decreasing kernicterus or in improving long-term neurodevelopmental outcomes remains unknown.



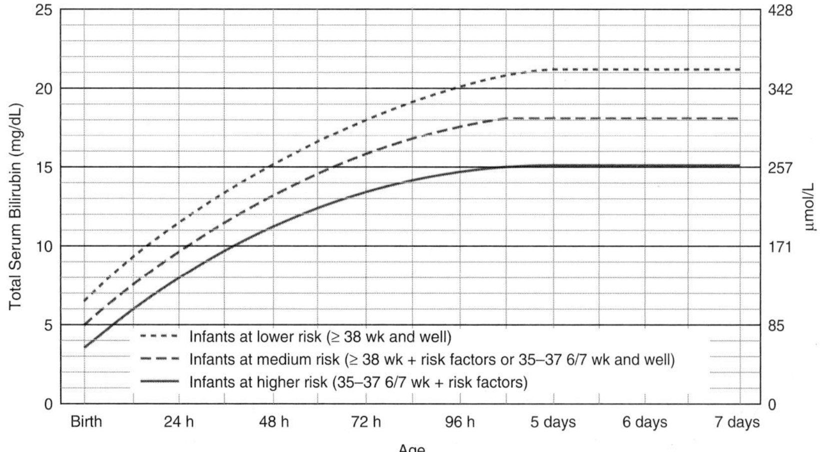


- Use total bilirubin. Do not subtract direct reacting or conjugated bilirubin.
- Risk factors = isoimmune hemolytic disease, G6PD deficiency, asphyxia, significant lethargy, temperature instability, sepsis, acidosis, or albumin < 3.0 g/dL (if measured).
- For well infants 35–37 6/7 wk can adjust TSB levels for intervention around the medium risk line. It is an option to intervene at lower TSB levels for infants closer to 35 wks and at higher TSB levels for those closer to 37 6/7 wk.
- It is an option to provide conventional phototherapy in hospital or at home at TSB levels 2–3 mg/dL (35–50 mmol/L) below those shown but home phototherapy should not be used in any infant with risk factors.

**FIGURE 56-2** Guidelines for phototherapy in hospitalized infants of 35 or more weeks' gestation. TSB, total serum bilirubin. (Reproduced with permission from American Academy of Pediatrics Subcommittee on Hyperbilirubinemia: Management of hyperbilirubinemia in the newborn infant 35 or more weeks of gestation, *Pediatrics*. 2004 Jul;114(1):297-316.)

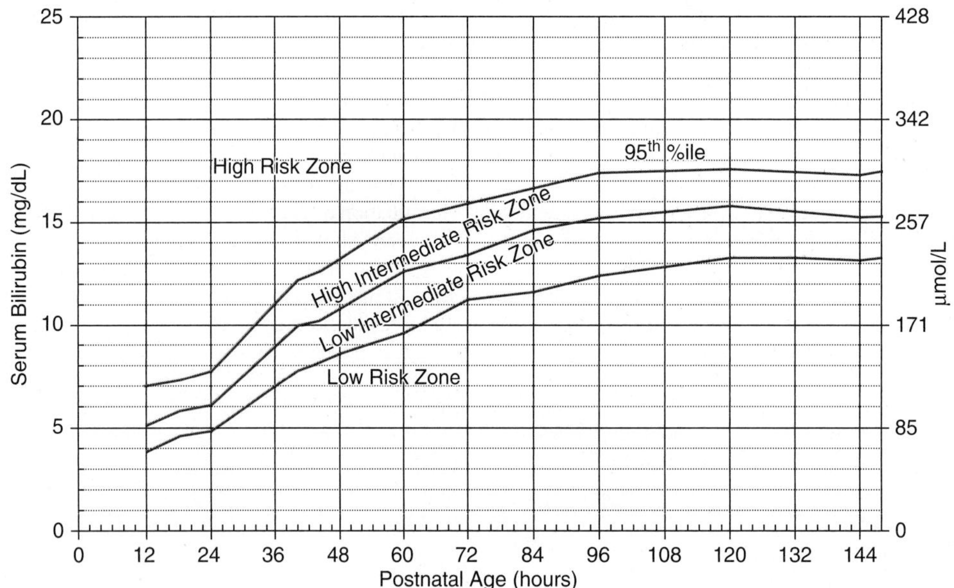


**FIGURE 56-3** Risk designation of term and near-term well newborns based on their hour-specific serum bilirubin values. The high-risk zone is designated by the 95th percentile track. The intermediate-risk zone is subdivided to upper- and lower-risk zones by the 75th percentile track. The low-risk zone has been electively and statistically defined by the 40th percentile track. (Reproduced with permission from American Academy of Pediatrics Subcommittee on Hyperbilirubinemia: Management of hyperbilirubinemia in the newborn infant 35 or more weeks of gestation, *Pediatrics.* 2004 Jul;114(1):297-316.)



#### Screening for and Prevention of Severe Hyperbilirubinemia in Healthy Full-Term and Late-Preterm Infants

Prompted by the recognition that, after hospital discharge, some apparently healthy term and late-preterm infants were developing severe hyperbilirubinemia and acute bilirubin encephalopathy, much emphasis has been placed on risk identification, ensuring appropriate postdischarge follow-up care, and prompt initiation of therapy for hyperbilirubinemia. Risk identification can be performed using either clinical risk factors, universal predischarge bilirubin screening, or both. If predischarge screening is performed, the bilirubin level should be interpreted according to the infant's age in hours by plotting it on available percentile curves of bilirubin levels, which allows stratification of risk into low, intermediate, and high levels (Fig. 56-3). Hemolytic disease confers a greater risk for the development of kernicterus, but there are numerous other risk factors. These include a previous sibling with jaundice, East Asian race, infant of a diabetic mother, male sex, bruising, cephalohematoma, gestational age less than 37 weeks, breastfeeding, excessive postnatal weight loss, visible jaundice before discharge, serum or transcutaneous bilirubin level above the 75th percentile for age in hours, G6PD deficiency, and short postnatal hospital stay. Some cases of kernicterus may be hard to prevent because of sudden, unpredictable, and marked increases in TSB concentrations (eg, in infants with G6PD deficiency that have been exposed to an environmental oxidant).

Parents should be appropriately educated about jaundice, preferably with supplemental written materials, and should be clear about how to seek medical help if they have concerns about the infant, especially jaundice. All infants should be discharged to the care of an identified primary care provider, and should be evaluated for jaundice, feeding, weight change, and urine and stool output by a qualified provider (in the office or at home) within 48 to 72 hours of discharge (or sooner if at high risk). Infants who are noticed to be jaundiced postdischarge should have a TSB level checked, and if this level exceeds the phototherapy threshold, then phototherapy should immediately be instituted, along with correction of hypernatremic dehydration (a common problem in such infants). Delays in initiation of phototherapy in infants with severe hyperbilirubinemia due to a long wait in the office or in the emergency room, or due to delays in obtaining the results of laboratory tests, should be avoided.

## SUGGESTED READINGS


Arnold C, Pedroza C, Tyson JE. Phototherapy in ELBW newborns: does it work? Is it safe? The evidence from randomized clinical trials. *Semin Perinatol.* 2014;38(7):452-464.

Bhutani VK, Wong RJ, Stevenson DK. Hyperbilirubinemia in preterm neonates. *Clin Perinatol.* 2016;43(2):215-232.

Darling EK, Ramsay T, Sprague AE, Walker MC, Guttmann A. Universal bilirubin screening and health care utilization. *Pediatrics.* 2014;134(4):e1017-e1024.

Dijk PH, Hulzebos CV. An evidence-based view on hyperbilirubinaemia. *Acta Paediatr.* 2012;101(464):3-10.

Götze T, Blessing H, Grillhösl C, Gerner P, Hoerning A. Neonatal cholestasis—differential diagnoses, current diagnostic procedures, and treatment. *Front Pediatr.* 2015;3:43.

Kaplan M, Hammerman C. The need for neonatal glucose-6-phosphate dehydrogenase screening: a global perspective. *J Perinatol.* 2009;29(Suppl 1):S46-S52.

Maisels MJ. Managing the jaundiced newborn: a persistent challenge. *CMAJ.* 2015;187(5):335-343.

Maisels MJ, McDonagh AF. Phototherapy for neonatal jaundice. *N Engl J Med.* 2008;358(9):920-928.

Maisels MJ, Bhutani VK, Bogen D, Newman TB, Stark AR, Watchko JF. Hyperbilirubinemia in the newborn infant ≥ 35 weeks' gestation: an update with clarifications. *Pediatrics.* 2009;124(4):1193-1198.

Murki S, Kumar P. Blood exchange transfusion for infants with severe neonatal hyperbilirubinemia. *Semin Perinatol.* 2011;35(3):175-184.

National Collaborating Centre for Women's and Children's Health (UK). *Neonatal Jaundice.* London: RCOG Press; 2010.

US Preventive Services Task Force. Screening of infants for hyperbilirubinemia to prevent chronic bilirubin encephalopathy: US Preventive Services Task Force recommendation statement. *Pediatrics.* 2009;124(4):1172-1177.

# 57 Respiratory Distress Syndrome

C. G. de Waal and A. H. van Kaam

## INTRODUCTION

Neonatal respiratory distress syndrome (RDS) is the most common cause of respiratory failure in preterm infants. Its incidence is inversely related to gestational age and increases to as high as 95% in infants born at 22 to 24 weeks of gestation. Over time, the outcome of infants suffering from RDS has changed dramatically. Forty years ago, approximately 50% of infants with RDS died. However, significant improvements in both prevention and treatment of RDS over the last 4 decades have markedly reduced mortality. As a consequence, the focus of improving outcome has now shifted from mortality to preventing (pulmonary) morbidity following RDS and its treatment.

## PATHOPHYSIOLOGY

The main feature of RDS is compromised lung function caused by both structural and biochemical immaturity of the lung.

### Structural Immaturity

Lung development during fetal life occurs in different stages. Following organogenesis in the first 2 stages (*embryonic* and *pseudoglandular*) of lung development, the *canalicular* stage, starting at approximately 16 weeks after conception, is the first step in lung differentiation, involving formation of an actual air-blood barrier. Differentiation continues in both the *saccular* and *alveolar* stages of lung development starting at 24 and 36 weeks' postconceptional age, respectively. This means that, at the time of birth, lung development of most preterm infants is still at the saccular stage, resulting in a reduced surface area for gas exchange and limited diffusion capacity due to thickened membranes at the air-blood interface.

### Biochemical Immaturity

The hallmark of RDS is a deficiency of *pulmonary surfactant*, a complex mixture of lipids (90%) and proteins (10%) that is synthesized in alveolar epithelial type II cells. Type II cells are 1 of the 2 epithelial cell types that line the alveolus. The most important function of surfactant is lowering of the alveolar surface tension, the force directed from the wall to the center of the alveolus at the air-liquid interface. This function is mainly attributed to the surfactant phospholipid dipalmitoylphosphatidylcholine and the surfactant hydrophobic proteins B and C. The hydrophilic surfactant proteins A and D play a role in innate host defense. Synthesis and storage of surfactant begins at about 16 weeks' gestation, and lung homogenates have high concentrations of surfactant by 20 weeks. However, surfactant is not secreted until later, appearing in amniotic fluid at approximately 28 weeks' gestation, although this may vary greatly among individuals. This explains why some infants with a gestational age of less than 30 weeks do not develop neonatal RDS while other infants, born at a more advanced gestation, do.

The high alveolar surface tension accompanying surfactant deficiency will increase the elastic recoil forces of the lung and decrease compliance of the respiratory system. As a result, preterm infants with RDS need to create large transpulmonary pressures to establish an adequate tidal volume. The absence of surfactant will also compromise lung volume stability, especially at the end of expiration. This makes the lung prone to a low end-expiratory lung volume and atelectasis, partly because the highly compliant chest wall is unable to counteract the increase in elastic recoil forces of the lung. A low end-expiratory lung volume may further compromise lung compliance and increase airway resistance and pulmonary vascular resistance. Due to the fact that the hypoxic pulmonary vasoconstriction response is often not functional in newborns, perfusion of collapsed sacculi-alveoli, also referred to as intrapulmonary right-to-left shunt, increases and results in (severe) hypoxemia.

## PATHOLOGY

At postmortem examination, the lungs from infants with RDS are firm and airless. Atelectasis is striking on gross inspection; when the lungs are fixed in inflation, only the airways and a few alveolar ducts are air filled (Fig. 57-1). Diffuse atelectasis and dilated terminal bronchioles and alveolar ducts lined with a homogenous hyaline-staining material characterize the microscopic picture (Fig. 57-2). The hyaline membranes are plasma clots containing fibrin, other plasma constituents, and cellular debris. The small pulmonary arterioles appear constricted. There is congestion of pulmonary capillaries and veins and an increase in pulmonary water with dilation of the lymphatics. Because of these histological features, RDS was initially named hyaline membrane disease.

Interstitial air leaks are common, and collections of air are often seen around small airways and vessels (Fig. 57-3). In some cases, the alveoli and hyaline membranes contain red cells. Electron microscopic examination shows degeneration of epithelial and endothelial cells and rupture of the basement membranes. If death occurs after 3 or 4 days of respiratory distress, the hyaline membranes are fragmented and numerous macrophages appear in the intra-alveolar spaces. The pulmonary interstitium is widened and filled with round cells and fibroblasts. After the first week, there is a proliferation of alveolar epithelial type II cells and capillaries. In severe cases, chronic changes occur, including metaplasia of the bronchiolar epithelium and interstitial fibrosis.

## PREDISPOSING FACTORS

As mentioned, the incidence of RDS is inversely related to gestational age. But there are also other factors that increase the risk of neonatal RDS. It is twice as common in males than in females at all gestational ages and is more common in white infants. Delivery by cesarean section, particularly if performed before the onset of spontaneous labor, is an independent risk factor as well. Infants of diabetic mothers are 5 times more likely to develop RDS than infants of nondiabetic mothers with the same gestational age, sex, and mode of delivery. A higher maternal age also predisposes for RDS. Finally, the second-born twin is more likely to be affected, and a family history of RDS increases the risk for any given premature infant.

On the other hand, complications of pregnancy, such as pregnancy-induced hypertension, chronic maternal hypertension, premature rupture of membranes, intrauterine infection, and subacute placental abruption, all decrease the incidence of RDS. Infants born to mothers addicted to narcotics are also at less risk for developing RDS.

### Predicting Lung Maturity and Respiratory Distress Syndrome

Lung fluid moves from the fetal lung into the amniotic cavity. Once surfactant begins to be secreted by the alveolar epithelial type II cells in the fetus, this lung fluid transports secreted surfactant from the alveoli to the amniotic fluid. The concentration of surfactant in amniotic fluid reflects the amount of surfactant available at the alveolar surfaces and thus the potential stability of the respiratory units and risk of RDS. The concentrations of the phospholipids lecithin and sphingomyelin are equal in amniotic fluid in midgestation, but after 34 weeks, there is twice as much lecithin as sphingomyelin. This knowledge led to the widespread use of the lecithin-sphingomyelin (L/S) ratio as an antenatal developmental index of biochemical maturity, to predict which fetuses will develop RDS when delivered.

Several other amniotic fluid tests for assessing lung maturity are now widely available, including the measurement of phosphatidylglycerol,

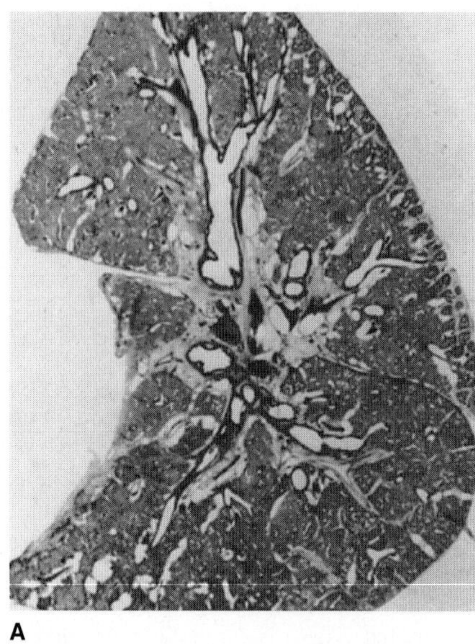
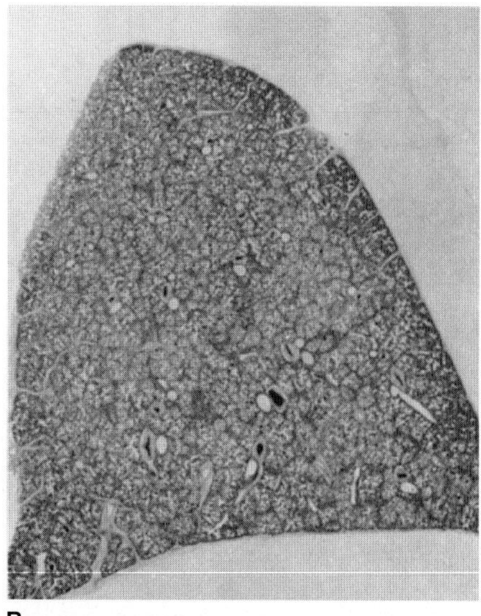

A B

**FIGURE 57-1** **A:** Longitudinal section of the left lung of a 1560-g infant, born at 30 weeks' gestation, who died at 2.5 days of age from neonatal respiratory distress syndrome. The lung was expanded with air to a pressure of 40 $cmH_2O$, then deflated to 10 $cmH_2O$ and fixed with the bronchus clamped. The airways are distended, and a few of the respiratory bronchioles are overinflated. Most of the alveolar ducts and alveoli are airless. **B:** Cross-section of the left upper lobe of a 1220-g infant, born at 29 weeks' gestation without lung disease, who died at 1 week of age after a sudden, massive intraventricular hemorrhage. Inflation and fixation were identical to those used for the lung in panel A. Almost all of the alveolar ducts are filled with air, and the airways are not overdistended.



a relatively surfactant-specific phospholipid, and the simple and rapid foam stability or shake test. Although these tests can provide very useful clinical guidance in certain situations, they are all limited by a high false-negative rate secondary to the accumulation of normal intracellular surfactant stores well before amniotic fluid levels of surfactant change. For this reason, amniotic fluid analysis for lung maturation are not routinely used in clinical practice.

Some investigators have also attempted to predict RDS during the first minutes *after* birth. At this time, gastric contents mainly comprise lung fluid or swallowed amniotic fluid. Several tests can assess the presence or absence of surfactant in the gastric aspirate: lamellar body count, stable microbubble test, and gastric aspirate shake test. Of these, the lamellar body count and the stable microbubble test seem most promising, with reported positive and negative predictive values ranging from 58% to 85% and 75% to 100%, respectively. However, there is currently only 1 randomized trial comparing surfactant treatment based on lamellar body count versus oxygen need, showing no difference in important clinical outcomes and the use of surfactant. The limited amount of prospective evidence is probably the most important reason why gastric content analysis to predict RDS has not found its way into clinical practice.

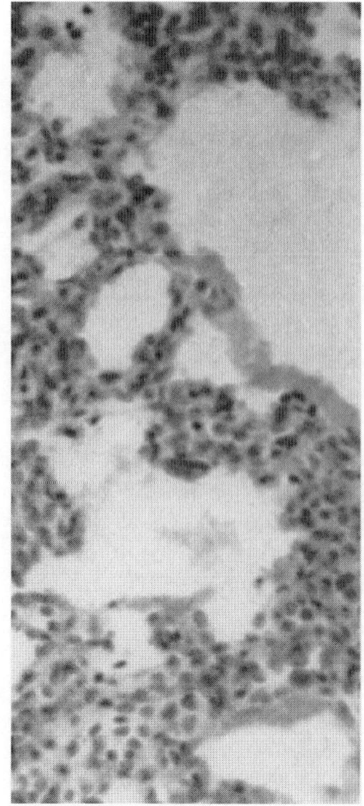
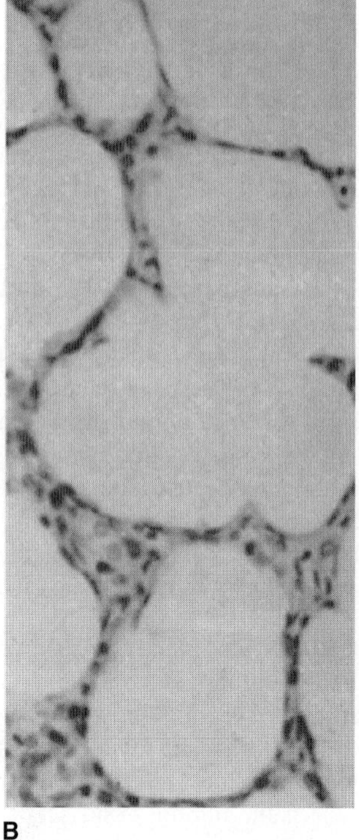

A B

**FIGURE 57-2** **A:** Magnified section (×100) of Fig. 57-1A. Some of the alveolar ducts are inflated, but there are no true alveoli. The cells of the interstitial tissue appear to be crowded, but no inflammatory cells are present. The homogenous staining material lining the walls of the alveolar ducts are plasma clots (ie, hyaline membranes). **B:** Magnified section (×100) of Fig. 57-1B. The interstitial tissue is thin. Although there are no true alveoli in this section, the total internal surface area is large, particularly compared with the lung in panel A.

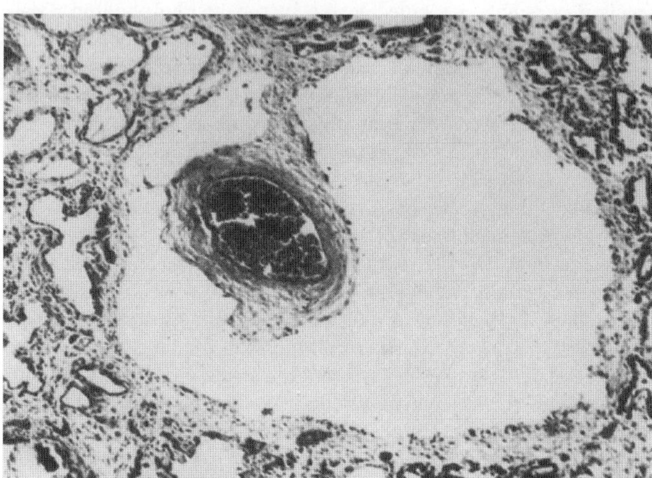

**FIGURE 57-3** Lung from an infant born after 25 weeks' gestation weighing 650 g who died at 40 hours of age. Note the immature respiratory units, some of which are lined with hyaline membranes. There is a large collection of interstitial air surrounding a small vessel (×100).

## CLINICAL FEATURES

Some infants with RDS fail to expand their lungs at birth despite vigorous inspiratory efforts, and have respiratory distress from delivery. Others initially inflate their lungs but develop progressive atelectasis and increasingly labored breathing in the first few hours of life. The characteristic clinical features of infants with neonatal respiratory distress are an expiratory grunt, tachypnea, intercostal and sternal retractions, and cyanosis. Grunting respiration is caused by a prolonged expiratory effort against a partially closed glottis. It is usually preceded by a strong inspiratory effort during which the intrathoracic pressure drops well below atmospheric pressure. During the prolonged expiration, intrathoracic pressure is maintained above atmospheric pressure. Infants do not grunt with every breath, and those with severe disease grunt most frequently. By maintaining a positive intrapulmonary pressure during most of the respiratory cycle, grunting probably helps to prevent atelectasis, which is 1 of the hallmarks of RDS.

Due to their decreased lung compliance, infants with RDS need to generate large transpulmonary pressures to establish an adequate tidal volume. The large negative intrathoracic pressures generated as the infant attempts to inflate its lungs cause the soft tissues of the chest cage to retract. These retractions are particularly notable in very small preterm infants as they have highly compliant chest walls. With severe respiratory distress, the lower sternum may be pulled in almost to the vertebral column by the forceful contraction of the diaphragm. Infants breathe primarily with the diaphragm and have very compliant chest walls; as a result they often have paradoxical breathing movements. Thus, as the chest caves in, its circumference becomes smaller while the abdominal circumference increases. As a result, breathing becomes less efficient and tidal volumes become smaller. By increasing their respiratory rate, the infants try to maintain an adequate minute volume as much as possible.

The combination of reduced alveolar ventilation and stability explains that breath sounds are often diminished in intensity and have a harsh, tubular quality. Occasionally, there are fine rales, particularly in those infants born by cesarean section who may have excessive lung liquid.

Cyanosis is an early sign of RDS and, as the disease progresses, may be present even when an infant breathes 100% oxygen. As the lungs become more difficult to ventilate, the work of breathing increases, the infant tires, and arterial carbon dioxide tension rises. At the same time, the hypoxemia and diminished peripheral blood flow cause metabolic acidosis as lactic acid accumulates. With the development of acidosis, potassium leaves the cells and its concentration in serum rises, in some instances to very high levels.

Urine output is usually diminished early in the course of the disease, and the infants may become progressively edematous. Some infants, especially very low–birth-weight infants, have systemic hypotension, peripheral pallor, slow capillary filling, and hypothermia when not treated in time with sufficient respiratory support and exogenous surfactant.

### Postnatal Lung Maturation

It takes only 1 to 2 days following birth for an immature lung to mature as it responds to the surge of glucocorticoids and β-adrenergic compounds released by the stress of delivery. Glucocorticoids increase surfactant synthesis, and β-adrenergic stimulation promotes its secretion. At the same time, structural changes occur in the lung. Thin-walled respiratory units develop, and the number of capillaries increases. With these changes, the signs and symptoms of respiratory distress usually subside after 48 to 72 hours of life. Recovery is usually heralded by diuresis. Clinical improvement is accompanied by a rapid fall in pulmonary vascular resistance and a rise in systemic arterial pressure. In some infants, particularly the least mature with birth weight less than 1500 g, this may permit development of a large shunt from the aorta through a patent ductus arteriosus to the pulmonary artery. In these infants, recovery may be interrupted by the development of pulmonary edema.

### Radiographic Features of Respiratory Distress Syndrome

The radiographic appearance of the lungs in infants with RDS is characterized by reduced aeration with a diffuse reticulogranular pattern of increased density, usually uniform in distribution (Fig. 57-4) but occasionally more marked in the bases or on 1 side. The densities are due to miliary atelectasis and interstitial edema. Lung volumes are small, and even radiographs taken after a maximal inspiration rarely show the diaphragm to be below the eighth or ninth interspace. The heart is usually normal in size, although it often appears large because of the large thymic shadow and decreased lung volume. The radiographic appearance of the lung can be altered by treatment with nasal continuous positive airway pressure (CPAP) or invasive mechanical ventilation with positive end-expiratory pressure. Later in the course of the disease, pulmonary edema, air leaks, or pulmonary hemorrhage can also affect the radiological appearance.

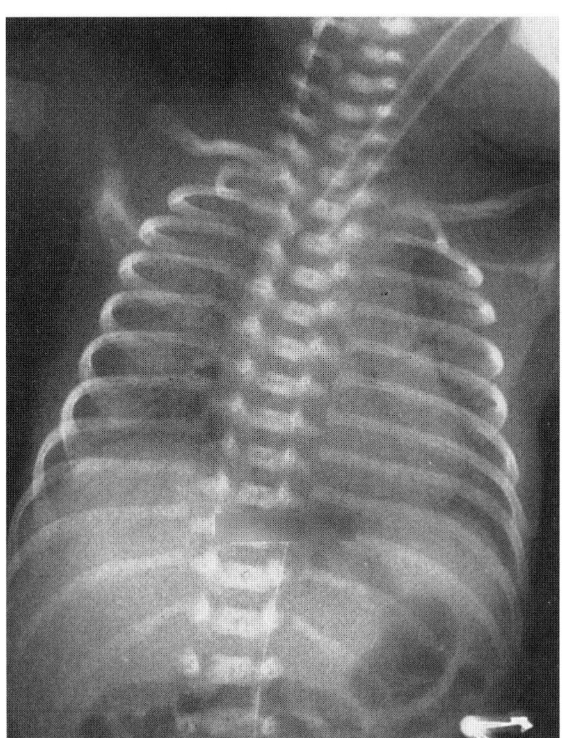

**FIGURE 57-4** Chest radiograph of an infant with respiratory distress syndrome. An endotracheal tube is present. Despite the application of positive pressure, the lung volume is reduced with the diaphragm at the eighth interspace. The lung parenchyma has a diffuse reticulogranular pattern, and air bronchograms are present.

## DIFFERENTIAL DIAGNOSIS

### Transient Tachypnea of the Newborn

It may be difficult to distinguish RDS from normal, physiological pulmonary transition after birth. During this transition, fluid needs to be cleared from the lung and an air-filled functional residual capacity need to be created. Preterm infants often show signs of respiratory distress, including grunting and retractions. Furthermore, some infants may be oxygen dependent. In some infants, pulmonary transition may take several hours, a condition also referred to as transient tachypnea of the newborn, or "wet lung." However, in contrast to RDS, these symptoms are usually not progressive but instead resolve within the first 24 to 48 hours. Furthermore, the chest x-ray shows hyperaeration of the lungs, perihilar streaking and fluid in the interlobar fissures.

### Congenital Pneumonia

Infants with congenital pneumonia, especially group B streptococcus, may also present with signs of respiratory distress that can be clinically and radiologically indistinguishable from RDS.

### Surfactant Dysfunction

Surfactant function also may be compromised by genetic disorders. For example, surfactant protein B deficiency and *ABCA3* mutations can have a striking resemblance to RDS. However, and in contrast to infants with RDS, signs of respiratory distress and cyanosis do not subside over the first 3 days of life and the response to exogenous surfactant treatment is only temporary.

## PREVENTION

Neonatal RDS is associated with incomplete development of the lung at the time of birth. Thus, premature delivery should be delayed, where possible. If this cannot be avoided, additional efforts should be made to accelerate lung maturation. Animal studies have shown that antenatal administration of glucocorticoids accelerates both structural and biochemical (surfactant) lung maturation.

In 1972, Liggins and Howie translated these findings to humans when they reported that administration of betamethasone to women in premature labor at least 2 days before delivery significantly reduced the incidence of respiratory distress. Numerous studies following this pivotal publication have confirmed that antenatal glucocorticoids reduce mortality and perinatal morbidities such as RDS, intraventricular hemorrhage, and necrotizing enterocolitis. Treatment consists of 2 doses of 12 mg of betamethasone given intramuscularly 24 hours apart, or 4 doses of 6 mg of dexamethasone given intramuscularly 12 hours apart. The benefits of antenatal steroid typically begin at around 24 hours after initiation of therapy and lasts 7 days. Current guidelines recommend treatment with antenatal glucocorticoids if preterm delivery is imminent between 24 and 34 weeks of gestation. Although observational cohort studies also suggest benefits of antenatal glucocorticoids between 22 and 26 weeks of gestation, the randomized evidence to support this is limited. In addition, a recent multicenter randomized trial found antenatal betamethasone of benefit for late preterm infants born between 34 and 37 weeks of gestation as well.

Repeated courses of antenatal glucocorticoids have been a matter of debate because of possible adverse effects on fetal growth. However, a systematic review of 10 randomized controlled trials clearly showed benefit of a repeated course of antenatal glucocorticoids without evidence for clinical relevant adverse effects on growth or long-term neurodevelopment. As a result, most clinicians have adopted a repeat course of antenatal glucocorticoids but only if preterm delivery is imminent.

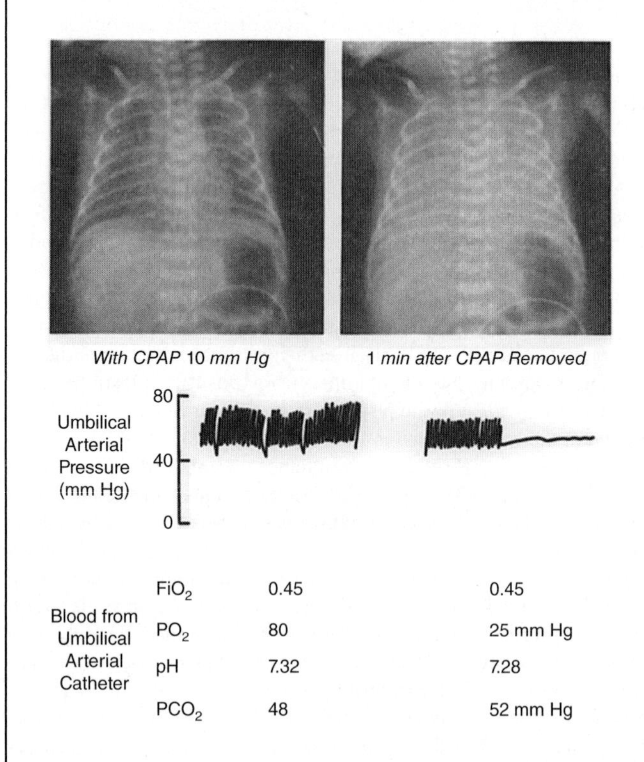


**FIGURE 57-5** Chest radiographs, aortic blood pressure, pH, and blood gases in an infant with neonatal respiratory distress during spontaneous breathing (*left*) and 1 minute after continuous positive airway pressure was temporarily removed (*right*). The marked fall in arterial oxygen tension from 80 to 25 mm Hg parallels the rapid development of atelectasis shown in the radiograph. CPAP, continuous positive airway pressure; $FiO_2$, inspired oxygen fraction; $PCO_2$, partial pressure of carbon dioxide; $PO_2$, partial pressure of oxygen.



## TREATMENT

### Assisting the Pulmonary Transition after Birth

At the time of birth, most of the lung is still fluid filled, and the infant clears the fluid by creating large expiratory pressures, also referred to as *expiratory braking*. Clinically, expiratory braking often presents itself as grunting and retractions. Due to the fact that fluid clearance takes time, most infants are cyanotic at birth and it takes them up to 10 minutes to attain an oxygen saturation ($SpO_2$) of 90% or more. It is clear that normal physiological pulmonary transition may be difficult to distinguish from RDS. For this reason, the initial treatment should be similar and consist of supporting the infant without causing injury to the vulnerable lungs.

### Respiratory Support

If the infant is spontaneously breathing, the expiratory phase of respiration should be supported with CPAP. If spontaneous breathing is absent or inadequate, positive-pressure ventilation should be initiated. There is insufficient evidence to support the use of a prolonged or sustained inflation. The fraction of inspired oxygen should be started between 0.21 and 0.30 and titrated according to the $SpO_2$ nomograms. If clinical signs of respiratory distress and cyanosis persist after the transitional phase, RDS is very likely and appropriate treatment should be started.

The primary aim in treatment of RDS is to restore lung function and gas exchange while avoiding treatment-induced injury to the vulnerable lungs of preterm infants. As low end-expiratory lung volume is the most prominent feature of RDS, stabilizing end-expiratory lung volume should be the first goal of treatment. In 1971, Gregory and colleagues showed the beneficial effects of CPAP on oxygenation. This improvement in oxygenation has been linked to a higher end-expiratory lung volume (Fig. 57-5). Recent studies have also shown that primary CPAP is the preferred mode of respiratory support after birth, as it reduces the need for invasive mechanical ventilation, surfactant treatment, and the risk of death or bronchopulmonary dysplasia. CPAP is usually administered via the nasal route using either a mask or prongs. Although the optimal level of CPAP still needs to be established, a continuous positive pressure of up to 6 to 10 $cmH_2O$ can be tolerated by the nasal route. Minimal invasive surfactant treatment (see below) and nasal intermittent positive-pressure ventilation might further enhance the success of CPAP in patients with RDS. However, there is insufficient evidence to support the use of humidified high-flow nasal cannula as an alternative primary mode for CPAP in infants with RDS.

In cases in which nasal noninvasive support is not effective in restoring lung function and gas exchange or if severe apnea occurs, intubation and mechanical ventilation should be started using either conventional modes or high-frequency ventilation. Again, maintaining an optimal lung volume should be the primary ventilation strategy when using these modes.

### Surfactant Replacement

Surfactant deficiency, 1 of the main features of RDS, can be treated by exogenous surfactant replacement. Administering exogenous surfactant into the lungs will lower the surface tension, improve lung compliance, and stabilize end-expiratory lung volume. Since the mid-1980s, a large number of carefully controlled clinical trials have been published showing that therapy with surfactant is safe, that it clearly reduces mortality from RDS, that it decreases the incidence of air leaks, and that in small infants it decreases the incidence of intracranial hemorrhage.

**Surfactant Products** Many different formulations of surfactant preparations are commercially available. Surfactant formulations fall into 3 major classes: (1) animal surfactants purified from animal lungs or bronchoalveolar lavage, (2) synthetic surfactants consisting primarily of phospholipids, and (3) synthetic surfactants that combine phospholipid mixtures with recombinant surfactant proteins or peptides based on surfactant protein structures. A recent systematic review of trials comparing animal-derived surfactant extract to synthetic surfactant consisting only of phospholipids showed that both are effective in the treatment and prevention of RDS. However, the benefits related to the need for ventilator support, the rate of pneumothoraces, and death were more pronounced when using animal-derived products. Although 2 trials of protein-containing synthetic surfactants compared to animal-derived surfactant extract showed no difference in death and chronic lung disease, further well-designed studies of adequate size and power are needed to confirm and refine these findings.

**Timing of Surfactant Therapy** There are 2 clearly defined treatment strategies for administration of surfactant: (1) prophylactic therapy, which requires the surfactant preparation to be instilled in the infant's trachea shortly after birth, preferably in the delivery room; and (2) rescue therapy, which is designed to treat infants with established RDS. The latter can be divided into early (< 2 hours after birth) or delayed (> 2 hours after birth) rescue treatment. It is important to acknowledge that most randomized controlled trials investigating the optimal timing of surfactant were performed in an era when antenatal corticosteroids were still being introduced in clinical care and primary intubation and mechanical ventilation (rather than the less invasive use of CPAP) was the preferred mode of respiratory support after birth. Under these circumstances, it was shown that mortality was lower in infants treated prophylactically compared with selective treatment, and in infants treated early compared with delayed rescue treatment.

More recent studies comparing invasive mechanical ventilation combined with prophylactic surfactant treatment to primary nasal CPAP and, if indicated, rescue surfactant treatment have shown that prophylactic treatment is associated with an increased risk of death or bronchopulmonary dysplasia (BPD). For this reason, prophylactic surfactant treatment is no longer recommended when using primary nasal CPAP at birth.

**Modes of Surfactant Delivery** Historically, surfactant was administered via an endotracheal tube during invasive mechanical ventilation. As the latter has been identified as a major risk factor for ventilator-induced lung injury and subsequent BPD, alternative, less invasive strategies of surfactant administration have been investigated. During the *Intubate SURfactant and Extubate* (INSURE) protocol, infants are intubated and surfactant is administered followed by immediate extubation to nasal CPAP. Compared with traditional surfactant treatment INSURE reduces the need for mechanical ventilation, but the effect on other clinical outcomes such as mortality and BPD at 36 weeks postmenstrual age is limited. With the aim of avoiding intubation altogether, some investigators explored the feasibility of administering surfactant during spontaneous breathing on nasal CPAP. Several studies have now shown that this route of administration, often referred to as *less-invasive surfactant application* (LISA) or minimally invasive surfactant therapy (MIST), reduces the need for invasive mechanical ventilation and death or BPD at 36 weeks postmenstrual age. Other modes of surfactant delivery, including the use of a laryngeal mask or nebulized surfactant administration, still need further evaluation.

### General Support of Infants with RDS

The infant should be cared for in a warm, neutral thermal environment. Initially, fluid intake should be restricted to 60 to 80 mL/kg and thereafter titrated on diuresis and serum sodium concentration. If the arterial pressure is low in the early course of the disease and if peripheral circulation is inadequate, as judged by poor capillary filling, the circulating volume may be increased with normal saline. Infusion of dopamine (5–10 μg/kg/min) may help maintain the circulation and avoid excessive fluid administration, especially in the very low–birth-weight infant. Given that the clinical presentation and radiographic findings of RDS and neonatal pneumonia—particularly secondary to *group B streptococcus*—may initially be indistinguishable, there should be a low threshold for starting antibiotics in infants presenting with respiratory distress after birth.

## COMPLICATIONS AND OUTCOMES

As a result of antenatal steroids, exogenous surfactant and gentler (noninvasive) modes of respiratory support, the majority of preterm infants nowadays survive the phase of early respiratory failure due to RDS. The most common short-term complication of RDS is pulmonary air leak. In the longer term, BPD can develop, especially if infants need a longer period of invasive mechanical ventilation. BPD itself results in prolonged need for supplemental oxygen, a higher incidence of respiratory illness with wheezing in the first years of life, and an increased risk of adverse neurodevelopmental outcome.

## SUGGESTED READINGS


Aldana-Aguirre JC, Pinto M, Featherstone RM, Kumar M. Less invasive surfactant administration versus intubation for surfactant delivery in preterm infants with respiratory distress syndrome: a systematic review and meta-analysis. *Arch Dis Child Fetal Neonatal Ed.* 2017;102(1):F17-F23.

Ardell S, Pfister RH, Soll R. Animal derived surfactant extract versus protein free synthetic surfactant for the prevention and treatment of respiratory distress syndrome. *Cochrane Database Syst Rev.* 2015;(5):CD000144.

Bahadue F, Soll R. Early versus delayed selective surfactant treatment for neonatal respiratory distress syndrome. *Cochrane Database Syst Rev.* 2012:CD001456.

Crowther CA, McKinlay CJ, Middleton P, Harding JE. Repeat doses of prenatal corticosteroids for women at risk of preterm birth for improving neonatal health outcomes. *Cochrane Database Syst Rev.* 2011;(5):CD003935.

Dawson JA, Kamlin CO, Vento M, et al. Defining the reference range for oxygen saturation for infants after birth. *Pediatrics.* 2010;125(6):e1340-e1347.

Engle WA; American Academy of Pediatrics Committee on Fetus and Newborn. Surfactant-replacement therapy for respiratory distress in the preterm and term neonate. *Pediatrics.* 2008; 121(2):419-432.

Gregory GA, Kitterman JA, Phibbs RH, Tooley WH, Hamilton WK. Treatment of the idiopathic respiratory-distress syndrome with continuous positive airway pressure. *N Engl J Med.* 1971;284(24): 1333-1340.

Gyamfi-Bannerman C, Thom EA, Blackwell SC, et al. Antenatal betamethasone for women at risk for late preterm delivery. *N Engl J Med.* 2016;374(14):1311-1320.

Liggins GC, Howie RN. A controlled trial of antepartum glucocorticoid treatment for prevention of the respiratory distress syndrome in premature infants. *Pediatrics.* 1972;50(4):515-525.

Meneses J, Bhandari V, Alves JG, Herrmann D. Noninvasive ventilation for respiratory distress syndrome: a randomized controlled trial. *Pediatrics.* 2011;127(2):300-307.

Pfister R, Soll R, Wiswell T. Protein-containing synthetic surfactant versus animal derived surfactant extract for the prevention and treatment of respiratory distress syndrome. *Cochrane Database Syst Rev.* 2007;(3):CD006069.

Rojas-Reyes M, Morley C, Soll R. Prophylactic versus selective use of surfactant in preventing morbidity and mortality in preterm infants. *Cochrane Database Syst Rev.* 2012;(3):CD000510.

Schmölzer GM, Kumar M, Pichler G, Aziz K, O'Reilly M, Cheung PY. Non-invasive versus invasive respiratory support in preterm infants at birth: systematic review and meta-analysis. *BMJ.* 2013;347:f5980.

Stevens TP, Harrington EW, Blennow M, Soll RF. Early surfactant administration with brief ventilation vs. selective surfactant and continued mechanical ventilation for preterm infants with or at risk for respiratory distress syndrome. *Cochrane Database Syst Rev.* 2007;(4):CD003063.

Verder H, Ebbesen F, Fenger-Grøn J, et al. Early surfactant guided by lamellar body counts on gastric aspirate in very preterm infants. *Neonatology.* 2013;104(2):116-122.

Wilkinson D, Andersen C, O'Donnell CP, De Paoli AG, Manley BJ. High flow nasal cannula for respiratory support in preterm infants. *Cochrane Database Syst Rev.* 2016;(2):CD006405.

Wyllie J, Bruinenberg J, Roehr CC, Rüdiger M, Trevisanuto D, Urlesberger B. European Resuscitation Council Guidelines for Resuscitation 2015. Section 7. Resuscitation and support of transition of babies at birth. *Resuscitation.* 2015;95:249-263.

# 58 Patent Ductus Arteriosus: From Bench to Bedside

Carl H. Backes, Claire Kovalchin, Brian K. Rivera, and Charles V. Smith



## INTRODUCTION

The ductus arteriosus (DA) is a vital component of the fetal circulation, when the placenta is the source of oxygen to the fetus. The DA provides a conduit for blood to bypass the high resistance pulmonary vascular bed and shunt toward the descending aorta and low-resistance placental circulation. At birth, the lungs are inflated and resistance in the pulmonary vascular bed decreases as the lungs become the source of oxygenation, rendering the DA no longer necessary. Over the first few days of life, the DA undergoes active constriction and occlusion; failure of this process results in a patent ductus arteriosus (PDA). In the majority (> 95%) of term infants and those born > 28 weeks of gestation, closure of the ductus occurs within hours. In contrast, PDAs occur in 70% of infants born prior to 28 weeks of gestation, with an incidence that is inversely proportional to gestational age (GA) at birth.

## BIOLOGICAL FACTORS

Closure of the DA involves a number of cellular and molecular processes that occur over 2 phases: (1) "functional" closure within hours after birth, characterized by ductal smooth muscle constriction; (2) "anatomic" occlusion over the next several days, characterized by ductal remodeling in response to hypoxia/ischemia of smooth muscle cells, resulting in permanent closure. Premature birth interrupts the normal maturation of ductal contractile mechanisms, increasing the likelihood of a PDA.

### PATHOPHYSIOLOGY AND FUNCTIONAL CLOSURE OF THE DA

In the fetus, most of the cardiac output from the right ventricle bypasses the lungs and flows from the main pulmonary artery (MPA) into the descending aorta via the DA. A number of factors regulate the magnitude of ductal shunting, including its size (diameter, length), pressure differences between the aorta and pulmonary artery, and systemic and pulmonary vascular resistances (SVR and PVR, respectively). If the diameter of the PDA is small, the diminutive cross-sectional opening offers a high resistance to flow; thus, shunting is minimal despite potentially large pressure differences. On the other hand, with a large ductal diameter, pressures tend to be similar, and the magnitude of the ductal shunting is determined primarily by a balance between SVR and PVR. The right-to-left ductal shunting in utero is due to the high PVR, which in combination with a low SVR, results in a low pulmonary blood flow during fetal life.

At birth, ventilation of the lungs triggers a large decrease in PVR, which coincides with an increase in SVR following removal of the placental circulation by clamping of the umbilical cord. These events result in a marked increase in pulmonary blood flow, and as PVR falls below SVR, there may be left-to-right ductal shunting through the DA from the aorta and into the pulmonary circulation (see also Chapter 45).

At birth, the dramatic, rapid rise in arterial oxygen content upon ventilation of the lungs triggers a cascade of events in which constriction of the DA would normally occur. With increasing gestational maturation, the amount of ductal constriction in response to increasing partial pressure of oxygen ($pO_2$) is greater, and the level of $pO_2$ required for initiation and maintenance of this process decreases.

The potential cellular mechanisms responsible for ductal constriction are summarized in Figure 58-1, and include the inhibition of voltage-dependent potassium channels by production of reactive oxygen species, the endothelin-1 constrictor pathway, and a fall in circulating prostaglandin $E_2$ ($PGE_2$) levels following clamping of the umbilical cord. $PGE_2$ is the most important prostanoid to regulate ductal patency in the fetus and neonate, and is produced by the placenta and ductus. In addition, the marked increase in pulmonary blood flow at birth promotes lung catabolism of circulating $PGE_2$, promoting ductal closure.

The mechanisms responsible for ductal constriction may be developmentally regulated. The formation of alveoli is believed to begin at approximately 28 weeks' gestation. Studies in preterm animal models have demonstrated an immaturity of both potassium and calcium channels. These impairments and other physiological consequences of preterm birth lead to ineffective oxygen-mediated constriction of the DA. The reduced pulmonary blood flow and metabolism among preterm infants contributes to increased circulating concentrations of $PGE_2$ and persistent ductal patency. Additionally, the sensitivity to $PGE_2$ is greater in preterm neonates than in more mature infants. Excessive fluid intake (> 170 mL/kg/day) has also been associated with increased risk of continued patency of the DA.

### ANATOMIC CLOSURE OF THE DA

Successful "functional" closure of the ductus results locally in ischemic hypoxia of the ductal wall. This results in cell death and production of hypoxia-mediated growth factors, which play a role in vascular remodeling and *permanent* ductal closure. Intimal thickening of the DA is also required for permanent ductal closure. Insufficient ductal smooth muscle constriction prevents the histological changes (intimal thickening, fragmentation of the internal elastic lamina) necessary for permanent closure of the DA.

Even minor alterations in the hypoxia-dependent mechanism may prevent anatomic DA closure. This potentially explains the proclivity of the ductus to "reopen" after echocardiographic evidence of its closure. The localized region of hypoxia within the ductal wall is promoted by the initial constriction of the ductus, which leads to cell death and ductal remodeling. It has been reported that, in DAs with no clinical signs of ductal patency after pharmacological therapy, those with residual luminal blood flow had a higher rate of reopening than did those with no luminal flow. The residual blood flow may provide sufficient oxygen to the luminal cells and tissues, preventing hypoxia-promoted closure. Mechanisms promoting ductal relaxation may then eventually lead to "reopening" of the ductus.

## DIAGNOSIS AND EVALUATION

### Clinical Assessment

The clinical features associated with shunting through the PDA depend on the magnitude of the ductal shunt and the compensatory ability of the immature myocardium to handle the additional volume load. The cardiac function of preterm infants (< 37 weeks) is more vulnerable to preload and afterload changes than those in their more mature counterparts.

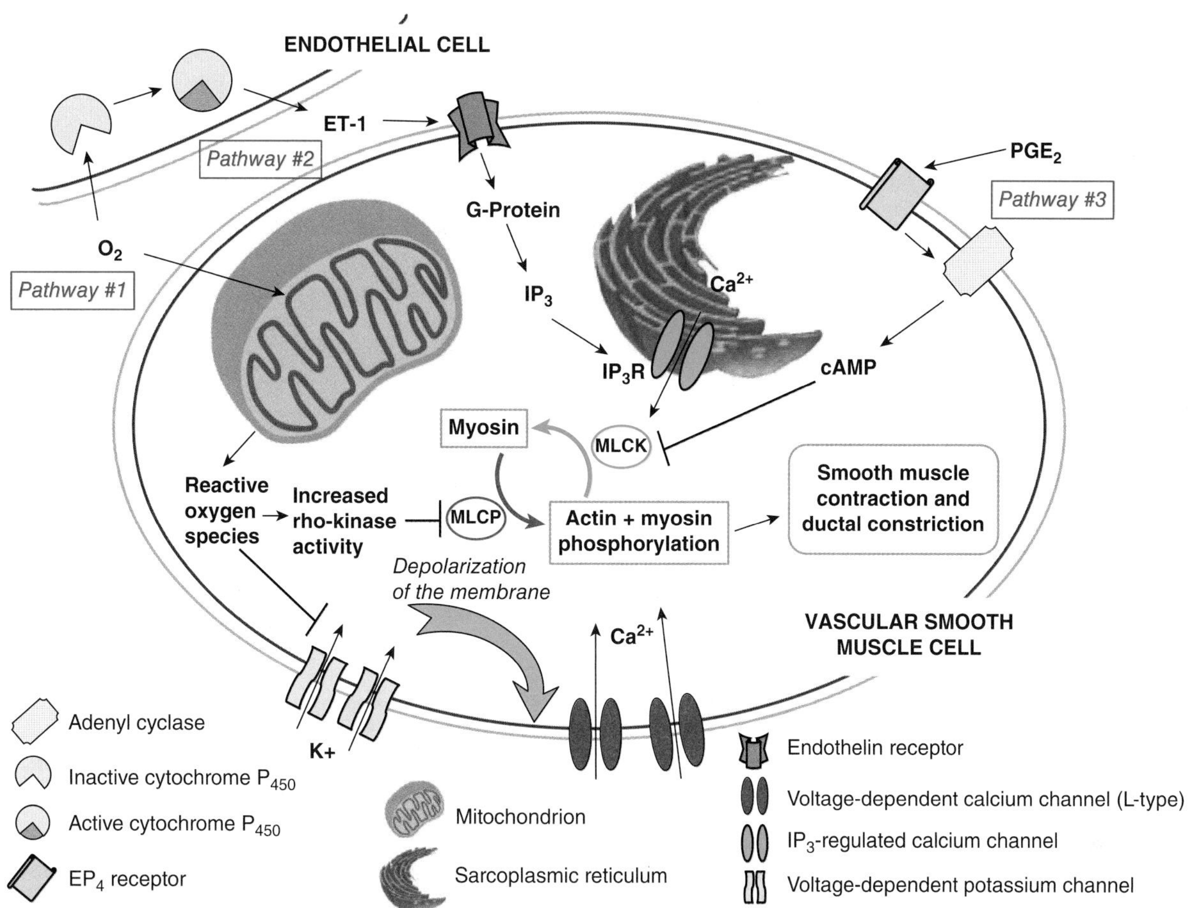


**FIGURE 58-1** A schematic model of mechanisms responsible for ductus arteriosis closure. $Ca^{2+}$, calcium ion; cAMP, cyclic adenosine monophosphate; $EP_4$ receptor, selective prostaglandin E receptor 4; ET-1, endothelin-1, ETA; G-protein, G-coupled receptor protein; $IP_3$, inositol triphosphate; $IP_3R$, $IP_3$ receptor; $K^+$, potassium ion; MLCK, myosin light chain kinase; MLCP, myosin light chain phosphatase; $O_2$, oxygen; $PGE_2$, prostaglandin $E_2$.

The murmur associated with a PDA is commonly heard best at the left sternal border in the second and third intercostal spaces. While older children may display the classic continuous, machinery murmur, very premature infants more commonly have a high frequency systolic murmur with a "rocky" quality. With increasing left-sided volume loading, a prominent second heart sound, mid-diastolic flow rumble at the apex, and a third heart sound may be present. As the left-to-right ductal shunt increases, the precordium becomes hyperactive, pulse pressure widens, and the peripheral pulses become more prominent. If the shunt becomes sufficiently large, evidence of left ventricular failure, including tachycardia, tachypnea, and rales on auscultation of the lung, may develop.

#### Usefulness of Clinical Assessment

Recent investigators have challenged the isolated use of clinical signs, with evidence of poor consistency and limited accuracy. During the first few days of life, preterm infants with large PDAs may have no clinical signs on physical examination due to a higher PVR, lower ductal shunt velocity, and compensatory increases in pulmonary lymph flow clearing the respiratory interstitum of excess fluid and protein. Thus, in most cases, even in the presence of a large PDA, pulmonary mechanics may not be adversely affected during the first 72 hours after birth. Following the expected drop in PVR over the first week of life, the murmur becomes apparent. After this time, the sensitivity and specificity of a murmur to diagnose a PDA are 79% and 94%, respectively. The left-to-right ductal shunt leads to tachycardia and increased stroke volume, which manifest clinically as hyperactive precordium, increased pulse volume, and wide pulse pressure. While these physical exam findings, alongside evidence of pulmonary overcirculation and left heart dilation on a chest radiograph, increase clinical suspicion for a PDA, the accurate diagnosis of ductal patency requires Doppler echocardiography.

#### Echocardiography

Echocardiography is the gold standard for PDA diagnosis. Two-dimensional echocardiography with Doppler flow studies provide accurate assessment of (1) ductal size (diameter), (2) pattern of ductal shunting, and (3) volume of ductal shunting. These echocardiographic indices can be used to define a hemodynamically significant PDA (HSPDA), discussed below (Figs. 58-2 to 58-6).

#### PDA Size

Ductal size is measured at the site of maximal constriction in end systole (Fig. 58-3). Traditionally, a ductal diameter > 1.5 mm is used define a HSPDA. However, this dimension cannot alone determine the need for PDA treatment or predict the likelihood of spontaneous closure. Alternatively, others have proposed indexing ductal diameter-to-body weight (in mm per kg) or left pulmonary artery (LPA) diameter (PDA:LPA ratio). The likelihood of spontaneous ductal closure during the first 3 days of life when there is a low PDA:LPA ratio (< 0.5) is 3-fold higher than if the ratio is large (≥ 1) or moderate (≥ 0.5–1). The relative benefits and limitations of different indices of PDA size remain incompletely characterized.

#### Flow Pattern

The primary direction and velocity of ductal shunting can be approximated using color Doppler; however, accurate determination of shunt velocity and directionality requires pulsed Doppler interrogation (Figs. 58-4 to 58-6). The pattern of Doppler shunting reflects the relative pressures (aortic and main pulmonary artery) at each end of the ductus in systole and diastole. For instance, when aortic pressure exceeds the pressure in the MPA, the shunt is left to right (positive tracing), but when MPA pressure exceeds aortic pressure, the shunt is right to left (negative tracing).

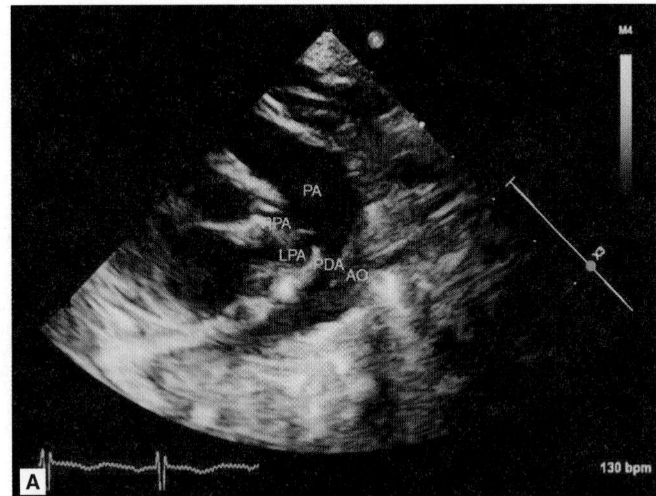


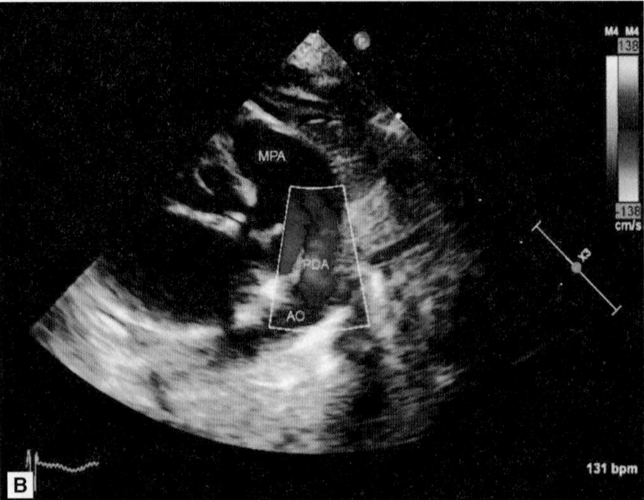


**FIGURE 58-2** **A:** Suprasternal ("ductal view") echocardiographic image showing the PDA connecting the pulmonary artery and aorta, as well as relationship to right and left pulmonary arteries. **B:** Similar image with color-flow Doppler indicating left-to-right ductal shunting (*red flow*). Ao, aorta; LPA, left pulmonary artery; MPA, main pulmonary artery; PA, pulmonary artery; PDA, patent ductus arteriosus; RPA, right pulmonary artery.

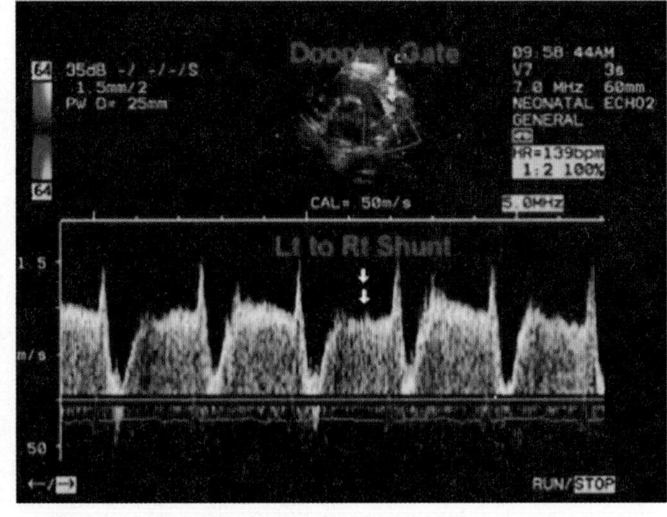


**FIGURE 58-4** Pulsed Doppler echocardiographic image of left-to-right flow through a patent ductus arteriosus. Note the positive (upward) trace.

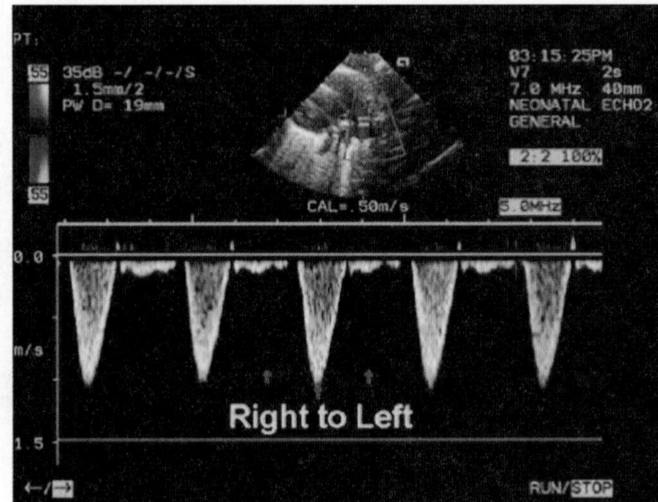


**FIGURE 58-5** Pulsed Doppler echocardiographic image of right-to-left flow through a patent ductus arteriosus in patient with severe pulmonary hypertension. Note the negative (downward) trace.

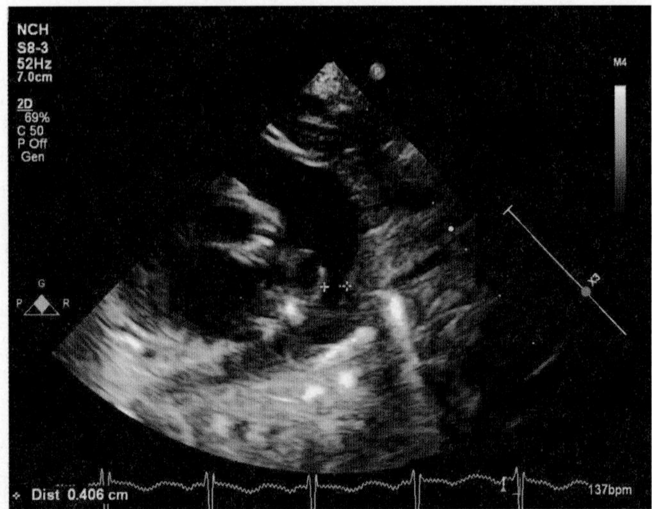


**FIGURE 58-3** Two-dimensional echocardiography from a high-parasternal ("ductal view"). The diameter of the ductus is ~4 mm measured at the site of maximal constriction.

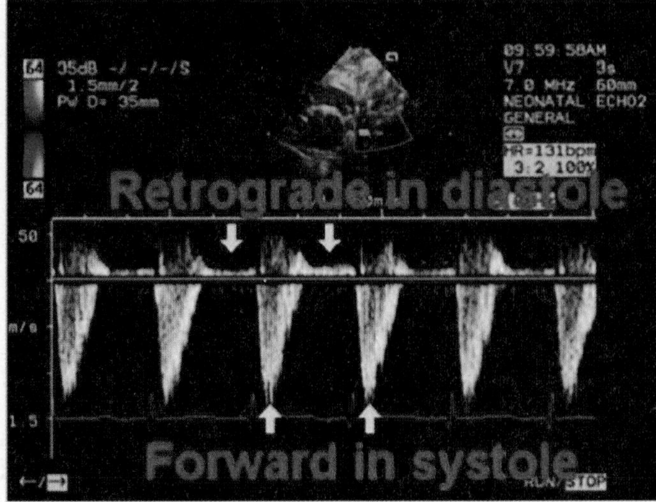


**FIGURE 58-6** Doppler image showing reverse (retrograde) flow in the descending aorta during diastole.

### Shunt Volume

The accurate measurement of the volume of ductal shunting requires cardiac catheterization, but the invasive nature of the procedure limits the feasibility of this in fragile neonates. A number of echocardiographic indices have been proposed to assess the volume of ductal shunting indirectly, including left atrial–to–aortic root ratios, left ventricular size, left ventricular output, and diastolic flow in the descending aorta. Retrograde diastolic blood flow in the descending aorta may represent the echocardiographic marker that best reflects the circulatory consequences of an HSPDA. The normal diastolic flow in the postductal descending aorta is low-velocity forward flow but as ductal shunting increases, the diastolic flow becomes progressively less and may become retrograde (Fig. 58-6).

## DEFINING A HEMODYNAMICALLY SIGNIFICANT PDA

Rather than an all-or-none approach in the determination and treatment of PDAs, efforts to define HSPDA according to the severity of echocardiographic criteria may provide a more selective approach to care and help to identify the subset of infants that are most likely to benefit from treatment (Table 58-1). Targeted use of PDA treatment in those with an HSPDA may enable healthcare providers to minimize risk and yield the greatest benefits.

An HSPDA has been defined based on ductal size or left heart dimensions (ratio of left atrium to aorta), and those echocardiographic indices are correlated to the likelihood of subsequent ductal closure or to a range of short or longer-term clinical outcomes. For instance, neonates with ductal diameters > 1.5 mm had the highest odds of an adverse outcome, whereas infants with PDA diameters ≤ 1.5 mm had outcomes similar to those with no PDA. Moreover, HSPDAs are less likely to close spontaneously than are small PDAs. However, marked heterogeneity in the criteria to define an HSPDA and the threshold for diagnosis or treatment of an HSPDA, limit equitable comparisons among studies. Despite widespread use of the term, consensus on the definition of HSPDA is lacking. More importantly, no studies have shown that treating, or not treating, an HSPDA improves longer-term outcomes. Recently, PDA scoring systems that take into account both clinical and echocardiographic data have been proposed and may provide more robust models for outcome prediction and allow further refinements in PDA management.

**TABLE 58-1 DEFINING A HEMODYNAMICALLY SIGNIFICANT PATENT DUCTUS ARTERIOSUS**

| Echocardiographic Parameter | Measure | HSPDA Cutoffs |
|---|---|---|
| Size | Minimum PDA diameter (mm) | ≥ 1.5 |
| | PDA/LPA | > 0.5 |
| | PDA diameter/kg weight (mm/kg) | ≥ 1.4 |
| Shunt pattern | End diastolic/peak systolic velocity across ductus | < 0.5 |
| Shunt volume | LA/aortic root[a] | ≥ 1.4 |
| | LV/aorta | > 2.1 |
| | Antegrade diastolic flow in MPA (pulsed-wave Doppler) | ≥ 0.5 |
| | Resistance index (cerebral Doppler) | ≥ 0.9 |
| | End-diastolic velocity in LPA (cm/s) | > 30–40 |
| | Left ventricular output, mL/min/kg | > 314 |
| | Diastolic flow pattern in systemic arteries[b] | Absent or retrograde flow |

[a]Ratio of diameters determined by M-mode echocardiography from parasternal long-axis view.

[b]Systemic arteries include descending aorta, middle cerebral, and superior mesenteric.

HSPDA, hemodynamically significant patent ductus arteriosus; LA, left atrium; LPA, left pulmonary artery; LV, left ventricle; MPA, main pulmonary artery; PDA, patent ductus arteriosus

## RISK FACTORS AND COMORBIDITIES ASSOCIATED WITH PDA

A ductal left-to-right shunt increases the pulmonary blood flow, which may eventually lead to pulmonary edema and decreased lung compliance. These changes in lung mechanics often require positive pressure and higher oxygen concentrations to maintain respiratory stability, but over time these contribute to the development of bronchopulmonary dysplasia (BPD).

Among preterm infants, persistent left-to-right shunting not only decreases lung function but also may lead to cardiac dysfunction, due to left-sided volume overload. These factors, coupled with a ductal steal phenomenon, may worsen systemic perfusion and contribute to a number of PDA-related morbidities. Although no causal link has been established, a PDA is considered by some to be a precursor to a number of morbidities, including BPD, neurological abnormalities, and necrotizing enterocolitis (NEC). Infants with a PDA have an 8-fold higher mortality than age-matched controls with a closed ductus.

### NEUROLOGICAL MORBIDITIES

Immediately after birth, preterm infants may lack cerebral autoregulation, placing them at risk for decreased cerebral perfusion in the setting of hypotension. This renders premature neonates vulnerable to neurological morbidities, including intraventricular hemorrhage (IVH). Because IVH typically occurs shortly after birth, prophylactic PDA treatment as a strategy to prevent IVH has gained considerable interest. Prophylactic indomethacin reduces IVH, but longer-term neurodevelopmental benefits at a corrected age of 18 months have not been observed.

### SUPPORTIVE THERAPY

Irrespective of the treatment approach, all neonates with PDA should receive supportive care to minimize symptoms related to ductal shunting.

### POSITIVE PRESSURE VENTILATION

Positive pressure ventilation (positive end-expiratory pressure, or PEEP) is intended to improve gas exchange and minimize the adverse effects of ductal shunting with pulmonary edema. However, the impact of prolonged positive pressure respiratory ventilation on feeding behavior and neurodevelopment remains poorly understood.

### FLUID RESTRICTION

Fluid restriction is widely recommended as a measure to limit the physiologic consequences of excessive volume load on the pulmonary circulation. Randomized studies and meta-analyses have demonstrated an association between higher fluid intake and PDA, and in turn between PDA and both congestive heart failure and NEC. Fluid restriction has been shown to reduce the risks of PDA, without increasing the risk of adverse consequences.

### DIURETICS

Diuretic therapy is intended to optimize lung compliance and oxygenation. However, furosemide (a loop diuretic) stimulates renal synthesis of $PGE_2$, and has been shown to increase the rate of ductal patency twofold when compared to chlorothiazide. In view of the evidence that furosemide may increase the prevalence of PDA, its routine use is not recommended.

### TREATMENT OF THE PATENT DUCTUS ARTERIOSUS

There exists consensus that a PDA should be closed by 2 years of age, to avoid the risks of pulmonary hypertension or bacterial endocarditis, but disagreement remains about the thresholds and strategies for PDA closure among extremely premature infants earlier in life. Some advocate closing PDAs aggressively, based on observational data showing

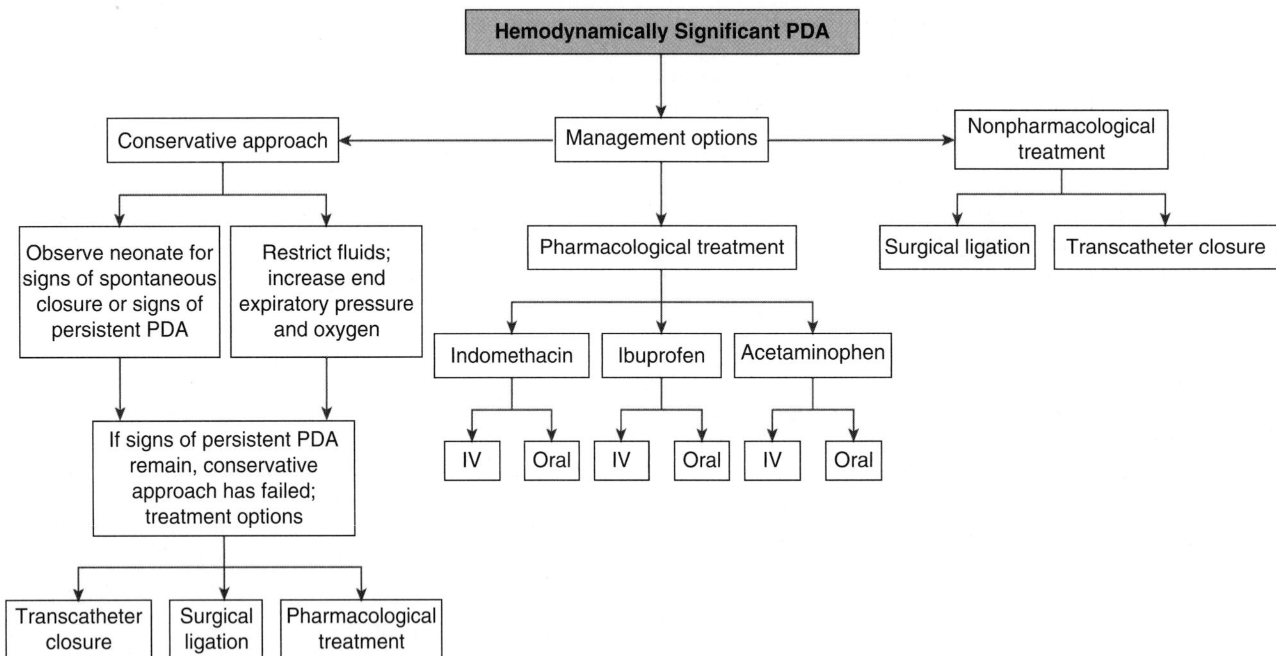


**FIGURE 58-7** Management algorithm for hemodynamically significant PDA. IV, intravenous; PDA, patent ductus arteriosus.



improved short-term outcomes following ductal closure. However, evidence for improved outcomes following treatment is not strong. Although *associated* with higher mortality and morbidity, PDA may not be causative. The treatment of PDA in preterm infants can be conservative, pharmacological (indomethacin, ibuprofen, acetaminophen), or nonpharmacological (catheter-based closure or surgical ligation), but the optimal approach has not been determined through prospective studies with long-term follow-up (Fig. 58-7).

## CONSERVATIVE MANAGEMENT

The conservative approach to the management of PDA through supportive therapy is aimed at reducing symptoms from the ductal shunt and providing the opportunity for spontaneous closure, thereby avoiding the risks of potentially unnecessary interventions. To date, the only randomized controlled trial (RCT) comparing treatment of an HSPDA versus conservative management was conducted over 30 years ago. In that study, the early surgical ligation group had lower rates of adverse outcomes than did the nonintervention group; however, the applicability of these findings in the setting of contemporary neonatal treatment (eg, antenatal corticosteroids, surfactant therapy) is controversial.

The rate of spontaneous ductal closure within the first 4 days of life is greater than 95% in neonates with birth weights > 1500 grams. In a single-center, prospective study of 122 infants with average birth weight of less than 800 grams, spontaneous permanent ductal closure occurred in 42 (34%), whereas the vast majority (80/122) had a persistent ductal shunt. Factors that predicted spontaneous closure included greater GA and absence of respiratory distress syndrome.

The natural history of the PDA in premature infants remains poorly characterized, though persistence beyond the first few days of life can still be associated with later closure. Spontaneous closure rates of around one-third have been observed by day 8 of life in infants with birth weights < 1000 grams, while closure by 165 days has been reported in approximately three-quarters of those born at 24 to 27 weeks of gestation. In a single-center, retrospective, observational study of infants with birth weights < 1500 grams, 21 infants were discharged home with an open ductus. Of those infants, 18 (86%) PDAs spontaneously closed at a mean post menstrual age of 48 weeks (51 days of life); none of the infants had evidence of heart failure secondary to prolonged PDA exposure.

Despite insufficient data on the risks associated with prolonged exposure to PDAs, recent evidence suggests a marked change among US providers away from traditional drug therapy and surgical ligation toward a conservative treatment approach. While conservative treatment may be a useful adjunct to ductal closure and may reduce unnecessary medical therapy or surgical ligation in an appreciable number of infants, the question remains as to what to do when PDAs fail to close following a period of conservative treatment, particularly if there are clinical and echocardiographic signs of an HSPDA or a need for continued respiratory support at a corrected age of 36 weeks.

## PHARMACOLOGICAL THERAPY

Among infants with a PDA warranting closure, 3 primary pharmacological options are available: indomethacin, ibuprofen, and acetaminophen (paracetamol) (Table 58-2). Studies have consistently shown that

**TABLE 58-2 PHARMACOLOGICAL TREATMENTS: TIMING AND DOSAGE**

| Treatment and Timing | Dosage |
|---|---|
| Indomethacin (IV)[a] | |
| Prophylactic treatment | 0.2 mg/kg, then 0.1 mg/kg at 12, 24, and 48 hours |
| Early symptomatic treatment (2–6 days) | 0.2 mg/kg, then 0.1 mg/kg at 12, 24, and 48 hours |
| Late symptomatic treatment (> 7 days) | 0.2 mg/kg at 0, 12, 24, and 48 hours |
| Ibuprofen (oral, 20 mg/mL)[b] | |
| Symptomatic treatment | 10 mg/kg, then 5mg/kg at 24 and 48 hours |
| Ibuprofen (IV) | |
| Prophylactic treatment | Not recommended |
| Symptomatic treatment | 10 mg/kg, then 5mg/kg at 24 and 48 hours |
| Acetaminophen/paracetamol (oral, IV) | |
| Symptomatic treatment | 15 mg/kg every 6 hours for 3 days |

[a]Indomethacin should always be infused over a period of at least 30 minutes.

[b]Commercial preparations of oral ibuprofen should be followed by 2 mL/kg of milk or water, as it is hyperosmolar.

Indomethacin and ibuprofen should not be used when renal impairment, thrombocytopenia, and active bleeding problems are evident. Exercise caution with hypotensive neonates or neonates who have been treated with postnatal corticosteroids.

IV, intravenous.

cyclooxygenase (COX) inhibitors, including indomethacin and ibuprofen, are more effective than placebo in closing the PDA in preterm infants. While indomethacin and ibuprofen are the only 2 US Federal Drug Administration–approved drugs for closure of a ductus in preterm babies, recent published experiences suggest that acetaminophen also may have a role. Data are not clear on which infants will respond to drug therapy. Some studies report no differences between responders and nonresponders, while other studies have suggested that failure is related to maturational factors (eg, birth weight, GA). The choice of 1 drug over the other also depends on local availability of the intravenous or enteral preparation.

### Indomethacin

Indomethacin mediates its effects, at least in part, by inhibiting local prostaglandin synthesis, and evidence exists to support its use. The potential timing of indomethacin varies according to whether a prophylactic, early, or late treatment is being considered.

The relative benefits of early versus late therapy have not yet been clearly established. Indomethacin therapy in the first 2 days of life is associated with higher rates of PDA closure than later treatment. Among 8 trials including 264 infants, early symptomatic treatment was associated with lower risks for BPD (odds ratio [OR], 0.39; 95% confidence interval [CI], 0.21–0.76) or NEC (OR, 0.24; 95% CI, 0.06–0.96), and need for surgical ligation (OR, 0.37; 95% CI, 0.20–0.68). On the other hand, in a large population-based cohort of infants born prior to 27 weeks of gestation, no differences in the rates of PDA surgery or death were observed following early (0–2 days), intermediate (3–6 days), or late (≥ 7 days) pharmacological treatment.

The optimal dosing strategy of indomethacin remains unknown. Although plasma drug concentrations correlate poorly with drug efficacy and side effects, some advocate for the potential value of obtaining plasma drug levels to titrate treatment regimens; however, data on optimal levels are not widely available and this approach is poorly characterized. A multicenter RCT that investigated the correlation between indomethacin levels and continued ductal patency showed that higher serum indomethacin concentrations were not associated with lower rates of patency, but were linked with higher rates of nephrotoxicity and retinopathy of prematurity.

Because indomethacin provides only transient suppression of prostaglandin synthesis, multiple courses of indomethacin are typically provided to achieve ductal constriction; however, data to support the provision of multiple courses of indomethacin are lacking, and prolonged treatment courses have been associated with an increased risk of NEC and renal impairment. These observations are consistent with a recent RCT that reported no difference in ductal closure rates but did report trends toward lower rates of NEC (1.4% vs 7%), following therapy with 3 versus 6 doses of indomethacin. These studies suggest that prolonged courses of indomethacin treatment should not be part of the routine management of the PDA during neonatal period.

### Ibuprofen

Among the COX inhibitors, it has been advocated that ibuprofen should be the preferred agent for PDA closure. Some studies have shown that while the rate of successful ductal closure with ibuprofen and indomethacin are similar, the rates of NEC and renal insufficiency, and the duration of mechanical ventilation are lower with ibuprofen. However, data on the safety of ibuprofen versus indomethacin are mixed. A recent study of over 6300 infants born at < 28 weeks of gestation reported similar short-term safety outcomes following exposure to indomethacin versus ibuprofen. Moreover, data shows that ibuprofen, but not indomethacin, interferes with binding of serum albumin at standard doses of the drugs, which would increase the risk of kernicterus among infants treated with ibuprofen.

Regarding the optimal route for administration, it has been shown that orogastric administration is as effective as intravenous administration. However, questions regarding the optimal dosing strategy, early versus expectant administration, and continuous versus intermittent dosing, remain unanswered. Data showing that prophylactic ibuprofen does not appear to be effective in preventing IVH, and may be associated with an increased risk of pulmonary hypertension, have led experts to recommend against the use of prophylactic ibuprofen.



**TABLE 58-3 CONTRAINDICATIONS TO USE OF INDOMETHACIN**

- Active gastrointestinal bleeding
- Necrotizing enterocolitis (NEC), active or suspected
- Creatinine ≥ 1.8–2.0 mg/dL
- Urine output < 1 mL/kg/h
- Platelet count < 50,000
- Active infection
- Suspected congenital heart disease
- Known gastrointestinal or renal anomaly

### Complications and Contraindications of COX Inhibitors

A number of studies have examined the short-term adverse effects of COX inhibitors in preterm infants. Indomethacin decreases gastrointestinal, renal, and cerebral blood flow. Consequently, treatment with indomethacin has been associated with spontaneous intestinal perforation, necrotizing enterocolitis, renal insufficiency, and altered cerebral perfusion. Importantly, healthcare providers should be aware of the high risk for isolated gastrointestinal perforation among preterm infants treated concurrently with indomethacin and dexamethasone. Despite the lack of consensus, a number of contraindications to COX inhibitors are shown in Table 58-3.

### Enteral Feeding during Therapy with COX Inhibitors

Indomethacin decreases intestinal blood flow and disrupts the gastrointestinal mucosal barrier function. While ibuprofen has less effect on gastrointestinal blood flow than does indomethacin, gastrointestinal permeability is altered following ibuprofen therapy. These findings have led to concerns that initiation or advancement of enteral feedings during PDA treatment with indomethacin or ibuprofen may increase the risk of adverse health outcomes in infants. However, a study of 177 infants born at < 31 weeks of gestation reported that infants randomized to trophic feeds (15 mL/kg/day) required less time to achieve the feeding goal (120 mL/kg/day) than did infants who remained nil per os (NPO) while receiving indomethacin or ibuprofen therapy. These observations are consistent with the growing body of literature on the safety and efficacy of enteral feeding during PDA treatment with COX inhibitors. Questions remain on optimal feeding regimens for high-risk subgroups of infants, including those with echocardiographic evidence of reversal or absence of perfusion in mesenteric arteries and those with intrauterine growth restriction. In these high-risk subgroups, a more judicious feeding regimen may be prudent.

### Failure to Respond to Initial Medical Management with COXI Inhibitors

Initial medical therapy with COX inhibitors will close the PDA in 50% to 75% of infants. Among infants failing to respond to initial therapy and with persistent HSPDA, a second course of treatment can be provided. Despite limited data, available evidence suggests a second course of pharmacological therapy results in closure rates of 40% to 56%. If a patient fails to responds to 2 courses of therapy, the success of additional drug treatment in closing the PDA is unlikely. In this clinical scenario, healthcare providers must reassess the indications for PDA closure and the potential hemodynamic consequences of the persistent ductus. In settings of a persistently small PDA, a recent study suggests that approximately 75% will spontaneously close on their own without pharmacological treatment.

### Acetaminophen

Data on the risks of indomethacin and ibuprofen have led to interest in alternative medical therapies for PDA closure, including acetaminophen (paracetamol). While small, observational reports suggest that acetaminophen may be an effective treatment for PDA, data on the risk/benefit profile of acetaminophen among preterm infants remain unknown. A recent Cochrane review identified only 2 RCTs involving acetaminophen for PDA closure in preterm infants. No differences in the rates of ductal closure between infants treated with acetaminophen versus oral ibuprofen were observed, but a lack of high-quality studies to guide evidence-based decision-making was recognized. A recent systematic review and meta-analysis included 16 studies, 14 of which were uncontrolled studies, comparing acetaminophen versus indomethacin, ibuprofen, or placebo. The authors reported ductal closure rates with acetaminophen of 49% (95% CI, 29–69%) and 76% (95% CI, 61–88%), respectively, following 3 and 6 days of treatment. Moreover, a recent study showed that, among infants born at < 32 weeks of gestation with a confirmed PDA, the ductus closed faster in the acetaminophen group than the placebo group (177 hours versus 338 hours for acetaminophen versus placebo, respectively) without detectable side effects. However, studies in animal models raise concerns that acetaminophen may have adverse effects on brain maturation, thus its routine use cannot be recommended prior to a more robust understanding of potential longer-term risks, including neurocognitive status.

## NONPHARMACOLOGIC INTERVENTION

### Surgical Ligation

Surgical ligation provides definitive PDA closure. While early surgical mortality is low, known risks of PDA ligation include pneumothorax, bleeding, and left vocal cord paralysis. Preterm infants are at risk for post-ligation cardiac syndrome (PLCS), characterized by hypotension requiring inotropic support and respiratory failure within 12 hours after surgery. Potential physiological mechanisms of PLCS include a sudden increase in SVR and reduction in cardiac preload, leading to decreased myocardial performance and compromised systemic and cerebral blood flow. Moreover, growing evidence of anesthesia-related long-term morbidities is concerning.

While no causal link has been established, infants undergoing surgical ligation have greater risk of short-term morbidities than do infants not treated surgically. While data on longer-term outcomes remain mixed, 2 large studies have shown that infants treated with surgical ligation had higher odds of neurodevelopmental impairment (NDI) at long-term follow-up. These observations have led to growing uncertainty on the safety and efficacy of surgical PDA ligation during infancy. In most contemporary settings, surgical ligation is reserved for infants with evidence of PDA-related morbidity (HSPDA) following failed drug therapy, or in clinical settings in which drug therapy is contraindicated.

A recent meta-analysis of 40 studies including 32,345 preterm infants < 32 weeks of gestation investigated the association of surgical ligation with the risks of short- and long-term morbidity and mortality, including NDI at 2 years of age, and compared these to alternative treatment strategies, including medical management. Surgical ligation was associated with greater risks of chronic lung disease, severe retinopathy of prematurity, and NDI than were observed with medical management, but also was associated with a lower mortality. The authors acknowledge that "sicker" infants, who may be at higher risk of NDI, may have been more likely to be assigned to surgical ligation. Of note, recent studies have reported no increase in mortality after moving away from an aggressive, early surgical approach to more conservative management.

### Catheter-Based PDA Closure

Catheter-based closure of the PDA is among the safest of interventional cardiac procedures and is considered by some to be the procedure of choice for PDA closure beyond the neonatal period. Although limited to observational and retrospective studies, more centers are reporting the safety and feasibility of catheter-based PDA closure in preterm infants. While data on short and longer-term outcomes of catheter-based PDA closure are limited, evidence of increased risk of vascular compromise (thrombus necessitating systemic anticoagulation) in lower weight infants is concerning. Although there are risks in any cardiac catheterization, certain technical challenges may be exaggerated in very low–weight infants; thus, the risks of catheter-based PDA closure in these patients have to be weighed against those associated with alternative surgical and medical management options. Presently, among infants who warrant PDA closure, the absence of studies comparing catheter-based versus surgical closure precludes determination of the optimal strategy for ductal closure.

## SCREENING AND PROPHYLAXIS

While some investigators have suggested that selective echocardiography among infants with PDA-related symptoms is more cost-effective without evidence of increased harm, others advocate for universal screening to provide early detection of a PDA prior to potential ductal sequelae. A recent population-based study among over 1500 preterm infants born at < 29 weeks of gestation reported that, compared to no PDA screening, early screening (first 3 days of life) was associated with lower in-hospital mortality (14.2% vs 18.5%; OR, 0.73) and lower incidence of pulmonary hemorrhage (5.7% vs 8.4%; OR, 0.60). However, the study was observational, and caution is warranted in the interpretation of findings. The optimal screening approach for the detection of a PDA in preterm infants has yet to be defined.

### PDA Prophylaxis with COX Inhibitors

In the Trial of Indomethacin Prophylaxis in Preterm Infants (TIPP), investigators randomized 1202 infants with birth weights of 500 to 1000 grams to receive prophylactic treatment (0.1 mg/kg of birth weight) or placebo intravenously, commencing within hours after birth, for 3 days. Infants receiving prophylactic indomethacin had a lower incidence of PDA (24% vs 50% in the placebo group; OR, 0.3) and of severe periventricular and IVH (9% vs 13% in the placebo group; OR, 0.6). There were no differences in the primary composite outcome of death or neurocognitive status at 18 months corrected age. These observations are consistent with a meta-analysis of 19 clinical trials including over 2800 infants that indicated that prophylactic indomethacin may have short-term benefits, including a reduction in the incidence of symptomatic PDA, the need for surgical ligation, and the incidence of severe IVH; however, these benefits did not translate into reductions in mortality or improvements in longer-term neurodevelopment. Thus, it could be argued that healthcare providers should not provide indomethacin prophylaxis with the expectation of increased survival or improved longer-term outcomes.

In a follow-up analysis of the TIPP trial, infants without a PDA who were treated with prophylactic indomethacin had a higher incidence of chronic lung disease (43%, 170/391) than did those given placebo (30%, 78/257; $P$ = 0.015). After adjusting for baseline prognostic factors, indomethacin prophylaxis among infants without a PDA was associated with a greater weight loss and need for supplemental oxygen. While prophylactic indomethacin decreases the incidence of a PDA, additional comorbidities of preterm birth (eg, BPD, NEC) remain unchanged or may, in fact, be increased following exposure.

## CONCLUSION

Medical and surgical interventions are effective in closing the PDA in most infants, but neither individual clinical trials nor meta-analyses have shown that closing the PDA results in improved long-term outcomes. Although many strategies for management of the persistent PDA have been proposed, none have been subject to systematic evaluation in RCTs that have been powered to detect differences in long-term outcomes. In the absence of clear data that adverse outcomes can be averted by closing the PDA, trials comparing closure to non-intervention are greatly needed. For a treatment to be the standard of care, the risks associated with a persistent PDA must outweigh the risks undertaken by the treatment; therefore, the primary endpoint for studies comparing PDA management strategies should not be successful closure, but rather mortality and longer-term outcomes.

## SUGGESTED READINGS

Backes CH, MD, Rivera BK, Bridge JA, et al. Percutaneous patent ductus arteriosus (PDA) closure during infancy: a meta-analysis. *Pediatrics*. 2017 January. http://pediatrics.aappublications.org/content/early/2017/01/11/peds.2016-2927. Accessed January 19, 2017.

Benitz WE. Patent ductus arteriosus: to treat or not to treat? *Arch Dis Child Fetal Neonatal Ed*. 2012;97(2):F80-F82.

Hamrick SE, Hansmann G. Patent ductus arteriosus of the preterm infant. *Pediatrics*. 2010;125(5):1020-1030.

Jain A, Shah PS. Diagnosis, evaluation, and management of patent ductus arteriosus in preterm neonates. *JAMA Pediatrics*. 2015; 169(9):863-872.

Kabra NS, Schmidt B, Roberts RS, Doyle LW, Papile L, Fanaroff A; Trial of Indomethacin Prophylaxis in Preterms Investigators. Neurosensory impairment after surgical closure of patent ductus arteriosus in extremely low birth weight infants: results from the Trial of Indomethacin Prophylaxis in Preterms. *J Pediatrics*. 2007;150(3):229-234, 234.e1.

Kluckow M, Evans N. Early echocardiographic prediction of symptomatic patent ductus arteriosus in preterm infants undergoing mechanical ventilation. *J Pediatrics*. 1995;127(5):774-779.

McNamara PJ, Sehgal A. Towards rational management of the patent ductus arteriosus: the need for disease staging. *Arch Dis Child Fetal Neonatal Ed*. 2007;92(6):F424-F427.

Perez KM, Laughon MM. What is new for patent ductus arteriosus management in premature infants in 2015? *Curr Opin Pediatrics*. 2015;27(2):158-164.

Roze JC, Cambonie G, Marchand-Martin L, et al; Hemodynamic EPIPAGE 2 Study Group. Association between early screening for patent ductus arteriosus and in-hospital mortality among extremely preterm infants. *JAMA*. 2015;313(24):2441-2448.

Schmidt B, Davis P, Moddemann D, et al; Trial of Indomethacin Prophylaxis in Preterms Investigators. Long-term effects of indomethacin prophylaxis in extremely-low-birth-weight infants. *N Engl J Med*. 2001;344(26):1966-1972.

Sellmer A, Bjerre JV, Schmidt MR, et al. Morbidity and mortality in preterm neonates with patent ductus arteriosus on day 3. *Arch Dis Child Fetal Neonatal Ed*. 2013;98(6):F505-F510.

Sosenko IR, Fajardo MF, Claure N, Bancalari E. Timing of patent ductus arteriosus treatment and respiratory outcome in premature infants: a double-blind randomized controlled trial. *J Pediatrics*. 2012;160(6):929-935.e1.

# 59 Neonatal Hemodynamics

Nicholas Evans

## INTRODUCTION

*Hemodynamics*, or the movement of blood, is necessary to delivery oxygen to the tissues of the body. *Oxygen delivery* is determined by several factors, and failure of any these can lead to organ injury and/or death. Oxygen delivery is determined by (1) the oxygen level and carrying capacity of the blood, both of which are easy to measure and monitor and (2) the flow rate of blood around the systemic and pulmonary circulations. Both the circulations are driven by the heart, and the flow is measured by the output of each of the ventricles. In a mature circulation, the right ventricular output (RVO) drives the pulmonary blood flow and the left ventricular output (LVO) drives the systemic blood flow. The efficiency with which each ventricle does this is determined by the volume of blood entering the ventricle (the preload), the health (or maturity) of the myocardium (contractility), and the resistance against which the ventricle is pumping (afterload).

In preterm infants, many of the morbidities, particularly the cerebral morbidities, are thought to have an ischemic origin, and the goal of circulatory support has always been prevention of neurological morbidity. It can be seen that there are many levels at which the delivery of oxygen to tissues can fail, and sorting out this complexity in a clinical scenario is an unresolved challenge. This chapter will focus specifically on the "movement of blood" component of this physiological cascade.



## THE TRANSITIONAL CIRCULATION

An understanding of neonatal circulatory pathology is intrinsically linked to an understanding of circulatory adaptation to extrauterine life. The right-sided dominance of the fetal circulation, with blood shunting right to left through the ductus arteriosus and foramen ovale to bypass the lungs, has to change rapidly to the left-sided dominance of the extrauterine circulation, with the whole cardiac output flowing through the lungs (see also Chapter 45).

At birth, this sequence must change in a very short timeframe. The lungs expand with the first breaths, the pulmonary arterioles dilate, right heart pressures fall, and blood pours into the pulmonary circulation to collect oxygen from the inhaled air. The removal of the low-resistance placenta from the systemic circulation increases resistance and pressure on the left side of the circulation, while the pulmonary blood flow increases the left heart preload. The result is a dramatic increase in the workload of the left heart. The muscle in the wall of the ductus arteriosus constricts powerfully in response to rising oxygen levels, closing functionally within the first 24 hours after birth and structurally after several days, to leave the ligamentum arteriosum, the fibrous ductal remnant that we all have.

During the last trimester of pregnancy, much of the fetal cardiopulmonary development is preparing for the major changes that accompany birth, so babies born prematurely have exquisite circulatory vulnerability during this period of the transitional circulation. More mature babies are also vulnerable if born in a compromised condition or if they become unwell shortly after birth.

## CLINICAL ASSESSMENT OF THE NEONATAL CIRCULATION

### Clinical Signs

Physical signs such as poor color, increased heart rate, prolonged capillary refill, low urinary output, and altered blood parameters such as low pH and rising lactate are some of the clinical signs that are typically used to assess the circulatory performance. All of these signs are useful in identifying the neonate with severe circulatory compromise, but have limited value for the early detection of circulatory compromise.

### Blood Pressure

If there is intra-arterial access, *blood pressure* (BP) can be accurately measured and continuously monitored. Because this is relatively easy, BP has traditionally featured very highly in neonatal circulatory assessment and many circulatory interventions have traditionally focused on increasing the BP. There exists good data on what is a normal range of BP but there is controversy within the field of neonatology as to what constitutes an "adequate" blood pressure, in other words, the BP below which organ injury can result. Further, there is an emerging body of evidence that challenges the accuracy of BP as a gold standard for circulatory well-being. There has been a common assumption in neonatology that BP equals blood flow, particularly cerebral blood flow (CBF), and this caused the early focus in diagnosis and treatment of circulatory problems in neonates to be directed solely at BP. Basic physiology tells us that this thinking must be flawed some of the time because pressure is the product of flow and resistance. Changes in either of these parameters can affect BP. This pressure-based thinking was always based on limited evidence. In very preterm babies, there are data showing an association between low early BP and ultrasound evidence of brain injury, such as intraventricular hemorrhage and periventricular leukomalacia. However, there are less data to support any relationship between hypotension in preterm babies with neurodevelopmental outcome, with several studies showing no association between them.

### Measurement of Blood Flow

Blood flow, rather than BP, provides a much more accurate marker of oxygen delivery. However, this is much more difficult to measure than BP. From a range of proposed methods, the 2 that are most widely used in both the research and clinical arena are Doppler cardiac ultrasound and near-infrared spectroscopy (NIRS).

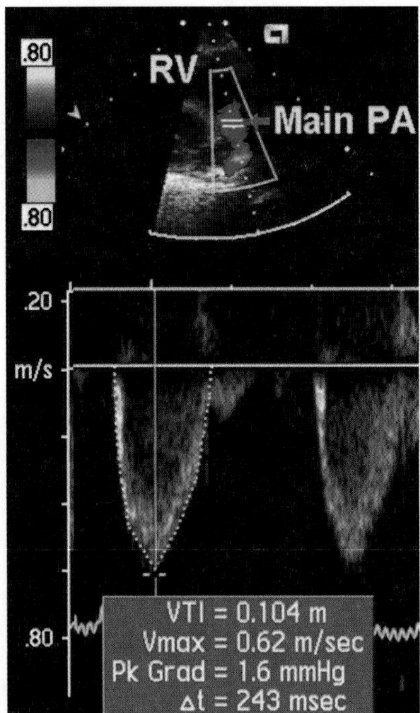


**FIGURE 59-1** Systolic Doppler velocity in the main pulmonary artery. The mean velocity is derived from the velocity time integral (VTI), which is the area under the Doppler velocity envelope. Δt, time differential; PA, pulmonary artery; Pk Grad, peak instantaneous Doppler gradient; RV, right ventricle; $V_{max}$, maximum velocity.

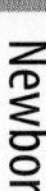


**Doppler Cardiac Ultrasound** Blood flow is the product of mean velocity and vessel cross-sectional area. Blood velocity can be measured with Doppler ultrasound (Fig. 59-1), and vessel size can be measured with 2-dimensional ultrasound (Fig. 59-2), as long as the vessel is of a reasonable size. This method in turn allows estimates of ventricular outputs and flow in other major vessels such as the superior vena

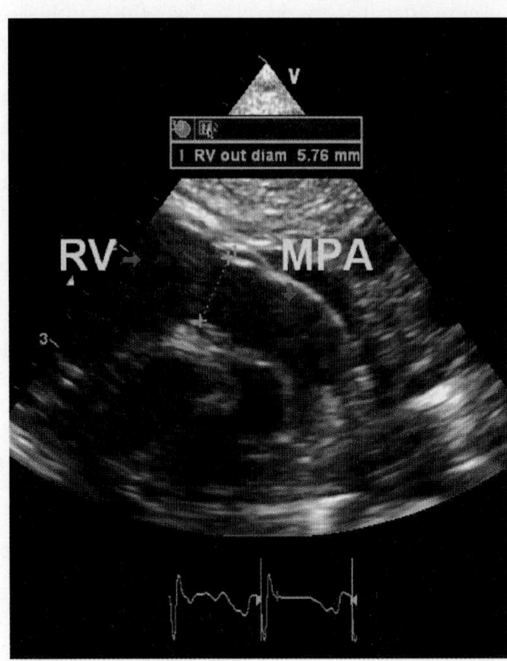


**FIGURE 59-2** Pulmonary artery dimensions. Measurement of the diameter (d) of the pulmonary valve ring in systole between the right ventricle (RV) and the main pulmonary artery (MPA). The cross-sectional area is derived from the equation $\pi \times (d^2/4)$. Stroke volume is VTI × cross-sectional area, and RV output is stroke volume × heart rate. VTI, velocity time integral.

cava (SVC). Because of this, Doppler ultrasound flow measurements in neonates are usually limited to the great vessels close to the heart: the main pulmonary artery for the RVO, the ascending aorta for the LVO and, for reasons that will be discussed below, measures of upper body and brain blood returning to the heart via the SVC. Because they are small, Doppler measures in the smaller organ blood vessels usually are limited to velocity and flow direction pattern, which may not accurately represent flow. The advantage of Doppler ultrasound is that it measures the hemodynamic variable that most closely represents oxygen delivery. The disadvantages are that it needs expensive equipment and a clinician with the skills to use it, and there are significant intrinsic errors, particularly in vessel size measurement. Further, because of the complexities of the shunts in the transitional circulation, ventricular outputs may not accurately represent systemic and pulmonary blood flows.

**Near-Infrared Spectroscopy** NIRS uses infrared light to measure oxygenated and deoxygenated hemoglobin and, from this, blood flow in the superficial tissues of the brain (and other organs). Organ blood flow is derived using the Fick principle from change in oxyhemoglobin in response to an increase inspired oxygen and indices of tissue oxygenation can be derived from the ratios between oxyhemoglobin and deoxyhemoglobin. In preterm babies, very low readings (< 50%) of regional cerebral oxygenation ($rScO_2$) during the first 1 to 3 days of life have been associated with poorer neurodevelopmental outcome and, in 1 of these studies, high $rScO_2$ saturation levels were also associated with poor outcome. Near-infrared spectroscopy also can be used in conjunction with BP to assess for loss of cerebral autoregulation. Infants who show high correlation between changes in mean blood pressure (MBP) and $rScO_2$ are more likely to have cerebral ultrasound abnormalities. However, in a moderate-sized pilot clinical trial, treatment directed on the basis of unblended $rScO_2$ reading did not improve clinical outcomes. Further trials are being planned to examine this more robustly.

## NEONATAL HEMODYNAMIC PATHOPHYSIOLOGY

The most commonly encountered hemodynamic disturbance is that seen in the transitional period in the very preterm infant. But there are also a variety of other clinical scenarios in which hemodynamic pathology is common. Given that the clinical recognition of neonatal circulatory compromise can be challenging, it is important to recognize that the following clinical situations are at high risk and to proactively exclude circulatory compromise.

### The Preterm Transitional Circulation

The preterm neonate is an exteriorized fetus, whose ventricular function is adapted to the low resistance of the placental circulation. The preterm myocardium is immature with fewer contractile components than a term neonate, so it may not adapt to the higher afterloads of extrauterine life. The fetal channels of the ductus arteriosus and foramen ovale also are less likely to close in preterm infants and the resultant left-to-right shunts may divert blood away from the systemic back into the pulmonary circulation. The circulation may be further compromised by the fact that preterm infants need positive pressure ventilation, and ventilation can also compromise cardiac performance. When an infant is born prematurely, the stage is set for circulatory compromise and, indeed, the intrapartum period and the first 24 hours after birth are a period of particular circulatory vulnerability for preterm neonates.

The intrapartum period is difficult to study, but in the early hours after birth, low BP, low systemic blood flow (SBF), and low CBF are all associated with ultrasound evidence of brain injury and adverse neurodevelopmental outcome. Thinking in this area has predominantly focused on autoregulation of the cerebral circulation or the ability of the circulation to maintain CBF through redistribution of blood flow once the BP drops below a critical value. Much of the study of CBF has focused on exploring this pressure/flow relationship. Although the results of these studies are somewhat inconsistent, NIRS studies suggest there is a subgroup of preterm infants in whom autoregulation is compromised and who, in turn, are at higher risk of ultrasound evidence of brain injury. It is unclear whether absent autoregulation is the primary problem or whether it is an intermediate response to another primary insult. These CBF data have tended to have little information about the system driving that blood flow, the cardiovascular system. This pressure-based thinking has been questioned by Doppler cardiac ultrasound studies that have focused on transitional hemodynamics in the heart and central measures of SBF. These studies showed that the usual measures of SBF, the ventricular outputs, can be confounded by left-to-right shunts through the fetal channels, which may be significant, even early after birth. These studies showed that, contrary to conventional thinking, shunts through the patent ductus arteriosus (PDA) could be quite large, even in the early postnatal hours, and these shunts were predominantly left-to-right. Further the patent foramen ovale may also be a site of significant left-to-right shunting. This impacts on the usual measure of SBF, the ventricular outputs. These will be confounded by these shunts, left-to-right ductal shunts increase LVO, and those through the foramen ovale increase RVO. For this reason, the Doppler measure of SVC flow was used to study the natural history of preterm SBF (upper body and brain) during the early postnatal period. These studies showed that low SVC flow occurs in about a third of babies born before 30 weeks, developing within a predictable timeframe of the first 12 hours after birth and is followed by improvement of flow by 24 to 48 hrs. There is a dose-dependent relationship between the severity of this low flow and grade of intraventricular hemorrhage (IVH), which develops as or after flow improves. There is also a significant association between lower average SVC flow in the first 24 hours and poor 3-year developmental outcome. The causes of this low-flow state are not completely clear but immaturity (lower gestational age) appears to be the main risk factor. Of note, at the time of measurement, a larger PDA (shunting blood away from the systemic circulation) and higher ventilatory pressures were also associated with lower flow, particularly in studies that were performed within 6 hours of birth.

Of clinical importance, there is only a weak relationship between BP and SBF, whether measured by SVC flow or ventricular outputs (Fig. 59-3), which is reflected by the close inverse relationship between flow and calculated vascular resistance. Although this could be compensatory, it may also be causative. There is consistent evidence that the preterm myocardium has a limited ability to respond to an increase in afterload, suggesting that the transition from the low-resistance intrauterine state to the high-resistance extrauterine state is the part of the primary problem. When this transition is compounded by large ductal shunts out of the systemic circulation (which are not uncommon in the early postnatal hours) and positive pressure ventilation, critically low blood flow to all organs of the body (not just the brain) results. This hypothesized model of preterm circulatory compromise has not yet been proven. However, these data emphasize that assessment of the neonatal circulation is more complicated than simply a measurement of BP.

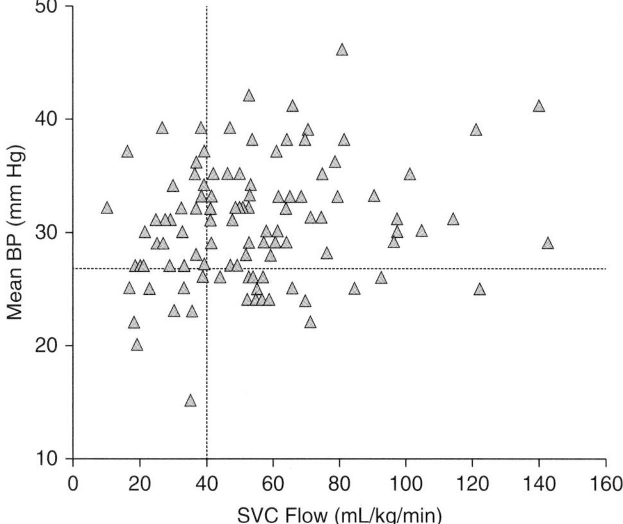


**FIGURE 59-3** Relationship between mean blood pressure and superior vena cava flow. The graph shows mean blood pressure (BP) versus superior vena cava (SVC) flow in 110 infants born before 30 weeks' gestation at a mean of 5 hours of age. The dotted lines represent possible lower limits of normal. For BP, this has been plotted at the mean gestation of the cohort, 27 weeks.

### Other Causes of Preterm Hypotension

The physics of fluid dynamics dictate that BP can be low because either flow or resistance, or both, are low, so hypotension is a symptom with many causes in preterm and more mature infants. After the period of circulatory transition, it is more usual that hypotension is associated with normal or high SBF; thus, the problem is more commonly loss of resistance. This has been best studied in neonatal sepsis; see below.

**Hypovolemia** *Hypovolaemia* is an uncommon cause of preterm circulatory compromise, and studies have demonstrated a lack of relationship between blood volume and BP. When seen as a primary pathology, hypovolemia is usually due to fetal blood loss and presents in the immediate postnatal period. These cases are usually associated with intrapartum blood loss from a vasa previa or fetoplacental transfusion, for example, after early clamping of a nuchal cord or from an acute fetomaternal hemorrhage. This is most often seen in term infants and can be clinically difficult to differentiate from the post resuscitation pallor that typically accompanies asphyxia. The clinician should be alert to the classic features of circulatory compromise with pallor, tachycardia, hypotension, low hematocrit, and a typical appearance on cardiac ultrasound of poorly filled ventricles.

**Patent Ductus Arteriosus** Patent ductus arteriosus during the first week is associated with both lower systolic and diastolic BPs, and hence mean BP. This association occurs because the PDA exposes the systemic circulation to the lower resistance of the pulmonary circulation throughout the cardiac cycle. Most PDAs are clinically silent during the first 3 postnatal days, so this needs to be considered in neonates with persistent hypotension. Diagnosis with cardiac ultrasound is quick and easy (Fig. 59-4). As discussed above, in the very early transitional period, a larger ductal diameter is significantly associated with lower SBF. After this time (and contrary to popular belief) our data suggests that many infants will protect their systemic circulation well in the presence of a significant PDA (see also Chapter 58).

**Sepsis** *Neonatal sepsis* can commonly present with signs of circulatory compromise. Little data exists about the hemodynamics of neonatal septic shock. In early onset sepsis, the problems are probably a combination of the transitional hemodynamics (described above)

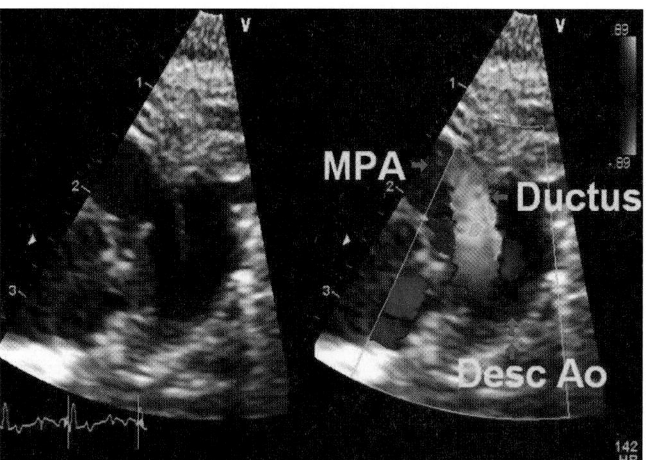


**FIGURE 59-4** Two-dimensional image and color Doppler mapping of a large patent ductus arteriosus. The red color Doppler mapping shows the left-to-right shunt through the patent ductus arteriosus (Ductus) from the descending aorta (Desc Ao) to the main pulmonary artery (MPA).

and pulmonary hypertension associated with pneumonia (described below). There are now studies that show that circulatory compromise associated with late onset sepsis in preterm infants is usually due to vasodilatory shock. These infants usually have normal or high SBF, indicating loss of vascular tone. In advanced septic shock, evidence of tissue ischemia can persist despite normalization of systemic hemodynamics. Although little studied in the newborn, this may be due to the microvascular dysfunction described in older subjects.

**Inotrope-Resistant Hypotension** Hypotension that is resistant to vasopressor support seems to be associated with poor adrenocortical function. However, blunted cortisol responses are not universally found in these infants, so the etiology is likely to be more complex than this. Our clinical observations and 1 more systematic study suggest that hypotension is associated with vasodilation, with the usual hemodynamic finding of normal or high SBF. The mechanistic complexity of vasodilatory shock has been described in older subjects. Whether these observations apply in the neonate is not known.

### The Term Infant with Asphyxia, Pulmonary Hypertension, or Severe Respiratory Distress

Term and near-term infants with *asphyxia, pulmonary hypertension, or severe respiratory distress* are a heterogenous group who also have a high risk of low SBF in the first 24 hours and, like the preterm infants, the incidence of low SBF becomes less with postnatal age. The causes of this are complex, and hemodynamic findings vary widely among infants. There is probably a varying degree of influence from all the factors already discussed, particularly the effect of high ventilatory pressures. In infants with perinatal asphyxia, hypoxic-ischemic damage to the myocardium is important in the etiology. One factor often not considered is the potential for high resistance in the pulmonary circulation to compromise the systemic circulation. The left ventricle can only pump into the systemic circulation what it receives from the pulmonary venous return. If pulmonary vascular resistance is high enough to restrict pulmonary blood flow and the ductus arteriosus and foramen ovale are closed or restricting (as they often are in these more mature infants), then the SBF will be similarly compromised. It has been suggested that myocardial contractility is poor in these infants but low left ventricular (LV) preload will also make the LV contractility appear poor. Therefore, this may be a secondary rather than a primary phenomenon. There can be quite dramatic increases in cardiac output in infants treated with nitric oxide (Fig. 59-5).

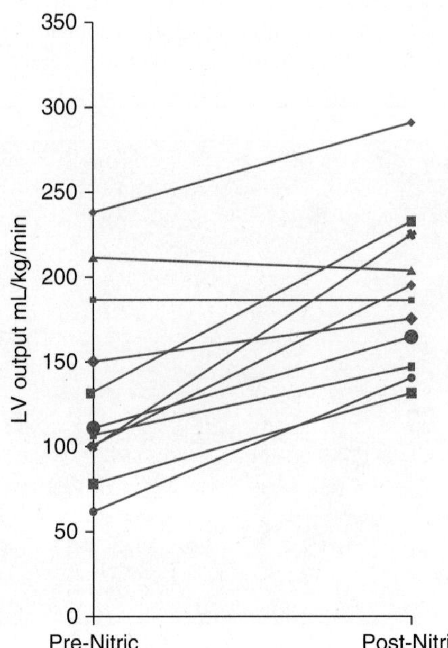


**FIGURE 59-5** Hemodynamic response to inhaled nitric oxide. The graph shows the change in left ventricular (LV) output in 11 term or near term infants before and within 30 minutes of commencing nitric oxide.

### Circulatory Collapse

Sudden circulatory collapse in infants is rare but catastrophic when it happens. It is characterized by rapid onset of all the typical clinical signs described above. Recognizing the problem is not typically difficult, but diagnosing the cause can be more problematic. Such infants are often assumed to be septic, and while sepsis should always be considered, it must never be assumed until other causes are excluded. Congenital heart lesions with ductal-dependent systemic circulations, such as critical coarctation or hypoplastic left heart syndrome, are the most important diagnoses to exclude. However, other rarities, such as cardiac tamponade resulting from a silastic long line catheter with the tip being left in the heart or acute viral myocarditis, can present unexpectedly in this way. Many of these diagnoses will be quickly apparent on cardiac ultrasound, thus emphasising the importance of ready access to point-of-care ultrasound in good neonatal care.

### Summary

Circulatory pathology is common during the first 24 hours in very preterm and sick term infants. The etiology is multifactorial but cardiac maladaptation to higher ex utero vascular resistance may be 1 factor. This can manifest as low BP and/or low Doppler-measured SBF, and the measurement of SBF together with BP will improve understanding of an infant's circulatory pathology. Low SBF is uncommon after 24 hours. Most infants with hypotension beyond the transitional period (and a few within the transitional period) have normal or high SBF, pointing to vasodilation as the dominant pathology. In some infants with persistent pulmonary hypertension of the newborn (PPHN), restricted pulmonary blood flow will in turn restrict systemic blood flow. Circulatory collapse may be due to sepsis, but this should not be assumed, and other primary cardiac causes should be looked for with cardiac ultrasound.

## CIRCULATORY SUPPORT IN THE PRETERM INFANT

Volume expansion, catecholamines, and increasingly, hydrocortisone are the main agents used in neonatal circulatory support. Empirically, each agent differs in its effect on the circulation: Volume expansion restores normovolemia in a hypovolemic infant and increases preload and hence cardiac output in a normovolemic infant. Inotropes increase SBF by increasing cardiac rate and myocardial contractility or by reducing afterload. Some inotropes have predominantly vasoconstrictive effects and modify preload and SBF by constricting the venous bed. Arterial constriction improves BP, but excessive constriction can reduce SBF by causing afterload compromise.

Dopamine and epinephrine are catecholamines, and have cardiac stimulant (inotropic) effects and predominantly pressor (vasoconstrictive) effects peripherally, particularly at higher doses. Dobutamine is primarily a β-adrenergic catecholamine with inotropic, chronotropic, and peripheral vasodilator effects Dopamine is a naturally occurring precursor to epinephrine and norepinephrine that has β, α, and dopaminergic effects. Each of these effects is more likely (in the order shown) to be stimulated as the dose increases. Over 10 mcg/kg/min, the α vasconstrictive effects on BP predominate, but in the very immature infant, these α effects may be apparent at lower doses. Epinephrine is an endogenous catecholamine and has broad α- and β-adrenergic effects and, like dopamine, vasoconstricts at higher doses. Hydrocortisone increases BP, but little data exists about how it does this in the neonate. The limited information there is suggests mixed central and peripheral effects with the latter probably dominating.

### The Evidence Base for Pharmacological Interventions

Clinical trials in this area have been mainly designed to look at changes in a physiological parameter (mainly BP) rather than effects on important clinical outcomes. These studies have demonstrated that routine early, or perinatal volume expansion does not change long-term preterm outcomes; that dopamine is better than dobutamine at increasing BP, but dobutamine may be better than dopamine for improving cardiac output; that epinephrine has similar effects to dopamine on BP and CBF; and that hydrocortisone will improve BP.

There is no evidence that supports an effect of any of these interventions on important clinical outcomes.

**Evidence for Inotrope Use** Dopamine is better than dobutamine at increasing BP, although this does not translate into better short-term outcomes. Epinephrine and dopamine have similar efficacy in increasing BP. None of the studies to date has been powered or designed to look at clinical outcomes. In most of these studies, infants were enrolled on the basis of BP below an intervention threshold, and change in BP was the main outcome measure. In a preterm infant study using Doppler measurement of LV output, an increase was shown with dobutamine, while LV output decreased with dopamine.

The author's group has, to their knowledge, performed the only randomized study of dopamine and dobutamine that enrolled preterm infants on the basis of low blood flow. Dobutamine produced significantly better increases in SBF (as measured by SVC flow) than dopamine, while dopamine produced better increases in BP. At 10 mcg/kg/min, there was no difference between the 2 drugs, but in those that needed to be increased to 20 mcg/kg/min, dobutamine produced more flow benefit, which was not seen in those on dopamine, even though BP continued to increase. However, these physiological differences did not translate into any significant differences in outcome. SVC flow will incorporate CBF, but the two are not interchangeable, so what effect do inotropes have on CBF? The effect of dobutamine on CBF in preterm infants has not been studied. Using the Xe clearance technique, it was shown that dopamine, while increasing LVO and MBP, did not increase CBF. Another study showed no effect on middle cerebral artery pulsatility index after dopamine in a group of preterm infants with normal BP but clinical evidence of poor perfusion. In an open label observational study, NIRS was used to show an increase in mean CBF after dopamine was given to a cohort of 12 preterm infants with an MBP of less than 30 mm Hg. In a double-blind randomized trial, also using NIRS, it was shown that both dopamine (at doses up to 10 mcg/kg/min) and epinephrine (at doses up to 0.5 mcg/kg/min) produced similar increases in regional cerebral intravascular oxygenation, which in turn was correlated with increases in MBP.

**Evidence for Volume Expansion (Including Delayed Umbilical Cord Clamping)** Systematic reviews have demonstrated that routine early volume expansion with an intravenous fluid bolus does not improve outcomes in preterm infants. There is likely no advantage in using a colloid compared to a crystalloid, and volume is not as good as dopamine at increasing BP. There is less data about the effect of volume on organ blood flows. Studies have shown increases in LV output or SVC flow with volume that did not translate to an increase in CBF. In all these studies, measurements were taken immediately after the volume expansion, so it is not known if these increases are sustained. There is some evidence that the fluid used in volume expansion redistributes quickly out of the vascular compartment.

The "natural" method to expand an infant's volume at birth is to delay the clamping of the cord to allow fetal blood in the placental compartment to drain back into the infant. The current evidence suggests that this is advantageous for the preterm infant, with systematic review showing delayed cord clamping associated with better circulatory stability, less IVH, and lower risk for necrotizing enterocolitis. The evidence is limited because it includes many small trials, and there are limited numbers of very preterm infants. In some parts of the world, delayed cord clamping is being introduced as a standard of care. A large prospective randomized trial to investigate the potential benefit of cord clamping in infants born before 30 weeks' gestation is under way to address this important question.

**Evidence for Hydrocortisone Administration** Much of the data on hydrocortisone is observational and relates to its use in inotrope-resistant hypotension. One randomized trial showed hydrocortisone at 2.5 mg/kg had similar efficacy to dopamine in improving BP in hypotensive preterm babies. There was no difference in other clinical outcomes. A Doppler ultrasound study has shown increases in BP, LV output, and systemic vascular resistance after 2 mg/kg of hydrocortisone in 14 infants with inotrope-resistant hypotension. However, the effects of hydrocortisone on CBF are not known.

#### Recommendations

There is no clinical outcome–based evidence on which to recommend therapeutic recommendations. No study has shown any improvement in any meaningful clinical outcome, short- or long-term, in response to a specific inotrope or other intervention. This lack of evidence for effect on clinical outcomes means that the approach to therapy therefore must be empirical and pragmatic. It is the author's view that many of the complexities of the transitional preterm circulation are not reflected in BP (or other commonly used clinical signs of circulatory compromise). Treatment targeted at BP alone will be appropriate in some infants, unnecessary in others, and miss (or deliver late therapy) in some who really need it. BP must be important, but it is the author's view that to target circulatory support requires measures of both pressure and flow. Despite this opinion, the reality is that measuring flow is difficult and many newborn intensive care units do not have access to appropriate equipment or skills and so will remain dependent on BP and other clinical parameters to guide therapy. Reflecting this reality, this chapter presents these clinical suggestions pragmatically in 3 parts: general measures and volume, a pressure-based approach, and a pressure- and flow-based approach.

**General Measures** Basic preventative strategies are important but are easily overlooked. Antenatal steroids mediate their effects on both the respiratory and cardiovascular systems. Infants born after maternal steroid treatment have higher BP and less need for inotropes, and are less likely to develop low systemic blood flow. There are few valid contraindications for administration of antenatal steroids and it remains probably the most effective therapeutic intervention in preterm neonatology. As discussed above, it is reasonable to consider delayed cord clamping in very preterm infants. Avoiding overventilation is also important both because of the direct negative effects on the circulation of high intrathoracic pressure but also because of the effects of low partial pressure of carbon dioxide ($pCO_2$) in reducing CBF.

Hypovolaemia is rare, but it does happen. It is difficult to diagnose clinically but easy to fix if it is present. For these reasons, volume expansion should be part of the initial approach to circulatory support with any inotrope strategy. The authors use normal saline at 10 mL/kg over 20 to 30 minutes but would not repeat that without a convincing response to treatment (falling heart rate and improving BP) or strong clinical and/or cardiac ultrasound evidence of hypovolemia. Overdoing volume expansion is as potentially harmful as underdoing it.

**A Blood Pressure Intervention Threshold** If treatment is being guided mainly by BP, then the first issue is determining what intervention threshold to use. In infants born before 30 weeks' gestation, most neonatologists would either aim to maintain MBP above 30 mm Hg or above the gestation (in weeks) of the infant. There is no outcome-based evidence to say which approach is correct. Empirically, because gestation is an important independent determinant of BP, it likely makes more sense to use the latter, in that it reflects the range of values in the population rather than using a "1 size fits all" approach.

Dobutamine increases the BP of many infants and seems better than dopamine at improving SBF. Therefore, within the first 24 hours after birth, when low SBF is common, there is an empirical logic in using dobutamine as a first-line treatment, with the pressor inotropes used as a second-line treatment in infants with an inadequate BP response. For a more consistent effect on BP, dopamine or epinephrine should be the first choice. Despite similar hemodynamic effects, there is more clinical experience with dopamine, so it would in general be used before epinephrine. When using a pressor inotrope in the first 24 hours, the risks of afterload compromise of SBF from vasoconstriction should be considered. Also, the principle that more BP may not necessarily be better was emphasised by studies that showed some infants with quite dramatic rises in estimated CBF in response to an increase in BP. Hyperperfusion after hypoperfusion seems important in the pathogenesis of IVH, so is probably best avoided. These risks can probably be minimized by starting at a low dose (5 µg/kg/min for dopamine or 0.01–0.02 µg/kg/min for epinephrine) and titrating in careful steps to a minimally acceptable BP. It is recommended to aim for MBP within 5 mm Hg of the therapeutic threshold and to be prepared to wean the infusion rate quickly in infants whose BP overshoots this level.

**Targeting Blood Pressure and Flow** A more complete understanding of the underlying cardiovascular hemodynamic state provides an effective basis for therapy, more than what BP alone can provide. This understanding requires point-of-care cardiac ultrasound, which should be targeted on the basis of postnatal age (3 to 9 hours of age is the highest risk time for low SBF in preterm babies) or clinical concern about the circulation (usually low BP). The 3 cardiac ultrasound measures, in order of importance, are (1) an indirect measure of systemic blood flow (SVC flow or RV output), (2) the size and direction of ductal shunt, and (3) assessment of degree of pulmonary hypertension. Intervention thresholds of 50 mL/kg/min for SVC flow and 150 mL/kg/min for RV output are recommended, and pathologically low measures of these 2 variables would be less than 40 and 120 mL/kg/min, respectively. Estimating blood flow requires measures of velocity and vessel size and can be time consuming to derive. Large atrial shunts are not common in the first 48 hours, so for clinical purposes, RV output is a reasonably accurate surrogate for SBF in the early postnatal period. Velocity in the main pulmonary artery is the dominant determinant of RV output and so measuring the maximum velocity in the pulmonary artery (PA $V_{max}$) provides a simple way to screen for low SBF (Fig. 59-6). If the PA $V_{max}$ is higher than 0.45 m/sec, low SBF is unlikely. If the PA $V_{max}$ is less than 0.35 m/sec, most infants have low SBF. Between 0.35 and 0.45 m/sec is a gray zone where discriminatory accuracy is not as good (Fig. 59-7). In practice, it is recommended to screen with PA $V_{max}$, followed by full RV output and/or SVC flow measures in those with a PA $V_{max}$ less than 0.45 m/sec.

In infants with large PDAs (> 2 mm in diameter) and predominantly left-to-right shunts, consideration should be given to closing the PDAs medically, particularly if there is low SBF or low MBP. Otherwise, infants with low SBF, as defined above, can be treated with volume and dobutamine, starting at 10 μg/kg/min and increasing to 20 μg/kg/min, depending on response and regardless of the MBP. However, if the MBP remained persistently below the number of weeks' gestation despite dobutamine, dopamine can be added at 5 μg/kg/min and titrated up to achieve a minimally acceptable MBP. It is rare to warrant escalating to doses of dopamine that are higher than 10 μg/kg/min, but if the SBF is known to be normal, higher doses than this could be considered.

After the first 24 hours, it is much more likely that the SBF will be normal or high. Hypotension that presents beyond this time frame

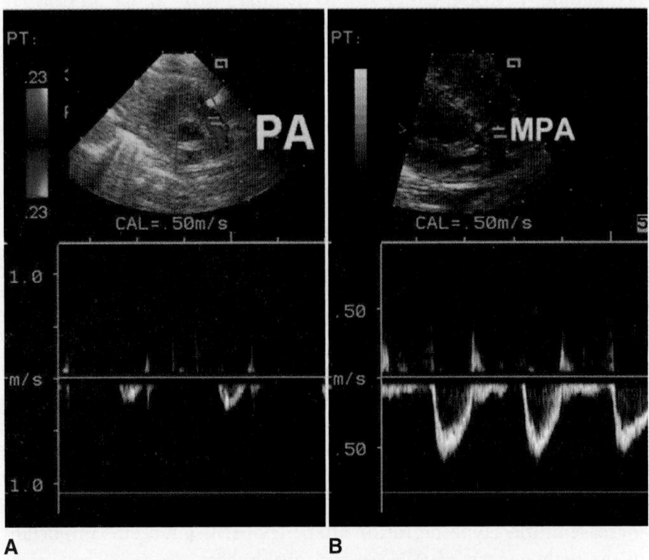


**FIGURE 59-6** Pulmonary artery flow. Echo-Doppler images show Doppler velocity in the pulmonary artery in 2 infants. **A:** The low $V_{max}$ of an infant with low systemic blood flow; **B:** a normal $V_{max}$. MPA, main pulmonary artery; PA, pulmonary artery.

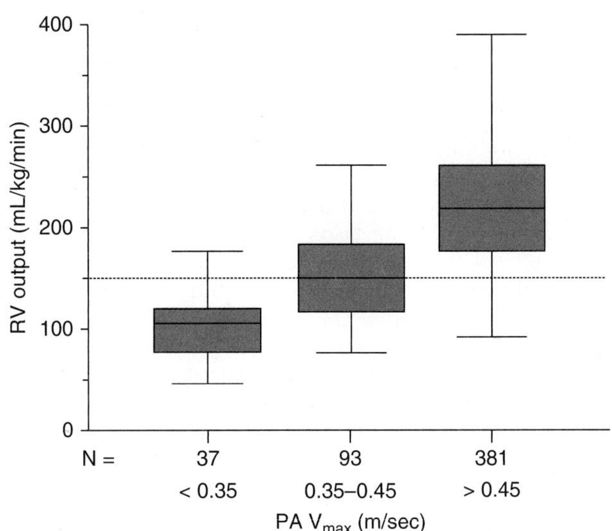


**FIGURE 59-7** Relationship between right ventricle output and pulmonary artery flow. The graph shows a box-and-whisker plot of right ventricle (RV) output against low, intermediate, and normal maximum velocity in the pulmonary artery (PA $V_{max}$). The dotted line denotes 150 mL/kg/min, the lower limit of normal.

typically indicates a loss of vascular tone and a pressor inotrope would be the logical therapeutic choice. Recommended treatment begins with dopamine at 5 μg/kg/min and titrating the dose up to achieve a minimally acceptable BP. There is no physiological reason why epinephrine should not be just as effective in this situation, though there is less clinical experience with it. Therefore, current recommendations are to use epinephrine as a second line to dopamine. If SBF is normal and other markers of circulatory status are satisfactory, clinicians can tolerate borderline low BPs (within 2 or 3 mm Hg of threshold). In infants where the BP drops lower than this or there are other clinical concerns, as long as the SBF was normal, dopamine should be titrated up to 20 μg/kg/min.

**Inotrope Resistance** There are 2 facets to *inotrope resistance*. The first is the resistant hypotension discussed above, and the second is the less well-recognized resistant low SBF, which may or may not be associated with hypotension. Inotrope resistance was observed in 40% of the low SBF infants enrolled in the authors' inotrope study and is not an uncommon finding in clinical practice. However, there is no reliable strategy that can be recommended to reverse the low SBF state in these infants. Neither epinephrine infusion nor hydrocortisone has been shown to be very effective for treating this. Systemic blood flow often increases gradually over the subsequent 12 to 36 hours.

Most infants with inotrope-resistant hypotension seem to be in a vasodilatory state, except in the first 24 hours when they overlap with a resistant low SBF group. The management of this resistant hypotension is empirical. Some would add in an epinephrine infusion, which can increase BP in infants already on maximum doses of dopamine. Increasingly, hydrocortisone (at doses of 1–2 mg/kg) is being used in this situation. While considerably more is known about the hemodynamic effects of epinephrine than of hydrocortisone, the association between low cortisol levels and resistant hypotension provides an empirical logic to using physiological doses of hydrocortisone in infants at risk of adrenal insufficiency. Our approach with resistant hypotension would depend on the clinical situation. Some would recommend that an epinephrine infusion be commenced before using hydrocortisone, but in the very premature infant it might be more effective to administer hydrocortisone. With the unresolved concerns about possible adverse neurological effects of early postnatal use of systemic corticosteroids, it seems wise to minimize the dose and duration of hydrocortisone when used in this way, starting with 1 to 2 mg/kg for 1 to 3 days, depending on the response. Septic shock is also often vasodilatory and can be very resistant to inotropes. Whether hydrocortisone should be used if there is suspected sepsis is open to question. This vasopressor-resistant loss of vascular tone (or vasoplegia) has been recognized as a feature of septic shock in older subjects and a variety of therapeutic strategies have been explored, including nitric oxide synthetase inhibitors and vasopressin. There is little evidence about these agents in resistant shock in newborns, although vasopressin has been tested in a small randomized trial as a primary inotrope against dopamine and has been found to have similar efficacy in improving BP.

## CIRCULATORY SUPPORT IN THE TERM INFANT

The early recognition of circulatory compromise is key to its subsequent management. Where possible, for example with hypovolemia, PPHN or ductal-dependent congenital heart lesions, treatment should be directed at the known cause. In general, the same principles should be applied in relation to pressure and flow, as discussed above. The effects of pulmonary vasoconstriction on systemic blood flow should always be considered in term infants. In infants with cardiac ultrasound–estimated pulmonary artery pressure above or similar to systemic pressure, there should be a low threshold for using inhaled nitric oxide (where available) as a circulatory support measure in this population. When using vasopressors in infants with severe lung disease and/or PPHN, it is important to consider that these drugs can constrict both the systemic and pulmonary vasculatures. This has not been explored in term infants, but in preterm infants, dopamine has a balanced effect on both circulations with quite wide interindividual variation. Therefore, the assumption that vasopressors will automatically squeeze blood into the pulmonary circulation may not be correct. For example, there is some observational data that norepinephrine may have a preferential pressor effect on the systemic circulation with some vasodilatory effect on the pulmonary circulation.

When the SBF appears low, it is recommended to use dobutamine as a first-line treatment, with dopamine or epinephrine as a back-up if the BP remains low, using a similar protocol to that described for preterm infants. When MBP is low and SBF is normal or oxygenation is borderline, dopamine or adrenaline are often better to use as a first-line treatment. The data described above suggests that norepinephrine may have advantages in this situation.

## FUTURE DIRECTIONS

This is an area of neonatology that is more defined by unknowns rather than by knowns. While it is important to show that circulatory support treatments actually produce the physiological effects according to their known mechanisms of action, unless studies can show that these effects improve clinical outcome, such research just becomes phenomenology. Circulatory support treatments have been in routine clinical practice for over 25 years, yet it is unknown whether they achieve the primary goal, which is to reduce neurological, neurodevelopmental, and neurobehavioral morbidities. Closing this knowledge gap is the challenge for the future.

## SUGGESTED READINGS


Barrington KJ. Common hemodynamic problems in the neonate. *Neonatology*. 2013;103(4):335-340.

Cox DJ, Groves AM. Inotropes in preterm infants—evidence for and against. *Acta Paediatr*. 2012;101(464):17-23.

El-Khuffash AF, McNamara PJ. Neonatologist performed functional echocardiography in the neonatal intensive care unit. *Semin Fetal Neonatal Med*. 2011;16:50-60.

Evans N. Which inotrope in which baby? *Arch Dis Child Fetal Neonatal Ed*. 2006;91(3):213-220.

Evans N. Functional echocardiography in the neonatal intensive care unit. In: Polin R, Kleinman CS, Seri I, eds. *Hemodynamics and Cardiology: Neonatology Questions and Controversies*. 1st ed. Philadelphia, PA: Saunders Elsevier; 2008: 83-109.

Evans N. Preterm patent ductus arteriosus: a continuing conundrum for the neonatologist? *Semin Fetal Neonatal Med*. 2015;20(4):272-277.

Noori S, Seri I. Evidence-based versus pathophysiology-based approach to diagnosis and treatment of neonatal cardiovascular compromise. *Semin Fetal Neonatal Med*. 2015;20(4):238-245.

Nuntnarumit P, Yang W, Bada-Ellzey HS. Blood pressure measurements in the newborn. *Clin Perinatol*. 1999;26(4):981-989.

Rabe H, Diaz-Rossello JL, Duley L, Dowswell T. Effect of timing of umbilical cord clamping and other strategies to influence placental transfusion at preterm birth on maternal and infant outcomes. *Cochrane Database Syst Rev*. 2012;(8):CD003248.

Sortica Da Costa C, Greisen G, Austin T. Is near-infrared spectroscopy clinically useful in the preterm infant. *Arch Dis Child Fetal Neonatal Ed*. 2015:100:F558-F561.




# 60 Necrotizing Enterocolitis

Ravi Mangal Patel and Josef Neu

## INTRODUCTION

Necrotizing enterocolitis (NEC) is a serious gastrointestinal disease that occurs primarily in preterm infants. The disease is characterized by the rapid onset of intestinal inflammation and, in severe cases, can lead to intestinal necrosis and multiorgan dysfunction that results in death. Since the 1950s, when neonatal intensive care was introduced at many centers around the world with survival of very low–birth-weight (VLBW) infants, NEC has been reported as a complication of premature birth. It remains the most common gastrointestinal complication in preterm infants, and is a major cause of morbidity and mortality in neonates, accounting for 10% of deaths in the neonatal intensive care unit (NICU). Reports from the United States, the United Kingdom, Sweden, and the Netherlands indicate that NEC is increasing as a cause of death, as survival from lung disease has improved for preterm infants.

## EPIDEMIOLOGY

### Incidence and Recent Trends

The incidence of NEC varies among studies, depending on the population studied, case definition, and geographic region. Among a large network of NICUs in the United States encompassing 58,555 infants weighing 500 to 1500 g, the combined incidence of medical and surgical NEC was 3.9% in 2013 (2.6% medical NEC, 1.2% surgical), which had significantly declined from 6.6% in 2007. Similarly, the incidence of NEC in the Neonatal Research Network for infants with birthweights between 401 and 1500 g and born at 22 to 28 weeks' gestation decreased from 13% in 2008 to 9% in 2012 ($P < 0.01$). This figure had previously increased between 1993 and 2008. The incidence of Bell stage 2 or 3 NEC for infants who survived for more than 12 hours after birth ranged from 15% at 23 weeks' gestation to 8% at 28 weeks' gestation. In a recent population-based cohort in the United Kingdom, the incidence of severe NEC was 3.2% (95% confidence interval [CI], 2.9–3.4; Fig. 60-1).

### Age at Onset

The age at onset of NEC varies depending on the gestational age of the infant. More immature preterm infants present later in the hospital course compared to more mature preterm or term infants. NEC in term infants typically presents early, with a reported mean age of onset of 4 days. This observation has suggested a potential developmental window of highest disease risk, although there is substantial variation in both the postnatal age and postmenstrual age (PMA) at onset, even among distinct gestational age subgroups. Among infants less than 32 weeks' gestation who required surgery for NEC, the PMA of onset was a median of 30.5 weeks (interquartile range 27.9–32.7 weeks) based on a large population-based study in the United Kingdom.

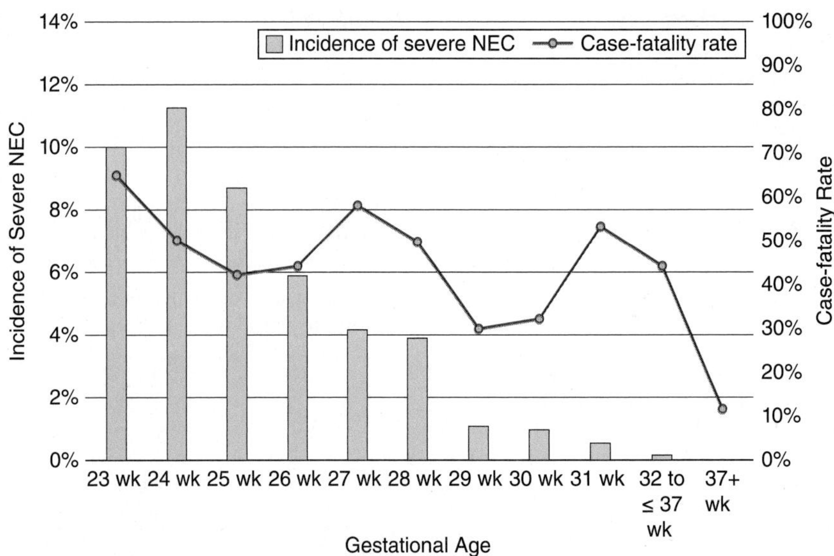


**FIGURE 60-1** Incidence and case-fatality rates of necrotizing enterocolitis (NEC) by gestational age. Data from a population-based cohort of 118,073 infants in the United Kingdom. No NEC cases observed for infants at 22 weeks' gestation ($n = 12$).



## CLINICAL PRESENTATION

### Signs and Symptoms

The clinical findings of NEC are variable and can involve both abdominal and systemic signs and symptoms. Infants can have rapid changes in findings within a short period of time and require close monitoring for deterioration if NEC is suspected. In 1978, Bell et al proposed a method to clinically stage the severity of NEC based on both clinical and radiographic findings (Table 60-1), and this staging system was subsequently expanded to a modified staging system. Although the *Bell staging* of NEC is commonly used, particularly in case definitions of NEC for clinical studies, there is no clear and universally utilized case definition of NEC. Hence, current definitions likely encompass heterogeneous clinical entities that share a similar clinical presentation. Recently, investigators from the United Kingdom proposed a gestational age–specific definition of NEC scored on clinical and radiographic findings. Non-gastrointestinal signs and symptoms include temperature instability, lethargy, apnea, and bradycardia, while more severe and progressive cases demonstrate instability of vital signs, respiratory failure, and shock. Gastrointestinal signs and symptoms include poor feeding, increases in pregavage residuals, emesis, abdominal distention, and bloody stools. As NEC worsens in severity, gastrointestinal symptoms become more pronounced with marked abdominal distention, gastrointestinal hemorrhage, and abdominal wall discoloration or erythema (Fig. 60-2). Abdominal wall discoloration is often an ominous sign, and a predictor of the severity of NEC. The differential diagnosis of NEC also requires consideration of spontaneous intestinal perforation, which presents with pneumoperitoneum. This is considered to be a distinct entity from NEC, and occurs earlier in the hospital course than NEC, often in the setting of no or minimal feeding; and is more common among extremely preterm infants (< 28 weeks' gestation). NEC in term infants accounts for approximately 10% of cases and these infants manifest symptoms similar to those of preterm infants, although they are likely to have a different pathophysiology of the disease, as discussed later.

### Radiographic Findings

The primary radiographic finding in NEC is *pneumatosis intestinalis*, a radiographic appearance of gas within the wall of the small or large intestine (Fig. 60-3). This is the hallmark of NEC and often establishes the diagnosis (Table 60-1). Other radiographic findings may include abdominal distention with evidence of ileus, portal venous gas, or pneumoperitoneum (Fig. 60-4). In addition, bowel loops that remain unchanged on serial radiographic films for 24 to 48 hours raise the concern for ischemic bowel. Infants with evidence of pneumoperitoneum require surgery. The presence of portal venous gas may be associated with a higher eventual need for surgery although its role as a prognostic marker for mortality is unclear.

**TABLE 60-1 DIAGNOSTIC FEATURES AND TREATMENT OF NEC**

| Staging of NEC | Clinical Signs and Symptoms | Radiographic Findings | Treatment |
|---|---|---|---|
| Suspected (Stage I) | Unexpected onset of feeding intolerance, abdominal distention, bloody stools, emesis, lethargy, apnea, bradycardia | Abdominal distention *without* radiographic evidence of pneumatosis intestinalis, portal venous gas, or free intraperitoneal air | Close clinical observation; consider bowel decompression, blood culture, short course of antibiotics, and brief discontinuation of feeding with monitoring of blood counts and abdominal radiographs for progression |
| Definite or medical (Stage II) | Unexpected onset of feeding intolerance, abdominal distention, bloody stools, emesis, lethargy, apnea, bradycardia | Abdominal distention *with* radiographic evidence of pneumatosis intestinalis, portal venous gas, or both; may also have dilated loops of bowel or ileus pattern | Bowel decompression and bowel rest for 7–10 days with broad-spectrum intravenous antibiotics; close monitoring of abdominal radiographs and blood counts |
| Surgical (Stage III) | Shock and disseminated intravascular coagulation; deteriorating laboratory values, including leukopenia, thrombocytopenia, acidosis, hyponatremia, and hyperkalemia | Free intraperitoneal air; in the setting of deteriorating clinical signs, infants with an ileus pattern, absence of bowel gas, or unchanging bowel gas pattern on serial abdominal radiographs may warrant surgery | Exploratory laparotomy or peritoneal drain placement |

NEC, necrotizing enterocolitis.
Data from Bell MJ, Ternberg JL, Feigin RD, et al. Neonatal necrotizing enterocolitis: therapeutic decisions based upon clinical staging, *Ann Surg.* 1978 Jan;187(1):1-7 and Walsh MC, Kliegman RM. Necrotizing enterocolitis: treatment based on staging criteria, *Pediatr Clin North Am.* 1986 Feb;33(1):179-201.

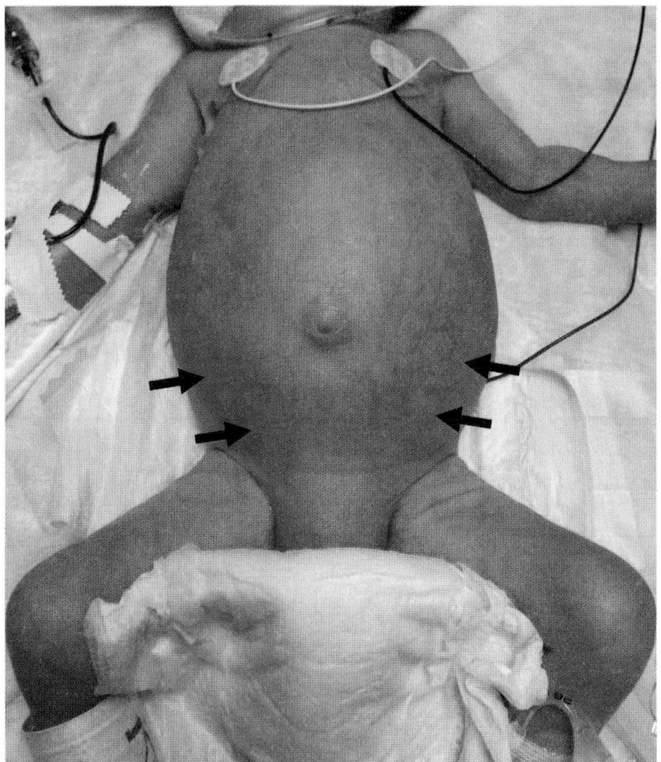

**FIGURE 60-2** Infant with surgical necrotizing enterocolitis demonstrating evidence of abdominal distention and abdominal wall erythema (*black arrows*).

**FIGURE 60-3** Chest and abdominal radiograph of an infant with necrotizing enterocolitis demonstrating diffuse pneumatosis intestinalis (*white arrows*).

## DIAGNOSTIC EVALUATION

The diagnostic evaluation of infants with suspected NEC includes evaluation for bloodstream infection, which can accompany NEC and is associated with worse outcome. Urine culture should also be obtained, as a urinary tract infection may precede the diagnosis of NEC. Patients with NEC should have a complete blood count with differential and serum chemistry monitored. Hematologic changes that occur with NEC include thrombocytopenia, coagulopathy, anemia, neutropenia or neutrophilia, eosinophilia, and lymphopenia; further, the presence of significant hematologic abnormalities is often associated with more severe disease. In addition, infants with NEC may develop hyponatremia, hyperkalemia, and metabolic acidosis.

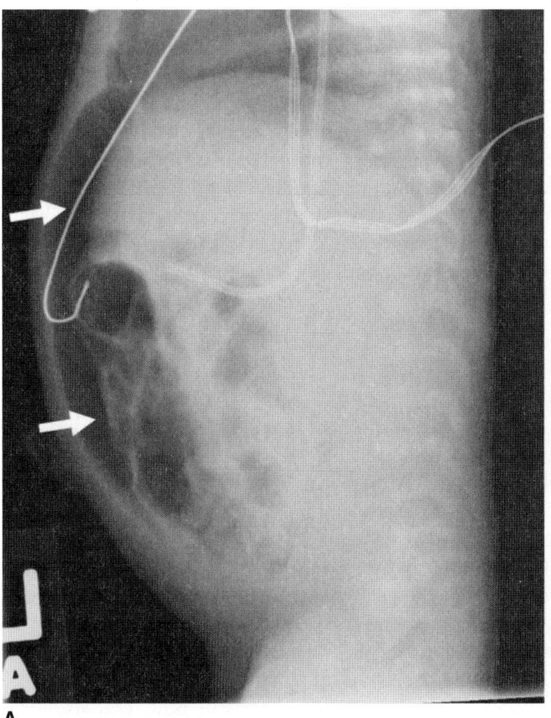


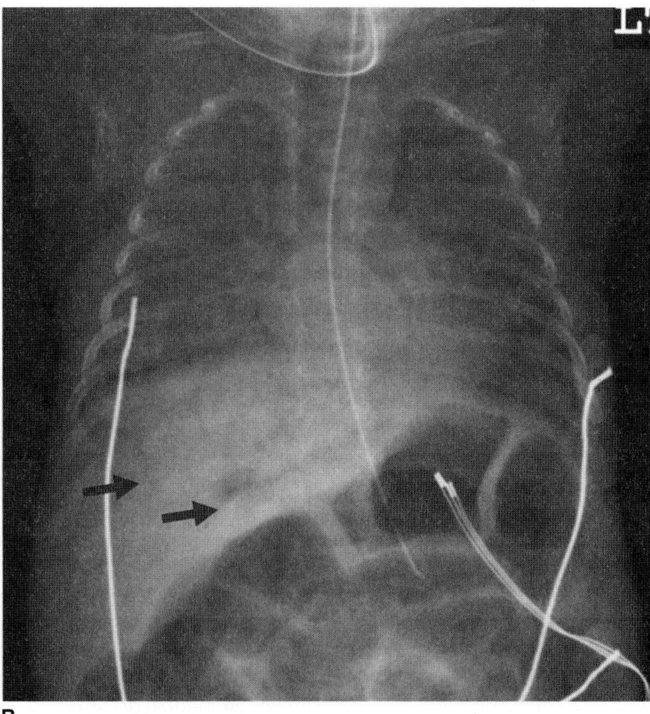


**FIGURE 60-4** **A:** Abdominal radiograph of an infant with pneumoperitoneum (*white arrows*). **B:** Radiograph of another infant with necrotizing enterocolitis and portal venous gas (*black arrows*).

Infants with suspected NEC should have abdominal radiographs taken that include both anteroposterior views and either left-lateral decubitus or cross-table images to evaluate for free intraperitoneal air (Fig. 60-4). Abdominal radiographs should be performed serially until the patient has demonstrated improvement in radiographic findings and clinical symptoms. Blood gas measurements should be performed at routine intervals to monitor for acidosis and respiratory deterioration. A lower serum pH (ie, metabolic acidosis) is associated with advanced disease. If infants appear likely to need surgery or demonstrate worsening clinical status, coagulation studies should be obtained, as disseminated intravascular coagulation is often present in advanced cases of NEC.

## TREATMENT

### Medical Management

The treatment of NEC is based on the severity and involves bowel decompression, bowel rest, antimicrobial therapy, and monitoring of serial abdominal radiographs and laboratory parameters (Table 60-1). Bloodstream infection develops in up to one-third of infants with NEC. Therefore, broad-spectrum antimicrobial therapy is indicated. Most bloodstream infections are caused by gram-negative bacteria, most commonly *Escherichia coli* and *Klebsiella.*

**Antibiotic Selection and Duration** There exists wide variation in the choice of antibiotic treatment for NEC, with a combination of vancomycin and gentamicin being the 2 most commonly used antibiotic agents in this population. Other commonly used antibiotics include ampicillin, cephalosporins, clindamycin, metronidazole, and carbapenems. In a small randomized controlled trial of 42 infants, the addition of anaerobic coverage with clindamycin to a standard regimen of ampicillin and gentamicin, compared to ampicillin and gentamicin alone, did not reduce the risk of intestinal perforation or death. However, surviving infants in the group receiving clindamycin, compared to ampicillin and gentamicin alone, had a higher incidence of intestinal stricture (40% vs 5.6%; $P = 0.02$). In a larger propensity-matched study of 2780 infants from 348 US NICUs, infants receiving initial anaerobic antimicrobial therapy at the onset of NEC, compared to those not exposed, had a higher risk of strictures (odds ratio [OR], 1.73; 95% CI, 1.11–2.72) but a lower risk of mortality (OR, 0.71; 95% CI, 0.52–0.95). In addition, this study found a decreasing use of clindamycin and increasing use of metronidazole during the study period, from 1997 to 2012. Therefore, the risks of intestinal stricture with anaerobic antimicrobial therapy should be balanced with the potential benefits in survival, particularly among infants with risk factors for high-case fatality (discussed in the next section). There is a paucity of data to guide the optimal duration of antibiotic treatment for NEC, although treatment for 7 to 10 days is common for definite NEC and often longer for surgical NEC or when specific pathogens are isolated (Table 60-1).

### Surgical Management

**Indications** Surgical treatment is necessary in 30% to 35% of infants with NEC, and mortality at 18 to 22 months of follow-up is as high as 50% among these infants. Pneumoperitoneum is the most frequent indication for surgery, although additional surgical criteria can include portal venous gas, abnormal paracentesis, abdominal wall erythema, palpable abdominal mass, or "fixed" intestinal loop on x-ray. A deterioration in clinical and laboratory parameters, as previously discussed, should also be considered when deciding whether surgery is indicated. Small studies have suggested that abdominal ultrasound may be useful in identification of bowel necrosis in infants with NEC, although this is currently not widely used.

**Surgical Approaches** The surgical treatment of NEC involves 1 of 2 approaches. Traditionally, management has involved an exploratory laparotomy with resection of affected bowel. However, especially in infants with a birth weight of less than 1000 g, peritoneal drainage has become a more commonly used method to provide abdominal decompression until the need for a definitive laparotomy can be reassessed. In a multicenter trial of 117 infants with perforated NEC, infants were randomized to primary peritoneal drainage or laparotomy with bowel resection. There was no difference in the 90-day postoperative mortality between laparotomy and primary peritoneal drainage treatment arms (35.5% vs 34.5%; relative risk, 1.03; 95% CI, 0.63–1.69), with similar findings in the subgroup of infants weighing less than 1000 g. In a multicenter observational study of 156 extremely low–birth-weight (ELBW) infants with either spontaneous intestinal perforation or severe NEC, 76% were treated with an initial peritoneal drain and did not need a subsequent laparotomy. However, of concern was a higher associated risk of death or neurodevelopmental impairment among infants receiving peritoneal drainage compared to initial laparotomy. Currently, a multicenter randomized trial is being conducted in the United States to compare these 2 surgical approaches with the primary outcome of death or neurodevelopmental impairment at 18 to 22 months of age.

## OUTCOMES

### Mortality

Cause-specific mortality from NEC is high and varies depending on the gestational age and birth weight of the infant, with case-fatality rates ranging from 65% at 23 weeks' gestation to 12% among term infants (Fig. 60-1). In a study of 7099 infants with NEC in a large multicenter cohort of NICUs, of whom 1505 died, factors associated with a higher risk of death included a lower gestational age, lower birth weight, treatment with assisted ventilation on the day of diagnosis, treatment with vasopressors at the time of diagnosis, and black race. The majority of deaths from NEC occur within 7 days of diagnosis.

### Long Term Outcomes

**Neurodevelopmental Impairment** Neurodevelopmental impairment is common among preterm infants with NEC, particularly those infants that required surgery or had a comorbid bloodstream infection. In a UK study that followed 119 (77%) of 157 infants with NEC until 7 years of age, and compared them to 6496 controls, those with a history of NEC had a higher incidence of cerebral palsy (6.8% vs 2.5%; unadjusted OR, 2.77; 95% CI, 1.33–5.77), attention-deficit/hyperactivity disorder (15.3% vs 7.3%; unadjusted OR, 2.24; 95% CI, 1.34–3.72), and decreased educational attainment. However, after adjusting for antenatal and neonatal factors, many of these differences were no longer significantly different between groups. If ELBW infants with NEC undergo surgery, they are at higher risk for significant long-term cognitive and motor impairment: 24% of these infants are diagnosed with cerebral palsy at 18 to 22 months corrected age and 57% have a degree of neurodevelopmental impairment, as compared to an incidence of impairment in 44% of infants with NEC not requiring surgery and 40% of infants without NEC. In addition, ELBW infants with sepsis and NEC have a similarly high incidence of neurodevelopmental impairment of 53% compared to an incidence of 29% among ELBW infants without infection. The highest risk of adverse outcomes appears to be in infants with both surgical NEC and late bacteremia, who were found to have 8-fold higher odds of cerebral palsy compared to infants without NEC or late bacteremia.

**Short-Bowel Syndrome** *Short-bowel syndrome* is the leading cause of intestinal failure in infants, accounting for 44% of cases. It results from the surgical resection of so much affected bowel that there remains insufficient intestinal mass to maintain growth, hydration, or electrolyte balance. The risk of short-bowel syndrome depends on the amount of bowel resected and the presence of an ileocecal valve. With bowel lengthening and tapering procedures, infants with only 35 cm of residual bowel have a 50% probability of being able to wean off of parenteral nutrition and achieve enteral autonomy. In a multicenter cohort of children with intestinal failure, each additional centimeter of residual bowel length was associated with higher odds of enteral autonomy (OR, 1.04; 95% CI, 1.02–1.06), as was having an ileocecal value present (OR, 2.80; 95% CI, 1.63–4.83). Even among children who remain on parenteral nutrition beyond 1 year of age, 64% are able to wean from it, and a diagnosis of NEC is associated with a greater probability of weaning off parental nutrition compared to other causes of short-bowel syndrome. However, among those infants unable to wean off parenteral nutrition, liver disease, sepsis, and re-hospitalization are common, and intestinal and liver transplantation may be necessary for survival. In the previously mentioned UK study with 7-year follow-up of infants with NEC, the incidence of gastrointestinal problems persisted for many infants. Compared to 3.2% of infants without NEC, 15.3% of infants with NEC reported ongoing bowel problems at 7 years of age and 5.1% had a bowel stoma present.

## PATHOGENESIS

The major underlying factor involved in the pathogenesis of NEC is prematurity, indicated by an increasing incidence and severity of NEC as gestational age falls (Fig. 60-1). Preterm infants have an immature epithelial barrier with a greater tendency for inflammation, a leakier gut, and decreased innate mucosal defenses. Studies of the intestinal microbiota have identified a number of differences in infants with NEC, compared to those without (discussed below). An important consideration is that NEC likely encompasses a spectrum of heterogeneous diseases that lead to intestinal injury and present with similar signs and symptoms. Therefore, the pathogenesis of "classical" NEC that predominately affects VLBW infants may differ from NEC in full-term infants, which typically presents earlier in the hospital course and predominately affects the colon. Multiple risk factors for NEC in term infants have been reported, including intrauterine growth retardation, birth asphyxia, congenital heart disease, gastroschisis, polycythemia, hypoglycemia, sepsis, exchange transfusion, blood transfusions, the use of umbilical catheters, milk-protein allergy, premature rupture of membranes, chorioamnionitis and gestational diabetes.

### Role of the Microbiome

The intestine must balance protection against harmful environmental antigens, such as pathogenic bacteria, while housing beneficial commensal bacteria. This balance is important in maintaining intestinal homeostasis. If disrupted, intestinal inflammation and injury may play a role in NEC. Commensal bacteria help protect against intestinal injury, maintain intestinal homeostasis and immune function, and support digestion of food. Preterm infants have delayed acquisition of beneficial commensal bacteria such as *Bifidobacterium* and are more likely to be colonized with virulent pathogens. A number of factors may influence this colonization. Decreased human milk feeding can result in decreased colonization of beneficial commensal bacteria such as *Bifidobacterium*, *Lactobacillus*, and *Bacteroides*. Prolonged empiric antibiotic therapy has been associated with an increased risk of NEC in several studies, and antibiotic treatment after birth results in decreased *Bifidobacterium* colonization. In addition, cesarean delivery may result in decreased *Bifidobacterium*, *Lactobacillus*, and *Bacteroides* colonization. Several studies have shown that infants who go on to develop NEC have changes in the prevalence of *Clostridium perfringens*, Firmicutes, Proteobacteria, and *Enterobacter* before the onset of NEC, as well as decreases in *Bifidobacterium*, with some changes occurring soon after birth. In a longitudinal study of 122 VLBW infants, those who went on to develop NEC had a relative abundance of Gram-negative facultative bacilli (Gammaproteobacteria) and a paucity of strict anaerobic bacteria, particularly Negativicutes. Additionally, changes in the microbiome that precede NEC may occur several weeks before NEC onset, and infants with NEC have lower microbial diversity. Finally, Toll-like receptors (TLRs) recognize microbial associated molecule patterns (MAMPs) such as lipopolysaccharide and peptidoglycan, which are part of the cell wall of bacteria. Toll-like receptor 4 activation has been implicated as a major pathway of NEC and can impair intestinal perfusion through changes in endothelial nitric oxide synthase signaling, which is ameliorated by administration of nitrate, a component of breast milk. In addition, commensal and probiotic bacteria have been shown to decrease TLR-mediated inflammation.

## PREVENTION

A number of systematic reviews and meta-analyses of randomized studies evaluating treatments that include NEC as either a primary or secondary outcome have been conducted, and are summarized in Table 60-2.

### Breast Milk



Breastfeeding of maternal milk has long been established as a key, if not most important, part of a strategy to prevent NEC. The risk of NEC is inversely related to the amount of breast milk exposure. There are a number of components of human milk, including oligosaccharides, lactoferrin, probiotics, epidermal growth factor, long-chain polyunsaturated fatty acids, platelet activating factor acetylhydrolase, immunoglobulins (IgA and IgG), arginine, and glutamine, that may mediate the benefits of breast milk in reducing NEC. When maternal breast milk is not available, donor human milk also reduces the risk of NEC in VLBW infants, as demonstrated in a large, multicenter randomized trial in Canada. In this trial, the incidence of NEC (Bell stage 2 or greater) was lower in infants fed donor milk using bovine-based fortifiers compared to infants fed preterm formula (1.7% vs 6.6%; $P = 0.02$). The trial showed no differences in the primary outcome of mean cognitive score at 18 months corrected age or in growth parameters. However, infants receiving donor milk, compared to infants receiving formula, were more likely to have a cognitive score less than 85 (27.2% vs 16.2%; $P = 0.02$) in analysis of secondary outcomes, raising potential concerns for the adverse long-term effects of donor human milk. Another randomized trial found an exclusive human milk diet with human milk–based fortifiers, compared to preterm formula, resulted in a decrease in the risk of severe NEC requiring surgery. Similar findings of a decrease in NEC with a human milk diet compared to a diet containing bovine products was reported in a multicenter observational study. In a systematic review completed before these studies, infants receiving donor milk demonstrated decreased weight, length, and head circumference compared to those receiving formula, although the comparisons were limited by inadequate fortification of donor milk. Another recent multicenter trial in the Netherlands found no significant effect of donor milk on severe infections or on mortality, and additional trials are ongoing.

### Probiotics

Given that an abnormal intestinal microbiome has been described in the pathogenesis of NEC, modifying the microbiome through the administration of bacteria that are contained in probiotic preparations or by administering prebiotics that support the growth of so-called health-promoting bacteria is a logical approach to prevention of NEC. Preclinical studies have shown that certain probiotics decrease proinflammatory mediators; increase anti-inflammatory mediators; support pathways important in growth, differentiation, and cytoprotection; decrease apoptosis; generate reactive-oxygen species important in regulating apoptotic, proliferative, and inflammatory signaling; and support intestinal barrier function.

Pooled results of randomized trials of probiotic supplementation in preterm infants show a decreased risk of NEC, mortality, and late-onset sepsis. However, questions regarding the optimal dose and preparation of probiotic therapy, lack of regulated commercial products, and risk of probiotic-associated sepsis have limited widespread use. A recent survey of 500 NICUs in the United States found that 14% were using probiotics in VLBW infants, with single-strain preparations being the predominant products utilized, many of which have not been extensively studied in preterm neonates. In addition, a recent large, multicenter trial found no effect of *Bifidobacterium breve* on the risk of NEC. This trial highlights the continued uncertainty regarding the effect of specific probiotic preparations on the risk of NEC. There is an inherent fallacy when one argues for the use of probiotics, encompassing a broad range of different preparations for the prevention of NEC. Each preparation should be considered individually rather than as a group. Caution in applying pharmacologic standards is needed when using these preparations in a vulnerable population such as preterm infants.

### Additional Strategies

**Feeding Strategies** There is limited evidence to support any single feeding strategy to reduce the risk of NEC, aside from the use of human milk, which is already a standard. Numerous studies in animals show that lack of enteral feeding leads to intestinal atrophy, exaggerated inflammatory responses, increased bacterial translocation, and risk

**TABLE 60-2 SYSTEMATIC REVIEWS AND META-ANALYSES OF EFFECT OF NEONATAL INTERVENTIONS ON NEC**

| Year | Enrolled *n*, (Trials) | Population | Intervention vs Placebo/Control | RR of NEC (95% CI) | Effect on NEC | Conclusion or Comment |
|---|---|---|---|---|---|---|
| 2016 | 1840 (3) | < 37 wk or < 2500 g | Oral IgA and/or IgG vs control | 0.84 (0.57–1.25) | None | No RCTs of oral IgA alone |
| 2015 | 949 (9) | Very preterm or VLBW | Slow (up to 24 mL/kg/d) vs faster (30–40 mL/kg/d) feeding advancement | 1.02 (0.64–1.62) | None | Further trials may be warranted |
| 2015 | 3462 (8) | Preterm infants | Animal vs synthetic surfactant preparation | 1.38 (1.08–1.76) | ↑ | Marginal decrease in risk of mortality |
| 2015 | 552 (2) | Preterm infants | Oral lactoferrin alone vs placebo | 0.30 (0.12–0.76) | ↓ | Moderate to low quality evidence; large trials ongoing |
| 2015 | 496 (1) | Preterm infants | Oral lactoferrin + probiotics vs placebo | 0.04 (0.00–0.62) | ↓ | Single trial |
| 2015 | 4929 (5) | < 28 wk | Oxygen saturation targets of 85–89% vs 91–95% | 1.24 (1.05–1.47) | ↑ | Moderate quality evidence |
| 2014 | 526 (4) | Preterm infants | Restricted vs liberal water intake | 0.43 (0.21–0.87) | ↓ | Also decreases risk of PDA |
| 2014 | 1070 (9) | < 37 wk or < 2500 g | Formula vs donor milk | 2.77 (1.40–5.46) | ↑ | Decreased growth with donor milk |
| 2014 | 1092 (8) | Very preterm or VLBW | Delayed enteral feeds (> 4 days after birth) vs earlier introduction | 0.93 (0.61–1.34) | None | Further trials may be warranted |
| 2014 | 5529 (20) | < 37 wk or < 2500 g | Probiotic supplementation vs placebo or no treatment | 0.43 (0.33–0.56) | ↓ | Evidence supports a change in practice |
| 2013 | 102 (3) | < 37 wk or < 2500 g | Dilute vs full strength formula | Not reported | Not reported | NEC was not reported as an outcome |
| 2013 | 748 (9) | Very preterm or VLBW | Early trophic feeding (up to 24 mL/kg/d) before 96 h of age vs enteral fasting | 1.07 (0.67–1.70) | None | Further trials may be warranted |
| 2013 | 130 (1) | < 37 wk PMA | Addition of lactase to milk vs placebo/no intervention | 0.32 (0.01–7.79) | None | Only 1 event of NEC |
| 2012 | 241 (5) | Preterm infants | Delayed cord clamping vs early clamping | 0.62 (0.43–0.90) | ↓ | Insufficient data for reliable conclusions |
| 2011 | 590 (3) | VLBW infants | Low vs high hemoglobin threshold for transfusion | 1.62 (0.83–3.13) | None | Further trials needed; large trials ongoing |
| 2011 | 465 (5) | VLBW infants | Continuous vs intermittent bolus tube feeding | 1.09 (0.58–2.07) | None | Insufficient data for reliable conclusions |
| 2008 | 84 (1) | ELBW infants | Prophylactic surgical ligation vs no intervention or cyclooxygenase inhibitor | 0.25 (0.08–0.83) | ↓ | Prophylactic surgical therapy not indicated given alternatives |
| 2007 | 310 (4) | Preterm infants with PDA | Prolonged (4+ doses) vs short (< 4 doses) course of indomethacin | 1.87 (1.07–3.27) | ↑ | Prolonged course cannot be recommended |
| 2007 | 152 (1) | Preterm infants | Arginine supplementation vs placebo | 0.24 (0.10–0.61) | ↓ | Data insufficient to support practice recommendation |
| 2006 | 1675 (8) | Preterm infants | Maternal treatment of antenatal corticosteroids vs placebo or no treatment | 0.46 (0.29–0.74) | ↓ | Treatment should be routine, with few exceptions |
| 2001 | 456 (5) | < 37 wk or < 2500 g | Enteral aminoglycoside vs control | 0.47 (0.28–0.78) | ↓ | Additional studies needed |

CI, confidence interval; ELBW, extremely low birth weight; Ig, immunoglobulin; NEC, necrotizing enterocolitis; PDA, patent ductus arteriosus; PMA, postmenstrual age; RCT, randomized controlled trial; RR, relative risk; VLBW, very low birth weight.



for intestinal damage. Total parenteral nutrition, delayed initiation of enteral feeding, and a longer duration to reach full enteral feeding are also associated with increased risk for late-onset sepsis in VLBW infants, which may be due, in part, to increased intestinal microbial translocation. A recent study suggests that later onset of feedings is associated with greater inflammatory response as well as increased adverse outcomes, such as chronic lung disease and retinopathy of prematurity. Meta-analysis of randomized trials found no benefit of early trophic feeding, compared to no feeding, or slow advancement of feeding, compared to rapid advancement of feeding, on the risk of NEC (Table 60-2). However, there was substantial clinical heterogeneity among the study populations with small sample sizes and imprecise estimates of treatment effects in the pooled estimates. The use of feeding protocols in observational studies is associated with a reduction in the incidence of NEC, although feeding protocols differ in approaches. The role of aspiration to evaluate gastric residuals as part of feeding is controversial, although larger volumes of gastric residuals have been associated with NEC in preclinical and clinical studies. A recent pilot trial that randomized 61 preterm infants to routine monitoring of gastric residuals versus no routine monitoring demonstrated no differences in NEC or other adverse outcomes.

**Avoidance of Acid Suppression Medications and Prolonged Antibiotic Exposure** Use of acid-suppression medications such as $H_2$ antagonists are associated with NEC, as is prolonged empiric antibiotic therapy in the setting of negative blood cultures. These $H_2$ antagonists reduce gastric pH and may lower bacterial diversity and increase the relative abundance of pathogenic bacteria by reducing the bactericidal effect of stomach acid on microbes entering the gastrointestinal tract. Of interest is that $H_2$ antagonist use is associated with increases in intestinal Proteobacteria, a phylum that has been shown to expand in abundance prior to NEC.

Similarly, antibiotic duration for greater than 3 days has been associated with a higher risk of colonization with pathogenic Gram-negative bacteria such as *Klebsiella*, *Enterobacter*, or *Citrobacter*. Although data from randomized trials are lacking, reducing the use of $H_2$ antagonists and other acid-suppression medications, and limiting prolonged empiric antibiotic therapy given negative cultures may help to decrease NEC. Use of quality improvement approaches can reduce the use of antibiotics and $H_2$ antagonists. Pragmatic randomized trials of the effects of shorter courses of antibiotics on the microbiome as well as short-term adverse outcomes are likely to provide important new information in this area.

**Delayed Cord Clamping, Oxygen Delivery, and Anemia** Additional potential risk factors for NEC include impaired intestinal oxygen delivery from anemia, abnormal regulation of intestinal blood flow, or lower oxygen saturation targets. The role of red blood cell transfusion in the pathogenesis of NEC is controversial and may be a marker of illness severity among infants who develop NEC rather than a causal factor. However, delayed clamping of the umbilical cord to allow for placental transfusion of blood may reduce the risk of NEC. However, more precise estimation of the effect of delayed cord clamping on NEC and longer-term data regarding safety in ELBW infants is needed.

**Biomarkers** Multiple biomarkers for NEC have been studied in the stool, serum, and urine in preterm infants. Some of the biomarkers that have been evaluated to date include urinary intestinal fatty acid–binding protein, urinary claudin-3, serum amyloid A, and fecal calprotectin. More recently an "electronic-nose" technique to detect fecal volatile organic compounds has been suggested as being potentially efficacious in the early diagnosis of NEC. All these techniques await rigorous validation prior to routine clinical use.

## CONCLUSION

Although recent studies suggest the incidence of NEC has been decreasing in the United States, it remains a major cause of death and serious morbidity in preterm infants. New approaches have provided insight into the role of the microbiome in the pathogenesis of NEC. Clinical studies have provided additional data to support the use of human milk and avoid harmful medications. However, additional studies are needed to better define and diagnose NEC and to identify biomarkers effective in identifying high-risk infants as well as safe, effective, and reliable prevention strategies in order to improve outcomes among infants who are diagnosed with NEC.

## SUGGESTED READINGS


AlFaleh K, Anabrees J. Probiotics for prevention of necrotizing enterocolitis in preterm infants. *Cochrane Database Syst Rev.* 2014;(4):CD005496.

Autmizguine J, Hornik CP, Benjamin DK Jr, et al. Anaerobic antimicrobial therapy after necrotizing enterocolitis in VLBW infants. *Pediatrics.* 2015;135(1):e117-e125.

Battersby C, Longford N, Costeloe K, Modi N; the UK Neonatal Collaborative Necrotising Enterocolitis Study Group. Development of a gestational age–specific case definition for neonatal necrotizing enterocolitis. *JAMA Pediatr.* 2017;171(3):256-263.

Battersby C, Longford N, Mandalia S, Costeloe K, Modi N. Incidence and enteral feed antecedents of severe neonatal necrotising enterocolitis across neonatal networks in England, 2012-13: a whole-population surveillance study. *Lancet Gastroenterol Hepatol.* 2017;2(1):43-51.

Clark RH, Gordon RH, Walker WM, Laughon M, Smith PB, Spitzer AR. Characteristics of patients who die of necrotizing enterocolitis. *J Perinatol.* 2012;32(3):199-204.

Costeloe K, Hardy P, Juszczak E, Wilks M, Millar MR; Probiotics in Preterm Infants Study Collaborative Group. *Bifidobacterium breve* BBG-001 in very preterm infants: a randomised controlled phase 3 trial. *Lancet.* 2016;387(10019):649-660.

Gordon PV, Clark R, Swanson JR, Spitzer A. Can a national dataset generate a nomogram for necrotizing enterocolitis onset? *J Perinatol.* 2014;34(10):732-735.

Neu J, Walker WA. Necrotizing enterocolitis. *N Engl J Med.* 2011;364(3):255-264.

O'Connor DL, Gibbins S, Kiss A, et al. Effect of supplemental donor human milk compared with preterm formula on neurodevelopment of very low-birth-weight infants at 18 months: a randomized clinical trial. *JAMA.* 2016;316(18):1897-1905.

Patel RM, Kandefer S, Walsh MC, et al. Causes and timing of death in extremely premature infants from 2000 through 2011. *N Engl J Med.* 2015;372(4):331-340.

Pike K, Brocklehurst P, Jones D, et al. Outcomes at 7 years for babies who developed neonatal necrotising enterocolitis: the ORACLE Children Study. *Arch Dis Child Fetal Neonatal Ed.* 2012;97(5):F318-F322.

Rao SC, Athalye-Jape GK, Deshpande GC, Simmer KN, Patole SK. Probiotic supplementation and late-onset sepsis in preterm infants: a meta-analysis. *Pediatrics.* 2016;137(3):e20153684.

Warner BB, Deych E, Zhou Y, et al. Gut bacteria dysbiosis and necrotising enterocolitis in very low birthweight infants: a prospective case-control study. *Lancet.* 2016;387(10031):1928-1936.

Yazji I, Sodhi CP, Lee EK, et al. Endothelial TLR4 activation impairs intestinal microcirculatory perfusion in necrotizing enterocolitis via eNOS-NO-nitrite signaling. *Proc Natl Acad Sci U S A.* 2013;110(23):9451-9456.




# 61 Intraventricular Hemorrhage

Brian H. Walsh and Terrie E. Inder

## INTRODUCTION

Neonatal germinal matrix hemorrhage/intraventricular hemorrhage (GMH/IVH) is the most common form of intracranial hemorrhage in preterm infants, and an important cause of long-term morbidities among survivors of neonatal intensive care. In its least severe form, the hemorrhage may be restricted to the germinal matrix area or subependymal zone. However, it frequently extends beyond the germinal matrix into the cerebral ventricles, following rupture of the germinal matrix hemorrhage into the ventricular space.

## INCIDENCE

Germinal matrix hemorrhage/intraventricular hemorrhage occurs most frequently among preterm infants. Its incidence decreases as gestational age and birth weight increase. Because of improvement in perinatal and neonatal care, the incidence of GMH/IVH has decreased over the past several decades. However, this decline is of a lesser extent than that in neonatal mortality. Approximately 3 decades ago, GMH/IVH was noted in 45% of very low–birth-weight (VLBW) infants and in greater than 60% of those with birth weight of 750 grams or less. By the early 1990s, the incidence of GMH/IVH decreased to 30% of VLBW infants, and to 40% among the extremely low–birth-weight (ELBW) survivors, and by the mid 1990s had decreased further to 24%. Since that time, however, the incidence has remained static, remaining about 25% among all VLBW infants based upon data from the Vermont Oxford Network database (Fig. 61-1A). The more severe hemorrhages, grades III and IV, occur in 12% to 17% of ELBW infants and in as high as 20% of those with birth weight of 750 grams or less (Fig. 61-1B). These severe hemorrhages occur in 17% to 28% of those born at 22 to 26 weeks' gestation and in 9% to 14% of those 27 to 32 weeks' gestation.

## PATHOGENESIS AND RISK FACTORS

The pathogenesis of GMH/IVH is complex and involves multiple risk factors and disorders, with biochemical, inflammatory, and hemodynamic alterations and predisposing to the development of hemorrhage. Ultimately, the mechanisms for predisposition to hemorrhage, and the relationship among GMH/IVH and white matter and neuronal injury may be linked to the generation of free radicals, reactive oxygen and nitrogen species, and gene-environment interactions.

Hemorrhage originates in the germinal matrix which is a prominent structure in the preterm brain during the second and early third trimesters that subsequently undergoes involution as gestation reaches term. The germinal matrix structure contains neuronal precursor cells prior to 20 weeks of gestation. As development progresses, the differentiating glioblasts give rise to oligodendroglial cells, which are important for myelination. The germinal matrix is supplied by a complex vascular network but is a low blood flow structure. The hemorrhage

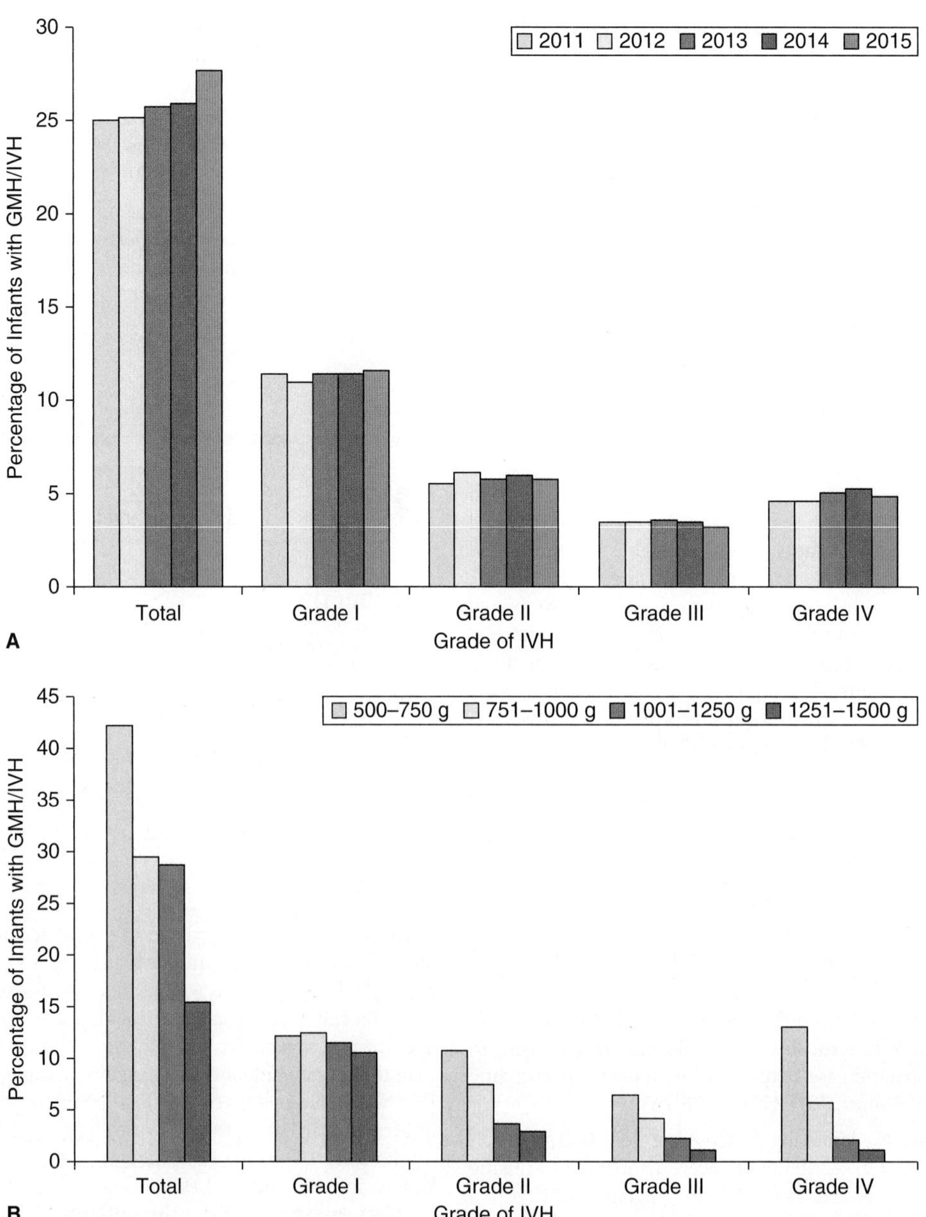


**FIGURE 61-1 A:** The incidence of all grades of IVH, and individual IVH grades, in the Vermont Oxford Network database from 2011 to 2015, stratified by year. **B:** The incidence of all grades of IVH, and individual IVH grades, in the Vermont Oxford Network database from 2011 to 2015, stratified by birth weight. GMH, germinal matrix hemorrhage; IVH, intraventricular hemorrhage.

appears to originate from the endothelial-lined vessels of the matrix, in particular, vessels in communication with the venous circulation, including capillary-venule junctions and small venules. These thin-walled germinal matrix capillaries are susceptible to rupture, for several potential reasons. Their large diameter offers lesser resistance to changes in intravascular pressure, to the immature endothelial cell tight junctions, and to low levels of structurally stabilizing proteins such as fibronectin and collagen in the extracellular matrix. Rupture of the capillaries results when the endothelial wall loses integrity and/or when there is imbalance of pressure between the intravascular lumen and the extravascular space.

Clinical risk factors associated with IVH include lower gestational age, lack of antenatal corticosteroids, clinical chorioamnionitis, male sex, significant delivery room resuscitation, mechanical ventilation, and hypotension requiring multiple inotropes. In Table 61-1, the predisposing cerebrovascular factors and alterations in cerebral hemodynamics that may result from a variety of antenatal and postnatal conditions are listed. As seen in the schematic diagram in Figure 61-2, a single factor or a combination of factors may disrupt the cerebral circulation, leading to GMH/IVH and its complications.

## CLINICAL MANIFESTATIONS AND DIAGNOSIS

Germinal matrix hemorrhage/intraventricular hemorrhage is usually detected in the first 4 to 5 days of life with approximately 40% to 50% occurring on the first day of life, and up to 90% within the first 72 hours. Approximately 20% of early-onset hemorrhage may evolve to become more severe, with the maximum extent typically seen within the first week of life. The majority of hemorrhages, in particular, small ones, are asymptomatic and are only detected by routine cranial ultrasound. However, larger cases of GMH/IVH may present with sudden clinical deterioration, especially when there is a significant blood loss. Other clinical manifestations include anemia or failure; seizures; tense, full, and/or bulging fontanels; split and wide sutures; apnea and bradycardia with desaturation episodes; poor perfusion; hypotension; severe metabolic acidosis; increase in oxygen requirement; and increase in ventilator support.

Imaging studies will establish the diagnosis of GMH/IVH. The current standard approach to diagnosis is the use of cranial ultrasonography. Findings on ultrasound have been interpreted with a high level of agreement among practitioners. Ultrasound can be performed at the

| TABLE 61-1 FACTORS THAT INFLUENCE THE PATHOGENESIS OF GMH/IVH | | |
|---|---|---|
| | **Factors in the Pathogenesis of GMH/IVH** | **Antenatal and Postnatal Conditions Leading to Vascular and Hemodynamic Alterations, Increasing Risks for GMH/IVH** |
| Intravascular | Increased cerebral blood flow | Systemic hypertension in the presence of a pressure-passive circulation |
| | | Rapid volume expansion |
| | | Hypercarbia |
| | | Reduced hematocrit |
| | | Hypoglycemia |
| | Fluctuating cerebral blood flow | Fluctuating systemic blood pressure (BP) in the presence of a pressure-passive circulation |
| | | Hypercarbia |
| | | Hypovolemia |
| | | Hypotension |
| | | Patent ductus arteriosus |
| | | High $FiO_2$ |
| | Decreased cerebral blood flow (resulting in reperfusion injury) | Systemic hypotension in presence of a pressure-passive circulation |
| | | Asphyxia |
| | Increased cerebral venous pressure | Asphyxia |
| | | Venous anatomic arrangement |
| | | Prolonged labor and vaginal delivery (some conflicting reports) |
| | | Respiratory management (high peak inspiratory pressure, tracheal suctioning, pneumothorax) |
| Vascular | Immature vasculature | Preterm birth and low birth weight |
| | Undergoing remodeling and involution | |
| | Simple endothelial-lined vessels without collagen or muscle | |
| | Immature tight junctions | |
| | Large diameter of germinal matrix vessels relative to cortical vessels | Conditions associated with $\downarrow PaO_2$, $\uparrow PaCO_2$, $\downarrow pH$ |
| | Vulnerability to hypoxemia-ischemia as located in vascular border zone | Hypoxia-ischemia reperfusion |
| | Vessel endothelial damage | Inflammation/infection |
| | | Hypotension/shock |
| | | Oxygen therapy, hyperoxia, generation of oxygen-reactive species and other free radicals |
| Extravascular | Deficient vascular and extracellular matrix support | Preterm birth and low birth weight |
| | Excessive fibrinolytic activity | Low factor XIII levels (conflicting reports of significance) |

$FiO_2$, fraction of inspired oxygen; GVH/IVH, germinal matrix hemorrhage/intraventricular hemorrhage; $PaCO_2$, arterial partial pressure of carbon dioxide; $PaO_2$, arterial partial pressure of oxygen.

bedside, thus avoiding the risks of transporting the infant for either computed tomography (CT) or magnetic resonance imaging (MRI) scans. Table 61-2 shows the grading of GMH/IVH, based on Papile criteria from CT scanning still employed by clinicians and researchers for cranial ultrasound findings. Others have added findings such as cystic periventricular leukomalacia (PVL) to indicate associated white matter injury and measurements of the lateral ventricles to define mild to severe ventriculomegaly. Volpe proposed a modification to the grading system for cranial ultrasound findings. This newer modified grading system takes into consideration the location of hemorrhage and the amount of blood detected in the ventricles (Fig. 61-3).



## COMPLICATIONS AND NEUROPATHOLOGICAL ASSOCIATIONS

Germinal matrix hemorrhage/intraventricular hemorrhage may cause the destruction of the germinal matrix, periventricular hemorrhagic infarction, ventriculomegaly or hydrocephalus, white matter injury, and loss of cerebellar volume—each of which may have implications for the prognosis of the infant.

During the second trimester, the ganglionic eminence and subventricular zone, which are part of and immediately associated with the germinal matrix, respectively, are rich locations for neuronal and glial proliferation. Therefore, destruction of the germinal matrix during this vulnerable period leads to a reduction in proliferation and migration of neuronal and glial precursor cells, which, in turn, may impact brain growth and, potentially, the developmental outcome of these infants.

Periventricular hemorrhagic infarction (PVHI) can be seen as large echodensities on cranial ultrasound within the parenchyma adjacent to the GMH/IVH. Papile initially described this as extension of the IVH into the parenchyma. However, subsequent study has indicated that while PVHI is strongly associated with IVH, it is not an extension of the IVH; rather, it occurs due to obstruction of venous drainage leading to a venous hemorrhagic infarct. The area of infarction evolves into tissue loss such that a porencephalic cyst may be noted on later follow-up cranial ultrasound.

*Periventricular leukomalacia* (PVL) is a form of white matter injury that is commonly associated with GMH/IVH. It occurs in the periventricular arterial border zones. Although the exact mechanism of injury is not fully defined, it is thought to occur secondary to ischemia and inflammation, with associated glial activation, and damage of the preoligodendrocytes.

PVL may be either focal or diffuse. Focal PVL is classically described as macroscopic areas of necrosis. These initially appear as echodense lesions in the periventricular area with or without blood in the ventricles. After several weeks, these echodense areas can become cystic, and are referred to as cystic PVL (Fig. 61-4). Cystic PVL occurs in less than 5% of very low–birth-weight infants, and represents the minority of PVL. More commonly, focal PVL consists of microscopic areas of necrosis, and is termed noncystic PVL. Diffuse PVL is characterized by a loss of preoligodendrocytes, rather than areas of necrosis. It leads to hypomyelination and is associated with ventriculomegaly due to decreased cerebral tissue volume. Cranial ultrasound has limited use in identifying noncystic and diffuse PVL, with MRI being a superior neuroimaging modality to screen for these types of injuries. The MRI findings among these infants include abnormalities on diffusion-weighted imaging and diffuse signal abnormalities.

About 2 to 3 weeks after the initial detection of GMH/IVH, some infants may present with increasing head circumference, separation of sutures, full and tense fontanels, and sun-setting appearance. A repeat cranial ultrasound in the presence of these manifestations of increased intracranial pressure will reveal prominence and enlargement of the cerebral ventricles (ventriculomegaly), and thus a diagnosis of posthemorrhagic hydrocephalus. Posthemorrhagic hydrocephalus results from a disturbance in cerebrospinal fluid (CSF) dynamics because of (1) the obstruction of the CSF pathway by blood clots in the posterior fossa cisterns, aqueduct of Sylvius, or foramen of Monro, and (2) postinflammatory changes in the arachnoid villi that may impair CSF absorption. Obstruction and delayed absorption of CSF leads to a progressive increase in ventricular size. Among those with GMH/IVH who survive for more than 14 days, 50% go on to develop ventricular dilation, which will progress in half of these infants. In 62% of those with progressive ventricular dilation, spontaneous arrest occurs, while the remaining 38% ultimately require nonsurgical or surgical

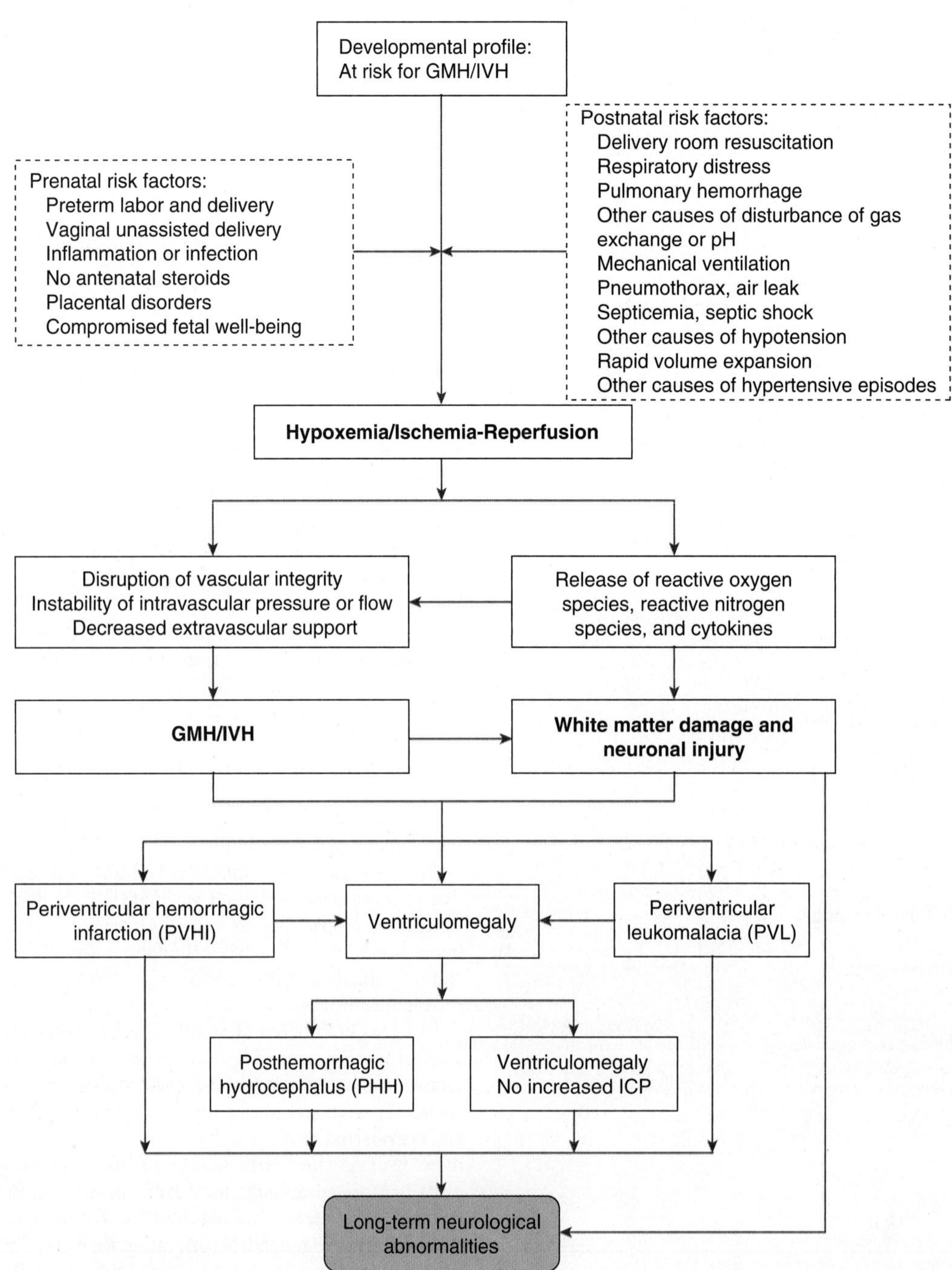


**FIGURE 61-2** Schematic diagram of the pathogenesis of germinal matrix hemorrhage/intraventricular hemorrhage (GMH/IVH) and its consequences. ICP, intracranial pressure.

treatment. Surgical intervention to relieve the increase in intracranial pressure and ameliorate associated clinical manifestations will be necessary for rapidly increasing head size, frequent apnea and bradycardia, and the need for increasing ventilatory support.

Ventriculomegaly may also occur without increased intracranial pressure (hydrocephalus ex-vacuo). This differs from posthemorrhagic hydrocephalus and may be a result of brain atrophy from periventricular white matter injury. It rarely requires surgical treatment.

**TABLE 61-2 CRANIAL ULTRASOUND FINDINGS AND GRADES OF HEMORRHAGES**

| Papile Criteria | Description | Volpe Criteria | Description |
|---|---|---|---|
| Grade I | Hemorrhage limited to the germinal matrix; may be unilateral or bilateral | Grade I | Blood in the germinal matrix area with or without minimal intraventricular hemorrhage (less than 10% of the ventricular space with blood) |
| Grade II | Blood noted within the ventricular system but not distending it | Grade II | Intraventricular hemorrhage with blood occupying 10–50% of the ventricular space (sagittal view) |
| Grade III | Blood in ventricles with distension or dilation of the ventricles | Grade III | Intraventricular hemorrhage with blood occupying greater than 50% of the ventricles with or without periventricular echodensities |
| Grade IV | Intraventricular hemorrhage with parenchymal extension | Separate notation of other findings | Periventricular hemorrhagic infarction<br>Cystic periventricular leukomalacia |

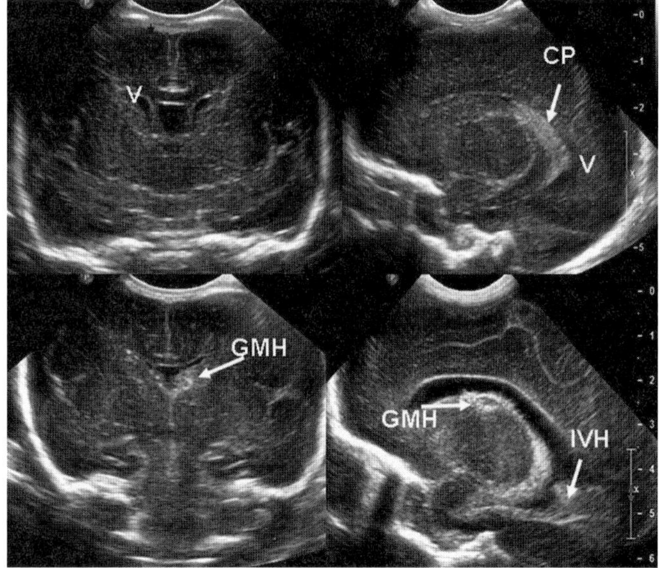


A

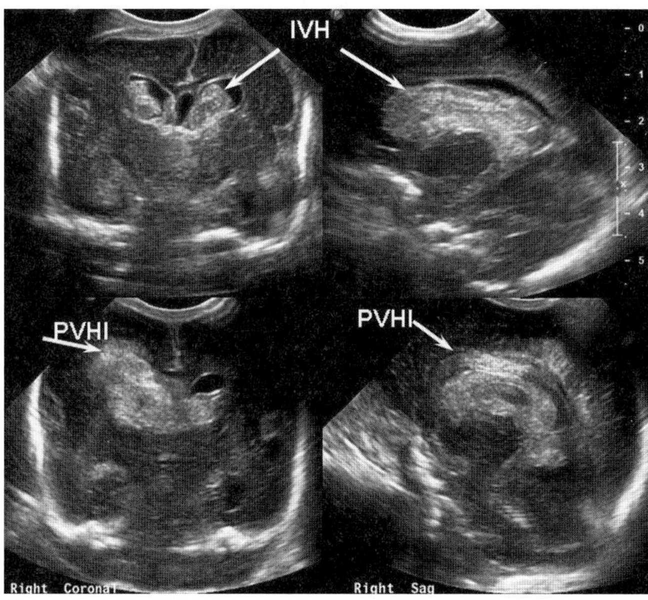


B

**FIGURE 61-3** **A:** The top panel shows coronal (*left*) and sagittal (*right*) views from a normal preterm brain. The bottom left panel shows a coronal view with a left germinal matrix hemorrhage (GMH), or grade I. The bottom right panel shows a sagittal section showing blood in the lateral ventricle (intraventricular hemorrhage [IVH]) filling less than 50% of the ventricular space; it is therefore a grade II germinal matrix hemorrhage/intraventricular hemorrhage. **B:** The top left panel shows a coronal view of bilateral hemorrhage (IVH) in the anterior ventricles, almost filling the ventricles. The top right panel shows a sagittal view of the hemorrhage or blood cast (IVH) filling and distending the lateral ventricle. This is a grade III hemorrhage. The bottom left panel shows a coronal view of hemorrhage with parenchymal involvement (arrows) representing periventricular hemorrhagic infarction (PVHI). The area of infarction is also noted in the sagittal view (arrow) in the bottom right panel. By Volpe criteria, the hemorrhage will be classified as a grade III with periventricular hemorrhagic infarction. V, ventricle; CP, choroid plexus.

Preterm infants with GMH/IVH without obvious parenchymal involvement may have evidence of white matter injury detected by MRI diffusion-weighted imaging at term postmenstrual age; diffuse, excessive, high signal intensity is noted in the cerebral white matter on T2-weighted images.

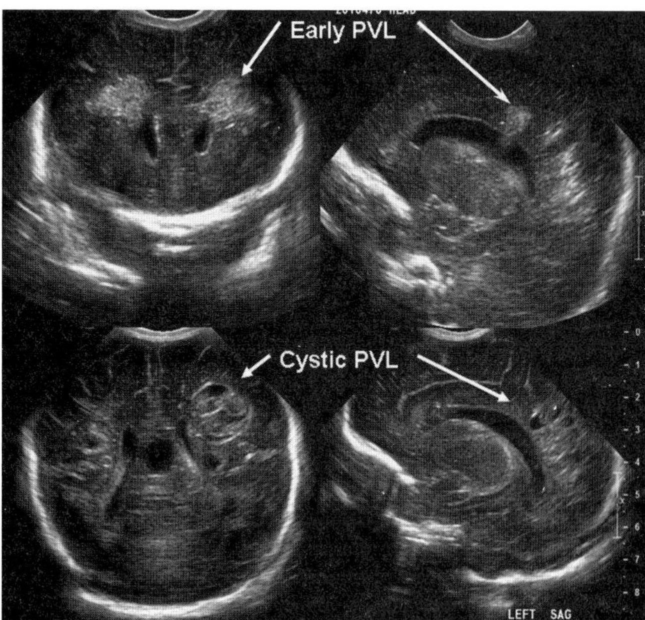


**FIGURE 61-4** The top panel shows the coronal and sagittal views of early periventricular leukomalacia (PVL), which appears echodense, as indicated by the arrows. A week later on the same child, the echodense areas have turned into multiples cysts in the periventricular area (cystic PVL).

Recent studies demonstrate that GMH/IVH is associated with reductions in cerebellar volume. This is thought to occur secondary to (1) a direct toxic effect of hemosiderin on the surface of the cerebellum, impairing the proliferation of the external granular layer, and (2) the loss of cortical neuronal inputs leading to underdevelopment of the cerebellum on the contralateral side from the site of the cortical injury (a maturation-distinctive form of diaschisis).

## MANAGEMENT

The treatment of GMH/IVH is primarily supportive. Management strategies include initiation of mechanical ventilation or increase in ventilatory support, and/or administration of oxygen in order to maintain optimal levels of the arterial partial pressure of carbon dioxide ($PaCO_2$) and the arterial partial pressure of oxygen ($PaO_2$); treatment of hypotension with slow volume expansion and then cautious use of pressors if unresponsive; blood transfusion to correct anemia from blood loss; correction of metabolic acidosis; anticonvulsant therapy for seizures; and administration of fresh frozen plasma, platelets, and other products if there is associated coagulopathy. Progression or evolution of GMH/IVH is monitored by serial cranial ultrasounds, especially for decision-making and parental counseling in the face of rapid clinical deterioration.

During early posthemorrhagic hydrocephalus, interventions such as diuretics and intraventricular fibrinolytic therapy have been trialed and shown to have no benefit in small randomized trials. The infants must be monitored with frequent cranial ultrasounds to examine changes in ventricular size. If there is increasing ventriculomegaly and raised intracranial pressure, the management is then directed at drainage of the CSF fluid to reduce the ventricular size. This can be done either by serial lumbar puncture or surgical intervention with the creation of a ventricular reservoir, or drainage of CSF by ventriculostomy. The optimum timing of intervention is unclear; however, retrospective data suggests that earlier intervention with serial therapeutic lumbar punctures may avoid the need for surgical intervention and improve neurodevelopmental outcome. A multicenter randomized trial of *early versus late ventricular intervention study* (ELVIS; ISRCTN43171322 or NCT00875758) is currently ongoing to validate this retrospective data.

Ventriculoperitoneal shunt is the definitive surgical treatment when there is continued progression of ventriculomegaly accompanied by increase in intracranial pressure. Shunt obstruction, malfunction, and infection can complicate shunt placement and long-term function. Endoscopic third ventriculostomy with choroid plexus cauterization may avoid the necessity for a shunt among those requiring surgical intervention. However, while the data is encouraging in hydrocephalus due to alternate etiologies, it has been less successful for the management of posthemorrhagic hydrocephalus in preterm infants, and ventriculoperioneal shunt remains the gold standard.

## PROGNOSIS AND LONG-TERM OUTCOMES

In severe GMH/IVH, sudden deterioration unresponsive to escalating support may be observed. Mortality in severe GMH/IVH, especially with associated periventricular hemorrhagic infarction, is 40%. Among those who survive for weeks after a hemorrhage with complicating progressive and persistent ventricular dilation, death occurs in 18%. In extremely low–birth-weight infants, after excluding deaths due to extreme immaturity, 7% to 9% of the deaths are attributable to hemorrhage.

Forty percent of ELBW infants who survive following a grade III or IV GMH/IVH have moderate-to-severe neurosensory impairments, including cerebral palsy, which occurs in 30% of survivors; severe neurodevelopmental impairment (developmental quotients 2 standard deviations below the mean) in 15% to 20%; bilateral deafness in 8%; and blindness in 2%. Among infants with lower grades of IVH (grade I and II), there is a 2-fold increase in the risk for neurodevelopmental impairment and a 2.6-fold increase in the risk of cerebral palsy, as compared to children of similar birth weight but normal cranial ultrasound. An alternate large cohort study of infants less than 29 weeks' gestation, reported that 20% of those with grade I or II IVH had moderate-to-severe neurosensory impairment, with 10% having cerebral palsy, and 8% having severe neurodevelopmental impairment (developmental quotients 2 standard deviations below the mean). However, even in the absence of abnormalities on cranial ultrasound, 10% of extremely low–birth-weight children are reported to have a moderate-to-severe neurosensory impairment at 18 to 22 months of age.



## PREVENTION

Several studies have addressed the prevention of IVH from the antenatal through the postnatal periods. Antenatal prevention is directed toward prevention of preterm birth through use of tocolytics, treatment of maternal complications (bleeding, chorioamnionitis, conditions that may predispose to preterm delivery), intrapartum fetal surveillance, the use of epidural rather than general anesthesia, controlled vaginal delivery, and administration of antenatal steroids. Antenatal steroids in particular have been repeatedly shown to significantly reduce the incidence of severe IVH. Data from the Neonatal Research Network finds the odds ratio for a severe IVH following a complete course of antenatal steroids is 0.39 (95% confidence interval, 0.27–0.57).

Postnatal preventive strategies include supportive measures, such as resuscitative measures at delivery with a goal of preventing hyperoxia; maintenance of optimal oxygenation and acid–base balance; gentle ventilation to prevent pneumothoraces and other air-leak syndromes; minimizing abrupt hemodynamic alterations, including slow volume expansion for low blood pressure and judicious use of inotropic agents (there are risks associated with sudden changes in systemic pressures in the presence of a pressure-passive cerebral circulation); and careful surfactant administration to improve respiratory status and oxygenation. Studies of pharmacologic agents such as pancuronium, ethamsylate, vitamin E, and phenobarbital do not demonstrate clear benefit.

Indomethacin, a prostaglandin H synthase inhibitor, inhibits generation of oxygen free radicals, promotes maturation of the germinal matrix, stabilizes cerebral blood flow, and attenuates the hyperemic response to hypoxia and hypercapnia. Indomethacin reduces the incidence of severe IVH, but despite this, its use has not resulted in an improvement in neurodevelopmental outcome. Additionally, administration of indomethacin has been associated with an increased risk of renal insufficiency, ileal perforation, and chronic lung disease. Therefore, despite the clear evidence for a reduction in severe IVH, due to the potential for adverse side effects and no clear impact on developmental outcome, the use of prophylactic indomethacin has remained limited. Recently, some groups have begun to explore a more targeted approach for prophylactic indomethacin, providing it to those at highest risk of a severe IVH, and therefore most likely to benefit.

## SUGGESTED READINGS


Bolisetty S, Dhawan A, Abdel-Latif M, Bajuk B, Stack J, Lui K. Intraventricular hemorrhage and neurodevelopmental outcomes in extreme preterm infants. *Pediatrics.* 2014;133(1):55-62.

Brouwer A, Groenendaal F, van Haastert IL, Rademaker K, Hanlo P, de Vries L. Neurodevelopmental outcome of preterm infants with severe intraventricular hemorrhage and therapy for post-hemorrhagic ventricular dilatation. *J Pediatr.* 2008;152(5):648-654.

Inder TE, Anderson NJ, Spencer C, Wells S, Volpe JJ. White matter injury in the premature infant: a comparison between serial cranial sonographic and MR findings at term. *AJNR American J Neuroradiol.* 2003;24(5):805-809.

Kadri H, Mawla AA, Kazah J. The incidence, timing, and predisposing factors of germinal matrix and intraventricular hemorrhage (GMH/IVH) in preterm neonates. *Childs Nervous Syst.* 2006;22(9):1086-1090.

Kidokoro H, Neil JJ, Inder TE. New MR imaging assessment tool to define brain abnormalities in very preterm infants at term. *AJNR American J Neuroradiol.* 2013;34(11):2208-2214.

Ment LR, Duncan CC, Ehrenkranz RA, et al. Intraventricular hemorrhage in the preterm neonate: timing and cerebral blood flow changes. *J Pediatr.* 1984;104(3):419-425.

Murphy BP, Inder TE, Rooks V, et al. Posthaemorrhagic ventricular dilatation in the premature infant: natural history and predictors of outcome. *Arch Dis Child Fetal Neonatal Ed.* 2002;87(1):F37-F41.

Papile LA, Burstein J, Burstein R, Koffler H. Incidence and evolution of subependymal and intraventricular hemorrhage: a study of infants with birth weights less than 1,500 gm. *J Pediatr.* 1978;92(4):529-534.

Payne AH, Hintz SR, Hibbs AM, et al. Neurodevelopmental outcomes of extremely low-gestational-age neonates with low-grade periventricular-intraventricular hemorrhage. *JAMA Pediatr.* 2013;167(5):451-459.

Schmidt B, Davis P, Moddemann D, et al; Trial of Indomethacin Prophylaxis in Preterms Investigators. Long-term effects of indomethacin prophylaxis in extremely-low-birth-weight infants. *N Engl J Med.* 2001;344(26):1966-1972.

Tam EW, Miller SP, Studholme C, et al. Differential effects of intraventricular hemorrhage and white matter injury on preterm cerebellar growth. *J Pediatr.* 2011;158(3):366-371.

Volpe JJ. Brain injury in premature infants: a complex amalgam of destructive and developmental disturbances. *Lancet Neurol.* 2009;8(1):110-124.


# 62 Bronchopulmonary Dysplasia

Erik A. Jensen, Huayan Zhang, and Haresh Kirpalani

## INTRODUCTION

Bronchopulmonary dysplasia (BPD) is the most common chronic complication associated with preterm birth. In the United States, it affects between 10,000 and 15,000 infants annually, including as many as 50% of extremely low–birth-weight (ELBW; birth weight < 1000 g) infants. BPD is a leading cause of mortality after the first month of life in extremely preterm infants and is a strong predictor of chronic respiratory and cardiovascular impairments, growth failure, and neurodevelopmental delay.

The first descriptions of BPD appeared in the literature soon after the advent of modern day neonatology. In the late 1950s and early 1960s, infant respiratory distress syndrome (RDS) was a leading cause of neonatal death among preterm infants. Increased use of mechanical ventilation improved survival rates for infants with severe RDS. However, prolonged treatment with invasive respiratory support and supplemental oxygen therapy was often necessary. These exposures contributed to chronic lung injury in surviving moderate preterm infants and the development of what Northway and colleagues first termed *bronchopulmonary dysplasia* in 1967.

As the use of antenatal corticosteroids, noninvasive continuous positive airway pressure (CPAP), and exogenous surfactant therapy increased during the subsequent decades, the epidemiology and pathophysiology of BPD evolved. It is now an infrequent complication among infants born with birth weights greater than 1500 g and gestational ages exceeding 32 weeks. In the presurfactant era, prominent airway injury, epithelial metaplasia, smooth muscle hypertrophy, and alternating parenchymal fibrosis and emphysema were the most common histological findings. This disease phenotype is often termed "old" BPD. The most common lung histology in BPD now commonly displays a homogenous disease pattern marked by reduced numbers of alveoli and pulmonary capillaries, and minimal areas of hyperinflation and focal collapse. This is termed "new" BPD. Importantly, the pathologic characteristics of both old and new BPD can develop in extremely preterm infants who require prolonged intubation and mechanical ventilation. Old and new BPD therefore likely represent a continuum of disease severity and may not be fully distinct disease entities.

## INCIDENCE

The incidence of BPD is highest among infants born with the lowest gestational ages and birth weights. The National Institutes of Child Health and Human Development's (NICHD) Neonatal Research Network (NRN) reported rates of supplemental oxygen use at 36 weeks postmenstrual age (PMA) among infants who survived to that time point. BPD rates ranged from 85% for those born at 22 weeks' gestation to 23% for those born at 28 weeks' gestation (Fig. 62-1). Among preterm infants born in Israel between 2000 and 2010, 31% of surviving ELBW infants received supplemental oxygen at 36 weeks PMA compared to 13.7% of very low–birth-weight (VLBW; birth weight < 1500 g) infants. BPD severity is also inversely proportional to gestational age and birth weight. Fifty-six percent of infants born at 22 weeks' gestation in the NRN cohort were diagnosed with severe BPD based on the National Institutes of Health (NIH) consensus definition, compared to only 8% of those born at 28 weeks' gestation (Fig. 62-1).

Finally, BPD rates vary depending on the definition of BPD applied to the cohort. The NRN compared 3 different definitions of BPD among infants with gestational ages between 22 and 28 weeks. Rates based on the NIH consensus definition were the highest (68%), as this includes infants who received supplemental oxygen for at least 28 days but were breathing in room air by 36 weeks PMA. Forty-two percent of the evaluated extremely preterm infants were diagnosed with BPD based on supplemental oxygen use at 36 weeks PMA and 40% by the physiologic definition.

## CURRENT DIAGNOSTIC CRITERIA

Along with the disease epidemiology, the diagnostic criteria for BPD have also evolved. The first widely used definition required supplemental oxygen exposure for at least 28 days and radiograph evidence of chronic lung injury. Subsequently, an oxygen requirement at 36 weeks PMA was shown to better predict adverse pulmonary outcomes at 2 years of life among VLBW infants. Many reports continue to define BPD using this criterion. In 2000, an NIH workshop recommended a graded diagnosis for BPD that incorporated both an oxygen requirement for greater than 28 days and the respiratory support utilized at 36 weeks PMA (Table 62-1). The presence of abnormal radiographic findings was not required. To address variability in target oxygen saturation ranges used in clinical practice, Walsh and colleagues proposed a "physiologic" definition for BPD to more objectively determine an infant's "need" for supplemental oxygen. This definition requires an oxygen reduction test to determine dependency at 36 weeks PMA among those receiving 30% or less supplemental oxygen. Unfortunately, the physiologic test is not consistently performed in clinical or research settings. Finally, recent data indicate that many former extremely preterm infants who do not meet the current diagnostic criteria for BPD experience deficits in respiratory health through childhood and into adulthood. These observations prompt continued



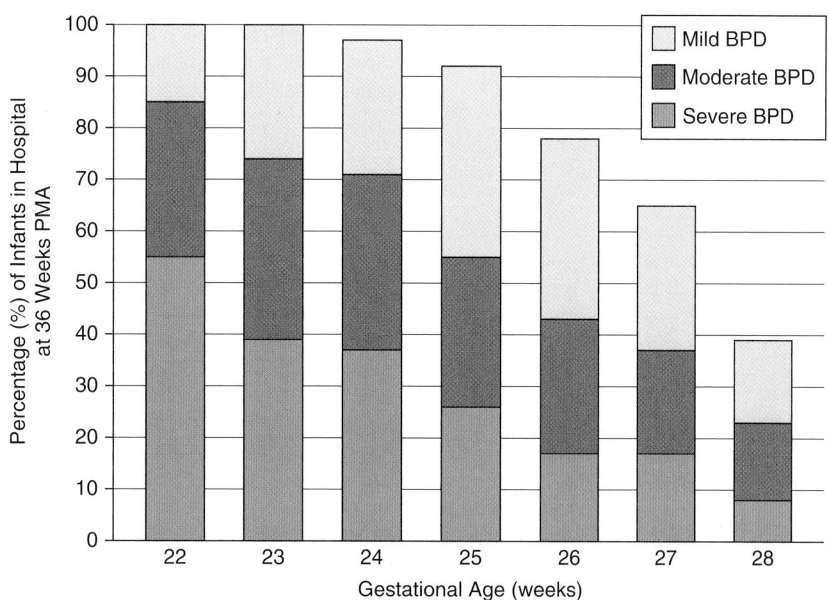


**FIGURE 62-1** Severity-based bronchopulmonary dysplasia (BPD) rates by gestational age for infants in hospital at 36 weeks postmenstrual age (PMA) or discharged/transferred at 33 to 36 PMA. (Figure generated from data published by the Eunice Kennedy Shriver National Institute of Child Health and Human Development Neonatal Research Network (NRN) in Stoll BJ, Hansen NI, Bell EF, et al; Eunice Kennedy Shriver National Institute of Child Health and Human Development Neonatal Research Network. Neonatal outcomes of extremely preterm infants from the NICHD Neonatal Research Network. *Pediatrics.* 2010;126(3):443-456. BPD severity classification based on Jobe AH, Bancalari E. Bronchopulmonary dysplasia. *Am J Respir Crit Care Med.* 2001;163(7):1723-1729.)

**TABLE 62-1 CURRENT DEFINITIONS OF BRONCHOPULMONARY DYSPLASIA**

| Definition | Criteria |
|---|---|
| **Shennan** (Originally defined for infants with BWs < 1500 g) | Treatment with supplemental oxygen at 36 weeks PMA |
| **2000 Workshop** (Originally defined for infants with GAs < 32 wk) | Treatment with supplemental oxygen for at least 28 d plus the following criteria to distinguish BPD severity: |
| Mild | Breathing in room air at 36 weeks PMA or discharge, whichever comes first |
| Moderate | Treatment with < 30% $O_2$ at 36 weeks PMA or discharge, whichever comes first |
| Severe | Treatment with ≥ 30% $O_2$ and/or positive airway pressure at 36 weeks PMA or discharge (whichever comes first) |
| **Physiologic** (Originally defined for infants with BWs 501–1500 g) | Infants treated with mechanical ventilation, continuous positive airway pressure or $O_2$ ≥ 30% at 36 weeks PMA diagnosed with BPD |
| | Infants treated with $O_2$ < 30% at 36 weeks PMA diagnosed with BPD if they failed a timed stepwise reduction to room air |

BW, birth weight; GA, gestational age; PMA, postmenstrual age.

**TABLE 62-2 EPIDEMIOLOGICAL RISK FACTORS FOR BRONCHOPULMONARY DYSPLASIA**

| | |
|---|---|
| **Prenatal risk factors** | • Maternal smoking<br>• Younger maternal age<br>• Intrauterine growth restriction<br>• Family history of asthma<br>• Genetic factors |
| **Risk factors at birth** | • Prematurity (lower gestational age and birth weight)<br>• Male gender<br>• Perinatal asphyxia<br>• Antepartum maternal hemorrhage<br>• Birth hospital level and premature infant birth volume<br>• Low Apgar scores<br>• Need for delivery room endotracheal intubation or cardiopulmonary resuscitation<br>• White race<br>• Presence of birth defects |
| **Postnatal risk factors** | • Invasive mechanical ventilation<br>• Longer duration of supplemental oxygen exposure<br>• Higher weight-adjusted fluid intake<br>• Patent ductus arteriosus<br>• Sepsis<br>• Necrotizing enterocolitis<br>• Grade III–IV intraventricular hemorrhage<br>• Gastroesophageal reflux<br>• Airway colonization or infection with *Ureaplasma urealyticum* and Gram-negative rod organisms |

efforts to develop more reliable means to diagnose and quantify chronic respiratory disease associated with extreme preterm birth.

## PATHOPHYSIOLOGY

In the presurfactant era, BPD was primarily attributed to chronic, postnatal lung injury from prolonged mechanical ventilation and supplemental oxygen therapy. In the current era, new BPD is increasingly recognized as a consequence of arrested lung alveolarization and pulmonary capillary formation following birth during the late canalicular or early saccular stages of lung growth. Although the terminal bronchial epithelium has sufficiently thinned to permit life-sustaining ex-utero gas exchange by this time, alveolar septation has not begun. Postmortem lung histology in extremely preterm infants with BPD demonstrates alveolar simplification, reduced secondary septation, and abnormal microvascular growth. In addition, multiple antenatal and postnatal factors, including infection, hyperoxia, and volu-/baro-/atelectrauma, contribute to the development of BPD by triggering inflammatory lung injury and cellular apoptosis. Abnormalities in extracellular matrix turnover and impaired structural remodeling follow these exposures and result in disordered elastin deposition, saccular wall fibrosis, and greater alveolar simplification.

## RISK FACTORS

Epidemiological studies have identified numerous individual risk factors for BPD (Table 62-2). However, BPD likely results from the combined effect of multiple perinatal and postnatal exposures on the developmentally immature lung rather than from a single risk factor.

### Perinatal Risk Factors

**Prematurity** Prematurity is the most important risk for BPD. Fewer than 5% of infants born at or beyond 30 weeks' gestation develop BPD compared to 50% or more of surviving infants born at 24 to 25 weeks' gestation. Fetal growth restriction and being small for gestational age further increase the risk for BPD. The odds of BPD are 2- to 3-fold higher among VLBW infants born with birth weights less than the 10th percentile for their gestational age. Finally, preterm male infants are twice as likely to develop BPD compared to female infants born at similar gestational ages and birth weights.

**Chorioamnionitis** Chorioamnionitis predisposes to preterm birth and is a proposed risk factor for BPD. In animal models, chorioamnionitis arrests lung alveolar and vascular development producing a BPD-like phenotype. However, the available evidence from large human studies is inconclusive as to whether chorioamnionitis is a true BPD risk factor. A 2011 meta-analysis found that preterm infants born to mothers with histologically but not clinically diagnosed chorioamnionitis were at increased risk for BPD. However, after adjusting for potential confounders, the association was no longer statistically significant. An important distinction may be the bacterial agent responsible for chorioamnionitis. A meta-analysis of 39 studies found that preterm infants with respiratory tract colonization by *Ureaplasma* spp, the most common bacterial organisms cultured in chorioamnionitis, were at increased risk for supplemental oxygen use at 28 days and 36 weeks PMA.

### Postnatal Risk Factors

**Mechanical Ventilation and Supplemental Oxygen Exposure** Mechanical ventilation and supplemental oxygen exposure are the best-described postnatal risk factors for BPD. Animal models show a clear link between mechanical ventilation and oxygen free-radical–induced lung injury that mimics human BPD. However, epidemiological evidence of a causal link between these exposures and BPD is less robust. Meta-analyses of randomized controlled trials show that the avoidance of mechanical ventilation in extremely preterm infants only leads to a small reduction in BPD risk. Importantly, BPD also develops in infants who have never required tracheal intubation and only had low supplemental oxygen requirements. Moreover, clinical trials have failed to demonstrate any impact of protective measures such as minimizing supplemental inspired oxygen during resuscitation, or targeting a lower saturation range, on the risk of BPD in extremely preterm infants.

**Patent Ductus Arteriosus** The presence of a patent ductus arteriosus (PDA) beyond the first days of life in preterm infants is another well-established risk factor for BPD. Whether this relationship is causal is unclear. Randomized controlled trials of prophylactic medical and/or surgical closure of a PDA showed no benefit for prevention of BPD. For example, the Trial of Indomethacin Prophylaxis in Preterms

(TIPP) found no reduction in BPD risk following prophylactic indomethacin despite a decrease in the incidence of PDA by more than 50%. In a small RCT, surgical ligation of a PDA within the first 24 hours of life compared to conservative management increased the risk for supplemental oxygen use and mechanical ventilation at 36 weeks PMA. Finally, a systematic review of all RCTs evaluating surgical and pharmacological methods of PDA closure at any time in the neonatal period found no reduction in BPD or the composite outcome of death or BPD with any therapy.

**Sepsis** Observational studies implicate postnatal sepsis as an independent risk factor for subsequently developing BPD. Although the direct role of infection is unclear, systemic inflammation and increased vascular permeability may cause immediate alveolar injury and long-term disruption of alveolarization. Of note, the risk for BPD may be further increased among infants diagnosed with postnatal sepsis who were exposed to chorioamnionitis in utero. Perinatal and postnatal airway colonization with *Ureaplasma* spp and Gram-negative rod bacteria are also associated with increased risk for BPD and later adverse respiratory outcomes.

## CLINICAL PRESENTATION

Exposure to invasive mechanical ventilation and supplemental oxygen during the first days and/or weeks of life is common among extremely preterm infants who develop BPD. However, some infants with minimal early respiratory support needs also develop BPD. The physical examination in BPD is highly variable and depends on the extent of pulmonary disease and the respiratory support. Classical signs of respiratory insufficiency such as tachypnea, chest wall retractions, and grunting or expiratory braking may be present. Auscultation may also reveal scattered areas of poor aeration, rales, crackles, and/or wheezing, depending on the presence and distribution of pulmonary edema, atelectasis, and airway narrowing. Importantly, the respiratory physical examination may also be largely normal in BPD, even in severe disease, when adequate lung aeration is achieved using positive airway pressure.

Radiographic findings in BPD vary according to the severity of the illness and the stage of the disease. Initial chest radiographs in extremely preterm infants commonly show low lung volumes with a homogenous fine granular or "ground glass" appearance consistent with RDS. With time, a more heterogeneous pattern marked by diffuse haziness, coarse interstitial densities, and small cyst-like structures may appear. In mild to moderate BPD, lung volumes appear normal or decreased depending on the presence and severity of atelectasis (Fig. 62-2). In contrast, the lungs of infants with severe BPD are often hyperinflated with larger cystic areas and coarse interstitial densities (Fig. 62-2). Acquired lobar emphysema and right ventricular enlargement from cor pulmonale may become apparent. The radiographic abnormalities seen in surviving infants with BPD often improve over time, although residual scarring can persist into adulthood.

Chest computed tomography (CT) is increasingly utilized to assess lung disease in BPD due to its greater sensitivity for identifying focal abnormalities such as acquired lobar emphysema and localized atelectatic or infectious consolidations. Chest CT with angiography can also complement echocardiography and cardiac catheterization assessment of pulmonary hypertension.

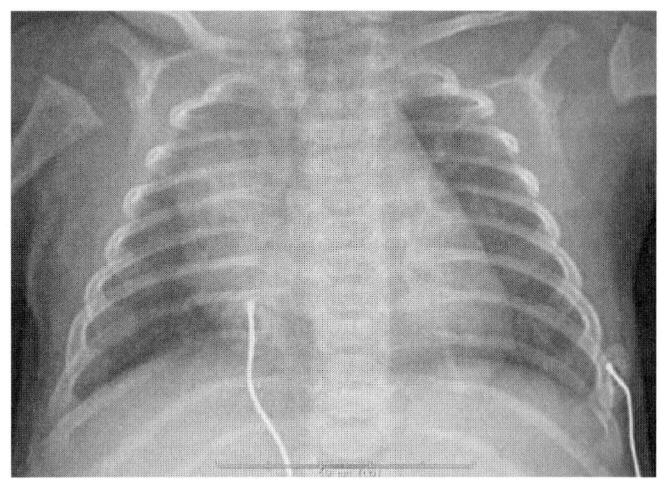
A

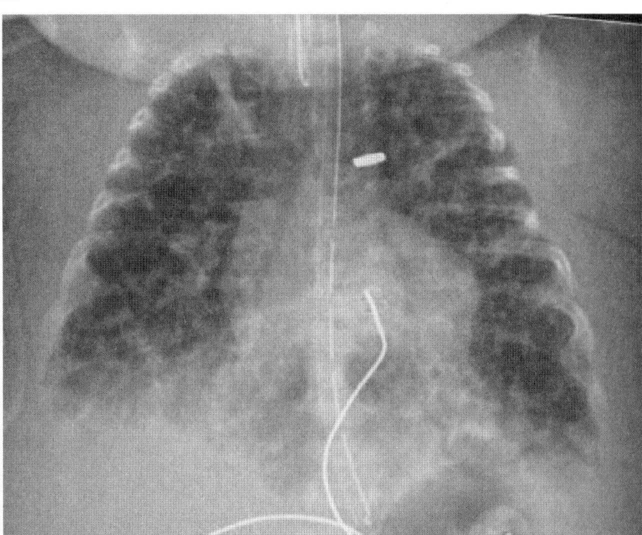
B

**FIGURE 62-2 A:** Chest radiograph from a 3-month-old female infant born at 28 weeks' gestation treated with 25% nasal cannula $O_2$ at 36 weeks postmenstrual age (moderate bronchopulmonary dysplasia [BPD]). The lungs show normal inflation with slightly coarsened lung markings and mild, mainly perihilar areas of subsegmental atelectasis. **B:** Chest radiograph from a 3-month-old male infant born at 23 weeks' gestation treated with invasive mechanical ventilation at 36 weeks postmenstrual age (severe BPD). The lungs are hyperinflated with severe, diffuse lung disease. There is a coarse honeycomb pattern throughout with cystic airspace disease, interstitial thickening, and scattered focal areas of atelectasis.

## PREVENTION

### Prematurity

It is unlikely that a single, postnatal intervention aimed at preventing BPD will be fully effective. As a result, any comprehensive effort to reduce BPD must include strategies to prevent extreme preterm birth. Although birth rates near the limits of viability improved slightly over the past decade in the United States, additional evidence-based interventions are needed to produce the substantial reductions in extreme preterm birth required to eradicate BPD.

### Avoidance of Mechanical Ventilation

Successful transition after birth requires lung aeration. Unfortunately, most extremely preterm infants are unable to independently clear fetal lung fluid and fully aerate the lungs. Weak respiratory muscles, a highly compliant chest wall, underexpression of transepithelial sodium channels, and deficient production of surfactant complicate this transition. Consequently, many require positive airway pressure and supplemental oxygen after birth. The optimal means to provide these potentially lifesaving interventions while minimizing lung injury remains an area of intense research.

Application of noninvasive CPAP immediately after birth facilitates lung recruitment while preventing stretch injury caused by the higher distending pressures often administered with invasive ventilation. Several large RCTs compared a strategy of early noninvasive CPAP to immediate intubation and surfactant administration. Meta-analyses of these trials found a small but statistically significant reduction in the risk for death or BPD at 36 weeks PMA among CPAP-treated infants. The 2 largest trials also showed a significant reduction in duration of mechanical ventilation and a trend toward shorter duration of oxygen exposure with early CPAP use.

### Less-Invasive Surfactant Administration

Less-invasive surfactant administration (LISA) is intended to provide the potential benefits of surfactant therapy without the harm of intubation. This instillation method utilizes a thin catheter (eg, an angiocatheter or small feeding tube) instead of a standard endotracheal tube to administer surfactant. Two meta-analyses of small RCTs and a Bayesian random-effects network meta-analysis suggest that LISA may be a more optimal approach than other early respiratory management strategies, such as CPAP alone, for preventing BPD.

### Pharmacological Therapy

**Caffeine** Caffeine stimulates breathing in preterm infants by increasing minute ventilation, $CO_2$ sensitivity, and diaphragmatic activity. The international Caffeine for Apnea of Prematurity (CAP) trial showed that caffeine reduced the risk for BPD and neurodevelopmental impairment. Caffeine is now the most commonly prescribed medication after antibiotics in the neonatal intensive care unit (NICU).

**Postnatal Corticosteroids** Dexamethasone, a synthetic corticosteroid and potent anti-inflammatory, is effective at reducing BPD. However, concerns for increased risk of neurodevelopmental impairment, particularly cerebral palsy, limit its use. Meta-analysis of available RCTs show that dexamethasone should not be used during the first week of life. Such "early" treatment increases the risk for gastrointestinal perforation, hypertrophic cardiomyopathy, cerebral palsy (CP), and major neurosensory disability. In contrast, dexamethasone use after the first week of life has not been found to increase the risk for CP. Adverse effects of this "late" dexamethasone therapy include transient hyperglycemia, glycosuria, and hypertension, as well as a possible increase in the risk for severe retinopathy of prematurity. Two meta-regressions by Doyle and colleagues highlight the importance of balancing the risks of neurodevelopmental impairment due to corticosteroids against those of BPD, itself a strong predictor of neurologic impairment. If the risk for BPD in the control population was less than approximately 33%, corticosteroid therapy significantly increased the risk for death or CP; whereas when the risk for BPD exceeded 60%, they reduced the risk for death or CP. Combined with the meta-analysis data, these results suggest that the adverse long-term effects of dexamethasone when used the first week of life and in infants at low risk for BPD, outweigh its benefits. However, among infants who continue to require invasive mechanical ventilation after the first 1 to 2 weeks of life, the balance may favor the use of corticosteroids. Importantly, the optimal dosing regimen and timing of initiation after the first week of life have not been determined.

Systemic hydrocortisone and inhaled budesonide have been studied as alternative anti-inflammatory therapies that may reduce lung disease and avoid the harmful long-term consequences of dexamethasone. Existing meta-analyses of RCTs evaluating these drugs failed to show clear benefit. More recently, 2 large multicenter RCTs reported reductions in BPD risk with these drugs. However, for inhaled budesonide, the risk for the composite outcome of death or BPD was of borderline statistical significance, owing to a trend toward higher rates of death in the steroid-treated infants. Long-term follow-up data and incorporation of the recent trial results into existing meta-analyses are necessary to fully assess the safety and efficacy of these 2 therapies.

**Vitamin A** Vitamin A is involved in a variety of processes in the human body, including growth of epithelial cells in the respiratory tract. Preliminary studies suggest that preterm infants who develop BPD have lower plasma vitamin A levels than infants who do not develop BPD. A multicenter RCT published in 1999 demonstrated reduced risk for BPD among ELBW infants who were treated with intramuscular injections of vitamin A during the first 4 weeks of life. Subsequently, 2 recent large observational studies reported similar rates of BPD among preterm infants treated with vitamin A and untreated controls. Although these observational results provide lower quality data than the RCT, they do raise questions about the efficacy of vitamin A to prevent BPD in the current era. Ongoing shortages of this drug limit its current clinical use. A planned international RCT of oral vitamin A supplementation in extremely preterm infants may provide important, contemporary data.

## MANAGEMENT OF ESTABLISHED BRONCHOPULMONARY DYSPLASIA

There are limited rigorous data to guide treatment during the chronic and resolution phases of BPD. This evidence gap, in turn, has led to considerable variation in the treatment of infants with established, severe BPD.

### Respiratory Management

The primary respiratory management strategy in RDS and evolving chronic lung disease is avoidance of mechanical ventilation by using noninvasive modalities (eg, nasal CPAP, high-flow nasal cannula) and permissive hypercapnia. For most infants with mild to moderate respiratory insufficiency secondary to established BPD, continued emphasis on noninvasive support with gradual weaning as permitted is appropriate. However, for some infants with severe lung disease, prolonged use of noninvasive modalities provides inadequate respiratory support. This may result in poor somatic and alveolar/vascular growth and persistent ventilation/perfusion (V/Q) mismatch, leading to the development of pulmonary hypertension. In this subset of infants, increased respiratory support and even invasive mechanical ventilation may be necessary to promote long-term recovery.

### Pharmacological Therapy

Medications such as corticosteroids, bronchodilators, and diuretics are commonly used in the management of established BPD. Unfortunately, RCTs evaluating the safety and efficacy of many of these are lacking. Several of the most common classes of drugs used in established BPD are listed in Table 62-3. When selecting a medication, including its dose and duration, clinicians should carefully consider the risks and benefits and be willing to discontinue therapies when clinical benefit is not observed.

### Diagnosis and Management of Pulmonary Arterial Hypertension

Pulmonary arterial hypertension (PAH) is a common cardiovascular complication in infants with BPD. Although the true incidence of PAH in BPD is unknown, several small retrospective reports estimate the rates to be between 25% and 45%, with a higher incidence among those with more severe lung disease. In a single center series, only 2% of infants with mild BPD had evidence of PAH on echocardiogram compared to 36% with moderate BPD and 50% with severe BPD. Infants diagnosed with BPD-related PAH have a higher risk of mortality than do those with BPD alone, however most survivors with BPD and PAH demonstrate improvement in PAH after the first 1 to 2 years of life.

There are no well-established, evidence-based guidelines to inform the appropriate diagnostic approach and management of PAH in BPD. At present, screening echocardiography performed at 36 weeks PMA in infants with severe BPD should be considered. A peak tricuspid valve regurgitant jet velocity > 2.8 m/s observed on Doppler echocardiography is diagnostic of PAH in BPD. When this measurement cannot be obtained, right atrial enlargement, interventricular septal flattening, right ventricular hypertrophy or dilation, and a short right ventricular ejection time are commonly used. Cardiac catheterization is used infrequently in BPD but is the gold standard to confirm the diagnosis of PAH and accurately assess its severity. Serum brain-type natriuretic peptide is also used to assess for PAH, but its validity in BPD needs confirmation.

The most common pharmacological therapies used in BPD related PAH are pulmonary vasodilators such as inhaled nitric oxide and systemic sildenafil. At present, only minimal published data support their efficacy in BPD, although survey data suggests that their use is common. As pulmonary vascular resistance can depend heavily on the degree of V/Q matching in the lung, ensuring adequate lung aeration is essential to the management of BPD-associated PAH. Reducing V/Q mismatch through effective ventilation may ameliorate the need for pharmacological PAH therapy.

**TABLE 62-3 COMMON MEDICATIONS USED IN THE TREATMENT OF ESTABLISHED BRONCHOPULMONARY DYSPLASIA**

| Drug Class and Example Agents | Potential Benefits | Concerns |
|---|---|---|
| Diuretics<br>Furosemide<br>Bumetanide<br>Thiazides<br>Spironolactone | • Decreases airway resistance, improves lung compliance and oxygenation<br>• May decrease extubation failure | • Electrolyte and acid–base imbalance, bone demineralization, nephrocalcinosis<br>• No data from large RCTs to define long-term safety and efficacy |
| Systemic steroids<br>Dexamethasone<br>Hydrocortisone | • Potent anti-inflammatory<br>• Reduces need for ventilatory support and supplemental oxygen<br>• Increases ability to successfully extubate | • Hyperglycemia, glycosuria, and hypertension<br>• Possible relationship with adverse neurodevelopment when used in the first week of life; no data for established BPD<br>• Optimal indication, dose, duration, and timing of initiation not established |
| Inhaled steroids<br>Budesonide<br>Fluticasone | • Decreases pulmonary inflammation | • Early use to prevent BPD may increase mortality risk<br>• Unclear efficacy in established BPD<br>• Paucity of data on adverse effects |
| Inhaled β-agonists<br>Albuterol<br>Levalbuterol | • Increases bronchodilation and decreases airway resistance<br>• Improves dynamic compliance | • Limited data on safety and efficacy in infants<br>• May exacerbate tracheobronchomalacia |
| Inhaled anticholinergics<br>Ipratropium | • Increases bronchodilation, decreases airway resistance, and improves lung compliance | • Limited data on safety and efficacy in infants |
| Pulmonary vasodilators<br>Inhaled nitric oxide<br>Sildenafil<br>Treprostinil<br>Bosentan<br>Iloprost | • Decreases pulmonary vascular resistance<br>• May decrease ventilation/perfusion mismatch | • Limited data on safety and efficacy in infants<br>• Increased mortality risk with high sildenafil doses observed in pediatric patients with PAH, unclear in patients < 1 year |

BPD, bronchopulmonary dysplasia; PAH, pulmonary hypertension; RCT, randomized controlled trial.



### Long-Term Mechanical Ventilation

Approximately 1% to 3% of extremely preterm infants who develop BPD ultimately require a tracheostomy to manage severe, persistent lung disease and/or associated airway abnormalities such as subglottic stenosis and tracheobronchomalacia. The appropriate timing of tracheostomy in this population remains controversial. However, among those infants in whom long-term invasive ventilation is highly likely, tracheostomy placement prior to approximately 4 months of life may improve neurodevelopment by facilitating earlier initiation of developmentally appropriate care. Following discharge from hospital, tracheostomy-dependent infants should ideally be followed-up within a multidisciplinary home ventilator program that includes otolaryngology, pediatric pulmonology, speech and nutrition therapy, as well as close neurodevelopmental monitoring.

## LONG-TERM OUTCOMES FOR INFANTS WITH BRONCHOPULMONARY DYSPLASIA

Broncopulmonary dysplasia is a strong predictor of several adverse health outcomes, including chronic cardiopulmonary impairment, growth failure, hearing and vision deficits, rehospitalization for respiratory illness in the first years of life, neurodevelopmental delay, and later mortality. Although most long-term follow-up data were obtained in patients from the presurfactant era, accumulating data indicate that new BPD also predisposes survivors to chronic morbidities that persist into adulthood.

### Respiratory Outcomes

Preterm infants diagnosed with BPD require hospital readmission for respiratory reasons during early childhood at approximately twice the rate of similar premature infants without BPD. Although rehospitalization rates decline after the second and third year of life, survivors remain at increased risk for respiratory-related hospitalizations well into adulthood. Lung function abnormalities and persistent respiratory symptoms, including exercise intolerance, dyspnea, cough, and wheeze, are also more common among children and adult survivors diagnosed with BPD during infancy.

### Neurodevelopmental Outcomes

A diagnosis of BPD is a strong predictor of future neurodevelopmental impairment (NDI) including deficits in psychomotor function, language, cognitive, behavior, vision, and hearing. In a Swiss national cohort of ELBW infants, a history of BPD increased the risk-adjusted odds of death or severe NDI at 2 years of life nearly 3-fold. The NRN found rates of NDI to be increased with greater severity of BPD, from 28.1% in ELBW infants without BPD to 61.9% in infants with severe BPD. Protracted mechanical ventilation beyond 36 weeks PMA is associated with an additional stepwise increase in the risk for both NDI and death among ELBW infants.

## SUMMARY

BPD is a multifactorial disease that results from a complex interaction between the developmentally immature lung and multiple perinatal and postnatal exposures. Since the first descriptions of BPD over 40 years ago, the epidemiology and pathophysiology of the disease evolved. New BPD primarily affects infants born less than 1500 g and 32 weeks gestation. Survivors with BPD are at increased risk for multiple chronic sequelae, including high rates of rehospitalization, prolonged deficits in pulmonary function, neurodevelopmental impairment, and postneonatal mortality. Emerging evidence indicates that many of these complications persist into adulthood. Unfortunately, BPD rates among infants born near the current limits of viability have not improved over past 2 to 3 decades. This demands new paradigms in BPD prevention and high quality, multicenter research to enable evidence-based strategies for the management of established BPD.

## SUGGESTED READINGS

Doyle LW, Halliday HL, Ehrenkranz RA, Davis PG, Sinclair JC. An update on the impact of postnatal systemic corticosteroids on mortality and cerebral palsy in preterm infants: effect modification by risk of bronchopulmonary dysplasia. *J Pediatr.* 2014;165(6): 1258-1260.

Ehrenkranz RA, Walsh MC, Vohr BR, et al; National Institutes of Child Health and Human Development Neonatal Research Network. Validation of the National Institutes of Health consensus definition of bronchopulmonary dysplasia. *Pediatrics*. 2005;116(6):1353-1360.

Gough A, Spence D, Linden M, Halliday HL, McGarvey LPA. General and respiratory health outcomes in adult survivors of bronchopulmonary dysplasia: a systematic review. *Chest*. 2012;141(6):1554-1567.

Hadchouel A, Franco-Montoya ML, Delacourt C. Altered lung development in bronchopulmonary dysplasia. *Birth Defects Res A Clin Mol Teratol*. 2014;100(3):158-167.

Isayama T, Iwami H, McDonald S, Beyene J. Association of noninvasive ventilation strategies with mortality and bronchopulmonary dysplasia among preterm infants: a systematic review and meta-analysis. *JAMA*. 2016;316(6):611-624.

Jensen EA, Foglia EE, Schmidt B. Evidence-based pharmacological therapies for prevention of bronchopulmonary dysplasia: application of the Grading of Recommendations Assessment, Development, and Evaluation (GRADE) methodology. *Clin Perinatol*. 2015;42(4):755-779.

Jensen EA, Schmidt B. Epidemiology of bronchopulmonary dysplasia. *Birth Defects Res A Clin Mol Teratol*. 2014;100(3):145-157.

Jobe AH, Bancalari E. Bronchopulmonary dysplasia. *Am J Respir Crit Care Med*. 2001;163(7):1723-1729.

Schmidt B, Roberts RS, Davis PG, et al; Caffeine for Apnea of Prematurity (CAP) Trial Investigators; Caffeine for Apnea of Prematurity CAP Trial Investigators. Prediction of late death or disability at age 5 years using a count of 3 neonatal morbidities in very low birth weight infants. *J Pediatr*. 2015;167(5):982-986.e2.

Shennan AT, Dunn MS, Ohlsson A, Lennox K, Hoskins EM. Abnormal pulmonary outcomes in premature infants: prediction from oxygen requirement in the neonatal period. *Pediatrics*. 1988;82(4):527-532.

Stoll BJ, Hansen NI, Bell EF, et al; Eunice Kennedy Shriver National Institute of Child Health and Human Development Neonatal Research Network. Neonatal outcomes of extremely preterm infants from the NICHD Neonatal Research Network. *Pediatrics*. 2010;126(3):443-456.

Subramaniam P, Ho J, Davis P. Prophylactic nasal continuous positive airway pressure for preventing morbidity and mortality in very preterm infants. *Cochrane Database Syst Rev*. 2016;6:CD001243.

Walsh MC, Wilson-Costello D, Zadell A, Newman N, Fanaroff A. Safety, reliability, and validity of a physiologic definition of bronchopulmonary dysplasia. *J Perinatol*. 2003;23(6):451-456.



# 63 Neonatal Emergencies

María Victoria Fraga

## INTRODUCTION

Several congenital anomalies presenting in the newborn period require immediate diagnosis and treatment. Certain conditions constitute medical and surgical emergencies in the delivery room and are best handled by anticipation and a multidisciplinary team approach to improve chances of successful outcomes. Basic principles of resuscitation should be applied in all cases by a team skilled in airway management and circulatory support. Recent advances in prenatal diagnostic technologies facilitate prenatal counseling as well as delivery room strategies and coordination of neonatal care.

## RESPIRATORY EMERGENCIES

The transition from fetus to newborn is the most complex physiologic adaptation that occurs in human life. Inadequate transition from fetal to neonatal life is one of the most common causes of cardiopulmonary insufficiency in the newborn.

### Airway Anomalies

Normal airway anatomy and patency are essential for a successful transition to extrauterine life. Bilateral choanal atresia is a life threatening condition. Since newborns are obligatory nose breathers, symptoms appear immediately after birth. It is often associated with other developmental anomalies such as *CHARGE* (coloboma, heart defects, choanal atresia, retarded growth and development, genitourinary abnormalities, and ear anomalies), Treacher Collins, and Tessier syndromes.

Micrognathia is usually associated with conditions such as Pierre Robin sequence. At birth, this can be severe enough to cause posterior displacement of the tongue with airway obstruction, and can be an airway emergency. In many cases, prone positioning and placement of an oral airway may relieve symptoms until surgical correction is possible, but in the extreme cases, even in the most experienced hands, intubation can be very challenging. Mandibular distraction osteogenesis has been increasingly used for neonates with this congenital anomaly.

Prenatal diagnosis has transformed the outcome of fetuses with airway obstruction. Thorough evaluation of prenatal imaging allows for categorizing fetuses with airway compromise into those who will require a special mode of delivery and those who can be delivered without any special resources. The ex utero intrapartum treatment (EXIT) approach allows accessing the airway while the fetus is still attached to placental support. This permits the fetal airway to be secured in an elective, controlled manner. Once adequate ventilation has been established, the fetus is taken off placental support. The indications for an EXIT procedure have grown over time and now include a myriad of conditions, including cervical lymphangiomas, cervical teratomas, large congenital lung malformations, and congenital high airway obstruction syndrome (CHAOS).

### Acute Hypoxemic Respiratory Failure

Neonatal hypoxemic respiratory failure (HRF) can be due to a variety of etiologies, including prematurity, perinatal insults or disorders of transition, and congenital lung abnormalities. Persistent pulmonary hypertension (PPHN) of the newborn refers to a failure of the normal fall in pulmonary vascular resistance that normally occurs during the first hours and days after birth. While PPHN can occasionally be an isolated problem with known obvious precipitant, it is more commonly associated with other causes of neonatal HRF.

**Respiratory Distress Syndrome** Respiratory distress syndrome (RDS) is the leading cause of respiratory insufficiency and respiratory failure in preterm infants, and its incidence increases with decreasing gestational age. It is caused by lung immaturity and surfactant deficiency. Clinical symptoms are grunting and retractions as well as progressive hypoxemia and hypercarbia. Severe cases require positive pressure ventilation and surfactant replacement therapy. In term infants, RDS most commonly presents as a result of delayed clearance of alveolar lung fluid and is most often seen with cesarean or precipitous deliveries. Other rare causes of neonatal RDS include congenital surfactant protein deficiencies.

**Congenital Lung Abnormalities** Large congenital lung lesions including congenital cystic adenomatoid malformation (CCAM), pulmonary sequestrations, bronchial atresias, foregut cysts, and congenital lobar emphysemas, may cause significant respiratory compromise by early compression of the tracheobronchial tree or by progressive air trapping, which may lead to a prompt surgical resection. They can also present with symptoms of pulmonary hypoplasia and pulmonary arterial hypertension.

Congenital diaphragmatic hernia (CDH) is a rare disorder in which a posterolateral diaphragmatic defect results in herniation of the abdominal contents into the chest and compression of the intrathoracic structures. Hypoplasia of the ipsilateral and contralateral lungs, severe PPHN, and left ventricular hypoplasia and dysfunction are present at birth and contribute to increased mortality. Prenatal imaging and several individual prenatal prognostic factors have been identified and can predict the clinical course after birth as well as long-term outcomes. Fetal interventions have become available but yet remain in an experimental phase. Optimal delivery room strategy and team assembly are essential and ideally, delivery at, or otherwise immediate transfer to a level III neonatal intensive care unit is warranted. After delivery, infants should be intubated with simultaneous placement of a suction catheter for gastric decompression. Early management focuses on treatment of HRF and PPHN. Surgical repair should ideally take place following a period of stabilization.

**Perinatal Asphyxia** Perinatal asphyxia is another well-known predisposing factor for PPHN. It can interfere with the circulatory transition during birth, impeding the decrease in PVR and increasing the risk for PPHN. There are various causes of respiratory failure in asphyxia, including fetal hypoxemia, ischemia, meconium aspiration, ventricular dysfunction, and acidosis.

**Air Leak** Air leaks such as pneumothorax and pneumomediastinum are collections of air that are located within the visceral and parietal pleura or in the mediastinal space. They can occur spontaneously, with an incidence of 1% in term infants after delivery, or they can be secondary to structural lung disease or meconium aspiration, and most often occur in patients receiving positive pressure ventilation. The clinical presentation depends upon the volume of air in the pleural space and/or mediastinum. Small pneumothoraces may be asymptomatic, whereas large air leaks may present with symptoms of tension pneumothorax with severe work of breathing, ipsilateral lung atelectasis, mediastinal shift, and cardiovascular instability due to impaired venous return. In this case, immediate intervention by needle aspiration/decompression followed by placement of a chest tube are required.

### The Role of Extracorporeal Membrane Oxygenation

Extracorporeal membrane oxygenation (ECMO) has been increasingly used to support infants with severe reversible respiratory and/or cardiac failure unresponsive to conventional medical interventions. Common diagnoses requiring ECMO in the neonatal population include meconium aspiration syndrome, CDH, sepsis, PPHN, RDS, and congenital lung abnormalities. Neonatal trials have demonstrated that ECMO is an effective treatment with acceptable cognitive and functional outcomes.

## CARDIOVASCULAR EMERGENCIES

### Congenital Heart Disease

Congenital heart disease is a common congenital disorder in newborns with a birth prevalence of approximately 1%. Delay in diagnosis may lead to devastating consequences. As pediatric cardiology has expanded greatly into fetal echocardiography, new surgeries and procedures have become available that carry significant improvement in long-term outcomes.

**Cyanotic Congenital Heart Disease** Cyanosis requires immediate attention and evaluation, and it is vitally important to distinguish between respiratory and cardiac causes as a matter of priority. Congenital heart diseases presenting with cyanosis in the newborn period include transposition of the great arteries (TGA), tricuspid atresia, tetralogy of Fallot, pulmonary atresia, critical pulmonary stenosis, and total anomalous pulmonary venous return (TAPVR). Newborns with TGA may present with inadequate mixing through the foramen ovale and an intact ventricular septum. This may require immediate intervention by transcatheter balloon atrial septostomy to improve mixing and oxygen delivery after birth. Obstructed TAPVR usually presents soon after birth with hypoxemic respiratory failure and radiographically commonly resembles RDS.

Early postnatal management of the cyanotic infant is greatly facilitated by a prenatal diagnosis with fetal echocardiography that helps to establish an appropriate management strategy (including optimal place for delivery). If a prenatal diagnosis has been made, then prenatal counseling as well as a coordinated multidisciplinary approach in the delivery room should already be in place. This would include, when indicated, immediate initiation of a prostaglandin infusion, and transfer to a cardiac unit for ongoing evaluation, including confirmatory postnatal echocardiography.

In the cyanosed infant without a prenatal diagnosis, if there is no access to echocardiography, a hyperoxia test may help. This determines whether the patient's cyanosis is due to lung disease or a fixed cardiopulmonary shunt that allows deoxygenated blood from the right atrium bypass the pulmonary circulation. A hyperoxia test is performed by measuring the arterial partial pressure of oxygen in the neonate breathing room air and then breathing 100% oxygen, each for 10 minutes. If the cause of the cyanosis is due to a cardiac defect, the arterial partial pressure of oxygen usually remains below 100 mm Hg. It is important to note that while it may help in the initial work-up, hyperoxia test does not completely rule out other causes for cyanosis, in particular PPHN or severe lung disease. Infants with suspected (but not yet confirmed) cardiac disease should be started on a prostaglandin E1 infusion to maintain ductal patency until additional diagnostic studies can be performed.

**Acyanotic Congenital Heart Disease** Critical acyanotic heart defects often present with symptoms of congestive heart failure or circulatory shock, within hours or days after birth. The timing of the onset of symptoms is often related to closure of the ductus arteriosus, in those infants whose systemic perfusion is dependent upon this. While many patients present very acutely within minutes or hours (eg, some newborns with critical aortic stenosis, coarctation of the aorta, or hypoplastic left heart syndrome), there may be a more gradual clinical decompensation when compared with cyanotic heart defects. Again, if a diagnosis of critical acyanotic congenital heart disease is suspected, then the immediate institution of prostaglandin infusion is recommended, until a confirmatory echocardiogram has been performed.

### Neonatal Shock

Shock or circulatory failure is defined as a physiologic state characterized by tissue hypoxia due to reduced oxygen delivery and/or increased oxygen consumption. It is manifested with physical findings of tissue hypoperfusion, hypotension, and metabolic acidosis. It is often reversible but it must be recognized and treated immediately to prevent progression to irreversible organ dysfunction.

Shock can be classified as hypovolemic, distributive, cardiogenic, and obstructive. Hypovolemic shock can be caused by fetomaternal hemorrhage, acute bleeding from umbilical cord rupture, or massive gastrointestinal or intracranial bleeding. Distributive shock secondary to sepsis is the most common cause of neonatal shock. Cardiogenic shock can present as a result of congenital heart diseases with obstructive left heart lesions (eg, critical aortic valve stenosis, critical coarctation, interrupted aortic arch) or as a result of cardiac arrhythmias and myocarditis. Lastly, obstructive shock occurs when extracardiac diseases lead to impaired cardiac output and is usually secondary to tension pneumothorax and cardiac tamponade. Bedside functional echocardiography or point-of-care echocardiography is a noninvasive tool that provides the neonatologist with a better understanding of the pathophysiology and allows a logical approach based on individualized hemodynamic findings. Increasingly, neonatologists perform serial echocardiographic assessments to target treatment and evaluate response.

## GASTROINTESTINAL EMERGENCIES

Emesis and feeding intolerance are frequent symptoms in neonates. These must be distinguished from pathological gastrointestinal processes that may require further and detailed evaluation.

### Intestinal Obstruction

Bilious emesis is synonymous with intestinal obstruction, either anatomical or functional. Any infant presenting with bilious emesis requires immediate evaluation. Malrotation with midgut volvulus is a time-sensitive neonatal emergency that requires urgent diagnosis performed by an upper gastrointestinal contrast study and prompt surgical intervention to prevent intestinal necrosis.

Congenital intestinal obstructions can affect the gastrointestinal (GI) tract from the esophagus to the rectum, and clinical symptoms are usually present within the first days of life. The classic triad of features of bowel obstruction are bilious emesis, constipation or failure to pass meconium within the first 48 hours of life, and abdominal distention. The initial management includes intravenous access to provide fluid resuscitation and the passage of a suitably sized nasogastric tube to achieve gastric decompression by continuous aspiration. Diagnosis is confirmed by x-ray and contrast studies, and surgical correction is indicated.

**Hirschsprung Disease** Hirschsprung disease is a motor disorder of the bowel that is caused by failure of enteric ganglion cell precursors to migrate during intestinal development. The resulting aganglionic segment of the colon fails to relax, causing a functional obstruction that presents clinically in the neonatal period with abdominal distention and failure to pass meconium. The diagnosis may be suspected clinically by obtaining intestinal decompression as a result of rectal examination and confirmed by rectal biopsy.

**Necrotizing Enterocolitis** Necrotizing enterocolitis (NEC) is the most common GI emergency in preterm infants that presents in the first 3 to 4 weeks of life. It is a multifactorial inflammatory disease of the bowel that leads to intestinal necrosis and perforation. Its incidence decreases with increasing gestational age. Although early recognition and aggressive treatment have improved clinical outcomes, NEC still accounts for substantial long-term morbidities and poor neurodevelopmental outcomes in survivors. Spontaneous intestinal perforation mostly occurs in extremely low–birth-weight infants and usually presents earlier than NEC, in the first few days of life. Once pneumoperitoneum is diagnosed, a surgical intervention, either laparotomy or peritoneal drain placement, is indicated.

**Omphalocele and Gastroschisis** Omphalocele and gastroschisis represent the most frequent congenital abdominal wall defects. Early detection of these malformations and associated anomalies allows multidisciplinary counseling and planning of delivery in a center equipped with high-risk pregnancy assistance, pediatric surgery, and neonatology. Early management involves immediate covering of herniated abdominal contents, nasogastric tube placement for gastric decompression, and surgical evaluation.



## NEUROLOGIC EMERGENCIES

### Seizures

Seizures are the most common neonatal neurological emergency and require prompt diagnosis and treatment. When present, they may reflect a potentially treatable etiology. Immediate evaluation is essential since prolonged seizures may precipitate hypoxemia, acidemia, alterations in glucose homeostasis, and hemodynamic changes in blood pressure and heart rate, all of which can contribute to further brain injury. Although most neonatal seizures are acute and reactive, some seizures occur without an identifiable cause and are termed idiopathic. Most neonatal seizures are focal in origin because of the delay in generalization of electrical activity secondary to lack of myelination and incomplete dendritic and synaptic formation in the immature brain. Neonatal seizures can be the result of a wide range of conditions: neonatal encephalopathy, intracranial hemorrhage, metabolic disturbances, central nervous system or systemic infections, inborn errors of metabolism, and structural brain lesions. Hypoxic ischemic encephalopathy secondary to perinatal asphyxia is the most common cause of neonatal seizures. Therapeutic hypothermia over a 72-hour period has been established as an effective neuroprotective strategy and has been demonstrated to significantly improve neurodevelopmental outcomes at 24 months of age. Treatment with anticonvulsants such as phenobarbital is indicated if seizure activity is suspected. Screening includes evaluation for electrolyte disturbances and glucose, cerebral spinal fluid studies, intracranial imaging, and electroencephalography.

### Neural Tube Defects

Neural tube defects must be emergently addressed unless completely covered by intact skin. The defect should be covered with a sterile, saline-soaked dressing and the infant should be placed in a prone or lateral position to avoid prolonged pressure over the lesion. Prompt neurosurgical evaluation and treatment are essential to optimize neurodevelopmental prognosis. Fetal surgery for myelomeningocele has become available over the past years. Its rationale is that early closure of the defect prevents further damage of the spinal cord and leakage of spinal fluid, which can therefore prevent or reverse herniation of the hindbrain (Chiari II malformation) and hydrocephalus. The Management of Myelomeningocele Study (MOMS) resulted in a decreased need for a cerebrospinal fluid shunt at 1 year of age and improvement in a composite score for mental developmental and motor function at 30 months of age. Fetal surgery for myelomeningocele is currently performed at highly specialized centers across North America and Europe.

## SUGGESTED READINGS


Adzick NS, Thorn EA, Spong CY, et al. A randomized trial of prenatal versus postnatal repair of myelomeningolcele. *N Engl J Med.* 2011;364(11):993-1004.

Araujo Barata, I. Cardiac emergencies. *Emerg Med Clin North Am.* 2013;31(3):677-704.

Breik O, Tivey D, Umapathysivam K, et al. Mandibular distraction osteogenesis for the management of upper airway obstruction in children with micrognathia: a systematic review. *Int J Oral Maxillofac Surg.* 2016;45(6):769-782.

Burge DM. The management of bilious vomiting in the neonate. *Early Hum Dev.* 2016;102:41-45.

Gamba P, Midrio P. Abdominal wall defects: Prenatal diagnosis, newborn management, and long-term outcomes. *Semin Pediatr Surg.* 2014;23(5):283-290.

Gien J, Kinsella JP. Management of pulmonary hypertension in infants with congenital diaphragmatic hernia. *J Perinatol.* 2016;36(2):s28-s31.

Laje P, Tharakan S, Hedrick H. Immediate operative management of the fetus with airway anomalies resulting from congenital malformations. *Semin Fetal Neonatal Med.* 2016:21(4):240-245.

Lakshminrusimha S, Saugstad OD. The fetal circulation, pathophysiology of hypoxemic respiratory failure and pulmonary hypertension in neonates, and the role of oxygen therapy. *J Perinatol.* 2016;36(2):s3-s11.

Parikh DH, Rasiah SV. Congenital lung lesions: postnatal management and outcome. *Semin Pediatr Surg.* 2015;24(4):160-167.

Wyllie J. Neonatal echocardiography. *Semin Fetal Neonatal Med.* 2015;20(3):173-180.


# 64 Developmental Outcomes of High-Risk Infants

Jennifer M. Brady and Sara B. DeMauro

## INTRODUCTION

Over the past half century, important advances in obstetric and neonatal intensive care have led to dramatic reductions in neonatal mortality at all gestational ages. However, prematurity remains a significant problem, and is associated with both mortality and important morbidities. According to the March of Dimes Report Card, 9.6% of children born in the United States in 2015 were preterm, or born at less than 37 weeks' gestation. In addition, perinatal events in full-term infants can also be associated with adverse outcomes. Children who are premature or critically ill at birth can have poor long-term medical outcomes as well as poor developmental and functional outcomes. This chapter addresses how and when to assess developmental outcomes of high-risk children, reviews the associations between specific risk factors and developmental outcomes, and finally briefly addresses future directions for the long term follow-up of high risk newborns.

## IDENTIFYING THE HIGH-RISK INFANT

Infants who are anticipated to be at high risk for developmental problems require close surveillance for developmental problems during the first few years of life. The American Academy of Pediatrics has defined high-risk infants as those infants who fall into 1 of 4 categories: "(1) the preterm infant; (2) the infant with special health care needs or dependence on technology; (3) the infant at risk because of family issues; and (4) the infant with anticipated early death." Such infants should be identified at the time of hospital discharge. Depending on the complexity of the child's medical needs, discharge planning should include a plan for ongoing management of medical problems; appointments with a primary care physician, developmental follow-up program, and any necessary medical specialists; identification of necessary home support services including home care or home nursing; and comprehensive education of the parents. Appropriate family counseling should be provided for as many caregivers as possible, and should include guidance for optimal medical and developmental care of the infant. In some situations, the follow-up program can also include care coordination and primary care in addition to addressing developmental needs. While there is evidence that such "medical homes" decrease resource utilization among children with complex medical conditions, the practicalities of setting up such programs have led to infrequent adoption of this model. Though all children with risk factors for developmental problems should be referred for routine surveillance at the time of hospital discharge, some are missed and some do not come immediately to attention. Therefore, it is essential for the general pediatrician or general practitioner to also provide basic screening in order to identify young children who may have delays and then to refer them for comprehensive evaluations.

## ASSESSING DEVELOPMENTAL OUTCOMES

Developmental outcomes evolve over the first several years of life. While some developmental outcomes can be measured in young infants, many important outcomes cannot be measured until school age. In general, surveillance should include multiple domains: motor, cognitive, language, behavior, and socioemotional skills. Assessment of outcomes serves several purposes: It provides parents with information about their children's development, alerts caregivers to the need for support services including early intervention for infants and toddlers and school services for older children, and provides outcomes for research studies that in turn inform parental counseling and future research. The assessment tools used for an individual child depend on that child's age and history, and the goals of the evaluation.

The earliest assessment of infant development includes a comprehensive neuromotor examination, a review of feeding and sleeping skills, and an evaluation of social interactions. Feeding is 1 of the first key skills for newborns; therefore, poor feeding skills may be an early marker of risk for slow attainment of developmental milestones. Structured motor evaluations such as the General Movements Assessment may be used to assess the risk for cerebral palsy (CP) in preterm infants.

The first few years of life represent an age range when developmental outcomes are most commonly assessed, and reported, in the context of large studies. Early developmental outcomes are most commonly assessed with the Bayley Scales of Infant and Toddler Development in the United States and many other countries. However, other assessments such as the Griffiths Mental Development Scales may also be used. Importantly, such assessments measure the extent to which the child can perform the developmental tasks typical for its age, but they are not intelligence tests. The key use of assessments during the infant and toddler years is to determine whether children would benefit from specific interventions, targeted to areas of developmental delay. For instance, emerging research suggests that early, targeted, and goal-oriented therapies may improve both motor outcomes and cognitive development among children at high risk for CP.

In children older than 2 years of age, multiple assessments are available to measure full-scale intelligence quotient (IQ) or developmental progress. Examples include the Differential Ability Scales (DAS), the Wechsler Preschool and Primary Scale of Intelligence (WPPSI), and the Wechsler Intelligence Scale for Children (WISC). By school age, assessments such as the Wechsler Individual Achievement Test (WIAT) can also be used to measure academic skills. School-age assessments of IQ generally correlate well with adult intelligence. However, it is critical to note that school-age assessments do not always correlate well with earlier developmental assessments. There are several possible explanations for children's shift in scores over time, including social class of parents and availability of educational and social supports. In addition, as described, the available assessments target different skill sets in infants and school age children. As time passes, neonatal events are less predictive of outcomes over time, and instead the child's sociodemographic environment becomes increasingly influential.

*Cerebral palsy* is defined as a disorder of movement and posture that involves abnormalities in tone, reflexes, coordination, and movement; delays in motor milestone achievement; and aberration in primitive reflexes that is permanent (although the presentation may evolve over time) It is caused by a nonprogressive interference, lesion, or abnormality of the developing immature brain. CP includes both an abnormality on physical examination and a corresponding functional limitation. The most common system for classification of motor abilities in CP is the Gross Motor Function Classification System (GMFCS). The GMFCS is useful because it is valid, reliable, and stable over time, particularly in children older than 2 years of age. The GMFCS allows clinicians and parents to plan appropriate therapies and frame expectations for how motor difficulties may evolve as children grow. Though it may not be possible to categorize severity of CP with confidence before 2 years of age, most children with CP present with muscle tone or movement abnormalities at far younger ages. Therefore, the clinician must be aware of the early signs of motor disorders and should, where possible, quickly provide access to essential therapies and resources so as to optimize outcomes.

High-risk children who do not have CP remain at increased risk for *developmental coordination disorder* (DCD), which is a problem of motor coordination and performance that impacts activities of daily living or academic achievement. The most common assessment tool for DCD is the Movement Assessment Battery for Children, but other equivalent tests are also used. The earliest age at which DCD can be diagnosed with confidence is 5 years. DCD is common in former preterm children and is associated with multiple concomitant developmental problems including speech and language, socioemotional, and behavior problems.

Children who were born preterm or were critically ill at birth have increased risk for behavioral, socioemotional and neuropsychiatric problems. Screening for behavioral or socioemotional problems in the early childhood years can be accomplished with multiple instruments; common choices are the Brief Infant and Toddler Social and Emotional Assessment (BITSEA) or the Child Behavior Checklist (CBCL). Importantly, children with a low IQ tend to have higher rates of behavior problems, making detection and concurrent management of both problems essential. Signs of *autism* can be detected with the Modified Checklist for Autism in Toddlers (M-CHAT), which is a validated screening instrument for children 16 to 30 months of age. Confirmation of the diagnosis of autism requires a full assessment by a child psychologist. Similarly, high-risk children have elevated rates of attention-deficit disorder.

As children progress through school age and enter adolescence, additional important aspects of development require assessment. High-risk children may experience executive function disorders, learning problems, poor academic achievement, decreased health-related quality of life, and functional problems. Most programs for surveillance of high-risk children end between 2 and 5 years of age, and state-mandated early intervention programs transition responsibility to school districts around the same time. Therefore, the burden of identifying and addressing such complex problems falls to the primary care physician and school districts. Primary care physicians must remain vigilant so as to identify these problems in a timely manner. It is important to note that higher-level neurobehavioral and cognitive problems lead to increased resource utilization and special education costs. These problems are likely to persist, influencing functional outcomes, including educational achievement, employment, wage-earning, marriage, and family building throughout the life spectrum.

## DEVELOPMENTAL OUTCOMES OF PRETERM INFANTS

*Prematurity* is the most common and well-recognized risk factor for poor outcomes in multiple developmental domains. The risk for most developmental outcomes is best described as a gradient, with risk increasing as gestational age decreases toward the limits of viability. In large studies, even "near term" birth at 37 to 38 weeks is associated with poor outcomes, when compared to birth at 39 to 40 weeks. Late-preterm–born children (34–36 weeks' gestation) do not routinely qualify for most developmental surveillance programs, yet they have increased risk for poor outcomes in multiple domains. These children deserve particular focus from primary care physicians, in whose hands the responsibility for detection and referral therefore falls. Most research into the outcomes of prematurity focuses on the very preterm and extremely preterm infants, in whom risk profiles are most elevated. Below, we briefly present results of several cohort studies that evaluated outcomes of large populations of extremely preterm infants.

In recent years, several large cohort studies have reported the early childhood developmental outcomes of extremely preterm infants. These study populations were heterogeneous, but generally included infants born at less than 27 weeks' gestational age, and were performed between 2004 and 2007. Follow-up evaluations completed between 2 and 3 years corrected age identified CP in 7% to 14% of the children in these cohorts. Severe neurodevelopmental impairment was generally defined as nonambulatory CP and/or developmental testing scores greater than 3 standard deviations below the mean. Blindness and deafness were not consistently included in the criteria for severe impairment. The overall rates of severe neurodevelopmental impairment ranged from 4% to 13%.

Premature infants who reach school age continue to experience increased risk for neurodevelopmental impairments. Nearly all those with severe impairments that were identified in early childhood continue to have moderate to severe impairments at school age. At school age, rates of CP of 9% to 10%, and cognitive disability rates of 4% to 36% have been reported in this population.

In addition to the risk of developmental delay associated with prematurity or low birth weight, additional postnatal morbidities further increase this risk. This section will discuss the impact on developmental outcomes of 6 postnatal morbidities: brain injury, bronchopulmonary dysplasia (BPD), necrotizing enterocolitis, retinopathy of prematurity, infection, and growth and nutrition. Although all of these factors increase the risk of developmental impairments, severe brain injury, severe retinopathy of prematurity, and BPD are most significantly associated with neurodevelopmental impairment, each contributing an additive increase in risk for adverse outcome. These relationships were first demonstrated at 18 months corrected age, and then validated in longer-term studies of several different cohorts.

It is also important to note that in addition to the above-mentioned biologic factors, socioeconomic factors and environment have an important impact on neurodevelopmental outcomes. Higher socioeconomic status has been suggested to be protective, improving cognitive development over the first few years of life, whereas adverse socioeconomic factors are associated with adverse developmental outcomes and behavior problems. Over time, as children get older, perinatal risk factors become less predictive and socioeconomic factors become more predictive of developmental trajectories.

### Brain Injury

Premature infants are at risk for many types of brain injury, including *intraventricular hemorrhage* (IVH), *intraparenchymal hemorrhage* (IPH), and *cystic periventricular leukomalacia* (PVL). Historically, IPH was referred to as grade IV IVH. Grade III IVH or IPH occurs in approximately 15% of infants born at less than 28 weeks' gestation, with PVL occurring in approximately 4%. It is well known that grade III IVH and IPH are associated with adverse developmental outcomes, whereas the impact of grade I and II IVH on developmental outcomes is still unclear, with some studies showing no impact and others demonstrating a small increase in risk for developmental delay. Presence of cystic PVL is associated with increased risk of CP. Infants with IVH or IPH, especially those with higher grade IVH, are at risk for *posthemorrhagic hydrocephalus* (PHH). Infants who experience PHH are at increased risk for developmental delays, with those who require ventriculoperitoneal shunt placement due to hydrocephalus at even further increased risk.

Cranial ultrasound (CUS) is the standard modality to evaluate for brain injury during the neonatal period. While early ultrasounds are helpful for acute decision-making, a near-term or 36-week corrected age CUS is more predictive of 2-year neurodevelopmental impairment or severe motor impairment. While many studies have explored the role of magnetic resonance imaging (MRI) for prediction of developmental outcomes, the diagnostic utility of this tool remains limited. Therefore, current guidelines do not recommend near-term MRI for routine preterm imaging due to insufficient evidence that the practice improves long-term outcomes. It is important to note that although IVH, IPH, and PVL are associated with increased risk of early developmental delays and CP, these findings are not as clearly diagnostic of later delays. Furthermore, a normal CUS during the neonatal period does not exclude future developmental delays, with 30% to 40% of those with "normal" CUS experiencing neurodevelopmental challenges at 18 to 30 months of age. Therefore, care must be taken when counseling parents on the impact of CUS findings in preterm infants, incorporating discussion of the predictive validity of CUS and potential impact of other known risk factors on future developmental outcomes.

### Bronchopulmonary Dysplasia

*Bronchopulmonary dysplasia* is the most common morbidity of prematurity, occurring in approximately half of all infants born less than 28 weeks' gestation. The most universally accepted definition of BPD requires oxygen dependence at 36 weeks' postmenstrual age. BPD is an independent predictor of adverse development at 2 and 5 years of age. Cognitive delays associated with BPD have been shown to present as late as 8 years of age.

Few therapies have been shown to both decrease the incidence of BPD and improve developmental outcomes. Vitamin A may reduce the composite outcome of BPD or death but has no effect on developmental outcomes. Postnatal steroids decrease risk for BPD but increase risk for CP if given within 4 days of life. Steroids given after 1 week of life have not been shown to increase the risk of CP. Surfactant improves the symptoms of respiratory distress but has not been associated with decreased rates of BPD. In addition, although surfactant may reduce mild disability at 1 year of age, this result does not seem to be sustained at 2 years of age. Antenatal corticosteroids reduce developmental impairment, but it is unclear if they decrease rates of BPD. Caffeine is the single treatment that has been shown to safely reduce BPD, death, or neurodevelopmental impairment at 18 to 21 months of age, and motor impairment until at least 5 years of age.

### Retinopathy of Prematurity

*Retinopathy of prematurity* (ROP) is a common morbidity of prematurity that results from abnormal retinal vascular growth after premature birth. Retinopathy of prematurity occurs in over half of infants born less than 28 weeks' gestation, with approximately 15% having more severe disease. Historically, blindness secondary to retinal detachment was the most feared complication of ROP. With improvements in surveillance and available treatments including cryotherapy, laser therapy, and anti–vascular endothelial growth factor treatment, blindness is now a rare outcome in developed countries. However, in the developing world, blindness is still a very real complication of untreated ROP.

Whether or not it requires treatment, ROP is associated with visual morbidities, including blindness, strabismus, and refractory errors. In addition, ROP is an independent risk factor for poor neurodevelopmental outcome. Retinopathy of prematurity has been associated with a strategy of targeting higher oxygen saturations for premature infants; however, this must be cautiously interpreted in the setting of increased risk of death associated with low oxygen saturation targeting strategies.

#### Necrotizing Enterocolitis

*Necrotizing enterocolitis* (NEC) occurs in 7% to 13% of infants born less than 28 weeks' gestational age. Although the precise etiology of NEC is unknown, it is thought to be an inflammatory process leading to necrosis of the bowel. Depending on the severity of disease, NEC can be treated either medically with antibiotics and bowel rest or surgically with drain placement or laparotomy.

Infants who experience NEC have increased rates of death, cognitive delay, CP, and developmental impairment at 18 months of age. In an observational study, surgical NEC, but not medical NEC, was most strongly associated with this increased risk of impairment. Both antenatal corticosteroid treatment and exclusive maternal milk nutrition have been associated with decreased risk of NEC in preterm infants.

#### Infection

Several factors, including immune system impairment, immaturity of the skin barriers, and the frequent need for invasive ventilations and lines, render premature infants at high risk for infection. Despite reduced rates of infection over the past few decades, with quality improvement efforts to reduce iatrogenic infections, approximately 25% of infants born less than 28 weeks' gestation still develop culture-positive sepsis during the neonatal hospitalization. Infection is associated with increased risk of cognitive delay, CP, and visual impairment at 18 to 22 months of age. Meningitis and fungal infections pose even higher risks of adverse developmental outcomes.

#### Growth and Nutrition

The importance of adequate growth and nutrition in premature infants has been increasingly recognized in recent years. This has led to early and more aggressive administration of total parenteral nutrition, early introduction of trophic enteral feedings, and more rapid increases in feeding volumes and fortification of feedings. Low growth velocity during the neonatal hospitalization is associated with increased risk for CP and developmental delays. Furthermore, slow postnatal head growth is highly predictive of later developmental disabilities during childhood. Despite recent interventions to improve nutrition and growth, evidence is still lacking to show that these interventions have a positive impact on developmental outcomes.

### OTHER GROUPS AT HIGH RISK FOR ADVERSE DEVELOPMENTAL OUTCOMES

Prenatal conditions and perinatal events can also increase risk for adverse developmental outcomes among infants born at or near term. Notable risk factors include intrauterine growth restriction (IUGR), congenital heart disease (CHD), hypoxic ischemic encephalopathy (HIE), and the need for extracorporeal membrane oxygenation (ECMO).

#### Intrauterine Growth Restriction

*Intrauterine growth restriction* refers to suboptimal fetal growth, with a lower-than-expected growth velocity in utero. Although placental insufficiency is a major contributor to IUGR, other factors, such as congenital infections, chromosomal abnormalities, and teratogen exposures, also can contribute to this. It has been associated with poor neurodevelopmental outcomes, including motor, cognitive, and language delays. While low birth weight and length are important, slow head growth seems to be the strongest predictor of poor outcomes.

#### Congenital Heart Disease

Advances in the surgical and medical management of children born with *congenital heart disease* have resulted in increased survival rates, creating an interest in the long-term outcomes of these children as they grow. Children with CHD are at increased risk for both motor and cognitive delays. On average, children with a history of CHD have developmental scores approximately 5 to 10 points lower than standardized norms.

Deficits in children with CHD do not appear to be attributable solely to intraoperative and postoperative events. Infants who are born with CHD often have brains that are more immature and smaller than expected for their gestational age. Brain MRI in this population has shown that brain injury, mainly white matter injury, is present both pre- and postoperatively. This suggests a pre-existing vulnerability in these infants, although the degree of white matter injury is yet to be correlated with developmental outcomes in this population.

#### Hypoxic-Ischemic Encephalopathy

*Hypoxic-ischemic encephalopathy* (HIE) results from a perinatal event that prevents an adequate blood or oxygen supply to the infant brain. The diagnosis of HIE generally requires history of an acute perinatal event (eg, cord prolapse or placental abruption), a standardized neurologic exam consistent with encephalopathy, low Apgar scores, and evidence of acidosis on umbilical cord or infant blood gas soon after birth. Infants with HIE have a significant risk of mortality and morbidity.

Numerous studies have shown a decreased risk of both mortality and survival with severe neurodevelopmental disability up to school age in children with moderate or severe HIE who undergo therapeutic hypothermia treatment, or "cooling." Yet, despite treatment with therapeutic hypothermia, these children are still at a high risk for significant impairments. Of those infants who receive therapeutic hypothermia, only about half survive without severe impairments, with approximately 20% of survivors being diagnosed with CP and 22% with developmental delay.

Early factors associated with more severe disability include a higher degree of encephalopathy on initial exam, requiring chest compressions for more than 1 minute, onset of breathing greater than 30 minutes after birth, or a base deficit of 16 or greater. An improving clinical examination during hypothermia with a normal discharge examination, as well as a normal brain MRI after hypothermia are associated with decreased risk for death or disability at 18 to 24 months of age. However, many children with a normal MRI still develop significant impairments, making follow-up of these children as they grow a necessity.

#### Extracorporeal Membrane Oxygenation

*Extracorporeal membrane oxygenation* (ECMO) is a lifesaving therapy that provides complete respiratory support with or without cardiac support for patients with severe respiratory and/or cardiac failure that is unresponsive to conventional medical treatments. It requires 1 or 2 large, surgically placed central catheters. The ECMO circuit, which includes a pump and oxygenator, then removes the patient's blood, artificially removes carbon dioxide and oxygenates the blood, and then returns the blood to the patient. Common conditions for which ECMO is used in neonates include meconium aspiration syndrome and congenital diaphragmatic hernia.

The risk of morbidity and mortality in infants requiring ECMO depends on a number of factors including comorbidities, the indication for ECMO, and complications experienced while on ECMO. Younger gestational age and lower birth weight are both associated with increased complications. (See also Chapter 108.)

### THE FUTURE OF NEONATAL DEVELOPMENTAL CARE

Despite the many well-recognized risk factors for developmental delay or impairment, no factor or combination of factors predicts with certainty the outcome of a vulnerable infant. Biologic, genetic, perinatal, postnatal, and sociodemographic factors all play critical roles in influencing a child's development. It is likely that early sensitive periods of heightened neuronal plasticity may provide opportunities to influence developmental trajectories. For example, as discussed above, a few early pilot trials have demonstrated that focused interventions, when delivered at the right time and with the right intensity, can improve motor outcomes of preterm-born infants at high risk for CP.

In future research, it will be essential to develop strategies to improve the neonatologist's and the pediatrician's ability to diagnose problems early, or to predict which children are at risk, and which specific outcomes (eg, cognitive, motor, behavioral, learning, coordination) are most likely to be affected. In-hand, focused interventions that target these risk profiles must be developed and tested. This would enable intervention *before* any evidence of pathology emerges. Often, children are at risk for several different types of poor outcomes; for example, children with cognitive problems are also at increased risk for behavior problems. At present, there are few proven interventions that target such mixed phenotypes.

The effects of prematurity and other high-risk conditions can influence not only childhood but also adult outcomes. Extremely preterm-born adults have higher rates of neuropsychiatric disorders, autism, and CP, and have less good functional outcomes including lower wage earning, lower rates of parenthood, lower marriage rates, and lower educational achievement. Strategies to mitigate these risks should begin during the postnatal period and continue at least through early childhood and school age. Clinicians should be acutely aware of their patients' risk profiles, and should pay attention to early signs of evolving problems, and quickly connect the patients with appropriate services and therapies, so as to optimize the developmental outcomes of these high-risk patients.

## SUGGESTED READINGS


American Academy of Pediatrics Committee on Fetus and Newborn. Hospital discharge of the high-risk neonate. *Pediatrics.* 2008;122(5):1119-1126.

American Academy of Pediatrics. Identifying infants and young children with developmental disorders in the medical home: an algorithm for developmental surveillance and screening. *Pediatrics.* 2006;118(1):405-420.

Bhutta AT, Cleves MA, Casey PH, et al. Cognitive and behavioral outcomes of school-aged children who were born preterm: a meta-analysis. *JAMA.* 2002;288(6):728-737.

de Jong M, Verhoeven M, van Baar AL. School outcome, cognitive functioning, and behaviour problems in moderate and late preterm children and adults: a review. *Semin Fetal Neonatal Med.* 2012;17(3):163-169.

Doyle LW, Anderson PJ. Adult outcome of extremely preterm infants. *Pediatrics.* 2010;126(2):342-351.

Hack M, Breslau N, Aram D, Weissman B, Klein N, Borawski-Clark E. The effect of very low birth weight and social risk on neurocognitive abilities at school age. *J Dev Behav Pediatr.* 1992;13(6):412-420.

Ho T, Dukhovny D, Zupancic JAF, et al. Choosing wisely in newborn medicine: five opportunities to increase value. *Pediatrics.* 2015;136(2):e482-e489.

Marlow N, Wolke D, Bracewell MA; EPICure Study Group. Neurologic and developmental disability at six years of age after extremely preterm birth. *N Engl J Med.* 2005;352(1):9-19.

Msall ME, Park JJ. The spectrum of behavioral outcomes after extreme prematurity: regulatory, attention, social, and adaptive dimensions. *Semin Perinatol.* 2008;32(1):42-50.

Roberts G, Anderson PJ, Davis N, et al; Victorian Infant Collaborative Study Group. Developmental coordination disorder in geographic cohorts of 8-year-old children born extremely preterm or extremely low birthweight in the 1990s. *Dev Med Child Neurol.* 2011;53(1):55-60.

Schmidt B, Asztalos EV, Roberts RS, et al. Impact of bronchopulmonary dysplasia, brain injury, and severe retinopathy on the outcome of extremely low-birth-weight infants at 18 months: results from the trial of indomethacin prophylaxis in preterms. *JAMA.* 2003;289(9):1124-1129.

Tagin MA, Woolcott CG, Vincer MJ, et al. Hypothermia for neonatal hypoxic ischemic encephalopathy: an updated systematic review and meta-analysis. *Arch Pediatr Adolesc Med.* 2012;166(6):558-566.

# 65 Somatic Growth and Development in Adolescence

Meghna R. Sebastian and Albert C. Hergenroeder

Puberty has been defined as the activation of the hypothalamic–pituitary–gonadal axis, which leads to gonadal maturation and the subsequent somatic manifestations associated with increased sex steroids and anabolic hormones. Adolescence refers to the development of adult social and cognitive behaviors. This is a period of intense physical and psychological changes. The sexual maturity rating (SMR) system described by Tanner and Marshall has been used to characterize the secondary sexual stages of puberty in boys based on pubic hair and genital development (PH1–5 and G1–5), and in girls based on breast and pubic hair development (B1–5 and PH1–5). Somatic changes observed during puberty correlate more closely with the SMR stage than with chronological age.

## GROWTH AND BODY COMPOSITION

Nearly 20% of the final adult height is achieved during puberty. The growth rate in childhood averages 5 to 6 cm per year. Prior to puberty there is a slight deceleration in growth rate. Pubertal growth is triggered by the pulsatile secretion of gonadotropin-releasing hormone, which leads to the release of gonadotropins and in turn sex steroids, which facilitate accelerated growth hormone secretion. Typically, both males and females begin their pubertal growth spurt when they reach SMR stage 2. However, boys most often reach their peak height velocity (PHV) at a later stage of genital development (G4 and PH4) compared to girls in relation to breast development (B3; Table 65-1). Linear growth in girls slows after menarche with an average of 7 cm of height increase after menarche. Height increases are usually complete by a bone age of 15 years in girls. In most boys, linear growth is complete at a bone age of 17 years. The average PHV in boys is 9.5 cm/year, while in girls is 8.25 cm/year. Thus, the longer period of growth and a higher height velocity contribute to a greater adult height in males compared to females. Final adult height is largely determined by the genetic potential, reflected in the mid-parental height.

Almost half of the final adult weight is achieved during puberty. In girls, the weight velocity usually peaks about 6 months after height velocity, at about 8.3 kg/year. Boys tend to show a peak in both height and weight velocity around the same time, with the peak average weight gain of 9 kg/year.

Besides changes in weight and height, pubertal changes are also observed in the proportions of fat, water, muscle, and bone. Body fat in healthy prepubertal girls is approximately 15% to 17% of body weight. At menarche, this increases to 22% to 24% because fat mass increases proportionately more than fat-free mass. Approximately 17% body fat is required for initiation of menstruation and 22% for maintenance of normal ovulatory menstrual cycles. In contrast, the percentage of body fat decreases in healthy males from approximately 14–15% to 10–11% during puberty as fat-free mass increases more than fat mass. Leptin is a principal mediator between body fat changes and pubertal neuroendocrine maturation.

## MUSCULOSKELETAL CHANGES

There is a 20-fold increase in the cross-sectional area of muscle fibers from birth to young adulthood. Glycogen and resting ATP stores increase in early adolescence. Adolescents have increased activity of muscle enzymes involved in oxidative activity, resulting in increased capacity for aerobic activity. These changes are associated with the increased strength seen during puberty. Puberty is also characterized by accumulation of the majority of adult peak bone mass. The rise in serum alkaline phosphatase concentration reflects this bone growth (Table 65-1). Most individuals accrue almost 50% of their final bone mass during puberty. Hence, optimizing bone mineral acquisition during puberty is essential to minimize the future risk of osteoporosis.

## HEMATOLOGIC CHANGES

Increases in hemoglobin concentration and red cell mass coincide with the adolescent growth spurt in boys. The average hemoglobin in early puberty is about 13.5 g/dL. Adult males achieve hemoglobin values of 13.5 to 17.5 g/dL. Hemoglobin values remain relatively stable in females between 12 and 15.5 g/dL (Table 65-1). Changes also occur in the serum concentrations of pro- and anticoagulant factors, with most factor levels being about 20% lower than adult values until the teenage years.

## CARDIORESPIRATORY CHANGES

Cardiac size increases in proportion to somatic growth in childhood and adolescence. Adolescent fat-free mass is predictive of left ventricular mass. While genetic and hormonal influences are the most important factors that determine fat-free mass and cardiac mass, aerobic training also affects heart mass. Blood pressure increases gradually in both sexes. Total cholesterol, low-density lipoprotein cholesterol, and triglyceride concentrations are higher in adolescents than in children. Serum high-density lipoprotein cholesterol levels fall in healthy males during puberty.

Respiratory rate is inversely proportional to body size. Adult values for respiratory rate are achieved in late childhood. The variability in awake and sleeping respiratory rates is high in infants and decreases to only 1 to 2 breaths per minute in adolescents. Though vital capacity increases, tidal volume per kilogram body weight is relative unchanged throughout life (6 mL/kg). Hence, the decrease in respiratory rate leads to a decline in minute ventilation with age from 250 mL/kg/min in newborns to 100 mL/kg/min in adolescents.

## NEUROLOGIC CHANGES

Adolescence has been associated with an increase in risk-taking behaviors. Sexual development and the more complex social environment that adolescents live in place high demands on central nervous system circuits that regulate emotional processes. The first 2 years of life are marked by an increase in brain volume of approximately 130%. In contrast, between 12 and 18 years the largest change in volume is about 14%. White matter volume increases more steeply in adolescent boys than girls. Gray matter decreases with age during adolescence. The prefrontal cortex, which is important for executive functioning, is thought to be the last region where the rate of decline of gray matter levels off. This happens in late adolescence and early adulthood. Unlike the atrophy that occurs in old age, this loss of gray matter is thought to be a result of synaptic pruning wherein redundant neuronal connections are eliminated. Thus, it is considered a process of developmental maturation. Adolescent psychological development is described in detail in Chapter 68.

## REPRODUCTIVE CHANGES

The functional maturation and growth of reproductive structures, as well as the development of secondary sexual characteristics, are the hallmarks of puberty. Secular trends have been observed over the last few decades with gradual lowering in the age of onset of puberty, particularly in girls. The age at menarche is 12.9 (± 1.2 years) in white

**TABLE 65-1 CLINICAL CORRELATES OF PUBERTAL MATURATION**

| | SMR 1 | SMR 2 | SMR 3 | SMR 4 | SMR 5 |
|---|---|---|---|---|---|
| **Girls** | | | | | |
| *Hematocrit (%)* | | | | | |
| White (mean) | 39.1 | 39.2 | 39.6 | 39.2 | 39.2 |
| (range) | 36.1–42.1 | 37.1–41.3 | 37.0–42.2 | 36.9–41.6 | 36.2–42.2 |
| Black (mean) | 37.3 | 38.9 | 39.0 | 38.4 | 38.7 |
| (range) | 34.6–39.9 | 35.7–42.1 | 35.2–42.6 | 34.9–42.8 | 35.9–41.5 |
| *Alkaline phosphatase (IU/L) (serum)* | | | | | |
| White (mean) | 70 | 89 | 76 | 33 | 38 |
| (range) | 51–90 | 49–134 | 36–108 | 16–60 | 23–76 |
| Black (mean) | 84 | 95 | 86 | 44 | 31 |
| (range) | 69–108 | 65–138 | 26–148 | 18–144 | 13–70 |
| Peak height velocity | | + | ++ | + | |
| Menarche | | + | ++ | ++ | |
| Slipped capital femoral epiphysis | | + | ++ | | |
| Acute worsening of scoliosis | | + | ++ | + | |
| Osgood-Schlatter disease | | + | ++ | | |
| Acne vulgaris | | + | ++ | ++ | |
| Physiological leucorrhea | | + | ++ | | |
| **Boys** | | | | | |
| *Hematocrit (%)* | | | | | |
| White (mean) | 39.5 | 39.8 | 40.9 | 42.3 | 43.8 |
| (range) | 37.1–41.8 | 36.7–42.8 | 38.2–43.5 | 39.7–44.8 | 41.1–46.4 |
| Black (mean) | 37.7 | 38.4 | 39.7 | 41.1 | 42.7 |
| (range) | 35.2–40.2 | 36.0–40.9 | 37.3–42.0 | 38.3–43.8 | 39.6–45.9 |
| *Alkaline phosphatase (IU/L) (serum)* | | | | | |
| White (mean) | 72 | 77 | 101 | 75 | 58 |
| (range) | 54–110 | 42–106 | 53–141 | 41–158 | 21–120 |
| Black (mean) | 77 | 94 | 122 | 116 | 75 |
| (range) | 43–130 | 53–204 | 46–240 | 32–228 | 23–228 |
| Peak height velocity | | | + | ++ | + |
| Ejaculation onset | | + | ++ | ++ | + |
| Ejaculation with fertility | | | + | ++ | ++ |
| Slipped capital femoral epiphysis | | + | ++ | + | |
| Acute worsening of scoliosis | | + | ++ | ++ | + |
| Osgood-Schlatter disease | | + | ++ | ++ | |
| Acne vulgaris | | + | ++ | ++ | + |
| Gynecomastia | | + | ++ | + | |

+ = May occur during this stage but is less likely than ++.

++ = Occurs most often during this sexual maturity rating.

SMR, sexual maturity rating.

Adapted with permission from Joffe A, Blythe MJ. Adolescent medicine: state of the art reviews. Handbook of adolescent medicine, *Adolesc Med State Art Rev* 2009 Aug;20(2):261-859.

girls and 12.1 (± 1.21 years) in African American girls. This typically occurs between SMR stages 3 and 4 (Table 65-1). Data suggests that the age at menarche has lowered by 2.5 to 4 months since the 1940s. The mean age of onset of male pubertal development is 11 years. The reproductive changes in adolescents are described in Chapters 66 and 67 for females and males, respectively. Chapter 533 describes the sequence of normal puberty.

## SUGGESTED READINGS

Armstrong N, Barker AR, McManus AM. Muscle metabolism changes with age and maturation: how do they relate to youth sport performance? *Br J Sports Med.* 2015;49(13):860-864.

Bordini B, Rosenfield RL. Normal pubertal development, II: clinical aspects of puberty. *Pediatr Rev.* 2011;32(7):281-292.

Chulani VL, Gordon LP. Adolescent growth and development. *Prim Care Clin Office Pract.* 2014;41(3):465-487.

Jaffray J, Young G. Developmental hemostasis: clinical implications from the fetus to the adolescent. *Pediatr Clin North Am.* 2013;60(6):1407-1417.

Janz KF, Dawson JD, Mahoney LT. Predicting heart growth during puberty: the Muscatine Study. *Pediatrics.* 2000;105(5):e63.

Luciana M. Adolescent brain development in normality and psychopathology. *Dev Psychopathol.* 2013;25(4, pt 2):1325-1345.

Marshall WA, Tanner JM. Variations in the pattern of pubertal changes in boys. *Arch Dis Child.* 1970;45(239):13-23.

Paus T. How environment and genes shape the adolescent brain. *Horm Behav.* 2013;64(2):195-202.

Rogol AD. Sex steroids, growth hormone, leptin and the pubertal growth spurt. *Endocr Dev.* 2010;17:77-85.

Ross KR, Rosen CL. Sleep and respiratory physiology in children. *Clin Chest Med.* 2014;35(3):457-467.

# 66 Reproductive Growth and Development in the Female Adolescent

Meghna R. Sebastian and Anna-Barbara Moscicki

Adolescence is a period of peak somatic as well as reproductive growth and development. The pattern of growth and functional maturation of various reproductive structures in females is described in this chapter. The stages of normal puberty are described in Chapter 533 and an overview of the hormonal influences that lead to these changes is in Chapter 513.

## BREAST

Breast development can be divided into four stages: a prepubertal period of quiescence; a pubertal period of rapid growth and lobular development; cyclic changes in stromal and epithelial elements during menstruation and pregnancy; and finally, involution of lobules, which starts after the age of 35. Breast buds may be appreciated in newborns due to the influence of maternal hormones. These buds typically regress within a few weeks of life, after which the mammary glands remain a rudimentary framework of glandular tissue and stroma through the rest of childhood. During puberty, estrogen is the predominant hormone responsible for an increase in adipose tissue, stromal growth, and ductal growth and branching in the developing breast tissue. Growth hormone and insulin-like growth factor 1 are also important in pubertal breast development. The role of progesterone is to promote the development of the lobules and alveoli—this being particularly important during pregnancy. Prolactin collaborates with progesterone to promote alveolar epithelial development as well as lactogenesis. Oxytocin, which is secreted by the supraoptic, paraventricular, and other accessory nuclei of the hypothalamus, causes contraction of myoepithelial cells and milk let-down in a lactating woman.

## VAGINA

In the newborn, the vagina is typically approximately 4 cm in depth. The vagina elongates throughout childhood commensurate with the growth of the child. Hence, unlike the uterus and the breast, which have a pubertal spurt in size, a drastic change in growth velocity of the vagina is not required. By menarche, the vagina reaches a mature depth of 5 to 7.5 cm anteriorly and 10.5 to 11.5 cm posteriorly. The prepubertal length of the vaginal orifice is about 10 mm. In addition to the increase in depth, the introitus increases in length during puberty to approximately 23 mm in an adult woman.

The effect of estrogen during puberty leads to a change in the appearance of the vaginal mucosa. Histologically, the vaginal epithelium consists of 4 layers of squamous cells—basal, parabasal, intermediate, and superficial. In early childhood, the epithelium is 2 to 8 layers thick and contains predominantly monomorphic-appearing basal and parabasal cells. During puberty, there is a transition to a thicker epithelium with several layers of superficial cornified squamous cells. To the naked eye, the mucosa appears pink rather than red, it develops a thick cobblestoned appearance, and the hymen appears thick with fimbriations.

With the onset of cyclic ovarian activity during puberty, many adolescents develop physiological leucorrhea due to the normal layer of desquamating superficial squamous cells. This is often noticed several months prior to menarche. The nature of the discharge varies with fluctuating hormone levels during the menstrual cycle. The amount of discharge is usually minimal immediately after menstruation, cloudy and sticky during the estrogenic phase of the cycle, thin and profuse during ovulation, sticky and thick under the influence of progesterone, and finally clear and watery again prior to ovulation. Vaginal discharge is a common reason for physician visits, and patients often need to be reassured of the physiological nature of the process.

The vaginal microbiome also changes with hormonal exposure during puberty. Older studies found a variety of nonpathogenic bacteria in the prepubertal vagina including diphtheroids, anaerobes, coagulase-negative staphylococci, *Escherichia coli*, and *Streptococcus viridans*. *Lactobacillus* species were infrequently observed in premenarcheal girls. These studies were limited by microbiological methods that relied on cultivating the organism. With new techniques, including gene sequencing of the 16S rRNA, scientists have been able to demonstrate that lactic acid–producing bacteria (LAB) colonize the vagina relatively early in puberty, much before the onset of menarche. LAB include *Lactobacillus*, *Streptococcus*, *Aerococcus*, *Facklamia*, *Atopobium*, and *Bifidobacterium*. Estrogen is thought to promote the production of glycogen in the vaginal epithelium, and this glycogen serves as an ideal substrate for LAB. The presence of LAB often leads to an acidic vaginal pH of 3.8 to 4.4. Besides, LAB produce enzymes and byproducts with an antibiotic effect, such as hydrogen peroxide and endopeptidase. This results in a vaginal milieu that is inhospitable to the growth of several pathogenic bacterial species. Besides LAB, through gene sequencing, *Gardenella vaginalis* has been found in healthy women as well as peripubertal girls with no history of sexual activity.

## UTERUS

The uterus consists of two portions: the cervix and the corpus, or body. The uterus appears tubular with a prominent cervix and smaller corpus in infancy and childhood. The corpus enlarges throughout late childhood and early puberty so that the uterus achieves the mature pear shape of an adult female by menarche. While the configuration is adult-like earlier in adolescence, the size of the uterus continues to increase well beyond menarche, and growth is often not complete until the age of 16 or 17.

The linings of the corpus and the cervix are distinct and different. Early in embryonic development, the cervix is lined by columnar cells of Müllerian origin. During fetal development, these cells are partly replaced by squamous cells from the urogenital sinus. The junction of the two types of cells is the squamocolumnar junction, and the area of the ectocervix that remains columnar is called ectopy. During puberty, the columnar region of the ectocervix starts to transform to squamous cells through a process referred to as squamous metaplasia. Uncommitted generative cells of the basal layer of the columnar epithelium transform this layer into squamous epithelium through replication and differentiation. This process results in a new squamocolumnar junction, which begins to move proximally. This area of transformation is referred to as the transformation zone. A major trigger for this change is the alteration in the vaginal pH from alkaline (>4.7) prior to puberty, to acidic (<4.5) after the onset of puberty. The transformation zone is where cervical cancers arise and is the prime target for the human papillomavirus due to the ongoing replication of the host cells. The columnar epithelium of the endocervix and the region of ectopy are targeted by *Chlamydia trachomatis* and *Neisseria gonorrhoeae*. Thus, an understanding of this process of cervical epithelial maturation helps explain the unique vulnerability of adolescents to certain infections.

The lining of the corpus is called the endometrium. It consists of a deeper stable basal layer of dense stroma and weakly proliferative glands and a superficial functional layer of epithelium, which is constantly changing during the menstrual cycle. After 20 weeks of gestation, a proliferation of glandular and stromal tissue is observed in the fetus. As the fetus approaches term, placental and maternal hormones cause the epithelial cells to appear tall and columnar. These cells are filled with glycogen and mucin. Soon after birth this peak period of secretory activity ceases and the endometrium regresses. Subsequently, throughout childhood, the endometrium is a thin, atrophic epithelial layer with minimal stroma. The hormonal changes that accompany puberty transform the endometrium into a dynamic tissue with a structure that varies with the phase of the menstrual cycle (Fig. 66-1). The phases of the menstrual cycle are an estrogen-dominated preovulatory phase, progesterone-dominated postovulatory phase, and a menstrual phase. During the preovulatory phase, estrogen leads to endometrial proliferation and thickening to approximately 0.65 cm (0.21–1.40). The glands and arteries elongate. The secretory phase, which is influenced by progesterone, follows. The endometrial thickness is about 1 cm (0.39–2.04) during this phase. The glands are

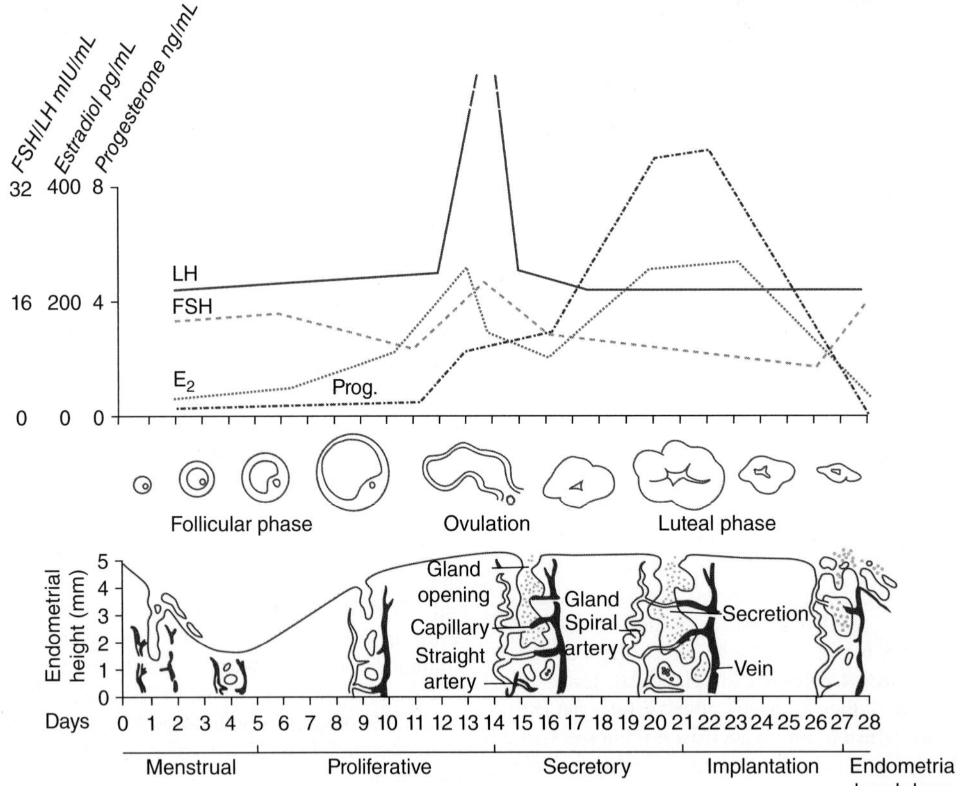


**FIGURE 66-1** Cyclic changes of the menstrual cycle. Hormone levels: luteinizing hormone (LH), follicle-stimulating hormone (FSH), estradiol ($E_2$), and progesterone (Prog.); follicle development and formation of the corpus luteum; and endometrial development. (Reproduced with permission from Speroff L, Fritz M: *Clinical Gynecologic Endocrinology and Infertility*. Baltimore, MD: Lippincott, Williams and Wilkins, 2005 (top image). Reproduced with permission from Moscicki AB, Shafer MA: Normal reproductive development in the adolescent female, *J Adolesc Health Care.* 1986 Nov;7(6 Suppl):41S-64S (bottom image).)

more tortuous and the arteries appear spiral. When fertilization and implantation do not occur, there is a decline in estrogen and progesterone concentrations. The fall in progesterone level triggers the breakdown of the endometrium due to ischemia from constriction of the arterioles, the release of proteolytic enzymes from lysosomes, and the disruption of basement membrane by matrix metalloproteinases. The endometrium is shed and menstruation results.

Until recently it was thought that the uterine cavity is sterile. Exploratory gene-sequencing studies have disproven this thought; and it is now known that the uterus is colonized by microbes different from those of the vagina. While *Bacteroides* species are most commonly found, *Lactobacilli*, *Prevotella spp*, *Atopobium vaginae*, and *Mobiluncus curtisii* have also been seen in the uterus. The gut microbiome, which has been extensively studied, has been found to play an essential role in human physiology. It is not unreasonable to postulate a similar role for the uterine microbiome. However, further research is needed to elucidate the role these microbes play in health and disease.

## OVARY

At birth the ovary is tiny and elongated and about the size of a small bean. It weighs about 1 g and the usual ranges of its dimensions are 0.5 to 1.5 cm in length, 0.3 to 0.5 cm in width, and 0.3 to 0.4 cm in thickness. It grows in size through childhood, but there is an intensification of this growth immediately prior to menarche. At menarche, the ranges of its dimensions are 2.7 to 3.5 cm in length, 1.5 to 2.4 cm in width, and 0.85 to 1.35 cm in thickness. It weighs about 6 g.

The number of ovarian follicles decline throughout the lifespan from a peak at 26 weeks of gestational age, to about 2 million at birth; 300,000 to 500,000 at menarche; and 100 at menopause. The hormonal changes during the menstrual cycle and the phases of follicle development are pictorially represented (Fig. 66-1). The process of maturation of the primordial follicle takes about 3 months. The first stage is for the oocyte in the primordial follicle to enlarge and the granulosa cells to proliferate. This leads to the formation of a primary follicle. In the next stage, a secondary follicle forms wherein the stroma differentiates into a theca interna and a theca externa. The theca interna cells express luteinizing hormone (LH) receptors and the granulosa cells express follicle-stimulating hormone (FSH) receptors. The initial stages of follicle development are gonadotropin independent, and the later stages are gonadotropin dependent. Stimulation by FSH makes the follicular granulosa cells produce estrogen. The growing follicle starts to develop an antral cavity, and as this cavity enlarges, a preovulatory follicle is formed. As estrogen production peaks, it reaches a level that provokes a suppression of FSH secretion and a surge in LH levels. The surge in LH levels is followed 16 to 24 hours later by the rupture of the follicle and the release of the ovum. The ruptured follicle then transforms into a corpus luteum. Estradiol levels decline and progesterone levels increase during the initial part of the luteal phase. The later part of the luteal phase is characterized by a slow rise in estrone and estradiol levels, in addition to the continuing increase in progesterone levels. This causes the suppression of FSH and LH secretion and involution of the corpus luteum. If fertilization and implantation occur, human chorionic gonadotropin (hCG) secreted by the placental tissue maintains the corpus luteum throughout pregnancy.

## SUGGESTED READINGS

Brosens I, Benagiano G. The endometrium from the neonate to the adolescent. *J Matern Fetal Neonatal Med.* 2016;29(8):1195-1199. doi: 10.3109/14767058.2015.1040756.

Colvin CW, Abdullatif H. Anatomy of female puberty: the clinical relevance of developmental changes in the reproductive system. *Clin Anat.* 2013;26(1):115-129. doi: 10.1002/ca.22164.

Duflos C, Plu-Bureau G, Thibaud E, Kuttenn F. Breast diseases in adolescents. *Endocr Dev.* 2012;22:208-221. doi: 10.1159/000326690.

Henriet P, Gaide Chevronnay HP, Marbaix E. The endocrine and paracrine control of menstruation. *Mol Cell Endocrinol.* 2012;358(2): 197-207. doi: 10.1016/j.mce.2011.07.042.

Hickey RJ, Zhou X, Settles ML, et al. Vaginal microbiota of adolescent girls prior to the onset of menarche resemble those of reproductive-age women. *mBio.* 2015;6(2). doi: 10.1128/mBio.00097-15.

Hwang LY, Ma Y, Benningfield SM, et al. Factors that influence the rate of epithelial maturation in the cervix in healthy young women. *J Adolesc Health.* 2009;44(2):103-110. doi: 10.1016/j.jadohealth.2008.10.006.

Macias H, Hinck L. Mammary gland development. *Wiley Interdiscip Rev Dev Biol.* 2012;1(4):533-557. doi: 10.1002/wdev.35.

Mancuso AC, Ryan GL. Normal vulvovaginal health in adolescents. *J Pediatr Adolesc Gynecol.* 2015;28(3):132-135. doi: 10.1016/j.jpag.2014.05.004.

Radivojevic UD, Lazovic GB, Kravic-Stevovic TK, et al. Differences in anthropometric and ultrasonographic parameters between adolescent girls with regular and irregular menstrual cycles: a case-study of 835 cases. *J Pediatr Adolesc Gynecol.* 2014;27(4):227-231. doi: 10.1016/j.jpag.2013.11.007.

Rojas J, Chavez-Castillo M, Olivar LC, et al. Physiologic course of female reproductive function: a molecular look into the prologue of life. *J Pregnancy.* 2015;2015:715735. doi: 10.1155/2015/715735.

Verstraelen H, Vilchez-Vargas R, Desimpel F, et al. Characterisation of the human uterine microbiome in non-pregnant women through deep sequencing of the V1-2 region of the 16S rRNA gene. *Peer J.* 2016;4:e1602. doi: 10.7717/peerj.1602.

# 67 Reproductive Growth and Development in the Male Adolescent

Meghna R. Sebastian and Albert C. Hergenroeder

Growth and functional maturation of the male reproductive organs occurs throughout childhood and adolescence with peak activity during puberty. This chapter will describe the pattern of this growth and maturation. The various stages of normal male puberty are described in Chapter 533 and testicular as well as scrotal masses are described in Chapter 78.

## EXTERNAL GENITAL ORGANS

External genitalia develop from a genital tubercle, which forms ventral to the cloaca. Early development is androgen independent and instead depends on transgenic pathways including *sonic hedgehog*. Once the genital tubercle is sexually dimorphic, further masculinization is dependent on androgen exposure. Elongation of the genital tubercle leads to the formation of a phallus, and closure of the urethral folds forms a penile urethra. The scrotum is formed by fusion of the labioscrotal swellings.

In infancy the average length and girth of the penis are 3.5 and 4.4 cm, respectively. While penile growth continues through childhood, a spurt in this growth is seen during stage 3 of the sexual maturity rating (SMR) system. The penis starts to increase in length prior to an increase in girth. During puberty, the scrotum enlarges, its skin darkens, and it develops rugae. Most external genital growth is complete within 5 years of entering SMR stage 2.

## EPIDIDYMIS, VAS DEFERENS, SEMINAL VESICLES, AND PROSTATE GLAND

The epididymis, vas deferens, and seminal vesicles develop from the wolffian duct under the influence of androgens. The epididymis has three regions: a caput, which is responsible for fluid resorption and secretion of glycopeptides; a corpus, where maturation of the sperm occurs; and a cauda, where sperm is stored. Its development follows a biphasic pattern with initial growth between 2 and 4 months of fetal life, followed by regression during infancy and then definitive development during childhood and puberty. When mature, it has a stretched length of 3 meters with the globular caput lying on the superior pole of the testis and the narrow cauda on its inferior pole.

The vas deferens starts where the cauda epididymis straightens out and, when fully grown, has a length of about 35 cm. Besides serving as a conduit to the ejaculatory duct, its complex epithelium has secretory and absorptive functions that contribute to the semen.

In the fetus, the seminal vesicle develops as a hook-like duct with side ducts from the distal wolffian duct. During puberty, the gland has increasing amounts of connective tissue and smooth muscle and its interior starts to appear septate. Its weight increases by a factor of 10. Functionally, the ampulla of the vas deferens, the seminal vesicle, and the ejaculatory duct can be considered a unit whose roles include secretion, resorption, and spermatophagy.

The prostate gland starts to develop at around 12 weeks of gestation. During childhood, there is progressive decline in the amount of smooth muscle and an increase in connective tissue. These proportions reverse during puberty and the gland enlarges to reach an adult size by the age of 20 to 25 years.

## TESTIS

The primitive gonads develop from the mesenchyme on the ventral surface of the mesonephric ridges (Fig. 67-1). The migration of germ cells from the yolk sac endoderm to the gonad is responsible for the differentiation of the sexually indifferent gonad to a testis at around 6 weeks of gestation. The fetal testis begins to develop columnar protrusions from the cortex to the medulla. These consist of primitive germ cells and pre-Sertoli cells, giving the appearance of a seminiferous cord by the 9th gestational week. After 10 to 15 weeks of gestation, testicular migration begins. The gubernaculum plays a vital role in this descent. It is thought that a relative swelling reaction is responsible for the transabdominal phase; and gubernacular remodeling and contraction leads to the inguinoscrotal phase of testicular descent. Insulin-like factor 3 (INSL3), which is secreted by fetal Leydig cells, and dihydrotestosterone are the main factors that contribute to the transabdominal phase of testicular descent. Pituitary gonadotropins, androgens, and possibly calcitonin gene-related peptide, which is a neurotransmitter released by the genitofemoral nerve, play an important role in the inguinoscrotal phase. Müllerian-inhibiting substance or anti-Müllerian hormone (AMH) is secreted by the Sertoli cells, and it causes regression of the Müllerian ducts. Persistent Müllerian duct syndrome results when this fails to occur. Males with persistent Müllerian duct syndrome have a uterus, fallopian tubes, and intra-abdominal testes. Testicular descent to the scrotal sac, though usually completed prior to birth, may at times be completed postnatally.

The neonatal testis has an average volume of 0.57 mL, while that of an adult is 15 to 25 mL. Testicular enlargement is typically the first sign of puberty, and a length of about 2.5 cm or a volume of about 4 mL indicates entry into puberty. The testis is lined by the tunica albuginea, which has three layers of connective tissue. The outermost layer is the tunica vaginalis and is made of superficial mesothelial cells. The middle layer is the thickest and consists of dense fibrous tissue, myoid cells, nerve fibers, and mast cells. The innermost layer is the tunica vascularis and is made of loose connective tissue with lymphatics, blood vessels, and nerves. This layer is continuous with the septa, which divide the testis into 250 to 300 lobules, each containing 2 to 4 seminiferous tubules.

### Seminiferous Tubules

The seminiferous tubules consist of Sertoli cells and germ cells. Until puberty, the seminiferous tubules are in reality solid cords that become convoluted tubules during puberty. In an adult, they have a diameter of 180 to 200 µm and length of 30 to 80 cm. The seminiferous tubules account for 90% of the testicular volume. The prepubertal germ cells

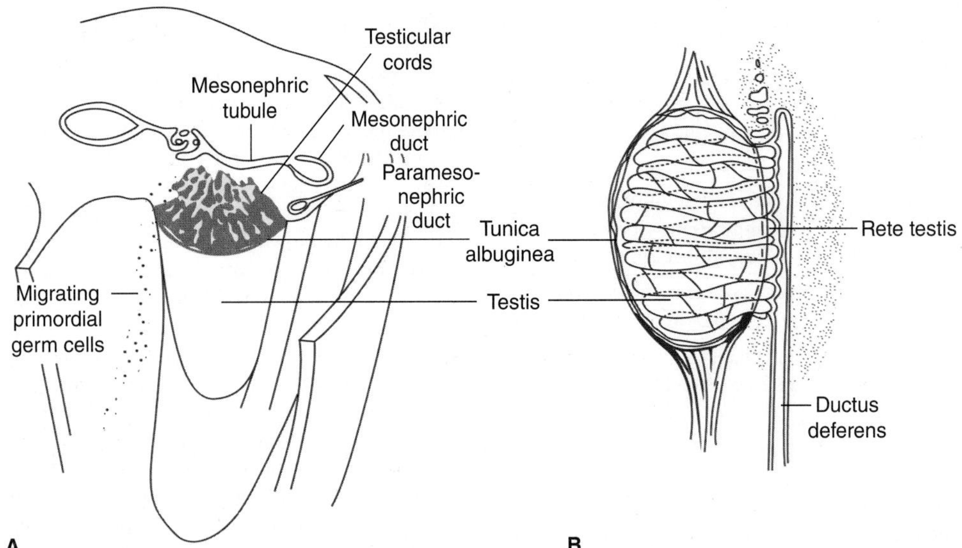


**FIGURE 67-1** Fetal testicular development. **A:** Transverse section through the lumbar section of a 6-week embryo. Note the primordial germ cells migrating to the primitive sex cords of the indifferent gonad. **B:** Testis and evolving ductus deferens in the fourth month of development.

include neonatal gonocytes, which are large cells near the center of the seminiferous cord. The more mature spermatogonia, spermatocytes, and spermatozoa are located at the periphery of the cord in contact with the basement membrane. Besides germ cells, there are 10 to 12 columnar Sertoli cells per tubule that rest on the basement membrane.

#### Sertoli Cells

In the prepubertal seminiferous cord, the Sertoli cells make up 93% to 97% of the cellular population, with germ cells accounting for only 5% to 7%. During puberty, the Sertoli cells gather in a single layer on the basement membrane between the spermatogonia and germ cells that have entered meiosis. A dramatic expansion of the germ cell population occurs with the onset of puberty. However, the total number of germ cells in an adult testis depends on the number of Sertoli cells, as each cell can only support the development of limited germ cells. The Sertoli cells form a blood–testis barrier that maintains the biochemical and immunological milieu of the seminiferous tubules. They also secrete AMH, whose role has been described earlier, and inhibin B, which is thought to play a role in spermatogenesis.

#### Leydig Cells

Typical Leydig cells develop around 6 weeks of gestation and disappear between 3 and 6 months after birth until puberty. During puberty, second-generation Leydig cells emerge. Leydig cells are located in the interstitium between seminiferous tubules. Testosterone from the Leydig cells is responsible for development of the wolffian duct structures, in utero masculinization, as well as pubertal maturation of the external genitalia, and it acts in a paracrine fashion to promote Sertoli cell maturation. Besides androgens, the Leydig cells secrete INSL3, which as described earlier is vital for testicular descent.

## SPERMATOGENESIS

During infancy, between 3 and 9 months, a process of "mini-puberty" causes the neonatal gonocytes to transform into adult dark spermatogonia. These mature further into adult pale spermatogonia, which are cells committed to spermatogenesis. In early childhood, between the ages of 3 and 4 years, these cells undergo mitotic division to form primary spermatocytes. Meiotic division and formation of a haploid chromosomal complement do not start until after puberty. Testosterone and adequate androgen receptors on the Sertoli cells are vital for meiotic division of the secondary spermatocyte. The secondary spermatocyte matures to form a spermatid and spermatozoa. The duration of spermatogenesis is usually about 60 days. Ejaculation is typically noted during SMR stage 3 and ejaculation with fertility in SMR stage 4.

## HYPOTHALAMIC–PITUITARY–GONADAL AXIS

In fetal life, the secretion of AMH by the Sertoli cells is independent of the pituitary. Leydig cells secrete INSL3 and testosterone under the influence of placental human chorionic gonadotropin. Pituitary gonadotropin secretion is low in the first week of life, after which it peaks between 3 and 6 months during the period of mini-puberty. Luteinizing hormone (LH) promotes Leydig cell function and the production of testosterone. Follicle-stimulating hormone (FSH) promotes Sertoli cell function and the production of AMH and inhibin B. Subsequently, during childhood the levels of gonadotropins and androgens fall, leading to a period of physiological hypogonadotropic hypogonadism. During puberty, pulsatile secretion of gonadotropin-releasing hormone (GnRH) occurs first during the night and later throughout the day. Pulsatile GnRH release leads to production of pituitary LH and FSH, which again induce the maturation of the Leydig cells and Sertoli cells. In contrast to the mini-puberty observed during infancy, during true puberty, Sertoli cells express androgen receptors. The androgen receptors allow intratesticular testosterone to promote spermatogenesis. Testosterone as well as inhibin exhibit a negative feedback effect on the pituitary. The hypothalamic-pituitary-testicular axis is illustrated in Fig. 67-2.

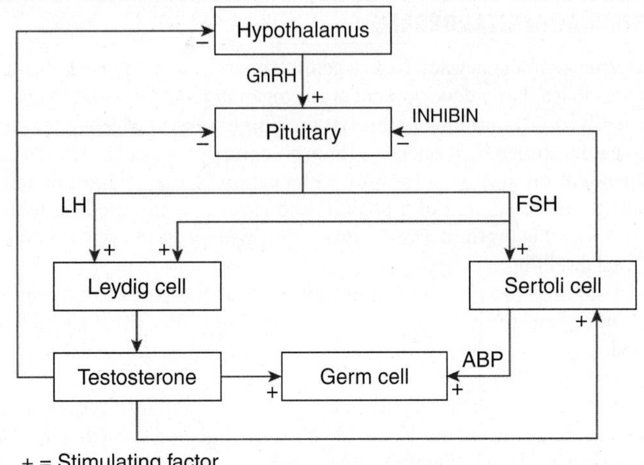


**FIGURE 67-2** The hypothalamic–pituitary–testicular axis. ABP, androgen-binding protein; FSH, follicle-stimulating hormone; GnRH, gonadotrophin-releasing hormone; LH, luteinizing hormone. (Adapted with permission from Fitzgerald PA: *Handbook of Clinical Endocrinology*, 2nd ed. Norwalk: Appleton & Lange; 1992.)

## SUGGESTED READINGS

Aumüller G, Riva A. Morphology and functions of the human seminal vesicle. *Andrologia*. 1992;24(4):183-196.

Chemes HE. Infancy is not a quiescent period of testicular development. *Int J Androl*. 2001;24(1):2-7.

Grinspon RP, Loreti N, Braslavsky D, et al. Sertoli cell markers in the diagnosis of paediatric male hypogonadism. *J Pediatr Endocrinol Metab*. 2012;25(1-2):3-11.

Grinspon RP, Rey RA. Anti-Müllerian hormone and sertoli cell function in paediatric male hypogonadism. *Horm Res Paediatr*. 2010;73(2):81-92.

Hutson JM, Southwell BR, Li R, et al. The regulation of testicular descent and the effects of cryptorchidism. *Endocr Rev*. 2013;5:725-752.

Nistal M, Paniagua R, González-Peramato P, Reyes-Múgica MY. Perspectives in pediatric pathology, chapter 4. Pubertal and adult testis. *Pediatr Dev Pathol*. 2015;18(3):187-202.

Nistal M, Paniagua R, González-Peramato P, Reyes-Múgica MY. Perspectives in pediatric pathology, chapter 3. Testicular development from birth to puberty: systematic evaluation of the prepubertal testis. *Pediatr Dev Pathol*. 2015;18(3):173-186.

Pitteloud N, Dwyer A. Hormonal control of spermatogenesis in men: therapeutic aspects in hypogonadotropic hypogonadism. *Ann Endocrinol (Paris)*. 2014;75(2):98-100.

Rey RA. Mini-puberty and true puberty: differences in testicular function. *Ann Endocrinol (Paris)*. 2014;75(2):58-63.

Rey RA, Grinspon RP, Gottlieb S, et al. Male hypogonadism: an extended classification based on a developmental, endocrine physiology-based approach. *Andrology*. 2013;1(1):3-16.

Tomava A, Deepinder F, Robeva R, Lalabonova H, Kumanov P, Agarwal A. Growth and development of male external genitalia. *Arch Pediatr Adolesc Med*. 2010;164(12):1152-1157.

# 68 Psychological Development

Elizabeth M. Ozer and Charles E. Irwin, Jr.

Psychological, physical, and social-role changes—shaped by social determinants and by other risk and protective factors—affect behavior during adolescence. Adolescence is a time of navigating new social challenges and adjusting to physical, cognitive, and emotional changes. Given the strong association between pubertal maturation and a wide array of social, behavioral, and emotional changes during adolescence, the psychosocial effects and opportunities associated with puberty are first briefly reviewed. This is followed by a discussion of psychological/psychosocial development during the stages of adolescence/young adulthood and, finally, an overview of changes in the social/environmental context during adolescence, with a primary focus on the healthcare system.

## PSYCHOSOCIAL EFFECTS OF PUBERTY

The onset of puberty creates hormonal changes—including dramatic increases in the secretion of adrenal androgens, gonadal steroids, and growth hormone. Androgens have been implicated as related to many of the behavior changes associated with the adolescent period. Increased levels of testosterone in adolescent boys are associated with aggression, risk-taking, and initiation of sexual intercourse; and during peak height velocity, boys tend to experience more conflict with their parents. Likewise, in pubertal girls, rising levels of estradiol are believed to be related to parental conflict, lessened behavioral inhibition, engaging in sexual activity, and increased risk-taking.

Specific psychosocial effects have been correlated with the timing of pubertal maturation. Earlier maturation for girls is associated with greater dissatisfaction with physical characteristics, lower self-esteem, and general unhappiness. Early-developing girls tend to associate with older adolescents. The early-maturing girl shows increased interest in sexuality, early identity crises, and more problem behavior in school with decreased interest in academic activities. Early pubertal maturation in boys is less consistently associated with adverse outcomes and may be advantageous in some respects. However, early puberty in boys has been found to be associated with hostility, aggression, risk-taking behavior, physical victimization, and early sexual intercourse. On the other hand, adolescent boys who perceive themselves to be developing later than their peers may be more prone to negative body image. In general, late-developing adolescents, both male and female, are less prone to risk-taking than those developing on time or early, perhaps because the social environment may provide greater support to later-developing adolescents.

Emerging evidence suggests that puberty and the broader period of adolescent brain development present a unique window of opportunity for social experiences to shape neural systems in enduring ways. Adolescence is a period of significant neural plasticity; thinking and learning transform the brain's physical structure and functional organization. As a result of developmental changes, adolescents experience new attractions, motivations, and desires for novel experiences. The neural changes that underpin the complex developmental processes of adolescence are leading to scientific advances at the nexus of cognitive neuroscience, social neuroscience, and developmental science. This increased understanding holds promise for addressing health risks and problems that emerge in adolescence, including increased rates of accidents and injuries, substance use, risky sexual activity, the onset of mental health disorders, and violence.

## PSYCHOSOCIAL DEVELOPMENT

While adolescence is often characterized as a period of psychological turmoil, most adolescents successfully navigate the important transitions of this period in the life cycle. The growing field of positive youth development has focused on developing personal, environmental, and social assets that enable successful transition from childhood through adolescence and into adulthood. Most adolescents are attached to their families and communities, succeed in school, and traverse their teen/emerging adult years without serious problems.

The adolescent is confronted with a series of psychological changes that, if mastered, allow for optimal functioning as an adult. An understanding of psychological development in adolescence enables the clinician to assess whether psychosocial development of the teenager is normal as well as helps the clinician to be an effective communicator with teenagers. Successful psychological development during adolescence involves developing competence in a number of realms: cognitive, moral, emotional, and social.

1. Cognitive development, or the changes in how adolescents think, reason, and understand, is dramatic. During the stages of adolescence, teenagers evolve from concrete thinkers to becoming able to think abstractly and apply hypothetical concepts (formal operational thinking). These changes are generally not complete until early adulthood. Becoming cognitively competent involves the ability to reason, problem-solve, think abstractly and reflect, and plan for the future.
2. Moral development refers to how adolescents construct right and wrong. Cognitive development helps lay the groundwork for the ability to engage in moral reasoning and prosocial behavior, such as caring for others and helping in the family and community.
3. Emotional development involves the development of a sense of identity, a central task of adolescence. A sense of identity involves an individual's self-concept, or beliefs about himself or herself, and self-esteem, how the individual feels about his or her self-concept.
4. Social development refers to how teens relate to others in their peer group, family, school, work, and community environments.

Normal development of the stages of adolescence and their associated impact on the adolescent and on delivery of health services are presented in Table 68-1.

**TABLE 68-1 NORMAL DEVELOPMENT OF THE STAGES OF ADOLESCENCE AND THEIR ASSOCIATED IMPACT ON THE ADOLESCENT AND ON DELIVERY OF HEALTH SERVICES**

| Characteristics | Impact on Adolescents | Impact on Health Service Delivery |
|---|---|---|
| **Early Adolescence (Ages 10–13 Years)** | | |
| Onset of puberty; becomes concerned with developing body | Major questions concerning normality of physical maturation; often concerned about the stages of sexual development and how the process relates to peers of same gender; occasional masturbation | Important to normalize differences and explain range of normal development |
| Begins to expand social relationships beyond family | Adolescents concentrate on relationships with peers; begin to become more interdependent with parents | Encourage teens to begin to take responsibility for their own health and contact with health professionals, in consultation with parents (eg, part of visit time alone with health provider) |
| Beginning of transition from concrete to abstract thinking; new attractions and desires; socioemotional competencies of self-regulation still developing | Risky attitudes and health behaviors may emerge; opportunity for excitement and motivation | Shift in health provider's focus from anticipatory guidance to parents to risk reduction and prevention education to adolescent; still address most health situations with adolescents in a concrete manner with simple language |
| **Middle Adolescence (Ages 14–16 Years)** | | |
| Pubertal development usually complete, and sexual drives emerge | Explores ability to attract others; sexual experimentation (same and opposite sex) begins; masturbation increases | Provide sexual health screening; establish clinician's office as safe place to ask questions and discuss sexuality |
| Peer group sets behavioral standards, although family values usually persist | Peer group influences engagement in positive and negative health behaviors; peers rather than parents may also offer key support | Important to emphasize role of teen in making good choices and taking responsibility; focus on navigating social relationships and peer pressure |
| Conflicts over independence | Increased assumption of independent action, together with continued need for parental support and guidance; able to discuss and negotiate changes in rules | Increased involvement of teen in setting health-related goals and being clear on how to handle health situations (eg, time to take medication); reinforce adolescents' growing competencies |
| Emergence of abstract thinking with new cognitive competencies | Increased ability to process information, see other perspectives, and reflect; often leads to questioning adult behavior; while adolescent may consider broader range of possibilities/options, may not yet be able to integrate into real life | Important to be clear that individual understands and knows what he or she needs to do regarding health concerns |
| **Late Adolescence/Emerging Adulthood (Ages 17–21 Years)** | | |
| Physical maturation complete; body image and gender role definition clearer | Begins to feel comfortable with relationships and decisions regarding sexuality and preference; individual relationships become more important than peer group | Affirm decisions regarding sexuality and gender |
| Individuals less egocentric and self-centered; better at understanding others' points of view; greater ability to self-reflect and be insightful | More open to questioning regarding their behavior; interdependence with shared power and responsibility and greater reciprocity | Adolescent more able to work with clinician on setting goals and changing behavior; clinicians can help adolescents make better health decisions by involving them in their own health management |
| Idealistic | Idealism may lead to conflict with family or authority figures | May have own/alternative ideas of how to take responsibility for their health; clinicians can help adolescents see that they have a range of options |
| Identity exploration/life roles begin to be defined | People most likely to be exploring options in their lives | Often interested in discussion of life goals; depending on health status (eg, chronic illness), may influence life goals |
| Cognitive development nearing completion | Most are capable of understanding a full range of options for health issues | Important to help adolescents/emerging adults become competent in negotiating the health care system; encourage parents, when appropriate, to decrease their monitoring of clinical management issues, yet remain engaged and available to their son or daughter |

During early adolescence (ages 10–13 years), teens are focused on their developing bodies, the peer group becomes increasingly important with concerns about acceptance and conformity, and individuals start to experiment with new behavior. Teens are transitioning from concrete to abstract thinking, and they have not yet developed the socioemotional competencies of self-regulation. The combination of these characteristics can lead to risky attitudes and behavior.

Middle adolescence (ages 14–16 years) is characterized by the emergence of formal operational thinking with new cognitive competencies such as changes in information processing, perspective taking, and reflection. Adolescents are now able to understand complex concepts, which often leads to a questioning of the thinking and behavior of adults. This is often the time of greatest conflict with parents, especially over independence, as adolescents and their parents are in the process of renegotiating the terms of their relationship as adolescents strive to gain autonomy.

There begins to be a shift from the egocentric world of the early adolescent to the more sociocentric world of the middle and late adolescent. Adolescents may contemplate more abstract concepts related to moral development, such as the law and justice. The ability to think abstractly also allows for reflection in the emotional realm, and focus shifts from same-sex friendships to dating/sexual relationships. While more mature thought processes begin to modulate impulsive behavior, risky health behaviors are of major concern in middle adolescence as peer norms to engage in certain risky behavior (eg, substances, sexual activity) increase and individuals make more independent choices.

Late adolescence has traditionally been defined as ages 17 to 21. A more recent concept in the development of late adolescence/young adults is the theory of emerging adulthood. This focuses on the years from about ages 18 to 25, recognizing those years as distinct from the preceding adolescent years as well as from the young adult years that follow. The phases of late adolescence/emerging adulthood are characterized by identity exploration—a time for exploring possibilities in life in many areas, including love and work. Consistent with this task, there is increased cognitive ability for self-reflection and insight. This is also the time when individuals begin to define a functional role in society. While the new emergence of a sociocentric view of the world with a strong sense of altruism may lead to conflict with family and society around moral and ethical issues rather than the egocentric issues of early adolescence, conflict between adolescents and their parents declines steadily in late adolescence and young adulthood. There is a shift in relationships toward interdependence, with shared power and responsibility, and greater reciprocity. While individuals continue to become less self-centered, late adolescence/emerging adulthood is a self-focused time of life when people often have few obligations to others and substantial autonomy in terms of their lives.

Within the health practice setting, clinicians can support these developmental processes through raising adolescents' awareness of their strengths across developmental realms and encouraging adolescents to take responsibility for the role they can play in their own health and well-being. Clinicians can help adolescents make better health decisions by involving them in their own health management; helping them see that they have a range of options; and encouraging parents, when appropriate, to decrease their monitoring of clinical management issues yet remain engaged and available to their son or daughter. Families play a critical role in successful development during adolescence by facilitating a graduated increase in independence, leading to interdependence and the associated responsibilities. Laying this groundwork becomes especially important in late adolescence/emerging adulthood when teens typically move out of their parents' home and begin to seek their own health care.

## CHANGES IN SOCIAL/ENVIRONMENTAL CONTEXT DURING ADOLESCENCE/YOUNG ADULTHOOD

The social/environmental context undergoes significant changes during adolescence. Middle and high schools are generally less structured and provide less support than elementary schools; work environments for older adolescents provide less supervision than schools and little guidance about career choices; and families provide less supervision and more freedom of choices, which increases the opportunity for initiation of health-risk behavior. At the same time, peers become highly influential in adolescents' health behavior decisions.

The context of health care also changes during adolescence. Access to health insurance for adolescents and young adults has improved markedly since the enactment of the Patient Protection and Affordable Care Act of 2010 (ACA); however, a significant number of young adults (ages 18–25 years) remain uninsured. In addition to expanding access to care, the ACA includes provisions for health services that include reimbursement for clinical preventive services that aim to reduce risky behavior, and reinforce healthy behaviors, strengths, and competencies in adolescents and young adults.

While health care for adolescents (up to 18 years) generally requires consent from a parent or guardian (as with younger children), in recognition of mature adolescents' capacity to understand the risk and benefits of treatment and adolescents' emerging autonomy, there are significant exceptions to the requirement of parental consent, largely governed by state law. Emancipated minors (as defined by living away from home, no longer subject to parental authority, economically self-sufficient, married, or members of the military service) may consent to their own health care. Some states permit all minors, minors above a certain age, or minors who are mature and/or capable of informed consent to give consent for general medical care. The requirement of parental permission is also waived for certain services delivered to adolescents age 12 years and older. In nearly every state, adolescents may receive care without parental permission for diagnosis and treatment of sexually transmitted infections. Also, many states allow adolescents to receive treatment without parental permission for other sensitive issues such as pregnancy, contraception, substance use disorders, and mental health problems treated on an outpatient basis.

Despite legal rights to access to services, adolescents' ability to accept care can be compromised by limits to the confidentiality of their care, with patient privacy an important concern for adolescents and young adults (AYAs). For example, even in situations where AYAs have the legal right to confidential care, when AYAs are covered on their parent's health insurance, the services they use can be exposed by explanation-of-benefits forms routinely sent to private insurance policy holders. Further, the increasing use of electronic medical record (EMR) systems poses threats to confidentiality with features such as automated insurance claim generation, facilitation of clinical information exchange, and online patient/parent access.

AYAs' nearly universal access to and facility with computers, mobile technology, and the Internet—coupled with burgeoning information technologies encompassing social networking tools and mobile and wearable devices—offer numerous options for improving and extending healthcare services, leveraging developmental windows during the AYA years. However, concerns about privacy and youths' ability to distinguish the quality and reliability of electronic information sources and advice suggest the importance of promoting AYA health and media literacy and safety, which could occur during clinical encounters or more broadly through health system–level endorsement of high-quality technology tools.

## SUGGESTED READINGS


An overview of minors' consent laws. Guttmacher Institute Web site. https://www.guttmacher.org/sites/default/files/pdfs/spibs/spib_OMCL.pdf. Published March 1, 2016. Accessed August 1, 2016.

Arnett JJ. A longer road to adulthood. In: *Emerging Adulthood: The Winding Road from the Late Teens Through the Twenties.* 2nd ed. New York, NY: Oxford University Press; 2015:1-29.

Coleman DL, Rosoff PM. The legal authority of mature minors to consent to general medical treatment. *Pediatrics.* 2013;131(4):786-793.

Crone EA, Dahl RE. Understanding adolescence as a period of social–affective engagement and goal flexibility. *Nat Rev Neurosci.* 2012;13(9):636-650.

Hollenstein T, Lougheed JP. Beyond storm and stress: typicality, transactions, timing, and temperament to account for adolescent change. *Am Psychol.* 2013;68(6):444-454.

Laursen B, Collins WA. Parent-child relationships during adolescence. In: Lerner RM, Steinberg L, eds. *Handbook of Adolescent Psychology,* vol 2. Hoboken, NJ: John Wiley & Sons, Inc; 2009:3-42.

Ozer EM, Urquhart JT, Brindis CD, et al. Young adult preventive health care guidelines: there but can't be found. *Arch Pediatr Adolesc Med.* 2012;166(3):240-247.

Peper JS, Dahl RE. Surging hormones: brain-behavior interactions during puberty. *Curr Dir Psychol Sci.* 2013;22(2):134-139.

Society for Adolescent Health and Medicine, American Academy of Pediatrics. Confidentiality protections for adolescents and young adults in the health care billing and insurance claims process. *J Adolesc Health.* 2016;58(3):374-377.

Steinberg L. Cognitive and affective development in adolescents. *Trends Cogn Sci.* 2005;9(2):69-74.


# 69 The Adolescent and Young Adult Visit

Charles E. Irwin, Jr. and Elizabeth M. Ozer

## INTRODUCTION

The pediatrician or child health practitioner has a formidable task in establishing herself or himself as the primary care clinician for an adolescent and young adult patient. A transition interview with patients and their families at approximately 10 years of age is an effective approach for developing a new relationship with the adolescent and the family. During this interview, the clinician must inform the parents and the patient about the changing nature of the relationship with the practitioner—the need for the clinician to have time alone with the patient and query the young person directly, and for the patient to be examined alone and be encouraged to generate his or her own questions for the clinician. These changes are best done through a discussion of normal adolescence and the need for adolescents to begin to make some decisions in a more independent manner with guidance and support from their families. During this transition interview, the clinician may want to provide the adolescent and family with some general information regarding the normal physiological and psychosocial changes of adolescence. Depending on the age and psychosocial functioning of the adolescent, the clinician may want to encourage the young person to come to the next visit alone. As the patient completes the second decade of life, the young adult needs to have developed the skills to assume primary responsibility for his or her own health care. At 18 years of age, young people have the legal right to assume full responsibility for their care even though they will often continue to receive significant emotional and financial support from their family. Given these changes, the clinician will need to have a discussion with the patient and family focusing on clarifying how the young adult wants health information shared with the family.

Confidentiality issues are fundamental to the delivery of health care to adolescents and young adults; they need to be able to seek the necessary care in a timely manner and give a candid and complete heath history when they do so. Some clinicians may feel uncomfortable with these principles and may want to clarify their position with the young person. From the first visit, the clinician must assure the young person of the confidentiality of all information within the confines of the legal system based upon the state or country in which the health care is being delivered. The clinician may need to restate this position on confidentiality during the gathering of information in sensitive areas (eg, gender identity, sexual behavior, substance use). In the areas of life-threatening disease or behavior (eg, suicidal behavior, homicidal intentions, or the management of chronic disease), the clinician always has the right to intervene on behalf of the patient's well-being, which generally involves identifying a parent, guardian, or supportive adult who can assist the young person with the problem.

## THE HISTORY

### The Clinical Interview

It is important to create an environment in which the young person is able to disclose information regarding his or her health habits. History taking should be guided by the developmental stage of adolescence and young adulthood (Table 69-1). The clinician also must recognize that many of the adolescent's or young adult's concerns may not be disclosed on the first visit and may unfold after a relationship has been established. A follow-up visit for a rather minor problem may be the visit at which other health concerns and risky behaviors are disclosed.

### Screening History

The screening history must focus on behavioral risk factors given that most of the morbidity and mortality during adolescence and young adulthood is related to risk-taking behaviors (eg, substance use, sexuality, recreational/motor vehicle use) and their associated risk factors; depression and its equivalents; and dietary intake. The clinician must distinguish between risk-taking behaviors that are developmentally adaptive, although often dangerous, and those that are pathologic. Using a biospychosocial model to screen enables the clinician to get a general assessment of the health and well-being of the adolescent and young adult. The Home, Education (or Employment), Eating, Activities, Drugs, Sexuality, Suicidality, Strengths (HEEADSSS) assessment tool is based on the biopsychosocial model (Table 69-1). This screening allows clinicians to assess the patient's well-being in a variety of domains. Over the past decade, there has been an increased emphasis on strength-based care, which encourages clinicians to ask about assets and the positive aspects of their patients' lives. This new paradigm is embedded in the last S of the HEEADSSS assessment.

**TABLE 69-1 HEEADSSS ASSESSMENT FOR PSYCHOSOCIAL CONCERNS: SCREENING HISTORY**

| Assessment Area | Questions |
|---|---|
| Home | How is the adolescent's home life? How are his/her relationships with family members? Where and with whom does the patient live? Is his/her living situation stable? |
| Education (or employment) | How is the adolescent's school performance? How is she/he doing in school? If adolescent is working, is he/she working full time or part time and what are his/her plans for the future? |
| Eating (incorporates body image) | Does the patient have a balanced diet? Is the adolescent trying to lose weight, and if so, is it in a healthy manner? How does the patient feel about his/her body? Has there been significant weight gain or loss recently? |
| Activities | How does the patient spend her/his time? Is he/she engaged in sports or other extracurricular activities? Is he/she engaging in dangerous or risky behaviors? Is the adolescent supervised during free time? With whom does the adolescent spend most of his/her time? Does he/she have a supportive peer group? |
| Drugs (including alcohol and tobacco) | Does the patient drink caffeinated beverages (including energy drinks)? Does the patient smoke or use electronic nicotine devices? Does the patient drink alcohol? If so, explore amount including frequency and context. Has the patient used other substances, including marijuana, over-the-counter drugs, or opioids? If there is any substance use, to what degree, and for how long? Consider using a screening tool (eg CRAFFT) if the patient endorses substance use to establish the severity. |
| Suicidality (including general mood assessment) | What is the patient's mood from day to day? Has he/she thought about or attempted suicide? Consider using the Patient Health Questionnaire-2 (PHQ-2) as a screening tool and advance to the Patient Health Questionnaire-9 (PHQ-9) for further assessment. |
| Strengths | Inquire about assets. What does the patient enjoy doing? What are the patient's life goals? |
| Sexuality | What is the patient's current gender identity? Is the patient attracted to males, females, or both? What is the patient's sexual orientation (heterosexual, homosexual, bisexual, or other)? Has the patient ever been sexually active and if so, with males, females, or both? Has the patient ever been tested for sexually transmitted infections? Is the patient using any contraception? Has the patient ever been pregnant or gotten someone pregnant? Has the patient ever been forced into having sex? Does the patient's family know about the patient's gender identity and sexual behavior? |

In addition to a detailed history, adolescents and young adults should have a comprehensive physical examination annually. Physical developmental progression during adolescence, including assessment of Tanner and Marshall sexual maturity rating (SMR), should be noted.

Behaviors that reflect possible involvement in risk behaviors include problems in family and peer relationships, a decrement in school functioning, legal problems, and behavioral problems reflective of substance use. Behaviors related to substance use may include unusual or dramatic mood swings, changes in personal habits, runaway behavior, depressive symptoms, and preoccupation with generating money. In addition to asking about risk behaviors, the clinician should query the adolescent and young adult about general mood and dietary behaviors. A 24-hour recall of dietary intake provides a general assessment of nutrient and caloric intake. Because many youth engage in risk behaviors, the clinician needs to have a brief office intervention for those engaging in such behaviors. One popular intervention based on the transtheoretical model developed by the National Cancer Institute is the 5 A's approach: asking, advising, assessing the willingness to change, assisting in behavior change, and arranging for follow-up (Table 69-2).

### Medical History

The critical components of the medical history include the current concern or presenting complaint of the young person and the family.

**TABLE 69-2 THE 5 A'S FOR BRIEF OFFICE-BASED INTERVENTIONS**

| | |
|---|---|
| Ask | Determine the presence of the behavior. |
| Advise | Deliver a clear, personalized message about the need to change the behavior. |
| Assess willingness to change | Determine whether the adolescent is prepared to change his or her behavior. |
| Assist the behavior change | Determine short-term, concrete actions to make the behavior change; set behavioral goals. Provide adjunct therapy as appropriate (eg, nicotine replacement for tobacco cessation). |
| Arrange follow-up | Schedule a follow-up visit or phone call soon after the date set for the behavior change, ideally within 1 week. |

Data from Manley M, Epps RP, Husten C, et al. Clinical intervention in tobacco control. A National Cancer Institute training project for physicians, *JAMA*. 1991 Dec 11;266(22): 3172-3173.

It is often beneficial to have both the parent and the adolescent in the room at the initiation of the appointment to gather the concerns of both because they may differ; the clinician wants to make certain that both are addressed during the visit. Past medical history, including family history, is often best gathered from both the parent and the adolescent through a questionnaire prior to or at the visit. Review of systems should be done in a targeted manner with specific questions about each system, especially during early adolescence, because of the increased somatization due to changes in the young person's body during this period of time.

## PHYSICAL ASSESSMENT

The extent to which each organ system is evaluated depends on whether the young person is coming for the annual well visit or for a specific complaint. The annual well visit is an opportunity for the clinician to assess growth and pubertal development during adolescence and instruct the young person in self-examination if indicated. Features related to risk behaviors (eg, substance use, sexuality, motor/recreational vehicle use) are outlined in Table 69-3. The following section identifies areas of the general adolescent and young adult examination that differ from that for the child. Parents of adolescents should be informed that the examination will include an examination of the genitalia with discussion of the SMR. The SMR is helpful in assessing some physical (eg, peak height velocity, menarche, changes in body habitus) and laboratory parameters (eg, BMI, hemoglobin).

### General Appearance

Particular attention should be directed to body posture, eye contact, dress, affect, mood, and energy level. Changes in body mass index may indicate the onset of a chronic medical disease, an eating disorder, depression, or substance abuse.

### Skin

Distribution of acne, hair, striae, ecchymoses, "needle tracks," and scars should be noted. The pubertal changes should be correlated with the appropriate stages of the SMR (see Chapter 65). Striae are common in areas of rapid growth, especially where subcutaneous fat is increasing (hips, breasts, buttocks, and lower abdomen). Check for warts, fungal infections, and exposure to excessive sun. Longitudinal scars on wrists may indicate suicide gestures or attempts or cutting behavior. Major scars or ecchymoses may indicate a history of unintentional injuries.

### Eyes

Visual acuity commonly changes, and astigmatism can appear during adolescence. If the adolescent cannot identify more than half the letters on the 20/40 line of the Snellen chart, a referral to an ophthalmologist or optometrist is indicated. Conjunctival injection and alterations in pupil reactivity may indicate substance use.

### Ears

Hearing is best checked by a pure-tone audiogram in early adolescence. The most common problem is high-tone sensorineural defects that may be related to listening to highly amplified music.

**TABLE 69-3 FINDINGS ASSOCIATED WITH RISK BEHAVIORS**

| |
|---|
| **Recreational/Motor Vehicle Use** |
| Skin |
| Abrasions |
| Ecchymoses |
| Lacerations |
| Musculoskeletal—fractures, sprains (acute and chronic) |
| **Sexual Activity** |
| Reproductive skin rash consistent with disease process |
| Adenopathy |
| Amenorrhea |
| Genital lesions |
| Vaginal/penile discharge |
| Cervical discharge, edema, friability |
| Uterine/adnexal tenderness |
| Enlarged uterus (pregnant) |
| **Substance Use** |
| General |
| Agitation, anxiety |
| Decreased general functional status—sleep disturbances, anorexia |
| Infection with HIV, hepatitis B, other STIs |
| Skin |
| Multiple bruises |
| Track marks |
| Abscesses |
| Central nervous system/mental status |
| Altered mental status |
| Decreased short-term memory |
| Decreased motivation |
| Decreased fine-motor movements |
| Diminished coordination |
| Head, eyes, ears, nose, oropharynx |
| Injected conjunctivae |
| Chronic nasal discharge, nasal mucosal irritation |
| Recurrent nosebleeds |
| Leukoplakia, gingival recession, dental caries |
| Mucosal inflammation (nasal passages, oropharynx) |
| Malodorous breath |
| Breast |
| Gynecomastia (males) |
| Cardiorespiratory |
| Tachycardia |
| Hypertension |
| Evidence of deconditioning |
| Chronic cough, recurrent bronchitis |
| Gastrointestinal |
| Abdominal pain and dyspepsia |
| Weight loss |
| Liver tenderness or enlargement |
| Musculoskeletal |
| Poor muscle tone/strength |

HIV, human immunodeficiency virus; STI, sexually transmitted infection.

### Nose

Constant erythema, trauma of the nose, or epistaxis may indicate substance use by inhalation. Trauma may also lead to a deviated septum.

### Teeth and Gums

Check for evidence of dental caries and gum infections. Look for signs of smokeless tobacco use. Enamel erosions may indicate the first sign of self-induced vomiting associated with some eating disorders.

Malocclusion occurs in approximately 50% of adolescents. Referral for dental services is often indicated.

#### Glands

Lymph nodes are generally palpable in the cervical, axillary, and inguinal areas. Lymph nodes greater than 1 cm and those that persist longer than 2 to 3 weeks should be investigated for infection or malignancy. Common infections associated with lymph node enlargement include infectious mononucleosis, pharyngitis, vaginitis, salpingitis, urethritis, and prostatitis.

#### Breasts

Examination of the breasts should be done for both males and females. In girls, assess SMR, symmetry, masses, and discharge. In boys, identify gynecomastia, a common finding in males beginning at SMR 2 in up to a third of males. Gynecomastia usually does not persist beyond SMR 4. Teaching self-breast examination is not critical during adolescence. Chapter 77 discusses breast abnormalities found during adolescence.

#### Cardiovascular System

The examination of the cardiovascular system is standard. Precordial activity may be somewhat increased because of a hyperdynamic state secondary to anemia, anxiety, pregnancy, or substance use. Congenital cardiac abnormalities will usually be diagnosed before adolescence. Prolapsed mitral valve and lesions secondary to rheumatic fever may first be diagnosed during adolescence. Increases in blood pressure are often secondary to anxiety or substance use. A re-check is often indicated during the visit.

#### Abdomen

Check for evidence of enlargement of the spleen, liver tenderness, and masses throughout the abdomen.

#### Rectal Examination

Rectal examinations of the adolescent are indicated with symptomatic genitourinary and gastrointestinal complaints including a history of receptive anal coitus.

#### Musculoskeletal System

Examination of the spine is undertaken to exclude scoliosis, especially in adolescents at SMR 2 to 3 (see Chapter 213). Check for overuse syndromes or osteochondroses. Muscle strength and joint flexibility should be checked.

#### Genitalia Examination

The examination of the male and female genitalia is a critical part of the examination for the adolescent. Males and females should have their genitalia inspected for normal development and SMR staging. The external examination of both males and females should include inspection for erythema, ulcerations, and discharge. See Chapters 79 and 228 for further discussion of assessment. Males who are uncircumcised should be assessed to see if their foreskin can be pulled back completely by the patient himself at SMR 5. Even though the US Preventive Services Task Force does not recommend teaching of self testicular examination for identification of testicular cancer, clinicians may find it a good tool for educating males about normal anatomical changes. Scrotal and testicular masses are discussed in Chapter 78. Pelvic examinations are indicated only if the patient presents with genitourinary or gastrointestinal symptoms that require the examination to establish a diagnosis. Cervical cancer screening (Pap) is only recommended for females starting at age 21 except in females with human immunodeficiency virus (HIV) or other immune deficiency.

#### Mental Status

Reading ability, comprehension, writing skills, and cognitive ability should be evaluated. Higher cognitive functioning may be measured through tasks that require sequencing, memory, spatial relationships, and organizational skills. Marked alterations in mood and energy are not consistent with normal adolescence. If the adolescent appears to have marked mood swings, the clinician must consider psychopathology, including substance use.

## LABORATORY SCREENING TESTS

All screening tests in adolescents and young adults are done based on risk assessment. There are no tests that are routine for adolescents and young adults at this point with the exception of Pap smears, which are recommended every 3 years beginning at 21 years.

#### Testing for Tuberculosis Infection

The purified protein derivative (PPD) skin test for tuberculosis (TB) is the most accessible screening test for TB. PPD should be considered based upon the risk factors of the patient, recommendations by the local/regional health department, or school/job requirements.

#### Complete Blood Count

Hematocrit or hemoglobin are the only components of the complete blood count (CBC) that should be considered if the patient has nutritional inadequacies associated with food insecurity, vegetarian/vegan diets, and disordered eating.

#### Metabolic Testing

Metabolic testing includes a lipid profile, diabetes screening, and liver enzymes. Patients who are overweight or obese should be screened. Other indications for screening include family history of cardiovascular disease, hyperlipidemia, hypertension, stroke, or diabetes; and history of hypertension, diabetes, or hyperlipidemia.

#### Sexually Transmitted Infections Screening

All sexually active adolescents should be screened annually for *Chlamydia trachomatis*. *Neisseria gonorrhea* screening is based on risk factors and local prevalence. All sexually active patients should be offered screening for HIV. If the patient has a history of a sexually transmitted infection (STI), he or she should be encouraged to have HIV testing.

#### Substance Use Screening

The role of substance use screening for comatose or combative youth in the emergency setting and with the onset of psychiatric symptoms is clear. There is considerable controversy regarding screening to confirm a suspicion of substance use in the routine office visit. There is little to be gained by screening adolescents who use substances unless they are engaged in a treatment program. Considerable problems exist with the sensitivity and specificity of urine screening for substance use. Testing indicates the presence or absence of use in the preceding few days and does not provide information about frequency, intensity, or chronicity of use. Ethical and legal issues must be addressed in obtaining the adolescent's consent in a nonemergency situation. Drug testing to confirm a history also conveys a message to the patient: The clinician does not believe the history. This statement may interfere with development of a long-term therapeutic relationship with the adolescent.

## IMMUNIZATIONS

There have been several recent changes in immunization schedules, and new vaccines have been developed that target adolescents and young adults. These factors make the adolescent and young adult period a crucial time for "catching up" on vaccines that were started and not finished and for consideration of the new adolescent and young adult–specific vaccines. It is recommended that clinicians refer to the Centers for Disease Control and Prevention Advisory Committee for Immunization Practices for recent updates on recommendations.

## PREVENTION

Over the past decade, a series of recommendations have been developed and modified (*Guidelines for Adolescent Preventive Services*, Bright Futures guidelines, and US Preventive Services Task Force recommendations) for preventive services and screening during adolescence. In Table 69-4, the recommendations for adolescence

**TABLE 69-4 US PREVENTIVE SERVICES TASK FORCE (USPSTF) A OR B RECOMMENDATIONS FOR ADOLESCENTS AND YOUNG ADULTS**

| Preventive Services | Recommendations for: Adolescents | Young Adults | Risk Factors and Other Notes |
|---|---|---|---|
| **Substance Use** | | | |
| Alcohol screening and counseling | | ✓ | |
| Tobacco education and brief counseling | ✓ | | |
| Tobacco screening and cessation help | | ✓ | |
| **Reproductive Health** | | | |
| HIV | + | ✓ | Test if <15 years at increased risk; everyone aged 15–65 |
| Syphilis | + | + | Anyone at increased risk |
| Chlamydia (females) | + | + | Test if ≤24 years and sexually active |
| Gonorrhea (females) | + | + | Test if ≤24 years and sexually active |
| STI (screening and counseling) | + | + | High-intensity counseling interventions |
| Cervical cancer screening | | ✓ | Test if ≥21 years |
| **Mental Health** | | | |
| Depression (screening and treatment) | ✓ | ✓ | Everyone ≥12 years when there are adequate systems in place to ensure accurate diagnosis, effective treatment, and follow-up |
| **Nutrition and Exercise** | | | |
| Lipid disorder | | + | Test if ≥20 with increased risk for coronary artery disease |
| Obesity/BMI screening and referral | ✓ | ✓ | |
| Hypertension | | ✓ | Test if ≥18 years |
| Healthy diet | | + | Anyone who is obese/overweight and has additional risk factors |
| **Safety/Violence** | | | |
| Intimate partner violence | ✓ | ✓ | Screen women of childbearing age |

✓ = All adolescents and/or young adults

+ = Applicable for those at risk

Guidelines as of 03/2016; subject to change.

For more information, visit the USPSTF Web site at http://www.uspreventiveservicestaskforce.org/.

**Additional Resources**: Adolescent and Young Adult Health National Resource Center. Summary of Recommended Guidelines for Clinical Preventive Services for Adolescents up to Age 18. 2016. http://nahic.ucsf.edu/wp-content/uploads/2016/04/Screening-Guidelines-4.26.16-ADOLS.pdf.

Adolescent and Young Adult Health National Resource Center. Summary of Recommended Guidelines for Clinical Preventive Services for Young Adults Ages 18-25. 2016. http://nahic.ucsf.edu/wp-content/uploads/2016/04/Screening-Guidelines-YA-4.26.16.pdf.

Data from USPSTF A and B Recommendations. U.S. Preventive Services Task Force. April 2017.

and young adulthood are highlighted. Many of the recommendations focus on health-promoting and health-damaging behaviors initiated during early adolescence. Sexual behavior, substance use, and vehicle use are often initiated during adolescence and continue to account for the major causes of morbidity and mortality through the fourth decade of life. Because intention to engage in a behavior is one of the most powerful predictors of initiation of a behavior, simple questions regarding intention should be a routine part of each clinical encounter beginning in late childhood. The identification of 1 risk behavior should alert the clinician to inquire about other risk behaviors. In addition, the clinician should query every adolescent about depressive symptomatology, eating behaviors, school functioning, and family interaction.

## SUGGESTED READINGS


Bonnie RJ, Stroud C, Breiner H, eds; Institute of Medicine; National Research Council. *Investing in the Health and Well-Being of Young Adults*. - Washington, DC: National Academy Press; 2015.

Committee on Adolescent Health Care Services and Models of Care for Treatment, Prevention, and Healthy Development. *Adolescent Health Services: Missing Opportunities*. Washington, DC: National Academies Press, 2009. http://www.ncbi.nlm.nih.gov/books/NBK215415/. Accessed February 9, 2017.

Neinstein LS, ed. *Neinstein's Adolescent and Young Adult Health Care: A Practical Guide*. 6th ed. Philadelphia, PA: Wolters Kluwer; 2016.

Patton GC, Sawyer SM, Santelli JS, et al. Our future: a Lancet commission on adolescent health and wellbeing. *Lancet*. 2016;387(10036):9-65.

US Preventive Services Task Force Web site. www.uspreventiveservicestaskforce.org/. Accessed September 2, 2016.


# 70 Healthcare Transition from Pediatric to Adult-Based Care for Youth and Young Adults with Special Healthcare Needs

Constance M. Wiemann, Albert C. Hergenroeder, and Beth H. Garland

Approximately 1 in 5 US families has a 6- to 21-year-old with a chronic illness. With advances in medicine that have improved the outcome for children with chronic illnesses, 90% of youth with special healthcare needs of a physical nature will enter adulthood, numbering one-half million annually. In addition to physical conditions, there are an estimated 600,000 16- to 17-year-olds in the United States with a serious mental illness. In fact, a number of chronic and severe mental health diagnoses (eg, schizophrenia, anxiety, eating disorders) present most often during this transition age period.

Healthcare transition (HCT) is defined as the purposeful planned movement of adolescents and young adults with chronic conditions from child-centered to adult-oriented healthcare systems. The American Academy of Pediatrics 2002 consensus statement identified multiple deficiencies in HCT, including youth and young adults with special healthcare needs (YYASHCN) not prepared for HCT; pediatric healthcare providers not prepared to assist in transition readiness for YYASHCN and their families; an adult healthcare system not adequately prepared to receive young adults with special healthcare needs; and inadequate communication between the subspecialty and medical home providers. As a result, increased morbidity and mortality have been reported in the post-transition period if the transition is poorly managed; those with complex conditions and neurocognitive disabilities tend to do worse. A single-center longitudinal cohort of children with sickle cell disease with 940 participants followed for 8857 patient-years demonstrated that the majority of deaths occurred after 18 years of age and transfer to adult care, with a mean of 1.2 years to death after transfer. In a group of adolescents and young adults with moderate to complex congenital heart disease, lapses in care of ≥2 years between the last pediatric and the first adult congenital heart disease visit occurred in 63% of patients, and were associated with a new, hemodynamically significant diagnosis at the time of their first adult congenital heart disease clinic visit. Moreover, increased morbidity and emergency department use as a result of foregone care during the transition from pediatric to adult healthcare have likely contributed to increased healthcare costs. These data indicate that HCT represents both a vulnerable period and clear opportunity to alter the trajectory of health outcomes.

Despite increased attention to the importance of HCT from pediatric to adult-based care, including the recognition by numerous professional medical organizations (eg, American Heart Association, American Academy of Pediatrics, American Diabetes Association) as to the need for comprehensive transition planning, progress in addressing these barriers has been slow and a strong evidence base is lacking. This chapter provides guidelines on how to initiate transition planning and how to build a transition planning program for YYASHCN. (Chapter 124 addresses HCT for medically complex patients, including those with a developmental disability.)

## THE TRANSITION PROCESS

It is helpful to think of HCT as occurring in three phases: transition preparation, active transfer between pediatric and adult healthcare systems, and engagement of the YYASHCN on the adult side. During *transition preparation*, often the longest phase, YYASHCN learn how to manage their disease and advocate for themselves both in and out of the healthcare system. During *active transfer between pediatric and adult healthcare systems*, YYASHCN make and keep a first appointment with an adult provider. YYASHCN are considered to have *engaged on the adult side* once they have attended more than one appointment with the same adult provider.

### Barriers to Successful Healthcare Transition

Numerous studies have identified barriers to successful HCT from the perspective of YYASHCN, caregivers, and pediatric and adult providers, as well as healthcare system-level factors. These are summarized in Table 70-1.

**TABLE 70-1 BARRIERS TO SUCCESSFUL HEALTHCARE TRANSITION**

**Youth and Young Adults**

- Are not adequately prepared to transition to adult-based care; many lack disease-specific knowledge as well as self-management and self-advocacy skills
- Are fearful about establishing relationships with new medical providers and bringing a new team "up to speed" on their illness
- Have difficulty finding an adult provider who is knowledgeable about their condition and willing to accept young adults with a childhood-onset disease
- View adult providers and the adult healthcare system as cold and uncaring

**Caregivers/Families**

- Resist leaving the pediatric setting and healthcare providers they have grown to trust, and are fearful that their child is being "kicked out" of pediatric care
- Often do not have a transition roadmap to follow and do not know what to expect from the adult healthcare system

**Pediatric Providers**

- Lack confidence in the ability of their adult colleagues to care for patients with conditions that originate in childhood
- Do not want to let go of patients they have cared for over many years
- Are not prepared to teach YYASHCN the skills needed to successfully engage in adult care
- Often report not being able to find adult providers to take their patients

**Adult Providers**

- Report young adult patients lack knowledge of their own chronic condition, lack self-efficacy about disease management, and lack an understanding of the adult healthcare system
- Are not comfortable treating childhood-onset chronic conditions
- May not be prepared to manage a young adult's viewpoint (eg, ambivalence to change) or style of disease management (eg, texting appointment reminders) or grapple with the management of a variety of changes during this time period (eg, YYASHCN's dating, peer, or educational struggles)

**System-Level**

- Gaps in care due to changes in health insurance as youth age into adulthood
- Inadequate communication between pediatric and adult providers and between primary care and subspecialist providers
- Once youth can legally consent for treatment (often at age 18), the caregiver role in transition is poorly defined

### Transition Preparation

For some YYASHCN and families, the expectation that youth will live into adulthood is new and requires a difficult adjustment at first. Realization that their pediatrician will no longer be their doctor and that they must navigate a new set of medical providers within a new system of health care can feel overwhelming. Many families express concern that they are being forced to leave a familiar and supportive healthcare system before being adequately prepared. Youth may also experience increased anxiety or depressive symptoms related to transition and to general development and changes during the transition to adulthood.

HCT is a partnership among providers, YYASHCN, and caregivers that ideally results in improvements in patient satisfaction, continuity of care, and adherence to care. Moreover, successful HCT is associated with maintenance of health after the transition, improved self-sufficiency and independence, prevention of secondary conditions related to forgone care and their associated costs, and decreased emergency department use. The best outcomes are more likely to occur when transition planning is purposeful and unfolds over a period of time.

HCT preparation is individualized in that one size does not fit all, with movement from one phase to the next depending on when the individual youth is developmentally ready, has stable disease, and is able to identify methods to pay for medical care. At times, HCT is precipitated by a major life event like attending college away from home or an unintended pregnancy.

**When Should Transition Planning Begin?** Young adults who have transitioned out of pediatric care often report wishing they had started having discussions with their pediatrician or primary care provider about transition planning at an earlier age. The AAP recommends initiating discussions about transition planning at age 14 years. Discussions should begin at least 2 years prior to the projected transfer out of pediatric care to give youth time to learn new healthcare management skills, and earlier for youth who are cognitively or developmentally delayed (see Chapter 124). In addition, for youth who will require adult providers from more than one subspecialty (eg, nephrologist and rheumatologist), it is best to stagger these individual transfers over a period of time.

**Shifting Responsibility** In the case of typical development and no severe cognitive impairment, family members or caregivers must learn to gradually shift responsibility for disease management to the young person. At each visit, there should be an opportunity for the provider to meet with the youth alone, without family members present. This can be facilitated by explaining to families that part of the youth taking on increasing responsibility for their health care includes being able to talk about their health to care providers by themselves. Families want a written transition plan or roadmap with tasks to be completed and timelines. This can help reduce the anxiety that occurs among some parents who are accustomed to directing their youth's health care, and also enables them to support the efforts of their YYASHCN.

**Improving Knowledge and Skills** The goal of transition planning is to ensure that patients have the knowledge and skills needed to manage their disease and advocate for their own health in the adult healthcare setting. Basic differences between pediatric and adult healthcare systems drive many of the skills that YYASHCN must learn in order to successfully engage on the adult side, where they will be making and keeping appointments, monitoring their own health, paying for their medical care, and possibly going to multiple doctors for their healthcare needs (Table 70-2).

Youth define successful transition as gradually assuming responsibility for self-management of their disease and having good quality of life on the adult side. Cultural beliefs about health and wellness should be taken into consideration. Essential healthcare self-management skills include scheduling appointments with healthcare providers, and therefore knowing which provider they are going to see and when; knowing what medication they are taking, why they are taking it, and when and how they take it; keeping records of medical appointments and outcomes, including bills; taking increasing responsibility for making medical decisions; being knowledgeable about their health condition and how it impacts them and the people around them; and being knowledgeable about insurance options. Table 70-3 contains a list of potential transition planning questions that may be asked by physicians or other healthcare providers to foster HCT discussions during the clinical encounter. It is helpful to use transition checklists and create customized, focused action plans and timelines for completion of all items.

Transition planning may also encompass skills related to broader psychosocial functioning and is important for youth with comorbid psychological diagnoses or high-risk behavior. Models of transition in mental health care focus on daily living needs and developmental milestones (eg, housing, education, employment) as well as education about mental health diagnosis, medication management, and accessibility of care. While a healthcare provider may not need or be able to address all of these areas, it is important to be aware how they all interact and recognize the need to partner with behavioral health specialists and social work.

Greater healthcare self-management skills promote greater self-confidence in managing one's disease, which has been associated with greater success in healthcare management on the adult side. Youth want to be part of the process and want providers who will listen and be sensitive to their needs. Encourage youth to practice advocacy skills by scheduling their own appointments and requesting medication refills. It may be helpful to have a care notebook that contains information about all doctors and specialists that provide medical and behavioral health care, and includes medical history, disability information, and important past records. One of the most important documents to help plan the transition process is a portable medical summary, which contains, at a minimum: (1) diagnosis, (2) problem list, (3) current medications, (4) doctors' names and phone numbers, (5) names and contact information for people who can help in the event of an emergency, (6) past surgeries, and (7) the most important laboratory results.

**TABLE 70-2 MAJOR DIFFERENCES BETWEEN PEDIATRIC AND ADULT HEALTHCARE SYSTEMS**

| Pediatric Health Care | Adult Health Care |
|---|---|
| One doctor or clinic provides almost all medical care related to the chronic illness | Different doctors for different healthcare needs |
| Warm, informal, and relaxed setting | Business-like, more formal setting |
| Scheduling is more flexible | Advanced planning for appointments required |
| Parents often schedule appointments | Patient schedules appointments |
| Patient is legally a minor | Patient is legally an adult |
| Family manages health needs | Patient monitors health and manages health needs |
| Family centered | Patient centered |
| Parents are responsible for paying for appointment; parents have insurance | Patient is responsible for paying for appointment; adult has own insurance |
| Support services are offered for financial and emotional issues | Patient must seek support for financial and emotional issues |

**TABLE 70-3 TRANSITION PREPARATION QUESTIONS TO HELP PATIENTS PREPARE TO TRANSITION FROM PEDIATRIC TO ADULT HEALTH CARE**

1. Tell me about your diagnosis and how it affects your body and your day-to-day life.
2. Tell me what signs you need to be aware of that indicate you are approaching an emergency situation with your diagnosis. How can you avoid the emergency? When do you call the doctor or go to the emergency room?
3. What number do you call in an emergency? Who are your doctors and how do you contact them? Do you have an ICE contact in your cell phone?
4. How do you schedule your doctor appointments?
5. Did you meet with your doctor without your parent and ask a question today?
6. What are the names of your medications? What are they for? When do you take them? How much do you take? Are there any foods, beverages, or other medications you should avoid when taking your prescriptions?
7. Do you take your medications and treatments by yourself?
8. What is the danger of mixing your medications with alcohol or drugs not prescribed by your doctor?
9. How do you fill and refill your prescriptions?
10. What questions do you have about sex and birth control?
11. What are the names of your medical/dental/vision insurance companies? Do you know your insurance identification numbers? Do you know the phone numbers for your insurance companies?
12. Will your current insurance benefits continue as you transfer to adult-based health care? If not, how will you get insurance?
13. When you transfer to adult-based health care, do you know who your doctor is going to be? If not, do you know how to find a doctor?

Health literacy, or the ability to obtain, process, and understand basic health information and services needed to make appropriate health decisions and follow instructions for treatment, is essential for YYASHCN in order to be able to manage their own health condition. Being able to ask questions is necessary to having healthy behaviors and is the key to informed decision-making. Youth want their pediatric doctors to talk to them, not their parents, and to ask about their opinions for their care. They should be encouraged to write questions down before each clinic visit. Good health and access to care depend largely on whether a patient can understand and remember the health information received.

**Motivational Interviewing and Transition Preparation** Equally important to the content delivered to the youth is the *process* by which the information is given. A youth's readiness and engagement help to determine if they are open to a provider's advice and education. Providers are encouraged to formally engage youth and young adults in this process. When the youth has some ownership of their plan, it increases the likelihood that they will follow through on the plan. Motivational interviewing has demonstrated efficacy for behavioral and lifestyle changes (eg, decreasing risk behaviors, exercise and diet changes, treatment adherence, making and keeping follow-up appointments), and suggests by its spirit of intervention that a healthcare provider *partners* with her/his patient for change, has general *acceptance* of the adolescent, demonstrates *compassion*, and *evokes* change talk from within the adolescent to increase the likelihood that change toward transition happens. Motivational interviewing or other forms of health behavior counseling promote a patient-centered approach by utilizing the young adult's motivation and reasons for continued positive health outcomes and supporting a model for youth engagement with medical providers.

**TABLE 70-4 NON–DISEASE-SPECIFIC HEALTHCARE TRANSITION READINESS, TRANSFER, AND SATISFACTION ASSESSMENTS**

| Tool | Completed By | Number of Items | Target Measures |
|---|---|---|---|
| **Readiness Assessments** | | | |
| Got Transition Readiness Assessment | Self-administered by patient and/or caregiver | Patient version: 24<br>Parent version: 27 | Transition importance, confidence, knowledge, and skills |
| Adolescent Assessment of Preparation for Transition (ADAPT) | Self-administered by patient | 26 | Quality of care received in (1) counseling on transition self-management; (2) counseling on prescription medication; and (3) transfer planning |
| Transition Readiness Assessment Questionnaire (TRAQ) | Self-administered by patient and/or caregiver | 20 | Skills |
| TRxANSITION Scale | Provider interviews patient and/or parent and scores responses | 32 | Knowledge and skills |
| STARx Questionnaire | Self-administered by patient and/or caregiver | 18 | Knowledge and skills |
| Am I ON TRAC? for Adult Care Questionnaire | Self-administered by patient and/or caregiver | 25 | Knowledge and behaviors |
| Transition-Q | Self-administered by patient | 14 | Skills |
| Self-Management Skills Assessment Guide | Self-administered by patient and/or caregiver | 21 | Healthcare awareness and decision-making |
| **Transfer Experience/Satisfaction Assessments** | | | |
| On Your Own Feet Transfer Experiences Scale | Self-administered by patient | 18 | Experience and satisfaction |
| Got Transition Health Care Transition Feedback Survey | Self-administered by patient and/or caregiver | 18 | Experience |

**HCT Resources** The volume and breadth of resources to evaluate and facilitate HCT preparation and readiness has grown substantially in recent years. An excellent resource for HCT materials and guidelines is Got Transition/Center for Health Care Transition Improvement (http://www.gottransition.org/). The overall aim of the center is to improve transition from pediatric to adult health care through the use of new and innovative strategies for health professionals and youth and families. In addition, Table 70-4 contains a list of peer-reviewed, published, HCT-related assessment tools that can be administered in the clinical setting.

**Active Transfer between Pediatric and Adult Healthcare Systems**

During this phase of transition, YYASHCN make and keep a first appointment with an adult provider. To reduce the risk of diminished health status during the transfer process, it is important to minimize the gap in time between the recommended and actual follow-up appointment with the adult provider. Youth are much more likely to make an appointment with an adult provider if they have been given specific contact information. Moreover, knowing which adult provider the youth is planning to see will facilitate future communication between pediatric and adult practices. Pediatric providers report that the lack of qualified adult healthcare providers to transition YYASHCN to is a barrier to HCT. There is not adequate capacity on the adult side; however, not having adult providers to refer to does not preclude the responsibility to do HCT planning. Pediatric providers should seek to establish relationships with adult providers who are willing to accept patients into their practice. Having a list of these adult providers to give to the patient/family with contact information can facilitate the patient and family taking an active role in planning their adult-based health care.

**Meeting an Adult Provider** Young adults who have an opportunity to meet an adult provider before transitioning out of pediatric care are more likely to successfully transfer to adult-based care. There are several models for facilitating this. Some practices instruct the YYASHCN to make an appointment with an adult provider, with a follow-up appointment in the pediatric practice before transitioning to the adult practice permanently. Some models support a period of planned parallel care, whereas others invite adult providers into the pediatric practice to meet patients while they are still under pediatric care. The latter is evidence-based to improve HCT. In most models, the patient initiates contact to make an appointment, although some pediatric providers send referrals directly to adult providers who then contact the patient to make her/his first appointment.

**Connecting Pediatric and Adult Healthcare Systems** Communication between pediatric and adult providers and a feedback loop that indicates the YYASHCN has kept a first appointment are ideal, but occur rarely. Routinely communicating with receiving care teams before and during the transfer process will increase the likelihood that adult providers have the information and guidance needed to safely care for these patients. YYASHCN with an identified medical home are more likely to transition successfully. It is important that the primary care providers on both the pediatric and adult sides work together to facilitate transition. Youth and families have reported better outcomes when they had a point of contact throughout the transition process. Care coordinators in both the pediatric and adult healthcare settings can be instrumental to ensuring a safe transfer between systems. Youth who have a transition "advocate" are more likely to obtain needed services. The advocate role can be performed by family members, healthcare or agency professionals, or the YYASHCN themselves. A portable medical summary sent to the adult provider ahead of the first visit will allow them to better engage the YYASHCN. This is important, as youth who perceive adult providers as unfamiliar with their medical past or do not demonstrate an interest in knowing them as individuals are less likely to return for a second visit. It is important to follow state and clinic-specific rules for the disclosure of health information between providers, making sure to obtain permission also of the young adult, unless they are transporting the summary to the new provider themselves.

In the absence of direct communication with an adult provider confirming that the YYASHCN attended a first adult clinic appointment, many pediatric providers call their former patients to verify transfer has occurred. It is helpful to gather detailed contact information prior to the last pediatric appointment, such as personal cell phone numbers and, with the young adult's permission, the names and numbers of friends or relatives who would know the youth's whereabouts over the next few years. Up to 50% of youth who transfer out of pediatric care are lost to this type of follow-up.

During the transfer process, it is not uncommon for youth who have not visited an adult provider to experience a health crisis and seek admittance to the pediatric emergency department or contact the pediatric service for continued care. In addition, there are times when YYASHCN who have transferred to an adult provider may need to be seen by a pediatric provider for a special service or procedure. To avoid confusing the YYASHCN and their families, the pediatric and adult providers should provide explicit instructions about which service will manage the patient's follow-up care.

#### Engagement on the Adult Side

The primary features of this stage of HCT are taking responsibility for managing one's own health within the adult healthcare system and attending more than one appointment with the same adult provider. It is not uncommon for YYASHCN to attend appointments with more than one adult provider before finding an adult doctor with whom they "connect." Common complaints are that adult providers are perceived as cold and uncaring and not accessible for questions outside of scheduled clinic hours. Due to the paucity of well-designed studies that evaluate transition outcomes, it is difficult to estimate how many youth remain with their first adult provider versus those who seek out alternatives. Thus, it is important to develop a feedback loop with adult providers to whom youth have transitioned until it is confirmed that they have attended at least two appointments. This feedback loop also facilitates the sharing of patient-specific health information (with patient permission), should questions about treatment arise.

**Factors That Increase or Decrease Gaps in Health Care** Factors that predict gaps in medical care during transition include living independently from parents; male gender; lower family income; greater travel distance to closest adult specialized clinic; public insurance; milder disease activity, severity, and complexity; fewer outpatient visits in pediatric care over the 3-year period before transfer; and history of at least one missed appointment. Factors that increase transfer to and engagement in adult care are greater disease complexity or more than one physical or mental health comorbidity; having a written referral to a specific professional who would provide follow-up care and attending the first or second outpatient visit in an adult clinic; greater independence in attending appointments; belief that follow-up should be continued in specialized adult care; and higher levels of self-efficacy.

### FINANCING HEALTHCARE TRANSITION PLANNING

Gaps in insurance coverage, which is more common for YYASHCN from lower socioeconomic levels, can lead to forgone care and adverse consequences. Insurance status is also a predictor of readiness for self-management. Fewer than 1 in 5 parents report having discussed with anyone how to obtain or keep some type of health insurance coverage as their adolescent becomes an adult. Having public insurance or switching from private to public insurance has been associated with higher rates of loss of insurance, which often occurs between 19 and 25 years of age. The 2010 Patient Protection and Affordable Care Act improved the health insurance coverage for YYASHCN through age 25 years, delaying the problem of lost medical insurance. However, this system may be challenging for young adults to navigate independently. As children and youth with multiple healthcare needs represent a major source of morbidity and resource utilization, accounting for 42% of all medical costs for children, and as these costs continue into adulthood, reimbursement for population-based management could encourage financing the critical period of transition from pediatric to adult care, when forgone care increases morbidity, mortality, and financial cost. The reader is referred to Got Transition/Center for Health Care Transition Improvement (http://www.gottransition.org/) for up-to-date information on coding for delivery of care related to HCT planning.

### BUILDING A CLINIC- OR SYSTEM-WIDE HCT PROGRAM

HCT preparation is more likely to occur if it is a priority of the clinical service and there are structures and processes in place to facilitate its incorporation into routine patient care. In the absence of evidence-based methods for HCT, the following are suggestions for how an individual clinic, service, or department could approach the development of an HCT program.

Got Transition/Center for Health Care Transition Improvement (http://www.gottransition.org/) has identified six core elements to help build an HCT planning program. They are (1) develop a formal transition policy with input from youth and families; (2) establish a patient registry to assist with tracking and monitoring; (3) conduct HCT readiness assessments beginning at age 14; (4) conduct regular transition planning; (5) manage the transfer of care between pediatric and adult care systems; and (6) confirm transfer completion.

For healthcare institutions with access to electronic medical records through Epic, there is an established transition planning tool to help facilitate discussions to prepare the YYASHCN for transition. Epic users can access this tool at the following link, using their username and password: https://galaxy.epic.com/?#Browse/page=1!68!600!1733006. Evidence that providers will use the tool, that they are satisfied with it, and that it increases HCT preparation activities has been reported.

#### Identify Current Practices and Processes

A first step in building an HCT program is to identify what processes are currently being used to prepare and transfer YYASHCN to adult-based care. This may involve developing a survey to be completed by all providers (eg, physicians, nurses, case workers) as within- and across-service variation in approaches to HCT are common. It is important to obtain information on how all three phases of HCT—transition preparation, active transfer between pediatric and adult health systems, and engagement of YYASHCN on the adult side—are currently being implemented. This process will help identify gaps and allow for prioritizing proposed solutions.

#### Build an Understanding of the Complexity of HCT

HCT is a complicated problem influenced by many factors, including the severity of the disease process, the cognitive level of the patient, the family/provider's capacity to facilitate transition, the knowledge and skills of the pediatric providers, medical insurance, differences between pediatric and adult health cultures, information technology, and the capacity of adult providers' care for pediatric onset conditions (also discussed in Table 70-1). It is important to build an understanding of this complexity and the need for clinic- or system-wide approaches to developing sustainable HCT structures and processes to ensure a successful transition to adult care. This will likely require meeting with those in decision-making positions and presenting findings on the health risks associated with transition that is poorly managed. It may help to engage testimony from YYASHCN and their families.

#### Focus on Medical Transition First

As HCT occurs at the same time as vocational, educational, housing, legal, and social transitions in a young adult's life, each with its own set of complexities, the medical team's primary focus should be on the transition of medical and behavioral health care. Communication between medical and behavioral health providers and the education system (high school, college) could facilitate both processes.

#### Employ Quality Improvement Methods and Identify Administrative Support

Quality improvement methods, such as Plan-Do-Study-Act (PDSA) cycles, can facilitate the implementation of strategies and evaluate their impact. Clinical services will have different starting points and degrees of commitment to improve their HCT processes. Personnel with dedicated time and effort to meeting with the clinic staff to discuss implementation and evaluation fidelity is needed, which in turn requires administrative support for the development of an HCT program.

### SUMMARY

Successful HCT requires a patient–family–provider partnership. The phases of HCT include planning, transfer, and engagement. Although providers prioritize the mechanics of HCT—ie, improving the patients' understanding their illness and self-management—the young adults see the highest priority outcome of HCT as its effect on their quality of life. Keeping this perspective in mind allows providers to support the patients' gaining confidence in their self-advocacy skills while offering a medical opinion on how the patients' decisions may impact the course of their illness.

Betz CL, O'Kane LS, Nehring WM, Lobo ML. Systematic review: health care transition practice service models. *Nurs Outlook.* 2016;64(3):229-243.

Bloom SR, Kuhlthau K, Van Cleave J, Knapp AA, Newacheck P, Perrin JM. Health care transition for youth with special health care needs. *J Adolesc Health.* 2012;51(3):213-219.

Cohen E, Berry JG, Camacho X, Anderson G, Wodchis W, Guttmann A. Patterns and costs of health care use of children with medical complexity. *Pediatrics.* 2012;130(6):e1463-e1470.

Hergenroeder AC, Wiemann CM, Bowman VF. Lessons learned in building a hospital-wide transition program from pediatric to adult-based health care for youth with special health care needs (YSHCN). *Int J Adolesc Med Health.* 2015. doi: 10.1515/ijamh-2015-0048.

Hergenroeder AC, Wiemann CM, Cohen MB. Current issues in transitioning from pediatric to adult-based care for youth with chronic health care needs. *J Pediatr.* 2015;167(6):1196-1201.

Lotstein DS, Ghandour R, Cash A, McGuire E, Strickland B, Newacheck P. Planning for health care transitions: results from the 2005–2006 National Survey of Children with Special Health Care Needs. *Pediatrics.* 2009;123(1):e145-e152.

The National Alliance to Advance Adolescent Health. Got Transition/ Center for Health Care Transition Improvement Web site. http:// gottransition.org/. Accessed March 19, 2018.

Quinn CT, Rogers ZR, McCavit TL, Buchanan GR. Improved survival of children and adolescents with sickle cell disease. *Blood.* 2010;115(17):3447-3452.

Reiss J, Gibson R. Health care transition: destinations unknown. *Pediatrics.* 2002;110(6, pt 2):1307-1314.

Rosen DS, Blum RW, Britto M, Sawyer SM, Siegel DM. Transition to adult health care for adolescents and young adults with chronic conditions: position paper of the Society for Adolescent Medicine. *J Adolesc Health.* 2003;33(4):309-311.

Singh SP, Paul M, Ford T, et al. Process, outcome and experience of transition from child to adult mental healthcare: multiperspective study. *Br J Psychiatry.* 2010;197(4):305-312. doi:10.1192/bjp.bp.109.075135.

Yeung E, Kay J, Roosevelt GE, Brandon M, Yetman AT. Lapse of care as a predictor for morbidity in adults with congenital heart disease. *Int J Cardiol.* 2008;125(1):62-65.

# PART 2 HEALTH PROBLEMS OF ADOLESCENTS

## 71 Mortality

Rebecca K. Erenrich and Elizabeth M. Ozer

Mortality rates for adolescents and young adults have decreased over the past decades globally and in the United States; however, adolescence and young adulthood remain risky periods of life. In the United States, after ages 5 to 9, the years with the lowest risk of death, the mortality rate increases. In 2014, the mortality rate was 14.0 per 100,000 population for early adolescents (10–14 years) and 45.5 per 100,000 population for late adolescents (15–19 years). The more than 200% increase in mortality across these intervals reflects the violent etiology of most deaths; increased access to motor vehicles and firearms, combined with use of substances, likely drives this increase. The trend continues to worsen in young adulthood: Young adults have 6 times the mortality rate of younger adolescents, with 83.8 deaths per 100,000 population (20–24 years).

The majority of adolescent and young adult deaths are due to preventable causes, with the top 3 causes of death in the United States—unintentional injury, suicide, and homicide—accounting for 70.6% of all deaths. Unintentional injuries account for the greatest number of adolescent deaths (39.7%); 12,586 young people died from unintentional injuries in 2014. Suicide, recently surpassing homicide, has become the second leading cause of death, accounting for 17.4% of adolescent and young adult deaths. Suicide has risen moderately for most groups, but tripled among girls ages 10 to 14 between 1999 and 2014, going from 0.5 per 100,000 to 1.5 per 100,000. Homicide, the third leading cause of death, accounts for 14.2% of all deaths among adolescents and young adults. Other frequent causes of mortality among adolescents and young adults ages 10 to 24 are malignant neoplasms (5.9% of deaths) and heart disease (3.2% of deaths).

Motor vehicle accidents are the leading cause of unintentional injury in the United States, accounting for 54.9% of fatal accidents (and 21.8% of all deaths) among adolescents and young adults. Inexperience, fatigue, failure to use seatbelts, alcohol use, high speed, and recklessness all contribute to motor vehicle accident mortality among adolescents. In order to mitigate these factors and the risk associated with 15- to 19-year-olds driving late at night, graduated driver licensing components, such as extended learners' permit holding periods, nighttime restrictions, and passenger restrictions that have been shown to be effective in reducing traffic mortality, have become widely accepted in the United States. Mortality rates for motor vehicle accidents among adolescents have decreased significantly in the past decade.

Firearms account for about 20% of deaths among US youth 10 to 24 years old. Gun death rates among 10- to 24-year-olds, currently 10.0 per 100,000 (about a third of the 1994 gun death rate), are at historic lows, mirroring the overall decline in gun crime in the general population. Still, firearms remain an important factor in adolescent mortality; they are the instrument of death in 88% of teen homicides and 41% of teen suicides, and almost 1 in 4 firearm injuries are fatal.

Alcohol and drug use are frequently directly linked to adolescent and young adult mortality globally; in the United States, they account for 13.0% of all deaths. However, this figure understates the extent to which drug and alcohol use contributes to other causes of adolescent and young adult mortality. For example, between 2006 and 2010, there were 4358 alcohol-attributable deaths among persons under age 21—1601 due to alcohol-related crashes, 1269 due to homicide, and 492 due to suicide.

While the disparities in adolescent and young adult death rates by socioeconomic status have declined significantly in the United States since 1990, substantial disparities in mortality by gender, race, and ethnicity persist. Males are more likely than females to die from the top 10 causes of death (except pregnancy and childbirth). The male–female disparity in suicide and homicide rates is particularly stark: males have consistently higher suicide and homicide rates than their female peers, averaging 3.7 times the suicide rate of females and 5.9 times the homicide rate. Black and American Indian/Alaska Native adolescents have the highest mortality, with 67.7 per 100,000 and 55.2 per 100,000 deaths, respectively. Asian/Pacific Islander adolescents have the lowest mortality (24.3 per 100,000); among adolescents of all races, those of Hispanic origin have lower mortality than those who are not Hispanic. Primary causes of death also differ by race. Homicide is the leading cause of death for black adolescents and young adults, accounting for 45.4% of all deaths among black, non-Hispanic males. Non-Hispanic American Indian/Alaska Native youth have the highest motor vehicle traffic mortality rate (more than double the rate of all other groups), followed by white, non-Hispanic youth.

## SUGGESTED READINGS

Centers for Disease Control and Prevention. Alcohol Related Disease Impact (ARDI) application, 2013. Available at: www.cdc.gov/ARDI. Accessed August 25, 2016.

Centers for Disease Control and Prevention, National Center for Health Statistics. Underlying Cause of Death 1999-2014 on CDC WONDER Online Database, released 2015. Available at: http://wonder.cdc.gov/ucd-icd10.html. Accessed August 25, 2016.

Currie J, Schwandt H. Inequality in mortality decreased among the young while increasing for older adults, 1990–2010. *Science*. 2016;352(6286):708-712.

Mokdad AH, Forouzanfar MH, Daoud F, et al. Global burden of diseases, injuries, and risk factors for young people's health during 1990–2013: a systematic analysis for the Global Burden of Disease Study 2013. *Lancet*. 2016;387(10036):2383-2401.

Mulye TP, Park MJ, Nelson CD, Adams SH, Irwin CE Jr, Brindis CD. Trends in adolescent and young adult health in the United States. *J Adolesc Health*. 2009;45(1):8-24.

Williams AF, Shults RA. Graduated driver licensing research, 2007–present: a review and commentary. *J Safety Res*. 2010;41:77-84.


# 72 Morbidity

Sharonda Alston-Taylor and Salina Mostajabian

## INTRODUCTION

According to the World Health Organization (WHO), there are about 1.2 billion adolescents ages 10 to 19 years worldwide, of whom more than 40 million live in the United States, based on the 2012 Census data. This population is growing in numbers as well as in racial-ethnic and socioeconomic status diversity, which presents unique challenges, such as inconsistent access to care and adverse effects related to poverty, unstable housing, and homelessness. These variables factor in to morbidity among adolescents and young adults, presenting opportunities through policies and programs to improve public health and health economics outcomes in youth. Measurements such as disability-adjusted life years (DALYs), which is the sum of years lived with disability (YLD) and years of life lost (YLL), are used in the field of public health to gain a better understanding of the burden of disease. These measures are particularly important when assessing morbidity in adolescents, since many chronic diseases of adulthood have their origin during the teen years.

## ADVERSE CHILDHOOD EXPERIENCES

Across the life course, adverse childhood experiences (ACEs) have been shown to impact adult morbidity. ACEs include abuse (psychological maltreatment, physical, or sexual), neglect, and household dysfunction (witnessing domestic violence; living with parents/adults who suffered from mental illness, alcohol abuse, or substance abuse; or loss of a parent, separated/divorced parents, or having an incarcerated household member). In addition to the aforementioned ACEs, other events such as bullying, neighborhood violence, and death of peers and family impact the health and well-being of youth. In the United States, more than 90% of 14-year-olds have experienced at least 1 ACE; those most affected are the poor, those with lower educational attainment, and racial-ethnic minorities. Adolescents with a greater number of and more recent ACEs have poorer health outcomes. Impaired health begins in early adolescence and progresses into adulthood. In fact, ACEs perpetuate chronic toxic stress, altering brain structure and metabolic responses, and increasing lifespan incidence of myocardial infarction, cerebrovascular disease, and stroke, in addition to other illness (eg, asthma).

## LEADING CAUSES OF MORBIDITY

### Risk Factors

Childhood and adolescent ACEs are linked to adolescent risky behaviors and increasing morbidity. Risky health behaviors, rather than infectious or chronic diseases, are the leading causes of morbidity among adolescents. ACEs increase the prevalence of risky behaviors and the onset of somatic complaints and poor health. Most morbidity results from 3 risky behaviors initiated in early to middle adolescence: substance use, sexual activity, and motor/recreational vehicle use. Many risk behaviors interrelate; for example, substance use plays a major role in motor vehicle crashes. The WHO recognizes alcohol use as the second leading cause of YLD among males ages 15 to 19 years old. For example, 21.9% of 9th through 12th graders rode with someone who was under the influence of alcohol, 10% drove while drinking, and 41.5% drove while texting or emailing. Use of substances is associated with sexual behavior, with a third of adolescents having used a substance prior to last sexual encounter, which often places adolescents at risk for acquisition of sexually transmitted infections (STIs) and unintended pregnancy. STIs are the most common reported infectious diseases in adolescents (see Chapter 228), and childbirth and complications related to pregnancy are the leading cause of inpatient hospitalizations for female adolescents (see Chapter 80). The Youth Risk Behavior Surveillance System of the Centers for Disease Control and Prevention provides valuable, ongoing data about adolescent risk behaviors in the United States.

The primary diagnosis for adolescent emergency room visits is injuries. Trauma-related disorders are also a leading reason for outpatient provider visits as well as inpatient hospitalization for both males and females.

### Chronic Disease and Morbidity

Chronic conditions or special healthcare needs are additional causes of morbidity. Although overall DALYs for adolescents have declined since 2000, the African region suffers the highest loss (300 per 1000 population) compared with wealthier western nations with 84 DALYs per 1000 population. HIV infection has been climbing up the ranks to 4th place among the other causes, which are depression, road injury, anemia, and self-harm. According to the WHO, other top causes of YLD are depression, iron deficiency anemia, asthma, neck and back pain, anxiety disorders, and alcohol use; these account for 50% of total YLD in this population. Depression, anxiety, attention deficit hyperactivity disorder, autism spectrum disorders, alcohol and substance abuse, and other mental health disorders affect between 13% and 20% of adolescents. Anxiety disorders are the most common diagnosis, followed by depression (see Chapter 94), though prevalence and incidence vary by demographics. Asthma is also a major chronic illness: About 16% of adolescents have lifetime asthma, and 8.7% report having current asthma. Diabetes (types 1 and 2) is another common chronic illness. The prevalence of both asthma and diabetes continue to increase, and obesity plays a major role. Obesity may be the most prevalent chronic illness in youth, affecting 17% of US adolescents, many of whom have morbid obesity. Increasing rates of worsening obesity complicate many other conditions including diabetes, asthma, depression, and overall quality of life into adulthood, as obese adolescents have a 70% chance of remaining overweight or obese as adults (see Chapter 24).

## ACCESS TO CARE

Morbidity from ACEs, risk behaviors, and chronic illnesses increases in those with limited access to care. Rates of uninsured children without a usual source of health care have decreased in the past 20 years. However, adolescents have higher rates than those under 6 years of age. Uninsured adolescents are less likely to see a healthcare provider. Data suggests that prolonged lack of insurance coverage contributes to a lapse in health care. Assessment by a provider and provision of anticipatory guidance are important for determining risk behaviors and reducing morbidity.

Centers for Disease Control and Prevention. Health, United States, 2015—special feature on racial and ethnic health disparities. http://www.cdc.gov/nchs/hus/special.htm. Accessed August 25, 2016.

Felitti VJ. Adverse childhood experiences and adult health. *Acad Pediatr*. 2009;9(3):131-132.

Flaherty EG, Thompson R, Dubowitz H, et al. Adverse childhood experiences and child health in early adolescence. *JAMA Pediatr*. 2013;167(7):622-629.

Gilbert LK, Breiding MJ, Merrick MT, et al. Childhood adversity and adult chronic disease. *Am J Prev Med*. 2015;48(3):345-349.

Kann L, McManus T, Harris WA, et al. Youth Risk Behavior Surveillance—United States, 2015. *MMWR Surveill Summ* 2016; 65(No. SS-6):1–174. http://dx.doi.org/10.15585/mmwr.ss6506a1. Accessed August 25, 2016.

Larkin H, Shields JJ, Anda RF. The health and social consequences of adverse childhood experiences (ACE) across the lifespan: an introduction to prevention and intervention in the community. *J Prev Interv Community*. 2012;40(4):263-270.

Mokdad AH, Forouzanfar MH, Daoud F, et al. Global burden of diseases, injuries, and risk factors for young people's health during 1990–2013: a systematic analysis for the Global Burden of Disease Study 2013. *Lancet*. 2016;387(10036):2383-2401.

World Health Organization. Adolescent health epidemiology. http://www.who.int/maternal_child_adolescent/epidemiology/adolescence/en/. Accessed August 25, 2016.

# 73 Sexual Behavior

Constance M. Wiemann and Erica B. Monasterio

While sexual behavior during adolescence includes the entire continuum of sexual expression, national data is sparse for any sexual behaviors other than heterosexual intercourse, which has decreased over the past 20 years. Currently, 79% of adolescents report using some form of contraception at first intercourse and 86% used a method to prevent pregnancy at last intercourse. These trends and the availability of long-acting reversible contraceptive methods and emergency contraception have resulted in substantial declines in rates of teenage pregnancy, births, and abortion.

A 2015 survey on sexual behavior of youth between the ages of 15 and 19 showed that 41.2% of high school students had experienced coitus at least once (43.2% of males and 39.2% of females). National data sets in the United States do not correlate socioeconomic status (SES) and coital activity in adolescents; thus, we are left only with data by race and ethnicity, an imperfect surrogate marker for SES and community characteristics. The percentages of youth reporting sexual intercourse vary by race and ethnicity: for blacks, 37.4% for female and 58.8% for male teenagers; for Hispanics, 39.8% for females and 45.1% for males; and for whites, 40.3% for females and 39.5% for males. Predictably, the higher the grade in school, the higher the percentage of students reporting sexual intercourse, with 9th graders at 24.1%, 10th graders at 35.7%, 11th graders at 49.6%, and 12th graders at 58.1%.

Data on other forms of partnered sexual behavior are limited. Data on oral sex from the 2013 National Survey on Family Growth showed that 49% of males and 45% of females ages 15 to 19 years old reported they had received oral sex. Smaller percentages (38% of males and 39% of females) reported having given oral sex. Again, reported engagement in these sexual behaviors increases with age and sexual experience, with higher percentages reporting both oral and vaginal sex than reporting solely oral sex. Reports of anal sex were equally common among males (10.2%) and females (10.5%) 15 to 19 years of age. Rates were much higher among 18- to 19-year-olds as compared to 15- to 17-year-olds for both genders (14.9% versus 7.0% among females and 16.6% versus 6.2% among males, respectively).

Among middle school students, rates of reported sexual intercourse are much lower, with 5.2% to 10.5% of students reporting ever having had intercourse (3.7% to 7.3% of girls and 5.6% to 13.5% of boys). Of note is the significant increase between 8th and 9th grades, which should encourage pediatricians to discuss sexual activity and risk reduction with their early adolescent patients.

Not all states include questions about sexual identity or same-sex sexual activity in the Centers for Disease Control and Prevention's Youth Risk Behavior Survey (YRBS), but data based on the 9 YRBS sites that do assess sexual identity show that high school youth who identified as gay or lesbian ranged from 1.0% to 2.6% (median, 1.3%), and as bisexual, from 2.9% to 5.2% (median, 3.7%), with 1.3% to 4.7% (median, 2.5%) reporting that they were unsure of their sexual identity. Data from the 12 sites that assessed same-sex sexual behavior showed that those who reported only same-sex sexual contact ranged from 0.7% to 3.9% (median, 2.5%), and those reporting both same-sex and opposite-sex sexual behavior ranged from 1.9% to 4.9% (median, 3.3%).

Pregnancy rates among 15- to 19-year-olds decreased 37%, from 83.8 per 1000 females in 2000 to 52.4 in 2011. The birth rate per 1000 females in the same age group declined 34% between 2000 and 2011, from 47.6 to 31.3 per 1000. Abortion rates also declined by nearly half, from 24.3 to 13.5 per 1000 females ages 15 to 19. Although pregnancy rates have decreased among all race/ethnic subgroups, pregnancy rates for black (93.8) and Hispanic (73.5) females, while demonstrating the steepest decline, have remained higher than for white (35.3) females aged 15–19 years. The highest rates of teen pregnancy in the United States continue to be found in states located in the South and Southwest, due a variety of factors, including differences in state demographic characteristics, the availability of comprehensive sexual health education, and knowledge about and availability of contraception.

An estimated 3 million adolescents are diagnosed with a sexually transmitted infection annually. Adolescents aged 15 to 19 years consistently demonstrate the highest age-specific rates of *Chlamydia trachomatis* and *Neisseria gonorrhoeae* in the United States. Youth tend to engage in sexual activity within sexual networks made up of their friends and community members, and due to the presence of these infections in specific sexual networks, sexually active black adolescents have much higher rates of chlamydia and gonorrhea than do American Indian/Alaska Native, Hispanic, white, or Asian/Pacific Islander adolescents.

## SUGGESTED READINGS

Boonstra HD. What is behind the declines in teen pregnancy rates? *Guttmacher Policy Review*. 2014;17(3):15-21. https://www.guttmacher.org/about/gpr/2014/09/what-behind-declines-teen-pregnancy-rates. Accessed August 25, 2016.

Centers for Disease Control and Prevention. Trends in the prevalence of sexual behaviors and HIV testing: national YRBS: 1991–2015. http://www.cdc.gov/healthyyouth/data/yrbs/pdf/trends/2015_us_sexual_trend_yrbs.pdf. Accessed August 25, 2016.

Child Trends Data Bank. Oral sex behaviors among teens. http://www.childtrends.org/?indicators=oral-sex-behaviors-among-teens. Accessed August 25, 2016.

Conklin K. Adolescent sexual health and behavior in the United States: positive trends and areas in need of improvement. Advocates for Youth Web site. http://www.advocatesforyouth.org/publications/publications-a-z/413-adolescent-sexual-behavior-i-demographics. Accessed August 25, 2016.

Kann L, Olsen EO, McManus T, et al. Centers for Disease Control and Prevention. Sexual identity, sex of sexual contacts, and health-risk behaviors among students in grades 9–12—Youth Risk Behavior Surveillance, selected sites, United States, 2001–2009. *MMWR Surveill Summ*. 2011;60(7):1-133.

National Center for Health Statistics. National Survey of Family Growth. Centers for Disease Control and Prevention Web site. http://www.cdc.gov/nchs/nsfg/. Accessed August 25, 2016.

# 74 Substance Use and Abuse

Chantay Banikarim

The leading causes of morbidity and mortality among adolescents and young adults are related to alcohol, smoking, and illicit drug use. According to 2015 data from Monitoring the Future (MTF), alcohol and tobacco use are at the lowest level in the survey's history, which dates back to 1975. From 1996 to the present, the 30-day prevalence of smoking declined by 83% and 79% in 8th and 10th graders, respectively. Seventy-five percent fewer students reported trying cigarettes in 2015 compared to 1997. Alcohol continues to be the most widely used substance in this population. In 2000, the prevalence of alcohol use in the past 30 days was 22%, 41%, and 50% among 8th, 10th, and 12th graders, respectively; the prevalence has now dropped to 10%, 22%, and 35%, respectively. Marijuana is the most widely used illicit drug with the highest prevalence rate among 12th graders at 35%; other illicit drug use declined across 8th through 12th grades from 34.1% in 1997 to 26.8% in 2015.

## CLINICAL PRESENTATION

Substance use often begins during adolescence or earlier. Adolescents use tobacco, alcohol, and illicit drugs to deal with problems, to enhance school performance, in response to peer pressure, or in response to desires for new experiences. Adolescents are more likely to use drugs if drugs are readily available in their community, if their peer group uses drugs, or if they have a mental health diagnosis such as depression or anxiety. Biologically, the adolescent brain is more vulnerable to substance use disorders, as the prefrontal cortex, which is responsible for judgment and impulse control, is not fully developed until the mid-20s. As there is no pathognomonic clinical presentation of substance use, clinical signs of substance use vary from behavioral and medical to a mental health complaint. The signs of substance use may be as subtle as appearing withdrawn, tired, or agitated. Secondary to substance use, a decline may be seen in school or athletic performance, and changes in peer groups, engagement in illegal activities, or other high-risk behaviors may occur.

## RISK FACTORS AND PROTECTIVE FACTORS

Known risk factors for the development of substance use disorder include male gender, gang involvement, academic failure, family history of a substance use disorder, use by peers, earlier age of onset, cognitive disability, and psychiatric comorbidities such as attention-deficit/hyperactivity disorder (ADHD) and depression. Many of these risk factors overlap with other problematic behaviors such as teen pregnancy, truancy, and violence. Protective factors against substance use include community involvement, healthy family and school relationships, and prosocial peers.

## SCREENING FOR DRUGS OF ABUSE

The American Academy of Pediatrics recommends annual screening of adolescents for tobacco, alcohol, and illicit drug use, including sports supplements and prescription drugs. Substance use screening should be incorporated into all healthcare visits for early identification of at-risk individuals. The healthcare provider, by creating a comfortable, trusting environment and using open-ended questions, may obtain an accurate substance use history from the adolescent patient. This portion of the history should take place without a parent in the room to help preserve patient confidentiality, which is necessary to obtain a complete psychosocial history. An effective opening question is: "During the past 12 months have you consumed alcohol, smoked marijuana, or used anything to get high?" If the response is "Yes" to drug use, proceed with asking the six CRAFFT questions to help further define the pattern of substance use.

C: Have you ever ridden in a CAR driven by yourself or someone who had been using alcohol or drugs?
R: Do you ever use alcohol or drugs to RELAX or feel better?
A: Do you ever use alcohol or drugs ALONE?
F: Do you ever FORGET things you did while using alcohol or drugs?
F: Do your family or FRIENDS ever tell you that you should cut down on your drinking or drug use?
T: Have you ever gotten into TROUBLE while you were using alcohol or drugs?

If the answer is "No" to use of drugs, complete the substance use screening by asking the "Car" question. A positive CRAFFT is defined as a score of 2 or more, indicating a high risk of having a substance use disorder. If the adolescent is using drugs, inquire about onset, duration, frequency, and route of drugs used. The CRAFFT screening tool is a validated developmentally appropriate tool that can be easily administered and scored by primary care physicians. Additional validated adolescent-specific substance use screening tools include the Alcohol Use Disorders Identification Test (AUDIT) and Problem Oriented Screening Instrument for Teenagers (POSIT). Through a careful history, the healthcare provider will be able to determine the impact of drug use on the adolescent's social life and academic performance, which are elements that can be incorporated into the treatment plan at the end of the visit. Red flags for a severe substance use disorder include daily use of a substance, CRAFFT score of 5 or higher, and memory lapses (drug-related blackouts) after substance use. A mood inventory and family history of substance use disorders are also part of the substance use history.

## TESTING FOR DRUGS OF ABUSE

The most commonly used tests for drugs of abuse are qualitative tests for screening purposes and quantitative tests for confirming test results. Most laboratories perform quantitative tests using either gas chromatography or mass spectrometry. The basic test screens for amphetamine, cocaine, marijuana, opioids, and phencyclidine. The period during which a drug may be detected after use varies according to the drug used and ranges from 1 to 7 days (Table 74-1). A positive drug test simply means the patient recently used this drug (within the past 1 to 7 days) but cannot be used to determine acute drug intoxication. Acute drug intoxication is a clinical diagnosis that can be supported by a positive drug screen. Clinicians ordering drug screens should be familiar with reasons for a false-positive drug test, such as taking a fluoroquinolone antibiotic, which can cross-react with an opiate screen. Similarly a patient taking an amphetamine for ADHD will test positive for amphetamines, which may be misinterpreted as abusing amphetamines. A false-negative result may occur if the urine sample is watered down or a masking substance was added to the urine such as soap, bleach, or ammonia. If clinical findings do not correlate with drug testing results, assistance from a laboratory should

**TABLE 74-1 URINE DRUG TESTING AND DURATION OF POSITIVITY**

| Drug | Duration of Positivity |
|---|---|
| Amphetamines | 48 hours |
| Barbiturates | 24–72 hours |
| Benzodiazepine | 72 hours |
| Cocaine | 48–72 hours |
| Ethanol | <12 hours (not routinely tested) |
| γ-Hydroxybutyrate | <12 hours |
| Heroin | 24 hours |
| Inhalant | Not routinely tested |
| LSD | Not detected in standard urine screens |
| Marijuana | Use of 1 dose (detectable for 48 hours); 4 times per week (5 days); daily use (10 days); chronic use (21–30 days) |
| Methadone | 3 days |
| 3,4- Methylenedioxymethamphetamine (MDMA) | Failure to detect MDMA unless large doses have been ingested |
| PCP | 8 days |

be sought for further help in interpretation of the test results. Accurate test results heavily depend on method of specimen collection; direct observation of specimen collection is the ideal method.

A drug screen should only be performed after obtaining the adolescent's consent, unless the patient is experiencing a life-threatening medical situation or there are legal reasons. The American Academy of Pediatrics opposes involuntary testing of adolescents for drugs of abuse. Prior to drug testing, a discussion with the patient regarding disclosure of test results to the guardian should take place. The drug test results may remain confidential if the patient chooses this route unless the drug use is posing an acute risk of harm to self or others. Home and school-based testing is not routinely recommended. Any information obtained from drug screening should be used for therapeutic rather than punitive purposes.

## ASSESSMENT

The *Diagnostic and Statistical Manual of Mental Disorders*, 5th edition (DSM-V), defines a substance use disorder as problematic use with the presence of 2 of 11 criteria over a 12-month period. The severity of use is further defined as mild, moderate, and severe, depending on the number of symptoms present. It is important to recognize that substance use can fluctuate with relapses and cycling back and forth in severity. Drug withdrawal is a clearly defined entity associated with prolonged use; the DSM-V specifically lists symptoms of withdrawal related to the drug used. Determining the impact of substance use on the adolescent's life is critical, as this information can help the adolescent understand the consequences of this use and the urgency and importance of participating in a treatment program as soon as possible.

## TREATMENT

Treatment recommendations for substance use disorders depend on several factors, including the presence of medical or mental conditions, developmental stage, age, gender, cultural background, readiness to change, and history of relapse. Patient and family engagement in treatment options is highly encouraged, as ultimately the adolescent must participate in the treatment program that is ideally supported by the family. Adolescents who are experimenting with drugs with no consequences or minor consequences may be briefly counseled on how to reduce and stop using drugs to avoid ongoing negative behavioral consequences utilizing motivational interviewing techniques and Prochaska and DiClemente's stages of change model. In addition to brief office-based interventions, outpatient treatment programs are available with varying intensities of therapy, individual and/or family-based sessions using cognitive behavioral therapeutic approaches, and motivational interviewing techniques. More severe substance use disorders require residential treatment programs followed by recovery support services, which can reduce the chances of relapse.

## COMMON DRUGS OF ABUSE

### Alcohol

Ethanol content is measured as "percent" (weight to volume) and in distilled beverages as "proof" units. In the United States, 1 proof means 0.5% ethanol, or twice the percent. The ethanol content varies depending on the beverage (from 3% to 60%).

Alcohol use increases through high school years. Adolescence is an entry point for developing an alcohol use disorder, given that earlier onset of using alcohol is associated with a greater risk of developing an alcohol use disorder.

Binge drinking is defined as having more than 4 to 5 drinks in one setting or achieving a blood alcohol level of 0.08% or higher. Binge drinking is increasing among high school students; two-thirds of high school students who currently drink report binge drinking more than 1 time in the past 30 days. Frequent binge drinkers are more likely to develop an alcohol or substance use disorder.

**Pharmacology** Ethanol is a central nervous system depressant with local and general anesthetic properties. Similar to other drugs of abuse, it causes the release of dopamine.

**Acute Effects** Symptoms of an acute intoxication occur at blood alcohol concentrations (BAC) between 50 and 150 mg/dL and include sleepiness, loss of social inhibitions, incoordination, depression, aggression, and euphoria. When BAC levels are above 150 mg/dL, the patient becomes lethargic, bradycardic, and hypotensive, and may have respiratory depression. Alcohol poisoning occurs with BAC around 450 mg/dL and may lead to stupor, coma, and death by respiratory depression. Adolescents who binge drink may experience a blackout, hangover, alcohol poisoning, or death. While under the influence of alcohol, adolescents experience poor judgment, which can translate into high-risk behaviors such as driving under the influence and having unprotected sex. Half of all head injuries among adolescents in the United States are associated with alcohol consumption, and a third of all fatal accidents among 15- to 20-year-olds involve alcohol.

**Long-Term Effects** Chronic binge drinking of alcohol can lead to liver disease, hypertension, heart disease, stroke, and various cancers including breast cancer. The adolescent brain, not being fully developed, is vulnerable to alcohol-induced brain damage and cognitive impairment. Binge drinking in this age group may lead to a reduction in brain volume, including the frontal regions, which are involved in executive function, impulsivity, and self-regulation.

**Treatment** In the acutely intoxicated patient, management depends on severity. Mild intoxication (<100 mg/dL of ethanol) can be managed with close observation, hydration, and analgesics. Moderate to severe intoxication (blood alcohol level [BAL] >300 mg/dL) requires provision of appropriate airway management and supportive care. Treatment for withdrawal symptoms depends on the degree of symptoms. In mild withdrawal, rest and hydration are sufficient. For severe symptoms, use of benzodiazepines may be helpful. Seizure management entails treatment with diazepam or phenytoin. Acute psychosis can be managed with haloperidol. Long-term management depends on the severity of the alcohol problem; treatment options range from brief office-based interventions to residential treatment programs.

**Prevention** Discussions about the hazards of alcohol use should begin in the doctor's office as early as 9 years of age, which is when children begin to think positively about alcohol use through exposure to alcohol advertising. Healthcare providers should encourage parents to have regular conversations regarding the hazards of drinking in high school and in college. These discussions can have a powerful impact on their future drinking behaviors. Young adults who had a conversation with their parent regarding the dangers of heavy drinking before entry into college were 20 times more likely to reduce their consumption of alcohol compared to those who did not receive the parental advice.

### Tobacco

The majority of adult smokers began smoking during adolescence. In addition to smoking cigarettes, many teens are also chewing tobacco and using hookahs and electronic nicotine delivery systems (ENDS). ENDS devices, including e-cigarettes, convert liquid nicotine into a vapor in a process known as "vaping." More teens are now using e-cigarettes than regular cigarettes, especially 8th graders, whose past-month reported use was 3.6% using cigarettes compared to 9.5% using e-cigarettes. Smoking e-cigarettes is strongly associated with later use of cigarettes, which may reverse the downward trend in smoking that has been observed over the last decade.

**Pharmacology** Nicotine is derived from the tobacco plant. It is a natural alkaloid that acts as a central nervous system stimulant by activating the dopamine system. A single cigarette delivers about 1 mg of nicotine while smoking. Given the highly addictive nature of nicotine, experimentation can lead to heavy smoking, and addiction can occur within a period of a few weeks.

**Risk Factors** Risk factors for initiation of adolescent smoking include availability of cigarettes, friend's smoking, smoking among family members, depression, and alcohol use.

**Acute Effect** The short-term consequences of nicotine use include euphoria, cough, bad breath, greater risk of infections, and addiction.

**Long-term Effects** Nicotine, tars, and other carcinogens in tobacco products are associated with malignancies of every organ of the body. Second-hand smoke exposure is associated with more frequent ear and respiratory infections, asthma attacks, and more missed days of school.

**Treatment** Tobacco use disorders can be further described as mild, moderate, or severe based on number of symptoms present. Determining the severity of the disorder as mild, moderate, or severe according to the DSM-V will help guide the intensity of the behavioral therapy. Tobacco cessation advice should be tailored to the patient's readiness to change, with the goal of moving the patient toward wanting to make a behavior change. The 5 A's model (Ask, Advise, Assess, Assist, and Arrange) may be used to guide the counseling sessions along with close follow-up. The 6 A's model adds anticipatory guidance to parents regarding smoking initiation and the impact of second-hand smoke in households during preventive care visits (Table 74-2). The healthcare provider should be prepared to devise a goal to reduce the frequency of smoking with a plan of action and close follow-up. Pharmacological agents such as the nicotine patch, nicotine gum, or bupropion, combined with psychological treatment, result in the highest long-term abstinence rates. During follow-up sessions, the patient should be assessed for withdrawal symptoms. Tobacco withdrawal symptoms occur in daily users who are cutting back or quitting. These symptoms include irritability, restlessness, trouble sleeping, and feeling anxious; withdrawal symptoms can cause the patient to resume smoking or revert back to the same intensity of smoking. Relapse is common, especially in the first few weeks, but diminishes considerably after 3 months of not smoking.

**TABLE 74-2 THE 5 A'S TO PREVENT SMOKING INITIATION OR SUPPORT SMOKING CESSATION AMONG ADOLESCENTS**

| Intervention | Technique |
|---|---|
| Ask | For all adolescents at every visit, ask about tobacco use without the parents in the room. For pre-teen children also inquire about tobacco use in an age-appropriate manner (eg, whether they have ever "tried" smoking or thought about trying). Also inquire about tobacco use among peers, as this may predict smoking initiation. |
| Advise | Strongly urge all tobacco users to quit in a clear, strong, personalized manner. Advise all nonusers to remain tobacco-free.<br>Advice should be<br>Clear: "I think it is important for you to quit smoking now, and I can help you." "Cutting down is not enough." "If you wait until you feel bad effects of smoking, it will be too late."<br>Strong: "As your doctor, I want you to know that quitting smoking is the most important thing you can do to protect your health now and in the future. I will help you quit."<br>Personalized: Tie tobacco use to current and future health and athletic performance, its social and economic costs, motivation level/readiness to quit, and the impact of tobacco use on siblings and others in the household. Remind parents of their responsibility as role models. |
| Assess | Determine the patient's willingness to quit smoking within the next 30 days.<br>If the patient is willing to make a quit attempt at this time, provide assistance.<br>If the patient will participate in an intensive treatment, deliver such a treatment or refer to an intensive intervention.<br>If the patient clearly states he or she is unwilling to make a quit attempt at this time, provide a motivation intervention.<br>If the patient is a member of a special population (eg, pregnant smoker, racial or ethnic minority), consider providing additional information relevant to this population. |
| Assist | Provide aid for the patient to quit (eg, set a quit date, provide counseling and self-help materials, refer to a quit line). |
| Arrange | Schedule follow-up contact, either in person or by telephone. Follow-up contact should occur soon after the quit date, preferably during the first week. A second follow-up contact is recommended within the first month. Schedule further follow-up contacts as indicated. |

Adapted with permission from Epps RP, Manley MW: *A Physician's Guide to Preventing Tobacco Use During Childhood and Adolescence*. Rockville: National Cancer Institute; 1990.

**Prevention** Healthcare providers are in a position to reduce the rate of initiation of tobacco products by screening their patients for tobacco use during every healthcare visit. Inquiring about the patient's incentive to smoke or stop smoking will provide a basis for effective counseling. At a minimum, tobacco screening is to be incorporated into routine preventive care visits. Engaging parents in this conversation is critical as parental smoking is a key factor for initiation of smoking during adolescent years. Educating the patient that there is no safe level of tobacco use is an integral part of the prevention counseling advice.

Stressing the importance of having a smoke-free home with the parent is helpful in prevention of not only the initiation of smoking but also exposure to second- and thirdhand smoke.

### Marijuana

Marijuana comes from the herbaceous plant *Cannabis sativa*, and tetrahydrocannabinol (THC) is the psychoactive ingredient. Marijuana preparations contain varying percentages of THC. Marijuana continues to be the most commonly used illicit drug, used mainly for recreational purposes, but there is growing interest in its medicinal uses for chronic pain and a few other gastrointestinal indications. Marijuana is still viewed as a "gateway drug" that may lead to other drug use during adolescence.

**Pharmacology** Marijuana may be inhaled or ingested. THC binds to two receptors, $CB_1$ and $CB_2$, located in the central and peripheral nervous systems. The binding of THC to these receptors releases dopamine, which is responsible for the psychoactive symptoms produced from using marijuana.

**Acute Effects** Daily users may experience hyperemesis syndrome characterized by nausea, vomiting, and abdominal pain. Shortly after using marijuana, the user will feel euphoria and an increase in heart rate, injected conjunctiva, and a dry mouth. Notable neurological symptoms from marijuana use include nystagmus, ataxia, decrease in reaction time, and short-term memory loss. As the drug wears off, the user becomes hungry and tired.

**Long-Term Effects** Daily users may experience a reduction in sperm count, gynecomastia, tolerance, a lack of motivation, cognitive impairments, reduction in IQ, poor school performance, and increased risk for acute adult-onset psychosis. Symptoms of chronic marijuana use are similar to a mood disorder with impairment in daily life activities.

**Treatment** An adolescent with a positive CRAFFT screen for marijuana should receive a brief counseling session; indications for more intense treatment are based on the duration and frequency of marijuana use. Drug treatment programs with motivational techniques and cognitive behavioral therapy have been effective in the adolescent population. The DSM-V also recognizes cannabis withdrawal, which occurs when frequent users abruptly stop using, leading to irritability, aggression, anger, and trouble sleeping.

Treatment with buspirone and gabapentin has been successful in addition to behavioral therapy. Given the high prevalence of marijuana use, healthcare providers will continue to be in a position to provide education on the short- and long-term health hazards of using marijuana to their adolescent patients.

### Prescription Pills

The most commonly abused prescription pills are opioids, central nervous system depressants, and stimulants. Young adults have the highest prevalence of abusing prescription pills at 5.9%, followed by adolescents at 3%. The majority of teens report getting the prescription pills from either a relative or friend. As the prescription rate for stimulants has increased, stimulant medication abuse has similarly increased over the past decade.

**Pharmacology** Opioids fall into a natural or synthetic category and have morphine-like properties. Natural opioids include morphine, heroin, and codeine, and synthetic opioids include hydromorphine and oxycodone. Depending on the opiate used, it may be ingested, smoked, or injected. Opioids exert their effect by binding to receptors in the gastrointestinal tract and central nervous system. The main sites of action in the central nervous system are the hypothalamus, thalamus, and limbic system. Stimulants acting on the central nervous system cause the release of dopamine, which creates a feeling of euphoria.

**Acute Effects** Stimulant users experience euphoria and an increase in energy levels, but agitation and anxiety may be felt, depending on the amount of stimulant consumed. Significant behavioral changes may occur, such as auditory hallucinations and paranoid ideation, depending on the amount used. Stimulants cause elevations in heart rate and blood pressure. In contrast to the effects of stimulant use, opiates and sedatives drop the heart rate and blood pressure, and depending on the amount used, respiratory depression and death may ensue.

**Long-Term Effects** Given the highly addictive nature of these drugs, withdrawal symptoms occur with abrupt cessation and are a diagnosable entity in the DSM-V. Chronic opiate users struggle with constipation, chronic rhinitis, and ulceration of nasal mucosa from snorting. From intravenous drug use, skin abscesses and cellulitis can occur. Females may experience irregular menses or amenorrhea. Extensive dental decay is a notable finding in chronic methamphetamine abusers and is referred to as "meth mouth."

**Treatment** The treatment for prescription pill abuse is similar to other substance use disorders and entails behavioral therapy with or without pharmacological treatment.

## SUGGESTED READINGS


Bright Futures/American Academy of Pediatrics. 2016 recommendations for preventive pediatric health care. Periodicity schedule. *Pediatrics*. 2016;137(1). http://pediatrics.aappublications.org/content/pediatrics/early/2015/12/07/peds.2015-3908.full.pdf. Accessed February 10, 2017.

Casey BJ, Jones RM, Hare TA. The adolescent brain. *Ann N Y Acad Sci*. 2008;1124:111-126.

Center for Adolescent Substance Abuse Research. CRAFFT Screen. http://www.ceasar-boston.org/CRAFFT/screenCRAFFT.php. Accessed February 10, 2017.

Farber HJ, Walley SC, Groner JA, Nelson KE; Section on Tobacco Control. Clinical practice policy to protect children from tobacco, nicotine, and tobacco smoke. *Pediatrics*. 2015;136(5):1008-1017.

Hadland SE, Harris SK. Youth marijuana use: state of the science for the practicing clinician. *Curr Opin Pediatr*. 2014;26(4):420-427.

Johnston LD, O'Malley PM, Miech RA, Bachman JB, Schulenberg JE. *Monitoring the Future: National Survey Results on Drug Use, 1975–2015: Overview: Key Findings on Adolescent Drug Use*. Ann Arbor, MI: Institute for Social Research; 2016. http://www.monitoringthefuture.org/pubs/monographs/mtf-overview2015.pdf. Accessed February 10, 2017.

Levy S, Siqueira LM; Committee on Substance Abuse, Ammerman SD, Gonzalez PK, Ryan SA, Siqueira LM, Smith VC. Testing for drugs of abuse in children and adolescents. *Pediatrics*. 2014;133(6):e1798-e1807.

Patrick ME, Schulenberg JE. Prevalence and predictors of adolescent alcohol use and binge drinking in the United States. *Alcohol Res*. 2013;35(2):193-200.

Pbert L, Farber H, Horn K, et al; American Academy of Pediatrics, Julius B. Richmond Center of Excellence Tobacco Consortium. State-of-the-art office-based interventions to eliminate youth tobacco use: the past decade. *Pediatrics*. 2015;135(4):734-747.

Silins E, Horwood LJ, Patton GC, et al; Cannabis Cohorts Research Consortium. Young adult sequelae of adolescent cannabis use: an integrative analysis. *Lancet Psychiatry*. 2014;1(4):286-293.

Substance Abuse and Mental Health Services Administration. Results from the 2013 National Survey on Drug Use and Health: summary of national findings, NSDUH Series H-48, HHS Publication No. (SMA) 14-4863. Rockville, MD: Substance Abuse and Mental Health Services Administration, 2014. http://www.samhsa.gov/data/sites/default/files/NSDUHresultsPDFWHTML2013/Web/NSDUHresults2013.pdf. Accessed February 10, 2017.

Turrisi R, Mallett KA, Cleveland MJ, et al. Evaluation of timing and dosage of a parent-based intervention to minimize college student's alcohol consumption. *J Stud Alcohol Drugs*. 2013;74(1):30-40.

U.S. Department of Health and Human Services. Preventing tobacco use among youth and young adults: a report of the Surgeon General. Atlanta, GA: US Department of Health and Human Services, Centers for Disease Control and Prevention, National Center for Chronic Disease Prevention and Health Promotion, Office on Smoking and Health, 2012. http://www.ncbi.nlm.nih.gov/books/NBK99237/. Accessed February 10, 2017.


# PART 3 MENTAL HEALTH DISORDERS IN THE ADOLESCENT

## 75 Depression, Anxiety, and Other Disorders in Adolescence

Rachel Wolfe, Amy Acosta, and Sindhu Idicula

Many adolescents experience worry from time to time, shifts in their moods, or times of dysphoria, including sadness or anger. Mood and anxiety disorders differ from normative concerns in that they can cause marked impairment, can produce changes in global functioning, and are pervasive. This chapter will provide an understanding of the epidemiology, clinical manifestations, diagnosis, treatment, and prevention of depression, anxiety, and other mental health disorders of children and adolescents.

The importance of recognizing and addressing mental health concerns not only is important for the individual patient, but also has a profound impact on public health. Suicide was the third leading cause of death for 10- to 24-year-olds in 2014. It followed only unintentional injury and homicide, and accounted for 5504 deaths in the United States. Significant risk factors for suicide include major depressive episodes and manic episodes.

Multiple factors play a role in mental health problems in youth. Risk factors for developing mental health problems, such as anxiety and depression, include family conflict, poverty, and school violence. Youth of color are more likely to experience greater barriers to care and higher prevalence of mental health concerns than their white peers. Heredity can be a risk factor for mood and anxiety disorders. In the case of major depression, youth with first-degree family members who are also depressed are 2 to 4 times more likely to have major depression.

Adolescence is a complicated period when individuals reach maturity in physical and sexual development, with a lag of maturity in other areas such as cognitive and emotional development. Biological changes, such as hormonal changes, may play a role in adolescents' vulnerability toward emotional and behavioral issues. Regions of the adolescent brain, such as the prefrontal cortex, which controls executive function, are still in the process of developing until the mid-20s. There is discussion that the changes that occur during adolescence are possibly linked to the vulnerability during adolescence of mood disorders, schizophrenia, and other conditions.

Initial screening for mood, anxiety, and other disorders may be done through the clinical screening during a medical visit (eg, HEADSS exam) and screening questionnaires. However, an extensive diagnostic interview to include self-report, caregiver report, history of symptoms, and other formal assessments are the ideal standard for the diagnosis of a mental health disorder.

## MOOD DISORDERS

## MAJOR DEPRESSIVE DISORDER AND PERSISTENT DEPRESSIVE DISORDER

Major depression and other depressive disorders are further discussed in Chapter 94. This discussion focuses on these disorders in the adolescent patient.

The clinical presentation of depression varies with age. Unlike school-aged children, adolescents are less likely to present with primarily somatic complaints, and unlike adults, adolescents are less likely to appear melancholic or sullen. More often, adolescents present with symptoms of irritable mood; anhedonia; boredom; hopelessness; sleep changes such as insomnia, hypersomnia, or day/night reversal; weight changes; and psychomotor retardation. Excessive feelings of guilt, shame, hopelessness, and helplessness are indicators of severity of depression and should prompt further screening for suicidal ideation, self-harm, and bullying. Adolescents with depression are more likely to engage in substance use and risky behaviors such as unsafe sex. Adolescents are more likely than children to experience suicidal ideation, act on suicidal feelings, and utilize more lethal means for suicide.

According to the *Diagnostic and Statistical Manual of Mental Disorders*, 5th edition (DSM-5), persistent depressive disorder (dysthymia) is characterized by depressed mood lasting at least 1 year in adolescents (compared to 2 years in adults). At least 2 of the following symptoms are present: changes in appetite, sleep difficulties, low energy, low self-esteem, poor concentration, and hopelessness. The adolescent may report having always felt this way, as symptoms are never absent for more than 2 months.

### EPIDEMIOLOGY AND ETIOLOGY

Lifetime prevalence of depressive disorders is approximately 12%. According to the Youth Risk Behavior Surveillance System, in 2015, 29.9% of youth reported feeling sad or hopeless, daily, for 2 or more weeks, in the past 12 months. According to the National Survey on Drug Use and Health, 11.4% (approximately 2.8 million) adolescents (ages 12–17 years) reported experiencing a major depressive episode in the past 12 months. Prevalence of major depression is higher for youth/young adults (18–29 years) than the rest of the adult population. Beginning in early adolescence, females are twice as likely as males to develop major depression, a trend that continues throughout adulthood. The DSM-5 indicates that the 12-month prevalence for persistent depressive disorder in the United States is approximately 0.5%. In addition, early onset, before age 21, is associated with a higher risk of personality disorders or substance use disorders.

The average length of a major depressive episode in children and adolescents ranges from 3 to 6 months for community samples and 5 to 8 months for referred samples. Length of episode is correlated positively with comorbidity of anxiety, dysthymic disorder, and substance abuse. The probability of recurrence is 40% in 2 years and 70% in 5 years. Between 20% and 40% of children and adolescents who experience an episode of major depression will go on to develop bipolar I disorder within 5 years. Depression has a high probability of recurrence that increases with each subsequent episode. Increase in time between episodes is correlated positively with recovery.

### DIAGNOSIS AND TREATMENT

The diagnosis of a depressive disorder requires consideration of severity, pervasiveness, and level of impairment in addition to gathering information on the presence of symptoms such as depressed mood, guilt, worthlessness, suicidal thoughts, irritability, decline in school performance, and withdrawal from social and other pleasurable activities. Diagnosis is best made by a thorough combined interview of the adolescent and caregivers. It is paramount to interview the adolescent separately, as it may be difficult for him/her to share certain thoughts, behaviors, or concerns in front of caregivers. In addition to clinical interviews, certain instruments such as the Children's Depression Inventory (CDI) for 8- to 13-year-olds and the Beck Depression Inventory for older adolescents may be useful in assessing symptoms. The Patient Health Questionnaire-9 (PHQ-9) can also be used to screen for depressive symptoms and additionally screens for difficulty of symptoms in daily life (eg, to do work at home). Clinicians should assess the extent to which symptoms are interfering with school, social, and family functioning, and assess for safety.

Early intervention for the treatment of adolescent depression is correlated with increased effectiveness. Given that depressive episodes may spontaneously resolve in adolescents, mild depressive episodes are typically treated with psychotherapy alone. Studies such as the Treatment for Adolescents with Depression Study (TADS) suggest that for moderate to severe depression, combination treatment with psychotherapy and medication are most effective, and if cognitive behavioral therapy (CBT) is added to psychotropic medication, recovery is accelerated.

There are 2 empirically supported psychotherapy approaches for depression in adolescents: CBT and interpersonal therapy (IPT). CBT focuses on improving mood by challenging, reframing, and restructuring negative self-beliefs. It can be administered in individual or group formats. Family involvement may also be helpful. IPT is a three-stage treatment that aims to improve the quality of the adolescent's interpersonal relationships, which is, in turn, thought to improve mood symptoms. Similar to CBT, family involvement may be helpful for adolescents involved in IPT.

The selective serotonin reuptake inhibitors (SSRIs) are the first line of treatment for depression. SSRIs with US Food and Drug Administration (FDA) approval for adolescents include fluoxetine and escitalopram and are typically recommended first-line treatments. Others, such as sertraline, fluvoxamine, and citalopram, have an evidence base in adults or for other disorders (such as anxiety disorders) in children and adolescents and may be used off-label for depression in adolescents. Typical side effects include gastrointestinal issues, headache, dry mouth, sedation, or insomnia. Medications that block both serotonin and norepinephrine—such as venlafaxine, mirtazapine, and duloxetine—may also be used off-label. Bupropion, a medication that targets norepinephrine and dopamine, is used often for depression as well as attention problems, but carries a risk of reducing the threshold for seizures.

In 2004, the FDA issued a black box warning regarding the use of antidepressants in children and adolescents, which was later expanded to include individuals under the age of 24 years. This was based on a meta-analysis reporting higher rates of suicidal ideation and attempts by those on antidepressants versus placebo (4% on antidepressants vs. 2% on placebo). There were relatively few suicide attempts, and no completed suicides. Studies subsequently have failed to demonstrate a consistent increased risk of suicidal ideation or attempts in youth or young adults taking antidepressants. Given this warning, the recommendation for physicians is continued use of antidepressants for patients who warrant treatment, with discussion of the warning with patients and families, and close follow-up (such as weekly visits or telephone check-in) for the first few months of treatment.



## BIPOLAR DISORDERS AND CYCLOTHYMIC DISORDER

Bipolar disorder manifests as depressive and manic or hypomanic episodes. There is controversy about how broadly or narrowly to apply criteria, leading to questions of whether bipolar disorder is overdiagnosed in childhood. Some of these concerns were addressed in the DSM-5 with the addition of disruptive mood dysregulation disorder (DMDD), characterized by persistent irritability and frequent episodes of behavior dysregulation. Although this pattern of symptoms may seem congruent with bipolar disorder due to the presence of outbursts, it has been found that as children mature, this symptom pattern usually manifests as a depressive or anxiety disorder.

The 4 most reported symptoms of bipolar disorder are increased energy, distractibility, pressured speech, and irritability. According to the DSM-5, a manic episode is defined as a discrete episode in which mood is abnormally elevated, expansive, or irritable. Adolescents with mania may also exhibit rapid speech, racing thoughts, highly goal-directed behaviors (eg, working on multiple projects or goals), grandiose self-esteem, and distractibility. Hypomanic episodes are characterized by elated or irritable mood and usually do not cause significant distress or impairment. Of note, in younger adolescents and children, mania may present as extreme silliness or happiness beyond what would be considered developmentally appropriate. Adolescents with bipolar disorders are more likely to experience rapid mood shifts between manic and depressive episodes (ie, rapid cycling). However, depressive episodes may last minutes, hours, or in some cases days.

According to the DSM-5, cyclothymic disorder is characterized by repeated periods of subsyndromal hypomanic and depressive symptoms that last for at least 1 year. Adolescents with cyclothymic disorder experience chronic changes or fluctuations in mood most days. The mood changes are not as severe as those seen in depressive or manic episodes, and symptoms would not meet criteria for full depressive episodes. However, symptoms still cause significant distress or impairment in the adolescent's ability to function in social or academic settings.

### EPIDEMIOLOGY AND ETIOLOGY

Bipolar and related disorders occur approximately twice as often in females as in males. The 12-month prevalence of all ages ranges from 0.0% to 0.6% globally, versus 0.6% prevalence in the United States. The lifetime prevalence is about 3% in adolescents, with females reporting slightly higher frequency of bipolar I and II disorder than males (3.3% in females versus 2.6% in males). The mean age of onset is 18 years for bipolar I disorder and the mid-20s for bipolar II disorder; however, both may be diagnosed earlier by a trained professional. Cyclothymic disorder usually develops in adolescence or early adulthood.

According to the DSM-5, family history of bipolar disorder is considered the strongest, most consistent risk factor for the diagnosis, with risk increasing according to degree of kinship. The prevalence of bipolar disorder in first-degree relatives of adults is increased eightfold to tenfold over what is expected of bipolar in community samples. In addition to genetic factors, environmental factors, including higher socioeconomic status, are also thought to increase risk.

### DIAGNOSIS AND TREATMENT

The diagnosis of a bipolar disorder or cyclothymic disorder is a clinical one, done through careful history, behavioral observation, and mental status examination showing characteristic mood changes, pressured speech, flight of ideas, and grandiosity. Collateral information from caregivers is critical in assessing bipolar disorders in children and adolescents. Scales may be helpful in assessment, such as the parent version of the Young Mania Rating Scale (YMRS) or the Child Mania Rating Scale for parents. Family history of bipolar disorder is supportive of the diagnosis.

One of the main challenges in the diagnosis of bipolar disease is that many symptoms of bipolar disease also overlap with other disorders. For example, both bipolar disorder and attention-deficit/hyperactivity disorder (ADHD) can show symptoms of irritability, accelerated speech, distractibility, and unusual energy. Thus, it is imperative that the evaluation is done thoughtfully and comprehensively with the patient's age and development in mind. For example, adolescents are developmentally prone to take risks, which may fit in the spectrum of normal adolescent behavior or may fit within the context of bipolar. When a diagnosis of bipolar disorder is entertained, it is helpful to develop a broad differential through careful and contextual reflection of the patient's presentation, and to utilize the consultation or referrals to child and adolescent psychiatrists to help with clarification of the diagnosis and management of the disorder.

Mood stabilization is the goal of treatment in bipolar disorder and cyclothymic disorder. Medications that have been utilized for mood stabilization in manic or mixed episodes include lithium, divalproex, carbamazepine, and atypical antipsychotic medications such as olanzapine, risperidone, quetiapine, ziprasidone, or aripiprazole. First-line treatment with monotherapy typically starts with lithium, an atypical antipsychotic, or divalproex, although a recent study called the Treatment of Early-Age Mania (TEAM) noted that risperidone was more effective than lithium or valproate for children or adolescents diagnosed with a manic or mixed bipolar disorder. Concerning side effects of lithium include tremor, nephrogenic diabetes insipidus, teratogenicity, and hypothyroidism. Notable side effects of divalproex include weight gain, sedation, teratogenicity, and hepatotoxicity. Both lithium and divalproex require monitoring of blood levels. Atypical antipsychotics, on the other hand, do not require blood monitoring, but are more commonly associated with metabolic syndrome, including weight gain and elevations in lipids and blood glucose.

Patients who do not tolerate 1 medication may need to switch to another medication. Patients who do not respond to monotherapy, particularly those with psychosis, may respond to a combination of a mood stabilizer and an atypical antipsychotic. Adjunctive use of benzodiazepines may be utilized to help with acute agitation or insomnia. For severe illness in adolescents resistant to treatment with pharmacotherapy, electroconvulsive therapy (ECT) may be utilized depending on whether it is legal in the state. For bipolar depressive episodes, the adult literature suggests the use of monotherapy with lithium, valproate, or atypical antipsychotics, or a combination of an SSRI with a mood stabilizer. Caution should be exercised with the use of SSRIs in patients with bipolar disorder, particularly without concurrent mood stabilization, as they may trigger episodes of mania, hypomania, mixed episodes, or rapid cycling. In cases of bipolar depression where SSRIs are used, mood stabilizing agents should be given.

Supportive psychotherapy may be included in treatment as an adjunct to psychopharmacological treatment approaches. Family psychoeducation with skill building currently has the most empirical support. Parents may also benefit from attending parent support groups.

## SUICIDE AND SUICIDAL BEHAVIOR

The most serious consequence of an adolescent mood disorder is suicide. Risk factors associated with suicide include nonsuicidal self-injury, a previous attempt or attempts, alcohol or substance abuse, the diagnosis of clinical depression, feelings of hopelessness, and isolation from others. Risk increases by gender (male), age (adolescents, older adults), isolation, and feelings of hopelessness. Protective factors include effective clinical care, family and community support, and support from mental and medical health workers. While some of the risk factors are unalterable (eg, family history of suicide), many protective factors can be initiated and employed through clinical treatment modalities (ie, access to care). The risk of suicide is highest during a major depressive episode. Therefore, targeted, proactive, preventive evidence-based treatments and support should be employed to reduce the risk of suicide for adolescents. For a complete discussion of this issue, see Chapter 94.

## ANXIETY DISORDERS

Anxiety disorders are the most commonly encountered mental health condition in adolescents, with lifetime prevalence estimated at 30%. Approximately half of all anxiety disorders in adults are present by early adolescence, and about half of all adolescents with anxiety disorders have another psychiatric disorder, most commonly depression. Fifty-eight percent of patients diagnosed with major depression have comorbid anxiety disorders, including 22.4% with a social phobia, 17.2% with generalized anxiety, and 9.9% with panic disorder. Anxiety disorders and their treatment are discussed further in Chapter 93.

Unifying features of anxiety disorders include excessive worries, fears, or anxieties that are extreme or out of context, and psychological (eg, fear of failure, fear of rejection), physiological (eg, dry mouth, sweating, accelerated heart rate), and behavioral (eg, procrastination, avoidance, rituals, impaired concentration) manifestations that persist over several months. All diagnosable anxiety disorders significantly interfere with school and/or social functioning. Both genetic and environmental factors are involved.

Anxiety disorders tend to run in families, and neuroimaging studies support a link among temperament, brain activity, and the development of anxiety disorders. Hardship and adversity, including poverty, witnessing or being a victim of trauma, living with chronic illness, and family disruption, including illness, death, and divorce, are risk factors for developing an anxiety disorder.

## SOCIAL ANXIETY DISORDER (SOCIAL PHOBIA)

Although more than half of all adolescents and adults identify themselves as shy, people with social anxiety disorder (SAD) experience persistent, overwhelming anxiety and extreme self-consciousness in everyday social situations. In adolescents, the fear of social situations is fairly broad. According to the DSM-5, patients with social anxiety have fears of being judged, embarrassed, or rejected because of perceived embarrassing behavior or displays of anxiety. They may be anxious for weeks prior to a dreaded event like a school dance. SAD may be specific, such as a fear of eating in public or of public speaking, or general, in which any or all social situations are painful. In addition to emotional distress, people with SAD can experience physical symptoms, including blushing, sweating, trembling, palpitations, nausea, lightheadedness or fainting, and stammering. People with SAD are more likely to have poor social skills, low self-esteem, and distorted body image. To receive a diagnosis of SAD, adolescents must experience an extended period of symptoms (about 6 months) and the symptoms must interfere significantly with their routine and/or cause significant distress.

### EPIDEMIOLOGY AND ETIOLOGY

SAD occurs approximately twice as frequently in females as in males. The 12-month prevalence of SAD in adolescents is about 7%, comparable to the prevalence in adults. Lifetime prevalence is approximately 9% in adolescents, with females reporting higher levels than males. The median age of onset is 13 years, with 75% of individuals having an onset between the ages of 8 and 15 years. Onset may be acute or gradual.

A genetic basis for developing SAD is supported by twin studies demonstrating a risk of developing SAD that is 2 to 3 times greater in adolescents who have at least 1 first-degree relative with this disorder. Single-photon emission tomography has shown that altered serotonin and dopamine activity may play a role in the development of SAD. However, parents with any kind of anxiety disorder or depression are more likely to raise anxious or socially phobic children, suggesting an epigenetic mechanism. Similarly, traumatic social experiences, such as being humiliated in the classroom, can trigger the onset or worsen the course of social phobia. Repetitive trauma, such as being bullied or excluded from social cliques, can also precipitate SAD.

### DIAGNOSIS AND TREATMENT

The diagnosis of SAD is based on history, usually collected through a psychodiagnostic interview, behavioral observation, parent-report measures, and child-report measures. The Social Phobia and Anxiety Inventory for Children (SPAI-C) is an example of a psychometrically sound instrument that includes both parent-report and child-report versions that can help quickly screen for symptoms and aid in the treatment planning for SAD.

Treatment studies consistently emphasize the importance of early diagnosis and treatment, with CBT and pharmacotherapy being the treatments of choice.

Two CBT approaches are supported by the American Psychological Association in the treatment of SAD in children and adolescents: 1) Social Effectiveness Training for Children and Adolescents (SET-C), and 2) the C.A.T. Project. SET-C incorporates group skills training and individualized behavioral exposure to treat SAD in 7- to 17-year-olds. This program has demonstrated superiority to pharmacological treatment. The C.A.T. Project, a cognitive-behavioral program designed specifically for adolescents with SAD, includes setting goals to overcome social fears through a "FEAR plan" and use of a workbook.

## SPECIFIC PHOBIA

Please refer to Chapter 93 for a discussion on specific phobias.

## GENERALIZED ANXIETY DISORDER

Generalized anxiety disorder (GAD) is characterized by inappropriate, excessive anxiety and worry about multiple events or activities. The worry is wide-ranging and difficult to control and results in clinically significant distress and/or impairment. Children and adolescents may tend to worry more about things such as competence or quality of performance on tasks.

### EPIDEMIOLOGY AND ETIOLOGY

GAD likely begins in childhood and early adolescence; however, median age of diagnosis is 30 years. Many individuals with GAD recall being anxious most of their lives, suggesting that onset may be younger but is considered as temperamental anxiety. The 12-month prevalence rates among adolescents is estimated at 0.9%, with 2.2% of adolescents reporting lifetime prevalence. The incidence increases with age, and females outnumber males 2–3 to 1. The etiology of GAD is multifactorial, with temperament and environment playing roles.

GAD is a classic example supporting the biopsychosocial model of understanding psychiatric illness. GAD runs in families, and thus genetic susceptibility and being raised by anxious, worried parents are risk factors. Childhood adversity, including poverty, witnessing trauma, and living with chronic illnesses such as asthma and diabetes, are also risk factors. Family disruptions, including parental illness, death, or divorce, may also contribute to the development of GAD. Children whose psychological needs are unmet and who are emotionally and/or physically neglected or abused are also at increased risk for developing GAD.

### DIAGNOSIS AND TREATMENT

Diagnosis is established by careful history that includes questions about emotions (eg, fear, worries), physical symptoms (eg, tachycardia, sweating, dizziness, lightheadedness), and behaviors (eg, procrastination, avoidance, poor concentration), and by ruling out other medical conditions (eg, hyperthyroidism, hypoglycemia, migraines, seizure disorders, lead intoxication), substance abuse (including excessive caffeine intake), and medication side effects. Primary care providers are aware that patients with GAD can present with somatic complaints such as stomachaches, headaches, or insomnia.

CBT is the treatment of choice for GAD. Treatment includes education to distinguish healthy from unhealthy worry; monitoring to increase awareness of triggers; cognitive restructuring to challenge negative, catastrophic, or magical thoughts; and exposure to anxiety-inducing situations or events. Mindfulness-based CBT approaches add strategies for controlling the physical effects of anxiety by teaching deep breathing and progressive relaxation exercises.

## PANIC DISORDER

Panic disorder is characterized by recurrent, unexpected panic attacks that consist of an acute sense of fear or distress that lasts for a few minutes. Attacks may be accompanied by a sense of dread or impending doom. Patients may believe they are about to die or are going crazy. Physical symptoms of hyperventilation, tachycardia, shortness of breath, dizziness, sweating, and trembling can be present. Patients with panic disorder are very worried about having future attacks and will change their behavior to avoid having attacks. As such, panic attacks are terrifying and can be disabling. They are frequently diagnosed in emergency departments where patients present believing they are dying of a heart attack or are going crazy. Patients are often afraid of having an attack in public, and agoraphobia is present in more than a third of cases.

### EPIDEMIOLOGY AND ETIOLOGY

The 12-month prevalence rate of panic disorder is 2% to 3% in adults and adolescents, with rates being about 2 times higher in females. Lifetime prevalence estimates are around 2.3%. Prevalence increases during adolescence. The symptoms of juvenile panic disorder are similar to those of adults and include heart palpitations, sweating, shortness of breath, trembling, faintness, nausea, and abdominal distress. Childhood panic disorder is associated with other anxiety disorders, including GAD and specific phobia, somatization disorder, major depression, dysthymic disorder, and bipolar disorder.

Anxiety disorders in parents place children at risk for the development of panic disorder, and separation anxiety in young children may be a precursor to the development of panic disorder in adolescents. Panic disorder may be viewed as a dysregulation of the fight-or-flight response wherein the response is turned on by a trigger, but the capacity to modulate and turn it off is diminished or lost. In addition to stimulants, panic attacks can be triggered by lactic acid, carbon dioxide, carbon monoxide (cigarette smoke), and cholecystokinin.

### DIAGNOSIS AND TREATMENT

Panic disorder is diagnosed through clinical interview with the patient and his/her parents. A psychometrically sound screening tool, such as the Revised Children's Anxiety and Depression Scale, may also be useful in gathering the appropriate data.

Panic disorder is treated with CBT and medication. CBT, particularly exposure-based intervention, has been shown to be an effective way to treat panic disorder. Exposure-based intervention is designed to inhibit a patient's avoidance response to induced panic symptoms while utilizing behavioral coping strategies (eg, deep breathing) to reduce the symptoms.

### PHARMACOLOGICAL TREATMENT OF ANXIETY DISORDERS

SSRIs and serotonin-norepinephrine reuptake inhibitors (SNRIs) are the first line of treatment for anxiety disorders, despite most of these medications not having an indication for the above anxiety disorders in the pediatric population. Duloxetine is the exception, as it has received an FDA indication for the treatment of GAD in adolescents, and can be titrated to a maximum dosage of 120 mg/day. Regardless of the lack of indication, SSRIs and SNRIs are readily utilized for anxiety disorders in pediatric patients, and have a solid evidence base that supports their efficacy and tolerability. A recent meta-analysis of all randomized, double-blind, placebo-controlled trials of SSRIs and SNRIs in pediatric patients with fear-based anxiety disorders showed modest effect size and did not show a statistically significant risk of suicidality.

While tricyclic antidepressants have been used for anxiety disorders and show efficacy, they have been greatly limited by severity of side effects. In addition to the antidepressants, other medications studied in anxiety disorders include benzodiazepines, buspirone, and atomoxetine. Benzodiazepines bind to the gamma-aminobutyric acid A ($GABA_A$) receptor and potentiate the inhibitory effects of gamma-aminobutyric acid (GABA). In randomized clinical trials of benzodiazepines versus placebo, there were no statistically significant differences in anxiety or clinical global improvement in patients treated with benzodiazepines, but notable side effects were drowsiness, irritability, and oppositional behavior. Additionally, benzodiazepines are highly addictive and may be abusable. Therefore, they are not the first-line medications for anxiety disorders. Buspirone, a $5\text{-HT}_{1A}$ agonist, was studied in a large, unpublished study, where it did not demonstrate statistically significant improvement over placebo. Atomoxetine was studied in a multicenter, double-blind, placebo-controlled trial for youth with ADHD and a comorbid anxiety disorder, and reductions in both anxiety and ADHD symptomatology were noticed, with limited side effects. Other medications that may be considered include gabapentin, pregabalin, tiagabine, hydroxyzine, beta blockers, and atypical antipsychotics. The recommendation for anxiety disorders is to start with an SSRI or SNRI, and to utilize other agents for switching or augmentation with failure of first-line treatments.

## OTHER DISORDERS

## OBSESSIVE-COMPULSIVE DISORDER

Obsessive thoughts and tendencies can be normal and adaptive. In obsessive-compulsive disorder (OCD), obsessions are intrusive and distressing, and persistent thoughts, images, or impulses may seem senseless and inconsistent with one's personal beliefs. Obsessions may involve fears of contamination, and intrusive thoughts may be aggressive, blasphemous, or sexual in content. Although the thoughts are rarely acted out, the fears are debilitating. Compulsions are repetitive, ritualistic mental acts or behaviors that the individual feels driven to perform in order to neutralize the obsessions and their associated fears. Examples of compulsions include hoarding, checking behavior, and hand washing. Obsessions and compulsions may change over time.

### EPIDEMIOLOGY AND ETIOLOGY

The median age of onset of OCD is 19.5 years, with a quarter of cases having their onset by the age of 14 years. The onset of OCD is bimodal with the first peak onset being around age 11 and the second occurring in early adulthood. Males have an earlier onset than females; however, by adolescence, rates of OCD are reported equally. Onset is usually gradual with a waxing and waning course. Twelve-month prevalence rates are estimated to be 1.2%.

A genetic basis for OCD is supported by twin studies and by the discovery of an OCD gene, a mutation in the human serotonin transporter gene *hSERT*. Animal models created by deleting certain genes in mice have produced offspring that obsessively groom until their fur falls off. Neuroimaging studies show abnormalities in brain activity, particularly in the anterior cingulate gyrus, and may differentiate hoarding from nonhoarding OCD. High-resolution magnetic resonance images show differences in the brain structures of individuals with OCD. Other risk factors include family history and stressful life events.

### DIAGNOSIS AND TREATMENT

The diagnosis of OCD requires a history taken with the parent and with the child. Behavioral observation and rating scales may also be useful in supporting a clinical interview. The Yale-Brown Obsessive-Compulsive Scale (Y-BOCS), a brief screening checklist, is widely used and has strong psychometric properties.

CBT and pharmacotherapy are the treatments of choice. The CBT technique used to treat OCD is exposure and response prevention (ERP). This technique inhibits the patient from engaging in his or her dysfunctional compulsion in response to anxiety, which allows the patient to learn more adaptive responses to cope with the anxiety.

For example, a patient who has to wash his or her hands immediately after touching a doorknob may not be allowed to do so for a period of time and instead is coached in breathing practices or other behavioral strategies for coping with the anxiety. ERP should only be performed by a trained clinician.

Treatment of OCD in adolescents typically consists of combination therapy with psychotherapy and psychopharmacology. Agents that block serotonin reuptake have resulted in improvement in symptoms. These medications must be titrated to sufficiently high doses for sufficient periods of time to constitute adequate trials. Blinded, placebo-controlled trials have studied clomipramine, fluoxetine, fluvoxamine, sertraline, and paroxetine. In adolescents, clomipramine has been studied most rigorously but is limited by problematic side effects such as dizziness, vision changes, tachycardia, and sedation. Given its impact on the heart and the liver, it is recommended that providers obtain electrocardiograms and liver function studies periodically throughout treatment. Fewer side effects are reported for SSRIs. Fluoxetine was superior to placebo in double-blind, placebo-controlled trials with a maximum dosage of 60 mg/day, and is now indicated by the FDA for the treatment of OCD in the pediatric population. Sertraline was found to be superior to placebo in a multisite, double-blind, placebo-controlled trial where the maximum dosage used was 200 mg/day, and also has earned an indication for the treatment of OCD in the pediatric population. Fluvoxamine also showed response in reducing symptoms in a double-blind, placebo-controlled trial with doses up to 200 mg/day, making it an indicated treatment for OCD in the pediatric population. In a head-to-head trial of clomipramine versus different SSRIs, clomipramine was significantly more effective than the SSRIs and the SSRIs performed similarly to each other and outperformed placebo. However, given the significant side effect profile of clomipramine, SSRIs are the first line for treatment of OCD.

## POST-TRAUMATIC STRESS DISORDER

Post-traumatic stress disorder (PTSD) is a cluster of symptoms that develop following exposure to 1 or more traumatic events. Examples of traumatic events that might result in PTSD include serious accidents (eg, car, train, and plane crashes); natural disasters (eg, floods, hurricanes, earthquakes); manmade atrocities (eg, terrorist attacks, random shootings, arson, war); violent personal attacks (eg, sexual assault, kidnapping, mugging, torture); physical, sexual, or emotional abuse; abandonment; and neglect. Chronic illnesses such as asthma, with suffocation as a near-death experience, and multiple surgeries in young children with congenital abnormalities can also lead to PTSD.

Following exposure to a traumatic event, individuals with PTSD experience intrusive symptoms such as recurrent dreams, distressing memories and/or flashbacks, and extreme distress when faced with reminders of the event. Individuals with PTSD will actively avoid anything associated with the trauma, including memories and external cues such as people, places, or objects that bring up memories of the event. Those who experience PTSD will also exhibit changes in their cognitive functioning and mood as associated with the trauma. For example, they may have difficulty remembering parts of the trauma, feel detached from others, experience exaggerated negative beliefs about themselves or others, or struggle to feel positive emotions. Lastly, individuals with PTSD will exhibit marked arousal symptoms such as hypervigilance, exaggerated startle response, and irritability.

PTSD patients may suffer from comorbid anxiety disorders and depression, and they may self-medicate with alcohol and drugs. A universal response to trauma is the experience of guilt and shame. Trauma victims, in an effort to feel control, will sacrifice self-image and self-esteem.

### EPIDEMIOLOGY AND ETIOLOGY

The lifetime prevalence rate of PTSD is estimated to be 9%. The National Comorbidity Survey Replication Adolescent Supplement states that the 12-month prevalence rate of PTSD among adolescents is approximately 5% with females reporting higher rates than males. More than two-thirds of Americans experience a significant trauma in their lives, and up to 20% experience such an event in any given year. Exposure to trauma is even higher in parts of the world ravaged by warfare, poverty, and famine. The likelihood of developing PTSD varies with the severity, duration, and proximity of the traumatic experience. Over half of all boys and girls in the general population are exposed to some form of trauma during their childhood and adolescence, including physical assault (47%), maltreatment (10%), sexual victimization (6%), and witnessing violence (25%).

Risk factors for the development of PTSD include female gender, previous exposure to trauma, previous psychiatric conditions, parental psychopathology, and low levels of social support. Neurobiological studies implicate deficiencies in the hypothalamic–pituitary–adrenal axis with lower-than-expected cortisol levels in PTSD patients. This may combine with higher-than-expected release of fight-or-flight response catecholamines that exacerbate the experience of trauma and intensify the creation of traumatic memories. Neuroimaging studies show differences between PTSD study participants with a preponderance of hyperarousal and those with more dissociative symptoms.

### DIAGNOSIS AND TREATMENT

Adolescents with PTSD resemble adults with PTSD. However, it is important to consider the critical developmental time period of adolescence, including identity development and possible consequences of experiencing trauma during this time; treatment of PTSD is critical.

The diagnosis of PTSD is established through a thorough, structured or semistructured clinical interview such as the Anxiety Disorders Interview Schedule (ADIS) for children and parents. Clinicians must be sensitive to the fact that children and adolescents may be unable to verbalize traumatic experiences or may be too afraid to disclose trauma. The clinical interview may be traumatizing, so clinicians must allow patients to disclose at their own pace. A brief screen for self-report symptoms with strong psychometric properties is the Child PTSD Symptom Scale (CPSS), which takes approximately 10 minutes to administer.

Trauma-focused CBT (TF-CBT) is the most comprehensively studied psychotherapeutic intervention and has the strongest evidence base to support its use in PTSD. TF-CBT incorporates exposure techniques (ie, encourages the patient to talk about the traumatic event), behavioral relaxation techniques, and cognitive restructuring to challenge false beliefs and distorted thoughts about the trauma. Caregiver psychoeducation and involvement are usually incorporated into TF-CBT.

There are limited studies looking at pharmacological intervention in PTSD. Most studies are done in adults, and conclusions are extrapolated for children and adolescents. Some studies have suggested that in the child and adolescent population the use of beta blockers immediately after trauma can prevent the development of PTSD, a finding that has been contradicted in the adult literature. However, the adult literature recommends the use of SSRIs as first-line treatment for PTSD. In addition, some studies show support for prazosin, an $alpha_1$ agonist, in overall symptom improvement and a decrease in nightmares and sleep disturbances. Preliminary studies suggest that venlafaxine may be efficacious in the treatment of adult PTSD, and that bupropion is not effective in reducing symptoms. Atypical antipsychotics have been useful in children and adolescents with PTSD, as well as $alpha_1$ agonists such as clonidine and guanfacine. Further research would be useful in guiding the diagnosis and treatment of PTSD in children and adolescents.

### SUGGESTED READINGS

American Academy of Child and Adolescent Psychiatry. Practice parameter for the assessment and treatment of children and adolescents with posttraumatic stress disorder. *J Am Acad Child Adolesc Psychiatry*. 2010;49:414-430.

American Psychiatric Association. *Diagnostic and Statistical Manual of Mental Disorders*. 5th ed. Washington, DC: American Psychiatric Association; 2013.

Brent D, Emslie G, Clarke G, et al. Switching to another SSRI or to venlafaxine with or without cognitive behavioral therapy for adolescents with SSRI-resistant depression: the TORDIA randomized controlled trial. *JAMA*. 2008;299:901-913.

Freeman J, Garcia A, Frank H, et al. Evidence base update for psychosocial treatments for pediatric obsessive-compulsive disorder. *J Clin Child Adolesc Psychol*. 2014;43:7-26.

Kendall PC, Compton SN, Walkup JT, et al. Clinical characteristics of anxiety disordered youth. *J Anxiety Disord*. 2010;24:360-365.

Kessler RC, Avenevoli S, Costello EJ, et al. Prevalence, persistence, and sociodemographic correlates of DSM-IV disorders in the National Comorbidity Survey Replication Adolescent Supplement. *Arch Gen Psychiatry*. 2012;69:372-380.

Klein DA, Goldenring JM, Adelman WP. HEEADSSS 3.0: The psychosocial interview for adolescents updated for a new century fueled by media. *Contemp Pediatr*. 2014:16-28.

March J, Silva S, Petrycki S, et al; Treatment for Adolescents with Depression Study (TADS) Team. Fluoxetine, cognitive-behavioral therapy, and their combination for adolescents with depression: Treatment for Adolescents with Depression Study (TADS) randomized controlled trial. *JAMA*. 2004;292(7):807-820.

Merikangas KR, He JP, Burstein M, et al. Lifetime prevalence of mental disorders in US adolescents: results from the National Comorbidity Survey Replication–Adolescent Supplement (NCS-A). *J Am Acad Child Adolesc Psychiatry*. 2010;49(10):980-989.

Mesa F, Beidel DC, Bunnell BE. An examination of psychopathology and daily impairment in adolescents with social anxiety disorder. *PLoS ONE*. 2014; 9(4):e93668. doi:10.1371/journal.pone.0093668.

National Center for Health Statistics. Adolescent Health. Centers for Disease Control and Prevention Web site. http://www.cdc.gov/nchs/fastats/adolescent-health.htm. Accessed July 6, 2016.

Parker GF. DSM-5 and psychotic and mood disorders. *J Am Acad Psychiatry Law*. 2014;42:182-190.

Pediatric OCD Treatment Study (POTS) Team. Cognitive-behavior therapy, sertraline, and their combination for children and adolescents with obsessive-compulsive disorder: the Pediatric OCD Treatment Study (POTS) randomized controlled trial. *JAMA*. 2004;292:1969-76.

Renk K, White R, Lauer B, McSwiggan M, Puff J, Lowell A. Bipolar disorder in children. *Psychiatry J*. 2014;2014:928685.

The Treatment for Adolescents with Depression Study (TADS): Long-term effectiveness and safety outcomes. *Arch Gen Psychiatry*. 2007;64:1132-1143.

Walkup JT, Albano AM, Piacentini J, et al. Cognitive behavioral therapy, sertraline, or a combination in childhood anxiety. *N Engl J Med*. 2008;359:2753-2766.

Youth.gov. Youth topics: Mental health: Risk and protective factors. Youth.gov Web site. http://youth.gov/youth-topics/youth-mental-health/risk-and-protective-factors-youth. Accessed July 6, 2016.

# 76 Disordered Eating

Andrea K. Garber and Sara M. Buckelew

## INTRODUCTION

Disordered eating describes a spectrum of abnormal eating behaviors with negative health impact. These behaviors often begin as a misguided attempt to control weight. In studies of school-based populations, about one-third of normal weight and three-quarters of overweight girls say that they are trying to lose weight. While they report attempting to make the positive lifestyle changes that we suggest in clinic, such as decreasing soda and exercising more, the majority are also engaging in disordered eating practices such as skipping meals and fasting. Of note, 10% of these normal weight girls and 18% of the overweight girls reported extreme behaviors including vomiting and laxative use. These disordered eating behaviors covary with other health damaging behaviors such as alcohol and tobacco use, negatively impact nutritional intake, predict significant weight *gain* over time, and increase the risk for development of an eating disorder.

Eating disorders represent the far end of the disordered eating spectrum in terms of severity and frequency of abnormal eating behaviors. Formerly considered relatively rare diagnoses, recent studies show that up to 8% of adolescents meet criteria for the range of eating disorders described in Tables 76-1 to 76-5, which will be the focus of this chapter. Such patients often present to clinic with acute medical consequences requiring hospitalization and/or intensive outpatient care. Thus, a large proportion of patients in any pediatric clinic will present with a range of disordered eating and associated health outcomes, which clinicians must be equipped to identify and address. Pica and rumination disorder are eating disorders as defined by the *Diagnostic and Statistical Manual of Mental Disorders*, 5th edition (DSM-5); however, they will not be discussed here, nor will feeding disorders.

Eating disorders diagnosed are according to the DSM-5. The changing demographic of eating disorders is in part due to revised diagnostic criteria in the DSM-5. In general, diagnostic criteria have been made more inclusive, which has improved the accuracy of diagnosis. Studies show that patients who were previously categorized as having an eating disorder not otherwise specified (EDNOS) by default

**TABLE 76-1 SUMMARIZED DSM-5 CRITERIA FOR ANOREXIA NERVOSA (AN)**

A. Restriction of energy intake relative to requirements, leading to low weight
B. Intense fear of weight gain or becoming fat, although underweight
C. Disturbance in the way in which one's body weight or shape is experienced, undue influence of body weight or shape on self-evaluation, or denial of the seriousness of the current low body weight.

**Subtypes of AN:**

1. Restricting type: During the last 3 months, the person has not regularly engaged in binge eating or purging behavior (ie, self-induced vomiting or the misuse of laxatives, diuretics, or enemas).
2. Binge eating/purging subtype: During the last 3 months, the person has regularly engaged in binge eating or purging behavior (ie, self-induced vomiting or the misuse of laxatives, diuretics, or enemas).

**TABLE 76-2 SUMMARIZED DSM-5 CRITERIA FOR BULIMIA NERVOSA (BN)**

A. Recurrent episodes of binge eating. An episode of binge eating is characterized by both of the following:
   1. Eating, in a discreet period of time (eg, within any 2-hour period), an amount of food that is definitely larger than most people would eat during a similar period of time and under similar circumstances.
   2. A sense of lack of control over eating during the episode (eg, a feeling that one cannot stop eating or control what or how much one is eating).
B. Recurrent inappropriate compensatory behavior to prevent weight gain, such as self-induced vomiting; misuse of laxatives, diuretics, enemas, or other medications; fasting; or excessive exercise.
C. The binge eating and inappropriate compensatory behaviors both occur, on average, at least once a week *for 3 months*.
D. Self-evaluation is unduly influenced by body shape and weight.
E. The disturbance does not occur exclusively during episodes of AN.

**Subtypes of BN:**

1. Purging type: During the current episode of BN, the person has regularly engaged in self-induced vomiting or the misuse of laxatives, diuretics, or enemas.
2. Non-purging type: During the current episode of BN, the person has used other inappropriate compensatory behaviors, such as fasting or excessive exercise, but has not regularly engaged in self-induced vomiting or the misuse of laxatives, diuretics, or enemas.

**TABLE 76-3 SUMMARIZED DSM-5 CRITERIA FOR BINGE EATING DISORDER (BED)**

A. Recurrent episodes of binge eating. An episode of binge eating is characterized by both of the following:
   1. Eating, in a discreet period of time (eg, within any 2-hour period), an amount of food that is definitely larger than most people would eat during a similar period of time and under similar circumstances.
   2. A sense of lack of control over eating during the episode (eg, a feeling that one cannot stop eating or control what or how much one is eating).

B. The binge eating episodes are associated with 3 or more of the following:
   1. Eating much more rapidly than normal;
   2. Eating until feeling uncomfortably full;
   3. Eating large amounts of food when not feeling physically hungry;
   4. Eating alone because of feeling embarrassed by how much one is eating;
   5. Feeling disgusted with oneself, depressed, or very guilty afterward.

C. There is marked distress regarding binge eating.

D. The binge occurs, on average, at least once a week for 3 months.

E. Binge eating is not associated with compensating behaviors as seen in BN.

**TABLE 76-5 SUMMARIZED DSM-5 FOR AVOIDANT/RESTRICTIVE FOOD INTAKE DISORDER**

A. An eating or feeding disturbance manifesting in persistent failure to meet nutritional and/or energy needs associated with one of the following:
   1. Significant weight loss (or growth failure);
   2. Significant nutritional deficiency;
   3. Dependence on enteral feeding or nutritional supplements;
   4. Marked interference with social functioning.

B. The disturbance is not explained by lack of food access or culturally sanctioned practice.

C. The disturbance does not exclusively occur during the course of AN or BN, and there is no evidence of body image disturbance.

D. The disturbance is not attributable to another medical or mental health diagnosis. When the condition does occur in the context of another condition or disorder, the severity of the eating disturbance exceeds that routinely associated with the condition or disorder and warrants additional clinical attention.

can now be diagnosed appropriately as having anorexia nervosa (AN) or bulimia nervosa (BN). In fact, the DSM-5 does not include EDNOS; rather the category of "other specified feeding and eating disorders" (OSFED) has been added. A new diagnostic category has come to the fore: avoidant/restrictive food intake disorder (ARFID). Patients in this category were formerly described as having "extreme picky eating."

AN is an eating disorder characterized by food restriction that typically results in extreme weight loss. As shown in Table 76-1, the diagnostic criteria for AN include low weight, distorted perception of body shape and size, and intense fear of weight gain. Notable changes in the DSM-5 are removal of the criteria requiring weight to be less than 85% of expected and the presence of amenorrhea. AN typically affects adolescent girls, with a lifetime prevalence of up to 1% in young women. However, the more inclusive DSM-5 criteria allow boys and a wider range of underweight individuals to be more readily included. As described below, a subcategory of "atypical AN" has been added to describe individuals with AN who present in a normal weight range. Such patients were often overweight prior to illness, and therefore this category includes an increasing number of boys and youth of lower socioeconomic status (SES). The diagnosis of AN is most often made in early to middle adolescence, with critical risk periods during developmental transition (eg, a transition to middle/junior high school, high school, or college) and a decision to embark on diets. Most of the complications associated with AN are due to malnutrition, and can be reversed with nutritional rehabilitation. However, a patient's denial about the seriousness of the illness and degree of weight loss is a barrier to recovery. Therefore, nutrition therapy in adolescents often begins with refeeding in a hospital or in outpatient therapy guided by parents (see "Treatment," below).

**TABLE 76-4 SUMMARIZED DSM-5 CRITERIA FOR OTHER SPECIFIED FEEDING AND EATING DISORDER (OSFED)**

1. **Atypical AN:** Meet all of the above criteria for AN but not underweight despite significant weight loss.
2. **BN (of low frequency and/or limited duration):** All criteria for BN are met except behaviors occur fewer than 1 time per week or for less than 3 months in duration.
3. **BED (of low frequency and/or limited duration):** All criteria for BED are met except behaviors occur fewer than 1 time per week or for less than 3 months in duration.
4. **Purging disorder:** Recurrent purging behavior to influence weight or shape in the absence of binge eating.
5. **Night eating syndrome:** Recurrent episode of night eating after waking or excessive eating after the evening meal; patient has awareness and recall of the episodes and they cause significant distress.

BN is characterized by binge and purge behavior and typically affects up to 4% of adolescent/young adult women. The word "bulimia" means a condition characterized by perpetual insatiable hunger with bouts of overeating. Table 76-2 shows the diagnostic criteria for BN. Episodes of binge behavior are followed by compensatory purging behavior, which may be vomiting, food restriction, use of laxatives, or compulsive overexercising. A notable change in the DSM-5 is the lower threshold of frequency of binge/purge episodes, making this diagnosis more inclusive. Patients with BN report anxiety about gaining weight; however, in contrast to individuals with AN, most individuals with BN are normal in weight. Therefore, it is critical to obtain a history of binging and purging behavior to establish the diagnosis. The mean age of onset of BN is 18 years, with most diagnoses made in middle to late adolescence and young adulthood. A history of childhood sexual abuse is more common in patients with BN as compared to AN.

Binge eating disorder (BED) was formerly considered a "research" diagnosis but is now recognized as a psychiatric diagnosis in the DSM-5. As shown in Table 76-3, BED is characterized by binging behavior without compensation by purging. Therefore, the majority of patients with BED are overweight. Among adolescents who are actively seeking clinical care for weight management, up to 35% meet the criteria for BED. Thus, while it is likely that BED contributes to overweight, studies suggest that overweight may *precede* the binge eating behavior.

OSFED replaces EDNOS to include atypical AN, subthreshold AN and BN, and other subcategories shown in Table 76-4. Patients with atypical AN meet all criteria of AN, but their weight is at or above normal despite significant weight loss. Subthreshold diagnoses describe patients with lower severity or frequency of behaviors. Subthreshold BN is defined as binge and purge behavior occurring fewer than 1 time per week or for less than 3 months in duration; subthreshold BED describes binge behavior occurring fewer than 1 time per week or for less than 3 months in duration. OSFED includes 2 additional subcategories. Purging disorder describes purging to lose weight or influence shape but without binge eating. Finally, night eating syndrome is characterized by episodes of eating after awakening from sleep or excessive eating after the evening meal resulting in significant distress.

ARFID is a new category that replaces and extends the former diagnosis of feeding disorder of infancy or early childhood, to describe individuals who persistently fail to meet appropriate nutritional and/or energy needs related to an eating or feeding disturbance (Table 76-5). ARFID is more than being a "picky eater"; patients may exhibit a lack of interest in food, or avoid foods based on various sensory characteristics, including appearance (color), smell, taste, texture, or temperature. Patients with ARFID may also have fears of choking or vomiting. The diagnosis of ARFID requires a careful differential because it may appear to overlap with other diagnoses characterized by food avoidance, including AN and autism spectrum disorder. However, ARFID is distinguished by 2 key features. First, an inability to meet nutritional needs results in weight loss, growth failure, dependence on nutritional supplements, or psychosocial problems. Second, unlike AN, there is no evidence of body image disturbance or drive for thinness in ARFID. Comorbid anxiety is more common than depression in these adolescents. Thus, the creation of this diagnostic category is an important step toward improving diagnosis, treatment, and research in this patient population.



## PATHOGENESIS AND ETIOLOGY

The etiology of eating disorders is multifactorial, including genetic, biological, psychological, and sociocultural influences. Eating disorders are highly heritable, with higher rates of concurrence among identical twins and/or first-degree relatives. Studies of twins estimate a heritability of 30% to 50% for AN. Genome-wide association studies are ongoing and have not implicated specific genes. The psychological factors associated with AN often include perfectionism, anxiety, obsessive behavior, and low self-esteem. BN is often associated with psychological factors including depression, anxiety, low self-esteem, personality disorders, disturbances in social functioning (eg, the inability to have meaningful interpersonal relationships, resulting in isolation from normal daily events), and substance abuse and self-harm/suicidal behavior. It is clear from several studies that levels of several hormones (such as leptin) and neuropeptides (such as serotonin) are altered in patients with eating disorders. Neuroimaging studies have furthered these findings by elucidating alterations in regional brain activity and neuroreceptor function. However, further research is needed to differentiate the traits that may predispose individuals to the development of an eating disorder, versus the state of altered brain functioning resulting from the eating disorder (including malnutrition). Insights from this line of research will assist with early detection and prevention as well as the development of potential drug targets for treatment. While it is clear that biological factors both contribute to the development of the eating disorder and result from the associated behaviors (namely, starvation and binging), the collective environment also plays an important role. Sociocultural factors that may facilitate the development of eating disorders in predisposed individuals include dieting, pressure to conform to an ideal weight/shape, media images, poor body image, peer pressure, and family/parental modeling.

## CLINICAL MANIFESTATIONS

An eating disorder should be suspected any time an adolescent loses significant weight, fails to gain appropriate weight, or develops food avoidance. The other general physical findings that an eating disordered patient may present with are shown in Table 76-6. Most of these physical findings and many of the initial alterations in cognitive functioning are related to the degree of malnutrition, while some result from purging behaviors. Since AN is often characterized by weight loss, other diagnoses such as diabetes mellitus should be ruled out. A diagnosis of BN requires consideration of additional medical conditions, including a range of gastrointestinal illnesses (eg, gastroesophageal reflux disease, gall bladder disease, ulcers).

The complications of eating disorders affect multiple biological systems, as shown in Table 76-7. For AN and restrictive eating disorders, complications are related to the degree of malnutrition; for BN or binge-purge AN, complications often arise from purging behavior. One acute complication that may emerge during treatment of a malnourished patient is refeeding syndrome. Refeeding syndrome describes the life-threatening electrolyte shifts that can occur when nutrition is reintroduced. In response to carbohydrate and protein feeding, insulin is released and facilitates the transport of nutrients into cells for metabolism. Electrolytes are drawn with the nutrients from the extracellular to the intracellular space, causing a shift in fluids and electrolytes. Dramatic changes in phosphorous, potassium, magnesium, and sodium can result in cardiac arrhythmias, breakdown of muscle, edema, delirium, and death. Thus, severely malnourished patients should be refed under close surveillance in a hospital to monitor for signs of refeeding syndrome.

| TABLE 76-6 GENERAL PHYSICAL FINDINGS IN THE EATING DISORDERED PATIENT |
|---|
| Hypothermia, complaints of feeling cold |
| Fatigue, weakness |
| Dizziness |
| Weight loss, lack of expected weight gain, or major weight fluctuations |
| Stunted height (if anorexia develops prior to the completion of the growth; this may be more common in males with anorexia, as their growth period is longer) |
| Delayed puberty |
| Oligo- or amenorrhea |
| Lanugo |
| Hair loss |
| Brittle hair and nails |
| Acrocyanosis |
| Edema, particularly lower extremity[a] |
| Tooth decay[a] |
| Gingivitis[a] |
| Russell's sign: calluses on the back of the hand secondary to abrasions from the teeth when the fingers are used to induce vomiting[a] |
| Swelling of the face and cheeks, including the lower eyelids, due to increased pressure of blood in the face during vomiting[a] |
| Enlargement of the salivary glands[a] |
| Dental erosions, tooth decay, and gingivitis[a] |
| Chest pain and heartburn[a] |
| Diarrhea, sometimes bloody, from laxative abuse[a] |

[a]More common in patients with BN (see Table 76-2) or AN-purging subtype (see Table 76-1).

## DIAGNOSIS

The diagnosis of an eating disorder is based on the clinical criteria established by the American Psychiatric Association and outlined earlier in the chapter and in Tables 76-1 to 76-5. The differential diagnosis for an eating disorder is shown in Table 76-8. Obtaining a complete history from the patient and the family is critical for establishing a diagnosis (Table 76-9). Physical evaluation of a patient suspected of an eating disorder includes determination of degree of malnutrition. In order to do this, measurement of height and weight, calculation of BMI, and plotting of these variables on gender-specific curves is necessary. These data points should be compared to prior growth history, if that information is available, to assess changes. If growth is normal, points should follow a curve that remains roughly within the same percentiles. In addition, comparing these points to reference populations using percent median BMI and amount of rate of weight loss can assist in determining degree of malnutrition. Lack of expected weight gain can be an early warning sign of malnutrition, while lack of expected height gain reflects longer-term malnutrition. Obtaining vital signs, including heart rate, blood pressure, and orthostatic changes, is necessary to determine the severity of malnutrition. Laboratory testing, including a comprehensive metabolic panel, a complete blood count, a pregnancy test, an erythrocyte sedimentation rate, liver function tests, thyroid hormone levels, and celiac screen may be needed at the time of assessment to help clarify a diagnosis. In patients with restricting-type anorexia, laboratory values are often normal, while in patients with purging, electrolyte changes such as significant hypokalemia can be seen. Further evaluation may include an electrocardiogram, particularly to look for arrhythmias and a prolonged QT interval.

## TREATMENT

The Society for Adolescent Health and Medicine (SAHM) highlights the needs for a multidisciplinary team knowledgeable in the care of patients with eating disorders. The team should include (1) a physician who can monitor weight, vital signs, and other consequences of malnutrition; (2) a nutritionist who can assist with meal planning and

**TABLE 76-7 COMPLICATIONS OF EATING DISORDERS, BY AFFECTED SYSTEM**

Fluids and electrolytes:
1. Dehydration
2. Hypokalemia, hypoglycemia, hypophosphatemia, hypomagnesemia
3. Hyponatremia, often due to water loading
4. Edema in hands and feet
5. Muscle cramping

Cardiovascular:
1. Hypotension
2. Orthostatic changes
3. Arrhythmias, bradycardia, prolonged QT
4. Mitral valve prolapse
5. Pericardial effusions
6. Enlargement and damage to the muscle of the heart secondary to the use of ipecac[a]

Skeletal: osteopenia, increased fracture risk

Laboratory values:
1. Anemia due to deficiency of iron, folate, and/or vitamin $B_{12}$
2. Low white blood cell count
3. Elevated liver function tests
4. Elevated amylase[a]

Gastrointestinal system:
1. Nausea
2. Constipation and abdominal bloating
3. Gastroesophageal reflux
4. Esophageal tear (due to persistent vomiting)[a]
5. Delayed gastric emptying
6. Swelling of the salivary glands (due to vomiting)[a]
7. Gastric dilatation and perforation[a]
8. Bloody diarrhea[a]

Endocrine:
1. Amenorrhea
2. Sick euthyroid syndrome
3. High cortisol levels
4. High cholesterol levels
5. Low testosterone levels (in males) leading to decreased libido

Respiratory
1. Aspiration pneumonia secondary to vomiting[a]
2. Pneumomediastinum, pneumothorax secondary to vomiting[a]

Brain
1. Delayed cognition

Psychological and behavioral:
1. Distortion in body shape and size
2. Anxiety, including obsessive behavior particularly around food
3. Depressive symptoms
4. Strict rituals around meal times and involving food
5. Social isolation particularly around meals, including avoiding meals with family and friends
6. Substance abuse[a]
7. Lack of impulse control, including cutting, shoplifting, stealing, and other risky behaviors[a]
8. Overly concerned with food, weight, and body shape
9. Eating in secret, hoarding and hiding of food

[a]More common in BN or anorexia purging subtype due to purging.

weight restoration; and (3) a therapist who is knowledgeable about treating eating disorders.

Returning to normal or healthy eating patterns is a goal for all patients, even for those who do not need to gain weight. Patients should be encouraged to consume regular meals and snacks throughout the day. A registered dietitian (RD) can educate parents and work with the therapy team to support the refeeding phase. In young adults or other youth living apart from parents, an RD may work directly with the patient to assist in developing meal plans and/or setting dietary calories, outlining healthy patterns such as increased variety or decreased food phobias.

Other important aspects of treatment for bulimia include regular moderate physical activity and dental care, as recurrent self-induced vomiting may cause dental erosions and caries. Meal skipping should be discouraged, and certain foods might be avoided because these may trigger subsequent binging or purging. Setting realistic weight goals may also be important.

Patients who are failing outpatient treatment may require a higher level of care, including intensive outpatient or partial hospitalization

**TABLE 76-8 DIFFERENTIAL DIAGNOSIS FOR EATING DISORDERS**

| |
|---|
| Pregnancy |
| Inflammatory bowel disease |
| Malabsorptive conditions, including celiac disease |
| Diabetes mellitus |
| Hyperthyroidism |
| Collagen vascular disease |
| Cancer and central nervous system tumors |
| Chronic infections such as tuberculosis and human immunodeficiency virus (HIV) |
| Obsessive-compulsive disorder |
| Anxiety disorders |
| Mood disorders |
| Psychosis |
| Substance abuse |

**TABLE 76-9 SCREENING AND HISTORY QUESTIONS WHEN AN EATING DISORDER IS SUSPECTED**

| |
|---|
| **Body Image History** |
| How do you feel about how you look? |
| How do your feelings about how you look/your body affect how you feel? |
| **Weight History** |
| How do you feel about your weight? |
| What is the most you ever weighed? How tall were you then? When was that? |
| What is the least you ever weighed since menarche? In the past year? How tall were you then? When was that? |
| How often do you weigh yourself? |
| What do you think you ought to weigh? |
| **Exercise History** |
| How often do you exercise? For how long? At what level of intensity? |
| How stressed are you if you miss a workout? |
| **Dietary Practice History** |
| What have you eaten in the last 24 hours? |
| Do you feel full after just starting to eat? |
| Do you skip meals? How often? |
| Do you count calories? Do you count fat grams? Do you have any taboo foods (foods you strictly avoid)? |
| Do you have any meal rituals? A set breakfast or lunch? |
| Do you frequently eat in secret or by yourself? |
| Do you have a history of any binging? How often? What types of foods? Are there any triggers to your binges? |
| Do you ever make yourself vomit? How often? Do you use laxatives or diet pills? |
| How much time do you spend thinking about food? Does it impact your concentration or other activities? |
| **Mental Health History** |
| Have you ever received therapy? Was it useful? |
| History of physical or sexual abuse |
| History of self-injurious behavior, eg, cutting |
| Use of cigarettes, drugs, or alcohol |
| **Family History** |
| Family history of obesity or eating disorders |
| Depression, substance abuse, suicide, or other mental illness |
| **Review of Systems** |
| Menstrual history |
| Gastrointestinal history, eg, history of constipation or diarrhea |

programs, or residential care programs. Hospitalization may be required as a first step for patients who are medically unstable. SAHM has published indications for hospitalization, including severe malnutrition, electrolyte disturbances, severe bradycardia or other cardiac dysrhythmias, orthostatic changes, acute food refusal, and uncontrollable binging and purging. Patients not meeting these criteria may still require close medical monitoring in the outpatient setting. For example, electrolytes should initially be monitored closely in patients who binge and purge, since purging-induced hypokalemia can lead to cardiac arrhythmias and sudden death.

For underweight patients, weight gain is crucial and the first few weeks of treatment appear to be critical in setting the long-term trajectory. In these cases, the early stages of both inpatient and outpatient treatment are largely focused on weight gain and may be referred to as the refeeding phase. For decades, refeeding was approached with extreme caution, using lower-calorie diets to avoid refeeding syndrome. Recently, clinical practice has begun shifting toward higher-calorie approaches since early weight gain has been identified as a predictor of full recovery. However, studies have yet to examine recovery rates using higher-calorie refeeding. Studies are also needed to define recovery goals in atypical AN and other cases where patients are not underweight. In addition to treating underlying deficiencies (such as iron and vitamin D), supplementation with a multivitamin is often recommended to maximize nutritional recovery. For those with low bone mineral density, 1300 mg calcium and 600 IU vitamin D are recommended.

Psychotherapy is crucial for full recovery from eating disorders. Patients may recover weight and other physiologic parameters (such as regular menses) but continue to have significant eating disorder cognitions. For adolescents with AN, family-based treatment (FBT) is now considered the first-line treatment. There is also evidence that FBT is efficacious for adolescents and young adults with BN. The first phase of FBT is focused on refeeding for weight restoration and enlists parents to take control of feeding. Studies show that 1.5 to 2 pounds of weight gain per week in the first 4 weeks of therapy predicts recovery at 1 year. This therapy is initiated in the outpatient setting once patients are medically stable. Cognitive behavioral therapy may be used in patients with BN and patients with AN who are young adults and/or living separately from parents. Initial therapeutic goals for BN are to break the binge/purge cycle and address co-occurring depression, substance abuse, and the tremendous shame that is often associated with the illness.

Patients with eating disorders have high rates of psychiatric comorbidities. Depression and anxiety most commonly co-occur in AN. There is a paucity of studies examining the benefits of psychotropic medication in patients with AN, including antidepressants and atypical neuroleptic medications. Antidepressant medications, particularly selective serotonin reuptake inhibitors (SSRIs), may be beneficial in treating coexisting symptoms of depression or obsessive-compulsive disorder, but have not been shown to be useful for AN. Malnutrition and chronic binging and purging may worsen symptoms of anxiety, depression, and obsessive behavior. If symptoms persist following weight restoration, medications may be more effective in treating those symptoms. For those with BN, SSRIs have demonstrated efficacy. It is important to reevaluate symptoms throughout the treatment and recovery process.

Recovery is typically defined at 1 year as a combination of weight restoration, cognitive recovery, and resumption of menses. Treatment outcomes are generally better in adolescents with eating disorders than in adults, possibly due to a shorter duration of illness. AN is recognized as a common and costly illness in adolescence because it requires intensive treatment and yet carries low recovery rates. Rates of clinical remission at 1 year are less than 50%, despite advances in treatment. The mortality rate in AN is 5%, which is the highest among all psychiatric diagnoses. The leading causes of death in patients with AN are suicide or medical complications of malnutrition/starvation. Mortality rates for BN are significantly lower. Good prognostic indicators for AN include adequate weight gain during the first several weeks of treatment; early identification and entry into treatment; short duration of symptoms; age less than 14; AN restricting subtype, rather than the binge/purge subtype; and no other mental health disorder (such as depression, anxiety, or substance abuse). Rates of recovery for BN are significantly higher than for AN. However, the course of recovery for all of the eating disorders can be long and marked by relapse: 43% of patients with AN will relapse in the first year after initial hospitalization. Currently, there is no evidence-based treatment for ARFID; however, clinically, exposure response prevention therapy is often used (similar to treatment for obsessive-compulsive disorder or simple phobias).

## PREVENTION

As discussed above, youth with disordered eating are at high risk for the development of a diagnosable eating disorder. The keys to successful treatment of eating disorders are early recognition of the problem and early intervention. Thus, primary prevention in the clinical setting must include screening for disordered eating or dieting behavior. Longitudinal studies have established dieting as a risk factor for both eventual weight gain and the development of an eating disorder. Therefore, practitioners should discourage unhealthy dieting practices while still striving to promote healthy habits in a society where a large proportion of the pediatric population in struggling with overweight. This requires a thoughtful and coordinated approach by all team members. For example, children and adolescents should be weighed at every medical appointment or at a minimum once a year to look for weight loss or growth failure, which are red flags for the development of an eating disorder. However, weighing at the start of the clinic visit can be stress- and shame-inducing for many adolescents and may undermine the goal of instituting healthy behavior changes. Therefore, clinical strategies such as blinded weights may be useful to shift the focus of the visit from weight to healthy behaviors. Outside of the clinic, peers, parents, and media are part of the collective environmental exposure that may trigger the onset of an eating disorder in those who are predisposed. Schools, communities, clinicians, and families can work to prevent eating disorders by promoting healthy eating and physical activity habits over weight or body shape. This can be accomplished by modeling healthy habits, avoiding diets and negative comments about body weight and shape, encouraging family meals, and exercising regularly. Media exposure including "pro-ana" Web sites that promote AN behaviors can be limited by parents and/or filtered with proper supervision in the home and clinic setting, where magazines and images depicting healthy body types can be selected.

## SUGGESTED READINGS


American Psychiatric Association. *Diagnostic and Statistical Manual of Mental Disorders*. 5th ed. Arlington, VA: American Psychiatric Association Publishing; 2013.

Bulik CM, Sullivan PF, Tozzi F, et al. Prevalence, heritability, and prospective risk factors for anorexia nervosa. *Arch Gen Psychiatry*. 2006;63(3):305-312.

Dold M, Aigner M, Klabunde M, Treasure J, Kasper S. Second-generation antipsychotic drugs in anorexia nervosa: a meta-analysis of randomized control trials. *Psychother Psychosom*. 2015;84:110-116.

Frank GK, Kaye WH. Current status of functional imaging in eating disorders. *Int J Eat Disord*. 2012;45(6):723-736.

Garber AK, Sawyer SM, Golden NH, et al. A systematic review of approaches to refeeding in patients with anorexia nervosa. *Int J Eat Disord*. 2016;49(3):293-310.

Golden NH, Katzman DK, Sawyer SM, et al. Update on the medical management of eating disorders in adolescents. *J Adolesc Health*. 2015;56(4):370-375.

Neumark-Sztainer D, Wall M, Eisenberg ME, et al. Overweight status and weight control behaviors in adolescents: longitudinal and secular trends from 1999 to 2004. *Prev Med*. 2006;43(1):52-59.

Norris ML, Spettigue WJ, Katzman DK. Update on eating disorders: current perspectives on avoidant/restrictive food intake disorder in children and youth. *Neuropsychiatr Dis Treat.* 2016;12: 213-218.

Society for Adolescent Health and Medicine; Golden NH, Katzman DK, Sawyer SM, et al. Position paper of the Society for Adolescent Health and Medicine: medical management of restrictive eating disorders in adolescents and young adults. *J Adolesc Health.* 2015; 56(1):121-125.

Swanson SA, Crow SJ, Le Grange D, Swendsen J, Merikangas KR. Prevalence and correlates of eating disorders in adolescents: results from the National Comorbidity Survey Replication Adolescent Supplement. *Arch Gen Psychiatry.* 2011;68(7):714-723.

Zerwas S, Bulik CM. Genetics and epigenetics of eating disorders. *Psychiatr Ann.* 2011;41(11):532-538.



# PART 4 REPRODUCTIVE HEALTH PROBLEMS

## 77 Breast Masses

Heather E. Needham and Jennifer C. Edman

The normal anatomy of the breast is shown in Figure 77-1. A variety of benign breast lesions occur in the female adolescent. The most typical presentation is a self-detected, asymptomatic mass. Complaints such as bloody discharge, nipple retraction, or skin dimpling are rare.

### ANATOMIC CHANGES AND CONGENITAL ABNORMALITIES

Breast asymmetry, a common condition in which one breast develops earlier or grows more rapidly than the other, usually occurs between sexual maturity rating (SMR) 2 and 4 and persists into adulthood in 25% of women. It is important to consider the age of the patient when assessing the etiology of a breast mass or enlargement. Normal thelarche usually occurs between 8 and 13 years of age. Rare congenital abnormalities of the breast include amastia (absent breast, associated with chest wall deformities such as pectus excavatum or Poland syndrome) and athelia (absent nipple). Polymastia (accessory breast tissue) and polythelia (accessory nipples) occur along the mammalian nipple line in 1% to 2% of girls and may be inheritable conditions. Breast atrophy developing after thelarche can be one sign of an eating disorder or other chronic illness such as scleroderma. The associated loss of both fat and glandular tissue in the breast results from significant weight loss. Virginal (juvenile) hypertrophy, the massive enlargement of one or both breasts caused by either increased tissue sensitivity to pubertal hormones or endogenous production of hormones from within breast cells, can be associated with a variety of problems, including headache, neck and back pain, dermatitis, embarrassment, and psychological difficulties. Reduction mammoplasty after completion of breast maturation may be indicated in female adolescents with severe virginal hypertrophy.

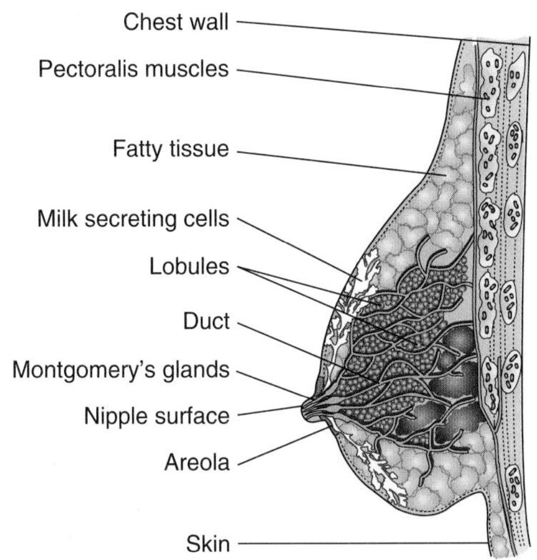


**FIGURE 77-1** Breast anatomy.

### CYSTS, FIBROCYSTIC CHANGE, AND FIBROADENOMAS

The most common breast masses in adolescents are solitary cysts, fibrocystic change, and fibroadenomas. Masses resulting from inflammation or trauma occur less frequently. Cancer is rare among female adolescents. A solitary cyst contains sterile fluid. Over half resolve spontaneously within 2 to 3 months, so fine-needle aspiration or biopsy is often unnecessary. Recurrent or multiple cysts in the adolescent may represent early fibrocystic change.

Fibrocystic change (benign proliferative breast change) is a physiological response of breast tissue to cyclic hormonal activity. The result is a dilation and proliferation of duct epithelium to form gross cysts. A benign condition more common during the third and fourth decades, fibrocystic change may occur during adolescence. Bilateral breast pain in the upper outer quadrants beginning in the premenstrual phase of the menstrual cycle and subsiding thereafter is the typical presentation. Adolescents tend to have dense breast tissue. Physical examination reveals areas of diffuse, cordlike thickening as well as discrete mobile lesions, which often increase in size during the premenstrual period. Supportive care, including nonsteroidal anti-inflammatory agents for pain and a well-fitting supportive bra, is the most common approach to treatment. Oral contraceptives reduce symptoms in 70% to 90% of cases.

The majority (70–90%) of adolescent breast masses that undergo biopsy are identified as fibroadenomas, which can be classified as simple fibroadenomas, juvenile fibroadenomas, and phyllodes tumor. A fibroadenoma is a benign proliferation of stromal elements, ducts, and acini. Physical examination reveals a rubbery, painless, well-demarcated mass, 1 to 3 cm in size, usually located in the upper outer quadrant of the breast. Fibroadenomas may regress spontaneously but usually persist and may require excisional biopsy. Peak incidence occurs during late adolescence, but fibroadenomas may present up to 2 years before menarche. Multiple and recurrent fibroadenomas may occur, but malignant potential has not been established.

Juvenile fibroadenoma, a histologically similar lesion but with less well-defined edges, presents as a rapidly enlarging breast mass that can reach immense proportions. Giant fibroadenomas are defined as being > 5 cm, and are found most commonly in young African American women. Complete excision is curative.

Phyllodes tumors are rare. These tumors are rapidly growing lesions that are usually large, are well demarcated, and have a small potential for malignancy. The large phyllodes tumor may cause overlying skin to become stretched and shiny with distended veins, erythema, and even ulceration. Intraductal papilloma, a slow-growing benign tumor located under the areola, often presents with a serous or bloody nipple discharge.

### BREAST CANCER

Primary breast cancer is rare in teenagers. Only 0.2% to 2% of all breast cancers occur before 25 years of age. The data from the Surveillance, Epidemiology, and End Results (SEER) Program of the National Cancer Institute (2009–2013) had 0% new cases for women < 20 years, and 1.8% of new cases in women 20 to 34 years of age. More than 60% of breast cancers in adolescents are not primary breast tumors but arise metastatically from distant sites (eg, lymphoma) or locally from nonbreast tissue (eg, angiosarcomas). Cancer, in contrast to benign breast disease, is characterized by a hard, fixed mass beneath the nipple. Approximately one-third to one-half of breast cancer cases have a positive family history. Only a small fraction of breast cancers (5–9%) are associated with breast cancer–associated genes (*BRCA1* or *BRCA2*). Risk factors for the development of adult breast cancer established during adolescence include menarche before age 12 years and cancer treatment–related radiation in the breast area (eg, for lymphoma). There is no clear association between use of oral contraceptives and later development of breast adenocarcinoma.

## OTHER BREAST MASSES

A contusion may present as a poorly defined tender mass, with or without overlying hematoma. Less than half of patients will give a history of antecedent trauma. Contusions usually resolve over several weeks but may persist for several months. Occasionally, scar tissue or fat necrosis develops, resulting in small areas of calcification. Treatment consists of local excision. Trauma may also draw attention to a preexisting lesion unrelated to the injury.

Mastitis, or breast infection, presents with the rapid onset of unilateral pain and localized inflammation. Infection is more common in newborns and lactating women but can occur in adolescents secondary to trauma, nipple piercing, ductal abnormalities, or reduced immune defenses. *Staphylococcus aureus* is the most common etiologic organism. The initial management of mastitis includes systemic antibiotics, warm compresses, and analgesia. Acute mastitis may lead to fluctuance and abscess formation. Circumareolar incision and drainage is then indicated. Abscess formation must be considered with persistent, unresponsive mastitis.

## ASSESSMENT

When assessing a breast mass, the history should identify previous trauma, fever, weight loss, nipple discharge, and medications. A family history of breast disease and the nature of any previous lesions should be obtained. A menstrual history of cyclic pain can be helpful in diagnosing fibrocystic changes. The history often elicits the use of oral contraceptive pills or other hormonal agents that can alter the breast. The physical examination includes assessment of SMR to avoid confusing the normal breast bud (especially if unilateral) with an abnormal mass. The size, location, and characteristics of the lesion should be described. Tenderness, warmth, and lymphadenopathy are consistent with infection. A hard, fixed lesion with overlying skin changes must be evaluated for cancer. Prolactin, thyroid, and gonadotropin levels are obtained to evaluate the symptom of galactorrhea.

Management of a suspected benign breast mass in an adolescent begins with reassurance and an observation period of 1 to 3 months. During this time, any change that occurs with the menstrual cycle should be noted. Masses that persist beyond this time should be referred for further evaluation. Fine-needle aspiration will distinguish a cystic from a solid lesion. Any aspirate obtained should undergo cytologic evaluation. A cyst will collapse after aspiration, yielding a clear yellow or brownish fluid, and the breast should be reexamined in 3 months. Breast core biopsy is a newer method to obtain tissue diagnosis. Excisional biopsy is indicated for a large solid or growing mass or one that yields an abnormal aspirate. The purpose of excision is to obtain a definitive diagnosis, avoid cosmetic deformity, and alleviate patient anxiety. Normal breast tissue can be spared because there is no need to remove a wide margin.

Mammography is rarely indicated in the evaluation of a palpable mass in an adolescent. The normally dense parenchymal tissue in the adolescent breast makes interpretation difficult. Mammography is not indicated for screening in this age group because of the low prevalence of malignancy. Ultrasonography is useful to differentiate between solid and cystic masses and to guide the fine-needle aspiration.

The value of teaching breast self-examination (BSE) to adolescents remains controversial. There is a lack of evidence of the benefits of a breast exam. The American Cancer Society's current recommendation is that "regular clinical breast exam and breast self-exam are not recommended." Some professionals argue that routine BSE in adolescents creates unnecessary anxiety and serves to identify a greater number of benign lesions. Teaching modified BSE may be a valuable educational component in the routine physical examination of the adolescent by leading to a discussion of normal development.

## ADOLESCENT GYNECOMASTIA

Pubertal gynecomastia, the glandular enlargement of breast tissue in males, is a common complaint (see Fig. 77-1). Gynecomastia, which occurs transiently in 40% to 60% of 10- to 16-year-old boys and peaks in incidence at SMR 2 to SMR 4 (age 14 years), results from a decreased ratio of androgen to estrogen and a change in end-organ receptor sensitivity. The breast tissue is frequently firm, tender, and often asymmetric. Spontaneous resolution occurs in 90% of boys within 2 years. Rare causes of gynecomastia include endogenous states of estrogen excess, such as testicular, adrenal, or pituitary tumors; hyperthyroidism and hypothyroidism; hepatic disorders; refeeding poststarvation; endogenous androgen deficiency states such as hypogonadism, Klinefelter syndrome, renal hemodialysis, and congenital adrenal hyperplasia; and specific drugs, including estrogen, testosterone, anabolic steroids, human chorionic gonadotropins, tricyclic antidepressants, insulin, alcohol, marijuana, amphetamines, methadone, cimetidine, digitalis, and cytotoxic agents, among others. Pseudogynecomastia (fatty tissue or muscle development), frequently confused with true gynecomastia (glandular enlargement), can be distinguished by comparing the consistency of the breast tissue with that of adipose tissue in the anterior axillary fold.

Diagnosis of gynecomastia is based on the typical history and examination and the exclusion of other causes of gynecomastia. The history includes a review of current medications and illicit drug use (eg, marijuana use has been associated with gynecomastia). Physical assessment should describe the SMR and findings of the testicular examination as well as the amount and quality of breast tissue present. If glandular tissue is less than 4 cm (eg, SMR 2–3 female breast), reassurance is the most appropriate treatment. In contrast, pubertal macrogynecomastia resembles female SMR 3 to SMR 5 breasts, extends more than 5 cm, and usually does not regress spontaneously. A surgical referral is indicated when pubertal gynecomastia has a prolonged course (> 2 years), when it causes psychological impairment, or if macrogynecomastia is present. Medications such as danazol, tamoxifen, and testolactone are not generally recommended for adolescents because of their side-effect profiles, lack of documented efficacy, and frequent return of breast tissue after the drug is discontinued.

## SUGGESTED READINGS


Amin AL, Purdy AC, Mattingly JD, Kong AL. Benign breast disease. *Surg Clin North Am.* 2013;93(2):299-308.

Breast cancer prevention and early detection. American Cancer Society Web site. http://www.cancer.org/cancer/breastcancer/moreinformation/breastcancerearlydetection/breast-cancer-early-detection-acs-recs. Published October 9, 2015. Revised October 20, 2015. Accessed June 20, 2016.

Dimitrakakis C, Tsigginou A, Zagouri F, et al. Breast cancer in women aged 25 years and younger. *Obstet Gynecol.* 2013;121(6):1235-1240.

DiVasta AD, Weldon C, Labow BI. The breast: examination and lesions. In: Emans SJ, Laufer MR, eds. *Pediatric and Adolescent Gynecology*. 6th ed. Philadelphia, PA: Lippincott, Williams & Wilkins; 2012:405-420.

Ladizinski B, Lee KC, Nutan FN, Higgins HW 2nd, Federman DG. Gyencomastia: etiologies, clinical presentations, diagnosis, and management. *South Med J.* 2014;107(1):44-49.

Lee M, Soltanian HT. Breast fibroadenomas in adolescents: current perspectives. *Adolesc Health Med Ther.* 2015;6:159-163.

Michala L, Tsigginou A, Zacharakis D, Dimitrakakis C. Breast disorders in girls and adolescents. Is there a need for a specialized service? *J Pediatr Adolesc Gynecol.* 2015;28:91-94.

# 78 Scrotal Masses

M. Brett Cooper and Mariam R. Chacko

## TESTICULAR TORSION

Testicular torsion is a surgical emergency, and clinicians caring for adolescent males must have a high index of suspicion given the short window for salvage of the testicle.

### ETIOLOGY

The exact etiology of torsion is unknown. However, the most common testicular anatomical abnormality, called the "bell clapper" deformity, can predispose to testicular torsion (Fig. 78-1). In this deformity, the tunica vaginalis completely surrounds the testicle, including the posterior aspect, and the absence of the normal posterior anchoring at the gubernaculum testis allows the testicle to twist freely.

### CLINICAL MANIFESTATIONS AND DIAGNOSIS

Common presentation includes abrupt onset of severe scrotal pain with associated nausea, vomiting, fever, and abdominal pain. Symptomatic males may describe prior transient episodes of scrotal pain consistent with intermittent torsion/detorsion. Typically, the adolescent presents later in the course with a scrotum that is swollen, tender, erythematous, and often difficult to examine. The cremasteric reflex is nearly always absent. Prehn's sign (ie, lessening of pain with scrotal elevation) had been used in the past to differentiate torsion from epididymitis, but it has since been found to be inferior to ultrasound. Diagnosis can be made on physical examination or with the assistance of color Doppler ultrasound, which has a sensitivity of 100% and a specificity of 75% (Fig. 78-2).

### TREATMENT

Treatment involves prompt surgical exploration and detorsion. Time is of the essence because testicular viability declines to 0 after 24 hours. Given the high incidence of retorsion, as well as torsion of the contralateral testis, the affected testis and the contralateral testis are fixed to the scrotum in a procedure called scrotal orchiopexy.

## TORSION OF TESTICULAR OR EPIDIDYMAL APPENDAGE

### ETIOLOGY

Both the testis and the epididymis have appendages (Fig. 78-3) that are remnants of the wolffian and müllerian ducts, respectively. The pedunculated shape of the appendages predisposes them to torsion.

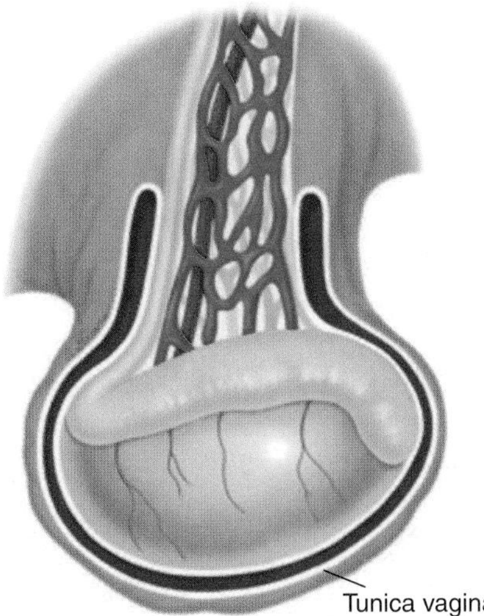


**FIGURE 78-1** Bell clapper deformity.

### CLINICAL PRESENTATION

The typical presentation of appendiceal torsion occurs in boys ages 7 to 12 years and includes pain that may be accompanied by nausea and vomiting. Palpation of the testis reveals tenderness over the superior or inferior pole of the testes with or without a palpable mass. The cremasteric reflex is usually present. The classic "blue dot" sign, if present, represents the infarcted appendage viewed through the scrotal skin.

### DIAGNOSIS

The diagnosis is usually made by clinical examination. If torsion of the testis cannot be ruled out, a color flow Doppler examination is indicated. Blood flow will be normal in appendiceal torsion.

### TREATMENT

Treatment is usually supportive, including analgesics, nonsteroidal anti-inflammatory drugs (NSAIDs), and scrotal elevation. If pain persists for longer than 5 days, consultation by a pediatric urologist is recommended.

## TRAUMA

Trauma may be a cause of pain and swelling of the scrotum. When the presentation includes an overlying hematocele, surgical exploration and repair may be required for testicular salvage.

## HYDROCELE

### ETIOLOGY

Hydroceles are related to congenital abnormalities in the inguinal canal. Communicating hydroceles develop when fluid tracks down the inguinal canal into the tunica vaginalis. Hydroceles may also form from trauma, infection (eg, epididymitis and orchitis), testicular torsion, or tumors.

### CLINICAL PRESENTATION AND DIAGNOSIS

Hydroceles are usually painless on exam. Communicating hydroceles may shift in size when the patient is upright or performs a Valsalva maneuver, whereas noncommunicating hydroceles will not. In most patients, a hydrocele will transilluminate, showing the presence of fluid. When palpated, it may feel like a supple, fluid-filled cyst.

### TREATMENT

Hydroceles are corrected electively, if at all. They are corrected if the patient is symptomatic with pain and/or pressure. Correcting the underlying cause of the hydrocele usually causes resolution.

## SPERMATOCELE

Spermatocele refers to the accumulation of sperm within the head of the epididymis (Fig. 78-4). Spermatoceles, which are benign cysts, are commonly found on routine physical examination or by the adolescent himself and usually do not require intervention unless symptomatic. On palpation, they are predominantly smooth, soft, well circumscribed, and found on the superior aspect of the testicle. They generally range in size from 2 to 5 cm. In addition, these cystic lesions may transilluminate. A spermatocele is corrected if the patient is symptomatic with pain and/or pressure.

## ORCHITIS

### ETIOLOGY

Orchitis rarely occurs in prepubertal males. The mumps virus is the most common cause of orchitis, but other viruses have been implicated (eg, coxsackievirus, echovirus, adenovirus, varicella).

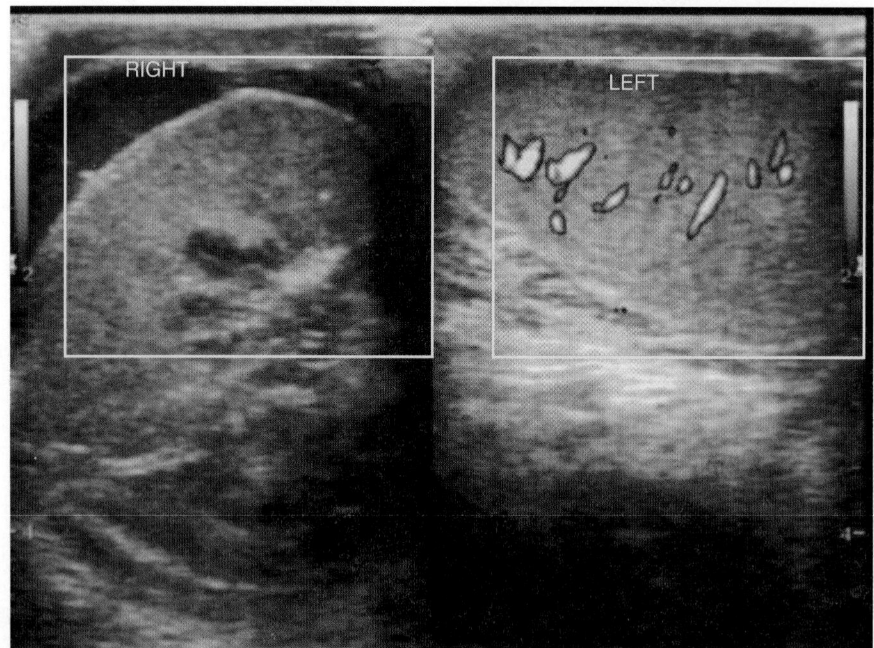


**FIGURE 78-2** Abnormal testicular ultrasound.

Bacterial orchitis is usually a consequence of contiguous spread from an epididymal infection. Mumps orchitis usually follows parotitis by about 4 to 8 days, but presentation up to 6 weeks later has been reported. In contrast, symptoms with other viruses occur commensurate with the other viral symptoms. There is also some evidence that these viruses cause post-viral inflammatory changes in the testicle.

### CLINICAL PRESENTATION AND DIAGNOSIS

The typical presentation includes edema, erythema, and tenderness of the testicle and may be associated with constitutional symptoms (eg, fever, nausea, lower abdominal pain). It is most often unilateral. The diagnosis is usually made by clinical examination.

### TREATMENT

Viral orchitis is treated supportively with rest and NSAIDs. Bacterial orchitis is treated with antibiotics and supportive care. Infertility is a rare complication of orchitis and most often results after bilateral cases.

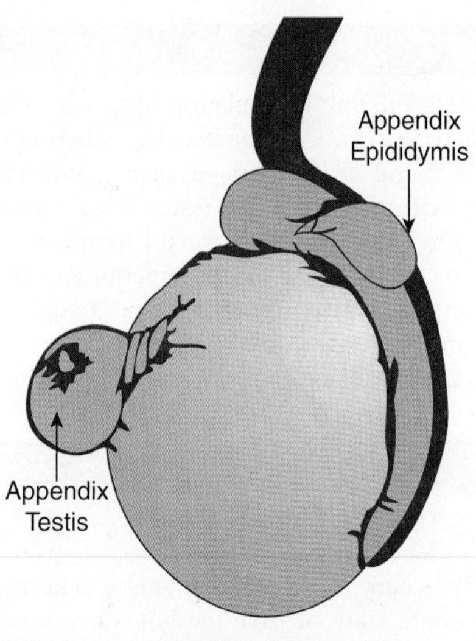


**FIGURE 78-3** Testicular and epididymal appendage.

## VARICOCELES

### ETIOLOGY

A varicocele is a dilatation of the pampiniform venous plexus within the scrotum. There are several theories as to the etiology of varicoceles. One theory involves the presence of incompetent valves within the veins along the spermatic cord, resulting in the backup of blood. Another theory is the "nutcracker effect," wherein the left renal vein is compressed between the aorta and superior mesenteric artery, resulting in an increase in pressure, which is then transmitted to the left testicular vein due to its right angle insertion. Support for this theory includes the fact that 85% to 95% of varicoceles are left-sided. Right-sided varicoceles can be associated with tumors and should always be investigated further using Doppler ultrasound to evaluate for inferior vena cava (IVC) obstruction. Varicoceles most often appear beginning at puberty. This is due to rapid growth of the testicles, with subsequent increased blood flow.

### CLINICAL PRESENTATION AND DIAGNOSIS

Varicoceles are usually asymptomatic in adolescents but occasionally may cause a dull ache after long periods of standing.

The diagnosis is usually made by clinical examination. Varicoceles may be graded on physical examination. A grade I (small) varicocele

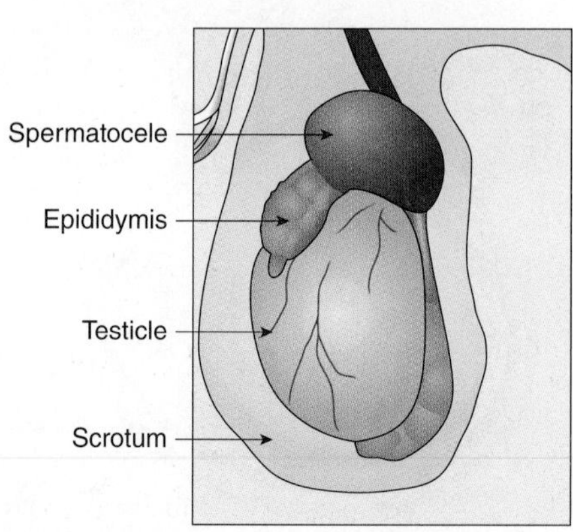


**FIGURE 78-4** Spermatocele.

is detectable only when the patient performs a Valsalva maneuver, a grade II (moderate) varicocele may be palpated while standing but is not visible on examination, and a grade III (large) varicocele is visible through the skin (ie, a "bag of worms").

### TREATMENT

The clinical relevance of asymptomatic varicoceles in adolescents is that they have been associated with both time-dependent testicular growth arrest and abnormal semen analyses in adolescents. Urologic referral to discuss surgical repair should be offered to adolescents with testicular growth arrest, bilateral varicoceles, and/or symptomatic (eg, painful) varicoceles, regardless of the grade of the varicocele. Semen analysis should be performed for all patients with high-grade varicoceles. However, there is no evidence that semen analysis is a direct correlate with future fertility when performed in adolescents.

## EPIDIDYMITIS

### ETIOLOGY

Epididymitis is an inflammatory disease of the epididymis. In prepubertal children, epididymitis may be caused by underlying genitourinary abnormalities, such as posterior urethral valves, ectopic ureters, and genitorectal fistulas. The causative organisms are often coliform bacteria, such as *Escherichia coli*. Among sexually active adolescents, most cases of epididymitis are attributed to the retrograde extension of *Chlamydia trachomatis* from the vas deferens; *Neisseria gonorrhoeae* is the second-most common organism.

### CLINICAL PRESENTATION

Patients may present with the gradual onset of scrotal pain and edema along with nausea, fever, abdominal or flank pain, and urethral discharge. On examination, the scrotum is often edematous and erythematous. Additionally, the epididymis is often tender to palpation. Fluctuance or fixation of the scrotal tissue around the epididymis is concerning for the presence of a scrotal abscess.

### DIAGNOSIS

The diagnosis is usually made by clinical examination. In contrast to testicular torsion, the cremasteric reflex should be intact and there should be a positive Prehn's sign. However, Prehn's sign has been found to be inferior to ultrasound to differentiate epididymitis from torsion.

### TREATMENT

Treatment includes appropriate antibiotic therapy for both the patient and his sexual partners. Patients who fail to improve during the initial 72 hours of outpatient management must be evaluated for the possibility of an abscess.

## TESTICULAR NEOPLASMS

### ETIOLOGY

According to the National Cancer Institute, testicular neoplasms represent the most common solid tumor in males age 15 to 34 years. Histologic types that occur most frequently in adolescence are germ cell tumors (95%) and include seminoma, embryonal carcinoma, teratoma, and choriocarcinoma. Leydig and Sertoli cell tumors are of stromal origin and may occur at any age, including adolescence.

### CLINICAL PRESENTATION

Patients often present with painless scrotal swelling of gradual onset. Adolescents with testicular cancer are more likely than other adolescents to have had cryptorchidism or testicular atrophy. Pain may be present if the tumor has hemorrhaged or become necrotic. When pain accompanies a tumor, it can lead to an erroneous diagnosis of an infectious or inflammatory process.

Physical examination usually reveals a firm, irregular mass that is opaque to transillumination, but cystic or necrotic areas of the tumor can be soft on palpation. Scrotal ultrasound may reveal intratesticular lesions. A hydrocele or varicocele may also be detected. The contralateral testis must be examined not only for comparison but also to rule out the presence of bilateral disease. The detection of cervical or supraclavicular lymph nodes may indicate an advanced stage of disease. Other possible findings include gynecomastia and breast tenderness. Because stromal tumors tend to produce androgens and/or estrogens, the prepubertal boy may present with early virilization, whereas the pubertal boy may present with feminization.

### DIAGNOSIS

Testicular tumor markers, most commonly beta human chorionic gonadotropin (hCG) and alpha-fetoprotein, are useful tests for certain histologic types and should be obtained before orchiectomy. The hCG level is elevated in choriocarcinoma, nonseminomatous mixed germ cell tumors, and seminoma with syncytiotrophoblasts. The alpha-fetoprotein level is elevated in nonseminomatous germ cell tumors, especially yolk sac tumors and embryonal carcinoma. However, these tumor markers should not be used for screening. Imaging of a scrotal mass is done using ultrasound or magnetic resonance imaging. Staging of a proven tumor requires chest and abdominal computed tomography.

### TREATMENT

Therapy is determined by staging and definitive histology and includes orchiectomy, retroperitoneal lymph node dissection, radiation, and chemotherapy. This results in an overall 5-year survival rate of more than 95%.

### SUGGESTED READINGS


Barbosa JA, Tiseo BC, Barayan GA, et al. Development and initial validation of a scoring system to diagnose testicular torsion in children. *J Urol.* 2013;189(5):1859-1864.

Blair RJ. Testicular and scrotal masses. *Pediatr Rev.* 2014;35(10):450-451.

Crawford P, Crop JA. Evaluation of scrotal masses. *Am Fam Physician*; 2014;89(9):723-727.

DaJusta DG, Granberg CF, Villanueva C, Baker LA. Contemporary review of testicular torsion: new concepts, emerging technologies and potential therapeutics technologies and potential therapeutics. *J Pediatr Urol.* 2013;9(6):723-730.

Diagnostic imaging pathways—scrotal mass. Department of Health, Government of Western Australia Web site. http://www.imaging-pathways.health.wa.gov.au/index.php/imaging-pathways/urological/scrotal-mass. Published August 2012. Accessed June 15, 2016.

Hameed A, White B, Chinegwundoh F, Thwaini A, Pahuja A. A review in management of testicular cancer: single center review. *World J Oncol.* 2011;2(3):94-101.

Montgomery JS, Bloom DA. Diagnosis and management of scrotal masses. *Med Clin North Am.* 2011;95(1):235-244.


# 79 Menstrual Problems

Sharonda Alston-Taylor, Sophie Remoue-Gonzales, and Jennifer C. Edman

Normal menstrual cycles during adolescence occur every 21 to 45 days, with duration of bleeding up to 7 days and blood loss of 20 to 60 mL (see Chapter 533). For those whose cycles are abnormal, the most common menstrual disorders in adolescents include amenorrhea, abnormal uterine bleeding, and dysmenorrhea, which are discussed in this chapter.

# AMENORRHEA

Amenorrhea, the absence of menses, can be either temporary or permanent. Traditionally, there are two categories: primary amenorrhea and secondary amenorrhea. Primary amenorrhea is defined as failure to menstruate either (1) by age 15 in the presence of breast development and normal growth, (2) within 3 years of thelarche, or (3) by age 13 with the absence of secondary sexual characteristics. Also, when delay in secondary sexual development and amenorrhea exists or cyclic pelvic pain accompanies primary amenorrhea, prompt evaluation should occur.

Secondary amenorrhea is cessation of menses for greater than 3 months or 90 days. While the etiologies of primary amenorrhea are typically genetic or anatomic, all causes of secondary amenorrhea may also present as primary amenorrhea. The evaluation of infrequent menses with cycle length longer than 6 weeks is the same as amenorrhea in this discussion. See Chapter 534 for further discussion on amenorrhea in the setting of delayed puberty.

## DIFFERENTIAL DIAGNOSIS

Do not overlook pregnancy, the most common cause of secondary amenorrhea, as a cause of primary amenorrhea. (See Chapter 80 for more information on the diagnosis of pregnancy.) Beyond pregnancy, the etiologies of primary and secondary amenorrhea include anatomic abnormalities or fall into three categories depending on the function of the pituitary gland in relation to the ovary: hypogonadotropic hypogonadism, hypergonadotropic hypogonadism, and eugonadotropic eugonadism. Another common classification system divides causes based on location of dysfunction within the hypothalamic–pituitary–adrenal (HPA) axis: hypothalamic, pituitary, ovarian, or other.

### Hypogonadotropic Hypogonadism

Hypogonadotropic hypogonadism indicates inadequate hypothalamic–pituitary stimulation of the ovary, and low levels of follicle-stimulating hormone (FSH), luteinizing hormone (LH), and estrogen characterize this state. Hypothalamic amenorrhea results from partial or complete inhibition of gonadotropin-releasing hormone (GnRH) release from the hypothalamus. See Table 79-1 for causes of amenorrhea characterized by hypogonadotropic hypogonadism. Excessive exercise and weight loss leading to amenorrhea may represent an eating disorder (see Chapter 76). Local lesions in the hypothalamus (eg, infiltrative processes, calcifications, gliomas, and germinomas), traumatic brain injury (TBI), and central nervous system radiation are all rare causes of GnRH deficiency. Isolated GnRH deficiency is associated with the absence (anosmia) or impairment (hyposmia) of the ability to smell (Kallman syndrome). Medications and illicit drugs may also result in amenorrhea.

Pituitary dysfunction and deficiencies or the inability to synthesize adequate amounts of gonadotropins may result from pituitary lesions, but panhypopituitarism and prolactinomas are more common. In panhypopituitarism, gonadotropin deficiency occurs before the development of changes in thyroid or adrenal function; isolated gonadotropin deficiency is rare.

The most common pituitary tumor causing amenorrhea is the prolactinoma. This type of tumor causes inhibition of the hypothalamic–pituitary–gonadal axis by secreting abnormally high levels of prolactin. Only 50% to 60% of females with adenomas have galactorrhea. The absence of galactorrhea does not eliminate suspicion for the tumor. Rarely, adenomas increase in size, causing symptoms such as vision change and headache associated with space-occupying lesions. Other causes of hyperprolactinemia include psychoactive drugs (eg, haloperidol, phenothiazines, amitriptyline, benzodiazepine, and cocaine), breastfeeding, and renal failure. Both hypercortisolism and hypothyroidism are associated with hyperprolactinemia and amenorrhea.

### Hypergonadotropic Hypogonadism

High levels of LH and FSH characterize hypergonadotropic hypogonadism. This ovarian dysfunction manifests clinically with menstrual irregularities. Such disorders include gonadal dysgenesis (abnormal ovarian development) and primary ovarian insufficiency (POI). There are multiple etiologies for POI (Table 79-1). Gonadal dysgenesis is

**TABLE 79-1 DIFFERENTIAL DIAGNOSES FOR PRIMARY AND SECONDARY AMENORRHEA, NEGATIVE PREGNANCY TEST**

| | Hypogonadotropic Hypogonadism | Hypergonadotropic Hypogonadism | Eugonadotropic Eugonadism |
|---|---|---|---|
| **Gonadotropin Levels** | Low FSH, normal/low LH, low estradiol | High FSH, normal/high LH | Normal FSH, LH, and estradiol |
| **Differential Diagnosis** | • Constitutional delay of puberty<br>• Chronic disease<br>  • Regional enteritis<br>  • Cystic fibrosis<br>  • Diabetes<br>• Anorexia nervosa/female athlete triad<br>  • Excessive exercise<br>• Stress<br>• Isolated GnRH deficiency (Kallaman Syndrome)<br>• Endocrinopathy<br>  • Hypothyroidism<br>  • CAH<br>  • Cushing disease<br>• Pituitary lesions<br>  • Craniopharyngiomas<br>  • Infiltrative processes<br>  • Infarction/Sheehan syndrome<br>• Pharmacologic agents/drugs<br>  • Contraceptives<br>  • Antiepileptics<br>  • SSRIs<br>  • Phenothiazine derivatives<br>  • Illicit (heroin, cocaine) | • Gonadal dysgenesis<br>• Primary ovarian insufficiency<br>  • Idiopathic<br>  • Infection<br>  • Hemorrhage<br>  • Compromised blood supply<br>  • Trauma<br>• Autoimmune<br>• Radiation<br>• Chemotherapy<br>• Turner syndrome (45,XO)<br>• Androgen insensitivity (46,XY)<br>• Abnormalities of ovarian FSH receptors<br>• Defects in estrogen biosynthesis | • Müllerian duct defects<br>• MRKH syndrome<br>• Uterine scarring<br>• PCOS<br>• Virilizing ovarian and adrenal tumors<br>• Pharmacologic agents/drugs |

CAH, congenital adrenal hyperplasia; FSH, follicle-stimulating hormone; GnRH, gonadotropin-releasing hormone; LH, luteinizing hormone; MRKH, Mayer-Rokitansky-Kuster-Hauser syndrome; PCOS, polycystic ovary syndrome; SSRIs, selective serotonin reuptake inhibitors.

seen in Turner syndrome (45,XO) (see Chapter 534) and fragile X, and in women with normal karyotype (46,XX) gonadal dysgenesis. Secondary amenorrhea is also associated with mosaic Turner syndrome.

Rarer causes of hypergonadotropic hypogonadal amenorrhea include pseudo-ovarian failure secondary to gonadotropin-resistant ovary syndrome (an abnormality of ovarian follicle-stimulating hormone receptors) and defects in estrogen biosynthesis, including 17-hydroxylase deficiency and 17-ketosteroid reductase deficiency. Late-onset congenital adrenal hyperplasia (CAH, 21-hydroxylase deficiency) may first present with secondary amenorrhea and signs of virilization (eg, clitoromegaly and hirsutism). Androgen insensitivity (46,XY) is the insensitivity of peripheral tissues to circulating androgens, external female phenotype, and amenorrhea.

#### Eugonadotropic Eugonadism

Normal FSH, LH, and estrogen levels characterize the eugonadotropic state. If primary amenorrhea occurs in this context, it is anatomic in origin. Defects in the development of the müllerian duct system are associated with primary amenorrhea resulting in imperforate hymen, vaginal atresia or absence, or other malformations of the cervix and the uterus. Except in cases of absence of the uterine cavity or endometrium, developmental genital tract obstructions present with painful swelling of the reproductive tract above the area of the blockage. These include hematocolpos (vaginal), hematometra (uterus), and hematoperitoneum (leakage of menstrual blood into the peritoneal cavity). The pain is cyclic in nature, coinciding with the timing of a menstrual cycle. Mayer-Rokitansky-Küster-Hauser syndrome is müllerian agenesis with primary amenorrhea resulting from absence or hypoplasia of the vagina, cervix, and/or uterus.

Secondary amenorrhea associated with normal FSH, LH, and estrogen levels has a wide differential diagnosis (Table 79-1), including uterine scarring and hyperandrogenic states. Uterine synechiae (Asherman syndrome) occurring after endometrial manipulation (eg, pregnancy, dilation and curettage) or infection (eg, pelvic inflammatory disease, tuberculous endometritis) can lead to secondary amenorrhea. Causes of amenorrhea and hyperandrogenism (eg, hirsutism and/or virilization) include polycystic ovarian syndrome (PCOS), virilizing ovarian or adrenal tumors, and drugs, including phenytoin, oral contraceptives, cocaine, and anabolic steroids.

**Polycystic Ovarian Syndrome** PCOS is the most common endocrine disorder in reproductive-aged women and a common cause of eugonadotropic secondary amenorrhea in adolescents. PCOS can also cause primary amenorrhea. Differing definitions and diagnostic criteria describe this clinically heterogeneous syndrome. The hallmarks of PCOS include ovulatory dysfunction and hyperandrogenism. Ovulatory dysfunction is clinical evidence of menstrual cycle irregularity or polycystic ovaries on ultrasound or other imaging. Hyperandrogenism is either (1) the clinical presence of hirsutism, inflammatory acne, or androgenic alopecia, *or* (2) biochemical elevations in serum testosterone and/or dehydroepiandrosterone sulfate (DHEAS). The hyperandrogenism is secondary to ovarian thecal cell proliferation and the resultant excess androgen production. The current hypothesis is that peripheral insulin resistance, which may or may not manifest as increased serum insulin levels, and an increase in serum LH relative to FSH contribute to thecal cell proliferation and further stimulation of androgen production. Although LH elevations and insulin resistance are common in women with PCOS, they are not required for diagnosis. Other clinical comorbidities include obesity, insulin resistance, glucose intolerance, and type II diabetes; mixed dyslipidemia (eg, low high-density lipoprotein, elevated triglycerides); metabolic syndrome; infertility; and endometrial cancer.

There are four accepted sets of diagnostic criteria. The National Institutes of Health criteria (1990) define PCOS by evidence of hyperandrogenism and chronic anovulation with exclusion of other causes of androgen excess. The Rotterdam criteria (2003) state that 2 of the following 3 findings are required for diagnosis: menstrual irregularity due to anovulation or oligo-ovulation, clinical and /or biochemical signs of hyperandrogenism, or polycystic ovaries (by ultrasound). The Androgen Excess and PCOS Society criteria (2006) specify that both androgen excess and ovulatory dysfunction must be present. Recent Pediatric Endocrine Society criteria for adolescent PCOS include the otherwise unexplained combination of abnormal uterine bleeding that persists for 1 to 2 years post-menarche and evidence of hyperandrogenism.

Since increased androgen levels may occur during normal pubertal development, confirmatory testing of hyperandrogenism is advisable. While PCOS accounts for up to 85% of adolescent hyperandrogenism, it is important to exclude other potential causes including CAH and other disorders of adrenal steroid metabolism, virilizing tumors, acromegaly, drugs such as valproic acid, and others. Routine ultrasound examination of the ovaries for diagnosing PCOS during adolescence is controversial since polycystic appearing ovaries may be a normal finding.

#### Evaluation of Amenorrhea

See Table 79-2 for a guide to history, physical examination, and evaluation.

**TABLE 79-2 HISTORY, PHYSICAL EXAMINATION, AND LABORATORY EVALUATION OF ADOLESCENT MENSTRUAL PROBLEMS**

| | |
|---|---|
| History | **Pubertal development**: age at pubarche and thelarche |
| | **Menstrual pattern**: age at menarche, cycle length, number of days bleeding, number of pads or tampons/day (PBAC), pain with menses |
| | **Sexual activity**: age at coitarche, partners (male and/or female), practices (vaginal, oral, anal, paraphernalia), past STI, pregnancy, protection (condoms, birth control) |
| | **Past medical and surgical**: premature birth, chronic illnesses (liver, kidney, bleeding disorders), known endocrinopathy, uterine procedures |
| | **Family**: pubertal delay, bleeding disorders, thyroidal illness, menstrual problems |
| | **Review of systems**: Weight changes, dieting and exercise habits, easy bruising and bleeding (epistaxis, frequent gum bleeding), galactorrhea, headaches, visual field defects, vaginal discharge, cyclic pelvic pain, dyspareunia, mental health (stress, anxiety, depression) |
| | **Medications and illicit drugs**: contraceptives, antiepileptics, SSRIs, haloperidol, phenothiazine, benzodiazepines, heroin, cocaine |
| Physical Examination | **Vital signs:** height, weight, body mass index, blood pressure, pulse, temperature |
| | **Thyroid**: assess for thyromegaly |
| | **Skin**: hirsutism (Ferriman-Gallwey score), inflammatory acne, bruising, acanthosis nigricans |
| | **Breast**: SMR, galactorrhea |
| | **Abdomen**: hepatomegaly, enlarged uterus |
| | **Pelvic**: SMR, clitoromegaly, vulva, introitus (hymen, color of vaginal mucosa, vaginal patency), vaginal discharge, cervical abnormalities such as polyps, hematocolpos, hematometra |
| | **Other**: Turner stigmata (webbed neck, shield chest, and wide-spaced nipples), anosmia |
| Laboratory Studies | Pregnancy test |
| | **Amenorrhea and AUB**: FSH, prolactin, TSH |
| | **Androgen excess:** testosterone (free and total), SHBG, DHEAS, 17-OHP |
| | **AUB/HMB**: PT/PTT, CBC, von Willebrand comprehensive panel |
| | **As indicated**: cortisol, estradiol, karyotype, expanded coagulopathy evaluation |
| Diagnostic Imaging | Pelvic ultrasound |

17-OHP, 17-hydroxyprogesterone; AUB, abnormal uterine bleeding; CBC, complete blood count; DHEAS, dehydroepiandrosterone sulfate; FSH, follicle-stimulating hormone; HMB, heavy menstrual bleeding; PBAC, pictorial blood assessment chart; PT, prothrombin time; PTT, partial thromboplastin time; SHBG, sex hormone–binding globulin; SMR, sexual maturity rating; SSRIs, selective serotonin reuptake inhibitors; STI, sexually transmitted infection; TSH, thyroid-stimulating hormone.

**History** The evaluation of amenorrhea requires a careful history and physical assessment. Taking a developmentally appropriate sexual history is essential. Exclude pregnancy via urine or serum pregnancy test before performing further workup. Constitutional delay is more common in boys and should be a diagnosis of exclusion. Inquire about family history of pubertal delay, stature in relation to family members, and presence of neonatal health problems including prematurity. Elucidate information suggesting additional causes of secondary amenorrhea, including symptoms of estrogen deficiency (eg, hot flashes, vaginal dryness) or risk factors for uterine scarring.

**Physical Examination** Neurologic examination is required to assess for increased intracranial pressure (papilledema) or expanding mass (bitemporal hemianopsia is one hallmark of pituitary tumors). If a complete pelvic examination is not possible for anatomic, cultural, or psychosocial reasons, an alternative is recto-abdominal examination. Patency and depth of the vagina can be determined by passing a lubricated cotton swab through the vaginal opening. If a pelvic examination cannot be completed or anatomic abnormalities are noted, a pelvic ultrasound or MRI should be performed.

**Screening Laboratory Tests** After ruling out pregnancy, initial tests should include serum FSH levels, prolactin, and thyroid function tests (TSH) (Fig. 79-1). If physical examination reveals hyperandrogenism, obtain serum testosterone (free and total) and DHEAS levels. Very high DHEAS levels are concerning for adrenal dysfunction. Prolactin levels of 20 to 60 μg/L may be difficult to interpret and need repeating while levels > 200 μg/L suggest macroadenoma. Some clinicians will also order a serum estradiol level. High FSH levels warrant a chromosomal evaluation.

### Management of Amenorrhea

**Management** Confirm any abnormal laboratory results. A progesterone challenge indirectly evaluates the presence of endogenous estrogen

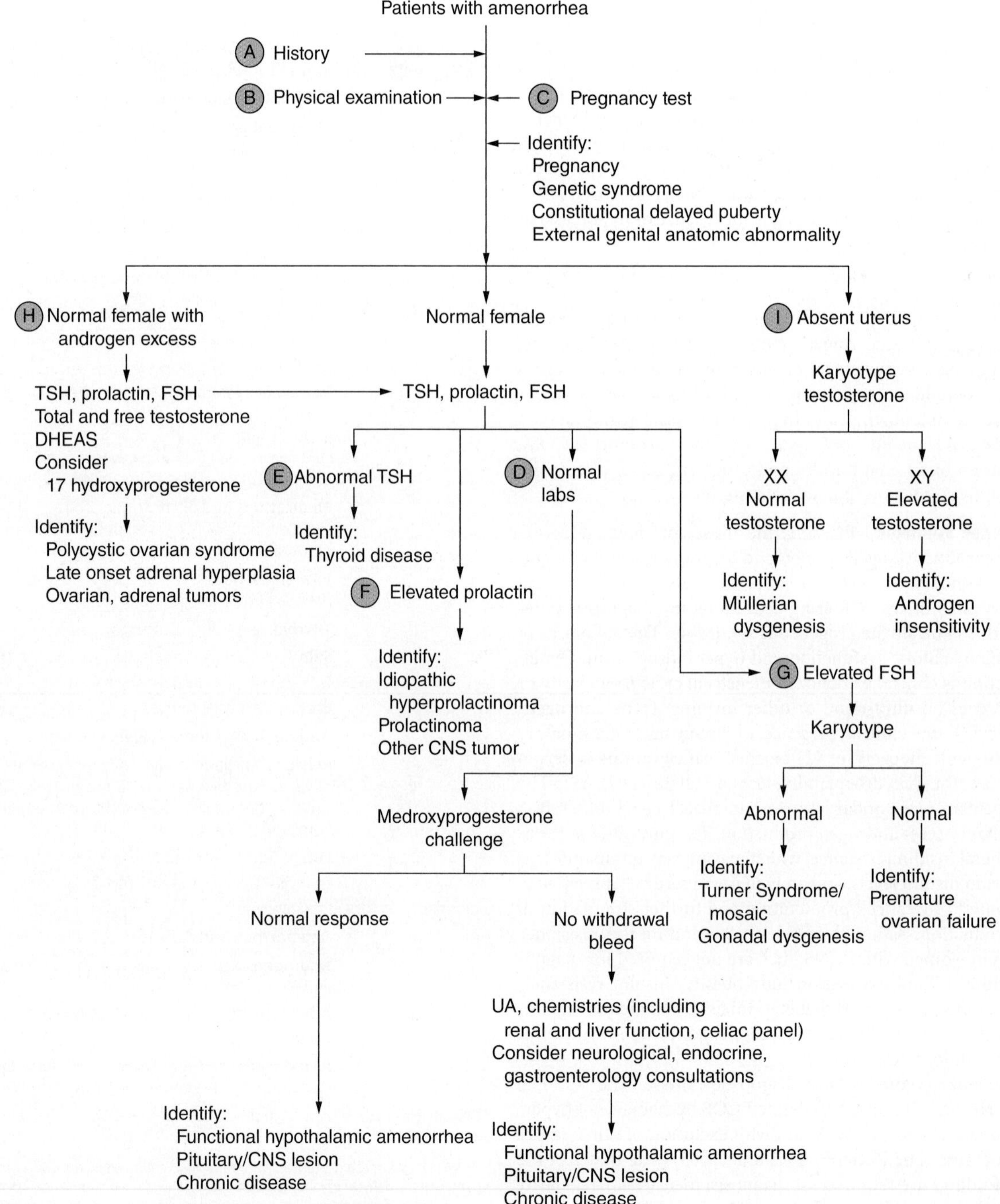


**FIGURE 79-1** Evaluation of primary and secondary amenorrhea. CNS, central nervous system; DHEAS, dehydroepiandrosterone sulfate; FSH, follicle-stimulating hormone; TSH, thyroid-stimulating hormone; UA, urinalysis.

and the competence of the reproductive outflow tract from uterus to vaginal opening. Prescribe medroxyprogesterone acetate 10 mg by mouth daily for 7 days; within 2 to 7 days of completion, uterine withdrawal bleeding should occur. Bleeding confirms competence of the hypothalamic–pituitary–gonadal axis and patency of the outflow tract. If no bleeding occurs after progesterone challenge, the reproductive outflow tract is abnormal or endogenous estrogen is inadequate. In such situations, the second step of the hormonal challenge test is to prime the endometrium: 2.5 mg of oral conjugated estrogen for 25 days with 10 mg of oral medroxyprogesterone acetate added from day 16 to day 25. It may be necessary to repeat this a second time if no bleeding is elicited. If no bleeding occurs after the second round, obtain pelvic sonography and further hormonal assays, including a serum estradiol level.

### TREATMENT

Suspected outflow obstruction of the reproductive tract necessitates appropriate imaging studies, further defining existing anatomy. Treatment of anatomic abnormalities is reconstructive surgery. Surgical correction of vaginal agenesis is appropriate prior to adulthood and before sexual debut.

Chapters 516 and 534 review the complete evaluation and treatment of hypothalamic-pituitary failure. Elevated prolactin levels in an asymptomatic patient suggest pituitary microadenoma; consider bromocriptine (a dopamine agonist) therapy. Treat ovarian failure with hormone replacement therapy, 0.3 to 0.625 mg of conjugated estrogen (the lowest amount to achieve the desired estrogen effect) on days 1 through 25 along with medroxyprogesterone acetate 10 mg on days 16 through 25 to avoid the effect of unopposed estrogen on the endometrium, which is linked to endometrial cancer. Counseling regarding bone health and calcium requirements is imperative. Provide appropriate counseling resources for those diagnosed with irreversible infertility of any cause.

PCOS treatment begins with lifestyle modification, emphasizing dietary adjustment and exercise. A 5% reduction in weight may regulate ovulation and improve cycle regularity. Combined oral contraceptives (or the combination patch or vaginal ring) is the first-line pharmacologic intervention since each provides cycle regulation and endometrial protection along with anti-androgenic effects mediated by increases in sex hormone-binding globulin. For women in whom estrogen is contraindicated, progesterone-only therapies (eg, the pill, monthly injection, subdermal implant, or IUD) will also provide endometrial protection but are limited in anti-androgenic effects. Anti-androgens such as spironolactone are effective against acne and hirsutism. Treatments for facial hirsutism include topical eflornithine and electrolysis. Metformin therapy improves insulin sensitivity and may decrease circulating androgen levels in women with PCOS, both decreasing hirsutism and improving ovulation and cycle regularity. Simultaneous use of metformin and combination oral contraceptives is beneficial. All patients with PCOS should be screened for dyslipidemia (fasting lipid profile) and glucose intolerance/type 2 diabetes (2-hour oral glucose tolerance test or hemoglobin A1C) regardless of body mass index or weight.

## ABNORMAL UTERINE BLEEDING

Abnormal uterine bleeding (AUB) is vaginal bleeding that occurs in cycles shorter than 21 days or longer than 45 days, lasts longer than 8 days, results in blood loss greater than 80 mL, and/or is associated with anemia. There are two general types: anovulatory and ovulatory dysfunctional uterine bleeding, with further classification by etiology: hormonal, local pathology (ie, vagina, cervix, and uterus), coagulopathy, and pregnancy related.

### DIFFERENTIAL DIAGNOSIS

The International Federation of Gynecology and Obstetrics (FIGO) recommends using the PALM-COEIN classification system to identify the etiology of AUB and heavy menstrual bleeding (HMB). PALM-COEIN stands for **p**olyp, **a**denomyosis, **l**eiomyoma, **m**alignancy and hyperplasia, **c**oagulopathy, **o**vulatory dysfunction, **e**ndometrial, **i**atrogenic, and **n**ot yet classified. Under this system, etiologies are written as AUB followed by the corresponding letter, eg, AUB-P (AUB caused by polyps). Multiple etiologies may exist in one patient; some conditions are uncommon in the adolescent population. The most common adolescent causes are AUB-C, AUB-O, and AUB-I.

**Polyp, Adenomyosis, Leiomyoma, Malignancy, and Endometrial** In general, polyps (AUB-P), adenomyosis (AUB-A), leiomyoma (AUB-L), and malignancies of the vagina and uterus (AUB-M) do not occur frequently in adolescents but should be included in the differential diagnosis when evaluating an adolescent with AUB and HMB. Cervical factors associated with bleeding include cervicitis, dysplasia, malignancy, hemangiomas, cervical polyps, and large fragile condylomas. Cervical and vaginal abnormalities are usually associated with light spotting or postcoital bleeding rather than frank vaginal bleeding. Endometritis (AUB-E) most commonly results from subclinical infections with sexually transmitted organisms such as *Chlamydia trachomatis*. Submucosal myomas, endometriosis, arteriovenous malformations, and uterine cancers are associated with irregular bleeding.

**Ovulatory Dysfunction** Ovulatory dysfunction (AUB-O) is the most common cause of AUB in adolescents, resulting from the immaturity or dysfunction of the hypothalamic–pituitary–gonadal axis. Anovulatory cycles are common during the first 1 to 2 years after menarche (75% are normal by year 1, 95% by year 5) and are characterized by oscillations in estrogen levels and lack of, or inadequate, progesterone production (see Chapters 66 and 533). This results in an abnormally thick and fragile endometrial lining that may slough in a disorderly and irregular fashion, leading to irregular menstrual bleeding and HMB. Bleeding secondary to anovulation is a diagnosis of exclusion and made only after a careful evaluation to eliminate other more serious causes. Potential hormonal causes of AUB include those previously described for secondary amenorrhea (Table 79-1).

**Iatrogenic** Iatrogenic (AUB-I) causes include common medications such as hormonal contraceptives (injectable, implants, oral contraceptive pills, IUD), antiepileptics, anticoagulants, chemotherapy, etc. Drug interactions with hormonal contraceptives and noncompliance can cause AUB.

**Coagulopathy** Coagulopathies (AUB-C) are the most common cause of HMB requiring hospitalization. AUB at the time of menarche may be the initial manifestation. Soiling clothes, soaking through double protection, or leaking onto the sheets at night indicates the need for further evaluation. The most common cause is von Willebrand disease, which has a prevalence of 1%; one should consider other primary and acquired coagulopathies and thrombocytopenias as well. The depletion of vitamin K–dependent clotting factors, fibrinogen, and plasminogen secondary to liver or mucosal bowel disease may also contribute to excessive bleeding. Patients with renal disease or hemodialysis might have AUB leading to HMB.

**AUB Not Yet Classified** Vaginal causes of AUB (AUB-N) include foreign bodies (eg, forgotten tampons or condoms), lacerations from either sexual abuse or intravaginal insertion of objects, and hymen tears. Ovarian cysts and malignant and benign tumors may also cause abnormal bleeding.

**Pregnancy-Related Causes** Complications of pregnancy may present as AUB (Chapter 80). Medical emergencies include ectopic pregnancy and threatened abortions.

### EVALUATION AND MANAGEMENT

The primary goals of clinical assessment are to determine the acuity, duration, and volume of blood loss as well as assess the need for medication, hospitalization, surgical intervention, or transfusion. First, exclude causes requiring immediate intervention. Table 79-2 outlines the pertinent history, physical examination, and laboratory evaluation. Women with vaginal bleeding, an acute abdominal complaint, and/or positive pregnancy test need immediate gynecologic consultation as this may indicate an ectopic pregnancy. Patients with significant blood loss resulting in anemia should be evaluated for both coagulopathies and thyroid disorders.

Stabilize patients with hemodynamic changes or an acute abdomen using appropriate fluid, electrolyte, and hemostatic stabilization. Stop acute HMB by administering conjugated estrogen, 25 mg intravenously every 6 hours for a total of 6 doses, with simultaneous use of combination oral contraceptives to stabilize the endometrium. If the patient is hemodynamically stable and only mildly anemic, prescribe a fixed-dose estrogen-progesterone combination oral contraceptive, one pill every 6 hours until bleeding stops. Taper the dose over the following 3 to 4 weeks, at which time a withdrawal bleed of 3 to 5 days is permitted, followed by cyclic combination oral contraceptive therapy. An antiemetic may be necessary with high-dose estrogen therapy. After 4 to 6 months, attempt to discontinue medication under close medical supervision. Other regimens include cyclic progesterone therapy; this regimen appears to be less efficacious in patients with primary AUB. Iron and folate replacement may be necessary for anemic patients (Hgb < 12 g/dL). For patients with mild breakthrough bleeding secondary to hormone use (eg, progesterone-only contraception), a trial of nonsteroidal anti-inflammatory drugs (NSAIDs) is recommended to decrease blood flow to the endometrium. Treatment of adolescents with AUB rarely requires dilation and curettage; it is contraindicated in patients with bleeding disorders.

Management strategies for AUB-O include decreasing the frequency of menstrual flow and/or inducing an atrophic endometrium. Options include continuous daily combined oral contraceptive use with a controlled withdrawal bleed every 3 to 4 months or induction of endometrial atrophy with either daily oral progesterone, intramuscular Depo-Provera every 3 months, or GnRH analogs such as leuprolide acetate. In addition to hormonal therapy, intranasal 1-deamino-8-D-arginine vasopressin (DDAVP) is an alternative therapy for individuals with von Willebrand disease or platelet dysfunction. Other therapies include antifibrinolytics (eg, tranexamic acid). An inherited bleeding disorder is a contraindication for the use of NSAIDs.

## DYSMENORRHEA

Dysmenorrhea, the experience of painful menstrual cramping and other menstruation-associated symptoms, remains one of the most common reproductive system complaints of menstruating female adolescents and is a leading cause of school and work absenteeism and decreased quality of life. The prevalence of dysmenorrhea approaches 50% to 93% during adolescence, peaking 1 to 2 years after menarche. This coincides with the establishment of ovulatory cycles. Most experience mild-to-moderate pain, but incapacitation occurs in 10% to 20% for 1 to 3 days each month; even more miss school and social activities.

### PATHOPHYSIOLOGY AND CLINICAL PRESENTATION

Alterations in four chemicals cause primary dysmenorrhea: prostaglandins, leukotrienes, prostacyclin, and vasopressin. Increased levels of prostaglandin ($PGF_{2\alpha}$) and leukotriene C4 and D4 stimulate uterine vasoconstriction, pain sensitization, and myometrium contractions. Prostacyclin is a vasodilator and muscle relaxant, but decreased levels occur in women with dysmenorrhea. Lastly, overproduction of vasopressin further increases uterine contractions. These four alterations lead to intense uterine contractions, vasoconstriction, and ischemic pain. During the first 36 to 48 hours of menses, prostaglandins increase within the endometrium, corresponding with the time of greatest discomfort. Beyond pain, systemic effects of the altered chemical milieu include nausea, vomiting, diarrhea, fatigue, headache, low back pain, thigh pain, dizziness, and syncope.

Secondary dysmenorrhea is associated with specific physiological and pathologic conditions, including pelvic infections (eg, endometritis, pelvic inflammatory disease), ectopic pregnancy, miscarriage, endometriosis, adhesions, IUD placement, uterine leiomyomas (rare in adolescence), ovarian cyst, cervical stenosis, and other anatomic abnormalities causing obstruction of the outflow tract. Nongynecologic causes include inflammatory bowel disease, irritable bowel syndrome, urinary tract problems, musculoskeletal conditions, and psychogenic (abuse).

### EVALUATION

A thorough history should detail age at menarche, date of onset of pain, relationship of onset and duration of pain to menses, date of last menstrual period, and impact of previous pain medications by type. A confidential interview should include the assessment of sexual activity and practices, history of abuse, use of contraceptives including condoms, sexually transmitted disease history, and previous pregnancies and outcomes. A review of systems will identify associated systemic symptoms. Evaluation includes a complete physical examination and pelvic examination with screening for secondary causes as described earlier in this chapter. If there is a secondary cause or there is minimal improvement after 6 months of treatment, proceed with additional laboratory studies, diagnostic imaging, and surgical procedures as necessary.

### MANAGEMENT

Therapy for primary dysmenorrhea focuses on inhibiting the synthesis or action of prostaglandins. Standard therapy includes appropriately dosed NSAIDs such as ibuprofen, naproxen sodium, or mefenamic acid begun 1 to 2 days before the expected onset of menses and continued through day 2 to 3 of bleeding. The 30% to 40% of females who do not respond to cyclooxygenase inhibitors (NSAIDs) potentially have dysmenorrhea mediated primarily through the lipoxygenase-dependent leukotriene pathway. Combination oral contraceptive pills (OCPs) improve symptoms in 90% of young women with primary dysmenorrhea, but it may take 3 cycles to achieve maximum therapeutic benefit. NSAIDs and OCPs used together can improve symptom relief. In addition, patients should be counseled to avoid smoking and caffeine. Alternative treatments noted to be effective include omega-3 polyunsaturated fatty acids, vitamin E, vitamin $B_1$, and minerals such as magnesium. Patients diagnosed with primary dysmenorrhea who do not improve with 6 months of adequate therapy should be evaluated for causes of secondary dysmenorrhea.

### SUGGESTED READINGS


Adams Hillard PJ. Menstruation in adolescents: what do we know? And what do we do with the information? *J Pediatr Adolesc Gynecol.* 2014;27(6):309-319.

American College of Obstetricians and Gynecologists. ACOG Committee Opinion No. 651: Menstruation in girls and adolescents: using the menstrual cycle as a vital sign. *Obstet Gynecol.* 2015;126(6):e143-e146.

Bradley LD, Gueye NA. The medical management of abnormal uterine bleeding in reproductive-aged women. *Am J Obstet Gynecol.* 2016;214(1):31-44.

Deligeoroglou E, Athanasopoulos N, Tsimaris P, Dimopoulos KD, Vrachnis N, Creatsas G. Evaluation and management of adolescent amenorrhea. *Ann N Y Acad Sci.* 2010;1205:23-32.

Harel Z. Dysmenorrhea in adolescents and young adults: an update on pharmacological treatments and management strategies. *Expert Opin Pharmacother.* 2012;13(15):2157-2170.

Ju H, Jones M, Mishra G. The prevalence and risk factors of dysmenorrhea. *Epidemiol Rev.* 2014;36:104-113.

Legro RS, Arslanian SA, Ehrmann DA, et al. Diagnosis and treatment of polycystic ovary syndrome: an Endocrine Society clinical practice guideline. *J Clin Endocrinol Metab.* 2013;98(12):4565-4592.

Munro MG, Critchley HO, Broder MS, Fraser IS; FIGO Working Group on Menstrual Disorders. FIGO classification system (PALM-COEIN) for causes of abnormal uterine bleeding in nongravid women of reproductive age. *Int J Gynaecol Obstet.* 2011;113(1):3-13.

Rosenfield RL. The diagnosis of polycystic ovary syndrome in adolescents. *Pediatrics.* 2015;136(6):1154-1165.

Sultan C, Gaspari L, Paris F. Adolescent dysmenorrhea. In: Sultan C, ed. *Pediatric and Adolescent Gynecology: Evidence-Based Clinical Practice.* 2nd ed. Basel, Switzerland: Karger; 2012:171-180.

# 80 Intrauterine and Ectopic Pregnancy

Fareeda Haamid and Erica B. Monasterio

## INTRAUTERINE PREGNANCY

### INTRODUCTION

Adolescent pregnancy is an important pediatric health concern. Pediatricians and general practitioners can play a vital role in the early diagnosis of pregnancy and promoting prenatal care. The World Health Organization reports a global average teenage birth rate among 15- to 19-year-olds of 49 births per 1000 females. Globally, the second leading cause of death in females aged 15 to 19 is complications occurring during pregnancy or delivery. The teenage birth rate in the United States has dramatically declined over the last 2 decades. The current preliminary rate of 22.3 per 1000 females aged 15 to 19 years is the lowest recorded rate.

### HISTORY

During any assessment of an adolescent female, it is advisable to record the date and normality of the last menstrual period. Once menarche is achieved, pregnancy should be ruled out any time a sexually active patient reports missing 1 or more menses. A history of unprotected intercourse since the last menses with or without amenorrhea or unusual vaginal bleeding should alert the physician to the possibility of pregnancy. The absence of historical information does not preclude pregnancy because the adolescent may be unwilling or unable to communicate a sexual history to the clinician for a variety of reasons. The typical symptoms associated with pregnancy (nausea, vomiting, intermenstrual spotting, breast tenderness, unexplained weight gain, urinary frequency, and fatigue, among others) may be present in any combination or may be absent early in pregnancy (Table 80-1).

### PHYSICAL EXAMINATION

A physical assessment, often including a pelvic examination, is critical to the evaluation of a possible pregnancy. Uterine size can be estimated based on a bimanual exam; in general, at 6 weeks, the uterus may be slightly softened but enlargement is difficult to appreciate, an 8-week uterus is about the size of an orange, and a 12-week uterus is the size of a grapefruit. As pregnancy progresses, the uterine fundus can be appreciated via an abdominal exam after 12 weeks, a 16-week uterus can be felt at the midpoint between the pubic symphysis and the umbilicus, and a 20-week uterus at the umbilicus.

**TABLE 80-1 SIGNS AND SYMPTOMS OF PREGNANCY**

| Common Signs and Symptoms of Early Pregnancy | Additional Signs and Symptoms of Pregnancy |
|---|---|
| Amenorrhea | Lightheadedness |
| Mild spotting | Nasal congestion |
| Breast tenderness | Dyspnea |
| Breast enlargement | Heartburn |
| Nausea | Increased appetite |
| Vomiting | Bloating |
| Fatigue | Constipation |
| Urinary frequency | Cramping (uterine) |
| | Skin findings: palmar erythema, hyperpigmentation, and spider angiomas |
| | Unexplained weight gain |
| | Mood changes |

### EVALUATION FOR PREGNANCY

The first day of the last menstrual period forms the basis of dating of pregnancy. The urine or serum pregnancy test confirms the presence of an early pregnancy, using detection of beta-human chorionic gonadotropin (β-hCG). Within 24 hours of implantation (which occurs 6 to 12 days after ovulation), the placenta produces hCG (≤ 5 IU/L) and concentrations double every 48 to 72 hours in a normal pregnancy. By 2 weeks, the level rises to more than 200 IU/L in a normal pregnancy, and concentration peaks at approximately 100,000 IU/L at 8 to 10 weeks gestation. Thereafter, the level drops to about 10,000 IU/L at 20 weeks and remains stable until term. Standard urine pregnancy tests are an accurate, sensitive, easy, and inexpensive diagnostic tool to detect early pregnancy with β-hCG sensitivities at levels of 20 to 50 IU/L. In contrast, the minimum serum β-hCG levels required for positive pregnancy tests are 5 to 10 IU/L for qualitative tests and 1 to 2 IU/L for ultrasensitive quantitative tests (Table 80-2).

### MANAGEMENT OF PREGNANCY

#### Options Counseling

Once an intrauterine pregnancy is confirmed, the provider is tasked with providing confidential counseling to the adolescent about her options. Outcome options include continuation of the pregnancy with subsequent parenting, adoption, or fostering of the child, or termination of the pregnancy. Based on her locale, an adolescent who desires to terminate a pregnancy should be made aware of whether or not she may provide consent independently or if parental notification and/or consent (or the legal alternative option of judicial bypass) is required. In addition, she should be advised of the legal restrictions related to the estimated gestational age and/or limited sources of care in some localities.

#### Prenatal Care

Ideally the adolescent should have an initial prenatal care visit within 1 to 2 weeks of diagnosis. Early prenatal care is associated with fewer adverse maternal, obstetrical, and neonatal outcomes in this high-risk population. The gold standard of adolescent prenatal care is utilization of a multidisciplinary, comprehensive, and adolescent-centered model. Prenatal care should include promotion and instruction regarding a healthy diet and appropriate weight gain. A daily prenatal vitamin and nutrition education pertaining to the developing fetus is important. Daily folic acid (folate) supplement (400 mg) included in prenatal vitamins is important in preventing neural tube defects, especially in the first 3 to 4 weeks of pregnancy.

All pregnant adolescents should be screened for chlamydia, gonorrhea, hepatitis B, HIV, and syphilis early during pregnancy, and repeat testing should occur in the third trimester (Table 80-3). Pregnancy is also a compelling motivator for adolescents to cease or at least reduce use of tobacco, alcohol, and other substances. Education about the risks of the aforementioned substances is an essential element of prenatal care. Positive screening should prompt a referral for treatment. Particular attention should be devoted to screening for depression. There is an association between untreated maternal depression and postpartum depression; both of which can lead to adverse maternal, neonatal, and childhood sequelae. Further evaluation and treatment should be initiated for those with positive depression screening. Intimate partner violence (IPV), either past or present, is associated with poor perinatal outcomes. A history of abuse within the last year is a prognostic indicator of violence during pregnancy. Brief screening tools and safety card–based guides to assessment and intervention are available. If child abuse or exploitation is suspected, the pediatrician should assure that the appropriate agencies/authorities are involved.

## ECTOPIC PREGNANCY

### EPIDEMIOLOGY

Ectopic pregnancy is a significant problem for young sexually active women, as reflected by a fourfold increase in incidence of the problem between 1970 and 1992, with 20 ectopic pregnancies reported per

**TABLE 80-2 DIAGNOSTIC PARAMETERS FOR DETERMINING THE VIABILITY OF A PREGNANCY**

| Diagnostic Modality | Viable Intrauterine Pregnancy | Nonviable Intrauterine Pregnancy | Ectopic Pregnancy |
|---|---|---|---|
| **Serum beta hCG quantitative** | Doubling hCG: every 36 hours (1.5 days), weeks 2–5; every 84 hours (3.5 days) after week 7 | Plateau or decreasing serial hCG | Abnormally slow-rising, plateau, or decreasing serial hCG |
| **Serum progesterone (less stable indicator)** | ≥ 22 ng/mL | < 5 ng/mL | < 5 ng/mL |
| **Transvaginal ultrasound** | Intrauterine gestational sac visualized (4.5–5 weeks gestation) | No intrauterine gestational sac visualized | Consistent with extrauterine pregnancy |
| **Fetal cardiac activity (Doppler ultrasound)** | Present (5–6 weeks gestation) | Absent | Absent |

Data from Alkatout I, Honemeyer U, Strauss A, et al. Clinical diagnosis and treatment of ectopic pregnancy, *Obstet Gynecol Surv.* 2013 Aug;68(8):571-581.

1000 pregnancies in 1992, the last time national data was reported by the CDC. Its incidence is difficult to estimate today. However, it remains the leading cause of maternal death in the first trimester of pregnancy and accounts for 4% to 10% of all pregnancy-related deaths annually. Overall, recent advances in determining early pregnancy coupled with the successful conservative management of early ectopic pregnancies have decreased mortality and morbidity while preserving fertility.

## PATHOPHYSIOLOGY

Approximately 97% of ectopic pregnancies conceived naturally occur in the fallopian tube itself. The most common factor that predisposes the young woman to tubal damage and therefore ectopic pregnancy is acute salpingitis, especially chlamydial infection. Other predisposing factors include congenital anomalies, previous pelvic or abdominal surgery, prior ectopic pregnancy, and endometriosis within the tube. When an adolescent with an IUD in place becomes pregnant, due to method failure, her risk for having an ectopic pregnancy is higher than the risk for ectopic in a non-contracepting adolescent. Cofactors linked to ectopic pregnancy include multiple sexual partners, cigarette smoking, vaginal douching, and early sexual debut. The outcome of an ectopic pregnancy depends on the location of implantation. A spontaneous "tubal abortion" is most likely to occur when the site of implantation is in the ampulla of the tube, whereas the more dangerous tubal rupture is most likely with implantation within the tube's isthmus.

## CLINICAL FEATURES

The common clinical presentation of an ectopic pregnancy includes lower abdominal pain (100%), amenorrhea (75%), intermenstrual spotting (75%), abdominal tenderness (90%), adnexal tenderness (85%), adnexal/pelvic mass (50%), and uterine enlargement mimicking early changes of pregnancy (most). Women with ectopic pregnancies have normal vital signs unless rupture occurs. When acute rupture into the peritoneum occurs, it is usually accompanied by acute hemorrhage, hypovolemia, and shock, resulting in a life-threatening situation.

## DIAGNOSIS

Key to the diagnosis of ectopic pregnancy are the assessment of presenting symptoms and physical findings, diagnostic features found on ultrasound examination, and laboratory test results. Laboratory tests helpful in differentiating between ectopic, intrauterine, and failing intrauterine pregnancies include serial quantitative hCG and serum progesterone levels (Table 80-2).

Ectopic pregnancy often produces hCG at a slower rate, although there is considerable overlap of concentrations in normal intrauterine and ectopic pregnancies early in gestation. If ectopic pregnancy is suspected, quantitative serum β-hCG should be obtained and repeated at 48 hours.

The differential diagnosis of the young woman presenting with abdominal pain, amenorrhea, and/or spotting includes a normal

**TABLE 80-3 2015 CDC[a] RECOMMENDATIONS FOR SEXUALLY TRANSMITTED INFECTION SCREENING IN PREGNANT ADOLESCENTS**

| Sexually Transmitted Infection (STI) | Population | Timing of Testing |
|---|---|---|
| *Chlamydia trachomatis* | All pregnant women | • 1st prenatal visit<br>• < 25 years: Retest in 3rd trimester even if prior negative<br>• Positive in 1st trimester: Retest in 3-6 months, preferably in 3rd trimester |
| *Neisseria gonorrheae* | All pregnant women < 25 years | • 1st prenatal visit<br>• Positive in 1st trimester: Retest in 3-6 months, preferably in 3rd trimester |
| Trichomonas vaginalis | • Asymptomatic pregnant women[b]<br>• Symptomatic pregnant women | • No routine testing<br>• At time of symptoms, treat if positive |
| Syphilis | All pregnant women | • 1st prenatal visit<br>• High risk: Retest in 3rd trimester and at delivery |
| HIV | All pregnant women | As early as possible |
| Hepatitis B | All pregnant women regardless of vaccination status | Early prenatal visit |
| Hepatitis C | All pregnant women at high risk (IDU past or present)[c] | 1st prenatal visit |
| Herpes simplex virus (HSV) | Undiagnosed prior to pregnancy | No routine testing |
| Bacterial vaginosis | • Asymptomatic pregnant women[b]<br>• Symptomatic pregnant women | • No routine testing<br>• At time of symptoms, treat if positive |

[a]Centers for Disease Control and Prevention.

[b]Pregnant adolescents may require more thorough evaluation for all STIs.

[c]Injection drug use.

intrauterine pregnancy (IUP), a failing IUP (spontaneous abortion), an ectopic pregnancy, pelvic inflammatory disease, chronic salpingitis, ovarian torsion or ruptured ovarian cyst, appendicitis, bladder/kidney disease, acute gastroenteritis, intra-abdominal inflammation, and vascular ischemic (bowel) or hemorrhagic (aorta or abdominal vessels) disease.

## TREATMENT

Management of ectopic pregnancy in adolescents frequently requires emergent surgical intervention such as laparotomy and salpingectomy on the affected side because of delayed diagnosis and rupture, with subsequent poor fertility prospects. With earlier recognition of the ectopic pregnancy before rupture, however, more conservative management can be employed, including expectant management, medical management with methotrexate, and salpingostomy by laparoscopy with comparable resolution of ectopic pregnancies and preservation of subsequent fertility. Expectant management is restricted to those adolescents who are asymptomatic with falling hCG levels who can understand and accept the potential risk of rupture and hemorrhage and adhere to follow-up recommendations. A good indication of potential for spontaneous reabsorption and resolution of an ectopic pregnancy is an initial hCG level under 200 IU/L. Candidates for medical management with single or two-dose methotrexate regimens include hemodynamically stable adolescents who are willing and able to comply with post-treatment monitoring, have a serum β-hCG level of < 5000 IU/L, and have no evidence of fetal cardiac activity on ultrasound and no contraindications to methotrexate use. For adolescents with hCG levels > 5000, fixed multidose methotrexate regimens may be appropriate if they meet all other criteria. Careful weekly follow-up is essential with β-hCG until the titer is less than 5 IU/L. Studies comparing treatment with methotrexate to tube-sparing laparoscopic surgery show no difference in overall tubal preservation, tubal patency, repeat ectopic pregnancy, or ability to conceive in the future. Management of ectopic pregnancy generally requires specialty consultation and co-management or referral.

## SUGGESTED READINGS


Alkatout I, Honemeyer U, Strauss A, et al. Clinical diagnosis and treatment of ectopic pregnancy. *Obstet Gynecol Surv.* 2013;68(8): 571-581.

American College of Obstetricians and Gynecologists. ACOG Practice Bulletin No. 94: Medical management of ectopic pregnancy. *Obstetr Gynecol.* 2008;111(6):1479-1485. Reaffirmed 2014.

Aruda MM, Waddicor K, Frese L, Cole JC, Burke P. Early pregnancy in adolescents: diagnosis, assessment, options counseling, and referral. *J Pediatr Health Care.* 2010;24(1):4-13.

Bachman EA, Barnhart K. Medical management of ectopic pregnancy: a comparison of regimens. *Clin Obstet Gynecol.* 2012;55(2):440-447.

The Center for Adolescent Substance Abuse Research. The CRAFFT screening tool for alcohol and other drug use disorders. http://www.ceasar-boston.org/CRAFFT/index.php. Accessed February 14, 2017.

Fleming N, O'Driscoll T, Becker G, et al. Adolescent pregnancy guidelines. *J Obstet Gynaecol Can.* 2015;37(8):740-759.

Futures without Violence. National Health Resource Center on Domestic Violence. Futures without Violence Web site. https://www.futureswithoutviolence.org/health/national-health-resource-center-on-domestic-violence/.

McCarthy FP, O'Brien U, Kenny LC. The management of teenage pregnancy. *BMJ.* 2014;349:g5887.

McCracken KA, Loveless M. Teen pregnancy: an update. *Curr Opin Obstet Gynecol.* 2014;26(5):355-359.

Pinzon JL, Jones VF, Committee on Adolescence, Committee on Early Childhood. Care of adolescent parents and their children. *Pediatrics.* 2012;130(6):e1743-e1756. American Academy of Pediatrics clinical report.

Trotman G, Chhatre G, Darolia R, Tefera E, Damle L, Gomez-Lobo V. The effect of Centering Pregnancy versus traditional prenatal care models on improved adolescent health behaviors in the perinatal period. *J Pediatr Adolesc Gynecol.* 2015;28(5):395-401.

US Department of Health and Human Services Office of Adolescent Health. Teen Pregnancy Prevention Program. https://www.hhs.gov/ash/oah/adolescent-health-topics/reproductive-health/teen-pregnancy/ttp-program.html. Accessed February 14, 2017.




# 81 Contraception


Heather E. Needham and Erica B. Monasterio


## INTRODUCTION

Contraception is a health behavior that often begins during adolescence and evolves throughout reproductive life. Approximately 80% of pregnancies in adolescents between 15 and 19 years of age in the United States are unintended. The Youth Risk Behavior Survey (2015) found that 30% of high school students had had sex within the last 3 months, and of those, 13.8% did not use a condom or any other form of contraception. This is significant in that more sexually active teens are utilizing contraceptive methods. Meanwhile, there was a decline in teen births in the United States to women between 15 and 19 years of age: 229,888 births in 2015 compared to 553,000 in 2011. This may be due in part to more teens remaining abstinent longer; more effective means of contraception, particularly long-acting reversible contraception (LARC); and the use of emergency contraception.

Discussions of sexual decision-making, abstinence, sexual activity, reproduction, and contraception occur frequently as a normal part of the well-adolescent visit for female adolescents. Females are more likely to seek out a contraceptive method if they perceive getting pregnant to be negative; they have long-term educational goals; and/or they have friends, family, and clinicians who promote the use of contraception. In contrast, male adolescents, who are not at risk for pregnancy and do not require prescriptive contraceptives, may have clinician contact only during a sports physical or treatment of an injury or acute illness. Although sexuality and contraceptives are not traditionally discussed during "the sports check," which often substitutes for the annual examination for male adolescents, clinicians should emphasize the need for such discussions because this visit may be the only contact between the male adolescent and a clinician.

## TYPE OF CONTRACEPTIVE

Common methods of contraception for male and female adolescents are reviewed in Table 81-1. Providers are encouraged to use an efficacy-based approach to discussing contraceptive options, starting with LARC methods, which have the highest efficacy for pregnancy prevention. Efficacy-based charts, such as those available from the CDC (https://www.cdc.gov/reproductivehealth/unintendedpregnancy/pdf/contraceptive_methods_508.pdf) or Bedsider (htpp://www.bedsider.org) can help providers explain and adolescents understand the effectiveness of different methods. Adolescents should be encouraged to choose a contraceptive method that they feel comfortable with, that they believe they can use successfully, and that meets their needs related to both pregnancy and sexually transmitted infection (STI) risk reduction. For some, the choice is condoms, which are relatively inexpensive, easily obtained, and highly effective for protection from pregnancy and STIs, but only when used consistently and correctly. For adolescents who choose to use a contraceptive method (LARC, Depo-Provera, or a combined hormonal method), it should be emphasized that when used correctly the methods are effective against pregnancy but do not protect against STIs. Counseling regarding emergency contraception and its effectiveness is imperative for individuals not using a LARC method in anticipation of method failure

**TABLE 81-1 METHODS OF CONTRACEPTION**

| Method | Mechanism of Action | Efficacy: Rate of Pregnancy First Year of Use[a] Perfect Use | Typical | Coital Dependence | Prescription Required | Protection from STIs/HIV | Complications | Comments |
|---|---|---|---|---|---|---|---|---|
| Abstinence | No intercourse | 0% | ? | No | No | +++ | None | |
| Combined hormonal contraceptive (pill, patch, ring) | Inhibits ovulation<br>Alters cervical mucus and endometrium | 0.3% | 9% | No | Yes | Some protection against pelvic inflammatory disease | Side effects, STIs (see text) | (See text) |
| Intrauterine contraception | Probably prevents implantation; thickens cervical mucous | < 1% | < 1% | No | Yes | No | (See text) | (See text) |
| Condom (female) | Barrier | 5% | 21% | Yes | No | ++ | Slippage | Expensive, difficult |
| Condom (male) | Barrier | 2% | 18% | Yes | No | ++ | Reaction to latex | Some dislike |
| Vaginal spermicides (foam, jelly, film, suppositories) | Spermicidal agent | 18% | 28% | Yes | No | No | Reaction to spermicide | Some describe as "messy" to use |
| Coitus interruptus | Withdrawal prior to ejaculation | 4% | 22% | Yes | No | No | None | Requires self-control; pre-ejaculatory semen contains sperm |
| Periodic abstinence | Abstinence during times of peak fertility | 2–5% | 12–22% | No | No | No | None | Requires monitoring menstrual cycle |
| Chance | Chance | 85% | 85% | Yes | No | No | Pregnancy | |
| Depot medroxyprogesterone | Suppresses ovulation, thickens cervical mucus | < 1% | 3% | No | Yes | No | (See text) | Requires intramuscular injection every 12 weeks; must comply with follow-up visits |
| Etonogestrel implant | Suppresses ovulation; thickens cervical mucus | 0.05% | 0.05% | No | Yes | No | (See text) | Requires implantation removal every 3 years |
| Emergency contraceptive pills | Suppresses ovulation and implantation | N/A | N/A | No | No—for Plan B One-Step | No | | Use within 72 hours of intercourse |

[a]*Theoretical efficacy* is defined as the best *estimate* of the accidental pregnancy rate during the first year of use among couples who initiated the use of a method (not necessarily for the first time) and who used it consistently and correctly. *Actual efficacy* is defined as a measure of the accidental pregnancy rate during the first year among "typical couples" who initiated the use of a method (not necessarily for the first time) if they did not stop use for any other reason.

+++Abstinence is the only method that is 100% effective in preventing STIs.

++Protective against STIs transmitted primarily in genital fluids.

Data from Hatcher RA TJ, Stewart F, Nelson AL, Cates W, Guest F, Kowal D. *Contraceptive Technology* 18th Revised Edition. 18th ed. New York: Ardent Media; 2004; Trussell J, Ellertson C, Stewart F, Raymond EG, Shochet T. The role of emergency contraception. *Am J Obstet Gynecol*. Apr 2004;190(4 Suppl):S30-S38.

or lapse in contraceptive use. Heterosexual adolescents, like adults, tend to decrease their use of condoms over time in a relationship, and higher relationship quality and more frequent intercourse are associated with less condom use.

## LONG-ACTING REVERSIBLE CONTRACEPTIVES

LARC methods are considered the most effective contraceptive methods because once they have been inserted they function independent of the adolescent. Both the American Academy of Pediatrics (AAP) and the American College of Obstetrics and Gynecology (ACOG) support LARC methods as first-line options. LARC includes the contraceptive implant (Nexplanon) and intrauterine devices (IUDs), which include progestin-only IUDs (Skyla and Mirena) that last between 3 and 5 years and a nonhormonal IUD (Paragard) that lasts for 10 years.

The single etonogestrel implant, Nexplanon, is an alternative delivery system for progestin-only contraception. Inserted under the skin in the upper arm, the implant is barely visible, long acting (3 years), and highly effective. As with depot medroxyprogesterone acetate (DMPA), menstrual side effects may limit the appeal of this method for some adolescents, but unlike DMPA, concerns about weight gain and bone mineral density are not an issue. Both DMPA and the etonogestrel implant may be excellent contraceptive methods for those adolescents who want long-term contraception not linked to coitus, are unable to use oral contraceptives, or cannot use estrogen-containing preparations.

Modern intrauterine contraceptive devices containing copper, such as Paragard (which impairs sperm function and prevents fertilization), or progestin, such as Mirena or Skyla (which thickens cervical mucus, induces reversible endometrial atrophy, and may suppress ovulation), can be an excellent choice for the adolescent seeking reliable long-term contraception, particularly if she has had a child. A few absolute contraindications for IUD insertion include current STI (eg, cervicitis or pelvic inflammatory disease), unexplained vaginal bleeding, and a uterine anomaly that could affect placement of the device. The use of intrauterine contraceptives requires careful consideration of the patient's history and current sexual risk. Although the risk of expulsion is slightly higher in women who have never had a child, nulliparity is not a contraindication to intrauterine contraceptive devices.

## ESTROGEN-PROGESTIN COMBINATION CONTRACEPTION

Combination hormonal methods, including oral contraceptive pills, the contraceptive patch, and the contraceptive ring, are the contraceptive methods of choice for many adolescents soon after their sexual debut because using these methods is independent of sexual intercourse. The mechanism of action for combined hormonal contraception, regardless of the mode of delivery of the estrogen and progestin, includes the inhibition of ovulation through the hypothalamic and pituitary effects of the exogenous hormones. A reduction of gonadotropin-releasing hormone (GnRH) pulses as well as decreased pituitary responsiveness to GnRH results in the suppression of luteinizing hormone and follicle-stimulating hormone production, inhibiting ovulation. The thickening of cervical mucus, which inhibits sperm transport and decreases sperm capacitation (the ability of the sperm to enter the egg), are additional mechanisms of action primarily attributable to progestins. Such hormonal methods are generally safe and highly effective, but because they afford essentially no protection against STIs including human immunodeficiency virus, the additional use of condoms is recommended. Dual-method (hormonal contraception plus condom) use, however, is reported by less than 10% of sexually active adolescents.

Combined hormonal contraceptives are associated with a number of minor side effects, including nausea, breast tenderness, occasional weight gain, and breakthrough bleeding, especially within the first 3 months of use. The United States Medical Eligibility Criteria for Contraceptive Use provides guidelines to counsel women on the safety of various methods in relation to numerous medical conditions. Please refer to the following for the complete listing: http://www.cdc.gov/reproductivehealth/unintendedpregnancy/usmec.htm. Conditions designated as 4 are considered unacceptable health risks in relation to the contraceptive method, and conditions designated as 3 represent risks that outweigh the benefits of using the contraceptive method. A few of the medical conditions within these categories include abnormal vaginal bleeding, liver disease, deep venous thrombosis, migraine with aura, and hypertension. Weight is also a factor to be considered when prescribing the contraceptive patch. For example, a patient who weighs over 198 pounds may have reduced contraceptive patch efficacy.

Constant advances are being made in combination hormonal contraception. New formulations, dosing regimens, and delivery methods have expanded the options for young women choosing these methods.

## PROGESTIN-ONLY CONTRACEPTION

The options for use of progestin-only contraception have also expanded. The mechanisms of action for progestin-only contraceptives include the inhibition of luteinizing hormone production and thus the inhibition of ovulation, thickening of cervical mucus to impact sperm capacitation, and an alteration in the endometrium including reversible endometrial atrophy. DMPA is given in a 150-mg intramuscular dose or a 104-mg subcutaneous dose every 13 weeks, providing reliable, highly effective injectable contraception. The subcutaneous formulation is newer, and an advantage is that it may allow for self-administration. DMPA use has been widely initiated by adolescents and is prescribed for over 1 million adolescent girls in the United States annually. DMPA appeals to adolescents because it is comparably long lasting, easy to use, and invisible to parents and partners. However, there are some significant concerns for adolescents and physicians. Primary among these concerns are weight gain, irregular bleeding/amenorrhea, and a reduction in bone mineral density associated with DMPA use. Weight gain is a common side effect, with an average weight gain of 5.4 pounds in the first year and 16.5 pounds after 5 years in adult women. For obese young women already struggling with their weight, this may be a significant deterrent to DMPA use. Irregular bleeding is a common reason for any method's discontinuance among adolescents, and amenorrhea, while a potentially beneficial side effect for adults, is often poorly tolerated by adolescents, who equate lack of menses with pregnancy. Of greatest concern to physicians is the black box warning related to decreased bone mineral density in DMPA users. In response to this concern, the Society for Adolescent Health and Medicine has issued a position paper on DMPA and bone density, recommending that providers continue to prescribe DMPA for patients who desire it, with an adequate explanation of benefits and potential risks. Bone density is most often regained after discontinuance of the method.

## EMERGENCY CONTRACEPTION

Clinicians play an important role in promoting the use of and providing prescriptions in advance for emergency contraception (EC). Adolescents have high failure rates of using contraceptive methods correctly, with the exception of LARC methods. Available EC methods in order of effectiveness are the copper IUD (pregnancy failure rate 0.09% and efficacy up to 5 days that is unaffected by the amount of time since unprotected sex or the patient's BMI), ulipristal acetate and mifepristone (pregnancy failure rate 0.9–2.1%, with decreasing efficacy over 5 days and appropriate for women with a BMI < 35), and levonorgestrel (pregnancy failure rate 0.6–3.1% with decreasing efficacy over 5 days and appropriate for women with a BMI < 26). The FDA approves ulipristal up to 5 days postcoitus, and levonorgestrel up to 3 days postcoitus. The Yuzpe regimen, which utilizes combined oral contraceptive pills, is least effective, but is an option if the previously mentioned methods are unavailable. All methods should be used within 5 days of unprotected sex. Indicated for use after unprotected or underprotected intercourse, EC reduces the risk of pregnancy by 88% to 99% with a primary mechanism of action of delaying or inhibiting ovulation for the oral methods, and the prevention of fertilization by inhibiting sperm motility and survival for the copper IUD. Despite the safety and efficacy of postcoital contraceptive methods, physicians may create barriers to adolescents' ability to use EC by limiting access based on timing in the menstrual cycle, requiring an office visit and a pregnancy test, and refusing to prescribe EC in advance due to concerns about overuse or that access to EC will discourage regular reproductive health care. EC efficacy is extremely time sensitive, with an increased risk of pregnancy as the time from unprotected intercourse to EC use increases. There are no contraindications to using EC except pregnancy. To facilitate quick and easy access to EC, physicians should educate all adolescents, male and female, sexually active and not, about EC and its use and consider providing a prescription for EC to female adolescents in advance so that it can be used as soon as possible when indicated.

## MEDICAL ASSESSMENT AT THE CONTRACEPTIVE VISIT

A complete medical and sexual history and limited physical assessment are recommended as a part of the first contraceptive visit to evaluate specific needs and eliminate serious contraindications to contraceptive use. Most methods of contraception can be initiated without a pelvic exam. Current recommendations to initiate Pap screening at age 21 years, combined with the ability to perform urine or vaginal self-swab screening for chlamydia and gonorrhea, have made it unnecessary to perform a pelvic examination in the asymptomatic adolescent requesting contraception. Follow-up may be individualized based on the adolescent's needs. A discussion of any side effects and difficulties in using the method and the need for continued contraception should be reviewed briefly with the patient at each visit. For the male adolescent, a brief review of need and type of contraceptive should be done at each well visit.

## METHOD INITIATION

Effective use of a contraceptive method is enhanced if the adolescent can initiate the method right away rather than waiting for her next menses. In the interest of enhancing the adolescent patient's ability to effectively prevent an unplanned pregnancy, the physician may opt for a "quick start" approach to initiating most contraceptive methods. The principles of the quick start approach include (1) immediate initiation of the method if it is 5 days or fewer since the onset of the last menstrual period; (2) a negative urine pregnancy test if it is greater than 5 days since the last menstrual period; (3) administration of emergency contraception if there has been unprotected sex in the prior 5 days, followed by initiation of the hormonal method the same day; (4) use of a backup method (condoms) for the next week; and (5) a follow-up pregnancy test in 2 weeks if the method was initiated after day 5 of the current menstrual cycle. Detailed instructions for the use of a quick start for method initiation (including LARC methods) can be found at http://www.rhedi.org/contraception/quick_start_algorithm.php.

Barral RL, Gold MA. Contraception. In: Neinstein LS, Katzman DK, Callahan ST, et al, eds. *Neinstein's Adolescent and Young Adult Health Care: A Practical Guide*. 6th ed. Philadelphia, PA: Wolters Kluwer; 2016:353-365.

Birth control methods. Bedsider Web site. http://www.bedsider.org/methods. Accessed June 24, 2016.

Cleland K, Zhu H, Goldstuck N, et al. The efficacy of intrauterine devices for emergency contraception: a systematic review of 35 years of experience. *Hum Reprod*. 2012;27:1994-2000.

Curtis KM, Tepper NK, Jatlaoui TC, et al. US Medical Eligibility Criteria for Contraceptive Use, 2016. *MMWR Recomm Rep*. 2016;65(No. RR-3):1-104.

Dayananda I, Emans SJ, Goldberg A. Contraception. In: Emans SJ, Laufer MR, eds. *Emans, Laufer, Goldstein's Pediatric and Adolescent Gynecology*. 6th ed. Philadelphia, PA: Lippincott Williams & Wilkins; 2012:447-473.

Eliscu AH, Burstein GR. Updates in contraceptive counseling for adolescents. *J Pediatr*. 2016;175:22-26.e1.

Finer LB, Zolna MR. Declines in unintended pregnancy in the United States, 2008–2011. *N Engl J Med*. 2016;374:843-852.

Hatcher RA, Trussel J, Nelson AL, et al. *Contraceptive Technology*. 20th ed. New York, NY. Ardent Media, Inc; 2012.

Kann L, McManus T, Harris WA, et al. Youth Risk Behavior Surveillance—United States, 2015. *MMWR Surveill Summ*. 2016;65(6):26-39.

Kumar N, Brown JD. Access barriers to long acting reversible contraceptives for adolescents. *J Adolesc Health*. 2016;59(3):248-53.

Society for Adolescent Health and Medicine. Emergency contraception for adolescents and young adults: guidance for health care professionals. *J Adolesc Health*. 2016;58(2):245-248.

# 82 Introduction to Developmental-Behavioral Pediatrics: Pediatric Developmental Assessment

Robert G. Voigt

## CHILD DEVELOPMENT: THE BASIC SCIENCE OF PEDIATRICS

Dr. Julius Richmond (1916–2008), a pediatrician, the first national director of Head Start, and the 12th Surgeon General of the United States (from 1977 to 1981), recognized child development as the basic science of pediatrics. The longitudinal process of child development distinguishes pediatric medicine from all other medical specialties, and child development and behavior have an impact on every pediatric healthcare encounter. In addition, developmental and behavioral concerns are the most prevalent concerns in pediatric medicine. For example, while congenital heart disease affects about 1% of the pediatric population, chronic developmental-behavioral disorders (such as learning disabilities and other learning problems, attention-deficit/hyperactivity disorder [ADHD], autism spectrum disorder, intellectual disabilities, and cerebral palsy) affect approximately 20% to 25% of the pediatric population. These numbers indicate that to provide subspecialty level care to all of these patients, board-certified developmental-behavioral pediatricians should outnumber board-certified pediatric cardiologists by at least 20 to 1. In actuality, pediatric cardiologists outnumber developmental-behavioral pediatricians by 4 to 1, resulting in a severe shortage of developmental-behavioral pediatricians and extremely long waiting lists at tertiary care developmental pediatric centers nationally. Thus, the majority of the pediatric population with developmental-behavioral concerns needs to be identified, diagnosed, and longitudinally managed by their primary care pediatric medical providers, reaffirming child development as the basic science of primary care pediatric practice.

## DEVELOPMENTAL SURVEILLANCE, SCREENING, AND EVALUATION

Because early intervention is critical in optimizing long-term developmental and behavioral outcomes, the American Academy of Pediatrics (AAP) has published policy statements to guide primary care pediatric medical providers in their identification and management of children with developmental delays. Current AAP policy describes three processes aimed at early identification of developmental delays: surveillance, screening, and evaluation. Developmental surveillance is a longitudinal clinical process that includes eliciting parental concerns, identifying medical and psychosocial risk and protective factors, documenting developmental histories provided by parents, and observing the developmental performance of the child. Developmental surveillance takes advantage of the clinical judgment and accumulated experience of pediatric medical providers, and it should be performed at every well-child encounter. Developmental screening involves the use of standardized questionnaires, which should be completed by parents at specified well-child visit ages (9 months, 18 months, 24 to 30 months, and prior to starting preschool or kindergarten). Developmental screening is designed to separate those who require further developmental evaluation from those who do not. If developmental concerns are identified through developmental surveillance or screening, children should be referred to their local early intervention (for children from birth to 3 years) or early childhood special education (for children from 3 to 5 years of age) programs. Developmental evaluation is a more complex process, including standardized developmental evaluation measures (rather than screens), and is aimed at making developmental diagnoses. AAP policy suggests that developmental evaluations can be performed by referral to pediatric subspecialists, such as developmental-behavioral pediatricians; however, given the prevalence of developmental-behavioral concerns in the general pediatric population, combined with the scarcity of developmental-behavioral pediatric subspecialists and long waiting lists at tertiary care child development centers nationally, it is essential that primary care pediatric medical providers include developmental evaluation and diagnosis as critical components of their clinical armamentarium.

## PEDIATRIC DEVELOPMENTAL ASSESSMENT

Pediatric medical providers undergo rigorous clinical training and develop a wealth of clinical experience through longitudinal pediatric practice. In pediatrics, as in all medical specialties, diagnoses are made via a combination of a thorough and detailed history that is confirmed by a direct examination. Thus, from a medical standpoint, chief complaints about developmental-behavioral concerns should be treated no differently than other common pediatric chief complaints. Developmental diagnoses can and should be made by primary pediatric medical providers through a pediatric developmental assessment process that includes a developmental history that is confirmed by a neurodevelopmental examination.

### Developmental History

Eliciting a developmental history from parents due to a chief complaint of a developmental-behavioral concern is no different from taking a medical history for any other common pediatric chief complaint. The developmental history is an elicitation of the temporal sequence of developmental milestone acquisition to date across the streams of development. Dr. Arnold Capute, who established developmental pediatric fellowship training at the Kennedy Krieger Institute at Johns Hopkins University School of Medicine, established a neurodevelopmental model involving 3 primary streams of neurodevelopment (Fig. 82-1): (1) neurocognitive, which includes the language and nonverbal/visual-motor problem-solving streams, which come together to form the social (primarily communicative; including social reciprocity and developing social relationships) and adaptive (primarily nonverbal/visual-motor problem solving; including activities of daily living, such as feeding and dressing); (2) neuromotor, which includes gross motor, fine motor, and oral motor development; and (3) neurobehavior, which includes attention and activity/impulsivity. A sample developmental milestone list across these streams of development to use in eliciting developmental histories from parents at typical well-child visit ages is shown in Table 82-1. More comprehensive developmental milestone lists to use in eliciting developmental histories from parents are widely available to pediatric clinicians, such as those included in the Learn the Signs, Act Early Web site from the Centers for Disease Control and Prevention.

When taking a developmental history, it is critical not just to document the attainment of a milestone, but to document the age of attainment of each milestone. For example, it is important information to know that a 2-year-old presenting with concerns about developmental

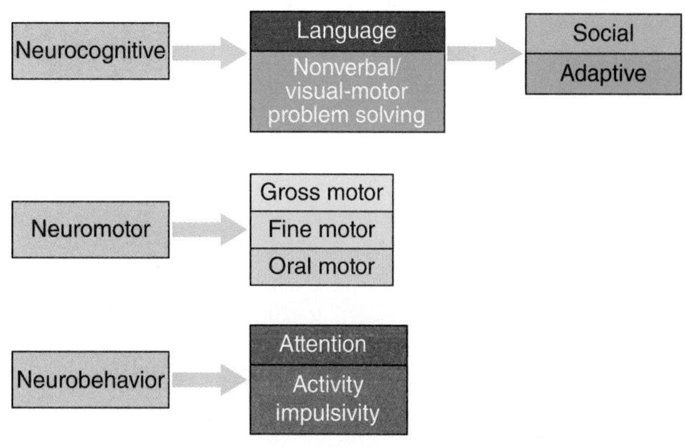


**FIGURE 82-1** Streams of development.

**TABLE 82-1 SAMPLE DEVELOPMENTAL MILESTONES TO CONSIDER WHEN ELICITING DEVELOPMENTAL HISTORIES FROM PARENTS AT WELL CHILD VISIT AGES**

| | Neurocognitive | | | | Neuromotor | | | Neurobehavior |
|---|---|---|---|---|---|---|---|---|
| **Age** | **Language** | **Social** | **Adaptive** | **Nonverbal/ Visual-Motor Problem Solving** | **Fine Motor** | **Gross Motor** | **Oral Motor/ Speech** | **Neurobehavioral Red Flags** |
| 1 mo | | Visually focuses on face | | | | Lifts head up in prone | | Extreme irritability or docility in infancy |
| 2 mo | | Social smile | | Visually tracks in horizontal and vertical planes | | Lifts chest up in prone | | Poor eye contact<br>Repetitive play (lining, sorting, spinning) |
| 4 mo | Coos (3 months); laughs (4 months) | | | Visually tracks through 360 degrees (3 months) | Hands unfisted | Supports weight with arms straight in prone; head steady in supported sitting | | Visual or verbal perseveration<br>Restricted interests |
| 6 mo | Babbles consonant sounds | Recognizes caregivers; exhibits stranger anxiety | | Reaches directly for objects; transfers objects from one hand to the other | | Rolls over both ways (5 months); sits without support | | Need for routine (picky eater who eats same food every day; upset with changes in usual car routes); upset with changes or transitions |
| 9 mo | Uses nonspecific "Mama/Dada" (at 8 months); uses specific "Mama/Dada" (at 10 months); uses gestured language (waves "bye-bye") | Plays imitative games ("peek-a-boo," "pat-a-cake"); follows a point; looks preferentially when name is called; exhibits separation anxiety | Finger feeds; holds own bottle | Looks after fallen toy (9 months); uncovers hidden toy (10 months) | Inferior pincer grasp | At 8 months: crawls, pulls to stand, comes to sit<br>At 9 months: cruises around furniture | | Motor stereotypies (hand flapping, toe walking)<br>Sensory hypo- or hyperresponsiveness |
| 12 mo | 2-word vocabulary; follows single-step gestured command ("give me") | Points to request; shares objects of interest with others; social referencing | Helps with dressing; drinks from a cup | Shows intentional release of objects | | Walks independently | | Low frustration tolerance<br>Emotional lability<br>Poor impulse control/ disinhibition |
| 15 mo | Uses immature jargon (inflection); follows single-step ungestured command (16 months) | Points to show/ share interest; shows affection | Feeds self with spoon | Scribbles in imitation | | Rarely falls with walking; walks up stairs with one hand held | | Hyperactivity<br>Inattention/easy distractibility |
| 18 mo | 10-word vocabulary; uses mature jargon (single words mixed with jargon); points to body parts | Pretend play; imitates household chores | | Scribbles spontaneously; stacks 3 blocks | | Runs; walks down stairs with one hand held | | |
| 24 mo | At least 50-word vocabulary; uses 2-word sentences (noun/verb); follows 2-step ungestured command | Parallel play | Unzips | Builds horizontal train of blocks | | Walks up and down stairs independently marking time (21 months); jumps up, getting both feet off the ground (24 months) | | |
| 30 mo | Differentiates just one item from a greater number; differentiates "on" from "under"; pronoun ("I/you") confusion ceases; echolalia ceases | | | Copies horizontal and vertical stroke in the appropriate orientation; copies circle as a circular motion | | Alternates feet up stairs; pedals tricycle | | |
| 3 y | 3-word sentences; identifies own name, gender, age | Interactive play; takes turns | Unbuttons | Copies a circle; recognizes colors | | Broad jumps; hops on one foot; alternates feet down stairs | Speech 75% understandable | |
| 4 y | Verbally relates experiences/tells stories | | Buttons | Copies a cross (3½ years) and square (4 years) | Handedness established; uses scissors | Gallops | Speech 100% understandable | |

(Continued)

**TABLE 82-1 SAMPLE DEVELOPMENTAL MILESTONES TO CONSIDER WHEN ELICITING DEVELOPMENTAL HISTORIES FROM PARENTS AT WELL CHILD VISIT AGES (CONTINUED)**

| | Neurocognitive | | | | Neuromotor | | | Neurobehavior |
|---|---|---|---|---|---|---|---|---|
| Age | Language | Social | Adaptive | Nonverbal/ Visual-Motor Problem Solving | Fine Motor | Gross Motor | Oral Motor/ Speech | Neurobehavioral Red Flags |
| 5 y | Follows 3-step commands; tells address, phone number; identifies coins | | Ties shoes | Copies a triangle; differentiates right and left; recognizes all letters of the alphabet (5½ years) | | Skips rhythmically | | |
| Red Flags | No gestured communication by 12 months; persistent echolalia beyond 30 months; pronoun ("I/you") confusion beyond 30 months | Flat facial expression/ no social smile; no pointing by 12 months; no response to name by 12 months | | Mouthing as primary means of exploration after 6 months | Fisting after 4 months; handedness before 1 year | Asymmetric movements; persistent primitive reflexes beyond 6 months; ↑ or ↓ muscle tone | Atypical/ monotonic speech prosody; stuttering after 5 years | |

delay can walk independently, but the developmental prognosis is very different if the child starting walking at 12 months of age (which would be considered age-appropriate attainment of this milestone) versus 21 months of age (which would be considered significantly delayed attainment of this milestone). While it is certainly difficult for parents to remember the age of attainment of every developmental milestone for their children, developmental histories that focus on developmental milestones that are most easily remembered by parents or that are temporally current (ie, milestones that have been recently attained) provide a wealth of information for the pediatric developmental assessment. For example, just about every parent remembers the age at which their child walked independently, but few can recall when their child first alternated their feet when walking up stairs, unless this milestone was just recently attained. Asking parents what their children were capable of doing at memorable events, such as their past birthday parties, also assists parents in their recall of developmental milestones.

An important concept to consider in taking a developmental history is the developmental quotient (DQ). The DQ can be calculated by dividing the developmental age of the child by his or her chronologic age and multiplying this by 100 to make it a percentage (DQ = [developmental age/chronologic age] × 100). For example, an 18-month-old child who has a language age of 9 months will have a developmental quotient in language development of 50% (developmental age of 9 months divided by chronologic age of 18 months times 100). While taking a developmental history, to determine a rate of developmental milestone acquisition over time, another way to calculate the DQ is to divide the age at which a milestone is expected to be attained by the age that it was actually attained and multiplying this by 100 to make it a percentage (DQ = [age milestone expected to be attained/age milestone is actually attained] × 100). For example, if a child did not wave "bye-bye," which is expected to occur around 9 months of age, until he or she was 18 months of age, the developmental quotient for the attainment of this milestone is 50% (age of expected milestone attainment of 9 months divided by the actual age of attainment of 18 months times 100). Tracking the DQ for each milestone reported in the developmental history across each developmental stream provides a slope for the developmental growth curve for each stream of development. For example, if parents report in a developmental history in the language stream that a 24-month-old child babbled consonant sounds at 12 months of age (expected at 6 months; DQ = 6 months/12 months × 100 = 50%), waved "bye-bye" at 18 months of age (expected at 9 months; DQ = 9 months/18 months × 100 = 50%), used a specific "Mama" and "Dada" at 20 months of age (expected at 10 months; DQ = 10 months/20 months × 100 = 50%), and just started to follow single-step gestured commands at 24 months of age (expected at 12 months; DQ = 12 months/24 months × 100 = 50%), the developmental history provides a historical slope that this child has acquired speech and language developmental milestones at 50% the expected rate. DQs between 85% and 115% are considered within age-appropriate limits, DQs between 70% and 85% are considered below average or at risk, and DQs less than 70% are considered delayed. All children with a DQ below 70% in any developmental stream, and all children with DQs between 70% and 85% in more than one developmental stream should be referred to their local early-intervention programs.

**Patterns of Developmental Delay** Information obtained from the developmental history provided by parents can be used to establish the slope of developmental milestone acquisition across time or the pattern of developmental delay. This pattern of developmental delay is critical both for guiding the most appropriate medical laboratory workup to pursue in an attempt to establish an etiologic diagnosis to account for the developmental delay and for direction regarding the intensity of therapeutic services to order for habilitative versus rehabilitative purposes. There are 3 primary patterns of developmental delay: static, progressive, and acute (Fig. 82-2).

In a static pattern of developmental delay, the developmental history suggests a consistent, albeit slower-than-expected, rate of developmental milestone acquisition over time. For example, in a 36-month-old with a static pattern of globally delayed developmental

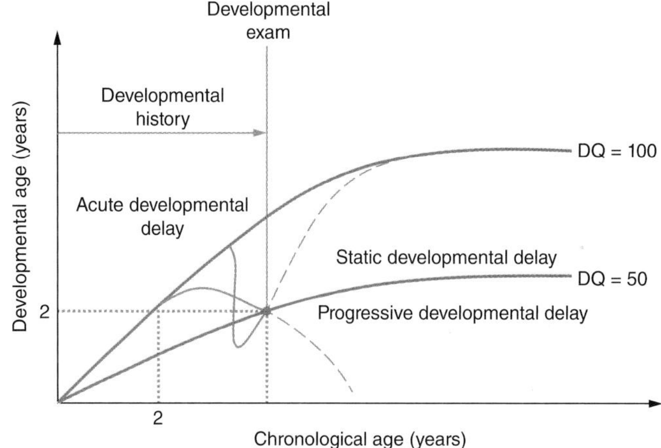


**FIGURE 82-2** Patterns of developmental delay.

milestones across developmental streams, parents may report in the developmental history that from a gross motor standpoint, the child walked at 18 months of age (expected at 12 months; DQ = 12 months/18 months × 100 = 67%) and just started jumping at 36 months of age (expected at 24 months; DQ = 24 months/36 months × 100 = 67%). From a nonverbal/visual-motor problem-solving standpoint, the parents may report that the child scribbled spontaneously between 24 and 30 months of age (expected at 18 months; DQ = 18 months/~27 months × 100 = 67%) and just started making horizontal trains of blocks about 1 month ago, at 35 months of age (expected at 24 months; DQ = 24/35 × 100 = 69%). From a language standpoint, the parents may report that the child waved "bye-bye" between 12 and 18 months of age (expected at 9 months; DQ = 9 months/~15 months × 100 = 60%), used a specific "Mama" and "Dada" at 18 months of age (expected at 10 months; DQ = 10 months/18 months × 100 = 55%), and just started using two-word sentences (expected at 24 months; DQ = 24 months/36 months × 100 = 67%) and following two-step commands (expected at 24 months; DQ = 24 months/36 months × 100 = 67%) at 36 months of age. Thus, the parents report a developmental history of globally delayed developmental milestones across developmental streams (with the DQs across streams being less than 70%), with a fairly consistent rate of delayed milestone acquisition both within each stream of development and across the different streams of development. Such a static pattern of developmental delay is by far the most common pattern of delayed developmental milestone acquisition observed in the pediatric population. In terms of medical laboratory workup, children with a static pattern of globally delayed developmental milestones should undergo a chromosome microarray analysis and DNA testing for fragile X syndrome. Extensive metabolic testing is generally not warranted in a child presenting with a static pattern of globally delayed developmental milestones, unless the child also has tonal or movement abnormalities, seizures, decompensation with mild illness, recurrent vomiting, unusual dietary preferences, failure to thrive, or other signs or symptoms of a metabolic disorder. Brain imaging can be considered with focal neurologic findings, macrocephaly, or microcephaly.

In a progressive pattern of developmental delay, the developmental history may include age-appropriate acquisition of early developmental milestones, but this is followed by plateauing of developmental milestone acquisition, followed by a loss of previously acquired developmental skills. For example, in the developmental history of a 24-month-old with a progressive pattern of delayed developmental milestones, parents may report that the child walked independently at 12 months of age (expected at 12 months; DQ = 12 months/12 months × 100 = 100%), ran at 18 months of age (expected at 18 months; DQ = 18 months/18 months × 100 = 100%), scribbled spontaneously at 18 months of age (expected at 18 months; DQ = 18 months/18 months × 100 = 100%), used a specific "Mama" and "Dada" and at least 2 other words by 12 months of age (expected at 12 months; DQ = 12 months/12 months × 100 = 100%), and was using at least 10 words by 18 months of age (expected at 18 months; DQ = 18 months/18 months × 100 = 100%). However, over the last 6 months, the parents report that the child stopped running, then stopped walking independently, and now can only walk with one hand held (expected at 10 months; DQ = 10 months/24 months × 100 = 42%). The parents also report that the child can no longer scribble and has stopped using any words, except for a specific "Mama" and "Dada" (expected at 10 months; DQ = 10 months/24 months × 100 = 42%). Thus, this developmental history indicates that this child has progressively lost developmental milestones over time across developmental streams. Such a progressive pattern of developmental delay is a classic pattern for children with inborn errors of metabolism. Thus, when a developmental history documents a progressive pattern of developmental delay, it is critical for a comprehensive metabolic workup to be pursued as soon as possible (plasma lactate, ammonia, amino acids, acylcarnitine profile; urine organic acids, urine purines/pyrimidines, urine mucopolysaccharides, etc.), as some inborn errors of metabolism are treatable, and the earlier the initiation of treatment, the better the developmental outcome.

In an acute pattern of developmental delay, the developmental history reports age-appropriate acquisition of early developmental milestones, followed by a sudden, acute drop in developmental milestone acquisition, followed by subsequent regain in developmental milestone acquisition. For example, in the developmental history of a 24-month-old with an acute pattern of developmental delay, parents may report that a child walked at 12 months of age (expected at 12 months; DQ = 12 months/12 months × 100 = 100%), ran at 18 months of age (expected at 18 months; DQ = 18 months/18 months × 100 = 100%), used a specific "Mama" and "Dada" and at least 2 other words by 12 months of age (expected at 12 months; DQ = 12 months/12 months × 100 = 100%), and pointed to body parts by 18 months of age (expected at 18 months; DQ = 18 months/18 months × 100 = 100%), but the child suddenly lost the ability to walk or to say any words shortly after turning 18 months of age. Subsequently, the child has just started to walk independently again at 24 months (expected at 12 months; DQ = 12 months/24 months × 100 = 50%) and has just started using a specific "Mama" and "Dada" and two other words again (expected at 12 months; DQ = 12 months/12 months × 100 = 50%). Thus, this developmental history indicates an acute loss of developmental milestones at 18 months of age followed by a period of recovery of previously acquired developmental skills. The medical etiology for such an acute pattern of developmental delay is usually obvious, as such a sudden acute drop in developmental milestone acquisition occurs in association with traumatic brain injuries, near-drownings, meningitis, encephalitis, etc. Thus, no further medical laboratory workup in an attempt to establish an etiologic diagnosis is typically indicated in children with acute patterns of developmental delay. However, it is critical to differentiate an acute pattern of developmental delay from a static pattern, as the intensity of therapeutic services to recommend differs between these two patterns of developmental delay. While therapeutic services for children with static patterns of developmental delay are habilitative in nature, in acute patterns of developmental delay, therapies are rehabilitative, as therapists work with children to regain the skills that they previously had acquired. As there is vast evidence to support the need for more intensive therapeutic interventions in rehabilitative settings, more intensive therapeutic interventions need to be ordered for children with acute patterns of developmental delay, in an attempt to guide their developmental trajectories back toward their original trajectory before the acute medical event that resulted in their acute loss of skills.

It is only the developmental history that can establish the pattern of developmental delay, which is required to guide pediatric medical providers in selecting the most appropriate medical laboratory workup to pursue in an attempt to determine the etiological diagnosis that accounts for the developmental delay and in ordering the most appropriate level of intensity of therapeutic interventions. An isolated failed developmental screen, or even a more comprehensive but isolated developmental evaluation, provides data for only one point in time, and thus provides no information whatsoever regarding the pattern of developmental delay (Figure 82-2). Thus, a comprehensive developmental history, which even in interdisciplinary developmental evaluation settings is typically performed only by the pediatric medical provider, is critical in the medical evaluation of children with developmental delays.

**Delay, Dissociation, and Deviation** The developmental history should identify three potential developmental problems: (1) developmental delay, (2) developmental dissociation, and (3) developmental deviation. Developmental delay is defined by a significant lag in acquisition of developmental milestones in one or more streams of development. As the most common causes of developmental delay in children tend to affect the brain diffusely, developmental delay is most commonly represented by a more global delay affecting all streams of development. For example, in children with Down syndrome, every neuron in the brain contains an extra copy of chromosome 21. Thus, most children with Down syndrome exhibit global delays across all developmental streams, rather than isolated delays in neurocognitive, neuromotor, or neurobehavioral development.

As an example of a child with developmental delay, consider the case of a 24-month-old boy who fails a developmental screen and whose parents are concerned that he is not talking. In the developmental history, from a gross motor standpoint, the parents report that the child sat independently at 12 months of age (expected at 6 months; DQ = 6 months/12 months × 100 = 50%), and he just started to take independent steps at 24 months of age (expected at 12 months; DQ = 12 months/24 months × 100 = 50%). From a nonverbal/visual-motor problem-solving standpoint, the parents report that the child began reaching for objects at 12 months of age (expected at 6 months; DQ = 6 months/12 months × 100 = 50%), he began uncovering hidden toys at 18 months of age (expected at 10 months; DQ = 10 months/18 months × 100 = 55%), and he just started showing an intentional release of objects at 24 months of age (expected at 12 months; DQ = 12 months/24 months × 100 = 50%). From a speech/language standpoint, the parents report that the child began babbling consonant sounds at 12 months of age (expected at 6 months; DQ = 6 months/12 months × 100 = 50%), he began using a specific "Mama" and "Dada" at 21 months of age (expected at 10 months; DQ = 10 months/21 months × 100 = 48%), and he just started to follow single-step gestured commands at 24 months of age (expected at 12 months; DQ = 12 months/24 months × 100 = 50%). This developmental history indicates that this child is showing globally delayed developmental milestones, and he has been acquiring developmental milestones at approximately 50% the expected rate both within and across developmental streams. Thus, despite the parents presenting concern about not talking, this child's language delay is actually a component of more globally delayed developmental milestones across developmental streams.

Developmental dissociation is defined by a difference in rates of development between developmental streams, with one stream discrepantly and disproportionately more delayed compared to the other streams. A 15% difference in DQ scores between two streams of development defines a developmental dissociation. As more global developmental delay is more commonly observed than dissociation, developmental dissociation can be considered a more atypical developmental pattern compared to global developmental delay, with larger dissociations being more atypical. Dissociation more often occurs in a setting of more globally delayed developmental milestones (eg, discrepant and disproportionate delays in language in a child with global cognitive delays), but it can occur and result in significant dysfunction even in a setting without any significant developmental delays (eg, as occurs in ADHD and learning disabilities). Examples of developmental dissociation include (1) cerebral palsy, where neuromotor development is discrepantly delayed compared to other developmental streams; (2) ADHD, where the neurobehavioral domains of attention, impulse control, and activity are discrepantly delayed compared to overall cognitive developmental level; and (3) learning disabilities, where there is either a dissociation between verbal and nonverbal cognitive abilities and/or where academic achievement is discrepantly delayed compared to cognitive expectations.

As an example of a child with developmental dissociation, consider another case of a 24-month-old boy who fails a developmental screen and whose parents are concerned that he is not talking. In the developmental history, from a gross motor standpoint, the parents report that the child sat independently at 6 months of age (expected at 6 months; DQ = 6 months/6 months × 100 = 100%), he walked independently at 12 months of age (expected at 12 months; DQ = 12 months/12 months × 100 = 100%), and he just started at 24 months to jump up, getting both feet off the ground (expected at 24 months; DQ = 24 months/24 months × 100 = 100%). From a nonverbal/visual-motor problem-solving standpoint, the parents report that the child began releasing objects intentionally at 12 months of age (expected at 12 months; DQ = 12 months/12 months × 100 = 100%), he scribbled spontaneously at 18 months of age (expected at 18 months; DQ = 18 months/18 months × 100 = 100%), and he just started aligning blocks to build horizontal trains at 24 months of age (expected at 24 months; DQ = 24 months/24 months × 100 = 100%). From a speech/language standpoint, the parents report that the child began babbling consonant sounds at 12 months of age (expected at 6 months; DQ = 6 months/12 months × 100 = 50%), he began using a specific "Mama" and "Dada" at 21 months of age (expected at 10 months; DQ = 10 months/21 months × 100 = 48%), and he just started to follow single-step gestured commands at 24 months of age (expected at 12 months; DQ = 12 months/24 months × 100 = 50%). This developmental history indicates that this child is evidencing age-appropriate acquisition of gross motor and nonverbal/visual-motor problem-solving skills (with acquisition of gross motor and nonverbal/visual-motor problem-solving skills at 100%, the expected rate), but his language development is discrepantly and disproportionately delayed (with acquisition of language skills at 50% of the expected rate). Thus, this child is exhibiting dissociation in his language development, and he can be described as exhibiting a language disorder. Note that while he is exhibiting dissociated delays in his language development, he has acquired language skills in the typical sequence of acquisition of language skills.

Developmental deviation is defined as a deviation in the usual sequential acquisition of developmental milestones within a developmental stream. When developmental deviation occurs, higher age-level developmental milestones are acquired before lower age-level developmental milestones within a developmental stream. This nonsequential developmental milestone acquisition observed with developmental deviation is more atypical than developmental dissociation or global developmental delay. Examples of developmental deviation include (1) cerebral palsy, where deviated motor milestone acquisition is often observed (eg, a child with a spastic diparetic form of cerebral palsy may be able to stand holding on to furniture, an 8-month-level skill, before he or she is able to sit independently, a 6-month-level skill, or roll over both ways, a 5-month-level skill, due to increased lower extremity muscle tone and a persistent positive support primitive reflex), and (2) autism spectrum disorders, where deviated language milestone acquisition is often observed (eg, a child with autism spectrum disorder may have a vocabulary of at least 50 words, a 24-month-level skill, before he or she uses a specific "Mama" and "Dada" to refer to his or her parents, a 10-month-level skill, or he or she may use multiword sentences, a 36-month-old level skill, but still be confusing pronouns and using echolalia, which are expected to cease by 30 months).

As an example of a child with developmental deviation, consider a final case of a 24-month-old boy who fails a developmental screen and whose parents are concerned that he is not talking. In the developmental history, from a gross motor standpoint, the parents report that the child sat independently at 6 months of age (expected at 6 months; DQ = 6 months/6 months × 100 = 100%), walked independently at 12 months of age (expected at 12 months; DQ = 12 months/12 months × 100 = 100%), and just started at 24 months of age to jump up, getting both feet off the ground (expected at 24 months; DQ = 24 months/24 months × 100 = 100%). From a nonverbal/visual-motor problem-solving standpoint, the parents report that the child began releasing objects intentionally at 12 months of age (expected at 12 months; DQ = 12 months/12 months × 100 = 100%), he scribbled spontaneously at 18 months of age (expected at 18 months; DQ = 18 months/18 months × 100 = 100%), and he just started building horizontal trains of blocks (expected at 24 months; DQ = 24 months/24 months × 100 = 100%), but he does not yet copy a circle as a circular motion (expected at 30 months). However, the parents report that he is able to recognize colors (expected at 36 months) and all the letters of the alphabet (expected at 5½ years of age). From a speech/language standpoint, the parents report that the child began babbling consonant sounds at 12 months of age (expected at 6 months; DQ = 6 months/12 months × 100 = 50%), and he currently has a 10-word vocabulary (expected at 18 months; DQ = 18 months/24 months × 100 = 75%), but he does not use a specific "Mama" or "Dada" (expected at 10 months; DQ less than 10 months/24 months × 100, or less than 42%), wave "bye-bye" (expected at 9 months; DQ less than 9 months/24 months × 100, or less than 38%), or follow single-step gestured commands (expected at 12 months; DQ less than 12 months/24 months × 100, or less than 50%). Thus, this developmental history indicates that this child is evidencing age-appropriate acquisition of gross motor developmental milestones (with acquisition of gross motor skills at 100% the expected rate). His acquisition of nonverbal/visual-motor problem-solving skills also appears age-appropriate (with acquisition of nonverbal/visual-motor problem-solving skills generally at 100% the expected rate) with upward developmental deviation to a 3-year-old to 5½-year-old level (given his ability to visually recognize colors and letters of the alphabet). However, this child's language development is discrepantly and disproportionately delayed compared to his acquisition of developmental milestones in other developmental streams; thus, he is exhibiting dissociation in his language development. In addition to this dissociation in his language development, he is also exhibiting significant developmental deviation in his acquisition of language milestones. While his parents report that he has a 10-word vocabulary, as expected at 18 months of age, he is not yet using a specific "Mama" or "Dada" to refer to his parents, as expected at 10 months, and he does not yet wave "bye-bye," as expected at 9 months. Thus, this child is exhibiting a very atypical developmental pattern, with age-appropriate gross motor development, age-appropriate nonverbal/visual-motor problem-solving development but with upward developmental deviation in his acquisition of nonverbal/visual-motor problem-solving skills, and dissociated delays and developmental deviation in his language development. As will be reviewed in Chapter 83, the more delayed, dissociated, and deviated a child's neurocognitive development is, the more atypical his or her neurobehavior is expected to be. Thus, the child in this example presents with an atypical developmental history that is characteristically accompanied by the atypical behaviors observed in children with autism spectrum disorders.

Three cases of a 24-month-old boy who fails a developmental screen and whose parents are concerned that he is not talking have been presented. Based on the medical process of history taking, the presence of developmental delay, dissociation, and/or deviation are identified in the developmental histories elicited, and 3 different diagnoses (global developmental delay, language disorder, autism spectrum disorder) are suspected, despite the same failed screen and the same parental chief complaint.



### Neurodevelopmental Examination

In a medical model, diagnoses for any chief complaint are made via a combination of a thorough and detailed history that is confirmed by direct examination. Thus, for a chief complaint of a developmental or behavioral concern, the first step is a thorough and detailed developmental history, which establishes the pattern of developmental delay (static, progressive, or acute) and identifies developmental delay, dissociation, and deviation. Then, a neurodevelopmental examination needs to be completed to confirm historical findings. The neurodevelopmental examination combines a traditional neurologic examination with direct developmental evaluation of the child. Confirmation of information gleaned from the developmental history can be made via the pediatric medical provider's completion of a standardized developmental evaluation instrument, several of which are available to pediatric medical providers, including the Capute Scales, the Parents' Evaluation of Developmental Status: Developmental Milestones (PEDS:DM) Assessment Level, and the Gesell Developmental Observation-Revised. With a tired, fussy, or otherwise uncooperative child, even an informal direct observation of a few developmental skills can often confirm estimates of a child's rate of developmental milestone acquisition based on the developmental history.

As an example of using a neurodevelopmental examination to confirm findings from the developmental history, consider another case of a 24-month-old boy who fails a developmental screen and whose parents are concerned that he is not talking. In this case, the developmental history documents that this child is presenting with delayed language milestones, but these language delays are occurring in the context of commensurate delays in motor and nonverbal/visual-motor problem-solving developmental milestones. The developmental history indicates that this child is acquiring developmental milestones globally in a static pattern at 50% the expected rate. On neurodevelopmental examination, from a gross motor standpoint, the child is directly observed to walk independently (expected at 12 months), but he is observed to frequently fall with walking (walking without frequent falling expected at 15 months), and he is not observed to be able to walk up stairs with one hand held (expected at 15 months). Thus, on neurodevelopmental examination, this child's gross motor development appears most secure at a 12-month level, for a corresponding DQ of 50% (12 months/24 months × 100). From a nonverbal/visual-motor problem-solving standpoint, the child is observed to show an intentional release (expected at 12 months), but he is not observed to scribble in imitation (less than 16 months). Thus, on neurodevelopmental examination, this child's nonverbal/visual-motor problem-solving development appears most secure at a 12-month level, for a corresponding DQ of 50% (12 months/24 months × 100). Finally, from a language standpoint, the child is observed to follow single-step gestured commands (expected at 12 months), but he is not observed to follow single-step ungestured commands (expected at 16 months). Thus, on neurodevelopmental examination, this child's language development also appears most secure at a 12-month level, for a corresponding DQ of 50% (12 months/24 months × 100). In this example, the developmental history indicated that this child was exhibiting a static pattern of globally delayed developmental milestones, with developmental milestone acquisition globally at 50% the expected rate, and the neurodevelopmental exam confirmed current globally delayed developmental milestones, with developmental quotients of 50% across all developmental streams. This neurodevelopmental examination confirmation of findings from the developmental history increases the validity of developmental conclusions.

## CONCLUSION

As child development is the basic science of pediatrics and developmental-behavioral concerns are the most prevalent chronic concerns in primary care pediatric practice, pediatric medical providers should consider the pediatric developmental assessment model described above as a routine component of primary care pediatric medical practice. This model is medically based, as chief complaints about developmental-behavioral concerns (such as a failed developmental screen) are evaluated through obtaining a developmental history and performing a neurodevelopmental examination. In this model, the developmental history establishes the pattern of developmental delay (critical for medical laboratory workup and therapeutic recommendations) and identifies developmental delay, dissociation, and deviation. The neurodevelopmental examination serves to confirm findings from the developmental history. Neurodevelopmental examination confirmation of information gleaned from the developmental history provides valid documentation of a child's current developmental status and proceeds toward making developmental-behavioral diagnoses.

## SUGGESTED READINGS

Accardo PJ, Capute AJ. *The Capute Scales: Cognitive Adaptive Test/Clinical Linguistic & Auditory Milestone Scale (CAT/CLAMS)*. Baltimore, MD: Paul H. Brookes Publishing Company; 2005.

American Academy of Pediatrics Council on Children with Disabilities, Section on Developmental-Behavioral Pediatrics, Bright Futures Steering Committee, Medical Home Initiatives for Children with Special Needs Project Advisory Committee. Identifying infants and young children with developmental disorders in the medical home: an algorithm for developmental surveillance and screening. *Pediatrics*. 2006;118:405-420.

Capute AJ, Accardo PJ. The infant neurodevelopmental assessment: a clinical interpretive manual for CAT-CLAMS in first two years of life, Part 1. *Curr Probl Pediatr*. 1996;26:238-257.

Capute AJ, Accardo PJ. The infant neurodevelopmental assessment: a clinical interpretive manual for CAT-CLAMS in the first two years of life, Part 2. *Curr Probl Pediatr*. 1996;26:279-306.

Centers for Disease Control and Prevention. Learn the signs. Act early: Developmental milestones. http://www.cdc.gov/ncbddd/actearly/milestones/. Accessed July 9, 2016.

Gesell Institute of Child Development. *Gesell Developmental Observation-Revised Examiner's Manual.* New Haven, CT: Gesell Institute of Child Development; 2011.

Glascoe FP, Robertshaw NS. *PEDS: Developmental Milestones, Professionals' Manual.* Nolensville, TN: Ellsworth & Vandermeer Press, LLC; 2011.

Richmond JB. Child development: a basic science for pediatrics. *Pediatrics.* 1967;39:649-658.

Shapiro BK, Gwynn H. Neurodevelopmental assessment of infants and young children. In: Accardo PJ, ed. *Capute and Accardo's Neurodevelopmental Disabilities in Infancy and Childhood.* 3rd ed. Baltimore, MD: Paul H. Brookes Publishing Company; 2008:367-393.





# 83 Developmental-Behavioral Pediatric Diagnosis

Robert G. Voigt

## INTRODUCTION

The previous chapter presented a medical model for pediatric medical providers to use to assess children presenting with chief complaints about development or behavior. In this model, a failed developmental screen or concerns identified through developmental surveillance function as a chief complaint, and this is followed by a comprehensive developmental history detailing the temporal acquisition of developmental milestones across developmental streams. The developmental history focuses on milestones that are easily remembered and those that are temporally current and provides data on the pattern of developmental delay (static, progressive, or acute) that helps guide decisions for medical laboratory workup and intensity of therapeutic services to order. The developmental history also identifies the three potential problems than can occur with development: developmental delay, developmental dissociation, and developmental deviation. Developmental delay represents a lag in the acquisition of developmental milestones compared to what is typically observed in children of similar chronologic age. Given that the majority of etiologies for developmental delay affect the brain diffusely (eg, chromosomal disorders), developmental delay more commonly presents as global delays across all streams of development. Developmental dissociation occurs when one stream of development is significantly more delayed than other streams. Since global developmental delay is a more commonly presenting scenario, developmental dissociation can be considered a more atypical presentation, and dissociations between developmental streams can be problematic, even in a setting without any significant developmental delay (as can be seen in learning disabilities or attention-deficit/hyperactivity disorder [ADHD]). Developmental deviation occurs when a child acquires developmental milestones in a nonsequential fashion; children with developmental deviation acquire higher-level developmental milestones within a developmental stream before acquiring lower-level developmental milestones within that stream. Thus, developmental deviation is defined by development or behavior that is atypical at any age. Once the developmental history has been completed, a neurodevelopmental examination, which includes a traditional neurologic examination and an extended developmental evaluation, is performed. In most cases, the neurodevelopmental examination should confirm findings from the developmental history, increasing the validity of the developmental conclusions drawn from this pediatric neurodevelopmental assessment process. Once the pediatric neurodevelopmental assessment has been completed, specific developmental-behavioral diagnoses can be made.

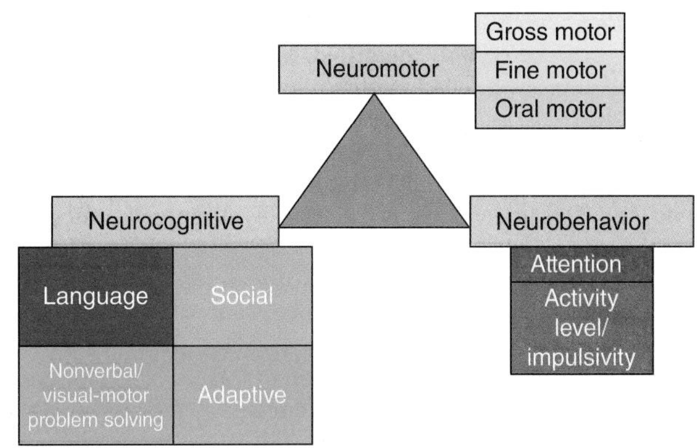


**FIGURE 83-1** Capute's Triangle (expanded).

## CAPUTE'S TRIANGLE

Dr. Arnold J. Capute (1923–2003), a pediatrician who was on the original staff of the John F. Kennedy Institute for Habilitation of the Mentally and Physically Handicapped Child (now the Kennedy Krieger Institute), and who established fellowship training in developmental pediatrics at the Johns Hopkins University School of Medicine in Baltimore, Maryland, is generally considered the "father" of the field of neurodevelopmental disabilities. Dr. Capute established a model for understanding the spectrum and continuum of developmental-behavioral diagnoses—from lower-incidence, higher-morbidity disorders such as intellectual disability, autism spectrum disorder, and cerebral palsy to higher-incidence, lower-morbidity disorders such as learning disability, ADHD, and motor incoordination (gross motor dyspraxia, fine motor dysgraphia, and speech articulation disorders). This model begins with a simple triangle that represents the three primary streams of neurodevelopment: the neurocognitive stream, the neuromotor stream, and the neurobehavioral stream (Fig. 83-1).

### Streams of Neurodevelopment

The different domains of neurodevelopment tend to be referred to as "streams," indicating that these domains of development have ongoing forward progression over time. The neuromotor stream of development includes gross motor, fine motor, and oral motor streams. The neurocognitive stream of development includes the language and nonverbal/visual-motor problem-solving streams, which come together to form the social (primarily communicative, including social reciprocity and developing social relationships) and adaptive (primarily nonverbal/visual-motor problem solving, including activities of daily living such as feeding and dressing) streams of development. The neurobehavioral stream might be considered to encompass all of child psychiatry, but this chapter will focus on the neurobehavioral streams of attention and hyperactivity/impulsivity.

## KEY NEURODEVELOPMENTAL PRINCIPLES

There are several key neurodevelopmental principles that guide developmental-behavioral diagnosis:

1. **There is a spectrum of disability within each neurodevelopmental stream, and mild disabilities predominate over severe disabilities.** In the neuromotor stream, mild disabilities such as gross motor dyspraxia, fine motor dysgraphia, and speech articulation disorders are more prevalent than cerebral palsy. In the neurocognitive stream, learning difficulties (both below average or slower learning and specific learning disabilities) are more prevalent than intellectual disability. In the neurobehavioral stream, ADHD is more prevalent than the more atypical behaviors observed in autism spectrum disorder.

2. **The more severe the developmental-behavioral disability, the earlier it can be reliably identified.** More severe disabilities, such as cerebral palsy, intellectual disability, and autism spectrum disorder, should in most cases be reliably diagnosed before 3 years of age (except for some cases of higher-functioning autism spectrum disorder), while more mild disabilities, such as learning disabilities and ADHD, can generally not be reliably diagnosed until a child reaches school age.
3. **There is a continuum of disability across neurodevelopmental streams: Delays in one stream of neurodevelopment are most likely to occur in association with delays in other streams of neurodevelopment.** Thus, the presenting developmental-behavioral chief complaint (eg, "He's not talking") often only represents the tip of the iceberg of more global underlying neurodevelopmental delays. In child development, diffuse/global developmental dysfunction across neurocognitive, neurobehavioral, and neuromotor streams is more prevalent than dissociated/deviated dysfunction. For example, in the neurocognitive stream of development, at the mild end of the spectrum, the more globally delayed pattern of slower learning (children with below-average to borderline intelligence, ie, IQs between 70 and 89) affects approximately 23% of the population, while the more dissociated pattern of learning disability affects only approximately 5% to 10% of the population. At the severe end of the neurocognitive spectrum, the more globally delayed developmental pattern of intellectual disability affects approximately 2% to 3% of the population, while the more dissociated and deviated social communication disorders occurring in children with autism spectrum disorder affect only about 1% of the population.
4. **Developmental delay, dissociation, and deviation reflect underlying central nervous system dysfunction.** Thus, children with more global central nervous system dysfunction (intellectual disability) are more likely to also exhibit developmental dissociation and deviation than are children without intellectual disability. For example, the dissociated neurobehavioral delays in attention and hyperactivity/impulsivity observed in ADHD and the more deviated neurobehavior observed in autism spectrum disorder are more commonly observed in children with intellectual disability (or more global central nervous system dysfunction) than in children without intellectual disability.
5. **In the continuum of neurodevelopmental disabilities, the more delayed, dissociated, and deviated the neurocognitive development, the more atypical the neurobehavior is likely to be.** Thus, children who have the most dissociated and deviated neurocognitive profiles (ie, a social communication disorder) are most likely to also have the most atypical neurobehavioral presentations. In this model, autism spectrum disorder results from the most dissociated and deviated neurocognitive profile (ie, a social communication disorder) in continuum with the most dissociated and deviated neurobehavioral profile (atypical inattention [poor sustained eye contact, perseveration, sensory hypo- or hyper-responsiveness] and stereotypic motor behaviors).

## DEVELOPMENTAL VERSUS ETIOLOGIC DIAGNOSIS AND IMPACT OF THE ENVIRONMENT

Before reviewing the spectrum and continuum of developmental-behavioral diagnoses, it is important to note that all developmental diagnoses, such as intellectual disability, autism spectrum disorder, cerebral palsy, learning disability, and ADHD, are descriptive in nature. Each child with a neurodevelopmental diagnosis has an underlying etiologic diagnosis that accounts for his or her neurodevelopmental disability. These etiologic diagnoses include genetic syndromes (eg, Down syndrome, fragile X syndrome), metabolic disorders (eg, inborn errors of metabolism, hypothyroidism), prematurity, teratogenic exposures (eg, in utero substance exposure, fetal alcohol syndrome), structural brain anomalies (eg, lissencephaly), infection/inflammation (eg, meningoencephalitis), hypoxia/ischemia, chronic illness/malnutrition, and traumatic brain injuries. The more severe the developmental delay, the more likely that an etiologic diagnosis will be uncovered. Unfortunately, as mild disabilities predominate over severe disabilities, a specific etiologic diagnosis is not determined in a majority of children with developmental disabilities. It is also critically important to acknowledge the impact of adverse childhood experiences and toxic stress (eg, abuse/neglect, caregiver substance abuse/mental illness, exposure to violence, poverty) as an etiology for impaired neurodevelopment. In addition, it is also essential to recognize the impact of environment and experiences on shaping neurodevelopmental outcomes, no matter the etiologic diagnosis.

## SPECTRUM OF GLOBAL DEVELOPMENTAL DELAY

Figure 83-2 illustrates the spectrum of global developmental delay. Starting from a child with age-appropriate neurocognitive, neurobehavioral, and neuromotor development, if a mild and global developmental delay occurs, then the mild end of this spectrum consists of children with mild neurocognitive delays, involving both language and nonverbal/visual-motor problem-solving developmental streams. In the school-aged population, the mild end of this spectrum includes children with below-average (IQ = 80–89) and borderline (IQ = 70–79) cognitive development, and these two groups of children, who experience significant difficulties with learning in a regular classroom environment, make up approximately 23% of the population. As the amount of developmental delay increases in children with global developmental delay, they will reach a level where they are described to have an intellectual disability. Children with intellectual disabilities possess cognitive and adaptive abilities more than 2 standard deviations below that expected for their chronologic ages, with IQs and adaptive behavior quotients below 70. Children with intellectual disability make up approximately 2% to 3% of the population. While some children with intellectual disability may exhibit age-appropriate acquisition of early motor milestones, in the spectrum of global developmental delay, children's neurobehavioral and neuromotor skills are generally commensurate with their levels of neurocognitive development. In other words, if a 6-year-old child has a cognitive age equivalent of 3 years, it is expected that his or her behavior and motor skills would be generally consistent with that of a 3-year-old.

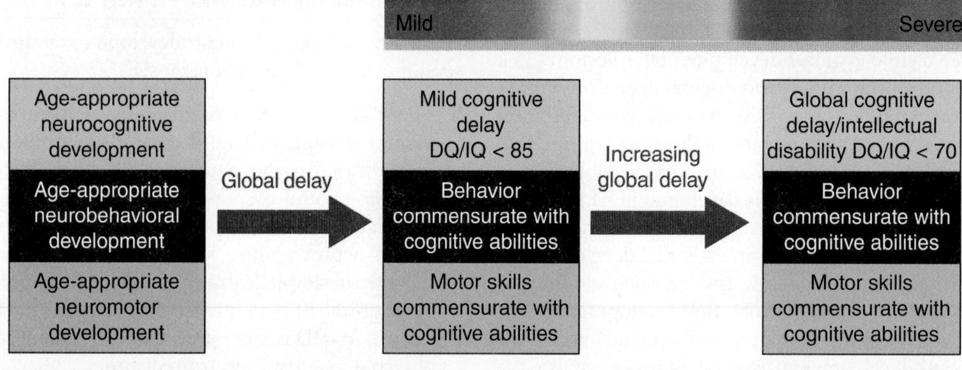


**FIGURE 83-2** Spectrum of global developmental delay.

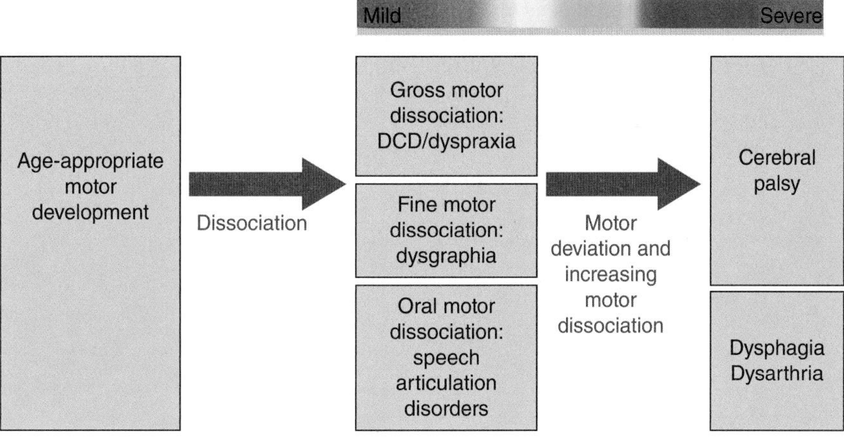


**FIGURE 83-3** Spectrum of motor dissociation and deviation.

## SPECTRUM OF NEUROMOTOR DISSOCIATION AND DEVIATION

Figure 83-3 illustrates the spectrum of neuromotor dissociation and deviation. In this spectrum, a child's motor skills are discrepantly and disproportionately delayed or dissociated from his or her skills in other developmental streams. At the mild end of this spectrum, children can evidence mildly discrepant delays in gross motor coordination (eg, dyspraxia or developmental coordination disorder) and/or fine motor coordination (eg, handwriting difficulties or dysgraphia) and/or speech articulation disorders. While these children at the mild end of the spectrum of motor dissociation and deviation do not generally exhibit "hard" neurologic signs (such as hypertonia, hypotonia, hyperreflexia, or ataxia), they often exhibit "soft" neurologic signs (such as mirror movements, dysdiadchokinesis, or posturing of the upper extremities with stressed gaits). As one moves across this spectrum from mild to severe, motor development becomes more dissociated and more deviated until one reaches the severe end of this spectrum, or cerebral palsy (with associated oromotor dysarthria and dysphagia). Children with cerebral palsy typically exhibit deviation in their motor development. For example, a child with spastic diparetic cerebral palsy may be able to stand against furniture (expected at 8 months) but not be able to sit independently (expected at 6 months) or roll over both ways (expected at 5 months). This deviated achievement of higher-level motor skills before achievement of lower-level motor skills is likely due to the child's increased lower-extremity muscle tone combined with a persistent positive support primitive reflex. In association with their dissociated and deviated motor development, children with cerebral palsy exhibit "hard" neurologic signs (eg, tonal abnormalities, hyperreflexia, persistent primitive reflexes, dyskinetic movements). Mild motor coordination difficulties (eg, dyspraxia, dysgraphia, speech articulation disorders) are far more prevalent than cerebral palsy, which has a prevalence of approximately 2 per 1000 children.

## SPECTRUM OF NEUROCOGNITIVE DISSOCIATION AND DEVIATION

Figure 83-4 illustrates the spectrum of neurocognitive dissociation and deviation. The neurocognitive stream of development consists of the language and nonverbal/visual-motor problem-solving streams of development, which come together to produce the social (primarily communicative) and adaptive (primarily nonverbal/visual-motor problem-solving) streams. In this spectrum, if a child exhibits mildly discrepant and disproportionate delays or dissociation in language development compared to nonverbal/visual-motor problem-solving development, he or she is at the mild end of a spectrum of dissociated and deviated language development, as illustrated across the top of Figure 83-4. In the preschool-aged population, such a child would be described as exhibiting a language disorder, but in the school-aged population, such a child would be described as exhibiting a language-based learning disability. In the school-aged population, a child's dissociated delays in language development can be very mild, as is observed in children with phonological processing deficits that result

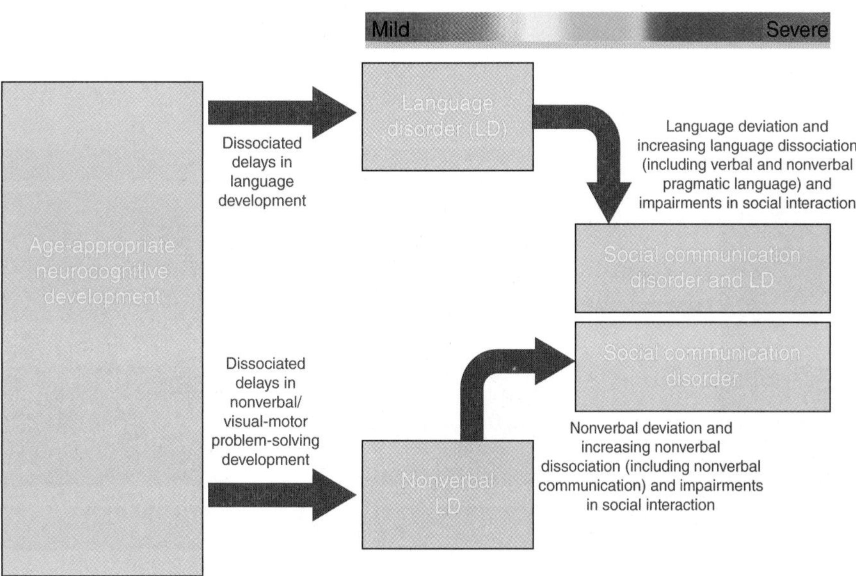


**FIGURE 83-4** Spectrum of neurocognitive dissociation and deviation.

in dysphonetic dyslexia. Such children at the mild end of a language-based learning disability spectrum would have difficulty with reading decoding, but they can visually memorize sight words (using their preserved nonverbal/visual-motor problem-solving abilities), comprehend what is read to them, and give oral answers to questions. However, as one moves across this spectrum from mild to moderate, more extensive language-based learning disabilities, resulting from dissociated delays in more diffuse aspects of receptive and expressive language, are encountered, which result in difficulties with reading comprehension, math word problems, written expression, oral expression, and listening comprehension. Moving further across this spectrum from moderate to severe, the dissociated delays in language involve even more diffuse aspects of language development, including verbal and nonverbal pragmatic language (the social use of language) and social interaction (including impairments in social reciprocity and developing social relationships), resulting in a social communication disorder. Children at the severe end of this spectrum of language dissociation and deviation also exhibit significant language deviation. For example, a child with this social communication disorder cognitive profile (and likely autism spectrum disorder [see below]) may have a 50-word vocabulary, as expected at 2 years of age, but not use a specific "Mama" or "Dada" to refer to his or her parents, as expected at 10 months of age. This inflated vocabulary is most often not used functionally and consists primarily of labels, rote memorization, or echolalia. In older children with this social communication disorder cognitive profile, language deviation may be observed by a vocabulary that is too numerous to count (greater than 3 years), use of multiword sentences (greater than 3 years), and an ability to label pictures, in combination with continued use of echolalia (echolalia usually ceases by 30 months of age) and continued pronoun confusion (pronoun confusion usually ceases by 30 months). Children at the severe end of this spectrum of language dissociation and deviation who do not have any associated restricted or repetitive behaviors are diagnosed with a social communication disorder. Children with autism spectrum disorder (and a language disorder) will have the social communication disorder cognitive profile at the severe end of this spectrum of language dissociation and deviation plus the atypical restricted, repetitive, and stereotypic behaviors at the severe end of the spectrum of neurobehavioral dissociation and deviation. While these children have discrepant delays in their language development, their nonverbal/visual-motor problem-solving skills remain relatively preserved (with the exception of their nonverbal pragmatic language). Thus, when these children with autism spectrum disorder perseverate, they tend to perseverate visually (eg, lining, sorting, spinning, exhibiting interest in flashing lights).

The bottom of Figure 83-4 illustrates the spectrum of dissociated and deviated nonverbal development. In this spectrum, a child exhibits discrepant and disproportionate delays (or dissociation) in nonverbal/visual-motor problem-solving development compared to language development. In the preschool-aged population, such a child would be described as exhibiting a visual-motor problem-solving disorder (also described as a visual perceptual, visual spatial, or visual motor deficit), but in the school-aged population, such a child would be described as exhibiting a nonverbal learning disability. In the school-aged population, a child's dissociated delays in nonverbal/visual-motor problem-solving development can be very mild, as is observed in children with orthographic processing deficits that result in dyseidetic dyslexia. Such children at the mild end of a nonverbal learning disability spectrum have difficulty with reading decoding, as they have trouble visually memorizing sight words, and they need to laboriously sound out most every word they try to decode (relying on their preserved language-based phonological processing). However, as one moves across this spectrum from mild to moderate, more-extensive nonverbal learning disabilities, involving more diffuse aspects of nonverbal/visual-motor problem-solving development, are encountered, which result in difficulties with writing, drawing, using scissors, shoe tying, right/left orientation, geometry, geography, and math. Moving further across this spectrum from moderate to severe, the dissociated delays in nonverbal development become more diffuse and extend to involve nonverbal aspects of social communication (eg, impaired understanding and use of facial expressions, trouble with staying on topic or taking turns in conversation, atypical speech prosody, lack of gestures, or trouble understanding figurative language, humor, or sarcasm), resulting in a social communication disorder, despite preserved language development relative to nonverbal development. Children at the severe end of this spectrum of nonverbal dissociation and deviation who do not have any restricted or repetitive behaviors are diagnosed with a social communication disorder. Children with autism spectrum disorder (with preserved language) will have the social communication disorder cognitive profile at the severe end of this spectrum of nonverbal dissociation and deviation plus the atypical restricted, repetitive, and stereotypic behaviors at the severe end of the spectrum of neurobehavioral dissociation and deviation. While these children have discrepant delays in their nonverbal/visual-motor problem-solving development (including nonverbal social communication), their language skills remain relatively preserved. Thus, when these children with autism spectrum disorder perseverate, they tend to perseverate verbally (eg, reciting facts about restricted areas of interest, such as train schedules, dinosaurs, baseball statistics).

## SPECTRUM OF NEUROBEHAVIORAL DISSOCIATION AND DEVIATION

Figure 83-5 illustrates the spectrum of neurobehavioral dissociation and deviation. In this spectrum, a child exhibits discrepant and disproportionate delays (or dissociation) in aspects of his or her neurobehavior compared to cognitive expectations. At the mild end of this spectrum, a child who exhibits developmentally inappropriate levels of inattention and hyperactivity (that are impairing his or her functioning across settings) is described as having ADHD. As one proceeds

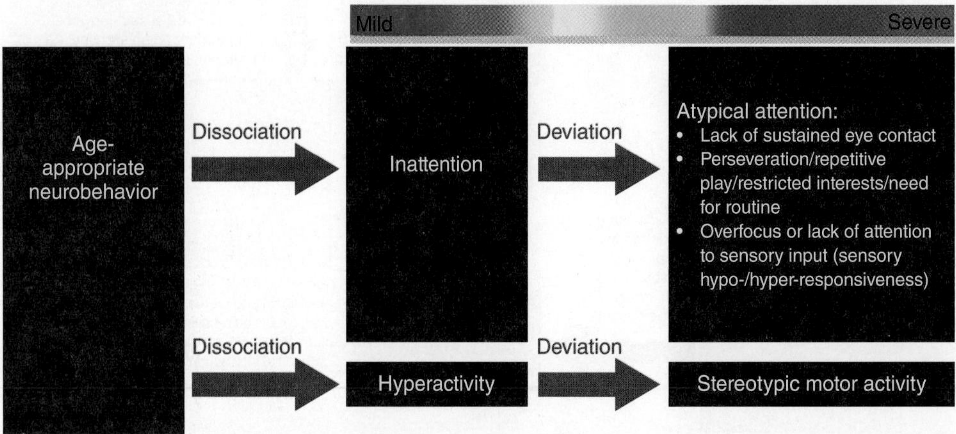


**FIGURE 83-5** Spectrum of neurobehavioral dissociation and deviation.

across this spectrum of neurobehavioral dissociation and deviation from mild to severe, increased neurobehavioral deviation is encountered. Rather than simple inattention, a more deviated or atypical pattern of attention is observed. While a child at this severe end of the neurobehavioral spectrum may lack the attention to sustain eye contact, he or she may overfocus or perseverate on restricted interests and routines and engage in repetitive play (eg, lining, sorting, spinning). He or she may also show atypicalities in attention to other sensory stimuli. For example, he or she may not react to painful stimuli but overreact to certain sounds or may overfocus on tight-fitting clothes, tags on shirts, or seams on socks. Rather than simple hyperactivity or fidgetiness as seen at the mild end of this spectrum, at the severe end of this spectrum of neurobehavioral dissociation and deviation, more atypical stereotypic motor activity (eg, hand flapping, body rocking or spinning, toe-walking) may be observed.

## CONTINUUM OF DEVELOPMENTAL-BEHAVIORAL DIAGNOSES

One of the key neurodevelopmental principles reviewed above is that there is a continuum of developmental-behavioral disability across neurodevelopmental streams. Thus, delays in one stream of neurodevelopment are most likely to occur in association with delays in other streams of neurodevelopment. This principle underlies the findings in children with global developmental delays, where all streams of development are fairly evenly delayed. However, the continuum of developmental disability can also be observed among children with dissociated and deviated development. Figure 83-6 illustrates the continuum of dissociated and deviated neurocognitive and neurobehavioral disability. At the mild end of this continuum, one encounters children with a combination of learning disabilities (from the spectrum of neurocognitive dissociation/deviation) and ADHD (from the spectrum of neurobehavioral dissociation/deviation). This comorbidity among learning disabilities and ADHD is widely recognized and may occur in up to 50% of children with either disorder. In addition, mild motor impairments from the spectrum of neuromotor dissociation and deviation, such as gross motor dyspraxia, dysgraphia, and speech articulation disorders, are also common comorbidities observed in children with learning disabilities and/or ADHD.

At the severe end of the continuum of dissociated and deviated neurocognitive and neurobehavioral disability, one encounters children with a combination of a social communication disorder (from the spectrum of neurocognitive dissociation/deviation) and the atypical attention (eg, lack of sustained eye contact, perseveration on restricted interests/need for routine, sensory hypo- or hyper-responsiveness) and stereotypic motor mannerisms observed at the severe end of the spectrum of neurobehavioral dissociation and deviation. Children with this combination of neurocognitive and neurobehavioral symptomatology (social communication disorders + atypical repetitive and stereotypic behavior) are described as having autism spectrum disorder.

## THE SPECTRUM AND CONTINUUM OF DEVELOPMENTAL-BEHAVIORAL DIAGNOSES

Figure 83-7 illustrates the entire spectrum and continuum of developmental-behavioral diagnoses. As shown in this figure, the continuum of developmental-behavioral diagnoses extends beyond those described above for learning disabilities + ADHD and social communication disorder + atypical attention/repetitive behaviors and stereotypic motor mannerisms (or autism spectrum disorder). For example, children with intellectual disability can also have autism spectrum disorder, if within their setting of more globally delayed developmental milestones, they exhibit dissociated delays and developmental deviation in social and language development (consistent with a social communication disorder) and associated atypical attention and repetitive/stereotypic behaviors. In fact, approximately one-half of children with autism spectrum disorders also have intellectual disability. These children have global (language and nonverbal/visual-motor problem-solving) cognitive delays, but their language is discrepantly delayed (dissociated) compared to their nonverbal/visual-motor problem-solving development. As also shown in this figure, children with intellectual disability can have ADHD. However, for children with intellectual disability to have ADHD, it must be proven that their levels of inattention and/or hyperactivity/impulsivity are dissociated from their underlying cognitive abilities. If a 10-year-old child with intellectual disability has the cognitive abilities of a 5-year-old, ADHD cannot be diagnosed if his or her levels of attention or activity are consistent with those of a 5-year-old. However, if his or her levels of attention or activity are consistent with those of a 3-year-old, then a dissociation would exist between neurocognitive and neurobehavioral domains, and ADHD could be appropriately diagnosed.

## CONCLUSION

Developmental-behavioral disorders are the most prevalent chronic medical problems encountered in primary care pediatrics. Rather than relying exclusively on developmental screening and referring on for further evaluation and diagnosis, particularly given the scarcity of developmental-behavioral specialists to whom to refer, pediatric medical providers are encouraged to take advantage of the skills attained via their rigorous medical training and adopt the medical model of pediatric developmental assessment described in Chapter 82. Once this assessment is completed and a pattern of developmental delay, dissociation, and deviation is established across neurocognitive, neurobehavioral, and neuromotor streams of development, with an understanding of the full spectrum and continuum of developmental-behavioral disorders, pediatric medical providers should feel confident in making developmental-behavioral diagnoses. The chapters to follow will review each of these diagnoses in more depth.



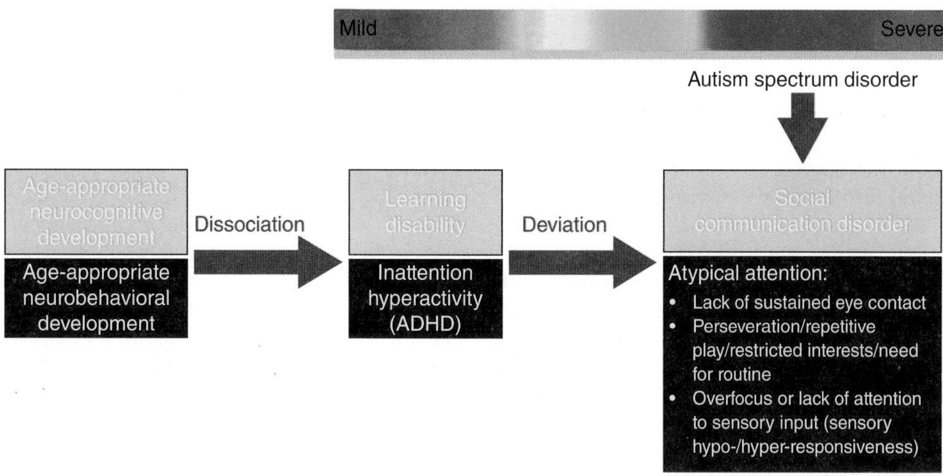


**FIGURE 83-6** Continuum of neurocognitive and neurobehavioral dissociation and deviation.

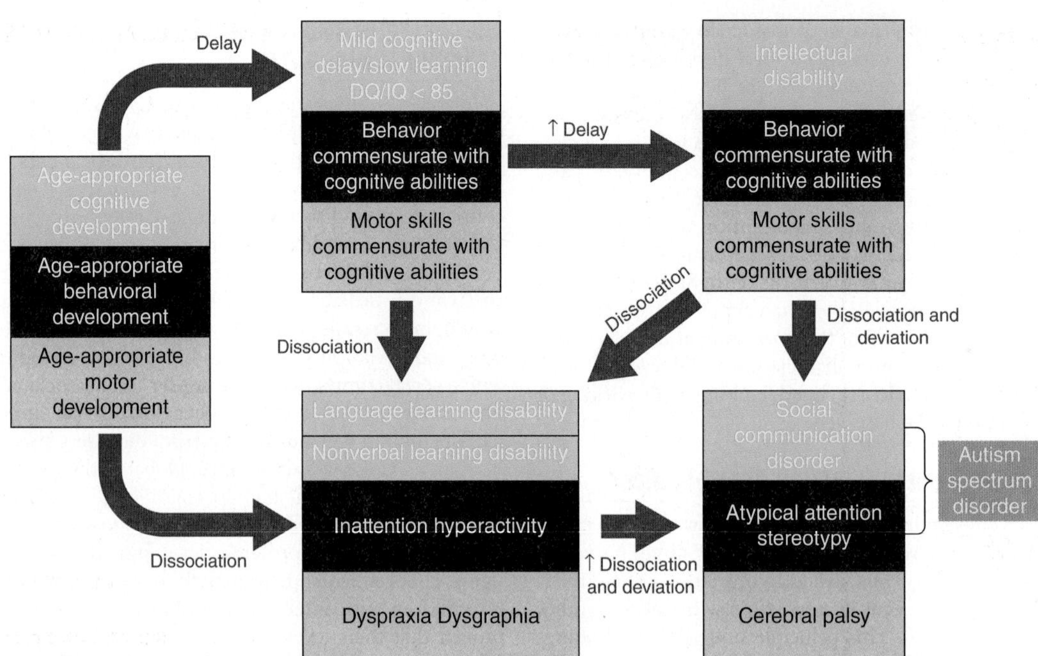


**FIGURE 83-7** Spectrum and continuum of developmental-behavioral diagnosis.



## SUGGESTED READINGS

Accardo PJ, Accardo JA, Capute AJ. A neurodevelopmental perspective on the continuum of developmental disabilities. In: Accardo PJ, ed. *Capute and Accardo's Neurodevelopmental Disabilities in Infancy and Childhood*. 3rd ed. Baltimore, MD: Paul H. Brookes Publishing Company; 2008:3-26.

Capute AJ. The expanded Strauss syndrome: MBD revisited. In: Accardo PJ, Blondis TA, Whitman BY, eds. *Attention Deficit Disorders and Hyperactivity*. New York, NY: Marcel Dekker, Inc; 1991:27-36.

Voigt RG. Developmental and behavioral diagnoses: the spectrum and continuum of developmental-behavioral disorders. In: Voigt RG, Macias MM, Myers SM, eds. *Developmental and Behavioral Pediatrics*. Elk Grove Village, IL: American Academy of Pediatrics; 2011:121-146.

# 84 Developmental and Behavioral Screening and Evaluation

Eboni Smith Hollier

## INTRODUCTION

Developmental-behavioral disorders are among the most common chronic medical problems encountered in primary care pediatric practice. In addition, the numbers of children with identified developmental-behavioral disorders have increased over time, and thus, so has the need for greater educational, therapeutic, and developmental-behavioral health supports. Primary pediatric medical providers are ideally positioned to identify developmental-behavioral problems at the earliest possible age, given their frequent and longitudinal contact with children and their families beginning at birth. While families rely on their primary care providers for their knowledge of diseases of childhood, they also consider primary pediatric medical providers as expert in all aspects of children's health, including development and behavior, and they typically first approach their primary pediatric medical providers about their concerns about their children's development or behavior before approaching any other professionals. This family reliance on their medical providers, combined with the prevalence of developmental-behavioral disorders, highlights the importance of routine developmental and behavioral surveillance, screening, and evaluation within the primary care medical home.

## DEVELOPMENTAL AND BEHAVIORAL SURVEILLANCE

The American Academy of Pediatrics (AAP) has published a policy statement on developmental surveillance, screening, and evaluation, and a clinical report on behavioral screening. Developmental and behavioral surveillance is a longitudinal process of developmental and behavioral monitoring over time within the primary care medical home. Developmental and behavioral surveillance should occur at every well child visit, and it helps to provide parent education, assists in supporting healthy development and behavior, and is useful in identifying children who may be at an increased risk of developmental and behavioral differences. Developmental surveillance relies on the clinical judgment and accumulated experience of pediatric medical providers, and it consists of five key components: (1) specifically asking about parental developmental-behavioral concerns, (2) identifying neurobiologic (eg, prematurity) and psychosocial (eg, maternal depression) risk and protective factors, (3) obtaining a developmental and behavioral history, (4) observing the child's development and behavior during the clinic visit, and (5) maintaining an accurate documentation of findings. If concerns are raised through developmental-behavioral surveillance, the child should be referred to his or her local early intervention (birth through 3 years of age) or early childhood special education (3 to 5 years of age) program.

## DEVELOPMENTAL AND BEHAVIORAL SCREENING

With the goal of identifying developmental and behavioral disorders as early as possible, so that interventions can begin at the youngest possible age when the central nervous system has increased capacity for plasticity, pediatric medical providers should implement developmental and behavioral screening during early childhood. Developmental and behavioral screening involves the administration of standardized and validated measures to parents/caregivers, as research has shown that parents reliably report on their children's development and behavior. Important screening test properties include sensitivity, specificity, predictive validity, reliability, and standardization sample. These screening tools are most commonly parent questionnaires, and

**TABLE 84-1 DEVELOPMENTAL SCREENING TESTS**

| |
|---|
| **General Screening:** |
| Ages and Stages Questionnaire (ASQ) |
| Parents' Evaluation of Developmental Status (PEDS) |
| Pediatric Symptom Checklist (PSC) |
| **Domain-Specific:** |
| Communication and Symbolic Behavior Scales (CSBS) |
| Ages and Stages Questionnaires: Social-Emotional (ASQ: SE) |
| Strengths and Difficulties Questionnaire (SDQ) |
| **Disorder-Specific (Autism):** |
| Modified Checklist for Autism in Toddlers (M-CHAT) |
| Screening Tool for Autism in Toddlers and Young Children (STAT) |
| Social Communication Questionnaire (SCQ) |

**TABLE 84-2 DEVELOPMENTAL EVALUATION TOOLS THAT CAN BE ADMINISTERED BY PEDIATRIC MEDICAL PROVIDERS**

| |
|---|
| Capute Scales: Cognitive Adaptive Test/Clinical Linguistic and Auditory Milestone Scale (CAT/CLAMS) |
| Parents' Evaluation of Developmental Status: Developmental Milestones, Assessment Level (PEDS:DM, Assessment Level) |
| Gesell Developmental Observation-Revised |
| Mullen Scales of Early Learning |
| Battelle Developmental Inventory |
| Peabody Picture Vocabulary Test |
| Expressive Vocabulary Test |
| Beery-Buktenica Developmental Test of Visual-Motor Integration |
| Kaufman Brief Intelligence Test (K-BIT) |
| Wide Range Achievement Test |

developmental and behavioral screening tests are designed to identify children at significant risk for a developmental or behavioral problem who require further evaluation. The AAP recommends, in addition to surveillance at every well-child visit, that all children be screened using a standardized screening tool during well-child visits at the specified ages of 9 months, 18 months, and 24 or 30 months. These specific ages were chosen at time points when specific developmental disorders are most likely to be identified. The AAP also recommends that all children be specifically screened for autism spectrum disorder (ASD) at the 18-month and 24-month well-child visits. Developmental-behavioral screening tests may be categorized as general, domain-specific, or disorder-specific screening tests. Examples of commonly used screening tools are presented in Table 84-1. When a screening test is positive, indicating that a child is at an increased risk for a developmental or behavioral problem, the child should be referred to their local early intervention or early childhood special education programs.

## DEVELOPMENTAL EVALUATION

For children who are identified as being at risk for developmental or behavioral differences through developmental-behavioral surveillance and screening, the AAP recommends that a diagnostic developmental evaluation be conducted in order to confirm the presence of a developmental disorder. Given the prevalence of developmental-behavioral disorders in the pediatric population and the scarcity of subspecialists (such as developmental-behavioral or neurodevelopmental disability pediatricians) to whom to refer, primary pediatric medical providers can perform developmental evaluations on all children determined to be at risk through surveillance or screening.

The developmental evaluation serves to confirm suspicions about possible developmental or behavioral disorders raised by surveillance or screening. The purpose of the developmental evaluation is to identify the presence of a specific developmental-behavioral diagnosis, to determine the severity and possible long-term prognosis, and to initiate specific therapeutic and/or educational interventions. If direct developmental evaluations are not completed by the primary pediatric medical provider to confirm concerns raised by surveillance or screening, the primary care provider needs to work closely with local early intervention or early childhood special education teams, who can perform the developmental evaluation. If the developmental evaluation performed by the early intervention or early childhood special education team confirms a developmental-behavioral disorder, the primary pediatric medical provider will need to proceed with further medical workup in an attempt to establish an etiologic diagnosis to account for the developmental-behavioral disorder.

Developmental evaluations may include direct evaluations of cognitive, communicative, adaptive, motor, and social skills. Developmental evaluations are accomplished through the use of standardized developmental evaluation tools that are validated and have acceptable psychometric properties. In developmental evaluation, multiple tests may be needed in order to obtain a thorough understanding of a child's developmental strengths and challenges. Factors such as examiner-child rapport and the child's level of interest, cooperation, and effort are also important to consider. Also, with very young children, having the caregiver present in the examination room may be important to help the child feel comfortable. In older children, it may be helpful to allow the child to determine whether he or she would like for the parent to remain in the examination room during the developmental evaluation. For infants, toddlers, and preschoolers, the developmental evaluation generally focuses on motor, nonverbal/visual-motor problem-solving, language, and social skills. For school-aged children, pediatric medical providers might consider brief standardized tests that evaluate visual-motor, language, and academic achievement to provide data to confirm the need for further school psychoeducational testing or to confirm findings from school psychoeducational testing. See Table 84-2 for examples of standardized developmental evaluation tools that can be administered by licensed primary pediatric medical providers.

## CONCLUSION

Given that developmental-behavioral disorders are among the most prevalent chronic medical problems in pediatrics, developmental surveillance, developmental screening, and developmental evaluation are important within the scope of primary care pediatric practice. Accumulated clinical experience and clinical judgment about typical and atypical child development and behavior, combined with knowledge and experience in administering and interpreting standardized developmental screening and evaluation measures, provides the best opportunity for earlier identification and earlier intervention, with the ultimate goal of improved long-term developmental-behavioral outcomes.

## SUGGESTED READINGS

American Academy of Pediatrics Council on Children with Disabilities, Section on Developmental-Behavioral Pediatrics, Bright Futures Steering Committee, Medical Home Initiatives for Children with Special Needs Project Advisory Committee. Identifying infants and young children with developmental disorders in the medical home: an algorithm for developmental surveillance and screening. *Pediatrics.* 2006;118:405-420.

Centers for Disease Control and Prevention. Developmental monitoring and screening. http://www.cdc.gov/ncbddd/childdevelopment/screening.html. Accessed July 15, 2016.

Boyle CA, Boulet S, Schieve LA, et al. Trends in the prevalence of developmental disabilities in US children, 1997–2008. *Pediatrics.* 2011;127(6):1034-1042.

Noritz GH, Murphy NA. Motor delays: early identification and evaluation. *Pediatrics.* 2013;131(6):e2016-e2027.

Weitzman C, Wegner L, Blum NJ, et al. Promoting optimal development: screening for behavioral and emotional problems. *Pediatrics.* 2015;135(2):384-395.

# 85 Basics of Management of Common Behavior Problems

Adiaha I. A. Spinks-Franklin



## INTRODUCTION

Behavior problems are among the most common presenting complaints that parents and caregivers have when seeking pediatric medical care, as up to 20% to 25% of the pediatric population may experience behavioral or emotional problems. Behavior problems can range from mild actions with minimal consequences to more significant behavior disorders with potentially severe outcomes. Evaluating behavior problems in children must take into account normal child development, temperament, parenting styles, and environmental circumstances.

## TEMPERAMENT, PERSONALITY, AND PARENTING STYLES

### Temperament

Temperament refers to the inborn, biologically based behavioral style with which an individual interacts with his or her environment. Drs. Alexander Thomas (1914–2003) and Stella Chess (1914–2007), who were American child psychiatrists, expanded upon the pioneering work of American pediatrician Dr. Herbert Birch (1918–1973) in the study of child temperament and behavior. Thomas, Chess, and Birch conducted a longitudinal study of child behavior and temperament and proposed nine behavior characteristics (Table 85-1). These nine characteristics (activity, rhythmicity, approach/withdrawal, adaptability, threshold of sensory responsiveness, intensity of reaction, quality of mood, distractibility, and attention/persistence) combine into three temperamental categories: easy, difficult, and slow to warm up.

Children with an easy temperament (40% of children) are described as having regular biological rhythms (eg, eating, sleeping, toileting), adapt easily to change and new environments, and are in a generally pleasant mood. These children do not become extremely agitated when they do not get their own way or their expectations are not met.

Children with a slow-to-warm-up temperament (15% of children) are often described as being shy. These children tend to adapt slowly to new people and environments. They will watch a group of children play while staying close to their parents. When given time, they will gradually join the group of children playing once they feel comfortable.

Children with difficult temperaments (10% of children) may be challenging for their parents to manage. Their biological rhythms are unpredictable, and they may not sleep, eat, or toilet at desired times. Children with difficult temperaments are more likely to have an irritable mood and react very negatively to unexpected changes in their routines or when their expectations are not met.

**TABLE 85-1 TEMPERAMENTAL BEHAVIOR CHARACTERISTICS**

| Behavior Characteristic | Description |
|---|---|
| Activity | The level and extent of motor activity |
| Rhythmicity | The degree of regularity of functions such as eating, elimination, and the cycle of sleeping and wakefulness |
| Approach or withdrawal | The response to a new object or person, in terms of whether the child accepts the new experience or withdraws from it |
| Adaptability | The adaptability of behavior to changes in the environment |
| Threshold of responsiveness | Sensitivity to a stimulus |
| Intensity of reaction | The energy level of responses |
| Quality of mood | The child's general mood or "disposition," whether cheerful or given to crying, pleasant or cranky, friendly or unfriendly |
| Distractibility | The degree of the child's distractibility from what he is doing |
| Attention span or persistence | The span of the child's attention and his persistence in an activity |

### Personality

Personality is the combination of temperament and life experience. Personality can be shaped by the influence of parenting styles, culture, environment, and underlying temperament.

### Goodness of Fit

*Goodness of fit* refers to how a particular trait or characteristic interacts with the environment and the people within the environment. Goodness of fit is based on an individual's temperamental characteristics and the specific aspects of the child's environment. The term is used to describe the interaction between the child's temperament and the parent's temperament.

### Parenting Styles

Parenting style refers to the manner in which a parent interacts and provides guidance to the child. The four most common parenting styles are authoritarian, passive, neglectful, and authoritative.

An authoritarian parenting style is also described as a strict parent. The parent tends to be demanding and does not respond to the individual needs of their children. There is little negotiation and dialogue between parent and child. Authoritarian parents do not offer warmth and nurturing to their children. The authoritarian parenting style is more likely to produce children who have low self-esteem, are insecure, are inappropriately shy, and have difficulty in social situations.

A passive parenting style is characterized by parents who are permissive toward their children. Rules and expectations are not clear, and there is often blurring of roles between the parent and child. The permissive parenting style can produce children who are insecure, have conflict with authority figures, have poor social skills, and are self-centered.

A neglectful parenting style is characterized by a parent who fails to meet the child's physical, emotional, and/or developmental needs. This is the most harmful parenting style. Children reared by neglectful parents are likely to have significant difficulty establishing appropriate trusting relationships with peers and others. This parenting style needs immediate intervention with mental health professionals and possibly child welfare authorities.

An authoritative parenting style is considered to be the healthiest parenting style. Authoritative parents tend to be flexible and nurturing toward their children. They offer rules and boundaries and discuss their expectations with their children. Authoritative parents are more willing to negotiate with their children when appropriate. The authoritative parenting style is more likely to produce confident, well-adjusted children.

## PRINCIPLES OF BEHAVIOR MANAGEMENT

Behavior management requires a systematic evaluation of (1) the description of the behaviors, (2) temperament and goodness of fit, (3) the developmental level of the child, (4) parental expectations and whether these are appropriate for the child's developmental abilities, (5) parenting styles, and (6) appropriate interventions to redirect the undesired behaviors. Anticipatory guidance and parent education about normal child development and behavior are important aspects of behavior management education for parents. Also important is the distinction between discipline and punishment. While these terms are often incorrectly used synonymously, there is an important difference between discipline and punishment. Discipline refers to a series of boundaries, rules, and guidance designed to encourage desired behaviors in children, while punishment is designed exclusively to reduce unwanted behaviors in children.

### Behavior Categories

When evaluating behaviors, it may be helpful to separate behaviors into categories. While there are a number of rubrics for evaluating behaviors, the following will explore one rubric involving three types of behaviors: internalizing behaviors, externalizing behaviors, and disruptive behaviors.

Internalizing behaviors generally refer to behaviors that may not be immediately noted by the parent but are experienced by the child. Internalizing behaviors may include feeling nervous or anxious, overwhelmed, or saddened. These behaviors may be exhibited in a variety of ways, such as resisting suggestions or directions from an adult, running away from an overwhelming situation, or isolating oneself from others.

Externalizing behaviors are easily observed by the parent or caregiver. Common externalizing behaviors include hyperactivity, poor impulse control, failure to follow directions, and becoming easily distracted. Externalizing behaviors can cause problems with how the child and/or the family function depending on where the behaviors occur and the circumstances around the behaviors. For example, the family may have a difficult time going on family outings because a child is impulsive and runs away from the parents in public places.

Disruptive behaviors are behaviors that may be potentially harmful or dangerous and more significantly interfere with how the child functions. Disruptive behaviors include aggression, self-injurious behaviors, destructive behaviors, and excessive tantrums.

#### Purpose of Behavior

Behavior has meaning. It is a form of communication. One purpose of a behavior may be for the child to avoid an aversive or painful experience. For example, an adolescent may have an algebra test at school and does not feel adequately prepared for the exam. The teen may feign an illness to stay home from school, thus avoiding taking the algebra test and possibly failing it.

Another purpose of behavior may be to escape an aversive stimulus. In this case, a child may engage in a behavior to get out of an unpleasant situation. For example, if it is a child's turn to wash dishes, and she does not like to wash dishes and does not want to do this chore, she may start a fight with a sibling or disobey a family rule. The parent reprimands the child and sends her to her bedroom as a punishment. Thus, the child escapes the aversive stimulus of having to wash the dishes.

Some children misbehave in order to gain attention from parents, caregivers, or teachers. When children gain attention by engaging in positive behaviors (eg, following instructions, completing an assignment), the child is more likely to continue to display the positive behavior. The positive behavior is positively reinforced by adding positive attention to the child when the child displays the desired behaviors. Conversely, some children only gain attention by engaging in inappropriate behaviors, such as throwing tantrums or breaking family rules. In this case, a parent may inadvertently ignore the child's good behaviors and preferentially give negative attention (eg, verbal reprimands, punishment) when the child engages in undesirable behaviors. As a result, the parent is reinforcing negative behaviors by inadvertently rewarding undesired behaviors with attention. In general, children seek the attention of the adults around them, whether good or bad, and parents need to make an effort to provide positive attention to desired behaviors and to ignore undesired, attention-seeking behaviors (that are not potentially harmful) in order to reinforce desired behaviors and extinguish undesired behaviors in their children.

#### Evaluating Behaviors

Evaluating a child's behavior requires a systematic approach. One way to evaluate behavior is to assess the ABCs of behavior: antecedents, behavior, and consequences.

**ABCs of Behavior: Antecedents, Behavior, and Consequences** Antecedents refer to the circumstances in the environment that occurred just before the child engaged in the behavior being observed. Antecedents can be triggers for undesirable behaviors. Clinicians should not ignore antecedents when taking a behavior history because many behavior problems can be addressed simply by understanding the circumstances that trigger a behavior. For example, a child is playing his favorite video game when a parent tells him to shut off the game and go complete his homework. The child throws a tantrum that includes crying, yelling at the parent, and refusing to comply with the command. In this case, the antecedent was engaging in a preferred activity that was unexpectedly interrupted and terminated.

Behaviors are the specific actions that the child displays that are undesirable to the parent. Behaviors should be described in detail because parents have different thresholds for what behaviors they consider to be problematic. For example, a "tantrum" may mean one thing to one parent and something completely different to another. The parent should describe the specific behaviors the child displays including verbal responses (eg, crying, screaming, name-calling, threatening), physical actions (eg, hitting, kicking, falling on the floor, self-injurious behaviors, running away), and what the child does with objects (eg, breaking toys, throwing objects, slamming doors). The clinician should also determine the frequency, duration, and location of the behavior outbursts.

Consequences are the circumstances that occur as a result of or reaction to the child's behaviors. Consequences may include any combination of reinforcers or punishments and can be natural or logical. A natural consequence occurs as an automatic result of the child's behavior. For example, if a child pulls a cat's tail and the cat scratches the child, this would be considered a natural consequence. Most natural consequences allow a child to learn from his own experiences. Some natural consequences may be dangerous (eg, the child rides his bike into the street and gets hit by a car), and such consequences should obviously be avoided.

Logical consequences are those that logically follow an undesired behavior. For example, if a student has a major temper tantrum at school that includes destroying school property, verbal aggression, and physical aggression, the other students in the class may ostracize the child and refuse to play with her because of her disruptive behaviors. This would be a logical consequence or punishment that is the result of the student's disruptive behaviors. If the child desires to make friends with her classmates, she will not engage in these disruptive behaviors, understanding that her behaviors can lead to being ostracized by peers. There are times when adults' responses to a child's behavior can reinforce the child's undesired behaviors. For example, when shopping at the grocery store, a parent walks down the toy aisle. The child screams and begs for a toy. The parent tells the child "no" and tries to distract the child. The child continues to scream and demand the toy. Customers in the grocery store begin to look at the parent and child. Embarrassed, the parent gives the child a toy to stop the tantrum. The child takes the toy and stops screaming. In this case, the parent positively reinforced tantrum behaviors on the toy aisle, so whenever the child wants a toy, he will have a tantrum to gain his desired object. Giving the child the toy acted as a negative reinforcer for the parent because giving the toy stopped the tantrum, which was aversive to the parent.

#### Behavior Rating Scales

There are times when behavior rating scales can be administered to a parent/caregiver or teacher to gain a better understanding of a child's behaviors. A number of behavior rating scales address behaviors such as symptoms of attention-deficit/hyperactivity disorder (ADHD), autism spectrum disorders (ASDs), anxiety, depression, and sleep, and there are also general behavior rating scales that evaluate a number of behaviors, such as attention, mood, adaptive behaviors, and resiliency. Research suggests that adults often accurately rate externalizing behaviors in children, while children are better able to rate their own internalizing symptoms. When children are 8 years old, they are capable of completing behavior rating scales that contain a Likert scale (ie, never, sometimes, often, always). A number of behavior rating scales have forms for parents/caregivers and teachers and a self-report form for the child (for ages 8 years and older). In order to gain a more comprehensive perspective of a child's behavior, it may be helpful for the clinician to have the parent, teacher, and child (if appropriate) complete behavior rating scales.

#### Behavior Management

Clinicians can offer parents guidance for addressing their child's behavior needs. Three principles to consider when evaluating behaviors and providing guidance for behavior management are the following: (1) behavior has meaning and is a form of communication,

(2) learned behaviors can be unlearned, and (3) people do what they do as long as it works.

**Behavior Has Meaning** Many times children engage in undesired behaviors as a way of communicating a thought or need to their parent/caregiver or teacher. Sometimes children may engage in inappropriate behavior when they desire the attention of an adult. At other times, a behavior may reveal the child is distressed or overwhelmed. Behaviors could also demonstrate that a child has difficulty regulating himself. It is important to note when inappropriate behaviors are a sign of more significant underlying psychopathology or psychosocial stress, such as abuse, anxiety disorders, mood disorders, neglect, or emerging psychoses.

**Learned Behaviors Can Be Unlearned** Parents train children and children train parents. There is generally a reciprocal give-and-take in a parent-child relationship. Effective parents adjust their parenting behaviors to meet the needs of their children. Children adjust their behaviors to meet parental expectations. As previously described, there are times when parents inadvertently reward and encourage undesired behaviors by reinforcing them. Over time, the child learns to engage in the undesired behavior more often than the desired behavior. Conversely, children learn to manipulate their parents by engaging in behaviors that are likely to give them what they want. A parent will need to unlearn ineffective parenting strategies in order to develop more effective parenting strategies. Children can unlearn inappropriate behaviors as they gain mastery of more appropriate behaviors.

**People Do What They Do as Long as It Works** It is common for people to engage in behaviors that meet their own needs. In most cases, these behaviors are appropriate. In some cases, these behaviors may be maladaptive and interfere with healthy interpersonal relationships. When children frequently engage in undesirable behaviors, they may continue to do so because a particular desire or need is being met by this negative behavior. As long as an undesired behavior is being rewarded or reinforced, the behavior is likely to continue. However, once the undesired behavior is no longer rewarded, it is likely to reduce in frequency and intensity. When the child learns that their inappropriate behavior is no longer effective in meeting their desires or needs, the child will need to learn a more appropriate way of behaving to meet their own needs. Therefore, people do what they do as long as it works; when it stops working, the behavior fades.

**Principles for Behavior Management** Children often function best when there is structure and routine, clear rules and expectations, and predictability and consistency in the home. Chaotic home environments can produce chaotic behaviors in children. Clinicians can encourage parents to develop structure in the home to include a basic routine and schedule, so the child can know what to expect and what his role is in the family. It is crucial that parents be consistent in how they establish rules and boundaries in the home. When parents are inconsistent in the way that discipline is applied in the home, the child is more likely to display inappropriate behaviors. Clinicians can encourage parents to sit down with their children to establish a few (3–5 maximum) basic, non-negotiable family rules (eg, Use your words; don't hit others. Sit on furniture; do not jump on it.). The family rules may need to be clearly displayed in the family home and reviewed on a regular basis in order to maintain family behavior expectations. Parents and children can establish agreed-upon rewards for following the rules and consequences for breaking the rules. When parents remove something from a child, it should be replaced with something else the parent prefers. For example, if the parent wants to reduce a child's TV time, replace it with outdoor play time. Parents should be encouraged to catch children being good by rewarding and reinforcing desired behaviors with praise, smiles, high-fives, hugs, and special attention. They should also be encouraged to ignore undesired attention-seeking behaviors, so as not to reinforce them. Consequences and punishments should be appropriate for undesired behavior that is potentially harmful and should encourage the child to learn self-control and self-regulation. A consequence of punishment should not injure a child's self-esteem or self-worth. If behavior concerns are more significant, parent behavior management training with a mental health professional may be warranted.

## COMMON BEHAVIOR PROBLEMS

Parents commonly seek pediatric care when they have concerns about their child's behavior problems. Behavior problems must be evaluated in the context of the setting, the child's developmental level, potential triggers, parenting style, the child's temperament, and parental expectations. Most behavior problems are benign and easily addressed. Some behavior problems are more significant and can be signs for diagnosable behavior disorders that require more extensive treatment and intervention. In this section, some common behavior problems will be reviewed.

### Temper Tantrums

Temper tantrums are outbursts of anger or frustration in a child. Temper tantrums are most common in children between the ages of 18 months and 3 years. Tantrums tend to occur more frequently in children with limited expressive language. Once language skills improve, and a child's ability to explain wants, needs, and opinions improves, tantrums tend to be reduced in frequency. Tantrums can take many forms, from quietly sulking to being physically and verbally aggressive with destruction of property or self-injurious behaviors.

When evaluating a child for temper tantrums, clinicians should take several factors into account, including a specific description of the tantrum behaviors (eg, crying, hitting, head banging, throwing objects), the antecedents or triggers (eg, being hungry or tired, being told "no," having a preferred activity interrupted, unexpected changes), the frequency (ie, how many times a day or week), the duration of the tantrums (eg, 15 minutes, 45 minutes), and the location where tantrums occur (eg, at home, at school, in the community). Taking a thorough history of behavior concerns sometimes requires a longer office visit (45–60 minutes). However, a few basic questions can provide a general idea of the characteristics of the tantrum behaviors:

- What are the potential triggers for the tantrums? Hunger or fatigue? Being denied his own way? Being told "no"? Being overstimulated or overwhelmed?
- What do the tantrums look like? Please describe a typical tantrum.
- Where do tantrums typically occur? At home? During family outings? At school or daycare? Are they more frequent in one setting than in others?
- How long does a typical tantrum last? Less than 5 minutes? Longer than 20 minutes?
- How frequently do they occur? Daily? Weekly?
- What makes the tantrum better or worse? Ignoring the behavior? Reprimanding the child? Walking away from the child? Trying to reason with the child?

Parents can be reassured that tantrums are common in children between the ages of 18 months and 3 years. The child's developmental level must also be taken into account. Behavior expectations should be appropriate for the child's developmental level, not necessarily the child's chronological age. A child who has developmental delays or intellectual disability may have a developmental level between 18 months and 3 years. In this case, tantrums may be expected in a child of this developmental level, despite the chronologic age of the child. Sometimes children with developmental delays have tantrums because adult expectations or demands are too complex for them to understand. In this case, adult expectations should be adjusted accordingly to meet the child's developmental level.

Tantrums can often be reduced by teaching a young child to communicate better to describe his or her feelings in simple words (eg, "I don't like it" or "I'm mad!"). An adult cannot reason with a child in the midst of a tantrum, but once the tantrum subsides, the child can be taught to describe his feelings with words rather than actions. Parents can ignore mild tantrums by avoiding eye contact with the child and walking away from the child in the midst of a tantrum (as long as the child is safe). Once the child realizes that no one is paying attention to his behavior, the tantrum will often subside, as the child runs after the parent. The parent can then compliment the child for using his words instead.

### Sleep Problems

Sleep behavior problems are one of the most common specific behavior problems parents report. When a child struggles to fall asleep or remain asleep, it can be quite disrupting to the functioning of the family. Behavior-related sleep problems can be divided into two main categories: sleep initiation and sleep maintenance problems. Problems with sleep initiation or maintenance can include inappropriate sleep associations, poor limit-setting, or delayed sleep phase.

**Inappropriate Sleep Associations** Sleep associations are the conditions needed for an individual to fall asleep. They are common because each individual prefers to fall asleep under different sets of conditions, such as temperature, lighting, or bedding, and can be inappropriate when the conditions are not sustained throughout the night. For children, sleep associations may involve a parent and accoutrements such as stuffed animals, music, lighting, and other items. The brain remembers the sleep environment as the person falls asleep. During the sleep cycle, the brain goes from deep sleep to light sleep and back. As the brain transitions from deep sleep to light sleep, the brain experiences a partial arousal, which is a break in the sleep cycle. The eyes may open to survey the environment. As long as the environment remains consistent, the person will immediately return to sleep. If the environment is different, the brain will awaken the person to re-create the environment that occurred at bedtime. A classic example is a 4-year-old child who likes for her father to read a book a bedtime, turn on a lamp in her room, and rub her back until she falls asleep. Once the child is asleep, the father turns off the light and leaves his daughter's bedroom. About 2 hours later, the child wakes up and notices that her bedroom is dark, and she is alone. The child calls out for a parent or gets out of bed and goes into her parents' room. Her father escorts her back to her bedroom, turns on the lamp, and rubs her back until she falls asleep again. This cycle continues throughout the night. To help children who have inappropriate sleep associations, the associations can be gradually reduced until a child learns to fall sleep without the "extras." One rule for bedtime success is to put a child to sleep when he is too sleepy to be awake and not too awake to go to sleep. When inappropriate sleep associations significantly impair the way a child sleeps, the child may be diagnosed with a sleep-onset association disorder and may require treatment with a sleep or behavior specialist.

**Poor Limit-Setting** Children with more difficult temperaments may have more problems with bedtime. Parents who do not consistently set limits and expectations may have difficulty getting a child to comply with any request, including mealtimes, bedtimes, and other activities. Poor limit-setting in the parent-child relationship can occur when the child refuses to go to bed and frequently makes demands on the parent, and the parent gives in to these demands. Inappropriate sleep associations may occur as a result of poor limit-setting. If a parent struggles with setting appropriate limits with their child, the parent may need help from a behavior psychologist, who can help re-establish natural parental authority in the parent-child relationship.

**Delayed Sleep Phase** Delayed sleep phase occurs when the natural circadian sleep rhythm shifts to a later time. This condition is common in children going through puberty because melatonin is secreted at a later time during puberty. Delayed sleep phases can also occur during weekends and school holidays, when the child's schedule is not as structured. For example, on weekends, a child may be allowed to stay awake until 11:00 PM and sleep until 9:00 AM the next morning. Then when school starts again on Monday, the child is expected to go to sleep by 9:00 PM and wake up for school at 6:00 AM. This would be a 3-hour shift in the child's sleep schedule, which can make it difficult for the child to awaken for school on Monday morning. Many cases of delayed sleep phase are more significant, where a child's sleep cycle is on a completely different time zone than the time zone in which the child lives (eg, going to sleep at 2:00 AM and waking up at noon). In order to address a delayed sleep phase, the child's weekend wake up time should be within 1 hour of the weekday wakeup time. It is important for the child to not sleep in on weekends and be allowed to take a short nap (less than 2 hours) in the middle of the day if needed on weekends. More significant sleep concerns can be addressed by a pediatric sleep specialist.

### Feeding Problems

Parents can become distressed when children do not eat as much or as often as the parent expects. It is estimated that 25% of typically developing children can have feeding problems. Feeding behaviors can range from mild sensory sensitivities to severe feeding disorders.

Many feeding and eating behaviors can be expected based upon normal child development. When children are toddlers, they are developing a sense of independence and may prefer to feed themselves. They will also refuse to eat nonpreferred foods. By preschool, children should be able to make themselves a simple meal (eg, a bowl of cereal, a sandwich). Preschoolers may prefer to eat the foods they can make for themselves, such as a peanut butter and jelly sandwich. By elementary school, a child should be able to help select the dinner menu, help pack his own lunch, and order his own food at a restaurant. The elementary school–aged child may refuse to take home-cooked meals to school for lunch, instead preferring to eat the cafeteria food that the other students are eating. By adolescence, a child is developing more independence from parents and establishing relationships outside the family. A teen may prefer to eat away from home with friends.

Some children refuse to try new foods. They prefer a select number of items and will not even taste a new food that is introduced. Some children do not like to try new foods because of the way the food looks, smells, or tastes. Others may be highly sensitive to certain food textures and are reluctant to put certain foods in their mouths. There are also situations where poor limit-setting may contribute to food refusals in a child who does not comply with adult requests. Finally, a child who is a bit anxious may be hesitant to try something new. The approach to helping a child try a new food should be based on the underlying reason for the refusal—sensory sensitivity, poor limit-setting, aversions, or anxieties. Treatment may include gradual introduction of very small portions (pea-sized) of the new food, with positive reinforcers provided when the child tolerates the new food. For example, if the child tolerates one green bean sitting on the side of his plate while he eats his other foods, the child earns one sticker. For children with more significant food aversions or severe sensory sensitivities, consultation with a pediatric occupational therapist or pediatric speech pathologist may be warranted.

## SUMMARY

Behavior problems are among the most common chief complaints in pediatric practice. Most behavior problems are mild and easily addressed through anticipatory guidance. Some behavior problems are more significant and begin to interfere with how a child functions and with the parent-child relationships. When evaluating behavior problems, clinicians should take into account normal development, child temperament, parenting styles, and environmental influences. Using a comprehensive approach to addressing common behavior problems is most effective. Consultation with a behavior specialist to address more severe behavior disorders may be warranted.

## SUGGESTED READINGS AND RESOURCES

### Suggested Readings

Barkley RA, Benton CM. *Your Defiant Child: Eight Steps to Better Behavior*. 2nd ed. New York, NY: Guilford Press; 2013.

Barkley RA. *Taking Charge of ADHD: The Complete and Authoritative Guide for Parents*. 3rd ed. New York, NY: Guilford Press; 2013.

### Suggested Resources

Empowering Parents: www.empoweringparents.com

Center on the Developing Child: http://developingchild.harvard.edu

Kids Health: www.kidshealth.org

National Institute of Mental Health (NIMH): www.nimh.nih.gov

Understood: www.understood.org

# 86 Early Intervention and Special Education

Dinah L. Godwin, Marcia Berretta, and Marie Turcich



## WHO REQUIRES EARLY INTERVENTION OR SPECIAL EDUCATION SERVICES?

This chapter will discuss the types of early intervention and special education services available, the referral process, and what pediatricians and other pediatric medical providers can do to help their families learn to navigate these important systems. Some red flags that should alert pediatric medical providers to the potential need for early intervention supports for infants and toddlers include high-risk neurobiologic (eg, prematurity) or psychosocial (eg, teenaged parents, maternal depression, poverty) conditions and failure to attain developmental milestones as expected. Red flags for preschool-aged children to alert pediatric medical providers to the potential need for special education preschool supports include high-risk neurobiologic or psychosocial conditions, new medical or developmental diagnoses, failure to attain developmental milestones as expected, and associated maladaptive behaviors. For school-aged children, red flags to alert pediatric medical providers to the potential need for special education supports include high-risk neurobiologic or psychosocial conditions, new medical or developmental diagnoses, failure to attain developmental milestones and academic skills (ie, school failure), and associated maladaptive behaviors.

### Role of Primary Care Pediatric Medical Providers

The role of primary care pediatric medical providers can be pivotal, not only in the medical outcomes for a child with special needs, but in the child's educational outcomes as well. The primary care pediatric medical provider can be both a source of information and advocacy for children and their families and an expert resource for educational staff to understand complex medical conditions, treatment plans, and their integration with educational services from preschool through adolescence. Children with neurodevelopmental disabilities, in particular, typically have chronic, lifelong conditions that will need varying degrees of intervention and treatment. The American Academy of Pediatrics (AAP) directs pediatricians to provide a medical home for these patients, to help coordinate medical care, and to act as a resource for families. While such patients may have ongoing needs for medical procedures or therapies, they are also likely to need additional educational services and supports.

Early intervention and special education are mandated by federal law to provide free, appropriate public education (FAPE) services to children with disabilities either through the Individuals with Disabilities Education Act (IDEA) or through Section 504 of the Rehabilitation Act of 1973. IDEA is the federal law that supports special education and related service programming for children and youth with disabilities. It was originally known as the Education of All Handicapped Children Act, passed in 1975, which provided special education services for children from 5 to 21 years of age. In 1986, this law was extended to include special education preschool support for children from 3 to 5 years of age. In addition, the 1986 law established the Grants for Infants and Families program (Part C of IDEA), which is a federal grant program that assists states in operating a comprehensive statewide program of early intervention services for infants and toddlers from birth through 3 years of age.

## EARLY INTERVENTION

### Key Concepts of Early Intervention Programs

Each state's Part C program establishes a statewide, family-centered, multidisciplinary interagency system of early intervention (EI) services for delivery in the local or regional area. Two categories of children are served by EI: (1) those with a diagnosed physical or mental condition with a high likelihood of developmental delays (eg, Down syndrome), or (2) those with a developmental delay in one or more of five developmental domains (cognitive, motor, communication, social/emotional, adaptive). Some states may also elect to serve infants at risk for delay because of biological or psychosocial/environmental factors.

Part C eligibility is determined by each state's definition of developmental delay and whether it includes children at risk for disabilities in the eligibility formula. States have been given some discretion for determining eligibility for entry into their programs. Each state can determine what the eligibility requirements are, as well as how much funding will be allotted to their program. An important part of the evaluation process for infants and toddlers (ages 0–36 months) includes informed clinical opinions of professionals experienced with the development of very young children. Although a referral from a pediatrician or other pediatric medical provider is not required, clinical information from pediatric medical providers may be helpful in determining a child's eligibility for EI services. There are a number of medically diagnosed conditions that will qualify an infant or toddler for EI services. A list of these conditions can be accessed by an online search using the term "early intervention" and the name of a state. The state's EI site will also provide information about the referral process and eligibility process for that specific state.

Some key principles of EI include: (1) infants and toddlers learn best through everyday experiences and interactions with familiar people in familiar contexts; (2) all families, with the necessary supports and resources, can enhance their children's learning and development; and (3) Individualized Family Service Plan (IFSP) outcomes must be functional and based on children's and families' needs and family-identified priorities.

### Early Intervention Referral Process

Pediatricians and other pediatric medical providers who identify that a child under the age of 3 years has a developmental delay or disability are legally mandated to make a referral to EI services. Federal regulations implementing Part C of IDEA require that children under 3 years of age be referred *no more than 7 days* after being identified as having a developmental delay or disability.

A referral to a state's EI program can be made by a physician or other healthcare provider, a family member, or a teacher. Referral forms are available through an online search using the term "early intervention" and the name of a state. An interdisciplinary team will conduct a comprehensive evaluation to determine a referred child's eligibility for EI. If this evaluation determines that a child is eligible for services, the interdisciplinary team, including the child's parents, develops an IFSP that focuses on involving the family in therapeutic interventions and builds on the settings and routines familiar to the child.

### Examples of Early Intervention Services

Early intervention services include licensed or credentialed professionals who provide (1) speech-language therapy, (2) physical therapy, (3) occupational therapy, (4) audiology and services for the hearing impaired, (5) services for the visually impaired, (5) nutrition services, (6) specialized skills training, and (7) case management. Part C of IDEA requires that eligible infants and toddlers with disabilities receive services in natural environments to the maximum extent appropriate. Natural environments include the family's home and/or community settings in which children without disabilities participate (such as childcare centers).

### Value of Early Intervention

Early intervention plans and services for infants and toddlers are based on research that demonstrates that learning occurs between intervention sessions. During a session, the EI provider utilizes his or her professional knowledge, skills, and expertise to share information with the child's regular caregivers. The caregivers then provide the intervention within the child's daily routines. Studies have found that children who participate in high-quality EI programs tend to have less need for special education and have greater language abilities, improved nutrition and health, and experience less child abuse and neglect. Economic analyses demonstrate that programs that intervene early to improve child outcomes have returns on investment (ROI) from $2.50 to $17.07 for every dollar spent on EI services.

#### How Are Early Intervention Services Funded?

Early intervention programs receive federal, state, and local funds, as well as collecting Medicaid, Children's Health Insurance Program (CHIP), private insurance, and payments from families. However, even though EI does collect payments from families, no family will be denied services due to an inability to pay.

#### Transition from Early Intervention Programs

When a child approaches the age of 3 years (no less than 3 months prior to the child's third birthday), the EI team works with the family to develop a plan for transition from EI services. There is a strong evidence base for children with and without special needs to participate in high-quality preschool programs, although preschool and even kindergarten are not mandatory in all states, and some families do opt to keep their children at home after EI services terminate. Options for children ages 3 years and up may include transitioning to a public school district's special education preschool program (for children from 3 to 5 years of age), a Head Start program, a private preschool, or a combination of public and private services. For the purposes of this chapter, we will focus on the public school programs for children with disabilities, as these services are mandated by federal law and are available to all children who meet eligibility criteria, regardless of variables such as geographic location or family income.

## SPECIAL EDUCATION

#### Key Concepts in Special Education

Children who have or are suspected of having developmental delays, learning problems, sensory deficits (such as hearing or visual impairment), or health conditions that affect their ability to learn may be eligible for special education services beginning at age 3 years. As with EI services, special education services are guided by IDEA, the federal law that delineates the requirements for school districts to provide educational services and supports to children with disabilities. The federal Office of Special Education and Rehabilitative Services (OSERS) oversees IDEA and funds special education programs to the states, with each state education agency responsible for administering IDEA in their state and distributing funds for special education programs. State boards of education and local school boards have some discretion in how services are provided, but every state, district, and individual school must comply with the mandates set forth in IDEA.

The underlying principle governing special education law is that all children, regardless of their disabilities, have the right to a "free and appropriate public education" in the "least restrictive environment." This terminology is important, as it underscores the expectations that children with disabilities have the right to be educated with their typically developing peers to the greatest extent possible.

The basic provisions of IDEA that relate to special education are as follows: (1) find and identify students who have a disability, (2) involve parents in decision making, (3) evaluate students in a nondiscriminatory way, (4) develop an individual education program (IEP) for each eligible student, (5) provide special instruction and supplementary aids and services, (6) provide services in the least restrictive environment, (7) maintain education records/files, and (8) provide processes for resolving parent complaints and grievances.

#### The Role of Pediatricians and Other Pediatric Medical Providers

Pediatricians and other primary care pediatric medical providers are often the first professionals to whom parents express their concerns about their child's development, learning, or behavior. Parents assume that pediatricians, in their role as child advocates, have expert knowledge about the educational system and can help guide them toward appropriate school-based services. Consequently, it is important for pediatricians and other pediatric medical providers to have a basic understanding of the process for accessing special education evaluations and services, so that they will be able to effectively advise families.

Pediatricians and other pediatric medical providers also have a critical role in early identification and referral for children whose families have not yet recognized a need for special services. When parents raise concerns about their child not making progress in school, having behavioral outbursts in the classroom, or experiencing difficulties with attention or focus, these are red flags that may indicate a need for evaluation for additional special educational services or supports. In addition to their medical evaluation and treatment recommendations, pediatricians and other medical providers should remember to address the child's school environment and to consider recommending a special educational evaluation as part of their treatment plan. Pediatricians and other pediatric medical providers should also be available to communicate with school district personnel to provide medical information and to discuss services, after obtaining parental consent as appropriate.

#### Brief Overview of Special Education Services

Beginning at age 3 years, children with known or suspected disabilities may be eligible for special education preschool services. This may include half-day or full-day preschool in a classroom setting with a low student-to-teacher ratio (usually no more than 4:1). Other services may be offered based on the child's evaluation and identified needs. These may include speech/language therapy, occupational therapy, physical therapy, behavioral therapy, transportation, and specialized services for children with visual and/or hearing impairments. Children with speech and language delays but with no other identified disabilities may qualify for speech/language therapy services through the school district, even if they are not enrolled in special education preschool or are attending a private preschool.

Special education preschool services are offered from age 3 years through kindergarten. For older children, special education services are offered in a variety of settings and formats, including self-contained special education classrooms, "resource" or specialized instruction classrooms for academic subjects, assistance from a paraprofessional in a mainstream classroom, or some combination of the above. The specific services provided will be based on the child's needs and, as noted above, should be offered in the least restrictive environment. Special education is available to children with disabilities through the age of 21 years, and for older adolescents, a plan for transitioning to postsecondary services that are appropriate for the adolescent's developmental level should be included in the IEP.

#### How to Request Special Education Services

Parents who have a concern about their child's development in one or more developmental domains or about their child's academic progress have the right under IDEA to request a full individual evaluation (FIE) of their child. Pediatricians and other pediatric medical providers should recommend that the parent request this FIE in writing to the school principal, who is responsible for ensuring that the campus is compliant with special education law. If a child is new to the school district and has not yet been enrolled in school, the parent should address the letter to the principal of the school to which the child is zoned. The family can contact their school district to obtain the contact information for their zoned school.

In the letter, parents should state the child's name and date of birth, their concerns and their reason for requesting the evaluation, and the contact information for the parents. The letter may include any supplemental information that may be helpful, such as the child's diagnosis or results from any outside evaluations that the child may have completed. Parents should keep a copy of the letter for their records. Parents may also wish to request a dated receipt from the school confirming that the letter was received. A sample letter for families to request a special education evaluation can be viewed at http://www.disabilityrightstx.org/resources/education.

#### The Evaluation Process

Once the school has received the parents' letter, the administration must respond to the parents within 15 school days. The school has the option to decline the parents' request, but they must decline in writing and state the reasons why they do not believe an evaluation is necessary. If the school does plan to evaluate the child, they must request that the parent sign consent forms giving them permission to complete an evaluation. Once these forms are received by the school, the testing process can begin, and the school has 45 school days in which to complete the FIE. Depending on the concerns identified, the evaluation may consist of any or all of the following: parent/caregiver interview, child interview, observation of the child, cognitive testing, speech and language evaluation, fine motor evaluation, gross motor evaluation, hearing testing, vision testing, psychological evaluation, and behavioral assessment.



### What Happens After Evaluation?

After the FIE has been completed, the school must provide a copy of the evaluation report to the parents and must convene a meeting of the evaluation team and the family in order to review the results and recommend services as appropriate. This meeting is usually called an Individualized Education Program (IEP) meeting; in some states, it may also be referred to as an Admission, Review, and Dismissal (ARD) meeting. This meeting may include the following individuals: school principal, school district diagnostician who completed the evaluation, special education or general education teachers, the EI specialist (if a child is transitioning from EI), school district personnel, the parents, and a language interpreter, if needed. At the IEP meeting, the results of the evaluations will be reviewed, and the school will inform the parents whether the child qualified for special education services and what services are being recommended. The parents will have an opportunity to ask questions and provide input. At the end of the meeting, all parties present will be asked to sign the meeting report to indicate agreement with the plan.

IEPs must be reviewed at a formal IEP meeting at least annually, but parents have the right to request an IEP meeting at any time, if they have concerns about their child's services. In addition, children receiving special education services must have a new FIE completed every 3 years.

Children may qualify for special education services under the following 13 educational classifications: (1) autism; (2) deafness; (3) deaf-blindness; (4) emotional disturbance; (5) hearing impairment; (6) intellectual disability; (7) multiple disabilities; (8) orthopedic impairment; (9) other health impaired (including attention-deficit/hyperactivity disorder [ADHD]; (10) specific learning disability (including dyslexia, dysgraphia, dyscalculia, nonverbal learning disability); (11) speech or language impairment; (12) traumatic brain injury; and (13) visual impairment.

## SECTION 504

Section 504 is a civil rights law with assistance and enforcement through the federal Office for Civil Rights (OCR). Section 504 is an antidiscrimination law that does not provide any type of funding; its purpose is to protect individuals with disabilities from discrimination in all federally assisted programs and activities. Section 504 prohibits recipients of federal funds, such as public school districts, from discriminating against individuals with disabilities. Students with disabilities are to be afforded the same opportunities to participate in academic, nonacademic, or extracurricular activities as non-disabled students.

Students who are identified as eligible for special education and related services under IDEA are included under provisions of Section 504. However, not all students who qualify for Section 504 are eligible for special education services under IDEA because Section 504 has a broader definition of the term "disability." Eligibility under 504 is not limited to certain disability categories, as it is under IDEA. Section 504, as a civil rights law, includes persons who have a "physical or mental impairment that substantially limits a major life activity," such as caring for oneself, performing tasks, walking, seeing, hearing, speaking, breathing, reading, writing, calculating math problems, concentrating, interacting with others, learning, or working. An impairment does not automatically mean that a student has a disability under Section 504; the impairment must substantially limit one or more major life activities in order to be considered a disability under Section 504. A student is not considered as an individual with a disability if the impairment is minor or transitory (ie, with an actual or expected duration of 6 months or less). An impairment that is episodic or in remission may be considered a disability if it substantially limits a major life activity when active. It is important for pediatricians and other pediatric medical providers to help families understand that a child's medical diagnosis does not automatically mean that the child is eligible to receive services under Section 504; an illness or impairment must cause a substantial limitation of the child's ability to learn or of another major life activity. Medical diagnoses are not sufficient to serve as an evaluation for the purposes of providing a "free and appropriate public education," but diagnoses may be considered among other sources of information in evaluating a student with an impairment. In addition to a medical diagnosis, other necessary sources of information include achievement/aptitude test results, teacher recommendations, physical condition, social/cultural background, and adaptive behavior.

Students with disabilities under Section 504 are eligible to receive accommodations, modifications, and supplementary aids and services in school, so that their individual educational needs are met as adequately as nondisabled peers. Students with disabilities under Section 504 must also be educated with their nondisabled peers "to the maximum extent appropriate." Placement in separate classrooms or special education programs can only occur following an individual evaluation that determines that a student cannot benefit from education in regular classes, even with the use of supplementary aids and services. Thus, services for students with disabilities under Section 504 regulations may include education in regular classrooms, education in regular classes with supplementary services, or special education and related services.

Primary care pediatric medical providers may advise parents to request Section 504 services when their patient has a chronic medical condition, such as diabetes or heart disease, which is not covered under IDEA. Section 504 may also be appropriate when a child with a disability is covered by IDEA—such as a child with ADHD, a mild emotional disorder, or an orthopedic impairment—but does not require IDEA/special education services to benefit from their school program and can remain in regular education with accommodations or modifications. Educational accommodations or modifications vary based on the child's specific needs; examples include shortened assignments, preferential seating, use of a tape recorder, or accessible building and transportation accommodations. Under IDEA, the ARD committee develops an IEP for the student, while a Section 504 committee develops a 504 plan for the student. There are some similarities between Section 504 and IDEA procedures that involve identification, evaluation, provision of services, and individual plan and procedural safeguards, although mandatory procedures are not identical, and school districts generally have greater flexibility under Section 504. It is important to keep in mind that although a child with a disability may be not eligible for special education services within the public school system, Section 504 accommodations or modifications, as well as supplementary aids and services, are available to ensure that the child's educational needs are met as adequately as those of nondisabled students.

## WHAT IF THE CHILD DOES NOT QUALIFY?

If a child does not meet eligibility criteria for IDEA or Section 504 services but nonetheless has difficulty meeting learning goals or passing benchmark examinations, he or she may receive other types of services that do not fall under the auspices of special education. Children who are struggling with academics may be offered Response to Intervention (RTI), a tiered system of evidence-based interventions for children who are not meeting grade-level expectations. RTI may involve supports such as tutoring, individual and group targeted instruction, or behavioral interventions. Children in RTI should be monitored frequently and consistently to ensure that the interventions are effective. RTI should not be implemented in lieu of a special education evaluation if a child appears to have a disability that may qualify them for special education services.

When disagreements arise between parents and school districts regarding eligibility and services under IDEA or Section 504, either party may use due-process hearing procedures to seek resolution. If a pediatric medical provider has a patient whose family has tried to obtain special education services or additional assistance for their child in school, but the school has not been responsive, the provider should recommend that the family seek help from community-based advocacy organizations, such as the Arc, which provides detailed educational advocacy and has chapters in all 50 states and the District of Columbia. Local chapters provide materials, training, and consultation to guide families through the special education system and to help families understand how to initiate complaints or grievances when their concerns are not resolved. For more information, families can contact their local Arc (http://www.thearc.org/find-a-chapter). There are also professional advocates, including attorneys and educational specialists, who are available for hire to help represent families in their conflicts with schools. State boards of education are also entrusted with the responsibility to ensure that local school districts and schools are in compliance with IDEA and other related laws, and each state board has established a process to investigate and respond to complaints and concerns.

## WHAT CAN PEDIATRIC MEDICAL PROVIDERS DO TO HELP FAMILIES WITH SCHOOL ISSUES?

Primary care pediatricians and other pediatric medical providers and parents of children with disabilities can obtain additional information about available services under Section 504 and IDEA by contacting their campus principal, district special education director, or the district 504 coordinator. These educators are knowledgeable about the federal laws and local school services that are available. Parents of students with special needs are often ill-equipped to navigate the complexities of the public school system and will benefit from healthcare professionals who have a knowledge base of the interplay of health care and children's educational programs.

Primary care pediatricians and other pediatric medical providers can have a significant positive impact on a child's educational services by providing personalized medical recommendations on behalf of their patient at an ARD or 504 committee meeting through written recommendations or participation in a conference call before or during the meeting. Pediatricians and other pediatric medical providers can also educate parents and school personnel regarding various medical conditions and their implications for educational programming and supports needed in the home and school environments. Opportunities for primary care pediatric medical providers to educate parents and teachers are widespread and can vary in complexity and duration, depending on the needs of the patient. Effective communication by healthcare professionals with parents and educators may involve brief phone calls or office visits or could include more extensive interactions, such as a series of community programs about a variety of common medical conditions found in schools, such as ADHD, neurological problems (eg, seizures), autism spectrum disorders, learning and intellectual disabilities, or adolescent health issues for students with special needs. Public school districts typically provide in-service training for their staff at scheduled times throughout the year and welcome presentations by medical professionals regarding children with developmental disabilities.

In its 2015 report on IDEA and children with special educational needs, the AAP strongly encourages pediatricians and other pediatric healthcare providers to develop an understanding of the laws governing early intervention and special education and to advise and support families whose children require these services. Through their advocacy, guidance, and support, pediatric medical providers can help ensure that children with disabilities have access to programs and services that will help to maximize their educational and functional potential.

## SUGGESTED READINGS AND WEB SITES

### Readings


Anderson W, Chitwood S, Hayden D, Takemoto C. *Negotiating the Special Education Maze.* 4th ed. Bethesda, MD: Woodbine House; 2008.

Lipkin PH, Okamoto J; Council on Children with Disabilities; Council on School Health. The Individuals with Disabilities Education Act (IDEA) for children with special educational needs. *Pediatrics.* 2015;136:e1650-e1662.

Wilmshurst, L, Brue AW. *The Complete Guide to Special Education: Expert Advice on Evaluations, IEPs, and Helping Kids Succeed.* 2nd ed. San Francisco, CA: John Wiley & Sons, Inc; 2010.

Wright P, Wright P. *From Emotions to Advocacy.* Hartfield, VA: Harbor House Law Press; 2002.


### Web Sites

The Arc (http://www.thearc.org/what-we-do/public-policy/policy-issues/education): An organization dedicated to the welfare of all children and adults with intellectual and developmental disabilities.

Center for Parent Information and Resources (http://www.parentcenterhub.org/): General information for parents of children with special needs, including links to state parent centers.

Council for Exceptional Children (http://www.cec.sped.org/): A professional organization dedicated to improving the educational success of individuals with disabilities.

International Dyslexia Association (https://dyslexiaida.org/)

LD Online (http://www.ldonline.org/): An educators' guide to learning disabilities and ADHD.

Understood (https://www.understood.org/en): Resources for parents of children struggling with learning and attention issues.

U.S. Department of Education – Information from the Office of Special Education and Rehabilitative Services – (http://www2.ed.gov/about/offices/list/osers/index.html?src=mr).

U.S. Department of Education Office of Special Education and Rehabilitative Services (http://www2.ed.gov/about/offices/list/ocr/504faq.html): Information from the Office of Civil Rights on Section 504.

Wrightslaw (http://www.wrightslaw.com/): Information about special education law, education law, and advocacy.

# 87 Global Developmental Delay and Intellectual Disability

Sarah Risen and Sherry Sellers Vinson

## NEURODEVELOPMENTAL STREAMS

Observation over centuries confirms that infants and children learn developmental skills in a predictable order within a predictable age range. These skills occur in the following neurodevelopmental streams: neuromotor (including gross motor, fine motor, and oral motor), neurocognitive (including language, social, nonverbal/visual-motor problem solving, and adaptive), and neurobehavior (including attention and activity/impulsivity). Gross motor skills include rolling over, crawling, and walking, and progressing to running, jumping, and skipping; fine motor skills include picking up an item, first with a full fist and then progressing to doing the same with a mature pincer grasp; oral motor skills include speech articulation and feeding. Nonverbal/visual-motor problem-solving skills include determining how to obtain an item that is out of reach or determining which of two containers is smaller. Expressive language skills include cooing, babbling, and progressing to saying words, phrases, and sentences. Receptive language skills include following a one-step command given with a gesture and progressing to following nongestured commands. Social skills include reciprocally smiling and progressing to interactive play with others.

One of the primary responsibilities of a primary care pediatric medical provider is the monitoring of each patient's skill attainment in each developmental stream to make certain that each patient acquires age-expected skills, which is considered meeting developmental milestones. Pediatric medical providers need to partner with their patients' parents and caregivers in this monitoring responsibility, since parents and caregivers observe their children daily, which allows them to report skill attainment, lack of skill attainment, or skill loss in a timely manner.

### Global Developmental Delay

Developmental delay occurs when a child gains a skill at an age beyond the expected age range for that skill's acquisition. Given that the most common etiologies for developmental delay tend to affect the brain diffusely (eg, chromosomal/genetic abnormalities), global developmental delay is more prevalent than focal or dissociated delay. Global developmental delay is defined by a significant delay in two or more developmental domains. While a mild or borderline delay is usually defined by developmental quotient, or DQ (developmental age/chronologic age × 100), below 85%, a significant delay is usually defined as a DQ of less than 70%. Thus, an 18-month-old child whose nonverbal/visual-motor problem-solving skills are at a 12-month level (DQ = 12 months/18 months × 100 = 67%) and whose language skills are at a 10-month level (DQ = 10 months/18 months × 100 = 56%) would be considered to have global developmental delay.

Infants and toddlers with global developmental delay who have delays involving both nonverbal/visual-motor problem solving and receptive language development are at significant risk for intellectual disability. The more severe the intellectual disability is, the younger the age a child is when it can be reliably identified. However, mild intellectual disability may be more difficult to confirm at early ages, particularly in children who have not received appropriate developmental stimulation. A hearing and seeing child with exposure to developmentally stimulating activities who has acquired developmental skills in nonverbal/visual-motor problem solving and receptive language at less than 70% the expected rate for age by 6 years of age would be predicted to score in a range of intellectual disability on a standardized intelligence test and on at least two adaptive behaviors on a standardized caretaker adaptive behavior questionnaire, with both of these measures using standard scores rather than DQs.

## STANDARD SCORES ON IQ TESTS

When considering intellectual disability and scores on standardized intelligence tests (which report intelligence quotient, or IQ scores) and measures of adaptive behavior, one must understand the meaning of standard scores. IQ tests are designed so that scores fall along a normal or bell-shaped curve for each age, with a mean IQ score of 100 and a standard deviation of 15 points. Intellectual disability is defined as intelligence that scores more than 2 standard deviations (ie, more than 30 IQ points) below the mean. IQ scores from 90 to 109 are considered average (accounting for 50% of the population), from 110 to 119 are considered high average (accounting for 16.1% of the population), from 120 to 129 are considered superior (accounting for 6.7% of the population), and scores of 130 and above are considered very superior (accounting for 2.2% of the population). IQ scores from 80 to 89 are considered low or below average (accounting for 16.1% of the population), from 70 to 79 are considered borderline (accounting for 6.7% of the population), and scores of 70 and below are considered in the range of intellectual disability (accounting for 2.2% of the population). To be diagnosed with an intellectual disability, in addition to scoring more than 2 standard deviations below the mean on IQ testing, the individual must also score more than 2 standard deviations below the mean on a standardized parent/caregiver completed questionnaire measuring adaptive behavior (which includes activities of daily living and other social/practical skills), and the onset of the disability must occur prior to 18 years of age. It is important to note that although they do not exhibit intellectual disability, children in the borderline and low average ranges of intelligence typically have significant difficulty keeping up in regular classrooms, and combined, they are often referred to as "slower learners." Such slower learners make up 22.8% of the population, and thus, slower learning is the most prevalent neurodevelopmental cause of school failure.

## LEVELS OF INTELLECTUAL DISABILITY

The levels of intellectual disability are (1) mild, with IQ scores between 50 and 69 (accounting for 85% of individuals with intellectual disability); (2) moderate, with IQ scores between 35 and 49 (accounting for 10% of individuals with intellectual disability); (3) severe, with IQ scores between 20 and 34 (accounting for 3% to 4% of individuals with intellectual disability); and (4) profound, with IQ scores less than 20 (accounting for 1% to 2% of individuals with intellectual disability). IQ tests generally provide a full-scale IQ score as well as IQ scores on subdomains of intelligence, such as verbal comprehension, nonverbal reasoning, working memory, and processing speed. Most commonly, individuals with intellectual disability score in the same range or adjacent ranges for each component of IQ and adaptive behavior testing. For example, an individual may score in the mild range of intellectual disability for all components of their IQ and adaptive behavior testing. Another individual may score in the moderate range of intellectual disability for verbal comprehension, working memory, and processing speed on IQ testing and in communication on adaptive behavior testing, but he or she may score in the mild range of intellectual disability for nonverbal reasoning on IQ testing and in daily living skills on adaptive behavior testing. However, a child with fine-motor incoordination accompanying the intellectual disability may have a processing speed standard score in the severe range of intellectual disability that drags down the child's other standard scores, which may be in the mild range. Knowing the standard scores for each component of the patients' IQ testing allows primary care pediatric medical providers to assist their patients' families to recognize their children's strengths to use when helping them learn in their weaker areas, determine appropriate assistive technology for circumventing significantly lower ability areas, and make lifespan plans.

## ADULT OUTCOMES

Years of evidence indicates that individuals with intellectual disability continue to gain new skills within the breadth of complexity of their learning abilities across their lifespans; however, the depth of the complexity of what they are able to learn plateaus in adulthood. The adult abilities of individuals with intellectual disability can be generally predicted as follows. The depth of complexity of learning of individuals with mild intellectual disability generally plateaus at an approximate 8- to 11-year-old level. This means that individuals with mild intellectual disabilities should have late 2nd- to early 6th-grade–level academic abilities as an adult, and most individuals with mild intellectual disability can live independently as adults, although they typically require intermittent support (such as when making financial decisions). The depth of complexity of learning for individuals with moderate intellectual disability generally plateaus at a 5- to 8-year-old level. Thus, individuals with moderate intellectual disability should have kindergarten to late 2nd-grade–level academic abilities, and individuals with moderate intellectual disabilities typically require limited support throughout the day (to navigate daily situations) as adults. The depth of complexity of learning for individuals with severe intellectual disability generally plateaus at a 2- to 5-year-old level; thus, individuals with severe intellectual disability typically require extensive support. Finally, the depth of complexity of learning for individuals with profound intellectual disability generally plateaus at less than a 2-year-old level; thus, individuals with profound intellectual disability typically require pervasive support. A single individual with intellectual disability usually has adult abilities scattering from the lowest age to the highest age in the predicted age range for his/her predicted adult ability range, with skills requiring more abstract reasoning being at the lowest age and skills requiring more concrete reasoning being at the highest age. Understanding these predicted adult outcomes allows primary care pediatric medical providers to help their patients' parents advocate for appropriate educational interventions to help their children reach their predicted adult outcomes and to plan for their children's transition to adulthood. Such advocacy and planning can begin early, since formal intellectual testing can be performed in a child's early years of elementary school.

## RESPONSIBILITIES OF THE MEDICAL HOME

Global developmental delay and intellectual disability are descriptive developmental diagnoses, and it is the primary care pediatric medical provider's role to attempt to determine an etiologic diagnosis to account for the global developmental delay or intellectual disability. The more severe the developmental delay or intellectual disability, the more likely an underlying etiologic diagnosis will be made. Unfortunately, since the vast majority (85%) of individuals with intellectual disability have mild intellectual disability, an etiologic diagnosis will not be discovered for the majority of individuals; however, recent advances in genetic testing are resulting in more etiologic diagnoses being made currently than ever before.

All individuals with global developmental delay or intellectual disability should undergo a chromosome microarray analysis and DNA testing for fragile X syndrome (the most common cause of inherited intellectual disability). Metabolic testing (eg, plasma amino acids, ammonia, lactate, acylcarnitine profiles; urine organic acids; mucopolysaccharides) should be considered in individuals with global developmental delay/intellectual disability who present with developmental regression, episodic encephalopathy, seizures, ataxia, involuntary movements, organomegaly, coarse facial features, decompensation with mild illness, episodic vomiting, or other metabolic signs. Other causes of intellectual disability include complications of prematurity, prenatal toxin exposure (eg, fetal alcohol syndrome), congenital infections, postnatal infections (encephalitis), hypoxia/ischemia, traumatic brain injury, and psychosocial deprivation.

Pediatric medical providers need to realize that the diagnosis of an intellectual disability is devastating to parents, as this diagnosis predicts that their child will need to live under some level of adult support across the lifespan. To provide an appropriate medical home for a child with an intellectual disability, pediatric medical providers and their staff should (1) assist parents in understanding public school special education law; (2) assist parents in recognizing appropriate expectations on which to base educational interventions/assistive technology requests; (3) monitor for mental health disorders (as all psychiatric disorders are more prevalent in individuals with intellectual disability compared to those without intellectual disability); (4) provide parents information about the availability of post-secondary job training and appropriate supervised jobs; (5) educate parents on the need for extracurricular/recreational activities and where to find them; (6) counsel parents on the importance of establishing adult guardianship before the child reaches 18 years of age and planning for the child's future past the parents' lives; (7) provide families information on Medicaid waivers and disability supports; and (8) transition their patients to adult medical/dental care.

It is critical for pediatric medical homes of children and adolescents with intellectual disability to be skilled in assisting parents in understanding their children's ability levels, so that they may establish developmentally appropriate expectations for their children, so as to avoid anxiety and frustration derivative of a mismatch between expectations and abilities, which may result in secondary social, emotional, or behavioral problems. If parents' expectations exceed a child's developmental abilities, in addition to frustrating the child and potentially causing low self-esteem, the parents will remain chronically disappointed in the child's inability to meet expectations and feel like a failure as a parent. On the other hand, if parents have appropriate expectations based on the ability level of the child, they can experience pride in their child's accomplishments, which validates their parenting skills.

## SUGGESTED READINGS


Acharya K, Msall ME. The spectrum of cognitive-adaptive developmental disorders in intellectual disability. In: Accardo PJ, ed. *Capute & Accardo's Neurodevelopmental Disabilities in Infancy and Childhood.* 3rd ed. Baltimore, MD: Paul H. Brookes Publishing Co; 2008:241-259.

American Psychiatric Association. Intellectual disability (intellectual developmental disorder). In: *Diagnostic and Statistical Manual of Mental Disorders.* 5th ed. Arlington, VA: American Psychiatric Association; 2013:33-41.

Fussell JJ, Reynolds AM. Cognitive development. In: Voigt RG, Macias MM, Myers SM, eds. *Developmental and Behavioral Pediatrics.* Elk Grove Village, IL: American Academy of Pediatrics; 2010:171-200.

Shapiro BK, Batshaw ML, Developmental delay and intellectual disability. In: Batshaw ML, Roizen NJ, Lotrecchiano GR, eds. *Children with Disabilities.* 7th ed. Baltimore, MD: Paul H. Brookes Publishing Co; 2013:245-263.






# 88 Delays in Motor Development and Motor Disabilities

Heidi Castillo, Jonathan Castillo, and Kathryn K. Ostermaier

## INTRODUCTION

Given that the most common causes of developmental delay affect the brain diffusely (eg, chromosomal/genetic syndromes), delays in motor development are most commonly a component of more globally delayed developmental milestones across neuromotor, neurocognitive, and neurobehavioral streams of development. Thus, when a child presents with a chief complaint of delays in motor development, a thorough developmental history is needed to uncover possibly more subtle delays in language, nonverbal/visual-motor problem-solving, social, or adaptive development. However, there is a spectrum of dissociated and deviated motor development, where motor development is discrepantly delayed compared to other domains in development, and in more severe cases, where motor skills are acquired in a developmentally deviated manner (see Chapter 83). This chapter will review the motor disabilities contained within this spectrum of discrepant (or dissociated and deviated) motor delay.

Embryologically, the neural system is one of the earliest to begin to develop and the last to be completed. This system develops in a predictable manner of progression from cephalad to caudal and proximal to distal, as do motor skills after birth. A deviation from this predicted pattern may represent the earliest signs of a future motor delay or disability. Motor disorders can be central or peripheral in origin. Understanding patterns of typical development will aid the clinician in appropriately diagnosing and treating the underlying condition.

Motor skills are not as correlated as other domains of development are to overall cognitive function, but when delayed, they are the most evident early on. When severe, these delays not only are obvious to clinicians but also are evident to family members. However, subtle differences in motor development may or may not predict an actual disorder. Therefore, it is important to remember that there is a wide range of normal variation in motor development, and even typically developing children may achieve motor milestones at different times. Since a motor delay can be particularly anxiety provoking to family members, it is imperative to approach these concerns in a caring manner, be able to explain the observations in family-centered language, and provide reassurance when appropriate.

In addition to identifying a discrepant delay (dissociation) or deviation in motor development, it is imperative that a clinician assess the nature of the disorder and evaluate for potential associated medical conditions and complications. Even when a definitive diagnosis cannot be obtained early on, timely identification of delays should prompt referrals to therapeutic services, which may improve the ultimate function and quality of life for children with motor disabilities.

## PATHOGENESIS AND EPIDEMIOLOGY

While motor development most often occurs in a predictable pattern, a delay, dissociation, or deviation from this pattern is most often, but not always, indicative of an underlying diagnosis. While motor delay is required for a motor disability diagnosis, deviation from the typical pattern of development does not always represent a problem (eg, walking before crawling). However, if the degree of this delay, dissociation, or deviation is severe, this usually represents an underlying motor disability. As motor pathways mature very rapidly in the first year of life, motor disabilities often present early on. These signs may be present, depending on severity, in utero (possibly leading to a difficult delivery) or at birth (eg, tone abnormalities and abnormal head growth). In mild cases, a deviation from the typical patterns may not present until later on and be most noticeable at school age. A clinician's familiarity with the sequence of typical motor development will aid in identification of an abnormality (see Chapter 82).

The progression of motor development includes the integration of primitive reflexes (eg, the asymmetric tonic neck reflex, the tonic labyrinthine extensor reflex, the positive support reflex) and the synchronous appearance of postural reactions, followed by the development of voluntary motor skills. This represents a shift from involuntary brain stem control to voluntary higher cortical control. The integration of most primitive reflexes occurs by 6 months of age. Early postural reactions are required prior to the appearance of other motor milestones, such as rolling. After this, motor development typically occurs in a stepwise progression from rolling to sitting, crawling, cruising, and ultimately to walking (Table 88-1). While it is important to be familiar with the typical timetable of motor milestones, it is also important to be familiar with the qualitative progression of motor coordination. For example, a 12-month-old child with left hemiparesis may show a voluntary release of objects (with his or her right hand) as expected at 12 months of age and thus does not exhibit a developmental delay in this skill, but careful observation will reveal that this child cannot accomplish this feat with either hand and tends to flex the left arm and fist the left hand. Thus, the best way to diagnose a motor disability is to carefully obtain and consider the developmental history and combine this with a full physical examination and detailed neurologic and neurodevelopmental examinations.

The spectrum of motor disabilities is wide and can be divided into central and peripheral in nature. Central motor disorders include a spectrum from the high-prevalence, low-morbidity developmental coordination disorders (eg, gross-motor dyspraxia and fine-motor dysgraphia) to the low-prevalence, high-morbidity presentation of cerebral palsy (CP). The estimated prevalence of CP is approximately 2 per 1000. CP is a static encephalopathy caused by a brain insult occurring in the prenatal, perinatal, or postnatal time periods, and it is nonprogressive. The most significant risk factor for CP is prematurity (< 32 weeks gestation, < 1500 g), and nearly half of children with CP are born preterm. Prenatal risk factors include genetic abnormalities and in utero strokes or exposure to viral infections, teratogens, or drugs. Perinatal risk factors include intrapartum asphyxia resulting in neonatal hypoxic-ischemic encephalopathy, which accounts for less than 10% of cases of CP. Postnatal risk factors include severe neonatal infections, strokes, trauma, or metabolic disease. Postnatal risk factors account for 10% of children with CP.

Peripheral causes of motor disability include both neuromuscular and structural defects. Peripheral causes of motor disability also represent a spectrum and include such disorders as spinal muscular atrophy, Charcot-Marie-Tooth disease, muscular dystrophy, and clubfoot.

**TABLE 88-1 MOTOR MILESTONES**

| Milestone (Gross Motor, Fine Motor) | Age Expected |
|---|---|
| Holds chin up in prone | 1 month |
| Holds chest up in prone | 2 months |
| Supports self on elbows in prone | 3 months |
| Rolls prone to supine; hands mostly open | 4 months |
| Rolls supine to prone; transfers objects | 5 months |
| Sits with anterior propping; rakes object with hand and grasps | 6 months |
| Crawls; holds one object in each hand | 8 months |
| Cruises; immature pincer | 9 months |
| Walks with one hand held; mature pincer | 11 months |
| Walks without assistance; voluntary release of objects | 12 months |
| Walks down stairs with one hand held; scribbles spontaneously | 18 months |
| Jumps off ground; imitates stroke | 24 months |
| Performs broad jump; draws circle | 36 months |

## CLINICAL MANIFESTATIONS

Motor disorders are not usually evident at birth, and therefore, children with identifiable risk factors should be closely monitored longitudinally. However, many children who will go on to be diagnosed with a motor disability will have a history of poor feeding in the neonatal period. Those with severe motor disabilities may be detected in the first year of life, while those with mild disabilities may not be noted until later ages, when more complex motor activities are expected.

### Cerebral Palsy

Children with CP most often present with delays and deviation in their acquisition of motor milestones combined with abnormalities in their neurological exams. Abnormalities in muscle tone may present as poor head control, opisthotonus, or scissoring of the lower extremities. Children with CP may exhibit persistence of primitive reflexes beyond the usual age of integration and brisk deep tendon reflexes or clonus.

CP is clinically described by the type and location of impaired motor function. Spastic CP presents with hyperreflexia and increased muscle tone due to muscle spasticity, and over time, children with spastic CP tend to develop muscle contractures. Spastic CP has been attributed to damage to the corticospinal or pyramidal tracts. Extrapyramidal CP includes dyskinetic and ataxic forms. Dyskinetic CP presents with uncontrolled, involuntary movements, such as dystonia or choreoathetosis, and it is related to damage to the basal ganglia. Ataxic CP presents with poor balance or coordination and gait instability, and it is related to damage to the cerebellum. CP is also described by the affected limbs: monoplegia (1 limb), hemiplegia (ipsilateral arm and leg), diplegia (bilateral lower extremities), triplegia (1 limb being unaffected or minimally affected when compared to the other 3; typically involves diplegia with a superimposed hemiplegia), and quadriplegia (all limbs affected, usually along with the trunk).

CP often presents with multiple medical comorbidities related to the underlying brain damage and poor motor control and coordination. Typically, the more severe the motor impairment, the more severe the comorbidities. Problems related to growth and feeding are attributable to oral-motor dysphagia, and 7% of children with CP require tube feeding. Gastroesophageal reflux is present in 50% and constipation in up to 70% of children with CP, and these gastrointestinal complications also contribute to poor feeding and growth. Orthopedic complications of spastic CP include joint dislocations, bone deformities, scoliosis, osteopenia, fractures, and muscle contractures. Sensory deficits are common, with visual impairments present in 30% and hearing deficits present in 10% to 20% of children with CP. Seizures occur in 25% to 40% of children with CP. Cognitive deficits or intellectual disability occur in 50% of children with spastic CP, with severity often correlated to the severity of the motor impairment. Children with CP without intellectual disability are at increased risk for learning disabilities. However, it is important to recognize that accurate cognitive testing is often challenging in children with limited motor control and verbal output.

### Progressive Neurodegenerative Disorders

Children with progressive neurodegenerative disorders present with motor impairments that worsen over time. Children in this category of disorders may have early typical motor development that is then noted to slow, plateau, and then regress or deteriorate. Duchenne muscular dystrophy (an X-linked disorder) will often be diagnosed at 4 to 6 years of age, when the child is noted to be clumsier than his peers, with difficulty running, jumping, and climbing stairs. A classic physical exam feature is Gowers' sign, which is seen when a child uses his hands to push off the floor in order to attain upright posture. Children with Duchenne muscular dystrophy often die in their early 20s.

Myotonic dystrophies often present in adulthood, but they can be quite severe and have congenital or juvenile presentations with poor prognosis. Spinal muscular atrophy types 2 to 4 have adult-onset muscle weakness; however, type 1 (Werdnig-Hoffmann disease) is the most common and the most severe. This type typically presents in the neonatal period with rapidly progressive weakness leading to respiratory failure and poor prognosis. Most children with this type of myotonic dystrophy often die by 2 to 3 years of age. Charcot-Marie-Tooth disease is a collection of hereditary peripheral neuropathies. These neuropathies primarily affect distal sensory and motor nerves, resulting in lower-extremity weakness, foot deformities such as pes cavus or hammer toes, and sensory deficits. Later changes include atrophy of intrinsic hand and foot muscles.

Although progressive neurodegenerative disorders are rare and represent a small number of children who present with motor delays, accurate diagnosis is crucial in order to predict the rate of progression, provide genetic counseling to family members, and deliver intervention for maximizing function and improving quality of life.

## DIAGNOSIS

The diagnosis of CP is often suggested by a child's clinical and neurological presentation, and evaluation should begin with detailed medical and developmental histories and physical and neurodevelopmental examinations. Particular attention should be paid to a child's prenatal and neonatal history to detect risk factors, age of attainment of developmental milestones and the presence of dissociated delays in motor development and deviated acquisition of motor milestones, review of the newborn screen, and careful review of the family history to look for relatives with neurological conditions that may suggest a genetic cause for CP. A detailed physical and neurologic exam that includes evaluation of tone, strength, balance, posture, and coordination will help to classify the type of CP. Regression or deterioration of milestones, atrophy or sensory changes, worsening of symptoms with illness, or hypotonia with weakness are suggestive of a neurodegenerative disease or a metabolic disorder.

Neuroimaging should be offered for all children with a new diagnosis of CP. Magnetic resonance imaging (MRI) is preferred over other imaging techniques, as it has been shown to have a higher diagnostic yield and can help determine etiology and timing of injury. MRI abnormalities can be seen in > 80% of children who present with an abnormal neurologic examination. Metabolic and genetic testing should be offered to those with atypical presentations, with suggestive family histories, or with normal neuroimaging or neuroimaging suggesting a developmental brain abnormality (such as lissencephaly/schizencephaly) or for those with no other etiologies identified by history. Metabolic testing should include serum concentrations of glucose, bicarbonate, creatine kinase (CK), ammonia, lactate, pyruvate, plasma amino acids, and urine organic acids. Genetic testing including chromosomal microarray analysis or whole-exome sequencing has been shown to determine a cause of CP in 15% to 30% of children who previously lacked an identifiable etiology. An electroencephalogram (EEG) may also be helpful if there is concern for seizures.

## TREATMENT

Treatment of a motor disability is tailored to the principal diagnosis. The core components of the longitudinal management of motor disabilities include (1) timely family-centered care; (2) family involvement in the therapeutic process; (3) maximization of functional independence; and (4) support of transition to adult medical care.

Primary care pediatric medical providers are key to timely family-centered care, as their early, frequent, and longitudinal relationship with children and their families allows for initial identification of parental concerns and early recognition of early signs of existent or evolving motor disorders. This prompt identification will allow for referral to appropriate therapy services and medical subspecialists as needed. In managing children with motor disabilities, the primary care pediatric medical provider should assume a leadership role of a multidisciplinary team (that starts with the child and his or her family and may also include physical therapists, occupational therapists, speech/language therapists, orthotists, dieticians, and medical subspecialists, including physiatrists, neurologists, developmental-behavioral pediatricians, neurosurgeons, and orthopedic surgeons) and assume coordination of care among the team members.

Throughout the duration of treatment, the focus should remain on optimizing developmental potential, decreasing medical comorbidities, and maximizing functional independence and quality of life. This is singularly important for those conditions expected to lead to significant lifelong disability or mortality (eg, muscular dystrophy, myotonic dystrophy, spinal muscular atrophy). From pharmacological, to physical, to surgical, there is a wide array of therapies to address issues associated with motor disabilities. Yet, regardless of the approach that the underlining condition may dictate, the family's active involvement in the therapeutic process is critical, significantly influencing the ultimate outcome. The primary care pediatric medical provider does not necessarily need to become an expert in every facet of care for all of the conditions that may lead to motor disability; however, having a basic understanding of the numerous aspects of care will allow mindful coordination of care and comanagement of comorbidities and complications with subspecialists.

In order to maximize functional independence over a lifetime, interventions must be commenced early on. These interventions can be initially provided through early intervention or early childhood special education programs and then through special education programs at school. Early intervention or school-based therapeutic services can be supplemented by additional private therapy services. Early intervention services may include feeding therapy, developmental therapy, speech therapy, occupational therapy, and physical therapy, and as the child ages, the need for more tailored therapies may emerge, such as augmentative communication therapy or robot-assisted walking therapy. Braces and splints to support positioning, sitting, or ambulation are often needed, as is ambulation equipment, such as walkers, standers, and wheelchairs. Adaptive modifications to bathrooms, bedrooms, access doorways, and automobiles may also be required.

At the center of an effective treatment approach for children with motor disabilities is the management of spasticity, pain, and musculoskeletal deformity. Spasticity can be isolated or generalized; such delineation will help guide management. Isolated spasticity may be treated with injections of onabotulinumtoxinA (Botox) directly into the affected muscle. Generalized spasticity can be addressed through the use of oral muscle relaxants such as dantrolene, diazepam, and baclofen or through neurosurgical implantation of an intrathecal baclofen pump.

Although surgical interventions have historically been aimed at diminishing muscle imbalance and preventing bony and soft-tissue deformity, recent advances in surgical approaches are providing innovative solutions to physiological drivers of motor disabilities. One treatment, dorsal rhizotomy, involves the selective separation of portions of the dorsal roots of the spinal cord, which can diminish lower-extremity spasticity.

No treatment algorithm is complete without a clear pathway to supporting patients through their transition to adult medical care. Rarely is a transition successful without providing the family with accurate information regarding community resources, adult healthcare providers, and information on patient and family support groups. Thus, the primary care office should have access to such information and help the family connect with these resources as part of comprehensive care.

## PREVENTION

While most cases of motor disabilities cannot be prevented currently, acquired cases of CP can be prevented. Measures to decrease meningitis (through appropriate immunizations), nonaccidental trauma, motor vehicle accidents, and stroke may contribute to a decrease in incidence of motor disability. Counseling families about unproven alternative therapies is also important in morbidity prevention. Clinicians should be prepared to discuss therapies for which no evidence base exists and to caution families when they are considering alternative therapies that may pose safety or financial burdens.



## SUGGESTED READINGS

Ashwal S, Russman BS, Blasco PA, et al; Quality Standards Subcommittee of the American Academy of Neurology; Practice Committee of the Child Neurology Society. Practice parameter: diagnostic assessment of the child with cerebral palsy: report of the Quality Standards Subcommittee of the American Academy of Neurology and the Practice Committee of the Child Neurology Society. *Neurology*. 2004;62(6):851-863.

Bushby K, Finkel R, Birnkrant DJ, et al; DMD Care Considerations Working Group. Diagnosis and management of Duchenne muscular dystrophy, part 1: diagnosis, and pharmacological and psychosocial management. *Lancet Neurol.* 2010;9(1):77-93.

Noritz GH, Murphy NA; Neuromotor Screening Expert Panel. Motor delays: early identification and evaluation. *Pediatrics.* 2013;131(6):e2016-e2027.

Quality Standards Subcommittee of the American Academy of Neurology; Delgado MR, Hirtz D, Aisen M, et al. Practice parameter: pharmacologic treatment of spasticity in children and adolescents with cerebral palsy (an evidence-based review): report of the Quality Standards Subcommittee of the American Academy of Neurology and the Practice Committee of the Child Neurology Society. *Neurology*. 2010;74(4):336-343.

Schultz MB, Blasco PA. Motor development. In: Voigt RG, Macias MM, Myers SM, eds. *Developmental and Behavioral Pediatrics*. Elk Grove Village, IL: American Academy of Pediatrics; 2011.

# 89 Delays in Speech/Language or Nonverbal Development and Learning Disabilities

Sonia Monteiro and Noel Mensah-Bonsu

## INTRODUCTION

Language and nonverbal/visual-motor problem solving are components of the neurocognitive stream of development. Because the most common causes of neurodevelopmental disability affect the brain diffusely (eg, genetic disorders), delays in language development are most commonly accompanied by delays in nonverbal/visual-motor problem-solving development and vice versa. Thus, the most prevalent mild neurodevelopmental difficulty that results in school failure is "slower learning," where both language and nonverbal/visual-motor problem solving are delayed, resulting in intelligence quotients in the borderline (IQ = 70–79) to low average (IQ = 80–89) range. The globally delayed pattern of slower learning occurs in 22.8% of the population, while the dissociated pattern of learning disabilities occurs in only approximately 5% to 10% of the population. In the dissociated pattern of learning disabilities, there is a discrepancy between cognitive abilities and academic achievement, typically with discrepant or dissociated delays in language relative to nonverbal/visual-motor problem-solving development (as observed in language-based learning disabilities) or discrepant or dissociated delays in nonverbal/visual-motor problem solving relative to language development (as observed in nonverbal learning disabilities). It is also important to note that inadequate academic instruction is a common cause of learning problems. This chapter will review the spectrum of dissociated delays in language and nonverbal/visual-motor problem-solving development, including specific language-based and nonverbal learning disabilities.

## DEFINITIONS OF SPEECH AND LANGUAGE

Language is defined as a method of both spoken and written communication. Language is made up of multiple components: phonology, morphology, syntax, semantics, and pragmatics. Phonology involves speech sounds (phonemes) that make up words, and morphology involves the units of language (morphemes) that make up words. Syntax is defined as the rules regarding how words can be combined into sentences, including verb tense, word order, and sentence structure. Semantics is defined as the meaning of words in context or when combined into sentences. Pragmatics is defined as the rules for social communication. Language is separated into expressive and receptive components. Expressive language refers to what a child is able to communicate verbally or through the use of signs or gestures. Receptive language refers to what a child is able to understand.

Speech includes the following components: articulation, fluency, and voice. Articulation involves the production of speech sounds and affects the intelligibility of speech. Fluency refers to the flow of sounds, syllables, and words together to form sentences. Voice includes the anatomical function of the vocal folds as well as airflow to produce sounds.

## SPEECH AND LANGUAGE DEVELOPMENT

Speech and language development can be divided into 3 periods during early childhood (birth to 2 years of age). The first is the *prespeech* period, which begins at birth. In the first few months of life, an infant will typically progress from alerting to sound to responding to and seeking familiar voices. An infant's cry will start to differentiate based on his or her needs. Cooing (the production of vowel sounds) occurs at around 3 months of age. The infant will begin to combine vowel sounds at around 5 months of age. This will be followed by the production of single consonant sounds, and by 6 months of age, vowel and consonant sounds will be combined together in the form of babbling. By 9 months of age, gestures including reaching to be picked up and waving "bye-bye" emerge.

The second period, known as the *naming* period, occurs between 10 and 18 months of age. It begins with the ability to identify caregivers and objects by name, and this ability progresses to the verbal expression of single words. Prior to 1 year of age, most children begin to use a specific "Mama" and "Dada" as their first words, and by 1 year of age, 1 or 2 additional single words will be used. Most children will start to comprehend words frequently used by caregivers (eg, "bath," "bottle") and will start to follow simple gestured commands by 12 months of age. By 14 months of age, a child may combine sounds or mimic conversational sounds with varying intonation in the form of immature jargon. By 18 months of age, a child may begin to mimic words that they hear (echolalia). Also by 18 months of age, a child should have a vocabulary of about 10 words. Gestures progress during this period with the emergence of pointing. By 12 months of age, a child will start pointing to indicate a want or need (protoimperative pointing), and by 14 months of age, the child will start pointing to obtain the attention of an adult to share something of interest (protodeclarative pointing).

Between 18 and 24 months of age, children will experience a dramatic increase in vocabulary, both receptively and expressively, which marks the *word combination* period. Total expressive language can include up to 50 to 100 words by the end of this period, and a child's receptive vocabulary is usually larger. Also by the end of this period, a child should be combining words into 2-word sentences. From a receptive language standpoint, by 18 months of age, children will also begin to identify body parts and point to pictures when named. By 2 years of age, a child's speech articulation should be at least 50% intelligible to others.

| TABLE 89-1 RED FLAGS FOR SPEECH AND LANGUAGE DELAY[a] | | |
|---|---|---|
| **Age** | **Receptive Language** | **Expressive Language** |
| 12 mo | Does not respond to name; does not gesture (wave, point) | Does not babble |
| 16 mo | | Does not use single words |
| 18 mo | Cannot follow simple commands ("give me," "come here") | Does not use at least 8–10 words |
| 24 mo | Does not follow a 2-step direction; cannot point to a picture | Does not use any 2-word combinations; speech is not at least 50% intelligible |
| 30 mo | | Continues to use echolalia; continues to confuse pronouns |
| 36 mo | Cannot answer "who/what/where" questions | Does not use 3- to 4-word sentences; speech is not 75% intelligible; leaves beginning or ending sounds off words |

[a]Loss of speech, babbling, or social skills is a red flag at any age.

By 30 months of age, echolalia should cease, children should be using pronouns appropriately, and they should be able to distinguish just 1 item from a greater number. By 3 years of age, a child should communicate in 3-word sentences, and their speech articulation should be 75% intelligible. Receptively, a 3-year-old child should be able to follow 2-step directions including prepositions and pay attention for longer periods of time when read to. At 3 years of age, children may begin to ask "what" and "where" questions. By 4 years of age, speech should be completely (100%) intelligible. A child at 4 years of age should be able to relate experiences verbally using complex syntax and speak fluently. Red flags for speech and language delay are shown in Table 89-1.

## PEDIATRIC ASSESSMENT OF SPEECH AND LANGUAGE

Speech and language milestones should be regularly assessed as part of routine developmental surveillance at every well child visit. Surveillance involves asking parents questions and documenting their responses regarding attainment of speech and language milestones, reviewing risk factors (including prematurity, previous concerns on prior evaluation, or concerns about appropriate environmental language stimulation). Parental concerns should be elicited and taken seriously. Surveillance also involves the provider's direct observation of the child's speech and language skills in the office visit.

Standardized screening tests, such as the Ages and Stages Questionnaire (ASQ) and Parents' Evaluation of Developmental Status (PEDS), are commonly used developmental screeners that assess multiple areas of development, including speech and language, and identify children who require further evaluation. Standardized screening tests should be regularly implemented at the 9-month, 18-month, and 24- or 30-month well child visits. Parents of older children should be asked if their child has any difficulty with verbal expression or with following directions.

Once a concern is identified (either through screening or surveillance), a referral for a speech and language evaluation should be made. This can be performed through early intervention or early childhood special education programs or by a private speech/language pathologist. In addition to referral for a speech and language evaluation, an audiology evaluation needs to be completed for every child with delayed speech and language skills to rule out hearing loss. Finally, it is important to note that boys with Klinefelter syndrome (XXY) tend to present with language disorders and language-based learning disabilities.

The differential diagnosis for a child presenting with concerns about delayed speech and language development includes language disorder, speech disorder, speech and language disorder, inadequate environmental stimulation, global developmental delay, social communication disorder, autism spectrum disorder, and hearing loss.

## PROMOTION OF LANGUAGE DEVELOPMENT



Developmental milestones in language cannot be attained without appropriate language stimulation in the environment. Previous research has emphasized the importance of exposing children to language from an early age. Parents are encouraged to speak frequently to their infants and describe what is going on around them. It is also critical that parents read to and share books with their children starting in infancy. It has been established that the number of words that children are exposed to can vary significantly based on socioeconomic factors. Children from lower-income homes hear far fewer words than children in middle- or high-income settings. In addition to these gaps, the quality of parent–child interaction in language development, regardless of socioeconomic status, is critically important to language development. Parents should respond to their infants' sounds and attempts at communication to encourage progression in language development. As their children become older, parents should be encouraged to have frequent conversations with their children.



## SPECTRUM OF DISSOCIATED SPEECH DELAY: SPEECH DISORDERS

Dissociated delays in speech development are defined as speech disorders. Speech disorders involve difficulties with sounds required in the production of speech and include voice disorder, speech fluency disorder, phonologic disorder, apraxia of speech, and dysarthria.

### Voice Disorder

Deficits in pitch, loudness, or vocal quality define a voice disorder. There may also be a hyper- or hyponasal quality to speech that may be secondary to anatomical differences (such as velopharyngeal insufficiency or adenoid hypertrophy).

### Fluency Disorder

In children with fluency disorders, the flow of speech is interrupted secondary to repetition of sounds or words and changes in the rate or rhythm of speech. Children between the ages of 2 and 3 years may have pauses, sound prolongations, or may repeat parts of words. This is considered to be a normal stage of language development and may be secondary to the dramatic increase in speech production during this time period. Usually these problems resolve without intervention by 4 years of age. If the dysfluency continues, stuttering is more likely, and referral for evaluation and treatment is indicated.

### Phonologic Disorder

Many children will make errors in pronunciation when using new words. Each speech sound has an age by which it should be mastered, and errors in the production or pattern of these sounds result in speech articulation that is difficult to understand. Simple consonant sounds (/b/, /p/, /m/) as well as all vowel sounds are usually mastered by 2 years of age. More complex consonant sounds (/j/, /r/, /s/) as well as blends (/ch/, /sh/) are mastered later on. Children should be able to produce all sounds in the English language by 8 years of age.

### Childhood Apraxia of Speech

Childhood apraxia of speech (CAS) is thought to be secondary to deficits in central nervous system mechanisms involved in organizing the motor movements necessary for the production of speech. It is not secondary to muscle weakness or paralysis. Children with CAS have difficulties with spontaneous production of sounds, syllables, and words. Most have a history of delayed cooing or babbling during infancy and delayed production of first words. Compared to children with a phonologic disorder who make consistent errors in speech production, children with CAS have irregular and inconsistent speech production.

### Dysarthria

Dysarthria is a motor disorder that is the result of impairment of muscles used in speech production. Muscles may be weak or paralyzed, or there may be problems with coordination. This limits jaw, lip, and tongue movement, resulting in a slow rate of speech, poor articulation, change in voice quality or pitch, and speech that sounds "mumbled" or "slurred." Dysarthria is most commonly observed in children with cerebral palsy (CP).

## SPECTRUM OF DISSOCIATED LANGUAGE DELAY

When children exhibit discrepant delays in their language development relative to their development in other developmental streams, they are described as exhibiting a dissociation in their language development. Of all the streams of development, the language stream is the best single predictor of cognitive potential. In addition, the ability to express and understand language has an impact on social functioning. Language ability predicts school readiness, and deficits in early language development are directly correlated to future language-based learning disabilities and decreased academic achievement.



### Language Disorders (Specific Language Impairment)

A language delay occurs when the progression of language development is occurring in the correct sequence, but at a rate slower than typical. Language delays occur more frequently in boys and when there is an established family history of language delay, speech/language disorders, or language-based learning disabilities. Additional risk factors include prematurity, lack of appropriate developmental stimulation, and lower socioeconomic status. Language delays should not be attributed to birth order (having siblings who "speak for" the child) or to the child being exposed to multiple languages. By 4 years of age, many children with a history of speech and language delays, especially those who have experienced a lack of appropriate language stimulation before receiving appropriate early intervention and early childhood special education services, will "catch up" and not have persistent language difficulties. However, many children will continue to exhibit persistent language delays. Preschool-aged children with dissociated delays in their language development currently meet DSM-5 criteria for a diagnosis of language disorder. However, children with persistent language delays as they enter school are at significant risk for developing language-based learning disabilities.

Children with a language disorder, also known as a specific language impairment, struggle to use language to express themselves and have difficulties understanding the messages of others. Children with language disorders can have discrepant delays in all or just 1 of the components of language (phonology, morphology, syntax, semantics, and pragmatics). These problems with language development are not secondary to hearing loss or to a language delay that is observed as a component of a global developmental delay. Children with language disorders by definition are not globally delayed, and most have typical nonverbal abilities, adaptive functioning, and social skills. Children with language disorders may initially present with a chief complaint of "delayed speech." However, once they start to use words, they may continue to struggle with following directions, being able to form sentences or use verb tenses correctly, or having a conversation.

Language disorders can involve both receptive and expressive language or just expressive language. They cannot involve only receptive language with spared expressive language, as a child can never express what he or she does not understand. A child with a receptive language disorder will have difficulty with understanding what is said and with following directions. Children with an expressive language disorder present with problems expressing their thoughts or needs. Their sentences may be shorter and less complex than what would be expected for their age or developmental level. They may mix up the order of words in sentences, leave words out, or make errors in verb tense. Most children with language disorders will have deficits in both expressive and receptive language. Children with a language disorder are at increased risk of language-based learning difficulties, even those children who appeared to have progressed to having typical spoken language. Children with both speech and language disorders are also at increased risk of emotional and behavioral problems.

### Language-Based Learning Disabilities

**Definitions of Learning Disability** A learning disability (LD) has been classically defined as an unexpected discrepancy in academic performance compared to intellectual potential; however, this definition has been challenged and remains controversial. The *Diagnostic and Statistical Manual of Mental Disorders*, 5th edition (DSM-5) characterizes "specific learning disorders" as being evidenced by academic skills that are substantially and quantifiably below those expected for an individual's chronologic age, which have persisted for at least 6 months despite the provision of targeted interventions, and that are not due to intellectual disability, uncorrected vision or hearing deficits, other mental or neurological disorders, psychosocial adversity, lack of proficiency in the language of academic instruction, or inadequate academic instruction. Thus, children with specific learning disorders must now show a lack of response to intervention before being considered to have a learning disability by many school districts. Previously, most children with slower learning (IQs between 70 and 90), who often struggled to keep up with average and above-average peers in regular classroom placements, did not qualify for any special education services. This is because the majority of children with slower learning, despite having academic achievement scores that are below grade level, have academic achievement abilities that are commensurate with their cognitive expectations, and thus show no discrepancy between cognitive abilities and academic achievement. However, the new DSM-5 definition qualifies students under the specific learning disorder diagnosis whose academic achievement is below that expected for chronologic age. Under this definition, a majority of children with slower learning may now qualify for special education services. Although these children do not have academic achievement that is below expected for their cognitive abilities, their academic achievement is certainly below that expected for their chronologic age. Hopefully, this change in definition will provide children who learn more slowly the same remedial special education services received by children with specific learning disabilities, particularly as research has shown these interventions to be effective in improving academic outcomes no matter whether an individual has a discrepancy between cognitive abilities and academic achievement or not.

**Spectrum of Language-Based Learning Disabilities** Children with preschool language disorders are at significant risk of developing language-based learning disabilities as they enter school. Children with language disorders can have discrepant delays in all or just 1 of the components of language (phonology, morphology, syntax, semantics, and pragmatics). Thus, the mild end of the spectrum of dissociated language delay would include discrepant delays in 1 component of language (eg, phonology), while the severe end would include discrepant delays in multiple components of receptive and expressive language, which is associated with discrepant verbal reasoning compared to nonverbal reasoning on IQ testing (Fig. 89-1).

Thus, the mild end of a spectrum of dissociated language delay includes individuals with dissociated difficulties in phonology, resulting in phonological processing disorders (Fig. 89-1). Children with difficulty with phonology have trouble learning to associate written symbols with the sounds they make, leading to dysphonetic dyslexia. Children with dysphonetic dyslexia have trouble sounding out words, and thus, they have difficulty with reading decoding, reading fluency, and encoding (spelling). However, children with dysphonetic dyslexia have intact nonverbal abilities, and they can memorize sight words. This skill may allow a child with dysphonetic dyslexia to compensate early on at school, but their reading disability becomes more apparent in advancing grades, when the focus shifts from "learning to read" to "reading to learn." In addition, despite their difficulties with phonology, children with dysphonetic dyslexia have otherwise intact language abilities. Thus, while they may not be able to obtain information through reading, they can understand and obtain information through being read to or through listening to books on tape. Similarly, while their difficulties with encoding negatively impact the written expression required of written reports, they can give oral reports without significant incident.

As more components of receptive and expressive language become dissociated, one moves toward the more severe end of the spectrum of dissociated language delay, and children experience language-based learning disabilities. These more severe delays—which may diffusely affect phonology, morphology, syntax, and semantics—negatively

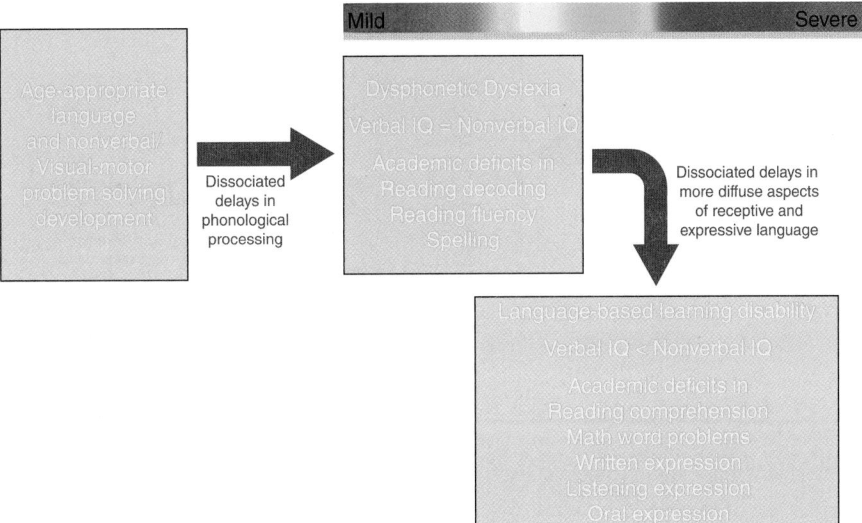


**FIGURE 89-1** Spectrum of language dissociation.

impact verbal reasoning, and children with language-based learning disabilities typically exhibit verbal IQ scores that are dissociated from nonverbal IQ scores. Rather than simply affecting reading decoding and encoding, language-based learning disabilities result in difficulties in reading comprehension, math word problems, written expression, listening comprehension, and oral expression. Children with language-based learning disabilities would have similar difficulties with comprehension whether attempting to read themselves or when being read to or listening to books on tape.

Children suspected of having dyslexia or language-based learning disabilities need to undergo a full and individual evaluation through their local public schools and be provided with direct language therapy services, remedial academic instruction, and maximal accommodations and modifications of all assignments, materials, texts, pacing, and grading when included in regular classroom settings.

## NONVERBAL/VISUAL-MOTOR PROBLEM-SOLVING DEVELOPMENT

Nonverbal/visual-motor problem-solving development involves the development of visual perceptual, visual-spatial, and visual-motor skills. In the first 3 months of life, this domain of development focuses on visual tracking, as children should be able to visually track through 360 degrees by 3 months of age. As this domain of development matures, skills include reaching for and transferring objects at 5 months, using an immature pincer grasp to pick up pellet-sized objects by 9 months, uncovering hidden toys by 10 months, and intentionally releasing objects into containers by 12 months. After 12 months, drawing and block construction skills emerge, with making a crayon mark at 12 months, scribbling spontaneously and stacking 3 blocks at 18 months, imitating a horizontal and vertical stroke and building a horizontal train of blocks at 24 months, and drawing a circle and building a 3-block bridge at age 3 years. Many adaptive skills also rely on nonverbal/visual-motor skill development, such as spoon feeding by 14 months, unzipping by 21 months, unbuttoning by 3 years, buttoning by 4 years, and tying shoes by 5 years.

## PEDIATRIC ASSESSMENT OF NONVERBAL/VISUAL-MOTOR PROBLEM SOLVING

Nonverbal/visual-motor problem-solving milestones should be regularly assessed as part of routine developmental surveillance at every well child visit. It may be more difficult to obtain a developmental history of nonverbal/visual-motor problem-solving skill acquisition from families; for example, they may not have exposed their children to crayons or blocks. Thus, the nonverbal/visual-motor problem-solving developmental history may need to focus on activities of daily living that rely on visual-motor problem-solving skills, such as feeding and dressing. Fortunately, while it may be difficult to elicit a developmental history in this domain, nonverbal/visual-motor problem solving is the domain that is easiest to observe in the office, as the items used in this domain are fun for children to complete (drawing, building with blocks, completing puzzles).

Standardized screening tests, such as the ASQ and PEDS, assess multiple areas of development, including nonverbal/visual-motor problem solving, and identify children who require further evaluation. Standardized screening tests should be regularly implemented at the 9-month, 18-month, and 24- or 30-month well child visit. Older children can be asked to draw pictures of a person or to provide a handwriting sample.

Once a concern is identified (either through screening or surveillance), a referral for an occupational therapy evaluation should be made. This can be performed through early intervention or early childhood special education programs or by a private occupational therapist. In addition to referral for an occupational therapy evaluation, a vision screen or ophthalmology evaluation needs to be completed for every child with delayed nonverbal/visual-motor problem-solving skills to rule out a vision impairment. Finally, children with specific medical diagnoses appear at higher risk for nonverbal/visual-motor problem-solving disorders and nonverbal learning disabilities, including children with Turner syndrome (XO), hydrocephalus/spina bifida, and velocardiofacial syndrome (deletion of chromosome 22q11.2).

## SPECTRUM OF DISSOCIATED NONVERBAL/VISUAL-MOTOR PROBLEM-SOLVING DEVELOPMENT

### Nonverbal/Visual-Motor Problem-Solving Disorders

Children may exhibit dissociated delays in nonverbal problem solving in multiple domains, including visual discrimination, visual figure-ground discrimination, visual sequencing, visual-motor processing, visual memory, visual closure, and visual-spatial relationships. Children with nonverbal/visual-motor problem-solving disorders will evidence dissociated delays in the milestones reviewed above. School-aged children with these delays will have difficulty with drawing, writing, right/left orientation, and completing puzzles, and may get lost in familiar places.

### Spectrum of Nonverbal Learning Disabilities

When children with persistent nonverbal/visual-motor problem-solving disorders enter school, they are at increased risk of developing nonverbal learning disabilities. At the mild end of the spectrum of nonverbal learning disabilities are children whose dissociated delays in nonverbal development involve primarily their orthographic processing (Fig. 89-2). Orthographic processing is the use of the visual system to form, store, and recall written letters and words and also involves using the visual system to process punctuation and capitalization. Children with orthographic processing deficits are at risk for

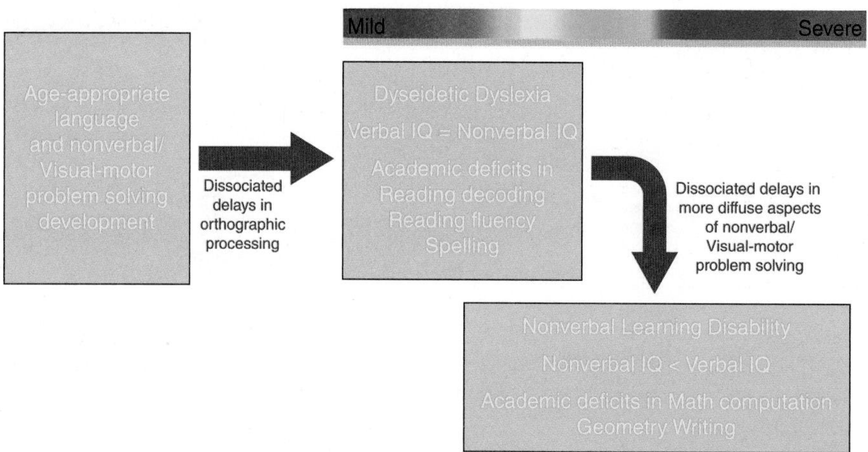


**FIGURE 89-2** Spectrum of nonverbal/visual-motor problem-solving dissociation.

developing dyseidetic dyslexia. Children with dyseidetic dyslexia have problems memorizing the pattern of letters (eg, they may confuse "b" and "d") and difficulty memorizing sight words. Given their preserved phonological processing, children with dyseidetic dyslexia need to laboriously sound out the same word over and over, and they tend to misspell phonetically.

As more components of nonverbal/visual-motor problem solving become dissociated, one moves toward the more severe end of the spectrum of dissociated nonverbal/visual-motor problem-solving delay, and children experience nonverbal learning disabilities. These more severe delays, which may diffusely affect visual discrimination, visual figure-ground discrimination, visual sequencing, visual-motor processing, visual memory, visual closure, and visual-spatial relationships, negatively impact nonverbal reasoning, and children with nonverbal learning disabilities typically exhibit nonverbal IQ scores that are dissociated from verbal IQ scores. Rather than simply having difficulty with reading sight words, nonverbal learning disabilities result in difficulties in writing (dysgraphia), drawing, right/left discrimination, completing puzzles, math computation and processing (dyscalculia), geometry, geography, and getting lost in familiar places, and may involve understanding spatial relations, including social reasoning. (The most severe end of the spectrum of nonverbal dissociation + deviation includes the social communication disorder typically observed in children previously described as having Asperger disorder, but currently described as having autism spectrum disorder without a language disorder; see Chapter 83 and Chapter 91.)

Children suspected of having dyseidetic dyslexia or nonverbal learning disabilities need to undergo a full and individual evaluation through their local schools and be provided with direct occupational therapy services, remedial academic instruction, and maximal accommodations and modifications of all assignments, materials, texts, pacing, and grading when included in regular classroom settings.

## COMORBIDITIES OF LEARNING DISABILITIES

In the continuum of developmental-behavioral diagnoses, dissociated delays in 1 stream of development are often associated with dissociated delays in other streams of development (see Chapter 83). Thus, children with the dissociated neurocognitive developmental profile of learning disabilities often also have the dissociated neurobehavioral developmental profile of attention-deficit/hyperactivity disorder (ADHD) and the dissociated neuromotor developmental profile of speech articulation disorders, handwriting difficulties (dysgraphia), and gross motor incoordination (dyspraxia). Up to 50% of children with ADHD have comorbid learning disabilities in reading (dyslexia), math (dyscalculia), or written expression.

Secondary social, emotional, or behavioral comorbidities are particularly concerning in children with learning disabilities. An unrecognized learning disability may result in school failure. Signs and symptoms of academic distress secondary to an unrecognized learning disability include increased time and effort to complete classroom assignments, anxiety or avoidance of school, acting out, failing grades, or grade retention. It is critical for primary care pediatric medical providers to know that grade retention has not been found to improve a child's educational outcome, and those who have been retained are more likely to have behavioral issues and to eventually drop out of school. Children who have been recognized by their schools to have learning disabilities require remedial special educational instruction in their areas of disability. However, just as importantly, they require maximal accommodations and modifications in order to be successfully included in regular classroom activities. Children with learning disabilities should not be expected to compete with similarly aged peers who do not share their specific learning disabilities in a regular classroom without maximal accommodations and modifications of all assignments, teaching materials, texts, testing, pacing, and grading. Children with learning disabilities should not be expected to attend to academic material that they do not understand or to complete assignments that are beyond their current level of ability. Maximal accommodations and modifications are required in order to ensure that demands and expectations for academic performance in the regular classroom are made commensurate with underlying abilities. Without such accommodations and modifications, demands for a child's performance will exceed his or her abilities, and this could produce secondary anxiety and frustration and lead to social, emotional, or behavioral difficulties, including low self-esteem, low self-confidence, school negativity, social withdrawal, task-avoidant and passively resistant behaviors (secondary inattention), and potentially school dropout. Such a mismatch between demands and expectations and performance also can result in attention-seeking, oppositional, or acting-out behaviors (that can be misperceived as secondary impulsivity or hyperactivity), which can lead to detention or school suspension. The regular classroom teachers of children with learning disabilities need to work very closely with their schools' learning disabilities specialists to ensure that maximal accommodations and modifications are being made in all regular classes. Examples of such accommodations and modifications may include being given extended time to complete shortened and maximally modified assignments, untimed tests, being provided audio textbooks or a calculator, and being allowed to give oral reports and oral answers to essay questions rather than written reports and essays. It is also very important for children with learning disabilities to participate in extracurricular activities that they enjoy, and in which they feel they are successful, in order to serve as a source of self-esteem building, socialization, and peer interaction. Extracurricular activities at school are particularly encouraged, so that school can remain a rewarding experience.

## SUGGESTED READINGS

American Speech-Language-Hearing Association. Child speech and language. http://www.asha.org/public/speech/disorders/ChildSand. Accessed June 10, 2016.

Accardo PJ, Capute AJ. *The Capute Scales: Cognitive Adaptive Test/Clinical Linguistic & Auditory Milestone Scale (CAT/CLAMS)*. Baltimore, MD: Paul H. Brookes Publishing Company; 2005.

American Psychiatric Association. Specific learning disorder. In: *Diagnostic and Statistical Manual of Mental Disorders*, 5th edition. Arlington, VA: American Psychiatric Association; 2013:66-74.

Centers for Disease Control and Prevention. Learn the signs. Act early. https://www.cdc.gov/ncbddd/actearly/. Accessed June 10, 2016.

Cortiella C, Horowitz SH. *The State of Learning Disabilities: Facts, Trends and Emerging Issues*. New York, NY: National Center for Learning Disabilities; 2014.

Council on Children With Disabilities; Section on Developmental Behavioral Pediatrics; Bright Futures Steering Committee; Medical Home Initiatives for Children With Special Needs Project Advisory Committee. Identifying infants and young children with developmental disorders in the medical home: an algorithm for developmental surveillance and screening [published correction appears in *Pediatrics*. 2006;118(4):1808-1809]. American Academy of Pediatrics Policy Statement. *Pediatrics*. 2006:118(1):405-420.

Learning Disabilities Association of America Web site. https://ldaamerica.org. Accessed August 17, 2016.

Macias MM, Twyman KA. Speech and language development and disorders. In: Voigt RG, Macias MM, Myers SM, eds. *Developmental and Behavioral Pediatrics*. Elk Grove Village, IL: American Academy of Pediatrics; 2010:201-219.

Wallace I, Berkman N, Watson L, et al. Screening for speech and language delay in children 5 years old and younger: a systematic review. *Pediatrics*. 2015;136:e448-e462.

# 90 Attention-Deficit/Hyperactivity Disorder

Renee S. Rodrigues-D'Souza

## INTRODUCTION

In the spectrum and continuum of developmental-behavioral diagnoses, attention-deficit/hyperactivity disorder (ADHD) represents a dissociation between cognitive abilities and the neurobehavioral domains of attention, impulse control, and motor activity. Individuals with ADHD have developmentally inappropriate levels of inattention and/or impulsivity/hyperactivity (ie, their levels of attention and impulse control/activity are discrepantly delayed or dissociated from their underlying cognitive abilities) that are impairing their functioning across settings.

ADHD is a frequently diagnosed but often misunderstood neurodevelopmental condition. The balance of the core features of inattention and/or hyperactivity and impulsivity combined with the complex array of socialization difficulties, impaired executive functions, and emotional dysregulation make ADHD a great masquerader for a variety of developmental/behavioral and psychiatric diagnoses. Therefore, understanding the many facets of this disorder can enhance diagnostic veracity and allow for a targeted approach to treatment.

## EPIDEMIOLOGY

ADHD is a disorder that begins in childhood, and symptoms are present from a young age. Several studies have been published on the prevalence of ADHD across populations and cultures, with most citing a prevalence between 4% and 12%. This relatively wide range reflects variations in diagnostic criteria, characteristics of the studied population, the number of sources used to establish the diagnosis, and the lack of biological markers for the disorder. Studies utilizing the diagnostic criteria of any edition of the *Diagnostic and Statistical Manual of Mental Disorders* have shown prevalence to be closer to 6% to 8%. ADHD is more prevalent in males than females, with a ratio of 3:1. Males are more likely to evidence the externalizing behaviors of hyperactivity and impulsivity (5:1 compared to females) and are therefore more likely to be identified early on, such as in preschool and early elementary school. Females tend to present with inattentive symptoms (2:1 male-to-female ratio) that may go undetected until later in childhood, such as middle to late elementary school. By early adolescence, hyperactivity mostly manifests as fidgetiness, restlessness, or impatience, while inattention persists.





## ETIOLOGY

Organic causes of ADHD can be found in 20% to 25% of cases and may include a history of very low birthweight (< 1500 grams), very preterm birth (gestational age < 32 weeks), fetal alcohol spectrum disorders, in utero drug exposure, environmental toxins (eg, lead, nicotine), and central nervous system trauma or infection. In the majority of cases, however, ADHD is thought to be multifactorial in etiology, drawing from genetic and environmental effects on neurobiology. Studies have found inherent differences in the structure and function of several areas of the brain, notably the basal ganglia (contributes to inhibition of automatic responses), the cerebellar vermis (contributes to regulation of motivation and coordination), and the prefrontal cortex of the frontal lobe. The latter in particular controls the executive functions of organization and regulation. Organization functions include attention, "filtering" (attending to relevant while blocking out irrelevant stimuli), planning, sequencing, rule acquisition, abstraction, and cognitive flexibility required for problem solving. Functions of regulation include initiation, inhibition, emotional regulation, monitoring (of internal and external stimuli), moral reasoning, and decision-making. Working memory and processing speed are 2 cognitive functions commonly measured on intelligence batteries that are used as surrogate indicators for executive function.

On a molecular basis, dopamine and norepinephrine imbalances have been implicated in the pathogenesis of ADHD. Both of these neurotransmitters may enhance the inhibitory effects of the frontal cortex on subcortical structures. Evidence also exists for a delay in cortical maturation (particularly in the lateral prefrontal cortex) in individuals with ADHD compared to the general population.

ADHD is polygenic with a significant component of heritability, as demonstrated in identical twin studies with > 50% concordance, and clinically by increased occurrence in first-degree relatives by 2- to 8-fold compared to the general population. Gene associations have been found with the dopamine transporter gene (*DAT1*), the D4 receptor gene (*DRD4*), and the human thyroid receptor-beta gene.

## CLINICAL MANIFESTATIONS

The hallmark characteristics of ADHD are developmentally inappropriate and persistent difficulties with inattention and/or hyperactive and impulsive behaviors that cause impairment in daily functioning across numerous settings. *Inattention* is characterized by a lack of focus, perseverance, or mental or physical presence for an expected, nonpreferred task or situation. Teachers may report that a student "stares off" in class or does not seem to know what is going on when called on. Inattentive students may be unable to filter out background noises to attend to the most salient stimulus (eg, the teacher). Socially, individuals with ADHD may be perceived as careless, disorganized, disinterested, or unmotivated.

Although *hyperactivity* is often equated with excessive motor activity (such as running about or climbing), it can also manifest as talkativeness or fidgetiness. Individuals may be perceived as being restless, "high-energy," "the class clown," or "a chatterbox." *Impulsivity* may refer to a predilection for rash decisions or actions, which may result in unintended harm to oneself or others. Parents may report younger children running off from them in a parking lot or acting out physically when they do not get their way. Socially, impulsive individuals may be perceived as intrusive (eg, interrupting conversations), attention-seeking, "bossy," short-sighted (ie, poor comprehension of both long-term rewards and consequences of decisions), and impatient.

Impulsive individuals may also have "no filter," meaning that they may make inappropriate remarks or say the first thing that comes to mind without regard for how the comments will be perceived. They may be labeled as "lacking common sense."

It is important to note that symptoms of ADHD can vary in intensity depending on the setting. Symptoms tend to be more apparent in unstructured settings or when the child is bored. A child who is engaged in a highly motivating activity (such as a videogame) may not display hyperactive, impulsive, or inattentive behaviors and may instead seem to "hyper-focus" on the game. This highlights the important point that ADHD is not a disorder of complete lack of attention; it is a disorder of *attention allocation*, ie, difficulty focusing for a nonpreferred task. Symptoms may also be diminished when receiving 1-on-1 attention and/or positive reinforcement for desired behaviors, when in a new setting, or when otherwise engaged in something of interest.



## DIAGNOSIS

The *Diagnostic and Statistical Manual of Mental Disorders*, 5th edition (DSM-5) lists the current clinical criteria for diagnosis of ADHD and its subtypes in children and adolescents younger than 17 years of age. The predominantly inattentive subtype of ADHD requires that at least 6 of 9 symptoms of inattention be present over a 6-month time span, while the hyperactive/impulsive subtype of ADHD requires at least 6 of 9 corresponding symptoms. The combined type presentation requires at least 6 in both categories of symptoms. The requirement of symptoms being present for at least 6 months is meant to eliminate or mitigate contributory effects of acute factors, such as life changes (eg, new school, divorce) or early stages of chronic illness. Although meant to be a list of essential diagnostic features, the DSM-5 checklist is certainly not a substitute for understanding a child's behavior in the broader context of developmental level, which represents the crucial clinical judgment piece necessary to make an ADHD diagnosis.

The DSM-5 specifies that symptoms of ADHD must be present to a significant degree prior to 12 years of age. This represents an expansion of the previous DSM-IV's age cutoff of 7 years to account for later detection of symptoms. The DSM-5 notes the importance of understanding a child's developmental level (ie, level of cognitive function) when considering a child's behavior. In other words, a 10-year-old child with a cognitive level of a 5-year-old will behave as a 5-year-old, even though that child might be perceived as hyperactive, impulsive, and inattentive for chronological age. Likewise, presenting a child with a challenge above that child's level of ability (eg, placing a "slower learner" in a typical classroom) may result in behaviors that can be misconstrued as symptoms of ADHD.

In order to make a diagnosis of ADHD, the presenting child should also experience a significant degree of impairment. Since the clinical and developmental histories are imperative to making the diagnosis, balancing perceptions against actual performance via feedback from multiple sources (eg, parents, teachers, therapists, report cards) can help assess this criterion. Several clinical tools exist to allow providers to collect data from several observers (eg, National Institute for Children's Health Quality [NICHQ] Vanderbilt Assessment Scales, online initial and follow-up versions available at http://www.nichq.org/childrens-health/adhd/resources/vanderbilt-assessment-scales). As a rule, symptoms must be developmentally inappropriate, persistent, pervasive, and impairing in order to meet criteria for ADHD.

Impairment due to ADHD symptoms is most often recognized when school performance diminishes, behavioral problems in the classroom interfere with the child's and with other students' learning, or when a child seems to be underperforming academically compared to his or her ability. Children with ADHD are more likely to be identified as "a behavior problem," leading to less time in the classroom and more time in the principal's office or at home due to suspension. Alternatively, a child may be placed in a behavior classroom where academics are emphasized less. Deficits in learning may result, even in the absence of a diagnosed learning disability, which may require special education intervention. Children with ADHD are also often made to repeat grades due to their behavioral immaturity and associated poor academic performance, and this further contributes to the increased rate of school attrition in teens with ADHD.

Social impairment due to rejection and neglect by peers may be less apparent, especially if the child with ADHD is blamed for lack of social acceptance due to intrusive or inconsiderate behaviors. Children with ADHD are at increased risk for teasing and bullying and may be targeted because of impulsive overreactions. Impairment in family function can occur if the child with ADHD has to constantly be redirected, prompted, reminded, or supervised. Medically, impairment may manifest as increased frequency of ER visits due to accidental injuries secondary to impulsive and hyperactive behaviors.

There may be some instances in which impairment is reported but is unsupported by feedback from other reporters. For instance, a cognitively average child in a high-achieving family may be viewed as "lazy" or "unmotivated." New parents may report that a toddler is too active and difficult to control. A teacher may report that a very bright child is inattentive in a typical classroom, when in fact the child is merely bored. In these instances, education of parents about developmentally appropriate behaviors, and discussion with educators about developmentally appropriate classroom demands and expectations, may be all that is needed. Cultural interpretations of behavior should also be explored.

## DIFFERENTIAL DIAGNOSIS AND COMORBIDITIES

Though the DSM-5 specifies that ADHD symptoms must not occur "solely as a manifestation of oppositional behavior, defiance, hostility or failure to understand tasks or instructions," all of these can occur as comorbidities. Table 90-1 lists comorbid conditions, many of which must also be considered in the differential when making a diagnosis of ADHD. For instance, children with learning disabilities and speech/language disorders may be misconstrued as having ADHD, when in fact they are struggling with language comprehension and/or language production. An unidentified intellectual disability or autism spectrum disorder may be incorrectly perceived as evidence of behavioral immaturity or defiance. Victims of neglect and/or violence may be perceived as inattentive and unmotivated in the classroom; conversely, children with ADHD are at increased risk of victimization. This again speaks to the importance of obtaining feedback from multiple reporters.

Common comorbid conditions with ADHD include oppositional-defiant disorder (up to 35%, though closer to 50% for combined type and 25% for predominantly inattentive type), conduct disorder (up to 25%), anxiety disorders (up to 25%), depressive disorders (up to 20%), and learning disorders (up to 50%). Motor coordination disorders (ranging from general "clumsiness" to dysgraphia) and tics also commonly co-occur with ADHD. Many children with ADHD also suffer from sleep disturbance, often due to an inability to calm their minds for sleep. Finally, children with ADHD may experience low self-esteem.

Difficulties with emotional regulation can result in overreactions to situations and then difficulty de-escalating. For instance, low frustration tolerance when a demand is placed on the child or when a desired object is denied can quickly lead to oppositional and defiant behaviors. Children with ADHD may be perceived as being "moody" or "irritable," even in the absence of a diagnosed mood disorder. Those with comorbid mood and/or conduct disorders, particularly in the context of substance abuse, are at increased risk for suicide attempts by early adulthood. Diagnostic surveys that include symptoms of common comorbidities, such as the NICHQ Vanderbilt Assessment Scale or the Conners 3rd Edition of the Comprehensive Behavior Rating Scales, can help identify co-existing conditions.

In-office evaluation should include vital signs, anthropometrics, hearing and vision screens, a comprehensive medical and developmental-behavioral history, a complete physical examination, a thorough neurological examination, and direct developmental evaluation. Further evaluation may include an audiological examination (or at least a hearing screen) to rule out a previously undetected hearing impairment and an ophthalmologic consultation (or at least a vision screen) to rule out a previously undetected visual impairment. A thorough medical history, including birth history, past medical history,

**TABLE 90-1 ADHD DIFFERENTIAL DIAGNOSIS AND POSSIBLE COMORBIDITIES**

| |
|---|
| **Medical** |
| Anemia |
| Chronic medical illness (multiple absences or fatigue) |
| Malnutrition/insufficient caloric intake |
| Medication side effects (antiepileptic drugs, antihistamines, antihypertensive drugs, bronchodilators) |
| Sleep disturbance (including sleep-disordered breathing) |
| Thyroid dysfunction (hypo- or hyperthyroidism) or thyroid medications |
| **Neurodevelopmental** |
| Autism spectrum disorder |
| Developmental coordination disorder |
| Epilepsy |
| Hearing impairment |
| Intellectual disability/global developmental delay |
| Learning disabilities or slow learning |
| Language disorders (including articulation and speech sound disorders) |
| Neurodegenerative disorders |
| Tourette syndrome/tic disorder |
| Visual impairment |
| **Behavioral/Mental Health** |
| Adjustment disorders/reactive emotional states |
| Anxiety disorders |
| Bipolar and related disorders |
| Conduct disorder |
| Depressive disorders |
| Dissociative disorders |
| Obsessive-compulsive and related disorders |
| Oppositional-defiant disorder/disruptive behavior disorder |
| Personality disorders |
| Post-traumatic stress disorder |
| Somatic disorders |
| Thought disorders (including schizophrenia and psychotic disorders) |
| **Psychosocial** |
| Inconsistent parenting practices (including lack of parenting due to parental psychopathology or mental health issues) |
| Lack of structure in the home/unregulated environment |
| Poor limit setting |
| Poverty |
| Substance abuse (including parental use) |
| Trauma (abuse, neglect, violence, victim of bullying) |

current medications, review of systems, family history, and social history can help guide any further medical testing. A history concerning for staring spells or other types of seizure activity would necessitate a sleep-deprived EEG and possibly brain MRI and neurological consultation, especially with any abnormal neurological exam findings. It is important to note that children with ADHD often evidence motor overflow and difficulty with rapid alternating movements (neurological "soft signs"). Dysmorphic features could indicate the potential need for genetic testing (such as chromosome microarray analysis and DNA testing for fragile X syndrome), as there are genetic syndromes that are highly associated with ADHD (eg, Klinefelter syndrome, Turner syndrome, 22q11.2 deletion [velocardiofacial] syndrome, neurofibromatosis 1) and with ADHD in a setting of intellectual disability (eg, fragile X syndrome, Williams syndrome, fetal alcohol syndrome). It is also important to consider inborn errors of metabolism, though medical history, developmental history, and review of newborn screening should help guide appropriate studies. In a primary care setting, several visits may be necessary to accomplish a full evaluation and to accumulate instrumental data.

Referral for psychological assessment or speech/language evaluation may be necessary to identify an underlying cognitive or learning disability. These assessments can be performed by school psychologists or through providers in the community. A mental health assessment is recommended for a suspected underlying or comorbid psychiatric disorder. Social work consultation can provide insight into the psychosocial situation and family dynamic within which the child is functioning.

## TREATMENT

Treatment of ADHD requires a multipronged, multidisciplinary approach. Demystifying the ADHD diagnosis and clarifying any misconceptions for families is the first step. ADHD is a neurodevelopmental (ie, brain-based) disorder and not the result of poor parenting or intentional misbehavior on the part of the child. Exploring mistaken beliefs about ADHD may help to relieve guilt, avoid blame, and alleviate stress and frustration, as well as increase the likelihood of adherence to a treatment plan. Anyone who has a role to play in any aspect of the child's daily functioning—family/caregivers, educators, the school's diagnostician or psychologist—needs to be a part of the treatment plan developed with the clinician. Treatment plans incorporating medication management, behavioral modification across settings, and development of life-long ADHD management strategies produce the best results.

Though medications can greatly decrease symptoms of ADHD, they are only effective when taken and are by no means curative. Many parents are wary of medications and would prefer a nonpharmacologic approach, making it all the more important to emphasize targeting the behavioral and cognitive aspects of ADHD, especially because this is what produces long-term benefits. The child with ADHD must learn coping strategies appropriate to developmental level at every stage of childhood and adolescence, so as to be well-prepared in adulthood. Early on, coping strategies will need to be modeled and provided externally until the child is able to internalize them. For instance, behavioral modification techniques, such as the use of praise, reward charts, and token economies (eg, earning stars that can be exchanged for tangible rewards), can help a child develop a new skill and reinforce a desired behavior until that behavior becomes routine. Praise should be frequent and specific, and it is highly effective when least expected (eg, "I like the way you are sitting quietly"). Understanding natural consequences (eg, not being able to watch a cartoon in the morning before school because it took too long to get dressed), losing privileges for undesired behaviors, and time-out also help modify behavior and are punctuated by maintaining a mostly positively reinforcing environment. Adults should model and help facilitate appropriate reactions to disappointment, problem-solving, and resolution of conflict. Having a daily report card that passes between home and school lets the child know that good behaviors are important across settings. Consistency within a setting and across settings is key for behavior management.

Parents and teachers need to be aware that they need the child with ADHD to look at them when giving directions; asking the child to repeat back the directions confirms what was heard. Keeping directions simple and brief, being clear about expectations and rules, and setting time limits for tasks can also be helpful. Breaking up large tasks into smaller tasks is imperative because of deficits in executive functions. For instance, making a calendar of what to accomplish week by week for an upcoming project, posting it in the child's room, and checking off accomplished items can avoid procrastination. Picture schedules for daily tasks (eg, steps for what to do in the shower), a checklist for chores, establishing a homework-only folder, and going through a child's backpack every day and getting it ready for the next day are all simple things that can be done to help a child function more successfully at home and school; these responsibilities can be passed on to the child as she or he gets older. Overall, behavior management can help to reduce oppositional and noncompliant behaviors, decrease internalizing symptoms (eg, feeling like a failure), increase positive self-image, and foster a feeling of being in control of symptoms—all of which may allow for lower doses of medication and long-lasting self-management benefits. Likewise, involvement in extracurricular activities that accentuate the child's strengths (eg, creativity, motoric abilities, intrepidness) and develop the child's natural interests can also help to build a positive self-concept and provide an outlet for energy that may not exist in the academic setting.

Parents should also be informed of Section 504 of the Rehabilitation Act of 1973, which addresses learning needs. Section 504 prohibits any program receiving federal funds from discriminating against an individual with a disability, defined as a "physical or mental impairment which substantially limits 1 or more major life activities, having a record of such an impairment, or regarded as having such an impairment." "Major life activities" are further defined as "caring for oneself, walking, seeing, hearing, speaking, breathing, working, performing manual tasks, and learning." Section 504 specifies that "reasonable accommodations" must be made. However, since schools do not receive extra funds to provide these services, 504 accommodations are not well-defined or regulated. What is offered may vary from district to district, school to school, and even classroom to classroom. Parents often report that the child's teacher for a new school year is not aware that the child is on a Section 504 plan, so it is important to encourage parents to establish good rapport with the classroom teacher early in the year, remind the teacher that the child is on a Section 504 plan, and follow up frequently with the teacher for feedback. Section 504 accommodations can include extra time for classwork and tests, shortened or reduced assignments, testing in a quiet environment, use of a study carrel, permission to stand while doing seat work, preferential seating close to the teacher, special cues the teacher gives the student to get attention, and "movement breaks," to name a few. It is important to emphasize that "extra time" for assignments and tests should not interfere with recess or lunch, as these are important socialization opportunities and built-in breaks that children with ADHD need to have as much as their peers. In fact, social skills groups at school, such as a "lunch bunch," can greatly help to address this area of deficit.

For children with moderate to severe symptoms of ADHD, it is recommended that the family seek services under the Individuals with Disabilities Education Act (IDEA). IDEA allows for services for individuals with ADHD under a designation of other health impairment (OHI), which accounts for "limited strength, vitality or alertness, including a heightened alertness to environmental stimuli, that results in limited alertness with respect to educational environment" and adversely affects the child's educational performance. Specific accommodations and modifications are then put into place via an individualized education program (IEP) and monitored over time according to established goals and objectives. The IEP is a legal document binding the school to these services and follows the student year to year. Although poor academic performance and a request for services under OHI should automatically initiate a full and individual evaluation (FIE), which includes cognitive, achievement, and speech/language testing in addition to behavioral assessment via observation and multi-rater checklists, this is not always the case, and private psychological assessment may be sought instead. Due to the high correlation between ADHD and learning disabilities and the susceptibility to mistake one for the other, a thorough psychological assessment is recommended.

### Medication

Though developing behavioral and cognitive strategies is an important part of ADHD management and may mitigate symptoms initially, medication is an important adjunctive therapy that oftentimes can help a child be more receptive to environmental modifications. Methylphenidate, mixed amphetamine salts, and dextroamphetamine all have US Food and Drug Administration (FDA) indications for treatment of ADHD in children. Atomoxetine, long-acting guanfacine, and long-acting clonidine are nonstimulant medications that also have FDA indications for treatment of ADHD.

**Stimulants** Stimulant medications are considered the first-line treatment of ADHD symptoms because they address all 3 of the core symptoms of ADHD, primarily by increasing dopamine and norepinephrine activity through inhibiting reuptake most notably in the caudate nucleus and prefrontal cortex. They have demonstrated safety and efficacy, with usage dating back to the 1930s, when amphetamines were prescribed to increase alertness in fighter pilots. Methylphenidate was released for general use in 1957 and was marketed for a number of conditions, including fatigue, narcolepsy, and to counteract the sedating effects of other drugs. Their role in treatment of "hyperkinesis" was not recognized until the 1960s.

Stimulants are effective in up to 70% to 80% of children at reducing the core symptoms of ADHD, when the medication is "on-board". By reducing impulsivity, stimulants can consequently also reduce oppositional/defiant and aggressive behaviors. Methylphenidates primarily block reuptake of dopamine and norepinephrine and secondarily facilitate their direct release from the neuron. Amphetamines, on the other hand, mostly increase the release of both of these neurotransmitters from storage sites into the synapse. This difference in principal mechanism of action may explain why some individuals respond better to 1 class of stimulant than the other.

Methylphenidate (best known under the trade name Ritalin but also including Metadate, Daytrana, and Quillivant) is racemic and only active in the dextro-isomer. The half-life is 2 to 3 hours, with a duration of action of generally 4 hours. Methylphenidate comes in short-acting (3- to 6-hour duration), intermediate-acting (6- to 8-hour duration), and long-acting (8- to 12-hour duration) preparations (see Tables 90-2 and 90-3). Dexmethylphenidate is marketed as Focalin and contains solely the active isomer, and it comes in a short-acting and long-acting version. Therefore, 10 mg of methylphenidate (Ritalin) is equivalent to 5 mg of dexmethylphenidate (Focalin). The methylphenidates have FDA approval for use in children as young as 6 years of age.

The mixed-amphetamine salts (Adderall and Adderall XR) and the dextroamphetamines (Dexedrine) have FDA approval for use in children as young as 3 years. Adderall has a duration of action of 3 to 6 hours, while the XR formulation can last up to 8 to 12 hours. While only the dextro-isomer is active, the levo-isomer converts to the dextro in vivo. This is important to know for converting doses from 1 class of stimulant to another. Dextroamphetamine has a 3- to 6-hour duration of action. Lisdexamfetamine, which is marketed as Vyvanse, is a long-acting preparation (lasting up to 12 hours). It is a pro-drug, which is broken down in vivo into lysine and dextroamphetamine.

**TABLE 90-2 STIMULANT PREPARATIONS**

| | MPH | D-MPH | MAS | D-AMPH | L-DAMPH |
|---|---|---|---|---|---|
| Short-acting (3–6 hours) | Ritalin<br>Methylin | Focalin | Adderall | Dexedrine<br>Dextrostat<br>ProCentra | |
| Intermediate-acting (6–8 hours) | Ritalin SR<br>Ritalin LA<br>Metadate CD | | | Dexedrine Spansules | |
| Long-acting (8–12 hours) | Concerta<br>Daytrana (patch)<br>Quillivant | Focalin XR | Adderall XR | | Vyvanse |

SECTION 6 Developmental and Behavioral Pediatrics

**TABLE 90-3 STIMULANT DOSING**

| Generic Name | Brand Name | Recommended Starting Dose | Prescribing Schedule | Maximum Daily Dose |
|---|---|---|---|---|
| MPH | Ritalin | 2.5–5 mg | 2.5–20 mg BID to TID | 60 mg |
| | Methylin | 2.5–5 mg | 2.5–20 mg BID to TID | 60 mg |
| | Ritalin SR | 10 mg | 10–60 mg daily | 60 mg |
| | Ritalin LA | 10 mg | 10–60 mg daily | 60 mg |
| | Metadate CD | 10 mg | 10–60 mg daily | 60 mg |
| | Concerta | 18 mg | 18–72 mg daily | 72 mg |
| | Daytrana | 10 mg | 10–30 mg daily | 30 mg |
| | Quillivant | 10 mg | 10–60 mg daily | 60 mg |
| D-MPH | Focalin | 2.5–5 mg | 2.5–10 mg BID or 2.5–5 mg TID | 20 mg |
| | Focalin XR | 5 mg | 5–30 mg daily | 30 mg |
| MAS | Adderall | 5 mg | 5–20 mg BID | 40 mg |
| | Adderall XR | 10 mg | 10–30 mg daily | 30 mg |
| D-AMPH | Dexedrine/Dextrostat | 5 mg | 5–20 mg BID or 5–10 mg TID | 40 mg |
| | ProCentra | 5 mg | 5–20 mg BID or 5–10 mg TID | 40 mg |
| | Dexedrine Spansules | 5 mg | 5–40 mg daily | 40 mg |
| L-DAMPH | Vyvanse | 10 mg | 10–70 mg daily | 70 mg |

BID, twice daily; D-AMPH, dextroamphetamine; D-MPH, dexmethylphenidate; L-DAMPH, lisdexamfetamine; MAS, mixed amphetamine salts; MPH, methylphenidate; TID, 3 times daily.

Stimulants are dosed by titrating to effect, not by a mg/kg model. Therefore, it is advisable to "start low and go slow"—ie, start at a low dose and titrate upward to maximize benefits and avoid side-effects. This underscores the need for frequent and reliable feedback from parents, caregivers, and teachers. Effects of stimulant medication can be seen within 20 to 60 minutes of taking the medication, although benefits may be modest initially before the dose is optimized. It is recommended that stimulant medication be taken after a meal or snack to avoid stomach upset and to provide calories before possible impending appetite suppression.

The most common side effects of stimulants in addition to appetite suppression and stomachache are headache, sleep disturbance, and jitteriness. Stomachache and headache typically abate after a week or so of initiating treatment. Appetite suppression may be substantial, so emphasizing a healthy but high-calorie diet is crucial. The higher the dose is and the longer the duration of action is, the greater the chance is for significant side effects. Higher doses also have the potential to create a "zombie" effect, which results from hyperfocusing and being perceived by parents as too quiet, sad, or having too much of a change in personality or typical vivaciousness. Twice-a-day or 3-times-a-day dosing of short-acting stimulant preparations allows the stimulant to nadir and appetite to return—eg, dosing the stimulant after breakfast, lunch, and late afternoon snack. However, this type of dosing does not allow for consistent coverage all day long, and troughs tend to occur during least-structured times of day (eg, bus ride to and from school, lunchtime, at daycare). Additionally, adherence to multiple doses can be an issue, and stigmatization among peers and school policies may make it difficult or impossible to take medications during the school day. Older children, who tend to have a significant amount of homework, studying, or extracurricular activities, as well as adolescents who may also have after-school jobs, may benefit most from 12-hour preparations, but they are at risk for sleep disturbance if taken too late in the day.

Understanding which medications can be opened and sprinkled versus which have to be swallowed whole is important when counseling families on options for stimulant medication treatment. Of the methylphenidate derivatives, Focalin XR, Ritalin LA, and Metadate CD are all capsules that can be opened and sprinkled on food (eg, applesauce). Focalin XR uses microbead technology, with 50% of the dose as immediate-release beads and 50% as enteric-coated for delayed release. Metadate CD has a biphasic release bead-delivery system, with 30% available for immediate release and 70% for delayed release. This differs from Ritalin LA, which has a bimodal release system, with 50% available for immediate release and 50% for delayed release. Methylphenidate ER (Concerta) utilizes an osmotic controlled-release oral delivery system (OROS) technology. The overcoat delivers an immediate release dose of methylphenidate, while the rest of the medication gradually permeates via osmotic pressure. It must be swallowed whole. Concerta 18 mg is equivalent in effect to Ritalin 5 mg TID. Quillivant XR (long-acting) is a liquid formulation, and Methylin (short-acting) is also available in liquid but also comes in a chewable formulation. The tablet versions of methylphenidate also can be crushed. Daytrana is a methylphenidate preparation that comes in a patch for children who will not take any form of medication by mouth. When applied for 9 hours, its effects last for 12 hours. Of the mixed amphetamine salts, Adderall XR uses bead technology with 50% immediate and 50% delayed release, and can be opened and sprinkled on food, while short-acting Adderall can be crushed. Of the dextroamphetamines, Dexedrine Spansules can be opened and sprinkled on food, ProCentra comes in a liquid, and Vyvanse can be opened and the powder dissolved in water. It is important that children not chew the beads of any of these stimulants, since they are differentially coated for immediate versus extended release. The *ADHD Medication Guide*, published by Dr. Andrew Adesman, is a free, downloadable chart that contains an updated listing of ADHD medications, how they can be administered, and their FDA indications (www.ADHD-MedicationGuide.com).

There is no evidence for development of tolerance to treatment with stimulant medication. There is also no evidence for increased risk of substance abuse; on the contrary, stimulant use has been correlated with reduced risk-taking behaviors, such as drug and alcohol abuse. However, short-acting stimulants have "street value" due to their potential for abuse when taken intranasally, and prescribers must be vigilant for drug diversion. There has been variable data about stimulants lowering the seizure threshold, but children with epilepsy are also at increased risk for ADHD. Communication with the managing neurologist is essential. Tics are another area of concern with stimulants, and although they do not cause tics, stimulants can unmask them in someone who is prone to tics. It is important to weigh the risks and benefits of stimulant use in children with tics, particularly given that tics naturally wax and wane.

Stimulants are considered to have minimal effects on vital signs and have not been found to increase the risk of adverse cardiac events in patients without cardiac disease. However, due to concerns over reports of sudden cardiac death and prolonged QT interval in patients with known cardiac conditions, a careful cardiac history and exam are required prior to starting treatment with stimulant medication. Before starting stimulants, patients should be screened for the following risk factors: history of congenital or structural heart abnormality, history of rheumatic fever, heart murmur, high blood pressure, chest pain, fainting, dizziness, unusual heart beat/racing heart, seizures, exercise intolerance, or use of medications or supplements known to prolong the QT interval or have cardiovascular effects. Likewise, family history should be screened for children or young adults with history of sudden cardiac death, sudden death of unknown origin, heart attack, or event requiring resuscitation; hypertrophic cardiomyopathy, dilated cardiomyopathy, long QT syndrome, cardiac arrhythmias (eg, Wolff-Parkinson-White syndrome), catecholaminergic paroxysmal ventricular tachycardia, Brugada syndrome, arrhythmogenic right ventricular dysplasia, or Marfan syndrome. Electrocardiography and possible cardiology referral should be considered for positive risk factors. Ongoing cardiovascular monitoring is advised for any patient taking stimulant medication.



**Nonstimulants** Some parents feel that nonstimulant medications are a "safer" option due to the vilification of stimulants in the media. However, it is important to review with families that none of the nonstimulants target all 3 of the core symptoms of ADHD, as the stimulants were designed to do. Furthermore, unlike stimulants, which can be used as needed because they only work when taken, nonstimulant medications need to be taken on a daily basis, including weekends, to maintain a therapeutic level. Atomoxetine (Strattera), long-acting guanfacine (Intuniv), and long-acting clonidine (Kapvay) all have FDA indications for treatment of ADHD in children as young as 6 years of age.

Atomoxetine is a selective norepinephrine reuptake inhibitor that acts by blocking the presynaptic norepinephrine transporter at the level of the prefrontal cortex. It is effective at addressing inattention. Dosing is recommended on a mg/kg basis, with an initial dose of 0.5 mg/kg/day that can then be titrated every 4 to 7 days to a maximum of 1.4 mg/kg/day. The capsule must be swallowed whole. Common side effects include appetite suppression (though not to the same extent as stimulants), gastrointestinal upset, sedation, and irritability. Atomoxetine has also been linked to elevated aminotransferases in a small percentage of patients (0.5%) that reversed upon stopping the medication and to acute liver failure in very rare instances. It can also potentially prolong the QT interval. Suicidal ideation has also been reported in some patients, usually within the first month of starting the medication, and atomoxetine carries an FDA black box warning. Its once-a-day dosing makes it convenient, though the dose can be delivered twice a day to minimize side effects. It can be given at night, which also helps to reduce side effects. Although its effect is less than that observed with stimulants, atomoxetine is an alternative for stimulant-wary parents and children prone to significant weight loss or tics on stimulants. Its main drawback is onset of effects, which may take weeks. Dosages are 10, 18, 25, 40, 60, 80, and 100 mg. Atomoxetine can be discontinued without weaning.

The alpha-2 adrenergic agonists are antihypertensives that have calming effects on the central nervous system. In fact, clonidine is often used to induce sleep. The alpha-2 adrenergic agonists mainly target hyperactivity and impulsivity and can be an option for children with ADHD and tics. Long-acting clonidine (Kapvay), which comes in 0.1- and 0.2-mg tablets, can be dosed every 12 hours, with a maximum dose of 0.4 mg/day. Long-acting guanfacine (Intuniv), which comes in 1, 2, 3, and 4 mg tablets, is meant to last 24 hours, with a maximum dose of 4 mg/day. Both of these medications must be swallowed whole. The "start low and go slow" principle applies here as well. The side-effect profile of the alpha-2 adrenergic agonists includes sedation, fatigue, anorexia, dry mouth, hypotension, and low mood. It is important to monitor orthostatic vital signs while titrating these medications. Since these medications may be used in conjunction with stimulants, it is imperative to ask about cardiac risk factors, as sudden cardiac death has been reported with combination treatment. These medications must also be weaned slowly due to risk of rebound hypertension.

**The MTA Study** In 1992, the National Institute of Mental Health and 6 teams of investigators began a multisite clinical trial known as the Multimodal Treatment of Attention Deficit Hyperactivity Disorder (MTA) study. Across 6 study sites, 579 children, aged 7 to 9+ years, were randomly assigned to 1 of 4 study groups for a 14-month intervention: (1) intensive medication management (MedMgt); (2) intensive behavioral treatments (Beh); (3) combined MedMgt and Beh (Comb); and (4) study diagnostic procedures followed by routine care in the community (CC). Medication management was initiated with short-acting methylphenidate; nonresponders were managed with an alternative stimulant or nonstimulant. The intensive behavioral treatments were based on known best practices at the time and involved the children, their parents, and their teachers.

MedMgt was found to be superior to routine CC in addressing core symptoms of ADHD, even though more than two-thirds of the children receiving CC were also being treated with stimulant medication. This was because the children in the MedMgt group were on significantly higher doses of the stimulant determined by optimum symptom control without limiting side effects. Though Comb treatment did not yield significantly greater benefits than MedMgt alone for core ADHD symptoms, similar outcomes could be achieved in the Comb group with lower medication doses. Comb treatment was also superior to MedMgt for many noncore ADHD symptoms, such as oppositionality, aggression, mood symptoms, social skills, parent-child relations, and aspects of academic functioning.

Benefits persisted across medication groups at 24 months but not at 36 months, regardless of original intervention group assigned. This was felt to reflect a possible age-related decline in ADHD symptoms, changes in intensity of medication management, starting or stopping medications altogether, or as yet unidentified reasons. Factors associated with worse outcomes at 36 months were severe symptoms, male gender, oppositional and disruptive behaviors, parent history of ADHD, and socioeconomic factors.

Follow-up studies at 6 to 8 years have shown that the type or intensity of the 14-month intervention did not predict subsequent functioning; rather, early ADHD symptom trajectory regardless of treatment type was prognostic. The implication is that children with behavioral and sociodemographic advantages, with the best response to any treatment, will have the best long-term prognosis. Long-term studies have found that stimulants are efficacious for at least 72 months and that children with the combined type presentation show the greatest impairment in adolescence. In summary, further studies are needed to understand the natural course of ADHD, but access to conscientious, responsive, and consistent medication management combined with ongoing behavioral interventions may produce the best long-term effects.

**Alternative "Treatments"** Often parents ask about over-the-counter supplements that can be used in lieu of medications. Popular supplements include essential fatty acids (linoleic and linolenic acids—omega-6 fatty acids), omega-3 fatty acids (eicosapentaenoic acid, docosahexaenoic acid), zinc, antioxidants, megavitamins, and herbs. There is no evidence that essential fatty acids or omega-3 fatty acids (marketed as "brain food") have direct benefit with regard to ADHD symptoms. Though nutrient deficiency (such as a diet poor in zinc, vitamins, or healthy foods in general) may produce sluggishness or conversely lack of attention due to hunger or related physical ailments, megadoses of vitamins and zinc supplementation in the absence of deficiency have not been proven to address symptoms of ADHD and may result in toxicity. Antioxidants (such as ginkgo biloba, ginseng, pycnogenol, carotenoids, and enzymatic and synthetic versions of the body's naturally occurring antioxidants) and herbs (such as chamomile, valerian root, water hyssop, wild oat extract, kava hops, lemon balm, and gotu kola) also have no clear medical evidence to support their use in the treatment of ADHD and may also cause toxicity. It is important to counsel parents that supplements are regulated by the FDA as "food," not "drugs," and are therefore not held to the same standard with regard to safety or efficacy, especially for children. Likewise, parents should be counseled against using drugs with no FDA indication for treatment of ADHD. For example, FDA-approved as antifungal treatments, nystatin and ketoconazole have also been recommended by some complementary and alternative medicine providers under the mistaken belief that yeast overgrowth in the gut causes disruptive behaviors. Instead of giving their children supplements, some parents may place their children with ADHD on elimination diets. Popular diets include those that eliminate refined sugars and added sugars, additives, preservatives, dyes, salicylates, gluten, and/or casein. Though none of these diets have proven efficacy in the reduction of ADHD symptoms, it is important to discuss healthy eating options and opportunities for physical activity/exercise with families.

## SUGGESTED READINGS


American Psychiatric Association. *Diagnostic and Statistical Manual of Mental Disorders,* 5th ed. Washington, DC: American Psychiatric Association; 2013.

Jensen PS, Arnold LE, Swanson JM, et al. 3-year follow-up of the NIMH MTA study. *J Am Acad Child Adolesc Psychiatry*. 2007; 46(8):989-1002.

Jensen PS, Hinshaw SP, Swanson JM, et al. Findings from the NIMH Multimodal Treatment Study of ADHD (MTA): implications and applications for primary care providers. *J Dev Behav Pediatr*. 2001; 22(1):60-73.

Lock TM, Worley KA, Wolraich ML. Attention-deficit/hyperactivity disorder. In: Wolraich ML, Drotar DD, Dworkin PH, Perrin EC, eds. *Developmental-Behavioral Pediatrics: Evidence and Practice*. Philadelphia, PA: Mosby, Inc; 2008:579-601.

Molina BS, Hinshaw SP, Swanson JM, et al; MTA Cooperative Group. The MTA at 8 years: prospective follow-up of children treated for combined-type ADHD in a multisite study. *J Am Acad Child Adolesc Psychiatry*. 2009;48(5):484-500.

Reiff MI, Stein MT. Attention-deficit/hyperactivity disorder. In: Voigt RG, Macias MM, Myers SM, eds. *Developmental and Behavioral Pediatrics*. Elk Grove Village, IL: American Academy of Pediatrics; 2011:327-348.

Thomas R, Sanders S, Doust J, Beller E, Glasziou P. Prevalence of attention-deficit/hyperactivity disorder: a systematic review and meta-analysis. *Pediatrics*. 2015;135(4):e994-e1001. doi: 10.1542/peds.2014-3482.

Subcommittee on Attention-Deficit/Hyperactivity Disorder; Steering Committee on Quality Improvement and Management; Wolraich M, Brown L, Brown RT, et al. ADHD: clinical practice guideline for the diagnosis, evaluation, and treatment of attention-deficit/hyperactivity disorder in children and adolescents. *Pediatrics*. 2011;128(5):1007-1022.


## HELPFUL WEBSITES AND RESOURCES

ADHD Medication Guide: www.ADHDMedicationGuide.com

ADD Warehouse: www.addwarehouse.com

Children and Adults with Attention-Deficit/Hyperactivity Disorder: www.chadd.org

National Institute for Children's Health Quality: www.nichq.org

# 91 Autism Spectrum Disorder

Robert G. Voigt

## AUTISM: IT'S NOT JUST A CHECKLIST

Children with autism spectrum disorder have impairments in reciprocal social interaction and social communication and restricted, repetitive interests and behaviors. The Centers for Disease Control and Prevention have reported that the estimated prevalence of autism spectrum disorder is 1 in 68 children aged 8 years; thus, autism spectrum disorder is 1 of the more common chronic medical conditions observed in pediatric medical practice. Unfortunately, rather than a focus on clinical judgment to diagnose and manage this common pediatric problem, in the era of the *Diagnostic and Statistical Manual of Mental Disorders* (DSM), which is periodically updated by the American Psychiatric Association, autism has become a checklist. Autism did not appear as a diagnosis in the DSM until the DSM-III was published in 1980. Subsequently, the DSM checklist criteria for autism have changed over time. In the DSM-IV-TR, which was published in 2000, to meet criteria for a diagnosis of "autistic disorder," a child had to meet at least 6 out of a total of 12 checklist symptoms, with at least 2 criteria from a checklist of impairments in social interaction, at least 2 criteria from a checklist of impairments in communication, and at least 1 criteria from a checklist of restricted, repetitive, and stereotyped behaviors. A separate diagnosis of "Asperger disorder" was added to the DSM-IV (published in 1994), which included the same checklists for impairments in social interaction and restricted, repetitive, and stereotypic behaviors, but not the checklist of impairments in communication, as individuals with Asperger disorder were felt to have no delays in language development. However, the diagnosis of Asperger disorder was deleted from the DSM-5 (published in 2013). Currently, in the DSM-5, there is a single diagnosis of "autism spectrum disorder." To meet DSM-5 criteria for "autism spectrum disorder," a child must meet all 3 criteria from a checklist of persistent deficits in social communication and social interaction and at least 2 out of 4 criteria from a checklist of restricted, repetitive patterns of behavior, interests, or activities. The DSM-5 also requires (1) specification as to whether the autism spectrum disorder occurs with or without a language disorder, with or without an intellectual disability, or whether it is associated with a known medical or genetic condition or environmental factor; and (2) a rating of the severity level for both the impairment in social communication and the restricted, repetitive behaviors (level 1: requiring support; level 2: requiring substantial support; level 3: requiring very substantial support).

While this checklist approach to diagnosing autism spectrum disorder is considered by some to be the state of the art, the goal of this chapter is for pediatric medical providers to understand autism spectrum disorder within the entire spectrum and continuum of developmental-behavioral diagnoses, not as a simplified checklist. While autism itself presents with a wide spectrum of symptom severity and comorbidity, ranging from individuals with superior intelligence and mildly autistic behaviors to those with intellectual disability and severe autistic behaviors, it also occurs in continuity within a broader spectrum of developmental-behavioral diagnoses. Autism spectrum disorder exhibits significant overlap with other developmental-behavioral diagnoses, including language disorder, language-based learning disability, nonverbal learning disability, social communication disorder, attention-deficit/hyperactivity disorder (ADHD), and intellectual disability. It is often difficult, for example, to determine whether the social skills exhibited by a child with a severe intellectual disability are commensurate with underlying cognitive abilities or whether the child has an intercurrent autism spectrum disorder. Similarly, it is often difficult to distinguish whether the social skills deficits exhibited by a child with a language disorder and associated ADHD are secondary to the language disorder (hesitance to interact due to language difficulties) and ADHD (inattention to social cues) or are better accounted for by an autism spectrum disorder diagnosis. In each of these difficult cases, clinical judgment and a knowledge of the entire spectrum and continuum of developmental-behavioral diagnoses, rather than a simple checklist approach, is required to make the appropriate diagnosis. A checklist approach implies that anyone armed with an autism checklist can be an autism expert. However, to truly understand autism spectrum disorder and its differential diagnosis, pediatric medical providers need the clinical judgment to appreciate the entire spectrum and continuum of developmental-behavioral diagnoses (see Chapter 83) and to recognize autism spectrum disorder's place within this spectrum and continuum.

In Chapter 82, a medical model for evaluating chief complaints about developmental-behavioral concerns is presented. If a family expresses concern that their child might have autism spectrum disorder, or if a child fails an autism screen (the American Academy of Pediatrics recommends autism screening at 24 and 30 months of age), pediatric medical providers should obtain a comprehensive and detailed developmental history of the temporal pattern of developmental milestone acquisition across developmental streams to identify developmental delay, dissociation, and deviation. Early warning signs of a possible autism spectrum disorder may include concerns about a child's poor eye contact; speech/language delay; deviation in acquisition of language milestones; lack of response to his or her name being called ("acting deaf"); lack of showing, pointing, or sharing interests; or any loss of language and/or social skills (a loss of language and/or social skills is reported by about one-third of parents with children with autism spectrum disorder).

In children with autism spectrum disorder, the developmental history typically uncovers a scattered, uneven, developmentally dissociated and deviated pattern of development. As reviewed in Chapter 83, in children with developmental delays, it is most common for the delays to be more global in nature; developmental dissociation (differences in rates of development between developmental streams) and/or deviation (nonsequential acquisition of developmental milestones within a developmental stream) are therefore considered atypical compared to more globally delayed developmental milestones. While it is certainly true that every individual, whether he or she exhibits developmental delays or has no developmental delays, exhibits unique strengths and weaknesses across developmental abilities, it is most common in the general population to have relatively evenly developed developmental abilities, and large discrepancies (or dissociations) between abilities in different developmental domains can be considered atypical. For example, any IQ test manual contains tables documenting the percentage of the population with differences between different IQ subscores (such as verbal and nonverbal IQ), and the greater the difference is between scores, the fewer people in the population there are who exhibit this difference. Thus, individuals with significant dissociations in their cognitive development can be considered to process information in an atypical way compared to the general population (who do not exhibit such dissociation in abilities). Contributing to this atypical information processing is developmental deviation, or nonsequential milestone acquisition, which is atypical at any age. It should follow from this that individuals with significant developmental dissociation and deviation, who process information in an atypical way compared to the majority of the population who do not exhibit dissociation or deviation, are more likely to exhibit atypical behavior.

A key neurodevelopmental principle presented in Chapter 83 is that the more delayed, dissociated, and deviated the neurocognitive development is, the more atypical the associated neurobehavior is expected to be. Thus, when using the popular checklist approach to autism diagnosis, the symptoms of autism derive from a "black box" without explanation; when using a pediatric developmental assessment process, the symptoms of autism may be better explained to families. When a developmental history indicates a scattered, uneven, atypical pattern of developmental dissociation and deviation in the neurocognitive stream of development (which includes social development), it is expected that such an atypical pattern of cognitive development would most likely be associated with a similarly atypical pattern of behavior.

## SPECTRUM OF NEUROCOGNITIVE DISSOCIATION AND DEVIATION

The neurocognitive stream of development includes the language and nonverbal/visual-motor problem-solving streams, which come together to form the social and adaptive streams of development (see Fig. 91-1 and Chapter 83). The social stream of development is primarily communicative and includes social reciprocity and developing social relationships; the adaptive stream of development primarily relies on nonverbal/visual-motor problem solving and includes activities of daily living, such as feeding and dressing. The developmental history obtained from parents of children with autism spectrum disorder typically includes a history of dissociation and deviation in the neurocognitive stream of development, and this dissociation and deviation is usually confirmed on neurodevelopmental examination.

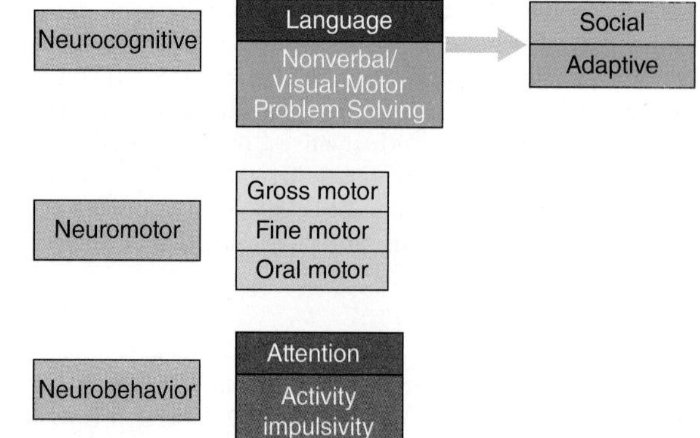


**FIGURE 91-1** Streams of development.

This dissociation in neurocognitive development may occur along the spectrum of dissociated/deviated language development or along the spectrum of dissociated/deviated nonverbal/visual-motor problem-solving development (Fig. 91-2). In either case, there is a significant discrepancy or dissociation between language and nonverbal abilities, and as reviewed above, such a discrepancy between these cognitive domains can be considered atypical compared to more global developmental delays. In addition, developmental deviation in acquisition of milestones within each of these streams adds to the atypicality in neurocognitive development observed in children with autism spectrum disorders.

In the past, autistic disorder and Asperger disorder were considered to be separate disorders. From a neurocognitive standpoint, children with autistic disorder and Asperger disorder both exhibited atypical, dissociated, and deviated developmental profiles. However, the dissociations in these 2 disorders were mirror images of one another: Children with autistic disorder generally exhibited a strength in nonverbal/visual-motor abilities and dissociated delays in language, while children with Asperger syndrome exhibited a relative strength in language abilities and dissociated delays in nonverbal/visual-motor abilities. However, as children with both of these disorders exhibited significant dissociation (and deviation) in their cognitive (including social) development, consistent with the continuum of developmental-behavioral diagnoses, their atypical neurocognitive profiles were associated with atypical neurobehavior. However, reflecting the difference in their underlying neurocognitive dissociations, the atypical repetitive behaviors exhibited by children with autistic disorder (who had discrepantly stronger nonverbal/visual-motor problem-solving development) tended to reflect their area of strength, with visual perseveration on spinning objects, flashing lights, lining up objects, etc. On the other hand, the atypical repetitive behaviors exhibited by children with Asperger disorder (who had discrepantly stronger language abilities) tended to reflect their area of strength, with verbal perseveration on factual information about restricted interests, such as train schedules, dinosaurs, or baseball statistics. However, with the elimination of the diagnosis of Asberger disorder in the DSM-5, a single category, autism spectrum disorder, was created. Those children who received an autistic disorder diagnosis in the DSM-IV are now diagnosed with autism spectrum disorder with a language disorder in the DSM-5, and those children who received a diagnosis of Asperger disorder in the DSM-4 are now diagnosed with autism spectrum disorder without a language disorder in the DSM-5. Despite these changes in DSM checklist diagnoses, in children with autism spectrum disorder, these atypical mirror image patterns of neurocognitive dissociation/deviation that are associated with social impairment continue

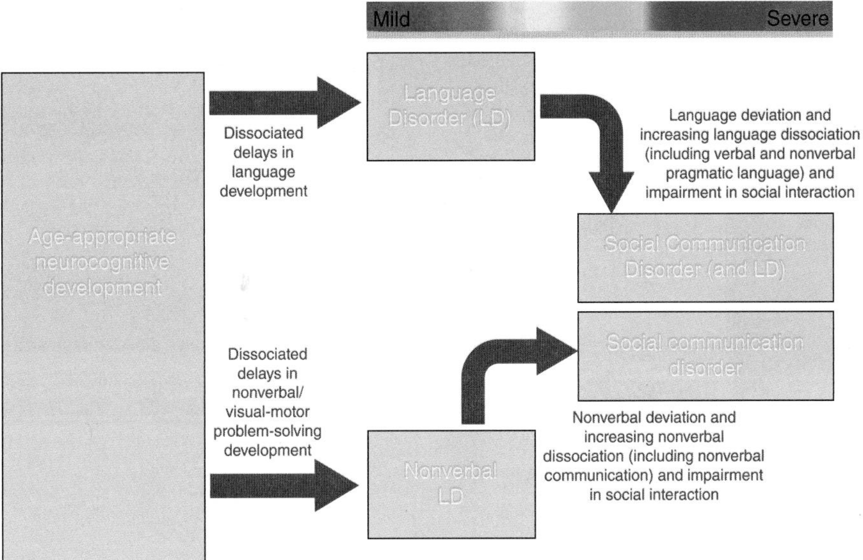


**FIGURE 91-2** Spectrum of neurocognitive dissociation and deviation.

to be associated with atypical neurobehavioral manifestations within the continuum of developmental-behavioral diagnoses.

Figure 91-2 illustrates the spectrum of neurocognitive dissociation and deviation. As reviewed in Chapter 83, there are 2 components to this spectrum, depending on whether the dissociated delays in development are due to language delays (the spectrum of dissociated and deviated language development, the top part of Fig. 91-2) or due to nonverbal/visual-motor problem-solving delays (the spectrum of dissociated and deviated nonverbal development, the bottom part of Fig. 91-2). At the mild end of the spectrum of dissociated language development, children have more mildly dissociated language delays, involving aspects of receptive and/or expressive language. In the preschool-aged population, these children are diagnosed with language disorders, and in the school-aged population, these children are diagnosed with language-based learning disabilities. However, as one proceeds to the more severe end of this spectrum of dissociated and deviated language development, more diffuse aspects of language/communication development (including both verbal and nonverbal pragmatic or social language development) and social interaction (including social reciprocity and developing social relationships) are impaired, and more deviation in the acquisition of language milestones is observed. This results in a neurocognitive diagnosis of a social communication disorder with an associated language disorder. The language deviation observed at this severe end of the spectrum of language dissociation and deviation is actually often an early red flag to suspect an autism spectrum disorder diagnosis. As an example of such language deviation in a younger child, parents might report in the developmental history that a child has a 50-word vocabulary, as expected at 2 years of age, but he or she does not yet use a specific "Mama" or "Dada" to refer to his or her parents, as expected at 10 months of age. This inflated vocabulary is most often not used functionally and consists primarily of labels, rote memorized scripts, or echolalia. In older children, language deviation may be observed by a vocabulary that is too numerous to count (> 3 years), use of multiword sentences (> 3 years), and an ability to label pictures, while at the same time, the child continues to use echolalia (echolalia usually ceases by 30 months of age) and to confuse pronouns (pronoun confusion usually ceases by 30 months). Children at this severe end of the spectrum of language dissociation and deviation who have autism spectrum disorder often also have developmentally deviated strengths or "splinter skills" in aspects of nonverbal/visual-motor problem solving. Consider as an example a 36-month-old child whose language development is at a 12-month level but who was able to visually recognize all the letters of the alphabet (5½-year-old–level skill) at 18 months of age, who recognizes shapes such as a pentagon and octagon, and who completes puzzles designed for 4-year-olds, but who does not yet draw a circle (a 36-month-old skill). More extreme dissociation, or "autistic savant skills," in art, math calculation, music, memory, or word reading (hyperlexia) also occur in approximately 10% of individuals with autism spectrum disorder.

The bottom part of Figure 91-2 illustrates the spectrum of nonverbal dissociation and deviation. In the mild end of this spectrum, children have more mildly dissociated nonverbal delays, involving aspects of visual perceptual, visual spatial, and/or visual motor abilities. In the preschool-aged population, these children are typically described as having a visual-perceptual, visual-spatial, and/or visual-motor deficit, and in the school-aged population, these children are diagnosed to have nonverbal learning disabilities. However, as one proceeds to the more severe end of this spectrum of dissociated nonverbal development, more diffuse aspects of nonverbal development, including nonverbal aspects of social communication and social interaction, are impaired, and more deviation in the acquisition of nonverbal milestones is observed. This again results in a neurocognitive diagnosis of social communication disorder, but without an associated language disorder.

Social communication disorder has been included in the DSM-5 as a stand-alone diagnosis. This diagnosis describes children who have pragmatic and social communication impairments similar to those observed in autism spectrum disorder, but they do not exhibit the associated restricted, repetitive, or stereotypic behaviors observed in children with autism spectrum disorder. Thus, a diagnosis of autism spectrum disorder is not made exclusively based on this atypical social communication disorder neurocognitive profile. To make a diagnosis of autism spectrum disorder within the continuum of developmental-behavioral diagnoses, this atypical neurocognitive profile must be accompanied by the atypical neurobehavioral profile observed at the severe end of the spectrum of neurobehavioral dissociation and deviation.

## SPECTRUM OF NEUROBEHAVIORAL DISSOCIATION AND DEVIATION

Figure 91-3 illustrates the spectrum of neurobehavioral dissociation and deviation. At the mild end of this spectrum, children exhibit dissociated delays in their attention spans and/or levels of impulse control and motor activity compared to their underlying cognitive abilities. In other words, they exhibit developmentally inappropriate levels of inattention and/or hyperactivity-impulsivity, and if these symptoms are impairing their functioning across settings, they are diagnosed as having ADHD. However, as one proceeds to the more severe end of this spectrum of dissociated and deviated neurobehavioral development,

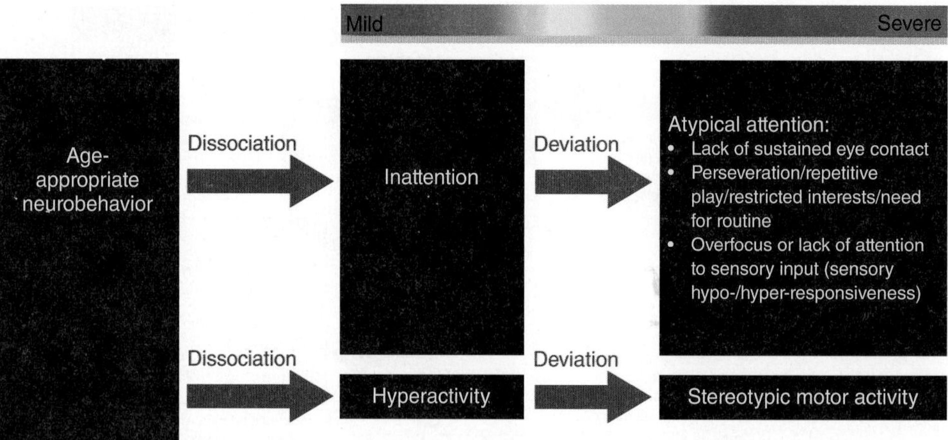


**FIGURE 91-3** Spectrum of neurobehavioral dissociation and deviation.

increased developmental deviation results in behaviors that are atypical at any age. Rather than simple inattention, children at the severe end of this spectrum exhibit atypical attention; while they may lack the attention (and social interest) to sustain eye contact, they may overfocus or perseverate on restricted interests and routines and engage in repetitive play (eg, lining, sorting, spinning). They may also show atypicalities in attention to other sensory stimuli. For example, they may not react to painful stimuli but overreact to certain sounds, or they may overfocus on tight-fitting clothes, tags on shirts, or seams on socks. Rather than the hyperactivity or fidgetiness observed at the mild end of this spectrum, at the severe end of this spectrum of neurobehavioral dissociation and deviation, more atypical stereotypic motor mannerisms (eg, hand flapping, body rocking or spinning, toe-walking) may be observed.

## CONTINUUM OF NEUROCOGNITIVE AND NEUROBEHAVIORAL STREAMS OF DEVELOPMENT

As discussed in Chapter 83, a key neurodevelopmental principle is that there is a continuum of developmental-behavioral disability across neurodevelopmental streams. Thus, delays in 1 stream of neurodevelopment are most likely to occur in association with delays in other streams of neurodevelopment. This continuum of developmental-behavioral disability can be observed among children with dissociated and deviated development and behavior, and it is the continuum between the severe end of the spectrum of neurocognitive dissociation and deviation (social communication disorder) and the severe end of the spectrum of neurobehavioral dissociation and deviation (restricted, repetitive, and stereotyped behavior) that defines autism spectrum disorder. Figure 91-4 illustrates this continuum of neurocognitive and neurobehavioral disability. At the mild end of this continuum, one encounters children with the common combination of learning disabilities (from the spectrum of neurocognitive dissociation/deviation) and ADHD (from the spectrum of neurobehavioral dissociation/deviation). As one proceeds across to the severe end of this continuum of neurocognitive and neurobehavioral disability, one encounters children with a combination of social communication disorders (from the spectrum of neurocognitive dissociation/deviation) and the atypical attention (lack of sustained eye contact, perseveration on restricted interests, need for routine, repetitive play, sensory hypo- or hyper-responsiveness) and stereotypic motor mannerisms observed at the severe end of the spectrum of neurobehavioral dissociation and deviation. Children with this combination of neurocognitive and neurobehavioral symptomatology (social communication disorders + atypical repetitive and stereotypic behavior) are diagnosed with autism spectrum disorder.

With an understanding of the entire spectrum and continuum of developmental-behavioral diagnoses, clinical judgment becomes the gold standard for autism spectrum disorder diagnoses. The developmental history and observations made during the neurodevelopmental examination should confirm that a child meets DSM-5 checklist criteria for an autism spectrum diagnosis. However, other standardized measures are necessary to confirm clinical concerns about autism spectrum disorder. These measures are more typically administered by psychologists or school district Child Study Teams, and include the Childhood Autism Rating Scale (CARS) and the Autism Diagnostic Observation Schedule (ADOS).

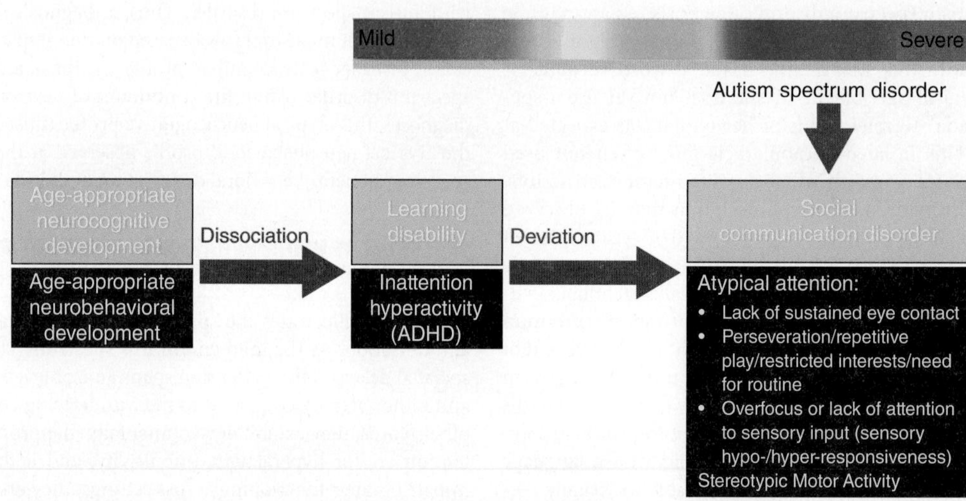


**FIGURE 91-4** Continuum of neurocognitive and neurobehavioral dissociation and deviation.

## DIFFERENTIAL DIAGNOSIS

Given that developmental-behavioral diagnoses exist along a spectrum and continuum, it is often difficult to make categorical diagnoses. The differential diagnosis for autism spectrum disorder includes social communication disorders, language disorder/language-based learning disabilities, nonverbal learning disabilities, ADHD, and intellectual disabilities. Children with social communication disorders share the social communication impairment observed in children with autism spectrum disorder, but they do not exhibit the restricted, repetitive, or stereotypic behaviors observed in autism spectrum disorder. Children with language disorders or language-based learning disabilities share the dissociated delays in language development observed in children with autism spectrum disorder (with an associated language disorder), and they may be hesitant to interact with other children due to their delayed language abilities. However, they tend not to exhibit the extent of dissociated verbal and nonverbal pragmatic language delays or the significant developmental deviation in language development observed in children with autism spectrum disorder. Children with language disorders also may attempt to communicate nonverbally to compensate for their verbal difficulties, and they do not exhibit the impairments in social reciprocity and development of social relationships nor the restricted, repetitive, and stereotypic behaviors observed in children with autism spectrum disorder. Similarly, children with nonverbal learning disabilities share the dissociated delays in nonverbal communication exhibited by children with autism spectrum disorder (without a language disorder) and may have difficulty with nonverbal communication and in "reading" social situations that negatively impact their social interactions, but they do not exhibit the severe impairments in social reciprocity and development of social relationships nor the restricted, repetitive, and stereotypic behaviors observed in children with autism spectrum disorder. Children with ADHD have deficits in attention and impulse control that impair their social interactions with peers, and they often have associated language-based or nonverbal learning disabilities, but they do not exhibit the impairments in social reciprocity and development of social relationships nor the restricted, repetitive, or stereotypic behaviors observed in autism spectrum disorder.

As a component of their globally delayed developmental milestones, children with intellectual disability often exhibit delays in their social skills. However, an additional diagnosis of autism spectrum disorder is given to children with intellectual disability only if their social communication and social interaction skills are discrepantly delayed (or dissociated) from their underlying cognitive abilities. Children with more severe to profound intellectual disability often engage in repetitive and stereotypic behaviors, but a diagnosis of autism spectrum disorder is given only if the child's social communication/social interaction is discrepantly delayed compared to his or her underlying cognitive abilities. In the continuum of developmental disabilities, the more delayed the development, the more frequently dissociation and deviation are also observed. Thus, children with intellectual disability are more likely to also have the developmentally dissociated and deviated developmental patterns observed in autism spectrum disorder. The Centers for Disease Control and Prevention reported that 32% of children with autism spectrum disorder also have intellectual disability and 56% of children with autism spectrum disorder have intellectual disability or borderline cognitive functioning.

Making a diagnosis of autism spectrum disorder is the first step for pediatric medical providers. Once a diagnosis is made, referral for early intervention or special education, medical laboratory workup, and longitudinal medical management, potentially including psychopharmacological management, remain the roles of the primary care pediatric medical provider.

## EARLY INTERVENTION AND SPECIAL EDUCATION

As early identification and early intervention are critical for optimizing long-term neurodevelopmental outcome, children should be referred to their local early intervention or special education programs as soon as a diagnosis of autism spectrum disorder is even suspected. Behavioral interventions based on applied behavior analysis (ABA) have the strongest empiric support for autism treatment. A report of the Surgeon General of the United States (1999) affirmed that 30 years of research has demonstrated the efficacy of ABA in reducing inappropriate disruptive and maladaptive behavior and in increasing communication, learning, and appropriate social behavior in children with autism spectrum disorder. Families can access a local certified behavioral therapist to provide ABA services through the Behavior Analyst Certification Board (http://www.bacb.com/).





Once children with autism spectrum disorders reach 3 years of age, they should qualify for an Individualized Education Program through their local public school districts under a primary categorical label of autism spectrum disorder. Children with autism spectrum disorder benefit from intensive direct and consultative language, behavioral, and social skills interventions aimed at maximizing functional communication and social interaction abilities and at modifying atypical and maladaptive behaviors. Children with autism spectrum disorder also benefit from very highly structured and supervised inclusion into regular classroom settings and activities for exposure to socially and communicatively appropriate role models with whom they can practice the communication and social interaction skills that they learn through their special educational and therapeutic services. The National Research Council has published comprehensive recommendations for the education of children with autism spectrum disorders. These guidelines recommend that a minimum of 25 hours per week of services be provided year round in which the child is engaged in individualized, highly structured, systematically planned, and developmentally appropriate educational activities. The guidelines further suggest that the priorities of focus of educational services for children with autism spectrum disorders should include functional spontaneous communication, social instruction delivered throughout the day in various settings, cognitive development, play skills, and proactive approaches to atypical and challenging behaviors. It is also important that parents be included as integral members of the intervention team and extend therapeutic goals to the home environment. Generalization and maintenance of newly learned skills in natural environments should be considered as important as the acquisition of new skills.

Children with autism spectrum disorder should receive intensive direct and consultative language therapy services that include a pragmatic language therapy component to address their delayed and deviated language development and social communication impairment. Augmentative communication strategies (eg, picture exchanges, visual schedules, manual signing, communication boards/devices) should be considered as a component of speech/language therapy in an attempt to improve functional communication and decrease frustration with communication breakdowns. Children with autism spectrum disorder who exhibit associated gross motor incoordination or delays in activities of daily living with a fine-motor component might also benefit from direct physical therapy and occupational therapy services.

Families with children with autism spectrum disorder should also benefit from all social and community services available to children with developmental disabilities and their families in their local communities. These services might include case management services, supplemental medical insurance or other financial assistance programs, educational advocacy services, parent support groups, functional behavioral analysis/in-home behavior management counseling services, respite care services, personal care attendant services, counseling regarding long-term legal and financial planning issues, summer camps, and other extracurricular activities.

The response to intervention for children with autism spectrum disorders can be extremely variable, with some children making rapid, substantial gains and others making very slow gains. It has been reported that up to 25% of children diagnosed with autism spectrum disorder may lose their autism spectrum disorder diagnosis over time. Although it is very difficult to predict, those more likely to respond to intervention are those with higher IQs and language abilities, those with milder autism symptoms, and those who are diagnosed early and receive more intensive intervention using behavioral techniques.

## MEDICAL LABORATORY WORKUP

As with all other children with delayed language development, all children with autism spectrum disorder with an associated language disorder need to undergo formal audiology evaluation to check their hearing status. In an attempt to establish an etiologic diagnosis to account for their autism spectrum disorder, all children with autism spectrum disorder should undergo a chromosome microarray analysis and DNA testing for fragile X syndrome. Further medical laboratory workup depends on the clinical presentation. If a child with autism spectrum disorder exhibits any metabolic signs or symptoms (eg, global developmental regression, decompensation with mild illness, tonal abnormalities, ataxia, recurrent vomiting), then a comprehensive metabolic workup to rule out inborn errors of metabolism would be indicated. If the physical examination reveals neurocutaneous findings (eg, tuberous sclerosis, neurofibromatosis), cleft palate and syndactyly (eg, Smith-Lemli-Opitz syndrome), or marked macrocephaly (eg, *PTEN* hamartoma syndromes), then targeted workup for these disorders should be pursued. In girls with deceleration of head growth, hand wringing, and loss of purposeful hand movements, testing for mutations in the *MECP2* gene should be pursued to rule out Rett syndrome.

## MEDICAL COMORBIDITIES

As a component of their restricted, repetitive behaviors, children with autism spectrum disorders are often very picky eaters, and this is associated with frequent complaints of constipation or loose stools. The workup and management of gastrointestinal complaints in children with autism spectrum disorders should proceed just as it would for children without autism spectrum disorder.

Children with autism spectrum disorders also frequently present with sleep difficulties, and lack of an appropriate amount of sleep can exacerbate daytime behavioral problems and increase family stress. While these sleep difficulties are often behavioral in nature, children with autism spectrum disorder can have medical problems resulting in sleep disruption (eg, gastroesophageal reflux, abdominal pain related to constipation, sleep apnea) or primary sleep disorders (eg, restless legs syndrome), and further workup and/or referral to a sleep specialist should be considered just as in children without autism spectrum disorders.

Approximately one-third of children with autism spectrum disorder will develop epilepsy, usually during adolescence. Electroencephalograms (EEGs) should be considered if seizures are suspected. If a child exhibits a significant isolated loss of language after 3 years of age (as opposed to the more typical autism regression, which involves regression in both language and social skills before 2 years of age), a sleep-deprived EEG may be indicated to rule out acquired epileptic aphasia or Landau-Kleffner syndrome.

## PSYCHOPHARMACOLOGY

There are no medications available to treat the core social communication/social interaction impairments or restricted/repetitive behaviors observed in children with autism spectrum disorders. However, children with autism spectrum disorders often present with secondary maladaptive behaviors, such as tantrums, aggression, and self-injury. Whenever there is an acute change in the behavior of a child with autism spectrum disorder, especially in children with limited verbal and nonverbal communication, it is important to rule out occult medical causes (eg, constipation, gastroesophageal reflux, lack of appropriate sleep, headaches, corneal abrasion, dental abscess, otitis media or externa, occult fractures) for the acute behavior change. Secondary maladaptive behaviors can also occur due to anxiety and frustration produced by demands and expectations for a child's performance at school or at home that are exceeding his or her underlying abilities. Such secondary maladaptive behaviors are also often inadvertently reinforced by parents or school personnel. Thus, behavioral interventions, including functional behavioral assessments and development of formal behavior management plans, along with parental behavior management training, should be considered the primary intervention for such maladaptive behaviors.

However, when maladaptive behaviors are preventing a child from taking advantage of therapeutic and educational interventions (tantrums), are causing significant harm to self (self-injurious behaviors) or others (aggression), or are becoming dangerous (elopement), then a careful trial of psychotropic medication can be considered. The only current medications with FDA approval for the treatment of irritability (including tantrums, aggressive behavior, and self-injury) in children with autism spectrum disorder are the atypical antipsychotics risperidone (for children > 5 years of age) and aripiprazole (for children > 6 years of age). As is true for children with intellectual disability, it is important to note that psychotropic medications for children with autism spectrum disorder typically are not as effective as when they are used in children without autism spectrum disorder, both in terms of the number of children with a positive response and in the magnitude of the positive response. In addition, children with autism spectrum disorder typically experience more psychotropic medication side effects compared to children without autism spectrum disorder. Thus, if a trial of psychotropic medication is being considered, it is important to start at a low dose and to increase the dose slowly to closely monitor both positive response and side effects.

## NONSTANDARD THERAPIES

Families with children with autism spectrum disorder need to be very careful with regard to their potential choices of nonstandard and non–evidence-based interventions that may be advocated for children with autism spectrum disorders. Families will likely learn of many nonstandard and unproven therapeutic interventions and explanations for autism with questionable scientific validity or evidence of their effectiveness. Given the lack of any biomedical treatments or cures for autism spectrum disorder offered by traditional, evidence-based medicine, parents are understandably desperate for any kind of biomedical treatment that might help their children. Unfortunately, a plethora of unproven (and often costly and potentially dangerous) interventions are widely available to exploit this parental sense of desperation. Families need to be very careful about considering any proposed intervention that is supported exclusively by personal testimonials rather than by data from double-blind, placebo-controlled clinical trials that are published in the peer-reviewed medical literature. Families need to be very careful that any intervention they may decide to proceed with is not potentially harmful to their children from a medical standpoint (such as potential impurities in unregulated nutritional supplements; potential toxic effects of megadoses of vitamins or minerals; potential nutritional deficiencies derivative of special diets; inappropriate use of and side effects from hyperbaric oxygen therapy; antifungal, antiviral, or antibiotic medications; chelating agents; immunotherapies; or withholding immunizations) and would be neither a financial nor time-consuming burden to the family (such as with "facilitated communication," "auditory integration," or other "sensory therapies") nor prevent them from taking advantage of the educational and behavioral interventions that have been shown to be most effective for children with autism spectrum disorders. Families can review information about scientifically supported interventions for autism spectrum disorder through the National Autism Center's National Standards Project (http://www.nationalautismcenter.org/national-standards-project/phase-2/) or through the Association for Science in Autism Treatment (http://www.asatonline.org/).

## CONCLUSION

Rather than the popular view of autism as a simple checklist of behaviors, given its prevalence in the pediatric population, pediatric medical providers need to understand autism within the entire spectrum and continuum of developmental disabilities. There is no such thing as an autism expert; autism and its differential diagnoses can only be understood through acquiring expertise across the entire spectrum and continuum of developmental-behavioral diagnoses. Concerns about autism should be treated no differently than any other chief complaint in pediatric medicine. The diagnosis of autism can be made through a comprehensive developmental history that is confirmed by observations made during a neurodevelopmental examination. This clinical approach will identify the delayed, dissociated, and deviated pattern of development observed in children with autism spectrum disorders, allowing pediatric medical providers to make the diagnosis; complete the medical laboratory workup in an attempt to establish an etiologic diagnosis; refer for evidence-based early intervention, special education, and therapeutic services; and longitudinally manage children with autism spectrum disorders and their families within their primary care medical home.

## SUGGESTED READINGS

American Psychiatric Association. Autism spectrum disorder. In: *Diagnostic and Statistical Manual of Mental Disorders*. 5th ed. Arlington, VA: American Psychiatric Association; 2013:50-59.

Ankenman K, Elgin J, Sullivan K, et al. Nonverbal and verbal cognitive discrepancy profiles in autism spectrum disorders: influence of age and gender. *Am J Intellect Dev Disabil*. 2014;119(1):84-89.

Christensen DL, Baio J, Braun KV, et al. Prevalence and characteristics of autism spectrum disorder among children aged 8 years—Autism and Developmental Disabilities Monitoring Network, 11 sites, United States, 2012. *MMWR Surveill Summ*. 2016:65(3):1-23.

Committee on Educational Interventions for Children with Autism, Division of Behavioral and Social Sciences and Education, National Research Council. *Educating Children with Autism*. Washington, DC: National Academy Press; 2001.

Department of Health and Human Services. *Mental Health: A Report of the Surgeon General* Rockville, MD: US Department of Health and Human Services, Substance Abuse and Mental Health Services Administration, Center for Mental Health Services, National Institutes of Health, National Institute of Mental Health; 1999.

Helt M, Kelley E, Kinsbourne M, et al. Can children with autism recover? If so, how? *Neuropsychol Rev*. 2008;18(4):339-366.

Johnson CP, Myers SM. Identification and evaluation of children with autism spectrum disorders. *Pediatrics*. 2007;120(5):1183-1215.

Joseph RM, Tager-Flusberg H, Lord C. Cognitive profiles and social-communicative functioning in children with autism spectrum disorder. *J Child Psychol Psychiatry*. 2002;43(6):807-821.

Klin A, Volkmar FR, Sparrow SS, Cicchetti DV, Rourke BP. Validity and neuropsychological characterization of Asperger syndrome: convergence with nonverbal learning disabilities syndrome. *J Child Psychol Psychiatry*. 1995;36(7):1127-1140.

Myers SM, Johnson CP. Management of children with autism spectrum disorders. *Pediatrics*. 2007;120(5):1162-1182.

# 92 Introduction to Pediatric Mental Health

Efrain Bleiberg, Amy Vyas, and Laurel Williams

Emotional and behavioral health is an integral component of children's health, lifetime well-being and adjustment, educational attainment, and ability to thrive in all functional domains. It is strongly associated with physical health and resilience in the face of psychosocial or biological adversity. By contrast, behavioral and emotional problems predict or negatively influence the course of pediatric illness.

The significance of emotional and behavioral health problems in pediatrics is underscored by the prevalence of mental health disorders in children. One in 5 children presents with a serious and persistent mental health disorder. The prevalence increases to one-third for the nearly 25% of children in the United States exposed to 2 or more adverse childhood experiences (ACEs), which include physical, emotional, or sexual maltreatment, or chronic or severe medical conditions. (For further discussion of ACEs, see Chapter 28.)

Suicide, the most tragic correlate of mental health disorders, is the second leading cause of death in youth ages 15 to 24 years, accounting for 3 times more deaths than all childhood malignancies or heart conditions combined and more than 20 times the deaths attributable to diabetes in this age group. More ominously, the number of completed suicides appears to be increasing in at least some pediatric populations. Between 1999 and 2014, completed suicides in girls 10 to 14 years old tripled, the largest percent increase in deaths by suicide in any age group.

Other mental health disorders also show increases in prevalence, notably autism, which according to the Centers for Disease Control and Prevention, has gone from 1 in 100 at the beginning of this decade to 1 in 68. Similar increases are noted in adolescent depression and anxiety disorders.

Even more significantly, there is a growing appreciation of the profound lifetime consequences and the cost to both the individual and to society of childhood mental disorders in terms of poor educational attainment and significantly increased risk for substance abuse and dependency, incarceration, violence toward both self and others, and poor health. Pediatric mental health disorders shape dysfunctional and maladaptive developmental and neurodevelopmental trajectories not only by impairing the acquisition of cognitive and social skills but also, more subtly, by negatively impacting caretakers' ability to provide the very developmental opportunities that underlie healthy adjustment and resilience.

Thus, pediatric mental health disorders lead to chronic lifetime psychopathology and poor health. For example, Winning et al showed that even after 50 years, mental health disorders in childhood were still associated with significantly increased cardiovascular morbidity and mortality. Not surprisingly, the Institute of Medicine's 2015 report stated that "in the United States, mental and behavioral disorders are the largest contributors to years lived with disability. They are also co-morbid with medical conditions and costly to the health care system and society." This report, however, noted a "quality chasm" between the number of individuals afflicted with mental health disorders and the availability and appropriateness of the care they receive.

Among youth with mental health disorders, less than 30% receive any form of treatment. For those who do receive treatment, their care is often fragmented, mostly focused on psychopharmacology, and, not infrequently, involves treatment interventions unsupported by evidence.

While geography, race, and socioeconomic status factor heavily in limiting access to treatment, an overall dearth of mental health professionals, particularly child and adolescent psychiatrists, is a major impediment to the provision of appropriate care. Clearly, innovative healthcare models are urgently needed to address the mental health needs of the pediatric population. These models largely focus on integrating mental health care with overall health care.

The passage of the Patient Protection and Affordable Care Act of 2011 placed increased emphasis on the development of medical homes designed to address, in a collaborative and coordinated fashion, the physical and mental health needs of patients. The Health Parity Law of 2012 requires parity in access to services for both physical and mental health disorders, further adding to the pressure on payers to address mental health problems together with other health conditions.

The pressure to integrate mental health into general healthcare places pediatricians in a position to play a key role in meeting the mental health needs of children. Yet studies consistently find that pediatricians feel unsure they possess the skills, knowledge, and tools needed to address mental health problems in their practices. A random sample of 1600 members of the American Academy of Pediatrics concluded that pediatricians feel both responsible and comfortable assessing and managing attention-deficit/hyperactivity disorder (70% of respondents). Yet less than one-third of those sampled felt equally comfortable managing other mental health conditions. A study of recently graduated pediatricians points out that additional training in mental health and developmental pediatrics could allow pediatricians to assume a larger role in identifying and providing first-line treatment for the most common mental health disorders in a variety of settings, from stand-alone pediatric practices to integrated care models.

In sum, mental health is key to health. Pediatricians need to possess the attitudes, skill, and knowledge required to assume a vital role in assessing and treating pediatric mental health disorders and in addressing the impact of mental health problems on medical conditions and of medical conditions on their patients' mental health.

## SUGGESTED READINGS

American Academy of Child and Adolescent Psychiatry. Child and adolescent psychiatry workforce crisis: solutions to improve early intervention and access to care. http://www.aacap.org/App_Themes/AACAP/docs/Advocacy/policy_resources/cap_workforce_crisis_201305.pdf. Accessed January 22, 2018.

American Academy of Pediatrics Ohio Chapter. Building mental wellness. http://ohioaap.org/projects/building-mental-wellness/. Accessed January 22, 2018.

Aupont O, Doerfler L, Conner DF, Stille C, Tisminetzky M, McLaughlin TJ. A collaborative care model to improve access to pediatric mental health services. *Adm Policy Ment Health.* 2013; 40(4):264-273.

Bethell CD, Newacheck P, Hawes E, Halfon N. Adverse childhood experiences: assessing the impact on health and school engagement and the mitigating role of resilience. *Health Aff.* 2014;33(12):106-115.

Curtin SC, Warner M, Hedegaard H. Increase in suicide in the United States, 1999–2014. http://www.cdc.gov/nchs/products/databriefs/db241.htm. Accessed January 22, 2018. National Center for Health Statistics Data Brief No. 241.

Freed GL, Dunham KM, Switalski KE, Jones MD Jr, McGuinnes GA; Research Advisory Committee of the American Board of Pediatrics. Recently trained general pediatricians: perspectives on residency training and scope of practice. *Pediatrics.* 2009;123(suppl 1): S38-S43.

Foy JM; American Academy of Pediatrics Task Force on Mental Health. Enhancing pediatric mental health care: algorithms for primary care. *Pediatrics.* 2010;125(suppl 3):S109-S125.

Martini R, Houston M, Chenven M, et al. ACOs & CAPs: preparing for the impact of healthcare reform on child and adolescent psychiatry practice. http://www.aacap.org/App_Themes/AACAP/docs/Advocacy/policy_resources/preparing_for_healthcare_reform_201303.pdf. Accessed January 22, 2018.

McCue Horwitz S, Storfer-Isser A, Kerker BD, et al. Do on-site mental health professionals change pediatricians' responses to children's mental health problems? *Acad Pediatr.* 2016;16(7):676-683.

National Alliance on Mental Illness. Mental health facts: children and teens. http://www.nami.org/getattachment/Learn-More/Mental-Health-by-the-Numbers/childrenmhfacts.pdf. Accessed January 22, 2018.

National Resident Matching Program. Results and Data: Specialties Matching Service: 2016 Appointment Year. Washington, DC: National Resident Matching Program; 2016:32.

Perou R, Bitsko RH, Blumberg SJ, et al. Mental health surveillance among children–United States, 2005–2011. *MMWR.* 2013;62(02): 1-35. http://www.cdc.gov/mmwr/preview/mmwrhtml/su6202a1.htm. Accessed January 22, 2018.

Prince M, Patel V, Saxena S, et al. No health without mental health. *Lancet.* 2007;370(9590):859-877.

Stein RE, Horwitz SM, Storfer-Isser A, Heneghan A, Olson L, Hoagwood KE. Do pediatricians think they are responsible for identification and management of child mental health problems? Results of the AAP periodic survey. *Ambul Pediatr.* 2008;8(1):11-17.

Winning A, Glymour MM, McCormick MC, Gilsanz P, Kubzansky LD. Psychological distress across the life course and cardiometabolic risk: findings from the 1958 British Birth Cohort Study. *J Am Coll Cardiol.* 2015;66(14):1577-1586.



# 93 Anxiety

Anthony C. Puliafico, Erica Chin, Alexandra Canetti, Paula Yanes-Lukin, Dylan Braun, and Moira Rynn

## DIAGNOSIS AND PREVALENCE

Anxiety disorders are common throughout childhood and adolescence, and the anxiety disorders observed throughout the life span often emerge during childhood. Prevalence rates for pediatric anxiety disorders are as high as 15% to 20%. Although some fears and anxieties are developmentally normative and even adaptive, they must be differentiated from anxiety disorders, which entail considerable impairment in academic, social, and family functioning. Unfortunately, anxiety disorders may go unnoticed, particularly when compared to the disruptive behavior disorders (eg, attention-deficit/hyperactivity disorder [ADHD] and oppositional defiant disorder) that are more frequently referred for treatment. Early identification and assessment of pediatric anxiety disorders require an evaluation that includes clinical interview, multi-informant report (parent, child, and teacher), careful attention to developmental level and ability, an evaluation of the family environment and the response of the caregivers to the child's anxiety, and an assessment of functional impairment in daily life. Pediatric anxiety disorders are highly comorbid with one another, and affected youth are likely to meet criteria for multiple anxiety disorders. Moreover, anxiety disorders may serve as a gateway to developing major depressive disorder, suicidal ideation and behavior, and substance abuse in adolescence. Fortunately, anxiety disorders are highly treatable conditions, particularly when identified early. In this chapter, we review the various types of anxiety disorders, approaches to screening and evaluation of anxiety, and evidence-based treatment approaches.

Listed below are descriptions of anxiety disorders observed in children and adolescents, including diagnostic criteria and prevalence rates. For all of these disorders, significant distress and/or impairment is required for a diagnosis.

### Separation Anxiety Disorder

Separation anxiety disorder is characterized by excessive anxiety or distress when anticipating or experiencing separation from caregivers or from home. Children suffering from separation anxiety disorder typically worry about harm befalling them or their caregivers when they are separated. They avoid attending social events or activities without their caregivers being present, and in severe cases, may try to avoid attending school to prevent separation. Children may also insist on sleeping near a caregiver and refuse to sleep away from home. Prevalence rates for separation anxiety disorder are estimated at 4%. Whereas some degree of separation anxiety is normative during the early toddler years, symptoms of separation anxiety disorder, interfering with the normal process of separation and individuation, may present as early as age 3. Initial onset is less common in adolescence.

### Social Anxiety Disorder

Social anxiety disorder involves excessive fear of being embarrassed and of being negatively evaluated or rejected by others. To meet criteria for a diagnosis of social anxiety disorder, children and adolescents must fear negative evaluation or rejection by their peers (not only adults). Youth with social anxiety disorder typically avoid feared social situations, including participating in class, speaking informally with peers, performing or speaking in front of others, or initiating social plans. Prevalence rates for social anxiety disorder in youth are estimated at 7%. Prevalence is most often noted during early to mid-adolescence, although social anxiety disorder frequently presents in childhood as well.

### Selective Mutism

Selective mutism is characterized by fear and unwillingness to speak with others. Youth suffering from selective mutism typically refuse to answer questions in class or speak when spoken to in informal settings, although they often feel comfortable speaking with parents, family members, or close friends. Selective mutism is highly comorbid with social anxiety disorder. Symptoms must persist for at least 1 month. Prevalence estimates are below 1% with median age of onset at 3 to 4 years of age. It is thought that selective mutism may represent an extension of early-onset social phobia.

### Generalized Anxiety Disorder

Generalized anxiety disorder (GAD) is characterized by excessive and often uncontrollable worry that persists more days than not for at least 6 months. Typical areas of worry in childhood include school and relations with peers, family health and relationships, personal and family safety, world affairs, and the future (eg, going to college, adult responsibilities, death). To meet criteria for GAD, youth must also experience at least 1 of the following associated symptoms: muscle tension/tightness, difficulty sleeping, impaired concentration, irritability, fatigue, and increased restlessness. Approximately 1% to 2% of children and 1% to 4% of adolescents suffer from GAD.

### Specific Phobia

A specific phobia is diagnosed when a child or adolescent exhibits an excessive fear of a particular situation or object. Common specific phobias in childhood and adolescence involve fear of certain animals, heights, injections, water, loud noises, vomiting, flying, choking, or dark areas. The fear must be considerably greater than would be expected of same-aged youth. Approximately 5% of children meet criteria for a specific phobia, with the prevalence rate increasing to at least 13% in adolescence. Phobias of animals and environmental situations, such as heights and water, have an earlier average age of onset, whereas situational phobias, including flights and elevators, are more common in adolescence.

### Panic Disorder

Panic disorder is characterized by the occurrence of panic attacks and anticipatory anxiety about subsequent panic attacks or avoidance of places or situations in which a panic attack is feared. At least 1 panic attack must be untriggered, or unprovoked by an anxiety-provoking situation or thought. That is, panic disorder would not be diagnosed if all panic attacks occurred within the context of a feared social situation or around an animal that the youth fears. A panic attack is defined as an episode of intense anxiety and at least 4 physical symptoms, such as pounding or racing heart, sweating, shortness of breath, dizziness, nausea, or feelings of choking. When experiencing a panic attack, youth may also experience feelings of de-realization or fear of dying or losing control. Panic disorder is uncommon in children, with prevalence rates estimated at less than 0.4%; prevalence rates gradually increase through adolescence. However, these low rates may reflect children being unable to communicate the specific physical experiences and consequent anxiety associated with panic disorder.

While obsessive-compulsive disorder and post-traumatic stress disorder are organized under separate sections of the DSM-V, they are often categorized as anxiety disorders.

#### Obsessive-Compulsive Disorder

Obsessive-compulsive disorder (OCD) is characterized by the presence of both obsessions, which are unwelcome and recurring thoughts, impulses, or images that increase anxiety, and compulsions, which are behaviors or mental actions that are completed repeatedly to reduce the anxiety caused by obsessions. These compulsions are often performed to avoid feared outcomes, but are usually excessive or unreasonable. Youth may also avoid known triggers in an effort to avoid or suppress their obsessive thoughts. The prevalence of OCD is thought to be between 1% to 2%, with 25% of patients developing the disorder before age 14.

#### Post-Traumatic Stress Disorder

Post-traumatic stress disorder (PTSD) affects some children and adolescents who have undergone, witnessed, or indirectly experienced a traumatic event. To meet criteria for PTSD, youth must exhibit at least 1 re-experiencing symptom, including intrusive memories or nightmares, "flashbacks" about the event, or distress and/or physiological reactivity. Youth must exhibit avoidance of people, places, or thoughts and feelings associated with the event. Finally, youth experience distorted perceptions and emotions, such as negative beliefs about their future, diminished interest in activities, failure to remember details of the event, hypervigilance, feeling detached from others, or constricted affect. A modified set of criteria were included for children ages 6 years and younger in the *Diagnostic and Statistical Manual of Mental Disorders*, 5th edition, with the major modification being that young children must experience either avoidance of stimuli associated with the trauma *or* distorted perceptions or emotions. These symptoms must persist for at least 30 days following the traumatic event. The prevalence of PTSD in children is thought to be less than 0.5%, while for adolescents, that rate may be as high as 5%.

## ETIOLOGY

Anxiety disorders result from the interaction of genetic predisposition and environmental effects. Research has suggested an association between the 5-HTTLPR polymorphism and avoidance, but genetic studies overall have been limited and mixed. There is strong familial aggregation for anxiety disorders. Anxiety disorders are more prevalent in first-degree relatives of children with anxiety disorders compared to those of children without an anxiety disorder, although the relative contributions of genes and environmental influence are unclear. With regard to environmental effects, parental factors including modeling of anxious behavior and high parental control have been identified as potential contributors to increased anxiety in childhood. Low perceived control, or the belief that one has little control over one's environment, has also been associated with increased anxiety. More specifically, low perceived control has been found to mediate the relationship between high parental behavioral control and increased anxiety. Future research is needed to understand more clearly the factors that contribute to the onset of anxiety disorders.

## APPROACHES TO SCREENING FOR CHILDHOOD ANXIETY DISORDERS

#### Identifying Symptoms of Anxiety Disorders

Identifying an anxiety disorder in a child or adolescent is often difficult because many hallmark symptoms of anxiety, including anxious cognitions, avoidance, and safety-related behaviors, are unobservable, completed privately, or understood by parents and other adults as "normal." Furthermore, young children often lack the capacity to identify and verbalize anxiety-related thoughts and feelings, and adolescents are frequently embarrassed to acknowledge symptoms of anxiety. As a result, pediatric anxiety disorders go unnoticed and untreated.

Often, the presence of physical symptoms may be the main indicator of a pediatric anxiety disorder. All anxiety disorders can present with a range of impairing physical symptoms (eg, headaches, gastric distress, insomnia, increased or decreased appetite, and increased activity). It is important that when these physical symptoms present themselves, and once medical causes are ruled out, a treating physician looks for the presence of an anxiety disorder. Parents and healthcare providers should consider potential signs, or "red flags" (Table 93-1), that may indicate the presence of each anxiety disorder in children and adolescents.

#### Normative Anxiety versus Anxiety Disorders

It is important for clinicians to distinguish between normal and pathological anxiety, keeping in mind that anxiety is an expected and typical part of development. Normal fear and anxiety follow a predictable course. It is largely understood that children's cognitive development serves to mediate the typical increase and decrease of certain fears and worries. In infancy, toddlerhood, and early childhood, fears may revolve around immediate and concrete threats. With infants exploring their world through direct sensory and motor contact, it follows that their fears may include loud noises and loss of physical contact from their caregivers. At 9 months of age, children are able to differentiate between familiar and unfamiliar faces and may present with typical stranger anxiety and separation concerns. As a child's cognitive and social capacities increase, their fears become more sophisticated and may incorporate anticipatory worries. Common preschool worries can include fears of thunder and lightning, the dark, or animals. Between the ages of 7 and 12, children develop an understanding of cause-and-effect relationships and anticipation of dangerous events. Concerns increasingly include health and harm as well as scrutiny and competence. Elementary school–aged children may present with worries about natural disasters, fears of traumatic events, school anxiety, and imaginary fears including ghosts and monsters. With adolescence, worries include fears of negative evaluations, rejection by peers, and anxiety about performance. Adolescents are also cognitively able to connect their physical symptoms to thoughts of anxiety. This may explain an increased awareness of panic cognitions for the adolescent, such as "fear of going crazy" when describing a panic attack.

Normative fears typically decrease with age and are relatively transient. Conversely, when anxiety becomes maladaptive, they are more persistent and typically interfere with a youth's academic, social, and/or family functioning. With regard to academic functioning, anxiety symptoms may lead to avoidance of schoolwork or even refusal to attend or stay in school. With regard to social functioning, anxiety symptoms may cause youth to avoid interacting with peers, attending social events, or stating their needs to others. With regard to family functioning, a youth's avoidance or need for reassurance may lead to family conflict or stress. Careful assessment of anxiety involves differentiating whether a child's fears are developmentally expected, and whether the worries present with increased frequency, severity, and persistent distress. Table 93-2 summarizes common normative fears and anxiety disorders associated with developmental levels.

#### Speaking with Children and Parents about Anxiety

When assessing for anxiety in youth, there are several factors to consider. First, as discussed earlier, it is important to obtain sufficient information to distinguish between normative fears and an anxiety disorder. The youth's developmental level and distress and impairment caused by anxiety in all areas of his or her life should guide this distinction. Also important to keep in mind is that youth with elevated anxiety often have difficulty describing their symptoms in detail, or may be embarrassed to share their symptoms with others. Providers should expect that youth may be reluctant to discuss anxiety, and will

**TABLE 93-1 OBSERVABLE SIGNS OF ANXIETY DISORDERS IN CHILDREN AND ADOLESCENTS**

| Disorder | Observable Signs |
|---|---|
| Separation anxiety disorder | • Child is overly "clingy" to parent<br>• Child struggles to separate from parents at school arrival or social event<br>• Child frequently calls parents when separated from them<br>• Child requires parents to sleep with him/her |
| Social anxiety disorder | • Child avoids participating in class and avoids certain classes<br>• Child sits alone at lunch, recess<br>• Child does not make or attend many social plans<br>• Child avoids speaking to unfamiliar people or attending events in which unfamiliar people will be present<br>• Child refuses to answer telephone or order food from a restaurant |
| Selective mutism | • Child avoids speaking to teacher or classmates<br>• Child does not answer questions asked of him/her<br>• Child speaks to family members at home, but not if less familiar people are present |
| Generalized anxiety disorder | • Child repeatedly asks parents or other adults for reassurance<br>• Child expresses worries that are not developmentally appropriate (eg, finances, terrorism)<br>• Child endorses frequent stomachaches, headaches, muscle tension, or difficulty sleeping |
| Specific phobia | • Child avoids situations that most same-aged peers typically face<br>• Child avoids eating due to fear of vomiting or choking<br>• Child refuses to visit pediatrician due to fear of injection<br>• Child refuses to sleep alone or attend movies due to fear of darkness<br>• Child becomes highly anxious when anticipating feared situations or objects |
| Panic disorder | • Child complains of episodes of intense anxiety or physical symptoms (e.g., racing heart, sweating, nausea, dizziness)<br>• Child avoids places in which he/she fears he/she will not be able to get help if anxious |
| Post-traumatic stress disorder | • Child exhibits marked change in mood or affect following a traumatic event<br>• Child avoids all reminders of a traumatic event he/she experienced or witnessed<br>• Child becomes more distant from family members or friends<br>• Child loses interest in activities<br>• Child demonstrates markedly increased vigilance or startle reflex |
| Obsessive-compulsive disorder | • Child expresses concerns that appear excessive or illogical, such as contracting germs from casual contact or causing harm to others<br>• Child engages in actions repeatedly, such as washing/cleaning, checking, arranging, repeating tasks, or seeking reassurance, and finds it difficult to stop<br>• Child becomes upset with parents or others who interrupt repeated actions, or who fail to assist in repeated actions |

often underreport anxiety symptoms. Furthermore, given the heritability of anxiety disorders, the provider should be mindful that parents may also suffer from anxiety, and that parental anxiety may impact the presentation of a youth's symptoms.

Providers should ask open-ended questions of the child and parents to increase the likelihood of accurate responses, and to build a sense of collaboration between provider and the child and family. It is further recommended that providers normalize the experience of anxiety by

**TABLE 93-2 COMMON NORMATIVE FEARS AND ANXIETY DISORDERS ASSOCIATED WITH AGE**

| Age | Common Fears | Anxiety Disorders |
|---|---|---|
| Infancy/toddlerhood, 0–3 years | Stranger anxiety<br>Separation anxiety<br>Fear of thunder, lightning, darkness, animals | Specific phobias<br>Separation anxiety disorder |
| Early childhood, 4–5 years | Fear of death and dying<br>Being kidnapped<br>Blood | Specific phobias<br>Separation anxiety disorder |
| Elementary school age, 5–10 years | Fear of specific objects (animals, monsters, ghosts)<br>Fear of natural disasters (accidents, traumatic events)<br>Germs, disease<br>School anxiety | Generalized anxiety disorder<br>Obsessive-compulsive disorder |
| Adolescence, 12–18 years | Rejection from peers | Social anxiety<br>Panic disorder |

explaining that all individuals experience anxiety, and that anxiety can often be helpful in keeping us safe from danger. A fire alarm analogy may benefit youth and parents: Just like a fire alarm may be set off by burning food or steam from the shower, our anxiety system can sometimes be set off by people or situations that are not actually dangerous. Finally, providers should keep in mind that pediatric anxiety disorders may manifest via physical symptoms, and they should consider an anxiety disorder if youth complain of physical symptoms that are not explained by a medical problem.

Providing basic psychoeducation to youth and families about anxiety can also aid discussion of anxiety symptoms and provide some relief to youth and parents. It is often helpful to share that (1) anxiety disorders are common among children and adolescents, (2) anxiety disorders are not the fault of the child or parents but instead are similar to a medical problem that requires appropriate treatment, and (3) there are helpful treatments for anxiety disorders, including psychosocial interventions and medication.

### Available Screening Measures

Early and routine screening during primary care visits can assist with early detection and intervention of anxiety disorders. Agreement between child- and parent-reports of anxiety symptoms are typically low, although agreement is higher for observable symptoms (eg, presence of compulsions) compared to nonobservable symptoms (eg, worry). As a result, the gold standard assessment includes multi-informant feedback from the child, parent/caregiver, and teachers, as appropriate. Self-report and caregiver rating scales for anxiety can assist clinicians in screening for anxiety symptoms at baseline and monitor response to treatment. Furthermore, self-reports are helpful in identifying anxiety in children who are less inclined to discuss their symptoms during the clinical examination. Follow-up discussions that elaborate on endorsed items on the self-report rating scale invite a youth to further elaborate on a symptom they may have otherwise minimized or downplayed during an interview. Table 93-3 provides a description of the most commonly used self-report and parent-report rating scales for assessment of anxiety symptoms in children and adolescents.

### Differential Diagnosis

Anxiety disorders have been reported to have a significant degree of inter-anxiety (homotypic) and heterotypic comorbidity. By late adolescence and young adulthood, comorbidity is common for youth affected with an anxiety disorder. With respect to heterotypic comorbidity, pediatric anxiety is a significant predictor of adult anxiety disorders, depression, and substance use problems. There is also an association between a higher number of anxiety disorders and an increased risk for heterotypic comorbidity later in life. In a 21-year

**TABLE 93-3 MEASURES TO ASSESS ANXIETY IN CHILDREN AND ADOLESCENTS**

*Anxiety: Questionnaires*

| Instrument (Author) | Construct(s) Assessed | Recommended Age Range | Time Period Assessed | Time to Complete | Version: Items (Long/Short) | Response Format | Scoring/Reports | Any Cost? |
|---|---|---|---|---|---|---|---|---|
| Revised Children's Manifest Anxiety Scale, Second Edition (RCMAS-2); Reynolds & Richmond, 2008 | Total anxiety; 3 subscales: physiological anxiety, worry, social anxiety; also assesses "defensiveness" (lie scale) and has "inconsistent reporting index" | 6–19 years | Not specified; current; "true of you" trait | 10–15 minutes | Youth: 49/10 | Each item rated true or not true | Sum of items; total scores with cutoff points | Yes; published by WPS |
| Multidimensional Anxiety Scale for Children (MASC); March et al., 1997 | Anxiety symptoms; 4 factors: physical symptoms, social anxiety, harm avoidance, separation anxiety | 8–19 years | "Recently" | < 15 minutes | Youth: 50/10<br>Parent: 50 | Each item rated on 4-point scale ranging from "never true about me" to "often true about me" | Sum of items; T-score cutoffs for different severity levels and for "caseness" | Yes; published by Multi-Health Systems |
| Screen for Child Anxiety Related Emotional Disorders (SCARED); Birmaher et al., 1999 | Anxiety disorder, including school avoidance | 9–19 years | Last 3 months | 10–15 minutes | Youth and parent: 41/5 | Each item rated on 3-point scale: "not true," "sometimes true," "very true" | Total scores with recommended cutoff points by age/gender | No; available at www.psychiatry.pitt.edu/research/tools-research/assessment-instruments |
| Spence Children's Anxiety Scale (SCAS); Spence, 1998 | Anxiety disorders | 7–17 years | Not specified; current (items written in present tense) | 10 minutes | Youth and parent: 38 | Each item rated on 4-point scale ranging from "never" to "always"; some items reverse scored | Sum of items; subscale scores for specific anxiety disorder given | No; available at www.scaswebsite.com |
| Revised Child Anxiety and Depression Scales (RCADS); Chorpita et al., 2000 | Anxiety disorder; depression | Grades 3–12 | Not specified; current (items written in present tense) | 10 minutes | Youth and parent: 47 | Each item comprises 4 statements of increasing intensity /severity (never to always) | Sum of items; T-score from appropriate grade level | No; available from authors, www.childfirst.ucla.edu |

*Anxiety: Clinician-Administered Measures*

| Instrument (Author) | Construct(s) Assessed | Age Range | Time Period Assessed | Time to Complete | Informant: Items (Long/Short) | Response Format | Scoring/Reports | Any cost? |
|---|---|---|---|---|---|---|---|---|
| Hamilton Anxiety Rating Scale (HAM-A); Hamilton, 1959 | Psychic anxiety (mental agitation and psychological distress) and somatic anxiety (physical complaints related to anxiety) | Children, adolescents, adults | Current (not specified) | 10–15 minutes | Youth only: 14 items | Each item has 4 statements of increasing intensity/severity (none to severe) | Sum of items; suggested cutoffs for different severity levels and for "caseness" | No, public domain |
| Pediatric Anxiety Rating Scale (PARS); RUPP Anxiety Study Group, 2002 | Anxiety symptoms and impairment for social phobia, separation anxiety, generalized anxiety disorder | 6–17 years | Last week | < 20 minutes | Youth and parent: 50 symptom items; 7 global items | Each symptom item scored as present or absent (yes/no); global ratings rated by clinician on 7 dimensions of severity using a 6-point scale of increasing severity | Total score is sum of 7 global severity items | No; obtain information and scale from Mark Riddle, MD, mriddle1@jhmi.edu |

DSM, *Diagnostic and Statistical Manual of Mental Disorders.*

longitudinal study in New Zealand, significant associations were found between the number of anxiety disorders reported and the risk for anxiety disorders, major depression, substance use, and suicidal behavior. Additionally, the authors found an association between the number of anxiety disorders and educational underachievement and teen pregnancy. As individuals present with a higher number of comorbid anxiety disorders, there is an increased risk for depression. Interestingly, however, earlier onset of anxiety disorders has not been found to confer an increased risk for depression. With respect to treatment response, comorbid anxiety and depression in children and adolescents is often associated with increased symptom severity and treatment resistance. With respect to behavioral disorders, 20% to 40% percent of children and adolescents with ADHD have comorbid anxiety. Anxiety disorders are often more challenging to identify in this population, as the disruptive behaviors are often the chief complaint and reason for referral. Parent reports may be skewed with respect to the more outward and disruptive observable behaviors. Children with comorbid anxiety and ADHD may also uniquely present with increased working memory deficits and with less hyperactivity. Continued careful assessment that includes self-report of internalizing symptoms for children is important in capturing the full picture of ADHD and potential mood or anxiety symptoms.



## TREATMENT APPROACHES

### Psychotherapy

The front-line evidence-based psychotherapy for anxiety disorders in children and adolescents is cognitive behavioral therapy (CBT). Numerous studies have noted the efficacy of CBT. Approximately two-thirds of children treated with CBT report significant relief and improvement. Cognitive behavioral therapy is time-limited, with treatment typically lasting for 16 to 20 weeks, followed by monthly booster sessions. Cognitive behavioral therapy involves the use of specific strategies and practices to reduce anxiety. The clinician focuses on restructuring maladaptive cognitions, reducing avoidant or anxiety-related behaviors, and guiding the child or adolescent in more consistently facing feared situations. Concepts and skills are taught through active instruction, role-playing, and both in- and out-of-session practice.

The components of CBT for childhood anxiety disorders include (1) psychoeducation; (2) self-monitoring of anxiety symptoms; (3) the examination and restructuring of cognitive errors that occur as a result of feeling anxious (eg, "black-and-white thinking," "catastrophizing," and "mind reading"); and (4) repeated exposure to people, places, or situations that are feared and avoided (eg, engagement in social situations, separating from primary caregiver). Additional strategies include relaxation techniques such as deep breathing, imagery, and progressive muscle relaxation. Problem-solving and communication skills may also be taught, depending on the presentation and needs of the child.

**Psychoeducation** Psychoeducation involves teaching youth and caregivers about anxiety disorders and their treatment. A therapist typically reviews the role of normative anxiety (eg, fight-or-flight response) and distinguishes between adaptive and maladaptive levels of and responses to anxiety. Children are further informed that anxiety disorders are common and treatable. A therapist often reviews the interrelationships between thoughts, feelings, and behaviors, and spells out that treatment will target each of these components to reduce anxiety. This component of treatment should also focus on the role of avoidance in maintaining anxiety, and should provide a rationale for repeated exposure to feared situations. Finally, the goals for treatment are discussed, which generally relate to the overarching goal of more consistently facing feared situations to reduce overall anxiety.

**Self-monitoring** The next stage of treatment involves information gathering via self-monitoring: (1) Which situations trigger anxiety? (2) How does the child respond to that trigger? (3) What physical symptoms does the child experience? (4) What thoughts does the child experience when anxious? The therapist works with the child to identify the cognitions and behaviors that contribute to anxiety maintenance.

**Cognitive Restructuring** Based on information gathered from self-monitoring, the therapist and child identify common thoughts that the child experiences when feeling anxious. The therapist and child then generate more realistic or alternative thoughts, either by examining the evidence for and against the thoughts (eg, the likelihood that the event will happen), determining the function of the thoughts and how to better manage them (eg, distancing oneself from the thoughts, talking back to the thoughts, seeing the thoughts as false alarms), or playing out the thoughts to the worst outcome (eg, using a "downward arrow" technique to identify a feared outcome). Often, coping statements or more rational responses are created and rehearsed in response to different situations. For younger children, cognitive restructuring may be limited to generating simple coping statements.

**Exposure to Feared Situations** To modify learned associations with feared and avoided situations, youth are encouraged to begin gradually and repeatedly facing feared and avoided situations. The facing of a feared situation is referred to as an *exposure*. In preparation for completing exposures, the therapist and the youth (and the caregiver, if appropriate) collaboratively create a list of anxiety-provoking situations and rate the child's anxiety in each proposed situations. With guidance and support from the therapist, the youth begins to engage in exposures both in and out of therapy sessions. For instance, a child with social anxiety disorder will practice facing feared social situations, such as initiating conversations with others, asking questions of unfamiliar people, or engaging in mildly embarrassing behavior. Cognitions experienced during the exposure are also reviewed and challenged as necessary, and coping statements may be used to help encourage the youth to successfully complete the exposure. As treatment progresses, the youth gradually and repeatedly faces all situations typically avoided due to anxiety, making sure to monitor and eliminate any behaviors that seek safety (eg, compulsions, reassurance seeking), as these behaviors reduce the efficacy of the exposures.

**Family Involvement** Treatment almost always involves the use of family/caregivers; the extent of caregiver involvement depends on the anxiety presentation and age of the youth, with caregiver involvement being essential with younger children. At minimum, psychoeducation is provided to family members (including siblings if needed) to (1) increase understanding of the child's anxiety; (2) increase support of the child, particularly as the child progresses through treatment; and (3) discuss appropriate ways in which the family can respond to the child's anxiety. The therapist may also need to work in greater depth with the child's family. Caregiver goals may be to minimize accommodations to anxiety, to model approach behavior versus avoidance, and to structure the parent's/caregiver's role of co-therapist in the home. Another common form of family involvement includes the use of reinforcement strategies, to reward exposure to feared situations, which helps to engage children in treatment and support their efforts.

### Medication

Well-delivered CBT is effective and recommended as a first-line treatment option for mild to moderate anxiety symptoms. However, it can be difficult to access CBT due to cost and/or lack of availability. Also, youth may be unable to successfully engage in CBT due to a number of factors, such as severity of symptoms, parental accommodation of anxiety symptoms, and comorbid diagnoses. Medication treatment, and specifically the class of antidepressants referred to as selective serotonin reuptake inhibitors (SSRIs), are considered first-line treatment as a monotherapy and in combination with CBT for pediatric anxiety disorders (Table 93-4). In cases of moderate to severe anxiety, CBT together with SSRI treatment is the optimal approach.

When a child begins a course of SSRI treatment, it is initially started at a low dose to assess tolerability. It is important for the provider to increase the dose to an adequate level to ensure treatment success while assessing carefully for adverse events. Dose increases should be made after the provider has assessed the child's level of response as well as tolerability of the medication. The adage "start low and go slow" is helpful to keep in mind when considering a course of SSRI treatment in youth. However, it is very important to achieve an

**TABLE 93-4 MEDICATIONS APPROVED FOR ANXIETY DISORDERS IN CHILDREN AND ADOLESCENTS**

| Generic Name (Brand Name) | Subclass | Dosing | FDA-Approved Uses | Ages | Additional Information |
|---|---|---|---|---|---|
| Fluoxetine (Prozac) | SSRI | 20–60 mg/d<br>Start 10 mg/d, increase to 20 mg/d on day 14 | OCD | 7 y and older | Long half-life (4–6 d)<br>Available in liquid form |
| Sertraline (Zoloft) | SSRI | 25–200 mg/d<br>Start at 25 mg/d and increase to 50 mg after 7 days; increase to 50 mg and then may increase every 4 weeks | OCD | 6 y and older | Available in liquid form |
| Fluvoxamine (Luvox) | SSRI | 50–200 mg/d<br>Oral daily dosing to twice/day<br>Start 25 mg at bedtime, increase by 25 mg/d q4–7 d; maximum dose is 200 mg/d up to 11 y, 300 mg/d for > 11 y | OCD | 8 y and older | |
| Duloxetine (Cymbalta) | SNRI | 30–60 mg/d<br>Start 30 mg/d; may increase by 30 mg/d after 2 weeks | GAD | 7 y and older | Used for treatment of neuropathic pain in adults |
| Clomipramine (Anafranil) | TCA | 100–200 mg at bedtime<br>Start 25 mg qd, increase by 25 mg/d q4–7 days; maximum 3 mg/kg/d up to 100 mg/d in first 2 wk and up to 200 mg/d maintainance | OCD | 10 y and older | |

GAD, generalized anxiety disorder; OCD, obsessive-compulsive disorder; q4–7, every 4 to 7; qd, once daily; SNRI, serotonin norepinephrine reuptake inhibitor; SSRI, selective serotonin reuptake inhibitor; TCA, tricyclic antidepressant.

adequate dose range, especially if the child remains symptomatic. It can be demoralizing for a child to be inadequately treated, leading to lack of response and delayed relief from symptoms. The most common adverse side effects associated with SSRI medications include headaches, upset stomach, diarrhea, and nausea. Weight gain is also a possible side effect, and weight should be monitored regularly. Adolescents should be made aware of the possibility of sexual side effects with SSRI treatment, and providers should inquire about sexual side effects during follow-up visits. Most side effects resolve over time, usually after 2 to 4 weeks, and it is helpful to maintain an inventory of physical symptoms that are reported at each visit. In addition, severity level of anxiety symptoms should be systematically assessed prior to medication initiation and subsequently at follow-up visits.

Family history of anxiety disorders may help guide medication choices based on treatment response by family members. Prescribers will also need to discuss the US Food and Drug Administration black box warning for antidepressants. It advises clinicians to monitor patients for increased risks of suicidality in children, adolescents, and young adults (under the age of 24 years) especially during the beginning of pharmacological treatment and during dose changes. It has been well documented that the benefits of treatment with antidepressant medications outweigh the risks. Another important recommendation is for the medication to be taken around the same time every day.

During the first 1 to 2 months of treatment with an SSRI, weekly or biweekly visits are recommended. If an actual visit is not possible, follow-up phone calls may be used. During follow-up visits, the prescriber should consider the following: (1) evaluate for side effects and medication tolerability, (2) assess for improvement and also signs of worsening, (3) assess adherence with medication and psychotherapy appointments, and (4) examine new and ongoing psychosocial stressors since last visit. The provider may also consider adjusting the timing of medication administration (eg, morning versus evening) based on side-effect occurrence, such as sedation or activation. Psychoeducation about developmentally normal fears and worries, anxiety disorders, and their treatment should be ongoing.

When the presenting anxiety is severe, or if insomnia due to anxiety is unresponsive to a behavioral sleep hygiene approach, youth may benefit from the short-term use of a low dose of diphenhydramine (Benadryl). If diphenhydramine is not effective, a benzodiazepine such as clonazepam is an alternative option, during the initial 4 to 6 weeks of treatment with an SSRI.

A therapeutic trial for SSRI medication is defined as a time frame of 8 to 16 weeks, during which treatment is provided at the maximum dose tolerated by the patient. If there is no improvement in symptoms after this time period, the provider should reassess for medication adherence, diagnosis, and comorbidities, and should consider the initiation of CBT if it has not been initiated previously. For patients who have not responded to an adequate medication trial, it is reasonable to consider a trial with a different SSRI. Another class of medications known as serotonin norepinephrine reuptake inhibitors (SNRIs; eg, duloxetine) are considered a third-line option following 2 adequate courses of an SSRI. For obsessive-compulsive disorder, clomipramine, which is a tricyclic antidepressant, is commonly used as a third-line option following 2 adequate trials of a SSRI. Clomipramine requires additional medical monitoring, including electrocardiograms at baseline, during titration, and at the maximum dose. Also, there is a therapeutic blood level that can be monitored.

It is recommended that an efficacious medication trial continue for 6 to 12 months after resolution of symptoms. Providers should consider delaying discontinuation if a youth is undergoing a life transition or potential stressor, such as a new academic year or moving away to college. Doses of SSRI medication should be tapered off gradually over several weeks to prevent discontinuation symptoms. Providers should schedule monthly follow-up visits for at least 1 to 2 months after the medication is discontinued in order to assess symptoms of discontinuation or relapse of symptoms.

## SUGGESTED READINGS

Beesdo K, Knappe S, Pine DS. Anxiety and anxiety disorders in children and adolescents: developmental issues and implications for DSM-V. *Psychiatr Clin North Am.* 2009;32(3):483-524.

Benjamin CL, Harrison JP, Settipani CA, Brodman DM, Kendall PC. Anxiety and related outcomes in young adults 7 to 19 years after receiving treatment for child anxiety. *J Consult Clin Psychol.* 2013;81(5):865-876.

Connolly SD, Bernstein GA. Practice parameter for the assessment and treatment of children and adolescents with anxiety disorders. *J Am Acad Child Adolesc Psychiatry.* 2007;46(2):267-283.

Essau C, Petermann F. *Anxiety Disorders in Children and Adolescents: Epidemiology, Risk Factors and Treatment.* 14th ed. New York, NY: Psychology Press; 2014:219-260.

Ginsburg GS, Drake KL, Tein JY, Teetsel R, Riddle MA. Preventing onset of anxiety disorders in offspring of anxious parents: a randomized controlled trial of a family-based intervention. *Am J Psychiatry.* 2015;172(12):1207-1214.

Ginsburg GS, Kendall PC, Sakolsky D, et al. Remission after acute treatment in children and adolescents with anxiety disorders: findings from the CAMS. *J Consult Clin Psychol.* 2011;79(6): 806-813.

Higa-McMillan CK, Francis SE, Rith-Najarian L, Chorpita BF. Evidence base update: 50 years of research on treatment for child and adolescent anxiety. *J Clin Child Adolesc Psychol.* 2015;45(2)91-113.

Pine DS, Klein RG. Anxiety disorders. In: Thapar A, Pine DS, Leckman JF, Scott S, Snowling MJ, Taylor EA, eds. *Rutter's Child and Adolescent Psychiatry.* 6th ed. London, UK: Wiley-Blackwell; 2015:822-840.

Rynn MA, Vidair H, Blackford J, eds. Anxiety disorders. *Child Adolesc Psychiatr Clin North Am.* 2012;21(3):457-702.

Walkup JT, Albano AM, Piacentini J, et al. Cognitive behavioral therapy, sertraline, or a combination in childhood anxiety. *N Engl J Med.* 2008;359:2753-2766.

Weisz JR, Chorpita BF, Palinkas LA, et al. Testing standard and modular designs for psychotherapy treating depression, anxiety, and conduct problems in youth: a randomized effectiveness trial. *Arch Gen Psych.* 2012;69(3):274-282.



# 94 Pediatric Depression and Bipolar Spectrum Disorders

Kirti Saxena, Rajniderpal Kaur, and Ajay Shah

## INTRODUCTION

Affect regulation is a developmental acquisition that is impacted by environmental factors. For clinicians caring for children and adolescents, it is important to differentiate between normal mood fluctuations and emotions and pervasive mood disorders that significantly impact the child's global functioning. A careful clinical assessment is necessary to make the diagnosis of mood disorders in children and adolescents, as there are no laboratory or neuroimaging tests that will ascertain the diagnosis. The clinical diagnosis of mood disorders is supported by research data obtained in epidemiological and longitudinal studies, as well as by clinical observations.

This chapter discusses how clinical diagnosis of both depressive and bipolar spectrum disorders is made based on the best available evidence. Additionally, this chapter provides an overview of both psychopharmacologic and psychotherapeutic treatments of depressive and bipolar spectrum disorders.

## EPIDEMIOLOGY

In the *Diagnostic and Statistical Manual of Mental Disorders*, 5th edition (DSM-V), the pediatric depressive disorders include disruptive mood dysregulation disorder (DMDD), major depressive disorder (MDD), persistent depressive disorder, and premenstrual dysphoric disorder. Within the DSM-V, the bipolar disorders include bipolar I disorder, bipolar II disorder, cyclothymic disorder, and unspecified bipolar disorder.

Prevalence of MDD in children ranges between 0.5% and 1.4% and increases to 11.4% in adolescents, with a male-to-female ratio of 1:1 during childhood and 1:3 during adolescence. The risk for MDD increases significantly after puberty, particularly in females. Disruptive mood dysregulation disorder is a relatively new diagnosis in the DSM-V; hence, the prevalence of this illness has not been clearly established. However, epidemiological studies that used criteria of DMDD retrospectively found the prevalence to range between 0.8% and 3.3%. The rate of DMDD is shown to be higher in males and school-aged children compared to females and adolescents. Studies have found the rate of bipolar spectrum disorders to be as high as 6.7%, with lifetime prevalence of mania to be between 0.1% and 1.7% among adolescents. Bipolar spectrum disorders have a male-to-female ratio of 1:1 throughout the life cycle.

## DIAGNOSING MOOD DISORDERS

### Presentation of Mood Disorder Symptoms

The DSM-V has clearly defined criteria for diagnosing depression and bipolar disorders in adults, children, and adolescents. There are no separate criteria for mood disorders in the pediatric population. However, the manifestations and presentation of mood symptoms in children and adolescents differ from those of adults. These differences likely result from the developmental and neurodevelopmental differences between adults and children in the emotional, cognitive, and physical domains. Therefore, although the DSM-V criteria are utilized to make a diagnosis of a mood disorder in a child or adolescent, clinicians must be aware of the impact of development on the presentation of mood disorders in the pediatric population.

For instance, when children experience depression, parents, caregivers, and schoolteachers may notice the child being more withdrawn; crying more easily and more than usual; complaining of stomachaches, headaches, or other somatic complaints; refusing to go to school; having significant changes in peer relationships; and having new behavioral problems. Children may have a decline in school performance, which may be due to difficulty concentrating related to depressed mood, and they may complain of boredom, which may suggest anhedonia. Also, children may view themselves in a negative light. Therefore, to make an evaluation of depression in a child, the clinician needs to be aware of the changes that have been and are occurring in the child's daily routine. This can assist the clinician in making a DSM-V diagnosis of a depressive disorder.

It is not uncommon for youth with mood lability, anger, and aggression to be considered for a diagnosis of bipolar disorder. Clinicians must explore the duration and quality of these symptoms while considering a diagnosis of a mood disorder in these youngsters.

### DSM-V Diagnostic Criteria for Depression and Bipolar Spectrum Disorders

**Criteria for Depressive Disorders** The criteria for a major depressive episode requires the presence of 5 or more of the following symptoms during a 2-week period: depressed mood, loss of interest/pleasure, changes in appetite or weight, sleep disturbance such as insomnia or hypersomnia, psychomotor retardation/agitation, diminished energy, diminished concentration, feelings of guilt or worthlessness, and recurrent thoughts of death or suicidal ideations. One of these symptoms must be either depressed mood or loss of interest/pleasure. The symptoms also must lead to significant impairment in important areas of functioning, and must not be related to the effects of a drug/substance or another medical condition.

Disruptive mood dysregulation disorder is classified as a depressive disorder in which children or adolescents have persistently irritable or angry mood nearly every day, and in which temper outbursts occur 3 or more times per week. These outbursts are disproportionate to the situation and developmental level of the child. The above characteristics must all be present for 12 months, and there cannot be a 3-month or longer duration in which these symptoms have not occurred. These characteristics must also occur in at least 2 different settings (eg, school and home), and the diagnosis can only be made for children between the ages of 6 and 18 years. These symptoms must be unrelated to that of a hypomanic, manic, or major depressive episode, and must not be better accounted for by another mental disorder or be related to the effects of a drug/substance or medical condition.

**Criteria for Bipolar I and II Disorders** For a diagnosis of bipolar I disorder, the child needs to have an elevated, expansive, or irritable mood and increased goal-directed activity or energy that lasts for at least 1 week and is present almost every day for most of the day. Together with the change in mood and energy, 3 of the following symptoms (or 4, if mood is irritable) need to be present: inflated self-esteem or grandiosity; decreased need for sleep; increased talkativeness; flight of ideas; distractibility; increased goal-directed activity (eg, at school, outside of school in the form of hypersexual behaviors) or psychomotor agitation (that is, purposeless non–goal-directed activity); or excessive involvement in activities that can lead to poor consequences (eg, spending too much money, being involved in behaviors of a sexual nature). These mood changes lead to significant disturbance in social and occupational functioning and may require hospitalization. The mood changes are not due to the effects of a drug of abuse, medications, or another medical illness.

To make a diagnosis of bipolar II disorder, the child or adolescent needs to have met criteria for a hypomanic episode. The symptoms of mania and hypomania are the same as noted above, except that a hypomanic episode lasts for at least 4 days. A manic episode must last for at least a week. In hypomania, the mood disturbance is not severe enough to lead to a marked impairment in overall functioning or to require hospitalization.

If psychotic symptoms are present during the mood changes, then the episode is defined as a manic episode with psychotic features.

#### Differential Diagnosis and Comorbidity

Both depression and bipolar disorders have symptoms that can overlap with other psychiatric disorders. These include oppositional defiant disorder, substance use disorders, post-traumatic stress disorder, adjustment disorder, and bereavement. Irritability is a symptom that is present across psychiatric illnesses. Therefore, whenever irritability is prominent in a child or adolescent, it is imperative to explore whether it is due to anxiety, substance use, a mood disorder, or another psychiatric disorder.

Mood disorders can occur due to medical conditions. Depression secondary to medical illnesses includes hypothyroidism, mononucleosis, anemia, and autoimmune diseases. Hyperthyroidism may mimic manic symptoms. Additionally, certain medications such as stimulants, corticosteroids, and contraceptives can cause side effects that overlap with symptoms of depression. Therefore, a complete medical evaluation is always necessary to rule out medical conditions as the cause of mood symptoms. However, chronic conditions such as juvenile diabetes, leukemia, and mood disorders (commonly depression) may need treatment with psychotherapeutic or psychopharmacological interventions.

When a child or adolescent presents with mood symptoms, it can be difficult to differentiate between a depressive disorder, a bipolar depressive disorder, or even mania/hypomania. It is important to gather information about the course of illness to assess the presence of manic/hypomanic episodes, family history of psychiatric illnesses, and the level of functional impairment. For instance, youth with bipolar disorder are more likely to have a strong family history of bipolar disorder, greater levels of dysfunction in family relationships and occupational functioning, and prior psychiatric hospitalizations. Other indicators for bipolar disorder include a history of psychotic symptoms or medication-induced mania. Several symptoms of attention-deficit/hyperactivity disorder (ADHD) overlap with bipolar symptoms, such as distractibility, increased talkativeness, and increased energy levels. In ADHD, these symptoms are persistently present during the course of the illness. However, since bipolar disorder is an episodic mood disorder, in youth with bipolar disorder, these symptoms are also episodic in nature. On the other hand, depressed youth may present with symptoms of inattentiveness, such as difficulty with sustaining attention, absent-mindedness, and avoidance of tasks that require mental effort. In such cases, it is important to ascertain whether the youth met criteria for ADHD prior to the onset of the depressive episode.

Most cases of MDD are associated with psychiatric comorbidity. It is estimated that up to 40% to 90% of youth with a diagnosis of MDD will have a comorbid psychiatric disorder. Anxiety and disruptive behavior disorders are commonly associated with MDD, with a 4-fold increased risk. Additionally, ADHD and substance use disorders are associated with MDD, with a 3-fold increased risk. The rate of comorbidity is extremely high in youth with DMDD, which is most commonly associated with oppositional defiant disorder. Bipolar disorder frequently co-occurs with ADHD, with risk being as high as 69%. Other disorders that are common comorbidities in adolescents with bipolar disorder include conduct disorder and substance abuse.

## PATHOGENESIS

The pathogenesis of affective illnesses is best conceptualized as an interaction between individual genetic vulnerabilities and exposure to adverse life events. The prevalence of a first-degree parent with depression is 30% to 50% in depressed youth, suggesting a strong genetic predisposition for this illness. Similarly, twin and family studies have shown high heritability of bipolar disorder. About 30% to 50% of patients with bipolar disorder have a first-degree relative with a bipolar spectrum illness. Other studies have suggested a heritability rate of 0.8.

Environmental factors, such as exposure to negative adverse childhood events, can influence the development of mood disorders. In fact, research has shown that genes are highly regulated by environmental signals throughout childhood development. Stressful events such as losses, abuse, neglect, and interpersonal conflict can moderate or mediate the onset and recurrence of depression. The effect of these stressors is an interplay between a child's negative attributional styles for interpreting and coping with stress, the availability of a caregiver's support, and genetic factors.

With the advances in brain imaging technology, there has been an increasing interest in the study of the neurobiological underpinnings of mood disorders. Studies conducted by Rao have shown that depressed adolescents and those at high risk for depression have significantly smaller left and right hippocampal volumes in comparisons to healthy controls. Furthermore, smaller hippocampal volumes were associated with higher levels of early-life adversity. Imaging studies conducted on bipolar youth have shown decreased total cerebral and smaller hippocampal volumes.

## ASSESSMENT OF YOUTH WITH MOOD DISORDERS

The assessment of a youth presenting with mood concerns can be summarized to include 3 main components. The first is screening for the presence of mood symptoms in a developmentally sensitive manner. When assessing the pediatric population for mental illness, it is important to obtain information from multiple sources to help develop an accurate picture of the illness and its course. The primary sources for information include (but are not limited to) the caretakers, the teachers, and the patient. Caretakers are better able to provide information pertaining to the onset of the illness and the external manifestations of mood disorders such as disruptive behaviors, sleep or appetite changes, decline in school performances, and increased isolation. It is important for the clinician to keep in mind the possibility that the caretaker's own psychopathology may influence their report of symptoms.

Adolescents should be interviewed alone to help develop rapport. Matters pertaining to confidentially should be discussed with adolescents at the beginning of the interview. Clinicians have the right to preserve confidentiality when working with the pediatric population as determined by state law. Children may have difficulty articulating their internal emotional state, reinforcing the importance that the clinician be attuned to the observable manifestations of mood disorders and the level of impairment.

Secondly, the diagnosis of mental illnesses is typically based on clinical presentation. Rating scales can be used to help assess the severity of symptoms and guide clinical management. Clinician-based rating scales include the Children's Depression Rating Scale, Revised, and the Young Mania Rating Scale. Parent-completed rating scales include the Child Behavior Checklist (which assesses for internalizing and externalizing disorders), the Child Mania Rating Scale, and the Quick Inventory of Depressive Symptoms. No laboratory tests are currently available to assist clinicians in making a diagnosis of a mood disorder.

Lastly, youth presenting with mood concerns should be assessed for the presence of suicidal ideation, self-injurious behaviors, and homicidal ideations (discussed further below). Preventing access to means of suicide is a vital suicide prevention strategy in adolescents.

Studies have shown that the presence of firearms in households increases the risk of adolescent suicide, and restricting the access to firearms reduces this risk. It is important to differentiate suicidal behavior from other forms of self-injurious behaviors. Youth who engage in self-injurious behaviors may do so with the intent to find relief from a negative affective state versus intent to end their life.

## TREATMENT OF DEPRESSION AND BIPOLAR SPECTRUM DISORDERS

Mental health disorders are among the leading causes of disability in the United States, making their recognition and treatment imperative. Approximately 20% of youth in America struggle with mental health concerns, and about 50% of all lifetime cases of mental health begin by age 14. Of note, mood disorders are a significant public health concern, as they account for extensive long-term morbidity. As primary care providers, pediatricians are required to screen for and address many issues within limited appointment times, often making mental health screening difficult. However, pediatricians are often the first line for families and patients struggling with mental health concerns, making it even more important for pediatricians to be well versed in recognizing depression and bipolar disorder, and knowing when to treat and when to refer.

Pediatricians may be hesitant to prescribe psychotropic medications to children and adolescents secondary to concerns over side effects or inexperience with treatment options, choosing instead to refer to a child and adolescent psychiatrist. However, due to the difficulty in accessing a child psychiatrist, it will be helpful for pediatricians to become familiar with the initial management of depressive and bipolar disorders in order to prevent delays of treatment and subsequent treatment resistance. Delays in treatment can lead to substantial sequelae such as worsening comorbid psychiatric issues, substance use, and decreased self-esteem. The content below provides guidelines for pediatricians aimed at the initial management of mood disorders.



### Depression

The management of depression in children and adolescents involves medications, psychosocial interventions such as psychoeducation for parents and school personnel, and psychotherapy. Selective serotonin reuptake inhibitors (SSRIs) are first-line medications for the treatment of depressive disorders. Their mechanism of action is thought to be primarily at the site of the serotonin transporter on the presynaptic terminal, inactivating it, thus preventing the reabsorption of serotonin back into the presynaptic terminal. This allows for higher levels of serotonin to bind to the postsynaptic serotonin receptor. There are 5 SSRIs used commonly in adults for depressive disorders; however, only 2 of them are approved for depression in children and adolescents. Fluoxetine, the oldest SSRI, is still considered the best initial choice for the treatment of depression in youth. Fluoxetine has Food and Drug Administration (FDA) approval for MDD in children and adolescents aged 8 to 18 years. Escitalopram has FDA approval for MDD in adolescents aged 12 to 17. Citalopram and sertraline have been shown to be helpful in pediatric depressive disorders but do not have FDA approval for this use. Paroxetine, although useful in adults, has had limited use in children and adolescents, as initial data regarding suicide risk led to an FDA statement proclaiming paroxetine to be unsafe in children and adolescents. Fluvoxamine, also an SSRI, is more commonly used for obsessive-compulsive disorder, for which it has a pediatric indication. Once a medication is started, pediatricians should be aware of potential side effects and the possibility of worsening thoughts (see below). The FDA recommends contact with patient and family on a weekly basis during the first 4 weeks of treatment, followed by biweekly assessments through week 12.

Psychosocial support plays a strong role in the treatment of depressed children and adolescents. Family support and education about the child's illness are a crucial aspect of treatment. As depression can impact social functioning and lead to symptoms such as lack of motivation, fluctuating energy, and decreased concentration, it is important to make school personnel such as teachers, daycare staff, and other adults involved in the child's life aware of the issues in order to allow for a better understanding of the child and enhanced support in those settings. Psychotherapy has an important role in the management of depression as well. For mild depressive disorders with time-limited stressors, psychotherapy is often the only treatment needed. Cognitive behavioral therapy (CBT) has robust evidence of effectiveness in the treatment of youth with depression. This therapeutic modality focuses on individuals' thoughts, feelings, and actions under the premise that changing maladaptive ways of thinking can change individuals' feelings and behavior patterns. Interpersonal therapy (IPT) is also effective in youth with depression, focusing on interpersonal issues and role transitions that are thought to lead to distress.

Studies have shown that combining medications with psychotherapy is the most effective way to treat pediatric depression. The Treatment for Adolescents with Depression Study (TADS) aimed to examine whether fluoxetine, CBT, or combination therapy was more efficacious. The 12-week data in this study showed response rates of 61% with fluoxetine monotherapy, 43% with CBT only, and 71% with combination therapy. The 36-week data showed that response rates were similar for all 3 interventions with 81% for fluoxetine monotherapy, 81% with CBT only, and 86% with combination therapy. These results suggest that intervention for depression in adolescents can be effective and that combination therapy may lead to a more rapid recovery than either medication or therapy alone. The Treatment of Resistant Depression in Adolescents (TORDIA) study enrolled adolescents aged 12 to 18 who had not responded to an initial trial with an SSRI. These subjects were then divided into the following 4 groups: switch to a different SSRI (paroxetine, citalopram, fluoxetine), switch to a different SSRI plus CBT, switch to venlafaxine, or switch to venlafaxine plus CBT. After 12 weeks, the combination of either an SSRI or venlafaxine with CBT showed the best response rate (54.8%), again providing evidence regarding the importance of combination treatment. The 24-week data from this study showed an overall remission rate of 38.9%, but more importantly, the data showed that the likelihood an adolescent would achieve remission of symptoms was based on how much improvement was noted within the first 12 weeks. This further illustrates the need for pediatricians to be able to detect depressive symptoms and initiate treatment while waiting for an appointment with a child psychiatrist. Treatment for depression can also be done in conjunction with consultation from a child psychiatrist.

### Bipolar Disorder

Bipolar disorder can be a difficult diagnosis to make in children and adolescents. A careful history includes drawing a timeline of mood episodes, demonstrating episodic hypomanic or manic episodes, which can help establish a diagnosis of bipolar disorder. For pediatricians, recognizing manic/hypomanic symptoms and subsequently referring the patient to a child and adolescent psychiatrist for further management is most appropriate. It is still important for pediatricians to be knowledgeable about the treatment options, as a referral may be difficult.

Until recently, pharmacologic treatment of pediatric bipolar disorder had been largely off-label. However, recent FDA-approved medications have expanded treatment options (Table 94-1). Antidepressants are not recommended as monotherapy in patients with bipolar disorder due to the emergence of manic/hypomanic symptoms in these patients. They should be used with caution in any bipolar spectrum patient. Strong therapeutic alliance and rapport between patient and provider also play a significant role in outcomes.

As with depression, psychotherapy in combination with medications is a key component in the treatment of pediatric bipolar spectrum disorders. Several therapies have been shown to be effective in bipolar youth. Family-focused treatment for adolescents (FFT-A), interpersonal social rhythm therapy (IPSRT), child- and family-focused cognitive behavioral therapy (CFF-CBT), multifamily psychoeducational psychotherapy (MF-PEP), and dialectical behavioral therapy (DBT) all have evidence for being helpful in youth with bipolar spectrum disorders.

**TABLE 94-1 FDA-APPROVED MEDICATIONS FOR TREATMENT OF BIPOLAR DISORDER**

| Medication | Indication | Monotherapy or Adjunct | Age Range |
|---|---|---|---|
| Lithium | Bipolar I mania | Monotherapy | 12–17 y |
| | Bipolar I maintenance | | 12–17 y |
| Asenapine | Bipolar I acute manic or mixed | Monotherapy | 10–17 y |
| Aripiprazole | Bipolar I acute manic or mixed | Monotherapy | 10–17 y |
| | Bipolar I acute manic or mixed | Adjunct to lithium or divalproex | 10–17 y |
| | Bipolar I maintenance (prevent recurrence of bipolar disorder) | Both | 10–17 y |
| Quetiapine ER | Bipolar I acute manic | Monotherapy | 10–17 y |
| | Bipolar I acute manic | Adjunct to lithium or divalproex | 10–17 y |
| Olanzapine | Bipolar I acute manic or mixed | Monotherapy | 13–17 y |
| | Bipolar I acute depressive in conjunction with fluoxetine | Note: not considered first line due to weight gain and metabolic concerns | 10–17 y |
| Risperidone | Bipolar I acute manic or mixed | Monotherapy | 10–17 y |

FDA, Food and Drug Administration.

#### Adverse Effects of Medications

Side effects for SSRIs include nausea, gastrointestinal discomfort, constipation/diarrhea, drowsiness, insomnia, akathisia (inner restlessness and inability to sit still), prolonged bleeding time, and sexual dysfunction. The most concerning side effect is the possibility of increased suicidal thinking and behavior, for which the FDA has implemented a black-box warning on all classes of antidepressant medications. It is important to understand that although this is a significant risk and requires close monitoring, far more children and adolescents have shown decreased suicidality following treatment with antidepressants. This was clearly depicted during the initial years following release of the black-box warning, which saw an increase in youth suicide rates.

In addition, SSRIs carry discontinuation-related side effects if medication is stopped abruptly. This can include nausea, headaches, dizziness, sleep dysregulation, agitation, and worsening depression and anxiety. All of the SSRIs should be decreased slowly. Fluoxetine, because it has the longest half-life, can theoretically be stopped without dose reduction, as it is thought to self-taper; however, many child psychiatrists still recommend step-wise dose reduction to minimize chances of discontinuation effects.

Side effects of lithium include nausea, vomiting, constipation, diarrhea, headache, dry mouth, weight gain, tremors, confusion, memory impairment, hypothyroidism, electrocardiogram changes, and nephrogenic diabetes insipidus. Lithium is also teratogenic, leading to an increase in the development of Ebstein anomaly. For this reason, a pregnancy test is recommended in all females of child-bearing age prior to initiation of lithium. Other baseline laboratory tests necessary prior to starting treatment with lithium include the ratio of blood-urea-nitrogen (BUN) to creatinine (Cr), and thyroid-stimulating hormone (TSH), which should also be assessed longitudinally every 3 months initially and approximately every 6 to 12 months once stable. Lithium also carries a very narrow therapeutic index and therefore requires close monitoring of levels, as doses are adjusted. It is recommended that lithium levels be checked 5 days following initiation and after each dose change. Afterward, lithium levels may be monitored every 3 to 6 months or when clinically indicated. A safe lithium level is generally 0.6 mEq/L to 1.2 mEq/L.

As a class, antipsychotic medications can lead to extrapyramidal side effects such as dystonia, akathisia, bradykinesia and parkinsonism, and tardive dyskinesia (irregular and involuntary jerky movements). These symptoms should be assessed at every visit. Antipsychotic medications also impact metabolic parameters such as weight gain, dyslipidemia, and glucose metabolism, and should be assessed at baseline and at scheduled intervals.

## SUICIDE

Suicide is the second leading cause of death in adolescents aged 15 to 19. According to the Youth Risk Behavior Surveillance System, the largest public health surveillance system in the United States, 17.7% of high school students had thoughts about suicide during the 12 months prior to the survey. During that same period, 14.6% of students had made a suicide plan, with 8.6% of students carrying out a suicide attempt.

Risk factors for suicide include previous attempt; witnessing or learning about a suicide attempt; mental health or substance use disorder; chronic medical disorder; family history of suicide; significant trauma, such as physical or sexual abuse; self-injurious behavior, such as cutting; and access to means, such as medications or firearms. Protective factors include family and peer support, cultural beliefs, access to and continued treatment, and positive coping skills. Pediatricians should make sure that parents are aware of local crisis hotlines and the nearest emergency rooms, and have done their best to remove means for suicide, such as access to medications and firearms.

Recent guidelines from the American Academy of Pediatrics have emphasized the importance of pediatricians being aware of warning signs that may signal suicidal thoughts, such as hopelessness, guilt, seeming withdrawn and isolated, being bullied, giving away valuables, substance use, and signs of self-harm, such as cutting. If these are noticed, it is important for the pediatrician to assess whether the child or adolescent is experiencing suicidal thoughts and/or behaviors. This sort of assessment may best be done with or without the parent/caretaker in the room. If the child or adolescent is assessed to be suicidal, the pediatrician must refer them to the nearest emergency room for an evaluation by a psychiatrist or send them directly to an inpatient psychiatric hospital for an evaluation. This same process must be followed if the pediatrician is unclear about the child's suicidal status.

## CONCLUSION

Depressive and bipolar spectrum disorders in children and adolescents carry significant long-term consequences, making recognition and prompt treatment a key component to decreasing morbidity and mortality for these patients. As these disorders can present similarly to other mental health diagnoses, it is important to know how to differentiate these conditions. Depression may present differently in children and adolescents compared to adults, and youth may not always directly report being depressed, making it important for pediatricians to be aware of warning symptoms/signs, especially when it comes to suicide. Although many medications are used to treat depression and bipolar disorder, only a few have been FDA approved for these indications in children and adolescents. Psychosocial interventions and adjunctive therapy performed by trained therapists are an additional key component to treatment. Due to the dearth of child psychiatrists in the United States and the fact that many families present initially to primary care physicians for mental health concerns, initial management strategies of depression are an essential component of the pediatrician's repertoire. More severe depression and bipolar spectrum disorders are ideally an indication for referral directly to child and adolescent psychiatrists.

American Diabetes Association; American Psychiatric Association; American Association of Clinical Endocrinologists; North American Association for the Study of Obesity. Consensus development conference on antipsychotic drugs and obesity and diabetes. *Diabetes Care*. 2004;27(2):596-601.

American Psychiatric Association. *Diagnostic and Statistical Manual of Mental Disorders*. 5th ed. Arlington, VA: American Psychiatric Association Publishing; 2013.

Birmaher B, Brent D, Bernet W, et al; AACAP Work Group on Quality Issues. Practice parameter for the assessment and treatment of children and adolescents with depressive disorders. *J Am Acad Child Adolesc Psychiatry*. 2007;46(11):1503-1526.

Chang KD, Howe M, Madaan V, Khanzode L. Bipolar disorder in children and adolescents. In: Steiner H, ed. *Handbook of Developmental Psychiatry*. Danvers, MA: World Scientific Publishing; 2011: 159-195.

Cipriani A, Zhou X, Del Giovane C, et al. Comparative efficacy and tolerability of antidepressants for major depressive disorder in children and adolescents: a network meta-analysis. *Lancet*. 2016;388(10047):881-890.

Compton SN, March JS, Brent D, et al. Cognitive-behavioral psychotherapy for anxiety and depressive disorders in children and adolescents: an evidence-based medicine review. *J Am Acad Child Adolesc Psychiatry*. 2004;43(8):930-959.

Copeland WE, Angold A, Costello EJ, Egger H. Prevalence, comorbidity, and correlates of DSM-5 proposed disruptive mood dysregulation disorder. *Am J Psychiatry*. 2013;170(2):173-179.

Dilillo D, Mauri S, Mantegazza C, Fabiano V, Mameli C, Zuccotti GV. Suicide in pediatrics: epidemiology, risk factors, warning signs and the role of the pediatrician in detecting them. *Ital J Pediatr*. 2015;41:49.

Dulcan MK. *Dulcan's Textbook of Child and Adolescent Psychiatry*. 2nd ed. Arlington, VA: American Psychiatric Association Publishing; 2016.

Miklowitz DJ, Axelson DA, Birmaher B, et al. Family-focused treatment for adolescents with bipolar disorder: results of a 2-year randomized trial. *Arch Gen Psychiatry*. 2008;65(9):1053-1061.

Shain B; American Academy of Pediatrics Committee on Adolescence. Suicide and suicide attempts in adolescents. *Pediatrics*. 2016;138(1):e20161420.

Wozniak J, Spencer T, Biederman J, et al. The clinical characteristics of unipolar vs. bipolar major depression in ADHD youth. *J Affect Disord*. 2004;82(suppl 1):S59-S69.



# 95 Disruptive Behavior Disorders and Psychotic Disorders

Chadi Calarge

Disruptive, problematic behavior is ubiquitous and an integral aspect of normal development. In fact, the natural drive of children to increasingly assert their autonomy as they grow older and more independent inevitably sets them on a path leading to disagreement and conflict with their caregivers. Of course, children vary greatly in their frustration tolerance, their overall self-regulation, and their need to assert themselves. Such interindividual differences interact with environmental responses, particularly in the caregiving environment, which itself may vary greatly in terms of sensitivity and responsiveness to children's developmental needs, capacity to promote trust and social learning, and ability to provide effective models in such areas as prosocial behavior; coping with frustration, stress, and conflict; and problem solving. This complex interaction between biologically based motivational dispositions and environmental responses shapes, organizes, and reinforces developmental trajectories in which normative conflict can turn into disruptive behavioral disorder.

## INDIVIDUAL DETERMINANTS OF BEHAVIOR

Temperament typically refers to the innate (ie, biological) aspects of one's personality. Children differ substantially in their temperamental traits, which can be observed as early as birth, although they are more reliably appreciated after the first few weeks of life. Traits include such characteristics as activity level, frustration tolerance, assertiveness, attention, emotional reactivity/intensity, impulsivity, fearfulness, and propensity to respond to soothing. A simple review of this list makes it apparent how temperament may play a key role in determining the child's inclination for engaging in behavior that could precipitate conflict. For instance, an impulsive, risk-taking child is more likely to break rules due to failure to plan his or her actions and consider their consequences. Of course, as executive functions are still developing during childhood, traits such as impulsivity must be evaluated in an age-appropriate manner.

## ENVIRONMENTAL DETERMINANTS OF BEHAVIOR

A complex process such as disruptive behavior is virtually never the product of a single factor. Instead, it results from the interaction of a number of factors that may contribute, in varying degrees, to different behaviors in the same child over time and across different children at the same developmental stage. Importantly, for a behavior to persist, it must be rewarded or "reinforced"; otherwise, it will more likely be extinguished. In behavioral terms (ie, operant conditioning), contingencies of reinforcement consist of 3 components: antecedents, behaviors, and consequences (referred to as the *ABCs of behavior*). Antecedents are stimuli, settings, and contexts that precede and influence the onset of a behavior, while consequences are the events that follow. Consequences could have no impact on the recurrence of a behavior, but they can also increase it or decrease it. Positive reinforcers are events that follow a behavior and make it more likely to recur. For instance, when an infant is comfortable (ie, antecedent) and smiles (ie, behavior), even if exhibiting a reflexive social smile, the parents feel excited and respond with increased attention to and engagement with the child (ie, consequences). This positive attention is enjoyed by the infant, prompting him or her to learn that a smile leads to more parental attention and positive emotions. As a result, the infant will smile more when he or she sees the parent. Thus, the smile is the behavior that gets reinforced, and the parents' attention is the reward or, technically speaking, the positive reinforcer. (Note here that the parents' increased attention to and engagement with the child is not only a reinforcer for the child but also a behavior that is reinforced by the child's enjoyment, leading to more engagement by the parent. This highlights the interactive nature of these transactions.) In contrast, an example of a maladaptive positive reinforcement pattern is when a child throws a temper tantrum and the parents seek to console him or her by giving in to a demand made by the child (eg, "I want a candy") or dropping a demand placed on the child (eg, "Please finish your homework"). As a result, the child will learn that tantrums allow her to get what she wants. This is not to be confused with negative reinforcement, which refers to a response or behavior being strengthened by stopping, removing, or avoiding a negative outcome or aversive stimulus. As an example, having to deal with a tantrum or fighting about homework is certainly an unpleasant experience for a parent. If conflicts occur often, the parent learns that not placing demands on the child allows him or her to avoid these aversive interactions. Importantly, using the term *learn* does not imply that the process is necessarily conscious or deliberate. Rather, it highlights the fact that the process is repetitive, leading to the establishment of patterns of behavior. These examples illustrate how the parent's response shapes the child's behavior. However, they are also meant to emphasize the bidirectional nature of the interaction, with the child's behavior shaping that of the parent as well.

Of course, in reality, the child is interacting with many more individuals in his or her life than a single parent. These different relationships will influence the child's conduct in various ways, depending on multiple factors, not the least of which is the emotional value attached by the child to each particular relationship. As the child develops, the meaning and salience of these relationships will change. In fact, although in a Western society parents are the primary role models for younger children, peer relationships take on increasing influence during the transition into adolescence.

## DETERMINANTS OF PATHOLOGICAL BEHAVIOR

Many individual and environmental factors have been implicated in the emergence of problematic disruptive behavior (Table 95-1). As noted earlier, significant impulsivity and emotional reactivity increase the risk for aggression. In addition, violent children exhibit deficits in social-cognitive or information-processing abilities (eg, they tend to interpret situations in a threatening and hostile manner). Intellectual disability and risk-taking behavior are additional risk factors, as is the presence of an anxiety or mood disorder, which may manifest in irritability, hostility, conflict, and even aggression. In utero exposure to alcohol, illicit drugs, malnutrition, or illness; perinatal complications; and lead toxicity have also been associated with disruptive behavior. Additionally, one's genetic endowment contributes to this risk not only through shaping temperamental traits but also by interacting with environmental factors, such as family-level risk factors that include poor family cohesion or high conflict, harsh or lax disciplinary practices, lack of positive parental involvement and supervision, and parental psychopathology.

**TABLE 95-1 EXAMPLES OF DETERMINANTS OF PATHOLOGICAL BEHAVIOR**

| |
|---|
| **Individual Level** |
| Genetic background (eg, variants of the monoamine oxidase A gene) |
| In utero exposure to alcohol, illicit drugs, malnutrition, or illness |
| Perinatal complications |
| Lead toxicity |
| Temperamental traits (eg, impulsivity, risk taking, emotional reactivity) |
| Intellectual disability |
| Language delays |
| Poor academic performance and low commitment to education |
| Deficits in social, cognitive, or information processing abilities (eg, tending to interpret situations in a threatening and hostile manner) |
| Comorbid psychopathology (eg, attention-deficit/hyperactivity disorder, depression, anxiety disorders) |
| **Family Level** |
| Poor family cohesion or high conflict |
| Divorce |
| Large family size |
| Harsh, lax, or inconsistent disciplinary practices |
| Lack of positive parental involvement and supervision |
| Poverty |
| Poor education |
| Parental substance use disorders or criminality |
| Parental mental illness |
| Teenage parenthood |
| **Peer Level** |
| Peer rejection |
| Association with delinquent peers |
| Involvement with gangs |
| **Society Level** |
| Enrollment in unsafe or failing schools |
| Harsh school suspension and expulsion policies |
| Severe punishment policies at schools |
| Neighborhoods with high levels of crime and poverty |
| Social disorganization in the community |

Although aggressive children bully others, they are also victims of bullying and peer rejection. This pattern further isolates them, depriving them from the social incentives to adopt more appropriate behavior. In adolescence, as peers' influence increases, association with delinquent peers and involvement with gangs further encourages individuals to engage in disruptive behavior.

## PROBLEMATIC BEHAVIOR

The spectrum of disruptive behaviors in childhood is broad and varies based on developmental stage. It ranges from the benign colic to more serious delinquency.

### Colic

Although all newborns cry, as this is their primary way of expressing distress, about 15% develop colic, defined as crying more than 3 hours a day, more than 3 days a week, for more than 3 weeks in a well-fed infant. Colic starts around age 2 weeks and almost always resolves by the fourth month of life. The presence of colic has not been consistently associated with particular risk factors or unfavorable outcomes. As such, no specific interventions are indicated, but pediatricians can help parents arrange access to support, providing respite and reducing stress. This would alleviate parental fatigue and reduce the risk of untoward outcomes (eg, shaken baby syndrome).

### Temper Tantrums

Temper tantrums are ubiquitous, reported by parents in as many as 80% of 2- to 4-year-old children. Tantrums occur daily in about 20% of 2-year-old children and 10% of 4-year-old children. Moderate to severe tantrums are reported in 5% of 3-year-old children. As would be expected, problem-solving skills are limited in toddlers. Therefore, they object to frustration with an emotional outburst, sometimes rising to the degree of a tantrum. Parents would be well-advised to avoid reinforcing the behavior, by doing the following:

1. Ensure the child is well-fed and rested, as hunger and sleep deprivation could contribute to irritability and noncompliance. In behavioral terms, hunger and sleep deprivation are a type of antecedents referred to as "setting events/establishing operations" because they increase the likelihood of engaging in behaviors to obtain or avoid consequences and alter the value of the reinforcer.
2. Identify triggers and establishing a routine that would give the toddler a sense of predictability.
3. Plan ahead by having access to activities that might engage the child and avoid triggering irritability (eg, having crayons or Play-Doh at a restaurant).
4. Distract the child to prevent initial frustration from escalating into a full-fledged temper tantrum. Many parents intuitively discover this technique and use it successfully.
5. Model for the child how to use words. Importantly, receptive language develops before expressive skills. Therefore, the parent can teach the child to use words like "I want," "tired," and "food." Teaching short phrases or words actually helps build adaptive skills, as opposed to getting angry with the child, which teaches him or her what behavior is not acceptable but not necessarily what is acceptable.
6. Allow the child to take part in the decision-making process by providing choices that are all acceptable to the parent. This gives the child a sense of control.
7. Promote adaptive and prosocial behavior by providing a labelled praise. "You sound like a big boy when you use your words." An unlabeled praise (eg, "good job") is useful but not as descriptive in terms of highlighting to the child the actual behavior to be encouraged and repeated.

The astute reader will notice that these suggestions are essentially based on identifying antecedents that precede the behavior and influence its emergence, and on helping the parent to set up more favorable ones. They also include teaching and promoting (ie, reinforcing) more appropriate behavior by setting up consequences that deliberately provide positive attention (ie, a positive reinforcer). Once these basic concepts are understood, many minor behavioral challenges can be addressed.

If the temper tantrums become problematic or perhaps include violence, parents may need to remove the child from the situation and enforce a time-out. The parent must specify a time-out spot (eg, a chair in the living room), make it clear that the child must remain in it, and end the time-out when the child has calmed down. This may be followed by a brief discussion about the behavior that precipitated the time-out, but the child must be reintegrated back into family life without laboring excessively over what had happened. It is important to select a place for time-out that is not engaging and to avoid areas that are dedicated for other functions, such as bedrooms. In fact, bedrooms are often filled with toys and distractions, undermining the purpose of a time-out. Moreover, using bedrooms could inadvertently associate them with aversive experiences, potentially leading to sleep problems. Also, it is important to remember that "time-out" is short for "time-out from positive reinforcement." This implies that during time-outs there must not be an interaction with the child. This also implies that, for time-outs to be effective, the child must feel that he or she is missing out on enjoyable time with the parent/family, while in time-out. In families in which the interactions between parent and child are minimal or mostly aversive, time-outs will not be very effective. As such, it is important when using time-outs to evaluate the overall nature of the parent-child interaction and address any deficiencies. Finally, it is also important to make time-outs a successful experience, with the child able to complete them in as brief a period of time as is reasonable. For instance, many recommend that time-outs last about 1 minute per year of age, although the evidence supporting this suggestion is in fact limited.



#### Breath-Holding Spells

Breath-holding spells usually appear in the second year of life, occurring at the initiation of a tantrum. Up to 5% of children develop at least 1 breath-holding spell. A positive family history for breath-holding or fainting is common. Two types have been described: (1) a cyanotic form, in which cyanosis of the face occurs until breathing resumes, and (2) a pallid type, in which the face is pale secondary to a vasovagal response. Syncope occasionally develops. Apnea is brief and without sequelae. A minority of these children will have symmetric tonic-clonic movements before fully recovering. Although benign and without long-term sequelae, breath-holding spells may be frightening to parents.

#### Oppositional Defiant Disorder

As disruptive behavior increases in intensity, frequency, and duration, and becomes entrenched, it may reach a level where clinical attention by mental health specialists becomes necessary. According to the *Diagnostic and Statistical Manual for Mental Disorders*, 5th edition (DSM-5), a diagnosis of oppositional defiant disorder (ODD) is made when the child exhibits an established pattern of disruptive behavior, characterized by irritability, temper tantrums, argumentativeness, defiance, behavioral noncompliance, being easily annoyed by and annoying to others, and vindictiveness. The difficulties must be present for at least 6 months and must interfere with the child's social, academic, or occupational functioning, hindering normal development.

#### Conduct Disorder

In conduct disorder, there is a persistent disregard of the rights of others and of societal norms and rules. Individuals with conduct disorder exhibit aggression (eg, bullying, threatening, initiating physical fights, cruelty, robbery, and rape), destructiveness (eg, deliberate destruction of property including by setting fires), deceitfulness (eg, breaking and entering, lying to obtain goods or avoid obligations, and theft), and serious violations of rules (eg, staying out past curfew and truancy, both starting before age 13 years, and running away from home). Again, the difficulties must be present for at least 6 months and impair the child's functioning (per DSM-5). Onset of conduct disorder before age 10 years (ie, childhood-onset type) is particularly pernicious, with a higher risk of delinquency and conversion into antisocial personality disorder in adulthood. In contrast, the adolescent-onset type appears more determined by peer influence, is time limited, and has a more favorable prognosis.

### ASSESSMENT OF DISRUPTIVE BEHAVIOR DISORDERS

Disruptive behavior disorders are relatively common, with the prevalence of ODD ranging between 1% and 11% (average 3.3%) and that of conduct disorder ranging between 2% and 10% (median 4%). Thus, pediatricians are bound to see children with these conditions, since parents will turn to them for guidance when the problems reach a significant level.

A thorough evaluation of the predisposing, precipitating, and persisting factors (3 Ps) is a key first step. Individual-, family-, peer-, and society-level risk factors (Table 95-1) must be identified. In addition, it is informative to query about the most typical antecedents and consequences related to problematic behavior. As discussed earlier, a behavior occurs within a context and is perpetuated by reinforcers. Therefore, evaluating for marital conflict, parental substance use, inconsistent or harsh discipline, stressors that the child and family are undergoing, and child maltreatment is absolutely necessary. Establishing the duration, context, and progression of the difficulties often provides clues to the nature of the problem. For instance, a worsening but long-standing disruptive behavior is more likely to be consistent with a disruptive behavior disorder compared to difficulties only a few weeks old. A behavior problem restricted to a particular environment (eg, only at home, or with 1 parent) should prompt the clinician to work with the parent(s) on identifying triggers. For example, a child who becomes disruptive only in math class may suffer from a specific learning disorder (ie, difficulties mastering number sense or number facts).

#### Nonpsychosocial Causes

Subsequently, efforts should be made to rule out medical conditions (eg, sleep apnea, visual problems), iatrogenic causes (eg, steroid treatment), unhealthy lifestyle habits (eg, poor sleep hygiene), and environmental toxins (eg, exposure to lead). Although a number of neurobiological markers, such as lower heart rate or skin conductance activity, reduced basal cortisol reactivity, and abnormalities in the prefrontal cortex and amygdala, have been described in children with disruptive behavior disorders, laboratory tests should be targeted, based on the clinical history, in order to rule out suspected medical conditions. To date, there is no test to establish a disruptive behavior disorder diagnosis.

### COMORBID PSYCHOPATHOLOGY

As noted earlier, temperamental traits and individual characteristics influence one's risk to develop disruptive behavior. When they reach an extreme, as is seen with attention-deficit/hyperactivity disorder (ADHD), impulsivity and disinhibition are associated with behavioral and emotional disinhibition. This accounts for the high comorbidity between ADHD and disruptive behavior disorders. For example, up to 95% of children with childhood-onset conduct disorder in clinical settings have ADHD. Determining what comorbid psychiatric conditions may be present is crucial to formulating a management plan. In fact, irritability is a nonspecific symptom that is part of the clinical presentation of virtually every psychiatric disorder in children (akin to fever in medical diseases). This includes major depressive disorder (in which irritability, rather than sadness or dysphoria, may be the sole affective symptom present), anxiety disorders, bipolar disorder, post-traumatic stress disorder, etc. Such comprehensive assessment is possible only when clinicians seek input from the child's teachers, daycare providers, or other care providers, in addition to the parents. This effort may be time-consuming but is necessary to establish the severity and pervasiveness of the symptoms and help determine the role comorbid conditions may be playing in the presenting problem. To that end, the use of rating scales (eg, National Institute for Children's Health Quality [NICHQ] Vanderbilt Assessment Scales, Pediatric Symptom Checklist-17, the Child Behavior Checklist) allows the clinician to collect this information from various informants in a reliable and time-efficient manner.

If the clinical picture appears complex, referrals to specialists may prove necessary. For instance, a referral for neuropsychological and academic testing may be indicated to evaluate for intellectual disability or specific learning disorders. A psychological evaluation may shed light on the inner emotional and psychological functioning of the child as well as on the family dynamics, and a psychiatric referral may also help determine the primacy of comorbid psychopathology, the presence of suicide risk, and whether pharmacotherapy is indicated.

## TREATMENT OF DISRUPTIVE BEHAVIOR DISORDERS

### Parent Management Training

Regardless of severity level, once the disruptive behavior reaches clinical attention, nonpharmacological interventions are a key component of the treatment. Mild forms may be successfully addressed with psychoeducation and self-help books on disruptive and problematic behavior. Many parents of younger children are capable of modifying the contingencies of reinforcement in their child's environment, leading to a resolution of the problem behavior. For chronic behavior problems, particularly as children become older, more formal professional help becomes necessary.

A variety of psychotherapeutic interventions and delivery methods (ie, group, family, individual settings) have been studied, some showing excellent efficacy. Most effective programs for disruptive behavior disorders are based on behavioral principles (ie, operant conditioning) and engage the parents directly in what is commonly referred to as *parent management training* (PMT). It must be made clear that the purpose of PMT is by no means to attribute the problematic behavior to inappropriate parenting. Many parents of children with disruptive behavior disorders are already burdened by guilt and a poor sense of self-efficacy. Rather, just as parents of a child with diabetes has to modify the diet to suit their child's special needs, parents of children with disruptive behavior are invited to try new methods to address their child's behavior challenges when the usual means are ineffective. The overarching goal of PMT interventions is to provide education about behavior principles (ie, ABCs of behavior), work with them on identifying antecedents (ie, triggers, contingencies, and reinforcers), encourage the use of rewards to reinforce adaptive behavior (eg, special time with parent, favorite activity, token economy), model prosocial behavior (eg, use words, complete chores, play gently), and withhold attention from (ie, ignoring) disruptive behavior. A common key component is promoting a positive, collaborative, warm parent-child relationship. The use of time-outs and withholding privileges may prove necessary but is not instrumental, and physical or aversive punishment is explicitly discouraged. The latter could impede the development of a healthy and warm parent-child relationship and serves as a poor model to help the child acquire adaptive behavioral skills.

### Additional Services

As discussed earlier, comorbid conditions may either present as disruptive behavior or contribute to it and attenuate treatment response. Therefore, when indicated, the treatment plan should include interventions to address these conditions. For instance, if neuropsychological testing reveals slow processing speed or academic testing shows specific learning disorders, the school should be petitioned to make the necessary accommodations available to the child (eg, longer time to complete an in-school assignment or exam, tutoring). It may be necessary to develop an individualized education plan or 504 plan, which are formal documents that lay out the challenges facing the child and the school's plan to address them. Children with language disorders may benefit from speech therapy and those with developmental coordination disorders may require occupational or physical therapy. The presence of ADHD or mood and anxiety disorders also would need to be addressed, as indicated.

### Pharmacotherapy for Disruptive Behavior Disorders

At times, the disruptive behavior reaches such a level of severity that it substantially interferes with the child's development (eg, academic failure, legal problems) or causes conflict with parents, caregivers, and peers (eg, school suspension, social isolation). Due to lack of access to effective psychotherapeutic interventions or limited response to them, or to address comorbid conditions, pharmacotherapy may prove necessary. A psychiatric referral or a consultation with a child and adolescent psychiatrist can be helpful to establish a treatment plan. Of course, any medication intervention will have to be tailored based on the child's needs, the family's preference, and the results of the assessment with regard to the presence of comorbid conditions and their contribution to the overall clinical picture. What follows will briefly describe some of the treatments available but is not meant to serve as an exhaustive summary.

**Psychostimulants** As noted earlier, ADHD is highly comorbid with disruptive behavior disorders, particularly when onset is in childhood. The impulsivity characteristic of ADHD contributes to behavioral and emotional disinhibition, associated with both ODD and conduct disorder. In fact, many studies have shown a substantial reduction in disruptive behavior when ADHD is successfully treated. A few studies have even shown a reduction in conduct problems with psychostimulants even in the absence of ADHD. The importance of treating comorbid ADHD cannot be overstated. Several studies in children with disruptive and aggressive behavior have shown that optimizing ADHD treatment obviates the need for any additional pharmacological interventions. Given that psychostimulants are the first-line medication treatment for ADHD, a trial may be indicated. While it may be cautious to initiate treatment with a short-acting formulation, particularly if the parents are nervous about adverse events, it is important to achieve symptom control in the evening and not simply during the school day in order to reduce conflict at home between the child and the parent. Importantly, children must be screened for cardiac abnormalities prior to initiating treatment and monitored for growth suppression and sleep disturbance afterwards.

**α-2 Agonists and Atomoxetine** Whether due to limited efficacy, intolerability, or parental objection, alternatives to psychostimulants may need to be considered. Guanfacine and clonidine are agonists of the presynaptic adrenergic α-2 receptor, and atomoxetine is an inhibitor of the presynaptic norepinephrine transporter. They are all approved by the United States Food and Drug Administration (FDA) for the treatment of ADHD and have been shown to reduce comorbid disruptive behavior. Guanfacine and clonidine may be particularly helpful if insomnia is problematic. Atomoxetine carries a black-box warning for emergence of suicidality.

**Antipsychotic Medications** A number of studies have found antipsychotic medications to be effective at controlling disruptive behavior, with a large effect size. In particular, risperidone and aripiprazole are 2 second-generation antipsychotics that are approved by the FDA for the treatment of irritability associated with autistic disorder. Over the last 2 decades, the newer second-generation antipsychotics have essentially replaced the older typical antipsychotics (eg, haloperidol or chlorpromazine). This was primarily due to concerns about irreversible movement disorders (ie, tardive dyskinesia) and the (unfounded) perception that they were more efficacious in psychotic disorders, as well as aggressive marketing practices. However, these newer medications are associated with substantial weight gain, insulin resistance, and dyslipidemia, as discussed later in this chapter. Therefore, while they may provide a fast and substantial reduction in aggression, clinicians must consider alternative options initially and reserve these drugs to more severe and treatment-resistant cases. Their initiation must be followed by close monitoring for cardiometabolic risk factors.

**Other Medications** Evidence also exists in support of antiepileptics, such as divalproex, in the treatment of aggression in children. Antidepressants, propranolol, buspirone, naltrexone, and many other medications, as well as supplements (eg, omega-3 fatty acids), have also been investigated with varying degrees of efficacy and evidence.

In summary, pharmacotherapy can be efficacious in the treatment of disruptive behavior, particularly reactive/impulsive (as opposed to premeditated or planned) aggression and disruptive behavior. However, nonpharmacological interventions should always be considered first and provided concurrently when pharmacotherapy proves necessary. In fact, studies have shown that, compared to pharmacotherapy alone, treatments combining pharmacotherapy with parent management training achieve better clinical response, use lower medication dosages, and are associated with higher parental satisfaction.

## PSYCHOSIS

Whereas aggression is perceived to be linked to mental illness, in general, and psychosis, in particular, less than 5% of patients with psychopathology are violent, and most violent acts are committed by individuals without identifiable psychiatric disorders. Nonetheless, it remains imperative for clinicians to have the necessary skills to screen patients for the presence of risk factors, including psychosis, which will be briefly reviewed here.

Psychosis is characterized by an alteration in reality testing, with patients experiencing any number of symptoms including hallucinations, delusions, or disorganized thinking/speech or behavior. These symptoms are further explained here:

- Hallucinations are perception-like experiences, occurring without an external stimulus. Hallucinations can impact all the sensory systems, but auditory and visual hallucinations are the most common. The presence of other types of hallucinations usually raises concerns about neurological conditions (eg, seizures, tumors).
- Delusions are false fixed beliefs that may be persecutory, referential (ie, when events or cues in the surroundings are believed to be directed at oneself), somatic, grandiose, or religious. Importantly, the beliefs must not be shared by others within the same cultural, social, or religious group. Some delusions may be bizarre or clearly implausible. Examples include thought insertion or withdrawal, when one's thoughts are believed to be put in or removed by outside forces.
- Disorganized thinking or speech refers to instances in which the individual is unable to maintain a train of thought or be coherent (eg, loose associations or word salad).
- Disorganized behavior may include immature or inappropriate behavior (eg, walking outside naked on a cold night) as well as catatonia, characterized by a marked decrease in reactivity to the environment.
- Primary psychotic disorders, like schizophrenia, are also often characterized by negative symptoms, which often account for much of the disease's morbidity. These are referred to as negative symptoms to capture the fact that the impacted area is subtracted from one's functioning or life. The 2 symptoms most prominent in schizophrenia are diminished emotional expressiveness affecting facial expressions, eye contact, intonation of speech, and body gestures, and avolition (ie, lack of desire to engage in activities, apathy). Additional negative symptoms include alogia (reduced speech output), anhedonia (reduced ability to experience pleasure), or asociality.

Of note, all psychotic symptoms may vary greatly in severity. Moreover, establishing the symptoms in children and adolescents can be particularly challenging, as hallucinations and delusions may not have become fully formed and crystallized. In addition, visual hallucinations, which occur more commonly in children, must be distinguished from normal fantasy play. This is especially true given that up to 15% of children may experience hallucinations, and while their presence is associated with a substantially increased risk for later psychosis, the vast majority resolve without sequelae.

# SCHIZOPHRENIA

The prototypical primary psychotic disorder is schizophrenia. It is referred to as childhood-onset schizophrenia when symptoms are established before 13 years of age and early-onset schizophrenia when onset is in adolescence (13–18 years old). While childhood-onset schizophrenia is fortunately rare, with a prevalence of about 1:10,000, up to 50% of cases of adult schizophrenia may have their onset in adolescence. Schizophrenia has been described in all countries and cultures, with estimates for its lifetime prevalence ranging between 0.3% and 0.7%, depending on race, ethnicity, geographic region, and sex. Cases with more negative symptoms and longer duration appear more common in males.

The diagnosis of schizophrenia is made based on criteria set in the DSM-5. According to the criteria, patients must exhibit 2 or more of the following: (1) delusions, (2) hallucinations, (3) disorganized thinking or speech, (4) grossly disorganized or catatonic behavior, or (5) negative symptoms. At least 1 of the symptoms must consist of 1 of the first 3. These symptoms must have been present for at least 1 month (less if successfully treated). In addition, continuous signs of the disturbance, including disruption of the child's or adolescent's developmental trajectory in interpersonal, academic, and occupational functioning, must persist for at least 6 months. Outside the periods of acute psychosis, participants may have prodromal or residual symptoms with the symptoms present in a more attenuated form. This is often the case in the initial stage of the disease, when delusions may simply be ideas that are overvalued but still disputable by facts (eg, feeling excluded by friends) and hallucinations merely consist of minor unusual perceptual experiences (eg, hearing one's name being called). As the condition progresses, symptom severity worsens (eg, feeling like friends are plotting against him or her or hearing voices making derogatory statements). The presence of symptoms for less than 6 months or the co-occurrence of mood disorders for a substantial period may lead to other diagnoses (eg, schizophreniform disorder or schizoaffective disorder) that would similarly require clinical attention but may have different prognoses.

## ETIOLOGY

Schizophrenia is a heterogeneous syndrome with no single etiology but, rather, the result of a complex interaction of multiple factors during development (ie, neurodevelopmental model). Genetic factors are certainly involved, as evidenced by the higher rate of schizophrenia among first-degree relatives of affected individuals and among monozygotic as opposed to dizygotic twins. Specific genes have in fact been identified, including the major histocompatibility complex, MIR137, and ZNF804a. Environmental factors include in utero exposure to maternal famine, paternal age, prenatal infections, obstetric complications, and immigrations. These are thought to cause direct cellular damage in the brain and alter genetic expression or induce epigenetic changes or de novo mutations in brain cells.

Of interest, recent research has focused on examining whether schizophrenia may be a manifestation of autoimmune encephalitis affecting the limbic system, caused by autoantibodies targeting the NR1 subunit of the N-methyl-D-aspartate receptor, the voltage-gated potassium channel, and the gamma aminobutyric acid receptor ($GABA_{B1}$), among others. However, the findings to date have been inconsistent.

## LABORATORY ABNORMALITIES

To date, no single laboratory, neuroimaging, or neuropsychological test is available to confirm or rule out the diagnosis of schizophrenia. However, a variety of structural and functional brain abnormalities have been associated with schizophrenia and include increased lateral ventricle volumes and decreases in hippocampus, thalamus, and frontal lobe volumes. Youth with childhood- and early-onset schizophrenia exhibit decreases in gray matter volumes and cortical folding that may plateau by early adulthood.

## PROGNOSIS

Onset of schizophrenia may be abrupt, but most children and adolescents exhibit an insidious course with symptoms gradually increasing in severity. Children with schizophrenia are more likely to have had psychopathology, including disruptive behavior, intellectual and language disabilities, and subtle motor delays, prior to disease onset. Earlier age of onset is associated with poorer prognosis, educational and cognitive achievement, and overall functioning. In addition, up to 20% of individuals with schizophrenia attempt suicide, with 5% to 6% of those attempts being successful. While suicide risk is elevated throughout life, it may be especially high for younger males with comorbid substance use disorders.

**TABLE 95-2 CONDITIONS OR SUBSTANCES ASSOCIATED WITH PSYCHOSIS**

| Conditions | Examples (Nonexhaustive List) |
|---|---|
| Central nervous system infections | Herpes encephalitis, human immunodeficiency virus infection, Lyme disease, syphilis |
| Hormonal abnormalities | Adrenocortical insufficiency, thyroid and parathyroid disease, panhypopituitarism |
| Electrolyte imbalances | Elevated or reduced concentrations of sodium, potassium, calcium, magnesium, phosphorus |
| Metabolic disorders | Hypoglycemia, lactic acidosis, liver failure and hepatic encephalopathy, porphyria |
| Vitamin deficiencies | Folate, niacin, vitamin $B_{12}$, vitamin D |
| Neurologic disorders | Seizures, encephalitis (including autoimmune encephalitis), traumatic brain injury, neoplasms, cerebrovascular disease, multiple sclerosis, Sydenham's chorea |
| Genetic | Velocardiofacial syndrome, Wilson disease, metachromatic leukodystrophy |
| Medications | Psychostimulants, dopamine receptor agonists, corticosteroids, anticholinergics, antiepileptics, antidepressants, antihypertensives, antihistaminergics, fluoroquinolone and cephalosporin antibiotics, procaine derivatives (procainamide, procaine, penicillin G), nonsteroidal anti-inflammatory drugs |
| Recreational substances | Alcohol (particularly delirium tremens), psychostimulants, hallucinogens, cannabinoids, opioids |
| Toxins | Contaminants in supplements and herbal remedies, anabolic steroids, heavy metal poisoning (eg, mercury, lead), carbon monoxide poisoning |

## DIFFERENTIAL DIAGNOSIS AND COMORBIDITY

The negative symptoms of schizophrenia overlap with depressive symptoms (eg, anhedonia, social withdrawal, psychomotor retardation, and concentration problems). Moreover, depressive disorders may be associated with psychosis, particularly when severe. In children, some schizophrenia symptoms may be characteristic of autism spectrum disorder, which is sometimes associated with mannerisms, bizarre behaviors, and social withdrawal. Obsessive compulsive disorder, eating disorder, and post-traumatic stress disorder all can be associated with perceptions or beliefs that may border on psychosis. Furthermore, several medical conditions and drugs of abuse, including psychostimulants, hallucinogens, and cannabinoids (whether it is marijuana or the increasingly used synthetic marijuana/cannabinoids), may be associated with psychosis. A thorough history with specific attention to developmental aspects as well as a thoughtful medical workup often helps establish the diagnosis.

Because multiple medical conditions may be associated with psychosis (Table 95-2), youth with suspected schizophrenia should be carefully evaluated with routine laboratory testing assessing blood counts, toxicology screen, and liver, kidney, and thyroid functions. A metabolic screen (lipid profile, glucose, insulin) is indicated at baseline to monitor treatment tolerability. More focused testing is based on the presence of specific indications (eg, neuroimaging studies or electroencephalogram in the presence of neurologic symptoms or seizures). Genetic testing is indicated if there are associated dysmorphic or syndromic features.

## TREATMENT OF SCHIZOPHRENIA

Antipsychotic medication is a primary treatment for schizophrenia. Even though several large-scale studies have failed to show any advantage of some of the newer, second-generation antipsychotics over the older, typical antipsychotics, the former are nevertheless used as first-line treatments. Several second-generation drugs, including risperidone, aripiprazole, quetiapine, paliperidone, and olanzapine, are approved by the FDA for use in youth with schizophrenia. Due to its propensity to cause significant weight gain without additional therapeutic advantage in youth, the FDA has advised against using olanzapine as first-line treatment in this age group. In treatment-resistant schizophrenia, clozapine has shown efficacy. However, it is associated with serious adverse events, including neutropenia, and requires mandatory monitoring.

Antipsychotics may cause a variety of adverse effects. Most notably, second-generation antipsychotics lead to substantial weight gain (several kilograms in 2 to 3 months) and cardiometabolic abnormalities. Therefore, recommendations for close monitoring of blood pressure, body mass index, waist circumference, lipids, and glucose/insulin have been made. Concerns about iron deficiency have also been recently raised. In addition, all antipsychotics may cause extrapyramidal side effects, including parkinsonian tremor, acute dystonia, and akathisia. Following long-term use, tardive dyskinesia could develop and may be irreversible, although the risk appears lower in children and adolescents than in adults. Nonetheless, patients should be periodically assessed while medicated.

Nonpharmacological interventions, such as psychoeducation, social skills training, and cognitive remediation, can help optimize the functioning of children and adolescents with schizophrenia, maintain high treatment adherence, and empower and support families. Due to the presence of cognitive and functional deficits, accommodations at school (eg, specialized educational programs) and vocational training may also be beneficial for some youth.

In summary, disruptive behavior is common in children, and pediatricians are uniquely positioned to guide families to seek and secure the necessary care. This is particularly true given that early interventions may improve long-term outcomes. While psychosis is fortunately rare in children, the limited access to mental health services due to the severe shortage of child psychiatrists and the emergence of cardiometabolic adverse events secondary to treatment also require pediatricians to lend their expertise to address the children's needs and minimize long-term sequelae.

## SUGGESTED READINGS

American Diabetes Association; American Psychiatric Association; American Association of Clinical Endocrinologists; North American Association for the Study of Obesity. Consensus development conference on antipsychotic drugs and obesity and diabetes. *Diabetes Care*. 2004;27(2):596-601.

American Psychiatric Association. *Diagnostic and Statistical Manual of Mental Disorders*. 5th ed. Washington, DC: American Psychiatric Publishing, Inc; 2013.

Calarge CA, Ziegler EE, Del Castillo N, et al. Iron homeostasis during risperidone treatment in children and adolescents. *J Clin Psychiatry*. 2015;76(11):1500-1505.

Epstein R, Fonnesbeck C, Williamson E, et al. *Psychosocial and Pharmacologic Interventions for Disruptive Behavior in Children and Adolescents*. Rockville, MD: Agency for Healthcare Research and Quality; 2015. https://www.ncbi.nlm.nih.gov/pubmed/26598779. Accessed January 25, 2018.

Eyberg SM, Nelson MM, Boggs SR. Evidence-based psychosocial treatments for children and adolescents with disruptive behavior. *J Clin Child Adolesc Psychol*. 2008;37(1):215-237.

Gurnani T, Ivanov I, Newcorn JH. Pharmacotherapy of aggression in child and adolescent psychiatric disorders. *J Child Adolesc Psychopharmacol*. 2016;26(1):65-73.

Kazdin AE. Parent management training: evidence, outcomes, and issues. *J Am Acad Child Adolesc Psychiatry*. 1997;36(10):1349-1356.

McClellan J, Stock S; American Academy of Child and Adolescent Psychiatry Committee on Quality Issues. Practice parameter for the assessment and treatment of children and adolescents with schizophrenia. *J Am Acad Child Adolesc Psychiatry*. 2013;52(9):976-990.

Robison SD, Frick PJ, Sheffield Morris A. Temperament and parenting: implications for understanding developmental pathways to conduct disorder. *Minerva Pediatr*. 2005;57(6):373-388.

Saylor KE, Amann BH. Impulsive aggression as a comorbidity of attention-deficit/hyperactivity disorder in children and adolescents. *J Child Adolesc Psychopharmacol*. 2016;26(1):19-25.

Stevens JR, Prince JB, Prager LM, Stern TA. Psychotic disorders in children and adolescents: a primer on contemporary evaluation and management. *Prim Care Companion CNS Disord*. 2014;16(2). doi:10.4088/PCC.13f01514.

Sukhodolsky DG, Smith SD, McCauley SA, Ibrahim K, Piasecka JB. Behavioral interventions for anger, irritability, and aggression in children and adolescents. *J Child Adolesc Psychopharmacol*. 2016;26(1):58-64.

# PART 1 THE PATHOPHYSIOLOGY OF ACUTE AND CRITICAL ILLNESS

# 96 Acute Respiratory Dysfunction

Bhushan Katira and Brian Kavanagh

## INTRODUCTION

Acute respiratory dysfunction in children warrants prompt diagnosis and management, particularly in neonates and infants, as decompensation can be fast and respiratory arrest is the most common cause of cardiac arrest in children. Their smaller airways, increased metabolic demands (relative to body mass), and decreased respiratory reserve may put children at a disadvantage compared to adults.

Severe respiratory dysfunction necessitates admission to the intensive care unit (ICU). Since the polio epidemic of the 1950s, ICUs have developed in parallel with our increasing understanding of respiration in health and disease. Respiratory support is now extensively used and has become progressively more sophisticated.

In this chapter, we will explore the approach to a child with acute respiratory dysfunction, the initial considerations about the differential diagnosis of those conditions, and the broad principles of management strategies. In order to provide perspective, we first review some essentials of normal respiratory function.

## NORMAL RESPIRATION

The principal purposes of respiration are to provide oxygen and remove carbon dioxide, and this normal function involves the following elements.

### Control of Respiration

*Respiratory centers* in the medulla receive stimulatory input from central respiratory pacer cells, central and peripheral chemoreceptors, upper airway receptors, and volitional pathways. These signals are integrated into a combined output to respiratory muscles in order to regulate breathing frequency, as well as the durations of inspiration and expiration.

### Neuromuscular Function

Central signals are carried by the cervical and thoracic nerves to the neck, thoracic muscles, and diaphragm. These signals maintain patency of the upper airway and drive the thoracic bellows to provide ventilation. Downward movement of the diaphragm and outward movement of internal intercostal muscles lead to negative intrathoracic pressure and movement of air into the lungs (inhalation). The relaxation of these muscles leads to passive recoil of the lung and moves the air out (exhalation). The more negative the intrathoracic pressure, the greater the tidal volume generated.

### Resting Lung Volume

At rest, *elastic recoil* tends to move the thoracic cage outward and the lung inward. The balance of these opposing forces, along with a surfactant in the alveoli that reduces the surface tension (ie, lessens the force required to distend the lung). Elastic recoil determines the resting volume of the lung at the end of expiration, also known as functional residual capacity (FRC). This is the effective volume available for gas exchange.

### Airflow in the Large and Small Airways

Airflow generated by mechanical movements passes through the airways. The nasal passages, nasopharynx, larynx, trachea, and mainstem bronchi constitute the large airways. The bronchial tree, from segmental to subsegmental bronchi and down to each alveolar unit, comprise the lower airways. Large airways offer less resistance and airflow is mostly laminar except at bifurcations and in the upper trachea near the glottis, where it tends to be turbulent. The airways humidify and warm the air.

### Alveoli

Air reaches the *alveoli*, which are small air-filled sacs covered with a surface-active agent called surfactant. Each alveolus is lined with epithelium and has an adjacent endothelial surface that lines the nearby capillaries. The interface is termed the alveolar-capillary membrane. Oxygen ($O_2$) and carbon dioxide ($CO_2$) are exchanged here along their respective concentration gradients. $CO_2$ moves from the pulmonary arterial blood (high concentration, endothelial) to the airspace (low concentration, epithelial), and oxygen moves in the reverse direction. Thus, adequate surfactant function and an intact alveolar-capillary membrane are keys to gas exchange.

### Pulmonary Vessels

The pulmonary artery brings blood rich in $CO_2$ and low in $O_2$ into contact with the alveoli, and the pulmonary veins deliver blood rich in $O_2$ and lower in $CO_2$ to the left atrium, for systemic distribution. Movement of blood flow along the capillaries is necessary for effective gas exchange. At alveolar level, the microvessels are either in the alveoli (alveolar) or in the interstitial space (extra-alveolar). At FRC, alveoli and vessels are optimally open.

### Ventricular Function

Normal ventricular function assures good pulmonary blood flow in the presence of enough preload. Low preload or suboptimal pump function leads to lower pulmonary blood flow and may affect gas exchange. The negative intrathoracic pressure also moves more blood into the lungs during inspiration and keeps it out of thorax during expiration, thus keeping a good balance throughout the respiratory cycle.

## RESPIRATORY FAILURE

The respiratory system can fail if any of the above components of respiration is dysfunctional. Infants and children are at increased risk of developing airways obstruction when compared with adults. This is in part due to anatomic differences, particularly of the upper airways (see Fig. 96-1), but also due to conditions that more frequently affect younger patients. Large (or upper) airway obstruction usually occurs in children because of inhalation of a foreign body or airway inflammation such as croup or epiglottitis; rare causes include external compression from tumours or vascular malformations. Usually, large airway obstruction causes inspiratory stridor; in contrast, peripheral airway obstruction from asthma or bronchiolitis causes expiratory wheezing. Bronchiolitis is caused by small airway inflammation and narrowing, leading to expiratory obstruction. If severe, it can lead to trapping of air in the alveoli and hyperinflation. Alveolar damage mostly occurs from infection, edema, alveolar collapse, or contusion or alveolar hemorrhage. Such alveoli have diminished ventilation but are perfused; thus, shunting of deoxygenated blood occurs from the pulmonary artery to the pulmonary vein. Hypercapnia and hypoxemia increase respiratory drive, which coupled with reduced compliance from an injured lung, increases the work of breathing.

*Chest wall restriction* (eg, circumferential burn scars, kyphoscoliosis) limits tidal volume and necessitates rapid, shallow breathing. Diaphragm paralysis results in the diaphragm being pulled up (passively) by the inspiratory effort, creating a paradoxical pattern of breathing and mechanical disadvantage.

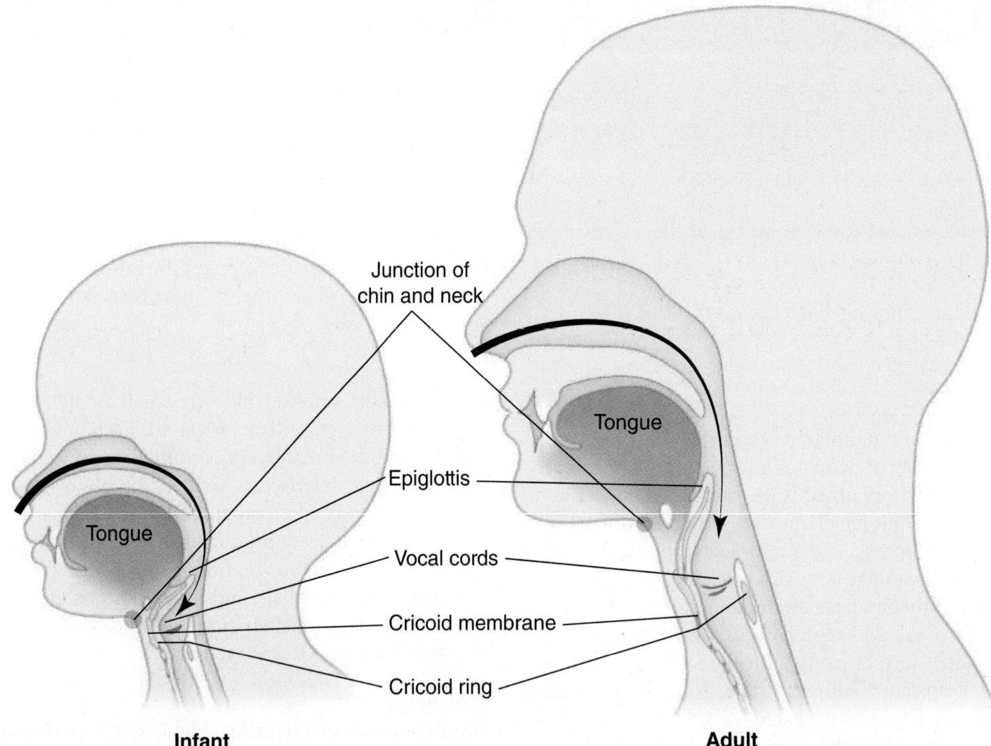


**FIGURE 96-1** Differences between infant and adult airways. (From Brown: *The Walls Manual of Emergency Airway Management*, 5th edition, Philadelphia, Wolters Kluwer, 2017 and The Difficult Airway Course [www.theairwaysite.com]. Used with permission.)



*Neurological dysfunction*, if severe or associated with elevated intracranial pressure, can depress respiration; in contrast, hyperventilation is characteristic of many congenital or acquired encephalopathies. Hyperventilation is also a typical finding as a compensation for metabolic acidosis (eg, ketoacidosis, salicylate ingestion). Sepsis increases utilization of oxygen, which elevates the work of breathing, and systemic inflammatory disorders (eg, systemic lupus erythematosus) can cause alveolar or pleural inflammation.

Finally, mechanical ventilation can damage the lungs; this is called ventilator-induced lung injury (VILI). Use of high tidal volume, suboptimal end-expiratory pressure, high driving pressure, and spontaneous breathing in injured lungs are some of the mechanisms that may contribute.

## ACUTE RESPIRATORY FAILURE

Based on the underlying pathophysiology, acute respiratory failure can be either hypoxemic or hypercapnic.

- Hypoxemic. Alveolar airspace disease (eg, acute respiratory distress syndrome, or ARDS) and/or pulmonary vascular disease (eg, persistent pulmonary hypertension, pulmonary embolism) result primarily in oxygenation failure.
- Hypercapnic. Airway obstruction and disordered control of breathing lead to low tidal volume or reduced flow, resulting in primary ventilation failure with elevation of $CO_2$.

## CHRONIC RESPIRATORY FAILURE

Chronic inflammation of alveoli, airways, or both (eg, cystic fibrosis, bronchopulmonary dysplasia), and chronic dysregulation of control of breathing (eg, central hypoventilation syndrome) can lead to long-term gas exchange failure, resulting in a baseline increase in $CO_2$ and ongoing $O_2$ dependence. Compensatory mechanisms of metabolic alkalosis to counter respiratory acidosis and re-establish a normal pH, and polycythemia to counter chronic hypoxemia become evident over time.

## EPIDEMIOLOGY OF RESPIRATORY FAILURE

The epidemiology of respiratory failure in children is complex because of developmental issues, variable severity of illnesses in the pediatric ICU, and classification based on syndromes (eg, ARDS, sepsis) versus disease entities.

### Croup

*Croup* is common in children aged 6 to 36 months, mostly in males. Family history is a risk factor, and it occurs most commonly in the fall and winter. Approximately 5% of children with croup in the emergency department (ED) are admitted to the hospital, and of those discharged home, approximately 5% return to the ED in 48 hours (see also Chapters 118 and 503).

### Respiratory Syncytial Virus

*Respiratory syncytial virus* (RSV) is typically seasonal, with outbreaks usually occurring between October and April in the northern hemisphere and April and September in the southern hemisphere. It is the most common cause of lower respiratory tract infection in children less than 1 year of age, and hospitalization is most common in those aged less than 3 months. The mortality from RSV is about 1% in children less than 4 years of age. Risk factors include age less than 6 months, daycare, older siblings, underlying lung disease, gestational age less than 35 weeks, congenital heart disease, secondhand smoke, and Down syndrome.

### Asthma Requiring ICU Admission

Sixty percent of asthmatic children have acute exacerbations, and the risk is greater in younger children or in those with inadequate interval asthma control. ICU admission is rare, but previous admission and exposure to multiple allergens are predictors (see also Chapter 505).

### Pneumonia

Approximately 156 million children under 5 years of age develop pneumonia each year worldwide, and about 20 million cases require hospital admission. Mortality in the developed world is low (1/1000) but high in the developing world. Risk factors include winter months, malnutrition, crowding, and chronic pulmonary, cardiac or neurologic conditions.

### Acute Respiratory Distress Syndrome

Acute respiratory distress syndrome in children is similar in its clinical, radiological, and pathological (see Fig. 96-2) characteristics

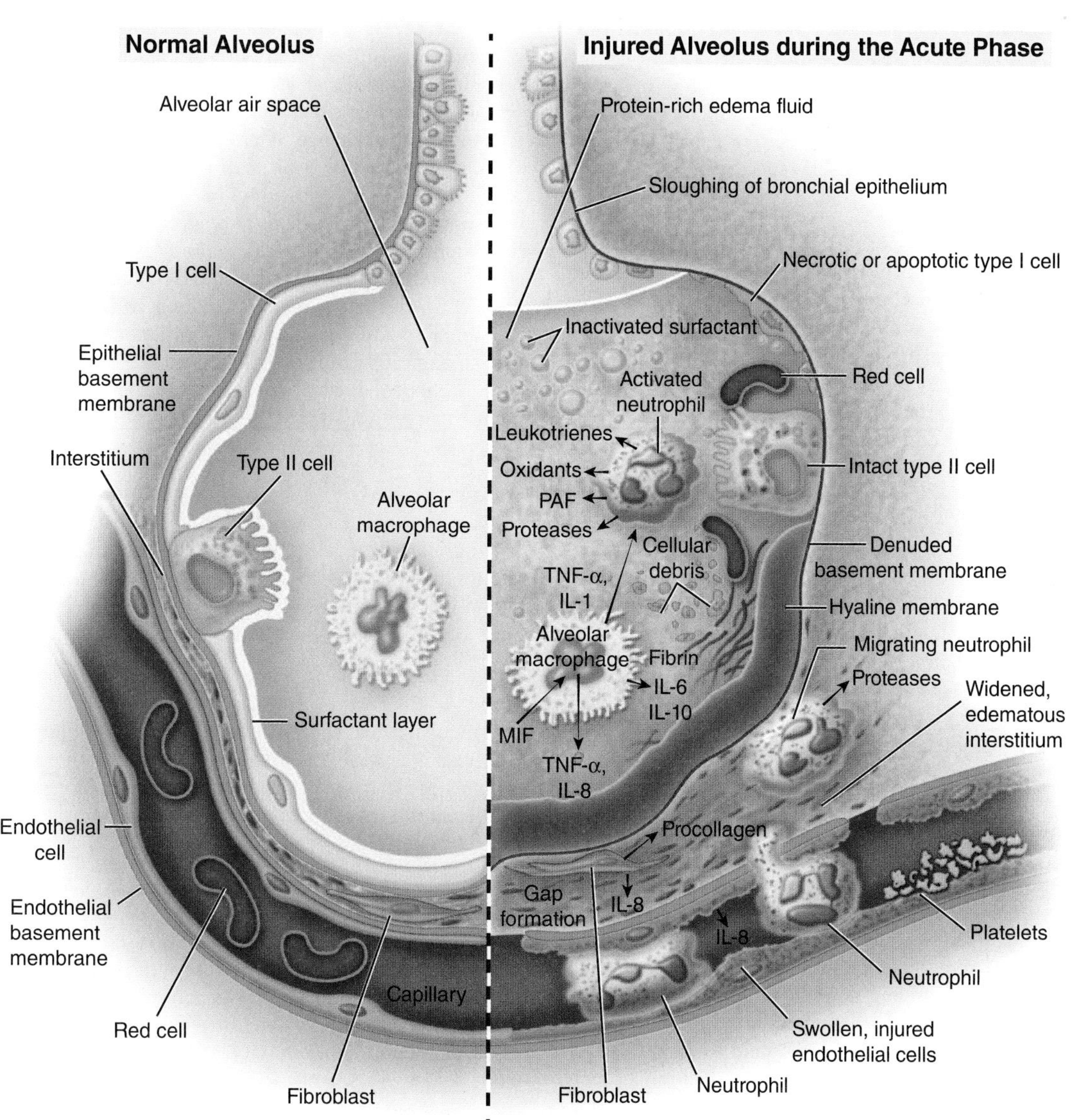


**FIGURE 96-2** Molecular biology and pathogenesis of ALI. (Reproduced with permission from Ware LB, Matthay MA. The acute respiratory distress syndrome, *N Engl J Med.* 2000 May 4;342(18):1334-1349.)

to ARDS in adults. However, the incidence (8 vs 15/1000 ICU admissions) and the mortality (less than 20%) are lower in children than in adults. In addition, death due to pediatric ARDS is usually due to hypoxemia, whereas in adults it is more commonly from multiorgan failure.

## INITIAL EVALUATION AND MANAGEMENT

A prompt evaluation can identify and facilitate the early stabilization of most sick children with respiratory failure. Hypopnea, severely increased work of breathing, dusky or mottled skin, pallor, and unresponsiveness can all herald imminent respiratory arrest.

### Airway

Immediate airway assessment is essential for any patient presenting in actual or pending respiratory failure. The airway is patent if there are good chest movements and no obstructive sounds. If necessary, airway patency can be achieved with suction to clear airway contents and mechanical maneuvers such as a jaw thrust or chin lift, repositioning, placement of an oropharyngeal airway, or endotracheal intubation.

### Breathing

Normal chest wall movement and breath sounds usually indicate adequate ventilation, although they cannot in themselves rule out hypercapnia or hypoxia. *Respiratory distress* is recognized by the use of accessory muscles, nasal flaring, subcostal and intercostal retraction. Severe distress is indicated by substernal, sternal, and suprasternal retraction. Auscultation may reveal crackles (airspace disease) or wheeze (airway disease), and the absence of cyanosis (confirmed by pulse oximetry) indicates adequate oxygenation. The unilateral absence of, or diminished, breath sounds indicates ipsilateral pneumothorax, major atelectasis, or pleural effusion.

## UNDERLYING DIAGNOSIS

### History

The history should include details of the course of the current symptoms, as well as any previous history of breathlessness, wheezing, cough or restricted activity, or failure to thrive. Access to or opportunities for ingestion of small objects, such as toys, or small pieces of food, should be specifically discussed with the caregivers, particularly if a foreign body is part of the differential diagnosis in a child with acute obstruction (see also Chapters 118 and 503).

### Investigations

Multiple investigations are available to help establish the underlying diagnosis, but the key lies in narrowing down the selection to a definitive test. A chest radiograph can confirm hyperinflation, consolidation, asymmetry, collapse, and pleural collections. Blood gas analysis will provide arterial $O_2$ and $CO_2$ tensions, and the pH may be useful as a guide to chronicity of a respiratory acidosis, or may determine whether there is a metabolic acidosis driving the process. Ultrasound of the chest is a useful tool to characterize pleural collections (single or loculated), to assist with drainage, or in recent years to confirm atelectasis or consolidation. Fiber-optic bronchoscopy can be used in the evaluation of central airway obstruction and sampling of alveolar fluid using the technique of bronchial alveolar lavage (BAL), and in children is usually conducted under general anesthesia.

#### Diagnosis of Specific Conditions

- *Croup.* The acute onset of stridor, fever, barking cough, and hoarseness in older children strongly suggest a diagnosis of croup. Throat pain, drooling, or swallowing difficulty may suggest *epiglottitis* rather than croup. Differential diagnoses in which the patients are typically toxic, with high fevers on presentation, include acute epiglottitis, retro- and parapharyngeal abscesses, paratonsillar abscesses, and bacterial tracheitis (see also Chapter 118). Additional possibilities include foreign body aspiration, acute angioneurotic edema, and upper airway injury from burns.
- *Bronchiolitis.* A 1- to 3-day history of upper respiratory infection–like symptoms followed by fever, cough, and respiratory distress (eg, tachypnea, retractions, wheezing, and rales) in children younger than 2 years of age suggest bronchiolitis. Cyanosis, lethargy, dehydration, or apnea would indicate severe bronchiolitis, and children presenting in this way should be hospitalized.
- *Asthma.* Acute exacerbations of asthma can be characterized by a dry cough with or without specific exposure (eg, cold air, pollens, dust). A history of atopy, positive family history for asthma, and seasonal symptoms indicate the diagnosis. Expiratory wheezes and hyperinflation are common. When severe, air entry may be almost absent with severe fatigue and altered sensorium (see also Chapter 505).
- *Pneumonia.* High-grade fever, cough, breathlessness, chest pain with increased work of breathing, presence of crackles, and bronchial breathing make a clinical diagnosis of pneumonia very likely. The chest radiograph typically shows patchy or homogenous consolidation. Hypoxemia usually is present, and hypercapnia also may be present if the pneumonia is severe or if the patient becomes fatigued. Elevated white counts, high inflammatory marks (eg, C-reactive protein and/or procalcitonin) point toward a bacterial etiology over viral. Nasal swab, sputum cultures, or bronchoscopic cultures are the most specific tests to identify the microbial etiology.
- *Pneumothorax.* Respiratory distress with unilateral absent air entry, a resonant percussion note, and a shift of the mediastinum (trachea and heart sounds) make the diagnosis, and chest x-ray is confirmatory.
- *Pleural effusion.* Reduced air entry with a dull percussion note, and bronchial breath sounds at the upper levels with a shift of the mediastinum to the opposite side (if ipsilateral atalecatsis is not marked) indicate pleural effusion. Chest x-ray is diagnostic in most cases and chest ultrasound provides additional confirmation and permits image-guided aspiration.

## RESPIRATORY SUPPORT

#### Supplemental Oxygen

*Supplemental oxygen* can be provided by nasal cannula or via a regular facemask or a nonrebreather mask. Oxygen flow is generally maintained at 3 to 4 times the minute ventilation so that all the inspiratory flow is provided by oxygen (100% $O_2$). Heated and humidified high-flow nasal cannula (HFNC) can also deliver high inspired $O_2$ with an additional component of positive pressure, which may assist with lung recruitment, though the level achieved is highly variable. The constant airflow displaces $CO_2$ from the anatomical dead space, thereby creating an oxygen reservoir. A HFNC also improves mucociliary function due to humidification and high flows.

#### Positive Pressure Ventilation

*Noninvasive ventilation* is routinely used to provide respiratory support in modern ICUs and can be applied in various ways. Continuous positive airway pressure (CPAP) opens the alveoli and increases FRC, thus improving oxygenation while the patient breathes spontaneously above this pressure to maintain ventilation. If efforts are inadequate, then bilevel positive airways pressure (BiPAP) can be applied. This provides an additional level of inspiratory support, as well as the option of providing mandatory breaths to further assist inspiratory effort and gas exchange. If problems persist or deteriorate, invasive ventilation should be instituted. In the case of a hypoxemic patient, an optimal positive end-expiratory pressure (PEEP) derived from a recruitment maneuver helps to open the alveoli and keep them open, thus increasing FRC. A tidal volume set at 6 mL/kg or adjusted to allow permissive hypercapnia (high $CO_2$ and pH > 7.2) reduces ongoing VILI. Adequate minute ventilation is achieved by adjusting the rate and providing good patient-ventilator synchrony. The inspiratory-to-expiratory time ratio is set such that it allows maximal oxygenation without reducing ventilation. High inspired $O_2$ concentrations are toxic to lung tissue and moderating the goals of oxygenation with a degree of permissive hypoxia might be beneficial.

#### Prone Positioning

*Prone positioning* has been used to improve oxygenation and ventilation in patients with ARDS. Prone positioning shifts the ventilation from nondependent to dependent parts of the lungs and moves abdominal contents away from the diaphragm, thus reducing impedance to ventilation in the injured area (Fig. 96-3).

**High-Frequency Oscillatory Ventilation** *High-frequency oscillatory ventilation* (HFOV) was designed with the goal of keeping the lungs open and reducing tidal shear stress. It ventilates the lungs at the optimal compliance and moves air/oxygen flow continuously in a central column instead of in bulk flow. It achieves ventilation directly in relation to the amplitude of the percussions and inversely in relation to the frequency applied.

**Inhaled Nitric Oxide** *Inhaled nitric oxide* (iNO) is a potent, selective pulmonary vasodilator. It is primarily indicated in pulmonary hypertension, especially in newborns. It is also used as an adjunct in hypoxic respiratory failure refractory to improve ventilation/perfusion matching, and therefore improve oxygenation. However, it is important to note that there is little evidence to support improved overall outcomes associated with the use of iNO in patients with ARDS. Inhaled nitric oxide delivery should be carefully monitored, as it can be toxic in high concentrations and may produce methemoglobinemia, though this is rare in the therapeutic dose range (usually up to 20 parts per million). It can also be cytotoxic to alveolar and vascular tissues.

#### Extracorporeal Membrane Oxygenation

Hypoxia unresponsive to all above therapies needs to be managed with extracorporeal life support. Use of venovenous extracorporeal membrane oxygenation (VV ECMO) helps the lungs rest and recover while oxygenation is achieved by an artificial membrane. Coexistent right heart failure or the presence of circulatory shock warrants the use of venoarterial (VA) ECMO. See also Chapter 108.

## SPECIFIC THERAPIES

#### Antimicrobials

Specific choices of primary or adjunctive antimicrobial agents are largely dictated by the disease severity; factors relating to the underlying host (immunocompetent or otherwise); whether the infection may have been nosocomial or community acquired; and local pathogens and likely susceptibility. Optimal broad-spectrum antibiotics, started early and narrowed by sensitivity results from culture, are the standard of care for the treatment of pneumonia. This may be achieved with single agents, or if specific organisms such as *Chlamydia*, *Mycoplasma*, or methicillin-resistant *Staphylococcus aureus* (MRSA) are potential pathogens, or in severe cases requiring ICU admission, then 2 or more empiric antibiotics should be used. Antiinfluenza therapy using oseltamivir should be considered for severe pneumonia needing ICU admission until influenza is ruled out.

#### Surfactants

Ongoing surfactant replacement in *primary surfactant deficiency* in neonates should be instituted if transplantation is an ultimate goal.

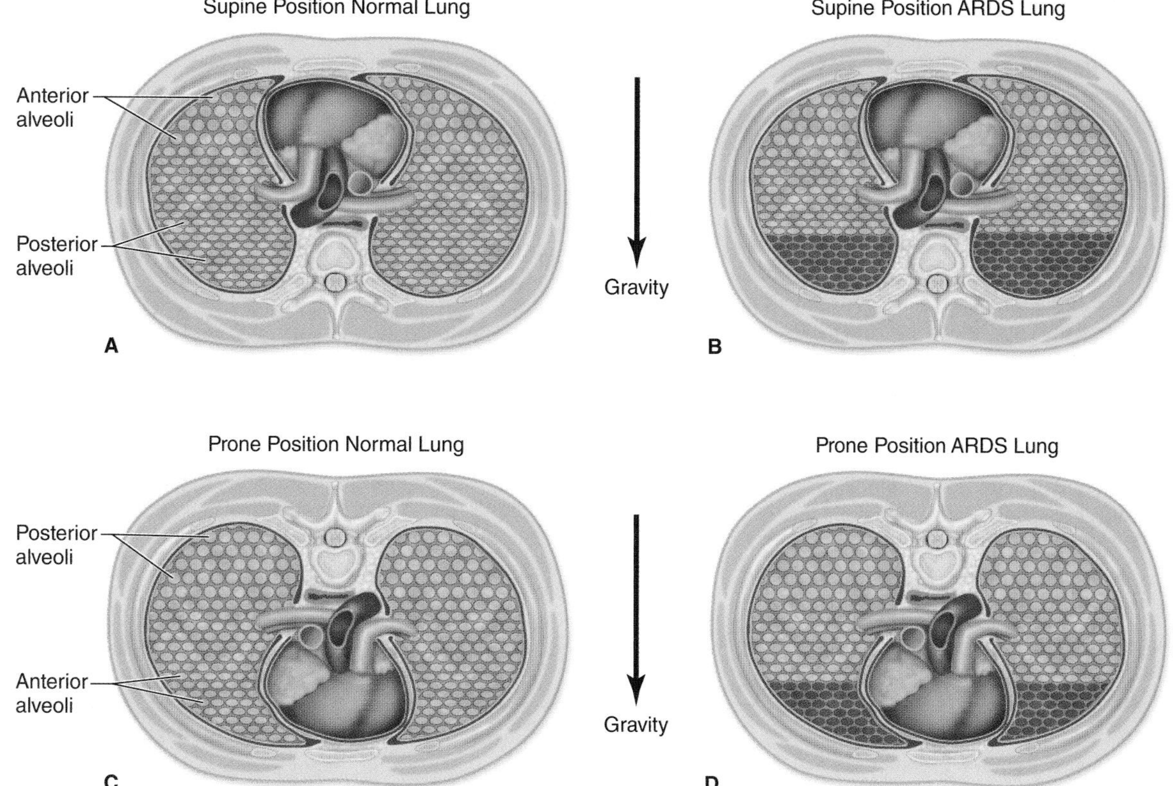


FIGURE 96-3 Physiologic benefits from prone positioning.

Outside of the newborn period, there is otherwise little evidence to support the use of surfactant in acute lung injury.

#### Bronchodilators

Rescue albuterol nebulization given continuously initially, and potentially followed by intravenous (IV) infusion in unresponsive cases of asthma, has become the standard of care. Magnesium sulphate and aminophylline are potential adjuncts to $\beta_2$-agonist therapy, and in the most severe cases, administration of inhalational anesthetic agents such as isoflurane or sevoflurane can be considered if appropriate delivery systems and monitoring exist.

#### Corticosteroids

Systemic steroids are strongly recommended in acute asthma exacerbations needing admission. Methylprednisolone 1 to 2 mg/kg/dose given every 6 to 8 hours either enterally or IV is the standard practice, though recent evidence suggests that a shorter course of dexamethasone may be a viable alternative. Steroids may also be useful to help reduce inflammation of the alveoli in cases of ARDS if given after a serious infection has been excluded.

## PREVENTION

Prevention is the key to reduce the burden of morbidity and mortality from childhood respiratory illnesses, and to prevent hospitalization.

#### Asthma

Outpatient stabilization and well-controlled, long-term treatment and action plans may prevent acute exacerbations from requiring hospital admissions, and from reaching the ICU. Prompt use of inhalers, allergen identification and control, and patient education and follow-up become keys to the management of childhood asthma (see also Chapter 505).

#### Viral and Bacterial Infections

Timely vaccinations, avoiding overcrowding, minimizing travel during the peak season, and early visits for timely diagnosis and management are important to avoid progression to severe illness and ICU admission.

#### Hospital-Acquired Infection

Adherence to strict protocols of hand hygiene, ventilator-associated pneumonia (VAP) prevention bundles, and ongoing healthcare team education are imperative to reduce hospital-acquired infections.

#### Minimizing Ventilator-Induced Lung Injury

Use of lung protective strategy, minimizing repeated opening and closing of alveoli, and judicious use of PEEP are some of the measures to reduce VILI.

## SUMMARY

Acute respiratory dysfunction is the most common cause for emergency and ICU visits in childhood. Preventive measures, prompt diagnosis, and early interventions with optimal respiratory support and diagnosis-driven therapies are all important mechanisms to reduce morbidity and mortality, in addition to potentially reducing healthcare costs.

## SUGGESTED READINGS

Avery ME, Mead J. Surface properties in relation to atelectasis and hyaline membrane disease. *AMA J Dis Child.* 1959;97(5, Pt 1): 517-523.

Bohn DJ. Acute hypoxic respiratory failure in children. In: Annich GM, Lynch WR, MacLaren G, Wilson JM, Bartlett RH. *ECMO: Extracorporeal Cardiopulmonary Support in Critical Care.* 4th ed. Ann Arbor, Michigan, USA: Extracorporeal Life Support Organization; 2012.

Bradley JS, Byington CL, Shah SS, et al; Pediatric Infectious Diseases Society; Infectious Diseases Society of America. The management of community-acquired pneumonia in infants and children older than 3 months of age: clinical practice guidelines by the Pediatric Infectious Diseases Society and the Infectious Diseases Society of America. *Clin Infect Dis.* 2011;53(7):e25-e75.

Bryan AC. Conference on the scientific basis of respiratory therapy. Pulmonary physiotherapy in the pediatric age group. Comments of a devil's advocate. *Am Rev Respir Dis.* 1974;110(6 Pt 2): 143-144.

Chameides L, Samson RA, Shexnayder SM, Hazinski MF. Recognition of respiratory distress and failure. In: *Pediatric Advanced Life Support Provider Manual.* Dallas, TX: American Heart Association; 2011:37.

National Heart, Lung, and Blood Institute; National Asthma Education and Prevention Program. Expert panel report 3: Guidelines for the diagnosis and management of asthma. Bethesda, MD: National Heart, Lung, and Blood Institute, 2007. NIH publication no. 08-4051.

Ralston SL, Lieberthal AS, Meissner HC, et al. Clinical practice guideline: the diagnosis, management, and prevention of bronchiolitis. *Pediatrics.* 2014;134:e1474-e1502.

Rudan I, Boschi-Pinto C, Biloglav Z, Mulholland K, Campbell H. Epidemiology and etiology of childhood pneumonia. *Bull World Health Organ.* 2008;86(5):408-416.

Tobin MJ, ed. *Principles and Practice of Mechanical Ventilation.* 3rd ed. New York, NY: McGraw-Hill Education; 2013.

Wing R, James C, Maranda LS, Armsby CC. Use of high-flow nasal cannula support in the emergency department reduces the need for intubation in pediatric acute respiratory insufficiency. *Pediatr Emerg Care.* 2012;28(11):1117-1123.

Wung JT, James LS, Kilchevsky E, James E. Management of infants with severe respiratory failure and persistence of the fetal circulation, without hyperventilation. *Pediatrics.* 1985;76(4):488-494.



# 97 Pathophysiology of Sepsis

Trung C. Nguyen and Joseph A. Carcillo

## INTRODUCTION AND EPIDEMIOLOGY

Sepsis continues to be the leading cause of death among children worldwide, accounting for more than 5.9 million deaths per year according to data from the World Health Organization and the United Nations Children's Fund. In the United States, sepsis poses a significant healthcare burden with approximately 75,000 children admitted annually to hospitals with severe sepsis and an associated cost of $4.8 billion. Understanding the pathophysiology of systemic inflammatory response syndrome (SIRS) and sepsis syndrome is essential for recognition and management of this deadly disease.

## PATHOGENESIS OF SIRS AND SEPSIS

In the 1990s, Bone and colleagues set forth the notion that systemic inflammation due to an infection can lead to SIRS, sepsis syndrome, multiple organ dysfunction syndrome (MODS), and multiple organ failure (MOF). Typically, after sensing an invading pathogen, the host's innate immune system is locally activated in order to eradicate the infection. This immune activation is mediated by pathogen-associated molecular patterns (PAMPS), such as lipopolysaccharides from bacterial cell walls that interact with the pattern recognition receptors (PRRS) such as toll-like receptors (TLRs), which are present on local immune cells. This initial interaction between PAMPS and PRRS will lead to a signaling cascade, resulting in inflammatory cytokine and chemokine synthesis and release. Injured and dying cells caused by this inflammation go on to release damage-associated molecular patterns (DAMPS) such as the intracellular protein high-mobility group box 1. DAMPS released from tissue injury amplify the cytokine response to PAMPS that can progress into a vicious cycle of tissue and organ injuries (Fig. 97-1). The inflammatory mediators synthesized and released during sepsis syndrome are meant to help the host in combating the invading pathogen. However, if unregulated, these inflammatory mediators can induce a pathologic state of shock in the host. Shock is defined as a state of cellular and tissue hypoxia due to reduced oxygen delivery and/or increased oxygen consumption or inadequate oxygen utilization. For example, the inflammatory cytokines tumor necrosis factor alpha (TNF-α) and interleukin-1beta can both (1) depress myocardial function and (2) pathologically vasodilate blood vessels partly through mechanisms of nitric oxide generation, both of which cause low blood perfusion to tissues. TNF-α also causes vascular leak syndrome by triggering the shedding of glycocalyx, which disrupts the endothelial cell lining. Glycocalyx, a multicomponent layer consisting of proteoglycans and glycoprotein that lines the luminal membrane of the endothelium, is essential in regulating vascular permeability and barrier function, hemostasis, vasomotor control, and immunological function. Thus, sepsis can cause significant disturbance in all organs, which can result in cardiovascular collapse, respiratory failure, immune dysregulation, acute kidney injury, coagulopathy, thrombotic microangiopathy, ischemic hepatitis, endotheliopathy, and mitochondrial dysfunction. The severity of these disturbances depends on many factors, including the genetic and environmental factors of both the host and the pathogen.

It is important to note that pathogenic microbes double every 30 minutes. Therefore, early source control with appropriate antibiotics and nidus removal is the key to stopping the progression from sepsis to severe sepsis or septic shock to MODS or MOF to death.

## DEFINITIONS

Bone and colleagues first proposed clinical definitions of SIRS, sepsis, severe sepsis, and septic shock. These definitions with modifications are still being used by pediatricians, though the term SIRS is no longer used in adults.

## CLINICAL MANIFESTATIONS OF SEPSIS AND SEPTIC SHOCK

Responding to the request from the Institute of Medicine for establishment of best practice guidelines across medicine, in 2002, the American College of Critical Care Medicine (ACCM) published its first guidelines, "Clinical Practice Parameters for Hemodynamic Support of Pediatric and Neonatal Patients in Septic Shock." This document reported the best clinical practices for pediatric sepsis that were associated with the best outcomes. By then, sepsis mortality had already decreased from 97% to 9% over past decades due to early recognition and innovations. The ACCM/PALS guidelines, were updated in 2007 and again in 2014. Many studies have evaluated the outcomes associated with implementation of the 2002 and 2007 guidelines. In resource-rich settings with intensive care units available, studies have found adherence to these ACCM/PALS guidelines have resulted in improved outcomes. The ACCM/PALS guidelines stress the importance of early sepsis recognition in order to implement the time-sensitive and goal-directed recommendations of septic shock resuscitation. Thus, a clear and easy clinical definition of septic shock is essential.

Septic pediatric patients can present to the doctor's office with a vague constellation of soft signs and symptoms including fever, runny nose, irritability, not eating well, not acting playful, and warm hands and feet. Others may present with overt septic shock with high fever, lethargy, and cold hands and feet, or with obvious vasodilatory shock with warm peripheries, bounding pulses and a high-output state. Table 97-1 lists the definition of clinical pediatric shock from the 2007 ACCM/PALS guidelines.

The ACCM/PALS guidelines suggest that septic shock should be diagnosed by clinical signs and symptoms including (1) hypothermia or hyperthermia; (2) altered mental status; and (3) peripheral vasodilation, bounding peripheral pulses, and wide pulse pressure (warm shock) or vasoconstriction with capillary refill > 2 seconds, diminished pulses, and mottled cool extremities (cold shock) before hypotension. Once the septic shock is recognized, shock resuscitation should be rapidly initiated with the goals of restoring normal (1) mental status, (2) threshold

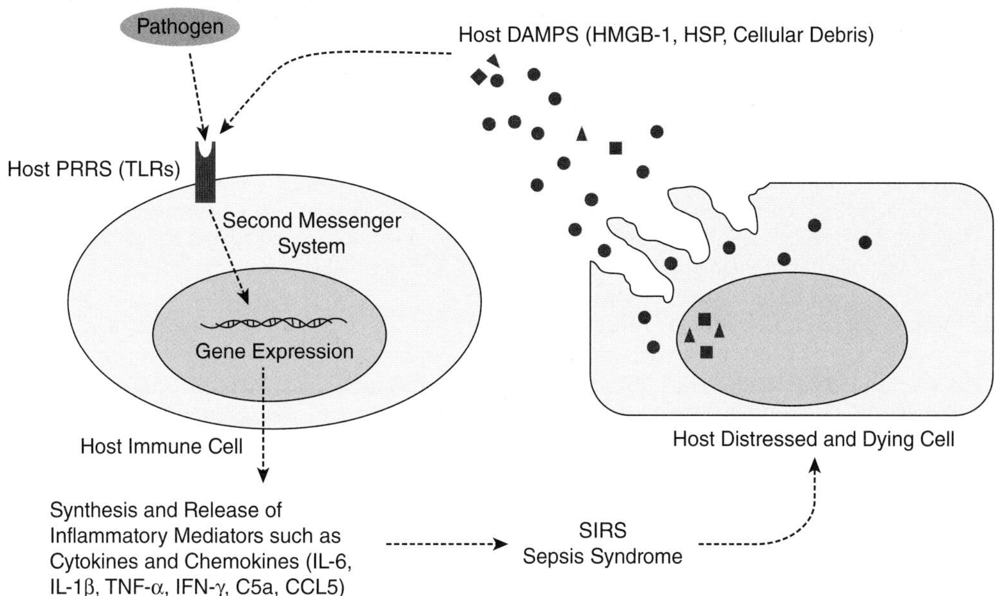


**FIGURE 97-1** Pathogen-associated molecular patterns (PAMPS) activate immune cells, and damage-associated molecular patterns (DAMPS) amplify the cytokine response to PAMPS via interaction with pattern recognition receptors (PRRS). These interactions lead to intracellular signal transduction cascades, synthesis and release of inflammatory mediators, and SIRS or sepsis syndrome. C5a, complement component C5; CCL5, chemokine ligand 5; HMGB-1, high-mobility group box 1; HSP, heat shock protein; IL-1β, interleukin-1beta; IL-6, interleukin 6; IFN-γ, interferon gamma; LPS, lipopolysaccharide; SIRS, systemic inflammatory response syndrome; TLR, toll-like receptor; TNF-α, tumor necrosis factor alpha.



heart rates, (3) peripheral perfusion (capillary refill < 3 seconds), (4) palpable distal pulses, and (5) blood pressure for age. The ACCM/PALS guidelines recommend implementing 5 key elements during the first hour of managing pediatric septic shock: (1) recognition, (2) establishing intravenous access, (3) starting intravenous fluids and resuscitation as needed, (4) administering antibiotics, and (5) starting vasoactive agents as needed (see also Chapter 106).

## WARM VERSUS COLD SHOCK

The majority (58%) of community-acquired fluid refractory pediatric septic shock presents as cold shock. On examination, the patient is difficult to arouse and exhibits cold hands and feet, weak peripheral pulses, and capillary refills delayed to > 2 seconds. In cold shock, the main defect is the significant reduction in oxygen delivery to tissues due to intravascular hypovolemia and/or myocardial dysfunction. The patient feels cold to the touch because the blood vessels vasoconstrict as a physiologic compensatory mechanism to maintain appropriate perfusion pressure and oxygen delivery to vital organs. If not appropriately resuscitated, the tissues will be starved of oxygen and energy substrates leading to tissue hypoxia, metabolic acidosis, and organ dysfunction. Thus, pediatric cold septic shock frequently responds well to volume resuscitation and to inotropic support, especially with peripheral epinephrine infusion being an excellent first choice for myocardial dysfunction. These patients commonly require mechanical ventilation to reduce cardiopulmonary work requirements.

In contrast, warm shock is the typical presentation in septic adults but only in 20% of septic children and is predominantly seen in older children or those with long-term central access. On examination, the patient again is difficult to arouse and has warm hands and feet, bounding peripheral pulses, and flash capillary refills. The main circulatory defect in warm shock is vasomotor paralysis (vasoplegia) with significant vasodilatation. Cardiac output is typically normal or increased though overall oxygen balance is deranged. Of note, adults with warm shock typically have a defect in oxygen extraction rather than oxygen delivery. Warm shock frequently responds to volume resuscitation and vasoconstrictor agents. Over time, a minority (10%) of patients may have a complete change in the hemodynamic state between warm and cold shock. In general, persistent pediatric septic shock will progress to cold shock with significant decrease in cardiac function.

**TABLE 97-1 DEFINITIONS OF SHOCK**

| | |
|---|---|
| Cold or warm shock | Decreased perfusion manifested by altered decreased mental status, capillary refills > 2 sec (cold shock) or flash capillary refill (warm shock), diminished (cold shock) or bounding (warm shock) peripheral pulses, mottled cool extremities (cold shock), or decreased urine output < 1 mL/kg/min |
| Fluid-refractory/dopamine-resistant shock | Shock persists despite ≥ 60 mL/kg fluid resuscitation (when appropriate) and dopamine infusion to 10 mcg/kg/min |
| Catecholamine-resistant shock | Shock persists despite use of the direct-acting catecholamines: epinephrine or norepinephrine |
| Refractory shock | Shock persists despite goal-directed use of inotropic agents, vasopressors, vasodilators, and maintenance of metabolic (glucose and calcium) and hormonal (thyroid, hydrocortisone, insulin) homeostasis |

Reproduced with permission from Brierley J, Carcillo JA, Choong K, et al: Clinical practice parameters for hemodynamic support of pediatric and neonatal septic shock: 2007 update from the American College of Critical Care Medicine, *Crit Care Med.* 2009 Feb;37(2):666-88.

## SEPSIS-INDUCED MULTIPLE ORGAN DYSFUNCTION SYNDROME AND FAILURE

Even with the best efforts in septic shock resuscitation and early control of the infective source, a subset of patients still progresses to significant tissue injury and MODS. Individual patients respond very differently from each other to septic shock resuscitation, and their response depends on the time to source control first and foremost, but also to the genetic makeup and environmental factors of both the host and pathogen. Current clinical and experimental evidence suggests that these genetic and environmental factors can impede the resolution of systemic inflammation in sepsis-induced MODS. Investigators propose that there is a spectrum of MODS pathobiology phenotypes such as thrombocytopenia-associated multiple organ failure (TAMOF), immunoparalysis, sequential MODS, hemophagocytic lymphohistiocytosis (HLH), macrophage activation syndrome (MAS), and others. The common denominator in these MODS phenotypes is immune dysregulation. Thus, understanding and recognizing these MODS pathobiology phenotypes may lead to better therapeutic strategies for the leading reversible cause of late death in sepsis.

TAMOF is a clinical syndrome characterized by new onset thrombocytopenia in a setting of evolving MODS. TAMOF represents a spectrum of mixed thrombotic microangiopathies and coagulopathies including thrombotic thrombocytopenic purpura, hemolytic uremic syndrome, and disseminated intravascular coagulation. The drop in platelet count in this syndrome suggests the pathologic involvement of platelets as they form disseminated microvascular thromboses in the vascular beds of tissues, which leads to ischemia and injury resulting in the observed MODS. Persistent SIRS in sepsis induces extensive endothelial and immunologic activation leading to a prothrombotic and antifibrinolytic state. In TAMOF, tissue factor, von Willebrand factor and platelets, and/or complement pathways are dysregulated. For example, patients with a genetic mutation in plasminogen activator inhibitor type 1, ADAMTS-13, or complement factors are at higher risk of developing TAMOF during sepsis.

Immunoparalysis is a state of impaired innate and/or adaptive immunity that occurs after the initial life-threatening proinflammatory insult in sepsis. The host immune system responds to the initial SIRS with a compensatory anti-inflammatory response syndrome (CARS) to prevent uncontrolled SIRS. If CARS persists, it will lead to a form of acquired immune deficiency. These patients are unable to clear the invading pathogens and will succumb to unresolved infection. Genetic predisposition such as an increase in anti-inflammatory cytokine production or other pathologic immune downregulation mechanisms places the patient at risk for immunoparalysis. Immunosuppressive medications such as steroids, antirejection drugs and chemotherapies can also induce a state of immunoparalysis.

Pathologic immune activation is an immune dysregulated state that leads to hyperinflammation. This occurs when the host immune system is unable to shut down the initial SIRS. The pathologic mechanism can be caused by a failure to shut down activated immune cells, such as a defect in the Fas/Fas ligand apoptotic pathway or in perforin or granzyme B-mediated cytolysis. Persistent presence of activated antigen presenting cells or persistent stimulation of TLR9 by pathogen can also lead to pathologic immune activation and hyperinflammation. Sequential MODS phenotypes have characteristic respiratory dysfunction followed by hepatic and renal failure evolving over the initial 3 days following sepsis presentation. These patients have an increased soluble Fas level, which inhibits apoptosis of activated immune cells after a viral infection. The clinical manifestations of this, HLH and MAS include a characteristic severe hepatitis and disseminated intravascular coagulation or TAMOF after an infection. HLH and MAS patients are typically found to have either an inherited or acquired defect in the ability of cytotoxic lymphocytes to induce cytolysis of target cells such as antigen presenting cells.

Currently, there is no single "magic bullet" agent to cure sepsis or abate the sequelae of septic shock. Nevertheless, in the United States, the overall sepsis mortality has significantly decreased over the past 4 decades thanks in part to early recognition and application of the best practice guidelines of septic shock resuscitation. However, sepsis-induced MODS is still the leading reversible cause of late death in pediatric sepsis with mortality increasing with each additional dysfunctional organ. Current active research is being directed at identifying common MODS pathobiology phenotypes and identifying therapeutic strategies for each pathologic mechanism. For example, anti–C5 monoclonal antibody and/or therapeutic plasma exchange are being studied to reverse TAMOF. Immune modulation therapies such as granulocyte-macrophage colony-stimulating factor are being studied to reverse immunoparalysis. Steroids, intravenous immunoglobulin, and interleukin-1 receptor antagonists are being studied to reverse MAS. Steroids, etoposide, and anti–interferon-gamma antibody therapies are agents that are currently being investigated in the treatment of HLH.

## CONCLUSION

Sepsis remains a healthcare burden worldwide with enormous human and economic toll. Significant progress has been made with septic shock resuscitation in the resource-rich developing and developed settings. National sepsis initiatives are in place to improve septic shock outcomes. Research targeting a role for personalized medicine strategies in pediatric sepsis-induced MODS and MOF is underway.

## SUGGESTED READINGS


Black RE, Cousens S, Johnson HL, et al. Global, regional, and national causes of child mortality in 2008: a systematic analysis. *Lancet.* 2010;375(9730):1969-1987.

Bone RC, Fisher CJ Jr, Clemmer TP, Slotman GJ, Metz CA, Balk RA. Sepsis syndrome: a valid clinical entity. Methylprednisolone Severe Sepsis Study Group. *Crit Care Med.* 1989;17(5):389-393.

Brierley J, Carcillo JA, Choong K, et al. Clinical practice parameters for hemodynamic support of pediatric and neonatal septic shock: 2007 update from the American College of Critical Care Medicine. *Criti Care Med.* 2009;37(2):666-688.

Brierley J, Peters MJ. Distinct hemodynamic patterns of septic shock at presentation to pediatric intensive care. *Pediatrics.* 2008;122(4): 752-759.

Carcillo JA, Han YY, Doughty L, Hall M, Nguyen TC, Aneja R. Inflammation and immunity: systemic inflammatory response syndrome, sepsis, acute lung injury, and multiple organ failure. In: Fuhrman BZ, Carcillo JA, Clark R, et al, ed. *Fuhrman and Zimmerman's Pediatric Critical Care.* 4th ed. Philadelphia, PA: Elsevier Mosby; 2011:1430-1438.

Ceneviva G, Paschall JA, Maffei F, Carcillo JA. Hemodynamic support in fluid-refractory pediatric septic shock. *Pediatrics.* 1998;102(2):e19.

Davis AL, Carcillo JA, Aneja RK, et al. American College of Critical Care Medicine Clinical Practice Parameters for Hemodynamic Support of Pediatric and Neonatal Septic Shock. *Crit Care Med.* 2017;45(6):1061-1093.

Goldstein B, Giroir B, Randolph A; International Consensus Conference on Pediatric Sepsis. International pediatric sepsis consensus conference: definitions for sepsis and organ dysfunction in pediatrics. *Pediatr Crit Care Med.* 2005;6(1):2-8.

Hickey MJ, Kubes P. Intravascular immunity: the host-pathogen encounter in blood vessels. *Nat Rev Immunol.* 2009;9(5):364-375.

Ince C, Mayeux PR, Nguyen T, et al. The endothelium in sepsis. *Shock.* 2016;45(3):259-270.

Matzinger P. The danger model: a renewed sense of self. *Science.* 2002;296(5566):301-305.

Matzinger P, Kamala T. Tissue-based class control: the other side of tolerance. *Nat Rev Immunol.* 2011;11(3):221-230.

Paul R, Melendez E, Stack A, Capraro A, Monuteaux M, Neuman MI. Improving adherence to PALS septic shock guidelines. *Pediatrics.* 2014;133(5):e1358-1366.

Singer M, Deutschman CS, Seymour CW, et al. The Third International Consensus Definitions for Sepsis and Septic Shock (Sepsis-3). *JAMA.* 2016; 23;315(8):801-810.

# 98 Acute Neurological Dysfunction

Ken Brady and John Beca

## ACUTE NEUROLOGICAL DYSFUNCTION

Altered consciousness can be a manifestation of a variety of disease processes. It is commonly indicative of life-threatening illness that requires urgent stabilization, diagnosis, and institution of disease-specific therapy to prevent ongoing neurologic injury and long-term neurodevelopmental disability. Although the anatomic structures related to consciousness have been defined, depressed consciousness is usually poorly localized to specific nervous system pathways, and often represents the consequence of a failed non-neurologic organ system.

The goals of this chapter are to review the pathophysiology and age-specific epidemiology of altered mental status, to delineate the current framework used to assess the presentation of depressed consciousness, to give a practical overview of its differential diagnosis, and finally to outline a strategy for stabilization, diagnostic evaluation, and emergent treatment options. A full discussion of the clinical approach to altered consciousness, including a comprehensive review of the interpretation of clinical signs, can be found in standard texts on coma.

## PATHOPHYSIOLOGY AND EPIDEMIOLOGY

Consciousness has 2 components, wakefulness and awareness (of self and of the surrounding environment). Awareness cannot occur without wakefulness but wakefulness can occur without awareness. Consciousness is dependent on the function of the reticular activating system (RAS) that promotes widespread cortical activation. The core areas for maintaining wakefulness are thought to be ascending glutamatergic and cholinergic neurons in the dorsal tegmentum of the midbrain and pons. These activate the central thalamus and basal forebrain, which in turn activate the cortex.

The level of arousal is a function of the overall state of activity of the brain. Awareness is a more complex and integrated process involving the cerebral cortex and thalamus. Coma is a state in which a child has eyes closed and is unaware and unresponsive to any external stimuli, except for reflex responses. It results from either damage to the RAS or profound global cortical dysfunction. While lesions of the RAS can result in coma, detailed knowledge of this anatomic pathway is generally not required as global cortical dysfunction is by far the most common cause of altered consciousness. Focal lesions that affect the RAS do occur, especially those that produce pressure in the posterior fossa.

### Regulation of Cerebral Blood Flow

Cerebral blood flow is tightly matched to the metabolic need of brain tissue, which is dependent on a continuous supply of oxygen and glucose for obligate-aerobic metabolism. Neither excessive nor inadequate cerebral blood flow can be tolerated for prolonged duration without causing brain injury. Multiple layers of adaptive mechanisms work simultaneously to adjust and constrain cerebral blood flow to an optimized level during disrupted physiological states such as shock or disturbed delivery of substrate.

**Systemic Vasoconstriction** The first adaptive mechanism to preserve cerebral blood flow is the systemic vasoconstrictor response to shock or hypotensive states, which is characteristically associated with neurohormonal activation. However, vessels in the brain have diminished responses to this neurohormonal state, so the net effect is to maintain arterial blood pressure with preserved cerebral blood flow and diminished blood flow to other systemic organ beds. This mechanism of cardiac output redistribution is highly relevant to the child in shock from low cardiac output. Vasoactive agents that modulate systemic vascular resistance will preserve cerebral perfusion pressure and cerebral blood flow in this setting, but do so at the expense of visceral perfusion.

**Pressure Autoregulation** When systemic vasoconstriction fails to maintain arterial blood pressure, vessels of the brain actively dilate to preserve cerebral blood flow. Modulation of cerebrovascular resistance in response to changes in arterial blood pressure is called *pressure autoregulation*, and is known to fail at a lower limit of arterial blood pressure. Although descriptions of autoregulation in hypertensive adults and women treated for pre-eclampsia suggested a lower limit of autoregulation at a mean arterial blood pressure of 50 mm Hg, lower limits of acceptable arterial blood pressure for pediatric patients are not known, but they are likely much lower and influenced by pathologic states, especially those that increase intracranial pressure.

**Neurovascular Coupling** When the global control of cerebral blood flow is at undisturbed, regional control is also active to provide heterogeneous distribution of flow to areas of high metabolic activity. This mechanism is called metabolic autoregulation or neurovascular coupling and is mediated by neurovascular units with astrocyte projections connecting neuronal synapses and resistance arterioles. Neurovascular coupling is useful clinically when it is desirable to reduce cerebral blood flow (and therefore blood volume and intracranial pressure). The induction of electrical silence with barbiturate coma reduces cerebral metabolism and cerebral blood flow by as much as 60% without causing a deficit of oxygen delivery.

**Carbon Dioxide Reactivity** Carbon dioxide diffuses freely into the cerebral spinal fluid, but bicarbonate buffers are unable to cross the blood-brain barrier. When minute ventilation and arterial carbon dioxide tension are normal, pH reactivity facilitates the regulation of constant carbon dioxide and pH levels in the spinal fluid. Acute hypercarbia lowers the pH of cerebrospinal fluid and this induces a profound vasodilatory effect on the resistance vessels of the brain. Acute hypocarbia raises the pH and induces a vasoconstrictive effect. These pathologic increases or reductions of cerebral blood flow are not necessarily matched to the metabolic activity of the brain and can cause significant injury. Hyperventilation to control intracranial pressure in children with traumatic brain injury is thought to cause ischemic injury and may be harmful outside of transient use to control acute spikes in intracranial pressure and impending herniation syndromes.

**Hypoxic and Hypoglycemic Vasodilation** Cerebral blood flow is increased (secondary to vasodilation) when oxygen or glucose delivery is reduced below the normal physiologic range. In patients with coma or acute brain injury, it is important to maintain hematocrit, systemic oxygenation, and blood glucose levels in the normal range.

### Herniation Syndromes

Brain herniation occurs if intracranial pressure is not controlled. There is displacement of part of the brain from 1 compartment in to another (see Chapter 105) and compression of adjacent structures. The syndromes of herniation include subfalcial, transtentorial, and tonsillar.

Subfalcial herniation is when unilateral hemisphere swelling leads to herniation of the cingulate gyrus under the falx. There is a direct relationship between the amount of midline shift and the degree of impaired consciousness. In adults, shift of 3 to 6 mm is associated with drowsiness, 6 to 9 mm with stupor, and > 9 mm with coma. This may lead to compression of branches of the anterior cerebral artery and infarction of the medial surface of the frontal lobes.

Transtentorial herniation occurs when there is downward displacement of the brain through the tentorial opening. It is classically divided into uncal herniation, in which the uncus of the temporal lobe herniates over the free edge of the tentorium compressing the 3rd cranial nerve, and central herniation, in which the diencephalon and brain stem are directly compressed. In earlier diencephalic stages, there is decorticate posturing with small, reactive pupils. As more rostral compression occurs, the midbrain–upper pons is compressed with decerebrate posturing and fixed mid-position pupils. As the lower pons and medulla are compressed, motor responses are lost and pupils become dilated and fixed.

Tonsillar herniation occurs when the cerebellar tonsils are forced into the upper spinal canal and there is compression of the caudal medulla. Respiratory and cardiovascular function may be impaired. Tonsillar herniation is commonly fatal.

### Epidemiology of Neurological Dysfunction

Traumatic brain injury is thought to be the leading cause of altered mental status in pediatrics. While the majority of cases are mild and do not result in hospital admission, the incidence of hospitalization for moderate to severe traumatic brain injury is close to 40 per 100,000. Hospitalization or death for nontraumatic pediatric coma occurs at an annual incidence of 30 per 100,000, with a reported mortality of nearly 50%. The incidence of this varies significantly with age: Children under 1 year of age have the highest incidence of nontraumatic coma, 160 per 100,000 per year. The most common causes of coma in children resulting in hospital admission or death are infection (38%), intoxication (10%), seizure (10%), complications of congenital malformations (8%), accidental causes such as inhalation or drowning (7%), and metabolic disorders (5%) (Fig. 98-1). The cause of coma was unknown in 15% of cases.

### Etiologies of Depressed Level of Consciousness

The full differential diagnosis of depressed consciousness in pediatrics is too large to list in this chapter, as neurologic dysfunction can be a common manifestation of any severe systemic illness, but key causes are listed in Table 98-1. They are commonly classified as those conditions with structural changes in the brain and those with a diffuse nonlocalizing etiology. In practice, the distinction is artificial because many of the pathologies may coexist in the same patient. For example, status epilepticus or electrolyte disorders may complicate most causes of coma. Trauma, stroke, poisoning, electrolyte (glucose, sodium, calcium, magnesium) disorders, and hypoxic ischemic encephalopathy will often have obvious features in the history, clinical presentation, or initial laboratory and head CT assessment, which lead promptly to the diagnosis. Some further considerations about less immediately obvious causes are discussed below.

**Infective Causes** The range of organisms (eg, bacteria, virus, fungus, protozoa) that can cause central nervous system (CNS) infection vary with geographic region, age, immune status (eg, immunizations, immunocompromise), season, and underlying comorbidities. CNS infection can be difficult to diagnose, and in up to 60% a causative agent is not identified. Commonly identified causes in developed economies include *Mycoplasma* pneumonia, herpes simplex virus 1 (HSV1), enterovirus, varicella, and bacterial meningoencephalitis. Arboviruses (eg, West Nile, eastern and western equine encephalitis) have occurred in seasonal outbreaks in parts of North America. In developing countries, tuberculous meningitis and vaccine preventable causes (eg, hemophilus influenza, measles, varicella, mumps, rubella) remain a frequent and important cause. Cerebral malaria, dengue, and Japanese encephalitis occur especially when mosquito populations are high. Cerebral abscess is associated with chronic sinus and middle ear infections and cyanotic congenital heart disease and is suggested by fever, focal neurological signs, and signs of raised intracranial pressure (ICP).

**Immune-Mediated and Demyelinating Causes** Acute demyelinating encephalomyelitis (ADEM) is 1 of the most common causes of encephalitis. It most commonly affects prepubertal children (mean age 5–8 years), is often preceded by infection, and typically involves the white matter tracts of the cerebral hemispheres, brain stem, optic nerves, and spinal cord. While ADEM typically has a monophasic course and a favorable prognosis, up to 20% to 25% of children have at least 1 relapse.

Immune-mediated encephalitides are increasingly being recognized in children. A now well-established example is anti- N-methyl-D-aspartate (NMDA) receptor encephalitis that is characterized by a mixture of psychiatric manifestations, seizures, hyperkinetic movement disorder, dysautonomia, and coma. In the California Encephalitis Project, anti-NMDA receptor encephalitis was more common than any single infectious cause. In about half of cases, it is associated with an ovarian teratoma. There is often an infectious prodrome, and an association with herpes virus as a trigger has been postulated.

Other conditions suspected of having an autoimmune basis are febrile infection-related epilepsy syndrome (FIRES) and acute necrotizing encephalopathy (ANE). Both typically follow a febrile illness. FIRES is an epileptic encephalopathy presenting with acute refractory status epilepticus, usually in previously well children. The seizures are

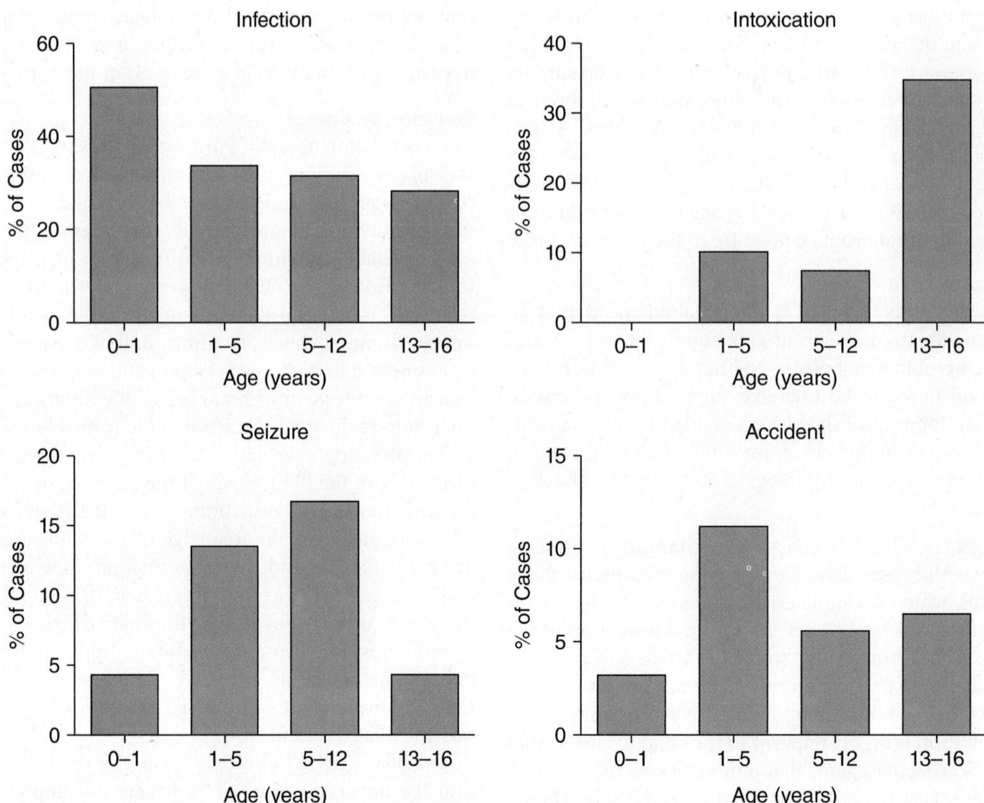


**FIGURE 98-1** Four common nontraumatic causes of depressed consciousness shown as a percentage of incidences by age. Infectious causes of coma are the most common at any age, with the highest incidence in infancy. Intoxication is most commonly seen in teenage populations. Seizures present with prolonged coma are mostly seen in the preteen and toddler years, and toddlers have the highest rates of accidents causing coma. Data from Wong CP, Forsyth RJ, Kelly TP, Eyre JA. Incidence, aetiology, and outcome of non-traumatic coma: a population based study. Archives of disease in childhood 2001;84:193-9.

**TABLE 98-1 ETIOLOGY OF ACUTE NEUROLOGICAL DYSFUNCTION**

| Category | Examples |
|---|---|
| Trauma | Diffuse axonal injury |
| | Hemorrhage (epidural/subdural/subarachnoid/parenchymal) |
| | Contusion |
| Infection | Bacterial, fungal, or viral meningitis/encephalitis |
| | Intracranial abscess |
| | Tuberculous meningitis/encephalitis |
| | Rickettsial encephalitis |
| Postinfectious/autoimmune | Acute disseminated encephalomyelitis (ADEM) |
| | Acute necrotizing encephalopathy (ANE) |
| | Multiple sclerosis |
| | Lupus cerebritis |
| Toxins | Common medications: narcotics, benzodiazepines, antidepressants, aspirin, acetaminophen, hypoglycemics |
| | Recreational drugs |
| | Environmental toxins |
| Seizure disorders | Febrile seizures |
| | Post-ictal state |
| | Secondary seizures |
| | Status epilepticus |
| | N-methyl-D-aspartate receptor–mediated epilepsy |
| Hypoxic encephalopathy | Shock |
| | Sepsis |
| | Drowning |
| | Cardiopulmonary arrest |
| Mass lesions | Neoplasms |
| | Hydrocephalus |
| | Hemorrhage |
| Electrolyte and endocrine disorders | Hypoglycemia |
| | Diabetic ketoacidosis |
| | Hyperosmolar nonketotic diabetes |
| | Hyponatremia and hypernatremia |
| | Uremia |
| | Hyperammonemia |
| Inborn errors | Urea cycle defects |
| | Amino and organic acidemias |
| | Mitochondrial disorders |
| Vascular | Vascular malformations |
| | Aneurysmal rupture |
| | Stroke, thrombosis |

commonly focal in onset and may have secondary generalization, and an EEG typically shows multiple bilateral frontal and temporal foci. ANE is characterized by altered consciousness and bilateral thalamic and external capsule lesions on MRI, which resolve between attacks. It is classically triggered by influenza A in children with an autosomal dominant mutation in *RANBP2*. The differential diagnosis includes Leigh Disease.

**Inborn Errors of Metabolism** Coma is an important and sometimes presenting feature of a number of inborn errors of metabolism (IEM). These include maple syrup urine disease, urea cycle enzyme defects, disorders of fatty acid oxidation, nonketotic hyperglycinemia, mitochondrial cytopathies, congenital lactic acidosis, and certain leukodystrophies. Minor preceding infections may precipitate decompensation and coma.

## CLINICAL MANIFESTATIONS AND DIAGNOSIS

### History

The initial history should be focused in nature, and a full history may be delayed by procedures to stabilize the patient. The goal of the initial history, therefore, is to efficiently gather sufficient preliminary information to direct immediate management, including rapid identification of elevated intracranial pressure or a structural lesion that requires urgent neurosurgical intervention. Knowledge of the timing of onset can be helpful: Sudden loss of consciousness is more likely with acute hemorrhage, seizure, and stroke, while a slower or fluctuating onset is more likely with hydrocephalus, an expanding intracranial mass, metabolic process, or infection. A history of vomiting, headache, fever, and seizures should be sought. Headache with positional changes or Valsalva maneuver suggest raised ICP. Fever suggests infection, although the absence of fever does not exclude it, especially in infants under 3 months of age or in immunocompromised children. A history of recent infectious illness is common in autoimmune and demyelinating conditions. A history of trauma may or may not be forthcoming if it was nonaccidental. Exposure to and availability of common toxins such as pesticides and prescription and recreational drugs can be rapidly assessed. Failure to thrive, developmental delay and parental consanguinity may each suggest an inborn error of metabolism in a young infant. Preexisting medical conditions, such as cancer, epilepsy, congenital heart defects, or metabolic or endocrine abnormalities, may also direct the workup. Recurrent coma may suggest recurrent nonconvulsive status epilepticus, inborn error of metabolism, or nonaccidental poisoning. A history of travel may indicate exposure to infections prevalent in specific areas.

### Examination

The goals of the physical examination are to (1) to identify, for immediate treatment, any compromise in airway, breathing, and circulation; (2) determine the level of consciousness; (3) assess for signs of raised intracranial pressure and/or localizing neurological signs; and (4) identify stigmata of any underlying cause.

The physical exam begins with basic vital signs to assess the status of oxygen delivery to the brain, including adequacy of ventilation and arterial oxygen saturation. Circulation is assessed with standard electrocardiogram (ECG) monitoring and findings should include an arterial blood pressure that is normal for age and extremities that are normothermic, without pallor or cyanosis, and without delayed capillary refill. Abnormalities of the basic vital assessment are addressed while further examination is performed, including a basic trauma survey.

Stereotypic patterns of spontaneous respiration may be observed while assessing vital signs, and these can help identify the etiology of the insult. A summary of stereotypic pathologic breathing patterns is given in Table 98-2.

### Quantifying the Level of Consciousness

Full consciousness has 2 components: wakefulness and awareness of self and the surrounding environment. *Coma* is a state of loss of wakefulness and complete lack of awareness. Between arousal and coma, the following terms have been applied in an inconsistent gradation: lethargy, obtundation, and stupor. *Lethargy* is a pathologic state of mild sleepiness and confusion. *Obtundation* is blunted alertness with diminished sensation of pain and diminished interaction with the environment. *Stupor* is a state of unresponsiveness but vigorous stimulation can produce some limited arousal. *Delirium* is also a type of impaired consciousness, both in wakefulness and awareness. The main characteristics are impaired attention, altered alertness, disorganized thinking and an acute onset with a fluctuating course. Other features such as disordered sleep-wake cycles, memory impairment, and hallucinations may also be present.

The most well-known scale that is used to quantify the arousal to stimuli is the Glasgow Coma Scale (GCS; Table 98-3). The GCS records the best response achieved during assessment, which includes efforts to arouse the patient with verbal, tactile, and painful stimuli. The GCS is the sum of scores in 3 simple domains: eye opening, verbal response, and motor response. It has been adapted for pediatric use, requiring mostly modifications in the verbal scoring. The individual components as well as the total score should be recorded. The motor response is the most powerful predictive component, so that particular care should be taken with performing and recording this accurately. In traumatic brain injury (TBI) in children, the predictive power of the motor score alone was as good as the full GCS and had a linear relationship with mortality.

**TABLE 98-2 BREATHING PATTERNS OBSERVED IN THE SETTING OF ACUTE NEUROLOGICAL DYSFUNCTION**

| Breathing Pattern | Definition | Possible Etiologies |
|---|---|---|
| Apnea | Absence of respiratory effort | Brain stem/spinal cord injury, brain death, neuromuscular blockade |
| Bradypnea | Decreased respiratory rate | Opioids, metabolic disorder, brain stem injury |
| Cheyne-Stokes | Alternating apnea and hyperpnea in a gradual crescendo-decrescendo pattern | Bilateral hemispheric or diencephalon injury |
| Biot's respiration (ataxic breathing) | Irregular rate and tidal volume | Medullary injury |
| Central neurogenic hyperventilation | Rapid and deep breathing | Pontine or midbrain injury |
| Apneustic respiration | Prolonged inspiration with a pause before a brief exhalation | Pontine injury |
| Kussmaul breathing | Tachypnea and hyperpnea | Systemic acidosis (eg, diabetic ketoacidosis, renal failure) |

### Presenting Neurological Signs Associated with Depressed Level of Consciousness

A targeted neurologic examination, focusing on cranial nerves and the motor system, can quickly identify signs of raised intracranial pressure and any focal signs. Core brain stem reflexes and the cranial nerves involved are the following: direct and consensual light reflex (II, III); oculocephalic ("doll's eyes") reflex (III, VI, VIII); oculovestibular ("caloric") reflex (III, VI, VIII); corneal reflex (V, VII); cough and gag reflexes (IX, X). Completely normal pupillary function and eye movements suggest that the lesion causing coma is above the midbrain. Pupillary abnormalities with correlates of the associated anatomic abnormalities are listed in Table 98-4. To properly assess the pupils, baseline pupil size is established in dim light and activity is assessed with a bright light directed at the eye. In the case of asymmetric pupils, the abnormality (constriction or dilation) is assigned from the baseline dim light assessment. When the pupils are more asymmetric in the dark, the smaller pupil is usually abnormal (Horner syndrome), while when they are more asymmetric in the light, the larger pupil is usually abnormal (3rd cranial nerve).

Conjugate lateral deviation of the eyes occurs with an ipsilateral hemisphere lesion, a contralateral hemisphere seizure focus, or a lesion of the contralateral pontine region. Tonic downward eye deviation occurs with injury or compression of the thalamus or dorsal midbrain (eg hydrocephalus), while tonic upward gaze has been associated with bilateral hemispheric damage. Ocular bobbing suggests a pontine lesion and rapid horizontal eye movements usually suggest seizures. Spontaneous roving eye movements indicate that the brain stem is intact.

The motor response is assessed in the awake child with a verbal command in the verbal child and spontaneous observation in the preverbal child. When consciousness is impaired, it is assessed by a painful stimulus. A sternal rub can be applied and the response observed. If there is any sort of flexion response, pain should be applied in the cranial nerve distribution (eg squeezing ear lobes, supraorbital pressure) as otherwise it is difficult to clearly distinguish flexor posturing, withdrawal, and localization. Elevated intracranial pressure is strongly suspected when abnormal flexion or extension or flaccidity is present. Lack of a motor response to painful stimulus with either increased or decreased tone is concerning for a low brain stem or spinal cord lesion. Flexion of the arms with extension of the legs has been classically labeled decorticate posturing, implying pathology above the tentorium, leaving the posterior compartment reflexes unopposed. Extension and internal rotation of the arms with leg extension has been similarly labeled decerebrate posturing, implying disruption of the infratentorial (brain stem) reflexes. These anatomic localizations, however, are not as clear-cut; flexor arm responses suggest less severe dysfunction, while extensor arm responses suggest more severe dysfunction but may still be supratentorial. Arm extension with leg flexion suggests pontine injury, and generalized flaccidity implies injury below the pontomedullary junction. At initial presentation, the distinctions are largely academic, as the presence of any of these abnormalities suggests life-threatening severity and prompts rapid evaluation with brain imaging. Asymmetries of motor response suggest lateralization and make a structural cause of altered consciousness more likely.

### Initial Management of a Child with Depressed Level of Consciousness

A depressed level of consciousness is a manifestation of either severe systemic disease or significant central nervous system disease and so requires urgent management. Coma is a medical emergency because of the potential for life-threatening complications and preventable

**TABLE 98-3 GLASGOW COMA SCORE**

| | Adult Glasgow Coma Score | Pediatric Glasgow Coma Score | Nonverbal Glasgow Coma Score |
|---|---|---|---|
| *Best eye-opening response* | | | |
| 1 | No eye opening | | |
| 2 | Eye opening to pain | | |
| 3 | Eye opening to speech | | |
| 4 | Spontaneous eye opening | | |
| *Best verbal response* | | | |
| 1 | No verbal response | No vocal response | No response to pain |
| 2 | Incomprehensible sounds | Occasional whimpers or moans | Mild grimace to pain |
| 3 | Inappropriate words | Cries inconsolably | Vigorous grimace to pain |
| 4 | Confused | Inappropriate interactions, cries but consolable | Less than usual ability or response to touch only |
| 5 | Oriented | Age-appropriate verbalization, smiles, orients to sound, tracks, interacts | Spontaneous facial and oromotor activity |
| *Best motor response* | | | |
| 1 | No motor response | | |
| 2 | Abnormal extension to pain | | |
| 3 | Abnormal flexion to pain | | |
| 4 | Withdraws from pain | | |
| 5 | Localizes pain or withdraws from touch | | |
| 6 | Obeys commands or performs spontaneous appropriate movement | | |

secondary brain injury. Initial management must be rapid and systematic with immediate priorities being (1) resuscitation and maintenance of cardiorespiratory stability, (2) treatment of reversible causes (eg, hypoglycemia), (3) treatment of complications (eg, intracranial hypertension, seizures), and (4) investigation and treatment of underlying causes. In practice, many of these can be achieved concurrently.

### Resuscitation and Immediate Treatment

Children with a depressed level of consciousness are at risk of airway obstruction and respiratory depression. Intubation and mechanical ventilation are indicated if any of the following is present (1) GCS < 9 or deteriorating, (2) signs of intracranial hypertension, (3) airway obstruction or loss of airway protection, (4) hypoxia ($SpO_2$ < 92% despite oxygen therapy), (4) hypoventilation, and (5) shock requiring ongoing fluid resuscitation and vasoactive therapy. The goals of mechanical ventilation are normal values for $PaO_2$ and $PaCO_2$. There is no indication for hyperventilation to reduce $PaCO_2$ below normal apart from the emergency management of life-threatening intracranial hypertension (until more definitive therapy is established). Immediate interventions should be aimed at correcting hypovolemia, hypoxemia, hypotension, hypoglycemia, and any other factors that may further exacerbate existing injury to the vulnerable brain. Hypotonic fluids can lead to hyponatremia and worsening of cerebral edema and should not be given; all intravenous fluids should be isotonic.

Early monitoring should include continuous ECG, oxygen saturation, and respiratory monitoring, and at least hourly measurement of blood pressure. If the child is critically ill, with shock or coma, an arterial line should be placed, for continuous blood pressure measurement and blood gas analysis.

**TABLE 98-4 PUPILLARY RESPONSES TO LIGHT**

| Size | Activity | Causes |
|---|---|---|
| Pinpoint | – | Pontine injury |
| Small (myosis) | Symmetric, reactive | Bilateral hemispheric dysfunction ("diencephalic pupils"), global metabolic disturbance, opiates, cholinergics |
| | Asymmetric | Horner's syndrome (sympathetic innervation of spinal cord, brachial plexus, and carotid) |
| Mid-dilation | Fixed | Midbrain lesion |
| Large (mydriasis) | Symmetric, reactive | Sympathomimetics, anticholinergics |
| | Symmetric, fixed, hippus (rhythmic spasm of the iris) | Dorsal midbrain lesion |
| | Asymmetric, fixed | Cranial nerve III, uncal herniation syndrome |

### Early Investigation

After initial stabilization, a head computed tomography (CT) scan will almost always be required, apart from children with known preexisting conditions having typical presentations of their illness (eg, epilepsy). This scan can detect intracranial hemorrhage, space-occupying lesions (eg, tumor, abscess), hydrocephalus, cerebral edema, and in some cases focal hypodensities (eg, infarct, ADEM, herpes simplex encephalitis). Contrast is rarely needed in the acute setting. Signs of raised ICP on CT scan include compression of sulci and lateral ventricles, loss of gray/white differentiation, lateral midline shift, and effacement of basal and quadrigeminal cisterns. However, a normal CT scan does not exclude intracranial hypertension, particularly if early in the clinical course. It is also less sensitive than a magnetic resonance imaging (MRI) scan for many pathologies. Once a patient has been stabilized and had initial investigations, an MRI scan is indicated if the cause of coma is still unclear or if there is a cause for which the MRI will provide significantly more information, particularly for injuries involving subcortical structures, the brain stem, and the spinal cord and for detecting ischemia (eg, stroke, early hypoxic ischemic encephalopathy), demyelinating diseases (eg, ADEM), hypertensive encephalopathy, metabolic brain disease, diffuse axonal injury, and venous thrombosis.

## TREATMENT OF COMPLICATIONS

Complications are discussed next as they may also need urgent management before further investigations and specific treatments are instigated.

### Intracranial Hypertension

Intracranial hypertension may be caused by mass lesions (eg, hemorrhage, tumor, abscess), hydrocephalus, or cerebral edema. Cerebral edema is common in trauma, infection, hepatic encephalopathy, inborn errors of metabolism, status epilepticus, and strokes and tumors. Intracranial hypertension should be considered in all children with impaired consciousness and especially those with a GCS < 9. Other suggestive signs are a bulging or tense fontanelle, a "setting-sun" sign (a persistent downward gaze), dilated pupils, and papilledema. Severe intracranial hypertension with impending herniation is suggested clinically by (1) hypertension with bradycardia and abnormalities of breathing pattern (Cushing's triad); (2) abnormalities of posture: decorticate, decerebrate, or flaccid (ie, motor response of the arms to pain is flexor posturing, extensor posturing, or absent, respectively); (3) abnormal pupils: unilateral or bilateral dilated or unreactive; (4) abnormal pattern of breathing; and (5) abnormal doll's eye (oculocephalic) or caloric (oculovestibular) reflexes. In addition, there are features on the head CT scan that suggest raised intracranial pressure (see above).

Severe intracranial hypertension is a medical emergency. Immediate treatment to lower ICP includes hyperosmolar therapy (hypertonic saline, mannitol), intubation and mechanical ventilation (if not performed already), and acute hyperventilation, together with anesthesia (narcotic and benzodiazepine, barbiturate) to reduce cerebral oxygen demand and muscle relaxation. Urgent CT scan may reveal pathology amenable to neurosurgical intervention to reduce ICP, including evacuation of mass lesions and diversion of cerebrospinal fluid (CSF) in hydrocephalus. Other therapies and neurosurgical interventions will be dictated by the underlying cause.

Standard neuroprotective measures should be undertaken in all patients with coma. These include a neutral head position; head of the bed elevated to 30° above horizontal; sedation and analgesia; maintenance of normal $PaO_2$, $PaCO_2$, and blood pressure/cardiac output; maintenance of normothermia (36°C–37.5°C); maintenance of normal to slightly high sodium (140–150 mmol/L); and avoidance of hyper or hypoglycemia. When intracranial pressure is known to be raised, either clinically, radiologically, or based on direct measurement, a tiered approach to reduction is taken. Additional interventions that have been considered include CSF drainage, hyperosmolar therapy, barbiturate coma, and decompressive craniectomy. Full discussion of these therapies can be found in Chapter 105.



#### Seizures

Seizures are common in comatose children. They may be the cause of the coma or they may be a complication of the underlying condition. If coma is persistent 1 hour after a seizure, the seizure should not be assumed to be the cause of the coma and management should be that of an unknown cause of coma. In children presenting with status epilepticus, an underlying acute condition is present in 30% to 50% of cases. For example, almost half of children with encephalitis will have at least 1 seizure. Prolonged seizures (> 30 minutes) may cause or exacerbate brain injury and can also increase ICP. They should therefore be treated aggressively and metabolic derangements (eg, low glucose, sodium, calcium, magnesium) should be rapidly identified and treated. The longer a seizure lasts, the less likely it is to resolve spontaneously, the harder it is to control, and the greater the risk is of morbidity and mortality. Most (80–92%) seizures that stop spontaneously do so within 5 minutes. Seizures should be treated with first-line agents if they have not stopped spontaneously after a maximum of 5 minutes (sooner if they are occurring secondary to an underlying condition or in the presence of raised ICP), and the cycle should be repeated after a further 5 minutes if the seizure does not stop. Intravenous lorazepam and diazepam are equally efficacious in terminating seizures acutely. If seizures do not stop after a second dose of 1 of these agents, a second-line agent should be used. Second-line agents include phenytoin or fosphenytoin, levetiracetam, and sodium valproate. Fosphenytoin is better tolerated than phenytoin and is preferred where it is available. Intravenous (IV) phenobarbital may also be used if other agents are not available, but it is more likely to cause respiratory depression. If the seizure persists beyond 30 to 40 minutes, options include another second-line agent or anesthetic doses of midazolam, pentobarbital, or propofol. In this setting, intubation and mechanical ventilation are typically required as hypoventilation or apnea will typically ensue. Where there is a severe underlying condition, especially if the child is in an intensive care unit, the treatment algorithm may be delivered faster.

An electroencephalogram (EEG) is indicated for any refractory seizures or when the cause of coma is unclear. EEG is principally useful to confirm the presence or absence of seizures, to exclude nonconvulsive seizures as a cause of persistent coma, and to differentiate nonconvulsive motor phenomena from electrographic seizures. Electroencephalogram patterns may also suggest a cause (eg, HSV encephalitis). Continuous EEG, where available, is indicated in children with refractory clinical or electrographic seizures, especially if intracranial hypertension is present or if muscle relaxant drugs are being used.

#### Investigation and Treatment of Underlying Causes

A lumbar puncture (LP) to test for infection should be performed if the patient has a fever, if meningitis or encephalitis is suspected, or if there is no clear cause of impaired consciousness. Cerebrospinal fluid should be analyzed for cell count, protein and glucose levels, Gram stain, viral polymerase chain reaction (PCR), bacterial culture, and other stains/PCR/culture (eg, tuberculosis, fungal) as indicated. The interpretation of CSF results is shown in Table 98-5. Additional CSF may be collected and stored for later testing for metabolic and immune mediated conditions as clinically indicated. The Gram stain may be negative in up to 60% of cases of bacterial meningitis; neither a normal Gram stain nor lymphocytosis excludes a bacterial cause. An abnormal CSF, even if typical for a viral infection, should be treated with antibiotics until culture results are known.

An LP is contraindicated or should be deferred in the presence of (1) shock, (2) clinical diagnosis of meningococcemia, (3) respiratory compromise, (4) coagulopathy or thrombocytopenia (platelets < 50,000), (5) local infection at the site where LP would be performed, (6) papilledema or clinical or CT signs of raised ICP, (7) focal neurological signs, (8) GCS < 9 or deteriorating, and (9) prolonged seizure and GCS ≤ 12. Opinions differ as to whether the last 3 of these are absolute contraindications. Decisions as to whether to perform an LP should be made by the most experienced clinician, taking into account the risks of herniation and benefits (making a definite diagnosis,

**TABLE 98-5 CEREBROSPINAL FLUID ANALYSIS**

| | White Cell Count | | Biochemistry | |
|---|---|---|---|---|
| | Neutrophils ($\times10^6$/L) | Lymphocytes ($\times10^6$/L) | Protein (g/L) | Glucose (CSF: blood ratio) |
| **Normal (> 1 month of age)** | 0 | ≤ 5 | < 0.4 | ≥ 0.6 (or ≥ 2.5 mmol/L) |
| **Normal term neonate** | 0 | < 20 | < 1.0 | ≥ 0.6 (or ≥ 2.5 mmol/L) |
| **Bacterial meninigitis** | 100–1000 (may be normal) | Usually < 100 | > 1.0 (may be normal) | < 0.4 (may be normal) |
| **Viral meningitis** | Usually < 100 | 10–1000 (may be normal) | 0.4–1.0 (may be normal) | Usually normal |
| **Tuberculous meningitis** | Usually < 100 | 50–1000 (may be normal) | 1–5 (may be normal) | < 0.3 (may be normal) |

knowing the antimicrobial sensitivity of an identified bacteria). If an LP is deferred, antibiotics that reflect the local sensitivity pattern of likely bacteria, and antiviral agents should be given. Herpes simplex encephalitis may be suggested by the presence of focal neurological signs, a fluctuating GCS of greater than 6 hours duration, and the presence of or contact with herpetic lesions.

A toxicology screen should always be performed if the cause of coma is unclear. Standard urine screens differ in terms of the drugs covered, so that knowledge of the local test is required. Additional blood or urine testing will be dictated by the clinical toxidrome (see Chapter 114). Drugs present in the house (especially in cases involving toddlers) and possible drugs of abuse (especially in cases involving teenagers) should be specifically sought out in the history.

Hypertension is common in the setting of coma and can be difficult to interpret. Impaired consciousness may be caused by hypertensive encephalopathy or hypertension may be a protective physiological response to raised intracranial pressure. The former requires urgent treatment to reduce blood pressure, while in the latter, such treatment may cause cerebral ischemia and exacerbate intracranial hypertension. Hypertensive encephalopathy may be caused by renal, cardiovascular (eg, coarctation of the aorta), vasculitic, and endocrine conditions (eg, pheochromocytoma) and also drugs (recreational and prescribed). It is suggested by a history of hypertension, headaches, visual disturbance, and seizures. It may be associated with posterior reversible encephalopathy syndrome (PRES) that has a typical pattern on CT/MRI scan with edema typically affecting the parietal-occipital regions, has most commonly been reported in children after hematopoietic stem cell and solid organ transplantation. PRES is thought to be caused by loss of autoregulation to rapid changes in blood pressure in the areas affected. However, 20% to 30% of children with PRES have normal or only slightly high blood pressure and it is speculated that endothelial dysfunction and inflammation may play an important role in the pathogenesis. Hypertensive encephalopathy should be managed with intravenous vasodilators and/or β-blockers with the goal of initial reduction in blood pressure of approximately 25% and then further reduction more slowly over 24 to 48 hours.

Metabolic emergencies such as diabetic ketoacidosis or severe hyperammonemia associated with acute liver failure or inborn errors of metabolism should be managed according to established guidelines that are disease specific. Demyelinating and autoimmune encephalopathies may be treated with steroids, immunoglobulin, or plasmapheresis (see Chapter 548).

*An extensive evidence-based guideline and an abbreviated algorithm for the investigation and management of a child with impaired consciousness have been published online by the Pediatric Accident and Emergency Research Group of the Royal College of Pediatrics and Child Health and the British Association of Emergency Medicine (http://www.nottingham.ac.uk/paediatric-guideline/index2.htm).*

## SUGGESTED READINGS


Alper G. Acute disseminated encephalomyelitis. *J Child Neurol.* 2012;27(11):1408-1425.

Bowman SM, Bird TM, Aitken ME, Tilford JM. Trends in hospitalizations associated with pediatric traumatic brain injuries. *Pediatrics.* 2008;122(5):988-993.

Chin RF, Neville BG, Peckham C, Bedford H, Wade A, Scott RC, Group NC. Incidence, cause, and short-term outcome of convulsive status epilepticus in childhood: prospective population-based study. *Lancet.* 2006;368(9531):222-229.

Coats B, Margulies SS. Material properties of human infant skull and suture at high rates. *J Neurotrauma.* 2006;23(8):1222-1232.

Czosnyka M, Brady K, Reinhard M, Smielewski P, Steiner LA. Monitoring of cerebrovascular autoregulation: facts, myths, and missing links. *Neurocrit Care.* 2009;10(3):373-386.

Fortune PM, Shann F. The motor response to stimulation predicts outcome as well as the full Glasgow Coma Scale in children with severe head injury. *Pediatr Crit Care Med.* 2010;11(3):339-342.

Glauser T, Shinnar S, Gloss D, et al. Evidence-Based Guideline: Treatment of Convulsive Status Epilepticus in Children and Adults: Report of the Guideline Committee of the American Epilepsy Society. *Epilepsy Curr.* 2016;16(1):48-61.

Paediatric Accident and Emergency Research Group of the Royal College of Paediatrics and Child Health and the British Association of Emergency Medicine. The management of a child with a decreased conscious level. http://www.rcpch.ac.uk/system/files/protected/page/the mgt of the child with decreased conscious level.pdf. Accessed May 15, 2017.

Seshia SS, Bingham WT, Kirkham FJ, Sadanand V. Nontraumatic coma in children and adolescents: diagnosis and management. *Neurol Clin.* 2011;29(4):1007-1043.

Tatman A, Warren A, Williams A, Powell JE, Whitehouse W. Development of a modified paediatric coma scale in intensive care clinical practice. *Arch Dis Child.* 1997;77(6):519-521.

Venkatesan A, Benavides DR. Autoimmune encephalitis and its relation to infection. *Curr Neurol Neurosci Rep.* 2015;15(3):3.

Wong CP, Forsyth RJ, Kelly TP, Eyre JA. Incidence, aetiology, and outcome of non-traumatic coma: a population based study. *Arch Dis Child.* 2001;84(3):193-199.




# PART 2 STABILIZATION AND MANAGEMENT OF THE ACUTELY ILL INFANT AND CHILD

# 99 Physiologic Monitoring

Fong Lam and V. Ben Sivarajan

## INTRODUCTION

Children with serious illness or injury with the potential for rapid deterioration invariably require close observation to detect changes in function or state. Careful bedside assessment provides the basis for appropriate triage and early awareness of clinical deterioration. Electronic monitoring complements this assessment by providing (1) repetitive or continuous assessment that does not disturb the patient, (2) a means for detecting the effectiveness of interventions, and (3) warning signals for physiological disturbances that permit staff to observe multiple patients simultaneously. The ideal monitoring system has been described by many as one that is accurate, able to predict deterioration, reproducible with a rapid response, operator independent, easy to use, safe, continuous, inexpensive, and integrative with other medical systems. To date, no such monitoring currently exists in clinical use.

## RESPIRATORY MONITORING

### Respiratory Rate

The respiratory rate (RR) and *tidal volume* ($V_T$; volume of each breath) together determine minute ventilation ($\dot{V}_E$; volume of air movement into and out of the lungs in 1 minute). Minute ventilation is product of RR × $V_T$. Since arterial blood carbon dioxide levels ($PaCO_2$) are inversely proportional to $\dot{V}_E$, decreases in RR and/or $V_T$ will lead to increases in $PaCO_2$. Therefore, determination of RR is an essential component for the evaluation of respiratory function.

There are several methods for determining RR, ranging from counting visual chest movement and auscultated breaths to using devices that measure changes in electrical bioimpedance, air movement at the nares, or inductance plethysmography. These methods each have advantages and limitations but none measure carbon dioxide ($CO_2$) levels. Auscultation provides the best estimation of RR and depth of breathing. It provides the practitioner the opportunity to listen for air movement within the lungs and to differentiate between problems related to airway obstruction (upper vs lower) and problems with poor lung/chest wall compliance. The drawback is that auscultation is time consuming and a static measure.

Transthoracic impedance monitoring is the technique most commonly used to continuously measure respiratory rate. A small current is passed between 2 electrodes across the chest (similar to those used for electrocardiography). During inhalation and chest rise, the electrodes move further apart, increasing the impedance between them. During exhalation, the electrodes move closer together and the impedance decreases. The sinusoidal changes in impedance are displayed as the RR. Transthoracic impedance monitoring is safe, relatively cheap, and readily available to all patients. It is important, however, to recognize its limitations. First and foremost, the interpreted signal is dependent on chest movement and not breathing, per se. Therefore, chest movement unrelated to breathing may be mistaken for breathing, overestimating RR. Next, chest movement may negate impedance measurements and also may result in the underestimation of RR. Finally, transthoracic impedance monitoring does not accurately measure the depth of breathing nor does it rely on actual air flow. Thus, patients who have airway obstruction may have significant chest movement but little to no ventilation of the lungs. This may lead to under-recognition of airway obstruction.

Other methods of monitoring RR are respiratory inductance plethysmography, airflow thermistor, and capnography (discussed below). Respiratory inductance plethysmography tends to be used in specialized settings, such as during polysomnography (sleep studies). This method utilizes elastic bands that encircle the chest and abdomen, and assumes that the thoracic cavity is a cylinder that expands and constricts circumferentially during inhalation and exhalation, respectively. Electrodes within the bands measure the changes in circumference of the chest and abdomen in order to determine a RR as well as to estimate a tidal volume. When used in conjunction with other measures of respiration, inductance plethysmography can be useful to differentiate different disorders of breathing, such as central versus obstructive sleep apnea. Caveats to using this device are the relatively specialized equipment needed for accurate measurement, correct placement of the bands, and tolerability of wearing the device.

Respiratory thermistors are devices that detect changes in air temperature at the nares in order to estimate RR. The thermistor is placed at the patient's nares and detects a difference between the warm gas breathed out during exhalation versus the cooler inhaled air. The changes in temperature are then used to determine RR. The relative changes in temperature do not relate to the volume of each breath, however; thus this device can only detect RR. Limitations in its use include inaccuracies during mouth breathing and underestimation of hypopnea.

## Capnography

$\dot{V}_E$ is inversely proportional to $PaCO_2$. Although RR is important, it is often inadequate to assess ventilation due to the inability to accurately take into account depth of breathing and physiologic changes within the lung including "dead space" ventilation ($\dot{V}_D$) which refers to air movement without the exchange of gases between the lung and the blood. Therefore, during situations in which accurate measurements of ventilation are desired, measurement of $CO_2$ levels may be necessary. The gold standard for measurement of ventilation is the arterial blood gas (discussed below). Although it is the truest measure of ventilation, it is invasive and is usually not continuous. In situations where continuous monitoring is necessary, capnography has become a standard of care, especially in the emergency department, intensive care units (ICUs), and operating rooms, and during procedural sedation.

Quantitative capnography is based on the ability of $CO_2$ to absorb infrared light. When gas is sampled within the path of airflow (mainstream) or from the side (sidestream), it passes through a detector that emits infrared light and detects the absorbance by $CO_2$. Alternatively, some devices use spectrometry to detect $CO_2$ levels. As the detector measures the exhaled $CO_2$ ($P_{ECO2}$), a tracing appears on the monitor (Fig. 99-1); this is the standard time-based capnograph. During a respiratory cycle, the partial pressure of carbon dioxide ($PCO_2$) of inhaled air is 0 mm Hg, accounting for the minimal amount of atmospheric $CO_2$ in relation to nitrogen and oxygen. This air enters the trachea, bronchi, and then the respiratory lung units (alveoli and respiratory bronchioles). Carbon dioxide quickly diffuses from the blood to the respiratory lung units, but not into the dead space. This dead space ventilation can be areas of normal, anatomic dead space (ie, trachea, mainstem bronchi, and nonrespiratory bronchioles) or pathologic areas of the lung that are poorly perfused (eg, pulmonary

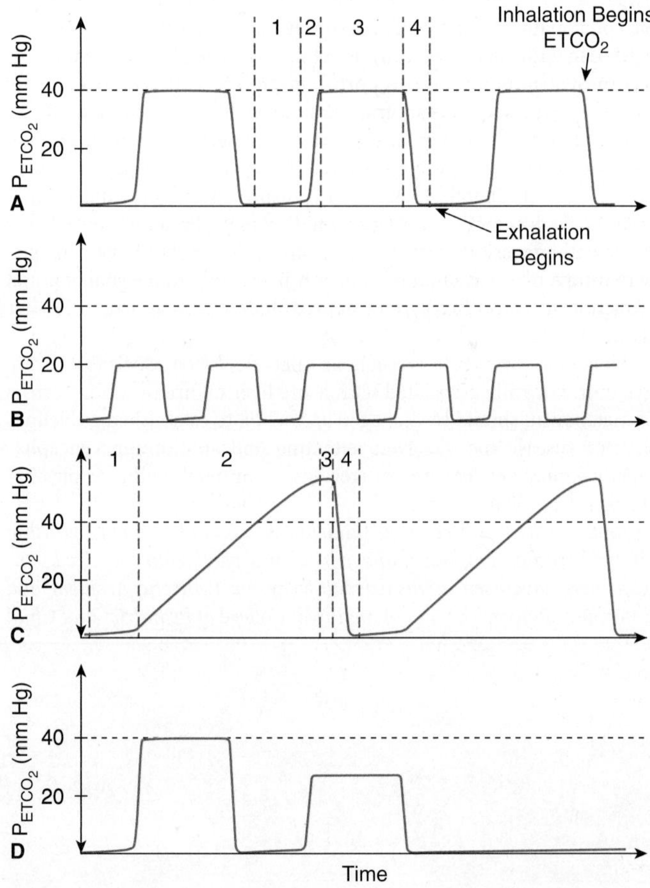


FIGURE 99-1 Quantitative capnography. **A:** In a normal capnograph, there is a prototypical square waveform for exhaled $CO_2$ ($P_{ECO2}$) that consists of 4 phases: (phase 1) exhalation of gas from the anatomic dead space; (phase 2, ascending phase) rapid addition of $CO_2$-containing alveolar gas; (phase 3, plateau phase) equalization of alveolar gas; and (phase 4, inhalation phase) rapid decline in $P_{ECO2}$. The intersection between phases 3 and 4 is where inhalation begins and is the point where the end-tidal $CO_2$ ($P_{ETCO2}$) is quantified. **B–D:** The waveform shape can provide insight to changes in the patient or equipment malposition. **B:** An increased respiratory rate with decreased $P_{ETCO2}$ may signify hyperventilation. **C:** Prolongation of phase 2 typically signifies bronchospasm. **D:** A previously normal waveform that quickly disappears may indicate detector dislodgement, complete airway obstruction, or cardiac arrest.

embolus and during cardiac arrest). During exhalation, the first volume of gas is from the anatomic dead space (trachea and bronchi); therefore, the $P_{ECO2}$ is 0 mm Hg (phase 1). As gas moves from the respiratory lung units into the larger airways, the $P_{ECO2}$ increases (phase 2). In normal lungs, this increase in expired $CO_2$ is rapid. In the latter phase of exhalation, the $P_{ECO2}$ plateaus (phase 3), resulting in the typical square-shaped waveform. At the end of exhalation, the end-tidal $CO_2$ ($P_{ETCO2}$) is quantified and displayed. As inhalation begins again (phase 4), the $P_{ECO2}$ quickly falls due to the movement of atmospheric $CO_2$ through the detector. Therefore, based on the capnograph waveform and $P_{ETCO2}$ value, the adequacy of ventilation can be continuously assessed in a reliable fashion.

Quantitative time-based capnography is used in situations where the adequacy of ventilation needs to be continuously monitored. The most common scenario includes one in which there may be disordered control of breathing, such as during procedural sedation and anesthesia or if patients have depressed sensorium or neuromuscular weakness. Additionally, capnography should routinely be used as a safety device in endotracheally intubated patients since disconnection from the ventilator, accidental extubation, or other mechanical problems will be detected by a loss of capnographic signal. To that end, qualitative (or colorimetric) capnography is used to quickly confirm endotracheal tube placement since the litmus paper within the device changes color when the expired $CO_2$ reaches a certain threshold. Capnography is also useful for making adjustments to a patient's ventilator settings, especially if rapid titration is necessary (such as to manage increased intracranial pressure) or if a blood gas measurement is not possible or warranted. Finally, an increasing recommendation is the use of quantitative capnography to assess the quality of chest compressions during cardiopulmonary resuscitation. Since the $P_{ETCO2}$ depends on blood flow through the lungs in addition to air flow, during cardiac arrest, $P_{ETCO2}$ will drop toward 0 due to lack of pulmonary blood flow. As chest compressions are instituted, $P_{ETCO2}$ will start to rise. As the effectiveness of chest compressions improve, the $P_{ETCO2}$ should also increase, given the same $\dot{V}_E$, due to improved pulmonary blood flow (Fig. 99-1E).

The utility of quantitative capnography lies not only in the $P_{ETCO2}$ value, but also with the shape of the waveform. Typically, the $P_{ETCO2}$ value is less than the $PaCO_2$ (~0–5 mm Hg) in normal lungs, owing to the anatomic dead space. In patients with higher degrees of lung disease, the difference between $PaCO_2$ and $P_{ETCO2}$ (dead space ventilation; $\dot{V}_D$) increases and can be followed to determine disease progression in critically ill patients, especially if they are tracheally intubated with a cuffed endotracheal tube. One of the most useful attributes of the capnographic waveforms is the ability to detect the degree of airway obstruction and bronchospasm. In patients with bronchospasm, $CO_2$ from the alveoli enters the large airways at variable rates due to increased resistance in the small airways. This is manifested as a slow, upward ramping of the capnographic waveform instead of the normal square waveform. If the obstruction is severe enough, the $P_{ETCO2}$ may never reach the true level of the $PaCO_2$ since inhalation begins prior to complete exhalation.

Capnography, like other devices, has its limitations and caveats. In nonintubated patients, capnography typically uses sidestream detectors via nasal cannula. In these cases, a decrease in $P_{ETCO2}$ may be caused by other environmental factors, such as dislodgement of the cannula, mouth breathing, or entrainment of atmospheric air (such as from the concomitant use of a high-flow nasal cannula for oxygenation). Additionally, appropriate interpretation of the capnographic waveform and $P_{ETCO2}$ can be confusing, at times. As an example, decreased ventilation will increase $P_{ETCO2}$, whereas decreased perfusion to areas of the lungs will decrease $P_{ETCO2}$. If a patient has both decreased ventilation and perfusion, then it will be difficult to interpret the true nature of the findings. The interpretation of changes in mainstream quantitative time-based capnography also assumes consistent (or no) breath-to-breath leaks in the system.

### Pulse Oximetry

Pulse oximetry is a mainstay in the monitoring of oxygen saturation. To recognize the benefits and limitations of pulse oximetry, it is important to understand the principles on which it is designed. Pulse oximetry depends on light absorption in a tissue bed, depending on the relative ratio of oxyhemoglobin ($HbO_2$) and deoxyhemoglobin (Hb) at 2 different wavelengths of light (Fig. 99-2). At red wavelengths, Hb has a higher light absorption than $HbO_2$; whereas at infrared wavelengths, $HbO_2$ has a higher light absorption than Hb. For standard pulse oximeters, light in the red and infrared wavelengths is emitted from a light emitting diode (LED) and travels through a tissue bed (eg, finger, earlobe, toe) to a detector on the opposite side. The ratio of the emitted (known) and the detected (measured) light intensities is calculated for each wavelength to determine the relative level of absorbance of each. Based on correlation curves using blood $O_2$ saturation levels from healthy human subjects, the $O_2$ saturation of the tissue is estimated. To estimate the arterial saturation, the pulse oximeter uses the pulsatility of blood in the tissue to its advantage. During systole, more blood is in the arterial system; therefore, more light is absorbed as there is more Hb and $HbO_2$ in the path of light. During diastole, there is less blood to absorb light in the pathway; therefore, the absorption of light is caused by the combination of tissue, venous blood, and non-pulsatile arterial blood. The difference in absorption during systole and diastole is then assumed to be caused by the contribution of arterial blood alone. The device then displays the oxygen saturation of pulsatile blood ($SpO_2$).

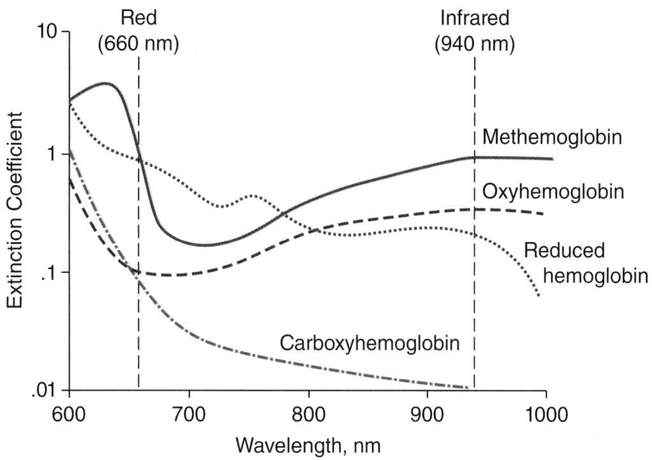


**FIGURE 99-2** Absorption of light by various types of hemoglobin. Note that at the 2 wavelengths used in standard pulse oximetry, the absorption of light of methemoglobin is equal. (Reproduced with permission from Jubran A: Pulse oximetry, *Crit Care.* 2015 Jul 16;19:272.)

An understanding of the basis of pulse oximetry helps clinicians to recognize its benefits and limitations as well as how to troubleshoot problems. Clearly, the main benefit of pulse oximetry is the ability to estimate arterial $O_2$ saturation in a continuous and noninvasive manner. For the vast majority of patients, $SpO_2$ measurements have replaced arterial oxygen saturation ($SaO_2$) measurements. Although newer devices have improved the reliability of $SpO_2$ measurements, there are still limitations to the accuracy of current pulse oximeters. It is important to remember that pulse oximeters average the signal over the preceding 20 beats; therefore, the displayed $SpO_2$ is actually reflective of changes that occurred up to 20 cardiac cycles ago. This is important during critical periods, such as during resuscitation or intubation. Since pulse oximetry relies on the device to distinguish between pulsatile blood and non-pulsatile blood, there are a number of conditions that may reduce the accuracy and/or reliability of measurement: patients with poor perfusion to the extremity used for pulse oximetry (eg, in severe shock, arterial occlusion, or hypothermia), excessive movement, and venous pulsation (eg, in severe tricuspid regurgitation). Since standard pulse oximeters typically rely on only the red and infrared wavelengths of light, certain dyshemoglobinemias, such as carboxyhemoglobinemia (overestimates $SpO_2$) and methemoglobinemia (overestimates $SpO_2$ and trends toward 85% as MetHb levels rise), may result in inaccurate measurements. In these instances, co-oximeters, which utilize multiple wavelengths of light, should be used in place of pulse oximeters. Finally, excessive ambient light interference or alterations in absorption (eg, from fingernail polish, dyes, pigments) can affect the accuracy of measurements. Another caveat is that there is a lower limit for accurate $SpO_2$ measurements with most devices. At lower $O_2$ saturations (below 80–85%), $SpO_2$ readings are considered to reflect a trend rather than an accurate saturation. This is of particular relevance in patients with cyanotic congenital heart disease, or in the setting of severe hypoxemic respiratory failure, when permissive hypoxia is a part of routine intensive care.

### Blood Gas Measurement

As described above, the gold standard to determine oxygenation and ventilation in patients is through the measurement of arterial blood gases (ABG), which characterizes efficiency of gas exchange and also disturbances in the metabolic and respiratory control of acid–base balance.

All modern blood gas analyzers take 4 measurements: sample temperature, pH, $PO_2$, and $PCO_2$. The pH, $PO_2$, and $PCO_2$ are directly measured, whereas most analyzers calculate the following using various equations and nomograms: bicarbonate ($HCO_3^-$), $O_2$ saturation ($SO_2$), and acid–base excess (ABE). This is important to take into consideration when there is a need for exact $SO_2$ values, such as in the presence of dyshemoglobinemias and when used to estimate cardiac output using the Fick principle. It is also important to understand the different areas of sampling available for blood gas determination. Although arterial sampling is the gold standard, blood gases can be obtained from the venous and capillary vessels, especially for outpatient monitoring of ventilation, but they cannot be used as a guide to adequacy of oxygenation. Blood venous samples tend to be approximately 0.05 to 0.1 pH units lower and have $PCO_2$ levels approximately 5 mm Hg higher than simultaneous arterial samples owing to the diffusion of $CO_2$ from the tissues into the capillary beds prior to returning to the venous system. In patients with poor perfusion due to shock, hypothermia, or the use of a tourniquet, these discrepancies may be greater. Therefore, when obtaining samples from these areas, it is important that the blood is free-flowing without the use of a tourniquet because restricted blood flow during sampling may artificially decrease the pH and increase the $PCO_2$. Venous $PO_2$ levels are a reflection of cellular $O_2$ uptake, and high levels may be indicative of impairment in mitrochondrial $O_2$ uptake from processes such as cyanide toxicity. The utility of capillary samples is entirely questionable, and many practitioners believe they do not have any role in blood gas monitoring. Finally, when obtaining any blood sample for blood gas analysis, it is important to ensure that there are no air bubbles in contact with the sample as this will affect the measurements, due to diffusion of gas between the blood and air.

The arterial pH (normal 7.35–7.45) reflects the acid-base balance within the system. If the arterial pH is less than 7.35, the blood is deemed *acidemic.* If the arterial pH is greater than 7.45, the blood is *alkalemic.* The 2 main determinants of pH in the blood are the $PCO_2$ (normal 35–45 mm Hg; a volatile acid released by the lungs) and serum bicarbonate levels ($HCO_3^-$; normal 22–26 mM beyond early postnatal life; primary buffering system), which are related to each other by the following chemical reaction:

$$CO_2 + H_2O \leftrightarrow H_2CO_3 \leftrightarrow H^+ + HCO_3^-$$

and are related to pH by the Henderson-Hasselbalch equation:

$$pH = 6.1 + \log\frac{[HCO_3]}{(0.03)(PCO_2)}$$

Other determinants are the levels of various proteins, ions, and other weak buffers within the blood and are out of the scope of this chapter. Since $PCO_2$ is a volatile acid that is exhaled by the lungs, as $PCO_2$ increases, the blood becomes more acidic and pH falls. For acute changes, if $PCO_2$ changes by 10 mm Hg, pH will change in the *opposite* direction by 0.08. Conversely, changes in $HCO_3^-$, a base, result in changes in pH in the *same* direction, such that an increase in $HCO_3^-$ by 10 mM increases the pH by 0.15. Of note, the $HCO_3^-$ result on standard blood gas analyzers is a *calculated* result based on the Henderson-Hasselbalch equation and the value should be compared to the serum total $CO_2$ ($tCO_2$; normal 23–30 mM) that is measured by serum chemistry. Taking these factors into account, basic acid–base disorders can be determined by proceeding in a step-wise fashion (Fig. 99-3), with more complex evaluations discussed in other resources.

The other component use of the arterial blood gas analysis is $PaO_2$ (normal 75–100 mm Hg). Although the majority of oxygen is carried by hemoglobin in the erythrocytes and reliably monitored using pulse oximetry, determination of $PaO_2$ is useful in patients with cyanotic heart disease in which $SpO_2$ is lower and less reliable, as well as when differentiating low $SpO_2$ in neonates using the hyperoxia test. Finally, $PaO_2$ levels are useful for characterizing the degree of lung injury in acute lung injury and acute respiratory distress syndrome for prognosis and research.

## CARDIOVASCULAR MONITORING

### Heart Rate and Rhythm

The heart rate and rhythm and their trends over a finite period of time are a fundamental part of the evaluation and treatment of critically ill patients. Electrocardiograms (ECGs) can be monitored continuously from electrodes placed on the chest, and a cardiotachometer determines heart rate from the frequency of the QRS signal. There are important sources of error to consider with these methods, however. When the signal is large, the T wave and QRS may both be detected, and the cardiotachometer may show a value that is twice normal. Failure to detect a signal can occur when the QRS amplitude changes—for example, with respiration, repositioning of the leads, or changes in posture. It is quite easy to misinterpret rhythm disturbances or misdiagnosis ST-segment abnormalities when reviewing a single lead rhythm or rhythm strip. Whenever a dysrhythmia or ECG abnormality is suspected based on the monitor, a 12 to 15-lead ECG should be obtained for true diagnostic purposes. Finally, one must remember that ECG only measures electrical activity and not actual cardiac muscle contractions, which is an important distinction in patients with pulseless electrical activity (PEA). Therefore, a pulse check is imperative in these patients to assess their systemic perfusion.

Bedside arrhythmia analysis and bed-to-bed switching (so that a central monitoring station was not required) allowed widespread use of electrocardiographic monitoring in adult ICUs in the 1960s and 1970s. Widespread adoption in pediatric ICUs did not occur until the late 1980s with the advent of modular units that allowed input from various devices. At this time, the potential for arrhythmia in postoperative cardiac surgical patients and other organ dysfunction states was becoming appreciated. Focused attention to ST-segment changes has been commonplace after operations that involve manipulation or reimplantation of the coronary origins such as the arterial switch operation and the Ross operation. The theoretical advantage of automated ST-segment analysis is balanced by the limitations of algorithms used by currently available software for this purpose in the pediatric populations.

### Blood Pressure

**Noninvasive Blood Pressure** Most commonly, noninvasive blood pressure assessment is performed using intermittent methods. Determining pressure using a sphygmomanometer with a cuff that occupies about two-thirds of the length and almost completely (80–100%) encircles the circumference of the limb segment remains the standard approach for initial patient assessment. The cuff is inflated to a pressure well above that occluding the arterial systolic pulse and is gradually deflated while listening for Korotkoff sounds. The first sound corresponds to arterial systolic pressure, and the muffling of the second sound corresponds to the arterial diastolic pressure. The systolic pressure can also be determined by palpating the artery distal to the cuff and noting the pressure at which the pulse is first felt when the cuff is deflated.

**Basic Algorithm for Acid-Base Disorders:**

1) Is the pH high (alkalemic), low (acidemic), or normal?
   a. *N.B.* If the pH is 7.40 but $pCO_2$ and/or $HCO_3^-$ are abnormal, the patient has a mixed acid-base disorder
2) What is the primary disorder: respiratory, metabolic, or mixed?
   a. Evaluate $pCO_2$ and $HCO_3^-$
      i. $pCO_2$ moves in the opposite direction as pH
      ii. $HCO_3^-$ moves in the same direction as pH
   b. If there is metabolic acidosis (low pH with low $HCO_3^-$), calculate the anion gap (AG)
      i. AG = s[$Na^+$] – s[$Cl^-$] – s[$tCO_2$], normal 12 ± 2 mM
         1. If elevated, think MUDPILES:
            a. Methanol
            b. Uremia
            c. Diabetic (or other) ketoacidosis
            d. Propylene glycol, paracetamol (acetaminophen) toxicity
            e. Iron, ibuprofen, isoniazid, inborn errors of metabolism
            f. Ethylene glycol
            g. Salicylates (aspirin)
         2. If normal, think renal or gastrointestinal losses using urinary electrolytes:
            UAG = u[$Na^+$] + u[$K^+$] – u[$Cl^-$]
            a. If UAG < 0, consider GI losses of bicarbonate
            b. If UAG ≥ 0, consider renal losses of bicarbonate
3) Is there compensation of the pH?
   a. Calculate the expected change in pH for abnormal $pCO_2$ and [$HCO_3^-$]
      i. Changes in $pCO_2$ by 10 mm Hg change pH by 0.08 in the **opposite** direction
      ii. Changes in [$HCO_3^-$] by 10 mM change pH by 0.15 in the **same** direction
   b. Calculate the expected compensation by $pCO_2$ or $HCO_3^-$:
      i. For primary metabolic disorders, $pCO_2$ should compensate as follows:
         1. Metabolic acidosis: $pCO_2 = (1.5 \times [HCO_3^-]) + 8 \pm 2$
         2. Metabolic alkalosis: $pCO_2 = (0.7 \times [HCO_3^-]) + 20 \pm 5$
      ii. For primary respiratory disorders, there are both acute and chronic compensatory mechanisms due to the changes in [$HCO_3^-$] by buffering in the blood versus by the kidneys:
         1. Respiratory acidosis:
            a. Acute: $[HCO_3^-] = 24 + \left(\frac{pCO_2 - 40}{10}\right)$
            b. Chronic: $[HCO_3^-] = 24 + 3.5 \times \left(\frac{pCO_2 - 40}{10}\right)$
         2. Respiratory alkalosis:
            a. Acute: $[HCO_3^-] = 24 - 2 \times \left(\frac{40 - pCO_2}{10}\right)$
            b. Chronic: $[HCO_3^-] = 24 - 4 \times \left(\frac{40 - pCO_2}{10}\right)$
   c. If the measured pH, $pCO_2$, and [$HCO_3^-$] are not as expected, the patient has a mixed acid-base disorder.

**FIGURE 99-3** Basic algorithm for arterial blood gas analysis. $pCO_2$, partial pressure of carbon dioxide; UAG, urinary anion gap.

Alternatively, most automated blood pressure cuffs utilize oscillometry to determine blood pressure. These devices detect pressure changes caused by turbulence in arterial blood flow as the cuff is deflated. These devices record the peak oscillations as the mean arterial blood pressures (MABP) and then extrapolate the systolic and diastolic blood pressure measurements. The most important factor that determines the accuracy of these oscillometric techniques in measuring MABP is cuff width–to–arm circumference ratio which ideally should be in the range of 0.44 to 0.55. A smaller cuff will overestimate the true MABP. It is also important to note that the mean bias of noninvasive methods become unreliable at both the higher and lower limits of physiologic blood pressure measured invasively (ie, severe hypertension or clinical shock, respectively).

**Principles of Invasive Pressure Monitoring** Briefly, once a vascular compartment of interest has been accessed by a catheter (eg, arterial, central venous, left atrial), the pulsations generated by the space are transmitted via a continuous column of fluid to a transducer that converts the analog signal into a digital one. When setting up a direct pressure monitoring system, it is important to ensure that the system has a baseline reference value; this is usually set to atmospheric pressure at the anatomic level of interest (such as the right atrium for vascular pressures). Other facets of calibration, such as damping, are important but out of the scope of this text.

### Central Venous Pressures and Atrial Pressures

*Central venous pressure* (CVP) is used as a proxy for central vascular volume. In general, as the volume in the vasculature increases, the CVP rises. More accurately, the measured CVP reflects the back pressure of venous return from the peripheries (this driving pressure from the peripheries is known as *mean circulatory filling pressure*). Changes in intravascular volume status, ventricular compliance, or intrathoracic pressure will affect the value of the CVP. The pressure from a catheter in the right atrium or a large central vein is used to monitor cardiac filling or, more precisely, right ventricular preload. Many assumptions are made when using CVP as a measure of intravascular volume, including lack of downstream obstruction, normal lung compliance, and a consistent relationship between pressure and volume (known as *ventricular elastance*). A more accurate measure of this is the *left atrial pressure*, which can be directly measured with a left atrial line, or indirectly using a Swan Ganz catheter with measurement of pulmonary artery wedge pressure. Left atrial lines are still placed in selected patients undergoing open heart surgery. However, the use of Swan Ganz catheters in pediatric patients, is now at most, rare and, in many units, obsolete.

With these constraints in mind, CVP can serve as a useful guide for determining how interventions are affecting cardiac filling in patients in whom responses are not very predictable (eg, the child with congestive circulatory failure in whom positive pressure ventilation is initiated or adjusted) or in patients in whom there is a narrow margin of safety (eg, the child with elevated intracranial pressure and low cardiac output). Normal values for CVP range from –3 to +3 mm Hg in the infant to 5 to 10 mm Hg in the child and young adult. These values, however, can be greatly affected by the use of positive-pressure breathing. Accordingly, it is usually more useful to judge relative changes rather than to rely on absolute targets for therapy. In addition to pressure monitoring, additional information regarding the adequacy of systemic oxygen delivery is provided by central venous saturations ($ScvO_2$) drawn from an appropriately

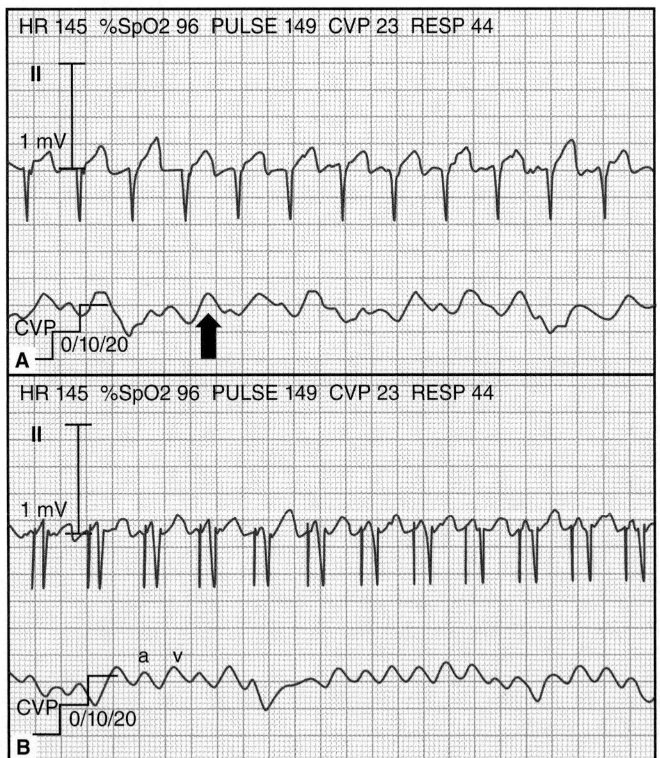


**FIGURE 99-4** Simultaneous electrocardiography and central venous pressure monitoring waveforms. **A:** The electrocardiogram has no easily discernible P-waves and the corresponding central venous pressure (CVP) trace shows canon *a*-waves (*arrow*), which is consistent with an atrioventricular (AV) dissociated rhythm and is mechanically reflective of atrial contraction against a closed AV valve apparatus. **B:** The same patient with atrial pacing demonstrates a CVP trace showing *a*- and *v*-waves related to coordinated atrial and ventricular contraction.



positioned central catheter with the tip in the superior vena cava–right atrial junction and without the confounding effects of a significant left-to-right atrial level shunt. By using the oxygen extraction ratio ($OER = [SaO_2 - ScvO_2/SaO_2]$; normal 0.2 – 0.3), an estimation of adequacy of cardiac output can be made, with OER > 0.3 as concerning for inadequate cardiac output for the current oxygen consumption state.

Continuous venous pressure tracings, and the appearance of its component *a*, *c*, and *v* waves, can also provide useful information as to nature of the underlying cardiac rhythm and changes therein (Fig. 99-4).

#### Arterial Pressures

The use of invasive arterial pressure monitoring is reserved for intraoperative, perioperative, or intensive care monitoring. The most common reasons for arterial line placement are for frequent blood gas measurement in patients with respiratory failure, for frequent blood sampling in unstable patients, and the need to monitor hemodynamic changes during periods of critical illness and in response to interventions and titrations of therapies. The choice of location of invasive arterial pressure monitoring is based on ease of access and limitation of complications, with important exceptions. These include not attempting catheterization of an artery that is known to have been completely or partially occluded, or in a circulation where there may already be compromised flow (a systemic-to-pulmonary shunt affecting flow to that arm, or dialysis fistula) or poor potential collateralization. In the case of surgery on the aortic arch, a right arm arterial line (typically radial) is used to guide cerebral perfusion both prior to and during cardiac surgery. In smaller infants and neonates, especially in the context of shock, cannulating peripheral arteries can be challenging. In these situations, the femoral artery may be the next choice. As a rule, the longer term consequences of vascular occlusion should always be considered when deciding on the optimal location of an arterial line, and the operator performing the procedure.

It is important to recognize that there are regional variations in blood pressure and that these can be accentuated in pathological states. Normally, mean blood pressures are equal throughout the large arteries, although systolic pressure is higher and diastolic is lower when comparing the large arteries of the legs to the brachial or radial artery. However, in states of low cardiac output, the systolic and mean blood pressures from a large central artery often are higher than values from more peripheral arteries depending on the degree of impairment of the perfusion, and peripheral vasoconstriction. The central systolic blood pressure may be sustained near normal levels even in the presence of shock, owing to severe vasoconstriction of peripheral arteries and arterioles.

### SUGGESTED READINGS


Berend K, de Vries APJ, Gans RO. Physiological approach to assessment of acid-base disturbances. *N Engl J Med.* 2014;371(15):1434-1445.

Corwin MJ, Lister G, Silvestri JM, et al; the Collaborative Home Infant Monitoring Evaluation (CHIME) Study Group. Agreement among raters in assessment of physiologic waveforms recorded by a cardiorespiratory monitor for home use. *Pediatr Res.* 1998;44(5):682-690.

Englehart MS, Schreiber MA. Measurement of acid-base resuscitation endpoints: lactate, base deficit, bicarbonate or what? *Curr Opin Crit Care.* 2006;12(6):569-574.

Hunt CE, Corwin MJ, Lister G, et al. Longitudinal assessment of hemoglobin oxygen saturation in healthy infants during the first 6 months of age. *J Pediatr.* 1999;135(5):580-586.

Jubran A. Pulse oximetry. *Crit Care.* 2015;19:272-278.

Nassar BS, Schmidt GA. Capnography during critical illness. *Chest.* 2016;149:576-585.

Ralston AC, Webb RK, Runciman, WB. Potential errors in pulse oximetry III: effects of interferences, dyes, dyshaemoglobins and other pigments. *Anaesthesia.* 1991;46(4):291-295.

Romagnoli S, Ricci Z, Quattrone D, Tofani L, Tujjar O, Villa G, Romano SM, De Gaudio AR. Accuracy of invasive arterial pressure monitoring in cardiovascular patients: an observational study. *Crit Care.* 2014;18(6):644.

Sackner MA, Watson H, Belsito AS, et al. Calibration of respiratory inductive plethysmograph during natural breathing. *J Appl Physiol.* 1989;66(1):410-420.

Sivarajan VB, Bohn D. Monitoring of standard hemodynamic parameters: heart rate, systemic blood pressure, atrial pressure, pulse oximetry, and end-tidal $CO_2$. *Ped Crit Care Med.* 2011;12(4 Suppl):S2-S11.

Takci S, Yigit S, Korkmaz A, Yurdakök M. Comparison between oscillometric and invasive blood pressure measurements in critically ill premature infants. *Acta Paediatr.* 2012;101(2):132-135.

Weese-Mayer DE, Corwin MJ, Peucker MR, Willinger M. Comparison of apnea identified by respiratory inductance plethysmography with that detected by end-tidal $CO_2$ or thermistor. *Am J Respir Crit Care Med.* 2000;162(2 Pt 1):471-480.


# 100 Vascular Access

Andreas A. Theodorou and Robert A. Berg

### INTRODUCTION

Rapid establishment of vascular access is necessary for aggressive fluid resuscitation and administration of medications such as catecholamines, antibiotics, narcotics, and sedatives during emergencies. However, attaining vascular access in a child during a life-threatening illness is difficult and often consumes precious time. An organized approach to vascular access can minimize this potentially life-threatening delay in treatment. This chapter discusses the priorities in vascular access during emergent, urgent, and stable situations. It also reviews various techniques for achieving vascular access and covers the relative indications and potential complications.

## PRIORITIES OF VASCULAR ACCESS

Time is critical when attaining vascular access in life-threatening emergencies such as cardiopulmonary arrest or shock. Of course, any pre-existing intravenous catheter should be utilized in the initial resuscitation efforts, regardless of how small such a catheter might be. If such access is not available during a life-threatening emergency, intraosseous access should be attained as rapidly as possible, especially in children under 6 years old. A practical approach is to pursue this and peripheral venous access simultaneously. Time should not be wasted waiting for attempts at peripheral venous catheterization before attempting intraosseous access, which can be attained more rapidly and more reliably. Similarly, skilled clinicians may attempt placing central venous catheters during life-threatening emergencies, but such attempts should not preclude simultaneous attempts at intraosseous access. After attaining intraosseous access for initial fluid resuscitation and infusion of emergency medications, peripheral or central venous catheterization is the next priority in order to ensure a more reliable, long-lasting vascular access.

For urgent situations, such as fluid resuscitation of a child with compensated shock or dehydration, the risk–benefit ratio shifts. Generally, it is most appropriate to initially insert a peripheral venous over-the-needle catheter. If multiple attempts are unsuccessful, or if the child requires fluids or medications that cannot be given safely in a peripheral vein, central venous catheterization should be attempted by a qualified individual. Of course, if the child's clinical condition deteriorates prior to achieving vascular access, priorities should be reassessed and it may be necessary to attain intraosseous access.

Relatively stable children may need vascular access for maintenance fluids or intravenous medications. Generally, peripheral venous cannulation with an over-the-needle catheter is adequate. If vascular access is necessary for more than 2 to 3 weeks, or if solutions to be infused can cause serious tissue injury if extravasated, a central venous catheter may be necessary. However, central venous catheterization entails added risks, and its inherent risks and benefits deserve consideration (Table 100-1).

## PERCUTANEOUS PERIPHERAL VEIN CANNULATION

Small-caliber plastic catheters have allowed for increasingly easy and reliable peripheral venous cannulation. Small over-the-needle catheters (22–24 gauge) are available to cannulate even the small veins of the hand, foot, or scalp of neonates and premature babies. Such peripheral venous catheters are generally all that are necessary for short-term delivery of intravenous fluids or medications.

The most common complication of peripheral venous cannulation is catheter displacement and infiltration of the tissues with the infusing fluid. Most intravenous solutions are isotonic or hypotonic and easily absorbed from the tissues. Infiltration with these solutions is generally treated by removing the catheter and elevating the limb. However, solutions that are very hypertonic (eg, those containing greater than 12.5% dextrose, 3% sodium chloride, or 8.4% sodium bicarbonate) or that contain irritating substances such as calcium or potassium salts, some antibiotics (eg, erythromycin), or medications with an extreme pH (eg, phenytoin) can cause substantial tissue injury leading to necrosis of the skin or subcutaneous tissues. Importantly, extravasation of vasoconstricting agents such as dopamine, epinephrine, and norepinephrine can result in profound local vasoconstriction and subsequent substantial tissue injury. Even without extravasation of the previously noted medications and fluids, local vascular injury can result in aseptic thrombophlebitis. This condition may serve as a nidus for suppurative thrombophlebitis. The risks of aseptic and suppurative thrombophlebitis increase with the duration of the indwelling catheter.

Selection of catheter size and peripheral venous site are important issues. For a patient in shock, the widest and shortest catheter is optimal, because longer, narrower catheters result in more resistance to flow. For the trauma victim, it is preferable to insert the catheter into an uninjured limb or at least a limb apparently free from major vascular trauma. The greater saphenous vein, median cubital vein, and external jugular vein are often used, because they are relatively large

**TABLE 100-1 VASCULAR ACCESS TECHNIQUES**

| Route | Indications | Benefits | Risks and Disadvantages |
|---|---|---|---|
| Peripheral | Short-term infusion of fluids or medications | Minimal training required<br>Minimal risk | Local<br>Hematoma, infiltrations, infections<br>Infection<br>Time-consuming (especially if vascular collapse) |
| Intraosseous | Emergent vascular access<br>Cardiac arrest<br>Hypotensive shock | Attained rapidly and reliably | Adverse effects *rare*<br>Osteomyelitis<br>Compartment syndrome<br>Fracture<br>Soft-tissue necrosis |
| Central venous—acute | Emergent vascular access<br>Hemodynamic monitoring<br>Infusion of:<br>Irritating medications and vesicants<br>Vasoactive agents | More secure then peripheral<br>Safer for certain infusions<br>Vasoactive agents | Advanced skills necessary<br>Often time-consuming<br>Pneumothorax<br>Chylothorax<br>Arrhythmia<br>Thrombosis<br>Embolus (air, catheter, wire)<br>Hemothorax<br>Hematoma<br>Malposition<br>Infection |
| Central venous—chronic (eg, Broviac, Hickman, peripherally inserted catheter) | Long-term parenteral nutrition<br>Prolonged or frequent administration of intravenous medications (eg, antibiotics, chemotherapy) | Compared to central venous—acute:<br>More secure<br>Lower infection risk<br>Lower thrombosis risk | Same as for central venous—acute |

and consistent in their anatomy. In older children, veins in the back of the hands and forearms are commonly used. Avoiding the dominant hand or the hand with the finger or thumb that the infant prefers to suck allows for improved patient comfort and function, although such choices are not always available.

Before the vein is cannulated, the operator should wash his or her hands well and use universal precautions, including protecting the operator's hands with gloves. The extremities should be adequately immobilized, and the site should be cleansed with alcohol or iodine-containing solutions and allowed to dry. A tourniquet should be applied in order to engorge and distend the vein. The skin can be stretched taut with the operator's nondominant hand in order to immobilize the vein. The operator should puncture the skin at a 15° to 30° angle, 5 to 10 mm distal to the expected entrance site into the vein. Next, the needle punctures the vein, usually resulting in blood return into the catheter hub. When this blood return occurs, the catheter is advanced a few millimeters to ensure that the catheter tip and the needle are in the lumen of the vein. The catheter is then advanced over the needle into the vein, and the needle is removed. The tourniquet is released, and saline is flushed intravenously to ensure patency of the catheter and vein. After the needle is removed, it should generally not be reinserted while the catheter is in the subcutaneous space or in the vein, because this could shear the tip of the catheter and generate a small plastic embolus.

Adequate immobilization of the extremity is an important aspect of successful peripheral vein cannulation. Moreover, it is important to adequately secure and protect the catheter after successful cannulation. Notably, ultrasound or devices using near-infrared have been used for difficult peripheral vein access.



## INTRAOSSEOUS INFUSION

Although emergency intraosseous (IO) infusions were common in the 1940s and 1950s, the arrival of butterfly needles and plastic catheters and the widespread use of venesection led to a virtual extinction of this technique for several decades. However, there has been a resurgence in the use of intraosseous infusions since the early 1980s. The principal value of intraosseous access is that it can be performed rapidly and reliably. Medical personnel can usually attain access in less than 1 minute during emergencies. The bone marrow cavity is effectively a noncollapsible vascular space, even in the setting of shock or cardiac arrest. Therefore, intraosseous access is the initial vascular access site of choice in patients with life-threatening problems such as cardiopulmonary arrest or decompensated shock.

Almost any medication that can be administered into a central or peripheral vein can be safely infused into the bone marrow, including crystalloid solutions, colloid solutions, blood products, and hypertonic solutions. In particular, all the medications the American Heart Association recommends for pediatric advanced life support can be safely and effectively administered via this route, including catecholamine infusions. Pharmacokinetic variables, such as onset of action and plasma concentrations, are similar with intraosseous or peripheral venous administration in cases of circulatory shock or cardiac arrest with cardiopulmonary resuscitation (CPR). Emergency medications should be followed by a saline flush to ensure rapid delivery into the circulation. In addition, the initial bone marrow aspirate is a reliable specimen for venous pH and $PCO_2$, blood typing and cross-matching, serum glucose, electrolytes, and blood cultures. Due to stasis in the bone marrow, the results of such studies may be less reliable after administering drugs through the intraosseous needle during CPR.

The greatest obstacle to successful intraosseous cannulation is psychological and originates from the natural reluctance by any inexperienced provider to force a needle into a child's bone. Experienced providers may at times wrongly forfeit this quick and reliable alternative to undertake venous cannulation via rapid percutaneous central venous catheterization or peripheral vein cutdown, sometimes resulting in dangerous delays in starting therapy. Intraosseous cannulation is generally a safe procedure but can result in complications, including osteomyelitis, fractures, subcutaneous or intramuscular extravasation of toxic medications (eg, epinephrine, calcium), and compartment syndrome. Compartment syndrome is easily avoided by monitoring the insertion site for swelling and discontinuing the infusion if significant swelling occurs. Microvascular pulmonary fat and bone marrow emboli have been demonstrated but do not appear to be a clinically significant problem. The risk of such complications is acceptable in the dire circumstances of hypotensive shock or cardiac arrest. Such risks, and the pain involved, may not be acceptable when the clinical indications are less stringent.

The most commonly utilized site for intraosseous access is the medial surface of the tibia, 1 to 3 cm below the tibial tuberosity (Fig. 100-1). Alternative sites include the distal tibia above the medial malleolus, the distal femur, and the anterior superior iliac spine. There are various styles of intraosseous needles. They are all designed to easily penetrate the bone cortex, and they all have a stylet to keep bone core from obstructing the needle during insertion. Aseptic technique and universal precautions should be followed. The needle should be twisted into, rather than pushed through, the bone marrow. Evidence for successful entrance into the marrow includes (1) the lack of resistance (or a "give") after the needle passes through the cortex, (2) the ability of the needle to remain upright without support, (3) aspiration of the bone marrow into a syringe, and (4) free flow of

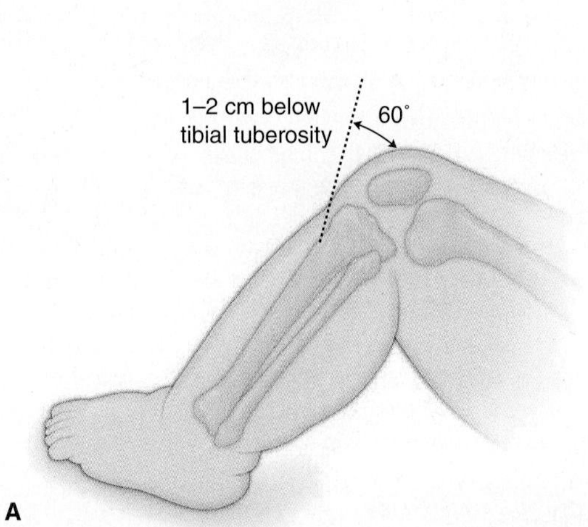


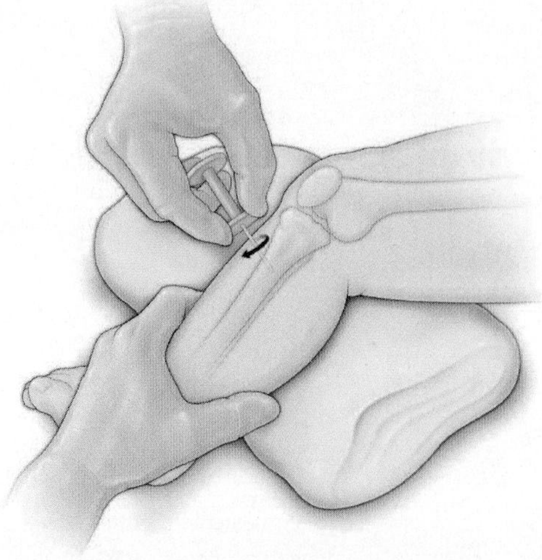


**FIGURE 100-1** Intraosseous cannulation. **A:** Preferred site for intraosseous cannulation in infants. **B:** Technique for insertion of the trocar. Note that the trocar is advanced with a twisting movement and in a caudal direction to avoid injuring the tibial growth plate.

the infusion without significant subcutaneous infiltration. Aspiration of bone marrow into the intraosseous needle is not always possible, especially in a very dehydrated patient. An alternative method of IO insertion involves using a battery-operated drill that allows for quick and effective insertion of the IO needle. Regardless of the insertion method used, infiltration of fluid into tissues around the bone is common when this route of infusion is used for a prolonged period of time or if the fluid is infused under great pressure. Infiltration will manifest as an enlarging leg circumference, fluid leaking out from the skin insertion site, or resistance to flow of the infusate.

## CENTRAL VENOUS CATHETERIZATION

Central venous catheterization provides more reliable and longer term vascular access than peripheral venous catheterization. In addition, central venous catheters permit hemodynamic monitoring and laboratory sampling of central venous blood. However, the convenience of central venous catheters must be balanced against the added risks.

Central venous cannulation is particularly suited for administering irritating or vasoconstrictive medications, which are diluted in the high blood flow of central veins, thereby limiting their contact with the vascular endothelium. Central venous cannulation may also offer a more expeditious alternative to peripheral venous access, particularly for patients who are in circulatory shock or cardiac arrest. Especially in these cases, a central venous catheter provides a means to monitor central venous pressure. In some circumstances, specialized central venous catheters may be used to monitor cardiac output, mixed venous oxygen saturation, pulmonary artery pressure, and pulmonary artery occlusion pressure.

In critically ill infants and children, polyurethane central venous catheters are generally inserted percutaneously through a large central vein such as the internal jugular, the subclavian, or the femoral vein. For chronic vascular access, particularly in patients requiring long-term chemotherapy, total parenteral nutrition, or antibiotics, Silastic catheters are often preferred, because they are less thrombogenic and have lower infection rates. It is now widely recommended that these catheters are placed using ultrasound guidance if this is available.

Peripherally inserted central catheters (PICC) have gained enormous popularity, because they can be inserted easily at the bedside, usually through a peripheral vein (eg, brachial vein), and advanced into a central location, using ultrasound and in some cases fluoroscopic guidance. The Broviac and Hickman catheters are placed in a central vein and tunneled out through a distant exit site in the skin. The Hickman catheters have Dacron cuffs that are very fibrogenic. The resultant fibrous scar around the Dacron allows for the catheter to be more securely anchored and decreases the risk of catheter infection from the skin. A last category of Silastic catheters is equipped with a proximal port that is embedded in the subcutaneous tissue (Port-A-Cath). These totally implantable venous access devices reduce the chance of microbial propagation through the catheter track and are most useful when only intermittent infusions are necessary.

There are unavoidable risks associated with all central venous catheters. During attempts to cannulate the internal jugular or subclavian veins, inadvertent needle puncture of the lungs can result in pneumothorax. Perforation of a large vessel with resultant leak into the pleural space can lead to hemothorax, and mechanical damage to the thoracic duct or thrombosis of the left brachiocephalic vein downstream from the insertion of the thoracic duct can lead to chylothorax. Central vein thrombosis and its attendant risks (venous congestion and edema, chylothorax) are particularly common in newborns and small infants because of the small size of their central vessels. In addition, injuries to nerves and arteries (including inadvertent cannulation) near the insertion site have been well documented.

When the central venous catheter is open to the atmosphere and the patient creates negative intravascular pressure with a spontaneous breath, it is possible for air embolism to occur. This can be minimized by keeping the needle or catheter exit site in a dependent position (eg, Trendelenburg position during internal jugular or subclavian catheterization). The Seldinger technique, or guidewire technique, is commonly used to simplify catheter placement. A needle or trocar is used to puncture the vessel, followed by passage of a wire through the trocar. The trocar is then removed, and the catheter is then introduced over the wire. This technique is convenient but is associated with both an increased risk of vessel perforation by the guidewire, and catheter malposition because of the potential for the guidewire to take an unexpected course in the vascular system.

The most significant risk of central venous catheterization is infection. The risks of both thrombosis and suppurative thrombophlebitis increases with time and is especially high in children who suffer from hypercoagulability and/or immune deficiencies. The possibility of a hypercoagulable state should be considered in critically ill children who develop catheter-related central venous thrombosis. Newer catheter materials (polyurethane, Silastic), heparin bonding, and low-dose heparin administration through the catheter may minimize the risks of thrombosis. Similarly, antibiotic bonding has been used to decrease the risk of infection. However, the most effective preventative measures are based on the conventional wisdom of placing central venous catheters only when indicated and removing them as soon as possible.

Local hemorrhage is common when removing the central venous catheters. Applying direct pressure as the catheter is removed can minimize the size of the hematoma. Air embolism is a rare, life-threatening complication associated with catheter removal. As during insertion, the risk of air embolism can be minimized by placing the patient in the Trendelenburg position, removing the catheter at the end of deep inspiration, and immediately covering the exit site with petroleum jelly gauze.

The most commonly used sites for central venous catheterization (Fig. 100-2) in acutely ill children are the internal jugular (less frequently, the external jugular vein is cannulated) or femoral veins. The subclavian veins are also often used by experienced clinicians, although the risk of pneumothorax or hemothorax is higher than with the other techniques. The femoral vein is the safest approach for less-experienced providers and, unlike in adults, does not seem to carry a higher risk of infection. Femoral cannulation offers clear anatomical landmarks, ease of hemostasis, and a safe distance from vital organs and sites of activity during resuscitation. Prior to catheterization of the neck veins, the child should be placed in the Trendelenburg. Conversely, if the femoral vein is used, a slight reverse Trendelenburg position will engorge the veins and improve the success rate.

Ultrasound-guided central venous access is now the preferred approach to clarify anatomy of nearby arteries and veins, identify the vein for cannulation, determine that the vein is patent, assure that the insertion needle tip is in the vessel prior to advancing a wire through the needle, and decrease the risk of complications, such as inadvertent arterial cannulation. The technique requires additional training and equipment but increases safety and effectiveness. The overall procedure is otherwise similar to the traditional approach utilizing landmark identification.

Local anesthesia with 1% lidocaine should be provided subcutaneously unless the patient is anesthetized. A syringe and needle are used to locate the vein and aspirate blood. For femoral vein catheterization, the vein is located immediately medial to the artery, 1 to 2 fingers' breadths below the inguinal ligament. The introducer needle is inserted into the vein at a 45° angle. When blood is aspirated freely, the syringe is removed and the hub of the needle is covered with the thumb of the nondominant hand. A guidewire is then placed through the needle, and the needle is removed (Seldinger technique). A dilator is advanced over the wire to dilate the subcutaneous space and the entrance into the vein. The dilator is then removed, and the catheter is placed over the guidewire. After the catheter is introduced into the vein, the guidewire is removed. The electrocardiogram should be monitored during the procedure, because the guidewire can trigger arrhythmias when advanced into the heart.

Once the procedure is complete, it is essential to aspirate all of the lumens of the line to check that blood flows freely, and then check the position of the central line using 1 or more of the following confirmatory tests (depending on availability): x-ray to confirm the position of the line tip; a blood gas to distinguish from an inadvertent arterial cannulation (although this can be confounded by the presence

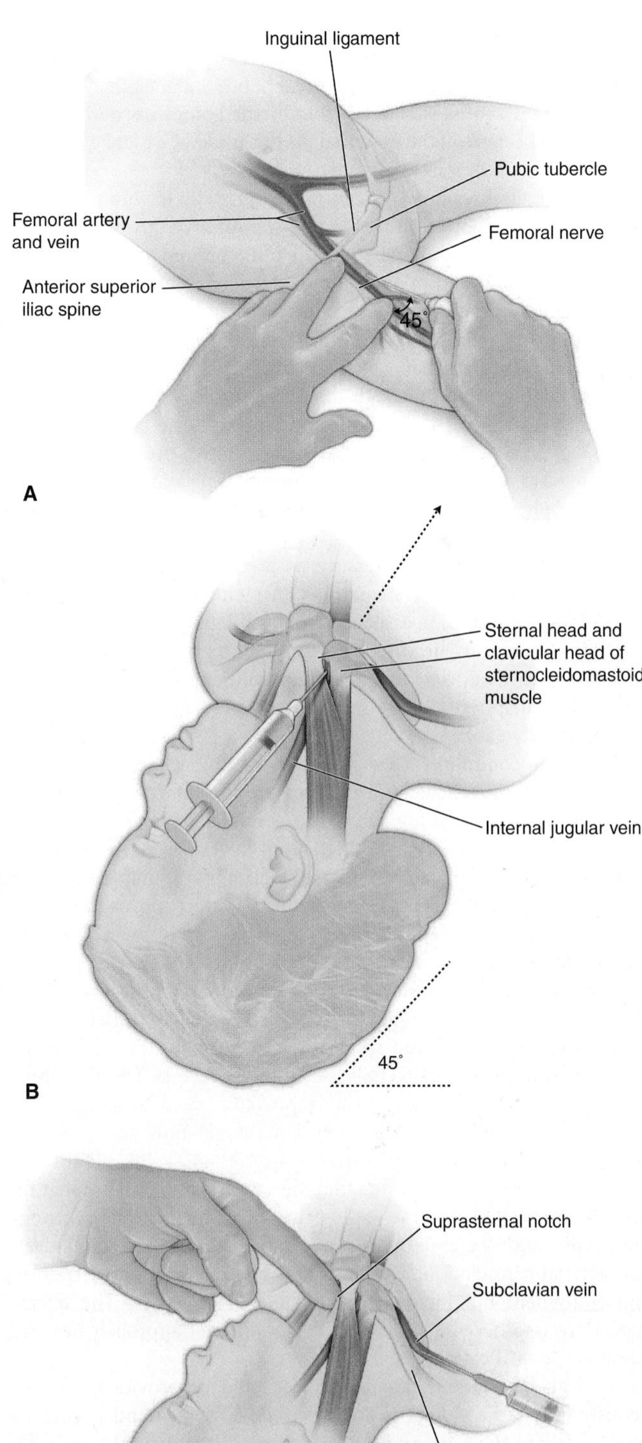


**FIGURE 100-2** Three commonly used sites for venous cannulation in children. **A:** Femoral vein. **B:** Internal jugular vein (the middle approach is shown here; the vein can be accessed via other alternative approaches). **C:** Subclavian vein.

of arterial hypoxemia); and observation of the pressure waveform of the cannulated vessel after zeroing the line (again, to rule out arterial cannulation). Continuous monitoring of the pressure during the procedure is essential in the setting of pulmonary artery catheterization.

Central line-associated bloodstream infections (CLABSI) are key quality indicators for not only intensive care units, but for hospitals as a whole and are associated with increased morbidity and increased mortality across multiple populations. Many institutions have central line checklists, or "bundles" that incorporate key interventions to minimize the risk of any adverse events related to central line insertion, in particular CLABSI. These include proper hand hygiene; preparing the skin with chlorhexidine; using a full-body sterile barrier, surgical masks, gowns, caps, and gloves for those performing the procedure; and removing unnecessary catheters. The introduction of central line bundles has been associated with a marked decrease in the rate of CLABSI.

Transduction of vascular pressure during the procedure provides a more effective means of confirmation and is essential if the catheter is to be inserted into the pulmonary artery. A radiograph can also be used to confirm position, but sometimes a single projection is insufficient to determine the precise distal site of the catheter (eg, distinguishing right atrium from right ventricle).

## ANALGESIA AND SEDATION FOR PROCEDURES

An important yet frequently neglected issue for any invasive procedure on a child is that of pain management and sedation. In the non-emergency situation, topical or local anesthetics should be used, and oral sucrose has been shown to lessen distress in younger infants. The psychological milieu during the procedure should also be optimized. Music, toys, and interaction with family members can be important tools for improving comfort, thereby increasing the likelihood of cooperation and technical success. Moreover, minimizing discomfort during the procedure generally encourages better cooperation during the next potentially painful procedure for that child. However, when sedation is provided, personnel qualified to handle sedation-induced respiratory failure or shock should be present.

## SUGGESTED READINGS


American Heart Association. *Emergency Cardiovascular Programs: Pediatric Advanced Life Support*. Dallas: American Heart Association; 2001.

Benkhadra M, Collignon M, Fournel I, et al. Ultrasound guidance allows faster peripheral IV cannulation in children under 3 years of age with difficult venous access: a prospective randomized study. *Paediatr Anaesth*. 2012;22(5):449-454.

Bruzoni M, Slater BJ, Wall J, St Peter SD, Dutta S. A prospective randomized trial of ultrasound- vs landmark-guided central venous access in the pediatric population. *J Am Coll Surg*. 2013;216:939-943.

Olaussen A, Williams B. Intraosseous access in the prehospital setting: literature review. *Prehosp Disaster Med*. 2012;27(5):1-5.

Pronovost P, Needham D, Berenholtz S, et al. An intervention to decrease catheter-related bloodstream infections in the ICU. *N Engl J Med*. 2006;355(26):2725-2732.

Reyes JA, Habash ML, Taylor RP. Femoral central venous catheters are not associated with higher rates of infection in the pediatric critical care population. *Am J Infect Control*. 2012;40(1):43-47.


# 101 Fluid Management of the Acutely Ill or Injured Child

Trevor Duke

## INTRODUCTION

Children with acute or critical illness may be hypovolemic, euvolemic, or hypervolemic. They may have lost blood (eg, hemorrhagic shock), plasma (eg, severe burns), extracellular fluid (eg, gastroenteritis or diarrhea), or electrolytes. They may have internal compartment fluid redistribution (eg, ascites or capillary leak from sepsis or Dengue shock syndrome) and despite being edematous may still have intravascular volume depletion. Children with acute or critical illness may have renal impairment or high antidiuretic hormone (ADH) levels that results in fluid retention. Decisions about fluid management need to be based on clinical features and understanding of pathophysiology, thus systematic and repeated clinical evaluations are essential to good quality care. In this chapter, several acute clinical syndromes that require careful fluid management will be discussed.

## SHOCK AND FLUID MANAGEMENT

Cells require oxygen for the production of adenosine triphosphate (ATP), the principal cellular energy source. In pathophysiological terms, shock occurs when cardiac output is insufficient to provide oxygen delivery to tissues for ATP production, leading to cellular dysoxia, with resulting anaerobic metabolism, lactic acidosis, and cellular dysfunction. The assumption behind fluid bolus therapy for shock is that it will improve cardiac output and in turn augment oxygen delivery to tissues. There are several clinical definitions of shock. Hypovolemic, low cardiac output shock manifests as "cold shock" with vasoconstriction, cold limbs, and tachycardia. This type of shock requires urgent fluid resuscitation. Cold shock occurs in severe dehydration (the classic examples being from cholera or gastroenteritis), hemorrhagic shock, and in some (generally late) stages of septic shock.

Fluid resuscitation for children with fever and signs of shock has been controversial. This is partly because many clinical definitions of shock encompass a continuum from adaptive physiological changes to fever, to states of severe hypotension and dysoxia. Fluid therapy for shock has also been controversial because fluid therapy alone will not deal with shock apart from that which occurs solely from extracellular fluid losses. Therefore, in settings where intensive care support is unavailable, fluid therapy alone in some forms of shock will be insufficient. Many children with fever and 1 or 2 clinical cardiovascular signs of shock do not have hypovolemia or dysoxia. They have high levels of adrenaline and renin-angiotensin, leading to tachycardia and vasoconstriction, and raised levels of ADH, which leads to fluid retention, thus protecting them from hypovolemia and shock. The assumption that fluid boluses will improve cardiac output and in turn augment oxygen delivery to tissues is not certain if the cardiac output is normal or the child is not hypovolemic. In this situation, the benefits of bolus fluid therapy are less and the costs of excess fluid will be tissue edema and perhaps a blunting of the adaptive cardiovascular responses. A transient increase in stroke volume after fluid bolus therapy, because of an increase in venous return and left ventricular end-diastolic (filling) pressure, is often accompanied by a reduction in heart rate. Thus, the effect on cardiac output, which is the product of the 2, in some circumstances will be small and transient. Large amounts of intravenous (IV) fluid will tend to accumulate in children with high ADH levels, and edema, reduced lung compliance, and other negative consequences may occur. The effect of fluid boluses on dampening adaptive responses like the hyperadrenergic state has been proposed but needs further study.

Revised guidelines for the management of shock, incorporating the World Health Organization's new fluid guidelines for shock, are in Appendix 101-1.

## SEVERE DEHYDRATION AND FLUID MANAGEMENT

Children with hypovolemic shock from severe dehydration should be given parenteral fluid immediately: administer 20 mL/kg of 0.9% sodium chloride (NaCl) or Ringer's lactate (or similar fluid) repeatedly until plasma volume is restored, and pulses are present (20–100 mL/kg may be required). Fluid can be given intravenously, or if an IV cannula cannot be inserted, into the bone marrow through an intraosseous needle. Nasogastric fluid is effective in severe dehydration, but once shock has developed, the splanchnic circulation is less able to absorb fluid. Intraperitoneal fluid is not effective in shock. Any child with shock who requires more than 40 mL per kg as a bolus should be urgently reviewed to consider the need for vasopressor or inotropic support, and to consider the adverse effects of more fluid on lung function, and where available intensive care review should be considered.

In calculating fluid requirements for children with dehydration, 3 fluid types need to be considered:

- Existing fluid deficit
- Ongoing fluid losses
- Maintenance fluid requirements

### Fluid Deficit

The fluid deficit is most reliably estimated from the loss of body weight if a recent pre-illness weight is available. The loss of weight is equal to the fluid deficit. (For example, if 600 grams have been lost, there is a fluid deficit of 600 mL, which represents 6% dehydration in a 10-kg child). The deficit may be overestimated in infants whose most recent weight was months ago, as the weight difference does not take account of normal growth, which may be 100 g to 150 g per week.

Clinical signs may be used to determine approximate fluid deficit. These are useful but not precise.

1. Mild dehydration (< 4%)
   - Usually no clinical signs; the child is thirsty
2. Moderate dehydration (4–6%)
   - Delayed capillary refill time
   - Increased respiratory rate
   - Mildly decreased tissue turgor
3. Severe dehydration (≥ 7%)
   - Very delayed capillary refill, > 3 seconds; cold, mottled skin
   - Other signs of shock (irritable or reduced consciousness level, hypotension, tachycardia)
   - Deep, acidotic breathing
   - Decreased tissue turgor

In children, hypotension is a late sign, but is often preceded by a narrowing of the pulse pressure from vasoconstriction. Other markers of mild to moderate dehydration include the following:

- A history of oliguria
- Lethargy
- Sunken eyes
- Dry mucous membranes
- Sunken fontanelle
- Absence of tears

In hypernatremic dehydration, the clinical signs of dehydration are less marked because the extracellular compartment is relatively preserved, and the degree of dehydration is underestimated. A child with hypernatremic dehydration may look only mildly unwell until they suddenly collapse with shock.

In severe dehydration, the existing deficit should be replaced over the first 12 to 24 hours, using the IV (or nasogastric) route. Faster deficit replacement has been shown to be safe in many children, but confers no advantage apart from earlier discharge from an emergency department. For replacement of deficit, an isotonic fluid should be used.

In severe dehydration electrolytes should be checked; hypokalemia is common in dehydration from diarrhea, but hyperkalemia can occur if there is prerenal failure resulting from hypovolemia, or severe metabolic acidosis. Hyper- and hyponatremia, hypoglycemia, and hypomagnesemia are commonly seen in children with severe dehydration.

Hypernatremic dehydration is most frequently caused by a water deficit (increased losses or reduced intake). In some cases, it is caused by an increase in total body sodium (such as ingestion of large quantities of sodium, incorrect preparation of milk formula, ingestion of hyperosmotic feeds in the setting of diarrhea). For hypernatremic dehydration, after the correction of shock if present, the aim is to lower the serum sodium slowly at a rate of no faster than 12 mmol/L in 24 hours (0.5 mmol/L per hour). This rate of normalization of serum sodium should be even slower if hypernatremia is chronic (weeks). If sodium is corrected too rapidly, cerebral edema, seizures, and permanent brain injury may occur. In moderate hypernatremic dehydration, $Na^+$ 150 to 169 mmol/L after initial resuscitation, replace the deficit plus maintenance over 48 hours. Nasogastric oral rehydration salts should be used whenever possible, remembering that these have a low sodium concentration (60–90 mmol/L). Monitor electrolytes every 4 to 6 hours. If requiring IV rehydration, then Ringer's lactate +5% dextrose, 0.9% NaCl + 5% dextrose, or PlasmaLyte with 5% dextrose should be given, adding maintenance potassium chloride once urine output has been established. In severe hypernatremic dehydration, $Na^+ > 169$ mmol/L, the child should be admitted to intensive care. After initial resuscitation from shock if present, the fluid deficit should be replaced using 0.9% NaCl + 5% dextrose over 72 to 96 hours. In severe hypernatremic dehydration, electrolytes and glucose should initially be checked hourly. If serum sodium is falling faster than 0.5 mmol/h, then the infusion rate should be slowed down by 20%, and the serum sodium should be rechecked after 1 hour. If, after 6 hours of rehydration therapy, the sodium is decreasing at a steady rate, then the electrolytes and glucose can be checked every 4 hours. If there are persistent neurological signs, cerebral imaging should be considered. Venous sinus thromboses can occur from severe hypernatremic dehydration.

#### Ongoing Losses

It is vitally important to document fluid balance carefully and, ideally, hourly in patients during active fluid resuscitation. Fluid balance charts should accurately record—whenever possible—output volumes, including urine, gastric aspirates, vomitus, diarrhea, drainage from fistulae, and other fluid losses. These will determine the volume and type of fluid and electrolyte replacement. In practice, it can be difficult to accurately measure all losses. A rule of thumb is to add 100 mL for every diarrheal stool in the previous 12 hours to make up the ongoing losses that are added to the total fluid intake for the next 12 hours.

#### Maintenance Fluid

For over 5 decades, the standard maintenance IV fluid for children in hospitals throughout the world was hypotonic saline and glucose. A commonly used solution was 4% dextrose and 0.18% NaCl (containing 30 mmol/L sodium and chloride), and another fluid used in some countries was 3.3% dextrose and 0.3% NaCl. The recommended flow rates of IV maintenance fluid followed the 100/50/20 rule: 100 mL/kg/day for the first 10 kg body weight, 50 mL/kg/day for the next 10 kg, and 20 mL/kg/day for each kg thereafter. This roughly equates with the 4/2/1 rule, which is in mL/kg per hour. This is approximately the amount of water that a well, active child who has a normal metabolism and normal renal function requires to excrete nitrogenous wastes in an isosmotic urine, that is, urine that is neither overly concentrated nor overly dilute. The composition of the recommended IV fluids was based on the calculation that, if a child receives "normal maintenance volumes" for weight using 4% dextrose and 0.18% NaCl, he or she would receive 2 to 3 mmol/kg/day sodium (the amount needed for metabolism and growth), and 3.5 mg/kg/min of glucose (enough to avoid hypoglycemia in a patient who is nil orally).

The problem lies in the assumptions underlying these recommendations. Sick children are not the same as well, active children. Hospitalized children with infectious processes, such as pneumonia, bronchiolitis, sepsis, or central nervous system infections, and those with other conditions including surgical emergencies and those who are postanesthesia, commonly have increased levels of ADH, which causes water retention. Depending on how sick they are, such children may also have impaired renal function, increased capillary permeability (including in the brain, lungs, and soft tissues), poor lung compliance, and hypoproteinemia. The retention of water by ADH is a protective physiological mechanism for fasting sick patients. However, the administration of "normal maintenance IV fluids" to a child who cannot excrete a free water load risks fluid overload and edema of tissues, lungs, brain, and other organs. The administration of an IV solution with a sodium content substantially lower than plasma in a child who has impaired ability to excrete free water leads to hyponatremia, and this can lead to brain cell edema. On an unknown number of occasions, this has resulted in seizures, cerebral edema, and death. While some risk factors for these complications are known, it is not easy to predict to which patients this will occur, and hyponatremia and cerebral edema can also occur in patients without known factors. Hyponatremia is not always preventable.

Probably even more frequent than neurological complications are those arising from excessive volumes of IV fluid relative to true requirements for fluid homeostasis. Tissue edema leads to poor lung compliance and worsening hypoxemia in children with respiratory infections, soft tissue edema, immobility and pressure areas in children in coma, and impaired kidney function. There are now many case series of iatrogenic hyponatremia and its consequences; patent safety alert warnings by national and coronial authorities from the UK, Northern Ireland, Canada, and elsewhere; and randomized trials showing a lower risk of hyponatremia in children who receive isotonic fluids.

In 2013, the World Health Organization (WHO) recommended that "children who require IV fluids for maintenance should be managed with Ringers lactate with 5% dextrose, or 0.9% normal saline with 5% dextrose or half-normal saline (0.45% NaCl) with 5% glucose."

Fluid management of critically ill children requires careful assessment of disease process, pathophysiology, hydration, and intravascular volume status and responses to administered fluid. Both standardized guidelines and an individualized approach are needed for optimal fluid management. Guidelines for prescribing maintenance fluid are detailed in Appendix 101-2, and the water and electrolyte contents of commonly used fluids are given in Table 101-1.

**TABLE 101-1 WATER AND ELECTROLYTE CONTENT OF COMMONLY USED IV FLUIDS**

| Fluid Type | $Na^+$ mmol/L | $K^+$ mmol/L | $Cl^-$ mmol/L | Other Anions mmol/L | Osmolality | Electrolyte-Free Water/L | Comments |
|---|---|---|---|---|---|---|---|
| **0.9% NaCl** | 154 | 0 | 154 | | 308 | 0 | |
| **0.45% NaCl** | 77 | 0 | 77 | | 154 | 500 | |
| **0.9% NaCl 5% dex** | 154 | 0 | 154 | | 560 | 0 | |
| **5% dex 0.45% NaCl** | 77 | 0 | 77 | | 406 | 500 | |
| **5% dex 0.2% NaCl** | 34 | 0 | 34 | | 321 | 780 | **Not safe to be used as maintenance fluid** |
| **4% dex 0.18% NaCl** | 31 | 0 | 31 | | 284 | 800 | |
| **5% dex** | 0 | 0 | 0 | | 252 | 1000 | |
| **Ringers lactate** | 130 | 4 | 109 | lactate 28 | 272 | 130 | **Suitable as IV maintenance fluids** |
| **Hartmann's solution** | 131 | 5.4 | 112 | lactate 28 | 274 | 100 | |
| **PlasmaLyte** | 140 | 5 | 98 | acetate 27, gluconate 23 | 294 | 60 | |
| **3% saline** | **513** | **0** | **513** | | **1027** | **0** | |

Cl, chloride; dex, dextrose; IV, intravenous; K, potassium; Na, sodium

## APPENDIX 101-1 GUIDELINES FOR THE FLUID MANAGEMENT OF CHILDREN WITH SIGNS OF IMPAIRED CIRCULATION OR SHOCK

**Children Who Have Some Signs of Circulatory Impairment but Do Not Have Shock**

Children with only 1 or 2 signs of impaired circulation, either cold extremities or a weak and fast pulse or capillary refill > 3 seconds, but who do not have the full clinical features of shock (ie, all 3 signs present together), should not receive any rapid infusions of fluids but should still receive maintenance fluids appropriate for age, weight, and disease process.

In the absence of shock, rapid IV infusions of fluids may be particularly harmful to children who have severe febrile illnesses, severe pneumonia, severe malaria, meningitis, severe acute malnutrition, severe anemia, congestive heart failure with pulmonary edema, congenital heart disease, or renal failure.

Children with any sign of impaired circulation (ie, cold extremities or weak and fast pulse or prolonged capillary refill), should be prioritized for full assessment and other treatments (treatment of the underlying cause and other possible treatments below), and reassessed within 1 hour.

**Children Who Have Shock**

Children who have shock (ie, who have all of the following signs: cold extremities and a weak and fast pulse and capillary refill > 3 seconds) should receive IV fluids and consideration for other treatment as follows:

- Give high-flow oxygen
- Give 10–20 mL/kg of isotonic crystalloid fluids over 30–60 min
- If severe anemia (severe palmar or conjunctival pallor), give blood as soon as possible and do not give other boluses of IV fluid
- Check blood glucose and correct if low
- Monitor the effect of fluid; fully assess to look for an underlying cause of shock

If the child is still in shock after initial fluid therapy, then consider a further infusion of 10 mL/kg over 30 min, and at the same time assess the need for other emergency treatments.

- Inotrope (adrenaline, dopamine) or vasoactive agent (noradrenaline) if hypotensive or persistent shock
- Antibiotics for bacterial sepsis +/− antimalarial if in malaria endemic area
- Diuretic (furosemide 1 mg/kg IV) if signs of fluid overload or heart failure
- Positive pressure respiratory support (such as continuous positive airway pressure) if hypoxemia or severe respiratory distress despite oxygen
- Hydrocortisone if hypotensive despite inotrope or vasopressor
- Adrenaline IV or intramuscular if any sign of anaphylaxis
- Antivenom if signs of snake bite
- Thiamine if beriberi is suspected, or if the child has severe malnutrition
- Echocardiogram to assess heart function and exclude tamponade
- Tranexamic acid and urgent blood transfusion if there is traumatic hemorrhage
- Surgical review if abdominal emergency or trauma

Reassess airway, breathing, circulation; monitor for the effects of emergency treatments; and further review the underlying cause of shock by history and examination.

If shock has resolved, then provide fluids to maintain normal hydration status only (maintenance fluids).

Decide on the best location of ongoing care and monitoring: intensive or high dependency area, pediatric unit. Order frequency of monitoring, reassessment, and other supportive care.

## APPENDIX 101-2 GUIDELINES FOR PRESCRIBING MAINTENANCE FLUID IN SICK CHILDREN

**Does This Child Need IV Fluid?**

Whenever possible, give enteral milk feeds to sick children, as this provides nutrition and reduces gastrointestinal complications and infections. If the child is too sick to take fluids orally, consider milk feeds via a nasogastric tube. Standard IV fluids provide no effective nutrition.

**Maintenance Fluid Composition**

For maintenance fluid in children older than 1 month of age, use isotonic fluids:

- Hartmann's solution with 5% dextrose (or Ringer's lactate with 5% glucose)
- PlasmaLyte with 5% dextrose where this is approved and available
- 0.45% NaCl with 5% dextrose
- 0.9% NaCl with 5% dextrose[a]

Do *not* use 0.18% NaCl, or 0.3% NaCl

**Fluid Volumes and Rates**

Calculate the total fluid intake (TFI) the child requires (oral, IV) for the day.

Full maintenance IV fluid:

- 100 mL/kg/day for first 10 kg of child's weight
- 50 mL/kg/day for each kg of child's weight between 10 and 20 kg
- 20 mL/kg/day for every kg of child's weight > 20 kg
- max: 2500 mL/day

This concept of full maintenance, based on the 100/50/20 (or 4/2/1 per hour) rule relates to the *maximum* volumes that are usually required for children receiving IV fluids. *For most sick children* less *IV fluid is required to maintain normal volume status.* It is generally best to start with no more than two-thirds of the calculated full maintenance IV fluid.

For children with central nervous system infections (meningitis, encephalitis, or coma) or acute lower respiratory infection (pneumonia or bronchiolitis), even less IV fluid may be required to maintain normal volume status. Correct dehydration if it is present, then continue with reduced TFI at approximately 50% to 70% maintenance and monitor closely.

(Continued)

**APPENDIX 101-2 GUIDELINES FOR PRESCRIBING MAINTENANCE FLUID IN SICK CHILDREN (CONTINUED)**

Infants on full enteral milk feeds often need more than this for optimal growth: up to 150 mL/kg/day.

As enteral/oral feeds increase, reduce IV fluids. If enteral feeds cease, increase IV fluids.

**Monitoring**

1. **Monitor the TFI.** Monitor the fluid the child actually receives, not just the volumes that are ordered or prescribed. Experience shows that the TFI is often in excess of the volumes that are prescribed.
2. **Children receiving IV fluids should be weighed every day.** An increase in weight of 5% or more over 24 hours indicates fluid overload. The IV fluids should be stopped and the serum sodium measured. A decrease in weight of 5% or more indicates dehydration. Weigh on the same scales in similar lightweight clothing for more accurate monitoring.
3. **Check for edema every day.** Check for puffy eyes and lower limb swelling. If either if these is present, stop IV fluids and reassess.
4. **Every child receiving 50% or more of maintenance volumes in IV fluids should have the serum electrolytes checked daily.** If the serum sodium is below 130 mmol/L, or has fallen by more than 5 mmol/L since admission, reassess the type and volume of IV fluid given. If the serum sodium is 150 mmol/L or above, or has risen by 5 mmol/L from the time of admission, review the possible causes (eg, dehydration, sodium excess).
5. **Measure blood glucose every 6 to 12 hours in infants under 6 months of age on IV fluid.** If the blood glucose is less than 3 mmol/L (54 mg/dL), change the IV fluid from that containing 5% to one containing 10% glucose, or feed the child.

[a]Normal saline (0.9% NaCl) is not ideal maintenance fluid for children, as it contains high chloride levels (150 mmol/L), which can lead to metabolic acidosis when large volumes are administered. Also, it may lead to sodium accumulation in children with malnutrition. Ringer's lactate, Hartmann's solution, and PlasmaLyte have lower chloride (110 mmol/L) and sodium (130–140 mmol/L) levels, and therefore are not likely to lead to hyperchloremic metabolic acidosis.

## SUGGESTED READINGS


Choong K, Arora S, Cheng J, et al. Hypotonic versus isotonic maintenance fluids after surgery for children: a randomized controlled trial. *Pediatrics.* 2011;128(5):857-866.

Duke T. New WHO guidelines on emergency triage assessment and treatment. *Lancet.* 2016;387(721):724.

Halberthal M, Halperin ML, Bohn D. Acute hyponatremia in children admitted to hospital: retrospective analysis of factors contributing to its development and resolution. *BMJ.* 2001;322:780-782.

Maitland K, Kiguli S, Opoka RO, et al. Mortality after fluid bolus in African children with severe infection. *N Eng J Med.* 2011;364: 2483-2495.

Maitland K, George EC, Evans JA, et al. Exploring mechanisms of excess mortality with early fluid resuscitation: insights from the FEAST trial. *BMC Med.* 2013;11:68.

McNab S, Duke T, South M, et al. 140 mmol/L of sodium versus 77 mmol/L of sodium in maintenance intravenous fluid therapy for children in hospital (PIMS): a randomised controlled double-blind trial. *Lancet.* 2016;385(9974):1190-1197.

Medicines and Healthcare Products Regulatory Agency. Intravenous 0.18% saline/4% glucose solution ("hypotonic saline") in children: reports of fatal hyponatraemia. https://www.gov.uk/drug-safety-update/intravenous-0-18-saline-4-glucose-solution-hypotonic-saline-in-children-reports-of-fatal-hyponatraemia. Published October 29, 2012. Accessed September 26, 2016.

Montañana PA, Modesto i Alapont V, Ocón AP, López PO, López Prats JL, Toledo Parreño JD. The use of isotonic fluid as maintenance therapy prevents iatrogenic hyponatremia in pediatrics: a randomized, controlled open study. *Pediatr Crit Care Med.* 2008;9(6): 589-597.

National Patient Safety Agency UK. *Reducing the Risk of Hyponatraemia When Administering Intravenous Infusions to Children.* National Health Service England; 2007. Patient Safety Alert 22. Report No.: NRLS-0409. http://www.nrls.npsa.nhs.uk/EasySiteWeb/getresource.axd?AssetID=60073&type=full&servicetype=Attachment. Accessed September 26, 2016.

World Health Organization. *Paediatric Emergency Triage, Assessment and Treatment:* Care of Critically Ill Children. Geneva: WHO; 2016.

World Health Organization. *Pocket Book of Hospital Care for Children: Guidelines for the Management of Common Illnesses with Limited Resources.* 2nd ed. Geneva: WHO; 2013.


# 102 Cardiopulmonary Resuscitation

Mary Fran Hazinski

## INTRODUCTION

Successful closed-chest cardiopulmonary resuscitation (CPR), the fundamental life-saving skill, was first reported in 1960, and the American Heart Association (AHA) has published pediatric and neonatal resuscitation guidelines since 1980. Although CPR has been widely taught to healthcare providers (HCPs) and the public, it is only recently that survival from cardiac arrest has improved. This improvement has occurred in association with an emphasis on teaching, monitoring, and improving CPR quality; widespread implementation of lay-rescuer CPR and automated external defibrillation (AED) programs; increased frequency of dispatcher-guided lay-rescuer CPR; and improvements in postcardiac arrest care, including targeted temperature management. Published studies from both out-of-hospital and in-hospital registries have provided additional information about the epidemiology, presentation, and outcome of pediatric cardiopulmonary arrest (CPA) at different ages and in different settings. The AHA Guidelines for Pediatric Basic Life Support (PBLS) and Pediatric Advanced Life Support (PALS) are now based on a continuous, structured international evidence-based review process. The reviews, sponsored by the AHA and the International Liaison Committee on Resuscitation (ILCOR), are posted on ILCOR's Web site (http://www.ilcor.org./home/), in the Systematic Evidence Evaluation and Review System.

Neonatal resuscitation guidelines are jointly created by the AHA and the American Academy of Pediatrics. These guidelines target resuscitation in the delivery room, emphasizing establishment of effective ventilation, because inadequate airway and ventilation are the most common problems requiring newborn resuscitation. Neonatal resuscitation guidelines are typically applied during the initial hospitalization of the newborn. The AHA infant Basic Life Support (BLS) and CPR guidelines typically apply to the infant after the initial hospitalization until 1 year of age. If a newborn remains hospitalized for treatment of heart disease, it is appropriate to apply infant CPR guidelines to provide a higher compression-to-ventilation ratio consistent with focus on establishment of adequate blood flow as well as oxygenation and ventilation. The AHA PBLS and CPR guidelines apply to children from 1 year of age to puberty. Adult BLS guidelines apply to adolescents. For ease of teaching and practice, providers in a unit such as a pediatric cardiovascular intensive care unit (ICU) may elect to apply the infant and child CPR guidelines to all patients in the unit.

In 2010, the AHA recommended a change in the initial sequence of CPR from ABC (airway, breathing, circulation/compressions) to CAB (circulation/compressions, airway, breathing). This change was made because the initial steps of opening the airway and delivering breaths are relatively complicated and often created long delays to initiating chest compressions. Although support of airway, oxygenation, and ventilation is especially important during pediatric cardiac arrest, this change in sequence should delay ventilation only by a few seconds, and is designed to shorten the overall time to initiation of CPR for all victims of cardiac arrest.

Every step in resuscitation is important, including treating prearrest conditions when possible; immediately identifying the arrest itself and providing high-quality CPR; and seamlessly integrating shock delivery with CPR when needed. Skilled, evidence- and protocol-supported postcardiac arrest care, including targeted temperature management is critical.

## PATHOGENESIS AND ETIOLOGY OF CARDIAC ARREST

The causes and types of cardiac arrest during infancy and childhood vary by age and arrest location and will affect the priorities of resuscitation. In the past, much of the evidence used to characterize pediatric cardiac arrest was based on extrapolation from adult series; however, in recent years, several pediatric cardiac arrest registries have provided a wealth of information about many characteristics of pediatric CPA.

### Data from Registries

Multiple large pediatric out-of-hospital cardiac arrest series have been published from registries such as the Cardiac Arrest Registry to Enhance Survival (CARES; https://mycares.net/), the Resuscitation Outcomes Consortium (ROC; https://roc.uwctc.org) registry, and the all-Japan Utstein Registry. In the United States, the Get with the Guidelines-Resuscitation (GWTG-R) registry, formerly the National Registry of Cardiopulmonary Resuscitation (http://www.heart.org/HEARTORG/Professional/GetWithTheGuidelines-Resuscitation/Get-With-The-Guidelines-Resuscitation_UCM_314496_SubHomePage.jsp) has published multiple pediatric series. These registries collect data based on the reporting templates known as the Utstein criteria. Publications from registries such as these contribute substantially to our knowledge of pediatric prearrest, arrest and postarrest conditions, further informing the emphasis of the AHA PBLS and PALS Guidelines.

### Asphyxial Versus Sudden Cardiac Arrest

There are 2 major types of CPA: those that occur secondary to progression of respiratory failure or shock (so-called *asphyxial* or *hypoxic* arrest) and those that occur as an abrupt cessation of cardiac function, called *sudden cardiac arrest* (SCA). These types of CPA can be further identified by the terminal cardiac rhythm. Bradycardia and pulseless electrical activity (PEA) are the most common terminal rhythms associated with asphyxial arrest; these rhythms are called "nonshockable" because shock delivery is not indicated to treat the arrest. Pulseless ventricular tachycardia (pVT) and ventricular fibrillation (VF) are the terminal rhythms associated with SCA; these rhythms are known as "shockable" rhythms because shock delivery is required. The incidence of each type of CPA varies with the age and condition of the child, and with the location and circumstances of the arrest. Resuscitation priorities vary with arrest type, the number of rescuers, and the location of the arrest.

At birth, approximately 5% to 10% of newborns require some resuscitation, ranging from simple stimulation or clearing of the airway to support of ventilation and occasionally to chest compressions. Most neonates in distress demonstrate bradycardia, and most will respond to the establishment of effective ventilation.

Asphyxial arrest is the most common type of CPA in infants and children. However, this type of arrest can occur in patients of any age with conditions such as respiratory failure, trauma, drowning, drug overdose, poisonings, metabolic disorders, and shock. In the United States, the most common causes of infant death include congenital malformations, disorders related to prematurity, sudden unexpected infant death (including sudden infant death syndrome [SIDS], suffocation, and strangulation) and injury. Injuries are the most common causes of childhood and adolescent death. See also Chapters 113 and 116.

The infant or child often develops bradycardia as a preterminal event after asphyxia arrest. Bradycardia in children may also result from vagal stimulation (eg, induced by suctioning or gagging), from other causes of hypoxia, or from heart block. In the minutes before an asphyxial or bradycardic arrest, oxygen delivery to the tissues is compromised by low arterial oxygen content, by inadequate blood flow, or both, and major organ ischemia is likely to be present even before the arrest occurs. Resuscitation requires conventional CPR because support of effective oxygenation and ventilation, and compressions are needed to support oxygen delivery.

The infant or child with SCA has pVT/VF that causes the abrupt cessation of cardiac function. This type of cardiac arrest is most common in adults but is less common in children, particularly before adolescence. SCA has been reported in young athletes following a blow to the chest (commotio cordis) and in infants and children with genetic anomalies of impulse formation and conduction (eg, channelopathies such as prolonged QT syndrome), congenital heart disease, coronary artery abnormalities, cardiac inflammation, cardiomyopathy, and drug toxicity. Because arterial oxygen content is normal at the time of SCA, immediate support of blood flow with chest compressions may maintain oxygen delivery for the first few minutes of the arrest. However, beyond the first minutes of arrest, arterial oxygen content declines rapidly, so conventional CPR is needed.

### Characteristics of Out-of-Hospital Arrest

Estimates of the incidence of asphyxial arrest versus SCA are based on extrapolation from mortality data collected by the Centers for Disease Control and Prevention and from published case series and registry data. In general, two-thirds of out-of-hospital pediatric cardiac arrests are asphyxial, about two-thirds of victims are infants who arrest at home, most are unwitnessed, and about half of the victims receive bystander CPR. These characteristics provide important information for exploring causes and prevention of CPR, targeting CPR education to parents and caregivers, and establishing resuscitation priorities for dispatcher-guided CPR.

Cardiac arrest in schools, particularly among student athletes, has stimulated grassroots efforts to establish CPR and AED programs in schools. Extrapolation from voluntary US databases suggests that approximately 1 per 100,000 high school athletes suffers from SCA annually, with the incidence higher in males and lower in females, and lower among nonathletes. In the United States, more than half of the SCA deaths in athletes are attributed to hypertrophic cardiomyopathy, commotio cordis (a blow to the chest that triggers ventricular tachycardia or fibrillation), or coronary artery anomalies. Some athletes or children with arrhythmias such as those caused by channelopathies may have syncopal episodes prior to the cardiac arrest event. Vigorous exercise can trigger lethal ventricular arrhythmias; many episodes of SCA in athletes occur during sporting events and are witnessed.

### Characteristics of In-Hospital Arrest

Publications from the nearly 10,000 pediatric arrests in the GWTG-R registry have enabled the characterization of in-hospital arrest in children. Most children with in-hospital cardiac arrest have prearrest respiratory insufficiency, shock, or congestive heart failure. The most common intermediate causes of arrest are hypotension, acute respiratory insufficiency, and arrhythmias. PEA or asystole is the terminal rhythm in two-thirds of the arrests. Of the children with initial pVT/VF, approximately half have a cardiac illness or surgical condition, and prearrest vasoactive infusions have been identified as proarrhythmic factors. Although pVT/VF is not a common initial arrest rhythm, VF is present at some time during resuscitation in approximately 25% of pediatric in-hospital arrests, so providers must be facile at integrating shock delivery with high-quality CPR.

## RESPIRATORY AND CARDIAC ARREST: CLINICAL MANIFESTATIONS

### Respiratory Arrest

*Respiratory arrest* is defined as the cessation of spontaneous respiratory activity in the presence of spontaneous circulation (palpable central pulses). The development of hypoxemia and tissue hypoxia will produce bradycardia and poor perfusion. Detection and immediate treatment of respiratory arrest and symptomatic bradycardia often prevent progression to CPA.

### Cardiopulmonary Arrest

*Cardiopulmonary arrest* is defined as the cessation of effective cardiac mechanical function and systemic perfusion. The victim is unconscious/unresponsive, with apnea or agonal gasps and with no palpable central pulses. Agonal gasps may be mistaken for effective spontaneous breathing, delaying the identification of cardiac arrest. They are much more common in the first minutes of SCA but are uncommon in children with asphyxial cardiac arrest. Agonal gasps can increase pulmonary gas exchange if the airway is patent. Gasps can also enhance venous return and create some coronary and carotid perfusion during the first minutes of arrest.

Once cardiac arrest develops, oxygen delivery ceases. Unless CPR is provided and spontaneous rhythm and perfusion are restored, the myocardium, brain, and all tissues will become progressively ischemic, and the likelihood of successful resuscitation diminishes with every passing minute. Generation of lactic acid, increased cell membrane permeability, production of free oxygen radicals, and activation of inflammatory mediators contribute to progressive organ and tissue destruction.

### Pulseless Electrical Activity and Asystole

*Pulseless electrical activity* is a term used to describe cardiac electrical activity that fails to produce sufficient mechanical function to generate a palpable central pulse. Although this term could encompass agonal (eg, bradyasystolic) rhythms, it is typically reserved for patients with narrow QRS complexes that fail to produce a palpable pulse. Reversible causes of PEA in children include tension pneumothorax, cardiac tamponade, hypovolemia, and, rarely, pulmonary embolus. If PEA is not promptly treated, the rhythm will ultimately deteriorate to asystole.

Asystole is the ultimate terminal rhythm, characterized by electrical silence. Asystole is likely to be present for any unwitnessed or prolonged arrest, and it is the most common rhythm reported in pediatric prehospital and in-hospital arrest. Although overall survival with asystole or PEA is poor, survival is higher among children than adults who present with these rhythms in in-hospital arrests.

### Ventricular Tachycardia and Fibrillation

Just as in adults, children in cardiac arrest who present with pVT/VF in the out-of-hospital or in-hospital setting typically have higher survival rates than those presenting with PEA or asystole. Untreated pVT will rapidly progress to VF, so treatment of these rhythms is identical and the rhythms are considered together in treatment algorithms.

During the first few minutes of VF, the amplitude of the VF will be high (so-called good VF), indicating that the myocardium initially has adequate oxygen and substrates. High-quality CPR can help maintain myocardial oxygenation and the amplitude and duration of VF (before it deteriorates to asystole). Rapid shock delivery is likely to result in elimination of the VF, enabling return of spontaneous cardiac rhythm and return of spontaneous circulation (ROSC). It is important to note that typically there is a delay between elimination of VF and ROSC, so CPR is needed until the shock can be delivered and after shock delivery until ROSC occurs.

If the VF remains untreated (ie, no CPR or shock delivery) for several minutes after arrest, the VF amplitude will gradually decrease (so-called bad VF), indicating severe myocardial ischemia. At this point, shock delivery is less likely to eliminate the VF; multiple shocks may be required. Even if VF is eliminated, return of spontaneous rhythm and return of spontaneous cardiac rhythm are less likely.

Untreated VF will ultimately progress to asystole. Once asystole is present, shock delivery will not be effective. High-quality CPR may result in the reappearance of VF (so-called secondary VF) that may respond to shock delivery, although the survival of patients who present with secondary VF is much lower than that of patients who present with VF as their initial rhythm.

## RESPIRATORY AND CARDIAC ARREST: MANAGEMENT

### Respiratory Arrest and Bradycardia

The child with respiratory failure, shock, or respiratory arrest typically develops bradycardia with poor perfusion before developing pulseless arrest. If rescuers detect and treat respiratory arrest and bradycardia before the development of pulseless arrest, survival is typically 75% or higher in both out-of-hospital and in-hospital settings.

Symptomatic bradycardia (ie, bradycardia with signs of poor perfusion) and respiratory arrest are both treated with support of airway, oxygenation, and ventilation through provision of bag-mask ventilation with oxygen. If the heart rate and perfusion improve but ventilation remains inadequate, mechanical ventilation is indicated. If the child's heart rate remains at or below 60 beats per minute with signs of poor perfusion despite support of adequate oxygenation and ventilation, chest compressions are added to the bag-mask ventilation (ie, CPR is provided).

When symptomatic bradycardia persists despite bag-mask ventilation and compressions, epinephrine is the drug of choice. Rescuers should consider using atropine for symptomatic bradycardia with increased vagal tone or when primary heart block is present. Cardiac pacing may also be needed.

Opiate overdose has emerged as a common cause of death in young adults. If the lay first responder or HCP encounters a victim of respiratory arrest with suspected drug overdose, naloxone administration is added to interventions such as bag-mask ventilation and CPR as indicated.

### Cardiopulmonary Arrest

Once *cardiopulmonary arrest* is present, immediate high-quality CPR is needed because CPR maintains a small but critical amount of blood flow (estimated at 10% to 33% of normal) and oxygen and substrate delivery to the heart, brain, and other organs. Performing CPR can prolong VF and can maintain or increase VF amplitude. This increases the window of opportunity for shock delivery and increases the likelihood that the shock delivery will be followed by return of spontaneous cardiac rhythm and ROSC.

### Cardiopulmonary Resuscitation Sequence

The appropriate sequence for pediatric resuscitation is determined by the type and location of the arrest and the type of rescuers and equipment available. A lone HCP must choose a sequence of actions, while multiple rescuers are able to accomplish several resuscitation steps simultaneously.

For the out-of-hospital arrest of a child or likely victim of asphyxial arrest, CPR focuses on initiation of high-quality conventional CPR. The lone HCP (with no nearby help or mobile phone) delivers about 5 cycles or about 2 minutes of CPR before leaving the victim to activate the emergency response system and retrieve an AED. The rescuer then returns to the victim to resume CPR and use the AED. If multiple bystanders are present during the out-of-hospital arrest, 1 rescuer remains with the victim to provide high-quality CPR while others activate the emergency response system and retrieve an AED.

During an in-hospital arrest, multiple rescuers are generally present to accomplish many tasks at the same time. The first HCP to identify cardiac arrest calls for nearby help and initiates resuscitation. As additional rescuers arrive with equipment, they will perform tasks such as providing bag-mask ventilation, attaching the adhesive defibrillator electrode pads and operating the defibrillator, establishing vascular access, serving as an alternate compressor, recording the resuscitation events, and functioning as team leader.

### High-Quality Cardiopulmonary Resuscitation Technique

The elements of *high-quality CPR* are compressions of adequate rate and depth, complete chest recoil after each compression, minimal number and duration of any interruptions in chest compressions, and avoidance of excessive ventilation.

During CPR, the child should be placed supine on a firm, flat surface. A backboard is generally used as this surface.

**Chest Compressions of Adequate Rate and Depth** *Chest compressions* create blood flow by increasing intrathoracic pressure and by directly compressing the heart. Myocardial blood flow is determined by the coronary perfusion pressure present between compressions. Coronary perfusion pressure is calculated as the difference between aortic end-diastolic pressure (during CPR, this is the aortic relaxation pressure) and the mean right atrial pressure; the mean CVP may be used as a surrogate for right atrial pressure. In adults with cardiac arrest, a coronary perfusion pressure greater than 15 mm Hg has been linked with ROSC. Although a similar threshold has not been established in children, if arterial and right atrial or central venous monitoring catheters are in place, rescuers should attempt to optimize coronary perfusion pressure by maximizing aortic relaxation pressure and minimizing right atrial and central venous pressure (see "Monitoring During Cardiopulmonary Resuscitation," below).

During CPR, blood flow, mean aortic relaxation pressure, and mean coronary perfusion pressure are increased by increasing the rate and force of chest compressions, and these variables are reduced when compressions are of either inadequate or excessive rate or inadequate depth. If the compression rate is too slow, blood flow generated by the compressions is inadequate. If the chest compression rate is too rapid, the depth of compressions may be compromised and chest recoil between compressions may be incomplete. The AHA-recommended chest compression rate for infants, children, and adults is 100 to 120 per minute.

The sternum is depressed approximately one-third the depth of the chest in the newborn and at least one-third the depth of the chest (about 1.5 in, or 4 cm) in the infant. The lone rescuer uses 2 fingers to compress the newborn or infant sternum, just below the intermammary line. When 2 HCPs are delivering CPR to the newborn or infant, the compressor uses the 2-thumb-encircling hands chest compression technique. The compressor's 2 thumbs are placed together on the sternum to depress the sternum (the thumbs can be placed side by side or they may overlap), while the fingers of both hands spread to encircle the thorax. The 2-thumb-encircling hands technique generates better coronary perfusion pressure and enables creation of more accurate depth of compression, and it may produce higher systolic and relaxation pressures with less rescuer fatigue than the 2-finger compression method.

Chest compressions in the child 1 year of age to puberty may be accomplished with 1 or 2 hands, whichever allows compression of the lower third of the sternum to a depth of at least one-third the depth of the chest and about 2 inches (5 cm). For chest compressions in the adolescent (after puberty) the traditional adult 2-hand technique is used to compress over the lower third of the sternum to a depth of 2 to 2.4 inches (5–6 cm). While excessive compression depth in adults can cause injuries such as rib fractures, inadequate compression depth is the more common problem and clearly reduces blood flow, coronary perfusion pressure, ROSC, and even survival from cardiac arrest.

Many CPR feedback devices are commercially available to provide visual and auditory indication and documentation of rate and depth of chest compressions and other resuscitation variables. These devices may be used for training and in actual resuscitations (see "Continuous Quality Improvement," below).

**Complete Chest Recoil after Each Compression** If rescuers fail to allow the chest wall to recoil completely after each compression, venous return to the heart is decreased, elevating right atrial pressure and reducing-coronary perfusion pressure. In addition, it prevents venous return to the heart and reduces the blood flow generated by the next compression. Rescuers who become fatigued while providing compressions are more likely to lean on the chest, failing to allow complete chest wall recoil. For this reason, during CPR, rescuers should rotate compressors about every 2 minutes (or more often if the compressor becomes fatigued or compression quality declines), and should monitor for and reduce leaning.

**Minimal Interruptions in Chest Compressions** Aortic relaxation pressure and coronary perfusion pressure fall whenever chest compressions are interrupted (eg, when breaths are provided or when compressions are interrupted to check rhythm or deliver a shock). Frequent or prolonged interruptions in chest compressions reduce mean coronary perfusion pressure, ROSC, and survival. Interruptions should, therefore, be minimized during CPR and rescuers should monitor the frequency and duration of any interruptions and strive to reduce them. The chest-compression fraction (CCF) is the total CPR time spent delivering compressions. The CCF should be at least 60% of total CPR time and the resuscitation team should strive for a CCF goal exceeding 80% of total CPR time.

**Avoid Excessive Ventilation** It is important to avoid excessive ventilation during CPR. When cardiac arrest is present, pulmonary blood flow, carbon dioxide delivery to the lungs, and oxygen uptake from the lungs are approximately 10% to 33% of normal, so victims need only a fraction of normal minute ventilation to match ventilation to perfusion during CPR. Excessive ventilation is harmful because it will reduce coronary perfusion pressure and blood flow during CPR. It will create positive intrathoracic pressure, reduce venous return to the heart, and reduce coronary perfusion and systemic and cerebral blood flow and survival.

The optimal compression-to-ventilation ratio for pediatric resuscitation is unknown. For pediatric CPR, the AHA recommends a 30:2 compression-to-ventilation ratio for single rescuers and a 15:2 ratio for 2 or more rescuers. Once an advanced airway is placed, rescuers should no longer deliver cycles of compressions and breaths. Instead, the rescuer performing compressions should deliver continuous chest compressions, and the rescuer providing ventilation should deliver approximately 10 breaths per minute (1 breath every 6 seconds).

**Continuous Chest Compressions versus Conventional CPR** Since 2008, the AHA has recommended Hands-Only/compression-only CPR for treatment of adult sudden witnessed cardiac arrest, particularly if the bystander is untrained or unwilling to provide mouth-to-mouth ventilation. The purpose of this recommendation was to increase the portion of victims of out-of-hospital cardiac arrest who receive some bystander CPR before the arrival of EMS providers. Because most pediatric cardiac arrest is asphyxial in origin, the AHA continues to recommend conventional CPR for infants and children with out-of-hospital cardiac arrest. This recommendation has been supported by pediatric data from out-of-hospital registries, with conventional CPR associated with higher survival than compression-only CPR, particularly in infants and particularly when asphyxial arrest is present.

### Advanced Cardiopulmonary Resuscitation Techniques

Open-chest CPR can produce nearly normal blood flow but is impractical for most resuscitation situations. This technique is often used in the immediate postoperative period for pediatric cardiovascular surgical patients, when the chest is left open or the sternotomy can be opened quickly.

Extracorporeal cardiopulmonary resuscitation (ECPR) is the use of extracorporeal membrane oxygenation (ECMO) during attempted resuscitation. Extracorporeal cardiopulmonary resuscitation has been successful for pediatric in-hospital resuscitation, particularly among children with heart disease (see Chapter 108). The timely implementation of ECMO may also be effective for preventing cardiac arrest among children with low cardiac output (eg, following cardiovascular surgery), septic shock, myocarditis, and cardiomyopathy.

### Monitoring during Cardiopulmonary Resuscitation

**Cardiopulmonary Resuscitation Feedback Devices** Several elements of CPR quality may be monitored and recorded, with devices that provide visual and auditory signals. These feedback devices range from relatively simple accelerometers to more complicated feedback defibrillators. The thresholds provided on the defibrillator screens and in recordings are typically consistent with a minimum 2-inch (5-cm) depth of acceptable chest compressions. These feedback defibrillators can be used to monitor the ECG, shock delivery, depth and rate of compressions, frequency and volume of breaths, and frequency and duration of any interruptions in chest compressions. This information is critical for team debriefing following every arrest as well as to set goals and monitor progress for improving CPR quality and survival in any resuscitation system.

**Exhaled or End-Tidal Carbon Dioxide Tension** Under normal conditions, the carbon dioxide tension in exhaled gas should be approximately equal to the carbon dioxide tension in both alveolar gas and pulmonary capillary blood. In very low flow states, if minute ventilation is fixed, the end-tidal carbon dioxide ($CO_2$) pressure ($P_{ETCO2}$) will vary with cardiac output. When cardiac arrest develops, blood flow to the lungs stops, so the $CO_2$ tension in the pulmonary capillaries, alveoli, and exhaled gas approaches zero. When effective chest compressions generate adequate pulmonary blood flow, the $CO_2$ delivered to the lungs and the partial pressure of $CO_2$ in exhaled gas should rise. ROSC is associated with a sharp and sustained rise in the $P_{ETCO2}$.

In intubated adult victims of cardiac arrest, a $P_{ETCO2}$ less than 10 mm Hg despite 20 minutes of resuscitation is associated with very low survival. Although a similar threshold has not been identified in children, if the $P_{ETCO2}$ remains less than 10 mm Hg, providers should make additional efforts to optimize CPR quality. Waveform capnography should be used for these measurements rather than intermittent colorimetric exhaled $CO_2$ monitors.

**Estimating Coronary Perfusion Pressure** Most hospitalized children who develop cardiac arrest are in the ICU (rather than in the general care ward), and invasive monitoring catheters may already be in place. If an intra-arterial and a central venous or right atrial catheter are in place, the coronary perfusion pressure can be estimated by subtracting the right atrial or central venous pressure from the aortic relaxation pressure (it will appear as the aortic diastolic pressure). The CPR technique should be optimized to maximize the estimated coronary perfusion pressure.

**Defibrillation** Because AED algorithms have been shown to be accurate in interpreting pediatric rhythms, the AHA recommends AED use for children ages 1 to 8 years in cardiac arrest, particularly for out-of-hospital arrest. Ideally, rescuers should use an AED with pediatric pads and a pediatric dose attenuator to deliver a shock dose appropriate for a small victim. However, if an AED with pediatric pads and dose attenuator is not available, rescuers should use an AED with adult pads. The pads should be placed according to the illustrations on the pads. They should not touch or overlap.

When an infant requires defibrillation, the use of a manual defibrillator is preferred to the use of an AED, because the dose can be more closely adjusted. If a manual defibrillator is not available, an AED with pediatric pads and a pediatric dose attenuator should be used. If such an AED is not available, an adult AED (one that administers an adult dose through adult pads) should be used.

When both pediatric and adult pads are available with the AED, it is important to use pediatric pads *only* for victims less than 8 years of age. If the pediatric pads are used for an older child, an adolescent, or an adult, they will likely attenuate the shock dose to one that is too small to eliminate VF in the larger victim.

For in-hospital manual defibrillation, rescuers should use infant pads or paddles for attempting defibrillation in infants up to 1 year of age and should use larger pads or paddles for patients 1 year of age and older. Rescuers should use the pads recommended by the defibrillator manufacturer.

Most commercially available defibrillators now use a biphasic waveform, while older defibrillators used a monophasic waveform. There are very limited data available regarding optimal manual biphasic waveform shock dose for defibrillation of children. In pediatric data from the GWTG-R in-hospital registry, an initial dose of 1 to 3 J/kg was associated with higher ROSC than a dose of more than 3 to 5 J/kg. The AHA recommends an initial shock of 2 J/kg. If the 2 J/kg initial dose fails to eliminate VF, rescuers should use a 4 J/kg dose for the second shock. For subsequent shocks, a dose of 4 J/kg is reasonable and a higher dose (up to a maximum of 10 J/kg) may be considered.

More research regarding the optimal defibrillation dose is needed. In general, weight-based defibrillation dosing may not be optimal, because the dose or current delivered to the myocardium is influenced not only by paddle or pad size and energy dose but also by transthoracic impedance, and transthoracic impedance is not linearly related to body weight. In the future, current-based defibrillation would make more sense than energy-based defibrillation.

### Organization of Pediatric Resuscitation

Resuscitation is organized around 2-minute periods of uninterrupted CPR. Once a defibrillator is attached, the rhythm is checked every 2 minutes and a shock is delivered if pVT/VF is present. When CPR is interrupted for shock delivery, rescuers should have the defibrillator charged and should deliver the shock within 10 seconds or less of the last chest compression, then should resume chest compressions immediately after shock delivery. Shock effectiveness (ie, likelihood of termination of VF and ultimate ROSC) decreases with every 10 seconds that elapse between the last compression and the shock delivery. When a shock eliminates VF, the most common rhythm for 30 to 60 seconds after shock delivery is asystole or PEA, so compressions are needed immediately after shock delivery.

### Advanced Airway

During resuscitation, the potential benefits of inserting an advanced airway should be weighed against the detrimental effects of the intubation attempt itself. Bag-mask ventilation for short periods may be as effective as ventilation through an advanced airway, but this form of ventilation requires training and frequent retraining. Inserting an advanced airway will enable delivery of uninterrupted chest compressions and may reduce gastric insufflation (and its attendant risks of regurgitation and aspiration), but it does require training and experience and will require interruption of chest compressions.

During resuscitation, the most experienced provider should perform intubation, with careful preparation and coordination of rescuer activities to minimize interruptions in chest compressions. Once the advanced airway is inserted, rescuers should also confirm placement using clinical examination plus a device such as a quantitative waveform capnography. If waveform capnography is not available, a qualitative colorimetric exhaled carbon dioxide detector may be used after several positive pressure breaths have been given. If the child weighs more than 20 kg, rescuers may use esophageal detector devices to confirm tracheal tube placement. These devices use suction to determine the ease with which gas can be withdrawn from the tube; the esophagus collapses easily under suction, preventing gas withdrawal, but the trachea is rigid and allows easy withdrawal of gas. Rescuers should verify correct tube position when the patient is transported and, during postcardiac arrest care, whenever the intubated child suddenly deteriorates.

### Drug Therapy

Although no drug has been shown to increase survival from pediatric cardiac arrest, the use of vasoconstrictors has been shown to increase blood pressure and coronary and cerebral blood flow and return of spontaneous cardiac rhythm in animals. Drugs with beta-adrenergic effects also increase spontaneous myocardial depolarization and contractility. The AHA recommends administering a standard dose of intravenous (IV) epinephrine (0.01 mg/kg) every 3 to 5 minutes during cardiac arrest.

During resuscitation, intravenous or intraosseous drug administration is preferable to endotracheal administration (see Chapter 100). Although lipid-soluble drugs can be administered by the endotracheal route, drug absorption is poor and unpredictable, and optimal drug doses for this route of administration are unknown. In fact, the lower blood concentrations of epinephrine resulting from endotracheal administration could produce undesirable vasodilatory β-2 adrenergic effects.

Intravenous high-dose epinephrine (HDE) is no longer recommended for routine use in pediatric resuscitation, because it is associated with decreased survival and neurological outcomes. Although HDE can increase the return of spontaneous cardiac rhythm, it can also increase postcardiac arrest myocardial oxygen consumption, myocardial dysfunction, and hemodynamic instability.

When shock-refractory VF is present, either amiodarone (5 mg/kg dose, to a maximum of 3 doses) or lidocaine (1 mg/kg dose) may be given as an antiarrhythmic. Because amiodarone can produce hypotension and arrhythmias, expert consultation is advised when the drug is considered for treatment of prearrest or postcardiac arrest arrhythmias.

Magnesium administration is indicated for treating *torsades de pointes* and when hypomagnesemia is documented or strongly suspected. However, it is no longer used routinely during resuscitation.

#### Termination of Resuscitation Efforts

There are no intra-arrest factors that reliably predict poor resuscitation outcomes. In the out-of-hospital setting, age less than 1 year, unwitnessed arrest, no bystander CPR, and nonshockable rhythm on EMS arrival are associated with poor outcome. In the in-hospital setting, age greater than 1 year and longer duration of cardiac arrest have been associated with poor outcome. However, no single factor predicts outcome, and recent emphases on CPR quality, and improved postcardiac arrest care could all have a significant positive impact on CPR outcomes.

#### Postcardiac Arrest Care

Following ROSC, ischemic and reperfusion injuries can cause cardiorespiratory instability, perfusion abnormalities, and organ dysfunction. *Reperfusion injury* is characterized by calcium entry into cells, activation of inflammatory mediators, and cell death. This inflammatory response includes the development of endothelial injury, capillary leak, neutrophil activation, platelet aggregation, and increases in mediators such as tumor necrosis factor and interleukins. Increased production of free oxygen radicals and decreased production of nitric oxide can cause vasoconstriction and further ischemic injury. Hyperglycemia is common in children after an arrest, and both extreme hyperglycemia and hypoglycemia have been linked with increased mortality in children.

Skilled postcardiac arrest care in adults has more than doubled neurologically intact survival to hospital discharge. Such care requires evidence-based and protocol-driven bundled care, including targeted temperature management and support of organ system function.

Following ROSC, rescuers must begin targeted temperature management, optimize hemodynamic support, titrate inspired oxygen administration, and support of ventilation to maintain normoxemia (unless cyanotic heart disease is present) and partial pressure of carbon dioxide ($PaCO_2$) appropriate for that patient, and support end-organ function. The use of protocols will support consistent care that can then be evaluated and modified as needed.

Children often demonstrate a brief period of spontaneous hypothermia followed by the development of hyperthermia after cardiac arrest. While hyperthermia is associated with worse neurological outcome, the recent Therapeutic Hypothermia to Improve Survival After Cardiac Arrest in Pediatric Patients (THAPCA, see http://www.THAPCA.gov) clinical trials network failed to show any benefit of induced hypothermia when compared to normothermia after out-of-hospital cardiac arrest. Results following in-hospital cardiac arrest are anticipated soon. Thus, at present, it is appropriate to recommend controlled normothermia and avoidance of hyperthermia in this at-risk population.

#### Continuous Quality Improvement

Every resuscitation program or setting must develop a process of continuous quality improvement. This process requires measurement of CPR quality, monitoring and review of resuscitation outcomes and techniques, and frequent opportunities for retraining. If the resuscitation team is not measuring performance, they cannot hope to improve it.

The availability of CPR courses for lay rescuers, including "CPR in schools" programs, can increase bystander CPR for out-of-hospital cardiac arrest. However, in addition to structured training programs, training opportunities must expand beyond the classroom. Opportunities to learn about CPR and to practice compressions are now offered to the lay public through kiosks in locations such as airports and through distribution of inflatable take-home manikins with instructions provided on a DVD.

All EMS dispatchers should use protocols to enable them to rapidly identify a likely cardiac arrest and guide untrained rescuers to initiate CPR; their effectiveness must be evaluated by documenting time to cardiac arrest identification and time to CPR initiation as part of the EMS system of continuous quality improvement. Voluntary registration of bystanders willing to perform CPR has enabled a type of "crowd sourcing" that has been effective in summoning rescuers to the scene of an out-of-hospital arrest. Smartphone programs are also available to guide rescuers through the steps of CPR by pacing compressions to the correct rate and reminding rescuers of CPR sequences and steps. These and other innovations are needed to increase the likelihood and quality of bystander CPR.

It is now clear that HCPs must regularly practice the skills and teamwork of resuscitation. However, the precise training duration and retraining interval needed to achieve and maintain resuscitation skills has not been established, and likely differs among HCPs who perform resuscitation frequently and those who rarely perform resuscitation. Providers need opportunities to refresh skills, particularly "just in time" training. Training with the use of realistic simulators holds promise to improve HCP skills and performance.

Team debriefing immediately following an attempted resuscitation is essential to team improvement in subsequent resuscitations. Such debriefing requires objective and professional discussion of team performance and identification of opportunities for improvement.

#### Prevention of Arrest

Ideally, successful treatment of prearrest conditions will prevent arrest or at least minimize potential organ ischemia before arrest ensues. In the in-hospital setting, a pediatric cardiac arrest outside of the ICU should be a rare event, and should trigger careful evaluation of the child's prearrest care and remediation of any shortcomings in assessment or treatment. Although rapid response or medical emergency teams may reduce the incidence of non-ICU pediatric arrests, the published success rates of these teams have varied widely.

## SUGGESTED READINGS


Cariou A, Nolan JP, Sunde K. Ten strategies to increase survival of cardiac arrest patients. *Intensive Care Med.* 2015;41(10):1820-1823.

Fukuda T, Ohashi-Fukuda N, Kobayashi H, et al. Conventional versus compression-only versus no bystander cardiopulmonary resuscitation for pediatric out-of-hospital cardiac arrest. *Circulation.* 2016;134(25):2060-2070.

Gupta P, Pasquali SK, Jacobs JP, et al; American Heart Association's Get with the Guidelines–Resuscitation Investigators. Outcomes following single and recurrent in-hospital cardiac arrests in children with heart disease: a report from American Heart Association's Get with the Guidelines Registry-Resuscitation. *Pediatr Crit Care Med.* 2016;17(6):531-539.

Hazinski MF, Nolan JP, Aickin R, et al. Part 1: Executive Summary: 2015 international consensus on cardiopulmonary resuscitation and emergency cardiovascular care science with treatment recommendations. *Circulation.* 2015;132(16 Suppl 1):S2-S39 (simultaneously published in *Resuscitation*).

Jacobs I, Nadkarni V, Bahr J, et al. Cardiac arrest and cardiopulmonary resuscitation outcome reports: update and simplification of the Utstein templates for resuscitation registries: a statement for healthcare professionals from a task force of the International Liaison Committee on Resuscitation (American Heart Association, European Resuscitation Council, Australian Resuscitation Council, New Zealand Resuscitation Council, Heart and Stroke Foundation of Canada, InterAmerican Heart Foundation, Resuscitation Councils of Southern Africa). *Circulation.* 2004;110(21):3385-3397.

Marino BS, Tabbutt S, MacLaren G, et al. Cardiopulmonary resuscitation in infants and children with cardiac disease: a scientific statement from the American Heart Association. *Circulation.* 2017;135:e1115-e1134.

Moler FW, Silverstein FS, Holubkov R, et al; THAPCA Trial Investigators. Therapeutic hypothermia after out-of-hospital cardiac arrest in children. *N Engl J Med.* 2015;372(20):1898-1908.

Naim MY, Burke RV, McNally BF. Association of bystander cardiopulmonary resuscitation with overall and neurologically favorable survival after pediatric out-of-hospital cardiac arrest in the United States: a report from the Cardiac Arrest Registry to Enhance Survival Surveillance Registry. *JAMA Pediatr*. 2017;171(2):133-141.

Neumar RW, Shuster M, Callaway CW, Part 1: Executive Summary: 2015 American Heart Association guidelines update for cardiopulmonary resuscitation and emergency cardiovascular care. *Circulation*. 2015;132(18 Suppl 2):S315-S367.

Tømte O, Andersen GØ, Jacobsen D, Drægni T, Auestad B, Sunde K. Strong and weak aspects of an established post-resuscitation treatment protocol—a five-year observational study. *Resuscitation*. 2011;82(9):1186-1193.

# 103 Stabilization and Transport

Anna C. Gunz and Niranjan Kissoon

## INTRODUCTION

In many countries, pediatric medical and surgical specialty services are regionalized to either community hospitals or tertiary and quaternary pediatric centers. Thus, critically ill children in need of these services may need to be transported considerable distances from their home communities in order to receive higher levels of care.

The main goal of successful patient transport is to transfer the patient to definitive care while preventing further deterioration. In order to achieve this goal, close monitoring, continued resuscitation, and time sensitive treatments may be necessary. However, there are inherent risks related to the transport, such as exposure to weather-related hazards, transport vehicle mishaps, and difficulties with patient monitoring and assessment due to the noisy, cramped, moving environment. In order to mitigate these risks and optimize patient care, there are many measures that can be taken. First, prompt telephone or video conferencing with specialized pediatric healthcare providers can guide patient management decisions and ensure that urgent medical interventions are initiated. Second, early discussion enables mobilization of resources and decisions on the appropriate mode of transportation. These discussions should address what equipment will be required in order to adequately and efficiently prepare for transport. Third, selecting the appropriate healthcare team to accompany the patient is imperative. The transport of critically ill children and neonates by specialized pediatric and neonatal transport teams has resulted in fewer adverse events and improved outcomes than those transported by providers without this specialized training. Given that most specialized teams are located in central areas, the time it takes for retrieval teams to reach the patient must be factored into the total transport time, and thus furthers the argument that prompt referral for transport is imperative. In the following, we will discuss important considerations of stabilization and transfer, including the timing of referral, who to refer, and how to mitigate the risk of transport.

## PATHOGENESIS AND EPIDEMIOLOGY

### When Is Patient Transport Necessary?

Generally, patients are transported from one facility to another to receive a higher level of care based on their medical diagnosis and on their diagnostic and treatment requirements. Decisions regarding when and where to transfer a patient are based on the local and regional resource availability, as well as patient acuity. Due to the centralization of specialized services, some children also may be transported electively for routine outpatient appointments. Patients that present to remote nursing stations or hospitals without the ability to admit pediatric patients may require semi-urgent transfer to seek general pediatric expertise. Other patients may require urgent and emergent transfer to tertiary or quaternary hospitals for specialized diagnostic or surgical services, subspecialty evaluation, or admission to a neonatal intensive care unit (NICU) or pediatric intensive care unit (PICU).

### Selecting the Optimal Mode of Transport

Local resources and infrastructure determine the mode of transport used to transfer children. In developing countries, patients may be transported by ambulance, as well as taxis, auto-rickshaws, bicycles, motorcycles, and even wheelbarrows. In developed countries, the discussion of patient transfer is usually limited to land and air ambulance, including fixed-wing and helicopters. Table 103-1 lists the characteristics of land and air transport. Appropriately triaging patients to a suitable mode of transport requires discussion of local resources, weather and traffic conditions, time of day, geography, and patient acuity. It is an area of ongoing research, particularly for trauma patients.

### Issues Related to Altitude

If the patient's location and/or acuity merit transport by helicopter or fixed-wing aircraft, there are a few physiologic considerations. At increased altitude, the barometric pressure decreases. Given that the partial pressure of oxygen ($PO_2$) is determined by the barometric pressure and fraction of inspired oxygen ($FiO_2$), at higher altitudes the $PO_2$ available at the alveolar level decreases. This causes mild desaturation in healthy individuals. In critically ill patients with significant oxygenation defects (such as those requiring 100% $FiO_2$), flying at high elevations is risky and efforts to improve oxygenation (eg, endotracheal intubation and effective ventilation) should be taken prior to transport.

Aeromedical transportation is subject to Boyle's law, which describes the inverse relationship between pressure and volume, such that as pressure decreases the volume increases. Thus, as barometric pressure decreases, volume-filled spaces will naturally expand. Therefore, during flight, pneumothoraces, intracranial air, air in abscesses, or gastric air bubbles may expand with deleterious consequences. Again, this should be anticipated, and efforts to prevent complications should be considered, including interventions (such as chest tube and nasogastric tube insertion) or selecting an alternate mode of transport. These considerations are more relevant when using fixed-wing air transport because of the greater altitude.

## CLINICAL MANIFESTATIONS

In order to successfully transport a patient from one facility to another, anticipation of care needs prior to catastrophic deterioration is needed. This involves some degree of clinical judgement and insight, and can sometimes be difficult to predict. However, there are some conditions that require direct admission to a PICU (such as meningococcemia or severe diabetic ketoacidosis) or evaluation at a pediatric center (such as significant pediatric trauma), and thus prompt referral should always be a priority. Regardless of the reason for patient presentation, given the logistical and geographic considerations of regional patient transfer, if a practitioner suspects the need for transfer, telephone consultation with the appropriate specialist is important to facilitate early activation of the appropriate transport team.

## DIAGNOSIS

Critically ill pediatric patients who require transport present with deranged physiology due to many disease states. Commonly, patients are transported after major trauma for treatment at a pediatric trauma center, or for other medical considerations such as cardiac disease (including congenital heart disease and myocarditis), respiratory illness (eg, bronchiolitis and pneumonia), infectious causes (eg, sepsis and meningitis), and neurological conditions (including seizures and traumatic brain injury). Newborns are transported for many reasons, including prematurity, transitional conditions requiring support (eg, respiratory distress syndrome, transient tachypnea of the newborn, and meconium aspiration), workup of congenital malformations, or other illnesses (eg, sepsis and hypoxic ischemic encephalopathy). The decision regarding when and whom to transfer will depend on a case-by-case discussion between the presenting and advising/receiving centers.

**TABLE 103-1 CHARACTERISTICS OF LAND AMBULANCE, HELICOPTER, AND FIXED-WING TRANSPORT**

| | Land Ambulance | Helicopter | Fixed-Wing Transport |
|---|---|---|---|
| **Mobility** | Rapid dispatch/deployment; restricted by traffic and other road conditions | Rapid deployment but restricted by need to refuel, reconfigure and pilot duty hours; not affected by ground traffic | Limited by flight plans, pilot duty hours and need for refueling/reconfiguring |
| **Destination** | Can reach any location with road service; often paired with other transport modality | Requires helipad/designated landing site/airport; access to on-scene calls in difficult terrain | Limited to airports and landing strips (often requires transfer to other modes of transport) |
| **Distance** | Can travel great distances but limited by speed | Need for refueling limits distances; varies with location but likely only cost effective if patient is > 45 miles from receiving facility | Long distances |
| **Speed** | Effective for short distances, urban areas | Relatively fast at covering great distances | Fastest modality |
| **Weather** | Rarely restricted by weather | Highly sensitive to weather conditions | Restricted in severe weather conditions (less so than for helicopters) |
| **Relative cost** | $ | $$$ (may be over-utilized) | $$$$$ |
| **Patient environment** | | | |
| Patient access | Most spacious; can stop vehicle to better access patient/perform intervention | Restrictive space; may not be configured for patient access when crew constrained | Often very restricted; may not be configured for patient access when crew constrained |
| Noise[a] | + (especially with sirens) | +++ | +++ |
| Vibrations[b] | Can stop vehicle to eliminate vibration | +++ | +++ |
| Effect of altitude | Not applicable | Unpressurized; dry air can dry secretions | Can pressurize and fly at low altitudes to mitigate |
| Risk of hypothermia | + | +++ | +++ |

[a]Complicates communication and patient evaluation, such as auscultation, and can be harmful to patients.

[b]Affects monitoring, such as oscillometric blood pressure measurement, and ability to perform procedures.

+ = present.

Data from Nichols DG, Schaffner DH: *Rogers Textbook of Pediatric Intensive Care Medicine*, 5th ed. Philadelphia: Lippincott Williams & Wilkins; 2015.

## TREATMENT

When an acutely ill pediatric patient presents in the community setting, the patient should be stabilized following a structured assessment and management process that focuses on airway, breathing, and circulation, as directed by the Pediatric Advanced Life Support or Advanced Trauma Life Support algorithms. Early telephone consultation with a consulting specialist is recommended. Prior arrangements and clinical needs may dictate who should be consulted and may include any of a general pediatrician, pediatric emergency physician, neonatologist, or pediatric intensivist. The consultation should include discussion of the appropriate treatment and diagnostic modalities that are required prior to transfer, and what the appropriate transport process should be. The processes by which these calls are initiated vary depending on local health system logistics and design, and all practicing clinicians should familiarize themselves with local transfer processes for their region.

The "scoop and run" philosophy (meaning achieving as rapid a turnaround as possible, often for the sickest and least stable patients) has long been seen as inadequate in the care of pediatric patients who require interfacility transport. Adequate preparation prior to transport is imperative. It has been well established that children are at risk of further physiologic deterioration during transport. In addition, system errors and equipment failure can complicate their transport and impact their care. Thus, adequate resuscitation prior to departure and anticipation of possible further deterioration is important and may necessitate aggressive, prophylactic interventions. Medical procedures are extremely challenging to perform in the transport environment where there is limited patient access, fewer medical personnel and less equipment available, environmental hazards (eg, temperature extremes), and other factors that make patient assessment and intervention challenging (eg, noise and vibration interference). Thus, decisions to perform interventions prior to transport are based on the risk of deterioration outweighing the risk of performing the intervention (including consideration of the time taken for these), even if less skilled personnel are available to perform them. These decisions should be made in conjunction with the receiving physician. For example, a patient with decreased and fluctuating level of consciousness or declining respiratory function from pneumonia may be endotracheally intubated for transport earlier than their clinical status would otherwise mandate it. Consideration of the mode of transport available should also be a factor when discussing prophylactic interventions. For example, a small pneumothorax may require a chest tube prior to aeromedical transfer given the risk of expansion en route.

Critically ill neonates and pediatric patients transported by providers with specialized training in neonatology or pediatrics, respectively, versus nonspecialized providers have repeatedly been shown to experience lower adverse event rates during transport, and have improved clinical outcomes. These specialized team members can also assist with the pretransport stabilization process and in any required interventions. Transport teams differ in provider composition, and involve a combination of nurse, paramedic, respiratory therapist, and physician providers, depending on patient acuity and local practices. Teams that have physician accompaniment on transport have not been demonstrated to be superior to those by trained non-physician transport providers with physician consultation, but studies restricted to severely ill children have not been done.

Prior to transfer, transport teams must ensure that they have adequate medication and equipment to monitor and manage a patient during transport, with reasonable provision for unexpected delays (eg, due to weather, mechanical issues, traffic). In addition, copies of all pertinent patient documentation, laboratory results, and diagnostic examinations should be prepared so that the receiving facility can continue, not reproduce, care. The use of checklists (Table 103-2) and protocols for sending facilities and transport teams can be helpful to standardize and streamline this process. Parental accompaniment on transport may improve the emotional well-being of the patient and the parent.

## PREVENTION

Transferring a patient between facilities can be resource intensive and can place the patient and the transport providers at significant risk. Thus, efforts to mitigate patient risk (as discussed above) should be employed. Early resuscitation and consultation with pediatric providers, as well as the possible institution of telemedicine, may aid in diagnostic evaluation of patients and in the triaging of patients who require transfer to the appropriate transport providers.

**TABLE 103-2 PRETRANSPORT CHECKLIST**

**Communication**

- ☐ Update receiving doctor of any status change
- ☐ Update receiving doctor of patient status immediately before transport
- ☐ Nurse-to-nurse handover (telephone)
- ☐ Discuss parent transfer options
- ☐ Provide family with receiving facility contact information

**Documentation**

- ☐ Discharge summary
- ☐ Copy of medical chart (including laboratory values)
- ☐ Copy of all diagnostic images

**Safety checks**

- ☐ Confirm position of ETT/central lines/NG/OG by CXR¥
- ☐ Resecure central/peripheral IVs and ensure function
- ☐ Resecure NG/OG tube
- ☐ Minimize infusion pumps and equipment
- ☐ Ensure monitoring equipment functioning, compatible, and adequate power, including battery back-up

**Preparation**

- ☐ Discuss most likely forms of patient deterioration and appropriate action plan on route
- ☐ Discuss any preventative interventions required
  - ☐ Intubation
  - ☐ Chest-tube insertion
  - ☐ NG/OG tube insertion
  - ☐ Adequate IV access

**During Transport**

- ☐ Ensure vehicle configuration allows monitoring of and access to patient and safely secures providers
- ☐ Active patient monitoring
- ☐ Call receiving facility to give updated time of arrival
- ☐ Notify receiving facility of any patient deterioration

**Medications**

- ☐ Prepare doses of all medications to be administered on route
- ☐ Prepare extra syringes of all infusions
- ☐ Prepare doses of relevant resuscitative drugs for critically ill
  - ☐ Epinephrine (bolus)
  - ☐ Atropine
  - ☐ Hypertonic saline
  - ☐ Mannitol
  - ☐ Extra bolus doses of sedative medications
  - ☐ NMBAs

**Ventilated Patient**

- ☐ Re-tape ETT
- ☐ Secure ventilator tubing draining away from patient
- ☐ Secure ventilator tubing to bed
- ☐ End-tidal $CO_2$
- ☐ Correlate end-tidal $CO_2$ to blood gas prior to discharge
- ☐ Stabilize on transport ventilator
- ☐ Consider neuromuscular blockade

**Airway/Ventilator Equipment**

- ☐ Working bag-mask ventilator (accessible)
- ☐ Appropriate-sized face mask available
- ☐ Select correct oral airway
- ☐ Have doses of intubating medication available
- ☐ Ensure adequate size and functioning of laryngoscope with 2 appropriate blades
- ☐ Ensure adequate size ETT available (size for patient and 1 size smaller)
- ☐ Ensure adequate oxygen/air supply
- ☐ Portable suction

Monitoring

ECG

$SaO_2$

$ETCO_2$

Temperature

Warming system

CXR, chest x-ray; ECG, electrocardiogram; $ETCO_2$, end-tidal carbon dioxide; ETT, endotracheal tube; IV, intravenous; NG, nasogastric; NMBAs, neuromuscular blocking agents; OG, orogastric tube; $SaO_2$, oxygen saturation.

## SUGGESTED READINGS


Allen CJ, Teisch LF, Meizoso P, et al. Prehospital care and transportation of pediatric trauma patients. *J Surg Res*. 2015;197(2):240-246.

Hansen ME, Hansen E. Left behind: caring for children in families experiencing patient transport. *Air Med J*. 2014;33(2):69-70.

King BR, King TM, Foster RL, et al. Pediatric and neonatal transport teams with and without a physician: a comparison of outcomes and interventions. *Pediatr Emerg Care*. 2007;23(2):77-82.

Kleinman ME, Donoghue AJ, Orr RA, Kissoon NT. Transport. In: Nichols DG, Schaffner DH, eds. *Rogers' Textbook of Pediatric Intensive Care Medicine* 5th ed. Philadelphia: Lippincott Williams & Wilkins; 2015:348-362.

Orr RA, Felmet KA, Han Y, et al. Pediatric specialized transport teams are associated with improved outcomes. *Pediatrics*. 2009;124(1):40-48.

Ramnarayan P, Thiru K, Parslow RC, et al. Effect of specialist retrieval teams on outcomes in children admitted to paediatric intensive care units in England and Wales: a retrospective cohort study. *Lancet*. 2010;376(9742):698-704.

Singh JM, Gunz A, Dhanani S, Aghari M, MacDonald RD. Frequency, composition, and predictors of in-transit critical events during pediatric critical care transport. Pediatr Crit Care Med. 2016;17(10):984-991.

Stewart CL, Metzger RR, Pyle L, et al. Helicopter versus ground emergency medical services for the transportation of traumatically injured children. *J Ped Surg*. 2015;50:347-352.

Stroud MH, Prodhan P, Moss MM, et al. Redefining the golden hour in pediatric transport. *Pediatr Crit Care Med*. 2008;9(4):435-437.

Weingart C, Herstich T, Baker P, et al. Making good better: implementing a standardized handoff in pediatric transport. *Air Med J*. 2013;32(1):40-46.

Woodward GA, Insoft RM, Pearson-Shaver AL, et al. The state of pediatric interfacility transport: consensus of the second National Pediatric and Neonatal Interfacility Transport Medicine Leadership Conference. *Pediatr Emerg Care*. 2002;18(1):38-43.

# 104 Respiratory Support

Sameer Kamath and Ira Cheifetz

## INTRODUCTION

Respiratory support is the mainstay in caring for children in respiratory failure (RF) and an integral part of pediatric critical care. Children, especially in the first few years of life, are more prone to RF than are adults, due to anatomic and physiologic differences and, thus, it continues to be a common indication for hospitalization in this age group.

*Respiratory failure* is defined as the failure to maintain adequate oxygenation (hypoxemia), ventilation (hypercarbia), or both (mixed). The etiology and pathophysiology of acute respiratory dysfunction and RF are discussed in Chapter 96. In this chapter, the fundamentals of respiratory physiology will briefly be addressed in order to understand the modes of respiratory support and their application in children with RF and will be followed by discussions of modes of respiratory support in children with RF.

## BASIC RESPIRATORY PHYSIOLOGY

The respiratory system must overcome elastic forces (lung and chest wall) and resistive forces (airways) to achieve gas flow. During spontaneous breathing, diaphragmatic contraction causes a drop in pleural and intrathoracic pressure resulting in air being "pulled" into the lungs, followed by passive recoil of the lungs and chest wall during exhalation. During positive-pressure ventilation (PPV), on the other hand, air is "pushed" into the lungs during inspiration, followed by passive recoil of the lungs and chest wall during expiration. Positive-pressure ventilation is, thus, by definition, nonphysiologic.

In healthy people, the work of breathing (WOB) is minimal, and the respiratory system works efficiently to meet the metabolic demands of the body. In disease states, however, the compliance and resistance of the respiratory system changes, causing increased demands on the respiratory system with resultant increased WOB. Elevated airway resistance in conditions such as bronchiolitis and asthma causes airflow limitation during expiration and hyperinflation with resultant hypercarbia due to increased pulmonary dead space; acute respiratory distress syndrome (ARDS) is associated with poor lung compliance with a tendency of alveolar units to collapse (atelectasis), contributing to ventilation-perfusion mismatch and intrapulmonary shunt, resulting in hypoxemia.

## MODES OF RESPIRATORY SUPPORT

The primary aim of respiratory support is to improve gas exchange while minimizing the patient's work of breathing. The full spectrum of commonly used respiratory support includes simple supplemental oxygen therapy; mechanical ventilation, including noninvasive positive pressure ventilation; invasive mechanical ventilation; and advanced and adjunct ventilator therapies. Extracorporeal membrane oxygenation (ECMO) is the therapy of choice when conventional respiratory support has failed (see Chapter 108) While mechanical ventilation can be achieved using negative or positive pressure, negative pressure ventilation (NPV), although appealing in concept and having inherent potential hemodynamic advantages, has failed to gain popularity as a practical mode of support in the intensive care unit (ICU), largely due to the disadvantages of limited physical access to the patient, lack of a protected airway, and challenges with secretion clearance. Thus, the discussion of MV in this chapter will focus on PPV.

### Supplemental Oxygen Therapy

**Nasal Cannula Oxygen** Nasal cannula oxygen is the most commonly used method to provide supplemental oxygen to patients in hypoxemic RF and is generally well tolerated. Standard nasal cannulas are limited by flow, and rates greater than 6 liters per minute (lpm) are generally not recommended due to limitations of the bubble humidification systems. The delivered fractional concentration of inspired oxygen ($FiO_2$) to the patient is variable due to entrainment of room air. While complications are infrequent, failure to provide humidification can result in erosion of the nasal septum and epistaxis.

**Face Mask Oxygen** Face mask oxygen is an effective and simple mode of delivering oxygen to patients but is not as well tolerated by children over longer time periods as is a nasal cannula. The mask limits the ability to eat and drink while receiving supplemental oxygen and in general is used for short time periods, such as in an emergency room or acute care clinics. The ability to achieve high $FiO_2$ delivery is again limited due to entrainment of room air. However, a nonrebreather version of the face mask with an oxygen-rich reservoir can be used when higher $FiO_2$ delivery is desired, as a temporizing measure until more definitive interventions can be implemented.

**High-Flow Nasal Cannula** A *high-flow nasal cannula* (HFNC) delivers a high flow of humidified and heated oxygen through nasal prongs. Depending on the gas delivery device and the cannula, flows up to 60 lpm can be attained for respiratory support. The HFNC was introduced as an alternative to nasal continuous positive airway pressure (CPAP) in neonates, but it is increasingly being used for patients with hypoxemic RF across all ages. Some of the postulated mechanisms of benefit include washout of anatomic dead space, subjective relief of dyspnea from meeting the inspiratory flow demand of patients, improved $FiO_2$ delivery by reducing the entrainment of room air as the delivered flow rates approach spontaneous demand, stenting of upper airways, and improved lung recruitment through generation of CPAP. However, HFNC should not be considered as noninvasive positive-pressure ventilation (NIPPV), and its use is generally discouraged in hypercarbic or severe hypoxemic RF.

HFNC support has been used in neonates to prevent endotracheal intubation, to support infants and children with bronchiolitis, to assist children and adults in hypoxemic RF, to provide increased oxygenation prior to intubation, and to reduce reintubation rates following extubation. HFNC support is generally well tolerated and has minimal complications. Frequent assessment of patients on HFNC is mandatory, and failure to detect clinical deterioration without timely interventions can result in poor outcomes. The decision to place infants and children on HFNC in non-ICU settings should, thus, be made carefully by the clinical care team.

### Noninvasive Positive-Pressure Ventilation

*Noninvasive positive-pressure ventilation* is the delivery of mechanical ventilation without an endotracheal tube or tracheostomy. It includes both CPAP and bilevel ventilation. It requires a patient interface, such as a mask, and a machine to deliver the support. The aim is to provide respiratory support while avoiding the perils of invasive ventilation, such as sedation and ventilation-associated pneumonia (VAP). It can be used to support both acute and chronic RF and is helpful in both hypoxemic and hypercarbic RF. Additionally, NIPPV can provide cardiopulmonary support for patients with acute, chronic, or acute-on-chronic heart failure. It can be safely delivered at home, for either continuous or intermittent (eg, nighttime) use, but this requires careful training of caregivers and appropriate adaptation of the home environment.

**Continuous Positive Airway Pressure** *Continuous positive airway pressure* is provided throughout the respiratory cycle while the patient is breathing spontaneously. Advantages include stenting of the upper airway and tracheobronchial tree, lung recruitment, and stenting of the lower airways in obstructive lung disease. CPAP is clinically used for patients with obstructive sleep apnea, tracheobronchomalacia, atelectasis, heart failure, and asthma with variable levels of supportive data and success. The keys to success are choosing an optimal interface based on patient tolerance and titration of pressure until the desired result is achieved.

**Bilevel Positive Airway Pressure** *Bilevel positive airway pressure* (BiPAP) provides CPAP throughout the respiratory cycle and, in addition, augments inspiration with volume or pressure support. Delivery of inspiratory support is triggered by the patient's respiratory effort to promote patient-ventilator synchrony. Difference between the

2 levels of pressure drives gas flow within the system. Tidal volume is determined by the driving pressure, extent of leak within the system, and compliance and resistance of the respiratory system. Bilevel positive airway pressure can be delivered using a variety of nasal prongs, or nasal or full-face masks, which interface with either regular ICU ventilators or dedicated NIPPV machines. Specialized machines tend to compensate better for system leaks and may have better patient-ventilator synchrony.

Bilevel positive airway pressure can be used effectively in a wide variety of clinical scenarios and has improved the ability to support neonates and children in RF without the need for intubation. Support with BiPAP can be effective and should be instituted early in patients failing nasal cannula or HFNC therapy. Early institution of positive pressure can prevent derecruitment and worsening hypoxemia.

Use of an oronasal or full-face mask is generally preferred in children, and heated humidification is strongly recommended. Sedation can be used with caution in appropriately monitored settings to enable tolerance of NIPPV and promote patient-ventilator synchrony. It is common to observe patients in RF with increased WOB subsequently (often rapidly) calm down and relax following initiation of BiPAP, as it improves their respiratory mechanics and unloads the respiratory muscles. Complications of BiPAP include skin breakdown and pressure ulcers due to the masks, gastric distension, emesis and aspiration, barotrauma/volutrauma, diminished venous return from positive intrathoracic pressure, and patient-ventilator asynchrony. In addition, continuous BiPAP creates challenges with verbal communication and oral feeding.



#### Invasive Mechanical Ventilation

*Invasive mechanical ventilation* can be delivered via an endotracheal tube or tracheostomy. Endotracheal intubation (orotracheal or nasotracheal) is routinely undertaken in emergency rooms, ICUs or operating rooms for children in whom NIPPV is not indicated or has failed. While use of cuffed endotracheal tubes was prohibited in the past, new low-pressure, high-volume cuffed tubes are safe and used routinely in pediatric ICUs. The key is to use appropriately sized tubes using the formula age/4 + 4 for uncuffed tubes and age/4 + 3 for cuffed tubes. Failure to pay attention to cuff pressures and/or leak and tube sizes can result in consequences to the subglottic space, including erosion, ulceration, and cartilage necrosis, with subsequent scarring and the potential need for airway reconstruction surgery and/or tracheostomy.

The intubation of children with RF is more challenging than intubation in well children in the operating room. The incidence of adverse events is higher in critically ill children and is being studied through the National Emergency Airway Registry for Children (NEAR4KIDS) initiative. Direct laryngoscopy remains the standard in most PICUs; however, use of videolaryngoscopy is gaining in popularity, as it provides the opportunity to educate learners and may improve intubation success rates in children with difficult airways.

**Intermittent Positive-Pressure Ventilation** Intermittent PPV involves provision of PPV via an endotracheal tube or tracheostomy. A wide variety of modes are available without data to support superiority of 1 mode over another. A detailed discussion of all modes of ventilation is beyond the scope of this chapter, but we will discuss basic principles and common modes of ventilation.

**Basic Principles of Invasive Ventilation** Modern ventilators are sophisticated machines with the ability to deliver high levels of support consistently. Despite several decades of research on this topic, no single mode of support has been noted to be superior; thus, in most cases, tailoring the mode of ventilator support to the physiologic needs of the patient, while at the same time using lung protective strategies, is the most appropriate approach.

In physics, force is measured as pressure (pressure = force/area), displacement as volume (volume = area × displacement), and the relevant rate of change as flow (average flow = Δ volume/Δ time). With respect to respiratory physiology, we are interested in the pressure necessary to achieve gas flow into the lungs. Pressure, volume, and flow are, thus, measurable variables in the respiratory cycle, and their relation is described by the equation of motion for the respiratory system:

$$\text{Transpulmonary pressure change (P)} = \text{elastance (E)} \times \text{tidal volume (V)} + \text{resistance (R)} \times \text{flow (F)}.$$

Elastance is the inverse of compliance, and, thus, the respiratory system equation of motion can be written as $P = V/C + R \times F$.

Modern positive-pressure ventilators typically support ventilation with the following principal variables:

- *Control* variable: Pressure, volume, or flow are called control variables. In modern ventilators, it is possible to switch from 1 control variable to another between, or even within, each breath.
- *Phase* variable: The time between breaths should be divided into 4 phases: the change from expiration to inspiration, inspiration, change from inspiration to expiration, and expiration. This convention helps to understand how a ventilator starts, what sustains and stops a breath, and what it does between inspirations. A particular variable is measured and used to start, sustain, and end each phase, and in this context, pressure, volume, flow, and time are referred to as phase variables.
- *Trigger* variable: While measuring 1 of the 3 variables within the equation of motion, a breath is initiated when 1 of the variables reaches a preset value. This is the trigger variable and can be pressure (inspiration starts when a drop in baseline pressure is detected), time (set the frequency to start breaths), or flow (detection of gas flow into the lungs triggers inspiration). The patient effort needed to trigger a breath is detected by the sensitivity settings, and, thus, the clinician can make it easier or harder for a patient to breathe based on the clinical situation by adjusting the trigger sensitivity.
- *Limit* variable: Limit refers to restricting the magnitude of a variable during inspiration. The limit variable is 1 that can reach and maintain a preset level (pressure, volume, or flow) before inspiration ends.
- *Cycle* variable: The variable that is measured and used to end inspiration is called the cycle variable. The cycle variable is generally flow or time but can be pressure or volume.
- *Baseline* variable: This variable is controlled during expiration and is measured and set relative to atmospheric pressure. While pressure, flow, and volume can serve as baseline variables, pressure is the most commonly applied baseline variable in the form of positive end-expiratory pressure (PEEP).

**Conventional Modes of Ventilation** Modes of ventilation can be characterized according to a particular pattern of mandatory (machine-triggered) or spontaneous (patient-triggered) breaths that are volume controlled or pressure controlled, or have elements of both (dual controlled). Pressure-controlled modes all set a peak inspiratory pressure (PIP) that is targeted during inspiration with rapid delivery of initial gas flow to attain that target, followed by deceleration of flow. Tidal volume attained is variable and depends on the respiratory system compliance and resistance, among other factors. In volume-controlled modes, the primary gas delivery target is tidal volume, and peak flow as well as flow waveform are set with a variable PIP from breath to breath. The differences between pressure- and volume-targeted modes are summarized in Table 104-1, and the ventilator variables are described below.

- *Fractional concentration of inspired oxygen* ($FiO_2$): In general, the lowest level of inspired oxygen concentration needed to maintain an oxygen saturations > 92% should be administered in order to avoid oxygen toxicity due to free radicals and denitrogenation. An $FiO_2$ < 60% is generally considered by most experts to be likely to be less injurious to lung tissue for the majority of patients, although patients with past exposure to medications such as bleomycin are at greater risk from oxygen toxicity.
- *Tidal volume* (VT) and *peak inspiratory pressure:* Large VT (> 10 mL/kg) results in alveolar overdistention and ventilator-induced lung injury (VILI). The ARDS network trial published in

**TABLE 104-1 VOLUME- VERSUS PRESSURE-TARGETED MODES**

| | Volume | Pressure |
|---|---|---|
| **Tidal volume** | Set | Variable |
| **Peak inspiratory pressure** | Variable | Set |
| **PEEP** | Set | Set |
| **Flow** | Set | Set but variable |
| **Inspiratory time** | Set | Set |
| **I:E ratio** | Set or variable | Set or variable |
| **$FiO_2$** | Set | Set |

$FiO_2$, fractional concentration of inspired oxygen; I:E, inspiratory-to-expiratory; PEEP, positive end-expiratory pressure.

2000 demonstrated a survival benefit in adults who were ventilated with low (6 mL/kg IBW) versus high VT (12 mL/kg IBW). While such a study has not been replicated in children, the practice of low VT in pediatric acute respiratory distress syndrome (PARDS) was endorsed by the Pediatric Acute Lung Injury Consensus Conference (PALICC). Most clinicians try to limit the PIP to less than 30 $cmH_2O$ in the absence of significant obstructive lung disease. Plateau pressure ($P_{plat}$) is the pressure measured during an inspiratory hold maneuver on the ventilator. It is more reflective of alveolar distending pressure and should ideally be less than 28 $cmH_2O$. Patients with obstructive lung disease often have a high PIP with $P_{plat} < 28$ $cmH_2O$, suggesting the alveolar distending pressures to be in the safe range.

- *Rate, inspiratory time* (Ti), and *inspiratory-to-expiratory* (I:E) ratio: The product of VT and rate constitute the patient's minute ventilation. The age of the patient and the underlying cause of RF should be considered when setting the rate. Neonates and infants will need faster rates than older children and adolescents. Patients with reduced respiratory compliance (lung units with short time constants) will likely need a faster rate compared to those with obstructive lung disease (lung units with long time constants). The effect of the rate and Ti on the I:E ratio should be closely monitored. As the set rate is increased without changes in Ti, the I:E ratio may become significantly prolonged, causing air trapping and subsequent patient-ventilator dysynchrony. A longer Ti with a faster rate will result in shorter exhalation times and will cause air-trapping, hyperinflation, and the presence of intrinsic PEEP. Patients with obstructive lung disease have prolonged exhalation times and, thus, may benefit from short Ti and low rates on the ventilator, while those with restrictive lung disease may benefit from short Ti and faster rates. In general, Ti between 0.4 and 0.8 seconds is appropriate in children and should be titrated based according to the needs of the individual patient.
- *Inspiratory flow:* Mean inspiratory flow is a ratio of VT and Ti, and, thus, one cannot change flow without affecting the timing variables. Changing from a decelerating flow to square-wave flow pattern may shorten Ti and the time required to deliver the VT. Inspiratory flow is usually preset in volume modes of ventilation and tends to be variable in pressure modes. As clinicians, it is important to realize the combined effects of flow, timing, and volume on end-expiratory lung volume (EELV).
- *Positive end-expiratory pressure:* End-expiratory lung volume is critical in patients with reduced respiratory system compliance and is maintained by the application of PEEP. Allowing the lungs to inflate and deflate from optimal EELV reduces cyclic opening and closing of lung units, thus limiting VILI. Identifying optimal PEEP, however, is challenging and should be determined by clinicians at the bedside based on the response at different levels of PEEP on oxygenation, lung mechanics, and hemodynamics. Excessive PEEP can result in lung overdistention, increased intrathoracic pressure with reduced cardiac output, and carbon dioxide retention; low PEEP can cause a reduction in EELV, increased low V/Q segments, and subsequent hypoxemia. The use of PEEP in patients with obstructive lung disease is controversial given an inherent tendency of such patients to air-trap and develop auto-PEEP (PEEPi). In this setting, some patients may benefit from the addition of extrinsic PEEP to overcome PEEPi, while others may benefit from no extrinsic PEEP.
- *Mean airway pressure* (MAP): Mean airway pressure is the integration of pressure over time and correlates with mean lung volume, alveolar ventilation, arterial oxygenation, hemodynamic performance, and potentially barotrauma. Inspiratory flow, ventilation rate, Ti, PEEP, and PIP/VT all have an effect on MAP, although the largest effects are from PEEP and Ti. It is common to characterize the level of ventilator support based on the MAP value needed to achieve adequate oxygenation.

***SYNCHRONIZED INTERMITTENT MANDATORY VENTILATION*** Synchronized intermittent mandatory ventilation (SIMV) is an intermittent mode of ventilation available with pressure (SIMV-PC) or volume (SIMV-VC) targeting. The breaths are delivered in synchrony with the patient's inspiratory effort. The gas supply is patient triggered during spontaneous breaths. If a patient inspiratory effort is sensed while the time window is open, a synchronized breath is delivered, and if no patient effort is detected at the time the window closes, a mandatory breath is delivered. This keeps machine inspiration or expiration in phase with the patient's respiratory cycle and avoids patient-ventilator dysynchrony due to "breath stacking." Pressure support is usually added to assist patient breaths. Pressure-targeted modes carry the risk of inadequate tidal volume and minute ventilation if lung compliance decreases, while volume-targeted modes maintain tidal volume but may contribute to barotrauma if rising airway pressures are not closely monitored.

***PRESSURE-REGULATED VOLUME CONTROL*** Pressure-regulated volume control (PRVC) provides dual control mode of ventilation with between-breath variability and combines features of volume and pressure ventilation. The target tidal volume and maximum pressure level are set. The machine attempts to achieve the volume target using a pressure-control gas delivery format using the lowest possible airway pressure. Over a series of breaths, the ventilator attempts to assess the pressure required to attain the set tidal volume with continuous adjustments between breaths based on a feedback mechanism. In patients with increased inspiratory demand, the delivered pressure may be inappropriately low, resulting in dyspnea, increased respiratory effort, and even cardiorespiratory collapse due to inadequate ventilatory support.

***AIRWAY PRESSURE RELEASE VENTILATION*** Airway pressure release ventilation (APRV) is often considered in patients with moderate to severe hypoxemic RF and maintains 2 levels of airway pressure (high and low) applied for defined periods of time. Spontaneous breathing is allowed at both levels. Inspiratory time or $T_{high}$ is much longer than expiratory time or $T_{low}$. $P_{high}$ is the airway pressure maintained during $T_{high}$, and $P_{low}$ is the CPAP maintained during $T_{low}$. Airway pressure release ventilation is generally well tolerated from a hemodynamic perspective. Maintenance of spontaneous breathing is essential for the success of this mode. Thus, oversedation and neuromuscular blockade should be avoided.

***PRESSURE SUPPORT VENTILATION*** Pressure support ventilation (PSV) is a pressure-targeted mode in which patient inspiratory effort is supported by the ventilator at a preset level of inspiratory pressure. Inspiration is triggered by the patient and terminated when inspiratory flow falls to a prespecified level (generally 25% of peak flow). Respiratory rate, inspiratory time, and tidal volume are patient determined, while the clinician controls the inspiratory pressure level. Pressure support ventilation is often used by clinicians when weaning from ventilator support or in conditions such as asthma so patients can control their own inspiratory and expiratory times. It is an inappropriate mode for patients with central hypoventilation or apnea.

As briefly mentioned at the start of this section, no mode of ventilation has shown clear benefit over another, and, hence, no specific recommendations can be made. Ventilator support should be tailored to the underlying disease process based on sound physiologic rationale. When constant minute ventilation is desired, such as in patients with traumatic brain injury to maintain $PaCO_2$ between 35 and 40 mm Hg, a volume-targeted mode may be appropriate, whereas when higher MAPs are desired to optimize EELV, APRV may be more appropriate. Given the complexity of teams involved in the care of critically ill children, standardization of practice and adherence to those standards is the key to achieve success with mechanical ventilation.

**Weaning of Ventilator Support and Tracheostomy** Extubation is the ultimate goal of ventilator management after recovery from RF for most patients; however, a few patients who are unable to wean undergo tracheostomies for continued long term ventilator support, if indicated. Tracheostomy offers the advantage of reduced need for sedation, lower risk of VAP, ability of the patient to mobilize and rehabilitate, and easy disconnection from ventilation for those needing only intermittent support. Timing of tracheostomy in the course of RF is a decision that should be made taking into consideration the trajectory of illness, comorbidities, age of the patient, and prognosis of the underlying disease process(es).

Intubated patients should be evaluated for readiness to extubate daily by use of a spontaneous breathing trial (SBT), using PSV, CPAP, or other techniques, if they meet readiness criteria. Those who pass an SBT should be extubated as soon as feasible to limit their time on invasive support. Several indices have been developed in an attempt to predict weaning and extubation success, but available literature suggests that these indices offer no improvement over clinical judgement. Extubation failure rates in children range from 2% to 20% with little relationship to duration of mechanical ventilation, with upper airway obstruction being the most common cause of extubation failure. Early extubation has several advantages that include limited exposure to sedatives, mitigation of ICU delirium, promotion of early mobility, and reducing ventilator-associated complications. Clinicians, however, should be wary of consequences of premature extubation, as extubation failure is associated with worse outcomes in children.

**High Frequency Ventilation** *High frequency ventilation* (HFV) is defined as a frequency that greatly exceeds the normal respiratory rate and has a delivered VT that is at or below anatomic dead space. There are 4 types of HFV: high frequency positive pressure ventilation (HFPPV); high frequency jet ventilation (HFJV); high frequency percussive ventilation (HFPV), and high frequency oscillatory ventilation (HFOV). High frequency modes by definition generate very small VT while maintaining EELV and, thus, have generated appeal by clinicians over time for patients with severe ARDS from the perspective of lung protection. Significant experience with HFV for RF in pediatrics is limited to HFOV. Thus, further discussion about HFV in this chapter will be limited to HFOV.

HFOV is the most commonly used form of high-frequency ventilation in neonates and pediatrics, and has been 1 of the mainstays of advanced ventilation of PARDS over the past 2 decades. While it has been widely used in all age groups, HFOV is falling out of favor in adults in the light of recent negative trials. It can be considered in children with PARDS with $P_{Plat}$ exceeding 28 $cmH_2O$ in the absence of reduced chest wall compliance. High-frequency oscillatory ventilation has the advantage of maintaining lung expansion through a constant MAP, with very low tidal volumes and is thus seen as a protective form of ventilation particularly in patients with air-leak, pulmonary interstitial emphysema, and high MAP requirements. It is important to note that HFOV is the only commonly used mode in which exhalation is active.

When initiating HFOV, by convention, MAP is initially set 4 to 6 $cmH_2O$ higher than conventional ventilator settings, and optimal lung volume is attained with stepwise increase or decrease in MAP while monitoring oxygenation and ventilation. Frequency is set based on the age and size of the patient, with neonates and infants being at higher frequencies (10–12 Hz) than older children (8–10 Hz) and adolescents (6–8 Hz). The amplitude is adjusted to achieve adequate chest "wiggle" and varies based on the extent of lung disease and size of the patient. Bias flow is typically set at 20 lpm and can be increased to help maintain MAP or to help meet spontaneous respiratory demand. Oxygenation improvement is achieved by stepwise increase in MAP and $FiO_2$, while ventilation is improved by increasing the amplitude or reducing the frequency. Generally, a small leak is required around the endotracheal tube to optimize ventilation, provided a stable MAP can be maintained.

Disadvantages of HFOV include the typically increased requirements for sedation or even neuromuscular blockade in children and adolescents, as well as the reduced ability to provide adequate pulmonary toilet and limited mobility due to a rigid ventilator circuit. Given that HFOV use in PARDS is associated with higher MAPs to increase EELV, hypotension from reduced venous return is often seen. Traditionally, patients on HFOV are weaned and transitioned to conventional ventilation prior to extubation. Extubation from HFOV after gradual reduction in support is possible but seldom practiced.

**Adjunct Therapies**

***INHALED NITRIC OXIDE*** Inhaled nitric oxide (iNO) is not recommended for routine use in PARDS. However, its use may be considered in those with documented pulmonary hypertension or right ventricular dysfunction, or in the presence of severe hypoxemic RF as a bridge to ECMO. If used, the response to iNO should be carefully monitored, and it should be discontinued if ineffective. If effective, it should be administered at the lowest effective dose to avoid toxicities such as methemoglobinemia.

***EXOGENOUS SURFACTANT*** While trials have suggested that a certain subset of pediatric RF patients may benefit from surfactant therapy, its routine use in patients with PARDS cannot be justified based on pediatric and adult data.

***FLUID MANAGEMENT*** Pediatric patients in RF should receive fluids to maintain adequate intravascular volume, end organ perfusion, and optimal oxygen delivery. Conservative or restricted fluid management strategy is superior to a liberal fluid strategy in ARDS. Conservative fluid strategy and appropriate use of diuretics help to reduce extravascular lung water and to improve gas exchange. Protocolized fluid management strategies are strongly encouraged to limit problems associated with fluid overload in RF.

***PRONE POSITIONING*** Prone positioning improves ventilation perfusion matching by recruitment of atelectatic posterior lung segments. While previous adult trials on prone positioning in ARDS showed improvements in oxygenation without any impact on survival, 1 recent adult study showed a 28- and 90-day survival advantage from early application of prolonged prone positioning in severe ARDS. The largest pediatric trial on prone positioning in acute lung injury did not reduce ventilator-free days or improve other relevant clinical outcomes. Prone positioning is, thus, not recommended for routine use in PARDS and needs further study.

***RECRUITMENT MANEUVERS*** Slow incremental and decremental PEEP steps can be used as a recruitment strategy in PARDS to improve oxygenation while closely monitoring hemodynamics. Sustained inflation maneuvers may contribute to barotrauma and should be avoided. Recruitment maneuvers (RM) in PARDS needs further study.

***AIRWAY CLEARANCE STRATEGIES*** Chest physical therapy has not been shown to be of benefit in RF. Closed suctioning systems are preferred to open ones to limit ventilator disconnection and loss of lung volumes in PARDS. Maintaining patency of the endotracheal tube and avoiding airway plugging is essential in patients with thick secretions. Thus, mucolytics may be used to enable mucus clearance in specific patient populations, although definitive data are lacking. Vest therapy, cough assist, and intermittent percussive ventilation (IPV) can help prevent the need for mechanical respiratory support or may facilitate weaning toward extubation in patients with ineffective cough.

***MONITORING*** The PALICC investigators have made recommendations for respiratory monitoring in patients with PARDS. These recommendations can be applied to all patients in RF and some are listed in Table 104-2. Other parameters such as ratio of dead space to tidal volume, esophageal manometry, flow-volume loops, dynamic pressure-volume curves, oxygenation index or oxygen saturation ($SaO_2$) index, and $PaO_2/FiO_2$ or $SaO_2/FiO_2$ can be used based on expertise of clinicians in their interpretation of the obtained data.

## SUMMARY

In summary, RF is a frequent cause of pediatric ICU admission, and the level of support needed can vary significantly among patients. Children in RF should be monitored closely with timely interventions to meet their respiratory demands. The mode of support should be titrated to optimize support while practicing lung-protective

**TABLE 104-2 MONITORING OF CHILDREN WITH RESPIRATORY FAILURE**

| Parameter Monitored | Clinical Information Obtained from Monitoring |
|---|---|
| Respiratory frequency, heart rate, pulse oximetry, and noninvasive blood pressure | Changes in clinical status |
| Exhaled tidal volume | Prevent VILI |
| Peak pressure | Level of support |
| Plateau pressure | |
| $FiO_2$, PEEP, mean airway pressure | Assessment of severity |
| Continuous carbon dioxide ($CO_2$) monitoring | Adequacy of ventilator support |
| Chest x-ray | Diagnosis, severity, equipment position |
| Arterial blood gas/capillary blood gas | Severity of lung disease<br>Adequacy of ventilator support |

$FiO_2$, fractional concentration of inspired oxygen; PEEP, positive end-expiratory pressure; VILI, ventilator-induced lung injury.

ventilation strategies and prevention of VILI. Adjunctive therapies should be used appropriately to limit time on mechanical ventilation, although supportive data are quite limited in pediatrics. Children failing conventional modes of support should be considered for nonconventional modes or initiated on ECMO support, if appropriate.

## SUGGESTED READINGS


Acute Respiratory Distress Syndrome Network; Brower RG, Matthay MA, Morris A, Schoenfeld D, Thompson BT, Wheeler A. Ventilation with lower tidal volumes as compared with traditional tidal volumes for acute lung injury and the acute respiratory distress syndrome. *N Engl J Med.* 2000;342(18):1301-1308.

Chatburn RL. Classification of mechanical ventilators. In: Tobin MJ, ed. *Principles and Practice of Mechanical Ventilation.* 2nd edition. McGraw-Hill Medical Publishing Division; 2006:37-52.

Corrêa TD, Sanches PR, de Morais LC, Scarin FC, Silva E, Barbas CS. Performance of noninvasive ventilation in acute respiratory failure in critically ill patients: a prospective, observational, cohort study. *BMC Pulm Med.* 2015;15:144.

Curley MA, Hibberd PL, Fineman LD, et al. Effect of prone positioning on clinical outcomes in children with acute lung injury: a randomized controlled trial. *JAMA.* 2005 Jul 13;294(2):229-237.

Curley MA, Wypij D, Watson RS, et al; RESTORE Study Investigators and the Pediatric Acute Lung Injury and Sepsis Investigators Network. Protocolized sedation vs usual care in pediatric patients mechanically ventilated for acute respiratory failure: a randomized clinical trial. *JAMA.* 2015;313(4):379-389.

Emeriaud G, Newth CJ; Pediatric Acute Lung Injury Consensus Conference Group. Monitoring of children with pediatric acute respiratory distress syndrome: proceedings from the pediatric acute lung injury consensus conference. *Pediatr Crit Care Med.* 2015;16(5):S86-S101.

Gajic O, Dara SI, Mendez JL, et al. Ventilator-associated lung injury in patients without acute lung injury at the onset of mechanical ventilation. *Crit Care Med.* 2004;32(9):1817-1824.

Kurachek SC, Newth CJ, Quasney MW, et al. Extubation failure in pediatric intensive care: a multiple-center study of risk factors and outcomes. *Crit Care Med.* 2003;31(11):2657-2664.

Lee JH, Rehder KJ, Williford L, Cheifetz IM, Turner DA. Use of high flow nasal cannula in critically ill infants, children and adults: a critical review of the literature. *Intensive Care Med.* 2013;39(2):247-257.

Maitra S, Bhattacharjee S, Khanna P, Baidya D. High-frequency ventilation does not provide mortality benefit in comparison with conventional lung-protective ventilation in acute respiratory distress syndrome: a meta-analysis of the randomized control trials. *Anesthesiology.* 2015;122(4):841-851.

Morley SL. Non-invasive ventilation in paediatric critical care. *Paediatr Respir Rev.* 2016;20:24-31.

Newth CJ, Venkatraman S, Wilson DF, et al; Eunice Shriver Kennedy National Institute of Child Health and Human Development Collaborative Pediatric Critical Care Research Network. Weaning and extubation readiness in pediatric patients. *Pediatr Crit Care Med.* 2009;10(1):1-11.

Nishisaki A, Ferry S, Colborn S, et al; National Emergency Airway Registry (NEAR); National Emergency Airway Registry for Kids (NEAR4KIDS) Investigators. Characterization of tracheal intubation process of care and safety outcomes in tertiary pediatric intensive care unit. *Pediatr Crit Care Med.* 2012;13(1):e5-e10.

Pediatric Acute Lung Injury Consensus Conference Group. Pediatric acute respiratory distress syndrome: consensus recommendations from the Pediatric Lung Injury Consensus Conference. *Pediatr Crit Care Med.* 2015;16(5):428-439.

Rehder KJ, Turner DA, Cheifetz IM. Extracorporeal membrane oxygenation for neonatal and pediatric respiratory failure: an evidence-based review of the past decade (2002–2012). *Pediatr Crit Care Med.* 2013;14(9):851-861.

Rimensberger PC, Cheifetz IM; Pediatric Acute Lung Injury Consensus Conference Group. Ventilatory support in children with pediatric acute respiratory distress syndrome: proceedings from the Pediatric Acute Lung Injury Consensus Conference. *Pediatr Crit Care Med.* 2015;16(5 Suppl 1):S51-S60.


# 105 Management of Acute Brain Injury

Charles Larson, Anne-Marie Guerguerian, and Warwick Butt



## INTRODUCTION

Primary etiologies of acute brain injury in children include traumatic brain injury (TBI), hypoxic-ischemic encephalopathy (HIE), stroke, cerebral hemorrhages, infections, inflammatory conditions, seizures, tumor or mass lesions, metabolic abnormalities, and toxins (Table 105-1). TBI is the leading cause of death and disability in both children older than 1 year of age and young adults. Following the primary injury, the tissues surrounding the injury and the entire brain are vulnerable to further secondary injuries. The purpose of the initial management, investigation, monitoring, and treatment of acute brain injuries is aimed at preventing this secondary injury.

### Pathophysiology of Secondary Injuries

Secondary injuries evolve in the minutes to days after the primary event and include both endogenous responses to the primary injury and secondary insults that occur in the field or during the course of care, such as hypoxemia or hypotension. Mechanisms involved in endogenous secondary injuries include energy failure, excitotoxicity and apoptosis, oxidative stress, mitochondrial dysfunction, inflammation, and multiple cell death pathways.

**Hypoxia-Ischemia, Energy Failure, Excitotoxicity, and Oxidative Stress** In severe injury with cessation of blood flow, as occurs in ischemic stroke or cardiac arrest, a characteristic pattern of injury ensues. Oxygen stores are depleted very rapidly (< 20 seconds), and adenosine triphosphate (ATP) stores are depleted within 5 minutes. No further ATP can be generated to fuel energy-dependent cellular processes, and cell membranes depolarize, resulting in influx of sodium and calcium, efflux of potassium, cellular swelling, oxygen free radical production, and release of excitatory neurotransmitters such as glutamate from astrocytes and neurons. The release of glutamate triggers further depolarization of adjacent cells, and this potent combination

**TABLE 105-1 ETIOLOGIES OF ACUTE BRAIN INJURY**

| |
|---|
| Trauma |
| Focal parenchymal contusion |
| Diffuse axonal injury |
| Intracranial hemorrhage |
| Hypoxic-ischemic encephalopathy |
| Severe shock |
| Cardiac arrest |
| Asphyxia (drowning, strangulation) |
| Cellular dysoxia (cyanide poisoning) |
| Central nervous system infection |
| Inflammatory, autoimmune, postinfectious |
| Mass lesions |
| Tumor |
| Hydrocephalus |
| Vascular |
| Arterial infarction |
| Cerebral venous thrombosis |
| Vasculitis |
| Status epilepticus |
| Toxins |
| Metabolic abnormalities |



of increased cellular metabolism and ischemia accelerates hypoxic injury. The same cellular dysfunction also occurs in situations of altered blood flow and is demonstrated in TBI, status epilepticus, and meningitis. In adult studies, cerebral blood flow (CBF) of less than 55 mL/100 g/min of brain tissue (at normothermia) led to inhibition of protein synthesis, key to the regeneration of injured tissues. CBF of less than 20 mL/100 g/min resulted in anoxic depolarization. These thresholds are likely higher in injured brain tissue, rendered vulnerable by excitotoxicity, seizures, and impaired oxygen utilization from mitochondrial dysfunction. Either globally or more focally, disturbance to the neurovascular unit that regulates CBF occurs in all forms of severe acute brain injury as a consequence of direct tissue disruption, edema, intracranial hypertension, vasospasm and loss of autoregulation. Much of the secondary injury in severe TBI and meningitis is hypoxic-ischemic in nature.

**Necrosis and Programed Cell Death** Energy failure, excitotoxicity, and oxidative stress are the principle mechanisms leading to cell death, which can take the form of necrosis or apoptosis. The age of the child (ie, maturity), the severity and duration of the primary and secondary insults, and the vulnerability of the brain region contribute differently to determining the vulnerability or the resilience of the tissue. In circumstances of severe injury, the most vulnerable brain regions are the watershed areas of the intervascular boundary zones and areas with the highest metabolic rate, such as the thalami, basal ganglia, and sensorimotor cortex.

Cerebral edema in acute brain injury peaks at 24 to 72 hours after the initial insult and can result from three mechanisms: astrocyte and neuronal swelling, vasogenic edema, and osmolar swelling. Vasogenic edema results from inflammation and disruption of the blood–brain barrier (BBB) with endothelial dysfunction, such as in meningoencephalitis. Osmolar swelling occurs when intracellular macromolecules degrade, thus increasing intracellular osmolarity and drawing in of water.

### Complications

The complications of acute brain injury can be focal and/or global. Focal neuroanatomical deficits are revealed on clinical examination with functional assessments (eg, Pediatric NIH Stroke Scale) or more globally with coma, with or without associated intracranial hypertension, seizures, or autonomic dysfunction. All of these factors can further exacerbate secondary injuries.

**Intracranial Compliance** According to the Monro-Kellie doctrine, intracranial pressure (ICP) relates to the intracranial volumes of three components: brain parenchyma, blood, and cerebrospinal fluid (CSF). Volume inside the developed cranium is fixed, therefore an increase in volume of one of the compartments or from a mass lesion will lead to an increase in pressure unless there is a corresponding decrease in one of the other compartments' volumes. Initially, the volume taken up by edema or a mass lesion such as an intracranial hemorrhage will be compensated for by an increase in CSF reabsorption with minimal increase in ICP. However, when the intracranial compliance is impaired as the lesion increases in size, and the capacity for further CSF displacement decreases, small increases in volume lead to significant increases in ICP. Intracranial hypertension will compromise CBF, which is proportional to the cerebral perfusion pressure (CPP; defined as the difference between the mean arterial pressure and the mean ICP or mean central venous pressure). This decrease in CBF impairs oxygen and substrate delivery, causing further ischemia and leading to a vicious cycle of secondary injury, edema, and intracranial hypertension. Ultimately, severe intracranial hypertension can lead to herniation of brain tissue through the foramen magnum, brain-stem compression, and death. Importantly, infants with unfused sutures, despite an increased capacity to accommodate changes in intracranial volume, are also at risk of increased ICP and herniation.

## INITIAL EVALUATION AND MANAGEMENT

Acute brain injury can present with altered level of consciousness, seizures, or focal neurologic deficits. The purpose of the initial evaluation is to identify and treat the acute injuries, and to preserve viable brain tissue by preventing secondary insults. The initial evaluation of acute neurologic dysfunction is discussed in detail in Chapter 98. Here, we will focus mainly on priorities in patient management.

The immediate management priorities in patients with acute brain injury are to maintain a patent airway, deliver adequate oxygenation, maintain a normal blood pressure, immobilize the cervical spine in patients with suspected trauma, avoid hypercarbia, and complete a focused neurologic assessment and rapid patient survey. Additionally, all investigations that will help dictate appropriate management (eg, measuring the blood glucose level and treating hypoglycemia promptly; Fig. 105-1) should be expedited.

### Stabilization of Airway, Breathing, and Circulation

Appropriate respiratory and cardiovascular support in the initial management of patients with severe head injuries is likely to profoundly impact their outcome. In a study of children with severe TBI from the National Pediatric Trauma Registry, those without hypotensive or hypoxic episodes fared best. The presence of hypotension tripled mortality, and the combination of both hypotension and hypoxia was associated with the worst outcomes. Indications for endotracheal intubation include upper airway obstruction or loss of upper airway reflexes, apnea, inadequate oxygenation or ventilation, coma with a Glasgow Coma Scale (GCS) score < 9, or signs of intracranial hypertension or impending herniation such as posturing or worsening coma scale score. Continuous cardiopulmonary monitoring should be commenced as early as possible. Rapid sequence intubation should be performed with manual axial in-line stabilization and neuroprotective measures. Nasotracheal intubation is relatively contraindicated in patients with suspected trauma until a base-of-skull fracture has been excluded on imaging. In intubated patients without signs of herniation, oxygenation and ventilation should target peripheral capillary oxygen saturation ($SpO_2$) ≥ 95% and normocapnia with end-tidal $CO_2$ monitoring used to titrate ventilation (partial pressure of $CO_2$ [$PaCO_2$] 35–45 mm Hg and pH 7.35–7.45). As a word of caution, rapid changes in $PaCO_2$ should be avoided unless there is an urgent need to treat intracranial hypertension. The reason for this is that CBF is greatly influenced by the pH of the CSF, which changes rapidly in response to sudden changes in $PaCO_2$. Sedation and analgesia should be given to prevent agitation and coughing, but agents particularly associated with hypotension should be avoided. In patients with signs of herniation, such as a fixed and dilated pupil or posturing, hyperventilation

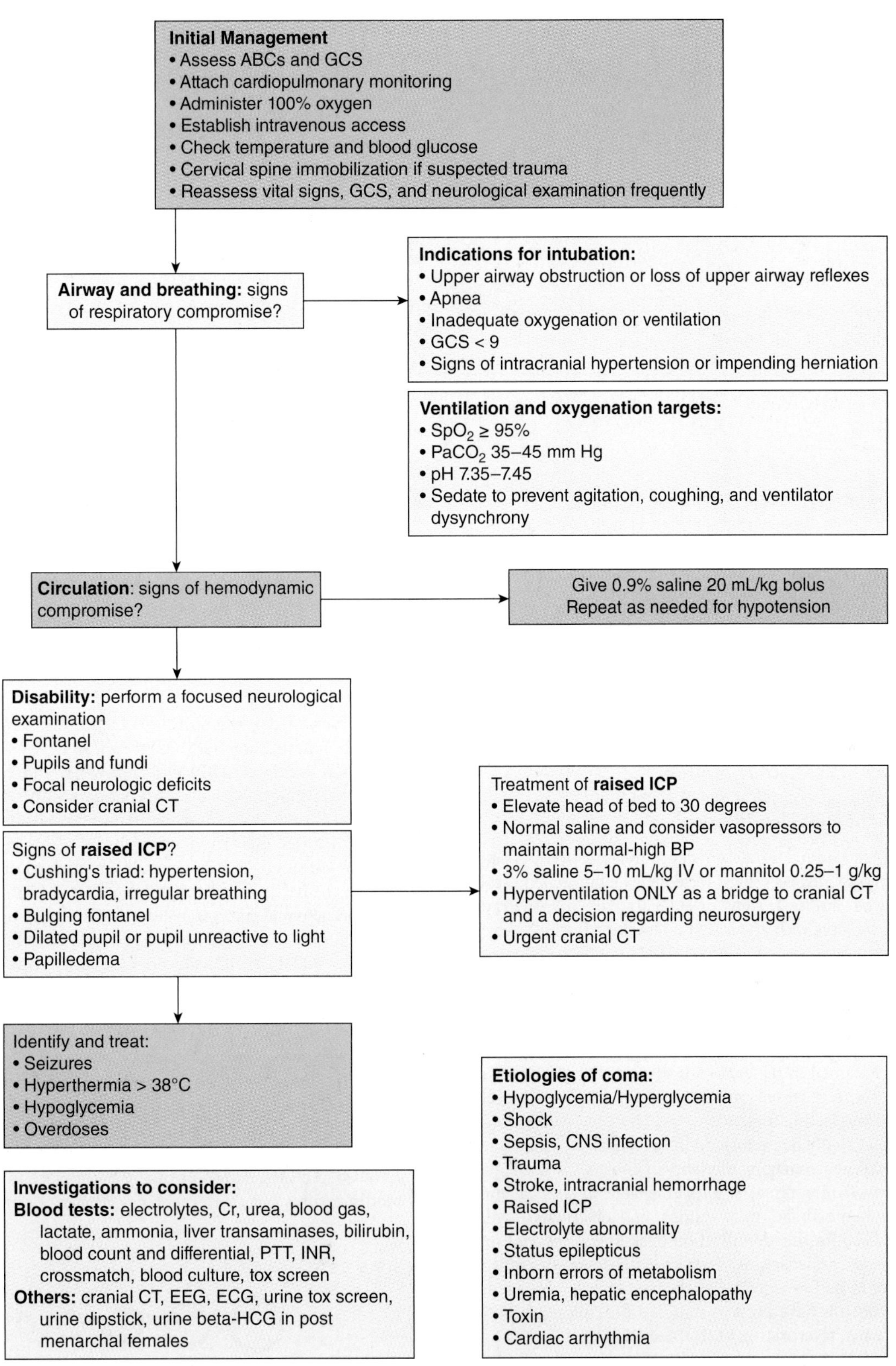


**FIGURE 105-1** Initial evaluation and management of acute brain injury. ABC, airway, breathing, circulation; CNS, central nervous system; Cr, creatinine; CT, computed tomography; EEG, electroencephalogram; GCS, Glasgow Coma Scale; HCG, human chorionic gonadotrophin; ICP, intracranial pressure; INR, international normalized ratio; $PaCO_2$, arterial partial pressure of carbon dioxide; PTT, partial thromboplastin time; $SpO_2$, oxygen saturation.

can be used as a bridge to prompt neuroimaging (computed tomography [CT]) and a decision regarding neurosurgical intervention. Hyperventilation is otherwise contraindicated because hypocapnea leads to cerebral vasospasm and a decrease in cerebral blood volume and CBF, increasing the risk of secondary ischemic injury, especially in the first 24 hours after injury when CBF is often at its lowest (Fig. 105-2).

Intravascular access should be obtained in patients with acute brain injury. Blood pressure is maintained with isotonic saline and vasoactive medications as needed. Glucose should be checked, and normoglycemia maintained. The patient should be exposed and log-rolled to avoid exacerbating any spinal injury. The temperature should be kept normal. While there is no evidence to support the routine use of deliberate hypothermia as a neuroprotective intervention, there is

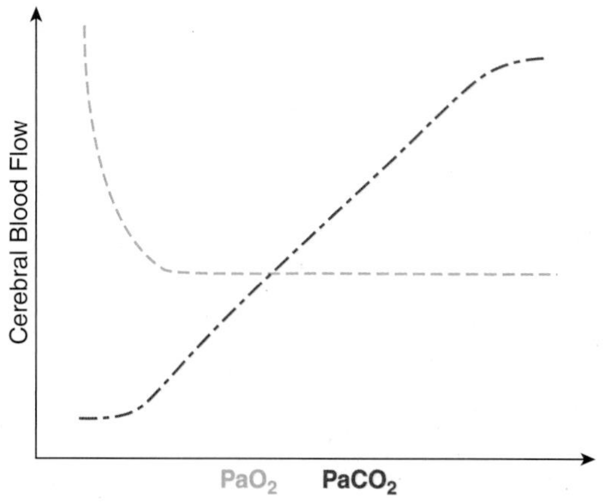


**FIGURE 105-2** Effect of arterial tensions of $O_2$ and $CO_2$ on cerebral blood flow.

good evidence that hyperthermia is detrimental through increases in cerebral metabolic rate. Fever or temperature swings are relatively common in the presence of brain injury and control of body temperature using a cooling blanket targeting normothermia can be useful in the early management of brain-injured patients.

#### Initial Investigations

The purposes of initial investigations (see Fig. 105-1) are threefold:

1) Identify and correct metabolic disturbances.
2) Identify and treat intracranial and spinal lesions that require emergent neurosurgical or medical intervention, such as a mass lesion, unstable cervical spine fracture, or stroke.
3) Identify and manage complications of acute brain injury, such as seizures and intracranial hypertension.

**Initial Neuroimaging** Indications for neuroimaging are persistent altered level of consciousness, new focal neurologic deficit, severe headache, vomiting, amnesia, signs of skull fracture or penetrating skull injury, and seizures with atypical or concerning features. Several decision-making rules for neuroimaging in TBI have been validated in the PECARN (Pediatric Emergency Care Applied Research Network), CATCH (Canadian Assessment of Tomography for Childhood Head injury), and CHALICE (Children's Head Injury Algorithm for the Prediction of Important Clinical Events) guidelines. Imaging of the spine should be obtained in patients with suspected trauma and tenderness over the spine, focal sensory or motor deficits, altered level of consciousness, or distracting injuries.

Cranial CT can rapidly be performed in the unstable patient and is generally the initial neuroimaging modality of choice. CT is adequate for identification of intracranial lesions amenable to surgical intervention, such as hemorrhage, mass lesions, and obstructive hydrocephalus, and is ideal for the identification of skull and cervical spine fractures. The major drawback of CT is radiation exposure and the theoretical risk of radiation-associated cancers; however, dose-reduction scanning protocols have become standard for children. Caution should be taken when interpreting a CT obtained in the first 24 hours, as some abnormalities may not be visible (eg, strokes or demyelination or global ischemia).

Magnetic resonance imaging (MRI) has advantages over CT but has the drawbacks of long image acquisition times that require immobility and limited access to the patient during the scan. MRI is the preferred modality for examining the spinal cord, and the posterior fossa, due to artifact from the dense temporal petrous bones on CT. It also can better demonstrate demyelination, infection, and inflammation. Diffusion-weighted MR imaging can demonstrate stroke (from ischemia to infarction) within hours, much earlier and better than can CT. It provides finer anatomic detail than CT, which may be required, for instance, to guide resection of a tumor. Therefore, although CT alone is generally adequate for initial neuroimaging to exclude intracranial blood, fractures, and hydrocephalus, early MRI may be required to diagnose and expedite treatment of stroke or demyelination, or to delineate a tumor for surgical planning. Due to the increased risk of upper cervical spine injury in young children and the lack of sensitivity of CT for cord and ligamentous injury, spinal MRI is performed in patients in whom the spine cannot be cleared on clinical grounds, even if the CT or plain radiographs are normal.

**Lumbar Puncture** A lumbar puncture to collect spinal fluid and to measure CSF pressure with manometry can assist in diagnosing infection, inflammatory and metabolic conditions, and subarachnoid hemorrhage, but should not be performed without excluding intracranial hypertension due to the risk of precipitating brain-stem herniation. A normal head CT does not exclude elevated ICP, and there are several documented cases of children with GCS 15 and raised ICP.

After initial stabilization, patients with severe brain injury should be transferred to a tertiary care facility with expertise in pediatric neurocritical care, neurosurgery, and neurology.

## MONITORING

Patients with moderate to severe brain injury should be managed in the intensive care unit. Close observation with continuous cardiopulmonary monitoring and constant reassessment with neurological examinations (eg, GCS score or Pediatric NIH Stroke Scale score) are key to track a patient's progress and monitor for complications. For critically ill children, multiple neuromonitoring modalities are available, with the greatest emphasis on ICP monitoring.

#### Intracranial Pressure Monitoring

The major aim of ICP monitoring is to prevent secondary hypoxic-ischemic injury from low CPP. CPP can be derived from the mean arterial blood pressure (ABP) and mean ICP and can be displayed with other continuous variables. All patients with severe TBI should be considered for ICP monitoring. Its use has not been shown to be beneficial in raised ICP from other forms of brain injury, such as asphyxia or infection. ICP is generally monitored either via a catheter placed in the lateral ventricle (an external ventricular drain) or an intraparenchymal microtransducer. The major advantages of an external ventricular drain are better accuracy and the ability to drain CSF to lower ICP. Microtransducers have lesser risks of infection and hemorrhage but cannot be recalibrated to 0 and tend to noticeably drift over the course of several days.

#### Pressure Reactivity and Pressure–Volume Compensatory Reserve

In health, the integrity of the neurovascular unit ensures that when arterial blood pressure (ABP) increases, pressure regulation leads to vasoconstriction in order to maintain a constant CBF, which in turn leads to a decrease in cerebral blood volume and a decrease in ICP (Fig. 105-3). Autoregulation normally takes place over a wide range of blood pressures but cerebrovascular reactivity can be deranged in

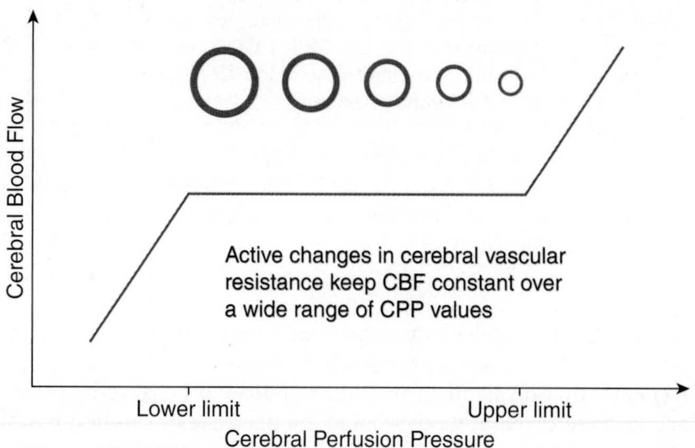


**FIGURE 105-3** Autoregulation of cerebral blood flow. CBF, cerebral blood flow; CPP, cerebral perfusion pressure.

the injured brain and can fail below a certain threshold CPP. With disturbed cerebrovascular reactivity or loss of cerebrovascular reserve, changes in ABP are directly transmitted to ICP.

Indices of cerebrovascular integrity can be derived from waveform and trend analysis of the ICP, ABP, and CPP. Examples include the pressure reactivity index (PRx), which captures the effect of slow changes in ABP on ICP when ICP is measured with a closed intracranial system (ie, no CSF drainage), and the pressure–volume compensation index (RAP), which is derived from small changes in intracranial volume throughout the cardiac cycle. Both the PRx and RAP indices have been shown to correlate with outcome in a limited number of adult and pediatric studies. Further studies are required to determine whether applying such measures in treatment algorithms can influence outcome.

#### Continuous Electroencephalogram

The use of continuous electroencephalogram (EEG) is increasing in the PICU. While the primary purpose is to detect and treat seizures, continuous EEG can also track the degree of encephalopathy over time, assist in prognostication, and monitor the achievement of burst suppression during the use of barbiturate therapy in severe TBI with refractory intracranial hypertension or refractory status epilepticus. Most commonly, a 20-lead EEG is used along with digital video recording, clinical event input from the bedside nurse, electromyography leads, and cardiopulmonary monitoring. Software detection algorithms are used to flag events suspicious for electrographic seizures but the output still requires review and interpretation by a neurologist or neurophysiologist, making this a resource-intensive form of monitoring. Recent studies of critically ill children report the prevalence of electrographic seizures to be around 30% in severe TBI, 35% in HIE secondary to cardiac arrest, 45% in CNS infection, and 60% in stroke. A shorter 1-hour EEG fails to identify half of children with seizures, one-third of which are exclusively subclinical. The yield increases to around 90% with 24 hours of monitoring.

The provision of a continuous EEG service is a resource-heavy undertaking and must be available on nights and weekends. While it is clear that continuous EEG adds information, more evidence is needed to determine whether treatment guided by this information will improve outcomes.

#### Transcranial Doppler

Transcranial Doppler (TCD) allows for the measurement of the velocity of blood in intracranial arteries, most commonly of the middle cerebral artery, and provides a repeatable surrogate for CBF. TCD-derived measures can also be used to estimate autoregulatory capacity or vasospasm.

#### Near-Infrared Spectroscopy

Near-infrared spectroscopy (NIRS) uses diode light sources to emit multiple wavelengths of near-infrared light (700–1000 nm) and measure tissue oxyhemoglobin and deoxyhemoglobin. Approximately 75% of the blood in the cerebral cortex is postcapillary, and NIRS provides a regional venous-weighted estimate of hemoglobin oxygen saturation. Cerebral NIRS has been increasingly applied in the monitoring of congenital heart surgery. While low cerebral NIRS saturations have been shown to predict adverse neurodevelopmental outcomes in some groups, prospective studies of algorithms incorporating NIRS in the intensive care unit are, in general, lacking.

#### Regional Brain Tissue Oxygenation ($PbtO_2$) or Microdialysis

For research purposes, catheters can be placed into brain parenchyma to measure regional oxygen tension, pH, and temperature. Microdialysis catheters are also available and can measure changes in glucose, lactate, pyruvate, neurotransmitters, and various amino acids. These catheters may be more sensitive to conditions of ischemia and their inclusion in management protocols has been associated with neurological outcomes, but pediatric experience is limited. A major drawback is that the measurements only reflect the metabolic conditions of a single brain region. Blood flow is known to be heterogeneous even in global injuries such as HIE after cardiac arrest, which begs the question of how best to use the information.

## TREATMENT



The management of severe acute brain injury requires input from multiple teams, including critical care, neurosurgery, neurology, and allied health, remembering that such injury often means a very long hospital course and subsequent rehabilitation for some patients. The general principles are prevention of secondary insults and treatment of complications, such as raised ICP. Specific treatments related to status epilepticus, stroke, and central nervous system infection are covered elsewhere in this book. We will focus on the treatment of raised ICP and the use of therapeutic targeted temperature management and hypothermia therapy.

#### Management of Raised Intracranial Pressure

The second edition of *Guidelines for the Acute Medical Management of Severe Traumatic Brain Injury in Infants, Children, and Adolescents* synthesizes the best evidence for the management of increased ICP in pediatric patients. Although there was insufficient evidence to support a specific treatment algorithm, we present a sensible approach to the management of raised ICP in intubated patients with ICP monitoring, the specifics and order of which may vary between centers. Although most of the evidence relates to severe TBI, the same approach can reasonably be applied to other forms of brain injury with cerebral edema and intracranial hypertension.

Measured ICP should be maintained below 20 mm Hg. CPP should be maintained above 40 mm Hg in children 0 to 5 years, above 50 mm Hg in children 6 to 17 years, and above 50 to 60 mm Hg in adults.

**First-Tier Therapies** Raised ICP in intubated patients should initially be treated with adequate sedation, analgesia, and neuromuscular blockade to prevent discomfort, agitation, coughing, and ventilator-patient dyssynchrony. The head of the bed should be elevated to 30 degrees with the head midline and no compression of the neck veins. Temperature should be kept normal. Peripheral capillary oxygen saturation ≥ 95% should be maintained, and blood gas targets include $PaCO_2$ 35 to 45 mm Hg and pH 7.35 to 7.45. Electrolytes should be monitored carefully, with special attention to sodium, which is often targeted at high-normal levels in the early phase of management.

In patients with a ventriculostomy catheter (external ventricular drain), CSF can be drained. This is often accomplished by setting the catheter to continuously drain at pressures above 15 mm Hg or by intermittent drainage to maintain ICP < 20 mm Hg.

If ICP remains elevated, hyperosmolar therapy, in the form of 3% saline 5 to 10 mL/kg or mannitol 0.25 to 1 g/kg can be given. Hypertonic saline is often preferred, as it avoids the osmotic diuresis and risk of hypotension induced by mannitol. However, sodium equilibrates across the BBB in a few hours and thus loses its effectiveness unless the serum sodium level is continuously increased. Furthermore, hypernatremia is associated with renal failure and ARDS in children treated for intracranial hypertension. Therefore, the use of hypertonic saline should be limited to the minimum amount required to maintain ICP < 20 mm Hg rather than used to target a certain serum sodium level.

**Second-Tier Therapies** In patients with persistently raised ICP despite optimization of these first tier therapies, mechanical problems or seizures should be ruled out. Due to the prevalence of subclinical seizures in acute brain injury, as previously described, seizure prophylaxis with phenytoin or levetiracetam should be considered in patients with severe acute brain injury. A repeat cranial CT should be considered to assess for surgical lesions. The following second-tier therapies are effective at reducing ICP but may be associated with adverse effects and have not been shown to improve outcomes and may cause harm in some.

Decompressive craniectomy releases ICP by removal of part of the skull with or without the dura. Despite effectively reducing ICP, its effect on patient outcomes is less clear. One small pediatric study found that it may improve functional outcomes. However, a large adult trial demonstrated no survival benefit and concerningly found a greater risk of unfavorable neurological outcome in those who underwent decompressive craniectomy. Results from another large trial are forthcoming.

High-dose barbiturate therapy can be titrated to produce electrophysiological burst suppression, which reduces cerebral metabolism, thereby reducing CBF and ICP. Barbiturate therapy has not been shown to improve outcome and is associated with an increased risk of infection.

**Therapeutic Hypothermia** Fever after any form of severe injury is associated with worse outcomes because of its impact on metabolism and cell death pathways. Mild hypothermia (32–34°C) does lower the ICP and has been used as a rescue therapy for raised ICP or as a first-line therapy for 24 to 72 hours to prevent secondary injury in severe TBI and HIE after cardiac arrest. Children are most often cooled using surface cooling. There have been multiple trials showing that the use of hypothermia therapy in severe TBI does not improve outcomes and may cause harm, including in pediatric patients. These trials have been criticized on the grounds that cooling was only achieved by 8 to 12 hours after injury, whereas animal models suggest that cooling within 4 to 6 hours is required for benefit. Cooled patients often need muscle relaxants to prevent shivering and should be observed for coagulopathy, electrolyte abnormalities, dysrhythmias, and altered drug metabolism. The ideal rate of rewarming is not known but should not exceed 0.5°C per hour and may need to be as slow as 0.7°C per 4 hours or may need to be titrated to systemic and cerebral hemodynamic endpoints. While therapeutic hypothermia has limited, if any, role after TBI in children, there is little doubt that fever is detrimental in this setting and that targeted normothermia should be part of all neuroprotective protocols for the first 48 to 72 hours after significant injury.

Mild hypothermia has been extensively studied in the management of HIE after cardiac arrest and has been shown to be beneficial in adults with ventricular tachycardia (VT) or ventricular fibrillation (VF) cardiac arrest. The 2 adult studies that showed benefit with therapeutic hypothermia both had ice-cold saline infused intravenously into the patients by paramedics in the ambulance, on the way to the hospital. However, targeted temperature normothermia has been recently shown to be equivalent to therapeutic hypothermia in adults after cardiac arrest. Cardiac arrest (mainly asystole compared to adults with VF) is different in children, with 80% to 90% being asphyxial in nature, and evidence for therapeutic hypothermia is lacking. A recent trial of therapeutic hypothermia in pediatric out-of-hospital cardiac arrest found that hypothermia did not confer any benefit in terms of survival when compared to controlled normothermia, and results from an in-hospital cardiac arrest cohort are forthcoming. By contrast, cooling in neonatal HIE is likely beneficial in terms of overall survival and functional outcome in survivors.



## OUTCOME PREDICTION

Prognostication can be helpful to discriminate between children who will recover to enjoy a reasonable quality of life and those who will certainly die or be dependent on others for all aspects of daily life. Prognostication in the ICU remains challenging and can be confounded by therapies such as sedation and neuromuscular blockade. Decisions are further complicated by differences in what families perceive to be a good or favorable outcome. High specificity and positive predictive value of tests used in prognostication are key to avoid forming an impression that leads to withdrawal of life supportive therapy in a child who would otherwise have enjoyed a good quality of life.

### Etiology and Circumstances

In children with return of spontaneous circulation (ROSC) after cardiac arrest, out-of-hospital location, younger age, longer duration of CPR, and asystole or pulseless electrical activity versus VT/VF as the initial rhythm are associated with poor outcome. In severe TBI, lower GCS score, particularly the motor score, after resuscitation; cerebral edema with unreactive pupils to light; and nonaccidental mechanism of injury portend a poorer prognosis.

### Physical Examination

The predictive value of clinical signs is better outside of 72 hours following injury and should be interpreted or delayed depending upon the level of sedation, neuromuscular blockade, and hypothermia. Absent pupillary responses, absent corneal reflexes and absent or extensor motor response after 24 hours carries a high predictive value for poor outcome in HIE after cardiac arrest. Interpretation requires more caution in severe TBI because of possible isolated injury to reflex arcs.

### Electrophysiology

Bilaterally absent somatosensory evoked potentials (SSEP) carry a greater than 90% specificity for poor outcome if performed outside of 24 hours from injury. Particularly in severe TBI, one must exclude structural abnormalities that can interfere with the test such as cord injury or subdural collection.

Burst suppression or a nonreactive EEG in the absence of sedation and metabolic abnormalities are strongly predictive of a poor outcome. Refractory status epilepticus on continuous EEG monitoring is associated with greatly increased odds of death or decline in functional status, but it lacks specificity.

### Neuroimaging

Normal head CTs are not helpful in predicting longer term outcomes, especially when done in the first 24 hours. MRI 3 to 5 days after injury is a better predictor, with the most useful sequences being diffusion-weighted imaging (DWI), diffusion tensor imaging (DTI), susceptibility-weighted imaging (SWI), and MR spectroscopy.

### Biomarkers

Several biomarkers have been studied in relation to outcomes after brain injury. These are ideally measured in the blood or urine, specific to brain tissue and elevated in proportion to the degree of brain damage. The most commonly studied biomarkers are neuron-specific enolase, s100b, and myelin basic protein. Some studies have reported impressive test characteristics but results between studies are inconsistent and no useful cutoff thresholds have emerged. At present, brain biomarkers cannot be recommended to guide clinical decisions, and should be considered in the context of research.

## SUGGESTED READINGS


Bayir H, Kochanek PM, Clark RS. Traumatic brain injury in infants and children: mechanisms of secondary damage and treatment in the intensive care unit. *Crit Care Clin*. 2003;19(3):529-549.

Brady KM, Shaffner DH, Lee JK, et al. Continuous monitoring of cerebrovascular pressure reactivity after traumatic brain injury in children. *Pediatrics*. 2009;124(6):e1205-e1212.

Figaji AA, Zwane E, Fieggen AG, Siesjo P, Peter JC. Transcranial Doppler pulsatility index is not a reliable indicator of intracranial pressure in children with severe traumatic brain injury. *Surg Neurol*. 2009;72(4):389-394.

Figaji AA, Zwane E, Graham Fieggen A, Argent AC, Le Roux PD, Peter JC. The effect of increased inspired fraction of oxygen on brain tissue oxygen tension in children with severe traumatic brain injury. *Neurocrit Care*. 2010;12(3):430-437.

Hutchison JS, Frndova H, Lo TY, Guerguerian AM; Hypothermia Pediatric Head Injury Trial Investigators; and Canadian Critical Care Trials Group. Impact of hypotension and low cerebral perfusion pressure on outcomes in children treated with hypothermia therapy following severe traumatic brain injury: a post hoc analysis of the Hypothermia Pediatric Head Injury Trial. *Dev Neurosci*. 2010;32(5-6):406-412.

Hutchison JS, Guerguerian AM. Cooling of children with severe traumatic brain injury. *Lancet Neurol*. 2013;12(6):527-529.

Hutchison JS, Ward RE, Lacroix J, et al. Hypothermia therapy after traumatic brain injury in children. *N Engl J Med*. 2008;358(23):2447-2456.

Ichord RN, Bastian R, Abraham L., et al. Interrater reliability of the Pediatric National Institutes of Health Stroke Scale (PedNIHSS) in a multicenter study. *Stroke*. 2011;42(3):613-617.

Kochanek PM, Carney N, Adelson PD, et al. Guidelines for the acute medical management of severe traumatic brain injury in infants, children, and adolescents—second edition. *Pediatr Crit Care Med*. 2012;13(Suppl 1):S1-S82.

Kochanek PM, Jackson TC, Ferguson NM, et al. Emerging therapies in traumatic brain injury. *Semin Neurol.* 2015;35(1):83-100.

Moler FW, Silverstein FS, Holubkov R, et al; THAPCA Trial Investigators. Therapeutic hypothermia after out-of-hospital cardiac arrest in children. *N Engl J Med.* 2015;372(20):1898-1908.

Topjian AA, French B, Sutton RM, et al. Early postresuscitation hypotension is associated with increased mortality following pediatric cardiac arrest. *Crit Care Med.* 2014;42(6):1518-1523.

Vavilala MS, Lee LA, Boddu K, et al. Cerebral autoregulation in pediatric traumatic brain injury. *Pediatr Crit Care Med.* 2004;5(3):257-263.

# 106 Early Management of Sepsis and Septic Shock

Mark J. Peters and Joe Brierley

## INTRODUCTION

*Sepsis* has been defined in adults and children in terms of changes in vital signs (heart rate, respiratory rate, temperature) and white cell count in the context of infection (Table 106-1). The *systemic inflammatory response syndrome* previously described the same response in the absence of confirmed infection (eg, after trauma or major surgery). Over the past decade, the Surviving Sepsis Campaign has made important efforts to develop consensus statements defining sepsis, sepsis syndrome, septic shock, and the SIRS in adults. The first set of guidelines were introduced in 2008 and were updated in 2012 and again in 2016 (Sepsis-3). These consensus statements included updated definitions for sepsis, sepsis syndrome, septic shock, and the systemic inflammatory response syndrome, as well as evidence-based guidelines and algorithms for the management of these conditions in adults. In this framework, sepsis is described as "a life-threatening organ dysfunction caused by a dysregulated host response to infection." Although new consensus definitions have not yet been developed for the pediatric population, this description can be applied to patients of all ages.

Regardless of how we define it, the early recognition of sepsis, resuscitation from shock, and control of the causative agent all have dramatic effects on survival, and delay in any of these steps is associated with an exponential increase in mortality. This is because the vast majority of deaths from sepsis in children occur in the first hours after diagnosis (Fig. 106-1). Recognition of the fact that the prehospital and emergency room management of patients with sepsis can determine their prognosis has been key in defining resuscitation priorities and timing of interventions for all those involved in their care.

## PATHOGENESIS AND EPIDEMIOLOGY

The pathogenesis of sepsis is not fully understood and there is no accepted gold standard to define the dysregulated response. However there exist 3 distinct (though sometimes overlapping) "phenotypes" of sepsis. The first phenotype is an overexuberant proinflammatory response, which at its extreme (eg, in the setting of meningococcal sepsis with purpura fulminans) includes widespread endothelial activation, disseminated intravascular coagulopathy, myocardial depression, and microvascular dysfunction. The second clinical manifestation is with multiple organ-system failure. Finally, for a subgroup of patients with sepsis that fail to respond adequately to an invading

**TABLE 106-1 CURRENT DEFINITIONS OF SEPSIS AND SEPTIC SHOCK FOR CHILDREN AND ADULTS**

| | Pediatric Definitions[a] | New Adult Definitions[b] |
|---|---|---|
| **SIRS** | The presence of at least 2 of 4 criteria, 1 of which must be abnormal temperature or leukocyte count:<br>• Core temperature of > 38.5°C or < 36°C<br>• Leukocyte count elevated or depressed for age (not secondary to chemotherapy-induced leukopenia) or > 10% immature neutrophils<br>• Tachycardia, defined as a mean heart rate > 2 SD above normal for age in the absence of external stimulus, chronic drugs, or painful stimuli; or otherwise unexplained persistent elevation over a 0.5- to 4-hr time period OR for children < 1 yr old: bradycardia, defined as a mean heart rate < 10th percentile for age in the absence of external vagal stimulus, β-blocker drugs, or congenital heart disease; or otherwise unexplained persistent depression over a 0.5-hr time period<br>• Mean respiratory rate > 2 SD above normal for age or mechanical ventilation for an acute process not related to underlying neuromuscular disease or the receipt of general anesthesia | Term no longer used |
| **Sepsis** | SIRS in the presence of or as a result of suspected or proven infection | Life-threatening organ dysfunction caused by a dysregulated response to infection<br>**Clinical criteria**<br>Suspected or documented infection and an acute increase of ≥ 2 SOFA points (a proxy for organ dysfunction) |
| **Severe sepsis** | Sepsis plus 1 of the following: cardiovascular organ dysfunction OR acute respiratory distress syndrome OR 2 or more other organ dysfunctions | Term no longer used |
| **Septic shock** | Sepsis and cardiovascular organ dysfunction | A subset of sepsis in which underlying circulatory and cellular metabolic abnormalities are profound enough to substantially increase mortality<br>**Criteria**<br>Sepsis and vasopressor therapy needed to elevate mean arterial pressure > 65 mm Hg, and lactate > 2 mmol/L despite adequate fluid resuscitation |

[a]From Goldstein B, Giroir B, Randolph A. International pediatric sepsis consensus conference: definitions for sepsis and organ dysfunction in pediatrics. *Pediatr Crit Care Med.* 2005;6(1):2-8.

[b]From Singer M, Deutschman CS, Seymour CW, et al. The Third International Consensus definitions for sepsis and septic shock (Sepsis-3). *JAMA.* 2016;315(8):801-810.

Note that the new Sepsis-3 definitions are based on nonspecific physiological derangement—an increased in a severity of illness score—rather than markers of sepsis, per se.

SD, standard deviation; SIRS, systemic inflammatory response syndrome; SOFA, sequential organ failure assessment score.

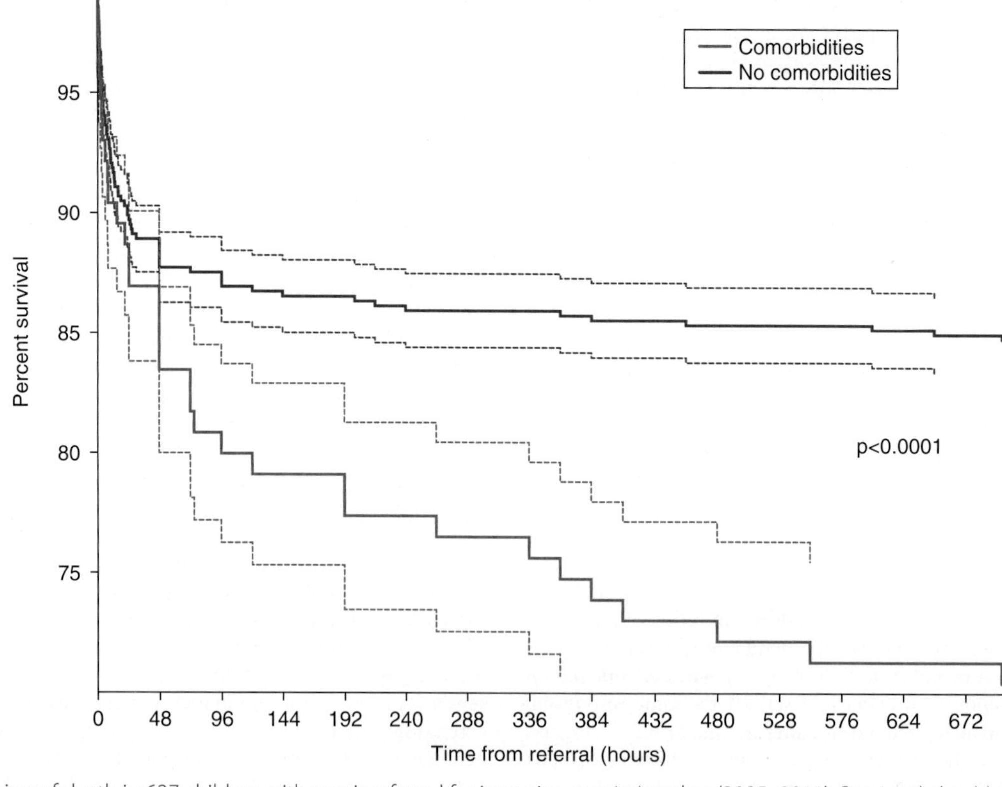


**FIGURE 106-1** Timing of death in 627 children with sepsis referred for intensive care in London (2005–2011). Previously healthy children who survived the first 48 hours of sepsis rarely die. However, sepsis frequently affects children with chronic diseases in whom the risk follows a different profile—not all of which can be attributed to sepsis. (Reproduced with permission from Cvetkovic M, Lutman D, Ramnarayan P, et al: Timing of Death in Children Referred for Intensive Care With Severe Sepsis: Implications for Interventional Studies, *Pediatr Crit Care Med.* 2015 Jun;16(5):410-417.)



microorganism, a state called "acquired immunoparalysis" or "monocyte deactivation" can be present. Increasingly there is a view that some of the more extreme phenotypes (eg, multiple organ failure with predominant hepatobiliary dysfunction and coagulopathy) may be considered as a form of hemophagocytic lymphohistiocytosis (HLH). This is an area of active investigation, and will undoubtedly be better characterized over coming years. At the time of writing, for most intensivists, care for sepsis includes treating the cause and providing organ support while awaiting recovery, rather than interventions specific to the phenotype.

The key pathological result of the inflammatory response that is relevant to early resuscitation is the net myocardial depressant effect. Importantly, however, the effect to which this myocardial depression can be compensated by other responses (eg, tachycardia, ventricular dilatation) and volume status varies widely between cases and results in a wide variety of hemodynamic presentations of septic shock that have only recently been defined in children (Fig. 106-2).

Sepsis rates are increasing in developed countries, perhaps in part reflecting a growing population of children living with chronic illness who are at greater risk, or reflecting more aggressive therapeutic immunosuppression for malignancy. A recent study estimated that around 1 in 20 pediatric intensive care unit (PICU) admissions are for sepsis or septic shock, though many more follow other serious infections. Newborns and infants have the highest rates of sepsis and septic shock and the worst outcomes. Serious comorbidities (including prematurity and congenital malformations), a history of complex surgical interventions, relatively immature immune systems, and greater difficulties in diagnosis all contribute to the vulnerability of this age group.

## PRESENTATION AND DIAGNOSIS

A single definition, tool, or biomarker to identify whether an individual patient has sepsis, or is at risk of developing septic shock, does not currently exist. However, pediatric resuscitation courses

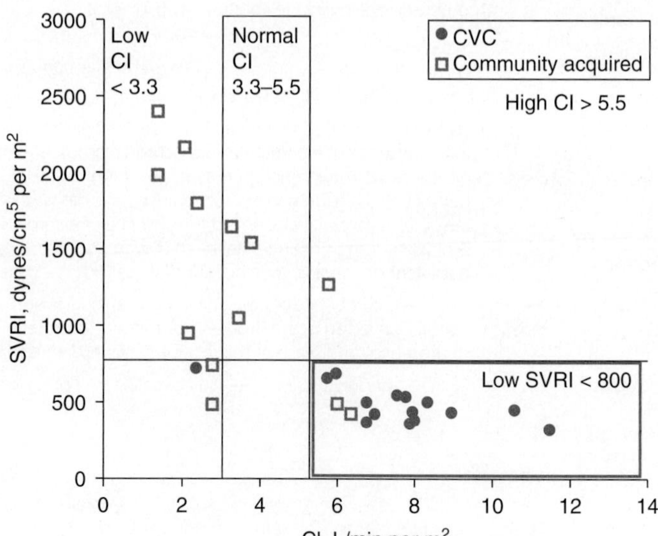


**FIGURE 106-2** Distribution of cardiac index and systemic vascular resistance index in 30 children with septic shock on PICU admission. Patients with central venous catheter–associated sepsis tended to have a warm shock pattern (high CI, low SVRI), whereas community-acquired sepsis was more typically cold shock (high SVRI). CI, cardiac index; CVC, central venous catheter; PICU, pediatric intensive care unit; SVRI, systemic vascular resistance index. (Reproduced with permission from Brierley J, Thiruchelvam T, Peters MJ: Hemodynamics of early pediatric fluid-resistant septic shock using non-invasive cardiac output (USCOM): Distinct profiles of CVC infection and community acquired sepsis, *Crit Care Med* 2005 Dec;33(12):A153-A153.)

(Pediatric Advanced Life Support [PALS] and Advanced Pediatric Life Support [APLS]) teach clinicians how to recognize a seriously ill child, and emphasize the importance of simultaneous assessment and resuscitation: "treating things that kill first." Additionally, more customized sepsis bundle guidance is now recommended, with a number of care steps to be delivered to achieve compliance (eg, the UK Sepsis Six bundle). If initial resuscitation does not reverse sepsis-associated shock, then more specific guidance, continuing into the ICU admission, advocates not only the reversal of the clinical features of shock, but also the importance of monitoring hemodynamic parameters and markers of oxygen delivery such as cardiac index, systemic vascular resistance index, and central venous oxygen saturation, taken from the superior vena cava. All such guidelines advocate steps within a specific timeframe and further action if initial steps are not effective.

Algorithms that identify high-risk features and mandate reassessment in case of uncertainty can be very effective. A recent review document by the National Institute for Clinical Excellence in the United Kingdom produced valuable algorithms for children and adults in various settings. The pediatric algorithm provides a pragmatic approach to the categorization of the risk (high, moderate, or low) of sepsis according to objective clinical features that include heart rate, respiratory rate, and level of consciousness.

The other key point to note is that because sepsis is a dynamic, exponential process, it is only rarely possible to exclude early sepsis, and the hallmark of sepsis is a rapid deterioration in the absence of appropriate treatment. Hence, a clinical assessment that concludes that sepsis is not *currently* present should include safety-net advice about what to do if things change. In the face of uncertainly, a planned reassessment is recommended.

## CLINICAL MANIFESTATIONS

There is no single symptom or sign that distinguishes sepsis from other causes of critical illness, nor is there a gold standard definition for sepsis. The threshold for a suspicion of sepsis must therefore consider the environment in which the assessment is taking place. In other words, a lower threshold would be appropriate for a bone marrow transplant recipient or others with immune dysfunction, or for younger children.

For the first responders, the overwhelming clinical priorities for a septic patient that has been resuscitated are continued observation for cardiorespiratory system failure (remembering that hypotension is a late sign), new organ system dysfunction, and source control (Fig. 106-3). Clinical practice surveys have consistently shown that the clinical care of children with sepsis is neither as prompt nor as reliable as staff or lay people would presume to be the case. This is of particular importance since the adherence to algorithms for assessment and intervention such as Surviving Sepsis or the Sepsis Six (Fig. 106-4), have been shown to improve both processes of care and outcomes. Most clinicians would plan to transfer a child with sepsis to the ICU prior to, or at the time when, fluid refractory shock is suspected, and certainly when vasoactive therapy is being considered.

## EARLY INTERVENTIONS FOR SUSPECTED SEPSIS

### Antibiotics

Without prompt and vigilant attention to source control, the outcomes of sepsis will inevitably be compromised. The recommendation from most sepsis care bundles is that appropriate antibiotics should be given within 60 minutes. The choice of antibiotics should be determined according to local policies with knowledge of the relevant pathogens and likely antibiotic resistances or sensitivities, as well as additional factors such as severe immunosuppression, chronic disease, or a semipermanent catheter for long-term parenteral nutrition.

### Fluid Resuscitation

The Starling relationship of increased stroke volume with increased end-diastolic filling is the basis for rapid intravenous volume expansion in septic shock. Current recommendations are for rapid administration of 20 mL/kg of crystalloid or colloid in the absence of signs of fluid overload (eg, hepatomegaly, lung crackles), repeated as necessary. While high-level evidence for this intervention is weak and subject to extensive debate, in an environment with ready access to positive pressure ventilation, early aggressive fluid resuscitation has been associated with substantially improved outcomes. We recommend this approach but wish to highlight that this is an *observed* trial of a fluid bolus, which might be curtailed if signs of fluid overload (eg, breathlessness, crepitations on chest auscultation, or increased liver size) occur, or repeated if it leads to clinical improvement but not reversal of shock. This is a dynamic situation needing the clinician to remain by the bedside to assess the physiological response to therapy.

The above principles of rapid fluid expansion for children with septic shock may not apply in all settings, particularly in developing nations. The Fluid Expansion as Supportive Therapy (FEAST) study, a large randomized study of early fluid resuscitation in children with sepsis presenting in a resource-poor area, demonstrated that not all children with sepsis respond similarly to early fluid administration. The study found that rapid and generous fluid resuscitation according to standard algorithms was associated with increased harm, and this led the World Health Organization (WHO) to adapt a different standard in resource-poor areas. The WHO has produced guidelines known as *Emergency Triage Assessment and Treatment* (ETAT) that specifically considers resource-limited environments and approaches to fluid resuscitation in children with malnutrition. The main differences for malnourished children being the cautious and more limited early fluid intravenous bolus administration, early blood transfusion in patients with severe anemia, and early introduction of nasogastric fluids rather than continued intravenous fluid therapy.

### Vasoactive Drug Infusions

If a child fails to respond to initial fluid and early inotrope resuscitation, then he or she is considered to be in a state of fluid-resistant septic shock. The early use of inotropes is recommended in patients with septic shock that do not respond promptly to fluid according to published consensus guidelines. Shock in children has been shown to have different manifestations compared to adults in whom vasoplegic high output or warm shock is usual. Children initially may present with this adult pattern—which some researchers have found more prevalent in hospital-acquired sepsis—but many present with cold shock, in which low cardiac output and high systemic vascular resistance predominate, often in community-acquired sepsis. Specific vasoactive medication to normalize this hemodynamic pattern is recommended: epinephrine for cold shock and norepinephrine for warm shock. However, this pattern changes over the period of resuscitation and stabilization. A child presenting in cold shock may transform to warm shock after a few hours, so frequent measurements of hemodynamic parameters and tailoring of vasoactive medication to achieve the hemodynamic parameter guideline goals is required. If this does not work, more aggressive treatment for catecholamine-resistance shock is mandated. Depending on shock morphology and response, aggressive treatment might include further inotrope titration, addition of inodilators, or extracorporeal membrane oxygenation (ECMO) support.

### Early Goal-Directed Therapy

*Early goal-directed therapy* refers to the resuscitation of patients according to specific hemodynamic targets beyond simple vital signs; examples being central venous oxygen saturation or the clearance of serum lactate. There is limited evidence to support this approach in populations with high predicted case fatality rate (≥ 40%). However, with the increasing adoption of aggressive early resuscitation bundles, the utility of this approach has been further questioned.

### Mechanical Ventilation

Early consideration of mechanical ventilation is recommended in septic shock. However, great care must be taken not to induce further myocardial depression with induction agents. Inhalational agents,

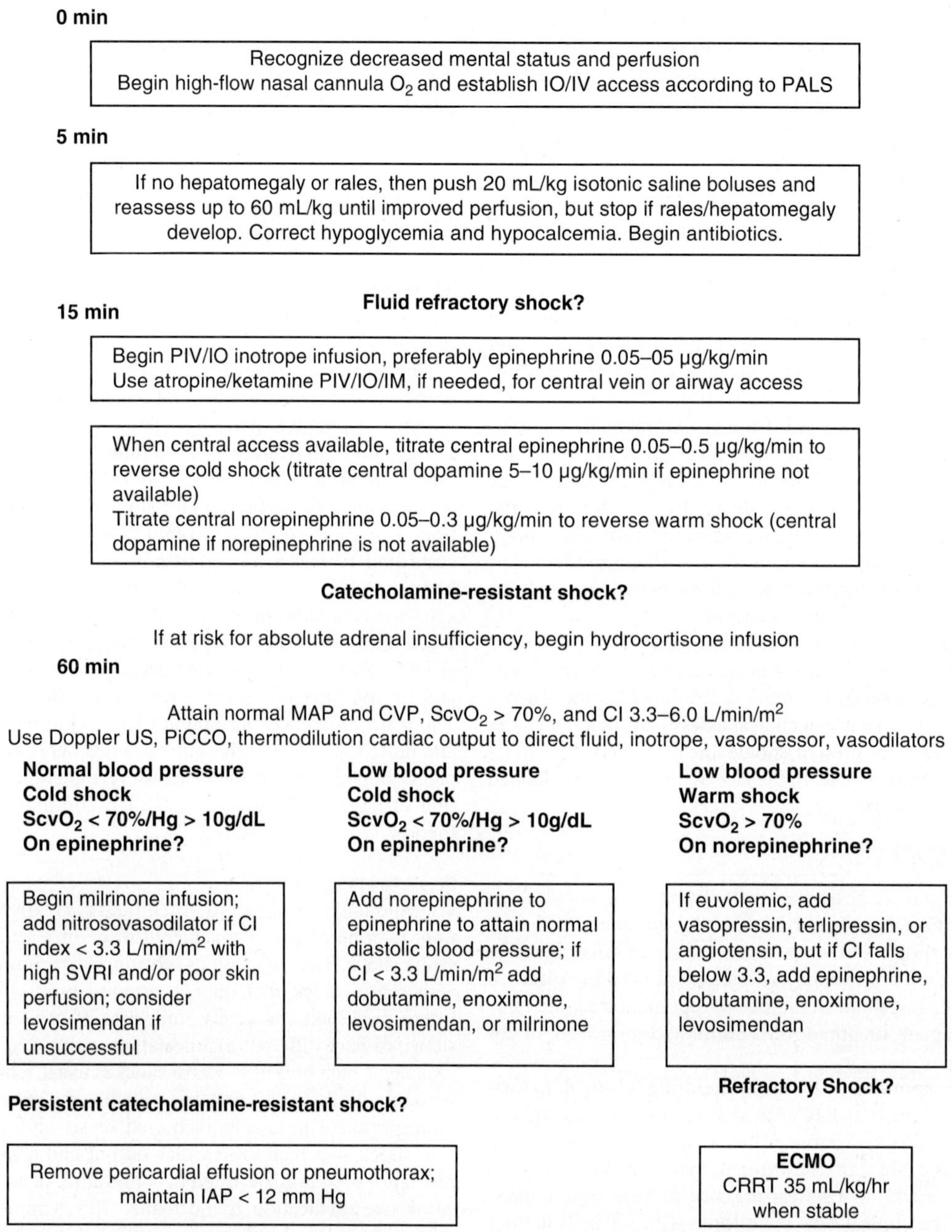

**0 min**

Recognize decreased mental status and perfusion
Begin high-flow nasal cannula $O_2$ and establish IO/IV access according to PALS

**5 min**

If no hepatomegaly or rales, then push 20 mL/kg isotonic saline boluses and reassess up to 60 mL/kg until improved perfusion, but stop if rales/hepatomegaly develop. Correct hypoglycemia and hypocalcemia. Begin antibiotics.

**15 min** **Fluid refractory shock?**

Begin PIV/IO inotrope infusion, preferably epinephrine 0.05–05 μg/kg/min
Use atropine/ketamine PIV/IO/IM, if needed, for central vein or airway access

When central access available, titrate central epinephrine 0.05–0.5 μg/kg/min to reverse cold shock (titrate central dopamine 5–10 μg/kg/min if epinephrine not available)
Titrate central norepinephrine 0.05–0.3 μg/kg/min to reverse warm shock (central dopamine if norepinephrine is not available)

**Catecholamine-resistant shock?**

If at risk for absolute adrenal insufficiency, begin hydrocortisone infusion

**60 min**

Attain normal MAP and CVP, $ScvO_2$ > 70%, and CI 3.3–6.0 L/min/m$^2$
Use Doppler US, PiCCO, thermodilution cardiac output to direct fluid, inotrope, vasopressor, vasodilators

| **Normal blood pressure**<br>**Cold shock**<br>**$ScvO_2$ < 70%/Hg > 10g/dL**<br>**On epinephrine?** | **Low blood pressure**<br>**Cold shock**<br>**$ScvO_2$ < 70%/Hg > 10g/dL**<br>**On epinephrine?** | **Low blood pressure**<br>**Warm shock**<br>**$ScvO_2$ > 70%**<br>**On norepinephrine?** |
|---|---|---|
| Begin milrinone infusion; add nitrosovasodilator if CI index < 3.3 L/min/m$^2$ with high SVRI and/or poor skin perfusion; consider levosimendan if unsuccessful | Add norepinephrine to epinephrine to attain normal diastolic blood pressure; if CI < 3.3 L/min/m$^2$ add dobutamine, enoximone, levosimendan, or milrinone | If euvolemic, add vasopressin, terlipressin, or angiotensin, but if CI falls below 3.3, add epinephrine, dobutamine, enoximone, levosimendan |

**Persistent catecholamine-resistant shock?**

Remove pericardial effusion or pneumothorax; maintain IAP < 12 mm Hg

**Refractory Shock?**

**ECMO**
CRRT 35 mL/kg/hr when stable

**FIGURE 106-3** Immediate management of septic shock. CI, cardiac index; CRRT, continuous renal replacement therapy; CVP, central venous pressure; ECMO, extracorporeal membrane oxygenation; FATD, femoral arterial thermodilution; IO, intraosseous; IV, intravenous; MAP, mean arterial pressure; PALS, Pediatric Advanced Life Support; PiCCO, pulse contour cardiac output; PIV, peripheral intravenous; $ScvO_2$, central venous oxygen saturation; SVRI, systemic vascular resistance index; US, ultrasound.

propofol, barbiturates, and high dose benzodiazepines should be avoided in this setting. In addition, etomidate should not be used, given the increased risk of adrenal suppression that has been associated with its administration in patients with sepsis. Once ventilation is established, recognition of the risk of acute lung injury or acute respiratory distress syndrome and adoption of a lung-protective strategy is recommended.

#### Extracorporeal Membrane Oxygenation

ECMO has been used successfully in refractory shock and severe acute respiratory distress syndrome in pediatric sepsis, with an overall survival to discharge of at least 50%. While there are no randomized trials of ECMO for septic shock, the typical physiology of shock, the often very elevated (supranormal) oxygen demands, and the need for high flows have led to the consideration of central cannulation (direct cannulation of the aorta and right atrium) as the approach of choice. While this approach does raise additional concerns for bleeding in patients who may already be coagulopathic, it provides the advantage of almost unlimited flows to meet the elevated metabolic demands of the hypoperfused tissues. When used early, ECMO runs are typically short (< 5 days) without long-term sequelae.

## PREVENTION

The value of immunization in preventing community-acquired infection is undisputed and is probably medicine's greatest influence on global health. Infection control measures in the hospital setting (eg, hand-washing, central venous line care, ventilator-associated pneumonia prevention, selective digestive decontamination) have been shown to have important benefits. The use of specific prophylaxis in immunosuppressed children also reduces the incidence of severe opportunistic infections.

## SUMMARY

Sepsis is a clinical syndrome that is vitally important to suspect, recognize, and treat early (even if the diagnosis is initially uncertain), with

Name:

Date of Birth:

Hospital No.:

*Affix Hospital Label if available*

THE UK SEPSIS TRUST

# Paediatric Sepsis 6

**Recognition of a child at risk:**

**If a child with suspected or proven infection AND has at least 2 of the following:**

- Core temperature < 36°C or > 38°C
- Inappropriate tachycardia (Refer to local criteria/APLS Guidance)
- Altered mental state (including: sleepiness/irritability/lethargy/floppiness)
- Reduced peripheral perfusion/prolonged capillary refill

Lower threshold of suspicion for: age < 3 months, chronic disease, recent surgery, or immunocompromised

**THINK: Could this child have SEVERE SEPSIS, SEPTIC SHOCK or RED FLAG SEPSIS*** - Ask for review by an experienced clinician.

High certainty of Sepsis
Respond with Paediatric Sepsis 6:

Complete all elements within 1 hour

| | Date/Time | Sign |
|---|---|---|
| **1. Give high flow oxygen:** | | |
| **2. Obtain IV/IO access & take blood tests:** | | |

a. Blood cultures
b. Blood glucose - treat low blood glucose
c. Blood gas (+ FBC, lactate/CRP as able)

| | Date/Time | Sign |
|---|---|---|
| **3. Give IV or IO antibiotics:** | | |

– Broad spectrum cover as per local policy

| | Date/Time | Sign |
|---|---|---|
| **4. Consider fluid resuscitation:** | | |

– Aim to restore normal circulating volume and physiological parameters
– Titrate 20 ml/kg Isotonic Fluid over 5 – 10 min and repeat if necessary
– Caution with fluid overload: Examine for crepitations & hepatomegaly

| | Date/Time | Sign |
|---|---|---|
| **5. Involve senior clinicians/specialists early:** | | |
| **6. Consider inotropic support early:** | | |

– If normal physiological parameters are not restored after ≥ 40 ml/kg fluids
– NB adrenaline or dopamine may be given via peripheral IV or IO access

Document reason(s) for variation overleaf

High certainty NOT Sepsis
or Unsure

| | Date/Time | Sign |
|---|---|---|
| Not Sepsis<br>Document reasons | | |
| Unsure | | |

Review within 1 hour

| | | |
|---|---|---|
| Not Sepsis<br>Document reasons | | |
| Sepsis<br>Start Sepsis 6 | | |
| Unsure | | |

Review within 1 hour

| | | |
|---|---|---|
| Not Sepsis<br>Document reasons | | |
| Sepsis<br>Start Sepsis 6 | | |
| Unsure | | |

Review within 1 hour

| | | |
|---|---|---|
| Not Sepsis<br>Document reasons | | |
| Sepsis<br>Start Sepsis 6 | | |
| Unsure | | |

Review within 1 hour

| | | |
|---|---|---|
| Not Sepsis<br>Document reasons | | |
| Sepsis<br>Start Sepsis 6 | | |

**FIGURE 106-4** The Paediatric Sepsis 6. An example of a bundle of care of early actions on suspicion of sepsis. Key elements are the time pressure to complete simple action (antibiotics, oxygen, intravenous or intraosseous access) and the requirement to involve senior staff. Note that uncertainty about a possible sepsis diagnosis requires repeated reassessment. (Reproduced with permission from Paediatric Sepsis 6 version 11.1 August 2015 in collaboration with the UK Sepsis Trust Paediatric Group.)

continued escalation if signs of shock persist. The application of sepsis bundles to guide clinical care is recommended, with the proviso that pediatric presentations, particularly in younger children, can differ from those of adults. However, early intervention and resuscitation, and source control remain the mainstay of the early management of sepsis and the most important determinants of outcome.

## SUGGESTED READINGS

Angus DC, Barnato AE, Bell D, et al. A systematic review and meta-analysis of early goal-directed therapy for septic shock: the ARISE, ProCESS and ProMISe Investigators. *Intensive Care Med.* 2005;41(9):1549-1560.

Brierley J, Thiruchelvam T, Peters MJ. Hemodynamics of early pediatric fluid-resistant septic shock using non-invasive cardiac output (USCOM): Distinct profiles of CVC infection and community acquired sepsis. *Crit Care Med.* 2005;33(12):A153-A153.

Cvetkovic M, Lutman D, Ramnarayan P, Pathan N, Inwald DP, Peters MJ. Timing of death in children referred for intensive care with severe sepsis: implications for interventional studies. *Pediatr Crit Care Med.* 2015;16(5);410-417.

Deep A, Goonasekera CDA, Wang Y, Brierley J. Evolution of haemodynamics and outcome of fluid-refractory septic shock in children. *Intensive Care Med.* 2013;39(9):1602-1609.

Goldstein B, Giroir B, Randolph A. International pediatric sepsis consensus conference: definitions for sepsis and organ dysfunction in pediatrics. *Pediatr Crit Care Med.* 2005;6(1):2-8.

MacLaren G, Butt W, Best D, Donath S, Taylor A. Extracorporeal membrane oxygenation for refractory septic shock in children: one institution's experience. *Pediatr Crit Care Med.* 2007;8(5): 447-451.

Maitland K, Kiguli S, Opoka RO, et al; FEAST Trial Group. Mortality after fluid bolus in African children with severe infection. *N Engl J Med.* 2011;364(26):2483-2495.

National Institute for Health and Care Excellence. Sepsis: recognition, diagnosis and early management. NICE guideline [NG51]. https://www.nice.org.uk/guidance/ng51. Updated July 2016.

Oliveira CF, Oliveira DSF, Gottschald AFC, et al. ACCM/PALS haemodynamic support guidelines for paediatric septic shock: an outcomes comparison with and without monitoring central venous oxygen saturation. *Intensive Care Med.* 2008;34(6):1065-1075.

Samuels M, Wieteska S, eds. *Advanced Paediatric Life Support: A Practical Approach to Emergencies.* 6th ed. Chichester, UK: John Wiley & Sons, Ltd; 2016.

Singer M, Deutschman CS, Seymour CW, et al. The Third International Consensus definitions for sepsis and septic shock (Sepsis-3). *JAMA.* 2016;315(8):801-810.

United Kingdom Sepsis Trust. Paediatric Sepsis 6. http://sepsistrust.org/wp-content/uploads/2015/08/Paediatric-Sepsis-6-version-11_1.pdf. Accessed March 17, 2017.

Ventura AMC, Shieh HH, Bousso A, et al. Double-blind prospective randomized controlled trial of dopamine versus epinephrine as first-line vasoactive drugs in pediatric septic shock. *Crit Care Med.* 2015;43(11):2292-2302.

World Health Organization. Emergency Triage Assessment and Treatment. Geneva, Switzerland: World Health Organization; 2005.



# 107 Cardiogenic Shock

Ronald A. Bronicki and Jack Price

The clinical syndrome of shock has great potential for significant morbidity and mortality and is one of the most challenging conditions to treat. In accordance with Barcroft's original construct for conceptualizing shock that was published nearly 100 years ago, shock results from 1 or more of the following mechanisms: impaired oxygenation or hypoxic hypoxia, reduced oxygen carrying capacity or anemic hypoxia, limited cardiac output or stagnant hypoxia, or impaired oxygen utilization or histotoxic hypoxia (eg, cyanide toxicity). Shock results from inadequate oxygen delivery relative to oxygen demand, and if the body's intrinsic compensatory mechanisms of increased cardiac output and oxygen extraction are insufficient, or left inadequately treated, this can rapidly result in organ dysfunction or failure. The etiologies of shock are broad, as are its manifestations, and in this review we will discuss the pathophysiology, assessment, and treatment of cardiogenic shock.

## PATHOPHYSIOLOGY

Shock results from inadequate oxygen delivery relative to oxygen demand. Shock is not necessarily a problem of blood volume, cardiac output, or blood pressure, but it is always a problem of inadequate tissue oxygen delivery:

$$DO_2 = CaO_2 \times CO,$$

where $DO_2$ is oxygen delivery, $CaO_2$ is arterial oxygen content, and CO is cardiac output.

Cardiogenic shock is due to low cardiac output, the causes of which can be classified according to the determinants of cardiac output: inadequate preload, excessive afterload, intrinsic muscle failure, or dysrhythmia.

## ETIOLOGY

Cardiogenic shock can result from a number of etiologies. Although not an exhaustive list, the most common categories and causes are listed below.

- Undiagnosed (or untreated) critical congenital heart disease: left heart obstructive lesions (critical coarctation, hypoplastic left heart syndrome, aortic stenosis); right heart obstructive lesions (critical pulmonary stenosis or pulmonary atresia); transposition of the great arteries
- Postoperative congenital heart disease: early low output syndrome; residual cardiac defects; late postoperative decompensation due to right, left, or bi-ventricular systolic or diastolic dysfunction; or pulmonary hypertension
- Primary myocardial disease: dilated, restrictive, hypertrophic cardiomyopathies
- Acute myocarditis
- Pericardial disease: acute tamponade or chronic pericardial constriction
- Arrhythmias: chronic untreated or undertreated arrhythmia resulting in cardiomyopathy, also pacemaker-induced cardiomyopathy can result from long term cardiac pacing
- Acute coronary syndromes
- Other etiologies of shock can manifest as cardiogenic shock

## CLINICAL RECOGNITION

The timely recognition of cardiogenic shock requires a high index of suspicion, an appreciation for high-risk groups (eg, patients with known underlying cardiac disease) and a comprehensive consideration of all available information, including the medical history, physical examination, laboratory tests, and hemodynamic parameters.

## HISTORY AND PHYSICAL EXAMINATION

Early markers of cardiogenic shock, from both the history and examination, may be subtle and easily missed or confused with other noncardiac causes of acute illness or shock leading to inappropriate interventions that may worsen the child's clinical condition. The most common misdiagnoses are hypovolemia as the cause for tachycardia (resulting in fluid administration that can lead to further decompensation), or asthma, pneumonia, or a combination leading to the common findings of respiratory distress, wheeze, rales, and clinical signs of lobar collapse.

Cardiogenic shock most typically presents with a history of lethargy, nausea, vomiting, and anorexia in a child, and decreased intake and tiring or sweatiness with feeds in an infant. Caregivers commonly report a history of cough and wheeze and other signs of respiratory distress (eg, tachypnea, labored breathing, grunting respirations, and intercostal and subcostal retractions). There may be a history of weight loss, though fluid retention may in extreme cases falsely counter this observation. A history of wheeze, also resulting from pulmonary edema, is very common in children with cardiogenic shock, and this finding may misdirect the unsuspecting clinician to an algorithm that involves the management of primary respiratory rather than cardiac disease. Examination may reveal a sternotomy or thoracotomy from previous cardiac surgery. On auscultation, there may be also be widespread crackles resulting from cardiogenic pulmonary edema, or reduced air entry to the left lung resulting from collapse of the lower lobe due to cardiomegaly. Tachycardia and a gallop may also be present, and there may be absent or diminished lower limb pulses raising the possibility of a coarctation of the aorta. Common abdominal findings include hepatomegaly and abdominal tenderness resulting from hepatic congestion. Decreased mentation, irritability, or altered mental status are late and ominous findings in patients with cardiogenic shock, suggestive of cerebral hypoperfusion. The perfusion exam may be abnormal and consist of decreased peripheral pulses, prolonged capillary refill and cool extremities. While the perfusion exam is an integral part of the assessment of any patient, it does have significant limitations, including a lack of correlation with measured hemodynamic indices such as cardiac output and systemic vascular resistance. Nonetheless, with this limitation in mind, it is essential to establish a baseline assessment of perfusion and to perform serial examinations in order to assess the response to interventions and for determining the clinical trajectory.

## HEMODYNAMIC MONITORING

Tachycardia is very common in patients with cardiogenic shock, and while this is most often a compensatory sinus tachycardia, it may also be an arrhythmia (supraventricular tachycardia, atrial flutter, or ectopic atrial tachycardia being most common, though ventricular tachycardia should also be excluded). Electrocardiogram (ECG) monitoring including a 12-lead should be routinely performed as soon as these are available. Patients may present with hypotension, so-called decompensated shock; however, it is not uncommon for the patient with cardiogenic shock to present with a normal if not elevated blood pressure due to a compensatory increase in systemic vascular resistance. Venous access should be established early in patients with cardiogenic shock, and when possible, central venous access should be obtained to assist with resuscitation as well as measurement of the central venous pressure (CVP) and central or mixed venous oxygen saturations ($SVO_2$). The CVP measures the right ventricular filling pressure and gives some indication of intravascular volume status and cardiac function. The CVP is often elevated in patients presenting with cardiogenic shock. The $SVO_2$ (normally 75% or greater) is an indirect measure of adequacy of cardiac output and status of tissue oxygen extraction, and a lower $SvO_2$ indicates higher oxygen extraction and therefore more precarious circulatory status.

## LABORATORY EVALUATION

All critically ill patients should have a comprehensive chemistry panel. Patients presenting with cardiogenic shock and acute kidney injury may initially have a normal serum creatinine, as changes in serum creatinine lag behind the acute insult and actual decrement in glomerular filtration rate. Indicators of hepatocellular injury, such as elevated transaminases, while not specific for hepatic injury may be elevated in a shock state. Similarly, in shock, the endothelium is activated, resulting in a prothrombotic phenotype and a consumptive coagulopathy. Hypocalcemia may be the cause of or contribute to the development of myocardial dysfunction. Other electrolyte abnormalities that may contribute to cardiac dysfunction include disturbances in potassium, magnesium, and phosphorous homeostasis. An arterial blood gas is indicated in the management of critically ill patients, allowing for the assessment of gas exchange, acid–base balance and serum lactate. An elevated anion gap may be an indication of a lactic acidosis and shock state, whereas a nonanion gap acidosis is generally due to a loss of bicarbonate or excessive chloride administration (due to diarrhea or renal tubular acidosis, or following volume expansion with normal saline). The anion gap is calculated as shown below:

$$([Na^+] + [K^+]) - ([HCO_3^-] + [Cl^-]), \text{ normally } 8\text{–}16 \text{ mmol/L}$$

It may seem evident, but it cannot be overemphasized that a patient with a normal lactate level may be in a state of impending shock. The use of venous oximetry and near infrared spectroscopy (NIRS) to assess the extent of oxygen extraction can help in providing a more timely assessment of impending and existing shock than a lactate level alone.

In the intubated patient, capnography (end-tidal carbon dioxide [$CO_2$] monitoring) should be used. In the absence of a significant leak, a normal arterial-to-end-tidal $CO_2$ gradient is consistent with hypoventilation (ie, gradient < 3–5 mm Hg), and an elevated gradient is due to wasted (or dead space) ventilation. A large gradient, indicative of a very low or zero end-tidal $CO_2$, is seen in patients with limited pulmonary perfusion or in cardiac arrest, and end-tidal $CO_2$ monitoring may be used to assess the effectiveness of chest compressions during cardiopulmonary resuscitation and the return of spontaneous circulation, which are indicated by an increase in end-tidal $CO_2$ and a narrowing arterial-to-end-tidal difference.

Serum troponin levels may provide some indication of the cause and severity of myocardial injury, and serial levels will indicate time course of an underlying insult, particularly if it is ischemic. Certain subtypes of troponin (I and T) are very sensitive and are specific biomarkers of the cardiomyocyte, and may be elevated due to hypoxic–ischemic injury, myocarditis/inflammatory processes, and trauma, and following cardiac surgery. Elevations in troponin are also seen in severe sepsis and pericarditis. Finally, the B-type natriuretic peptide (BNP), which is indicative of cardiac distension, is a useful biomarker in the presence of cardiogenic shock. While this cannot distinguish among the multitudes of underlying pathophysiologies, it can provide a surrogate for the progression of the clinical course.

### Ancillary Investigations

**Chest Radiograph** A chest radiograph typically shows cardiomegaly and may also provide additional information, such as congenital heart disease, that may contribute to the diagnosis. Pulmonary edema may be present and is typically limited to the interstitium, and thus oxygenation is minimally if at all impacted. In more severe cases, alveolar edema is present, in which case oxygenation is impaired. Importantly, the chest radiograph will help to distinguish primary respiratory from cardiac disease. It is important to appreciate that, in longstanding heart failure, chronic pulmonary venous hypertension leads to functional and structural adaptive changes within the lung, and interstitial edema may be absent or minimal despite the presence of significant heart failure. The accumulation of interstitial edema in the bronchovascular sheath may compress small airways, leading to airway obstruction, hyperinflation, and flattened diaphragms.

**Echocardiography** An echocardiogram should be obtained in any child presenting with cardiogenic shock, or in a situation in which it may be in the differential diagnosis. This will be key to distinguish between systolic and diastolic disease, assess for pericardial fluid and tamponade, and in the diagnosis of any structural heart disease or residual defects in children with operated congenital heart disease. Additionally, echocardiography can be used to assess the degree of dysfunction and also may help assess response to therapy. It is important to note, however, that symptomatic improvement typically predates objective echocardiographic improvement, and indeed the latter may never normalize despite the child returning to baseline after appropriate interventions.

## PRINCIPLES OF MEDICAL MANAGEMENT: OPTIMIZING THE RELATIONSHIP BETWEEN OXYGEN DELIVERY AND CONSUMPTION

For patients at risk for or in a state of shock, all strategies that optimize the relationship between oxygen delivery and demand should be considered. These include adequate hemoglobin (to maximize the oxygen carrying capacity and delivery) as well as other measures that target intravascular volume, contractility, and loading conditions to optimize cardiac output. Strategies that minimize oxygen consumption should also be considered and include mechanical ventilation, elimination of anxiety with sedation, and the avoidance of hyperthermia, as elevated body temperature increases the metabolic rate and therefore global oxygen demand.

### The Role of Mechanical Ventilation

While under normal conditions, the respiratory pump consumes less than 3% of total body oxygen consumption and receives less than 5% of total CO, in patients with cardiogenic shock, the diaphragmatic oxygen demands alone may increase to 50% of total cardiac output. Thus, one of the basic tenets of managing a critically ill patient in an impending or existing shock state is to mechanically unload the respiratory pump, allowing for a redistribution of a limited CO to other vital organs, including the brain. This may be accomplished with noninvasive continuous or bi-level positive airway pressure (CPAP or BiPAP, respectively) or invasively with endotracheal positive pressure ventilation. An additional benefit of positive airway pressure and the resulting increase in intrathoracic pressure is that it "mechanically" unloads the left ventricle by creating a pressure gradient between intra- and extrathoracic arterial vessels. Furthermore, mechanical ventilation eliminates labored breathing, and in doing so leads to a partial withdrawal of adrenergic activity and the associated increase in systemic vascular resistance, contributing to a reduction in left ventricular afterload, which is particularly beneficial to patients with left ventricular systolic failure.

#### Determinants of Preload and Afterload and Their Pharmacological Manipulation

The optimal management of the patient in impending or existing cardiogenic shock requires a thorough understanding of circulatory physiology and determinants of cardiac output, the pathophysiology of cardiogenic shock, an assessment and determination of each patient's hemodynamic profile, and the careful selection of vasoactive agents that are best suited for each patient.

Systemic venous return, which is a determinant of right heart filling or preload, results from the pressure gradient between the systemic venous reservoirs (the mean systemic pressure) and the right atrium. Increased intravascular volume increases the mean systemic venous pressure, systemic venous return, right atrial pressure, right ventricular diastolic pressure (ie, filling pressure), and ultimately right ventricular diastolic volume (ie, preload). Venoconstrictors increase systemic venous return by decreasing venous capacitance and increasing the mean systemic pressure, whereas venodilators decrease the effective intravascular volume by increasing venous capacitance and sequestering intravascular volume within the venous reservoirs. A diuretic such as furosemide decreases the mean systemic pressure acutely by inducing venodilation and over time by decreasing intravascular volume.

Impaired systolic ventricular function leads to increased sensitivity to changes in afterload. Ventricular afterload may be reduced pharmacologically by arterial vasodilators, or mechanically (eg, positive pressure ventilation). Arterial vasodilators decrease vascular impedance, increasing stroke volume and cardiac output and reducing end-systolic volume but have no appreciable effect on preload or ventricular filling pressures. Inotropes increase stroke volume and cardiac output by augmenting contractility without changing filling pressures, and almost all inotropes produce a dose-dependent increase the heart rate that may actually contribute to an increase in cardiac output. However, tachycardia can also increase myocardial oxygen consumption and may compromise coronary filling, as well as increasing the risk of tachyarrhythmias, all of which can further exacerbate the depressed stroke volume and cardiac output.

Vasodilators, inotropes, inodilators, and diuretics are in an important minority. Prostaglandins are the mainstay of pharmacological management of cardiogenic shock. While deciding the optimal approach to vasoactive therapy, it is essential to have a clear understanding of the underlying etiology and pathophysiology, and of the desirable and unwanted effects of potential agents. The vasoactive management of a ductal-dependent lesion presenting with cardiogenic shock would be completely different to that of a child presenting with acute myocarditis. Another example would be the almost contradictory management approaches for acute or end-stage systolic vs diastolic heart failure. The mechanisms of action of specific pharmacological agents are discussed in detail in Chapter 111.

#### Intravascular Volume

In patients with cardiac dysfunction/failure, an understanding of the nature of the dysfunction (ie, systolic vs diastolic) as well as a determination of the optimal ventricular filling pressure are indicated because ventricular compliance (the relationship between pressure and volume

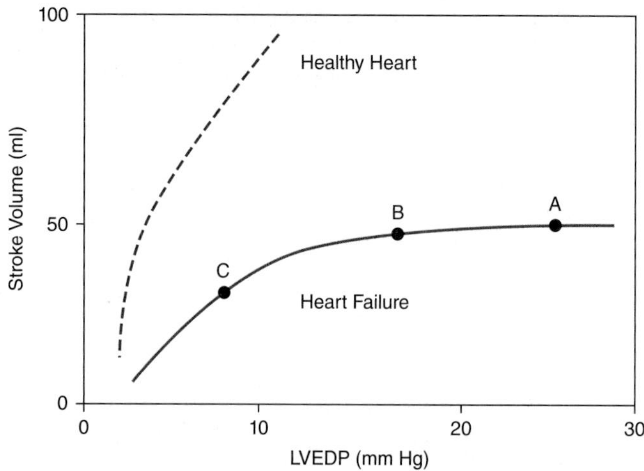


**FIGURE 107-1** Relationship between left ventricular end-diastolic pressure (LVEDP) and stroke volume (SV) in the healthy and failing heart.

for a distensible structure) is highly variable and what generates stroke volume is not the diastolic pressure per se but rather the extent to which the myocardium is stretched (ie, ventricular end diastolic *volume*). Further confounding the interpretation of the CVP is the fact that in the presence of cardiac and or pulmonary disease there may be only limited correlation between the CVP/right ventricular diastolic pressure and left ventricular diastolic pressure. By using a CVP, or in some postoperative patients a left atrial pressure, the optimal ventricular filling pressure can be determined by administering volume and monitoring the hemodynamic response. A favorable response is objectively reflected in a prompt rise in arterial blood pressure and fall in heart rate (ie, preload reserve is present). With a favorable response. it can be inferred that the ventricle is positioned on the ascending portion of its pressure–stroke volume curve (Fig. 107-1). A lack of response is consistent with the ventricle residing on the flat portion, or even on a potential downturn of its pressure–stroke volume curve (ie, preload reserve has been exhausted), in which case inotropy and/or afterload-reducing therapies are indicated to improve cardiac output. Diuretics and/or venodilators may be prudent in order to decrease systemic venous return and ventricular filling pressures (ie, preload), ameliorating pulmonary and systemic venous congestion.

Unlike in patients with systolic dysfunction, volume expansion may be indicated in patients with ventricular diastolic dysfunction/decreased ventricular compliance where an elevated ventricular filling pressure is needed in order to adequately generate sufficient diastolic filling to produce an adequate stroke volume. Significant diastolic dysfunction/decreased ventricular compliance is seen in patients with ventricular hypertrophy (eg, resulting from an obstructive lesion, such as semilunar valve stenosis or systemic hypertension, and hypertrophic cardiomyopathy) and restrictive cardiomyopathy, and in some patients after right heart surgery or following the Fontan procedure. The extent to which a pericardial effusion impacts ventricular compliance and filling depends on the amount and rate of fluid accumulation. With time, the compliance of the pericardium increases, allowing for a greater amount of fluid accumulation without necessarily a commensurate increase in pressure. In any case, once stroke volume and CO begin to wane, the situation becomes urgent, as the ventricle is now operating on the steep portion of its pressure–volume (compliance) curve. Volume is indicated as a temporizing measure until the fluid can be removed.

#### Mechanical Circulatory Support

In patients with cardiogenic shock in whom conventional medical management has failed, those who are rapidly decompensating, and those in whom definitive surgical management is not part of the early treatment algorithm, mechanical cardiac support—either extracorporeal membrane oxygenation (ECMO) or a ventricular assist device (VAD)—should be considered (see Chapter 108). Both ECMO and VAD provide temporary circulatory support, ensuring adequate systemic oxygen delivery and end-organ perfusion while minimizing myocardial oxygen consumption. Both ECMO and VAD support allow the myocardium a period of rest and recovery, and in some cases provide a window of stability for further diagnostic assessment.

#### Special Considerations for Infants

When managing cardiogenic shock, it is important to remember that infants have less cardiopulmonary reserve than do children and adults, which is an important consideration that cannot be overemphasized. The cardiomyocyte of the newborn/infant possesses relatively few, poorly organized contractile proteins, and the immature sarcoplasmic reticulum leads to inefficient calcium handling. As a result, the myocardium is less responsive to fluid and inotropes, and is more susceptible to increases in afterload. The mechanics of the lungs, chest wall, and diaphragm are also immature, with more chest wall compliance and reduced diaphragmatic contractile reserve, resulting in higher oxygen consumption by the respiratory unit in health. This is significantly exaggerated in the presence of cardiogenic shock which is characterized by tachypnea and increased respiratory effort.

## TARGETED MANAGEMENT OF CARDIOGENIC SHOCK

#### Systolic Heart Failure

The optimal first-line strategy for treating systolic heart failure is to alter ventricular loading conditions, resulting in the desired hemodynamic effects of an increase in stroke volume and cardiac output without any unwanted effects on myocardial oxygen delivery and demand. This is typically achieved with a combination of vasodilators or inodilators and diuretics, and on occasions, the careful use of inotropes, in order both to reduce load and to improve contractility. When selecting the right agent or agents, it is important to focus on the desirable and unwanted effects that are often dose dependent, as well as the onset and duration of action and half-life of agents. A note of caution should also be introduced for drugs with a longer half-life, such as milrinone, which is commonly used to support patients in established end-stage heart failure. Milrinone is an ideal drug in terms of its hemodynamic effects that combine vasodilation with improved diastolic performance and some improvement in contractility, but its vasodilator effects may manifest with hypotension in an already marginal patient with acute cardiogenic shock. Unlike many other vasoactive agents, milrinone has a relatively long half-life, further prolonging its effects in the presence of renal dysfunction, which often coexists in patients with cardiogenic shock. As an alternative, in the acute phase where hypotension is present or may be manifested with vasodilation, epinephrine in low doses provides some afterload reduction while providing significantly greater inotropic support than dobutamine, dopamine, or milrinone. It may be prudent to initiate therapy with epinephrine in order to establish the desired clinical trajectory with the subsequent addition of or transition to vasodilators or inodilators.

#### Diastolic Heart Failure

Diastolic heart failure is characterized by a low stroke volume and cardiac output that is due to inadequate ventricular filling despite an elevated ventricular end diastolic pressure. As discussed, determining the optimal filling pressure (adequate preload) is essential. In these patients, diuretics and vasodilators will reduce the systemic venous return and decrease pulmonary venous pressure and the formation of pulmonary edema, but may compromise stroke volume and cardiac output by reducing filling. In the absence of systolic dysfunction, inotropes are generally deleterious, as they typically cause an increase in heart rate, which may compromise ventricular filling while increasing myocardial oxygen consumption and the propensity for developing tachyarrhythmias. In general, the primary approach in this setting is careful support of intravascular volume and control of heart rate.

#### Postoperative Cardiac Dysfunction

There are several intraoperative factors that may contribute to postoperative cardiovascular dysfunction after cardiopulmonary bypass. The systemic inflammatory response to cardiopulmonary bypass and myocardial ischemia reperfusion injury can lead to elevated systemic vascular resistance and left ventricular afterload as well as myocardial systolic and diastolic dysfunction. Furthermore, pulmonary ischemia reperfusion injury leads to pulmonary endothelial dysfunction and heightened pulmonary vascular reactivity and elevated right ventricular afterload. Similarly, neurohormonal activation is often present postoperatively, contributing to increases in left ventricular afterload, which may compromise cardiac output and systemic oxygen delivery if left ventricular systolic function is impaired.

#### Congenital Heart Disease

Cardiogenic shock may be the presenting feature of several types of unoperated congenital heart diseases, regardless of ventricular function. Important examples that merit discussion are ductal-dependent lesions with obstruction to systemic or pulmonary blood flow. In any critically ill–appearing newborn with or without cyanosis, a ductal-dependent lesion should be considered and prostaglandin $E_1$ ($PGE_1$) should be initiated without delay if it is in the differential diagnosis. Maintaining patency of the ductus is essential for systemic perfusion in newborns with left-sided obstructive lesions, or for maintaining pulmonary perfusion in newborns with right-sided obstructive lesions. Prostaglandin $E_1$ may also be indicated in transposition of the great arteries to provide adequate intercirculatory mixing. Important dose-dependent side effects include apnea, irritability, fever, and hypotension. Additional vasoactive agents may be indicated to provide further afterload reduction or inotropic support during the resuscitative and perioperative periods.

In newborns with single ventricle physiology, the systemic and pulmonary circulations are in parallel, with the respective vascular resistances determining the distribution of cardiac output to the systemic and pulmonary circulations. These infants are at significant risk of cardiogenic shock due to systemic hypoperfusion (and often, pulmonary overcirculation). Optimization of systemic perfusion in these precarious patients can be achieved by avoiding factors that excessively dilate the pulmonary vasculature (eg, hyperoxia, alkalosis, and hypocarbia) as well as careful control of afterload on the systemic ventricle. Achieving this critical balance requires meticulous attention to ventilation, with very careful use of systemic vasodilators, inodilators, or very low doses of epinephrine.

**Critical Aortic Stenosis** Critical aortic stenosis is characterized by afterload-induced heart failure, with neurohormonal activation, and typically presents in the newborn period as cardiogenic shock with pallor, globally diminished pulses, end-organ dysfunction, and acidosis. For these patients, the therapy of choice is to urgently address the obstruction through the surgical or transcatheter approach. The clinical condition can be temporarily ameliorated through mechanical ventilation (to reduce afterload as well as the work of breathing) and the very careful use of short-acting vasodilators or inodilators, or very-low-dose inotropes and diuretics. Additionally, it is worthwhile considering maintaining ductal patency with $PGE_1$. In this situation, the addition of $PGE_1$ provides increased systemic perfusion (with deoxygenated blood) through a right-to-left ductal shunt.

**Severe Aortic and Mitral Regurgitation** Heart failure due to mitral and/or aortic regurgitation is associated with marked activation of neurohormonal pathways and elevations in systemic vascular resistance. In these situations, the careful use of a combined veno- and arterial vasodilator, such as nitroprusside, has been shown to provide significant acute hemodynamic benefit by increasing the forward stroke volume while reducing ventricular filling pressures. Aortic regurgitation causes diastolic hypotension that falls further with afterload reduction, which may compromise coronary perfusion. Nonetheless, the fall in diastolic pressure appears to be well tolerated, as the relationship between myocardial oxygen delivery and demand improves substantially as a result of a significant increase in forward stroke volume and a reduction in ventricular diastolic and systolic loads. Inotropes with afterload-reducing properties may also provide significant hemodynamic benefit.

## CONCLUSION

An understanding of the pathophysiology of cardiogenic shock, circulatory physiology, and therapeutic strategies that improve the relationship between global and myocardial oxygen supply and demand are necessary for optimizing the outcomes of patients at risk for or in a state of shock. Essential to this exercise is the timely and accurate assessment of cardiac function, cardiac output, and tissue oxygenation.

## SUGGESTED READINGS

Artman M, Graham TP Jr. Guidelines for vasodilator therapy of congestive heart failure in infants and children. *Am Heart J.* 1987; 113(4):994-1005.

Blatchford JW 3rd, Barragy TP, Lillehei TJ, Ring WS. The effects of cardioplegic arrest on left ventricular systolic and diastolic function of the intact neonatal heart. *J Thorac Cardiovasc Surg.* 1994;107(2): 527-535.

Bronicki RA. Shock states. In: Perkin R, Anas N, Swift J, eds. *Pediatric Hospital Medicine.* 1st ed. Philadelphia, PA: Lippincott Williams & Wilkins; 2007:192-208.

Bronicki RA, Anas NG. Cardiopulmonary interaction. *Pediatr Crit Care Med.* 2009;10(3):313-322.

Chaturvedi RR, Herron T, Simmons R, et al, Passive stiffness of myocardium from congenital heart disease and implications for diastole. *Circulation.* 2010;121(8):979-988.

Graham Jr, TP. Ventricular performance in congenital heart disease. *Circulation.* 1991;84(6):2259-2274.

Hoffman GM, Tweddell JS, Ghanayem NS, et al. Alteration of the critical arteriovenous oxygen saturation relationship by sustained afterload reduction after the Norwood procedure. *J Thorac Cardiovasc Surg.* 2004;127(3):738-745.

Nichols DG. Respiratory muscle performance in infants and children. *J Pediatr.* 1991;118(4 Pt 1):493-502.

Reddy VM, Liddicoat JR, McElhinney DB, et al. Hemodynamic effects of epinephrine, bicarbonate and calcium in the early postnatal period in a lamb model of single-ventricle physiology created in utero. *J Am Coll Cardiol.* 1996;28(7):1877-1883.

Romero T, Friedman WF. Limited left ventricular response to volume overload in the neonatal period: a comparative study with the adult animal. *Pediat Res.* 1979;13(8):910-915.

Roussos C, Macklem PT. The respiratory muscles. *New Engl J Med.* 1982;307(30):786-797.

Viires N, Sillye G, Aubier M, Rassidakis A, Roussos C. Regional blood flow distribution in dog during induced hypotension and low cardiac output. *J Clin Invest.* 1983;72(3):935-947.



# 108 Extracorporeal Membrane Oxygenation

Patricia Bastero and James A. Thomas

## BACKGROUND

Extracorporeal membrane oxygenation (ECMO) is used to provide temporary mechanical support for severe cardiac, respiratory, or cardiorespiratory failure that is unresponsive to conventional therapies. While the principles of ECMO and cardiopulmonary bypass are similar in that they both support the cardiorespiratory system, ECMO is a bedside technology in the ICU that is used for much longer periods of support, and ideally should be a less complex and invasive procedure in terms of cannulation and perfusion techniques, durability of equipment, patient monitoring, and troubleshooting. ECMO cannulation is ideally extrathoracic (although for cardiac ECMO, direct cardiac cannulation is often used), and the miniaturized circuitry efficiently pumps blood through the extracorporeal circuit and provides excellent gas exchange through the membrane oxygenator, while minimizing complications of red cell trauma, embolization, clot, and mechanical failure.

The first reported successful outcome of ECMO support in the ICU was in 1971, in an adult trauma victim with severe acute respiratory distress syndrome who was supported for 75 hours on a custom-built ECMO circuit. Perhaps the most famous "first" in the history of ECMO was in 1975, when a newborn girl named Esperanza, who was dying of meconium aspiration syndrome, was rescued with the assistance of a research ECMO circuit. Esperanza (meaning *hope* in Spanish) became the symbol of the promise of this new therapy.

During the 1970s, there were a number of reports of the anecdotal use of ECMO in adults, in individual patients or small cohorts with variable outcomes, and then in 1979, a single randomized clinical trial from Zapol and colleagues demonstrated no benefit from ECMO over conventional treatment. ECMO was largely abandoned in adults for the next 2 decades.

The early pediatric and neonatal experience was different, and as a result of small but encouraging trials in neonates and children, pediatricians and pediatric surgical specialists continued to develop ECMO. The landmark UK Collaborative ECMO Trial in the early 1990s demonstrated improved survival in newborns with hypoxemic respiratory failure randomized for ECMO support compared to conventional therapy. The worldwide use of ECMO for neonatal acute hypoxemic respiratory failure continued to increase until the mid-1990s, with a decline over the past decade. The use of cardiac ECMO however began to take off in the late 1990s, and continues. The pandemic H1N1 influenza outbreak of 2009 resulted in a rapid surge in the international experience with ECMO to support respiratory failure in adults with encouraging outcomes reported at experienced ECMO centers in Australia, New Zealand, and the United Kingdom. Since then, the numbers of adults cannulated for ECMO has overtaken the annual number of pediatric (non-neonatal) cases worldwide. To date, since its inception in the mid-1980s, the Extracorporeal Life Support Organization (ELSO) registry (a voluntary international registry for pediatric and adult ECMO centers) reports more than 78 000 ECMO cases, with annual adult cardiac and respiratory ECMO numbers now exceeding their pediatric counterparts.

## OVERALL GOALS OF ECMO

ECMO is a supportive, not curative, therapy, and offers a period of rest and recovery of the failing heart and/or lungs, and an opportunity for underlying diseases to be treated. Additionally, the initiation of ECMO should prompt a thorough reappraisal of the patient's illness, aggressive diagnostic clarification, and implementation of a comprehensive treatment plan that will (1) help reverse the disease, and (2) maximize the patient's chances of weaning from ECMO. Often before cannulation, ECMO patients are so unstable and are treated empirically without a full diagnostic workup. ECMO provides a relative physiologic stability that enables further evaluation using imaging techniques (eg, computed tomography [CT], echocardiography [echo], angiography), lung biopsy, or other interventions as needed, which then help inform prognosis and guide therapy.

The physiologic goals of ECMO are straightforward. ECMO must provide oxygenation and $CO_2$ removal and must adequately support the cardiac output and satisfy systemic oxygen delivery as needed. Current generation ECMO oxygenators are highly efficient at achieving gas exchange, as long as blood flow is adequate, and most ECMO pumps can provide supranormal blood flow that is fast enough to satisfy even the highest metabolic demands, such as in the setting of septic shock.

Most patients are cannulated for ECMO because they have a reversible condition and for these patients, ECMO serves as a "bridge to recovery." Patients with acute hypoxemic respiratory failure with ARDS, or those with post-cardiopulmonary bypass myocardial stun are examples of common indications for ECMO in whom a period of organ rest is expected to be followed by recovery. Other patients are cannulated with the goal of supporting them until a transplantable organ (eg, lung or heart) or long term mechanical device (eg, ventricular assist device) can be placed. The therapeutic goal of ECMO for these patients is often referred to as "bridge to transplant," "bridge to device," or "bridge to decision."

## THE PHYSIOLOGY OF ECMO SUPPORT

ECMO, regardless of the mode, involves drainage of systemic venous blood to an external oxygenator that performs $CO_2$ removal and oxygenation, with subsequent delivery of oxygenated blood to the patient. While providing cardiorespiratory support, the introduction of the ECMO circuit inevitably disrupts the body's natural equilibrium. This happens through a number of mechanisms. First, there is a need for active anticoagulation to prevent thrombosis caused by blood exposure to artificial surfaces. Second, the blood must be warmed in the extracorporeal circuit. Third, the contact of blood with exogenous surfaces and circuitry leads to an inflammatory response akin to the systemic inflammatory response. Last, in some cases, ECMO provides a portal for other physiology-altering therapies, such as continuous renal replacement therapy or plasmapheresis.

### Carbon Dioxide Clearance

Carbon dioxide exchange depends on the gradient between the partial pressures of $CO_2$ ($PCO_2$) on either side of the membrane: the blood (venous) phase (PvCO2) versus gas phase ($PgpCO_2$), as well as the overall membrane surface area, the material and geometry of the membrane, and the gas flow rate through it. The gas that flows through the oxygenator, known as the *sweep gas*, has a $PCO_2$ of 0 mmHg. Since the oxygenator surface area, material, and geometry are fixed, the sweep gas controls $CO_2$ elimination, and the higher the sweep is, the greater the $CO_2$ removal is.

### Oxygenation

Oxygen exchange depends on the gradient of $O_2$ partial pressures between the gas ($PgpO_2$) and blood ($PvO_2$) phases in the oxygenator, the surface area, and the $O_2$ permeability of the membrane, as well as the $O_2$ diffusion capacity in blood. The sweep fraction of inspired oxygen ($FiO_2$) determines the $PO_2$ gradient in the oxygenator, and sweep flow rate has little impact on blood oxygenation (except at the lowest sweep flow rates). Oxygenation determines the total $O_2$ content of blood ($CaO_2$), which itself depends on red blood cell (RBC) hemoglobin concentration and $O_2$ saturation.

### Oxygen Delivery

Tissue oxygen delivery ($DO_2$) is a function of both blood $O_2$ content ($CaO_2$) and cardiac output (CO). The extracorporeal circuit generates continuous nonpulsatile flow, but the net circulatory support is very different depending on the mode of ECMO. The circulatory contribution of venovenous (VV) ECMO is in general secondary to the improvements in oxygenation of pulmonary and systemic blood, cardiopulmonary interactions due to reduced ventilatory settings, and right ventricular afterload on cardiac function. In contrast, venoarterial (VA) ECMO can support some or all of the cardiac output, or in some cases can provide even supranormal circulatory support depending on the flows and underlying condition. At higher flow rates, more blood is directed through the extracorporeal circuit and diverted from the native heart resulting in less pulsatility, as evidenced on the pulse contour of the arterial blood pressure trace.

## MODES OF ECMO SUPPORT

The site of post-oxygenator blood return (vein, atrium, artery) determines the ECMO mode: thus for VV ECMO, oxygenated blood is returned to the systemic venous system (central vein or right atrium), and for VA ECMO, oxygenated blood is returned to the systemic arterial system (aorta, carotid artery, or femoral artery). Both modes involve drainage of systemic venous blood from large central veins or the right atrium. VA ECMO provides full or partial cardiopulmonary support for cardiac, respiratory, or cardiorespiratory failure, whereas VV ECMO primarily provides respiratory support with some secondary beneficial circulatory effects for patients with severe hypoxemic and/or hypercarbic respiratory failure.

### Venovenous ECMO support

**Indications** In general, VV ECMO is indicated for single organ (respiratory) failure, for pulmonary hypertension in the newborn, or in multisystem diseases with associated respiratory failure where cardiac function is relatively preserved. The list of conditions that can be supported with VV ECMO is extensive and continues to grow (Table 108-1), and this is due to many factors, including increased familiarity with the therapy, potential for rehabilitation on ECMO, and a readiness to offer longer ECMO runs (often exceeding 3–4 weeks) with a low complication rate in order to offer a realistic chance of lung recovery. Over the past decade there has been a philosophical shift in considering ECMO as a more standard therapy, which may be preferable to aggressive and potentially destructive ventilator strategies, rather than one of last resort.

**TABLE 108-1 COMMON INDICATIONS FOR VENOVENOUS ECMO**

| Isolated Respiratory Disease | Multisystem Disease with Respiratory Failure |
|---|---|
| Pneumonia (viral, bacterial, aspiration) | Congenital diaphragmatic hernia |
| Acute lung injury/ARDS | Meconium aspiration syndrome with PPHN |
| Status asthmaticus | Neonatal sepsis with PPHN |
| Sickle cell acute chest syndrome | Pulmonary embolism |
| Air leak syndromes | Primary or secondary pulmonary hypertension |
| Pulmonary interstitial disease | Sepsis with hypoxemic respiratory failure |
| Airway obstruction by foreign body | Malignancy with respiratory failure |
| Mediastinal mass (extrinsic obstruction) | |
| Blunt/penetrating thoracic trauma | |

ARDS, acute respiratory distress syndrome; ECMO, extracorporeal membrane oxygenation; PPHN, persistent pulmonary hypertension of the newborn.

**Cannulation** Cannulation location and type are determined by patient factors as well as by institutional practice and preference for cannula type. Anatomic considerations include apparent vessel sizes and courses (assessed by precannulation imaging), presence of adjacent stomata or injuries that might contaminate a cannulation site, and likelihood of the need for patient mobility while on ECMO support. VV ECMO support can be achieved using 2 separate cannulae: 1 for drainage that is typically introduced to the femoral vein with the tip lying in the inferior vena cava, and a separate return cannula typically introduced to the jugular vein with the tip in the right atrium. Alternatively, a double-lumen cannula can be used that has the advantage of only using a single site, typically the internal jugular or subclavian vein. While more convenient, double-lumen VV cannulae are more challenging to position optimally, with not only the cannula tip but the orientation being important determinants of successful support. They can also be flow limited, particularly by venous drainage at higher flow rates.

**Management Goals** VV ECMO management revolves around ensuring adequate tissue $O_2$ delivery and *adequate* and *appropriate* respiratory support, while of course providing meticulous general intensive care with careful attention to fluid balance, nutrition, sedation toxicity, infection control, and patient positioning, and providing physical rehabilitation as appropriate. Determining adequate tissue oxygenation in patients is an inexact science, but most intensivists have developed a sense of sufficiency using clinical and laboratory markers. Since tissue $O_2$ delivery depends on adequate hemoglobin concentration, arterial $O_2$ saturation, and cardiac output, these must be constantly assessed. For most VV ECMO patients, hemoglobin concentrations of 10 to 12 g/dL with $SaO_2$ in the 75% to 80% range are adequate. The reason for targeting (or accepting) lower saturations is that they are generally adequate to meet the body's metabolic demands, and given that the oxygenated blood is returned to the right (not the left) side of the heart and that lung injury is severe in the early phase, higher saturations are often unachievable.

Without direct invasive measurement, the assessment of cardiac output is imprecise, but a combination of poor pulses, cool distal extremities, low mixed venous saturations, rising lactate concentrations, and declining near-infrared spectroscopy saturation trends may point to inadequate tissue oxygenation and inadequate cardiac output. The causes may be related to the adequacy of the ECMO support, and if such a situation arises acutely, it is essential to look for other contributory factors including sepsis, bleeding, tachycardia, or cardiac dysfunction, as well as mechanical reasons. In order to better support the cardiac output on VV ECMO, assuming that any acute mechanical issues have been ruled out, the options are to introduce inotropes and/or vasodilators to support the heart, or to convert to VA ECMO.

A factor that may have contributed to the dismal results of early ECMO trials in adults was that aggressive ventilation was often continued after cannulation. This practice gave way to the notion of *rest settings*, which are typically much lower than precannulation settings but aim to maintain lung inflation with a positive mean airway pressure, thus avoiding complete atelectasis. Some adult and pediatric centers have explored extubating VV ECMO patients, which also provides the potential advantage of avoidance of ongoing sedation, thus enabling some rehabilitation and spontaneous airway clearance while on ECMO.

**Duration of Support** The anticipated duration of VV ECMO support will be related to the underlying disease. Typically, the duration is 1 to 3 days for pediatric asthma, less than 7 days for newborns with acute hypoxemic respiratory failure and pulmonary hypertension (eg, meconium aspiration), 10 to 14 days for congenital diaphragmatic hernia, and significantly longer—up to several weeks—for other pediatric respiratory indications (eg, infective, parenchymal, or interstitial).

**Weaning** The actual practice of weaning a patient from VV ECMO is relatively straightforward, assuming that it is being done in a controlled, planned manner. More challenging is the timing of the decision of *when* to wean, and *what are the respiratory goals* for the transition off circuit. In some cases (eg, when a patient is having uncontrolled bleeding), the respiratory goal will have to be any ventilator settings that can keep a patient alive, including advanced strategies and the use of nitric oxide. Ideally however, intensivists will time the weaning based upon clinical and radiological signs of pulmonary improvement (eg, chest x-ray, tidal volumes, improving oxygen saturations, and good $CO_2$ clearance on reduced or no sweep gas flow). Most patients will transition from ECMO to low levels of positive pressure ventilation if still intubated on ECMO, and those that have been extubated on ECMO would generally be decannulated on noninvasive respiratory support.

An advantage of VV over VA ECMO is that a clinical trial off ECMO can be done with the circuit flowing and cannulae in position for any period of time, by disconnecting the sweep gas and capping the oxygenator, allowing the blood and gas phases inside to equilibrate over the course of 30 to 60 minutes, with ventilator or respiratory support being titrated according to the patient's blood gases. If the support required with the oxygenator capped is on target, generally after a trial of at least 2 to 4 hours, the ECMO cannulae are removed. If the patient's ventilator support requirements exceed the desired target, decannulation is postponed until a successful trial off is achieved.

**Outcomes** Survival following VV ECMO varies according to the underlying pathology. For Neonatal respiratory ECMO, according to the ELSO registry 2015 International Summary, cumulative survival-to-discharge rates range from 75% to 84%, being highest among those patients cannulated for meconium aspiration syndrome (90%) and respiratory distress syndrome (84%) and lowest among those with congenital diaphragmatic hernia (51%). Beyond the neonatal period, survival is lower but closely grouped among all VV ECMO categories, between 64% and 69%. Highest survival rates occurred in patients cannulated for aspiration pneumonia (68%) and viral pneumonias (65%) and lowest for *Pneumocystis* pneumonia (51%). Since these numbers represent cumulative survival, they are slow to reflect recent improvements in VV ECMO technology and management, which routinely exceed 80% in many high-volume centers.

### Venoarterial ECMO (Fig. 108-1)

**Indications** VA ECMO provides pulmonary and circulatory support. While it can be used in isolated respiratory disease (and historically was the mainstay for respiratory support), the need to cannulate a large artery that will either need to be ligated or repaired at the end of the ECMO course, and the higher complication rate of VA ECMO, make it a less desirable mode than VV ECMO for this application. VA ECMO is most appropriately deployed for either isolated severe cardiovascular disease (eg, dysrhythmia, severe contractile dysfunction post-cardiotomy, or cardiogenic shock), after cardiac arrest (eg, extracorporeal cardiopulmonary resuscitation, or ECPR), or in patients with combined respiratory and cardiovascular disease poorly responsive to inotropic or vasopressor support (Table 108-2). One important note of caution warrants mentioning: ECMO support in general is ineffective in the presence of aortic regurgitation, as a significant proportion of the postoxygenator arterial blood flows back to the left ventricle, resulting in inadequate cardiac output, coronary flow, and volume overload of the left ventricle.

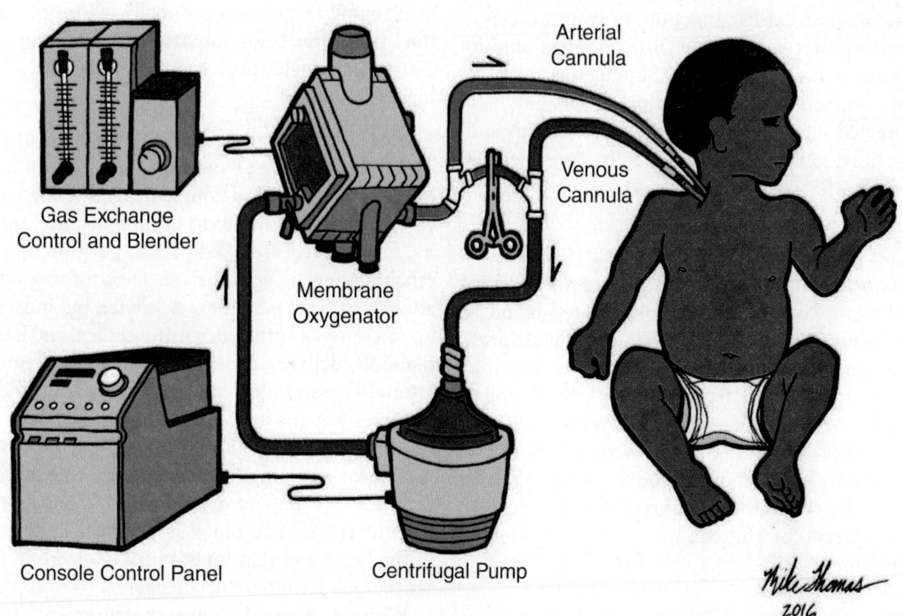


**FIGURE 108-1** The Extracorporeal Circuit. Peripheral venoarterial ECMO with cannulation of the carotid artery and internal jugular vein, illustrating standard components of the ECMO circuit.

**TABLE 108-2 INDICATIONS FOR VENOARTERIAL ECMO**

| Isolated Cardiovascular Disease | Multisystem Disease with Cardiovascular Failure |
|---|---|
| Myocarditis/dilated cardiomyopathy | ECPR |
| Malignant dysrhythmias | Septic shock with biventricular or high-output heart failure |
| ECPR | PPHN with right heart failure |
| Myocardial stun after surgery for congenital heart disease | Pulmonary embolism with right heart failure |
| Cardiac allograft failure (primary and delayed rejection) | Primary pulmonary hypertension |
| Preoperative CHD presenting in cardiogenic shock | |
| Shunt obstruction in shunt-dependent lesions | |
| Pericardial disease, including tamponade | |

CHD, congenital heart disease; ECMO, extracorporeal membrane oxygenation; ECPR, extracorporeal cardiopulmonary resuscitation; PPHN, persistent pulmonary hypertension of the newborn.

**Cannulation Strategies** Generally, the patient's diagnosis and flow requirements drive the cannulation approach in VA ECMO. Patients with normal metabolic requirements need normal or mildly increased ECMO flows—typically 75% to 110% of their estimated cardiac output (eg, patients after cardiac surgery with a biventricular circulation or patients with a dysrhythmia)—whereas patients with increased metabolic needs may need flows that exceed 150% of normal cardiac output (eg, patients with single ventricle physiology or high-output septic shock). Patients requiring high-flow ECMO support, and a high proportion of those placed on ECMO after cardiac surgery, will typically undergo central cannulation in which short, wide-bore cannulae are placed via a sternotomy directly in the right atrium and ascending aorta to enable higher flow rates. Patients not requiring high flows, those without existing sternotomies, or those in the setting of cardiac arrest will typically be placed on VA ECMO through peripheral cannulation via the right internal jugular vein or a femoral vein, with blood returning to the right carotid artery or femoral artery. Femoral access is more commonly used in older children, adolescents, and adults.

**Management Goals** VA ECMO aims to optimize tissue $DO_2$ to meet local metabolic demands and decrease myocardial work so the heart can rest and recover from the antecedent insult. Alternatively, in patients with end-stage cardiac failure, VA ECMO may provide temporary cardiac support as a bridge to a long-term cardiac ventricular assist device. VA ECMO helps with myocardial recovery by "unloading" the heart. This is accomplished by decreasing ventricular end-diastolic pressures, which optimizes coronary perfusion pressure, decreases wall stress, and decreases myocardial work. Cardiac output provided by VA ECMO usually approximates 80% of the total cardiac output, and there is always some blood return to the left ventricle, from the bronchial vessels for example, and at least minimal ejection through the aortic valve. This residual endogenous cardiac output helps prevent blood stasis and inappropriate cardiac loading. Sometimes, to achieve aortic valve opening, inotropic agents and/or vasodilators to decrease systemic vascular resistance (SVR) may be required. In situations with inadequate oxygen delivery, increasing ECMO flow, optimizing intravascular volume augmenting oxygen-carrying capacity by increasing hemoglobin concentrations to > 10 g/dL, and controlling the SVR may all help to improve tissue $DO_2$.

Achieving proper oxygenation and ventilation is generally straightforward with VA support, as the lungs (whether or healthy or diseased) are mostly bypassed by the extracorporeal circuit and as a consequence, there is less functional right-to-left shunting than in VV ECMO. As in VV ECMO, low ventilator settings (ie, rest settings) are typically used for most patients on VA ECMO, with the proviso that in patients on femoral ECMO support with cardiac ejection of pulmonary venous returning blood, the upper body oxygen saturation should be monitored to ensure adequate cerebral oxygenation. As in VV ECMO, the sweep gas flow controls $CO_2$ clearance, with higher flow increasing $CO_2$ removal. Oxygenation is managed by titrating the sweep gas $FiO_2$ and blood flow rate. High blood flow rates, however, may result in transit times through the oxygenator that exceed the system's ability to maximally oxygenate the blood, especially if the venous blood is severely hypoxemic. Placement of a second oxygenator in parallel to the first cuts the transit time in half and doubles the amount of time the system has to oxygenate the blood prior to returning it to the patient.

**Duration of VA ECMO Support** The anticipated duration of VA ECMO support depends on the underlying disease. If the indication is a low cardiac output or difficulty separating from cardiopulmonary bypass after cardiac surgery, then the ECMO run would generally be less than 1 week, with survival being much reduced beyond 10 days of support. Inability to achieve any weaning after 3 to 5 days should prompt the use of echo, CT, or cardiac catheterization to search for an additional cause (eg, residual cardiac lesion). In the setting of septic shock, assuming that high flows are achieved early in the disease course, a relatively short course (less than 5 days) would be anticipated. If VA ECMO support is a bridge to a long-term ventricular assist device, then this conversion is generally performed once the full assessment of transplant candidacy, and other organ system recovery, has occurred.

**Weaning** Weaning patients from VA ECMO requires there to be improved cardiovascular function as evidenced by return of heart rate variability, control of dysrhythmias, decreased vasoactive medication requirements, and improving pulse pressure, suggesting ejection. It is important to prepare the patient for a successful wean. To that end, it is essential to optimize ventilator support, institute appropriate inotropic therapy before weaning to give the vasoactive medication time to work, optimize hematocrit level (> 30%), and minimize excess oxygen consumption with adequate sedation and analgesia, and neuromuscular blockade if required.

A preliminary assessment of weaning readiness may involve decreasing ECMO flows to 30% to 50% of predicted cardiac output, in a sufficiently loaded heart, potentially with a modest degree of inotropic support. If a patient becomes tachycardic or hypotensive and/or develops lactic acidosis, then he/she may not be ready to wean from ECMO. Contractile function can also be assessed by echocardiogram on decreased ECMO flows to help predict how the heart will perform off mechanical support (Table 108-3).

**Outcomes** According to the latest ELSO International Summary, overall survival in VA ECMO for cardiac disease ranges between 41%

**TABLE 108-3 WEANING FROM VENOARTERIAL ECMO**

**Preparation**

1. Perform echo assessment of cardiac function/recovery
2. Sedate patient
3. Adjust ventilator to achieve appropriate blood gas values for the cardiac lesion
4. Ensure adequate pulmonary toilet
5. Initiate inotropic/vasodilator support
6. Optimize intravascular volume and hematocrit
7. Control arrhythmia

**Weaning**

1. Reduce circuit flow rate over 24 hours (faster tapering may be possible, at the discretion of the medical team)
2. Monitor for signs and symptoms of appropriate cardiac output (urine output, lactate, $SvO_2$, blood pressure, NIRS).
3. Consider stopping the wean if cardiac output is suboptimal and give more time for recovery. Reassess.
4. Consider echo to guide weaning process (assess ventricular function, filling status, residual lesions)

echo, echocardiogram; ECMO, extracorporeal membrane oxygenation; NIRS, near infrared spectroscopy; $SvO_2$, mixed venous oxygen saturation.

**TABLE 108-4 COMMON COMPLICATIONS OF ECMO**

| Class | Examples |
|---|---|
| Mechanical | Oxygenator failure, tubing rupture, pump malfunction, clots in circuit |
| Hemorrhagic | GI hemorrhage, cannula site bleeding, hemolysis, DIC |
| Neurologic | Seizures, CNS infarction, CNS hemorrhage, brain death |
| Renal | Creatinine 1.5–3, creatinine > 3.0, requirement for renal replacement |
| Cardiovascular | CPR required, myocardial stun, arrhythmia, hypertension, tamponade |
| Pulmonary | Pneumothorax requiring treatment, pulmonary hemorrhage |
| Infectious | Culture-proven infection, WBC < 1500 |
| Metabolic | Glucose < 40, > 240; pH < 7.20, > 7.60; bilirubinemia (> 2 direct, or > 15 total) |
| Limb | Ischemia, compartment syndrome, fasciotomy, amputation |

Extracorporeal Life Support Organization Registry. http://www.elso.org/Registry.aspx.
CNS, central nervous system; CPR, cardiopulmonary resuscitation; ECMO, extracorporeal membrane oxygenation; DIC, disseminated intravascular coagulation; GI, gastrointestinal; WBC, white blood count.

and 51% in neonatal and pediatric patients, respectively, and is 41% for ECPR. These results represent an average of survival rates from centers with different expertise and resources. Centers with lower patient volumes and less experience likely experience lower overall survival (and likely higher morbidity) than higher-volume ECMO centers, whose outcomes are more favorable.

## COMPLICATIONS

ECMO is a low-volume, high-risk therapy that includes complex circuitry, multiple connections and access points, and systemic anticoagulation, and therefore represents a rich source of potential complications. Key players include bleeding and clotting (see below), sepsis, additional organ failure, or mechanical complications. Indeed, mortality related to complications is as important a consideration as mortality related to the underlying disease or lack of recovery from ECMO. The ELSO registry tracks 9 classes of complications (Table 108-4).

## ANTICOAGULATION

Finding the proper balance between blocking the natural tendency for blood exposed to thrombogenic surfaces to clot and preventing uncontrolled bleeding within the body is critical to a successful ECMO run. An ideal anticoagulation regimen would achieve these dual goals and would also be easy to monitor and titrate. Not surprisingly, neither the ideal anticoagulant nor the ideal monitoring system exists. Unfractionated heparin remains the preferred drug for anticoagulation while on ECMO and is given as a bolus during cannulation, and then as an infusion throughout the period of support. Most ECLS programs monitor the anticoagulation effect using the activated clotting time (ACT) as the primary endpoint, with therapeutic ranges varying from 150 to 220 seconds, depending on the specific assay and the type of heparin (porcine or bovine). Other tests of heparin's anticoagulation activity include partial thromboplastin times, heparin or anti-factor Xa levels, and other standard coagulation tests to monitor the blood's innate ability to clot. Some units monitor the whole blood clotting tendencies using the thromboelastogram or similar technologies. Collaboration between the ECMO and coagulation teams is an indispensable method to optimize the anticoagulation regimen for individual patients, speed the diagnosis of the frequent complications of systemic heparinization (eg, bleeding, heparin resistance, thrombophilia), and prompt their rapid and specific correction.

## FUTURE DIRECTIONS

Over the past four decades, ECMO has evolved from a therapy of last resort with an almost unacceptably high mortality rate to a more routine consideration in the management of severe cardiopulmonary disease. While inroads against the major complications associated with ECMO have been made, more work needs to be done. Nonetheless, there is cause for optimism, and as ECMO approaches its 50th anniversary, the prospects for routine integration into critical care have never been brighter. The field has started to solve some of the major problems that have resulted in lethal complications for patients supported for more than a few days, and technology has become both highly sophisticated and less beset with risk, while at the same time becoming simpler to manage. Over time, it is likely that ECMO will continue to become a more routine therapy that replaces more hazardous frontline treatments for severe cardiopulmonary diseases.

## SUGGESTED READINGS


Annich G, Lynch W, MacLaren G, Wilson J, Bartlett R, eds. *ECMO: Extracorporeal Cardiopulmonary Support in Critical Care*, 4th ed. Ann Arbor, MI: Extracorporeal Life Support Organization; 2012.

Anton-Martin P, Thompson MT, Sheeran PD, Fischer AC, Taylor D, Thomas JA. Extubation during pediatric extracorporeal membrane oxygenation: a single-center experience. *Pediatr Crit Care Med.* 2014;15(9):861-869.

de Caen AR, Berg MD, Chameides L, et al. Part 12: pediatric advanced life support. 2015 American Heart Association Guidelines Update for Cardiopulmonary Resuscitation and Emergency Cardiovascular Care. *Circulation.* 2015;132(18 Suppl 2):S526-S542.

Langer T, Santini A, Bottino N, et al. "Awake" extracorporeal membrane oxygenation (ECMO): pathophysiology, technical considerations, and pioneering. *Crit Care.* 2016;20(1):150.

Pediatric Acute Lung Injury Consensus Conference Group. Pediatric acute respiratory distress syndrome: consensus recommendations from the Pediatric Acute Lung Injury Consensus Conference. *Pediatr Crit Care Med.* 2015;16(5):428-439.

Peek GJ, Mugford M, Tiruvoipati R, et al. Efficacy and economic assessment of conventional ventilatory support versus extracorporeal membrane oxygenation for severe adult respiratory failure (CESAR): a multicentre randomised controlled trial. *Lancet.* 2009;374(9698):1351-1363.

UK Collaborative ECMO Trial Group. UK collaborative randomised trial of neonatal extracorporeal membrane oxygenation. *Lancet* 1996;348(9020):75-82.

Zamora IJ, Shekerdemian L, Fallon SC, Olutoye OO, Cass DL, Rycus PL, Burgman C, Lee TC. Outcomes comparing dual-lumen to multisite venovenous ECMO in the pediatric population: the Extracorporeal Life Support Registry experience. *J Pediatr Surg.* 2014; 49(10):1452-1457.


# 109 Perioperative Care

R. Blaine Easley and Desmond B. Henry

The term *perioperative care* refers to all the clinical activities that take place around a surgical intervention, from the preoperative assessment to the postoperative discharge. In modern institutions, perioperative care is performed in a defined physical area that usually accommodates scheduling, admission, preoperative preparation, the procedure itself (the operating room or a procedural suite), recovery from the procedure (phase I and II), and discharge. Support services—including sterile processing, materials management, the pharmacy, the laboratory, pathology, and diagnostic imaging—are frequently adjacent. The success and subsequent demand for new procedures such as cardiac catheterization or endoscopy, which are not strictly surgical but require expertise and equipment similar to surgery, have created a need to duplicate existing perioperative resources in other areas. The same principles that are detailed here for surgical procedures apply to these procedural areas.

## PREOPERATIVE ASSESSMENT AND CARE

Nearly all parents and children experience anxiety at the prospect of surgery. Preparing children for their surgical and operating room experience should begin before the patient makes contact with their anesthesiologist. The surgeon or primary care provider should be the first ones to ensure that the child receives the best perioperative care possible and to assure the child's family that this will be the case, answering their questions or facilitating access to someone who can answer them.

Many institutions arrange orientation and a preoperative tour days before surgery to instruct and educate the child and parent on what to expect. As part of the preoperative program, most of these institutions have developed child-friendly environments, with coloring books, tours, videos, and the invaluable help of a child-life specialist who can help reduce the level of anxiety. Allowing children to take a favorite toy or blanket into the operating room provides great comfort to many children.

The primary goal of preoperative assessment and care is preparing a patient for surgery, and ensuring that a full assessment of risk has been performed. This involves the following points: (1) screening for conditions that may require consultation workup or treatment, (2) optimizing any pre-existing medical conditions, and (3) counseling patients and parents about the expected course of anesthesia and surgery. The anesthesiologists should make every effort to see the child and the family to understand their needs and expectations and to perform a complete preoperative evaluation. The anesthetic, postoperative pain management, and discharge plans can all be explained to the child, if appropriate, and to the family at this time. This is also a good opportunity to obtain informed consent.

The preoperative evaluation usually consists of a careful history and an targeted physical examination aimed at establishing surgical risk and designing anesthetic planning and postoperative care. The physical examination should be sufficiently complete to detect any major problems and should be informed by the medical history (Table 109-1).

### Laboratory Evaluation

Because of low predictive value and cost-effectiveness, many centers no longer perform routine laboratory screening tests in otherwise healthy children scheduled for minor elective surgery. However, important baseline values (eg, hemoglobin level determination) in anticipation of major blood loss or specific diagnostic tests to rule out major organ-specific pathology are still performed. At present, there are no universal guidelines concerning preoperative laboratory testing; many anesthesiologists follow institutional protocols or their own personal preferences.

Mild anemia (hemoglobin [Hb] ≤ 9.5 g/dL) has been reported in up to 2% of pediatric patients undergoing elective surgery. No studies to date have shown justification to modify the perioperative management in otherwise healthy children who have a borderline low hemoglobin concentration, and therefore routine hemoglobin determinations are usually not necessary. However, it is reasonable to obtain preoperative hemoglobin values in (1) former preterm infants (postoperative apnea), (2) patients with chronic illness, (3) children with sickle cell disease (including sickle cell anemia, sickle Hb C disease, and the sickle thalassemias), and (4) those instances where having a baseline hemoglobin value may be useful (along with blood typing and cross-matching) in anticipation of significant surgical loss. In patients with sickle cell disease, the optimal level of sickle Hb and the role of transfusion to avoid perioperative complications in different categories of surgery and anesthesia (regional vs general) is still unknown. Perioperative evaluation and management of patients with this disease is best performed in conjunction with the patient's hematologist and surgeon.

Routine coagulation screening also has a weak predictive value for assessing the risk of surgical bleeding in patients with no history of abnormal bleeding. Screening is only advisable in patients in whom a hemostatic defect is suspected either by history or physical examination, patients in whom minimal postoperative bleeding could be critical (eg, neurosurgical interventions), or when the surgical procedure is likely to cause perioperative coagulation dysfunction (eg, cardiopulmonary bypass).

The value of routine preoperative pregnancy testing in women of childbearing age, particularly in adolescent females, is controversial. There is no scientific evidence that short-term exposure to anesthetics can induce spontaneous abortions or congenital malformations. However, surgery involves physical and psychological stresses, and exposure to x-rays and nonanesthetic medications may result in finite fetal risk.

Arguments against preoperative pregnancy testing are based on lack of demonstrated cost-effectiveness and on confidentiality and consent issues.

### Perioperative Surgical Home

Efforts to improve quality, efficiency and safety of perioperative care have led to the development of the *perioperative surgical home*. This concept involves more than a preoperative or preanesthesia assessment clinic; it seeks to integrate the preoperative evaluation of the patient and preparation of the family and patient for the entire course of perioperative care. This includes coordination of medical and surgical specialists and developing a plan for the preparation and intra-hospital care that allows the patient to safely transition into the surgical home and back into the care of their primary medical specialist. "Roadmaps" not only establish expectations for the family and perioperative team, but they allow for the development of procedural dashboards that can assist in monitoring the patient's progress throughout the course of care. In pediatrics, the use of roadmaps has been proposed as a method of safely managing medically complex medical patients outside of their medical home. The focus of this approach is family- and patient-centered care and utilizes the electronic medical record to improve communication between providers to deliver safe, high-quality, and efficient care.

## SPECIFIC ISSUES THAT INFLUENCE ANESTHETIC MANAGEMENT

### Obstructive Sleep Apnea

Several studies have indicated that there is an increased risk of postoperative respiratory difficulty in patients with moderate to severe obstructive sleep apnea, and a majority of anesthesiologists will hospitalize these patients for postoperative respiratory monitoring. Children older than 3 years of age and who have mild obstructive sleep apnea uncomplicated by comorbid conditions do not routinely require admission and often have their surgery performed in day surgery centers.

### Preoperative Fasting

Preoperative fasting is recommended to prevent aspiration of particulate material and liquids into the lungs while the airway-protective reflexes are suppressed under an anesthetic. However, fasting is eminently difficult to enforce with children, not only because the child is unlikely to see the benefits, but also because prolonged fasting is ill advised in small infants or debilitated children who may have reduced glycogen stores. Any attempt to implement unreasonable fasting criteria is an invitation for violation, which may happen without family knowledge if the child is old enough. Several studies have confirmed the safety of having clear liquids (apple juice, glucose-electrolyte solutions) up to 2 to 4 hours preoperatively in healthy infants and children (Table 109-2).

### Upper Respiratory Infection

Anesthesiologists and surgeons often face decisions regarding children who are experiencing respiratory symptoms at the time of a scheduled surgery. Upper respiratory infections (URIs) are very common in children, averaging 5 to 10 episodes per year, especially in those under the age of 2 years. The prevalence is even higher in children with chronic illnesses and those who attend day-care centers; therefore, sometimes the scheduling of elective surgery is a gamble. Some studies indicate significant risk for laryngospasm, bronchospasm, arterial $O_2$ desaturation, and postextubation stridor in children who are suffering from a

**TABLE 109-1 THE PREANESTHETIC HISTORY, SYSTEMIC REVIEW, AND RELATED ANESTHETIC IMPLICATIONS**

| System | History | Anesthetic Considerations |
|---|---|---|
| Central nervous and neuromuscular | Seizures | Adequacy of seizure control |
| | | Type of medications and preoperative serum levels (if appropriate) |
| | | Interactions between anticonvulsants and anesthetic agents (eg, phenytoin increases fentanyl and nondepolarizing muscle relaxant requirements) |
| | Head injury | Concern for raised intracranial pressure (some anesthetics increase cerebral blood flow and can worsen intracranial hypertension) |
| | | Risk of aspiration |
| | CNS tumor | Elevated intracranial pressure (same as head injury) |
| | | Steroid use |
| | | Chemotherapeutic agents and interactions with other drugs |
| | Neuromuscular disease | Aspiration risk secondary to bulbar dysfunction and swallowing incoordination |
| | | Risk of hyperkalemia from depolarizing muscle relaxant. |
| | | Risk of malignant hyperthermia from anesthetic gases and succinylcholine |
| | | Altered response to nondepolarizing muscle relaxants |
| Cardiovascular | Cyanotic heart defect | Right-to-left cardiac shunt creates a high risk for paradoxical embolus |
| | Other congenital or acquired heart disease | Consider hemodynamic response to different anesthetic agents |
| | | Antibiotic prophylaxis for bacterial endocarditis |
| Respiratory | Prematurity | Elevated risk of postoperative apnea and anemia |
| | Bronchopulmonary dysplasia | Reactive airway disease resulting in acute intrathoracic airway obstruction intraoperatively |
| | | Impaired gas exchange, particularly during induction and recovery from anesthesia |
| | | Increased pulmonary vascular resistance resulting in right ventricular dysfunction |
| | | Airway strictures from prolonged tracheal cannulation |
| | Asthma | Consider timing and dose of bronchodilators and steroids in perioperative management |
| | Croup | Subglottic narrowing |
| | URI/bronchiolitis | Possible reactive airway disease |
| | | Lower respiratory infection |
| | Cystic fibrosis | Recent acute infection and antibiotic treatment |
| | | Anesthetic- or ventilation–induced bronchorrhea, reactive airway disease, or pulmonary hemorrhage |
| | | Pulmonary hypertension and cor pulmonale |
| | | Risk of pneumothorax |
| | | Nutritional status |
| | Obstructive sleep apnea/ sleep-disordered breathing | Risk of perioperative airway obstruction |
| | | Avoid narcotics |
| | | Pulmonary hypertension and cor pulmonale |
| Gastrointestinal/ hepatic | Vomiting, diarrhea | Dehydration and electrolyte imbalances |
| | Gastroesophageal reflux | Risk of aspiration (full stomach) |
| | | Reactive airway disease |
| | Growth failure and malnutrition | Hypoglycemia |
| | | Hypoglycemia and hemorrhage |
| | Liver dysfunction | Altered drug metabolism |
| | | Risk for coagulopathy |
| | | Immunosuppression |
| | Short-gut syndrome/ malabsorption | Nutritional deficiencies |
| | | Anemia |
| | | Hypoalbuminemia and altered drug metabolism |
| Genitourinary | Bladder exstrophy and neurogenic bladder | Risk of latex allergy |
| | Renal failure | Hypervolemia and arterial hypertension |
| | Dialysis | Anemia |
| | | Uremic coagulopathy |
| | | Electrolyte abnormalities and acid–base disorder |
| | | Altered drug metabolism and clearance |
| | | Serum potassium must be known before administering succinylcholine |
| Endocrine/ metabolic | Diabetes | Current status and insulin requirement |
| | | Intraoperative hyper- or hypoglycemia |
| | Adrenal disease | Steroid replacement therapy needs to be altered to accommodate operative stress |

*(Continued)*

**TABLE 109-1 THE PREANESTHETIC HISTORY, SYSTEMIC REVIEW, AND RELATED ANESTHETIC IMPLICATIONS (CONTINUED)**

| System | History | Anesthetic Considerations |
|---|---|---|
| Hematologic | Bruising, excessive bleeding | Undiagnosed coagulopathy |
| | Sickle cell disease | Anemia is likely |
| | | Perioperative avoidance of dehydration, hypoxemia, acidosis, hypothermia |
| | Human immunodeficiency virus infection | Susceptibility to infection; infectious risk to medical personnel; antiretroviral medications and possible drug interactions |

CNS, central nervous system; URI, upper respiratory infection

URI, whereas other studies did not show major increased risk. There is still controversy among pediatric anesthesiologists on whether to proceed with surgery in the presence of a current or recent URI. The decision often depends on the experience of the anesthesiologist and the type and urgency of the surgery. Most anesthesiologists postpone elective surgery if the patient exhibits 1 or more of the following: fever, ill appearance, purulent rhinorrhea, tachypnea, or involvement of the lower respiratory tract. More severe viral respiratory infections such as laryngotracheobronchitis (croup) and respiratory syncytial virus (RSV) will almost always lead to a delay in surgery, typically for 2 or more weeks, and in the case of RSV and cardiac surgery requiring cardiopulmonary bypass, typically for more than 4 weeks.

### Central Apnea of the Neonate

Infants born prior to 37 weeks gestational age who are less than 56 weeks postconceptional age at the time of surgery are at greater risk of anesthetic complications than full-term infants. Apnea, periodic breathing, and bradycardia are common during and after general anesthesia or sedation. As a rule, these patients should be admitted overnight for cardiopulmonary monitoring or at least undergo in-hospital prolonged observation (typically > 8 hours) prior to discharge. Limited data suggest that spinal anesthesia may offer a lower risk of respiratory depression in young infants, but data in the literature are in conflict. Full-term infants (gestational age greater than 37 weeks) require overnight admission or extended observation if they are less than 44 weeks postconceptional age at the time of surgery. Most centers will defer elective, outpatient procedures (whether surgical or diagnostic) requiring anesthesia to be done until after 50 weeks postconceptual age to avoid apnea risk.

### Bronchopulmonary Dysplasia

Preoperative evaluation in children with bronchopulmonary dysplasia should include an assessment of the severity of their mechanical and gas-exchange abnormalities (see Chapter 62). Hypercapnia, metabolic alkalosis (elevated serum bicarbonate), hypochloremia, and hypokalemia are common in patients with severe disease and are often aggravated by the chronic use of loop diuretics. Hepatomegaly may indicate the presence of right ventricular dysfunction and suggests a limited cardiac reserve. A preoperative echocardiogram will confirm the presence of right-atrial and ventricular hypertrophy and enlargement and affords the opportunity to estimate the right-ventricular pressures.

Infants and children with bronchopulmonary dysplasia may have recently been treated with opioids and benzodiazepines and may therefore exhibit tolerance to these medications when used as part of the perioperative regime. Growth failure, chronic malnutrition, and the ensuing hypoproteinemia may affect the pharmacology of anesthetic drugs. Patients with hepatic congestion may also suffer from impaired hepatic clearance of drugs. Prolonged diuretic therapy may cause calcium wasting, nephrocalcinosis, and impaired renal function. Infants treated with long-term corticosteroids require treatment with "stress" corticosteroid doses in the perioperative period.

**TABLE 109-2 AMERICAN SOCIETY OF ANESTHESIOLOGISTS FASTING GUIDELINES**

| Ingested Material | Minimum Fast[a] |
|---|---|
| Clear liquids[b] | 2 hours |
| Breast milk | 4 hours |
| Infant formula | 6 hours |
| Nonhuman milk | 6 hours |
| Light meal[c] | 6 hours |

[a]Fasting times apply to all ages.

[b]Water, fruit juice without pulp, carbonated beverages, clear tea, and black coffee

[c]Dry toast and clear liquid. Fried or fatty foods may prolong gastric emptying time. Both amount and type of food must be considered.

The guidelines recommend no routine use of gastrointestinal stimulants, gastric acid secretion blockers, or oral antacids.

### Asthma

It is important for anesthesiologists to recognize the various presentations of asthma before surgery is undertaken. Active wheezing or decreased breath sounds indicate active airway obstruction and, if possible, should prompt a deferral of surgery until the airway obstruction is relieved. Preoperative pulmonary function testing is not necessary unless it is used to optimize the drug regimen in the patient with severe disease. It is usually recommended that all preoperative treatments be continued through the morning of surgery. In addition, some anesthesiologists routinely administer a nebulized beta-adrenergic agonist before inducing anesthesia. Patients who have received chronic steroid therapy, either systemically or at high doses via aerosol, should be treated with stress corticosteroid doses. Anesthetic induction can be accomplished by any route. At present, sevoflurane is the inhalational agent of choice, because it does not irritate the airways and has bronchodilatory effects. Among the intravenous anesthetics, ketamine has been proposed as a last resort adjuvant in the treatment of status asthmaticus, because it causes bronchodilation. Propofol has a weaker histamine-releasing effect than other rapid-acting sedatives and therefore is often preferred to etomidate or thiopental for induction or short anesthetic courses in asthmatic patients. A slow, smooth emergence from anesthesia minimizes the risk of bronchospasm. Unless contraindicated, many anesthesiologists proceed with extubation under deep anesthesia to minimize airway irritation during emergence, when airway reflexes may be enhanced.

### Sickle Cell Disease

Appropriate preoperative evaluation and preparation are mandatory in children who suffer from the various forms of sickle cell disease. Children who have experienced frequent crises, including acute chest syndrome, or who require multiple transfusions represent a particularly high anesthetic risk.

Although there is no ideal anesthetic technique, perioperative complications may be minimized by vigilant observation, adequate pain control, and careful avoidance of dehydration or any other circumstances that lead to decreased tissue perfusion or arterial oxygenation. The choice of transfusion strategy before surgery depends on the patient's history and should be carefully planned in conjunction with the patient's pediatrician, hematologist, and surgeon.

## ANESTHETIC RISK ASSESSMENT

The risk of anesthesia during surgery depends to a large extent on the child's health and the complexity of the surgery. The most common classification often used to determine the relative risk is the American Society of Anesthesiologists (ASA) Physical Status Classification (Table 109-3); it is important to note that the ASA classification does not account for the risk of the surgery itself or for the existence of multiple diseases.

**TABLE 109-3 AMERICAN SOCIETY OF ANESTHESIOLOGISTS PHYSICAL STATUS CLASSIFICATION**

| ASA Category | Preoperative Health Status | Comments, Examples |
|---|---|---|
| ASA I | Normal healthy patient | No organic, physiological, or psychiatric disturbance; excludes the very young and very old; healthy with good exercise tolerance |
| ASA II | Patients with mild systemic disease | No functional limitations; history of well-controlled disease states; controlled non–insulin-dependent diabetes mellitus, controlled hypertension, epilepsy, asthma, or thyroid conditions; ASA I with active allergies, mild respiratory condition, pregnancy, mild obesity |
| ASA III | Patients with severe systemic disease | Disease state limits activity but is not incapacitating; no immediate danger of death |
| | | Examples: controlled congestive heart failure of more than 6 months' duration, controlled insulin-dependent diabetes mellitus, controlled hypertension, stable angina, bronchospastic disease with intermittent symptoms, chronic renal failure, morbid obesity |
| ASA IV | Patients with severe systemic disease that is a constant threat to life | Significant perioperative risk that may lead to death because of existing medical problem of greater importance than the planned surgery; has severe disease, severe congestive heart failure, moderate to severe obstructive pulmonary disease, unstable angina pectoris, hepatorenal syndrome, poorly controlled or any end-stage disease state |
| ASA V | Moribund patients who are not expected to survive without the operation | Terminally ill patients with imminent risk of death, multiorgan failure, sepsis syndrome with hemodynamic instability |
| ASA VI | A declared brain-dead patient whose organs are being removed for transplantation | |
| ASA E | Emergency operation of any variety | Useful for modification of any of the above classifications (ie, ASA II-E) |

ASA, American Society of Anesthesiologists; CHF, congestive heart failure; COPD, chronic obstructive pulmonary disease; IDDM, insulin-dependent diabetes mellitus.



## INDUCTION AND MAINTENANCE OF ANESTHESIA

Intraoperative management requires complex skills beyond the scope of this chapter. However, pediatricians should have some familiarity with the various components of this management, especially those that may affect the postoperative course or that may raise questions by the family.

### Induction of Anesthesia

The main goal of the induction phase is to achieve surgical anesthesia in a manner that is fast, smooth, and least distressing for the patient. In children, this is usually best accomplished by using inhalational rather than intravenous agents. Ultimately, the choice of anesthetic induction technique is determined by the patient risks, the state of health, and the circumstances of the moment. For instance, in a child at risk for aspiration, a rapid intravenous sequence results in safer tracheal intubation and is preferable to an inhalational induction.

In a typical induction, the child is brought to the operating room area, often accompanied by a parent and a favorite toy. Monitoring equipment, including a pulse oximeter, electrocardiographic electrodes, and a blood pressure cuff, is placed gently on the child. Next, a facemask carrying oxygen and frequently mixed with nitrous oxide is carefully placed on the child's face. One to 2 minutes of inhaling nitrous oxide induces a state of euphoria. At this point, an inhalational induction with a volatile anesthetic such as sevoflurane is introduced into the inhaled gas mixture. Once the child is unconscious, an intravenous line is started and more comprehensive intraoperative monitoring is applied if appropriate. Alternatively, a child can undergo an intravenous induction using a hypnotic agent. Using either induction technique, surgical anesthesia can be maintained by spontaneous ventilation with a mask and inhaled anesthetic gas. However, it is usually safer to secure the airway either with a supraglottic device (like a laryngeal mask airway) or an endotracheal tube.

### Choice of Anesthetic

There is a wide choice of inhalational (volatile) anesthetics, but sevoflurane, desflurane, and isoflurane are the ones most commonly used in the United States. Dosing with these agents is defined by the minimum alveolar concentration (MAC), which is the alveolar concentration that provides sufficient depth of anesthesia for surgery in 50% of patients. For most potent inhalational agents, the alveolar concentration reflects the arterial concentration of anesthetic in the blood perfusing the brain. Thus, the MAC is an indication of anesthetic potency analogous to the median effective dose ($ED_{50}$). Inhalational anesthetics have the advantage of producing both a rapid onset and a rapid offset of anesthesia. The less soluble the agent is in the blood (ie, the lower the blood/gas partition coefficient of the anesthetic), the faster the induction and the emergence from anesthesia will be. Inhalational agents are also convenient to administer (as they do not require special access) and provide profound amnesia and excellent analgesia. However, among their disadvantages, they cause airway irritation (thus rendering the patient more likely to cough or develop laryngospasm, bronchospasm, or breath-holding) and nausea and vomiting.

Intravenous anesthetics belong in several pharmacological families, including but not limited to barbiturates, narcotics, and benzodiazepines. They have the advantage of speed—generally inducing anesthesia more rapidly than inhalational agents—without some of the complications. On the other hand, they require intravenous access, which is threatening to a usually already apprehensive child. All intravenous agents have some effect on cardiorespiratory function, usually including some degree of respiratory depression, apnea, and hypotension. In infants and children, combinations of intravenous agents and infusions of propofol, dexmedetomidine, and/or ketamine have been used to provide total intravenous anesthesia (TIVA). While typically less associated with nausea and vomiting and emergence delirium, the disadvantages are cost and prolonged duration of recovery from TIVA.

### Maintenance of Anesthesia

During surgery, the obvious expectation is that the patient remain asleep, unaware of pain, unresponsive without motion, and hemodynamically stable. Anesthesia is usually maintained with nitrous oxide, an inhalational anesthetic, and an opioid to increase intraoperative and postoperative analgesia. Benzodiazepines are often given as premedication or intraoperatively to supplement hypnosis and amnesia. A nondepolarizing muscle relaxant (vecuronium or rocuronium) provides neuromuscular blockade if needed. Some of the medications used in pediatric anesthesia, along with their most common side effects, are listed in Table 109-4.

## INTRAOPERATIVE MONITORING

Standard monitoring equipment used in pediatric anesthesia includes pulse oximeter, electrocardiogram (EKG), invasive or noninvasive

**TABLE 109-4 ANESTHETIC IMPLICATIONS OF FREQUENTLY USED MEDICATIONS**

| Drugs | Anesthetic Implications |
|---|---|
| **Analgesics** | |
| Non-steroidal anti-inflammatory drugs (NSAIDs; ketorolac, ibuprofen) | Altered platelet function and prolonged bleeding time |
| | Increased risk of renal dysfunction, especially in newborns and dehydrated patients |
| | May precipitate asthma/bronchospasm in susceptible individuals |
| Opioids | "Gold standard" for providing analgesia |
| | Increased incidence of postoperative nausea and vomiting |
| | May cause respiratory depression that can last longer than analgesic effect, especially infants < 3 months of age |
| Morphine | Inexpensive with longer duration of action |
| | Metabolites have neurotoxic effect and may cause myoclonus |
| | Histamine release (pruritus, hypotension, asthma) |
| | May cause SIADH |
| Fentanyl | More potent with faster onset of action than morphine |
| | Minimal hemodynamic effects, chest wall rigidity in high dose or rapid administration, bradycardia |
| **Antibiotics** | |
| Aminoglycosides | May potentiate neuromuscular blockade |
| | Nephrotoxicity and irreversible ototoxicity |
| Clindamycin | Cardiac arrest (with rapid IV administration) |
| | Arrhythmia due to $QT_C$ prolongation |
| Vancomycin | Red man syndrome: hypotension and cardiac arrest with rapid infusion |
| | Necrosis and tissue sloughing with extravasation |
| | May cause nephrotoxicity and ototoxicity |
| **Anticonvulsants** | |
| Phenytoin | May cause increased requirements of nondepolarizing relaxants and fentanyl |
| | Pain and thrombophlebitis on injection into small vein |
| | Hypotension, arrhythmia, bradycardia, cardiovascular collapse (especially with rapid IV administration) |
| | May cause sedation/drowsiness |
| | Peripheral neuropathy and bone marrow toxicity |
| | Hepatoxicity especially in children < 2 years of age |
| Valproic acid | Inhibition of platelet aggregation, thrombocytopenia, and bleeding |
| **Sedative-Anxiolytics** | |
| Benzodiazepines | May cause sedation, anxiolysis, or hypnosis |
| | Respiratory depression |
| | Antegrade amnesia |
| | Raise seizure threshold |
| Midazolam | Use frequently for premedication (rapid onset and short acting) |
| | Unique advantage of many routes of administration (oral, intranasal, intravenous, buccal) |
| **Muscle Relaxants** | |
| Succinylcholine | Rapid onset with short duration of action; used in rapid sequence induction |
| | Initial fasciculation may cause elevated intracranial and intraocular pressure and postoperative myalgia |
| | Metabolized by plasma cholinesterase; may cause prolonged effect in patients with cholinesterase deficiency |
| | May trigger malignant hyperthermia (MH) in susceptible patients |
| | Contraindicated in patients with myotonia, hyperkalemia |
| Rocuronium | Utilized for rapid sequence, routine endotracheal intubation, and maintenance of muscle relaxation |
| | Metabolized by the liver and excreted in bile |
| Vecuronium | Routine endotracheal intubation and maintenance of muscle relaxation |
| | Metabolized by both liver and kidney |
| Cisatracurium | Metabolized rapidly by nonenzymatic degradation (Hofmann elimination) Useful in hepatic or renal disease |
| | Mild histamine release with minimal and transient cardiovascular effects |
| **Intravenous Anesthetic Agents** | |
| Propofol | Rapid-acting hypnotic and amnestic agent |
| | Rapid emergence, useful for short procedures |
| | Increases seizure threshold and has antiemetic properties |
| | No analgesic and anxiolytic properties |
| | Painful when injected into small vessels |
| | May cause hypotension, vasodilation, respiratory depression |

*(Continued)*

**TABLE 109-4 ANESTHETIC IMPLICATIONS OF FREQUENTLY USED MEDICATIONS (CONTINUED)**

| Drugs | Anesthetic Implications |
|---|---|
| Dexmedetomidine | Mild anxiolytic and sedative |
| | Central action via alpha receptors |
| | Decreased heart rate |
| | Increased blood pressure |
| | Minimal effect on myocardial function |
| | Augments the effect of other agents (opioids and benzodiazepines) |
| Etomidate | Rapid-acting hypnotic |
| | Rapid emergence |
| | Cardiovascular stability with induction doses |
| | Respiratory depression |
| | Pain on injection |
| | No analgesic or anxiolytic properties |
| | Adrenocortical suppression |
| | Associated with myoclonus |
| Ketamine | Produces "dissociative anesthesia" |
| | Analgesic properties |
| | Causes endogenous catecholamine release, resulting in tachycardia, elevated BP, and bronchodilatation |
| | Significant sialorrhea |
| | Increases intracranial and intraocular pressure |
| | Emergence delirium |
| **Inhalational Agents** | |
| Potent vapors (sevoflurane, desflurane, isoflurane, enflurane, halothane, etc) | Complete anesthetics |
| | Vasodilation and hypotension |
| | Myocardial depressant properties |
| | May trigger MH in susceptible individuals |
| Nitrous oxide | Amnesia and mild analgesia |
| | Danger of hypoxic mixture with low oxygen concentration |

BP, blood pressure; IV, intravenous; MH, malignant hyperthermia; SIADH, syndrome of inappropriate antidiuretic hormone secretion



blood pressure monitor, end-tidal $CO_2$ monitor, and thermometer. Other continuous routine measurements include the fraction of inspired oxygen, and the concentrations of air, anesthetic vapors, and nitrous oxide are often monitored as a routine. Rarely, additional monitoring is needed; however, there is growing use of adjunct monitoring devices, specifically awareness monitors and cerebral oxygenation monitors, that is growing in anesthetic and critical care of infants and children.

### Bispectral Index Monitoring

The bispectral index (BIS) monitor is a neurophysiological monitoring device that uses processed electroencephalogram (EEG) signals to continually assess the level of consciousness during general anesthesia or deep sedation. The BIS is based on bispectral processing of various EEG frequencies from cortical and subcortical brain regions calculated with Fourier's analysis. It correlates the patient's sedation depth by comparing EEG signals obtained from that patient with EEG traces stored in its database. The saved database is derived from almost 1000 healthy adult volunteers at specific clinically important end points during anesthesia. A BIS value of 0 equals isoelectric EEG, while 100 is the expected value for a fully awake patient (0, coma; 40–60, general anesthesia; 60–90, sedated; 100, awake). The deeper the level of anesthesia or sedation is, the lower the BIS is.

BIS monitoring provides an assessment to the depth of anesthesia and is therefore useful in reducing the likelihood of the recall phenomenon. It also allows safe titration of anesthetic or sedating agents to a specific bispectral index in the operating room or procedural units, thereby ensuring that potent agents are used according to patient need. BIS monitoring also has been found to be useful in quantifying the depth of nondissociative procedural sedation and analgesia in children.

Conversely, the BIS index monitor may not be entirely reliable in infants younger than 12 months of age because of the differences in EEG patterns that the BIS algorithm utilizes. It is also prone to artifacts, and therefore cannot be relied upon in situations such as brain death, hypothermia, and circulatory arrest. The BIS index has a poor correlation during dissociative anesthesia with ketamine and opioids.

### Cerebral Oxygenation Monitoring

The use of near infrared spectroscopy (NIRS) cerebral oximetry monitoring has increased over the past decades in both anesthesiology and critical care practices as a surrogate for cerebral perfusion during the care of critically ill patients, both inside and outside the operating room. While infants and children undergoing cardiac surgery represent the largest population for application of this technology, usage occurs in other operative situations, such as spine surgery, vascular surgery, and transplantation. The use of near infrared spectroscopy (NIRS) cerebral oximetry monitoring has increased over the past decades in both anesthesiology and critical care practices as a surrogate for cerebral perfusion during the care of critically ill patients, both inside and outside the operating room. Infants and children undergoing cardiac surgery represent the largest population for application of this technology, but NIRS monitoring is also used in other operative situations, such as during spine surgery, vascular surgery, and transplantation. While NIRS values and trends have been associated with clinical and neurodevelopmental outcomes in selected cardiac subgroups, the overall utility and application of this technology remains under investigation. Normal cerebral oxygen saturation in adults and children is > 60%.

## POSTOPERATIVE CARE

The main goal of postoperative care is to ensure smooth return (or emergence) from anesthesia and surgery to the patient's baseline state. The initial recovery period is critical; up to 13% of all reported

| TABLE 109-5 MODIFIED ALDRETE RECOVERY SCORE (> 9 REQUIRED FOR DISCHARGE) | |
|---|---|
| **Criterion** | **Score** |
| **Activity** | |
| Moves 4 extremities voluntarily or on command | 2 |
| Moves 2 extremities voluntarily or on command, or moves weakly | 1 |
| Does not move any extremities voluntarily or on command | 0 |
| **Respiration** | |
| Able to deep-breathe, cough, and/or cry | 2 |
| Dyspneic or limited in breathing | 1 |
| Apneic | 0 |
| **Circulation** | |
| BP within 20 mm Hg of preanesthetic value | 2 |
| BP within 20–50 mm Hg of preanesthetic value | 1 |
| BP within 50 mm Hg of preanesthetic value | 0 |
| **Consciousness** | |
| Fully awake and oriented | 2 |
| Wakes to stimuli | 1 |
| Unresponsive | 0 |
| **Oxygen Saturation ($SpO_2$)** | |
| $SpO_2$ > 92% on room air | 2 |
| Supplemental oxygen to maintain $SpO_2$ > 92% | 1 |
| $SpO_2$ < 92% | 0 |

adverse events occur at this time. Therefore, it is essential that every facility where children undergo surgery has a well-equipped postanesthesia care unit (PACU) with dedicated nursing staff able to detect and manage immediate postoperative problems. Following arrival at the unit and proper briefing by the anesthesiologist, staff should maintain a constant surveillance of airway patency, ventilation, and circulatory function. Common problems experienced in children are emergence delirium, sore throat, shivering, nausea/vomiting, and pain. A patient is usually deemed stable enough for discharge when consciousness is fully recovered, postoperative nausea and vomiting are controlled, and pain is relieved. There are several scoring systems for determining discharge readiness in the PACU (see Tables 109-5 and 109-6). After an appropriate period of observation, patients will be discharged from the operative area to home, to a postoperative inpatient area, or on occasion to a critical care unit. It is important that clear instructions are given to parents or caregivers, and a structured sign-out is given to receiving clinicians regarding postoperative analgesia and sedation where appropriate (see Chapter 110) and intravenous fluid therapy with particular attention to the avoidance of hypotonic fluids (see Chapter 101).

| TABLE 109-6 POSTANESTHESIA CARE UNIT DISCHARGE READINESS SCORE (SCORE OF 6 REQUIRED FOR DISCHARGE) | |
|---|---|
| **Criterion** | **Score** |
| **Consciousness** | |
| Awake | 2 |
| Responding to stimuli | 1 |
| Not responding | 0 |
| **Airway** | |
| Coughing on command or crying | 2 |
| Maintaining good airway | 1 |
| Airway requires maintenance | 0 |
| **Movement** | |
| Moving limbs purposefully | 2 |
| Nonpurposeful movements | 1 |
| Not moving | 0 |

## SUGGESTED READINGS




Brady M, Kinn S, Ness V, O'Rourke K, Randhawa N, Stuart P. Preoperative fasting for preventing perioperative complications in children. *Cochrane Database Syst Rev.* 2009;4:CD005285.

Coté CJ. Anesthesiological considerations for children with obstructive sleep apnea. *Curr Opin Anaesthesiol.* 2015;28(3):327-332.

Ferrari LR, Antonelli RC, Bader A. Beyond the preoperative clinic: considerations for pediatric care redesign aligning the patientfamily-centered medical home and the perioperative surgical home. *Anesth Analg.* 2015;120(5):1167-1170.

Kasman N, Brady K. Cerebral oximetry for pediatric anesthesia: why do intelligent clinicians disagree? *Paediatr Anaesth.* 2011;21(5):473-478.

Kern D, Fourcade O, Mazoit JX, et al. The relationship between bispectral index and endtidal concentration of sevoflurane during anesthesia and recovery in spontaneously ventilating children. *Paediatr Anaesth.* 2007;17(3):249-254.

Lerman J. A disquisition on sleep-disordered breathing in children. *Pediatr Anesth.* 2009;19(Suppl 1):100-108.

Malviya S, Galinkin JL, Bannister CF, et al. The incidence of intraoperative awareness in children: childhood awareness and recall evaluation. *Anesth Analg.* 2009;109(5):1421-1427.

Mani V, Morton NS. Overview of total intravenous anesthesia in children. *Paediatr Anesth.* 2010;20(3):211-220.

Maxwell LG, Yaster M. Perioperative management issues in pediatric patients. *Anesthesiol Clin North Am.* 2000;18(3):601-632.

O'Connor ME, Drasner K. Preoperative laboratory testing of children undergoing elective surgery. *Anesth Analg.* 1990;70(2):176-180.

Section on Anesthesiology and Pain Medicine. Critical elements for the pediatric perioperative anesthesia environment. *Pediatrics.* 2015;136(6):1200-1205.

von Ungern-Sternberg BS, Boda K, Chambers NA, et al. Risk assessment for respiratory complications in paediatric anaesthesia: a prospective cohort study. *Lancet.* 2010;376(9743):773-783.


# 110 Pain and Sedation

Stuart R. Hall and Dean B. Andropoulos

## PAIN

From the dark years when medicine taught that neonates feel no pain, we have emerged into an era when, finally, pain and sedation assessment have become as important as any other vital sign in every patient. Sedation and pain management can present challenges for the pediatric practitioner: Many patients are too young to verbalize their discomfort. Practically, there are no truly objective measures of pain: It is a personal, often emotional, experience unique to each patient. Pediatric patients range from the articulate to the noncommunicative, providing unique challenges in the management of their pain.

### THE PATHOPHYSIOLOGY OF PAIN

Pain has been defined by the International Association of Pain as "an unpleasant sensory and emotional experience associated with actual or potential tissue damage, or described in terms of such damage." Pain can be both an expected physiologic response to a noxious stimulus or an abnormal, pathologic response, as might be the case in chronic pain syndromes.

The classic pain pathway involves nociceptive neurons that respond to painful chemical, mechanical, and thermal stimuli. They are found in their greatest numbers in the skin but are present in many tissues throughout the body. Once stimulated, they transmit signals along peripheral nerve fibers to the lower and midbrain; pain is perceived in the cerebral cortex. Faster A-delta fibers elicit "sharp" initial sensations, while signals along C fibers are perceived as burning, aching sensations of a more chronic nature.

Stimulation of nociceptive neurons causes the release of many local mediators, including histamine, bradykinins, substance P, prostaglandins, growth factors, and $H^+$ and $K^+$ ions. The mere perception of pain, then, is in itself an inflammatory process. Repeated stimulation of peripheral nociceptors, causing repetitive firing of the involved A-delta and C fibers, can lead to hypersensitization of the afferent pathway. This can transform the experience of pain into a neuropathic process, leading to hyperalgesia, an exaggerated response to painful stimuli, or even allodynia, a pain response to otherwise nonpainful stimulation in the tissues surrounding the injury. Factors that predispose patients to the development of neuropathic pain are not well understood.

As defined, pain has an emotional component. Individual patients will have different, yet valid, responses to similar painful stimuli. The assessment and management of pain needs to be tailored to the patient's level of development, ability to communicate, and ability to tolerate discomfort.

## THE DIAGNOSIS OF PAIN

The experience of pain is subjective and its assessment can be challenging, particularly in the young. Adults and mature younger patients can be asked to rank their pain on a scale of 0 to 10, with 10 being the worst imaginable pain. It is important to calibrate both the patient's and the caregiver's expectations: Sometimes, a 5 is tolerable, whereas sometimes a 3 is intolerable. Treating pain begins with assessment, and there is therapeutic value in patients simply knowing that their physicians are interested in treating their pain. Younger patients present more of a challenge. In the case of children in the early stages of verbal development, behavioral changes can indicate a level of discomfort. Some children become withdrawn, and others may act out. If pain is a possibility in a given clinical situation, it must be part of the differential when diagnosing a change in the patient's usual behavior.

Patients unable to communicate verbally present a greater challenge. Several scales, which translate the numerical values of the pain scale into visual stimuli, are widely available. These might show a happy face to correspond with no pain, a grumpy face for moderate pain, and a crying face for more severe pain. Children can indicate which face corresponds to how they feel. There are published, well-designed systems for scoring pain in nonverbal patients; the FLACC (Face, Legs, Activity, Cry, Consolability) scale is shown in Table 110-1. In situations in which patients may be unable to cooperate at all with such an assessment, such as in an intubated and sedated patient, clinical judgment comes into play: Tachycardia, hypertension, tachypnea, or any sign of sympathetic nervous system stimulation may indicate the patient is feeling pain.

## THE TREATMENT OF PAIN: PHARMACOLOGICAL INTERVENTIONS

### Simple Analgesics: Acetaminophen and Nonsteroidal Anti-Inflammatory Drugs

Acetaminophen (paracetamol), a highly-selective cyclooxygenase-2 (COX-2) inhibitor, is an important first-line analgesic (Table 110-2). At recommended doses, acetaminophen is well-tolerated. Generally, it is given enterally, within the maximum daily dose recommendations, but is also highly effective in its intravenous form in patients. The chief concern with acetaminophen administration is its potential for hepatic toxicity by its potential to deplete stores of glutathione in the liver. It also has antipyretic effects, as do the nonsteroidal anti-inflammatory drugs (NSAIDs), so bear in mind that scheduled acetaminophen may mask an underlying fever.

NSAIDs are highly effective analgesics and have anti-pyretic properties. They are, in general, nonselective COX inhibitors. As such, they have the potential for various toxicities and side effects. The following is not an exhaustive list:

- Gastric: Direct irritation by acidic molecules (enteral administration); indirect irritation by decreased prostaglandin production
- Renal: Decreased renal blood flow
- Platelets: Inhibition of platelet aggregation

NSAIDs, while very effective analgesics, may be contraindicated in the immediate postoperative period or in any patient in whom bleeding is a concern, and are contraindicated in patients with compromised renal function.

### Opioids

Opioid medications make up the cornerstone of treatment for moderate-to-severe pain. Opioids, originally derived from opium poppies, include a wide range of natural, semi-synthetic, and synthetic compounds (Table 110-3). Opioid receptors are found in the central and peripheral nervous systems and the gastrointestinal (GI) tract. Stimulation of these receptors causes analgesia, cough suppression (a desirable result), and pruritus, respiratory depression, and decreased GI motility (undesirable results). Most centers will, by protocol, recommend a bowel regimen for patients in whom opioids will be used for more than a few days. Additionally, it is good practice to be prepared to treat the potentially life-threatening side effect of opioid respiratory depression in any patient receiving parenteral opioids. Some institutions, by protocol, will have an opioid antagonist, naloxone, available for any such patient, particularly if the opioids are being administered intravenously.

Choice of individual opioid should be guided by personal preference and patient response. Some patients might report excessive itching with morphine, for example, but will tolerate hydromorphone well. Periprocedural analgesia is perhaps best achieved with longer-acting medications like morphine and hydromorphone, rather than shorter-acting medications like fentanyl. Once patients resume oral intake, and pain has been well controlled with intravenous (IV) medications, opioids are available in many oral (PO) formulations, the most common of these being codeine sulfate. Usually, the

**TABLE 110-1 FLACC NONVERBAL SEDATION SCALE**

| | Appropriate for Preverbal Patients Younger Than 3 Years and for Older, Nonverbal Patients | | |
|---|---|---|---|
| | 0 | 1 | 2 |
| FACE | No particular expression or smile | Occasional grimace or frown, withdrawn, disinterested | Frequent to constant quivering chin, clenched jaw |
| LEGS | Normal position or relaxed | Uneasy, restless, tense | Kicking or legs drawn up |
| ACTIVITY | Lying quietly, normal position, moves easily | Squirming, shifting back and forth, tense | Arched, rigid, or jerking |
| CRY | No cry (awake or asleep) | Moans or whimpers, occasional complaint | Crying steadily, screams or sobs, frequent complaints |
| CONSOLABILITY | Content, relaxed | Reassured by occasional touching, hugging, or being talked to; distractible | Difficult to console or comfort |

Each of the 5 categories—face, legs, activity, cry, consolability (FLACC)—is scored from 0 to 2, which results in a total score between 0 and 10.

Reproduced with permission from Voepel-Lewis T, Merkel S, Tait AR, et al: The Reliability and Validity of the Face, Legs, Activity, Cry, Consolability Observational Tool as a Measure of Pain in Children with Cognitive Impairment, *Anesth Analg*. 2002 Nov;95(5):1224-1229.

**TABLE 110-2 NONOPIOID ANALGESICS, SEDATIVES, AND HYPNOTICS**

| Medication | Route | Dose/Interval | Comments |
|---|---|---|---|
| **ADJUVANTS** | | | |
| **CLONIDINE** | IV | 1–2 μg/kg every 6–8 hours | Potential for hypotension |
| **KETAMINE** | IV | 0.2–0.5 mg/kg every 30 minutes to 1 hour | In critical care settings |
| | IV continuous infusion | 200 μg/kg/hr | In critical care settings |
| **ACETAMINOPHEN AND NSAIDs** | | | |
| **ACETAMINOPHEN** | IV, PO | 15 mg/kg, every 4–6 hours, not to exceed 3 g/24 hours in adolescents, 4 g/24 hours in adults | Often dosed by institutional protocol; caution in concomitant administration of opioid + acetaminophen combination preparations |
| **KETOROLAC** | IV | 0.5–1 mg/kg initial dose, followed by 0.5 mg/kg every 6 hours | Do not exceed 30 mg/dose or 120 mg/day |
| | PO | Typical adult dose 20 mg followed by 10 mg every 6 hours | |
| **IBUPROFEN** | PO | 4–10 mg/kg dose every 6–8 hours, not to exceed 40 mg/kg/day | Often dosed by institutional protocol |
| **NAPROXEN** | PO | 5–7 mg/kg/dose every 8–12 hours | Analgesia in children |
| | PO | 200 mg every 12 hours | OTC labeling |
| | PO | Initial dose 500 mg, then 250 mg twice a day | Adult analgesic dose |
| **BENZODIAZEPINES** | | | |
| **MIDAZOLAM** | IV continuous infusion | 0.01–0.03 mg/kg/hr initial dose | Titrate to effect; assumes an intubated monitored patient |
| **LORAZEPAM** | IV | 0.03–0.05 mg/kg/dose every 4–8 hours | Initial dose, titrated as needed; usual single dose maximum 1–2 mg |
| | IV | 1–2 mg every 4–8 hours | Adult dose |
| | PO | 0.03–0.05 mg/kg/dose every 4–8 hours | For benzodiazepine withdrawal, titrated as needed based on last scheduled interval dosing |
| **DIAZEPAM** | PO | 0.5–1 mg every 3–4 hours | Titrate as necessary, typical starting dose for muscle spasm |
| **OTHER SEDATIVE INFUSIONS** | | | |
| **DEXMEDETOMIDINE** | IV | 0.3 μg/kg/hour, titrated by 0.1 μg/kg/hour not to exceed 0.7 μg/kg/hour | Patients needing short-term (less than 24 hours) sedation; monitor for bradycardia |
| **PROPOFOL** | IV | 50–150 μg/kg/min | Limited use in critical care setting, clinically useful doses can be much higher |

IV, intravenous; OTC, over the counter; PO, by mouth

PO forms are compounded with acetaminophen, and it is important to keep the maximum dose of acetaminophen in mind when titrating oral doses. Many institutions also have protocols to simplify the safe administration of oral opioids with doses standardized to patient weight ranges.

Methadone is a synthetic opioid with a very long and variable half-life, ranging in individual patients from 12–15 hours to 60 or more hours. In the hands of pain specialists, it is sometimes used for the acute management of very painful conditions or procedures, but the variability in its metabolism and elimination make it unsuitable for more general use as an analgesic. Its long half-life, however, makes it very useful in a slow weaning and detoxification process for patients who have become habituated to opioids. In this situation, calculations can be made to determine the methadone dose equivalent to parenteral infusion or oral opioids. Clinical pharmacists and institutional protocols can help guide this transition.

Tramadol, a synthetic opioid-like drug with some serotonin- and norepinephrine-reuptake blockade, has affinity for the μ-receptor. It is available both alone and in combination with acetaminophen for the treatment of moderate to severe pain. In the United States, it is not frequently used in children other than for postoperative pain, but it may be appropriate for the older teenager. While tramadol clinically has not shown as much respiratory depression in older children as traditional opioids, there are reports of this important adverse effect in younger patients. Additional common side effects are nausea and vomiting.

### Multimodal Analgesia

Multimodal analgesia, using a combination of medications, has several advantages. Using different classes of medications together can target different mechanisms of the experience of pain. A combination of acetaminophen and an opioid, for example, affects both the COX pathway and the opioid receptors in the central nervous system (CNS). In patients with low risk of bleeding, NSAIDs can be of great help, in adding to the attack on the inflammatory mechanism of pain. Sometimes, however, it might seem that no combination of medications is effective, or that the side effects of 1 of the medications are unsatisfactory. Consultation with a pain specialist may be helpful in cases where both patient and caregiver become frustrated with inadequate analgesia.

### Clonidine

Clonidine is a centrally acting $\alpha_2$ and imidazoline agonist that has had extensive use in pediatrics as a medication for attention-deficit/hyperactivity disorders, in addition to its original indication as an antihypertensive. Clinically, it is not US Food and Drug Administration (FDA) labelled for use in pain, but it has been effective as an adjuvant analgesic, particularly in patients who have used opioid medications for extended periods of time.

### Ketamine

Ketamine is an N-methyl-D-aspartate (NMDA)-receptor antagonist which may also have some activity on opioid receptors and the monoamine oxidase system. Administered as an intramuscular or intravenous agent, it is intensely analgesic in very small doses; however, even commonly prescribed doses can induce a dissociative state that can be very unpleasant for the patient. Nystagmus and hypersalivation are common, as are tachycardia and transient increases in blood pressure. Use of ketamine as an analgesic infusion is not recommended in patients not continuously monitored in a critical care setting, and it is not labeled for this use in the United States.

**TABLE 110-3 OPIOID MEDICATIONS**

| Medication | Route | Dose | Clinical Duration | Morphine Equivalence (To 1 Mg Morphine Iv) | Comments |
|---|---|---|---|---|---|
| **MORPHINE** | IV | 0.05–0.1 mg/kg/dose; typical adult starting dose, 2 mg | 1–4 hours | 1:1 | Monitor for respiratory depression, especially with PCA |
| | PO | 0.2–0.5 mg/kg dose | 1–4 hours | 3 mg | Start with lower doses; 0.3 mg/kg typical starting dose for moderate–severe pain |
| **FENTANYL** | IV | 1 μg/kg | 30–60 minutes | 10 μg | Not appropriate outside ICU without specialist input; high risk of respiratory depression |
| **HYDROMORPHONE** | IV | 0.01–0.015 mg/kg; typical adult starting dose, 0.2 mg | 3–4 hours | 0.15 mg | Monitor for respiratory depression, especially with PCA |
| | PO | 0.03–0.08 mg/kg; typical adult starting dose, 2 mg | 3–4 hours | 0.75 mg | Moderate to severe pain |
| **METHADONE** | IV | 0.1 mg/kg | 4–8 hours | Variable | Not recommended for most acute pain situations |
| | PO | 0.2 mg/kg | 4–8 hours | Variable | Again, not recommended for most acute pain situations |
| **HYDROCODONE + ACETAMINOPHEN** | PO | 0.135 mg/kg hydrocodone | 3–4 hours | 3 mg | Acetaminophen dose should not exceed lower of 15 mg/kg/day or 2.6 g/day |
| **OXYCODONE + ACETAMINOPHEN** | PO | 0.05–0.15 mg/kg oxycodone | 3–4 hours | 3 mg | Acetaminophen dose should not exceed lower of 15 mg/kg/day or 2.6 g/day |
| **TRAMADOL** | PO | 1–2 mg/kg | 4–6 hours | 2–3 mg | Not to exceed 100 mg/dose or 400 mg/day, not for young children |

ICU, intensive care unit; IV, intravenous; PCA, Patient-controlled analgesia; PO, by mouth



## SEDATION

Sedation generally refers to the depression of the level of consciousness. It can describe, in varying degree, anything from mild anxiolysis to full unconsciousness. Sedation in the critical care unit often means "relaxing" a patient to the point where he or she can tolerate the many invasions of confinement: endotracheal tubes, mechanical ventilation, drains, invasive catheters, and even physical restraints. It is important to remember that while euphoria is a common side effect of opioid medications, opioids alone do not generally depress consciousness enough for a patient to be comfortable in every situation. For the most part, patients will need a combination of an analgesic plus a sedative (see Table 110-2) to tolerate long periods of intubation in the intensive care unit (ICU).

### Benzodiazepines

Benzodiazepines act at the gamma-aminobutyric acid (GABA) receptor. They produce anxiolytic, sedative, hypnotic, and anticonvulsant effects, in addition to a degree of muscle relaxation, though they are not paralytic agents. They can be administered by mouth, submucosally (intranasally or buccally), or as intravenous boluses or infusions. Benzodiazepines cause dose-dependent respiratory depression, likely through a combination CNS depression and muscle relaxation. The combination of benzodiazepine with opioids, then, has the very real potential to cause apnea. This may not be a problem in a patient who is intubated and ventilated and monitored in the ICU, but can become an issue as the patient becomes ready to wean from ventilation, or in a patient requiring light or moderate anesthesia as procedural sedation outside of an ICU setting.

Although benzodiazepines do not inherently have analgesic properties, there are situations in which they will aid pain relief. For example, patients experiencing significant anxiety with regard to their pain relief might benefit from treatment with benzodiazepines; additionally, patients who have had procedures associated with significant postop muscle spasm, such as after scoliosis surgery, may experience significant discomfort from muscle spasm, which can be very effectively alleviated with benzodiazepines.

Intravenous benzodiazepines, combined with intravenous opioids, have for decades been the sedative/analgesic combinations of choice used in critical care units. With short-term use (ie, over the span of hours or several days), they are easily titratable, and they can make patients very comfortable and able to tolerate the anxiety of invasive procedures, pain, and the presence of an endotracheal tube. However, with more prolonged requirements, practitioners often find themselves having to increase infusions of both medications and patients develop tachyphylaxis and concomitant habituation to these medications, as patients fail to respond to the given dose. Tachyphylaxis develops at a rate directly proportional to the half-life of the administered drug. Patients in whom intermediate or long-term use of such infusions is likely may benefit from initiation of therapy with longer-acting medications from the beginning. Tachyphylaxis to morphine, for example, develops at a slower rate than does tachyphylaxis to fentanyl. However, a longer half-life means less ease of titration. Giving a dose of a medication with a long half-life is a commitment to its effect, and potential side effects, for a longer period of time. Tachyphylaxis and habituation can be mitigated to a point using intermittent dosing, lowest necessary doses for the shortest possible time, and the daily interruption of sedating and analgesic infusions.

### Dexmedetomidine

Dexmedetomidine is a central $\alpha_2$ agonist, similar to clonidine, that has promise as a sedative/analgesic infusion in the critical care unit in patients with cardiopulmonary monitoring. As for many other agents, there is no FDA-approved indication for dexmedetomidine in pediatrics. Although it is a sedative, it is often combined with opioids and/or benzodiazepines for infusions lasting a short term (ie, days). It is not recommended for long-term infusion. Patients can develop tachyphylaxis to its effects rapidly because of its short distribution half-life (6 minutes) and rapid elimination half-life (2 hours), and they can develop a rebound phenomenon (typically tachycardia and agitation) if it is acutely discontinued after several days of use. It is not associated with a decrease in respiratory drive. The prescriber must be mindful, however, that in combination with a benzodiazepine or opioids, the depression of consciousness from dexmedetomidine can augment the risk of apnea from other drugs. The most concerning side effect of dexmedetomidine is bradycardia, usually clinically insignificant, but which may be profound in patients already prone to slow heart rates (eg, trisomy 21). Hypertension can occur with higher-dose infusions, sometimes potentiated by the concomitant administration of vagolytic agents to counteract bradycardia. Dexmedetomidine should be avoided in children with bradyarrhythmias and in children with hepatic impairment. Although sedated, patients can be aware of their surroundings, and amnesia is not usually reported with dexmedetomidine infusions. It is most commonly administered intravenously, but other routes (eg, intranasal) have also been used. Outside of the operating room, dexmedetomidine is perhaps most suited for either monitored procedural sedation or short periods of sedation in the ICU.

#### Propofol

Propofol is a general anesthetic drug that is very short acting and has the ability to cause deep depression of consciousness and anterograde amnesia. It can produce profound respiratory depression and may produce systemic vasodilation and hypotension, which are somewhat dose dependent. Propofol has been associated with propofol infusion syndrome, a potentially lethal metabolic syndrome that can lead to lactic acidosis, rhabdomyolysis, and cardiac, renal, and hepatic failure following prolonged propofol use. It would appear that, while this is an unpredictable phenomenon, at-risk patients are those with a significant inflammatory state (eg, sepsis, severe acute respiratory distress syndrome). Propofol is often used for induction and maintenance of intravenous anesthesia, or for procedural sedation, and can be used for short periods in the ICU in intubated patients with cardiopulmonary monitoring who have stable hemodynamics, and who do not have any concern for underlying shock, sepsis, or severe respiratory disease. Its exact mechanism of action is not known, but it may potentiate GABA-A receptors and have some action as a sodium channel blocker. Propofol is not currently FDA licensed for use as a sedating agent in the pediatric ICU.

### MONITORING PATIENTS

What constitutes appropriate monitoring depends on the patient and the context. Sedation, especially procedural sedation, is usually accompanied by continuous monitoring of all vital signs: heart rate, blood pressure, oxygen saturation, respiratory rate, and temperature. Continuous infusions of benzodiazepines and narcotics, within the context of the critical care unit, are often used in patients already monitored for these signs for other reasons. Respiratory depression in a patient on mechanical ventilation not in the process of a ventilator wean is not an issue, but it can become an issue as the patient is prepared for extubation.

Any continuous infusion of a narcotic should be accompanied by pulse oximetry, at the very least. Some institutions restrict continuous infusions to monitored units where all patients are on such monitoring. Patient-controlled analgesia, when it does not include a basal rate of infusion of narcotics, has an inherent measure of safety in that if a patient becomes sleepy, he or she will not push the button to receive another dose of medication. Consider using pulse oximetry in any patient who needs frequent administration of narcotics, or concomitant narcotic–benzodiazepine administration, at least until the patient's response to the medication has been assessed or the patient's recovery allows for weaning doses. Pulse oximetry, with limits tailored to an individual's physiology, is perhaps more reliable than chest-wall impedance monitoring of respiratory rate, which can fail to appreciate respirations in the older patient with a large thorax.

Another caveat that bears repeating is that combining medications can have a synergistic effect on respiratory depression; the combination of benzodiazepines and narcotics a classic example. Drugs such as dexmedetomidine, which may possess no inherent direct respiratory depression, do contribute to depressed levels of consciousness and can potentiate the direct respiratory depression of other medications. It is important to remember that combinations of medications should be used with caution.

### CONCLUSION

Analgesia in the postoperative setting, or in patients with acute injury, usually starts with simple oral agents such as scheduled acetaminophen and/or NSAIDs. The next step will often be the addition of an opioid medication, often provided in combination with acetaminophen. Patients who cannot tolerate oral opioids can benefit from parenteral therapy; those old enough, or mature enough, can feel some measure of control over their own care through the use of a patient-controlled analgesia pump. When these measures fail, a pain management specialist can help with more complicated therapeutic interventions, or can even help optimize conventional therapy.

In the critical care environment, many patients will need sedation and analgesia, particularly those who are mechanically ventilated. Benzodiazepine and opioid infusions are the mainstay of therapy, either alone or combined with the more recent inclusion of dexmedetomidine infusions. Weaning these therapies is often a slow process, and patients receiving these infusions for weeks (or longer) will often need a long-term taper of long-acting enteral benzodiazepines and opioids, such as oral lorazepam and methadone. Remember that the experience of both pain and anxiety are, by definition, personal and emotional, and not all patients will respond to the same therapy. Cognitive-based therapies can be of great assistance to helping any patient deal with both chronic pain and chronic exposure to the healthcare environment.

### SUGGESTED READINGS


Barnes S, Yaster M, Kudchadkar SR. Pediatric sedation management. *Pediatr Rev.* 2016;37(5):203-212.

Committee on Psychosocial Aspects of Child and Family Health; Task Force on Pain in Infants, Children, and Adolescents. The assessment and management of acute pain in infants, children, and adolescents. *Pediatrics.* 2001;108(3):793-797.

Hsu DC, Cravero JP. Selection of medications for procedural sedation outside of the operating room. http://www.uptodate.com/contents/selection-of-medications-for-pediatric-procedural-sedation-outside-of-the-operating-room. Accessed September 16, 2016.

Mason K, ed. *Pediatric Sedation Outside of the Operating Room.* 2nd edition. New York: Springer; 2015.

O'Donnell FT, Rosen KR. Pediatric pain management: a review. *Mo Med.* 2014;111(3):231-237.

Verghese ST, Hannallah RS. Acute pain management in children. *J Pain Res.* 2010;3:105-123.


# 111 Vasoactive Medications

Javier J. Lasa and Brady S. Moffett

### INTRODUCTION

The use of vasoactive medications in the management of critically ill pediatric patients is common, with formal recommendations for their use in pediatric advanced life support algorithms first published over 30 years ago. Vasoactives are utilized throughout all pediatric age ranges and disease processes and continue to serve an important therapeutic role in the resuscitation of critically ill children. An understanding of the physiologic and pharmacologic underpinnings of each vasoactive class and subtype is absolutely necessary for the pediatric acute care provider. The provision of timely and effective therapy in the critical care or emergency room setting also requires an understanding of the wide variety of etiologies that contribute to hemodynamic instability in children: septic, cardiogenic, distributive, and hypovolemic shock states, in addition to cardiogenic shock related to acute heart failure or decompensated chronic heart failure. This chapter will describe the various medical therapies that modulate cardiovascular physiology, often termed *vasoactives*, while comparing and contrasting their pharmacologic properties, indications, and current practice in the pediatric population. The pharmacological properties, mechanisms of action, and cardiovascular effects are summarized in Tables 111-1 to 111-4.

**TABLE 111-1 DOSING AND MONITORING OF COMMON INTRAVENOUS VASOPRESSOR, VASODILATOR, AND INOTROPIC AGENTS**

| Drug | Dosing | Effects | Potential Adverse Events |
|---|---|---|---|
| Dobutamine | IV infusion: 2–20 μg/kg/min | Contractility, peripheral vasodilation | Tachycardia, arrhythmias |
| Dopamine | IV infusion: 2.5–20 μg/kg/min | Systemic vasodilation (low doses)<br>contractility, dose-dependent vasoconstriction | Hypertension, arrhythmias |
| Enalaprilat | IV bolus: 5–10 μg/kg/dose every 8–24 hours | Vasodilation | Hypotension, AKI |
| Epinephrine | IV infusion: 0.01–1 μg/kg/min | Myocardial contractility, dose-dependent peripheral vasoconstriction | Arrhythmias, hyperglycemia |
| Esmolol | IV bolus: 100–500 μg/kg<br>IV infusion: 50–1000 μg/kg/min | Vasodilation, SA node and AV conduction slowing (class II antiarrhythmic) | Hypotension, bradycardia, hypoglycemia |
| Fenoldopam | IV infusion: 0.01–0.3 μg/kg/min | Peripheral vasodilation; may increase urine output when used at low doses | Hypotension |
| Hydralazine | IV bolus: 0.1–0.6 mg/kg/dose every 6–8 hours | Vasodilation | Hypotension; reflex tachycardia |
| Labetalol | IV bolus: 0.2–1 mg/kg/dose; maximum: 40 mg<br>IV infusion: 0.25–3 mg/kg/hour | Vasodilation; minimal effect on heart rate, cardiac output, or stroke volume | Hypotension, bradycardia, hypoglycemia |
| Milrinone | IV infusion: 0.375–0.75 μg/kg/min | Myocardial contractility, vasodilation | Hypotension, arrhythmia, thrombocytopenia |
| Nesiritide | IV infusion: 0.01–0.03 μg/kg/min | Vasodilation | Hypotension, arrhythmia, AKI |
| Nicardipine | IV infusion: 0.5–5 μg/kg/min | Vasodilation | Hypotension |
| Nitroprusside | IV infusion: 0.2–4 μg/kg/min | Vasodilation | Hypotension (start very low dose in neonates), cyanide toxicity |
| Nitroglycerin | IV infusion: 0.5–4 μg/kg/min | Vasodilation | Hypotension |
| Norepinephrine | IV infusion: 0.05–1 μg/kg/min | Peripheral vasoconstriction, contractility | Arrhythmias, peripheral ischemia |
| Phenylephrine | IV bolus: 5–20 μg/kg/dose every 10–15 minutes as needed<br>IV infusion: 0.1–0.5 μg/kg/min | Peripheral vasoconstriction | Peripheral ischemia |
| Prostaglandin $E_1$ | IV infusion: 0.005–0.25 μg/kg/min | Vasodilation | Hypotension, apnea (dose related) |
| Vasopressin | IV infusion: 0.0003–0.001 unit/kg/min | Vasoconstriction, water retention | Peripheral, splanchnic, and coronary vasoconstriction, dilutional hyponatremia |

*All IV infusions should be given continuously unless bolus dosing indicated.*

AKI, acute kidney injury.

Data from Lexicomp. *Drug Information Handbook*. Hudson, OH: Lexi-Comp; 2016.

**TABLE 111-2 DOSING AND MONITORING OF COMMON ENTERAL VASOACTIVE MEDICATIONS**

| Drug | Dosing | Effects | Potential Adverse Events |
|---|---|---|---|
| Amlodipine | Enteral: 0.1 mg/kg/day; max: 10 mg/day | Peripheral vasodilation, coronary vasodilation | Hypotension, peripheral edema |
| Atenolol | Enteral: 0.5–2 mg/kg/day given 1–2 times daily; max: 100 mg/day | Reduced heart rate, antihypertensive effects | Bradycardia, hypotension, hypoglycemia |
| Candesartan | Enteral: 0.2 mg/kg/day divided 1–2 times per day; max: 0.4 mg/kg/dose or 32 mg/day | Peripheral vasodilation | Hypotension, acute kidney injury, angioedema |
| Captopril | Enteral: 0.01–6 mg/kg/day divided 3 times daily; max: 150 mg/day; (Note: Neonates should start at the lower doses to prevent hypotension and AKI) | Peripheral vasodilation | Hypotension, AKI, angioedema |
| Clonidine | Enteral: 5–10 μg/kg/day in divided doses every 8–12 hours; max: 0.9 mg/day | Peripheral vasodilation | Hypotension, rebound hypertension, sedation |
| Enalapril | Enteral: 0.1–0.5 mg/kg/day divided twice daily; max: 40 mg/day | Peripheral vasodilation | Hypotension, AKI, angioedema |
| Lisinopril | Enteral: 0.07–0.6 mg/kg/day given once daily; max: 40 mg/day | Peripheral vasodilation | Hypotension, AKI, angioedema |
| Losartan | Enteral: children 6–16 years: 0.7 mg/kg/day 1–2 times per day; max dose: 1.4 mg/kg/day or 100 mg/day | Peripheral vasodilation | Hypotension, acute kidney injury, angioedema |
| Metoprolol | Enteral: immediate release: 0.1–0.2 mg/kg/dose given 1–2 times a day; max: 200 mg/day | Reduced heart rate, antihypertensive effects | Bradycardia, hypotension, hypoglycemia |
| Nifedipine | Immediate release: enteral: 0.1–0.25 mg/kg/dose; maximum single dose: 10 mg<br>Extended release: enteral: initial: 0.25–0.5 mg/kg/day given once daily or divided in 2 doses per day; max: 120 mg/day | Peripheral vasodilation, coronary vasodilation | Hypotension |
| Propranolol | Enteral: immediate release: 1–4 mg/kg/dose 3–4 times per day; max: 640 mg/day | Reduced heart rate, antihypertensive effects | Bradycardia, hypotension, hypoglycemia |
| Valsartan | Enteral: 0.4–3.4 mg/kg/dose once daily; max: 160 mg/day (max dose varies on patient weight) | Peripheral vasodilation | Hypotension, acute kidney injury, angioedema |

Data from Lexicomp. *Drug Information Handbook*. Hudson, OH: Lexi-Comp; 2016.

**TABLE 111-3 MECHANISM OF ACTION AND PHARMACOKINETICS OF COMMON INTRAVENOUS VASOACTIVE MEDICATIONS**

| Drug | Mechanism of Action | Pharmacokinetics |
|---|---|---|
| Dobutamine | $\beta_1$, $\beta_2$ agonist | Onset: rapid; half-life: 2 min<br>Metabolism: tissues and liver to inactive metabolites<br>Elimination: urine (as metabolites) |
| Dopamine | DA agonist (2–5 μg/kg/min)<br>$\beta_1$ (5–10 μg/kg/min)<br>α (10–20 μg/kg/min) | Onset: rapid; half-life: 2 min<br>Metabolism: renal, hepatic, plasma; 75% to inactive metabolites; 25% to norepinephrine<br>Elimination: urine (as metabolites) |
| Enalaprilat | ACE inhibitor | Onset: ≤15 min; half-life: 11.9 h<br>Metabolism: none<br>Elimination: urine |
| Epinephrine | $\beta_1$, $\alpha_1$, $\beta_2$ agonist (more $\beta_1$ and less $\alpha_1$ at lower doses) | Onset: rapid; half-life: < 5 min<br>Metabolism: COMT and MAO<br>Elimination: urine (inactive metabolites) |
| Esmolol | Selective $\beta_1$ antagonist | Onset: 2–10 min; half-life: 2–5 min<br>Metabolism: red blood cell esterases<br>Elimination: urine |
| Fenoldopam | $DA_1$-receptor agonist | Onset: rapid; half-life: 3–5 min<br>Metabolism: hepatic<br>Elimination: urine (90%); GI (10%) |
| Hydralazine | Direct arteriolar vasodilator | Onset: 10–80 min; half-life: 3–7 h<br>Metabolism: hepatic acetylation<br>Elimination: urine (as metabolites) |
| Labetalol | $\alpha_1$ antagonist<br>Nonselective $\beta_1$, $\beta_2$ antagonist | Onset: 2–5 min; half-life: ~5.5 h<br>Metabolism: hepatic, extensive first-pass effect<br>Elimination: urine |
| Milrinone | Phosphodiesterase-3 inhibitor | Onset: 5–15 min; half-life: 1–5 h (dependent on renal function)<br>Metabolism: majority is excreted unchanged<br>Elimination: urine |
| Nesiritide | B-type natriuretic peptide | Onset: 15 min; half-life: ~18 min<br>Metabolism: vascular endopeptidases<br>Elimination: primarily eliminated by metabolism; some urinary excretion |
| Nicardipine | Inhibits calcium influx into vascular smooth muscle | Onset: rapid; half-life: 45 mins<br>Metabolism: hepatic with extensive first-pass effect<br>Elimination: urine; GI |
| Nitroprusside | Direct action on venous and arteriolar smooth muscle | Onset: rapid; half-life: 2 min<br>Metabolism: rhodanase-mediated conversion of cyanide to thiocyanate<br>Elimination: urine (as thiocyanate) |
| Nitroglycerin | Direct action on primarily venous smooth muscle, coronary artery vasodilation | Onset: rapid; half-life: 1–4 min<br>Metabolism: hepatic, extensive first-pass effect<br>Elimination: urine |
| Norepinephrine | $\alpha_1$, $\beta_1$ agonist | Onset: rapid; half-life: 1–2 min<br>Metabolism: COMT and MAO<br>Elimination: urine (inactive metabolites) |
| Phenylephrine | $\alpha_1$ agonist | Onset: rapid; half-life: 2–3 h<br>Metabolism: hepatic<br>Elimination: urine (mostly as inactive metabolites) |
| Prostaglandin $E_1$ | Direct vasodilatory effect on vascular and ductus arteriosus smooth muscle | Onset:15 min to many hours; half-life: 30 s to 10 min<br>Metabolism: ~70% to 80% by oxidation in the lungs<br>Elimination: primarily urine (90% as metabolites) |
| Vasopressin | $V_{1a,b}$ and $V_2$ receptors | Onset: within 15 min; half-life: 10–20 min<br>Metabolism: hepatic, renal<br>Elimination: urine |

ACE, angiotensin-converting enzyme; COMT, catechol-O-methyl transferase; DA, dopaminergic receptor; MAO, monoamine oxidase.

Data from Lexicomp. *Drug Information Handbook*. Hudson, OH: Lexi-Comp; 2016.

## VASOPRESSORS

Medications that primarily target receptors on peripheral arterial vasculature with resulting vasoconstriction and increased systemic arterial blood pressure are classified as vasopressors. Myocardial and peripheral adrenergic receptors present on cell surfaces play vital roles in the mechanistic action of vasopressors. In particular, α-adrenergic receptors function as excitatory triggers for vasoconstriction with multiple subtypes (eg, $\alpha_{1A}$, $\alpha_{1B}$, $\alpha_{1C}$, $\alpha_2$) identified with unique properties in their respective tissue distributions. These receptors belong to the

**TABLE 111-4 MECHANISM OF ACTION AND PHARMACOKINETICS OF COMMON ENTERAL VASOACTIVE MEDICATIONS**

| Drug | Mechanism of Action | Pharmacokinetics |
|---|---|---|
| Amlodipine | Inhibits calcium influx into vascular smooth muscle | Onset: 24–48 h after first dose; half-life: 30–50 h<br>Metabolism: hepatic<br>Elimination: urine |
| Atenolol | Selective $\beta_1$ antagonist | Onset: ≤ 1 h; half-life: 3.5–7 h<br>Metabolism: limited hepatic<br>Elimination: urine and GI, largely unchanged |
| Candesartan | Angiotensin II blocker | Onset: 2 h; half-life: 4–6 h<br>Metabolism: unidentified enzyme<br>Elimination: urine and GI |
| Captopril | ACE inhibitor | Onset: < 15 min; half-life: 1–2.3 h<br>Metabolism: hepatic<br>Elimination: urine |
| Clonidine | $\alpha_2$ agonist | Onset: 0.5–1 h; half-life: 8–72 h (longer in younger children)<br>Metabolism: extensively hepatic with enterohepatic recirculation<br>Elimination: urine |
| Enalapril | ACE inhibitor | Onset: ~1 h; half-life: 2–13 h (longer in younger children)<br>Metabolism: prodrug, undergoes hepatic biotransformation to enalaprilat<br>Elimination: urine |
| Hydralazine | Direct effect on vascular smooth muscle | Onset: 1–2 h; half-life: 3–7 h<br>Metabolism: hepatic acetylation, extensive first-pass effect (oral)<br>Elimination: urine (as metabolites) |
| Metoprolol | Nonselective β-receptor antagonist | Onset: ≤1 h; half-life: 3–10 h (dependent on enzymatic expression)<br>Metabolism: extensively hepatic with significant first-pass effect<br>Elimination: urine |
| Nifedipine | Inhibits calcium influx into vascular smooth muscle | Onset: immediate release: ~20 min; half-life: 2–5 h<br>Metabolism: hepatic<br>Elimination: urine (inactive metabolites) |
| Lisinopril | ACE inhibitor | Onset:1 h; half-life: 12 h<br>Metabolism: none<br>Elimination: urine (unchanged) |
| Losartan | Angiotensin II blocker | Onset: 6 h; half-life: ~2 h<br>Metabolism: hepatic to active metabolite with extensive first-pass effect<br>Elimination: urine and GI |
| Propranolol | Nonselective β-receptor antagonist | Onset: 1–2 h; half-life: 3–6 h (may be longer in neonates)<br>Metabolism: hepatic with extensive first-pass effect<br>Elimination: urine |
| Valsartan | Angiotensin II blocker | Onset: 2 h; half-life: 4–6 h<br>Metabolism: unidentified enzyme<br>Elimination: urine and GI |

ACE, angiotensin-converting enzyme; GI, gastrointestinal

Data from Lexicomp. *Drug Information Handbook*. Hudson, OH: Lexi-Comp; 2016.

G protein–coupled superfamily of receptors, which utilize intracellular signals to regulate the release of calcium in peripheral smooth muscle cells. An alternative mechanism for vasoconstriction can be found in the activation of dopaminergic receptors. The $DA_1$ receptor, a postsynaptic receptor located in the renal, splanchnic, coronary, and cerebral vascular beds, produces smooth muscle relaxation on stimulation.

### Phenylephrine

Phenylephrine is a pure $\alpha_1$ agonist resulting in peripheral arterial vasoconstriction with no inotropic effect. It is metabolized by oxidative deamination and glucuronidation and is renally eliminated as inactive metabolites. The intravenous onset of action is rapid and half-life is short (15–20 minutes). It has been used in patients with tetralogy of Fallot with hypercyanotic spells to increase pulmonary blood flow during acute episodes of desaturation. It can be administered as a bolus in acute situations or as a continuous infusion. Afterload, with associated increases in myocardial oxygen consumption, is often increased due to the profound vasoconstriction that occurs with use, and therefore should be avoided in patients with heart failure.

### Vasopressin

Vasopressin is also known as antidiuretic hormone. When given intravenously, the half-life is short (~10 minutes) and it is hepatically metabolized. The effect desired of vasopressin therapy is dependent on clinical indication and dose. Dosing of vasopressin can vary widely, with low doses used for treatment of diabetes insipidus, mid-range doses used for catecholamine refractory hypotension, and higher doses used for splanchnic bed vasoconstriction. The vasopressor effect occurs by assisting α- and β-adrenergic agents and does not occur due to direct action of vasopressin. Activation of the $V_{1a}$ receptor opens voltage-gated $K^+$ channels, which releases $H^+$ ions from adrenergic receptors, allowing a catecholamine effect. Additional mechanisms, consisting of decreased generation of nitric oxide and increased intracellular concentrations of calcium in the periphery are also theorized to provide benefit. Vasopressin also acts on the $V_2$ receptor, reducing free water excretion.

Vasopressin has been used in vasodilatory shock (eg, due to sepsis) and in postoperative cardiac surgical patients. Caution is warranted in patients already receiving high doses of peripherally acting α-adrenergic agents, as profound peripheral vasoconstriction and tissue necrosis can occur. The use of vasopressin may increase the risk of splanchnic ischemia and necrotizing enterocolitis, particularly in neonates and infants. Serum sodium values should be monitored during vasopressin therapy to avoid dilutional hyponatremia.

## VASOPRESSORS WITH INOTROPIC EFFECTS

Catecholamines produce increased contractility (inotropic effects) and heart rate (chronotropic effects) through activation of $\beta_1$-adrenergic receptors, with minimal vasoconstriction. The effects are mediated by G-protein coupling, which in turn leads to increased cyclic adenosine monophosphate (cAMP) with subsequent increases in intracellular calcium. In contrast, stimulation of $\beta_2$-adrenergic receptors induces smooth muscle relaxation with vasodilation, as well as bronchodilation. Some vasoactive agents exert adrenergic effects across receptor subtypes as well as in a dose-response fashion, exhibiting primary activity with 1 receptor but also acting upon other receptor subtypes at larger doses.

### Dopamine

The mechanism of action and clinical effects of continuous infusion dopamine are dose dependent. Lower doses will activate dopaminergic receptors in the kidney inducing vasodilation, while increasing doses agonize $\beta_1$ receptors and $\beta_2$ receptors (increasing inotropy and mild peripheral vasodilation), and at the highest doses, $\alpha_1$ receptors (increasing peripheral vasoconstriction). The lower doses of dopamine have been thought to increase renal blood flow and improve urine output, but the clinical effect of this is questionable. Dopamine is primarily metabolized into inactive forms by renal and hepatic mechanisms (~75%) while approximately 25% is changed into active norepinephrine. Neonates and infants have been shown to have nonlinear dopamine pharmacokinetics, and clearance may increase with increasing dose. Dopamine also inhibits thyroid stimulating hormone (TSH) and prolactin release from the anterior pituitary gland, making thyroid function testing challenging for patients on dopamine infusions. Dopamine is used in many different areas of intensive care as an inotropic and vasopressor agent and is frequently used in the neonatal population as treatment for hypotension. Additional adverse effects include arrhythmias and hyperglycemia.

### Epinephrine

Epinephrine exerts its primary physiologic effects through stimulation of $\beta_1$- (inotropic) and $\alpha_1$- (vasoconstrictor) adrenergic receptors. Other effects include stimulation of $\beta_2$ and $\alpha_2$ receptors, though the clinical effect of these is overshadowed by the primary mechanisms. Low doses of continuous infusion epinephrine can be used to elicit inotropic effects through $\beta_1$ stimulation without the $\alpha_1$-mediated peripheral vasoconstriction. Epinephrine has a short half-life (~5 minutes) and is metabolized in the adrenergic neuron by catechol-O-methyltransferase, monoamine oxidase, and various hepatic metabolic routes.

Epinephrine is used in a variety of intensive care settings to increase inotropy and vasoconstriction. Current cardiopulmonary resuscitation guidelines recommend the use of epinephrine for cardiac arrest to improve blood flow through the coronary arteries. Unwanted effects of epinephrine include hyperglycemia (from hepatic $\beta_2$ receptor stimulation, producing gluconeogenesis and glycogenolysis), tachycardia, and arrhythmias.

### Norepinephrine

Norepinephrine exhibits its primary cardiovascular effects through stimulation of $\alpha_1$-adrenergic receptors, producing peripheral vasoconstriction. It is also a weak $\beta_1$ receptor agonist, though the $\alpha_1$ effect is much more pronounced than the $\beta_1$ effect. In practice, it is most often administered with the aim of increasing systemic vascular tone with modest inotropy in the setting of severe hypotension or vasodilatory shock. The onset of action when given intravenously is nearly immediate and norepinephrine has a short half-life (1–2 minutes). Catechol-O-methyltransferase and monoamine oxidase metabolize norepinephrine into inactive metabolites, which are eliminated in the urine. Potential adverse events include peripheral tissue necrosis due to profound peripheral vasoconstriction, arrhythmias, and hyperglycemia.

## VASODILATORS

### Angiotensin-Converting Enzyme Inhibitors/Angiotensin Receptor Blockers

Angiotensin-converting enzyme (ACE) inhibitors (eg, captopril, enalapril, lisinopril) exhibit their clinical effects of vasodilation by inhibiting the conversion of angiotensin I to angiotensin II, which is a potent vasoconstrictor that triggers the release of norepinephrine and aldosterone. Enalapril is a prodrug metabolized to enalaprilat. Enalapril and captopril are metabolized hepatically and metabolites are excreted, to varying degrees, in the urine and feces. Conversely, lisinopril is not hepatically metabolized but is excreted unchanged in the urine.

Angiotensin receptor blockers (ARBs; eg, valsartan, losartan, candesartan) work by direct blockade of angiotensin II at the receptor site, resulting in vasodilation. Both also have vasodilatory effects on the efferent arteriole of the glomerulus, reducing intraglomerular pressure. The onset of action for oral ACE inhibitors ranges from 1 to 2 hours after administration. The duration of action is prolonged in neonates and infants as compared to children and adults, and can be prolonged in patients with severe heart failure. The ARBs have similar onset and durations to the ACE inhibitors and are metabolized hepatically and excreted in the urine and feces.

Typical uses of ACE inhibitors and ARBs include treatment of hypertension, reduction of afterload in heart failure, and reduction of proteinuria in patients with hypertension and diabetes. Enalapril and captopril have had reported uses in patients with congenital heart disease to reduce afterload, treat heart failure, and reduce intracardiac shunting. Enalaprilat is the only intravenous ACE inhibitor, and typically is used to treat acute hypertension. There is limited data relating to the use of ARBs in pediatrics, but these agents are most often used to treat chronic hypertension in patients intolerant of ACE inhibitors. Adverse events associated with ACE inhibitors and ARBs include hypotension and acute kidney injury, particularly in the neonatal and infant population. Angioedema is a rare but serious adverse event that has been reported in children after ACE inhibitor administration.

Esmolol is available in intravenous form and has been used as a continuous infusion in the treatment of hypertension after cardiac surgery, as well as for heart rate or arrhythmia control. Labetalol, in intravenous and oral formulations, is commonly used as an antihypertensive in the acute setting, such as during hypertensive crisis. Other β-blockers (eg, atenolol, metoprolol, and propranolol) are most often utilized in the long-term treatment of hypertension.

Potential adverse events with β-blockers include hypotension, fatigue, and cognitive difficulties. Hypoglycemia can occur due to the blockade of the $\beta_2$ receptors on the liver and the inhibition of glycogenolysis and gluconeogenesis.

### Calcium Channel Antagonists

Calcium channel blockers can be divided into 2 classes. The dihydropyridines (eg, amlodipine, nifedipine, nicardipine, clevidipine) all act peripherally, and the non-dihydropyridines (eg, verapamil and diltiazem) act on the myocardium. Amlodipine has a long half-life (30–50 hours) and is hepatically metabolized. Nifedipine has a shorter half-life and a rapid onset of action (~5 minutes) and is also hepatically metabolized (by cytochrome P450 3A4). Similarly, nicardipine has a rapid onset of action when given intravenously and is extensively metabolized by cytochrome P450 3A4.

Amlodipine, nifedipine, and nicardipine are currently available as oral formulations, and nicardipine and clevidipine are only available as intravenous formulations. Amlodipine has been used in pediatric patients for long-term treatment of hypertension, while nifedipine has been used for long-term and acute treatment of hypertension. Nicardipine has been used in the cardiac and non-cardiac postsurgical setting. Verapamil and diltiazem are infrequently used in the pediatric population as vasodilators.

Potential adverse events with peripherally acting calcium channel blockers include hypotension and lower extremity edema with long-term use. Immediate-release nifedipine has been noted to cause profound hypotension when used in patients with autonomic dysfunction, such as patients with neurologic injury. Verapamil and diltiazem cannot be recommended in patients less than 1 year of age due to reports of cardiovascular collapse after administration.

#### Venous and Arteriolar Vasodilators

Nitroprusside, nitroglycerin, and hydralazine have direct arteriolar and venous dilating activities, with nitroprusside having a stronger effect on arteriolar vessels, and nitroglycerin on the venous capacitance vessels. Hydralazine has direct action on the arterioles only. Nitroprusside has been commonly used as an antihypertensive agent in a variety of settings. Nitroglycerin has the added effect of coronary vasodilation and has been used in cases where myocardial ischemia may be present. Nitroglycerin is hepatically metabolized to di- and mononitrate metabolites, which are renally eliminated or further metabolized by blood esterases. Hydralazine is available as intravenous and oral formulations, and is a useful antihypertensive in an acute crisis but has the disadvantage of rapid onset tachyphylaxis. Hydralazine may also be ineffective in patients who are rapid acetylators and metabolize the drug quickly.

The metabolism of nitroprusside is catalyzed by the enzyme rhodanase. Nitroprusside releases cyanide molecules on metabolism, which are bound by endogenous thiosulfate into the less toxic and renally excreted form of thiocyanate. Cyanide toxicity occurs when capacity for the production of thiocyanate is overwhelmed and excess cyanide binds to hemoglobin, forming cyanomethemoglobin. Risk factors for cyanide toxicity include high doses (> 2 μg/kg/min), long duration of therapy (> 48 hours), and diminished kidney function. The concomitant use of nitroglycerin may also increase the risk of cyanide toxicity. Thiosulfate, often mixed in the same syringe as the nitroprusside, can be used to prevent or mitigate cyanide toxicity in patients at risk. Other potential adverse events include hypotension.

#### Nesiritide

Nesiritide is a recombinant B-type natriuretic peptide that produces peripheral vasodilation and diuresis, and has been used for heart failure and after cardiac surgery. It is metabolized by proteolytic cleavage by vascular endopeptidases and then internalized into the cell, with a small amount of metabolites renally excreted. Adverse events associated with nesiritide include hypotension, electrolyte imbalances (through natriuresis), and acute kidney injury.

### INODILATORS: DRUGS WITH MIXED VASODILATOR AND INOTROPIC EFFECTS

#### Milrinone

Milrinone is a phosphodiesterase-3 inhibitor that inhibits the breakdown of cAMP, leading to increased L-type calcium channel production and intracellular calcium release, ultimately leading to increased inotropy. Peripheral vasodilation is theorized to occur as a result of generation of nitric oxide by the inhibition of cAMP breakdown in the periphery. Milrinone is renally eliminated without undergoing metabolism. It is widely used after cardiac surgery and has been used to increase cardiac output in patients with acute decompensated heart failure, and in patients with septic shock. Hypotension is the primary adverse event, and it can be mitigated with careful titrations of dose. Arrhythmias and thrombocytopenia have also been reported.

#### Dobutamine

Dobutamine was the first synthetic catecholamine. It is a pure β ($\beta_1$ and $\beta_2$) agonist, which produces increased contractility, heart rate, and peripheral vasodilation. Dobutamine is primarily metabolized in the tissues to inactive metabolites. It is used in post–cardiac surgical patients, patients with heart failure, and other patients in states of low cardiac output. Dobutamine has been shown in some models to increase myocardial oxygen consumption due to significant increases in heart rate that is not met by an adequate increase in oxygen delivery, which has introduced the need for caution in some patient populations.

### MISCELLANEOUS CARDIOVASCULAR DRUGS

#### β-Blockers

β-Blockers are typically classified into selective ($\beta_1$ antagonism) or nonselective ($\beta_1$ and $\beta_2$ antagonism) subclasses and are often used to lower or control systemic blood pressure. Metabolism of β-blockers is varied. Esmolol is metabolized by blood esterases, labetalol is metabolized by glucoronide conjugation in the liver, atenolol has limited hepatic metabolism, and metoprolol is extensively hepatically metabolized by cytochrome P450 2D6. Elimination is drug specific and occurs via the kidney and feces.

#### Clonidine

Clonidine has a unique mechanism of action in that it is an $\alpha_2$ agonist, which works to inhibit the effect of catecholamines on $\alpha_1$ receptors, thus producing vasodilation. It can be used as an antihypertensive agent, a sedating drug, or a mild analgesic. Clonidine is metabolized via extensive hepatic metabolism into inactive metabolites, which are renally eliminated. Clonidine is available in oral, intravenous, and transdermal patch formulations. Potential adverse events include hypotension or rebound hypertension when therapy is rapidly discontinued.

#### Fenoldopam

Fenoldopam is a $DA_1$-receptor antagonist that primarily acts locally at the kidney as a weak vasodilator with natriuretic and diuretic effects. Fenoldopam is metabolized via hepatic methylation, sulfation, and glucuronidation to inactive metabolites that are eliminated through the kidney. Fenoldopam has been used most frequently in the treatment of postsurgical hypertension. Lower doses of fenoldopam have been reported to increase urine output in the presence of diuretics. Few adverse events are associated with fenoldopam, the most frequent being hypotension.

#### Prostaglandin $E_1$

Prostaglandin $E_1$ is primarily used in neonatal patients to maintain patency of the ductus arteriosus. Prostaglandin $E_1$ has a rapid onset of action and is primarily metabolized via oxidation in the lung. Adverse events with prostaglandin $E_1$ include hypotension (through systemic vasodilation) as well as fever, irritability, and apnea.

### SUGGESTED READINGS


Blowey DL. Update on the pharmacologic treatment of hypertension in pediatrics. *J Clin Hypertens (Greenwich)*. 2012;14(6):383-387.

Gaies MG, Gurney JG, Yen AH, et al. Vasoactive–inotrope score as a predictor of morbidity and mortality in infants after cardiopulmonary bypass. *Pediatr Crit Care Med*. 2010;11(2):234-238.

Kearns GL, Abdel-Rahman SM, Alander SW, Blowey DL, Leeder JS, Kauffman RE. Developmental pharmacology—drug disposition, action, and therapy in infants and children. *N Engl J Med*. 2003; 349(12):1157-1167.

Klugman D, Goswami ES, Berger JT. Pediatric Cardiac Intensive Care Society 2014 consensus statement: pharmacotherapies in cardiac critical care antihypertensives. *Pediatr Crit Care Med*. 2016; 17(3 Suppl 1):S101-S108.

Momma K. ACE inhibitors in pediatric patients with heart failure. *Paediatr Drugs*. 2006;8(1):55-69.

Robinson RF, Nahata MC, Batisky DL, Mahan JD. Pharmacologic treatment of chronic pediatric hypertension. *Paediatr Drugs*. 2005;7(1):27-40.

Rossano JW, Cabrera AG, Jefferies JL, Naim MP, Humlicek T. Pediatric Cardiac Intensive Care Society 2014 consensus statement: pharmacotherapies in cardiac critical care chronic heart failure. *Ped Crit Care Med*. 2016;17(3 Suppl 1):S20-S34.

Tume SC, Schwarts SM, Bronicki RA. Pediatric Cardiac Intensive Care Society 2014 consensus statement: pharmacotherapies in cardiac critical care treatment of acute heart failure. *Pediatr Crit Care Med*. 2016;17(3 Suppl 1):S16-S19.

# 112 Simulation-Based Team Training

Jennifer Arnold, Patricia Bastero, and Daniel Spencer Lemke

## INTRODUCTION

Simulation is an effective educational technique that not only improves learning for medical trainees and providers, but also leads to improved patient care delivery and outcomes. When simulation-based medical education (SBME) is implemented by experienced educators and integrated into educational curricula and systems, it allows for safe experimentation, learning from mistakes, deliberate practice, and standardized assessment of learners' competency.

Simulation-based training has been used for several decades to improve safety in high-risk industries such as aviation, where human error can lead to significant loss of life. Simulation-based training has contributed to the safety and reliability of the aviation industry through both technical skill training, where pilots practice the mechanics of how to fly a plane in a cockpit simulator and, more recently, in behavioral skill training during which the entire flight crew practices effective teamwork skills called crew resource management (CRM). Healthcare, like aviation, has identified that deficiencies in effective teamwork and communication account for up to 70% of medical errors. Based on the CRM skills identified as critical for safety in aviation, David Gaba, a founder of modern healthcare simulation and an anesthesiologist, adapted these skills for anesthesiology and termed them anesthesia crisis resource management (ACRM). There are 15 skills in total that are now identified as critical for effective healthcare teams (see Table 112-1).

Research has shown that these skills not only apply to the anesthesia field but can be applied to all of healthcare and are a key learning component of SBME. Although CRM is not yet a required component of medical education, medical and nursing schools, hospitals, and academic centers are increasingly incorporating SBME programs to train and improve the use of these critical skills.

## SIMULATION AS A TOOL BEYOND EDUCATION

Simulation, often used as an educational methodology, can be utilized for very different purposes, such as for improving quality and patient safety, as a method to assess competency, for introducing innovation or process change into healthcare, and for research. The implementation of simulation must be adapted to the specific goal desired.

Implementation of simulation with an intent to improve quality and patient safety is becoming more common in hospitals and academic institutions. The major sources of medical errors include latent safety threats and potential errors in hospital environments and systems of care that go unrecognized until they result in patient harm. To improve patient safety, simulation experts and learners can replicate high-risk clinical situations in actual patient care settings (known as *in situ simulation*) in order to identify and ameliorate latent safety threats in new and existing hospital environments and systems of care before they adversely affect a patient.

Simulation activities aimed at assessing healthcare providers' competency in either technical and/or behavioral skills represent a growing opportunity for healthcare and educational institutions. These activities involve the use of validated scenarios, checklists, and other assessment tools to evaluate clinicians' competency as related to the specific cognitive, technical, and behavioral skills being evaluated. As of today, this is most commonly done for high-risk skill sets such as the management of difficult airways and resuscitation (eg, Pediatric Advance Life Support training and certification).

Research activities can advance the science of healthcare simulation and ultimately improve healthcare delivery. SBME research can occur in 3 formats. First, simulation can be a safe "laboratory" test bed to assess healthcare interventions, techniques, or tools, such as the effectiveness of video laryngoscopy versus traditional laryngoscopy in neonatal intubations. Second, investigators often perform studies to evaluate the effectiveness of SBME and related interventions, such as a comparison of traditional education versus SBME training for medical students. Finally, investigation of the best methodologies and strategies for implementing SBME is an important endeavor to identify the optimal and the most cost-effective ways to utilize SBME for healthcare education.

## KEY CONCEPTS IN SIMULATION-BASED MEDICAL EDUCATION

Simulation offers learners the experience of providing actual patient care in a safe environment where mistakes can be made and learned from, consistent with adult learning. Andragogy, or the method and practice of adult learning, emphasizes the fact that adult learners are autodidacts whose own experiences affect their learning. They must want to learn, the learning must be of value to them and their work, and they prefer to focus on problems, which must be realistic. Kolb's experiential learning circle describes adult learning with 4 critical elements as applied in simulation:

1. *Experience.* The learners are exposed to a simulated scenario close to a real-life situation, and they perform based on previous learning.
2. *Reflection.* During the debriefing phase, learners are guided through an exploration of their thought processes by the debriefer to analyze why they did what they did.
3. *Conceptualization.* After analyzing their paradigms, adult learners adopt new perspectives and define optimal performance and "take-home" points.
4. *Experimentation.* Participants apply new or modified behaviors and/or skills to future simulations and real-life situations.

SBME provides an ideal framework for education and learning that correlates well with adult learning theory (Table 112-2).

There are 3 main phases to simulation: *introduction* to the simulated environment, *participation* in a simulated scenario, and *debriefing*. During the introduction, the instructors create a comfortable and safe environment in which to learn. They acknowledge that

**TABLE 112-1 FIFTEEN ANESTHESIA CRISIS RESOURCE MANAGEMENT SKILLS**

| | | |
|---|---|---|
| Know the environment | Communicate effectively | Re-evaluate repeatedly |
| Anticipate and plan | Use all available information | Use good teamwork |
| Call for help early | Prevent and manage fixation errors | Allocate attention wisely |
| Exercise leadership and followership | Use cognitive aids | Set priorities dynamically |
| Distribute workload | Cross (double) check | |
| Mobilize all available resources | | |

Data from Gaba DM, Fish KJ, Howard SK. *Crisis Management in Anesthesiology.* New York: Churchill Livingston; 1994.

**TABLE 112-2 CORRELATION OF SIMULATION-BASED EDUCATIONAL PRINCIPLES AND ADULT LEARNING THEORY**

| Simulation Curriculum Principle | Adult Learning Principle |
|---|---|
| Provides immediate, on-demand practice | Adults prefer to learn by doing |
| Introduction and presimulation coursework presents educational concepts before simulation | Adults prefer learning concepts and principles |
| Provides deliberate practice | Adults prefer to apply what they learn soon after learning it and at their own pace |
| Learner-focused debriefings allow for self-reflection | Adults like to set their own learning objectives |
| Debriefing allows for immediate learning | Adults like to receive immediate feedback |

Adapted with permission from Arnold J. The neonatal resuscitation program comes of age, *J Pediatr.* 2011 Sep;159(3):357-358.e1.

all participants are intelligent and are willing to give their best and improve (a basic principle). It is during this phase that the participants are familiarized with the simulated environment where they will work, and where the instructor "requests" buying in of realism. The simulated scenario in which they will participate should be relevant to what the adult learners are interested in, should focus on problems they would like to solve, and should be as close to the real-life situation as possible. Still, participants go through an unfreezing stage (according to Lewin's adult learning theory) as they are suddenly introduced to an unknown situation, the clinical case, in a new environment—the simulation room. In the scenario, learners are able to manage a clinical situation as they would in actual patient care. Although they may be naturally conscious that their performances might have been suboptimal, the learners are reminded that their actions have no actual consequences in simulation, and are reassured that there would be no repercussions. These reassurances should provide them with a psychologically safe environment which will then maximize the learning opportunity.

Each scenario is followed by a debriefing, during which the adult learners reflect on their actions, exploring what went right or wrong and, more importantly, what were the triggers for their actions and how to either reinforce or modify those perspectives to improve their future performances. Applying the components of adult learning described by Bloom's taxonomy, the simulated scenario asks for the participants to remember, understand, and apply previous learning and skills that are analyzed and evaluated later during debriefing.

## SIMULATION-BASED MEDICAL EDUCATION CURRICULUM DESIGN

### Educational Goals and Objectives

Medical education seeks to translate expert knowledge and best practices, as determined by outcomes-based research, into improved patient outcomes by changing the performance of medical practitioners. Simulated experiences for learners should be designed around specific goals and objectives. Learning objectives will drive how the simulation will be implemented. These objectives can be cognitive, technical, and/or behavioral, and can be targeted at individuals or teams.

Curriculum design starts with identification of clear learning objectives. For example, SBME can improve technical aspects of procedures, such as suturing, placement of intravenous catheters, or splinting extremity fractures through the use of practice on task trainers. Also, SBME can improve learners' ability to manage complex clinical situations such as a cardiac arrest or intraoperative complications such as fire in the operating room, or provide an opportunity to improve communication techniques such as delivery of bad news or disclosure of medical error in time-sensitive or emotionally stressful situations. SBME allows learners adequate time to practice these skills in a safe environment without risking patient safety, up to a level of mastery, before performing the skills in situations with actual patients. For noneducational simulation activities, such as quality- and safety-based activities, the simulation encounter should be designed to answer specific questions and identify latent safety threats in our systems of care. The approach to development and implementation of SBME should vary based on the specific objectives of the simulation activity.

### Target Learners

SBME should vary based on the experience and background of the learners. Identification of the target learners is critical when developing SBME. Novice learners may benefit from simple working models to demonstrate the use of the equipment and mechanics of a procedure. A more advanced learner may benefit from higher fidelity models to add to the immersion in the simulation. Advanced learners may also benefit from embedding a simple procedure into a complex clinical scenario to challenge multiple types of skills simultaneously. For a course on splinting extremities, for example, the curriculum should be different for an introductory course for medical students compared with a refresher course for senior clinicians. Different professions will require different training models at first, but ultimately, multidisciplinary teams will require interprofessional training. Training can be focused on critical CRM skills, such as speaking up from a position lower on the team hierarchy or, for leaders, using techniques to encourage all members of the team to speak up.

### Methodology

The key benefit of SBME is the opportunity for practice of a skill or clinical situation as needed to achieve competency. Deliberate practice involves the repetition of a skill, while focusing on specific elements critical for effective skill performance, receiving expert feedback, and allowing sufficient time to improve. Technical skills may require short episodes of deliberate practice distributed over a long period of time. Team activities that are time-sensitive and depend on complicated choreography may benefit from deliberate practice akin to theater rehearsals or team-sport drills. The ideal frequency of SBME for optimal performance has yet to be determined, but distributed learning over time has been shown to be better for many technical, cognitive, and behavioral skills than a single longer session. Debriefing and feedback can be interspersed during the simulation or immediately after and are critical for learning.

### Simulation Implementation

After identification of clear learning objectives, implementation of simulation activities requires the following steps: evidence-based curriculum and scenario design, identification of appropriate simulator technology, achievement of optimal fidelity or realism (according to available resources), and effective debriefing preparation and expertise.

Development of a simulation scenario requires a detailed description of the patient and the medical history, the clinical context, any changes in status of the patient, and ultimately, the expected interventions and actions of the target learners during the simulation. Often, the best scenarios are based on actual cases. In order to recreate a realistic scenario, details must be considered so that the case is realistic to learners but also so that it can be reproduced for subsequent learners. There are many templates available to help guide the simulation educator in development of an effective scenario.

Choosing appropriate simulation technology requires an understanding of the types of simulators available and the learning objectives. The nature of the learning objectives informs the type of simulation experience that should be used. To teach an individual a technical skill such as suturing a wound, a low-tech skills trainer can be used. To train a healthcare team in CRM, a highly interactive and technical manikin (high-fidelity manikin), if available, will allow the team to actually care for a patient and focus the learning on behavioral skills. By immersing a team in an environment with a high-fidelity manikin, the instructor can simulate the time-pressure and stress, which makes the use of closed-loop communication, shared mental modeling, and other CRM skills essential for the team to perform well. As a final example, to foster empathy and enhance listening skills, use of an actor or standardized patient will be essential to allow for immersed learning of difficult conversations.

Fidelity of a simulation is another aspect to be considered. Manikins and task-trainers are not real, which makes the training or testing environment safe. However, using manikins or task trainers could get in the way of learning if the participants are forced to translate skills or steps into a clinical setting. The less the simulation environment differs from the clinical environment, the greater the usefulness of the simulation is. Using the equipment actually used in the learner's work setting will help to transfer skills learned in simulation to real life. Providing the appropriate auditory, tactile, visual, and even olfactory cues should be considered to allow the learners to share the instructors' same mental model of the situation. Similarly, in simulation-based quality and safety encounters, such as testing a new operating room layout, it is important that the dimensions of the room and equipment match the space of the actual room. For team training or team-testing, having the complete multidisciplinary team present during the simulation is an important part of realism. For each simulation encounter, optimal realism should be a goal. Debriefing preparation is key for all simulation-based activities. For SBME, developing the debriefing skills of the instructors is essential. It is imperative that all debriefers participate in some form of training on effective debriefing and facilitation techniques. Clinical knowledge, while important, may not be as critical as debriefing expertise, and can be augmented by including a content expert for a particular case. For quality and safety types of simulations, debriefing checklists should be developed to focus on identifying latent safety threats in the clinical system being evaluated as opposed to identifying performance gaps by the clinicians.

## EXAMPLES OF THE APPLICATION OF SIMULATION

### Status Epilepticus with Airway Compromise

The learning objectives for this SBME activity may include effective airway management skills, seizure treatment, effective teamwork, and communication during a crisis. The target learners would include the minimal number of healthcare providers that would care for a patient in this situation: nurses, respiratory therapist, and physician(s). A simulation scenario would be scripted to include the expected progression of the case. It would be useful to have a high-fidelity manikin capable of showing abnormal movements or seizures with auditory signs of upper respiratory tract obstruction. The debriefing preparation would include a checklist of proper evaluation of a patient in respiratory distress including ABCs (airway, breathing, and circulation), as well as the medical management of the seizure and examples of effective teamwork and communication skills.

### Evaluation of Latent Safety Threats Related to the Design of a New Operating Room

The critical objectives of this example of quality improvement and patient safety simulation activity focus on identifying possible patient latent safety threats (LSTs) related to physical layout, accessibility of emergency equipment and supplies, and care workflows and processes. A high-risk operating room (OR) simulated case, such as massive hemorrhage or fire in the OR, might be scripted to test the new environment. The reproduction of the space, such as a mock-up in a warehouse, should replicate, as closely as possible, the architectural drawings. The debriefing checklist should include questions to uncover LSTs, such as accessibility and visibility to patient and patient information, adequate lighting, accessibility to emergency equipment, and ease of personnel flow within the space, among others.

## EVALUATION OF SIMULATION-BASED MEDICAL EDUCATION CURRICULUM

All simulation-based curricula must themselves be evaluated and adapted. Many layers of testing may be needed to provide a complete picture of how a particular curriculum works. Knowledge testing, self-efficacy surveys, assessment of learner satisfaction, observation of skills in patient care scenarios, and ultimately, patient outcomes may be examined to determine the best method for educating learners.

## CONCLUSION

Times are changing, new rules arise, and the old ways of learning through trial and error, near-misses, or anecdotes from others are no longer acceptable. Society now has higher standards for healthcare education and patient safety. Technology has made incredible advances, and the public is aware of them. Now apprentices can learn and practice utilizing new technologies, such as surgical and resuscitation task trainers, before they have achieved mastery, helping them improve without the risks associated with actual patient exposure. Not only that, time for exposure to rare and/or high-risk clinical situations is significantly reduced as trainee working hours are decreasing. This is where simulation plays a key role, providing learners with realistic clinical situations on demand and where the errors made which have no real implication other than the lessons learned by the learners.

## SUGGESTED READINGS


Bryan RL, Kreuter MW, Brownson RC. Integrating adult learning principles into training for public health practice. *Health Promot Pract.* 2009;10(4):557-563.

Cheng A, Auerbach M, Hunt EA, et al. Designing and Conducting Simulation-based Research. *Pediatrics.* 2014;133(6):1091-1101.

Gaba DM, Fish KJ, Howard SK. *Crisis Management in Anesthesiology.* New York: Churchill Livingston; 1994.

Helmreich RL, Davies JM. Anaesthetic simulation and lessons to be learned from aviation. *Can J Anaesth.* 1997;44(9):907-912.

Issenberg SB, McGaghie WC, Hart IR, et al. Simulation technology for health care professional skills training and assessment. *JAMA.* 1999;282(9):861-866.

Issenberg SB, McGaghie WC, Petrusa ER, Gordon DE, Scalese RJ. Features and uses of high-fidelity medical simulations that lead to effective learning: a BEME systematic review. *Med Teach.* 2005;27(1):10-28.

Knowles MS. Application in continuing education for the health professions: chapter five of "Andragogy in Action." *Mobius.* 1985;5(2):80-100.

Kohn LT, Corrigan JM, Donaldson MS. *To Err is Human—Building a Safer Health System.* Washington: National Academy Press; 1999.

McGaghie WC, Draycott TJ, Dunn WF, Lopez CM, Stefanidis D. Evaluating the impact of simulation on translational outcomes. *Simul Healthc.* 2011;6(Suppl):S42-S47.

McGaghie WC, Issenberg SB, Petrusa ER, Scalese RJ. Effect of practice on standardized learning outcomes in simulation-based medical education. *Med Educ.* 2006;40(8):792-797.

McGaghie WC, Issenberg SB, Petrusa ER, Scalese RJ. A critical review of simulation-based medical education research: 2003–2009. *Med Educ.* 2010;44(1):50-63.




# PART 3 INJURIES AND UNTOWARD EVENTS

# 113 Caregiver-Reported Acute Infant Events

Michael J. Corwin

## INTRODUCTION

The assessment and management of infants who are described, by a parent or other caregiver, as having had a frightening, perhaps life-threatening, event is a challenging problem for clinicians. The fear that the infant may experience additional episodes, perhaps a fatal one, heightens the anxiety level of both families and medical professionals.

## DEFINITION

Prior to 1986, parent/caregiver-reported acute events in infants were commonly referred to as an *aborted crib death* or *near-miss sudden infant death syndrome* (SIDS). However, in 1986, a National Institutes of Health (NIH) Consensus Development Conference on Infantile Apnea and Home Monitoring recommended use of a newly defined term: *apparent life-threatening event* (ALTE). The consensus conference defined an ALTE as "an episode that is frightening to the observer and that is characterized by some combination of apnea (central or occasionally obstructive), color change (usually cyanotic or pallid but occasionally erythematous or plethoric), marked change in muscle tone (usually limpness), choking, or gagging." In addition, it was recommended that previously used terminology such as *aborted crib death* or *near-miss sudden infant death syndrome* be abandoned to avoid implication of a causal association between this type of spell and SIDS.

Apparent life-threatening events were described in the Consensus Development Conference statement as a "chief complaint that describes a general clinical syndrome." Although the definition of an apparent life-threatening event appeared straightforward, in practice, determining whether or not an infant experienced an ALTE has been extraordinarily difficult for clinicians, and it has frequently led to hospital admissions and testing of questionable value. In response to this dilemma, in 2016, a clinical practice guideline was published by the American Academy of Pediatrics (AAP), which suggested using event characteristics, rather than the term ALTE, to describe events and suggested new terminology, *brief resolved unexplained events* (BRUE), be used for events that met specific characteristics. The definition of a BRUE is a sudden, brief (ie, < 1minute), and now resolved episode with at least 1 of the following: cyanosis or pallor; absent, decreased, or irregular breathing; marked change in tone (hyper- or hypotonia); and altered responsiveness. In addition, criteria were provided to risk stratify infants having events that met the BRUE criteria, and management guidelines were provided for infants who met criteria to be considered low risk.

## INCIDENCE

Since the terminology is newly developed, there are no data on the incidence of BRUE. Data regarding the incidence of ALTEs are also limited, due to the imprecise manner in which this terminology has been applied. However, the incidence of ALTE was estimated to be 0.05% to 1% in population-based studies. Some perspective on the occurrence of idiopathic ALTE can be obtained from the Collaborative Home Infant Monitoring Evaluation (CHIME study), which was conducted at 5 medical centers (located in Cleveland, Toledo, Chicago, Los Angeles, and Honolulu) during the mid-1990s. This study included a systematic review of infants who presented with diagnoses consistent with ALTE and found that a typical urban medical center hospital provides care for about 1 case of possible ALTE each week and that approximately 20% of such cases will be considered an idiopathic ALTE.

## CLINICAL PRESENTATION

Most commonly, infants are no longer experiencing respiratory or circulatory dysfunction by the time they are first seen by medical professionals. Even in cases in which an emergency medical team has been called, the signs commonly have resolved by the time emergency medical technicians arrive. In some cases, during a routine well-child visit, a parent may describe an event that was witnessed days or weeks in the past.

Among the most difficult tasks for the clinician is to identify the events that the infant actually experienced. The ability of the caretakers to provide an accurate history is diminished by the fact that they may have been frightened to the point of panic. The situation may be further confounded by circumstances such as a dark room, clothes or covers obscuring the view of the infant, or inexperience evaluating infant behavior.

If the infant has current symptoms or abnormal vital signs (eg, cough, respiratory symptoms, or fever), or if there is a likely diagnosis suggested by the history and physical (eg, gastroesophageal reflux, feeding difficulties, or airway abnormality), then the event is not a BRUE and the evaluation and management should be guided by the specific findings. If the infant is well appearing, and meets the criteria provided above, then the event should be considered a BRUE, and evaluation and management should be based on risk stratification criteria. Infants experiencing an event meeting the BRUE criteria are considered at lower risk if there are no specific concerns raised by the history and physical (eg, family history of sudden cardiac death or subtle, nondiagnostic social feeding or respiratory problems) and they meet the following low-risk criteria: age > 60 days, at least 32 weeks' gestation and corrected gestational age at least 45 weeks, no CPR given by a trained medical provider, event lasted < 1 minute, first-time event.

## EVALUATION

### Infants Meeting Lower-Risk BRUE Criteria

For infants who meet the BRUE criteria and are in the lower-risk category, the AAP clinical practice guideline should be followed. Caregivers should be educated about BRUE and engaged in shared decision-making to guide evaluation, disposition, and follow-up, and resources for CPR training should be offered to the caregiver. Depending on the circumstances, it may be appropriate to obtain pertussis testing or a 12-lead electrocardiogram (ECG). The guideline recommends that clinicians should not obtain laboratory studies such as white blood cell (WBC) count, blood culture, cerebrospinal fluid (CSF) analysis or culture, serum electrolytes, blood urea nitrogen (BUN), creatinine, ammonia, blood gasses, urine organic acids, plasma amino acids or acylcamitines, chest radiograph, echocardiogram, electroencephalogram (EEG), or studies for GER. Clinicians also should not initiate home cardiorespiratory monitoring and should not prescribe acid suppression therapy or antiepileptic medications. In addition, the guidelines states that clinicians need not obtain viral respiratory tests, urinalysis, blood glucose, serum bicarbonate, serum lactic acid, laboratory evaluation for anemia, or neuroimaging, and need not admit the patient to the hospital solely for cardiorespiratory monitoring.

### Infants Meeting Higher-Risk BRUE Criteria, with Persistent Symptoms or With Findings Suggesting A Diagnosis

The relatively small number of infants who meet higher-risk BRUE criteria or who have symptoms or other findings suggesting an underlying explanation for the event should receive a careful investigation, directed by the specific findings to identify a cause. Recognizing that most of the signs potentially relate to disturbed breathing, the initial focus in an evaluation is often directed at assessing respiratory function unless there are other cues in the history. Examples include respiratory infection, especially respiratory syncytial virus; seizures; tumors of the central nervous system; gastroesophageal reflux; drug-induced respiratory depression; poisoning; postanesthetic depression; upper airway obstruction; arrhythmias; inborn errors of metabolism; and child abuse (eg, Munchausen syndrome). Based on the results of the history and physical examination, clinicians should identify those conditions that require further investigation. Table 113-1 lists the tests commonly used in the evaluation of these infants. Diagnoses may include infections, gastroesophageal reflux, and seizures. In addition,

**TABLE 113-1 DIAGNOSTIC TESTING FOR INFANTS MEETING HIGHER-RISK BRUE CRITERIA**

**Initial assessment appropriate in most infants requiring evaluation**

- Complete blood count with differential (evidence of infection)
- Plasma concentrations of glucose, electrolytes, BUN, calcium, and magnesium (evidence of $CO_2$ retention or bicarbonate loss, hyponatremia, hypoglycemia)
- Cardiorespiratory monitoring (evidence of dysrhythmia or irregular breathing)

**Tests occasionally indicated based on other findings**

- Neurologic testing (EEG, brain imaging)
- Cardiac evaluation (chest radiograph, ECG, echocardiogram, Holter monitoring)
- Infectious disease evaluation (bacterial and viral screening, lumbar puncture, chest radiograph)
- Metabolic analyses (arterial blood gases, lactate, pyruvate, $NH_4$, urine amino and organic acids, aminotransferases)
- Polysomnography (simultaneous recordings of multiple physiological signals, usually for at least 8 hours, with channels selected based on nature of symptoms)
- Esophageal pH and impedance monitoring with simultaneous polysomnography (pH probe alone is not useful for evaluation of ALTE)
- Child abuse investigation (skeletal survey, video surveillance)

ALTE, apparent life-threatening event; BRUE, brief resolved unexplained event; BUN, blood urea nitrogen; ECG, electrocardiogram; EEG, electroencephalogram among infants who were born prematurely, while no specific etiology may be identified, BRUE episodes may be attributable to persistent apnea of prematurity. In some cases, it may be possible to document features that suggest an immature respiratory control based on physiological recordings; however, no prognostic value of these recordings has been demonstrated.

## PROGNOSIS

For infants in whom a cause for the event is identified, the prognosis is determined by the particular diagnosis and by the ability to successfully provide treatment. In those cases in which the event is associated with prematurity, no further episodes are usually observed beyond the 43 to 44 weeks postconception age. Although premature infants have a higher rate of sudden unexpected death than do term infants, the occurrence of apnea has not been shown to add to this risk.

Among infants with an event meeting the lower-risk BRUE criteria, the prognosis is believed to be very good, with little data to suggest that subsequent episodes are likely to occur or that an underlying diagnosis might have been missed due to limiting the observation period or testing performed. However, outcome data based on use of the newly published AAP clinical practice guideline are not yet available. Among infants with a BRUE that falls into the higher-risk category, data from studies among the heterogeneous group of infants considered to have had an ALTE do not provide convincing evidence that these infants are at increased risk for neurodevelopmental problems. Controlled follow-up studies have reported a slight increase in subtle neurologic abnormalities at 1 to 3 years post-ALTE and an increased frequency of breath-holding spells; however, no differences were observed at 10 years. The rate of recurrent ALTE episodes or subsequent death is not well studied but appears to be less than 5%. One common problem in understanding the prognosis of recurrent ALTE is the difficulty in disentangling child abuse from other causes. Although, the proportion of ALTE cases that may be attributable to child abuse is unknown, such cases have been well documented. Factors that increase the suspicion of child abuse include recurrent ALTE requiring cardiopulmonary resuscitation, history of SIDS or ALTE in siblings, and episodes that occur only in the presence of a single caretaker. Infants who have ALTE features suggestive of child abuse are at particularly high risk of recurrent episodes or death.

## MANAGEMENT

In the majority of cases that meet the lower-risk BRUE criteria, the AAP clinical practice guideline should be followed: Families need reassurance with a clear explanation of why no further intervention is needed and, if appropriate, need advice regarding childcare practices that will decrease the likelihood of recurrence (eg, proper feeding technique to reduce choking). Although there is often reluctance on the part of both families and clinicians to accept simple reassurance and counseling, there is no evidence that these episodes are associated with increased risk of morbidity or mortality. In this setting, undertaking an extensive workup that may be both intrusive and expensive has little justification and may heighten, rather than reduce, anxiety. Alternatively, when the event meets the higher-risk BRUE criteria, or the suspected underlying diagnosis warrants it, hospitalization is appropriate, and the results of the inpatient evaluation, as described above, along with the ongoing clinical course will dictate subsequent management strategies.

Home cardiorespiratory monitoring is a potential management option that is controversial. Standard home cardiorespiratory devices detect when the heart rate falls below or above a preset range or when there is no chest wall movement for a preset length of time. Most currently used monitors also record waveforms during events (documented monitoring), which can facilitate diagnosis and decisions about when to stop monitoring. Oxygen saturation measurements can be included on some monitors if specifically requested. Although there have not been studies demonstrating a therapeutic benefit from home cardiorespiratory monitoring, in selected cases, monitor recordings may provide some diagnostic value, or may provide reassurance that clinically important events are not occurring. It should be noted that standard cardiorespiratory monitoring typically detects only chest wall movement and heart rate, and there may be circumstances (eg, suspected obstructive apnea) in which monitoring oxygen saturation by pulse oximetry may be more appropriate than cardiorespiratory monitoring. The decision regarding potential use of a home cardiorespiratory monitor should be made on a case-by-case basis after considering with the family the potential benefits, uncertainties, and stresses involved. Circumstances in which home cardiorespiratory monitoring may be considered would include premature infants with recurrent episodes of apnea and bradycardia, or infants with unstable airways or chronic lung disease.

Infants who experience multiple events are at very high risk for substantial morbidity, including death. In such cases, it is critical to identify the underlying cause, so that appropriate intervention can be initiated. The most common causes of recurrent events include infections, seizures, gastroesophageal reflux, and child abuse. Of these, the most difficult and the most important to diagnose is child abuse. However, an appropriate index of suspicion and a careful look for features consistent with abuse can be lifesaving. In cases of multiple events, where a specific diagnosis cannot be identified, use of a home monitor with memory may be of value in determining whether the events described are in fact genuine and, if they are genuine, to define physiologic changes that occur during the event.

## SUGGESTED READINGS


Brand DA, Altman RL, Purtill K, Edwards KS. Yield of diagnostic testing in infants who have had an apparent life-threatening event. *Pediatrics.* 2005;115(4):885-893.

Fu LY, Moon RY. Apparent life-threatening events: an update. *Pediatr Rev.* 2012;33(8):361-368.

Kaji AH, Claudius I, Santillanes G, et al. Apparent life-threatening event: multicenter prospective cohort study to develop a clinical decision rule for admission to the hospital. *Ann Emerg Med.* 2013;61(4):379-387.

Kant S, Fisher JD, Nelson DG, Khan S. Mortality after discharge in clinically stable infants admitted with a first-time apparent life-threatening event. *Am J Emerg Med.* 2013;31(4):730-733.

McGovern MC, Smith MB. Causes of apparent life threatening events in infants: a systematic review. *Arch Dis Child.* 2004;89(11):1043-1048.

Mittal MK, Donda K, Baren JM. Role of pneumography and esophageal pH monitoring in the evaluation of infants with apparent life-threatening event: a prospective observational study. *Clin Pediatr (Phila).* 2013;52(4):338-43.

Mittal MK, Sun G, Baren JM. A clinical decision rule to identify infants with apparent life-threatening event who can be safely discharged from the emergency department. *Pediatr Emerg Care.* 2012;28(7):599-605.

National Institutes of Health Consensus Development Conference on Infantile Apnea and Home Monitoring, Sept 29 to Oct 1, 1986. *Pediatrics.* 1987;79:292-299.

Putnam-Hornstein E, Schneiderman JU, Cleves MA, Magruder J, Krous HF. A prospective study of sudden unexpected infant death after reported maltreatment. *J Pediatr.* 2014;164(1):142-148.

Ramanathan R, Corwin MJ, Hunt CE, et al; Collaborative Home Infant Monitoring Evaluation (CHIME) Study Group. Cardiorespiratory events recorded on home monitors: comparison of healthy infants with those at increased risk for SIDS. *JAMA.* 2001;285(17):2199-2207.

Tieder JS, Altman RL, Bonkowsky JL, et al. Management of apparent life-threatening events in infants: a systematic review. *J Pediatr.* 2013;163(1):94-99.

Tieder JS, Bonkowsky JL, Etzel RA, et al; Subcommittee on Apparent Life-Threatening Events. Brief resolved unexplained events (formerly apparent life-threatening events) and evaluation of lower-risk infants: executive summary. *Pediatrics.* 2016;137(5):e20160591.

# 114 Toxic Ingestions and Exposures

Sing-Yi Feng and Collin S. Goto

## MANAGEMENT OF THE INTOXICATED PATIENT

Morbidity and mortality from childhood poisoning have decreased in the last few decades. This decrease can be credited to the development of poison control centers with a sophisticated poison management database, new governmental regulations, widespread use of child-resistant enclosures for medications, safer packaging for consumer products, public education and anticipatory guidance, and a growing understanding of the environmental and pharmacologic foundations of toxicology.

In particular, poison control centers, if available, provide immediate and expert advice from trained specialists in poison information to aid the practitioner in the management of poisoned patients, with particular reference to decontamination, antidotes, or other medical treatment; selection of appropriate laboratory tests; and enhanced drug elimination.

### POISON PREVENTION

The goal of poison prevention programs is to prevent pediatric poisoning through legislation and educational strategies; medication safety, such as parental anticipatory guidance regarding medication; and household safety during well-child visits. Brochures and other poison prevention materials can be obtained from local poison centers or through national bodies and legislative initiatives, such as the Poison Prevention Packaging Act (in the United States) have been instrumental in decreasing the impact of childhood poisoning.

### EPIDEMIOLOGY

Young children usually have little difficulty finding toxic substances, which can result in accidental poisoning. Personal-care products and cleaning substances are the most common agents involved in household intoxications, although pharmaceutical products are responsible for the majority of fatalities. Analgesics are the most common pharmaceutical exposure.

There are fewer adolescent exposures reported to poison centers compared with younger children, but most adolescent poisonings are intentional and involve greater amounts of toxins, often with multiple agents, and with delayed presentation for medical attention. As a consequence, adolescent poisonings often result in more serious toxicity.

### EVALUATION OF THE POISONED PATIENT

A presumptive diagnosis can often be made using information from the history, vital signs, and physical examination before extensive laboratory results are available. The type of toxin, timing, amount, and route of exposure are ascertained by asking the patient, family members, or other sources, and are critical to guiding therapy. The circumstances of the exposure and history of psychiatric illness help determine the risk for intentional harm. Potentially toxic household products such as automotive and cleaning products should not be overlooked. Paramedics and first responders provide important information about the scene of exposure and progression of the patient's signs and symptoms.

#### Discussion with the Poison Center

The value of a discussion with the local poison center cannot be overstated in terms of identification of substances through diagnostic tests, but also in piecing together the puzzle of unusual toxidromes and, equally importantly, in guiding immediate and longer term investigations and therapeutic interventions.

#### Toxidromes

Toxidromes or "toxic syndromes," are characteristic physical findings that indicate the presence of a specific category of toxins (Table 114-1). Toxidromes are especially helpful when the patient has been exposed to a single toxin. Exposure to multiple substances can obscure the clinical diagnosis, whereas other disease processes may mimic the toxidromes. Stimulation or inhibition of specific central or autonomic receptors results in the classic toxidromes (Fig. 114-1).

#### Laboratory Evaluation

Basic laboratory evaluation provides valuable information for the diagnosis and management of the poisoned patient. An arterial blood gas demonstrating an acid–base disturbance, and calculation of the anion gap ($Na^+ - [Cl^- + HCO_3^-]$) can narrow the differential diagnosis (Table 114-2). An elevated anion gap suggests the presence of an unidentified negatively charged molecule in the serum, which may represent a toxin or a byproduct of the intoxication, such as lactate.

If there is an unexplained metabolic acidosis, obtaining serum osmolarity, electrolytes, blood urea nitrogen (BUN), and glucose, and then calculating the osmolar gap (measured serum osmolarity – calculated serum osmolarity; normal is less than 10) can aid in diagnosis. The calculated osmolality is estimated by

$$2[\text{Na}]+\frac{[\text{Glucose}]}{18}+\frac{[\text{BUN}]}{2.8}.$$

An elevated osmolar gap indicates the presence of a low-molecular-weight and osmotically active substance such as methanol or ethylene glycol in the blood. An elevated anion gap metabolic acidosis accompanied by an elevated osmolar gap suggests toxic alcohol poisoning. A normal osmolar gap does not eliminate the possibility of toxic alcohol poisoning if the alcohol has already been converted into toxic metabolites.

Quantitative blood tests are ordered for specific drugs or toxins whose serum concentration can guide therapy or predict toxicity. In cases of unknown ingestions, serum acetaminophen and salicylate levels are obtained because these poisonings are common and early diagnostic clues may be absent.

**TABLE 114-1 COMMON TOXIDROMES**

| Mechanism | Classes of Drugs | Toxidrome |
|---|---|---|
| Anticholinergic | Antidepressants, antiparkinson medications, atropine, antihistamines, antipsychotics | Delirium, dry skin, flushing, hyperthermia, mydriasis, tachycardia, urinary retention, ileus |
| Cholinergic muscarinic | Organophosphates, carbamates, pilocarpine | Diarrhea, diaphoresis, urination, miosis, bradycardia, bronchorrhea, bronchospasm, emesis, lacrimation, lethargy, salivation |
| Cholinergic nicotinic | Organophosphates, carbamates, pilocarpine | Miosis, tachycardia, weakness, hypertension, fasciculations |
| Sympathomimetic | Cocaine, amphetamines, etc | Agitation, diaphoresis, hypertension, hyperthermia, seizures, tachycardia |
| Sedative-hypnotic withdrawal | Ethanol, benzodiazepines, barbiturates | Anxiety, diaphoresis, hypertension, mydriasis, cardiovascular failure, convulsions, delirium, tachycardia |
| Opioid withdrawal | Opioids | **Psychological:** anxiety, agitation, cravings, insomnia, hallucinations, dysphoria<br>**Physical:** tachycardia, hypertension, tachypnea, diaphoresis, piloerection, vomiting, diarrhea, mydriasis, tremors, seizures |

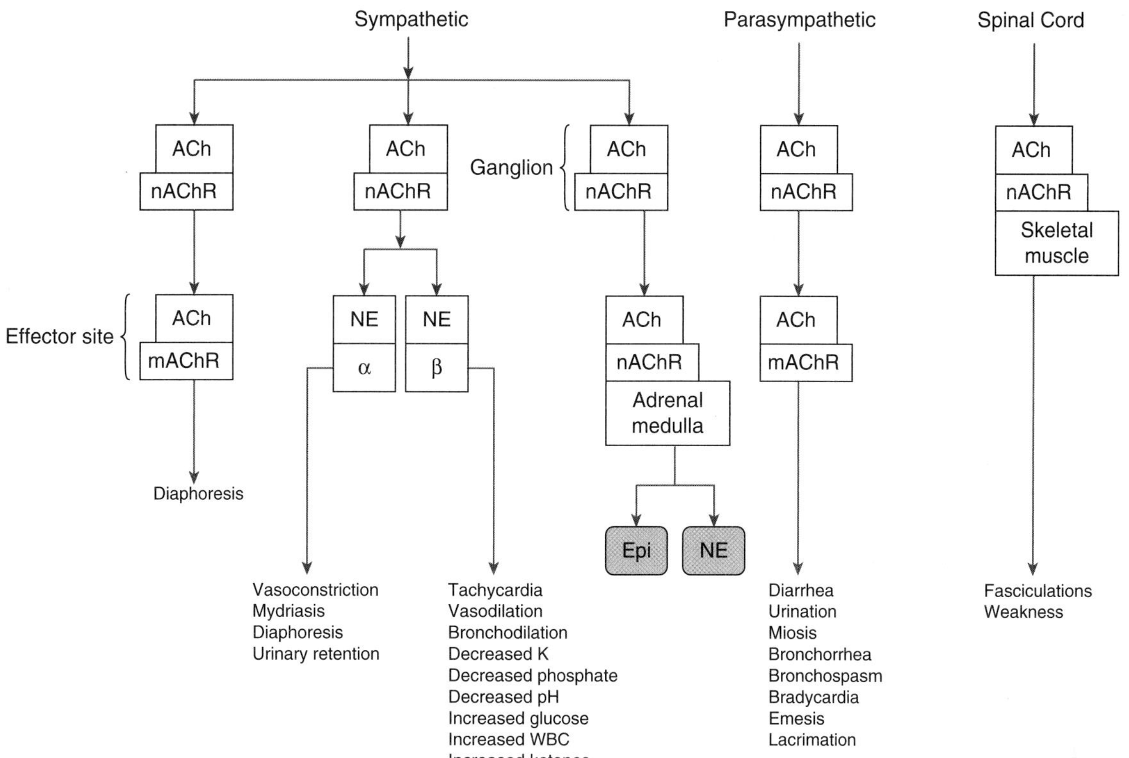


**FIGURE 114-1** Toxidromes. Stimulation or inhibition of specific receptors in the autonomic and somatic nervous systems results in the classic toxidromes, manifested by specific symptoms. α, α-adrenergic receptor; ACh, acetylcholine; β, β-adrenergic receptor; Epi, epinephrine; mAChR, muscarinic acetylecholine receptor; nAChR, nicotinic acetylcholine receptor; NE, norepinephrine; WBC, white blood cells.

Toxicology screens should only be ordered when the result is expected to influence patient management. The history and clinical toxidrome are usually adequate to narrow the differential diagnosis and guide management decisions. Comprehensive blood or urine toxicology screens have a longer turnaround time and qualitatively detect only 40 to 100 specific drugs. They will not affect emergency management but may be helpful to the admitting physicians when the patient's diagnosis remains unclear and the clinical course is complicated.

### Radiology

Abdominal radiographs aid in the visualization of radio-opaque substances such as bezoars, radio-opaque medications (ie, ferrous sulfate pills), metals, and drug-filled packets. Serial abdominal radiographs may be useful to assess adequacy of gastrointestinal decontamination in such patients.

**TABLE 114-2 CAUSES OF HIGH ANION GAP METABOLIC ACIDOSIS**

| Lactic Acidosis | Non–Lactic Acid Metabolic Acidosis |
|---|---|
| Acetaminophen (levels > 600 mg/dL) | Exogenous organic and mineral acids |
| β-Adrenergic receptor agonists | Formaldehyde (formic acid) |
| Biguanides (metformin/phenformin) | Ibuprofen (propionic acid) |
| Carbon monoxide | Ketoacidosis (alcoholic, diabetic, starvation) |
| Cyanide | Metaldehyde |
| HAART (highly active antiretroviral therapy) | Salicylates (salicylic acid) |
| Hydrogen sulfide | Toxic alcohols (methanol/ethylene glycol) |
| Hypoxia | Valproic acid |
| Iron | |
| Isoniazid | |
| Methylxanthines (caffeine, theophylline) | |
| Salicylates | |
| Sodium azide | |

### Resuscitation and Stabilization

Initial treatment follows the same principles applied to other life-threatening conditions. Decreased respiratory effort, airway obstruction, and severe respiratory distress are indications for endotracheal intubation and mechanical ventilation. If there is suspicion of opioid intoxication, judicious use of an opioid antagonist may restore normal breathing, precluding the need for endotracheal intubation. Intravenous access should be obtained promptly, and cardiovascular dysfunction corrected with intravenous fluids and pharmacologic support. Appropriate monitoring includes measurement of temperature, respiratory rate, oxygen saturation, heart rate, blood pressure, and serial electrocardiograms.

## DECONTAMINATION

The goals of decontamination are to prevent the absorption of a toxin into the systemic circulation either internally from the gastrointestinal tract or externally from the skin or eyes, and this should be performed as early as possible.

### Ocular and Dermal Decontamination

Immediate and thorough irrigation with tap water or normal saline may ameliorate injury following ocular and dermal exposures. Contact lenses should be removed and irrigation of the eyes performed rapidly to prevent ocular damage. The patient's clothing, jewelry, and other items should be removed for dermal decontamination, and care is required to protect healthcare staff from secondary toxin exposure.

### Syrup of Ipecac

This is a potent emetic that is no longer recommended as a home remedy for ingestions. The efficacy of syrup of ipecac in improving clinical outcomes remains unproven, and its use may delay the use of other decontamination techniques such as activated charcoal.

### Activated Charcoal

Activated charcoal administered into the gastrointestinal tract binds most toxins, decreasing systemic absorption. It is ineffective for iron and other metals, lithium and other small ions, cyanide, alcohols, and most caustics. The dose of activated charcoal is 1 g/kg by mouth or via nasogastric tube for children and 50 to 100 g for adolescents and adults. If a nasogastric tube is necessary, consideration must be given as to whether the expected benefit exceeds the risk. Patients with protracted vomiting are not candidates for activated charcoal, and those with decreased consciousness or undergoing sedation should not receive charcoal unless the airway has been protected with an endotracheal tube, to protect from life-threatening aspiration.

### Gastric Lavage

Orogastric lavage can be considered in patients who present to medical attention within 1 to 2 hours after ingestion of a potentially lethal toxin. It is not routinely recommended for all overdose patients due to the risk of complications, including visceral perforation, tracheal placement of the orogastric lavage tube, and aspiration of vomit. This should not be performed in patients with depressed mental status and an unprotected airway and ingestion of a caustic or hydrocarbon. A large-bore lavage tube (pediatrics, 16–28 Fr; adults, 36–40 Fr) is placed orogastrically with the patient in the left lateral decubitus position to optimize gastric decontamination and reduce the risk of aspiration. The stomach is lavaged with 50 to 250 mL aliquots of water or saline until clear of residual toxin.

### Whole Bowel Irrigation

Whole bowel irrigation reduces the absorption of ingested toxins by decreasing gastrointestinal transit time. Polyethylene glycol electrolyte solution is administered via nasogastric tube at rates of 25 to 40 mL/kg/hour for children and 1.5 to 2 L/hour for adults until rectal effluent is clear. This should be stopped if no rectal effluent occurs after several hours. Indications include ingestion of delayed-release medications, substances not adsorbed by charcoal, or drug-filled packages in drug smugglers ("body packers").

## ENHANCED ELIMINATION

Enhanced elimination procedures hasten the excretion of toxins from the systemic circulation at a rate greater than endogenous clearance.

### Multiple-Dose Activated Charcoal

Multiple-dose activated charcoal enhances elimination and decontaminates the gastrointestinal tract by (1) disrupting enterohepatic recirculation of the toxin, (2) utilizing the intestinal mucosa as a dialysis membrane ("gut dialysis") to draw the toxin from the bloodstream into the intestinal lumen, and (3) binding any toxin present in the gut. It enhances elimination of substances that undergo enterohepatic recirculation such as phenobarbital, quinidine, theophylline, carbamazepine, and dapsone as well as substances that can form bezoars such as salicylates. The dose of activated charcoal without cathartic administration is 0.5 to 1 g/kg by mouth or via nasogastric tube every 4 hours. It should be discontinued if ileus develops. Complications include charcoal aspiration, formation of charcoal bezoars, and intestinal obstruction.

### Urinary Alkalinization

Urinary alkalinization enhances the elimination of drugs that are weak acids (ie, salicylates) by trapping the ionized drug in the renal tubule, where it is subsequently excreted in the urine (Fig. 114-2). Sodium bicarbonate is administered in a dose of 1 to 2 mEq/kg intravenously followed by a continuous infusion titrated to a urinary pH of 7.0 to 8.0. Hypokalemia must be corrected because it impedes urinary alkalinization as potassium is reabsorbed in exchange for hydrogen ions.

### Extracorporeal Methods

Extracorporeal methods of removing toxins include hemodialysis, continuous hemofiltration, and hemoperfusion, and are typically used in severe cases; in patients in whom there is impairment of the natural mechanism of elimination, who are deteriorating despite maximal supportive care; in toxins with delayed effects; or if a blood level of the toxin is associated with severe toxicity or death.

Hemodialysis is effective for toxins with small volumes of distribution (< 1.0 L/kg), low molecular weight, and low protein binding (eg, salicylates, theophylline, methanol, barbiturates, ethylene glycol, and lithium). Continuous hemofiltration techniques such as continuous venovenous hemofiltration (CVVH) and continuous venovenous hemodiafiltration (CVVHD) can be used for the removal of molecules up to 40 kDa. The advantages of CVVH and CVVHD are that they can be performed in hemodynamically unstable patients and can be performed over a prolonged period of therapy. Hemoperfusion is similar to hemodialysis except for substitution of the dialysis membrane by a cartridge containing an adsorbent material such as charcoal, and is more effective for larger molecules because there is no ultrafiltration. Despite these advantages, the use of hemoperfusion has declined in recent years due to the short shelf life of the cartridges and the technical difficulty of the procedure. Hemoperfusion does not correct acid–base or fluid balance, or electrolyte abnormalities.

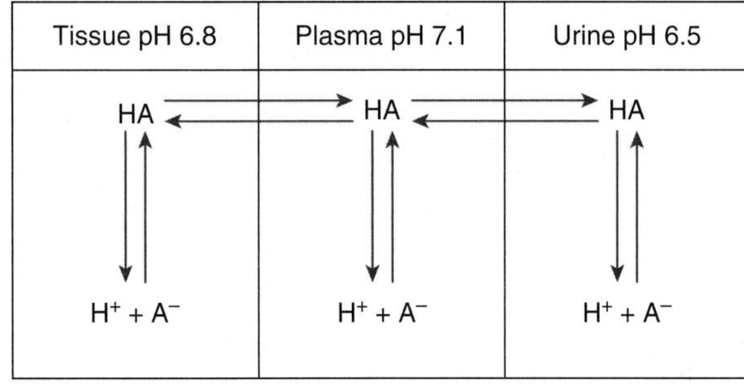


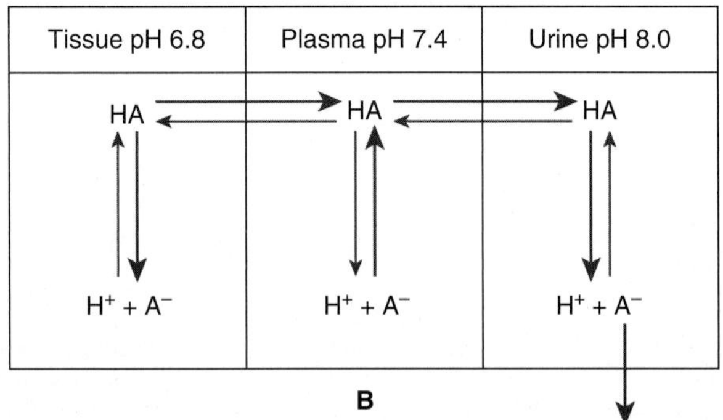


**FIGURE 114-2** Urinary alkalinization. Urinary alkalinization (ion trapping) is used to enhance the urinary excretion of weak acids, especially salicylates. Most drugs are partially dissociated at physiologic pH in a proportion that is determined by the drug's dissociation constant (pKa) and the pH of the medium in which the drug is dissolved. Cell membranes are more permeable to substances that are in the nonionized form. The ionization of a weak acid (HA) is increased in an alkaline environment. An increase in urine pH increases the proportion of drug in the ionized form, thereby reducing the drug's rate of diffusion from the renal tubule lumen back into the blood. This causes the weak acid to be trapped in the urine and excreted from the body.

### Antidotes

Antidotes prevent or reverse the effects of poisoning. Most are dispositional antidotes that decrease toxicity by altering absorption, distribution, metabolism, or elimination. Competitive antagonists interfere with the toxin binding to receptor sites. Physiologic antagonists alter the physiologic effect of the toxin. Antidotes are available for a very limited number of poisonings and do not replace meticulous supportive care and good clinical judgment. The risks and benefits of each antidote must be carefully considered.

## DISPOSITION AFTER TOXIN EXPOSURE

Asymptomatic patients with a potential toxic exposure are observed for at least 4 to 8 hours from the time of exposure. If symptoms develop, the patient is admitted to the hospital for further evaluation and management. Any patient with severe toxicity will require admission to an intensive care unit. A longer observation period is required for toxins with delayed onset of action, such as sustained-release products, agents with toxic metabolites, and drugs with delayed distribution into the tissue compartment. Cellular injury may begin early with delayed onset of overt symptoms, such as with acetaminophen.

All pediatric exposures require social evaluation to determine home safety and provide poison prevention education. Patients may have been intentionally poisoned as a form of physical abuse or for purposes of sexual exploitation. Any intentional overdose warrants psychiatric evaluation of suicidal intent. Patients with chemical dependency should be referred to an appropriate treatment program.

# PHARMACEUTICAL AGENTS

## ACETAMINOPHEN

Acetaminophen (*N*-acetyl-*p*-aminophenol, or APAP), a widely used analgesic and antipyretic agent, is responsible for 10% of all calls to poison control centers. After therapeutic dosing, acetaminophen undergoes glucuronidation and sulfation in the liver prior to urinary and bile excretion (Fig. 114-3). A small percentage is oxidized in the hepatocytes by the cytochrome P450 system of CYP oxidases to produce *N*-acetyl-*p*-benzoquinoneimine (NAPQI), a highly reactive 2-electron species that can act as an oxidant and thus is highly cytotoxic. *N*-acetyl-*p*-benzoquinoneimine is eliminated by conjugation to the reduced form of glutathione (GSH), and the resulting APAP-GSH conjugate is eliminated as mercapturic acid and cysteine conjugates. After an overdose, however, the amount of NAPQI generated can exceed the capacity of this detoxification mechanism. *N*-acetyl-*p*-benzoquinoneimine then accumulates in the hepatocytes and toxicity ensues. Acute ingestion of more than 150 to 200 mg/kg in children or 7.5 g in adults is potentially hepatotoxic. Chronic or subacute overdose also results in liver injury.

The clinical presentation of acute acetaminophen toxicity is described in 4 phases. Phase 1 occurs during the first few hours after ingestion and is characterized by gastrointestinal symptoms of nausea, vomiting, and abdominal pain, but some patients are asymptomatic. Phase 2 is known as a quiescent phase and occurs within 24 hours, as the acute gastrointestinal symptoms subside. The onset of hepatotoxicity is manifested by upper-right quadrant abdominal tenderness and elevation of laboratory markers of liver injury such as transaminases and prothrombin time (PT). Phase 3 is the period of maximal hepatotoxicity, usually occurring within 72 to 96 hours. In mild cases, spontaneous recovery occurs. In severe cases, fulminant hepatic failure is manifested by coagulopathy, encephalopathy, and coma. Fatalities typically occur between 3 and 5 days because of multiorgan failure, hemorrhage, respiratory failure, sepsis, and cerebral edema. Phase 4 is the period of hepatic recovery, which may take a week or longer, depending on the severity of the liver injury.

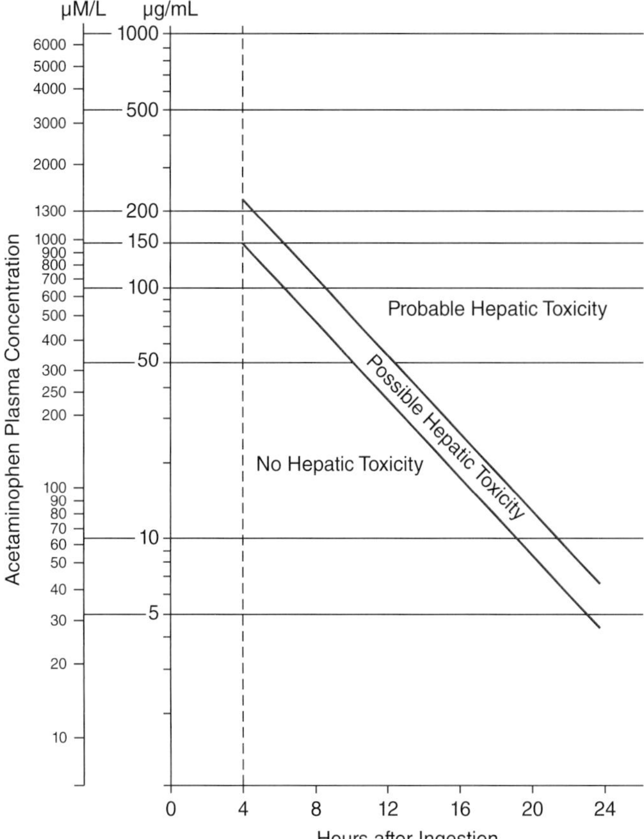


**FIGURE 114-4** Rumack-Matthews nomogram of hepatotoxicity after acetaminophen ingestion. The Rumack-Matthews nomogram shows the risk of hepatotoxicity based on the relationship between plasma acetaminophen concentration and time after ingestion. The range between the red lines represents a 25% chance of clinically significant disease.

Treatment decisions are guided by plotting the serum acetaminophen concentration on the Rumack-Matthew nomogram (Fig. 114-4) at 4 hours or more after a single acute ingestion. The nomogram is not used to predict toxicity after subacute overdose or multiple ingestions over a prolonged time period. Antidotal therapy with *N*-acetylcysteine (NAC) is initiated if the acetaminophen level is above the lower (possible hepatotoxicity) line on the nomogram, and should be started

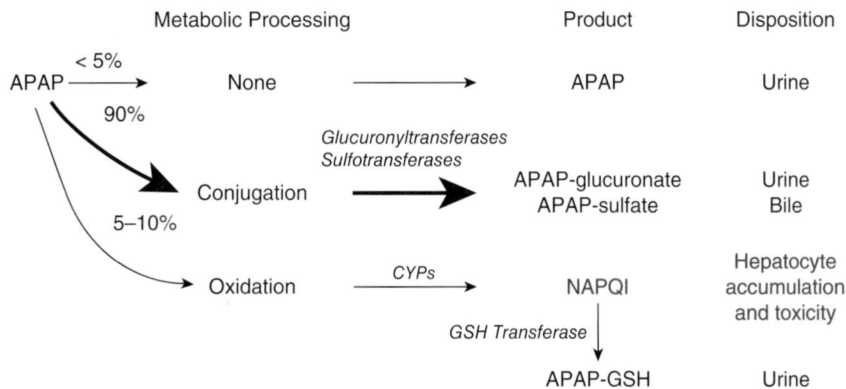


**FIGURE 114-3** Mechanism of acetaminophen (*N*-acetyl-*p*-aminophenol, or APAP) toxicity. See text for details. CYP, cytochrome P450; GSH, glutathione; NAPQI, *N*-acetyl-*p*-benzoquinoneimine.

within 8 to 10 hours of drug ingestion because its efficacy for preventing fulminant hepatic failure diminishes thereafter.

NAC functions both as a glutathione precursor to replenish depleted glutathione stores and as a glutathione substitute that directly binds to NAPQI. In addition, NAC facilitates the sulfation pathway of acetaminophen metabolism. NAC comes in both oral and intravenous preparations. The United States Food and Drug Administration's (FDA) approved oral NAC protocol consists of a loading dose of 140 mg/kg followed by 17 subsequent doses of 70 mg/kg administered every 4 hours over a 72-hour period. Treatment may be discontinued at 24 hours if there has been no elevation of liver transaminases and acetaminophen is no longer detectable in the serum. There are several intravenous NAC regimens that have been utilized, including 21-, 36-, and 48-hour protocols. The commonly used 21-hour protocol consists of a loading dose of 150 mg/kg administered over 1 hour, followed by an additional 50 mg/kg over the next 4 hours, and a subsequent 100 mg/kg over the next 16 hours. Repeated 100 mg/kg doses over 16 hours can be administered if the patient continues to have significantly elevated liver transaminases.

Laboratory monitoring includes measuring the serum acetaminophen level, liver transaminases, electrolytes, BUN, creatinine, and PT. Patients with severe hepatotoxicity require early evaluation for liver transplantation.

## ANTICOAGULANTS

Warfarin was initially used as a rodenticide before its therapeutic applications were recognized. These compounds inhibit vitamin K, a cofactor required for the synthesis of coagulation factors II, VII, IX, and X. The typical clinical scenario for warfarin ingestion would be a toddler who has ingested a small amount of rodenticide. In this situation, no significant anticoagulation is expected, and no interventions are required. In contrast, larger ingestions with suicidal intent or chronic exposures may result in poisoning. The anticoagulant effect will not be seen until the circulating clotting factors have been degraded, which may take 1 to 2 days. Excessive anticoagulation results in ecchymoses, bleeding gums, subconjunctival hemorrhage, hematemesis, melena, or hematuria. In severe cases, intracranial hemorrhage or gastrointestinal bleeding is life threatening. The duration of effect after a single dose of warfarin is 2 to 7 days, whereas coagulopathy from superwarfarin poisoning often persists for months due to an extremely long elimination half-life.

Laboratory monitoring includes evaluation of coagulation, in particular the PT and international normalized ratio (INR). A normal PT 48 hours after ingestion rules out poisoning. Severe hemorrhage is treated with fresh-frozen plasma, packed red blood cells, and other blood products, as needed. Administration of vitamin $K_1$ (phytonadione), often as repeated doses for prolonged coagulopathy, allows regeneration of clotting factors, but peak effect may take 24 hours or longer. Vitamin $K_1$ is recommended for documented coagulopathy but should not be administered prophylactically because it will mask the development of toxicity and make the end point of treatment difficult to assess.

## ANTICONVULSANTS

Carbamazepine, phenobarbital, phenytoin, and valproic acid are frequently responsible for acute intoxications and are discussed here because serum concentrations are available rapidly from the laboratory to aid in patient management. Newer anticonvulsants are becoming more common. However, serum concentration measurements are not rapidly available, and overdoses are typically managed with nonspecific supportive care.

### Carbamazepine

Carbamazepine is a central nervous system sodium channel inhibitor. Toxic manifestations after an overdose are similar to those produced by tricyclic antidepressants (TCAs), with which carbamazepine is structurally related, resulting in central nervous system depression, anticholinergic effects, and myocardial sodium channel inhibition. Induction of vasopressin secretion may result in the syndrome of inappropriate secretion of antidiuretic hormone. Carbamazepine toxicity is characterized by neurologic abnormalities, including nystagmus, ataxia, dysarthria, myoclonus, and dystonia, and at higher levels (above 40 mg/dL) results in coma, respiratory depression, and seizures. Cardiovascular disturbances include tachycardia, hypotension, myocardial depression, and cardiac conduction abnormalities, such as prolongation of the QRS complex and QT interval. Mydriasis, hyperthermia, ileus, and other signs of cholinergic inhibition may occur.

Monitoring after a significant ingestion should include obtaining a serum carbamazepine level every 4 to 6 hours until a downward trend is established. Serum electrolytes should be checked for hyponatremia, and electrocardiogram monitoring helps detect cardiotoxicity. Treatment is supportive. Enhanced elimination procedures may be considered in patients with severe toxicity that is not responsive to standard supportive care.

### Phenobarbital

Barbiturates depress central nervous system function by enhancing the neuronal inhibition mediated by γ-aminobutyric acid (GABA). Supratherapeutic serum phenobarbital levels are associated with progressive ataxia, dysarthria, nystagmus, sedation, coma, hypothermia, and respiratory depression. Decreased sympathetic tone results in bradycardia and hypotension. Serial phenobarbital levels should be obtained until they are decreasing and the patient's symptoms are improving. Treatment is supportive. Enhanced elimination may benefit patients with severe toxicity refractory to supportive care.

### Phenytoin

Phenytoin and fosphenytoin are nonsedating at therapeutic doses. Phenytoin decreases the activity of neuronal voltage-dependent sodium channels, resulting in suppression of seizures. Excessive doses result in ataxia, nystagmus, diplopia, dysarthria, confusion, coma, and respiratory depression. Cardiotoxicity has not been reported following oral overdoses of phenytoin, although rapid intravenous administration may cause bradycardia and hypotension.

Phenytoin is poorly water soluble, and the intravenous preparation requires a solution of 40% propylene glycol and 10% ethanol at a pH of 12. Rapid infusion (> 50 mg/min phenytoin) results in myocardial depression and decreased systemic vascular resistance largely caused by the propylene glycol. Local irritation and tissue damage may be caused by the propylene glycol and the alkaline pH of the intravenous formulation. Fosphenytoin is a water-soluble product that is converted to phenytoin following intravenous administration. It is buffered to a pH of 8 to 9 and does not contain propylene glycol, allowing rapid intravenous administration (up to 150 mg/min of phenytoin equivalents). However, excessive doses of fosphenytoin have been reported to cause myocardial depression.

Serial serum phenytoin levels should be obtained until a downward trend is documented. Management is supportive. Multiple-dose activated charcoal may enhance the elimination of phenytoin, but is usually not necessary because of the success of supportive care alone.

### Valproic Acid

Valproic acid inhibits voltage-gated sodium channels and increases GABA levels in the central nervous system, resulting in central nervous system depression. In addition, valproic acid interferes with fatty acid metabolism by causing carnitine deficiency, impaired mitochondrial β-oxidation, and disruption of the urea cycle.

Patients with valproic acid toxicity can present with confusion and lethargy that may progress to coma, cerebral edema, and respiratory failure. Severe toxicity includes hypotension, metabolic acidosis, hypernatremia, hypocalcemia, pancreatitis, hepatic injury, hyperammonemia, renal insufficiency, and bone marrow suppression. Elevated ammonia levels result in valproate-induced hyperammonemic encephalopathy, characterized by altered mental status, focal neurologic abnormalities, and seizures.

Serial valproate levels should be obtained until a downward trend is established and the patient's symptoms are improving. Other useful laboratory studies include blood gas analysis, complete blood count, serum electrolytes, glucose, BUN, creatinine, calcium, liver transaminases, bilirubin, PT, lipase, amylase, lactate, ammonia, and carnitine. Treatment with carnitine is recommended if hyperammonemia, hepatotoxicity, or carnitine deficiency is present. Enhanced elimination techniques may be considered in patients with severe toxicity.

### Antipsychotics

The antipsychotic medications are classified as typical or atypical. The typical antipsychotics (eg, haloperidol, thioridazine, promethazine, mesoridazine, and chlorpromazine) were introduced in the 1950s but were associated with serious adverse effects, including extrapyramidal syndromes (particularly dyskinesia in children), tardive dyskinesia, and neuroleptic malignant syndrome (NMS). The atypical antipsychotics were developed to overcome these shortcomings. Examples of atypical agents include aripiprazole, olanzapine, clozapine, quetiapine, ziprasidone and risperidone.

The clinical presentation of mild intoxication with atypical antipsychotics includes confusion, sedation, vagolysis, and orthostatic hypotension with reflex tachycardia. Severe overdoses result in coma, seizures, respiratory arrest, and hypothermia or hyperthermia. Cardiovascular effects include hypotension due to impaired myocardial contractility and peripheral vasodilation, as well as widened QRS complex and QTc interval prolongation resulting in ventricular arrhythmias including torsade de pointes.

Extrapyramidal dystonic reactions include tremor, rigidity, bradykinesia, and spasms of the muscles of the eyes (oculogyric crisis), face, tongue, lips, jaw, neck (torticollis), abdomen (tortipelvis), and spine (opisthotonus). NMS is a life-threatening condition characterized by altered mental status, muscular rigidity, hyperthermia, and autonomic dysfunction.

Diagnosis is based on the clinical presentation. Quantitative blood levels are not routinely available. Comprehensive urine toxicology screens may detect only phenothiazines. Continuous electrocardiogram monitoring is essential to detect cardiac conduction abnormalities and dysrhythmias.

Management is primarily supportive. Specific interventions include sodium bicarbonate for treatment of myocardial sodium channel blockade and QRS interval prolongation, and magnesium infusion and cardioversion or defibrillation for ventricular arrhythmias. Dystonic reactions are treated with diphenhydramine or benztropine. Management of NMS requires aggressive cooling measures, intravenous hydration, advanced airway management as indicated, and intravenous benzodiazepines for sedation and muscle relaxation. Dantrolene (a muscle relaxant) may be of benefit if there is severe malignant hyperpyrexia, particularly in the setting of pending or actual rhabdomyolysis.

## β-BLOCKERS AND CALCIUM CHANNEL BLOCKERS

β-Adrenergic blocker (BB) and calcium channel blocker (CCB) medications are discussed together because of similarities in clinical presentation and management after overdose. Many of these similarities are due to their common effect of inhibiting the influx of calcium into myocardial cells, where it participates in physiologic signaling and other critical processes. Severe poisoning is difficult to treat and is associated with significant morbidity and mortality.

β-Blockers inhibit the binding of catecholamines to β-adrenergic receptors. Blockade of cardiac $\beta_1$-adrenergic receptors results in decreased chronotropy and inotropy, and the blockade of noncardiac $\beta_2$-adrenergic receptors antagonizes bronchial and smooth muscle relaxation, and also causes hypoglycemia by inhibition of glycogenolysis and gluconeogenesis.

Calcium channel blockers inhibit the influx of calcium through the L-type calcium channels of myocardial cells, resulting in decreased chronotropy and inotropy. Antagonism of similar vascular smooth muscle calcium channels results in coronary and peripheral vasodilation. Additionally, calcium-mediated insulin release from pancreatic β-islet cells is inhibited, preventing myocardial cells from utilizing glucose as an energy source, resulting in further myocardial dysfunction. The resulting shock state resembles diabetic ketoacidosis, with hyperglycemia and acidemia.



The hallmark of BB and CCB poisoning is cardiovascular depression and shock, with bradycardia, heart block, impaired cardiac contractility, and hypotension. Altered mental status is usually caused by cerebral hypoperfusion, but in the case of β-blockers may also be caused by hypoglycemia. β-Blockers that cross the blood-brain barrier and have membrane-depressant effects, such as propranolol, may cause coma, convulsions, and respiratory arrest. Noncardiac effects of CCBs include nausea, vomiting, and hyperglycemia. Global hypoperfusion may result in angina or myocardial infarction, cerebral ischemia, hepatic dysfunction, renal failure, and metabolic acidosis.

Diagnosis of BB and CCB poisoning is based on the history and clinical presentation, especially bradycardia and hypotension. β-Blocker poisoning may cause hypoglycemia, whereas CCB poisoning typically results in hyperglycemia. Studies that are helpful in assessment and management include electrolytes, glucose, BUN, creatinine, blood gas analysis, and electrocardiogram monitoring. A rapid bedside cardiac echocardiogram is useful to assess myocardial function. Patients with severe poisoning may require invasive monitoring to guide management.

Gastric lavage and administration of activated charcoal may be helpful early in patients with large recent ingestions. If the patient already has significant bradycardia, hypotension, or altered mental status, resuscitative procedures take precedence. Whole-bowel irrigation and multiple-dose activated charcoal should be considered in patients with ingestion of sustained-release preparations. General supportive measures include atropine for bradycardia and intravenous fluids for hypotension. Calcium and catecholamines should be used initially but may be ineffective after calcium channels and β-adrenergic receptors are inhibited. Glucagon is a specific antidote for β-blocker poisoning and has been used with some success in calcium channel blocker overdose as well. Glucagon produces positive inotropic and chronotropic effects by stimulating adenyl cyclase and opening calcium channels independent of the β-adrenergic receptor activation. Vasopressin improves blood pressure and increases the response to catecholamines. Hyperinsulinemia/euglycemia therapy improves myocardial contractility in calcium channel blocker overdose, often when other pharmacologic therapy has failed. It is postulated that this therapy corrects the impaired myocardial substrate utilization caused by calcium channel blocker–induced hypoinsulinemia, resulting in improved carbohydrate metabolism and increased myocardial contractility. Intravenous fat emulsion (IFE) therapy has been recently used to manage severe calcium channel blocker overdose. Although the mechanism is not well understood, it has been theorized that IFE sequesters lipophilic toxins such as CCBs in an intravascular lipid channel. This may decrease the distribution of the CCB into the tissue and result in the redistribution of the toxic drug back into the lipid channel. When pharmacologic therapy has failed, cardiopulmonary bypass or extracorporeal membrane oxygenation may be lifesaving.



## CLONIDINE

Clonidine is a centrally acting antihypertensive that is also prescribed for conditions such as attention-deficit/hyperactivity disorder and drug withdrawal. Clonidine binds to inhibitory presynaptic $\alpha_2$-adrenergic receptors in the medulla, resulting in decreased sympathetic outflow from the central nervous system.

The hallmark of intoxication is generalized sympathetic depression. Neurologic manifestations are similar to the opioid toxidrome and include pinpoint pupils, hypotonia, sedation, coma, hypothermia, respiratory depression, and apnea. Cardiovascular toxicity is manifested by bradycardia, decreased cardiac output, and hypotension.

Although clonidine poisoning mimics the opioid toxidrome, it does not reliably respond to naloxone. Sinus bradycardia does not require treatment unless it is associated with hypotension and poor perfusion. Atropine will often improve heart rate and cardiac output. Persistent hypotension is treated with intravenous fluids and catecholamine infusion. Coma and respiratory depression may require advanced airway management. Gastrointestinal decontamination is usually not indicated because of rapid onset of symptoms and good outcome with supportive care.

## CYCLIC ANTIDEPRESSANTS

TCAs were developed to treat depression in the 1950s, but TCA overdoses caused severe toxicity, resulting in many poisoning deaths. The selective serotonin reuptake inhibitors (SSRIs) were introduced in the 1980s and have a better safety profile than the TCAs. TCAs inhibit the reuptake of biogenic amine neurotransmitters in the central nervous system, including norepinephrine, dopamine, and serotonin. In overdose, other mechanisms result in toxicity, including antagonism of muscarinic cholinergic receptors, $\alpha_1$-adrenergic receptors, serotonin receptors, histaminic $H_1$ and $H_2$ receptors, $GABA_A$ receptors, and myocardial fast sodium channels.

Patients with significant TCA ingestions usually manifest symptoms within 30 to 60 minutes, and life-threatening toxicity within 6 hours. The most common cause of death is cardiovascular toxicity. Inhibition of myocardial fast sodium channels causes slowed phase 0 ventricular depolarization, decreased contractility, widened QRS and QT intervals, and ventricular arrhythmias including torsades de pointes. Severe hypotension is caused by norepinephrine depletion, $\alpha_1$-adrenergic receptor blockade, myocardial depression, and dysrhythmias. Muscarinic cholinergic receptor blockade results in sedation, coma, myoclonus, and seizures. Other anticholinergic effects include tachycardia, hyperthermia, mydriasis, ileus, urinary retention, diminished sweating, and dry mucus membranes. Seizures are also caused by inhibition of $GABA_A$ receptors.

SSRIs do not usually cause severe toxicity except in large overdoses. However, excessive serotonergic activity may result in the life-threatening serotonin syndrome. Some SSRIs cause additional toxicity via inhibition of dopamine and norepinephrine reuptake and antagonism of $\alpha_1$-adrenergic receptors. Some agents also have sodium and potassium channel inhibition causing QRS and QTc prolongation. Significant SSRI overdose results in nausea, ataxia, and sedation. Coma and respiratory depression may occur, particularly when alcohol or other sedating drugs are also involved. Some agents, such as buproprion, may cause tremor, agitation, and seizures. Cardiovascular effects include sinus tachycardia, hypotension, and cardiac conduction disturbances, but are usually not life threatening.

Serotonin syndrome is caused by excessive stimulation of serotonin $5\text{-}HT_{2A}$ and possibly $5\text{-}HT_{1A}$ receptors. This often occurs when an SSRI is combined with another drug with serotonergic activity, but it has been reported in patients taking single or multiple SSRIs. Its manifestations include agitation, altered mental status, coma, incoordination, myoclonus, hyperreflexia, tremor, muscle rigidity, diarrhea, diaphoresis, and hyperthermia. Patients may only exhibit a few of the symptoms, making the diagnosis challenging. Deaths are caused by hyperthermia, rhabdomyolysis, lactic acidosis, disseminated intravascular coagulation, and multiorgan failure.

Diagnosis of cyclic antidepressant poisoning is based on the history and clinical presentation. In the patient with an unknown ingestion, the combination of anticholinergic signs, coma, seizures, hypotension, and a widened QRS interval strongly suggests TCA poisoning. Because of the potential lethality of TCA poisoning, gastrointestinal decontamination procedures are considered for patients who present early after an overdose. Patients presenting later with severe symptoms are unlikely to benefit from such procedures.

The management of cyclic antidepressant poisoning is mainly supportive. Intravenous access and cardiac monitoring should be immediately established. Endotracheal intubation is indicated if significant central nervous system depression is present. Hypotension should be treated with rapid crystalloid infusion and pharmacologic support. Norepinephrine is recommended because of its predominant $\alpha_1$-mediated vasoconstrictive effects. Seizures are treated aggressively, and anticonvulsants that enhance GABA, such as benzodiazepines or barbiturates, are usually effective. It is important to monitor the QRS interval, and prolongation is associated with seizures (> 100 ms) and ventricular arrhythmias (> 160 ms). Ventricular dysrhythmias and hypotension are treated with serum alkalinization and sodium loading. Increasing the extracellular sodium concentration helps overcome the sodium channel blockade caused by TCAs, and serum alkalinization diminishes drug binding to the fast sodium channel. A QRS interval greater than 100 milliseconds, ventricular dysrhythmias, or intractable hypotension should be treated with intravenous sodium bicarbonate in a dose of 1 to 2 mEq/kg, aiming for a pH between 7.45 and 7.55. Use of hypertonic saline (3% NaCl) to increase the extracellular sodium concentration may also be considered in difficult cases. Ventricular dysrhythmias that fail to respond to sodium bicarbonate may be treated with lidocaine, a class IB antiarrhythmic agent. Although lidocaine theoretically can worsen ventricular dysrhythmias, it has been used safely in TCA poisoning. Phenytoin (another class IB antiarrhythmic agent) should not be used and may worsen ventricular dysrhythmias. Patients with cardiogenic shock who fail to respond to maximal therapeutic interventions are candidates for extracorporeal life support, such as cardiopulmonary bypass or extracorporeal membrane oxygenation to support the patient until the TCA is eliminated and cardiotoxicity abates.

Serotonin syndrome is diagnosed when characteristic symptoms occur in the setting of serotonergic medication use and other etiologies are excluded. Treatment consists of immediate withdrawal of any offending drugs and supportive care that focuses on decreasing hyperthermia and muscular rigidity. Effective measures include external cooling, intravenous hydration, and benzodiazepines or neuromuscular blockade to achieve muscle relaxation. Case reports support cyproheptadine to treat serotonin syndrome owing to its inhibitory effects at $5\text{-}HT_{1A}$ and $5\text{-}HT_{2A}$ serotonin receptors.

## DIGOXIN AND CARDIAC GLYCOSIDES

Digoxin is still used at times to treat congestive heart failure (CHF) and control ventricular rate in supraventricular tachydysrhythmias. The narrow therapeutic index of digoxin increases the risk of toxicity during therapeutic administration. Other sources of exposure include unintentional and intentional overdose, as well as ingestion of plants (ie, foxglove, oleander, and lily of the valley) and other natural sources of cardiac glycosides.

Digoxin produces its therapeutic effects through inhibition of the sodium-potassium–adenosine triphosphatase ($Na^+/K^+$-ATPase) pump, resulting in an increase in intracellular sodium and an increase in extracellular potassium. The increased intracellular sodium inhibits efflux of calcium through the $Na^+/Ca^{2+}$ antiporter at the cell membrane. The result is an increase in intracellular calcium that results in improved inotropy. Digoxin also enhances vagal tone, decreasing the rate of depolarization and conduction through the sinoatrial and atrioventricular nodes, and increasing the refractory period. Digoxin poisoning results in excessive increases in intracellular calcium with oscillatory disturbances of membrane potential, resulting in ectopy and tachydysrhythmias.

The clinical presentation of acute digoxin poisoning includes cardiac and noncardiac features. The noncardiac effects include gastrointestinal manifestations such as nausea, vomiting, and diarrhea; neurologic manifestations such as confusion, headaches, weakness, and seizures; and visual manifestations such as blurred vision, scotoma, and xanthopsia. The cardiac effects of digoxin poisoning are the primary, potentially fatal concern. Prolongation of the PR interval, with bradycardia and varying degrees of atrioventricular block can result in life-threatening bradyarrhythmias. Additionally, increased myocardial automaticity and excitability can result in atrial, junctional, and ventricular ectopy, and tachyarrhythmias.

The serum digoxin level must be interpreted with caution. The correlation between clinical effects and digoxin level is based on the steady state concentration, so the level is more helpful in predicting chronic rather than acute toxicity. Although the therapeutic range for serum digoxin is usually between 0.5 and 2 ng/mL, up to 10% of patients in this range may demonstrate toxicity. Digoxin demonstrates a biphasic distribution pattern following acute overdose. Serum levels will initially be elevated without clinical toxicity because distribution into the tissues occurs over many hours. Digoxin levels 10 times greater than the therapeutic serum concentration can be seen in patients during the first few hours after acute overdose without apparent toxicity. Similar concentrations in a patient with chronic toxicity would be fatal. Serum digoxin concentrations then decline as the drug is distributed into the tissues and eliminated by the kidneys, and it is during this phase that toxicity may begin.

Management of digoxin poisoning begins with standard supportive care and continuous electrocardiogram monitoring. Intravenous access is obtained, and blood is analyzed for serum digoxin, electrolyte, creatinine, calcium, and magnesium concentrations.

The treatment of choice for serious digoxin poisoning is intravenous administration of digoxin-specific Fab antibody fragments. Indications include life-threatening dysrhythmia, conduction delay, hyperkalemia (> 5 mmol/L), cardiogenic shock, or cardiac arrest due to digoxin overdose. Other indications include a high likelihood of progression to life-threatening digoxin toxicity, such as ingestion of more than 4 mg or 0.1 mg/kg in a child, ingestion of more than 10 mg in an adult, serum digoxin level greater than or equal to 15 ng/mL at any time or greater than or equal to 10 ng/mL 6 hours after ingestion, or rapidly progressive signs and symptoms of digoxin poisoning. Dosing of digoxin-specific Fab, in theory, is dose dependent, but relies on accurate knowledge of amount ingested and cannot be guided by blood levels. It is more practical to administer an empiric dose of 10 to 20 vials of digoxin-specific Fab for acute overdose, repeating as needed to reverse life-threatening toxicity. A lower dose is recommended for chronic digoxin poisoning to reduce the toxic effects by neutralizing a fraction of the digoxin while maintaining therapeutic benefits in the patient with underlying cardiac disease. Empiric dosing of digoxin-specific Fab for chronic poisoning is 1 to 2 vials for children and 3 to 6 vials for adults, titrated to clinical effect. Following administration of digoxin-specific Fab, total serum digoxin levels increase dramatically because digoxin is pulled from the tissue compartment into the intravascular space, where it is bound by the Fab fragments and inactivated. The kidneys then excrete this complex. Measurement of free serum digoxin levels may be helpful in guiding further therapy.

A crucial aspect in the treatment of digoxin poisoning is the management of electrolyte homeostasis. Hyperkalemia is a consequence of digoxin poisoning and may be treated with sodium bicarbonate or dextrose and insulin but the use of calcium is contraindicated, as this can further increase dysrhythmias. Although digoxin initially causes an elevated extracellular potassium concentration, serum potassium concentrations often fall precipitously following digoxin-specific Fab and must be checked frequently. Hypokalemia is especially dangerous in digoxin poisoning because it exacerbates cardiotoxicity. A fall in serum potassium concentration from 3.5 mEq/L to 3 mEq/L increases cardiac sensitivity to digoxin by approximately 50%. Patients with chronic digoxin toxicity are often hypokalemic because of concomitant treatment with diuretics. Significant hypokalemia should be corrected cautiously, especially in the patient with renal insufficiency.

Magnesium is a cofactor for the $Na^+/K^+$-ATPase pump. Hypomagnesemia potentiates digoxin-induced cardiotoxicity and inhibits correction of hypokalemia. Patients who are on chronic digoxin therapy may be hypomagnesemic because of concurrent diuretic use. Intracellular magnesium depletion may be present despite a normal serum magnesium concentration. Magnesium replacement is indicated for patients with digoxin-related cardiotoxicity, hypokalemia, and documented hypomagnesemia. Caution is again advised in the patient with renal insufficiency.

Gastrointestinal decontamination may be considered for recent acute ingestions. Activated charcoal binds to digoxin, decreasing gastrointestinal absorption. Digoxin poisoning results in conduction delays and increased vagal tone, and therefore induced emesis and gastric lavage are avoided because vagal stimulation may induce bradydysrhythmias.

## IRON

Iron is an important cause of severe childhood poisoning. Its toxic effects are mediated primarily by free-radical production, resulting in multiorgan injury.

**TABLE 114-3 ESTIMATION OF IRON-POISONING SEVERITY BASED UPON AMOUNT INGESTED AND PEAK LEVELS AFTER 4 HOURS**

| Elemental Iron Ingested (mg/kg) | Peak Iron Levels (μg/dL) | Severity of Iron Poisoning |
|---|---|---|
| < 20 | < 300 | Asymptomatic to mild |
| 20–60 | 300–500 | Mild to moderate |
| > 60 | > 500 | Severe to lethal |

The first stage of iron poisoning results from direct gastrointestinal toxicity and is characterized by nausea, vomiting, diarrhea, and abdominal pain. Hematemesis and hematochezia may also occur. The second stage is the latent stage, which usually occurs 6 to 24 hours after ingestion and is characterized by lethargy, tachycardia, and metabolic acidosis. The third stage is shock and systemic toxicity, with circulatory collapse, hypovolema and gastrointestinal bleeding, lethargy, seizures, or coma, which can occur very rapidly after a massive ingestion or up to 24 hours after a moderate ingestion. The fourth stage is acute hepatic failure, which can occur 2 to 3 days after ingestion. The fifth stage refers to later mechanical complications resulting from the initial corrosive gastrointestinal injury, such as gastric outlet obstruction and small intestinal strictures. These may manifest 2 to 8 weeks following ingestion.

Diagnosis is based on a history of iron ingestion and the presence of consistent signs and symptoms, especially gastrointestinal distress or shock. The absence of symptoms within the first 6 hours excludes serious iron toxicity. The amount of elemental iron ingested and peak levels 4 hours after ingestion correlate with toxicity (Table 114-3). Concomitant investigations should include blood gas analysis, electrolytes, glucose, renal and liver functions, and coagulation studies. Abdominal radiographs may identify iron tablets, concretions, or free air in the abdomen.

Intravenous chelation with deferoxamine should be considered for any patient with a serum iron level greater than 500 μg/dL or signs of significant toxicity such as metabolic acidosis and hypoperfusion. Deferoxamine binds iron with high affinity, forming ferrioxamine (deferoxamine-iron) that is eliminated by the kidneys. The classic vin rosé coloration of the urine does not always occur despite significant iron toxicity. Therapy may be discontinued when systemic toxicity resolves and serum iron levels return to normal.

Whole bowel irrigation is recommended when iron tablets are seen on radiographs of the gastrointestinal tract. Serial abdominal radiographs are obtained to document elimination of the iron tablets. Surgery may be required to excise adherent iron concretions that cannot be removed with whole bowel irrigation. Although hemodialysis does not enhance elimination of iron, it may be necessary to remove the ferrioxamine complex in patients with renal failure.

## OPIOIDS

Opioids are categorized as natural opiates derived from the *Papaver somniferum*, the opium poppy (ie, morphine, codeine), semisynthetic opioids (ie, heroin, hydrocodone), and synthetic opioids (ie, fentanyl, meperidine). Opiate receptor activation results in analgesia, euphoria, sedation, respiratory depression, miosis, gastrointestinal dysmotility, and pruritus.

The classic opioid toxidrome consists of coma, respiratory depression, and miosis. Other effects include bradycardia, hypotension, hypothermia, ileus, decreased muscle tone, and hyporeflexia leading to apnea, cardiovascular collapse, and death. Noncardiogenic pulmonary edema occurs, especially with heroin overdoses. Seizures are associated with certain opioids such as meperidine, propoxyphene, and tramadol.

Diagnosis should not be difficult when the opioid toxidrome is present and improvement occurs with administration of the opioid antagonist naloxone. Urine toxicology screens can confirm recent use of certain opioids. Serum acetaminophen and salicylate levels should be obtained because many prescription opioids are combined with these analgesics.

Initial management is focused on support of the airway and ventilation. Early administration of naloxone may obviate the need for definitive airway management. The primary goal is reversal of respiratory depression, which usually improves rapidly after naloxone. High-potency opioids such as fentanyl may require higher doses. Altered mental status and respiratory depression will not be effectively reversed if other sedative-hypnotic drugs are also contributing to toxicity.

A useful starting dose of naloxone for the opioid-dependent patient is 0.1 mg intravenously followed by escalating doses every 1 to 2 minutes as needed to a maximum of 10 mg. Isolated opioid toxicity is unlikely if there is no improvement after 10 mg of naloxone.

Patients who initially respond to naloxone must be closely monitored for several hours because its duration of action is shorter than that of many opioids. Return of respiratory depression requires additional doses or continuous infusion of naloxone and hospital admission.

## SALICYLATES

The primary therapeutic mechanism of action of salicylates is decreased biosynthesis of prostaglandins via inhibition of cyclooxygenase, which results in their analgesic, antipyretic, and anti-inflammatory properties. The pathophysiology of salicylate poisoning is complex because of the multiple mechanisms of toxicity (Table 114-4).

Acid–base disturbances are characteristic of salicylate toxicity. Stimulation of the medullary respiratory center results in hyperpnea and primary respiratory alkalosis. However, an elevated anion gap metabolic acidosis also begins early and worsens as the poisoning progresses. Blood gas analysis demonstrates early respiratory alkalosis, followed by mixed respiratory alkalosis and metabolic acidosis. The respiratory alkalosis may be blunted if the patient also has salicylate-induced pulmonary edema, severe central nervous system toxicity, or coingestion of another agent that results in respiratory depression.

Fluid and electrolyte abnormalities are always present with significant salicylate poisoning. Dehydration results from vomiting, hyperventilation, hyperthermia, diaphoresis, and diuresis associated with obligatory excretion of $Na^+$, $K^+$, and $HCO_3^-$ as a response to the respiratory alkalosis. Hyperglycemia is often present early as increased energy demand promotes glycolysis and gluconeogenesis. Later, increased metabolic demands exceeding the supply of glucose result in hypoglycemia. Neuroglycopenia may occur even in the presence of a normal serum glucose concentration.

Central nervous system toxicity is manifested by lethargy, delirium, seizures, coma, and respiratory depression. Acidemia contributes to central nervous system toxicity because it decreases salicylate dissociation and promotes the ingress of salicylate into the brain. Hyperthermia, cerebral edema, respiratory failure, and cardiovascular collapse ultimately result in death.

Diagnosis is based on the history of salicylate exposure as well as characteristic laboratory and clinical findings, and is confirmed by serum salicylate levels. Blood gases, electrolyte, renal function, and glucose levels should be monitored closely. Measurement of the serum salicylate concentration confirms the diagnosis and helps predict severity of toxicity but must be evaluated in the context of the patient's clinical examination and laboratory results as well as other factors such as time elapsed since ingestion, formulation of the salicylate, and adequacy of decontamination. Serial salicylate levels are needed because of the possibility of delayed absorption from sustained-release products or tablet concretions in the gastrointestinal tract.

Treatment of salicylate poisoning begins with meticulous correction of fluid, electrolyte, and acid–base disturbances. Dehydration requires fluid resuscitation to restore adequate circulating volume, tissue perfusion, and urine output. Excessive hydration should be avoided as it increases the risk of pulmonary and cerebral edema. Potassium is added to maintenance fluids to replace ongoing losses. Dextrose is provided even if the patient is normoglycemic, because increased metabolic demands often result in neuroglycopenia.

Sodium bicarbonate is a specific treatment for salicylate poisoning for 2 main reasons. First, sodium bicarbonate increases the serum pH and favors movement of salicylate from the central nervous system and other organs into the serum compartment. Second, alkalinization of the urine favors excretion and enhanced elimination of salicylate. Intravenous sodium bicarbonate is indicated when the patient is symptomatic and the serum salicylate level is greater than 40 mg/dL. Hypokalemia must be corrected to achieve urinary alkalinization. The goal of sodium bicarbonate therapy is a urinary pH of 7.5 to 8 and a serum pH of 7.4 to 7.5. Frequent salicylate, blood gas, electrolyte, and urine pH determinations guide therapy.

In cases of severe intoxication (levels > 100 mg/dL), or if there is renal failure, profound acid–base imbalance, or progressive clinical deterioration, hemodialysis can be used to eliminate salicylate and correct fluid, electrolyte, and acid–base disturbances. Gastrointestinal decontamination with activated charcoal binds salicylate, preventing systemic absorption. Multiple-dose activated charcoal is recommended in salicylate poisoning because of delayed absorption from sustained-release preparations or salicylate concretions. The end points of therapy are resolution of symptoms, normalization of electrolyte and acid–base disturbances, and serial salicylate levels that remain less than 25 mg/dL after sodium bicarbonate therapy has been discontinued.

**TABLE 114-4 PATHOPHYSIOLOGY OF SALICYLATE POISONING**

| Toxicity | Physiologic Effect |
|---|---|
| Vasoconstriction of auditory microvasculature | Tinnitus |
| Stimulation of medullary respiratory center | Hyperpnea, respiratory alkalosis |
| Stimulation of medullary chemoreceptor trigger zone | Vomiting, fluid, and electrolyte loss |
| Local gastric irritation | Gastritis, vomiting, fluid and electrolyte loss |
| Uncoupling of oxidative phosphorylation | Decreased ATP production, increased $CO_2$ production, increased $O_2$ consumption, increased glucose demand, hyperthermia, hyperpnea, increased insensible fluid loss |
| Inhibition of Krebs cycle enzymes | Metabolic acidosis (increased lactate, pyruvate) |
| Inhibition of amino acid metabolism | Metabolic acidosis, aminoacidemia, aminoaciduria |
| Altered glucose metabolism | Increased glycolysis and gluconeogenesis, hyperglycemia, hypoglycemia, decreased CSF glucose concentration |
| Altered fatty acid metabolism | Ketoacidosis (increased β-hydroxybutyrate, acetoacetate, acetone) |
| Inhibition of platelet cyclooxygenase | Decreased platelet function |
| Decreased prothrombin formation | Thrombocytopenia |
| Increased capillary fragility | Hypoprothrombinemia, increased prothrombin time and bleeding time |
| Increased permeability of pulmonary vasculature | Noncardiogenic pulmonary edema |

ATP, adenosine triphosphate; CSF, cerebrospinal fluid.

## SULFONYLUREAS

Sulfonylureas can cause prolonged and severe hypoglycemia following an acute overdose. The sulfonylurea family includes acetohexamide, carbutamide, chlorpropamide, glibornuride, gliclazide, glimepiride, glipizide, gliquidone, glyburide, tolazamide, and tolbutamide. They bind to receptors on pancreatic β cells, stimulating release of insulin. They also enhance peripheral insulin sensitivity and reduce gluconeogenesis.

Early signs and symptoms of hypoglycemia are secondary to the associated catecholamine release and include anxiety, tremor, diaphoresis, tachycardia, and vomiting. Neuroglycopenia results in confusion, lethargy, coma, and seizures. Permanent brain injury or death is the consequence of severe and prolonged hypoglycemia.

The diagnosis of sulfonylurea poisoning is based on history of ingestion and clinical manifestations of hypoglycemia. Serum concentrations are not rapidly available. Supportive care, immediate treatment with intravenous dextrose, and hospitalization are indicated for significant hypoglycemia. The agent of choice for treating sulfonylurea overdose is octreotide, a semisynthetic long-acting analog of somatostatin that inhibits the release of insulin from the pancreas, reduces dextrose requirements, and prevents rebound hypoglycemia in patients with sulfonylurea poisoning. The starting dose is 4 to 5 μg/kg/day divided every 6 hours intravenously or subcutaneously in children and up to 50 to 100 μg every 6 hours in adults. Persistent hypoglycemia may necessitate more frequent dosing or continuous infusion. Most significant sulfonylurea poisonings will require 24 hours of octreotide therapy and another 24 hours of observation after therapy is discontinued to monitor for recurrent hypoglycemia.

Blood glucose should be monitored frequently in asymptomatic patients who may have ingested a sulfonylurea. The patient should be allowed normal access to food and liquids. Patients who do not develop hypoglycemia within 8 hours of ingestion are probably safe to discharge home, although some experts recommend 24-hour hospital observation for all patients. Intravenous dextrose is not indicated in euglycemic patients because it masks the onset of hypoglycemia, makes it difficult to ascertain whether the patient is dependent on intravenous dextrose, and prolongs the observation period. Excessive dextrose stimulates release of insulin, which results in rebound hypoglycemia.

## ENVIRONMENTAL AND HOUSEHOLD TOXINS

### CARBON MONOXIDE

Carbon monoxide (CO) is an odorless gas produced by incomplete combustion of carbon-containing material. Common sources of exposure include house fires, automobile exhaust, and improperly ventilated water heaters, stoves, furnaces, fireplaces, and space heaters. Inhalation of CO is the leading cause of poisoning death in the United States.

CO causes cellular hypoxia via several mechanisms. First, CO binds to hemoglobin with an affinity 250 times greater than that of oxygen, forming carboxyhemoglobin (COHb). This results in decreased oxyhemoglobin saturation and oxygen delivery to the tissues. Second, the formation of COHb shifts the oxyhemoglobin dissociation curve to the left, further diminishing release of oxygen to the tissues. Third, CO binds to cytochrome oxidase, impairing cellular respiration and oxidative metabolism. In addition, CO binds to myoglobin, resulting in myocardial depression, hypotension, dysrhythmias, and cardiac arrest.

The diagnosis of CO poisoning is readily suspected in the patient found unconscious in a house fire or running automobile. However, the diagnosis is difficult when the patient presents with nonspecific symptoms after an unrecognized exposure. Mild to moderate CO exposures present with malaise, nausea, vomiting, dyspnea, headache, dizziness, and confusion. Such patients are often misdiagnosed with influenza or gastroenteritis. Severe poisoning is characterized by syncope, seizures, coma, cardiorespiratory depression, and death.

Once suspected, the exposure can be confirmed by determining the COHb level from a blood gas sample using co-oximetry. There is a correlation between COHb levels and clinical presentation (Table 114-5). However, if significant time has elapsed since exposure, the COHb level will underestimate the initial severity of the poisoning. Metabolic acidosis is an indicator of the severity of cellular hypoxia and ischemia. In cases of CO poisoning, arterial co-oximetry should be performed, which directly measures oxygen saturation and specifically detects COHb. Routine blood gas analysis may reveal a normal partial pressure of oxygen ($PO_2$) because dissolved oxygen is unaffected by COHb and transcutaneous pulse oximeters give false normal readings because they do not distinguish between oxyhemoglobin and COHb.

In addition to general supportive measures, the treatment of CO poisoning is aimed at reducing the amount of CO bound to hemoglobin, cytochrome oxidase, and myoglobin by administering the highest possible oxygen concentration to the patient as this reduces the half-life from approximately 4 hours in room air (21% oxygen) to 1 hour when the patient is on 100% oxygen. Hyperbaric oxygen treatment at 2 to 3 atm pressure can further decrease the COHb half-life to 20 to 30 minutes. Although the utility of hyperbaric therapy remains controversial because of conflicting research design and results, it should be considered for patients with significant CO poisoning (COHb levels > 25%, acute neurological symptoms or metabolic acidosis with pH < 7.20) if practical. The regional poison control center and hyperbaric chamber can help guide this decision, which is also based on distance from a hyperbaric center and the patient's stability.

**TABLE 114-5 SYMPTOMS AND SIGNS OF CARBON MONOXIDE POISONING AND METHEMOGLOBINEMIA**

| Carboxyhemoglobin (%) | Symptoms and Signs |
|---|---|
| 0–10 | None |
| 10–20 | Headache |
| 20–40 | Increasing headache, nausea, vomiting, dyspnea, fatigue, lightheadedness, impaired judgment |
| 40–60 | Tachypnea, tachycardia, confusion, syncope, seizure, coma |
| 60–70 | Hypotension, dysrhythmias, coma, death |
| > 70 | Rapidly fatal |
| **Methemoglobin (%)[a]** | |
| 0–15 | Cyanosis |
| 20–40 | Dyspnea, headache, tachypnea, tachycardia |
| 40–50 | Confusion, lethargy, metabolic acidosis |
| > 50 | Coma, dysrhythmias, seizures |
| > 70 | Lethal |

[a]In the absence of anemia.

### CAUSTICS

Caustic agents are found in household products such as drain cleaners, oven cleaners, rust removers, toilet bowl cleaners, tile cleaners, and hair straighteners. They are capable of causing serious injury on contact with the skin, eyes, and gastrointestinal tract.

The most commonly encountered caustic agents are acids and alkalis. Acids denature proteins (coagulation necrosis), producing a firm coagulum that may limit tissue penetration. Acids often have a strong odor and cause immediate pain, which can limit the amount ingested. Alkalis dissolve proteins and saponify fats (liquefaction necrosis), resulting in deeper tissue penetration. Alkalis are often odorless and do not cause immediate pain on contact, which may allow ingestion of larger volumes. Strong acids (very low pH) and strong alkalis (very high pH) cause the greatest damage, but the severity of tissue injury is also determined by other factors such as duration of contact, volume of exposure, and physical state of the caustic substance.

Ingestion is the most common route of exposure. The complete absence of signs and symptoms after several hours usually indicates that significant injury has not occurred. However, the absence of oropharyngeal burns on physical examination does not completely rule out the possibility of esophageal or gastric injury. Patients with caustic burns usually report pain of the mouth, throat, chest, or abdomen. Young children manifest pain by crying, drooling, and refusing to swallow. Esophageal perforation usually causes severe mediastinitis. Gastric injury may result in hematemesis and epigastric or upper-left quadrant abdominal pain. Peritonitis and metabolic acidosis are ominous signs, correlating with severity of tissue necrosis, esophageal or gastrointestinal perforation, and sepsis.

Respiratory tract injury may occur via direct extension of esophageal burns or secondary to aspiration of the caustic while swallowing or vomiting. Upper airway edema may result in hoarseness, stridor, and catastrophic upper airway obstruction. Pulmonary involvement includes bronchospasm and pneumonitis.

Ocular exposure to caustic agents, especially strong alkalis, often results in severe damage. Initial findings include eye pain, blepharospasm, lacrimation, conjunctival injection, and edema. Necrosis and opacification of the cornea, lens, and anterior chamber lead to blindness. Dermal contact results in localized pain, erythema, blistering, and deeper necrosis when the exposure is severe.

The caustic substance should be identified with respect to pH, concentration, amount, and time of exposure. Immediate decontamination is of the utmost importance. Patients should be undressed, inspected for dermal exposures, and washed thoroughly with tepid water. In the case of ocular exposures, the eyes should be immediately irrigated. Tap water is usually readily available, and the eyes should be flushed under running water for a minimum of 15 minutes. In the emergency department, local anesthetic drops may be applied and each eye irrigated with at least a liter of saline. After thorough ocular decontamination, the pH of the tears should be checked with litmus paper or a urine dipstick. Further irrigation is indicated if the pH has not returned to approximately 7.4. Following irrigation, a Wood lamp and fluorescein dye are used to evaluate for corneal and conjunctival injuries. Ophthalmologic consultation should be obtained for all ocular caustic injuries.

Following ingestion of a caustic substance, gastrointestinal decontamination is of limited utility. The mouth should be rinsed thoroughly in patients with oral burns. Some experts recommend diluting the gastric contents by having the patient drink small volumes of water or milk. The placement of a small nasogastric tube to suction the stomach may be considered in recent and large intentional ingestions. Activated charcoal does not bind caustics and obscures endoscopy.

Imaging for serious caustic ingestions may include lateral neck, chest, and abdominal radiographs. Patients with respiratory distress require laryngoscopy to assess for airway burns. Immediate surgical consultation is required if esophageal or gastrointestinal perforation is suspected based on hypotension, mediastinitis, abdominal rigidity, sepsis, metabolic acidosis, and radiographic or endoscopic evidence.

Gastroenterology consultation is required for all caustic ingestions with signs and symptoms of injury. If the patient is stable, endoscopy should ideally be performed within the first 24 hours after ingestion to evaluate full progression of the burn. Endoscopic grading of the severity of esophageal injuries helps to guide subsequent management (Table 114-6). Antibiotics should not be administered prophylactically for mild injuries, but are indicated for patients with gastrointestinal perforation or signs of infection.

## HYDROCARBONS

Hydrocarbons are found in many common household and automotive products. They are derived from petroleum distillation and other sources, including coal tar, plant oils, and animal fats. Hydrocarbon exposures are a frequent cause of pediatric morbidity and mortality. Common clinical scenarios include toddlers who aspirate a liquid hydrocarbon and recreational inhalation of volatile hydrocarbons by adolescents.

Most hydrocarbons are poorly absorbed from the gastrointestinal tract after ingestion and lack systemic toxicity. The chief concern is pulmonary aspiration resulting in chemical pneumonitis. The risk for aspiration is determined by the hydrocarbon's physical properties of viscosity and surface tension. Viscosity is the tendency to resist flow and is the best predictor of aspiration. Hydrocarbons with low viscosity have the highest risk for aspiration, while those with high viscosity are less likely to be aspirated. Surface tension is the cohesive force between molecules and defines the ability of the liquid to move along a surface. Hydrocarbons with low surface tension have a higher risk for aspiration. Volatility is the ability of a liquid to vaporize into a gas. Volatile hydrocarbons can displace alveolar oxygen, resulting in hypoxia. These compounds are easily absorbed across the alveolar-capillary membrane, resulting in systemic effects such as central nervous system depression.

The respiratory injuries caused by hydrocarbon aspiration are multifactorial. Irritation of the larynx and trachea results in coughing, choking, and laryngospasm. Spread of the hydrocarbon to the lower airways results in bronchospasm, bronchial inflammation, and necrosis. When the hydrocarbon reaches the alveoli, changes in pulmonary dynamics occur due to lipid solubilization and disruption of the surfactant layer, resulting in alveolar collapse and decreased compliance. Direct injury to lung parenchyma results in alveolar edema, exudates, and hemorrhage, with interstitial inflammation and necrosis leading to a further ventilation-perfusion mismatch and decreased compliance.

Cardiovascular toxicity is unusual after hydrocarbon ingestion or aspiration but is well described with inhalational abuse of halogenated or aromatic hydrocarbons. Sensitization of the myocardium to endogenous catecholamines results in ectopy, tachydysrhythmias, ventricular fibrillation, and sudden death. The term *sudden sniffing death syndrome* has been used to describe this phenomenon associated with inhalational solvent abuse.

Central nervous system depression following hydrocarbon aspiration is most commonly caused by hypoxia secondary to pulmonary injury. Systemic absorption of volatile hydrocarbons following inhalation or ingestion can result in central nervous system depression because of disruption of neuronal membranes. It is this alteration of mental status that is sought by the inhalant abuser. Chronic inhalational abuse of volatile hydrocarbons can result in irreversible white matter degeneration and dementia. Certain hydrocarbons, including camphor, halogenated hydrocarbons, aromatic hydrocarbons and hydrocarbons containing metals or pesticides, have systemic toxicities that may require consultation with a poison control center.

Most patients with hydrocarbon aspiration will have immediate symptoms of coughing, gagging, and choking. In mild cases, these symptoms may be transient, but patients with significant aspiration will have persistent coughing and tachypnea. Patients with severe aspiration present with severe respiratory distress, including coughing, grunting, bronchospasm, tachypnea, intercostal retractions, use of accessory muscles, cyanosis, agitation, and somnolence. Other patients may have more gradual development of respiratory distress.

Patients who remain asymptomatic for 6 hours after ingestion are unlikely to have pulmonary aspiration and may be safely discharged

**TABLE 114-6 GRADING OF ESOPHAGEAL BURNS**

| Esophageal Burn Grade | Endoscopic Description | Complications | Management |
|---|---|---|---|
| Grade I | Superficial erythema and edema | None | Resume normal diet as tolerated<br>Steroids not indicated |
| Grade II | Partial-thickness injuries with ulceration extending into the submucosa | Grade IIb burns are at greater risk for acute perforation and subsequent stricture formation after healing | Grade II burns usually require total parenteral nutrition until healing occurs |
| | Grade IIa burns are noncircumferential<br>Grade IIb burns are near or fully circumferential | Grade II burns are at increased risk of carcinoma development after decades | It is controversial whether steroids are of benefit for grade IIb burns to decrease stricture formation |
| Grade III | Full-thickness injuries with necrosis extending to periesophageal tissues | Greatest risk for acute perforation, subsequent stricture formation, and carcinoma development | Surgical intervention for perforation<br>Total parenteral nutrition until healing occurs<br>Steroids do not decrease stricture formation |

home with careful follow-up instructions. Symptomatic patients are admitted to the hospital for further observation and management. Persistent cough or tachypnea should be evaluated with a chest radiograph, which usually demonstrates pneumonitis. Pneumatoceles are a late finding, appearing on radiographs a week or 2 after the initial necrotizing pneumonitis. In patients with more significant respiratory distress, blood gas analysis may demonstrate hypoxemia and hypercarbia with a combined respiratory and metabolic acidosis. Empiric antibiotics are usually not recommended unless fever and leukocytosis develop later, suggesting bacterial superinfection. Corticosteroids are not helpful in limiting the pulmonary injury.

Patients with severe respiratory distress require immediate endotracheal intubation with mechanical ventilation and oxygenation. Decreased lung compliance necessitates increased positive end-expiratory pressures. Patients who fail these interventions may be candidates for extracorporeal membrane oxygenation to allow time for the lungs to heal.

The use of gastrointestinal decontamination following hydrocarbon ingestion is controversial because the primary risk is pulmonary aspiration. For these agents, gastric decontamination is not indicated because of the increased risk of aspiration. Some experts recommend gastric emptying for hydrocarbons with serious systemic toxicity, especially large intentional ingestions. However, the benefit of gastric emptying must be weighed against the risk of aspiration pneumonitis. Most ingestions occur in young children and are unintentional, resulting in smaller volumes ingested, reducing the need for gastric decontamination. Activated charcoal has poor adsorptive capacity for most hydrocarbons.

## METHANOL AND ETHYLENE GLYCOL

Methanol and ethylene glycol are found in many consumer products. Ingestion of these toxic alcohols results in significant morbidity and mortality, but outcomes can be improved with early diagnosis and treatment.

Both alcohols derive their toxicity from the fact that they are metabolized by alcohol and aldehyde dehydrogenases into more toxic metabolites. The parent alcohol initially causes an elevated osmolar gap, followed by the gradual development of an elevated anion gap metabolic acidosis as toxic metabolites are formed. Later, the osmolar gap normalizes and severe anion gap metabolic acidosis predominates.

The toxic metabolite of methanol is formic acid, which causes metabolic acidosis as well as optic nerve and brain injury. The principal toxic metabolites of ethylene glycol are glycolic and oxalic acid. Glycolic acid is primarily responsible for the metabolic acidosis. Oxalic acid causes calcium oxalate precipitation in the kidney, leading to renal failure, and in the brain, resulting in altered mental status, coma, seizures, and cerebral edema. Widespread calcium oxalate precipitation may lead to severe hypocalcemia with seizures, prolonged QT interval on electrocardiogram, and ventricular dysrhythmias.

Suspected methanol and ethylene glycol ingestions must be taken with extreme caution because the lethal dose is very low. Initial symptoms include ataxia, altered mental status, and vomiting. Patients will subsequently exhibit Kussmaul respirations as metabolic acidosis develops. Both poisonings can result in coma, seizures, myocardial depression, and hypotension. Visual disturbances and blindness are specific to methanol, whereas renal failure, calcium oxalate formation, and hypocalcemia are specific to ethylene glycol poisoning.

The diagnosis of methanol or ethylene glycol poisoning is based on a careful history and interpretation of physical examination and laboratory data. Measurement of blood methanol and ethylene glycol levels confirms the diagnosis and guides therapy, but results may not be immediately available. Other helpful laboratory studies include serum osmolality, blood gas analysis, BUN, creatinine, electrolytes, calcium, glucose, and lactate. Elevated anion gap metabolic acidosis not due to lactate suggests toxic alcohol poisoning. Urinalysis may reveal calcium oxalate crystals due to ethylene glycol poisoning.

The treatment of methanol and ethylene glycol poisoning is aimed at preventing formation of toxic metabolites by blocking the activity of alcohol dehydrogenase. Two therapeutic options are available for the blockade of alcohol dehydrogenase: ethanol and fomepizole. The newer antidote fomepizole has many advantages over ethanol: It does not have the risk of inebriation or hypoglycemia, it can be intermittently dosed, and it does not require monitoring of serum concentrations or monitoring in the ICU setting, which make it the antidote of choice for toxic alcohol poisoning. The indications for fomepizole in the setting of suspected methanol or ethylene glycol poisoning are outlined in Table 114-7. Because the turnaround time for methanol and ethylene glycol levels may be long, the decision to start treatment with fomepizole must often be made based on clinical presentation, an elevated osmolar gap, or an elevated anion gap metabolic acidosis. The loading dose of fomepizole is 15 mg/kg intravenously (up to 1 g), followed by maintenance doses of 10 mg/kg every 12 hours for 4 doses, then 15 mg/kg every 12 hours thereafter.

**TABLE 114-7 TREATMENT OF SUSPECTED METHANOL OR ETHYLENE GLYCOL POISONING**

| **Indications for Fomepizole Treatment** |
|---|
| Methanol or ethylene glycol level > 20 mg/dL |
| Osmolar gap > 10 mOsm/L not accounted for by ethanol or other alcohols |
| Serum bicarbonate < 20 mEq/L |
| Arterial pH < 7.3 |
| Oxalate crystals in the urine (ethylene glycol) |
| **Indications for Hemodialysis** |
| Methanol or ethylene glycol level > 50 mg/dL (or osmolar gap > 10 mOsm/L not accounted for by ethanol or other alcohols) *and* therapy with fomepizole or ethanol not immediately available to block formation of toxic metabolites |
| Significant metabolic acidosis (pH < 7.25–7.3) |
| Renal failure |
| Visual disturbances or severe neurologic abnormalities |

Hemodialysis eliminates the toxic alcohol and its metabolites, and corrects fluid, electrolyte, and acid–base disturbances. The indications for hemodialysis are outlined in Table 114-7. Early nephrology consultation for hemodialysis is critical for seriously poisoned patients. Treatment with fomepizole and dialysis should be continued until serum methanol or ethylene glycol levels are negligible, the increased osmolar gap and anion gap metabolic acidosis are resolved, and the patient is clinically improved.

## METHEMOGLOBINEMIA

Methemoglobinemia occurs when hemoglobin is oxidized to form methemoglobin (MetHb) as a result of exposure to oxidizing drugs, nitrate-contaminated well water, or other oxidative stress, as well as to inhaled nitric oxide without an appropriate controlled delivery system. MetHb is unable to bind and transport oxygen, and the oxyhemoglobin dissociation curve is shifted to the left, further reducing oxygen delivery to the tissues. These effects are exacerbated when anemia is present. Many oxidizing agents also cause hemolysis secondary to oxidative effects on the cell membrane, especially in patients with glucose-6-phosphate dehydrogenase (G6PD) deficiency.

Two enzyme systems are responsible for reducing MetHb back to normal hemoglobin (Fig. 114-5). The primary enzyme is nicotinamide adenine dinucleotide (NADH)-dependent MetHb reductase that utilizes NADH generated from glycolysis and performs 95% of this activity. The secondary enzyme is nicotinamide adenine dinucleotide phosphate (NADPH)-dependent MetHb reductase that relies on the G6PD-dependent hexose monophosphate shunt. This second enzyme system accounts for only 5% of normal activity but can be induced to rapidly reduce MetHb to hemoglobin. The antidote methylene blue increases the activity of this second NADPH-dependent pathway.

The signs and symptoms of methemoglobinemia result from cellular hypoxia. Clinical severity correlates with increasing MetHb levels as shown in Table 114-5. For a given MetHb level, the clinical effects will be more severe if the patient has concomitant anemia. Diagnosis depends on a high index of suspicion and history of exposure to oxidizing agents. Methemoglobinemia should be suspected in the

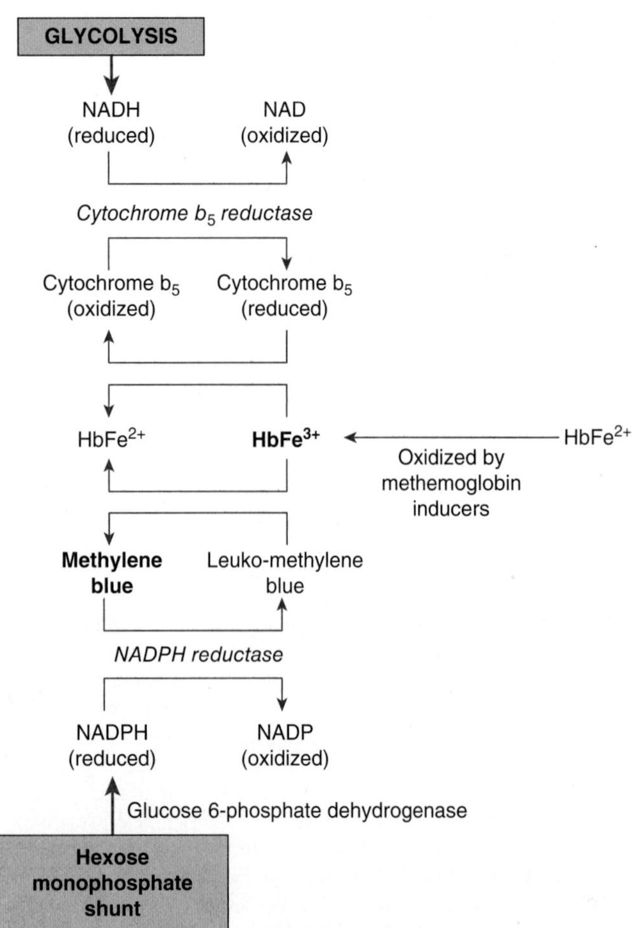


**FIGURE 114-5** Formation and reduction of methemoglobin. Methemoglobin inducers oxidize ferrous hemoglobin ($HbFe^{2+}$) to methemoglobin ($HbFe^{3+}$). Nicotinamide adenine dinucleotide (NADH) from glycolysis aids the reduction of methemoglobin back to ferrous hemoglobin via the NAD-dependent cytochrome $b_5$ reductase enzyme system. The antidote methylene blue reduces methemoglobin via nicotinamide adenine dinucleotide phosphate (NADPH) reductase and NADP from the hexose monophospate shunt.

cyanotic patient with no obvious cardiac or respiratory disease, whose cyanosis does not improve with oxygen and is out of proportion to the degree of respiratory distress. Infants presenting with gastroenteritis and methemoglobinemia may have severe metabolic acidosis and shock that is out of proportion to degree of dehydration.

The patient's blood has a characteristic chocolate brown color. The diagnosis is confirmed by sending a blood sample to the laboratory for measurement of the MetHb level and blood gas analysis on a co-oximeter. Routine blood gas analysis does not detect MetHb, and as for COHb, incorrectly calculates normal oxygen saturation based on the measured $PO_2$ (which is normal). With significant cellular hypoxia, blood gas analysis demonstrates metabolic acidosis, and serum lactate is elevated secondary to anaerobic metabolism. The absorption spectrum of MetHb causes transcutaneous pulse oximeters to measure oxygen saturation incorrectly.

Patients with MetHb levels less than 20% usually improve simply with supportive care and removal of the oxidizing agent. More severely affected patients require treatment with methylene blue. A lower threshold for treatment is indicated in patients with anemia or cardiopulmonary disease. Methylene blue is a thiazine dye that increases the reduction of MetHb to Hb and ultimately reduces MetHb to Hb (Fig. 114-5). This pathway requires G6PD, and therefore, methylene blue may cause hemolysis in patients with G6PD deficiency. The dose of methylene blue is 1 to 2 mg/kg intravenously over 5 minutes, repeated in 30 minutes if the response is inadequate. Methylene blue will transiently cause a false decrease in oxygen saturation measured by transcutaneous pulse oximetry. Excessive doses of methylene blue (> 7 mg/kg) may actually cause methemoglobinemia. If the patient has not responded to a second dose of methylene blue, consider other problems such as G6PD deficiency or NADPH-dependent MetHb reductase deficiency. Exchange transfusion may be considered in patients with severe methemoglobinemia if methylene blue has failed or is contraindicated.

## ORGANOPHOSPHORUS AND CARBAMATE INSECTICIDES

Organophosphorus and carbamate insecticides prevent the breakdown of acetylcholine in the synaptic cleft by inhibiting the acetylcholinesterase (AChE) enzyme, resulting in continued stimulation of muscarinic, nicotinic, and central nervous system receptors. Carbamates form reversible bonds with AChE that undergo spontaneous hydrolysis with full return of AChE activity by 24 hours in most cases. Carbamate toxicity is shorter and less severe compared to organophosphorus compounds, which can permanently inhibit AChE, resulting in prolonged toxicity. The "aging" process during which the reversible bond becomes a stable covalent bond may take 24 to 72 hours. Infants are at increased risk of toxicity because they have decreased AChE activity compared to adults.

Organophosphorus and carbamate poisoning results in signs and symptoms of cholinergic excess, which are summarized in the cholinergic muscarinic and nicotinic toxidromes. The primary cause of death is respiratory failure. The pulmonary muscarinic effects include bronchorrhea and bronchospasm, whereas the nicotinic effects on skeletal muscle result in weakness, muscular incoordination, and fasciculations. The respiratory compromise is compounded by central nervous system cholinergic effects, including coma and seizures.

Diagnosis is based on history of exposure and clinical presentation consistent with cholinergic excess (muscarinic and nicotinic toxidromes). Plasma cholinesterase and red blood cell (RBC) cholinesterase activity are both decreased after organophosphorus poisoning. Plasma cholinesterase activity is a more readily available and sensitive measure of organophosphorus poisoning. A plasma cholinesterase level 20% to 50% of normal correlates with mild poisoning, 10% to 20% indicates moderate poisoning, and less than 10% is severe. Red blood cell cholinesterase activity is a more specific test for organophosphorus poisoning, but is not readily available in most hospitals. Plasma cholinesterase and RBC cholinesterase levels are not helpful with initial management and diagnosis of organophosphorus compound toxicity but aid management of prolonged toxicity. Cholinesterase measurements are not helpful after carbamate poisoning because the inhibition of cholinesterase activity is usually mild and transient.

The first priority of treatment is decontamination of the victim and protection of healthcare providers from secondary exposure. Resuscitation is focused on correcting respiratory dysfunction. Atropine is the initial antidote for organophosphorus and carbamate poisoning because it is a competitive antagonist of muscarinic acetylcholine receptors. The goal of atropinization is the reduction of pulmonary secretions, reversal of bronchospasm, and improvement in respiratory distress. The initial dose of atropine is 0.02 mg/kg intravenously up to 0.5 to 2 mg in adults, doubling the dose every 5 minutes until adequate oxygenation is achieved. Extremely high doses are required to overcome the cholinergic excess, and severely poisoned patients require frequent dosing or continuous intravenous infusion. Atropine has no effect at nicotinic receptors, and will not reverse nicotinic toxicity.

The second antidote for organophosphorus poisoning is pralidoxime chloride (2-PAM), which reactivates AChE, reverses both muscarinic and nicotinic effects, and reduces atropine requirements. Pralidoxime must be administered early for organophosphorus poisoning because the inhibition of AChE becomes irreversible over time. Pralidoxime is not necessary for carbamate poisoning because of rapid hydrolysis of the carbamate–AChE complex. The dose of 2-PAM is 25 to 50 mg/kg intravenously in children, up to 1 to 2 g in adults, over 15 to 30 minutes, repeated if there is no improvement in muscle weakness or fasciculations. Severely poisoned patients require repeat dosing or continuous infusion, which may be necessary for several days.

## SUGGESTED READINGS


Bateman DN, Page CB. Antidotes to coumarins, isoniazid, methothrexate and thyroxine, toxins that work via metabolic processes. *Br J Clin Pharmacol.* 2016;81(3):437-445.

Blackford MG, Felter T, Gothard MD, Reed MD. Assessment of the clinical use of intravenous and oral N-acetylcysteine in the treatment of acute acetaminophen poisoning in children: a retrospective review. *Clin Ther.* 2011;33(9):1322-1330.

Calello DP, Henretic FM. Pediatric toxicology: specialized approach to the poisoned child. *Emerg Med Clin North Am.* 2014;32(1):29-52.

Campbell C, Osterhoudt KC. Prevention of childhood lead poisoning. *Curr Opin Pediatr.* 2000;12(5):428-437.

Chang TP, Rangan C. Iron poisoning: a literature-based review of epidemiology, diagnosis, and management. *Pediatr Emerg Care.* 2011;27(10):978-985.

Graudins A, Lee HM, Druda D. Calcium channel antagonist and beta-blocker overdose: antidotes and adjunct therapies. *Br J Clin Pharmacol.* 2016;81(3):453-461.

King AM, Aaron CK. Organophosphate and carbamate poisoning. *Emerg Med Clin North Am.* 2015;33(1):133-151.

Klein-Schwartz W, Stassinos GL, Isbister GK. Treatment of sulfonylurea and insulin overdose. *Br J Clin Pharmacol.* 2016;81(3):496-504.

McMartin K, Jacobsen D, Hovda KE. Antidotes for poisonings by alcohols that form toxic metabolites. *Br J Clin Pharmacol.* 2016;81(3):501-515.

Park KS. Evaluation and management of caustic injuries from ingestion of acid or alkaline substances. *Clin Endosc.* 2014;47(4):301-307.

Rasimas JJ, Liebelt EL. Adverse effects and toxicity of the atypical antipsychotics: what is important for the pediatric emergency practitioner. *Clin Pediatr Emerg Med.* 2012;13(4):300-310.

Roderique JD, Josef CS, Feldman MJ, Spiess BS. A modern literature review of carbon monoxide poisoning theories, therapies and potential targets for therapy advancement. *Toxicology.* 2015;334:45-48.

Star K, Edwards IR, Choonara I. Valproic acid and fatalities in children: a review of individual case safety reports in VigiBase. *PLoS One.* 2014;9(10):e108970.

Tormoehlen LM, Tekulve KJ, Nañagas KA. Hydrocarbon toxicity: a review. *Clin Toxicol (Phila).* 2014;52(5):479-489.


# 115 Submersion Injuries


Rohit P. Shenoi


## INTRODUCTION

Drowning is defined as a process resulting in primary respiratory impairment from submersion or immersion in a liquid medium. For drowning to occur, the face and airway must be immersed. Drowning is a major public health problem. According to the World Health Organization (WHO), there are 372,000 deaths per year worldwide attributed to drowning. More than 90% of these deaths occur in low- and middle-income countries. It is 1 of the 10 leading causes of death worldwide among people between 1 and 24 years of age. The full extent of the world's drowning problem is underreported since statistics exclude intentional drowning and drowning deaths resulting from flood disasters, tsunamis, and water transport incidents.

In the United States, drowning is the leading cause of unintentional injury-related death among children 1 to 4 years of age, with a death rate of 2.4 per 100,000. Approximately 1 in 5 people who die from drowning are children aged 14 and younger. In 2014, there were 7701 emergency department visits for nonfatal unintentional submersions and 892 unintentional drowning deaths in US children 0 to 18 years of age. Fortunately, the death rate due to drowning in children is decreasing. The crude death rate due to unintentional drowning in children decreased from 1.17 per 100,000 in 2009 to 1.06 per 100,000 in 2014. Rates are highest in the southern United States. Most victims of nonfatal drowning do well, but about 5% to 10% of these incidents result in severe neurologic damage secondary to cardiac arrest. These are even more common when drowning occurs in open bodies of water.



Key risk factors for drowning are: a lack of barriers controlling exposure to bodies of water; lack of adequate, close supervision for infants and young children who are a drowning risk; poor swimming skills; low awareness of water dangers; and high-risk behavior, including consuming alcohol while engaging in water-related activities, especially among adolescents and young adults. Other risk factors include the failure to wear life jackets and seizure disorders. In low- and middle-income countries, transport on water and water crossings, lack of safe water supply, and flood disasters are additional risk factors. Drowning victims involved in natural disasters may also have associated traumatic injuries.

There are 2 peaks of incidence of drowning in children: The first is in the infant/toddler age group and occurs in bathtubs and swimming pools, and the second is in the adolescent age group and is frequently related to risk-taking behavior in swimming pools and during recreational water sports in natural bodies of water. Drowning rates are influenced by factors such as access to swimming pools, the motivation to learn how to swim, and participation in water-related recreational activities, as well as demographics. African-American children are at between 3- and 5-fold increased risk of drowning than children of similar ages of other racial or ethnic groups.

Among all US residents between the years 1999 and 2010, natural water was the most frequent drowning location, accounting for 47.2% of all unintentional drowning deaths (including deaths while boating), followed by other/unspecified places (26.8%), swimming pools (16.3%), and bathtubs (9.7%). Age is an important determinant of where a child drowns. Most infant drownings occur in bathtubs and large buckets, largely when children are left unsupervised. Most deaths due to drowning in toddlers occur in swimming pools. School-age children and adolescents are more likely to drown in natural water than swimming pools, and fatal submersions in boating accidents usually occur when individuals do not wear a personal flotation device or wear it improperly. Inadequate marine training and the use of alcohol also contribute to fatal boating incidents. Alcohol increases the risk of drowning by impairing judgment and performance and by causing disorientation and hypothermia, and although data is lacking, illicit drugs would likely have similar effects. Above ground pools without barrier fencing (they are outside the purview of local building codes) and entrapment in a drain of a swimming pool (particularly with hair being entangled or a body part "sucked in") are also high-risk settings. Another dangerous situation may occur when swimmers hyperventilate before swimming underwater or try to hold their breath for long periods of time. This can render a swimmer unconscious ("shallow water blackout"), leading to drowning. Hyperventilation or breath-holding before diving or swimming decreases the body's stores of $CO_2$ and the arterial partial pressure of carbon dioxide ($PaCO_2$), delaying the cerebral response to come to the surface to breathe. The blackout is caused by the drop in the arterial partial pressure of oxygen ($PaO_2$) in arterial blood gas, resulting in hypoxia and loss of consciousness under water. Underlying conditions such as epilepsy and autism increase the risk of drowning. No study has specifically studied developmental disabilities or attention-deficit/hyperactivity disorder as drowning risk factors. Undiagnosed malignant cardiac arrhythmias or propensity for these (eg, long QT syndrome), cardiomyopathy, or other subclinical cardiac diseases may lead to sudden cardiac events or cardiac arrest leading to drowning.

The relationship between swimming ability and drowning is complex and important. The ability to swim may or may not decrease drowning risk and does not completely protect against drowning. A proficient swimmer may have an elevated risk of drowning due to increased aquatic exposure and participation in potentially dangerous aquatic situations. Similarly, a good swimmer may suffer an immersion accident, which then becomes submersion due to fatigue, particularly in cold water. Even a strong swimmer may succumb rapidly due to hypothermia in icy water. Nevertheless, swimming lessons do reduce drowning risk in small children and it is possible for preschool-aged (24–42 months) children to develop the water-safety skills necessary to survive a fall into a home swimming pool after training.

## TERMINOLOGY

Confusion exists around the terminology used to describe drowning events. Terms such as *near-drowning*, *wet* or *dry drowning*, *active* or *passive drowning*, *silent drowning*, or *secondary drowning* should be avoided. Instead, the Utstein style for classifying submersion injuries is recommended. The term *drowned* should be used to describe a person who has died from drowning. Drowning outcomes should be classified as *death*, *no morbidity*, or *morbidity* (further categorized as *moderately disabled*, *severely disabled*, *vegetative state/coma*, and *brain dead*).

## PATHOPHYSIOLOGY

When a person begins to drown, water first enters the victim's mouth and is either swallowed or spat out. The victim then voluntarily holds his/her breath. If water enters the oropharynx or larynx, there may be laryngospasm. The breath-holding and laryngospasm prevent respiration, and hypoxia, hypercarbia, and acidosis ensue. As the hypoxia worsens and laryngospasm abates, victims actively breathe in and aspirate water. Ultimately, there is loss of consciousness and apnea. The cardiovascular response begins with initial tachycardia followed by bradycardia, pulseless electrical activity, and finally, asystole. This whole process may take a few minutes but may be more protracted in hypothermic conditions. Drowning in cold or icy water confers protective effects on many organ systems, including the brain, through reductions in consumption, resulting in delayed cellular anoxia and adenosine triphosphate (ATP) depletion in a temperature-dependent manner. Cerebral oxygen consumption falls at least 5% for each 1°C reduction in temperature when the range of ambient temperature is between 37°C and 20°C. Cold water drowning results in a rapid fall in core temperature, particularly if there is associated aspiration, and this is the reason that seemingly miraculous anecdotal accounts exist of intact survival after hypothermic submersion accidents. Importantly, these conditions—even in the absence of vital signs—warrant prolonged resuscitative efforts (see also Chapter 102), though it is important to note that a recent study and meta-analysis did not observe a protective effect of colder water in drowning victims.

Aspiration of water into the alveoli leads to surfactant dysfunction and washout. Salt-water and fresh-water aspiration cause similar degrees of injury, although there may be differences in osmotic gradients. Regardless, there is disruption of the delicate alveolar-capillary membrane with attendant shifts in fluids, plasma, and electrolytes. The clinical picture is that of pulmonary edema with reduced lung compliance, ventilation-perfusion mismatch, atelectasis, and bronchospasm. Submersion victims may swallow large amounts of water. During resuscitation, they may vomit their stomach contents and aspiration into the lungs may occur, predisposing them to aspiration pneumonia.

Depending on when rescue occurs, and the timing of appropriate resuscitative measures, the patient may recover with or without subsequent therapy with resolution of hypoxia, hypercarbia, and acidosis. If the patient is not ventilated (or does not resume spontaneous effective respiration) soon enough, then profound hypoxemia will ensue and ultimately will lead to organ hypoperfusion and cardiopulmonary arrest. The most common organ failures within the first 24 hours of drowning are respiratory, followed by neurologic, cardiovascular, gastrointestinal, hematological, and least commonly, renal. Severely injured victims of submersion are at risk of multiorgan dysfunction due to severe hypoxia and hypoxic-ischemic brain injury or even brain death, as well as acute respiratory distress syndrome or sepsis syndrome attributable to aspiration pneumonia or nosocomial infections. Posthypoxic encephalopathy with or without cerebral edema is the most common cause of death in hospitalized drowning victims.

While brain injury is 1 of the most common sequelae of drowning, it is also important to investigate the possibility of concurrent trauma or neurologic disease (eg, seizures resulting in loss of consciousness before drowning) as factors associated with this.

## MANAGEMENT

The response to a drowning victim involves a multilevel approach from the initial water rescue and on-scene resuscitation to hospital transport to emergency room and in-patient resuscitation and care and rehabilitation. A universal Drowning Chain of Survival comprising 5 links that serve as a guide informing important lifesaving steps for lay and professional rescuers has been proposed. This chain of survival has the potential to greatly improve the chances of prevention, survival, and recovery from drowning. The 5 steps of the chain are prevent drowning, recognize distress, provide flotation, remove from water, and provide care as needed. A classification of the severity of submersion injuries, based on a retrospective review of 1831 adult cases of submersions of predominantly seawater rescues, has been proposed (Fig. 115-1). The clinical findings of the victims and interventions that were administered at the submersion scene were evaluated, and a treatment algorithm was developed. Patients are categorized into 6 subgroups based upon the severity of respiratory compromise at the submersion site. The grading is as follows:

- Grade 1 (normal lung auscultation with coughing) survival = 100%;
- Grade 2 (abnormal lung auscultation with rales in some lung fields) survival = 99%;
- Grade 3 (auscultatory evidence of acute pulmonary edema without arterial hypotension) survival = 95% to 96%;
- Grade 4 (evidence of acute pulmonary edema with arterial hypotension) survival = 78% to 82%;
- Grade 5 (isolated respiratory arrest) survival = 31% to 44%; and
- Grade 6 (cardiopulmonary arrest); survival = 7% to 12%.

It is uncertain whether this classification that was developed for adults would be applicable for children and infants, or whether similar results would be obtained if this scale were to be validated prospectively, although it does provide clinicians with a helpful prognostic guide.

### Prehospital Management

Bystander rescue and resuscitation of drowning victims play an important role in positive outcome. The victim should be removed rapidly and safely from the water without placing the rescuer at undue risk. The potential rescuer should, if possible, instruct someone else to call for help while staying on-scene to provide assistance. He or she must watch where the victim is in the water, or ask a bystander to keep constant watch. If possible, the rescuer should provide some form of flotation to prevent submersion. Staying out of the water reduces the rescuer's risk of drowning. Prompt resuscitation by safely removing the victim from the water as rapidly as possible is encouraged. Rescue breathing may begin while the victim is still in the water if doing so will not delay removing the victim from the water. Administering chest compressions in the water is not advised. Water does not act as an obstructive foreign body, so attempts to remove it by abdominal or chest thrusts or placing the person head down should be avoided. Doing so only delays the initiation of ventilation and increases the chances of vomiting. Upon removal of the victim from the water, cardiopulmonary resuscitation (CPR) is commenced if the victim is unresponsive or not breathing. For the lone rescuer, 5 cycles (about 2 minutes) of compressions and ventilations are administered before activating the emergency response system and getting an automated external defibrillator (AED). If 2 rescuers are present, the second rescuer is instructed to activate the emergency response system immediately and prepare the AED while the first rescuer performs CPR. Coexisting cervical spine injuries are in general rare, and so immobilization of the cervical spine is only recommended if there is a high-risk mechanism, such as diving into shallow water or an accident involving boating, waterskiing, or surfing. In an unwitnessed

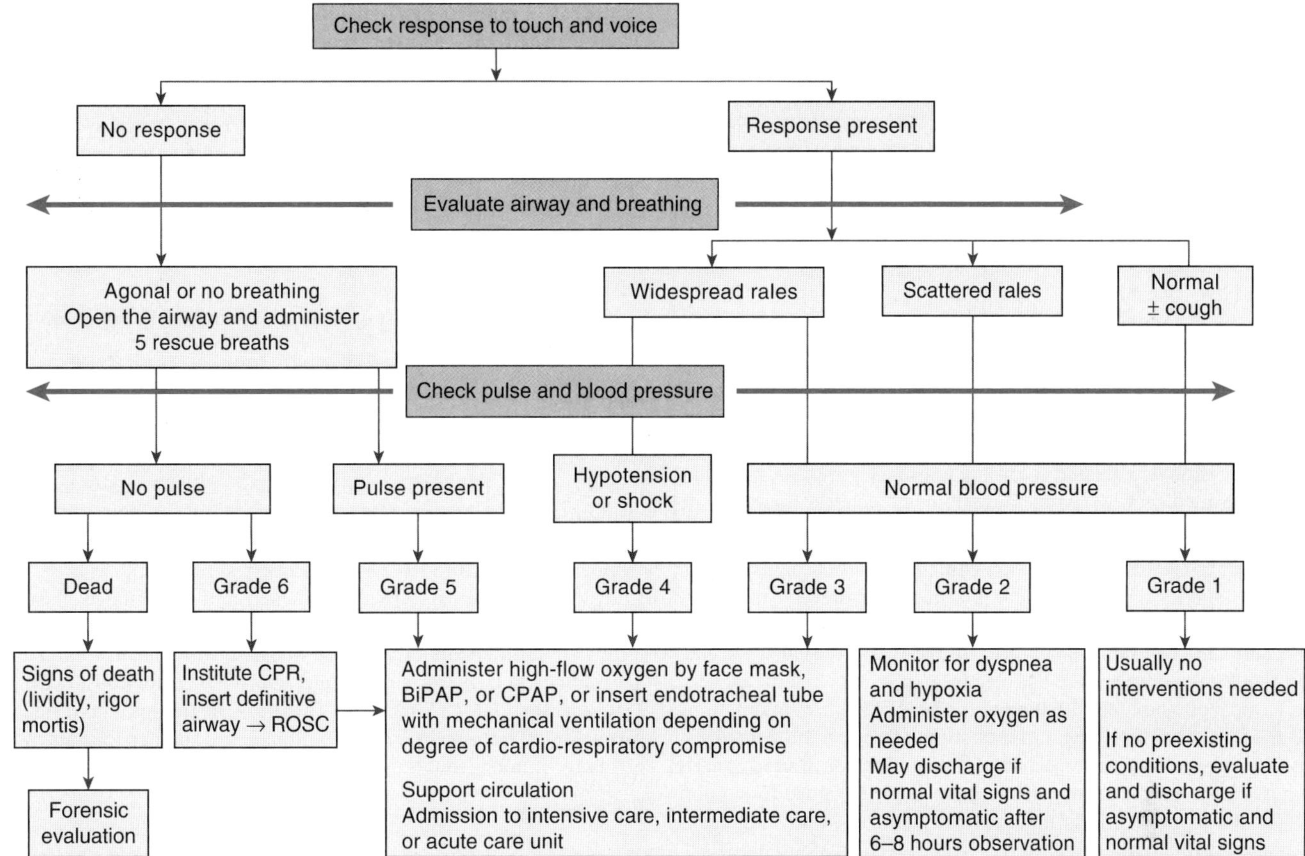


**FIGURE 115-1** Classification of submersion severity and management of submersion victims. BiPAP, bilevel positive airway pressure; CPAP, continuous positive airway pressure; CPR, cardiopulmonary resuscitation; ROSC, return of spontaneous circulation.

event, depending on depth of water and the age/abilities of the child, responders will often err on the side of caution with cervical spine protection. Regurgitation of stomach occurs in more than 65% of persons who require rescue breathing alone and in 86% of those who require CPR with chest compressions. Most patients will need suctioning of the oral cavity as soon as this is available.

#### Emergency Department

A majority of submersion victims recover spontaneously and fewer than 6% of all persons who are rescued by lifeguards need medical attention in a hospital. Successful resuscitation requires close attention to oxygenation, ventilation, circulation, and the prevention and treatment of hypothermia. For the spontaneously breathing patient with respiratory distress, 100% oxygen should be administered by a nonrebreathing mask or high-flow oxygen by nasal cannula, bilevel positive airway pressure (BiPAP), or continuous positive airway pressure (CPAP). Because of atelectasis, pulmonary edema, and intrapulmonary shunting, positive airway pressure can increase the functional residual capacity and improve lung compliance. Bronchospasm should be treated with nebulized or inhaled β-agonists such as albuterol or levalbuterol. Pulmonary edema and reduced lung compliance in severe cases will necessitate endotracheal intubation with positive pressure ventilation and positive end-expiratory pressure. Criteria for intubation are the presence of neurologic deterioration or an inability to protect the airway, the inability to maintain a $PaO_2$ above 60 mm Hg or oxygen saturation ($SpO_2$) above 90% despite supplemental oxygen, or a $PaCO_2$ above 50 mm Hg—all of which indicate actual or pending acute respiratory failure. If tracheal intubation is performed, this should be done as a rapid sequence procedure, avoiding bag-mask ventilation, and an orogastric tube should be placed to relieve stomach distension.

Survival after prolonged submersion and cardiac arrest in cold water is possible, so it is imperative that resuscitation continues until the patient has been warmed adequately. All wet clothing should be removed. A hypothermic patient will require rewarming using passive and active external rewarming (eg, application of warm blankets, heating pads, radiant heat, forced warm air), or active internal core rewarming (eg, warmed humidified oxygen via tracheal tube, irrigation of peritoneal and pleural cavities with warm fluids).

Antibiotics or steroids are not routinely indicated in victims of drowning. If the person remains unresponsive without an obvious cause, a toxicologic investigation and computed tomography of the head and neck should be considered. The administration of naloxone may be considered if opioid intoxication is suspected. In the acute phase, measurements of electrolytes, blood urea nitrogen, creatinine, and hematocrit are rarely helpful. Criteria for hospitalization include persistent dyspnea or hypoxia beyond 8 hours postsubmersion, and severe submersion injuries with unconsciousness, respiratory failure, and hypothermia.

#### Intensive Care Management

**Respiratory System** The pathologic features are acute lung injury with acute respiratory distress syndrome, generally necessitating mechanical ventilation, as in the treatment of other types of acute lung injury. The manifestations of lung injury, pulmonary edema, and aspiration often progress over the first 24 hours, so weaning is generally withheld during this period. The patient should be monitored daily for fever, leukocytosis, persistent or new lung infiltrates, and a leukocyte response in the bronchoalveolar lavage. Early-onset pneumonia can occur due to aspiration of polluted water, endogenous flora, or gastric contents. Aspiration of swimming-pool water rarely results in pneumonia, whereas drowning in ponds or lakes significantly increases the risk of this. The risk of pneumonia increases during prolonged mechanical ventilation and may be detected by the third or fourth day of hospitalization, or later, when pulmonary edema has nearly resolved. A secondary pneumonia is often related to nosocomial pathogens. Empirical therapy should initially include broad-spectrum antibiotics, covering the most predictable Gram-negative and

Gram-positive pathogens. Later, antibiotic therapy should be guided by the results of culture and sensitivity testing of bronchial secretions. There is no evidence supporting the use of steroids or exogenous surfactant for reducing pulmonary injury in victims of drowning.

In the most severe cases of acute lung injury with refractory hypoxemia, hypercarbia, or both, extracorporeal membrane oxygenation (ECMO) may be considered as it would for other etiologies of acute respiratory failure, in patients with predominantly single-organ (pulmonary) failure. ECMO also has been used as a temporizing measure with absence of early cardiac recovery after drowning associated with profound hypothermia.

**Circulatory System** In most submersion victims, adequate oxygenation, crystalloid boluses, and measures to correct hypothermia lead to a stable hemodynamic status. Cardiac dysfunction may occur in severely injured victims, particularly those who have suffered significant cardiopulmonary arrest requiring CPR. In these patients, circulatory failure should be treated according to usual algorithms, including vasoactive medications, potentially utilizing echocardiography to assess function and fluid status, as well as response to interventions.

**Neurologic System** Victims who are comatose or show signs of neurological injury should be closely monitored to prevent secondary neurologic injuries due to cerebral ischemia and edema, hypoxemia, fluid and electrolyte imbalance, acidosis, seizures, and postresuscitation rise in temperature. Usual protective measures to reduce elevated intracranial pressure (eg, elevation of the head of the bed, maintaining the head midline, avoiding noxious stimulation, careful blood gas, glucose and electrolyte control) should be routinely instituted as early as possible in this situation. While there is no evidence to support therapeutic hypothermia in these patients, controlled normothermia without allowing core temperature to increase to greater than 37.5°C should be a part of routine management, as hyperthermia is known to worsen preexisting anoxic brain injury. Placing the patient on a cooling blanket targeting normothermia will avoid unwanted swings in temperature in these vulnerable patients.

**Other Systems** Sepsis and disseminated intravascular coagulation may occur during the first 72 hours after resuscitation. Renal insufficiency or failure is rare but can occur as a result of anoxia, shock, myoglobinuria, or hemoglobinuria. These sequelae will all require specific interventions, although in general are not primary determinants of prognosis.

## OUTCOMES AFTER DROWNING: PROGNOSTIC INDICATORS

The longer term outcomes after drowning are largely determined by the degree of neurological injury, and this, in turn, is typically related to whether or not there has been a cardiac arrest. Victims who arrive at a hospital without a perfusing cardiac rhythm who are subsequently successfully resuscitated are highly likely to have neurological injury unless they have been submerged in icy water. Neurological injury that is associated with cardiac arrest after submersion is typically severe and may progress to brain death or be otherwise unsurvivable. By contrast, other organ failures that occur are generally reversible.

Factors influencing survival and long-term morbidity include duration of submersion, water temperature, how promptly and effectively CPR was provided, and the subsequent interval prior to return of a perfusing cardiac rhythm. The issue of hypothermia in submersion accidents is an important one in northern climates. There are many case reports of intact neurological survival in children who have been submerged in icy water (below 5°C). This, of course, is biased literature, but is relevant when deciding when to terminate CPR in a drowned hypothermic patient because there may be a neuroprotective effect of rapidly induced hypothermia.

The strongest predictor of outcome in victims of drowning is the duration of submersion victims is submersion duration. However, time estimates of the duration of submersion are notoriously inaccurate. Many of the events are unwitnessed, so the time between the actual submersion and being found is often unknown. Additionally, a caregiver may minimize the time because of feelings of guilt that may be related to lack of supervision of the victim at a vulnerable time. With that in mind, a meta-analysis revealed that favorable outcome was associated with shorter compared to longer submersion durations. For submersion duration of less than 5 to 6 minutes, the risk ratio was 2.9; for less than 10 to 11 minutes, it was 5.1; and for less than 15 to 25 minutes, it was 26.9. Favorable outcomes were also seen with shorter emergency medical service response times (risk ratio = 2.8) and salt water versus fresh water submersion (risk ratio = 1.16). No differences in outcomes have been observed with the age of the victim, water temperatures, or witnessed versus unwitnessed drownings.

### Long-Term Outcomes in Survivors

A good health-related quality of life is achieved in a majority of submersion victims who survive long term after a submersion event. However, as already stated, the overall quality of life is dependent on submersion time. Mean quality-of-life scores were significantly lower in victims for whom the submersion time exceeded 10 minutes compared to patients with shorter submersion times. Additionally, neurological dysfunction and a lower full-scale intelligence quotient (FSIQ) may occur long term in seriously injured submersion victims. In a study, cognitive or neurologic deficits were detected in 17 of 21 subjects, although 11 of them were reported to have a full recovery at hospital discharge. The study revealed that 57% of the drowned and resuscitated children had neurological dysfunction and 40% had a low FSIQ. The median estimated submersion time of the subjects with normal FSIQ was 3.5 minutes, which was significantly shorter than for those with an FSIQ less than 80, 12.5 minutes. Therefore, neurological and neuropsychological long-term follow-up of pediatric submersion victims is highly recommended.

## PREVENTION

The prevention of drowning is the mainstay in reducing the burden of injuries associated with submersions. Safety interventions are grouped based on their ability to change the environment, the individual at risk, or the agent of injury (water).

### Water Safety

Recommended water safety measures include:

1. Adult supervision of young children around any body of water is vitally important. Because drowning occurs quickly and quietly, adults should not be involved in any other distracting activity (such as reading, playing cards, talking on the phone or texting, or mowing the lawn) while supervising children, even if lifeguards are present. A responsible adult should be designated to be a "water watcher" to monitor young children while in the bath and when children swim or play in or around water. For preschool children, "touch supervision," which involves an adult being close enough to reach the child at all times, is recommended. Older children should use the buddy system. Swimming with a friend and selecting swimming sites that have lifeguards when possible are recommended.
2. Since epilepsy is a known risk factor for drowning, these patients should have one-on-one supervision around water, including swimming pools, take showers instead of bathing in a tub, and wear life jackets when boating. Children with autism spectrum disorders and developmental delay should be closely supervised around water.
3. All children should learn to swim. While formal swimming lessons can begin at age 4 years of age, water survival skills could be taught to toddlers between 1 and 4 years of age. More research is needed to determine which types of swimming instruction and water-survival skills are most effective in preventing drowning in young children of various ages. Nevertheless, constant and careful supervision of children who are in and around water should always occur.
4. Immediate CPR at the site of a submersion incident can be lifesaving. Parents and caregivers should be trained in basic life support.
5. Approved personal flotation devices (PFDs) should be used. Air-filled or foam toys, such as water wings, noodles, or inner tubes are not life jackets and are not designed to keep swimmers safe.

6. The consumption of alcoholic beverages should be avoided before or during swimming, boating, or water skiing or while supervising children. Swimmers should not hyperventilate before swimming underwater or try to hold their breath for long periods of time.
7. Knowledge of the local weather conditions is important prior to swimming or boating. Strong winds and thunderstorms with lightning strikes can be dangerous.
8. Lifeguards at swimming pools and beaches serve to make them safer by monitoring the aquatic environment, enforcing rules and regulations, and educating swimmers about safety and injury prevention.

#### Home Swimming Pools

The best method to prevent submersions in unsupervised young children is to install fencing that completely isolates the pool area from the house and yard; this type of fencing has been shown to decrease the rate of pool-immersion injuries among young children by more than 50%. Fences should be at least 4 feet high, and no opening under the fence should be more than 4 inches. Vertical members of the fence should be less than 4 inches apart to keep a child from squeezing through them, and there should be no footholds or handholds that could help a young child climb the fence. Self-closing and self-latching gates that open outward with latches that are out of reach of children are also required. The latch should be placed at least 54 inches above the bottom of the gate. It is also advisable to remove floats, balls, and other toys from the pool and surrounding area immediately after use so that children are not tempted to enter the pool area unsupervised. Additional barriers, such as automatic door locks and alarms to prevent access to the pool area, are helpful. Pool covers and pool alarms are not recommended as a substitute for isolation pool fencing. In order to prevent drain entrapments and entanglement in swimming pools and spas, the use of special drain covers, safety vacuum-release systems, filter pumps with multiple drains, and a variety of other pressure-venting filter-construction techniques are required.

#### Natural Bodies of Water

When boating in natural bodies of water, it is essential to use life jackets approved by the US Coast Guard or an equivalent. This is important regardless of the distance to be traveled, the size of the boat, or the swimming ability of the boater. Life jackets can reduce risk for weaker swimmers, too. At the beach, bathers should know the meaning of and obey warnings represented by colored beach flags. These may vary from 1 beach to another. Water that is discolored and choppy, foamy, or filled with debris and moving in a channel away from shore may indicate a rip current. If caught in a rip current, the swimmer should first swim parallel to shore and then, once free of the current, should swim diagonally toward the shore.

### SUGGESTED READINGS


Berg MD, Schexnayder SM, Chameides L, et al. Part 13: pediatric basic life support: 2010 American Heart Association guidelines for cardiopulmonary resuscitation and emergency cardiovascular care. *Circulation*. 2010;122(18 Suppl 3):S862-S875.

Burke CR, Chan T, Brogan TV, et al. Extracorporeal life support for victims of drowning. *Resuscitation*. 2016;104:19-23.

Centers for Disease Control. Home & recreational safety. Water-related injuries. http://www.cdc.gov/HomeandRecreationalSafety/Water-Safety/index.html. Updated May 2, 2016.

Conn AW, Miyasaka K, Katayama M, et al. A canine study of cold water drowning in fresh versus salt water. *Crit Care Med*. 1995;23(12):2029-2037.

Idris AH, Berg RA, Bierens J, et al; American Heart Association. Recommended guidelines for uniform reporting of data from drowning: the "Utstein style." *Circulation*. 2003;108(20):2565-2574.

Quan L, Bierens JJ, Lis R, Rowhani-Rahbar A, Morley P, Perkins GD. Predicting outcome of drowning at the scene: a systematic review and meta-analyses. *Resuscitation*. 2016;104:63-75.

Suominen PK, Sutinen N, Valle S, Olkkola KT, Lönnqvist T. Neurocognitive long term follow-up study on drowned children. *Resuscitation*. 2014;85(8):1059-1064.

Suominen PK, Vähätalo R, Sintonen H, Haverinen A, Roine RP. Health-related quality of life after a drowning incident as a child. *Resuscitation*. 2011;82(10):1318-1322.

Szpilman D, Bierens JJ, Handley AJ, Orlowski JP. Drowning. *N Engl J Med*. 2012;366(22):2102-2110.

Szpilman D, Webber J, Quan L, et al. Creating a drowning chain of survival. *Resuscitation*. 2014;85(9):1149-1152.

Venema AM, Groothoff JW, Bierens JJ. The role of bystanders during rescue and resuscitation of drowning victims. *Resuscitation*. 2010;81(4):434-439.

Weiss J; American Academy of Pediatrics Committee on Injury, Violence, and Poison Prevention. Prevention of drowning. *Pediatrics*. 2010; 126(1):e253-e262.

World Health Organization. Global report on drowning: preventing a leading killer. Geneva, Switzerland: World Health Organization; 2014.


# 116 Trauma, Burns, and Bites

Adam C. Alder and Robert P. Foglia



Trauma is the number 1 cause of mortality and morbidity for children even in the developed world, and major resources are still needed to prevent and treat traumatic injuries. Between 1 month and 18 years of age, one-half of all deaths in children are the result of a traumatic injury. Trauma accounts for more deaths in children in this age range than all forms of cancer, heart disease, and infections combined. The objectives of this chapter will be to review the differences between adults and children in regard to mechanism of injury and physiologic response; discuss pathophysiology and the initial management of the trauma victim; and outline common injuries involving various organ systems.

Most infants and children with traumatic injuries are seen in the emergency department with nearly half of the facilities being adult centers rather than pediatric-specific trauma facilities. This underscores the importance of education of community emergency department, family, and pediatric specialists. Not surprisingly, the significantly injured child requires evaluation and management skills that may not be available in every emergency department. Caregivers may have less experience with their care and an understanding of the initial management and stabilization of these patients and their safe and timely transfer to the higher level of care needed for definitive management.

## CHILDHOOD TRAUMA

The often invoked maxim that children, and especially infants and young children, are not small adults applies also to understanding and treating traumatic injuries. The differences involve anatomical and physical characteristics, physiological and psychological responses, and even the very mechanisms by which trauma occurs. Adult practitioners often need to be reminded that, for instance, children have greater surface ratio of area to mass than do adolescents or adults. This results in greater dissipation of heat and water, which may compound the effects of other traumatic injuries. The head of an infant or small child encompasses a much larger percentage of the total body than that of adults and subjects children to higher rates of brain and skull injuries. The child's skeleton exhibits greater elasticity than that of the adult and is therefore more likely to tolerate compression and visceral injury without fractures. A vast majority of childhood injuries are passive and result from blunt trauma and thus tend to involve multiple organs. Yet children tend to experience better outcomes compared to adults with the same mechanism of injury because of factors such as the occurrence of fewer bone fractures and the lack of comorbid disorders. It is important to remember that, while a recovery of function and quality of life after blunt injury is common, physical function tends to remain lower than age-matched norms at 6 months postinjury, and often the childhood trauma victim and his or her family bears the consequence of that injury for a lifetime.

### Trauma Scores

A common language that objectively describes injuries and their consequences is very useful in the frenzied circumstances that are the norm in the trauma management process. The Glasgow Coma Scale (GCS) and Injury Severity Scale (ISS) have been mainstays in the assessment and subsequent review of outcomes in pediatric trauma patients. Additional scoring systems are used widely for pediatric trauma and include the Pediatric Trauma Score (used for triage of new patients), the Abbreviated Injury Score (primarily used for classification of the patient for research and comparison purposes), and the Trauma and Injury Severity Score (allows an estimation of the probability of survival).

### Trauma Management

The evaluation and management of the injured child is best performed using a standard protocol. The Advanced Trauma Life Support (ATLS) protocol is widely used and establishes 3 sequential events: the primary Survey, the secondary survey, and a definitive care phase.

### Primary Survey

The primary survey is performed immediately on arrival to the emergency department and may be completed in the first several minutes (Table 116-1). Seminal to this phase is the rapid assessment of vital functions followed by the appropriate resuscitation measures without progression until that portion of the primary survey has been confirmed or corrected.

The reality of trauma assessment and management is that it is frequently a team effort with multiple parallel actions, but it is meaningful to consider the actions as a series of single steps. It is critical not to progress from 1 of the steps until you have completed the assessment and any needed interventions. As an example, when assessing the airway (A), if the patient does not have a secure airway and the patient needs to be intubated, this must occur before moving on to breathing (B), and so on. The assessments and interventions related to the primary survey must identify life-threatening conditions and provide the needed emergent therapies. Thus, these must be rapid and decisions must be made with the available evidence. This does not allow at time for definitive treatment or diagnosis, but rather limited assessment and stabilizing treatment for life-threatening conditions.

**Assessment of Vital Functions** Early on in the primary survey, there must be assessment of vital functions, including declaration of a working weight. The airway and breathing are first in line in the primary survey. In children, inadequate oxygenation and ventilation are the most common causes of cardiac arrest after trauma. In every case, the mouth should be opened and the pharynx examined for foreign material or loose teeth. Secretions should be cleared and, if the child is unconscious, a jaw thrust maneuver or insertion of an oral airway may be used to prevent upper airway obstruction. Supplemental oxygen should be given. The presence of persistent respiratory distress or insufficient respiratory effort is usually an indication for tracheal intubation, which should be performed efficiently by the most experienced individual. Bag and mask ventilation can often provide adequate ventilation even in the most difficult circumstances and is preferable to unskilled tracheal intubation, particularly if laryngeal or tracheal injuries are suspected. Additional specialty aids for intubation include video-assisted direct laryngoscopy, such as the glide scope, or applying a laryngeal mask airway. These devices, when used by experienced providers, can be lifesaving for the difficult airway.

**TABLE 116-1 ELEMENTS OF THE PRIMARY SURVEY FOR TRAUMA VICTIMS**

| |
|---|
| **A**irway |
| **B**reathing |
| **C**irculation with hemorrhage control |
| **D**isability: neurologic status |
| **E**xpose: completely undress patient |

If intubation has failed and adjuncts have only partially supported delivery of oxygen, a surgical airway may be necessary. If the patient has a suspected injury and no stridor but apparent upper airway obstruction, after several unsuccessful attempts of endotracheal intubation, a cricothyroidotomy is the next step. A tracheostomy attempted outside of the operating room (OR), particularly in a small child, can be a very difficult procedure, and is not the treatment of choice in this situation. Rarely, in the circumstance where there is a suspected laryngeal crush injury and stridor, consideration should be given to proceeding directly to a cricothyroidotomy without attempted endotracheal intubation because of the risk of creating a false passage in placing the airway via an endotracheal route.

After airway patency is assured, attention should move to other aspects of respiratory function. Palpation and auscultation are used to determine whether the trachea is in the midline. Auscultation for breath sounds should be completed and they should be heard well bilaterally. A tracheal shift or a decrease of breath sounds on 1 side of the chest may indicate a pneumothorax or hemothorax. If the patient is stable, a chest radiograph should be obtained to establish the origin of the findings.

If there is a shift of the trachea away from the side of absent breath sounds in the setting of hemodynamic instability, then a tension pneumothorax is suspected and emergent treatment is indicated. This can be carried out by simply placing a needle into the pleural space through the second intercostal space at the midclavicular line. This allows relief of the tension and provides an opportunity to place a chest tube for continued evacuation of air. Chest tube placement or tube thoracostomy is the appropriate treatment for a traumatic accumulation of gas or liquid in the pleural space. In a small infant, a 12- to 14-French chest tube is appropriate. In an older child, an 18- to 24-French chest tube is preferable. A larger-bore chest tube is more appropriate if a hemothorax is suspected. A pigtail-type catheter may both allow for adequate evacuation of air and fluid and provide some improved comfort associated with smaller-diameter tubes. Prior to placing the chest tube, clinicians should consider the level of the diaphragm on that side of the chest to avoid injuring abdominal organs. Placement of the chest tube should be anterior to the midaxillary line at the level of the fourth intercostal space. It is best placed in this location to prevent the patient from lying on the tube. The use of a metal obturator with a very sharp, pointed end should be avoided because of the high risk of injury to the lungs or vascular organs. The chest tube should be placed to suction using a Pleur-evac chamber to measure output and assess for air leak. A chest film should be obtained to confirm evacuation of the pneumothorax and assess for position of the tube. Regular reassessment of chest tube positioning, patency, and drainage or bubbling are extremely important aspects of management of these patients.

Rib fractures are less frequently seen in the young child compared to older children and adults. Typically, they require little treatment aside from pain control and assessment of the respiratory effort. However, a child with several contiguous rib fractures may have a flail chest, a condition characterized by a paradoxic inward movement of a portion of the chest during inspiration. This reduces both the functional residual capacity and the tidal volume, requiring positive pressure ventilation if the respiratory effort is inadequate.

A sucking chest wound involves a penetrating injury that allows air to enter the chest during inspiration. The resulting pneumothorax can be prevented from becoming larger by placing a flap valve dressing over the injury until a chest tube can be inserted and the chest wall can be subsequently repaired.

The next step in the primary survey is assessing the adequacy of tissue perfusion (see Chapter 107). A number of physical signs, including tachycardia, pallor, cool extremities, confusion, combativeness, or a decreased blood pressure, can reflect inadequate perfusion. The presence of poor perfusion should raise the suspicion of hypovolemic shock. After hemorrhage, blood pressure is usually maintained until the child loses 20% of the blood volume; thus, hypotension is a late manifestation of a significant injury. The capillary refill time provides a quick assessment of perfusion, provided that the patient is not cold. Initial management of shock includes infusion of crystalloid in the amount of 20 mL/kg as a bolus. Rapid assessment for the location of blood loss should be completed and initial attempts at hemorrhage control may include direct pressure on a wound or open fracture, placement of a pelvic binder or sheet to stabilize a bleeding pelvic fracture, or surgical assessment or consideration of transfer for large volume hemorrhage from a chest tube or evidence of an intra-abdominal injury. In the child with severe shock (hypotension, tachycardia, poor perfusion), consideration for early blood transfusion or utilization of a massive transfusion protocol has been associated with less coagulopathy.

Completion of the primary survey requires a rapid assessment of the entire patient, including neurologic function. The cervical collar, which is often applied prior to arrival, should be temporarily removed to carry out the neck examination. An examination of the back and all other locations that are difficult to see (eg, armpits and perineum) must be completed. It is necessary to remove all clothing to complete this assessment. It is particularly important to establish at this point whether the child has any lateralizing neurological signs that suggest an intracranial space-occupying lesion or spinal cord injury.

A critical consideration of the pediatric trauma patient is the rapid loss of body heat and susceptibility to hypothermia, which can be associated with coagulopathy, physiologic dysfunction, and death. Thus, the critically injured child and the environment may require active interventions to prevent heat loss and cooling, including environmental temperature control, avoiding unnecessary exposure, warm forced air or warming blankets, and active warming through the infusion of warm fluids.

### Intravenous Access

It has become the norm that any child with a significant traumatic injury should have 2 intravenous (IV) lines. If there is an injury involving the abdomen, then at least 1 of the lines should be in an upper extremity or neck. The ideal IV access is a large-bore peripheral IV placed in the upper extremity. Attempts should first be made to place an ideal IV, although this may be challenging in the young child, particularly if hypovolemic. In such conditions, successful placement of a small-bore peripheral intravenous line may gain precious time for the initial resuscitation. A larger-gauge catheter can be inserted later under less pressing circumstances. If peripheral intravenous access cannot be achieved within several minutes, alternative methods of access should be attempted (see Chapter 100) including intraosseous access and, if skilled personnel are available, insertion of a central venous catheter either percutaneously or by surgical venotomy. Subclavian vein access in the trauma patient, particularly in one who is hypotensive or hypovolemic, can be particularly challenging if the clinician has not had significant experience in placing these lines. Additionally, it carries the potential consequence of an iatrogenic pneumothorax or hemothorax. Also, central venous pressure monitoring in the emergency department is unnecessary in the majority of pediatric trauma victims.

After vascular access is established, fluid resuscitation can be initiated accompanied by frequent reassessment of hemodynamic function (heart rate, blood pressure, state of alertness, capillary refill). A urinary catheter can be a valuable measure of organ perfusion, and consideration of placement in a major trauma patient after assessment for urethral injury is mandatory.

### Secondary Survey

The secondary survey includes a history and a complete head-to-toe examination of the child with a focus on specific organ systems. The mnemonic AMPLE assists in obtaining a rapid and complete history by focusing on **A**llergies, **M**edications, **P**ast illnesses, **L**ast meal, and **E**vents and environment involved with the injury. In the secondary survey, the evaluation, testing, and interventions should be individualized for each patient. Every part of the body should be palpated, the chest and abdomen auscultated, and the patient log rolled to examine the back and to perform a rectal examination.

**Head and Neck** The presumption that every patient may have suffered a cervical spine injury has become integral to initial trauma management. Cervical stabilization is thus 1 of the first steps of stabilization and must be continued until cervical injury can be adequately excluded. Immobilization of the cervical spine is usually carried out by prehospital personnel and can be achieved with appropriately sized Philadelphia or Aspen collars or by using sandbags on either side of the head and applying tape over the sandbag and the forehead of the patient. A foam cervical collar will not adequately stabilize the neck. A caregiver can stabilize the cervical spine by holding both mastoids and mandibles in a manner that prevents flexion–extension and lateral movements. If the child is awake and cooperative, the absence of pain or other findings upon careful, full-range mobilization of the neck is usually sufficient to exclude injury. However, physical examination alone cannot exclude a spinal injury in (1) a patient who is uncooperative or unresponsive, (2) the young child unable to give a meaningful or reliable response to questions, or (3) the patient with a significant distracting painful injury elsewhere. Pain with neck movement, tenderness to palpation of the cervical vertebrae, a detectable cervical spine deformity, or a neurologic abnormality referable to the neck are all good reasons to continue immobilization and protection of the cervical spine and to obtain specialized imaging studies and neurosurgical consultation if available.

The assessment and management of acute neurological injuries are discussed elsewhere. Inspection and palpation of the head focuses on the detection of eye and ear injuries, and craniofacial fractures. Crepitus usually indicates a communication between the sinuses and the subcutaneous tissue through a facial bone fracture. Tenderness over the maxilla and mandible, and malocclusion also indicate facial bone fractures. Rhinorrhea or otorrhea suggest a spinal fluid leak through a fracture at the base of the skull.

Examination of the neck and cervical spine includes palpation to identify tenderness, mobilization to assess range of motion, a motor and sensory examination, evaluation of reflexes, and appropriate imaging studies. Difficulty in carrying out this examination is most commonly the result of an altered level of consciousness and/or lack of ability to cooperate because of the patient's age, or the distracting effects of other injuries. Signs of airway obstruction, hoarseness, stridor, crepitus, or significant soft tissue swelling are alerts for a possible airway injury.

In patients who have undergone stabilization of the neck with a collar, examination of the cervical spine requires the removal of the collar. This may require manual stabilization of the neck during the exam in patients who are unconscious or uncooperative. After inspecting for injury, the cervical spine is palpated. Selecting which patients should undergo evaluation of the cervical spine using imaging has been evaluated in a multicenter study under the direction of the Pediatric Emergency Care Applied Research Network (PECARN). They identified 8 factors that were predictive of cervical spine injuries in children: altered mental status, focal neurologic deficits, complaint of neck pain, torticollis, substantial torso injury, predisposing condition, diving, and high-risk motor vehicle crash. These factors should be considered when deciding which patients should be cleared without imaging. In the author's experience, if there is pain on palpation or if there is a deformity or swelling, the cervical collar is reapplied and an imaging study should be performed, especially when there is substantial torso injury or high-energy injury mechanism. If no abnormality on examination is noted and no pain elicited, the patient is asked to rotate the head and neck to each side, move it laterally, and then flex and extend it. If movement is limited or pain occurs, the collar is reapplied and imaging studies are indicated. If again no pain or abnormality is noted, the patient's cervical spine has been "cleared" and no diagnostic imaging is needed. As above, the decision process is more difficult if, for any reason but usually for loss of consciousness or lack of cooperation, the cervical spine cannot be "cleared" using these criteria. Because of the differences in the body habitus of children, a plain cervical spine series may be all that is required in the awake patient with cervical pain or in a child unable to cooperate with an exam as a way to exclude major cervical anomalies in the initial evaluation. Computerized tomography (CT) examination is infrequently needed but may provide a practical method to assess for neck injuries in children. It is important to recognize, however, that a normal neck CT scan does not eliminate the need to perform a functional examination of the neck once it is possible to obtain patient cooperation. Magnetic resonance imaging (MRI), without CT, may eventually be required to exclude an injury in the patient with persistent pain.

**Chest** More than 80% of thoracic injuries in children are caused by blunt trauma. The incidence decreases to slightly less than 60% in adolescents. In the patient with blunt chest injuries, the most common cause of death is a head injury; in patients with penetrating chest injury, the death is most often caused by the chest injury itself.

The majority of thoracic injuries can be handled well with supplemental oxygen, tube thoracotomy, and analgesia. Approximately 5% to 10% of all blunt chest injuries may require a thoracotomy. Immediate life-threatening conditions, which should be identified and stabilized during the primary survey, include complete airway obstruction, tension pneumothorax, massive hemothorax, cardiac tamponade, and penetrating cardiac injury. Also potentially life-threatening conditions include pulmonary contusion, myocardial contusion, aortic disruption, diaphragmatic rupture, tracheobronchial disruption, and esophageal perforation. Indications for emergent thoracotomy in the OR include a penetrating wound to the heart or aorta, continued significant intrathoracic bleeding from other source (≥ 3–4 mL/kg/hour), an imaging study indicating an injury to the aorta or other large vessel, a pneumothorax with an open chest wall injury, a large continuing air leak indicative of a bronchial injury, cardiac tamponade, impalpable pulses with closed chest compression, diaphragmatic rupture, and esophageal perforation. Emergent thoracotomy in the emergency department (ER thoracotomy) has an exceedingly low survival rate and very few indications, especially in the patient who is the victim of blunt trauma. This therapy should only be considered if one has the skills, experience, and ability to definitively manage any identified injuries.

**Abdomen** The secondary survey of the abdomen includes inspection, palpation, percussion, auscultation, and the use of imaging studies as needed. Abdominal blunt trauma carries an increased risk of injuring multiple organs. The presence of a "seat belt" sign, a linear abdominal wall ecchymosis, is indicative of a rapid deceleration mechanism of injury. This deceleration can often cause significant intra-abdominal injuries. The combination of a seat belt injury and significant tenderness on palpation should cause a high degree of suspicion for injuries of the abdominal viscera.

A nasogastric tube should be placed to decompress the stomach if distended. If there is any evidence of a mid-face fracture, the tube should be placed via an orogastric route to avoid the possibility of the tube being misplaced into the cranial cavity. Distention of the stomach alone can cause pain and even respiratory compromise.

The presence of a pelvic fracture should raise suspicions of a concomitant retroperitoneal or urethral injury. Urethral injury is common in males and should be suspected if there is blood in the urethral meatus or a high-riding prostate on rectal examination. If there is a significant suspicion to a urethral injury, a retrograde urethrogram should be performed before inserting a Foley catheter. Contemporary evaluation of the abdomen often includes an abdominal and pelvic computerized tomography scan. With the new generation of helical scanners, a full abdominal examination can be carried out in minutes. Radiological assessment should only be performed, however, once the patient is sufficiently stable. Peritoneal lavage is now used in very limited circumstances, because the presence of free blood in the abdominal cavity is no longer considered an automatic indication for surgery. For the same reason bedside ultrasound or the focused assessment with sonography for trauma (FAST) exam is of limited value in the stable pediatric patient.

The spleen and the liver are 2 of the abdominal organs most commonly injured. The conservative management of childhood splenic and liver injuries is common practice today. A multicenter study of pediatric level I trauma centers conducted by the pediatric research consortium ATOMAC+ has provided an evidence-based guideline that was validated in a prospective review of patients with blunt liver and spleen injuries (Fig. 116-1). This guideline is based on the assessment of the hemodynamic stability of patients regardless of injury grade. This is in contrast to previous guidelines that were grade based. Major decision points include initial assessment of the patient's hemodynamic stability and normal values, response to volume resuscitation, and measurement of blood counts. Intervention is indicated for patients with ongoing blood loss and hemodynamic stability. Use of interventional radiology techniques for control of hepatic or splenic sources of bleeding are becoming more common, but frequently are only available at specialized pediatric trauma centers. Indications for surgery include unstable hemodynamics unresponsive to blood transfusion and interventional control techniques for hemorrhage.

Injuries to the pancreas are often the result of a blunt injury, such as those caused by the handlebar of a bicycle, rapid deceleration in a motor vehicle accident, a fall, or intentional child abuse. Penetrating pancreatic injuries are rare and most commonly associated with gunshot injuries. Because of the location of the pancreas and regardless of mechanism, there are often coexisting injuries to the stomach, duodenum, kidneys, or spine. The diagnosis is made on the basis of laboratory studies (elevation in amylase and lipase) and imaging studies (a CT scan demonstrating pancreatic edema, hematoma, or disruption). A penetrating injury of the abdomen with a pancreatic injury requires laparotomy. A blunt injury with stable vital signs and no peritonitis should undergo dedicated cross-sectional imaging. Injuries with a high likelihood of disruption of the pancreatic duct are better managed operatively if the injury can be characterized within the first 24 to 48 hours from injury. This approach reduces the number of interventions, shortens the length of stay, and decreases the time to complete resolution of the injury. The decision to defer operation is usually prompted by a blunt injury, lack of peritonitis, and imaging showing no obvious pancreatic disruption. Nonoperative treatment consists of bowel rest, intravenous nutrition, and administration of octreotide as needed to decrease pancreatic exocrine secretions. A decision to change from nonoperative management to operative intervention is based on the development of peritonitis, persistent amylase/lipase elevations, and fever. A pancreatic pseudocyst is a known later complication of pancreatic trauma, often associated with an elevation in lipase and amylase. The pseudocyst is initially managed nonoperatively, but if still present for over 6 weeks, consideration should be given to internal drainage to the stomach or small bowel.

Intestinal injuries can occur throughout the bowel. The ligament of Treitz and the ileocecal valve are 2 vulnerable points because shear forces tend to tear the bowel at the points where it is tethered to the abdominal wall. Additional mechanisms that can cause a tear in the mesentery or perforation of the small bowel are related to compression against the spine by a force against the anterior abdominal wall. This type of injury may be associated with a Chance fracture of the spine, a fracture along a transverse plane in the vertebral body. The duodenum is also often injured when compressed between the abdominal wall and the spine. A duodenal hematoma can be diagnosed by an upper gastrointestinal (GI) contrast study or an abdominal CT scan and in older children is generally managed conservatively. A duodenal injury in children younger than 5 years of age is highly associated with inflicted injury and should raise suspicion by providers. These inflicted injuries have a higher likelihood of requiring operative intervention (53% of all cases).

Microscopic hematuria in a patient with a normal CT scan does not itself warrant admission, and outpatient follow-up is reasonable. An abnormal CT scan or macroscopic hematuria are indications for hospital admission. If the CT scan shows a major blood extravasation or nonvisualization of renal flow, arteriography is indicated. If the vasculature is normal, the renal injury can be managed as with other solid organ injuries. However, operative intervention is required if hypertension or hemodynamic instability occurs. Bladder rupture can be identified on cystogram and CT scan and requires operative

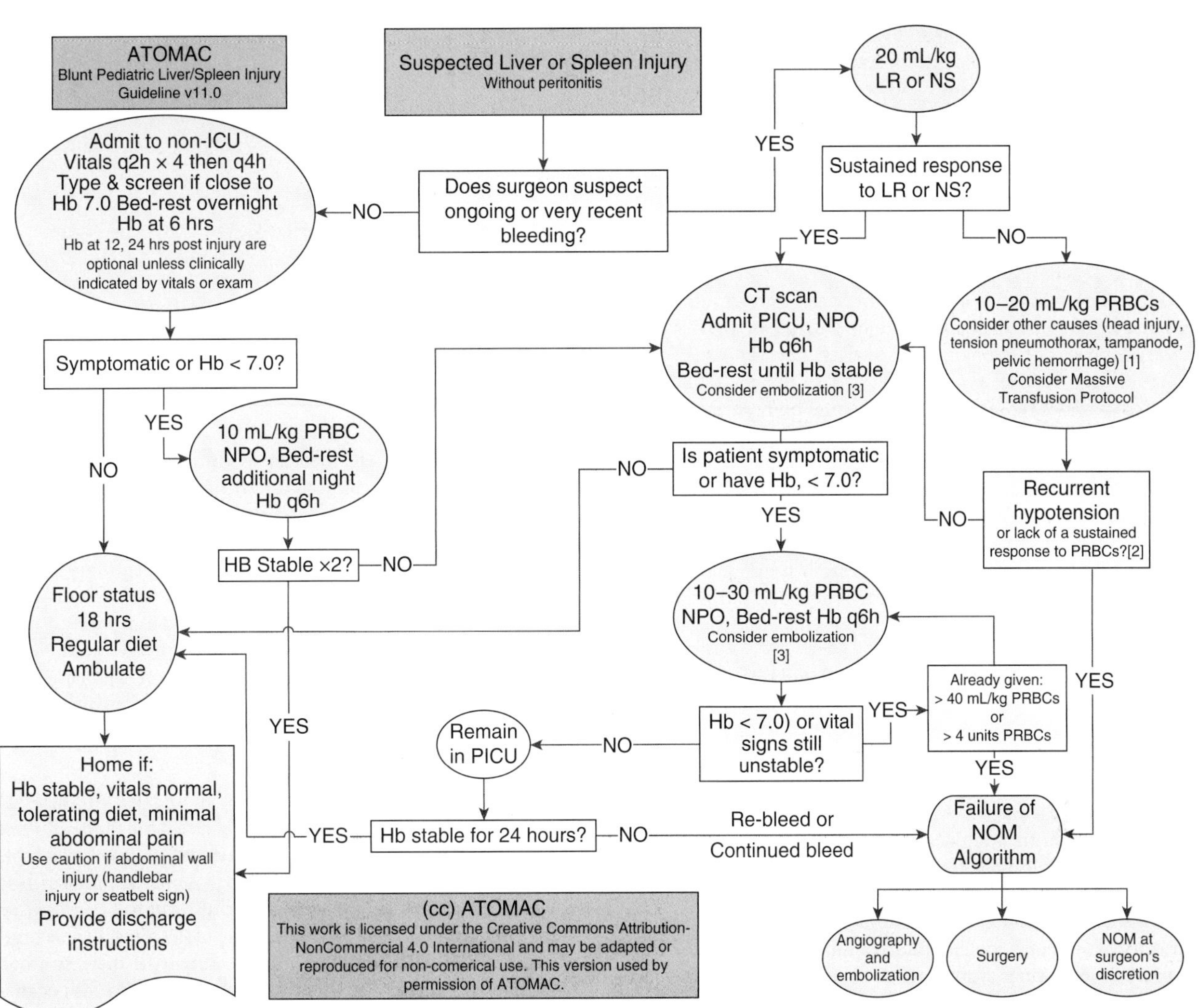


**FIGURE 116-1** ATOMAC guideline for management of BLSI. BLSI, blunt liver/spleen injury; CT, computed tomography; Hb, hemoglobin; LR, lactated ringers; NOM, non-operative management; NPO, non per os, or nothing by mouth; NS, normal saline; PICU, pediatric intensive care unit; PRBC, packed red blood cell; q6h, every 6 hours; SBP, systolic blood pressure.

[1]More than 50% of injured children with hypotension have no significant intra-abdominal bleeding but do have severe traumatic brain injury.

[2]Recurrent hypotension within the first hour because of intra-abdominal bleeding or an SBP of less than 50 mmHg after transfusion is an ominous sign, and strong consideration should be given to operative or angiographic intervention.

[3]Embolizing CT blush may be considered, but more than 80% of children with blush do not require angiography for successful NOM.

[4]Interventional modalities such as ERCP, laparoscopy, angiography, or percutaneous drainage may be required to manage complications of bile leak or hemobilia.

intervention if the perforation is intraperitoneal. Extraperitoneal bladder ruptures can be managed with transurethral catheter drainage.

### Nonaccidental Trauma

This subject is covered extensively elsewhere. In the evaluation of the trauma patient, the suspicion of child abuse should be kept in mind. This is particularly true if any or several of the following are noted: (1) a discrepancy between the history and the degree of injury, (2) a prolonged interval from injury to treatment, (3) a history of repeated similar injuries, (4) an inappropriate parental response, or (5) a changing history given by the caretaker.

## BURNS

Burn injuries are the third most common cause of death due to trauma in children in the United States, accounting for 2500 deaths and over 10,000 cases of severe, permanent disability annually. Many of these injuries are preventable. The majority of hospital admissions of pediatric burn patients are children younger than 2 years of age. Burns are often caused by hot liquids in younger children, particularly those under 3 years of age, and by fire in older children and adults. The initial resuscitation has a fundamental role, particularly in the case of large–surface-area burns. The outcome for the burned patient is related to the magnitude of the injury, and is influenced substantially by the quality of the care provided. Patients with significant burn injuries are best cared for in a burn center. Survival rates in pediatric burn victims with 40% to 60% body surface area (BSA) burns have been reported to be as high as 100%, and with 60% to 100% BSA, burn survival is 86%.

Burns can be categorized as the result of thermal, electrical, chemical, or radiation injury. The majority of burns in children have a thermal mechanism. Developmental differences in BSA-to-body mass ratio and thickness of the skin account for most differences in the response to a burn injury between infants, children, and adults. The child has a larger BSA-to-body mass ratio in comparison to an adult. A 1-year-old weighing 10 kg has one-seventh the body mass of an adult and one-third the BSA of an adult. Accordingly, the child has a larger evaporative fluid loss and greater difficulty maintaining temperature regulation. The child's skin is not as thick as the adult's, and thus can burn more deeply after the same duration of contact with a comparable heat source.

The severity of tissue damage after a burn is related to several factors: (1) temperature of the heat source responsible for the burn,

(2) duration of exposure, (3) area of the body burned, and (4) age of the patient. Burns to the palms of the hand and soles of the feet tend to be less deep than similar burns to other parts of the body because of the relative thickness of the epidermis in those areas. Likewise, while a shoulder burn may require a skin graft because of the depth of burn, a facial burn after a similar exposure may heal spontaneously, because the rich blood supply of the face limits the injury by dissipating heat more rapidly from that area.

### The Assessment of Burn Surface and Depth

The accurate determination of the burned surface area is an integral part of burn-wound management. In adults, the rule of nines is a simple and accurate way of estimating this surface. Each upper extremity and each of the anterior or posterior surfaces of the chest, abdomen, and lower extremities represents 9% of the total body surface. Unfortunately, the same rule is not applicable to children. The head and neck of a child younger than 1 year of age accounts for 21% of the BSA. The modified Lund and Browder BSA chart (Fig. 116-2) can be used to estimate the percent of the BSA involved in a burn. Except in "stocking-glove" burns that extend from the tip of an extremity to the trunk, it is often necessary to approximate the magnitude of involvement of a body part. Especially in the case of irregular burns, it is also useful to know that the palm of a child represents approximately 1% of the BSA.

Burn depth is categorized as either partial or full thickness. *Partial-thickness burns* involve the epidermis and portions of the dermis. This corresponds to the older nomenclature of first-degree burns, which are exemplified by sunburn, and second-degree burns, which are characterized by a red or mottled appearance, blisters, edema, and a weeping, moist surface. Because of involvement of the dermal nerve endings, they are both painful to the touch and sensitive to cold air. Partial-thickness burns are subclassified as superficial or deep partial-thickness burns. Superficial partial-thickness burns tend to heal spontaneously over 7 to 14 days postinjury. Deep partial-thickness burns may heal spontaneously, but over a longer period of time, and may require tangential excision and skin grafting. Full-thickness or third-degree burns involve all skin layers. Their color can be variable. The tissue appears dry and inelastic, and the area is insensitive. Full-thickness burns will not heal spontaneously. As a rule, they require excision and skin grafting. Small full-thickness burns may heal by wound contracture. In some burns, the central portion is full thickness and the peripheral portion is partial thickness. In rare cases, the burns may extend into the deep tissues underneath the skin. These deep burns are associated with increased resuscitative needs and complications.



**TABLE 116-2 BURN CENTER TRANSFER CRITERIA**

| |
|---|
| Partial thickness > 10% BSA |
| Any full-thickness burn |
| Inhalation injury |
| Circumferential burn |
| Chemical burn |
| Involvement of face, hands, feet, genitalia, perineum, or major joint |
| Burned children in hospitals without qualified personnel or equipment for pediatric care |
| Burn injuries in children with preexisting medical conditions that could complicate management or recovery or affect mortality |

### Management of the Burned Patient

**Immediate Treatment** The first step of immediate burn care is to make sure that there is no ongoing injury. If there is any clothing or object that may still be a significant source of heat, it should be immediately removed from the patient. Jewelry should also be removed from the area and the burn should be wrapped with a clean, dry cloth. Cold liquids should not be applied to burns larger than 1% or 2% of the BSA because the cold can result in diminished local perfusion, which may worsen the injury. Instead, the burns should be dressed with clean, moist dressings and the patient kept warm. The patient should be made as comfortable as possible, and rapid transport should be arranged to a local hospital for immediate resuscitation and stabilization. Criteria for transfer to a burn center are given in Table 116-2.

**Fluid Resuscitation** Intravenous access should be obtained in any patient with a burn greater than 10% BSA, and fluid resuscitation should be initiated. If needed, the IV may be placed through burned tissue. A calculated burn resuscitation volume has shown benefits. However, the guideline is to achieve a urine output of 1 mL/kg/hour in young children and 30 to 50 mL/hour in adolescents. A Foley catheter should be inserted to monitor urinary output. If there is a perineal burn, bladder catheterization should be performed before edema formation makes this difficult.

**Airway and Lung Injuries** Any patient with a potential for a smoke-inhalation injury requires a rapid physical examination with special attention to the integrity of the airway and to gas exchange. Carbonaceous material in the oropharynx, nasopharynx, or sputum should be noted. Pharyngeal burns, stridor, significant bronchorrhea, dyspnea, or decreased arterial oxygen saturation are indications of airway or

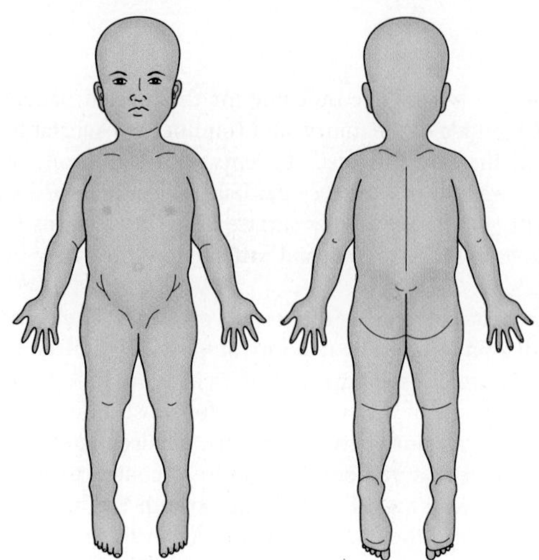

| Area | Age–Years | | | | | % 2° | % 3° | % Total |
|---|---|---|---|---|---|---|---|---|
| | 0–1 | 1–4 | 5–9 | 10–15 | Adult | | | |
| Head | 19 | 17 | 13 | 10 | 7 | | | |
| Neck | 2 | 2 | 2 | 2 | 2 | | | |
| Ant. Trunk | 13 | 13 | 13 | 13 | 13 | | | |
| Post. Trunk | 13 | 13 | 13 | 13 | 13 | | | |
| R. Buttock | 2–1/2 | 2–1/2 | 2–1/2 | 2–1/2 | 2–1/2 | | | |
| L. Buttock | 2–1/2 | 2–1/2 | 2–1/2 | 2–1/2 | 2–1/2 | | | |
| Genitalia | 1 | 1 | 1 | 1 | 1 | | | |
| R. U. Arm | 4 | 4 | 4 | 4 | 4 | | | |
| L. U. Arm | 4 | 4 | 4 | 4 | 4 | | | |
| R. L. Arm | 3 | 3 | 3 | 3 | 3 | | | |
| L. L. Arm | 3 | 3 | 3 | 3 | 3 | | | |
| R. Hand | 2–1/2 | 2–1/2 | 2–1/2 | 2–1/2 | 2–1/2 | | | |
| L. Hand | 2–1/2 | 2–1/2 | 2–1/2 | 2–1/2 | 2–1/2 | | | |
| R. Thigh | 5–1/2 | 6–1/2 | 8–1/2 | 8–1/2 | 9–1/2 | | | |
| L. Thigh | 5–1/2 | 6–1/2 | 8–1/2 | 8–1/2 | 9–1/2 | | | |
| R. Leg | 5 | 5 | 5–1/2 | 6 | 7 | | | |
| L. Leg | 5 | 5 | 5–1/2 | 6 | 7 | | | |
| R. Foot | 3–1/2 | 3–1/2 | 3–1/2 | 3–1/2 | 3–1/2 | | | |
| L. Foot | 3–1/2 | 3–1/2 | 3–1/2 | 3–1/2 | 3–1/2 | | | |
| | | | | Total BSA Burn | | | | |

Modified from Lund and Browder

• Hand Method for nonuniform burns—palm of child's hand approximates 1 percent of child's total BSA burn.

**FIGURE 116-2** Modified Lund and Browder body surface area chart.

lung injuries. Supplemental oxygen should be given. Any concern about airway patency should be addressed by cannulating the trachea before edema makes endotracheal intubation difficult. Bronchoscopy can confirm the presence of carbonaceous material below the vocal cords. Arterial blood gas and carboxyhemoglobin levels should be determined.

Three important complications are associated with smoke-inhalation injuries: carbon monoxide poisoning, thermal injury to the upper respiratory tract, and chemical injury by combustion products to the lower respiratory tract. Carbon monoxide intoxication should be suspected in any patient who has been exposed to combustion products, especially if the exposure occurred in a closed environment and if the patient has an altered state of consciousness or signs of poor oxygen delivery, such as a metabolic acidosis.

Thermal burns can affect the pharynx, the nasopharynx, and the upper airway, causing edema and mucosal sloughing. Direct thermal injuries are rare below the glottis, although steam may carry sufficient heat to cause burns in the trachea and bronchi. Inhalational injuries in the subglottic airways are almost invariably due to chemical damage to the lower respiratory tract, including the bronchi, terminal bronchioles, and alveoli. Their severity varies from bronchial irritation causing cough, increased mucus production, and bronchospasm to more serious alveolar-capillary disruption resulting in respiratory failure.

In patients with burns greater than 25% to 30% of their BSA, pulmonary edema is a common complication, independent of smoke inhalation. Its mechanism involves fluid overload, hypoalbuminemia, and systemic inflammation initiated by the burn. Infection of the respiratory tract is common and carries a high morbidity and a significant mortality risk. Respiratory failure resulting from any of the aforementioned mechanisms occurs in more than half of the children who die as a result of their burns.

**Fluid Resuscitation** Fluid resuscitation within the first 24 hours can be done with crystalloid alone, crystalloid and colloid, or hypertonic saline. Each regimen has its rationale and proponents. The majority of burn centers favor a crystalloid resuscitation based on an initial intravenous infusion of 4 mL of Ringer lactate solution per kilogram of body weight per percent of BSA burned. In addition, the patient should receive maintenance fluid. Half of the calculated resuscitation fluid is given in the first 8 hours of the resuscitation and the remaining half in hours 9 through 24. In the course of the treatment, the volume of Ringer lactate infusion is adjusted to maintain urine output at 1 mL/kg/hour. The initial fluid calculation is a guide to fluid management. The adequacy of fluid resuscitation is manifested by an appropriate urine output. In this manner, the patient's homeostatic mechanisms are used to guide the therapy and to avoid over- and underhydration. Patients who are unable to attain a rate of 1 mL/kg/hour despite increasing the volume of resuscitation should have a deeper injury suspected. Tissue edema of the burn wound, although unavoidable, can cause complications of its own. A partial-thickness burn of the back may progress to a full-thickness burn because of dependent edema. This is particularly true if the patient is resuscitated with excessive amounts of fluid.

In patients with myoglobinuria or hemoglobinuria, a larger urine output is desirable and consideration should be given to the administration of sodium bicarbonate to raise urine pH. The use of a diuretic during the resuscitative phase is rarely indicated and should be avoided.

A number of metabolic disturbances can occur with fluid resuscitation. Metabolic acidosis is most often due to inadequate perfusion and is best treated by increasing fluid volume. Hyperkalemia can be seen in patients with electrical burns and is a consequence of red blood cell breakdown. Moderate hyponatremia can occur at all stages of stabilization due to intracellular shift of sodium and natriuresis, and can be partly attributed to crystalloid resuscitation. If the patient is symptomatic, the judicious use of hypertonic saline may be indicated in experienced hands.

**Circumferential Burns** Circumferential burns deserve specific attention because they have a potential to cause additional vascular or respiratory derangements. In the case of an extremity injury, burned skin and subcutaneous tissue do not expand to accommodate swelling in the extremity, limiting venous outflow. Continued arterial inflow causes edema in the distal portion of the extremity, eventually occluding the arterial vessels. Arterial inflow is then compromised. Cyanosis, paresthesia, weakness, or a decreased or absent pulse can be observed and are indications for escharotomy involving both sides of the fingers, toes, feet, hands, arms, or legs. For circumferential burns to the chest, a limited tidal volume or chest rise and blood–gas exchange abnormalities should prompt similar action. The chest escharotomy consists of bilateral vertical incisions in the midaxillary line and a transverse costal incision. The escharotomy can be done at the bedside because these burns are full thickness in nature and the skin is insensitive.

**Burn-Wound Management** Initial treatment consists of debridement of the wound injury and application of a topical silver-containing antimicrobial such as silver sulfadiazine (Silvadene). Daily wound care involves either whirlpooling and wound debridement of the burn eschar or applying a silver salt product and leaving it on the burns for several days. After this, the burn is assessed for signs of spontaneous re-epithelialization and formation of capillary buds, followed by the reapplication of the antimicrobial, assessment of mobility, and wrapping. Sedation facilitates aggressive wound debridement and alleviates the anxiety and discomfort associated with this type of repetitive care.

The use of split-thickness skin grafting is often indicated in full-thickness and deep partial-thickness burns. An early decision to carry out tangential excision of the burn and split thickness skin grafting has the advantage of a lower risk of infection, shorter hospitalization, and improved outcome. After several days of burn-wound assessment, a determination of whether the burn will heal spontaneously can usually be made.

**Nutrition** Burn patients have perhaps the largest caloric needs of any single group of pediatric patients. In a child who has suffered a large BSA burn, the caloric needs may be 50% greater than the calculated basal needs for body weight or surface area. Additionally, the protein requirements are increased to nearly 2 g/kg/day due to significant loss through the affected tissues. Many patients will not ingest a sufficient amount of calories orally. In addition, because of the need for daily burn-wound debridement and procedural sedation, the patient may not ingest nutrients for a number of hours before or after the debridement procedure. The use of enteral feeding via a nasogastric tube is an excellent method for supplying the appropriate caloric needs and carries a much lower risk of morbidity when compared to intravenous nutrition. Enteral feedings can be started as soon as 24 hours after the burn. If enteral feedings cannot be used, central parenteral nutrition is indicated. Central intravenous access can be challenging if the areas typically used for access are burned. Rotating intravenous access for total parenteral nutrition is a common technique with variable success in reducing the risk of bacteremia. A central line bundle and dressing protocol should be followed and the catheters removed as soon as possible to reduce the risk of bacteremia.

### Infections

Infections are the major cause of death and a major cause of morbidity in burn patients. The infections can be divided into 3 types: (1) primary wound or graft infection; (2) bacteremia and catheter-related sepsis; and (3) infections at other sites (lung, urinary tract). In children, risk of infection is increased in inhalation injuries, burns greater than 30% BSA, and full-thickness burns.

The type of bacterial flora that colonizes burn injuries changes with time. In the first week, Gram-positive organisms predominate. By week 2, Gram-negative organisms increase in frequency and number. By week 3, infections due to fungal organisms and antibiotic-resistant organisms are often found. There has been no proven benefit of using prophylactic intravenous antibiotic therapy in burn patients.

In contrast, the use of topical antimicrobials is well documented to be efficacious in burn-wound management. Almost all of the topical antimicrobial agents have silver as the antimicrobial agent. There has been an evolution over the past 40 years in the use of various topical agents for burn care. Silver nitrate was associated with a marked decrease in burn-wound infection and improved survival with its use. However, difficulty with dressing changes, staining, and metabolic complications were noted. For the past 3 decades, silver sulfadiazine is the topical agent used most frequently throughout the United States because it affords good Gram-positive and Gram-negative coverage and it is relatively easy to apply. A disadvantage to its use is the development of leukopenia in a small number of patients. It is often unclear whether this is the result of using the silver sulfadiazine or infection. Sulfamylon is an alternative agent that has the advantage of better penetration of the burn eschar. It is of particular benefit in ear burns, where the cartilage may be involved. Its disadvantages are that it acts as a carbonic anhydrase inhibitor and that it may be painful for the patient. More recently, a series of silver impregnated products, for example Aquacel Ag (Convatec) and Acticoat (Smith and Nephew) have become available and have been associated with excellent results in burn-wound care. This family of topical agents often has greater ease of use than silver sulfadiazine. They come in sheets, are easier to apply, and can be left in place for a number of days. This decreases both the amount of caregiver time needed for wound care and the number of times the patient must be sedated and exposed to discomfort with dressing changes.

A major principle in burn care is to obtain coverage of the burn wound. This can be achieved by spontaneous re-epithelialization or by graft coverage. Most superficial partial-thickness burns heal spontaneously and do not require skin grafting for a satisfactory cosmetic result. Tangential excision of the burn eschar and split-thickness skin grafts are indicated in children with full-thickness burns and deep partial-thickness burns. Tangential excision removes the dead burn tissue to the point that capillary bleeding is identified. The recipient bed is then usually covered with a meshed graft (1.5:1, 3:1, or 6:1) of approximately 14/1000-inch thickness. The meshing allows for expansion of the skin graft, an important consideration in the patient with an extensive burn. In addition, it prevents the accumulation of fluid between the native tissue base and at the graft, which would hinder graft adherence. The cosmetic result declines as more widely meshed grafts are used.

A major research interest for decades in the field of burn injury has been in the area of biological dressings. Ideally, the patient's own skin would and should be used. However, in large–surface-area burns, there is often not enough skin. The use of cultured epidermal autografts began in 1985. This technique consists of taking a portion of skin from a patient and growing that tissue in culture. Large sheets of autograft can be harvested and applied to a recipient bed on the patient. However, the tissue is very fragile and the cost of producing the cultured autografts is high. Another technique is to place a combination of a thinner (6/1000 to 7/1000 inch) split-thickness skin graft and a donor dermal base (AlloDerm) on the recipient site. This allows for earlier reharvesting of a graft from the same donor site of the burn patient and affords good coverage for a deep burn.

In patients where there is a clear need for wound coverage but not enough tissue available for skin grafting, cadaveric homograft or porcine xenograft can be used as a temporary biological dressing. These types of grafts would typically be recognized as foreign tissue by an immunocompetent recipient and rejected in 4 to 5 days. In patients with significant burns, there often is a degree of immune dysfunction and these grafts may last for up to 10 to 14 days. Biological dressings decrease the risk of infection based on the same principle as do grafts. They also decrease fluid loss and discomfort with dressing changes, while allowing spontaneous epithelialization of the native skin. They can be used in patients in whom (1) there is not enough native skin to cover a burn and coverage is needed until sufficient skin is available for grafting, (2) there is a burn-wound infection and a split-thickness skin graft is likely to become infected, and (3) there is a reasonable likelihood that the wound will epithelialize spontaneously and thus will not require a skin graft, but prompt coverage is desirable.

### Prevention of Burns

As with other injuries in children, there are ample opportunities for avoidance of burn injuries through educational processes. Burn injuries in children younger than 3 years of age are often caused by hot liquids, and not fires. This age group compromises the majority of pediatric burn injuries. Therefore, prevention in this population could potentially significantly decrease the number of burns seen in children.

In children younger than 6 months of age, burns due to hot liquids often occur because of a parent carrying both a child and a cup containing hot liquids such as coffee or tea. As the child becomes a toddler, their curiosity can lead to burn injuries because of the home not being "burn safe." Parents are often well educated in terms of child proofing various rooms in the house, so that the child does not tumble down a flight of stairs or pull a lamp off of a table. The 2 rooms that carry the highest risk or burns in children are the kitchen and bathroom. Any electrical cord hanging off a counter affords the opportunity for the child to pull on the cord and thus pull the coffee pot, electric fryer, or electric slow cooker, and its contents, onto himself or herself. Likewise, allowing a bathtub to be filled with warm or hot water with an unsupervised child carries significant risk of burn injury. During the summer months, the child is at risk for injuries in the area of outdoor cooking appliances such as barbecue grills and campfires. Fortunately, the incidence of electrical burns has markedly decreased over the past 30 years with the use of much better insulation for electrical wiring of home products.

In children older than 5 years of age, burn wounds are more commonly caused by fire. Again, there are excellent educational opportunities. Fire-related injuries are often due to children playing with matches or other combustible products. These types of injuries are very predictable, with burn injuries from fireworks being a common example. Suspicion of abuse is also necessary in the when there are delays to seeking care or the pattern of injury does not fit the provided history.

## ANIMAL AND HUMAN BITES

Between 80% and 90% of all bites are inflicted by dogs and 5% to 15% by cats. The remainder involve humans or a variety of species including rodents, bats, and other wild animals. Bites merit consideration either because they involve substantive tissue injuries or because of the potential for the transmission of zoonosis to the victim.

### Dog Bites

Approximately 5 million dog bites occur in the United States annually. Of these, approximately 800,000 require medical attention. More than half occur in children and the incidence is highest in 5- to 9-year-old boys, decreasing with age and severity thereafter. Over 75% of the dogs causing the injury either belong to the child's family or a neighbor.

All pediatric dog bite victims should be treated as trauma patients. The force of a dog's bite not only may result in soft tissue laceration or puncture, but also may cause bone fractures. The upper extremity is the most commonly injured area, particularly in older children, whereas the head and neck are more frequently involved in children younger than 4 years of age. Facial and neck wounds can be associated with mandibular fractures, intracranial injuries, and cervical spine injuries.

After a bite, the wounds should be thoroughly cleaned, debrided of devitalized tissue, and copiously irrigated. Tetanus toxoid should be administered when immunization status is unknown or out of date. Options regarding wound management include primary, delayed, and secondary closure. The decision is based on the amount of wound contamination, the degree of tissue loss, and the length of time since the injury. Particularly in wounds involving the face, the infectious risks of early closure need to be weighed against the potential for a poor cosmetic result if the wound is allowed to close without suture repair. Infection occurs in one-third of pediatric hand wounds, despite appropriate initial therapy, prompting the recommendation of antibiotic prophylaxis in most cases. Amoxicillin/clavulanate provides good coverage for many of the organisms isolated.

Education has been shown to decrease the number of dog bite injuries. Common recommendations rooted in common sense include avoiding contact with strange dogs; not leaving young children alone at home with a dog; and teaching children, if they are old enough, of the need to respect a dog's territory, particularly while the dog is feeding or protecting her pups.

### Cat Bites

Although cat bites are less common than dog bites, they appear to carry a higher risk of infection. *Pasteurella multocida* is the most common organism; it is isolated from 20% to 80% of all infected cat bites and from the mouth of 90% of the cats tested. Cat scratch fever is caused by *Bartonella henselae,* which can be transmitted by a cat bite or scratch from the cat's claw and is discussed in detail elsewhere (see Chapter 252).

The injured area is typically much smaller than in a dog bite. Treatment principles, however, are the same in regard to initial management, assessment, and infection prevention and treatment. Since the vast majority of cat bites are not deep or associated with tissue loss, wounds are typically left open. A significant index of suspicion is appropriate for the patient who develops subsequent fever or lymphadenopathy. This may be indicative of an abscess or cat scratch disease.

### Human Bites

Human bites are considered to be the third most common bite wound following dog and cat bites. The true incidence is unknown; many cases are not reported because they involve only minor injury or because the patient or family does not wish to admit the mechanism of injury. The bite can be either accidental or purposeful, and can range from minor to serious. Some wounds do not involve an occlusive bite and result from an accidental or purposeful impact against another person's teeth. Over one-half of bite wounds occur in the upper extremity and 10% to 20% involve the head and neck area. Human oral flora includes potentially infectious species of both aerobic and anaerobic organisms, and the overall risk of infection is at least as high as with dog bites.

### Bite Wound Evaluation and Care

Evaluation of bite injuries includes a history of the event; a pertinent medical history; assessment of the vulnerability of the patient to infection, very particularly for tetanus and rabies (see Chapters 284 and 316); and a detailed examination of the wound. In cases where presentation is delayed, there often is an increased likelihood of infection. The initial evaluation should note and document the following: wound size and depth; type of wound (eg, abrasion, puncture, avulsion, laceration) and whether there is any tissue loss; where appropriate, motor and sensory function of the affected area; and signs of infection, such as pain, swelling, erythema, drainage, red streaking, or fever.

Bite wounds resulting in a superficial abrasion or contusion need no further treatment after cleaning and evaluation. With more extensive wounds, if exploration appears appropriate or if there is any concern regarding neurovascular abnormalities, a surgical consultation should be obtained. Potential complications include abscess formation, joint penetration, fracture, tendon disruption, tenosynovitis, osteomyelitis, and a paronychia. A decision to close the wound is best made by an experienced clinician and should consider factors such as the degree of contamination, length of time since the injury, signs of infection, the location of the wound, the degree of tissue loss, and whether the patient is immunocompromised. For example, a facial wound with tissue loss may be best treated with wound closure or approximation and an antibiotic therapy, while a hand wound that is 24 hours old with signs of infection may be better treated by leaving the wound open, elevating the extremity, and administering parenteral antibiotics.

## SUGGESTED READINGS

Alemayehu H, Tsao K, Wulkan ML, et al. Multi-institutional experience with penetrating pancreatic injuries in children. *Pediatr Surg Int.* 2014;30(11):1107-1110.

Blot S, Hoste E, Colardyn F. Acute respiratory failure that complicates the resuscitation of pediatric patients with scald injuries. *J Burn Care Rehabil.* 2000;21(3):289-290.

Demetriades D, Karaiskakis M, Velmahos GC, Alo K, Murray J, Chan L. Pelvic fractures in pediatric and adult trauma patients: are they different injuries? *J Trauma.* 2003;54(6):1146-1151.

Gilchrist J, Sacks JJ, White D, Kresnow MJ. Dog bites: still a problem? *Inj Prev.* 2008;14(5):296-301.

Iqbal CW, St Peter SD, Tsao K, et al; Pancreatic Trauma in Children (PATCH) Study Group. Operative vs nonoperative management for blunt pancreatic transection in children: multi-institutional outcomes. *J Am Coll Surg.* 2014;218(2):157-162

Kaye AE, Belz JM, Kirschner RE. Pediatric dog bite injuries: a 5-year review of the experience at the Children's Hospital of Philadelphia. *Plast Reconstr Surg.* 2009;124(2):551-558.

Leonard JC, Kuppermann N, Olsen C, et al. Factors associated with cervical spine injury in children after blunt trauma. *Ann Emerg Med.* 2011 Aug;58(2):145-155.

Notrica DM, Eubanks JW 3rd, Tuggle DW, et al. Nonoperative management of blunt liver and spleen injury in children: evaluation of the ATOMAC guideline using GRADE. *J Trauma Acute Care Surg.* 2015;79(4):683-693.

Ott R, Kramer R, Martus P, Bussenius-Kammerer M, Carbon R, Rupprecht H. Prognostic value of trauma scores in pediatric patients with multiple injuries. *J Trauma.* 2000;49(4):729-736.

Sheridan RL, Remensnyder JP, Schnitzer JJ, Schulz JT, Ryan CM, Tompkins RG. Current expectations for survival in pediatric burns. *Arch Pediatr Adolesc Med.* 2000;154(3):246-249.

Sowrey L, Lawson KA, Garcia-Filion P. Duodenal injuries in the very young: child abuse? *J Trauma Acute Care Surg.* 2013;74(1):136-141.

Stylianos S; APSA Trauma Committee. Evidence-based guidelines for resource utilization in children with isolated spleen or liver injury. *J Ped Surg.* 2000;35(2);164-169.

# 117 Envenomation*

James Tibballs and Kenneth D. Winkel

## INTRODUCTION

Numerous terrestrial and marine animals may envenomate humans, with children overrepresented among the victims. Treatment, in some cases, may include mechanical ventilation and intensive cardiovascular support, as well as the application of specific therapies and, in some cases, the administration of antivenom. This chapter describes some of the more common animals, their toxins, and the injuries that they cause, and outlines treatment appropriate for each. Snakebites and scorpion stings cause most deaths and morbidity. Envenomation is, for most clinicians, rarely encountered, but if missed, may have catastrophic effects on the victims. It is therefore important to have a high index of suspicion for envenomation, when circumstances and clinical presentation would suggest that this is a possibility, and also to seek advice early from experts in the field when treating these patients.

## SNAKEBITE

Snakebite is most common among highly populated rural communities in tropical developing countries. The annual incidence of snakebites, according to the World Health Organization, is 5 million bites leading to 2.5 million envenomations and 100,000 to 200,000 deaths, of which about 50,000 occur in India. Many more survivors have

*Portions of this chapter previously appeared in a different format in *Rogers' Textbook of Pediatric Intensive Care, Fifth Edition*, published by Lippincott Williams & Wilkins.

significant handicaps. A worldwide lack of antivenoms contributes to this neglected public health problem.

Medically significant venomous snakes are from 2 major families: the *Elapidae* and *Viperidae*. Elapids are front-fanged terrestrial snakes, including dangerous Australian snakes (taipan, brown, death adder, tiger, and black snakes); the cobras, mambas, and kraits of Asia and Africa; and the coral snakes of the Americas. Elapid venoms are highly neurotoxic with an additional cytotoxicity in some species, such as spitting cobras. Vipers, including the rattlesnakes of the Americas and vipers, have large front-folding fangs and venom that is, generally, less systemically toxic than that of the elapids, but is notable for inducing bite-site swelling and local tissue destruction.

## VENOM

Snake venoms are complex mixtures of toxic and nontoxic substances, mostly proteins, that have neurotoxic, myotoxic, procoagulant, anticoagulant, cytotoxic, and hemolytic properties. Many are metalloproteinases and phospholipases.

## DIFFERENTIAL DIAGNOSIS

The diagnosis may be unclear in young children or others unable to give a clear history (eg, those found unconscious) or bitten at night or in dense scrub where snakes may not be seen. The differential diagnoses of venomous snakebite include nonvenomous snakebite or a bite or sting by another venomous creature, stroke or head injury, neuropathy (eg, Guillain-Barré syndrome), metabolic disturbance, allergic reaction, toxin ingestion, or sepsis.

## DIAGNOSIS OF ENVENOMATION

There should be a high index of suspicion for a diagnosis of envenomation when children become suddenly unwell in areas where snakes exist, alongside a constellation of localized and generalized clinical signs that may or may not include obvious puncture marks (Table 117-1).

### Clinical Signs and Symptoms

Symptoms and signs of envenomation follow a predictable time sequence but may vary enormously according to body weight, amount of venom injected, age and state of health of the patient, time since the bite, prior bite history, and allergy status, as well as the site of the bite (Table 117-2). The effects of envenomation are specific to snake genera and species but biogeographical variation in venom within a species with some variation in clinical presentation is well known. Coagulation disturbances are common after many elapid and viper bites, although severe hemorrhage is infrequent. Myolysis is particularly prominent in envenomations from South American pit vipers, sea snakes, and Australian black snakes, whereas death adder and king cobra envenomations are specifically neurotoxic. Renal failure may result from myolysis or may be a primary effect after Russell's viper and *Bothrops* envenomations. Bite-site swelling and tissue necrosis may be severe after Asian cobra and pit viper bites and may lead to a compartment syndrome and may even require limb amputation.

**TABLE 117-1 EXPECTED SEQUENCE OF MAJOR SYSTEMIC SYMPTOMS AND SIGNS AFTER ENVENOMATION BY ELAPID SNAKE SPECIES[a]**

| |
|---|
| **< 1 h after Bite** |
| Headache |
| Nausea, vomiting, abdominal pain |
| Transient hypotension associated with confusion or loss of consciousness |
| Coagulopathy (laboratory testing or whole blood clotting time) |
| Regional lymphadenitis |
| **1–3 h after Bite** |
| Paresis/paralysis of cranial nerves (eg, ptosis, double vision, external ophthalmoplegia, dysphonia, dysphagia, myopathic facies) |
| Hemorrhage from mucosal surfaces and needle punctures secondary to disseminated intravascular coagulation (DIC) |
| Tachycardia, hypotension |
| Tachypnea, shallow tidal volume |
| **> 3 h after Bite** |
| Paresis/paralysis of truncal and limb muscles |
| Paresis/paralysis of respiratory muscles (respiratory failure) |
| Peripheral circulatory failure (shock), hypoxemia, cyanosis |
| Rhabdomyolysis |
| Dark urine (due to myoglobinuria or hemoglobin) |
| Renal failure secondary to combinations of shock, hypoxemia, DIC, rhabdomyolysis, and hemolysis |
| Coma secondary to cerebral hypoxemia or ischemia, occasionally due to hemorrhage |

[a]A more rapid illness may develop after multiple bites or in a small child.

### Investigations

A snake venom detection kit (SVDK) can be used to detect venom at either the bite site or in the urine or blood. However, this kit is only clinically applicable in Australia and Papua New Guinea. Significant morbidity can result from disseminated intravascular coagulopathy (DIC), rhabdomyolysis, primary or secondary renal impairment, and electrolyte imbalance after envenomation. Thus, routine laboratory investigations should include full coagulation and DIC studies (or, if unavailable, a 20-minute whole blood clotting test), renal function, urinalysis, and careful monitoring of electrolytes. A full blood count may reveal a mildly elevated white cell count as well as thrombocytopenia, which may occur in isolation or as part of DIC or microangiopathic hemolytic anemia. Cardiotoxicity (either primary or secondary to hyperkalemia associated with rhabdomyolysis) may also be present, and an electrocardiogram (ECG) should be performed and cardiac troponin measured if this is suspected.

## TREATMENT OF VENOMOUS SNAKEBITE

### First Aid

First aid is important prehospital and in-hospital, and all snakebites should be pre-emptively managed as potentially serious envenomations from the moment of first suspicion. While a significant number of venomous snakebites do not result in systemic envenomation because the snake injected no venom or only a small amount, the severity of envenomation cannot be predicted at the time of the bite. Since at least 95% of bites occur on the limbs and approximately 60% involve a lower limb, they are easily treated with first aid.

Some of the earlier, traditionally applied first-aid practices may have no benefit or may even be harmful. Venom may be injected quite deeply, and consequently, little venom is removed by incision or excision (cutting or sucking). These practices are not recommended, and indeed may be dangerous, particularly in the coagulopathic patient. The use of arterial tourniquet, especially for prolonged periods, may also be dangerous and is not recommended for any type of venomous bite or sting.

**Pressure-Immobilization** Pressure-immobilization first aid was developed for Australian elapid envenomation. Immobilization without pressure remains a routine first-aid recommendation for crotalid and viper bites. In the pressure-immobilization technique (Fig. 117-1), a continuous, ideally elasticized, bandage is applied, as tightly as binding a sprained ankle, to the whole limb and then a splint applied to further prevent movement. Compression of lymphatic channels and inactivation of the muscle pump delays venom reaching the circulation and buys time for the victim to reach a hospital. Compression without immobilization is ineffective. If applied correctly, pressure-immobilization first aid may be safely left in situ for several hours.

The timing of removal of a pressure-immobilization bandage is important. Once an asymptomatic patient has reached a hospital stocked with appropriate antivenom, first-aid measures may be removed. If, on removal of first aid, the patient's condition deteriorates, the bandages can be reapplied while antivenom is administered. If a patient arrives at a hospital with obvious envenomation but without pressure-immobilization, it should be applied.

**TABLE 117-2 THE CLINICAL FEATURES OF VARIOUS MEDICALLY SIGNIFICANT VENOMOUS SNAKES OF THE WORLD**

| | Clinical Features | | | | |
|---|---|---|---|---|---|
| **Region and Species** | **Neurotoxic** | **Coagulopathic** | **Local Cytotoxic** | **Myotoxic** | **Other** |
| **South America** | | | | | |
| *Bothrops* spp (lance-headed vipers) | – | ++ | ++ | + | Shock, renal failure |
| *Crotalus durissus terrificus* (pit vipers) | ++ | ++ | – | +++ | Renal failure |
| **North America** | | | | | |
| *Crotalus* spp (pit vipers) | + | ++ | ++ | + | Shock, renal failure |
| *Micrurus* spp (coral snakes) | ++ | | | ++ | |
| **Australia and Papua New Guinea** | | | | | |
| *Oxyuranus* spp (taipan) | +++ | +++ | | + | Renal failure |
| *Acanthophis* spp (death adder) | +++ | | | | |
| *Notechis* spp (tiger) | +++ | +++ | + | ++ | Renal failure |
| *Pseudechis* spp (black) | + | ++ | + | +++ | Renal failure |
| *Pseudonaja* spp (brown) | ++ | +++ | | | Renal failure |
| **Asia** | | | | | |
| *Daboia russelii* (Russell's viper) | –/+ | +++ | ++ | +++ | Shock, renal failure |
| *Naja* spp (cobras) | +++ | | +++ | | Shock |
| *Naja philippinensis* (Philippine cobra) | +++ | – | + | – | Shock |
| *Ophiophagus hannah* (king cobra) | +++ | | | | |
| *Echis carinatus* (saw-scaled viper) | – | ++ | +++ | – | Shock, renal failure |
| *Bungaris* spp (kraits) | ++ | | – | – | |
| *Calloselasma rhodostoma* (Malayan pit viper) | | +++ | +++ | | Shock, renal failure |
| **Europe** | | | | | |
| *Vipera* spp (European adders) | +/– | + | + | | Shock, renal failure |
| **Africa** | | | | | |
| *Cerastes cerastes* (Saharan horned viper) | | +++ | ++ | | Shock |
| *Echis ocellatus* (carpet viper) | | +++ | ++ | | Shock, renal failure |
| *Naja* spp (African spitting cobras) | | | +++ | | |
| *Bitis gabonica* (Gaboon viper) | + | +++ | +++ | | Cardiotoxic |
| *Bitis arietans* (puff adder) | | ++ | +++ | | Cardiotoxic |
| *Dendroaspis* spp (mambas) | +++ | | +/++ | | |
| **Indo-Pacific** | | | | | |
| Hydrophids (sea snakes) | +++ | | | ++/+++ | Renal failure |

The symbols represent subjective degrees of severity: – = little clinical effect; + = mild effect of envenomation; ++ = moderate effect; +++ = severe effect. It is an only an approximate guide, as the extent of the envenomation syndrome varies with the species or subspecies.

Data from Meier J, White J. *Clinical Toxicity of Animal Venoms and Poisons.* Boca Raton, Fla: CRC Press; 1995 Clinical Toxinology Resource Web site (http://www.toxinology.com/).

### Medical Treatment of Envenomation

The management principles are resuscitation, antivenom administration, and treatment of specific effects of venom. A careful history and examination should be undertaken with reference to the features of envenomation described above, as well as to any previous envenomations and allergies to antivenoms or to other venoms, and with reference to allergic illnesses and asthma. Samples for venom detection and for investigations should be obtained where appropriate and an attempt made to identify the genus of snake. The key question is whether or not to give antivenom, an issue that should be regularly reassessed, as envenomation is a highly dynamic situation reflecting ongoing absorption of venom (see "Choice of Antivenom," below).

If the patient has not developed any symptoms or signs of envenomation, nor any indication of coagulopathy or myolysis by 4 to 6 hours after bite or removal of first aid, then it is unlikely that significant envenomation has occurred. However, the delayed onset of symptoms, particularly relating to neurotoxicity and rhabdomyolysis, may occur up to 24 hours after the bite or removal of first aid. Particular care is required if a neurotoxic elapid bite is suspected, as few early signs may be present. Overnight observation is highly desirable, especially if the victim is a young child or comes from a remote area. Envenomated patients should ideally be admitted to a hospital and observed for a period of at least 24 hours, depending on the clinical circumstances. Frequent neurological observations should be performed and pathology studies repeated regularly to monitor progression of the illness.

### Local Effects

Viper envenomation causes local effects such as skin blistering, limb swelling, and tissue necrosis. Although progressive limb swelling is an indication for antivenom use, its effectiveness at reducing local venom effects remains controversial. The role of fasciotomy in North American crotaline (pit viper) envenomation causing limb swelling is controversial. Fasciotomy is generally considered unnecessary when crotaline antivenom has been administered but intracompartment pressures should be carefully monitored to guide surgical intervention. Local blistering may progress to full thickness skin necrosis over 3 to 7 days and is prone to infection.

### Management of Coagulopathy and Hematologic Abnormalities

Envenomation can lead to a procoagulant state and thrombotic microangiopathic renal failure (for example, with Australian elapid venoms and Russell's viper venom). In other cases, a consumptive coagulopathy and DIC-like state can result. Antivenom per se does not correct coagulopathy. After circulating venom has been neutralized, it may be 4 to 6 hours or longer before the hepatic production of intrinsic plasma clotting factors can normalize coagulation tests.

Whether to give or withhold coagulation factors—for example, in the form of fresh frozen plasma (FFP)—is a controversial question. While it does hasten the restoration of coagulation after antivenom in the treatment of Australian snake envenomation, the administration of FFP may exacerbate the effects of coagulopathy in the continued

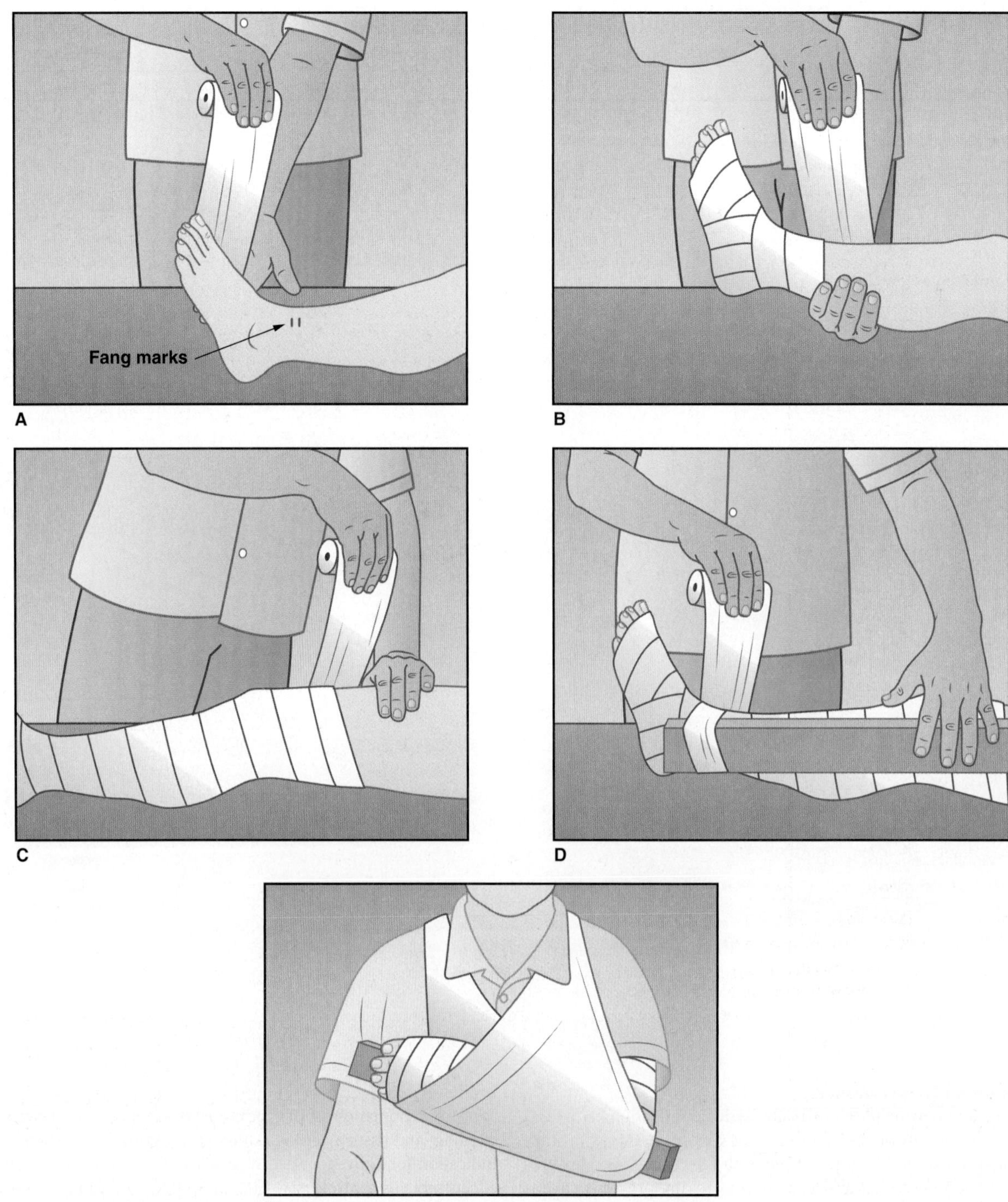


FIGURE 117-1 First-aid pressure-immobilization for elapid snakebite.

presence of venom. A lack of improvement in a victim's clotting times on retesting may represent either insufficient antivenom or insufficient time for hepatic regeneration of clotting factors, while improvement in coagulation may represent the efficacy of antivenom or natural hepatic regeneration of clotting factors. While it is reasonable to withhold FFP unless coagulation restores itself within approximately 6 hours after antivenom administration, active bleeding or the risk for this according to coagulation studies, despite adequate quantities of antivenom, is an indication for factor replacement. Whole blood transfusion is reserved for significant anemia and hypovolemia. In North America, extrapolation from other hematologic conditions suggests that coagulopathy with parameters exceeding critical thresholds (international normalized ratio [INR] > 3, activated partial thromboplastin time [aPTT] > 50 seconds, platelets < 50,000/mm$^3$, and fibrinogen < 75 mg/dL) is associated with a major bleeding risk of 1% over a few days and thus warrants coagulation factor replacement.

#### Neurotoxicity

Descending paralysis, starting with ptosis and external ophthalmoplegia and progressing to respiratory failure, are typical neurotoxic signs of envenomation. In severe cases resulting in respiratory failure, supplemental oxygen and endotracheal intubation with mechanical ventilation are indicated. If antivenom is delayed or if inadequate doses are given, recovery may take days or weeks.

#### Rhabdomyolysis and Renal Failure

Many factors, including circulatory shock, which can be, a direct toxic effect of venom, rhabdomyolysis, and coagulopathy, may contribute to the development of renal failure. Hyperkalemia secondary to rhabdomyolysis may be treated with calcium, insulin and glucose, salbutamol (albuterol), or ion-exchange resins. Hemodialysis may occasionally be required, particularly if there has been a delay in treatment with antivenom. In some cases, long-term renal morbidity may occur.

### Shock and Cardiotoxicity

The etiology of shock may vary with the snake species and includes fluid sequestration into necrotic tissue, altered vascular permeability, autopharmacological phenomena, acute reactions to venom or antivenom, and cardiotoxicity that is either direct or secondary to hypoxemia or hypotension. The procoagulant state may be associated with myocardial ischemia and pulmonary hypertension. Acute systemic hypotension associated with procoagulopathy after Australian brown snakebite may be lethal.

### Other Considerations

Spitting cobras of Asia and Africa and the South African rinkhals spray venom from their fangs into a victim's eyes, potentially causing blindness (*venom ophthalmia*) with painful chemical conjunctivitis, corneal ulceration, anterior uveitis, and possible secondary infection. The eyes should be irrigated immediately with generous volumes of water followed by other treatment, such as cycloplegics, topical antibiotics, and analgesia.

All victims should receive appropriate tetanus prophylaxis, but antibiotic prophylaxis is only routinely warranted if the bite wound is contaminated. Other treatments include analgesia (though it is advisable to avoid sedating agents such as morphine, if possible), and early intervention with mobilization, splinting, and occupational and physical therapy are recommended to prevent secondary complications associated with immobility.

### Antivenom

Presently, antivenom is the only specific clinical treatment for venomous snakebite. However, it does not immediately reverse the effects of venom and may not neutralize all effects, particularly if administration is delayed. Antivenoms are immunoglobulins or their fragments derived from plasma of animals immunized with venom. The choice of antivenom is determined by the genus or species of snake or by geographic location if unknown.

**Indications** Antivenom should not be given for a positive result from a venom detection kit or for only the presence of bite marks, unless there are signs of systemic envenomation (neurological signs, abdominal symptoms, abnormal bleeding, coagulopathy, rhabdomyolysis, hematuria, or myoglobinuria) or progressive limb swelling and/or necrosis. If pressure-immobilization first aid is in place, the symptoms or signs of envenomation, including laboratory signs, may only become rapidly apparent when this is removed.

**Choice of Antivenom** The correct choice is crucial. Antivenoms only neutralize the venoms used in their production. Generally, they provide little or no neutralization of other snake venoms. The correct antivenom should be based on unequivocal morphological identification of the snake, use of an SVDK (only available for Australia and Papua New Guinea), or on geographical location, combined with a specific clinical syndrome.

Identification of the snake aids with the selection of the appropriate antivenom and forewarns clinicians of expected effects. Formal identification by a highly experienced professional herpetologist is ideal. Sometimes, the snake is not seen, or is only glimpsed in retreat, rendering identification impossible or unreliable. In addition, especially concerning young children, a history may be vague or lacking. In all these circumstances, a contingency plan for choice of antivenom should be based on knowledge of local species. Bites by exotic snakes (ie, snakes from other countries or regions kept in zoos or private collections) are very problematic and hospitals should have contingency plans to urgently obtain an appropriate antivenom from local poison information centers.

The SVDK is a rapid 2-step enzyme immunoassay that uses antibodies to the venoms of major Australian snake genera. Venom from a bite-site swab or a blood or urine sample reacts with specific antibodies in different reaction wells, resulting in a rapid color change that indicates the snake group involved and thus helps to select the antivenom required. Bite-site swabs are the most reliable samples for use in an SVDK, provided the bite site has not been washed. Blood and urine samples are less reliable, although urine may be useful when presentation is delayed, or if the bite site cannot be identified. Although a positive SVDK test of blood or urine confirms that envenomation has occurred, it is not per se an indication to give antivenom. The information should be used in conjunction with clinical presentation, knowledge of snakes in the geographic area, and identification of snakes to determine whether to use an antivenom and, if so, which to use.



If a reliable identification of the snake cannot be made, then polyvalent antivenom or a selection of monovalent antivenoms that cover likely local species should be used. For example, in Australia, a combination of brown and tiger snake antivenoms is satisfactory for all snake envenomation in the state of Victoria, whereas tiger snake antivenom alone is satisfactory for the state of Tasmania. Elsewhere, polyvalent antivenom containing tiger, brown, black, death adder, and taipan antivenoms is required.

**Administration of Antivenom** Snake antivenoms are given intravenously and should be administered with the guidance of experts. Antivenoms should be diluted in at least 100 mL of normal saline, 5% dextrose, or Hartmann (Ringer lactate) solution. The administration and dosing of antivenoms may vary according to the severity of the envenomation rather than the size of the patient, and should be guided by regional poison experts. Initial administration should be slow, while the patient is observed for signs of allergic reaction. If no reaction is observed, the infusion may be run over 15 to 30 minutes. Acute (within minutes or hours) and delayed (days to weeks) hypersensitivity can occur with antivenom administration. If the patient reacts to the antivenom, the rate may be slowed or the infusion ceased temporarily. If the reaction is severe, treatment with epinephrine, antihistamines, corticosteroids, or plasma volume expanders should be undertaken, as required. The decision to recommence antivenom should be based on the clinical state of the patient. A prior allergy to antivenom is not an absolute contraindication to subsequent administration. In the case of the patient with a known allergy to antivenom or to horse serum, the decision to withhold antivenom should be based on the severity of envenomation and availability of resuscitation facilities and skills.



**Premedication for Antivenom** Premedication to reduce adverse reactions to antivenom is recommended. Premedication with subcutaneous (not intravenous or intramuscular) epinephrine is particularly recommended for polyvalent antivenom in a low-resource setting and for higher risk patients, such as those with equine allergy and asthma. Antihistamines are not recommended due to the ineffectiveness of promethazine in a randomized placebo-controlled trial in Brazil. Additionally, antihistamines may confound the effects of venom through their sedative and hypotensive actions.

**Serum Sickness** Serum sickness, due to the deposition of immune complexes, is a recognized complication of the administration of foreign protein solutions such as antivenoms. Symptoms include fever, rash, arthralgia, lymphadenopathy, and a flu-like illness. It usually occurs 7 to 10 days after antivenom administration. The possibility of serum sickness, and the usual symptoms and signs, should be discussed with a patient prior to discharge, so that it may be recognized and treated early. It is common after administration of Australian snake antivenoms, irrespective of volumes or type of antivenom. Accordingly, prophylactic corticosteroids should be considered in all cases (eg, prednisolone 1–2 mg/kg daily for 5 days) and especially if the patient has a past history of exposure to equine protein.

### Anticholinesterase Treatment

Anticholinesterase inhibitors such as neostigmine may assist in the emergency management of predominantly postjunctional neurotoxic envenomations, such as by the Philippine cobra and Papuan death adder, due to the curare-like actions of their neurotoxins.

## SCORPION STINGS

Of approximately 1900 known species of scorpions, about 30 cause serious and life-threatening illness. Scorpion stings are the second most frequent cause of envenomation deaths, with about 3250 deaths annually from more than 1.2 million stings (0.27%). Scorpions are nocturnally active creatures in warm or hot dry climates within 45° latitudes of the equator.

## VENOM

Scorpion venom is a complex mixture of mucopolysaccharides, hyaluronidase, serotonin, histamine, protease inhibitors, histamine releasers, and protein neurotoxins. In addition, the venom of some species contains potassium channel inhibitors, ryanodine-type calcium channel modulators, and inhibitors of the inactivation of voltage-gated sodium channels, resulting in a massive release of transmitters at sympathetic, parasympathetic, and neuromuscular receptors.

## ENVENOMATION

Distinctive syndromes of severe envenomation are caused by members of a scorpion genera in 7 principal world regions: Mexico, southern American states (Texas, Arizona, New Mexico), South America (Brazil, Venezuela, Colombia, Argentina), India, Near and Middle East, north-Saharan Africa, Sahelian Africa, and South Africa (Table 117-3).

The principal life-threatening effects are cardiovascular and neurotoxic in most species; some species may also cause coagulopathy that is usually mild, and in some (eg, *Centruroides sculpturatus*), the effects are essentially confined to neurotoxicity. A systemic inflammatory response with cytokine release, kinin release, and complement activation may lead to multiorgan failure. Mortality is variable; for example, it has been reported in 8.9% of 685 child victims in Tunisia, 1.3% of 1212 child victims in Morocco, and 12.5% of 41 child victims in Egypt.

**TABLE 117-3 GENERA, SPECIES, AND DISTRIBUTION OF DANGEROUS SCORPIONS**

| Genus | Species | Distribution |
|---|---|---|
| *Androctonus* | *aeneas* | North Africa, Saharan oases, African Sahel |
| | *australis* | North Africa, Saharan oases |
| | *crassicauda* | North Africa, Saudi Arabia, Turkey |
| | *mauretanicus* | Morocco |
| | *hoggarensis* | Saharan mountains |
| *Hottentotta* | *franzwerneri* | Morocco |
| | *tamulus* | India |
| *Buthus* | *occitanus* | East Mediterranean rim, African Sahel |
| *Leiurus* | *quinquestriatus* | Africa, Middle East |
| *Parabuthus* | *granulatus* | South Africa |
| | *transvaalicus* | South Africa, Zimbabwe |
| | *villosus* | South Africa, Namibia |
| | *liosoma* | Saudi Arabia |
| *Hemiscorpius* | *lepturus* | Iran, Iraq |
| *Mesobuthus* | *eupeus* | Turkey, Caucasus, Iran, Afghanistan |
| *Centruroides* | *sculpturatus* | Southern United States |
| | *infamatus* | Southern United States, Mexico |
| | *elegans, noxius, suffusus, limpidus* | Mexico |
| | *gracilis* | Columbia |
| *Tityus* | *pachyurus* | Columbia |
| | *trinitatis* | Trinidad |
| | *bahiensis, brazilae, discrepans, cambridgei, serrulatus, stigmurus* | Brazil |
| | *caripitensis, surorientalis, grellanoparrai* | Venezuela |
| | *trivittatus* | Argentina |

Adapted with permission from Chippaux JP, Goyffon M: Epidemiology of scorpionism: a global appraisal. *Acta Trop.* 2008 Aug;107(2):71-79.

Envenomation by Australian and European species are limited to local pain and mild systemic effects.

### Neurotoxicity

Although pain is the universal feature of envenomation, usually requiring systemic or topical analgesia (lidocaine), a wide variety of other neurological symptoms and signs constitutes species-specific syndromes. Generally, envenomation may cause coma, convulsions, cerebral edema, external ophthalmoplegia, mydriasis, meiosis, agitation, rigidity, tremor, twitching, tongue and muscle fasciculation, respiratory failure, gastric and pancreatic hypersecretion, bradycardia, tachycardia, salivation, sweating, abdominal pain, vomiting, and priapism. Some species cause lethal cardiovascular failure. Rhabdomyolysis and renal toxicity are infrequent.

### Cardiotoxicity

Acute biventricular failure occurs in 2 clinical phases due to combined catecholamine stress-induced, sudden (takotsubo-like) cardiomyopathy and direct cardiotoxicity. An early vascular phase is caused by profound vasoconstriction with increased ventricular afterload, impeded ventricular emptying, and increased ventricular filling pressures. Systemic hypertension and pulmonary edema are evident. A subsequent myocardial phase ensues due to coronary artery spasm or increase in coronary resistance, with consequent low cardiac output and systemic hypotension. Cardiac creatine kinase (CK-MB) enzymes and troponin levels are raised.

## TREATMENT

### Antivenom Therapy

The efficacy of scorpion antivenoms is variable and is related in part to the species of scorpion. Although antivenom reduces the levels of free circulating venom antigen, the clinical relevance of this is questionable. Moreover, the incidence of reactions to a specific antivenom may be significant, and therefore, its administration must be weighed against the degree of envenomation, local knowledge of species, and their effects and duration since envenomation.

### Supportive Therapy

Supportive cardiovascular therapy is necessary in severe envenomation. Intensive monitoring and titration of vasoactive agents, along with judicious mechanical ventilation, are required. In early envenomation, catecholamine release causes hypertension, but this later culminates in cardiac failure and hypotension. A titratable vasodilator is desirable at least in the hypertensive phase of the syndrome and possibly later, in conjunction with an inotropic agent. When peripheral circulatory failure and pulmonary edema are present, mechanical ventilation and infusion of dobutamine markedly improve cardiac output, systemic arterial pressure, and right ventricular ejection fraction, while decreasing pulmonary artery occlusion pressure. Extracorporeal support of cardiac output may be necessary. Hydrocortisone does not improve outcome.

# SPIDER BITE

Thousands of species of spiders exist in nearly all global environments. Consequently, spider bites are 1 of the most common problems in toxinology. Fortunately, in most cases, only transient local or radiating pain, bite-site redness, swelling, and itchiness occur. Since virtually nothing is known about the venom of the majority of spiders, the most appropriate approach to medical management is symptomatic. Few antivenoms exist. The most dangerous spiders include funnel-web spiders (*Atrax* or *Hadronyche* species), comb-footed spiders (*Latrodectus* species), *Phoneutria*, and the necrotizing species, the most important of which are the recluse or violin spiders (*Loxosceles* species). These require specific treatment.

# FUNNEL-WEB SPIDER

More than 30 species of highly dangerous funnel-web spiders inhabit the eastern seaboard of Australia. Funnel-web spiders can cause death within 2 hours. Fortunately, severe envenomation is uncommon and no fatalities have occurred since the introduction of an antivenom in 1980. Identification of funnel-webs may be difficult because some resemble less dangerous trapdoor spiders. Any dark-colored or brown spider with a body length of 2 to 3 cm on the eastern seaboard of Australia should be regarded as a funnel-web. Capture and formal identification of the spider is helpful.

### VENOM

While the venoms have many components, the key polypeptide neurotoxins of around 42 amino acids are the γ-atracotoxins (γ-ACTXs), which act by slowing sodium current inactivation. These toxins cause spontaneous repetitive generation of action potentials, triggering the release of excessive catecholamines and eventual exhaustion of predominantly sympathetic neurotransmitters and leading to a characteristic biphasic clinical syndrome. Acetylcholine is also released at neuromuscular junctions and in the autonomic nervous system.

### ENVENOMATION

#### Local Effects

Funnel-web spider bites are painful—lasting for days to weeks because of direct trauma and acidity—and accompanied by local swelling and erythema. Although most bites by funnel-web spiders are confined to local effects, a severe systemic syndrome may ensue.

#### Systemic Effects

The cardiovascular effects are due to catecholamine excess and direct cardiac toxicity. The latter may not be reversed with antivenom. The syndrome of envenomation occurs in 2 phases:

- Phase 1 is characterized by perioral numbness; nausea and vomiting; gastric dilation; sweating, salivation, and lacrimation; and dyspnea, hypertension, and local and generalized muscle fasciculation or spasm.
- Phase 2 is characterized by hypotension, hypoventilation and apnoea, acute pulmonary edema, coma, and eventually irreversible cardiac arrest.

### TREATMENT

Treatment should include appropriate respiratory and circulatory support, as well prompt application of a pressure-immobilization bandage to the affected limb, as for neurotoxic elapid snakebite. The bandage should only be removed when appropriate resuscitation can be given and antivenom is available. If available, antivenom should be given. If antivenom is not available, the pressure-immobilization bandage should be kept in place, because venom may be inactivated at the bite site. Specific additional therapies include atropine for excessive salivation and bronchorrhea, as well as muscle relaxants for muscle fasciculation and spasm. Asymptomatic patients may be discharged 4 hours after a bite or removal of first aid. Antitetanus status should be updated. Follow-up is needed for potential secondary infection.

## COMB-FOOTED (WIDOW) SPIDERS

Comb-footed spiders of the family Theridiidae exist worldwide. The *Latrodectus* genus, including the widow, button, koppie, and redback spiders, are the most important causes of spider bites, but mortality is rare. Antivenoms are available. In Australia, more redback spider (*L hasselti*) antivenom is used than any other antivenom.

### VENOM

The exact mechanism(s) by which the toxins of *Lactrodectus* spiders exert their clinical effects are poorly understood, as is the precise cause of rare fatalities. The key toxin, α-latrotoxin, forms calcium-permeable pores in presynaptic membranes and stimulates the release of catecholamines from sympathetic nerves and acetycholine from motor nerve endings.

### ENVENOMATION

Bites by *Lactrodectus* spiders produce a recognizable syndrome called *latrodectism* that may necessitate antivenom. The untreated syndrome may persist for weeks or months. The bite is usually, although not always, painful. Visible puncture marks and local swelling are uncommon. The onset of symptoms and signs is highly variable, but progression is generally slow. Effects may persist for weeks or even months after an untreated bite. Signs and symptoms include local pain, swelling and lymphadenopathy, and local or generalized sweating. Systemic features include rash, fever, myalgia, neck spasm, migratory arthralgia, hypertension, tachycardia, nausea and vomiting, abdominal pain, headache, lethargy, and insomnia. Rare but lethal complications include myocarditis, rhabdomyolysis, and paralysis.

### TREATMENT

Indications for antivenom include pain unrelieved by simple analgesia (eg, local application of ice or oral analgesics) and/or systemic symptoms or signs of envenomation such as vomiting, severe headache, abdominal pain and collapse, hypertension, arthralgia, or myalgia. When the clinical findings are atypical but the history is suggestive, a trial of antivenom may be helpful both diagnostically and therapeutically. Typically, antivenom is effective within the first 2 hours, but symptoms can reappear necessitating a further dose. Unlike most other antivenoms, the administration of widow or redback spider antivenom may be effective even several weeks after a bite. In general, premedication for acute hypersensitivity or steroids for delayed hypersensitivity are not recommended unless there is a history of horse allergy or prior exposure to equine immunoglobulin, which may predispose to acute or delayed allergic reactions.

## BEE, WASP, AND ANT (HYMENOPTERA) STINGS

Most stings by Hymenoptera (bees, wasps, and ants) are mild and self-limiting. However, a life-threatening immediate hypersensitivity reaction (anaphylaxis) may occur for which the same treatment protocol should be adopted regardless of the responsible creature. In Australia, annual deaths from anaphylactic reactions to insect stings are approximately 0.1 per million population, approximately equal to snakebite deaths. By contrast, in the United States, annual deaths from Hymenoptera stings are 0.26 per million, which is 7 to 8 times more frequent than snakebite deaths.

The location of a single sting may cause a significant problem. For example, a pharyngeal sting may obstruct the airway, while a corneal sting may threaten vision. Multiple stings may also cause massive envenomation.

### BEE STINGS

Within the superfamily Apoidea, subfamilies include the social bumble bees (Bombinae) and honey bees (Apinae). The common honeybee (*Apis mellifera ligustica*) is well established throughout the world and is an important cause of Hymenopteran stings. It does not tend to attack in a swarm, unlike the aggressive Africanized honey bee (*Apis mellifera scutellata*) that is responsible for mass envenomations in the Americas. Cases of massive bee envenomation (venom toxicity) are rare outside of those areas where the Africanized strain is endemic. While the majority of bee stings are trivial, rapid death may follow either mass stings or from anaphylactic reactions in hypersensitive individuals (even after a single sting). Most bee sting–related deaths occur in outdoor workers, especially farmers, truck drivers, and beekeepers (and their families, including children).

### WASP STINGS

The majority of social wasps belong to 1 of the 2 subfamilies of Vespidae: Vespinae and Polistinae. The subfamily Vespinae includes 4 genera: *Dolichovespula* (yellow jackets), *Vespula* (common social wasps), *Vespa* (hornets, large potentially very dangerous wasps that inject more toxic venom, in larger quantities, than bees and smaller wasps), and *Provespa*. The subfamily Polistinae includes some species of the paper wasps of the genus *Polistes*. Vespinae are found in Eurasia, North America, and North Africa. The United States has 17 native species of yellow jackets, the exotic European hornet (*Vespa crabro*), and the European wasp (*Vespula germanica*). *Vespula* yellow jackets have spread and become well established in non-native regions such as Australia, New Zealand, South America, and South Africa. In northern Australia, serious wasp stings are generally due to native paper wasps. In Asia, deaths frequently occur in children and young adults from stings of Oriental and tropical *Vespa* wasps. Like bees, wasps are colony insects that construct large nests, often among the lower tree branches where they can be accidentally disturbed, provoking an aggressive swarm attack.

## ANT STINGS

Ants (family Formicidae) are widespread, with approximately 8800 species worldwide. Relatively few species are medically important and these can be divided into 2 major groups, distinguished by the development of a venom injection apparatus. The first group gives an irritating bite, which is then sprayed with secretions from their abdominal glands. The second group causes painful true stings, injecting allergenic venom. These are typified by the jumper ants (*Myrmecia* species) in Australia and the fire ants (*Solenopsis* species) in the Americas. Other groups also cause occasional allergic reactions.

The red fire ant, *S invicta*, is of particular clinical significance. It forms super-colonies and is an aggressive, territorial species that swarms onto an intruder. Stings are multiple, usually in the tens or hundreds. Approximately one-quarter of patients stung will develop some degree of allergy. Numerous fatalities, but rarely among children, have occurred in the United States, where fire ants have become widespread since their introduction in the 1930s. They also now are established in Australia. Fire ant venom contains alkaloids known as piperidines, which produce a very painful burning sensation and cause a characteristic urticarious pustule at the sting site. Jumper ants inject enzymes, pharmacologically active substances, and allergenic proteins.



## VENOMS

A typical wasp sting contains 2 to 20 μg of venom, which consists of active amines (serotonin, histamine, tyramine, catecholamines); histamine-releasing peptides or mastoparans; wasp kinins, which are pain-inducing molecules; and antigen 5 (the most active allergen). In addition, venoms contain several enzymes, including phospholipases, hyaluronidases, and cholinesterases that also contribute to the allergic response. The venom of some wasp species contain neurotoxins and acetylcholine. The potency of the venom varies greatly among species. Hornets have potent venom that can deliver lethal doses in as few as 50 to 200 stings. Social wasps have less potent venom and deliver smaller quantities.

In contrast, a single bee sting typically contains about 50 μg of venom consisting of enzymes, small proteins, and peptides and amines. Melittin, which hydrolyzes cell membranes, changing cell permeability and inducing pain, is the primary component of bee venom, making up 50% of the venom. Phospholipase $A_2$, a major allergen that also causes pain and hemolysis, is another component of bee venom. Additional components are hyaluronidase (a "spreading factor" that allows venom components to permeate tissue), amines (histamine, dopamine, norepinephrine), and peptide 401 (a mast cell degranulating peptide that triggers the inflammatory cascade). An estimated 500 to 1500 bee stings would deliver a lethal dose. Africanized honeybees deliver slightly less (but equally toxic) venom than European honeybees. Deaths due to venom toxicity have occurred within 4 hours but may be delayed until 7 to 9 days after stinging.

## ENVENOMATION BY BEE, WASP, AND ANT STINGS

Simple bee, wasp, and ant stings in nonallergic individuals produce immediate burning pain, redness, and swelling at the sting site. Pain usually subsides over some hours, while redness and swelling resolve more slowly. With multiple stings, the effects are dramatically amplified, and systemic effects include headache, vomiting, thirst, pain, edema, discolored urine (hematuria and/or myoglobinuria), jaundice, and confusion. Rhabdomyolysis, intravascular hemolysis, coagulopathy, thrombocytopenia, metabolic disturbances, encephalopathy, liver dysfunction, and myocardial damage have also been reported. The inflammatory response may precipitate an acute coronary syndrome. Deaths from venom toxicity have been recorded in many countries, generally when there are more than 200, and usually approximately 500, bee stings but may also occur after as few as 25 to 30 wasp or hornet stings. Hospitalization is mandatory for victims receiving more than 10 stings. It is important to remember that children are at greater risk of toxicity due to the higher dose of venom per unit of body mass.

### Systemic Allergy

Children with hypersensitivity to bee, wasp, or ant stings may develop rapid catastrophic anaphylaxis, causing death within minutes. Severe systemic reactions are less common in children than adults but the risk of recurrence persists for decades.

### Large Local Reactions

In some patients, venom allergy may cause large local reactions. These may involve the swelling of the whole limb within 24 hours.

## TREATMENT FOR BEE, WASP, AND ANT STINGS

### Simple Stings

The stinger should be removed as soon as possible (by any effective method) to limit the amount of venom injected. The majority of single bee stings do not require treatment, although cold packs and oral analgesia are valuable. Wasps and ants do not leave their stinger behind; therefore, each individual insect may sting multiple times.

### Large Local Reactions

Large local reactions usually respond well to symptomatic treatment with nonsteroidal anti-inflammatory agents and topical steroid creams. Oral steroids and antihistamines are often used.

### Anaphylaxis

Treatment is based on administration of epinephrine (adrenaline) as definitive therapy supported by oxygen, β-agonists for bronchoconstriction, steroids, and intravenous fluid for hypotension. Individuals at risk of anaphylaxis from insect stings must carry and be taught to use autoinjectable intramuscular epinephrine available in numerous proprietary preparations. Most mortalities occur in victims with a known insect sting allergy. Patients with a history of anaphylaxis to bee or wasp venom and a positive skin test should also have maintenance immunotherapy (injection of small quantities of pure bee or wasp venom) for at least 3 to 5 years.

### Multiple Stings

Patients with serious systemic effects may require resuscitation with circulatory support. In particular, renal function should be closely monitored, and in some cases, hemofiltration or long-term hemodialysis is necessary. As for other etiologies, tetanus status should be checked. In cases of multiple wasp stings, septicemia should be anticipated and antibiotic prophylaxis considered.

# JELLYFISH STINGS

All 4 classes of the phylum Cnidaria (Hydrozoa, Scyphozoa, Cubozoa, Anthozoa) have nematocysts (stinging cells) and cause human envenomation. Three of the classes are described as jellyfish because of their gelatinous free-floating medusal life-cycle stage. Of these, Scyphozoa are true jellyfish, Cubozoa are box jellyfish, and Hydrozoa are hydroids. Large chirodropid (multi-tentacled) cubozoan jellyfish have killed or seriously injured numerous victims, while small carybdeid (single-tentacled) cubozoan jellyfish and some species of hydroids have caused occasional deaths.

## CHIRODROPIDS

These large jellyfish have a box-shaped white or translucent bell, 20 cm by 30 cm weighing more than 6 kg, from whose 4 corners arise bundles of up to 15 translucent, extensile tentacles. The most prominent, or notorious, is *Chironex fleckeri* (Australian box jellyfish), which inhabits the waters of northern Australia and the Indo-Pacific region, including Vietnam, the Philippines, Malaysia, Thailand, and likely Indonesia. It has caused approximately 80 deaths in Australia.

The tentacles of mature specimens stretch 3 meters. The wide, ribbon-like tentacles are covered with millions of nematocysts, which discharge toxins via a penetrating everting thread or tube upon contact, much like a spring-loaded syringe. The threads have denticles that enable them to drill 1 mm into the dermis of human skin. As the tube everts and penetrates the skin, it releases venom directly into any transfixed capillaries, thus ensuring rapid toxicity.

### VENOM

Toxic components of *C fleckeri* venom include hemolysins (causing hyperkalemia), dermatonecrotic factors, and protein components with probable direct cardiotoxicty as the result of membrane pore formation (porination).

### ENVENOMATION

*C fleckeri* are rarely noticed by a victim before contact with tentacles, usually while wading or swimming in shallow water. The tentacles are easily torn from the jellyfish by the encounter and, in adhering to the victim's skin, resemble earthworms of a pink, gray, or bluish hue. During the first 15 minutes, pain increases in mounting waves, despite removal of the tentacles. The victim may scream and become irrational. The lesions are distinctive and resemble marks made by a whip 8 to 10 mm wide, on which is a frosted ladder pattern that matches the bands of nematocysts on the tentacles. Whealing is prompt and massive. Edema, erythema, and vesiculation soon follow, and when these subside (after approximately 10 days), patches of full-thickness necrosis leave permanent scars. The severity of injury is related to size of the jellyfish and the extent of tentacle contact. Most stings are quite minor. The mechanism of death in humans is not known with certainty but case reports suggest a consequence of combined cardiovascular and respiratory failure.

### ANTIVENOM

*C fleckeri* antivenom is the only jellyfish antivenom manufactured worldwide. It is concentrated immunoglobulin derived from the serum of sheep injected with *C fleckeri* venom. Each vial contains sufficient activity to neutralize 20,000 intravenous $LD_{50}$ mouse doses. Antivenom is used in about 10% of envenomations.

### TREATMENT OF ENVENOMATION

The severity and rapidity of envenomation necessitate decisive action:

- Immediate first aid involves retrieval of victim from the water to avoid further contact with the creature(s) and to prevent drowning, basic life support, and inactivation of undischarged nematocysts by pouring vinegar (4–6% acetic acid) over adhering tentacles to prevent further envenomation. (Alcohol in any form, which discharges nematocysts, must not be used this purpose.)
- Advanced cardiopulmonary resuscitation should be performed on the beach, during transportation, and at the hospital, where extracorporeal life support and treatment for hyperkalemia may be required.
- Administer antivenom (3 vials of 17% ovine whole Ig).

#### Indications for Antivenom

Antivenom should be administered as soon as possible in the following circumstances:

- unconsciousness, cardiorespiratory arrest, hypotension, dysrhythmia, hypoventilation, difficulty swallowing, or speaking;
- severe pain (parenteral analgesia is also usually required), and
- possibility of significant skin scarring.

The initial dose is 3 vials infused intravenously, diluted 1 in 10 with a crystalloid solution.



### LABORATORY DIAGNOSIS

The simplest and quickest way to confirm *C fleckeri* envenomation is to identify characteristic nematocysts on microscopic examination of a piece of ordinary transparent sticky tape approximately 4 to 8 cm long that has been applied to the sting site. The tape is applied to a lesion, stroked several times, removed, and with its sticky side up, affixed onto a glass slide. Microscopic examination of skin scrapings is an alternative. Nematocysts of *C fleckeri* and *Chiropsella bronzie* are difficult to distinguish.

### PREVENTION

Swimming and wading should be restricted to the safe months of the year and to beaches enclosed by jellyfish-resistant nets ("stinger enclosures"). Protective "stinger suits" offer additional protection for swimmers.

## CARYBDEIDS

Carybdeids are also box jellyfish: The bell is cubic but small, and from each of the 4 corners arises an arm (pedalium), usually bearing only a single tentacle. About 25 species exist in tropical Australian, Indo-Pacific, and Caribbean waters.

### IRUKANDJI SYNDROME

Numerous small Carybdeid jellyfish cause a distinct syndrome that was initially observed in northern Australian waters but is now recognized worldwide. The syndrome was initially attributed to the sting of a near invisible jellyfish called *Carukia barnesi.* Its squarish bell is barely 12 mm wide with 4 tentacles up to 35 cm. Irukandji syndrome, attributed to other carybdeids, has been reported from many other regions including the Pacific Islands, Papua New Guinea, Hawaii, Fiji, Japan, China, Qatar, Thailand, Malaysia, and the Caribbean.



### VENOM AND ENVENOMATION CAUSING IRUKANDJI SYNDROME

*C barnesi* venom contains a potent neuronal sodium channel modulator that releases high levels of catecholamines, causing tachycardia, increased cardiac output, and systemic and pulmonary hypertension. This hyperadrenergic state may explain some clinical features of *Irukandji syndrome.* The victim rarely sees the offending jellyfish but is often aware of a slight sting to the upper body. Although the sting may be unnoticed, the onset of symptoms forces the victim to leave the water. The sting is merely an oval area of barely perceptible erythema measuring about 5 cm by 7 cm. Irregularly spaced papules ("goose pimples") up to 2 mm in diameter develop within 20 minutes and then fade but erythema may last several days.

From 5 minutes to 2 hours after the sting, but usually after about 30 minutes, a distinctive severe syndrome develops. Severe low back pain, cramping muscle pains, nausea, vomiting, profuse sweating, headache, restlessness, and agitation almost invariably occur, sometimes with hypertension. Abdominal pain is associated with spasm of the muscles of the abdominal wall, and cramps occur in limb muscles. Occasionally, cerebral edema causes loss of consciousness and acute cardiac failure occurs and manifests as pulmonary edema, poor contractility, low cardiac output, and raised cardiac enzymes. The onset of pulmonary edema is delayed, occurring after several to many hours. The mechanism of cardiac failure is probably secondary to hypertension and direct myocardial depression. Although hypertension may have been brief, it may cause an acute "stress" cardiomyopathy (Takotsubo cardiomyopathy) secondary to catecholamine release. Additionally, toxins may cause membrane poration with disruption of membrane function and accompanying rises in serum troponin levels.

Most stings do not cause serious illness but 2 fatalities have been attributed to unseen jellyfish causing Irukandji syndrome in northern Australia. In both, intracerebral hemorrhage was associated with severe hypertension.

### TREATMENT

Pain relief is important. Repeated doses of intravenous or intramuscular opiates may be required, with care not to cause hypotension. Among victims of Irukandji syndrome, intravenous magnesium salts provide pain relief and a reduction in blood pressure. Otherwise, treatment is oxygen, diuretics, vasodilators, inotropic support, and mechanical respiratory support. Antihypertensive therapy may be required initially. Although infusions of phentolamine have been used successively, a more titratable nitrate infusion would be preferable.

## OTHER JELLYFISH

*Carybdea rastoni* is a small jellyfish often found in swarms, with a very wide distribution in the western Pacific Ocean and most Australian and Japanese waters. The bell is approximately 2 to 3 cm in diameter and its tentacles trail 30 cm. Its purified protein toxins cause vasoconstriction (perhaps by release of catecholamines), release of prostaglandins, and contraction of smooth muscle. Tentacles bear ovoid nematocysts. Stings cause immediate pain with 4 linear lesions 10 to 20 cm in length and may blister. No specific management exists.

*Alatina alata*, or the Hawaiian box jellyfish, has a bell approximately 8 cm high and 5 cm wide and tentacles about 0.5 m long. Stinging causes moderate pain and may cause Irukandji syndrome. Immersion of the sting in hot water is analgesic. The venom causes poration of red cells and release of potassium with cardiovascular collapse.

*Physalia physalis* and *Physalia utriculus* (Portuguese Man-of-War, Blue Bottle) are found in all hot and temperate waters. They are easily identifiable jellyfish and are the most frequent cause of significantly painful jellyfish stings. Most stings are minor, and immersion of a stung limb in hot water provides pain relief. The main lethal toxin, physalitoxin, is a glycoprotein that causes cardiorespiratory collapse, and no antivenom exists. Three deaths have been attributed to the Atlantic *P physalis* on the southeast coast of the United States but no fatalities have been attributed to the Pacific *P utriculus* in Australia. In the few deaths that have been reported worldwide, victims were in cardiac arrest within minutes of contact with the tentacles.

## FISH STINGS

Numerous fish have dorsal or pectoral spines that may inflict a traumatic wound made worse by deposition of venom.

## STONEFISH

Species of the stonefish genus *Synanceia* are found throughout the whole Indo-Pacific region, including the north of Australia. Stonefish may easily be mistaken for a piece of rock or dead coral encrusted with marine growth. The venom apparatus is purely defensive, and plays no role in the capture of prey. Stonefish have 13 dorsal spines, each of which carries 2 basal venom glands. When disturbed, the spines become erect. When trodden upon, venom is forced out the tips of the spines into the victim's foot.

### VENOM

Venoms of all 3 species (*S verrucosa*, *S horrida*, and *S trachynis*) depress the cardiovascular and neuromuscular systems and have a direct effect on muscle. Less dangerous effects are hemolysis, an increase in vascular permeability, and effects due to a host of enzymes, including hyaluronidase. Experimentally, venom injected intravenously causes hypotension, respiratory distress and paralysis by direct myotoxicity. Various protein toxins have been isolated and been determined to be cytotoxins, to release acetylcholine and other transmitters, to cause myolysis, and to cause cardiovascular collapse by negative inotropic actions and vasodilation.

### ENVENOMATION

Stings are extremely painful, which causes the victim to become irrational. The severity of the signs and symptoms is usually in direct proportion to the depth of penetration of the spine(s) and the number of spines involved. As well as local swelling and pain, muscle weakness and paralysis may develop in the affected limb, and shock may occur. Fatalities have occurred in Indo-Pacific regions, and a single death has been reported in Australia.

### ANTIVENOM

Stonefish antivenom, an equine $Fab'_2$ preparation, neutralizes the venoms of *S trachynis*, *S verrucosa*, and *S horrida*. Vials contain approximately 2 mL, which will neutralize 20 mg of venom in vitro.

### TREATMENT

The initial priority is pain relief. Relief in minor cases may be achieved by bathing or immersing the sting with warm to hot water. In severe cases, pain relief may only be obtained by the combined use of antivenom and opiate drugs. A local anaesthetic may be injected into the track of the sting and the surrounding area, but regional nerve block should be considered.

Antivenom, usually given intramuscularly (not in the region of the sting), is recommended for all cases, except those involving only a single puncture wound with only moderate discomfort. The initial dose of antivenom is determined by the number of spines and depth of penetration. One vial (2000 units of antivenom in 2 mL) is sufficient for every 1 to 2 spine punctures. In very severe cases, 3 or more vials may be required and the use of the intravenous route should be considered, particularly if the pain is widespread or the patient is in circulatory shock. Stonefish stings require fastidious wound toilet, regional analgesia, and appropriate antibiotics. Delayed presentation and suboptimal care may be associated with poor wound healing and problematic infection.

The injured limb should be comfortably immobilized. Administration of an antibiotic (eg, trimethoprim-sulfamethoxazole, third-generation cephalosporins, imipenem) that is active against pathogens found in salt or brackish water (*Vibrio* spp, *Aeromonas* spp, *Plesiomonas* spp) is recommended. Tetanus prophylaxis should be updated. Severe injuries may require early surgical debridement of dead tissue and drainage. Skin grafting may be necessary when antivenom has been delayed and when considerable ulceration exists. Sometimes a sting remains painful for months, or recurrent inflammation or discharge occurs. This is usually due to an embedded spine fragment, which is semitransparent and may be deeply embedded, and therefore, may be undetectable except by ultrasound examination and subsequent surgical exploration.

## OTHER STINGING FISH

Numerous other fish with stinging spines of the families Scorpaenidae (scorpionfish), Synanceiidae, and Trachinidae exist in the world's oceans and fresh waters. The mechanical penetration or laceration by their spines is painful and many also envenomate. Examples are the butterfly cod or lionfish (*Pterois volitans*), waspfish (*Apistops caloundra*), scorpion cod (*Scorpaena cardinalis*), South Australian cobbler (*Gymnapistes marmoratus*), fortescue (*Centropogon australis*), bullrout (*Notesthes robusta*), gurnard perch (*Neosebastes pandus*), goblinfish (*Glyptauchen panduratus*), ghoul (*Inimicus caledonicus*), and numerous catfish, weeverfish, rabbitfish, and spinefeet (*Siganus lineatus* and *S spinus*). Many envenomations occur among amateur collectors of *Pterois volitans*.

### TREATMENT

Little is known about the nature of the venoms associated with the dorsal spines of the many stinging fish. There are no specific antivenoms for these, except for the possibility of using stonefish antivenom for lionfish and other closely related Scorpaenidae based on analogous venom pharmacology. Otherwise, the management of a wound is the same as for stonefish.

## STINGRAYS

Stingrays have barbed tails that may inflict serious leg, abdominal, or chest wounds. Direct damage by penetration of the stinging barb is usually of greater importance than the introduction of the venom or a marine pathogen. A swimmer cruising the ocean floor is at risk of a serious chest wound when disturbing settled rays, as is the occupant of an open small boat when a ray leaps from the water surface.

Significant wounds require exploratory surgery because the wound track may contain a trail of glandular and integumentary sheath material as well as necrotic tissue. Penetrating wounds to the chest or abdomen, even when apparently minor, should be imaged or explored, because of likely damage to internal organs. Tetanus prophylaxis should be updated. The introduction of marine bacterial infection is possible after penetrating injury.

### SUGGESTED READINGS


Abroug F, Ouanes-Besbes L, Ouanes I, et al. Meta-analysis of controlled studies on immunotherapy in severe scorpion envenomation. *Emerg Med J*. 2011;28(11):963-969.

Abroug F, Souheil E, Ouanes I, Dachraoui F, Fekih-Hassen M, Ouanes Besbes L. Scorpion-related cardiomyopathy: clinical characteristics, pathophysiology, and treatment. *Clin Toxicol (Phila)*. 2015;53(6):511-518.

Aksel G, Guler S, Dogan NO, Corbacioglu SK. A randomized trial comparing intravenous paracetamol, topical lidocaine, and ice application for treatment of pain associated with scorpion stings. *Hum Exp Toxicol*. 2015;34(6):662-667.

Bush SP, Ruha AM, Seifert SA, et al. Comparison of F(ab')2 versus Fab antivenom for pit viper envenomation: a prospective, blinded, multicenter, randomized clinical trial. *Clin Toxicol (Phila)*. 2015;53(1):37-45.

Dart RC, Bogdan G, Heard K, et al. A randomized, double-blind, placebo-controlled trial of a highly purified equine F(ab)2 antibody black widow spider antivenom. *Ann Emerg Med*. 2013;61(4):458-467.

Gershwin LA, Richardson AJ, Winkel KD, et al. Biology and ecology of Irukandji jellyfish (Cnidaria: Cubozoa). *Adv Mar Biol*. 2013;66:1-85.

Habib AG. Effect of pre-medication on early adverse reactions following antivenom use in snakebite: a systematic review and meta-analysis. *Drug Saf*. 2011;34(10):869-880.

Isbister GK, Buckley NA, Page CB, et al. A randomized controlled trial of fresh frozen plasma for treating venom-induced consumption coagulopathy in cases of Australian snakebite (ASP-18). *J Thromb Haemost*. 2013;11(7):1310-1318.

Isbister GK, Maduwage K, Scorgie FE, et al. Venom concentrations and clotting factor levels in a prospective cohort of Russell's viper bites with coagulopathy. *PLoS Negl Trop Dis*. 2015;9(8):e0003968.

Isbister GK, Page CB, Buckley NA, et al. Randomized controlled trial of intravenous antivenom versus placebo for latrodectism: the second Redback Antivenom Evaluation (RAVE-II) study. *Ann Emerg Med*. 2014;64(6):620-628.

León G, Herrera M, Segura Á, Villalta M, Vargas M, Gutierrez JM. Pathogenic mechanisms underlying adverse reactions induced by intravenous administration of snake antivenoms. *Toxicon*. 2013;76:63-76.

Miller M, O'Leary MA, Isbister GK. Towards rationalisation of antivenom use in funnel-web spider envenoming: enzyme immunoassays for venom concentrations. *Clin Toxicol (Phila)*. 2016;54(3):245-251.

Ryan NM, Kearney RT, Brown SG, Isbister GK. Incidence of serum sickness after the administration of Australian snake antivenom (ASP-22). *Clin Toxicol (Phila)*. 2016;54(1):27-33.

Sutherland SK, Coulter AR, Harris RD. Rationalisation of first-aid measures for elapid snakebite. *Lancet*. 1979;1(8109):183-185.

Wilcox CL, Yanagihara AA. Heated debates: Hot-water immersion or ice packs as first aid for cnidarian envenomations? *Toxins (Basel)*. 2016;8(4):97.




# 118 Acute Upper Airway Obstruction

Thuy L. Ngo and M. Douglas Baker

## INTRODUCTION

Acute upper airway obstruction is a common pediatric problem caused by a variety of disorders (Table 118-1). The degree of severity of obstruction is variable, depending upon the underlying problem and the size of the airway.

Acute respiratory failure involving the upper airways can be a life-threatening emergency that requires emergent action. Failure to rapidly assess and properly manage acute upper airway obstruction may lead to cardiopulmonary arrest in pediatric patients, who have less pulmonary reserve compared to adults. In this chapter, we will review pediatric upper airway anatomy and discuss the causes, presentation, evaluation, and management of acute upper airway obstruction.

## PEDIATRIC AIRWAY CONSIDERATIONS

Compared to adults, pediatric patients have a larger occiput, larger tongue, shorter mandible, and prominent adenoids and tonsils (Fig. 118-1). These differences combine with a relatively smaller airway, lower functional residual capacity, higher peripheral airway resistance, and higher oxygen consumption to put infants and young children at higher risk for decompensation from an upper airway obstruction.

During inspiration, loose supraglottic tissues collapse inward due to negative inspiratory pressures and then freely enlarge on expiration. This yields characteristic inspiratory stridor in children with supraglottic disorders such as laryngomalacia and supraglottic stenosis. By comparison, the subglottic region is completely encircled by the cricoid cartilage, giving it a fixed size essentially unaffected by airway pressure. Thus, disorders in the subglottic region resulting in

**TABLE 118-1 DIFFERENTIAL DIAGNOSIS OF UPPER AIRWAY OBSTRUCTION**

| |
|---|
| **Supraglottic Disorders** |
| Anatomic abnormalities |
| Angioedema |
| Cervical adenitis |
| Foreign body impaction |
| Peritonsillar abscess |
| Retropharyngeal abscess |
| Epiglottitis |
| Tonsillar/adenoidal enlargement |
| Trauma (mechanical/chemical) |
| **Subglottic Disorders** |
| Anatomic abnormalities |
| Angioedema |
| Bacterial tracheitis |
| Croup |
| Diphtheria |
| Foreign body aspiration |
| Trauma (mechanical/chemical) |
| **Central Nervous System Disorders** |
| Loss of airway protective mechanism |

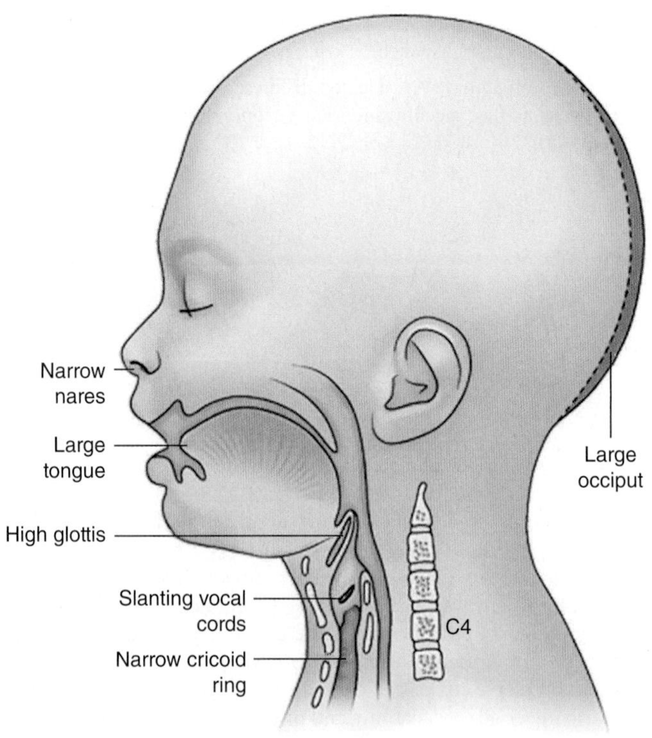


**FIGURE 118-1** Anatomical differences in pediatric airways.

decreased lumen size typically produce biphasic stridor, as seen in croup or foreign body aspiration.

# INFECTION

## CROUP

### ETIOLOGY

*Laryngotracheobronchitis*, commonly known as croup, is a viral infection resulting in inflammation of the glottis and subglottis. This inflammation or edema produces a characteristic barking cough. Croup is both the most common cause of stridor and infectious cause of upper airway obstruction, affecting up to 5% of all children. The vast majority of cases occur between 6 months and 3 years of age, although croup can afflict older children. Croup has been associated with a number of different viruses, many of which are given in Table 118-2.

### CLINICAL PRESENTATION

The clinical presentation of croup may vary. Generally, the illness begins with a prodrome of nasal congestion and rhinorrhea, similar to other viral upper respiratory infections (URI). Fever usually occurs during the first 24 hours of illness. Within 12 to 48 hours, signs and symptoms of upper airway obstruction such as inspiratory stridor and the classic "barking seal" cough develop, with hoarseness appearing later. The illness may last 3 to 14 days, depending on the severity of the case.

Spasmodic croup typically affects children between 3 months and 3 years of age who are afebrile and previously well or had mild URI symptoms. This disorder usually has nighttime onset and is a noninfectious variant of croup. Affected children awake with sudden dyspnea, barking cough, and inspiratory stridor. Symptoms rapidly resolve, yet recurrence is common. Both allergens and gastroesophageal reflux have been implicated as potential etiologies.

### DIAGNOSIS

*Croup* is a clinical diagnosis based on the presence of a barking cough, stridor, and preceding viral URI. Laboratory assessment is typically not indicated. Radiographic examination of the soft tissues of the neck may assist in distinguishing between other causes of upper airway obstruction. In croup, the anteroposterior radiograph will show both subglottic narrowing and progressive tracheal narrowing as it reaches the subglottis. This is referred to as the "steeple sign," and is due to mucosal edema below the vocal cords (Fig. 118-2).

### MANAGEMENT

Croup is often a mild and self-limiting illness. Mild cases typically present with the barking cough, hoarseness, and stridor, only when agitated. One dose of oral corticosteroids, such as dexamethasone, and humidified air are recommended for these cases. However, there is some evidence to suggest that higher humidity air offers no benefit over lower humidity air. More severe cases may present with biphasic stridor, agitation, and increased work of breathing, even at rest. In

**TABLE 118-2 INFECTIOUS AGENTS CAUSING CROUP**

| Etiologic Agents | Frequency | Severity of Symptoms |
|---|---|---|
| Parainfluenza (1, 2, 3) | ++++ | + to +++ |
| Influenza (A + B) | ++ | + to ++++ |
| Respiratory syncytial virus | ++ | + to ++ |
| Adenovirus (1–3, 5–7) | ++ | + to ++ |
| Rhinovirus | + | + |
| Mycoplasma | + | + |
| Coxsackie (A9, B4, 5) | + | + |
| Enteric cytopathic human orphan (ECHO) virus (4, 11, 21) | + | + |
| Herpes simplex virus | + | + |
| Reovirus | + | + |

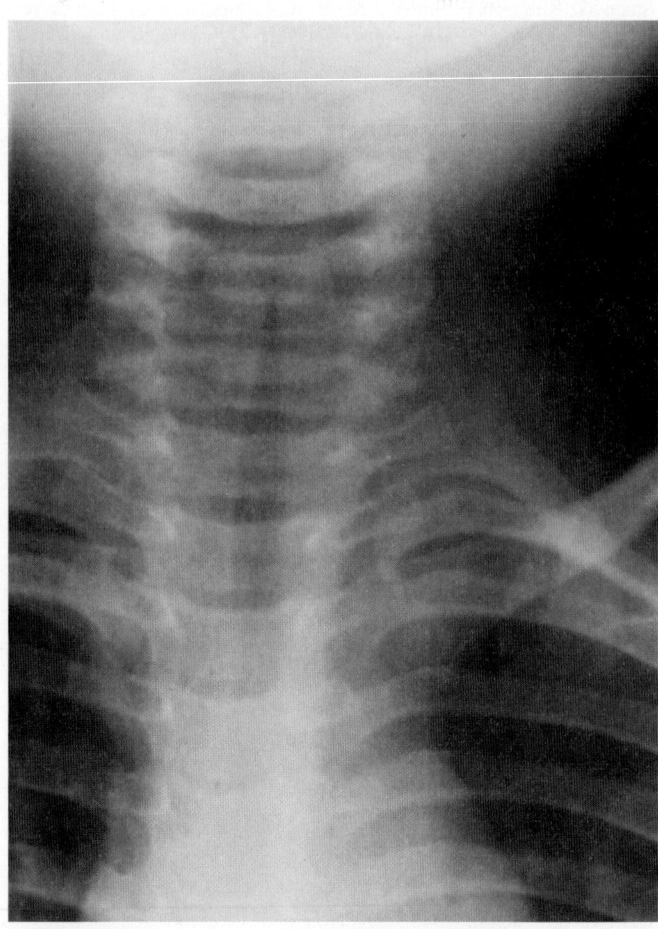

**FIGURE 118-2** Croup. Classic "steeple" sign seen on an anterioposterior radiograph of the neck showing narrowing of the subglottic tracheal narrowing.

addition to corticosteroid therapy, these patients may require inhaled racemic epinephrine, which has been shown to effectively decrease signs and symptoms of airway obstruction. The effects of racemic epinephrine are short-lived, therefore the possibility of recurrence of swelling and symptoms must always be considered. Patients who are administered inhaled epinephrine should be observed for a minimum of 2 to 3 hours after treatment in case of recurrence of airway symptoms. Patients who require repeated doses of racemic epinephrine may require hospitalization. The most severe cases cause significant upper airway obstruction, resulting in oxygen desaturations, cyanosis, and subsequent respiratory failure if not managed appropriately. In these cases, an advanced airway may be indicated if other less invasive interventions are unsuccessful in alleviating symptoms. As tracheal intubation may lead to subglottic stenosis after extubation, it must be performed judiciously.

## EPIGLOTTITIS (SUPRAGLOTTITIS)

### ETIOLOGY

Infection of the epiglottis may rapidly cause airway obstruction and is a true life-threatening emergency. Epiglottitis is described as an infectious process of the epiglottis and/or its associated structures and is more accurately termed supraglottitis. This process is classically caused by *Haemophilus influenzae* type B (HIB), leading to edema and inflammation and producing a swollen, cherry-red epiglottis. Since the advent of the HIB vaccine, the incidence of supraglottitis due to *H influenzae* type B has declined remarkably. Other infectious etiologic agents include *Streptococcus*, *Staphylococcus*, and *Pseudomonas* species.

### CLINICAL PRESENTATION

Supraglottitis most commonly affects children between 2 and 6 years of age, but can occur at any age. The classic presentation of supraglottitis is an anxious, toxic-appearing, febrile young child who quietly sits upright, leaning forward with his/her chin forward and neck extended, drooling, and with obvious inspiratory stridor and labored breathing. This position is known as the tripod position. In contrast to croup, cough and hoarseness are often not present. Unfortunately for the diagnostician, the tripod position and the other findings are often absent. Given the variable presentation and infrequent occurrence of supraglottitis, it is essential for the physician to maintain a high index of suspicion for this disease.

### DIAGNOSIS

Care should be taken as to not upset the child during the examination or perform painful procedures such as blood tests, as this can precipitate significant respiratory distress. During evaluating of the oropharynx, visualization of an edematous and erythematous epiglottis may be possible. Gentle *external* manipulation of the laryngotracheal area may produce pain. Any manipulation of the oropharynx of a child with supraglottitis can be unsafe, potentially leading to significant respiratory compromise from airway obstruction and possible respiratory failure. A lateral neck radiograph may reveal the classic "thumb sign," depicting a swollen epiglottis (Fig. 118-3). An often present finding on lateral neck radiograph is the obliteration of the vallecula, which should otherwise be open and visible. If a radiograph is to be obtained, it should be performed in an unobtrusive manner, under direct observation by a healthcare provider.

### MANAGEMENT

For children with supraglottitis, expedient care of the airway is the most important priority. Airway management in supraglottitis should involve experienced individuals under controlled conditions. While awaiting definitive airway management, preferably in the operating room by skilled anesthesiologists and otolaryngologists, it is imperative to handle the patient gently, and to administer oxygen in an unobtrusive manner. Blood collection and intravenous (IV) access should occur only after the airway is secured. Early intubation and intravenous parenteral antibiotics to eliminate the causative bacteria have reduced mortality significantly. Appropriate antibiotic choices include ampicillin/sulbactam, cefotaxime, ceftriaxone, or clindamycin. If methicillin-resistant *Staphylococcus aureus* is suspected, then addition of vancomycin is warranted.

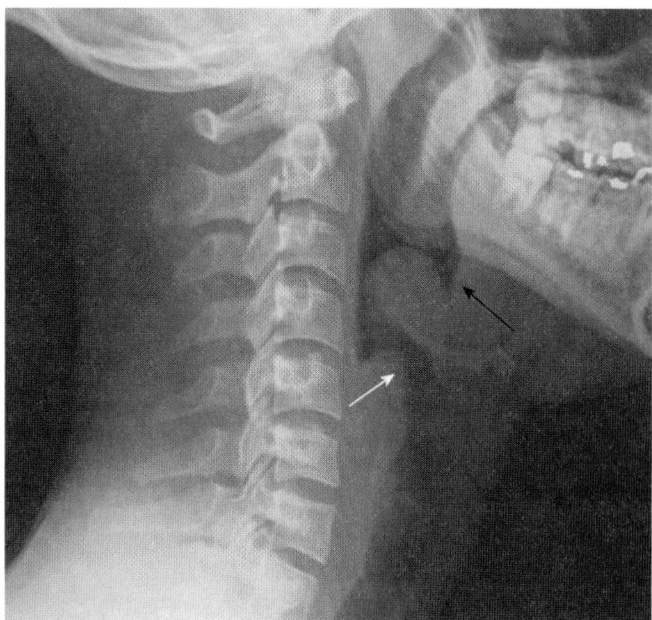

**FIGURE 118-3** Epiglottitis. Classic thumbprint sign seen on a lateral radiograph of the neck revealing enlargement of the epiglottis with amputation of the vallecula (*black arrow*) and thickening of the aryepiglottic folds (*white arrow*).

## BACTERIAL TRACHEITIS

### ETIOLOGY

The incidence of *bacterial tracheitis* is far lower than that of uncomplicated viral croup. Bacterial tracheitis can occur as a primary bacterial infection or may follow viral croup as a secondary bacterial infection. This disease's symptoms are similar to croup, but with copious purulent tracheal secretions and positive bacterial cultures. *S aureus* is the most commonly implicated bacteria. *H influenzae* and streptococcal species are less commonly isolated. Bacterial tracheitis can cause airway edema, purulent secretions, and development of a pseudomembrane, which may cause severe airway obstruction.

### CLINICAL PRESENTATION

Affected children may present with mild URI symptoms, followed by sore throat, fever, stridor, and a "brassy" cough. These symptoms may be present for up to a week prior to initial presentation. However, the progression of respiratory obstruction and distress can be more rapid and significant than in patients with croup. On initial presentation, patients with bacterial tracheitis are often highly febrile, appear ill, and have more severe symptoms than patients with croup. About 50% of children will also have a concomitant pneumonia. Of note, children with tracheostomy tubes are at higher risk for bacterial tracheitis.

### DIAGNOSIS

Although a peripheral white blood cell count might not be elevated, an obvious left shift with high band count is noted most often. Blood cultures are usually negative. Lateral neck radiographs may demonstrate subglottic edema, and chest radiographs may demonstrate focal infiltrates, although there are no pathognomonic radiographic signs of bacterial tracheitis. While the aforementioned studies may suggest bacterial tracheitis, airway endoscopy can confirm the diagnosis by visualization of an inflamed trachea and subglottis as well as a pseudomembrane.

### MANAGEMENT

Children with bacterial tracheitis must be managed in an intensive care setting. The most important aspect of therapy is maintenance of a patent airway. Copious purulent secretions and subglottic space narrowing are common causes of airway obstruction and children may require an advanced airway. While the child is intubated, aggressive and frequent pulmonary and tracheal toilet should be performed, and endoscopy may be required for deeper suctioning. Broad spectrum antibiotics such as third-generation cephalosporins and vancomycin should be initiated until cultures results and sensitivities are available.

## RETROPHARYNGEAL ABSCESS

### ETIOLOGY

The retropharyngeal space is located on both sides of the pharyngeal midline, immediately posterior to the pharynx, larynx, and trachea, and extending from the base of the skull to the level of the seventh cervical and first thoracic vertebrae. Contained within this space are lymph nodes that drain the nose, paranasal sinuses, nasopharynx, and ears. The majority of these lymph nodes atrophy in later childhood, reducing the likelihood of abscess formation in older children. *Retropharyngeal abscess* (RPA) usually affects children between the ages of 6 months and 6 years, with the mean age being 3 to 5 years. Infections are often polymicrobial, but common isolated organisms include anaerobes, streptococcal species, and *S aureus*. Retropharyngeal abscess is rarely reported in infants younger than 3 months of age. In those instances, *Escherichia coli* and group B *Streptococcus* are often the identified pathogens.

### CLINICAL PRESENTATION

The clinical presentation can mimic epiglottitis; however, the onset of RPA is less abrupt. Typically, a several day–long prodrome (eg, URI symptoms, pharyngitis) precedes the onset of bacterial infection. Following extension of infection to the retropharyngeal space and lymph node suppuration, more serious signs and symptoms develop. Thus, the most common presenting complaints include fever, sore throat, and neck pain. The collection of purulent material can act as a mass lesion, extrinsically compressing or distorting upper airway structures and leading to stridor, drooling, and a toxic appearance. The abscess can also cause meningismus; thus, RPA should be considered in the child with nuchal rigidity but without cerebrospinal fluid (CSF) pleocytosis.

### DIAGNOSIS

Diagnosis is often made by clinical examination from the constellation of signs and symptoms, including ill appearance, neck swelling and pain with movement, torticollis, muffled "hot potato" voice, dysphonia, drooling, and trismus. If RPA is suspected, but physical findings are equivocal, radiographic studies can help confirm the diagnosis. Although sometimes interpreted as normal or nonconfirmatory, a lateral neck radiograph can be helpful. A positive film demonstrates an increase in the width of the soft tissues anterior to the upper cervical vertebrae. With proper neck extension, this space normally measures less than one-half the adjacent vertebral body width in a child older than 1 year, and less than the full adjacent vertebral body width in younger infants. Computed tomography (CT) of the neck with IV contrast can identify both abscess extension to neighboring spaces and its location relative to sensitive structures such as the internal jugular veins and carotid arteries. CT can also distinguish RPA from cellulitis and is often used when determining the course of treatment.

### MANAGEMENT

A child with RPA should be managed in consultation with an otolaryngologist and hospitalized for intravenous antibiotic therapy. Initial antibiotic management can include ceftriaxone, ampicillin/sulbactam, or clindamycin. Intubation is indicated for airway compromise. Surgical intervention may be necessary in order to drain abscesses that are large, cause airway compromise, or are refractory to antibiotics.

## PERITONSILLAR ABSCESS

### ETIOLOGY

*Peritonsillar abscesses* are caused by an infection between the palatine tonsils and the capsule. It is the most common deep infection of the throat in adults and therefore is seen more commonly in adolescents. Depending on the size of the abscess, airway obstruction is a potential complication. Chronic tonsillitis can predispose patients to peritonsillar abscesses and this is often preceded by an acute streptococcal pharyngitis. Peritonsillar abscesses are often polymicrobial, consisting of both aerobic and anaerobic bacteria. The most common aerobic isolates include *Streptococcus pyogenes*, *S aureus*, *H influenzae*, and *Neisseria* species. There is no evidence of person-to-person transmission of infection, with the exception of those resulting from human bites.

### CLINICAL PRESENTATION

The adolescent often presents highly febrile and ill-appearing, complaining of worsening sore throat, and a "hot potato" or muffled voice. They may also complain of referred ear pain and odynophagia. On exam, patients will often exhibit trismus, along with palate edema on the same side as the abscess, with uvular deviation to the contralateral side.

### DIAGNOSIS

Peritonsillar abscess can be difficult to distinguish from cellulitis. While advanced radiographic imaging such as ultrasound or CT can be performed, the gold standard for diagnosis is needle aspiration by a trained physician. Due to the polymicrobial nature of this infection, aspirated fluid should be sent for both aerobic and anaerobic cultures.

### MANAGEMENT

Initial antibiotic therapy should be broad spectrum to cover both aerobic and anaerobic species until the results of the culture from the needle aspiration become available. Broad-spectrum penicillins and clindamycin would cover the most common species; however, some resistance has been reported, particularly with anaerobes such as *Bacteroides*. Many otolaryngologists recommend 10 to 14 days of antibiotic therapy.

## FOREIGN BODIES

### ETIOLOGY

According to the National Safety Council, choking is one of the leading causes of unintentional deaths in infants and young children. Choking is also responsible for a high number of emergency department visits. The most common items include food (peanuts, seeds, popcorn, grapes) and nonfood items (coins, balloons, marbles). Round items are particularly dangerous, as they can become lodged and completely obstruct the airway.

### CLINICAL PRESENTATION

The initial presentation varies depending on the age of the child, the object aspirated, where the object is located in the airway, and how long the foreign body has been present. Patients with marked respiratory distress and cyanosis are true airway emergencies. More commonly, in the acute presentation, patients have sudden onset of choking or coughing, followed by wheezing, dyspnea, and/or stridor. Decreased air entry on auscultation, wheezing, and fever are more commonly observed with bronchial foreign bodies, while stridor and hoarseness are more often associated with laryngotracheal foreign bodies. It is important to understand that the symptoms associated with upper airway obstruction due to the presence of foreign bodies can be highly variable, and sometimes nearly absent. Thus, a continued high degree of suspicion should be maintained when a patient's history suggests this possibility.

## DIAGNOSIS

In the absence of an observed acute choking episode, the diagnosis of foreign body aspiration can be delayed. In fact, as many as 15% to 20% of foreign body aspirations are diagnosed more than a month after aspiration. Patients with a chronic, unexplained cough, wheezing, or recurrent pneumonias should raise suspicion for a foreign body aspiration. Chest radiography may not be helpful as most aspirated foreign bodies are radiolucent. Some children with documented foreign body aspiration have completely normal chest radiographs, both upright and decubitus views. There can be secondary signs of obstructive emphysema with hyperinflation of one lobe of the lungs compared to the other. This is caused by a partial airway obstruction with subsequent air trapping, and is most apparent when images are captured during exhalation. CT imaging can also be useful to identify an otherwise radiolucent foreign body.

## MANAGEMENT

Foreign body aspirations leading to airway compromise need emergent management to protect the airway, prior to determining the presence or absence of a foreign body. Blind finger sweeps should be avoided as the foreign body could be pushed back into the airway, causing further obstruction. In the young child who is unable to control his or her actions, this maneuver also puts the rescuer at risk for injury. In the unconscious, nonbreathing child, following failed chest or abdominal thrusts, a tongue-jaw lift should be performed by grasping both the tongue and lower jaw between the thumb and finger, and lifting. This draws the tongue away from the back of the throat and might partially relieve the obstruction. If the foreign body is visualized, it should be removed.

When there is a strong suspicion for a foreign body aspiration, rigid bronchoscopy can be both diagnostic and therapeutic. This method permits control of the airway and of any subsequent bleeding of the mucosa, as well as object visualization and removal. Flexible bronchoscopy can also be performed, but is less preferred as providers run the risk of dislodging the object, and there is less airway control.

# TRAUMA

## BLUNT AND PENETRATING INJURIES

Trauma to the airway causing obstruction can occur from both blunt and penetrating injuries. Given the aforementioned pediatric airway anatomy considerations, as well as less cartilaginous support, pediatric airways are more susceptible to obstruction from trauma. In addition to the traumatic injury, the airway can be obstructed by foreign bodies, loose teeth, secretions, bleeding, compression from external forces, or subcutaneous air (Fig. 118-4). According to Advanced Trauma Life Support guidelines, a trauma patient's airway must be secured prior to proceeding with the primary and secondary surveys. This may require placement of an advanced airway or aggressively suctioning secretions to assist with the oxygenation and ventilation, thus preventing cardiopulmonary demise. Further evaluation with CT imaging may assist in determining the extent of injuries in a hemodynamically stable patient. Consultation with trauma surgery and/or otolaryngology may be necessary, especially for the unstable patient who requires operative management.

## THERMAL INJURIES

The tissues of the upper airway are subject to injury when exposed to extremely high or low temperature substances, such as hot drinks or frozen foods. Case reports of thermal epiglottitis and uvulitis have been published sporadically. When such injuries occur, the management of the injured airway should follow usual guidelines. In the absence of secondary infection, antibiotics are not indicated for these injuries.

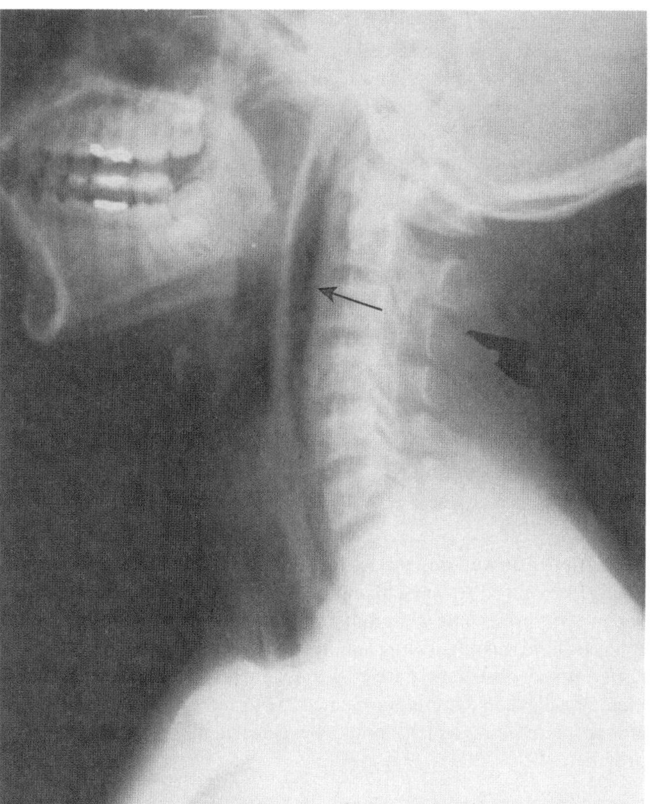

**FIGURE 118-4** Soft-tissue neck x-ray of an adolescent who sustained a laryngeal fracture resulting in subcutaneous emphysema of the neck. Note the obvious soft-tissue air tracking along the fascial planes (*arrow*). (Reproduced with permission from Cho TJ, Kim H: Unusual presentation of spontaneous pneumomediastinum, *Lung India*. 2010 Oct;27(4):239-241.)

# ANAPHYLAXIS

*Anaphylaxis* is an acute, life-threatening immuonoglobulin E (IgE)-mediated systemic reaction to an allergen that requires immediate attention and effective management. Symptom onset occurs suddenly and involves 2 or more organ systems. Such symptoms include urticaria, angioedema, flushing, lip or tongue swelling, throat tightness/swelling, retropharyngeal or laryngeal edema, cough, wheezing, respiratory distress, abdominal pain, vomiting, syncope, or dizziness. Patients may also present in anaphylactic shock and be hypotensive, in addition to the above symptoms. The most common identified causes include insect bites or stings, ingested foods or medications, vaccinations, or contact with an offending agent. Often the etiologic agent is not determined. Intramuscular (IM) epinephrine is the initial treatment of choice and significantly decreases morbidity and mortality. Additional supportive therapies include corticosteroids, $H_1$ antihistamines, and $H_2$ antihistamines. Patients who have significant airway obstruction require multiple doses of IM epinephrine, and those who have refractory hypotension should be admitted for further management.

Patients and families should be counseled about potential exposures and when to administer IM epinephrine. Given the severity of anaphylaxis, it is prudent to refer patients to a pediatric allergist who can assist the family in identifying the allergen and initiating long-term therapies (anti-IgE therapy, desensitization) as indicated.

# INGESTION OF CAUSTIC SUBSTANCES

Over 200,000 exposures to cleaning substances are reported to the US Poison Control Center annually. Many of these are caustic agents, including acid, alkali, or oxidizing agents. These substances include laundry detergents, toilet bowel cleaners, floor cleaners, oven cleaners, ammonia, bleaches, and all-purpose cleaners. Approximately 80% of caustic ingestions occur in children younger than 5 years of age and are often unintentional. These products may appear attractive to a young child because of color, texture, scent, or packaging in alternate "safe" containers such as soft drink bottles.

Caustic agents can burn the skin, tongue, throat, esophagus, and stomach. Children may present with drooling, dysphagia, stridor, and/or wheezing. Upon presentation, it is imperative to determine the substance ingested and consult the Poison Control Center. If the patient has respiratory compromise, an advanced airway should be considered to prevent cardiopulmonary collapse. A chest radiograph should be obtained to rule out mediastinitis or aspiration pneumonitis. Occasionally, endoscopy is needed to assess the extent of injuries in a persistently symptomatic child. Treatment involves supportive care as the mucosa heals, as there is no antidote for caustic substances. Poison prevention and anticipatory guidance are necessary to prevent future ingestions and injuries.

## SUMMARY

Acute upper airway obstructions can be life-threatening and require quick recognition to prevent morbidity and mortality. Management depends on presenting symptoms and physical exam findings. Understanding and distinguishing among the various etiologies of acute upper airway obstruction are critical for instituting effective management to alleviate symptoms. Some cases may necessitate advanced airway placement, which should be performed by an experienced provider.

## SUGGESTED READINGS


Bjornson CL, Klassen TP, Williamson J, et al; Pediatric Emergency Research Canada Network. A randomized trial of a single dose of oral dexamethasone for mild croup. *New Engl J Med.* 2004;351(13):1306-1313.

Darras KE, Roston AT, Yewchuk LK. Imaging of acute airway obstruction in infants and children. *Radiographics.* 2015;35(7):2064-2079.

Harless J, Ramaiah R, Bhananker S. Pediatric airway management. *Int J Crit Ill Inj Sc.* 2014;4(1):65-70.

Mandal A, Kabra SK, Lodha R. Upper airway obstruction in children. *Indian J Pediatr.* 2015;82(8):737-744.

National Safety Council. *Injury Facts 2016.* Itasca, IL: National Safety Council; 2016.

Richards AM. Pediatric respiratory emergencies. *Emerg Med Clin North Am.* 2016;34(1):77-96.

Russell KF, Liang Y, O'Gorman K, Johnson DW, Klassen TP. Glucocorticoids for croup. *Cochrane Database Syst Rev.* 2011;(1):CD001955.

Simons FE, Ardusso LR, Bilò MB, et al. 2012 Update: World Allergy Organization Guidelines for the assessment and management of anaphylaxis. *Curr Opins Allergy Clin Immunol.* 2012;12(4):389-399.

Virbalas J, Smith L. Upper airway obstruction. *Pediatr Rev.* 2015;36(2):62-72.




# 119 Temperature Dysregulation

Rohit P. Shenoi and Daniel M. Rubalcava

## PHYSIOLOGY OF TEMPERATURE REGULATION AND HEAT TRANSFER

Healthy humans are able to self-regulate their body temperature within a narrow range (37±0.4°C or 98.6±0.8°F), despite wide variations in ambient temperature. Temperature regulation is performed by the thermoregulatory center in the preoptic anterior hypothalamus, which integrates impulses transmitted by the peripheral warm and cold receptors of the skin and the central thermoreceptors located in the hypothalamus, spinal cord, viscera, and great veins. Normally, the body maintains a balance between the heat generated by the muscles and liver and the heat lost through the skin and lungs. During exercise, there may be as much as a 4-fold increase in heat production. In febrile states, homeostatic mechanisms such as vasoconstriction and shivering raise the body temperature by increasing heat production and decreasing heat dissipation until a new elevated set point is reached. When the illness abates, the set point returns to the original lower level. Lowering of the body temperature is heralded by the onset of sweating.

There are 4 methods of heat transfer to and from the body: conduction, radiation, convection, and evaporation. Conduction helps transfer heat from the body to a solid or liquid medium that is in contact with it, and is the primary mechanism of cooling during ice or water immersion, which, if prolonged, can lead to hypothermia, especially in cold climates. In the lungs, heat is lost by conduction to water vapor and air. Radiation transfers heat from a warmer body to a colder body via electromagnetic waves, and is a principal mechanism of heat elimination in temperate environments. The amount of heat transferred through conduction or radiation is dependent on the temperature gradient between the skin and surroundings, as well as skin blood flow and insulation characteristics (adiposity, hair, clothing). In convection, heat is transferred from the body to the surrounding air, according to the ambient air temperature and wind speed. Evaporation removes heat from the body when sweat (or water that is in contact with the body) vaporizes from its liquid state, and the rate of evaporation is dependent on the relative humidity, ambient air temperature, wind velocity, and degree of sweat production. The evaporation of sweat is a principal mechanism for heat elimination through body heat production or when the ambient temperature rises.

The adaptation to heat stress relies on both a greater rate of sweating at a lower degree of exercise and a lower electrolyte content of sweat. Sweating and subsequent evaporation are very effective mechanisms of temperature control, provided that the environmental humidity is low enough to permit evaporation. This does not occur when the air becomes saturated with water vapor at humidity levels of 90% to 95% and is reduced at humidity levels greater than 75%. In addition, sweating can cause a substantial water and electrolyte loss occurring at up to 1 L/hour/m$^2$ of body surface area.

When the ambient temperature drops, cold-sensitive neurons in the skin are stimulated, sending impulses to the hypothalamus to cause piloerection and heat generation by shivering. Piloerection traps an insulating layer of air around the body in order to minimize heat loss. Shivering is not a compensatory mechanism in neonates; instead, they generate heat independent of muscle contraction in their brown adipose tissue through the oxidation of fatty acids being mediated by the sympathetic nervous system. The role of brown adipose tissue beyond the neonatal period is unclear, though it has been suggested that an adaptive conversion from white to brown adipose tissue may occur as a response to cold stress beyond this age. In addition to the above metabolic responses, cold temperature leads to peripheral vasoconstriction and shunts blood away from the periphery to the core. Additionally, cold temperatures lead to antidiuretic hormone antagonism, resulting in increased urine output and hemoconcentration.

## HEAT-RELATED ILLNESS

*Hyperthermia* is an uncontrolled elevation of the core body temperature that outpaces the body's ability to lose heat. Fever is distinct from hyperthermia in that inflammation-induced cytokine activation leads to a reset of the hypothalamic thermostat set-point, resulting in an elevation of body temperature that exceeds the normal daily variation. Heat-related illnesses occur when an elevated body temperature caused by endogenous heat production and ambient heat exposure together exceed heat dissipation mechanisms in the body. The differential diagnoses of heat related illness are given in Table 119-1.

**TABLE 119-1 DIFFERENTIAL DIAGNOSIS OF HYPERTHERMIA**

| Condition | Symptoms |
|---|---|
| Sepsis and/or meningitis | Presentation includes high fever, seldom exceeding 41°C, with altered mental status. There is usually a focus of infection, such as meningitis or pneumonia. |
| Drug overdose | Causative drugs include amphetamines, MDMA, cocaine, salicylates, anticholinergics, and bath salts. Search for a history of drug ingestion and toxidromes with hyperpyrexia and seizures. Measure serum drug levels and send urinary drug screens. |
| Status epilepticus | There is usually a history of prolonged seizures before the onset of hyperthermia. Rhabdomyolysis may occur. |
| Serotonin syndrome | This occurs after excessive stimulation of the 5-$HT_{1A}$ subtype serotonin receptor. It is characterized by hyperthermia with increased muscle tone, tremors, gastrointestinal upset, restlessness, and changes in level of consciousness. It occurs due to drug interactions with SSRIs, dextromethorphan, meperidine, L-tryptophan, amphetamines, and sumatriptan, or when MAOIs are combined with tricyclic antidepressants. |
| Neuroleptic malignant syndrome | Presentation includes muscle rigidity, autonomic dysfunction, and altered mental status, and usually follows administration of antipsychotics or withdrawal of dopaminergic agents. Temperature elevation and alteration of mental status occur after the onset of "lead pipe" muscle rigidity. There is marked elevation of creatine phosphokinase (CPK) and leukocytosis, which are nonspecific findings. |
| Malignant hyperthermia | A congenital disorder of calcium regulation in striated muscle. It occurs after exposure to general anesthesia, depolarizing muscle agents, or rarely after severe exertion. The typical scenario is muscle rigidity and hyperthermia following the administration of general anesthesia. |
| Thyroid storm | Though rare in children, it can manifest with hyperpyrexia, tachycardia, and heart failure with agitation and delirium. It is seen in the setting of thyroid surgery, trauma, or infection. |
| Hemorrhagic shock with encephalopathy | Presentation includes hyperpyrexia with mental status changes and multiorgan failure in previously well young children. The cause is unknown. |

MAOI, monoamine oxidase inhibitor; MDMA, 3,4-methylenedioxymethamphetamine; SSRI, selective serotonin reuptake inhibitor.

## EPIDEMIOLOGY

There are 2 groups of children who are at risk for heat-related illness or heat stress. The first group includes infants who are left bundled in their cribs and young children who are left unattended in closed automobiles. Even with moderate ambient temperatures, the temperature inside closed vehicles can rise dangerously high causing significant morbidity or death. Studies show a greater than 14°C (40°F) temperature increase in the first hour inside the car for all ambient temperatures between 22°C (72°F) and 36°C (95.5°F). During the 13-year period from 1998 through the end of 2012, there were 556 child vehicular hyperthermia deaths in the United States, of which more than half resulted from the child being left unattended by the caregiver. In addition, there are approximately 1000 heat stroke injuries annually from vehicular hyperthermia.

The other at-risk group includes youth engaged in athletic activities and children exposed to excessive environmental heat (eg, during border crossings through the harsh desert environment in the southern United States). Heat-related illness is a common reason for missed athletic activities, and is highest among football players, with rates peaking in August. This is more prevalent in overweight or obese individuals.

Heat-related illnesses can exacerbate existing medical conditions, and death from heat exposure can be preceded by various symptoms, which makes the absolute rate or incidence of heat-related death difficult to determine. Additionally, the criteria used to determine heat-related causes of death vary across states in the United States. These factors can lead to underreporting heat-related deaths or to reporting heat as a factor contributing to death rather than the underlying cause.

## PATHOPHYSIOLOGY

In hyperthermia, the body temperature is elevated above normal because the heat-dissipating homeostatic mechanisms activated at temperatures above the set point are overwhelmed. Contrary to earlier thinking, children do not have less effective thermoregulatory ability, insufficient cardiovascular capacity, or lower physical exertion tolerance compared to adults when they exercise in the heat and maintain adequate hydration. The main modifiable risk factors for exertional heat-illness risk related to sports and other physical activities in a hot environment include poor hydration status, undue physical exertion, lack of time to recover from repeated exercise bouts, closely scheduled same-day training or sports competition, and clothes, uniforms, and protective equipment that do not allow heat dissipation.

## CLASSIFICATION

The spectrum of heat-illness spans minor conditions such as heat cramps, heat edema, and heat syncope to the more serious heat exhaustion and life-threatening heatstroke. In heat cramps, there are painful, involuntary muscle contractions during or immediately after exercise. This resolves after rest, cooling off, and drinking an electrolyte-carbohydrate mixture. *Heat edema*, caused by interstitial fluid pooling in the dependent extremities, is treated by elevation of the extremities and use of compression stockings. *Heat syncope* is characterized by a brief loss of consciousness in relation to heat exposure with rapid recovery to baseline. It is usually precipitated by peripheral vasodilation, orthostatic pooling of blood in the dependent areas, prolonged standing, and dehydration. The victim usually recovers after a period of rest and rehydration and after being moved to a cooler area.

*Heat exhaustion* is a moderately severe heat illness characterized by muscle cramps, fatigue, headache, nausea, vomiting, dizziness, or fainting. The skin is often cool and moist, indicating that body sweating is still intact. The pulse rate is typically fast and weak, and breathing is rapid and shallow. The core temperature may be normal or slightly elevated but less than 40°C (104°F). If untreated, heat exhaustion can progress to heatstroke.

*Heatstroke* is a life-threatening condition that occurs in patients who are exposed to excessive environmental heat when the core body temperature reaches or exceeds 40°C. It is accompanied by tachycardia, headache, and central nervous system dysfunction such as dizziness, headache, confusion, seizures, or coma. This can progress to rhabdomyolysis, encephalopathy, liver and kidney failure, coagulopathy, and multiple organ system failure. Sweating is usually absent in heatstroke, though its absence is not essential to make a diagnosis.

Heatstroke is classified as classical (nonexertional) or exertional. Nonexertional heatstroke is most commonly seen during heat waves and affects people who are least able to tolerate heat, such as the chronically ill, the very young, and the aged. The exertional form is seen in people who are actively exercising or those with convulsive status epilepticus or prolonged agitation. The prodrome may consist of nonspecific complaints such as lethargy, vomiting, nausea, weakness, or headache, and may go unrecognized. Risk factors include poor conditioning, recent illness, lack of rest or sleep, poor acclimatization, or dehydration.

## CLINICAL EFFECTS

Hyperthermia initially causes an increase in cellular metabolism with an increase in heat production. There is cutaneous vasodilatation, tachypnea, and increased cardiac output. At further elevations in body temperature, as in heatstroke, cardiac output and oxygen delivery cannot keep pace with the accelerated metabolic rate. Heat stress induces an acute inflammatory reaction mediated by interleukins, cytokines, and proteins that cause an increase in mucosal permeability. Together with endotoxemia, alterations in the microcirculation occur, with resultant endothelial and tissue injury. Common complications of hyperthermia include acute respiratory distress syndrome, disseminated intravascular coagulation, acute renal injury, hepatic injury, and rhabdomyolysis. Rhabdomyolysis, which is the uncontrolled breakdown of skeletal muscle, is an important and life-threatening consequence of heatstroke.

## LABORATORY FINDINGS

Early in the disease, hypokalemia, hypophosphatemia, and respiratory alkalosis (due to stimulation of the respiratory center) occur. Serum lactate dehydrogenase will be elevated as a consequence of cellular injury, and elevated transaminases, usually peaking at 48 hours, indicate hepatic damage. As the disease advances, patients will have metabolic acidosis with elevation in the serum lactate. If significant skeletal muscle injury has occurred, rhabdomyolysis ensues and can be diagnosed by elevated creatine kinase levels and myoglobinuria, hyperkalemia, and acidosis with derangements of renal function. Rhabdomyolysis requires aggressive proactive management with hydration, maintenance of normal to alkaline blood pH, and, potentially, dialysis. Myocardial injury may occur during heatstroke, resulting in an increase in cardiac enzymes and ST-segment changes on the electrocardiogram (ECG).

## MANAGEMENT

The principles of management include cooling, airway protection, supporting cardiorespiratory function, repleting intravascular volume, and pre-emptive management and early intervention to minimize complications. For milder forms of heat injury, reducing the level of physical activity, transport to a cooler environment, and oral rehydration are usually sufficient, and when heat cramps are present, salt as well as water may be replaced using a simple 0.1% to 0.2% salt solution (~ 1/4 teaspoon of table salt per 8 oz of water).

Heatstroke, however, is a medical emergency, and rapid temperature reduction is of paramount importance. First aid should involve removing the patient's clothes and cooling the body by applying wet towels, drenching the victim with water, and maintaining a cool environment during transport. Victims will need basic or advanced life support measures, based on the severity of the heatstroke. On arrival in the emergency department, the patient's airway, breathing, and circulation should be assessed and supported as necessary. Patients will need intravenous or intraosseous access and resuscitation using isotonic fluids at room temperature. Most will need at least 20 to 40 mL/kg of normal saline, and those with exertional heat stroke require more fluids. After initial fluid resuscitation, fluid administration should be guided by central venous pressure monitoring to avoid circulatory overload. Since cardiac function may be reduced in victims of heatstroke, vasopressors may be required. To ensure rapid cooling, ice should be placed in the neck, axillae, and groin, and water-soaked sheets and cooling fans utilized; in severe cases, the patient should be placed on a cooling blanket, targeting normothermia. Additional measures for active cooling include the administration of cold intravenous fluids or nasogastric fluids, as well as instillation of cooled fluids to the peritoneum. The use of cardiopulmonary bypass and extracorporeal membrane oxygenation have both been used in the most refractory cases and to support those with multiorgan failure. Benzodiazepines and potentially neuromuscular blockade may be administered for agitation and shivering during active cooling in order to minimize oxygen consumption in intubated patients. Patients with heatstroke, and those with any organ system dysfunction or failure, and those requiring continued active cooling should be monitored in an intensive care unit (ICU).

## PROGNOSIS

The prognosis of pediatric victims of heatstroke is not well described, most likely because there is a broad spectrum of manifestations and degrees of severity. However, factors associated with a poor prognosis include the magnitude of temperature elevation, refractoriness to initial measures, and the number of organ systems involved. Survivors may manifest neurocognitive deficits of varying degrees.

## PREVENTION

Acclimatization of athletes and educating participants and coaches involved in sporting activities are primary methods of prevention of heat-related illness. Current National Athletic Trainers' Association (NATA) recommendations suggest a 14-day acclimatization period for all warm weather conditioning. Additionally, the education of participants and caregivers on the dangers of heat-related illness and the importance of proper hydration before, during, and after strenuous activity are key factors in prevention. Fluid replacement should approximate sweat and urine losses so that athletes lose no more than 2% body weight per day on average. This equates to an older child consuming 200 to 300 mL fluid every 10 to 20 minutes during exercise.

To prevent hyperthermia related to automobiles, caregivers should never leave a child unattended in a vehicle, even if the windows are partially open or the engine is running and the air conditioning is turned on. Absentee child-care policies requiring parent and caregiver notification if a child does not arrive to daycare, as well as physical reminders (written, electronic, or visual) that their child is in the vehicle, may also help avoid a caregiver inadvertently leaving a child in the vehicle. Finally, parents should teach children that a vehicle is not a play area, ensure all vehicles remain locked when not in use, and store keys out of a child's reach.

Secondary prevention is crucial to prevent progression. A child exhibiting nausea, vomiting, headache, dizziness, or mental status change after heat exposure should be removed from the activity, rehydrated, and immediately evaluated for potential heat exhaustion or heatstroke by a healthcare professional trained in the assessment of this condition, so that active measures can be instituted to prevent further complications of heat exhaustion and heatstroke.

## NONENVIRONMENTAL HYPERTHERMIA

### Malignant Hyperthermia

*Malignant hyperthermia* (MH) is an autosomal-dominant disorder with an estimated prevalence of 1:3000. The principal defect is a mutation in the gene for the skeletal muscle ryanodine receptor (*RyR1*), which is a calcium channel found in the sarcoplasmic reticulum. Malignant hyperthermia is a rare event and is most commonly triggered by the use of volatile inhalation anesthetic agents or the muscle-depolarizing agent succinylcholine.

In the appropriate setting, the early signs of MH include an inappropriately elevated $CO_2$ production and $O_2$ consumption, a mixed metabolic and respiratory acidosis, profuse sweating, and mottling of the skin. Other clinical features include tachycardia, cardiac arrhythmias and blood pressure instability, masseter spasm (if succinylcholine is used), and generalized muscle rigidity. Later in the illness, hyperkalemia, a rapid increase in body temperature, very elevated serum creatine kinase and myoglobin levels, myoglobinuria, and disseminated intravascular coagulation occur, terminating in cardiac arrest.

The important management goals are to avoid the use of triggering agents in at-risk individuals (by using total intravenous anesthesia), and to have a high index of suspicion if clinical signs could indicate the onset of this.

The treatment of MH begins with stopping the trigger agent, hyperventilating the patient, using nontrigger anesthesia, and terminating the surgery. Intravenous (IV) dantrolene 2.5 mg/kg should be administered. Additional doses or an infusion of dantrolene should be administered until cardiac and respiratory systems stabilize. Immediate additional supportive care involves the treatment of hyperthermia with IV fluids and cooling measures; anticipatory management; early intervention for hyperkalemia, metabolic acidosis, and arrhythmias; and maintaining a urine output of > 2 mL/kg/hour.

### Drug-Induced Hyperthermia

Patients who are intoxicated from using illicit drugs such as cocaine, amphetamines, synthetic cathinone ("bath salt"), and MDMA

(3,4-methylenedioxymethamphetamine) present with signs of sympathetic overactivity, such as hypertension, tachycardia, and hyperthermia. Hyperthermia results from the direct drug effects on the central nervous system, prolonged physical exertion, and hot environmental conditions. Patients are diaphoretic and agitated, and may have delirium. This condition is differentiated from anticholinergic toxicity in that patients with anticholinergic toxicity generally present with reduced or absent sweating, whereas patients with MDMA toxicity are usually diaphoretic. The pattern of speech is clear but pressured for MDMA and resembles a "mouthful of marbles" with anticholinergic toxicity.

The management consists of cardiorespiratory support, fluid resuscitation, management of hyperthermia and hypertension, and the use of sedatives for psychomotor agitation.

## HYPOTHERMIA

Hypothermia, which is defined as a core body temperature less than 35°C (95°F), is caused by exposure to cold but can also occur in warm climates when the victim is exposed to wet and windy conditions. Every year, there are about 1300 hypothermia deaths in the United States, with rates being highest among those with advanced age, male sex, drug intoxication, homelessness, and mental illness. In the United States, the highest death rates are observed in areas with mild climates that experience rapid temperature changes or at higher elevations where a significant drop in nighttime temperature can occur.

Other conditions associated with hypothermia include major trauma with blood loss and/or exposure, sepsis, extensive burns, hypothalamic dysfunction such as in traumatic brain injury, drug overdose from sedatives, hypnotics or opiates, adrenal insufficiency, anorexia nervosa, and malnutrition. Rarely, it may be a manifestation of child maltreatment due to cold bathing or submersion.

### PATHOPHYSIOLOGY

Children, especially young infants, are at increased risk for hypothermia because of their larger body surface area relative to mass and their inability to recognize low ambient temperature as a danger. Very young children also have limited glycogen stores to augment heat production and are unable to shiver. Though children are more likely to experience hypothermia than adults, severely hypothermic children can have better neurological outcomes, especially if severe cooling rapidly occurs before circulatory arrest.

### CLASSIFICATION

Hypothermia is classified as mild, with a core temperature of 32°C to 35°C (90°F–95°F); moderate, with a core temperature of 28°C to 32°C (82°F–90°F); or severe, with a core temperature below 28°C (82°F). Mild hypothermia causes shivering, cutaneous vasoconstriction, and increased metabolic rate. Behavioral responses include seeking a warm environment and putting on protective clothing. As hypothermia progresses, these compensatory mechanisms begin to fail and victims are unable to generate enough heat. Circulatory insufficiency and manifestations of inadequate cerebral oxygen delivery with altered mental status occur, with apathy, ataxia, slurred speech, confusion, lethargy, and odd behavior such as "paradoxical undressing," which occurs due to perceived warmth caused by changes in peripheral blood flow. In severe hypothermia, all body systems begin to fail. Bradycardia, ventricular arrhythmias, fixed and dilated pupils, cardiorespiratory arrest, coma, and muscle rigidity ensue. Victims of severe hypothermia may lack detectable vital signs, thus all patients with hypothermia should be rewarmed and vital signs and brain stem activity should be reassessed before being declared dead.

### CLINICAL EFFECTS

For every 1°C (1.8°F) drop in body temperature, metabolic activity decreases by 7%. Hypothermia has membrane depressant effects with resultant ionic and electrical conduction disturbances of the brain, heart, peripheral nerves, and other organs and systems. The most important changes include decreased cerebral metabolism and cardiorespiratory depression and failure. The initial exposure to cold induces a release of catecholamines, which results in increased cardiac output, peripheral vasoconstriction, and respiratory drive. As hypothermia progresses, there is a decrease in myocardial depolarization, resulting in bradycardia and decreased cardiac output. Circulatory collapse may occur due to hypovolemia, depression of myocardial function, sludging of blood, bradycardia, or malignant arrhythmias such as ventricular fibrillation. Altered respiratory drive is first manifested by shallow, slow, irregular respirations and, eventually, apnea. Specific neurological signs range from altered mental status to coma and include lack of pupillary and corneal reflexes and global areflexia. Clinically, the skin is mottled, and there may be concurrent frostbite. Cold-induced diuresis, failure of the renal concentrating mechanism and vascular-leak–induced interstitial extravasation of fluids contribute to hypovolemia. Hypothermia can cause reduced gastrointestinal motility, which results in gastric dilatation and ileus. Cardiac arrest may occur in patients with severe hypothermia during their extrication and transport. This is termed *rescue collapse* and is attributed to a combination of factors including circulatory collapse caused by hypovolemia, malignant arrhythmias associated with moving the patient, or further cooling. *Afterdrop*, defined as a continued drop in body temperature after rescue, has been described in experimental models. However, with the use of active external and minimally invasive rewarming and concurrent esophageal temperature measurement, afterdrop has not been reported in hypothermia victims.

### LABORATORY FINDINGS

Hypoglycemia should be ruled out in all victims of hypothermia. Hypokalemia may occur in mild hypothermia, although in severe cases, hyperkalemia occurs due to cell death and renal dysfunction. Coagulopathy, thrombocytopenia, leukopenia, and deranged liver and renal function are often present; creatine kinase may be elevated due to rhabdomyolysis. The hematocrit increases 2% for every 1°C drop in body temperature. A chest radiograph may reveal pulmonary aspiration or pulmonary edema, the latter often seen during rewarming, likely due to reperfusion injury.

The effect of cold on arterial pH and blood gases may lead to confusion in the interpretation of arterial blood gas results. Blood pH increases with cooling due to the inhibition of dissociation of water molecules, and the partial pressures of $CO_2$ and $O_2$ decrease with cooling, although the blood content of these gases remain unchanged. Since blood is warmed to 37°C (98.6°F) in blood gas analyzers, the measured values (uncorrected) represent what the blood gas parameters would have been if the patient were normothermic. Actual in vivo values in the hypothermic patient (corrected) are derived mathematically. If the clinician acts on the corrected values, there is a risk of inducing hypoventilation and alveolar collapse. Therefore, pH and the partial pressure of carbon dioxide ($PCO_2$) should be left uncorrected after the sample has been warmed in the machine, and the test should be interpreted just as in a normothermic patient.

#### Electrocardiogram

Hypothermia first results in prolongation of PR, QRS, and QT intervals, with sinoatrial node depression and bradycardia. As core body temperature decreases, sinus bradycardia progresses to atrial fibrillation, then ventricular fibrillation, and finally cardiac asystole. Artifacts in the ECG may occur due to shivering. The Osborn wave (J point deflection at the junction of the QRS and ST segment) may be present when the body temperature drops below 30°C (86°F), though it is of no prognostic value.

### MANAGEMENT

The principles of management include support of the airway, breathing, and circulation; institution of effective rewarming techniques; and assessment for and treatment of comorbidities such as trauma, medical illness, and intoxication. When assessing patients with hypothermia, it is important to use a low-reading thermometer to measure accurate core body temperature, as standard clinical thermometers do not read under 34°C (93°F). Temperature should be monitored centrally.

The intensity of treatment depends on the length of cold exposure and the victim's body temperature, but rewarming should commence immediately. Victims should be moved to a warm environment, wet clothing removed, and all exposed body surfaces covered with anything at hand, including blankets, clothing, newspapers, etc. This method of passive external rewarming protects the patient from further heat loss and uses the patient's own endogenous heat for rewarming. Additionally, these patients will benefit from active external rewarming, such as forced-air heating blanket, radiant heat lamp, or a water heating pad. The administration of warm oral fluids is beneficial. Most patients with mild hypothermia can be treated in the nearest emergency department.

Patients with moderate and severe hypothermia should be transported to a medical center for advanced rewarming measures and critical care. Supplemental oxygen administration with warm, humidified 100% oxygen via a nonrebreather mask is essential, as the oxygen–dissociation curve shifts leftward with hypothermia. Aggressive fluid resuscitation with warm intravenous fluids at 38°C to 42°C is recommended, and concurrent hypoglycemia should be treated with intravenous dextrose. Severe hypothermia leads to hypoventilation or respiratory arrest, so these patients will require bag-valve mask ventilation and endotracheal intubation. Rarely, cold-induced trismus may preclude orotracheal intubation and necessitate fiberoptic intubation or placement of a surgical airway. A severely hypothermic patient may have a very weak and irregular pulse, making the assessment for a pulse difficult. Cardiopulmonary resuscitation (CPR) should be initiated if no vital signs or cardiac activity are detected. Defibrillation and pharmacologic therapy based on advanced pediatric life support protocols will be necessary for the treatment of ventricular fibrillation or pulseless ventricular tachycardia. Unfortunately, these patients may be refractory to conventional therapy until they are rewarmed. Toxic accumulation of drugs may occur due to altered metabolism at very low temperatures. It is reasonable to administer 1 to 3 doses of vasopressors during CPR while actively rewarming to 30°C. Patients should be placed in a horizontal position and all maneuvers should be performed gently to avoid inducing malignant arrhythmias such as ventricular fibrillation.

In the hospital, more aggressive or "active" rewarming should be instituted, ideally through the use of forced-air rewarming and warmed intravenous fluids. A rate of rewarming of 1°C to 1.5°C pr hour can be achieved in patients with a perfusing rhythm. More invasive rewarming techniques may be necessary for severe hypothermic patients with limited or absent circulation. These include gastric, peritoneal, pleural, or bladder lavage with warmed fluids at 40°C and extracorporeal rewarming. Extracorporeal support is reserved for patients with severe hypothermia with cardiac arrest or absent circulation or who are refractory to other methods of increasing body temperature. If the patient does not regain mental status when the temperature reaches 32°C, a search for metabolic, toxic, or CNS causes should be undertaken. Termination of CPR should be considered if there is no return of cardiac activity once a core temperature of 32°C has been achieved. Additionally, potassium levels greater than 12 mmol/L, a marker of cell death and possible prehypothermia hypoxia, should prompt a consideration of termination of resuscitation.

## FROSTBITE

Victims of hypothermia may also suffer from frostbite, typically affecting exposed body parts such as the ears, nose, cheeks, chin, fingers, and toes. In the early stages, the affected areas become very painful and the skin becomes cold and numb. Later in the illness, blisters develop, and in severe frostbite, the skin may turn black. Patients should be moved to a warm environment and wet clothing removed. The affected extremity should be placed in a basin of warm water (38°C–42°C or 100°F–108°F) for 30 minutes. The temperature of the water should be continually adjusted. Affected areas should not be rubbed, and analgesics may be required. Patients' tetanus immunization status should be assessed and prophylaxis administered accordingly.

## PROGNOSIS

Hypothermia decreases cerebral oxygen requirements, so survival without neurologic impairment is possible, even when these patients may require prolonged CPR. It is very difficult to accurately prognosticate outcome at the initial presentation in the setting of severe hypothermia. The lowest initial temperature in a surviving child and adult with hypothermia were 14.2°C (57.6°F) and 13.7°C (56.7°F), respectively, and survival without neurologic impairment in patients with severe hypothermia treated with cardiac bypass or extracorporeal membrane oxygenation can range from 47% to 63%.

## DIFFERENTIAL DIAGNOSIS

The diagnosis is straightforward in exposure-related hypothermia. However, one should consider other conditions as a cause or contributing factor in mild hypothermia. Increased heat loss may occur from iatrogenic causes, such as administration of cold fluids; overdose from sedatives, hypnotics, or opiates; dermatologic conditions with skin desquamation; or burns. Decreased heat production can occur in very young or old patients, hypoglycemic states, malnutrition, endocrinopathies such as adrenal insufficiency or profound hypothyroidism, diabetic or alcoholic ketoacidosis, or stress or trauma states. Impaired thermoregulation can result from other etiologies, such as traumatic brain or spine injury, stroke, or cerebral hemorrhage.

## PREVENTION

Parents and caregivers should be aware of the risks of cold weather and plan accordingly. Children should be supervised and those who are exposed to cold weather should be adequately clothed in layers with additional insulation, and in water-resistant clothing when appropriate, and should always be well hydrated.

## SUGGESTED READINGS

Bergeron MF, Devore C, Rice SG; Council on Sports Medicine and Fitness and Council on School Health; American Academy of Pediatrics. Policy statement—climatic heat stress and exercising children and adolescents. *Pediatrics*. 2011;128(3):e741-e747.

Brown DJ, Brugger H, Boyd J, Paal P. Accidental hypothermia. *N Engl J Med*. 2012;367(20):1930-1938.

Casa DJ, DeMartini JK, Bergeron MF, et al. National Athletic Trainers' Association position statement: exertional heat illnesses. *J Athl Train*. 2015;50(9):986-1000.

Centers for Disease Control and Prevention (CDC). Heat illness among high school athletes—United States, 2005–2009. *MMWR Morb Mortal Wkly Rep*. 2010;59(32):1009-1013.

Centers for Disease Control and Prevention (CDC). Nonfatal sports and recreation heat illness treated in hospital emergency departments—United States, 2001–2009. MMWR Morb Mortal Wkly Rep. 2011;60(29):977.

Guard A, Gallagher SS. Heat related deaths to young children in parked cars: an analysis of 171 fatalities in the United States, 1995–2002. *Inj Prev*. 2005;11(1):33-37.

Lipman GS, Eifling KP, Ellis MA, Gaudio FG, Otten EM, Grissom CK; Wilderness Medical Society. Wilderness Medical Society practice guidelines for the prevention and treatment of heat-related illness: 2014 update. *Wilderness Environ Med*. 2014;25(4 Suppl):S55-S65.

McIntosh SE, Opacic M, Freer L, et al; Wilderness Medical Society. Wilderness Medical Society practice guidelines for the prevention and treatment of frostbite: 2014 update. *Wilderness Environ Med*. 2014;25(4 Suppl):S43-S54.

Mulcahy AR, Watts MR. Accidental hypothermia: an evidence-based approach. *Emerg Med Pract*. 2009;11(1):1-26.

Nelson NG, Collins CL, Comstock RD, McKenzie LB. Exertional heat-related injuries treated in emergency departments in the U.S., 1997–2006. *Am J Prev Med*. 2011;40(1):54-60.

Rischall ML, Rowland-Fisher A. Evidence-based management of accidental hypothermia in the emergency department. *Emerg Med Pract*. 2016;18(1):1-18.

Soar J, Perkins GD, Abbas G, et al. European Resuscitation Council Guidelines for Resuscitation 2010 Section 8: cardiac arrest in special circumstances: electrolyte abnormalities, poisoning, drowning, accidental hypothermia, hyperthermia, asthma, anaphylaxis, cardiac surgery, trauma, pregnancy, electrocution. *Resuscitation.* 2010;81(10):1400-1433.

Tansey EA, Johnson CD. Recent advances in thermoregulation. *Adv Physiol Educ.* 2015;39(3):139-148.

Zafren K, Giesbrecht GG, Danzl DF, et al; Wilderness Medical Society. Wilderness Medical Society practice guidelines for the out-of-hospital evaluation and treatment of accidental hypothermia: 2014 update. *Wilderness Environ Med.* 2014;25(4 Suppl):S66-S85.

# 120 Complex Care

James A. Feinstein, Mark Brittan, and Christopher J. Stille

## DEFINITION OF CHILDREN WITH MEDICAL COMPLEXITY

In 1997, the Maternal Child Health Bureau adopted the term *children with special healthcare needs* (CSHCN) to identify children who have, or are at risk of having, a chronic physical, developmental, behavioral, or emotional condition that requires health and related services of a type or amount beyond that generally required by children. The prevalence of CSHCN ranges from 12% to 19%. Children with special healthcare needs use more resources and have greater unmet healthcare needs (both primary and specialty care), higher costs, and inadequate insurance. Compared to those without special healthcare needs, there is an increase in healthcare costs borne by families of CSHCN, particularly those who have private insurance. Among CSHCN, poor and minority children are at higher risk for inadequate insurance, as are children with higher levels of functional disability.

A small, but growing, subset of CSHCN can be described as *children with medical complexity* (CMC), who have medical fragility and intensive care needs that are not easily met by existing healthcare models. Common characteristics of the CMC population include chronic conditions requiring multiple hospital and office-based medical and nonmedical services; a reliance on medical equipment and technology, multiple medications, specialized surgeries, and other therapies; and the need for effective care coordination. While there is not yet 1 commonly accepted operational definition of CMC, they likely comprise approximately 5.8% of all US children insured by Medicaid and account for 34% of Medicaid spending for all children. Common frameworks for clinical and research definitions include the World Health Organization's framework for classifying impairments, disabilities, and handicaps; the International Classification of Diseases (ICD)-based complex chronic condition classification system; and the proprietary Clinical Risk Groups maintained by 3M Health Information Systems. The level of and time involved in care coordination for CMC depend both on the medical complexity and fragility, and on a variety of nonmedical factors that impact access to needed services. This chapter presents an approach to care coordination for medically complex and fragile children with chronic conditions.

## THE CHALLENGES OF ORGANIZING CARE FOR CHILDREN WITH MEDICAL COMPLEXITY

Medical complexity and fragility caused by chronic disease affect the children themselves, families, communities, the healthcare system, and society at large. Families, providers, and organizations seeking to improve health care have identified multiple barriers in providing effective care coordination for CMC. Caregivers face constant stress as they try to balance work and family life with the needs of their sick child. A child's tenuous health status often means frequent inpatient and outpatient healthcare visits; in order to remain home, families and home healthcare workers often must maintain a home medical environment akin to an intensive care unit (eg, ventilator equipment, monitoring devices, suction equipment, oxygen supplies). Identifying and negotiating the maze of community- and hospital-based services, obtaining insurance coverage, and accessing social entitlement programs present a Herculean task.

Community services are often uncoordinated, underutilized, fragmented, or even nonexistent. This is particularly true in both small rural communities and inner cities, where inadequate funding and the lack of trained personnel make it difficult to deliver federally or state-mandated services, such as timely health maintenance visits or certification for home health services. Children with medical complexity require multiple medical services and frequent admissions, but care is often partitioned with limited communication among providers, contributing to duplicative or unnecessary investigations and therapies, the potential for costly medical errors, and frustration for families. Families complain that they are often excluded from decision-making and lack the information needed to care for their children at home. Society is impacted by the disproportionately high healthcare costs of CMC and by the loss of productivity because of parents taking time off from work and siblings missing school.

## THE MEDICAL HOME MODEL AND APPROACH TO COORDINATING CARE

### The Medical Home Model

The medical home model, a coordinated approach to care involving multiple team members (including primary care clinicians [PCCs], specialty clinicians, therapists, nutritionists, home care providers, etc), has been put forward as the ideal model for caring for CMC. The American Academy of Pediatrics and others advocate the medical home, a concept of accessible, continuous, comprehensive, family-centered, coordinated, compassionate, and culturally effective care, to meet the needs of all children. For most children, the primary care practice is the ideal setting in which to implement the medical home. However, in the current healthcare system in the United States, many PCCs have difficulty managing the multiple uncommon diagnoses, treatments, and technologies characteristic of CMC, as well as coordinating their many nonmedical services (eg, education, out-of-home care, family support, insurance) by themselves. Many PCCs also do not have the time or expertise to manage long and frequent hospitalizations or arbitrate among multiple tertiary center specialists who may espouse competing diagnoses and treatments.

### An Approach to Care Coordination

In response to the complex management needs of CMC, many tertiary centers in the United States have developed disease- or condition-specific programs that provide care coordination for CMC (eg, diabetes programs, tracheostomy/ventilator programs). More recently, disease- or condition-independent care coordination programs have been developed to address the needs of CMC whose conditions cross multiple specialty areas. Some provide care coordination for specific populations (eg, recipients of services from Title V, the Maternal and Child Health Services Block Grant Program). Others offer a predominantly outpatient or hospitalist-based inpatient complex care service, in which direct primary and/or consultative care is provided by physician-led teams, some of whom also provide comanagement with community PCCs. Finally, a few programs offer integrated inpatient and outpatient services. Many of these models have shown a decrease in hospital days, increase in family satisfaction, and decrease in costs after enrollment in their program, but the lack of standardized definitions of the populations served makes comparisons among these models difficult. It is also important to underscore that, because of capacity, access, and cost considerations, only a small subset of CMC will ever have contact with these tertiary care coordination programs, although the lessons learned from these specialized models are broadly applicable. Building capacity for community-based primary care practices to provide care for CMC, either independently or in comanagement arrangements with tertiary care programs, is essential.

Regardless of the model, a team approach that incorporates the concepts of the medical home with the child and family at the center is key to meeting the needs of CMC. Close collaboration and good communication ensure the expertise needed to access resources and benefits while minimizing the burden on each team member. A leader of the team who can serve as the point person for the family, often a PCC or complex care clinician, should be identified. The leader is unlikely to be expert in all domains of the child's care but must know how to access (and be accessible to) the others. Initially, the tertiary center program physician or nurse care coordinator may take the leadership role. As the child stabilizes and the disease trajectory becomes more defined, the PCC may take on the role. Over time, the family often achieves such a level of expertise in both the child's medical management and coordination that they take the lead, with input as needed from the PCC and tertiary center program. Such programs have demonstrated better quality outcomes and improved healthcare utilization.

A recent, parent-led innovation that highlights the value of such a team approach is illustrated by *care mapping*, a parent-led process in which the child's needs are grouped and color-coded into the various sectors of caregivers, such as medical, therapies, education, and family supports. A care map places the family and child at the core of a care team flanked by a primary care practice and a tertiary center program that have together assumed responsibility for care coordination, and highlights the many other needs that might be coordinated by the medical home. The primary care practice ensures routine and acute care for the child, particularly if the child lives far away from the tertiary hospital center, and local care coordination services to the extent they are able. The tertiary center program providing care coordination may be disease or condition specific, although tertiary programs typically function better if they are able to coordinate care for a broad range of diseases and conditions. It may be a formal care coordination program or an ad hoc group of providers who have come together to serve a particular child. Ideally, the care team includes an invested physician, nurse, and social worker as well as other providers and advocates, if available. Other care coordination team members play a vital but potentially intermittent role in their work to coordinate and connect the many other members of a child's care team.

## CARE COORDINATION FOR THE CHILD WITH MEDICAL COMPLEXITY

### Care Coordination Needs Assessment

There is ample literature describing the differences in perceptions, needs, and goals of families and providers, as well as tools to assess and document needs. The first step in identifying care coordination needs is to identify and harmonize the goals of the family and care team. In addition to the traditional "problem list" and care plans familiar to most healthcare professionals, listening as the family tells the child's story and describes their hopes and dreams for the child generally provides an appreciation for their medical sophistication, understanding of the medical condition(s), cultural and religious values, and general approach to the challenges that they will likely encounter. It is important to learn what, if any, limits to invasive interventions the family wishes to put on the child's care and to understand why they feel as they do. After learning of the family's goals, it is important to determine what resources exist and are needed to meet the goals. What is truly known of the child's diagnoses and prognosis? Are other studies or consultations needed? This information is crucial to appropriately advising the family about invasive interventions or alternative code status. Care coordinators must also recognize how their own values may influence their opinions and should seek input from others who may have differing views.

### Initial Care Coordination Services

Tertiary center programs providing care coordination often have more resources than do PCCs and their practices. After the role of each program is clarified, care coordination personnel can assist the family in identifying and obtaining the insurance, social benefits, and community services needed. Recreational programs, community-based therapies, and parent-to-parent organizations can be identified. For families without experience navigating the healthcare system, it is helpful if the program providing care coordination actually makes the initial connections for the family (eg, calls the local rehabilitation or developmental service coordinator, helps fill out insurance forms) rather than simply providing a list of names and numbers to the family.

After needs and resources are identified, regardless of the format chosen, a comprehensive care plan should be developed to serve as a "road map" for the patient, family, and care team. It should include relevant medical and nonmedical information that will assist the family and team members in meeting the goals established for the child. One very useful purpose of the plan is to provide a synopsis of the child's medical history and plan of care for each of several issues. Careful documentation of active diagnoses and past problems, as well as relevant testing (particularly when a diagnosis is uncertain), enhances communication among providers, improves consultations, minimizes unnecessary testing, and provides the primary care physician with a comprehensive overview. Synthesizing information may identify conflicts between plans proposed by different specialists and enhance a unified approach to the child's care. Developing the summary with the family will identify missing or erroneous information and help focus the plan on their goals. It also serves to educate the family and enhance their ability to participate in care and develop skill as advocates and coordinators. A well-prepared and updated care plan can speed and ease subsequent emergency room visits and hospital admissions. The description of a child's diagnoses, a list of providers and medications, a baseline exam, and an overview of the child's care as well as an emergency plan may also enhance the child's safety. It is vital to revise and update the care plan frequently as conditions and plans change. Parents and other providers must advise the coordinators who update the plan of medication and other therapeutic changes that may have occurred. Moreover, care plans can become quite unwieldy if used to document all care coordination issues, and must be brief enough to be understood and used quickly.

### Hospital-to-Home Care Coordination Services

Ensuring a seamless transition from hospital to home for CMC requires involvement of the care coordination team and enormous attention to detail. This is particularly true when the child is going home for the first time after a diagnosis of a chronic condition has been made, but the principles remain the same with each discharge. Prior to discharge, the child's medical and nonmedical needs must have been addressed; caregiver education must have been completed; and needed home renovations, transportation, and community services put in place. Insurance and social benefits must have been identified and accessed as much as possible. An emergency plan, often a simple algorithm, for dealing with nonacute, urgent, and emergent problems should have been developed and integrated into the overall care plan. In small communities or in the case of a child with unusual or unstable conditions, it may be helpful to provide the local emergency medical services and emergency room with details about the child and his or her common problems and usual therapies. Most important, the PCC's practice must be involved in the discharge planning. Ideally, the PCC should participate in a discharge planning conference in person or by telephone and, at a minimum, the care coordination summary should be provided to him or her. Prior to discharge, the family, PCC, and tertiary center program should agree on their respective care coordination roles and responsibilities and a list of contact numbers should be provided to the family and PCC.

Initially after discharge, it may be helpful to families and PCCs if the tertiary center program providing care coordination acts as a single point of contact for all tertiary center services. This is particularly true when the child's conditions cross multiple specialty boundaries, because the tertiary center program is often better able to identify and locate the appropriate consultant. As the family and the PCC become more familiar with the child and more confident in managing his or her problems, they will be better able to decide when the PCC should see the child for acute illness and follow-up, and whether a particular specialist at the tertiary center should be contacted. Indeed, families often develop sufficient expertise to direct the child's care coordination needs themselves. Electronic communication between the PCC, specialists, and families may be a helpful and efficient use of time.

Over time, the tertiary center program providing care coordination remains a useful backup to the family, the PCC practice, and other members of the care coordination team. Changes in disease trajectory, the particular expertise of the tertiary program, or admission to a hospital often necessitate the input of the tertiary center program providing care coordination. Such a program knows the child, family, and primary care physician and thus often reduces hospital stays, decreases unnecessary studies or failed therapies, and facilitates introduction of new resources (eg, at times of transition, when traveling). Finally, maintaining an extended-care coordination team can facilitate assessment of and documentation for needed technology supports.

## REIMBURSEMENT FOR CARE COORDINATION SERVICES

Care coordination is time and resource intensive, yet payment strategies are inconsistent and often insufficient. In the current, prevalent fee-for-service system in the United States, time-based Current Procedural Terminology (CPT) codes can be used to charge for services if more than 50% of the time in an outpatient visit is spent in counseling and coordination. Private and public payers generally pay for office and hospital visits billed accordingly. Prolonged face-to-face services are also billable, although care coordination is not often included in these. Services other than face-to-face occupy more time and are less frequently paid. It is therefore essential when providing care coordination to enlist the help of the most expert team members to provide services efficiently and to document carefully all of these services in the hope that payers will recognize their importance and reimbursement will improve in the future.

Recent developments in the United States, promoted by the Affordable Care Act and led by the Centers for Medicare and Medicaid Services as well as some commercial payers, are beginning to shift payment models away from traditional fee-for-service and toward value-based care. These models are often hybrids that include payment incentives, such as pay-for-performance components, and prospective payments, such as care coordination stipends and risk-adjusted per-member capitation. These innovations have great potential to recognize the critical role and value of care coordination in the care of CMC, and enable primary care and specialty practices to provide care coordination among their suite of services. They are currently only in their beginning stages, and their impact on the care and health of CMC will take time to be realized.

## SUGGESTED READINGS


Ader J, Stille CJ, Keller D, Miller BF, Barr MS, Perrin JM. The medical home and integrated behavioral health: advancing the policy agenda. *Pediatrics*. 2015;135(5):909-917.

Berry JG, Hall M, Neff J, et al. Children with medical complexity and Medicaid: spending and cost savings. *Health Aff (Millwood)*. 2014;33(12):2199-2206.

Cohen E, Kuo DZ, Agrawal R, et al. Children with medical complexity: an emerging population for clinical and research initiatives. *Pediatrics*. 2011;127(3):529-538.

Council on Children with Disabilities; Medical Home Implementation Project Advisory Committee. Patient- and family-centered care coordination: a framework for integrating care for children and youth across multiple systems. *Pediatrics*. 2014;133(5):e1451-e1460.

Kuo DZ, Cohen E, Agrawal R, Berry JG, Casey PH. A national profile of caregiver challenges among more medically complex children with special health care needs. *Arch Pediatr Adolesc Med*. 2011;165(11):1020-1026.

McPherson M, Arango P, Fox H, et al. A new definition of children with special health care needs. *Pediatrics*. 1998;102(1, pt 1):137-140.

Medical Home Initiatives for Children with Special Needs Project Advisory Committee, American Academy of Pediatrics. The medical home. *Pediatrics*. 2002;110(1, pt 1):185-186.

Toomey SL, Chien AT, Elliott MN, Ratner J, Schuster MA. Disparities in unmet need for care coordination: the national survey of children's health. *Pediatrics*. 2013;131(2):217-224.

Van Cleave J, Okumura MJ, Swigonski N, O'Connor KG, Mann M, Lail JL. Medical homes for children with special health care needs: primary care or subspecialty service? *Acad Pediatr*. 2016;16(4): 366-372.

Wise PH, Huffman LC, Brat G. *A Critical Analysis of Care Coordination Strategies for Children with Special Health Care Needs*. Technical Review No. 14. AHRQ Publication No. 07-0054. Rockville, MD: Agency for Healthcare Research and Quality; 2007.




# 121 Managing Technology in Children with Medical Complexity

James A. Feinstein, Mark Brittan, and Christopher J. Stille

## INTRODUCTION

In 1987, the former US Office of Technology Assistance defined the medically fragile, technology-dependent child as "one who needs both a medical device to compensate for the loss of a vital body function and substantial ongoing nursing care to avert death or further disability." The continued growth of medical knowledge and technology over the years has led to an increase in the number of children with medical complexity (CMC) who, through the use of technological assistance, live longer and at home, yet still have frequent hospital admissions. While no newer standard definition of medical complexity and fragility has been established, a number of definitions exist with the most common unifying theme being a reliance on medical technology devices, such as the use of a tracheostomy, mechanical ventilation, an enteral feeding tube, or a vascular access device. Some have incorporated the use of assistive devices associated with communication or mobility impairments into the definition of technology assistance. In this chapter, we will review select technology devices and supports, examine the role of specialized therapists to address functionality, and discuss assistive devices and home modifications needed to improve the child's mobility, transportation, and activities of daily living. Educational and communication devices are beyond the scope of this chapter due to their complexity and rapid change (see Chapter 89).

## ASSESSING TECHNOLOGY NEEDS

A child's diagnosis and prognosis should guide the shared decision-making process between the family and the care team about whether to pursue the use of certain medical technologies. The child's family is integral to deciding whether a particular technology support is consistent with their overall goals for their child. Simply because a particular intervention or technology is available rarely means it *must* be performed or acquired, especially if it will not significantly alter the course of a child's ability to meet a goal.

If assistive technology is desired, the choice of support or device requires input from the family and multiple members of the coordination team. The primary care physician and tertiary center program providing care coordination must be able to advise the family on the potential benefits and possible limitations of a certain technology support, particularly if they have specialized expertise (eg, a tracheostomy and ventilator program). Frequently, input from other specialists, therapists, teachers, technology vendors, durable medical equipment companies, and insurers is required to ensure that the technology is appropriate. When assistive technology devices are first placed or revised in the hospital setting, case management should be involved to review and coordinate appropriate home health services for the family.

All technology should maximize the child's participation in developmentally appropriate physical, cognitive, adaptive, and social activities. Thus, it is important to consider child-centered factors (eg, size; growth; anticipated medical, physical, and developmental needs; play) when deciding on the type of support. It is also critical to consider caregiver factors (physical and cognitive) and the environment in which the device will be used (school, home, community), because it will not be used if the family, teachers, and therapists find it unacceptable. Durability, repair services, and expenses must also be considered, particularly when considering high-technology electronic assistive devices. All attempts should be made to prescribe the most appropriate device the first time, because many insurers limit the number of replacements that will be covered over a given period.

Letters of medical necessity justifying prescription of a technology support should document the medical condition, anticipated medical and functional course, the patient goals, and the reasons why less-expensive alternatives are not acceptable. Letters of medical necessity may need to be submitted well in advance of the anticipated need for some items, particularly some of the higher technology and expensive equipment. Should denials of coverage occur, the prescriber must be prepared to write additional letters, place phone calls to the insurer's medical director, and otherwise advocate for reconsideration of authorization. Specialists and therapists experienced with the equipment can be invaluable in this appeal process.

## SELECTED TECHNOLOGY SUPPORTS

### Enteral and Parenteral Nutrition

Children with medical complexity who have swallowing disorders and other gastrointestinal problems often require supplemental or complete enteral or parenteral feeding. It is important to recognize that these children may have very different nutritional needs from healthy children of the same age or size. For example, an oxygen-dependent child with chronic lung disease may have increased caloric needs due to increased work of breathing, and those caloric needs may suddenly decrease if chronic ventilator support is initiated. Monitoring body weight and length and head circumference is necessary in deciding on the individualized nutritional plan. Periodic assessment of trace elements, minerals, and electrolyte balance is also important, particularly when caloric needs are low enough that standard enteral formulas must be diluted. A nutritionist or gastroenterologist is often essential in guiding nutritional management (See Chapters 23 and 25).

A number of technologies support the delivery of enteral nutrition, including nasogastric feeding tubes, gastrostomy tubes (G tubes), or gastrojejunostomy tubes (GJ tubes). Children with medical complexity who require long-term enteral feeding most frequently benefit from G- or GJ-tube placement; this procedure may be combined with a Nissen fundoplication for children at high risk of aspiration. Both G and GJ tubes allow for the controlled delivery of nutrition, fluids, and medications. G-tube feedings can be administered by gravity or with a feeding pump; GJ-tube feedings require a feeding pump. Once out of the postoperative period, parents and caregivers with appropriate training can manage and replace G tubes, including dislodged G tubes, in the home setting. However, GJ tubes must be replaced under x-ray guidance, usually by an interventional radiologist. Families should develop a plan with their provider regarding what to do in the event of a dislodged or malfunctioning tube. Additional complications associated with G and GJ tubes may include irritations or infections of the ostomy site, as well as granulomas at the ostomy site; these complications are best managed by a provider with G- and GJ-tube experience.

### Intravenous Access

Indications for chronic central venous access in CMC include continuous or intermittent intravenous nutrition, chronic intravenous medications or immunotherapy, and assured venous access in precarious children with poor peripheral access. Chronic central venous access can be obtained with a peripherally inserted central catheter (PICC), a tunneled central venous catheter (CVC), or a subcutaneously implanted reservoir and catheter port. Each option is available as either a single lumen or a double lumen device and CVCs are available with 3 lumens. PICCs tend to be used when relatively short periods of access are needed. They pose little danger of pneumothorax or bleeding, but their length and small diameter make clotting of the catheter more frequent and can limit the infusion rate. PICCs are not tunneled under the skin before entering the vein, so there is a greater potential for infection and accidental removal. CVCs are often chosen when frequent or continuous long-term access is needed. Although the collar of a tunneled CVC provides some protection, CVCs may be damaged or dislodged by pulling on the catheter. Ports are used when intermittent but secure chronic central access is required. The reservoir is relatively large and must be accessed with a needle through the skin, making it less attractive for young children. Most providers allow swimming in patients with ports, but discourage it in patients with CVCs despite a lack of evidence that swimming increases infections. Problems with ports include subcutaneous infiltration when the needle is dislodged and surgical removal when infected.

Several problems can arise with chronic central venous access, although evidence-based recommendations for preventing complications are available. Good hand-washing, skin antisepsis, and catheter site dressing are essential. Specialized "central access teams" reduce catheter-related infections, complications, and costs, and these teams are helpful in teaching providers and families how to maintain and troubleshoot problems with the catheter. Antibiotic "lock" or "flush" techniques, in which a vancomycin–heparin solution is instilled in the catheter, are also effective. The "lock" (ie, allowing the solution to dwell in the catheter) may be more effective than simply flushing the solution through the catheter, but concern about vancomycin-resistant organisms has led many to reserve the use of locks for patients with repeated infections. Other approaches to infection in chronic central venous access include the use of antiseptic or antimicrobial-impregnated lines.

Clotting is another major complication of central catheters. Prophylaxis against clots within the catheter is provided by heparin-containing flushes when accessed frequently or by instilling a heparin solution when deaccessing a subcutaneously implanted reservoir and catheter, and monthly thereafter. If blood cannot be withdrawn and a clot is suspected, tissue plasminogen activator may be effective. The high frequency of large vein thromboses associated with central lines is of concern, particularly in children who are dependent on long-term central venous access for survival. Thus, several groups recommend the use of low doses of warfarin or low–molecular-weight heparin, although support for this practice is limited.

### Respiratory Monitoring

**Pulse Oximetry** Many CMC receive supplemental oxygen or ventilator support at home and may benefit from pulse oximetry to maintain safety and provide guidance in adjusting the level of support. The pulse oximeter alarms should be set at levels that alert the caretaker to assess the child and potentially intervene. Setting limits too close to the child's baseline range will result in multiple alarms and decrease use of the monitor. Instructions for the caregivers should include specific parameters for when supplemental oxygen should be initiated (eg, when blood saturation of oxygen [$SpO_2$] is less than 90%) and when the physician should be called.

**Apnea Monitors** Apnea monitors are generally used when CMC with a tracheostomy or mechanical ventilator are asleep or not directly observed by a caregiver. The monitor settings are typically based on the child's age and set in conjunction with the child's pulmonologist and respiratory therapist. Although positive-pressure home ventilators are equipped with high- and low-inspiratory pressure alarms, an apnea alarm can be an important adjunct safety device. For example, the ventilator's low-pressure alarm is designed to alert caregivers to ventilator circuit disconnection, leakage within the ventilator circuit, or tracheostomy tube decannulation. However, the low-pressure alarm may not be triggered after decannulation because of the high resistance of small tracheostomy tubes or after circuit disconnection because the tubing may be obstructed by clothing or bedding.

### Airway Clearance

**Suctioning and Cough-Assist Devices** Airway clearance techniques loosen mucus and clear it from the lungs and upper airway structures. Suctioning is required intermittently in children with tracheostomy tubes and in other conditions (eg, severe cerebral palsy, spinal muscular atrophy) that cause copious secretions and decreased airway clearance. Portable suction machines are typically used for travel, and stationary machines are used in the home. A mechanical cough-assist device (insufflator-exsufflator) is used to stimulate a cough in individuals with neuromuscular weakness. The cough-assist device gradually applies a positive pressure to the airway via a mask or mouthpiece, then rapidly shifts to a negative pressure. In children with muscular dystrophy, insufflator-exsufflator has been shown to be safe, well-tolerated, and effective in preventing pulmonary complications.

**High-Frequency Chest Compression** High-frequency chest compression (HFCC) is indicated for assistance with airway clearance in patients with cystic fibrosis and is increasingly used for other conditions that result in difficulty mobilizing pulmonary secretions and lead to recurrent pneumonia or atelectasis. The HFCC device consists of 2 components: an air delivery device with a motor-driven valve and an inflatable vest. The air delivery device creates oscillating air pressure that is delivered to the vest via hoses. This action produces high-frequency chest compressions that create an oscillatory effect within the airways to help mobilize bronchial secretions. Generally, the frequency and pressure of the HFCC are set at 10 to 15 Hz and 4 to 6 cm of water, respectively, for 20 minutes 2 to 3 times per day.

### Oxygen

Supplemental oxygen is commonly prescribed for home use in CMC who have chronic lung disease, congenital heart disease, neuromuscular weakness, or chronic respiratory insufficiency (with or without mechanical ventilation). A general guideline is that the child must require a fraction of inspired oxygen ($FiO_2$) less than or equal to 0.35 to be discharged from the hospital, and caregivers should contact the physician when a higher $FiO_2$ is required to maintain saturations at a predefined acceptable level at home. In the hospital, blenders and mechanical ventilators are capable of delivering a specific $FiO_2$. At home, 100% oxygen is generally delivered and the desired $FiO_2$ is achieved by varying the flow rate via nasal cannula, mask, tracheostomy collar, or ventilator. The amount of air entrained with each breath determines the actual $FiO_2$ received by the child. As a general rule, the $FiO_2$ likely exceeds 0.35 when oxygen flow through a nasal cannula exceeds 2 liters per minute in infants or 3 to 4 liters per minute in older children, when Venturi-type valves calibrated for greater than 35% $O_2$ are used, when nonrebreather masks are used, and when flow exceeds 4 liters per minute on a home ventilator. It may be helpful to measure the relationship between flow and $FiO_2$ on a home ventilator prior to discharging the child from the hospital.

Oxygen is supplied in liquid form, as a compressed gas, or from an oxygen concentrator. Liquid oxygen is more portable, and lightweight liquid oxygen tanks can be refilled from a large reservoir tank kept at home. However, liquid oxygen may cost more and may not last as long as compressed oxygen because it evaporates. Moreover, liquid oxygen is cold and can burn if it comes into contact with the skin. Compressed oxygen is available in cylinders, ranging in size from small portable tanks to large stationary tanks for home use. An oxygen concentrator is an electric machine that can deliver approximately 4 liters per minute of 100% oxygen. The percentage decreases at higher flow rates. It is recommended that families using a concentrator have a backup cylinder of compressed oxygen in case of a power failure. All families should be reminded never to smoke or allow others to smoke when oxygen is being used.

### Tracheostomy

Children require tracheostomy tubes for indications including upper airway obstruction (eg, anatomic abnormalities), airway protection (eg, aspiration risk), and long-term ventilation (eg, chronic lung disease). The tracheostomy tube is placed surgically, after which the child is generally monitored in the intensive care unit until the first tracheostomy tube change in 5 to 7 days. "Stay sutures" are placed on each side of the tracheal incision to facilitate reinsertion of the tube if it becomes dislodged before the stoma has matured. Complications in the early postoperative period include accidental decannulation, obstruction of the tube, infection, hemorrhage, and creation of a false passage if the tube is improperly replaced. In general, 25% to 50% of children with tracheostomy tubes will eventually have complications (typically infections and obstruction), but death from a complication is rare.

The selection of the tracheostomy tube is based on several factors. The tube should be at least 1 to 2 cm above the carina and the diameter should be selected to avoid pressure on the tracheal wall, minimize work of breathing, and, if possible, promote translaryngeal airflow in order to facilitate vocalization. Pediatric tracheostomy tubes are generally composed of silicone, which is quite flexible, or polyvinyl chloride, which may be either flexible or rigid. They are characterized by internal diameter, outer diameter, and cannula length, but are usually referred to by their internal diameter. A neonatal tracheostomy tube has a shorter cannula and neck flange. The tracheostomy tube may have an inflatable cuff to reduce the risk of aspiration and/or help reduce the "leak" when requiring ventilator support. Depending on the manufacturer, the cuff should be inflated with either air or sterile water.

Adequate humidification of the trachea to minimize thick secretions in the tracheostomy tube is accomplished by using a tracheostomy collar with humidified oxygen or air when sleeping and when ill. During travel and other activities, the tracheostomy tube can be covered with a heat and moisture exchanger (HME), speaking valve, or cap. The speaking valve is a 1-way valve that allows air to pass into the tube on inspiration, but forces air back through the vocal cords on expiration. Children with tracheostomies generally require suctioning at least 3 to 4 times per day and more frequently during times of respiratory illness. Signs that a child needs suctioning include rattling mucus sounds, tachypnea, secretions pooling at the opening of the tracheostomy tube, or signs of respiratory distress. Normal saline drops instilled prior to suctioning help loosen the thick secretions or elicit a cough. The size of the suction catheter depends on the size of the tracheostomy tube. Shallow suctioning removes secretions at the opening of the tracheostomy. Suctioning just past the tip of the tracheostomy tube allows complete clearance. The desired depth of the suction catheter can be calculated as tracheostomy length + adapter length + up to 5 mm. Suctioning until the catheter meets resistance from the carina should generally be avoided, as this may injure the lining of the airway. Applying suction pressure both on insertion and on withdrawal of the suction catheter facilitates removal of the secretions. Following suctioning, many children with tracheostomy tubes may benefit from a few manual ventilation breaths to rerecruit the lung.

The child with a tracheostomy tube must be attended at all times by a trained adult caregiver who knows emergency tracheostomy management. A "to-go" bag containing a suction machine with suction catheters, extra tracheostomy tubes (1 of the same size and 1 a size smaller), ties, gloves, saline vials, a water-soluble lubricant, an extra HME, a manual resuscitation device, and any inhaled respiratory medications must accompany the child when outside the home.

### Mechanical Ventilation

**Noninvasive Mechanical Ventilation** Noninvasive mechanical ventilation is accomplished without an endotracheal airway using either positive- or negative-pressure support. Improved pediatric-appropriate masks and portable ventilators designed for home use have helped make intermittent noninvasive positive-pressure mechanical ventilation a reasonable therapeutic option for an increasing number of CMC who have chronic upper airway obstruction or progressive respiratory insufficiency. Cognitively intact CMC can be managed with continuous noninvasive mechanical ventilation using a combination of mask and positive-pressure ventilation at night and a positive-pressure ventilator attached to a small mouthpiece that the child can intermittently trigger to receive a full ventilator breath ("sip and puff") during the day. The use of noninvasive mechanical ventilation has been shown to reduce pneumonia or atelectasis, improve gas exchange, reduce hospitalizations, and improve sleep quality.

**Invasive Mechanical Ventilation** Long-term invasive ventilation refers to the application of positive-pressure ventilation through a tracheostomy tube. There are no specific guidelines for inducing invasive mechanical ventilation. In general, this mode is chosen when noninvasive ventilation interfaces are not accepted or tolerated, when the need for ventilatory support exceeds a major part of the day and the child cannot cooperate with the "sip and puff" device, or when bulbar function is impaired and a tracheostomy tube is required for airway hygiene. Children with medical complexity who require invasive mechanical ventilation can be safely cared for at home and successfully reintegrated into the community. Caregivers (including nurses and respite caregivers) should be formally trained in how to provide care for these children. In general, medical cost comparisons between hospital and home care reveal that for most children, care at home was less expensive than in a hospital, although this is somewhat dependent on the complexity of the child's care, the amount of nursing care required at home, the number and duration of readmissions to the hospital, and the ability of parents to provide unpaid care.

### Functionality and Mobility

Chronic illness and significant injury in childhood usually result in impairment, defined by the World Health Organization (WHO) as any loss or abnormality of psychological, physical, or anatomic structure or function. Disability is the limitation in activity caused by impairment. Handicap exists when an impairment or disability limits or prevents participation in a role that is normal for age and gender, within the social and cultural milieu. Goals of management of pediatric chronic disease and disability include minimizing the impairment and maximizing activity and participation in age-appropriate life roles (school, play, work). The approach to care is often interdisciplinary and should be coordinated, comprehensive, and family-centered.

The major objective in disability management is to facilitate independent function in the particular areas—referred to as domains—that are affected. Function is promoted in mobility, self-care, communication, cognition, and/or psychosocial domains. In each area, efforts are initially directed toward assisting the child to accomplish skills independently. This is accomplished through treatment strategies that enhance the functional capacity either of the affected system, when skills can be restored or developed, or through compensatory strategies using systems unaffected by the pathologic condition. Secondary disability should be prevented to the extent possible. When necessary, prescription of equipment or modifications to the physical or social environment may provide the child with greater independence. Psychological and educational techniques may also enhance patient performance. Prescriptions for therapy programs, adaptive equipment, orthoses, and prostheses should be age appropriate and include consideration of the child's ongoing growth and development.

**Specialized Therapists** Because of their role in coordinating care, physicians (whether in the tertiary center or primary care setting) must clearly understand the roles and functions of the specialized therapists who have relevant expertise. Care teams for CMC may include physical and occupational therapists, speech language pathologists, nutritionists, respiratory therapists, pharmacists, child-life specialists, and nurse case managers, all of whom play a critical role in planning and delivering appropriate care for CMC. Many or all of these specialized therapists are simultaneously involved when providing care for the most complex CMC, and frequent communication between the entire care team is necessary to ensure coordinated care.

Most commonly, physical therapists, occupational therapists, and speech pathologists are involved with CMC. Physical therapy addresses problems associated with neuromuscular dysfunction and gross motor delay as they influence the child's ability to be mobile within the environment. Occupational therapy addresses problems with neuromuscular dysfunction, sensory perception, psychosocial competence, and fine motor delay as they influence the child's ability to participate in self-care, play, and school activities. In practice, there is often considerable overlap in the methods and techniques used by the 2 disciplines, especially with very young children. In general, children should be referred for physical therapy evaluation when there is a delay in gross motor development or concern about the child's quality of movement. Children should be referred for occupational therapy evaluation when there is reason to suspect impairment in the performance of age-appropriate daily tasks or routines, including self-care, play, or social interaction, or in the execution of school-related activities that have a perceptual-motor component. Referral should include a complete diagnosis, information about relevant precautions (eg, allergies, weight-bearing status, exercise tolerance), and the reason for referral. In addition, copies of previous evaluations help the therapist avoid repeating unnecessary interviews pertaining to the child's medical background or developmental history.

Speech-language pathologists are professionals who are educated in the study of human communication, including normal development and communication disorders. Speech-language pathologists are also trained to recognize neurologic and upper aerodigestive disorders that affect speech and swallowing. By evaluating the speech, language, cognitive-communication, and swallowing skills of children with disabilities, the speech-language pathologist can determine specific deficits, the severity of the disorder (often based on age-level norms), and possible etiologic and contributing factors. This information forms the basis of a treatment plan for the child. The recommendations may include formal therapy or parent training and consultation with periodic rechecks. Depending on the type of disorder, therapy may include exercises to improve oral-motor skills, exercises to develop appropriate articulation placement, or activities to develop functional language skills. Some children lack the basic prerequisites for verbal communication for a variety of causes (ie, tracheostomy, significant hearing loss, neuromuscular disorder). For those children, augmentative or alternative communication systems are developed. Regardless of the type of therapy, parent involvement is a key component of the treatment process. Therefore, parents are encouraged to observe the therapy sessions whenever possible and are given instructions for working with the child at home. It is important to note that early intervention is critical for the best long-term prognosis.

**Orthoses** Orthoses can be defined as custom-fitted devices applied to or around a body segment that are designed to meet specific musculoskeletal goals, such as (1) prevention of movement because of abnormal tone or movement that is involuntary, (2) maintenance of joint alignment to facilitate body mechanics, and (3) stabilization of a joint. Acronyms used to describe orthoses generally refer to the body part (eg, *AFO* is the acronym for *ankle-foot orthosis*). The family and child should meet with a specialist skilled in functionality (eg, rehabilitation, neurodevelopmental pediatrics, or orthopedics) and the child's therapists to establish the goals and appropriate use and care of an orthosis before it is prescribed. Orthoses should be simple, durable, strong, easy to use, lightweight, and cosmetically pleasing. They must fit well and be used as prescribed to be effective. The child's condition and the purpose of the orthosis should be indicated on the prescription and consultation with an orthotist considered. Shoes for use with orthotics should have a wide toe box with an upper of soft leather, canvas, synthetic, or nylon fabric and a tongue that goes far down into the toe box. Specialty shoes are expensive, but insurers may reimburse the family if a prescription and letter of medical necessity are presented. Skin breakdown is the most common complication of orthoses. Skin should be checked daily, and if an area of redness lasts longer than 20 to 30 minutes, the orthotist or physician should be notified. The goals, fit, and use of the orthoses should be reviewed at least every 6 months until growth stabilizes and each time the child experiences therapist transitions (eg, when starting school).

**Wheeled Mobility and Seating** A child's inability to master the environment independently may lead to decreased socialization, learned helplessness, and delayed development. Therefore, wheeled mobility should be considered as early as necessary to facilitate developmentally appropriate independence and functional activity (Table 121-1). Because poor positioning and restriction of movement can result in pressure areas and musculoskeletal deformity, mobility devices are often combined with customized positioning or seating systems when the child needs assistance to maintain appropriate position and use of the trunk, head, or limbs. Multiple physical impairments may lead to the need for wheeled mobility (eg, weakness, low endurance, movement disorders, abnormal tone, or pain syndromes). The type of wheeled mobility should be based on the child's immediate and anticipated needs and goals (eg, duration of need, ability to self-propel, other assistive technology, surgery, ability to partially ambulate), family issues (eg, transportation, access, lifting restrictions), and the proposed environment in which the device will be used. Although 12- to 18-month-old children with normal cognition have been demonstrated to use powered mobility safely, evaluation for motorized options requires detailed assessment of sensory, motor, cognitive, and behavioral status, as well as consideration of accessibility.

**Car Restraints and Transportation** Most CMC will be safest when positioned facing rearward in the back seat of the car for as long

**TABLE 121-1 WHEELED MOBILITY**

| | Types | Indications | Advantages | Limitations | Comments |
|---|---|---|---|---|---|
| **Passive** | Strollers | Mild to moderate impairment | Lightweight<br>Easily transported and stored | Does not accommodate other assistive technologies<br>Uncomfortable with limited custom seating options | Good for quick transport short distances |
| | Manual upright wheelchairs | Functionally nonambulatory in some settings | Frame allows custom seating<br>Facilitates self-mobility goals | Heavier and more expensive than a stroller<br>Limited insurance coverage for needed replacement due to growth or other factors<br>Must tolerate prolonged upright positioning | Avoid unnecessary restraint of head or limbs during activity |
| | Manual tilt-in-space wheelchairs | Significantly impaired head and trunk control | Accommodates position changes and respiratory impairment | Heavier than manual wheelchair<br>Larger turning radius and may not fit in small car trunks<br>Cannot be easily and efficiently self-propelled | Minitilt of the back can facilitate self-propulsion |
| **Active** | Manual upright wheelchairs | Nonambulatory or partially ambulatory with good trunk control | Lightweight and portable<br>Good for learning self-propulsion | When endurance is low, the chair can maneuver only level surfaces and considerable energy may be expended | Wheelchairs for sports and 1-arm drive are available |
| | Power wheelchairs | Nonambulatory with cognitive level 2–3 years and insufficient motor control/endurance for a manual chair | Multiple seating and positioning options<br>Increased control over environment<br>Accommodates assistive technology | Heavy and generally requires vehicle lift<br>Repairs may be costly<br>Must have the ability to store, operate, and maintain a complex device | Emotional and behavioral challenges must be considered |
| | Scooters | Impaired lower extremity strength and/or need to conserve energy | Less expensive and lighter than power wheelchair | Minimal seating options for poor tone | Progressive neuromuscular disorders should be excluded prior to purchase |

as possible (Table 121-2). Others will require alternative restraints. Commercially available car beds are designed to accommodate infants in the 1.8 to 9 kg range. Car beds are indicated for low–birth-weight infants (less than 2.3 kg) who failed conventional car seat testing prior to discharge and infants with other selected conditions. Padding must not be placed between the infant and the car bed or the harness system because it may interfere with the effectiveness of the restraint system. Safety vests are designed for children at least 2 years old, weighing between 9 and 76 kg. These children cannot sit safely in a conventional car seat or wear appropriate lap belt or shoulder harness because of motor, behavioral, or positioning problems. The safety vest is applied prior to placing a child in the car and then it is anchored to the vehicle by a tether strap and seatbelt.

Specialized car seats are designed for children between 10 and 48 kg who require more physical support than is provided by conventional seats. The Federal Motor Vehicle Safety Standard status of the particular model should be verified before prescribing or advising a family on its purchase. Parents should be trained in appropriate application of necessary tethers and harness fit, since problems with restraints usually arise from inappropriate application and fit of tether and harness.

**TABLE 121-2 VEHICLE RESTRAINTS**

| Types | Indications | Conditions | Advantages | Limitations | Comments |
|---|---|---|---|---|---|
| Car beds | Infant who cannot sit in car seat | < 2.3 kg body weight<br>Instability in sitting position<br>Risk of fractures<br>Casts or surgery | Infant may ride on back, front, or right side | For babies < 10 kg<br>More vulnerable during side impact | Place head toward center of vehicle to protect in case of side impact |
| Travel vests | Child > 2 to < 9 years of age and < 76 kg unable to sit safely in conventional car seat | Severe motor, behavioral, or positioning problems due to casts, contractures, or respiratory compromise | Variety of models<br>Optional crotch strap<br>Child can be semireclined | Must be used in the backseat<br>Tether required for installation | Child should be in rear seat and fitted by specialist |
| Safety vests | Child 10–40 kg unable to sit upright | Reclined need for child with cast, contracture, or small hips | Can be used upright, supine, prone, or side lying | Child must fit on bench seat, must be > 2 yr | Requires 2 seatbelts if child > 30 lb |
| Wheelchair restraints | Child in wheelchair, but travel safer in properly fitted car seat | | Eliminates need for mechanically difficult transfers | Injuries more likely if belts, harnesses, headrest not configured for travel restraint | If wheelchair travel is necessary, use crash-tested model with 4-point tie-down system in forward-facing position<br>Secure child with 3-point belts |

Additional consideration in the use of car restraints applies to selected populations. Children with tracheostomies should avoid restraint systems that may impair ventilation or risk impact to the tracheostomy tube in an accident. They should be kept facing the rear in a convertible, well-fitting car seat. When the seat is turned forward, one must ensure that the chin does not cover the tracheostomy. Pulse oximetry can be used to verify appropriate saturations while seated in the car seat. Children with seizure disorders should be in restraints that will provide appropriate support of airway during and after a seizure. A specialized car seat restraint may be necessary for a child weighing more than 20 kg who has frequent seizures, because this is the usual upper weight limit for commercial car seats with harness straps. Children with hypotonia and/or risk for high cervical subluxation (eg, Down syndrome, achondroplasia) or fractures (eg, osteogenesis imperfecta) should use a rear-facing car seat as long as possible. A standard convertible child safety seat allows children weighing up to 15 kg to face rearward.

Children who use wheelchairs should ride in a properly fitting car seat rather than in the wheelchair whenever possible. If transport in the wheelchair is necessary, it should be secured in a forward-facing position with 4-point tie-downs for the chair and a separate 3-point belt restraint for the child. Trays must be removed and head support is strongly advised. Other medical equipment should be anchored to the floor, if possible. There are no tethers made specifically for medical equipment in a private vehicle. Thus, options include placing the equipment under the vehicle seat or wedging it in place with pillows, foam, or blankets. Unused seat belts may also be used to ensure that the equipment will remain secured in the event of a crash. Batteries for equipment should be dry cell or gel cell to limit flammability.

**Transfer Aids and Lifts** Many medically fragile and complex children with special healthcare needs will attain close to adult size and weight. Some are able to bear weight but need assistance to move from 1 surface to another. Safe and efficient transfers require skill and practice. Therapists can instruct caregivers in appropriate techniques. A full-lift transfer is required if the child bears no weight when being transferred. Transfer aids should be considered for any child who weighs more than 25 kg and cannot be safely transferred by 1 caregiver alone. Aids should also be considered for children with inconsistent ability to assist in transfers (eg, frequent seizures, behavioral issues, variable endurance) or when caregivers cannot safely lift a child. There is no single transfer aid that accomplishes full-lift transfers in all settings from all surfaces. If possible, the family should try the equipment before buying it; if the mechanical aid is not easy and efficient, they will likely revert to lifting the child manually. Some insurers consider transfer aids medically necessary only for transfers between bed and chair, wheelchair, or commode. Reimbursement for toilet lifts and ceiling lifts mounted on tracks will often require strong advocacy. Bathing a baby is relatively easy compared with transferring and positioning a slippery child, particularly when the child has poor head control or severely affected muscle tone. When children have episodic emergencies (eg, seizures or mucus plugs in a tracheostomy), bathing equipment that allows the caretaker use of both hands is essential. Bathing equipment should provide comfortable restraint and positioning while ensuring safety during medical emergencies. Anticipated growth, changes in medical condition, limitations of the bathroom space, and the need to accommodate other family members should all be considered when evaluating bathroom equipment.

As with much durable medical equipment, it is often best to test equipment prior to purchase or purchase from a vendor that allows exchanges in case it does not meet family and child goals. Low-technology options for the child with good head and trunk control, but with poor balance, include waterproof upright corner chairs with anterior trunk supports and pelvic belts. Medium-technology systems restrain the child in a semireclining position and are made for the child who cannot sit or maintain head control. Features include adjustable seat and back, trunk and pelvic harness, leg straps, and adjustable frame height for easier transfers. High-technology systems include a battery-operated, push-button lift for individuals from ages 3 years old to adult.

**Access to and in the Home** Remodeling should be considered when access to the home or living spaces limits caregiving, the child's anticipated acquisition of independence skills, or the safety of child and caregiver. Home adaptations also can improve the child's ability to perform activities of daily living (eg, eating, dressing, hygiene) and participate in social and avocational activities within both the family unit and the community. Input from developmental and rehabilitation specialists and therapists can help families develop realistic goals and plan environmental modifications. Leveling thresholds and investing in automatic power door openers can improve access through the front door. External doorways should be widened to 36 in if possible. The majority of homes have at least 1 or 2 steps leading up to the external door. Building codes require that wheelchair ramps be 12 in long for every 1 in rise. Ramps should be a minimum of 36 in wide, have enclosed handrails, and have a 5-ft-square level area for maneuvering on the landing. Vertical platform lifts consist of a platform attached to a tower that houses an electric motor and drive mechanism. They have a lifting height of 12 ft and require 30 sq ft of space. Porch lifts are similar to vertical platform lifts but have a maximum lifting height of about 6 ft. They are especially useful when space is limited. Chair lifts enable the user to be carried up the stairs and can be used both inside and outside and on straight or curved stairways, but are not appropriate for children who use a wheelchair full time. All renovations are relatively expensive and may not be reimbursed by insurance companies. Families should be aware that many state programs offer financial assistance for any necessary home remodeling if the home is owned, but often not for rental homes. Alternative solutions for moving the child during an emergency must be considered.

Bathrooms are often the smallest rooms in the house, with a narrow doorway and turning radius that limits easy access to the toilet, sink, and bath and shower. Low-tech solutions include installing a hand shower in the bathtub, using single-lever faucets, and modifying the toilet by raising or lowering the toilet seat height. The use of a bath or shower chair and a commode with needed supports is often helpful. Minor modifications to the bathroom include using nonskid tile and removing counter cabinets to increase wheelchair accessibility. Call buttons and intercoms can be installed for emergency assistance. High-technology solutions include ceiling-mounted lift, power bathtub lift, electronic faucets, self-flushing toilets, and walk-in baths or showers.

Access to the bedroom is also essential. Low-technology modifications include simply adjusting the bed height for ease of transfer; changing from swinging to sliding doors to increase space and visibility within closets, and lowering closet shelves so that a child, short adult, or seated person can choose clothing. A bedside compact refrigerator is often useful for fluids or medications, and an emergency button or intercom to request assistance is essential. Higher-tech solutions include power beds. Similar accommodations throughout the home (eg, kitchen and living room) can make it possible for the child to reach different rooms and participate to the best of his or her abilities.

## EMERGENCY PREPAREDNESS

Because CMC and the technologies they rely upon require access to basic services like power, water, heat, cooling, communication, and transportation, parents and caregivers must have an emergency preparedness plan should an environmental emergency disrupt these services. The Federal Emergency Management Agency (FEMA) provides detailed information on preparing for an emergency for individuals with special healthcare needs (https://www.ready.gov/individuals-access-functional-needs). The FEMA information recommends that parents make a written plan, and that they also (1) keep a disaster supply kit of emergency supplies at home, including basic supplies for survival, as well as the child's health information, extra medical supplies, equipment, and health provider contact numbers; (2) create a support network, including relatives, friends, caregivers, and neighbors, who can provide coordinated assistance during an emergency; (3) develop a communication plan with the support network to send and receive updates on the situation; and (4) alert local police, fire, and utility (water, electricity) companies that a child with medical complexity lives in the home so that each can prioritize their rescue efforts or restoration of services in the event of an emergency.

## SUGGESTED READINGS


Alexander MA, Matthews DJ. *Pediatric Rehabilitation: Principles and Practice.* 4th ed. New York, NY: Demos Medical; 2009.

Berry JG, Hall DE, Kuo DZ, et al. Hospital utilization and characteristics of patients experiencing recurrent readmissions within children's hospitals. *JAMA.* 2011;305(7):682-690.

Bull M, Agran P, Laraque D, et al. American Academy of Pediatrics. Committee on Injury and Poison Prevention. Transporting children with special health care needs. *Pediatrics.* 1999;104(4, pt 1):988-992.

Center for Universal Design, NC State University College of Design. Residential rehabilitation, remodeling and universal design. 2006. https://www.ncsu.edu/ncsu/design/cud/pubs_p/docs/residential_remodelinl.pdf. Accessed January 22, 2018.

DeLegge MH. Consensus statements regarding optimal management of home enteral nutrition (HEN) access. *JPEN J Parenter Enteral Nutr.* 2006;30(1 Suppl):S39-S40.

Fox D, Brittan M, Stille C. The Pediatric Inpatient Family Care Conference: a proposed structure toward shared decision-making. *Hosp Pediatr.* 2014;4(5):305-310.

Haffner JC, Schurman SJ. The technology-dependent child. *Pediatr Clin North Am.* 2001;48(3):751-764.

Norregaard O. Noninvasive ventilation in children. *Eur Respir J.* 2002;20(5):1332-1342.

O'Neil J, Bull MJ, Sobus K. Issues and approaches to safely transporting children with special healthcare needs. *J Pediatr Rehabil Med.* 2011;4(4):279-288.

Sherman JM, Davis S, Albamonte-Petrick S, et al. Care of the child with a chronic tracheostomy. This official statement of the American Thoracic Society was adopted by the ATS Board of Directors, July 1999. *Am J Respir Crit Care Med.* 2000;161(1):297-308.

Spratling R. Defining technology dependence in children and adolescents. *West J Nurs Res.* 2015;37(5):634-651.

Zhu H, Das P, Roberson DW, et al. Hospitalizations in children with preexisting tracheostomy: a national perspective. *Laryngoscope.* 2015;125(2):462-468.


# 122 Managing Children with Intellectual and Developmental Disabilities

Heather Moore and Carl D. Tapia

## INTRODUCTION

Childhood development occurs in biological, psychological, social, and emotional domains, and progresses from complete dependence to autonomy. Development—while predictable and linear—does not progress synchronously for each individual. Disparities in the progression of abilities should be recognized early and intervention started as soon as possible.

Intelligence is the ability to learn, reason, problem solve, and navigate the world independently. Adaptive behavior refers to the skills to successfully function in the community. It is comprised of conceptual skills such as language and literacy; social skills such as interpersonal interactions, self-awareness, and self-esteem; and practical skills such as activities of daily living, instrumental activities of daily living, and occupational skills. Global developmental delay describes delay in children less than 5 years of age in 2 or more developmental domains noted above. This delay is thought to be a predictor of future intellectual disability (ID), but not all children with global developmental delay progress to the diagnosis of ID. ID is a neurodevelopmental disorder described as deficits in both cognitive intelligence and adaptive skills occurring before the age of 18 years. ID is anticipated to be lifelong. It is estimated that 1% to 3% of the general population is affected with ID. Many conditions are associated with ID, and so the presentation is variable. Therefore, treatment strategies must be flexible and individualized.

Individuals with ID, particularly those with higher severity disabilities, have less frequent receipt of recommended preventive care and a greater mortality rate compared to the general population. Routine care as well as treatment of associated limitations and concurrent disorders is therefore crucial. The current emphasis of treatment for ID is habilitation, or promoting function to achieve the highest capability and minimizing or preventing deterioration. Most systems prioritize keeping children in their homes or communities and not in institutions. It should be stressed that the sooner the recognition of developmental delay and the initiation of treatment occur, the better the outcome will be. This chapter focuses on the evaluation and management of intellectual and developmental disabilities for children with medical complexity.

## EVALUATION OF INTELLECTUAL AND DEVELOPMENTAL DISABILITY

Preventive care is the backbone of clinical services for children. Well-child visits occur frequently in the first 2 years and provide an excellent opportunity for surveillance of developmental progression and detection of delays. Developmental delays in the older child may present as behavior concerns or school failure. Once an abnormality is detected, the clinician can then evaluate the types and degree of delay and begin to consider differential diagnoses.

A general approach should begin with a thorough history and physical examination. Complete prenatal and birth histories should be reviewed for factors associated with genetic or metabolic disorders, birth trauma, or substance abuse. The past medical history should be reviewed for developmental milestones, abnormalities in newborn screening, established or suspected diagnoses, healthcare utilization patterns, and previous concern for developmental disorder. The family history (at least 3 generations) may reveal important information with respect to inheritable disorders. A detailed physical examination should include growth parameters, attention to dysmorphisms, and a careful neurologic evaluation.

Further screening that uses a number of validated and standardized tools may be completed. If an underlying genetic syndrome is present or suspected, evaluation for associated comorbidities (such as thyroid disorders in children with Down syndrome) should be considered. While referral to a developmental or neurological specialist may be warranted, it should not delay initiation of treatment (for further details, see Chapter 87).

## CARING FOR CHILDEN WITH INTELLECTUAL AND DEVELOPMENTAL DISABILITY

### The Medical Home

The American Academy of Pediatrics highly recommends that health care of infants, children, adolescence, and young adults be accessible, continuous, comprehensive, family centered, coordinated, compassionate, and culturally effective; this is the definition of the medical home approach to care. Access to a medical home is of particular importance for the infant/toddler with global developmental delay or the child/adolescent with ID.

The initial step in the management of a child with developmental delay or ID is establishment of care within a family-centered medical home and with a well-trained clinician able to provide ongoing high-quality care to the patient. The clinician should review previous clinical evaluations and prescribed interventions and therapies, and discuss with the family the effectiveness of the interventions. A multidisciplinary team that can provide preventive care, developmental and behavioral evaluation, clinical supervision of associated conditions, care coordination, referrals to community resources, and support for the family is optimal. The team should also give consideration to the goals and preferences of the family and plan accordingly. A special-needs patient registry should be maintained within the practice, and any child with developmental delay or ID should be included on the list and reviewed at regular intervals to ensure regular follow-up and completion of referrals and recommended care. A review of specialist care and healthcare utilization is helpful to assess barriers to progress. A care summary and care plan should reflect current interventions, medications, therapies, procedures, and future planned care. Early referral for developmental support—such as early intervention services under Part C of the Individuals with Disabilities Education Act or speech, occupational, and physical therapy—is critical.

#### Comorbidities in Children with Intellectual and Developmental Disability

A considerable percentage of children with ID have other chronic conditions. The clinician should be aware of the most common comorbidities, ready to guide parents with recommendations and provide specialty referrals as needed (see Chapter 126). Behavioral concerns, academic advancement, and social interactions may all worsen in the face of unrecognized comorbidities. It is estimated that 60% to 70% of children with ID present with significant behavioral concerns. Approximately 10% to 60% of children with ID also have diagnosed behavioral health conditions, much higher than in the general population. The presence of cooccurring behavioral health conditions is predictive of limitations in academic advancement, occupational accomplishment, and social inclusion, and is often more important than the severity of the ID alone. Early detection of behavioral health comorbidity is essential, as these disorders often persist across the lifespan for children with ID. It is estimated that only 10% of children and adolescents with ID receive appropriate specialized behavioral health services.

Feeding disorders often coincide with the presence of ID and often lead to malnutrition, vitamin deficiency, and micronutrient deficiency. Oral dysphagia, food aversions, and textural issues interfere with the eating experience of some children with ID and can impact caloric intake. Clinicians should probe for very prolonged eating times, loss of oral skills, food refusal, repetitive emesis, coughing/choking with meals, irritability with feeding time, drooling, and food hoarding in the mouth. Gastroesophageal reflux is notably more common in children with ID but may be unrecognized in the child with communication deficits. Parents may overestimate eating skills or caloric intake. Examination by a speech pathologist, occupational therapist, or gastrointestinal specialist may be warranted for concerns of dysphagia, refractory poor growth, or concern for recurrent aspiration. Particular importance should be paid to the oral health of children with ID, as often they are resistant to oral care and therefore prone to gingivitis, dental caries, and periodontitis. Dental interventions by a team familiar with ID may be needed. Vitamin and micronutrient replacement should be considered, along with supplemental feedings, if the child exhibits significant malnutrition. In more severe cases, gastrostomy tube placement may be necessary.

Children with ID are more likely to suffer from sleep disturbances. Poor sleep may be present in up to 85% of children with ID. Symptoms of poor sleep include excessive daytime sleepiness, hyperactivity, and aggressive behavior—all of which can lead to a decline in overall functioning. A sleep study should be considered if there is concern for obstructive sleep apnea or other sleep disorders. Attention to good sleep hygiene is important, but may be complicated by behavior disturbances and altered sleep–wake cycles (for further information, see Chapter 502).

#### The Education System

Every child over 3 years of age with a diagnosis of ID should have a full diagnostic evaluation completed within the public school system. The clinician should be familiar with the rights of families and responsibilities of the school system for special education services (see Chapter 86). The goal is optimal education of the child in the least restrictive environment. The clinician and team should advocate for necessary related services, such as therapies, psychological counseling, therapeutic physical education activities, and social work assistance. The clinician and/or other team members should assist the family and school in setting appropriate but challenging goals. For children with medical comorbidities, the clinician should guide the plan of care for medical interventions during the school day and must be accessible to school personnel for changes in medical status.

Some families—perhaps concerned about previous experiences in the school system, exposure to viral illnesses, or harm from other children—may request homebound services or choose not to enroll their child in school. The clinician should be sensitive to these concerns but should help advocate for the best placement that suits the child's developmental and educational needs.

#### Family Support

Caregivers of children with ID suffer more stress compared to matched caregivers of children without ID, which may lead to worse health outcomes. Disruptive behaviors may emerge as young as 2.5 to 3 years of age, adding to the cumulative stress of caring for a child with a disability and functional delays. The healthcare team should screen for caregiver burnout and caregiver stress, and provide encouragement, regular follow-up, and referrals for respite care, attendant services, parent support groups, faith-based organizations, advocacy associations, and financial resources.

Siblings of intellectually disabled children may exhibit behavior concerns. Clinicians can assist by explaining the child's diagnosis and answering questions at an appropriate developmental level, and promoting good communication and normalization of feelings such as guilt, jealousy, anger, and shame. As children with disabilities may outlive their parents, it is important to include older siblings in long-term planning. Caregivers should be encouraged to pursue therapy or counseling when necessary.

#### Community Inclusion

The child with ID may have barriers to forming emotional connections and healthy attachments with peers. They may also spend more time with adults, be less likely to participate in group activities, and be more likely to experience bullying. However, friendships are associated with better quality of life and improved socioemotional development. Attention should be given to fostering peer relationships and encouraging involvement in peer-based social encounters and physical activities.

When children with ID are integrated into general classrooms, studies show no disruption to the academic achievements of others in the class. Children with delays have been shown to gain communication abilities and motor skills through interactions with typically developing classmates. Students with cognitive delays demonstrate higher levels of engaged behavior, spend less time alone or solely with adults, and devote a greater amount of time to academic work.

### SUMMARY

Several factors are critical in the care of the child with developmental or ID. It is important to establish care in a medical home experienced in caring for children with disabilities. Comorbidities should be identified and addressed. Early intervention for developmental support is crucial. Advocacy within the education system may be needed to ensure the appropriate placement and provision of services. Caregiver and sibling support is vital. Community activities and opportunities for peer interaction and meaningful friendships allow for greater quality of life and achievement.

### SUGGESTED READINGS

American Academy of Pediatrics Committee on Children with Disabilities. The pediatrician's role in development and implementation of an Individual Education Plan (IEP) and/or an Individual Family Service Plan (IFSP). *Pediatrics.* 1999;104(1, pt 1):124-127.

American Academy of Pediatrics Council on Children with Disabilities; Cartwright JD. Provision of educationally related services for children and adolescents with chronic diseases and disabling conditions. *Pediatrics.* 2007;119(6):1218-1223.

Dessemonte SR, Bless G. The impact of including children with intellectual disability in general education classrooms on the academic achievement of their low-, average-, and high-achieving peers. *J Intellect Dev Disabil.* 2013;38(1):23-30.

Einfeld SL, Ellis LA, Emerson E. Comorbidity of intellectual disability and mental disorder in children and adolescents: a systematic review. *J Intellect Dev Disabil.* 2011;36(2):137-143.

Gregory AM, Sadeh A. Annual Research Review: Sleep problems in childhood psychiatric disorders—a review of the latest science. *J Child Psychol Psychiatry.* 2016;57(3):296-317.

Moeschler JB, Shevell M; American Academy of Pediatrics Committee on Genetics. Comprehensive evaluation of the child with intellectual disability or global developmental delays. *Pediatrics.* 2014;134(3):e903-e918.

Munir KM. The co-occurrence of mental disorders in children and adolescents with intellectual disability/intellectual developmental disorder. *Curr Opin Psychiatry.* 2016;29(2):95-102.

Murphy NA, Carbone PS; American Academy of Pediatrics Council on Children with Disabilities. Parent-provider-community partnerships: optimizing outcomes for children with disabilities. *Pediatrics.* 2011;128(4):795-802.

Myers SM, Johnson CP; American Academy of Pediatrics Council on Children with Disabilities. Management of children with autism spectrum disorders. *Pediatrics.* 2007;120(5):1162-1182.

Ptomey LT, Wittenbrook W. Position of the Academy of Nutrition and Dietetics: nutrition services for individuals with intellectual and developmental disabilities and special health care needs. *J Acad Nutr Diet.* 2015;115(4):593-608.

Solish A, Perry A, Minnes P. Participation of children with and without disabilities in social, recreational and leisure activities. *J Applied Res Intellect Disabil.* 2010;23:226-236.

# 123 Ethical Issues in Pediatric Patients with Medical Complexity

Jill Ann Jarrell and Carl D. Tapia

## INTRODUCTION

Caring for children with medical complexity (CMC) requires substantial time, effort, knowledge, and commitment on the part of families and healthcare professionals, and also involves a willingness to grapple with unique and complex ethical issues. It is important for general pediatricians and practitioners who work with children with disabilities to understand these ethical issues and develop skills in problem solving and ethical analysis. Here, we present a brief review of the basic principles of medical ethics as they relate to CMC and a discussion of specific or unique ethical issues in CMC and models for ethical problem solving.

## PRINCIPLES OF MEDICAL ETHICS IMPORTANT IN CARING FOR CMC

The basic principles of medical ethics are autonomy, beneficence, nonmaleficence, and justice. The relative importance of these principles varies based on source and situation, and also on the addition of the principles of veracity and fidelity. There are some caveats to these principles that are particular to pediatrics and even more so to CMC, as many in this population have a variable between chronological age and developmental or cognitive ability.

### Autonomy

Autonomy literally means "self-rule" and refers to the patient's right to make decisions and act on them freely and without interference. An important qualification to the right to autonomy is that the decision-maker have *capacity*, which is not typically present in CMC. However, autonomy and capacity should be viewed on a spectrum and relevant to the decision to be made. For example, a patient who has the developmental level of a 6-year-old likely does not have the capacity to make complex treatment decisions, but he or she can indicate a preference for cherry- or grape-flavored medication.

Parents usually assume the role of surrogate decision-maker for children and are given parental authority, which does not replace patient autonomy. For example, if a mother wishes to pursue tracheostomy in a patient who is deemed inappropriate for surgery by the medical team, the ethics committee is consulted to help determine the next steps. The ethics committee would need to balance issues of parental authority, not patient autonomy, with other ethical principles in advising the medical team.

Common topics in pediatric care are issues of parental consent for a procedure or treatment plan as well as pediatric assent. The 2 can and should coexist when applicable. Consider, for example, a situation in which the parents of a patient with severe scoliosis wish to pursue spinal surgery, but the patient has the cognition to understand that this surgery will inflict pain and does not wish to proceed. In this scenario, we have parental consent but do not have patient assent, so further discussion and mediation should occur.

### Beneficence and Nonmaleficence

Beneficence underscores the moral obligation to act for the benefit of others. In medicine, beneficence requires the physician to act in the patient's best interest, thus recommending therapies that maximize benefit and minimize burden. Nonmaleficence means not harming or inflicting as little harm as possible to reach a beneficial outcome.

### Justice

The principle of justice is the moral obligation to act on the basis of fair adjudication between competing claims. In healthcare ethics, this can be subdivided into 3 categories: fair distribution of scarce resources (distributive justice), respect for people's rights (rights-based justice), and respect for morally acceptable laws (legal justice).

### Veracity and Fidelity

Veracity, often referred to as *truth telling*, is a legal and ethical principle that states that healthcare professionals should be honest and give full disclosure to the patient, abstain from misrepresentation or deceit, and report known lapses in the standard of care. Fidelity requires loyalty, fairness, truthfulness, advocacy, and dedication to patients. Fidelity refers to the concept of keeping a commitment and is based upon the virtue of caring.

## ETHICAL ISSUES FACED BY FAMILES AND CAREGIVERS OF CMC

### Caregeiver Fatigue and Medicalization of Parenting

Because of the intense time and emotional commitment required to care for CMC, parents often become consumed with their role as caregiver. Additionally, parents of CMC are often asked to take on complex medical roles in caring for their children in the hospital and in the home. This level of immersion in the care of another can be physically, mentally, and emotionally taxing for the parents. They may also experience guilt in balancing the role of nurturing versus medical caregiver.

Clearly, this phenomenon is not in the patient's best interest and should be avoided. It is recommended that providers intervene by screening for caregiver fatigue and stress at well-child visits or as clinically indicated and by offering resources for counseling, support, and respite services.

### Compromised Duties and Obligations

The entire family is affected by the presence of a CMC. Time and attention given to typical siblings, spouses, elderly family members, or extended family may be inadequate. Caregiver work or educational advancement opportunities may be limited, as might be caregiver and family rest and recreation.

These stresses may lead to behavior concerns in siblings, relationship strain or divorce, and financial stressors or even bankruptcy. Providers should inquire about the health of the family unit at well-child visits or as clinically indicated, and actively involve other members of the care team—such as social work and child life—in problem-solving these issues.

#### Social and Legal Ramifications

Because CMC need to have multiple support services in the home, the families may feel their privacy has been invaded. This population's need to be geographically close to primary, subspecialty, and emergency medical services can necessitate the family moving away from a known community, which can be expensive and socially isolating.

Families are held responsible for adhering to complex medication, therapy, pulmonary toilet, and positioning regimens, as well as attending multiple primary and subspecialty care appointments. Failure to do so can be interpreted as medical neglect, for which the family can face legal consequences.

*Care coordination*, discussed in detail elsewhere in this section, is essential in CMC for assisting families with navigating home care, travel, therapies, and appointments and can help deal with social or legal challenges.

### ETHICAL ISSUES FACED BY THE HEALTHCARE TEAM

#### Balancing Parental Authority with the Patient's Best Interest

Throughout the course of the child's life, the parents and caregivers become the experts in their child, as they are more familiar with the daily patterns and needs. While it is important for the provider to respect this role of parents as experts, it is essential that the provider also help preserve their role as parent/family member.

It is difficult in CMC to discern where the patient ends and the caregiver and family begin. Thus, the patient-centered model of care has given way to the family-centered model of care, whereby the family is treated as an extension of the patient. Implicit in this model is balancing patient autonomy with parental authority in determining the patient's best interests.

Providers for CMC should recognize that conflict between the healthcare team and family may be due to frustration over losing control. A useful strategy is acknowledging caregiver authority and concerns and working with them in a collaborative approach.

Many families seek complementary and alternative medicine, utilize or request unproven therapies, or decline recommended therapies. In this case, the role of the healthcare team is to assess the risk of harm and impact on the family. In cases where benefit is unlikely, the possibility of harm is great, or significant secondary effects likely (such as financial strain), the provider must balance parental authority with beneficence and nonmaleficence. Some practices develop policies to set the expectation that persistent dissonance may result in the discharge of families. An example is vaccine-refusal policies. An alternate approach is to listen to the family concerns and expectations, remain honest about harm, and negotiate a compromise that maximizes safety and minimizes harm.

#### Provider Role Fidelity

Because of the increase in time and intensity required to care for CMC, home healthcare nurses, providers, and other members of the healthcare team can become emotionally invested in their patients and families to the point of compromising their objectivity. This may hinder their ability to discern what is in the patient's best interest and even cause them to violate professional boundaries.

A best practice is working with colleagues, ancillary staff, and home-care services to develop accountability in this area. For example, it may be good for the home healthcare nurse, and the patient and family if the nurses are rotated on a scheduled basis, to cross-check the care plan and orders and to give all parties an emotional break. Likewise, provider holidays in the clinic setting, whereby the provider who typically cares for the patient steps back for a visit or a certain time allotment and allows a different provider to assume care for the patient, can provide a fresh perspective on the care plan and some emotional distance.

*Self-care*, the intentional practice by healthcare providers to provide and promote physical, emotional, psychological, and spiritual health and balance for themselves and their colleagues, is essential to the success and stability of teams caring for CMC and should be recognized and encouraged.

#### Inadequate Work Force

Healthcare professionals lack education and experience in diagnosing, treating, and counseling CMC and their families. Meanwhile, the CMC population continues to grow in scope and complexity. Thus, it is imperative to advocate for policies that develop an able and adequate workforce to care for CMC, and to develop and promote best practices and guidelines for their care.

#### Justice: Equitable Resource Distribution and Reimbursement

Healthcare professionals are sometimes asked to approve services that are not medically necessary or seem to be primarily for the convenience of the family. An example is a family requesting extended private-duty nursing for a child with very few skilled-nursing needs, because it is a benefit of the family's health plan. In this case, the provider must balance issues of parent autonomy, distributive justice, and veracity. It is ideal to have written policies that justify the medical decision and clearly explain the relevant criteria. The provider must then negotiate the needs of the family with his or her professional judgment to deny the care, seek an alternative strategy, or consider a second opinion. In the case of private-duty nursing, for example, the provider could refer the family for respite resources or attendant services (if available), or refer to a peer for a second opinion.

Healthcare teams caring for CMC spend an inordinate amount of time responding to e-mails, writing letters, filling out forms, and participating in meetings or calls with families, other healthcare providers, support services, and legal entities. In addition to interrupting routine work flows, there are insufficient benchmarks for coding and billing and fair reimbursement for these services. Persistent advocacy is necessary to disseminate best practices in novel reimbursement and support of these non–face-to-face clinical activities.

## COMMON ETHICAL DILEMMAS IN CARING FOR CMC

### DIAGNOSIS AND PROGNOSIS

Children with medical complexity often have a constellation of diseases or manifestations of 1 disease affecting multiple organ systems. Some CMC have undiagnosed diseases or even newly discovered diagnoses. Additionally, CMC may have very rare diseases that manifest differently in every child. In short, the name of a child's disease or syndrome may not be helpful in guiding prognosis or treatment, given the rarity of the disease or the number and complexity of the comorbidities.

Closely related to diagnosis is prognosis, literally meaning *foreknowledge*, which refers to the provider anticipating, communicating, and preparing for the likely disease course or courses. Because CMC have such varied, complicated, and compounded diseases, projecting the disease course can be exquisitely difficult. These projections have potential ethical impacts if a provider is not careful and complete in communicating a particular diagnosis. For example, sending the family of an infant with trisomy 18 home from the nursery with hospice may be appropriate for infants with significant functional limitations and severe comorbid conditions, but doing the same for infants with very few sequelae (given growing evidence of infants and young adults with trisomy 18 who are doing well and gaining milestones) is less clear. This may lead some families to feel abandoned by the health system. The advisable action of the provider in this scenario is to make a disposition recommendation based on clinical status and not diagnosis, educate the family about possible outcomes, and ensure coordination with an experienced provider who can provide close follow-up.

In another example, consider a patient who has a neurologic condition characterized by progressive weakness and debility but has unrevealing genetic tests. Although the disorder may resemble a muscular atrophy or other progressive neuromuscular disease, the diagnosis is potentially devastating. This puts 2 ethical tenets—veracity and beneficence—at odds. The practitioner may be in conflict, balancing the need to disclose the worst-case scenario versus the risk of distress and confusion for the patient and family.

In disclosing prognostic information, the provider should consider the best interests of the child, parental surrogate decision-making, and, if possible, pediatric assent. Experience has been that veracity leads to increased autonomy, which is in the patient's best interest. Some patients or families may wish to not discuss specifics of prognoses at certain times, and prognostic information should then be disclosed incrementally.

In some situations, caregivers may not recognize a child's disease course despite repeated discussions, perhaps due to grief and denial. For example, consider a patient with a terminal or degenerative disease process, who endures repeated hospitalizations, intensive care unit (ICU) stays, intubations, and other invasive interventions. Multiple physicians recognize that aggressive interventions are causing pain and recommend a palliative approach. If the caregivers do not agree or seek to escalate care further, the provider may feel conflict between supporting the wishes of the family versus futility and causing harm. The provider may need assistance in communicating the prognosis to the caregivers in the form of repeated discussions involving a multidisciplinary team. Ancillary providers, such as chaplaincy and social work, can help address barriers to caregiver understanding and acceptance and facilitate discussions with subspecialty services to reinforce prognosis. In rare cases where parental authority continually conflicts with the patient's best interest as determined by the care team, an ethics committee consult may be helpful to establish institutional boundaries and to consider legal intervention to protect the child.

## TREATMENTS AND INTERVENTIONS

Providers have an ethical obligation to advise caregivers on the options they believe to be most appropriate, rather than laying out all available options and leaving the parents to choose with little guidance. Knowing specifically what each intervention can and cannot do (Table 123-1) is essential. It is also important to take into account the complexity of these patients and know that there are multiple issues contributing to 1 problem that may only partially be solved or addressed with an intervention. For example, consider a child with a congenital high-airway obstruction syndrome (CHAOS), who may have 100% of his or her problems solved with a tracheotomy. However, a child with CHAOS and Townes-Brocks syndrome may only have 25% overall improvement with a tracheotomy. Table 123-2 provides some self-reflective questions that providers and care teams can use to help them formulate recommendations in challenging or complicated cases.

**TABLE 123-2 QUESTIONS TO AID IN FORMULATING AN ETHICAL RECOMMENDATION FOR INTERVENTIONS AND TREATMENTS IN CHILDREN WITH MEDICAL COMPLEXITY**

| |
|---|
| What specific symptom or condition is being targeted with this intervention? |
| Is there a reasonable chance this problem/symptom will be ameliorated with this treatment? Fully or partially? |
| Is it within the institutional and population "norm"? |
| Does the intended outcome support the family's values and goals? |
| Is this intervention in the child's best interest? |
| Do the patient and family understand the risks, benefits, and all potential long-term outcomes of this treatment? |

**Utilizing a Shared Decision-Making Model** The consideration and implementation of assistive technology in CMC are value-sensitive decisions and necessitate a shared decision-making approach, where families express their goals and values and the provider offers medical recommendations so that a plan can be negotiated.

Consider Ariel, a 16-year-old with Lennox-Gastaut syndrome with progressive seizures, encephalopathy, and dysphagia with several episodes of aspiration pneumonia and failure to thrive, for which she has been hospitalized multiple times for enteral nutrition, hydration, and antibiotics. She enjoys eating, even though it isn't enough to sustain her caloric need, and the family is frustrated with the repeated hospitalizations and time away from home. The care team recommended a spectrum of ethical care plan options, ranging from placement of gastrostomy and addition of a pediatric surgeon, gastroenterologist, and dietitian to the care team with intensified outpatient follow-up, to not placing a gastrostomy and implementing hospice, which would enable Ariel to eat, spend more time at home, and have outpatient follow-up appointments as desired. Because the latter option was more in line with the family's values and goals, hospice was initiated at home and the gastrostomy was not pursued.

**Advance Care Planning** Rarely do children with medical complexity have an advance directive or an advance care plan, despite the recommendation for pediatric patients with a life-limiting illness to have such documents and discussions with their care teams and families. It is important to reiterate that having advance care plans in CMC promotes patient autonomy, parental authority, beneficence, nonmaleficence, and justice (see Chapter 128).

## SUMMARY

Caring for children with medical complexity is wrought with ethical challenges for the caregiver, provider, healthcare team, institutions, and society at large. Working collaboratively with families and multidisciplinary care teams can help alleviate caregiver and provider burden, promote communication, and optimize patient care. More research and policy work is anticipated in this area.

**TABLE 123-1 COMMON INTERVENTIONS CONSIDERED IN CHILDREN WITH MEDICAL COMPLEXITY WITH INDICATIONS FOR TREATMENT, BENEFITS, AND RISKS**

| Intervention | Treats | Does Not Treat | Benefits | Risks |
|---|---|---|---|---|
| Gastrostomy | Unable to meet caloric needs by mouth | Aspiration, respiratory tract infections | Removable, amenable to home care | Infection, bleeding, pain |
| Nissen fundoplication | Vomiting, esophagitis, hematemesis | Aspiration, respiratory tract infections | Can be very effective | Invasive procedure, can be ineffective |
| Salivary duct ligation/injection/removal | Excessive secretions | Aspiration, respiratory tract infections | Injection is temporary, ligation/removal is permanent | Variable success rate |
| Tracheotomy | Airway obstruction | Secretion management, aspiration | Amenable to home care, removable | Bleeding, mucous plug/obstruction, increased respiratory infections |
| Laryngotracheal separation | Secretions, aspiration | – | Effective | Eliminates ability to vocalize, lack of long-term evidence for respiratory outcomes |
| Spinal surgery | Scoliosis | Respiratory tract infections | Effective | Invasive, painful, lack of long-term evidence for respiratory outcomes |

Courageous Parents Network Web site. https://courageousparentsnetwork.org. Accessed December 12, 2016.

Ethics Committee of the American Board of Pediatrics. Bioethics bibliography. https://www.abp.org/sites/abp/files/pdf/bioethics.pdf. Accessed December 12, 2016.

Hauer JM. *Caring for Children Who Have Severe Neurological Impairment: A Life with Grace*. Baltimore, MD: Johns Hopkins University Press; 2013.

McCullough LB, Brothers KB, Chung WK, et al, on behalf of the Clinical Sequencing Exploratory Research (CSER) Consortium Pediatrics Working Group. Professionally responsible disclosure of genomic sequencing results in pediatric practice. *Pediatrics*. 2015;136(4):e974-e982.

Nelson KE, Mahant S. Shared decision-making about assistive technology for the child with severe neurologic impairment. *Pediatr Clin North Am*. 2014;61(4):641-652.

Okun A. Ethics for the pediatrician. *Pediatr Rev*. 2010;31(12):514-517.

Schwantes S, O'Brien HW. Pediatric palliative care for children with complex dhronic medical conditions. *Pediatr Clin North Am*. 2014;61(4):797-821.



# 124 Transition for Children with Medical Complexity

Elisha Acosta and Cynthia Peacock

The transition process and appropriate transfer of care are particularly important for children with complex medical care needs. The American Academy of Pediatrics, American Academy of Family Physicians, and American College of Physicians-American Society of Internal Medicine highlighted this in their original consensus statement on healthcare transitions for young adults with special healthcare needs, published in *Pediatrics* in 2002, which stated the goal of transition as "maximiz[ing] lifelong functioning and potential through the provision of high-quality, developmentally appropriate health care services that continue uninterrupted as the individual moves from adolescence to adulthood." Cooperation between various healthcare practitioners in the pediatric and adult spheres is needed to accomplish the goal of healthcare transition in a way that is family-centered, compassionate, coordinated, and comprehensive.

Children and youth with special healthcare needs (CYSHCN) are broadly defined in the United States as "those who have 1 or more chronic physical, developmental, behavioral, or emotional conditions and who also require health and related services of a type or amount beyond that required by children generally." The population of CYSHCN continues to grow as scientific advances for many pediatric chronic conditions increases longevity for even the most complex and medically fragile childhood conditions. Today, an estimated 18.4% of US youth ages 12 to 18 meet this broad definition of CYSHCN, with approximately 90% currently reaching adulthood. The need for structured transition planning of this high-risk population has been a focus of federal agencies for over a decade, and is specifically addressed in the Healthy People 2020 campaign. Despite this attention, the most recent National Survey of Children with Special Health Care Needs in 2009–2010 found no discernible improvements in transition outcomes since the 2005–2006 national survey. The survey utilizes a composite of 4 measures: transition to an adult provider, changing healthcare needs, maintaining health insurance coverage, and taking increased responsibility for self-care.

Certainly, medical advancements over the last century have increased the survival into adulthood of individuals with various chronic conditions, such as congenital heart disease, sickle cell disease, cystic fibrosis, and insulin-dependent diabetes mellitus. Regrettably, these same populations have been noted to experience increased morbidity and mortality at the time of transition from pediatric to adult care. A small subset of CYSHCN, children with medical complexity (CMC), account for up to one-third of overall healthcare spending for children and an increasing percentage of pediatric hospitalizations and recurrent hospital admissions. Yet very little is known about this population once they arrive in the adult healthcare system. Currently, a consistent definition for this heterogeneous subgroup does not exist, but it is clear that CMC have numerous ongoing and complex medical care services that go unmet.

## DEFINING TRANSITION FOR CHILDREN WITH MEDICAL COMPLEXITY

The transition of a child with medical complexity includes various factors that should be considered and addressed by the medical home, a concept that embraces the foundation of patient- and family-centered care and supports a collaborative partnership with shared decision-making. The transition process can take years and ideally starts no later than early adolescence. Children with medical complexity require special consideration in regard to the child's ability to gain medical and legal independence. Traditional transition planning and processes focus on increasing an adolescent's participation in their medical care, including knowledge of disease, medication management, and healthcare utilization planning. Based on the degree of developmental delay, as well as physical or intellectual disability, an individual's ability to transition to an independent medical care plan may be limited and therefore may require the participation of caregivers and other representatives.

In addition to the transition of primary care, many CMC will undergo transition of multiple subspecialists. Ideally, each of these transitions should be done with participation from multidisciplinary teams from both the pediatric and internal medicine domains. Specialty care continues to be vital for the youth with medical complexity as they age into the adult healthcare system, and a single provider or care coordinator to help the youth and their families navigate each of these transitions is helpful.

Of note, a child with intellectual disabilities may require the assistance of a legal guardian to make informed medical decisions even after they reach the legal age of consent. Practitioners should be aware of the laws and legal process surrounding guardianship, assisted medical decision-making, and advanced directives in their state. A guardian is generally someone who is appointed to make legal decisions, which could include medical or financial, for another person who is unable to make those decisions because they are determined to be incapacitated. The process of being granted guardianship often requires physician involvement to describe capacity, and can be costly and time consuming for families. Pediatric providers will have to become familiar with their state-specific guardianship process or least restrictive alternatives depending on the youth's decision-making ability and guide families regarding where to go for assistance with the process. Numerous healthcare systems across the nation have established medical-legal partnerships to help CYSHCN and their families address guardianship and other issues that will help keep them healthy and safe in their communities. (More information and resources can be found at http://medical-legalpartnership.org/.)

There are multiple funding considerations in terms of insurance coverage, as well as the establishment of dedicated funds, that may be needed to cover an individual's living and medical expenses should their parent or caregiver pass away. The Affordable Care Act signed into law in 2010 expands the ability for all young adults to remain on their parent's private insurance through age 26. Some adult dependents with disabilities can apply through the parent's employer-provided health plans to continue to receive coverage even beyond their 26th birthday. While these avenues for retaining private insurance funding are important, the majority of children and young adults with severe disabilities utilize Medicaid for their health insurance. Ensuring continued coverage requires additional work, as all 18-year-olds on SSI (Supplemental Security Income) must go through a redetermination process under the adult criteria. The adult criteria depend on the applicant's inability to work. As a result of this difference, approximately 30% of those who had SSI as a youth will lose it when this redetermination process takes place at 18 years of age. Consequently, many of these young adults who lose their SSI eligibility are no longer eligible for Medicaid coverage, which will affect ability to purchase or obtain medications and supplies, and to follow-up with healthcare providers. Medicare coverage is possible if a parent or caregiver has become disabled, retired, or died, and the adult child receives benefits as a dependent of the parent. Finally, special trusts may be necessary to protect eligibility for the government programs described above. This may be the case if the death of a relative or settlement of a legal case has resulted in income.

Maximizing lifelong function and potential includes meaningful transition from the school system to the workforce, if possible, or to an appropriate secondary education setting. The US Department of Labor's Office of Disability Employment Policy sets forth 5 guideposts to help attain this outcome: school-based preparatory experiences, career preparation and work-based learning, youth development and leadership, connecting activities, and family involvement and supports. Vocational training and job support may be available through waiver programs, state disability programs, and systems for individuals with intellectual disability. Another consideration may include day habilitation, or "day hab," which is a community-based program designed to help people with developmental disabilities lead more independent and productive, fulfilling lives. Finally, adult day care centers are designed to provide care and companionship for adults who are older or more severely disabled and need assistance or supervision during the day. These programs also have the benefit of providing respite to family members and caregivers.

Ensuring a safe transition into the adult healthcare system for CMC means preserving as many of the services and resources that the patient and his or her family receive in the pediatric sphere and will continue to require as he or she moves to adult care. Skilled nursing services; occupational, physical, and speech therapies; and durable medical equipment may need a different funding mechanism such as waiver programs that offer long-term services and supports. These supports are designed to keep in the community an individual who otherwise might require placement in a nursing home, institution, or hospital. State-specific information about waivers can be found at www.medicaidwaiver.org.

## BARRIERS TO TRANSITION

Numerous barriers continue to exist surrounding the transition process. Importantly, adult healthcare systems historically have a "disease-centered approach" compared to the "family-centered approach" central to pediatric healthcare. This change in the approach to care can be disconcerting to both providers and families. In addition, difficulty may be experienced in finding adult providers comfortable with the diagnoses of and devices used for pediatric patients. Another significant barrier is the additional time it takes for providers across disciplines to discuss transition with one other, review new diagnoses, and counsel patients and families. New funding mechanisms are emerging to help pediatric providers find reimbursement for healthcare coordination. Health insurances, both commercial and government, are recognizing reimbursement procedures for non–face-to-face care coordination. Medicare currently reimburses monthly for care coordination that exceeds 20 minutes outside of the office visit.

There also exist youth, family, community, and system-wide characteristics that contribute to the barriers experienced. Having an emotional, behavioral, or developmental condition has been identified as a risk factor for not receiving adequate transition preparation and higher health utilization. Limitations in mental health resources and availability of adult providers/therapies, as well as affordable, developmentally appropriate day activities, are major barriers to comprehensive and successful transition.

## BEST PRACTICES IN TRANSITION



Certain systems of care are associated with better transition outcomes. In the 2009–2010 national survey, CYSHCN who identified receiving healthcare within a medical home were more likely to indicate that they also received transition healthcare services. One best practice is coordinating care beyond the medical home and into the medical neighborhood. Medical neighborhoods or health neighborhoods consist of a diverse collection of healthcare providers and institutions that provide comprehensive care, resources, and support to patients and their families, including services that address numerous social determinants. The use of a dedicated transition coordinator is another best practice. Some model transition programs utilize dedicated transition clinics—usually based in a children's hospital—to provide expert assistance and promote active involvement of the youths and their caregivers. Handoffs between pediatric and adult providers are an important aspect of effective transition. Summarizing the medical history into a more concise form is a best practice, as is direct communication with the adult provider and, if possible, utilization of a condition fact sheet that details the young adult's condition and suggested care. Evidence suggests that meeting adult providers before transfer is especially helpful and effective. Transition readiness is another critical component. Transition readiness includes building transition skills and identifying areas for readiness training.

## SUMMARY

The transition process and transfer planning for CMC has unique considerations in regard to medical and legal independence, appropriate funding, and participation in appropriate post-schooling activities. This process should, whenever possible, be planned, be structured, and start early. Pediatricians are encouraged to engage their adult healthcare colleagues in transition planning, while preparing their patients and families in a developmental way to transfer out of the pediatric healthcare system.

## SUGGESTED READINGS


American Academy of Pediatrics; American Academy of Family Physicians; American College of Physicians-American Society of Internal Medicine. A consensus statement on health care transitions for young adults with special health care needs. *Pediatrics*. 2002;110(6, pt 2): 1304-1306.

American Academy of Pediatrics; American Academy of Family Physicians; American College of Physicians; Transitions Clinical Report Authoring Group. Clinical report—supporting the health care transition from adolescence to adulthood in the medical home. *Pediatrics*. 2011;128(1):182-200.

Cohen E, Kuo DZ, Agrawal R, et al. Children with medical complexity: an emerging population for clinical and research initiatives. *Pediatrics*. 2011;127(3):529-538.

Davis AM, Brown RF, Taylor JL, Epstein RA, McPheeters ML. Transition care for children with special health care needs. *Pediatrics*. 2014;134(5):900-908.

HealthyPeople.gov. Healthy People 2020: Adolescent Health. https://www.healthypeople.gov/2020/topics-objectives/topic/Adolescent-Health. Originally published 2014; updated November 27, 2016. Accessed November 28, 2016.

McManus MA, Pollack LR, Cooley WC, et al. Current status of transition preparation among youth with special needs in the United States. *Pediatrics*. 2013;131(6):1090-1097.

White PH. Access to health care: health insurance considerations for young adults with special health care needs/disabilities. *Pediatrics*. 2002;110(6, pt 2):1328-1335.

# 125 Palliative and Hospice Care for Children

Shih-Ning Liaw, Barbara L. Jones, and Julie Hauer

## INTRODUCTION

Palliative care is a model of interprofessional care that seeks to improve the quality of life of patients with serious illnesses and their families. This care includes the prevention and relief of suffering by promptly identifying and treating pain and other sources of distress, whether they are physical, psychosocial, or spiritual. Pediatric palliative care teams may include clinicians from a variety of professional backgrounds, including physicians, nurses, social workers, chaplains, and child life specialists. While hospice care in the United States represents a service delivery model for patients nearing the end of life, palliative care can provide longitudinal support throughout a patient's life. Hospice and Palliative Medicine is a recognized medical subspecialty with board certification and accredited fellowship training programs, and pediatric palliative care programs are in various stages of development throughout the country. Palliative care for children with serious illness encompasses a broad range of approaches and interventions with variances depending on individual patient circumstances. However, certain goals and functions of palliative care remain common regardless of specific illness or disease trajectory. This chapter is focused on providing a general overview of palliative care through describing one of its primary functions, which is the development of a care plan.

## DEVELOPING A PALLIATIVE CARE PLAN

### HEALTH TRAJECTORIES AND TIMING OF PALLIATIVE CARE

Different health trajectories guide the timing of incorporating the principles of palliative care into clinical management. Patients who may benefit from palliative care consultation have conditions that can be categorized by the following: (1) those where treatment is possible but may ultimately be unsuccessful, such as malignancies not responding to conventional protocols or advanced disease awaiting organ transplantation; (2) those where intensive long-term treatment is aimed at optimizing health and function but may ultimately lead to life-threatening complications, such as muscular dystrophy or cystic fibrosis; and (3) those where severe disability causes vulnerability to recurrent illness, hospitalizations, and decline in function. There is considerable overlap in these categorizations, and Figure 125-1 illustrates a conceptual model of potential health trajectories that demonstrate the hope of benefit from various medical and surgical interventions, as well as the potential worsening of the clinical course despite these interventions.

Palliative care consultation can be useful for counseling and symptom management at any time in a child's trajectory: from the time of diagnosis, in conjunction with disease-directed treatment, through end-of-life care, and into bereavement. Families of children with a diagnosis in which cure may not be possible are ideally introduced to palliative care at the time of diagnosis in order to establish a supportive relationship for longitudinal care. Changes in clinical status or decision points for medical or surgical interventions often represent opportunities for palliative care referral. Palliative care is a resource that can be introduced to families by acknowledging the shared hope that their child will have the intended benefit of treatment available while honestly reflecting that not every child receives the hoped-for benefit. A brochure highlighting information about palliative care can be included along with the other materials that teams provide to families. Palliative care teams can also be integrated into medical teams providing care for oncology patients, patients awaiting transplantation, and other children with complex chronic conditions. For additional details related to children with chronic illness, refer to Chapter 126.

### BENEFIT OF EARLY INTEGRATION

Early initiation of palliative care facilitates attention to communication, symptom management, medical decision making, psychosocial support, and quality of life. Randomized controlled trials evaluating early integration of palliative care in adult patients with advanced cancer demonstrate that palliative care consultation can lead to meaningful improvements in quality of life, symptom burden, and mood. In addition, early integration of palliative care leads to better documentation of a patient's treatment preferences, higher-quality end-of-life care, fewer deaths in intensive care settings, and even prolonged survival in certain patient populations.

Uncertainty of prognosis has been identified as a common barrier to integration of palliative care and optimal end-of-life care for seriously ill children. Yet, evidence suggests that families of children with serious illness benefit most from palliative care during these times of uncertainty. Early introduction of palliative care assures use of interventions to address physical and emotional distress and is considered helpful by parents even when that information is upsetting. Although medical teams often worry that families are not ready, studies demonstrate that integration of palliative care does not lessen parents' hope.

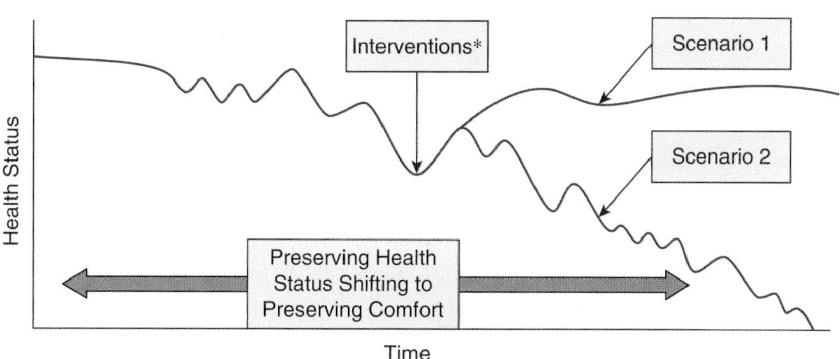


**FIGURE 125-1** Health trajectories for children with serious illness.

Clinicians of all levels of experience report that initiating conversations about poor prognosis is challenging. Yet the majority of parents of children with cancer and those with children in the intensive care unit say they want honest prognostic information. Families identify that high-quality medical care includes caring and sensitive physician communication about what to expect as a child nears the end of life. Discussions that allow families to prepare for death provide positive benefit to later bereavement. Families who are not well prepared tend to choose more intensive care at the end of life. In retrospect, most bereaved family members indicated that palliative care was provided too late in the disease course, whereas fewer than 5% thought palliative care referrals occurred too early.

## COMMUNICATION TOOLS IN PALLIATIVE CARE

Defining goals of care is a critical part of guiding decision making by identifying interventions that meet identified goals rather than treat a medical problem in isolation. Palliative care recognizes that families and clinicians alike experience distress when they encounter the limits of medicine. Ensuring the care team is experienced in communicating with patients and families compassionately, clearly, and honestly is essential. At such times, medical decisions are often made out of a sense that something more needs to be done. Palliative care helps to identify other care priorities, such as symptom management and location of care, that may be important to patients and their families. Disease-directed treatment and palliative care are not mutually exclusive and should be provided concurrently for children with serious illnesses. Areas of assessment in palliative care include eliciting a patient's and family's understanding of the disease course and exploring unmet emotional, psychosocial, and spiritual needs. This chapter discusses many of the concepts and tools used to engage with a family in the creation of a plan of care. A systematic approach to this process is described below. Communication tools used for this purpose are reviewed in Table 125-1.

## THE INTERPROFESSIONAL TEAM

Palliative care is only possible with an interprofessional team. An interprofessional team approach enables collaboration among disciplines and enhances the holistic care that is provided to the child and family. Among hospital-based pediatric palliative care programs and community-based hospice programs, the most common disciplines on staff are physicians, nurses, social workers, and chaplains. Child life specialists also serve a unique role in pediatric palliative care. These individual areas of expertise are critical to managing the multidimensional needs encountered by children and families.

- **Physicians and nurses** bring expertise in symptom management, treatment planning, and bedside care.

**TABLE 125-1 COMMUNICATION TOOLS USED IN PALLIATIVE CARE**

| Objectives | Suggested Language |
|---|---|
| Getting to know child and family | Tell us about your child before he or she became ill. |
| | What makes your child happy? Sad? |
| | What is your understanding of your child's illness/condition and its likely course? |
| | In light of your understanding of your child's illness, what is most important to you and your family? |
| | What are your hopes? What are your worries? |
| Determine goals of care as a guide to decision making | We will always review how the interventions available meet the goals you've identified. |
| | Goals commonly include comfort and quality of life along with hope for life extension, although they may shift to providing care at home when less benefit or greater burden is seen from care in the hospital, may shift to comfort only when limited benefit is identified from the treatment available, and can be focused on a specific activity such as maintaining current health status for a family trip. |
| Focus on parental expertise | Although I will honestly reflect on changes in your daughter's health and functional status, you are the expert in how these changes look and affect her quality of life. |
| | Although we bring expertise in evaluating and managing health problems in children, you are the expert in how such problems look in your daughter. |
| Anticipate worries | We know that worries of parents at such times often include: Is my child suffering? Will my child get better? Is there more we can do? We will talk through these worries. |
| | We can talk through some of the "what ifs" so as to address any worries you may have, so you know what to expect, to assure that we have a care plan in place, and to allow you to focus on spending time with your daughter. |
| Reflect on the past as a guide to the future | I wonder if we are seeing less recovery and less time between each illness. |
| | Do you think we are seeing fewer good days now compared to 6 and 12 months ago? |
| | Your child's story will guide us along the way. Our job as parents and care providers is to watch, listen, and reflect honestly on what the story is telling us. |
| Acknowledge the limits of interventions | I cannot imagine how hard it is to be seeing fewer good days. I wish we had interventions that could reverse this. |
| | Your child continues to receive exceptional care at home. My observation is that we are seeing fewer benefits from the treatment we have available. What have you observed? |
| Limiting treatment does not mean limiting care | I worry that your child's body is getting tired despite the best treatment available. |
| | It might make sense to identify what we won't do if her body becomes too tired to sustain adequate breathing. We won't limit treatments that have reasonable benefit but will protect her from interventions that may harm or prolong suffering. |
| | We will always provide care that maximizes comfort throughout her life. |
| Hope for the best; prepare for the rest | We know families often hold simultaneously their hope for the best possible outcome with their realistic understanding of the severity of the problem. |
| Offer continuity with a safety net | We might not know when your child will have more problems, but you will always have a team available to help guide and support you on this journey. |
| Identify decision making as a dynamic process | What might seem like the "right" decision today could change. Your decisions can change as the clinical course changes. |
| | Stopping a medical intervention is ethically and legally the same as not starting an intervention but can feel very different emotionally. |

- **Social workers** provide psychosocial assessment and supportive counseling for the child and family adjusting to changes, skill in exploring hopes and worries of a patient and family, and expertise in identifying community resources.
- **Chaplains** support faith traditions and spiritual values that promote hope and support families as they face change, loss, or grief.
- **Child life specialists** facilitate communication with children through activities that assist with emotional distress, can also explore a deeper understanding of patients' fears and wishes, and enhance psychosocial supports for siblings.

Palliative care teams can also assist members of the healthcare team in managing the distress that comes with caring for a child with a serious illness. Interprofessional teams can assure that the physical, emotional, spiritual, and practical needs of children and families are addressed and that a supportive environment is provided for members of the healthcare team.

## CREATING A PLAN OF CARE

Identifying shared goals is a beneficial place to start. For parents of children with serious illness at a time of uncertainty, this can include acknowledgment that everyone continues to hope for the best outcome possible. From there, parents can often guide physicians and team members by sharing their story. Team members can then reflect on what has been communicated and explore deeper with the family:

- Please share with me what the past few weeks or months have been like and what you understand about your child's health status.
- What are you anticipating? What are you worrying about?
- Can you share what this has been like for you?

Parents often feel they need to focus on how well their child will do so they do not appear to be giving up. This can give the impression of not understanding how serious things are. However, parents often understand what the team is saying but find it hard to talk about the possibility of ongoing decline or death.

The best guide to future decisions includes defining what can be expected from current treatment available (eg, continued chemotherapy with a goal of controlling the disease for as long as possible and improving the quality of life) and a reflection on the benefit of past treatment (eg, sharing the observation of seeing declining benefit from chronic treatment and treatment during each acute illness exacerbation). It allows physicians to consider what is likely to happen (probable) and what may happen (possible). Questions to consider and review to assist with this reflection include the following:

- Have goals of care been identified as a guide to decisions?
- Have options that meet these goals been offered?
- Will the intervention benefit the whole patient, or does it manage a problem in isolation?
- How will the course look with or without the treatment available?
- Will an intervention bridge to the identified goals, such as maintaining or improving comfort and quality of life?
- Will an intervention provide sufficient recovery or prolong a process?
- Do we continue to see a benefit from chronic and acute treatment options with maintenance or return of health and functional status?
- Are we seeing less benefit from chronic and acute treatment over time with less return to prior baseline, longer periods of illness, or a shorter time between each illness?
- What percentage of each day or week is "good" or "quality" time, and how does that compare to 1 year ago, 6 months ago, 1 month ago, and today?
- Will the interventions being considered maintain or improve health, or will they prolong a process of decline or suffering?
- How much is the child able to enjoy relationships and activities and engage with loved ones?

In the process of decision making and defining a care plan, certain steps can help determine how to proceed if the benefit hoped for from an intervention does not occur:

- Define with the family the goals that you intend to meet.
- Identify the likelihood of an intervention meeting these goals.
- Know the evidence for the possible benefit and harm for the interventions available.
- Define a time period in which the intervention would be expected to meet the goal.
- Discuss a plan if the hoped-for benefit does not occur in this time period.

### Advance Care Planning

Advance care planning plays an important role in helping patients and families think through elements of their care as they live with serious illness and approach the end of life. Patients, families, and healthcare team members often find these discussions difficult to have. Trusted clinicians with long-term relationships with a patient and family are in a privileged position to have these conversations. Ideally, advance care planning takes place during times of relative stability and before moments of crisis. Advance care planning tools are available specifically for children and can assist the clinician in guiding discussions about care preferences. *My Wishes*, for pediatric patients, and *Voicing My Choices*, for adolescents, use developmentally appropriate language and medical terms to cover the following themes:

- How I want people to treat me
- How I want to be comforted
- What I want my family and friends to know
- What I want my doctors and nurses to know

### Resuscitation Status

Discussing resuscitation status requires an honest assessment of the likelihood of benefit and possible harm. Resuscitation status is a shared medical decision that incorporates both the medical assessment of benefit and the goals of care of the patient and family. The clinician's responsibility for this assessment is to discuss anticipated life-threatening events and to consider whether an intervention (intubation, chest compressions, defibrillation) will reverse the primary problem or whether the event is a result of a problem that cannot be reversed or improved. Understanding the broader goals of care allows the clinician to discuss resuscitation in the context of what is most important to the patient and family. Rather than asking whether to perform resuscitative efforts, which implies offering something that would benefit the child, clinicians should recommend pursuing or limiting resuscitative interventions based on the goals of care. During these discussions, clinicians can remind families that the child's decline in health is not a result of any decisions made to limit interventions or care but rather a result of the underlying disease process. Clinicians can continue to offer reassurance that the patient will be cared for with treatments that are consistent with the goals of care.

### Appointing a Healthcare Proxy

Appointing a healthcare proxy allows a patient over 18 years of age to designate another person to make medical decisions if the patient is unable to make or communicate those decisions. A social worker or other trusted team member involved with the patient can assist with the process of identifying someone whom the patient trusts. They can help identify the appropriate form that allows this information to be documented. In addition, the process of appointing a healthcare proxy provides an opportunity to discuss goals of care, facilitate decision making, and assure knowledge of the patient's preferences.

### Communicating the Plan of Care

Great care is only possible when critical information is determined, documented, and communicated to those involved in the child's care. Areas of need discussed throughout this chapter that are an important part of this process include:

- **Locations** of care: this includes the location of medical care (clinics, hospitals, and emergency service systems) and the community in which the child lives (home, respite care, school, and times of community-based transportation)

- **Individuals** involved in the child's care: family, healthcare proxy (often a family member), home care nurses, providers of care in foster care or group homes, school nurses and teachers, respite care providers, bus drivers, healthcare teams (primary care providers, specialty physicians, other members of these medical team), and palliative care/hospice teams
- **Information** to include in documentation: goals of care and how these goals guide decisions, healthcare and symptom management plans that meet these goals, location of health care for acute illness, resuscitation status, care plans for home and school in the event of a life-threatening event, contact information for individuals with expertise and availability to assist at times of acute events (designated physician, palliative care clinicians, and/or hospice team)

Most families find that preparing for the "what-if" scenarios with a trusted provider is helpful and does not lessen hope. Documenting and communicating this information can assure that previously defined care plans are carried out, including protecting the child from interventions that are anticipated to cause potential harm without long-term benefit. This process also requires a dialogue to take place about how these plans can be supported in different settings, such as school or group homes. In addition to communicating plans of care to school nurses, teachers, home nurses, and group home providers, sharing information, with parental agreement, that helps illuminate the medical decision-making process enables others to understand why certain interventions should be pursued and why some have been limited. This can help minimize moral distress and help direct others involved in the child's care to know that there is always care to provide.



## SYMPTOM MANAGEMENT IN PEDIATRIC PALLIATIVE CARE

Among all children receiving palliative care, the most common problems encountered are cognitive and speech impairments, feeding difficulties, seizures, sleep disturbances, and pain. These symptoms are often sequelae of conditions that cause severe neurologic impairment, and they are best managed in the context of multispecialty care. Pediatric palliative care clinicians may serve in a collaborative role as they coordinate care across multiple specialties to ensure that these sources of discomfort are fully addressed.

Among children with cancer, the most common symptoms identified near the end of life are fatigue, pain, dyspnea, gastrointestinal problems (anorexia, nausea, vomiting, constipation, diarrhea), delirium, depression, and anxiety. Medications commonly used for treatment of these symptoms are shown in Table 125-2.

## PAIN ASSESSMENT AND MANAGEMENT

The assessment and management of pain is discussed in Chapter 110. The discussion below is focused on the management of pain in the child with a complex chronic condition.

### Pain Assessment in Children with Complex Chronic Conditions

Pain is assessed through either self-report or observational assessment. Assessment that utilizes reporting and rating of pain must be appropriate to the child's cognitive level. Parents and caregivers often have the best understanding of the child's functional level and manifestations of pain-related behaviors. Clinicians should use a validated pain rating system appropriate for the level of intellectual function.

Pain assessment tools involve the concept of placing and understanding things in order of magnitude. Children from age 5 or 6 are developing the ability to create a series in order of size but only through trial and error. Pain rating tools appropriate for this functional age include poker chips and Oucher. Children from ages 7 to 10 can more reliably use tools to quantify pain, such as the Wong-Baker faces pain rating scale. Adolescents develop the ability to use a numerical rating scale, such as a 0 to 10 scale, to rate their pain without the use of a tool.

Depending on their developmental age and functional status, younger children or children with developmental disabilities may be able to indicate the presence, location, and severity of pain. Observational tools have been developed for use in nonverbal children or those unable to report pain. Pain assessment must be performed in the context of other sources of distress, such as hunger or anxiety.

### Observational Tools

Observational tools assess vocalizations, facial expression, consolability, interactivity, mood, eating and sleeping, protective actions, movement, tone and posture, and physiologic measures. The *FLACC* (Face, Legs, Activity, Cry, Consolability) assessment tool provides a simple, consistent method of pain assessment in nonverbal or preverbal children. The FLACC tool was revised (r-FLACC) to include behaviors specific to children with neurologic impairment. The *Non-Communicating Children's Pain Checklist–Revised (NCCPC-R)* is a validated pain assessment tool for children with severe cognitive impairment, but it is cumbersome for use in the clinical setting. The *Pediatric Pain Profile (PPP)* is a 20-item behavioral rating scale designed to assess pain in children with severe neurologic impairment, and the *Individualized Numeric Rating Scale (INRS)* is designed to incorporate parents' knowledge of their child's unique expression of pain.

### Characterization of Pain

Pain is usually classified as either nociceptive or neuropathic. Nociceptive somatic pain is caused by stimulation of nociceptors in skin, soft tissue, skeletal muscle, and bone. It is well localized and usually described as sharp, aching, squeezing, stabbing, or throbbing. Nociceptive visceral pain is caused by stimulation of nociceptors and stretch receptors in the viscera, and it is poorly localized and often described as dull, crampy, or achy. Neuropathic pain is caused by stimulation or abnormal functioning of damaged sensory nerves and is usually described as burning, shooting, or tingling.

Disease-related sources of pain may include nociceptive somatic pain from bone metastases or tumor; nociceptive visceral pain, such as from cholelithiasis or bowel distension; and neuropathic pain from tumor infiltration of peripheral nerves. Treatment-related pain may include mucositis and neuropathic pain.

The degree of pain experienced following a stimulus varies markedly within and among individuals. Previous pain exposure modulates responses such that one can either increase or decrease the subsequent pain response to a specific stimulus. The mechanisms controlling individual pain responses include differences in central pain processing functions that vary with previous life events, descending inhibition of pain transmission within the spinal cord and periphery, and a host of other factors. Thus, in one individual, the same stimulus may result in varied responses at different times.

Children with neurologic impairment experience pain more frequently than the general pediatric population. Identifying a source of pain in a nonverbal child with a developmental disability poses a unique and significant challenge. Commonly recognized pain sources in these children include acute etiologies, such as fracture, urinary tract infection, or pancreatitis; and chronic etiologies, such as gastroesophageal reflex, constipation, feeding difficulties, positioning, spasticity, hip pain, or dental pain. Table 125-3 outlines etiologies of acute and chronic pain to consider.

Underlying central nervous system dysfunction poses the potential for altered pain modulation pathways in the brain, which may in turn alter the response to both noxious and nonpainful stimuli. In children with severe neurologic impairment who exhibit persistent pain-related behaviors, extensive diagnostic workup may not yield a definitive nociceptive source of pain. As a diagnosis of exclusion, the term "neuro-irritability" can be used to describe this scenario.

One etiologic hypothesis for chronic pain in children with severe neurologic impairment is the gastrointestinal tract. Literature suggests that children with a gastrostomy tube and those taking medications for feeding, gastroesophageal reflux, or gastrointestinal motility experience higher rates of pain. This association may include a component of hyperalgesia (increased sensitivity to painful stimuli) or allodynia (pain induced by nonpainful stimuli), and

**TABLE 125-2 MEDICATIONS COMMONLY USED IN PALLIATIVE CARE (MAXIMUM WEIGHT 50 kg)**

| Symptoms | Medications | Usual Starting Dose |
|---|---|---|
| Dyspnea | Morphine (or opioid equivalent) | 0.05–0.1 mg/kg PO or 0.015–0.03 mg/kg SQ/IV q 3–4 h prn |
| | Lorazepam | 0.02–0.05 mg/kg PO/SL/SQ/IV q 6 h prn (max dose 2 mg) |
| Respiratory secretions | Glycopyrrolate | 0.04–0.05 mg/kg PO q 4–8 h or 0.004–0.005 mg/kg IV q 3-4 h |
| | Scopolamine | Adolescents: 1.5 mg by transdermal patch q 72 h |
| | Hyoscyamine | *0.125 mg/mL solution* |
| | | 3–4 kg: 4 drops PO q 4 h prn (0.125 mg/mL) |
| | | 10 kg: 8 drops PO q 4 h prn (0.125 mg/mL) |
| | | 50 kg: 1 mL PO q 4 h prn |
| | | *0.125 mg/5 mL elixir* |
| | | 10 kg: 1.25 mL PO q 4 h prn |
| | | 20 kg: 2.5 mL PO q 4 h prn |
| | | 40 kg: 3.75 mL PO q 4 h prn |
| | | 50 kg: 5 mL PO q 4 h prn |
| | Atropine | 1–2 drops SL q 4–6 h prn (1% ophthalmic drops) |
| Fatigue | Methylphenidate | 0.05–0.1 mg/kg PO q AM and q noon |
| Anorexia/weight loss | Megestrol acetate | Use in children > 10 years old: 100 mg PO BID |
| | | If no effect in 2 weeks, increase to 200 mg BID |
| Constipation | Polyethylene glycol | 0.7–1.5 g/kg (8.5–17 g) PO daily |
| | Senna liquid | 2–6 years: 2.5–3.75 mL PO daily |
| | | > 6–12 years: 5–7.5 mL PO daily |
| | Lactulose | 15–30 mL PO BID or 5–10 mL PO q 2 h until stool |
| | Bisacodyl suppository | 1 suppository PR daily prn |
| | Sodium phosphate enema | 1 PR every other day as needed |
| | Methylnaltrexone | 0.15 mg/kg SQ daily |
| Nausea/vomiting | Metoclopramide | 0.1–0.2 mg/kg PO/IV q 6 h |
| | Ondansetron | 0.15 mg/kg PO/IV q 8 h prn |
| | Haloperidol | 0.01–0.02 mg/kg PO q 8 h prn |
| | Diphenhydramine | 1 mg/kg PO/IV q 6 h prn |
| | Scopolamine | Adolescents: 1.5 mg by transdermal patch q 72 h |
| | Lorazepam | 0.02–0.05 mg/kg PO/SL/SQ/IV q 6 h prn (max dose 2 mg) |
| | Dexamethasone | 0.1 mg/kg PO/IV q 6 h |
| | Dronabinol | 0.05–0.1 mg/kg PO q 12 h |
| | Aprepitant | Adolescents: 125 mg PO 1 hour prior to chemotherapy, then 80 mg q day on days 2 and 3 |
| Fever | Acetaminophen | 15 mg/kg PO/PR q 4–6 h as needed |
| | Ibuprofen | 10 mg/kg PO q 6–8 h as needed |
| Insomnia | Melatonin | 2–3 mg PO qhs |
| | Trazodone | 0.75–1 mg/kg PO qhs |
| | Clonidine | 0.002 mg/kg PO qhs |
| Anxiety | Lorazepam | 0.02–0.05 mg/kg PO/SL/SQ/IV q 6 h prn (max dose 2 mg) |
| | Clonazepam | 0.005–0.01 mg/kg PO q 8–12 h |
| Agitation/delirium | Haloperidol | 0.01–0.02 mg/kg PO q 8 h prn |
| | | For acute agitation: 0.025–0.05 mg/kg PO, may repeat 0.025 mg/kg in 1 h prn |
| | Risperidone | 0.25–0.5 mg PO daily or divided BID |
| | Olanzapine | 1.25–2.5 mg PO daily |
| | Quetiapine | 25 mg PO BID |
| Muscle spasm | Diazepam | 0.03–0.05 mg/kg PO/IV q 6–8 h prn |
| | Baclofen | 2.5–5 mg PO q 8 h |
| Seizures | Lorazepam | 0.1 mg/kg PO/SL/PR, may repeat in 15 minutes |
| | Midazolam | 0.2 mg/kg SL/intranasal |
| | Diazepam rectal gel | 2–5 years: 0.5 mg/kg q 15 minutes × 3 doses |
| | | 6–11 years: 0.3 mg/kg q 15 minutes × 3 doses |
| | | > 12 years: 0.2 mg/kg q 15 minutes × 3 doses |
| | | (Round dose to 2.5, 5, 10, 15, or 20 mg/dose) |
| Neuropathic pain | Gabapentin | Day 1–3: 2 mg/kg PO TID or 5 mg/kg PO qhs |
| | | Day 4–6: 4 mg/kg PO TID or 2.5 mg/kg q AM and midday and 5 mg/kg qhs |
| | | Day 7–9: 6 mg/kg PO TID or 2 mg/kg q AM and midday and 10 mg/kg qhs |
| | | Day 10–12: 8 mg/kg TID or 5 mg/kg q AM and midday and 10 mg/kg qhs |
| | Amitriptyline or nortriptyline | Day 1–4: 0.2 mg/kg PO qhs |
| | | Day 4–8: 0.4 mg/kg PO qhs |

IV, intravenous; PO, oral; PR, per rectum; prn, as needed; SL, sublingual; SQ, subcutaneous.

Adapted from Hauer J, Duncan J, Scullion BF. *Pediatric Pain and Symptom Management Guidelines* 2014. Dana Farber Cancer Institute/Boston Children's Hospital Pediatric Advanced Care Team. 

**TABLE 125-3 ETIOLOGY OF PAIN/IRRITABILITY IN CHILDREN WITH SEVERE NEUROLOGIC IMPAIRMENT**

| |
|---|
| **Head, Eyes, Ears, Nose, Throat** |
| Acute otitis media, pharyngitis, sinusitis, dental abscess/gingival inflammation, corneal abrasion, glaucoma, ventriculoperitoneal shunt malfunction |
| **Chest** |
| Pulmonary aspiration/pneumonia, esophagitis, pericardial effusion, supraventricular tachycardia, cardiac ischemia |
| **Abdomen** |
| Gastrointestinal: gastroesophageal reflux disease, gastritis/gastric ulcer, peptic ulcer disease, food allergy, appendicitis, intussusception, constipation, delayed/impaired motility, rectal fissure, visceral hyperalgesia |
| Liver/gallbladder: hepatitis, cholecystitis |
| Pancreas: pancreatitis |
| Renal: urinary tract infection, nephrolithiasis, neuropathic bladder, obstructive uropathy |
| Genitourinary: inguinal hernia, testicular torsion, ovarian torsion/cyst, menstrual cramps |
| **Skin/Extremities** |
| Pressure sore/decubitus ulcer |
| **Psychosocial** |
| Loss of caregiver, change in home environment, nonaccidental trauma |
| **General** |
| Medication toxicity, sleep disturbance |

these patients could potentially benefit from treatments used for neuropathic pain.

### Management of Pain

The World Health Organization (WHO) developed a tool in 1986 to guide medication selection for pain treatment, referred to as the analgesic ladder. It was revised in 2012 for children with chronic illnesses from a 3-step ladder to a 2-step approach, eliminating the category of moderate pain and the recommendation for weak opioids. Evidence has shown that codeine is not as effective or safe as was once thought, and it is no longer recommended for routine use. Codeine is ineffective in over one-third of individuals due to variability in conversion of codeine into its active metabolite, and ibuprofen has been demonstrated to achieve equivalent analgesia with fewer side effects than codeine. Furthermore, genetic variability in the metabolism of codeine places some individuals at higher risk for serious side effects, such as respiratory depression, at routine doses. Tramadol was also eliminated in the updated 2-step approach due to the lack of safety and efficacy data in the pediatric population.

The first step of the 2-step approach is used for mild pain and includes the use of nonopioid analgesics, including acetaminophen, ibuprofen, and ketorolac. The second step is used for moderate to severe pain and includes the use of opioid analgesics, starting with a lower dose for moderate pain and a higher dose for severe pain. Adjuvant medications can be used at either step, especially for neuropathic pain. Integrative medicine offers approaches such as guided imagery, meditation, hypnosis, storytelling, music, art therapy, and acupuncture that may be useful (see Chapter 13). Acupuncture, hypnosis, and mind-body therapies have proven to be efficacious interventions for pain and anxiety in children. Hypnosis specifically has been effective in lessening procedural distress, reducing procedural time, and reducing procedural pain and anxiety for children.

### Safe and Effective Use of Opioids

Commonly used opioid medications are shown in Table 110-3. Opioids are the most effective agents for management of pain and dyspnea. However, fear of respiratory depression or addiction remains a barrier to the effective use of opioids, even at the end of life. This is unwarranted as opioid-induced respiratory depression is unlikely when dosed appropriately, adjusted for renal or hepatic impairment, and titrated in a standardized manner. The association of opioid use with end-of-life care can result in the misconception that opioid use either hastens death or indicates that someone is dying. When used effectively, opioids do not hasten death and are the mainstay of management for pain and dyspnea throughout the course of illness.

For optimal treatment of persistent, moderate-to-severe pain, opioid administration should be scheduled around the clock based on the duration of analgesic effect of the specific opioid. Once the opioid requirement is determined, it can be converted to a sustained-release formulation given 2 or 3 times daily, with immediate-release doses as needed for breakthrough pain. A reasonable trial dose for breakthrough pain is 10% of the 24-hour opioid requirement. It can be given as often as every 1 to 2 hours to achieve pain relief. Based on the patient's response and the requirement for breakthrough analgesia, the daily dose of analgesics may be increased by 25% to 50% per day until adequate analgesia is achieved or until there are intolerable or unmanageable side effects. For most opioids, there is no fixed upper limit for the effective dose. In renal impairment, fentanyl and methadone are considered the safest, oxycodone and hydromorphone should be used with caution, and morphine should be avoided.

Opioid side effects are common (Table 125-4), and management of these is important to assure continued use of necessary analgesics. Stimulant laxatives, such as senna or bisacodyl, should be initiated when opioids are prescribed to prevent constipation. For many other side effects, such as sedation and nausea, symptom improvement may occur without dose adjustment after several days.

Use of sustained-release options in children is often limited by route of administration and required dosage. For example, sustained-release morphine is only available as a capsule or tablet, and the smallest dose is 10 mg. Methadone is an important long-acting option given its availability as a liquid. However, titration of methadone can be complicated given its rapid distribution phase (half-life 2–3 hours) followed by slow elimination phase (half-life 4.2–130 hours). This extended elimination phase may result in drug accumulation and toxicity 2 to 5 days after starting or increasing methadone.

When switching from one opioid to another, the calculated equianalgesic dose should be decreased by 25% to 50% to account for incomplete cross-tolerance. Subsequent dosing can then be adjusted

**TABLE 125-4 MANAGEMENT OF OPIOID SIDE EFFECTS**

| |
|---|
| **Respiratory Depression** |
| Breathing will become less labored once pain is controlled, but significant opioid-induced respiratory depression is unlikely with appropriate dosing |
| May occur with rapid titration or at high doses in opioid-naive patients |
| Dose reduction by 20% if analgesia is satisfactory |
| Opioid rotation |
| **Sedation and Hypersomnolence** |
| Mild sedation is common |
| Patients generally become tolerant over days to this effect of opioids |
| **Constipation** |
| Opioid-induced constipation is very common, but it can be effectively prevented and treated with agents such as laxatives (Table 125-2) |
| **Urinary Retention** |
| Opioid rotation |
| **Nausea and Vomiting** |
| Patients generally become tolerant |
| Can be effectively treated with one of the antidopaminergic antiemetics, such as metoclopramide or haloperidol (Table 125-2) |
| **Pruritus** |
| Antihistamines (diphenhydramine, hydroxyzine) are of limited efficacy |
| Naloxone and naltrexone may be more effective |
| **Myoclonus** |
| Clonazepam, baclofen |
| **Delirium** |
| Neuroleptics (Table 125-2) |
| **Hyperalgesia** |
| Opioid rotation (consider methadone) |

**TABLE 125-5 OPIOID DOSING FOR CHILDREN OVER 6 MONTHS OF AGE (MAXIMUM WEIGHT 50 kg)**

| | Equianalgesic Dose | | Usual Oral Dose | Usual IV dose |
|---|---|---|---|---|
| Drug | Oral (mg) | IV (mg) | Oral (mg) | IV (mg) |
| Morphine | 30 | 10 | 0.2–0.3 mg/kg q 3–4 h | 0.05–0.1 mg/kg q 2–4 h |
| Hydromorphone | 6–8 | 1.5–2 | 0.04–0.06 mg/kg q 3–4 h | 0.015 mg/kg q 2–4 h |
| Oxycodone | 15–20 | N/A | 0.1–0.2 mg/kg q 4–6 h | N/A |
| Fentanyl | N/A | 0.1 (100 μg) | N/A | 0.5–2 μg/kg/h continuous |
| Methadone[a] | | | 0.1 mg/kg q 6–8 h | 0.05–0.1 mg/kg q 6–8 h |

IV, intravenous; N/A, not applicable.

[a]Dose-dependent potency, requires expertise in use.



depending on clinical response. Equivalent dosing information is shown in Table 125-5.

For a systematic approach to management of escalating symptoms, see Table 125-6.

## MANAGEMENT OF OTHER SYMPTOMS

### Dyspnea

Dyspnea is the experience of shortness of breath, difficulty breathing, or painful breathing. It is a common symptom of numerous medical disorders, including pulmonary parenchymal and obstructive disorders, neuromuscular disease, congestive heart failure, and chest wall disorders (see Chapter 512). Measures of respiratory rate, oxygen saturation, blood gas levels, and family perception do not necessarily correlate with the patient's perception of breathlessness.

Treating dyspnea is typically focused on identifying and treating the underlying cause. If dyspnea persists despite maximal medical management of identified causes, interventions include an oxygen trial, cool air from a fan or open window, repositioning, hypnosis, lorazepam for associated anxiety, and morphine sulfate. A recent review by the American College of Physicians concluded that treating adults with dyspnea with short-term opioids is beneficial, resulting in improvement of refractory dyspnea without significant sedation or respiratory depression. A suggested starting dose for an opioid-naïve patient is 25% to 30% of the dose used for pain, or if the patient is already on an opioid, the dose can be increased by 30%.

In a child with cancer, dyspnea can be due to airway obstruction from tumor, pleural effusion, pulmonary fibrosis from chemotherapy, superior vena cava syndrome, pulmonary edema, and anemia. Interventions include radiotherapy for tumor-related airway obstruction, thoracentesis for pleural effusion, diuretics to decrease pulmonary edema, and transfusion for significant anemia. Treatment decisions are guided by their ability to achieve comfort and whether the intervention requires hospitalization.

In children with severe neurologic impairment, recurrent respiratory problems may lead to respiratory insufficiency and life-threatening complications. As in adults with chronic respiratory disorders, these children require symptom management that incorporates elements used for both chronic and acute respiratory management. Table 125-7 outlines chronic and acute home care strategies for individuals with severe neurologic impairment who experience aspiration of oral secretions. Note that the table includes consideration of use of morphine sulfate as goals shift from medical treatment to comfort when a decline in health status is observed. Further study is needed to determine when best to integrate morphine sulfate into the care plans of patients who have chronic aspiration and recurrent distressing respiratory exacerbations.

**TABLE 125-6 GENERAL GUIDELINES FOR MANAGEMENT OF ESCALATING PAIN**

| |
|---|
| Bedside titration with intravenous (IV) bolus every 15 minutes until pain is relieved |
| If on opioids, initial bolus will be 10–20% of the 24-hour opioid dose |
| Increase opioid bolus by 30–50% every third dose if pain continues |
| Once patient has obtained adequate pain relief, calculate the new 24-hour opioid dose including rescue doses |
| Determine route for around-the-clock dosing that is best suited to patient's ongoing analgesic needs (oral, IV, transdermal) |
| Consider adding an adjuvant or co-analgesic (eg, a nonsteroidal anti-inflammatory drug, benzodiazepine, corticosteroids, or ketamine) |
| If the patient has significant opioid adverse effects *with* adequate pain control, rotate opioids and reduce the equianalgesic dose (Table 125-5) of the new opioid by 25–50% |
| If the patient has significant opioid adverse effects *without* adequate pain control, rotate opioids without a reduction in the equianalgesic dose |
| Reduce the dose of the opioid by 20% *if* there has been a reduction in pain |

**TABLE 125-7 RESPIRATORY HOME MANAGEMENT: MEDICAL TREATMENT AND COMFORT STRATEGIES**

| | |
|---|---|
| **Chronic Interventions** | |
| Suctioning | As needed for comfort |
| Oxygen | Assessed by appearance of patient or by oximeter |
| Nebulized albuterol | Every 3–4 hours for coughing, wheezing, congestion |
| Nebulized ipratropium | Every 3–4 hours for coughing, wheezing, congestion |
| Nebulized saline | Every 3–4 hours for coughing, wheezing, congestion |
| Chest physiotherapy or vest | 2 times/day, increase to 4 times/day with increased symptoms[a] |
| Nebulized budesonide | 2 times/day, increase to 4 times/day with increased symptoms[a] |
| Salmeterol | Family history of atopy or benefit from daily albuterol |
| **Acute Interventions** for respiratory exacerbations from chronic aspiration | |
| Clindamycin, amoxicillin/clavulanate, or levofloxacin/moxifloxacin[b] | 10–14 days |
| Systemic corticosteroids[c] | 5 days |
| **Additional Interventions** for symptom management and end-of-life care | |
| Fan on face | Relieves sensation of breathlessness |
| Morphine sulfate | Use for discomfort or respiratory distress |
| | Starting dose 0.1 mg/kg/dose PO/SL/G-tube |
| | May increase by 30% until comfortable |
| Glycopyrrolate, scopolamine, or atropine | Might contribute to mucous plugging |
| | Decreases oral and respiratory secretions in end-of-life care |

[a]Symptoms include increased coughing, secretions, congestion, respiratory rate, and breathing effort.

[b]Use in children with aspiration problems when symptoms persist despite an increase in chronic interventions.

[c]Include with third or fourth exacerbation, or sooner if symptoms return within 2 months of antibiotic course.

Reproduced with permissions from Hauer JM. Respiratory symptom management in a child with severe neurologic impairment, *J Palliat Med.* 2007 Oct;10(5):1201-1207.

### Nausea and Vomiting

Nausea, vomiting, and retching are commonly encountered in oncology patients, in children with severe neurologic impairment, and at the end of life. An understanding of the pathophysiology of nausea and vomiting and the neurotransmitters involved can guide evaluation and selection from the management options available (see Chapter 377). In children with neurologic impairment, retching and vomiting are commonly attributed to gastroesophageal reflux disease (GERD), but stimulation of the emetic reflex is likely an underreported source of symptoms in these patients. Management options other than treatment of GERD should also be considered.

Symptom management strategies based on involved receptors and origin of symptoms are outlined in Table 125-8. As with pain, management of nausea and vomiting includes evaluating for treatable causes in addition to using medications that block involved receptors.

### Constipation and Bowel Obstruction

Constipation is a common cause of discomfort and pain at the end of life. Multiple factors may contribute to constipation, including decreased physical mobility, decreased fluid and nutritional intake, and opioid use. Patients receiving scheduled opioids should always have a bowel regimen consisting of a stimulant laxative, such as senna or bisacodyl. Osmotic laxatives, such as polyethylene glycol, and stool softeners, such as docusate, may provide benefit as additional agents. Methylnaltrexone, a peripherally acting opioid antagonist, blocks the effects of opioids in the gastrointestinal tract and is available as a subcutaneous injection for opioid-induced constipation refractory to standard therapies.

In some patients, spinal cord compression or bowel obstruction may result from tumor. Malignant bowel obstruction may cause refractory vomiting and painful abdominal distention. Medical management of the obstruction consists of systemic corticosteroids and antisecretory medications, such as anticholinergics, proton pump inhibitors, and somatostatin analogues, while treatment with opioids for pain and antiemetics for nausea provides symptomatic relief. Metoclopramide, an antiemetic with a prokinetic effect, is contraindicated in complete obstruction. Surgical placement of a venting gastrostomy tube is an option and should be considered in the context of the patient's goals of care and overall prognosis.

### Cachexia and Anorexia

Cachexia is a common finding in patients with advanced cancer. Poor nutritional intake and increased metabolic demands, impaired taste, and depression may all contribute to weight loss. Treatment should be directed at identifiable causes.

Severe cancer-related wasting is associated with poor outcomes in adult cancer patients, and increasing caloric intake does not improve outcomes. Clinicians can address concerns about starvation by explaining that the cancer itself is responsible and that increasing nutrition, particularly through artificial means, cannot halt or reverse this process. Goals for management should instead focus on associated symptoms and maintenance of function.

When considering enteral or parenteral nutrition, discussion should include anticipated benefits and the potential for complications as the child's cancer progresses. This allows the team and family to define a plan to reassess after a period of time whether the interventions are helpful. Discussion at the time of initiation of supplemental nutrition may make reconsideration of this intervention less distressing for families as the child's illness progresses.

Pharmacologic interventions include corticosteroids, which can produce a short-term increase in appetite for up to 4 weeks, megestrol acetate, and cannabinoids, such as dronabinol. Megestrol acetate should be used with caution as it is associated with severe adrenal suppression in children with cancer, and its use has not been associated with improvements in morbidity or mortality in adults with serious illness.

### Artificial Nutrition and Hydration

Discussing nutrition and hydration can be difficult given the instinctive need for parents to provide nutrition to their children and the association of nutrition as a source of nourishment and comfort. Understandably, this makes it difficult for families to consider that artificially provided nutrition may not provide benefit or may actually cause harm. As mentioned earlier, providing enteral and parenteral nutrition does not reverse the severe cancer-related wasting that is associated with poor outcomes in adult cancer patients. Discussion should focus on strategies that meet the child's goals of care.

Certain patients, such as those with brain stem involvement of a central nervous system tumor or with a progressive neurologic disease, may develop swallowing impairment, and can be evaluated as discussed in Chapter 23. Symptoms of coughing or choking when eating or drinking should be considered signs of aspiration. A swallowing study can be considered to evaluate the risk of aspiration with solids and liquids of different consistencies. Liquids can be thickened to the appropriate consistency if needed. Nasogastric or gastrostomy tube

**TABLE 125-8 TREATMENT OF NAUSEA AND VOMITING**

| Central Sites | Causes | Receptors/Mechanisms | Therapeutic Agents |
|---|---|---|---|
| Vomiting center (VC) | Final common pathway with numerous inputs | Histamine ($H_1$) | Antihistamines (diphenhydramine, promethazine) |
| | | Acetylcholine (Ach) | Anticholinergics (scopolamine, hyoscyamine) |
| | | Neurokinin 1 ($NK_1$) | $NK_1$ antagonists (aprepitant) |
| Chemoreceptor trigger zone (CTZ) | Medications (chemotherapy, opioids, antibiotics, anticonvulsants) | Dopamine ($D_2$) | Butyrophenones (haloperidol, droperidol) |
| | Metabolic imbalance (hyponatremia, hypercalcemia, uremia, ketoacidosis) | | Phenothiazines (prochlorperazine, chlorpromazine) |
| | Toxins (ischemic bowel) | Serotonin ($5\text{-}HT_3$) | Serotonin antagonists (ondansetron, granisetron) |
| Vestibular | Disorders of the vestibular nucleus and cranial nerve VIII | Histamine ($H_1$) | Antihistamines (diphenhydramine, promethazine) |
| | | Acetylcholine (Ach) | Anticholinergics (scopolamine, hyoscyamine) |
| Meningeal mechanoreceptors | Increased intracranial pressure, tumor, infection | Stimulation of the VC | Corticosteroids |
| Cortex | Anxiety | Stimulation of CTZ and VC | Relaxation techniques |
| | | | Benzodiazepines, dronabinol |
| **Gastrointestinal Sites** | **Causes** | **Receptors/Mechanisms** | **Therapeutic Agents** |
| Mechanoreceptors and chemoreceptors | Stasis (anticholinergics, opioids), constipation, autonomic neuropathy, mucositis, gastritis, radiation, chemotherapy, tumor, hepatic distention | Vagal afferents (cranial nerve X) | $H_2$-blockers, proton pump inhibitors (ranitidine, omeprazole) |
| | | | Prokinetic agents (metoclopramide) |
| | | Histamine ($H_1$) | Antihistamines (diphenhydramine, promethazine) |
| | | Serotonin ($5\text{-}HT_3$) | Serotonin antagonists (ondansetron, granisetron) |

placement for nutrition can be considered as an option for provision of fluid and nutrition while minimizing food-related aspiration risks. This choice may be most appropriate in patients who are expected to live and have a reasonable quality of life for some time. Even with a gastrostomy tube, patients remain at risk for aspiration of oropharyngeal secretions.

For some children, placement of a gastrostomy tube may undermine the identified goals of care. When eating provides significant pleasure to the patient, choosing to maintain oral feeding may positively impact quality of life despite the risks of aspiration. Some may choose to use a gastrostomy tube to meet nutritional goals and provide tastes of food for pleasure by mouth. As a patient nears the end of life, nutritional strategies can be discussed and reassessed.

#### Feeding Intolerance

Feeding intolerance can be a source of distressing symptoms for children with severe neurologic impairment receiving nutrition through a feeding tube. As with recurrent respiratory exacerbations as a result of chronic pulmonary aspiration, the initial benefit from treatment interventions may lessen over time. At such times, it can be beneficial to integrate medical and symptom management strategies.

Management includes treating contributing problems such as constipation and delayed gastric emptying. Experience shows that some children may benefit from an empiric trial of medications used for nausea and vomiting, being mindful of which medication targets which receptor to avoid duplication. Unfortunately, there is no evidence to guide physicians in such patients. One must be careful not to introduce too many trial options when there is no evidence to support benefit from any one medication. Other intervention strategies include adjustment of feeding schedules, an empiric trial of an elemental formula, an empiric trial of metronidazole for small bowel bacterial overgrowth, and replacing a gastrostomy feeding tube with a jejunostomy feeding tube.

Unfortunately, some children will have persistent discomfort with enteral feeds despite using these intervention options. At such times, some children may benefit from a decrease by 25% to 30% or greater in the total amount of formula provided by feeding tube. Certain observations may suggest benefit of such a trial: Has feeding intolerance occurred or worsened as there has been a decline in the overall functional status? Is weight gain out of proportion to the linear growth on the same nutrition? Does the child appear puffy or edematous at times? Families again benefit at such times from a reflection on goals of care and determining approaches that meet these goals.

#### Fatigue

Fatigue is identified by parents as the most common symptom in the last month of life and the source of greatest distress for children with cancer. It is also the least likely to be treated successfully.

Fatigue is a multidimensional symptom with both physical elements (muscle weakness, decreased energy) and cognitive or affective elements (difficulty concentrating, difficulty maintaining attention, lack of motivation and interest). Younger children and adolescents with cancer define fatigue differently. Younger children emphasize the physical aspects of the symptom, whereas adolescents describe multiple dimensions and distinguish between mental and physical fatigue.

Parents of children with cancer note that physical and emotional dimensions of fatigue create significant disruptions for the entire family. Parents describe mood changes in the child and also report delays around the household and family activities because of the need to accommodate the fatigued child. Fatigue also limits children who wish to attend school.

Opioid analgesics may contribute to diminished levels of energy and decreased ability to concentrate. Coexisting or contributing factors include anemia, infection, pain, deconditioning, sleep disturbance, depression, and anxiety. Assessment instruments used to assess fatigue in children measure onset, course, severity, duration, and distress, and concurrently assess other associated symptoms.

Multimodal approaches to treatment may be most effective. Psychostimulants such as methylphenidate can be used to increase wakefulness, particularly when patients have opioid-related somnolence. Because of the short duration of action, patients can control the timing of doses to coincide with important events during the day, such as time with family and friends. Other interventions include treatment of depression, anxiety, and sleep disturbance, as well as psychosocial interventions, blood transfusions, exercise programs, acupuncture, rest, and relaxation (including playing/socializing).

#### Psychological Distress, Depression, and Anxiety

Pain, anxiety, distress, and suffering in children are best thought of as interrelated symptoms; addressing each is important to the relief of the others. Children with cancer commonly encounter symptoms of worrying, sadness, nervousness, and irritability. Such symptoms can be difficult for children to separate out from physical symptoms; an example is a child who describes, "I am hurting; my heart is sad." Screening for psychosocial distress among children with cancer remains inconsistent and varies based on institutional size and resources. Levels of distress in a family can be stratified into three levels: a universal level that applies to all families, a targeted level that presents with acute needs, and a clinical level that is persistent and/or escalating. At the universal level, children and families often experience resilience and engage family and social support systems to ameliorate their distress. At the targeted level, acute distress requires more targeted interventions and close monitoring. At clinical levels of distress, consultation with behavioral health specialists, such as social workers or psychologists, can develop a plan of care that more fully addresses their risk factors.

Children with cancer commonly experience situational symptoms of depression and anxiety, ranging from feeling sad and anxious to meeting diagnostic criteria for psychiatric treatment. Mood disorders experienced during initial diagnosis often persist and may even exacerbate during treatment. Intervention at the onset of depression and anxiety may help reduce the risk for continued emotional distress.

Psychological well-being has as much of an impact as physical well-being on quality-of-life measures in children with chronic progressive diseases such as cystic fibrosis. As seen in children with cancer, a variety of emotional symptoms were identified in children with cystic fibrosis and Duchenne muscular dystrophy, including feelings of isolation, minor depressive symptoms, insecurity, and a high level of anxiety. Symptoms of depression and anxiety may escalate as the underlying disease progresses and becomes severe.

Children with serious illness who experience psychological distress can benefit from a multidimensional approach to treatment. Psychotherapeutic and psychopharmacologic treatment options should be considered. Guided imagery, mindfulness-based interventions, and hypnosis can be effective tools. Social workers, child life specialists, child psychologists, or other trained experts are essential members of the team to assist children with expressing emotional symptoms of distress through age-appropriate activities. Supportive interventions for depression and anxiety for the child include normalization of their experiences, supportive counseling, introduction to support groups or other children, and provision of psychoeducational resources. Clinical interventions range from psychotherapeutic counseling, mindfulness-based interventions, support groups, art therapy, problem-solving skills, and bibliotherapy.

Psychopharmacologic treatment can be considered for symptoms of depression and anxiety that persist despite nonpharmacologic interventions. Medications should always be used in conjunction with ongoing supportive counseling and psychosocial interventions. Selective serotonin reuptake inhibitors (SSRIs) have some safety data in medically ill children, although efficacy has been difficult to demonstrate. The following considerations should be kept in mind when using SSRIs:

- Therapeutic benefit may not be seen until 2 to 4 weeks after initiation.
- Side effects can occur within a few days of initiation and include dry mouth, constipation, urinary retention, sedation, anxiety, agitation, insomnia, irritability, impulsivity, akathisia, and hypomania.
- Suicidal thoughts may develop, recognizing that worsening symptoms such as agitation and irritability may be precursor signs.

- Drug–drug interactions are possible, including serotonin syndrome, which presents with mental status changes, autonomic hyperactivity (hypertension, hyperthermia), and neuromuscular abnormalities (tremor, myoclonus).
- Consideration of off-label use should be discussed with the family.
- Discontinuation syndrome occurs when SSRIs are stopped abruptly (more common with paroxetine), and symptoms include anxiety, irritability, dizziness, nausea, fatigue, myalgias, and chills.

Methylphenidate has been used for the treatment of depression in adults receiving palliative care and can be considered for a child with depressive symptoms and fatigue. An improvement in mood may be seen more rapidly than with SSRIs, which can be an advantage if the patient is nearing the end of life. However, methylphenidate may exacerbate anxiety and anorexia and should be used with caution.

Benzodiazepines are commonly used to treat symptoms of anxiety and provide rapid-onset, short-term relief. They should be used cautiously chronically given the lack of evidence to indicate long-term benefit and the development of dependence.



#### Delirium and Agitation

Delirium is a disturbance of consciousness with an acute onset over hours to days. Associated features include a fluctuating course, disordered thinking, change in cognition, inattention, altered sleep–wake cycle, perceptual disturbances, and psychomotor disturbances. Delirium can be described as 3 subtypes: hyperactive, hypoactive, or mixed. Hyperactive delirium is characterized by psychomotor agitation, whereas a patient with hypoactive delirium may seem withdrawn or disinterested. A patient may also fluctuate between these 2 subtypes. Causes of delirium include medications (opioids, anticholinergics, benzodiazepines), metabolic disturbances (infection, dehydration, renal, liver, electrolyte, brain metastases), and psychosocial contributors (emotional distress, intensive care). When compared to adults, delirium in children tends to have a more acute onset with greater agitation, mood lability, and irritability. Adults are more likely to have impaired memory and cognitive deficits. Delirium is an important consideration for children in the intensive care unit, and assessment tools have been developed for use with children.

In contrast, agitation is considered an unpleasant state of arousal that may represent an appropriate response to an underlying stressor. It is a nonspecific behavioral response in a variety of clinical situations, including pain, delirium, and anxiety. In children with severe neurologic impairment, these diagnoses may be difficult to distinguish. Management of delirium and agitation first involves evaluating for treatable medical causes, including medications, metabolic disturbances, and sources of discomfort (pain, dyspnea, muscle spasms, position, constipation). It is also helpful to consider conditions that mimic the appearance of agitation, such as akathisia (an unpleasant state of motor restlessness) from antidopaminergic medications, myoclonus or withdrawal from opioids, and paradoxical reactions. First-line treatment of delirium consists of environmental modifications that help to orient and calm the patient. If delirium is persistent or severe, pharmacologic treatment with neuroleptics, such as haloperidol, olanzapine, and quetiapine, may be considered. Benzodiazepines and opioids may worsen delirium, and decreasing exposure to these medications should be considered.

#### Sleep Disturbance

Sleep disturbance in children with serious illness can include difficulties in falling asleep, trouble staying asleep, early morning awakening, nonrestorative sleep, and periods of too much sleep. A review of records of children who died from cancer identified that twice as many children reported "too much sleep" as a problem in the last month of life. A comparison of quality of sleep identified that children with human immunodeficiency virus (HIV) had more nightmares and more general sleep problems. Children with sickle cell disease slept significantly less on nights when they were experiencing pain compared with nights that were pain-free. Predictors of sleep disturbance among patients with cancer include pain, breathing difficulty, headaches, hot flashes, limb movements, frequent urination, nausea, vomiting, and greater amounts of radiation.

Consequences of impaired sleep include fatigue, impaired daytime functioning, mood disturbances, negative impact on quality of life, reduced social/emotional well-being, reduced ability to cope, and impaired perception of illness severity. Sleep disturbances may worsen symptoms of depression, anxiety, and pain.

There are 2 general approaches for treatment of sleep problems. Pharmacologic treatments include melatonin, antidepressants such as tricyclic antidepressants and trazodone, clonidine, and neuroleptics (especially for patients with delirium). Benzodiazepines tend to be overused, leading to dependency and tolerance, and should only be used in a time-limited manner. Psychological and behavioral interventions include stimulus control, sleep restriction, sleep education, and relaxation training. When sleep problems are linked to symptoms or correlated with a disorder, treatment of the underlying condition may improve sleep.

#### Anemia and Bleeding

For a child with fatigue, dyspnea, or significant dizziness, a red blood cell transfusion may help improve well-being and quality of life. As time progresses, the symptomatic benefit from blood transfusions may decrease as the disease progresses, offsetting the benefit with the risk of transfusion-related complications.

Mucosal bleeding can sometimes be controlled with aminocaproic acid given orally or intravenously to inhibit fibrinolysis. Topical options include fibrin sealants. The tannins present in black teas can also help to stop bleeding. At home, patients can press a wet tea bag onto bleeding gums.

Profuse bleeding in the setting of thrombocytopenia at the end of life can be terrifying if family members are not prepared for this possible event. Most often, platelet transfusions are not possible in the home setting. Therefore, careful planning and consideration are necessary so as not to disrupt the child's last days. Preparing a plan for families can allow them to remain with their child. This can include having dark sheets and towels readily accessible to mask the color and quantity of blood. Management plans for potentially distressing symptoms should also be defined, including medication doses for opioids and benzodiazepines, with medications and syringes readily available. The possibility of intracranial bleeding should also be anticipated and managed symptomatically, including a medication plan if a seizure occurs.

#### Fever and Infection

Parents of children with cancer are well aware of the consequences of fever and neutropenia during the child's treatment course. As a child nears the end of life, the role of hospitalizations and intravenous antibiotics can be guided by the goals of care. Discussions with the child and family can help guide decisions for investigative measures and treatment.

#### Seizures

Seizures can be highly distressing for families and caregivers to witness. Seizures may occur near the end of life as a result of central nervous system disease, intracranial hemorrhage, electrolyte abnormalities, fever, or hypoxia. Management options for acute seizures in the absence of intravenous access include rectal diazepam or midazolam given sublingually or intranasally.

#### Increased Intracranial Pressure

Children with intracranial tumors are at risk for experiencing symptoms of increased intracranial pressure as the disease progresses. Symptoms include headache, vomiting, and somnolence. Although ventricular shunting can be considered, tumor growth can quickly block a shunt or lead to recurrence of elevated pressure. Dexamethasone can be effective in alleviating symptoms, and dosing can be titrated as new symptoms arise or if initial symptoms wane. Corticosteroid-associated side effects, including mood changes and a cushingoid appearance, should be part of ongoing discussion about dose titration.

#### Spinal Cord Compression

Early diagnosis and management of spinal cord compression maximizes the chances of preservation of function. Presenting symptoms include sensory and motor changes as well as bowel and bladder function abnormalities. Prompt imaging, typically with magnetic resonance imaging, should be provided when cord compression is suspected. Dexamethasone is used to decrease edema at the site of compression, thereby reducing symptoms and preserving neurologic function. Decompressive surgery plus radiation therapy is the mainstay of treatment and increases the chances of recovery to ambulation. As always, the specific intervention recommended should take the patient's overall functional status and goals of care into consideration.

## MANAGEMENT OF SYMPTOMS AT END OF LIFE

Symptoms that may present when death is imminent include pain, dyspnea, agitation, and oral secretions. Management of escalating pain is outlined in Table 125-6. Algorithms or templated orders can improve management of pain, dyspnea, or agitation. In addition to opioids for pain and dyspnea, adjuvants for agitation and anxiety should include a benzodiazepine (intermittent lorazepam or continuous midazolam) or a neuroleptic (haloperidol).

Ketamine has been identified as a beneficial adjuvant with opioids. In conjunction with opioids, it reduces opioid tolerance and provides greater coverage for neuropathic pain. Ketamine's *N*-methyl-D-aspartate (NMDA) receptor antagonist property has been identified as the mechanism for these observed benefits. The dosing for ketamine as an adjuvant analgesic is significantly lower than anesthetic doses. It can be initiated at 0.05 to 0.1 mg/kg/h as a continuous intravenous infusion, and it is also available in oral formulations for intermittent use.

### Palliative Sedation

Palliative sedation is the practice of sedating a patient to the point of unconsciousness and is used as a last resort when all other methods of controlling suffering have proven unsuccessful. Refractory symptoms identified as leading to palliative sedation include agitation, pain, respiratory distress, and myoclonus. Although rarely needed, when a child's refractory symptoms cannot be managed with opioids, benzodiazepines, and other adjuvants, palliative sedation may be warranted. The most common medications used are benzodiazepines, barbiturates, and neuroleptics, and propofol and ketamine may have a role as well.

A summary of points to consider and to review with the family and healthcare providers include the following:

- The child has a terminal illness and is experiencing an unbearable symptom that is refractory to other interventions.
- Evaluation and management of symptoms has used the expertise of palliative care and/or pain specialists.
- Palliative sedation is ethically and legally acceptable and is distinguished from active euthanasia.
- The ethical principle of double effect justifies that the intended benefits (comfort) outweigh possible unintended but foreseeable consequences (sedation to unconsciousness and death).
- The decision and principles involved must be discussed with all staff involved.
- After agreement is reached with the child's healthcare team, the information is shared with the family with all questions and concerns addressed.
- Consent is obtained and documented.
- Families are prepared that their child may live "hours to days."
- An appropriate level of nursing care and monitoring is ensured.
- A peaceful, quiet setting, with a minimum of intrusions is created.
- A detailed plan is developed, including drugs, doses, and criteria for increasing medication by boluses or increased hourly infusions.
- The procedure is documented in the medical record.
- Orders not contributing to comfort are discontinued (eg, vital sign monitoring, laboratory studies, certain medications).
- The team should continue to elicit and respond to concerns, questions, and suggestions.
- After the patient's death, arrange follow-up discussions with the family and with the healthcare team.

When managing escalating symptoms at the end of life, the ethical principle of double effect is often cited. This principle includes the following:

- The action must not be immoral in itself.
- The action must be undertaken with the *intention* of achieving only the good effect. Possible bad effects may be *foreseen* but must not be *intended.*
- The action must not achieve the good effect by means of a bad effect.
- The action must be undertaken for a proportionally grave reason.
- All medical treatments have both intended benefit and unintended risk, including death.

### Forgoing Artificial Nutrition and Hydration

Forgoing artificial nutrition and hydration (ANH) remains one of the more difficult areas of consideration given the symbolic significance of nutrition, the myths about "starvation" and dehydration, and underrecognition of the complications of ANH. The American Academy of Pediatrics recognizes in a policy statement that "Life-sustaining medical treatment encompasses all interventions that may prolong the life of patients," including routinely used medical interventions such as antibiotics, insulin, chemotherapy, and ANH. Like other medical interventions, ANH should be evaluated by weighing its benefits and burdens in light of the clinical circumstances and goals of care. It is ethically and legally permissible to discontinue ANH when it is prolonging or contributing to suffering.

Forgoing ANH can lessen discomfort at the end of life as a result of decreased oral and airway secretions, resulting in decreased choking and dyspnea. Mouth dryness can be relieved with moistened swabs, ice chips, petroleum jelly on the lips, and careful oral hygiene. Chronically ill individuals often do not experience hunger when ANH is discontinued, and the resulting ketosis produces a sense of well-being, analgesia, and mild euphoria. Individuals at the end of life without ANH naturally eat and drink less as physiology, including intestinal function, slows down. Those who continue to receive enteral feeds or intravenous hydration are at risk for vomiting, pulmonary secretions, and edema when the body is no longer able to process the same quantity of nutrition or hydration. Clinical monitoring for feeding intolerance, respiratory difficulties, and signs of fluid overload should prompt recommendations to decrease or discontinue fluid intake during the end-of-life period.

When considering the discontinuation of ANH, clinicians should counsel families that death is likely to ensue in the range of days to weeks. Typically, death occurs 3 to 14 days after discontinuation of fluids. This can be shorter when there is a preceding decline in the function of other organs and can be longer when small amounts of water are used to flush an enteral tube after medication administration. As they near death, patients become less aware of their surroundings and become increasingly somnolent. Families should be assured that their care teams, particularly their palliative care and hospice providers, will work with them to ensure that their child's death is as peaceful and comfortable as possible.

### Preparing Families for the End of Life

Issues not related to the management of specific symptoms that are central to providing quality palliative care include preparing the family for the end of life, planning the location of death, preparation of home care and/or hospice services, and issues such as autopsy, organ bank donation, and any desired tissue banking. Most hospitals and home hospice programs have specific documentation requirements and processes to assist families with these issues.

## SUGGESTED READINGS

Feudtner C, Kang TI, Hexem KR, et al. Pediatric palliative care patients: a prospective multicenter cohort study. *Pediatrics*. 2011; 127:1094-1101.

Friebert S, Williams C. *NHPCO's Facts and Figures: Pediatric Palliative & Hospice Care in America*. 2015 ed. Alexandria, VA: National Hospice and Palliative Care Organization; 2014. Available at: http://www.nhpco.org/sites/default/files/public/quality/Pediatric_Facts-Figures.pdf. Accessed September 8, 2016.

Hauer JM. *Caring for Children Who Have Severe Neurological Impairment: A Life with Grace*. Baltimore, MD: Johns Hopkins University Press; 2013.

Levetown M. Communicating with children and families: from everyday interactions to skill in conveying distressing information. *Pediatrics*. 2008;121:e1441-e1460.

Morrison W, Kang T. Judging the quality of mercy: drawing a line between palliation and euthanasia. *Pediatrics*. 2014;133(suppl 1):S31-S36.

Steele AC, Mullins LL, Mullins AJ, Muriel AC. Psychosocial interventions and therapeutic support as a standard of care in pediatric oncology. *Pediatr Blood Cancer*. 2015;62:S585-S618.

Temel JS, Greer JA, Muzikansky A, et al. Early palliative care for patients with metastatic non-small-cell lung cancer. *N Engl J Med*. 2010;363:733-742.

Wolfe J, Grier HE, Klar N, et al. Symptoms and suffering at the end of life in children with cancer. *N Engl J Med*. 2000;342:326-333.

Wolfe J, Hinds PS, Sourkes BM. *Textbook of Interdisciplinary Pediatric Palliative Care*. Philadelphia, PA: Elsevier Saunders; 2011.

World Health Organization. *WHO Guidelines on the Pharmacological Treatment of Persistent Pain in Children with Medical Illnesses*. Geneva, Switzerland: WHO Press; 2012.



# 126 Palliative Care for Children with Chronic Diseases

Lisa Humphrey, Amy Trowbridge, and Jill Ann Jarrell

## INTRODUCTION

Caring for a child with a chronic illness from which he or she is not likely to recover is one of the most difficult challenges we face as healthcare providers. Children with medical complexity (CMC) comprise an increasing proportion of the pediatric population, and although the overall number of pediatric deaths has declined recently in the United States, this population is living longer with numerous and unique healthcare needs. CMC account for a large percentage of technology utilization in pediatrics as well as inpatient hospitalizations. When hospitalized, they face a much higher risk of mortality than non-CMC pediatric patients. Given the increasing disease burden in and the fragility of CMC, there are palliative care issues and needs unique to this population that warrant an in-depth discussion.

Although a multitude of descriptors and definitions exist for and within this patient population, this chapter will exclusively use the CMC designation. For a discussion of these varying terminologies, please refer to Section 9 of this textbook titled "Children with Medical Complexity."

## PROGNOSTICATION IN CHILDREN WITH MEDICAL COMPLEXITY

The term *prognosis* comes from the Greek meaning "for knowledge" and is used in medicine to communicate expected disease course among members of the healthcare team or to the patient and family, often for decision-making and planning purposes. Prognostication is always a difficult task to perform and difficult to communicate, but it is especially challenging in CMC.

### CHALLENGES

It is well established that physicians are poor prognosticators and typically overestimate survival. The length of the physician's relationship with the patient has been suggested to be inversely proportional to the physician's prognostic accuracy. This is important in CMC as healthcare teams often care for patients from birth through adolescence and even into adulthood and thus may be less accurate in their ability to provide meaningful and precise prognostic information.

CMC often have numerous problems involving multiple organ systems and sometimes very rare diseases or conditions, leaving providers with little or no precedent to predict disease trajectory. Additionally, every patient has a unique set of social and environmental circumstances that influence how their diseases manifest and how they respond to stressors and treatment over time.

Existing prognostic models are largely disease specific and based on functional status or laboratory values. Feudtner and colleagues suggest that disease severity, age, previous hospitalizations, and certain chronic conditions can be predictive of mortality 1 year after hospitalization.

For children diagnosed with a disease that has a typical clinical course (Huntington disease, spinal muscular atrophy type 1), Schwantes and colleagues advise creating a road map with the patient and family that includes the disease course as well as benefits and risks of potential interventions along the way. They use the example of a young boy presenting with asymptomatic Duchenne muscular dystrophy and advise discussing what to expect early in the course, including medical technology such as assisted ventilation and artificial hydration and nutrition.

In cases where the underlying disease is unknown or multifactorial, it can be helpful to use the patient as his or her own benchmark and compare the patient's ability to participate in activities such as playing, walking, or feeding over time to establish a clinical and functional trajectory. For example, "Jeremy was able to play with his rattle a couple of hours a day last month, now he doesn't play with it at all and he is having trouble tolerating his feeds. If the disease follows its natural course, we expect this decline to continue."

### COMMUNICATING PROGNOSIS

Communicating an uncertain prognosis can be confusing for patients and families as they witness potentially many ups and downs in the clinical course. The patient–family–provider relationship can be damaged if there are misunderstandings or unfulfilled expectations. For example, a patient experiences an acute decompensation and the family receives counsel regarding advancing palliative goals or initiating hospice services, the patient then stabilizes or improves slightly and the family loses trust in the provider's ability to anticipate the clinical course or mistrusts the motive of the healthcare team.

One helpful strategy is to use graphics to articulate the patient's waxing and waning to emphasize the overall downward disease trajectory (Fig. 126-1). It is important to emphasize to families that planning for alterations in care is a flexible process that can and should change with the patient's clinical status.

Families of CMC have high information needs, and most families want to know as many details as possible about what to expect with their child. It is recommended that prognosis for length of life be shared in ranges such as minutes to hours or weeks to months to allow families to plan and prepare and also to allow for variability in the patient's course.

## ADVANCE CARE PLANNING FOR CHILDREN WITH MEDICAL COMPLEXITY

### BENEFITS OF ADVANCE CARE PLANNING

High-quality advance care planning provides benefits to patients, families, and healthcare providers. When parents have the opportunity to discuss their child's end-of-life care plan, they feel more control over the situation, are more certain in their decisions, report improved communication with their child's healthcare team, and have more confidence that their child received the best care possible. Effective advance care planning increases the likelihood that a child will die in the family's preferred location and can decrease levels of complicated grief after death. Many families are having these discussions privately but do not feel able to have them with their physicians or other members of the healthcare team.

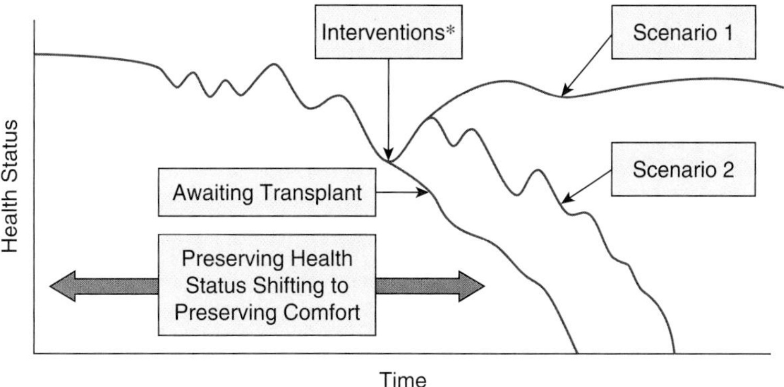


**FIGURE 126-1** Children with cancer awaiting organ transplant or with severe developmental impairment. Hope for the best, but prepare for the rest.



## BARRIERS TO EFFECTIVE ADVANCE CARE PLANNING

Parents and providers admit that there are numerous barriers to having these difficult conversations. Families note their hesitancy comes from fear of death or fear of losing hope, uncertainty, a preference to focus on being alive, feeling like "it's not time yet" (child not sick enough), feeling too "stressed out," fear that care will change, or denial of severity of illness.

Providers often cite their own lack of training and the lack of a dedicated palliative care team as reasons why advance care planning does not occur sooner. They also note difficulties inherent in the medical system, including time constraints, language barriers, or feeling like they do not know the patient or family well enough. Several providers note that uncertain prognoses make advance care planning even more challenging. Many providers also admit that they delay advance care planning conversations because they are afraid to take away a family's hope.

## UNIQUE CHALLENGES OF ADVANCE CARE PLANNING

Discussing advance care planning topics with the families of CMC presents unique challenges. The concept of "quality of life" is paramount to these discussions. First, families and practitioners have personal beliefs and experiences that influence their definition of quality of life; thus, it can be difficult to agree on what is in the patient's best interest. Second, many parents of CMC have a reconfigured role, one in which they are not only the parent, but also the nurse, respiratory therapist, aide, etc., for their child. For many parents, their own lives begin to revolve around the care of their child. The death of their child not only comes with the unimaginable grief of losing a child, but also with the loss of their identity as caregiver. This dual role of the parent can affect decision making.

## TOOLS FOR ADVANCE CARE PLANNING

### Explore Personal Beliefs

All providers have their own beliefs, religious backgrounds, political affiliations, or personal or professional experiences that may be affecting the way they are approaching the care of a sick child or the counsel of a family. Recognizing the impact of one's own beliefs and potential biases is an important first step toward approaching care and communication in an objective fashion.

### Help Families Create a "Philosophy of Care"

Advance care planning is often thought of as a series of specific decisions regarding what a family does not want for their child (eg, cardiac resuscitation, intubation). This narrow focus is provider centric and is not intuitive to families. Instead, the focus of conversations should be on what a family does want for their child. Providers should work with families to develop a general philosophy of care that can be broadly applied to specific decisions. These conversations ideally should happen during periods of relative stability. When specific decisions need to be made, both the family and the provider can draw on their mutually developed philosophy of care.

### Hope for Benefit Versus Risk of Harm

For a child who is chronically ill in whom cure is not the goal, every intervention is essentially palliative. If providers talk about each new intervention in the life of these children, even the small ones, in the context of hope for benefit versus risk of harm all along, families can and will have an easier time understanding this framework when bigger decisions arise and when stabilization is no longer an option. Medical culture carries a strong bias toward intervention, feeling that "doing something" is better than "doing nothing." Providers are prone to referring to proposed interventions as "treatments," which implies assumed benefit, such as life prolongation or cure. When results of procedures or medications are unknown, this should be reflected in the description. Using language like "we will choose to use this intervention because of the hope we have of its ability to improve quality of life" or "we will protect our child from this intervention so that we can avoid potential harm" removes language bias and allows the family to participate in the patient's care, no matter what choice they make. Too often, interventions are chosen with minimal discussion of their intended goals or whether that goal aligns with the patient's overarching philosophy of care.

### Decision Making Is Not Black and White

Families of CMC are constantly searching for a balance between the suffering or burden that may come with a particular intervention and the hope for a perceived improvement in quality of life or a prolonged duration of life. This can result in seemingly paradoxical care plans that include some "restorative" interventions and some "palliative" interventions. In addition, perceived suffering and quality of life may change daily, and for this reason, families may change their minds regarding what types of care will help them achieve their goals for their child. For some, this means they may not be able to make a decision about a particular intervention in advance; they need to wait and see what the balance of suffering and quality is at that time. Providers should respect this process and avoid pressuring future decisions by instead focusing on what can be done today to make the child's life better and the broader philosophy of care. Providers too should avoid labeling a family's overall intentions as *curative* versus *palliative*; they are almost always both.

### The Role of Hope

Hope has an integral role in palliative and end-of-life care and should not be confused with denial. Although many hope for a miracle, most possess other hopes for themselves or their child such as hope for time, hope for comfort, hope for companionship, hope to die at home, or a hope that loved ones do not suffer. To have hopelessness is to risk demoralization, which is sense of failure. Expert palliative care should mitigate hopelessness by being agents of hope-identifying strategies for patients and their caregivers. Palliative care seeks to foster hope through open dialogue regarding prognosis, interventions, and goals of care. Studies support that such tasks increase caregiver hope and expressed goals of care when end of life approaches.

#### Advance Care Planning Is a Process, Not a Single Conversation

Advance care planning cannot and does not occur all at once. Providers should aim to strike a balance with families between not addressing these crucial topics often or early enough and overwhelming parents with too frequent discussion about end of life. Providers can work with families to develop agreed-upon intervals to review the family's goals of care and the care team's success at achieving them.



### DISCUSSING DO NOT RESUSCITATE ORDERS

By discussing resuscitation in the context of a family's broader goals of care, we can avoid surprising families with this topic, and it can be presented as another tool to achieve their goals for their child. Some key communication tactics for this specific discussion include the following:

- Avoid dichotomies such as "doing everything" or "doing nothing." ("Do you want us to do everything for your child if her heart stops?") This implies that interventions could be helpful and can make parents feel as though they are "refusing" care for their child.
- Discuss a do not resuscitate (DNR) order as a tool to *protect* a child from interventions that will not be helpful and may harm the child. Do not overemphasize the harm.
- It is not necessary to discuss every single item that is included in a DNR order. This can be overwhelming for parents and may lead to decisions that are inconsistent.
- Use the word "die": "If your child's heart stops, that would mean your child has died. The team could attempt to restart their heart . . ."
- Give legitimacy to both sides of a decision: "Some loving parents choose to allow cardiac resuscitation, in the hopes that it would lead to more good time for the child down the road, while other loving parents choose to protect their child from cardiac resuscitation, valuing the opportunity to hold their child at the end of his or her life."
- Consider making a recommendation if the family has expressed clear goals and the medical circumstances are clear. "Based on what you have told me about Jonny, I recommend we use this order to protect him from XYZ."
- Remind families that they can change their mind at any time and that in an out-of-hospital setting, it is always up to them when, where, and with whom they choose to share a completed out-of-hospital DNR form.

### DOCUMENTING ADVANCE CARE PLANNING

Each healthcare system's electronic medical record has a unique location and format for in-hospital DNR orders. Most need to be completed or co-signed by an attending physician; however, providers of any level can initiate these conversations.

Each state uses its own form to document physician orders for out-of-hospital resuscitation. Some examples are Out-of-Hospital DNR, Physician Orders for Life-Sustaining Treatment (POLST), and Medical Orders for Scope of Treatment (MOST). These forms are completed and signed by a healthcare professional and, thus, must be honored by in-home emergency personnel and in emergency rooms. It is important for physicians to research the specific legal document in the state in which they practice in order to provide the most accurate counsel to patients and families.

Advanced directives are meant for use in the event that a previously competent patient can no longer make his or her own healthcare decisions. Synonyms and types of advance directives vary by state but may include living will, directive to physician, and medical power of attorney.

Children should be included in these decisions to the extent that they are neurologically and developmentally capable. The Aging with Dignity Organization has created several useful family- and patient-friendly documents. "Five Wishes" is appropriate for mature teens or young adults and meets the requirements to serve as a legal advanced directive. "Voicing My Choices" and "My Choices" are planning documents for adolescents and children, respectively, that are not legal documents, but can be used by both families and healthcare providers to discuss and understand a child's or young adult's wishes for the end of his or her life. These documents are written in everyday language and allow patients to express their wishes in the spiritual, emotional, and personal realms in addition to giving medical direction.

## CARE COORDINATION AND PALLIATIVE CARE IN CHILDREN WITH MEDICAL COMPLEXITY

### CARE COORDINATION DEFINITION

*Care coordination* refers to the intentional oversight, coordinating, and streamlining of services for CMC including primary, specialty, and consult medical providers and teams; support services such as therapies, equipment companies, and private duty nursing companies; and other entities such as social, legal, or community partners. Although everyone on the healthcare team should divide and share care coordination responsibilities, there is often a specific person or group within the healthcare team that leads care coordination efforts for CMC (care coordinators). Care coordination should not only be concerned with the medical decisions at hand but should also involve the child's care team consistently forward thinking to create and execute plans that will fulfill the child's healthcare needs and manage and treat future health problems that the child could experience.

### CARE COORDINATION IN PALLIATIVE CARE

Implicit in palliative care is an emphasis on transdisciplinary care that focuses on enhanced communication efforts among healthcare providers and between the healthcare team and patient and family. Although sometimes not explicitly called care coordination, this is indeed part of the function of a palliative care team (including hospice teams), and some care coordination efforts may be duplicative with those provided by the patient's medical home. Hence, roles in care coordination among the healthcare team members should be discussed and defined clearly. It may be helpful for the primary care provider (PCP) or PCP's care coordinator to participate in the palliative care interdisciplinary team meeting or conferences when discussing shared patients.

### CONCURRENT CARE

One common misconception in this area is that a patient has to choose between curative and palliative services. Traditionally, palliative care services can and should be provided in conjunction with any disease-directed treatments. However, in the past, patients who engaged hospice services were required to forego curative or disease-directed therapies. For the CMC population specifically, patients and families often fear they must forego their private duty nursing (PDN) hours for home care if they pursue hospice services. The Patient Protection and Affordable Care Act (ACA) of 2010 requires all state Medicaid programs and state children's health insurance programs (SCHIPs) to pay for both curative and hospice services for children under 21 who meet hospice qualifications. This means that, currently, patients with Medicaid or SCHIP can have PDN, continue to see their doctors, and receive potentially curative therapies while they are on hospice.

### ETHICAL CONSIDERATIONS

Children who have a chronic illness can have surprising insight into their disease based on their personal experience, which may have granted some a precocious ability to understand death and potentially a greater capacity to participate in decision making than a same-aged healthy peer. As such, they should be afforded the right to assent to therapies and also the voice to actively participate in decisions affecting their health or end-of-life care. The healthcare provider can assess capacity on a case-by-case basis and seek assent from the pediatric patient when appropriate. Conversely, CMC may have associated intellectual limitations rendering them not competent, even when greater than 18, to make decisions for themselves as they lack the capacity to understand the ramifications of their decision making. In these cases, courts determine competency and grant legal guardianship when warranted.

For further discussion on patient-related ethical issues or ethical issues specific to the family or provider in caring for CMC, please refer to Section 9 of this textbook titled "Children with Medical Complexity."

## TALKING WITH CHILDREN ABOUT DEATH

This topic is one that is important for pediatric providers to understand and address with family members and other members of the healthcare team. Although it is important for all children and young adults with serious illness or healthy children with ill family members, it is discussed here to highlight the need to understand comprehension of death across developmental spectrums given the long nature of illness in CMC.

### DEATH COMPREHENSION AND STAGES OF DEVELOPMENT

Death comprehension requires acquisition of its four subconcepts: universality, inevitability, irreversibility, and nonfunctionality. It takes time to acquire these associations, and children do so in an orderly fashion influenced by many factors in the cultural and family environment, as well as the child's own psychological and cognitive makeup. For additional discussion, refer to Chapter 127, Supporting the Grieving Child and Family.

For typically developing children, prior to age 2, all interactions with the outside world are sensory and motor, and there is likely no intellectual concept of death. Starting in early childhood, at ages 2 to 7, orientation is self-centered, and the outside world is considered only from the child's personal and subjective point of view. To children, imaginary and magical things are important determinants of occurrences. At this stage, dead things should be able to eat and feel and breathe. Parents can be immortal, and dying animals should be able to return.

From ages 7 to 11, thinking is less egocentric and more concrete. Reasoning is based on direct observation, and concepts of death are in the present tense. They feel the pain of separation and may not be concerned with afterlife and its abstractions. After age 12, full intellectual capacities develop and with them the ability to deal in abstractions. However, this often clashes with the developmental milestones of adolescence: the need for peer support, the desire to fit in, and the drive to question all as one forms their own thoughts and identity. Thus, adolescents often struggle with the morality of death, especially in disenfranchised causes of death (eg, suicide), and often seek to mourn separate from their parents, preferring instead the company of their peers and to appear "normal."

### TALKING WITH CHILDREN ABOUT THEIR OWN DEATH

Under age 2, no discussion of death will be understood, and therefore, no discussion is needed. Symptom relief, comfort care, holding, and hugging are the requirements as death approaches. For children ages 2 to 7, death is seen as temporary, sleep-like, reversible, and, perhaps, a result of magical actions originating within the child. It often is necessary to attempt to correct misperceptions and feelings of guilt and self-blame. Feelings of separation and abandonment are also major concerns that parents and healthcare teams should monitor. At about age 7, children begin to understand that animals and people do not die because of a magical spell they or others cast, but perceive reality as they grasp universality and inevitability. They often ask repetitive questions secondary to their need to know the details of the dying experience. Truthfulness is paramount, and description of details that adults might take for granted is necessary, for example, explaining that in death there is no pain or hunger or coldness. Adolescents' concerns about their changed physical appearance, hair loss, and weakness need to be acknowledged, and they must be given the opportunity to express their anger.

It is important to talk with a child about his or her death at his or her developmental level so that the child's concerns, questions, and fears can be adequately assessed and addressed. A team-based approach should be used, drawing on the expertise of physicians, nurses, psychologists, art therapists, child life specialists, social workers, and chaplains.

Questions about death should be answered honestly and directly, presenting an opportunity to explore the subject. Ask open-ended questions to generate conversation: "How do you think your treatment is going?" "What do you think will happen to you?" "Do you think you will be able to go back to school?" "Do you want to keep taking your medicines?" "What do you think would happen if you stopped your medicines?" Patients desire to be heard, not necessarily for their stressors to be ameliorated.

It is not as common as one might think that a seriously ill child asks, "Am I going to die?" If they do, it is almost certainly because they know they are and they are probing to see if it is safe to talk about it. False, overly reassuring answers are only evasive and certain to stop meaningful conversation. Rather, responses such as, "I'm worried for you because the last medications, as you know, did not work" or "It's possible, but I am not sure. What do you think?" are better. Generally, because there is often uncertainty, it is best to help others find their own answers, rather than to provide one for them.

### HOW WILL I DIE?

Like adults, children with full death conceptualization worry not only about whether they will die but also how they will die. Children seldom ask for information for fear of breaking the mutual pretense that they and their caregivers have shared and thus causing the eruption of difficult emotions for all. However, the consequence of this reticence is a child's imagination running rampant and painting a picture worse than reality. It is therefore incumbent upon healthcare providers to encourage and support conversations between patients and their caregivers to ensure correct information and support of these difficult emotions. Such discussions can also identify hopes that a child or caregiver has (eg, no pain), and consequently, a more robust healthcare plan can be devised.

### LAST GOODBYES

Like adults, children need time for their last goodbyes and to put their affairs in order. To whom they would give their favorite toys, computer, or clothes is as important to children as putting financial affairs in order and saying goodbye to spouses and friends are to adults. Verbalization is difficult for some children, and art therapy, puppet play, and music are alternatives to talking. Child life specialists are especially well trained in such techniques and should be called on to help. Care providers must understand that it is necessary to set aside time for these discussions and that they are every bit as important as anything else in the therapeutic armamentarium.

Like all things related to caring for children, all of the above must take into consideration the cultural context in which the patient and family exist. It is vital for healthcare teams to have open conversations with the family to better understand cultural and religious norms and preferences for discussing death and grief.

## BEREAVEMENT

Although bereavement is discussed elsewhere in this textbook, the grief of a medical caregiver when one loses a chronic patient is a distinct aspect of caring for CMC and warrants discussion.

### BEREAVED MEDICAL PROFESSIONALS

Healthcare professionals, not unlike the patients and families they treat, are subject to the great emotional pain that accompanies death. Repeat exposure to such tragedy can make the burdens or providing care even more difficult. Professionals may experience frustration, a prolonged sense of failure, helplessness, sadness, and depression.

Healthcare providers frequently minimize their own grief because they feel it does not compare to that of the families they serve or is not valid. Moreover, there is usually no one on the treatment team whose purpose it is to monitor or support the team's grief work. Where, then, do the professionals find help?

## INDIVIDUAL GRIEF WORK

Healthcare professionals need to see themselves as a help agent in their own grief work, both from a proactive and reactive perspective. Proactively, identification and implementation of a self-care plan are integral parts of being a whole physician seeking longevity and job satisfaction. Integral to self-care is the acknowledgement that it is individualistic and can/should change over time as the individual changes. Examples include exercising, prayer, dinner with friends, mindfulness, or a ritual deployed with each and every death. At times, these self-care practices will be insufficient to the level of grief present. Healthcare practitioners should educate themselves on identifying within themselves when they are struggling and have an action plan in place to reach out to colleagues for help.



## COLLEAGUES

Important sources of support also come from other members of the treatment team. As for patients, it is important that team members have this opportunity to express their frustrations and release their own burdens. A well-functioning team is of great help. When difficult discussions are occurring or end-of-life care is being provided, encourage team members to perform their work in pairs, allowing a shared experience between teammates that can then facilitate debriefings and support. Periodic team meetings focused on open discussions regarding the dilemmas of treatment choices, angry families, social injustices, and the apparent inhumanity of God are another opportunity provided by a functional team. Additionally, many hospitals are recognizing the need to promote and support staff wellness and have resources available. Such programs can include the critical incident management programs, second victims programs, and when needed, confidential counseling with mental health specialists.

## SUGGESTED READINGS

Aging with Dignity. Five wishes: changing the way we talk about and plan for care at the end of life. Available at: https://www.agingwithdignity.org/five-wishes/about-five-wishes. Accessed September 9, 2016.

Davies B, Sehring SA, Partridge JC, et al. Barriers to palliative care for children: perceptions of pediatric health care providers. *Pediatrics.* 2008;121(2):282-288.

Dellon E, Shores M, Nelson K, et al. Caregiver perspectives on discussions about the use of intensive treatments in cystic fibrosis. *J Pain Symptom Manage.* 2010;40(6):821-828.

Durall A, Zurakowski D, Wolfe J. Barriers to conducting advance care discussions for children with life-threatening conditions. *Pediatrics.* 2012;129(4):e975-e982.

Dussel V, Kreicbergs U, Hilden J, et al. Looking beyond where children die: determinants and effects of planning a child's location of death. *J Pain Symptom Manage.* 2009;37:33-42.

Feudtner C, Carroll KW, Hexem KR, Silberman J, Kang TI, Kazak AE. Parental hopeful patterns of thinking, emotions, and pediatric palliative care decision making: a prospective cohort study. *Arch Pediatr Adolesc Med.* 2010;164(9):831-839.

Feudtner C, Hexem K, Shabbout A, et al. Prediction of pediatric death in the year after hospitalization: a population-level retrospective cohort study. *J Palliat Med.* 2009;12(2):160-169.

Hauer J. *Caring for Children Who Have Severe Neurologic Impairment.* Baltimore, MD: Johns Hopkins University Press; 2013.

Hunter S, Smith D. Predictors of children's understandings of death: age, cognitive ability, death experience and maternal communicative competence. *Omega.* 2008;57:143-161.

Klick J, Ballantine A. Providing care in chronic disease: the ever-changing balance of integrating palliative and restorative medicine. *Pediatr Clin North Am.* 2007;54(5):799-812.

Liberman D, Pham P, Nager A. Pediatric advance directives: parents' knowledge, experience, and preferences. *Pediatrics.* 2014;134(2):e436-e443.

Nielson D. Discussing death with pediatric patients: implications for nurses. 2012. *J Pediatr Nurs.* 2012;27(5):e59-e64.

Nyborn JA, Olcese M, Nickerson T, Mack JW. "Don't try to cover the sky with your hands": parents' experiences with prognosis communication about their children with advanced cancer. *J Palliat Med.* 2016;19(6):626-631.

Schwantes S, O'Brien HW. Pediatric palliative care for children with complex chronic medical conditions. *Pediatr Clin North Am.* 2014;61(4):797-821.

# 127 Supporting the Grieving Child and Family

David J. Schonfeld

## INTRODUCTION

Virtually all children experience the death of a family member or friend. Approximately 1 of every 20 children experiences the death of a parent by 16 years of age. Although a normative and universal experience, bereavement can cause significant adjustment difficulties for children and adolescents, at least temporarily impact their ability to learn, and result in feelings and behaviors that may concern parents and other adults as well as the children themselves. Pediatricians and other pediatric healthcare providers can play a vital role by building on their preexisting relationship with the child and family to ensure that the child understands accurately what has occurred, provide advice to families on how to help promote adjustment and coping, identify misconceptions and reactions (eg, unwarranted fears, guilt, somatization, depression) that would benefit from clarification or additional services, and assist the child and family in identifying supportive resources within the community.

Children and adolescents who are actively grieving may be reluctant to disclose their feelings and concerns to parents and other adults and give the false impression that they are disinterested, unaffected, or fully adjusted to the loss. Some young children may not understand what has occurred or the implications of the death, while other children and adolescents may sense accurately that the topic is uncomfortable for adults, worry that their reactions are somehow abnormal, and/or be reluctant to burden further their parents who appear already overwhelmed with their own grief. Indeed, the egocentrism of children may lead them to conclude that they are personally hurting their parents if they initiate a conversation that seems to prompt signs of distress, such as crying, in their parents (ie, that they are upsetting their parents by talking about the death rather than simply prompting their parents' expression of the distress caused by the death; in a similar manner, many healthcare providers are reluctant to initiate conversations with children out of concern that such discussions may upset them). For this reason, it is helpful to offer to speak with children and adolescents alone so that they can talk freely and share their reactions without concern about upsetting their parents. Parents, in turn, who are grieving themselves, may wish to believe that their children are spared the pain they are experiencing and/or be less attentive to their children's reactions and needs. Since children have difficulty sustaining strong emotions for extended periods of time, they may conduct the work of mourning in "spurts," employ denial or other means to delay or limit their engagement in the process, or use play or behavior to communicate and process their feelings. Therefore, for many reasons, adults, including pediatric healthcare providers and parents, may underestimate the impact of a death on children and adolescents and miss important opportunities to offer support and assistance.

Pediatricians can begin by creating an environment where children and adolescents feel it is safe and where they are welcome to discuss their thoughts and feelings related to the death. Physicians often worry, though, that they do not know what to say that will be helpful and do not wish to make matters worse by raising the topic. Approaches to initiate discussion by adults that may be *less* helpful include (1) trying to "cheer up" those who are actively grieving (eg, "I'm sure you will feel better soon" or "At least your father is no longer in pain"); (2) encouraging people to be strong or to hide or minimize their expressions of distress (eg, "You don't want to have your son see you cry" or "You are the man of the house now that your father has died"); and (3) telling people how they should or do feel rather than asking them about their own feelings (eg, "You must be angry" is often not helpful, whereas stating "I have the sense you may be angry—is that the case?" or "I wonder if you are angry" is more likely to be well received). Much can be accomplished by a genuine and empathic statement of concern (eg, "I'm sorry to hear that your brother died"), a willingness to be with the individual who is actively grieving without trying to change his or her feelings immediately, active listening, and an offer to provide assistance now and in the future.

## MISCONCEPTIONS, LITERAL MISINTERPRETATIONS, AND GUILT

Adjustment requires that the children first understand what has occurred and its implications. There are 4 basic concepts about death that children must come to understand: (1) death is irreversible—very young children may equate death with separation and await the deceased's return; (2) all life functions end completely at the time of death (termed *nonfunctionality* or *finality*)—if this is not understood, children may worry about the physical suffering of the deceased; (3) all living things eventually die—if children do not understand the inevitability of death, they may question what the deceased individual or the child himself or herself did that was responsible for this person being selected to die; and (4) a realistic understanding of the cause of death, which helps to minimize the attribution of the cause to unrelated thoughts or actions of the victim or the child. While most children, on average, come to learn these concepts by the age of 5 to 7 years, personal experience and educational interventions can accelerate comprehension. For this reason, children with a terminal condition generally have a precocious understanding of these concepts and an appreciation of their own mortality. For additional discussion about talking to children about death, refer to Chapter 126.

Young children's limited conceptual understanding, coupled with a tendency for adults to withhold relevant information, often results in misconceptions and misunderstandings. The magical thinking and egocentrism of children prompt them to assume guilt related to the death for some thought, action, or failure to act. Often, this guilt is illogical (eg, "My father had a heart attack because I upset him that morning" or "If only I had stayed home from school that day, I would have been able to get help for my mother earlier") and too often remains fully unknown to others but may cause a great deal of distress for children; similar guilt feelings are common among adolescents and adults as well.

While religious explanations can be shared with children at any age, they are generally rather abstract and prone to literal misinterpretations and, especially for young children, should be accompanied by explanations about the physical realities of death (eg, "When people die, their body is no longer working; the person doesn't move, breathe, see, or feel pain"). Simply stating that the person "went to heaven" or "was chosen by God to be at His side" may lead to questions about how to get to or from heaven or worries that others close to the child (or the child himself or herself) may be chosen next.

## RISK FACTORS FOR DIFFICULTY ADJUSTING

Rando outlines a number of factors associated with complicated mourning that relate to the nature of the death or factors associated to relationships and support. Risk factors include deaths that are sudden or unexpected, especially when they are random, violent, mutilating, or traumatic; deaths that occur after a very lengthy illness; deaths that the bereaved individual perceives could have been prevented; a relationship with the deceased characterized by ambivalence, dependency, or anger prior to the death; lack of sufficient social support after the death; or prior or concurrent losses, stressors, or mental health problems to which the bereaved is still trying to adjust.

When the death of a family member is due to a long-standing illness, children may experience graduated feelings of loss as the illness progresses. Such anticipatory grieving allows children to "practice" grieving at a time when they can comfort themselves by the realization that their family member is still alive whenever the feelings become overwhelming. Problems may arise when one family member's course of grieving is not in synchrony with that of others, such as when one individual becomes resigned to the acceptance of the death and communicates or visits less and is perceived by other family members as abandoning the individual who is critically ill. Anticipatory grieving is a painful process, and children (and adults) may find themselves hoping for the dying process to end and may experience excessive guilt for wishing for the death of a seriously ill family member.

The death of a family member is often compounded by subsequent losses, such as the decreased availability of surviving family members secondary to the need for the surviving parent to begin or increase the hours of working outside of the home, the surviving parent dating or otherwise establishing a new relationship with another adult outside the home, or parental depression that may lead the surviving parent(s) to withdraw from interactions with the child. Financial pressures, relocations prompted from a need or desire to move to a new home, and similar stressors add to the challenge already presented by the task of bereavement.

## FUNERAL ATTENDANCE

Especially when the death is sudden or unexpected, parents must make decisions quickly under very stressful conditions about whether or not to include the children in funerals and other memorial activities. Children who have been excluded from such events miss an opportunity to benefit equally from the support of family members and friends, may have more difficulty understanding or accepting what has occurred, and often wonder what could be done to their family member or friend that is so horrifying that they are not permitted to view. In general, it is helpful instead to explain to the child in clear and direct terms what is expected to occur at the funeral and to invite the child to participate to the level of his or her comfort, without any attempt to force or coerce participation. In addition, an adult who is not personally grieving but is well known to the child (eg, a sitter, daycare provider, or neighbor) can accompany the child and monitor and address his or her needs and reactions, allowing the child to titrate the level of involvement. Even if children stand in the lobby of a funeral home and hand out mass cards to arriving guests, without stepping into the viewing room, they may benefit from feeling that they contributed to honoring the deceased family member and from sharing the support of relatives and family friends.

## ENSURING FOLLOW-UP AND OFFERING RESOURCES

Pediatricians and other pediatric healthcare providers play an important role in helping adults identify and attend to their children's needs around the time of the death and during the period of readjustment, which often lasts months to years (the duration depending in large part on the closeness of the child's relationship to the deceased and whether or not risk factors for complicated mourning are present). Referral for additional support or counseling should be considered, especially when the death involves a close family member (eg, sibling or parent) or close friend (especially for older children and adolescents), when risk factors for complicated mourning are anticipated (eg, death from suicide, parents' inability to talk to the child about the death, when child or parent is experiencing guilt associated with the death), when the initial reactions seem intense (eg, child appears markedly depressed or suicidal) or unusual (eg, failure to show any distress after the death of a parent), or when intensive grieving is prolonged and associated with impairments in daily function (eg, sleep or eating problems or deterioration in school performance). Children who are grieving should be expected to have at least some transient difficulties with school work secondary to problems with attention, sleeping, and sadness; parents should be encouraged to contact the school to help arrange for support services prior to academic failure, which can otherwise become an additional stressor for the grieving child. Pediatricians and other pediatric healthcare providers should be aware of local bereavement support groups and counseling services for children and families and offer these resources, and they should schedule periodic follow-up appointments in order to answer questions and monitor adjustment rather than simply inviting the family to call as needed. Contact can be made around the time of anniversaries of the death or birthday of the deceased or around the time of special occasions and holidays, which may be particularly stressful. Adjusting to a significant loss is a lifelong process; children will reprocess the experience at each new stage in their life, applying new cognitive and emotional insights to try and reach a more satisfying explanation or justification for the death. Parents should be prepared that new developmental stages or significant milestones (eg, graduation, marriage, birth of first child) may stimulate new questions and renewed feelings about the death. Siblings of children who have died too often are overlooked and may require active outreach. It is particularly challenging for pediatricians to know what role they can play in supporting families when the individual who has died is the family's only child. Ongoing communication and offers to meet for follow-up can be very helpful to the family in this setting. Adults often underestimate the significant impact on children of the death of a peer. Pediatricians can also play an important role in not only providing consultation to schools related to the needs of their patients but also in advising on how to provide support to others in the school community.

The Coalition to Support Grieving Students was established to develop a set of resources approved by 10 of the leading professional organizations of school professionals to guide educators and other school personnel in supporting and caring for their grieving students. Pediatricians can ensure that schools in their community are aware of these resources, which are available at no charge to the public at www.grievingstudents.org. The video training modules include expert commentary, school professionals who share their observations and advice, and bereaved children and family members who offer their perspective on adjusting to loss. Handouts and reference materials oriented for classroom educators, principals/administrators, and student support personnel that summarize the training videos, as well as a range of additional resources, can be downloaded from the Web site. Although developed for use by educators, the materials are appropriate for the professional development of pediatric healthcare providers as well.



## IMPACT ON THE HEALTHCARE PROVIDER

Being with a child who is actively grieving is uncomfortable for many healthcare providers who have devoted their careers to decreasing the suffering of children. The death of a child patient is a particularly stressful personal and professional experience faced by pediatric healthcare providers. Healthcare providers should reflect on their personal feelings about death in order to be more available to provide support to children and families and in order to ensure adequate help for themselves.

## SUGGESTED READINGS

Adams D, Deveau E. When a brother or sister is dying of cancer: the vulnerability of the adolescent sibling. *Death Stud.* 1987;11: 279-295.

Clunies-Ross C, Lansdown R. Concepts of death, illness, and isolation found in children with leukemia. *Child Care Health Dev.* 1988;14:373-386.

Ewalt P, Perkins L. The real experience of death among adolescents: an empirical study. *J Contemp Soc Work.* 1979;60:547-551.

Rando T. *Treatment of Complicated Mourning.* Champaign, IL: Research Press; 1993.

Schonfeld D. Talking with children about death. *J Pediatr Health Care.* 1993;7:269-274.

Schonfeld DJ, Demaria T; Committee on Psychosocial Aspects of Child and Family Health; Disaster Preparedness Advisory Council. Supporting the grieving child and family. *Pediatrics.* 2016;138(3):e20162147.

Schonfeld D, Kappelman M. The impact of school-based education on the young child's understanding of death. *J Dev Behav Pediatr.* 1990;11(5):247-252.

Schonfeld D, Lichtenstein R, Kline M, Speese-Linehan D. *How to Respond to and Prepare for a Crisis.* 2nd ed. Alexandria, VA: Association for Supervision and Curriculum Development; 2002.

Schonfeld D, Quackenbush M. *The Grieving Student: A Teacher's Guide.* Baltimore, MD: Brookes Publishing; 2010.

Speece M, Brent S. Children's understanding of death: a review of three components of a death concept. *Child Dev.* 1984;55:1671-1686.

Spinetta J. The dying child's awareness of death: a review. *Psychol Bull.* 1974;81:256-260.

Wender E; American Academy of Pediatrics Committee on Psychosocial Aspects of Child and Family Health. Supporting the family after the death of a child. *Pediatrics.* 2012;130(6):1164-1169.

# 128 Ethics, Law, and Medical Care Near the End of Life

Theodore E. Schall, Pamela G. Nathanson, Annemarie Boyan, Wynne Morrison, and Chris Feudtner

As in all of pediatric care, providing care near the end of life to pediatric patients is best done in a collaborative manner, with patients, parents, and other family members working with members of the clinical team to assure the highest quality of care for the patient. While in most cases medical care decisions can be made in a mutually agreeable manner, in some cases of care near the end of life, difficult questions, disagreements, or conflict can arise. In this chapter, we focus on several challenges that can arise in these difficult cases.

## WHO HAS THE AUTHORITY TO PROVIDE CONSENT FOR TREATMENT AND MAKE MEDICAL DECISIONS?

As a general rule, children under the age of majority are governed by their parents or legal guardians, and the rights of parents include consenting to treatment and making medical decisions for the minors under their care. However, there are some limited exceptions to this rule. Many state laws contain exceptions for minors to make their own medical decisions, and there are also circumstances in which parental rights to refuse care are limited by state public policy (eg, no right of refusal of low-risk, life-saving treatments for a child due to a parent's own religious reasons). Parents found by the courts to be abusive or neglectful may also lose the legal authority to make medical decisions for their children.

The general rule of parental authority has 3 exceptions that allow for minors to make their own medical decisions, the legal details of which vary state by state. First, a majority of (but not all) states grant full medical decision-making authority to emancipated minors (although the criteria for emancipation also differ across states, with, for example, some states requiring that a female patient have given birth to a child, whereas in other states having been pregnant is sufficient). Second, some states allow minors to consent to treatment for specific "carved-out" conditions and needs, including sexually transmitted infections, reproductive health care, and mental health care, without parental knowledge. Finally, in some states without consent statutes, courts have recognized a "mature minor" doctrine, which allows minors who have the maturity level to understand the risks and benefits of a treatment to consent to that treatment.

Until recently, courts held that although minors were sometimes able to refuse medical care, they could not refuse life-saving treatment. Courts in a few recent cases have held that minors who clearly understand the consequences of refusing treatment may do so even when the consequence is death. Although not every state allows minors to make these decisions, the values and perspectives of minor patients should nonetheless be discussed with the authorized decision maker and documented by the medical provider.

## DOES THE AUTHORIZED PERSON HAVE CAPACITY?

Determining capacity to consent to treatment is a challenge faced in every domain of medicine, yet capacity determination presents uniquely in pediatric settings and especially at the end of life. Although infants and young children are always developmentally incapable of consent, their parents or guardians may also temporarily or permanently lack capacity. In adolescents and young adults treated in pediatric hospitals, questions of capacity arise as a result of both the law and the usual development of capacity over time. Even when a minor is permitted by law to consent to care, the provider must still determine whether that minor has the capacity to make the decision the law permits him or her to make.

No universally accepted standard exists for defining decisional capacity. Nonetheless, patients and family members enter the healthcare arena with varying degrees of ability to understand and make complex medical decisions. In the overwhelming context of end-of-life care of a child, even ordinarily capable adults may experience fluctuations in their capacity to make medical decisions. Providers should understand that "capacity" describes a decision-making process, not the conclusion that a parent or guardian reaches. Some providers have a tendency to question and apply a much higher degree of scrutiny to the capacity of a patient or parent who disagrees with the medical team than one who agrees, especially when the stakes are high, as is the case with difficult end-of-life decisions. This tendency should be avoided, as capacity is not judged based on agreement or disagreement with medical advice. Providers must also distinguish between determinations of capacity and the diagnosis of physical or mental health conditions: parents and guardians are generally not the patients of pediatricians, and clinicians should not attempt to diagnose nonpatients.

Determination of capacity should follow a standard protocol that reveals a surrogate's ability to come to a complete understanding of risks, benefits, and alternatives to the medical decision being requested. Some parents' or legal guardians' capacity may be enhanced with the use of decision aids, written materials, or, if the surrogate has limited English proficiency, additional language services. If a parent's barrier to understanding cannot be overcome, that person cannot be relied on to consent to a minor's care, and resort to the other parent, social service agencies, or the courts might be necessary.

The stresses inherent in end-of-life care for a child may compromise parental capacity in both healthy parents and those with an underlying mental health problem. Increased depression and anxiety may arise from changing family dynamics, bearing witness to a child's suffering, or the impending loss of a loved one. Psychosocial support of parents and families through interdisciplinary care teams may help to relieve some of the burden experienced by parents facing a child's death. Both typically healthy parents and those with a previous mental health diagnosis may benefit from a referral to counseling, pastoral care, or other therapeutic support.

## HOW TO PROCEED IN THE ABSENCE OF CAPACITY?

Finding that a parent or guardian lacks capacity to consent to treatment does not give medical staff the right to make medical decisions for the patient. In the absence of an adult capable of giving consent for a minor patient, a surrogate must be selected. Depending on local statutes and the specific situation, surrogate selection may be made by the incapacitated parent, a standardized legal process, or the court system. Many states have systems for identifying a default surrogate, based on the level of relationship with the patient (eg, parent, spouse, adult sibling), and others allow a parent/guardian to appoint such surrogates by completing a simple document.

Additionally, patients who are over the age of majority and whose capacity periodically changes or is likely to decline are encouraged to select a surrogate ahead of time to make medical decisions on their behalf if they become incapacitated. This surrogate may be a parent or close family member, or the surrogate may be any other adult with capacity. Neither hospital staff nor other outpatient medical providers should be selected as surrogates, but they are often key in identifying this potential problem, initiating a discussion with patients, and providing forms to identify surrogates.

## DID AN ADULT PATIENT ISSUE AN ADVANCE DIRECTIVE?

Patients who have attained the legal right to make their own medical decisions should be encouraged to complete and regularly update advance directives. While there is controversy over the effectiveness of advance directives, they provide some basis for proxy decision making informed by substituted judgment and an opportunity to address subjects that may previously have been avoided.

## ENGAGING CHILDREN AND ADOLESCENTS IN DECISION MAKING

Both children and adolescents should be included in conversations about their fears, hopes, and wishes at the end of life. Parents and patients often try to protect one another from upsetting or painful information that both may already know, which only creates tension and a sense of isolation for the child at a time when the child most needs connection. Even when young patients lack the legal right to make choices for themselves, earnest efforts should be made to gain their perspectives and to support their wishes. The push to give older children and adolescents more control over the circumstances of their own deaths reflects respect for both the progressive development of capacity and the special circumstances of pediatric life-limiting illness.

Devastating illness often has a profound effect on a young patient's ability to understand medical choices, dying, and illness itself. Children who have been living with serious illness and medical treatment may attain a greater maturity level and capacity for understanding their treatment choices based on their lengthy experience of illness. Serious illness and its treatment may also impact decision-making capacity in patients, either permanently or temporarily, due to reduced cognitive functioning, medication effects, or other impediments to communication that limit the ability to express a choice. Clinicians should assess capacity on an ongoing basis.

Although minors generally cannot consent, care providers can nonetheless seek assent, although the utility of this concept remains controversial. Assent generally involves tailoring information to the minor's stage of development and making a clinical assessment about the appropriateness of the minor's understanding as well as the impact of outside factors. Unlike the consent process, assent seeking often includes a disclosure that the treatment will be provided with or without agreement from the patient. Although assent may not be an appropriate model for all dying children and young adults, the underlying notion of respect for young patients argues for including them whenever possible in the decision-making process. Assent of older children is required for participation in most research studies and may thus become necessary if families are considering experimental trials near the end of life.

Adolescents and young adults with typical cognitive development are able to make complex, well-reasoned decisions at a fairly young age. Yet their use of these skills is inconsistent and vulnerable to social pressure, so even mature teens often need support in their decision-making processes. The sensitive nature of medical care and changing relationships with parents over time make the provision of care to teens transitioning to adulthood legally and ethically fraught. As patients develop through adolescence, there is generally more of a need for an independent relationship with healthcare providers.



## REQUESTS TO WITHHOLD INFORMATION FROM PATIENTS

Parents or guardians may ask the medical team to withhold information, such as a diagnosis or prognosis, from the patient or other extended family. Nondisclosure of this kind can be burdensome for members of the care team, who already are responsible for a complex system of interprofessional communication, and they may find the supplemental task of concealment stressful. Beyond (or because of) its psychological effects on the medical team, nondisclosure of diagnosis or prognosis may be ethically inappropriate.

While parents and guardians may have the legal and procedural right to control the information given to patients, the choice not to disclose information about current or future circumstances can impose a significant burden, particularly when the patient is an older child or adolescent. In practical terms, staff will encounter difficulties in fully engaging with patients if they are unable to answer questions truthfully or to provide a coherent explanation or justification for the care being provided.

In terms of emotional burden, hiding information related to a child's diagnosis or prognosis can increase the stress level of the patient, family members, and staff. Providers must explore the reasons behind the parents' decision to withhold this information, which are often based on fear. Parents who are trying to protect their child from painful and scary information need to be reassured that their child probably understands more than they realize about their illness and that having an honest, age-appropriate conversation may provide the child with desperately needed reassurance and support.

## CONFLICTS ABOUT LIFE-SUSTAINING THERAPIES

Medical teams struggle to clearly distinguish between which choices are appropriate to offer to patients and parents and which, if chosen, impose an undue burden on either families or patients. The boundaries of parent or guardian discretion are particularly difficult to clarify in a medical model of shared decision making. Providers have an ethical obligation to advise parents on the options they believe to be most appropriate, rather than laying out all available options and leaving the parents to choose with little guidance.

Disagreement between patients and families can be traumatic to patients and ethically troubling to the medical team, particularly frontline staff. One common scenario involves a young patient who is tired and wishes to stop aggressive treatment and focus on comfort, in conflict with parents or family members who want to "do everything." Providers in these circumstances are challenged to engage the patient and parents in open dialogue, ensuring that each party's message is heard by the other. In these circumstances, providers must be careful to ensure that the patient's preferences are taken into consideration, even though the parents have ultimate decision-making authority. Providers may also take this opportunity to limit the options that are offered to the parents to those that they truly feel will benefit the patient without significant burden.

Because feeding, especially the feeding of children, is seen as a basic element of caring, withdrawal and withholding of artificially routed nutrition and hydration (ARNH) often raise powerful emotional and social concerns. Importantly, ARNH is distinct from orally consumed food and drink; ARNH is a medical treatment that, like other medical treatments, can be both harmful and beneficial for patients. Stopping medically provided ARNH, while common in the terminal care of children, has been deemed ethically acceptable only in limited circumstances in which the child will not derive a net benefit from the treatment. Sometimes there is conflict over the feeling of taking something away; although there is broad consensus among ethicists that withholding and withdrawing a medical treatment are ethically equivalent, parents and providers may find one more difficult than the other. In other circumstances, conflict may arise when teams and families disagree over the appropriateness of introducing or removing ARNH, on the basis of religious or philosophical positions. Parents or providers may hold fears that withholding or withdrawing ARNH will cause a patient to suffer from thirst or starvation. Comprehensive palliative care measures should be provided to the patient to ensure the child's comfort and ease the medical team's and the family's concerns.

## CONFLICTS ABOUT COMFORT-PROMOTING THERAPIES

Introducing the idea of palliative care or hospice can be challenging for patients, family members, and caretakers who may feel unprepared to confront the reality of a patient's suffering or eventual death. While pediatric programs have led the charge for the early incorporation of palliative therapies in medical care, patients and families nonetheless are often hesitant to work with palliative care professionals because to do so can be seen as "giving up." In addition, although palliative care is increasingly integrated into the treatment of chronic conditions, hospice remains in the public imagination devoted only to the care of the terminally ill, and therefore, for some families, it can be symbolic of an unacceptably grim prognosis.

Staff may feel particularly distressed when parents and guardians refuse pharmacologic management of their children's pain. Some parents view pain medicines as morally unacceptable or inappropriate for use in pediatric patients or worry about addiction. Conflicts with or erosion of trust in medical teams might also be a cause for parents and guardians to refuse pain medications. Some parents and guardians ask to reduce doses of opioids given to their children to allow for periods of wakefulness as death approaches, putting the medical team in the difficult position of weighing a patient's suffering against the family's process of making meaning of the death. In all of these situations, providers must remember that, even in models of family-centered care, the primary duty is to the patient. While the parent or guardian has the legal right to refuse interventions, the provider has an ethical obligation to advocate for appropriate pain management.

Many parents and guardians express concern that sedating medications may shorten life and that use of such agents may lead to thoughts that the parent/guardian or the medical team was responsible for the child's death. There is an ethically important difference between treating pain and killing, even when the provision of pain medication has the potential to reduce the life span. This distinction is often called the "doctrine of double effect." Although the difference may be difficult to discern in clinical practice, the "double effect" situation is common, and it is ethically appropriate for clinicians to err on the side of keeping patients comfortable. Taking the family's values and goals into account, a clinician should feel confident that aggressively treating symptoms including pain is appropriate, even when that treatment may indirectly bring a quicker death. Furthermore, some studies suggest that pediatric patients whose pain and other symptoms are appropriately managed may actually live longer.

## CONFLICTS ABOUT BRAIN DEATH STATUS

The classification of brain stem death as death is a relatively recent event in the history of human dying and remains controversial with the public. In several highly publicized recent cases, parents have objected to brain death determinations and to the cessation of interventions that support the cardiovascular and respiratory functioning of their deceased children. While there are some states that give parents legal standing to object to brain death determinations, most states reserve for clinicians and institutions the right to cease medical interventions for patients determined to be dead. Clinical staff should aim to be respectful of family goals and values even in the midst of ethical disagreement over the disputed death of a patient. Chaplaincy services, social workers, and other clinical team members with psychosocial expertise are ideally suited to support families through such difficult transitions.

## SUGGESTED READINGS


Bernat JL. Controversies in defining and determining death in critical care. *Nat Rev Neurol.* 2013;9(3):164-173.

Coleman DL, Rosoff PM. The legal authority of mature minors to consent to general medical treatment. *Pediatrics.* 2013;131(4): 786-793.

Diekema DS. Parental refusals of medical treatment: the harm principle as threshold for state intervention. *Theor Med Bioeth.* 2004;25(4):243-264.

Diekema DS, Botkin JR; American Academy of Pediatrics Committee on Bioethics. Clinical report: forgoing medically provided nutrition and hydration in children. *Pediatrics.* 2009;124(2):813-822.

Durall A, Zurakowski D, Wolfe J. Barriers to conducting advance care discussions for children with life-threatening conditions. *Pediatrics.* 2012;129.(4):e975-e982.

Feudtner C. Collaborative communication in pediatric palliative care: a foundation for problem-solving and decision-making. *Pediatr Clin North Am.* 2007;54(5):583-607.

Katz AL, Webb SA; American Academy of Pediatrics Committee on Bioethics. Informed consent in decision-making in pediatric practice. *Pediatrics.* 2016;138:20161485.

Lane SH, Kohlenberg E. Emancipated minors: health policy and implications for nursing. *J Pediatr Nurs.* 2012;27(5):533-548.

Morrison W, Kang T. Judging the quality of mercy: drawing a line between palliation and euthanasia. *Pediatrics.* 2014;133(suppl 1): S31-S36.

Nakagawa TA, Ashwal S, Mathur M, et al. Clinical report: guidelines for the determination of brain death in infants and children: an update of the 1987 task force recommendations. *Pediatrics.* 2011;128(3):e720-e740.

Rosenberg AR, Wolfe J, Wiener L, Lyon M, Feudtner C. Ethics, emotions, and the skills of talking about progressing disease with terminally ill adolescents: a narrative review. *JAMA Pediatr.* 2016;170(12):1216-1223.

Van der Heide A, van der Maas PJ, Van der Wal G, Kollée LA, de Leeuw R. Using potentially life-shortening drugs in neonates and infants. *Crit Care Med.* 2000;28(7):2595-2599.

Weidner NJ, Plantz DM. Ethical considerations in the management of analgesia in terminally ill pediatric patients. *J Pain Symptom Manage.* 2014;48(5):998-1003.

Wiener L, Zadeh S, Battles H, Baird K, Ballard E, Osherow J. Allowing adolescents and young adults to plan their end-of-life care. *Pediatrics.* 2012;130(5):897-905.

# PART 1 INTRODUCTION

## 129 Principles of Inborn Errors of Metabolism

Jean-Marie Saudubray, William J. Craigen, and Angela Garcia Cazorla

### INTRODUCTION

Over 800 human diseases that are due to inborn errors of metabolism (IEM) are now recognized, and this number is constantly increasing. However, the incidence of inborn errors may well be underestimated because diagnostic errors are frequent. Despite the relative abundance of new case reports, there is considerable evidence, including that based on the recent introduction of next-generation sequencing, that many of these disorders remain undetected or misdiagnosed. More than 300 "new" disorders have been described in the past 5 years, 85% of which present with predominantly neurologic manifestations. Several factors conspire to make the clinical diagnosis of IEM difficult.

IEM are individually rare but collectively numerous. The application of tandem mass spectrometry (tandem MS) to newborn screening and prenatal diagnostic testing has enabled presymptomatic diagnosis for some IEMs. However, for many IEM disorders, neonatal screening tests are either too slow, too expensive, or too unreliable; consequently, a simple method of clinical screening is mandatory before initiating sophisticated biochemical investigations. The clinical diagnosis of IEM relies upon a limited number of principles:

- Consider IEM in parallel with other more common conditions; for example, sepsis or anoxic-ischemic encephalopathy in neonates, and intoxication, encephalitis, and brain tumors in older patients.
- Be aware of symptoms that persist and remain unexplained after the initial treatment and the usual investigations have been performed.
- Collect blood and urine samples at the right time in relation to an acute illness.
- Suspect that any neonatal death may be due to an IEM, particularly deaths that are attributed to sepsis.
- Carefully review all autopsy findings.
- Do not confuse a symptom (eg, peripheral neuropathy, retinitis pigmentosa, cardiomyopathy) or a syndrome (eg, Reye syndrome, Leigh syndrome, sudden infant death) with etiology.
- Remember that an IEM can present at any age, from fetal life to old age.
- Know that although most genetic metabolic errors are hereditary and transmitted as recessive disorders, the majority of individual cases appear sporadically.
- Initially consider inborn errors that are amenable to treatment (mainly those that cause intoxication). **Do not miss a treatable disorder**.
- In acute emergency situations, undertake first those few investigations that are able to diagnose treatable IEM: **First take care of the patient (emergency treatment) and then the family (genetic counseling)**.

In this section, inborn errors amenable to treatment are printed in bold. Additional information and diagnostic checklists are available online.

### CLASSIFICATION

The vast majority of IEMs involve abnormalities in enzymes and transport proteins. However, all the metabolic disorders can be divided into the following 2 large clinical categories.

#### Category 1

This category includes disorders that either involve only 1 functional system (eg, the endocrine system, immune system, coagulation factors, or lipoproteins) or affect only 1 organ or anatomic system (eg, the intestine, renal tubules, erythrocytes, or connective tissue). Presenting symptoms are uniform (eg, a bleeding tendency in coagulation factor defects or hemolytic anemia in defects of glycolysis), and the correct diagnosis is usually easy to establish even when the basic biochemical lesion gives rise to systemic consequences. These disorders are usually well known and identified by organ-specific specialists (eg, cardiologists, endocrinologists, immunologists, hematologists).

#### Category 2

This category includes diseases in which the basic biochemical lesion either affects 1 metabolic pathway common to a large number of cells or organs (eg, storage diseases due to lysosomal disorders, energy deficiency in mitochondrial disorders) or is restricted to 1 organ but gives rise to humoral and systemic consequences (eg, hyperammonemia in urea cycle defects, hypoglycemia in hepatic glycogenosis). The diseases in this category have a great diversity of presenting symptoms. The specific disorders mentioned are discussed later in this section.

From a pathophysiologic perspective, metabolic disorders from category 2 can be divided into 3 diagnostically useful groups.

**Group 1: Disorders That Cause Intoxication** This group includes inborn errors of intermediary metabolism (IEIM) that lead to acute or progressive intoxication from the accumulation of toxic compounds proximal to the metabolic block. In this group are inborn errors of amino acid catabolism (eg, phenylketonuria, maple syrup urine disease, homocystinuria, tyrosinemia), most organic acidurias (eg, methylmalonic, propionic, isovaleric), congenital urea cycle defects, sugar intolerances (eg, galactosemia, hereditary fructose intolerance), and metal intoxication (eg, Wilson, Menkes, hemochromatosis, porphyrias). All the conditions in this group share clinical similarities: They do not interfere with embryonic and fetal development, and they present with a symptom-free interval and clinical signs of "intoxication" that may be acute (eg, vomiting, coma, liver failure, thromboembolic complications) or chronic (eg, failure to thrive, developmental delay, ectopia lentis, cardiomyopathy, epilepsy).

Conditions that can provoke acute metabolic attacks include catabolism, fever, intercurrent illness, and ingestion of specific foods. Clinical expression is often both late in onset and intermittent. The diagnosis is straightforward and most commonly relies on plasma and urine amino acid, organic acid, or acylcarnitine chromatography. Most of these disorders are treatable and require the emergency removal of the toxin by special diets, extracorporeal procedures, or "cleansing" drugs (eg, carnitine, sodium benzoate, penicillamine).

Although the pathophysiology is somewhat different, the inborn errors of neurotransmitter synthesis and catabolism (monoamines, γ-aminobutyric acid [GABA], and glycine) and the inborn errors of amino acid synthesis (serine, glutamine, proline/ornithine, and asparagine) can also be included in this group because they share many characteristics: They are IEIMs; their diagnosis relies on plasma, urine, and cerebrospinal fluid (CSF) investigations (eg, amino acid, organic acid analyses); and some are amenable to treatment even when the disorder is present in utero—for example, 3-phosphoglycerate dehydrogenase deficiency.

**Group 2: Disorders Involving Energy Metabolism** These consist of IEMs with symptoms due, at least in part, to a deficiency in energy production or utilization within the liver, myocardium, muscle, brain, or other tissues. This group can be divided into mitochondrial and cytoplasmic energy defects. Mitochondrial defects are the most severe and are generally untreatable. They include the congenital lactic acidemias (eg, defects of the pyruvate transporter, pyruvate carboxylase, pyruvate dehydrogenase, and the Krebs cycle), mitochondrial respiratory chain disorders, and fatty acid oxidation (FAO) and ketone body defects. Only the latter are partly treatable. Cytoplasmic energy defects are generally less severe. They include disorders of glycolysis, glycogen metabolism and gluconeogenesis, hyperinsulinism, and glucose transporter defects (all treatable disorders); the more recently described disorders of creatine metabolism (partly treatable); and the new inborn errors of the pentose phosphate pathways (untreatable). Common symptoms in this group include hypoglycemia, lactic acidemia, hepatomegaly, acute recurrent crises, severe generalized hypotonia, myopathy, cardiomyopathy, failure to thrive, cardiac failure, circulatory collapse, sudden unexpected death in infancy, and brain involvement. Some of the mitochondrial disorders and pentose phosphate pathway defects can interfere with embryonic and fetal development and can cause dysmorphism, dysplasia, and malformations. Diagnosis is difficult and relies on function tests, enzymatic analyses requiring biopsies or cell culture, and molecular analyses.

**Group 3: Disorders Involving Complex Molecules** This group involves cellular organelles (lysosomes, peroxisomes, endoplasmic reticulum, Golgi apparatus, mitochondria, and intracellular trafficking) and includes diseases that disturb the synthesis, remodeling, recycling, trafficking, and catabolism of complex molecules. Symptoms are most often permanent, progressive, independent of intercurrent events (even if an acute crisis may have occurred in the course of a disorder), and unrelated to food intake. All lysosomal storage disorders (LSDs), peroxisomal disorders (PBDs), disorders of intracellular trafficking and processing (eg, $\alpha_1$-antitrypsin), and congenital disorders of glycosylation (CDG) belong to this group. Besides these well-known disorders, a novel and rapidly expanding group of IEMs involving the synthesis, remodeling, and recycling of complex lipids and fatty acids has recently been described. This biochemical group encompasses metabolic defects of phospholipids, triglycerides, sphingolipids, isoprenoids, cholesterol, ubiquinone, dolichol, plasmalogens, and non–mitochondrial complex long-chain fatty acid metabolism (very-long-chain fatty acids [VLCFA], fatty alcohol, branched chain fatty acids, eicosanoids derived from arachidonic acid, prostaglandins, and leukotrienes).

Almost none of these are treatable acutely; however, enzyme replacement therapy is now available for several lysosomal disorders. Intracellular localization of all these disorders is presented in Figure 129-1.

The newly described metabolic disorders affecting cytoplasmic and mitochondrial tRNA synthetases, autophagy, and other factors related to cytoplasmic protein synthesis, transporters, channels, and enzymes implicated in the logistics and regulation of the cell challenge our



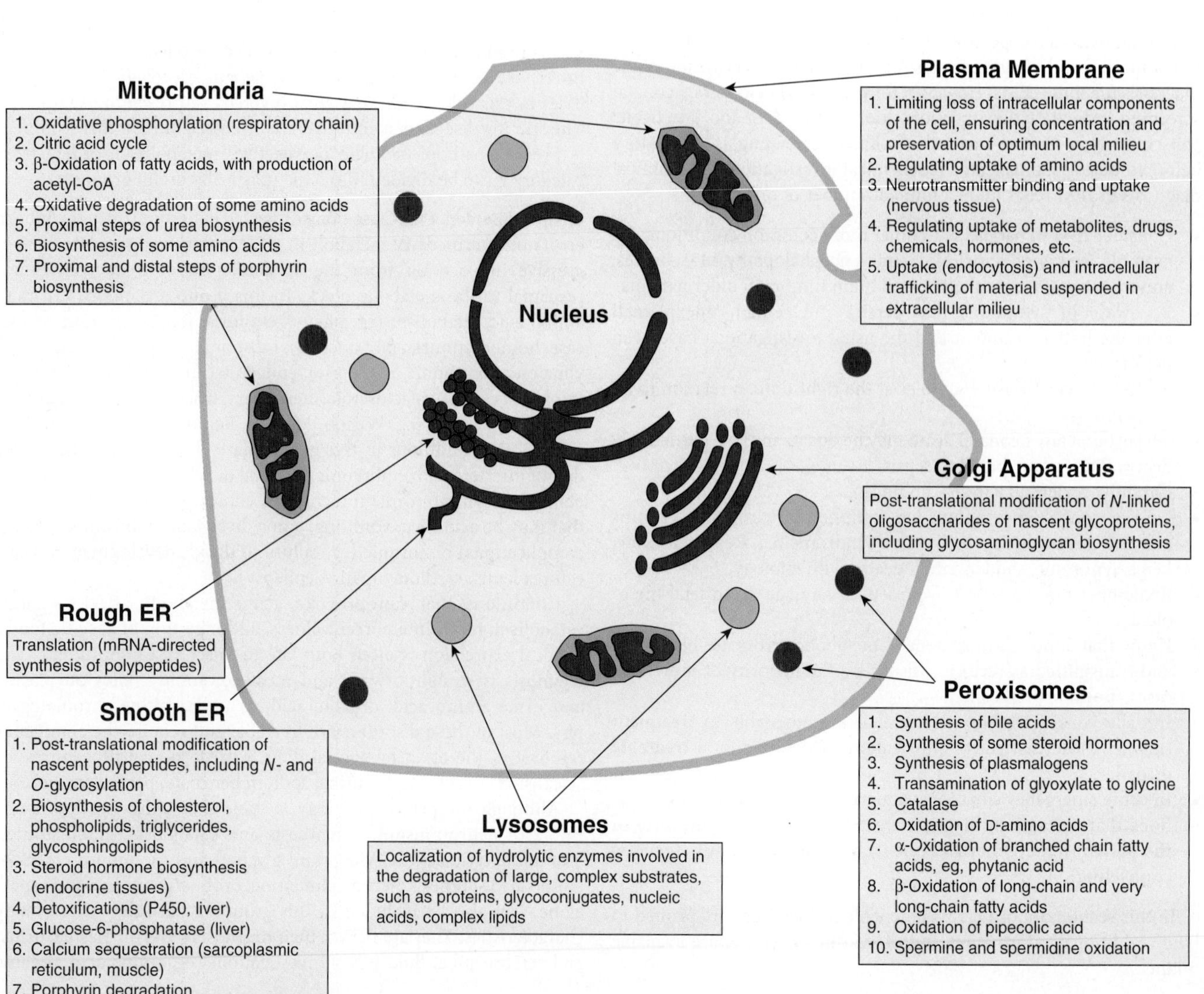


**FIGURE 129-1** Cartoon showing intracellular localization of inborn errors of metabolism.

current classification based on organelles and form a bridge between "classic" metabolic diseases with metabolic markers and those caused by structural proteins mutations without such markers and that are most often diagnosed by molecular techniques.

## GENETICS

Although most of these disorders are inherited as autosomal recessive conditions, a significant minority are transmitted as X-linked recessive disorders and a few as dominant diseases. Many cases appear to be sporadic given the small size of sibships in developed countries. Consanguinity is rare, and thus many affected patients are compound heterozygotes. In these cases, the phenotype is generally driven by the less severe mutation. Mutations in the mitochondrial genome, which is maternally inherited, make up a rapidly growing subgroup of IEMs; these disorders exhibit unique genetic and clinical characteristics. Compared to many other genetic diseases in which the gene product is unknown or not fully recognized, almost all IEMs were primarily identified because of a suggestive biochemical profile and confirmed by an enzymatic defect. These biochemical methods remain the basis of diagnostic procedures and assessment of management, although a growing number of IEMs are henceforth identified by molecular techniques (gene panels and next-generation sequencing). Antenatal diagnosis is available for most of these conditions.

## CLINICAL PRESENTATION

A few metabolic disorders are recognized by newborn screening of the general population (eg, phenylketonuria) or through at-risk families. Apart from these, there are 5 groups of clinical circumstances in which a metabolic disorder is possible:

1. Antenatal period
2. Acute or chronic neonatal period (birth to 1 month)
3. Later-onset acute and recurrent attacks of symptoms such as coma, ataxia, vomiting, and acidosis (crisis)
4. Chronic and progressive generalized symptoms that can be mainly gastrointestinal (eg, chronic vomiting), failure to thrive, hypotonia, recurrent infections, or muscular or neurologic symptoms (eg, myopathy, developmental delay, neurologic deterioration, epilepsy)
5. Specific and irreversible presentations that can involve any organ or system (eg, heart, liver, intestine, kidney, lungs, endocrine, immune and hematologic systems, bone, collagen, skin); many IEMs can present with specific isolated symptoms, such as cardiomyopathy, hepatomegaly, lens dislocation, renal tubulopathy, hyperkeratotic plaques, and so on

### Antenatal Symptoms

These can be classified in 3 major clinical categories:

1. True malformations such as skeletal malformations, congenital heart disease, visceral aplasias, and neural tube defects
2. Dysplasias (eg, cortical heterotopias, cortical cysts, posterior fossa abnormalities, polycystic kidneys, liver cysts)
3. Functional signs such as intrauterine growth retardation, hydrops fetalis, hepatosplenomegaly, microcephaly, coarse facies, or facial dysmorphism

According to this classification, true irreversible malformations are only observed in *O*-glycosylation disorders, primary or secondary to manganese transporter *SLC39A8* mutations (Chapter 164), in cholesterol synthesis defects (Chapter 159), in amino acid synthesis disorders such with glutamine and asparagine synthetase deficiency (lissencephaly) (Chapter 140), and rarely in severe energetic defects such as glutaric aciduria type II (Chapter 145), some respiratory chain disorders, and the mitochondrial thiamine pyrophosphate carrier defect (*SLC25A19*) responsible for the Amish lethal microcephaly (Chapter 144). Notably, the congenital microcephaly observed in serine synthesis defects is partly reversible upon early treatment with serine in its mild form, but not in the severe Neu-Laxova presentation (Chapter 135). Lysosomal, peroxisomal, and *N*-glycosylation defects are responsible for dysplasia and functional abnormalities that are variably reversible. The vast majority of "true intoxication" disorders (amino acid and organic acid catabolism disorders) do not interfere with the embryo-fetal development and do not give rise to dysmorphism and antenatal symptoms (although some severe organic acidurias may present with subtle congenital signs).



### Neonatal and Early Infancy Period

**Acute Encephalopathy and Metabolic Crash** The neonate has a limited repertoire of responses to severe illness. IEMs may present with nonspecific symptoms such as respiratory distress, hypotonia, a poor sucking reflex, vomiting, lethargy, or seizures—problems that can easily be attributed to sepsis or some other common cause. Prior death of a sibling from a similar IEM may have been attributed to sepsis, cardiac failure, or intraventricular hemorrhage.

Group 1 disorders are illustrated by an infant born full term who, after a normal pregnancy and delivery and an initial symptom-free period, relentlessly deteriorates for no apparent reason and does not respond to symptomatic therapy. The interval between birth and clinical symptoms may range from hours to weeks. Investigations that are routinely performed in sick neonates include a chest x-ray, CSF examination, bacteriologic studies, and cerebral ultrasound examination, and all yield normal results. This unexpected and "mysterious" deterioration after a normal initial period is the most important indication for this group of IEMs. Careful reevaluation of the child's condition is then warranted.

In group 2 disorders (energy deficiencies), the clinical presentation is often less striking and displays variable severity. A clinical algorithm for screening for treatable IEMs in neonates is presented in Figure 129-2.

**Neurologic Deterioration (Coma, Lethargy)** This is the most frequent presenting sign in "intoxication" disorders. Typically, the first reported sign is poor sucking and feeding, after which the child sinks into an unexplained coma despite supportive measures. At a more advanced state, neurovegetative problems with respiratory abnormalities, hiccups, apnea, bradycardia, and hypothermia can appear. In the comatose state, characteristic changes in muscle tone and involuntary movements appear. Generalized hypertonic episodes with opisthotonus, boxing, or pedaling movements and slow limb elevations are observed in **maple syrup urine disease (MSUD)**. As most nonmetabolic causes of coma are associated with hypotonia, the presence of "normal" peripheral muscle tone in a comatose child reflects a relative hypertonia. In **organic acidurias**, axial hypotonia and limb hypertonia with fast, large-amplitude tremors and myoclonic jerks (often mistaken for convulsions) are typical. An abnormal urine and body odor is present in some diseases in which volatile metabolites accumulate; for example, a maple syrup odor in MSUD and a sweaty-feet odor in **isovaleric acidemia (IVA)** and **glutaric acidemia type II**.

In energy deficiencies, the clinical presentation is less obvious and displays a more variable severity. In many conditions, there is no symptom-free interval. The most frequent findings are a severe generalized hypotonia, rapidly progressive neurologic deterioration, and possible dysmorphism or malformations. In contrast to the intoxication group, lethargy and coma are rarely initial signs. Lactic acidemia with or without metabolic acidosis is frequent. Cardiac and hepatic involvement are also commonly associated with energy deficiencies.

In the neonatal period, only a few lysosomal storage disorders present with neurologic deterioration. By contrast, many peroxisomal biogenesis defects present at birth with dysmorphism and severe neurologic dysfunction. Severe forms of CDG involving *N*- and *O*-glycosylation, glycosylphosphatidylinositol anchor, and dolichol phosphate biosynthesis may also present with acute congenital neurologic dysfunction, although they more often present with hypotonia, seizures, dysmorphism, malformations, and diverse visceral involvement.

**Seizures** Always consider the possibility of an IEM in a neonate with unexplained and refractory epilepsy. Neonatal metabolic seizures are often a mixture of partial, erratic myoclonus of the face and extremities, or tonic seizures. Classically the term **early myoclonic encephalopathy (EME)** has been used if myoclonic seizures dominate the clinical pattern. The electroencephalogram (EEG) often shows a

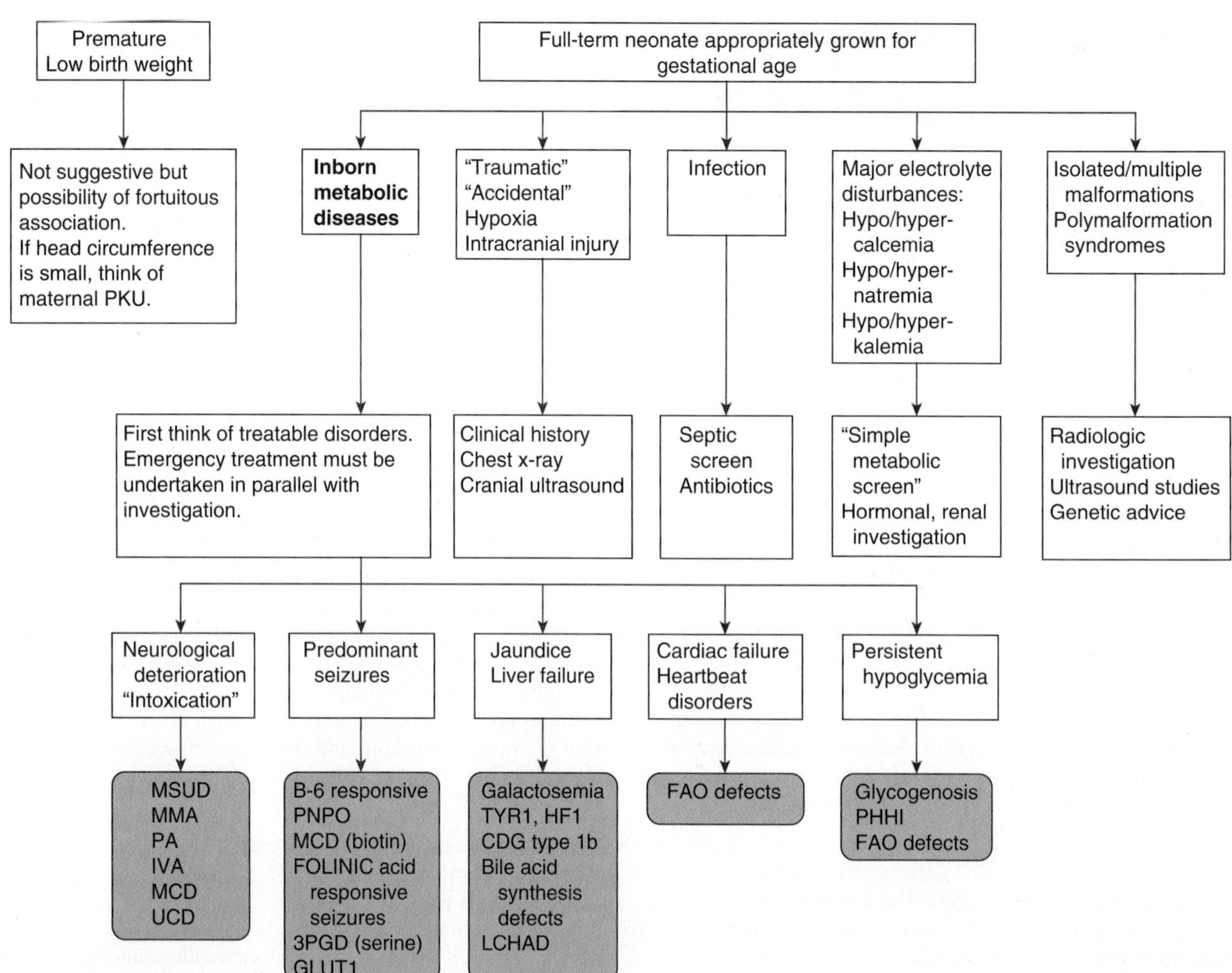


**FIGURE 129-2** The "sick" neonate: An algorithm for screening for treatable inborn errors of metabolism (IEMs). 3PGD, 3-phosphoglycerate dehydrogenase; CDG, congenital disorders of glycosylation; FAO, fatty acid oxidation disorders; HFI, hereditary fructose intolerance; IVA, isovaleric acidemia; LCHAD, 3-hydroxy long-chain acyl-CoA dehydrogenase; MCD, multiple carboxylase deficiency; MMA, methylmalonic aciduria; MSUD, maple syrup urine disease; PA, propionic acidemia; PHHI, primary hyperinsulinemic hypoglycemia of infancy; PKU, phenylketonuria; PNPO, pyridox(am)ine-5′-phosphate oxidase; TYR-1, tyrosinemia type 1; UCD, urea cycle defects.

burst-suppression pattern; however, myoclonic jerks may occur without EEG abnormalities.

Five treatable disorders can present in the neonatal period predominantly with intractable seizures: **pyridoxine-responsive seizures, folinic acid–responsive epilepsy (both allelic to antiquitin deficiency), pyridox(am)ine-5′-phosphate oxidase deficiency, 3-phosphoglycerate dehydrogenase deficiency** responsive to serine supplementation, and persistent **hyperinsulinemic hypoglycemia**. Also, biotin-responsive **holocarboxylase synthetase deficiency** may rarely present predominantly with neonatal seizures. **GLUT1 deficiency** (brain glucose transporter), which is responsive to a hyperketotic diet, and biotin-responsive **biotinidase deficiency** can also present in the first months of life as epileptic encephalopathy.

Many other untreatable inherited disorders can present in the neonatal period with severe epilepsy: nonketotic hyperglycinemia, D-glyceric aciduria, and mitochondrial glutamate transporter defect (all 3 presenting with myoclonic epilepsy and a burst-suppression EEG pattern), peroxisomal biogenesis defects, respiratory chain disorders, sulfite oxidase deficiency, and Menkes disease. In all these conditions, epilepsy is severe; has an early onset; and can present with spasms, myoclonus, and partial or generalized tonic-clonic crises.

**Hypotonia** Severe hypotonia is a common symptom in sick neonates. It is more generally observed in nonmetabolic severe fetal neuromuscular disorders (Chapter 560). Only a few IEMs present with isolated hypotonia in the neonatal period, and very few are treatable. The most severe metabolic hypotonias are observed in hereditary lactic acidemia, respiratory chain disorders, **urea cycle defects**, nonketotic hyperglycinemia (NKH), sulphite oxidase deficiency, peroxisomal disorders, Lowe syndrome, and trifunctional enzyme deficiency. Severe forms of Pompe disease (α-glucosidase deficiency) can initially mimic respiratory chain disorders or trifunctional enzyme deficiency when generalized hypotonia is associated with cardiomyopathy. However, Pompe disease does not strictly start in the neonatal period. Prader-Willi syndrome, one of the most frequent causes of isolated neonatal hypotonia at birth, can mimic hypotonia-cystinuria syndrome. Severe global hypotonia and hypomotility mimicking neuromuscular diseases can appear in some treatable IEMs such as **biogenic amine defects, primary carnitine deficiency** (not strictly in the neonatal period), **fatty acid oxidation (FAO) defects** (Chapter 145), **genetic defects of riboflavin transport**, and **primary coenzyme Q10 defects** (Chapter 153). A **pyridostigmine-responsive congenital myasthenic syndrome** can be a presenting sign in ALG2, ALG14, DPAGT1, GFPT1, and GMPPB CDGs (Chapter 158).

These 3 neurologic presentations are summarized in Table 129-1.

**Hepatic and Gastrointestinal Presentation** Seven main clinical groups of hepatic symptoms can be identified:

1. Hepatomegaly with hypoglycemia and seizures without liver failure suggest **glycogenosis type I** or **III** (typically massive hepatomegaly), **gluconeogenesis defects**, or **severe hyperinsulinism** (with moderate hepatomegaly).
2. Liver failure (jaundice, coagulopathy, hepatocellular necrosis with elevated serum transaminases, and hypoglycemia with ascites and edema) suggests **fructosemia due to hereditary fructose**

**TABLE 129-1 NEUROLOGIC PRESENTATIONS IN NEONATES AND IN EARLY INFANCY**

| Predominant Clinical Symptom | Main Clinical Signs | Biological Signs | Best Diagnoses (Disorder/ Enzyme Deficiency) |
|---|---|---|---|
| Neurologic deterioration: mostly metabolic and treatable | Lethargy, coma, hiccups | Ketosis, acidosis | **MSUD** (odor) |
| | Poor sucking, hypothermia | Hyperlactacidemia | **MMA, PA, IVA** (odor) |
| | Hypotonia, hypertonia | Hyperammonemia | **MCD** |
| | Abnormal movements | Bone marrow suppression | **Urea cycle defects** |
| | Large-amplitude tremor | Characteristic changes of AAC or OAC | **CAVA deficiency** |
| | Myoclonic jerks | | **GA type II** (odor) |
| | Burst suppression | | |
| | Abnormal odor | | |
| Seizures: sometimes metabolic, sometimes treatable | Isolated | Metabolic ketoacidosis | **MCD** |
| | Generalized | Typical OAC profile | |
| | | None | **Pyridoxine responsive, folinic acid responsive (antiquitin deficiency)** |
| | | Hypocalcemia with hypomagnesemia | **Congenital magnesium malabsorption** |
| | | Severe hypoglycemia | **PHHI** |
| | Generalized hypsarrhythmia | Low serine (plasma/CSF) | **3-PGD** |
| | Major microcephaly | | |
| | Severe hypotonia | Low HVA, 5-HIAA in CSF, vanillactic acid (urine) | **PNPO** (pyridoxamine phosphate responsive) |
| | Myoclonic jerks | Hyperglycinemia | NKH |
| | Burst suppression | None | Glutamate transporter |
| | | S-Sulfocysteine | Sulfite oxidase |
| | Facial dysmorphia | VLCFA, phytanic, plasmalogen | Peroxisomal defects |
| | Malformations | Glycosylated transferrin | CDG syndrome |
| | Severe hypotonia | Sterols in plasma | Cholesterol biosynthesis |
| Severe hypotonia: rarely metabolic, many not treatable | Isolated | None | Prader-Willi syndrome |
| | | Massive cystinuria | Hypotonia cystinuria syndrome |
| | Predominant dysmorphia | VLCFA, phytanic, plasmalogen | Peroxisomal defects |
| | Malformations | Sterols in plasma | Cholesterol defects |
| | | Glycosylated transferrin | Glycosylation defects |
| | | APO-B glycosylation | Polymalformation syndromes with muscular dystrophy (Walker-Warburg syndrome, with muscle, eye, brain, and other anomalies) |
| | Cataract | Lactic acidemia | Lowe syndrome |
| | Tubulopathy | Enzyme/DNA analyses | Respiratory chain |
| | Cardiomyopathy | Vacuolated lymphocytes | **Pompe disease** |
| | Abnormal movements (dystonia-parkinsonism, oculogyric crises), feeding difficulties, temperature instability | Abnormal CSF<br>Biogenic amines/pterines, glycine | **Neurotransmitter disorders** |
| | **Pyridostigmine-responsive congenital myasthenic syndrome** | Serum transferrin IEF type 1 pattern in some | **ALG2, ALG14, DPAGT1, GFPT1, and GMPPB CDGs** |
| | | Normal CK | |
| | Macroglossia | Lactic acidemia | Respiratory chain |
| | Hepatopathy | Acylcarnitine | **Trifunctional enzyme (FAO)** |
| | | | **Carnitine transporter** |
| | | | **Riboflavin transporter** |
| | | COQ10 fibroblasts, muscle | **Primary COQ10 defects** |

3-PGD, 3-phosphoglycerate dehydrogenase; 5-HIAA, 5-hydroxy indole acetic acid; AAC, amino acid chromatography; CDG, congenital disorders of glycosylation; CAVA, carbonic anhydrase VA isoform; COQ10, coenzyme Q10; GA II, glutaric aciduria type II; HVA, homovanillic acid; IVA, isovaleric acidemia; MCD, multiple carboxylase deficiency; MMA, methylmalonic aciduria; MSUD, maple syrup urine disease; NKH, nonketotic hyperglycinemia; OAC, organic acid chromatography; PA, propionic acidemia; PHHI, primary hyperinsulinemic hypoglycemia of infancy; PNPO, pyridox(am)ine-5′-phosphate oxidase; VLCFA, very-long-chain fatty acids.

**intolerance** (now rare because infant formulas are fructose free); **galactosemia; tyrosinemia type I** (after 3 weeks); neonatal hemochromatosis; respiratory chain disorders (and notably mitochondrial DNA depletion syndromes); and transaldolase deficiency, a disorder of the pentose phosphate pathway that can present with hydrops fetalis. Severe fetal growth retardation, lactic acidosis, failure to thrive, hyperaminoaciduria, very high serum ferritin concentrations, hemosiderosis of the liver, and early death suggest GRACILE syndrome (Finnish lethal neonatal metabolic syndrome). Investigating patients with severe hepatic failure is difficult, with many pitfalls. At an advanced state, nonspecific abnormalities secondary to liver damage can be present. Mellituria (galactosuria, glycosuria, fructosuria), hyperammonemia, lactic acidemia, hypoglycemia after a short fast, hypertyrosinemia (> 200 μmol/L), and hypermethioninemia (sometimes > 500 μmol/L) are encountered in all cases of advanced hepatocellular disease.

3. The recently described mutations in *IARS* and *LARS* (coding for cytoplasmic isoleucyl- and leucyl-tRNA synthetases, respectively) present with hypoalbuminemia, recurrent acute infantile liver failure (RALF), anemia, seizures, and encephalopathic crisis. Recently, *NBAS* (neuroblastoma amplified sequence; involved in Golgi vesicular transport) mutations were also identified as a new cause of fever-dependent episodes of RALF with onset in infancy.
4. Cholestatic jaundice with failure to thrive is a predominant finding in $\alpha_1$-antitrypsin deficiency, Byler disease, **inborn errors of bile acid metabolism**, peroxisomal disorders, Niemann-Pick type C disease, CDG syndromes, **citrin deficiency**, and hepatocerebral syndrome due to mitochondrial DNA depletion. **Long-chain 3-hydroxyacyl-CoA dehydrogenase** (LCHAD) deficiency can present early in infancy as cholestatic jaundice, liver failure, and hepatic fibrosis. **Cerebrotendinous xanthomatosis**, **citrin deficiency**, **arginase deficiency**, and Niemann-Pick C can present as a transient asymptomatic jaundice before neurologic signs appear later in life. Two new complex lipid synthesis disorders, the MEGDEL syndrome (*SERAC* mutations) that can mimic Niemann-Pick type C disease with a positive filipin test and the spastic paraparesis type 5 due to oxysterol 7-hydroxylase deficiency, may also present with such a transient cholestatic liver disease.
5. Liver steatosis: Hepatic presentations of **FAO disorders** and **urea cycle disorders (UCDs)** consist of acute steatosis or Reye syndrome–like with normal bilirubin rather than true liver failure. **LCHAD** deficiency is an exception that may present early in infancy (but not strictly in the neonatal period) as cholestatic jaundice, liver failure, and hepatic fibrosis (Chapter 145). Chanarin-Dorfman syndrome (*ABHD5* mutations) presents early in infancy with liver steatosis, cataracts, deafness, congenital ichthyosis, and myopathy while the newly described cytoplasmic glycerol-3-phosphate dehydrogenase 1 deficiency displays an asymptomatic early infantile hepatomegaly and steatosis with transient hypertriglyceridemia.
6. Hepatosplenomegaly (HSM) with other signs of storage disorders (coarse facies, macroglossia, hydrops fetalis, ascites, edema, dysostosis multiplex, vacuolated lymphocytes) is observed in lysosomal diseases. HSM with inflammatory syndrome, including hematologic or immunologic features, may be observed in lysinuric protein intolerance (macrophage-activating syndrome), mevalonic aciduria and leukopenia (inflammatory syndrome and recurrent severe anemia), and transaldolase deficiency (hydrops fetalis with severe anemia).
7. Congenital diarrheal disorders (CDDs) may be caused by mutations in genes related to disaccharidase deficiency or an ion or nutrient transport defect like *SLC26A3* mutations causing congenital secretory chloride diarrhea, pancreatic insufficiency, lipid trafficking, or **PMI-CDG(Ib)** and ALG8-CDG(Ih). A disorder presenting with CDD linked to *DGAT1* mutations involved in triglyceride synthesis has recently been described. Affected neonates present with vomiting, colicky pain, nonbloody, watery diarrhea, protein-losing enteropathy, hypoalbuminemia, and hyperlipidemia.

**Cardiac Presentation** Some metabolic disorders can present predominantly with cardiac disease. Heart failure and a dilated or hypertrophic cardiomyopathy, most often associated with hypotonia, muscle weakness, and failure to thrive, suggest FAO disorders, respiratory chain disorders, or Pompe disease. **Carnitine-uptake defect (systemic carnitine defect)** responds dramatically to carnitine administration. Some respiratory chain disorders are tissue specific and expressed only in the myocardium. CDG syndrome (PMM-CDG) can sometimes present in infancy with cardiac failure due to pericardial effusion, cardiac tamponade, and cardiomyopathy. Dolichol kinase 1 deficiency (DOLK-CDG) may present with progressive dilated cardiomyopathy resulting in death within 1 year. Other clinical manifestations include microcephaly; "parchment-like" ichthyosis with loss of hair, eyebrows, and eyelashes; intractable seizures; severe hypotonia with elevated creatine kinase (CK); and severe liver dysfunction (Chapter 158). Many defects of **long-chain FAO** can present with cardiomyopathy, arrhythmias, or conduction defects (atrioventricular block, bundle branch block, ventricular tachycardia), which may lead to cardiac arrest.

**Initial Approach to the Investigation** If clinical assessment suggests an IEM, general supportive measures and laboratory investigations should be undertaken concurrently (Table 129-2). Abnormal urine odor can be diagnostic.

Ketonuria (2–3+) in a newborn is always abnormal and is an important sign of a metabolic disease. Hypocalcemia and elevated or reduced blood glucose concentrations are frequently present in metabolic diseases. The physician should be wary of attributing marked neurologic dysfunction purely to these findings.

The metabolic acidosis of organic acidurias is usually accompanied by an elevated anion gap. Urine pH should be below 5; otherwise, renal acidosis is a possibility. A normal blood pH does not exclude a moderate lactic acidemia, which is significant in the absence of infection or tissue hypoxia. Blood ammonia and lactic acid concentrations should be determined systematically in at-risk newborns. Hyperammonemia with ketoacidosis suggests an underlying organic acidemia. However, isolated hyperammonemia can occur in organic acidemias, and an elevated ammonia level alone can induce respiratory alkalosis. Moderately elevated lactate concentrations (3–6 mmol/L) are often observed in organic acidemias and in the hyperammonemias; levels > 10 mmol/L are frequent in hypoxia. With hypoxic lactic acidosis, the lactate-to-pyruvate ratio is > 20, and ketosis is absent. Propionic, methylmalonic, and isovaleric acidemias frequently present with granulocytopenia and thrombocytopenia, which may be mistaken for sepsis. Transaldolase deficiency and early-onset forms of mevalonate kinase deficiency present with severe recurrent hemolytic anemia. Adequate amounts of plasma, urine, blood on filter paper, and CSF should always be stored, because they may later be important in

**TABLE 129-2 PROTOCOL FOR EMERGENCY INVESTIGATIONS (NEONATAL AND LATE-ONSET SITUATIONS)**

| | Immediate Investigations | Storage of Samples |
|---|---|---|
| Urine | Smell (special odor)<br>Look (special color)<br>Acetone (Acetest, Ames)<br>Reducing substances (Clinitest, Ames)<br>pH (pHstix Merck)<br>Sulfitest (Merck)<br>Electrolytes (Na, K), urea, creatinine<br>Uric acid | Urine collection: collect fresh sample and put it in the refrigerator<br>Freezing: freeze samples collected before and after treatment at −20°C, and collect an aliquot 24 h after treatment<br>Metabolic investigation: OAC, AAC, orotic acid, porphyrins |
| Blood | Blood cell count<br>Electrolytes (search for anion gap)<br>Glucose, calcium<br>Blood gases (pH, $P_{CO_2}$, $HCO_3$, H, $P_{O_2}$)<br>Uric acid<br>Prothrombin time<br>Transaminases (and other liver tests)<br>Creatine kinase (CK)<br>Ammonia<br>Lactic, 3-hydroxybutyrate<br>Free fatty acids | Plasma (5 mL) heparinized at −20°C<br>Blood on filter paper: 2 spots (as "Guthrie" test)<br>Whole blood (10–15 mL) collected on EDTA and frozen (for molecular biology studies)<br>Major metabolic investigations: Total homocysteine, AAC, acylcarnitine (tandem MS), OAC, porphyrins, neurotransmitters |
| Miscellaneous | Lumbar puncture<br>Chest x-ray<br>Cardiac ultrasound, ECG<br>Cerebral ultrasound, EEG | Skin biopsy (fibroblast culture)<br>CSF (1 mL), frozen (neurotransmitters, AA)<br>Postmortem: liver, muscle biopsies |

AA, amino acid; AAC, amino acid chromatography; CSF, cerebrospinal fluid; ECG, electrocardiogram; EDTA, ethylenediaminetetraacetic acid; EEG, electroencephalogram; MS, mass spectrometry; OAC, organic acid chromatography.

establishing a diagnosis. Using these precious samples should be carefully planned after advice from specialists in IEM.

After obtaining clinical and laboratory data, a process that should be completed within 2 to 4 hours, specific therapeutic recommendations can be made; this avoids long delays associated with waiting for the results of sophisticated diagnostic investigations. On the basis of this evaluation, most patients can be classified into 1 of 5 types (Table 129-3; see also earlier section on hepatic and



**TABLE 129-3 CLASSIFICATION OF INBORN ERRORS REVEALED IN THE NEONATAL PERIOD AND EARLY IN INFANCY WITH NEUROLOGIC DETERIORATION**

| Types | Clinical Type | Acidosis/Ketosis | Other Signs | Most Usual Diagnosis (Disorder/Enzyme Deficiency) | Elective Methods of Investigation |
|---|---|---|---|---|---|
| I | **Neurological deterioration**, "intoxication" type<br>Abnormal slow movements (boxing)<br>Limb hypertonia | Acidosis 0<br>DNPH +++<br>Acetest 0/± | $NH_3$ N or ↑ ±<br>Lactate N or ↑<br>Glucose N, Calcium N | **MSUD** (special odor) | Amino acid chromatography (plasma, urine)<br>Blood spot for tandem MS-MS |
| II | **Neurological deterioration**,<br>"Intoxication" type<br>Fast large tremors<br>Dehydration | **Acidosis ++**<br>**Acetest ++**<br>DNPH 0/± | $NH_3$ ↑ +/++<br>Lactate N or ↑<br>± leukopenia, thrombopenia<br>Glucose N or ↑ +<br>Calcium N or ↓ + | **Organic acidurias (MMA, PA, IVA, MCD)**<br>**Ketolysis defects**<br>**CAVA defect** | OAC by GLCMS (urine, plasma)<br>Carnitine (plasma)<br>Carnitine esters by tandem MS (urine, plasma)<br>Blood spot for tandem MS |
| | **Neurological deterioration**,<br>"energy deficiency" type,<br>with liver or cardiac symptoms | Acidosis ++/±<br>**Acetest 0**<br>DNPH 0 | $NH_3$ ↑ ±/++<br>Lactate ↑ ±/++<br>**Glucose** ↓ +/++ | **Fatty acid oxidation (FAO), ketogenesis defects** (**GA II, CPT II, CAT, VLCAD, MCKAT, HMGCoA lyase**) | Idem above<br>Tolerance test, fasting test, fatty acid oxidation studies on lymphocytes or fibroblasts<br>Molecular studies |
| III | **Neurological deterioration**,<br>"energy deficiency" type<br>Polypnea, hypotonia<br>Lactic acidosis,<br>sometimes well tolerated | Acidosis +++/+<br>Acetest ++/0<br>**Lactate +++/+** | $NH_3$ N or ↑ ±<br>Blood count: anemia or N<br>Glucose N or ↓ ± | Congenital lactic acidoses (pyruvate carrier, PC, **PDH**, Krebs cycle, RCD **MCD)** | Plasma redox states ratios (L:P, 3 OHB: AA)<br>OAC (urine), AAC (plasma)<br>Enzyme, molecular assays |
| IV (a) | **Neurological deterioration**, "intoxication" type<br>Moderate hepatocellular disturbances<br>Hypotonia, seizures, coma | Acidosis 0 (alkalosis)<br>Acetest 0/+<br>DNPH 0 | **$NH_3$** ↑ +/+++<br>Lactate N or ↑ +<br>Glucose N | **Urea cycle defects**<br>**Triple H**<br>**FAO** defects (**GAII, CPTII, VLCAD, LCHAD, CAT**)<br>**PA, MMA, IVA (with leukothrombopenia)** | AAC, OAC (plasma, urine)<br>Carnitine esters by tandem MS (urine, plasma)<br>Orotic acid (urine)<br>Liver or intestine enzyme studies (CPS, OTC)<br>Molecular studies |
| (b) | **Neurological deterioration**<br>Seizures<br>Myoclonic jerks<br>Severe hypotonia | Acidosis 0<br>Acetest/DNPH 0<br>No major metabolic disturbance | $NH_3$ N<br>Lactate N or ↑ +<br>Blood count N<br>Glucose N | NKH, SO plus XO<br>**3-PGD**<br>**B6-dependency/PNPO and neurotransmitter defects**<br>Peroxisomal defects<br>Trifunctional enzyme<br>CDG syndrome<br>Cholesterol biosynthesis<br>Respiratory chain | AAC (plasma, CSF)<br>AAC (plasma, CSF)<br>OAC, neurotransmitters (plasma, urine, CSF)<br>VLCFA, phytanic acid in plasma<br>Acylcarnitine profile, OAC<br>Glycosylated transferrin (plasma)<br>Sterols (plasma)<br>Lactate and molecular studies |
| V (a) | **Recurrent hypoglycemia with hepatomegaly**<br>No liver failure | Acidosis ++/0<br>Acetest +/0 | Lactate ↑ +/++<br>$NH_3$ ↑ +/0 | **Glycogenosis type I** (acidosis, acetest ±)<br>**Glycogenosis type III** (acetest ++)<br>**Fructose Bi Pase**<br>**FAO defects** (acetest –)<br>**PHHI** (acetest –) intractable hypoglycemia | Fasting test, loading test<br>DNA analyses, enzyme studies<br>Lactic acidosis and ketosis<br>Organic acids, acylcarnitine<br>Insulin plasma levels |
| (b) | **Hepatomegaly**<br>Jaundice<br>**Liver failure**<br>Hepatocellular necrosis | Acidosis +/0<br>Acetest +/0 | $NH_3$ N or ↑ +<br>Lactate +/++<br>Glucose N or ↓ ++ | **Galactosemia, HFI**<br>**Tyrosinemia type I (tubulopathy)**<br>NN hemochromatosis<br>TALDO (with anemia)<br>RCD (mito DNA depletion) | DNA analyses, enzyme studies<br>Organic acids (succinyl acetone)<br>Molecular analysis<br>Polyols (tandem MS)<br>Lactate, molecular studies |

*(Continued)*

**TABLE 129-3 CLASSIFICATION OF INBORN ERRORS REVEALED IN THE NEONATAL PERIOD AND EARLY IN INFANCY WITH NEUROLOGIC DETERIORATION (CONTINUED)**

| Types | Clinical Type | Acidosis/Ketosis | Other Signs | Most Usual Diagnosis (Disorder/Enzyme Deficiency) | Elective Methods of Investigation |
|---|---|---|---|---|---|
| (c) | **Hepatomegaly**<br>**Cholestatic jaundice**<br>**+ Failure to thrive**<br>**+ Chronic diarrhea**<br>**+ Osteoporosis**<br>**+ Rickets** | Acidosis 0<br>Ketosis 0 | $NH_3$ N<br>Lactate N<br>Glucose N | **Alpha1-antitrypsin**<br>**Bile acid defects**<br>**Peroxisomal defects**<br>**CDG syndrome**<br>**Niemann-Pick C**<br>**MEGDEL syndrome**<br>**LCHAD**<br>**Cholesterol metabolism and CTX**<br>**Mevalonic aciduria**<br>**Citrin and Arginase deficiency** | Protein electrophoresis<br>Bile acids (plasma, urine, bile)<br>VLCFA, phytanic, and bile acids<br>Glycosylated transferrin<br>Plasma sterols, Filipin test<br>Filipin test, molecular studies<br>OAC, acylcarnitine profile<br>Plasma sterols<br>OAC<br>AAC (citrulline can be normal) |
| (d) | **Hepatosplenomegaly**<br>**"Storage" signs (coarse facies, ascites, hydrops fetalis, macroglossia, bone changes, cherry-red spot, vacuolated lymphocytes)**<br>**+ Failure to thrive**<br>**+ Chronic diarrhea**<br>**+ Hemolytic anemia** | Acidosis 0<br>Acetest 0<br>DNPH 0 | $NH_3$ N<br>Lactate N or ↑<br>Glucose N<br>Hepatic signs +/++ | **Congenital erythropoietic porphyria**<br>GM1 gangliosidosis<br>ISSD (sialidosis type II)<br>I-cell disease<br>Niemann-Pick type A<br>MPS VII<br>Galactosialidosis<br>CDG syndrome<br>Mevalonic aciduria<br>TALDO (with anemia) | Porphyrins<br>Oligosaccharides, sialic acid<br>Mucopolysaccharides<br>Enzyme, molecular studies<br>Glycosylated transferrin<br>OAC<br>Polyols (tandem MS) |

±, slight; +, moderate; ++, marked; +++, significant/massive; ↑ elevated; ↓ decreased; 0, absent (acidosis) or negative (acetest, dinitrophenylhydrazine, DNPH); AA, acetoacetate; AAC, amino acid chromatography; CAT, carnitine acylcarnitine translocase; CAVA, carbonic anhydrase VA isoform; CPS, carbamyl phosphate synthetase; CPT II, carnitine palmitoyltransferase II; CTX, cerebrotendinous xanthomatosis; DNPH, dinitro phenyl hydrazine test (detects alpha-keto acids); GA II, glutaric aciduria type II; GLCMS, gas liquid chromatography mass spectrometry; HMGCoA, 3-OH-3-methylglutaryl coenzyme A; ISSD, infantile sialic acid storage disease; IVA, isovaleric acidemia; L, lactate; LCHAD, 3-OH long-chain acyl-CoA dehydrogenase; MCD, multiple carboxylase; MCKAT, medium-chain 3-ketoacyl-CoA A thiolase; MMA, methylmalonic acidemia; MPS VII, mucopolysaccharidosis type VII; MSUD, maple syrup urine disease; N, normal (normal values = $NH_3$ < 80 μM; lactate < 1.5 mM; glucose 3.5–5.5 mM); NKH, nonketotic hyperglycinemia; OAC, organic acid chromatography; 3-OHB, 3-hydroxybutyrate; OTC, ornithine transcarbamylase; P, pyruvate; PA, propionic acidemia; PC, pyruvate carboxylase; PDH, pyruvate dehydrogenase; 3-PGD, 3-phosphoglycerate dehydrogenase; PNPO, pyridox(am)ine-5′-phosphate oxidase; SO, sulfite oxidase; TALDO, transaldolase; VLCAD, very-long-chain acyl-CoA dehydrogenase; VLCFA, very-long-chain fatty acids; XO, xanthine oxidase.

Reproduced with permission from Scriver CR, Sly WS, Childs B, et al: *The Metabolic and Molecular Basis of Inherited Disease*, 8th ed. New York: McGraw-Hill; 2002.

gastrointestinal presentations). Some significant symptoms (eg, metabolic acidosis and especially ketosis) can be moderate and transient, largely depending on the symptomatic therapy. Conversely, at an advanced state, many nonspecific abnormalities (eg, respiratory acidosis, severe lactic acidemia, secondary hyperammonemia) can disturb the original metabolic profile. This applies particularly to IEM with a rapid fatal course, such as urea cycle disorders, in which the initial characteristic presentation of hyperammonemia with respiratory alkalosis shifts rapidly to a rather nonspecific picture of acidosis and lactic acidemia as respiratory effort is lost due to encephalopathy.

We have found that more than 80% of newborns with IEM have **MSUD (maple syrup urine disease), organic acidurias, urea cycle defects**, nonketotic hyperglycinemia, mitochondrial respiratory chain disorders, or **fatty acid oxidation disorders**.

**Approach to Therapy** Immediate therapy of acute encephalopathy due to any of the likely IEMs involves measures to decrease the production of offending metabolites and to increase their excretion. Treatment should include the following:

1. Ensure adequate cardiorespiratory function to allow removal of any accumulating metabolites. Adequate hydration is essential to maintain good urine output, because many of the offending diffusible metabolites are freely filtered at the glomerulus.
2. Reverse the catabolic state and reduce exposure to the offending nutrients. Neonates with severe ketoacidosis present with intracellular dehydration that is often underestimated. In this situation, aggressive rehydration with hypotonic fluids and alkalization may cause or exacerbate preexisting cerebral edema. Therefore, rehydration should be planned over a 48-hour period, with an infusion of less than 150 mL/kg/24 hours that contains an average concentration of 75 to 150 mmol/L of $Na^+$ (4.5–9 g/L of NaCl), 30 to 40 mmol/L of $K^+$ (2–3 g/L of KCl), and 5% glucose. Acidosis can be partially corrected with intravenous bicarbonate, especially if it does not improve with the first measures applied for toxin removal. However, aggressive therapy with repeated boluses of intravenous bicarbonate may induce hypernatremia, cerebral edema, and even cerebral hemorrhage. In mildly affected patients, hydration can be performed using a standard 5% to 10% glucose solution containing 75 mmol/L of $Na^+$ (4.5 g/L of NaCl) and 20 mmol/L of $K^+$ (1.5 g/L of KCl). High-calorie, protein-free nutrition should be started in parallel, using carbohydrates and lipids to provide 100 kcal/kg/d. Initially, for the 24- to 36-hour period needed to test gastric tolerance, parenteral and enteral nutrition are used together.
3. After these measures have been instituted, and even before a precise biochemical diagnosis has been made, begin hemodialysis or hemofiltration to remove the offending small molecule as quickly as possible if the patient is comatose or semicomatose.
4. Provide therapy specific to the disease; for example:
   a. Whatever the disease, nutrition is extremely important, and both the method of administration and the composition of feeds must be rapidly determined. Briefly, 4 types of diet can be considered: normal, low-protein, carbohydrate-restricted, and high-glucose, with or without lipid restriction.
   b. Cofactor administration, which will sometimes improve the function of a genetically defective enzyme (eg, vitamin $B_6$ in recurrent intractable seizures, $B_{12}$ in some cases of methylmalonic aciduria because $B_{12}$ is a cofactor for methylmalonyl-CoA mutase).

c. Metabolic manipulation and cleansing drugs such as administering sodium benzoate and phenylacetate in hyperammonemias or carnitine in organic acidurias to divert a toxic substrate to a benign excretable form.

**Later Onset, Acute, and Recurrent Attacks (Late Infancy and Beyond)**

In about 50% of the patients with IEM, onset of symptoms is delayed. The symptom-free period is often longer than 1 year and may extend into late childhood, adolescence, or even adulthood. Each attack can follow a rapid course ending either in spontaneous improvement, permanent disability, or unexplained death despite supportive measures. Between attacks, the patient may appear normal. Onset of acute disease may occur without overt cause but may be precipitated by an intercurrent event related to excessive protein intake, prolonged fasting, prolonged exercise, infection, or any condition that enhances protein catabolism. Recurrent crisis in a context of chronic encephalopathy or neurologic deterioration is an important sign of an IEM.

**Coma, Strokes, and Attacks of Vomiting with Lethargy** Acute encephalopathy is a common problem in children and adults with IEM. All types of coma may be indicative of an IEM, including those presenting with focal neurologic signs (Table 129-4). Age at onset, accompanying clinical signs (eg, hepatic, gastrointestinal, neurologic, psychiatric), mode of evolution (improvement, sequelae, death), and routine laboratory data do not allow an IEM to be ruled out a priori. Two categories can be distinguished:

1. *Metabolic coma without focal neurologic signs.* The main varieties of metabolic coma may be observed in these late-onset, acute diseases, such as predominant metabolic acidosis, predominant hyperammonemia, predominant hypoglycemia, or combinations of these 3 abnormalities. A rather confusing finding in some organic acidurias and ketolytic defects is ketoacidosis with hyperglycemia and glycosuria that mimics diabetic coma. The diagnostic approach to these metabolic derangements is discussed below. Many late-onset ornithine transcarbamylase patients are first diagnosed as viral encephalitis and treated with acyclovir (Zovirax). Our aphorism to our residents was "Write on the Zovirax box: Did you measure ammonia?"
2. *Neurologic coma with focal signs, seizures, severe intracranial hypertension, strokes, or stroke-like episodes.* Although most recurrent metabolic comas are not accompanied by neurologic signs other than encephalopathy, some patients with organic acidemias and urea cycle defects present with focal neurologic signs or cerebral edema. These patients can be mistakenly diagnosed as having a cerebrovascular accident or cerebral tumor. In these disorders, stopping the protein intake, infusing large amounts of glucose, and giving "cleansing drugs" (eg, carnitine, sodium benzoate) can be lifesaving. **Biotin-responsive basal ganglia disease** is a treatable condition that presents in childhood with a subacute encephalopathic picture of undefined origin, including confusion, vomiting, and a vague history of febrile illness. **Pyruvate dehydrogenase (PDH) and biotinidase deficiency** are other treatable causes that may present in a similar manner. Arterial tortuosity syndrome (*GLUT10* mutations) characterized by generalized tortuosity and elongation of all major arteries may result in acute infarction due to ischemic strokes or an increased risk of thrombosis.

All severe forms of **homocystinuria** (total homocysteine > 100 μM/L) can cause an acute cerebrovascular accident from early childhood to adulthood. These forms include **cystathionine-β-synthase deficiency** (usually $B_6$-responsive in late-onset presentations), severe **methylenetetrahydrofolate reductase (MTHFR) defects** (folate responsive), and **cobalamin defects CblC and CblD** (hydroxycobalamin responsive). Patients with **methylmalonic acidemia (MMA)** may, after first presenting with metabolic decompensation, have acute extrapyramidal and corticospinal tract involvement caused by destruction of the globus pallidus bilaterally. Glutaric acidemia (GA) type I frequently presents with an encephalopathic episode, mimicking encephalitis. Mitochondrial encephalopathy, lactic acidosis, and stroke-like episodes (MELAS) syndrome is another important diagnostic consideration in such late-onset and recurrent comas. Early episodic central nervous system problems, possibly associated with liver insufficiency or cardiac failure, have been the initial findings in some cases of congenital disorders of glycosylation (CDG) syndrome. **Wilson disease** can rarely present with an acute episode of encephalopathy with extrapyramidal signs. **Monocarboxylate transporter type 1 deficiency** (MCT1) has been reported as a cause of recurrent episodes of severe ketoacidosis often associated with cycling vomiting but without reduced consciousness. **Riboflavin transporter defects** can present as brainstem encephalitis since the symptoms can be triggered by viral infections followed by progressive weakness and cranial nerve involvement, including bulbar palsy. Depending on the underlying genetic defect, treatment with riboflavin reverts the clinical picture. Mutations in *TANGO2* (transport and Golgi organization 2) causing infancy-onset recurrent metabolic crises with encephalocardiomyopathy have been recently described.

In summary, all these disorders should be considered in the differential diagnosis of strokes or stroke-like episodes. Vaguely defined or undocumented diagnoses such as encephalitis, basilar migraine, intoxication, poisoning, or cerebral thrombophlebitis should therefore be questioned, particularly when even moderate ketoacidosis, lactic acidemia, or hyperammonemia is present. In fact, these apparent initial acute manifestations are frequently preceded by other premonitory symptoms, such as acute ataxia, persistent anorexia, chronic vomiting, failure to thrive, hypotonia, and progressive developmental delay—all symptoms that are often observed with urea cycle disorders (eg, **ornithine transcarbamylase deficiency [OTC]** and **argininosuccinic aciduria**), mitochondrial respiratory chain defects, **late MSUD**, and **organic acidurias**. Late-onset forms of **PDH** deficiency can present in childhood with recurrent attacks of ataxia, sometimes described by the patient as recurrent episodes of pain or muscular weakness (due to dystonia or to peripheral neuropathy). **Hartnup disease** is a classical but rare cause of acute recurrent ataxias.

When coma is associated with hepatic dysfunction, Reye syndrome secondary to disorders of **fatty acid oxidation** or **the urea cycle** should be considered. Hepatic coma with liver failure and lactic acidemia can be the presenting sign of respiratory chain disorders and is a fairly common presentation of late-onset OTC. Hepatic coma with cirrhosis, chronic hepatic dysfunction, hemolytic jaundice, and various neurologic signs (psychiatric, extrapyramidal) is a classic but underdiagnosed manifestation of Wilson disease. A similar clinical scenario can be found at advanced stages of **manganese transporter deficiency** characterized by dystonia/parkinsonism, hypermanganesemia, polycythemia, and chronic liver disease.

**Acute Psychiatric Symptoms** Late-onset forms of congenital hyperammonemia, mainly partial **OTC deficiency**, can present late in childhood or in adolescence with psychiatric symptoms. Because hyperammonemia and liver dysfunction can be mild even at the time of acute attacks, these intermittent late-onset forms of urea cycle disorders can easily be misdiagnosed as hysteria, schizophrenia, or alcohol or drug intoxication. **Acute intermittent porphyria** and **hereditary coproporphyria** present classically with recurrent attacks of vomiting, abdominal pain, neuropathy, and psychiatric symptoms. Patients with **homocysteine remethylation defects** may present with schizophrenia-like episodes that are responsive to folate. In view of these possible diagnoses, **it is justified to systematically measure ammonia, porphyrins, and plasma homocysteine in every patient presenting with unexplained acute psychiatric symptoms.**

**Reye Syndrome and Sudden Infant Death Syndrome (SIDS)** Within the past decade, an increasing number of IEMs have been described that produce episodes fulfilling the criteria originally used to define Reye syndrome. There is now considerable evidence that many of the disorders (mostly **fatty acid oxidation and urea cycle defects**) responsible for Reye syndrome were misdiagnosed in the past because of inadequate investigations for IEM. Another important reason for this underestimation is that blood and urine specimens for metabolic investigations must be collected at an appropriate time in relation to the illness, because most conditions affecting the mitochondrial

**TABLE 129-4 DIAGNOSTIC APPROACH TO RECURRENT ATTACKS OF COMA AND VOMITING WITH LETHARGY**

| Clinical Presentation | Laboratory Studies | Other Features | Most Frequent Diagnosis (Disorder/ Enzyme Deficiency) | Differential Diagnosis |
|---|---|---|---|---|
| Metabolic coma (without focal neurological signs) | Acidosis (metabolic)<br>**(pH < 7.20,**<br>$CO_3H < 10$ mmol,<br>$pCO_2 < 25$ mm)<br>+/–Hyperammonemia<br>($NH_3 > 100$ μmol/L) | Ketosis + | **Organic acidurias, MSUD**<br>**MCD**, PC, RCD<br>**Ketolysis defects, MCT1**<br>**Gluconeogenesis defects**<br>**CAVA defect**<br>**TANGO II** | Diabetes<br>Intoxication<br>Encephalitis |
| | | Ketosis – | **PDH, Ketogenesis defects**<br>**FAO, FDP**, EPEMA<br>**Riboflavin transporter** | |
| | Hyperammonemia<br>($NH_3 > 100$ μmol/L)<br>Respiratory alkalosis<br>(pH > 7.45, $pCO_2 < 25$) | Normal glucose | **Urea cycle defects**<br>**Triple H, LPI**<br>**TANGO II** | Reye syndrome<br>Encephalitis<br>Intoxication |
| | | Hypoglycemia | **FAO (MCAD)**<br>**HMG-CoA lyase** | |
| | Hypoglycemia<br>(< 2 mmol/L) | Acidosis + | **Gluconeogenesis defects**<br>**MSUD** (ketosis +)<br>**HMG-CoA lyase**<br>**FAO** (ketosis –) | Drugs and toxin<br>Ketotic hypoglycemia<br>Adrenal insufficiency<br>GH deficiency<br>Hypopituitarism |
| | Lactic acidemia<br>(> 4 mmol/L) | Normal glucose | PC, **MCD**, Krebs cycle<br>Respiratory chain<br>**PDH** (without ketosis)<br>EPEMA syndrome<br>TANGO II | |
| | | Hypoglycemia | **Gluconeogenesis defects** (ketosis variable)<br>**FAO** (moderate lactic acidemia, no ketosis) | |
| Neurological coma (with focal signs, seizures, or intracranial hypertension) | Biological signs are very variable, can be absent or moderate; see above "Metabolic coma" | Cerebral edema | **MSUD, OTC** | Cerebral tumor<br>Migraine<br>Encephalitis |
| | | Hemiplegia (hemianopsia) | **MSUD, OTC, MMA, PA**, PGK | Moyamoya syndrome |
| | | Extrapyramidal signs | **MMA, GA I, Wilson disease**<br>**Homocystinuria** | Vascular hemiplegia |
| | | Basal ganglia necrosis | **BGBRD (caudate and putamen necrosis)**<br>**Leigh syndrome** | Cerebral thrombophlebitis<br>Infectious acute necrotizing encephalitis |
| | | Stroke and stroke like | **UCD, MMA, PA, IVA**<br>Respiratory chain (MELAS)<br>**Homocystinurias**<br>CDG syndrome<br>**Thiamine-responsive megaloblastic anemia**<br>**Fabry** (rarely presenting sign)<br>Maltase acid (rare)<br>GLUT 10 | Cerebral tumor<br>Reye syndrome |
| | Abnormal coagulation<br>Hemolytic anemia | Thromboembolic accidents | **Homocystinurias (all kinds)**<br>CDG, PGK | |
| Hepatic coma (hepatomegaly cytolysis or liver failure) | Normal bilirubin<br>Slight elevation of transaminases | Steatosis and fibrosis | **FAO, UCD** | Hepatitis<br>Reye syndrome |
| Reye syndrome | Lactic acidemia<br>Hemolytic jaundice | Liver failure<br>Cirrhosis | Respiratory chain defects<br>**Wilson** disease<br>**Manganese transporter deficiency** | |
| | Hypoglycemia | Exudative enteropathy | Hepatic fibrosis with enteropathy (**CDG Ib**) | |

BGBRD, biotin-responsive basal ganglia disease; CDG, carbohydrate-deficient glycoprotein syndrome; EPEMA, encephalopathy, petechiae, ethylmalonic aciduria syndrome; FAO, fatty acid oxidation; FDP, fructose 1-6 diphosphatase; GA, glutaric aciduria; GLUT 10, glucose transporter 10; GH, growth hormone; HMG-CoA, 3-hydroxy-3-methylglutaryl coenzyme A; IVA, isovaleric acidemia; LPI, lysinuric protein intolerance; MCD, multiple carboxylase deficiency; MCT, monocarboxylic acid transporter; MELAS, mitochondrial encephalopathy lactic acidosis stroke-like episodes; MMA, methylmalonic acidemia; MSUD, maple syrup urine disease; OTC, ornithine transcarbamylase; PA, propionic acidemia; PC, pyruvate carboxylase; PDH, pyruvate dehydrogenase; PGK, phosphoglycerate kinase; RCD, respiratory-chain defects; TANGO II, transport and Golgi organization 2; UCD, urea cycle disorders; bold type, treatable disorders.

Adapted with permission from Scriver CR, Sly WS, Childs B, et al: *The Metabolic and Molecular Basis of Inherited Disease*, 8th ed. New York: McGraw-Hill; 2002.

pathway and urea cycle and fatty acid oxidation (FAO) disorders may produce only intermittent abnormalities. In addition, a normal or nonspecific urinary organic acid and acylcarnitine pattern, even at the time of an acute attack, does not exclude an inherited FAO disorder. However, true SIDS due to an IEM is a rare event despite the large number of publications on the topic and despite the fact that at least > 30 metabolic defects are possible causes. This assertion is not true in the first week of life, in which SIDS may be due to a fatty acid oxidation disorder, and investigations for these disorders is mandatory. The recently described *IARS* and *LARS* (coding for isoleucine and leucine tRNA synthetetases, respectively) and *NBAS* mutations (the latter triggered by fever) presenting with recurrent episodes of acute liver failure may have been mistaken for Reye syndrome.

**Exercise Intolerance and Recurrent Myoglobinuria** Many IEMs may present with exercise intolerance and recurrent myoglobinuria syndrome (myalgias, cramping, and/or limb weakness associated with elevated serum levels of creatine phosphokinase [CK is usually > 100 times upper limit of normal], recurrent pigmenturia, and sometimes acute renal failure). In the last instance, or when the patient is in a comatose state, clinical muscular symptoms can be missed. An important rule is to check serum CK and for myoglobinuria in such conditions. The disorders of muscle energy metabolism present in 2 ways.

First, in the glycogenosis disorders, exercising muscle is most vulnerable during the initial stages of exercise and during intense exercise. A "second-wind" phenomenon sometimes develops. Clinically, the glycogenosis disorders are mostly observed in late childhood, adolescence, or adulthood. The CK level remains elevated in most patients. The most frequent and typical disorder in this group is McArdle disease due to myophosphorylase deficiency (Chapter 149).

Second, in the FAO disorders, attacks of myoglobinuria occur typically after mild to moderate prolonged exercise and are particularly likely when patients are additionally stressed by fasting, cold, or infection. This group is largely dominated by muscle **carnitine palmitoyltransferase (CPT) II, very-long-chain acyl-CoA dehydrogenase, LCHAD, and trifunctional protein (TFP)** deficiencies, which may occur in childhood, in adolescence, or later (Chapter 145).

Mutations in *TANGO2* encoding transport and Golgi organization 2 homolog have been recently described in infants and children with episodic rhabdomyolysis, hypoglycemia, hyperammonemia, and susceptibility to life-threatening cardiac tachyarrhythmias mimicking an FAO defect. Mutations in *RYR1* encoding the ryanodine receptor present with muscle rigidity and rhabdomyolysis when affected individuals are exposed to general anesthesia from infancy (recessive mutations) to adulthood (dominant mutations).

*Lpin1* mutations have recently been found in 60% of a series of patients presenting with unexplained recurrent myoglobinuria triggered by fever after exclusion of a primary FAO disorder. This suggests that lpin1 deficiency should be regarded as a major cause of severe myoglobinuria in infants and toddlers in an inflammatory context.

Adenylate deaminase deficiency has been suspected to cause exercise intolerance and cramps in a few patients, but the relationship between clinical symptoms and the enzyme defect is uncertain. Respiratory chain disorders (RCDs) can present with recurrent muscle pain and myoglobinuria from the neonatal period to adolescence. RCD should be suspected when lactic acidemia is accompanied by an elevated lactate-to-pyruvate ratio, either permanently or after meals. Sometimes the lactate abnormality will be found only after an exercise test. In RCD, muscle symptoms are often associated with cardiomyopathy or diverse neurologic signs (encephalomyopathy).

**Initial Approach to and Protocol for Investigation of Acute Late-Onset Encephalopathy** As with the approach to acute neonatal distress, the initial approach to these disorders is based on the appropriate use of a few screening tests. As with neonates, the laboratory data listed in Table 129-2 must be collected simultaneously during the acute attack and before and after treatment.

***METABOLIC ACIDOSIS AND KETOSIS*** Metabolic acidosis can be observed in a large variety of acquired conditions, including infections, severe catabolic states, tissue anoxia, severe dehydration, and intoxication, all of which should be ruled out. However, these can also trigger acute decompensation of an unrecognized IEM. Metabolic acidosis resulting from IEM may develop as result of accumulation of an anion (lactate, ketone bodies, organic acid, or a combination of both) or loss of bicarbonate, which is usually due to renal tubular dysfunction. In metabolic acidosis resulting from a fixed anion, the plasma chloride concentration is normal, and the anion gap, a reflection of the concentration of unmeasured anions, is increased. In patients with metabolic acidosis caused by loss of bicarbonate, the plasma chloride is elevated, and the anion gap (the difference between the plasma sodium and the sum of the chloride and bicarbonate) is generally normal (ie, 10–15 mmol/L). In metabolic acidosis with a high anion gap, the presence or absence of ketonuria is the major clinical clue to the diagnosis.

When metabolic acidosis is not associated with ketosis, **pyruvate dehydrogenase (PDH)** deficiency, **FAO disorders**, and some **disorders of gluconeogenesis** should be considered, particularly when there is moderate to severe lactic acidemia. All these disorders except PDH deficiency have concomitant fasting hypoglycemia. When metabolic acidosis occurs with a "normal" anion gap and without lactic acidemia or hypoglycemia, the most frequent cause is **renal tubular acidosis (RTA)**, but **pyroglutamic aciduria** can be mistaken for RTA type II.

A number of IEMs cause metabolic acidosis with an associated ketosis. They can be classified according to blood glucose concentration—high, normal, or low (Fig. 129-3). With hyperglycemia, the first diagnosis is diabetic ketoacidosis. However, organic acidurias such as **propionic, methylmalonic, or isovaleric acidemia** and **ketolytic defects** can also be associated with hyperglycemia and glycosuria, mimicking diabetes. Monocarboxylic transporter-1 (MCT1; encoded by *SLC16A1*), involved in lactate, pyruvate, and ketone transport, and TANGO II (involved in transport and Golgi organization) are 2 newly described disorders presenting as recurrent crisis of ketoacidosis with variable levels of glucose, lactate, and ammonia.

With hypoglycemia, the **gluconeogenesis defects** are most probable (**glucose-6 phosphatase: glycogenosis type I** and **fructose-1,6-biphosphatase deficiency**), all with hepatomegaly and lactic acidemia. Rarely, respiratory chain defects can also mimic this presentation. When there is no significant hepatomegaly, late-onset forms of MSUD and organic acidurias should be considered. A classic differential diagnosis is **adrenal insufficiency**, which can cause a ketoacidotic attack with hypoglycemia.

If the glucose level is normal, congenital lactic acidosis must be considered in addition to the disorders discussed above. According to this schematic approach to inherited ketoacidotic states, a simplistic diagnosis of fasting ketoacidosis or ketotic hypoglycemia should be questioned when there is a concomitant severe metabolic acidosis.

***KETOSIS*** While ketonuria should always be considered abnormal in neonates, it is a physiologic result of catabolism in late infancy, childhood, and even adolescence. However, as a general rule, hyperketosis that produces metabolic acidosis is not physiologic. Ketosis that is not associated with acidosis, lactic acidemia, or hypoglycemia is likely to be a normal physiologic reflection of the nutritional state (fasting, catabolism, vomiting, or medium-chain triglyceride-enriched or other ketogenic diets). Of interest are ketolytic defects (**succinyl-CoA transferase** and **3-ketothiolase** deficiencies) that can present with permanent moderate ketonuria occurring mainly after eating at the end of the day.

Significant fasting ketonuria without acidosis is often observed in **glycogenosis type III** in childhood (with marked hepatomegaly) and in the rare **glycogen synthase** defect in infancy (with normal liver size). In both disorders, there is fasting hypoglycemia and postprandial lactic acidemia and hyperglycemia (Fig. 129-4).

Ketosis without acidosis is observed in ketotic hypoglycemias of childhood (a frequent condition) and is associated with hypoglycemias due to **adrenal insufficiency**. Absence of ketonuria in hypoglycemic states, as well as in fasting and catabolic circumstances, is an important observation, suggesting an inherited disorder of **fatty acid oxidation or ketogenesis disorder**. It can also be observed in **hyperinsulinemic states** at any age and in **growth hormone deficiency** in infancy.

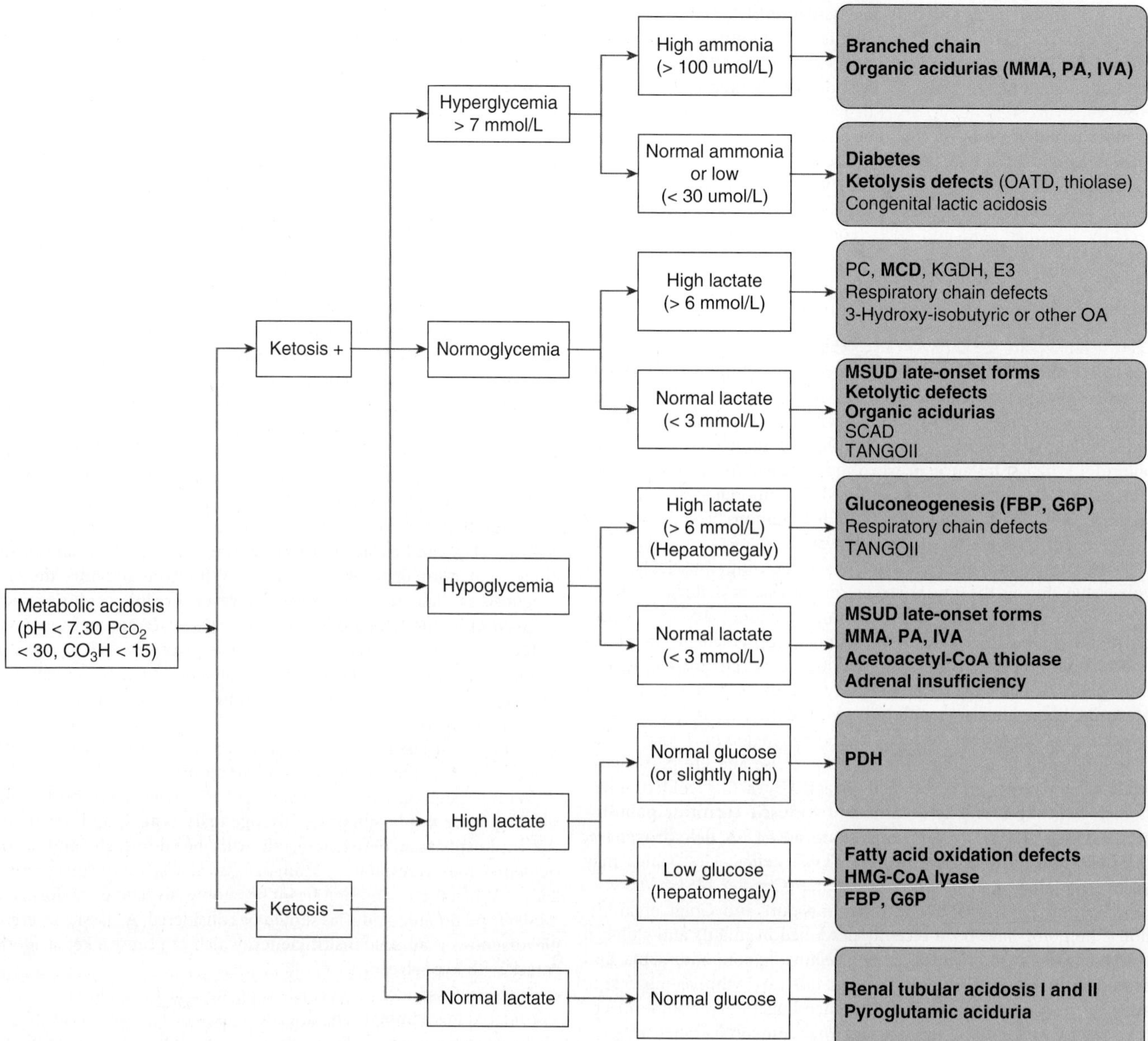


**FIGURE 129-3** Metabolic acidosis and ketotic states. E3, lipoamide oxidoreductase; FBP, fructose bisphosphatase; G6P, glucose-6-phosphatase; GS, glycogen synthetase; HMG-CoA, 3-hydroxy-3-methylglutaryl coenzyme A; IVA, isovaleric acidemia; KGDH, α-ketoglutarate dehydrogenase; MCAD, medium-chain acyl-CoA dehydrogenase; MCD, multiple carboxylase deficiency; MCT, monocarboxylate transporter; MMA, methylmalonic aciduria; MSUD, maple syrup urine disease; OATD, oxoacid CoA transferase; PA, propionic acidemia; PC, pyruvate carboxylase; PDH, pyruvate dehydrogenase; SCAD, short-chain acyl-CoA dehydrogenase; SCHAD, hydroxy short-chain acyl-CoA dehydrogenase; TANGO II, transport and Golgi organization 2. Bold type indicates treatable disorders.

***HYPOGLYCEMIA*** The diagnostic approach to hypoglycemia is based on 4 major clinical criteria: (1) characteristic timing of hypoglycemia (unpredictable, only postprandial, or after exposure, and only after fasting), (2) liver size, (3) association with lactic acidemia (after eating or in fasting state), and (4) association with hyperketosis or hypoketosis (see Fig. 129-4). Other clinical findings of interest are hepatic failure; vascular hypotension; dehydration; short stature; neonatal body size (head circumference, weight, and height); and evidence of encephalopathy, myopathy, or cardiomyopathy.

Erratic and postprandial hypoglycemias are observed in hyperinsulinism and in Munchausen syndrome by proxy. Most patients with hepatic failure display short-term postprandial hypoglycemia.

Fasting hypoglycemias can be classified into 2 groups based on the liver size:

1. *Fasting hypoglycemia with permanent hepatomegaly.* Hypoglycemia associated with permanent hepatomegaly is usually due to an IEM. When hepatomegaly is the most prominent feature without liver insufficiency, gluconeogenesis defects with **fasting** lactic acidosis (**glucose-6-phosphatase deficiency:** glycogenosis type I, **fructose-1,6-bisphosphatase deficiency**) and glycogenolysis defects with **postprandial** lactic acidemia (glycogenosis types III, VI, and IX) are the most likely diagnoses. **FAO defects** and respiratory chain disorders can also present with hepatomegaly at the time of acute fasting hypoglycemia mimicking gluconeogenesis enzyme defects. **CDG syndrome type Ib** (**phosphomannose isomerase deficiency**) with hepatic fibrosis and exudative enteropathy can cause hypoglycemia early in infancy.
2. *Fasting hypoglycemia without permanent hepatomegaly.* It is important to assess the presence of metabolic acidosis and ketosis when the patient is hypoglycemic. **Absence of or only mild ketonuria in concomitant fasting hypoglycemia (or in catabolic context) is almost diagnostic of a fatty acid oxidation disorder (FAO).** Adrenal insufficiency should also be considered, especially when vascular hypotension, dehydration, and hyponatremia are

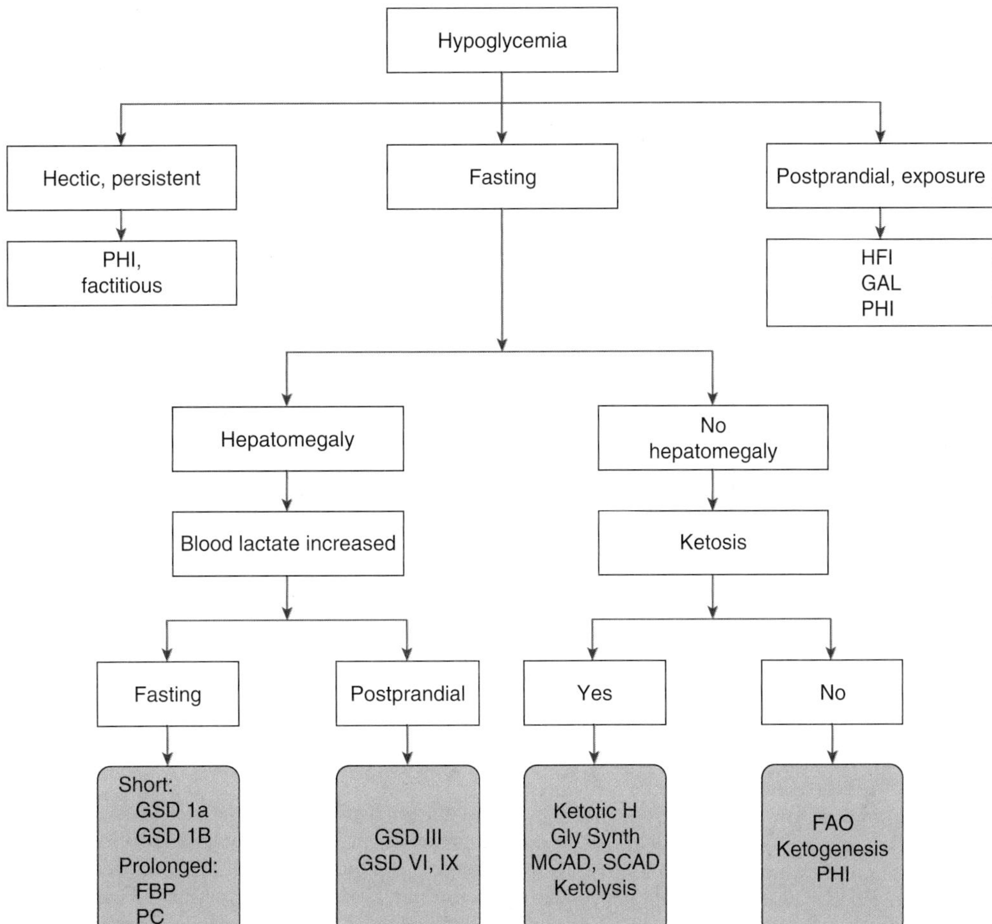


**FIGURE 129-4** Clinical approach to inborn errors in hypoglycemias. CK, creatine kinase; FAO, fatty acid oxidation disorders; FBP, fructose-1, 6-biphosphatase; Gal, galactosemia; Gly Synth, glycogen synthetase; GSD, glycogenosis; HFI, hereditary fructose intolerance; MCAD/SCAD, medium-/short-chain acyl-CoA dehydrogenase; PC, pyruvate carboxylase; PHI, persistent hyperinsulinism.



present. Severe hypoglycemia with metabolic acidosis and absence of ketosis, in the context of Reye syndrome, suggests **HMG-CoA lyase deficiency, HMG-CoA synthetase deficiency, or FAO disorders**. Fasting hypoglycemia with ketosis occurring mainly in the morning and in the absence of metabolic acidosis suggests recurrent functional ketotic hypoglycemia, which presents mostly in late infancy or childhood in those who were small for gestational age or those with macrocephaly. Patients with all types of adrenal insufficiency (peripheral or central) and glycogen synthetase deficiency can share this presentation, as can the rare patients with distal blocks of FAO and ketolysis defects.

In summary, fasting hypoglycemia with at least 1 of the 3 following features is a priori due to an IEM: (1) permanent **hepatomegaly**, (2) **metabolic acidosis**, and (3) **absence of ketonuria concomitant with hypoglycemia**. Hypoketotic hypoglycemias encompass several groups of disorders, including **hyperinsulinemic states**, **growth hormone deficiency**, **inborn errors of FAO**, and **ketogenesis defects** (see the previous "Ketosis" section).

***HYPERAMMONEMIA*** Many IEMs can give rise to hyperammonemia. In the context of acute neonatal encephalopathy, severe hyperammonemia (> 500 μmol/L) is generally caused either by a **UCD** (with respiratory alkalosis, no ketosis, and no bone marrow suppression) or an **organic acidemia (OA; propionic acidemia [PA], MMA, IVA** with metabolic acidosis, ketosis, and leukothrombocytopenia) (Chapter 132). Plasma glutamine is generally elevated in **UCD** (> 1000 μmol/L) **and LPI**, whereas it is close to normal or low (< 500 μmoles/l) in **OAs**. Plasma citrulline levels further allow the distinction between mitochondrial and cytoplasmic **UCDs** (Chapter 141). Severe neonatal forms of ornithine aminotransferase defect may mimic ornithine transcarbamylase deficiency, before ornithine elevation occurs. Hyperammonemia with hyperornithinemia and homocitrullinuria is diagnostic for the mitochondrial ornithine transporter defect (**HHH syndrome**) (Chapter 141).

Neonatal hyperammonemia associated with lactic acidosis (> 6 mmol/L) and hyperketosis suggests pyruvate carboxylase (with low glutamine and high citrulline) (Chapter 154), **multiple carboxylase** or carbonic anhydrase VA deficiencies both with characteristic organic acid profile.

In a context of severe hypoketotic hypoglycemia, hyperammonemia (in general $NH_3$ < 250 μmol/L) suggests a **hyperinsulinism/hyperammonemia syndrome** linked to activating mutations in the glutamate dehydrogenase gene or a **fatty oxidation defect** with cardiac involvement (Chapter 145). Transient hyperammonemia with hypoglycemia may also be observed in premature babies with respiratory distress syndrome. A low plasma lysine level with low ornithine and arginine in the face of a high urinary excretion of these dibasic amino acids is diagnostic for lysinuric protein intolerance (Chapter 139). Mild elevations of $NH_3$ (< 150 μmol/L) may also be a concomitant finding in **MSUD, PDH deficiency**, and patients treated with sodium valproate (the latter with hyperglycinemia).

***LACTIC ACIDEMIA*** Lactate and pyruvate are normal metabolites. Their plasma levels reflect the equilibrium between their cytoplasmic production from glycolysis and their mitochondrial consumption by different tissues. Lactic acidemia (> 2.5 mmol/L) can be due to an elevation of pyruvate (> 0.30 mmol/L), the NADH/NAD ratio (> 20), or $H^+$ (severe acidosis: pH < 7:20), or all of these.

Blood lactate accumulates due to elevation of the NADH/NAD ratio in circulatory collapse, in hypoxia, and in other conditions involving failure of cellular respiration and all severe acidotic states. These conditions must be excluded before an inborn error of lactate-pyruvate oxidation is sought. Persistent lactic acidemias can also result from many acquired conditions, such as diarrhea, persistent infections (mainly of the urinary tract), hyperventilation, and hepatic failure. Ketosis is absent in most lactic acidemias secondary to tissue hypoxia, while it is a nearly constant finding in most IEMs (except in **PDH deficiency**, **GSD type I**, and **FAO disorders**). On the other hand, the level of lactate is not discriminating; some acquired disorders are associated with very high levels, whereas lactate is only moderately raised in some inborn errors of lactate-pyruvate metabolism. Nutritional state also influences the levels of lactate and pyruvate.

Four types of IEM can be considered: The cytoplasmic defects present in a context of hypoglycemia with hepatomegaly: **disorders of liver glycogen metabolism** and **liver gluconeogenesis**. The mitochondrial defects present in a context of neurologic deterioration: lactate-pyruvate oxidation defects (mitochondrial pyruvate transporter [MPC], **PDH**, pyruvate carboxylase [PC], and Krebs cycle defects) and deficient activity in 1 of the components of the respiratory chain (Chapter 153).

The diagnosis of lactic acidemia is further based on 2 metabolic criteria:

- *Time of occurrence of lactic acidemia relative to feeding:* in **glycogenosis (GSD) type 1a (glucose-6-phosphatase deficiency) and in gluconeogenesis** defect (**fructose bisphosphatase**), lactic acidemia reaches its maximum level (up to 15 mmol/L) when the patient is fasting, acidotic, and hypoglycemic. By contrast, in **GSD types III and VI** and in **glycogen synthetase deficiency**, lactic acidemia is observed only in the postprandial period in patients on a carbohydrate-rich diet. Here, lactic acidemia never exceeds 6 mmol/L, and therefore, there is no acidosis (bicarbonate > 18 mmol/L). In PC deficiency severe lactic acidemia (> 7 mmol/L) is present in both the fed and the fasted states but tends to decrease in the postprandial period. In disorders of MPC, **PDH**, α-ketoglutarate dehydrogenase, and respiratory chain function, maximum lactate levels are observed in the fed state (although all lactic acidemias exceeding 7 mmol/L appear more or less persistent). In these disorders, there is a real risk of missing a moderate (although significant) lactic acidemia if the level is checked only before breakfast after an overnight fast (as is usual for laboratory investigations).
- *Determination of lactate-to-pyruvate (L/P) and ketone body ratios before and after meals.* These ratios are useful only in "mitochondrial" lactic acidemias in a neurologic context. They indirectly reflect cytoplasmic (L/P) and mitochondrial (3OHB/AA) redox potential states. They must be measured in carefully collected blood samples.
    - When pyruvic acidemia (> 0.3 mmol/L) is associated with a normal or low L/P ratio (< 12) without hyperketonemia, **PDH deficiency** or MPC is highly probable, regardless of the lactate level.
    - When the L/P ratio is very high (> 30) and is associated with a paradoxical postprandial hyperketonemia and with a normal or low 3OHB/AA ratio (< 1.5), a diagnosis of PC deficiency is virtually certain. In severe PC deficiency, there is also a very characteristic AA profile with hyperammonemia, high citrulline, and low glutamine.
    - When both L/P and 3OHB/AA ratios are elevated and associated with a significant postprandial hyperketonemia, RCD should be suspected.
    - All other situations, especially when the L/P ratio is high without hyperketonemia, are compatible with RCD, but acquired anoxic conditions should also be ruled out (see above).

#### Chronic and Progressive General Symptoms

Many late-onset acute presentations of IEM are actually preceded by premonitory symptoms that may have been ignored or misinterpreted. These symptoms fall schematically into 3 categories: gastrointestinal, muscular, or neurologic.

**Gastrointestinal Involvement, Failure to Thrive, Anemia, and Recurrent Infections** Gastrointestinal (GI) nonspecific findings (anorexia, failure to thrive, chronic vomiting) and osteoporosis occur in a wide variety of IEMs. Unfortunately, their cause often remains unrecognized, thus delaying the diagnosis. Persistent anorexia, feeding difficulties, chronic vomiting, failure to thrive, frequent infections, osteopenia, generalized hypotonia in association with chronic diarrhea, anemia, and bone marrow suppression are frequent presenting symptoms and signs in IEM. They are easily misdiagnosed as cow's milk protein intolerance; celiac disease; chronic ear, nose, and throat infections; late-onset chronic pyloric stenosis; and so on. Congenital immunodeficiencies (CIDs) are also frequently considered, although only a few CIDs present early in infancy with this clinical picture. Faced with these presentations with no definitive diagnosis despite extensive gastroenterological, hematologic, and immunologic investigation, it is mandatory to seriously consider conditions such as **organic aciduria-methylmalonic aciduria (MMA), propionic acidemia (PA), isovaleric acidemia (IVA), urea cycle defects, lysinuric protein intolerance**, and respiratory chain defects. Appropriate studies should be carried out (Table 129-5).

**Muscle Involvement** Many IEMs present with severe hypotonia, muscular weakness, and poor muscle mass. These include most of the late-onset forms of **urea cycle defects** and many **organic acidurias.** Severe neonatal generalized hypotonia and progressive myopathy, with or without an associated nonobstructive idiopathic cardiomyopathy, can be the presenting features of mitochondrial respiratory chain disorders and other congenital lactic acidemias, **FAO defects**, peroxisomal disorders, muscular glycogenolysis defects, **Pompe disease**, some other lysosomal disorders, and complex lipids synthesis/remodeling defects.

**Neurologic Involvement** Neurologic symptoms are frequent and encompass progressive psychomotor retardation, seizures, several neurologic abnormalities in both the central and peripheral system, sensorineural defects, and psychiatric symptoms.

However, some aminoacidopathies and urine organic acidopathies that were identified in children with intellectual disabilities in the late 1970s, when urine and plasma amino acid chromatography was first systematically measured, are now recognized to be of similar frequency in unaffected populations, such that their causative relationship with intellectual disability is uncertain. These include histidinemia, hyperlysinemia, some types of hyperprolinemia, α-amino-adipic aciduria, saccharopinuria, and acetyl amino aciduria due to amino acylase I deficiency, adenylosuccinase deficiency, dihydropyrimidine dehydrogenase deficiency, 4-hydroxybutyric aciduria, D-2-hydroxyglutaric aciduria, and late-onset NKH. Several other inborn errors are now known to rarely, if ever, cause true developmental arrest. Rather, repeated episodes of subacute metabolic crises result in progressive developmental delay. In the 21st century, many new disorders involving the nervous system were revealed by a genome-wide next-generation sequencing (NGS) approach, in patients in whom clinical suspicion of an IEM was low prior to the genetic testing. This is mostly true for the mitochondrial disorders (> 300 new defects), the congenital disorders of glycosylation (> 100 new defects), and the new category of complex lipid and fatty acid synthesis and remodeling defects (> 60 new disorders).

A highly simplified general approach to identification of IEMs associated with chronic encephalopathy is shown in Figure 129-5.

Neurologic signs of IEM can be classified according to age at presentation, the presence or absence of associated extraneurologic signs, and the neurologic presentation itself. IEMs with neurologic signs presenting in the neonate (birth to 1 month) and those presenting intermittently as acute attacks of coma, lethargy, ataxia, or acute psychiatric symptoms were discussed earlier (see Tables 129-1, 129-3, and 129-4).

#### Early Infancy

***DISORDERS ASSOCIATED WITH EXTRANEUROLOGIC SYMPTOMS*** Visceral signs appear in lysosomal disorders. Cardiomyopathy (associated with early neurologic dysfunction, failure to thrive, and hypotonia), sometimes responsible for cardiac failure, is suggestive of respiratory chain disorders, D-2-hydroxyglutaric aciduria (with atrioventricular block), or CDG syndrome. Abnormal hair and cutaneous signs appear in Menkes disease, Sjögren-Larsson syndrome, biotinidase deficiency,

**TABLE 129-5 DIAGNOSTIC APPROACH TO INBORN ERRORS OF METABOLISM WITH CHRONIC DIARRHEA, POOR FEEDING, VOMITING, AND FAILURE TO THRIVE**

| Leading Symptoms | Other Signs | Age of Onset | Diagnosis (Disorder/Enzyme Deficiency) |
|---|---|---|---|
| Severe watery diarrhea | Nonacidic diarrhea | Congenital to infancy | **Congenital chloride diarrhea** |
| Attacks of dehydration | Hypochloremic alkalosis | | |
| | Acidic diarrhea, reducing substances in stools | Neonatal | **Glucose-galactose malabsorption** |
| | | | **Lactase deficiency** |
| | Acidic diarrhea, reducing substances in stools after weaning | Neonatal to infancy | **Sucrase isomaltase** |
| | Skin lesions, alopecia | Neonatal or postweaning | **Acrodermatitis enteropathica** |
| Protein-losing enteropathy | Nonbloody, watery diarrhea | Neonatal | DGAT1 deficiency |
| | Cholangitis crisis +/ hypoglycemia | Infancy | **PMI-CDG (Ib)**, ALG8- CDG (Ih), ALG6-CDG (Ic) |
| | Hypoglycemia | Infancy | PMM-CDG (1a) |
| Fat-soluble vitamin malabsorption | Cholestatic jaundice | Neonatal to infancy | **Bile acid synthesis defects** |
| Severe hypocholesterolemia | Ichthyosis, keratodermia, deafness, mental retardation | | Infantile Refsum |
| Osteopenia | | | MEDNIK |
| Steatorrhea | Hepatomegaly, hypotonia, retinitis pigmentosa, deafness | Infancy | Infantile Refsum |
| | | | PMM-CDG (1a) |
| | Abdominal distension, ataxia, acanthocytosis, peripheral neuropathy, retinitis pigmentosa | Infancy | **Abetalipo I and II** (no acanthocytes, no neurologic sign in type II) |
| | Pancreatic insufficiency, neutropenia, pancytopenia | Early in infancy | Pearson syndrome |
| | | | Shwachman syndrome |
| Severe failure to thrive, anorexia, poor feeding, with predominant hepatosplenomegaly | Severe hypoglycemia, inflammatory bowel disease, neutropenia | Neonatal to early infancy | **Glycogenosis type Ib** (no splenomegaly) |
| | Hypotonia, vacuolated lymphocytes, adrenal gland calcifications | Neonatal | **Wolman** |
| | Recurrent infections, inflammatory bowel disease | Infancy | **X-linked chronic granulomatosis** |
| | Megaloblastic anemia, neuropathy, homocystinuria, MMA | 1–5 years | **Intrinsic factor** |
| | Leukoneutropenia, osteopenia, hyperammonemia, interstitial pneumonia, | Infancy | **Lysinuric protein intolerance** |
| | Recurrent fever, inflammatory bowel syndrome, hyper-IgD, recurrent hemolytic anemia | Infancy | Mevalonate kinase |
| Severe failure to thrive, anorexia, poor feeding, with megaloblastic anemia | Oral lesion, neuropathy, infections, pancytopenia, homocystinuria, MMA | 1–2 years | **TCII** |
| | | | **Intrinsic factor** |
| | Stomatitis, peripheral neuropathy, infections, intracranial calcifications | Infancy | **Congenital folate malabsorption** |
| | Severe pancytopenia, abnormal marrow precursors, lactic acidosis | Neonatal | Pearson syndrome |
| Severe failure to thrive, anorexia, poor feeding, no hepatosplenomegaly, no megaloblastic anemia | Severe hypoproteinemia, putrefaction diarrhea | Infancy | **Enterokinase** |
| | Diarrhea after weaning, cutaneous lesion (periorificial), low plasma zinc | Infancy | **Acrodermatitis enteropathica** |
| | Ketoacidotic attacks, vomiting | Infancy | **Organic acidurias** (MMA, PA), mito. DNA deletions |
| | Intestinal pseudo-obstruction with peripheral neuropathy | Childhood to adulthood | MNGIE syndrome |
| | Vomiting, lethargy, hypotonia, hyperammonemia | Infancy | **Urea cycle defects** (mainly OTC) |
| | Frequent infections, lymphopenia | Infancy | **Adenosine deaminase** |
| | Developmental delay, relapsing petechiae, orthostatic acrocyanosis | Infancy | EPEMA syndrome |
| | Skin laxity, pili torti, hypothermia, hypotonia, seizures, facial dysmorphism | Infancy | Menkes disease |

Bold font indicates treatable disorders.

CDG, carbohydrate-deficient glycoprotein syndrome; DGAT1, acyl-CoA:diacylglycerol acyltransferase 1; EPEMA, ethylmaloic encephalopathy; MMA, methylmalonic acidemia; MEDNIK, acronym for a syndrome caused by mutations in *AP1S1* presenting with a low serum copper and ceruloplasmin, in combination with mental retardation, variable intestinal pseudo-obstruction, deafness, ichthyosis, and raised transaminases; MNGIE, myoneurogastrointestinal encephalopathy secondary to thymidine kinase deficiency; OTC, ornithine transcarbamylase; PA, propionic acidemia; TCII, transcobalamin II.

and respiratory chain disorders. Peculiar fat pads on the buttocks, thick and sticky skin, and inverted nipples are highly suggestive of CDG syndrome. Generalized cyanosis unresponsive to oxygen, suggesting methemoglobinemia and associated with severe hypertonicity, indicates cytochrome-b5-reductase deficiency. Orthostatic acrocyanosis, relapsing petechiae, pyramidal signs, intellectual disability, and recurrent attacks of lactic acidosis suggest ethylmalonic encephalopathy (EPEMA syndrome). The presence of megaloblastic anemia suggests an inborn error of folate and cobalamin (Cbl) metabolism. Ocular abnormalities, such as cherry-red spot, optic atrophy, nystagmus, abnormal eye movements, and retinitis pigmentosa, can be extremely helpful diagnostic signs.

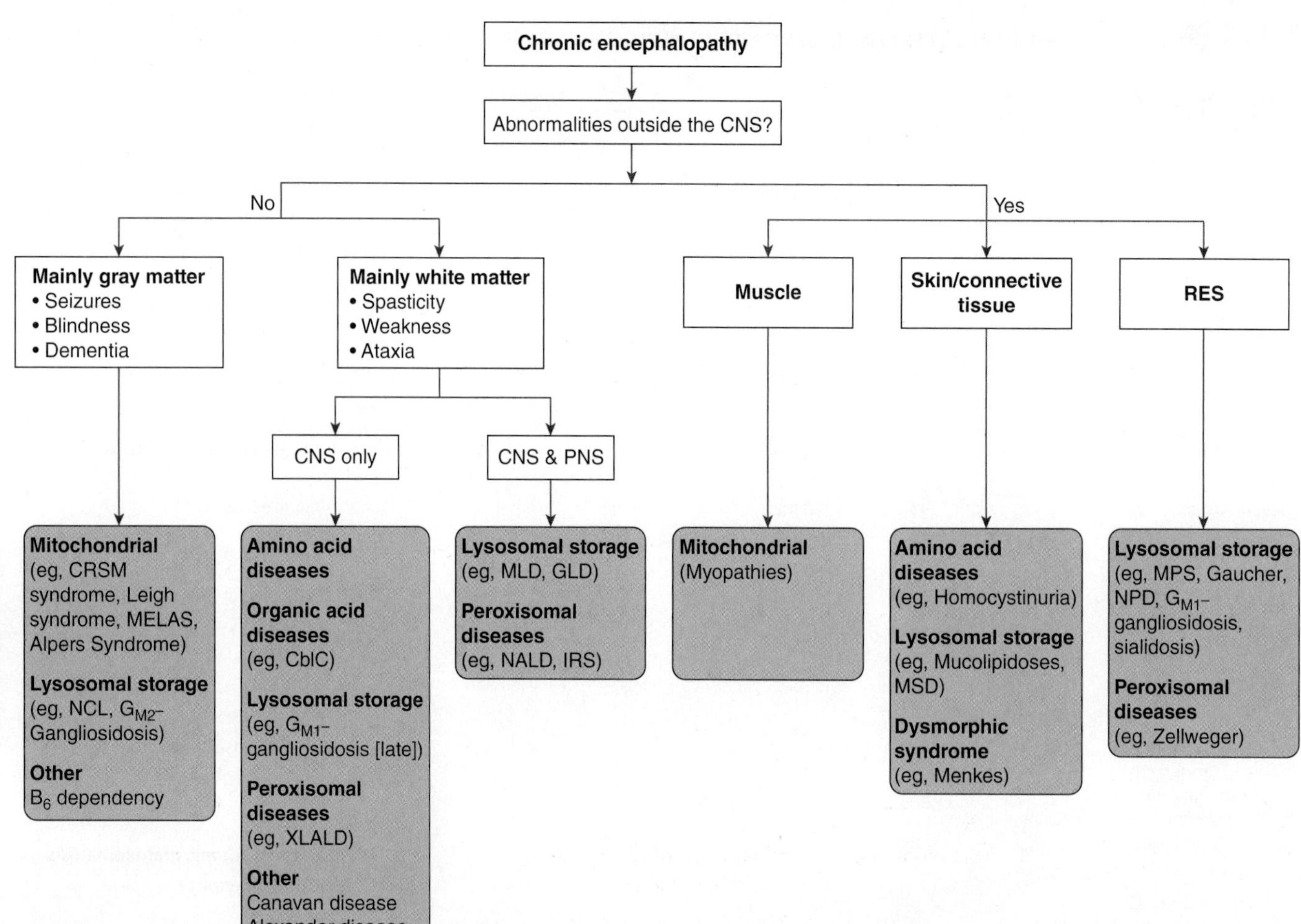


**FIGURE 129-5** An approach to the identification of inborn errors of metabolism causing chronic encephalopathy. CblC, cobalamin C disease; CNS, central nervous system; CRSM, cherry-red spot myoclonus; GLD, globoid cell leukodystrophy; IRS, infantile Refsum syndrome; MELAS, mitochondrial encephalomyopathy, lactic acidosis, and stroke-like episodes syndrome; MLD, metachromatic leukodystrophy; MPS, mucopolysaccharide storage disorder; MSD, multiple sulfatase deficiency; NALD, neonatal adrenoleukodystrophy; NCL, neuronal ceroid lipofuscinosis; NPD, Niemann-Pick disease; PNS, peripheral nervous system; RES, reticuloendothelial system; XLALD, X-linked adrenoleukodystrophy.



***DISORDERS WITH SPECIFIC OR SUGGESTIVE NEUROLOGIC SIGNS*** (Table 129-6) Predominant extrapyramidal symptoms are associated with inborn errors of biopterin and aromatic amino acid metabolism, pyridox(am)ine-5′-phosphate oxidase deficiency, Lesch-Nyhan syndrome, cytochrome-b5-reductase deficiency, Crigler-Najjar syndrome, the early-onset form of glutaric acidemia (GA) type I, and **cerebral creatine deficiency.** Dystonia can also be observed as a subtle but presenting sign in X-linked Pelizaeus-Merzbacher syndrome. It can be also associated with psychomotor retardation, spastic paraplegia, and ataxia in cerebral **folate deficiency syndrome.** Epileptic encephalopathy, neurologic regression, ocular symptoms, and recurrent attacks of neurologic crises are also useful symptoms that lead one to suspect the diagnosis.

Macrocephaly with a **startle response to sound, incessant crying,** and irritability occur in Tay-Sachs, Sandhoff, Canavan, and Alexander diseases, vacuolating leukoencephalopathy, and hydroxyglutaric aciduria and respiratory chain disorders (RCD) due to complex I deficiency in which hypertrophic cardiomyopathy may also be observed.

Recurrent attacks of neurologic crisis associated with progressive neurologic and mental deterioration suggest Leigh syndrome, which is really a clinical phenotype of a number of mitochondrial disorders. Recurrent stroke-like episodes, often associated with anorexia, failure to thrive, and hypotonia, can be presenting symptoms in urea cycle defects (mostly ornithine transcarbamylase [OTC] deficiency), late-onset MSUD, organic acidurias, GA type I, CDG syndrome, and RCD. Thromboembolic events later in life can be the presenting sign of **classical homocystinuria**, CDG syndrome, and Fabry disease.

***DISORDERS WITH NONSPECIFIC DEVELOPMENTAL DELAY*** Many IEMs present with nonspecific early progressive developmental delay, poor feeding, hypotonia, some degree of ataxia, frequent autistic features, and seizures. They can masquerade as cerebral palsy by presenting as a permanent impairment of movement or posture. Consequently, it is mandatory to systematically screen such children for the following IEMs, which are at least partly treatable: late-onset subacute forms of hyperammonemia (usually OTC deficiency in girls) and inborn errors of neurotransmitter synthesis, especially dopa-responsive dystonia due to cyclohydrolase deficiency, tyrosine hydroxylase deficiency, and aromatic-L-amino-acid-decarboxylase deficiency. Recurrent seizures that are unresponsive to anticonvulsants are the presenting symptom of the blood-brain barrier glucose-transporter (GLUT-1) defect. The treatable cerebral folate deficiency syndrome (improved by folinic acid) should also be subject to systematic screening.

**Late Infancy to Early Childhood (1–5 Years)** In this age group, establishing a diagnosis becomes easier. Seven general categories that encompass almost all pediatric neurology can be defined according to the accompanying signs and leading symptom: (1) with prominent extraneurologic symptoms, (2) spastic or flaccid paraplegia, (3) unsteady gait including ataxia and dyspraxia or myoclonia, (4) epilepsy, (5) arrest of development or regression, (6) dystonia/abnormal movements, and (7) behavioral disturbances.

**Progressive paraplegia and spasticity** are presenting signs in many IEMs. A growing number of so-called hereditary spastic paraplegias (SPG) linked to mutations of genes implicated in phospholipid synthesis and remodeling have very recently been elucidated. Of the potentially treatable disorders, a rapidly progressive flaccid paraparesis resembling subacute degeneration of the cord can be the presenting sign of inherited **cobalamin-synthesis defects.** Spastic paraparesis is

**TABLE 129-6 PROGRESSIVE NEUROLOGIC AND MENTAL DETERIORATION WITH SUGGESTIVE NEUROLOGIC SIGNS (1–12 MONTHS)**

| Leading Symptoms | Other Signs | Diagnosis (Disorder/Enzyme Deficiency) |
|---|---|---|
| **With Suggestive Neurologic Signs** | | |
| Extrapyramidal signs | Major parkinsonism | **Inborn errors of biopterin metabolism** |
| | Abnormal neurotransmitters | **Aromatic amino acid decarboxylase** |
| | | **Tyrosine hydroxylase, PNPO** |
| | Choreoathetosis, self-mutilation | Lesch-Nyhan (X-linked) hyperuricemia |
| | Bilateral athetosis, hypertonicity | Cytochrome b5 reductase |
| | Dystonia, stridor | Pelizaeus-Merzbacher (X-linked) |
| | Kernicterus syndrome | Crigler-Najjar |
| | Acute-onset, pseudoencephalitis | **Glutaric aciduria type I** |
| | Low cerebral creatine | **Creatine deficiency** (GAMT) |
| | Spastic paraplegia, ataxia, epilepsy | **Cerebral folate deficiency** |
| | Leigh syndrome | **PDH**, RCD |
| Painful pyramidal hypertonia | Opisthotonos | Krabbe, Gaucher III, Niemann-Pick type C |
| Early epilepsy | Spasticity | NKH, SO, **untreated MSUD and OA** |
| Infantile spasm | | **MCD**, Menkes |
| Macrocephaly, startle response to sound | Cherry-red spot, myoclonic jerks | Tay-Sachs, Sandhoff, Canavan, Alexander |
| | | Vacuolating leukoencephalopathy |
| Ocular symptoms | Optic atrophy, incessant crying | Krabbe (infantile) |
| | Dystonia, choreoathetosis | **GA I**, L-2-hydroxyglutaric aciduria |
| | Progressive irritability | Respiratory chain, peroxisomal defects |
| Recurrent attacks of neurological crises | Failure to thrive, hyperventilation attacks | Leigh syndrome (PC, PDH, respiratory chain, MAMEL syndrome) |
| | Stroke-like episodes | **Urea cycle defects, MSUD, OA, GA I** |
| | | CDG syndrome, respiratory chain |
| | Thromboembolic accidents | **Homocystinurias**, CDG syndrome |
| **Without Suggestive Neurologic Signs** | | |
| Evidence of developmental arrest | Infantile spasms, hypsarrhythmia, autistic features | **Untreated PKU, biopterin defects** |
| | | Peroxisomal defects, Rett syndrome |
| Nonspecific symptoms | Frequent autistic feature | **Hyperammonemia** (late-onset subacute) |
| Apparently nonprogressive disorder | Poor feeding, failure to thrive | 4-OH-butyric, L2-OH-, D2-OH-glutaric acidurias |
| | Hypotonia, seizures | Mevalonic aciduria |
| | With diverse neurologic findings simulating cerebral palsy | Adenylosuccinase, pyrimidine defects |
| | | 3-Methylglutaconic, fumarase |
| | | Other OA, **creatine deficiency** |
| | | **3-PGD**, 3-phosphoserine phosphatase |
| | | **Homocystinurias**, Salla disease |
| | | **Neurotransmitter defects**, |
| | | **Cerebral folate deficiency** |
| | | Angelman, **GLUT-1** |

Bold font indicates treatable disorders.

CDG, congenital disorder of glycosylation; GAI; glutaric aciduria type I; GAMT, guanidinoacetate methyltransferase; MAMEL, methylmalonic aciduria mitochondrial encephalopathy Leigh-like; MCD, multiple carboxylase deficiency; MSUD, maple syrup urine disease; OA, organic acidemias; PC, pyruvate carboxylase; PDH, pyruvate dehydrogenase; 3-PGD, 3-phosphoglycerate dehydrogenase; PKU, phenylketonuria; PNPO, pyridox(am)ine-5′-phosphate oxidase; RCD, respiratory chain disorders.

an almost constant finding in **HHH syndrome** and can be the leading symptom in **dopaminergic synthesis defects** and **biotinidase deficiency**. **Arginase deficiency** is a rare disorder that presents early in infancy to childhood (2 months to 5 years) with progressive spastic diplegia, scissoring or tiptoe gait, and developmental arrest.

**Unsteady gait and uncoordinated movements** (when standing, walking, sitting, reaching for objects, speaking, and swallowing) may be due to cerebellar ataxia, dyspraxia, or myoclonia. Several groups of disorders must be considered. A careful investigation of organic acid and amino acid metabolism is always mandatory, especially during episodes of metabolic stress. Disorders with disturbances of OA and AA and/or other metabolic biomarkers are numerous, and some are potentially treatable, including **PDH**, **creatine deficiency due to guanidinoacetate-methyltransferase deficiency**, **PA, MMA, GLUT1, LCHAD, and vitamin E–responsive ataxias**.

**Predominant epilepsy and myoclonus with progressive deterioration** are frequent presenting signs in many untreatable IEMs (eg, ceroid lipofuscinosis and sphingolipidosis and the emerging group of GPI-anchor biosynthesis defects). Some of the most representative treatable IEMs leading to refractory seizures as a major symptom without clear neurologic deterioration are **creatine defects**, **GLUT1** deficiency, and late-onset **pyridoxine-dependent epilepsy**.

Only a few disorders present between 1 and 5 years of age with an **isolated developmental arrest or regression** of cognitive and perceptual abilities without other significant neurologic or extraneurologic signs. Sanfilippo disease is one, although regression of high-level achievements, loss of speech, and agitation usually begin after 5 years of age. Although nonmetabolic, Rett syndrome is another such disease; it should be considered when a girl, without a family history, presents between 1 and 2 years of age with autistic behavior, developmental regression, typical stereotyped hand movements, and acquired microcephaly.

Extrapyramidal symptoms observed in IEM include dystonia, parkinsonism, chorea, and tremor; however, dystonia is predominant in this age category (from 1–5 years of life) and until late infancy. Although usually associated with other neurologic symptoms, some IEMs can initially present as an isolated dystonia, eg, **neurotransmitter defects (in particular Segawa disease**, pantothenate kinase–associated neurodegeneration [PKAN], Leigh syndrome, Lesch-Nyhan disease, **PDH deficiency**, and **homocystinurias**). However, in general, in intermediary and energy metabolism defects, dystonia tends to be abrupt, develops rapidly, and is generalized and postural from the very first stages of the disease. Some illustrative examples are **GA1, PDH deficiency, thiamine transporter 2 deficiency due to *SLC19A3* mutations (biotin-thiamine basal ganglia responsive disorder), and homocystinurias. GLUT1** deficiency can cause paroxysmal exercise-induced dyskinesia and other paroxysmal complex movement disorders. Most IEMs with extrapyramidal symptoms exhibit abnormal brain magnetic resonance imaging patterns; however, brain image is usually normal in neurotransmitter defects, GLUT1 deficiency, and genetic primary dystonias.

Marked hyperactivity and agitation are very common in Sanfilippo disease (even before regression), whereas autistic behavior may be striking in creatine transporter defect, succinate semialdehyde dehydrogenase, untreated phenylketonuria (PKU), mild forms of Smith-Lemli-Opitz, and a rare disease recently described due to inactivating mutations in ***BCKDK* (branched chain ketoacid dehydrogenase kinase)** that is associated with low plasma branched chain amino acids. This disorder should be potentially treatable by branched chain amino acid supplementation.

**Late Childhood to Adolescence (5–15 Years)** Some conditions affect primarily cognitive function, whereas others present with more extensive neurologic involvement with normal or subnormal intellectual functioning

There are 6 clinical categories:

- **With predominant extrapyramidal signs** (parkinsonian syndrome, dystonia, choreoathetosis). In fact, almost all neurometabolic disorders can cause dystonia at some stage, which is frequently a combined dystonia (with associated symptoms). At this period of life, IEMs that produce dystonia as a major sign include disorders that have been also included from 1 to 5 years of age; however, **Wilson disease**, **Segawa disease (dominant GTPCH)**, **GLUT1 deficiency**, and neurodegeneration with brain iron accumulation (NBIA) syndrome are among the most relevant at this period of life. Some IEMs can also initially present as pure dystonias such as PKAN deficiency, **PDH**, Lesch-Nyhan syndrome, and juvenile metachromatic leukodystrophy. Although more common in older age groups, lysosomal disorders can also begin in childhood with parkinsonism as the leading sign. Special consideration should be given to ceroid lipofuscinosis (CNL), GM1 gangliosidosis, and Niemann-Pick disease type C.
- **Severe neurologic and mental deterioration and diffuse central nervous system involvement.** Patients have in common severe neurologic dysfunction with pyramidal signs, incoordination, seizures, visual failure, impaired school performance, and dementia. In association with splenomegaly or hepatomegaly, these signs suggest Niemann-Pick disease type C or Gaucher disease type III. When visceral signs are absent, they may indicate juvenile metachromatic leukodystrophy, X-linked adrenoleukodystrophy, Krabbe disease, juvenile GM1 and GM2 gangliosidoses, or mitochondrial disorders. Peroxisomal biogenesis defects can also present in the second decade of life with peripheral neuropathy initially mimicking Charcot-Marie-Tooth type II disease.
- **Polymyoclonus and epilepsy.** These are often present in the juvenile form of ceroid lipofuscinosis, Lafora disease after puberty, and some sphingolipidoses and respiratory chain disorders.
- **Predominant cerebellar ataxia.** This can be the presenting feature of peroxisomal disorders, CDG syndrome, **Refsum disease** (these 3 can also manifest peripheral neuropathy and retinitis pigmentosa), Lafora disease, **cerebrotendinous xanthomatosis (CTX)**, late-onset forms of sphingolipidoses, and RCD. Some forms of **coenzyme Q10 (CoQ10) synthesis defects** can respond to idebenone supplementation. Other forms of treatable ataxia are **GLUT1 deficiency, vitamin E–responsive ataxias, and Hartnup disease.**
- **Predominant polyneuropathy.** Porphyrias and tyrosinemia type I can present with an acute attack of polyneuropathy that mimics Guillain-Barré syndrome. Many other disorders can present with late-onset progressive polyneuropathy that can mimic hereditary ataxia, such as Charcot-Marie-Tooth disease, lysosomal and peroxisomal diseases, energy metabolism defects (**PDH, LCHAD**), abetalipoproteinemia, and CDG syndrome.
- **Behavioral disturbances**. Behavioral disturbances (personality and character changes), loss of speech, scholastic failure, mental regression, dementia, psychosis, and schizophrenia-like syndrome may be presenting signs of treatable IEMs. **OTC deficiency** can present with episodes of abnormal behavior and character change until hyperammonemia and coma reveal the true situation. **Homocystinuria** due to MTHFR deficiency has presented as isolated schizophrenia. Searching for these treatable disorders is mandatory, including also **CTX** and **Wilson disease**.

### Recommended Laboratory Tests in Neurologic Syndromes

- Patients are motivated by the hope of a potentially effective treatment, understanding about the prognosis, and availability of genetic counseling.
- IEMs are attractive diagnoses because (1) in many cases, simple blood and urine tests (many of them available in an emergency) can be diagnostic; (2) knowing the biochemistry can (theoretically) point toward a treatment; (3) for some diagnoses, treatment is indeed available; and (4) if recognized early during a pregnancy, antenatal testing is possible for at-risk families.
- In this context, beware of the following attitudes: (1) ignorant or slow ("Oh, metabolic disease are too rare; I didn't see any in my practice!"), with the risk of missing an opportunity to make a diagnosis and start a life-saving therapy; (2) too naïve (lack of familiarity with metabolic disease) with the risk of ordering tests for the wrong situations; and (3) too systematic (the overly detailed approach: "Too much thought, not enough thinking") with the risk of ordering inappropriate tests. All 3 attitudes have a high cost-benefit ratio.
- Metabolic testing is mandatory in 3 situations: (1) in **urgent situations:** rule out treatable disorders: test, treat, then think! (see Table 129-2); (2) **the unexpected pregnancy (in families at risk):** test according to the proband's phenotype; rush in case prenatal diagnosis is important and available; and (3) **symptoms are persistent, progressive, and unexplained**: think (and get help from specialized centers) and then test; use diagnostic algorithms for help and prioritize treatable disorders. Avoid ordering long lists of tests for potential possibilities. **Otherwise, monitor and reevaluate.**
- Nonmetabolic differential diagnoses are numerous: Nutritional phenocopies, toxic ingestions, infections, endocrinopathies, many unexplained or vaguely defined neurologic and psychiatric conditions, and Munchausen or Munchausen-by-proxy are the most frequent.
- Table 129-7 lists a tentative metabolic approach to neurologic syndromes focusing on treatable IEMs.

### Storage Syndrome and Conditions with Dysmorphic Physical Findings

A diagnostically challenging group of IEMs are those associated with somatic dysmorphism. These disorders present a challenge because (1) they are rare; (2) they often involve the metabolism of large, water-insoluble metabolites that are technically difficult to isolate and analyze; (3) the defect is often in a relatively inaccessible subcellular organelle (eg, peroxisomes, mitochondria, lysosomes, Golgi, endoplasmic reticulum); (4) the techniques required to demonstrate the presence of the specific biochemical abnormality are difficult to master and often still at an experimental/research step (metabolomics, lipidomics); (5) the basic defect often impairs the synthesis or remodeling of some compound so that substrate accumulation does not occur and therefore cannot help in making a diagnosis; and

**TABLE 129-7 RECOMMENDED LABORATORY TESTS IN NEUROLOGIC SYNDROMES FOCUSED ON TREATABLE INBORN ERRORS OF METABOLISM**

| Predominant Neurologic Syndrome | Laboratory Tests (Rational Approach Based on Associated Clinical Signs and Treatable Disorders) | Treatable Disorders |
|---|---|---|
| Isolated developmental delay/ intellectual disability (ID) | Basic laboratory tests[a]: blood glucose, acid-base status, blood counts, liver function, creatine kinase, uric acid, thyroid function, alkaline phosphatase<br>Plasma: lactate, ammonium, amino acids, total homocysteine, folate, biotinidase activity<br>Urine: creatine metabolites, organic acids (including 4-hydroxybutyric acid), amino acids, glycosaminoglycans (GAGs), purines, pyrimidines<br>Consider maternal phenylalanine | **Phenylketonuria (PKU), homocystinurias, urea cycle defects**, amino acid synthesis defects, **thyroid defects, biotinidase deficiency, Hartnup disease** |
| With dysmorphic features | Consider also plasma sterols, peroxisomal studies (very-long-chain fatty acids, phytanic acid, plasmalogens), transferrin isoelectric focusing for glycosylation studies (CDG), mucopolysaccharides and oligosaccharides in urine<br>For the study of ID +/– dysmorphic features, genetic tests (cytogenetic studies, microarrays, NGS, and targeted DNA studies have the highest diagnostic yield) | Smith-Lemli-Opitz (SLO) syndrome, peroxisomal diseases (only partially by some supplements)<br>Mucopolysaccharidosis |
| Behavioral and psychiatric manifestations including autistic signs | Basic laboratory tests[a]<br>Plasma: ammonium, amino acids, total homocysteine, folate, sterols (including oxysterols), copper, ceruloplasmin<br>Urine: GAGs, organic acids (4-hydroxybutyric acid), amino acids, purines, creatine, creatinine, and guanidinoacetate<br>Depending on additional clinical signs and brain MRI pattern: peroxisomal studies, lysosomal studies | **PKU, urea cycle disorders, homocystinurias, folate metabolism defects, Wilson disease**, BCKDH kinase deficiency, CTD, mild forms of SLO, Niemann-Pick disease type C, X-ALD (at some stages), Hartnup disease |
| Epilepsy | Basic laboratory tests[a] adding calcium, magnesium<br>Plasma: lactate, ammonium, amino acids, total homocysteine, folate, biotinidase activity, copper and ceruloplasmin, VLCFA<br>Urine: organic acids, creatine, creatinine and guanidinoacetate, sulphite test, purines and pyrimidines, pipecolic acid, and 5-AASA<br>CSF: glucose, lactate, amino acids, 5-methyltetrahydrofolate (5-MTHF), pterines, biogenic amines, GABA<br>Consider lysosomal studies and targeted tests if PME<br>Consider genetic tests for GPI-anchor biosynthesis pathway defects and other defects of complex lipid synthesis (FA2H, ELOVL4, GM3 synthase) | **GLUT-1, homocystinurias, IEM of folate metabolism, organic acidurias, biotinidase deficiency**, creatine synthesis defects, serine biosynthesis defects, Menkes disease (only partially treatable), **late-onset forms of pyridoxine-dependent epilepsy, pterin defects (DHPR), AADC deficiency**, MoCo deficiency (cyclic pyranopterin monophosphate: treatment recently introduced) |
| Ataxia | Basic laboratory tests[a] adding albumin, cholesterol, triglycerides, and α-fetoprotein<br>Plasma: lactate, pyruvate, ammonium, amino acids, biotinidase activity, vitamin E, sterols (including oxysterols), ceruloplasmin, peroxisomal studies (including phytanic acid), coenzyme Q10, transferrin electrophoresis<br>Urine: organic acids (including 4-hydroxybutyric and mevalonic acids), amino acids, purines<br>CSF: glucose, lactate, pyruvate<br>Consider lysosomal/mitochondrial/NBIA studies depending on the clinical and brain MRI signs<br>Consider lipidome studies (plasma, CSF)<br>Consider genetic panels of inherited ataxias and other NGS techniques | **PDH deficiency (thiamine-responsive; ketogenic diet), biotinidase deficiency, GLUT-1**, abetalipoproteinemia, CTX, Refsum disease, coenzyme Q10 deficiencies, Hartnup disease, Niemann-Pick disease type C |
| Dystonia-parkinsonism | Basic laboratory tests[a]<br>Plasma: lactate, pyruvate, ammonium, amino acids, biotinidase activity, sterols (including oxysterols), copper, ceruloplasmin, uric acid, manganese<br>Urine: organic acids, uric acid, creatine, creatinine and guanidinoacetate, purines, GAGs, oligosaccharides<br>CSF: glucose, lactate, pyruvate, amino acids, 5-methyltetrahydrofolate, pterines, biogenic amines, GABA<br>Consider lysosomal/mitochondrial/NBIA studies depending on the clinical and brain MRI signs<br>Consider genetic panels of inherited dystonias, parkinsonism, and other NGS techniques | **Neurotransmitter defects, GLUT-1 deficiency, thiamine transport defects (TBBGDs), PDH defects, organic acidurias, homocystinurias, IEM of folate metabolism**, defects of creatine biosynthesis, **Wilson disease, biotinidase deficiency**, Niemann-Pick disease type C, CTX, manganese defects |
| Chorea | Basic laboratory tests[a]<br>Plasma: lactate, pyruvate, ammonium, amino acids, total homocystinuria, folate, biotinidase activity, sterols (including oxysterols), copper, ceruloplasmin, uric acid, galactose 1 P, transferrin electrophoresis<br>Urine: organic acids, uric acid, creatine, creatinine and guanidinoacetate, purines, galactitol, sulphite test<br>CSF: glucose, lactate, pyruvate, amino acids, 5-methyltetrahydrofolate, pterines, biogenic amines, GABA<br>Consider NCL studies and GPI-anchor synthesis defect genetic tests<br>Consider genetic panels of inherited choreas and other NGS techniques | Glutaric aciduria I and other classic organic acidurias (MMA, PA), GAMT, GLUT-1, homocystinurias, pterin and neurotransmitter defects, Niemann-Pick disease type C, Wilson disease, galactosemia, cerebral folate deficiency due to *FOLR* mutations, MoCo deficiency, NKH |

(*Continued*)

**TABLE 129-7 RECOMMENDED LABORATORY TESTS IN NEUROLOGIC SYNDROMES FOCUSED ON TREATABLE INBORN ERRORS OF METABOLISM (CONTINUED)**

| Predominant Neurologic Syndrome | Laboratory Tests (Rational Approach Based on Associated Clinical Signs and Treatable Disorders) | Treatable Disorders |
|---|---|---|
| Spasticity | Basic laboratory tests[a]<br>Plasma: lactate, pyruvate, ammonium, amino acids, total homocystinuria, folate, biotinidase activity, vitamin E, triglycerides, cholesterol, sterols, peroxisomal studies<br>Urine: organic acids, amino acids, GAGs, oligosaccharides, sialic acid<br>CSF: biogenic amines, pterines, and 5-MTHF<br>Consider lysosomal/mitochondrial/NBIA studies depending on clinical and MRI findings<br>Consider genes related to HSP and plasma, CSF lipidome | HHH, arginase deficiency, ornithine aminotransferase deficiency, homocysteine remethylation defects, biotinidase deficiency, cerebral folate deficiencies, dopamine synthesis defects (atypical TH), CTX, vitamin E deficiency |
| Peripheral neuropathy | Basic laboratory tests[a]<br>Plasma: lactate, pyruvate, ammonium, amino acids, folate, vitamin E, triglycerides, cholesterol, acylcarnitines, sterols, peroxisomal studies, transferrin electrophoresis<br>Urine: amino acids, GAGs, oligosaccharides, thymidine, porphyrins<br>Consider lysosomal/mitochondrial/NBIA studies depending on clinical and MRI findings | Refsum disease, X-ALD (treatable at some stages), homocysteine remethylation defects, CTX, abetalipoproteinemia, LCHAD, trifunctional protein, PDH, vitamin E malabsorption, ornithine aminotransferase, serine deficiency |

[a]These basic laboratory tests should be considered as a routine screening in every neurologic syndrome.

Disorders that must be treated as an emergency are set in bold type.

AADC, amino acid decarboxylase; 5-AASA, 5-aminoadipic semialdehyde; BCKDH, branched chain ketoacid dehydrogenase; CTX, cerebrotendinous xanthomatosis; DHPR, dihydropteridine reductase; FOLR, folate receptor; GA1, glutaric aciduria type 1; GAG, glycosaminoglycan; GAMT, guanidinoacetate methyltransferase; GTPCH, GTP cyclohydrolase I; HHH, hyperammonemia, hyperornithinemia, homocitrullinuria; HSP, hereditary spastic paraparesis; LCHAD, long-chain 3-hydroxyacyl-CoA dehydrogenase; MMA, methylmalonic aciduria; MoCo, molybdenum cofactor deficiency; MRI, magnetic resonance imaging; NGS, next-generation sequencing; NKH, nonketotic hyperglycinemia; PA, propionic academia; PDH, pyruvate dehydrogenase deficiency; PME, progressive myoclonus epilepsy; X-ADL, x-linked adrenoleukodystrophy; TH, tyrosine hydroxylase.

Data from Saudubray JM, Baumgartner M, Walter J: *Inborn Metabolic Diseases*. 6th ed. Berlin, Germany: Springer Verlag; 2016.



(6) there are few screening tests that are useful for ruling out entire classes of disorders, such as amino acid analysis for aminoacidopathies. Although the dysmorphism associated with IEM may be severe, with some prominent exceptions, it generally involves disturbances of shape (distortions) rather than fusion or cellular migration defect (disruptions) or abnormalities of number, such as polydactyly (true malformations). The dysmorphism tends to become more pronounced with age, and histologic and ultrastructural abnormalities obtained by tissue biopsy are often prominent.

### Symptoms Specific to an Organ or System

IEM can involve any organ or system, in any scenario, at any age. Some of these phenotypes are rare and very distinctive (eg, lens dislocation and thromboembolic accidents in homocystinuria or palmoplantar hyperkeratosis with keratitis in tyrosinemia type II), whereas others are common and rather nonspecific (eg, hepatomegaly, seizures, intellectual disability).

### How Does Laboratory Investigation Help?

The definitive diagnosis of IEM is based on a wide range of biochemical studies, many of which are not readily available in community hospitals or in routine diagnostic laboratories. In recent years, biochemical testing has been supplemented by molecular genetic studies, including gene panels and NGS of exomes and genomes. Although molecular testing has undeniably enhanced the investigation of these disorders, the biochemical phenotype remains central to identifying the primary metabolic defect and confirming the pathogenicity of DNA variants. The pattern and extent of tissue involvement often provide important clues to the underlying nature of the condition. Imaging studies, electrophysiologic testing (eg, nerve conduction velocities, brainstem auditory-evoked responses, EEG, electromyography), and histopathologic, histochemical, and ultrastructural studies on biopsied tissue are all useful. Analysis of various metabolic intermediates—such as amino acids, organic acids, acylcarnitines, free fatty acid profile including VLCFA, sterols, neurotransmitters, creatine, purines and pyrimidines, and isoelectrofocusing of serum sialotransferrin—in plasma, urine, and CSF may also provide critical leads to a diagnosis. At this stage of investigation, it is often helpful to consider whether the condition is more likely to be an inborn error of small-molecule metabolism, such as an aminoacidopathy or organic acidopathy, or an organelle disease. This distinction is useful, because the investigation of each group differs, especially with respect to the analysis of metabolic intermediates. In small-molecule diseases, analysis of water-soluble metabolites, such as amino acids and organic acids, is helpful. It is also technically easier than analyzing the high-molecular-weight, often water-insoluble metabolites that accumulate in organelle diseases, such as the lysosomal storage disorders. With amino acid and organic acid defects, a single laboratory test often covers a wide range of diseases and has some of the characteristics of metabolic screening. Recent (and accelerating) progress in metabolomics and lipidomics (still not readily available in current practice) will allow the identification in the near future of many more metabolic signatures, including those of organelle diseases in which secondary accumulation of other high-molecular-weight compounds is common and diagnostically confusing. The diagnostic value of analyzing metabolic intermediates is greatly enhanced in children with small-molecule diseases (intoxication and energy disorders) by provocative physiologic testing such as carefully monitored prolonged fasting. However, this type of investigation is inherently dangerous, and it should only be undertaken under carefully monitored circumstances in a hospital. Ultimately, identifying the biochemical phenotype in children with IEM requires specific analysis of the activity of the mutant gene product, the catalytic protein such as the enzyme or transporter involved. This is particularly true of the organelle diseases in which clinical overlap often creates diagnostic confusion. For example, type 1 Gaucher disease is easily confused clinically with type B Niemann-Pick disease. Confident differentiation requires measurement of the relevant lysosomal enzyme activities in an appropriate tissue, such as leukocytes or cultured skin fibroblasts.

As with all genetic diseases, the highest level of definition of IEM is demonstration of disease-causing mutations in the relevant genes. However, because locus and allelic heterogeneity is often enormous, mutation analysis has been only rarely useful as a first line of investigation. However, mutation analysis does provide powerful confirmation of defects identified on the basis of biochemical data, and the more recent ability to perform whole-exome analysis in an ever shorter time frame (days to weeks) has the potential to have a major impact on patient diagnosis and management. After a mutation is identified as causing disease within a family, testing for the molecular defect provides a relatively simple and reliable method for carrier detection and prenatal diagnosis.

## NEWBORN SCREENING

Robert Guthrie pioneered newborn screening in the early 1960s when he developed a test for phenylketonuria (PKU) using a novel bacterial-inhibition assay. Guthrie was also responsible for introducing the use of a dried blood sample on filter paper (the "Guthrie test"). This was followed by further bacterial-inhibition assays to detect other aminoacidopathies (eg, maple syrup urine disease, homocystinuria, urea cycle disorders), but initially, only screening for PKU was widely adopted. In 1975, Jean Dussault described screening for congenital hypothyroidism, and since then, other disorders covered in screening programs have included congenital adrenal hyperplasia, the galactosemias, cystic fibrosis, biotinidase deficiency, glucose-6-phosphate dehydrogenase deficiency, aminoacidopathies, fatty acid oxidation disorders, various lysosomal storage disorders, and most recently peroxisomal disorders. The application of tandem mass spectrometry to newborn screening was first described in 1990, allowing for the quantitation of certain amino acids. Further technical advances led to the use of acylcarnitines as a means for detecting certain organic acidurias and fatty acid oxidation disorders. This new technology has greatly improved both newborn screening and the diagnosis of many IEM.

### Aims and Criteria of Newborn Screening

The initial aim of newborn screening was to identify infants who had serious but treatable disorders so as to facilitate interventions to prevent or ameliorate the clinical consequences of the disease. In recent years, with the advent of tandem mass spectrometry—which can detect many disorders at one time, providing the ability for early detection of currently untreatable disorders (see below)—there has been discussion about how screening might benefit families, rather than just individual neonates. The World Health Organization has published guidelines, as has the United States. In the United States, national guidelines, termed Recommended Uniform Screening Panel (RUSP), are established by Secretary's Advisory Committee on Heritable Disorders in Newborns and Children (SACHDNC) in conjunction with the Department of Health and Human Services. Recommended testing can be divided into "core" and "secondary" conditions, with the latter being disorders identified unintentionally in the course of screening for core disorders. Core disorders are defined as fulfilling the following criteria: there is a specific and sensitive test available, the health outcomes of the condition are well understood, there is an available and effective treatment, and identification of the condition could affect the future reproductive decisions of the family. In reality, the criteria can be reduced to 2 main considerations that would justify screening for any specific disorder: (1) There should be a benefit from neonatal detection, and (2) the overall benefit should be reasonably balanced by the costs of all kinds—the financial costs and the cost of harm, if any, to individuals by early detection of the disorder or by false assignment of a positive or negative result. It is important to remember that newborn screening covers the whole process, from sampling to the appropriate referral of an affected baby for the start of treatment and assessment of overall outcome. Currently, the RUSP is limited to 34 recommended core conditions and 24 secondary conditions. However, individual states define which conditions will be subject to newborn screening, and although the majority of conditions are included in all state programs, there are differences in implementing newer tests such as X-linked adrenoleukodystrophy and various lysosomal storage disorders such as Pompe, Fabry, and Krabbe disease. This in part reflects the advocacy system used by states in defining their screened conditions, where motivated lay groups may influence legislative mandates and competing financial needs and priorities may affect implementation. Online information on each state's program is available (http://genes-r-us.uthscsa.edu/resources/newborn/newborn_menu.htm).

### Cutoff Values for Screening Labs



Determining the cutoff point for each analyte is always a compromise between the aim for perfect sensitivity (detecting all the cases) and keeping the false-negative rate as low as possible. It is important for the laboratory to establish age-dependent cutoff values, as these can vary greatly. Physicians must bear in mind that no screening test is perfect, although some may be close. If clinical presentation suggests a disorder that is included in newborn screening, a diagnostic test should be done, even if the screening test was negative.

### Classification of IEM Detected by Newborn Screening

Newborn screening has opened new perspectives in preventive medicine. Disorders of amino acid, organic acid, and fatty acid metabolism are now often detected in the newborn screening laboratory, rather than by the clinical metabolic service. Early detection provides 4 possibilities.

1. The disorder may present in the first days of life, before any newborn screening result is likely. Disorders in this category include neonatal presentations of urea cycle defects; organic acidemias such as methylmalonic acidemia; classic galactosemia; and, less commonly, almost any of the fatty acid oxidation defects. Detection by newborn screening is unlikely to directly benefit most cases in this category. However, it seems appropriate to include these early presenting disorders in the screening suite, as some may have delayed diagnosis or onset of symptoms. On occasion, a diagnosis may never be made, with the baby having been thought to have died from sepsis.
2. The disorder may be later presenting, and an effective treatment can beneficially alter the natural history. Cases in this category include the less severe urea cycle disorders; most aminoacidopathies, such as maple syrup urine disease (MSUD); tyrosinemias; homocystinuria; phenylketonuria (PKU); some organic acidemias; and most fatty acid oxidation disorders. The recent possibility to screen for most of the lysosomal disorders from a blood spot now raises the question of whether to extend the newborn screening to those disorders in which a preventive therapeutic effectiveness has been shown, and screening these disorders is being implemented or subjected to pilot studies. This possibility raises many practical, organizational, financial, and ethical questions.
3. The disorder may be benign, or largely so, and most cases will have no benefit from early diagnosis. It is hard to know yet which cases will fit into this category, but newborn screening, if carefully and sensitively conducted, provides an excellent opportunity for elucidating the natural history of disorders that might fall into this category. Such conditions include 3-methylcrotonyl CoA carboxylase and 2-methylbutyryl CoA dehydrogenase deficiency. Mild forms of several disorders will readily be detected by newborn screening but will not need treatment.
4. The disorder may be severe and progressive, starting late in life and not being treatable, like many sphingolipidoses. With a few exceptions, these defects are not screened despite the benefits of genetic counseling for at-risk parents.

### Screening for Individual Inborn Errors of Metabolism

Well over 50 IEMs can now be detected by newborn screening, with varying degrees of certainty. Only the most frequent IEIM are cited below.

**Phenylketonuria** Screening for phenylketonuria (PKU) has been implemented in most developed countries since the late 1960s. The initial test first reported in 1963 was the "Guthrie test," a bacterial-inhibition assay. Alternative methods that were subsequently developed include fluorimetry and colorimetry. More recently, PKU screening has been done by tandem mass spectrometry (MS), where this is available. Screening in the United States may take place after 24 hours, but elsewhere, testing after at least 48 hours is more typical. Patients under good control of phenylalanine levels by 3 to 4 weeks along with maintenance of good average control have good neuropsychological outcomes. There are still minor deficits, in particular in those with poor dietary compliance, and maternal PKU remains a persistent problem.

**Galactosemia** Galactose-1-phosphate uridyl transferase (GALT) deficiency, galactokinase deficiency, and galactose epimerase deficiency can all be detected by newborn screening. Methods used in screening include measuring metabolites, galactose, and galactose-1-phosphate, or measuring enzyme activity directly. Enzyme screening for GALT deficiency is the most common approach, but the use of galactose has the advantage of identifying other defects of the Leloir pathway. Moderate metabolite elevations and severely reduced but not absent GALT activity are seen in compound heterozygosity for a severe mutation in the transferase GALT gene and a common "Duarte" mutation. The differentiation is important, as a Duarte/galactosemia compound heterozygotes need no treatment. Despite early identification and treatment, the long-term outcome for severe GALT deficiency ("classic galactosemia") is not good, with at least half of affected children having early intellectual problems and long-term educational and health complications. There is no evidence that presymptomatic treatment alters outcome, although death may be avoided in neonates who are prone to sepsis. The poor outcomes seen in treated patients reflects the biological complexity of galactose and glycoprotein metabolism, and as a result, not all developed countries screen for the galactosemias.

**Aminoacidopathies**

***DISORDERS OF THE UREA CYCLE*** Citrullinemia and argininosuccinic aciduria, either severe or delayed onset, can be diagnosed with high sensitivity by measuring citrulline, although the test will also detect mild, asymptomatic citrullinemia. *N*-Acetylglutamate synthetase, carbamyl phosphate synthetase, and ornithine transcarbamylase deficiencies cannot be so easily detected due to the fundamental problem of using low concentrations of metabolites to identify disorders. Low citrulline is an indicator of a proximal urea cycle disorder, but a low cut-off for citrulline overlaps with the lower end of normal ranges, especially when citrulline may be low in sick neonates in general. In addition, patients may be well into the disease course before screening results are available.

***OTHER AMINOACIDOPATHIES*** Problems in the identification of the tyrosinemias reflect the limitations of particular analytes. In tyrosinemia type 1 (fumarylacetoacetate hydrolase deficiency), the blood tyrosine level in newborns is often initially not high, and there is considerable overlap with transient tyrosinemia seen in a significant fraction of newborn. Hence this disorder is usually not detectable by tandem MS without an unacceptable false-positive rate when using tyrosine as the primary analyte. However, combining tyrosine with the disease-specific analyte succinylacetone markedly improves the positive predictive value. Tyrosinemia type 2 is readily detectable but lacks the attendant second metabolite and thus may be missed. Classical MSUD can readily be detected, but milder variant forms may be missed. A result indicating classic MSUD needs to be handled as an emergency since outcomes depend heavily on the early institution of appropriate therapy. Cystathionine β-synthase deficiency (homocystinuria) is currently detected by an elevated methionine level, but there may be a delay in the rise in methionine. Direct detection of homocysteine is a better analyte for identifying both homocystinuria and cobalamin disorders but is not currently achievable due to the fact that the majority of homocysteine is protein bound.

**Organic Acid Disorders** Organic acids that form acylcarnitines can be detected by tandem MS, and a number of organic acid disorders have been so detected. The classic organic acid disorders, methylmalonic (MMA), propionic (PA), and isovaleric acidemias, can readily be detected, although the baby may be symptomatic before newborn screening results are available. An elevation of propionyl carnitine (C3) may indicate PA, MMA, vitamin $B_{12}$ deficiency secondary to maternal deficiency, or a defect in the formation of adenosylcobalamin such as cobalamin C, D, or F defects. Newborn screening has uncovered an unexpected frequency of cases of 3-methylcrotonyl-CoA carboxylase (3MCC) deficiency, previously thought to be rare. This disorder is 1 of several that appear to be benign in most instances. Biotinidase deficiency can be detected by a specific enzyme assay on dried blood spots that is more sensitive than tandem MS testing, whereas holocarboxylase synthetase deficiency, previously thought to be a more severe early-onset disorder, can be detected based on elevated C3 and C5-OH, and this has led to the recognition of milder and intermittent forms of the disorder. Disorders that do not accumulate acylcarnitines such as the hydroxyglutaric acidurias cannot currently be detected by tandem MS testing.

**Fatty Acid Oxidation (FAO) Disorders** Disorders of carnitine uptake, the carnitine cycle, and mitochondrial β-oxidation can be detected by tandem MS testing of acylcarnitine. For several disorders, newborn screening programs have detected more cases than have historically presented clinically. While some of these subjects might never have experienced episodes of decompensation, it is currently not possible to distinguish who is most at risk; by definition, all have a functional defect in oxidation rates. This is especially true of medium-chain acyl-CoA dehydrogenase (MCAD) deficiency, the most frequently occurring FAO disorder, in which the detection rate improved considerably with the inclusion into newborn screening programs, and importantly, the death rate and long-term complications dropped precipitously.

Other disorders often tested for in various combinations in newborn screening programs, but of more importance for general pediatricians or those with other specialties, are congenital hypothyroidism, cystic fibrosis, congenital adrenal hyperplasia (CAH), glucose-6-phosphate dehydrogenase deficiency, hemoglobinopathies, and immunodeficiencies. Newborn screening for critical heart lesions using pulse oximetry and screening for congenital hearing loss are also being broadly adopted.

## SUGGESTED READINGS


Collardeau-Frachon S, Cordier MP, Rossi M, et al Antenatal manifestations of inborn errors of metabolism: autopsy findings suggestive of a metabolic disorder. *J Inherit Metab Dis*. 2016;39:597-610.

Garcia-Cazorla A, Mochel F, Lamari F, Saudubray JM. The clinical spectrum of inherited diseases involved in the synthesis and remodeling of complex lipids. A tentative overview. *J Inherit Metab Dis*. 2015;38:19-40.

Jansen ME, Lister KJ, van Kranen HJ, Cornel MC. Policy making in newborn screening needs a structured and transparent approach. *Front Public Health*. 2017;5:53.

Lamari F, Mochel F, Saudubray JM. An overview of inborn errors of complex lipid biosynthesis and remodelling. *J Inherit Metab Dis*. 2015;38:3-18.

Millington DS, Kodo N, Norwood DL, Roe CR. Tandem mass spectrometry: a new method for acylcarnitine profiling with potential for neonatal screening for inborn errors of metabolism. *J Inherited Metab Dis*. 1990;13(3):321-324.

Morava E, Rahman S, Peters V, et al. Quo vadis: the re-definition of "inborn metabolic diseases." *J Inherit Metab Dis*. 2015;38:1003-1006.

Peake RW, Bodamer OA. Newborn screening for lysosomal storage disorders. *J Pediatr Genet*. 2017;6(1):51-60.

Saudubray JM, Garcia Cazorla A. Clinical approach to inborn errors of metabolism in paediatrics. In: Saudubray JM, Baumgartner M, Walter J (eds). *Inborn Metabolic Diseases*. 6th ed. Berlin, Germany: Springer Verlag; 2016:3-69.

van Rijt WJ, Koolhaas GD, Bekhof J, et al. Inborn errors of metabolism that cause sudden infant death: a systematic review with implications for population neonatal screening programmes. *Neonatology*. 2016;109:297-302.

Vaz FM, Pras-Raves M, Bootsma AH, van Kampen AH. Principles and practice of lipidomics. *J Inherit Metab Dis*. 2015;38:41-52.

Villoria JG, Pajares S, López RM, Marin JL, Ribes A. Neonatal screening for inherited metabolic diseases in 2016. *Semin Pediatr Neurol*. 2016;23(4):257-272.

Walterfang M, Bonnot O, Mocellin R, Velakoulis D. The neuropsychiatry of inborn errors of metabolism. *J Inherit Metab Dis*. 2013;36:687-702.

# 130 Hyperphenylalaninemias and Phenylketonuria

Bernd Christian Schwahn

## INTRODUCTION

Hyperphenylalaninemia causes chronic toxic encephalopathy, depending on the timing, extent, and length of exposure to increased phenylalanine concentrations. Severe hyperphenylalaninemia leading to phenylketonuria (PKU) has a distinct role in the field of inherited metabolic disorders: PKU is the first genetic disease that could be treated exclusively by dietary manipulation and that could be entirely prevented by universal newborn screening and presymptomatic dietary intervention. This has had a huge impact on pediatric medicine, on the evolution of neonatal screening, and on the concept of gene-environment interaction. Genetic defects associated with hyperphenylalaninemia can be regarded as a strong risk factor for neurodisability, but the clinical outcome is more determined by the quality of metabolic treatment than by genetic variability.

## PATHOGENESIS AND EPIDEMIOLOGY

### Metabolic Derangement

Hyperphenylalaninemia is caused by impaired hydroxylation of phenylalanine to tyrosine (Fig. 130-1). The enzyme phenylalanine 4-hydroxylase (PAH) is predominantly expressed in the liver and

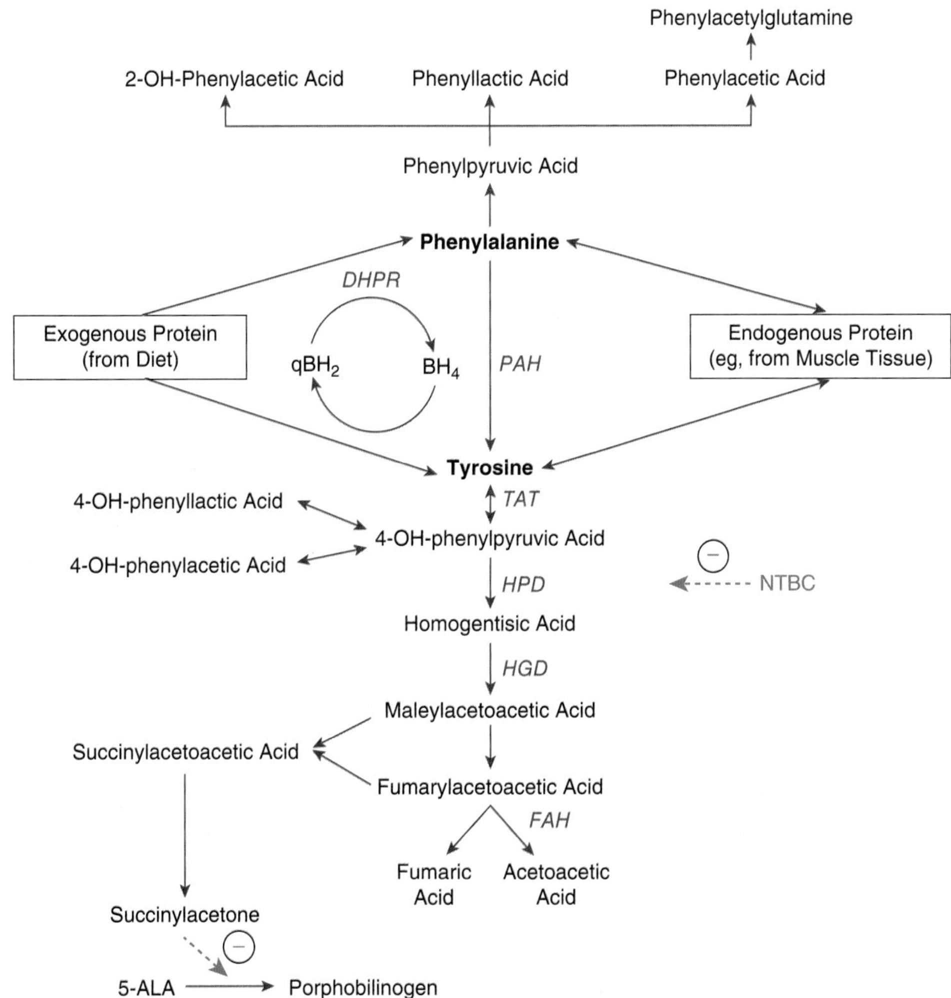


**FIGURE 130-1** Pathway of phenylalanine and tyrosine degradation. Phenylalanine from dietary protein or endogenous proteolysis is hydroxylated by phenylalanine hydroxylase (PAH) using tetrahydrobiopterin ($BH_4$) as a cofactor. $BH_4$ is thereby oxidized in 2 steps to dihydrobiopterin ($qBH_2$). $BH_2$ needs to be reduced back to $BH_4$ by dihydropterin reductase (DHPR). In severe PAH deficiency, phenylalanine accumulates and is deaminated to phenylpyruvic acid, which can be further metabolized. Phenylalanine and its alternative metabolites can then be found in urine.

Tyrosine stems from dietary protein or endogenous proteolysis or is synthesized from phenylalanine. The first and rate-limiting step is its deamination to 4-OH-phenylpyruvic acid by the enzyme tyrosine aminotransferase (TAT). This step is reversible. 4-OH-phenylpyruvic acid is then oxidized via 4-OH-phenylpyruvic dioxygenase (HPD) to homogentisic acid. Deficiency of TAT and deficiency or inhibition of HPD both lead to accumulation of tyrosine. Homogentisic acid is further oxidized by homogentisate dioxygenase (HGD) to maleylacetoacetic acid (MAA) and fumarylacetoacetic acid (FAA). Fumarylacetoacetate hydrolase (FAH) cleaves FAA to fumaric acid and acetoacetic acid. In FAH deficiency, MAA and FAA accumulate and are converted to succinylacetoacetate, which is decarboxylated to succinylacetone. Succinylacetone inhibits both HPD, causing hypertyrosinemia, and porphobilinogen synthase, causing symptoms of acute intermittent porphyria. 2(2-Nitro-4-trifluoromethylbenzoyl)-1,3-cyclohexane dione (NTBC) is a strong inhibitor of HPD and is used to avoid accumulation of MAA and FAA in FAH deficiency.

requires tetrahydrobiopterin ($BH_4$) as a cofactor. A lack of PAH activity leads to accumulation of phenylalanine, with levels usually exceeding 20 mg/dL (1200 μmol/L); increased excretion of its metabolites phenylacetate and phenylpyruvate; and decreased availability of the product tyrosine, which is needed for synthesis of protein, neurotransmitters, and melatonin. The phenylalanine pool is a function of dietary intake and losses through excretion, residual metabolic activity, and net protein synthesis.

The damage to the brain is believed to result from direct toxicity of phenylalanine and depletion of tyrosine, tryptophan, and other large neutral amino acids that compete with phenylalanine for uptake into the brain compartment.

Individuals with moderate hyperphenylalaninemia between 10 and 20 mg/dL when untreated (mild PKU) have residual activities of 1% to 5%, and an activity of > 5% may require no or only minor dietary modification.

#### Genetics

Phenylalanine hydroxylase deficiency (Mendelian Inheritance in Man [MIM] no. 261600) is one of the most common inherited metabolic disorders, affecting approximately 1 in 15,000 people in the United States. It has a higher incidence in whites and Native Americans and a lower incidence in blacks, Hispanics, and Asians. In North America, about 75% of individuals with PAH deficiency identified by newborn screening have the severe form and require treatment. All forms are transmitted in an autosomal recessive manner. The gene for phenylalanine hydroxylase has been mapped to chromosome 12q24.1, and more than 950 mutations have been identified (PAH mutation database; http://www.biopku.org). Most individuals are compound heterozygotes, and certain PAH alleles are associated with PKU and others with non-PKU hyperphenylalaninemia. However, the relationship between the clinical phenotype and the genotype is not always constant. Mutation analysis and genotype determination may be helpful for genetic counseling.

## CLINICAL MANIFESTATIONS

There is a continuous clinical spectrum of severity that ranges from malformation and intellectual disability to asymptomatic mild hyperphenylalaninemia. Symptoms depend on the extent and ontogenetic timing of an organism's exposure to elevated phenylalanine concentrations.

#### Maternal PKU Syndrome

Intrauterine exposure of an unborn child to elevated phenylalanine concentrations due to maternal hyperphenylalaninemia can cause a disruption of embryo-fetal development. This syndrome, called maternal phenylketonuria (mPKU), has been consistently observed with maternal hyperphenylalaninemia above 20 mg/dL (1200 μmol/L) and includes intrauterine dystrophy; facial dysmorphism resembling fetal alcohol syndrome; microcephaly and intellectual disability; and malformations, especially of the heart and great vessels. The risk for mPKU increases when maternal plasma phenylalanine concentrations rise above 6 mg/dL (360 μmol/L). The relatively low threshold for embryo-fetal toxicity can be explained by an increased vulnerability of the unborn child and by the adverse effects of high maternal phenylalanine concentrations on transplacental transport of other amino acids.

#### Early Treated Child after Diagnosis by Newborn Screening

Affected children born to heterozygous mothers experience a steep postnatal rise in phenylalanine, but they have no symptoms at birth: fetal phenylalanine accumulation is effectively prevented by high demands and possibly transplacental clearance. Clinical manifestations of hyperphenylalaninemia can be completely prevented by initiation of treatment within the first 2 weeks of life. Upon testing, however, affected children may display subtle neurocognitive deficits in comparison to unaffected siblings despite optimal treatment.

Inadequacy or discontinuation of early dietary treatment before the age of 8 years is associated with poorer performance on IQ measures and can lead to attention deficit and mood disorders. Exposure to high phenylalanine concentrations beyond puberty causes decreased performance on measures of attention and speed of processing and can be associated with behavioral disorders but only rarely with irreversible neuropsychiatric disease. Many affected adults experience a lack of energy and concentration, mood swings, and fatigue when off treatment.

#### Clinical Manifestation and Late Diagnosis

Affected children may become lethargic or appear irritable and have feeding difficulties during the first weeks of life, but this does not usually prompt investigation and diagnosis. In early infancy, they can develop a peculiar mousy smell due to the excretion of phenylacetic acid, and approximately one-third will develop an eczematoid rash or infantile spasms. A clinical diagnosis of PKU is usually only made in the second half of the first year of life, after seizures or delayed psychomotor development lead to further biochemical investigation. At this time, affected infants appear less pigmented compared to their unaffected siblings and exhibit microcephaly due to decreased brain growth, which is reflected by cortical atrophy on brain imaging. The majority have behavioral disturbances such as restlessness, anxiety, aggression, repetitive behavior, and sleep disturbance. Approximately 90% of individuals with untreated PKU will have severe intellectual disability with intelligence quotients of under 30 on psychometric assessment. Untreated, PKU does not seem to shorten the life span, apart from complications associated with severe neurodisability.

Up to 10% of untreated individuals with severe hyperphenylalaninemia escape the PKU phenotype. It has been hypothesized that their brain may have been protected from high phenylalanine concentrations by alterations in amino acid transport across the blood-brain barrier.

## DIAGNOSIS

#### Newborn Screening

Hyperphenylalaninemia can be diagnosed at any age by measuring plasma amino acid concentrations but is usually identified through routine newborn screening programs between the second and seventh day of life. It is not necessary to delay testing until milk feeding has started. The screening threshold varies depending on timing of testing, but endogenous protein catabolism after birth will lead to increased phenylalanine concentrations > 2 to 2.5 mg/dL (120–150 μmol/L) and a ratio of phenylalanine over tyrosine > 3 in affected children. Dried blood spot (DBS) phenylalanine concentrations in affected babies are usually in a range of 400 to 900 μmol/L. Due to a rapid postnatal rise, they often reach 1200 to 2000 μmol/L in confirmatory plasma samples, and tyrosine levels are within the normal range. Diagnostic evaluation of hyperphenylalaninemia is shown in Figure 130-2.

#### Differential Diagnosis and Confirmatory Testing

In healthy term newborns, screening for PKU using phenylalanine concentrations in DBS is fairly specific, whereas it will often be falsely positive in premature or sick babies. Abnormal screening results need to be confirmed by quantitative analysis of plasma amino acids to exclude a secondary increase of phenylalanine due to liver dysfunction (eg, caused by immaturity, sepsis, hypoxic multiorgan failure, or galactosemia), where tyrosine and methionine are elevated as well.

One to 2% of newborns identified by screening have hyperphenylalaninemia secondary to a deficiency of the PAH cofactor $BH_4$ due to a genetic defect in $BH_4$ synthesis (PTPS, PCD, or GCPDH deficiency) or recycling (dihydropterin reductase [DHPR] deficiency). These children are not clinically distinguishable from those with primary hyperphenylalaninemia but they require a completely different treatment. Therefore, every newborn with persistent isolated

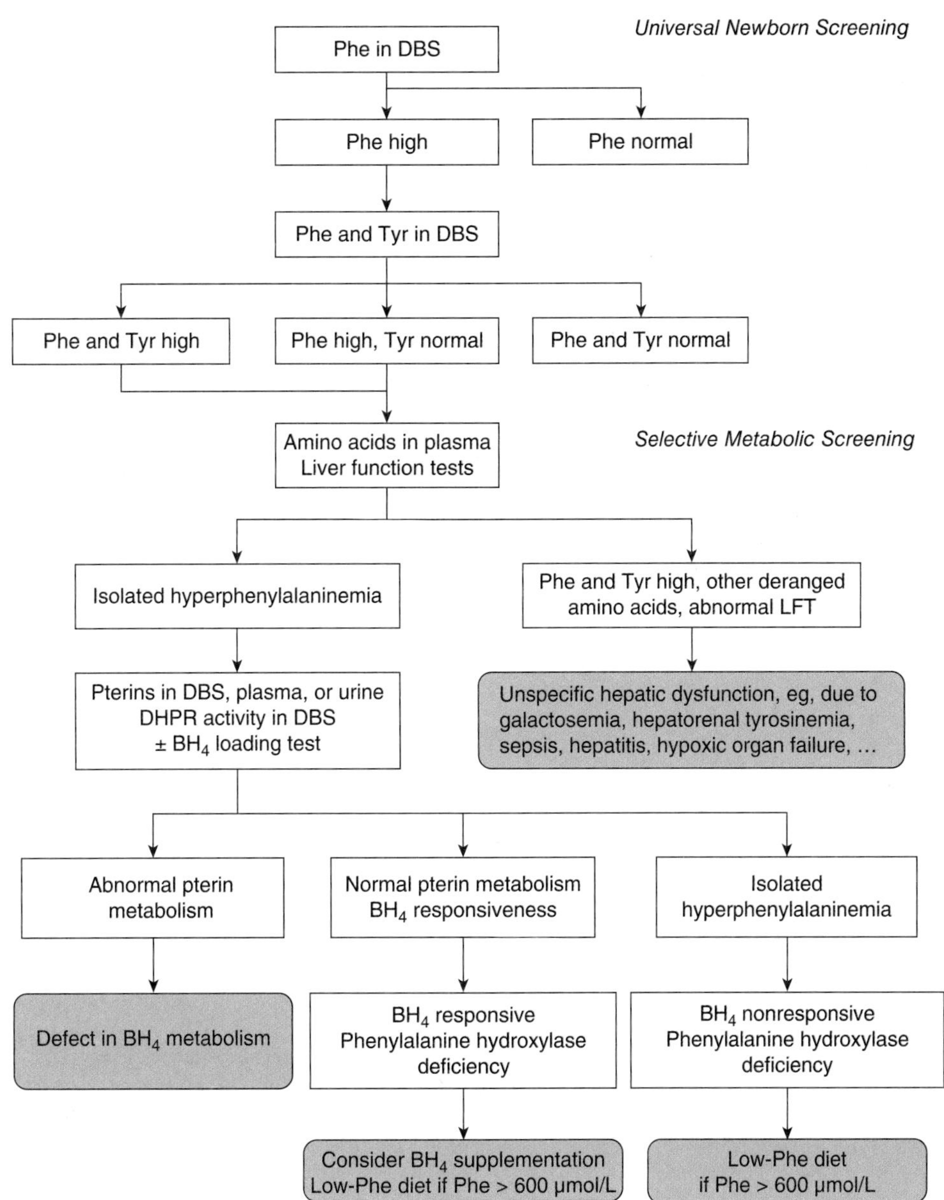


**FIGURE 130-2** Diagnostic algorithm for evaluation of hyperphenylalaninemia in newborns. $BH_4$, tetrahydrobiopterin; DBS, dried blood spot; DHPR, dihydropterin reductase; LFT, liver function tests; Phe, phenylalanine; $qBH_2$, dihydrobiopterin; Tyr, tyrosine.

hyperphenylalaninemia must be tested for total biopterin concentration in blood or urine and for DHPR activity in a DBS. Several countries use a $BH_4$ loading test with a single dose of 20 mg $BH_4$ per kg body weight and monitor phenylalanine concentrations for 24 hours to determine whether a cofactor deficiency is present. Km variants of PAH may also respond to $BH_4$ supplementation.

## TREATMENT AND PREVENTION

### Dietary Restriction of Phenylalanine Intake

Dietary restriction of phenylalanine is achieved by reducing the intake of protein from natural sources to a few grams per day and adjusted according to results. Nutritional needs are met by commercially available mixtures of phenylalanine-free amino acids and micronutrients, special low-protein medical foods, and free foods such as fruit and most vegetables. Treatment is guided by phenylalanine concentrations in plasma or DBS as a marker for phenylalanine accumulation within the body. Target concentrations differ slightly between different countries, but it is generally accepted that during the most vulnerable period of life (the first 5 years), plasma phenylalanine should not fall below 1- to 2-fold the normal mean (1 mg/dL or 60 μmol/L; standard deviation 0.25 mg/dL or 15 μmol/L) and should not exceed 4- to 6-fold normal (4–6 mg/dL or 240–360 μmol/L). Most guidelines recommend target blood phenylalanine concentrations of 2 to 6 mg/dL for patients until 12 years of age and 2 to 10 mg/dL for those over 12 years. However, treatment targets depend on personal objectives and individual susceptibility to adverse effects toward high phenylalanine concentrations.

Other goals for successful treatment are to avoid malnutrition (especially protein malnutrition due to overrestrictive diet and insufficient substitution with amino acids) or deficiency of micronutrients such as calcium, phosphate, vitamin $B_{12}$, long-chain polyunsaturated fatty acids, and selenium, and also to promote normal psychosocial development despite the highly artificial and controlled diet.

To meet treatment targets, it is mandatory to closely monitor phenylalanine concentrations, growth, and psychomotor development. Nutritional parameters in blood and psychometric testing are required as clinically indicated. Expert dietetic input is important to appropriately advise parents, caregivers, and teachers about the treatment, and early psychosocial intervention should be offered to families who struggle to adhere to dietary recommendations.

Supplementation with $BH_4$ can improve PAH activity by acting as chemical chaperone to stabilize the defective enzyme and to protect it against premature proteasomal degradation. Doses of 5 to 20 mg/kg body weight per day have been used and can variably improve phenylalanine tolerance in up to 50% of treated individuals with missense mutations affecting the catalytic, regulatory, oligomerization, and $BH_4$-binding domains, and especially in those with moderate hyperphenylalaninemia.

The orally or subcutaneously administered plant enzyme phenylalanine ammonia lyase can assist in reducing the phenylalanine pool and therefore increase the dietary allowance of natural protein. Parenteral treatment is complicated by the high immunogenic potential of this nonhuman enzyme and frequent allergic reactions. Research continues on liver transplant and other gene delivery systems.

#### Late Diagnosed PKU

Dietary treatment should be considered even if the diagnosis of hyperphenylalaninemia is made after infancy and irreversible brain injury has already occurred. Even untreated adolescents and adults with PKU can benefit from lowering plasma phenylalanine to alleviate psychiatric symptoms and facilitate their care. Patients and caregivers may decide after a 6-month diet trial whether the burden of treatment is balanced by improvements in the clinical condition and treatment should be continued.

#### Pregnancy in Women with Hyperphenylalaninemia

Primary prevention of maternal PKU syndrome starts with early advice about contraception in teenage girls with hyperphenylalaninemia. Contraceptive measures are recommended for every sexually active woman whose plasma phenylalanine concentrations exceed 10 mg/dL (600 μmol/L). Phenylalanine target concentrations prior to conception and throughout pregnancy are 2 to 6 mg/dL (120–360 μmol/L). Phenylalanine requirements increase considerably from the third trimester of pregnancy onward. Twice-weekly phenylalanine measurements and at least monthly nutritional blood tests are required to allow frequent adjustments of the intake of phenylalanine, protein substitute, and additional tyrosine.

## SUGGESTED READINGS


Camp KM, Parisi MA, Acosta PB, et al. Phenylketonuria Scientific Review Conference: state of the science and future research needs. *Mol Genet Metab.* 2014;112:87-122.

Følling I. The discovery of phenylketonuria. *Acta Paediatr Suppl.* 1994;407:4-10.

Lindegren M, Krishnaswami S, Fonnesbeck C, et al. Adjuvant treatment for phenylketonuria (PKU). Comparative effectiveness review No. 56. Rockville, MD: Agency for Healthcare Research and Quality; Feb 2012; AHRQ Publication No 12-EHC035-EF.

Ney DM, Blank RD, Hansen KE. Advances in the nutritional and pharmacological management of phenylketonuria. *Curr Opin Clin Nutr Metab Care.* 2014;17:61-68.

Singh RH, Cunningham AC, Mofidi S, et al. Updated, web-based nutrition management guideline for PKU: an evidence and consensus based approach. *Mol Genet Metab.* 2016;118:72-83.

Van Spronsen FJ, van Wegberg AMJ, Ahring K, et al. Key European guidelines for the diagnosis and management of patients with phenylketonuria. *Lancet Diabetes Endocrinol.* 2017;5:743-756.

Vockley J, Andersson HC, Antshel KM, et al. Phenylalanine hydroxylase deficiency: diagnosis and management guideline. *Genet Med.* 2014;16:188-200.

Waisbren SE, Noel K, Fahrbach K, et al. Phenylalanine blood levels and clinical outcomes in phenylketonuria: a systematic literature review and meta-analysis. *Mol Genet Metab.* 2007;92:63-70.




# 131 Disorders of Tyrosine Metabolism

Markus Grompe

## INTRODUCTION

The tyrosine degradation pathway consists of 5 enzymes, and inherited disorders have been described for 4 of these. Importantly, not all defects are characterized by hypertyrosinemia, and disease pathologies are not all caused by elevated tyrosine levels. Furthermore, hypertyrosinemia is not specific for disorders of the tyrosine degradation pathway. It can also be found in other conditions such as transient tyrosinemia of the preterm newborn, scurvy, and many diseases that cause hepatocellular injury.

## HEPATORENAL TYROSINEMIA (HEREDITARY TYROSINEMIA TYPE 1)

### CLINICAL PRESENTATION

Hereditary tyrosinemia type 1 (HT1) is the most severe disorder of the pathway and causes early hepatic failure as well as renal injury. Symptoms are not present at birth, and early therapy can completely prevent severe disease manifestations. In untreated patients, liver failure may begin early in infancy and result in vomiting, jaundice, hypoglycemia, ascites, and bleeding. In later onset cases, the manifestations include failure to thrive, hepatosplenomegaly, a tendency to bleed, and hypophosphatemic rickets due to renal tubular dysfunction of the Fanconi type. Intellectual disability is not a primary feature. Acute attacks of peripheral neuropathy, resembling acute porphyria, with severe abdominal pain, vomiting, and paralysis, may occur. The risk of cirrhosis and hepatocellular carcinoma is significantly elevated in this disorder, and late-presenting individuals have a high risk of cancer.

#### Metabolic Derangement and Pathophysiology

Deficiency of the last enzyme in tyrosine catabolism, fumarylacetoacetate hydrolase (FAH), leads to the accumulation of fumarylacetoacetate, a metabolite that causes hepatic and renal cellular damage (Fig. 131-1). Fumarylacetoacetate can be reduced to succinylacetoacetate, which is decarboxylated to succinylacetone, the pathognomonic hallmark metabolite of this disorder. Secondary inhibition of 4-hydroxyphenylpyruvate dioxygenase (HPD) leads to elevated concentrations of tyrosine, and accumulating tyrosine metabolites such as 4-hydroxyphenylpyruvate, -lactate, and -acetate are excreted in urine, a phenomenon known as *tyrosyluria.* Succinylacetone is a potent inhibitor of porphobilinogen synthase and thus causes secondary acute intermittent porphyria (see Chapter 162). Complete absence of FAH leads to early infantile disease, but milder cases with much later onset can exist even within the same sibship.

### GENETICS

Tyrosinemia type 1 (MIM no. 276700) is inherited in an autosomal recessive manner. The *FAH* gene is located at chromosome 15q23-q25. More than 100 mutations have been reported, the most common of which is IVS12,G-A,+5, which is found in one-quarter of all alleles in the United States. Due to a founder effect, this mutation has a very high carrier frequency and disease incidence in the French Canadian population. A clear genotype-phenotype correlation has not been established. Antenatal testing can be accomplished by molecular methods. Somatic reversion and self-induced mutation correction occur in over 50% of cases. Rare hepatocytes revert the mutation, reacquire FAH activity, and then expand to large nodules of healthy and functional tissue. This phenomenon explains the milder clinical course of some patients, as well as the large phenotypic differences within sibships.

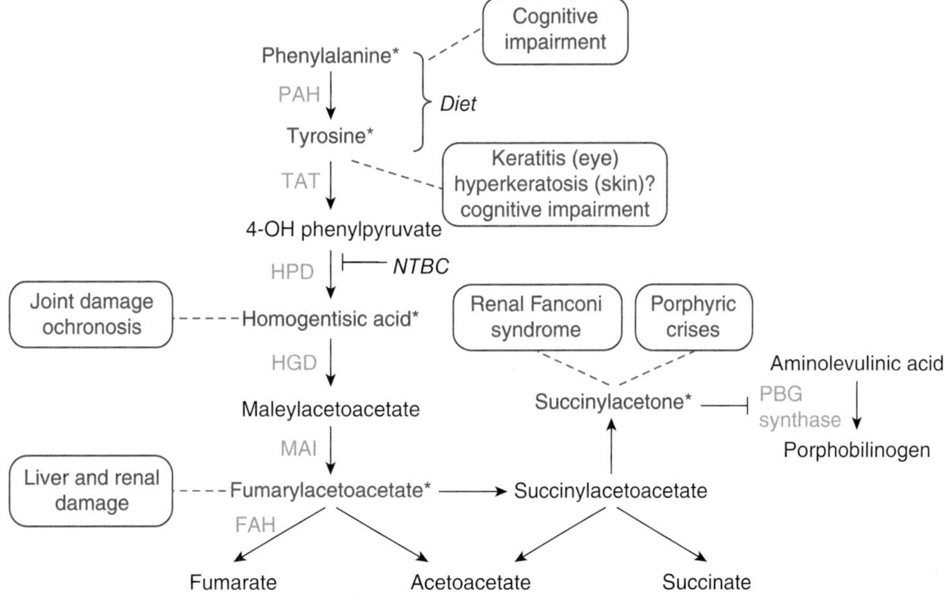


**FIGURE 131-1** Phenylalanine-tyrosine catabolic pathway.

## DIAGNOSTIC TESTS AND DIFFERENTIAL DIAGNOSES

Succinylacetone is now assayed by most newborn screening programs in North America, which leads to the early detection of most cases. Highly elevated concentrations of α-fetoprotein (AFP) are usually seen even in neonates. If the diagnosis is not made by newborn screening, patients will present with hepatic dysfunction. Importantly, transaminase elevations are relatively mild, and synthetic functions (bilirubin, coagulation factors) are disproportionately impaired. Tyrosine and often methionine are elevated. However, all biochemical abnormalities apart from elevated succinylacetone are not HT1 specific and can be found in other liver diseases. Children with suspected tyrosinemia should have their blood or urine evaluated for an elevation of succinylacetone, which is diagnostic. The diagnosis should then be confirmed by mutation analysis.

## TREATMENT, PROGNOSIS, AND LONG-TERM OUTCOME

Nitisinone [2(2-nitro-4-trifluoromethylbenzoyl)-1,3-cyclohexanedione; NTBC] is US Food and Drug Administration (FDA) approved for HT1 therapy. The drug effectively treats the liver failure and renal Fanconi syndrome of HT1 in almost all affected infants. Nitisinone inhibits the second step of tyrosine catabolism, 4-OH phenylpyruvic dioxygenase (HPD), and thus prevents the accumulation of toxic metabolites (see Fig. 131-1). The largest treated patient cohort was reported from Québec and unambiguously demonstrated the therapeutic efficacy of the drug. If started before 6 months of age, the prognosis is very good and hepatocellular carcinoma is extremely rare. The risk of long-term complications, including cancer, increases significantly if drug therapy is delayed. The inhibition of HPD with NTBC leads to iatrogenic tyrosinemia type 3 with elevated tyrosine levels. Hence, drug therapy needs to be combined with a diet low in phenylalanine and tyrosine to keep plasma tyrosine below 400 μmol/L to prevent keratitis, hyperkeratosis, and possible cognitive decline. Suggested guidelines for management have been proposed. Routine measurements of plasma succinylacetone and NTBC blood levels are recommended to assure effective dosing. Plasma tyrosine and phenylalanine should be monitored to ensure adequate dietary management. In addition, liver function tests and AFP levels must be monitored, and regular imaging tests are recommended to detect early signs of liver tumors. Liver transplantation is the only other therapeutic option if NTBC therapy fails or if hepatocellular carcinoma develops. The latter has been observed in only a few patients, mostly in those with preexistent significant liver damage from delayed therapy.

# OCULOCUTANEOUS TYROSINEMIA (TYROSINEMIA TYPE 2)

## CLINICAL PRESENTATION

The characteristic features of this disease are bilateral corneal ulcers or dendritic keratitis, presenting with photophobia, pain, and lacrimation, and erythematous papular or hyperkeratotic painful lesions on pressure areas of the palms and soles. The liver and kidney are not affected. About 60% of patients display intellectual disability, but it is unclear whether this is the result of elevated tyrosine or reflects an ascertainment bias. Symptoms usually start in the first year of life but may occur at any age and in any combination.

## METABOLIC DERANGEMENT, INCLUDING PATHOPHYSIOLOGY

Tyrosine aminotransferase (TAT), the first enzyme in tyrosine degradation, is deficient in oculocutaneous tyrosinemia. Tyrosine itself is not toxic to the liver or the kidney. Plasma concentrations of tyrosine are higher than in other forms of tyrosinemia, and the urine contains large amounts of tyrosine metabolites. The lesions on the palms and soles and in the eyes are believed to result from local crystallization of tyrosine, which is poorly soluble. A causal relation between high tyrosine levels and intellectual disability has not been established.

## GENETICS

Tyrosinemia type 2 (MIM no. 276600) is inherited in an autosomal recessive manner. The *TAT* gene is located at chromosome 16q22.1-q22.3. More than 15 mutations have been identified.

Newborn screening programs may detect the illness by using tyrosine as a screening parameter. In symptomatic cases, plasma amino acid analysis reveals tyrosine concentrations that usually exceed 1200 μmol/L. In less pronounced hypertyrosinemia, a diagnosis of tyrosinemia type 3 should be considered. Molecular testing is used to confirm the diagnosis.

### TREATMENT, PROGNOSIS, AND LONG-TERM OUTCOME

Oculocutaneous tyrosinemia responds to a diet low in phenylalanine and tyrosine. This diet is similar to the diet for severe hyperphenylalaninemia and needs to be supplemented with a commercially available phenylalanine- and tyrosine-free protein substitute, with micronutrients, and with special low-protein staple foods. Treatment aims to keep plasma tyrosine below 800 μmol/L to prevent oculocutaneous manifestations. Safe tyrosine concentrations to prevent brain damage have not been defined and may be lower. Maternal tyrosinemia may have an adverse effect on the developing fetus in women with tyrosinemia type 2, indicating the need for strict dietary control during pregnancy.

## TYROSINEMIA TYPE 3

### CLINICAL PRESENTATION

Several patients with this disorder have been identified, and most suffer from neurologic symptoms such as mild to severe intellectual disability and, less frequently, seizures. No other organ systems are involved. It is unclear whether elevated tyrosine levels cause neurologic dysfunction or whether an ascertainment bias (metabolic testing in patients with developmental delay) explains the reported association.

### METABOLIC DERANGEMENT, INCLUDING PATHOPHYSIOLOGY

Tyrosinemia type 3 is caused by a deficiency of 4-hydroxyphenylpyruvate dioxygenase (HPD), the same enzyme inhibited by nitisinone used in the treatment of HT1. Tyrosine levels are elevated but usually not to levels that cause corneal ulcers or hyperkeratosis.

### GENETICS

Deficiency of HPD (MIM no. 276710) is inherited in an autosomal recessive manner. The *HPD* gene is located at chromosome 12q24-qter, and a few mutations have been identified.

### DIAGNOSTIC TESTS, INCLUDING DIFFERENTIAL DIAGNOSES

Plasma tyrosine concentrations of 500 to 1200 μmol/L suggest tyrosinemia type 3. Tyrosyluria is usually observed, and the diagnosis can be confirmed by mutational analysis.

### TREATMENT, PROGNOSIS, AND LONG-TERM OUTCOME

Treatment is similar to that for oculocutaneous tyrosinemia is recommended, although the benefit of dietary treatment has not been demonstrated.

## HAWKINSINURIA

### CLINICAL PRESENTATION

The few patients who have been identified with this disorder suffer from failure to thrive and, sometimes, severe metabolic acidosis during infancy, which seems to be precipitated by weaning from breastfeeding. Further development seems to be normal, and asymptomatic individuals have been described.

### METABOLIC DERANGEMENT, INCLUDING PATHOPHYSIOLOGY

Normally, HPD (EC 1.13.11.27) converts 4-OH phenylpyruvate into homogentisic acid. In hawkinsinuria, however, the enzyme functions abnormally and catalyzes formation of 2 unusual metabolites of 4-hydroxyphenylpyruvate, hawkinsin and 4-hydroxycyclohexylacetate. This process is thought to lead to a depletion of glutathione, which is associated with 5-oxoprolinuria and metabolic acidosis.

### GENETICS

Hawkinsinuria (MIM no. 140350) is allelic to tyrosinemia type 3 and is transmitted as an autosomal dominant trait with variable penetrance. Mutations within the *HPD* gene cause a hyperactive, abnormally functioning enzyme.

### DIAGNOSTIC TESTS, INCLUDING DIFFERENTIAL DIAGNOSES

The identification of hawkinsin and 4-hydroxycyclohexylacetate in urine by gas chromatography–mass spectrometry allows a diagnosis. Moderate tyrosinemia, tyrosyluria, and 5-oxoprolinuria have been observed during infancy.

### TREATMENT, PROGNOSIS, AND LONG-TERM OUTCOME

Treatment consists of mild dietary phenylalanine and tyrosine restriction. *N*-Acetylcysteine therapy has been reported. Symptomatic infants have developed normally.

## ALKAPTONURIA

In 1902, Garrod was the first to suggest that this disorder results from an inherited absence of the liver enzyme that catalyzes the oxidation of homogentisic acid (see Fig. 133-1). This hypothesis gave rise to the 1-gene, 1-enzyme hypothesis and the field of biochemical genetics.

### CLINICAL PRESENTATION

Persons with alkaptonuria are usually asymptomatic in childhood, but oxidation of urinary homogentisic acid may lead to deposition of a dark pigment in an infant's diaper ("black nappy" disease). After the third decade, deposition of brownish or bluish pigment is seen, particularly in the ears and sclerae. This pigmentation may be extensive in fibrous tissues, including heart valves, and is referred to as *ochronosis*. Ochronotic arthritis, which occurs in adulthood, produces symptoms resembling rheumatoid arthritis or osteoarthritis, with limitation of motion; complete ankylosis is common.

### METABOLIC DERANGEMENT, INCLUDING PATHOPHYSIOLOGY

Alkaptonuria results from defective activity of the enzyme homogentisate 1,2-dioxygenase (HGD), the third enzyme in tyrosine degradation. The disorder is characterized by the excretion of dark-colored urine containing large amounts of homogentisic acid, which causes a positive test result for reducing substances. Fresh urine appears normal, but on standing and particularly after alkalinization, oxidation of homogentisic acid to benzoquinone proceeds, and a dark brown or black pigment appears; this is believed to act as a chemical irritant and can damage the cartilage. Blood tyrosine levels are not elevated.

### GENETICS

Alkaptonuria (MIM no. 203500) is an autosomal recessive disorder. A few hundred patients have been reported. The *HGD* gene is located on chromosome 13q21-q23, and several mutations have been described.

### DIAGNOSTIC TESTS, INCLUDING DIFFERENTIAL DIAGNOSES

Homogentisic acid can be measured in urine by gas chromatography–mass spectrometry once the condition is suspected. The diagnosis is usually first made in adult life during routine urinalysis or during investigation of arthritis.

### TREATMENT, PROGNOSIS, AND LONG-TERM OUTCOME

Treatment of alkaptonuria has not been successful so far. Strict dietary restriction of phenylalanine and tyrosine is usually not accepted by adults. Nitisinone therapy represents a hopeful new approach, but proper clinical trials have not yet been reported. Moderate doses can completely block the accumulation of homogentisic acid and likely would prevent disease progression. Therapy cannot reverse the symptoms related to ankylosing arthritis or aortic or mitral valvulitis (Table 131-1).

**TABLE 131-1 OTHER RARE DISORDERS OF TYROSINE METABOLISM**

| Disorder | Clinical Presentation | Metabolic Derangement | Genetics | Diagnostic Tests | Treatment |
|---|---|---|---|---|---|
| Tyrosinemia 2 (tyrosine aminotransferase deficiency) | Corneal ulcers, palmar and plantar keratosis, (mental retardation) | Plasma tyrosine > 1200 μmol/L | Autosomal recessive, *TAT* gene at 16q22.1-q22.3 | Plasma amino acid analysis, mutation analysis | Dietary restriction of phenylalanine and tyrosine |
| Tyrosinemia 3 (4-hydroxyphenylpyruvate dioxygenase deficiency) | Mental retardation | Plasma tyrosine > 500–1200 μmol/L | Autosomal recessive, *HPD* gene at 12q24-qter | Plasma amino acid analysis, mutation analysis | Dietary restriction of phenylalanine and tyrosine |
| Hawkinsinuria (4-hydroxyphenylpyruvate dioxygenase deficiency) | Infantile failure to thrive, metabolic acidosis | Moderate hypertyrosinemia and 5-oxoprolinuria | Autosomal dominant, *HPD* gene at 12q24-qter | Plasma amino acid analysis, organic acids in urine | Dietary restriction of phenylalanine and tyrosine; *N*-acetylcysteine |
| Alkaptonuria (homogentisate 1,2-dioxygenase deficiency) | Dark urine, adult-onset ochronosis and arthritis | Excretion of homogentisic acid in urine | Autosomal recessive, *HGD* gene at 13q21-13q23 | Analysis of urinary organic acids, mutation analysis | Nitisinone |

## SUGGESTED READINGS


De Jesus VR, Adam BW, Mandel D, Cuthbert CD, Matern D. Succinylacetone as primary marker to detect tyrosinemia type I in newborns and its measurement by newborn screening programs. *Mol Genet Metab.* 2014;113:67-75.

Demers SI, Russo P, Lettre F, Tanguay RM. Frequent mutation reversion inversely correlates with clinical severity in a genetic liver disease, hereditary tyrosinemia. *Hum Pathol.* 2003;34:1313-1320.

Gomez-Ospina N, Scott AI, Oh GJ, et al. Expanding the phenotype of hawkinsinuria: new insights from response to N-acetyl-L-cysteine. *J Inherit Metab Dis.* 2016;39:821-829.

Grompe M, St-Louis M, Demers SI, et al. A single mutation of the fumarylacetoacetate hydrolase gene in French Canadians with hereditary tyrosinemia type I. *N Engl J Med.* 1994:331;353-357.

Holme E, Lindstedt S. Tyrosinaemia type I and NTBC (2-(2-nitro-4-trifluoromethylbenzoyl)-1,3- cyclohexanedione). *J Inherit Metab Dis.* 1998;21:507-517.

Kvittingen EA, Rootwelt H, Berger R, Brandtzaeg P. Self-induced correction of the genetic defect in tyrosinemia type I. *J Clin Invest.* 1994;94:1657-1661.

Larochelle J, Alvarez F, Bussieres JF, et al. Effect of nitisinone (NTBC) treatment on the clinical course of hepatorenal tyrosinemia in Quebec. *Mol Genet Metab.* 2012;107:49-54.

Mitchell GA, Grompe M, Lambert M, Tanguay RM. Hypertyrosinemia. In Valle D, Beaudet AL, Vogelstein B, et al (eds): *The Online Metabolic and Molecular Bases of Inherited Disease.* New York, NY: McGraw-Hill; 2014.

Ranganath LR, Timmis OG, Gallagher JA. Progress in alkaptonuria: are we near to an effective therapy? *J Inherit Metab Dis.* 2015;38:787-789.

Schiff M, Broue P, Chabrol B, et al. Heterogeneity of follow-up procedures in French and Belgian patients with treated hereditary tyrosinemia type 1: results of a questionnaire and proposed guidelines. *J Inherit Metab Dis.* 2012;35:823-829.


# 132 Disorders of Branched Chain Amino and Organic Acid Metabolism

Jerry Vockley

## CATABOLISM OF BRANCHED CHAIN AMINO ACIDS

The 3 essential branched chain amino acids (BCAAs), leucine, isoleucine, and valine, encompass about 25% of human protein. They are metabolized in mitochondria. The first 2 catabolic steps are common to the 3 BCAAs (Fig. 132-1). The first reaction, which occurs primarily in muscle, involves reversible transamination to 2-oxo (or keto) acids and is followed by oxidative decarboxylation to coenzyme A (CoA) derivatives by branched chain oxo (or keto) acid dehydrogenase (BCKD). BCKD is similar in structure to pyruvate dehydrogenase (and shares a common subunit), is also highly regulated by a kinase/phosphatase system, and plays a key role in nitrogen metabolism.

Subsequently, the degradative pathway of BCAAs diverges. Leucine is catabolized to acetoacetate (making it a ketogenic amino acid) and acetyl-CoA, which enters the Krebs cycle. The final step in the catabolism of isoleucine involves cleavage into acetyl-CoA and propionyl-CoA, the latter of which enters the Krebs cycle via conversion to succinyl-CoA. Valine is also ultimately catabolized to propionyl-CoA.

The most frequent inborn errors affecting the BCAA catabolic pathway are maple syrup urine disease (MSUD) and the isovaleric, propionic, and methylmalonic acidemias (or acidurias). These 4 disorders can present with neonatal metabolic collapse, as a late-onset acute intermittent form, or as a chronic progressive form. Many other rarer defects have also been described in this catabolic pathway. All of these disorders can be diagnosed by identifying acylcarnitines and organic compounds in plasma and urines by gas chromatography (CG)–mass spectrometry (MS) or tandem MS, and all can be detected by newborn screening using tandem MS.

## MAPLE SYRUP URINE DISEASE

In MSUD (branched chain ketoaciduria), major cerebral symptoms appear early in the newborn period, and the urine has an odor reminiscent of maple syrup. The BCAAs are present in high concentration in the blood and urine, and the ketoacid analogues are found in the urine. Alloisoleucine, an alternative metabolite of isoleucine, accumulates in blood in this disorder and is generally diagnostic, although it may also be detected in isovaleric acidemia.

### CLINICAL FINDINGS

Infants with MSUD appear well at birth. In the typical patient, symptoms begin after 3 to 5 days of age, and patients progress rapidly to death within 2 to 4 weeks if untreated. Early manifestations include feeding difficulties, irregular respirations, progressive loss of the Moro reflex, and lethargy. Severe hypoglycemia may occur due to leucine being an insulin secretagogue. Characteristically, these patients develop convulsions, opisthotonos, and generalized muscular rigidity, and boxing and pedaling movements with or without intermittent flaccidity. Death usually occurs after decerebrate rigidity develops. Cortical atrophy may be seen on computed tomography (CT) or magnetic resonance imaging (MRI) scan, and the myelin is usually hypodense. This is consistent with the defective myelinization that has been observed at autopsy. The feature that distinguishes any form of branched chain ketoaciduria from other cerebral degenerative diseases of infancy is the characteristic maple syrup, or caramel, odor of the urine, skin, cerumen, or hair. The odor may become evident 1 or 2 days after birth and may persist, but varies

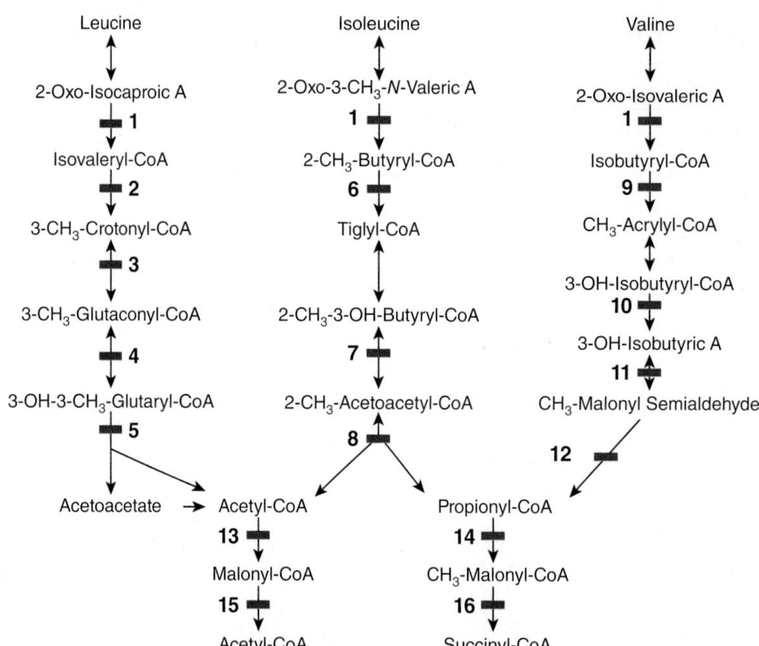


**1**. Branched-chain 2-keto acid dehydrogenase complex. **2**. Isovaleryl-coenzyme A (CoA) dehydrogenase. **3**. 3-Methylcrotonyl-CoA carboxylase. **4**. 3-Methylglutoconyl-CoA hydratase **5**. 3-Hydroxy-3-methylglutaryl-CoA lyase. **6**. Short/branched chain acyl-CoA dehydrogenase (2-methyl-butyryl-CoA dehydrogenase). **7**. 2-Methyl-3-hydroxybutyryl-CoA dehydrogenase **8**. 2-Methylacetoacetyl-CoA thiolase. **9**. Isobutyryl-CoA dehydrogenase **10**. 3-Hydroxyisobutyryl-CoA deacylase. **11**. 3-Hydroxyisobutyric acid dehydrogenase **12**. Methylmalonic semi-aldehyde dehydrogenase. **13**. Acetyl-CoA carboxylase (cytosolic) **14**. Propionyl-CoA carboxylase. **15**. Malonyl-CoA decarboxylase. **16**. Methylmalonyl-CoA mutase

**FIGURE 132-1** Metabolism of leucine, isoleucine, and valine. The enzymes involved in the stages of metabolism are numbered.

in intensity and may not be detected in some specimens. Identification by newborn screening has resulted in more patients surviving to childhood and even early adulthood. In these patients, there is an ongoing risk for episodes of metabolic decompensation during times of physiologic stress and illness. Central nervous system hyperleucinosis, the result of uncontrolled leucine release largely from skeletal muscle during periods of catabolism, leads to cerebral edema and can lead to catastrophic brain damage or death. In older children and adults, care must be taken to avoid excess intravenous fluids that can precipitate uncal herniation.

Milder forms of the disease occur that are known as intermittent branched chain aminoaciduria; they represent variant mutations in the same enzyme complex as in classic MSUD. Ataxia and repeated episodes of lethargy with ketoacidosis progressing to coma occur without mental retardation; these episodes may be precipitated by infection or anesthesia. Recently, a novel disorder reflecting overactivity of BCKD due to loss of BCKD kinase activity that normally inhibits BCKD was described. This overactivity leads to reduced levels of plasma BCAAs, autism, epilepsy, and intellectual disability.

## BIOCHEMICAL FINDINGS AND GENETICS

Increased quantities of isoleucine, leucine, and valine (and perturbation of the normal 1:2:3 ratio) and their ketoacid derivatives are found in the plasma and urine. The presence of an abnormal amino acid, alloisoleucine, is typically diagnostic for MSUD. The catabolism of BCAAs is initiated by a transamination reaction to generate the respective ketoacids, which then undergo decarboxylation to CoA derivatives. The defect in MSUD is in the oxidative decarboxylation of the ketoacids, catalyzed by a mitochondrial multienzyme complex similar to pyruvate dehydrogenase and to α-ketoglutarate dehydrogenase. For this reason, autosomal recessive mutations in 4 different genes can cause MSUD. Patients have been identified with defects in the E1α, E1β, E2, and E3 subunits of the complex. The E3 subunit is shared by all 3 complexes, and patients with defects in this gene have simultaneous deficiency of branched chain ketoacid dehydrogenase, pyruvate dehydrogenase, and α-ketoglutarate dehydrogenase. MSUD is rare in most populations, with an incidence of approximately 1 in 150,000; however, it is common in the Mennonite population in the United States due to a founder effect.

## THERAPY

Experience has now been accumulated with prolonged use of special diets in which the intake of leucine, isoleucine, and valine are closely controlled. Concentrations of the BCAAs in plasma can be maintained within normal limits, but this therapy is difficult. Many patients have had permanent brain injury before treatment is started. Commercial products are available that are useful in management. Intravenous solutions of amino acids that exclude the BCAAs take advantage of protein synthesis to reduce concentrations of leucine and the other amino acids and reverse coma in acute episodes of metabolic imbalance. Rare patients have a thiamine-responsive form of MSUD, and therefore, this vitamin should be tried in all patients. Experience with siblings of previous patients, in whom very early diagnosis is possible, and with patients detected by neonatal screening programs, indicates that a normal IQ may be achieved, although many still have suboptimal intellectual and neurologic outcomes. As a result, liver replacement has gained in popularity as a treatment in countries where it is available. Liver transplantation is essentially curative, and patients no longer require a protein-restricted diet and are no longer at risk of metabolic decompensation during catabolic events. Livers explanted from MSUD patients can even be transplanted into patients with other indications for transplant (a so-called domino transplant) since BCKD activity is abundant in the recipient's skeletal muscle. Use of sodium phenylbutyrate, known to inhibit the inhibitory BCKD kinase, has been proposed as a means for enhancing any residual BCKD activity.

# ISOVALERIC ACIDEMIA

Isovaleric acidemia was the first condition recognized as an organic acidemia when the odor of "sweaty feet" in an infant with episodic encephalopathy was shown to be caused by isovaleric acid that accumulated due to a defect in isovaleryl-CoA dehydrogenase, the mitochondrial enzyme in the leucine catabolic pathway that converts isovaleryl-CoA to 3-methylcrotonyl-CoA.

### CLINICAL FINDINGS

Isovaleric acidemia may present in the newborn period with encephalopathy, metabolic acidosis, and the characteristic odor of sweaty feet; however, it more often presents in infancy or childhood with episodes of encephalopathy, hepatomegaly, and odor, brought on by infections or increased protein intake. Severe hyperammonemia is rare. If untreated, the condition is often fatal, and intellectual disability is common. Patients identified through newborn screening are typically of normal intelligence if supported appropriately though intermittent episodes of metabolic decompensation.

### DIAGNOSIS

Characteristic metabolites on organic acid analysis include isovalerylglycine and 3-hydroxyisovaleric acid; isovaleric acid itself is not detected by most analytic methods. All accumulated isovaleryl-CoA is normally excreted as nontoxic isovalerylglycine, but during infection or after a protein load, the increased concentration of isovaleryl-CoA exceeds the capacity of the liver to esterify it, and it appears as isovaleric and 3-hydroxyisovaleric acids. Acylcarnitine analysis will identify the accumulation of isovalerylcarnitine (a C5 acylcarnitine). The enzyme defect can be demonstrated in many tissues, including leukocytes and cultured fibroblasts. The disorder is effectively diagnosed by newborn screening, although nearly half of such infants have a variant allele that leads to increased metabolite production but little or no risk of clinical disease.

### GENETICS

The disorder is inherited as an autosomal recessive trait. The gene encoding isovaleryl-CoA dehydrogenase is on chromosome 15 (15q15.1), and many disease-causing mutations have been identified. Prenatal diagnosis can be based on enzyme assay of cultured amniocytes or chorionic villus cells or, in families in which the mutations are known, molecular analysis. Isovalerylglycine is also increased in the amniotic fluid surrounding an affected fetus but is difficult to detect by standard methods. A common variant accounts for approximately half of the mutant alleles identified in patients identified by newborn screening.

### TREATMENT

Acute episodes of acidosis may require treatment with intravenous glucose and bicarbonate. Long-term treatment involves restricting leucine intake to amounts necessary for normal growth and development and providing exogenous carnitine to increase excretion of isovaleryl-CoA as isovalerylcarnitine. Using glycine to increase excretion of the carbon skeleton as isovalerylglycine has become less common. Supplementation with an amino acid–restricted protein source is often necessary to support normal growth in childhood.

## PROPIONIC ACIDEMIA

Propionic acidemia was first described, albeit unknowingly, when ketotic hyperglycinemia was noted as a syndrome of intellectual disability and episodic ketoacidosis, neutropenia, thrombocytopenia, osteoporosis, and hyperglycinemia were induced by protein intake or infection. The discovery that propionic acidemia (as well as methylmalonic acidemia and mitochondrial β-ketothiolase deficiency) could cause the condition was made only when methods to examine and identify organic acids became available.

The disorder is due to a defect in propionyl-CoA carboxylase (PCC), a biotin-dependent enzyme that converts propionyl-CoA (an intermediate in the oxidation of isoleucine, threonine, valine, and methionine and odd chain fatty acids) to D-methylmalonyl-CoA (Fig. 132-2). Biotin deficiency due to biotinidase or holocarboxylase synthase deficiency (see Chapter 143) can lead to a secondary PCC deficiency. About one-third of the propionic acid is derived from the amino acids isoleucine, valine, methionine, and threonine; one-third is from the catabolism of cholesterol and odd chain fatty acids; and one-third is produced by bowel flora and absorbed into the bloodstream.

### CLINICAL FINDINGS

Like many other organic acidemias, propionic acidemia can present in the neonate with severe and life-threatening ketoacidosis, hyperammonemic encephalopathy, and bone marrow suppression. An equally common and more chronic course presents later in infancy with episodes of vomiting, ketoacidosis brought on by infections, failure to thrive, and osteoporosis severe enough to cause pathologic fractures. Acute striatal damage may occur, usually, but not always, during an episode of ketoacidosis, leading to a movement disorder. Developmental delay may be present and is probably caused more by newborn hyperammonemia or recurrent illness in infancy than by the disease itself. Recurrent pancreatitis can be seen in conjunction with vomiting and ketoacidosis. Cardiomyopathy is an increasingly recognized finding, especially in patients with a common mutation found in the Amish population in the United States. Patients identified by newborn screening may be asymptomatic at birth but are at risk for metabolic decompensation with physiologic stress or illness.

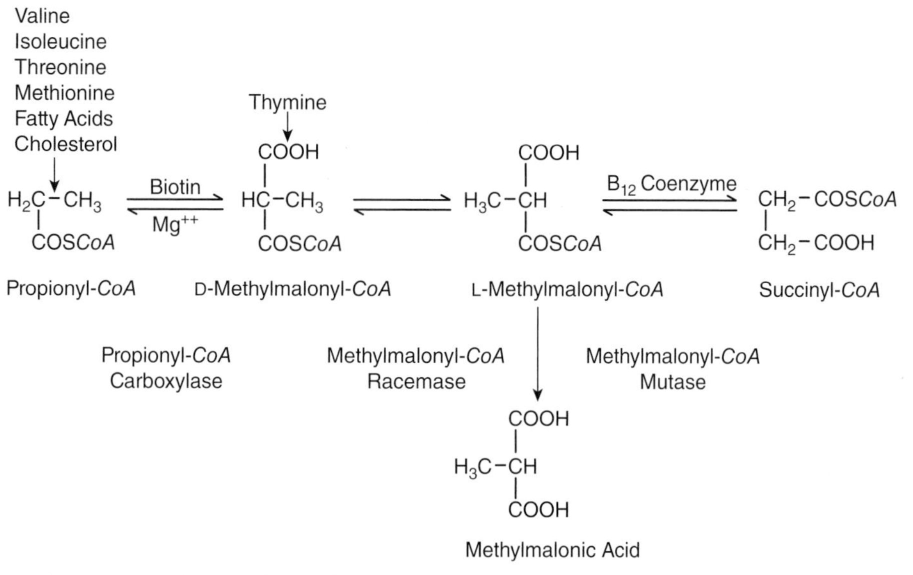

**FIGURE 132-2** Metabolism of propionic acid. Sites of the defect in propionic acidemia and methylmalonic acidemia are in propionyl-CoA carboxylase and methylmalonyl-CoA mutase or its cofactor adenosylcobalamin.

## DIAGNOSIS

Urine organic acid analysis typically shows large amounts of 3-hydroxypropionic and methylcitric acids, often with propionylglycine, tiglylglycine, and the abnormal ketone bodies made when propionyl-CoA is incorporated instead of acetyl-CoA. Acylcarnitine analysis shows increased propionylcarnitine (C3 carnitine), and glycine levels in blood and urine are often elevated. The defect in PCC can be demonstrated in many tissues, including leukocytes and cultured fibroblasts. Confirmation of the diagnosis is now more commonly obtained through DNA sequencing of the *PCCA* and *PCCB* genes. Propionic acidemia is effectively identified by newborn screening using tandem MS.

## GENETICS

The disorder is inherited as an autosomal recessive trait. PCC is a dodecamer of 6 α and 6 β subunits, which are encoded on chromosomes 13 and 3, respectively. Prenatal diagnosis of an affected fetus can be made by demonstrating enzyme deficiency in cultured amniocytes or chorionic villus cells, by demonstrating elevated methylcitric acid in amniotic fluid, or by DNA analysis.

## TREATMENT

Dietary restriction of protein or propiogenic amino acids to amounts necessary to support normal growth and development is indicated, typically with protein intake of less than 1 g/kg per day in older children. Supplementation with an amino acid–restricted protein source is often necessary to support normal growth in childhood. Treatment with carnitine is useful in secondary carnitine deficiency and may increase excretion of propionyl-CoA as propionylcarnitine. Attacks of ketoacidosis that complicate infections should be treated with fluid and electrolytes. Intermittent administration of an oral, nonabsorbable antibiotic, such as neomycin or metronidazole, can reduce propionic acid production by bowel flora. Biotin is usually tried but is rarely effective. Therapy often reduces the frequency and severity of attacks of ketoacidosis, and some patients treated in this manner do well and have normal intelligence; many, however, die in early childhood. In those children with hyperammonemia, treatment with carglumic acid ("carbaglu") can relieve the inhibition of the urea cycle and reduce ammonia levels. Liver transplantation increasingly is being used to treat propionic acidemia. It appears to reduce the frequency and severity of episodes of metabolic decompensation and increase dietary protein tolerance, but patients remain at some risk (albeit lower) for acute neurologic events. Liver transplantation paradoxically also usually reverses even severe cardiomyopathy when present.

# METHYLMALONIC ACIDEMIAS

Accumulation of methylmalonic acid in inherited methylmalonic acidemias is due to deficiency of methylmalonyl-CoA mutase, the enzyme that converts L-methylmalonyl-CoA to succinyl-CoA (see Fig. 132-2), or its required adenosylcobalamin cofactor. In some patients, mutase deficiency is caused by mutations in the mutase gene, but in others, it is caused by a defect in the biosynthesis of adenosylcobalamin from vitamin $B_{12}$. If this defect also blocks synthesis of methyl-$B_{12}$ (which is required by *N5*-methyltetrahydrofolate: homocysteine methyltransferase for the remethylation of homocysteine to methionine), homocystinuria accompanies accumulation of methylmalonic acid.

Before the enzyme and gene defects were known, patients with defects in $B_{12}$ metabolism were classified by genetic complementation. Table 142-1 shows the enzyme defect responsible for each complementation group. The cblC, cblD, cblF, and cblJ defects reduce synthesis of adenosyl- and methyl-$B_{12}$, and the cblA and cblB defects limit synthesis only of adenosyl-$B_{12}$. CblX is a consequence of mutations in the X-linked transcription factor HCFC1 that directs transcription of the *cblC* gene. In addition, atypical forms of moderate to mild methylmalonic acid (MMA) excretion have been recently observed in several genetic disorders not directly involved in the main methylmalonate catabolic pathway. Mitochondrial DNA depletion is associated with loss of subunits of the succinyl-CoA synthetase complex (SUCLA2, SUCLG1, and SUCLG2; see Chapter 153), and MMA is elevated in association with succinylcarnitine ester excretion. Malonyl-CoA decarboxylase deficiency exhibits mild MMA increases and is associated with very high malonic acid excretion, yet is likely a benign metabolic phenotype.

## CLINICAL FINDINGS

As in propionic acidemia, patients with methylmalonic acidemia due to mutase deficiency can present with life-threatening hyperammonemia, ketoacidosis, and thrombocytopenia in the first weeks or months of life; they can also present later, with the more chronic course of ketotic hyperglycinemia, with vomiting, intermittent attacks of life-threatening ketoacidosis, and failure to thrive. As a rule, patients with defects in adenosyl-$B_{12}$ biosynthesis have somewhat milder disease. Acute striatal damage may occur often, but not always during an episode of ketoacidosis. Interstitial nephritis is common, recurrent pancreatitis occurs, and optic atrophy has been described. Patients identified by newborn screening may be asymptomatic at birth but are at risk for metabolic decompensation with physiologic stress or illness.

Patients with both homocystinuria and methylmalonic aciduria usually present during the first months of life with failure to thrive, macrocytic anemia, megaloblastosis, nonspecific neurologic manifestation such as hypotonia, and, unexpectedly, hemolytic-uremic syndrome. Thromboembolism and episodes of ketoacidosis are rare. Even when identified through newborn screening, the clinical outcome may be poor.

## DIAGNOSIS

Urinary organic acid analysis shows increased methylmalonic acid and, especially in patients with mutase defects, tiglylglycine, 3-hydroxypropionic and methylcitric acids, and the same abnormal ketone bodies found in propionic acidemia. Acylcarnitine analysis shows increased propionylcarnitine (although typically not as high as in propionic acidemia), and glycine levels are often elevated in blood and urine. Blood concentrations of vitamin $B_{12}$ are normal. When homocystinuria is present, amino acid analysis also shows low methionine and high cystathionine, but since most homocysteine is bound to protein, routine plasma amino acid studies do not readily detect homocysteine and it must be quantified by another means. In addition, methylmalonic acid excretion in cobalamin defects is usually lower than in mutase deficiency. The defect in methylmalonyl-CoA mutase can be demonstrated in many tissues, including leukocytes and cultured fibroblasts, and complementation analysis is available in a few centers. Confirmation of the diagnosis is now more commonly obtained through DNA sequencing of the appropriate gene. Methylmalonic acidemia is effectively identified by newborn screening using tandem MS, with elevated C3-carnitine as the relevant analyte.

## GENETICS

With the exception of cblX, all forms of methylmalonic acidemia are inherited as autosomal recessive traits. The gene encoding methylmalonyl-CoA mutase is on chromosome 6 (6p.12-21.1), and a number of disease-causing mutations have been identified. Prenatal diagnosis of mutase deficiency can be established by performing an enzyme assay on cultured amniocytes or chorionic villus cells; by demonstrating increased methylmalonic and methylcitric acids in amniotic fluid; or, if the mutations in the family are already known, by molecular analysis.

See Chapter 142 for prenatal diagnosis of cbl defects.

## TREATMENT

As in propionic acidemia, treatment of mutase-deficient methylmalonic acidemia relies on restricting dietary protein (or propiogenic amino acids) to amounts necessary to support normal growth and development and intermittent treatment with nonabsorbable antibiotics. Carnitine is useful to treat secondary carnitine deficiency, and attacks of ketoacidosis should be treated with fluid and electrolytes. Some patients treated in this way do well, but many die in early childhood. Liver transplantation may be curative, and successful outcomes after combined liver-kidney transplantation in patients with chronic renal failure have been reported. However, MMA levels remain elevated after transplantation and may necessitate continued dietary restrictions to avoid injuring the renal graft. Large doses of vitamin $B_{12}$ lower methylmalonic acid excretion only in patients with defects of adenosyl-$B_{12}$ biosynthesis.

Patients with methylmalonic aciduria and homocystinuria are treated with betaine, another methyl donor for the conversion of homocysteine to methionine, and intramuscular or subcutaneous vitamin $B_{12}$. These measures reduce excretion of methylmalonic acid and homocysteine, but often without appreciable clinical response. Many patients succumb during childhood because of hemolytic-uremic syndrome or cardiorespiratory arrest, but long-term survival, often with neurologic sequelae, can occur.

## OTHER RARE ORGANIC ACIDEMIAS

## ISOLATED 3-METHYLCROTONYL-CoA CARBOXYLASE DEFICIENCY

The biotin-containing enzyme 3-methylcrotonyl-CoA carboxylase (MCC) converts 3-methylcrotonyl-CoA, an intermediate in leucine oxidation, to 3-methylglutaconyl-CoA. MCC deficiency can exist alone or, in multiple carboxylase deficiency, together with deficiency of carboxylases for propionyl-CoA, pyruvate, and acetyl-CoA. It has become increasingly recognized due to newborn screening by tandem MS.

### CLINICAL FINDINGS

Most enzyme-deficient individuals do not develop symptoms: however, individuals rarely may develop metabolic decompensation due to physiologic stress or illness, and secondary carnitine deficiency can be observed.

### DIAGNOSIS

Urine organic acid analysis shows increased 3-hydroxyisovaleric acid and 3-methylcrotonylglycine, but the amounts of the latter can be small and hard to detect. Tandem MS shows increased 3-hydroxyisovalerylcarnitine. Serum carnitine levels may be very low, probably as a consequence of 3-hydroxyisovalerylcarnitine excretion. MCC deficiency can be demonstrated in several tissues, including leukocytes and cultured fibroblasts; however, confirmation of diagnosis is now typically through DNA sequencing of the appropriate genes. MCC deficiency is effectively identified through newborn screening using tandem MS, although it may also represent placental transfer from an unrecognized, affected mother.

### GENETICS

Isolated MCC deficiency is usually inherited as an autosomal recessive trait due to mutations in the *MCCC1* and *MCCC* genes encoding the alpha and beta subunits of the enzyme, although rare dominant negative alleles have been reported. The genes encoding the alpha and beta subunits are on chromosomes 3 and 5, respectively, and a variety of pathogenic mutations have been described. Prenatal diagnosis can be established by enzyme assay in cultured amniocytes or chorionic villus cells or by demonstrating increased 3-methylcrotonylglycine in amniotic fluid.

### TREATMENT

Most affected individuals require no chronic treatment other than monitoring for secondary carnitine deficiency. If an episode of acute metabolic decompensation occurs, it should be treated with fluids, glucose, and electrolytes.

## 3-METHYLGLUTACONIC ACIDURIAS

The 3-methylglutaconic acidurias (3-MGA) are a group of disorders with excretion of a common metabolite due to multiple different causes. Five types have been recognized, although a more recent classification divided the disorder into primary versus secondary. Type I (3-MGA type I), or primary 3-MGA is a rare disorder identified in patients who present a wide spectrum of neurologic symptoms ranging from no symptoms at 2 years, to mild developmental delay to severe encephalopathy with basal ganglia involvement, quadriplegia, athetoid movement disorder, and leukoencephalopathy in a 61-year-old woman.

There is a high excretion in urine of 3-methylglutaconic (3-MGC) and 3-methylglutaric, which derive from accumulation of 3-MGC-CoA proximal to the block. There is also a high excretion of 3-hydroxyisovaleric acid with a normal amount of 3-hydroxy-3-methylglutaric acid. The deficient enzyme activity is 3-MGC-CoA hydratase encoded by the *AUH* gene, which can be measured in fibroblasts. Several pathogenic variants have been identified.

3-MGA type I must be distinguished from other conditions associated with secondary 3-MGA including Barth syndrome (*TAZ* gene) (see Chapter 153), Costeff optic atrophy syndrome (*OPA3* gene), MEGDEL syndrome (*SERAC1* gene), dilated cardiomyopathy with ataxia syndrome (*DNAJC19* gene), defects in the *TMEM70* gene, and disorders of unknown origin summarized as 3-MGA type IV. The clinical features and age of onset are remarkably variable, including cardiomyopathy, optic atrophy, Leigh syndrome, hyperammonemia, and lactic acidemia.

## 2-METHYL-3-HYDROXYBUTYRYL-CoA DEHYDROGENASE DEFICIENCY

This rare disorder affects males and typically is characterized by a progressive neurodegenerative course with retinopathy and cardiomyopathy, although there is broad clinical heterogeneity. Onset may be neonatal, but often it occurs in early childhood, with rigidity, dystonic posturing, spastic diplegia, dysarthria, choreoathetoid movements, cortical blindness, myoclonic seizures, brain atrophy, and periventricular white matter and basal ganglia abnormalities—features resembling the sequelae of neonatal hypoxic-anoxic brain injury. This typical presentation differs from other branched chain catabolic disorders and particularly from 2-methyl-acetoacetyl-CoA thiolase deficiency, the next step on the isoleucine catabolic pathway, which generally present with acute severe ketoacidosis attacks (see Chapter 147). Although rare, patients may have an acute metabolic decompensation with hypoglycemia and hyperammonemia, and yet remain neurologically intact.

2-Methyl-3-hydroxybutyryl-CoA dehydrogenase (MHBD) deficiency, also known as HSD10 disease, is characterized by elevations of urinary 2-methyl-3-hydroxybutyrate and tiglylglycine without elevation of 2-methylacetoacetate. MHBD activity can be measured in fibroblasts and lymphocytes. MHBD deficiency is caused by mutations in the *HSD17B10* gene encoding the HSD10 protein located on the X chromosome. The clinical variability is likely due to the dual functions for the protein in intermediary metabolism and mitochondrial RNA processing. There is currently no effective treatment. Heterozygous females may exhibit intellectual disability. Newborn screening may reveal elevated C5-OH, but the condition may be missed by screening.

## SHORT/BRANCHED CHAIN ACYL-CoA DEHYDROGENASE (SBCAD) AND ISOBUTYRYL-CoA DEHYDROGENASE (IBD) DEFICIENCIES

Isolated 2-methylbutyrylglycinuria with 2-methylbutyrylcarnitine (2-MBC) caused by SBCAD deficiency at the third step of isoleucine catabolism pathway was originally described in a patient with brain lesions and neonatal hypoglycemia. Many asymptomatic individuals with this defect have been found in newborn screening programs based on elevated C5-acylcarnitine (2-MBC), as a result of a founder mutation in the Hmong population. The disorder is now considered to be a benign biochemical phenotype.

Mitochondrial IBD catalyzes the third step of valine degradation and is encoded by the *ACAD8* gene. Originally identified in a patient with cardiomyopathy likely due to a pronounced secondary carnitine deficiency, the disorder is now routinely detected on the basis of elevated butyryl-carnitine/isobutyrylcarnitine (C4-acylcarnitine) concentration in newborn blood spots analyzed by tandem MS. Most patients thus identified have remained asymptomatic, although a nonspecific picture of mild hypotonia and developmental delay is still reported in some patients.

## SUGGESTED READINGS


Alfardan J, Mohsen AW, Copeland S, et al. Characterization of new ACADSB gene sequence mutations and clinical implications in patients with 2-methylbutyrylglycinuria identified by newborn screening. *Mol Genet Metab.* 2010;100:333-338.

Forsyth R, Vockley CW, Edick MJ, et al. Outcomes of cases with 3-methylcrotonyl-CoA carboxylase (3-MCC) deficiency: report from the inborn errors of metabolism information system. *Mol Genet Metab.* 2016;118:15-20.

Grunert SC, Wendel U, Lindner M, et al. Clinical and neurocognitive outcome in symptomatic isovaleric acidemia. *Orphanet J Rare Dis.* 2012;7:9.

Grunert SC, Mullerleile S, De Silva L, et al. Propionic acidemia: clinical course and outcome in 55 pediatric and adolescent patients. *Orphanet J Rare Dis.* 2013;8:6.

Knerr I, Weinhold N, Vockley J, Gibson KM. Advances and challenges in the treatment of branched-chain amino/keto acid metabolic defects. *J Inherit Metab Dis.* 2012;35:29-40.

Manoli I, Myles JG, Sloan JL, Shchelochkov OA, Venditti CP. A critical reappraisal of dietary practices in methylmalonic acidemia raises concerns about the safety of medical foods. Part 1: isolated methylmalonic acidemias. *Genet Med.* 2016;18:386-395.

Novarino G, El-Fishawy P, Kayserili H, et al. Mutations in BCKD-kinase lead to a potentially treatable form of autism with epilepsy. *Science.* 2012;338:394-397.

Strauss KA, Wardley B, Robinson D, et al. Classical maple syrup urine disease and brain development: principles of management and formula design. *Mol Genet Metab.* 2010;99:333-345.

Wortmann SB, Duran M, Anikster Y, et al. Inborn errors of metabolism with 3-methylglutaconic aciduria as discriminative feature: proper classification and nomenclature. *J Inherit Metab Dis.* 2013;36:923-928.

Zschocke J. HSD10 disease: clinical consequences of mutations in the HSD17B10 gene. *J Inherit Metab Dis.* 2012;35:81-89.


# 133 Disorders of Sulfur-Containing Amino Acid Group Metabolism

Bernd C. Schwahn

## INTRODUCTION

Sulfur-containing amino acids have various important roles: They mediate the transfer of methyl groups for virtually all transmethylation reactions; they provide reactive thiol groups that are needed for detoxification of endogenous and exogenous substances; they help maintain the intracellular redox potential; and they are a source of sulfate. More than 20 disorders of sulfur-containing amino acid metabolism have been described.

Severe hyperhomocysteinemia, defined when plasma total homocysteine (tHcy) concentration is above 100 µmol/L, is generally caused by single-enzyme deficiencies of homocysteine metabolism. When concentrations of free homocysteine exceed the plasma protein binding capacity, the disulfide homocysteine forms nonenzymatically and is excreted in urine, hence causing homocystinuria. The term *homocystinuria* is sometimes used to indicate the most common form of the disease, which is caused by defective activity of the enzyme cystathionine β-synthase (CBS). Homocystinuria, however, also results from defects in the folate- and cobalamin-dependent remethylation cycle (see Chapter 142), of which 5,10-methylenetetrahydrofolate reductase (MTHFR) deficiency and the cobalamin C defect are by far the most common. Severe nutritional deficiency of cobalamin or folate can also cause hyperhomocysteinemia and homocystinuria and should always be ruled out first.

## CLASSICAL HOMOCYSTINURIA (CBS DEFICIENCY)

### PATHOGENESIS, EPIDEMIOLOGY, AND GENETICS

The disturbance in metabolism resulting in homocystinuria is shown in Figure 133-1. CBS initiates the first step of homocysteine elimination. As a consequence of CBS deficiency, homocysteine, *S*-adenosylhomocysteine (SAH), *S*-adenosylmethionine (SAM), and methionine accumulate when methionine intake exceeds the residual transsulfuration and total remethylation activity. Moreover, high SAH inhibits many transmethylases, which increases accumulation of SAM and methionine. Increased homocysteine facilitates remethylation, which leads to further accumulation of methionine. The intermediate metabolites cystathionine and cysteine are decreased. The pathophysiology of CBS deficiency is not completely understood, but accumulation of homocysteine plays a major role in the development of vascular damage and thromboembolic complications. Classic tests of clotting function are normal, but elevated homocysteine causes increased platelet adhesiveness, damage to endothelial cells, and proliferation of smooth muscle and fibrous tissue within the vessel wall. Defective cross-linking of collagen fibrils contributes to the connective tissue dysplasia, and structural alterations of fibrillin structures in zonular fibers cause lens dislocation.

The real incidence of CBS deficiency is not known but may vary between 1:20,000 and 1:200,000. CBS deficiency (MIM No. 236200) is an autosomal recessive trait. The CBS gene has been mapped to chromosome 21q22.3, and more than 100 different mutations have been identified, most of them being private. However, 2 mutations, p.I278T and p.G307S, account for 25% to 50% of all affected alleles, depending on the population. p.I278T and a few other mutations are usually associated with pyridoxine responsiveness. Antenatal diagnosis has been performed by assaying CBS activity in cultured amniocytes or cultured chorionic villi. Mutational analysis can be used for prenatal diagnosis once the mutation(s) of the index case is known.

### CLINICAL PRESENTATION

Classical homocystinuria presents as a multisystemic disease with a dysplasia of connective tissue, a predisposition to arterial and venous thromboembolism, and often with intellectual disability. Clinical variability is wide, but the development of signs and symptoms usually occurs in the first decade, with the exception of embolism, which occurs later. Homocystinuria is one of the few disorders of amino acid metabolism in which the clinical manifestations tend to be progressive in adulthood because of arteriosclerosis and thrombotic complications.

The most characteristic feature of this disorder is subluxation of the ocular lens, which occurs in almost all untreated individuals by adulthood. Most patients have osteoporosis and skeletal abnormalities similar to those seen in Marfan syndrome, including tall stature, scoliosis, genu valgum, pes cavus, arachnodactyly, and pectus carinatum or excavatum. In homocystinuria, however, the joints tend to have restricted mobility rather than hypermobility. Intellectual disability is common, although often mild, and many individuals have psychiatric disturbances.

### DIAGNOSIS AND DIFFERENTIAL DIAGNOSIS

Once hyperhomocysteinemia, usually in the range of 80 to 300 µmol/L, has been identified, plasma amino acid chromatography can be used to search for hypermethioninemia and low cystine, cystathionine, and serine concentrations. Defects of folate- and cobalamin-dependent remethylation can be differentiated by a low or normal plasma methionine concentration and increased cystathionine. Increased urinary methylmalonic acid excretion and megaloblastic anemia suggest either concomitant cobalamin deficiency or a defect in cobalamin transport

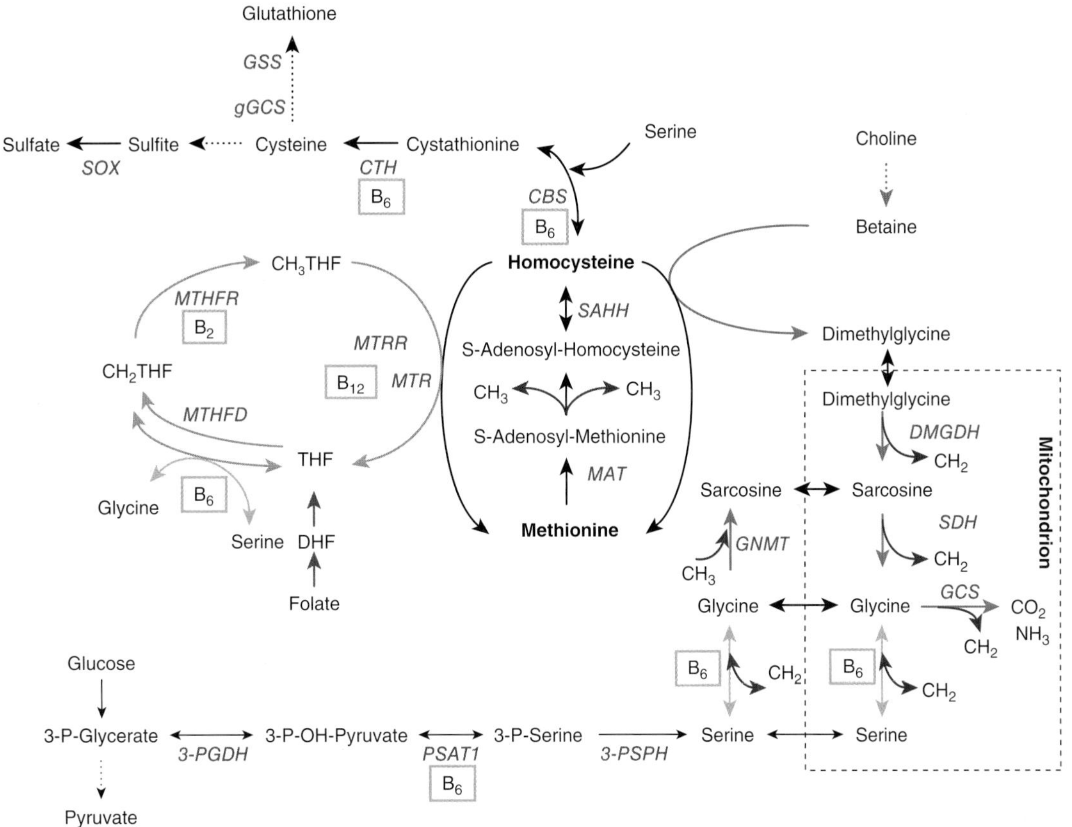


**FIGURE 133-1** Pathways of sulfur amino acids and methyl group metabolism in man. Methionine adenosyltransferase (MAT) activates methionine to *S*-adenosylmethionine (SAM), the universal methyl group donor for numerous methylation reactions. These "transmethylation" reactions yield a methylated product and demethylated *S*-adenosylhomocysteine (SAH), which is readily hydrolyzed to homocysteine by SAH-hydrolase (SAHH). Excessive homocysteine is removed by condensation with serine, catalyzed by cystathionine beta synthase (CBS), an enzyme requiring pyridoxal phosphate (vitamin $B_6$) as cofactor. Cystathionine is catabolized to cysteine by cystathionase (CTH), another $B_6$-dependent enzyme, and eventually to sulfite. Highly reactive sulfite is oxidized to sulfate by sulfite oxidase (SOX). Cysteine is a precursor for the synthesis of glutathione via gamma-glutamylcysteine synthetase (gGCS) and glutathione synthetase (GSS). A considerable proportion of homocysteine is recycled by remethylation to methionine via the cobalamin (vitamin $B_{12}$)–dependent enzyme methionine synthase (MTR). This reaction needs 5-methylfolate ($CH_3THF$) as a methyl donor, which is provided by 5,10-methylenetetrahydrofolate reductase (MTHFR) from 5,10-methylenetetrahydrofolate ($CH_2THF$), thus diverting 1-carbon units from nucleotide synthesis to methylation. MTHFR requires riboflavin (vitamin $B_2$) as a cofactor. The choline metabolite betaine provides a methyl group for an alternative remethylation reaction of homocysteine in liver and kidney. Apart from exogenous methyl groups that are ingested with methionine, choline, or betaine, the main endogenous source of 1-carbon units is from serine. Serine is synthesized from glucose in a series of enzyme reactions involving 3-phosphoglycerate dehydrogenase (3-PGDH), phosphoserine aminotransferase 1 (PSAT1), and 3-phosphoserine phosphatase (3-PSPH). Serine is converted to glycine by serine hydroxymethyltransferase (SHMT), forming methylenetetrahydrofolate ($CH_2$). An excess of $CH_3$ groups can be buffered by formation of sarcosine via glycine-*N*-methyltransferase (GNMT). Sarcosine is also a product of betaine catabolism to dimethylglycine, which is further demethylated by dimethylglycine dehydrogenase (DMGDH). Sarcosine can be converted to glycine by sarcosine dehydrogenase (SDH). GNMT and SDH form the sarcosine-glycine cycle, which regulates the ratio of SAM to SAH and thereby the flux through transmethylation reactions that use SAM as methyl donor.

or metabolism. Severe folate or cobalamin deficiency should be ruled out by measuring serum vitamin concentrations (Fig. 133-2; see Chapter 142). The diagnosis can be confirmed by molecular genetic testing or by measuring enzyme activity in fibroblasts or lymphocytes.

## TREATMENT, PROGNOSIS, AND LONG-TERM OUTCOME

Approximately half of all CBS-deficient individuals respond to supplementation with large doses of pyridoxine with clear biochemical improvement. Responsiveness is determined by the properties of the mutant apoenzyme and should be tested in every patient by administration of pyridoxine for at least a week (500 mg daily in children and 1000 mg daily in adults). Medical treatment aims to control the biochemical abnormalities to prevent complications or halt the progression of symptoms. Early treatment and maintenance of tHcy below 50 μmol/L prevents exposure to excessive concentrations of free homocysteine and appears to be associated with a near-normal risk for thromboembolic events, improvement in behavior and IQ, and avoidance of lens dislocation. Those who do not respond sufficiently to pyridoxine supplementation need to be treated with a diet low in methionine and supplemented with L-cystine. In addition, the methyl donor betaine should be added to enhance remethylation. Individuals who do not restrict their methionine intake may develop extreme hypermethioninemia while taking betaine and are at risk for brain edema if plasma methionine exceeds 1000 μmol/L.

Nutritional cobalamin and folate deficiency must be avoided. Platelet aggregation inhibitors such as acetylsalicylate or dipyridamole may have a place in secondary prevention of thromboembolic events. Successful pregnancies of women with CBS deficiency have been reported. There is an increased risk for thromboembolic events around pregnancy but no adverse outcome in the infants.

# METHYLENETETRAHYDROFOLATE REDUCTASE DEFICIENCY

## PATHOGENESIS, EPIDEMIOLOGY, AND GENETICS

5,10-Methylenetetrahydrofolate reductase (MTHFR) provides 5-methylfolate for the remethylation of homocysteine, a reaction that is catalyzed by the enzyme methionine synthase and requires cobalamin.

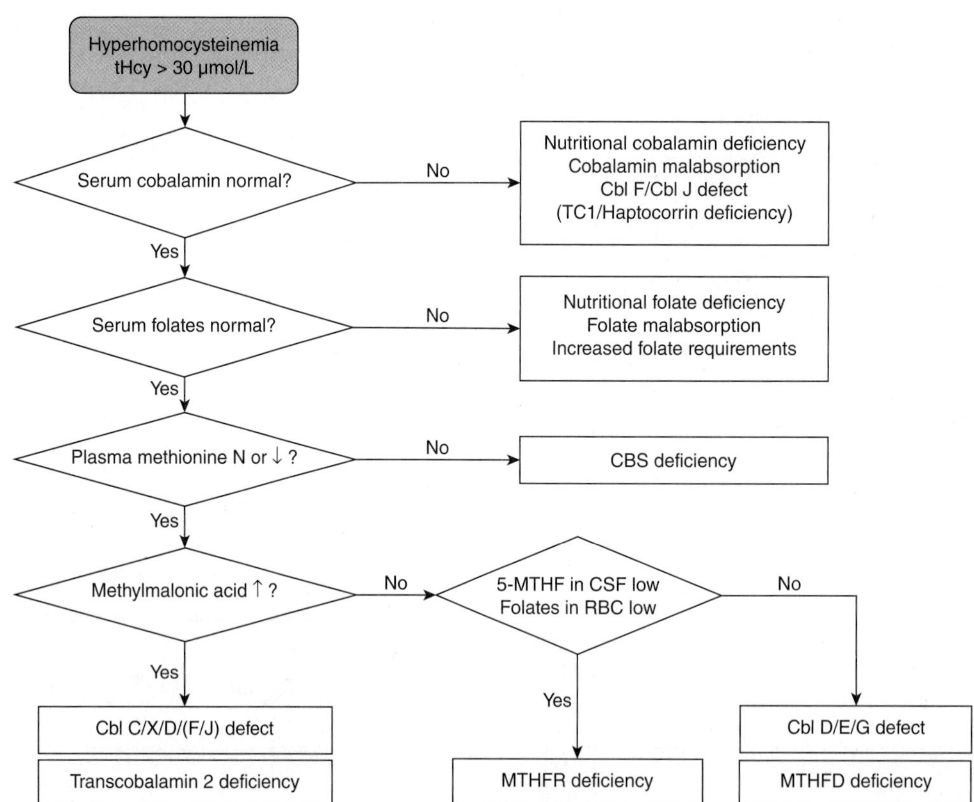


**FIGURE 133-2** Biochemical differentiation of hyperhomocysteinemia. Hyperhomocysteinemia of moderate (> 30 µmol/L) or severe (> 100 µmol/L) extent can be caused by genetic defects of homocysteine metabolism or by severe folate or cobalamin deficiency. Low serum cobalamin or folate concentrations are usually caused by nutritional deficiency or malabsorption but can also be found in the very rare cobalamin (Cbl) F or J defects. Lack of a response to parenteral cobalamin substitution requires further in vitro or genetic studies. Normal or elevated plasma methionine concentrations point to cystathionine beta synthase (CBS) deficiency. Low or decreased levels suggest a defect of remethylation. This can be further differentiated by measuring methylmalonic acid (MMA). Increased MMA reveals functional cobalamin deficiency, which is not found in disorders involving folate-dependent remethylation, such as 5,10-methylenetetrahydrofolate reductase (MTHFR) deficiency, 5,10-methylenetetrahydrofolate dehydrogenase (MTHFD) deficiency, or deficiencies of methionine synthase (MTR) or MTR reductase (MTRR), known as Cbl G or E defects, respectively. The latter 2 conditions are associated with intracellular accumulation of 5-methylfolate, which is decreased in MTHFR deficiency in erythrocytes or cerebrospinal fluid (CSF). Increased MMA together with increased plasma homocysteine and normal serum cobalamin points to a defect in intracellular cobalamin processing (Cbl C, D, and X defects) or transcobalamin 2 deficiency. RBC, red blood cell.

MTHFR diverts 1-carbon units from nucleotide synthesis to remethylation. A lack of MTHFR causes homocysteine accumulation in many extrahepatic tissues, including the brain. Alternative hepatic remethylation using betaine is enhanced, leading to betaine depletion. Transsulfuration is enhanced and cystathionine accumulates, while methionine and SAM are decreased. The latter may be responsible for the dysmyelination, resembling that seen in cobalamin deficiency.

MTHFR deficiency (MIM no. 236250) is an autosomal recessive trait caused by biallelic pathogenic, and mostly private, mutations in the *MTHFR* gene on chromosome 1p36.3. The real incidence has not been established, but there have been a few hundred patients described worldwide. The common polymorphism c.665C>T (formerly known as c.677C>T) does confer a thermolabile variant, and homozygotes have a decreased MTHFR activity when their folate status is poor. They may have mild to moderate hyperhomocysteinemia but no clinical symptoms. The c.665C>T polymorphism has gained much interest in the past as a potential risk factor for cardiovascular disease and other multifactorial conditions in the general population.

## CLINICAL PRESENTATION

Like individuals with CBS deficiency, those with MTHFR deficiency are at risk for arteriosclerosis and thromboembolism. They have, however, fewer skeletal symptoms, and lens dislocation has not been reported. Many suffer from ataxia or neuropathic gait disturbance and a dysmyelinating chronic encephalopathy associated with apnea, seizures, and intellectual disability. Psychiatric disturbances are very common. The phenotype of severe MTHFR deficiency ranges from early neonatal death to nearly asymptomatic adults and is dependent on genetic and environmental modifiers. The 2 genetic defects affecting methionine synthase (MTR) and MTR reductase (MTRR) share similarities with MTHFR deficiency, as do 5 other primary defects in cobalamin metabolism (see Chapter 142). These are, however, much less common and are associated with hematologic abnormalities, in particular megaloblastic anemia, due to methylfolate trapping, which is not a feature of MTHFR deficiency.

## DIAGNOSIS AND DIFFERENTIAL DIAGNOSIS

Severe MTHFR deficiency can be suspected in the presence of moderate or severe hyperhomocysteinemia in combination with low-normal methionine and increased cystathionine in the absence of methylmalonic aciduria, megaloblastic anemia, and folate and cobalamin deficiency. The diagnosis must be confirmed with direct enzyme assay in fibroblasts or molecular genetic testing.

## TREATMENT AND PROGNOSIS

There is no dietary treatment for MTHFR deficiency, but methionine supplementation can be beneficial. For alternative remethylation, an increased supply of betaine can partly compensate for the lack of folate- and cobalamin-dependent remethylation. Betaine supplementation was highly effective in preventing disease-associated symptoms when started early in an animal disease model and in a few prospectively treated children. Late-diagnosed patients show an improvement of myelination and neuropsychiatric symptoms on treatment with betaine, but their prognosis is generally poor.

## MOLYBDENUM COFACTOR DEFICIENCY AND ISOLATED SULFITE OXIDASE DEFICIENCY

### PATHOGENESIS, EPIDEMIOLOGY, AND GENETICS

The terminal step in the oxidative degradation of cysteine and methionine, the conversion of sulfite to sulfate, is catalyzed by the molybdenum-containing enzyme sulfite oxidase. Sulfite oxidase deficiency can be caused by a defect in the gene for the apoenzyme itself or by 1 of 3 defects in the synthesis of the molybdenum cofactor (MoC) required for its function. MoC is required for 3 more enzymes, namely aldehyde oxidase, mitochondrial amidoxime-reducing component (mARC), and xanthine dehydrogenase. The brain pathology is believed to result from defective sulfite oxidase activity. In MoC deficiency (MoCD), xanthinuria may also lead to xanthine stones.

MoCD (MIM no. 252150) may result from defects in 3 different genes: (1) *MOCS1* (6p21.3), which encodes 2 enzymes for the synthesis of the precursor; (2) *MOCS2* (5q11), which encodes molybdopterin synthase that converts the precursor into the organic moiety of molybdenum cofactor; and (3) *GEPH* (14q24), which encodes the gephyrin gene. Gephyrin catalyzes the insertion of molybdenum into molybdopterin. Approximately two-thirds of patients have biallelic pathogenic variants in *MOCS1* and one-third in *MOCS2*. Defects in *GEPH* are extremely rare. Isolated sulfite oxidase deficiency (MIM no. 272300) is also an autosomal recessive trait that seems to be rarer than MoCD. The *SUOX* gene is located on chromosome 12q13.2.

### CLINICAL PRESENTATION

The classical presentation is that of a severe, early, myoclonic epileptic encephalopathy, muscular hypo- or hypertonia, progressive microcephaly, and developmental arrest. Lens dislocation is an early finding. Death during childhood is commonly seen. Milder presentations have been described with developmental delay, seizures, and slowly progressive dystonic and choreoathetotic movement disorder.

### DIAGNOSIS AND DIFFERENTIAL DIAGNOSIS

Increased urinary sulfite can be detected in fresh urine using commercial strip tests normally used in the food industry. This test is readily available at the bedside of an encephalopathic child but has a poor reliability. Increased *S*-sulfocysteine can be detected in body fluids by amino acid chromatography, and affected children have reduced plasma cystine concentrations. In MoCD, hypoxanthine and xanthine concentrations are increased in body fluids and uric acid is very low within a few days after birth. The diagnosis of all defects can be confirmed in cultured fibroblasts or liver tissue, but molecular genetic testing is indicated in most cases to facilitate prenatal diagnosis in future pregnancies.

### TREATMENT AND PROGNOSIS

MoCD due to *MOCS1* defects can now be successfully treated with substitution of the lacking enzymatic product cyclic pyranopterin monophosphate (cPMP). However, clinical outcomes are poor unless treatment is initiated at a presymptomatic stage. There is no effective treatment available for the other 2 forms of MoCD or sulfite oxidase deficiency.

## GLUTATHIONE SYNTHASE DEFICIENCY (PYROGLUTAMIC ACIDURIA)

### PATHOGENESIS, EPIDEMIOLOGY, AND GENETICS

The synthesis and recycling of the sulfur-containing tripeptide glutathione involve a series of 6 enzymatic reactions termed the γ-glutamyl cycle. Glutathione has various important biological functions, such as transport of amino acids, reduction and detoxification of free radicals and drugs, and synthesis of other biomolecules. Defects in 4 of the enzymes of the gamma-glutamyl cycle are associated with disease (Table 133-1), 2 of which manifest with hemolytic anemia. The most frequently recognized and most severe disease is glutathione synthetase deficiency.

### CLINICAL PRESENTATION

Two clinically distinct forms of glutathione synthetase deficiency are known: a rare erythrocytic form that manifests as mild hemolytic anemia and that can be associated with splenomegaly, and a more frequent generalized form that is associated with a variable degree of early neonatal metabolic acidosis, jaundice and hemolytic anemia, and central nervous system symptoms such as ataxia, dystonia, intellectual disability, and retinopathy.

**TABLE 133-1 OTHER RARE DISORDERS OF SULPHUR-CONTAINING AMINO ACIDS**

| Disorder | Clinical Presentation | Metabolic Derangement | Genetics | Diagnostic Tests | Treatment |
|---|---|---|---|---|---|
| Methionine adenosyltransferase deficiency | Neurologic symptoms and demyelination possible | Isolated hypermethioninemia; low SAM; mild hyperhomocysteinemia | AR, *MAT1A* gene on 10q22 | Analysis of amino acids, total homocysteine, and SAM in plasma; mutational testing | SAM supplementation in symptomatic individuals |
| Methionine synthase (MS) and MS reductase deficiency | Dysmyelination; retinopathy; megaloblastic anemia; intellectual disability | Hyperhomocysteinemia; low methionine; secondary disturbance of folate cycle | AR, *MTR* gene (1q43) or *MTRR* gene (5p15.3-15.2) | Amino acids and total homocysteine in plasma; enzyme assay; mutation testing | Supplementation with cobalamin, betaine, and possibly methionine |
| SAH hydrolase deficiency | Hepatitis with neonatal cholestasis; poor synthetic liver function; (cardio)myopathy; intellectual disability | Mild hyperhomocysteinemia; gross elevation of SAH; mild increase of methionine and SAM | AR, *AHCY* gene on 20cen-q13.1 | Amino acids, total homocysteine, SAM and SAH in plasma; enzyme assay; mutation testing | Supplementation with creatine and phosphatidylcholine; methionine restriction |
| Cystathioninuria (cystathionase deficiency) | Asymptomatic | Accumulation of cystathionine in plasma and urine | AR, *CTH* gene on 1p31.1 | Amino acids and total homocysteine in plasma; urinary amino acids | No specific treatment |
| Gamma-glutamylcysteine synthetase deficiency | Hemolytic anemia; neurologic symptoms possible | Low glutathione and gamma-glutamylcysteine in erythrocytes | AR, 2 genes for 2 subunits, *GCLM* on 1p.22.1 and *GCLC* on 6p12 | Glutathione and gamma-glutamylcysteine in RBC; enzyme assay; mutation analysis | Avoidance of drugs known to induce hemolysis in glucose-6-phosphate dehydrogenase |
| Glutathionuria (gamma-glutamyl transpeptidase deficiency) | Mental retardation or seizures possible | Increased glutathione in plasma and urine | AR, 4 genes at 22q11.1-q11.2 are involved | Amino acids in plasma; glutathione in RBC, enzyme assay; mutation analysis | No specific treatment |
| 5-Oxoprolinase deficiency | No consistent symptoms | Gross urinary excretion of 5-oxoproline; no metabolic acidosis | AR, at least 2 genes code for 2 subunits | Urinary organic acids; enzyme assay; mutation analysis | No specific treatment |

AR, autosomal recessive; RBC, red blood cell; SAH, *S*-adenosylhomocysteine; SAM, *S*-adenosylmethionine.

Urinary organic acid analysis can readily detect 5-oxoproline (pyroglutamic acid) in newborns with metabolic acidosis without ketosis, hypoglycemia or hyperlactic acidemia. The diagnosis can be confirmed by assay of enzyme activity in blood cells or cultured fibroblasts. Oxoprolinuria secondary to severe depression of glutathione levels has been described in various other conditions such as intoxication with acetaminophen, primary or secondary hyperhomocysteinemia, or a decompensated urea cycle defect.

### TREATMENT

Correction of acidosis is required in severe cases. Early enteral administration of radical scavengers such as vitamin E or C can help to prevent central nervous system injury. Patients should avoid drugs that can induce hemolysis in glucose-6-phosphate dehydrogenase deficiency.

### SUGGESTED READINGS

Atwal PS, Scaglia F. Molybdenum cofactor deficiency. *Mol Genet Metab.* 2016;117:1-4.

Froese DS, Huemer M, Suormala T, et al. Mutation update and review of severe methylenetetrahydrofolate reductase deficiency. *Hum Mutat.* 2016;37:427-438.

Huemer M, Diodato D, Schwahn B, et al. Guidelines for diagnosis and management of the cobalamin-related remethylation disorders cblC, cblD, cblE, cblF, cblG, cblJ, and MTHFR deficiency. *J Inherit Metab Dis.* 2017;40(1):21-48.

Kumar T, Sharma GS, Singh LR. Homocystinuria: therapeutic approach. *Clin Chim Acta.* 2016;458:55-62.

Mudd SH. Hypermethioninemias of genetic and non-genetic origin: a review. *Am J Med Genet C Semin Med Genet.* 2011;15:3-32.

Mudd SH, Skovby F, Levy HL, et al. The natural history of homocystinuria due to cystathione beta-synthase deficiency. *Am J Hum Genet.* 1985;37:1-31.

Ristoff E, Larsson A. Inborn errors in the metabolism of glutathione. *Orphanet J Rare Dis.* 2007;2:16.

Schwahn BC, Van Spronsen FJ, Belaidi AA, et al. Efficacy and safety of cyclic pyranopterin monophosphate substitution in severe molybdenum cofactor deficiency type A: a prospective cohort study. *Lancet.* 2015;386:1955-1963.

Strauss KA, Morton DH, Puffenberger EG, et al. Prevention of brain disease from severe 5,10-methylenetetrahydrofolate reductase deficiency. *Mol Genet Metab.* 2007;91:165-175.

# 134 Disorders of Glycine Metabolism

Johan L. K. Van Hove

### INTRODUCTION

Formation and elimination of glycine occur through many pathways. One precursor of glycine is choline, which can be oxidized to betaine and sequentially demethylated to dimethylglycine, sarcosine, and glycine, which is finally degraded to $CO_2$ and $NH_3$. Different defects in glycine metabolism lead to distinct biochemical or clinical phenotypes.

### DISORDERS OF GLYCINE METABOLISM

## NONKETOTIC HYPERGLYCINEMIA (GLYCINE ENCEPHALOPATHY)

Nonketotic hyperglycinemia (NKH), also known as glycine encephalopathy (GCE), is an inherited metabolic disorder defined by deficient activity of the glycine cleavage enzyme, the main catabolic enzyme for the amino acid glycine. This results in large amounts of glycine in body fluids, often without further metabolic abnormalities. The term *nonketotic hyperglycinemia* reflects the history of organic acid disorders, where prior to the development of techniques to identify abnormal organic acids such as propionic acid, children who suffered from extreme acidosis and ketosis were found to have elevated plasma glycine. Subsequently, children who had increased glycine but lacked the ketosis were identified. Classic NKH is caused by mutations in protein components of the glycine cleavage enzyme. Variant NKH is caused by defects in a cofactor of the enzyme lipoic acid and encompasses a subset of the lipoate deficiency syndromes.

## CLASSIC NONKETOTIC HYPERGLYCINEMIA

### CLINICAL PRESENTATION

Two clinical variants of classic NKH are recognized: severe NKH and attenuated NKH.

Patients with severe NKH typically present as neonates or, more rarely, in the early infancy with a severe epileptic encephalopathy. Neonates appear normal at birth but develop muscular hypotonia, lethargy developing into a deep comatose state, myoclonic seizures and epileptic hiccups, and apnea within the first days of life. The hypopnea and apnea necessitate ventilator support in 85% of patients but spontaneously resolve within the first 3 weeks. The electroencephalogram (EEG) in the neonate shows a typical burst-suppression pattern, which in later infancy develops into hypsarrhythmia and multifocal epilepsy. Infants develop progressive spasticity with central hypotonia, develop therapy-resistant epilepsy, and gain no developmental skills beyond that of young infants. Orthopedic problems of scoliosis and hip problems and recurrent bronchopneumonitis are common complications in long-term survivors. Survival varies from months to decades.

An attenuated form of NKH is present in 1 of 6 affected children and is characterized by developmental progress, an absence of seizures or therapy-responsive epilepsy, and mild to absent spasticity. Half of the patients with attenuated NKH present similarly in the neonatal period, whereas others present in infancy, with those presenting after 4 months of age tending to have a better outcome. Patients with attenuated NKH make variable developmental progress, varying from a severely affected individual who only learns to sit, grasp, and communicate and who has a readily treatable epilepsy, to a patient with only mild to moderate developmental delay without epilepsy. Most patients have severe attention-deficit/hyperactivity disorder, many have chorea, and some may have intermittent episodes of severe lethargy and ataxia.

Brain magnetic resonance imaging (MRI) shows a characteristic pattern of diffusion restriction in the posterior limb of the internal capsule, brain stem corticospinal tract, central tegmental tracts, and cerebellar white matter, which during infancy extends to the entire corticospinal tract in the cerebrum and brain stem. Children with severe NKH develop variable atrophy of the cerebrum and cerebellum, which is less present in attenuated NKH. The corpus callosum is short and becomes thin over time. Brain malformations, including agenesis of the corpus callosum or hydrocephalus with retrocerebellar cysts, are present in 7% of patients with severe NKH. Magnetic resonance spectroscopy with long echo time (135 milliseconds) can identify elevated brain glycine.

### METABOLIC DERANGEMENT, INCLUDING PATHOPHYSIOLOGY

NKH is caused by defects in the mitochondrial glycine cleavage system (GCS), a multiprotein complex that catalyzes the degradation of glycine to $CO_2$ and $NH_3$, thereby transferring a 1-carbon unit onto tetrahydrofolate to form 5,10-methylenetetrahydrofolate (MeTHF). A block in the GCS leads to accumulation of glycine and a lack of MeTHF, which promotes further production of glycine from serine, via serine hydroxymethyl transferase (see Chapter 133, Fig. 133-1). Glycine modulates *N*-methyl-D-aspartate (NMDA)–mediated neurotransmission, and excess glycine overstimulates these receptors. The accumulation of glycine in NKH is most pronounced in the cerebral compartment. The pathophysiology of NKH is currently not well understood. Spongiosis due to splitting at the intraperiod line of formed myelin is the main feature of neuropathology.

## GENETICS

All forms of NKH (OMIM no. 605899) are inherited as autosomal recessive traits. The enzyme is multimeric with 4 distinct protein components: P protein (a pyridoxal phosphate–dependent glycine decarboxylase, 9p22, gene *GLDC*), T protein (a tetrahydrofolate-requiring aminomethyltransferase, 3p21.2-p21.1, gene *AMT*), H protein (a lipoic acid–containing protein, 16q24, gene *GCSH*), and L protein (a dihydrolipoamide dehydrogenase, gene unknown). Mutations in the *GLDC* gene account for 80% of patients, and mutations in the *AMT* gene account for 20% of patients, with no mutations to date identified in *GCSH*. Up to 20% of the disease alleles in *GLDC* consist of exonic deletions or duplications. Combined sequencing and deletion duplication testing of *GLDC* and *AMT* identifies mutations in 98% of patients.

## DIAGNOSTIC TESTS AND DIFFERENTIAL DIAGNOSES

Hyperglycinemia on plasma amino acid analysis in the absence of ketoacidosis often is the first indication of NKH but has low specificity. A more specific result in NKH is the finding of elevated glycine in the cerebrospinal fluid (CSF; > 60 μM; normal < 20 μM), with an increased CSF-to-plasma glycine ratio (> 0.02). For accurate diagnosis, the CSF must be without blood and without increased protein and with CSF and plasma amino acids obtained simultaneously. Confirmation of the diagnosis by enzyme assay in liver of by molecular genetic studies is essential.

Transient NKH is a phenocopy of an epileptic encephalopathic presentation in a neonate with raised glycine levels, not caused by a genetic defect in GCS. The most common cause is hypoxic ischemic injury. Acute neonatal herpes infection can also mimic NKH with very elevated glycine levels. Valproate inhibits the GCS and can cause raised glycine levels in both plasma and CSF, with an increased CSF-to-plasma ratio. Analysis of organic acids in urine helps to differentiate it from hyperglycinemia secondary to an organic acidemia. Specifically, methylmalonic acid and homocysteine should be measured in infants to exclude cobalamin X disorder. The P protein uses pyridoxal-phosphate as a cofactor, and disorders of pyridoxine activation (*PNPO*) cause glycine elevation; hence CSF pyridoxal-phosphate levels should be measured. For variant NKH, see below.

Prenatal diagnosis and preimplantation genetic diagnoses have been done successfully by molecular analysis if the genetic cause is known. Prenatal diagnosis is also possible by enzyme assay in uncultured fresh chorionic villus sample biopsies, but rare false-negative results have been reported.

## TREATMENT, PROGNOSIS, AND LONG-TERM OUTCOME

Current treatment consists of reducing glycine levels and inhibiting the effect of excessive glycine at the NMDA receptor. Benzoate conjugates with glycine to form hippurate, which is excreted in the urine resulting in removal of glycine. The dose of benzoate, divided in at least 3 or 4 doses per day, is individually adjusted to provide a normal plasma glycine level, identified as < 300 μM taken 1 to 2 hours after a benzoate dose. Excessive benzoate dosing, which depletes the glycine pool, is toxic and should be avoided. Most common dosing is 250 to 450 mg/kg/d in attenuated NKH and 500 to 750 mg/kg/d in the severe form, but individual titration is essential. Dextromethorphan, 3 to 10 mg/kg/d, is used as a mild NMDA receptor antagonist, with ketamine as an alternative. Therapy with applied behavior analysis (ABA therapy) has been most effective for attenuated NKH children, particularly with attention-deficit/hyperactivity symptoms. Valproate and vigabatrin must be avoided. The impact of treatment on severe NKH is limited to increased alertness and decreased seizures but is ineffective at preventing the very poor prognosis. Given the dismal prognosis in severe NKH, withdrawal of intensive care during the apneic phase in the neonatal period is an ethical consideration for some families. In contrast, in attenuated NKH, early treatment improves developmental outcome, reduces epilepsy, improves chorea, and avoids episodic lethargy.

Genetics is the dominant prognostic factor, and presence of a single allele with residual enzymatic activity is necessary for the attenuated phenotype. High levels of CSF glycine, brain malformations, early development of spasticity, and persistent burst suppression on EEG predict a severe phenotype, whereas a low CSF-to-plasma glycine ratio and late onset predict an attenuated phenotype.

# LIPOATE DEFICIENCY SYNDROMES (INCLUDING VARIANT NKH)

Lipoate is a cofactor of several mitochondrial enzymes including GCS and pyruvate dehydrogenase. It is synthesized within mitochondria in a complex biosynthetic pathway, and its deficiency causes variable elevations of glycine and lactic acidosis.

## CLINICAL PRESENTATION

The clinical presentation of this group of disorders is heterogeneous and involves either a single feature or a combination of the following clinical presentations. Some patients present with severe epileptic encephalopathy with burst-suppression pattern and cortical involvement (all genes). In contrast, some patients only exhibit mild and stable developmental delay and well-controlled epilepsy (*LIAS*, *LIPT1*). Leigh disease and progressive cerebral atrophy or cerebellar atrophy are common presentations (all genes). Cavitating leukodystrophy with episodic worsening can cause severe brain dysfunction (*BOLA3*, *NFU1*, *ISCA2*). Pulmonary hypertension and cardiomyopathy can be fatal complications in a subset of patients (*NFU1*, *LIPT1*, *BOLA3*). Spastic paraplegia, optic atrophy, and peripheral neuropathy with preserved cognition form the milder end of the spectrum (*GLRX5*, *IBA57*).

## METABOLIC DERANGEMENT, INCLUDING PATHOPHYSIOLOGY

Lipoate is synthesized on the H protein from the fatty acid octanoate, received by lipoyltransferase 2 (*LIPT2*) from intramitochondrial fatty acid synthesis, by insertion of sulfur atoms of the iron sulfur cluster of the enzyme lipoate synthase (*LIAS*), and then transferred to the recipient enzymes by lipoyltransferase 1 (*LIPT1*). The iron sulfur cluster is synthesized in a complex multistep process that involves up to 20 genes. Iron sulfur clusters are also present in respiratory chain enzymes and in Krebs cycle enzymes such as aconitase. Lipoate is a catalytic intermediate for the following enzymes: pyruvate dehydrogenase, 2-ketoglutarate dehydrogenase, branched chain amino acid dehydrogenase, 2-ketoadipate dehydrogenase, and the glycine cleavage enzyme system. Disorders affecting the biosynthesis of lipoate cause variably deficient activities of these enzymes, with the most extensive deficiencies in patients with mutations in *NFU1* and the least deficiencies in patients with mutations in *GLRX5*. Most commonly observed is a combination of elevated glycine levels similar to NKH; however, with the exception for *LIPT1*, the CSF glycine levels tend to be lower. Lactate concentrations can vary from severely elevated to near normal. A presentation without lactic acidosis but with elevated glycine levels constitutes a variant NKH presentation, which is responsible for 4% of NKH cases.

## GENETICS

Mutations have been reported in each of the 3 genes of lipoate metabolism: lipoyltransferase 2 (*LIPT2*), lipoate synthase (*LIAS*), and lipoyltransferase 1 (*LIPT1*). In addition, mutations in genes affecting the synthesis of the iron sulfur cluster of lipoate synthase can be causative, including *GLRX5*, *BOLA3*, *NFU1*, *IBA57*, and *ISCA2*. All are inherited in an autosomal recessive manner.

## DIAGNOSTIC TESTS AND DIFFERENTIAL DIAGNOSES

All patients have mild to pronounced elevations of glycine, more so in plasma than in the CSF. Many patients have intermittent elevations of lactic acid. Elevated 2-ketoglutarate and, rarely, 2-ketoadipate can be observed in the urine organic acid analysis. The enzyme assay of pyruvate dehydrogenase has been shown to be deficient in fibroblasts in all patients. A Western blot of lipoylation of mitochondrial enzymes shows reduced lipoylation. Molecular genetic testing is commonly used to establish the diagnosis. If identified by untargeted molecular screening, such as whole-exome sequencing, then functional confirmation in fibroblasts is recommended.

### TREATMENT, PROGNOSIS, AND LONG-TERM OUTCOME

There is currently no specific treatment for these disorders. Provision of exogenous lipoate is not transferred to the deficient proteins and is generally ineffective. Maintenance of anabolism is indicated, particularly for intermittent relapsing disorders such as BOLA3 deficiency. A ketogenic diet for the pyruvate dehydrogenase deficiency caused by lipoate disorders is contraindicated because it can cause severe 2-ketoglutaric acidosis.

### SUGGESTED READINGS


Ajit Bolar N, Vanlander AV, Wilbrecht C, et al. Mutation of the iron-sulfur cluster assembly gene IBA57 causes severe myopathy and encephalopathy. *Hum Mol Genet.* 2013;22:2590-2602.

Baker PR II, Friederich MW, Swanson MA, et al. Variant non ketotic hyperglycinemia is caused by mutations in LIAS, BOLA3 and the novel gene GLRX5. *Brain.* 2014;137:366-379.

Cameron JM, Janer A, Levandovskiy V, et al. Mutations in iron-sulfur cluster scaffold genes NFU1 and BOLA3 cause a fatal deficiency of multiple respiratory chain and 2-oxoacid dehydrogenase enzymes. *Am J Hum Genet.* 2011;89:486-495.

Coughlin CR II, Swanson MA, Kronquist K, et al. The genetic basis of classic nonketotic hyperglycinemia due to mutations in *GLDC* and *AMT*. *Genet Med.* 2017;19(1):104-111.

Hennermann JB, Berger J-M, Grieben U, et al. Prediction of long-term outcome in glycine encephalopathy: a clinical survey. *J Inherit Metab Dis.* 2012;35:253-261.

Hoover-Fong JE, Shah S, Van Hove JL, Applegarth D, Toone J, Hamosh A. Natural history of nonketotic hyperglycinemia in 65 patients. *Neurology.* 2004;63:1847-1853.

Maio N, Rouault TA. Iron-sulfur cluster biogenesis in mammalian cells: new insights into molecular mechanisms of cluster delivery. *Biochim Biophys Acta.* 2015;1853:1493-1512.

Mayr JA, Feichtinger RG, Tort F, et al. Lipoic acid biosynthesis defects. *J Inherit Metab Dis.* 2014;37:553-563.

Swanson MA, Coughlin CR II, Scharer GH, et al. Biochemical and molecular predictors for prognosis in nonketotic hyperglycinemia. *Ann Neurol.* 2015;78:606-618.

Van Hove JLK, Vande Kerckhove K, Hennermann JB, et al. Benzoate treatment and the glycine index in nonketotic hyperglycinaemia. *J Inherit Metab Dis.* 2005;28:651-663.


# 135 Disorders of Amino Acid Synthesis: Serine, Proline, Ornithine, and Glutamine

Bernd C. Schwahn

### INTRODUCTION

Almost all disorders of amino acid metabolism are caused by defects in catabolic pathways. However, a few genetic disorders of the biosynthesis of nonessential amino acids have been identified. Deficient endogenous production of serine, proline, ornithine, or glutamine each leads to a deficiency of the respective amino acid and to distinct diseases. The diagnosis requires recognizing a decrease of amino acid concentrations below the reference range. Children with disorders of synthetic pathways are not prone to decompensation under catabolic stress. However, they share signs of compromised intrauterine development and central nervous dysfunction and, if severely affected, suffer from dysmorphism and congenital malformations.

## DISORDERS OF L-SERINE SYNTHESIS

De novo synthesis of L-serine from glucose (see Fig. 133-1) is necessary to provide the organism with sufficient quantities of serine required for protein synthesis, modification of complex lipids, and as a donor of transferable 1-carbon units for the synthesis of the nucleotide bases adenine, guanine, and thymine. Genetic defects in each of the 3 steps of serine synthesis are associated with neurologic disease comprised of a global developmental disorder, microcephaly, seizures, and progressive polyneuropathy. Severe deficiency of any of the 3 enzymes is one of the main causes for the genetically heterogenous Neu-Laxova syndrome (NLS), which is characterized by intrauterine growth failure, facial dysmorphism (shortened eyelids, proptosis, round gaping mouth), microcephaly, hyperkeratosis or even ichthyosis, flexion deformities, peripheral edema, and malformations of central nervous system (CNS) and limbs, with an often fatal outcome.

Each of the 3 defects is very rare, but diagnosis is important, as children affected with attenuated forms benefit from L-serine supplementation, and each has an autosomal recessive risk of recurrence.

## 3-PHOSPHOGLYCERATE DEHYDROGENASE (3-PGDH) DEFICIENCY

### PATHOGENESIS, EPIDEMIOLOGY, AND GENETICS

A biallelic disruption of the *PHDGH* gene on chromosome 1p12 is responsible for 3-PGDH deficiency (Online Mendelian Inheritance in Man [MIM] no. 601815). 3-PGDH catalyzes the first step in L-serine biosynthesis, and deficient enzyme activity leads to serine deficiency. At least 100 cases of Neu-Laxova syndrome have been described, and significantly fewer children have attenuated forms.

### CLINICAL MANIFESTATIONS

Attenuated 3-PGDH deficiency is a neurometabolic disease characterized by intrauterine growth failure, congenital microcephaly, intractable seizures, and later, a global developmental disorder and spasticity. Cataracts and hypogonadism have also been observed. Brain magnetic resonance imaging (MRI) shows severe atrophy and hypomyelination. Mild forms may manifest with isolated late-onset seizures and signs of polyneuropathy.

### DIAGNOSIS INCLUDING DIFFERENTIAL DIAGNOSIS

Amino acid analysis in cerebrospinal fluid (CSF) or preprandial plasma reveals decreased serine and moderately low glycine concentrations. 5-Methylfolate in CSF can be decreased. Postprandial amino acid levels may be normal. The diagnosis can be confirmed by enzyme assay in fibroblasts or by DNA-based testing.

### TREATMENT AND PROGNOSIS

Early supplementation with high enteral doses of L-serine and possibly glycine can have a dramatic effect on seizures and psychomotor development. Antenatal treatment has been attempted to avoid prenatal developmental injury.

## PHOSPHOSERINE AMINOTRANSFERASE 1 (PSAT1) DEFICIENCY

### PATHOGENESIS, EPIDEMIOLOGY, AND GENETICS

Phosphoserine aminotransferase 1 is encoded by the *PSAT1* gene located on chromosome 9q21.2 and is composed of 9 exons that generate 2 alternatively spliced mRNAs (*PSAT1α* and *PSAT1β*). PSAT1 deficiency (OMIM no. 610992) is very rare. Fewer than 10 patients have been identified, most of them presenting with Neu-Laxova syndrome. Underdiagnosis of attenuated forms is likely.

## CLINICAL MANIFESTATIONS

The presentation is similar to 3-PGDH deficiency.

## DIAGNOSIS INCLUDING DIFFERENTIAL DIAGNOSIS

Amino acid analysis in CSF reveals decreased serine and moderately low glycine concentrations. Plasma amino acids can be normal, especially if not obtained in a preprandial state. The diagnosis can be confirmed by enzyme assay in fibroblasts but has been ascertained retrospectively in most cases by mutation analysis after genome-wide screening.

## TREATMENT AND PROGNOSIS

Successful treatment with immediate postnatal supplementation of L-serine in a neonate with attenuated PSAT1 deficiency has been reported.

# PHOSPHOSERINE PHOSPHATASE (PSP) DEFICIENCY

## PATHOGENESIS, EPIDEMIOLOGY, AND GENETICS

Phosphoserine phosphatase (PSP) catalyzes the last step in the biosynthesis of serine from carbohydrates, the hydrolysis of O-phosphoserine. PSP deficiency (MIM no. 614023) is caused by a biallelic disruption of the *PSPH* gene, which is located on chromosome 7p11.2. The inheritance is autosomal recessive. At least 10 patients have been identified.

## CLINICAL MANIFESTATIONS

One patient presented with pre- and postnatal growth retardation, moderate psychomotor retardation, and facial dysmorphism, but was also affected with Williams Beuren syndrome. Another patient presented with NLS, and a further 7 patients from 1 family were described that mainly presented with microcephaly and intellectual disability.

## DIAGNOSIS INCLUDING DIFFERENTIAL DIAGNOSIS

The diagnosis can be suspected by finding low serine concentrations in CSF and plasma and confirmed by enzyme assay in fibroblasts or mutation analysis.

## TREATMENT AND PROGNOSIS

Children with attenuated forms have clinically benefited from L-serine supplementation.

# DISORDERS OF PROLINE AND ORNITHINE BIOSYNTHESIS

Proline and the nonproteinogenic amino acid ornithine are synthesized from glutamate via the intermediate Δ1-pyrroline-5-carboxylate (P5C) (Fig. 135-1). The synthesis of P5C is catalyzed by aldehyde dehydrogenase 18 family member A1, also known as Δ1-pyrroline-5-carboxylate synthase (P5CS). P5C can be reduced to proline by pyrroline-5-carboxylate reductase 1 (P5CR1) or aminated to ornithine by the enzyme ornithine aminotransferase (OAT). Proline is an important constituent of proteins, especially of collagens, whereas ornithine is required as a precursor for the synthesis of polyamines and, crucially, as an acceptor of carbamoyl phosphate in the urea cycle. Proline deficiency leads to a disruption of connective tissue at various levels, and a lack of ornithine leads to hyperammonemia and neurologic disease.

# P5CS DEFICIENCY

## PATHOGENESIS, EPIDEMIOLOGY, AND GENETICS

P5CS is encoded by the *ALDH18A1* gene, located at 10q24.3. P5CS deficiency (MIM no. 138250) is inherited as a recessive trait and causes an insufficient synthesis of both proline and ornithine. The consequent relative deficiency of the urea cycle intermediates ornithine, citrulline, and arginine leads to hyperammonemia, which is aggravated by fasting. Proline deficiency leads to structural defects in connective tissue matrix proteins and congenital multisystem disease. P5CS deficiency has only been described in a few individuals.

## CLINICAL MANIFESTATIONS

This disorder is difficult to diagnose. Affected children have microcephaly and global developmental disorder. Some show spastic paraplegia, retinopathy, or seizures. Signs of connective tissue dysplasia are usually found, including joint hypermobility, skin laxity, hernias, and sometimes cataract formation.

## DIAGNOSIS INCLUDING DIFFERENTIAL DIAGNOSIS

Plasma amino acid analysis can show low concentrations of proline, ornithine, arginine, and citrulline. Plasma ammonia rises with fasting and paradoxically falls after protein feeding. The diagnosis can be confirmed by mutation analysis. Direct enzyme assay is not possible. The differential diagnosis includes other cutis laxa syndromes and disorders of copper transport (Menkes disease) or protein glycosylation.

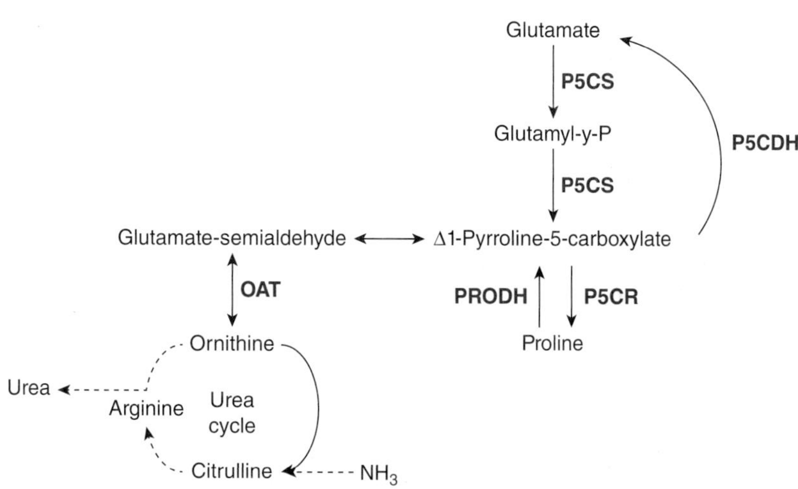


**FIGURE 135-1** Proline is synthesized in 3 steps from the precursor glutamate involving the enzymes Δ1-pyrroline-5-carboxylate (P5C) synthase (P5CS) and P5C reductase (P5CR). The intermediate P5C has a tautomeric form, glutamate γ-semialdehyde, which can be transaminated to ornithine by the enzyme ornithine aminotransferase (OAT). Ornithine can thus be a source of proline but is mainly required for the function of the urea cycle and the endogenous production of arginine. Proline dehydrogenase (PRODH) catalyzes the catabolism of proline back to P5C, which can be further converted to glutamate by Δ1-pyrroline-5-carboxylate dehydrogenase (P5CDH).

Treatment aims at supplementing L-proline and L-citrulline.

## P5C REDUCTASE (P5CR) DEFICIENCY

### PATHOGENESIS, EPIDEMIOLOGY, AND GENETICS

The *PYCR1* gene is located on chromosome 17q25.3 and is composed of 9 exons that generate 5 alternatively spliced mRNAs that encode 4 different isoforms of the mitochondrial enzyme P5CR. P5CR deficiency is inherited as a recessive trait. An increasing number of patients with a diagnosis of one of the cutis laxa syndromes such as De Barsy syndrome have been diagnosed with P5CR deficiency (MIM no. 614438).

### CLINICAL MANIFESTATIONS

Patients present with mild facial dysmorphism and signs similar to P5CS deficiency. However, they have no lack of ornithine and are not prone to hyperammonemia.

### DIAGNOSIS INCLUDING DIFFERENTIAL DIAGNOSIS

Plasma amino acid concentrations may be normal. The diagnosis can be confirmed with genetic testing. Outcomes or treatment attempts have not been reported.

## GLUTAMINE SYNTHASE DEFICIENCY

### PATHOGENESIS, EPIDEMIOLOGY, AND GENETICS

Glutamine synthase deficiency (MIM no. 610015) is a rare disease caused by biallelic genetic defects in the *GLUL* gene on chromosome 1q25.3. It has only been described in a few patients. The insufficient production of glutamine leads to a disruption of fetal development and to postnatal hyperammonemia and a severe developmental disorder.

### CLINICAL MANIFESTATIONS

The original patients presented at birth with necrotizing erythema, severe enteropathy, brain malformation, encephalopathy, and intractable seizures and died from multiorgan failure. A purely neurologic presentation with seizures and a global developmental disorder has also been described.

### DIAGNOSIS INCLUDING DIFFERENTIAL DIAGNOSIS

The diagnosis can be suspected upon finding moderate hyperammonemia with low glutamine and glutamate concentrations in plasma and CSF amino acids. It can be confirmed by enzyme activity measurements in lymphocytes and genetic testing.

### TREATMENT AND PROGNOSIS

Severe glutamine synthase deficiency is not compatible with survival. Attenuated cases may benefit from L-glutamine supplementation.

### SUGGESTED READINGS


Acuna-Hidalgo R, Schanze D, Kariminejad A, et al. Neu-Laxova syndrome is a heterogeneous metabolic disorder caused by defects in enzymes of the L-Serine biosynthesis pathway. *Am J Hum Genet.* 2014;95:285-293.

Baumgartner MR, Hu CA, Almashanu S, et al. Hyperammonemia with reduced ornithine, citrulline, arginine and proline: a new inborn error caused by a mutation in the gene encoding delta(1)-pyrroline-5-carboxylate synthase. *Hum Mol Genet.* 2000;9:2853-2858.

Coutelier M, Goizet C, Durr A, et al. Alteration of ornithine metabolism leads to dominant and recessive hereditary spastic paraplegia. *Brain.* 2015;138:2191-2205.

Haberle J, Gorg B, Rutsch F, et al. Congenital glutamine deficiency with glutamine synthetase mutations. *N Eng J Med.* 2005;353:1926-1933.

Haberle J, Shahbeck N, Ibrahim K, et al. Natural course of glutamine synthetase deficiency in a 3 year old patient. *Mol Genet Metab.* 2011;103:89-91.

Lin D-S, Chang J-H, Liu H-L, et al. Compound heterozygous mutations in PYCR1 further expand the phenotypic spectrum of de Barsy syndrome. *Am J Med Genet.* 2011;155A:3095-3099.

Reversade B, Escande-Beillard N, Dimopoulou A, et al. Mutations in PYCR1 cause cutis laxa with progeroid features. *Nat Genet.* 2009;41:1016-1021.

Shaheen R, Rahbeeni Z, Alhashem A. Neu-Laxova syndrome, an inborn error of serine metabolism, is caused by mutations in PHGDH. *Am J Hum Genet.* 2014;94:898-904.

van der Crabben SN, Verhoeven-Duif NM, Brilstra EH, et al. An update on serine deficiency disorders. *J Inherit Metab Dis.* 2013;36:613-619.

Skidmore D L, Chitayat D, Morgan T, et al. Further expansion of the phenotypic spectrum associated with mutations in ALDH18A1, encoding delta-1-pyrroline-5-carboxylate synthase (P5CS). *Am J Med Genet.* 2011;155A:1848-1856.


# 136 Disorders of Metabolism of Lysine and Related Compounds

David M. Koeller

### INTRODUCTION

Lysine is an essential amino acid that can be degraded via 2 alternative pathways. The predominant route is via the saccharopine pathway, with the peroxisomal pipecolic acid pathway playing a relatively minor role. Degradation of lysine through either pathway leads to the formation of α-aminoadipic semialdehyde, which is catabolized to acetyl-coenzyme A (CoA) and enters the tricarboxylic acid (TCA) cycle.

## HYPERLYSINEMIA TYPES I AND II

The first 2 steps in the saccharopine pathway of lysine degradation are catalyzed by α-aminoadipic semialdehyde synthase (AASS), a bifunctional enzyme with both lysine-ketoglutarate reductase and saccharopine dehydrogenase activities. Mutations in the *AASS* gene that affect both activities result in hyperlysinemia type 1, whereas mutations that primarily affect saccharopine dehydrogenase activity result in hyperlysinemia type 2. Types 1 and 2 hyperlysinemia are both associated with a marked elevation of serum lysine and significant lysinuria. Type 2 patients also have elevated urinary saccharopine. Another biochemical feature of hyperlysinemia is elevation of serum and urinary pipecolic acid. Elevation of pipecolic acid also occurs in disorders of peroxisome biogenesis, but in those disorders, there is no associated elevation of lysine. Hyperlysinemia was first identified in patients being evaluated for neurodevelopmental problems but has subsequently been observed in asymptomatic family members and other normal individuals, leading to a consensus that isolated hyperlysinemia does not cause symptoms.

## 2-AMINOADIPIC, 2-OXOADIPIC ACIDURIA

The degradation pathways for lysine, hydroxylysine, and tryptophan converge with the formation of 2-oxoadipic acid, which is converted to glutaryl-CoA by 2-oxoadipic acid dehydrogenase. Mutations in the gene for 2-oxoadipic acid dehydrogenase (*DHTKD1*) result in the accumulation of 2-oxoadipic acid and its transamination product 2-aminoadipic acid. The diagnosis is based on the presence of both 2-oxoadipic and 2-aminoadipic acid in the urine, which are normally present in only trace amounts. It is a very rare disorder, with only 20 to 30 patients reported. Some patients were reported to have significant neurodevelopmental impairment, but the majority have been developmentally normal, suggesting that it is a biochemical abnormality that, like hyperlysinemia, does not cause symptoms.

## GLUTARIC ACIDEMIA TYPE I

Glutaric acidemia type I (GA-I) is an autosomal recessive disorder of lysine, hydroxylysine, and tryptophan metabolism that can result in significant neurologic impairment. GA-I results from mutations in the *GCDH* gene that encodes glutaryl-CoA dehydrogenase (GCDH), a mitochondrial matrix enzyme that catalyzes the conversion of glutaryl-CoA to crotonyl-CoA. The loss of GCDH activity in GA-I results in the accumulation of the neurotoxic metabolites glutaric acid and 3-OH glutaric acid in the blood, urine, and cerebrospinal fluid.

### CLINICAL FEATURES

Patients with GA-I are often macrocephalic at birth and initially show nearly normal achievement of early developmental milestones. However, untreated patients usually develop progressive dystonia and dyskinesia within the first 3 years of life. Symptoms may have a gradual onset and progression, but most commonly, there is an acute onset associated with striatal injury that occurs during a metabolic crisis resulting from a febrile illness, a febrile reaction to a vaccination, or other metabolic stresses. Degeneration of the caudate and putamen of the basal ganglia, widening of the Sylvian fissures, and frontotemporal atrophy are commonly demonstrable by brain imaging. Pathologically the most characteristic feature of GA-I is a loss of neurons in the caudate and putamen. Severe spongiform change in the white matter is also commonly observed. Following the implementation of tandem mass spectrometry (MS/MS)-based newborn screening, allowing for the presymptomatic identification and treatment of affected infants, the neurologic outcome of patients with GA-I has markedly improved. The majority of infants identified by newborn screening never experience an acute metabolic crisis and avoid the striatal damage that results in dystonia and other dyskinesia.

### TREATMENT

GA-I is an intoxication-type inborn error of metabolism, a group of diseases that includes urea cycle disorders, organic acidurias, and maple syrup urine disease. Common features of these disorders include a risk for metabolic decompensation with the accumulation of toxic metabolites, and a high risk for neurodevelopmental impairments. Treatment is with a low-protein diet. The primary goal of dietary treatment for GA-I is to reduce the intake of lysine, which is the predominant source of the neurotoxic glutaric and 3-OH glutaric acids that accumulate in affected patients. This is typically accomplished using specialized infant formula lacking lysine and tryptophan that is then supplemented with standard infant formula to provide adequate lysine and tryptophan for growth. Carnitine is also used in order to prevent secondary carnitine depletion and to promote the detoxification of glutaric acid via the formation nontoxic glutaryl-carnitine. Increased formation of glutaryl-carnitine may also prevent intracellular CoA deficiency resulting from the accumulation of glutaryl-CoA. Another key aspect of the treatment of GA-I is aggressive emergency management during periods of increased risk for catabolism, typically during childhood infections. This includes providing intravenous (IV) glucose, reduction of protein intake but maintenance of adequate caloric intake, and fluid therapy to maintain normal hydration and electrolyte balance. Several international studies have shown that this approach to treatment is highly effective when started prior to the onset of neurologic symptoms. It has been argued that arginine intake should be increased to compete with lysine uptake into the brain through their shared transporter, but this remains unsettled.

A peculiar feature of GA-I is that the characteristic acute striatal injury rarely occurs after 3 years of age and has never been reported after age 6. As a result, current treatment guidelines allow for a relaxation of the strict dietary lysine restriction after age 6 years. Due to concern that episodes of catabolism even after age 6 could may cause subclinical neurologic damage, aggressive emergency management with IV glucose may be beneficial, although currently there is no evidence in support of this approach.

### DIAGNOSIS

Elevation of glutaryl-carnitine (C5DC) in newborn blood spots can be detected by MS/MS-based newborn screening. However, some patients, known as low excretors, may have normal or only intermittent elevation of C5DC, which can make ascertainment by newborn screening difficult. For the same reason, measuring serum or urine glutaric and 3-OH glutaric acid levels may not be relied on for confirmation of a positive newborn screen. Definitive diagnosis can be obtained via either DNA analysis of the *GCDH* gene or measurement of GCDH activity in cultured fibroblasts or white blood cells.

Patients with GA-I rarely develop a metabolic acidosis or other biochemical abnormalities that typically lead to testing for disorders of organic acid metabolism. Therefore, recognition of the characteristic clinical signs and symptoms of GA-I is critical in order to make the diagnosis. Urinary organic acid analysis and quantitation of serum acylcarnitines can be used to screen patients suspected to have GA-I based on clinical symptoms. Most have elevation of urinary glutaric and 3-OH glutaric acid, as well as increased serum glutaryl-carnitine. However, these tests may miss low excretors, particularly when in a well state; therefore, DNA and/or enzyme testing can be done if the clinical suspicion is high.

Prenatal diagnosis of an affected fetus can be made by measuring enzyme activity in cultured amniocytes or chorionic villus cells, or by demonstrating increased glutaric acid in amniotic fluid. However, DNA testing is the preferred method for prenatal diagnosis when the familial mutations are known.

### D- AND L-2-HYDROXYGLUTARIC ACIDEMIAS

The neurologic damage that occurs in patients with GA-I results from the toxic effects of glutaric and 3-OH glutaric acids. A related compound, 2-hydroxyglutaric acid, accumulates in 4 inherited metabolic disorders that are also associated with neurologic damage. There are 2 enantiomers of 2-hydroxygluturate (D-2-hydroxyglutarate and L-2-hydroxyglutarate), which are both derived from 2-ketogluturate, a TCA cycle intermediate with no direct link to lysine metabolism.

### CLINICAL MANIFESTATIONS

L-2-Hydroxyglutaric aciduria (L-2HG) is an autosomal recessive disorder resulting from mutations in the gene for L-2-hydroxyglutarate dehydrogenase (*L2HGDH*). Patients typically present with neurodevelopmental impairment and/or seizures during childhood. Symptoms are progressive and may also include macrocephaly and signs of extrapyramidal and cerebellar dysfunction. Brain imaging is highly characteristic and includes predominantly subcortical cerebral white matter changes and abnormalities of the basal ganglia. In later stages, the cerebral white matter and basal ganglia abnormalities become more diffuse, and there is atrophy of the cerebral white matter. Patients have an increased risk for brain malignancies, particularly gliomas, indicating that hydroxyglutaric acid functions as an oncometabolite when elevated.

There are 2 types of D-2-hydroxyglutaric aciduria (D-2HG). Type 1 is an autosomal recessive disease caused by mutations in the D-2-hydroxyglutarate dehydrogenase gene (*D2HGDH*). Type 2 is an autosomal dominant disorder associated with gain-of-function mutations in the *IDH2* gene that encodes the mitochondrial TCA cycle enzyme isocitrate dehydrogenase. Type 1 patients usually present within the first 6 years of life with developmental delay, hypotonia, and seizures. Type 2 patients have similar symptoms but typically have an earlier onset (≤ 2 years), with a more severe and progressive course. Cardiomyopathy is a unique feature of type 2. There is significant variability in the severity of symptoms in type 1 patients, including within families. Neuroimaging features include enlargement of the lateral ventricles and frontal subarachnoid spaces, subdural effusions, subependymal pseudocysts, signs of delayed cerebral maturation, and multifocal cerebral white matter abnormalities.

Mutations in the gene for the mitochondrial citrate carrier (*SLC25A1*) result in the accumulation of both D- and L-2-hydroxyglutarate.

This autosomal recessive disorder has a neonatal onset with symptoms that may include profound psychomotor retardation, hypotonia, seizures, microcephaly, sensorineural hearing loss, agenesis of the corpus callosum, and optic atrophy. Early death (< 2 years) is typical.

## DIAGNOSIS

Both L- and D-2-hydroxyglutaric acid can be measured in the blood, urine, and cerebrospinal fluid by organic acid analysis using gas chromatography–mass spectrometry. However, differentiation between the D and L isomers of 2-hydroxyglutaric acid requires special techniques available only in a few referral labs. Levels of 2-hydroxyglutarate are highest in patients with type 2 D-2HG, but overlap in the other 3 disorders. A unique finding in L-2HG is a modest (2–5-fold) elevation of lysine in the plasma and cerebrospinal fluid. Patients with combined D- and L-2HG have abnormalities of Krebs cycle intermediates in the urine, including reduced citrate and isocitrate, and elevated fumarate, succinate, and 2-ketoglutarate. The definitive diagnosis of all 4 disorders can be made by DNA testing.

## SUGGESTED READINGS


Boy N, Mühlhausen C, Maier EM, et al. Proposed recommendations for the diagnosis and management of individuals with glutaric aciduria type I – second revision. *J Inherit Metab Dis*. 2017;40(1):75-101.

Danhauser K, Sauer SW, Haack TB, et al. DHTKD1 mutations cause 2-aminoadipic and 2-oxoadipic aciduria. *Am J Hum Genet*. 2012;91(6):1082-1087.

Edvardson S, Porcelli V, Jalas C, et al. Agenesis of corpus callosum and optic nerve hypoplasia due to mutations in SLC25A1 encoding the mitochondrial citrate transporter. *J Med Genet*. 2013;50(4):240-245.

Houten SM, Te Brinke H, Denis S, et al. Genetic basis of hyperlysinemia. *Orphanet J Rare Dis*. 2013;8:57.

Houten SM, te Brinke H, Denis S, et al. Genetic basis of hyperlysinemia. *Orphanet J Rare Dis*. 2013;8(1):1-8.

Kranendijk M, Struys EA, van Schaftingen E, et al. IDH2 mutations in patients with D-2-hydroxyglutaric aciduria. *Science*. 2010;330(6002):336.

Sacksteder KA, Biery BJ, Morrell JC, et al. Identification of the alpha-aminoadipic semialdehyde synthase gene, which is defective in familial hyperlysinemia. *Am J Hum Genet*. 2000;66(6):1736-1743.

Steenweg ME, Salomons GS, Yapici Z, et al. L-2-Hydroxyglutaric aciduria: pattern of MR imaging abnormalities in 56 patients. *Radiology*. 2009;251(3):856-865.

Struys EA, Salomons GS, Achouri Y, et al. Mutations in the D-2-hydroxyglutarate dehydrogenase gene cause D-2-hydroxyglutaric aciduria. *Am J Hum Genet*. 2005;76(2):358-360.

Vilarinho L, Cardoso ML, Gaspar P, et al. Novel L2HGDH mutations in 21 patients with L-2-hydroxyglutaric aciduria of Portuguese origin. *Hum Mutat*. 2005;26(4):395-396.


# 137 Disorders of Metabolism of Neurotransmitter Amino Acids

Brett H. Graham and Eva Morava Kozicz

## INTRODUCTION

This chapter describes inherited disorders affecting the catabolism of γ-aminobutyric acid (GABA), those affecting receptors for neurotransmitters (GABA and glycine), and those affecting the metabolism of monoamines. Other disorders that impinge on metabolism of neurotransmitter amino acids are described elsewhere in the textbook. (Glutamine synthase deficiency is discussed in Chapter 135, pyridoxine responsive disorders in Chapter 144, and glycine/serine disorders in Chapters 134 and 135).

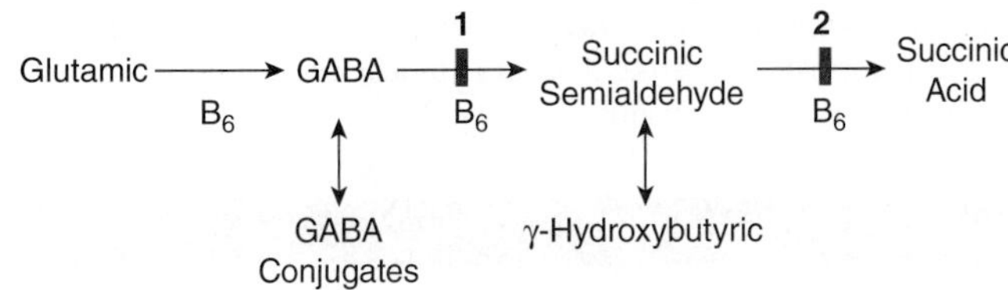


**FIGURE 137-1** Brain metabolism of γ-aminobutyric acid (GABA). 1 = GABA transaminase; 2 = succinic semialdehyde dehydrogenase. Enzyme defects are indicated by solid red bars. $B_6$, pyridoxal phosphate coenzyme.

Two genetic defects are known in GABA catabolism (Fig. 137-1): GABA transaminase deficiency and succinic semialdehyde dehydrogenase (SSADH) deficiency.

Hyperekplexia, characterized by neonatal hypertonia and excessive startle responses, is caused by defects in glycerinergic neurotransmission and is genetically heterogeneous. Mutations in genes encoding various $GABA_A$ receptor subunits cause various types of epilepsy.

Nine defects have been reported in the metabolism of monoamines (Figs. 137-2 and 137-3): five in the synthesis of the cofactor tetrahydrobiopterin, tyrosine-hydroxylase (TH) deficiency, aromatic amino acid decarboxylase (AADC) deficiency, dopamine β-hydroxylase (DBH) deficiency, and monoamine oxidase A (MAO-A) deficiency. In addition, 2 disorders affecting monoamine transport have been described: dopamine transporter deficiency syndrome (DTDS) and vesicular monoamine transporter disease (VMAT2). All are associated with neurologic symptoms except DBH deficiency (orthostatic hypotension). With the exception of MAO-A deficiency, most disorders can be at least partially ameliorated with pharmacotherapeutic approaches.

## DEFECTS OF GABA CATABOLISM

## GABA TRANSAMINASE DEFICIENCY

### CLINICAL PRESENTATION

GABA transaminase deficiency was first reported in 1984 in a Flemish family in association with severe neonatal/early infantile epileptic encephalopathy and growth acceleration. The extremely rare disease

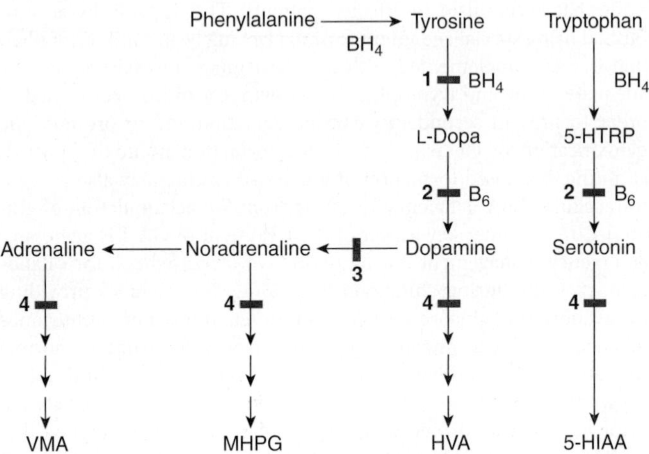


**FIGURE 137-2** Monoamine metabolism. 1 = tyrosine hydroxylase; 2 = aromatic L-amino acid decarboxylase; 3 = dopamine β-hydroxylase; 4 = monoamine oxidase. Enzyme defects are indicated by solid red bars. $B_6$, pyridoxal phosphate coenzyme; $BH_4$, tetrahydrobiopterin; 5-HIAA, 5-hydroxyindole acetic acid; 5-HTRP, 5-hydroxytryptophan; HVA, homovanillic acid; MHPG, 3-methoxy-4-hydroxyphenylglycol; VMA, vanillylmandelic acid.

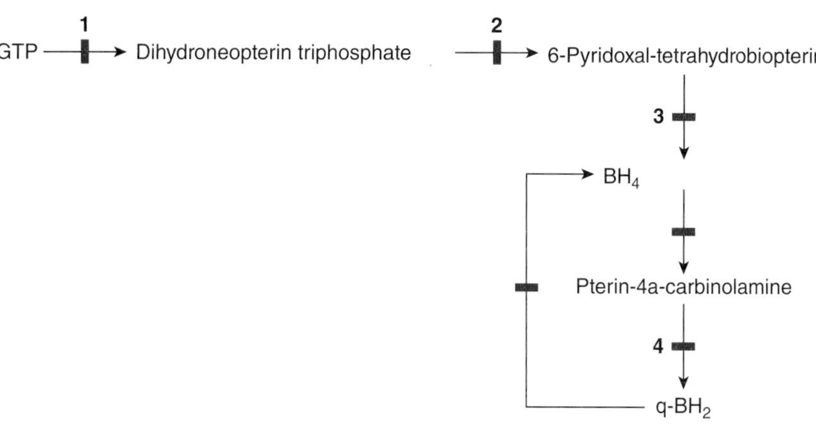


**FIGURE 137-3** Tetrahydrobiopterin metabolism. 1 = GTP cyclohydrolase (GTPCH); 2 = 6-pyruvoyl tetrahydropterin synthase (PTPS); 3 = sepiapterin reductase (SR); 4 = pterincarbinolamine reductase (PCBD); 5 = dihydropterin reductase (DHPR). Enzyme defects are indicated by solid red bars. $BH_4$, tetrahydrobiopterin; GTP, guanosine triphosphate; q-$BH_2$, quinonoid dihydrobiopterin.

has been confirmed in 3 unrelated patients and an older sibling of 1 of these patients who died at the age of 1 year. The siblings also showed feeding difficulties from birth, often necessitating gavage feeding; profound axial hypotonia; and generalized convulsions. Hyperreflexia was present during the first 6 to 8 months. Psychomotor development was nearly absent. Growth acceleration was present from birth, due to hypersecretion of growth hormone. Postmortem examination of the brain showed spongiform leukodystrophy.

### METABOLIC DERANGEMENT

Deficiency of GABA transaminase is associated with decreased catabolism of GABA (see Fig. 137-1) and perturbation of mitochondrial nucleotide salvage. The concentrations of GABA, GABA conjugates, and β-alanine in the cerebrospinal fluid (CSF) and plasma are increased. β-Alanine is an alternative substrate for GABA transaminase, which explains its increase in this disease. Disruption of mitochondrial nucleotide salvage disrupts efficient synthesis of mitochondrial DNA (mtDNA) and causes its depletion (leading to a secondary defect in mitochondrial oxidative phosphorylation), which has been demonstrated in primary fibroblasts derived from a patient with GABA transaminase deficiency.

### GENETICS

GABA transaminase deficiency (Mendelian Inheritance in Man [MIM] no. 137150) is an autosomal recessive disease, and GABA transaminase is encoded by *ABAT* on chromosome 16p13.3.

### DIAGNOSIS

Biochemical diagnosis requires analysis of amino acid in the CSF. Since levels of free GABA in the CSF are low, sensitive techniques must be used, such as ion-exchange chromatography with fluorescence detection, a stable isotope dilution technique, or magnetic resonance spectroscopy. Enzymatic confirmation is obtained using lymphocytes, lymphoblasts, or liver tissue. Prenatal diagnosis is possible by enzymatic analysis of chorionic villus tissue, but not of amniocytes, or by molecular testing when pathogenic variants have been identified. Molecular diagnosis is now often the primary diagnostic test, predominantly through whole-exome sequencing given the high degree of genetic locus heterogeneity of early infantile epileptic encephalopathy.

### TREATMENT

No effective treatment is available. Pyridoxine (up to 3 × 1 g/d) and picrotoxin (up to 0.12 mg/kg/d) have been used in the index case of GABA-T deficiency without evidence of improvement. The siblings died at the ages of 1, 2, and 7 years.

## SUCCINIC SEMIALDEHYDE DEHYDROGENASE DEFICIENCY

### CLINICAL PRESENTATION

Succinic semialdehyde dehydrogenase (SSADH) deficiency was first reported in 1981 and has been documented in hundreds of patients. The clinical picture ranges from mild to severe and usually comprises psychomotor retardation, delayed speech development, cognitive impairment, hypotonia, and ataxia. Less frequent features are convulsions, aggressive behavior, oculomotor apraxia, choreoathetosis, and nystagmus. Neuropsychiatric features (hyperkinetic behavior, aggression, self-injurious behaviors, and hallucinations), epilepsy, and sleep disturbances are present in approximately 50% of patients. Ataxia may resolve with age. Brain magnetic resonance imaging (MR) may demonstrate abnormalities of the basal ganglia, delayed myelination, and cerebellar atrophy.

### METABOLIC DERANGEMENT

SSADH converts succinic semialdehyde (the product of GABA transaminase) to succinic acid (see Fig. 137-1). SSADH deficiency results in an increase of γ-hydroxybutyrate (4-hydroxybutyric acid) in body fluids and is the biochemical hallmark of the disease. This accumulation tends to decrease with age. Other compounds such as metabolites of the α- and β-oxidation of γ-hydroxybutyrate are variably increased. The latter (glycolic acid, which is converted to glycine) is a pharmacologically active compound, which may explain at least part of the symptomatology.

### GENETICS

SSADH deficiency is an autosomal recessive disease, and SSADH is encoded by *ALDH5A1* (MIM no. 610045) on chromosome 6p22.

### DIAGNOSIS

Biochemical diagnosis is made by analysis of organic acids in bodily fluids. One must consider that γ-hydroxybutyrate is unstable in urine and that, in some patients, the excretion of this compound is only modestly increased. The enzyme deficiency can be demonstrated in lymphocytes and lymphoblasts. Prenatal diagnosis can be performed by isotope-dilution mass spectrometry to measure γ-hydroxybutyric acid levels in amniotic fluid and determination of SSADH activity in amniocytes or chorionic villus tissue (or by molecular testing when pathogenic variants have been identified). Molecular diagnosis is now often the primary diagnostic test, predominantly through whole-exome sequencing given the high degree of heterogeneity of the genetic loci for neurodevelopmental disorders.

### TREATMENT

No clearly effective therapy is available for SSADH deficiency. The major goal of current treatment is partial amelioration of the most disabling symptoms (ie, seizures and neurobehavioral disturbances, especially obsessive-compulsive and anxiety disorders in SSADH deficiency). Novel treatment strategies including targeting of oxidative damage and $GABA_B$ receptor antagonism are currently under investigation.

## DEFECTS OF NEUROTRANSMITTER RECEPTORS

## HYPEREKPLEXIA

### CLINICAL PRESENTATION

Hyperekplexia (startle disease) is characterized by 3 main symptoms: (1) generalized stiffness immediately after birth, which gradually normalizes during the first years of life; (2) an excessive startle reflex to unexpected, particularly auditory, stimuli; and (3) short-lived generalized stiffness preventing voluntary movements following the startle response. There may be associated features such as periodic limb movements in sleep and hypnagogic (occurring when falling asleep) myoclonus.

### METABOLIC DERANGEMENT

Hyperekplexia is associated with perturbations of glycinergic neurotransmission. Most patients show a defect in the $\alpha_1$ subunit of the glycine receptor. Others have a defect in the β subunit, in receptor-associated proteins, or in the presynaptic glycine transporter. A hypothesis for the underlying pathogenic mechanism for hyperekplexia is that an elevated intracellular chloride concentration late in neuronal development ablates α1β glycinergic synapses but spares GABAergic synapses.

### GENETICS

Hyperekplexia can be inherited in an autosomal dominant, autosomal recessive, or X-linked pattern. The genes for the $\alpha_1$ subunit (*GLRA1*, MIM no. 138491) and the β subunit (*GLRB*, MIM no. 138492) are on chromosome 5q33 and chromosome 4q31.3, respectively. The genes encoding the receptor-associated proteins gephyrin (*GPHN*, MIM no. 603930) and Rho guanine nucleotide exchange factor 9 (*ARHGEF9*, MIM no. 300429) are on chromosomes 14q23.3-q24.1 and Xq11.1, respectively. The gene encoding the presynaptic sodium- and chloride-dependent glycine transporter 2 (*SLC6A5*, MIM no. 604159) is on chromosome 11p15.1.

### DIAGNOSIS

The diagnosis can be made through molecular testing (eg, gene panels or whole-exome sequencing given the genetic heterogeneity) and the response to treatment: clonazepam reduces the frequency and magnitude of startle responses. It binds to the benzodiazepine site of the $GABA_A$ receptor.

### TREATMENT

The stiffness decreases during the first years of life, but the excessive startle responses remain. The favorable effect of clonazepam on the startle response is mentioned under "Diagnosis" above.

## $GABA_A$ RECEPTOR DEFECT

### CLINICAL PRESENTATION

Mutations in a $GABA_A$ receptor subunit were first reported in 2001 in 2 large families, 1 with febrile seizures and generalized tonic-clonic seizures and the other with febrile seizures, childhood absence epilepsy, and other forms of epilepsy. It is a rare form of dominantly inherited epilepsy. The associated phenotypes range from early infantile to childhood absence epilepsy and juvenile myoclonic epileptic encephalopathy.

### METABOLIC DERANGEMENT

Mutations of $GABA_A$ receptor subunits disturb assembly and intracellular trafficking of intact $GABA_A$ receptors to the plasma membrane at synapses, thereby causing seizures by disrupting GABA-dependent fast inhibitory synaptic transmission, predominantly in the gray matter of the central nervous system.

### GENETICS

There is a superfamily of 19 proteins that can comprise subunits of the $GABA_A$ receptor. Heterozygous pathogenic variants in genes encoding 6 of these subunits have been associated with epilepsies to date, making $GABA_A$ receptor–related epilepsy an autosomal dominant disorder. The affected genes include *GABRA1* (MIM no. 137160, chromosome 5q34), *GABRB1* (MIM no. 137190, chromosome 4p12), *GABRB2* (MIM no. 600232, chromosome 5q34), *GABRB3* (MIM no. 137192, chromosome 15q12), *GABRG2* (MIM no. 137164, chromosome 5q34), and *GABRD* (MIM no. 137163, chromosome 1p36.33).

### DIAGNOSIS

The diagnosis is based on molecular analysis of the receptor genes, typically by whole-exome sequencing or multigene panel testing given the genetic heterogeneity of epilepsy.

### TREATMENT

Patients often respond to benzodiazepines. The prognosis is largely determined by the type of epilepsy and febrile seizures.

## MONOAMINE METABOLISM DEFECTS

Among the 11 known defects in monoamine metabolism, only tyrosine hydroxylase deficiency will be described in detail; the others are summarized in Table 137-1.

## TYROSINE HYDROXYLASE DEFICIENCY

### CLINICAL PRESENTATION

Tyrosine hydroxylase (TH) deficiency results in a broad phenotypic spectrum that can manifest as mild (TH-deficient dopa-responsive dystonia), moderately severe (TH-deficient infantile parkinsonism), and very severe (TH-deficient progressive infantile encephalopathy) forms. Most patients with TH-deficient dopa-responsive dystonia present between 1 and 12 years of age with lower limb dystonia and difficulty walking, with diurnal fluctuations of symptoms that are worse at night and with improvement in the morning following sleep. With TH-deficient infantile parkinsonism, patients typically present in their first year of life with truncal or generalized hypotonia and delayed motor development that, in combination with the hypotonia, may mimic a primary neuromuscular disorder. Classical extrapyramidal signs also generally appear during infancy. A hypokinetic-rigid parkinsonian syndrome can develop. Patients with TH-deficient progressive infantile encephalopathy present before 6 months of age with severe motor delay, hypokinesia, truncal hypotonia, and limb hypertonia. Encephalopathy often persists and progresses into intellectual disability.

### METABOLIC DERANGEMENT

TH converts tyrosine into L-dopa, the direct precursor of catecholamine biosynthesis (see Fig. 137-2). It is a rate-limiting step in this biosynthesis pathway. The enzyme is expressed in the brain and in the adrenal glands, and tetrohydrobiopterin ($BH_4$) is an essential cofactor. The biochemical hallmarks of the disease are low levels of homovanillic acid (HVA) and 3-methoxy-4-hydroxyphenylethyleneglycol (MHPG), the catabolites of dopamine and norepinephrine, respectively, in the CSF. In addition, 5-hydroxyindoleacetic acid (5-HIAA) levels are normal, and serotonin metabolism is unaffected.

**TABLE 137-1 DEFECTS OF MONOAMINE METABOLISM**

| | Clinical Presentation | Metabolic Derangement | Genetics | Diagnostic Tests | Treatment |
|---|---|---|---|---|---|
| GTPCH-I defect | Dopa-responsive dystonia | Defective biosynthesis of serotonin and catecholamines | AR/AD; MIM: 600225 | Amines and pterines in CSF; enzyme activity in fibroblasts; mutation analysis | Low-dose L-dopa + dopa-decarboxylase inhibitor + 5-OH-tryptophan |
| PTPS defect | Psychomotor retardation, abnormal tone and movements, irritability, lethargy, seizures, poor temperature control, microcephaly | Defective biosynthesis of serotonin and catecholamines | AR; MIM: 261640 | Amines and pterines in CSF; enzyme activity in fibroblasts; mutation analysis | Low-dose L-dopa + dopa-decarboxylase inhibitor + 5-OH-tryptophan, eventual folinic acid supplement |
| SR defect | Psychomotor retardation, abnormal tone and movements, irritability, lethargy, seizures, poor temperature control, microcephaly | Defective biosynthesis of serotonin and catecholamines | AR; MIM: 182125 | Amines and pterines in CSF; enzyme activity in fibroblasts; mutation analysis | Low-dose L-dopa + dopa-decarboxylase inhibitor + 5-OH-tryptophan |
| DHPR defect | Psychomotor retardation, abnormal tone and movements, irritability, lethargy, seizures, poor temperature control, microcephaly | Defective biosynthesis of serotonin and catecholamines | AR; MIM: 261630 | Amines and pterines in CSF; enzyme activity in blood; mutation analysis | Low-dose L-dopa + dopa-decarboxylase inhibitor + 5-OH-tryptophan + folinic acid supplement |
| PCBD defect | Mild and transient neurologic symptoms | Defective biosynthesis of serotonin and catecholamines | AR; MIM: 126090 | Amines and pterines in CSF, enzyme activity in fibroblasts; mutation analysis | < 1 y: BH4; > 1 y: no effective treatment |
| AADC defect | Psychomotor retardation, abnormal tone and movements, epilepsy, autonomic dysfunction | Deficient biosynthesis of serotonin and catecholamines; increased L-dopa and 5-OH-tryptophan | AR; MIM: 608643 | Amines in CSF, enzyme activity in plasma; mutation analysis | Bromocriptine + trihexyphenidyl + tranylcypromine |
| DBH defect | Orthostatic hypotension, variable other symptoms | Deficient biosynthesis of noradrenaline | AR; MIM: 609312 | Noradrenaline and dopamine in plasma; enzyme activity in plasma; mutation analysis | L-Dihydrophenylserine |
| MAO-A defect | Borderline intellectual disability, psychiatric symptoms | Deficient catabolism of serotonin and catecholamine metabolites | X-linked MIM: 309850 | Amines in urine | No treatment |
| DTDS | Irritability, axial hypotonia, hypokinetic parkinsonism-dystonia | Defect in dopamine transporter that reuptakes dopamine from synapse | *SLC6A3*; AR; MIM: 126455 | Elevated HVA:5-HIAA ratio (> 5, normal range 1.3–4) in CSF | No effective treatment |
| VMAT2 | Severe parkinsonism, dystonia, and oculogyric crisis | Defect in packaging of dopamine and serotonin into vesicles for synaptic transmission | *SLC18A2*; AR; MIM: 193001 | Elevated HVA and 5-HIAA in urine; low norepinephrine and dopamine in urine | Pramipexole (dopamine agonist) |

AADC, aromatic amino acid decarboxylase; AD, autosomal dominant; AR, autosomal recessive; BH4, tetrahydrobiopterin; CSF, cerebrospinal fluid; DBH, dopamine beta hydroxylase; DHPR, dihydropterine reductase; DTDS, dopamine transporter deficiency syndrome; GTPCH-1, guanosine triphosphate cyclohydrolase; 5-HIAA, 5-hydroxyindole acetic acid; HVA, homovanillic acid; MAO, monoamine oxidase; MIM, Mendelian Inheritance in Man; PCBD, pterin-4 alpha-carbinolamine dehydratase; PTPS, protein tyrosine phosphatase; SR, sarcoplasmic reticulum; VMAT2, vesicular monoamine transporter 2.

## GENETICS

TH (*TH*, MIM no. 191290) is located on chromosome 11p15.5, and the deficiency is inherited in an autosomal recessive fashion. Founder (common) pathogenic variants have been reported for the Dutch (c.698G>A; p.Arg233His) and Greek (c.707T>C; p.Leu236Pro) populations.

## DIAGNOSIS

The most important biochemical diagnostic test is the measurement of HVA, MHPG, and 5-HIAA in the CSF. Urinary measurements are not reliable in the diagnosis of this disorder. Tyrosine and phenylalanine levels are usually normal in the bodily fluids of these patients. Enzyme measurement is not a diagnostic option as there is no enzyme activity detectable in bodily fluids, blood cells, and fibroblasts. Molecular diagnosis can be obtained by single gene testing, multigene panel testing, or whole-exome sequencing.

## TREATMENT

In most cases, TH deficiency can be treated with low-dose L-dopa in combination with an L-dopa decarboxylase inhibitor. However, the response is variable and ranges from complete remission to no improvement, with the milder deficiency being responsive. Therapy should be started with low-dose L-dopa (initial dose 0.5–3 mg/kg/d in 3 divided doses), since these patients are very prone to significant side effects even on low doses (mainly irritability, dyskinesia, and ballism), particularly for the more severe forms.

## SUGGESTED READINGS


Besse A, Wu P, Bruni F, et al. The GABA transaminase, ABAT, is essential for mitochondrial nucleoside metabolism. *Cell Metab.* 2015;21:417-427.

Furukawa Y, Kish S. Tyrosine hydroxylase deficiency. In: Pagon RA, Adam MP, Ardinger HH, et al, eds. *GeneReviews*. Seattle, WA: University of Washington; 2017.

Hirose S. Mutant GABA(A) receptor subunits in genetic (idiopathic) epilepsy. *Prog Brain Res.* 2014;213:55-85.

Lachance-Touchette P, Brown P, Meloche C, et al. Novel alpha-1 and gamma-2 GABA-A receptor subunit mutations in families with idiopathic generalized epilepsy. *Eur J Neurosci.* 2011;34:237-249.

Malaspina P, Roullet JB, Pearl PL, et al. Succinic semialdehyde dehydrogenase deficiency (SSADHD): pathophysiological complexity and multifactorial trait associations in a rare monogenic disorder of GABA metabolism. *Neurochem Int.* 2016;99:72-84.

Marecos C, Ng J, Kurian MA. What is new for monoamine neurotransmitter disorders? *J Inherit Metab Dis.* 2014;37:619-626.

Parviz M, Vogel K, Gibson KM, Pearl PL. Disorders of GABA metabolism: SSADH and GABA-transaminase deficiencies. *J Pediatr Epilepsy.* 2014;3:217-227.

Thomas RH, Chung SK, Wood SE, et al. Genotype-phenotype correlations in hyperekplexia: apneas, learning difficulties and speech delay. *Brain.* 2013;136:3085-3095.

Zhang Y, Bode A, Nguyen B, Keramidas A, Lynch JW. Investigating the mechanism by which gain-of-function mutations to the α1 glycine receptor cause hyperekplexia. *J Biol Chem.* 2016;291:15332-15341.

# 138 Disorders of Creatine and Ornithine Metabolism

Sylvia Stockler-Ipsiroglu



## CREATINE METABOLISM

Creatine is both ingested in the diet and synthesized mainly in the liver and pancreas by the action of arginine:glycine amidinotransferase (AGAT) and guanidinoacetate methyltransferase (GAMT), with arginine, glycine, and *S*-adenosyl methionine as essential substrates (Fig. 138-1). AGAT catalyzes the first of the two reactions involved in the de novo synthesis of creatine. This reaction uses arginine and glycine as substrates and yields guanidinoacetate and ornithine as products. Guanidinoacetate is further converted to creatine by the action of GAMT, using *S*-adenosylmethionine as a methyl group donor, with this reaction consuming a significant fraction of all methyl groups. Creatine reaches muscle and brain via an active transmembrane creatine transport system (CRTR). Creatine is then used in the cellular pool of creatine/creatine-phosphate, which together with creatine kinase and adenosine triphosphate (ATP)/adenosine diphosphate (ADP) provides a high-energy phosphate buffering system. Intracellular creatine and creatine phosphate are nonenzymatically converted to creatinine, with a daily turnover rate of 1.5%. Creatinine is excreted in urine, and the daily urinary creatinine excretion is directly proportional to total body creatine.

Creatine deficiency syndromes represent a group of inborn errors of metabolism, including disorders of creatine synthesis (AGAT; Mendelian Inheritance in Man [MIM] no. 602360) and GAMT (MIM no. 601240) deficiency and disorders of creatine transport, including the X-linked transmembrane creatine transporter (X-CRTR; MIM no. 300036) deficiency. Inheritance of GAMT and AGAT deficiency is autosomal recessive, whereas the gene for X-CRTR deficiency (*SLC6A8*) is located on the X chromosome. GAMT and AGAT deficiency are rare disorders, whereas X-CRTR deficiency has been diagnosed in up to 2% of patients who have X-linked intellectual disability. This frequency is comparable to the frequency of fragile X syndrome, which constitutes a rather frequent cause of X-linked intellectual disability.

### CLINICAL PRESENTATION

The main symptoms observed in all 3 creatine deficiency syndromes are intellectual disability with pronounced speech delay, autistic behavior, and seizures. To date, 16 patients have been described with AGAT deficiency. The presenting features included poor growth, delayed psychomotor and language development, and occasional seizures. Patients with GAMT deficiency may exhibit a more complex clinical phenotype, including intractable epilepsy, extrapyramidal movement disorder, and abnormal signal intensities of the basal ganglia. The clinical phenotype of X-CRTR deficiency varies from mild to severe intellectual disability associated with speech delay and seizures. Dysmorphic features, microcephaly, and moderate brain atrophy have been described in some patients. Heterozygote females may have learning difficulties. Skewed X-inactivation may cause pronounced

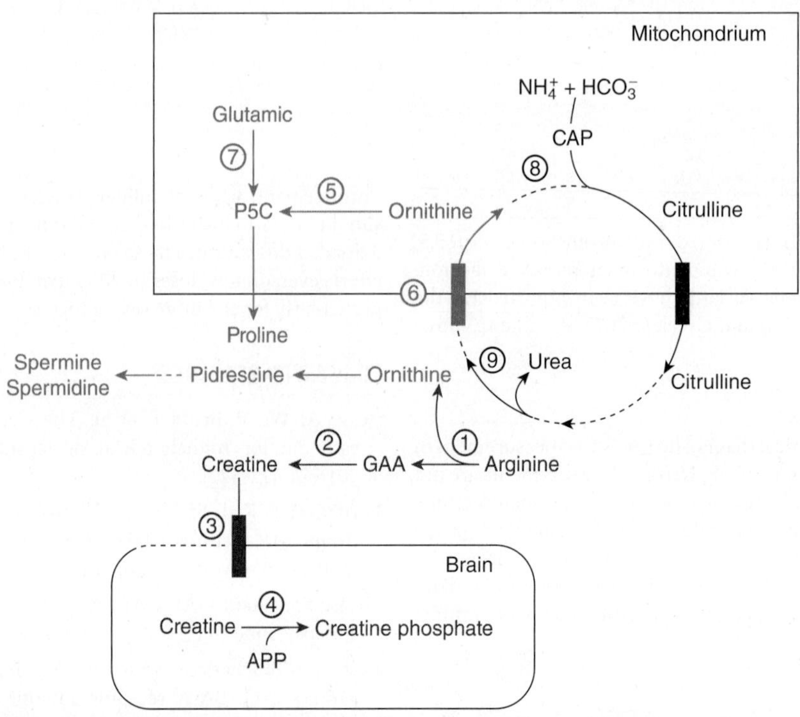


**FIGURE 138-1** Metabolic pathways of creatine and ornithine. 1 = AGAT (arginine:glycine aminotransferase); 2 = GAMT (guanidinoacetate methyltransferase); 3 = X-CRTR (X-linked creatine transporter deficiency, SLC6A8); 4 = CK (creatine kinase); 5 = OAT (ornithine aminotransferase); 6 = ORNT1 (ornithine transporter 1, SLC25A15); 7 = P5CS (pyrroline-5-carboxylate synthase); 8 = OTC (ornithine transcarbamylase); 9 = Arginase. ATP, adenosine triphosphate; CAP, carbamyl phosphate; P5C, pyrroline-5-carboxylate; GAA, guanidinoacetate.

clinical manifestations in these cases similar to the male phenotype. Interestingly, patients with disorders of creatine synthesis and creatine transport do not have signs of cardiomyopathy or significant skeletal myopathy, although muscle tissue appears to be another site of creatine depletion.

## PATHOPHYSIOLOGY

Patients with disorders of creatine synthesis have systemic depletion of creatine and creatine phosphate due to impairment of de novo creatine biosynthesis. Patients with X-CRTR deficiency have an intact de novo synthesis of creatine, but due to impairment of transmembrane creatine transport, they have intracellular depletion of creatine and creatine phosphate, while extracellular (urinary) creatine concentrations are normal or even elevated. The brain is the major site of creatine depletion in all these disorders. Patients with GAMT deficiency have accumulation of guanidinoacetate in addition to creatine deficiency. As guanidinoacetate is neurotoxic in high concentrations, this compound is presumed to play a major role in the pathophysiology of GAMT deficiency.

## DIAGNOSIS

The typical biochemical abnormality of creatine deficiency syndromes is cerebral creatine deficiency, which is demonstrated *by in vivo* proton magnetic resonance spectroscopy. Creatine has a prominent proton magnetic spectrum in the brain, and its deficiency cannot be overlooked (Fig. 138-2).

Guanidinoacetate accumulates in GAMT deficiency and is deficient in AGAT deficiency. Thus, in the face of creatine deficiency, measurement of guanidinoacetate in bodily fluids may discriminate GAMT deficiency (high concentration) from AGAT deficiency (low concentration). In patients with X-CRTR deficiency, the urinary creatine excretion relative to the creatinine excretion is elevated, and an elevated urinary-creatine-to-creatinine ratio can be used as an initial biochemical diagnostic marker for the disease. The diagnosis of all these disorders is confirmed by molecular genetic analysis of the respective genes and by studies of enzyme activities and, in the case of X-CRTR deficiency, creatine uptake. In particular, GAMT and AGAT deficiency is confirmed enzymatically by determining the respective enzyme activities in fibroblasts or virus-transformed lymphoblasts. X-CRTR deficiency is confirmed by creatine uptake studies in cultured fibroblasts.

## TREATMENT

Cerebral creatine deficiency, as caused by disorders of creatine synthesis (GAMT and AGAT deficiency), can be corrected by oral supplementation of creatine monohydrate (400 mg/kg body weight/d). Treatment of GAMT deficiency also requires therapeutic measures to reduce the accumulation of guanidinoacetate. This is mainly achieved by dietary restriction of arginine, which is the rate-limiting substrate to the synthesis of guanidinoacetate. Substitution of ornithine, which competitively inhibits AGAT activity and thus reduces the synthesis of guanidinoacetate, may enhance this effect. Treatment leads to substantial clinical benefit, including significant

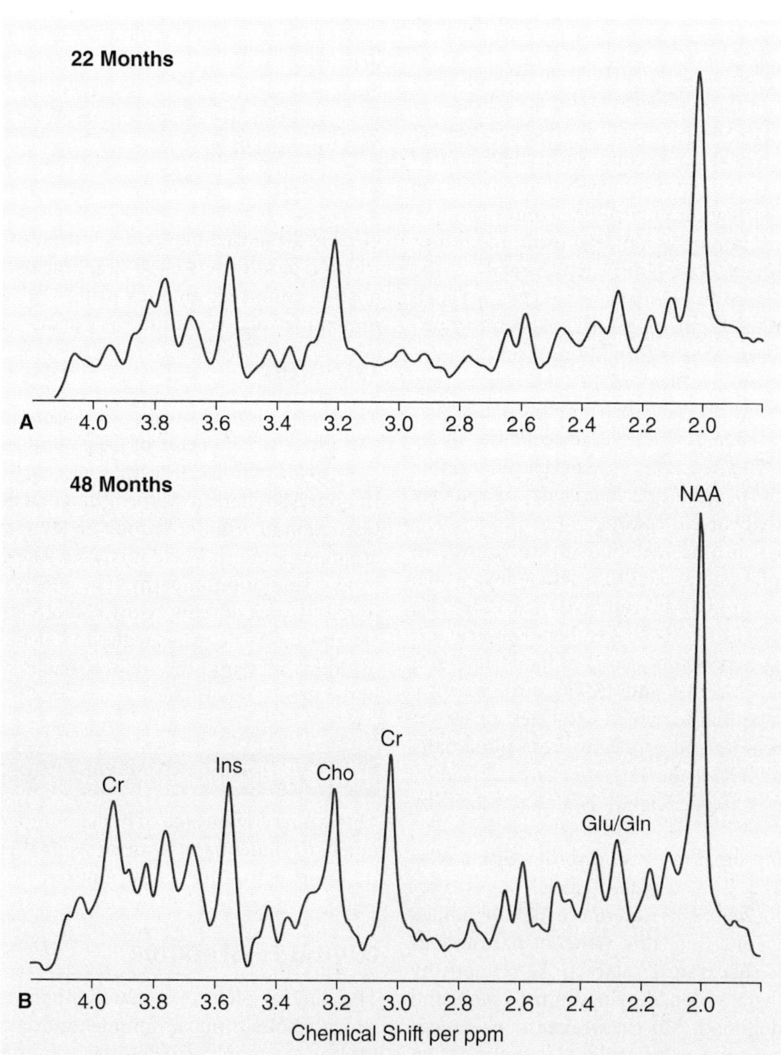


**FIGURE 138-2** In vivo proton magnetic resonance spectroscopy (1H MRS) of the brain of a patient with cerebral creatine deficiency due to guanidinoacetate methyltransferase (GAMT) deficiency. **A:** Complete lack of creatine resonance. **B:** Normalization of creatine spectrum after 6 months of treatment with oral creatine monohydrate.

**TABLE 138-1 CLINICAL, BIOCHEMICAL, AND DIAGNOSTIC FEATURES AND TREATMENT OF CREATINE DEFICIENCY SYNDROMES**

| Creatine Deficiency Syndrome | Main Clinical Features | Additional Clinical Features | Main Diagnostic Features | Additional Diagnostic Features | Treatment |
|---|---|---|---|---|---|
| AGAT deficiency | | | | Low urinary excretion of guanidinoacetate | Oral supplementation of creatine monohydrate |
| GAMT deficiency | Mental retardation, speech delay, autistic behavior, seizures | Extrapyramidal movement disorder, basal ganglia changes, intractable epilepsy | Cerebral creatine deficiency | High urinary excretion of guanidinoacetate | Oral supplementation of creatine monohydrate and dietary reduction of arginine together with oral substitution of ornithine |
| X-CRTR deficiency | | Dysmorphic features, growth retardation | | High urinary-creatine-to-creatinine ratio | None available |

AGAT, arginine:glycine amidinotransferase; GAMT, guanidinoacetate methyltransferase; X-CRTR, X-linked creatine transporter deficiency.

developmental progress in AGAT deficiency and improvement of epilepsy and any movement disorder in GAMT deficiency. Early recognition and treatment in the newborn period might prevent major symptoms and signs of both disorders. Unfortunately, in X-CRTR deficiency, oral creatine substitution does not result in an increase in creatine levels in the brain and no alternative causal treatment is available for this disorder, although the use of *S*-adenosyl methionine as adjuvant therapy has been reported. (For an overview of clinical, biochemical, and diagnostic features and treatment of creatine deficiency syndromes, see Table 138-1.)

## ORNITHINE METABOLISM

Ornithine is a nonprotein amino acid that has various functions (see Fig. 138-1). First, it is a key intermediate in the urea cycle. There, it is produced from arginine via the arginase reaction, yielding ornithine and urea. This reaction occurs in the cytoplasm. Second, ornithine is transported via the ornithine transporter (ORNT1 or *SLC25A15* gene) into mitochondria, where it serves as an essential substrate for ornithine transcarbamylase (OTC) in the intramitochondrial part of the urea cycle. OTC catalyzes the formation of citrulline from ornithine and carbamyl phosphate. Third, intramitochondrial ornithine is also a substrate for ornithine aminotransferase (OAT), which catalyzes the conversion of ornithine to $\Delta^1$-pyrroline-5-carboxylate (P5C), which is an essential substrate for proline synthesis. Fourth, extramitochondrial ornithine is the key substrate for the formation of polyamines, spermine, and spermidine, which are involved in DNA packaging. Fifth, ornithine is derived from a reaction that arginine undergoes with glycine in order to form guanidinoacetate, an essential intermediate in creatine synthesis. This reaction is catalyzed by arginine amidinotransferase (AGAT), and ornithine plays a regulatory role (via allosteric inhibition) in the activity of this enzyme.

Three disorders affecting ornithine metabolism are known in humans: (1) ornithine aminotransferase (OAT) deficiency, which causes gyrate atrophy of the choroid and retina (MIM no. 258870); (2) ornithine transporter (ORNT1 or *SLC25A15* gene) deficiency, which causes hyperornithemia-hyperammonemia-homocitrullinuria (HHH) syndrome (MIM no. 238970); and (3) a more recently described deficiency of P5C synthetase, which catalyzes an essential step in the synthesis of proline and ornithine from glutamate. Whereas OAT deficiency and HHH syndrome are characterized by hyperornithinemia, P5C synthetase deficiency is characterized by hypo-ornithinemia.

OAT deficiency is a rare autosomal recessive disorder with a relatively high prevalence in Finland. Clinically, OAT deficiency is characterized by ocular manifestations: patients experience night blindness in early childhood as a first sign of retinopathy. Other ocular findings include myopia and posterior subcapsular cataract. As retinopathy progresses, patients lose peripheral vision, develop tunnel vision, and become virtually blind by adulthood. Muscle weakness, electroencephalography changes, brain atrophy, and peripheral nervous system involvement have been described as additional complications in single patients.

Pathophysiologically, OAT catalyzes the transfer of an amino group from ornithine to α-ketoglutarte, forming glutamate and glutamyl-5 semialdehyde; the latter subsequently cyclizes to P5C. Normally the equilibrium of the reaction is directed toward the production of P5C. Thus, in OAT deficiency, hyperornithinemia is the biochemical hallmark. Urinary excretion of ornithine is also high, and due to competitive inhibition of tubular reabsorption, urinary concentrations of lysine, arginine, and cystine may also be elevated. Hyperornithinemia results in inhibition of creatine synthesis. Therefore, patients with OAT have moderately decreased creatine levels in the muscles and brain. It is not known whether low creatine levels contribute to the pathophysiology of the disease, but intellection disability, epilepsy, and behavioral problems are seem in a subset of patients. Interestingly, in neonates, the equilibrium of the reaction of OAT is directed toward synthesis of ornithine from P5C. Thus, neonates with OAT deficiency have low levels of ornithine rather than hyperornithinemia. A lack of ornithine results is depletion of substrates for the urea cycle and thus results in low levels of citrulline and arginine and in hyperammonemia.

### DIAGNOSIS

OAT is diagnosed by demonstration of high plasma ornithine levels, which typically are 5 to 20 times higher than the normal range. Diagnosis is confirmed by measuring OAT activity in fibroblasts and by mutational analysis of the OAT gene.

### TREATMENT

Treatment aims to correct the amino acid abnormalities. Pyridoxal phosphate is a cofactor of OAT, and some patients respond to high dosages of pyridoxine with some correction of the ornithine levels. In nonresponders, hyperornithinemia is partially corrected by dietary restriction of arginine through a low-protein diet supplemented with arginine-free amino acid mixtures. The goal of treatment is to slow the progression of retinopathy. The effects of this treatment on the long-term outcome of retinopathy and other disease manifestations are not yet known. As neonates with OAT deficiency have decreased levels of ornithine and arginine, an arginine-restricted diet is contraindicated in the neonatal period.

## HHH SYNDROME

This is a rare syndrome of hyperammonemia, hyperornithinemia, and homocitrullinemia; it is an autosomal recessive disorder of ornithine transport across the mitochondrial membrane (ORNT1, *SLC25A15* gene).

### CLINICAL PRESENTATION

The clinical picture is mainly characterized by hyperammonemia, which results from intramitochondrial ornithine depletion and thus insufficient supply of ornithine as substrate for the urea cycle. Dietary protein loads and catabolism lead to intermittent hyperammonemia associated with vomiting, ataxia, lethargy, irritability, confusion, and

**TABLE 138-2 CLINICAL, BIOCHEMICAL, AND DIAGNOSTIC FEATURES AND TREATMENT OF DISORDERS AFFECTING THE METABOLISM OF ORNITHINE**

| Disorder Affecting Ornithine Metabolism | Main Clinical Features | Diagnostic Features | Treatment |
|---|---|---|---|
| OAT deficiency | Retinopathy, cataract<br>Muscular weakness, brain atrophy, peripheral nervous system involvement<br>Neonatal hyperammonemia | Hyperornithinemia<br>Neonatal hypo-ornithinemia, hypocitrullinemia, hypoargininemia | Dietary reduction of arginine<br>Pyridoxine<br>Arginine restriction contraindicated in neonates |
| HHH syndrome | Intermittent hyperammonemia associated with vomiting, lethargy, psychiatric symptoms, ataxia<br>Progressive spastic paraparesis, developmental delay, mental retardation | Hyperornithinemia, hyperammonemia, homocitrullinuria | Protein restriction<br>Avoidance of catabolic states<br>Citrulline supplementation |
| P5C synthetase deficiency | Muscular hypotonia, progressive spasticity, failure to thrive<br>Cutis laxa, hyperextensible joints, cataracts | Hypo-ornithinemia, hypocitrullinemia, hypoargininemia | Substitution of ornithine and proline |

OAT, ornithine aminotransferase; HHH, hyperornithinemia, hyperammonemia, homocitrullinuria syndrome; P5C, pyrroline-5-carboxylate.

other psychiatric manifestations. Neonatal onset and lethal hyperammonemic coma have been described in single cases. In the long term, patients may develop chronic neurologic deficits (eg, progressive spastic paraparesis), developmental delay, and intellectual disability. Although extramitochondrial levels of ornithine are high, patients are not likely to develop retinopathy as one would expect from hyperornithemia caused by OAT deficiency.

In addition to hyperornithinemia and hyperammonemia, the disorder is characterized by homocitrullinuria, which arises from alternative metabolism of carbamyl phosphate via lysine. Orotic aciduria, which is a common feature of various urea cycle defects, is also present in HHH syndrome as a sign of carbamyl phosphate accumulation.

## DIAGNOSIS

The diagnosis of HHH syndrome is established by the characteristic combination of elevated ornithine levels in blood and elevated excretion of homocitrulline in urine, along with intermittent hyperammonemia. Confirmation of the diagnosis is possible by ornithine incorporation assays in fibroblasts and by mutational analysis of the *SLC25A15* gene.

## TREATMENT

Treatment is directed toward preventing increased ammonia production through a protein-restricted diet and avoidance of catabolic states. Citrulline supplementation helps to reduce the ammonia load as it consumes additional nitrogen via its conversion to arginine.

# P5C SYNTHETASE DEFICIENCY

P5C synthetase is encoded by the *ALDH18A1* gene, and enzyme deficiency (MIM no. 138250) leads to a complex clinical phenotype involving both the nervous system and connective tissues. Manifestations included muscular hypotonia, frequent vomiting, failure to thrive, cutis laxa, hyperextensible joints, developmental delay, seizures in infancy, cataracts, progressive spasticity, and severe intellectual disability. Because P5C synthetase acts at the interface between ornithine and proline synthesis, both hypoprolinemia and hypo-ornithinemia are characteristic diagnostic features. As a consequence of hypoprolinemia, citrulline and arginine are also low, and hyperammonemia may occur as a result of an insufficient supply of these substrates to the urea cycle. Treatment with ornithine and proline has not been effective in preventing the clinical manifestations. More recently, autosomal dominant spastic paraparesis type 9 (MIM no. 601162) has been found to be caused by heterozygous missense substitutions in the *ALDH18A1* gene. Finally, de novo heterozygous mutations in *ALDH18A1* affecting the highly conserved amino acid Arg138 of P5CS leads to a progeroid cutis laxa phenotype termed De Barsy syndrome (ARCL3A; MIM no. 219150), with cataracts or corneal clouding, thin skin with visible veins and wrinkles, moderate intellectual disability, clenched fingers, and pre- and postnatal growth retardation. Since the enzyme forms a dimer of dimers, the heterozygous variants potentially have a significant effect on enzyme activity. (For an overview of the clinical, biochemical, and diagnostic features and treatment of disorders affecting ornithine metabolism, see Table 138-2.)

## SUGGESTED READINGS


Battini R, Alessandrì MG, Casalini C, Casarano M, Tosetti M, Cioni G. Fifteen-year follow-up of Italian families affected by arginine glycine amidinotransferase deficiency. *Orphanet J Rare Dis.* 2017;12(1):21.

Baumgartner MR, Rabier D, Nassogne MC, et al. Delta-pyrroline-5-carboxylate synthase deficiency: neurodegeneration, cataracts and connective tissue manifestations combined with hyperammonaemia and reduced ornithine, citrulline, arginine and proline. *Eur J Pediatr.* 2005;164:31-36.

Coutelier M, Goizet C, Durr A, et al. Alteration of ornithine metabolism leads to dominant and recessive hereditary spastic paraplegia. *Brain.* 2015;138:2191-2205.

Fischer-Zirnsak B, Escande-Beillard N, Ganesh J, et al. Recurrent de novo mutations affecting residue Arg138 of pyrroline-5-carboxylate synthase cause a progeroid form of autosomal-dominant cutis laxa. *Am J Hum Genet.* 2015;97(3):483-492.

Jaggumantri S, Dunbar M, Edgar V, et al. Treatment of creatine transporter (SLC6A8) deficiency with oral S-adenosyl methionine as adjunct to L-arginine, glycine, and creatine supplements. *Pediatr Neurol.* 2015;53(4):360-363.

Mercimek-Mahmutoglu S, Salomons GS. Creatine deficiency syndromes. In: Pagon RA, Adam MP, Ardinger HH, eds. *GeneReviews.* Seattle, WA: University of Washington; 1993-2017.

Mercimek-Mahmutoglu S, Stockler-Ipsiroglu S, Adami A, et al. GAMT deficiency. Features, treatment and outcome in an inborn error of creatine synthesis. *Neurology.* 2006;67:480-484.

Stockler-Ipsiroglu S, Apatean D, Battini R, et al. Arginine: glycine amidinotransferase (AGAT) deficiency: clinical features and long term outcomes in 16 patients diagnosed worldwide. *Mol Genet Metab.* 2015;116(4):252-259.

Stockler-Ipsiroglu S, van Karnebeek CD. Cerebral creatine deficiencies: a group of treatable intellectual developmental disorders. *Semin Neurol.* 2014;34(3):350-356.

# 139 Disorders of Amino Acid Transport Across Cell Membranes

Kirsti Näntö-Salonen, Harri Niinikoski, and Manuel Schiff

## TRANSEPITHELIAL TRANSPORT OF AMINO ACIDS

Epithelial cells in renal tubules and intestinal mucosa use several different transport systems to move amino acids through the luminal (apical) and the antiluminal (basolateral) membranes of the cell, using sodium-dependent symporters, proton-motive forces, and concentration gradients of other amino acids. Each transporter system prefers groups of amino acids with certain physicochemical properties, but most individual amino acids can use more than 1 transporter. The transport activities have been classified into 5 main groups: (1) the "basic system" for cystine and the structurally related dibasic cationic amino acids lysine, arginine, and ornithine; (2) the "neutral system" for neutral amino acids; (3) the "acidic system" for glutamate and aspartate; (4) the "iminoglycine system" for proline, hydroxyproline, and glycine; and (5) the "β-amino acid system."

Inherited defects in amino acid transport at the cell membrane (Fig. 139-1 and Table 139-1) are expressed as selective renal aminoaciduria (ie, the concentration of the affected amino acids is high in the urine while it is normal or low in plasma). Intestinal absorption of these amino acids is almost always impaired. The symptoms of these disorders result from an excess of certain amino acids in the urine or a lack of them in the tissues.

The principal selective aminoacidurias, cystinuria, lysinuric protein intolerance, and Hartnup disorder, are caused by defects of the luminal cystine/dibasic amino acid transporter, the antiluminal (basolateral) dibasic amino acid transporter, and the neutral amino acid transporter, respectively. Other rare transport defects include autosomal dominant dibasic aminoaciduria type I, isolated lysinuria, isolated cystinuria, iminoglycinuria, and dicarboxylic aminoaciduria.

## CYSTINURIA

### INTRODUCTION

Defective reabsorption of cystine in the renal tubuli leads to high urinary concentrations of poorly soluble cystine. Cystinuria (Mendelian Inheritance in Man [MIM] no. 220100) causes 1% to 2% of kidney stones in adults and up to 8% in children. In a patient with severe neurologic symptoms or marked hypotonia, cystinuria suggests a contiguous gene deletion on chromosome 2p16 or 2p21. Transient cystinuria may occur in infancy due to immature transport mechanisms.

### PATHOGENESIS AND EPIDEMIOLOGY

Cystine and dibasic amino acids are transported across the apical surface of the epithelial cells in the jejunal mucosa and the proximal renal tubule by a high-affinity luminal transporter (system $b^{0+}$). Normally 99% of the filtered cystine is reabsorbed in the kidney.

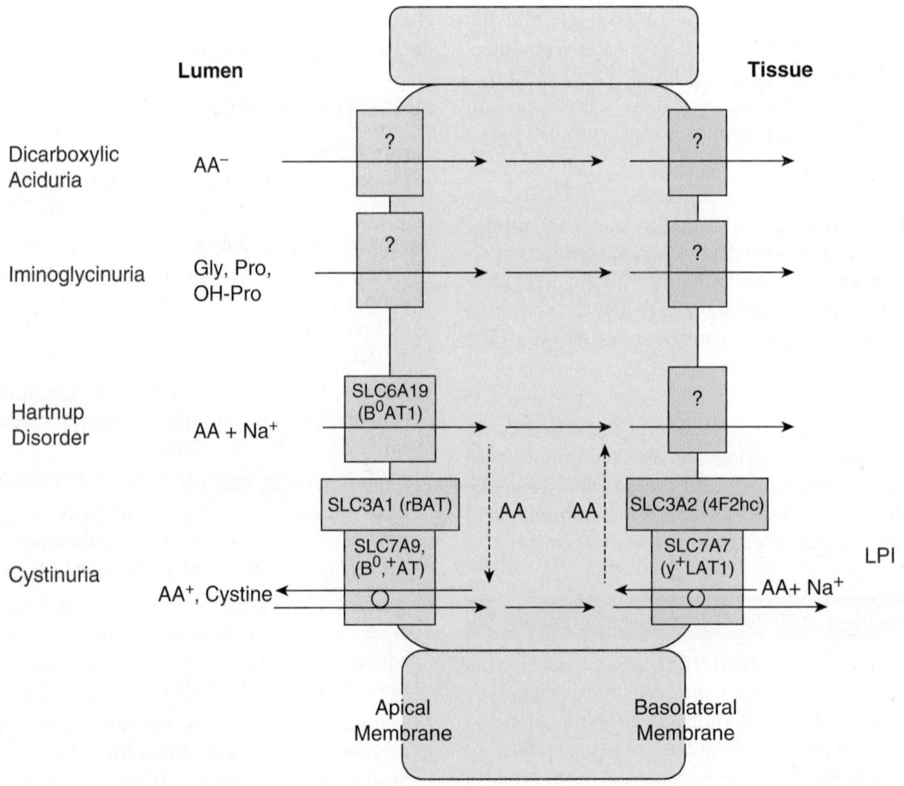


**FIGURE 139-1** Simplified schematic representation of amino acid transport in proximal tubular epithelial cell including transport systems for negatively charged dicarboxylic amino acids (AA⁻), imino acids, (glycine, proline, and hydroxyproline); neutral amino acids (AA); and cystine and positively charged dibasic amino acids (AA⁺). The sites of the presently known molecular transporter defects are indicated in red.

Cystine and the dibasic amino acids are transported into the epithelial cells by a luminal transporter (in exchange for neutral amino acids), and further from the epithelial cell into tissues by an antiluminal (basolateral) transporter (in exchange for neutral amino acids and sodium). Both these transporters are heteromers of a heavy subunit (*N*-glycosylated type 2 membrane glycoprotein) and a light subunit (nonglycosylated polytopic membrane protein) linked by a disulfide bridge. The light subunit $b^{0,+}$AT I and the heavy subunit rBAT of the luminal transporter are encoded by the genes *SLC7A9* and *SLC3A1*, and the light subunit $^{+}$LAT1 and the heavy subunit 4F2hc of the basolateral transporter by the genes *SLC7A7* and *SLC3A2*, respectively.

The neutral transporter system ($b^{0,+}$ATI encoded by the gene *SLC6A19*) is expressed only at the luminal border of the epithelial cells. It transports alanine, asparagine, citrulline, glutamine, histidine, isoleucine, leucine, phenylalanine, serine, threonine, tryptophan, tyrosine, and valine into the epithelial cells. Dicarboxylic amino acids are transported by *SCL1A1* and proline, hydroxyproline, and glycine by *SLC36A2*.

**TABLE 139-1 TRANSPORT DEFECTS OF AMINO ACIDS AT THE CELL MEMBRANE**

| Aminoaciduria | Gene | Chromosome | Affected Protein | Urinary Amino Acids | Plasma Amino Acids | Clinical Presentation | Incidence |
|---|---|---|---|---|---|---|---|
| Cystinuria A | *SLC3A1* | 2p21 | rBAT | Cys, Lys, Arg, Orn (↑) | Cys, Lys, Arg, Orn (normal) | Urolithiasis | 1:7000; varies between populations |
| Cystinuria B | *SLC7A9* | 19q13.11 | $b^{0,+}AT$ | | | | |
| Lysinuric protein intolerance (LPI) | *SLC7A7* | 14q11.2 | y+LAT1 | Lys, Arg, Orn (↑) Ala, Gln, Gly, Ser (↑) | Lys, Arg, Orn (↓) | Protein intolerance hyper-ammonemia after protein load; failure to thrive, hepatomegaly; multisystem manifestations | Very rare (in Finland 1:60,000; local conglomerates in, eg, Italy and Japan) |
| Hartnup disorder | *SLC6A19* | 5p15.33 | $B^0AT1$ | Neutral amino acids (↑) | Neutral amino acids (↓) | Mostly asymptomatic on adequate protein intake; pellagra-like dermatitis on sun-exposed areas; intermittent ataxia; neuropsychiatric symptoms | 1:14,000–1:45,000 |
| Iminoglycinuria | ? | ? | ? | Pro, Hypro, Gly (↑) | Pro, Hypro, Gly (↓) | Asymptomatic? | 1:10,000 |
| Dicarboxylic aciduria | *SLC1A1* | 9p24 | EAAT3 | Asp, Glu (↑) | Asp, Glu (↓) | Asymptomatic? Neuropsychiatric symptoms? | 1:35,000 |

Neutral amino acids: alanine, serine, threonine, valine, leucine, isoleucine, phenylalanine, tyrosine, tryptophan, histidine, citrulline, and the monoamino-dicarboxylic amides asparagine and glutamine.

Ala, alanine; Arg, arginine; Asp, aspartic acid; Cys, cystine; Gln, glutamine; Glu, glutamic acid; Hypro, hydroxyproline; Lys, lysine; Orn, ornithine; Pro, proline.

If the transporter is defective, large amounts of cystine are excreted in the urine. When the intratubular cystine concentration exceeds the threshold of solubility, crystals and stones will form. Sufficient amounts of cystine and dibasic amino acids are apparently absorbed from the intestine via alternative mechanisms (eg, in oligopeptide form), since no signs of deficiency of these amino acids have been described in these patients.

The average incidence of cystinuria is 1:7000, but it varies considerably between populations. Cystinuria type A (former type I) is caused by over 150 mutations in the *SLC3A1* gene on chromosome 2p16, and cystinuria type B (former non-type I) by over 100 mutations in the *SLC7A9* gene on chromosome 19q13. These genes encode the heavy subunit rBAT and the light subunit $b^{0,+}AT$ of the amino acid transporter, respectively. Cystinuria type A represents 60% of cases and is a true autosomal recessive disorder, while type B is inherited in an apparently dominant mode (as far as cystine urinary excretion is concerned) but with very incomplete penetrance. Thus, individuals harboring 1 mutation in *SLC7A9* may exhibit an abnormal urinary cystine excretion but they may generally remain free of clinical symptoms, as opposed to clinically symptomatic individuals who harbor 2 *SLC7A9* mutations. Individuals with the rare type AB cystinuria have 2 mutated alleles in the same gene in addition to a mutated allele in the other gene and so are actually AAB or ABB. Most of the mutations have been detected only in individual patients. There seems to be no reliable genotype-phenotype correlation.

Three distinct syndromes with cystinuria and neurologic symptoms are caused by homozygous contiguous gene deletions involving the *SLC3A1* gene: hypotonia-cystinuria syndrome, atypical hypotonia-cystinuria syndrome, and 2p21 syndrome. Recessive contiguous gene deletions in chromosome 2p16 cause a combination of cystinuria and mitochondrial disease.

## CLINICAL MANIFESTATIONS

Some patients never develop symptomatic kidney stones, but others suffer from recurrent acute "stone episodes" from early childhood, often clustered between long asymptomatic periods. The symptoms include abdominal or lower back pain, hematuria, pyuria, or spontaneous passing of stones. Cystine crystals may cause inflammation and renal injury. Urinary tract obstruction, recurrent infections and, ultimately, renal failure are possible complications.

## DIAGNOSIS

Cystine stones can usually be seen in radiographs and are also visible by ultrasonography. Mixed stones are not uncommon, and chemical analysis of the stones may be unreliable. Hexagonal cystine crystals can be detected in urinalysis. A positive nitroprusside test and amino acid analysis of the urine lead to the diagnosis. Patients with cystinuria generally excrete more than 400 mg (1.7 mmol) of cystine/1.73 m²/d into the urine compared to normal values of less than 50 to 60 mg (0.26 mmol)/1.73 m²/d. However, the excretion varies markedly, and a cut-off value of 150 μmol/mmol creatinine has been suggested. Plasma concentrations of cystine and the dibasic amino acids are normal or slightly decreased. Molecular genetic analysis is available. A hyperechogenic colon in fetal ultrasound has led to prenatal diagnosis in some cases.

## TREATMENT

The aim of the treatment of cystinuria is to prevent the formation of crystals and stones within the kidney and urinary tract. High fluid intake to dilute the urine and permanent alkalinization of the urine to improve cystine solubility are essential. The recommended fluid intake for adults is up to 4000 to 5000 mL/24 h (1.75–2 L/m²/24 h), 500 mL of this before bedtime and, if possible, 500 mL during the night. Amounts of at least 1000 mL/m²/24 h up to 3000 mL/d have been suggested for children. As cystine is much more soluble in alkaline urine, the goal is to keep the urinary pH constantly between 7 and 8. This is best achieved with potassium citrate, 2 to 4 mEq/kg/d in 2 to 4 doses, adjusted by monitoring of urinary pH. Restriction of dietary animal protein to limit endogenous cystine synthesis from methionine may be helpful, and moderate sodium restriction decreases cystine excretion.

If the standard therapy fails to dissolve and prevent the formation of new stones, a thiol derivative is added. Thiol drugs decrease urinary free cystine concentration by splitting cystine into 2 cysteine molecules that form soluble drug-cysteine disulfide compounds that are excreted in the urine. The dose of D-penicillamine is 30 mg/kg/d up to 3 to 4 g/d in 3 doses; for children, an initial dose of 5 mg/kg/d increased up to 20 to 40 mg/kg/d has been recommended. Penicillamine has many side effects such as hypersensitivity reactions, bone marrow suppression, liver and kidney problems, trace metal deficiencies and disturbances in taste. Pyridoxine supplementation is needed. Mercaptopropionylglycine (tiopronin) is better tolerated. The dose (10–20 mg/kg/d up to 1000 mg/d in 3 doses) is increased gradually and adjusted individually. Captopril has fewest side effects but may not be as effective as the other thiol compounds. It may have a role as alternative therapy. Alkaline pH increases the efficacy of the thiols. Careful monitoring of liver enzymes, complete blood count, zinc and copper levels, and urinary protein excretion is mandatory.

Percutaneous nephrolithotomy and extracorporeal shock-wave lithotripsy may not be able to destroy the extremely hard cystine stones. New, minimally invasive techniques minimize the need for open surgery for stone removal. Surgical procedures should always be combined with conservative preventive therapy.

It is essential to monitor renal function and to detect developing stones early. Regular follow-up also supports adherence to the treatment. Weekly home monitoring of urinary pH and specific gravity, regular measurement of free cystine concentration (with a target of < 100 μmol/mmol creatinine), determination of cystine crystal volume in morning urine, and direct assessment of urinary supersaturation are useful.

### PROGNOSIS

Cystinuria patients frequently develop stones during the first decade of life and should perhaps be treated prophylactically from an early age. Recurrent urinary tract infections, urinary tract obstruction, and renal insufficiency are possible complications. Early detection of the disease by screening the family members is valuable.

## LYSINURIC PROTEIN INTOLERANCE

### INTRODUCTION

In lysinuric protein intolerance (LPI; MIM no. 222700), the transport defect for the dibasic cationic amino acids leads to poor intestinal absorption and urinary loss of arginine, ornithine, and, particularly, lysine. Lack of the urea cycle intermediates arginine and ornithine leads to hyperammonemia and protein intolerance, and insufficient supply of lysine affects growth and the immune system. Many patients develop severe renal, hematologic, and pulmonary complications.

### PATHOGENESIS AND EPIDEMIOLOGY

Hyperammonemia after protein ingestion and protective aversion to high-protein foods make LPI resemble urea cycle enzyme disorders (see Chapter 141). Fewer than 200 patients have been reported, with the highest incidence in Finland (1:60,000), but there are also clusters of families in Italy and Japan and sporadic cases on all continents.

The transport of the dibasic cationic amino acids lysine, arginine, and ornithine is defective at the basolateral membranes of epithelial cells in the renal tubules and small intestine. Limited intestinal absorption of these amino acids and massive urinary loss of particularly lysine result in low plasma concentrations, while the concentrations of neutral amino acids in plasma are slightly increased. Glutamine and alanine concentrations are often more clearly elevated due to the malfunction of the urea cycle. It is unclear if the transport defect is expressed in any nonepithelial cells. The possibility of abnormal cationic amino acid transport between various intracellular compartments has been speculated.

The pathogenic mechanisms for the variable multiorgan involvement in LPI are still unknown. The malfunction of the urea cycle in LPI is best explained by a "functional deficiency" of the intermediates arginine and ornithine in the hepatocytes. A deficiency of arginine, the rate-limiting precursor of nitric oxide synthesis, may result in persistently low nitric oxide concentrations that potentially influence vascular endothelial and immunologic functions. A similar mechanism has been suggested to impair the function of alveolar macrophages, contributing to the development of alveolar proteinosis, a potentially fatal complication of LPI. However, other investigators have found evidence for increased nitric oxide synthesis, mediated, in theory, by increased intracellular arginine concentrations and subsequent arginine trapping within the cell that may result from the transport defect.

A deficiency of the essential amino acid lysine is thought to contribute to the poor growth and in the skeletal and immunologic manifestations of LPI. Occasional patients have severe carnitine deficiency due to dietary deficiency. The principal dietary source of carnitine is red meat, consumed in very small amounts by most patients with LPI. Chronic lysine deficiency also limits endogenous carnitine biosynthesis, and low plasma levels of dibasic amino acids may diminish growth hormone secretion. IGF1 expression is downregulated in the mouse model of LPI, leading to fetal growth restriction.

### CLINICAL MANIFESTATIONS

The full natural history of LPI remains to be characterized, as most of the oldest diagnosed patients are still in their 60s. Postprandial episodes of hyperammonemia, with poor feeding, vomiting, stupor, and unconsciousness, usually begin when the infants start receiving formula or other foods with higher protein content than breast milk. Tube feeding may be fatal. Strong aversion to high-protein foods with failure to thrive is evident by the age of 1 year, aggravating the protein malnutrition and amino acid deficiencies. Children present with growth failure, hepatosplenomegaly, muscular hypotonia, and occasional bone fractures. Neurologic development is normal if severe or prolonged hyperammonemia has been avoided. Bone maturation is retarded, and there is often a marked delay of puberty. In adults, the clinical heterogeneity of LPI is striking. Most affected adults are of moderately short stature, with abundant subcutaneous fat on a square-shaped trunk and thin extremities. They have marked hepatomegaly with or without splenomegaly. Two-thirds have skeletal changes (eg, osteopenia), but pathologic fractures seldom occur. Radiologic signs of pulmonary fibrosis are common, but few patients suffer from symptomatic interstitial lung disease. Mental capacity depends on the prior history of hyperammonemia. Most patients have mild normochromic or hypochromic anemia, leukopenia, and thrombocytopenia, and their reticulocyte count is often slightly elevated. Combined hyperlipidemia with elevated low-density lipoprotein cholesterol and triglycerides is a common finding. High serum immunoglobulin G concentrations and abnormalities in the distribution of lymphocyte subpopulations and in humoral immune responses have been reported.

### DIAGNOSIS

The diagnosis is based on the combination of increased urinary excretion and low plasma concentrations of the cationic amino acids, especially lysine. The concentrations of plasma lysine, arginine, and ornithine are usually less than 80 μmol/L, 40 μmol/L, and 30 μmol/L, respectively. If plasma amino acid concentrations are exceptionally low due to very limited protein intake, urinary cationic amino acid excretion may sometimes be within the reference range. Hyperammonemia and orotic aciduria typically develop after protein-rich meals. Nonspecific but consistent findings include elevated serum lactate dehydrogenase activity and increased serum concentrations of ferritin, which in association with high triglyceride levels represent the hallmark of a secondary macrophage activation syndrome typical of LPI. In addition, serum zinc is elevated. The mode of inheritance is autosomal recessive, and the diagnosis can be confirmed by mutation analysis. At least 50 different mutations have been reported in the *SLC7A7* gene on chromosome 14q, encoding the light subunit of the dibasic amino acid transporter. All Finnish patients share the same founder mutation 1181-2A>T that causes abnormal splicing, leading to a translational frame shift and a premature stop codon. The phenotypic variability is wide among the genetically homogeneous Finnish patients and among homozygous patients with other mutations, and no genotype/phenotype correlation has been established.

### TREATMENT

The principal aims of treatment are to prevent hyperammonemia and to provide sufficient protein (1–1.5 g/kg/d in children and 0.6–1.0 g/kg/d in adults) and essential amino acids for normal metabolism, growth, and development. As a neutral amino acid, L-citrulline is readily absorbed in LPI and can be used to improve the function of the urea cycle where it is converted to arginine and ornithine. Approximately 50 to 100 mg/kg/d of L-citrulline is given in 3 to 5 doses with protein-containing meals. For patients with constantly highly elevated glutamine and glycine levels, sodium benzoate and/or sodium phenylbutyrate may help to diminish the nitrogen load. There is marked interindividual variation in the protein tolerance, and infections, pregnancy, and lactation may alter protein tolerance significantly. Frequent follow-up of urinary orotic acid excretion and the amino acid profile is necessary. Correction of lysine deficiency in LPI is complicated by its poor intestinal absorption and the resulting osmotic diarrhea if given in too high doses. However, moderate oral L-lysine-HCl supplementation (20–30 mg/kg/d in 3 divided doses) elevates plasma lysine concentration to low-normal range without gastrointestinal or other side effects. Carnitine supplementation is indicated in case of overt carnitine deficiency. Due to the protein-restricted diet, patients need supplementary calcium, vitamins, and trace elements. Growth hormone therapy has been successfully given to children with LPI whose severe growth retardation has not responded to improved nutrition and metabolic control. Statins are safe and effective in treatment of hypercholesterolemia.

The rare hyperammonemic crisis is treated following the guidelines for urea cycle disorders. All protein- and nitrogen-containing substances should be removed from the diet and sufficient energy supplied as intravenous glucose and lipid. Intravenous infusion of ornithine, arginine, or citrulline, beginning with a priming dose of 0.5 to 1.0 mmol/kg in 5 to 10 minutes and continuing with 0.5 to 1.0 mmol/kg/h, will rapidly clear the hyperammonemia. Sodium benzoate and sodium phenylbutyrate may also be used to promote alternate pathways of ammonia elimination.

Varicella infections are usually severe and can be fatal, and patients should be immunized and treated with acyclovir. Other complications include systemic lupus erythematosus, bone marrow involvement with hemophagocytic lymphohistiocytosis (HLH), and interstitial pulmonary disease with alveolar proteinosis, in some cases progressing to fatal multiorgan failure. The treatment with immunosuppression or intravenous immunoglobulin is still experimental. In alveolar proteinosis, bronchoalveolar lavage and steroid therapy have shown some effect; in addition, granulocyte-macrophage colony-stimulating factor therapy has recently been proposed for idiopathic alveolar proteinosis but with unclear effects. One child with alveolar proteinosis went through an initially successful heart-lung transplantation, but died later after recurrence of the disease.

Several recent reports indicate that variable degrees of renal dysfunction are common in LPI, with Fanconi-type tubular problems (mild proteinuria, glucosuria, phosphaturia, tubular acidosis, and microscopic hematuria) and slowly deteriorating glomerular filtration that has led to end-stage renal disease and renal transplant in several cases. A recent survey detected such problems in approximately 50% of the Finnish patients. Urinary $\beta_2$-microglobulin may serve as an early tubular marker of renal involvement. Pregnancies in LPI patients have been complicated by toxemia, anemia, or bleeding during delivery, but many have completed pregnancy successfully.

### PROGNOSIS

With early diagnosis, a low-protein diet, and medical therapy, the outcome in most patients is fairly good. However, although hyperammonemia and the associated intellectual disability can be avoided with current therapy, several other complications may develop. The accumulating knowledge of the multisystem manifestations of LPI, the pathogenesis of which probably rely on immune dysfunction and HLH, is changing the previous concept that LPI is usually a fairly benign and easily treatable condition.

## HARTNUP DISEASE

### INTRODUCTION

The classical symptoms of Hartnup disease (MIM no. 234500), pellagra-like dermatitis, intermittent ataxia, and neuropsychiatric impairments, closely resemble those of nutritional niacin (nicotinic acid and nicotinamide) deficiency. Since the first description of the syndrome in several members of the Hartnup family in 1956, an extensive number of subjects who fulfil the biochemical diagnostic criteria have been reported, mostly detected in newborn screening programs. However, most of those identified remain asymptomatic.

### PATHOGENESIS AND EPIDEMIOLOGY

The molecular defect involves a sodium-dependent and chloride-independent neutral amino acid transporter, B(0)AT1 (*SLC6A19*) in the apical brush border membrane of the renal proximal tubule and intestinal epithelial cells. Mutations in *SLC6A19* impair intestinal uptake and tubular reabsorption of all the neutral amino acids (ie, alanine, serine, threonine, valine, leucine, isoleucine, phenylalanine, tyrosine, tryptophan, histidine, and citrulline) and the monoamino-dicarboxylic amides asparagine and glutamine. The transporter associates with partner proteins that are necessary for its expression, namely collectrin (Tmem27) in the kidney and angiotensin-converting enzyme 2 (ACE2) in the intestine, both components of the renin–angiotensin system.

As a consequence of the dysfunctional transport system, the affected amino acids are readily absorbed in the intestine as short oligopeptides but not as free amino acids. They are excreted in 5- to 20-fold excess into the urine, leading to decreased or low-normal plasma concentrations. The stools of patients contain increased amounts of free amino acids, closely reflecting the urinary excretion pattern. The unabsorbed amino acids in the colon are exposed to bacterial degradation. Degradation of tryptophan produces large amounts of indole compounds, which are then excreted in the urine.

Systemic tryptophan deficiency plays a central role in the development of clinical symptoms including neuropsychiatric, as tryptophan is the precursor of the neurotransmitter serotonin. Most importantly, tryptophan deficiency leads to reduced availability of nicotinic acid, the precursor of NAD(P)H. Subsequent deficiency of nicotinic acid (or niacin) and its amide, nicotinamide, may explain the pellagra-like lesions that are ascribable to nutritional niacin deficiency. The wide phenotypic variability of Hartnup disease may be explained by nutritional factors and genetic differences owing to the high frequency of compound heterozygotes. The previously mentioned tissue-specific partner proteins may also play a role in the clinical variability.

The reported incidence of Hartnup disease in newborns screened for aminoaciduria varies from 1 in 14,000 to 1 in 45,000. Hartnup disease is an autosomal recessive disorder caused by mutations in *SLC6A19*. The most common allele, D173N, does not completely inactivate the transport mechanism.

### CLINICAL MANIFESTATIONS

In the few patients exhibiting clinical symptoms, the skin lesions and neurologic problems usually appear in early childhood and tend to spontaneously ameliorate with age. Exposure to sunlight, fever, diarrhea, inadequate diet, or psychological stress may precipitate the symptoms. Pellagra-like skin changes are found on light-exposed areas. The skin rash may mimic those seen in zinc deficiency, and the rare combination of celiac disease and Hartnup disease has led to severe skin issues, intermittent cerebellar ataxia, attacks of headache, muscle pain, and weakness. Occasionally, patients present with intellectual disability, seizures, or psychosis-like symptoms. Maternal Hartnup disease appears to be harmless to the fetus.

### DIAGNOSIS

The characteristic urinary excretion of neutral amino acids and their low-normal plasma concentrations are keys to the diagnosis. Urinary excretion of indole compounds may be within the normal range if the patient consumes normal or low amounts of dietary protein, but an oral load of L-tryptophan in most cases leads to a supranormal increase in indole excretion. Genetic testing of *SLC6A19* is available.

### TREATMENT AND PROGNOSIS

Clinical symptoms may be prevented by sufficient dietary intake of niacin or adequate supply of high-quality protein that allows the necessary amount of tryptophan to be absorbed in oligopeptide form. Skin and neurologic symptoms usually disappear with oral nicotinamide (50–300 mg/d). Tryptophan ethyl ester has been successfully used to circumvent the transport defect. Oral neomycin reduces intestinal degradation of tryptophan and decreases indole production; however, the causative role of the indole compounds in the disease is not well understood. Early recognition of the condition in newborn screening programs allows adequate follow-up and prevention of symptomatic disease.

Camargo SMR, Bockenhauser D, Kleta R. Aminoacidurias: clinical and molecular aspects. *Kidney Int*. 2008;73:918-925.

Claes DJ, Jackson E. Cystinuria: mechanisms and management. *Pediatr Nephrol*. 2012;27:2031-2038.

Eggerman T, Venghaus A, Zerres K. Cystinuria: an inborn cause of urolithiasis. *Orphanet J Rare Dis*. 2012;7:19.

Ogier de Baulny H, Schiff M, Dionisi-Vici C. Lysinuric protein intolerance (LPI): a multi organ disease by far more complex than a classic urea cycle disorder. *Mol Genet Metab*. 2012;106:12-17.

Pereira DJ, Schoolwert AC, Pais VM. Cystinuria: current concepts and future directions. *Clin Nephrol*. 2015;83:138-146.

Sumorok N, Goldfarb DS. Update on cystinuria. *Curr Opin Nephrol Hypertens*. 2013;22:427-431.

Tanner LM, Näntö-Salonen K, Venetoklis J, et al. Nutrient intake in lysinuric protein intolerance. *J Inherit Metab Dis*. 2007;30:716-721.

Tringham M, Kurko J, Tanner L, et al. Exploring the transcriptomic variation caused by the Finnish founder mutation of lysinuric protein intolerance (LPI). *Mol Genet Metab*. 2012;105:408-415.



# 140 Other Disorders of Amino Acid Metabolism

Bernd C. Schwahn

## INTRODUCTION

The introduction of amino acid analysis to clinical diagnostic practice during the 1960s led to the discovery of multiple disorders of amino acid catabolism, transport, and synthesis. Most have been described in detail in the preceding chapters. A few remaining disorders of amino acid modification or salvage are presented in Table 140-1.

Amino acid analysis was initially targeted to subjects with unexplained symptoms, often neurologic in nature. Due to this ascertainment bias, a few of the newly described disorders were initially believed to cause disease before their benign nature was recognized. The most prominent example is histidinemia, which is relatively common and was included in universal newborn screening programs for many years. Other examples of apparently benign biochemical phenotypes are listed in Table 140-2.

## MISCELLANEOUS DISEASE-CAUSING DISORDERS OF AMINO ACID METABOLISM

Two disorders of the N-terminal modification of amino acids are associated with neurometabolic disease. Aminoacylase-1 deficiency (ACY1D) is a rare metabolic disorder that affects salvage of a group of acetylated amino acids and may also impair detoxification of exogenous small molecules such as benzoate. Most identified children do exhibit neurologic abnormalities such as intellectual disability, seizures, hypotonia, and motor delay, but there are asymptomatic individuals as well. Deficiency of aminoacylase 2 is known as Canavan disease. This is a severe neurodegenerative disease with onset in early infancy. Severe truncal hypotonia, hyperextension of legs and flexion of arms, blindness, severe intellectual disability, and death during toddler age are commonly seen. Macrocephaly and megalencephaly are typical, with demyelination and leukodystrophy on imaging and spongy degeneration and astrocytic swelling with normal neurons on histopathology.

Two peptidase defects impair the salvage of L-proline. Prolidase is involved in the final stage of degradation of endogenous and dietary proteins, in particular of collagen. Prolidase deficiency leads to a lack of L-proline with subsequent skin ulcers and compromised immune defense, probably due to impaired complement function. Cleavage of L-proline from dipeptides is impaired in carnosinemia and homocarnosinosis, 2 biochemical manifestations of a defect in carnosinase dipeptidase 1. Affected individuals accumulate endogenous and exogenous carnosine and poultry-derived anserine, but increased

**TABLE 140-1 MISCELLANEOUS DISEASE-CAUSING GENETIC DISORDERS OF AMINO ACID METABOLISM**

| Disorder | Clinical Presentation | Metabolic Derangement | Genetics | Diagnostic Tests |
|---|---|---|---|---|
| Aminoacylase 1 deficiency (OMIM 609924) | Unspecific neurologic abnormalities (intellectual disability, seizures, hypotonia, motor delay) in many but not all affected individuals | Increased urinary excretion of *N*-acetylated amino acids (methionine, glutamic acid, alanine, leucine, glycine, valine, isoleucine) | AR, *ACY1* gene on 3p21.2 | Urinary organic acids; genetic testing |
| Aminoacylase 2 deficiency (Canavan disease, OMIM 271900) | Infantile-onset dystonia, blindness, intellectual disability, seizures macrocephaly, early death | Increased excretion of *N*-acetyl-aspartate (NAA) in urine | AR, *ASPA* gene on 17p13.2 | Urinary organic acids; high NAA peak in NMR spectroscopy; enzyme analysis; genetic testing |
| Prolidase deficiency (OMIM 170100) | Variable inflammatory and ulcerative skin lesions, mainly on legs; recurrent airway infections during childhood; intellectual impairment; and mild facial dysmorphism | Massive excretion of imidodipeptides (with C-terminal proline or hydroxyproline, particularly alanylproline and glycylproline) | AR, *PEPD* gene on 19q13.11 | Special laboratory dipeptide analysis in urine; enzyme analysis; genetic testing |
| Carnosinemia and homocarnosinosis (carnosine dipeptidase 1 deficiency, OMIM 236130) | Inconsistent association with developmental disorder, spastic diplegia, and neurodegeneration | Increased plasma and urine concentration of the histidine dipeptides carnosine and anserine; in severe cases, also of homocarnosine | AR, *CNDP1*, gene on 18q22.3 | Amino acids in plasma and urine; carnosinase activity; genetic testing |
| Glycine *N*-methyltransferase deficiency (OMIM 606664) | Mild hepatomegaly, transaminasemia | Isolated accumulation of methionine and SAM | AR, *GNMT* gene on 6p21.1 | Amino acids, homocysteine, and *S*-adenosylmethionine in plasma |
| Hyperprolinemia type 2 (delta-1-pyrroline-5-carboxylate dehydrogenase deficiency, OMIM 239510) | Global developmental disorder, seizures | Defect in catabolism of proline leads to gross accumulation of proline and its precursor pyrroline-5-carboxylate | AR, *ALDH4A1* gene on 1p36.13 | Amino acids and pyrroline-5-carboxylate in plasma or urine, enzyme assay, genetic testing |

AR, autosomal recessive pattern of inheritance; NMR, nuclear magnetic resonance; OMIM, Online Mendelian Inheritance in Man database.

**TABLE 140-2 GENETIC DISORDERS OF AMINO ACID METABOLISM WITH DOUBTFUL CLINICAL SIGNIFICANCE**

| Disorder | Remarks | Metabolic Derangement | Genetics | Diagnostic Tests |
|---|---|---|---|---|
| Histidinemia (histidase deficiency) | Relatively frequent (up to 1 in 10,000) | High histidine in blood, urine, and CSF; low urocanic acid | AR, *HAL* gene on 12q.23.1 | Amino acids in plasma or urine; enzyme activity in fibroblasts; genetic testing |
| Urocanic aciduria (urocanase deficiency) | Very rare | Inconsistent elevation of histidine; high urocanic acid excretion in urine | AR, *UROC1* gene on 3q21.3 | Specific methods to measure urocanic acid or uroglucanoylglycine; genetic testing |
| Sarcosinemia (sarcosine dehydrogenase deficiency) | Secondary sarcosinemia found in folate deficiency or multiple acyl-CoA dehydrogenase deficiency (MADD) | Accumulation of sarcosine in body fluids | AR, *SARDH* gene on 9q34.2 | Plasma amino acids; serum folate; urinary organic acids to exclude MADD |
| Hyperprolinemia type 1 (proline dehydrogenase deficiency) | Part of 22q11 microdeletion syndromes | Moderate accumulation of proline in body fluids, normal P5C | AR, *PRODH* gene on 22q11.21 | Amino acids in plasma or urine; genetic testing |
| Hyperhydroxyprolinemia | Moderate elevation of hydroxyproline also seen with increased collagen turnover | Accumulation of hydroxyproline | AR, *PRODH2* gene on 19q13.12 | Amino acids in plasma or urine; genetic testing |
| Hyperlysinemia and saccharopinuria (2-aminoadipic semialdehyde synthase [AASS] deficiency) | Partial AASS deficiency leads to isolated saccharopinuria | Accumulation of saccharopine and lysine in body fluids | AR, *AASS* gene on 7q31.32 | Amino acids in plasma or urine; genetic testing |
| Trimethylaminuria (flavin-containing monooxygenase 3 deficiency) | Fish-odor syndrome, common | Accumulation of trimethylamine (TMA) and TMA oxide (TMAO) with increased ratio of TMA/TMAO | AR, *FMO3* gene on 1q24.3 | TMA/TMA-*N*-oxide in urine by NMR or tandem mass spectrometry; genetic testing |
| Dimethylglycine dehydrogenase deficiency | Fish-odor syndrome, very rare | Accumulation of dimethylglycine (DMG) | AR, *DMGDH* gene on 5q14.1 | Organic acids in urine to exclude MADD; plasma betaine and DMG; genetic testing |

AR, autosomal recessive pattern of inheritance; CSF, cerebrospinal fluid; NMR, nuclear magnetic resonance.

homocarnosine is only found in individuals with very low residual enzyme activity. Not all known cases show neurologic symptoms; however, there is more recent evidence indicating a role of carnosinase-1 in neurodegeneration.

Glycine-*N*-methyltransferase deficiency impairs the interconversion of glycine to sarcosine and leads to a disruption of the regulation of 1-carbon-unit metabolism (see Chapter 134). It manifests as mild liver disease and is a rare cause of isolated hypermethioninemia.

Hyperprolinemia type 2 is a neurometabolic disease caused by a defect in the second step of L-proline catabolism with subsequent accumulation of pyrroline-5-carboxylate (P5C) and 3-OH-pyrroline-5-carboxylate (see Fig. 135-1). Inactivation of pyridoxal phosphate by P5C and other aldehyde toxicity has been hypothesized to explain the neurotoxicity of P5C.

## GENETIC AMINO ACID DISORDERS OF QUESTIONABLE CLINICAL SIGNIFICANCE

Other amino acid disorders that have questionable clinical relevance are detailed in Table 140-2, together with their enzyme defects, genes, and required investigations to confirm an accidental diagnosis.

Two disorders are known to cause fish-odor syndrome, a persistent and unpleasant body odor similar to decaying fish. Trimethylaminuria is caused by the accumulation of malodorous trimethylamine (TMA) due to high dietary intake or increased bacterial intestinal production of TMA from its precursors carnitine, choline, or phosphatidylcholine (lecithin), on the background of impaired oxidation of TMA to the odorless TMA oxide. There are no physical symptoms, and mild forms are relatively common (prevalence of up to 1 in 400). Severe forms are found in up to 1 in 40,000 individuals who can experience marked psychosocial distress due to the persistent smell and subsequent social isolation. Dietary modification and antibiotic treatment can be helpful.

Only a few individuals have been described who emanate a fish-like odor due to accumulation of dimethylglycine (DMG). In one case, this was accompanied by muscular fatigue and elevated creatine kinase levels. Dimethylglycine dehydrogenase is involved in the metabolism of choline, converting dimethylglycine to sarcosine (see Chapter 134).

## SUGGESTED READINGS


Bellia F, Vecchio G, Rizzarelli E. Carnosinases, their substrates and diseases. *Molecules*. 2014;19:2299-2329.

Brosco JP, Sanders LM, Dharia R, et al. The lure of treatment: expanded newborn screening and the curious case of histidinemia. *Pediatrics*. 2010;125:417-419.

Espinos C, Pineda M, Martinez-Rubio D, et al. Mutations in the urocanase gene UROC1 are associated with urocanic aciduria. *J Med Genet*. 2009;46:407-411.

Hoshino H, Kubota M. Canavan disease: clinical features and recent advances in research. *Pediatr Int*. 2014;56:477-483.

Houten SM, Te Brinke H, Denis S, et al. Genetic basis of hyperlysinemia. *Orphanet J Rare Dis*. 2013;8:57.

Lupi A, Tenni R, Rossi A, et al. Human prolidase and prolidase deficiency: an overview on the characterization of the enzyme involved in proline recycling and on the effects of its mutations. *Amino Acids*. 2008;35:739-752.

Mudd SH, Cerone R, Schiaffino MC, et al. Glycine N-methyltransferase deficiency: a novel inborn error causing persistent isolated hypermethioninaemia. *J Inherit Metab Dis*. 2001;24:448-464.

Sommer A, Christensen E, Schwenger S, et al. The molecular basis of aminoacylase 1 deficiency. *Biochim Biophys Acta*. 2011;1812:685-690.

Summitt CB, Johnson LC, Jonsson TJ, et al. Proline dehydrogenase 2 (PRODH2) is a hydroxyproline dehydrogenase (HYPDH) and molecular target for treating primary hyperoxaluria. *Biochem J*. 2015;466:273-281.

Tondo M, Calpena E, Arriola G, et al. Clinical, biochemical, molecular and therapeutic aspects of 2 new cases of 2-aminoadipic semialdehyde synthase deficiency. *Mol Genet Metab*. 2013;110:231-236.

van de Ven S, Gardeitchik T, Kouwenberg D, et al. Long-term clinical outcome, therapy and mild mitochondrial dysfunction in hyperprolinemia. *J Inherit Metab Dis*. 2014;37:383-390.

Zhou J, Shephard EA. Mutation, polymorphism and perspectives for the future of human flavin-containing monooxygenase 3. *Mutat Res*. 2006;612:165-171.

# 141 Urea Cycle Disorders

Lindsay C. Burrage, Brendan Lee, and Sandesh C.S. Nagamani

## THE UREA CYCLE

Animals excrete excess nitrogen in 3 major forms: ammonia, uric acid, and urea. Mammals are ureotelic organisms, which means that they are dependent on the synthesis and excretion of urea to maintain nitrogen balance. The urea cycle (also called the ornithine cycle), first described in 1932 by Hans Krebs and Kurt Henseleit, converts waste nitrogen derived from dietary protein and amino acid catabolism into urea. The urea cycle consists of a cofactor synthesizing enzyme (*N*-acetylglutamate synthase [NAGS]), 5 catalytic enzymes (carbamoyl-phosphate synthase 1 [CPS1], ornithine transcarbamylase [OTC], argininosuccinate synthase 1 [ASS1], argininosuccinate lyase [ASL], and arginase 1 [ARG1]), and 2 transporters (mitochondrial aspartate/glutamate carrier SLC25A13 or citrin and mitochondrial ornithine transporter ORNT1 or SLCA15) that facilitate the transfer of nitrogen from ammonia and aspartate to urea (Fig. 141-1). The initial 2 catalytic reactions occur within the mitochondria, whereas the remaining reactions, including the generation of urea, occur in the cytosol. The complete urea cycle exists only in the liver, although certain enzymatic components of the urea cycle (eg, ASS1 and ASL) are also expressed in a variety of other tissues.

NAGS synthesizes *N*-acetylglutamate, a cofactor required for the allosteric activation of CPS1 that catalyzes the first and rate-limiting step of the urea cycle. CPS1 synthesizes carbamoyl-phosphate from ammonia and bicarbonate, and in this step, the first atom of waste nitrogen enters the urea cycle (see Fig. 141-1). Carbamoyl-phosphate and ornithine are converted to citrulline by the enzyme OTC, and citrulline is actively transported out of the mitochondria by the ornithine transporters (ORNT1 or SLC25A15 and ORNT2 or SLC25A2). The second atom of waste nitrogen enters the urea cycle in the form of aspartate. Citrin, the mitochondrial aspartate/glutamate carrier, transports aspartate across the mitochondrial membrane into the cytosol. ASS1 conjugates citrulline and aspartate to form argininosuccinic acid, which is cleaved by ASL into fumarate and arginine. In the final step of the urea cycle, ARG1 hydrolyzes arginine into urea and ornithine. The ornithine is transported back into the mitochondria by ORNT1.

More than 90% of nitrogen derived from dietary sources and protein catabolism is not used for anabolic processes and must be excreted as urea. Deficiency of one of the urea cycle enzymes or transporters leads to a urea cycle disorder (UCD). UCDs are a group of inborn errors of metabolism characterized by inability to excrete waste nitrogen and accumulation of ammonia and glutamine (Table 141-1). Effective ureagenesis is not only dependent on the primary components of the urea cycle but also on the availability of substrates, intermediate metabolites, and adenosine triphosphate. Consequently, decreased flux through the urea cycle and hyperammonemia are observed in metabolic disorders like carbonic anhydrase VA deficiency (deficiency of $HCO_3^-$), lysinuric protein intolerance (decreased availability of arginine and ornithine), and fatty acid oxidation disorders (decreased availability of adenosine triphosphate [ATP]).

## HYPERAMMONEMIA: A HALLMARK OF UREA CYCLE DISORDERS

Hyperammonemia (elevated levels of $NH_3$ and $NH_4^+$ in the tissues and blood) is a feature common to severe forms of all UCDs. The exact mechanism by which ammonia causes neurotoxicity is unclear. However, elevations of glutamine in the brain leading to cerebral edema, altered blood-brain barrier function, excitotoxicity due to increased extracellular glutamate, altered glucose and energy metabolism, and increased oxidative stress have been proposed as pathogenic mechanisms.

The clinical presentation of individuals with hyperammonemia is variable and nonspecific. In infancy, the presentation may mimic sepsis with symptoms such as lethargy, poor feeding, vomiting, seizures, coma, and even death if untreated. In older children and adults, the clinical presentation of hyperammonemia may include avoidance of dietary protein, headache, altered mental status, confusion, cyclic vomiting, behavioral abnormalities, and psychosis, which, without

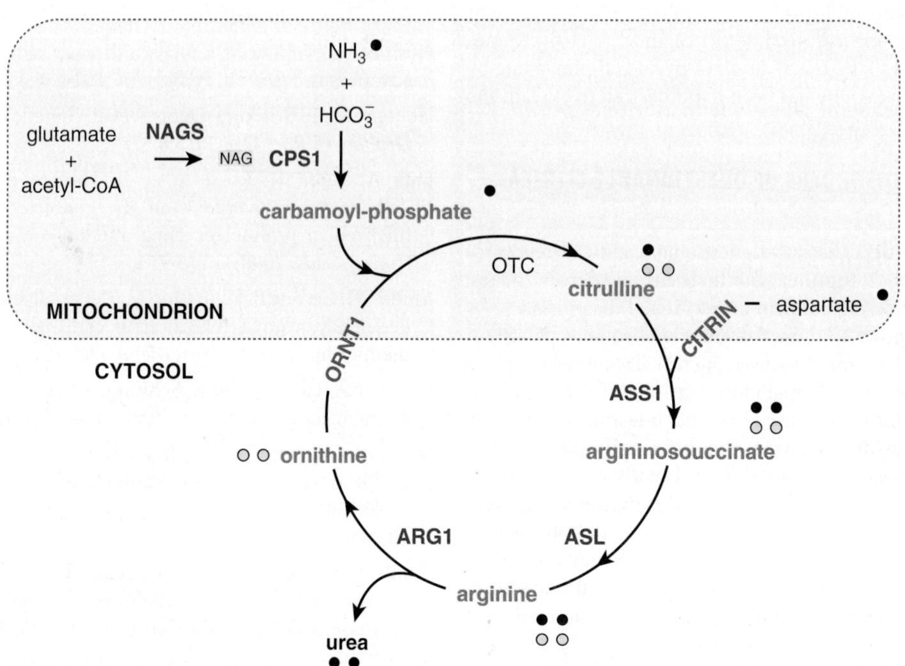


**FIGURE 141-1** The urea cycle. The nitrogen from ammonia and aspartate (*black circles*) is transferred to urea via the enzymes (depicted in *blue*) and transporters (depicted in *red*) of the urea cycle. Ornithine that contains 2 nitrogen atoms (*yellow circles*) is recycled, and hence, the urea cycle is also called the ornithine cycle. ARG1, arginase 1; ASL, argininosuccinate lyase; ASS1, argininosuccinate synthase 1; citrin, mitochondrial aspartate/glutamate carrier; CPS1, carbamoyl-phosphate synthase 1; NAGS, *N*-acetylglutamate synthase; ORNT1, mitochondrial ornithine transporter; OTC, ornithine transcarbamylase.

**TABLE 141-1 UREA CYCLE DISORDERS**

| Disorder | Inheritance | Enzyme or Transporter | Clinical Manifestations | Biochemical Markers[a] |
|---|---|---|---|---|
| *N*-acetylglutamate synthase deficiency | Autosomal recessive | *N*-acetylglutamate synthase | Encephalopathy, neurobehavioral | Hyperammonemia, elevated plasma glutamine, low citrulline |
| Carbamyl phosphate synthetase deficiency | Autosomal recessive | Carbamyl phosphate synthetase | Encephalopathy, neurobehavioral | Hyperammonemia, elevated plasma glutamine, low citrulline |
| Ornithine transcarbamylase (OTC) deficiency | X-linked semi-dominant | Ornithine transcarbamylase deficiency | Encephalopathy, neurobehavioral, liver disease (infrequently) | Hyperammonemia, elevated plasma glutamine, low citrulline, elevated urine orotic acid |
| Citrullinemia type I | Autosomal recessive | Argininosuccinate synthetase | Encephalopathy, neurobehavioral | Hyperammonemia, elevated plasma citrulline |
| Argininosuccinic aciduria | Autosomal recessive | Argininosuccinate lyase | Encephalopathy, neurobehavioral, liver disease (frequently), trichorrhexis nodosa | Hyperammonemia, elevated plasma citrulline, and argininosuccinic acid |
| Argininemia | Autosomal recessive | Arginase | Spastic diplegia, neurobehavioral | Elevated plasma arginine, elevated urine orotic acid |
| Hyperornithinemia-hyperammonemia-homocitrullinuria (HHH) | Autosomal recessive | Ornithine mitochondrial transporter | Encephalopathy, neurobehavioral, spastic diplegia, retinal disease | Hyperammonemia, elevated plasma ornithine, elevated urine homocitrulline, elevated urine orotic acid |
| Citrullinemia type II | Autosomal recessive | Citrin (aspartate/glutamate transporter) | Neuropsychiatric, neonatal cholestatic hepatitis | Hyperammonemia, elevated plasma citrulline, and arginine |
| Hyperdibasic aminoaciduria, (lysinuric protein intolerance) | Autosomal recessive | Dibasic amino acid transporter | Protein intolerance, vomiting, pulmonary alveolar proteinosis, glomerulonephritis, immune deficiency | Hyperammonemia, elevated urine lysine, ornithine, and arginine |

[a]The biochemical features illustrate the typical features observed with each disorder. The typical features are not always found, and thus, clinical judgment should be used in interpretation of results. Hyperammonemia, hyperalaninemia, and hyperglutaminemia may be found in individuals with suboptimal control.

AR, autosomal recessive; ARG1, arginase 1; ASL, argininosuccinate lyase; ASS1, argininosuccinate synthase 1; CPS1, carbamoyl-phosphate synthase 1; HHH, hyperornithinemia-hyperammonemia-homocitrullinuria; NAGS, *N*-acetylglutamate synthase; OTC, ornithine transcarbamylase; RBC, red blood cell; SLC25A13, mitochondrial aspartate/glutamate carrier; SLCA15, mitochondrial ornithine transporter ORNT1; UCD, urea cycle disorder.



treatment, may progress to seizures, coma, and death. In adolescents and adults, the presentation may mimic intoxication or psychiatric disorders. Hyperammonemia can have devastating consequences, and even a single episode, if severe or prolonged, can lead to significant neurocognitive deficits, intellectual disability, or even coma and death.

The diagnosis of hyperammonemia is dependent on reliable and timely measurement of blood ammonia. To accurately measure ammonia in the blood, a free-flowing sample should be collected, placed on ice, and processed within 30 minutes. Typically, automated analyzers that use a colorimetric method for detection are available in large hospital laboratories, which facilitates the reporting of a result in a timely manner.

The differential diagnosis for hyperammonemia is broad and, in addition to UCDs, includes liver failure, portosystemic shunts, treatment with valproic acid or certain forms of chemotherapy, herpes simplex virus infection, hyperammonemia-hyperinsulinism syndrome, and other inborn errors of metabolism such as fatty acid oxidations disorders, mitochondrial disorders, and organic acidemias. Typically, a low blood urea nitrogen and respiratory alkalosis in a severely ill child are clues that a UCD is the potential cause for the hyperammonemia. Metabolic acidosis, ketoacidosis, or lactic acidosis may indicate that organic aciduria or mitochondrial disorders are causes for the hyperammonemia. Low ketones and hypoglycemia may indicate a fatty acid oxidation disorder. Urine organic acids and plasma acylcarnitine profiling can be helpful in the diagnosis of organic acidurias and fatty acid oxidation disorders. Urine orotic acid, arising from the accumulation of carbamoyl-phosphate due to a defect in one of the later steps of the urea cycle, may help identify where the potential block is occurring. Transient hyperammonemia of the newborn (THAN), a disorder more common in premature infants, may also present with severe hyperammonemia in the neonatal period. Interestingly, although the exact etiology of THAN remains unclear, children who survive THAN typically do not have further episodes of hyperammonemia.

## CLINICAL DESCRIPTION OF UREA CYCLE DISORDERS

The UCDs have been traditionally classified into proximal disorders (NAGS, CPS1, and OTC deficiencies), distal disorders (ASS1, ASL, and ARG1 deficiencies), and transporter deficiencies (hyperornithinemia-hyperammonemia-homocitrullinuria [HHH] syndrome and citrin deficiency due to ORNT1/SLC25A15 and SLC25A13 deficiencies, respectively). All UCDs are transmitted in an autosomal recessive manner except OTC deficiency, which is X-linked.

The classic presentation of a severe form of UCD is that of a neonate who develops symptoms within the first week of life that include poor suck, vomiting, tachypnea, and altered mental status. If not recognized and treated early, the lethargy can progress to coma and death. Findings associated with severe encephalopathy include papilledema, increased reflexes, and decerebrate or decorticate posture. The laboratory testing typically shows respiratory alkalosis (until encephalopathy leads to depressed breathing and a respiratory acidosis), elevated plasma ammonia, and hyperglutaminemia. Neuroimaging typically reveals features of cerebral edema including effacement of sulci and ventricles and flattening of the cerebral gyri. The electroencephalogram may reveal low-voltage slow waves and burst suppression pattern. In individuals with partial enzymatic deficiencies, hyperammonemia may develop later during childhood or be delayed until the adult years. These individuals may present with behavioral abnormalities, ataxia, headaches, dysarthria, and other neurologic symptoms.

### *N*-Acetylglutamate Synthase Deficiency

NAGS deficiency results in decreased synthesis of the cofactor *N*-acetylglutamate, which leads to reduced activity of CPS1. Although NAGS deficiency is a rare UCD, it is likely to be underdiagnosed as the clinical manifestations are variable and the biochemical profile is not specific. Severe NAGS deficiency can present with neonatal hyperammonemia. Patients with milder enzymatic deficiency can present with headaches, ataxia, altered mental status, or neuropsychiatric syndromes, and the diagnosis may be delayed until adulthood. Plasma amino acid analysis usually demonstrates hyperglutaminemia (a marker of decreased nitrogen disposal) and low levels of citrulline. Urinary orotic acid levels are not elevated. The diagnosis can be established by molecular genetic testing that includes tests to detect sequence and copy number variants in *NAGS*. An accurate diagnosis is important because of the availability of a specific treatment, carglumic acid (*N*-carbamoyl-L-glutamate), a synthetic analogue of *N*-acetylglutamate, which can prevent hyperammonemia in this disorder.

#### Carbamoyl-Phosphate Synthase 1 Deficiency

CPS1, a mitochondrial enzyme, catalyzes the synthesis of carbamoyl-phosphate from bicarbonate and ammonia, which is the rate-limiting step of the urea cycle. This enzyme is distinct from CPS2, which is a part of a larger enzymatic complex required for synthesis of the pyrimidines in the cytosol. CPS1 deficiency can present with hyperammonemic crises in the newborn period or later during childhood or adulthood. The biochemical findings on plasma amino acid analysis are similar to that of NAGS deficiency and include elevated glutamine and reduced levels or absence of citrulline. Urinary orotic acid levels are not elevated. The diagnosis can be confirmed by molecular genetic testing of *CPS1* or by enzymatic testing from a liver biopsy specimen.

#### Ornithine Transcarbamylase Deficiency

Ornithine transcarbamylase (OTC) deficiency is the only X-linked UCD. Because males are hemizygous, they typically present with a more severe phenotype as compared to heterozygous females. Males with OTC deficiency typically present with severe neonatal hyperammonemia. However, late-onset presentations in males have also been reported. In females, the severity of presentation ranges from symptomatic early-onset hyperammonemia to late-onset hyperammonemia, and many carrier females are asymptomatic. Overall, estimates suggest that approximately 15% of female carriers for OTC deficiency will have symptoms at some point during their lifetime. Some females may only present with hyperammonemia in the setting of certain stressors such as a high protein load, prolonged fasting, severe gastrointestinal illness, and following surgery or childbirth. This wide phenotypic variability in females has been attributed to skewed X-inactivation. In addition to hyperammonemia, acute hepatic failure, liver dysfunction, and hepatocellular injury are known to be presenting features in OTC deficiency. Liver abnormalities, when present, may delay the identification of OTC deficiency as the cause of hyperammonemia, as elevated ammonia may be attributed to liver dysfunction.

The diagnosis of OTC deficiency is suspected based on low plasma levels of citrulline and arginine along with elevations in urinary orotic acid. This elevation in urinary orotic acid classically distinguishes OTC deficiency from NAGS and CPS1 deficiencies. The diagnosis of OTC deficiency in asymptomatic females or in patients with intermittent symptoms can be challenging because the metabolite levels are typically normal. Although the diagnosis can be confirmed by pursuing molecular genetic testing (sequencing and analysis for copy number variants involving the *OTC* gene), such testing does not reveal a pathogenic variant in approximately 15% of patients suspected of having OTC deficiency. Assessing OTC enzyme activity in a specimen from a liver biopsy may aid the diagnosis. The allopurinol challenge has also been used as a diagnostic tool in females suspected of having OTC deficiency.

#### Argininosuccinate Synthase 1 Deficiency

ASS1 deficiency (also known as citrullinemia type 1) can present with hyperammonemia in the neonatal period or later during childhood. A marked elevation in plasma citrulline is the biochemical hallmark of the disorder. The citrulline elevation in ASS1 deficiency is typically significantly higher than the more mild elevations observed in citrin deficiency (citrullinemia type 2). The diagnosis can be confirmed by molecular genetic testing or by assessing ASS1 enzyme activity in fibroblasts. Newborn screening can help identify neonates with citrullinemia.

#### Argininosuccinate Lyase Deficiency

ASL deficiency leads to accumulation and excretion of argininosuccinic acid, and thus, this disorder is also called argininosuccinic aciduria. The abundant urinary excretion of argininosuccinate provides a means for the excretion of excess nitrogen, but can also lead to loss of citric acid cycle intermediates and hypokalemia. Whereas ASL deficiency can present with early-onset hyperammonemia, patients with mild enzymatic deficiencies rarely decompensate, and a subset of patients never develops hyperammonemia. A specific hair abnormality characterized by brittle and coarse hair, trichorrhexis nodosa, is a characteristic but not universal finding in children. Hepatomegaly, chronic hepatic injury, and cirrhosis have been described in the disorder. A subset of individuals with ASL deficiency can develop neurocognitive deficits and hypertension even in the absence of documented hyperammonemia. Recently, it has been shown that ASL is required for synthesis of nitric oxide (NO) and that NO deficiency may be responsible for the hypertension. The diagnosis is made by detection of argininosuccinic acid in the plasma and urine. Plasma amino acid analyses typically demonstrate mildly elevated citrulline levels and low arginine levels. The diagnosis can be suspected based on newborn screening and confirmed by molecular genetic testing or by assessment of ASL activity in fibroblasts or red blood cells.

#### Arginase 1 Deficiency

Prior to the introduction of newborn screening, the typical presentation of individuals with ARG1 deficiency included spastic diplegia, intellectual disability or developmental delay, and seizures. Other manifestations of the disorder include self-restriction of protein in the diet, growth deficiency, and liver dysfunction including hepatic fibrosis and cirrhosis. Although hyperammonemia is very rare in the neonatal period, patients may develop hyperammonemia during childhood or adulthood. The biochemical hallmark of the disorder is the elevated levels of plasma arginine. ARG1 enzyme activity testing in red blood cells and molecular genetic testing can be performed to confirm the diagnosis. Treatment includes dietary protein restriction and alternate pathway therapy. The goal of therapy is to reduce plasma arginine to near-normal levels, a target that is often challenging to achieve. Despite standard treatment, many patients still develop the spastic diplegia and intellectual disability characteristic of this disorder. Newborn screening for this disorder is not yet universal.

### DEFICIENCY OF TRANSPORTERS

#### Citrin Deficiency

Deficiency of the mitochondrial aspartate/glutamate carrier (SLC25A13, citrin) leads to a decreased availability of aspartate for conjugation with citrulline, which can result in decreased flux through the urea cycle. Citrin deficiency can manifest with neonatal cholestasis or failure to thrive in children, and liver failure has been described in some children. Children with failure to thrive caused by citrin deficiency typically prefer protein-rich and/or lipid-rich foods and are averse to carbohydrate-rich foods. In adults, citrin deficiency can present with neuropsychiatric symptoms including irritability, delusions, hyperactivity, aggression, and disorientation, along with dysarthria, muscle weakness, and altered mental status. Adults with citrin deficiency are at risk for developing pancreatitis, hyperlipidemia, fatty liver, and hepatocellular carcinoma. The biochemical findings vary with age and the type of presentation. For instance, young infants with neonatal intrahepatic cholestasis can have hypoproteinemia, elevated alpha-fetoprotein, and elevated plasma levels of citrulline, arginine, methionine, threonine, and tyrosine. Adults with citrin deficiency typically have mildly elevated citrulline and arginine levels. Newborn screening may detect elevated citrulline, and the diagnosis can be confirmed by molecular genetic testing.

#### Hyperornithinemia-Hyperammonemia-Homocitrullinuria Syndrome

SLC25A15 or ORNT1 transports ornithine across to the mitochondrial membrane. Deficiency of this transporter results in decreased availability of ornithine for ureagenesis, thus causing hyperammonemia. HHH syndrome has a wide spectrum of clinical presentations, varying from neonatal hyperammonemia and coma to a slowly progressive spastic diplegia, intellectual disability, myoclonic epilepsy, and behavioral abnormalities. Whereas the majority of individuals are diagnosed during infancy or childhood, a significant fraction are only diagnosed during adulthood. The classic biochemical findings include hyperammonemia, homocitrullinuria (lysine plus carbamoylphosphate), hyperornithinemia, low plasma creatine, and orotic aciduria. Complications can include hepatic abnormalities, coagulopathy, and retinal degeneration. Treatment involves protein-restricted diet, citrulline supplementation, and nitrogen-scavenging agents as needed. Newborn screening may identify affected individuals, but ornithine may not be elevated to diagnostic levels in newborns. The diagnosis can be established by molecular genetic testing.

## OTHER GENETIC DISORDERS THAT RESULT IN DECREASED UREA PRODUCTION

The efficient flux of nitrogen through the urea cycle is intricately linked to the availability of substrates, intermediates, ATP, and the interconnectedness of the urea cycle with other metabolic pathways. Deficiencies in enzymes or transport proteins that are involved in the synthesis or transport of substrates or intermediates can result in a secondary deficiency of the urea cycle.

### Carbonic Anhydrase VA Deficiency

A more recently described cause of severe neonatal or infantile hyperammonemia is carbonic anhydrase VA deficiency, an autosomal recessive disorder. In addition to hyperammonemia, patients present with encephalopathy, hypoglycemia, and lactic acidemia. Carbonic anhydrase VA generates bicarbonate for at least 4 enzymes: CPS1, pyruvate carboxylase, 3-methylcrotonyl carboxylase, and propionyl-CoA carboxylase. Decreased flux through reactions catalyzed by these enzymes is proposed to explain the biochemical and clinical features. Patients with this disorder require a sick-day diet (eg, increased calories, decreased protein intake) during intercurrent illnesses that increase the risk for metabolic decompensation. Given the secondary deficiency of CPS1, *N*-carbamoyl-L-glutamate has been used in the management.

### Lysinuric Protein Intolerance

Lysinuric protein intolerance (LPI) is caused by a deficiency of SLC7A7, a transporter of cationic amino acids including lysine, arginine, and ornithine across the epithelial cell membranes. The intracellular deficiency of arginine and ornithine in LPI results in hyperammonemia due to a secondary dysfunction of the urea cycle. This disorder has been described in Chapter 139.

### Organic Acidemias and Fatty Acid Oxidation Disorders

Methylmalonic acidemia, propionic acidemia, and fatty acid oxidation disorders can result in accumulation of acyl-CoA intermediates, which can interfere with urea production by different mechanisms including decreased synthesis of *N*-acetylglutamate. Hyperammonemia is typically a secondary phenomenon observed during metabolic crises in these disorders. Heterozygous hypermorphic mutations in glutamate dehydrogenase lead to hyperammonemia from the excess generation of ammonia and α-ketoglutarate from glutamate, with α-ketoglutarate also leading to hyperinsulinism and hypoglycemia. The hyperammonemia appears to be asymptomatic with no evidence for impaired ureagenesis or elevations of glutamine.

## DIAGNOSIS OF UREA CYCLE DISORDERS

When a UCD is suspected, plasma amino acid analysis and urine orotic acid measurements should be performed on an emergent basis. Generally, metabolites upstream of the defect are elevated, while those distal to the enzymatic defect are low. If a transporter deficiency is being considered, urinary amino acid analysis may also be helpful. The typical metabolite signatures of the various UCDs are presented in Table 141-1. Enzymatic analyses are available for diagnosis, but these tests are only available at specialized centers and have generally been superseded by more widely available molecular genetic testing. Molecular genetic testing includes methods to assess sequence variants, as well as copy number variations (eg, deletions or duplications that disrupt a gene). Sanger sequencing of single genes as well as panel testing that simultaneously interrogates multiple genes using next-generation sequencing technologies are clinically available. Copy number variation is assessed using array comparative genomic hybridization or multiplex ligation-dependent probe amplification or, in the case of next-generation sequencing, read depth analysis.

More recently, newborn screening for a subset of UCDs (eg, ASS1, ASL, ARG1, and citrin deficiencies) has been used to facilitate early diagnosis and initiation of treatment in the presymptomatic period. Currently, newborn screening cannot reliably detect the proximal disorders (NAGS, CPS1, and OTC deficiencies).

## TREATMENT

The main goal of management during metabolic crises is to rapidly reduce ammonia levels in the blood while the long-term management is focused on preventing hyperammonemia. Dietary modification, supplementation with urea cycle intermediates such as citrulline and arginine, and use of alternate pathway therapies are the cornerstones of treatment of UCDs. Hepatic transplantation may be considered in individuals with severe or recurrent metabolic decompensations or in individuals who develop progressive liver disease.

### Management of Hyperammonemic Crises

The management of hyperammonemic episodes is best performed in the setting of a critical care unit. Precipitating causes for hyperammonemia such as infections, catabolic states, noncompliance with diet or medications, and gastrointestinal bleeding should be actively sought and addressed. Decreasing nitrogen load by temporary elimination of protein, promoting anabolism, and preventing protein breakdown by intravenous infusion of dextrose and insulin are critical in reducing the blood ammonia levels. Intravenous administration of sodium benzoate/sodium phenylacetate and arginine can facilitate nitrogen disposal through alternate pathways and may be required for reducing blood ammonia. In patients with hyperammonemic coma, significantly elevated ammonia levels, and ammonia levels that do not decrease with intravenous alternate pathway therapy, hemodialysis should be promptly instituted. If hemodialysis is unavailable, hemofiltration is an acceptable alternative. Provision of small amounts of essential amino acids within 24 to 36 hours of admission may be needed to avoid rebound hyperammonemia from essential amino acid deficiency.

### Long-Term Management

**Dietary Therapy** Except in citrin deficiency, dietary management in all UCDs includes some form of protein restriction. In patients with severe UCDs, the intake of protein is typically limited to the minimal daily requirement for age, and restriction beyond this is often needed to maintain nitrogen homeostasis. Half of the protein allowance is typically provided as an essential amino acid supplement. Supplementing with nonprotein formulae may be required to provide age-appropriate calories. The dietary restrictions in patients with mild forms of UCDs are typically less stringent. Citrin deficiency is an exception because a diet rich in lipids and protein and low in carbohydrates is recommended for patients with this disorder.

The supplementation of urea cycle intermediates not only provides deficient metabolites but can also facilitate excretion of nitrogen. Citrulline has only 1 waste nitrogen and, when used in CPS1 or OTC deficiencies, can facilitate the disposal of nitrogen from aspartate as urea. In ASS1 and ASL deficiencies, supplementation with arginine can enable excretion of nitrogen in the form of citrulline and argininosuccinic acid, respectively (Table 141-2).

**Alternate Pathway Therapy** Benzoate and phenylacetate conjugate with glycine (which has 1 atom of nitrogen) and glutamine (which has 2 atoms of nitrogen) to form hippuric acid and phenylacetylglutamine, respectively. These nitrogenous waste products can be excreted in the urine and thus serve as an alternative pathway for nitrogen disposal (see Table 141-2). Sodium phenylbutyrate has an odor and unpalatable taste. Thus, recently, 2 formulations of phenylbutyrate that are tasteless and odorless have been developed. Pheburane is a formulation containing sodium

**TABLE 141-2 UREA CYCLE INTERMEDIATES AND ALTERNATE PATHWAY THERAPY FOR THE LONG-TERM MANAGEMENT OF UCDs[a]**

| UCD | L-Citrulline | L-Arginine (free base) | Sodium Phenylbutyrate | Glycerol Phenylbutyrate[a] | Sodium Benzoate | *N*-Carbamoyl-L-Glutamate |
|---|---|---|---|---|---|---|
| NAGS deficiency | — | — | — | | — | ~100 mg/kg$^{-1}$/d$^{-1}$ |
| CPS1 and OTC deficiency | 100 mg/kg$^{-1}$/d$^{-1}$ or 3.8 g/m$^{-2}$/d$^{-1}$ | — | 450–600 mg/kg$^{-1}$/d$^{-1}$ if < 20 kg<br>9900–13,000 mg/m$^{-2}$/d$^{-1}$ if > 20 kg | 4.4–11.2 mL/m$^{-2}$/d$^{-1}$ | 250 mg/kg$^{-1}$/d$^{-1}$ or 5500 mg/m$^{-2}$/d$^{-1}$ | — |
| ASS1 deficiency | — | 400–700 mg/kg$^{-1}$/d–$^{1}$ or 8800–15,400 mg/m$^{-2}$/d$^{-1}$ | 450–600 mg/kg$^{-1}$/d$^{-1}$ if < 20 kg<br>9900–13,000 mg/m$^{-2}$/d$^{-1}$ if > 20 kg | 4.4–11.2 mL/m$^{-2}$/d$^{-1}$ | 250 mg/kg$^{-1}$/d$^{-1}$ or 5500 mg/m$^{-2}$/d$^{-1}$ | — |
| ASL deficiency | — | 400–700 mg/kg$^{-1}$/d$^{-1}$ or 8800–15,400 mg/m$^{-2}$/d$^{-1}$ | 450–600 mg/kg$^{-1}$/d$^{-1}$ if < 20 kg<br>9900–13,000 mg/m$^{-2}$/d$^{-1}$ if > 20 kg | 4.4–11.2 mL/m$^{-2}$/d$^{-1}$ | 250 mg/kg$^{-1}$/d$^{-1}$ or 5500 mg/m$^{-2}$/d$^{-1}$ | — |
| ARG1 deficiency | — | — | 450–600 mg/kg$^{-1}$/d$^{-1}$ if < 20 kg<br>9900–13,000 mg/m$^{-2}$/d$^{-1}$ if > 20 kg | 4.4–11.2 mL/m$^{-2}$/d$^{-1}$ | 250 mg/kg$^{-1}$/d$^{-1}$ or 5500 mg/m$^{-2}$/d$^{-1}$ | — |

[a]The dose ranges depicted are those that are typically used in individuals with UCDs. The safety and efficacy of phenylbutyrate doses greater than 20 g/d are not known. The dose of glycerol phenylbutyrate depicted is the recommended initial dose in phenylbutyrate-naïve patients. When switching from sodium phenylbutyrate, the total daily dosage of glycerol phenylbutyrate (mL) = total daily dosage of sodium phenylbutyrate (g) × 0.86. The maximal daily dose for benzoate is 12 g. The dose for *N*-carbamoyl-L-glutamate was determined from a small cohort of individuals with NAGS deficiency. When prescribing doses in the upper ranges of the recommended dosing, toxicity should be monitored.

ARG1, arginase 1; ASL, argininosuccinate lyase; ASS1, argininosuccinate synthase 1; CPS1, carbamoyl-phosphate synthase 1; NAGS, *N*-acetylglutamate synthase; OTC, ornithine transcarbamylase; UCD, urea cycle disorder.



phenylbutyrate, and glycerol phenylbutyrate comprises 3 molecules of phenylbutyrate attached to a glycerol backbone. Hydrolysis of glycerol is needed for release of the phenylbutyrate, leading to improved pharmacokinetics and a more stable ammonia profile. Alternate pathway therapies are useful for prevention of hyperammonemic episodes.

***N*-Carbamoyl-L-Glutamate** The mitochondrial membrane is impermeable to *N*-acetylglutamate. Thus, a structural analog, carglumic acid (*N*-carbamoyl-L-glutamate), that crosses the mitochondrial membrane has been developed for the treatment of NAGS deficiency. In several patients, treatment with carglumic acid has been reported to be useful in the treatment and prevention of hyperammonemia. Organic acidurias (methylmalonic, propionic, and isovaleric acidurias) can present with hyperammonemia due to inhibition of NAGS by the accumulated organic acids. Treatment with carglumic acid has been hypothesized to be beneficial in these conditions and in carbonic anhydrase VA deficiency.

**Monitoring Long-Term Management** Height, weight, body mass index, and laboratory indices of nutritional status should be monitored on a regular basis. Tests to assess hepatic inflammation and synthetic function should be considered at regular intervals, especially in individuals who have evidence for ongoing hepatic inflammation or fibrosis. The diet, urea cycle intermediates, and the alternate pathway therapies should be titrated to promote adequate nutrition and prevent hyperammonemic episodes. Plasma amino acids analyses and blood ammonia levels are typically used to assess metabolic control in UCDs. Elevated plasma glutamine level has been considered as a surrogate marker for the risk of hyperammonemia and likely is a major contributor to encephalopathy. Blood ammonia concentrations can fluctuate considerably during each day. Recent evidence from controlled trials shows that early morning fasting ammonia levels correlate strongly with daily ammonia exposure and with the risk for future hyperammonemic episodes. Thus, whenever possible, early morning ammonia should be measured to assess metabolic control. Quantifying drug metabolites in plasma may be of value in monitoring the safety of phenylbutyrate therapy; however, such testing is not widely available. A ratio of plasma phenylacetate to phenylacetylglutamine has been proposed as a useful biomarker.

### Liver Transplantation

Liver transplantation has been an increasingly used strategy for patients with severe UCDs as replacement of the liver effectively "cures" the hepatic enzymatic deficiency and prevents hyperammonemia. Moreover, reports indicate improved quality of life and normalization of diet. However, liver transplantation is not without inherent risks, and according to one recent study, the 5-year survival rate for pediatric patients with UCDs after liver transplantation is approximately 89%. Liver transplantation is not expected to treat the extrahepatic manifestations of disorders such as ASL deficiency, and its efficacy in ARG1 deficiency has not been determined. In addition, in proximal UCDs, plasma citrulline levels remain low following transplantation, reflecting the primary contribution of intestinal citrulline to the plasma citrulline pool, although the consequences of this metabolic abnormality in the setting of a normal hepatic urea cycle function remain unclear. The timing of transplantation is challenging as the technical difficulties of hepatic transplantation in very small infants need to be balanced with the risk for sequelae associated with repeated hyperammonemia episodes that occur over time as a child grows older.

### Practical Aspects of Treatment

Practical aspects of management for patients with all UCDs include education regarding avoidance of prolonged fasting, large protein loads, ensuring adequate fluid intake, provision of letters that could be of use in emergent situations, and recommendation of use of an emergency bracelet. Precautions should be taken during the pre- and perioperative periods to prevent catabolic stress that could lead to hyperammonemia. Patients require close monitoring and possibly hospitalization during intercurrent illnesses which may increase risk for hyperammonemia. Appropriate genetic counseling should be provided so that patients and families have a clear understanding of recurrence risks for their particular disorder, and testing should be offered to other family members at risk. Efforts should be made to connect those affected and their families with family organizations and support groups, which often are very useful resources of information.

## OUTCOMES

Prior to the availability of alternative-pathway therapy, few patients with severe UCD survived infancy. In the 1980s, the 5-year survival was estimated to be approximately 25%, and nearly all of the children who survived the hyperammonemic episodes had neurocognitive deficits and intellectual disability. With the implementation of newborn screening programs across all 50 states in the United States, availability of alternative-pathway therapy and dialysis, and increased awareness of these disorders, the outcome has improved. It is estimated that 66% of children with neonatal-onset disease and 89% with later-onset disease survive the initial hyperammonemic crisis; however, the morbidity still remains high. A study by the Urea Cycle Disorder Consortium reported that two-thirds of children with neonatal-onset disease and one-quarter of children with late-onset UCDs have intellectual disability, behavioral challenges, and deficits in attention and executive function.


## ACKNOWLEDGMENT

This work was supported by the Urea Cycle Disorders Consortium (UCDC; U54HD061221), which is a part of the National Institutes of Health (NIH) Rare Disease Clinical Research Network (RDCRN), supported through collaboration between the Office of Rare Diseases Research (ORDR), the National Center for Advancing Translational Science (NCATS), and the Eunice Kennedy Shriver National Institute of Child Health and Human Development (NICHD). This work was also supported by the Clinical Translational Core of Baylor College of Medicine IDDRC (U54 HD083092) from the NICHD. The content is solely the responsibility of the authors and does not necessarily represent the official views of the NICHD or NIH.


## SUGGESTED READINGS




Ah Mew N, Lanpher BC, Gropman A, et al. Urea cycle disorders. In: Pagon RA, Adam MP, Ardinger HH, et al, eds. *GeneReviews®* [Internet]. Seattle, WA: University of Washington, Seattle; 1993-2016; 2003 Apr 29 [updated 2015 Apr 9].

Batshaw ML, Tuchman M, Summar M, Seminara J, Members of the Urea Cycle Disorders Consortium. A longitudinal study of urea cycle disorders. *Mol Genet Metab.* 2014;113:127-130.

Gropman AL, Summar M, Leonard JV. Neurological implications of urea cycle disorders. *J Inherited Metab Dis.* 2007;30:865-879.

Krebs HA, Henseleit K. Studies on urea formation in the animal organism. *Hoppe-Seylers Z Physiol Chem.* 1932;210:33-66.

Krivitzky L, Babikian T, Lee HS, Thomas NH, Burk-Paull KL, Batshaw ML. Intellectual, adaptive, and behavioral functioning in children with urea cycle disorders *Pediatr Res.* 2009;66:96-101.

Singh RH. Nutritional management of patients with urea cycle disorders. *J Inherited Metab Dis.* 2007;30:880-887.

Yu L, Rayhill SC, Hsu EK, Landis CS. Liver transplantation for urea cycle disorders: analysis of the united network for organ sharing database. *Transplant Proc.* 2015;47:2413-2418.




# PART 3 VITAMINS

# 142 Vitamin $B_{12}$ and Folic Acid

Oleg A. Shchelochkov and Charles P. Venditti

## VITAMIN $B_{12}$

Cobalamin (vitamin $B_{12}$) is a complex organometallic molecule that is synthesized by many bacteria and is obtained in the human diet from meat, fish, and dairy products. It is not present in plant foods, so strict vegetarians are at risk for dietary deficiency. Derivatives of cobalamin are required for the activity of 2 enzymes: methylcobalamin and 5′-deoxyadenosylcobalamin. Methylcobalamin is generated during the catalytic cycle of methionine synthase, a cytoplasmic enzyme that catalyzes methylation of homocysteine to methionine (see Chapter 133). 5′-Deoxyadenosylcobalamin (AdoCbl) is required for the mitochondrial enzyme methylmalonyl-coenzyme A (CoA) mutase to catalyze the conversion of methylmalonyl-CoA, formed during catabolism of branched-chain amino acids and odd-chain fatty acids, to succinyl-CoA (see Chapter 132). Therefore, inborn errors of cobalamin metabolism result in isolated methylmalonic aciduria, isolated homocystinuria, or combined methylmalonic aciduria and homocystinuria, depending on which step in cobalamin metabolism is affected. Without treatment, hyperhomocysteinemia is usually accompanied by hypomethioninemia. Significantly elevated homocysteine levels may be associated with an increased risk of thrombosis. Decreased methionine is associated with abnormalities of the white matter of the nervous system. Elevated levels of methylmalonic acid can lead to metabolic acidosis.

### METABOLISM OF COBALAMIN

Cobalamin consists of a planar corrin ring with a central cobalt atom, a 5,6-dimethylbenzimidazole base, and an upper axial ligand attached to the cobalt atom that varies in different forms of cobalamin. Physiologically important cobalamins include hydroxycobalamin (OHCbl), methylcobalamin (MeCbl), and adenosylcobalamin (AdoCbl). The most common commercially available form of vitamin $B_{12}$ contains a cyano group in the upper axial position (CNCbl). The central cobalt can exist in the oxidized $Co^{3+}$ state (cob[III]alamin), the $Co^{2+}$ state (cob[II]alamin), or the fully reduced $Co^{1+}$ state (cob[I]alamin). Converting exogenous cobalamin, typically in the form of cob(III)alamin, to its biologically active coenzyme forms involves reducing the central cobalt to cob(I)alamin and then adding the appropriate upper axial ligand (Fig. 142-1).

Absorption of dietary cobalamin is a complex process that is dependent on several cobalamin-binding proteins. Cobalamin is released from food in the acidic environment of the stomach, where it becomes bound to transcobalamin I (TCN1) found in saliva and gastric juice. Transcobalamin I is broken down in the intestine by proteolytic enzymes, and cobalamin binds the gastric intrinsic factor (GIF). The GIF-cobalamin complex is taken up by enterocytes in the distal ileum in a process mediated by a receptor, cubam, composed of 2 proteins, cubilin (CUBN) and amnionless (AMN). After uptake by enterocytes, cobalamin is released into the circulation, where it binds the transport protein transcobalamin II (TCN2).

In blood, transcobalamin II–bound cobalamin is available for uptake by most cell types. Following endocytosis, mediated by the transcobalamin receptor (TCBLR encoded by *CD320*), the cobalamin–transcobalamin II complex dissociates in lysosomes, and free cobalamin is transferred to the cytoplasm with the participation of at least 2 proteins LMBRD1 (cblF) and ABCD4 (cblJ). Upon egress of the cobalamin from the lysosome, the vitamin begins the cytosolic pathway of metabolism. This process involves MMACHC (cblC), which removes axial cobalamin moieties, reduces $Co^{3+}$ to $Co^{2+}$, and facilitates the transfer of cobalamin to MMADHC (cblD). Subsequently, cobalamin becomes associated with methionine synthase in the cytoplasm, or it may be further transported to the mitochondria, where it is converted to 5′-deoxyadenosylcobalamin, the active cofactor for methylmalonyl-CoA mutase. The steps of cellular cobalamin metabolism common to synthesis of both coenzyme derivatives remain under study.

The catalytic cycle of methionine synthase involves transfer of a methyl group from 5-methyl-THF to an enzyme-bound cob(I)alamin molecule, forming methylcobalamin (MeCbl). The methyl group is then transferred from MeCbl to homocysteine, forming

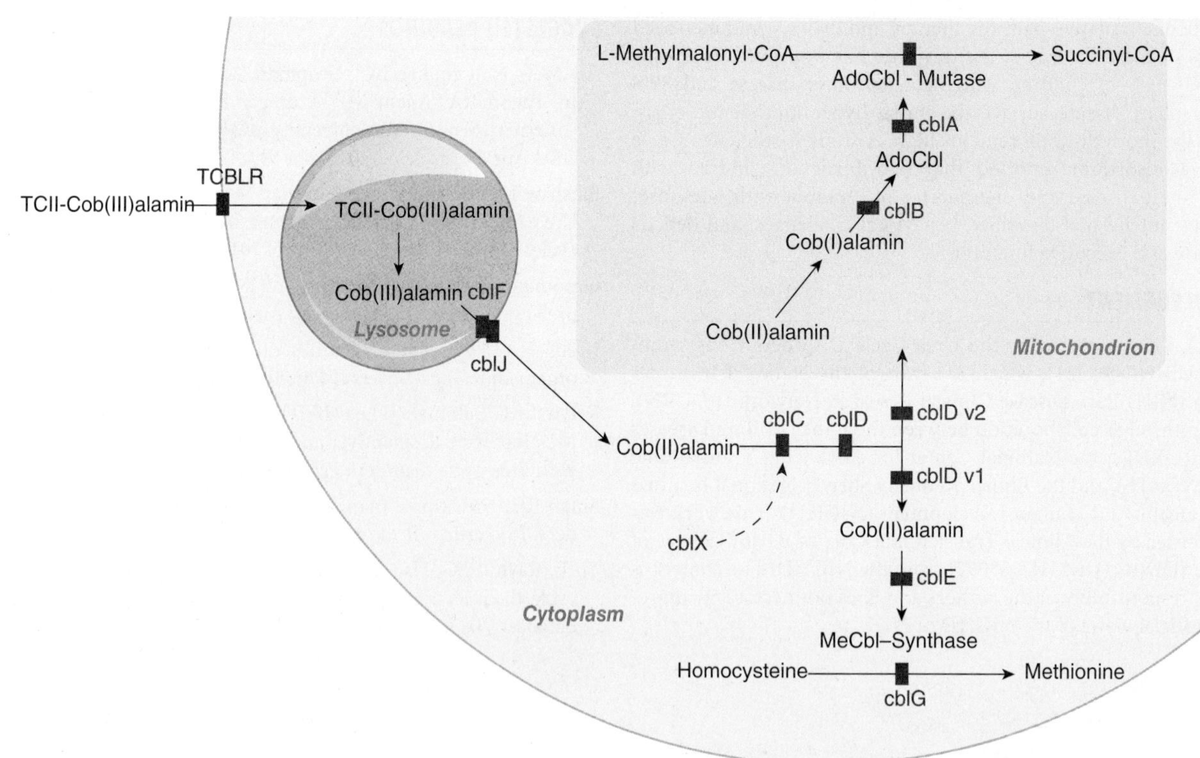


**FIGURE 142-1** Metabolic pathway of cobalamin. The steps affected by inborn errors of cobalamin metabolism are shown by the red bars. AdoCbl, 5′-deoxyadenosylcobalamin; cblA, cobalamin A deficiency; cblB, cobalamin B deficiency; cblC, cobalamin C deficiency; cblD, cobalamin D deficiency; cblD v1, cobalamin D deficiency variant 1; cblD v2, cobalamin D deficiency variant 2; cblE, cobalamin E deficiency; cblF, cobalamin F deficiency; cblG, cobalamin G deficiency; cblJ, cobalamin J deficiency; cblX, cobalamin X deficiency; MeCbl, methylcobalamin; mutase, methylmalonyl-CoA mutase; synthase, methionine synthase; TCII, transcobalamin; TCBLR, transcobalamin receptor.

methionine and regenerating cob(I)alamin. Occasionally the cob(I) alamin is oxidized to cob(II)alamin; when this occurs, regeneration of MeCbl requires the activity of a second protein, methionine synthase reductase, which uses adenosylmethionine as its methyl group donor. Remethylation of homocysteine to form methionine thus requires the activity of both methionine synthase (cblG) and methionine synthase reductase (cblE).

The system by which cobalamin enters the mitochondria is unknown, as is the form of cobalamin that crosses the mitochondrial membrane. Mitochondrial reductases that can support reduction of cob(II)alamin to cob(I)alamin have been identified in vitro, but the enzyme that catalyzes this reaction in vivo is not yet known. Cob(I)alamin receives the adenosine base from ATP to form 5'-deoxyadenosylcobalamin (AdoCbl) in a reaction catalyzed by cob(I)alamin adenosyltransferase, encoded by the *MMAB* gene (cblB). Another protein, the product of the *MMAA* gene (cblA), appears to play a role in supporting the formation of holo-methylmalonyl-CoA mutase and in maintaining the enzyme-bound cobalamin in its active form. The presence of methylmalonyl-CoA mutase, cobalamin adenosyltransferase, and the MMAA protein, possibly in association with a cob(II)alamin reductase, is required for conversion of methylmalonyl-CoA to succinyl-CoA in vivo.

## ISOLATED METHYLMALONIC ACIDURIA

### METABOLIC DERANGEMENT

Isolated methylmalonic aciduria is seen in patients with methylmalonyl-CoA mutase deficiency (Online Mendelian Inheritance in Man [OMIM] no. 251000), cblA deficiency (OMIM no. 251100), cblB deficiency (OMIM no. 251110), and cblD deficiency variant 2 (OMIM no. 277410). Methylmalonyl-CoA mutase deficiency, also referred to as the *mut* disorder is caused by mutations in the *MUT* gene on chromosome 6p12.3. The *mut* disorder has been subdivided into 2 classes: (1) in *mut*$^0$, there is no stimulation of mutase activity in cultured cells on incubation with hydroxycobalamin (OHCbl), and there is often no detectable mutase protein; (2) in *mut*$^-$, mutase activity is stimulated by addition of OHCbl. Deleterious mutations in the *MMAA* gene on chromosome 4q31.21 result in decreased synthesis of adenosylcobalamin (cblA deficiency). The cblB deficiency is caused by mutations in the *MMAB* gene on chromosome 12q24.11. Patients with mutations resulting in the loss of function of cblD required for the AdoCbl synthesis also experience isolated methylmalonic aciduria and are referred to as having cblD deficiency variant 2.

### CLINICAL PRESENTATION

Patients with isolated methylmalonic aciduria are prone to episodes of life-threatening acidosis, often in response to infection or to increased protein intake. Initial presentation is most frequently during infancy, with vomiting, hypotonia, irritability, and lethargy, which can progress to coma and death if not treated. In the most severely affected individuals, there may be intractable acidosis during the neonatal period that leads to death, but in many patients, the disorder is characterized by recurrent acidotic crises characterized by high anion gap metabolic acidosis, ketoacidosis, lactic acidosis, and hyperammonemia. Anemia, neutropenia, thrombocytopenia, failure to thrive, optic nerve atrophy, acute and chronic kidney disease, pancreatitis, and basal ganglia injury occur variably, but are well-recognized complications of the disorder. Studies of a series of patients have shown that presentation is typically most severe in individuals with *mut*$^0$. The clinical course of patients with cblB deficiency may resemble that of *mut*$^0$ patients. cblA, cblD variant 2, *mut*$^-$, and rare OHCbl-responsive cblB patients have the least severe presentation and the best prognosis. Clinically unstable patients with severe methylmalonic acidemia may be candidates for an elective liver transplantation. Progression to end-stage renal failure will necessitate kidney or combined liver-kidney transplantation.

## DIAGNOSTIC TESTS

Analysis of urinary organic acids from these patients reveals elevated levels of methylmalonic acid and propionyl-CoA derived metabolites such as methylcitric acid, 3-hydroxypropionic acid, and tiglylglycine. Amino acid analysis usually reveals elevated glycine in blood and urine, while the acylcarnitine carnitine profile shows elevated propionylcarnitine and methylmalonylcarnitine. Accumulation of CoA conjugates may result in secondary carnitine deficiency necessitating carnitine supplementation.

Elevation of methylmalonic acid levels may also be seen in individuals with methylmalonyl-CoA epimerase (racemase) deficiency and in patients with mutations affecting either subunit of succinyl-CoA ligase; however, in these orders, the levels are lower than in *mut*, cblA, and cblB patients. Mild elevations of methylmalonic acid need to be distinguished from dietary vitamin $B_{12}$ deficiency and other forms of abnormal cobalamin absorption in the gastrointestinal tract. Elevations of both malonic and methylmalonic acids on the urine organic acid assay can be seen in the combined malonic and methylmalonic aciduria (CMAMMA; OMIM no. 614265) due to mutations in *ACSF3*. Differentiation between the different forms of methylmalonic aciduria depends on molecular and biochemical methods. DNA-based molecular genetic testing has become the initial confirmatory step. If DNA analysis does not reveal the diagnosis, cellular biochemical testing using cultured fibroblasts becomes necessary.

## GENETICS

All 4 disorders are inherited as autosomal recessive traits. Mutations in most families are private, but several mutations are relatively common within a specific ethnic group. Most pathogenic variants are missense or nonsense mutations, but copy number variants (deletions and insertions) have also been described. Genotype-phenotype correlations are difficult, but in general, patients with 2 nonsense, larger copy number variants and known severe missense mutations have a more severe course of the disease and should be considered for transplantation sooner. Patients with cblD deficiency variant 2 appear to have mutations in exon 3 and 4 of the *MMADHC* gene encoding a protein domain required for the AdoCbl synthesis.

## TREATMENT

Patients with isolated methylmalonic aciduria require life-long monitoring and management. Episodes of acute metabolic decompensation are treated with intravenous fluids containing glucose, appropriate electrolytes, and if necessary, bicarbonate replacement. Dietary goals include a brief restriction of protein intake and supplementation of calories through carbohydrate and lipids. OHCbl responsiveness needs to be established in all patients. Acute mental status changes and new neurologic findings, even in the absence of acidosis, should be treated as metabolic emergencies. Chronic dietary management may require the judicious use of medical foods deficient in amino acids (ie, isoleucine, valine, threonine, and methionine), the precursors of methylmalonic acid. Due to poor palatability of protein-modified diet, frequent nausea, vomiting, and poor appetite, most patients need a gastrostomy tube to facilitate enteral feeding. Carnitine supplementation is used to prevent and treat secondary carnitine deficiency. Patients who experience frequent and severe decompensations may need to be evaluated for liver or combined liver-kidney transplantation. Liver and liver-kidney transplantation helps stabilize patients metabolically and reduce the number of hospitalizations secondary to acidotic decompensations and hyperammonemia. Even after liver and liver-kidney transplantation, patients need to continue a protein-restricted diet and should be monitored for secondary carnitine deficiency. Any changes in the neurologic status should prompt proactive management of metabolic status, as vision loss and brain injury can occur even after liver transplantation. The decision to undergo organ transplantation requires a consideration of many factors including the severity of the disorder, organ availability, rate of surgical complications, and the need for life-long immunosuppression.

# ISOLATED HOMOCYSTINURIA



## METABOLIC DERANGEMENT

Homocystinuria in the absence of methylmalonic aciduria is seen in patients with the cblE (OMIM no. 236270), cblG (OMIM no. 250940), and cblD variant 1 (OMIM no. 277410) deficiencies. In all 3 disorders, methionine synthase function is impaired; in the cblG deficiency, synthase-specific activity in cell extracts is decreased under all assay conditions, while in cblE deficiency, specific activity is decreased only in the presence of limiting concentrations of exogenous reducing agent. The cblG deficiency is caused by mutations affecting the *MTR* gene on chromosome 1q43, which encodes methionine synthase. The cblE deficiency is caused by mutations of the *MTRR* gene on chromosome 5p15.31, which encodes methionine synthase reductase. cblD variant 1 deficiency is caused by deleterious mutations in the gene *MMADHC* on chromosome 2q23.2 encoding a protein that participates in the intracellular conversion of cobalamin to adenosylcobalamin (AdoCbl) and methylcobalamin (MeCbl).

## CLINICAL PRESENTATION

Patients with these disorders manifest with megaloblastic anemia and neurologic problems, including developmental delay, cerebral atrophy, hypotonia, microcephaly, and seizures. Some patients may present with hemolytic-uremic syndrome, renal artery thrombosis, and pulmonary hypertension. In some patients, total plasma homocysteine can be as high as in patients with homocystinuria due to cystathionine β-synthase deficiency. Presentation is typically within the first 2 years of life, but it can also present in adulthood.

## DIAGNOSTIC TESTS

Decreased methionine synthase activity results in increased total plasma homocysteine and in homocysteine in the urine, as well as reduced levels of methionine and elevated cystathionine. Serum cobalamin levels are normal. These disorders can be differentiated from homocystinuria due to cystathionine β-synthase deficiency, which presents with generally higher levels of homocysteine, elevated methionine, and decreased cystathionine levels (see Chapter 133). The diagnosis is confirmed either by DNA analysis of the implicated genes or by biochemical studies of patient's fibroblasts. Affected fibroblasts are characterized by decreased methyl-THF incorporation with normal propionate incorporation and by decreased methylcobalamin synthesis with normal adenosylcobalamin synthesis. The disorders can be differentiated by the response of methionine synthase–specific activity to the titration of a reducing agent, but more typically, they are differentiated by complementation analysis.

## GENETICS

All 3 disorders are inherited as autosomal recessive traits. Genotype-phenotype correlations are difficult to establish. Most described mutations are missense or nonsense. Patients with CblD variant 1 defect tend to have mutations in exons 6 and 8 of the *MMADHC* gene encoding a protein domain responsible for the MeCbl synthesis.

## TREATMENT

Affected individuals can tolerate the recommended daily allowance of protein and need to avoid dietary methionine deficiency. For this reason, medical foods deficient in methionine are not recommended in this group of disorders. Patients respond to OHCbl injections. Supplementation with betaine (250 mg/kg/24 h) facilitates the conversion of homocysteine to methionine through an alternative pathway independent of methionine synthase, via hepatic betaine-homocysteine methyltransferase. To support remethylation reactions, patients with hyperhomocysteninemia are supplemented with folic or folinic acid. In patients with significant hyperhomocysteinemia, attention should be given to the management of risk factors predisposing to hypercoagulability.

# COMBINED METHYLMALONIC ACIDURIA AND HOMOCYSTINURIA

## METABOLIC DERANGEMENT

Five inborn errors of metabolism that affect early steps in cobalamin metabolism result in combined methylmalonic aciduria and homocystinuria. The cblC disorder (OMIM no. 277400) is caused by mutations in *MMACHC* on chromosome 1p34.1. The cblD disorder (OMIM no. 277410) is caused by mutations in *MMADHC* on chromosome 2q23.2. Products of these genes participate in the conversion of $Co^{3+}$ to $Co^{2+}$ and removal of the axial ligand. Although the original patients with the cblD disorder had combined methylmalonic acid and homocystinuria, additional patients with isolated homocystinuria (cblD variant 1) and isolated methylmalonic aciduria (cblD variant 2) have subsequently been recognized. The cblF (OMIM no. 277380) deficiency and cblJ (OMIM no. 614857) deficiency result in the inability to transfer endocytosed cobalamin from the lysosome to the cytoplasm. cblX deficiency (OMIM no. 309541) is a unique form of combined methylmalonic acidemia and homocystinuria. It is caused by mutations in the gene *HCFC1* on chromosome X, which encodes a transcriptional coregulator involved in expression of *MMACHC* (cblC).

## CLINICAL PRESENTATION

Most patients with combined methylmalonic aciduria and homocystinuria belong to the cblC class. Without treatment, individuals with this disorder typically present during the first year of life with megaloblastic anemia, failure to thrive, developmental delay, hypotonia, seizures, macrocephaly, and cerebral atrophy. Other patients present later in life or in adulthood with ataxia, dementia, or psychosis. Most patients with cblC deficiency develop a bull's eye maculopathy and then optic nerve pallor. Retinal degeneration in cblC deficiency can be seen as early as 2 months of age and appears to be resistant to treatment with OHCbl. Noncompaction cardiomyopathy can be present in some patients, necessitating life-long surveillance of the cardiac function. Despite the presence of methylmalonic aciduria, metabolic decompensations are infrequent.

Presentation in classic cblD deficiency is similar to that of cblC. cblF and cblJ deficiencies are clinically variable but tend to show better response to treatment with parenteral hydroxocobalamin. Frequent findings have included feeding difficulties, failure to thrive, growth retardation, and persistent stomatitis. Due to the likely role of LMBRD1 (cblF) and ABCD4 (cblJ) in the intestinal uptake of dietary cobalamin, patients may present with low plasma cobalamin levels. The clinical picture of cblX disorder is dominated by developmental delays, intellectual disability, and intractable epilepsy.

## DIAGNOSTIC TESTS

Patients with these disorders have the biochemical characteristics of both methylmalonic aciduria and homocystinuria, although methylmalonic acid levels are generally lower than in patients with isolated methylmalonic aciduria. Fibroblasts show decreased function of both methylmalonyl-CoA mutase and methionine synthase, and decreased synthesis of both adenosylcobalamin and methylcobalamin (Table 142-1). Fibroblasts from patients with the cblC or cblD disorder are unable to accumulate cobalamin in cells, reflecting the inability of cells to retain cobalamin that is not bound to one of the cobalamin-dependent enzymes. In cblF and cblJ disorder, fibroblasts accumulate large amounts of cobalamin, but most of this is unmetabolized cobalamin that is trapped within the lysosomes.

## GENETICS

cblC, cblD, cblF, and cblJ deficiencies are inherited as autosomal recessive traits. Over 40 mutations in the *MMACHC* gene have been identified. The most common of these is a c.271dupA mutation that represents 40% of identified mutant alleles, primarily in patients of European or western Asian origin. It is associated with early-onset severe disease when homozygous. Several other mutations show evidence of clustering in specific ethnic groups, and genotype-phenotype correlations have been observed. A small number of mutations in the *MMADHC* gene have been identified in patients with the much rarer cblD disorder. The classical cblD disorder is associated with truncating mutations, while mutations at the C-terminal domain are associated with isolated homocystinuria (variant 1), and mutations in the N-terminal domain are associated with isolated methylmalonic aciduria (variant 2). Most known mutations in cblF are truncating, resulting in the loss of function of it respective protein. cblJ deficiency is very rare, and the full spectrum of mutations is under study. The *HCFC1* gene implicated in the cblX disorder is located on the distal subband of chromosome Xq28 and is inherited as an X-linked trait. *HCFC1* encodes a chromatin-associated protein playing a role in the transcriptional regulation of gene expression. Impaired function of *HCFC1* results in dysregulated expression of *MMACHC* (cblC) and likely genes encoding components of the glycine cleavage complex, which may explain biochemical findings and intractable epilepsy observed in these patients.

## TREATMENT

Patients with combined methylmalonic aciduria and homocystinuria are treated with large doses of cobalamin (up to 0.35 mg/kg/24 h, up to the maximum dose of 30 mg/24 h) administered subcutaneously or intramuscularly. Higher doses require concentrated forms of OHCbl to reduce the volume. Hydroxycobalamin is recommended

**TABLE 142-1 CLINICAL AND LABORATORY FINDINGS IN INBORN ERRORS OF METABOLISM**

| Class | MMA | Hcy | Propionate Incorporation | Methyl-THF Incorporation | Cellular Cobalamin Uptake | AdoCbl Synthesis | MeCbl Synthesis |
|---|---|---|---|---|---|---|---|
| mut | ↑ | N | ↓ | N | N | ↓ | N |
| cblA | ↑ | N | ↓ | N | N | ↓ | N |
| cblB | ↑ | N | ↓ | N | N | ↓ | N |
| cblC | ↑ | ↑ | ↓ | ↓ | ↓ | ↓ | ↓ |
| cblX | ↑ | ↑ | ↓ | ↓ | ↓ | ↓ | ↓ |
| cblD | ↑ | ↑ | ↓ | ↓ | ↓ | ↓ | ↓ |
| cblDv1 | N | ↑ | N | ↓ | N | N | ↓ |
| cblDv2 | ↑ | N | ↓ | N | N | ↓ | N |
| cblE | N | ↑ | N | ↓ | N | N | ↓ |
| cblF | ↑ | ↑ | ↓ | ↓ | ↑ | ↓ | ↓ |
| cblJ | ↑ | ↑ | ↓ | ↓ | ↑ | ↓ | ↓ |
| cblG | N | ↑ | N | ↓ | N | N | ↓ |

↑, the value is increased compared to control; ↓, the value is decreased compared to control; AdoCbl, conversion of [$^{57}$Co]CNCbl to adenosylcobalamin by cultured fibroblasts; Cobalamin Uptake, uptake of [$^{57}$Co]CNCbl by cultured fibroblasts; Hcy, homocystinuria/hyperhomocysteinemia; MeCbl, conversion of [$^{57}$Co]CNCbl to methylcobalamin by cultured fibroblasts; Methyl-THF incorporation of label from [$^{14}$C]methyl-THF into cellular macromolecules by cultured fibroblasts (methionine synthase function); MMA, methylmalonic aciduria/acidemia; N, the value is unchanged from control; Propionate incorporation of label from [$^{14}$C]propionate into cellular macromolecules by cultured fibroblasts (methylmalonyl-CoA mutase function).

over more widely available CNCbl; this may be true for other cobalamin disorders as well. Patients can tolerate the recommended daily allowance of protein. Medical foods deficient in methionine are not recommended in these patients. Carnitine supplementation is used to treat secondary carnitine deficiency. Supplementation with betaine, which supports conversion of homocysteine to methionine by the liver enzyme betaine-homocysteine methyltransferase, has proved effective in patients with homocystinuria. In patients with persistent hyperhomocysteinemia, attention should be given to the management of risk factors predisposing to hypercoagulability.

## INBORN ERRORS OF COBALAMIN UPTAKE AND TRANSPORT

Combined methylmalonic aciduria and homocystinuria is also seen in patients with defects affecting intestinal uptake of cobalamin, its transport in the serum, and cellular uptake. Decreased uptake occurs in individuals with intrinsic factor deficiency (OMIM no. 261000), caused by mutations in the *GIF* gene on chromosome 11q12.1, and in those with Imerslund-Gräsbeck syndrome (IGS; OMIM no. 261100). The latter disorder is the result of dysfunction of the vitamin $B_{12}$ receptor in the distal ileum, which can be caused by mutations at the *CUBN* gene on chromosome 10p13 or the *AMN* gene on chromosome 14q32, which encode cubilin and amnionless, the respective components of the cubam complex. Additional IGS families are not linked to either chromosome and represent further genetic heterogeneity in this disorder. Patients with these disorders usually present between 1 and 5 years of age with decreased serum cobalamin levels, megaloblastic anemia, and neurologic impairment. IGS patients often have proteinuria as well since cubilin and amnionless also mediate protein homeostasis in renal tubules. These disorders show an autosomal recessive inheritance. Clusters of IGS have been identified in Finland (*CUBN* mutations), Norway (*AMN* mutations), and the eastern Mediterranean (both genes). In the absence of readily available clinical tests to assess cobalamin uptake, specific diagnosis in these patients depends on molecular analysis of the *GIF*, *CUBN*, and *AMN* genes. Intrinsic factor deficiency and IGS require life-long treatment with parenteral hydroxocobalamin.

Patients with transcobalamin II deficiency (OMIM no. 275350) usually present in the first months of life with megaloblastic anemia, failure to thrive, weakness, and, frequently, immunologic dysfunction. Without treatment, neurologic impairment develops. Most cobalamin circulating in blood is bound to transcobalamin II. Cobalamin bound to transcobalamin II is not available for uptake by most types of cells; rather, transcobalamin II is the primary transporter of vitamin $B_{12}$ to peripheral tissues. Thus, total serum cobalamin levels may be normal, while the unsaturated vitamin $B_{12}$ binding capacity is reduced. The disorder is inherited as autosomal recessive trait. Mutations in the *TCN2* gene on chromosome 22q12 have been identified in a small number of patients. Treatment involves maintaining very high serum levels of cobalamin by intramuscular route.

The uptake of cobalamin bound to transcobalamin II is mediated by the transcobalamin receptor (*CD320*, OMIM no. 606475). Known patients were identified on the newborn screen based on elevated propionylcarnitine (C3) in blood spots. Patients tend to have mildly elevated methylmalonic acidemia with normal total plasma homocysteine at birth and readily respond to hydroxocobalamin injections. Plasma vitamin $B_{12}$ levels can be elevated even without cobalamin supplementation. Studies of cellular vitamin $B_{12}$ metabolism using fibroblasts reveal normal propionate and methyltetrahydrofolate metabolism, normal conversion of cyanocobalamin to adenosylcobalamin and methylcobalamin, but reduced cobalamin binding and uptake. Methylmalonic acidemia appears to be transient; however, the long-term outcome and natural history of this condition are poorly understood.

## FOLIC ACID

The folates are a class of molecules comprising folic acid and its derivatives. Biologically active folates consist of folic acid reduced to a tetrahydrofolate (THF) derivative through the attachment of 1-carbon groups to $N^5$ and $N^{10}$ of the pterin ring, and by addition of up to 6 additional glutamate residues by γ-peptide linkage. Folate is synthesized by many types of bacteria and is obtained in the diet from both plant and animal foods.

Within cells, folates accept 1-carbon units from various sources, primarily serine (via the reaction catalyzed by serine hydroxymethyltransferase) but also from glycine (the glycine cleavage system), formate (formyl-THF synthetase), and histidine (breakdown mediated by glutamate formiminotransferase and formiminotetrahydrofolate cyclodeaminase). Several reactions utilize 1-carbon units derived from folates (Fig. 142-2). Methyl-THF is required for methylation of homocysteine to form methionine, catalyzed by methionine synthase (described in the section on vitamin $B_{12}$; see also Chapter 133). Catalytic conversion of uridylate to thymidylate requires 5,10-methylene-THF for

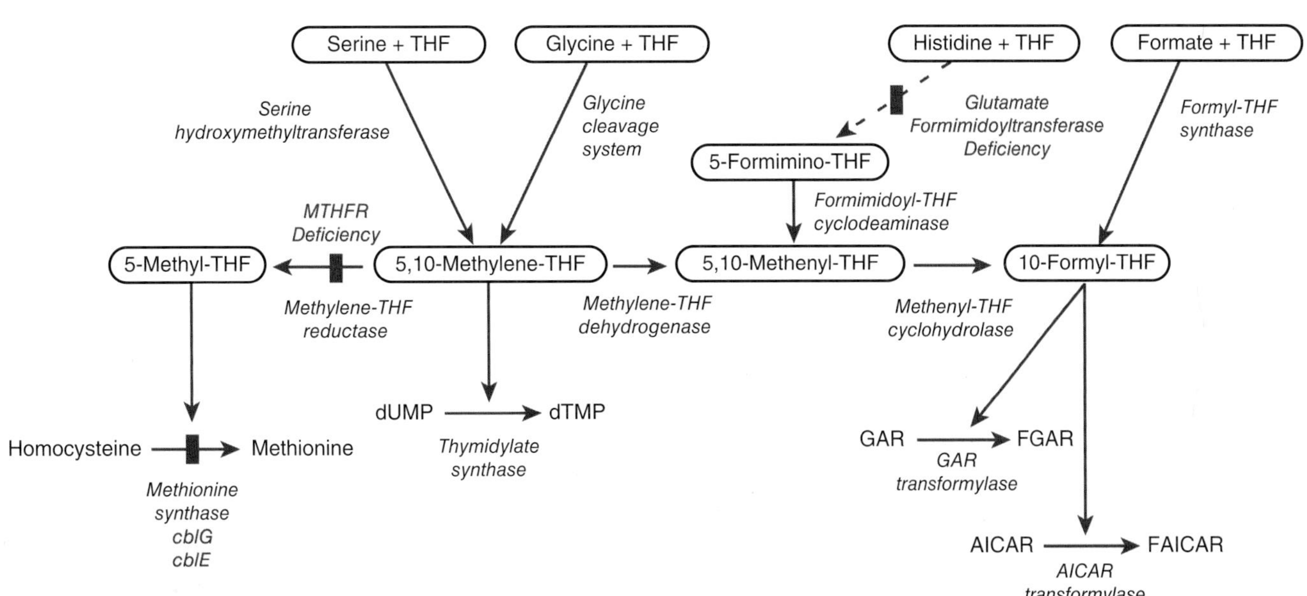


**FIGURE 142-2** Metabolic pathway of folate. The steps affected in known inborn errors of cobalamin metabolism are shown by red bars. Note that the cblE and cblG disorders were discussed earlier in the section on inborn errors of cobalamin. AICAR, amino-4-imidazolecarboxamide ribonucleotide; dTMP, thymidylate; dUMP, deoxyuridylate; FAICAR, formamido-4-imidazolecarboxamide ribonucleotide; FGAR, formylglycinamide ribonucleotide; GAR, glycinamide ribonucleotide; THF, tetrahydrofolate.

the activity of thymidylate synthase. Carbons 2 and 8 of the purine ring are added by the folate-dependent enzymes GAR transformylase and AICAR transformylase, both of which use 10-formyl-THF as a 1-carbon donor. Thus, synthesis of both purines and 1 of 2 pyrimidines required for DNA synthesis is dependent on folates.

Interconversion of 1-carbon substituted folates is an important aspect of cellular metabolism. 5,10-Methylene-THF can be reduced to 5-methyl-THF by the enzyme methylene-THF reductase (MTHFR). Alternatively, it can be oxidized to form 10-formyl-THF by sequential reactions catalyzed by methylene-THF dehydrogenase and methenyl-THF cyclohydrolase. The 2 activities are catalyzed by a single multifunctional protein called C1-THF synthase (OMIM no. 172460). The reaction catalyzed by MTHFR is irreversible under physiologic conditions. This means that when activity of methionine synthase, the only reaction that utilizes methyl-THF, is impaired (as in cobalamin deficiency or in the cblC, cblD, cblF, cblJ, cblE, and cblG disorders), cellular folate is trapped in its methylated form, resulting in deficiency of other folate coenzyme forms.

## MTHFR DEFICIENCY

The most common inborn error of folate metabolism is MTHFR deficiency (OMIM no. 236250) due to mutations of the *MTHFR* gene on chromosome 1p36.22 (see Chapter 133). Decreased MTHFR activity results in deficiency of methyl-THF, the source of the methyl group used by methionine synthase. Thus, biochemically, MTHFR deficiency is characterized by hyperhomocysteinemia and homocystinuria with hypomethioninemia. Clinical presentation varies, but patients usually show symptoms during infancy or early childhood that include feeding difficulties, lethargy, hypotonia, developmental delay, and seizures. Cerebral atrophy and demyelination are often present. Patients with later onset may have intellectual disability, ataxia, or psychiatric problems. Unlike patients with inborn errors of cobalamin metabolism, in which methionine synthase activity is impaired, patients with MTHFR deficiency do not have megaloblastic anemia. Cultured fibroblasts have decreased incorporation of label from [$^{14}$C]formate into cellular macromolecules, but incorporation of label from [$^{14}$C] methyl-THF is normal. Diagnosis depends on molecular DNA analysis revealing deleterious mutations or enzyme assay of cell extracts demonstrating reduced MTHFR-specific activity.

MTHFR deficiency is inherited as an autosomal recessive trait. Almost all mutations have been restricted to 1 or 2 families—an exception is a c.1129C>T mutation that is present at a high frequency among the Old Order Amish.

Patients with MTHFR deficiency have been treated with a variety of agents, including methyl-THF and other folates, methionine, pyridoxine, cobalamin, carnitine, betaine, and riboflavin, individually and in various combinations. Of these, betaine appears to be the most effective. Treatment is most successful when the disease is diagnosed at an early stage, before irreversible neurologic damage occurs.

MTHFR deficiency needs to be differentiated from common polymorphism in the *MTHFR* gene Common polymorphisms of the *MTHFR* gene result in decreased enzyme activity less severe than that seen in patients with severe MTHFR deficiency. The most well studied of these is a c.665C>T (formerly c.677C>T) variant that results in "thermolability" of the enzyme. Homozygosity for the c.665C>T variant is associated with increased serum homocysteine levels in individuals with low folate intake, but the clinical significance of this variant is doubtful.

## GLUTAMATE FORMIMINOTRANSFERASE DEFICIENCY

A small number of patients have been identified who have deficiency of the bifunctional enzyme that catalyzes the transfer of the formimino group from formiminoglutamate (FIGLU), generated during histidine catabolism, to THF to form 5-formimidoyl-THF, which is then converted to 10-formyl-THF. Patients with glutamate formiminotransferase deficiency (OMIM no. 229100) are characterized by elevated FIGLU levels either constitutively or in response to a histidine load. Because the affected enzyme is expressed only in liver and kidney, using enzyme assay to confirm the diagnosis is performed using molecular DNA analysis. Two classes of patients have been reported: one was characterized by intellectual disability, physical retardation, and cortical atrophy, while the second showed no intellectual disability but massive FIGLU excretion. Therefore, it has been suggested that the severe manifestations in the first group of patients were the result of ascertainment bias.

The gene encoding the bifunctional enzyme, *FTCD*, has been identified on chromosome 21q22.3, and causative mutations have been identified in several patients. It remains unclear whether there is any clinical phenotype beyond FIGLU excretion in this disorder. The disorder is inherited as autosomal recessive trait and is amenable to newborn screening.

## HEREDITARY FOLATE MALABSORPTION

Mutations in a proton-coupled folate transporter result in reduced intestinal folate uptake (OMIM no. 229050), impaired transport across the blood-brain barrier, and ultimately intracellular folate deficiency. Therefore, presentation typically occurs in the first months of life with diarrhea, failure to thrive, developmental delay, megaloblastic anemia, and neurologic deterioration. Serum and cerebrospinal fluid folate levels are reduced. Patients with this autosomal recessive disorder have mutations in the *SLC46A1* gene on chromosome 17q11.2. Optimal treatment involves maintaining adequate levels of folate in the central nervous system to avoid neurologic impairment; the appropriate level must be determined for each patient individually and may involve administration of very large doses of folate.

## SUGGESTED READINGS


Baumgartner MR, Hörster F, Dionisi-Vici C, et al. Proposed guidelines for the diagnosis and management of methylmalonic and propionic acidemia. *Orphanet J Rare Dis.* 2014;9:130.

Carrillo N, Adams D, Venditti CP. Disorders of intracellular cobalamin metabolism. GeneReviews® 2013; Available from: https://www.ncbi.nlm.nih.gov/books/NBK1328/. Accessed June 24, 2017.

Carrillo-Carrasco N, Sloan J, Valle D, et al. Hydroxocobalamin dose escalation improves metabolic control in cblC. *J Inherit Metab Dis.* 2009;32(6):728-731.

Fraser JL, Venditti CP. Methylmalonic and propionic acidemias: clinical management update. *Curr Opin Pediatr.* 2016;28(6):682-693.

Hickey SE, Curry CJ, Toriello HV. ACMG Practice Guideline: lack of evidence for MTHFR polymorphism testing. *Genet Med.* 2013; 15(2):153-156.

Manoli I, Myles JG, Sloan JL, et al. A critical reappraisal of dietary practices in methylmalonic acidemia raises concerns about the safety of medical foods. Part 1: isolated methylmalonic acidemias. *Genet Med.* 2016;18(4):386-395.

Manoli I, Myles JG, Sloan JL, et al. A critical reappraisal of dietary practices in methylmalonic acidemia raises concerns about the safety of medical foods. Part 2: cobalamin C deficiency. *Genet Med.* 2016;18(4):396-404.

Manoli I, Sloan JL, Venditti CP. Isolated methylmalonic acidemia. GeneReviews® [Internet] 2016. https://www.ncbi.nlm.nih.gov/books/NBK1231/. Accessed June 24, 2017.

Quadros EV, Lai SC, Nakayama Y, et al. Positive newborn screen for methylmalonic aciduria identifies the first mutation in TCblR/CD320, the gene for cellular uptake of transcobalamin-bound vitamin B(12). *Hum Mutat.* 2010;31(8):924-929.

Rutsch F, Gailus S, Miousse IR, et al. Identification of a putative lysosomal cobalamin exporter altered in the cblF defect of vitamin B12 metabolism. *Nat Genet.* 2009;41(2):234-239.

Sloan JL, Johnston JJ, Manoli I, et al. Exome sequencing identifies ACSF3 as a cause of combined malonic and methylmalonic aciduria. *Nat Genet.* 2011;43(9):883-886.

Yu HC, Sloan JL, Scharer G, et al. An X-linked cobalamin disorder caused by mutations in transcriptional coregulator HCFC1. *Am J Hum Genet.* 2013;93(3):506-514.

# 143 Biotin Responsive Disorders

William J. Craigen and Eva Morava Kozicz



## INTRODUCTION

Biotin (vitamin $B_7$ or vitamin H) is a water-soluble vitamin that functions as a carboxyl carrier in carboxylation, decarboxylation, and transcarboxylation reactions, and is attached to a lysine residue in a highly conserved domain common to all biotin-dependent carboxylases. The 5 biotin-dependent carboxylases in humans are mitochondrial propionyl-coenzyme A (CoA), β-methylcrotonyl-CoA, pyruvate carboxylases, and mitochondrial and cytosolic forms of acetyl-CoA carboxylase, with each carboxylase having specific roles in fatty acid, glucose, and amino acid metabolism. Biotin is covalently attached to carboxylases by the enzyme holocarboxylase synthetase (HLCS) encoded by the *HLCS* gene, while biotinidase, encoded by the *BTD* gene, provides free biotin following proteolysis of the carboxylase protein. Hence, biotinidase deficiency (Mendelian Inheritance in Man [MIM] no. 253260) reflects an inability to hydrolyze biocytin (biotinyllysine) or small biotin-containing peptide fragments from carboxylases, leading to a lack of free biotin, while holocarboxylase synthetase deficiency (MIM no. 253270) reflects a failure to incorporate biotin into the apoenzymes. The activity of HLCS involves a 2-step, adenosine triphosphate (ATP)-dependent reaction in which biotin is first activated to biotinyl-5'-adenosine monophosphate (AMP) and then transferred to the apocarboxylase substrate, with release of AMP. Failure to attach or recycle biotin leads to significantly reduced activity of these biotin-dependent carboxylases and results in multiple carboxylase deficiency. Humans cannot synthesize biotin, and they obtain it from exogenous sources via intestinal absorption. Absorption of biotin and transport of the vitamin into a variety of cell types occurs via a saturable, $Na^+$-dependent, carrier-mediated mechanism that involves the human sodium-dependent multivitamin transporter, hSMVT, encoded by the *SLC5A6* gene, which has been shown to also transport pantothenate and lipoate.

More recently, HLCS has also been shown to have an additional role as a nuclear protein that may catalyze the binding of biotin to distinct lysine residues in chromatin proteins such as histones, although the specific mechanisms at play remain under debate. HLCS-dependent epigenetic marks are reported to be abundant in genomic regions that are subject to transcriptional repression. HLCS has been proposed to be a member of a multi-protein gene repression complex that directs its localization within chromatin. HLCS has also been linked to the regulation of histone deacetylases in a biotin-independent manner and to the regulation of heat shock proteins and inflammatory cytokines. Hence, HLCS appears to be a multifaceted protein involved in intermediary metabolism, as a transcriptional repressor, and in gene regulation of biotin-dependent and independent pathways.

## BIOTINIDASE AND HOLOCARBOXYLASE SYNTHETASE DEFICIENCY

Deficiencies of biotinidase and HLCS are autosomal recessive disorders with considerable clinical variability. Newborn screening for biotinidase deficiency has been carried out since the 1980s using direct enzyme testing. HLCS deficiency is screened for by tandem mass spectroscopy using elevated propionylcarnitine (C3) and hydroxypentanoylcarnitine (C5-OH) on dried blood spots. The urine organic acid profile may demonstrate elevated lactic, 3-OH isovaleric, 3-OH propionic, 3-methylcrotonyl, methylcitric, and tiglylglycine consistent with loss of function of the above carboxylases.

Prior to the advent of universal newborn screening in the United States, the age of onset of symptoms was used in the initial diagnostic evaluation to differentiate between HLCS deficiency and biotinidase deficiency, with biotinidase generally presenting after 3 months. However, milder forms of HLCS deficiency are now recognized, and this distinction is not so clear. The typical triad of multiple carboxylase deficiency is of alopecia, dermatitis, and encephalopathy. Clasically HLCS deficiency presents in the neonatal period with emesis, hypotonia, lethargy, seizures, metabolic ketolactic acidosis, hyperammonemia, developmental delay, skin rash, and alopecia. Left untreated, infants will progress to profound metabolic acidosis, cerebral edema, coma, and death. However, milder cases have been observed, with ketolactic acidemia associated with infections. Untreated, biotinidase deficiency usually presents later in infancy with periorificial dermatitis resembling acrodermatitis enteropathica, patchy alopecia, and neurologic abnormalities such as ataxia, neurosensory defects, developmental delay, and epilepsy. Cerebral calcifications may be seen. In both conditions, the rash may be complicated by superinfection with monilia.

## DIAGNOSIS

Two forms of biotinidase deficiency are recognized: profound biotinidase deficiency with enzymatic activity below 10% of control values, and partial biotinidase deficiency with activity between 10% and 30% of control values. Treatment is universally accepted for profound deficiency; however, the need to treat partial deficiencies with biotin remains unsettled, with only anecdotal reports of a rash, hypotonia, and hair loss in untreated patients. The potential benefits of avoiding any ectodermal complications and preventing potential seizures can be discussed with parents; however, partial biotinidase patients generally have no biochemical abnormalities in blood and urine and have a benign natural course. The carrier frequency in European populations for a partial loss of function missense variant p.D444H is about 4%, and partial deficiency cases typically have this variant in conjunction with a severe allele. Biochemical testing in symptomatic patients with profound biotinidase or HLCS deficiency by urinary organic acid analysis shows increased 3-methylcrotonylglycine and 3-hydroxyisovaleric acid, often with methylcitric, 3-hydroxypropionic, and lactic acids. Acylcarnitine analysis by tandem mass spectroscopy shows propionyl- and 3-hydroxyisovalerylcarnitine, along with lactic acidemia. Holocarboxylase synthetase deficiency can be demonstrated in fibroblasts or leukocytes by measuring individual carboxylase activities. Biotinidase activity is typically assayed in serum, although the enzyme is labile, and this may lead to falsely reduced activity. DNA testing can confirm the diagnosis.

## TREATMENT

The mainstay of treatment for both biotinidase and HLCS deficiency is biotin supplementation in an effort to alleviate the symptoms of the enzyme deficiency or prevent symptoms from developing in asymptomatic individuals. The former responds promptly to 5 to 10 mg of biotin, whereas much higher doses may be required for the latter disorder. Effectiveness can be monitored by acylcarnitine profiling, determining lactate concentrations, and analysis of urinary organic acids.

## BIOTIN-RESPONSIVE BASAL GANGLIA DISEASE

Biotin-responsive basal ganglia disease (BBGD), also known as biotin-thiamine–responsive basal ganglia disease (BTBGD), is an autosomal recessive disorder that presents in early childhood with confusion, dysarthria, external ophthalmoplegia, and dysphagia, often in conjunction with intercurrent febrile illness and, if untreated, progresses to dystonia, quadriplegia, and eventual death. Cerebral magnetic resonance imaging shows bilateral central necrosis of the caudate head with variable involvement of the putamen. In the initial reports, although symptoms disappeared within a few days of biotin administration (5–10 mg/kg/d) and reappeared within 1 month if biotin was discontinued, it has subsequently been reported that one-third of patients who were initially responsive to biotin alone subsequently relapsed, but when thiamine was added, further improvement was observed, with no further episodes of decompensation. A recent comparison of thiamine-only (40 mg/kg/d) versus thiamine plus biotin treatment observed minimal difference in outcome. The basis for biotin responsiveness is currently unknown. To date, almost 90 patients have been described, many from consanguineous Middle Eastern families. The defect is in a thiamine transporter (hTHTR2) on the cell surface encoded by the *SLC19A3* gene that has no demonstrated involvement with biotin transport. It has been speculated that the higher level of biotin after administration may increase the activity of biotin-dependent enzymes, resulting in an overall improvement of energy production, which is impaired in thiamine deficiency.

Finally, a single child has been described with biallelic variants in the human sodium-dependent multivitamin transporter, hSMVT, encoded by the *SLC5A6* gene. The child exhibited failure to thrive, microcephaly and brain anomalies, spasticity, developmental delay, variable immunodeficiency, osteoporosis, and pathologic bone fractures.

## SUGGESTED READINGS


Algahtani H, Ghamdi S, Shirah B, Alharbi B, Algahtani R, Bazaid A. Biotin-thiamine-responsive basal ganglia disease: catastrophic consequences of delay in diagnosis and treatment. *Neurol Res.* 2017;39(2):117-125.

Donti TR, Blackburn PR, Atwal PS. Holocarboxylase synthetase deficiency pre and post newborn screening. *Mol Genet Metab Rep.* 2016;7:40-44.

Haagerup A, Andersen JB, Blichfeldt S, Christensen MF. Biotinidase deficiency: two cases of very early presentation. *Dev Med Child Neurol.* 1997;39:832-835.

Ozand PT, Gascon GG, Al Essa M, et al. Biotin-responsive basal ganglia disease; a novel entity. *Brain.* 1998;121:1267-1279.

Subramanian VS, Constantinescu AR, Benke PJ, Said HM. Mutations in SLC5A6 associated with brain, immune, bone, and intestinal dysfunction in a young child. *Hum Genet.* 2017;136(2):253-261.

Tabarki B, Alfadhel M, AlShahwan S, Hundallah K, AlShafi S, AlHashem A. Treatment of biotin-responsive basal ganglia disease: open comparative study between the combination of biotin plus thiamine versus thiamine alone. *Eur J Paediatr Neurol.* 2015; 19(5):547-552.

Touma E, Suormala T, Baumgartner ER, et al. Holocarboxylase synthetase deficiency: report of a case with onset in late infancy. *J Inherited Metab Dis.* 1999;22:115-122.

Wolf B. Biotinidase deficiency. In: Pagon RA, Adam MP, Ardinger HH, et al, eds. *GeneReviews.* Seattle, WA: University of Washington; 2016.


# 144 Vitamin $B_1$ and Vitamin $B_6$ Responsive Disorders

Brett H. Graham

## VITAMIN $B_1$ (THIAMINE)

### INTRODUCTION

Thiamine has long been recognized as an essential nutrient. Its minimal essential requirement is about 0.5 mg/1000 kcal, which is usually obtained through a normal, well-balanced diet (recommended daily thiamine intake ranges from 0.2 mg in neonates to 1–1.2 mg in adults). However, requirements are variable and increase in parallel with carbohydrate intake and during pregnancy, lactation, and hypermetabolic states. Thiamine is physiologically active in its phosphorylated form, thiamine pyrophosphate (TPP), which is a coenzyme for pyruvate dehydrogenase (PDH), α-ketoglutarate dehydrogenase, and branched-chain α-ketoacid dehydrogenase (BCKDH) in the mitochondrion; 2-hydroxyacyl-CoA lyase in the peroxisome; and transketolase (pentose phosphate pathway) in the cytosol. Being placed at these highly regulated enzymatic steps, thiamine plays a crucial role in carbohydrate metabolism and in the metabolic switch from the fed to the fasting state.

Acute acquired thiamine deficiency states (as occurs with total parenteral nutrition without thiamine supplementation or beriberi) are life-threatening emergencies and present with cardiac failure, Gayet-Wernicke encephalopathy, and/or lactic acidosis. Metabolic markers include elevated serum lactate and pyruvate with normal lactate-to-pyruvate ratio, slight elevations of branched-chain amino acids in plasma, the presence of α-keto acids (ketoglutarate, pyruvate, branched-chain keto acids) in urine with a positive dinitrophenylhydrazine (DNPH) reaction, and low transketolase activity in red blood cells. However, these markers are rarely available in an emergency, and the diagnosis relies on the primary care or emergency physician recognizing the disorder and administering the lifesaving therapeutic test of thiamine 5 mg/kg/d. There is no significant risk of adverse effects from supplementation.

### METABOLISM

Through the diet, thiamine is consumed as phosphate derivatives and converted into free thiamine by phosphatases present in the lumen of the small intestine. The epithelia of the small intestine contain two thiamine transporters, THTR1 and THTR2, which are localized to the basal and apical membranes of the polarized cell, respectively (these transporters are variably expressed in other tissues). Within the cell, free thiamine is converted into TPP in the cytosol by thiamine pyrophosphokinase (TPK). A mitochondrial TPP carrier (TPC) imports TPP from the cytosol into the mitochondrion, allowing TPP to associate with mitochondrial dehydrogenases.

### GENETICS

Thiamine-dependent inborn errors of metabolism are rare. They can be caused by: (1) mutations in subunits of PDH or BCKDH that directly or indirectly interfere with the binding of TPP and thus activation of the apoenzyme, (2) a defect of conversion of thiamine into TPP, or (3) defects of specific cellular or mitochondrial transporters of thiamine and TPP, respectively. THTR1 is encoded by *SLC19A2* (chromosome 1q24.2; Mendelian Inheritance in Man [MIM] no. 603941). THTR2 is encoded by *SLC19A3* (chromosome 2q36.3; MIM no. 606152). TPK is encoded by *TPK1* (chromosome 7q35; MIM no. 606370). TPC is encoded by *SLC25A19* (chromosome 17q25.1; MIM no. 606152). Pathogenic variants in each of these genes cause autosomal recessive syndromes with predominant neurologic signs and symptoms (deficiency of THTR1 also causes thiamine-responsive megaloblastic anemia) as summarized in Table 144-1.

## VITAMIN $B_6$ (PYRIDOXINE)

### INTRODUCTION

Vitamin $B_6$ is present in the human body as 6 vitamers that all share a 2-methyl-3-hydroxypyridine structure but differ in the nature of their C4 and C5 functional groups. The C4 carbon bears a $CH_2OH$ group in pyridoxine, a CHO group in pyridoxal, and a $CH_2NH_2$ group in pyridoxamine. All 3 of these C4 variants can exist with the C5 substituent esterified to phosphate: the pyridoxal 5′-phosphate (PLP) is a highly reactive chemical. The requirement for $B_6$ is primarily related to the fact that PLP is the cofactor for over 160 enzyme-catalyzed reactions that occur in humans. PLP is required for the metabolism of many amino acids and neurotransmitters including decarboxylation of aromatic amino acid, glutamate, and histidine; transamination of branched-chain amino acid, tyrosine, and γ-aminobutyric acid (GABA); the glycine cleavage system; threonine and serine dehydratase; cystathionine β-synthase; and aminolevulinate synthase. Consequently, there are many biochemical markers for $B_6$ deficiency or dependency states.

**TABLE 144-1 VITAMIN $B_1$ AND $B_6$ DISORDERS**

| Vitamin | Defect (Mechanisms) | Disorder/Clinical Features | Biochemical Markers and Diagnostic Tests | Reported Dose(s) |
|---|---|---|---|---|
| **Thiamine (vitamin $B_1$)** | Dietary deficiency | Total parenteral nutrition without $B_1$ supplement | High plasma lactate | 2–4 mg/d (20 mg in emergency) |
| | | Breastfed babies from mothers who eat $B_1$-deficient food; beriberi; Gayet-Wernicke encephalopathy | Urinary α-keto acids (DNPH positive)<br>Low transketolase in erythrocytes | |
| | Defective binding of coenzyme (TPP) to enzyme or role of TPP in assisting protein folding: chaperone molecule? | Maple syrup urine disease (branched-chain α-keto acid dehydrogenase) (see Chapter 132) | High leucine, isoleucine, valine, alloisoleucine with plasma amino acids | 10–1000 mg/d |
| | | Pyruvate dehydrogenase deficiency (see Chapter 154) | High lactate and pyruvate with normal lactate/pyruvate ratio | 20–800 mg/d |
| | Thiamine transporter THTR1 (*SLC19A2*) deficiency | Thiamine-responsive megaloblastic anemia with diabetes and deafness | Megaloblastic anemia<br>No biochemical marker<br>*SLC19A2* DNA testing | 20–300 mg/d (1–4 mg/kg/d) |
| | Thiamine transporter THTR2 (*SLC19A3*) deficiency | Biotin-responsive basal ganglia disease; Leigh syndrome; Wernicke encephalopathy; infantile spasms | High lactate in plasma and CSF; elevated α-ketoglutarate with urine organic acids; low free thiamine in CSF and fibroblasts<br>*SLC19A3* DNA testing | Thiamine: 30–1500 mg/d (10–40 mg/kg/d)<br>Biotin: 2–10 mg/d |
| | Mitochondrial thiamine pyrophosphate transporter (TPP, *SLC25A19*) deficiency | Amish microcephaly; Bilateral striatal necrosis with progressive axonal polyneuropathy | High lactate in plasma or CSF; elevated α-ketoglutarate with urine organic acids<br>*SLC25A19* DNA testing | Not thiamine responsive, but ketogenic diet may be helpful |
| | Thiamine pyrophosphokinase (*TPK1*) deficiency | Ataxia, psychomotor retardation, and progressive dystonia | High lactate in plasma or CSF; elevated α-ketoglutarate with urine organic acids<br>*TPK1* DNA testing | 100–200 mg/d |
| Pyridoxine (vitamin $B_6$) | Defective intake or malabsorption of $B_6$ vitamers | Celiac disease and other malabsorption syndromes | Xanthurenic acid in urines | Pyridoxine: 8 μg/kg |
| | | Dietary deficiency of vitamin $B_6$ | High threonine, glycine, and serine levels in plasma | |
| | Inborn errors of vitamin $B_6$ metabolism: defective metabolism of pyridoxine, pyridoxal, and pyridox(am)ine to its active metabolic form, pyridoxal phosphate (PLP) | Pyridox(am)ine phosphate oxidase defect: neonatal seizures, myoclonic jerks, burst suppression pattern at EEG, severe hypotonia, typically responsive to pyridoxal phosphate (PLP) and not to pyridoxine | Low HVA and 5HIAA in CSF; high vanillacetic acid (VLA) in urine<br>*PNPO* DNA testing | PLP: 30 mg/kg/d |
| | | *PROSC* deficiency: neonatal seizures, myoclonic jerks, burst suppression pattern at EEG, encephalopathy, and intellectual disability, typically partially responsive to pyridoxine and PLP | Low PLP in CSF and elevated CSF levels of 3-ortho-methyldopa, L-dopa, and/or 5-hydroxytryptophan<br>*PROSC* DNA testing | Pyridoxine: 50–500 mg/d (5–30 mg/kg/d)<br>PLP: 30 mg/kg/d |
| | | Hypophosphatasia: alkaline phosphatase deficiency: tissue-nonspecific alkaline phosphatase is required for the dephosphorylation of PLP to form pyridoxal, which can then enter the brain and other tissues (neonatal convulsions with burst suppression on EEG and rickets, or infantile spasms with hypsarrhythmia) | Paradoxically low levels of serum alkaline phosphatase<br>High PLP and low pyridoxal in plasma | For acute management of seizures: pyridoxine 100 mg IV |
| | Inborn errors causing accumulation of metabolites and drugs that inactivate PLP | Pyridoxine-responsive epilepsy (PDE) (seizures of perinatal onset refractory to all anticonvulsants that respond dramatically to pyridoxine and recur soon after pyridoxine is stopped): α-amino-adipic acid dehydrogenase (ALDH7A1) is an enzyme of pipecolic acid metabolism that is deficient in PDE and responsible for the accumulation of δ-1-piperideine-6-carboxylic acid (P6C) that inactivates PLP | Elevated pipecolic acid and P6C in CSF and plasma; elevated α-amino-adipic acid (AASA) in CSF and urines that persists despite $B_6$ treatment<br>*ALDH7A1* DNA testing | Pyridoxine: 50–500 mg/d (5–30 mg/kg/d) |

(Continued)

**TABLE 144-1 VITAMIN $B_1$ AND $B_6$ DISORDERS (CONTINUED)**

| Vitamin | Defect (Mechanisms) | Disorder/Clinical Features | Biochemical Markers and Diagnostic Tests | Reported Dose(s) |
|---|---|---|---|---|
| | | Hyperprolinemia type II (δ-1-pyrroline-5-carboxylic acid [P5C] dehydrogenase deficiency); this block causes accumulation of P5C, which inactivates PLP; features of this disorder include seizures and intellectual disability | Elevated proline and P5C in plasma and urine; elevated hydroxyproline and glycine in urine<br>*ALDH4A1* DNA testing | Pyridoxine: 50–100 mg/d |
| | Inborn errors affecting PLP-dependent enzymes (mutations impairing the binding of PLP to the enzyme or possible role of PLP in assisting protein folding: chaperone molecule?) | Pyridoxine-responsive anemia (or X-linked sideroblastic anemia) is caused by a defect in the erythroid-specific form of δ-aminolevulinate synthase (presents in the second decade of life with a microcytic, hypochromic anemia with a sideroblastic marrow and other problems caused by iron overload); 90% of patients are $B_6$ responsive | Enzyme assay in RBC<br>*ALAS2* DNA testing | Pyridoxine: 75–300 mg/d |
| | | Classical homocystinuria due to cystathionine β-synthase deficiency (see Chapter 142); about 50% of patients are fully or partially responsive | Total homocysteine > 100 μmol/L<br>Presence of free homocysteine<br>Methionine > 30 μmol/L | Pyridoxine: 200–750 mg/d |
| | | Ornithine δ-amino transferase (OAT) deficiency: gyrate atrophy of the choroid and retina (see Chapter 138); only 10% are responsive | Ornithine > 500 μmol/L in plasma | Pyridoxine: 500 mg/d |

CSF, cerebrospinal fluid; DNPH, 2,4-dinitrophenylhydrazine; EEG, electroencephalogram; 5HIAA, 5-hydroxyindoleacetic acid; HVA, homovanillic acid; PLP, pyridoxal 5′-phosphate; RBC, red blood cell; TPP, thiamine pyrophosphate.

## METABOLISM

The phosphorylated $B_6$ vitamers in the diet are thought to be hydrolyzed by intestinal phosphatases before absorption. The absorbed vitamers are rapidly cleared by uptake into the liver, where they are phosphorylated by pyridoxal kinase. Pyridoxine phosphate and pyridoxamine phosphate are then converted to PLP by pyridox(am)-5′-phosphate oxidase (PNPO). PLP reenters the circulation bound to the lysine-190 residue of albumin. Delivery of PLP to the tissues requires hydrolysis of circulating PLP to pyridoxal by the ectoenzyme tissue nonspecific alkaline phosphatase. Only pyridoxal is able to cross the blood-brain barrier and enter other tissues, but intracellularly, pyridoxal needs to be rephosphorylated by pyridoxal kinase to regenerate active cofactor PLP.

## GENETICS

There are several mechanisms that can lead to an increased requirement for pyridoxine or PLP: (1) inborn errors affecting the pathways of $B_6$ vitamer metabolism (PNPO and alkaline phosphatase defects); (2) inborn errors that lead to accumulation of small molecules that react with PLP and inactivate it (hyperprolinemia type II and pyridoxine-responsive epilepsy); (3) inborn errors affecting specific PLP-dependent enzymes (X-linked sideroblastic anemia, classical homocystinuria, and gyrate atrophy of the choroid); (4) celiac disease, which is thought to lead to malabsorption of $B_6$ vitamers, or renal dialysis, which leads to increased losses of $B_6$ vitamers from the circulation; and (5) drugs that affect the metabolism of $B_6$ vitamers (enzyme-inducing anticonvulsants, methyl xanthines) or that react with PLP. Thus isoniazid inhibits pyridoxine phosphokinase and isoniazid metabolites bind to and inactivate $B_6$ vitamers; therefore, isoniazid can induce a pyridoxine-dependent peripheral neuropathy in patients who are slow isoniazid inactivators or who have renal insufficiency. Pyridoxine-dependent inborn errors are summarized in Table 144-1. Pyridoxine-dependent epilepsy is an autosomal recessive disorder caused by biallelic pathogenic variants in *ALDH7A1* (chromosome 5q23.2; MIM no. 107323). *ALDH7A1* encodes α-amino-adipic acid dehydrogenase, an enzyme of lysine and pipecolic acid metabolism. A deficiency of this enzyme results in the accumulation of δ-1-piperideine-6-carboxylic acid (P6C), which reacts with PLP and inactivates it. Treatment involves provision of large amounts of pyridoxine (10–30 mg/kg/d), along with a lysine-restricted diet supplemented with arginine (300–400 mg/kg/d) to compete with lysine uptake at the blood-brain barrier. PLP-responsive epilepsy is an autosomal recessive disorder caused by pyridoxal 5′-phosphate oxidase (PNPO) deficiency due to biallelic pathogenic variants in *PNPO* (chromosome 17q21.32; MIM no. 610090). Historically, it was thought that treatment of this disorder requires provision of PLP; however, it is clear that a subset of patients respond to pharmacologic doses of pyridoxine. Another disorder associated with a functional reduction in PLP is a defect in the enzyme $\Delta^1$-pyrroline 5-carboxylate dehydrogenase (P5CDh), which normally converts $\Delta^1$-pyrroline 5-carboxylate (P5C) into glutamate as part of a proline degradation pathway; hence, this disorder is known as hyperprolinemia type II, with high concentrations of both proline and P5C. This is a complex neurometabolic disorder caused by biallelic mutations in the gene *ALDH4A1* (chromosome 1p36, MIM no. 606811), but it has been shown that, much like the condensation of P6C with PLP, P5C can similarly react with PLP and create a PLP deficiency state. Finally, a more recently described form of pyridoxine-dependent epilepsy is an autosomal recessive disorder caused by biallelic pathogenic variants in *PROSC* (chromosome 8p11.23, MIM no. 604436). The role of PROSC in pyridoxine metabolism is not yet fully understood, but it is thought to be involved in intracellular homeostatic regulation of PLP levels as it binds PLP. Disorders reviewed in more detail in other chapters that may respond to pyridoxine are listed in Table 144-1.

## SUGGESTED READINGS


Brown G. Defects of thiamine transport and metabolism. *J Inherit Metab Dis.* 2014;37:577-585.

Cazzola M, Malcovati L. Diagnosis and treatment of sideroblastic anemias: from defective heme synthesis to abnormal RNA splicing. *Hematology Am Soc Hematol Educ Program.* 2015;2015:19-25.

Cellini B, Montioli R, Oppici E, et al. The chaperone role of the pyridoxal 5′-phosphate and its implications for rare diseases involving B6-dependent enzymes. *Clin Biochem.* 2014;47:158-165.

Coughlin CR 2nd, van Karnebeek CD, Al-Hertani W, et al. Triple therapy with pyridoxine, arginine supplementation and dietary lysine restriction in pyridoxine-dependent epilepsy: neurodevelopmental outcome. *Mol Genet Metab.* 2015;116(1-2):35-43.

Darin N, Reid E, Prunetti L, et al. Mutations in *PROSC* disrupt cellular pyridoxal phosphate homeostasis and cause vitamin-B(6)-dependent epilepsy. *Am J Hum Genet.* 2016;99:1325-1337.

Fraccascia P, Casteels M, De Schryver E, et al. Role of thiamine pyrophosphate in oligomerisation, functioning and import of peroxisomal 2-hydroxyacyl-CoA lyase. *Biochim Biophys Acta.* 2011;1814:1226-1233.

Gospe SM Jr. Pyridoxine-dependent epilepsy. In: Pagon RA, Adam MP, Ardinger HH, et al, eds. *GeneReviews®*. Seattle, WA: University of Washington; 2017.

Manzetti S, Zhang J, van der Spoel D. Thiamin function, metabolism, uptake, and transport. *Biochemistry.* 2014;53:821-835.

Mayr JA, Freisinger P, Schlachter K, et al. Thiamine pyrophosphokinase deficiency in encephalopathic children with defects in the pyruvate oxidation pathway. *Am J Hum Genet.* 2011;89:806-812.

Ortigoza Escobar JD, Pérez Dueñas B. Treatable inborn errors of metabolism due to membrane vitamin transporters deficiency. *Semin Pediatr Neurol.* 2016;23:341-350.

Plecko B, Paul K, Mills P, et al. Pyridoxine responsiveness in novel mutations of the PNPO gene. *Neurology.* 2014;82(16):1425-1433.

Van de Ven S, Gardeitchik T, Kouwenberg D, Kluijtmans L, Wevers R, Morava E. Long-term clinical outcome, therapy and mild mitochondrial dysfunction in hyperprolinemia. *J Inherit Metab Dis.* 2014;37:383-390.

# 145 Disorders of Fatty Acid Oxidation

Jerry Vockley

## INTRODUCTION

Mitochondrial fatty acid oxidation provides the main source of energy for heart and skeletal muscle and, through generation of acetyl-coenzyme A (CoA), for tricarboxylic acid (TCA) cycle function and ketone body production; it also provides energy for other tissues when the supply of glucose is limited. Long-chain fatty acids entering the cell are esterified with carnitine before being transported across the mitochondrial membrane through a series of steps known as the carnitine cycle. The free CoA esters then undergo β-oxidation in the mitochondrial matrix (Fig. 145-1). Disorders that interfere with any of these steps limit energy production in heart and skeletal muscle at rest and reduce the ability of other tissues, including the brain, to tolerate a low-glucose milieu during times of increased energy demand.

Disorders of long-chain fatty acid oxidation (FAO) include defects in the cellular carnitine transporter, carnitine palmitoyltransferase (CPT) I and II, carnitine-acylcarnitine translocase (CACT), very-long-chain acyl-CoA dehydrogenase (VLCAD), mitochondrial trifunctional protein (TFP), and isolated long-chain 3-hydroxyacyl-CoA dehydrogenase (LCHAD). They can present at any age, largely dependent on the residual activity of the defective enzyme. Complete deficiencies typically manifest in infancy or early childhood; about 25% in the first week of life. Neonates may present with cardiac arrhythmias or sudden death, and occasionally with facial dysmorphism and malformations, including renal cystic dysplasia. Infants and young children may show involvement of liver, heart, or skeletal muscle, with life-threatening fasting- or stress-related hypoketotic hypoglycemia or Reye-like syndrome. Conduction abnormalities, arrhythmias, or dilated or hypertrophic cardiomyopathy and muscle weakness or fasting- and/or exercise-induced rhabdomyolysis are common findings. Onset in adolescence and early adulthood is usually with episodes of recurrent rhabdomyolysis without hypoglycemia. Cardiomyopathy may be present. Medium-chain acyl-CoA dehydrogenase (MCAD) deficiency historically presented with hypoketotic hypoglycemia with or without hyperammonemia or sudden death with fasting or illness. Most patients with recurrent Reye syndrome ultimately proved to have MCAD deficiency. Once the disease is identified in a patient (possibly by newborn screening), the outlook is excellent as long as care is taken during times of illness. Short-chain acyl-CoA dehydrogenase (SCAD) deficiency has been reported in a wide variety of clinical settings but is now generally recognized as a benign biochemical phenotype rather than a disease. Short-chain 3-hydroxyacyl-CoA dehydrogenase (SCHAD/ACADSB) deficiency is anomalous in this group of disorders in that it typically presents as an insulin hypersensitivity syndrome with hypoglycemia.

The diagnosis of an FAO disorder is straightforward when a patient is clinically symptomatic, with characteristic metabolites easily identifiable in blood and urine by tandem mass spectrometry (MS-MS) and urine organic acid analysis by gas chromatography–mass spectrometry (GC-MS). However, in many cases, these metabolites may disappear when a patient is well. Probably the most important single diagnostic test is analysis of the acylcarnitine ester profile in serum or plasma by MS-MS, which identifies characteristic esters in most disorders, even when patients are symptom-free. Confirmation of the diagnosis is most often accomplished through gene sequencing. Other tests that may be useful include analysis of urine organic acids, free and total carnitine in serum and urine, and enzyme assays or acylcarnitine profiling in leukocytes or fibroblasts. Newborn screening by MS-MS is an effective tool for early detection of FAO disorders in asymptomatic infants and is now routinely performed in the United States and many other countries. Combined, approximately 2 to 3 per 10,000 newborns in the United States have an FAO disorder.

Treatment of acute symptoms including encephalopathy associated with hypoketotic hypoglycemia is with 10% glucose (usually with electrolytes) given intravenously to deliver at least 8 mg/kg/min. Intravenous L-carnitine may be helpful if low and is lifesaving in carnitine transporter deficiency. Long-term therapy involves replenishing carnitine stores with oral L-carnitine and preventing hypoglycemia. This may be accomplished by providing a snack before bedtime, but continuous intragastric feeding may be required. Supplementation with medium-chain triglycerides in long-chain FAO disorders provides a fat source that patients can metabolize. Except for MCAD deficiency and carnitine transporter defect, the long-term prognosis for most of these conditions remains guarded even when identified by newborn screening, with sudden death often occurring due to a conduction defect, arrhythmias, and cardiomyopathy.

## CARNITINE UPTAKE DEFECT (PRIMARY CARNITINE DEFICIENCY)

This disorder is caused by a defect in the sodium-dependent high-affinity carnitine transporter (OCTN2) in the cellular plasma membrane, which ultimately limits β-oxidation by reducing entry of long-chain acyl-CoA esters into mitochondria (see Fig. 145-1). The resultant absorptive defect of carnitine in the kidney and intestine leads to very low levels of free carnitine in serum, and the disorder responds dramatically to L-carnitine. It is inherited as an autosomal recessive trait.

### CLINICAL FEATURES

The condition may present in early infancy or in late childhood, usually with dilated cardiomyopathy or recurrent episodes of encephalopathy and hypoketotic hypoglycemia. Skeletal muscle involvement may be apparent as hypotonia or proximal limb weakness. Conduction defects and arrhythmias are rare. Sudden death is observed, with autopsy showing fat in the heart, liver, renal tubules, and skeletal muscle. Adult presentations with cardiomyopathy and arrhythmias have been reported, as has identification of asymptomatic affected females identified through a carnitine deficiency in a newborn.

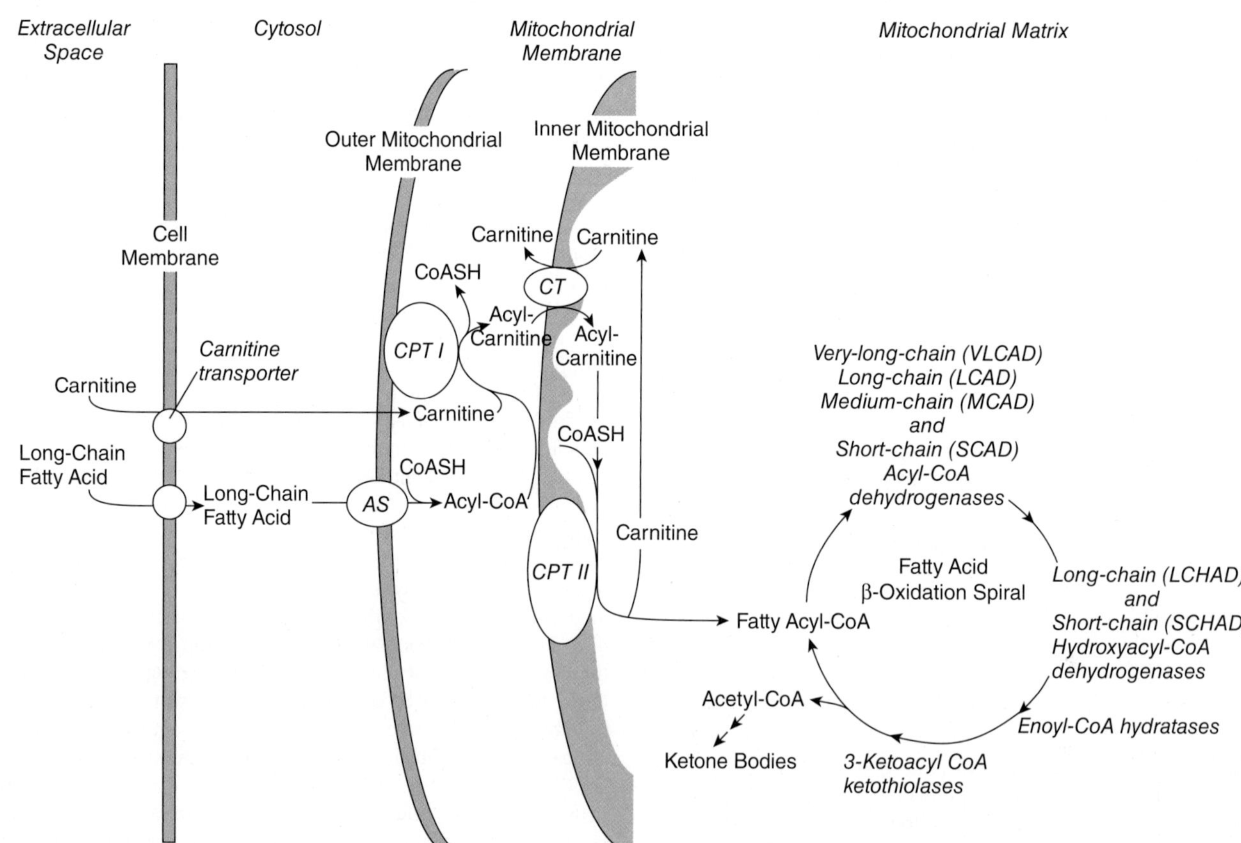


**FIGURE 145-1** Transport and metabolism of fatty acids. To cross the mitochondrial membrane, long-chain fatty acids must be covalently attached to carnitine by carnitine palmitoyltransferase I (CPT I) of the mitochondrial outer membrane and transferred by the carnitine-acylcarnitine translocase (CACT) within the inner membrane. Carnitine palmitoyltransferase II (CPT II), also within the inner membrane, releases the fatty acyl-CoA from carnitine into the mitochondrial matrix. Medium- and short-chain fatty acids can freely enter the mitochondria and do not require the carnitine cycle. Fatty acids are oxidized in a cycle that removes 1 acetyl-CoA moiety per turn. Dehydrogenases specific to long-, medium-, and short-chain fatty acids catalyze the first reaction. As described in the text, defects have been found in each of the transporters and enzymes shown. Ketone bodies are formed in the liver from acetyl-CoA. All defects of fatty acid oxidation are inherited as autosomal recessive diseases. AS, acyl-CoA synthetase.



### DIAGNOSIS

The diagnosis is based on finding extremely low levels of carnitine in serum and tissues; serum carnitine may be 1 μmol/L or undetectable (normal 30–70 μmol/L). Organic acid and acylcarnitine analysis are usually normal. The gene encoding the carnitine transporter is localized to chromosome 5 (5q31), and many disease-causing mutations have been described. Diagnosis is most easily confirmed through gene sequencing. Carnitine transport may also be demonstrated to be deficient in fibroblasts, and fetal diagnosis is possible based on the same assay on amniocytes.

### TREATMENT

The response to L-carnitine supplementation is dramatic and lifesaving; 100 to 300 mg/kg per day can be given intravenously in emergency situations and then administered orally chronically.

## DEFECTS OF THE CARNITINE CYCLE

Short- and medium-chain fatty acids can enter mitochondria directly, but fatty acids longer than $C_{12}$ must be esterified with coenzyme A and transported across the mitochondrial membrane by CPT I, CPT II, and carnitine-acylcarnitine translocase (see Fig. 145-1). CPT I in the mitochondrial outer membrane first transfers the acyl moieties from CoA to carnitine, the translocase moves the carnitine esters across the inner membrane, and CPT II on the matrix side of the inner membrane transfers the carnitine esters to CoA and releases the CoA esters, which enter the β-oxidation spiral. Defects of CPT I, CPT II, and translocase are inherited as autosomal recessive traits.

### CLINICAL FEATURES

CPT I deficiency usually presents in infancy with episodes of fasting-induced hypoketotic hypoglycemia. There are 2 distinct phenotypes of CPT II deficiency, dictated by residual enzyme activity. The more common muscular form presents with exercise-induced muscle pain and rhabdomyolysis in adolescence or early adult life. More rarely, a severe hepatocardiomuscular presentation occurs in infants and children. Those who present as neonates die in 1 to 2 weeks with hepatomegaly, cardiomyopathy, and encephalopathy, and they often have renal cystic dysplasia. Those presenting later usually exhibit hypoketotic hypoglycemia, cardiomyopathy, and muscle disease and are at risk for sudden death due to conduction defects or arrhythmias.

CACT deficiency usually presents as a life-threatening disease in the newborn period, with hypoglycemia, hyperammonemia, conduction defects, arrhythmias, and evidence of skeletal muscle involvement, with high creatine phosphokinase (CPK) values. The ultimate prognosis of this condition is good if the child survives the neonatal period, although cardiomyopathy remains a chronic problem in some patients.

### DIAGNOSIS

The serum acylcarnitine profile is usually normal in CPT I deficiency, although the concentrations of all species may be relatively low, and free carnitine may be high. $C_{16}$ esters are usually elevated in CPT II and CACT deficiency. There are no changes in amino acids (eg, high or low citrulline) to indicate a urea cycle defect as the cause of the hyperammonemia in translocase deficiency, and urine organic acids are normal or show only mild dicarboxylic aciduria. Free carnitine concentration in serum is 2 to 3 times normal in CPT I deficiency and is typically very low in CPT II and translocase deficiency.

All 3 enzymes can be assayed in fibroblasts and leukocytes, and while prenatal diagnosis by enzyme assay on amniocytes should be possible in all of these disorders, it has been accomplished only in CPT II and translocase deficiency. In some instances, a prenatal diagnosis of CPT II can also be made by ultrasonography that shows enlarged echogenic kidneys. Gene sequencing is now the easiest way to confirm a diagnosis. Disease-causing mutations have been identified in all the genes. All 3 diseases can be identified through newborn screening with acylcarnitine profiling, but milder, late-onset forms are usually missed.

### TREATMENT

Acute episodes of hypoketotic hypoglycemia should be treated with intravenous glucose-containing fluids, and treatment of hyperammonemia may require dialysis. Preventing fasting may be sufficient in CPT I deficiency, but continuous nighttime intragastic feeding may be necessary in CPT II and translocase deficiency. Carnitine should be given when the serum carnitine level is low to avoid secondary carnitine deficiency.

## DEFECTS OF β-OXIDATION

Once in the mitochondrial matrix, acyl-CoA esters enter the β-oxidation spiral, where a series of 4 reactions remove the 2-carbon compound acetyl-CoA. Flavin adenine dinucleotide (FAD)-containing acyl-CoA dehydrogenases oxidize the acyl-CoA to 2,3-enoyl-CoA, which then becomes hydrated to a 3-hydroxyacyl-CoA by hydratases. Oxidation to a 3-ketoacyl-CoA by nicotinamide adenine dinucleotide (NAD)-requiring hydroxyacyl-CoA dehydrogenases and removal of acetyl-CoA by 3-ketothiolases follow, and the acyl-CoA, now 2 carbons shorter, reenters the spiral.

All these reactions are catalyzed by enzymes with distinct (but often overlapping) chain-length specificities. For example, different FAD-containing acyl-CoA dehydrogenases act on very-long-chain ($C_{12-24}$), long-chain ($C_{6-20}$), medium-chain ($C_{4-14}$), and short-chain ($C_{4-6}$) acyl-CoAs. Similar specificities exist for the hydratases, hydroxyacyl-CoA dehydrogenases, and thiolases.

Inherited disorders in most of these enzymes have been described. As a rule, defects in long-chain–specific enzymes block β-oxidation more completely and cause more severe clinical disease. Most of these conditions are rare, but VLCAD deficiency, MCAD deficiency, and LCHAD deficiency are relatively common and therefore merit further discussion. All 3 are inherited as autosomal recessive traits. Short-chain acyl-CoA dehydrogenase deficiency is frequently suspected on neonatal screening on the basis of ethylmalonic and butyryl carnitine accumulation, but the relevance is questionable, as many individuals remain asymptomatic without treatment.

## VERY-LONG-CHAIN ACYL-CoA DEHYDROGENASE (VLCAD) DEFICIENCY

### CLINICAL FEATURES

VLCAD deficiency can present in the newborn period with arrhythmias and sudden death, or with hepatic, cardiac, or muscle presentations later in infancy or childhood. The hepatic presentation is characterized by fasting-induced hypoketotic hypoglycemia, encephalopathy, and mild hepatomegaly, often with mild acidosis, hyperammonemia, and elevated liver transaminases. Some patients present with arrhythmias or dilated or hypertrophic cardiomyopathy in infancy or childhood, and a few patients present with exercise-induced muscle pain, rhabdomyolysis, elevated CPK levels, and myoglobinuria. Cardiomyopathy may present (or recur) at any age. Adolescent- or adult-onset episodes of recurrent rhabdomyolysis have been described. Patients are at greatest risk of hypoglycemia in the first few years of life, with a transition to predominantly muscular symptoms thereafter.

### DIAGNOSIS



Analysis of serum acylcarnitines by MS-MS usually reveals elevations of saturated and unsaturated $C_{14-18}$ esters, even between episodes. Urine organic acid analysis during acute illness often shows increased $C_6$ (adipic), $C_8$ (suberic), and $C_{10}$ (sebacic) dicarboxylic acids. However, because very similar changes can be seen in resolving ketosis and after ingesting medium-chain triglycerides, this will not raise suspicion of disease unless $C_{12}$ and $C_{14}$ dicarboxylic acids are also present. Serum concentration of free carnitine is usually low. Newborn screening is possible by MS-MS and routine in the United States and many other countries. The incidence of VLCAD deficiency is approximately 1:40,000 live births.

VLCAD deficiency and accumulation of characteristic acylcarnitines can be demonstrated in fibroblasts or leukocytes, and enzyme assay in cultured amniocytes can be used for prenatal diagnosis. The gene encoding the enzyme has been cloned and localized to chromosome 17p13. Many disease-causing mutations have been described. Confirmation of the diagnosis is now most commonly obtained by DNA sequencing.

### TREATMENT

Treatment of acute episodes includes institution of a high glucose intravenous (IV) infusion rate (8–10 mg/kg/min) and addressing any underlying intercurrent illnesses. Chronic management involves avoidance of fasting and supplementation with medium-chain triglycerides as a souce of fatty acid derived energy. Carnitine supplementation may be helpful if blood free carnitine level is low. Continuous intragastric feeding may be necessary. Fasting in the first year of life should be limited to 4 hours up to age 6 months, 6 hours up to age 12 months, and 8 hours thereafter.

## MEDIUM-CHAIN ACYL-CoA DEHYDROGENASE (MCAD) DEFICIENCY

### CLINICAL FEATURES

MCAD deficiency is the most common FAO defect, with a frequency of 1:10,000 to 1:20,000 in individuals of western European ancestry. It is much less common in Asian and African populations. When identified through newborn screening, MCAD deficiency is an easily treated disorder that nonetheless can still be life threatening. In countries in which MCAD deficiency is not screened for at birth, symptoms usually develop between 18 and 36 months of life with episodes of fasting-induced vomiting, lethargy progressing to coma and seizures, hypoketotic hypoglycemia, and hepatomegaly, often with mild hyperammonemia. The liver may appear fatty by imaging. Misdiagnosis as Reye syndrome or, because the initial episode is fatal in about 25% of patients, sudden infant death syndrome is common. Levels of uric acid, liver transaminases, and CPK are often elevated during the acute episode, and liver biopsy shows microvesicular steatosis. Autopsy shows fatty infiltration of the liver, renal tubules, and heart and skeletal muscle. Enzyme-deficient individuals may not develop symptoms.

### DIAGNOSIS

Analysis of serum acylcarnitines by MS-MS shows elevations of $C_8$, $C_{8:1}$, $C_{10}$, and $C_{10:1}$ esters, even between episodes. Urine organic acids during acute illness often show increased $C_6$ (adipic), $C_8$ (suberic), and $C_{10}$ (sebacic) dicarboxylic acids, together with hexanoylglycine, suberylglycine, and phenylpropionylglycine. The dicarboxylic aciduria also occurs during resolving physiologic ketosis and after ingestion of medium-chain triglycerides. It will not be perceived as abnormal unless the glycine esters, or unsaturated or longer-chain dicarboxylic acids, are also present. Free carnitine level in serum is usually low.

The enzyme defect can be demonstrated in several tissues, including fibroblasts and leukocytes, but molecular diagnosis is often more readily available. The gene encoding MCAD has been localized to chromosome 1p31. Many disease-causing variants have been identified, but the K304E mutation, which changes the lysine residue at position 304 of the mature enzyme to glutamic acid, accounts for 90% of mutant alleles found in Caucasian populations. Ninety percent of affected Caucasians have at least 1 copy of this mutation (81% are homozygous and 18% are compound heterozygous), and analysis for this mutation will confirm the diagnosis in many patients. MCAD deficiency can be identified through newborn screening with MS-MS.

### TREATMENT

Acute episodes should be treated with IV glucose at an infusion rate of 8 to 10 mg/kg/min. Long-term treatment consists of avoiding fasting, usually by providing carbohydrate snacks at bedtime. Oral carnitine (50–100 mg/kg/d) is used by some, but not all, clinicians. Developmental delay, behavioral problems, and other chronic central nervous system problems may occur if there are episodes of hypoglycemia, but if such an injury does not occur, prognosis is quite good. As a rule, fasting should be avoided, especially in younger children.

## LONG-CHAIN 3-HYDROXYACYL-CoA DEHYDROGENASE (LCHAD) DEFICIENCY



NAD-dependent 3-hydroxyacyl-CoA dehydrogenases catalyze oxidation of 3-hydroxyacyl-CoA esters to their 3-keto analogues. LCHAD, the long-chain-specific enzyme, acts on acyl groups longer than $C_8$ and exists in mitochondria as part of a protein complex with 3 activities. This mitochondrial trifunctional protein (MTP) is an $\alpha_4\beta_4$ octamer, with the α subunit harboring LCHAD and long-chain enoyl-CoA hydratase activities, and the β subunit bearing long-chain β-ketothiolase activity. LCHAD deficiency can exist alone or with deficiency of the other 2 enzymes. Isolated LCHAD deficiency occurs in 1:40,000 to 1:80,000 newborns.

### CLINICAL FEATURES

Patients with isolated LCHAD deficiency often present in infancy with fasting-induced hypoketotic hypoglycemia; however, patients may also present with neonatal cardiomyopathy or, later in life, with exercise-induced rhabdomyolysis. A clinical history often reveals a pregnancy complicated by acute fatty liver or HELLP (*h*emolysis, *e*levated *l*iver enzymes, and *l*ow *p*latelets). Unlike most other fatty acid oxidation disorders, severe and progressive cholestatic liver disease is common, and many patients develop retinopathy with hypopigmentation or focal pigmentary aggregations. Many patients die in early childhood. The presentation of individuals with MTP deficiency is similar to that of isolated LCHAD deficiency, but it is usually earlier and more severe.

### DIAGNOSIS

Acylcarnitine analysis by MS-MS is usually diagnostic and shows elevated saturated and unsaturated $C_{16}$ and $C_{18}$ hydroxyacylcarnitines. Organic acid analysis often shows elevated $C_{6-14}$ 3-hydroxydicarboxylic acids, but the same abnormalities can be seen in patients with respiratory chain defects and glycogenoses and are not specific. The enzyme defect can be demonstrated in fibroblasts and leukocytes and, for prenatal diagnosis, in amniocytes. The genes encoding the α and β subunits are localized to chromosome 2p23.3. The E510Q mutation, which changes the glutamic acid residue at position 510 to glutamine, accounts for nearly 90% of mutant alleles in Europeans. LCHAD and MTP deficiency can be identified through newborn screening with MS-MS.

### TREATMENT

Therapy is much the same as that for VLCAD, CPT, and CACT deficiencies. As in VLCAD deficiency, it may be necessary to completely eliminate fasting by continuous intragastric feeding, and medium-chain triglycerides may be used to provide calories. Carnitine may be useful to prevent depletion of stores. Oral supplements of docosahexaenoic acid, a polyunsaturated $C_{20}$ acid, appear useful in slowing the progression of retinopathy.

## GLUTARIC ACIDEMIA TYPE II

Electrons from the acyl-CoA dehydrogenases involved in fatty acid and amino acid oxidation are transferred from their FAD coenzymes into the respiratory chain via redox centers in electron transfer flavoprotein (ETF) and ETF:ubiquinone oxidoreductase (ETF:QO). Recessively inherited defects in ETF and ETF:QO cause glutaric acidemia type II (GA2), also known as multiple acyl-CoA dehydrogenase deficiency (MADD). Several additional gene defects presenting with a biochemical pattern of GA2 have recently been described, including defects of cellular riboflavin transport and FAD synthesis. Historically, prior to the molecular characterization of the disorders, they were clinically described as Brown-Vialetto-Van Laere syndrome and Fazio Londe syndrome—progressive neuromuscular disorders with variable features of myopathy, hearing loss, optic atrophy, and ataxia. Treatment with high-dose riboflavin can be lifesaving.

### CLINICAL FEATURES

GA2 may present in the neonatal period with severe hypoglycemia, metabolic acidosis, hyperammonemia, and the odor of sweaty feet typical of isovaleric acidemia, often with cardiomyopathy, facial dysmorphism, and severe renal cystic dysplasia. Most such patients die within the first days or weeks of life, often of conduction defects or arrhythmias. Fatty infiltration of the liver, renal tubules, and heart and skeletal muscle are consistent autopsy findings. Milder disease, sometimes called ethylmalonic adipic aciduria, may present with episodic vomiting, hypoketotic hypoglycemia, and hepatomegaly in childhood, or simply as hypoglycemia in adult life. Leukodystrophy and cardiomyopathy may also be present, along with an elevated CPK.

### DIAGNOSIS

Acylcarnitine analysis by MS-MS shows glutarylcarnitine, isovalerylcarnitine, and straight-chain esters of chain lengths $C_4$, $C_8$, $C_{10}$, $C_{10:1}$, and $C_{12}$. Urine organic acids show increased ethylmalonic, glutaric, 2-hydroxyglutaric, and 3-hydroxyisovaleric acids, together with $C_6$, $C_8$, and $C_{10}$ dicarboxylic acids and isovalerylglycine. The serum carnitine concentration is usually low. Elevated serum sarcosine on amino acid analysis is common in patients with mild disease.

Assays using fibroblasts show that some GA2 patients are deficient in ETF and, more commonly, that others are deficient in ETF:QO. Disease-causing mutations in the 3 genes encoding ETF:QO and the α and β subunits of ETF have been identified in many patients. Additional molecular defects in the cellular riboflavin transporter and FAD synthesis have recently been described; thus, gene sequencing of all of these genes is typically the easiest way to make a diagnosis when a metabolite pattern is suggestive of GA2. GA2 is identifiable through newborn screening by MS-MS.

### TREATMENT

Patients with complete defects die during the first weeks of life, usually of conduction defects or arrhythmias, but those with incomplete defects can survive well into adult life. As in other fatty acid oxidation disorders, treatment relies on the avoidance of fasting, sometimes with continuous intragastric feeding, and carnitine to replenish lost stores. High-dose riboflavin supplementation can benefit a subset of patients, and the use of D/L-3-hydroxybutyrate has been shown to be effective in reversing the leukodystrophy in a few patients not responsive to riboflavin.

### SUGGESTED READINGS

Derks TG, van Spronsen FJ, Rake JP, van der Hilst CS, Span MM, Smit GP. Safe and unsafe duration of fasting for children with MCAD deficiency. *Eur J Pediatr*. 2007;166:5-11.

Gallant NM, Leydiker K, Tang H, et al. Biochemical, molecular, and clinical characteristics of children with short chain acyl-CoA dehydrogenase deficiency detected by newborn screening in California. *Mol Genet Metab*. 2012;106(1):55-61.

Gillingham MB, Connor WE, Matern D, et al. Optimal dietary therapy of long-chain 3-hydroxyacyl-CoA dehydrogenase deficiency. *Mol Genet Metab.* 2003;79:114-123.

Houten SM, Violante S, Ventura FV, Wanders RJ. The biochemistry and physiology of mitochondrial fatty acid β-oxidation and its genetic disorders. *Annu Rev Physiol.* 2016;78:23-44.

Iafolla AK, Thompson RJ, Roe CR. Medium-chain acyl-coenzyme A dehydrogenase deficiency: clinical course in 120 affected children. *J Pediatr.* 1994;124:409.

Olsen RK, Konarikova E, Giancaspero TA, et al. Riboflavin-responsive and non-responsive mutations in FAD synthase cause multiple acyl-CoA dehydrogenase and combined respiratory-chain deficiency. *Am J Hum Genet.* 2016;98:1130-1145.

Pena LD, van Calcar SC, Hansen J, et al. Outcomes and genotype-phenotype correlations in 52 individuals with VLCAD deficiency diagnosed by NBS and enrolled in the IBEM-IS database. *Mol Genet Metab.* 2016;118:272-281.

Spiekerkoetter U. Mitochondrial fatty acid oxidation disorders: clinical presentation of long-chain fatty acid oxidation defects before and after newborn screening. *J Inherit Metab Dis.* 2010;33:527-532.

Spiekerkoetter U, Lindner M, Santer R, et al. Management and outcome in 75 individuals with long-chain fatty acid oxidation defects: results from a workshop. *J Inherit Metab Dis.* 2009;32:488-497.

Therrell BL, Lloyd-Puryear MA, Camp KM, Mann MY. Inborn errors of metabolism identified via newborn screening: ten-year incidence data and costs of nutritional interventions for research agenda planning. *Mol Genet Metab.* 2014;113:14-26.

# 146 Disorders of Ketogenesis

Jerry Vockley

## INTRODUCTION

Hepatic biosynthesis of ketone bodies involves the condensation of acetyl-coenzyme A (CoA) and acetoacetyl-CoA to hydroxymethylglutaryl-CoA (HMG-CoA) by HMG-CoA synthase, followed by hydrolysis of HMG-CoA to acetyl-CoA and acetoacetic acid (AcAc) by HMG-CoA lyase as the final step in leucine degradation. AcAc is reduced to 3-hydroxybutyric acid (3HB), and extrahepatic tissues use the 2 ketone bodies as energy sources during fasting (ketolysis). Recessively inherited defects of HMG-CoA synthase (HMGCS2) and HMG-CoA lyase (HMGCL) cause hypoketotic hypoglycemia during fasting, and defects of ketolysis cause persistent or episodic ketoacidosis.

## HYDROXYMETHYLGLUTARYL-CoA SYNTHASE DEFICIENCY

Deficiency of HMG-CoA synthase (MIM no. 605911) causes hypoketotic hypoglycemia, typically during intercurrent illnesses, along with encephalopathy and hepatomegaly. Serum free fatty acids are very elevated, urine and serum ketones are inappropriately low or absent, transaminases are elevated, urine organic acid analysis shows severe dicarboxylic aciduria with unsaturated and 3-hydroxy derivatives, and serum acylcarnitines are normal. When the deficiency is suspected, mutation analysis can confirm the diagnosis. Treatment involves avoiding fasting and administering glucose during episodes of hypoglycemia, along with bedtime carbohydrates such as uncooked cornstarch.

## HYDROXYMETHYLGLUTARYL-CoA LYASE DEFICIENCY

Deficiency of 3-hydroxy-3-methylglutaryl-CoA lyase (MIM no. 246450) can present in the newborn period with severe hypoketotic hypoglycemia, elevated transaminases, metabolic acidosis, and hyperammonemia, or later with episodes of hypoglycemia, hepatomegaly, and encephalopathy following intercurrent infection. The latter form of the disease is often mistaken for Reye syndrome. If not promptly treated, cerebral atrophy, neurologic effects, and developmental disabilities may follow. Adolescent- and adult-onset patients have been described and may also have a leukoencephalopathy. It is a common organic aciduria in the Saudi population but is otherwise rare.



### DIAGNOSIS

Urine organic acid analysis shows increased 3-hydroxy-3-methylglutaric, 3-methylglutaconic, and 3-methylglutaric acids, and tandem mass spectrometry (MS/MS) shows increased 3-hydroxy-3-methylglutarylcarnitine. The disorder can also be identified by MS/MS on newborn screening blood spots with elevations typically reported as "C5-hydroxyacylcarntine," a designation shared by several other isobaric metabolites. Due to the possibility of a catastrophic presentation, rapid additional diagnostic testing by urine organic acids is necessary. Liver function tests may be abnormal at times of acute illness. The enzyme defect is apparent in many tissues, including fibroblasts and peripheral leukocytes, but is usually not necessary to measure due to the availability of DNA testing. Fetal disease can be diagnosed by enzyme assay on cultured amniocytes or chorionic villus samples, by demonstrating the characteristic organic acids in amniotic fluid, or by DNA analysis if a familial mutation is known.

### TREATMENT

Acute management requires intravenous fluids, electrolytes, and glucose. Long-term management is directed at avoiding fasting and the resulting hypoglycemia, and bedtime carbohydrates may be warranted. The possible life-threatening consequences of fasting make it imperative that parents bring the child to the hospital as soon as possible when oral intake is compromised.

### SUGGESTED READINGS

Bakker HD, Wanders RJA, Schutgens RBH, et al. 3-Hydroxy-3-methylglutaryl-CoA lyase deficiency: absence of clinical symptoms due to a self-imposed dietary fat and protein restriction. *J Inherit Metab Dis.* 1993;16:1061-1062.

Fukao T, Mitchell G, Sass JO, Hori T, Orii K, Aoyama Y. Ketone body metabolism and its defects. *J Inherit Metab Dis.* 2014;37:541-551.

Ramos M, Menao S, Arnedo M, et al. New case of mitochondrial HMG-CoA synthase deficiency. Functional analysis of eight mutations. *Eur J Med Genet.* 2013;56:411-415.

Sass JO. Inborn errors of ketogenesis and ketone body utilization. *J Inherit Metab Dis.* 2012;35:23-28.

Zschocke J, Penzien JM, Bielen M, et al. The diagnosis of mitochondrial HMG-synthase deficiency. *J Pediatr.* 2002;140:778-780.

# 147 Disorders of Ketolysis

Jerry Vockley

## INTRODUCTION

Ketolysis involves esterification of acetylacetate (AcAc) to AcAc-coenzyme A (CoA) by succinyl-CoA:3-oxoacid transferase (SCOT, *OXCT1* gene) and hydrolysis of AcAcCoA by mitochondrial acetoacetyl-CoA thiolase (T2, *ACAT1* gene) to form acetyl-CoA. Inherited disorders of ketolysis involve these 2 enzymes and cause persistent or episodic ketoacidosis. If SCOT is entirely lacking, ketolysis is completely blocked, but if functional T2 is completely absent, some ketolysis is still possible, likely due to the presence of another mitochondrial enzyme, medium chain 3-ketoacyl-CoA thiolase, that has some activity for hydrolyzing AcAcCoA. This latter enzyme may explain in part why permanent ketosis is often observed in SCOT deficiency but not in T2 deficiency. Ketone body production is regulated by the hormones glucagon and catecholamines, which induce free fatty acid (FFA) mobilization from adipose tissue, fatty acid oxidation, and ketogenesis in the liver, while insulin suppresses these steps. Ketogenic stresses including fasting, prolonged exertion, febrile illnesses, and vomiting and diarrhea, leading to both FFA oxidation and ketone body synthesis. The enzymes of ketogenesis (see Chapter 146); hydroxymethylglutaryl-CoA synthase and lyase, generate AcAc, which is then reduced by mitochondrial D-β-hydroxybutyrate (D-βOHB)-dehydrogenase (BDH1) in the liver to D-βOHB. Ketone bodies then circulate to peripheral tissues, where BDH1 regenerates AcAc, allowing SCOT and T2 to generate acetyl-CoA in order to maintain cellular energy production via the tricarboxylic acid (TCA) cycle and spare glucose utilization.

## SUCCINYL-CoA TRANSFERASE DEFICIENCY

SCOT deficiency (Online Mendelian Inheritance in Man [MIM] no. 245050) is characterized by persistent or exaggerated episodic ketoacidosis, often beginning in infancy, with increased levels of ketone bodies in the blood even in the fed state. A diagnosis can be established by enzyme assay in fibroblasts or by mutation analysis, and prenatal diagnosis can be accomplished in the same manner.

## BETA-KETOTHIOLASE DEFICIENCY

Mitochondrial 3-ketothiolase releases acetyl-CoA from AcAcCoA and from 2-methylacetoacetyl-CoA, an intermediate in isoleucine oxidation (see Chapter 132). Mitochondrial 3-ketothiolase deficiency (MIM no. 203750) can present in infancy with hypoglycemia, elevated transaminases, hyperuricemia, metabolic acidosis, and severe ketosis, or later with fasting- or protein-induced episodes of vomiting, hepatomegaly, ketoacidosis, and encephalopathy.

### DIAGNOSIS

In SCOT deficiency, levels of ketones in the blood may be persistently elevated or show episodic increases during illness. Urine organic acid analysis shows increased 3-hydroxybutyrate and acetoacetate levels. In beta-ketothiolase deficiency, urine organic acid analysis shows increased 2-methyl-3-hydroxybutyric acid, 2-methylacetoacetic acid, and tiglylglycine levels, but they may be obscured during acute illnesses by 3-hydroxybutyrate (3HB) and AcAc and may be detectable only between episodes or after an oral load of isoleucine. Glycine levels are often elevated in blood and urine. In blood acylcarnitine analysis, C5:1 acylcarnitine (tiglylcarnitine) and C5-OH acylcarnitine (2-methyl-3-hydroxybutyrylcarnitine) may be elevated, but this is not a consistent finding, and the disorder is not readily detectable by newborn screening. While usually not necessary to establish a diagnosis, the enzyme defects can be demonstrated in fibroblasts and leukocytes, and in amniocytes for prenatal diagnosis. Disease-causing mutations can be identified by clinically available DNA sequencing.

### TREATMENT

Treatment of acute episodes in SCOT deficiency is supportive, providing IV fluids and glucose for hydration and calories until normal caloric intake can be re-established. Chronic bicarbonate administration may be necessary if chronic ketosis is present. Anecdotally, long-term outcomes appear good, but formal longitudinal studies have not been performed. Beta-ketothiolase deficiency should be treated with intravenous glucose and sodium bicarbonate. A low-protein/isoleucine-restricted diet, coupled with avoidance of fasting, decreases the frequency and severity of acute episodes and permits normal growth and development if irreversible neurologic damage has not already occurred.

### SUGGESTED READINGS


Fukao T, Mitchell G, Sass JO, Hori T, Orii K, Aoyama Y. Ketone body metabolism and its defects. *J Inherit Metab Dis.* 2014;37:541-551.

Fukao T, Scriver CR, Kondo N. The clinical phenotype and outcome of mitochondrial acetoacetyl-CoA thiolase deficiency (beta-ketothiolase or T2 deficiency) in 26 enzymatically proved and mutation-defined patients. *Mol Genet Metab.* 2001;72:109-114.

Sass JO. Inborn errors of ketogenesis and ketone body utilization. *J Inherit Metab Dis.* 2012;35:23-28.

Saudubray JM, Specola N, Middleton B, et al. Hyperketotic states due to inherited defects of ketolysis. *Enzyme.* 1987;38:80-90.


# 148 Disorders of Leukotriene Synthesis and Degradation

William B. Rizzo

### INTRODUCTION

Leukotrienes (LTs) are inflammatory lipid mediators synthesized from arachidonic acid (C20:4), a 20-carbon polyunsaturated fatty acid that is present in membrane phospholipids. LTs consist of several biochemically distinct forms ($LTA_4$, $LTB_4$, $LTC_4$, $LTD_4$, $LTE_4$) that act through interactions with specific cellular receptors. $LTC_4$, $LTD_4$, and $LTE_4$ are distinct from the other LT species because they are formed by the incorporation of cysteine into their structures and are referred to as cysteinyl-LTs. These lipid mediators are biologically active in allergic and immune reactions, bronchoconstriction, neutrophil and macrophage chemotaxis, and T-cell differentiation. Emerging data also implicate their involvement in neurologic processes.

### PATHOGENESIS AND EPIDEMIOLOGY

Several rare disorders of LT metabolism have been identified. They can be classified into those that either block LT synthesis or prevent its degradation (Fig. 148-1). All are rare and have an unknown incidence.

#### Disorders of Leukotriene Synthesis

The biosynthesis of LT begins with 5-lipooxygenase acting on arachidonic acid to produce the short-lived $LTA_4$, which is the metabolic precursor for the other LTs. $LTA_4$ is enzymatically converted to $LTB_4$, a potent proinflammatory mediator, and is also acted on by $LTC_4$ synthase, which uses glutathione as a co-substrate, to generate $LTC_4$ and the subsequent series of cysteinyl-LTs ($LTD_4$ and $LTE_4$). Deficient $LTC_4$ synthase activity has been described in 2 children who had severely reduced levels of $LTC_4$, $LTD_4$, and $LTE_4$. Since glutathione is a co-substrate for this enzyme, patients with genetic defects in the production of glutathione (eg, glutathione synthetase deficiency) also exhibit reductions of all cysteinyl-LT species. $LTC_4$ is converted to $LTD_4$ by γ-glutamyl transpeptidase, and patients with deficiency of this enzyme accumulate $LTC_4$ and have profound reductions in $LTD_4$ and $LTE_4$. The subsequent metabolic step uses dipeptidase to convert $LTD_4$ to $LTE_4$. One 15-year-old patient with suspected dipeptidase deficiency accumulated $LTD_4$ and had undetectable $LTE_4$.

#### Disorders of Leukotriene Degradation

The degradation of $LTB_4$ (and $LTE_4$) proceeds by ω-oxidation, which adds a hydroxyl group to the C20-carbon of $LTB_4$. This reaction is catalyzed by the P450 enzyme CYP4F3A. 20-Hydroxy-$LTB_4$ is subsequently oxidized via an aldehyde intermediate to 20-carboxy-$LTB_4$ (see Fig. 148-1). Patients with Sjögren-Larsson syndrome have deficient fatty aldehyde dehydrogenase and cannot carry out this alcohol-acid conversion and thus accumulate $LTB_4$ and 20-hydroxy-$LTB_4$. In neutrophils, CYP4F3A can also catalyze this alcohol-acid conversion, but its overall contribution to LT degradation is comparatively minor

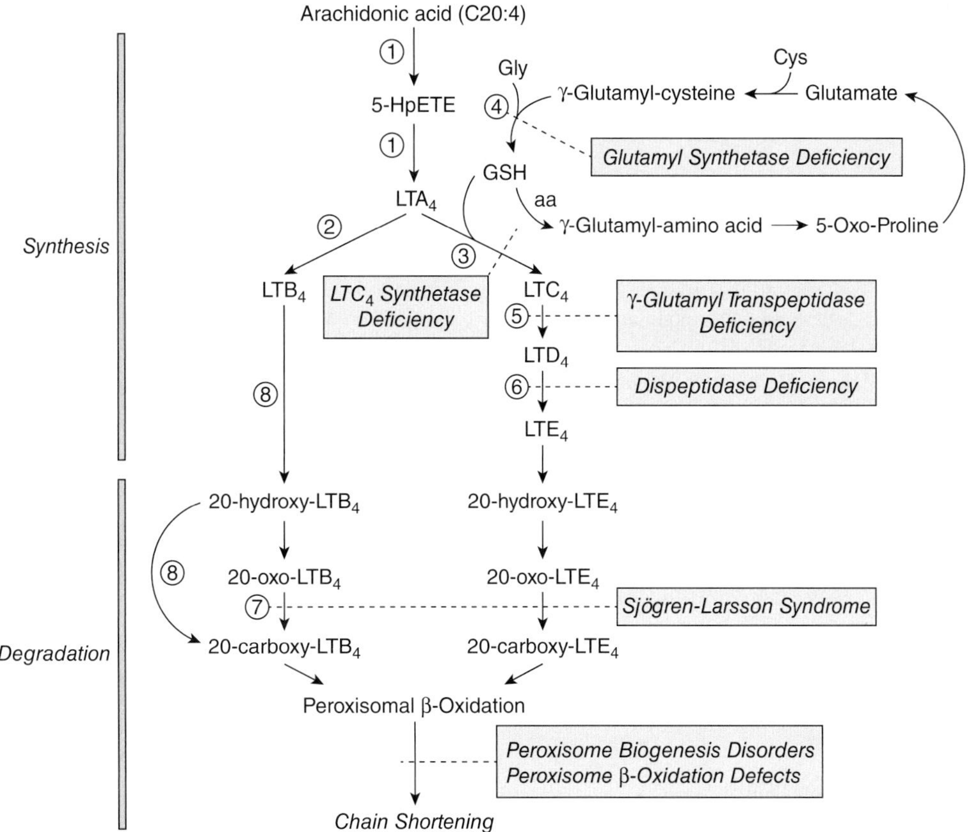


**FIGURE 148-1** Metabolic pathway for leukotriene synthesis and degradation. Enzymes catalyzing reactions are indicated as circled numbers: 1 = 5-lipoxygenase; 2 = $LTA_4$ hydrolase; 3 = $LTC_4$ synthase; 4 = glutathione synthetase; 5 = γ-glutamyl transpeptidase; 6 = dipeptidase; 7 = fatty aldehyde dehydrogenase; and 8 = CYP4F3A. Disorders are enclosed in rectangles. aa, amino acid; GSH, glutathione; 5-HpETE, 5-hydroperoxy-eicosatetraenoic acid.

in other tissues. Subsequent catalytic steps in 20-carboxy-$LTB_4$ require peroxisomal β-oxidation to shorten the carbon chain. Consequently, patients with peroxisome biogenesis disorders (Zellweger spectrum disorders) and isolated defects in peroxisomal β-oxidation exhibit increased $LTB_4$ (and $LTE_4$) metabolites (see Fig. 148-1).

How these biochemical abnormalities contribute to the pathogenesis of the LT diseases is not known. Since all of the disorders with impaired synthesis of the cysteinyl-LTs have significant neurologic symptoms, it is likely that these LTs are critical for normal brain function. Moreover, the disorders of LT degradation (Sjögren-Larsson syndrome and peroxisomal disorders) have additional biochemical abnormalities and exhibit multiorgan involvement, which complicates identifying the specific contributions of LTs to the total phenotype. Symptoms of inflammation, asthma, and immune dysfunction are not prominent among the LT disorders. Curiously, animal studies indicate that $LTB_4$ can induce pruritus when administered subcutaneously.

## CLINICAL MANIFESTATIONS

Clinical features of the LT disorders vary widely, but most patients have serious neurologic symptoms. Hypotonia, psychomotor retardation, microcephaly, and failure to thrive are reported in $LTC_4$ synthase deficiency. Patients with γ-glutamyl transpeptidase deficiency have exhibited variable intellectual disability, seizures, behavior problems, poor coordination, and/or dysmorphisms. The patient with suspected dipeptidase deficiency had intellectual disability, mild motor deficits, and hearing impairment. Diseases of glutathione production are associated with hemolytic anemia, metabolic acidosis, intellectual disability, and progressive neurologic symptoms. Sjögren-Larsson syndrome has a characteristic triad of pruritic ichthyosis, intellectual disability, and spasticity. Peroxisome biosynthesis disorders and isolated peroxisome β-oxidation defects share features of hypotonia, psychomotor retardation, seizures, deafness, and visual impairment.

## DIAGNOSIS

LT disorders are undoubtedly underrecognized. In light of very limited knowledge of their clinical phenotype, the suspicion of a cysteinyl-LT disorder should arise after eliminating more common neurologic diseases. Unfortunately, diagnostic testing is problematic. Although screening urine, cerebrospinal fluid, or blood for LT metabolites is feasible in a research setting, the analytical method is demanding, and a diagnostic test is not yet universally available for the practicing physician. Consequently, genetic testing is probably the most convenient, but still unproven, method for diagnosis, since disease-causing mutations in most of the primary disorders of LT biosynthesis are still unknown. In contrast, disorders of LT degradation (Sjögren-Larsson syndrome, peroxisome defects) are readily diagnosed using conventional biochemical and molecular tests.

## TREATMENT

Effective therapy for the LT biosynthetic disorders has not been developed. Zileuton, which inhibits 5-lipooxygenase and lowers $LTB_4$ levels, was anecdotally reported to improve the pruritus in several patients with Sjögren-Larsson syndrome, but no convincing benefit was seen in a recent double-blind clinical trial. No reports have been published on the use of cysteinyl-LT receptor antagonists (eg, montelukast) in the LT synthetic disorders.

## PREVENTION

As suspected genetic diseases, prevention of LT disorders can theoretically be achieved by prenatal diagnosis.

## SUGGESTED READINGS

Liu M, Yokomizo T. The role of leukotrienes in allergic diseases. *Allergol Int.* 2015;64:17-26.

Mayatepek E. Leukotriene C4 synthesis deficiency: a member of a probably underdiagnosed new group of neurometabolic diseases. *Eur J Pediatr*. 2000;159:811-818.

Mayatepek E, Flock B. Leukotriene C4-synthesis deficiency: a new inborn error of metabolism linked to a fatal developmental syndrome. *Lancet*. 1998;352:1514-1517.

Mayatepek E, Flock B. Increased urinary excretion of LTB4 and omega-carboxy-LTB4 in patients with Zellweger syndrome. *Clin Chim Acta*. 1999;282:151-155.

Mayatepek E, Hoffmann GF, Carlsson B, Larsspm A, Becker K. Impaired synthesis of lipoxygenase products in glutathione synthetase deficiency. *Pediatr Res*. 1994;35:307-310.

Mayatepek E, Lindner M, Zelezny R, Lindner W, Brandstetter G, Hoffmann GF. A severely affected infant with absence of cysteinyl leukotrienes in cerebrospinal fluid: further evidence that leukotriene C4-synthesis deficiency is a new neurometabolic disorder. *Neuropediatrics*. 1999;30:5-7.

Mayatepek E, Okun JG, Meissner T, et al. Synthesis and metabolism of leukotrienes in γ-glutamyl transpeptidase deficiency. *J Lipid Res*. 2004;45:900-904.

Murphy RC, Gijón MA. Biosynthesis and metabolism of leukotrienes. *Biochem J*. 2007;405:379-395.

Rizzo WB. Sjögren-Larsson syndrome: molecular genetics and biochemical pathogenesis of fatty aldehyde dehydrogenase deficiency. *Mol Genet Metab*. 2007:90:1-9.

Willemsen MAAP, Rotteveel JJ, de Jong JGN, et al. Defective metabolism of leukotriene B4 in the Sjögren-Larsson syndrome. *J Neurol Sci*. 2000;183:61-67.




# PART 4 CARBOHYDRATES

## 149 Disorders of Glycogen Metabolism

Priya S. Kishnani and Yuan-Tsong Chen

### GLYCOGEN STORAGE DISEASE

Glycogen, the storage form of glucose in animal cells, is composed of glucose residues joined in straight chains by α-1,4 linkages and branched at intervals of 4 to 10 residues with α-1,6 linkages. The tree-like molecule can have a molecular weight of many millions and may aggregate to form structures recognizable by electron microscopy. In muscle, glycogen forms β particles, which are spherical and contain up to 60,000 glucose residues. Each β particle contains a covalently linked protein called *glycogenin*. Liver contains β particles and rosettes of glycogen called α particles, which appear to be aggregated β particles.

The primary function of glycogen varies in different tissues. In skeletal muscle, stored glycogen is a source of fuel that is used for short-term, high-energy consumption during muscle activity; in the brain, the small amount of stored glycogen is used during brief periods of hypoglycemia or hypoxia as an emergency supply of energy. In contrast, the liver takes up glucose from the bloodstream after a meal and stores it as glycogen. When blood glucose levels start to fall, the liver converts glycogen back into glucose and releases it into the blood for use by tissues such as brain and erythrocytes that cannot store significant amounts of glycogen.

Glycogen storage diseases (GSDs) are inherited disorders that affect glycogen metabolism. Disorders in virtually every enzyme involved in the synthesis or degradation of glycogen and its regulation cause some type of GSD. Excluded from this section are those conditions in which tissue glycogen accumulation is secondary, such as overtreatment of diabetes mellitus with insulin or administration of pharmacologic amounts of glucocorticoids.

There are more than 12 forms of glycogenosis (Fig. 149-1). The glycogen found in these disorders is abnormal in quantity or quality or both. Historically, the GSDs were categorized numerically in the order in which the enzymatic defects were identified. This section classifies the diseases by the organs involved and the clinical manifestations.

Liver and muscle have abundant glycogen and are the most commonly and seriously affected tissues. The GSDs that principally affect the liver (see Fig. 149-1) include glucose-6-phosphatase deficiency (type I), debranching enzyme deficiency (type III), branching enzyme deficiency (type IV), liver phosphorylase deficiency (type VI), phosphorylase kinase deficiency (type IX), liver glycogen synthase deficiency (type 0), and glucose transporter-2 defect (type XI). Because carbohydrate metabolism in the liver affects plasma glucose levels, the disorders of hepatic glycogen degradation and glucose release typically cause fasting hypoglycemia and hepatomegaly. Some GSDs are associated with liver complications; for example, hepatic adenomas with risk for malignant transformation in GSD type I and liver cirrhosis with risk for progression to end-stage liver failure or malignancy (types III, IV, and some forms of type IX). Other organs besides liver may also be involved; for example, renal dysfunction in GSD type I; cardiac involvement in types I, II, III, IV, and adenosine monophosphate (AMP)-activated protein kinase gamma-2 (PRKAG2); myopathy in types 0, II, III, IV, and PRKAG2; and some rare forms of phosphorylase kinase deficiency.

The role of glycogen in muscle is to provide substrates for the generation of sufficient adenosine triphosphate (ATP) for muscle contraction. The muscle GSDs can be divided into 2 groups (see Fig. 149-1). The first group is a muscle-energy disorder due to a block in glycolysis and is characterized by muscle pain, exercise intolerance, myoglobinuria, and susceptibility to fatigue. This group includes type V (McArdle disease), a muscle phosphorylase deficiency, and deficiencies of phosphofructokinase (type VII), phosphoglycerate kinase, phosphoglycerate mutase (type X), lactate dehydrogenase, fructose 1,6-bisphosphate aldolase A, and pyruvate kinase. Some of these enzyme deficiencies are associated with a compensated hemolysis, suggesting a more generalized defect in glucose metabolism. The second group is characterized by progressive skeletal myopathy and/or cardiomyopathy and is represented by a lysosomal enzyme deficiency (acid α-glucosidase, type II). This group also includes muscle glycogen synthase deficiency, lysosomal associated membrane protein 2 (LAMP2) deficiency, and PRKAG2 defect. Deficiency of glycogenin-1 due to *GYG1* mutations has been recently shown to result in accumulation of polyglucosan, leading to a polyglucosan body myopathy.

The overall frequency of all forms of GSD is approximately 1 in 10,000 live births. Most of the GSDs are inherited as autosomal recessive traits, but PRKAG2 is autosomal dominant, and phosphoglycerate kinase deficiency and a common form of phosphorylase kinase deficiency are X-linked disorders. The most common childhood disorders are glucose-6-phosphatase deficiency (type I), lysosomal acid α-glucosidase deficiency (type II), debrancher deficiency (type III), and liver phosphorylase kinase deficiency (type IX). The most common adult disorders are myophosphorylase deficiency (type V or McArdle disease) and the late- or adult-onset form of GSD type II (Pompe disease). In the past, the prognosis for many GSDs was guarded; however, early diagnosis and better management have improved the survival rates, and many affected children are now adults. Consequently, the natural history of these disorders continues to unfold.

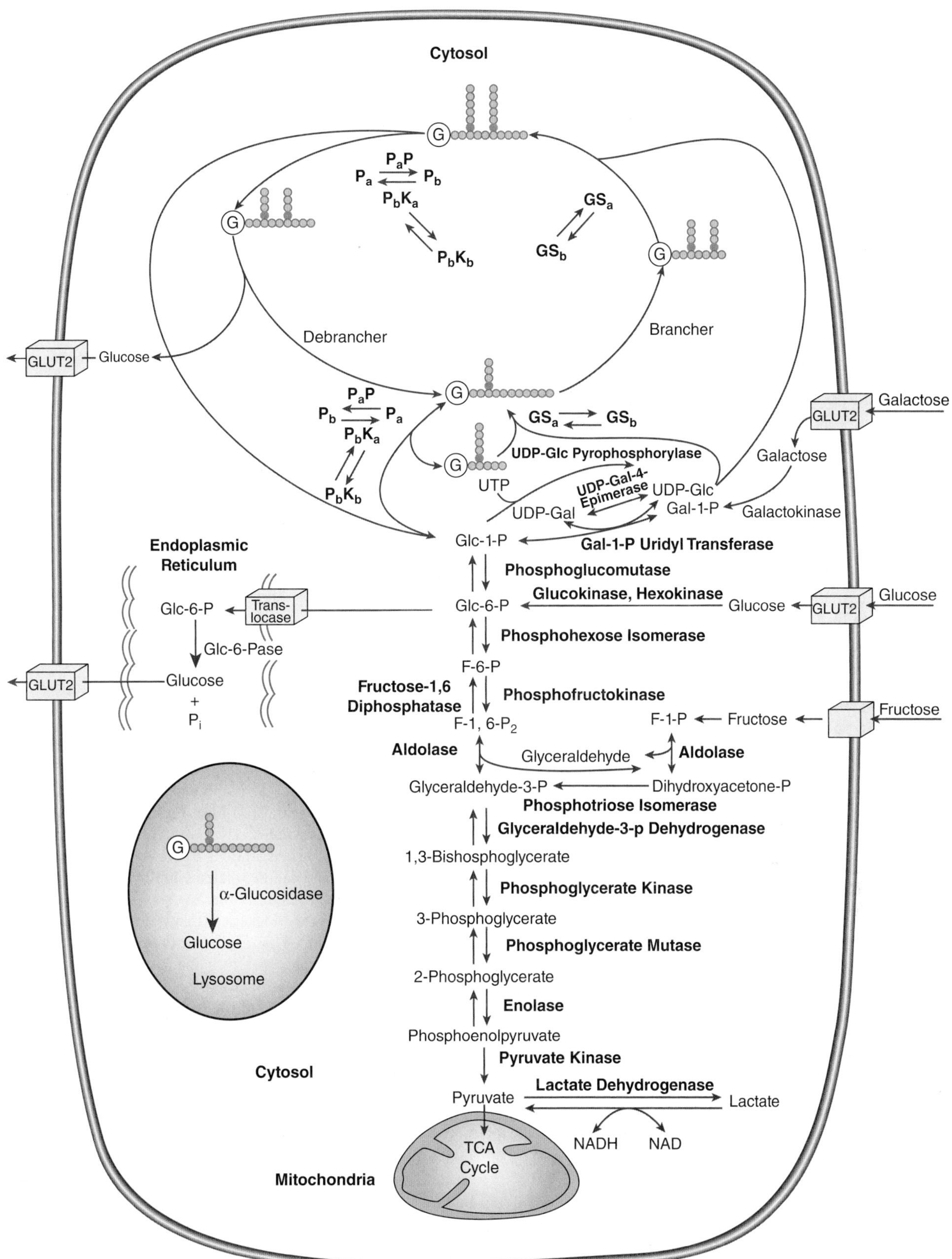


**FIGURE 149-1** Metabolic pathways related to glycogen storage diseases and to galactose and fructose disorders. Nonstandard abbreviations are as follows: G, glycogenin, the primer protein for glycogen synthesis; GSa, active glycogen synthase; GSb, inactive glycogen synthase; Pa, active phosphorylase; Pb, inactive phosphorylase; PaP, phosphorylase a phosphatase; pbKa, active phosphorylase b kinase; PbKb, inactive phosphorylase b kinase. (Modified with permission from Isselbacher KJ, Martin JB: *Harrison's Principles of Internal Medicine*, 13th ed. New York: McGraw-Hill; 1994.)

## TYPE I GLYCOGEN STORAGE DISEASE (GLUCOSE-6-PHOSPHATASE OR TRANSLOCASE DEFICIENCY, VON GIERKE DISEASE)

### CLINICAL PRESENTATION

Type I GSD is due to a defect in glucose-6-phosphatase in liver, kidney, and intestinal mucosa. It can be divided into 2 subtypes: type Ia, in which the glucose-6-phosphatase enzyme is defective, and type Ib, which is caused by a defect in the translocase that transports glucose-6-phosphate across the microsomal membrane. Patients with type I disease may develop hypoglycemia and lactic acidosis during the neonatal period but more commonly present at 3 to 4 months of age with hepatomegaly or hypoglycemia. These children often have doll-like faces with fat cheeks, relatively thin extremities, short stature, and a protuberant abdomen that is the result of massive hepatomegaly; the kidneys are enlarged, but the spleen and heart are of normal size.

The biochemical hallmarks of the disease are hypoglycemia, lactic acidosis, hyperuricemia, and hyperlipidemia. Hypoglycemia and lactic acidosis can develop after a short fast. Hyperuricemia is present in young children, but gout rarely develops before puberty. Despite hepatomegaly, liver enzymes are usually normal or near normal. Intermittent diarrhea may occur; the mechanism is not clear. In GSD type Ib, this could be attributed to inflammation of the bowel. Easy bruising, epistaxis, and menorrhagia are associated with a prolonged bleeding time as a result of impaired platelet aggregation/adhesion.

Hypertriglyceridemia may cause the plasma to appear "milky," and cholesterol and phospholipid concentrations are also elevated. The lipid abnormality resembles type IV hyperlipidemia and is characterized by increased levels of very-low-density lipoprotein (VLDL) and low-density lipoprotein (LDL); increased levels of apolipoproteins B, C, and E; and normal or reduced levels of apolipoproteins A and D. The hepatocytes are distended by glycogen and fat with large and prominent lipid vacuoles. There is no associated liver fibrosis.

All these findings apply to both type Ia and Ib GSDs, but in type Ib, recurrent bacterial infections due to neutropenia and impaired neutrophil function can occur. Oral and intestinal mucosa ulcerations are common, and inflammatory bowel disease may occur.

### METABOLIC DERANGEMENT

The block in GSD type I is at a critical step in glucose metabolism, with inability to make glucose via either glycogenolysis or gluconeogenesis. The defects in both type Ia and Ib lead to inadequate conversion of glucose-6-phosphate to glucose in the liver; thus, affected individuals are susceptible to fasting hypoglycemia and a complete dependence on exogenous glucose to maintain normal blood glucose levels.

### GENETICS

Type I GSD (Online Mendelian Inheritance in Man [OMIM] no. 232200) is an autosomal recessive disorder. The structural gene for glucose-6-phosphatase (type Ia) is located on chromosome 17q21. There are some common mutations repeatedly seen in different ethnic groups. A few examples are R83C (Caucasian 32%, Jewish 93–100%), R83H (Chinese 38%), 727 G>T splicing mutation (Japanese 88%, Chinese 36%), 35X, G188R, and Q347X (Caucasian 21%).

The structural gene for glucose-6-phosphate translocase (type Ib; *SLC37A4*) is located on chromosome 11q23. Two common mutations associated with GSD Ib in different ethnic groups are G339C (Caucasian 15%, German 29%) and c.1042delCT (Caucasian 31%, German 32%). Carrier detection and prenatal diagnosis using targeted genetic mutation analysis are possible if family mutations are known.

### DIAGNOSTIC TESTS

Type I GSD can be suspected on the basis of clinical presentation and the hallmark laboratory findings of hypoglycemia, lactic acidosis, hyperuricemia, and hyperlipidemia. Neutropenia is noted in GSD Ib patients, typically after the first couple years of life. Administration of glucagon or epinephrine causes little or no rise in blood glucose but increases lactate levels significantly. This test is dangerous during fasting and should not done to make a diagnosis of GSD I. Gene-based mutation analysis via single-gene sequencing or gene panels now provides a noninvasive way to diagnose the disorder for the majority of type Ia and Ib patients; a liver biopsy to demonstrate a deficiency is now rarely required.

### TREATMENT

Treatment is designed to maintain normal blood glucose levels and is achieved by continuous nasogastric infusion of glucose or oral administration of uncooked cornstarch. Nasogastric drip feeding in early infancy may consist of an elemental enteral formula or may contain only glucose or a glucose polymer to maintain normoglycemia during the night; frequent meals containing a high-carbohydrate content are given during the day.

Uncooked cornstarch acts as a slow-release form of glucose and can be given at a dose of 1.6 g/kg of body weight every 4 hours for children under the age of 2 years. As the child grows older, the cornstarch regimen can be changed to every 6 hours, and it can be given by mouth as a liquid (1:2 weight:volume) at a dose of 1.75 to 2.5 g/kg of body weight. Because fructose and galactose cannot be converted to free glucose, dietary intake should be restricted, and dietary supplements of multivitamins, calcium, and vitamin D are required to prevent nutritional deficiencies. Dietary therapy improves glucose control, lactic acidosis, hyperuricemia, hyperlipidemia, and renal function. In some individuals, this therapy fails to completely normalize blood uric acid and lipids levels despite good metabolic control; this is typically noted after puberty. In such situations, hyperuricemia can be controlled with allopurinol, a xanthine oxidase inhibitor. Hyperlipidemia can be managed with lipid-lowering drugs such as 3-hydroxy-3-methylglutaryl–coenzyme A (HMG-CoA) reductase inhibitors and fibrate. Microalbuminuria is an early indicator of renal dysfunction in GSD type I disease and can be treated with low doses of angiotensin-converting enzyme (ACE) inhibitors, such as captopril and lisinopril, or angiotensin receptor blockers. At low doses, these medications improve renal perfusion. Thiazide diuretics can help to manage hypercalciuria and nephrocalcinosis by enhancing renal reabsorption of filtered calcium and decreasing urinary calcium excretion. Individuals with GSD I can have hypocitraturia. In such situations, citrate supplements may be beneficial in preventing or ameliorating nephrocalcinosis and development of urinary calculi. Anemia can develop secondary to chronic kidney disease in GSD I disease. Erythropoietin therapy can be initiated if hemoglobin decreases to 10 g/dL to prevent the need for repeated blood transfusions. There are several other causes of anemia in GSD I including nutritional causes from dietary restrictions; poor intake of iron, vitamin $B_{12}$, and folic acid; chronic lactic acidosis; chronic renal involvement; platelet dysfunction leading to a bleeding diathesis; and irritable bowel disease. Large hepatic adenomas have shown an association with anemia in GSD I.

In patients with GSD type Ib, granulocyte and granulocyte-macrophage colony-stimulating factors (G-CSF) have been used to correct the neutropenia, to decrease the severity of bacterial infection, and to improve the chronic inflammatory bowel disease. Vitamin E supplements have also been reported to improve the neutropenia and reduce the frequency of infection. Derivatives of 5-aminosalicylic acid (5-ASA) may be a helpful adjunct for treating gastrointestinal complaints in GSD Ib patients provided renal function is monitored. For patients with GSD-associated inflammatory bowel disease who have not responded to G-CSF and 5-ASA therapy, adalimumab may be an effective therapeutic option.

Some groups advocate orthotopic liver transplantation as a potential cure of type I GSD, but the inherent short- and long-term complications leave this as a treatment of last resort, usually for patients with liver malignancy, multiple liver adenomas, metabolic derangements refractory to medical management, or liver failure. Large adenomas (> 2 cm) that increase rapidly in size or number may require partial hepatic resection. Smaller adenomas (< 2 cm) may be treated with percutaneous ethanol injection or transcatheter arterial embolization.

Prior to surgery, the patient's bleeding status should be evaluated, and good metabolic control should be established. Prolonged bleeding time can be corrected with a constant intravenous glucose infusion for 24 to 48 hours prior to surgery. Use of 1-deamino-8-D-arginine vasopressin (DDAVP) can be given during surgery to reduce bleeding complications, and normal glucose levels should be maintained throughout and after surgery.

Several newer approaches have emerged in the management of GSD I. Modified cornstarch preparations, which are more palatable and can maintain euglycemia for longer periods of time than uncooked cornstarch, are available. Extended-release waxy maize starch has demonstrated significant reduction in insulin release and reduced starch use in some patients. Medium-chain triglyceride (MCT) supplementation can lead to lowering of lactate, triglyceride, and uric acid levels in the blood of GSD I patients. MCT supplementation may lead to better metabolic control and growth in children. Gene therapy is being explored as a treatment modality. Animal models treated with adeno-associated virus (AAV) vectors containing a human G6Pase regulatory cassette/promoter have shown efficacy in regulating G6Pase expression appropriately.

### LONG-TERM COMPLICATIONS

Although type I GSD mainly affects the liver, multiple organ systems are also involved. Gout usually becomes symptomatic around puberty as a result of the long-term hyperuricemia. Puberty is often delayed; affected females can have ultrasound findings consistent with polycystic ovaries. However, the other features of polycystic ovary syndrome such as acne and hirsutism are not seen. Despite the ovarian findings, fertility appears to be normal, and there have been several reports of successful pregnancy in this population. Hypertriglyceridemia causes an increased risk of pancreatitis, but premature atherosclerosis has not been documented. Impaired platelet aggregation and increased antioxidative defense to prevent lipid peroxidation may function as a protective mechanism to help reduce the risk of atherosclerosis. Another reason could be due to lack of a cohort of patients who have reached the age to manifest these complications.

By the second or third decade, some patients with type I GSD develop hepatic adenomas that can hemorrhage and may become malignant. Other complications include iron refractory anemia, pulmonary hypertension, and osteoporosis.

Renal disease is a late complication, and almost all patients older than age 20 years have proteinuria. Many affected individuals have hypertension, kidney stones, nephrocalcinosis, and altered creatinine clearance. Glomerular hyperfiltration, increased renal plasma flow, and microalbuminuria can occur before the onset of gross proteinuria. In young patients, hyperfiltration and hyperperfusion may be the only signs of renal abnormalities. With advanced renal disease, focal segmental glomerulosclerosis and interstitial fibrosis are evident on biopsy. In some individuals, renal function deteriorates and progresses to failure, requiring dialysis or transplantation. Other abnormalities in renal function include amyloidosis, Fanconi-like syndrome, and a distal renal tubular acidification defect. During pregnancy, the increases in renal perfusion and maternal blood volume that normally occur can exacerbate renal problems. In addition, hypoglycemia may also become more difficult to control.

### PROGNOSIS

In the past, many patients with type I GSD died, and the prognosis was guarded for those who survived. The long-term complications occur mostly in adults whose disease was not adequately treated during childhood. Early diagnosis and effective treatment have improved the outcome; however, renal disease and formation of hepatic adenomas with potential risk for malignant transformation remain as serious complications.



## TYPE III GLYCOGEN STORAGE DISEASE (DEBRANCHER DEFICIENCY, LIMIT DEXTRINOSIS)

Type III GSD is caused by a deficiency of glycogen debranching enzyme. Debranching and phosphorylase enzyme are responsible for complete degradation of glycogen; when debranching enzyme is defective, glycogen breakdown is incomplete, and an abnormal glycogen that has short outer chains and resembles limit dextrin accumulates.

### CLINICAL PRESENTATION

Deficiency of glycogen-debranching enzyme causes hepatomegaly, hypoglycemia, short stature, variable skeletal myopathy, and cardiomyopathy. The disorder usually involves both liver and muscle and is termed *type IIIa GSD*. However, in about 15% of patients, the disease appears to involve only the liver and is classified as *type IIIb*.

During infancy and childhood, the disorder may be at a first glance similar to type I disease, because hepatomegaly, hypoglycemia, hyperlipidemia, and growth retardation are common features of both. However, a more marked elevation of liver enzymes (aspartate aminotransferase [AST] and alanine aminotransferase [ALT]); an increased creatine kinase in patients with a myopathy; and, especially, an absence of lactic acidosis when fasting are biochemical findings that can separate GSD III from GSD I. Splenomegaly may be present, but kidneys are not enlarged in type III. Remarkably, hepatomegaly and hepatic symptoms in type III patients improve with age and usually disappear after puberty. However, progressive liver fibrosis and liver cirrhosis with failure may occur, especially later in life. It is thus important to follow these patients closely as liver disease can progress later in life after an apparent quiescent period.

Hepatocellular carcinoma has also been reported, more typically in patients with progressive liver cirrhosis. The frequency of hepatic adenomas reported in individuals with GSD III is far less compared to GSD I.

In patients with muscle involvement (type IIIa), muscle weakness is usually less pronounced during childhood but can become severe during the third or fourth decade of life, as evidenced by slowly progressive weakness and muscle wasting in both proximal and distal muscle groups. Electromyographic (EMG) changes are consistent with a widespread myopathy, and nerve conduction may be abnormal. Cardiomyopathy with an asymmetric septal hypertrophy is often noted in individuals with GSD IIIa, but overt cardiac dysfunction is rare. There have been infrequent reports of cardiac conduction abnormalities with resultant death. Myocardial fibrosis requiring a cardiac transplant has also been reported in a few cases. In rare instances, hepatic symptoms may be so mild that the diagnosis is not made until adulthood, when neuromuscular disease becomes manifest. Polycystic ovaries appear to be a common finding in female patients; fertility, however, does not seem to be affected, and successful pregnancy outcome has been reported in many.

Hypoglycemia, hyperlipidemia, and elevated liver transaminases occur in childhood. In contrast to type I disease, fasting ketosis is prominent, and fasting blood lactate and uric acid concentrations are usually normal. The administration of glucagon 2 hours after a carbohydrate meal causes a normal rise of blood glucose levels, but after an overnight fast, glucagon may provoke no change in blood glucose, the latter timing of administration being potentially dangerous. Serum creatine kinase levels can sometimes be used to identify patients with muscle involvement, but normal levels do not rule out muscle enzyme deficiency.

The histology of the liver is characterized by a universal distention of hepatocytes by glycogen and by the presence of fibrous septa, which is often noted early in the disease. The fibrosis and the paucity of fat distinguish type III from type I GSD. The fibrosis can range from minimal periportal fibrosis to micronodular cirrhosis.

The type III glycogenoses (MIM no. 232400) are inherited as autosomal recessive traits. The disease has been reported in many different ethnic groups, and the frequency is relatively high in non-Ashkenazi Jews of North African descent, inhabitants of the Faroe Islands, and some Inuit populations. The gene for debranching enzyme (*AGL*) is located on chromosome 1p21. At least 130 different mutations that cause type III disease have been identified in the *AGL* gene. These mutations include commonly seen missense and nonsense mutations, some splicing, and small insertion/deletion mutations. Two mutations (17delAG and Q6X), both located in exon 3 at amino acid codons 5 and 6, are exclusively found in the subtype GSD IIIb. DNA-based targeted mutation analysis can detect carriers and make a prenatal diagnosis if disease-causing family mutations are already known.

## DIAGNOSTIC TESTS

In GSD type IIIa, deficient debranching enzyme activity can be demonstrated in liver, skeletal muscle, and heart. In contrast, type IIIb patients have debranching enzyme deficiency in the liver but not in muscle. In the past, definitive assignment of subtype required enzyme assays in both liver and muscle. DNA-based analyses now provide a noninvasive way of subtyping in the majority of patients.

## TREATMENT

Dietary management of type III disease is less demanding than in type I. If hypoglycemia is present, small, frequent feeds with complex carbohydrates with cornstarch supplements or nocturnal gastric drip feedings are usually effective. Addition of a high-protein diet during the daytime plus overnight protein enteral infusion is very effective in preventing hypoglycemia and in keeping the overall starch needs down. Overtreatment with cornstarch can result in excessive glycogen buildup, which is detrimental. Exogenous protein can be used as a substrate for gluconeogenesis, a pathway that is intact in type III GSD. It also has an added benefit in patients with a myopathy, as it prevents endogenous protein breakdown. The nutritional goal is to achieve a sustained normal level of blood glucose. Excess intake of cornstarch or excessively large meals should be avoided because they can lead to excess glycogen storage in the liver and muscle, insulin resistance, and in turn, excess weight gain. MCT-enriched diet is being explored as an alternative source of energy. Submaximal aerobic exercise is also important in individuals with GSD IIIa. Patients do not need to restrict dietary intake of fructose and galactose, as do those with type I disease; however, simple sugars should be avoided as they result in sudden increases in blood glucose levels. Cardiac symptoms are usually minimal and do not require pharmacologic intervention; β-adrenergic blockers may be indicated in cases of asymmetric septal hypertrophy and left ventricular outflow tract obstruction. Caution with the use of β-blockers is needed as it can result in hypoglycemia. Liver and cardiac transplantation has been performed in patients with end-stage cirrhosis or hepatic carcinoma and cardiac failure or fibrosis.

## PROGNOSIS

Liver symptoms improve with age and usually disappear after puberty. Cirrhosis of the liver may occur later in life, and this needs close monitoring. In type IIIa disease, muscle weakness and atrophy worsen during adulthood. Some patients have significant cardiac involvement, requiring routine monitoring.

# TYPE IV GLYCOGEN STORAGE DISEASE (BRANCHING ENZYME DEFICIENCY, AMYLOPECTINOSIS, POLYGLUCOSAN DISEASE, OR ANDERSEN DISEASE)

Deficiency of branching enzyme activity results in accumulation of an abnormal glycogen with poor solubility. The disease is referred to as *type IV GSD*, or *amylopectinosis*, because the abnormal glycogen has fewer branch points, more (1–4) linked glucose units, and longer outer chains, resulting in a structure resembling amylopectin or polyglucosan. Polyglucosan, which is positive on periodic acid-Schiff (PAS) and partially resistant to diastase digestion, accumulates in all tissues of patients but to different degrees.

## CLINICAL PRESENTATION AND LABORATORY FINDINGS

This disorder is clinically variable. The typical presentation of GSD IV, originally described by Andersen in 1956, is characterized by failure to thrive, hepatosplenomegaly, and progressive liver cirrhosis leading to death in early childhood. Some patients can develop hepatic adenomas and hepatocellular carcinoma. Patients usually present in the first 18 months of life with hepatosplenomegaly and failure to thrive. The cirrhosis progresses to cause portal hypertension, ascites, esophageal varices, and liver failure that leads to death by age 5 years. There can be extrahepatic manifestations in these cases, involving the central and peripheral nervous systems and musculoskeletal manifestation mainly involving cardiac and skeletal muscles. A milder, nonprogressive hepatic form is less frequent.

The neuromuscular presentation of GSD IV is heterogeneous, and 4 main variants can be distinguished on the basis of age at onset. The perinatal form presents as fetal akinesia deformation sequence (FADS) and is characterized by multiple congenital contractures (arthrogryposis multiplex congenita), hydrops fetalis, and perinatal death. The congenital form includes hypotonia, muscle wasting, neuronal involvement, inconsistent cardiomyopathy, and death in early infancy. The childhood form is dominated by myopathy or by cardiomyopathy. There are other systemic manifestations in this form of disease. The adult form, known as adult polyglucosan body disease (APBD), can present as an isolated myopathy or as a multisystem disorder with central and peripheral nervous system dysfunction characterized by neurogenic bladder, peripheral neuropathy, and leukodystrophy. Mild cognitive impairment has also been noted in patients with APBD; dementia is reported less consistently.

Tissue deposition of amylopectin-like materials can be demonstrated in liver, heart, muscle, skin, intestine, brain, spinal cord, and peripheral nerve. The histologic findings in the liver are characterized by both micronodular cirrhosis and faintly stained basophilic inclusions in the hepatocytes. The inclusions consist of coarsely clumped stored material that is positive on PAS and partially resistant to diastase digestion. Electron microscopy shows an accumulation of fibrillar aggregations typical of amylopectin, in addition to the conventional glycogen particles. Definitive diagnosis requires demonstration that branching enzyme activity is deficient in liver, muscle, cultured skin fibroblasts, or leukocytes, or requires genetic testing of the *GBE1* gene.

Definitive diagnosis of the adult disease requires an assay of branching enzyme in leukocytes or nerve biopsy or DNA testing.

## GENETICS

Type IV GSD (MIM no. 232500) is a rare autosomal recessive disorder. The glycogen-branching enzyme gene (*GBE1*) is located on chromosome 3p12. One of the common mutations seen in Ashkenazi Jews with APBD is homozygosity for the c.986A>C (p.Y329S) mutation in the *GBE1* gene. All forms of the disease are caused by mutations in the same branching enzyme gene; its characterization in individual patients may be useful in predicting the clinical course. It has been shown that GBE deficiency resulting in perinatal death or in fatal infantile hypotonia is invariably associated with severe mutations. Conversely, milder nonlethal neuromuscular cases harbored at least 1 mild missense mutation. There is a recent observation of a deep intronic mutation previously not identified in individuals who appeared heterozygous for a known mutation yet were affected. For the hepatic form, some mutations are associated with a good prognosis and lack of liver disease progression. Prenatal diagnosis is available by using cultured amniocytes or chorionic villi to measure the level of enzymatic activity. Identification of specific mutations is possible by DNA sequencing.

## TREATMENT

There is no specific treatment for type IV GSD. For progressive hepatic failure, liver transplantation has been performed. Caution should be taken in selecting patients for liver transplantation, as a nonprogressive hepatic form of the disease exists. Furthermore, in some patients, extrahepatic manifestations of the disease such as cardiomyopathy and central nervous system (CNS) involvement may occur after transplantation.

# TYPE VI GLYCOGEN STORAGE DISEASE (LIVER PHOSPHORYLASE DEFICIENCY OR HERS DISEASE)

The number of patients with enzymatically documented liver phosphorylase deficiency is small. This is likely due to an under- or misdiagnosis of cases. Regulation of the liver phosphorylase occurs through phosphorylation of the enzyme by phosphorylase kinase, which converts the inactive glycogen phosphorylase b form to the active a form.

## CLINICAL PRESENTATION AND LABORATORY FINDINGS

It was previously thought that patients with liver phosphorylase deficiency have a benign course. Clinical heterogeneity has recently been reported with the clinical symptoms observed in affected individuals. These have varied presentations, from hepatomegaly and subclinical hypoglycemia to severe hepatomegaly with recurrent severe ketotic hypoglycemia Affected individuals may present with ketotic hypoglycemia after overnight fasting or hypoglycemia after prolonged fasting. Patients with the mild phenotype typically present with hepatomegaly and growth retardation early in childhood; however, developmental delay is uncommon. The heart and skeletal muscles are not involved. The hepatomegaly and growth retardation improve with age and usually disappear around puberty, yet the long-term complications of this disease are not well studied.

Lactic acid and uric acid concentrations are normal. Liver transaminases tend to be usually elevated. Plasma ketone levels can be elevated during episodes of hypoglycemia. Hepatic glycogen phosphorylase can be measured in frozen liver biopsy tissue. Liver biopsy shows distended hepatocytes due to excessive granular glycogen accumulation. Electron microscopy shows granular glycogen accumulation with a normal structure. Noninvasive diagnostic methods, which may be preferred over invasive liver biopsy, include DNA analysis using Sanger sequencing and next-generation sequencing panels.

## GENETICS

GSD VI (MIM no. 232700) is an autosomal recessive disease. Diagnosis rests on enzyme analysis of the liver biopsy or DNA sequencing of the liver phosphorylase gene. The gene *PYGL* has been mapped to chromosome 14q21-22 and has 20 exons. Many mutations are known in this gene; they are mostly missense. A splice site mutation in intron 13 has been identified in the Mennonite population.

## TREATMENT AND PROGNOSIS

Treatment is symptomatic. Main goals of nutritional management are to prevent hypoglycemia and provide adequate nutrition. Small frequent feeds and avoiding fasting will help to prevent hypoglycemic episodes. A high-protein diet is recommended due to intact gluconeogenesis. Long-term follow-up of these patients is needed to better understand the natural history. Prognosis is very good from a hypoglycemia perspective.

# TYPE IX GLYCOGEN STORAGE DISEASE (LIVER PHOSPHORYLASE KINASE DEFICIENCY)

This disorder represents a heterogeneous group of glycogenoses. Phosphorylase, the rate-limiting enzyme of glycogenolysis, is activated by a cascade of enzymatic reactions involving adenylate cyclase, cyclic adenosine monophosphate–dependent protein kinase (protein kinase A), and phosphorylase kinase. Phosphorylase kinase has 4 subunits (α, β, γ, δ), each encoded by different genes on different chromosomes (X chromosome and autosomes) and differentially expressed in various tissues. The cascade of reactions to activate phosphorylase (from b to a form) is stimulated primarily by glucagon. A glycogenosis could result from an enzyme deficiency along this pathway; the most common is phosphorylase kinase deficiency.

The clinical heterogeneity of type IX GSD results from the complexity of the phosphorylase kinase holoenzyme, with its 4 subunits. Based on the gene/subunit involved, the tissues that are primarily affected, and the mode of inheritance, phosphorylase kinase deficiency can be divided into several subtypes: (1) an X-linked recessive liver disease of infancy or childhood, (2) an autosomal recessive liver and muscle disease, (3) a pure myopathy affecting both sexes but predominantly men, (4) an autosomal recessive severe liver disease associated with cirrhosis, and (5) a fatal infantile cardiomyopathy.

# X-LINKED LIVER PHOSPHORYLASE KINASE DEFICIENCY CAUSED BY *PHKA2* MUTATIONS

X-linked liver phosphorylase kinase deficiency (MIM no. 306000) is one of the most common liver glycogenoses. The X-linked gene (*PHKA2*) is located on Xp22.2-p22.1 and encodes the liver isoforms of the α subunit. Defects in *PHKA2* give rise to X-linked liver phosphorylase kinase deficiency, characterized by hypoglycemia, hepatomegaly, chronic liver disease, growth retardation and delayed motor development, hypercholesterolemia, hypertriglyceridemia, elevated liver enzymes, and hyperketosis after fasting. Lactate and uric acid levels are normal. The rise in blood glucose concentration following the administration of glucagon is normal. Although initially thought to be a benign condition, a wide range of clinical manifestations have been observed in affected individuals, with some having a very extreme phenotype. Being an X-linked condition, it is seen more in males, although some female carriers also exhibit a broad spectrum of clinical symptoms. Typically, children present between the ages of 1 and 5 years with the above symptoms, which usually ameliorate during puberty. Most adults achieve a normal final height and are practically asymptomatic despite a persistent phosphorylase kinase deficiency. The true natural history of this disorder is being uncovered, and it is now recognized that the condition is not benign as previously thought; in fact, some patients can have a more severe phenotype with long-term sequelae such as liver cirrhosis.

X-linked phosphorylase kinase deficiency is further subclassified into XLG1, with no detectable activity of phosphorylase kinase in liver and erythrocytes, and XLG2, with normal activity in erythrocytes and deficiency in liver.

Liver histology shows glycogen-distended hepatocytes. The accumulated glycogen has a frayed or burst appearance that is less compact than in type I or type III GSD. Fibrous septae and low-grade inflammatory changes may be present.

# AUTOSOMAL LIVER AND MUSCLE PHOSPHORYLASE KINASE DEFICIENCY CAUSED BY *PHKB* MUTATIONS

Autosomal liver and muscle phosphorylase kinase deficiency (MIM no. 261750) is inherited in an autosomal recessive manner. This form of phosphorylase kinase deficiency is caused by mutations in the β subunit of the gene *PHKB*, located on chromosome 16q12-13. As in the X-linked form of the disorder, hepatomegaly and growth retardation are the predominant symptoms in early childhood. Some patients also exhibit muscle hypotonia and have reduced activity of phosphorylase kinase in muscle.

# AUTOSOMAL LIVER PHOSPHORYLASE KINASE DEFICIENCY CAUSED BY *PHKG2* MUTATIONS

This form of the phosphorylase kinase deficiency is due to mutations in the testis/liver isoform of the γ subunit of the gene (γTL, *PHKG2*) located on chromosome 16p12.1. Patients with this autosomal recessive form of liver phosphorylase kinase deficiency (MIM no. 172471) typically have a more severe clinical course characterized by marked hepatomegaly, recurrent fasting hypoglycemia, impaired glucagon response, and fibrosis, which in the majority of reported cases progressed to frank liver cirrhosis and progressive hepatic failure. Hepatic adenomas have been seen in some individuals. Other reported manifestations include bile duct proliferation, cholestasis, esophageal varices, splenomegaly, renal tubular damage, muscle weakness, and delayed motor milestones. Patients tend to have very low liver phosphorylase kinase activity and elevated liver transaminases. The spectrum of severity has a wide variation and continues to evolve as more cases come to light.

## MUSCLE-SPECIFIC PHOSPHORYLASE KINASE DEFICIENCY CAUSED BY *PKHA1* MUTATIONS

Muscle-specific phosphorylase kinase deficiency (MIM no. 172470) could be inherited in an X-linked or autosomal recessive manner. The structural gene for the muscle-specific (*PHKA1*) α subunit is located at Xq12. Defects in *PHKA1* result in X-linked deficiency of phosphorylase kinase in muscle. Symptoms include exercise intolerance, cramps, myalgia, weakness, atrophy, and myoglobinuria. The activity of the enzyme is decreased in muscle but, when tested, has been normal in liver and blood cells. There is no hepatomegaly or cardiomegaly.

The gene for the muscle γ subunit (γM, *PHKG1*) has been localized to chromosome 7p12. No mutations in this gene have been reported so far.

## CARDIAC-SPECIFIC PHOSPHORYLASE KINASE DEFICIENCY

Several sporadic cases of cardiac-specific phosphorylase kinase deficiency (MIM no. 261740) have been reported. All affected individuals died during infancy from cardiac failure due to massive glycogen deposition in the myocardium. However, a recent study showed that the existence of cardiac-specific primary phosphorylase kinase deficiency is questionable, because no mutations in the 8 genes encoding the phosphorylase kinase subunits were found. Instead, a recurrent activating R531Q mutation in the γ-2 subunit of the AMP-activated protein kinase (*PRKAG2*) gene was the cause in most patients. This condition is discussed further in the section on PRKAG2 deficiency.

### GENETICS

The structural gene for the liver isoform (*PHKA2*) of the phosphorylase kinase α subunit is located on chromosome Xp22.2-p22.1, and mutations of this gene have been found in the disorder. Several missense, nonsense, and splice site mutations in this gene have been identified in familial and sporadic cases of liver phosphorylase kinase deficiency. A unique, large deletion of the *PHKA2* gene was attributed to unequal homologous recombination between Alu repeats in introns 19 and 26 in a Japanese boy.

Mutations in the *PHKB* gene located on chromosome 16q12-13 result in deficiency of phosphorylase kinase in both liver and muscle. There is a predominance of null mutations (nonsense, frameshift, and splice site mutations).

Mutations in the testis/liver isoform of the γ subunit of the gene (γTL, *PHKG2*) located on chromosome 16p12.1 are responsible for the severe liver form of GSD IX, which causes recurrent hypoglycemia and liver fibrosis.

There still is not a complete understanding of genotype and phenotype in GSD IX, and severe cases are noted in patients with all forms of the disease.

### DIAGNOSIS

The diagnosis of GSD type IX is complicated by the highly complex nature of phosphorylase kinase. Defects in 3 of the 4 different subunits that make up the holoenzyme, including both isoforms of the α subunit, result in disease with a spectrum of severity of clinical symptoms involving the liver, blood cells, bone, and cardiac muscle. Diagnosis of phosphorylase kinase deficiency requires the enzymatic defect be present in affected tissues; the diagnosis can be missed without studies of the liver, muscle, or heart in certain instances. Furthermore, phosphorylase kinase activity in blood cells has been shown, in some cases, not to accurately reflect its activity in liver. The enzyme assay is also unable to differentiate between deficiency of the α subunit, with consequent X-linked inheritance, and deficiency of the β or γ subunits, with an autosomal recessive pattern of inheritance. Thus, in many instances, mutation analysis is needed.

### TREATMENT

The treatment for liver phosphorylase kinase deficiency is based on symptoms. A complex carbohydrate diet and frequent meals are effective in preventing hypoglycemia. High dietary protein is recommended as it provides precursors for gluconeogenesis, provides direct fuel for muscles, and may reduce glycogen storage. Prognosis for the X-linked and certain autosomal forms is good; adult patients have normal stature and minimal hepatomegaly. Individuals with mutations in the γ subunit typically have a more severe clinical course with progressive liver disease; however, long-term follow-up is needed across all patients with phosphorylase kinase deficiency. Hepatic status may be monitored by liver enzyme levels and abdominal ultrasound/magnetic resonance imaging every 6 to 12 months, or as clinically indicated.

## TYPE 0 GLYCOGEN STORAGE DISEASE (LIVER GLYCOGEN SYNTHASE DEFICIENCY)

Glycogen synthase normally catalyzes the formation of α-1,4-linkages that elongate chains of glucose molecules to form glycogen. In GSD 0, only glycogen synthesis in the liver is impaired.

Strictly speaking, this is not a type of GSD, as the deficiency of the enzyme leads to decreased glycogen stores.

### CLINICAL PRESENTATION

Patients present in early infancy with early morning drowsiness and fatigue, and sometimes convulsions associated with hypoglycemia and hyperketonemia. There is no hepatomegaly, prominent muscle symptoms, or hyperlipidemia. Most children are cognitively and developmentally normal. Short stature and osteopenia are common features, but other long-term complications, common in other types of GSD, have thus far not been reported in GSD 0.

Because a substantial fraction of dietary carbohydrate is normally stored in the liver as glycogen, inability to synthesize hepatic glycogen causes postprandial hyperglycemia after ingesting a carbohydrate-containing meal. Prolonged hyperglycemia, lactic acidosis, and hyperalaninemia with normal insulin levels after glucose administration suggest a possible glycogen synthase deficiency. Definitive diagnosis requires a liver biopsy to measure the enzyme activity or to identify mutations in the liver glycogen synthase gene.

### GENETICS

GSD 0 (MIM no. 240600) is caused by mutations in the *GYS2* gene located on chromosome 12p12.2 and is inherited in an autosomal recessive manner. To date, approximately 15 different mutations have been documented, the majority of which are unique within particular families. The only common mutation is in exon 4 (R246X) and has been found in patients of Italian descent both in Europe and in North America. Cases of GSD 0 have been identified throughout Europe and North and South America.

### TREATMENT

Treatment is symptomatic and involves frequent meals rich in protein and a nighttime supplement of uncooked cornstarch to alleviate hypoglycemia. Prognosis seems good, as patients survive to adulthood with resolution of hypoglycemia except during pregnancy.

## TYPE XI GLYCOGEN STORAGE DISEASE (HEPATIC GLYCOGENOSIS WITH RENAL FANCONI SYNDROME, FANCONI-BICKEL SYNDROME)

Type XI GSD (MIM no. 227810) is a rare autosomal recessive disorder caused by defects in the facilitative glucose transporter 2 (*GLUT2*), which transports glucose in and out of hepatocytes, pancreatic beta cells, and the basolateral membranes of intestinal and renal epithelial cells. (*GLUT2* is described in Chapter 152.)

## MUSCLE GLYCOGENOSES: GLYCOGENOSIS WITH MUSCLE ENERGY IMPAIRMENT

## TYPE V GLYCOGEN STORAGE DISEASE (MUSCLE PHOSPHORYLASE DEFICIENCY, OR MCARDLE DISEASE)

Deficiency of muscle phosphorylase is the prototype muscle-energy disorder. Deficiency of this enzyme in muscle limits ATP generation by glycogenolysis and results in glycogen accumulation.

### CLINICAL PRESENTATION AND LABORATORY FINDINGS

Most patients are diagnosed in the second or third decade of life, but many report weakness and lack of endurance since childhood. Symptoms are characterized by exercise intolerance with episodic muscle cramping and pain; about 35% report permanent pain that impacts general activities and sleep. Two types of activity tend to cause symptoms: (1) brief exercise of great intensity, such as sprinting or carrying heavy loads, and (2) less intense but sustained activity, such as climbing stairs or walking uphill. Moderate exercise, such as walking on level ground, can be performed by most patients for long periods. Many patients experience a characteristic "second wind" phenomenon; if they rest briefly at the first sign of muscle pain, they can resume exercise with more ease. About half report burgundy-colored urine after exercise, which is the consequence of myoglobinuria secondary to the rhabdomyolysis. Intense myoglobinuria after vigorous exercise may cause renal failure. Later in adult life, persistent weakness and muscle wasting may develop with fatty replacement. Some cases have presented as late as the eighth decade of life. Rarely, patients present in infancy with progressive weakness, hypotonia, respiratory distress, and early death. This has to be considered in the differential diagnosis of the floppy baby syndrome, but this is a rare presentation. Thus, there can be a broad, heterogeneous spectrum of clinical presentation with the neonatal form, which is rapidly fatal at one extreme, with the benign classical form with myalgia, cramps, and dark-colored urine at the other. Despite disability, longevity does not appear to be affected, except in the neonatal form.

The level of serum creatine kinase is usually elevated at rest and increases more after exercise. Exercise also increases the levels of blood ammonia, inosine, hypoxanthine, and uric acid. The latter abnormalities are attributed to accelerated recycling of muscle purine nucleotides in the face of insufficient ATP production.

### GENETICS

Type V GSD (MIM no. 232600) is an autosomal recessive disorder that does not appear to have ethnic predilection. In most cases, heterozygous carriers are clinically unaffected; however, there are reports of heterozygotes manifesting with this disease. The gene for muscle phosphorylase (*PYGM*) is located on chromosome 11q13. The most common mutation noted in 90% of North American patients is a nonsense mutation that changes an arginine to a stop at codon 49 (R49X), and the most common mutation found in about 60% of Japanese patients is deletion of a single codon (F708). Other common Caucasian mutations (G204S in exon 5 and K542T in exon 14) make DNA-based diagnosis and carrier testing for McArdle disease possible for the 2 populations. Overall, an array of mutations in the *PYGM* gene have been identified with no phenotype/genotype correlation.

### DIAGNOSIS

Previously, McArdle disease was diagnosed through an ischemic forearm exercise test, with a lack of an increase in blood lactate levels and exaggerated blood ammonia elevations. However, this was associated with severe complications and often confused with false-positive test results. A nonischemic forearm exercise test was developed and determined to be indicative of muscle glycogenosis. This noninvasive test has high sensitivity, is easy to perform, and is cost-effective; however, the abnormal exercise response is not limited to type V disease and can occur with other defects in glycogenolysis or glycolysis, such as deficiencies of muscle phosphofructokinase or debranching enzyme (noted when the test is done after fasting). Definitive diagnosis is made by enzymatic assay in muscle tissue or by mutation analysis of the myophosphorylase gene.

### TREATMENT

In general, avoidance of strenuous exercise can prevent a major attack of rhabdomyolysis and myoglobinuria-induced renal damage. Aerobic training and oral administration of sucrose can augment exercise tolerance. A high-protein diet may increase exercise endurance in some patients. Vitamin $B_6$ supplementation can reduce exercise intolerance and muscle cramps and increase general well-being. Low-dose creatine supplementation at a dose of 10 to 20 g daily is thought to improve muscle function by permitting exercise to continue to a level of greater energy depletion. Creatine may also lessen the effects of extracellular potassium on membrane excitability that induces fatigue in both normal individuals and those with McArdle disease.

## TYPE VII GLYCOGEN STORAGE DISEASE (MUSCLE PHOSPHOFRUCTOKINASE DEFICIENCY, OR TARUI DISEASE)

Type VII disease is caused by a deficiency of muscle phosphofructokinase, which catalyzes the conversion of fructose-6-phosphate to fructose-1,6-diphosphate and is a key regulatory enzyme of glycolysis.

Phosphofructokinase is composed of 3 isozyme subunits (M, muscle; L, liver; and P, platelet), which are encoded by different genes and are differentially expressed in tissues. Skeletal muscle contains only M-subunit isozymes, and red blood cells contain a hybrid of L and M forms. Type VII disease is due to defective M isoenzyme, which causes complete enzyme deficiency in muscle and partial deficiency in red blood cells.

### CLINICAL PRESENTATION AND LABORATORY FINDINGS

The features are similar to those in type V disease, namely fatigue and pain with exercise. Vigorous exercise causes severe muscle cramps and myoglobinuria. Several features of type VII disease are distinctive: (1) Exercise intolerance is usually evident in childhood, is more severe than in type V disease, and may be associated with nausea and vomiting; (2) a compensated hemolysis occurs as evidenced by an increased level of serum bilirubin and reticulocyte count; (3) hyperuricemia is common and becomes more marked after exercise; (4) an abnormal glycogen-resembling amylopectin is present in muscle fibers; it is PAS positive and resistant to diastase digestion; (5) there is no spontaneous second-wind phenomenon because of the inability to metabolize blood glucose; and (6) exercise intolerance is particularly acute following meals rich in carbohydrate because the ingested glucose inhibits lipolysis, thereby depriving muscle of fatty acid and ketone substrates. In contrast, patients with type V disease can metabolize glucose derived from either liver glycogenolysis or exogenous glucose.

Rare type VII variants have also been reported: (1) presentation in infancy with hypotonia and limb weakness and a rapidly progressive myopathy leading to early death (by age 4); (2) presentation in adulthood characterized by a slowly progressive, fixed muscle weakness rather than by cramps and myoglobinuria; (3) manifestation in infancy as congenital myopathy and arthrogryposis with fatal outcome; (4) presentation in infancy with hypotonia, mild developmental delay, and seizures; and (5) presentation with acute renal failure.

Type VII GSD (MIM no. 232800) is inherited in an autosomal recessive manner; the gene for the M isoenzyme is located on chromosome 12q13.3. It exhibits a strong male predominance, and most reported patients are either Japanese or Ashkenazi Jews. Multiple mutations, including splicing defects, frameshifts, and missense mutations, have been identified. There is no obvious genotype-phenotype correlation. Ashkenazi Jewish patients share 2 common mutations in the gene; the more frequent is an exon 5 splicing defect, which accounts for about 68% of mutant alleles in this population.

### DIAGNOSIS

Molecular genetic testing including mutation analysis and gene sequencing can identify common pathogenic variants. The diagnosis can also be based on biochemical or histochemical demonstration of the enzymatic defect in the muscle. The M-isoenzyme defect must be demonstrated in muscle, red blood cells, or cultured skin fibroblasts.

### TREATMENT

There is no specific treatment for this condition. Avoiding strenuous exercise is advisable to prevent acute attacks of muscle cramps and myoglobinuria. Ingestion of simple carbohydrates before strenuous exercise has shown some benefit in improving exercise tolerance. Clinical benefit of a ketogenic diet has been reported in an infant with infantile phosphofructokinase deficiency with arthrogryposis. In general, avoiding drugs such as statins and taking malignant hyperthermia precautions for patients undergoing anesthesia are appropriate for the muscle GSDs.



## TYPE X GLYCOGEN STORAGE DISEASE (PHOSPHOGLYCERATE MUTASE DEFICIENCY)

Phosphoglycerate mutase (PGAM) deficiency (MIM no. 261670) is a rare and usually benign muscle glycogenosis. The *PGAM2* gene encodes the PGAM enzyme involved in terminal glycolysis. Mutations in this gene lead to reduced activity of PGAM, which is involved in glycolytic pathways in skeletal muscles. Patients are usually asymptomatic except for bouts of exercise-induced cramps and myoglobinuria triggered by strenuous exercise. Elevated serum creatine kinase levels are seen, and muscle biopsies may show tubular aggregates in type 2 muscle fibers.

## OTHER MUSCLE GLYCOGENOSES WITH MUSCLE-ENERGY IMPAIRMENT

Five additional enzyme defects produce muscle glycogenoses, namely deficiencies in phosphoglycerate kinase, lactate dehydrogenase, fructose 1,6-bisphosphate aldolase A, and pyruvate kinase. All 5 enzymes affect terminal glycolysis, and deficiency causes muscle-energy impairment similar to that in type V and VII disease. The failure of blood lactate to increase in response to exercise can be used to separate muscle glycogenoses from disorders of lipid metabolism, such as carnitine palmitoyl transferase II deficiency and very-long-chain acyl-coenzyme A dehydrogenase deficiency, which also cause muscle cramps and myoglobinuria. Muscle glycogen levels may be normal in the disorders affecting terminal glycolysis, and definitive diagnosis is made by assaying the enzymatic activity in muscle. Molecular testing, including DNA sequence analysis, is available for most of these disorders.

## GLYCOGENOSES WITH PROGRESSIVE SKELETAL OR CARDIAC MYOPATHY

## GLYCOGEN STORAGE DISEASE TYPE II (ACID α-1,4-GLUCOSIDASE DEFICIENCY, ACID MALTASE DEFICIENCY, OR POMPE DISEASE)

GSD type II, or Pompe disease, is caused by a deficiency of lysosomal acid α-1,4-glucosidase (GAA), the enzyme responsible for degrading glycogen in lysosomal vacuoles. Deficiency of GAA results in lysosomal glycogen accumulation in multiple tissues and cell types, with cardiac, skeletal, and smooth muscle cells being the most seriously affected. This disease is thus characterized by accumulation of glycogen in lysosomes as opposed to its accumulation in cytoplasm in the other glycogenoses. With disease progression, cytoplasmic glycogen is often noted; this reflects rupture or leakage from the lysosomes.

### CLINICAL PRESENTATION AND LABORATORY FINDINGS

The disorder is broadly categorized into infantile and late-onset forms. The disorder encompasses a range of phenotypes, including extent of myopathy, cardiomyopathy, respiratory muscle involvement, and clinical severity. At the most severe end of the disease spectrum is the classic infantile form with massive cardiomegaly, hypotonia, and death prior to 1 year of age. Infants may appear normal at birth but soon develop generalized muscle weakness with feeding difficulties, macroglossia, hepatomegaly, and congestive heart failure due to a rapidly progressive hypertrophic cardiomyopathy. Electrocardiographic findings include high-voltage QRS complexes and a shortened PR interval. Death usually occurs from cardiorespiratory failure.

Late-onset Pompe disease (juvenile or late childhood form and adult form) is characterized by skeletal and respiratory muscle manifestations and a more slowly progressive course but with significant morbidity. In the juvenile form, some patients present with delayed motor milestones (if age of onset is early enough) and difficulty in walking, proximal muscle weakness, and respiratory muscle involvement; swallowing difficulties; variable extent of cardiac involvement; and death before the end of the second decade. Adults present with a slowly progressive myopathy, and in some cases, cardiac involvement is noted, with onset between the second and seventh decades. The clinical picture is dominated by slowly progressive proximal muscle weakness with truncal involvement and greater involvement of the lower than the upper limbs. Pelvic girdle, paraspinal muscle, and diaphragm are the most seriously affected. With disease progression, patients become confined to a wheelchair and require artificial ventilation. Respiratory symptoms are manifested by somnolence, morning headache, orthopnea, and exertional dyspnea, which eventually lead to sleep-disordered breathing and respiratory failure. Respiratory failure is the cause of significant morbidity and mortality in this form of the disease. In rare instances, respiratory insufficiency with minimal to no muscle weakness is the presenting symptom. Multisystem involvement is common in Pompe disease. Urinary tract and bowel involvement may present with urinary incontinence, weak urine stream, dribbling, or bowel incontinence. Gastrointestinal system involvement is not uncommon and may manifest as swallowing difficulty, chronic diarrhea, postprandial bloating, abdominal pain, and irritable bowel syndrome. Small-fiber neuropathy, which presents with painful paresthesia or pin-and-needles sensations, is also seen in adult cases. The age of death in late-onset Pompe disease varies from early childhood to late adulthood, depending on the rate of disease progression and the extent of respiratory muscle involvement.

Laboratory findings include elevated levels of serum creatine kinase, aspartate transaminase, and lactate dehydrogenase. Urine glucose tetrasaccharide, a breakdown product of glycogen, is a good biomarker for disease severity and also for monitoring progression and treatment response. Vacuolated lymphocytes may be observed on a blood smear. Chest x-ray and electrocardiography are useful in infantile cases; massive cardiomegaly is noted on chest x-ray and often provides the first clue. Electrocardiographic findings include a high-voltage QRS complex and a shortened PR interval. Echocardiography may reveal thickening of both ventricles or of the intraventricular septum or may reveal left ventricular outflow tract obstruction. Muscle biopsy shows the presence of vacuoles that stain positively for glycogen, and muscle acid phosphatase is increased, presumably from a compensatory increase of lysosomal enzymes. Electron microscopy reveals the membrane-bound glycogen accumulation. EMG reveals myopathic features with irritability of muscle fibers and pseudomyotonic discharges. Serum creatine kinase concentration is not always elevated in adults, and, depending on the muscle biopsied or tested, muscle histology or EMG may not be abnormal. It is prudent to examine affected muscle for enzymology if the clinical diagnosis is suspected.

### GENETICS

Pompe disease (MIM no. 232400) is an autosomal recessive pan-ethnic disorder. The infantile-onset form has an apparent higher incidence among African Americans and Chinese, whereas the late-onset adult form has a higher incidence in the Netherlands. The gene for acid-α-glucosidase is on chromosome 17q25. More than 500 mutations and numerous variants in the *GAA* gene have been identified. The mutations are spread across the gene. Among the recurrent mutations in the infantile-onset cases is a single base pair deletion, Δ525T, which is seen in 9% of US cases. This same mutation accounts for 34% of Dutch cases. The exon 18 deletion mutation is seen in infantile-onset cases and accounts for about 25% of Dutch and Canadian cases but only about 5% of US cases. The leaky IVS1(-13T>G) splice site mutation accounts for about 36% to 90% of late-onset cases in Caucasian populations. The R854X mutation is found in many African American and African cases; D645E is seen in many Chinese infantile cases; c.2238G>C (p.W746C) is the most common in late-onset cases in mainland China.

### DIAGNOSIS

The diagnosis can be established by demonstrating absence or reduced levels of acid-α-glucosidase activity in muscle, cultured skin fibroblasts, and blood cell–based assays such as leukocytes, mononuclear cells, or dried blood spot, using maltose, glycogen, or 4-methylumbelliferyl-alpha-d-glucopyranoside (4MUG) as a substrate. Deficiency is usually more severe in the infantile form than in late-onset Pompe disease. Prenatal diagnosis using amniocytes or chorionic villi is available. Carrier detection and prenatal diagnosis, using DNA-based targeted mutation analysis, are also possible if disease-causing family mutations are already known. Sanger gene sequencing, next-generation sequencing, and whole-exome sequencing strategies allow identification of causative mutations.

### TREATMENT

Until 2006, there was no effective treatment for Pompe disease, and treatment options were limited to supportive or palliative care. Enzyme replacement therapy (ERT) with alglucosidase alfa, which provides recombinant human acid-α-glucosidase, is currently available as the first effective treatment for this once devastating and lethal disease. Data from various clinical trials have shown that recombinant acid-α-glucosidase improves cardiac function and skeletal muscle function in individuals with Pompe disease across the disease spectrum. Early diagnosis and initiation of ERT as soon as possible have been shown to lead to better outcomes, especially in infantile cases. Studies from Taiwan, where newborn screening has been available for a number of years now, have shown that newborns with infantile Pompe disease achieve better clinical outcomes and might have better immune tolerance when started on ERT very early in their life. A pilot newborn screening program implemented in Missouri showed that newborns could be diagnosed as early as the second day of life, potentially leading to early treatment initiation and improved outcomes. This study estimated the prevalence of Pompe disease to be 1 in 5436. Patients who are negative for cross-reacting immunologic material (CRIM) develop a high titer antibody against the infused enzyme and respond to the ERT less favorably. Treatment using immunosuppressive agents such as methotrexate, rituximab, and intravenous immunoglobulin have demonstrated efficacy in preventing the development of an immune response to ERT. For patients with the late-onset form of the disease, a high-protein diet may be beneficial. Respiratory muscle strength training, when given with ERT, has demonstrated improvements in respiratory parameters. Submaximal exercise regimens have been beneficial in improving muscle strength, pain, and fatigue. Ventilatory support, when indicated, should be used. It improves the patient's quality of life and is particularly beneficial during a period of respiratory decompensation. A multidisciplinary team approach is needed for successful treatment of Pompe disease.

Newer therapies are being explored to improve the safety and efficacy of ERT. Studies are under way to enhance response to ERT through focusing on targeting and uptake of GAA via the addition of mannose 6-phosphate residues to the engineered alpha-glucosidase and simultaneous administration of pharmacologic chaperones to enhance delivery of ERT to the lysosomes. Gene therapy is another approach to treating patients with Pompe disease.

## MUSCLE GLYCOGEN SYNTHASE DEFICIENCY

GSD due to muscle glycogen synthase (glycogen synthase I [GYS1]) deficiency (MIM no. 138570) should not be confused with liver glycogen synthase deficiency (GSD 0), discussed earlier. Muscle glycogen synthase deficiency is extremely rare, with only a handful of cases reported in the scientific literature. The first characterization of the disease was reported in 3 children of consanguineous parents of Syrian origin. The oldest brother died from sudden cardiac arrest at age 10.5 years; the younger brother at age 11 showed muscle fatigue, hypertrophic cardiomyopathy, an abnormal heart rate, and hypotension while exercising; and a 2-year-old sister had mildly impaired cardiac function at rest. Muscle biopsies showed lack of glycogen, predominantly oxidative fibers, and mitochondrial proliferation. Glucose tolerance was normal. Molecular study revealed a homozygous stop mutation R462X in *GYS1* in 3 siblings and homozygous 2-base deletion in exon 2 of *GYS1* as present in another case of sudden cardiac death in an 8-year-old child.

## DANON DISEASE

Deficiency of lysosomal-associated membrane protein 2 (LAMP2; also called Danon disease; MIM no. 300257) is an X-linked semi-dominant disorder that results in accumulation of glycogen in the heart and skeletal muscle, leading to cardiomyopathy, skeletal myopathy, and intellectual disability. Clinically, these patients present primarily with hypertrophic cardiomyopathy but can be distinguished from the usual causes of hypertrophic cardiomyopathy due to defects in sarcomere protein genes by their electrophysiologic abnormalities, particularly ventricular preexcitation and conduction defects. The onset of the disorder varies from infancy to young adulthood, with females having similar, albeit less frequent and later onset, complications. Underrecognized clinical manifestations in Danon disease include peripheral pigmentary retinopathy, lens changes, and an abnormal electroretinogram. The prognosis for LAMP2 deficiency is poor, with progressive end-stage heart failure early in adulthood. Treatment is mainly symptomatic and involves management of heart failure, correction of conduction abnormalities, and physical therapy, among others. Cardiac transplantation has been tried successfully in some cases.

## AMP-ACTIVATED PROTEIN KINASE GAMMA 2 DEFICIENCY (PRKAG2 DEFICIENCY)

PRKAG2 deficiency (MIM no. 602743) is caused by mutations in the *PRKAG2* gene mapped to chromosome 7q36. The *PRKAG2* gene encodes the γ2 subunit of AMP-activated protein kinase (AMPK), which regulates many cellular ATP metabolic pathways. Affected individuals present with cardiac abnormalities including hypertrophic cardiomyopathy and conduction system abnormalities, particularly Wolff-Parkinson-White syndrome. Cardiac manifestations are variable and include supraventricular tachycardia, sinus bradycardia, left ventricular dysfunction, and even sudden cardiac death in some cases. In addition to cardiac involvement, there is a broad spectrum of clinical problems including myalgia, myopathy, and seizures. Cardiomyopathy due to *PRKAG2* mutations is compatible with long-term survival except for a congenital form that presents in early infancy with a rapidly fatal course. PRKAG2 syndrome should be considered in the differential diagnosis in infants presenting with severe hypertrophic cardiomyopathy. In rare instances, PRKAG2 cases maybe misdiagnosed as infantile Pompe disease due to clinical similarities.

## LATE-ONSET POLYGLUCOSAN BODY MYOPATHY DUE TO GYG1 DEFICIENCY

Mutations in the *GYG1* gene affecting glycogenin-1-dependent glycogen biosynthesis cause an autosomal recessive slowly progressive skeletal myopathy, with a reduced or complete absence of glyogenin-1. The most common clinical symptom is adult-onset proximal muscle weakness prominently affecting hip and shoulder girdles. Cardiac symptoms are uncommon. In contrast to GSD IV APBD, nervous system involvement has not been reported, although both disorders lead to polyglucosan deposition. Muscle biopsies show PAS-positive diastase-resistant storage material in around 30% to 40% of muscle fibers. Electron microscopy reveals the typical polyglucosan structure. Management includes symptomatic support for gait abnormalities, bladder dysfunction, and periodic surveillance to monitor for new neurologic deficits. Effects on life expectancy are unknown; however, supportive care may play an important role in determining longevity.

## POLYGLUCOSAN BODY MYOPATHY DUE TO RBCK1 DEFICIENCY

Mutations in the E3 ubiquitin ligase *RBCK1* cause a childhood or juvenile onset of myopathy, with a progressive cardiomyopathy that may require heart transplantation in a subset of patients. Patients have extensive polyglucosan accumulation in skeletal muscle and in the heart in cases of cardiomyopathy. Different mutations in the *RBCK1* gene may cause either an immune disorder or myopathy/cardiomyopathy. This clinical diversity may be explained by the nature and location of the *RBCK1* mutations.

### SUGGESTED READINGS


Akman HO, Aykit Y, Amuk OC, et al. Late-onset polyglucosan body myopathy in five patients with a homozygous mutation in GYG1. *Neuromuscul Disord.* 2016;26(1):16-20.

D'Souza RS, Levandowski C, Slavov D, et al. Danon disease: clinical features, evaluation, and management. *Circ Heart Fail.* 2014;7(5):843-849.

Hogrel JY, van den Bogaart F, Ledoux I, et al. Diagnostic power of the non-ischaemic forearm exercise test in detecting glycogenosis type V. *Eur J Neurol.* 2015;22(6):933-940.

Hopkins PV, Campbell C, Klug T, Rogers S, Raburn-Miller J, Kiesling J. Lysosomal storage disorder screening implementation: findings from the first six months of full population pilot testing in Missouri. *J Pediatr.* 2015;166(1):172-177.

Kishnani PS, Austin SL, Abdenur JE, et al. Diagnosis and management of glycogen storage disease type I: a practice guideline of the American College of Medical Genetics and Genomics. *Genet Med.* 2010;12(7):446-463.

Kishnani PS, Beckemeyer AA, Mendelsohn NJ. The new era of Pompe disease: advances in the detection, understanding of the phenotypic spectrum, pathophysiology, and management. *Am J Med Genet C Semin Med Genet.* 2012;160c(1):1-7.

Kishnani PS, Austin SL, Arn P, et al. Glycogen storage disease type III diagnosis and management guidelines. *Genet Med.* 2010;12(7):446-463.

Kollberg G, Tulinius M, Gilljam T, et al. Cardiomyopathy and exercise intolerance in muscle glycogen storage disease. *N Engl J Med.* 2007;357(15):1507-1514.

Pagon RA, Adam MP, Ardinger HH, et al. Glycogen storage disease type V. GeneReviews(R). Seattle, WA: University of Washington, Seattle; 2014.

Porto AG, Brun F, Severini GM, et al. Clinical spectrum of PRKAG2 syndrome. *Circ Arrhythm Electrophysiol.* 2016;9(1):e003121.

Quinlivan R, Martinuzzi A, Schoser B. Pharmacological and nutritional treatment for McArdle disease (glycogen storage disease type V). *Cochrane Database Syst Rev.* 2014;11:Cd003458.

Yang CF, Yang CC, Liao HC, et al. Very early treatment for infantile-onset Pompe disease contributes to better outcomes. *J Pediatr.* 2016;169:174-80.e1.


# 150 Disorders of Galactose and Fructose Metabolism and Gluconeogenesis

Priya S. Kishnani and Yuan-Tsong Chen

## DISORDERS OF GALACTOSE METABOLISM

Galactosemia denotes the elevated level of galactose in the blood and, among other reasons, is found in 3 distinct inborn errors of galactose metabolism involving 1 of the following enzymes that comprise the Leloir pathway: galactose-1-phosphate uridyl transferase (GALT), galactokinase (GALK), and uridine diphosphate galactose-4-epimerase (GALE). The term *galactosemia,* although adequate for the deficiencies of any of these three disorders, generally designates the transferase deficiency that is by far the most prevalent form, and when completely deficient the disorder is called *classical galactosemia.*

### GALACTOSE-1-PHOSPHATE URIDYL TRANSFERASE (GALT) DEFICIENCY GALACTOSEMIA

Galactose is a disaccharide made up of glucose and galactose. Classical galactosemia due to a complete GALT deficiency is a serious disease, with an incidence of approximately 1 in 30,000 to 60,000. Symptoms typically appear by the second half of the first week of life, when the newborn receives high amounts of lactose (up to 40% of calories in breast milk and certain formulas). Without the transferase activity, the infant is unable to metabolize galactose-1-phosphate (see Chapter 149, Fig. 149-1), the accumulation of which is associated with injury to parenchymal cells of the kidney, liver, and brain.

### CLINICAL PRESENTATION

The diagnosis of GALT deficiency should be considered in newborns, older infants, or children with any of the following clinical manifestations: jaundice, hepatomegaly, vomiting, hypoglycemia, convulsions, lethargy, irritability, feeding difficulties, poor weight gain, amino aciduria, nuclear cataracts, vitreous hemorrhage, hepatic cirrhosis, ascites, splenomegaly, or intellectual disability. Patients with galactosemia are at an increased risk of *Escherichia coli* neonatal sepsis. Importantly, the onset of sepsis often precedes the diagnosis of galactosemia. Pseudotumor cerebri may occur and may cause a bulging fontanel.

When the diagnosis is not made at birth, damage to the liver (cirrhosis) and brain (intellectual disability) becomes increasingly severe and may be irreversible. Symptoms are milder and improve when milk is temporarily withdrawn and replaced by lactose-free nutrition.

Partial transferase deficiency may be due to the Duarte variant and is generally asymptomatic. It is more frequent than classical galactosemia and is often diagnosed by newborn screening because of moderately elevated blood galactose or low transferase activity.

### GENETICS

GALT deficiency galactosemia (Online Mendelian Inheritance in Man [MIM] 230400) is inherited as an autosomal recessive disorder and leads to accumulation of galactose-1-phosphate. The gene for GALT is located on chromosome 9p13. There are several enzymatic variants of galactosemia depending on the residual enzyme activity. Duarte variant is the most common abnormal allele and has a carrier frequency of 12% in the general population, with the allele being designated D. Individuals who are homozygous for the Duarte variant have diminished red cell enzyme activity (50% of normal) but no clinical manifestations. The most common complete loss of function variant leading to classical galactosemia is Q188R, and the allele is designated G. Individuals with Duarte galactosemia (D/G) who are compound heterozygous for the classical allele and the Duarte variant have 25% of the enzyme activity, and the red blood cell (RBC) galactose-1-phosphate level is often elevated. These children are generally asymptomatic, but many physicians restrict lactose intake when the erythrocyte galactose-1-phosphate levels are elevated. Evidence for the need for dietary intervention in D/G is lacking, with more recent reports indicating no difference in outcome whether or not affected children are treated. Some African American patients have milder symptoms despite absence of measurable transferase activity in erythrocytes. These patients retain 10% of wild-type enzyme activity in liver and intestinal mucosa, while most Caucasian patients have no detectable activity in any of these tissues when harboring the Q188R allele in the homozygous state. In African Americans, 48% of disease alleles are represented by the S135L mutation, a mutation that may be responsible for the milder disease. In the white population, 70% of complete loss of function alleles are represented by the Q188R missense mutation. Hence, a variety of genotypes can be seen, and treatment should be directed at more severe loss of function variants. Carrier testing and prenatal diagnosis can be carried out by direct enzyme analysis of amniocytes or chorionic villi, and testing can be DNA based.

## DIAGNOSIS

A preliminary diagnosis of galactosemia is suggested by demonstrating a reducing substance in urine specimens collected while the patient is receiving human or cow's milk or another formulas containing lactose. The reducing substance found in urine by Clinitest can be identified by chromatography or by an enzymatic test specific for quantifying galactose. Galactosuria is present provided the last milk feed has not occurred more than a few hours prior and the child is not vomiting excessively. Caution is needed in choosing the kind of test used for reducing substances. Clinistix urine test results are negative, because the test materials rely on the action of glucose oxidase, which is specific for glucose and does not react with galactose. However, owing to a proximal renal tubular syndrome, the acutely ill baby may also excrete glucose together with amino acids. In the past, diagnostic challenge tests dependent on administering galactose orally or intravenously were used. These should be avoided because galactose is injurious to persons with galactosemia. Light and electron microscopy of hepatic tissue reveals fatty infiltration, the formation of pseudoacini, and eventual macronodular cirrhosis. These changes are consistent with a metabolic disease but do not indicate the precise defect.

Definitive diagnosis can be made by direct enzyme assay using erythrocytes or other tissues that also exhibit increased concentrations of galactose-1-phosphate (Paigen assay). The gold standard for diagnosing classical galactosemia is measuring GALT activity in erythrocytes (isolated from either heparin or ethylenediaminetetraacetic acid whole blood; Beutler assay). It is important to confirm that the patient did not receive a blood transfusion prior to collecting the blood sample, as a diagnosis of galactosemia could be missed.

## TREATMENT

Because of widespread newborn screening for galactosemia, patients are being identified early and treated early (see Chapter 129). The most important step in the initial management of patients with classical galactosemia is immediately removing all galactose from the diet as soon as the condition is suspected. Additional therapies may be indicated in the case of complications such as sepsis, liver failure with clotting abnormalities, or hyperbilirubinemia. For long-term management, individuals need to be on a soy-based formula and a formula based on casein hydrolysates and dextrin maltose, as these are carbohydrate sources with very little galactose. However, some galactose will inevitably be introduced into the diet, as many foods, such as fruits and vegetables, bread, and legumes, contain trace amounts of galactose. There are controversies concerning the daily allowance of galactose during long-term treatment with a very strict diet; one extreme restricts galactose-containing fruits and vegetables, and the other extreme advises only a lactose-free diet. Calcium and vitamin D supplements are needed when receiving the restricted diet to reduce the risk of osteopenia and osteoporosis.

Elimination of galactose from the diet reverses growth failure and renal and hepatic dysfunction. Cataracts regress, and most patients have no impairment of eyesight. Early diagnosis and treatment have improved the prognosis of galactosemia; on long-term follow-up, however, patients still manifest ovarian failure with primary or secondary amenorrhea, developmental delay, and learning disabilities, which increase in severity with age. In addition, most will manifest speech disorders, such as speech apraxia, while a smaller number demonstrate poor growth and impaired motor function and balance (with or without overt ataxia). The relative control of galactose-1-phosphate levels does not always correlate with long-term outcome, leading to the belief that other factors such as UDP-galactose deficiency (a donor for galactolipids and proteins) may be responsible. Other factors could include ongoing damage due to endogenous galactose synthesis, with some damage likely occurring in utero. However, it appears that a substantial part of the long-term complications originates from continuous toxicity during life.

## GALACTOKINASE (GALK) DEFICIENCY

GALK deficiency is generally considered to be rare when compared to classical galactosemia.

## CLINICAL PRESENTATION

In contrast to the multiple systems that are affected in GALT deficiency galactosemia, cataract and, rarely, pseudotumor cerebri caused by galactitol accumulation are the only consistently reported abnormalities in this disorder, and the affected infant is otherwise asymptomatic. A high incidence of this disorder is found among the Romani population coming from some regions of East Europe. The high incidence is attributable to a founder effect, as demonstrated by the segregation of a single missense mutation (P28T) that is present in about 5% of the Romani population.

## GENETICS

Two genes have been reported to encode GALK: *GK1* on chromosome 17q24 and *GK2* on chromosome 15. Mutations causing GALK deficiency (MIM no. 230200) have been identified only in *GK1*. A majority of these mutations are missense variants that cause amino acid changes of conserved residues that have an active role in the enzyme's stability and activity. It is now known that human GK2 is a highly efficient GalNAc kinase with GALK activity when this sugar is present at high concentrations. Thus, GALK deficiency is not genetically heterogeneous.

## DIAGNOSIS

Affected patients have an increased concentration of blood galactose levels, provided they have been fed a lactose-containing formula. A final diagnosis is made by demonstrating normal transferase activity and an absence of GALK activity in erythrocytes. Since many newborn screening programs directly measure GALT activity and do not measure galactose levels directly, the diagnosis of GALK deficiency often relies on clinical suspicion.

## TREATMENT

Treatment is dietary restriction of galactose intake. As patients with GALK deficiency have minimal complications aside from cataracts, inhibition of GALK activity by a selective inhibitor may be a promising approach for controlling damage in classical galactosemia in GALT-deficient patients.

## URIDINE DIPHOSPHATE (UDP) GALACTOSE-4-EPIMERASE (GALE) DEFICIENCY

In this deficiency, the abnormally accumulated metabolites are very much like those seen in GALT deficiency; however, there is also an increase in cellular UDP-galactose.

## CLINICAL PRESENTATION

In general, 2 forms of epimerase deficiency have previously been recognized. A benign, peripheral form may be discovered incidentally through a neonatal screening program. Affected persons in this case are healthy and without problems; the enzyme deficiency is limited to leukocytes and erythrocytes, without deranged metabolism in other tissues, and no treatment is required. The second form of epimerase deficiency is more severe and generalized, with clinical manifestations that resemble GALT deficiency. Patients typically develop cataracts within the first few months of life; these are followed by liver, kidney, and brain damage. Affected individuals have additional symptoms of hypotonia and sensorineural hearing loss. The enzyme deficiency is generalized, and clinical symptoms respond to restriction of dietary galactose. However, in GALE deficiency, there is a range of metabolic derangements observed in patients, suggesting there may exist a spectrum of disease severity.

## GENETICS

The gene for epimerase, *GALE*, is located on chromosome 1p35-36, and mutations responsible for both forms of the epimerase deficiency (MIM no. 606953) have been identified.

## DIAGNOSIS

Although this form of galactosemia is rare, it must be considered in a symptomatic patient with measurable galactose-1-phosphate who has normal GALT activity. Diagnosis is confirmed by the assay of epimerase in erythrocytes.

## TREATMENT

Infants with the benign form of epimerase deficiency do not require treatment. Patients with the severe form of epimerase deficiency cannot synthesize galactose from glucose and are therefore galactose dependent. Because galactose is an essential component of many nervous system structural proteins, patients are placed on a galactose-restricted diet rather than a galactose-free diet.

# DISORDERS OF FRUCTOSE METABOLISM

## DEFICIENCY OF FRUCTOKINASE (BENIGN FRUCTOSURIA)

Benign fructosuria (MIM no. 229800) is not associated with any clinical manifestations. It is an incidental finding usually made through the detection of fructose as the reducing substance in the urine. No treatment is necessary.

## DEFICIENCY OF FRUCTOSE-1-PHOSPHATE OR FRUCTOSE 1,6-BISPHOSPHATE ALDOLASE (ALDOLASE B, OR HEREDITARY FRUCTOSE INTOLERANCE)

This severe disease of infants develops following the ingestion of fructose-containing foods and is caused by deficiency of aldolase B (fructose 1,6-bisphosphate aldolase) activity in the liver, kidney, and intestine. The enzyme catalyzes the hydrolysis of fructose-1-phosphate and fructose 1,6-bisphosphate into the 3-carbon sugars dihydroxyacetone phosphate, glyceraldehyde 3-phosphate, and glyceraldehyde. Deficiency of this enzyme activity causes a rapid accumulation of fructose-1-phosphate and initiates severe toxic symptoms when infants or children ingest fructose.

## CLINICAL PRESENTATION

Patients with fructose intolerance are healthy and asymptomatic until fructose or sucrose (table sugar) is ingested (usually from fruit, fruit juice, or sweetened cereal). Current infant formulas rarely contain sucrose. Clinical manifestations may resemble those of galactosemia and include jaundice, hepatomegaly, vomiting, lethargy, irritability, and convulsions. Laboratory findings include prolonged clotting time, hypoalbuminemia, elevation of bilirubin and liver transaminase levels, and proximal tubular dysfunction (Fanconi type with hyperphosphaturia). If the disease is not diagnosed and intake of the noxious sugar persists, postprandial hypoglycemic episodes recur, and liver and kidney failure progress, eventually leading to death.

Older patients usually develop an aversion to fructose-containing foods after experiencing recurrent abdominal pain, anorexia, and nausea while consuming these foods. Despite their self-imposed dietary restriction, some patients develop chronic fructose intoxication and present with growth failure and hepatomegaly. Others may be asymptomatic into adulthood, with significant absence of dental caries and a positive family history as the only indicators of disease. Some patients have suffered iatrogenic death or life-threatening events during fructose infusions.

## GENETICS

The true incidence of hereditary fructose intolerance (MIM no. 229600) is not known but may be as high as 1 in 23,000. The gene encoding aldolase B is on chromosome 9q22.3. Several mutations causing hereditary fructose intolerance have been identified. A single missense mutation, a G-to-C transversion in exon 5 that results in the alanine at position 149 being replaced by a proline (A149P), is the most common mutation identified in northern Europeans. This mutation plus 2 other mutations, A174D and N334K, account for approximately 80% to 85% of hereditary fructose intolerance in Europe and the United States. The diagnosis of hereditary fructose intolerance can thus be made by screening for these mutations in the majority of patients. Prenatal diagnosis is possible by either amniocentesis or chorionic villi sampling using DNA sequencing.

## DIAGNOSIS

Suspicion of the enzyme deficiency is fostered by the presence of a reducing substance in the urine during an attack. Laboratory studies show evidence of hepatic impairment, with increased blood bilirubin, methionine, and tyrosine, and abnormal coagulation tests. A proximal renal tubular acidosis develops with renal Fanconi syndrome, producing amino aciduria and hypokalemia. Metabolic abnormalities include hypoglycemia, hypophosphatemia from inorganic phosphate trapping and renal tubular loss, metabolic acidosis from increased lactate and renal bicarbonate losses, and hyperuricemia due to inhibition of adenosine monophosphate deaminase. Anemia and thrombocytopenia are also common.

Definitive diagnosis is typically made by mutation analysis. If no mutations are found, and when the clinical diagnosis is highly probable, an intravenous fructose tolerance load can be performed, which is more reliable and less dangerous than an oral load. It first results in a rapid fall of serum phosphate, then of blood glucose, and a subsequent rise of uric acid and magnesium concentrations. Alternatively, aldolase B activity can be measured on a liver biopsy sample.

## TREATMENT

Treatment consists of completely eliminating all sources of sucrose, fructose, and sorbitol from the diet, preferably with the help of a dietician familiar with metabolic disorders, as many foods contain these ingredients. Formula-fed infants with hereditary fructose intolerance who cannot tolerate lactose-based formulas must be given sucrose-free soy or elemental formulas. Whereas commonly used formulas that contain corn syrup (glucose polymer) solids are safe for patients with hereditary fructose intolerance, foods with "high fructose corn syrup solids" must be avoided. Medications must be carefully screened for the presence of sorbitol and sucrose sweeteners, and water-soluble vitamin supplements should be given.

With treatment, liver and kidney dysfunction improve, and catch-up growth is common. Intellectual development is usually unimpaired. As the patient matures, symptoms become milder even after fructose ingestion, and the long-term prognosis is good. Owing to dietary avoidance of sucrose, affected patients have few dental caries.

## DISORDERS OF GLUCONEOGENESIS

Gluconeogenesis is an important means of maintaining adequate glucose levels during fasting or stressful conditions by converting 3-carbon compounds derived from triglyceride hydrolysis (glycerol), lactate, and gluconeogenic amino acids to glucose via pyruvate. Three enzymes are central to gluconeogenesis: pyruvate carboxylase, phosphoenolpyruvate carboxykinase (PEPCK), and fructose 1,6-diphosphatase, with the remaining steps catalyzed by reversible glycolytic enzymes. Human diseases in all 3 enzymes are now recognized, with both a cytoplasmic and mitochondrial isoform of PEPCK present, but only the former is currently associated with disease.

### PYRUVATE CARBOXYLASE DEFICIENCY

Pyruvate carboxylase deficiency (MIM no. 266150) is an autosomal recessive disorder caused by mutations in the *PC* gene located on chromosome 11q13.2. The carboxylation of pyruvate to oxaloacetate in the mitochondrial matrix is important in maintaining the redox state of the cell, in replenishing tricarboxylic acid (TCA) cycle intermediates, and in generation of glucose via gluconeogenesis. The accumulation of pyruvate leads to elevated levels of lactic acid and alanine. Increased ketone body production reflects an increased pool of acetyl CoA from fatty acids and pyruvate due to diminished oxaloacetate available to form citrate via citrate synthase. Pyruvate carboxylase is 1 of 4 biotin-dependent carboxylases (see Chapter 143) and is considered "anaplerotic" in that it replenishes TCA cycle intermediates lost to biosynthetic pathways.

#### CLINICAL PRESENTATION

Historically, pyruvate carboxylase deficiency was categorized as type A, B, or C, depending on the severity of the clinical course. A lethal neonatal disease associated with metabolic acidosis, lactic acidosis, hyperammonemia, and elevated alanine and citrulline constitutes type B, with hyperammonemia and hypercitrullinemia a consequence of impaired ureagenesis due to a secondary aspartate deficiency, since transamination of oxaloacetate is a leading source of aspartate. A cystic periventricular leukomalacia seen on cerebral ultrasound in association with congenital lactic acidosis is suggestive of the disorder, as is the presence of a renal tubular acidosis. Type A has been reported with a more mild yet still often severe disease course, but without hyperammonemia or hypercitrullinemia. Onset is in the neonatal period or infancy and is clinically characterized by frequent lactic acidosis, severe developmental delay, failure to thrive, hypotonia, pyramidal tract signs, ataxia, nystagmus, convulsions, and occasional hypoglycemia. Brain imagining can reveal a Leigh disease pattern of necrotizing encephalopathy. Survival to young adulthood can be seen, and this form is often found in Canadian Native American populations. The group C form is the mildest, with periodic episodes of ketosis and lactic acidosis, but better preservation of cognitive and motor development.

#### DIAGNOSIS

Depending on the form of the disorder, the diagnosis is suggested by the finding of elevated lactate and pyruvate with or without increased ammonia and citrulline. Pyruvate carboxylase is a broadly expressed enzyme, and the diagnosis can typically be established by demonstrating an enzyme deficiency in either the liver or skin fibroblasts or by DNA testing. In patients with known mutations, carrier detection and prenatal diagnosis are possible using a DNA-based test. Type A patients generally have missense substitutions, while type B patients often harbor more severe truncating mutations. Several type C patients have been found to harbor somatic mosaic mutations.

#### TREATMENT

The more common forms of the disease are severe and generally refractory to interventions, while for the mild form of the disorder, the goal of therapy is to avoid induction of gluconeogenesis by frequent feeding. There is no specific intervention beyond supportive care during an episode of lactic acidosis, with use of intravenous glucose, bicarbonate, citrate salts, and a trial of biotin. Use of anaplerotic therapy with the odd chain triglyceride triheptanoin, designed to replenish TCA cycle intermediates by its metabolism to succinate via propionate, has been reported but remains to be established as a viable therapy.

### FRUCTOSE 1,6-DIPHOSPHATASE DEFICIENCY

Fructose 1,6-diphosphatase deficiency (MIM no. 229700) is a defect in gluconeogenesis. The gene encoding fructose 1,6-diphosphatase (*FBP1*) is located on chromosome 9q22.

#### CLINICAL PRESENTATION

The disease is characterized by life-threatening fasting episodes of lactic acidosis, hypoglycemia, hyperventilation, convulsions, and coma. Hepatomegaly is present during acute episodes. These episodes are triggered by a decrease in oral food intake during febrile illness or gastroenteritis. Laboratory findings include low blood glucose, high lactate and uric acid concentrations, glyceroluria, and metabolic acidosis. In contrast to hereditary fructose intolerance, there is usually no aversion to sweets, and renal tubular and liver functions are normal.

#### DIAGNOSIS

The diagnosis is established by demonstrating an enzyme deficiency in either the liver or an intestinal biopsy specimen or by DNA testing. The enzyme defect may sometimes be demonstrated in leukocytes. In patients with known mutations, carrier detection and prenatal diagnosis are possible using a DNA-based test.

#### TREATMENT

Treatment of acute attacks consists of correcting hypoglycemia and acidosis by intravenous infusion, and the response is usually rapid. Later, avoiding fasting and eliminating fructose and sucrose from the diet prevent further episodes. For long-term prevention of hypoglycemia, a slowly released carbohydrate such as cornstarch is useful. Patients who survive childhood appear to develop normally. In some women managed with an appropriate diet, successful pregnancies have been reported.

### PHOSPHOENOLPYRUVATE CARBOXYKINASE DEFICIENCY

PEPCK deficiency (MIM no. 261680) to date has been reported only for the cytosolic form of PEPCK encoded by the gene *PCK1* located on chromosome 20q13.31. The mitochondrial isoform encoded by *PCK2* has yet to be unequivocally associated with disease. The enzyme converts oxaloacetate into phosphoenolpyruvate, removing a TCA cycle intermediate, and is thus "cataplerotic."

#### CLINICAL PRESENTATION

There have been less than 10 reported cases of either the mitochondrial or cytosolic forms. Most cases were diagnosed through enzymatic activity, and only 3 have been confirmed through DNA sequencing of the *PCK1* gene. Enzymatic activity is determined through liver, fibroblast, or lymphocyte samples; however, fibroblasts and lymphocytes are not suitable for diagnosing the cytosolic form because these tissues possess only mitochondrial PEPCK.

The clinical features are heterogeneous but frequently include hypoglycemia, lactic acidemia, liver failure, hepatomegaly, hypotonia, developmental delay, and failure to thrive. More recently, 2 families have been described with molecularly confirmed cytoplasmic PEPCK deficiency. One family had 2 affected sisters with recurrent hypoglycemia, lactic academia, and ketonuria, while the second family had an infant who presented at 9 months of age with acute liver failure, extremely high blood transaminases, hypoalbuminemia, a coagulopathy, and mild hypoglycemia and hyperammonemia, following an episode of gastroenteritis. In the latter case, a very elevated glutamine, low citrulline and arginine, and a modest orotic aciduria suggested a urea cycle disorder, while urine organic acid analysis revealed an abundance of TCA cycle intermediates fumarate, succinate, malate, and α-ketoglutarate but no glycerol. Liver biopsy revealed diffuse macrosteatosis, and the child's symptoms resolved with intravenous glucose and supportive care, and liver functions returned to normal within a few weeks.

## DIAGNOSIS

The clinical diagnosis of PEPCK deficiency is challenging given the nonspecific metabolic perturbations, but recurrent hypoglycemia and lactic acidosis suggest a defect in gluconeogenesis. Since the utilization of glycerol as a substrate for glucose formation is intact in PEPCK deficiency, hypoglycemia appears to be a less prominent feature. The apparent dysfunction of the urea cycle may reflect an accumulation of TCA cycle intermediates, with α-ketoglutarate shunting into glutamate and hence glutamine, leading to increased ammonia production, while stalling of the TCA cycle may account for liver failure. As noted, diagnosis by enzyme testing is limited by the presence of 1 or both isoforms in differing tissues and cell types. The recent cases depended on the availability of whole-exome sequencing, an increasingly important diagnostic tool for metabolic disorders.

## TREATMENT

Like other gluconeogenic disorders, acute treatment is supportive and directed at correcting acidosis and hypoglycemia. Long-term treatment is focused on avoiding fasting to reduce dependence on gluconeogenesis, and cornstarch may be a useful supplement.

## SUGGESTED READINGS

Asberg C, Hjalmarson O, Alm J, Martinsson T, Waldenstrom J, Hellerud C. Fructose 1,6-bisphosphatase deficiency: enzyme and mutation analysis performed on calcitriol-stimulated monocytes with a note on long-term prognosis. *J Inherit Metab Dis*. 2010;33(Suppl 3): S113-121.

Bosch AM. Classical galactosaemia revisited. *J Inherit Metab Dis*. 2006;29(4):516-525.

Bouteldja N, Timson DJ. The biochemical basis of hereditary fructose intolerance. *J Inherit Metab Dis*. 2010;33(2):105-112.

Fridovich-Keil JL, Gubbels CS, Spencer JB, Sanders RD, Land JA, Rubio-Gozalbo E. Ovarian function in girls and women with GALT-deficiency galactosemia. *J Inherit Metab Dis*. 2011;34(2):357-366.

Hennermann JB, Schadewaldt P, Vetter B, Shin YS, Monch E, Klein J. Features and outcome of galactokinase deficiency in children diagnosed by newborn screening. *J Inherit Metab Dis*. 2011;34(2):399-407.

Marin-Valencia I, Roe CR, Pascual JM. Pyruvate carboxylase deficiency: mechanisms, mimics and anaplerosis. *Mol Genet Metab*. 2010;101(1):9-17.

Openo KK, Schulz JM, Vargas CA, et al. Epimerase-deficiency galactosemia is not a binary condition. *Am J Hum Genet*. 2006;78(1):89-102.

Santra S, Cameron JM, Shyr C, et al. Cytosolic phosphoenolpyruvate carboxykinase deficiency presenting with acute liver failure following gastroenteritis. *Mol Genet Metab*. 2016;118(1):21-27.

Timson DJ. The structural and molecular biology of type III galactosemia. *IUBMB Life*. 2006;58(2):83-89.

# 151 Disorders of Pentose Phosphate Pathway

Priya S. Kishnani and Yuan-Tsong Chen

## DISORDERS OF PENTOSE METABOLISM

About 90% of glucose metabolism in the body occurs via the glycolytic pathway and the remaining 10% via the hexose monophosphate pathway. The hexose monophosphate shunt leads to formation of pentoses and generates NADH. One of the metabolites, ribose-5-phosphate, is used in the biosynthesis of ribonucleotides and deoxyribonucleotides. Through the transketolase and transaldolase reactions, the pentose phosphates can be converted back to fructose-6-phosphate and glucose-6-phosphate. The congenital abnormalities in pentose metabolism include a benign pentosuria and 2 recently described enzyme deficiencies: transaldolase deficiency and ribose-5-phosphate isomerase deficiency.

## ESSENTIAL PENTOSURIA

Essential pentosuria (Online Mendelian Inheritance in Man [MIM] no. 260800) is a benign disorder encountered mainly in Ashkenazi Jews and is inherited as an autosomal recessive trait. The urine contains L-xylulose, which is excreted in increased amounts because of a block in the conversion of L-xylulose to xylitol due to xylitol dehydrogenase deficiency. The condition is usually discovered accidentally following a urine test for reducing substances. No treatment is required.

## TRANSALDOLASE DEFICIENCY

Transaldolase deficiency (MIM no. 606003) affects the nonoxidative branch of the hexose monophosphate pathway. This rare, multisystemic disease has been reported in the literature in less than 30 patients. Patients present in early infancy with various degrees of hepatic, cardiac, and renal involvement. Hepatosplenomegaly and liver dysfunction, along with pancytopenia, are the most common clinical features. Patients also exhibit cutis laxa and dysmorphic facial features. Occasionally, antenatal symptoms of hydrops fetalis and oligohydramnios are present as well. In the most recently reported case, antenatal ultrasound revealed hyperechogenic bowel, and the patient required surgical intervention for intestinal obstruction at birth.

Transaldolase deficiency is detected through the listed clinical features and biochemical abnormalities. Urine and plasma biochemistry reveals elevated levels of D-arabitol, ribitol, and erythritol, among others. Enzyme assay of low transaldolase activity in the lymphoblasts/fibroblasts and DNA sequencing confirm the diagnosis. Currently, there is no treatment available for this deficiency; however, there is ongoing investigation of *N*-acetylcysteine therapy in a mouse model.

## RIBOSE-5-PHOSPHATE ISOMERASE DEFICIENCY

To date, only 1 case of ribose-5-phosphate isomerase deficiency (MIM no. 608611) has been reported. The affected male had psychomotor retardation from early in life and developed epilepsy at 4 years of age. Thereafter, a slow neurologic regression developed with prominent cerebellar ataxia, some spasticity, optic atrophy, and a mild sensorimotor neuropathy. Magnetic resonance imaging of the brain at ages 11 and 14 years showed extensive abnormalities of the cerebral white matter. Proton magnetic resonance spectroscopy of the brain revealed elevated levels of ribitol and D-arabitol. These pentitols were also increased in urine and plasma, which is similar to the patient with transaldolase deficiency, and there is a notable accumulation of pentitols in the central nervous system; however, the pathophysiology of the disorder is not understood. Enzyme assays in cultured fibroblasts showed deficient ribose-5-phosphate isomerase activity, which was confirmed by a molecular study.

## SUGGESTED READINGS

Eyaid W, Al Harbi T, Anazi S, et al. Transaldolase deficiency: report of 12 new cases and further delineation of the phenotype. *J Inherit Metab Dis*. 2013;36(6):997-1004.

Pierce SB, Spurrell CH, Mandell JB, et al. Garrod's fourth inborn error of metabolism solved by the identification of mutations causing pentosuria. *Proc Natl Acad Sci*. 2011;108(45):18313-18317.

van der Knaap MS, Wevers RA, Struys EA, et al. Leukoencephalopathy associated with a disturbance in the metabolism of polyols. *Ann Neurol*. 1999;46(6):925-928.

# 152 Disorders of Glucose Transporters

René Santer

## GENERAL CONSIDERATIONS

D-Glucose and other monosaccharides are hydrophilic substances that cannot easily cross the lipophilic bilayer of the cell membrane. Since carbohydrates are important for supplying energy to essentially all cell types, specific transport mechanisms have evolved. While vesicle-associated glucose transport has been described fairly recently, transporter proteins have been known for years. Such proteins are embedded into the cell membrane and function as hydrophilic pores that allow cellular uptake and release and transcellular transport of monosaccharides.

Glucose transporter proteins can be divided into 2 groups: (1) sodium-dependent glucose transporters (SGLTs; symporter systems, secondary "active" transporters), which are members of the solute carrier family 5 (SLC5) and couple sugar transport to the electrochemical gradient of sodium, and hence can transport glucose against its own concentration gradient (Fig. 152-1); and (2) facilitative glucose transporters (GLUTs, uniporter systems, "passive" transporters), which are members of the SLC2 family that can transport monosaccharides only along an existing gradient (Fig. 152-2). To date, 5 congenital defects of monosaccharide transport are known (Fig. 152-3). Their clinical picture is the consequence of tissue-specific expression and substrate specificity of the affected transporter.

## CONGENITAL GLUCOSE-GALACTOSE MALABSORPTION

### PATHOPHYSIOLOGY AND GENETICS

A congenital defect of the sodium-dependent monosaccharide transporter SGLT1 at the apical membrane of enterocytes is the basic defect of congenital glucose-galactose malabsorption (GGM; Mendelian Inheritance in Man [MIM] No. 182380). Shortly after suggestions were first published that the principal mechanism for glucose absorption at the intestinal brush border is co-transport with sodium, the first descriptions of monosaccharide malabsorption in pediatric patients were published. Insights into the physiology of intestinal glucose absorption were dramatically advanced in the 1980s after cloning a gene for an SGLT, which also opened the field to molecular genetic studies in humans. This work led to a model with 6 conformational states (Fig. 152-4) and that describes SGLT1 as a sodium-dependent glucose carrier transporting sodium and glucose with a stoichiometry of 2:1.

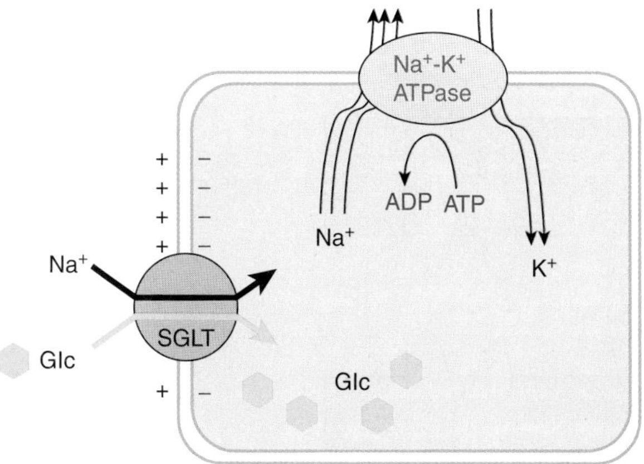


**FIGURE 152-1** Schematic of transport mediated by a sodium-dependent glucose transporter (SGLT) protein. Energy for this process is provided by the action of the sodium/potassium ATPase located at the basolateral side of the cell membrane exporting 3 sodium ions for the influx of 2 potassium ions and thus generating an electrical and chemical gradient. Transport of glucose (or other monosaccharides) at the apical membrane is coupled to the transport of sodium (for details, see Fig. 152-4). While sodium ions here are transported because of the low concentration and the negative charge within the cell, glucose can be transported against its own gradient. Transport for glucose is therefore termed *secondary active.*

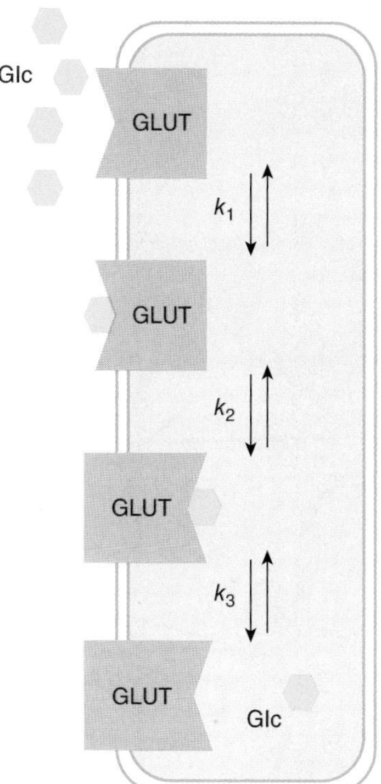


**FIGURE 152-2** Schematic of transport mediated by a facilitative glucose transporter (GLUT) protein. GLUT proteins are embedded into the cell membrane, where they can be found in 2 conformations, with an open side directed to either the outside or the inside of the cell. Affinity of glucose (or other monosaccharides) to the transporter on both sides can be characterized by specific equilibrium constants. Net transport is possible only in the direction of the lower concentration of the sugar.

SGLT1 may also act as a sodium transporter in the absence of glucose, and it transports about 200 to 300 molecules of water per cycle of the transporter, which suggests that the 250,000 copies of SGLT1 that can be found on each enterocyte are responsible for approximately 50% of the water transport of the intestine.

Examination of SGLT1 provides a simplified model of glucose transport at the apical membrane of enterocytes. Glucose transport largely depends on the luminal glucose concentration. In addition to SGLT1, there is a diffusive component, and facilitative transporters are expressed there depending on luminal glucose concentration. At a low concentration of glucose, SGLT1—with its ability to transport glucose against a concentration gradient—acts as a scavenger, recovering any glucose that might escape from enterocytes via the small number of facilitative transporters that are present there under these conditions. At intermediate glucose concentrations, SGLT1 is the major transporter but acts in "passive" mode. Postprandially, however, glucose transporter-2 (GLUT2)-mediated diffusive transport is the major route of glucose absorption, with SGLT1 acting as a regulator, triggering the passive component so that GLUT2 expression matches dietary intake of carbohydrates.

This concept explains many of the observations on kinetic data of brush border membrane glucose transport. However, in view of this model, it is surprising that both GLUT2 knockout animals and patients with a congenital defect of GLUT2 (Fanconi-Bickel syndrome) do not show an impairment of intestinal glucose absorption. One may speculate that SGLT1 is upregulated under these circumstances and may compensate for a deficiency of the diffusive component of brush border membrane glucose transport.

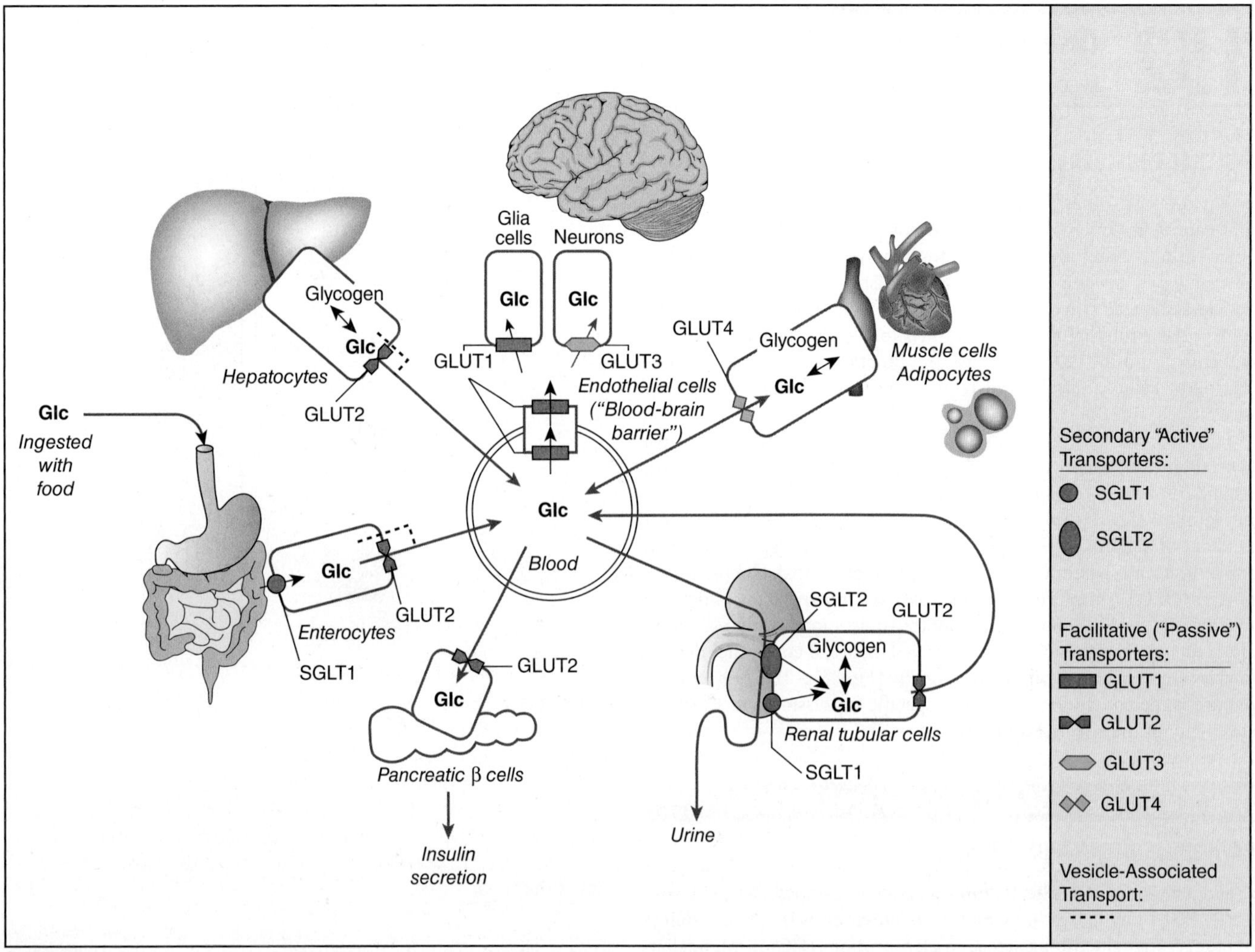

**FIGURE 152-3** Overview of glucose transporters in humans. Transport across cell membranes is depicted by arrows, and specific transporters are shown as symbols: rounded symbols are used for sodium-dependent, secondary "active" transporters (SGLTs); angular symbols are used for facilitative, "passive" transporters (GLUTs). Red symbols represent the known defects of SGLT1 (glucose-galactose malabsorption), SGLT2 (familial renal glucosuria), GLUT1 (glucose transporter-1 deficiency), and GLUT2 (Fanconi-Bickel syndrome). GLUT10 deficiency (arterial tortuosity syndrome) is not depicted here (see text for more details).

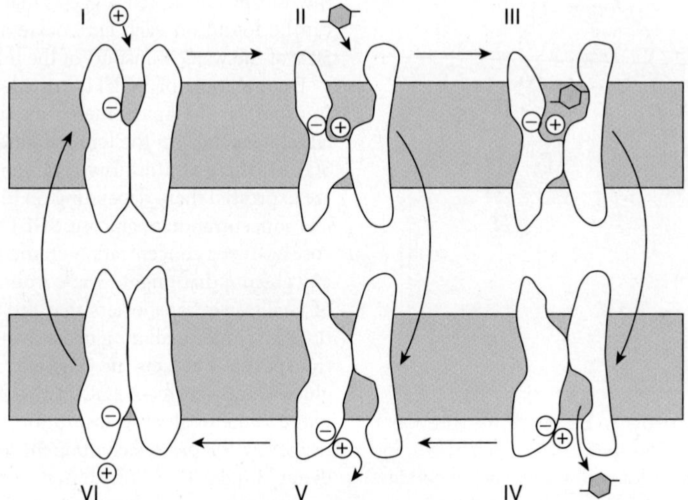


**FIGURE 152-4** Schematic of transport mediated by a sodium-dependent glucose transporter (SGLT) protein. SGLT proteins are embedded in the apical membrane of enterocytes and renal tubular cells. Binding of positively charged sodium ions first occurs at a region formed by the N-terminal sequence of the protein (stage I). This induces a conformational change of the transporter (II) and facilitates sugar binding (III) and sodium and sugar transport to the inner face of the protein against the glucose concentration gradient. The sugar first disassociates from the inner face of the carrier (IV), followed by sodium (V), which disassociates due to the low intracellular sodium concentration. The ligand-free carrier resumes its original configuration (VI→I) as a consequence of the negative membrane potential and the high external sodium gradient. Note that the cycle can also function without glucose binding, allowing sodium and water transport (II→V).

SGLT1 contributes to the transcellular transport of glucose and galactose, which is completed by the transport out of the cell at the basolateral membrane by facilitative diffusion or by a membrane vesicle-associated transport. Malabsorption of the 2 monosaccharides results in osmotic effects with massive fluid loss into the intestine. Fructose is not a substrate for SGLT1; it can be absorbed by facilitative diffusion mediated by GLUT5 and GLUT2, both on the apical and basolateral side, and is thus well tolerated by these patients. Both truncating and missense mutations of the SGLT1 gene *SLC5A1* have resulted in the absence of a functioning transporter protein within the apical enterocyte membrane. The fact that patients with GGM show mild glucosuria points to a physiologic role of this transporter in renal glucose reabsorption.

GGM is a relatively rare autosomal recessive disorder, but the exact prevalence is unknown. *SLC5A1*, located on chromosome 22q13, comprises 15 exons and encodes a protein of 664 amino acids that forms 14 transmembraneous loops. To date, approximately 60 different mutations have been found scattered all over the gene; the existence of a mutational hotspot is controversial.

### CLINICAL PRESENTATION

In general, children with GGM present within days after a normal pregnancy and birth. First clinical signs are bloating and profuse watery diarrhea. Stools are so loose that they may be mistaken for urine. Typically, polyhydramnios is not observed. Both breast- and bottle-fed infants are affected, and symptoms may even begin when newborns are given only small amounts of glucose or polymers of glucose. As a result, patients develop severe hypertonic dehydration with fever, which may be misinterpreted as a sign of an intestinal infection. If the correct diagnosis is missed and glucose and galactose are not eliminated from the diet, and if parenteral fluid administration is not available, patients die from hypovolemic shock. In typical cases, the diagnosis is considered after repeated frustrating attempts to switch from parenteral fluids to oral feeds. Chronic dehydration might be responsible for nephrolithiasis and nephrocalcinosis that develop in many cases.

### DIAGNOSTIC EVALUATION

Due to its life-threatening character, GGM must be suspected clinically, and treatment must be initiated before an ultimate diagnosis is established. The clinical stabilization on parenteral nutrition with no foods given by mouth or on a fructose-based formula suggests the diagnosis. The finding of an acidic stool and reducing substances in the stool can be a clue to diagnosis, and most patients have mild intermittent glucosuria. Oral monosaccharide tolerance tests (measuring stool pH and reducing substances, and blood glucose) combined with a hydrogen breath test can be performed. In these tests, glucose and galactose (but not fructose) may evoke severe clinical symptoms in affected infants, but some of the test parameters may be unreliable due to antibiotics, which are frequently given to sick neonates. Glucose and galactose uptake studies on intestinal biopsies are possible, but they are invasive and time consuming. Molecular genetic studies on genomic DNA are recommended early if clinical signs are suggestive, particularly if prenatal diagnosis is likely to be requested in a future pregnancy.

### TREATMENT AND PROGNOSIS

Whenever GGM is considered, glucose and galactose should be omitted from the diet. A formula containing fructose as the only carbohydrate is easily prepared by adding monosaccharide to commercially available carbohydrate-free dietary products. The preparation of the diet becomes more complicated when additional foods are introduced, but glucose tolerance improves with age by an as yet unknown mechanism. To date, there are no long-term studies on the outcome of GGM patients, and it is not clear how strictly patients should adhere to the glucose- and galactose-restricted diet to avoid an increased risk of nephrolithiasis. Likewise, there is no information on long-term sequelae of a high-fructose diet on liver function.



## RENAL GLUCOSURIA

### PATHOPHYSIOLOGY AND GENETICS

Renal glucosuria (MIM No. 233100) is an isolated defect of tubular glucose reabsorption at the proximal tubules and does not affect any other glomerular or tubular kidney functions. A large number of individuals with renal glucosuria carry mutations in the SGLT2 gene *SLC5A2*, located on chromosome 16p11. Its product is a low-affinity carrier that transports glucose (but not galactose) across the apical membrane of proximal renal tubulus cells.

Transcellular transport is carried out by GLUT2, which is expressed at the basolateral membrane. Homozygosity or compound heterozygosity for *SLC5A2* mutations results in severe renal glucosuria, generally in the range of 10 to more than 100 g/1.73 m$^2$/d, whereas heterozygosity is associated with milder glucosuria of 0.4 to 5.0 (up to 10) g/1.73 m$^2$/d. Since glucosuria has not been observed consistently in all heterozygous carriers of mutations, inheritance of renal glucosuria is best characterized as a codominant trait with variable penetrance. To date, approximately 50 SGLT2 mutations have been described, which are scattered throughout the gene. Most mutations affect only single pedigrees; only a splice mutation (IVS 7 +5 G>A) was found in several kindreds of different ethnic backgrounds.

### CLINICAL PRESENTATION

Mild renal glucosuria, generally considered a "nondisease," is relatively common. Individuals with a higher glucose excretion or even virtual absence of tubular glucose reabsorption (termed *renal glucosuria type 0*) are extremely rare. Only a small number of patients present with polyuria or enuresis. Most individuals with renal glucosuria are detected during a routine urine examination when a positive test for glucose is found. All other tubular functions are normal; there are no signs of renal tubular acidosis or rickets due to tubular phosphate loss. Also, mild hyperaminoaciduria is generally not present but can occasionally be a secondary phenomenon in individuals with massive glucosuria. Renal glucosuria must be distinguished from diabetes mellitus, which can be easily excluded by the observation of normal blood glucose concentrations.

Only individuals with massive glucose excretion have occasionally been reported to develop a propensity to hypovolemia and hypoglycemia. A temporary delay in somatic maturation due to calorie loss and/or the activation of counterregulatory hormones has been described. In this context, as an alternative approach to treating diabetes, inhibitors of SGLT2 have been developed. They result in a similar biochemical profile as found in individuals with renal glucosuria, with a daily glucose loss of 30 to 60 g/1.73 m$^2$/d. Their use in type 2 diabetes has been shown to significantly reduce elevated hemoglobin A1c, and side effects such as weight loss, volume depletion, and a reduction in blood pressure have been considered quite helpful in patients who frequently suffer from "metabolic syndrome." Therefore, despite a seemingly benign course in individuals who daily lose high amounts of glucose with their urine, almost no studies on long-term effects in renal glucosuria patients exist, and long-term outcome has not been systematically evaluated.

### DIAGNOSTIC EVALUATION

Diagnosis is straightforward in patients with glucosuria and normoglycemia who do not show any other evidence of renal tubular dysfunction.

### TREATMENT AND PROGNOSIS

For most cases, dietary treatment is not necessary, and the prognosis, even in individuals with type 0 glucosuria, is excellent.

## GLUCOSE TRANSPORTER-1 DEFICIENCY SYNDROME

### PATHOPHYSIOLOGY AND GENETICS

Glucose transporter-1 (GLUT1) is a membrane-spanning, glycosylated protein that provides basal glucose entry across most blood-tissue barriers. This protein exclusively facilitates glucose transport across the luminal and abluminal membranes of brain capillaries that represent the blood-brain barrier created by the impermeable tight junctions between these cells. Consequently, GLUT1 deficiency (MIM No. 606777) results in a low glucose concentration in the cerebrospinal fluid (CSF), termed *hypoglycorrhachia*. Thus, GLUT1 is important for glucose transport to glial cells and neurons.

Unlike astrocytes and oligodendrocytes that mainly use GLUT1 for glucose transport, the carrier responsible for glucose uptake by neurons is GLUT3, for which a congenital defect has not been described in humans. Interestingly, it has recently been shown that GLUT3 is also an important glucose carrier in the trophoblast and that mice homozygous for GLUT3 die during embryogenesis. Heterozygous animals, however, survive but are born with severe fetal growth retardation. Since glucose is the principal fuel for cerebral energy metabolism, GLUT1 deficiency with its effects on glia cells and the blood-brain barrier results in impaired energy supply to the brain.

The majority of patients with GLUT1 deficiency carry heterozygous de novo mutations in the GLUT1 gene *SLC2A1*, which is located on chromosome 1p. Mutations are distributed randomly and are of various types (missense, nonsense, and splice-site mutations, and large deletions). Phenotype-genotype correlation is yet unclear, but missense mutations may cause a milder phenotype than haploinsufficiency. Autosomal dominant GLUT1 deficiency has been identified in a few unrelated families. The fact that heterozygosity for a GLUT1 mutation is sufficient to cause GLUT1 deficiency highlights the importance of glucose for the developing brain; presumably, homozygosity for a GLUT1 mutation is lethal in utero.



### CLINICAL PRESENTATION

GLUT1 deficiency syndrome typically presents as an early-onset epileptic encephalopathy. For unknown reasons, fetal development is undisturbed; pregnancy, delivery, and the neonatal period are uneventful. The majority of patients develop epilepsy within the first year of life as cerebral glucose demand increases. Occasionally, patients without epilepsy have been identified; others develop only paroxysmal dyskinesia. Seizures are of various types and frequency, are often refractory to anticonvulsants, and are sometimes aggravated by fasting. In infants, peculiar eye movements, staring spells, drop attacks, and cyanotic spells are the most frequent symptoms. Older children present predominantly with epilepsy absences, myoclonus, and grand mal seizures. Interictal electroencephalograms (EEGs) in GLUT1 deficiency may be normal regardless of age. Occasionally, EEG recordings may show an improvement after glucose intake. In a study of ictal EEG features in 20 patients, focal slowing or epileptiform discharges were most prevalent in infants, and generalized 2.5- to 4-Hz spike-wave patterns were most prevalent in older children. No structural brain abnormalities are detected by neuroimaging, but positron emission tomography studies may show a diminished cortical uptake, with a more severe reduction in metabolism in the mesial temporal regions and thalami, accentuating a relative signal increase in the basal ganglia.

No dysmorphic features are observed. In early childhood, global developmental delay and a complex motor disorder become apparent. Motor milestones are delayed, and speech is often significantly slurred and slowed, but all patients acquire speech and mobility. Hypotonia and ataxia result in a broad-based, unsteady gait. A substantial number of patients display additional dystonic features and elements of spasticity. GLUT1 deficiency is not a degenerative disorder, although individuals with severe cases develop secondary microcephaly.

### DIAGNOSTIC EVALUATION

GLUT1 deficiency should be suspected in any patient with hypoglycorrhachia if hypoglycemia or a central nervous system (CNS) infection is absent. In affected individuals, absolute values for CSF glucose concentrations are generally less than 45 mg/dL, but for accurate diagnosis, the CSF-to-blood-glucose ratio is superior to the absolute concentration. This should be obtained in a nonictal, metabolic steady state following a 4- to 6-hour fast with blood glucose determined before the lumbar puncture to avoid stress-related hyperglycemia. Hypoglycorrhachia with a ratio less than 0.46 together with a low to normal CSF lactate is diagnostic, but the numeric value of this ratio does not correlate with clinical severity.

GLUT1 deficiency should be confirmed by molecular genetic methods or by glucose uptake studies in erythrocytes (in which 5% of their membrane protein is GLUT1). In such studies, glucose uptake is reduced to about half of the control values. Again, transport kinetics do not correlate with disease severity.

### TREATMENT AND PROGNOSIS

GLUT1 deficiency syndrome can be successfully treated with a high-fat, low-carbohydrate ("ketogenic") diet. Ketone bodies derived from dietary fat restore brain energy metabolism since the transport route into the CNS is not dependent on GLUT1. Such a diet can effectively control seizures, but anticonvulsant medication may be necessary in the later course of the disease, and neurologic function and movement usually remain impaired. In contrast to intractable epilepsy, for which such a diet was originally developed, it is recommended that patients with GLUT1 deficiency remain on a ketogenic diet throughout childhood and into adolescence, by which time the cerebral glucose demands decrease to adult levels.

Inhibitors of GLUT1 such as anticonvulsants (phenobarbital, chloral hydrate, diazepam), methylxanthines (theophylline, caffeine), alcohol, and green tea should be avoided. If treatment with anticonvulsants is necessary (eg, due to noncompliance with the diet or incomplete seizure control on diet), carbamazepine or phenytoin, which do not interfere with GLUT1 function, should be considered as an add-on medication. Dietary antioxidants such as α-lipoic acid (600–1800 mg/d in 3 divided doses) have been recommended in GLUT1 deficiency.

## FANCONI-BICKEL SYNDROME

### PATHOPHYSIOLOGY AND GENETICS

Fanconi-Bickel syndrome (FBS; MIM No. 227810) is caused by a congenital deficiency or impaired function of GLUT2, a high $K_m$ monosaccharide carrier that transports glucose and galactose. The main clinical features of FBS can be explained by the fact that this facilitative carrier is expressed both in hepatocytes and at the basolateral membrane of reabsorbing cells of the renal proximal tubules. GLUT2 is also found at the apical and basolateral membranes of enterocytes and within the cell membrane of pancreatic β cells.

Intestinal uptake of glucose and galactose appears unimpaired in FBS; this has been explained by additional transport systems for glucose. Postprandial hyperglycemia and hypergalactosemia are caused by impaired hepatic uptake of these 2 monosaccharides. To date, it remains unclear if hyperglycemia in FBS is further exaggerated by a diminished insulin response due to an impairment of glucose sensing of β cells. In hepatocytes, GLUT2 seems to function as a glucose sensor. In the fasting state, when extracellular glucose concentration declines, the concentrations of glucose and glucose-6-phosphate within hepatocytes are inappropriately high in FBS patients. This stimulates glycogen synthesis and inhibits gluconeogenesis and glycogenolysis, which ultimately predisposes the individual to hypoglycemia and hepatic glycogen accumulation. Impaired transport of glucose out of renal tubular cells results in the accumulation of glycogen and free glucose within these cells. This impairs other transport functions and results in a generalized tubulopathy with disproportionately severe glucosuria. The extreme amounts of glucose lost with the urine (even at times when blood glucose is low) may contribute to the propensity to develop hypoglycemia.

FBS is a very rare autosomal recessive condition caused by mutations of the GLUT2 gene *SLC2A2*. More than 70% of cases come from consanguineous families. The human gene, mapped to chromosome 3q26, encodes a 524 amino acid protein with 55% amino acid identity to GLUT1. In contrast to SGLTs, all GLUT proteins form 12 transmembranous loops within the cell membrane. The genomic structure of *SLC2A2* encompasses 11 exons, and to date,

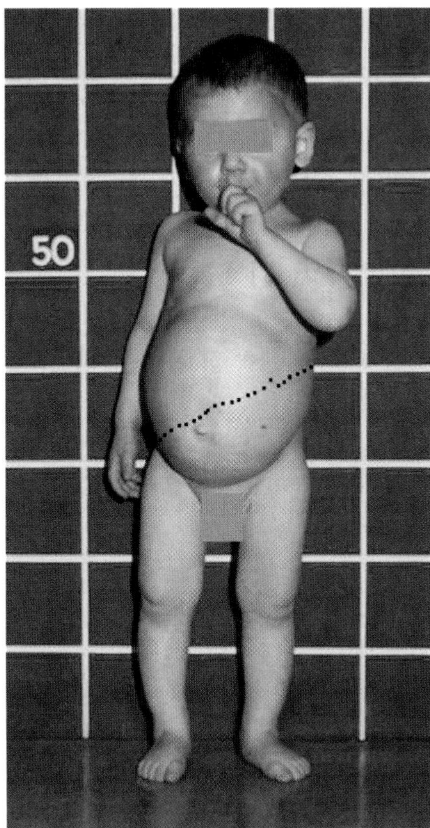


**FIGURE 152-5** Two-year-old Turkish boy with typical signs of Fanconi-Bickel syndrome due to homozygosity for an *SLC2A2* (GLUT2) mutation. Note the short stature, the distended abdomen due to hepatomegaly, and bowing of the legs because of renal phosphate loss due to generalized tubulopathy.

approximately 70 different mutations scattered throughout the gene have been detected.

## CLINICAL PRESENTATION

Patients with FBS typically present at 3 to 10 months with hepatomegaly, a Fanconi-type nephropathy, a propensity to hypoglycemia in the fasting state, and glucose and galactose intolerance in the fed state. A few cases have presented during neonatal screening with hypergalactosemia, and cataracts have occasionally been observed in infants with FBS. At an early age, hepatomegaly, which is caused by massive accumulation of glycogen, may not yet be present, and nonspecific symptoms such as fever, vomiting, chronic diarrhea, and failure to thrive may predominate. With increasing age, the clinical presentation of a protuberant abdomen, moon-shaped face, and short stature becomes more and more similar to other hepatic glycogen storage diseases (Fig. 152-5). The kidneys accumulate glycogen, and their enlargement can be detected by ultrasound. Hypophosphatemic rickets is the major manifestation of tubular dysfunction, which results in joint swelling, bowing of legs, and pathologic fractures. FBS patients have an entirely normal mental development, but growth and puberty are severely retarded. A case of hepatocellular carcinoma has been reported in a 6-year-old child, as is seen in other glycogen storage disorders.

## DIAGNOSTIC EVALUATION

The diagnosis of FBS is suggested by the characteristic combination of an altered glucose homeostasis, hepatic glycogen accumulation, and the typical features of a Fanconi-type tubulopathy. Fasting hypoglycemia and impaired glucose and galactose tolerance may be documented during oral loading tests. Laboratory findings include mildly elevated transaminases without signs of any impairment of synthetic or secretory function. Plasma lipids, uric acid, and lactate may be elevated. If a liver biopsy is performed, both histologic and biochemical methods show an increased glycogen content; however, enzymatic studies of all glycogenolytic enzymes are normal. Hyperaminoaciduria, hyperphosphaturia, hypercalciuria, renal tubular acidosis, mild tubular proteinuria, and polyuria are indicative of a generalized proximal tubular dysfunction. A hallmark of FBS is the relatively severe glucosuria. The calculated tubular glucose reabsorption is dramatically reduced or even zero in most patients. The diagnosis of FBS is ultimately confirmed by the detection of homozygosity or compound heterozygosity for *SLC2A2* mutations.

## TREATMENT AND PROGNOSIS

Only symptomatic treatment is available. Measures are directed toward improving glucose homeostasis and ameliorating the consequences of renal tubulopathy. FBS patients should receive a diet with adequate caloric intake to compensate for the renal glucose losses. Frequent feeds using slowly absorbed carbohydrates are recommended. Continuous carbohydrate supply by oligosaccharide solutions provided via a tube feeding during the night may be indicated. Uncooked cornstarch has a beneficial effect on metabolic control, particularly on growth.

For the tubulopathy, water and electrolytes have to be replaced in appropriate amounts. Administration of alkali may be necessary to compensate for renal tubular acidosis. Hypophosphatemic rickets requires supplementation with phosphate and vitamin D. With these measures, the prognosis is fairly good, and some of the originally described pediatric patients have reached adulthood. The main problems for adult patients are short stature and orthopedic problems caused by hypophosphatemic rickets and osteomalacia. Metabolic decompensation with severe acidosis or renal insufficiency similar to diabetic glomerulosclerosis has been a rare complication that causes death in childhood.

# ARTERIAL TORTUOSITY SYNDROME

Deficiency of the facilitative glucose transporter GLUT10—encoded by *SLC2A10*, which is located on chromosome 20q13.1—has been shown to be the cause of arterial tortuosity syndrome (MIM No. 208050). Patients with this autosomal-recessive disorder have tortuosity and elongation of all major arteries and aorta, multiple pulmonary artery stenoses, telangiectasias of the cheeks, stretchable skin, and laxity of joints. Some patients have diaphragmatic, gastric, and inguinal hernias; intestinal elongation; and keratoconus. Soft nasal cartilage and micrognathia are noted in some. The mechanism by which the defect of a glucose transporter causes these symptoms is not understood, but recent evidence suggests that the substrate for GLUT10 is dehydroascorbic acid. This condition is also associated with upregulation of the transforming growth factor (TGF)-β pathway, reminiscent of the perturbed signaling seen in the connective tissue disorders Loeys-Dietz and Marfan syndrome.

# RENAL HYPOURICEMIA

Renal hypouricemia is characterized by impaired uric acid reabsorption at the apical membrane of proximal renal tubule. The disorder is not lethal and may be asymptomatic. However, nephrolithiasis and exercise-induced acute renal failure are observed in 10% to 20% of patients. Two forms are recognized: renal hypouricemia-1 (RHUC1) is caused by homozygous or compound heterozygous mutations in URAT1 encoded by the *SLC22A12* gene located on chromosome 11q13 and is not part of the glucose transporter superfamily; and renal hypouricemia-2 (RHUC2) is caused by homozygous or compound heterozygous mutations in GLUT9 encoded by the *SLC2A9* gene located on chromosome 11q13. It was initially believed to be involved in fructose and deoxyglucose transport; however, uric acid is now known to be the primary metabolite that is transported. Hence, similar to GLUT10, GLUT9 is primarily involved in transporting molecules that are not carbohydrates.

Chedane-Girault C, Dabadie A, Maurage C, et al. Neonatal diarrhea due to congenital glucose-galactose malabsorption: report of seven cases. *Arch Pediatr*. 2012;19(12):1289-1292.

Gras D, Roze E, Caillet S, et al. GLUT1 deficiency syndrome: an update. *Rev Neurol (Paris)*. 2014;170(2):91-99.

Lindquist B, Meeuwisse GW. Chronic diarrhoea caused by monosaccharide malabsorption. *Acta Paediatr*. 1962;51:674-685.

Martin MG, Turk E, Lostao MP, et al. Defects in Na(+)/glucose cotransporter (SGLT1) trafficking and function cause glucose-galactose malabsorption. *Nat Genet*. 1996;12:216-220.

Németh CE, Marcolongo P, Gamberucci A, et al. Glucose transporter type 10-lacking in arterial tortuosity syndrome-facilitates dehydroascorbic acid transport. *FEBS Lett*. 2016;590(11):1630-1640.

Santer R, Schneppenheim R, Dombrowski A, et al. Mutations in GLUT2, the gene for the liver-type glucose transporter, in patients with Fanconi-Bickel syndrome. *Nat Genet*. 1997;17:324-326.

Shima Y, Nozu K, Nozu Y, et al. Recurrent EIARF and PRES with severe renal hypouricemia by compound heterozygous SLC2A9 mutation. *Pediatrics*. 2011;127(6):e1621-e1625.

Thorens B. GLUT2, glucose sensing and glucose homeostasis. *Diabetologia*. 2015;58(2):221-232.

Turk E, Zabel B, Mundlos S, et al. Glucose/galactose malabsorption caused by a defect in the Na(+)/glucose cotransporter. *Nature*. 1991;350:354-356.

Vallon V, Thomson SC. Targeting renal glucose reabsorption to treat hyperglycaemia: the pleiotropic effects of SGLT2 inhibition. *Diabetologia*. 2017;60(2):215-225.

Wright EM, Loo DD, Hirayama BA. Biology of human sodium glucose transporters. *Physiol Rev*. 2011;91(2):733-794.

Zoppi N, Chiarelli N, Cinquina V, Ritelli M, Colombi M. GLUT10 deficiency leads to oxidative stress and non-canonical αvβ3 integrin-mediated TGFβ signalling associated with extracellular matrix disarray in arterial tortuosity syndrome skin fibroblasts. *Hum Mol Genet*. 2015;24(23):6769-6787.



# PART 5 DISORDERS OF OXIDATIVE PHOSPHORYLATION AND PYRUVATE OXIDATION

## 153 Respiratory Chain Disorders

Juan M. Pascual and Salvatore DiMauro

### INTRODUCTION

The respiratory chain (RC) is the terminal pathway of mitochondrial metabolism, where most energy is produced as adenosine triphosphate (ATP). It is also the only metabolic pathway under dual genetic control: Of the approximately 80 subunits of the RC, 13 are encoded by mitochondrial DNA (mtDNA) and the rest by nuclear DNA (nDNA). Defects of the RC cause an extremely heterogeneous group of disorders that affect both children and adults, often involving multiple tissues and resulting in characteristic syndromes but sometimes affecting single tissues. Disorders due to mutations in mtDNA are especially challenging for the clinician because the rules of mitochondrial genetics make for intrafamilial variability, including often elusive maternal inheritance, syndromic or nonsyndromic multisystem involvement, and variably severe laboratory abnormalities. Disorders due to mutations in nDNA are inherited as Mendelian traits and include "direct hits," or mutations directly affecting subunits of the RC; "indirect hits," or mutations in proteins needed for the proper assembly of individual RC complexes; and defects of intergenomic signaling, such as mutations in proteins needed for the maintenance of mtDNA (translation, replication, repair). The central disorder of pediatric interest is Leigh syndrome (LS), which reflects the consequences of impaired energy metabolism on the developing brain and is characterized clinically by psychomotor regression and signs of brain stem dysfunction; radiologically, it is characterized by bilateral, symmetrical lesions in the basal ganglia and the brain stem. LS is associated with both mtDNA- and nDNA-related disorders and with defects of pyruvate metabolism (see Chapter 154).

### HISTORY

The first pathogenic mutations in mtDNA were reported 1988, when Holt and colleagues described large-scale deletions in patients with mitochondrial myopathies and Wallace and colleagues described a point mutation in the gene encoding subunit 4 of complex I (ND4) in a family with Leber hereditary optic neuropathy (LHON). However, these 2 papers opened up a veritable Pandora's box: the "morbidity map" of mtDNA has gone from the 1-point mutation of 1988 to over 200 pathogenic point mutations in 2008 (Fig. 153-1). In 1995, Bourgeron and colleagues described the first "direct hit" mutation in nDNA in 2 sisters with LS and complex II deficiency; the first "indirect hit" also caused LS and was due to mutations in SURF1, a protein needed to assemble cytochrome c oxidase (COX, complex IV of the RC); 2 papers, 1 published in 1989 and the other in 1991, suggested that mutations in nDNA-encoded maintenance proteins were responsible for multiple mtDNA deletions in patients with autosomal dominant progressive external ophthalmoplegia (PEO) and for mtDNA depletion in 2 infants with myopathic or hepatocerebral presentations. Multiple specific nuclear genes have since been associated with defects of intergenomic communication.

### MITOCHONDRIAL GENETICS

Given the importance of mtDNA-related diseases, all practicing pediatricians ought to be familiar with the rules of mitochondrial genetics, which differ from those of Mendelian genetics in the following ways:

1. *Heteroplasmy and threshold effect.* Each cell contains hundreds or thousands of mtDNA copies, which, during cell division, distribute randomly among daughter cells. In normal tissues, all mtDNA molecules are identical (homoplasmy). Most deleterious mutations of mtDNA usually affect some but not all mtDNAs within a cell, a tissue, or an individual (heteroplasmy), and the clinical expression of a pathogenic mtDNA mutation is largely determined by the relative proportion of normal and mutant genomes in different tissues. A minimum critical number of mutant mtDNAs is required to cause mitochondrial dysfunction in a particular organ or tissue and mitochondrial disease in an individual (*threshold effect*).
2. *Mitotic segregation.* At cell division, the proportion of mutant mtDNAs in daughter cells may shift, and the phenotype may change accordingly. This phenomenon, called *mitotic segregation*, explains how certain patients with mtDNA-related disorders may actually shift from one clinical phenotype to another as they grow older.

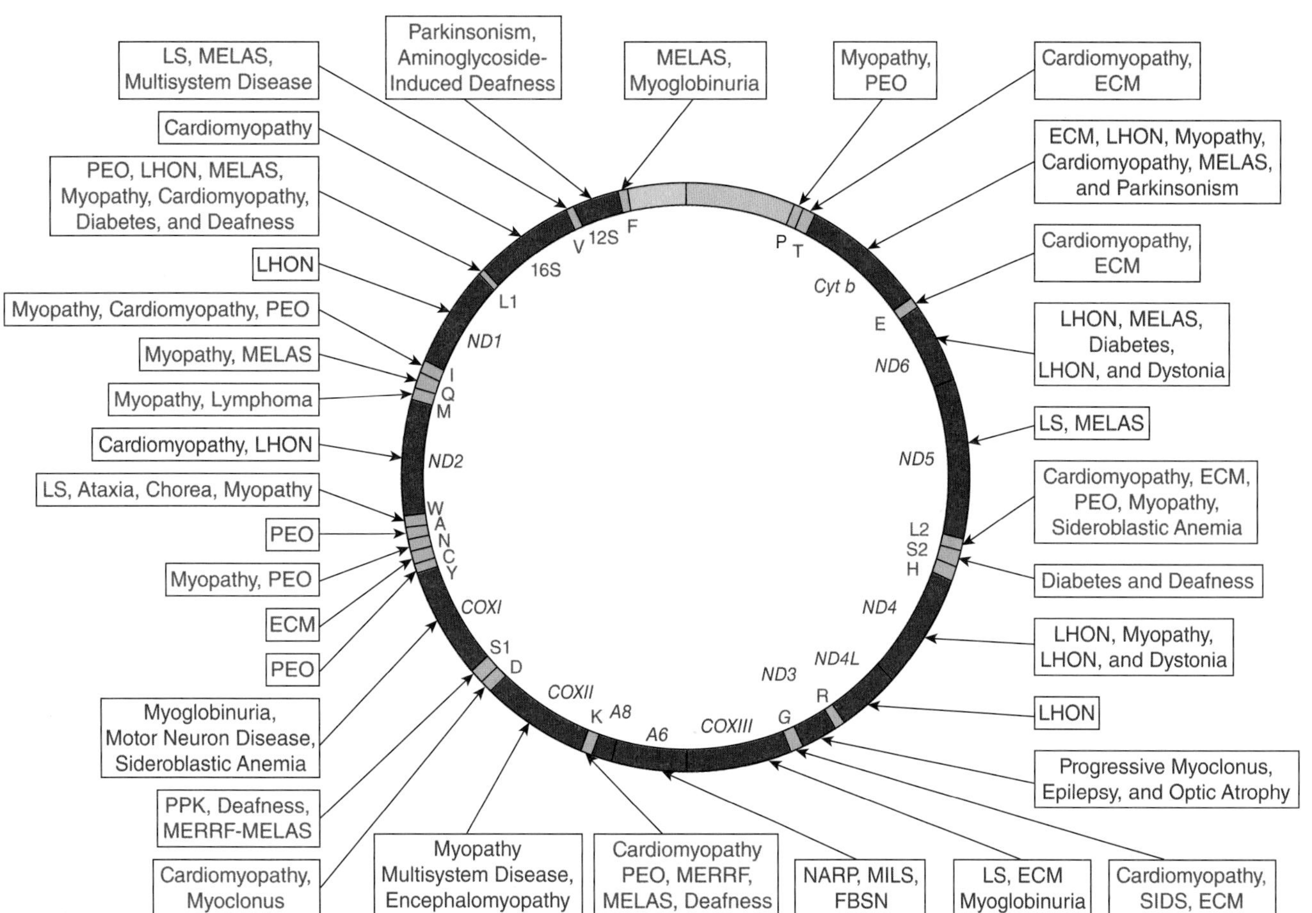


**FIGURE 153-1** Morbidity map of the human genome. Differently shaded areas in the 15.5-kb mtDNA map represent the protein-coding genes for the 7 subunits of complex I (ND), 3 subunits of complex IV (COX), cytochrome b (Cyt b), 2 subunits of ATP synthetase (ATPase 6 and 8), 12S and 16S rRNA, and the 22 trNAs. One-letter codes represent the corresponding amino acids. FBSN, familial bilateral striatal necrosis; KSS, Kearns-Sayre syndrome; LHON, Leber hereditary optic neuropathy; MELAS, mitochondrial encephalomyopathy, lactic acidosis, and stroke-like episodes; MERRF, myoclonic epilepsy with ragged red fibers; MILS, maternally inherited Leigh syndrome; NARP, neuropathy, ataxia, retinitis pigmentosa; PEO, progressive external ophthalmoplegia.



3. *Maternal inheritance.* At fertilization, all mtDNA derives from the oocyte. Therefore, the mode of transmission of mtDNA and of mtDNA point mutations (single deletions of mtDNA are usually sporadic events) differs from Mendelian inheritance. A mother carrying an mtDNA point mutation will pass it on to all her children (males and females), but only her daughters will transmit it to their progeny. A disease expressed in both sexes in a family but with no evidence of paternal transmission is strongly suggestive of an mtDNA point mutation.

Over 200 point mutations and innumerable large-scale rearrangements have been associated with a bewildering variety of diseases (Figs. 153-1 and 153-2). This is not surprising when one considers that mitochondria are ubiquitous organelles and that all human tissues, in isolation or in various combinations, can be affected by mtDNA mutations. This concept is illustrated in Table 153-1, which summarizes the symptoms and signs described in mitochondrial encephalomyopathies due to single rearrangements (Kearns-Sayre syndrome [KSS], Pearson syndrome [PS], and progressive external ophthalmoplegia [PEO]); due to point mutations in genes affecting protein synthesis in toto (mitochondrial encephalomyopathy, lactic acidosis, and stroke-like episodes [MELAS]; myoclonus epilepsy and ragged red fibers [MERRF]); and due to mutations affecting a protein-coding gene (neuropathy, ataxia, retinitis pigmentosa [NARP] and maternally inherited Leigh syndrome [MILS]). This table highlights the clinical features of the most common syndromes, which are difficult to miss in typical patients. However, it also serves to remind the astute clinician that any combination of these symptoms and signs should raise the suspicion of an mtDNA-related disorder.

## CLINICAL PRESENTATIONS

### Disorders due to mtDNA Mutations

Among the maternally inherited encephalomyopathies, 4 syndromes are more common. The first is MELAS (mitochondrial encephalomyopathy, lactic acidosis, and stroke-like episodes), which usually presents in children or young adults after normal early development. Symptoms include recurrent vomiting; migraine-like headaches; and stroke-like episodes causing cortical blindness, hemiparesis, or hemianopia. Magnetic resonance imaging (MRI) of the brain shows "infarcts" that do not correspond to the distribution of major vessels, raising the question of whether the strokes are vascular or metabolic in nature. The most common mtDNA mutation is A3243G in the *tRNA*$^{Leu(UUR)}$ gene, but about a dozen other mutations have been associated with MELAS.

The second syndrome is MERRF (myoclonus epilepsy with ragged red fibers), characterized by myoclonus, seizures, mitochondrial myopathy, and cerebellar ataxia. Less common signs include dementia, hearing loss, peripheral neuropathy, and multiple lipomas. The typical mtDNA mutation in MERRF is A8344G in the *tRNA*$^{Lys}$ gene, but other mutations in the same gene have been reported.

The third syndrome comes in 2 subtypes. The first is NARP (neuropathy, ataxia, retinitis pigmentosa), which usually affects young adults and causes retinitis pigmentosa, dementia, seizures, ataxia, proximal weakness, and sensory neuropathy. The second is a maternally inherited form of Leigh syndrome (MILS). NARP and MILS can affect maternal relatives in the same family (NARP with ~79% mutant load; MILS with ~90% mutant load).

The fourth syndrome, Leber hereditary optic neuropathy (LHON), is characterized by acute or subacute loss of vision in young adults,

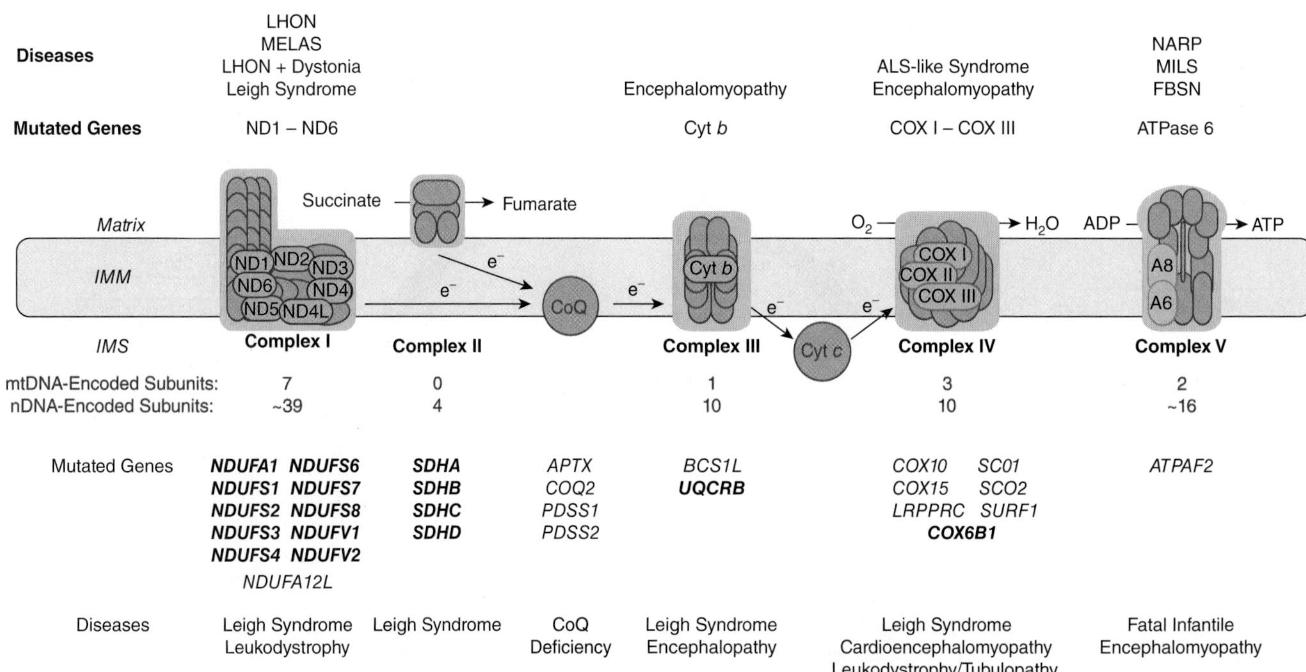


**FIGURE 153-2** Schematic representation of the mitochondrial respiratory chain (RC), showing nDNA-encoded subunits (blue) and mtDNA-encoded subunits in different colors. Protons are pumped from the matrix to the intermembrane space (IMM) through complexes I, III, and IV and are pumped back to the matrix through complex V to produce ATP. Coenzyme Q (CoQ) and cytochrome c (Cyt c) are electron (e-) transfer carriers. Diseases due to mutations in mtDNA (above the CR) or to mutations in nDNA (below the RC) are listed according to the correspondingly affected RC complex. Mutant genes shown in bold encode subunits of RC complexes ("direct hits"); mutant genes shown in plain font encode assembly factors. ALS, amyotrophic lateral sclerosis; FBSN, familial bilateral striatal necrosis; LHON, Leber hereditary optic neuropathy; MELAS, mitochondrial encephalomyopathy, lactic acidosis, and stroke-like episodes; MILS, maternally inherited form of Leigh syndrome; NARP, neuropathy ataxia retinitis pigmentosa; SDH, succinate dehydrogenase; TCA, tricarboxylic acid.



more frequently males, due to bilateral optic atrophy. Mutations in 3 genes of complex I (ND genes) have been associated with LHON: G11778A in *ND4*, G3460A in *ND1*, and T14484C in *ND6*.

Three sporadic conditions are associated with mtDNA single deletions: Kearns-Sayre syndrome (KSS), progressive external ophthalmoplegia (PEO), and Pearson syndrome (PS). KSS is a multisystem disorder with onset before age 20; symptoms include impaired eye movements (PEO), pigmentary retinopathy, and heart block. Frequent additional signs include ataxia, dementia, and endocrine problems (diabetes mellitus, short stature, hypoparathyroidism). Lactic acidosis and markedly elevated cerebrospinal fluid (CSF) protein (> 100 mg/dL) are typical laboratory abnormalities.

PEO is a relatively benign disorder characterized by ptosis, PEO, and proximal myopathy. Sideroblastic anemia and exocrine pancreatic dysfunction characterize PS, a commonly fatal disorder of infancy.

Two mtDNA genes encoding subunits of complex I (*ND3* and *ND5*) have to be considered when confronted with patients with LS or MELAS, even if maternal inheritance is absent or not obvious, if ragged red fibers are not abundant, and if lactic acidosis is not severe.

It is often stated that any patient exhibiting multiple organ involvement and evidence of maternal inheritance should be suspected of harboring a pathogenic mtDNA mutation until proven otherwise. While this rule of thumb has some practical value, it is also important to remember that the reverse is not true—that is, patients with involvement of a single tissue and no evidence of maternal inheritance can still harbor pathogenic mutations in their mtDNA. This is especially true for skeletal muscle. We have mentioned previously how isolated myopathy with PEO can be due to single large-scale mtDNA deletions. Isolated myopathy without PEO has been associated with point mutations in several tRNA genes. In addition, exercise intolerance, myalgia, and myoglobinuria can be the sole presentation of RC defects due to mutations in protein-coding genes.

### Disorders Due to Mutations in nDNA

"Direct hits" refer to mutations in genes encoding subunits of the RC. Until very recently, only pathogenic mutations in subunit A of complex II and in a handful of complex I subunits have been associated with disease, usually LS and leukoencephalopathy (see Fig. 153-2). A mutation in the ubiquitously expressed COX6b1 subunit has now been associated with cystic leukoencephalopathy, the first direct hit affecting complex IV.

"Indirect hits" are mutations that alter proteins that are not subunits of the RC but that are indispensable for the correct assembly of RC complexes. These have been described for all complexes except complex II (see Fig. 153-2). They cause a variety of multisystemic syndromes, often characterized by encephalopathy (LS or LS-like) and the selective involvement of another organ or tissue, which can offer a diagnostic clue (eg, cardiomyopathy in patients with *SCO2* mutations). For practitioners, mutations in the *SURF1* gene are especially important, because they are the most common causes of COX-deficient LS, which in turn is one of the most common forms of LS. Neuroradiologic LS-like lesions are also present in infants with congenital lactic acidosis; renal tubulopathy; liver failure with hepatosiderosis; and encephalopathy with psychomotor retardation, a devastating syndrome labeled GRACILE (growth retardation, aminoaciduria, cholestasis, iron overload, lactic acidosis, and early death) due to mutations in an assembly protein (BCS1L) for complex III (see Fig. 153-2).

A relatively recent addition to this group of disorders is coenzyme $Q_{10}$ ($CoQ_{10}$) deficiency, which can cause 4 major autosomal recessive syndromes. The first is a predominantly myopathic form, with exercise intolerance and recurrent myoglobinuria, as well as central nervous system involvement, with seizures, ataxia, or mental retardation. The second is a predominantly ataxic form, mimicking spinocerebellar ataxia, with prominent cerebellar atrophy and a variety of inconsistently associated features, including seizures, mental retardation, pyramidal signs, and peripheral neuropathy. The third syndrome is

**TABLE 153-1 CLINICAL FEATURES IN MITOCHONDRIAL DISEASE DUE TO mtDNA MUTATIONS**

| | | Δ-mtDNA | | tRNA | | ATPase | |
|---|---|---|---|---|---|---|---|
| **Tissue** | **Symptom/Sign** | **Kearns-Sayre Syndrome (KSS)** | **Pearson Syndrome** | **Myoclonic Epilepsy and Ragged Red Fibers (MERRF)** | **Mitochondrial Encephalomyopathy, Lactic Acidosis, and Stroke-Like Episodes (MELAS)** | **Neuropathy, Ataxia, Retinitis Pigmentosa (NARP)** | **Maternally Inherited Leigh Syndrome (MILS)** |
| **Central Nervous System (CNS)** | Seizures | – | – | + | + | – | + |
| | Ataxia | + | – | + | + | + | ± |
| | Myoclonus | – | – | + | ± | – | – |
| | Psychomotor retardation | – | – | – | – | – | + |
| | Psychomotor regression | + | – | ± | + | – | – |
| | Hemiparesis/hemianopia | – | – | – | + | – | – |
| | Cortical blindness | – | – | – | + | – | – |
| | Migraine-like headaches | – | – | – | + | – | – |
| | Dystonia | – | – | – | + | – | + |
| **PNS** | Peripheral neuropathy | ± | – | ± | ± | + | – |
| **Muscle** | Weakness/exercise intolerance | + | – | + | + | + | + |
| | Ophthalmoplegia | + | ± | – | – | – | – |
| | Ptosis | + | – | – | – | – | – |
| **Eye** | Pigmentary retinopathy | + | – | – | – | + | ± |
| | Optic atrophy | – | – | – | – | ± | ± |
| | Cataracts | – | – | – | – | – | – |
| **Blood** | Sideroblastic anemia | ± | + | – | – | – | – |
| **Endocrine** | Diabetes mellitus | ± | – | – | ± | – | – |
| | Short stature | + | – | + | + | – | – |
| | Hypoparathyroidism | ± | – | – | – | – | – |
| **Heart** | Conduction block | + | – | – | ± | – | – |
| | Cardiomyopathy | ± | – | – | ± | – | ± |
| **Gastrointestinal** | Exocrine pancreatic dysfunction | ± | + | – | – | – | – |
| | Intestinal pseudo-obstruction | – | – | – | – | – | – |
| **ENT** | Sensorineural hearing loss | – | – | + | + | ± | – |
| **Kidney** | Fanconi syndrome | ± | ± | – | ± | – | – |
| **Laboratory** | Lactic acidosis | + | + | + | + | – | ± |
| | Muscle biopsy: ragged red fibers | + | ± | + | + | – | – |
| **Inheritance** | Maternal | – | – | + | + | + | + |
| | Sporadic | + | + | – | – | – | – |

ENT, ear, nose, and throat; PNS, peripheral nervous system.

a pure myopathy, with exercise intolerance and proximal limb weakness. The fourth presentation is a mitochondrial encephalomyopathy associated with nephrosis. This association is an important clue to the correct diagnosis, because other RC disorders are often associated with renal tubular dysfunction but rarely with glomerular disease. As has long been suspected, mutations in several genes directly or indirectly involved in $CoQ_{10}$ biosynthesis have been identified, and more will undoubtedly be discovered. Diagnosing $CoQ_{10}$ deficiency has practical importance, because many patients respond, some very effectively, to $CoQ_{10}$ supplementation.

### Disorders Due to Defects in Intergenomic Signaling

In these disorders, mutations in nuclear genes cause qualitative (multiple deletions) or quantitative (depletion) alterations of mtDNA. Multiple deletions and depletion often coexist, because they are commonly due to altered control of the intramitochondrial nucleotide pool, which is essential for maintaining mtDNA.

The most common clinical feature of patients with multiple mtDNA deletions in skeletal muscle is PEO, which can be inherited as an autosomal dominant or recessive trait (Table 153-2). Autosomal dominant PEO has been associated with mutations in 4 genes that

**TABLE 153-2 SYNDROMES, GENES, AND PROTEINS ASSOCIATED WITH MULTIPLE mtDNA DELETIONS**

| Syndrome | nDNA Gene | Protein |
|---|---|---|
| MNGIE | *TYMP* | Thymidine phosphorylase (TP) |
| AD-PEO | *ANT1* | Adenine nucleotide translocator (ANT) |
| AD-PEO | *PEO1* | Helicase (twinkle) |
| AD-PEO/AR-PEO | *POLG* | Polymerase γ |
| AD-PEO, hearing loss | *POLG2* | Polymerase γ accessory subunit |
| AD-PEO, visual and hearing loss | *OPA1* | Dynamin-related GTPase |

AD, autosomal dominant; AR, autosomal recessive; MNGIE, mitochondrial neurogastrointestinal encephalopathy; PEO, progressive external ophthalmoplegia.

encode proteins involved in mitochondrial nucleotide metabolism: *ANT1*, encoding an isoform of the adenine nucleotide transporter; *PEO1* (formerly known as *Twinkle*), encoding a helicase; and *POLG*, encoding the mitochondrial γ polymerase. Autosomal dominant PEO with visual and hearing loss can also be due to mutations in *OPA1*, which encodes a dynamin-related GTPase essential for mitochondrial motility and is more often associated with dominant optic atrophy (DOA), the Mendelian counterpart of the maternally inherited LHON (see above).

Mutations in *POLG* are especially interesting for many reasons. First, they appear to be the most common causes of Mendelian PEO. Second, they can cause both dominant and recessive forms of PEO. Third, they have been associated with a striking variety of clinical features, including sensory ataxic neuropathy, dysarthria, and ophthalmoplegia (SANDO), mitochondrial recessive ataxic syndrome (MIRAS), deafness, hypogonadism, seizures, myoclonus, affective disorders, and gastrointestinal dysmotility. Fourth, and crucially important for pediatricians, *POLG* mutations are the most common causes of Alpers syndrome, a disorder of childhood characterized by liver insufficiency and gray matter involvement (poliodystrophy) and accompanied by mtDNA depletion (see below). This clinical heterogeneity is largely explained by the complexity of the enzyme, which comprises an exonuclease domain with proofreading function, and a polymerase domain with mtDNA-replicating function, connected by a "linker" domain. A fifth noteworthy feature of *POLG* mutations is that they can also affect the gene (*POLG2*) encoding the accessory rather than the catalytic subunit and can cause autosomal recessive PEO.

A special autosomal recessive form of PEO that combines multiple deletions and depletion of mtDNA in muscle is MNGIE (mitochondrial neurogastrointestinal encephalomyopathy), a disorder of young adults characterized by PEO, peripheral neuropathy, leukoencephalopathy, and severe gastrointestinal dysmotility leading to cachexia and early death. The gene (*TYMP*) responsible for MNGIE encodes the enzyme thymidine phosphorylase (TP); although extramitochondrial, mutated TP alters the homeostasis of the intramitochondrial nucleotide pool.

Two main syndromes have been associated with mtDNA depletion, one dominated by myopathy and the other by liver and brain dysfunction. Myopathic mtDNA depletion can be fatal in infancy or later in childhood due to mutations in *TK2* (encoding thymidine kinase 2), with respiratory failure, but it may also affect the central nervous system (CNS) and mimic spinal muscular atrophy. The hepatocerebral form of mtDNA depletion usually manifests in infancy or early childhood and has been attributed to mutations in *POLG* (see above), *DGUOK* (encoding deoxyguanosine kinase), *SUCLA2* (encoding the b subunit of succinyl-CoA-synthase [SCS-A]), *SUCLG1* (encoding the a subunit of SCS-A), or *RRM2B* (encoding a p53-controlled ribonucleotide reductase subunit [p53R2]). Autosomal recessive hepatocerebral syndrome was also attributed to mutations in 2 genes that are not directly involved in nucleotide metabolism: *MPV17* (encoding an inner mitochondrial membrane protein) and *PEO1* (mutations in this gene can also cause autosomal dominant PEO and multiple mtDNA deletions, as described above). A homozygous mutation (R50Q) in *MPV17* causes a distinctive severe disorder dominated by peripheral neuropathy and liver failure in children of the Navajo Nation (Navajo neurohepatopathy [NNH]).

Defects of mtDNA translation have been associated with mutations in various nucleus-encoded factors needed for mitochondrial protein synthesis, including mitoribosomal proteins (MRPS16; MRPS22, resulting in multisystemic disease); mRNA-specific translation factors (LRPPRC, resulting in LS, Canadian type); general translation factors (EFG1, resulting in hepatocerebral syndrome; TSFM, resulting in encephalomyopathy or cardiomyopathy); tRNA processing and base-modification enzymes (pseudouridine synthetase; PUS1, resulting in myopathy, lactic acidosis, and sideroblastic anemia [MLASA]); and aminoacyl-tRNA synthetases (Arg-tRNA synthetase, resulting in pontocerebellar hypoplasia; Asp-tRNA synthetase, resulting in leukoencephalopathy; Gly-tRNA synthetase, resulting in Charcot-Marie-Tooth type 2 [CMT2] or in spinal muscular atrophy type V [SMA V]). As rare as these disorders are—at least until now—they should be considered in the differential diagnosis of more common pediatric neurology disorders, such as LS, leukodystrophy, and hepatocerebral syndrome.

#### Defects of the Lipid Milieu

The inner mitochondrial membrane (IMM) is essential for RC function. Thus, alterations of the phospholipid composition of the IMM may result in RC defects. This appears to be the case in Barth syndrome, an X-linked disorder of childhood manifesting as myopathy, cardiomyopathy, leukopenia, and growth retardation. The gene responsible for Barth syndrome (initially dubbed *G4.5* and now called *TAZ*) encodes a family of proteins called *tafazzins*, which share conserved regions with acyltransferases of diverse organisms. It has been documented in Barth syndrome that mutant tafazzins lead to impaired or altered synthesis of cardiolipin, the major phospholipid component of the IMM, which may impair the function of multiple RC complexes, including their ability to assemble in "supercomplexes."

#### Defects of Mitochondrial Dynamics

In most tissues, including the CNS, mitochondria are extremely dynamic organelles, which move constantly, split by fission, and fuse with one another. This gives mitochondria the ability to travel very long distances (eg, from the soma of a spinal cord motor neuron to the neuromuscular junction of a motor nerve in the toe), to spread energy in different areas of the cell, and to regulate their survival through mitophagy.

Although the RC may be affected only indirectly, disorders of mitochondrial dynamics are being described with increased frequency and generally affect the optic nerve (dominant optic atrophy due to mutations in *OPA1*), the peripheral nerve (CMT2 due to mutations in *MFN2*), or the long tracts in the CNS (hereditary spastic paraplegia [HSP]). In addition, there is also evidence that defects of mitochondrial motility may play a role in the pathogenesis of common neurodegenerative disorders.

## DIAGNOSTIC EVALUATION

The striking clinical heterogeneity of mitochondrial disorders poses a diagnostic challenge. The following 5 criteria may be of some help (Table 153-3).

#### Clinical Presentation

As noted earlier, the complexity of the clinical presentation can direct attention to mutations in mtDNA, especially when certain telltale symptoms coexist: short stature, neurosensory hearing loss, PEO, axonal neuropathy, diabetes mellitus, hypertrophic cardiomyopathy, or renal tubular acidosis. On the other hand, it is equally important not to exclude mtDNA mutations in patients who have involvement of a single tissue, such as myopathy, cardiomyopathy, or renal disease. If the renal involvement affects glomerular rather than tubular function, the possibility of $CoQ_{10}$ deficiency should be considered, as many $CoQ_{10}$ deficiencies are associated with nephrosis.

**TABLE 153-3 SYNDROMES, GENES, AND PROTEINS ASSOCIATED WITH mtDNA DEPLETION**

| Syndrome | nDNA Gene | Protein |
|---|---|---|
| Myopathy-plus | *TK2* | Mitochondrial thymidine kinase |
| | *RRM2B* | p53-controlled ribonucleotide reductase subunit |
| Hepatocerebral | *DGUOK* | Deoxyguanosine kinase |
| Alpers | *POLG* | Polymerase γ |
| | *SUCLA2* | β subunit of succinyl-CoA synthase (SCS-A) |
| | *SUCLG1* | α subunit of SCS-A |
| | *PEO1* | Helicase (twinkle) |
| | *MPV17* | IMM protein |
| MNGIE | *TYMP* | Thymidine phosphorylase |

MNGIE, mitochondrial neurogastrointestinal encephalomyopathy.

#### Inheritance

Because most mtDNA-related disorders are maternally inherited but clinical expression is extremely variable, it is crucially important to collect a meticulous family history, with special attention to soft signs in maternal relatives, such as short stature, migraines, deafness, and diabetes. However, lack of maternal inheritance does not exclude the diagnosis (such as in cases of KSS and myopathy, discussed previously). In children with LS, inheritance is an important initial discriminator across mtDNA-related forms (MILS; mutations in *ND5* or *ND3*) and Mendelian forms (complex I subunits, COX assembly factors, $CoQ_{10}$ deficiency, defects of mtDNA translation).

#### Laboratory Findings

Lactic acidosis is a common finding in defects of the RC, and the lactate-to-pyruvate ratio is usually elevated (50:1 to 200:1, compared to a normal ratio of 25:1). Information about CSF lactate and pyruvate is important because CSF values can be increased in children with encephalopathy and normal blood lactate. However, lack of lactic acidosis does not exclude the diagnosis. For example, in patients with NARP or MILS, blood lactate and pyruvate can be normal or only mildly elevated. Serum creatine kinase (CK) levels are usually normal or modestly increased except in patients with myopathy during episodes of myoglobinuria. As another exception to this rule and as a useful diagnostic clue, serum CK values can be markedly elevated in children with the myopathic form of mtDNA depletion, such as those with mutations in the gene (*TK2*) encoding thymidine kinase. Another important laboratory test is serum thymidine, which is greatly increased in patients with MNGIE (see Table 153-3).

#### Neuroradiology

Bilateral signal hyperintensities in the basal ganglia on magnetic resonance imaging are typical of LS. Stroke-like lesions in the posterior cerebral hemispheres are typically seen in patients with MELAS. Diffuse signal abnormality of the central white matter is characteristic of KSS, whereas basal ganglia calcifications are common in both MELAS and KSS. Leukodystrophy, sometimes cavitating, has been associated with mutations in an assembly protein of complex I, with a newly described mutation in *COX VIB1*, and in defects of mtDNA translation. Proton magnetic resonance spectroscopy reveals lactate accumulation in the CSF and in specific areas of the brain, where lactate concentration can be compared to the concentration of *N*-acetyl-L-aspartate (NAA), an indicator of neuronal viability.

#### Exercise Physiology

Impaired oxygen extraction by exercising muscle can be detected by near-infrared spectroscopy, which measures the degree of deoxygenation of hemoglobin. A simpler test is based on measuring the partial pressure of oxygen ($PO_2$) in cubital venous blood after forearm aerobic exercise. $PO_2$ rises paradoxically in patients with mitochondrial myopathy or PEO, and the degree of rise reflects the severity of oxidative impairment. By $^{31}$P-magnetic resonance spectroscopy, the ratio of phosphocreatine to inorganic phosphate (PCr to Pi) can be measured in muscle at rest, during exercise, and during recovery. In patients with mitochondrial dysfunction, PCr-to-Pi ratios are lower than normal at rest, decrease excessively during exercise, and return to baseline more slowly than normal.

## PATHOLOGY

Muscle biopsy plays a central role in diagnosing mitochondrial disorders. Abnormal mitochondrial proliferation, a hallmark of mitochondrial dysfunction, can be revealed with the modified Gomori trichrome stain ("ragged red fibers" [RRF]) or, better, with the succinate dehydrogenase (SDH) reaction ("ragged blue fibers"). RRF are present in muscle biopsies taken from patients with most disorders due to mtDNA mutations, in which—because of heteroplasmy—they show a "checkerboard" pattern. Rare exceptions to this rule include NARP/MILS and LHON, given the high percentage of heteroplasmy or homoplasmy in these disorders. RRF are also present in Mendelian mitochondrial diseases, especially in those due to defects of intergenomic signaling.

The cytochrome c oxidase (COX) histochemical reaction typically reveals scattered COX-negative fibers, which usually correspond to—but are not confined to—RRF. RRF are COX positive in 2 main conditions: (1) typical MELAS syndrome and (2) mutations in mtDNA genes encoding cytochrome b or complex I subunits. To confirm the pathogenicity of an mtDNA mutation, single fibers can be dissected out of thick cross-sections of muscle and used to determine the levels of a given mutation by polymerase chain reaction (PCR). Finding higher levels of the mutation in affected (RRF or COX-negative fibers) than in unaffected (non-RRF, COX-positive fibers) fibers is strong evidence that the mutation in question is pathogenic.

A simple and elegant stratagem to reveal COX-deficient (as opposed to COX-negative) fibers is to superimpose the SDH and COX stain. In normal conditions, the brown COX stain prevails in all fibers, whereas the blue SDH stain "shines through" in COX-deficient fibers. When the COX stain is uniformly decreased in all fibers (rather than in a mosaic pattern), this points toward nucleus-encoded defects of complex IV, such as *SURF1* mutations in LS.

Electron microscopy has lost much of its historical diagnostic value, but it can reveal focal accumulations of mitochondria or mitochondrial with paracrystalline inclusions in cases in which histochemical results are equivocal.

The neuropathology in mitochondrial encephalomyopathies consists of 4 basic histologic lesions: spongy degeneration, neuronal loss, gliosis, and demyelination. While these lesions are nonspecific, their distribution patterns vary in patients with different mtDNA-related disorders. Thus, the neuropathology of KSS is characterized by spongiform degeneration, which is usually generalized and affects both gray and white matter. In MELAS, multifocal necrosis predominates, affecting the cerebral cortex or the subcortical white matter, and the cerebellum, thalamus, and basal ganglia. Calcification of basal ganglia is also common. In MERRF, neuronal degeneration, astrocytosis, and demyelination affect preferentially the cerebellum (especially the dentate nucleus), the brain stem (especially the olivary nucleus), and the spinal cord. In LS, there are symmetrical, bilateral foci of necrosis in the basal ganglia, thalamus, midbrain, and pons. Microscopically, the lesions show vascular proliferation, gliosis, neuronal loss, demyelination, and cystic cavitation.

## BIOCHEMISTRY

All 13 proteins encoded by mtDNA are components of the mitochondrial RC. Seven (ND1–ND5, ND4L, and ND6) are subunits of complex I, 1 (cytochrome b) is part of complex III, 3 (COX I, COX II, and COX III) are subunits of complex IV, and 2 (ATPase 6 and ATPase 8) are subunits of complex V (see Fig. 153-2). Therefore, disorders caused by mutations of mtDNA (regardless of whether they are primary or secondary to defects of intergenomic communication) are usually associated with biochemical defects of oxidative phosphorylation. Skeletal muscle is the preferred tissue for biochemical analysis, because it is rich in mitochondria, it is invariably affected in multisystem disorders (mitochondrial encephalomyopathies), and it is the most common tissue affected in isolation (mitochondrial myopathies). There is some controversy about whether fresh muscle tissue is needed or if frozen tissue suffices. It is our view that—except for the rare cases in which freshly isolated mitochondria for polarographic analyses are required—frozen specimens provide adequate biochemical information. Because mitochondrial proliferation in muscle (RRF) is a common occurrence, activities of RC complexes should be referred to the activity of citrate synthase, a nuclear-encoded enzyme of the mitochondrial matrix that is a good marker of mitochondrial abundance.

Biochemical studies in muscle extract from patients with mitochondrial disorders yield 2 main types of results. The first pattern consists of partial defects in the activities of multiple complexes containing mtDNA-encoded subunits (I, III, and IV), contrasting with normal or increased activities of SDH (complex II) and citrate synthase. The second pattern is a severe deficiency in the activity of one specific respiratory complex. As a rule, the first pattern is found in patients with single or multiple mtDNA deletions (eg, KSS, SANDO), mtDNA depletion (eg, Alpers syndrome), or mutations in tRNA genes (eg, MELAS, MERRF), because these genetic errors impair mitochondrial protein synthesis in toto. The second pattern is also typical of mutations in mtDNA protein-coding genes. For example, mutations in the cytochrome b gene cause isolated complex III deficiency, or mutations in *SURF1* cause isolated COX deficiency. However, mutations in ND genes, which are encountered with increasing frequency in patients with MELAS, LS, LHON, or overlap syndromes, cause inconsistent and often modest impairment of complex I activity.

## MOLECULAR GENETICS

Human mtDNA is a 16,569-base pair circle of double-stranded DNA. It is highly compact and contains only 37 genes: 2 genes encode ribosomal RNAs (rRNAs), 22 encode transfer RNAs (tRNAs), and 13 encode polypeptides. Over 200 pathogenic mutations have been identified in mtDNA (see Fig. 153-1).

However, a large—and steadily increasing—number of mutations have been found in nuclear DNA that affect subunits of the RC directly or indirectly (assembly proteins, mtDNA integrity, translation or replication, and IMM lipid milieu). Thus, the "menu" for the molecular definition of an RC disease has become very long, and it is impossible (and prohibitively expensive) to sample every item in the list. The first decision is to consider whether the mutation is more likely to be in mtDNA or in nDNA. Although MitoChips, which allow sequencing of mtDNA in its entirety, are becoming accessible, it is still more rational to decide—on the basis of the criteria outlined above—whether the mutation affects mtDNA protein synthesis in toto or if it affects individual mtDNA-encoded proteins. If the mutation is more likely to affect the nuclear DNA, clinical and biochemical data will help one decide which nuclear genes to sequence. For example, an infant who is the product of a consanguineous union and has a severe mitochondrial myopathy with multiple RC defects and markedly decreased content of mtDNA in muscle should be screened for a *TK2* mutation. With the implementation of whole-exome and whole-genome next-generation DNA sequencing, it is increasingly likely that patients affected with a mitochondrial disorder will be diagnosed in this fashion, where the challenge will be to assess the clinical importance of DNA variants of uncertain significance in known or potential disease genes. Accurate molecular diagnosis is of practical importance, because it offers the parents of children with lethal diseases the option of prenatal diagnosis for future pregnancies and insights into the natural history of any specific disorder.

## TREATMENT

Treatment of mitochondrial diseases is still woefully inadequate. Besides palliative pharmacologic and surgical interventions directed at alleviating symptoms, approaches to therapy include (1) removing toxic products, especially lactic acid; (2) administering artificial electron acceptors, such as vitamin $K_3$ and vitamin C; (3) administering metabolites and cofactors, such as L-carnitine and coenzyme $Q_{10}$ ($CoQ_{10}$); and (4) administering oxygen radical scavengers, such as $CoQ_{10}$. A simple and effective therapeutic approach is aerobic exercise, which prevents muscle deconditioning and improves functional and biochemical features of muscles harboring pathogenic mtDNA mutations.

Gene therapy is daunting in these conditions. However, if we could cause even a small shift in the relative proportion of mutant and normal mtDNAs, thus lowering the mutant load below the pathogenic threshold, we might significantly improve the clinical expression. Various strategies are being considered, including using peptide nucleic acids (PNAs) to inhibit the replication of complementary mutant mtDNAs or using pharmacologic approaches directed to eliminate mitochondria with high proportions of mutations. The observation that myoblasts often contain lesser amounts of pathogenic mtDNA mutations than mature muscle fibers has led to the use of myotoxic agents or isometric exercise to induce limited muscle damage, which is followed by regeneration of muscle fibers harboring lower mutational loads. Although these therapies have met with mixed results, they show our ability to affect mutational loads, at least in skeletal muscle.

Treatment of Mendelian mitochondrial disorders is also very limited. It is encouraging, however, that allogeneic bone marrow transplantation (the first stem cell therapy in this field) in a patient with MNGIE has resulted in steady clinical, laboratory, and biochemical improvement over 2 years.

## SUGGESTED READINGS

Chung WK, Martin K, Jalas C, et al. Mutations in COQ4, an essential component of coenzyme Q biosynthesis, cause lethal neonatal mitochondrial encephalomyopathy. *J Med Genet.* 2015;52:627-635.

DiMauro S, Hirano M, Schon EA. Approaches to the treatment of mitochondrial diseases. *Muscle Nerve.* 2006;34:265-283.

DiMauro S, Quinzii C, Hirano M. Mutations in coenzyme Q10 biosynthetic genes. *J Clin Invest.* 2007;117:587-589.

DiMauro S, Schon EA, Carelli V, Hirano M. The clinical maze of mitochondrial neurology. *Nat Rev Neurol.* 2013;9:429-444.

El-Hattab AW, Craigen WJ, Scaglia F. Mitochondrial DNA maintenance defects. *Biochim Biophys Acta.* 2017;1863(6):1539-1555. doi:10.1016/j.bbadis. 2017.02.017.

Holt IJ, Harding AE, Morgan Hughes JA. Deletions of muscle mitochondrial DNA in patients with mitochondrial myopathies. *Nature.* 1988;331:717-719.

Mayr JA. Lipid metabolism in mitochondrial membranes. *J Inherit Metab Dis.* 2015;38:137-144.

Mishra P, Chan DC. Mitochondrial dynamics and inheritance during cell division, development and disease. *Nat Rev Mol Cell Biol.* 2014;15:634-646.

Oskoui M, Davidzon G, Pascual J, et al. Clinical spectrum of mitochondrial DNA depletion due to mutations in the thymidine kinase 2 gene. *Arch Neurol.* 2006;63:1122-1126.

Spinazzola A, Viscomi C, Fernandez-Vizarra E, et al. MPV17 encodes an inner mitochondrial membrane protein and is mutated in infantile hepatic mitochondrial DNA depletion. *Nature Genet.* 2006; 38:570-575.

Wallace DC, Singh G, Lott MT, et al. Mitochondrial DNA mutation associated with Leber's hereditary optic neuropathy. *Science.* 1988;242:1427-1430.

Zhu Z, Yao J, Johns T, et al. SURF1, encoding a factor involved in the biogenesis of cytochrome c oxidase, is mutated in Leigh syndrome. *Nat Genet.* 1998;20:337-343.

# 154 Disorders of Energy Metabolism

Juan M. Pascual and Salvatore DiMauro

## INTRODUCTION

Surprisingly, the number of energy metabolism disorders compatible with life is still expanding, and their manifestations are reaching truly pleomorphic proportions. Collectively, these disorders spare no organ or tissue and can mimic many of the diseases routinely encountered by primary care clinicians. In addition to the well-known role of energy metabolism enzymes in balancing the flux of high-energy bonds inside cells and the supply of fuels to them, some also seem to serve multiple roles. For example, mutations in some pyruvate metabolism enzymes impair axonal migration and can also alter craniofacial configuration. Many mutations are linked to selective neuronal necrosis and apoptosis and to edema (spongiosis) of the cerebral white matter; paradoxically, most cause enhanced excitation and epilepsy and result in increased neuronal energy demands. These unexpected manifestations probably occur because flux through energy metabolism pathways sustains the synthesis and recycling of neurotransmitters and other signaling molecules by groups of neural cells. Consequently, the brain usually bears the full burden of these diseases, but cardiac and skeletal muscles, liver, and kidney are also frequently involved.

## PYRUVATE DEHYDROGENASE DEFICIENCY

Defects in the pyruvate dehydrogenase (PDH) complex are a frequent cause of lactic acidosis. PDH is a large mitochondrial matrix enzyme complex that catalyzes the oxidative decarboxylation of pyruvate to form acetyl-CoA, nicotinamide adenine dinucleotide (NADH), and carbon dioxide ($CO_2$). Symptoms vary considerably in patients with PDH complex deficiency, and almost equal numbers of males and females are affected, despite the location of the PDH E1 alpha subunit gene (*PDHA*) in the X chromosome, a paradox explained by selective female X-inactivation. Thus, the phenotype of PDH deficiency is dictated by mutation severity (especially in males) and by the pattern of X-inactivation in females. Dozens of *PDHA1* mutations have been identified. In addition, there are patients harboring mutations in the E1 beta subunit, the E2 dihydrolipoyl transacetylase segment of the complex, the E3 (dihydrolipoamide dehydrogenase) subunit, the E3-binding protein, the lipoyl-containing protein X, lipoyltransferase, and the PDH phosphatase (Table 154-1).

**TABLE 154-1 PYRUVATE METABOLISM DISORDERS**

| Disease | Biochemical Variants | Inheritance | Manifestations |
|---|---|---|---|
| Pyruvate dehydrogenase deficiency | E1a | X-linked | Lactic acidosis |
| | E1b | AR | Episodic ataxia |
| | E2 | AR | Cerebral dysgenesis |
| | E3 | AR | Infantile epilepsy |
| | Pyruvate dehydrogenase phosphatase | AR | Leigh syndrome |
| | X protein | AR | Alternating hemiplegia |
| | Lipoyltransferase | AR | Lactic acidosis |
| Pyruvate carboxylase deficiency | A (infantile) | AR | Lactic acidosis |
| | B (neonatal) | AR | Hyperammonemia |
| | C (benign) | AR | Hypercitrullinemia |
| | | | Basal ganglia necrosis |
| | | | Infantile epilepsy |

AR, autosomal recessive



Neonates with pyruvate dehydrogenase complex (PDC) defects may present with severe acidosis caused by progressive lactate and pyruvate accumulation, hypotonia, microcephaly, partial, or total agenesis of the corpus callosum (Fig. 154-1), and dysmorphic features similar to those seen in fetal alcohol syndrome. The acidosis is

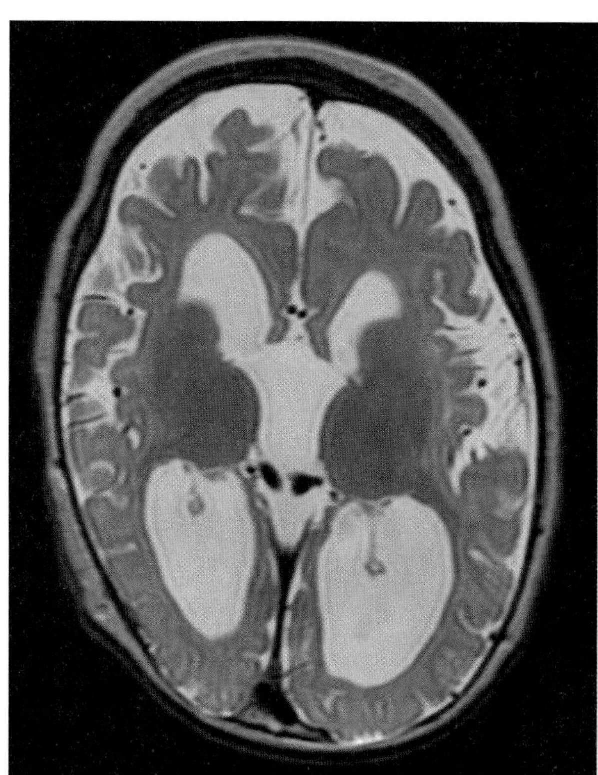

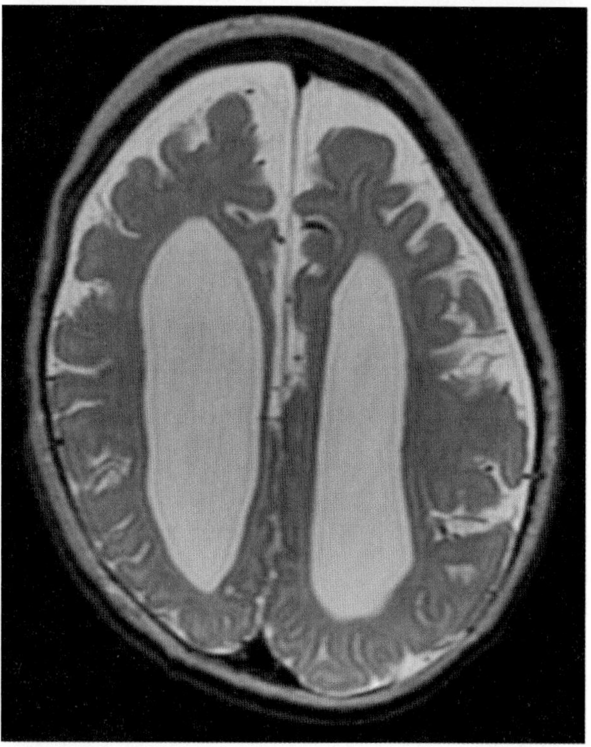

**FIGURE 154-1** Pyruvate dehydrogenase deficiency in a 10-month-old girl. T2-weighted magnetic resonance images showing axial sections at the level of the thalamus (top) and of the centrum semiovale (bottom). Severe cortical atrophy (predominantly in the frontal lobes and Sylvian opercula), white matter underdevelopment (more pronounced in the occipital lobes) and increased water content, and agenesis of the corpus callosum are characteristic features.

refractory to treatment, but thiamine pyrophosphate and dichloroacetate are often administered. If these infants survive this initial phase, they have severe neurologic impairment and often die by about 3 years of age. Some children present later during the first year of life with Leigh syndrome (LS). The clinical manifestations can be indistinguishable from forms caused by respiratory chain disorders (see Chapter 153).

Milder variants can present during infancy, childhood, or even adulthood with episodic cerebellar ataxia, which may occur spontaneously, be precipitated by carbohydrate intake, or occur in conjunction with otherwise mild infections. Dystonic attacks and progressive peripheral neuropathy may occur. Lactic acidosis is usually not found during testing of these patients, but mild postprandial hyperlactatemia may occur. The diagnosis of these disorders requires measurements of lactate and pyruvate in plasma and cerebrospinal fluid (lactate-to-pyruvate ratio <15); analysis of amino acids in plasma (hyperalaninemia) and of organic acids in urine (lactic, pyruvic acids); and neuroradiologic investigations, including magnetic resonance spectroscopy to detect lactate. Enzymatic analysis of fibroblast PDH activity is usually performed, and molecular diagnosis is available. A ketogenic diet together with thiamine supplementation can afford substantial benefit in responsive cases. Dichloroacetate is sometimes temporarily used to enhance lactate clearance.



## PYRUVATE CARBOXYLASE DEFICIENCY

Pyruvate carboxylase (PC) deficiency is an autosomal recessive disease due to mutation of the PC gene, which is located in chromosome 11. PC catalyzes the conversion of pyruvate to oxaloacetate when abundant acetyl-CoA is available, thus replenishing Krebs cycle intermediates in the mitochondrial matrix. The enzyme is bound to biotin. PC is involved in gluconeogenesis, lipogenesis, and neurotransmitter synthesis. PC deficiency presents with 3 degrees of phenotypic severity:

1. An infantile form (A) with moderate lactic acidosis, mental and motor deficits, hypotonia, pyramidal tract dysfunction, ataxia, and seizures leading to death in infancy. Episodes of vomiting, acidosis, and tachypnea can be triggered by metabolic imbalance or infection.
2. A severe neonatal form (B), presenting as severe lactic acidosis, hypoglycemia, hepatomegaly, depressed consciousness, and severely abnormal development. Abnormal limb and ocular movements are common findings. Brain magnetic resonance imaging reveals cystic periventricular leukomalacia. Hyperammonemia with mild hypercitrullinemia, high lactate-to-pyruvate ratio, paradoxical postprandial ketosis, and low glutamate comprise a very suggestive metabolic profile, mostly due to depletion of intracellular aspartate and oxaloacetate. Early death is common.
3. A rare benign form (C), presenting with episodic acidosis and moderate mental impairment compatible with survival and near-normal neurologic performance. A variety of mutations have been identified, some of which significantly impair PC activity. Enzymatic analysis of fibroblast PC activity can be performed, followed by genotyping. Dietary modification with triheptanoin (an odd chain triglyceride) supplementation has been attempted to increase acetyl-CoA and anaplerotic propionyl-CoA. Liver transplantation has also been performed.

## DISORDERS OF THE KREBS CYCLE

Several tricarboxylic acid enzymes are susceptible to mutations that cause severe mitochondrial dysfunction inherited as autosomal recessive traits. Autosomal recessive defects of aconitase, the E3 component of the α-ketoglutarate dehydrogenase complex (also shared by the pyruvate dehydrogenase complex); succinate dehydrogenase (SDH, also part of the mitochondrial respiratory chain and known as *complex II*); and fumarase (fumarate hydratase [FH]) are collectively associated with profound encephalopathy and excretion of specific metabolic precursors and by-products. The manifestations are pleomorphic. In the case of SDH, autosomal recessive mutations of subunit A cause LS (or optic atrophy in the elderly), while germline heterozygous mutations in subunits B, C, and D are associated with paraganglioma, and mutations in subunits B and D are associated with pheochromocytoma and severely reduced tumor SDH activity. Autosomal recessive FH mutations, which cause structural brain malformations, dysmorphic facial features, and neonatal polycythemia, are independently associated with uterine and cutaneous leiomyomas and with papillary renal cell cancer in germline carriers. Hence, the SDH- and FH-related tumors are inherited in an autosomal dominant fashion. E3 (dihydrolipoamide dehydrogenase) deficiency, a "crossroads" disorder, causes accumulation of pyruvate and branched-chain amino acids in plasma and excretion of branched-chain α-keto acids in urine. Succinyl-CoA synthetase complex defects presenting early in life as LS associated with mitochondrial depletion have been described recently. These patients present with an accumulation of succinyl carnitine and mild methylmalonic aciduria.

Mutations in *ACO2*, the gene encoding aconitase 2, the mitochondrial enzyme that interconverts citrate to isocitrate, cause severe infantile cerebellar-retinal degenerative syndrome or mild neurodegenerative symptoms with truncal ataxia and distal hypotonia.

## MITOCHONDRIAL TRANSPORTER DISORDERS

Mitochondria store and use a variety of energetic compounds that travel the outer and inner organelle membranes through specific transporters. The adenosine nucleotide (adenosine triphosphate and adenosine diphosphage) translocator (ANT1), the malate/aspartate shuttle, the voltage-dependent anion channels (VDAC), the carnitine translocase, and the recently identified pyruvate transporter are important representatives of an expanding class of molecules increasingly implicated in human disease states. For example, autosomal dominant *ANT1* mutations destabilize mitochondrial DNA maintenance, causing multiple mitochondrial DNA (mtDNA) deletions that manifest as progressive external ophthalmoplegia and facioscapulohumeral muscular dystrophy, whereas recessive mutations cause congenital heart defects, cataracts, and lactic acidosis.

## SUGGESTED READINGS


Briere JJ, Favier J, Gimenez-Roqueplo AP, Rustin P. Tricarboxylic acid cycle dysfunction as a cause of human diseases and tumor formation. *Am J Physiol Cell Physiol.* 2006;291(6):C1114-1120.

De Vivo DC. Complexities of the pyruvate dehydrogenase complex. *Neurology.* 1998;51(5):1247-1249.

Lissens W, De Meirleir L, Seneca S, et al. Mutations in the X-linked pyruvate dehydrogenase (E1) alpha subunit gene (PDHA1) in patients with a pyruvate dehydrogenase complex deficiency. *Hum Mutat.* 2000;15(3):209-219.

Maj MC, MacKay N, Levandovskiy V, et al. Pyruvate dehydrogenase phosphatase deficiency: identification of the first mutation in two brothers and restoration of activity by protein complementation. *J Clin Endocrinol Metab.* 2005;90(7):4101-4107.

Mochel F, DeLonlay P, Touati G, et al. Pyruvate carboxylase deficiency: clinical and biochemical response to anaplerotic diet therapy. *Mol Genet Metab.* 2005;84(4):305-312.

Nissenkorn A, Michelson M, Ben-Zeev B, Lerman-Sagie T. Inborn errors of metabolism: a cause of abnormal brain development. *Neurology.* 2001;56(10):1265-1272.

Roe CR, Mochel F. Anaplerotic diet therapy in inherited metabolic disease: therapeutic potential. *J Inherited Metab Dis.* 2006; 29(2-3):332-340.

Rustin P, Bourgeron T, Parfait B, Chretien D, Munnich A, Rotig A. Inborn errors of the Krebs cycle: a group of unusual mitochondrial diseases in human. *Biochim Biophys Acta.* 1997;1361(2):185-197.

Tein I. Carnitine transport: pathophysiology and metabolism of known molecular defects. *J Inherited Metab Dis.* 2003;26(2-3):147-169.

# 155 Mucopolysaccharidosis, Glycoproteinosis, and Mucolipidosis

Laurie A. Robak and V. Reid Sutton

## MUCOPOLYSACCHARIDOSES

### INTRODUCTION

The mucopolysaccharidoses (MPS) are a family of rare, progressive, multisystem lysosomal storage disorders that are caused by defects in the enzymes that catabolize glycosaminoglycans (GAGs). These disorders are clinically heterogeneous, but some common features include coarse facial features, hepatosplenomegaly, developmental delay/regression, umbilical/inguinal hernias, and a constellation of radiographic bone abnormalities known as dysostosis multiplex. There are 7 clinically defined MPS syndromes (MPS I, II, III, IV, VI, VII, and IX), which are caused by pathogenic variants in 1 of 11 genes (Table 155-1). Within each disorder, there is a wide spectrum of clinical effects ranging from mild to severe (phenotypic heterogeneity) depending on the degree of residual enzymatic activity. Intravenous enzyme replacement therapy is available for many of the MPS and is aimed at reducing the progression of non–central nervous system (CNS) symptoms. Hematopoietic stem cell transplantation (HCST), which is associated with substantial risks, may preserve cognitive function if performed early during the course of the disease.

### PATHOGENESIS AND EPIDEMIOLOGY

With the exception of MPS II (Hunter syndrome; X-linked), MPS are inherited in an autosomal recessive manner. In affected individuals, 1 or more specific GAGs—dermatan sulfate (DS), heparan sulfate (HS), keratan sulfate (KS), and chondroitin-6-sulfate—accumulate within the lysosomes, interfering with recycling of cellular material (Fig. 155-1). GAGs build up in the lysosome over time, affecting cellular function. Different GAGs are expressed in different tissues, leading to the variable manifestations seen in each of the MPS disorders. The estimated prevalence of MPS in the United States is approximately 1 in 25,000, although prevalence estimates vary in different parts of the world. Prevalence varies by disease and ethnicity.

### CLINICAL PRESENTATION

MPS disorders, like all lysosomal storage diseases, are progressive conditions. Infants typically do not manifest signs or symptoms at birth, and the disease is suspected as the phenotype evolves over time.

MPS disorders tend to present in 1 of 3 ways:

- With "coarse" facial features (eg, MPS IH, MPS II)
- With learning difficulties, behavioral disturbances, and developmental delay/regression (eg, MPS III)
- As a skeletal dysplasia (eg, MPS IV, VI)

When an MPS is suspected from clinical, laboratory, and radiologic findings, the diagnosis can be confirmed by enzyme assay on white blood cells or skin fibroblasts or by the identification of biallelic pathogenic variants in the particular gene. While qualitative or quantitative demonstration of increased urinary GAG excretion is supportive evidence of an MPS, urinary screening tests for MPS disorders have reduced sensitivity, particularly with dilute specimens and in individuals with mild disease. False-negative results, especially in MPS III and IV, are well recognized; therefore, a negative screening test should not dissuade the clinician from pursuing a diagnosis of an MPS disease when the clinical suspicion is high. Although algorithms aimed at helping the diagnostic process have been developed, their use in clinical practice is limited by the clinical heterogeneity in this group of disorders.

If urinary GAG analysis is normal and enzyme and molecular testing has not yielded a diagnosis of an MPS, other diagnostic possibilities should be considered. Urine oligosaccharide and sialic acid analysis should be undertaken to exclude oligosaccharidoses and other glycoproteinoses. White cell and plasma lysosomal enzyme studies should be performed to confirm abnormalities and to exclude galactosialidosis, mannosidosis, and related disorders. Radiographs should be reviewed to confirm the presence of dysostosis multiplex (Fig. 155-2), and abnormal lysosomal storage should be confirmed by examining a skin biopsy under electron microscopy. If all these investigations are normal, it is important to remember that some non-lysosomal disturbances can mimic storage diseases (eg, geleophysic dysplasia, Coffin-Lowry syndrome, Williams syndrome, and Costello syndrome).

There is a tendency to classify the individual MPS disorders into "mild" and "severe" subtypes, based either on survival or on the presence or absence of CNS disease. This is in reality a gross oversimplification; it is preferable to consider the disorders on a clinical spectrum. Although many are compatible with prolonged survival, for the majority of individuals, these are not benign conditions.

#### Mucopolysaccharidosis Type I

MPS I is traditionally divided into 3 different disorders: Hurler (MPS IH; Mendelian Inheritance in Man [MIM] no. 607014), Scheie (MPS IS; MIM no. 607016), and Hurler-Scheie (MPS IH-S; MIM no. 607015). Hurler is considered the most severe, with onset in the first few years of life, and Scheie the least severe, with onset in the second or third decade. With Hurler-Scheie, the age of onset and severity of symptoms are intermediate between Hurler and Scheie. All 3 diagnostic entities are caused by enzymatic deficiency of α-L-iduronidase, which is encoded by the *IDUA* gene. The diagnosis can be suggested by the finding of dermatan and heparan sulfate in the urine. Infants with Hurler syndrome appear normal at birth. Early manifestations may include inguinal/umbilical hernias, frequent upper respiratory infections, and otitis media. Coarsening of the facial features, caused by infiltration of GAGs in the soft tissues and dysostosis of the facial bones, emerges during the first 2 years of life and results in thickened lips, ear lobules, nose, and tongue (Fig. 155-3). Although growth for the first 12 to 18 months of life is normal, the skeletal deformities eventually lead to severe growth restriction. Although initially development may be normal, developmental delay is usually present by age 18 months, which may be followed by developmental plateauing and/or developmental regression. Upper respiratory tract obstruction may occur secondary to midface hypoplasia, enlarged tongue, and infiltration of the respiratory tract by accumulating GAGs. Obstructive sleep apnea is usual, and affected children require ear, nose, and throat (ENT) assessment. Hearing loss is common due to GAG accumulation, frequent otitis media, and damage to the eighth cranial nerve. A number of patients will have a large head circumference, and communicating hydrocephalus will develop in up to 40% of patients. The abdomen may become protuberant secondary to hepatosplenomegaly. Diarrhea is also a frequent complication of Hurler syndrome. Corneal deposition of GAGs becomes clinically apparent as corneal clouding during the second year of life (Fig. 155-4). Individuals may have a dysplastic odontoid process and are at risk of sudden and severe spinal cord damage secondary to atlantoaxial subluxation (Fig. 155-5). Carpal tunnel syndrome is frequent. Cardiac involvement, which includes progressive thickening of cardiac valves, is nearly universal and may lead to mitral/aortic regurgitation and cardiomyopathy. Prognosis depends on the severity of cardiac and respiratory involvement. Death typically occurs within the first 10 years of life due to cardiorespiratory complications.

**TABLE 155-1 THE MUCOPOLYSACCHARIDOSES (MPS)**

| Disease (Eponym) | Gene | Inheritance | Enzyme Deficiency | Airway Obstruction | Behavioral Problems | Cardiac Valve Disease | Cardio-myopathy | Carpal Tunnel | Coarse Facies | Corneal Clouding | Develop-mental Delay | Develop-mental Regression |
|---|---|---|---|---|---|---|---|---|---|---|---|---|
| MPS IH (Hurler) | *IDUA* | AR | α-L-iduronidase | +++ | +/– | +++ | + | +++ | +++ | + | +++ | +++ |
| MPS IH/S (Hurler-Scheie) | *IDUA* | AR | α-L-iduronidase | – | – | +++ | | +++ | +/– | + | – | +/– |
| MPS IS (Scheie) | *IDUA* | AR | α-L-iduronidase | – | – | +++ | | +++ | – | + | – | – |
| MPS II (Hunter) | *IDS* | XL | Iduronidate-2-sulfatase | + | + | + | + | + | + | – | + | + |
| MPS IIIA (Sanfilippo A) | *SGSH* | AR | Heparan-*N*-sulfatase | +/– | +++ | +/– | +/– | – | + | – | +++ | +++ |
| MPS IIIB (Sanfilippo B) | *NAGLU* | AR | *N*-Acetylglucosa-minidase | +/– | +++ | +/– | +/– | – | + | – | ++ | ++ |
| MPS IIIC (Sanfilippo C) | *HGSNAT* | AR | Acetyl-CoA: α-glucosaminide acetyltransferase | +/– | ++ | +/– | +/– | – | + | – | ++ | ++ |
| MPS IIID (Sanfilippo D) | *GNS* | AR | *N*-Acetylglucos-amine 6-sulfatase | +/– | +++ | +/– | +/– | – | + | – | ++ | ++ |
| MPS IVA (Morquio A) | *GALNS* | AR | Galactose-6-sulfatase | ++ | – | + | + | – | + | + | – | – |
| MPS IVB (Morquio B) | *GLB1* | AR | β-Galactosidase | ++ | – | + | + | – | + | + | – | – |
| MPS VI (Maroteaux-Lamy) | *ARSB* | AR | *N*-Acetylgalactos-amine-4-sulfatase | + | – | ++ | ++ | – | + | + | – | – |
| MPS VII (Sly) | *GUSB* | AR | β-Glucuronidase | +/– | +/– | + | +/– | – | + | +++ | + | +/– |
| MPS IX (Natowicz) | *HYAL1* | AR | Hyaluronidase | – | – | – | – | – | – | – | – | – |

At the other end of the clinical spectrum from Hurler syndrome are patients diagnosed in late childhood or early adult life with Scheie syndrome, usually because of orthopedic or ophthalmologic problems. In MPS IS, cognition is normal, and individuals may have a normal life span. Some patients require cardiac valve surgery, but the clinical picture tends to be dominated by bone and joint involvement. Carpal tunnel syndrome is almost universal. In some patients, corneal clouding limits vision to such a degree that corneal transplantation is necessary. Most patients tolerate this procedure well, and the transplanted cornea remains clear. However, before a patient undergoes this surgery, a careful assessment of retinal function is necessary to ensure that the visual loss is not secondary to retinopathy, which also occurs in MPS IS. Hearing loss is also common.

Between these 2 extremes is a continuous clinical spectrum that is often labeled Hurler-Scheie syndrome (Fig. 155-6). Symptoms typically develop between 3 and 10 years of age. These patients may develop late-onset neurologic deterioration, but most of the active clinical problems relate to progressive joint stiffness and degenerative bone disease. Hepatosplenomegaly may occur, but is less common than in Hurler syndrome. Spondylolisthesis of L5/S1 is very common and may require surgical repair (Fig. 155-7). Progressive visual loss due to a combination of corneal clouding and retinal disease is common, and many patients will develop progressive cardiac disease. Frequent chest infections, limited chest expansion, and upper respiratory obstruction are known complications. Sleep apnea can be troublesome, and routine pulse oximetry overnight during sleep should be performed annually. Some require continuous positive airway pressure (CPAP) via a nasal mask. In patients who cannot tolerate the tight-fitting mask or the noise of the machine, tracheostomy remains the only alternative. In general, this is poorly tolerated in MPS disorders, as it is often associated with an increase in airway secretions that requires frequent suction.

Enzyme replacement therapy (laronidase) is available for the non-neuronopathic manifestations of MPS I via a weekly infusion of 0.58 mg/kg over 4 hours. Laronidase does not cross the blood-brain barrier; therefore, it is thought that any apparent effect on neurologic function occurs through improvement in the patient's general condition. In most treated patients, there is a rapid reduction in urinary GAGs, followed by a much slower decline after the first 6 months of treatment. After 6 years of treatment, there is continued improvement in growth, shoulder flexion, and sleep apnea. Early treatment is essential to prevent some complications such as cardiac valve lesions. Most infusion-associated reactions have been mild and easily managed either by slowing the rate of infusion or premedicating with an antihistamine or corticosteroid. Anaphylaxis has been reported in a few patients. HSCT is recommended only for severe MPS I (Hurler) given the morbidity and mortality associated with this procedure.

#### Mucopolysaccharidosis Type II

The enzyme deficiency in MPS II is iduronidate 2-sulfatase, which is encoded by the *IDS* gene. In contrast to MPS I, MPS II (MIM no. 309900) is X-linked, meaning that males are typically affected, while females are carriers; however, a few cases have been described in females. Lack of significant corneal clouding distinguishes MPS II from MPS I. Like MPS I, there is significant heterogeneity in the age of onset as well as in severity and progression of symptoms. In severely affected patients, the diagnosis is usually established in the second year of life. The diagnosis can be suggested by the finding of dermatan and heparan sulfate in the urine. Symptoms include coarse facial appearance, hepatosplenomegaly, and joint contractures, particularly of the phalangeal joints. A nodular ivory rash around the scapulae and on the extensor surfaces is considered pathognomonic of the disorder but is rare in childhood. Most patients have short stature and macrocephaly. Additional findings include frequent upper respiratory infections, umbilical/inguinal hernias, and frequent otitis media. Dysostosis multiplex may develop over time. Developmental delay and/or regression may be present in more severe forms of the disease. The behavioral phenotype includes sleep disturbance, challenging behavioral problems, and attention deficit disorder. Diarrhea is common in the early-onset form of the disease. Cardiac valvar disease and cardiomyopathy may cause early morbidity and mortality. Carpal tunnel syndrome is frequent. It should be routinely screened for using a nerve conduction velocity test, and release should be performed when identified.

| Dysostosis Multiplex | Diarrhea | Frequent Otitis Media | Hearing Loss | HSM | Hernias | Joint Contractures | Macrocephaly | Restrictive Respiratory Disease | Seizures | Short Stature | Sleep Disturbance | Soft Tissue Swelling | Synovitis |
|---|---|---|---|---|---|---|---|---|---|---|---|---|---|
| +++ | +++ | +++ | + | +++ | + | +++ | +++ | +++ | – | +++ | – | – | – |
| + | + | | | + | | | | | – | ++ | – | – | – |
| + | + | | | | | | | | – | + | – | – | – |
| + | ++ | + | + | +++ | + | +++ | + | + | – | + | + | – | – |
| + | +++ | + | + | + | + | +/– | +/– | – | + | + | +++ | – | – |
| + | +++ | + | + | + | + | +/– | +/– | – | + | + | +++ | – | – |
| + | +++ | + | + | + | + | +/– | +/– | – | + | + | +++ | – | – |
| + | +++ | + | + | + | + | +/– | +/– | – | + | + | +++ | – | – |
| + | + | + | + | +/– | – | – | – | ++ | – | +++ | – | – | – |
| + | + | + | + | +/– | – | – | – | ++ | – | +++ | – | – | – |
| + | + | + | ++ | + | – | – | – | + | – | +++ | – | – | – |
| +++ | – | + | + | +++ | + | +++ | + | ++ | – | +++ | + | – | – |
| – | – | – | – | – | – | – | – | – | – | +/– | – | + | + |

In individuals with less severe forms of MPS II, intelligence may be preserved into adulthood. Cervical cord compression due to hyperplasia of the dura and ligamentum flavum can lead to a progressive cervical myelopathy (Fig. 155-8). This usually presents with decreasing exercise tolerance that can be mistaken for progression of joint stiffness. From the age of 10 years, these patients should have the craniocervical junction routinely evaluated by magnetic resonance imaging (MRI), and posterior decompression should be performed in those with cervical compromise. Atlantoaxial instability is usually not a feature of MPS II, as the odontoid process is usually well developed; therefore, spinal fusion in addition to the decompression is usually not required. Most adults with MPS II develop upper respiratory obstruction and sleep apnea. Many benefit from the use of nasal CPAP devices, although the masks often have to be shaped individually because of the abnormal facial anatomy.

Idursulfatase is approved for enzyme replacement therapy for MPS II at 0.5 mg/kg/wk. Treatment results in improvements in the 6-minute walk test, reductions in the degree of hepatosplenomegaly, decreased urinary GAG excretion, improved hearing, and improved joint range of motion. Like laronidase, it does not cross the blood-brain barrier and thus has no effect on cognitive function. HCST has shown promise in smaller studies, but requires further study to determine long-term efficacy in this group of patients.

#### Mucopolysaccharidosis Type III

MPS III, or Sanfilippo syndrome, is a clinically identical but biochemically heterogeneous group of 4 conditions all associated with an inability to catabolize heparan sulfate. MPS IIIA (MIM no. 252900) is the most common, caused by variants in the gene *SGSH*, which encodes for heparin-*N*-sulfatase. The next most frequent is MPS IIIB (*NAGLU*, *N*-acetylglucosaminidase; MIM no. 252920). Types IIIC (*HGSNAT*, acetyl-CoA:α-glucosaminide acetyltransferase; MIM no. 252930) and IIID (*GNS*, *N*-acetylglucosamine 6-sulfatase, MIM no. 252940) are very rare. In contrast to other MPS diseases, the hallmark of MPS III is prominent CNS involvement in the presence of a mild somatic phenotype. Because of this combination, the diagnosis is usually established much later in life (4–5 years) compared to other disorders. The diagnosis can be suggested by the finding of heparan sulfate in the urine. In a typically affected patient, the initial presentation is usually with developmental delay and mildly coarse facial features with dry, coarse hair, usually without hepatosplenomegaly. Somatic features are usually mild (Fig. 155-9). There is often a history of recurrent upper respiratory infections and hernias, and most patients have troublesome diarrhea. Sleep disturbance can present early in life and, in its extreme form, produces a reversal of the normal sleep/wake cycle.

Gradually, the behavioral phenotype evolves into severely challenging behaviors with extreme hyperactivity, aggression, and temper tantrums. During this phase, the diagnosis is established in the majority of individuals. As the disease advances, developmental milestones are lost and increasing spasticity leads to a progressive loss of motor skills. Behavioral problems and sleep disturbance require attention, although both are resistant to treatment. The challenging behavior responds poorly to a psychological or behavioral approach. In some individuals, benzodiazepines are used to modify aggressive or destructive behavior. Environmental modification within the home is an essential part of management. It is preferable to try improving the child's sleep pattern first, as the parents are better able to deal with the challenging behavior if fully rested. The use of melatonin has been encouraging, with a positive response obtained in at least 75% of those treated. Regular respite care is essential to allow the parents time for themselves and for normal siblings.

In the early teenage years, patients may progressively lose more skills and experience swallowing dysfunction. Seizures are common in the later stages in some patients and can be difficult to control, while other patients develop a severe movement disorder resistant to treatment. Mood disturbances with prolonged crying can be extremely distressing for the parents of affected children. Eventually, the disorder culminates in a vegetative existence in the mid-to-late teens. Death usually occurs around the second decade for patients with MPS IIIA, although patients with MPS IIIB-D may have a more attenuated course and can survive into the third or fourth decade. The disorder is probably underdiagnosed at the less severe end of the clinical spectrum, as these individuals may have only mild learning difficulties until the age of 20 to 30 years.

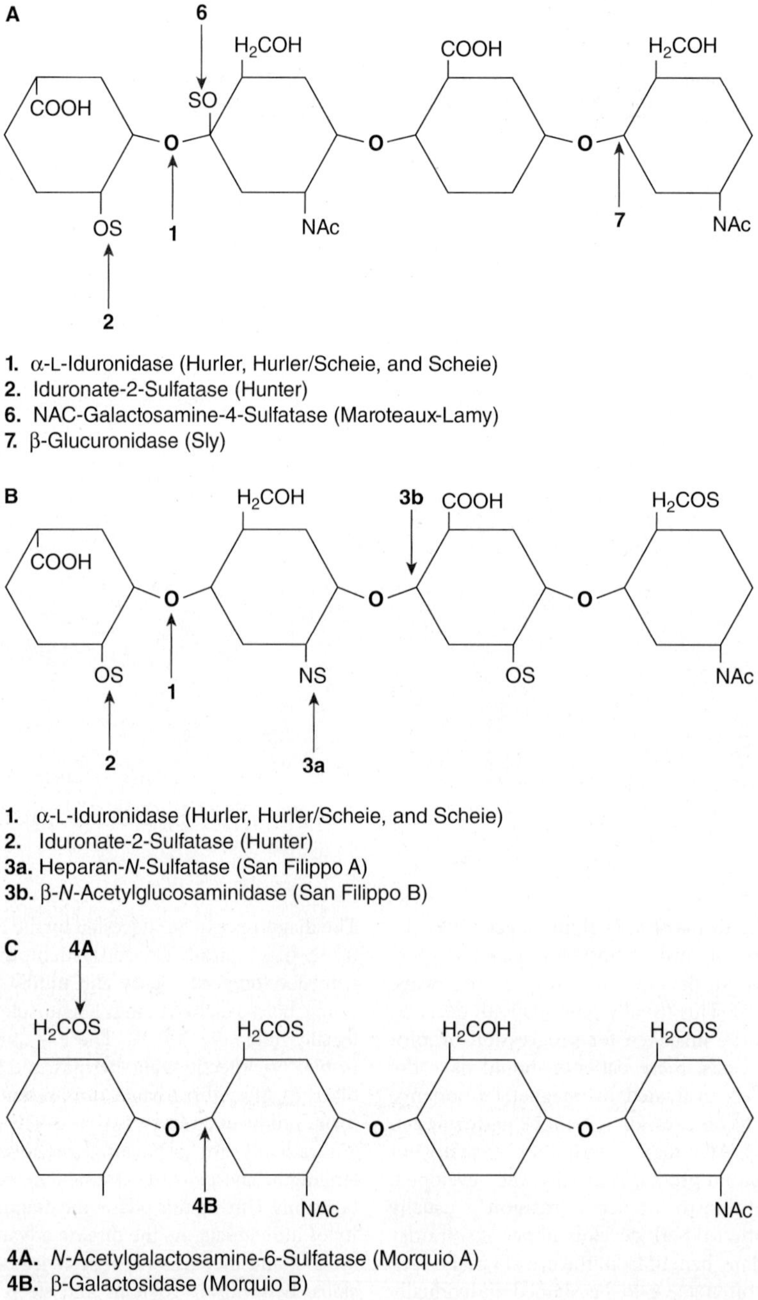
A
6
H2COH
COOH
H2COH
COOH
SO
O
O
O
OS
1
NAc
7
NAc
2
1. α-L-Iduronidase (Hurler, Hurler/Scheie, and Scheie)
2. Iduronate-2-Sulfatase (Hunter)
6. NAC-Galactosamine-4-Sulfatase (Maroteaux-Lamy)
7. β-Glucuronidase (Sly)
B
H2COH
3b
COOH
H2COS
COOH
O
O
O
OS
1
NS
OS
NAc
2
3a
1. α-L-Iduronidase (Hurler, Hurler/Scheie, and Scheie)
2. Iduronate-2-Sulfatase (Hunter)
3a. Heparan-N-Sulfatase (San Filippo A)
3b. β-N-Acetylglucosaminidase (San Filippo B)
C
4A
H2COS
H2COS
H2COH
H2COS
O
O
O
4B
NAc
NAc
4A. N-Acetylgalactosamine-6-Sulfatase (Morquio A)
4B. β-Galactosidase (Morquio B)

**FIGURE 155-1** **A:** The catabolism of dermatan sulfate. **B:** The catabolism of heparan sulfate. **C:** The catabolism of keratan sulfate.

Enzyme replacement therapy has not been approved in MPS III by the US Food and Drug Administration (FDA), as it does not cross the blood-brain barrier. There are several ongoing clinical trials involving intrathecal administration of enzyme and intrathecal gene therapy. Intravenous enzyme products that are able to cross the blood-brain barrier are also being investigated. HCST does not ameliorate the neurologic outcomes in patients with MPS III.

#### Mucopolysaccharidosis Type IV

Individuals with MPS IV, or Morquio syndrome, present primarily with a severe skeletal dysplasia. MPS IVA (galactose-6-sulfatase, *GALNS*; MIM no. 253000) accounts for 95% of cases, and MPS IVB (β-galactosidase; MIM no. 612222) accounts for 5%; they are clinically indistinguishable. Individuals with MPS IV appear normal at birth. Like other MPS, there is a wide range of phenotypic variability ranging from severe early-onset to mild, slowly progressive disease. Unlike other MPS, these individuals do not have coarse facial features, and developmental delay/intellectual disability does not occur. Instead, the clinical course includes severe bone disease and short stature. Affected individuals have loose peripheral joints (especially the wrists) with some limitation in range of motion in large joints; this joint phenotype distinguishes individuals with MPS IV from patients with other MPS diseases. The diagnosis can be suggested by the finding of keratan and chondroitin-6-sulfate in the urine. The severe form of the disease is diagnosed between 1 and 3 years of life, and initial presentation includes kyphoscoliosis, genu valgum, severe pectus carinatum, and decreased growth velocity. The radiologic abnormalities are different from the classic dysostosis multiplex seen in MPS I, II, VI, and VII and are characterized by vertebral platyspondyly and other features of a generalized spondyloepiphyseal dysplasia (Fig. 155-10). Severely affected males have an average adult height of 123 cm and females 117 cm. The greatest immediate danger is the inevitable odontoid dysplasia that is present in all severely affected patients (Fig. 155-11). Without treatment, MPS IV patients may suffer irreversible neurologic deficits. Care must be taken not to hyperextend the neck, especially during intubation for surgical procedures. Chronic cervical myelopathy presents with an insidious loss of motor function and evolves into a slowly

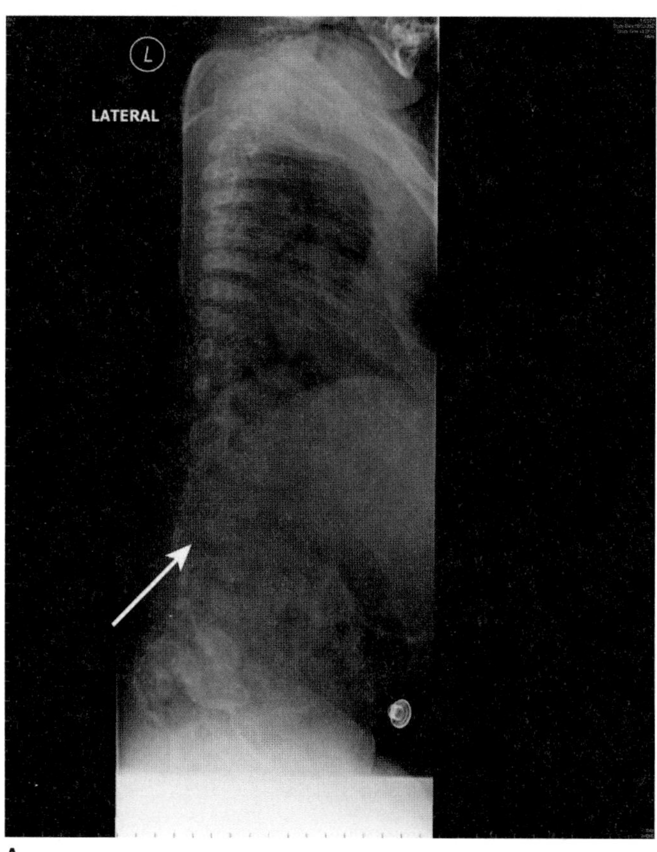


A

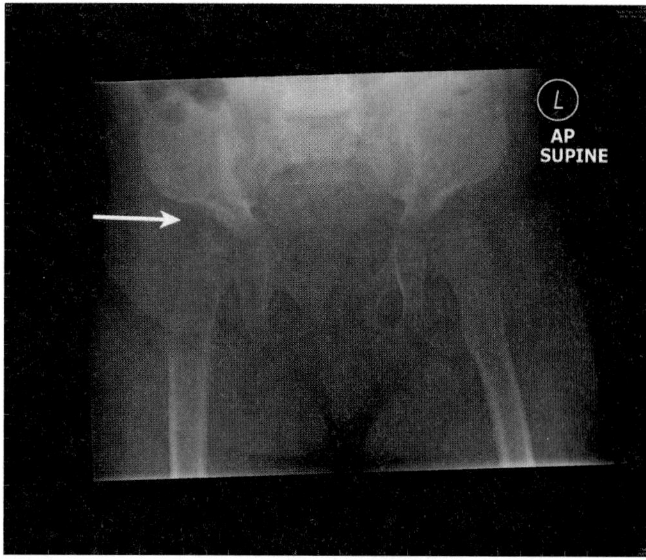


B

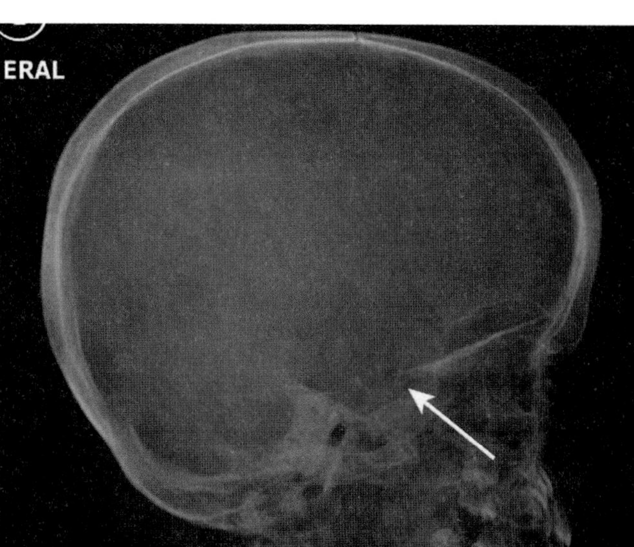


C

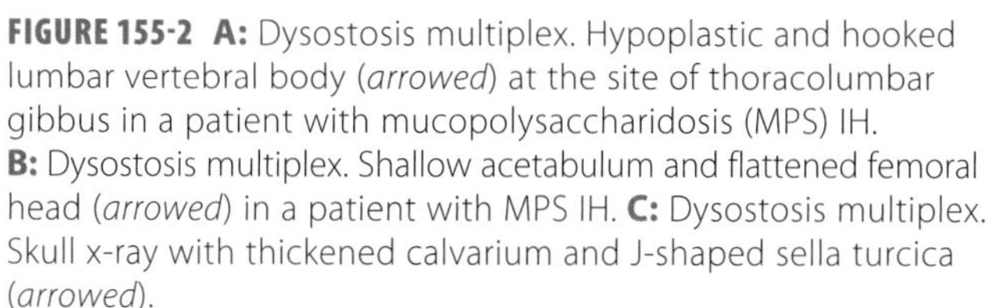

**FIGURE 155-2** **A:** Dysostosis multiplex. Hypoplastic and hooked lumbar vertebral body (*arrowed*) at the site of thoracolumbar gibbus in a patient with mucopolysaccharidosis (MPS) IH. **B:** Dysostosis multiplex. Shallow acetabulum and flattened femoral head (*arrowed*) in a patient with MPS IH. **C:** Dysostosis multiplex. Skull x-ray with thickened calvarium and J-shaped sella turcica (*arrowed*).



progressive tetraparesis unless the instability in the cervical region is detected and corrected. Flexion/extension radiographic views of the cervical spine are helpful in identifying patients likely to benefit from early spinal fusion. MRI scanning of the cervical region will demonstrate the degree of cervical involvement and should be performed at regular intervals. The timing of cervical fusion remains controversial, with some recommending prophylactic fusion in patients whose radiographs show atlantoaxial subluxation, while others would not recommend intervention until there are clinical signs or symptoms. The situation requires continual vigilance, as instability may develop farther down the vertebral column. Very little else can be done for the bone deformities present in this condition. Corrective surgery for genu valgum often produces only a temporary cosmetic improvement and does not greatly improve mobility. Most adults with the severe form of this disease prefer to use a motorized wheelchair, and because of their lack of mobility, obesity is a major problem (Fig. 155-12).

Individuals with MPS IV have a high risk of respiratory complications due to GAG accumulation in the upper respiratory tract, leading to tissue hypertrophy, airway obstruction, and obstructive sleep apnea. Restrictive lung disease results from a small thorax and thoracic spinal anomalies, which can lead to respiratory failure, and is the most common cause of death in adulthood. Cardiac complications, including valvar regurgitation or stenosis and ventricular hypertrophy, may occur. Dental decay is common, secondary to enamel hypoplasia, and the teeth are generally pointed and widely spaced. A number of patients will develop mild corneal haze as adults, but this rarely needs treatment. Mild to moderate hearing loss is common.

Enzyme replacement therapy (elosulfase alfa) is available for MPS IVA. It is administered at a dose of 2 mg/kg weekly and leads to an improvement in the 6-minute walk test and quality of life. Serious adverse events are not common, but as with other forms of enzyme replacement therapy, premedication with an antihistamine and antipyretic may help reduce infusion-associated reactions.

*[MPS V was originally Scheie disease, but when it was recognized that this was a milder form of MPS I, it was renamed MPS IS; therefore, there is no MPS V.]*

### Mucopolysaccharidosis Type VI

MPS VI, also known as Maroteaux-Lamy disease (MIM no. 253200), is due to pathogenic variants in the gene *ARSB* that encodes the enzyme *N*-acetylgalactosamine-4-sulfatase. Like other MPS conditions, MPS VI is associated with considerable clinical heterogeneity. In the typical or severe form of the disease (sometimes referred to as "rapidly progressing"), the clinical phenotype includes short stature, coarse facial features, hepatosplenomegaly, dysostosis multiplex, corneal clouding, and cardiac abnormalities. Other associated features include upper respiratory obstruction, middle-ear disease, corneal clouding, and progressive joint stiffness. Cardiac involvement is universal and can be severe and is a leading cause of death in rapidly progressing

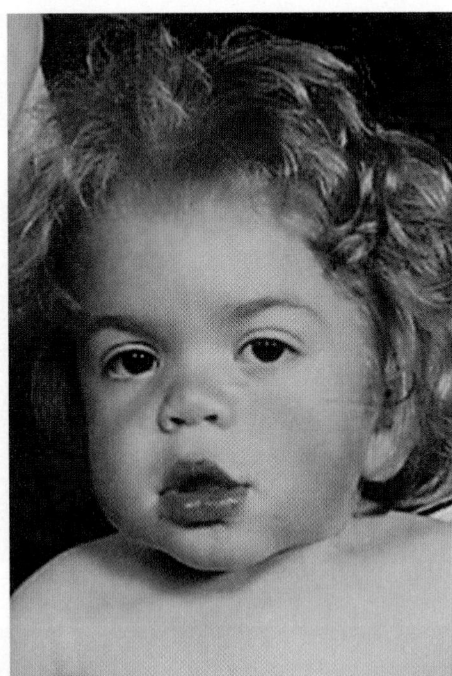

**FIGURE 155-3** Facial features in mucopolysaccharidosis (MPS) IH at diagnosis, age 12 months: mid-face hypoplasia, "button" nose, and thick lips.

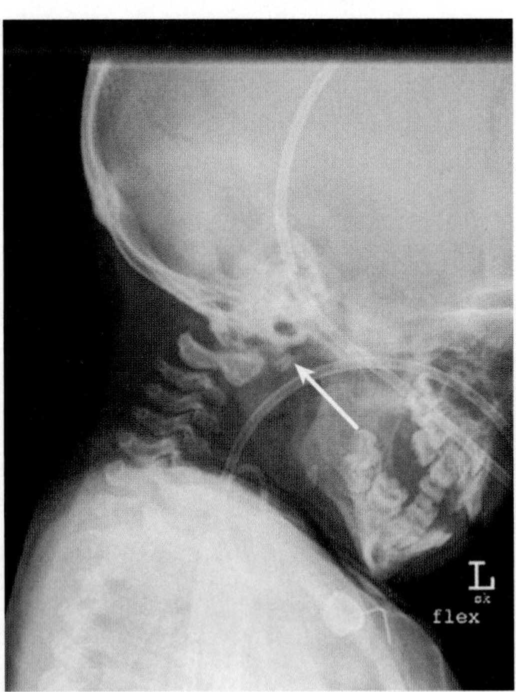


**FIGURE 155-5** Lateral x-ray of the cervical spine taken in flexion. The first cervical vertebra (*arrowed*) has slipped anteriorly over the top of C2 because of odontoid dysplasia and subsequent instability at the craniocervical junction.



MPS VI in the second or third decade of life. The diagnosis can be suggested by the finding of dermatan and chondroitin-6-sulfate in the urine. In severely affected individuals, diffuse airway narrowing can lead to cor pulmonale over time. All individuals, even those at the less severe end of the clinical spectrum ("slowly progressing" form of the disease), are at risk of cervical myelopathy secondary to dural and ligamentous hyperplasia. Atlantoaxial subluxation is variable, and it is often not possible to predict whether cervical fusion will be necessary in addition to decompression in individuals with cervical cord disease until the time of operation. People with MPS VI are at risk of 2 complications that are seen particularly in this MPS: sudden blindness due to optic nerve compression and intracranial venous hypertension secondary to the compression at the craniocervical junction. Regular ophthalmologic assessments are mandatory.

Figure 155-13 illustrates 2 patients of approximately the same age, one with rapidly progressing disease (Fig. 155-13A) and the other with a more slowly progressing variant (Fig. 155-13B).

Prior to the advent of enzyme replacement therapy, patients with MPS VI were successfully treated with HCST. However, galsulfase is approved for enzyme replacement therapy for Maroteaux-Lamy disease and is administered intravenously at a dose of 1 mg/kg weekly and results in significant improvements in endurance.

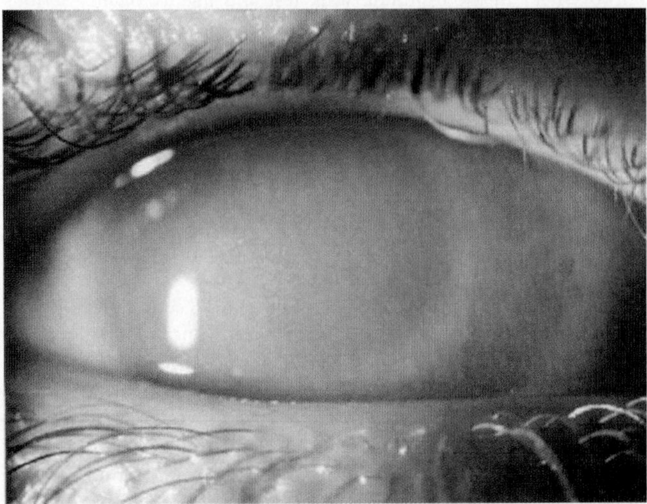

**FIGURE 155-4** Mucopolysaccharidosis (MPS) I corneal clouding.

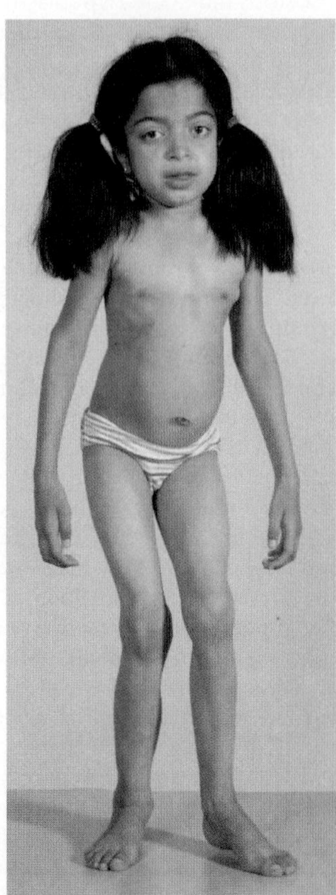

**FIGURE 155-6** An individual with an intermediate form of mucopolysaccharidosis (MPS) I (MPS IH/S, Hurler-Scheie disease). Note joint stiffness and relatively normal facial appearance.

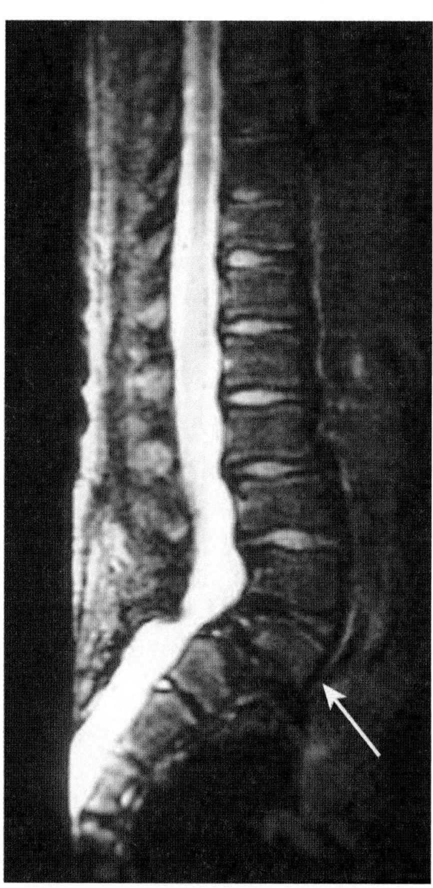

**FIGURE 155-7** Lateral magnetic resonance imaging scan of the lumbar-sacral spine in a patient with mucopolysaccharidosis (MPS) I H/S. The fifth lumbar vertebra (*arrowed*) has slipped anteriorly over the top of the sacrum.

### Mucopolysaccharidosis Type VII

MPS VII, or Sly syndrome (MIM no. 253220), is due to pathogenic variants in the gene *GUSB* (β-glucuronidase deficiency). This disorder is very rare, occurring in < 1 in 250,000 live births. Because one of the main modes of presentation is nonimmune hydrops fetalis, affected individuals are few in number. Infants with hydrops fetalis surviving delivery have a wide spectrum of disease severity. MPS VII can also present in the absence of hydrops fetalis, and in these individuals, the initial presenting symptoms are short stature, coarse facial features, cognitive impairment, hepatosplenomegaly, and dysostosis multiplex. Other common features can include corneal clouding, restrictive lung disease, cardiac valvar disease, and joint contractures. Visual impairment, sleep apnea, and cardiomyopathy occur in approximately one-third of patients. Spinal stenosis may occur. A diagnosis can be suggested by the finding of dermatan, heparan,

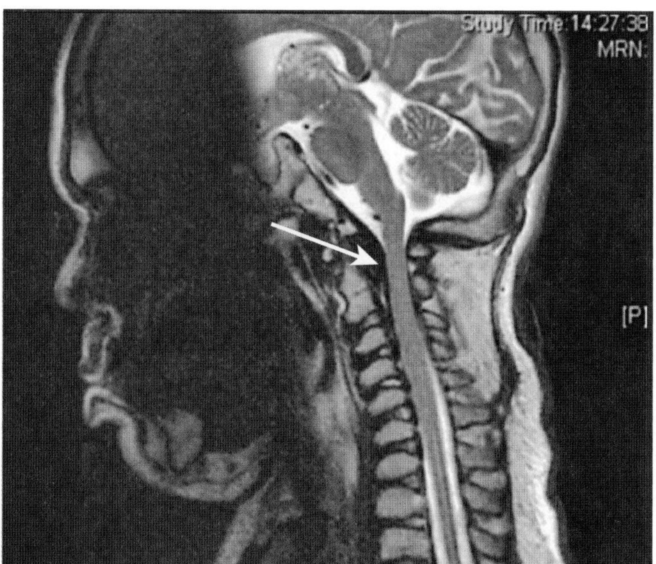


**FIGURE 155-8** A lateral magnetic resonance imaging scan of the craniocervical junction in a patient with mucopolysaccharidosis (MPS) II. Notice the lack of cerebrospinal fluid around the cervical cord (*arrowed*) due to thickening of ligaments and dura. The odontoid is also dysplastic.

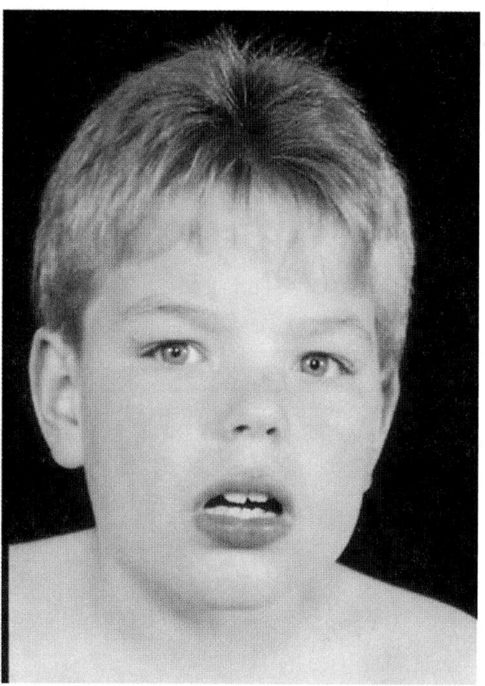

**FIGURE 155-9** Facial features in a 7-year-old boy with mucopolysaccharidosis (MPS) III at diagnosis.

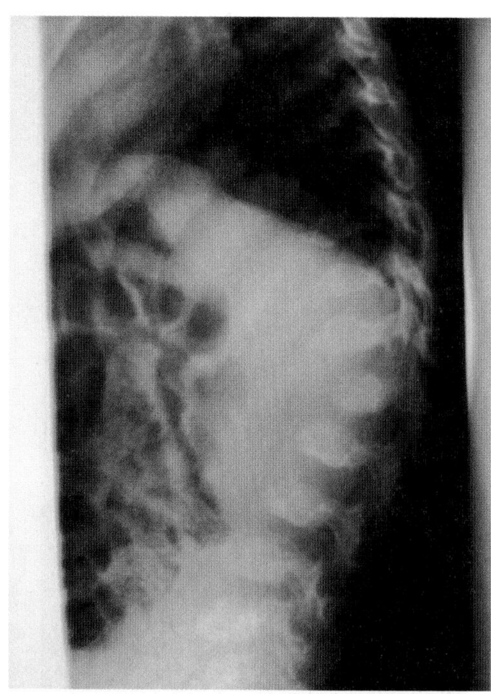

**FIGURE 155-10** Lateral spine x-ray of mucopolysaccharidosis (MPS) IV. Generalized vertebral abnormality (platyspondyly) is present in contrast to the single vertebral anomaly seen in MPS IH (Fig. 155-2).

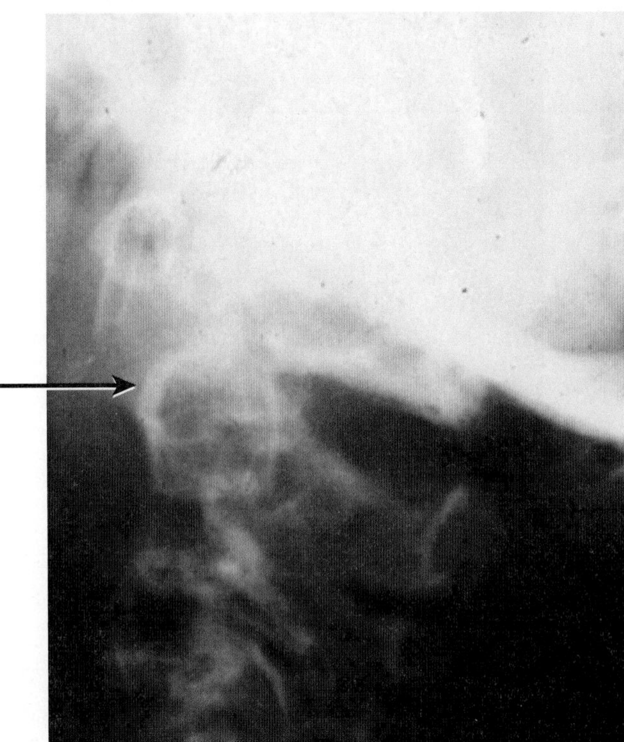

**FIGURE 155-11** Odontoid dysplasia (*arrowed*) in a patient with mucopolysaccharidosis (MPS) IV.

and chondroitin-6-sulfate in the urine. There are no treatments for MPS VII approved by the FDA; however, a recombinant human β-glucuronidase (rhGUS) is in phase III clinical trials at the time of the writing of this chapter.

#### Mucopolysaccharidosis Type IX

MPS IX (MIM no. 601492), or Natowicz disease, is vanishingly rare. Thus far, only 4 patients from 2 families have been described with *HYAL1* variants leading to deficiency of hyaluronidase. The first was a 14-year-old girl with mild short stature and multiple periarticular soft tissue masses. There was no other visceral or CNS involvement, although synovial histology revealed abundant lysosomal storage and abundant GAGs in the extracellular matrix. A second family with 3 affected children was later described as having joint pain, swelling, and proliferative synovitis with normal stature and no soft tissue masses. The diagnosis can be suggested by the finding of hyaluronic acid in the urine. No FDA-approved treatment exists for MPS IX.

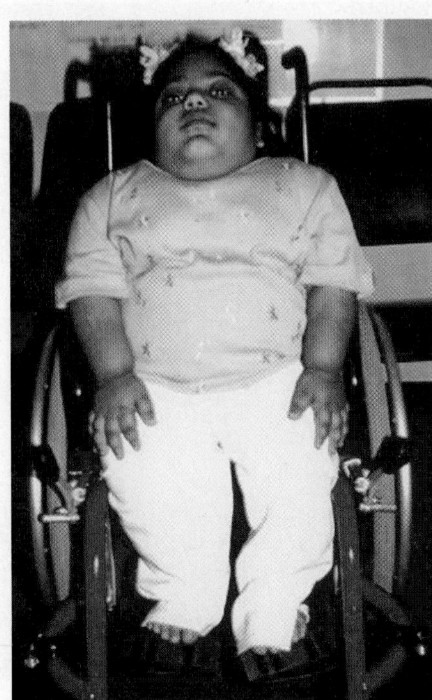

**FIGURE 155-12** A 10-year-old girl with mucopolysaccharidosis (MPS) IV. The immobility leads to obesity in many affected children.

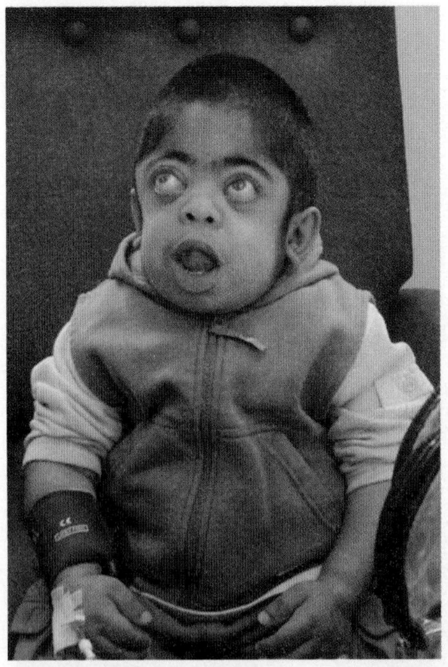

A

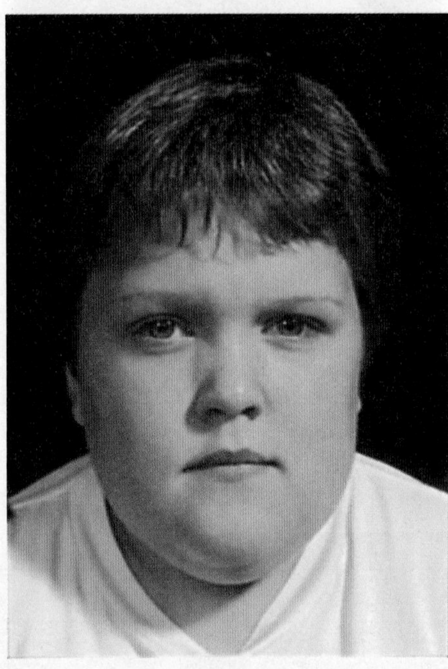

B

**FIGURE 155-13** **A:** A 14-year-old boy with rapidly progressive mucopolysaccharidosis (MPS) VI. **B:** A 15-year-old girl with slowly progressive MPS VI.

## MANAGEMENT OF MPS

Despite recent advances, definitive or curative treatment for most disorders affecting the brain is still not possible. However, enzyme replacement therapy and HSCT can slow or halt the progression of disease in some patients. Even in the most severely affected patients, careful attention to palliative therapies can have a beneficial effect on quality of life, and all patients should be under regular specialist care.

### Hematopoietic Stem Cell Transplantation (HSCT)

Since 1980, bone marrow transplantation (BMT) has been used as a cell-based form of "gene therapy" in patients with MPS. Initially, many different types of MPS disease were treated, but it is now generally accepted that the therapy is of no benefit in MPS III and IV, and there remains considerable doubt about its efficacy in severe MPS II. In carefully selected patients with MPS IH and VI, BMT alters the course of the disease, although the indications for treatment in both disorders differ. In addition, now that recombinant enzyme replacement therapy is available for MPS VI, transplantation is typically reserved for patients with severe MPS IH alone. In MPS IH, the primary objective is to avoid intellectual deterioration; consequently, BMT must be performed at an early age (< 18 months). Following successful BMT, urinary GAG excretion quickly increases and then falls to the normal range after 3 to 6 months. Organomegaly resolves, and there is partial clearing of the cornea. Cardiomyopathy, if present, is also successfully reversed. In MPS IH, developmental progress is maintained in the majority of patients who receive BMT earlier than 18 months of age, and the final DQ (developmental quotient) is usually identical to the DQ at the time of BMT. The skeletal disease, however, is very resistant to correction. Although remodeling of the facial bones can change the coarse facial appearance and growth of long bones is improved, the vertebral bodies are not significantly improved, and marked spinal deformity can result over time. Almost all patients with MPS IH who have had a successful BMT require complex corrective spinal surgery. Despite this, the majority of successfully transplanted patients have a good quality of life, and this therapy can no longer be regarded as experimental. For many patients, it offers their only chance of long-term survival. Figure 155-14 depicts MPS IH patients after HSCT.

Recent advances in transplantation for MPS disorders have included enzyme replacement therapy (ERT) as an adjunct to transplant; the increasing use of alternative donor cell sources, especially umbilical cord blood cells (UCB); and new, less toxic induction regimens. The major barriers to success following HSCT in MPS are the high rate of graft rejection and the toxicity associated with the treatment. There is some evidence that using ERT before transplant may lessen this risk. Experience suggests that the combination of ERT and HSCT is safe, and in some patients, pretreatment with ERT can be life-saving and can allow the patient to then go on to successful HSCT. The early results of using UCB as a cell source for HSCT seem promising. UCB is usually rapidly available from UCB banks. Characteristics of this cell source are delayed engraftment, better reconstitution of progenitors, higher thymic function, and a lower incidence of graft-versus-host disease. When a choice is available, most centers transplanting many MPS I patients are using UCB over matched unrelated bone marrow donors.

### Enzyme Replacement Therapy (ERT)

ERT replaces the deficient enzyme via weekly intravenous infusions. Clinical trials in MPS I, II, IV, and VI have resulted in improvements in organomegaly, endurance, and respiratory function. The best results are obtained when treatment is started early in the course of the disease. However, ERT has some limitations; none of the products can cross the blood-brain barrier, and some patients have immune-mediated reactions to the protein infusion. Anaphylaxis is an uncommon but serious complication in some individuals. The treatments are very expensive and are therefore not readily available in countries that have other pressing health care needs. Table 155-2 gives an overview of the available therapies.

**Future Developments with ERT** It is likely that further studies will be done in MPS I, II, and III to determine whether ERT can offer effective delivery to the CNS. This may include direct convective delivery to the brain, injection into the ventricles or lumbar space with or without increases in dosage, or the addition of an immunosuppressant. Clinical trials are already under way for intrathecal administration in the case of MPS IIIA.

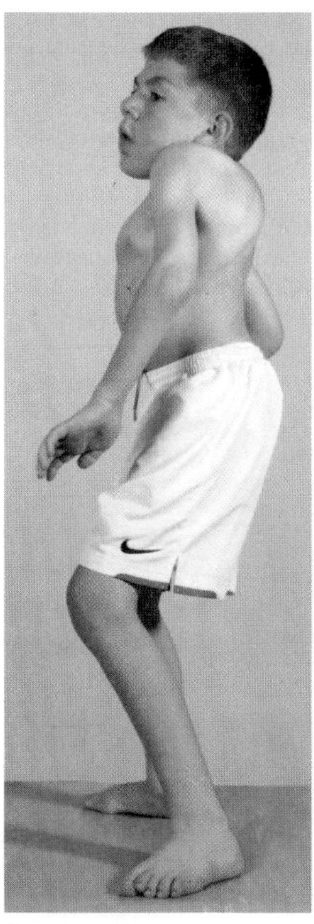
A

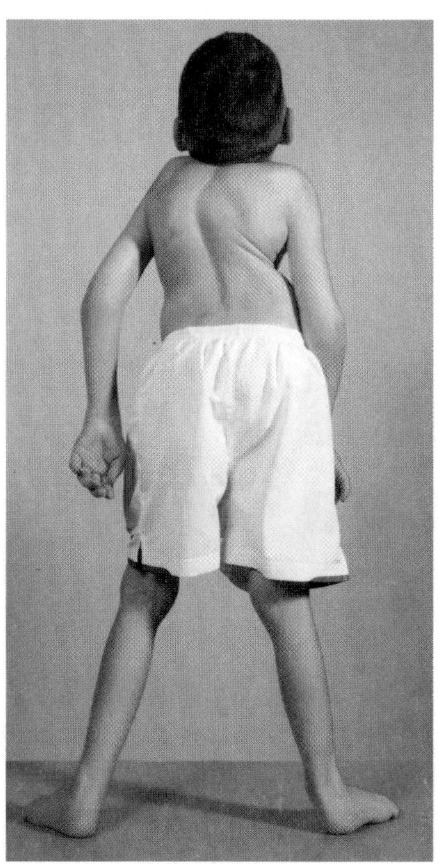
B

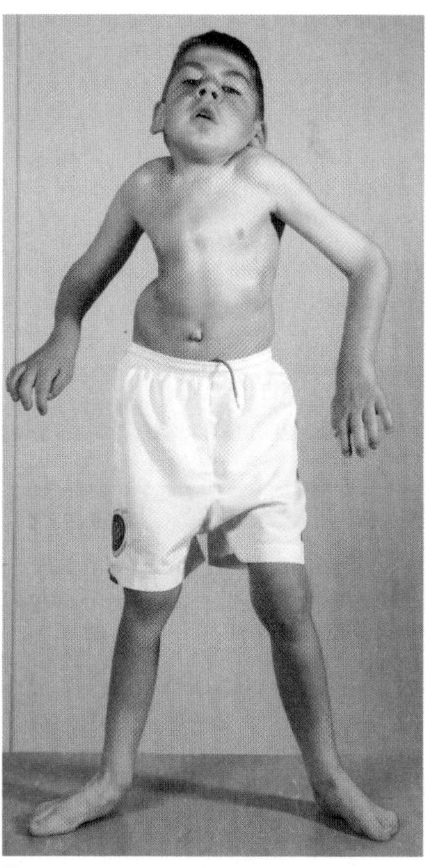
C

**FIGURE 155-14 A, B,** and **C:** An 8-year-old male patient with mucopolysaccharidosis (MPS) IH. Severe spinal deformity after hematopoietic stem cell transplantation.

**TABLE 155-2 ENZYME REPLACEMENT THERAPY FOR MUCOPOLYSACCHARIDOSES**

| Disorder | Product | Dosage per Week by Intravenous Infusion |
|---|---|---|
| MPS I | Laronidase | 0.58 mg/kg |
| MPS II | Idursulfase | 0.5 mg/kg |
| MPS IVA | Elosulfase alpha | 2 mg/kg |
| MPS VI | Galsulfase (Naglazyme) | 1 mg/kg |

#### Substrate Reduction Therapy

Substrate reduction therapy (SRT) using an inhibitor of glycosphingolipid synthesis (by inhibiting glucosylceramide synthase) is a licensed treatment for managing a different lysosomal storage disorder, type 1 Gaucher disease (see Chapter 156). The approved drug miglustat (Zavesca, Actelion) is active orally, and because it is a small molecule, it can cross the blood-brain barrier. As a result, trials of miglustat are under way in several other lysosomal storage disorders that affect the brain, including MPS III; however, it has not ameliorated neurologic symptoms in individuals with neuronopathic Gaucher disease.

Genistein, an isoflavone found to be abundant in soybeans, has many important potential cellular effects. One of these is to inhibit the function of the epidermal growth factor receptor, which is required for full expression of genes coding for enzymes involved in GAG production; in turn, this leads to an inhibition of the synthesis of GAGs within the cell. However, clinical trials of genistein supplementation in MPS IIIA have yielded conflicting results about efficacy.

#### Supportive Therapy

Appropriate education, speech therapy, physiotherapy, and occupational therapy should be offered to all patients, and parents should be given help with regard to appropriate financial support, aids, and adaptation. When dysfunctional swallowing is suspected, a formal assessment from a speech-language pathologist should be undertaken and videofluoroscopy performed if appropriate. If the child is at risk from aspiration, nonoral feeding should be instituted; most parents prefer a surgically placed gastrostomy tube rather than a nasogastric tube for this purpose.

ERT can be used as a symptomatic therapy in several situations. Intravenous ERT can rapidly reduce the size of the liver and spleen of affected patients and can improve joint stiffness. This leads to an improved quality of life and may be considered a justifiable reason for prescribing ERT in this group of patients, even though this therapy will not improve CNS disease. A clinical trial of ERT in patients under age 5 with MPS I (most of whom had the Hurler variant) describes a wide range of clinical effects across many organ systems.

# MUCOLIPIDOSES, GLYCOPROTEINOSES, AND RELATED DISORDERS

## MUCOLIPIDOSES

### INTRODUCTION

The mucolipidoses are a rare group of disorders originally named because they were clinically intermediate between MPS and lipidoses. However, mucolipids do not exist in nature. Mucolipidoses (ML) I and IV are very different conditions from ML II and III. The conditions are considered together for simplicity, but it is important to note that the enzymatic basis and the clinical phenotype are very different in these conditions despite the common use of the term *mucolipidosis*.

### PATHOGENESIS AND EPIDEMIOLOGY

All ML are inherited in an autosomal recessive manner. Prevalence varies with ethnicity; ML IV is more common in individuals of Ashkenazi Jewish ancestry. Males and females are equally affected.

### CLINICAL PRESENTATION

#### Mucolipidosis Type I (ML I, Sialidosis)

ML I (sialidosis; MIM no. 256550) is a very rare, heterogeneous disorder caused by pathogenic variants in *NEU1*, leading to deficiency of the neuraminidase enzyme. Classically, there are 2 major phenotypes described: sialidosis type I, or cherry-red spot myoclonus syndrome (CRSM), and sialidosis type II, which is more severe. CRSM usually presents toward the end of the first decade of life with myoclonus and ataxia associated with a cherry-red spot in the macula. In the second decade of life, affected individuals typically develop ataxia, myoclonic epilepsy, and progressive vision loss. Macular cherry-red spots are always present, and in addition, small punctate opacities in the anterior and posterior subcapsular regions are usually found on ocular examination. Hepatosplenomegaly may occur. Action myoclonus can be exacerbated by excitement, stress, lack of sleep, and other factors. It may be very disabling and respond very poorly to treatment. If present, dysostosis multiplex is typically mild. There is no cognitive impairment. Eventually, affected individuals become wheelchair-bound and unable to use their hands. Feeding is disrupted, and dysarthria eventually makes communicating very difficult. Despite these profound abnormalities, patients survive well into middle age. A milder phenotype, with adult-onset myoclonus with or without mild ataxia and without cherry-red spots, has been described. The more common presentation is sialidosis type II, which may present with hydrops fetalis or after birth with cherry-red spots, coarse facial features, hepatosplenomegaly, dysostosis multiplex, short stature, and severe intellectual disability. Seizures and hearing loss may occur. Death usually occurs in the late teenage years. Currently, there is no treatment for ML I.

#### Mucolipidosis Type II (ML II, I-Cell Disease, Leroy Disease)

ML II (I-cell disease; MIM no. 252500) is caused by pathogenic variants in *GNPTAB*, which encodes for the enzyme *N*-acetylglucosamine 1-phosphotransferase. I-cell disease refers to inclusions observed in affected cells by microscopy. The basic biochemical defect involves an abnormality in the posttranslational modification of lysosomal enzymes in which a targeting sequence (mannose-6-phosphate) fails to be added to the maturing enzyme. Consequently, lysosomal enzymes are not routed to the lysosome but are lost to the extracellular spaces and are not able to degrade material that accumulates in lysosomes. As a result, plasma levels of several lysosomal hydrolases, including β-D-hexosaminidase, β-D-glucuronidase, β-D-galactosidase, α-L-fucosidase, and arylsulfatase A are elevated in ML II and III.

In contrast to other lysosomal storage disorders, symptoms of I-cell disease are often present at birth. Patients may have low or low-normal birth weight with poor postnatal growth. Coarse facial features may occur in infancy and progress over time. Hyperplastic gums are an important clue to diagnosis and are often noted at birth or soon after (Fig. 155-15). Otitis media occurs frequently, and the cry/voice is hoarse. Periosteal new bone formation is often prominent. Cardiac

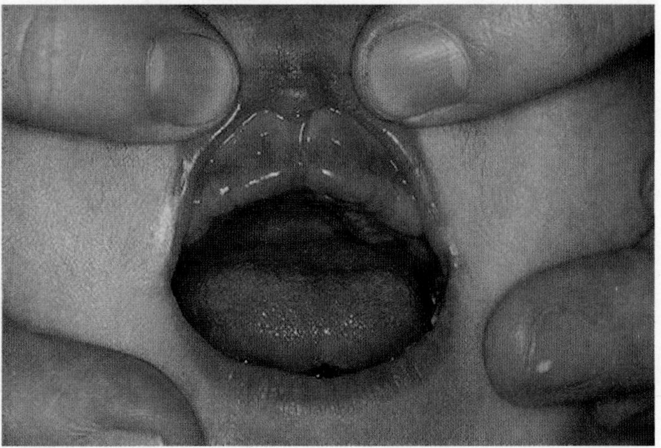

**FIGURE 155-15** Hyperplasia of the gums in a neonate with mucolipidosis II (I-cell disease).

valvar disease affecting the mitral and, less frequently, aortic valves is common. Affected individuals have developmental delay, involving motor more often than speech deficits, and exhibit poor feeding. Hepatosplenomegaly is not common. In contrast to other storage disorders, the head circumference in patients with ML II is usually small, and premature sutural synostosis can occur. Death usually occurs in infancy due to cardiac failure or infection. Pulmonary hypertension may occur in individuals with longer survival.

#### Mucolipidosis Type III (ML III α/β, Pseudo-Hurler Polydystrophy)

Like ML II, ML III (MIM no. 252600) is a recessive disorder caused by pathogenic variants in *GNPTAB*. The *GNPTAB* gene encodes α and β subunits, which can lead to either ML II or a ML III clinical phenotype. The *N*-acetylglucosamine 1-phosphotransferase enzyme has a multisubunit structure with an $\alpha2\beta2\gamma2$ structure. In contrast to ML II, ML III may also be due to pathogenic variants in *GNPTG*.

ML III, also known as pseudo-Hurler polydystrophy, is a slowly progressive disorder with onset in early childhood. Clinical features include short stature, slow growth, and mild-moderate dysostosis multiplex, which characteristically has the greatest impact on the ball-and-socket joints. Other features include course facial features, mild hepatosplenomegaly, and mild developmental delay. The disorder produces severe orthopedic problems secondary to progressive joint stiffness. Affected individuals are unable to raise their arms above their heads, and progressive hip dysplasia (Fig. 155-16) often leads to severe problems with mobility by early adult life. Most have carpal tunnel syndrome, and cardiac valvar lesions (typically leading to aortic incompetence) can develop later in life, requiring surgical repair.

#### Mucolipidosis Type IV (ML IV)

ML IV (MIM no. 252650) is due to defects in the *MCOLN1* gene, which encodes for mucolipin 1. Affected individuals present in the first year of life with corneal opacity and severe developmental delay, and they generally reach a maximum developmental age of around 18 months for verbal and motor skills. Affected individuals experience difficulties with speech, chewing, and swallowing. Hypotonia is usually present. Although vision is usually normal at birth, severe progressive visual loss occurs due to a combination of dystrophic retinopathy and corneal opacity. Production of stomach acid may be impaired (achlorhydria), and anemia may occur due to poor gastric absorption. Progressive renal failure has been observed beginning in the third decade. There is no organomegaly or dysostosis. Affected individuals may survive into adulthood, although survival is usually attenuated. Some individuals with an attenuated phenotype have been described. Typically, they have a much slower progression of the disease and prolonged survival; clinical features include mild developmental delay and mild progressive visual loss. Management consists of physical therapy and iron supplementation to prevent iron deficiency anemia, secondary to achlorhydria.

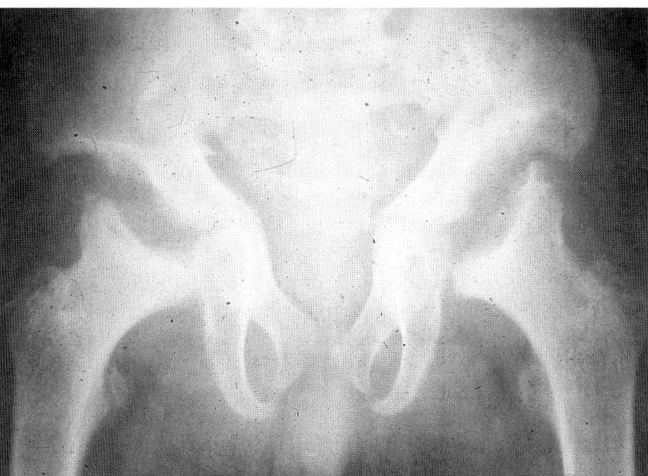

**FIGURE 155-16** X-ray of hips and pelvis in a patient with mucolipidosis type III (pseudo-Hurler polydystrophy). The femoral heads have been completely eroded.

### MANAGEMENT

Unfortunately, there currently is no effective cure or treatment for any of the mucolipidoses, and supportive care is all that can be offered. Some individuals with ML have received HSCT treatment, although this has not been associated with an improvement in cognitive abilities.

## GLYCOPROTEINOSES AND OTHER RELATED DISORDERS

### CLINICAL PRESENTATION

#### Mannosidoses (α-Mannosidase Deficiency, α-Mannosidosis; β-Mannosidase Deficiency, β-Mannosidosis)

**α-Mannosidosis** α-Mannosidosis (MIM no. 248500) is caused by pathogenic variants in *MAN2B1* and, like many lysosomal storage disorders, has a range of clinical presentation from severe to mild. Most individuals have the moderate form, diagnosed before the age of 10 years, which is characterized by coarse facial features, hearing loss, ataxia, intellectual disability, immunodeficiency, skeletal abnormalities, and rarely a beaten copper appearance to the skull x-ray. In the severe form, early death results from progressive nervous system dysfunction. In the mild form, diagnosis occurs after age 10, lacks skeletal abnormalities, and is more slowly progressive. The diagnosis can be suggested by oligosaccharide analysis of the urine. HCST has been used as a therapy in the severe and moderate forms in a few cases.

Figure 155-17 shows the characteristic clinical phenotype of a child with α-mannosidosis at presentation.

**β-Mannosidosis** The clinical phenotype is not well characterized, as there have been very few reported cases. The first patients described with an isolated deficiency of β-mannosidase were adults who presented with angiokeratoma and mild learning difficulties. A severe presentation with infantile epileptic encephalopathy has also been reported.

#### Fucosidosis (a-Fucosidase Deficiency)

Fucosidosis (MIM no. 230000) is a rare autosomal recessive disorder due to pathogenic variants in *FUCA*. Neurologic characteristics

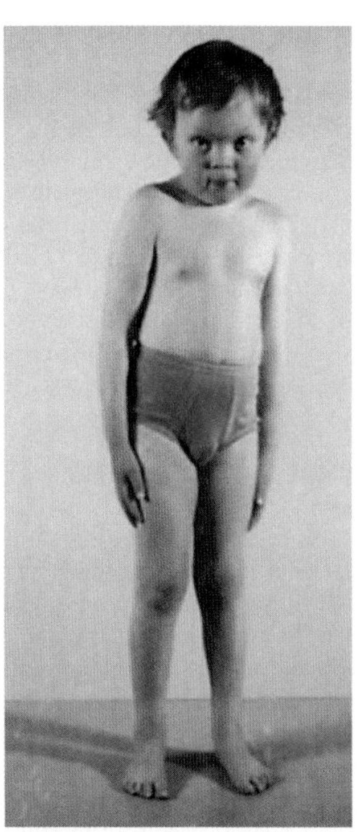

**FIGURE 155-17** A 6-year-old boy with mannosidosis at presentation.

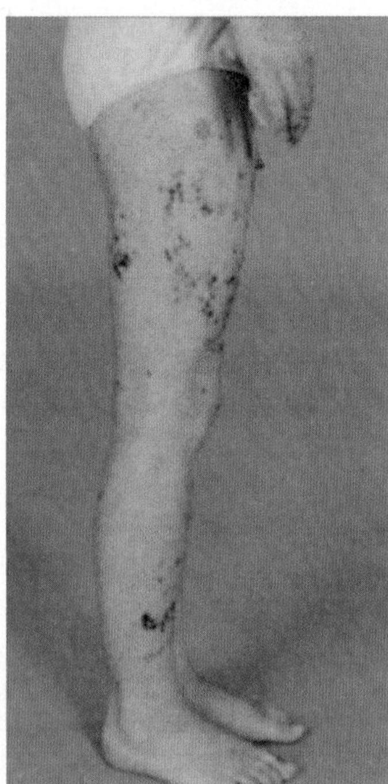

**FIGURE 155-18** Extensive angiokeratomas on the leg of a patient with fucosidosis.

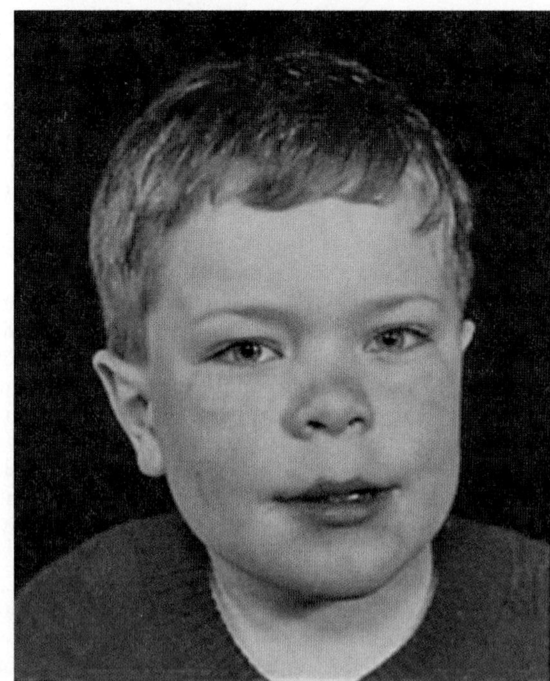

**FIGURE 155-19** Facial features of aspartylglucosaminuria at diagnosis, age 4 years.

include developmental delay, intellectual disability that may progress to dementia, spasticity, and seizures. Other features include dysostosis multiplex and angiokeratomas (Fig. 155-18).

#### Schindler Disease (α-*N*-Acetylgalactosaminidase Deficiency)

Although only a few patients with this disorder have been reported, a wide clinical spectrum has been described. Schindler disease (MIM no. 609241) is autosomal recessive, due to pathogenic variants in *NAGA*. The condition was first described in infants with severe neurologic involvement, including developmental regression, myoclonus, spasticity, and rapidly progressive dementia. Subsequent patients have been described with a mild disorder, also known as Kanzaki disease (MIM no. 609242) consisting of adult-onset angiokeratomas, hearing loss, and mild cognitive impairment. An intermediate phenotype, with cardiomyopathy and hepatomegaly, has also been described.

#### Aspartylglucosaminuria (Aspartylglucosaminidase Deficiency)

Although this disorder occurs in all ethnic groups, it is more common in the Finnish population. Aspartylglucosaminuria (MIM no. 208400) is an autosomal recessive disorder due to pathogenic variants in the *AGA* gene. Initially, development is usually normal and patients present in early childhood with speech delay. Intellectual disability worsens over time, and seizures or movement disorders may occur. Other associated features are angiokeratomas, dysostosis multiplex, joint hypermobility, osteoporosis, short stature, and dysmorphic facial features (ocular hypertelorism, small ears, sagging cheeks, full lips, short nose; Fig. 155-19).

#### Galactosialidosis (Sialidosis Type II, Combined Neuraminidase and β-Galactosidase Deficiency)

Galactosialidosis (MIM no. 256540) is an autosomal recessive disease due to pathogenic variants in *CTSA*, encoding the protective protein/cathepsin A (PPCA). In the neonatal form, individuals may present with hydrops fetalis, hepatosplenomegaly, inguinal hernia, coarse facial features, macular cherry-red spots, cardiomegaly, and kidney failure. The infantile form includes short stature, hepatosplenomegaly, cherry-red spots, inguinal hernia, coarse facial features, and cardiac valvular disease. In contrast, the juvenile and adulthood forms are characterized by ataxia, myoclonus, and progressive cognitive impairment. Angiokeratomas, coarse facial features, and vision/hearing loss may also be present.

#### Multiple Sulfatase Deficiency (MSD)

MSD (MIM no. 272200) is a very rare disorder that results from a deficiency of all lysosomal sulfatases. It is to a deficiency of the formylglycine modifying enzyme, encoded by the *SUMF1* (sulfatase-modifying factor-1) gene, that converts a specific cysteine thiol residue to an aldehyde, an essential factor for the activity of all sulfatases. Most of these sulfatases are enzymes responsible for other lysosomal storage disorders. As a result, the clinical features of MSD are a heterogeneous combination of several disorders, including metachromatic leukodystrophy, Maroteaux-Lamy syndrome, X-linked ichthyosis, Hunter syndrome, Sanfilippo A syndrome, and Morquio syndrome. Consequently, individuals may have developmental delay/regression, coarse facial features, dysostosis multiplex, ichthyosis, and hepatosplenomegaly. Corneal clouding, hearing loss, and cardiac abnormalities may occur. MRI shows evidence of white matter changes similar to metachromatic leukodystrophy. Biochemical testing reveals accumulation of GAGs, sulfatides, and gangliosides. The severity of the condition can vary from a neonatal form, with death occurring in the first few years of life, to a rare adult-onset disease with attenuated symptoms.

#### Free Sialic Acid Storage Disorders (Salla Disease and Infantile Sialic Acid Storage Disease [ISSD])

ISSD (MIM 269920) and Salla disease (sialuria, Finnish type; MIM no. 604369) are allelic autosomal recessive disorders due to a defect in the transport of free sialic acid across the lysosomal membrane caused by mutations in *SLC17A5*. Salla disease is considered to be milder than ISSD, and both conditions exhibit excessive free sialic acid in the urine. In ISSD, neonatal presentation includes hydrops fetalis, hypopigmentation, recurrent severe infection, and failure to thrive (Fig. 155-20). Dysostosis multiplex, vacuolated lymphocytes, and cardiac disease are usual features, and the facial appearance is often coarse. Most affected patients die in the first year of life. Salla disease is characterized by progressive neurologic symptoms including developmental delay or regression, spasticity, seizures, and athetosis. Progression is slower than for ISSD, and patients may survive to adulthood.

## MANAGEMENT OF GLYCOPROTEINOSES AND RELATED DISORDERS

For the majority of disorders, treatment is symptomatic only. ERT has not yet been developed for these disorders. HCST has been performed in α-mannosidosis, fucosidosis, and aspartylglucosaminuria and may be a useful therapy in carefully selected patients.

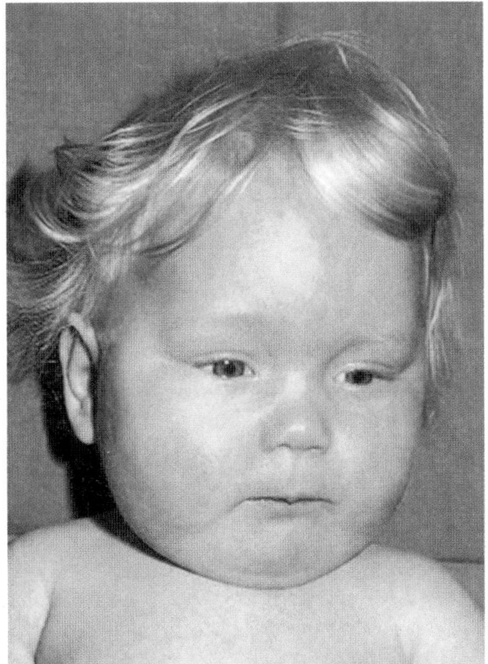

**FIGURE 155-20** An infant with infantile sialic acid storage disease. Note mild facial dysmorphism and fair hair.

## GENETIC COUNSELING AND PRENATAL DIAGNOSIS

All of the conditions discussed in this chapter are genetic, and diagnosis within a family should be followed by referral for appropriate genetic counseling. Prenatal diagnosis is possible for all the disorders. In some conditions, this can be done by direct enzyme assay on uncultured chorionic villus material at an early stage in pregnancy (10–12 weeks). In others, cultured cells or analysis of amniotic fluid may be more diagnostic. Genetic testing for known pathogenic variants may be performed as well. Preimplantation genetic diagnosis is also a possibility. Because of the clinical overlap between these disorders, it is imperative that an accurate diagnosis be established in the index case, before embarking on prenatal testing during subsequent pregnancies.

### SUGGESTED READINGS


Boustany RM. Lysosomal storage diseases—the horizon expands. *Nat Rev Neurol.* 2013;9:583-598.

Filocamo M, Morrone A. Lysosomal storage disorders: molecular basis and laboratory testing. *Hum Genomics.* 2011;5:156-169.

Parenti G, Andria G, Ballabio A. Lysosomal storage diseases: from pathophysiology to therapy. *Annu Rev Med.* 2015;66:471-486.


# 156 Sphingolipidoses

Laurie A. Robak and V. Reid Sutton

## INTRODUCTION

The sphingolipidoses are a group of rare, multisystemic, clinically heterogeneous lysosomal storage disorders characterized by defects in the breakdown of complex lipids. Clinical findings may include hepatosplenomegaly, bone involvement, macular cherry red spots, interstitial lung disease, hematopoietic abnormalities, and neurologic disease. Because the affected enzymes are expressed in different tissues and the degree of enzymatic impairment may vary, clinical manifestations are quite variable. There is a wide range in age of onset from prenatal nonimmune hydrops to slowly progressive adult-onset disease. All but one of the sphingolipidoses are autosomal recessive conditions; Fabry disease is inherited as an X-linked disorder.

A diagnosis of sphingolipidosis requires a high index of clinical suspicion. Either the demonstration of a deficiency of lysosomal enzyme activity or gene sequencing can establish a specific diagnosis of most sphingolipidoses. Histopathologic studies on bone marrow aspirates or on tissue obtained by biopsy often show the presence of storage cells; however, the changes are generally not specific enough (except in the case of Gaucher disease) to make the diagnosis of a specific sphingolipidosis. Prenatal diagnosis of all the sphingolipidoses is possible through molecular genetic studies on chorionic villus samples or cultured amniotic fluid cells.

The sphingolipidoses, with their corresponding gene(s) gene and enzymatic defects, are shown in Table 156-1.

**TABLE 156-1 BIOCHEMICAL CLASSIFICATION AND GENETICS OF THE SPHINGOLIPIDOSES**

| Disorder | Enzyme Defect | Gene |
|---|---|---|
| Gaucher disease, types 1, 2, and 3 | Glucocerebrosidase (β-glucosidase) | *GBA* |
| Gaucher disease with normal glucocerebrosidase | Saposin C | *PSAP* |
| Fabry disease | α-Galactosidase A | *GLA* |
| Niemann-Pick disease, types A and B | Acid sphingomyelinase | *SMPD1* |
| Niemann-Pick disease, type C | Intracellular cholesterol trafficking defect | *NPC1* |
| Metachromatic leukodystrophy | Arylsulfatase A | *ARSA* |
| Metachromatic leukodystrophy with normal arylsulfatase A | Saposin B | *PSAP* |
| Krabbe disease | Galactocerebrosidase | *GALC* |
| GM1 gangliosidosis | β-Galactosidase | *GLB1* |
| Tay-Sachs disease | β-Hexosaminidase A | *HEXA* |
| GM2 activator deficiency | GM2 activator protein | *GM2A* |
| Sandhoff disease | β-Hexosaminidase A and B | *HEXB* |
| Farber lipogranulomatosis | Ceramidase | *ASAH* |

Treatments available for the sphingolipidoses include enzyme replacement therapy, substrate reduction therapy, hematopoietic stem cell transplantation, and symptomatic care.

## PATHOGENESIS AND EPIDEMIOLOGY

The normal stepwise degradation of glycosphingolipids occurs in lysosomes. Sphingolipidoses are due to the accumulation of compounds containing a large lipophilic core called *ceramide* and either a hydrophilic oligosaccharide (glycosphingolipid) or a phosphorylcholine (sphingomyelin) (Fig. 156-1). Each step in the catabolism of the sphingolipids is catalyzed by one of a series of hydrolytic enzymes that requires the presence of activator proteins (Fig. 156-2).

The prevalence of sphingolipidoses range from 1 in 100,000 (Gaucher disease) to less than 100 cases reported (Farber lipogranulomatosis). Some populations have a higher frequency of certain sphingolipidoses (eg, increased prevalence of Niemann-Pick type C in the French Acadian population and high carrier frequency for Gaucher and Tay-Sachs diseases in individuals of Ashkenazi Jewish ancestry).

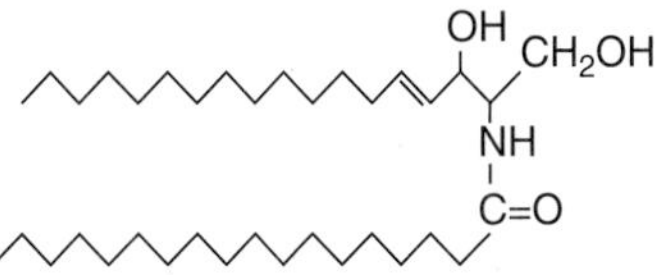

OH $CH_2OH$
NH
C=O

**FIGURE 156-1** Structure of ceramide (*N*-acylsphingenine).

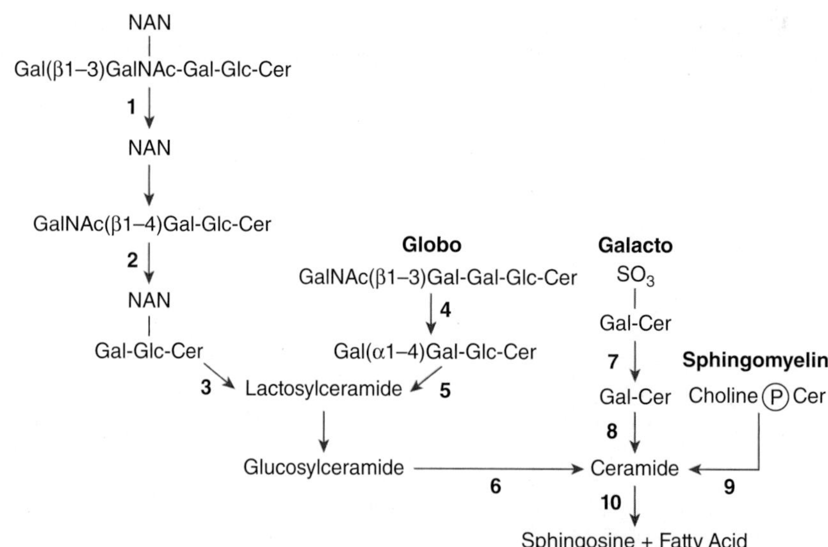


**FIGURE 156-2** Summary of the structure and catabolism of sphingolipids. 1, β-galactosidase; 2, β-hexosaminidase A + GM2 activator protein; 3, α-neuraminidase (sialidase) + saposin B; 4, β-hexosaminidase A; 5, α-galactosidase + saposin B; 6, glucocerebrosidase + saposin C; 7, arylsulfatase A; 8, galactocerebrosidase; 9, acid sphingomyelinase; 10, acid ceramidase + saposin D and C.



## CLINICAL PRESENTATION

### Gaucher Disease

Gaucher disease, the most common of the sphingolipidoses, is caused by biallelic pathogenic variants in the *GBA* gene, which encodes the enzyme glucocerebrosidase. The most common presentation, found in 95% of individuals with Gaucher disease, is so-called type 1 (generally considered the nonneuronopathic form; Mendelian Inheritance in Man [MIM] no. 230800). The most common presenting symptoms are hepatomegaly, splenomegaly, and bone pain. Patients may also come to clinical attention as a result of a history of excessive bleeding due to thrombocytopenia caused by hypersplenism. The majority of individuals with Gaucher disease have bone disease, manifested as acute/chronic bone pain, pathologic fractures, and avascular necrosis of the femoral head(s). Acute bone pain, or "bone crises," resembling sickle cell crises may be clinically indistinguishable from osteomyelitis. Chronic bone pain, especially in the legs, is typically worst at night. Cytopenias, such as anemia, leukopenia, and thrombocytopenia, are another common manifestation. Individuals may also have pulmonary involvement, including interstitial lung disease, pulmonary hypertension, and lobar consolidations. Although type 1 is generally considered the nonneuronopathic form of Gaucher, more recent studies have shown that individuals with Gaucher and unaffected carriers of *GBA* variants have an increased risk of Parkinson disease.

Individuals with type 2 and type 3 disease have the neuronopathic form of Gaucher disease. With type 2 (MIM no. 230900), the age of onset is usually before 2 years and the clinical course is rapidly progressive. Type 3 (MIM no. 231000) is characterized by an onset after 2 years and a clinical course that is more slowly progressive. However, this is a spectrum rather than 2 distinct diseases, and there are individuals with onset before the age of 2 years who may have a more slowly progressive course.

In type 2 disease, developmental delay and feeding difficulties typically present by 2 to 4 months of age. Other associated features include failure to thrive, strabismus, difficulty swallowing, and opisthotonic posturing. Type 2 is associated with a protuberant abdomen (due to massive hepatosplenomegaly) and macular cherry-red spots. Anemia, leukopenia, and marked thrombocytopenia are prominent.

Gaucher disease type 3 is clinically heterogeneous. Affected individuals may present at 2 to 3 years of age with massive hepatosplenomegaly that may lead to cirrhosis. Infiltration of the lungs with storage cells causes restrictive pulmonary disease. The first sign of neurologic involvement is often oculomotor apraxia. Skeletal involvement is often severe, with chronic bone pain, multiple bone crises, fractures, and avascular necrosis of large joints. In some patients, severe thoracic kyphoscoliosis is a prominent feature of the disease. Individuals may also present in early to middle childhood with myoclonus, dementia, ataxia, and slowing of horizontal saccadic eye movements. Smooth-pursuit eye movements may initially be normal. The spleen and liver are usually enlarged. Treatment-resistant generalized tonic-clonic seizures and spasticity may develop later. Skeletal lesions, like those seen in patients with type 1 disease, occur in most patients. Ultimately, death may occur in the second or third decade of life.

The perinatal-lethal form of Gaucher disease (MIM no. 608013) is characterized by severe generalized ichthyosis, multiple congenital anomalies (arthrogryposis, dysmorphic facial features), hepatosplenomegaly, pancytopenia, and severe central nervous system (CNS) impairment. CNS manifestations include marked paucity of spontaneous movement, hypertonicity and hyperreflexia, neck retraction, and poor suck. In some cases, nonimmune hydrops may occur and is severe. Survival beyond a few weeks is rare.

The cardiovascular form of Gaucher disease (type 3C; MIM no 231005) is associated exclusively with homozygosity for p.D409H. The main presenting feature is cardiovascular disease with calcification of both the mitral and aortic valves. Affected individuals may also have mild hepatosplenomegaly and corneal opacities in addition to supranuclear gaze palsy, but typically lack many of the other features of type 1 Gaucher disease.

There are several modes of treatment for Gaucher disease, including enzyme replacement therapy, substrate reduction therapy, and hematopoietic stem cell transplantation (HSCT). Further details can be found under the "Management" section.

### Fabry Disease

Fabry disease (MIM no. 301500) is an X-linked sphingolipidosis due to pathogenic variants in the *GLA* gene, which encodes the enzyme α-galactosidase A. This enzyme breaks down globotriaosylceramide, and in Fabry disease, globotriaosylceramide accumulates in the blood vessels, kidney, skin, and nervous system. Although classically described as primarily affecting males, females carriers are usually also symptomatic. The reason carrier females for Fabry disease have symptoms at such a high rate compared with other X-linked inborn errors of metabolism is that in Fabry disease there is no cell complementation, meaning that cells that have the normal allele active do not correct the defect in other cells where the mutant allele is active. Fabry disease usually presents late in the first decade of life with acroparesthesia, which is episodic, severe, burning pain in the hands and feet. These episodes may be precipitated by extremes of temperature, physical exertion, fever, and/or psychological stress. Pain in the joints may be clinically indistinguishable from pauciarticular arthritis, and abdominal pain may resemble an acute abdomen or chronic inflammatory bowel disease. Abnormalities of sweating, including anhydrosis, hypohydrosis, and even hyperhidrosis, are common. By the mid to late teens, increasing numbers of tiny red to black papular lesions (angiokeratomas) develop around the umbilicus and on the skin of the buttocks, scrotum, penis, and buccal mucosa. Angiokeratomas occur less frequently in females. Corneal and lenticular opacities are common. Renal function deteriorates over time, resulting in proteinuria, azotemia, and renal insufficiency. End-stage renal disease occurs in the third to fifth decade of life, limiting life expectancy unless dialysis or renal transplantation is performed. Cardiac disease may include mitral valve insufficiency and electrocardiographic changes (ST-segment changes, T-wave inversions, short PR interval). Progressive hypertrophic cardiomyopathy is a major cause of morbidity and mortality in patients with treated renal disease. Small vessel involvement in the CNS may lead to transient ischemic attacks or stroke. Life expectancy is shortened due to renal disease, cardiac involvement, and stroke. Affected females typically have a milder course than affected males, but there is a broad spectrum of severity. Enzyme replacement therapy is available for Fabry disease and will be discussed in the "Management" section.

### Niemann-Pick Type A/B

Niemann-Pick disease types A and B are due to pathogenic variants in *SMPD1*, which encodes the enzyme acid sphingomyelinase. A deficiency of this enzyme leads to the accumulation of sphingomyelin within the lysosome. There are 2 types: Niemann-Pick A is associated with neurologic findings, whereas Niemann-Pick B is not associated with neurologic symptoms. Children with Niemann-Pick A (MIM no. 257200) typically present in the first few months of life with failure to thrive, developmental delay, and marked hepatosplenomegaly. Gastrointestinal symptoms, such as diarrhea, constipation, vomiting, and feeding problems, may occur. Later, they may develop generalized muscle wasting, weakness, and hypotonia. Many affected infants have a macular cherry-red spot, and there may be interstitial lung disease. Death usually occurs in the second or third decade. Niemann Pick B (MIM no. 607616) typically presents later than type A and symptoms are more slowly progressive. The initial presenting symptom is usually hepatosplenomegaly, which is progressive and associated with elevated serum levels of transaminase. Interstitial lung disease, hyperlipidemia, osteopenia, and thrombocytopenia are also associated with type B. Some individuals will have a macular cherry-red spot. Despite type B being labeled as "nonneuronopathic," up to a third of patients can have neurologic symptoms such as peripheral neuropathy, extrapyramidal symptoms, intellectual disability, and psychiatric illness. Individuals with type B usually survive through adulthood. No specific management exists, but enzyme replacement therapy is currently under investigation.

### Niemann-Pick Type C

Niemann-Pick type C (MIM no. 257220) is due to pathogenic variants in *NPC1* (95%) or *NPC2* (5%), leading to impaired cholesterol esterification, which adversely affects cholesterol transport from the lysosome and causes an accumulation of sphingomyelin. The estimated population prevalence is 1 in 150,000, and it occurs more frequently in individuals of French-Acadian descent from Nova Scotia. Previously, the disease affecting this population was called Niemann-Pick D; however, the affected individuals have mutations in *NPC1*, and this designation is no longer used.

Niemann Pick C can present throughout the lifespan, including prenatally. Affected infants may present with neonatal ascites and hyperbilirubinemia with the histologic characteristics of giant-cell hepatitis. Rarely, neonatal liver involvement progresses to acute hepatic necrosis and early death. In most infants, the hepatopathy resolves spontaneously over several days. Lung infiltrates may also be present or may be the only initial presenting symptom. Surviving infants may have hypotonia and developmental delay within the first few months of life, or these may not present until later in life.

Individuals may also present without ascites in the first 1 to 3 years of life with developmental or psychomotor delay, then with slowly progressive regression, ataxia, dysarthria, dystonia, and hepatosplenomegaly. Vertical supranuclear gaze palsy is often present, and seizures and cataplexy are common. Death usually occurs by 3 to 10 years of age.

The childhood presentation includes clumsiness, learning disabilities, dystonia, and difficulties with gait progressing to ataxia. Vertical supranuclear palsy may be present. Speech may later be affected (dysarthria/dysphonia). Seizures, peripheral neuropathy, and sleep disturbance may also occur. Niemann-Pick C may also present in adolescence or adulthood with cognitive deterioration, dysarthria, dystonia, and gait difficulties. Psychiatric disease may be a prominent symptom in adult-onset presentations. The disease progresses more slowly than in other sphingolipidoses. No specific US Food and Drug Administration (FDA)-approved therapy exists for Niemann-Pick C.

### Metachromatic Leukodystrophy

Metachromatic leukodystrophy (MLD) (MIM no. 250100) is due to deficiency of the arylsulfatase A enzyme, caused by pathogenic variants in the *ARSA* gene. A few cases have been described with pathogenic *PSAP* variants that encode a protein (saposin B) that is required for the activation of the enzyme arylsulfatase A. The most common form is late infantile, in which individuals present between 1 and 2 years of age after normal development. Presenting symptoms include weakness, hypotonia, developmental delay, clumsiness, toe-walking, falls, and slurred speech. Developmental regression may occur, with loss of walking and other motor milestones. Individuals may have also have seizures, increased muscle tone, optic atrophy, and peripheral neuropathy. Ophthalmoscopic examination may show the presence of atypical cherry-red spots. Progression is initially slow but soon becomes more rapid with the development of generalized spasticity, developmental regression, and ultimately decerebrate posturing. Nerve conduction velocities are slow, and cerebrospinal fluid (CSF) protein concentrations are elevated. Computed tomography (CT) studies show progressive attenuation and loss of periventricular white matter, followed by marked demyelination throughout the CNS. For a detailed review of neuroimaging in MLD, please see Chapter 566. Survival for some years in a quasi-vegetative state is not uncommon. The life expectancy is typically 3 to 4 years after symptom onset but is variable.

The juvenile form of MLD generally presents at 4 to 10 years of age with a history of deteriorating school performance. It may be associated with personality changes, including obsessiveness, emotional lability, and social withdrawal, as well as ataxia and dysarthria. Progression of the disease is typically slow, and seizures generally occur later during the disease. Survival into the late teens or later is common.

Adult MLD usually presents with personality changes and problems in job or school performance. Emotional lability, substance abuse, inappropriate affect, seizures, peripheral neuropathy, and auditory hallucinations may occur. Adult MLD is progressive, and toward the end of the disease course, affected individuals may lose speech, motor, and visual function. There is no specific therapy for metachromatic leukodystrophy.

### Krabbe Disease

Krabbe disease (MIM no. 245200) is due to pathogenic variants in the *GALC* gene, which encodes the enzyme galactocerebrosidase. In the classic infantile form of Krabbe disease, affected individuals present before 6 months of age with developmental delay, spasticity, and irritability. Irritability is characterized by frequent crying without apparent cause and hypersensitivity to touch, sound, and sight; this is fairly universal and unique and should be a good clue to the diagnosis. Affected infants may also have seizures and feeding difficulties. As the disease progresses, neurologic deterioration continues, manifested as developmental regression, hypertonicity, seizures, and optic atrophy. Hepatosplenomegaly does not occur. The CSF protein is elevated. Eventually, vision is lost, and there is no voluntary movement. Affected individuals typically die by 2 years of age. The later-onset forms are more rare. There is an early childhood form with onset between age 6 months and 3 years. Symptoms are similar to the classic infantile form, with extreme irritability, hypersensitivity to sensory stimuli, developmental delay/regression, ataxia, and vision loss. Death results a few years after symptom onset. In the juvenile form (ages 3–8), developmental regression, ataxia, vision loss, and hemiparesis occur. The course is more indolent than the infantile and early childhood forms, but survival is attenuated. Finally, Krabbe disease may present in adolescence/adulthood with weakness, paresthesias, and progressive loss of gait and cognition. For a detailed review of neuroimaging findings in Krabbe disease, please see Chapter 566. There is no specific therapy for Krabbe disease.

### GM1 Gangliosidosis (Isolated β-Galactosidase Deficiency)

GM1 gangliosidosis is an autosomal recessive disease due to pathogenic variants in the *GLB1* gene that encodes the enzyme β-galactosidase. There is a range of phenotypes from infantile to adult onset, being divided into types I, II, and III, depending on age of onset. The most severely affected present in the newborn period (type I; MIM no. 230500) with a rapidly progressive course characterized by hepatosplenomegaly, coarse facial features, cardiac involvement, dysostosis multiplex, and spasticity. Most severely affected infants make little or no developmental progress and die in infancy from progressive neurodegeneration. Half of the patients with this early-onset variant will have macular cherry-red spots.

Individuals with late infantile or juvenile disease (type II; MIM no. 230600) present between ages 1 and 10 with motor delay or developmental regression. Other symptoms may include hepatosplenomegaly, dysostosis multiplex, and cardiac involvement. Corneal clouding is usually present later during the illness, but cherry-red spots are typically absent. Brain imaging shows progressive atrophy. Life expectancy is limited. In contrast, adult GM1 gangliosidosis (type III; MIM no. 230650) is a very different disorder, with a presentation often delayed until the second or third decade of life. The initial presentation with a movement disorder is followed by progressive pyramidal and extrapyramidal disease resulting in dysarthria, ataxia, and prominent dystonia. Symptoms may initially be diagnosed as Parkinson disease. Skeletal changes are minimal and consist essentially of minor radiologic abnormalities, and there is no hepatosplenomegaly or cognitive impairment. Most survive into middle age. No specific treatment exists for this disease.

### Tay-Sachs Disease

Tay-Sachs disease (GM2 gangliosidosis type I; MIM no. 272800) is an autosomal recessive disorder caused by deficiency of the α subunit of hexosaminidase A, which leads to accumulation of lysosomal GM2 gangliosides. The affected gene is *HEXA*. Biochemically, this disease is diagnosed by low to absent levels of hexosaminidase A enzyme activity. In the classic form of Tay-Sachs disease, affected infants appear normal at birth. Beginning at 3 to 5 months of age, motor weakness develops and is often associated with an exaggerated startle response. By 6 to 10 months of age, affected infants have progressive hypotonia, poor head control, and failure to achieve gross motor skills. Ophthalmologic examination typically reveals the presence of macular cherry-red spots. Hepatosplenomegaly is usually absent. Progressive macrocephaly begins by 18 months of age. Over time, symptoms evolve into progressive neurologic deterioration, seizures, spasticity, and blindness. The course of the disease is relentlessly progressive, with death occurring by age 3 to 5 years.

In the juvenile/subacute form of the disease, age of onset is later and disease progression slower than in the classic form. The age of onset is between 2 and 10 years of age. Presenting symptoms include ataxia and incoordination. Over time, speech and cognition deteriorate. Seizures and spasticity are also present. Cherry-red spots may be observed but are not universal. Visual loss may occur. Death is due to progressive neurologic deterioration, typically in the early teens.

In the adult-onset form, individuals present with slowly progressive neurodegeneration, and the clinical course is much more variable. Presenting symptoms include muscle weakness and dysarthria. Muscle fasciculations and wasting may also be present. Individuals may have dementia and psychiatric disease.

There is no specific treatment for Tay-Sachs disease.

### GM2 Activator Deficiency (GM2 Gangliosidosis, AB Variant)

Like Tay-Sachs disease, GM2 activator deficiency (MIM no. 272750) is characterized by accumulation of GM2 gangliosides within the lysosome. In contrast to Tay-Sachs disease, the affected gene is *GM2A*, which encodes the GM2 activator protein that is required for the activation of the enzyme β-hexosaminidase A. This disorder is extremely rare, and the phenotype is identical to Tay-Sachs disease. GM2 activator deficiency may be distinguished from Tay-Sachs disease biochemically due to *normal in vitro* activity of the enzyme hexosaminidase A. Unfortunately, no therapy is available for GM2 activator deficiency.

### Sandhoff Disease

This disorder (GM2 gangliosidosis type II; MIM no. 268800) is due to biallelic pathogenic variants in *HEXB*, which encodes the β subunit, which is required for both hexosaminidase A and B enzyme function. As a consequence, GM2 gangliosides accumulate in lysosomes. In most cases, Sandhoff disease is clinically indistinguishable from Tay-Sachs disease. In some, however, mild-to-moderate enlargement of the liver and spleen may occur, and radiographs may show subtle evidence of dysostosis multiplex. Specific treatment does not exist for this disease.

### Farber Lipogranulomatosis

Farber disease (MIM no. 228000) is due to deficiency of the enzyme acid ceramidase, encoded by the *ASAH1* gene. As with other lysosomal storage disorders, its severity varies, with onset ranging from prenatal fetal hydrops to adulthood. Affected individuals typically present with progressive painful, swollen joints and a hoarse cry. Subcutaneous nodules may be present over the joints, and contractures may develop. The other main feature is progressive neurologic deterioration. Other associated features include respiratory problems, dysphagia, recurrent vomiting, pulmonary consolidation, and fever. Hepatosplenomegaly is present. Death from progressive neurologic deterioration and chronic pulmonary disease usually occurs within several months of the onset of the disease. There is no FDA-approved therapy for this disease.

## MANAGEMENT

Management of sphingolipidoses may include enzyme replacement therapy, substrate reduction therapy, and hematopoietic stem cell transplantation (HSCT). Enzyme replacement therapy (ERT) has emerged as one of the most important advances in the treatment of sphingolipidoses (Table 156-2).

ERT is available for Gaucher and Fabry disease and is given as biweekly intravenous infusions. For type 1 Gaucher disease, ERT has been demonstrated to reduce hepatosplenomegaly, skeletal manifestations, hematologic abnormalities, and quality of life. However, lung parenchymal disease is not improved by ERT. There are 3 different forms of ERT available, distinguished by the method of production. All appear similarly effective; however, no study has directly compared efficacy in treatment-naive patients. The neurologic manifestations of type 2 and type 3 diseases do not respond to ERT because the enzyme does not cross the blood-brain barrier; however, ERT may be helpful for the somatic changes of Gaucher disease, particularly in relief of bone pain. It is important to note that that safety of imiglucerase is not

**TABLE 156-2 ENZYME REPLACEMENT THERAPY OF THE SPHINGOLIPIDOSES**

| Disease | Enzyme Preparation | Dosage Regimen |
|---|---|---|
| Gaucher disease | Imiglucerase | 30–60 units/kg every 2 weeks |
| | Velaglucerase alfa | 30–60 units/kg every 2 weeks |
| | Taliglucerase alfa | 30–60 units/kg every 2 weeks |
| Fabry disease | Agalsidase beta | 1 mg/kg every 2 weeks |
| | Agalsidase alfa[a] | 0.2 mg/kg every 2 weeks |

[a]Not approved for use in the United States.

established for individuals less than age 2; the safety of velaglucerase and taliglucerase is not established in those under 4 years of age. The most common adverse effect of ERT is immune-mediated sensitivity/infusion reaction, which can include headaches, dizziness, hypotension, fatigue, nausea, and fever. This may be managed by pretreatment antihistamines and/or corticosteroids as well as decreasing the rate of infusion.

There are 2 different forms of ERT available for Fabry disease; however, only agalsidase beta is approved for use in the United States. The effect of ERT in preventing cardiac disease, strokes, and renal failure is unproven. The most common adverse effect is an infusion reaction. In addition, symptomatic management of acroparesthesias (with carbamazepine, gabapentin, or diphenylhydantoin) and proteinuria (angiotensin-converting enzyme inhibitors or angiotensin receptor blockers) can be helpful. Hemodialysis and kidney transplantation may be offered to those with end-stage renal disease.

ERT is not currently available for other sphingolipidoses, but this is an active area of investigation. A phase II/III clinical trial is ongoing for Niemann-Pick A/B and a phase I trial for Niemann-Pick C. A phase I trial examining enzymatic replacement through intrathecal administration of umbilical cord blood cells is ongoing for metachromatic leukodystrophy, Tay-Sachs disease, and Sandhoff disease.

Substrate reduction therapy (SRT) inhibits synthesis of the storage product that builds up in lysosomes. Individuals with residual enzymatic activity may more effectively clear storage material. An advantage of SRT is that, unlike ERT, it may be taken orally. However, there may be increased side effects compared to ERT. There are 2 forms of SRT available for Gaucher disease. Miglustat (100 mg 3 times a day) inhibits glucosylceramide synthase, which reduces glycosphingolipid production, allowing residual glucocerebrosidase to function. It is approved for those over the age of 18. Benefits include reductions in liver/spleen volume and improvements in hemoglobin and platelet counts similar to imiglucerase. Adverse effects include peripheral neuropathy and tremor, which usually resolve in a few months, gastrointestinal distress, diarrhea, weight loss, and low platelet counts. Another substrate reduction therapy, eliglustat, is approved for monotherapy of Gaucher disease (84 mg once or twice daily, depending on metabolizer status) in individuals age 18 years or older. Prior to initiation, CYP2D6 genotype status needs to be assessed, because ultra-rapid metabolizers may not see a benefit and the frequency of dosing is based on metabolizer status. Benefits include reductions in liver/spleen volume and improvements in hemoglobin and platelet counts similar to ERT. Adverse effects include fatigue, headache, nausea, diarrhea, back pain, pain in extremities, and upper abdominal pain. Miglustat is under investigation for Niemann-Pick C, as it can cross the blood-brain barrier. A small study has shown improvements in saccadic eye movements, swallowing capacity, and hearing, and a slower deterioration in ambulation. However, this therapy is not yet approved in the United States.

With HSCT, stem cells repopulate the bone marrow and differentiate into different hematopoietic lineages and then migrate into tissues. The enzyme is then secreted and taken up by surrounding cells. This method may reduce or halt the progression of CNS disease in some sphingolipidoses. However, there is significant morbidity and mortality associated with this procedure. HCST was previously performed in Gaucher disease types 1 and 3, but has been largely supplanted by ERT and SRT due to morbidity and mortality associated with HSCT. HSCT does not improve outcomes in type 2 Gaucher disease. For Krabbe disease, HSCT may be performed in individuals with mild or no symptoms and improves cognitive function, but a slow peripheral nervous system decline may still occur. Variable results have been reported for Niemann-Pick A, but no improvements in CNS disease have been reported. Small studies have shown some improvement in neurologic symptoms for individuals with metachromatic leukodystrophy if performed prior to the onset of or in the presence of mild CNS disease. HCST is under investigation as a therapy for Niemann-Pick C. Information regarding investigational therapies may be found on the ClinicalTrials.gov Web site (www.clinicaltrials.gov).

For individuals with sphingolipidoses, efforts should be made to reduce pain and discomfort. Adequate nutrition and hydration should be provided. Seizures should be managed with antiepileptic agents. Psychiatric symptoms should also be managed by a psychiatrist familiar with sphingolipidoses. Physical, occupational, and speech therapy may decrease the loss of skills in some individuals with CNS disease. Education and supportive care should be made available to family members of those with sphingolipidoses.



## SUGGESTED READINGS


Boustany RM. Lysosomal storage diseases—the horizon expands. *Nat Rev Neurol.* 2013;9:583-598.

Filocamo M, Morrone A. Lysosomal storage disorders: molecular basis and laboratory testing. *Hum Genomics.* 2011;5:156-169.

Migeon BR. X inactivation, female mosaicism, and sex differences in renal diseases. *J Am Soc Nephrol.* 2008;19:2052-2059.

Parenti G, Andria G, Ballabio A. Lysosomal storage diseases: from pathophysiology to therapy. *Annu Rev Med.* 2015;66:471-486.




# 157 Peroxisome Disorders

Michael Wangler, William B. Rizzo, and Nancy Braverman

## INTRODUCTION TO PEROXISOME BIOLOGY AND METABOLISM

Peroxisomes are single membrane-bound organelles present in virtually all eukaryotic cells that number between hundreds to a few thousand per cell. Peroxisomes appear on electron micrographs as spherical organelles (Fig. 157-1) and contain a dense proteinaceous matrix composed of over 50 enzymes. Peroxisomes are involved in a diverse list of metabolic processes, but the most well characterized are the enzymatic β-oxidation of very-long-chain fatty acids and other substrates, biosynthesis of plasmalogens and bile acids, α-oxidation of branched chain fatty acids (phytanic acid), and glyoxylate and lysine degradation. Furthermore, catalase and other antioxidant enzymes in

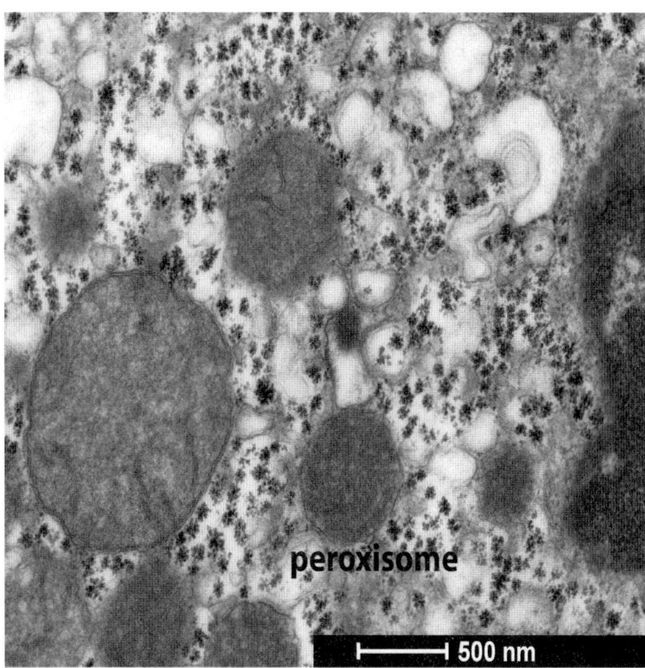


**FIGURE 157-1** Electron micrograph of human liver hepatocytes showing peroxisomes, spherical electron dense granules approximately 500 nm in diameter. Also seen are the mitochondria and glycogen granules. (Used with permission from Milton Finegold, MD, Professor of Pathology and Immunology, Baylor College of Medicine.)

**TABLE 157-1 HUMAN GENES INVOLVED IN PEROXISOMAL BIOGENESIS**

| Human Gene Symbol | Gene/Locus OMIM No. | Chromosome Location | Disease Phenotype |
|---|---|---|---|
| *PEX1* | 602136 | 7q21.2 | PBD-ZSD |
| *PEX2* | 170993 | 8q21.13 | PBD-ZSD |
| *PEX3* | 603164 | 6q24.2 | PBD-ZSD |
| *PEX5* | 600414 | 12p13.31 | PBD-ZSD<br>PBD-RCDP[a] |
| *PEX6* | 601498 | 6p21.1 | PBD-ZSD |
| *PEX7* | 601757 | 6q23.3 | PBD-RCDP |
| *PEX10* | 602859 | 1p36.32 | PBD-ZSD |
| *PEX11B* | 603867 | 1q21.1 | PBD-ZSD |
| *PEX12* | 601758 | 17q12 | PBD-ZSD |
| *PEX13* | 601789 | 2p15 | PBD-ZSD |
| *PEX14* | 601791 | 1p36.22 | PBD-ZSD |
| *PEX16* | 603360 | 11p11.2 | PBD-ZSD |
| *PEX19* | 600279 | 1q23.2 | PBD-ZSD |
| *PEX26* | 608666 | 22q11.21 | PBD-ZSD |

Note. See text for abbreviations.

[a]Baroy T, Koster J, Stromme P, et al. A novel type of rhizomelic chondrodysplasia punctata, RCDP5, is caused by loss of the PEX5 long isoform. *Hum Mol Genet*. 2015;24(20):5845-5854.

peroxisomes play a role in regulating the cellular redox balance. Peroxisomes form through the concerted action of an evolutionarily conserved protein machinery encoded by the *PEX* genes (Table 157-1). The *PEX* gene products orchestrate a process of de novo peroxisome biogenesis that begins with designation of membrane compartment, derived from the endoplasmic reticulum. In addition to de novo peroxisome biogenesis, peroxisomes can form from existing peroxisomes through fission, and recent studies have suggested that fission may play at least as important a role in creating new peroxisomes as de novo biogenesis.

Peroxisome biogenesis begins with membrane derived from the endoplasmic reticulum. The membrane designation step underlying de novo biogenesis of peroxisomes is a process that requires the *PEX3*, *PEX16*, and *PEX19* genes (Fig. 157-2A). While PEX3 and PEX16 proteins associate with the early peroxisome membrane, PEX19 is a cytosolic protein involved in targeting membrane proteins to the peroxisome. The resulting pre-peroxisomal vesicle is populated with additional peroxisomal membrane proteins by PEX19 protein and others, and eventually becomes competent to import matrix enzymes. The import of peroxisomal enzymes starts with the translation of these proteins on free ribosomes in the cytosol. The translated proteins contain 1 of 2 peroxisome-targeting signals. Peroxisome-targeting signal 1 (PTS1) is a C-terminal tripeptide (-SKL or conservative variants thereof) and is used by more than 90% of peroxisome enzymes or matrix proteins. Peroxisome-targeting signal 2 (PTS2) is a structural motif located close to the N-terminus and utilized by a few enzymes, including one involved in β-oxidation (peroxisomal thiolase 1), α-oxidation (phytanoyl-CoA hydroxylase), and plasmalogen biosynthesis (alkyl-glycerone phosphate synthase). The import of enzymes into the peroxisome requires that these PTS1 or PTS2 sequences be bound by their cytosolic receptors encoded by *PEX5* and *PEX7*, respectively. In addition, PEX7 and its PTS2 cargo require binding to the long isoform of PEX5, in order to be carried to the peroxisome membrane (Fig. 157-2B). Docking of the PEX5-PEX7 receptor complex is mediated by binding to specific peroxisome membrane proteins (PEX13, PEX14). The newly synthesized matrix enzymes are then translocated into the organelle. A group of membrane proteins, PEX2, PEX10, and PEX12, are involved in the ubiquitination of PEX5 protein. Mono-ubiquitinated PEX5 (and presumably PEX7) is recycled to the cytosol for additional rounds of import by the PEX1-PEX6-PEX26 proteins using the energy from adenosine triphosphate (ATP) hydrolysis. PEX1 and PEX6 proteins form a unique hexameric double-ring structure allowing this process to proceed. Peroxisomal fission (Fig. 157-3) requires *PEX11* genes, thought to encode relatively specific peroxisome fission proteins as well as additional genetic machinery, including *DNM1L* and *FIS1* genes that encode proteins

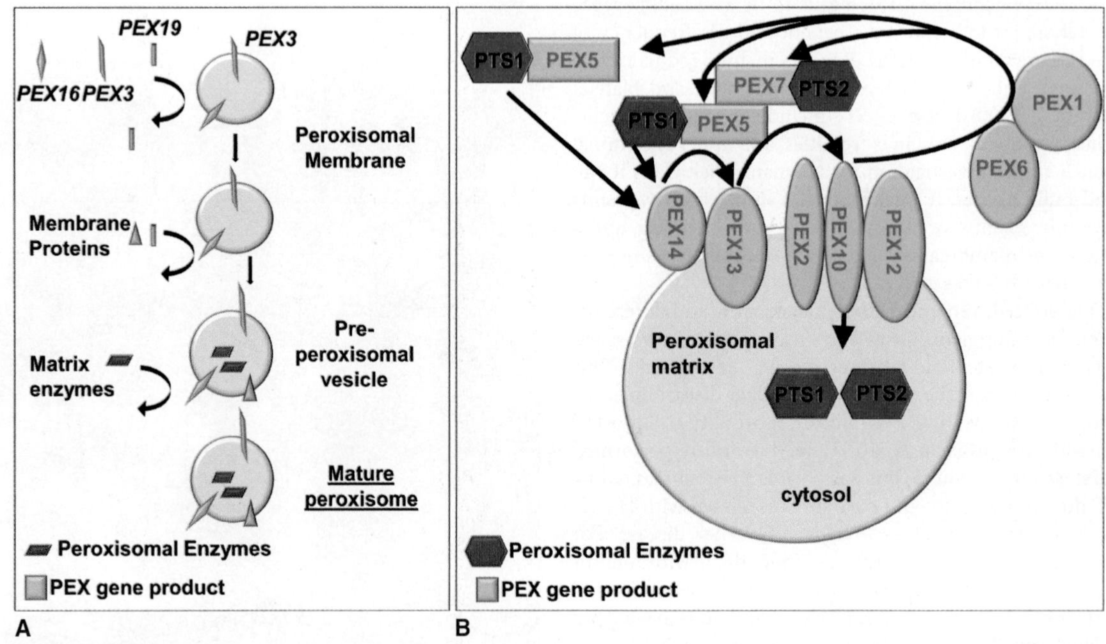


**FIGURE 157-2** Peroxisome biogenesis. **A:** Early factors encoded by PEX3, PEX16, and PEX19 are required for membrane biogenesis. PEX19, which is a cytosolic protein, continues to populate the pre-peroxisomal vesicle with peroxisome membrane proteins; after the addition of membrane proteins, the pre-peroxisomal vesicle can take on matrix enzymes, and a mature peroxisome is produced. Mature peroxisomes can undergo fission (Fig. 157-3), a process that may be equally as important for providing new peroxisomes in a cell. **B:** The process of matrix protein internalization or import involves the recognition of cytosolically translated peroxisome enzymes (*red rhomboids*); these are bound by receptors encoded by *PEX5* and *PEX7* depending on the targeting signal. The receptor cargo complex docks with the peroxisome membrane, and the cargo is shuttled to the matrix while the receptor is recycled, a process requiring *PEX14*, *PEX13*, and ubiquitination machinery encoded by *PEX2*, *PEX10*, and *PEX12*. Recycling also depends on *PEX1* and *PEX6*.

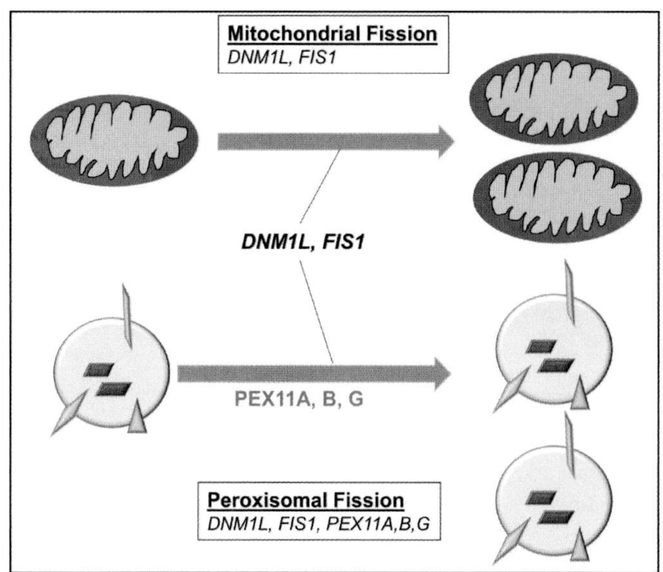


**FIGURE 157-3** Shared organelle fission factors encoded by *DNM1L* and *FIS1* are responsible for peroxisome and mitochondrial fission. *PEX11* genes (*PEX11 A, B, G*) encode factors specifically involved in peroxisome but not mitochondrial fission. DNM1L has been implicated in a number of encephalopathy cases (OMIM no. 614388).

shared between mitochondria and peroxisomes. The *PEX* genes thus encode machinery that is responsible for the systematic formation of peroxisomes within the cell.

Once the peroxisomal enzymes are internalized, the mature peroxisome carries out its biochemical function. The β-oxidation systems of peroxisomes and mitochondria have distinct but overlapping substrate specificities, with peroxisomes preferentially oxidizing very-long-chain ($C_{22}$–$C_{26}$) fatty acids to $C_{18}$–$C_{16}$, and then delivering these to mitochondria for further oxidation. β-Oxidation enzymes also differ; in peroxisomes, the first step is catalyzed by acyl-coenzyme A (CoA) oxidase, which produces $H_2O_2$, whereas the analogous enzymes in mitochondria (acyl-CoA dehydrogenases) transfer their electrons to the respiratory chain via electron transport flavoprotein (ETF) and ETF-dehydrogenase. In peroxisomal β-oxidation, the $H_2O_2$ produced is efficiently eliminated by catalase, another peroxisome matrix enzyme. Additional oxidase enzymes are present in peroxisomes and function in various biochemical pathways.

## PEROXISOME DISORDERS CLASSIFICATION

Understanding how peroxisomes form and function aids in dividing the clinical disorders into 2 main classes: (1) peroxisome biogenesis disorders (PBD), which are characterized by deficiency of multiple peroxisome functions due to mutations in the *PEX* genes leading to dysfunctional organelle biogenesis, and (2) single-enzyme disorders in which only 1 peroxisome function is deficient due to loss of 1 enzyme or a single peroxisome component (Table 157-2). Biogenesis disorders can be further divided into Zellweger spectrum disorders (ZSDs), which are more generalized and involve mislocalization of all peroxisome enzymes, and rhizomelic chondrodysplasia punctata (RCDP) types 1 and 5, which are specific for PTS2 localization defects (*PEX7* or *PEX5*). The mutations in the type 5 RCDP subtype have recently been described and involve unique mutations in the *PEX5* gene predicted to disrupt only the PEX5-PEX7 protein complex but not PEX5-PTS1 import (see Fig. 157-2B). Many of the single-enzyme defects mimic features of PBD, and around 10% of PBD cases diagnosed clinically are found to be due to single-enzyme defects.

Classifying PBD has changed over time from a group of named seemingly clinically distinct disorders to the realization of a clinical spectrum due to a common etiology—*PEX* gene defects. The ZSD accounts for the majority of PBD patients and includes at least 3 phenotypes originally thought to represent discrete disorders but that are now recognized as segments of a continuous spectrum (Table 157-3). Patients with PBD-ZSD of different severities, previously designated Zellweger syndrome (ZS), neonatal adrenoleukodystrophy (NALD), and infantile Refsum disease (IRD), are now classified as having severe, intermediate, or mild PBD-ZSD. The PBD-ZSD are a genetically heterogeneous set of disorders with 13 causative loci to date (*PEX1, PEX2, PEX3, PEX5, PEX6, PEX10, PEX11B, PEX12, PEX13, PEX14, PEX16, PEX19*, and *PEX26*). These genes underlie the earlier 13 complementation groups determined by somatic cell hybridization studies in which the cellular defect in one patient's cells was tested for complementation by another patient's cells. All PBD-ZSD are inherited as autosomal recessive traits and have an aggregate incidence estimated at 1 in 50,000, although milder cases diagnosed by DNA sequencing may not have always been detected in the past. Newborn screening for X-linked adrenoleukodystrophy, which was recently approved at the federal level in the United States, will also detect most PBD-ZSD cases and is expected to provide more accurate estimates of disease incidence in the future. Genetic defects in *PEX* genes generally exhibit significant locus heterogeneity as the ZSD phenotype is similar across the majority of cases involving any of the *PEX* loci. However, the type of mutation does have significant predictive value, with a number of milder missense mutations associated with milder ZSD phenotypes. Therefore, for most *PEX* loci, there is a strong genotype-phenotype correlation between the mutation, its effect on the encoded PEX protein, the downstream biochemical defects, and severity of the clinical phenotype. Thus, patients with biallelic loss-of-function alleles (eg, premature stop codons, frameshifts, or splice site mutations) are likely to exhibit more severe biochemical defects and clinical disease than patients with hypomorphic missense or in-frame alleles. Patients with hypomorphic alleles particularly in *PEX2, PEX10*, and *PEX16* have been reported with later onset ataxia phenotypes.

**TABLE 157-2 CLASSIFICATION OF DIFFERENT GROUPS OF PEROXISOME DISORDERS**

| | Peroxisome Biogenesis Disorders | | Selected Peroxisome Single Enzyme Defects[a] | | |
|---|---|---|---|---|---|
| **Diagnostic Studies** | **PBD-ZSD** | **RCDP Type 1 and 5** | **X-ALD** | **D-BP Deficiency, Acyl-CoA Oxidase Deficiency, Other β-Oxidation Defects[a]** | **RCDP Types 2, 3, and 4** |
| VLCFAs | ↑ | N | ↑ | ↑ | N |
| Phytanic acid | N[b]-↑ | N-↑ | N | N-↑ | N |
| Pristanic acid | N[b]-↑ | N | N | N-↑ | N |
| RBC plasmalogens | ↓ | ↓ | N | N | ↓ |
| Catalase solubility in fibroblasts | ↑ | N | N | N | N |
| Gene(s) | *PEX1, 2, 3, 5, 6, 10, 11B, 12, 13, 14, 16, 19, 26* | *PEX7, PEX5* (in the PEX7 binding region) | *ABCD1* | *HSD17B4, ACOX1, ACBD5* | *GNPAT, AGPS, FAR1* |

Note. See text for abbreviations.

[a]See Table 157-4.

[b]Normal levels can be seen in mild PBD-ZSD phenotypes; fibroblast enzyme studies can assist in detecting enzymatic defects in these cases.

**TABLE 157-3 THE CLINICAL SPECTRUM OF PBD-ZSD**

| System | Finding | Severe | Intermediate | Mild |
|---|---|---|---|---|
| Neurologic | Neuronal migration defect | Present | Absent | Absent |
| | Seizures | Present | Variable | Absent |
| | Demyelinating leukodystrophy | Absent | Variable | Variable |
| | Hearing loss | Present | Progressive | Progressive |
| Ocular | Cataracts | Variable | Variable | Variable |
| | Retinal degeneration | Present | Progressive | Progressive |
| Hepatic | Hepatobiliary disease | Present | Present early on, improves over time | Variable early on, improves over time |
| Craniofacial | Dysmorphology | Classic | Less severe | Less severe |
| Renal | Cysts | Present | Absent | Absent |
| | Calcium oxalate stones | Absent | Variable | Variable |
| Adrenal | Insufficiency | Absent | Variable | Variable |
| Skeletal | Chondrodysplasia punctata | Present | Absent | Absent |
| | Osteopenia | Absent | Variable | Variable |
| Dentition | Amelogenesis imperfecta | Absent | Secondary teeth | Secondary teeth |
| Survival | | Less than 1 year | Into at least childhood | Into at least second decade, slower evolution of disease |



Also, patients with the *PEX1* p.G843D allele exhibit a milder PBD phenotype. The p.G843D allele is the most common disease-causing allele in European populations. Other milder phenotypes include the recently reported mild ZSD syndrome (Heimler syndrome), which has the common features of hearing loss, retinal degeneration, and tooth enamel hypoplasia, but emphasizes that normal intellect is part of the spectrum, and in this case results from *PEX1* or *PEX6* hypomorphic alleles.

In addition, given that some peroxisome fission proteins are shared with mitochondria, some patients have been described with defects affecting both mitochondria and peroxisomes. In particular, autosomal recessive loss-of-function and dominant de novo missense variants in the middle domain of the *DNM1L* gene with dominant-negative activity are implicated in cases of infantile encephalopathy that affect both mitochondria and peroxisomes.

The single-enzyme peroxisome disorders include at least 11 different disorders inherited as autosomal recessive traits, except for X-linked adrenoleukodystrophy (ALD), nearly all of which are uncommon, with incidences of less than 1 in 50,000 (Table 157-4). X-linked ALD (X-ALD) is a neurologic disorder with abnormal accumulation of very-long-chain fatty acids (VLCFA) and an incidence in males of about 1 in 18,000. At the cellular level, peroxisomes in the single-enzyme defects typically appear cytologically normal and have normal import of matrix proteins, although there are exceptions.

## PEROXISOME BIOGENESIS DISORDERS (PBD)

### ZELLWEGER SPECTRUM DISORDERS (ZSD)

#### Clinical Aspects

PBD-ZSD have severe, intermediate, and mild forms. In the severe cases of PBD-ZSD, the *PEX* gene defects are null or strong hypomorphic alleles, and these infants are recognized in the neonatal period by having classic neuronal migration defects in the brain causing neonatal seizures and a characteristic facial dysmorphology. Affected infants have a high forehead, shallow supraorbital ridges, epicanthal folds, a small nose with a broad flat nasal bridge, anteverted nares, and micrognathia (Fig. 157-4A–B). The anterior fontanelle is large. Cataracts and a pigmentary retinopathy are common. Profound hypotonia, feeding problems, and growth failure are present. Hearing impairment is common, and some infants fail their newborn hearing screen. Liver function is abnormal, with conjugated hyperbilirubinemia and elevated transaminases. Radiologic examination reveals punctate calcifications ("calcific stippling") in the hips and knees. Multiple small renal cysts are common but may not be detected by ultrasound examination. Infants with the severe form rarely live beyond 1 year of age, largely because the brain malformations are not compatible with life.

In the intermediate and milder forms of PBD-ZSD, dysmorphic facial features are less severe or may even be absent (Fig. 157-4C–D). These patients are not born with malformations but instead have a progressive disorder of peroxisome dysfunction over time. The majority of intermediate patients will develop adrenal insufficiency, and some will develop leukodystrophy. Hypotonia and seizures are common. Because of their flat facial features, single transverse palmer creases, and hypotonia, a few patients were thought to have Down syndrome. Survival can range through childhood, to even older patients, but all have cognitive defects, sensorineural hearing loss, and retinopathy.

Milder ZSD patients may have minimal dysmorphic features and hypotonia (see Fig. 157-4D). The predominant manifestations may be hepatomegaly, cholestasis, and failure to thrive in early infancy. Liver disease usually improves, but can progress to liver failure later on in a few patients. Decreased bone mineral density may be seen, which can require treatment with bisphosphonates. As they get older, virtually all patients develop sensorineural hearing loss and pigmentary retinopathy. The degree of cognitive deficiency can vary from moderate delays to normal intellect. In addition, atypical phenotypes with later onset ataxia, resembling autosomal recessive spinocerebellar ataxias, have been noted in patients with mild mutations in *PEX* genes such as *PEX2*, *PEX10*, and *PEX16*.

#### Biochemical and Molecular Aspects

The most frequently used diagnostic laboratory tests for PBD detect abnormalities of peroxisome metabolic processes, including elevated plasma VLCFA and pristanic acid (substrates for peroxisomal β-oxidation), phytanic acid (substrate for peroxisomal α-oxidation), and decreased red blood cell (RBC) plasmalogens (product of peroxisomal plasmalogen synthesis). Plasma VLCFA (C26:0 and C26:1) levels are increased in PBD-ZSD to an extent roughly correlating with clinical severity (Table 157-5). Compared to control levels, VLCFAs are elevated about 10-fold in the severe form, 5-fold in the intermediate form, and 3-fold (or even normal) in the milder forms. Similarly, plasma phytanic acid is increased 10- to a 100-fold in severe PBD-ZSD patients who are old enough to ingest dietary precursors of this compound. Erythrocyte plasmalogens are reduced by 10-fold or more, yet they can be normal in milder ZSD. Other blood and urine laboratory abnormalities in PBD-ZSD due to defective peroxisomal β-oxidation include increased medium- and long-chain dicarboxylic acids, pipecolic acid, and bile acid precursors such as dihydroxy-cholestanoic acid (DHCA) and trihydroxy-cholesanoic acid (THCA), and deficient docosahexaenoic acid (DHA) and mature bile acids (cholic acid and chenodeoxycholic acid).

**TABLE 157-4 OVERVIEW OF SINGLE PEROXISOMAL ENZYMES/PROTEIN DEFECTS**

| Disorder | OMIM No. | Phenotype(s) | Gene | Abnormalities | Peroxisomal Enzyme Pathways |
|---|---|---|---|---|---|
| X-linked adrenoleukodystrophy | 300100 | Childhood cerebral form (ccALD), adult adrenomyeloneuropathy (AMN) | *ABCD1* | ↑ VLCFA | Fatty acid β-oxidation |
| Acyl-CoA-binding protein 5 deficiency | —[a] | Leukodystrophy, ataxia and retinal dystrophy | *ACBD5* | ↑ VLCFA | |
| Peroxisomal acyl-CoA oxidase deficiency | 264470 | Similar to PBD-ZSD | *ACOX1* | ↑ VLCFA | |
| D-bifunctional protein deficiency | 261515<br>233400 | Similar to PBD-ZSD "pseudo-Zellweger spectrum" | *HSD17B4* | ↑ VLCFA and branched chain (pristanic and phytanic acids) | |
| Leukoencephalopathy with dystonia and motor neuropathy | 184755 | Dystonia; combined peripheral motor and sensory neuropathy | *SCP2* | ↑ Pristanic acid, abnormal bile alcohol in urine | |
| Alpha-methylacyl-CoA racemase deficiency | 614307 | Peripheral motor and sensory neuropathy, hepatobiliary disease | *AMACR* | ↑ Pristanic acid<br>↑ C27 bile acid intermediates | |
| Bile acid synthesis defect, congenital, 5 | 616278[b] | Progressive liver failure, coagulopathy | *ABCD3* | ↑ VLCFA<br>↑ C27 bile acid intermediates | |
| Refsum disease | 266500 | Peripheral motor and sensory neuropathy with retinal degeneration | *PHYH* | ↑ Phytanic acid | Fatty acid α-oxidation |
| RCDP, type 2 | 222765 | Similar to RCDP1 | *GNPAT* | ↓ Plasmalogens | Ether phospholipid biosynthesis |
| RCDP, type 3 | 600121 | Similar to RCDP1 | *AGPS* | ↓ Plasmalogens | |
| RCDP, type 4 (peroxisomal fatty acyl-CoA reductase 1 disorder) | 616154 | Absence of skeletal dysplasia | *FAR1* | ↓ Plasmalogens | |
| Acatalasemia | 614097 | Oral ulcers catalase | *CAT* | | Hydrogen peroxide degradation |
| Primary hyperoxaluria type 1 | 259900 | Nephrocalcinosis, end-stage renal failure | *AGXT* | Hyperoxaluria calcium-oxalate renal stones | Glyoxylate detoxification |

Note. See text for abbreviations.

[a]Ferdinandusse S, Falkenberg KM, Koster J, et al. ACBD5 deficiency causes a defect in peroxisomal very-long-chain fatty acid metabolism. *J Med Genet.* 2016; doi:10.1136/jmedgenet-2016-104132.

[b]Ferdinandusse S, Jimenez-Sanchez G, Koster J, et al. A novel bile acid biosynthesis defect due to a deficiency of peroxisomal ABCD3. *Hum Mol Genet.* 2015;24:361-370.

Traditionally, confirmation of diagnoses was made based on clinical phenotype and enzymatic assays of peroxisome β-oxidation and plasmalogen synthesis in cultured skin fibroblasts. These assays were often supplemented by immunohistochemical studies localizing PTS1- and PTS2-targeted matrix proteins and peroxisome membrane proteins, and complementation analysis was used to identify the responsible *PEX* gene. Currently, with advances in next-generation DNA sequencing technology, patients with clinical and biochemical

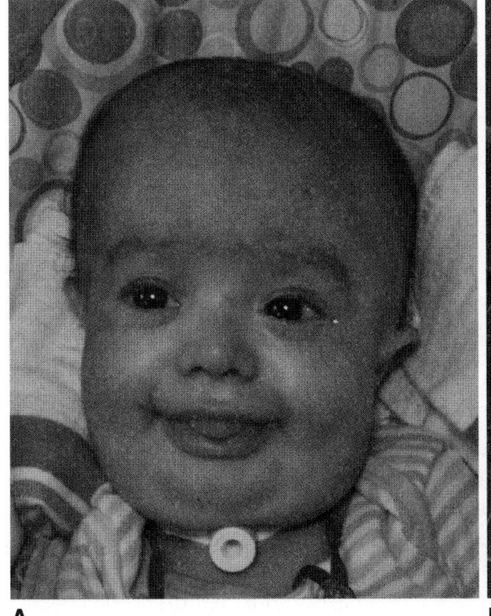
A

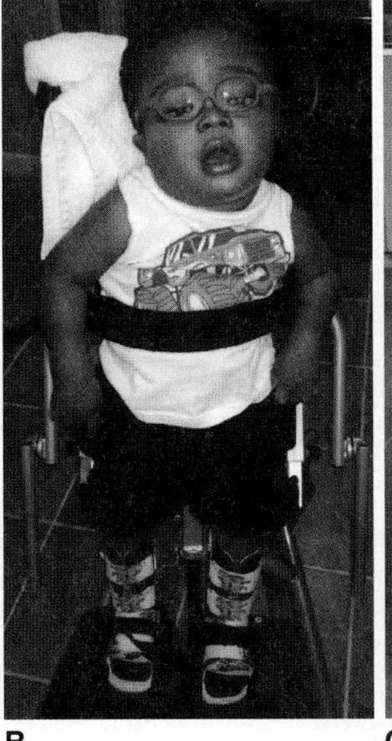
B

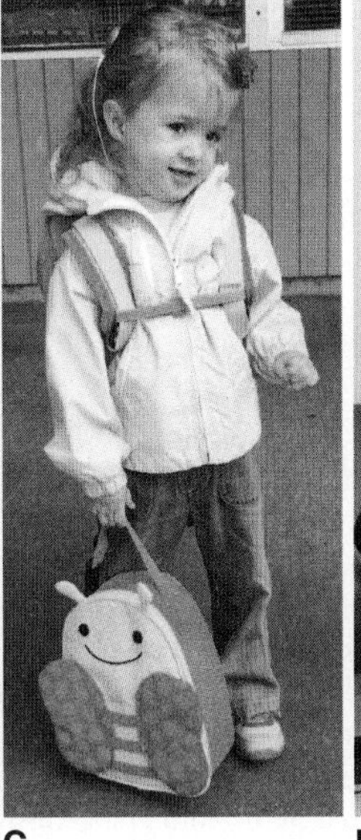
C

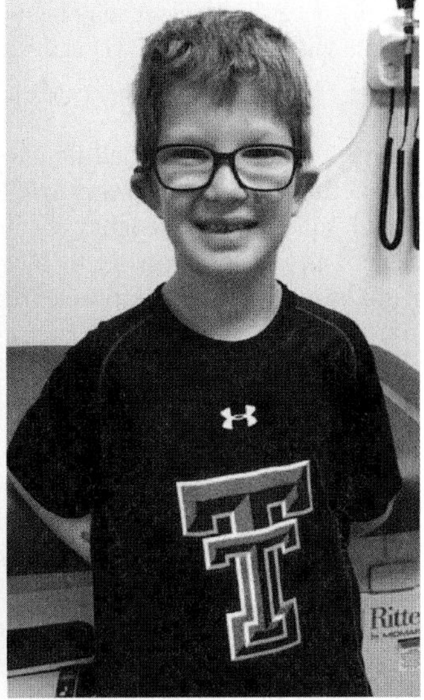
D

**FIGURE 157-4** Facial appearances of peroxisome biogenesis disorder (PBD) patients with the PBD-Zellweger spectrum disorder (ZSD). **A:** Infant with severe PBD (Zellweger syndrome). **B:** Child with intermediate to severe form. **C:** School-age child with mild-intermediate form. **D:** School-age child with mild form. (Reproduced with permission from the Global Foundation for Peroxisomal Disorders [GFPD].)

**TABLE 157-5 PLASMA TOTAL VERY-LONG-CHAIN FATTY ACIDS IN CONTROLS SUBJECTS AND PEROXISOME DISORDERS**

| Analyte | Normal | Zellweger Syndrome | X-Linked Adrenoleukodystrophy (affected male) |
|---|---|---|---|
| C22:0 (comparison analyte) | 21.0 ± 6.3 | 8.7 ± 5.0 | 18.5 ± 5.1 |
| C24:0 | 17.6 ± 5.4 | 17.5 ± 8.6 | 32.3 ± 8.2 |
| C26:0 (hexacosanoic) | 0.23 ± 0.09 | 3.9 ± 1.5 | 1.30 ± 0.45 |
| C24/C22 | 0.84 ± 0.10 | 2.07 ± 0.28 | 1.71 ± 0.23 |
| C26/C22 | 0.01 ± 0.004 | 0.50 ± 0.16 | 0.07 ± 0.03 |

Data from Moser AB, Kreiter N, Bezman L, et al. Plasma very-long-chain fatty acids in 3,000 peroxisome disease patients and 29,000 controls, *Ann Neurol*. 1999 Jan;45(1):100-110.



features of PBD-ZSD are increasingly being diagnosed molecularly by sequencing panels that quickly identify *PEX* gene mutations. Increasingly, reports of milder cases are emerging based on whole-exome sequencing, and in these cases, comprehensive biochemical and enzymatic studies are useful for functional validation of sequence variants and phenotype correlations.

## MANAGEMENT

Treatment is palliative in severe ZSD where disease begins prenatally and largely supportive in the intermediate and milder forms. Supplementation with dietary omega-3 fatty acids (DHA) has been used in some patients, although little objective evidence exists for its efficacy to improve neurovisual function. In older individuals, plasma phytanic acid concentrations should be monitored and dietary phytanic acid restriction can be considered, although the benefits have not been conclusively demonstrated. Regular monitoring of growth and nutrition is required. In general, feeding difficulties are common, and placement of a gastrostomy tube may be required to improve nutrition and to facilitate care. Liver dysfunction due to cholestasis can cause steatorrhea, fat-soluble vitamin deficiency with concomitant rickets, and coagulopathy, requiring vitamin D and K supplementation. Supplements of all lipid-soluble vitamins (K, A, D, and E) are often administered. Liver function studies and abdominal ultrasound can be useful to diagnose and monitor hepatic dysfunction in PBD-ZSD. A recent systematic study of cholic acid supplementation in a cohort of ZSD patients showed this can improve the cholestasis, but whether it improves the overall clinical outcome is not known.

Given the high risk for adrenal insufficiency, regular evaluation of adrenal function is required, and early evidence of adrenal insufficiency requires adrenal hormone replacement therapy. Anticonvulsant medications are indicated to control seizures. Hearing loss typically requires hearing aids, and cochlear implants have been successfully used. Eye glasses may help correct visual acuity. In addition, patients with mild PBD-ZSD can experience significant dental issues due to the lack of normal tooth enamel and require specialized dental care.

Genetic counseling for all families is imperative. All known PBD are inherited as autosomal recessive traits, with a 25% recurrence risk for each subsequent pregnancy of couples who have had 1 PBD infant. Prenatal diagnosis is possible by biochemical methods and molecular methods, and preimplantation genetic diagnosis is possible by DNA studies of isolated blastocysts.

## RHIZOMELIC CHONDRODYSPLASIA PUNCTATA (RCDP)

The second PBD phenotypic spectrum, accounting for about 20% of PBD patients, is RCDP. Although both disorders involve defects in peroxisome biogenesis, RCDP is clinically and genetically distinct from PBD-ZSD. RCDP is characterized by severe bone dysplasia, postnatal growth deficiency, intellectual disability, epilepsy, and cataracts. As in ZSD, there is a spectrum of phenotypes, from severe to mild. Most patients have mutations in *PEX7*, the gene encoding the receptor for PTS2 proteins leading to a peroxisome biogenesis defect characterized by mislocalization of enzymes encoded by the genes *AGPS*, *PHYH*, and *ACAA1*. A few RCDP patients (<10%) have single-enzyme defects in 1 of the 3 peroxisome matrix enzymes necessary for plasmalogen synthesis (encoded by *FAR1, GNPAT, AGPS*), or a defect in the PEX5 protein region that binds to PEX7 protein (a peroxisome biogenesis defect).

Patients with classic RCDP have severe skeletal involvement at birth distinct from PBD-ZSD (Fig. 157-5). There is rhizomelia with shortening of the proximal limbs (Fig. 157-5A–B) and limited range of movement of the large joints of the extremities. Radiologic examination shows coronal clefts of the vertebral bodies apparent on lateral spine films (Fig. 157-5C) and extensive calcific stippling that involves the epiphyses of long bones (Fig. 157-5D); it is most prominent in the knees, elbows, hips, and shoulders. RCDP patients also have a flat face with frontal bossing.

In RCDP, diagnostic testing of peroxisome functions show a different pattern than that seen in typical PBD-ZSD. RCDP patients have very low levels of erythrocyte plasmalogens, typically more severely reduced than in PBD-ZSD. In RCDP, including the biogenesis subtypes (1 and 5), plasma VLCFA levels are normal, possibly because PTS1-targeted peroxisomal thiolase 2 (sterol carrier protein X) substitutes for the lack of the PTS2-targeted peroxisomal thiolase 1.

Management is largely supportive for patients with RCDP. The consequences of the severe skeletal involvement should be carefully assessed in RCDP patients with complete skeletal surveys. Orthopedic interventions may be needed for cervical spine stenosis and hip and shoulder dysplasia, as needed for each child and their expected clinical trajectory. Ophthalmologic exams are recommended as cataracts are universal. Cardiac malformations are common, and a renal evaluation should be undertaken at diagnosis. Severe growth and psychomotor retardation is present, and most classical patients die by late childhood. However, there are patients with milder disease who have better survival. Growth curves for classical and nonclassical RCDP are now available. The more mildly affected patients have improved growth and mild intellectual defects but little or no rhizomelia. Thus far, oral plasmalogen supplementation has not been shown to have significant clinical benefit.

# PEROXISOME SINGLE-ENZYME DEFECTS

## X-LINKED ADRENOLEUKODYSTROPHY

### Clinical Aspects

X-ALD is a neurodegenerative disorder related to defective peroxisomal oxidation of VLCFA. There are multiple phenotypic presentations for males with X-ALD. The most severe is childhood cerebral X-ALD (ccALD), which is a rapidly progressive, inflammatory, central demyelinating disease that begins between ages 3 and 10. About 35% of X-ALD males manifest this phenotype with progressive behavioral, cognitive, and neurologic abnormalities that lead to total disability within 3 years and eventually to death. Nearly all of these patients have adrenal insufficiency. The onset of neurologic symptoms for patients with ccALD is usually insidious with declining school performance, staring spells, and behavior problems that progress to gait disturbances, visual impairment, incoordination manifesting as poor handwriting, loss of spoken language, and dementia. Some boys with ccALD manifest initially as a new-onset attention deficit disorder. At the time of diagnosis, nearly all of these patients have adrenal insufficiency, which can even develop years prior to the onset of neurologic symptoms. Brain magnetic resonance imaging (MRI) in patients with

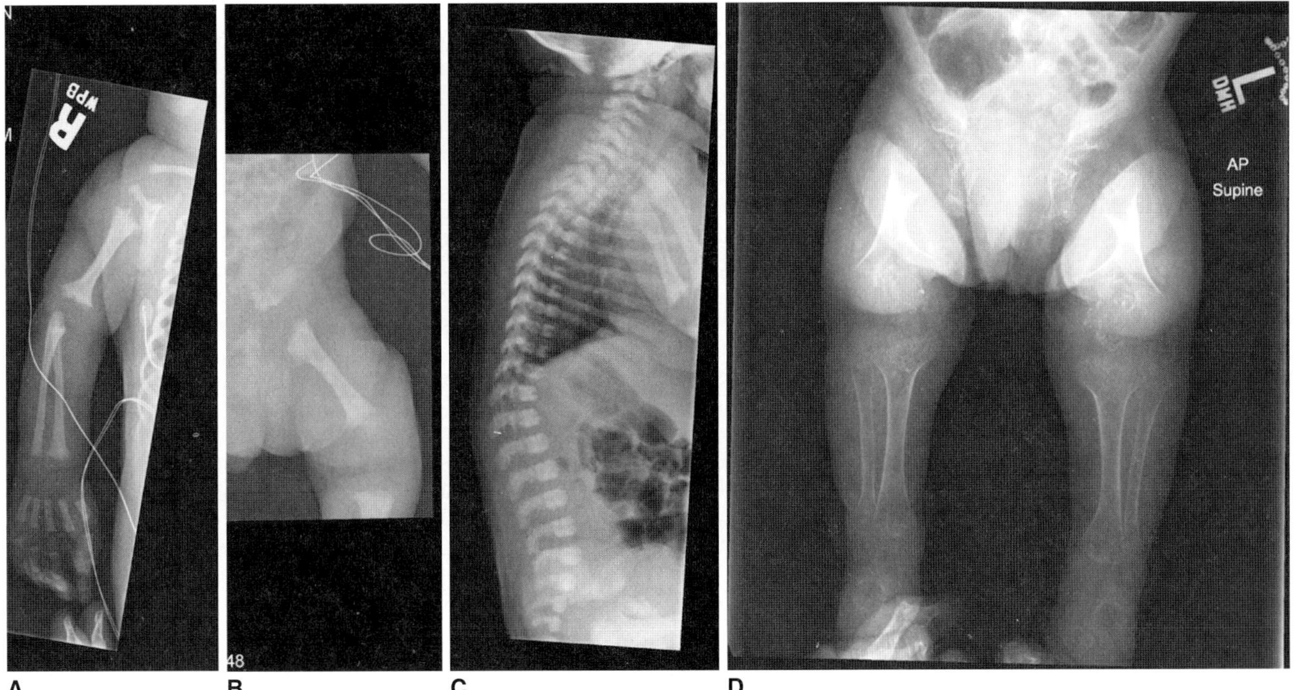


**FIGURE 157-5** Radiographs of an infant with rhizomelia chondrodysplasia punctata (RCDP). **A.** Forearm showing extreme rhizomelia and punctate calcifications. **B.** Upper leg showing rhizomelia. **C.** Lateral spine showing coronal clefts of the vertebral bodies. **D.** Lower extremities showing punctate calcifications.



cerebral disease will show T2-weighted symmetric areas of increased signal in the parieto-occipital region, although about 10% of patients with prominent behavioral symptoms present with frontal demyelination (see Chapter 566).

A second, distinct phenotype, known as adrenomyeloneuropathy (AMN), usually begins in the third to fourth decade and is characterized by a distal axonopathy, mainly involving the spinal cord and long tract nerves. AMN patients manifest a slowly progressive gait disturbance and progressive urinary sphincter dysfunction. About two-thirds of AMN patients develop adrenal insufficiency, and about 40% eventually manifest cerebral demyelination. This and other evidence has led to the suggestion that AMN may be the "default" disease phenotype for individuals with X-ALD but that additional triggers of inflammatory changes can produce childhood cerebral forms.

Other phenotypic presentations include adults with isolated adrenal involvement or "Addison disease only," but many of these men eventually develop AMN symptoms. Although X-ALD is X-linked, female carriers can develop progressive lower extremity dysfunction, similar to AMN, depending on the pattern of lionization in a female carrier.

#### Biochemical and Molecular Aspects

This highly variable, X-linked, neurodegenerative disorder is caused by mutations in *ABCD1*, the gene encoding ALDP, an ATP-binding cassette (ABC) transporter located in the peroxisome membrane. ALDP function is postulated to be required for VLCFA to enter peroxisomes, where they are degraded by peroxisomal β-oxidation. When the diagnosis of X-ALD is considered, the combination of plasma VLCFA levels and molecular analysis can identify all X-ALD hemizygotes and heterozygotes. Regardless of their phenotype, X-ALD patients have a marked elevation of plasma VLCFA, particularly C26:0. In cultured skin fibroblasts, β-oxidation of VLCFA is impaired. Plasma VLCFAs are elevated prior to the onset of neurologic disease, which allows identification of presymptomatic boys. Although most (85%) of female heterozygotes have elevated plasma VLCFA, DNA mutation analysis is the most reliable method for detecting X-ALD carriers. Most mutations in *ABCD1* are private, and over 750 different mutations have been reported. There is no correlation between the nature of the *ABCD1* mutation and phenotypic severity. In fact, multiple affected members in a single family, all with the same mutant *ABCD1* allele, may manifest the extremes of phenotypic expression; individuals with the childhood cerebral form occur in the same family as individuals with only AMN or isolated adrenal insufficiency. This provides strong evidence for the presence of modifier genes or environmental factors that affect phenotypic expression of the disease.

Prenatal diagnosis is possible by measuring VLCFA (in males) in amniocytes and chorionic villi cells or by molecular analysis of *ABCD1*. Newborn screening for X-ALD is possible using tandem mass spectrometry to detect accumulation of C26:0-lyso-PC in dried blood spots, and screening has been initiated in a few state newborn screening programs in the United States.

ALDP, the protein product of ABCD1, is a peroxisome membrane transporter that functions either as a homodimer of 2 ALDP subunits or a heterodimer of ALDP with 1 of 3 other related ABC transporters found in the peroxisomal membrane. The ligands for these transporters are not known with certainty but are likely to be long-chain fatty acids, fatty acyl-CoAs, or other lipid molecules. The ALDP homodimer is probably limited to transporting VLCFA or VLCFA-CoA. In X-ALD, VLCFAs that cannot be degraded by peroxisomal β-oxidation are incorporated into other lipids including cholesterol esters, sphingolipids, cerebrosides, and phospholipids. Accumulation of these VLCFA-containing lipids seems to be a necessary factor for symptom expression, but the precise pathogenic mechanisms leading to neurologic and adrenal disease are unclear. Nevertheless, evidence is emerging from the *Abcd1* gene knockout mouse model that oxidative stress may be a key contributor to the slowly progressive myeloneuropathy of AMN. In postmortem ccALD brain, microglial cells are activated and undergo apoptosis in regions of demyelination, which can be recapitulated in mice by intracerebral injection of VLCFA-containing lyso-phosphatidylcholine (VLCFA-lyso-PC).

## MANAGEMENT

Most X-ALD males will develop adrenal insufficiency at some point in life. Therefore, all males should be monitored for adrenal function, at the time of diagnosis and then yearly, by measuring 8:00 AM cortisol and adrenocorticotropic hormone. Adrenal hormone replacement with hydrocortisone is usually sufficient, although some patients may require mineralocorticoid supplementation in addition. The highly variable neurologic phenotypic manifestations of X-ALD make evaluating any therapy that is initiated at a presymptomatic stage difficult. Reducing VLCFA by dietary measures does not arrest cerebral disease once established. Reducing VLCFA as a preventative therapy with dietary measures such as "Lorenzo's oil" can be accomplished, but there is no unambiguous clinical trial evidence that this is effective. Reducing VLCFA by dietary measures does not arrest cerebral disease after it is established. In contrast, performing hematopoietic stem cell transplantation (HSCT) in boys who are in the early stages of the childhood cerebral phenotype arrests progression of the brain disease. Therefore, young presymptomatic boys should be monitored with regular brain MRIs every 6 to 12 months to detect the onset of cerebral disease and allow HSCT at the earliest possible time, since demyelination can continue for several months after transplantation. The decision about whether to undergo HSCT is based on demonstrating very early white matter disease on MRI and minimal neuropsychological impairment. Once cerebral disease is well established in boys, care is palliative. Successful gene therapy using genetically corrected bone marrow–derived stem cells has recently been reported with initial outcomes that are comparable to those seen with HSCT and is currently in clinical trials.

Given the wide phenotypic variation in X-ALD and its inherited nature, all families require genetic counseling.



## ADDITIONAL SINGLE-ENZYME DEFECTS

### Disorders of Peroxisome Fatty Acid β-Oxidation

In addition to X-ALD, at least 7 inherited disorders of peroxisomal fatty acid β-oxidation have been identified. After X-ALD, D-bifunctional protein deficiency is the most common. Deficiency of acyl-CoA oxidase enzymes (ACOX1), peroxisomal thiolases (pTH1 and pTH2) and 2-methylacyl-CoA racemase (AMACR), ATP-binding cassette transporter 3 (ABCD3), and Acyl-CoA binding domain-containing protein 5 (ACBD5) are considerably more rare. Interestingly, the clinical phenotype of several of these enzyme deficiencies, particularly ACOX1 and D-bifunctional protein, in the β-oxidation pathway resembles that of ZSD patients, suggesting that disruption of peroxisomal β-oxidation plays a major role in the pathophysiology of PBD. Some patients with isolated peroxisomal fatty acid oxidation defects, such as AMACR deficiency, may present in late child or adulthood as isolated peripheral neuropathy mimicking Charcot-Marie-Tooth disorder.

Diagnosing these patients depends on detecting peroxisomal β-oxidation defects (increased VLCFA and/or increased pristanic acid and bile acid precursors) with other peroxisome functions and normal peroxisomal assembly. All of these disorders are inherited as autosomal recessive traits, and prenatal diagnosis is available.

### Refsum Disease

This disorder in the peroxisomal α-oxidation of phytanic acid typically presents in the second decade of life but can occur in children, as a third of patients experience their first symptoms before 10 years of age. Virtually all patients develop retinitis pigmentosa, with night blindness as an initial symptom. Progressive combined sensory and motor neuropathy affecting mainly the lower extremities is a later symptom, as are cerebellar dysfunction and ataxia. Other less uniform symptoms include early-onset anosmia, cardiomyopathy with arrhythmias, and ichthyotic skin rash.

The primary defect is deficiency of phytanoyl-CoA hydroxylase caused by mutations in the *PHYH* gene in 90% of patients and *PEX7* gene in 10%. Refsum disease is an autosomal recessive disorder, and prenatal diagnosis by biochemical and/or molecular methods is possible. Plasma phytanic acid levels are markedly elevated (100- to 1000-fold), which affords a simple diagnostic test. The enzymatic defect can be demonstrated in cultured skin fibroblasts.

Phytanic acid and its metabolic precursor, phytol, are solely derived from the diet and found in fat from ruminant animals (meat and dairy products from cow, sheep, and other ruminants) and some fatty fishes. Diets restricted in these substances produce a gradual but dramatic decline in plasma and tissue phytanic acid. This can be hastened by plasmapheresis. Patients who maintain their phytanic acid at near normal levels often improve clinically. For these reasons, dietary treatment should be instituted as soon as possible and maintained for life.

### Primary Hyperoxaluria Type I

Primary hyperoxaluria type I (PH1) is characterized by an accumulation of calcium oxalate leading to renal failure and is due to deficiency of the peroxisomal enzyme alanine-glyoxylate aminotransferase. The age of onset ranges from infancy to adulthood. PH1 is caused by mutations in the *AGXT* gene, which lead to impaired transamination of glyoxylate. Oxidation of glyoxylate to oxalate results in massive calcium oxalate accumulation, eventually producing nephrocalcinosis and renal failure. The diagnosis of HP1 is based on demonstrating increased oxalate and glycolate in urine. DNA studies identify autosomal recessive mutations in the *AGXT* gene. One of the common mutations (p.G170R) in combination with an *AGXT* polymorphism (p.P11L) leads to mistargeting of the enzyme to mitochondria rather than peroxisomes. In PH1 patients who have some residual AGT enzyme activity, approximately one-third will show a biochemical and clinical response to pharmacologic doses of pyridoxine, which is a cofactor for the enzyme. The lack of AGT activity in the liver underlies the oxalate accumulation so that organ transplantation of liver prior to renal failure or combined renal and liver transplantations are definitive therapies.

## SUGGESTED READINGS

### Peroxisomal Biogenesis Disorders

Braverman NE, Chen L, Lin P, et al. Mutation analysis of PEX7 in 60 probands with rhizomelic chondrodysplasia punctate and functional correlations of genotype with phenotype. *Hum Mutat.* 2002;20(4):284-297.

Braverman NE, Raymond GV, Rizzo WB, et al. Peroxisome biogenesis disorders in the Zellweger spectrum: an overview of current diagnosis, clinical manifestations and treatment guidelines. *Mol Genet Metab.* 2016;117(3):313-321.

Moser AB, Kreiter N, Bezman L, et al. Plasma very long chain fatty acids in 3,000 peroxisome disease patients and 29,000 controls. *Ann Neurol.* 1999;45(1):100-110.

Rush ET, Goodwin JL, Braverman NE, Rizzo WB. Low bone mineral density is a common feature for Zellweger spectrum disorders. *Mol Genet Metab.* 2016;117(1):33-37.

Steinberg S, Dodt G, Raymond GV, Braverman NE, Moser AB, Moser HW. Peroxisome biogenesis disorders. *Biochim Biophys Acta.* 2006;1763(12):1733-1748.

Steinberg SJ, Raymond GV, Braverman NE, Moser AB. Peroxisome biogenesis disorders, zellweger syndrome spectrum. In: Pagon RA, Adam MP, Ardinger HH, eds. GeneReviews® [Internet]. Seattle, WA: University of Washington, Seattle; 1993-2015.

Waterham JR, Koster J, van Roermund CWT, et al. A lethal defect in mitochondrial and peroxisomal fission. *N Engl J Med.* 2007;356:1736.

Weller S, Gould SJ, Valle D. Peroxisome biogenesis disorders. *Ann Rev Genomics Hum Genet.* 2003;4:165.

### Single-Enzyme Disorders

Berger J, Gärtner J. X-linked adrenoleukodystrophy: clinical, biochemical and pathogenetic aspects. *Biochim Biophys Acta.* 2006;1763:1721.

Cochat P, Groothoff J. Primary hyperoxaluria type 1: practical and ethical issues. *Pediatr Nephrol.* 2013;28(12):2273-2281.

Cartier N, Aubourg P. A successful stem cell gene therapy using lentiviral vector. *Hum Gene Ther.* 2007;18:941.

Wanders RJA, Waterham HR. Peroxisomal disorders: the single peroxisomal enzyme deficiencies. *Biochim Biophys Acta.* 2006;1763:1707.

# 158 Congenital Disorders of Protein Glycosylation

Jaak Jaeken

## INTRODUCTION

Glycosylation is an important posttranslational protein modification occurring in the cytoplasm, the endoplasmic reticulum, and the Golgi apparatus. A rapidly growing family of genetic diseases is due to defects in protein and lipid glycosylation (congenital disorders of glycosylation [CDG]). Most CDGs are severe, multisystem diseases with prominent neurologic involvement. Nearly 100 CDGs have been identified. This chapter is limited to the protein glycosylation defects (some 80 disorders). Twenty-five CDGs are due to an *N*-glycosylation defect (Table 158-1). Twenty disorders have been identified in *O*-glycosylation, including some long-known diseases such as hereditary multiple exostoses (Table 158-2). Thirty-four disorders have a combined *N*- and *O*-glycosylation defect, including dolichol metabolism defects (Table 158-3). Important tools in the diagnosis are serum transferrin (Tf) isoelectric focusing (IEF), serum apolipoprotein C-III (apo C-III) isoelectrofocusing, protein-linked glycan analysis, and genetic analysis. In this text, we use the nomenclature introduced in 2009, namely the official gene symbol (not in italics) followed by "-CDG."

## PROTEIN GLYCOSYLATION

CDGs are a rapidly growing family of genetic diseases caused by defects in the synthesis of the glycan moiety of glycoconjugates (glycoproteins and glycolipids). There are 2 main types of protein

**TABLE 158-1 CONGENITAL DISORDERS OF PROTEIN *N*-GLYCOSYLATION**

| | Clinically Affected Organs | Metabolic Defect | Biochemical Findings | Phenotype MIM No. |
|---|---|---|---|---|
| GMPPA-CDG | Autonomic nerve fibers of distal esophagus and lacrimal glands, neurons of brain, and visual and hearing systems | Guanosine diphosphate (GDP) mannose pyrophosphorylase A | Normal Tf, apo C-III, IgG, and total protein IEF; increased GDP-mannose in lymphoblasts | 615510 |
| GMPPB-CDG | Brain, skeletal muscles, eyes, heart | GDP mannose pyrophosphorylase B | Increased serum creatine kinase; normal Tf IEF; hypoglycosylation of α-dystroglycan | 615350 |
| DPAGT1-CDG | Brain, neuromuscular junction | UDP-GlcNAc: Dol-P-GlcNAc-P transferase | Type 1 Tf IEF; accumulation of Dol-P in fibroblasts | 608093 |
| ALG13-CDG | Brain, eyes, liver | UDP-GlcNAc: Dol-PP-GlcNAc transferase | Type 1 Tf IEF; accumulation of GlcNAc-PP-Dol in fibroblasts | 300884 |
| ALG2-CDG | Brain, eyes, skeletal muscles, neuromuscular junction | Mannosyltransferase 2 | Decrease of factor XI; type 1 Tf IEF; accumulation of ManGlcNAc$_2$-PP-Dol and Man$_2$GlcNAc$_2$-PP-Dol in fibroblasts | 607906 |
| ALG14-CDG | Neuromuscular junction | UDP-GlcNAc:Dol-PP-GlcNAc transferase | Type 1 Tf IEF; accumulation of GlcNAc-PP-Dol in fibroblasts | 616227 |
| ALG11-CDG | Brain, hearing system | Mannosyltransferase 4/5 | Type 1 Tf IEF; accumulation of Man$_3$GlcNAc$_2$-PP-Dol and Man$_4$GlcNAc$_2$-PP-Dol in fibroblasts | 613661 |
| RFT1-CDG | Brain, hearing system | Flippase of Man$_5$GlcNAc$_2$-PP-Dol (or cofactor of this flippase) | Type 1 Tf IEF; accumulation of Man$_5$GlcNA$_2$-PP-Dol in fibroblasts | 612015 |
| ALG3-CDG | Brain, skeleton | Mannosyltransferase 6 | Type 1 Tf IEF; accumulation of Man$_5$GlcNAc$_2$-PP-Dol in fibroblasts | 601110 |
| ALG9-CDG | Brain, liver, kidneys, and variable involvement of adipose tissue, heart, skeleton, intestine | Mannosyltransferase 7/9 | Type 1 Tf IEF; accumulation of Man$_6$GlcNAc$_2$-PP-Dol and Man$_8$GlcNAc$_2$-PP-Dol in fibroblasts | 608776<br>263210 |
| ALG12-CDG | Brain, skeleton, heart, genitalia, immune system | Mannosyltransferase 8 | Variable decrease of serum IgG; type 1 Tf IEF; accumulation of Man$_7$GlcNAc$_2$-PP-Dol in fibroblasts | 607143 |
| ALG8-CDG | Brain, and variable involvement of eyes, gastrointestinal system, liver, heart, skeleton | Glucosyltransferase 1 | Type 1 Tf IEF; accumulation of Glc$_1$Man$_9$ GlcNAc$_2$-PP-Dol in fibroblasts | 608104 |
| TUSC3-CDG | Brain | Component of oligosaccharyl-transferase TUSC3 | Normal Tf IEF | 611093 |
| DDOST-CDG | Brain, eyes, liver | Component of oligosaccharyl-transferase DDOST | Type 1 Tf IEF | 614507 |
| STT3A-CDG | Brain, gastrointestinal tract | Component of oligosaccharyl-transferase STT3A | Type 1 Tf IEF | 615596 |
| STT3B-CDG | Brain, optic nerve, gastrointestinal tract | Component of oligosaccharyl-transferase STT3B | Type 1 Tf IEF | 615597 |
| SSR3-CDG | Brain, lungs, gastrointestinal system | Signal sequence receptor 3 of TRAP complex | Type 1 Tf IEF | |
| SSR4-CDG | Brain, respiratory system, skeleton | Signal sequence receptor 4 of TRAP complex | Type 1 Tf IEF | 300934 |
| MOGS-CDG | Brain, skeleton, immune system | Mannosyl-oligosaccharide glucosidase | Normal Tf IEF; tetrasaccharide [Glc(α1-2) Glc(α1-3)Glc(α1-3)Man] in urine | 606056 |
| MAN1B1-CDG | Brain, cranial skeleton, fat tissue | Golgi α1-2 mannosidase 1 | Type 1 Tf IEF; Man$_5$ on Tf glycan analysis | 614202 |
| MGAT2-CDG | Brain, skeleton, intestine | *N*-Acetylglucosaminyltransferase 2 | Increased serum GOT but normal GPT; type 2 Tf IEF; Tf glycan analysis: accumulation of monoantennary *N*-acetyllactosamine type glycan | 212066 |

IEF, isoelectric focusing; Tf, transferrin. See text for other abbreviations.

**TABLE 158-2 CONGENITAL DISORDERS OF *O*-GLYCOSYLATION**

| | Clinically Affected Organs | Metabolic Defect | Biochemical Findings | Phenotype MIM No. |
|---|---|---|---|---|
| XYLT1-CDG | Brain, skeleton, articulations, fat | Xylosyltransferase 1 | | 615777 |
| XYLT2-CDG | Brain, eyes, heart, hearing system, bones | Xylosyltransferase 2 | | |
| B4GALT7-CDG | Brain, skeleton, articulations, skin | B-1,4-galactosyltransferase 7 | | 130070 |
| B3GALT6-CDG | Skeleton, joints, skin | B-1,3-galactosyltransferase 6 | | 615349 |
| B3GAT3-CDG | Brain, aorta, heart, skeleton, joints, skin, teeth | B-1,3-glucuronyltransferase 3 | | 606374 |
| CHSY1-CDG | Brain, teeth, skeleton, hearing system | Chondroitin synthase 1 | | 605282 |
| EOGT-CDG | Skin, skeleton | EGF domain-specific *O*-GlcNAc transferase | | 615297 |
| GALNT3-CDG | Subcutaneous tissue | UDP-*N*-acetyl-α-D-galactosamine:polypeptide *N*-acetylgalactosaminyltransferase 3 | Hyperphosphatemia | 211900 |
| SLC35D1-CDG | Skeleton (generalized) | Solute carrier family 35 (UDP-glucuronic acid/UDP-*N*-acetylgalactosamine dual transporter) member D1 | | 269250 |
| POMT1-CDG | Brain, eyes, skeletal muscles, heart | Protein *O*-mannosyltransferase 1 | Increased serum creatine kinase | 236670<br>609308<br>613155 |
| POMT2-CDG | Brain, eyes, skeletal muscles | Protein *O*-mannosyltransferase 2 | Increased serum creatine kinase | 613150<br>613156<br>613158 |
| POMGNT1-CDG | Brain, eyes, skeletal muscles | Protein *O*-mannose β-1,2-N-acetylglucosaminyltransferase | Increased serum creatine kinase | 253280<br>613151<br>613157 |
| B3GALNT2-CDG | Brain, eyes, skeletal muscles | B-1,3-*N*-acetylgalactosaminyltransferase 2 | Increased serum creatine kinase | 615181 |
| LARGE-CDG | Brain, eyes, skeletal muscles | Acetylglucosaminyltransferase-like protein | Increased serum creatine kinase | 608840 |
| POFUT1-CDG | Skin | Protein *O*-fucosyltransferase 1 | | 615327 |
| LFNG-CDG | Axial skeleton, associated muscles | *O*-Fucose–specific β-1,3-*N*-acetylglucosaminyltransferase | | 609813 |
| B3GALTL-CDG | Eyes, skeleton, and variable involvement of other organs | O-Fucose–specific β-1,3-glucosyltransferase | | 261540 |
| POGLUT1-CDG | Skin | Protein *O*-glucosyltransferase 1 | | 615696 |



glycosylation: *N*-glycosylation and *O*-glycosylation. *N*-glycosylation (*N*-glycans attached to an amino group of asparagine of proteins) comprises an assembly part and a processing part and extends over 3 cellular compartments: the cytosol, the endoplasmic reticulum (ER), and the Golgi.

The assembly part of the *N*-glycosylation starts on the cytosolic side of the ER, with the transfer of N-acetylglucosamine (GlcNAc) phosphate from UDP-GlcNAc to membrane-bound dolichyl monophosphate (Dol-P), forming GlcNAc-pyrophosphate-dolichol (GlcNAc-PP-Dol). One GlcNAc and 5 mannose (Man) residues are subsequently attached to this lipid-linked monosaccharide in a stepwise manner (Fig. 158-1). The donor of these mannoses is a nucleotide-activated sugar, GDP-Man, which is synthesized from fructose 6-phosphate, an intermediate of the glycolytic pathway (Fig. 158-2). The lipid-linked heptasaccharide $Man_5GlcNAc_2$ is translocated by a flippase across the ER membrane and is elongated at the lumenal side by the attachment of 4 mannose residues and subsequently of 3 glucose residues. The 3 mannosyltransferases and 3 glucosyltransferases involved require dolichyl-phosphate-bound monosaccharides (Dol-P-Man and Dol-P-Glc). The completed $Glc_3Man_9GlcNAc_2$ oligosaccharide is then transferred to selected asparagine residues of the nascent proteins by the oligosaccharyltransferase complex.

The processing part of the *N*-glycosylation starts in the ER by trimming the glucose residues (catalyzed by glucosidases I and II) and 1 mannose (catalyzed by α-mannosidase I). The residual glycoprotein intermediate is directed to the cis-Golgi, where the processing pathway branches. A minor branch targets glycoproteins to the lysosomes (after the action of a GlcNAc-phosphotransferase and removal of the GlcNAc residues, leaving high-mannose glycoproteins capped with Man 6-P). The main branch leads to further trimming of mannoses (leaving a trimannosyl core) and the addition of GlcNAc, galactose, and, eventually, sialic acid in the medial- and trans-Golgi. Another modification of many *N*-glycoproteins in the Golgi is the attachment of fucose to the GlcNAc residue that is linked to asparagine.

*O*-glycosylation (*O*-glycans attached to the hydroxyl group of threonine or serine of proteins) has no processing part and thus consists only of assembly. Unlike *N*-glycosylation, this assembly mainly occurs in the Golgi. *O*-glycan structures show a greater diversity than *N*-glycans. Examples of important *O*-glycans are *O*-*N*-acetylgalactosaminylglycans (mucin-type glycans), *O*-xylosylglycans (glycosaminylglycans), *O*-mannosyl glycans, and *O*-fucosylglycans.

## GENETIC DISEASES OF PROTEIN *N*-GLYCOSYLATION

Twenty-five diseases are known in protein *N*-glycosylation: 22 assembly defects (CDG-I group) and 3 processing defects (CDG-II group). Here we discuss only the most frequent disorders, PMM2-CDG, ALG1-CDG, ALG6-CDG, and MPI-CDG, in some detail, since all the other diseases are very rare. The latter are summarized in Table 158-1.

## PHOSPHOMANNOMUTASE 2 DEFICIENCY (PMM2-CDG)

### CLINICAL PRESENTATION

PMM2-CDG (Online Mendelian Inheritance in Man [MIM] no. 212065) is by far the most frequent protein *N*-glycosylation disorder (> 700 patients are known worldwide). The clinical spectrum is

**TABLE 158-3 CONGENITAL DISORDERS OF *N*- AND *O*-GLYCOSYLATION**

| | Clinically Affected Organs | Metabolic Defect | Biochemical Findings | Phenotype MIM No. |
|---|---|---|---|---|
| DHDDS-CDG | Retina | Dehydrodolichyl diphosphate synthase | Normal Tf IEF; normal dolichol-linked oligosaccharides in fibroblasts | 613861 |
| NUS1-CDG | Brain, eyes, skeleton | Nogo-B receptor (subunit of *cis*-prenyltransferase) | Serum Tf IEF? | 617082 |
| SRD5A3-CDG | Brain, eyes, heart, skin, joints | Steroid 5 α-reductase 3 | Type 1 Tf IEF; normal or low levels of normal dolichol-linked oligosaccharides in fibroblasts | 617379 |
| DOLK-CDG | Brain, heart, skin | Dolichol kinase | Type 1 Tf IEF; normal or low levels of normal dolichol-linked oligosaccharides in fibroblasts | 610768 |
| DPM1-CDG | Brain, eyes, skeletal muscles | GDP-Man: Dol-P-mannosyltransferase 1 (Dol-P-Man synthase 1) | Increased serum creatine kinase; type 1 Tf IEF; accumulation of $Man_5GlcNAc_2$-PP-Dol in fibroblasts | 608799 |
| DPM2-CDG | Brain, skeletal muscles | GDP-Man: Dol-P-mannosyltransferase 2 (Dol-P-Man synthase 2) | Increased serum creatine kinase; type 1 Tf IEF; accumulation of $Man_5GlcNAc_2$-PP-Dol in fibroblasts | 615042 |
| DPM3-CDG | Skeletal and cardiac muscles | GDP-Man: Dol-P-mannosyltransferase 3 (Dol-P-Man synthase 3) | Increased serum creatine kinase; type 1 Tf IEF; accumulation of $Man_5GlcNAc_2$-PP-Dol in fibroblasts | 612937 |
| MPDU1-CDG | Brain, eyes, skin | Man-P-Dol utilization 1 | Type 1 Tf IEF; accumulation of $Man_5GlcNAc_2$-PP-Dol in fibroblasts | 609180 |
| SEC23B-CDG | Red cell lineage; secondary involvement of heart, liver, beta cells | Coat protein complex II (COPII) component SEC23B | Positive HEMPAS (hereditary erythroblastic multinuclearity with acidified serum test) | 224100 |
| GFPT1-CDG | Neuromuscular junction, skeletal muscles | Glutamine:fructose 6-phosphate amidotransferase 1 | Increased serum creatine kinase (inconstant); Tf IEF?; tubular aggregates in myofibers | 610542 |
| PGM3-CDG | Brain, immune system, skeleton | Phosphoglucomutase 3 | T- and B-cell deficiency; hyper-IgE (inconstant); normal Tf and apo C-III IEF | 615816 |
| GNE-CDG | Skeletal muscles (with sparing of quadriceps muscles), rarely cardiac muscles | UDP-GlcNAc 2-epimerase/ Man-NAc kinase | Normal or mildly increased serum creatine kinase | 269921<br>600737<br>605820 |
| NANS-CDG | Brain, skeleton | *N*-Acetylneuraminic acid synthase | Normal Tf IEF | |
| B4GALT1-CDG | Face, eyes | B-1,4-galactosyltransferase | Increased serum creatine kinase (mild) and AST; type 2 Tf IEF | 607091 |
| ST3GAL3-CDG | Brain | B-galactoside α-2,3-sialyltransferase 3 | | |
| CPS2-CDG | Brain, intestine, kidneys, erythrocytes | Carbamylphosphate synthetase 2 deficiency | Mild increase of blood ammonia; abnormalities in peripheral blood smear | 616457 |
| SLC35A1-CDG | Brain, heart, kidneys, platelets | CMP-sialic acid transporter | Type 2 Tf IEF | 603585 |
| SLC35A2-CDG | Brain, skeleton, eyes, gastrointestinal system | UDP-galactose transporter | Type 2 Tf IEF (in 50%) | 300896 |
| SLC35A3-CDG | Brain, skeleton | UDP-GlcNAc transporter | Tf IEF? | 615553 |
| SLC35C1-CDG | Brain, cranial skeleton, neutrophils | GDP-fucose transporter | Persistent neutrophilia; Bombay blood group (inconstant) | 266265 |
| COG1-CDG | Brain, skeleton | COG component 1 | Type 2 Tf IEF; apo C-III IEF: hyposialylation | 611209 |
| COG2-CDG | Brain, liver | COG component 2 | Type 2 Tf IEF | |
| COG4-CDG | Brain, face | COG component 4 | Type 2 Tf IEF; apo C-III IEF: hyposialylation | 613489 |
| COG5-CDG | Brain, liver, hearing system, vision, bladder | COG component 5 | Type 2 Tf IEF; apo C-III IEF: hyposialylation | 613612 |
| COG6-CDG | Brain, liver, gastrointestinal system, immune system | COG component 6 | Type 2 Tf IEF; apo C-III IEF: hyposialylation | 614576 |
| COG7-CDG | Brain, skeleton, skin, heart, liver, intestine, thermoregulation | COG component 7 | Type 2 Tf IEF; apo C-III IEF: hyposialylation | 608779 |
| COG8-CDG | Brain, eyes, peripheral nervous system | COG component 8 | Type 2 Tf IEF; apo C-III IEF: hyposialylation | 611182 |
| ATP6V0A2-CDG | Skin, brain, eyes, neuromuscular system, skeleton | V0 subunit of V-ATPase | Type 2 Tf IEF (can be normal in first months of life); apo C-III IEF: hyposialylation | 219200<br>278250 |
| ATP6AP1-CDG | Brain, B cells, liver, (muscles, hearing system) | Accessory protein Ac45 of the V-ATPase | Type 2 Tf IEF | |
| TMEM165-CDG | Brain, skeleton | Transmembrane protein 165 | Increased serum AST, ALT (mild), creatine kinase, LDH (mild); type 2 Tf IEF; apo C-III IEF: hyposialylation | 614727 |

*(Continued)*

**TABLE 158-3 CONGENITAL DISORDERS OF *N*- AND *O*-GLYCOSYLATION (CONTINUED)**

| | Clinically Affected Organs | Metabolic Defect | Biochemical Findings | Phenotype MIM No. |
|---|---|---|---|---|
| PGM1-CDG | Uvula (palate, lips), heart, liver, muscles, endocrine organs | Phosphoglucomutase 1 | Hypoglycemia, increased serum transaminases and creatine kinase, growth hormone deficiency, type 2 Tf IEF, Tf glycan analysis: CDG-I/II | 612934 |
| TMEM199-CDG | Liver | Transmembrane protein 199 | Increased serum transaminases, alkaline phosphatase, and LDL cholesterol; decreased serum ceruloplasmin; type 2 Tf IEF; apo C-III IEF: hyposialylation | 616829 |
| CCDC115-CDG | Liver, spleen, brain | Coiled-coil domain containing 115 | Increased serum transaminases and LDL cholesterol; decreased serum ceruloplasmin; type 2 Tf IEF; apo C-III IEF: hyposialylation | 616828 |
| SLC39A8-CDG | Brain, skeleton, immune system | Solute carrier family 39 (zinc transporter), member 8 | Decreased serum Mn and Zn; type 2 Tf IEF; apo C-III IEF: hyposialylation | 616721 |

COG, conserved oligomeric Golgi complex; Tf, transferrin. See text for other abbreviations.

very broad. The nervous system is affected in all patients, and most other organs are involved in variable ways. The neurologic picture comprises alternating internal strabismus and other abnormal eye movements, axial hypotonia, psychomotor disability, ataxia, and hyporeflexia. After infancy, symptoms include retinitis pigmentosa, stroke-like episodes, and sometimes epilepsy. During the first year(s) of life, there are variable feeding problems (anorexia, vomiting, diarrhea) that can result in severe failure to thrive. Other features are a variable dysmorphism (large, hypoplastic/dysplastic ears, abnormal subcutaneous adipose tissue distribution [fat pads, inverted nipples]), mild to moderate hepatomegaly, skeletal abnormalities (including atlantoaxial subluxation), and hypogonadism. Some infants develop pericardial effusion or cardiomyopathy. At the other end of the clinical spectrum are patients with a very mild phenotype (no dysmorphism, mild psychomotor disability). Patients often have an extroverted and happy appearance. There is a substantially increased mortality in the first years of life due to vital organ involvement or severe infection.

## METABOLIC DERANGEMENT

PMM2-CDG is a (cytosolic) defect in the second step of the mannose pathway (transforming mannose-6-phosphate into mannose-1-phosphate), which normally leads to the synthesis of guanosine diphosphate (GDP)-mannose (see Fig. 158-2). This nucleotide sugar is the donor of mannose used in the ER to assemble the dolichol-pyrophosphate oligosaccharide precursor. Deficiency of GDP-mannose causes hypoglycosylation of numerous glycoproteins, including serum proteins, lysosomal enzymes, and membranous glycoproteins.

## GENETICS

PMM2-CDG is an autosomal recessive disease due to mutations of *PMM2* on chromosome 16p13. Some 100 mutations have been identified (mainly missense mutations), the most frequent being the R141H mutation. Prenatal diagnosis is possible by enzymatic analysis of amniocytes and chorionic villus cells; this should be combined with mutation analysis of the *PMM2* gene.

## DIAGNOSTIC TESTS

The diagnosis of PMM2-CDG (and of congenital disorders of *N*-glycosylation in general) is usually made by IEF and immunofixation of serum transferrin (see Fig. 158-1). Normal serum transferrin is mainly composed of tetrasialotransferrin and small amounts of mono-, di-, tri-, penta-, and hexasialotransferrins. The partial deficiency of sialic acid (a negatively charged and end-standing sugar) in CDG causes a cathodal shift. Two main types of cathodal shift can be recognized: Type 1 is characterized by an increase of both disialo- and asialotransferrin and a decrease of tetrasialotransferrin; in type 2, there

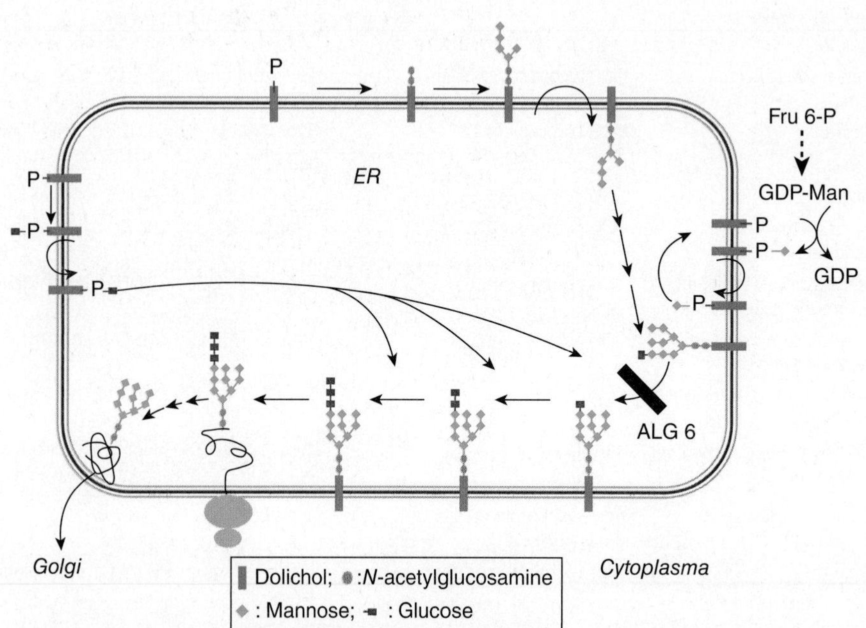


**FIGURE 158-1** Scheme of the endoplasmic reticulum part of the *N*-glycosylation pathway (see text for explanation). The *black bar* beside *ALG6* indicates the defect in ALG6-CDG.

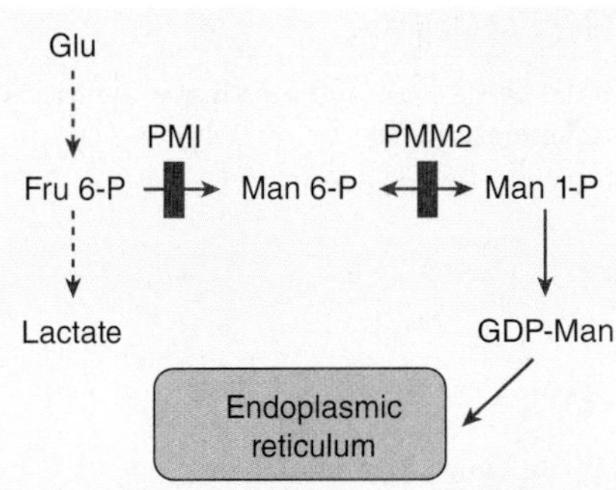


**FIGURE 158-2** Scheme of the synthesis of guanosine diphosphate (GDP)-mannose from fructose 6-phosphate. *Vertical red bars* indicate defects in PMM2-CDG and in MPI-CDG.

is also an increase of the tri- and/or monosialotransferrin bands (Fig. 158-3). In PMM2 deficiency, a type 1 pattern is found. Recently, capillary zone electrophoresis of total serum has been introduced for the diagnosis of CDG (see Fig. 158-1). In addition to the previously mentioned serum glycoprotein abnormalities, laboratory findings include elevation of serum transaminase levels, hypoalbuminemia, hypocholesterolemia, and renal tubular proteinuria. To confirm the diagnosis, the activity of PMM2 should be measured in leukocytes or fibroblasts.

## PHOSPHOMANNOSE-ISOMERASE DEFICIENCY (MPI-CDG)

### CLINICAL PRESENTATION

Some 25 patients with MPI-CDG (MIM no. 602579) have been reported with this mainly hepatic-intestinal disease. Together with ALG8-CDG, it is the only known *N*-linked CDG without (or with only minor) neurologic involvement. Symptoms start in the first year of life and consist of various combinations of recurrent vomiting, abdominal pain, protein-losing enteropathy, recurrent thromboses, gastrointestinal bleeding, liver disease, and symptoms of hypoglycemia. Several patients have died.

### METABOLIC DERANGEMENT

The defect is in the first step in the biosynthesis of the nucleotide sugar GDP-mannose (see Fig. 158-2). The substrate of the enzyme, fructose 6-phosphate, does not accumulate, since it is an intermediate of the glycolytic pathway. The blood biochemical abnormalities are indistinguishable from those found in PMM2-CDG.

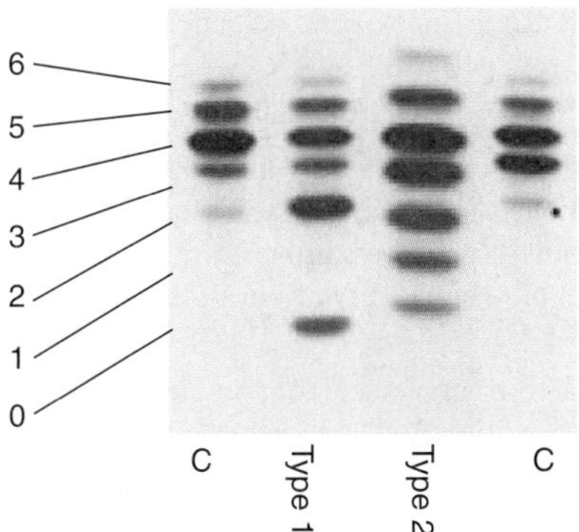


**FIGURE 158-3** Isoelectrofocusing of serum transferrin showing controls (C), a type 1 pattern, and a type 2 pattern (see text for explanation). The figures on the left indicate the number of sialic acid residues on each sialotransferrin fraction.

### GENETICS

Inheritance of MPI-CDG is autosomal recessive. The gene (*PMI*) has been localized to chromosome 15q22, and several (missense) mutations have been identified. Prenatal diagnosis is possible.

### DIAGNOSTIC TESTS

The diagnosis is confirmed by finding a decreased activity of phosphomannose isomerase in leukocytes or fibroblasts and/or mutation(s) in the *MPI* gene.

### TREATMENT

This is the only known CDG that can be effectively treated. The treatment is simple and consists of oral mannose (1 g/kg body weight per day, divided in 4–6 doses). The rationale for this treatment is that hexokinases phosphorylate mannose to mannose 6-phosphate, thus bypassing the defect.

## GLUCOSYLTRANSFERASE I DEFICIENCY (ALG6-CDG)

### CLINICAL PRESENTATION

Fifty-four patients have been reported with ALG6-CDG (MIM no. 603147). As in PMM2-CDG, patients show hypotonia, strabismus, and seizures, but psychomotor development is less affected, there is less dysmorphism, and there is usually no retinitis pigmentosa or cerebellar hypoplasia. In 1 patient, idiopathic intracranial hypertension and optic atrophy were reported.

For an unknown reason, some of the glycoproteins have unusually low blood levels (particularly factor XI and coagulation inhibitors such as antithrombin and protein C). The reason why the clinical picture in these patients is milder than that of PMM2-deficient patients may be because a deficiency in glucosylation of the dolichol-linked oligosaccharides does not affect the biosynthesis of GDP-mannose; therefore, it does not affect the biosynthesis of GDP-fucose or of glycosylphosphatidylinositol-anchored glycoproteins.

### METABOLIC DERANGEMENT

Glucosyltransferase I deficiency is a defect in the attachment of the first glucose (of 3) to the dolichol-linked mannose$_9$-*N*-acetylglucosamine$_2$ ER intermediate. It causes hypoglycosylation of serum glycoproteins because nonglucosylated oligosaccharides are a suboptimal substrate for oligosaccharyltransferase.

### GENETICS

ALG6-CDG is an autosomal recessive disease. The gene has been localized to chromosome 1p22.3. Prenatal diagnosis is possible.

### DIAGNOSTIC TESTS

This disease illustrates that even in cases of mild psychomotor disability without any specific dysmorphism, IEF of serum sialotransferrins should be performed. When a type 1 pattern is found, PMM2 and PMI deficiency must be considered first. If these enzymes show normal activities, the next step is genetic analysis (CDG panel analysis or whole-exome sequencing).

## MANNOSYLTRANSFERASE 1 DEFICIENCY (ALG1-CDG)

### CLINICAL PRESENTATION

Fifty-seven patients with ALG1-CDG (MIM no. 608540) have been reported. Its phenotype is predominantly neurologic involvement. Constant features are developmental disabilities and hypotonia. A majority of patients show dysmorphism, microcephaly, intractable seizures, visual disturbances, tremor, ataxia, severe infections, and cerebral abnormalities. Survival of the reported patients ranged from 2 days to over 20 years.

### METABOLIC DERANGEMENT

ALG1 attaches the first of 9 mannoses to $GlcNAc_2$-PP-Dol at the outside of the ER membrane. Laboratory abnormalities comprise decreased levels of serum low-density lipoprotein (LDL) cholesterol, factor XI, and antithrombin and increased serum transaminases.

### GENETICS

Inheritance is autosomal recessive. Thirteen variants have been reported in the *ALG1* gene.

### DIAGNOSTIC TESTS

Serum Tf IEF shows a type 1 pattern. The diagnosis has to be confirmed by mutation analysis of *ALG1*.

## GENETIC DISEASES OF PROTEIN *O*-GLYCOSYLATION

Twenty genetic diseases have been identified in protein O-glycosylation. The most frequent is hereditary multiple exostoses, which is one of the 3 known CDGs with autosomal dominant inheritance. The others are summarized in Table 158-2.

## HEREDITARY MULTIPLE EXOSTOSES (EXT1/EXT2-CDG)

### CLINICAL PRESENTATION

This disease is characterized by osteochondromas of the ends of long bones. These tumors are often present at birth; their growth slows during adolescence and stops in adulthood. Malignant degeneration is present in only a small percentage of the lesions. Complications may result from compression of peripheral nerves and blood vessels. Treatment is only necessary when there are complications or (rare) malignant degeneration. Prognosis is usually good.

### METABOLIC DERANGEMENT

The basic defect is in the Golgi-localized EXT1/EXT2 complex, which has both glucuronyltransferase and *N*-acetyl-D-hexosaminyltransferase activities involved in the polymerization of heparan sulfate.

### GENETICS

Transmission of hereditary multiple exostoses (MIM no. 608177 and 608210) is autosomal dominant.

### DIAGNOSTIC TESTS

The diagnosis is based on mutation analysis of the *EXT* genes.

## GENETIC DISEASES OF PROTEIN *N*- AND *O*-GLYCOSYLATION

Thirty-four genetic diseases have been identified with a combined *N*- and O-glycosylation defect. The most frequent is hereditary inclusion body myopathy. The others are summarized in Table 158-3.

## RECESSIVE HEREDITARY INCLUSION BODY MYOPATHY

### CLINICAL PRESENTATION

The disease is characterized by adult-onset, progressive distal and proximal muscle weakness. Patients eventually become wheelchair-bound in 2 to 3 decades, but remarkably, the quadriceps muscles are spared.

### METABOLIC DERANGEMENT

The defect is in the first 2 steps of the sialic acid synthesis catalyzed by UDP-GlcNAc epimerase/kinase.

### GENETICS

Inheritance of recessive hereditary inclusion body myopathy (MIM no. 600737) is autosomal recessive.

### DIAGNOSTIC TESTS

The diagnosis is confirmed by mutation analysis.

## TREATMENT OF CONGENITAL DISORDERS OF PROTEIN GLYCOSYLATION

An effective treatment is available only for MPI-CDG (oral mannose; see above). There is a partial treatment for PIGM-CDG (oral butyrate controls seizures), SLC35C1-CDG (oral fucose controls infections), PGM1-CDG (galactose improves liver function and endocrine abnormalities and reduces hypoglycemic episodes), PGM3-CDG (hematopoietic stem cell transplantation corrects neutropenia and lymphopenia), and the CDGs that can present as a congenital myasthenic syndrome, namely DPAGT1-CDG, ALG2-CDG, ALG14-CDG, GFPT1-CDG, and GMPPB-CDG (cholinesterase inhibitors).

### SUGGESTED READINGS


Boycott KM, Beaulieu CL, Kernohan KD, et al. Autosomal-recessive intellectual disability with cerebellar atrophy syndrome caused by mutation of the manganese and zinc transporter gene SLC39A8. *Am J Hum Genet.* 2015;97:886-893.

Freeze HH, Chong JX, Bamshad MJ, Ng BG. Solving glycosylation disorders: fundamental approaches reveal complicated pathways. *Am J Hum Genet.* 2014;94:161-175.

Jaeken J, Lefeber D, Matthijs G. Clinical utility gene card for phosphomannomutase 2 deficiency. *Eur J Hum Genet.* 2014;22:8.

Jaeken J, Vanderschueren-Lodeweyckx M, Casaer P, et al. Familial psychomotor retardation with markedly fluctuating serum proteins, FSH and GH levels, partial TBG-deficiency, increased serum arylsulphatase A and increased CSF protein: a new syndrome? *Pediatr Res.* 1980;14:179.

Jaeken J, Van Eijk HG, van der Heul C, et al. Sialic acid-deficient serum and cerebrospinal fluid transferrin in a newly recognized genetic syndrome. *Clin Chim Acta.* 1984;144:245-247.

Jansen JC, Cirak S, van Scherpenzeel M, et al. CCDC115 deficiency causes a disorder of Golgi homeostasis with abnormal protein glycosylation. *Am J Hum Genet.* 2016;98:310-321.

Jansen JC, Timal S, van Scherpenzeel M, et al. TMEM199 deficiency is a disorder of Golgi homeostasis characterized by elevated aminotransferases, alkaline phosphatase and cholesterol, and abnormal glycosylation. *Am J Hum Genet.* 2016;98:322-330.

Matthijs G, Rymen D, Millón MB, Souche E, Race V. Approaches to homozygosity mapping and exome sequencing for the identification of novel types of CDG. *Glycoconj J.* 2013;30:67-76.

Matthijs G, Schollen E, Pardon E, et al. Mutations in PMM2, a phosphomannomutase gene on chromosome 16p13, in carbohydrate-deficient glycoprotein type I syndrome (Jaeken syndrome). *Nat Genet.* 1997;16:88-92.

Morava E. Galactose supplementation in phosphoglucomutase 1 deficiency: review and outlook for a novel treatable CDG. *Mol Genet Metab.* 2014;112:275-279.

Park JH, Hogrebe M, Gruneberg M, et al. A disorder of manganese transport and glycosylation. *Am J Hum Genet.* 2015;97:894-903.

Van Schaftingen E, Jaeken J. Phosphomannomutase deficiency is a cause of carbohydrate-deficient glycoprotein syndrome type I. *Febs Lett.* 1995;377:318-320.

# 159 Disorders of Cholesterol Synthesis

Shibani Kanungo and Robert D. Steiner

## INTRODUCTION

Cholesterol is an essential lipid, available through diet but also synthesized endogenously from acetyl-coenzyme A, formed as a byproduct of glucose and fatty acids through glycolysis and β-oxidation pathways, respectively. Cholesterol is a major end product of the isoprenoid and sterol biosynthetic pathway involving numerous enzymatic steps. Enzymatic defects in the pre-squalene cholesterol synthesis pathway are responsible for inherited sterol disorders such as mevalonic aciduria (MVA) and hyper-immunoglobulinemia D and periodic fever syndrome (HIDS). In the descending post-squalene pathway, enzymatic defects are responsible for disorders such as Antley-Bixler syndrome with genital anomalies and disordered steroidogenesis (ABS1), congenital hemidysplasia with ichthyosiform nevus and limb defects (CHILD) syndrome, CK syndrome, sterol C4 methyl oxidase deficiency (SC4MOL), X-linked dominant chondrodysplasia punctata 2 (CDPX2)/Conradi-Hünermann syndrome, lathosterolosis, desmosterolosis, and the widely known Smith-Lemli-Opitz syndrome (SLOS). Hydrops-ectopic calcification–moth-eaten (HEM)/Greenberg skeletal dysplasia was earlier thought to be a disorder of sterol metabolism but more recently has been shown to be a laminopathy.

## PATHOGENESIS AND EPIDEMIOLOGY

Cholesterol has numerous essential functions as a major component of cell membranes and myelin in the nervous system, cellular signal transduction and expression (eg, activation of hedgehog proteins), and as a precursor of bile acid and steroid hormone synthesis; thus, it has perhaps a unique influence on both embryonic and postnatal development.

The isoprenoid synthesis pathway (Fig. 159-1) leads to the synthesis of cholesterol (an important constituent of cell membranes and a precursor of steroid hormones and bile acids), haem A (a component of complex IV of the respiratory chain), ubiquinone (an electron carrier in the respiratory chain), dolichol (which is required for glycosylation of proteins), farnesyl-pyrophosphate, and geranylgeranyl-pyrophosphate (which are important for prenylation of proteins). Prenylation of proteins is important in many signaling cascades in the cell.

The cholesterol synthesis pathway is tightly regulated. When cholesterol levels in the cell are low, transcription of the HMG-CoA reductase gene (*HMGR*), and probably the transcription of every other gene involved in the cholesterol synthesis pathway, is upregulated by sterol regulatory element binding proteins, particularly SREBP-2. In contrast, high levels of sterols reduce the activity of the cholesterol-synthesizing enzymes via reduced SREBP-2 activity. High levels of sterols in the cell also lead to increased production of oxysterols, which act on the liver X receptor (LXR); this, in turn, drives the disposal of the excess cholesterol. LXR may also reduce cholesterol synthesis by downregulating SREBP-2.

Maternal dietary sources of cholesterol are the primary source for the developing fetus prior to formation of the embryonic blood-brain barrier (BBB) at around 12 to 18 weeks of gestation. However, after the BBB is formed, brain tissue is completely dependent on endogenous cholesterol synthesis within the brain. Thus, all enzyme defects in the cholesterol biosynthesis pathway, with the exception of HIDS, lead to clinical findings of dysmorphic features, organ malformation during embryonic development, and frequently neurocognitive deficits.

The mode of inheritance, location of corresponding gene for mutation analysis testing, biochemical enzyme defects, and abnormal/diagnostic metabolites for each sterol disorder in descending order in the cholesterol synthesis pathway are presented in Table 159-1.

Of all the disorders of cholesterol synthesis, epidemiologic data have been most extensively reported in SLOS and in the milder clinical version of mevalonate kinase deficiency (MKD), HIDS, as summarized in Table 159-2.

MVA, CDPX2, CHILD syndrome, CK syndrome, SC4MOL deficiency, desmosterolosis, lathosterolosis, and Antley-Bixler syndrome are all considered extremely rare. Thus, the incidence and prevalence of these disorders are unknown.

## CLINICAL MANIFESTATIONS, DIAGNOSIS, TREATMENT, AND PREVENTION

### Smith-Lemli-Opitz Syndrome (SLOS)

SLOS (Online Mendelian Inheritance in Man [OMIM] no. 270400) is an autosomal recessive disorder caused by mutations in the *DHCR7* gene (OMIM no. 602858) on chromosome 11q13.4, resulting in deficiency of the enzyme 7-dehydrocholesterol $\Delta^7$-reductase (DHCR7). SLOS was originally described by Smith and colleagues in 1964 as a multiple malformation syndrome and includes a wide spectrum of characteristic central nervous system (CNS) malformations, limb defects, facial dysmorphism, and urogenital and other anomalies. Typical features on the severely affected end of the spectrum include in utero or neonatal demise due to major congenital midline organ malformations and/or multiple organ failure; at the milder end of the spectrum, clinical features include only minor physical, developmental, and behavioral manifestations. Typical SLOS facial features include microcephaly, ptosis, midface hypoplasia, a small upturned nose, and micrognathia (Fig. 159-2). Consistent with midline involvement during embryogenesis (as discussed earlier), cleft palate, submucosal clefts, and/or bifid uvula frequently are observed. Genital malformations can range from varying degrees of hypospadias to complete gender reversal (46,XY phenotypic females; Fig. 159-3). Gastrointestinal symptoms are common, including feeding difficulties, gastroesophageal reflux, formula intolerance, recurrent vomiting, constipation, pyloric stenosis, malrotation, and colonic aganglionosis/Hirschsprung disease. Liver disease has also been reported with 2 main patterns of liver involvement: progressive cholestasis and stable isolated hypertransaminasemia. Cardiac involvement can include congenital heart defects such as atrioventricular canal, hypoplastic left heart sequence, septal defects, and other defects. Hypertension without structural defects has also been reported. Abnormal neural crest development is considered the putative cause of colonic aganglionosis/Hirschsprung disease and endocardial cushion defects. Limb anomalies include variably short proximally placed thumbs, single palmar creases, postaxial polydactyly, rarely ectrodactyly, and nearly universally syndactyly of the second and third toes (a classic SLOS finding; Fig. 159-4). Other anomalies reported include cataracts, skin photosensitivity, blepharoptosis, optic nerve hypoplasia or atrophy, and adrenal insufficiency.

Neurodevelopmental and behavioral abnormalities are frequent and highly variable in SLOS. A behavioral profile includes intellectual disability, sensory hyperreactivity, irritability, language impairment, sleep-cycle disturbance, self-injurious behavior, syndrome-specific motor movements, repetitive movements, tactile hypersensitivity, and autism spectrum behaviors.

The differential diagnosis can include trisomy 13 and trisomy 18 syndromes, Pallister-Hall syndrome, Dubowitz syndrome, Noonan syndrome, and Meckel-Gruber syndrome, among others. The features of mild SLOS can be very subtle, and a delay in establishing a diagnosis is not uncommon. At the same time, severely affected individuals may have profound cardiac and/or brain malformations, including holoprosencephaly, dominating the clinical picture and may die in the neonatal period without a unifying diagnosis identified.

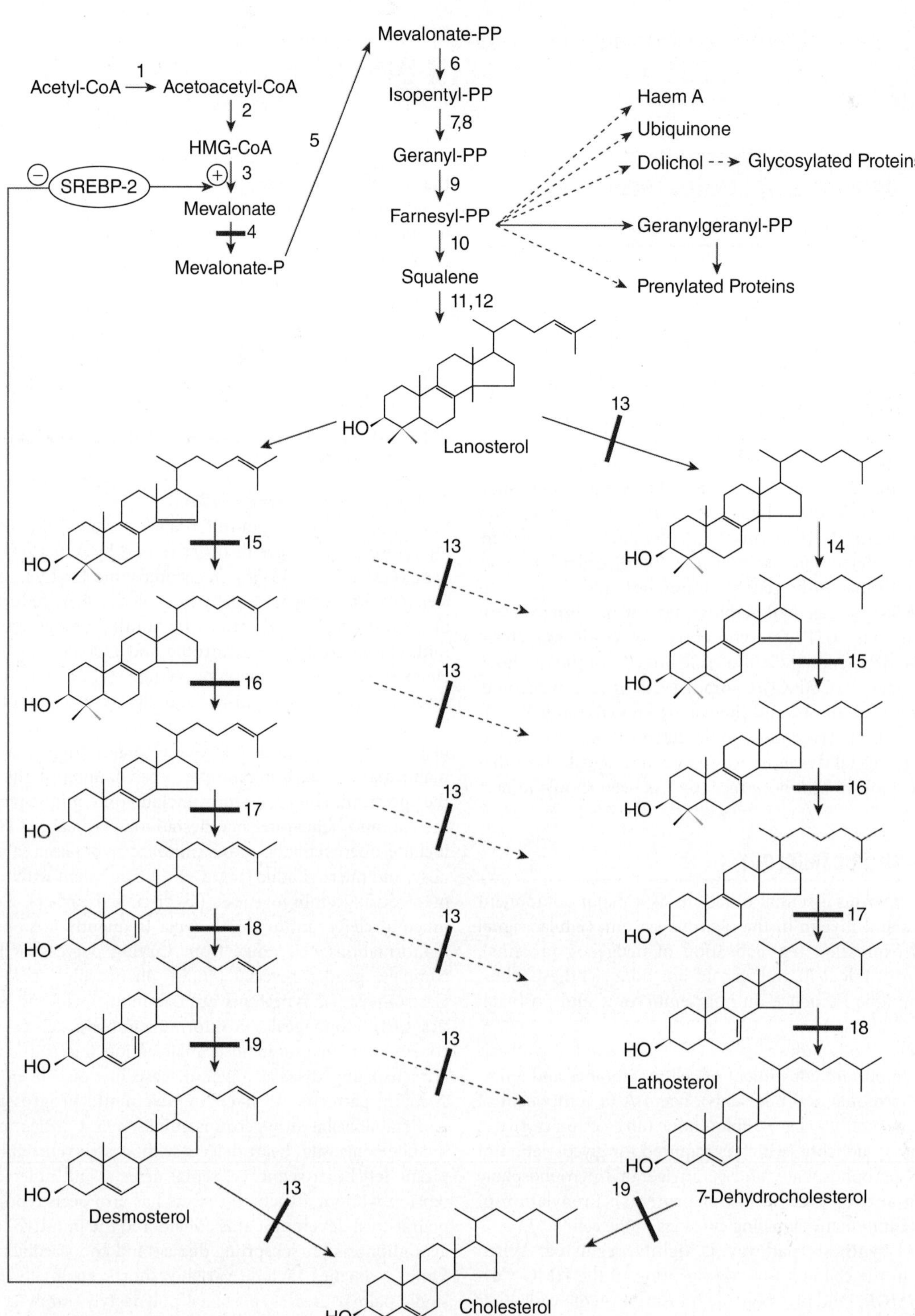


**FIGURE 159-1** Pathway for synthesis of isoprenoids and cholesterol. CoA, coenzyme A; HMG, 3-hydroxy-3-methylglutaryl; P, phosphate; PP, pyrophosphate; SREBP, sterol responsive element binding protein. Numbered enzymatic steps (bar across *arrow* indicates deficiency disorder known): 1, acetyl-CoA acetyl transferase; 2, HMG-CoA synthase; 3, HMG-CoA reductase; 4, mevalonate kinase; 5, mevalonate-P kinase; 6, mevalonate-PP decarboxylase; 7, isopentenyl-PP isomerase; 8, geranyl-PP synthase; 9, farnesyl-PP synthase; 10, squalene synthase; 11, squalene epoxidase; 12, 2,3-oxidosqualene sterol cyclase; 13, sterol $\Delta^{24}$-reductase (deficient in desmosterolosis); 14, sterol C14-demethylase; 15, sterol $\Delta^{14}$-reductase; 16, sterol C4-demethylase complex (3β-hydroxysteroid dehydrogenase component deficient in CHILD syndrome); 17, sterol $\Delta^{8}\Delta^{7}$-isomerase (deficient in Conradi-Hünermann syndrome); 18, sterol $\Delta^{5}$-destaurase (deficient in lathosterolosis); 19, sterol $\Delta^{7}$-reductase (deficient in Smith-Lemli-Opitz syndrome).

Diagnostic testing, as noted in Table 159-1, includes blood sterol profiling through gas chromatography/mass spectrometry (GC/MS), which shows an accumulation of 7-dehydrocholesterol (7DHC) and 8-dehydrocholesterol (8DHC) with reduced or low-normal cholesterol levels in patient plasma, amniotic fluid, or chorionic villi (in the setting of prenatal diagnosis), cultured skin fibroblasts, and other tissues. If needed in atypical cases, sterols in cultured lymphoblasts can be measured, and enzyme analysis has been useful on occasion. Diagnostic confirmation is by *DHCR7* gene mutation analysis.

There is no proven effective therapy for SLOS. Dietary cholesterol supplementation is often provided; however, most recent reports indicate that it does not improve developmental outcome or behavior, probably due to poor access of cholesterol to the CNS. Circulating cholesterol likely does not cross the BBB, and the brain depends

**TABLE 159-1 GENETIC AND BIOCHEMICAL CHARACTERISTICS IN DISORDERS OF CHOLESTEROL SYNTHESIS**

| Disorders in Descending Order of Cholesterol Synthesis Pathway[a] (Phenotype MIM#) | Inheritance | Chromosome Location | Mutation Gene (OMIM #) | Enzyme Defect | Diagnostic Testing/Metabolites[a,b] (Preferred Lab Specimen) |
|---|---|---|---|---|---|
| Mevalonic aciduria (610377)<br>HIDS (260920) | Autosomal recessive | 12q24 | *MVK*[c] (251170) | Mevalonate kinase | Mevalonic acid /mevalonolactone (urine organic acids)<br>*(may be normal in HIDS especially if not collected during febrile episode)* |
| Antley-Bixler syndrome (ABS1) (201750) | Autosomal recessive | 1q11.2 | *POR* (124015) | Cytochrome P450 oxidoreductase | Lanosterol (blood sterol profile) |
| Sterol C4 methyl oxidase deficiency (SC4MOL/MCCPD) (616834) | Autosomal recessive | 4q32-q34 | *MSMO1* (607545) | Sterol C-4 methyl oxidase | 4,4′-Dimethylsterols and 4-monomethylsterols (blood and skin flake sterol profile) |
| CHILD syndrome (308050) | X-linked | Xq28 | *NSDHL* (300275) | 3β-Hydroxysterol dehydrogenase | 4-Carboxylsterols (transformed lymphoblast sterol profile) |
| CK syndrome (XLID) (300831) | X-linked | Xq28 | *NSDHL* (300275) | 3β-Hydroxysterol dehydrogenase | 4-Carboxylsterols (transformed lymphoblast sterol profile) |
| CDPX2/Conradi-Hunermann Syndrome (302960) | X-linked | Xp11.22-11.23 | *EBP* (300205) | 3β-Hydroxysterol $\Delta^{7,8}$-reductase | Cholesta-8(9)-en-3-ol (blood and skin fibroblast sterol profile) |
| Lathosterolosis (607330) | Autosomal recessive | 11q23.3 | *SC5DL*[c] (602286) | 3β-Hydroxysterol $\Delta^{5}$-desaturase | Lathosterol (blood sterol profile) |
| Desmosterolosis (602398) | Autosomal recessive | 1p31.1-p33 | *DHCR24*[c] (606418) | 3β-Hydroxysterol $\Delta^{24}$-reductase (24DHC reductase) | Desmosterol (blood sterol profile) |
| SLOS (270400) | Autosomal recessive | 11q12-13 | *DHCR7* (602858) | 3β-Hydroxysterol $\Delta^{7}$-reductase (7DHC reductase) | 7-Dehydrocholesterol and 8-dehydrocholesterol (blood sterol profile) |

[a]Phenotypic and diagnostic metabolite changes may be subtle and difficult to detect so additional diagnostic testing may be indicated if clinical suspicion high.

[b]These tests/metabolites may not accurately identify all cases.

[c]Molecular genetics testing is available in the United States for all the respective genes except *MVK*, *SC5DL*, and *DHCR24* and is useful to confirm diagnosis for most sterol metabolism disorders. Enzymatic testing for most sterol disorders is difficult and at present limited to research laboratories in the United States.

MIM, Mendelian Inheritance in Man; OMIM, Online Mendelian Inheritance in Man; XLID, X-linked Intellectual disability. See text for other abbreviations.

primarily on de novo synthesis. Adjunctive use of bile acids along with cholesterol was previously tested in very limited studies, but there is insufficient evidence for their use. Administration of HMG-CoA reductase inhibitors (simvastatin) in conjunction with dietary cholesterol supplementation is investigational. Stress steroid coverage for adrenal insufficiency is debated. Surgical intervention as needed for structural malformations should be considered as clinically indicated. Given the common finding of intellectual disability, supportive therapy and educational intervention with close monitoring of developmental and educational progress are essential. Prenatal maternal supplementation with dietary cholesterol in pregnancies affected with an SLOS infant is debated, as is administration of high-dose cholesterol, for example in the form of fresh frozen plasma in the setting of serious illness or pending surgery.

#### Mevalonic Aciduria (MVA)

MVA (OMIM no. 610377) is a rare autosomal recessive disorder caused by mutations in the *MVK* gene (OMIM no. 251170) located on chromosome 12q24.11, resulting in deficiency of mevalonate kinase (MVK), a key peroxisomal enzyme involved in the biosynthesis of cholesterol and isoprenoids in the pre-squalene pathway. The disorder can also manifest as a milder form, HIDS (OMIM no. 260920). MVA and HIDS represent 2 ends of a phenotypic spectrum caused by MVK enzyme deficiency, and are often referred to together as the MKD disorders. HIDS, a milder variant of MVK deficiency, can be a lifelong disorder with recurring episode of fever occurring every 4 to 6 weeks. Symptoms typically present before the end of the first year of life and can be triggered by vaccination, minor trauma, surgery, or other metabolic stressors, although they often occur without obvious inciting factors. Fever lasts 4 to 6 days and is accompanied by a high sedimentation rate, cervical lymphadenopathy, abdominal pain with vomiting, diarrhea, hepatosplenomegaly, headache, arthralgias and sometimes arthritis of large joints, erythematous maculopapular rash, and sometimes painful aphthous ulcers in the mouth or vagina. Unlike patients with more severe MVA, children with HIDS have no neurodevelopmental impairment or dysmorphism and enjoy a relatively

**TABLE 159-2 DISORDERS OF CHOLESTEROL SYNTHESIS EPIDEMIOLOGY**

| Disorder (country/region/ethnic group) | Incidence (source) | Carrier Frequency |
|---|---|---|
| **SLOS** | | |
| United States | 1 in 20,000 to 1 in 40,000 live births (birth prevalence) | — |
| United States | 1 in 50,000 (biochemical testing) | — |
| (Canada) | 1 in 26,500 (biochemical testing) | 1 in 30 |
| (Pacific Northwest of United States) | 1 in 1590 to 1 in 13,500 (newborn blood spots) | 1 in 30 |
| IVS8-1G>C mutation (US African American) | 1 in 75,061 (newborn blood spots) | 1 in 42 to 100 |
| **HIDS** | | |
| V377 Imutation (Dutch) | 1 in 5196 | 1 in 153 |
| Any *MVK* mutation | 1 in 53,656 | 1 in 65 |
| Pediatric mevalonate kinase deficiency cases | 1 in 771,400 | — |

Data from Kanungo S, Soares N, He M, et al: Sterol metabolism disorders and neurodevelopment: an update, *Dev Disabil Res Rev.* 2013;17(3):197-210.

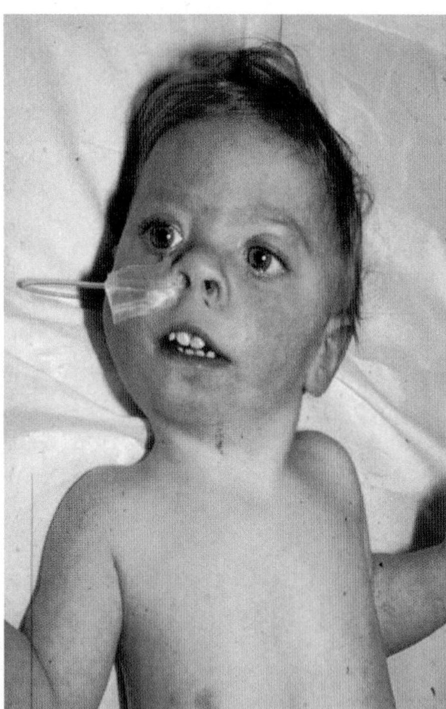

**FIGURE 159-2** Infant with Smith-Lemli-Opitz syndrome showing prominent central forehead, anteverted nares, small chin, and low-set ears.



normal adult life span. Although both HIDS and MVA are caused by mutations in the same *MVK* gene, a consistent genotype-phenotype correlation has not been demonstrated. Deficiency of MVK enzyme and subsequently cholesterol results in loss of feedback inhibition on the rate-limiting enzyme HMG-CoA reductase (see Fig. 159-1), leading to massive MVA production and excretion in the urine.

Diagnostic testing, as noted in Table 159-1, includes urine organic acid analysis, especially during febrile episodes, and *MVK* gene mutation analysis.

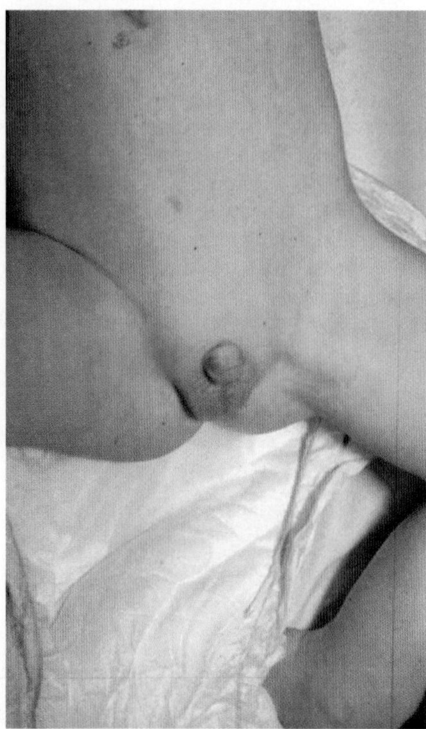

**FIGURE 159-3** Infant with Smith-Lemli-Opitz syndrome showing cryptorchidism.

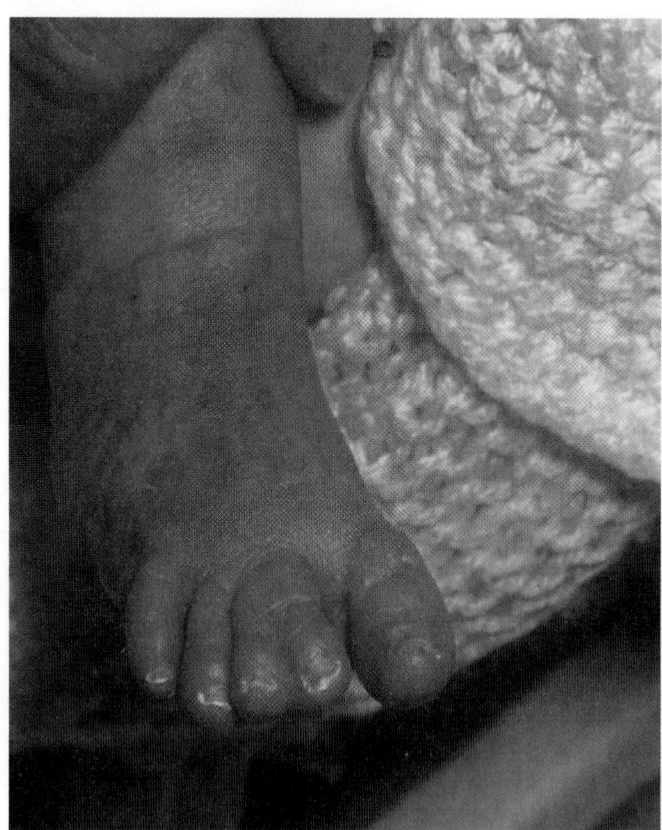

**FIGURE 159-4** Neonate with Smith-Lemli-Opitz syndrome showing 2/3 syndactyly of toes.

Treatment for MVA is primarily supportive, and the prognosis remains poor. Corticosteroid therapy can help diminish the severity of an MVA crisis but does not prevent the overall poor prognosis. Allogeneic bone marrow transplantation reported in 2 MVA patients normalized all biologic markers of inflammation, improved language skills, and was associated with resolution of febrile episodes. The mainstay of therapy for HIDS has been supportive with antipyretics and analgesics use. In HIDS, there have been some benefits seen from use of anakinra (an interleukin-1 receptor antagonist), but as on-demand therapy during crises, and etanercept.

#### Antley-Bixler Syndrome with Genital Anomalies and Disordered Steroidogenesis (ABS1)

ABS1 (OMIM no. 201750) is a rare autosomal recessive craniosynostosis syndrome caused by homozygous or compound heterozygous mutations in the *POR* gene encoding cytochrome P450 oxidoreductase (POR) (OMIM no. 124015), located on chromosome 7q11.2. This disorder affects the initial steps of the post-squalene pathway (see Fig. 159-1), affecting C-14 lanosterol demethylase and resulting in POR deficiency. There is another form of Antley-Bixler syndrome, ABS2 (Antley-Bixler syndrome without genital anomalies or disordered steroidogenesis); ABS2 is caused by *FGFR2* gene mutations and is not a sterol disorder and thus will not be further considered here.

Signs and symptoms include characteristic perinatal onset of radiohumeral synostosis, a wide spectrum of midface hypoplasia, choanal stenosis or atresia, multiple joint contractures, genitourinary anomalies, and impaired steroidogenesis. Mortality is high in the neonatal period secondary to airway compromise. Apart from craniosynostosis, other neurologic abnormalities noted include hydrocephalus and Arnold-Chiari malformation.

Diagnostic testing, as noted in Table 159-1, includes blood sterol profiling, which may show elevated lanosterol, but *POR* gene mutation analysis is needed for confirmation.

Treatment for individuals with ABS1 includes steroid hormone supplementation for adrenal insufficiency and addisonian crisis, especially during severe febrile illness or major surgery.

### Sterol C4 Methyl Oxidase (SC4MOL) Deficiency/Microcephaly, Congenital Cataract, and Psoriasiform Dermatitis (MCCPD)

SC4MOL deficiency/MCCPD (OMIM no. 616834) is a rare, recently reported disorder described in 2 patients. Some of the clinical features reported include severe ichthyosiform erythroderma affecting the entire body, congenital cataracts, microcephaly, delayed skeletal and sexual maturation, developmental delay, inflammatory joint disease, and an abnormal immunocyte phenotype with significant increase of activated granulocytes.

Diagnostic testing, as noted in Table 159-1, includes sterol profiling of skin flakes, skin fibroblasts, or transformed lymphocytes (if such analysis is available), with elevations of 4,4′-dimethylsterols and 4α-monomethylsterols in plasma, along with confirmatory *MSMO1* gene mutation analysis. There is no known treatment for many of the clinical manifestations; however, the psoriasiform dermatitis improved significantly with statin and cholesterol treatment.

### X-Linked Sterol Disorders

CHILD syndrome, CK syndrome, and X-linked dominant chondrodysplasia punctata 2 (CDPX2) are X-linked disorders, and the clinical characteristics are noted in Table 159-3. Diagnostic testing, as noted in Table 159-1, includes sterol profiling, with confirmation with corresponding gene mutation analysis.

**TABLE 159-3 CLINICAL CHARACTERISTICS AND TREATMENT IN DISORDERS OF CHOLESTEROL SYNTHESIS**

| Disorders | Clinical Presentation Spectrum | Reported Therapies[a] |
|---|---|---|
| SLOS | Central nervous system anomalies: Microcephaly to frank holoprosencephaly, enlarged ventricles, partial or complete agenesis of the corpus callosum, dysplastic cerebral gyri, cerebralheterotopias, cerebral and cerebellar defects such as white matter hypoplasia, cerebellar hypoplasia with severe hypoplasia or aplasia of the vermis, spinal cord defects, disturbed cerebral neuronal migration, dysplasia of the medial olivary nuclei and ectopic Purkinje cells, seizures<br>Neuro logic and developmental-behavioral: Hypotonia, irritability, lethargy, sensorineural hearing loss, autism spectrum disorder, mild to severe intellectual disability or even normal IQ; sensory hyper reactivity, language impairment, sleep-cycle disturbance, self-injurious behavior<br>Cardiac: Endocardial cushion defects, atrioventricular canal, hypoplastic left heart sequence and septal defects, hypertension<br>Ear, nose, and throat: Cleft palate, submucosal clefts, and/or bifid uvula<br>Gastrointestinal: Failure to thrive, feeding difficulties, gastrointestinal reflux, formula intolerance, recurrent vomiting, constipation, pyloric stenosis, gut malrotation; progressive cholestasis, stable isolated elevated liver transaminase, intestinal aganglionosis/Hirschsprung disease<br>Genitourinary: Hypospadias, ambiguous genitalia or gender reversal<br>Extremities: Syndactyly of the second and third (2/3) toes; variably short proximally placed thumbs, single palmar creases, postaxial polydactyly, rarely ectrodactyly<br>Other: Cataracts, skin photosensitivity, blepharoptosis, optic nerve hypoplasia or atrophy; and adrenal insufficiency | Dietary cholesterol supplementation, HMG-CoA reductase inhibitors, supportive with surgery for malformations, early intervention services |
| Mevalonic aciduria (MVA)[b] | Progressive cerebellar ataxia, dysmorphic features, and progressive visual impairment with development of cataracts, uveitis worsening episodically, hepatosplenomegaly, lymphadenopathy, anemia, diarrhea and malabsorption, death in infancy to the less severely affected patients with severe intellectual disability, hypotonia, myopathy, and retinitis pigmentosa. Virtually all patients have recurrent crises characterized by fever, lymphadenopathy, hepatosplenomegaly, arthalgia, edema, and morbilliform rash. These patients also have progressive cerebellar atrophy. | Primarily supportive with antipyretics, analgesics, corticosteroids; allogeneic bone marrow transplantation; combined orthotopic liver transplantation (OLT) and allogeneic bone marrow transplantation |
| HIDS (milder form of MVA) | Lifelong disorder, recurring attacks every 4-6 week of fever starting typically before the end of the first year of life. Vaccination, minor trauma, surgery, or stress are trigger, high fever lasting 4–6 days with accompanying high erythrocyte sedimentation rate, cervical lymphadenopathy, abdominal pain with vomiting, diarrhea, hepatosplenomegaly, headache, arthralgias and sometimes arthritis of large joints, erythematous maculopapular rash, and sometimes painful, aphthous ulcers in the mouth or vagina.<br>No neuro-developmental impairment or dysmorphism, relatively normal adult life span. | Primarily supportive with antipyretics, analgesics, corticosteroids; anakinra, entanercept |
| Antley-Bixler syndrome (ABS1)[b] | Severe craniosynostosis, brachycephaly with high broad forehead, hydrocephalus and Arnold-Chiari malformation, perinatal onset of radiohumeral synostosis; a wide spectrum of midface hypoplasia, choanal stenosis or atresia, multiple joint contractures, genitourinary anomalies, and impaired steroidogenesis; possible adrenal insufficiency and addisonian crisis especially during severe febrile illness or major surgery | Steroid hormone supplementation for addisonian crises |
| Sterol C4 methyl oxidase deficiency (SC4MOL)[b] | Severe ichthyosiform erythroderma, congenital cataracts, microcephaly, delayed skeletal and sexual maturation, mild to moderate developmental delay, abnormal immunocyte phenotype, and apparent inflammatory joint disease | No known; supportive |
| CHILD syndrome | Inflammatory nevus with wax-like scaling and a marked affinity for skin folds, unique lateralization and strict midline demarcation, hypoplasia of internal organs such as brain, lung, heart, kidney, and skeletal structures with shortness or absence of limbs, ipsilateral/neurosensory hearing loss, cerebral hypoplasia with cortical polymicrogyria, ventriculomegaly, absent corpus callosum, ipsilateral cerebellar dysplasia with completely normal contralateral side of the brain; normal intelligence in females | No known; supportive |
| CK syndrome[b] | Microcephaly, large ears, mild to severe cognitive impairment, seizures beginning in infancy, cerebral cortical malformations, hypotonia, behavioral problems with self-mutilatory tendencies, speech delay and oro-facial dysmorphism, scoliosis, kyphosis, and lordosis, and arachnodactyly and hyperextensible joints, mild to severe intellectual disability in males, possible psychopathology in carrier females | No known; supportive |
| CDPX2 Conradi-Hunermann syndrome | Pattern of abnormal punctate calcification of dystrophic epiphyseal cartilage and other cartilaginous structures, prenatal and postnatal growth retardation, rhizomelic or rhizomesomelic limb shortening, ichthyosis, craniofacial appearance with frontal bossing, midface hypoplasia, flat nasal bridge, midline orofacial defects, agenesis or hypoplasia of corpus callosum; congenital cataracts, microphthalmia, microcornea; sensorineural hearing loss, tethered cord, Dandy-Walkermalformation, cervical myelopathy, normal intelligence in females | No known; supportive |

(Continued)

**TABLE 159-3 CLINICAL CHARACTERISTICS AND TREATMENT IN DISORDERS OF CHOLESTEROL SYNTHESIS (CONTINUED)**

| Disorders | Clinical Presentation Spectrum | Reported Therapies[a] |
|---|---|---|
| Lathosterolosis[b] | Microcephaly, neural tube defects, bitemporal narrowing, congenital cataracts, type II Arnold-Chiari malformation, brain atrophy (hydrocephalus "ex vacuo"), demyelination and dystrophic calcification, intrauterine and postnatal growth retardation, seizures, intellectualdisability, "butterfly vertebrae", postaxial polydactyly, bilateral soft tissue syndactyly; horseshoe kidneys, bilobate gallbladder, and progressive intrahepatic cholestasis, progressive hepatosplenomegaly, gingival hypertrophy, corneal clouding | No known; supportive |
| Desmosterolosis[b] | Dysmorphic facial features, severe developmental delay, retrognathia, mild to severe arthrogryposis involving upper limbs, failure to thrive, microcephaly and macrocephaly, seizures, agenesis of corpus callosum, hydrocephalus and ventriculomegaly with thinning of white matter in both cerebrum and cerebellum, rhizomesomelic shortening of extremities, nystagmus, strabismus, downslanting palpebral fissures, cleft palate, cutis aplasia, soft tissue 2–4 toe syndactyly, osteosclerosis, clubfeet, cardiac defects, and ambiguous genitalia | No known; supportive |

[a]None of the reported therapies have been definitively proven effective in controlled clinical trials.

[b]Very few cases reported to date; full phenotypic spectrum not known.

There are no known specific treatments for these disorders, but supportive surgical treatment of cataracts and/or scoliosis or other malformations may be indicated, and early intervention for developmental disabilities is recommended.

### Rare Sterol Disorders

Lathosterolosis and desmosterolosis malformation syndrome clinical characteristics are noted in Table 159-3. It is important to note that too few cases of these conditions have been reported for the phenotypic spectrum to be well understood. Diagnostic testing, as noted in Table 159-1, includes sterol profiling and confirmatory corresponding gene mutation analysis.

There are no known specific treatments or prevention for these disorders; supportive treatment is recommended, as is early intervention for developmental disabilities.

## SUGGESTED READINGS


Desvergne B, Michalik L, Wahli W. Transcriptional regulation of metabolism. *Physiol Rev.* 2006;86(2):465-514.

Drenth JP, van der Meer JW. Hereditary periodic fever. *N Engl J Med.* 2001;345:1748-1757.

Goldstein JL, Brown MS. Regulation of the mevalonate pathway. *Nature.* 1990;343(6257):425-430.

He M, Smith L, Chang R, Li X, Vockley J. The role of sterol-C4-methyl oxidase in epidermal biology. *Biochim Biophys Acta.* 2014;1841(3):331-335.

Herman GE, Kelley RI, Pureza V, et al. Characterization of mutations in 22 females with X-linked dominant chondrodysplasia punctata (Happle syndrome). *Genet Med.* 2002;4(6):434-438.

Kanungo S, Soares N, He M, Steiner RD. Sterol metabolism disorders and neurodevelopment-an update. *Dev Disabil Res Rev.* 2013;17(3):197-210.

Kostjukovits S, Kalliokoski L, Antila K, Korppi M. Treatment of hyperimmunoglobulinemia D syndrome with biologics in children: review of the literature and Finnish experience. *Eur J Pediatr.* 2015; 174:707-714.

Neven B, Valayannopoulos V, Quartier P, et al. Allogeneic bone marrow transplantation in mevalonic aciduria. *N Engl J Med.* 2007;356:2700-2703.

Porter FD, Herman GE. Malformation syndromes caused by disorders of cholesterol synthesis. *J Lipid Res.* 2011;52:6-34.

Preiksaitiene E, Caro A, Benušienė E, et al. A novel missense mutation in the NSDHL gene identified in a Lithuanian family by targeted next-generation sequencing causes CK syndrome. *Am J Med Genet A.* 2015;167(6):1342-1348.

Rossi M, D'Armiento M, Parisi I, et al. Clinical phenotype of lathosterolosis. *Am J Med Genet A.* 2007;143A:2371-2381.

Zolotushko J, Flusser H, Markus B, et al. The desmosterolosis phenotype: spasticity, microcephaly and micrognathia with agenesis of corpus callosum and loss of white matter. *Eur J Hum Genet.* 2011;19:942-946.


# 160 Disorders of Bile Acid Synthesis

William J. Craigen

## INTRODUCTION

Bile (gall) is a greenish yellow secretion produced by hepatocytes and actively pumped into the bile duct tree to be passed to the gallbladder, where it is concentrated, stored, and subsequently released into the duodenum under hormonal and neural control. Bile is a mildly alkaline liquid composed of electrolytes, bile acids and salts, cholesterol, phospholipids, heme breakdown products such a bilirubin and biliverdin that provide color, and water. Bile acids are derived from cholesterol and act as detergents important in keeping cholesterol in solution in bile and in the digestion and absorption of fats and fat-soluble vitamins in the intestine. The detergent properties of bile acids are determined by the number and orientation of the hydroxyl groups and the presence or absence of an amino acid moiety. The conversion of cholesterol to bile acids and the secretion of cholesterol into bile constitute a major route for the elimination of excess cholesterol. Bile acids have also been identified as important transcriptional activators as natural ligands for transcription factor farnesoid X receptor (FXR; also known as bile acid receptor or nuclear receptor subfamily 1 group H member 4) and by modulating energy metabolism through signaling via the membrane-bound, G-protein–coupled bile acid receptor 1 (Gpbar-1, also known as TGR5). The expression of a number of genes that encode proteins involved in bile acid synthesis, transport, and metabolism is directly controlled by bile acids via activation of FXR and Gpbar-1, as are other genes involved in lipid and glucose metabolism. Hepatic FXR inhibits bile acid synthesis by a feedback mechanism requiring small heterodimer partner (SHP)-mediated CYP7A1 repression. SHP, an unusual nuclear receptor lacking a DNA-binding domain, exhibits transcriptional repression upon dimerization with several transcription factors. Additionally, ileal FXR induces FGF19 secretion into the portal circulation in response to bile acid absorption, which in turn represses hepatic CYP7A1 through FGFR4-mediated signaling, a pathway requiring the interaction of FGFR4 and the cell surface single-pass transmembrane protein β-Klotho. Activation of FXR interferes with glycolytic glucose metabolism, directing glucose to glycogen storage. FXR activation also represses de novo lipogenesis via inhibition of lipogenic enzymes such as acetyl-CoA carboxylase-1 and fatty acid synthase, leading to a reduced hepatic very-low-density lipoprotein output. Hence, bile acids act as metabolic integrators that are particularly active postprandially, promoting glycogen accumulation and inhibiting lipid synthesis.

Individuals with disorders of bile acid synthesis may exhibit liver disease due to impaired bile secretion (cholestasis), along with symptoms of fat-soluble vitamin deficiency, gallstones, steatorrhea due to fat malabsorption, and the accumulation of cholesterol in tissues leading to cutaneous xanthomata and atherosclerosis. The major bile acids produced in the liver are the taurine and glycine conjugates (amidates) of chenodeoxycholic acid (CDCA) and cholic acid (CA), the 2 primary bile acids. CA is a trihydroxy-bile acid with hydroxyl groups at positions C-3, C-7, and C-12, whereas CDCA is a dihydroxy-bile acid with hydroxyl groups at C-3 and C-7. Secretion of these conjugated bile acids into the canaliculi via the bile salt export pump encoded by the *ABCB11* gene (defective in progressive familial intrahepatic cholestasis [PFIC] type 2 [PFIC2]) is required for clearance of bile acids from the liver, and its expression is induced by FXR. The ABC transporters MDR3/ABCB4 (PFIC3), the ABCG5/ABCG8 heterodimer, and MRP2/ABCC2, responsible for hepatobiliary transport of phospholipids, cholesterol, and hydrophilic organic anions such as divalent bile acid conjugates, respectively, are also subject to FXR-mediated upregulation. Co-secretion of bile acids and these lipids allows for mixed micelle formation in bile and is essential for protection of the biliary system from the cytotoxic detergent properties of high bile acid concentrations. Within the micelles, the polar bile acids surround the insoluble hydrophobic fatty acids and monoglycerides and deliver the hydrophobic fat to the enterocyte brush border membrane of the small intestine for degradation and absorption.

A fraction of the bile salts are modified and/or deconjugated by colonic bacteria resulting in the secondary bile acids: deoxycholic acid (DCA) from CA and lithocholic (LCA) acid from CDCA, and free primary bile acids after deconjugation. Other secondary bile acids are ursodeoxycholic acid (UDCA), hyodeoxycholic acid (HDCA), and hyocholic acid (HCA). Both primary and secondary bile acids are reabsorbed in the terminal ileum and in the large intestine followed by transport back to the liver via the portal circulation. In the ileum, the reabsorption of bile acids is dependent on the apical sodium-dependent bile salt transporter (ASBT; SLC10A2) at the brush border. In the enterocyte, bile acids are transported through the cytoplasm via cytosolic intestinal bile acid-binding protein (IBABP) to the basolateral membrane, where the heterodimeric organic solute transporter Ostα/Ostβ releases bile acids into the portal circulation. At the basolateral membrane of hepatocytes, the sodium taurocholic acid cotransporting polypeptide (NTCP, SLC10A1) has a substrate specificity limited to conjugated bile acids. Members of the superfamily of organic anion transporter polypeptides (OATP), OATP1A2, OATP1B1, and OATP1B3, share overlapping substrate specificities for conjugated and unconjugated bile acids, as well as for neutral steroids, steroid sulfates, and selected organic cations. Expression of ASBT on the apical surface of cholangiocytes suggests there is a bile acid shunt from the biliary tract to the liver. The enterohepatic circulation maintains a bile acid pool of about 2 to 4 g that goes through approximately 4 to 12 cycles per day, with considerable individual variability. Fecal loss constitutes about 5% of the total pool per day, and the pool is maintained by hepatic bile acid synthesis, thus maintaining bile acid homeostasis. A failure to reabsorb bile acids leads to bile acid diarrhea (BAD), a relatively common disorder due to either malabsorption of intestinal bile acids and/or excess hepatic production. In a subset of patients, genetic variants in Gpbar-1, FGF19, FGFR4, and β-Klotho affect bile acid production and homeostasis, while the gut microbiome alters enterohepatic circulation via variation in the production of naturally occurring FXR bile acid agonists and antagonists. FGF19 and 7-α-hydroxy-4-cholesten-3-one serve as biomarkers of disease activity.

The conversion of cholesterol to bile acids involves the enzymatic modification to the sterol nucleus and the sterol side chain. The major pathway for bile acid synthesis, the neutral or classic pathway, begins with the conversion of cholesterol to 7α-hydroxycholesterol. A second pathway, the acidic or alternative pathway, starts with the conversion of cholesterol to 27-hydroxycholesterol. The neutral and acidic pathways share several enzymes; hence, inborn errors can potentially disrupt both routes for the synthesis of bile acids. A simplified version of the major bile acid synthesis pathways is shown in Figure 160-1.

Bile acids become cytotoxic at abnormally high concentrations, and the degree of cytotoxicity is dependent on their physicochemical properties. CA is the most hydrophilic bile acid with 3 hydroxy groups and hence is less cytotoxic, whereas DCA and CDCA are more cytotoxic because they only have 2 hydroxyl groups. LCA is the most cytotoxic naturally occurring bile acid, with only 1 hydroxyl group. UDCA, present in humans only in trace amounts (and abundant in bears), is devoid of cytotoxic properties. UDCA is relatively hydrophilic despite being a dihydroxy-bile acid due to the hydroxyl group at C-7 being in the β rather than the α configuration, as in CDCA. Along with the primary bile acids, UDCA is used as a therapeutic agent in a variety of disorders complicated by cholestasis.

There are at least 17 enzymes involved in the synthesis of bile acids, which involves the addition of hydroxyl groups to the ring structure of cholesterol and oxidation and shortening of the side chain. The modifications to the cholesterol side chain involve 27-hydroxylation, further oxidation to a C27 bile acid, alteration of the stereochemistry of the C27 bile acid coenzyme A (CoA) ester (racemization), and then β-oxidation in peroxisomes to produce a C24 bile acid CoA ester that is then conjugated to glycine or taurine prior to excretion. Since bile acids are potentially cytotoxic, the expression of selected enzymes in the biosynthesis pathway is tightly regulated by feedback inhibition and feed-forward induction mechanisms.

Disorders of bile acid synthesis that affect transformation of the cholesterol nucleus produce hepatobiliary disease; those that affect the oxidation of the cholesterol side chain often also cause extrahepatic disease, in particular neurologic manifestations. This is probably because the early steps of the acidic pathway for bile acid synthesis play an important role in controlling cholesterol concentrations in extrahepatic tissues. Unusual bile acids and bile alcohols in plasma, feces, or urine are detected by fast atom bombardment mass spectrometry (FAB-MS) or, more commonly, electrospray ionization tandem mass spectrometry (ESI-MS/MS).

## CHOLESTEROL 7α-HYDROXYLASE DEFICIENCY

### CLINICAL PRESENTATION

This disorder has not yet been detected in symptomatic children. Homozygous cholesterol 7α-hydroxylase deficiency has been detected in adults with hypercholesterolemia, hypertriglyceridemia, and premature gallstone disease. Their low-density lipoprotein (LDL) cholesterol levels are resistant to treatment with inhibitors of 3-hydroxy-3-methylglutaryl (HMG)-CoA reductase (statins). A study of family members revealed that individuals heterozygous for the mutation were also hyperlipidemic, consistent with this being a codominant disorder.

### METABOLIC DERANGEMENT AND PATHOPHYSIOLOGY

A block at the level of cholesterol 7α-hydroxylase prevents the neutral pathway from synthesizing bile acids. However, this is likely compensated for by an upregulation of the acidic pathway, leading to an increase in the synthesis of CDCA. In 1 homozygote, the cholesterol content of a liver biopsy was increased. Fecal bile acid output was reduced, and the ratio of CDCA-derived fecal bile acids to CA-derived fecal bile acids was increased.

### GENETICS

Cholesterol 7α-hydroxylase deficiency is a codominant disorder caused by mutations in the *CYP7A1* gene on chromosome 8q11-q12. The only mutation described to date is a frameshift mutation (L413fs*414) that results in loss of enzyme function.

### DIAGNOSIS

There is no simple blood or urine test for cholesterol 7α-hydroxylase deficiency. Analysis of CYP7A1 can be undertaken in a patient with statin-resistant hypercholesterolemia.

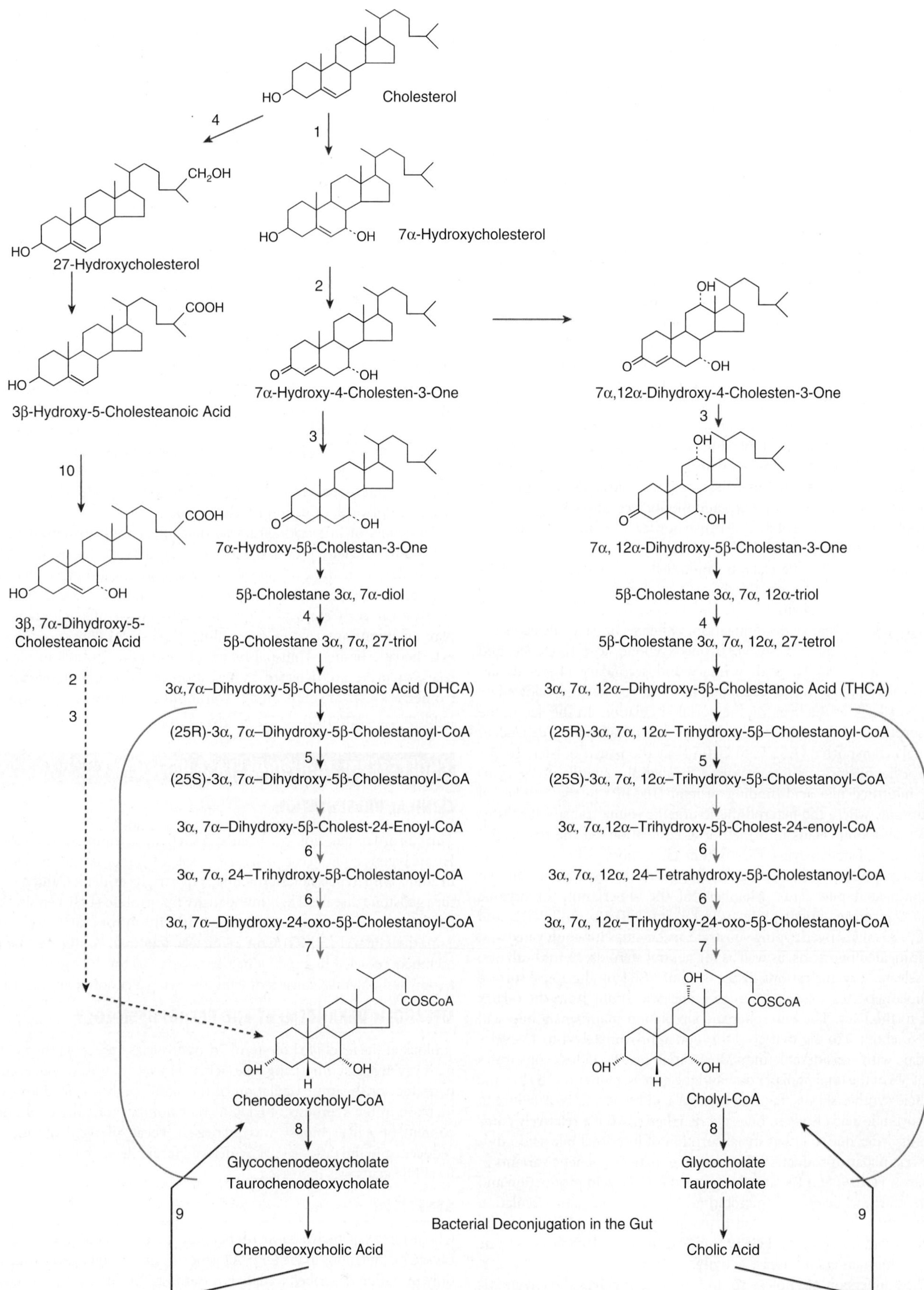


**FIGURE 160-1** Simplified representation of 2 major pathways for the synthesis of bile acids from cholesterol—the acidic pathway on the left, starting with formation of 27-hydroxycholesterol, and the neutral pathway(s) on the right, starting with formation of 7α-hydroxycholesterol. Several enzymes participate in both pathways. Deficiencies have been described in cholesterol 7α-hydroxylase (1); 3β-hydroxy-$\Delta^5$-C27-steroid dehydrogenase/isomerase (2); $\Delta^4$-3-oxosteroid-5β-reductase (3); sterol 27-hydroxylase (4); α-methyl-acyl-CoA racemase (5); peroxisomal D-bifunctional protein (6); peroxisomal sterol carrier protein X (thiolase) (7); bile acid CoA:amino acid *N*-acyltransferase deficiency (8); bile acyl-CoA synthetase (9); and oxysterol 7α-hydroxylase (10). Reactions thought to occur predominantly in the peroxisomes are included in the green brackets. Disorders of peroxisome biogenesis affect many steps, including the reactions of peroxisomal β-oxidation, which is depicted by *blue arrows*.

## TREATMENT AND LONG-TERM OUTCOME

Control of plasma cholesterol and triglyceride levels requires treatment with a combination of a powerful HMG-CoA reductase inhibitor (atorvastatin) and niacin. The variability of the disorder and long-term prognosis are not known.

# 3β-HYDROXY-$\Delta^5$-$C_{27}$-STEROID DEHYDROGENASE DEFICIENCY

## CLINICAL PRESENTATION

Deficiency of 3β-HSD (congenital bile acid synthesis defect type 1 [CBAS1]; Mendelian Inheritance in Man [MIM] no. 607764) typically manifests in the neonatal period with conjugated hyperbilirubinemia, elevated transaminases, and a normal γ-glutamyl transpeptidase (GGT). There is often associated steatorrhea, and a liver biopsy shows a giant-cell hepatitis with evidence of cholestasis (retained bile pigment). Fat-soluble vitamin malabsorption may become evident as rickets (or even severe symptomatic hypocalcemia), vitamin K–responsive coagulopathy, or low plasma concentrations of vitamin E or vitamin A. If left untreated, the liver disease progresses with hepatomegaly, splenomegaly, and evidence of increasing fibrosis on a liver biopsy resembling PFIC, although pruritus is less common in 3β-HSD deficiency than in PFIC. Occasionally, the disorder is detected in a patient with chronic hepatitis in the second decade or beyond.

## METABOLIC DERANGEMENT AND PATHOPHYSIOLOGY

3β-HSD is involved in both the neutral and acidic pathways of bile acid synthesis, so a loss of enzyme activity leads to marked impairment of CDCA and CA synthesis. The accumulating 3β-hydroxy-$\Delta^5$ intermediates (such as 7α-hydroxycholesterol) can undergo the other reactions required for conversion to C24 bile acids. Affected individuals synthesize considerable amounts of bile acids that resemble CDCA and CA, except that they retain the 3β-hydroxy-$\Delta^5$ configuration of cholesterol. These bile acids are readily sulfated, so the major urinary bile acids are sulfated 3β,7α-dihydroxy-5-cholenoic acid, sulfated 3β,7α,12α–trihydroxycholenoic acid, and their glycine conjugates. The bile acids that are produced in large amounts are not substrates for the bile salt export pump and may in fact inhibit it. Thus, transport of bile acids into bile is very much reduced, leading to cholestasis. Bile acid deficiency in the gut contributes to malabsorption of fat and fat-soluble vitamins.

## GENETICS

3β-HSD deficiency is an autosomal recessive disorder caused by reduced or absent activity of 3β-hydroxy-$\Delta^5$-$C_{27}$-steroid dehydrogenase, which is encoded by the *HSD3B7* gene on chromosome 16p11.2-12. Prenatal diagnosis by DNA analysis is possible; however, this is a treatable disease.

## DIAGNOSIS

Urine bile acid analysis shows peaks attributable to the sulfates and glycine-conjugated sulfates of 3β,7α-dihydroxy-5-cholenoic acid and 3β,7α,12α-trihydroxy-5-cholenoic acid, whereas plasma bile acid analysis demonstrates the presence of these 2 bile acids and C27 analogues, particularly 3β,7α-dihydroxy-5-cholestenoic acid. The plasma concentrations of CDCA and CA are strikingly low for a child with cholestasis. The activity of 3β-HSD is reduced in cultured skin fibroblasts, and mutations can be found in the *HSD3B7* gene.

## TREATMENT AND LONG-TERM OUTCOME

Severe coagulopathy requires intravenous vitamin K. Seizures and tetany due to hypocalcemia require intravenous calcium and correction of vitamin D deficiency. Both of these problems will not recur once bile acid replacement has been started. The first patients were treated with CDCA at a dose of 12 to 18 mg/kg/d for 2 months, followed by 9 to 12 mg/kg/d for maintenance. This led to resolution of symptoms and rapid normalization of liver function tests, with improvement in the appearances in the liver biopsy. Treatment with CDCA controls the disease into adult life, whereas untreated children with 3β-HSD deficiency may die from the complications of cirrhosis before age 5. Some children with severe liver disease have shown an initial rise in transaminases with CDCA treatment. In such patients, changing to a combination of cholic acid (7 mg/kg/d) plus CDCA (7 mg/kg/d) has produced a gradual normalization of liver function tests.

# $\Delta^4$-3-OXOSTEROID 5β-REDUCTASE DEFICIENCY

$\Delta^4$-3-Oxosteroid 5β-reductase deficiency (congenital bile acid synthesis defect type 2 [CBAS2]; MIM no. 235555) leads to increased urinary excretion of bile acids with a 3-oxo-$\Delta^4$ structure, principally the glycine and taurine conjugates of 7α-hydroxy-3-oxo-4-cholenoic acid and 7α,12α-dihydroxy-3-oxo-4-cholenoic acid. However, patients who excrete these 3-oxo-$\Delta^4$ bile acids as the major urinary bile acids can be divided into 2 groups: individuals with mutations in SRD5B1 (*AKR1D1*, the gene encoding the 5β-reductase enzyme) and those in whom mutations in the gene have been excluded. In the second group, the cause of excretion of 3-oxo-$\Delta^4$ bile acids remains uncertain but is associated with fulminant liver failure due to conditions such as neonatal hemochromatosis, and because this pattern of urinary bile acid excretion can be a nonspecific consequence of severe liver disease, the description in this chapter will be limited to patients with proven *AKR1D1* mutations. However, it has been reported that the 2 types can be distinguished through urinary steroid analysis by gas chromatography–mass spectrometry (GC-MS) of both cortisol and cortisone compounds, such as 5β-tetrahydrocortisol and 5β-tetrahydrocortisone.

All known patients presented as neonates with cholestatic jaundice and raised transaminases but normal GGT, low vitamin E, and a coagulopathy that improved with parenteral vitamin K. Their liver biopsies showed giant cell transformation, canalicular and hepatocellular cholestasis, portal inflammation, septal fibrosis, occasional necrotic foci, and in some cases, increased extramedullary hematopoiesis. Cholestasis persisted in all cases. One infant progressed to liver failure, failed to respond to treatment with UDCA or CDCA, and required a liver transplant at 19 weeks. One child failed to respond to UDCA treatment but responded well to treatment with CDCA and CA (started at 8 months) and was asymptomatic at the age of 10 years. One patient showed an initial response to CDCA plus CA but then deteriorated and required transplantation. A pair of twin patients responded to treatment with CA started at 8 months and remained well at age 5 years.

## METABOLIC DERANGEMENT AND PATHOPHYSIOLOGY

$\Delta^4$-3-Oxosteroid 5β-reductase is thought to be involved in both the neutral and the acidic pathways of bile acid synthesis and in a pathway needed for the degradation of steroid hormones with a 3-oxo-$\Delta^4$ structure (including glucocorticoids, mineralocorticoids, testosterone, and progesterone). The impaired function of the bile acid synthetic pathways results in very markedly reduced synthesis of CDCA and CA. These bile acids are present at unusually low concentration in the plasma and urine (for a child with cholestasis). The bile acid precursors with a 3-oxo-$\Delta^4$ structure undergo side chain oxidation to produce 7α-hydroxy-3-oxo-4-cholenoic acid and 7α,12α-dihydroxy-3-oxo-4-cholenoic acid. The glycine and taurine conjugates of these bile acids are prominent in plasma and are the major bile acids in urine. Bile acids with a 3-oxo-$\Delta^4$ structure are not substrates for the bile salt export pump and may inhibit it, leading to reduced bile flow (cholestasis).

Accumulating 3-oxo-$\Delta^4$ intermediates (such as 7α-hydroxy-cholest-4-en-3-one) can be converted by a 5α-reductase enzyme to 5α(H) derivatives (eg, 7α-hydroxy-5α-cholestan-3-one) and hence to 5α(H)- or allo-bile acids (eg, allochenodeoxycholic acid, 3α,7α-dihydroxy-5α-cholanic acid). In one patient, although 3-oxo-$\Delta^4$ bile acids were the major bile acids in infancy, by age 11, the major plasma bile acids were allo-bile acids. At the age of 11, the child had no evidence of liver disease or malabsorption despite having stopped treatment with CDCA and CA for a year. This suggests that, as childhood progresses, the formation of allo-bile acids may actually compensate for the 5β-reductase deficiency. The same patient was shown to have only trace amounts of 5β-reduced steroid metabolites in the urine. Despite the impaired degradation of 3-oxo-$\Delta^4$ steroid hormones, there was no evidence of cushingoid features, hypertension, or sex hormone accumulation, again suggesting that the 5α-reductase pathway can compensate.

### GENETICS

Some patients with a urine bile acid profile suggestive of 5β-reductase deficiency harbor biallelic mutations in the *AKR1D1* gene (MIM no. 604741), while others lack detectable mutations in the gene.

### DIAGNOSIS

Urine bile acid analysis shows that the main bile acids in the urine are 3-oxo-$\Delta^4$ bile acids and that excretion of the corresponding saturated bile acids is markedly reduced. Plasma bile acid analysis in infancy shows markedly elevated concentrations of 7α-hydroxy-4-cholenoic acid and 7α,12α-dihydroxy-4-cholenoic acid. In an older child, the major plasma bile acids were allo-bile acids.

### TREATMENT AND LONG-TERM OUTCOME

Treatment of a bleeding diathesis with parenteral vitamin K may be required. Vitamin D may be needed for rickets. Deficiency of 5β-reductase can progress rapidly to liver failure. However, treatment with bile acid replacement therapy can normalize liver function and lead to good long-term health. Successful treatment regimens include CDCA and CA (8 mg/kg/d of each) and CA alone. It is currently unknown whether there is spontaneous improvement with age, which would make continued bile acid replacement unnecessary. Any such tendency for spontaneous resolution will make assessments of long-term bile acid replacement strategies difficult.

## OXYSTEROL 7α-HYDROXYLASE DEFICIENCY

### CLINICAL PRESENTATION

The first case of oxysterol 7α-hydroxylase deficiency (congenital bile acid synthesis defect type 3 [CBAS3]; MIM no. 613812) was described in 1998 by Setchell and colleagues. The infant was born to consanguineous parents and, beginning at 8 weeks of life, had severe cholestatic liver disease but normal GGT. He did not respond to CA replacement therapy, required liver transplantation, and died of complications of the transplant.

Mutations in the *CYP7B1* gene encoding oxysterol 7α-hydroxylase have been shown in patients with hereditary spastic paraplegia type 5 (HSP5; MIM no. 270800) Affected patients have lower extremity weakness and spasticity, posterior column sensory impairment (demonstrated by diminished vibration sensation and proprioception), and some degree of bladder dysfunction. The age of onset varies from infancy to 40 years. Thus, this seems to be another disorder that can cause cholestasis in the neonate and neurologic disease later in life.

### METABOLIC DERANGEMENT AND PATHOPHYSIOLOGY

In the liver, oxysterol 7α-hydroxylase is essential for the acidic pathway of bile acid synthesis. Deficiency of the enzyme leads to synthesis of 3β-hydroxy-5-cholenoic acid, which has cholestatic and hepatotoxic properties. In extrahepatic tissues, oxysterol 7α-hydroxylase contributes to a pathway for cholesterol degradation, and it provides the primary metabolic route for the modification of dehydroepiandrosterone neurosteroids in the brain. Loss of 1 or both of these functions may explain the neurologic disease.

### GENETICS

Oxysterol 7α-hydroxylase deficiency is an autosomal recessive disorder caused by mutations in the *CYP7B1* gene on chromosome 8q21.3. A child with liver disease was homozygous for an R388X nonsense mutation, as was 1 patient with HSP5. Other patients with HSP5 have had missense mutations.

### DIAGNOSIS

In the reported neonatal case, FAB-MS analysis of urine revealed major peaks of m/z ratio 453 and 510 attributable to 3β-hydroxy-5-cholenoic acid 3-sulfate and its glycine conjugate. GC-MS analysis of plasma indicated that the main bile acids were 3β-hydroxy-5-cholenoic acid and 3β-hydroxy-5-cholestenoic acid; the concentration of 27-hydroxycholesterol in plasma was very markedly increased.

### TREATMENT AND LONG-TERM OUTCOME

The 1 reported patient who presented with cholestatic liver disease in infancy showed a deterioration with UDCA therapy and no improvement with cholic acid, and required a liver transplant for hepatic failure at 4 months. The fact that homozygous mutations have been found in patients with HSP5 suggests that some individuals with oxysterol 7α-hydroxylase deficiency either do not develop cholestatic liver disease or have mild and self-limiting liver dysfunction. No specific treatment has been described.

## CEREBROTENDINOUS XANTHOMATOSIS (STEROL 27-HYDROXYLASE DEFICIENCY)

### CLINICAL PRESENTATION

Cerebrotendinous xanthomatosis (CTX) has a range of clinical presentations, including cholestatic jaundice in early infancy, diarrhea and cataracts in the preschool child, learning difficulties in childhood, dementia in young adult life, and the development of tendon xanthomata and early atherosclerosis. The early liver disease can be fatal, and the early-onset dementia can progress to severe neurologic dysfunction. These devastating outcomes are preventable with bile acid replacement therapy. Hence, early diagnosis, based on a high index of suspicion and appropriate tests, is extremely important.

It is important to recognize that the neurologic deterioration is highly variable. For example, some patients are intellectually normal but suffer from a neuropathy or mild spastic paraparesis; others have no neurologic signs but present with psychiatric symptoms resembling schizophrenia. Motor dysfunction (spastic paraparesis, ataxia, expressive dysphasia) develops in approximately 60% of patients in the second or third decade of life.

Tendon xanthomata may be detectable during the second decade of life but usually appear in the third or fourth decade. The Achilles tendon is the most common site; other sites include the tibial tuberosities and the extensor tendons of the fingers and the triceps. Premature atherosclerosis leading to death from myocardial infarction occurs in some patients. In others, death is caused by progression of the neurologic disease with increasing spasticity, tremor and ataxia, and pseudobulbar palsy.

Magnetic resonance imaging (MRI) of the brain may show diffuse cerebral atrophy and increased signal intensity in the cerebellar white matter on T2-weighted scans. Osteoporosis is also common in CTX and is associated with low plasma concentrations of 25-hydroxy-vitamin D and 24,25-dihydroxy-vitamin D, predisposing to pathologic fractures.

### METABOLIC DERANGEMENT AND PATHOPHYSIOLOGY

Sterol 27-hydroxylase is present in the liver and in extrahepatic tissues. It is the first step in the acidic pathway for bile acid synthesis and provides a route for removing cholesterol from extrahepatic tissues. In CTX, accumulating cholesterol partly is converted to cholestanol. Sterol 27-hydroxylase also participates in the neutral pathway of bile acid synthesis. 5β-Cholestane-3α,7α,12α-triol cannot be hydroxylated in the C27 position and accumulates in the liver. Consequently, it is metabolized by an alternative pathway, starting with hydroxylation in the C25 position, a process that occurs in the endoplasmic reticulum. Further hydroxylation (eg, in the C22 or C23 position) results in the synthesis of the characteristic bile alcohols that are found (as glucuronides) in the urine. Bile acid precursors other than 5β-cholestane-3α,7α,12α-triol also accumulate. Some of these (eg, 7α-hydroxy-cholest-4-en-3-one) are likely converted to cholestanol by a pathway involving 7α-dehydroxylation. Because patients with CTX have a reduced rate of bile acid synthesis, the normal feedback inhibition of cholesterol 7α-hydroxylase by bile acids is reduced. This further enhances the production of bile alcohols and cholestanol from bile acid precursors. Disruption of bile acid synthesis is likely responsible for the cholestatic liver disease of infancy, but the major symptoms of CTX in older children and adults are produced by accumulation of cholesterol and cholestanol in almost every tissue of the body, particularly in the nervous system, atherosclerotic plaques, and tendon xanthomata.

## GENETICS

CTX (MIM no. 213700) is an autosomal recessive disorder caused by deficiency of sterol 27-hydroxylase, which is encoded by the *CYP27A1* gene located on chromosome 2q33-qter. Many mutations have been described; prenatal diagnosis is typically undertaken by DNA testing.

## DIAGNOSIS

Analysis of cholanoids (bile acids and bile alcohols) in urine shows a suggestive pattern dominated by the excretion of cholestane-tetrol glucuronides, and cholestane-pentol glucuronides. This pattern must be distinguished from a normal pattern in some infants in which the major cholanoids in urine, albeit at much lower concentration, are nor-cholestane pentol glucuronides and cholestane-pentol glucuronides. Analysis of plasma shows that at all ages the concentration of 5β-cholestane-3α,7α,12α,25-tetrol is increased. In adults, the plasma concentration of cholestanol is typically increased, but this is not a reliable diagnostic marker. The full sterol profile shows increased concentrations of several cholesterol precursors. 27-Hydroxylation of C27 sterols can be measured in cultured skin fibroblasts, and the enzyme activity is virtually absent in fibroblasts from patients with CTX.

## TREATMENT AND LONG-TERM OUTCOME

Without treatment, the neonatal-onset liver disease can be fatal. Adults with untreated CTX usually die from progressive neurologic dysfunction or myocardial infarction between the ages of 30 and 60 years. The treatment for CTX that has been thoroughly evaluated is CDCA, with the results of this treatment first reported in 1984. The rates of cholestanol and cholesterol synthesis were reduced, and plasma cholestanol concentrations fell. A significant fraction of patients showed reversal of their neurologic disability, with improved cognition and orientation and enhanced strength and independence. In contrast, the MRI findings do not show obvious improvement. Urinary excretion of bile-alcohol glucuronides is markedly suppressed. CDCA almost certainly works by suppressing cholesterol 7α-hydroxylase activity. UDCA, which does not inhibit the enzyme, is ineffective. Adults are generally treated with a dose of 750 mg/d of CDCA. Other treatments include HMG-CoA reductase inhibitors (statins such as lovastatin) and LDL apheresis. The osteoporosis seen in patients with CTX appears to be resistant to CDCA therapy. Cholestatic liver disease in infancy may be self-limiting, but in those children in whom it is not, bile acid treatment has been successful, with CA therapy preferable to CDCA.

# α-METHYL-ACYL-CoA RACEMASE DEFICIENCY

## CLINICAL PRESENTATION

α-Methyl-acyl-CoA racemase (AMACR) deficiency (congenital bile acid synthesis defect type 4 [CBAS4]; MIM no. 214950) was first described in a child in 2001. An infant with AMACR deficiency presented with a coagulopathy due to vitamin K deficiency, and a sibling had died from bleeding with the same cause. The infant had mild cholestatic jaundice with elevated aspartate aminotransferase and, in contrast to 3β-HSD deficiency, 5β-reductase deficiency, and CTX, a raised GGT. Liver biopsy showed a mild nonspecific lymphocytic portal infiltrate and abundant giant cell transformation. AMACR deficiency may also present with developmental delay in childhood and with epilepsy and encephalopathy, which may result in permanent neurologic deficits (eg, blindness, cognitive decline). Adult patients have developed an insidious pigmentary retinopathy, spastic paraparesis, tremor, and a demyelinating sensory motor neuropathy. MRI scans have revealed high signal in the pons, basal ganglia, thalami, cerebral peduncles, and subcortical white matter.

## METABOLIC DERANGEMENT AND PATHOPHYSIOLOGY

The neutral bile acid synthesis pathway produces the 25R isomers of 3α,7α-dihydroxy-5β-cholestanoic acid (DHCA)-CoA and 3α,7α,12α-trihydroxy-5β-cholestanoic acid (THCA)-CoA. AMACR is required to convert these to the 25S isomers, which are the substrates for peroxisomal β-oxidation. In patients with AMACR deficiency, the 25R isomers of DHCA and THCA accumulate as the free acids and taurine conjugates. AMACR is also required for converting the 2R isomer of pristanoyl-CoA to the 2S isomer, which is the substrate for β-oxidation. Plasma concentrations of pristanic acid can be grossly elevated. High levels of phytanic acid cause neurologic damage in Refsum disease, and it is quite likely that the very high levels of the (structurally similar) pristanic acid contribute to the neurologic disease in AMACR deficiency.

## GENETICS

AMACR deficiency is an autosomal recessive disorder caused by mutations in the *AMACR* gene on chromosome 5p13.2-q11.1. One particular mutation (c.154T>C) has been found in 4 patients, including those with neonatal cholestasis and adult-onset neurologic disease.

## DIAGNOSIS

Analysis of urinary bile acids in a cholestatic infant reveals major peaks attributable to taurine conjugated THCA and mono- and dihydroxylated derivatives. Analysis of plasma bile acids by GC-MS reveals increased concentrations of DHCA and THCA and the C29-dicarboxylic acid. High-performance liquid chromatography (HPLC)-ESI-MS/MS is used to demonstrate that it is the (25R) isomer of THCA that is accumulating. GC-MS analysis of plasma fatty acids shows an elevated concentration of pristanic acid with a mildly elevated to normal plasma phytanic acid concentration and normal very-long-chain fatty acids.

## TREATMENT AND LONG-TERM OUTCOME

The outcome for patients with AMACR deficiency has varied considerably from neonatal death caused by hemorrhage due to vitamin K deficiency to difficulty in walking in the sixth decade. Parenteral vitamin K may be lifesaving in the neonatal period. One patient who presented with neonatal cholestasis was treated with CA, leading to improved liver function tests. Reduction of plasma pristanic acid levels appears advisable and can be achieved with a low-phytanic-acid diet, which involves, in particular, restriction of dairy products, beef, and lamb. It is unclear whether bile acid replacement therapy has a role in preventing the neurologic disease.

# ABCD3 DEFICIENCY

## CLINICAL PRESENTATION

A female, born of consanguineous Turkish parents, presented with hepatosplenomegaly, severe iron-deficient anemia, and coagulopathy at 18 months of age. Cognitive and motor development were normal, but transaminases were elevated, and liver biopsy showed fibrosis and hepatocellular regeneration. The liver disease was progressive, and she underwent liver transplantation at age 4 but died of respiratory complications.

### GENETICS

Deficiency of ABCD3, encoded by the *ABCD3* gene located on chromosome 1.21.3, causes congenital deficiency of bile acid synthesis type 5 (CBAS5; MIM no. 616278). ABCD3 is one of three ATP-binding cassette transporters present in the peroxisomal membrane that catalyze ATP-dependent transport of substrates for metabolic pathways localized in peroxisomes; hence, this autosomal recessive disorder is a transporter deficiency. The child harbored a 1.7-kbp deletion leading to protein truncation p.Y635Nfs*.

### DIAGNOSIS

Laboratory studies showed marked accumulation of the peroxisomal C27 bile acid intermediates DHCA and THCA. Very-long-chain fatty acids were also increased, but phytanic and pristanic acid levels were normal in plasma. Patient fibroblasts showed reduced numbers of abnormally enlarged peroxisomes as well as reduced β-oxidation of pristanic acid.



## ACYL-CoA OXIDASE 2 DEFICIENCY

### CLINICAL PRESENTATION

To date, 2 families have been reported. The index case was an 8-year-old Turkish male from a consanguineous family who presented at 8 months of age with intermittently moderately elevated transaminase levels and a normal GGT. He had hypolipidemia and low vitamin D, with evidence of fat malabsorption. At 6 years of age, the liver showed fibrosis, and he exhibited mild ataxia and cognitive impairment. A second family with 2 affected adolescent siblings has also been reported with isolated elevation of transaminases, normal liver histology, and a characteristic bile acid profile.

Acyl-CoA oxidase 2 (ACOX2) is a branched-chain acyl-CoA oxidase, a peroxisomal enzyme believed to be involved in the metabolism of branched-chain fatty acids and bile acid intermediates.

### GENETICS

Deficiency of ACOX2 causes congenital bile acid synthesis defect type 6 (CBAS6; MIM no. 617308). In the Turkish child, exome sequencing revealed a homozygous premature termination mutation (p.Y69*) in ACOX2, encoded by the *ACOX2* gene on chromosome 3p14, whereas the second family had the missense substitution p.R225W.

### DIAGNOSIS

Plasma and urine bile acid analysis revealed elevated levels of the C27 intermediate bile acids DHCA and THCA, principally as taurine conjugates, consistent with defective peroxisomal β-oxidation of DHCA-CoA and THCA-CoA. Notably, the levels of long-chain, branched-chain fatty acids (phytanic and pristanic acids) were both normal, and there was no elevation of very-long-chain fatty acids in the plasma, consistent with their metabolism by straight-chain acyl-CoA oxidase (ACOX1).

### TREATMENT AND LONG-TERM OUTCOME

No treatment was described for this child, but since he had low CA levels, a trial with CA supplementation was anticipated.

## PEROXISOMAL D-BIFUNCTIONAL PROTEIN DEFICIENCY

### CLINICAL PRESENTATION

Peroxisomal D-bifunctional protein (DBP) deficiency usually presents in the neonatal period with profound hypotonia and seizures. Other typical features include visual impairment, severe developmental delay, and a characteristic appearance of high forehead, high-arched palate, enlarged fontanel, long philtrum, epicanthic folds, hypertelorism, macrocephaly, retrognathia, and low-set ears. Brain imaging may show gross ventricular dilatation, neocortical dysplasia, cerebral demyelination, and cerebellar atrophy. Liver dysfunction is present in a quarter of patients, and nearly half have hepatomegaly. Postmortem examination of 11 patients showed polymicrogyria in two-thirds of cases, while renal cysts and adrenal cortical atrophy were seen in a third of autopsied cases. Less common features include delay of bone maturation, skeletal malformations, and epiphyseal stippling.

### METABOLIC DERANGEMENT AND PATHOPHYSIOLOGY

DBP catalyzes the second and third steps of peroxisomal β-oxidation of fatty acid derivatives. The enzyme name derives from the 2 activities; a hydroxyacyl-CoA dehydrogenase unit and an enoyl-CoA hydratase unit. It is involved in the β-oxidation of very-long-chain fatty acids, pristanic acid, and DHCA and THCA. Thus, the concentrations of all these substrates are often elevated in plasma, although the accumulation of pristanate depends on the dietary intake of phytanate.

DBP-deficient patients can be classified into 3 types: one deficient in both the hydratase and the dehydrogenase components, a second deficient in only the hydratase unit, and a third type that is deficient in only the dehydrogenase unit. The 3 types can be distinguished by bile acid analysis.

### GENETICS

DBP deficiency is an autosomal recessive disorder caused by mutations in the *HSD17B4* gene on chromosome 5q2.

### DIAGNOSIS

Sometimes the urine bile acid profile is abnormal, showing the presence of taurine-conjugated tetrahydroxy cholestanoic acid and taurine-conjugated tetrahydroxy cholestanoic acid. Analysis of plasma bile acids may show unconjugated varanic acid (3α,7α,12α, 24-tetrahydroxy-5β-cholestanoic acid) as a major component. This can distinguish patients with DBP deficiency from those with peroxisome biogenesis defects. THCA and DHCA are elevated in plasma in three-fourths of patients with DBP deficiency. Nearly all patients have elevated very-long-chain fatty acids, while fewer patients have elevated pristanic acid. The diagnosis of DBP deficiency is achieved by measuring a range of peroxisome functions in cultured skin fibroblasts followed by DNA analysis. These tests distinguish patients with DBP deficiency from patients with disorders of peroxisome biogenesis, who can be similar both clinically and biochemically.

### TREATMENT AND LONG-TERM OUTCOME

Most infants with DBP deficiency die before age 2 years. However, 12 reported patients survived beyond 2 years, and 5 of these patients survived beyond 7.5 years. Biochemical analysis showed a clear correlation between peroxisomal β-oxidation activity and survival.

## PEROXISOMAL STEROL CARRIER PROTEIN X DEFICIENCY

### CLINICAL PRESENTATION

Only 1 patient has been described with this disorder, a 45-year-old man who started stuttering at age 7 and who developed spasmodic torticollis and a dystonic head tremor in stressful situations at age 17. At age 29, he was diagnosed with hypergonadotropic hypogonadism and azoospermia. Dystonia became progressively worse, and at age 44, brain MRI showed bilateral hyperintense signals in the thalamus, butterfly-like lesions in the pons, and lesions in the occipital region. Neurologic examination revealed hyposmia, pathologic saccadic eye movements, and a slight hypoacusis. A brother was similarly clinically affected.

### METABOLIC DERANGEMENT AND PATHOPHYSIOLOGY

Sterol carrier protein X (SCPx) is a thiolase active on branched-chain CoA esters in the peroxisomes. It is involved in the β-oxidation of C27 bile acids and pristanic acid. Thus, it converts

3α,7α,12α-trihydroxy-24-oxo-5β-cholestanoyl-CoA and CoA to cholyl-CoA and propionyl-CoA. In SCPx deficiency, accumulating 3α,7α,12α-trihydroxy-24-oxo-5β-cholestanoic acid is thought to undergo decarboxylation to 3α,7α,12α-trihydroxy-27-nor-5β-cholestan-24-one. This in turn is thought to be hydroxylated 2 or 3 times to generate pentahydroxy-27-nor-5β-cholestan-24-one glucuronides and hexahydroxy-27-nor-5β-cholestan-24-one glucuronides. Reduction of the 24-oxo group likely generates 27-nor-5β-cholestane pentol and hexol glucuronides.

### GENETICS

Peroxisomal sterol carrier protein X deficiency is caused by mutations in the *SCP2* gene on chromosome 1p32, leading to leukoencephalopathy with dystonia and motor neuropathy (LKDMN; MIM no. 613724). The *SCP2* gene encodes 2 proteins, SCPx and sterol carrier protein 2 (SCP2), as a result of transcription initiation from 2 independently regulated promoters. The longer protein is SCPx, with the 2 proteins sharing a common C-terminus. The SCPx protein is a peroxisome-associated thiolase that is involved in the oxidation of branched-chain fatty acids, whereas the SCP2 protein appears to be an intracellular lipid transfer protein. The 1 patient described was homozygous for a 1-nucleotide insertion (545_546insA).

### DIAGNOSIS

The plasma concentrations of DHCA and THCA were slightly elevated in plasma, while pristanate was considerably more elevated. Given the rarity of patients, care should be taken when interpreting the results from analysis of urinary cholanoids by electrospray/FAB-MS.

### TREATMENT AND LONG-TERM OUTCOME

In the 1 described case, onset of neurologic disease was in childhood, but progression was slow. No treatment has been attempted, but dietary control of high pristanate levels would seem warranted.

## FAMILIAL HYPERCHOLANEMIA (INCLUDING BILE ACID-CoA:AMINO ACID *N*-ACYLTRANSFERASE DEFICIENCY)

### CLINICAL PRESENTATION

Familial hypercholanemia is characterized by elevated serum bile acid concentrations, itching, and fat malabsorption. Patients who have proven mutations in the bile acid-CoA:amino acid *N*-acyltransferase (BAAT) gene have had cholestatic jaundice, vitamin D deficiency, and mild portal and focal lobular hepatitis in liver biopsies. Among the Amish population, the presentation is with failure to thrive, sometimes with pruritus and occasionally with coagulopathy but not jaundice.

### METABOLIC DERANGEMENT AND PATHOPHYSIOLOGY

In BAAT deficiency, the liver produces unconjugated (nonamidated) bile acids instead of the usual glycine and taurine conjugates of CA and CDCA. The major urinary bile acid is unconjugated CA. CA and CDCA are also excreted as sulfate and glucuronide conjugates.

### GENETICS

Familial hypercholanemia (FHCA; MIM no. 607748) is genetically heterogeneous. BAAT deficiency is an autosomal recessive disorder caused by mutations in the *BAAT* gene on chromosome 9q22.3. The disorder in the Amish is caused by homozygosity for a missense mutation (c.226A>G; p.M76V) in the *BAAT* gene. In the same population, a second locus was identified, the *TJP2* locus. The *TJP2* gene, located on chromosome 9q21.11, encodes tight junction protein-2, which belongs to a family of membrane-associated guanylate kinase homologs involved in the organization of epithelial and endothelial intercellular junctions via binding to Claudin proteins. A missense variant, p.V48A, was observed in Amish pedigrees. There was reduced penetrance in some homozygous individuals, and other symptomatic family members were also heterozygous for the founder mutation in *BAAT*, reflecting complex genetic interactions. Another case of a girl born to consanguineous parents of Pakistani origin who presented in infancy with jaundice, failure to thrive, and rickets was shown to have an amidation defect and was found to be homozygous for a c.415C>T (p.R139X) mutation in *BAAT* gene. More recently, other patients have been described with progressive familial intrahepatic cholestasis type 4 (PFIC4; MIM no. 615878) caused by homozygous or compound heterozygous mutation in the *TJP2* gene. This appears to be associated with increase risk for hepatocellular carcinoma. Another enzyme, epoxide hydrolase encoded by the *EPHX1* gene on chromosome 1q42.12, has also been associated with familial hypercholanemia in a single Chinese pedigree. Finally, the sodium taurocholate co-transporting polypeptide SLC10A1 (NTCP), encoded by the *SLC10A1* gene on chromosome 14q24.1, a key transporter of conjugated bile salts from the portal circulation into the hepatocyte, has been associated with hypercholanemia in a single patient. Besides hypercholanemia, the child was clinically characterized by mild hypotonia, growth retardation, and delayed motor milestones.

### DIAGNOSIS

Analysis of urine by negative ion FAB-MS or ESI-MS shows that the major urinary bile acid is an unconjugated trihydroxycholanoic acid, and GC-MS shows that it is unconjugated CA. Other bile acids that may be detected include sulfated dihydroxycholanoic acids, trihydroxycholanoic acids, and dihydroxycholanoic acids.

### TREATMENT AND LONG-TERM OUTCOME

Treatment of vitamin K deficiency may be lifesaving, and treatment of rickets may require 1α-hydroxycholecalciferol or 1,25-dihydroxycholecalciferol. The Amish patients appear to show improvement in symptoms with UDCA, but it is important to reiterate that familial hypercholanemia of the Amish can be caused by defects both in the gene responsible for integrity of tight junctions (*TJP2*) and in the *BAAT* gene.

### BILE ACYL-COA LIGASE DEFICIENCY

To date, a single case of bile acyl-CoA ligase (BACL) deficiency has been identified in an infant of consanguineous Pakistani parents. The child was born premature and had persistent cholestasis unresponsive to UDCA. Liver biopsy showed inconspicuous bile ducts, portal-portal bridging fibrosis, parenchymal nodularity, and slight hepatocellular cholestasis. This led to an investigation into heritable forms of cholestasis. Bile acid analysis was performed at 8 months of age, and at that time, the child not jaundiced and serum transaminase values were within the normal ranges.

### DIAGNOSIS

C24 bile acids that have been deconjugated by gut bacteria are returned to the liver in the enterohepatic circulation and are amidated with either glycine or taurine prior to being secreted into bile by the bile salt export pump. Two separate enzymes catalyze this conjugation, the first is BACL, which converts CDCA, CA, and bile acids produced by bacteria, such as deoxycholic acid, to their CoA thioesters, followed by BAAT, which catalyzes the amidation of the bile acid-CoA thioester to form the glycine or taurine conjugate. Urine ESI-MS/MS identified unconjugated CA and unconjugated CDCA, while sulphate and glucuronide conjugates of dihydroxy- and trihydroxycholanoic acids were present. The glycine and taurine conjugates of CDCA and CA were absent, consistent with a defect in amidation. Similarly, the plasma subjected to GC-MS contained a high proportion of unconjugated bile acids.

BACL is encoded by the *SLC27A5* gene located on chromosome 19q13.43. The child harbored a homozygous mutation (c.1012C>T; H338Y) in the *SLC27A5* gene; however, she was also found to have a homozygous variant c.1772A>G (p.N591S) in *ABCB11*, the cause of PFIC2. Bile acid analysis was similarly consistent with an amidation defect in the child's sister, and that child was also homozygous for the *SLC75A5* variant and heterozygous for the *ABCB11* variant. At the time of the report, both siblings were healthy without any therapeutic interventions.

## PEROXISOME BIOGENESIS DISORDERS

Disorders of peroxisome biogenesis are discussed in Chapter 157. As inborn errors affecting bile acid synthesis, they can be detected in infancy by analysis of urinary bile acids; this usually shows substantial excretion of taurine-conjugated tetrahydroxy cholestanoic acids. Analysis of plasma bile acids is a useful test for diagnosing an older child with a suspected peroxisomal disorder; the plasma typically contains the C27 bile acids, THCA and DHCA, and the C29-dicarboxylic acid. The analysis of plasma bile acids and pristanate in a child with normal very-long-chain fatty acids may reveal a peroxisome biogenesis defect, emphasizing the importance of considering bile acid analysis in children suspected of having a peroxisomal defect.



### SUGGESTED READINGS


Berginer VM, Salen G, Shefer S. Long-term treatment of CTX with chenodeoxycholic acid therapy. *N Engl J Med.* 1984;311:1649-1602.

Camilleri M. Bile acid diarrhea: prevalence, pathogenesis, and therapy. *Gut Liver.* 2015;9(3):332-339.

Carlton VE, Harris BZ, Puffenberger EG, et al. Complex inheritance of familial hypercholanemia with associated mutations in TJP2 and BAAT. *Nat Genet.* 2003;34:91-96.

Chong CP, Mills PB, McClean P, Gissen P, Bruce C, Stahlschmidt J, Knisely AS, Clayton PT. Bile acid-CoA ligase deficiency: a new inborn error of bile acid metabolism. *J Inherit Metab Dis.* 2012;35(3):521-530.

Ferdinandusse S, Denis S, Clayton PT, et al. Mutations in the gene encoding peroxisomal alpha-methylacyl-CoA racemase cause adult-onset sensory motor neuropathy. *Nat Genet.* 2000;24(2):188-191.

Ferdinandusse S, Jimenez-Sanchez J, Koster J, et al. A novel bile acid biosynthesis defect due to a deficiency of peroxisomal ABCD3. *Hum Mol Genet.* 2015;24(2):361-370.

Gonzales E, Cresteil D, Baussan C, Dabadie A, Gerhardt MF, Jacquemin E. SRD5B1 (AKR1D1) gene analysis in delta(4)-3-oxosteroid 5-beta-reductase deficiency: evidence for primary genetic defect. *J Hepatol.* 2004;40:716-718.

Juřica J, Dovrtělová G, Nosková K, Zendulka O. Bile acids, nuclear receptors and cytochrome P450. *Physiol Res.* 2016;65:S427-S440.

Lefebvre P, Cariou B, Lien F, Kuipers F, Staels B. Role of bile acids and bile acid receptors in metabolic regulation. *Physiol Rev.* 2009;89:147-191.

Pullinger CR, Eng C, Salen G, et al. Human cholesterol 7alpha-hydroxylase (CYP7A1) deficiency has a hypercholesterolemic phenotype. *J Clin Invest.* 2002;110(1):109-117.

Vaz FM, Paulusma CC, Huidekoper H, et al. Sodium taurocholate cotransporting polypeptide (SLC10A1) deficiency: conjugated hypercholanemia without a clear clinical phenotype. *Hepatology.* 2015;61(1):260-267.

Vilarinho S, Sari S, Mazzacuva F, et al. ACOX2 deficiency: a disorder of bile acid synthesis with transaminase elevation, liver fibrosis, ataxia, and cognitive impairment. *Proc Natl Acad Sci U S A.* 2016; 113(40):11289-11293.


# 161 Disorders of Lipid and Lipoprotein Metabolism

Luis A. Umana and William J. Craigen

## INTRODUCTION

Disorders of lipid and lipoprotein metabolism are characterized by dyslipidemia, which is defined as either elevated or low levels of 1 or more of the major lipoprotein classes: chylomicrons, very-low-density lipoproteins (VLDLs), low-density lipoproteins (LDLs), and high-density lipoproteins (HDLs). Dyslipidemia can result from a mutation in a single gene that plays an important role in lipoprotein metabolism. However, more commonly, dyslipidemia reflects the influence of multiple genes. Environmental influences such as excessive dietary intake of fat and calories and limited physical activity, particularly when associated with obesity, can also contribute significantly to dyslipidemia. Much of what has been learned about dyslipidemia derives from studies of rare single-gene disorders. This chapter presents a theoretical and practical approach to the diagnosis and treatment of dyslipidemia in infants, children, and adolescents. The major clinical complication of dyslipidemia is a predilection to atherosclerosis starting early in life and leading to cardiovascular disease (CVD) in adulthood. At the extremes of dyslipidemia, where inherited disorders of lipid and lipoprotein metabolism are more likely to occur, premature CVD is more frequent and can be accompanied by deposition of lipid in various tissues. Conversely, certain single-gene loss-of-function mutations may also protect the individual from CVD, providing insights into novel therapies. Children with profound hypertriglyceridemia are at high risk of pancreatitis.

## BACKGROUND

A number of clinical, epidemiologic, metabolic, genetic, and randomized clinical trials strongly support the tenet that the origins of atherosclerosis and CVD risk factors begin in childhood and adolescence and that treatment should begin early in life. Several longitudinal pathologic studies from the general population have found that early atherosclerotic lesions of fatty streaks and fibrous plaques in children, adolescents, and young adults who died from accidental causes are significantly related to higher antecedent levels of total cholesterol (TC) and LDL cholesterol (LDL-C); to lower levels of HDL cholesterol (HDL-C); and to other CVD risk factors such as obesity, higher blood pressure, and cigarette smoking. The effect of these risk factors on coronary lesion severity is multiplicative rather than additive.

Four major prospective population studies from the Coronary Artery Risk Development in Young Adults (CARDIA) and the Special Turku Coronary Risk Factor Intervention Project (STRIP) trials showed that CVD risk factors in children and adolescents, particularly LDL-C and obesity, predicted clinical manifestations of atherosclerosis in young adults, as judged by coronary artery calcium, carotid intima-medial thickness (IMT), or brachial flow-mediated dilatation.

Hyperlipidemias have historically been classified by the type of lipoprotein particle that is elevated or reduced in those thought to have primary dyslipidemia, also known as the Fredrickson classification. Studies have also been performed in high-risk youth who were selected because 1 parent had CVD or because they have inherited a known metabolic disorder of lipoprotein metabolism that produces premature CVD. Half of the children of men who had CVD before age 50 had 1 of 7 dyslipidemic profiles: elevated LDL-C alone (type IIa) or combined with high triglycerides (TG; type IIb); elevated TG alone (type IV); low HDL-C alone (hypoalpha); and type IIa, type IIb, or type IV also accompanied by low HDL-C. Elevated levels of apolipoprotein B (apoB), in the presence of normal LDL-C (hyperapobetalipoproteinemia or hyperapoB), were prevalent in young offspring of adults with premature CVD and hyperapoB. The levels of apoB and apolipoprotein A-I (apoA-I), the major apolipoproteins of LDL and HDL, respectively, and the ratio of apoB to apoA-I in young offspring were stronger predictors of premature coronary artery disease (CAD) in their parents than LDL-C and HDL-C levels.

Examples of inherited lipoprotein disorders that often present in youth at high risk of future CVD include familial hypercholesterolemia (FH; which is caused by a defect in the LDL receptor, LDLR), familial combined hyperlipidemia (FCHL) and its metabolic cousin hyperapoB, the prototypes for hepatic overproduction of VLDL, which is often accompanied by insulin resistance and the dyslipidemic triad of hyper-TG, increased small, dense LDL particles (LDL-P), and low HDL-C (see below).

## LIPOPROTEIN CLASSIFICATION AND PROPERTIES

Plasma lipoproteins are spherical particles consisting of a core of nonpolar lipids—TG and cholesteryl ester—surrounded by a surface coating consisting of proteins (apolipoproteins) and more polar lipids, phospholipids, and unesterified (free) cholesterol. Plasma lipoproteins are classified by their density and electrophoretic mobility into 4 major groups: chylomicrons, VLDL, LDL, and HDL (Table 161-1). After electrophoresis, chylomicrons remain at the origin, and VLDL, LDL, and HDL migrate in the same positions as pre-β-, β-, and α-globulins, respectively. The hydrated density of the lipoproteins is related to their chemical composition and the relative content of lipid and apolipoprotein. Chylomicrons are 99% lipid, most of it being TG (see Table 161-1). After plasma has stood overnight, these large particles (80–500 nm) will rise to the top, where they appear as a creamy layer. VLDL is about 90% lipid, the majority of it being TG, with lesser amounts of cholesterol. When present in plasma in increased amounts, VLDL are large enough (30–80 nm) to create a cloudy or turbid appearance to plasma. LDL are the major carriers of cholesterol in plasma, and about 50% of their weight is cholesteryl ester and cholesterol. HDL comprise about equal amounts of apolipoprotein and lipid, principally phospholipids and cholesterol.

### Apolipoproteins

Lipoproteins are associated with several apolipoproteins (Table 161-2). Nomenclature for the apolipoproteins follows an alphabetical scheme. The characteristics of the 10 major apolipoproteins and their functions are summarized in Table 161-2.

## ORIGIN AND FATE OF PLASMA LIPIDS AND LIPOPROTEINS

The transport of plasma lipids by lipoproteins may be divided into exogenous (dietary) and endogenous systems (Fig. 161-1).

### Exogenous Lipid Transport

Most dietary lipid is in the form of neutral fat or TG (75–150 g/d). The amount of cholesterol in the diet is typically about 300 mg/d but varies from 100 to 600 mg/d. In addition to dietary cholesterol, about 1100 mg of biliary cholesterol is secreted each day from the liver into the intestine (see Fig. 161-1). In the small intestine, lipids are emulsified by bile salts and hydrolyzed by pancreatic lipases. The bile acids are then reabsorbed by the intestinal bile acid transporter (IBAT) for return to the liver through the enterohepatic pathway (see Fig. 161-1). TG is broken down into fatty acids and 2-monoglycerides; cholesteryl ester is hydrolyzed into fatty acids and unesterified cholesterol. These components are then absorbed by the intestinal cells. The absorption of cholesterol occurs in the jejunum, through the high-affinity uptake of dietary and biliary cholesterol by the Niemann-Pick C-1L-1 (NPC1L1) protein (see Fig. 161-1). Normally, about half the dietary and biliary cholesterol is absorbed daily. Excessive cholesterol absorption is prevented by the ABCG5/ABCG8 transporters, which act together to pump excess cholesterol and plant sterols from the intestine back into the lumen for excretion into the stool (see Fig. 161-1). Lack of 1 of these transporters causes sitosterolemia (also known as phytosterolemia, Mendelian Inheritance in Man [MIM] No. 210250).

In intestinal cells, monoglycerides are reesterified into TG, and cholesterol is esterified by acyl cholesterol acyltransferase (ACAT).

**TABLE 161-2 CLASSIFICATION AND PROPERTIES OF MAJOR HUMAN PLASMA APOLIPOPROTEINS**

| Apolipoprotein | Molecular Weight | Chromosomal Location | Function |
|---|---|---|---|
| ApoA-I | 29,016 | 11 | Cofactor LCAT |
| ApoA-II | 17,414 | 1 | Inhibits HL and VLDL hydrolysis |
| ApoA-IV | 44,465 | 11 | Activates LCAT |
| ApoB-100 | 512,723 | 2 | Secretion of triglyceride from liver; binding ligand to LDL receptor |
| ApoB-48 | 240,800 | 2 | Secretion of triglyceride from intestine |
| ApoC-I | 6630 | 19 | Inhibits apoE |
| ApoC-II | 8900 | 19 | Cofactor LDL |
| ApoC-III 0–2 | 8800 | 11 | Inhibits apoC-II activation of LPL |
| ApoD | 19,000 | 3 | Reverse cholesterol transport |
| ApoE | 34,145 | 19 | Facilitates uptake of chylomicron and IDL |

HL, hepatic lipase; IDL, intermediate-density lipoprotein; LCAT, lecithin cholesteryl acyltransferase; LDL, low-density lipoprotein; LPL, lipoprotein lipase; VLDL, very-low-density lipoprotein.

**TABLE 161-1 CLASSIFICATION AND PROPERTIES OF THE MAJOR HUMAN PLASMA LIPOPROTEINS**

| | Chylomicrons | Very-Low-Density (Pre-β) Lipoprotein | Low-Density (β) Lipoprotein | High-Density (α) Lipoproteins |
|---|---|---|---|---|
| Hydrated density ranges (g/mL) | < 0.95 | 0.95–1.006 | 1.019–1.063 | 1.063–1.21 |
| Electrophoretic migration | Origin | Pre-β | β | α |
| Average composition (%) | | | | |
| Cholesterol[a] | 3 | 22 | 50 | 20 |
| Triglyceride | 90 | 55 | 5 | 5 |
| Phospholipid | 6 | 15 | 25 | 25 |
| Protein | 1 | 8 | 20 | 50 |
| Major apoproteins | ApoB-48 | ApoB-100 | ApoB-100 | ApoA-I, II |
| | ApoC-I, II, III | ApoC-I, II, III | | ApoC-I, II, III |
| | ApoC-I, II, IV, apoE | ApoE | | ApoE |
| Origin | Intestine | Liver, intestine | Metabolic product of VLDL catabolism | Liver, intestine |
| Function | Transport dietary triglycerides | Transport hepatic triglycerides | Provide cholesterol to cells | Reverse cholesterol transport |

[a]Includes the mass cholesterol ester and unesterified cholesterol.

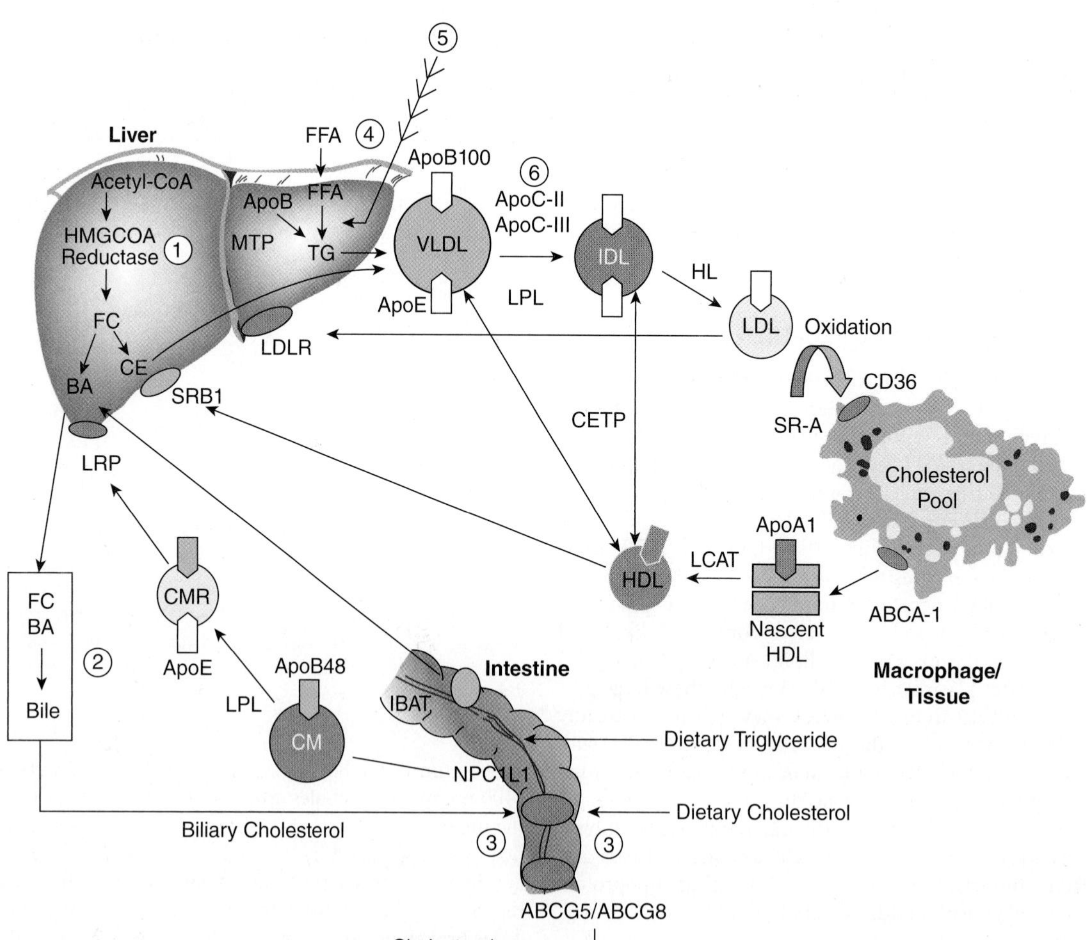


**FIGURE 161-1** Overview of lipoprotein metabolism. Three major pathways of plasma lipoprotein metabolism are shown: transport of dietary (exogenous) fat (left); transport of hepatic (endogenous) fat (center); and reverse cholesterol transport (bottom). A detailed description appears in the text. The sites of action of the 6 major lipid-altering drugs on exogenous and endogenous pathways of lipoprotein metabolism are (1) inhibition of hydroxymethylglutaryl (HMG)–coenzyme A (CoA) reductase by statins; (2) binding of bile acids by sequestrants, interfering with their reabsorption by the ileal bile acid transporter (IBAT); (3) binding of a cholesterol absorption inhibitor to the Niemann-Pick C1L1, decreasing the absorption of dietary and biliary cholesterol; (4) decreased mobilization of free fatty acids (FFA) by nicotinic acid, leading to decreased uptake of FFA by liver and reduced very-low-density lipoprotein (VLDL), intermediate-density lipoprotein (IDL), and low-density lipoprotein (LDL) production; (5) inhibition of triglyceride (TG) synthesis by omega-3 fatty acids; and (6) upregulation of lipoprotein lipase (LPL) and decreased production of apoC-III, an inhibitor of LPL, by a fibric acid derivative, leading to decreased VLDL-TG. The hepatic cholesterol pool is decreased by the agents at steps 1, 2, and 3, each leading to an upregulation of the LDLR.

Both lipids are packaged into chylomicrons, along with apolipoproteins apoA-I, apoA-II, apoA-IV, and apoB-48 (the intestine-specific short form of apoB generated by RNA editing of the apoB mRNA). Chylomicrons are secreted into the thoracic duct; from there, they enter the peripheral circulation, where they acquire apoC-II and apoE from HDL. Chylomicrons are too large to cross the endothelial barrier, and apoC-II, a cofactor for lipoprotein lipase (LPL), facilitates the hydrolysis of TG near the endothelial lining of blood vessels. The fatty acids that are released are taken up by muscle cells for energy utilization or by adipose cells for re-esterification into TG. As a result, a chylomicron remnant is produced that is enriched in cholesteryl ester and apoE. This remnant is rapidly taken up by the liver by receptor-mediated endocytosis of remnants through the interaction of apoE with the chylomicron remnant receptor (LRP) or the LDLR on the surface of parenchymal cells (see Fig. 161-1).

The uptake of dietary and biliary cholesterol is part of a process that reduces the pool of hepatic cholesterol by downregulating the LDLR and by inhibiting the rate-limiting enzyme of cholesterol biosynthesis, hydroxymethylglutaryl (HMG)–coenzyme A (CoA) reductase (see also below).

#### Endogenous Lipid Transport

In the fasting state, most TG in plasma is transported by VLDL. TG is synthesized in the liver, packaged into VLDL with other lipids and apolipoproteins (see Table 161-1)—primarily apoB-100, apoE, apoC-I, apoC-II, and apoC-III—and secreted into plasma. VLDL TG is subsequently hydrolyzed by LPL and its cofactor apoC-II to produce VLDL remnants and then intermediate-density lipoproteins (IDLs; density, 1.006–1.019 g/mL). TG can be transferred from VLDL and IDL to HDL and LDL in exchange for cholesteryl ester by the cholesterol ester transfer protein (CETP) (see Fig. 161-1). Compared with VLDL, IDLs are relatively enriched in cholesteryl ester and depleted in TG. Some IDLs are taken up directly by the liver, but others are hydrolyzed by hepatic lipase (HL) to produce LDL, the final end product of VLDL metabolism (see Fig. 161-1).

The apoB-100 (the full-length protein synthesized in the liver) component of the cholesteryl ester–rich LDL is recognized and bound by the high-affinity LDLR either in the liver or in extrahepatic cells (see Fig. 161-1). The bound LDLs are internalized by absorptive endocytosis. In lysosomes, apoB-100 is broken down into amino acids, cholesteryl esters are hydrolyzed, and unesterified cholesterol is released. Cholesterol mediates the proteolytic release of a transcription factor, the sterol regulatory element binding protein (SREBP), from the endoplasmic reticulum (ER). This effect occurs through the SREBP cleavage-activating protein (SCAP), which is both a sensor of sterols and a binding partner of SREBP. For example, when hepatocytes are depleted of cholesterol, SCAP transports SREBP from the ER to the Golgi, where 2 proteases—site-1 protease and site-2 protease—act in sequence to release the NH2-terminal of SREBP from the membrane. The NH2-terminal of SREBP containing the bHLH-zip domain of SREBP enters the nucleus and binds to a sterol response element (SRE) in the promoter area of the LDLR and HMG-CoA reductase genes, increasing their transcription. As the cholesterol content of the hepatocyte increases, the SREBP/SCAP complex is not incorporated into the ER, SREBP cannot reach the Golgi, the NH2-terminal domain of SREBP cannot be released from the membrane for transport into the nucleus, and the transcription of the LDLR and HMG-CoA reductase genes decreases.

This pathway has important clinical implications. For example, excess dietary and biliary cholesterol leads to the downregulation of the LDLR and HMG-CoA reductase and an increase in LDL-C. Dietary saturated fat content has an even more profound effect on LDL-C than dietary cholesterol. When cholesterol is reesterified by ACAT, SCAP senses a decrease in hepatic cholesterol, leading to the upregulation of the LDLR and HMG-CoA reductase genes by SREBP, promoting both synthesis and uptake of cholesterol. However, the preferred substrate for ACAT is oleic acid. Thus, excess saturated fatty acids decrease ACAT activity and thereby increase unesterified cholesterol, which inhibits the proteolysis and release of SREBP and thereby downregulates the LDLR and HMG-CoA reductase genes, followed by an increase in LDL-C. Decreasing dietary cholesterol and saturated fatty acids or decreasing the hepatic cholesterol content with drugs, such as cholesterol absorption inhibitors (CAIs) and the bile acid sequestrants (BAS) (see Fig. 161-1), leads to an upregulation of LDLR and HMG-CoA reductase genes and lower LDL-C. Inhibitors of HMG-CoA reductase (the statins) also reduce the liver's cholesterol content, leading to an upregulation of LDLR and import of cholesterol from the plasma, but without the concomitant increase in HMG-CoA reductase activity (see Fig. 161-1).

When plasma LDL-C exceeds 100 mg/dL, the capacity to process LDL through the LDLR pathway is exceeded. Increased numbers of LDL particles cross the endothelial barrier; LDLs are trapped in the vascular wall by proteoglycans and are then modified by either oxidation or glycation. Such modified LDL binds to the scavenger receptors CD36 and SRA (see Fig. 161-1) and enters cells such as macrophages by a low-affinity, LDLR-independent mechanism. This alternate pathway is not subject to feedback inhibition of LDLR synthesis by LDL-derived cholesterol. Thus, LDL continues to be taken up in an unregulated fashion, leading to excess deposition of cholesterol and cholesteryl ester in macrophages (see Fig. 161-1). Dyslipidemias that favor an increased uptake of LDL through the scavenger pathway promote the production of foam cells and the associated atherosclerosis and xanthomas.

#### Reverse Cholesterol Transport

HDLs are synthesized as nascent particles primarily in the liver but also in the intestine. After entering plasma, HDL participates in 2 important reactions. In the process of lipolysis by LPL, apoA-I is transferred from chylomicrons to HDL; in exchange, apoC-II and apoE on HDL are transferred to the TG-rich lipoproteins. ApoA-I is a cofactor for the enzyme lecithin cholesterol acyltransferase (LCAT; see Tables 161-1 and 161-2). Unesterified cholesterol is removed from peripheral cells through the ATP-binding cassette (ABC) protein ABCA1 and esterified through the action of LCAT and apoA-I (see Fig. 161-1). These cholesteryl esters are then transferred from HDL to the apoB-containing lipoproteins by CETP, from which they are taken up by LDLR and LRP (see Fig. 161-1). Cholesteryl ester may also be delivered directly to the liver through an HDL receptor (SRB1). These reactions reflect a process called reverse cholesterol transport and may explain the protective effect that HDL and apoA-I have against the development of atherosclerosis. Conversely, factors that impede this process appear to promote atherosclerosis.

## SCREENING FOR DYSLIPIDEMIA IN YOUTH

Two major approaches have been considered to detect dyslipidemia in youth, namely screening in the general population or in a selected population. The extensive literature related to these 2 screening approaches has been reviewed in detail in 2 publications from 2016 cited below.

Traditionally, screening for dyslipidemias in high-risk children was recommended, because they have multiple CVD risk factors or a family history of premature CVD and/or hypercholesterolemia. LDL-C has been the main focus of diagnosis and treatment. Less attention has been paid to HDL-C and TG. Now, with obesity and the metabolic syndrome evident in children, the focus of screening will likely include other factors such as obesity, low HDL-C, non-HDL-C (TC minus HDL-C), elevated TG, elevated apoB (reflecting increased small dense LDL-P), glucose intolerance and insulin resistance, and higher blood pressure levels.

#### Who to Screen

**Selective Screening** In 1992, the National Cholesterol Education Program (NCEP) Expert Panel on Blood Cholesterol Levels in Children and Adolescents recommended that selective, not general, screening be performed, as follows:

1. A lipoprotein profile in youth whose parents and/or grandparents required coronary artery bypass surgery or balloon angioplasty prior to age 55 years.
2. A lipoprotein profile in those with a family history of myocardial infarction, angina pectoris, peripheral or cerebral vascular disease, or sudden death prior to age 55.
3. A TC in those whose parents have high TC levels (> 240 mg/dL).
4. A lipoprotein profile if the parental/grandparental family history is not known, and the patient has 2 or more other risk factors for CAD, including obesity (body mass index [BMI] > 30), hypertension, cigarette smoking, low HDL-C, physical inactivity, and diabetes mellitus.

**Universal Screening** Universal lipid screening of all children has been controversial. Some of the arguments in favor of universal screening propose that recommendations based on family history of CVD or hypercholesterolemia will fail to detect substantial numbers of children who have elevated lipid levels. Universal screening might be performed to detect those with undiagnosed heterozygous FH or more marked FCHL; these patients will require more intensive treatment, including possible drug therapy. Identifying children and adolescents affected with hypercholesterolemia through universal screening may bring to attention their adult relatives who will have greater coronary mortality than relatives of children with normal cholesterol levels. If universal lipid screening is combined with an assessment of obesity and high blood pressure, it can also lead to detecting additional relatives from families at high risk for CVD.

It is clear that CVD risk factors cluster in childhood and persist into adulthood. While it is known that offspring of parents with CVD generally have higher LDL and TG and lower HDL-C in childhood and in young adulthood, the majority of children with dyslipidemia and multiple risk factors will be missed by selective screening.

Ideally, each child and adolescent should have an assessment of their plasma lipids and lipoproteins. But what are some of the concerns about universal lipid screening in childhood? Using TC in childhood to predict TC or LDL-C in young adults that is sufficiently high to warrant treatment is often associated with less-than-optimal sensitivity, specificity, and predictive power of a positive test. Several longitudinal studies have found that when the 75th percentile for TC in young children is used as a screening cut point, about half the individuals who will require treatment as adults are identified by universal lipid screening. However, in 1 report, the sensitivity was much lower when screening occurred during adolescence, presumably reflecting the temporary shift of LDL-C to lower values during this period of rapid growth and development.

#### What to Measure

For selective screening, a lipoprotein profile after an overnight fast is measured for children who have a positive family history of premature CVD or dyslipidemia, obesity, or multiple CVD risk factors and for those suspected of having secondary dyslipidemia. Such a

**TABLE 161-3 ACCEPTABLE, BORDERLINE, AND HIGH PLASMA LIPID, LIPOPROTEIN, AND APOLIPOPROTEIN CONCENTRATIONS (MG/DL) FOR CHILDREN AND ADOLESCENTS[a]**

| Category | Acceptable | Borderline | High[b] |
|---|---|---|---|
| Total cholesterol | < 170 | 170–199 | ≥ 200 |
| LDL cholesterol | < 110 | 110–129 | ≥ 130 |
| Non-HDL cholesterol | < 123 | 123–143 | ≥ 144 |
| Apolipoprotein B | < 90 | 90–109 | ≥ 110 |
| Triglycerides | | | |
| 0–9 years | < 75 | 75–99 | ≥ 100 |
| 10–19 years | < 90 | 90–129 | ≥ 130 |
| **Category** | **Acceptable** | **Borderline** | **Low[b]** |
| HDL cholesterol | > 45 | 35–45 | < 35 |
| Apolipoprotein A-I | > 120 | 110–120 | < 110 |

[a]Values for plasma lipid and lipoprotein levels are from the National Cholesterol Education Program (NCEP) Expert Panel on Cholesterol Levels in Children. Values for plasma apolipoprotein B and A-I are from the National Health and Nutrition Examination Survey III (NHANES III).

[b]The cut points for a high or low value represent approximately the 95th and 5th percentiles, respectively.



profile includes TC, TG, LDL-C, HDL-C, and non–HDL-C. Levels of lipoproteins are typically measured and expressed in terms of their cholesterol content. LDL-C is calculated from the Friedewald equation: LDL-C = TC − HDL-C − (TG/5). Total TG in the fasting state divided by 5 is used to estimate the levels of VLDL-C. If the TG is > 400 mg/dL, this formula cannot be used, and a direct LDL-C should be measured. If the patient is nonfasting, TC HDL-C and non–HDL-C levels can be measured.

ApoB and apoA-I might also be determined, using well-standardized immunochemical methods. Such measurements might provide additional useful information, particularly in children whose parents have premature CAD. Age-, sex-, and race-specific cut points for apoB and apoA-I, empirically derived from the National Health and Nutrition Education Survey (NHANES) sample, are available and provide cut points that might be used to define elevated apoB and low apoA-I (Table 161-3). ApoB provides an assessment of the total number of apoB-containing lipoprotein particles.

#### Non–HDL-C

Non–HDL-C is determined by subtracting HDL-C from TC and can be measured in plasma from nonfasting patients. Non-HDL-C reflects the amount of cholesterol carried by the "atherogenic" apoB-containing lipoproteins (VLDL, IDL, LDL, and Lp[a]). In adults, non–HDL-C appears to be a better independent predictor of CVD than LDL-C. In children, non–HDL-C is at least as good a predictor as LDL of future dyslipidemia in adulthood. Percentiles for non–HDL-C in children are available from the Bogalusa study (see Table 161-3).

#### Summary

For universal screening, the simplest approach is measuring TC, HDL-C, and non-HDL in nonfasting patients. However, treatment algorithms in pediatrics are usually focused on fasting LDL-C. Hyper-TG is usually assessed as part of the dyslipidemic triad and is often elevated in obesity and the metabolic syndrome. Thus, in an ideal screening program, TC, TG, LDL-C, HDL-C, and non–HDL-C would be assessed by performing a lipoprotein profile in the fasting state. With regard to recommendations for universal and selective screening, the US Preventive Services Task Force (USPSTF) released recommendations on lipid screening in children and adolescents in 2016, updating the 2007 recommendations. The 2016 recommendation statement was accompanied by 2 companion evidence reports on screening for detection of FH and multifactorial dyslipidemia (cited in Suggested Readings). The conclusion of the task force was unchanged from 2007: "The current evidence is insufficient to assess the balance of benefits and harms of screening for lipid disorders in children and adolescents younger than 20 years." This reflects the continued uncertainty concerning preventative screening. Nonetheless, in 2011, the National Heart, Lung, and Blood Institute Expert Panel on Integrated Guidelines for Cardiovascular Health and Risk Reduction in Children and Adolescents (https://www.nhlbi.nih.gov/health-pro/guidelines/current/cardiovascular-health-pediatric-guidelines/summary#chap9) recommended universal and selective screening for all children and those at increased risk, and these guidelines are endorsed by the American Academy of Pediatrics (AAP) and the American Heart Association (AHA).

#### When to Sample for Dyslipidemia

Human plasma cholesterol levels are lowest during intrauterine life. At birth, the mean (1 standard deviation [SD]) plasma levels (mg/dL) are TC 74, LDL-C 31, HDL-C 37, and TG 37. TC and LDL-C increase rapidly in the first weeks of life. The lipids and lipoproteins continue to increase gradually until 2 years of age, during which time the kind and source of the milk in the infant's diet can markedly influence these levels. Therefore, screening for dyslipidemia is not generally recommended before 2 years of age. After 2 years of age, the levels of the lipids and lipoproteins become quite constant up to adolescence.

Ten years of age has been proposed as a good time to obtain a lipoprotein profile. Children this age are able to fast easier, the values are predictive of future adult lipoprotein profiles, and adolescence has not yet altered their lipid profile. Since TC and LDL-C may fall 10% to 20% (or more) during adolescence, it is preferable to screen children at risk for familial dyslipidemias before adolescence, between ages 2 and 10. Even in FH heterozygotes, there is a significant fall in lipid levels in adolescence. If sampling occurs during adolescence and the results are abnormal, then they are likely to be even higher after adolescence. If the results during adolescence are normal, then sampling will need to be repeated toward the end of adolescence (for girls, age 16 and, for boys, age 18).

The complete phenotypic expression of some disorders, such as FCHL, can be delayed until adulthood, so the continued evaluation of such subjects from high-risk families with FCHL should occur well into adulthood. However, elevated apoB is the first expression of FCHL in adolescents and young adults. Age-related factors, such as increased BMI and lifestyle changes, contribute to the degree of dyslipidemia in such youth.

## DEFINITION OF DYSLIPIDEMIA

Cut points to define elevated TC, LDL-C, apoB, non–HDL-C, and TG and low HDL-C and apoA-I in children and adolescents are found in Table 161-3. Dyslipidemia is present if 1 or more of these lipid, lipoprotein, or apolipoprotein factors are abnormal. As noted earlier, in offspring of men who had CVD before 50 years of age, 7 different dyslipidemic profiles were present. Such results emphasize the importance of evaluating a lipoprotein profile in the fasting state.

#### Primary Versus Secondary Dyslipoproteinemia

Before considering a dyslipoproteinemia to be a primary disorder, secondary causes must be excluded (Table 161-4). Each child with dyslipidemia should have routine blood tests to help rule out secondary causes of the disease. These include fasting blood sugar and tests of kidney, liver, and thyroid function. In secondary dyslipidemia, the associated disorder producing the dyslipidemia should be treated first in an attempt to normalize lipoprotein levels; however, if the dyslipidemia persists—for example, as it often does in type 1 diabetes and the nephrotic syndrome—the patient will require dietary treatment and, if indicated, drug therapy using the same guidelines as in primary dyslipidemias.

## GUIDELINES FOR TREATING DYSLIPIDEMIA IN CHILDREN AND ADOLESCENTS

General guidelines for the dietary and pharmacologic treatment of primary and secondary dyslipidemias in youth are presented here. Specific guidelines germane to each inherited disorder of dyslipidemia are provided as necessary in subsequent sections of this chapter.

| TABLE 161-4 | CAUSES OF SECONDARY DYSLIPIDEMIA IN CHILDREN AND ADOLESCENTS |
|---|---|
| **Exogenous** | |
| Alcohol | |
| Oral contraceptives | |
| Prednisone | |
| Anabolic steroids | |
| 13-*cis*-Retinoic acid | |
| **Endocrine and Metabolic** | |
| Acute intermittent porphyria | |
| Type 1 and type 2 diabetes | |
| Hypopituitarism | |
| Hypothyroidism | |
| Lipodystrophy | |
| Pregnancy | |
| **Renal** | |
| Chronic renal failure | |
| Hemolytic-uremic syndrome | |
| Nephrotic syndrome | |
| **Hepatic** | |
| Benign recurrent intrahepatic cholestasis | |
| Congenital biliary atresia | |
| Alagille syndrome | |
| **Storage Diseases** | |
| Cystinosis | |
| Gaucher disease | |
| Glycogen storage disease | |
| Juvenile Tay-Sachs disease | |
| Niemann-Pick disease | |
| Tay-Sachs disease | |
| **Acute and Transient** | |
| Burns | |
| Hepatitis | |
| **Others** | |
| Anorexia nervosa | |
| Cancer survivor | |
| Heart transplantation | |
| Idiopathic hypercalcemia | |
| Kawasaki disease | |
| Klinefelter syndrome | |
| Progeria (Hutchinson-Gilford syndrome) | |
| Rheumatoid arthritis | |
| Systemic lupus erythematosus | |
| Werner syndrome | |

### Dietary Therapy

The first form of therapy for children with dyslipidemia is a diet containing decreased amounts of total fat, saturated fat, cholesterol, and simple sugars, but containing increased complex carbohydrates. No decrease in total protein is recommended. Calories are sufficient to maintain normal growth and development. The NCEP pediatric panel recommended diet treatment after 2 years of age. Recent data from randomized clinical trials in general populations, such as STRIP, indicate that a diet low in total fat, saturated fat, and cholesterol may be instituted safely and effectively under medical supervision at 6 months of age.

**When to Initiate Treatment with Diet** If the first lipoprotein profile indicates that TC, LDL-C, non–HDL-C, or TG is elevated, or if the HDL-C is low (see Table 161-3), then another confirmatory profile is obtained at least 3 weeks later. If dyslipidemia persists, secondary causes (see Table 161-4) are ruled out and dietary treatment begun. A fat-restricted diet, previously termed the Step-One diet and now referred to as Cardiovascular Health Integrated Lifestyle Diet (CHILD 1), is usually started and the lipoprotein profile repeated in 6 to 8 weeks. If the dyslipidemia persists, then a more restrictive diet, previously termed the Step-Two diet and now referred to as CHILD 2, is initiated. Both diets require dietary counseling and physician monitoring. The CHILD 1 diet calls for less than 10% of total calories from saturated fatty acids, no more than 30% of calories from total fat, and less than 300 mg/d of cholesterol. The CHILD 1 diet is evaluated for at least 3 months before prescribing the CHILD 2 diet. The CHILD 2 diet entails further reduction of the saturated fatty acid intake to less than 7% of calories and reduced cholesterol intake to less than 200 mg/d.



**Safety and Efficacy of Dietary Therapy in Infants, Children, and Adolescents** The efficacy and safety of diets to treat dyslipidemia in youth have been demonstrated across the age spectrum of pediatric patients—for example, from age 7 months to 7 years and from age 7 to age 11 in STRIP and from ages 8 to 10 throughout adolescence in the Dietary Intervention Study in Children (DISC). In some studies, there were lower intakes of calcium, zinc, vitamin E, and phosphorus on low-fat diets. Therefore, although normal growth is maintained on low-fat diets, attention needs to be paid to ensure adequate intake of these key minerals and vitamins.

Owen and colleagues analyzed 37 publications on the effect of breastfeeding versus formula feeding on TC in adolescents and adults. While TC was higher in breastfed versus formula-fed infants, this did not persist in childhood and adolescence, where there was no relationship of TC to infant feeding. In adults, TC of breastfed infants was actually lower than TC of formula-fed infants. Hence, human milk remains the gold standard for infant feeding.

Using margarines (about 3 servings daily) high in either plant stanol esters or plant sterol esters can reduce LDL-C an additional 10% to 15% when added to a low-fat diet. Water-soluble fibers such as psyllium can lower LDL-C an additional 5% to 10%.

Consuming a soy protein beverage does not appear to lower LDL-C but does lower VLDL-C and TG and increases HDL-C. Compared with placebo, supplementing a low-fat diet with an omega-3 fatty acid (docosahexaenoic acid, 1.2 g/d) did not lower LDL-C but changed the distribution between the LDL subclasses with a significant 91% increase in the largest LDL subclass and a 48% decrease in the smallest LDL subclass 3. Garlic extract therapy does not lower LDL-C in hyperlipidemic children.

Overall, a diet low in fat for children with dyslipidemia appears both safe and effective. Medical and nutritional support is necessary to reinforce good dietary behaviors and to ensure nutritional adequacy.

**Effect of a Low-Fat Diet in Childhood on Future CVD in Adulthood** That a low-saturated-fat, low-cholesterol diet in childhood will prevent CVD in adulthood can only be inferred from epidemiological studies. Obesity already promotes insulin resistance in childhood. In that regard, a low-saturated-fat dietary counseling program starting in infancy in STRIP improved insulin sensitivity in 9-year-old healthy children. Further, in STRIP, a low-saturated-fat diet introduced in infancy and maintained during the first decade of life was associated with enhanced endothelial function in boys, but not in girls, and was mediated in part by the diet-induced reduction in TC. In the same Finnish study, at 10 years of age, 10% of the intervention girls were overweight compared with 19% of the control girls, but this significant difference was not seen in the boys. Most recent results from the same study cohort demonstrates a reduced rate of metabolic syndrome in adolescents and young adults exposed to early dietary intervention.

### Pharmacologic Therapy

There are 6 main classes of lipid-altering drugs (see Fig. 161-1): (1) inhibitors of HMG-CoA reductase (the statins), (2) BAS, (3) CAI, (4) niacin (nicotinic acid), (5) fish oils as omega-3 fatty acids (eicosapentaenoic acid and docosahexaenoic acid), and (6) fibric acid derivatives. More recently, biologicals have been developed that have a significant impact on LDL-C. A humanized monoclonal antibody that inhibits the LDLR modulator proprotein convertase subtilisin-kexin type 9 (PCSK9) has been shown, either as monotherapy or in conjunction with a statin, to significantly reduce LDL-C by on an average 60%, with attendant reduction in cardiovascular events. Other novel therapies include the apoB-100 antisense molecule mipomersen, and a microsomal triglyceride transfer protein (MTP) inhibitor lomitapide. ApoB antisense and MTP inhibitor therapies are currently approved for patients with homozygous familial hypercholesterolemia.

**Guidelines for Instituting Drug Therapy** The primary use of drugs in pediatrics is to lower significantly elevated LDL-C levels, primarily but not exclusively in those from families with premature CVD or significant dyslipidemia. Drug treatment to lower LDL-C is initiated when the post-dietary LDL-C is greater than 190 mg/dL and there is a negative or unobtainable family history of premature CVD. If the post-dietary LDL-C is greater than 160 mg/dL and there is a family history of premature CVD, 2 or more risk factors for CVD, or the metabolic syndrome is present, drug treatment is started after 10 years of age.

The statins and the BAS are the 2 main classes of pharmaceutical agents currently used in children over 10 years of age who have sufficiently elevated LDL-C. Ezetimibe, a CAI that blocks the absorption of cholesterol and plant sterols through the NPC1L1 protein (see Fig. 161-1), is also effective but is not yet approved by the US Food and Drug Administration (FDA) for use in children except in those rare children with homozygous FH or sitosterolemia (see below). The statins, BAS, and CAI act by reducing hepatic cholesterol, leading to release of SREBP from the cytoplasm into the nucleus, where SREBP binds to the SRE element of the LDLR gene promoter, increases the number of LDLR, and decreases LDL-C. Since SREBP also upregulates the gene for HMG-CoA reductase, the BAS and CAI are both associated with a compensatory increase in cholesterol biosynthesis, limiting their efficacy (see Fig. 161-1). Therefore, both classes of agents might effectively be used in conjunction with the statins, which reduce hepatic cholesterol by inhibiting HMG-CoA reductase and decreasing cholesterol biosynthesis.

Niacin is not routinely used in pediatrics, although some FH homozygotes respond well to it (55–87 mg/kg/d in divided doses) due to the significant reduction of VLDL production, leading to a decreased synthesis of LDL. Since aspirin is not used in children because of Reye syndrome, ibuprofen can be used if necessary to prevent flushing. The fibrates (48, 96, or 145 mg/d) are also not routinely used in pediatrics, except in the adolescent with a TG level of 500 mg/dL or higher who may be at increased risk of pancreatitis (see also below). Fish oils (1–2 g/d) may also be used to treat marked hyper-TG in children and adolescents by decreasing the biosynthesis of TG (see Fig. 161-1).

**Bile Acid Sequestrants** BAS are the only class of pharmacologic agents recommended by the NCEP for lipid-lowering therapy because of their extensive track record of safety over 3 decades. In fact, the sequestrants have never been approved by the FDA for use in children. These agents suffer from significant tolerability issues and provide only a modest LDL-C reduction of about 15%. A 16.9% decrease in LDL-C was reported when cholestyramine (8 g) was used to treat boys and girls with FH. However, Liacouras and others found that 52 of 63 children discontinued cholestyramine treatment after an average of 21.9 months because of gritty taste and gastrointestinal complaints. The second-generation sequestrant colesevelam (625-mg tablets) has a greater affinity for bile salts and therefore can be used in a lower total dose (3–6 tablets daily). In comparison with the first-generation BAS, colesevelam is associated with less annoying side effects such as constipation and gritty taste and does not interfere with the absorption of other drugs.

In randomized clinical trials, cholestyramine did not affect height velocity. Fat-soluble vitamins were maintained, except in 1 study, where the BAS group had significantly lower 25-hydroxyvitamin D levels than the placebo group. Low folate and high homocysteine levels have been reported.

**HMG-CoA Reductase Inhibitors (Statins)** The statins are widely used to lower TC and LDL-C in adults. Numerous randomized controlled trials have demonstrated the safety and efficacy of the statins in male and female adolescents with FH. A meta-analysis of 6 trials showed high efficacy for LDL-C and apoB lowering and no increase in side effects compared with placebo. Atorvastatin, lovastatin, pravastatin, and simvastatin are approved by the FDA for use in adolescents with FH. Starting doses are atorvastatin, 10 mg/d; lovastatin, 40 mg/d; pravastatin, 40 mg/d; and simvastatin, 20 mg/d. All are available generically.

Using carotid IMT as a surrogate marker for atherosclerosis, Wiegman and colleagues demonstrated that a 24% reduction in LDL-C in FH heterozygote children and adolescents (8–15 years of age) using pravastatin produced a significant decrease in carotid IMT, compared to those on placebos. A follow-up study of this Dutch cohort showed that younger age at statin initiation was an independent predictor of the treatment's effect on carotid IMT. Statin therapy also restores endothelial function in children with FH. Thus, early intervention with statins appears likely to reduce future atherosclerosis and CVD in those with FH.

The statins may also be useful in adolescents with FCHL and metabolic syndrome, whose LDL-C is greater than 160 mg/dL after diet and weight control and who have multiple risk factors or a family history of premature CVD. Even in young women with polycystic ovarian syndrome (PCOS; see also below), there is increased carotid IMT, again suggesting that greater attention be paid to managing dyslipidemia and other CVD risk factors early in life.

**Side Effects of the Statins in Children and Adolescents**

***LIVER AND MUSCLE*** Increases in liver enzymes up to 3× the upper limit of normal levels have been reported in several adolescents treated with higher doses of simvastatin (40 mg/d) and atorvastatin (20 mg/d). In a meta-analysis, the prevalence of elevated alanine aminotransferase in the statin group was 0.66% (3 per 454 patients). Instances of asymptomatic increases (> 10-fold) in creatine kinase (CK), while unusual, have been reported in adolescents receiving statin therapy. Such adolescents are monitored for elevations in hepatic transaminases and CK concentrations. Liver function tests are monitored at each clinic visit 2 to 3 times per year. CK is measured at baseline and is repeated if myalgias develop.

***SPECIAL ISSUES IN YOUNG FEMALES*** Adult women with FH and CVD may be more responsive to LDL-C-lowering therapy than similarly affected men, as assessed by regression of coronary plaques and tendon xanthomas. Statin therapy in adult women with CVD has an overall favorable safety profile, but fewer studies have been performed in adolescent girls. Nevertheless, there has been no adverse effect on growth and development or on adrenal and gonadal hormones.

Statins are contraindicated during pregnancy because of the potential risk to a developing fetus. Statins should be administered to adolescent girls only when they are highly unlikely to conceive. Birth control is mandatory for those who are sexually active. Because of the above concerns and the long-term commitment to therapy and because CAD often occurs after menopause, the use of statins to treat adolescent females has been debated.

Although treating adolescent patients with FH appears clearly indicated, especially in those with a strong family history of premature CAD, additional studies are needed to document the long-term safety of statin therapy and to determine its potential effects on the prevention of adult atherosclerosis and coronary events.

**Metabolic Syndrome Beyond Dyslipidemia** Statin therapy is recommended in patients whose LDL-C level is greater than 160 mg/dL. For most patients, however, LDL-C will be lower than 160 mg/dL, and a low-fat diet, exercise, and weight reduction are paramount. Metformin has been used in several studies of obese adolescents who have metabolic syndrome and hyperinsulinemia.

**Treatment of Dyslipidemia Secondary to Other Diseases**

**Type 1 Diabetes** Children with type 1 diabetes often have a dyslipidemia, the severity of which is related to diabetic control. The American Diabetes Association (ADA) recommends optimizing glucose control and dietary intervention as the first step in treating these children. However, if the LDL-C is greater than 160 mg/dL after such treatment, the ADA strongly recommends using statins. This recommendation is based on the high risk of CVD in affected adults and on the abnormal carotid IMT in children with type 1 diabetes.

**TABLE 161-5 LEVELS OF LIPIDS, LIPOPROTEINS, AND APOLIPOPROTEIN B IN CHILDREN WITH THE MOST COMMON LIPOPROTEIN ABNORMALITIES**

| | | Plasma Concentrations (mg/dL) | | | | | |
|---|---|---|---|---|---|---|---|
| **Lipoprotein Disorder** | **Age (Years)** | **TC** | **Triglycerides** | **HDL-C** | **LDL-C** | **ApoB** | **LDL-C/ApoB** |
| FH (n = 20) | 8.0 ± 4.7 | 323 ± 44 | 86 ± 36 | 44 ± 8 | 262 ± 45 | 219 ± 42 | 1.22 ± 0.22 |
| FCHL (n = 65) | 9.3 ± 4.7 | 220 ± 51 | 120 ± 91 | 45 ± 11 | 149 ± 48 | 153 ± 39 | 0.98 ± 0.19 |
| HyperapoB (n = 11) | 7.8 ± 4.6 | 200 ± 20 | 91 ± 35 | 52 ± 7 | 130 ± 16 | 138 ± 21 | 0.95 ± 0.10 |
| Normals (n = 110) | 8.7 ± 1.8 | 162 ± 31 | 70 ± 39 | 51 ± 10 | 97 ± 27 | 85 ± 20 | 1.15 ± 0.20 |

apoB, apolipoprotein B; FCHL, familial combined hyperlipidemia; FH, familial hypercholesterolemia; HDL-C, high-density lipoprotein cholesterol; LDL-C, low-density lipoprotein cholesterol. HyperapoB, hyperapobetalipoproteinemia; TC, total cholesterol;

**Nephrotic Syndrome** The dyslipidemia in children with nephrotic syndrome can be marked. LDL-C is close to that in FH heterozygotes (Table 161-5). TG can approach 300 mg/dL. Twenty percent of patients with nephrotic syndrome are unresponsive to steroids, and most of these cases can be attributed to focal segmental glomerulosclerosis. Such individuals with an LDL-C greater than 160 mg/dL may be at an increased risk for developing atherosclerosis and CVD and may warrant treatment with a statin.

## METABOLIC DISORDERS OF DYSLIPIDEMIA IN YOUTH

### DISORDERS AFFECTING LDL RECEPTOR ACTIVITY

There are 5 disorders expressed in pediatrics that result from mutations in the LDLR or from mutations in other genes that impact LDLR activity (Fig. 161-2). Elevated LDL-C can vary considerably in these 5 conditions (see also below), but each disorder causes early atherosclerosis and premature CVD. These 5 disorders include FH; familial defective apoB-100 (FDB); autosomal recessive hypercholesterolemia (ARH); sitosterolemia; and mutations in proprotein convertase subtilisin-like kexin type 9 (PCSK9). Each disorder warrants diet and drug therapy in childhood to decrease atherosclerosis and subsequent CVD.

### FAMILIAL HYPERCHOLESTEROLEMIA

#### FH Heterozygotes

FH (MIM No. 143890) is the prototype for the diagnosis and treatment of dyslipidemia in children. Heterozygous FH, an autosomal dominant disorder, presents at birth and early in life with a 2- to 3-fold elevation in TC and LDL-C (see Table 161-5). It is a codominant disorder in which half the children of an FH parent and a normal parent will have FH; in such families, the cut point for LDL-C that minimizes misclassification is 160 mg/dL. FH affects about 1 in 300 people and

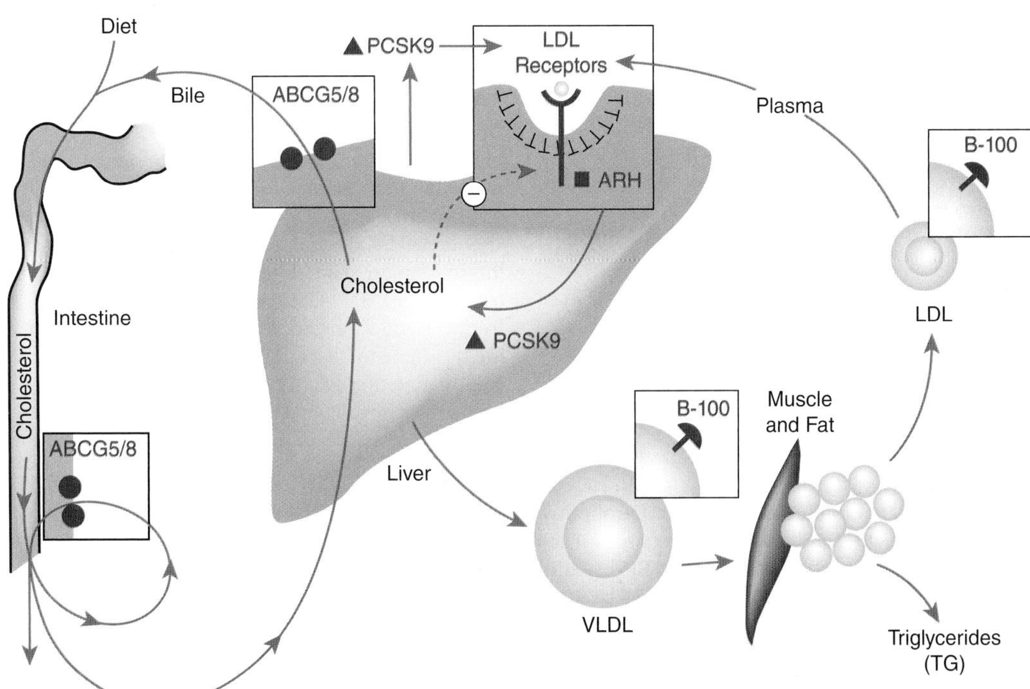


**FIGURE 161-2** Schema depicting 5 inherited disorders of lipoprotein metabolism that present in childhood with marked elevations of low-density lipoproteins (LDL), leading to premature atherosclerosis. Apolipoprotein B (apoB), the major apolipoprotein of very-low-density lipoproteins (VLDL) and LDL, is necessary for the secretion of VLDL and the uptake of its catabolic product, LDL, by the LDL receptor (LDLR). Defects in the structure of apoB (defective ApoB-100) or in the LDLR (familial hypercholesterolemia, FH) affect the normal binding, internalization, or recycling of the LDLR. Autosomal recessive hypercholesterolemia (ARH) results from a defect in the ARH protein that normally interacts with the cytoplasmic component of the LDLR, allowing the tyrosine phosphorylation and internalization of the LDLR. The proprotein convertase subtilisin-like kexin type 9 (PCSK9) is a serine protease that promotes the degradation of the LDL receptor. Gain-of-function mutations that increase PCSK9 activity decrease LDLR activity. Proposed mechanisms include targeting of the LDLR in the Golgi for degradation in the lysosome, interfering with the recycling of the LDLR after secreted PCSK9 binds to the LDLR at the cell surface, or directing the LDLR to the lysosome to be degraded. The molecular defects responsible for sitosterolemia are caused by mutations in 2 genes that encode the half-transporters, *ABCG5* and *ABCG8*, preventing their normal dual functions of limiting the absorption of cholesterol and plant sterols and promoting their excretion from liver into bile.

is due to 1 of more than 900 different mutations in the LDLR gene that can affect the normal synthesis, transport, LDL-binding ability, and clustering (in coated pits) of the LDLR (see Fig. 161-2). FH heterozygous children and adolescents manifest increased carotid IMT, decreased brachial endothelial reactivity, but rarely overt CAD. Less than 10% of FH adolescent heterozygotes develop tendon xanthomas. HDL-C is below average in FH children (see Table 161-5). In FH adults, about half of untreated male heterozygotes and 25% of untreated female heterozygotes will develop CVD by 50 years of age.

Treatment of FH heterozygotes includes a diet low in cholesterol and saturated fat that can be improved by supplements with plant stanol esters or plant sterol esters and water-soluble fiber. BAS are safe and moderately effective in FH heterozygotes, but compliance is an issue. The dose of BAS required to achieve an LDL-C below 160 mg/dL is related to the baseline LDL-C level and not to body weight; an adult dose is usually required. FH heterozygous children respond well to statins, which are well tolerated. However, adding a BAS or CAI (see also above) to a statin is often necessary to achieve LDL-C goals. Niacin is generally not used to treat FH heterozygous children, unless LDL-C is persistently elevated or unusual hyper-TG, low HDL-C, or elevated Lp(a) lipoprotein is present.

#### FH Homozygotes

About 1 in a million children inherit a mutant allele for FH from both parents, leading to a 4- to 8-fold elevated LDL-C that often leads to precocious atherosclerosis and death from CVD in the second decade. Atherosclerosis also often affects the aortic valve, leading to life-threatening supravalvular aortic stenosis. Virtually all FH homozygotes have planar xanthomas by the age of 5 years, notably in the webbing of fingers and toes and over the buttocks. The seminal studies of such FH homozygous children led to the discovery of the LDLR, which is absent or functionally deficient in such children.

FH homozygotes respond somewhat to high doses of potent statins and to niacin. Since FH homozygotes have markedly diminished, if any, LDLR activity, the statins and niacin both work by decreasing hepatic VLDL production, leading to decreased LDL production. A CAI also lowers LDL in FH homozygotes, especially in combination with a more potent statin. In the end, however, FH homozygotes will require LDL apheresis every 2 weeks to further lower LDL into a less atherogenic range. Newer interventions with PCSK9 inhibition or antisense molecules can have dramatic effects, but optimal therapies are still under investigation.

### FAMILIAL DEFECTIVE APOB-100

FDB (also known as autosomal dominant hypercholesterolemia type B; MIM No. 144010) results from mutations in the gene encoding apoB-100, resulting in an impaired ability of the apoB-100 ligand on LDL to bind to the LDLR; decreased clearance of LDL; and elevated LDL-C of mild, moderate, or marked degree (see Fig. 161-2). Heterozygotes for FDB are relatively common (eg, 1 per 1000 in Europeans). About 1 in 20 patients with FDB has tendon xanthomas, and the condition appears clinically similar to adult heterozygous FH patients. Some adult patients with FDB develop premature CAD, but FDB itself is not a common cause of premature CAD. Treatment of FDB is similar to that for heterozygous FH.

### AUTOSOMAL RECESSIVE HYPERCHOLESTEROLEMIA

Children with ARH (MIM No. 603813) are clinically similar to those with homozygous FH, although LDL-C is not usually as elevated (between 350 and 550 mg/dL). Both parents of an ARH child usually have a normal lipoprotein profile. The ARH protein, LDLR adaptor protein 1 (LDLRAP1) normally interacts with the cytoplasmic component of the LDLR and other cell surface–oriented molecules, allowing their tyrosine phosphorylation. The deficiency of the ARH protein prevents the normal internalization of the LDLR, leading to marked elevations of LDL-C (see Fig. 161-2). Patients with ARH manifest a dramatic response to statins alone or when combined with the CAI ezetimibe.

### SITOSTEROLEMIA

Sitosterolemia (MIM No. 210250, also known as phytosterolemia) is a rare autosomal recessive disorder expressed in childhood and characterized by markedly elevated (> 30-fold) plasma levels of plant sterols. This is due to hyperabsorption and inefficient excretion of plant sterols. TC and LDL-C can be normal, moderately elevated, or markedly elevated, depending on the dietary content of cholesterol and plant sterol. Sitosterolemia patients absorb a higher percentage of dietary cholesterol than normal, and they secrete less cholesterol into bile, which decreases LDLR activity and, in turn, increases LDL-C (see Fig. 161-2).

The diagnosis of sitosterolemia is considered and plant sterols measured in any child or adolescent who has xanthomas despite disproportionately low LDL-C. In addition, previously undiagnosed adults can mimic FH heterozygotes. Patients with sitosterolemia may develop aortic stenosis as do those with homozygous FH. CVD can present in the first or second decade of life but is usually delayed until early to middle adulthood.

The molecular defects responsible for sitosterolemia are caused by mutations in 2 genes that encode the half-transporters ABCG5 and ABCG8, which are located on chromosome 2p in a head-to-head orientation. ABCG5 and ABCG8 are expressed exclusively in human liver and intestine, the sites of the 2 metabolic abnormalities in sitosterolemia (see Fig. 161-2). The dual functions of ABCG5 and ABCG8 are to limit the absorption of cholesterol and plant sterols and to promote their excretion from liver into bile.

The dietary treatment of sitosterolemia is important, and both cholesterol and plant sterols must be markedly reduced by avoiding high-fat animal and plant products. Saturated fats are also restricted. Statins are less effective in this disorder, since the high sterol content in the liver reduces cholesterol production. BAS are quite effective, as is ezetimibe.

### MUTATIONS IN PROPROTEIN CONVERTASE SUBTILISIN-LIKE KEXIN TYPE 9 (PCSK9)

PCSK9 is a serine protease that facilitates the degradation of LDLR. Gain-of-function mutations that increase PCSK9 activity decrease LDLR activity, producing a phenotype similar to FH. Loss-of-function mutations that decrease PCSK9 activity increase LDLR activity, leading to a lifetime of low LDL-C and a markedly reduced incidence of CVD.

Secreted PCSK9 binds to the LDLR at the cell surface, leading to the internalization of an LDLR/PCSK9 complex in conjunction with ARH (see Fig. 161-2). PCSK9 may interfere with the recycling of LDLR from the endosome back to the cell surface, or it may direct LDLR to the lysosome to be degraded. Patients with hypercholesterolemia and gain-of-function PCSK9 mutations respond well to treatment similar to that used for FH heterozygotes.

## DISORDERS OF OVERPRODUCTION OF VLDL AND LDL

### FAMILIAL COMBINED HYPERLIPIDEMIA

FCHL is an autosomal dominant disorder with variable lipid phenotypic expression: elevated LDL-C level alone (type IIa); elevated LDL-C with hyper-TG (type IIb); or normal LDL-C with hyper-TG (type IV). The expression of FCHL can be delayed until adulthood, but it is not unusual to see FCHL children in families with premature CAD. Total apoB can also be elevated in normolipidemic adolescents and young adults with FCHL before the combined dyslipidemia expresses itself. The mean TC and LDL-C in children with FCHL is about 100 mg/dL lower than in those with FH, and TG is elevated (see Table 161-5). The ratio of LDL-C to apoB is low in FCHL, indicating the presence of small, dense LDL particles, in contrast to FH, where the LDL-C/apoB ratio is high, reflecting the underlying large LDL particles (see Table 161-5). In a pediatric lipid clinic population, FCHL is 3 times as prevalent as FH. Tendon xanthomas are not present in children or adults with FCHL. Adolescents with FCHL are at risk for developing glucose intolerance, insulin resistance, visceral obesity, hypertension, and CVD as adults.

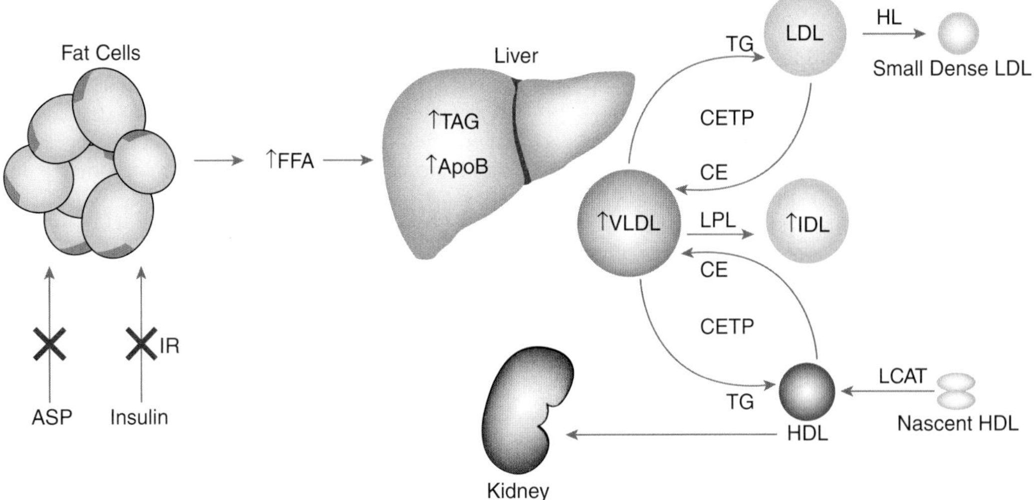


**FIGURE 161-3** Pathophysiology of the dyslipidemic triad. The dyslipidemic triad is often present in familial combined hyperlipidemia (FCHL), hyperapoB, and metabolic syndrome. In the dyslipidemic triad (high very-low-density lipoprotein [VLDL]-triglycerides [TG], increased numbers of small dense low-density lipoprotein particles [LDL-P], and decreased high-density-lipoprotein cholesterol [HDL-C]), increased flux of free fatty acids (FFA) from adipose tissue, often due to insulin resistance or defects in the action of the acylation stimulatory protein (ASP), enhances hepatic uptake of FFA, leading to increased production of TG, apolipoprotein B (apoB), and VLDL. The increased secretion of VLDL-TG promotes a greater exchange of TG (triglyceride) in VLDL for cholesteryl esters (CE) in LDL and HDL by cholesterol ester transfer protein (CETP). This results in CE-depleted but TG-enriched LDL and HDL. When TG in LDL and HDL is hydrolyzed by hepatic lipase (HL), smaller, denser LDL and HDL are produced. Such HDL is more likely to be excreted by the kidneys, resulting in low HDL-C levels.

#### Metabolic Basis of FCHL, HyperapoB, and Other Small Dense LDL Syndromes

The abnormal free fatty acid (FFA) metabolism in FCHL (MIM no. 144250) and other small dense LDL syndromes may reflect the primary defect in these patients (Fig. 161-3). Impaired insulin-mediated suppression of hormone-sensitive lipase in adipocytes leads to an elevation in FFA (Fig. 161-3). Elevated FFA may drive hepatic overproduction of TG and apoB, leading to a 2- to 3-fold increased production of VLDL and the dyslipidemic triad (Fig. 161-3). Insulin resistance also interferes with insulin-dependent normal upregulation of LPL, leading to decreased lipolysis of TG in VLDL and in intestinally derived TG-rich lipoproteins. This paradigm may also result from a cellular defect that prevents the normal effect of acylation stimulatory protein (ASP; Fig. 161-3), namely, stimulation of incorporating FFA into TG in the adipocyte. Insulin resistance may also occur in the liver, leading to an increase rather than a normal decrease in hepatic gluconeogenesis. Finally, FFA and glucose compete as oxidative fuel sources in muscle, such that increased concentrations of FFA inhibit glucose uptake and result in insulin resistance.

#### Genetic and Molecular Defects

This group of disorders is clearly genetically heterogeneous, and several genes (oligogenic effect) may influence the expression of increased small dense LDL, low HDL-C, FCHL, and the other small dense LDL syndromes. Pajukanta and coworkers provided strong evidence that the gene underlying the linkage of FCHL to chromosome 1q21–23 is the upstream transcription factor-1 (*USF-1*) gene, which regulates many important genes in lipid metabolism, including HL (see Fig. 161-3), and is linked to type 2 diabetes mellitus.

#### Metabolic Syndrome

Obesity is of critical importance in the development of metabolic syndrome. There is no current consensus regarding the definition of metabolic syndrome in youth; one proposal for children age 12 to 17 years was presented by Cook and colleagues in the third NHANES survey. An adolescent is considered to have metabolic syndrome if 3 or more of the following factors are present: (1) TG ≥ 110 mg/dL; (2) HDL-C ≤ 40 mg/dL; (3) waist circumference ≥ 90th percentile; (4) fasting glucose ≥ 110 mg/dL; and (5) blood pressure ≥ 90th percentile for age, sex, and height. One alternative to waist circumference may be a BMI greater than the 95th percentile for age and gender.

The prevalence of metabolic syndrome in adolescents increases with the severity of obesity and insulin resistance, as does the dyslipidemic triad, elevated highly sensitive C-reactive protein (hsCRP), and decreased adiponectin. Higher LDL-C levels and obesity and higher blood pressure levels in such adolescents increase carotid IMT as in adults. Of note, metabolic syndrome in childhood predicts adult metabolic syndrome and CVD 2 to 3 decades later. The finding of acanthosis nigricans is a sign of the underlying insulin resistance.

### TREATMENT OF DISORDERS OF VLDL OVERPRODUCTION

A diet reduced in total and saturated fat and simple sugars, regular aerobic exercise (1000 calories per week), and reaching an ideal body weight are critical factors for reducing VLDL and for improving insulin resistance. Two classes of drugs, fibric acids and niacin acid, lower TG and increase HDL-C in adults and may also convert small dense LDL to larger LDL. However, fibrates and niacin are not ordinarily used in pediatric patients. The statins are the most effective in lowering LDL-C and the total number of atherogenic, small dense LDL particles and are reserved for adolescents with FCHL or the metabolic syndrome who have an elevation of LDL-C greater than 160 mg/dL. Cholestyramine can be used to treat pediatric patients with FCHL with sufficiently elevated LDL-C.

#### Use of Metformin in Metabolic Syndrome

Metformin has been used to treat obese hyperinsulinemic adolescents with metabolic syndrome. Metformin can enhance insulin sensitivity and can reduce fasting blood glucose, insulin levels, plasma lipids, FFA, and leptin.

#### Polycystic Ovarian Syndrome

PCOS often presents in adolescence with menstrual disorders, acne, and hirsutism. Insulin resistance, considered an important underlying cause of PCOS, puts more adolescent girls at risk for PCOS and its complications, including dyslipidemia. After diet and weight control, the majority of endocrinologists use an estrogen/progesterone combination for treating PCOS, and almost 70% use metformin in obese teenagers with PCOS. Increased carotid IMT has been detected in young adults with PCOS, and earlier diagnosis and treatment of this disorder in adolescence may prevent its full-blown expression and CVD complications in adulthood.

## FAMILIAL METABOLIC DISORDERS OF TG-RICH LIPOPROTEINS

Metabolic disorders involving the TG-rich lipoproteins—chylomicrons, VLDL, and their remnants—are heterogeneous. Hypertriglyceridemia may result from increased synthesis or decreased catabolism of 1 or more of these lipoprotein classes or from a combination of enhanced synthesis and suppressed catabolism. Most hypertriglyceridemia in children and adolescents is due to VLDL overproduction, often accompanied by obesity or overweight and other components of metabolic syndrome (see above). The focus here is on inherited disorders of marked hypertriglyceridemia.

### DISORDERS OF MARKED HYPERTRIGLYCERIDEMIA

Most hypertriglyceridemia in children and adolescents is due to VLDL overproduction that results in 1 of the small dense syndromes (see above). There are a few rare disorders that are expressed as marked hypertriglyceridemia: LPL deficiency (MIM No. 238600); defects in apoC-II (MIM No. 207750), the cofactor for LPL; HL deficiency (MIM No. 614025), and GPIHBP1 deficiency (MIM No. 615947). Glycosylphosphatidylinositol-anchored high density lipoprotein-binding protein 1 (GPIHBP1) is a capillary endothelial cell surface protein that provides a platform for LPL-mediated processing of chylomicrons. Combined lipase deficiency (MIM No. 246650), due to mutations in lipase maturation factor 1 (*LMF1*), an ER chaperone protein required for proper maturation of lipases, is associated with loss of both LPL and HL activities. Mutations in *APOA5* (MIM No. 145750) cause type V hyperlipoproteinemia and are inherited in a codominant form. Finally, a transient infantile form of hypertriglyceridemia (MIM No. 614480) has been reported with biallelic mutations in glycerol-3-phosphate dehydrogenase 1 (GPD1).

Once triglyceride levels exceed 1000 mg/dL, pancreatitis is a major concern, and eruptive xanthomas, lipemia retinalis, and creamy blood can also be found. The diagnosis requires a determination of lipolytic activity in plasma after the intravenous injection of heparin (60 U/kg) or alternatively DNA-based testing. LPL deficiency presents at birth or in the first year of life, whereas the expression of the other 2 disorders is usually delayed until adulthood. HL deficiency is associated with premature CAD, whereas LPL and apoC-II defects are not.

Treatment of each of these disorders includes a very-low-fat diet (10–15% of calories) that can also benefit from supplementation with medium-chain triglycerides (MCTs). Portagen, a soybean-based formula enriched in MCT, is available for infants with LPL deficiency. Lipid-lowering drugs are ineffective in the LPL and apoC-II disorders. HL deficiency responds to treatment with statins and, to a lesser extent, fibrates. A gene therapy approach using adeno-associated virus (Glybera) was approved for use in LPL deficiency in the European Union; however, it was removed from the market do to limited interest and high cost.

### DYSBETALIPOPROTEINEMIA (TYPE III HYPERLIPOPROTEINEMIA)

Dysbetalipoproteinemia is a disorder that usually exhibits about equally elevated TC and TG levels (> 300 mg/dL). The more common recessive form (MIM No. 617347) has a delayed penetrance until adulthood and is due to the combination of an E2/E2 genotype in the *APOE* gene (these amino acid variants promote slower uptake of TG-rich lipoproteins by the LDLR) and overproduction of VLDL (see Fig. 161-3). The more rare dominant form of the disorder is expressed as dyslipidemia starting in adolescence. A low-fat diet and treatment with fibrates, niacin, or statins are very effective. Tendon, tuberous, and planar (especially in the palms) xanthomas; CVD; and glucose intolerance often occur in adulthood.

### INHERITED DISORDERS OF HDL METABOLISM

Usually low levels of HDL-C, associated with increased CVD, are secondary to VLDL overproduction (see above) and are expressed as a component of the dyslipidemic triad. There are, however, primary HDL disorders associated with low HDL-C levels and CVD termed familial HDL deficiency (MIM No. 604091) caused by apoA-I mutations, leading to hypoalphalipoproteinemia, or mutations in the *ABCA1* transporter that cause a secondary reduction in apoA1 levels. The rarer disorder Tangier disease (corneal clouding, orange tonsils, peripheral neuropathy) (MIM No. 205400) is a more severe allelic disorder due to mutations in *ABCA1*, a cholesterol efflux pump in the cellular lipid removal pathway. Low HDL-C is a feature of LCAT deficiency (Norum disease; MIM No. 245900), with clinical features of corneal opacities, target cell hemolytic anemia, and proteinuria with renal failure. A similar deficiency in HDL-C is seen in fish eye disease (MIM No. 136120), a loss of HDL LCAT activity. α-LCAT, deficient in fish eye disease, is specific for HDL, whereas β-LCAT, deficient in Norum disease, is specific for combined VLDL and LDL. The clinical and chemical characteristics of these disorders are summarized in Tables 161-6 and 161-7. Conversely, CETP transfers cholesterol

**TABLE 161-6 CLINICAL FINDINGS IN HYPOLIPOPROTEINEMIA DUE TO DEFICIENCIES IN HDL**

| Familial Disorders[a] | Neurologic | Gastrointestinal | Hematologic | Ophthalmologic | Cardiologic | Biopsy Findings | Other Findings |
|---|---|---|---|---|---|---|---|
| Tangier disease | Relapsing peripheral neuropathy | Moderate splenomegaly, mild hepatomegaly | Normal; stomatocytosis | Corneal infiltration (adults) | CAD | Foam cells in bone marrow, skin, small nerves, and rectum | Enlarged orange tonsils |
| LCAT deficiency | Usually absent (occasionally peripheral neuropathy; sensorineural hearing loss) | Normal | Normochromic anemia; platelet environment disorder | Diffuse corneal opacities (childhood); normal visual acuity; corneal arcus | Premature atherosclerosis (peripheral) | Foam cells in bone marrow and renal glomeruli; sea-blue histiocytes in spleen and bone marrow | Proteinuria with late renal insufficiency; genetic linkage with haptoglobin |
| Fish eye disease | Normal | Normal | Normal | Dense corneal opacities; reduced visual acuity | Atherosclerosis at old age | Not performed | |
| Apolipoprotein A-I and C-III deficiency | Normal | Normal | Normal | Corneal clouding; normal visual acuity | Premature CAD | Lipid-laden histiocytes in skin | Planar and tendon xanthomas |
| HDL deficiency with planar xanthomas | Normal | Hepatomegaly | Normal | Corneal opacity | Premature CAD | Foam cells in skin and rectal tumors | Planar xanthomas; xanthelasma |

[a]Clinical findings in hypoalphalipoproteinemia confined to premature CAD; patients with apolipoprotein A-I variants are clinically normal.

CAD, coronary artery disease; HDL, high-density lipoprotein; LCAT, lecithin cholesterol acyltransferase.

**TABLE 161-7 LABORATORY FINDINGS IN HYPOLIPOPROTEINEMIA DUE TO DEFICIENCIES IN HDL**

| | Plasma Lipids | | Plasma Lipoproteins | | | |
|---|---|---|---|---|---|---|
| Familial Disorder | Cholesterol (mg/dL) | Triglyceride (mg/dL) | VLDL | LDL | HDL | LCAT Activity |
| Hypoalphalipo-proteinemia | Normal | Normal | Normal | Normal | Low (< 5th percentile) | Normal |
| Apolipoprotein A-I variants ApoA Milano | Normal (184–231) | Elevated (181–319) | Normal | Normal or elevated; increased triglyceride content | Low (< 1st percentile); enlarged particles; ApoA-I-cysteine variant | Normal |
| Tangier disease | Low (38–112) | Normal or high (116–332) | Beta mobility on electrophoresis; ApoC apolipoproteins low | Low (< 10th percentile); increased triglyceride content | Barely detectable amounts of mutant HDL | Decreased (half-normal) |
| LCAT deficiency | Low, normal, or high (42–565) | Normal or high (105–900) | Beta mobility on electrophoresis | Low amounts of abnormal, large LDL | Low amounts of abnormal HDL | Marked decreased (0–10% of normal) |
| Fish eye disease | Normal | Elevated | Elevated | Normal level by increased triglyceride content; large particles | Low (< 5th percentile) | Partial decrease |
| Apolipoprotein A-I and C-III deficiency | Normal | Normal | Reduced; ApoC-III apolipoprotein absent | — | Trace amounts | Decreased (half-normal) |
| HDL deficiency with planar xanthomas | Normal | Normal or high | Elevated; broad beta band on electrophoresis; ApoC-III apolipoprotein increased | Normal level (increased triglyceride and ApoA-II content) | Trace amounts | Normal |

HDL, high-density lipoprotein; LCAT, lecithin cholesterol acyltransferase; LDL, low-density lipoprotein; VLDL, very-low-density lipoprotein.

from HDL particles to other lipoproteins, and the lipoprotein phenotype of CETP deficiency (MIM No. 143470) is characterized by both increased levels of HDL and decreased levels of LDL. It often presents as high HDL-C and may be associated with reduced risk of CVD. A low-fat diet is also indicated in children with inherited disorders of low HDL. Drugs, including niacin, are rarely used in such children.

## ELEVATED LEVELS OF LP(A) LIPOPROTEIN

Lp(a) lipoprotein is a very large lipoprotein ($M_r$ 3 × $10^6$) found in the density range of 1.050 to 1.080 g/mL. Its lipid composition is similar to LDL, but Lp(a) contains 2 proteins, apoB-100 and a large glycoprotein called apo(a). The latter is attached to apoB-100 through a disulfide bond. Apo(a) is homologous to plasminogen and has a variable number of repeats of the kringle 4 region, which are under genetic control. An inverse relationship exists between the size of apo(a) (based on the number of kringle repeats) and the levels of Lp(a). Lp(a) is measured by immunochemical methods. Elevated Lp(a) appears to be inherited and is often strongly associated with premature CVD in some families. Lp(a) levels should be measured in a child who has had a stroke. Niacin is the only lipid-altering drug that reduces Lp(a). It is not known if treatment of elevated Lp(a) will prevent future or recurrent CVD.

## DEFICIENCIES IN APOB-CONTAINING LIPOPROTEINS

The clinical and chemical findings associated with inherited disorders of deficiencies in apoB-containing lipoproteins—abetalipoproteinemia, heterozygous hypobetalipoproteinemia, homozygous hypobetalipoproteinemia (either null alleles in the apoB gene or compound heterozygotes for truncated apoB)—are summarized in Tables 161-8 and 161-9.

Abetalipoproteinemia (MIM No. 200100) is a rare autosomal recessive disorder characterized by hypocholesterolemia and malabsorption of fat-soluble vitamins leading to retinal degeneration, neuropathy, coagulopathy, and hepatic steatosis. The underlying pathology of both disorders is improper packaging and secretion of apoB-containing particles (see Table 161-8). The diagnosis is based on the demonstration of large intracellular fat particles in biopsy specimens of the jejunum, on the failure to form chylomicrons following a meal, and on the absence of apoB in plasma. Abetalipoproteinemia is not caused by a defect in the *APOB* gene. The defect in the synthesis and secretion of apoB is secondary to the absence of the MTP from the liver and intestine.

Hypobetalipoproteinemia can be secondary to anemia, dysproteinemias, hyperthyroidism, intestinal lymphangiectasia with malabsorption, myocardial infarction, severe infections, and trauma. Children or

**TABLE 161-8 CLINICAL FINDINGS IN HYPOLIPOPROTEINEMIA CAUSED BY DEFICIENCIES IN APOLIPOPROTEIN B (APOB)–CONTAINING LIPOPROTEINS**

| Familial Disorders | Neurologic | Gastrointestinal | Hematologic | Ophthalmologic | Cardiologic | Biopsy Findings | Other Findings |
|---|---|---|---|---|---|---|---|
| Abetalipoproteinemia | Cerebellar ataxia | Severe fat malabsorption | Acanthocytes | Atypical retinitis pigmentosa | Arrhythmias | Gross intracellular fat in jejunal cells | Myopathy (occasionally) depleted adipose mass |
| Heterozygous hypobetalipoproteinemia | Usually absent[a] | Minimal fat malabsorption | Acanthocytes (occasionally) | Usually absent[b] | None | None | — |
| Homozygous hypobetalipoproteinemia[c] | Ataxia | Severe fat malabsorption | Acanthocytes | Atypical retinitis pigmentosa | — | Gross intracellular fat in jejunal cells | — |
| Homozygous hypobetalipoproteinemia[d] | Usually absent | Minimal to mild fat malabsorption | Mild acanthocytes | Usually absent | None | None | — |

[a]Spinocerebellar degeneration and peripheral neuropathy have been described in some patients.

[b]Atypical retinitis pigmentosa has been reported in some patients.

[c]Homozygotes for "null alleles" in apoB gene.

[d]Usually compound heterozygotes for truncated apoB.

**TABLE 161-9 LABORATORY FINDINGS IN HYPOLIPOPROTEINEMIA DUE TO DEFICIENCIES IN APOLIPOPROTEIN B (APOB)–CONTAINING LIPOPROTEINS**

| | Plasma Lipids | | Plasma Lipoproteins | | | | |
|---|---|---|---|---|---|---|---|
| **Familial Disorder** | **Cholesterol (mg/dL)** | **Triglyceride (mg/dL)** | **Chylomicrons** | **VLDL** | **LDL** | **HDL** | **LCAT Activity** |
| Abetalipoproteinemia | Low (35–70) | Very low (1–10) | Absent | Absent | Absent | Low apoC-$III_{0,1}$; both absent | Decreased |
| Heterozygous hypobetalipoproteinemia | Low (55–146) | Low or normal (20–146) | Low | Low | Low (10–50% of normal) | Normal | — |
| Homozygous hypobetalipoproteinemia[a] | Low | Very low | Absent | Absent | Absent | Low | — |
| Homozygous hypobetalipoproteinemia[b] | Low (25–75) | Normal | Low | Low | Very low (0–21) | Low to high (20–77) | — |

[a]Homozygotes for "null alleles" in apoB gene.

[b]Usually compound heterozygotes fro truncated apoB.

adults have few clinical symptoms (see Table 161-8). Like familial hyperalphalipoproteinemia, primary hypobetalipoproteinemia may confer a decreased risk for CVD. One form of the disorder, familial hypobetalipoproteinemia-1 (FBHL1; MIM No. 615558), is inherited as an autosomal codominant disorder; almost all of the mutations are heterozygous nonsense mutations or frameshift mutations that create a premature stop codon in *APOB*. A truncated apoB protein is usually found in the plasma.

The clinical and chemical presentation of homozygous hypobetalipoproteinemia in children depends on whether they are homozygous for null alleles in the apoB gene (ie, make no detectable apoB) or homozygous (or compound heterozygotes) for other alleles and whether their lipoproteins contain small amounts of apoB or a truncated apoB (see Tables 161-8 and 161-9). Null-allele homozygotes are similar phenotypically to those with abetalipoproteinemia; however, their parents are heterozygous for hypobetalipoproteinemia.

Another form of hypobetalipoproteinemia is termed chylomicron retention disease (Anderson disease; MIM No. 246700), an autosomal recessive disorder caused by mutations of the gene *SAR1B*, which belongs to the Sar1-ADP-ribosylation factor family of small GTPases that govern the intracellular trafficking of proteins in coat protein (COP)-coated vesicles and are needed for the release of chylomicrons from intestinal enterocytes. It typically presents in infancy with failure to thrive and steatorrhea, complicated by malabsorption of fat-soluble vitamins, although it is generally milder than abetalipoproteinemia. Peripheral neuropathy due to vitamin deficiency can be seen and creatine kinase may be elevated. Heterozygotes have reduced HDL-C and apoA1 but are otherwise asymptomatic.

A more recently described form of hypobetaliproteinemia, referred to as familial hypobetalipoproteinemia-2 (FBHL2) (MIM No. 605019), with low apoB, total cholesterol, LDL-C, and HDL-C, is caused by heterozygous, compound heterozygous, and homozygous variants in the *ANGPTL3* gene as a codominant trait. This disorder likewise reduces the risk of CVD.

## TREATMENT OF HYPOLIPOPROTEINEMIAS

Patients with abetalipoproteinemia and those who are null-allele homozygotes for hypobetalipoproteinemia (see Table 161-8) require similar treatment approaches. Steatorrhea can be controlled by reducing the intake of fat to 5 to 20 g/d. This measure alone can result in marked clinical improvement and growth acceleration. In addition, the diet should be supplemented with linoleic acid (eg, 5 g of corn oil or safflower oil per day). MCT as a caloric substitute for long-chain fatty acids may produce hepatic fibrosis; thus, MCT should be used with caution, if at all. Fat-soluble vitamins should be added to the diet. Rickets can be prevented by normal quantities of vitamin D, but 200 to 400 IU/kg/d of vitamin A may be required to raise the level of vitamin A in plasma to normal. Enough vitamin K (5–10 mg/d) should be given to maintain a normal prothrombin time. Most importantly, large doses (150–200 mg/kg/d) of vitamin E must be given. Neurologic and retinal complications may be prevented or ameliorated through oral supplementation with vitamin E.

In Tangier disease, a low-fat diet diminishes the abnormal lipoprotein species that are believed to be remnants of abnormal chylomicron metabolism. The large LDL species found in LCAT deficiency is also thought to be a remnant of abnormal chylomicron metabolism. Its disappearance on a low-fat diet may have a beneficial effect, because large LDL may be involved in the pathogenesis of renal disease. Patients with other syndromes associated with deficiencies of HDL and premature atherosclerosis are also treated with a diet modified in total fat, saturated fat, and cholesterol.

## SUGGESTED READINGS


Bachorik PS, Lovejoy KL, Carroll MD, Johnson CL. Apolipoprotein B and AI distributions in the United States 1988–1991: results of the National Health and Nutrition Examination Survey III (NHANES III). *Clin Chem*. 1997;43:2364-2378.

Chang Y, Robidoux J. Dyslipidemia management update. *Curr Opin Pharmacol*. 2017;33:47-55.

Chiang J, Kirkman MS, Laffel L, Peters AL. Type 1 diabetes through the life span: a position statement of the American Diabetes Association. *Diabetes Care*. 2014;37(7):2034-2054.

Haney EM, Huffman LH, Bougatsos C, Freeman M, Steiner RD, Nelson HD. Screening and treatment for lipid disorders in children and adolescents: systematic evidence review for the US Preventive Services Task Force. *Pediatrics*. 2007;120:e189-e214.

Li S, Chen W, Srinivasan SR, et al. Childhood cardiovascular risk factors and carotid vascular changes in adulthood: the Bogalusa Heart Study. *JAMA*. 2003;290(17):2271-2276.

Lozano P, Henrikson NB, Morrison CC, et al. Lipid screening in childhood and adolescence for detection of multifactorial dyslipidemia: evidence report and systematic review for the US Preventive Services Task Force. *JAMA*. 2016;316(6):634-644.

Lozano P, Henrikson NB, Dunn J, et al. Lipid screening in childhood and adolescence for detection of familial hypercholesterolemia: evidence report and systematic review for the US Preventive Services Task Force. *JAMA*. 2016;316(6):645-655.

Magnussen CG, Raitakari OT, Thomson R, et al. Utility of currently recommended pediatric dyslipidemia classifications in predicting dyslipidemia in adulthood: evidence from the Childhood Determinants of Adult Health (CDAH) study, Cardiovascular Risk in Young Finns Study, and Bogalusa Heart Study. *Circulation*. 2008;117:32-42.

Morrison JA, Friedman LA, Wang P, Glueck CJ. Metabolic syndrome in childhood predicts adult metabolic syndrome and type 2 diabetes mellitus 25 to 30 years later. *J Pediatr*. 2008;152:201-206.

Nupponen M, Pahkala K, Juonala M, et al. Metabolic syndrome from adolescence to early adulthood: effect of infancy-onset dietary counseling of low saturated fat: the Special Turku Coronary Risk Factor Intervention Project (STRIP). *Circulation*. 2015;131(7):605-613.

Sabatie MS, Giugliano RP, Keech AC, et al. Evolocumab and clinical outcomes in patients with cardiovascular disease. *N Engl J Med*. 2017;376(18):1713-1722.

Youngblom E, Pariani M, Knowles JW. Familial Hypercholesterolemia. In: Pagon RA, Adam MP, Ardinger HH, et al, eds. *GeneReviews®*. Seattle, WA: University of Washington, Seattle; 2016.

# 162 Disorders of Heme Biosynthesis: The Porphyrias

Robert J. Desnick and Manisha Balwani

## INTRODUCTION

The porphyrias are a group of inherited and acquired metabolic disorders, each resulting from the deficient or increased activity of a specific enzyme in the heme biosynthetic pathway. These enzyme alterations are inherited as autosomal-dominant or -recessive and X-linked traits, with the exception of porphyria cutanea tarda (PCT), which usually is sporadic. These disorders are classified as either hepatic or erythropoietic, depending on the primary site of overproduction and accumulation of the porphyrin precursor(s) or porphyrin(s) (Table 162-1). Clinically, they are classified as acute and cutaneous, although some have overlapping features. Manifestations of the acute hepatic porphyrias are primarily neurologic, including severe abdominal pain, neuropathy, and secondary mental symptoms, whereas the erythropoietic porphyrias characteristically cause cutaneous phototoxicity.

## PATHOGENESIS AND EPIDEMIOLOGY

The neurologic involvement in the hepatic porphyrias, which typically presents after puberty, results from the hepatic overproduction of a neurotoxic metabolite(s). Certain steroid hormones, porphyrinogenic drugs, and dieting influence the production of porphyrin precursors and porphyrins, thereby precipitating acute attacks. In the cutaneous porphyrias, sensitivity to sunlight may occur in infancy or childhood because of the excitation of excess porphyrins in the skin by long-wave ultraviolet light, which can lead to cell damage, scarring, and deformation.

These disorders are rare. The acute hepatic porphyrias have a prevalence of 3 to 5 per 100,000 and occur more frequently in Scandinavia, South Africa, and the United Kingdom. Recent estimates of the prevalence suggest that 1 in approxiamately 1700 Caucasians have pathogenic mutations for the most common acute hepatic porphyria, acute intermittent porphyria (AIP). However, the penetrance may be as low as 1%, indicating the importance of environmental and genetic precipitating/preventative factors. PCT is the most common porphyria, and its estimated prevalence is approximately 5 to 10 per 100,000 in Caucasians. Erythropoietic protoporphyria is the most common erythropoietic porphyria and is the most common porphyria in children. Aminolevulinic acid (ALA) dehydrogenase-deficient porphyria (ADP), congenital erythropoietic porphyria, and X-linked protoporphyria all are extremely rare with 10, more than 200, and approximately 50 patients, respectively, reported in the literature.

Rare homozygous variants of the autosomal dominant hepatic porphyrias have been identified and usually manifest clinically before the patient reaches puberty. The symptoms in these patients usually are more severe and occur earlier than those of patients with the respective autosomal-dominant porphyria (see below). Thus, the porphyrias are actually ecogenic disorders in which environmental, physiologic, and genetic factors interact to cause disease.

Many symptoms of the porphyrias are nonspecific, and diagnosis often is delayed. Laboratory testing can confirm or exclude the diagnosis of a porphyria. Table 162-1 summarizes the major metabolites that accumulate in each porphyria. Urinary 5′-ALA and porphobilinogen (PBG) are easily quantitated by chemical methods, and the urinary porphyrin isomers can be separated and quantitated by high-performance liquid chromatography. However, a definite diagnosis requires demonstration of the specific enzyme or gene defect. The isolation and characterization of the genes encoding all the heme biosynthetic enzymes have permitted the identification of the molecular lesions that cause each porphyria. Such mutation analyses provide

**TABLE 162-1 CLINICAL, METABOLIC, AND GENETIC CHARACTERISTICS OF THE HUMAN PORPHYRIAS**

| | | | | | | Porphyrin Excretion | |
|---|---|---|---|---|---|---|---|
| Type/Porphyria | Deficient Enzyme | Inheritance | Photosensitivity | Neurovisceral Symptoms | Increased Erythrocyte Porphyrins | Urine | Stool |
| **Hepatic Porphyrias** | | | | | | | |
| ALA dehydratase deficiency (ADP) | ALA dehydratase | AR | — | + | PROTO | ALA, COPRO III | — |
| Acute intermittent porphyria (AIP) | HMB-synthase | AD | — | + | — | ALA, PBG | — |
| Porphyria cutanea tarda (PCT) | URO-decarboxylase | AD | +++ | — | — | URO I, 7-carboxylate porphyrin | ISOCOPRO |
| Hepatoerythropoietic porphyria | URO-decarboxylase | AR | +++ | +/− | | | |
| Hereditary coproporphyria (HCP) | COPRO-oxidase | AD | + | + | — | ALA, PBG, COPRO III | COPRO III |
| Variegate porphyria (VP) | PROTO-oxidase | AD | + | + | — | ALA, PBG, COPRO III | PROTO IX, 5-carboxylate porphyrin |
| **Erythropoietic Porphyrias** | | | | | | | |
| Congenital erythropoietic porphyria (CEP) | URO-synthase | AR | +++ | — | URO I | URO I | COPRO I<br>URO I |
| Erythropoietic protoporphyria (EPP) | Ferrochelatase | AR | + | — | PROTO IX | — | PROTO |
| X-linked protoporphyria (XLP) | ALA-synthase 2 (overexpressed) | XL | + | — | PROTO IX | — | PROTO |

AD, autosomal dominant; ALA, aminolevulinic acid; AR, autosomal recessive; COPRO I, coproporphyrin I; COPRO III, coproporphyrin III; ISOCOPRO, isocoproporphyrin; PBG, porphobilinogen; PROTO, protoporphyrin; PROTO IX, protoporphyrin IX; URO I, uroporphyrin I; URO III, uroporphyrin III; XL, X-linked.

precise heterozygote or homozygote identification and prenatal diagnosis in families with known mutations.

The American Porphyria Foundation (www.porphyriafoundation.com) and the European Porphyria Initiative (www.porphyria-europe.org) sponsor informative and up-to-date Web sites. An extensive list of unsafe and safe drugs for individuals with porphyria is given at the Drug Database for Acute Porphyrias (www.drugs-porphyria.org).

## HEME BIOSYNTHESIS

Heme biosynthesis involves 8 enzymatic steps in the conversion of glycine and succinyl-coenzyme A (CoA) to heme (Fig. 162-1 and Table 162-2). The first and last 3 enzymes in the heme biosynthetic pathway occur in the mitochondrion, whereas the other 4 occur in the cytosol (see Fig. 162-1). The first enzyme, ALA-synthase, catalyzes the condensation of glycine, activated by pyridoxal phosphate and succinyl-CoA, to form ALA. Hepatic ALAS1 can be induced in the liver by a variety of drugs, steroids, and other chemicals. Distinct housekeeping and erythroid-specific forms of ALA-synthase are encoded by separate genes located on chromosome 3p21.1 (*ALAS1*) and Xp11.2 (*ALAS2*). The deficient activity of the X-linked erythroid-specific ALAS2 enzyme causes X-linked sideroblastic anemia (mutations in the X-linked *ALAS2* gene that result in deficient ALAS2 activity cause sideroblastic anemia; see Chapter 144), whereas *ALAS2* mutations in the last exon cause its overexpression, resulting in X-linked protoporphyria (XLP; see below).

The second enzyme, ALA-dehydratase (ALAD), catalyzes the condensation of 2 molecules of ALA to form PBG. Four molecules of PBG

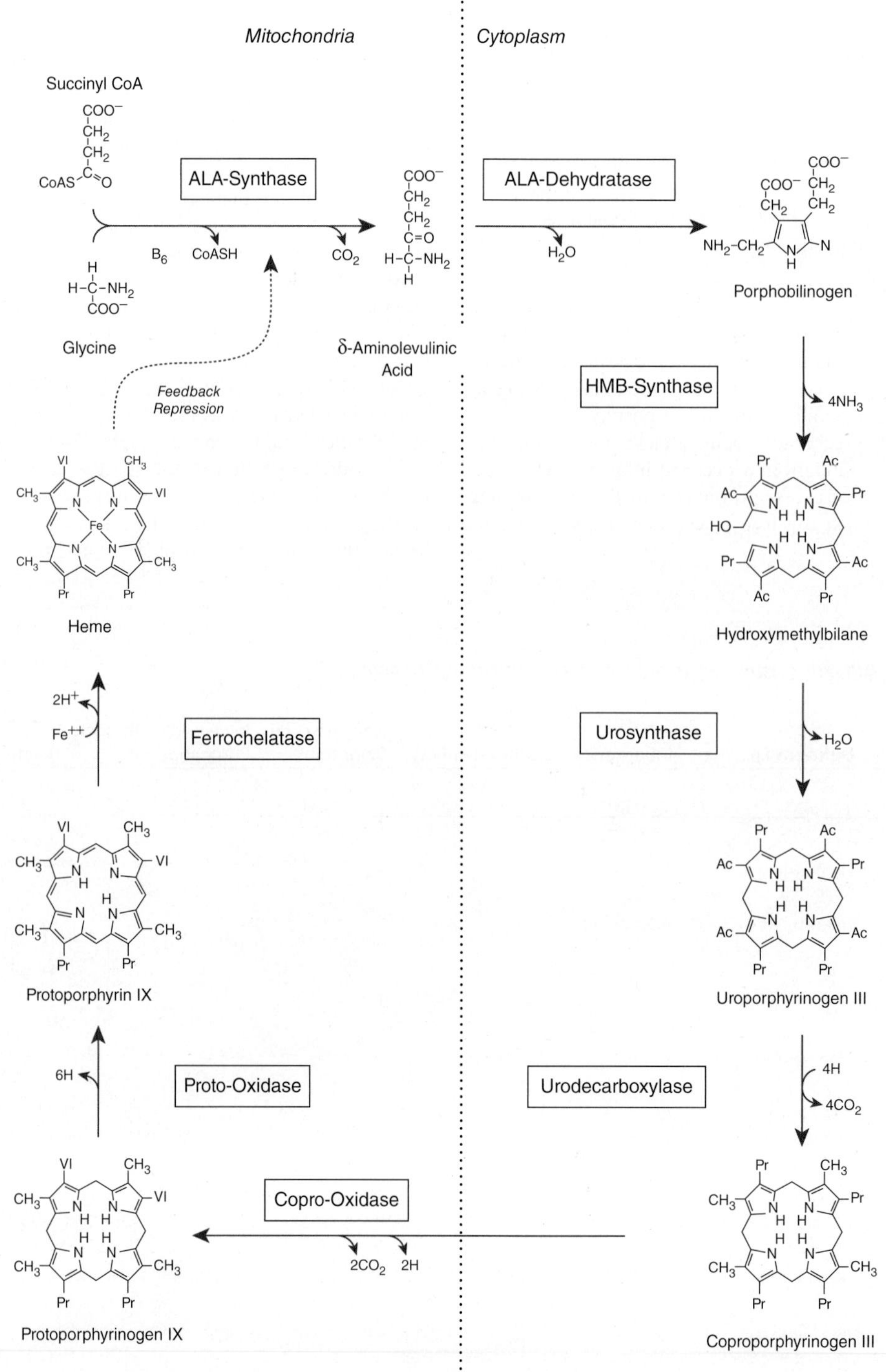


**FIGURE 162-1** The human heme biosynthetic pathway.

**TABLE 162-2 THE HUMAN HEME BIOSYNTHESIS GENES[a]**

| Gene | Chromosome Location | cDNA/Protein | Genomic Organization Length/No. of Exons |
|---|---|---|---|
| ALA-synthase | | | |
| Housekeeping (*ALAS1*) | 3p21.1 | 2199 bp/640 aa | 17 kb/11 exons |
| Erythroid-specific (*ALAS2*) | Xp11.21 | 1937 bp/587 aa | 22 kb/11 exons |
| ALA-dehydratase (*ALAD*) | | | |
| Housekeeping | 9q34 | 1149 bp/330 aa | 15.9 kb/exons 1A, 2–12 |
| Erythroid-specific | 9q34 | 1154 bp/33 aa | 15.9 kb/exons 1B, 2–12 |
| HMB-synthase (*HMBS*) | | | |
| Housekeeping | 11q23.3 | 1086 bp/361 aa | 11 kb/exons 1, 3–15 |
| Erythroid-specific | 11q23.3 | 1035 bp/344 aa | 11 kb/exons 2–15 |
| URO-synthase (*UROS*) | | | |
| Housekeeping | 10q25.2→q26.3 | 1296 bp/265 aa | 34 kb/exons 1, 2B–10 |
| Erythroid-specific | 10q25.2→q26.3 | 1216 bp/265 aa | 34 kb/exons 2A, 2B–10 |
| URO-decarboxylate (*UROD*) | 1p34 | 1104 bp/367 aa | 3 kb/10 exons |
| COPRO-oxidase (*CPOX*) | 3q12 | 1062 bp/354 aa | 14 kb/7 exons |
| PROTO-oxidase (*PPOX*) | 1q23 | 1431 bp/477 aa | 5.5 kb/13 exons |
| Ferrochelatase (*FECH*) | 18q21.3 | 1269 bp/423 aa | 45 kb/11 exons |

[a]cDNA base pairs (bp), number of encoded amino acids (aa), genomic length in kilobases (kb), and number of exons are indicated.

condense to form the tetrapyrrole uroporphyrinogen III by a 2-step process catalyzed by the third enzyme in the pathway, hydroxymethylbilane (HMB)-synthase (HMBS, also known as *PBG-deaminase*). HMBS catalyzes the head-to-tail condensation of 4 PBG molecules by a series of deaminations to form the linear tetrapyrrole HMB. Uroporphyrinogen (URO)-synthase (UROS), the fourth pathway enzyme, then catalyzes the rearrangement and rapid cyclization of HMB to form the asymmetric, physiologic, octacarboxylate porphyrinogen uroporphyrinogen III isomer (see Fig. 162-1).

The fifth enzyme in the pathway, URO-decarboxylase (UROD), catalyzes the sequential removal of the 4 carboxyl groups from the acetic acid side chains of URO III to form coproporphyrinogen (COPRO) III, a tetracarboxylate porphyrinogen. This compound then enters the mitochondrion via a membrane transporter, whereas COPRO oxidase (CPOX), the sixth enzyme, catalyzes the decarboxylation of 2 of the 4 propionic acid groups. This then forms the 2 vinyl groups of protoporphyrinogen (PROTO) IX, a dicarboxylate porphyrinogen. Next, PROTO-oxidase (PPOX) oxidizes PROTO IX to protoporphyrin IX by removing 6 hydrogen atoms. The product of the reaction is a porphyrin (oxidized form), in contrast to the preceding tetrapyrrole intermediates, which are porphyrinogens (reduced forms). Finally, ferrous iron is inserted into protoporphyrin IX to form heme, a reaction catalyzed by the eighth enzyme in the pathway, ferrochelatase (FECH, also known as *heme synthetase*).

### REGULATION OF HEME BIOSYNTHESIS

Regulation of heme synthesis differs in the 2 major heme-forming tissues, the liver and erythron. Approximately 85% of the heme produced in the body is synthesized in erythroid cells to provide heme for hemoglobin; most of the remainder is produced in hepatocytes, primarily for synthesizing cytochromes, P450 enzymes, and other hemoproteins. In the liver, the biosynthetic pathway is under negative feedback control. "Free" heme in the liver regulates the synthesis and mitochondrial translocation of the housekeeping form of ALA-synthase (ALAS1). Heme represses the synthesis of the *ALAS1* mRNA and interferes with the transport of the enzyme from the cytosol into mitochondria. Hepatic *ALAS1* is inducible by many of the same chemicals that induce the cytochrome P450 enzymes in the liver's endoplasmic reticulum. Because most hepatic heme is used for synthesizing cytochrome P450 enzymes, hepatic ALAS1 and the cytochrome P450 enzymes are regulated in a coordinated fashion.

Different regulatory mechanisms control production of heme for hemoglobin. The erythroid-specific ALA-synthase gene (*ALAS2*) on the X chromosome is expressed at higher levels than that of the hepatic enzyme, and an erythroid-specific control mechanism regulates iron transport into erythroid cells. During erythroid differentiation, the activities of the heme biosynthetic enzymes are increased.

## THE HEPATIC PORPHYRIAS

The acute hepatic porphyrias are characterized by the rapid onset of neurovisceral manifestations. During the acute attack, individuals have markedly elevated plasma and urinary concentrations of the porphyrin precursors, ALA and PBG, which originate in the liver.

## ALA-DEHYDRATASE–DEFICIENT PORPHYRIA (ADP)

### PATHOGENESIS AND EPIDEMIOLOGY

*ADP* is a rare autosomal-recessive trait (MIM no. 612740) that has been described in only a few patients. The onset and severity of the disease are variable, presumably depending on the amount of residual ALA-dehydratase activity. All patients had significantly elevated levels of plasma and urinary ALA and markedly decreased ALA-dehydratase activity. Treatment and prevention of neurologic complications are the same as for other acute porphyrias (see below).

### CLINICAL FEATURES

The first reported cases were in 2 unrelated German men who had clinical onset during adolescence of abdominal pain and neuropathy, resembling AIP. A Swedish infant presented with failure to thrive and required transfusions and parenteral nutrition. Presumably, the earlier age of onset and more severe manifestations reflect a more severe enzyme deficiency. At age 63, a Belgian man developed an acute motor polyneuropathy that was associated with a myeloproliferative disorder. This patient was heterozygous for an ALA-dehydratase mutation that presumably was present in erythroblasts, which underwent clonal expansion due to the bone marrow malignancy.

### DIAGNOSIS

Patients have increased urinary levels of ALA and coproporphyrin. ALA-dehydratase activity in erythrocytes is less than 5% of normal. Lead or succinylacetone (which accumulates in hereditary tyrosinemia and is structurally similar to ALA) can inhibit ALA-dehydratase and increase urinary excretion. It may cause manifestations that resemble those of the acute porphyrias, lead intoxication (see Chapter 10), and hereditary tyrosinemia (fumarylacetoacetase deficiency; see Chapter 131). These conditions should, therefore, be considered in the differential diagnosis of ADP. DNA analysis revealed different mutations (see the Human Gene Mutation Database, www.hgmd.org).

Heterozygotes are clinically asymptomatic and do not excrete increased levels of ALA, but they can be detected by demonstrating intermediate levels of erythrocyte ALA-dehydratase activity or by demonstrating a specific ALA-dehydratase gene mutation. Prenatal diagnosis is possible by determining the ALA-dehydratase activity or the family's specific gene mutation(s) in cultured chorionic villi or amniocytes.

### TREATMENT

Treatment is similar to that of AIP (see below).

## ACUTE INTERMITTENT PORPHYRIA (AIP)

*AIP* is an autosomal-dominant condition resulting from half-normal HMB-synthase activity. The disease is pan-ethnic but is especially common in Scandinavia and Great Britain. The enzyme deficiency can be demonstrated in most heterozygous individuals, but clinical expression is highly variable. Activation of the disease is related to ecogenic factors, such as porphyrinogenic drugs, dieting, and certain steroid hormones, which can precipitate the manifestations. Attacks can be prevented by avoiding known precipitating factors. Rare cases of homozygous AIP have been reported in children.

### CLINICAL FEATURES

There are 3 AIP subtypes (MIM no. 176000). (1) Most heterozygotes remain clinically asymptomatic (latent) unless exposed to factors that increase production of porphyrin. Common precipitating factors include endogenous and exogenous gonadal steroids, porphyrinogenic drugs, ingestion of alcohol, and low-calorie diets (usually instituted for weight loss). (2) "Asymptomatic high excreters" (ASHE) are heterozygotes who have high ALA and PBG levels but are clinically asymptomatic. These individuals often had an attack previously and are presumably more susceptible to acute attacks. (3) Another subtype is heterozygotes who have recurrent attacks (> 4 per year), with high levels of urine PBG and ALA. Most of them are women, many of whom have attacks in the luteal phase of their menstrual cycles.

Table 162-3 lists the major drugs that are harmful in AIP (and in hereditary coproporphyria [HCP] and variegate porphyria [VP]) and some drugs and anesthetic agents known to be safe. More extensive lists of drugs considered harmful or safe are available at the Drug Database for Acute Porphyrias (www.drugs-porphyria.org) and at www.porphyriafoundation.com and www.porphyria-europe.com, but information is incomplete for many drugs. Attacks also can be provoked by infections and by surgery.

**TABLE 162-3 CATEGORIES OF UNSAFE AND SAFE DRUGS IN AIP, HCP, AND VP**

| Unsafe | Safe |
|---|---|
| Barbiturates | Narcotic analgesics |
| Sulfonamide antibiotics | Aspirin |
| Meprobamate | Acetaminophen |
| Glutethimide | Phenothiazines |
| Methyprylon | Penicillin and derivatives |
| Ethchlorvynol | Streptomycin |
| Mephenytoin | Glucocorticoids |
| Succinimides | Bromides |
| Carbamazepine | Insulin |
| Valproic acid | Atropine |
| Pyrazolones | |
| Griseofulvin | |
| Ergots | |
| Synthetic estrogens and progestogens | |
| Danazol | |
| Alcohol | |

AIP, acute intermittent porphyria; HCP, hereditary coproporphyria; VP, variegate porphyria.

Because the neurovisceral symptoms rarely occur before puberty and often are nonspecific, a high index of suspicion is required to make the diagnosis. The disease can be disabling but is rarely fatal. Acute abdominal pain, the most common symptom, usually is severe and poorly localized.

Ileus, abdominal distention, and decreased bowel sounds are common manifestations. However, increased bowel sounds and diarrhea may occur. Abdominal tenderness, fever, and leukocytosis usually are absent or mild because the symptoms are neurologic rather than inflammatory. Nausea; vomiting; constipation; tachycardia; hypertension; mental symptoms; muscle weakness; sensory loss; dysuria; urinary retention; and pain in the limbs, head, neck, or chest are characteristic. Tachycardia, hypertension, restlessness, tremors, and excess sweating are due to sympathetic overactivity.

The peripheral neuropathy is the result of axonal degeneration (rather than demyelination) and affects primarily motor neurons. Significant neuropathy does not occur with all acute attacks; abdominal symptoms usually are more prominent. Motor neuropathy initially affects the proximal muscles, more often in the shoulders and arms. The course and degree of involvement vary. Deep tendon reflexes may be normal or hyperactive but usually are decreased or absent with advanced neuropathy. Motor weakness can be asymmetric and focal and may involve cranial nerves. Sensory changes such as paresthesias and loss of sensation are less prominent. Progressive muscle weakness can lead to respiratory and bulbar paralysis and death when diagnosis and treatment are delayed. Sudden death may result from sympathetic overactivity and cardiac arrhythmia.

Mental symptoms, such as anxiety, insomnia, depression, disorientation, hallucinations, and paranoia, can occur in acute attacks. Seizures can be caused by neurologic effects or by hyponatremia. Treating seizures is difficult because virtually all antiepileptic drugs (except bromides) may exacerbate AIP (clonazepam may be safer than is phenytoin or barbiturates). Hyponatremia results from hypothalamic involvement and inappropriate secretion of an antidiuretic hormone or from electrolyte depletion due to vomiting, diarrhea, poor intake, or excess renal sodium loss. Persistent hypertension and impaired renal function may occur. When an attack resolves, abdominal pain may disappear within hours, and paresis begins to improve within days and may continue to improve over the course of several years, although the neuropathy can be persistent.

### DIAGNOSIS

ALA and PBG levels are increased in plasma and urine during acute attacks. Although the diagnosis of an acute attack is based on clinical findings and not the absolute level of these porphyrin precursors, the increase is expected to be substantial. Excretion of PBG usually ranges from 50 to 200 mg/24 h (220–880 mmol/24 h; normal, 0–4 mg/24 h [0–18 mmol/24 h]), and urinary excretion of ALA ranges from 20 to 100 mg/24 h (150–760 mmol/24 h; normal, 1–7 mg/24 h [8–53 mmol/24 h]). The excretion of these compounds generally decreases with clinical improvement, particularly after administration of hematin infusions. A normal urinary PBG level effectively excludes AIP as a cause for current symptoms. Fecal porphyrins usually are normal or minimally increased in AIP, in contrast to HCP and VP. Most asymptomatic ("latent") heterozygotes with HMB-synthase deficiency have normal urinary excretion of ALA and PBG. Therefore, screening asymptomatic family members by target sequencing of the family's *HMBS* mutation is required.

The enzyme deficiency is detectable in erythrocytes from most AIP heterozygotes (classic AIP). The activity is higher in young erythrocytes and may increase into the normal range in AIP when erythropoiesis is increased due to a concurrent condition. However, patients with the rare erythroid form of AIP (erythroid or variant AIP) have normal enzyme levels in erythrocytes and deficient activity in nonerythroid tissues. The erythroid and housekeeping forms of HMB-synthase are encoded by a single gene that has 2 promoters. One promotes transcription of a messenger RNA for the housekeeping enzyme found in all tissues, and the other promoter encodes the erythroid-specific transcript found only in erythroid cells. More than 400 mutations causing AIP have been identified (see the Human Gene Mutation Database, www.hgmd.org). Mutations that cause erythroid AIP variants with half-normal enzyme in nonerythroid tissues but normal activity in erythrocytes include point mutations in the initiation methionine codon (which prevent translation) or in the 5'-donor splice site of intron 1 (which causes abnormal splicing of the HMB-synthase transcript). Identifying the HMB-synthase gene mutation in an index case enables detection of latent family members and establishment of a prenatal diagnosis, which is seldom done because the prognosis of individuals with HMB-synthase mutations generally is favorable.

### TREATMENT

During acute attacks, narcotic analgesics usually are required for abdominal pain, and phenothiazines are useful for nausea, vomiting, anxiety, and restlessness. Benzodiazepines in low doses are probably safe if a minor tranquilizer is required. Intravenous hemin should be used initially for attacks requiring hospitalization. A trial of intravenous dextrose (300–400 g/d) is no longer recommended for mild attacks if hemin is available. The standard regimen is 3 to 4 mg/kg of heme in the form of lyophilized hematin (Recordati Rare Diseases), heme albumin (hematin reconstituted with human albumin), or heme arginate (Orphan Europe), infused daily for 4 days. Heme arginate and heme albumin are chemically stable and are less likely than hematin to produce phlebitis or an anticoagulant effect. The rate of recovery from an acute attack depends on the degree of neuronal damage and may be rapid (1–2 days) with prompt therapy. Recovery from severe motor neuropathy may continue for months or years. Identifying and avoiding inciting factors can hasten recovery from an attack and prevent future attacks. Numerous inciting factors may contribute to a symptomatic episode. Recurrent attacks often occur during the menstrual cycle in some women and can be prevented with a gonadotropin-releasing hormone analogue (which prevents ovulation and production of progesterone). Patients with recurrent attacks without an identifiable trigger can also be managed with prophylactic hemin as a single outpatient dose given weekly, biweekly, or monthly. Hemin can also be given prophylactically as an outpatient treatment during the prodromal phase of an acute attack before patients develop severe symptoms.

In the rare patient with recurrent attacks who does not respond to the above therapy, orthotopic liver transplantation has proven to be effective. After transplantation, the elevated urinary ALA and PBG levels return to normal in 24 hours. Liver transplantation is a high-risk procedure and should be considered only in patients refractory to medical treatment. Currently, RNA interference and gene therapy approaches to treat and/or prevent acute attacks are in clinical trials.

## HOMOZYGOUS DOMINANT AIP

*Homozygous-dominant AIP* is a rare form of porphyria presenting in infancy. Patients inherit HMB-synthase mutations from each of their heterozygous parents; therefore, they have very low (< 2%) enzyme activity. In these homozygous-affected patients, manifestations of disease include failure to thrive, developmental delay, bilateral cataracts, or hepatosplenomegaly. Acute attacks do not occur, and urinary ALA and PBG are markedly elevated. Studies of brain magnetic resonance imaging scans of children with homozygous AIP suggested damage primarily in white matter that was myelinated postnatally, whereas tracks that myelinated prenatally were normal. These findings suggest that ALA or PBG present in large amounts postnatally cause damage to nerve tissue. Prenatally, excess amounts of ALA and PBG cross the placenta and are excreted in the mother's urine. Most children with homozygous AIP die at an early age.

## HEREDITARY COPROPORPHYRIA (HCP)

*Hereditary coproporphyria (HCP)* is an autosomal-dominant hepatic porphyria that results from half-normal COPRO-oxidase activity. Photosensitivity may occur. Cases of homozygous-dominant HCP have been reported.

### CLINICAL FEATURES



HCP is influenced by the same factors that cause attacks in AIP. The disease is latent before puberty, and symptoms occur more frequently in women. Neurovisceral symptoms and other manifestations are virtually identical to those of AIP. Photosensitivity may resemble that in PCT and VP. Cutaneous lesions may begin in childhood in the rare homozygous-dominant cases.

## HOMOZYGOUS-DOMINANT HCP AND HARDEROPORPHYRIA

Individuals with mutations in both their COPRO-oxidase alleles and markedly decreased COPRO-oxidase activities have been described; these mutations cause homozygous-dominant HCP or a rare variant form called *harderoporphyria* (MIM no. 121300). Homozygous HCP presents early in childhood with symptoms of growth retardation, hypertrichosis, and skin hyperpigmentation. Later, these patients can have acute porphyric attacks.

Individuals with harderoporphyria, which is a biochemical and clinical variant form of HCP in which hemolysis and erythropoietic features are prominent, usually present in early childhood with jaundice, hemolytic anemia, hepatosplenomegaly, and skin photosensitivity. However, the symptoms may be variable; acute attacks do not occur.

### DIAGNOSIS

Concentrations of coproporphyrin are markedly increased in the urine and feces of patients with HCP when the disease is symptomatic and sometimes when there are no symptoms. Urinary ALA and PBG levels are increased during acute attacks but may return to normal when symptoms resolve. Although the diagnosis can be confirmed by measuring COPRO-oxidase activity, these assays are not widely available and require cells other than erythrocytes. COPRO-oxidase (*CPOX*) gene mutations are diagnostic, and more than 60 have been reported (see www.hgmd.org). Patients with homozygous HCP have markedly increased fecal COPRO III due to markedly deficient (< 10%) COPRO-oxidase activity. In patients with harderoporphyria, urinary COPRO III, fecal porphyrins (66–90% harderoporphyrin), and zinc protoporphyrin are increased. Most reported patients with harderoporphyria are either homoallelic or heteroallelic for the K404E missense mutation.

### TREATMENT

Neurologic symptoms are treated as in AIP. Phlebotomy and chloroquine are ineffective when cutaneous lesions are present.

## VARIEGATE PORPHYRIA (VP)

*Variegate porphyria (VP)*, an acute hepatic porphyria resulting from the deficient activity of PROTO-oxidase, is inherited as an autosomal-dominant trait (MIM no. 176200) and can present with neurovisceral symptoms, photosensitivity, or both. Homozygous VP is rare and presents in early childhood.

### CLINICAL FEATURES

Neurovisceral signs and symptoms develop after puberty and are similar to those of AIP or HCP. Attacks are provoked by the same drugs, steroids, and nutritional factors that are detrimental in AIP. Skin manifestations are more common than in HCP but usually occur apart from the neurovisceral symptoms. Because the skin lesions in VP, HCP, and PCT are not distinguishable by clinical examination or biopsy, these conditions must be diagnosed by assay of porphyrins and porphyrin precursors in blood, urine, and feces or by demonstration of PROTO-oxidase gene mutations.

VP is particularly common in South Africa, where every 3 in 1000 whites have the disorder. Most are descendants of a couple who emigrated from Holland to South Africa in 1688. Homozygous-dominant VP is associated with photosensitivity, neurologic symptoms, and developmental disturbances, including growth retardation in infancy or childhood; all cases had increased erythrocyte levels of zinc protoporphyrin, a characteristic finding in all homozygous porphyrias so far described.

## HOMOZYGOUS DOMINANT VP

Affected individuals with homozygous-dominant VP have mutations affecting both PROTO-oxidase alleles, resulting in very low enzyme activity levels. These patients generally develop cutaneous symptoms, including photosensitivity and hypertrichosis, before the age of 2 years. Scarring and deformities of the face and digits may be prominent. Most patients do not have acute attacks. Neurologic symptoms in some patients include intellectual disabilities, epilepsy, growth retardation, and nystagmus. Laboratory findings include elevated erythrocyte zinc protoporphyrin levels, as in other homozygous-dominant porphyrias. Mutations have been identified in most patients with homozygous VP. Expression studies have indicated that these mutations have very low residual activity.

### DIAGNOSIS

Urinary ALA and PBG levels are increased during acute attacks but may return to normal more quickly than in AIP. Increases in fecal protoporphyrin and coproporphyrin III and in urinary coproporphyrin III are more persistent. Plasma levels of porphyrins are increased, particularly when there are cutaneous lesions. VP can be distinguished rapidly from all other porphyrias by examining the fluorescence emission spectrum of porphyrins in plasma at neutral pH. This test is particularly useful for differentiating VP from PCT.

Assays of PROTO-oxidase activity in cultured fibroblasts or lymphocytes are not widely available. Some latent cases of VP can be diagnosed by measuring fecal porphyrins in relatives of patients with VP. The diagnosis can be established by demonstrating a PROTO-oxidase (*PPOX*) gene mutation.

### TREATMENT

As in AIP, acute attacks are treated with hematin. Other than avoiding sun exposure, there are few effective measures for treating the skin lesions. Beta-carotene, phlebotomy, and chloroquine are not helpful.

## PORPHYRIA CUTANEA TARDA (PCT)

*PCT*, the most common of the porphyrias (MIM no. 176100), can be sporadic (type I) or familial (types II and III) and can develop after exposure to halogenated aromatic hydrocarbons. Hepatic URO-decarboxylase is deficient in all types of PCT and for clinical manifestations must be substantially reduced (< 20% of normal). Generation of a URO-decarboxylase inhibitor, specifically in the liver in the presence of iron and under conditions of oxidative stress, presumably causes this decrease. In type I PCT, URO-decarboxylase activity is normal in erythrocytes. In type II PCT, an autosomal-dominant trait, the enzyme is systemically deficient. In type III PCT, which clusters in families, deficiency of the enzyme activity is limited to the liver. Deficient hepatic URO-decarboxylase and a porphyrin pattern resembling PCT can be produced by exposure of normal individuals to a number of halogenated aromatic hydrocarbons.

Hepatoerythropoietic porphyria (HEP) is an autosomal-recessive form of this porphyria, as affected individuals inherit an URO-decarboxylase mutation from each parent and have a severe systematic deficiency of URO-decarboxylase activity. HEP usually presents in childhood.

### CLINICAL FEATURES

Cutaneous photosensitivity is the major clinical feature. Neurologic manifestations are not observed. Fluid-filled vesicles and bullae develop on sun-exposed areas such as the face, the dorsa of the hands and feet, the forearms, and the legs. The skin in these areas is friable, and minor trauma may lead to the formation of bullae. The appearance of small white plaques, termed *milia*, may precede or follow formation of vesicles. Bullae and denuded skin heal slowly and are subject to infection. Other features include hypertrichosis and hyperpigmentation, especially of the face, and thickening, scarring, and calcification resembling the cutaneous changes of systemic sclerosis.

Several factors contribute to the development of hepatic URO-decarboxylase deficiency and include excess alcohol use, iron overload, and use of estrogens. Recently, the importance of excess hepatic iron as a precipitating factor was documented by finding an increased prevalence of the common hemochromatosis-causing mutations, *HFE* C282Y and H63D, patients with types I and II PCT. PCT is strongly associated with hepatitis C in southern Europe and the United States. PCT also can be induced by various chemicals; an epidemic of PCT occurred in eastern Turkey in the 1950s from the consumption of wheat contaminated with the fungicide hexachlorobenzene. This chemical produces a disorder similar to PCT and induces hepatic URO-decarboxylase deficiency in animals. PCT in humans has occurred after exposure to other chemicals, including di- and trichlorophenols and 2,3,7,8-tetrachlorodibenzo-(*p*)-dioxin (TCDD, dioxin). Patients with PCT characteristically have liver damage and are at risk for development of hepatocellular carcinoma (see Chapter 454). These carcinomas do not produce porphyrins.

HEP resembles congenital erythropoietic porphyria (CEP) and usually presents with blistering skin lesions, hypertrichosis, scarring, and red urine in infancy or childhood.

### DIAGNOSIS

Porphyrin levels are increased in the liver, plasma, urine, and stool. The urinary ALA level may be slightly increased, but the PBG level is normal. Urinary porphyrins consist mostly of uroporphyrin and 7-carboxylate porphyrin, with lesser amounts of coproporphyrin and 5- and 6-carboxylate porphyrins. Plasma porphyrins also are increased in a pattern that resembles that in urine. Isocoproporphyrins are increased in feces and sometimes in plasma and urine. The finding of increased isocoproporphyrins is diagnostic for a deficiency of hepatic URO-decarboxylase.

Type II PCT and HEP can be diagnosed by finding decreased URO-decarboxylase activity in erythrocytes or by identifying mutations in the URO-decarboxylase gene. URO-decarboxylase activity in liver, erythrocytes, and cultured skin fibroblasts in type II PCT is approximately 50% of normal in affected individuals and in family members with latent disease. In HEP, the URO-decarboxylase activity is markedly deficient, with typical levels of 3% to 10% of normal. More than 120 mutations have been identified in the URO-decarboxylase (*UROD*) gene from unrelated patients with type II PCT and HEP (see the Human Gene Mutation Database, www.hgmd.org).

### TREATMENT

Alcohol, estrogens, iron supplements, and, if possible, any drugs that may exacerbate the disease should be discontinued, but this step does not always lead to improvement. A complete response can almost always be achieved by repeated phlebotomy to reduce hepatic iron. A unit (450 mL) of blood can be removed every 1 to 2 weeks. Because iron overload is not marked in most cases, remission may occur after only 5 or 6 phlebotomies. Patients with PCT and hemochromatosis may require many more phlebotomies. Hemoglobin levels or hematocrits and serum ferritin should be followed closely to prevent development of iron deficiency and anemia. After remission, continued phlebotomy may not be needed, even if ferritin levels return to normal. Relapses are treated again by phlebotomy.

PCT also can be treated with chloroquine or hydroxychloroquine, both of which complex with the excess porphyrins and promote their excretion. Small doses (eg, 125 mg of chloroquine phosphate twice weekly) should be given, because standard doses can induce transient, sometimes marked, increases in photosensitivity and hepatocellular damage. Hepatic imaging can diagnose or exclude complicating hepatocellular carcinoma. Treating PCT in patients with end-stage renal disease is facilitated by administering erythropoietin.

## HEPATOERYTHROPOIETIC PORPHYRIA (HEP)

*HEP*, which is the homozygous form of familial (type II) PCT, resembles CEP clinically. Excess porphyrins originate mostly from the liver, with a pattern consistent with severe URO-decarboxylase deficiency. There also is a substantial increase in erythrocyte zinc protoporphyrin in HEP, as in homozygous-dominant forms of the acute porphyrias, ADP, and some cases of CEP.

HEP usually presents with blistering skin lesions, hypertrichosis, scarring, and red urine in infancy or childhood. Sclerodermoid skin changes are sometimes prominent. Unusually mild cases have been described. Concurrent conditions that affect liver function may alter the severity of the disease. For example, hepatitis A caused the disease to manifest in a 2-year-old child and then improved with recovery from this viral infection.

HEP is readily distinguished from CEP by increases in both uroporphyrin and heptacarboxyl porphyrin in urine and in isocoproporphyrins in stool. In most cases of CEP, the excess erythrocyte porphyrins are predominantly URO I and COPRO I rather than zinc protoporphyrin. Erythropoietic protoporphyria is readily distinguished by its nonblistering photosensitivity and normal urine porphyrins and by demonstration that the excess erythrocyte protoporphyrin is free and not complexed with zinc. As in CEP, avoiding sunlight is most important in managing this disease. The outlook depends on the severity of the enzyme deficiency and may be favorable if sunlight can be avoided. Phlebotomy has shown little or no benefit.

## THE ERYTHROPOIETIC PORPHYRIAS

In the erythropoietic porphyrias, porphyrins from bone erythroid cells, erythrocytes, and plasma are deposited in the skin vessels and lead to cutaneous photosensitivity.

## CONGENITAL ERYTHROPOIETIC PORPHYRIA (CEP)

*CEP* is an autosomal-recessive disorder also known as *Gunther disease* (MIM no. 263700). It results from the markedly deficient activity of URO synthase and the accumulation of uroporphyrin I and coproporphyrin I isomers and is manifested by hemolytic anemia and severe cutaneous photosensitivity.

### CLINICAL FEATURES

Severe cutaneous photosensitivity can begin from the first days of life. The disease may be recognized in utero as a cause of nonimmune hydrops fetalis. The skin over sun-exposed areas is friable, and bullae and vesicles are prone to rupture and infection. Skin thickening, focal hypo- and hyperpigmentation, and hypertrichosis of the face and extremities are characteristic. Secondary infection of the cutaneous lesions can disfigure the face and hands. Porphyrins are deposited in teeth and bones. Consequently, the teeth are reddish brown and fluoresce on exposure to long-wave ultraviolet light. Hemolysis likely is caused by the marked increase in erythrocyte porphyrins and leads to splenomegaly. Adults with a milder form of the disease have been described.

### DIAGNOSIS

Uroporphyrin and coproporphyrin (mostly type I isomers) accumulate in the bone marrow, erythrocytes, plasma, urine, and feces. The diagnosis should be confirmed by demonstration of markedly deficient URO-synthase activity and/or URO-synthase gene mutations. The disease can be detected in utero by measuring porphyrins in amniotic fluid and URO-synthase activity or demonstrating the family's URO-synthase (*UROS*) mutations in cultured amniotic cells or chorionic villi. Approximately 50 URO-synthase mutations have been reported (see the Human Gene Mutation Database, www.hgmd.org).

### TREATMENT



Protection from sunlight is essential, and minor skin trauma should be avoided. Beta-carotene may be of limited value. In transfusion-dependent patients, periodic transfusions of fresh packed erythrocytes can suppress erythropoiesis effectively but can result in iron overload. Complete or partial splenectomy may reduce hemolysis and decrease transfusion requirements, if necessary. Complicating bacterial infections should be treated promptly. Recently, bone marrow or cord blood transplantation has proven effective in several transfusion-dependent children, providing the rationale for stem cell gene therapy. Recently, afamelanotide, a synthetic peptide agonist of melanocortin receptors, has been approved in the European Union for the treatment of erythropoietic protoporphyria and may be useful in patients with CEP.

## ERYTHROPOIETIC PROTOPORPHYRIA (EPP)

*Erythropoietic protoporphyria (EPP)* is an autosomal-recessive inherited disorder (MIM no. 177000) resulting from the markedly deficient (< 30% of normal) FECH activity, the last enzyme in the heme biosynthetic pathway. EPP is the most common erythropoietic porphyria and is the most common porphyria in children and the second most common in adults. Patients with EPP have FECH activities as low as 15% to 25% in lymphocytes and cultured fibroblasts. In most patients, a disabling (ie, causative) mutation in 1 *FECH* allele is combined with a relatively common intron 3 (IVS3-48T>C) single nucleotide alteration in the other allele, which results in decreased amounts of the normal enzyme. The C allele results in expression of an aberrantly spliced mRNA that is degraded by a nonsense-mediated decay mechanism, thus decreasing the steady-state level of normal FECH mRNA transcribed from the C allele. The low-expression allele is found in approximately 10% of the general Caucasian population. In several studies, more than 90% of patients with symptomatic EPP had a causative *FECH* mutation and the common low-expression allele. Individuals having only 1 or 2 IVS3-48T>C alleles usually are asymptomatic.

### CLINICAL FEATURES

Skin photosensitivity usually begins in childhood. The skin manifestations differ from those of other porphyrias. Redness, swelling, burning, and itching can develop within minutes of exposure to sun and can resemble angioedema. Symptoms (eg, excruciating pain) may seem out of proportion to the visible skin lesions. Sparse vesicles and bullae occur in 10% of cases. Chronic skin changes may include lichenification, leathery pseudovesicles, labial grooving, and nail changes. Severe scarring is rare, as are pigment changes, friability, and hirsutism.

The primary source of excess protoporphyrin is the bone marrow reticulocyte. Erythrocyte protoporphyrin is mostly free (not complexed with zinc) and is mostly bound to hemoglobin. In plasma, protoporphyrin is bound to albumin. Hemolysis and anemia are usually absent or mild.

Liver function usually is normal, but as many as 20% of patients with EPP may have minor abnormalities of liver function, and in some patients (~5%), accumulation of protoporphyrin causes chronic liver disease that can progress to liver failure and death. The hepatic complications often are preceded by increasing levels of erythrocyte and plasma protoporphyrin and probably result, in part, from accumulation of protoporphyrin in the liver. Protoporphyrin is insoluble; it forms crystalline structures in liver cells and can decrease hepatic bile flow. Some patients have gallstones that are at least partially composed of protoporphyrin.

### DIAGNOSIS

A substantial increase in erythrocyte protoporphyrin, which is predominantly free and not complexed with zinc, is the hallmark of this disease. Protoporphyrin levels are also variably increased in bone marrow, plasma, bile, and feces. Plasma and fecal porphyrins are less increased than in most other cutaneous porphyrias and occasionally are normal. Therefore, measuring erythrocyte protoporphyrin is important for diagnosis. Because erythrocyte protoporphyrin concentrations are increased in other conditions, it is important to confirm the diagnosis by an assay that distinguishes free and zinc-complexed protoporphyrin. Erythrocytes in EPP exhibit red fluorescence when examined by fluorescence microscopy at 632 to 634 nm. Urinary levels of porphyrins and porphyrin precursors (ALA and PBG) are normal. FECH enzyme activity assays are not widely available. *FECH* mutation analysis is recommended to detect the causative mutation and, in most affected families, the presence of the IVS3-48T>C alteration in the other *FECH* allele. To date, more than 185 mutations have been identified in the *FECH* gene (see the Human Gene Mutation Database; www.hgmd.org).

### TREATMENT

Avoiding exposure to sunlight and wearing clothing designed to provide protection for individuals with chronic photosensitivity are essential. Recent clinical trials of afamelanotide, an α-melanocyte-stimulating hormone analogue, showed that patients could tolerate increased exposure to sun without pain. Long-term studies showed an improvement in the quality of life of patients and that the drug was well tolerated with minor adverse events. This drug is now approved by the European Medicines Agency and available to patients in the European Union.

Treating hepatic complications is difficult. However, cholestyramine and other porphyrin absorbents, such as activated charcoal, may interrupt the enterohepatic circulation of protoporphyrin and promote its fecal excretion, leading to some improvement. Complete or partial splenectomy may be helpful when the disease is accompanied by hemolysis and significant splenomegaly or secondary hypersplenism. Restriction of calories and drugs or hormones that may induce the heme pathway or impair hepatic excretory function should be avoided. Iron deficiency should be prevented or treated. Transfusions or intravenous heme therapy may suppress production of erythroid and hepatic protoporphyrin and occasionally are beneficial. Liver transplantation has been performed in some patients with severe liver complications. However, liver disease often eventually recurs in the transplanted liver because of continued bone marrow production of excess protoporphyrin. Posttransplantation treatment with hemin and plasmapheresis may help prevent recurrence of this complication. Bone marrow transplantation, which has been successful in human EPP and has prevented liver disease in a mouse model, should be considered after the liver transplantation if a suitable donor can be found.

## X-LINKED PROTOPORPHYRIA (XLP)

*X-linked protoporphyria (XLP)*, an X-linked form of erythropoietic porphyria, was first described in 2008 (MIM no. 300752). This disease results from gain-of-function mutations in the erythroid-specific ALA-synthase 2 (*ALAS2*) gene that increase the activity of ALA-synthase 2 approximately 2- to 3-fold, thereby increasing heme biosynthesis and resulting in the accumulation of protoporphyrin IX in erythroid cells, plasma, and vascular endothelium. Analogous to the erythroid release of protoporphyrin into the circulation and deposition in the skin vasculature, exposure to sunlight triggers activation of protoporphyrin.

### CLINICAL FEATURES

The clinical manifestations in affected males resemble those of patients with EPP. Manifestations in heterozygous females range from clinically asymptomatic to as severe as those in affected males, depending on the extent of random X chromosome inactivation.

### DIAGNOSIS

Patients with typical EPP manifestations who do not have a *FECH* mutation should be tested for *ALAS2* mutations, which cause XLP.

### TREATMENT

The treatment for XLP is the same as that for EPP.

## ACKNOWLEDGMENT

This work was supported in part by the Porphyrias Consortium (U54 DK083909), which is a part of the NCATS Rare Diseases Clinical Research Network (RDCRN). RDCRN is an initiative of the Office of Rare Diseases Research (ORDR), NCATS, funded through a collaboration between NCATS and the National Institute of Diabetes and Digestive and Kidney Diseases. M.B. is supported in part by the National Institutes of Health Career Development Award (K23 DK095946).

### SUGGESTED READINGS

Anderson KE, Bloomer JR, Bonkovsky HL, et al. Recommendations for the diagnosis and treatment of the acute porphyrias. *Am Intern Med.* 2005;142:439-450.

Anderson KE, Sassa S, Bishop D, Desnick RJ. Disorders of heme-biosynthesis; X-linked sideroblastic anemia and the porphyrias. In: Valle D, Beaudet AL, Vogelstein B, et al, eds. *The Metabolic and Molecular Bases of Inherited Disease.* 8th ed. New York, NY: McGraw-Hill; 2014.

Balwani M, Desnick RJ. The porphyrias: advances in diagnosis and treatment. *Blood.* 2012;120:4496-4504.

Balwani M, Doheny D, Bishop DF, et al. Loss-of-function ferrochelatase and gain-of-function erythroid-specific 5-aminolevulinate synthase mutations causing erythropoietic protoporphyria and X-linked protoporphyria in North American patients reveal novel mutations and a high prevalence of X-linked protoporphyria. *Molec Med.* 2013;19:26-35.

Biolcati G, Marchesini E, Sorge F, et al. Long-term observational study of afamelanotide in 115 patients with erythropoietic protoporphyria. *Br J Dermatol.* 2015;172:1601-1612.

Bonkovsky HL, Maddukuri VC, Yazici C, et al. Acute porphyrias in the USA: features of 108 subjects from Porphyrias Consortium. *Am J Med.* 2014;127:1233-1241.

Desnick RJ, Astrin KH. Congenital erythropoietic porphyria: advances in pathogenesis and treatment. *Br J Haematol.* 2002;117:779-795.

Langendonk JG, Balwani M, Anderson KE, et al. Afamelanotide for erythropoietic protoporphyria. *N Engl J Med.* 2015;373:48-59.

Phillips JD, Bergonia HA, Reilly CA, et al. A porphomethene inhibitor of uroporphyrinogen decarboxylase causes porphyria cutanea tarda. *Proc Natl Acad Sci USA.* 2007;104:5079-5084.

Puy H, Gouya L, Deybach JC. Porphyrias. *Lancet.* 2010;375:924-937.

Solis C, Martinez-Bermejo A, Naidich TP, et al. Acute intermittent porphyria: studies of the severe homozygous dominant disease provides insights into the neurologic attacks in acute porphyrias. *Arch Neurol.* 2004;61:1764-1770.

Yasuda M, Erwin AL, Liu LU, et al. Liver transplantation for acute intermittent porphyria: biochemical and pathologic studies of the explanted liver. *Molec Med.* 2015;21:487-495.

# 163 Disorders of Purine and Pyrimidine Metabolism

Ayman W. El-Hattab and Fernando Scaglia

### INTRODUCTION

Purines (adenine and guanine) and pyrimidines (thymine, cytosine, and uracil) are nitrogenous bases that are essential components of nucleotides. The addition of pentose monosaccharide (ribose or deoxyribose) to a base results in a nucleoside, which can be a ribonucleoside (adenosine, guanosine, cytidine, and uridine) or a deoxyribonucleoside (deoxyadenosine, deoxyguanosine, deoxycytidine, and thymidine). Nucleotides result from the binding of nucleosides to phosphate. The binding of a nucleoside to 1, 2, or 3 phosphate groups produces nucleoside mono-, di-, or triphosphate, respectively. Nucleotides are essential for all cells. In addition to their vital role as building blocks for DNA and RNA, they serve as carriers of activated intermediates in the synthesis of a variety of complex molecules, structural components of several essential coenzymes, messengers in signal transduction pathways, regulatory components for many of the metabolic pathways, and currency for energy transfer in cells.

Purine and pyrimidine bases are synthesized de novo or can be obtained through salvage pathways that allow the reuse of bases provided by food or normal cell turnover. The degradation of purine and pyrimidine occurs through catabolic pathways (Figs. 163-1 and 163-2). Disorders of purine and pyrimidine metabolism result from defects in any of the 3 metabolic processes: de novo synthesis, salvage pathways, and catabolism.

## DISORDERS OF PURINE METABOLISM

The de novo biosynthetic pathway of purines starts with ribose phosphate that is first converted to phosphoribosylpyrophosphate (PRPP) by the action of phosphoribosylpyrophosphate synthetase (PRPS), which is necessary for both the de novo and salvage pathways of purine and pyrimidine biosynthesis. PRPP then passes through a number of enzymatic reactions to synthesize inosine monophosphate (IMP), which is then converted to adenosine monophosphate (AMP) or guanosine monophosphate (GMP). There are 10 enzymatic steps in de novo purine synthesis to generate IMP carried out by 6 distinct enzymes, and these assemble into a multiprotein complex termed the purinosome in response to a need for purines. Because the metabolite intermediates in the biosynthetic process have significant biologic properties, there is tight regulation of purine synthesis. Adenylosuccinate lyase deficiency (Mendelian Inheritance in Man [MIM] no. 103050) and AICA-ribosiduria (MIM no. 608688) are severe neurologic defects in this pathway, with the latter due to AICAR transformylase/IMP cyclohydrolase (ATIC) deficiency.

The purine salvage pathway utilizes the purine bases adenine, guanine, and hypoxanthine and reconverts them to AMP, GMP, and IMP, respectively. Defects in this pathway include hypoxanthine-guanine phosphoribosyl transferase (HPRT) deficiency (Lesch-Nyhan syndrome), adenine phosphoribosyl transferase (APRT) deficiency, and deoxyguanosine kinase (DGK) deficiency.

The catabolic pathway allows the breakdown of AMP, GMP, and IMP to uric acid. Disorders of purine catabolism include muscle adenosine monophosphate deaminase (AMPD) deficiency, adenosine deaminase (ADA) deficiency, purine nucleoside phosphorylase (PNP) deficiency, and xanthine oxidase deficiency (see Fig. 163-1).

## PHOSPHORIBOSYLPYROPHOSPHATE SYNTHETASE DEFICIENCY

While PRPP is necessary for both pyrimidine and purine metabolism, the clinical problems associated with PRPP synthetase deficiency appear to be due to reduced purine and, in particular, reduced guanosine triphosphate (GTP) production. Although PRPP is a substrate necessary for pyrimidine metabolism, pyrimidine nucleotides would not be expected to be affected as severely as purine nucleotides because, unlike for purine salvage, PRPP is not essential for pyrimidine salvage. The gene encoding PRPS is on the X chromosome; hence, most patients are typically male, but affected females are also observed. Three distinct but clinically overlapping conditions have been described due to loss of PRPS activity: X-linked Charcot-Marie-Tooth disease-5 (CMTX5; MIM no. 311070), Arts syndrome (MIM no. 301835), and isolated X-linked sensorineural deafness (DFNX1; MIM no. 304500). A fourth condition associated with increased PRPS activity (superactivity) is associated with purine overproduction and hyperuricemia leading to gout, along with neurodevelopmental problems and hearing loss. The cause of the superactivity is loss of allosteric feedback inhibition of the enzyme.

### CLINICAL PRESENTATION

Charcot-Marie-Tooth disease-5 exhibits early-onset hearing loss, lower leg weakness and atrophy beginning in childhood, and progressive loss of vision associated with optic atrophy, although the latter finding is variable; progressive retinitis pigmentosa may occur in some cases. Electrophysiologic studies demonstrate a sensorimotor peripheral neuropathy. Females may be similarly affected depending on the degree of skewing of X-inactivation. Neurocognitive development is intact in most patients. Hypouricemia is observed, and creatine kinase may be elevated.

Arts syndrome is characterized by intellectual disability, hypotonia, early-onset ataxia, delayed motor development, hearing loss, optic atrophy, and susceptibility to respiratory tract infections. Nerve conduction studies may show an axonal sensorimotor neuropathy, consistent with CMTX5, reflecting the overlapping clinical features.

Isolated X-linked sensorineural deafness may manifest as congenital profound sensorineural hearing loss in males, with female carriers exhibiting a mild to moderate hearing loss. Other families have been described with an older age of onset of hearing loss in males and symmetric or asymmetric hearing loss in adult females.

### DIAGNOSIS

The diagnosis is suggested by the finding of low serum uric acid and a family pedigree suggestive of X-linked inheritance. Other purines and pyrimidines may be normal, although hypoxanthine can be similarly reduced. PRPS activity can be measured in any number of cell types, including erythrocytes and fibroblasts, and DNA sequencing of the *PRPS1* gene is available.

### TREATMENT

There is no specific intervention other than supportive care. It has been proposed that purine deficiency can be ameliorated by provision of *S*-adenosylmethionine (SAM) since SAM is readily absorbed and can be hydrolyzed to adenosine, which can subsequently be salvaged.

## ADENYLOSUCCINATE LYASE AND AICAR TRANSFORMYLASE/IMP CYCLOHYDROLASE DEFICIENCY

Adenylosuccinate lyase (adenylosuccinase; ADSL) catalyzes 2 steps in purine nucleotide synthesis: the conversion of succinylaminoimidazole carboxamide ribotide (SAICAR) into aminoimidazole carboxamide ribotide (AICAR) and the formation of AMP from adenylosuccinate (S-AMP) (see Fig. 163-1). ADSL deficiency is an autosomal recessive disease that results in loss of the conversion of the substrates AICAR and S-AMP to the 2 succinylpurines succinylaminoimidazole carboxamide (SAICA) riboside and succinyladenosine, respectively. The accumulation of these succinylpurines is believed to have toxic effects, particularly on the nervous system, although the exact disease mechanism is unknown. The incidence of ADSL deficiency is not known. It has been reported in approximately 80 individuals.

### CLINICAL PRESENTATION

ADSL deficiency (MIM no. 103050) is associated with a broad clinical spectrum of variable severity and an age of onset ranging from prenatal to childhood. The severity ranges from prenatal onset, a fatal neonatal form, a severe form (type I), to a mild to moderate form (type II). Prenatal manifestations include impaired intrauterine growth, microcephaly, and fetal hypokinesia. The fatal neonatal presentation is characterized by encephalopathy, severe hypotonia and weakness, intractable seizures, and respiratory failure. The severe childhood presentation (type I) is the most common phenotype and is typically associated with moderate to severe psychomotor retardation, epilepsy

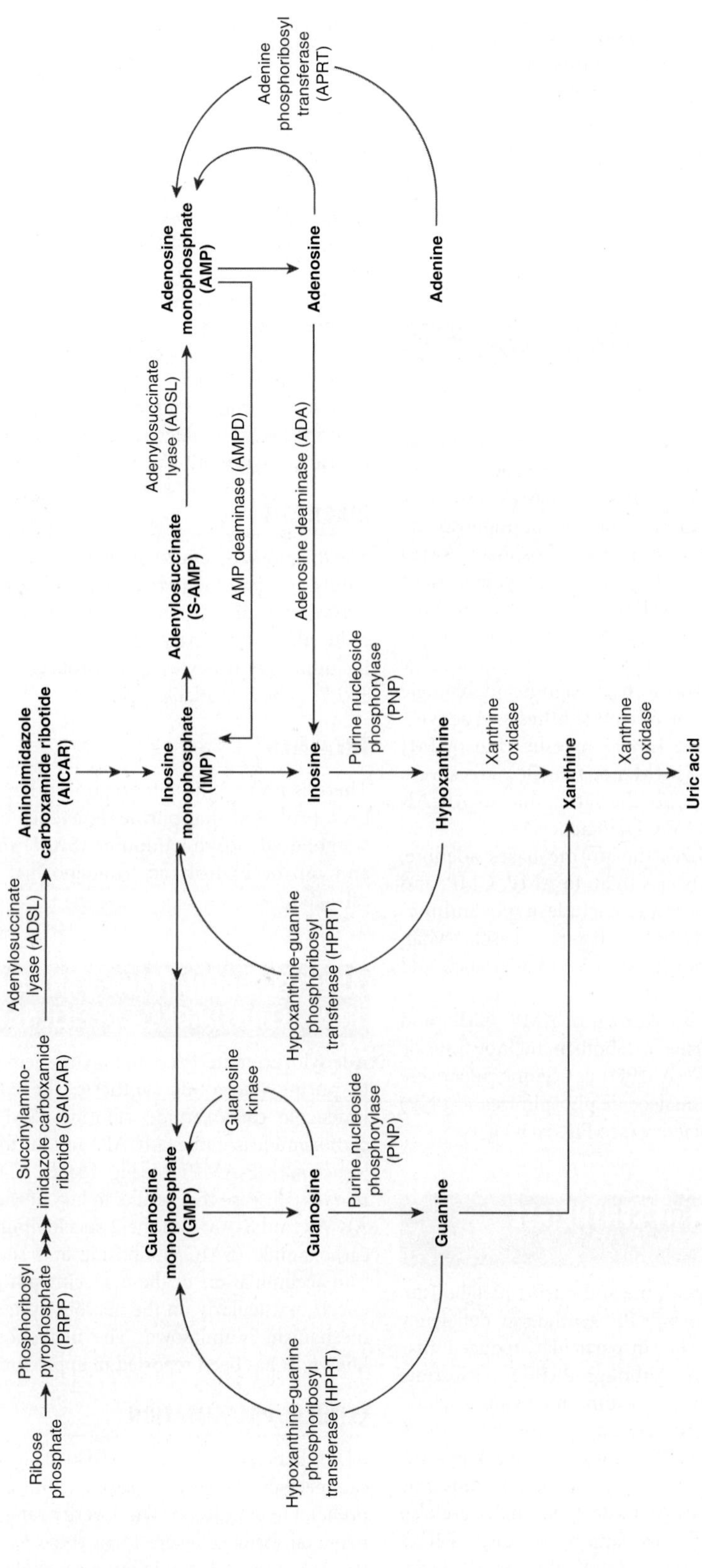


**FIGURE 163-1** Purine metabolic pathways.

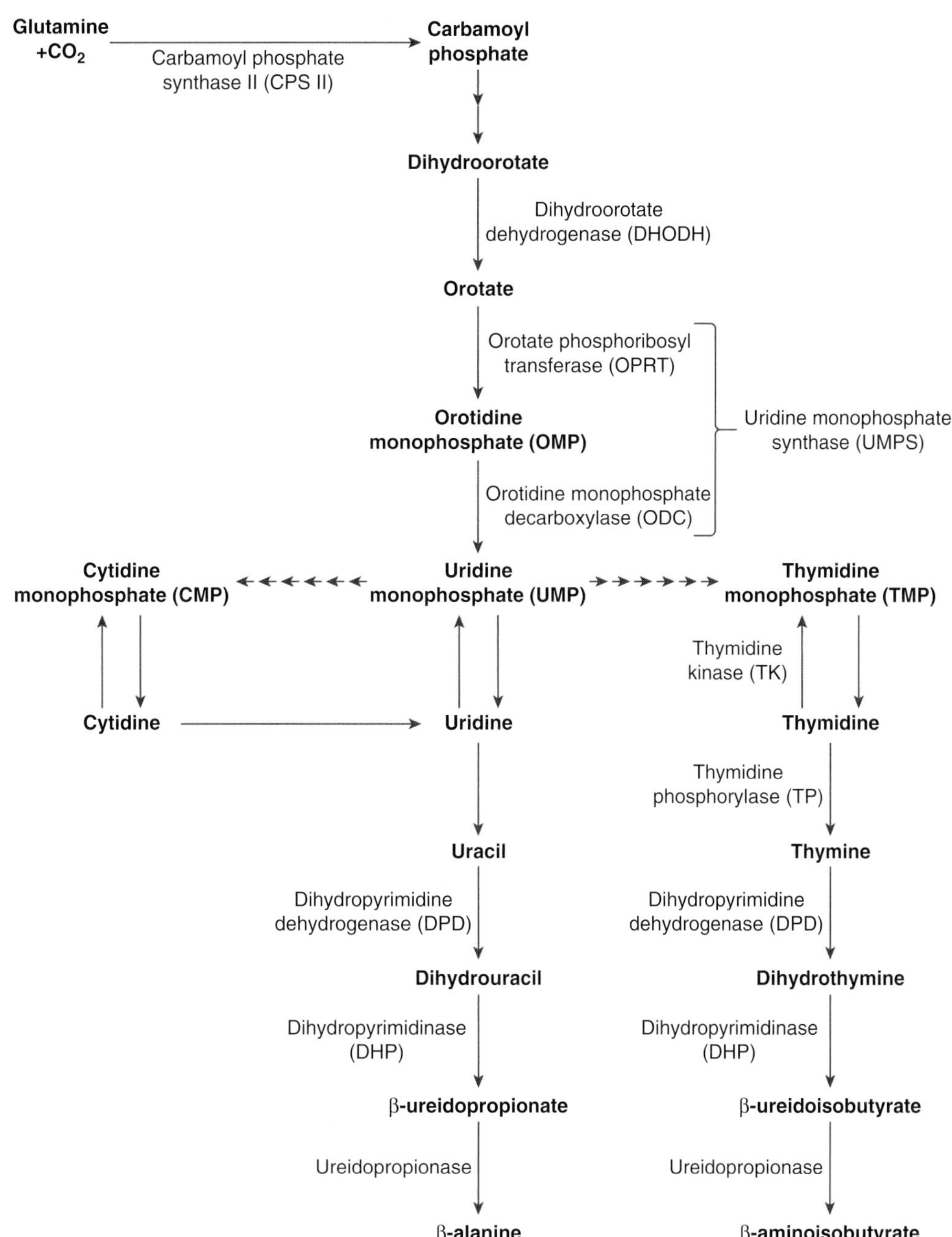


**FIGURE 163-2** Pyrimidine metabolic pathways.



starting after the first year, muscular hypotonia and wasting, feeding difficulties, growth failure, microcephaly, and various behavioral disturbances including autistic features, agitation, temper tantrums, and self-mutilation. Children with the milder form (type II) can present with mild to moderate psychomotor retardation, hypotonia, ataxia, and autistic features. Neuroimaging often shows brain atrophy, hypomyelination, and atrophy of the cerebellum, particularly of the vermis.

## DIAGNOSIS

In ADSL deficiency, the succinylpurines SAICA riboside and succinyladenosine accumulate in urine, cerebrospinal fluid (CSF), and to a minor extent plasma. The marked clinical heterogeneity of ADSL deficiency justifies systematic screening for the disorder in unexplained psychomotor delay, particularly when accompanied by behavioral problems, and in neurologic diseases with convulsions or hypotonia. The diagnosis is based on the presence of SAICA riboside and succinyladenosine in urine and CSF, which are normally undetectable. A diagnosis can be confirmed by measuring the ADSL enzyme activity in liver, kidney, blood lymphocytes, or cultured fibroblasts or by molecular sequencing of the *ADSL* gene encoding the ADSL enzyme.

## TREATMENT AND PROGNOSIS

The treatment is largely symptomatic, and there is no effective treatment available for the metabolic disease. The prognosis for survival of children with ADSL deficiency varies greatly. Those with the fatal neonatal presentation typically die within the first months of life, whereas those with the mild form (type II) can reach adult age. In children with the severe presentation (type I), further evolution is characterized by absent or minimal progression of psychomotor development and persistence of autistic behavior.

AICA-ribosiduria (MIM no. 608688) is a more recently described disorder identified in a single case and caused by a defect in the final steps of purine de novo biosynthesis of AICAR-transformylase/IMP-cyclohydrolase (ATIC). The single case was a 4-year-old who exhibited dysmorphic features, epilepsy, severe developmental delay, and congenital blindness. ATIC is a bifunctional enzyme; AICAR-TF catalyzes the transformylation of AICAR and 10-formyl-tetrahydrofolate to produce formyl-AICAR (FAICAR) and tetrahydrofolate, while the IMP cyclohydrolase (IMP-CH) moiety cyclizes FAICAR to IMP. The C-terminal domain of the protein is responsible for the AICAR-TF activity, whereas the IMP-CH activity resides in the N-terminal domain. The condition is inherited in an autosomal recessive manner, and no specific therapies are currently available.

## HYPOXANTHINE-GUANINE PHOSPHORIBOSYL TRANSFERASE DEFICIENCY (LESCH-NYHAN SYNDROME)

Hypoxanthine-guanine phosphoribosyl transferase (HPRT) uses PRPP as a source of ribose phosphate to be transferred to hypoxanthine resulting in IMP and to guanine resulting in GMP (see Fig. 163-1). HPRT deficiency results in the X-linked recessive disease termed Lesch-Nyhan syndrome (MIM no. 300322). The deficiency of HPRT results in the accumulation of its substrates (hypoxanthine, guanine, and their product xanthine) and of PRPP and depletion of its products (GMP and the other guanine nucleotides and IMP). The accumulation of PRPP leads to an enhancement of the purine synthesis rate and excessive production of uric acid. The pathogenesis of the neurologic symptoms of Lesch-Nyhan syndrome is still not fully understood. However, a number of studies showed abnormalities of the dopaminergic neurotransmitter system in this disease. Autopsy studies showed a reduction in the basal ganglia of dopamine and tyrosine hydroxylase, the dopamine synthetizing tetrahydrobiopterin-dependent enzyme. Whereas positron emission tomography studies of the brains of subjects with Lesch-Nyhan syndrome have revealed large reductions in dopaminergic terminals not only in the basal ganglia but also in other brain areas, depletion of guanine or adenine nucleotides is proposed as an explanation for the neurologic complications of HPRT deficiency. ATP depletion might result in impairment of energy production, DNA repair, and metabolic defense against oxidant stress. GTP depletion has been proposed to interfere with the function of G proteins and the formation of tetrahydrobiopterin. The prevalence of Lesch-Nyhan syndrome is approximately 1:380,000. It appears to occur in all populations with relatively equal frequency.



### CLINICAL PRESENTATION

Lesch-Nyhan syndrome is an X-linked disorder that affects males and is characterized by neurologic dysfunction, behavioral disturbances, cognitive impairment, and uric acid overproduction.

Children with Lesch-Nyhan syndrome typically have a normal prenatal and perinatal course and appear entirely normal at birth. Most infants show normal development during the first 3 to 6 months of life. The most common presenting feature is developmental delay during the first year of life, with hypotonia and delayed motor skills usually evident by age 3 to 6 months. Within the first few years of life, abnormal involuntary extrapyramidal movements emerge, including dystonia, choreoathetosis, opisthotonos, and sometimes ballismus. They also develop signs of pyramidal involvement including an increase in muscle tone, spasticity, hyperreflexia, sustained ankle clonus, scissoring of the lower extremities, and extensor plantar reflexes. The neurologic picture closely resembles athetoid cerebral palsy. Therefore, many affected children may initially be diagnosed as having cerebral palsy. The motor disability is so severe that virtually all children with Lesch-Nyhan syndrome never walk and are confined to a wheelchair. An increased incidence of dislocation of the hips and club feet may be related to the early hypotonia. About half of affected individuals have seizures.

Almost all affected individuals eventually develop persistent self-injurious behavior, a hallmark of the disease. Some children develop self-injurious behavior during the first year of life, most develop it between ages 2 and 3 years, and some have delayed presentation of these behaviors until early adolescence. Self-injury most often involves biting of the lips, tongue, cheeks, fingers, and hands. Biting can be highly variable, with affected children going through periods when they show extensive self-mutilation and other periods when this is no longer a problem. Self-injurious behavior tends to be correlated, at least in some cases, with emotional stress. In addition, some older children develop opisthotonic spasms, laryngeal spasm, and stridor that sometimes produces a temporary cyanosis. Others bang their heads or limbs against hard objects, throw themselves from the bed, or injure themselves on sharp edges of wheelchairs that are left unpadded. Other compulsive behaviors may include aggressiveness, vomiting, and coprolalia. Aggressive acts against others can take the form of biting, hitting, spitting, or kicking.

Affected children may have attention deficits. Most affected individuals are cognitively impaired, although cognitive function is difficult to assess because of the behavioral disturbances, motor deficits, and attentional problems. Nonverbal intelligence can be preserved, and some affected individuals display normal intelligence.

The overproduction of uric acid is present at birth. Overproduction of uric acid may lead to deposition of uric acid crystals, sodium urate, or calculi in the kidneys, ureters, or bladder. Crystals appear as an orange sandy material; calculi may be multiple tiny stones or discrete large stones that are difficult to pass. The stones may cause hematuria and increase the risk for urinary tract infections. Stones may be the presenting feature of the disease, but often go unrecognized for months or years. During early infancy, the first indication of the disease may be the presence of brownish to red-orange sand in the diapers, particularly when the baby becomes dehydrated. Some of the infants are very irritable, with episodes of screaming, suggesting the possibility of renal colic. Another potential consequence of untreated hyperuricemia is gouty arthritis caused by uric acid crystal deposition in articular cartilage. Gout is uncommon in children with Lesch-Nyhan syndrome and typically develops long after other symptoms present.

Other manifestations include growth and puberty delays, testicular atrophy in affected males, megaloblastic anemia, electroencephalogram changes with slowing or disorganization, and brain atrophy with reduced cerebral volume and reduced caudate nucleus volume in neuroimaging. End-stage renal disease, which prior to the availability of allopurinol was the rule in this disease, is less common now but still occurs.

Partial HPRT deficiency has rarely been reported in individuals with gout. Most of those affected have a normal neurologic examination, but occasionally, spasticity, dysarthria, and a spinocerebellar syndrome are found. Whereas most subjects with Lesch-Nyhan syndrome do not develop gouty arthritis, this finding is common in partial HPRT deficiency. Partial HPRT deficiency can also present with isolated dystonia, mild cognitive impairment, and behavioral problems.

Although female carriers are generally asymptomatic, they may have increased uric acid excretion, and some may develop symptoms of hyperuricemia in later years. A few females with Lesch-Nyhan syndrome were reported. These females had nonrandom X chromosome inactivation (skewed inactivation) resulting in the inactivation of the X chromosome carrying the normal allele.

### DIAGNOSIS

Affected children excrete excessive amounts of uric acid, ranging from 25 to 140 mg (normal < 18 mg/kg/24 h) or 0.15 to 0.85 mmol/kg/24 h (normal 0.1 mmol/kg/24 h). Determination of the ratio of uric acid to creatinine (mg/mg) in morning samples of urine provides a screening test. This ratio is much higher in affected children when compared to the normal upper limit of 2.5, 2.0, 1.0, and 0.6 for infants, 2-year-old children, 10-year-old children, and adults, respectively. Increased ratios are also found in other disorders with uric acid overproduction, including glycogen storage disease type I and lymphoproliferative diseases. The overproduction of uric acid is generally accompanied by an increase of serum uric acid. However, a normal uric acid level does not exclude Lesch-Nyhan syndrome because around 5% to 10% may have uric acid in the normal or high-normal range, particularly before puberty. Female carriers may have elevated uric acid excretion. Hypoxanthine and xanthine are also elevated in body fluids of affected individuals. Measuring HPRT enzyme activity can be performed in erythrocytes or skin fibroblasts. Individuals with Lesch-Nyhan syndrome display absent or nearly undetectable HPRT activity. In partial deficiencies, similar low or higher values may be found. Molecular confirmation requires DNA sequencing of the *HPRT1* gene.

### TREATMENT AND PROGNOSIS

Treatment comprises controlling uric acid overproduction and the neurobehavioral manifestations. The overproduction of uric acid must be reduced to lower the risk for nephrolithiasis, urate nephropathy, and gouty arthritis. Overproduction of uric acid can be controlled with allopurinol, which blocks the conversion of hypoxanthine and xanthine into uric acid catalyzed by xanthine oxidase. The dose of allopurinol is adjusted to maintain the uric acid level within normal limits and can approach 20 mg/kg/d if needed. Allopurinol therapy results in the accumulation of hypoxanthine and xanthine; xanthine may also form stones. Therefore, affected individuals need to take in enough fluids to avoid periods of relative dehydration. This higher intake will diminish the occurrence of urinary concretions composed of xanthine that have been noted occasionally in children treated with allopurinol. Renal stones that form despite allopurinol may require lithotripsy or surgery. Unfortunately, control of the serum concentration of uric acid even from birth using allopurinol has no effect on behavioral and neurologic symptoms.

There is no uniformly effective intervention for managing the neurobehavioral aspects of the disease. Self-injurious and other deleterious behaviors are best managed by a combination of physical, behavioral, and medical interventions. To prevent self-injury, all affected individuals require physical restraints. Affected individuals should be made more comfortable by appropriate restraints. Hands can be kept away from the mouth and yet be left free for use by constructing loose-fitting wraparound fabric splints for the elbows. Lip guards and occasionally tooth extraction are needed to avoid self-injury through biting. Although children with the Lesch-Nyhan syndrome seem to be incapable of learning from punishment, they do respond to positive experiences. Partial improvement in self-mutilation has also been reported from using both positive and negative conditioning programs. Despite trials with a variety of agents, no successful pharmacologic treatment for the neurobehavioral manifestations has yet been found. Baclofen or benzodiazepines can improve spasticity, and haloperidol and barbiturates may sometimes improve choreoathetosis. Adequate nutrition should also be prescribed, since many of these children take a very long time to eat and may develop malnutrition.

If management of symptoms is effective, most individuals survive into the second or third decade of life. There may be slow progression of disease in adulthood. Sudden death is increasingly being recognized. Sudden death appears to be more common in older individuals, often with no discernable cause. Respiratory abnormalities have been implicated, and forceful opisthotonos may result in atlantoaxial subluxation, leading to sudden death.

## ADENINE PHOSPHORIBOSYL TRANSFERASE DEFICIENCY

Adenine phosphoribosyl transferase (APRT) uses PRPP as a source of ribose phosphate to be transferred to adenine, resulting in AMP (Fig. 163-1). APRT deficiency (MIM no. 614723) is an autosomal recessive disease resulting from the loss of adenine salvage. Consequently, adenine is oxidized by xanthine oxidase into dihydroxyadenine, which is very poorly soluble, and symptoms are caused by the urinary precipitation of this compound. Approximately 300 individuals have been diagnosed worldwide.

### CLINICAL PRESENTATION

Approximately half of individuals with APRT deficiency are asymptomatic. The deficiency may clinically manifest in childhood, even from birth, but may also remain silent for several decades. Symptoms include urinary passage of gravel, small stones, and crystals, frequently accompanied by abdominal colic, dysuria, hematuria, and urinary tract infections. Some affected individuals may present with acute anuric renal failure, while others may develop chronic renal failure requiring dialysis and transplantation. The urinary precipitates are composed of dihydroxyadenine, which can form radiotranslucent stones.



### DIAGNOSIS

The presence of brownish spots on diapers or the finding of round, brownish crystals in urine under a light microscope suggests the presence of dihydroxyadenine. APRT enzyme activity can be measured in erythrocytes. Molecular confirmation can be obtained by DNA sequencing of the *APRT* gene.

### TREATMENT AND PROGNOSIS

In symptomatic individuals, allopurinol can be used to inhibit the formation of dihydroxyadenine. In addition, dietary purine restriction and a high fluid intake are recommended for both symptomatic and asymptomatic individuals. The ultimate prognosis depends on renal function at the time of diagnosis. Late recognition may result in irreversible renal insufficiency requiring chronic dialysis, whereas early treatment may result in prevention of stones. Kidney transplantation has been followed by recurrence of microcrystalline deposits and subsequent loss of graft function.

## DEOXYGUANOSINE KINASE DEFICIENCY

Guanosine kinase converts guanosine to GMP. Deoxyguanosine kinase (DGK) converts the deoxy- form of guanosine to deoxy-GMP. DGK is a mitochondrial enzyme that plays an essential role in supplying nucleotide precursors through a salvage pathway. The synthesis of mitochondrial DNA (mtDNA), which is continuous throughout the cell cycle, is heavily dependent on the salvage pathway for the supply of deoxynucleotides. Therefore, deficiency of DGK results in depletion of DNA building blocks in mitochondria, leading to decreased levels of mtDNA (mtDNA depletion). DGK deficiency (MIM no. 251880) results in a hepatocerebral mtDNA depletion syndrome termed mtDNA depletion syndrome-3, which is an autosomal recessive disease that has been reported in over 100 individuals.

### CLINICAL PRESENTATION

DGK-related hepatocerebral mtDNA depletion syndrome mainly presents in 2 forms: multiorgan disease in neonates and isolated hepatic disease later in infancy or childhood. The majority of affected individuals have a neonatal-onset multiorgan illness that presents with lactic acidosis and hypoglycemia in the first week of life. Within weeks of birth, infants develop hepatic disease and neurologic dysfunction. Severe myopathy, developmental regression, and a typical rotary nystagmus evolving into opsoclonus are also seen. Cholestasis is prominent early in the clinical course. Liver involvement may cause neonatal- or infantile-onset liver failure that is generally progressive with ascites, edema, and coagulopathy. A minority of affected individuals present initially in infancy or childhood with isolated hepatic disease, occasionally following a viral illness. Affected individuals with this later onset form may develop mild hypotonia and renal involvement manifesting as proteinuria and aminoaciduria. Other rare manifestations include neonatal hemochromatosis with liver mtDNA depletion, adult-onset myopathy with mtDNA multiple deletions in skeletal muscle, and infantile- or childhood-onset noncirrhotic portal hypertension.

### DIAGNOSIS

The majority of affected newborns with the multiorgan form of the disease exhibit an elevated serum concentration of tyrosine or phenylalanine on the newborn screening. Findings of intrahepatic cholestasis typically include elevations in serum concentrations of liver transaminases, gamma-glutamyltransferase (GGT), and conjugated hyperbilirubinemia. An increased serum concentration of ferritin is observed in a large number of affected infants. Lactic acidosis and hypoglycemia are common findings. Electron transport chain (ETC) activity in liver typically shows a combined deficiency of complexes I, III, and IV, with preservation of complex II activity due to the fact that only complex II contains no mtDNA-encoded proteins. Liver histopathology typically reveals microvesicular cholestasis, but may show bridging fibrosis, giant cell hepatitis, or cirrhosis. Liver electron microscopy may reveal an increase in the number of mitochondria and is commonly associated with abnormal cristae. The diagnosis of mtDNA depletion is confirmed by demonstrating reduced mtDNA content in liver and muscle. The molecular confirmation of DGK deficiency is based on DNA sequencing of the *DGUOK* gene.

### TREATMENT AND PROGNOSIS

Treatment is largely supportive. Hepatic dysfunction is progressive in the majority of individuals with both forms of DGK-related hepatocerebral mtDNA depletion syndrome and is the most common cause of death. Hepatocellular carcinoma is also a potential complication in long-term survivors. To date, survival after liver transplantation has been low, and the benefits of liver transplantation are controversial because of the often severe neurologic involvement.



## MUSCLE ADENOSINE MONOPHOSPHATE DEAMINASE DEFICIENCY

AMP deaminase (AMPD) catalyzes the conversion of AMP into IMP and ammonia (see Fig. 163-1). Muscle, liver, and erythrocytes contain different isoforms of AMPD. The muscle AMPD isoform, also called myoadenylate deaminase, is closely associated with the contractile apparatus and is nearly inactive in resting muscle but becomes highly active during contraction. Muscle AMPD is important for energy production during muscle contraction as the conversion of AMP to IMP helps in removing AMP formed during exercise to favor the regeneration of ATP from ADP and in releasing IMP, which stimulates glycolysis and hence energy production. Myoadenylate deaminase deficiency (MIM no. 615511) is an autosomal recessive disease that has been found in 1% to 2% of the Caucasian population, but most enzyme-deficient individuals are asymptomatic. It has been suggested that the muscle dysfunction observed in myoadenylate deaminase deficiency is caused by impairment of energy production required for muscle contraction. However, the identification of numerous asymptomatic individuals with this deficiency suggests that deficiency might have a synergistic effect in association with other disorders, and the myoadenylate deaminase deficiency in and by itself may not necessarily cause disease.

### CLINICAL PRESENTATION

As stated, most individuals with myoadenylate deaminase deficiency are asymptomatic. When symptomatic, the disease typically presents in early adulthood, but onset can range from infancy to late adulthood. Typical manifestations include muscle weakness, fatigue, cramps, or myalgia following moderate to vigorous exercise, sometimes accompanied by an increase in serum creatine kinase and minor electromyographic abnormalities. Rhabdomyolysis and myoglobinuria may also occur. Muscular wasting and histologic abnormalities are usually absent. Other less frequent manifestations include hypotonia and cardiomyopathy. In addition to the primary enzyme deficiency, secondary myoadenylate deaminase deficiency has been reported in several neuromuscular disorders, including amyotrophic lateral sclerosis, facioscapulohumeral myopathy, Kugelberg-Welander syndrome, Werdnig-Hoffmann disease, and polyneuropathies.

### DIAGNOSIS

Screening for this disease can be performed by an exercise test in which the several-fold elevation of venous plasma ammonia recorded in normal subjects is absent in myoadenylate deaminase deficiency. In affected individuals, AMPD enzyme activity in muscle tissue is generally below 2% of normal. DNA sequencing of the *AMPD1* gene encoding the muscle AMPD is available for molecular confirmation.

### TREATMENT AND PROGNOSIS

Symptomatic individuals may display a gradual worsening of their symptoms, which may lead to marked debility. Patients should be advised to exercise with caution to prevent rhabdomyolysis and myoglobinuria. Administration of ribose (2–60 g/d orally in divided doses) has been reported to improve muscular strength and endurance in some patients. After ribose is converted into ribose phosphate, it could increase the synthesis of purine nucleotides, which could explain the improvement associated with its supplementation.

## ADENOSINE DEAMINASE DEFICIENCY

Adenosine deaminase (ADA) catalyzes the deamination of adenosine and deoxyadenosine (see Fig. 163-1). ADA deficiency (MIM no. 102700) is an autosomal recessive immune deficiency disease that results from the accumulation of adenosine, deoxyadenosine, and their derivatives, notably deoxy-ATP. These compounds induce the premature death of lymphoid progenitor cells, resulting in impairment of the generation of T cells, B cells, and NK lymphocytes. The disorder and its treatment are discussed in Chapter 184.

## PURINE NUCLEOSIDE PHOSPHORYLASE DEFICIENCY

Purine nucleoside phosphorylase (PNP) catalyzes the dephosphorylation of inosine, deoxyinosine, guanosine, and deoxyguanosine (see Fig. 163-1). PNP deficiency (MIM no. 613179) is an autosomal recessive immune deficiency disease that results from the accumulation of deoxy-GTP, formed from deoxyguanosine, which results in the inhibition of ribonucleotide reductase, the enzyme that catalyzes the formation of deoxyribonucleotides from ribonucleotides. This leads to an impairment of DNA synthesis and subsequent cell division. This enzyme is ubiquitously expressed, which may explain the presence of neurologic symptoms in about two-thirds of children with PNP deficiency.

## XANTHINE OXIDASE DEFICIENCY AND MOLYBDENUM COFACTOR DEFICIENCY

Xanthine oxidase (also called xanthine dehydrogenase or xanthine oxidoreductase) catalyzes the conversion of hypoxanthine into xanthine and xanthine into uric acid (see Fig. 163-1). It is composed of 2 subunits, each of which contains molybdenum cofactor. Xanthine oxidase deficiency (MIM no. 278300) is an autosomal recessive disease that results from the inability to convert hypoxanthine and xanthine into uric acid and is characterized by xanthinuria. Xanthinuria can be divided into xanthinuria type I and type II, with the former due to loss of xanthine oxidase activity and the latter due to loss of both xanthine oxidase and aldehyde oxidase activities (MIM no. 603592). The clinical features of these 2 disorders are very similar and are a consequence of xanthine accumulation. A distinguishing feature is that type I patients can metabolize allopurinol, whereas type II patients cannot. Xanthine has very limited solubility; therefore, when it accumulates, it forms renal stones and deposits in muscles leading to myositis. Xanthine oxidase deficiency can also occur in combination with the deficiency of the other molybdenum cofactor–dependent enzyme sulfite oxidase. The combined deficiency of xanthine oxidase and sulfite oxidase is caused by molybdenum cofactor deficiency, resulting from defects in molybdenum cofactor biosynthesis, whereas xanthinuria type II reflects a defect in molybdenum cofactor sulfurase (MOCOS). MOCOS specifically sulfurates the molybdenum cofactor of xanthine oxidase and aldehyde oxidase. Sulfite oxidase deficiency results in the accumulation of neurotoxic sulfite and other sulfur-containing metabolites.

### CLINICAL PRESENTATION

Individuals with xanthinuria can be completely asymptomatic, although in about one-third of the cases, kidney stones form. Most often, they are radiotranslucent, and they may appear at any age and cause a variety of symptoms, including hematuria, renal colic, and even acute renal failure. Myopathy with myalgia and stiffness may be present, caused by crystalline xanthine deposits in muscle and precipitated by strenuous exercise. In isolated sulfite oxidase or combined xanthine oxidase and sulfite oxidase deficiencies (molybdenum cofactor deficiency), the clinical picture of sulfite oxidase deficiency supersedes that of xanthine oxidase deficiency. The symptoms include neonatal hypotonia, feeding difficulties, intractable seizures, microcephaly, and severe psychomotor retardation.

### DIAGNOSIS

The deficiency of xanthine oxidase results in the near total replacement of uric acid by hypoxanthine and xanthine as the end products of purine catabolism. This alteration is clearly manifested in urine, in which uric acid is reduced and xanthine and hypoxanthine accumulate. In plasma, the uric acid concentration is also low and the xanthine concentration is high. However, plasma hypoxanthine is not elevated or is minimally elevated due to the efficient reutilization by HPRT. In combined xanthine oxidase and sulfite oxidase deficiency or in isolated sulfite oxidase deficiency, there is additional excessive excretion of sulfite and other sulfur-containing metabolites such as *S*-sulfocysteine, thiosulfate, and taurine. The accumulated sulfites react with homocysteine, leading to notably low plasma homocysteine. The enzymatic diagnosis of xanthine oxidase deficiency requires liver or small intestine mucosa, the only human tissues that normally contain substantial amounts of xanthine oxidase. Sulfite oxidase and the molybdenum cofactor can be assayed in liver and fibroblasts. A molecular diagnosis can be confirmed in xanthine oxidase deficiency by DNA sequencing of the *XDH* gene and in isolated sulfite oxidase deficiency by DNA sequencing of the *SUOX* gene. Molybdenum cofactor deficiency can be confirmed molecularly by sequencing the *MOCS1* (MIM no. 252150), *MOCS2* (MIM no. 252160), and *GPHN* (MIM no. 615501) genes encoding the enzymes of molybdenum cofactor biosynthesis. In a survey of 82 cases of molybdenum cofactor deficiency, the initial clinical presentation in 72% of patients was seizures, followed by poor feeding in 25%, and hypotonia in 11%. Mortality was approximately 50% in the cohort, with a median age of onset the first day of life and a median survival of 36 months.

### TREATMENT AND PROGNOSIS

Xanthine oxidase deficiency is mostly benign, but in order to prevent renal stones, a low-purine diet should be prescribed and fluid intake increased. The prognosis for combined xanthine oxidase and sulfite oxidase deficiency (molybdenum cofactor deficiency) and isolated sulfite oxidase deficiency is very poor. The treatment is largely symptomatic, and there is no effective treatment that affects the course of the disease. A sulfur amino acid–restricted diet does not appear to alter the course of disease. Although cPMP (cyclic pyranopterin monophosphate) is a promising investigational therapy for molybdenum cofactor deficiency caused by defects in *MOCS1*, which is required for the initial step of molybdenum cofactor synthesis catalyzing the conversion of GTP in cPMP, it remains unproven.

## DISORDERS OF PYRIMIDINE METABOLISM

The pyrimidine de novo biosynthetic pathway starts with the formation of carbamoyl phosphate by the cytosolic carbamoyl phosphate synthase (CPSII). This enzyme is different from mitochondrial CPSI, which catalyzes the first step of the urea cycle. Formation of carbamoyl phosphate is followed by the synthesis of the nucleoside monophosphates uridine monophosphate (UMP), cytidine monophosphate (CMP), their deoxy counterparts, and thymidine monophosphate (TMP). Disorders in this pathway include dihydroorotate dehydrogenase (DHODH) deficiency (Miller syndrome) and uridine monophosphate synthase (UMPS) deficiency (hereditary orotic aciduria). The pyrimidine salvage pathway converts cytidine, uridine, and thymidine into CMP, UMP, and TMP, respectively. A disorder of this salvage pathway is thymidine kinase 2 (TK2) deficiency. The pyrimidine catabolic pathway starts with CMP, UMP, and TMP, and yields β-alanine and β-aminoisobutyrate, which are converted into intermediates of the citric acid cycle. Disorders of this pathway include thymidine phosphorylase (TP) deficiency, dihydropyrimidine dehydrogenase (DPD) deficiency, dihydropyrimidinase (DHP) deficiency, and ureidopropionase deficiency (see Fig. 163-2).

## DIHYDROOROTATE DEHYDROGENASE DEFICIENCY (MILLER SYNDROME)

Dihydroorotate dehydrogenase (DHODH) converts dihydroorotate to orotic acid (see Fig. 163-2). DHODH deficiency results in a rare autosomal recessive multiple malformation disorder called Miller syndrome or postaxial acrofacial dysostosis. The mechanism by which DHODH deficiency causes Miller syndrome is unclear. This syndrome has been reported in about 30 cases.

### CLINICAL MANIFESTATIONS

Miller syndrome (MIM no. 263750) is characterized by postnatal growth retardation, cleft lip and palate, choanal atresia, eyelid coloboma, ectropion, distinctive facial features (downslanting palpebral fissure, malar hypoplasia, micrognathia, and cup-shaped low-set ears), limb defects (ulnar hypoplasia, radial hypoplasia, in-curving forearms, radioulnar synostosis, syndactyly, thumb hypoplasia, and absent fifth finger and toe), other skeletal deformities (rib defects, pectus excavatum, supernumerary vertebrae, and congenital hip dislocation), gastrointestinal abnormalities (pyloric stenosis and midgut malrotation), genital defects (micropenis and cryptorchidism), renal malformation, accessory nipples, conical teeth, and hearing impairment.

### DIAGNOSIS

The clinical diagnosis of Miller syndrome is based on the constellation of the clinical features listed above. A molecular diagnosis is achieved by sequencing the *DHODH* gene.

### TREATMENT

Treatment is symptomatic and aims to correct the malformations. Affected children typically have normal intelligence.

## URIDINE MONOPHOSPHATE SYNTHASE DEFICIENCY (OROTIC ACIDURIA)

UMP synthase (UMPS) is a bifunctional enzyme that catalyzes 2 reactions in pyrimidine biosynthesis. In the first, orotate phosphoribosyl transferase (OPRT) converts orotate to orotidine monophosphate (OMP). In the second reaction, OMP decarboxylase (ODC) converts OMP to UMP (see Fig. 163-2). UMP synthase deficiency results in accumulation of orotic acid and impaired synthesis of pyrimidine nucleotides. The deficiency of pyrimidine nucleotides leads to abnormal cell division, which results in megaloblastic anemia and growth failure. Orotic aciduria (MIM no. 258900) is a rare autosomal recessive disease that has been reported in about 20 cases.

### CLINICAL MANIFESTATIONS

The first manifestation of orotic aciduria is usually megaloblastic anemia, which appears a few weeks or months after birth. Anisocytosis, poikilocytosis, and hypochromia are often seen in the blood smear. Bone marrow examination reveals erythroid hyperplasia and numerous megaloblastic erythroid precursors. The anemia does not respond to folic acid or vitamin $B_{12}$. T-cell dysfunction can be seen in some affected children. Failure to thrive and growth failure occur, and psychomotor development is delayed in some.

### DIAGNOSIS

Orotic acid is massively excreted in urine. Occasionally orotic acid crystalluria is observed. The enzyme activity can be assessed in erythrocytes. The diagnosis can be confirmed by DNA sequencing of the *UMPS* gene.

### TREATMENT AND PROGNOSIS

The enzyme defect can be bypassed by the administration of uridine, which is converted to UMP by uridine kinase. An initial dose of 100 to 150 mg/kg/d induces a prompt hematologic response and acceleration of growth. The dosage should then be adjusted to obtain the lowest possible level of orotic acid. In some cases, normal psychomotor development has been achieved, but not in others, possibly owing to delayed onset of therapy. Recently, uridine triacetate has been approved by the US Food and Drug Administration (FDA) to treat orotic aciduria. The recommended starting dosage is 60 mg/kg once daily, and the dose can be increased to 120 mg/kg once daily if urine orotic acid levels increase or remain above normal or for worsening disease.

## THYMIDINE KINASE 2 DEFICIENCY

Thymidine kinase 2 (TK2) is a mitochondrial deoxyribonucleoside kinase that phosphorylates thymidine, deoxycytidine, and deoxyuridine into TMP, deoxy-CMP, and deoxy-UMP, respectively (see Fig. 163-2). This enzyme is essential in the supply of nucleotide precursors for mitochondrial DNA synthesis. TK2 deficiency (MIM no. 609560) results in a myopathic mtDNA depletion syndrome termed mtDNA depletion syndrome-2, which is an autosomal recessive disease that has been reported in approximately 60 individuals.

### CLINICAL PRESENTATION

The clinical presentation of TK2-related mtDNA depletion syndrome is variable, with a phenotypic continuum that ranges from severe to mild. The most typical presentation is the infantile or childhood-onset isolated myopathy in which the prenatal and perinatal histories are usually unremarkable, and onset is typically in the first 2 years of life. Initial development is normal, followed by gradual onset of hypotonia. Subsequently, generalized fatigue, decreased physical stamina, proximal muscle weakness, and feeding difficulties develop, and muscle atrophy becomes evident. Some children develop bulbar weakness including dysarthria and dysphagia. Previously acquired motor skills are lost; however, cognitive function is typically spared. Less frequent manifestations include early severe muscle weakness with encephalopathy and intractable epilepsy, myopathy with liver involvement, a spinal muscular atrophy–like presentation, late-onset proximal muscle weakness, adult-onset progressive myopathy, chronic external ophthalmoplegia, and sensorineural hearing loss. Inheritance is autosomal recessive.

### DIAGNOSIS

Serum creatine phosphokinase concentration is usually elevated, and electromyography (EMG) usually shows nonspecific myopathic changes. Histopathologic findings in skeletal muscle include prominent variation in fiber size, sarcoplasmic vacuoles, and increased connective tissue. Ragged red fibers are present, and succinate dehydrogenase activity (complex II) is increased, whereas cytochrome c oxidase activity is low or absent. Electron microscopy shows abnormal mitochondria with circular cristae. mtDNA content is typically severely reduced in muscle tissue. ETC activity assays in skeletal muscle typically show decreased activity of multiple complexes, with complex I, I + III, and IV being the most affected. The diagnosis is confirmed by DNA sequencing of the *TK2* gene.

### TREATMENT AND PROGNOSIS

Treatment is largely supportive. Typically, muscle weakness rapidly progresses, leading to respiratory failure and death within a few years after onset. Most children succumb to complications of respiratory muscle weakness; several affected children were ventilator dependent before age 6 years. The most common cause of death is pulmonary infection.

## THYMIDINE PHOSPHORYLASE DEFICIENCY

Thymidine phosphorylase (TP) catalyzes the phosphorolytic cleavage of thymidine and deoxyuridine to thymine and uracil, respectively (see Fig. 163-2). TP deficiency results in mitochondrial neurogastrointestinal encephalomyopathic (MNGIE) mitochondrial DNA depletion syndrome termed mtDNA depletion syndrome-1 (MIM no. 603041). The enzyme deficiency results in marked accumulation of thymidine, which provokes an imbalance of the mitochondrial nucleotides and hence compromises the replication of mtDNA leading to mtDNA depletion. MNGIE is an autosomal recessive disease, with more than 120 affected individuals being reported.

### CLINICAL PRESENTATION

MNGIE is characterized by gastrointestinal dysmotility and cachexia, progressive external ophthalmoplegia with ptosis, peripheral neuropathy, myopathy, and leukoencephalopathy. The onset of the disease is usually between the first and fifth decades with the majority presenting before the age of 20 years. Progressive gastrointestinal dysmotility, caused primarily by enteric myopathy, occurs in all affected individuals, and symptoms include early satiety, nausea, dysphagia, gastroesophageal reflux, postprandial emesis, episodic abdominal pain, episodic abdominal distention, and diarrhea. Weight loss and cachexia coincide with the onset of gastrointestinal symptoms, and affected individuals invariably have a thin body habitus and reduced muscle mass. Ptosis and ophthalmoplegia are common findings. In addition, all affected individuals have peripheral neuropathy that is demyelinating in all cases, and about half also have axonal neuropathy. The symptoms of neuropathy include paresthesias that occur in a stocking-glove distribution and weakness that is usually symmetric and distal. Lower extremities are more prominently affected than upper extremities. Unilateral or bilateral foot drop, as well as clawed hands, may occur. Leukoencephalopathy is another common feature; however, it is usually asymptomatic. Intellectual disability is described in some individuals, and dementia can be a rare late feature of the disease. Other variable manifestations include anemia, hepatic cirrhosis with increased liver enzymes and macrovesicular steatosis, sensorineural hearing loss, diverticulitis, and hypogonadism.

### DIAGNOSIS

Affected individuals can have elevated CSF protein and plasma lactate, and thymidine and deoxyuridine are increased in plasma. EMG and nerve conduction velocity testing show myopathic changes and decreased motor and sensory nerve conduction velocities. Neuroimaging typically demonstrates diffuse white matter abnormalities. mtDNA depletion, mitochondrial proliferation, and smooth cell atrophy are observed in the external layer of the muscularis propria in the stomach and in the small intestine. Skeletal muscle generally shows histologic abnormalities of a mitochondrial myopathy including ragged red fibers and defects in the activities of single or multiple ETC complexes, with the most common being a defect in complex IV (cytochrome c oxidase). Enzyme activity of TP can be assessed in leukocytes, and the diagnosis can be confirmed by DNA sequencing of *TYMP*, the gene encoding TP.

### TREATMENT AND PROGNOSIS

Treatment is largely symptomatic. The disease is progressive with a poor prognosis, and the mean age of death is approximately 35 years. Allogeneic stem cell transplantation was shown to produce nearly full biochemical correction of the deoxythymidine and deoxyuridine imbalances in plasma, and clinical improvements after successful engraftment of donor cells; however, high morbidity and mortality prevent the general use of this therapy for MNGIE disease.

## DIHYDROPYRIMIDINE DEHYDROGENASE DEFICIENCY

Dihydropyrimidine dehydrogenase (DPD) catalyzes the conversion of uracil and thymine into dihydrouracil and dihydrothymine, respectively (see Fig. 163-2). DPD deficiency is an autosomal recessive neurologic disease. The DPD deficiency (MIM no. 274270) results in the accumulation of uracil and thymine and depletion of the end products β-alanine and β-aminoisobutyrate. The mechanism responsible for the neurologic symptoms in this disease remains unknown; however, the reduction of β-alanine, a neuromodulator that can block the reuptake of γ-aminobutyric acid, may play a role.

### CLINICAL PRESENTATION

DPD deficiency is associated with a highly variable phenotype, with some affected individuals being asymptomatic. In symptomatic disease, the onset is usually in infancy, although a later onset may occur. Most affected children display epilepsy and psychomotor delay, often accompanied by generalized hypertonia, hyperreflexia, growth retardation, microcephaly, autistic features, ocular abnormalities (microphthalmia, coloboma, nystagmus, and optic atrophy), and cerebral atrophy and white matter abnormalities on neuroimaging. Affected individuals and carrier (heterozygous) adults who receive the pyrimidine analog 5-fluorouracil, a classic treatment of various cancers, including breast, ovary, and colon, can develop severe life-threatening toxicity. The marked potentiation of the action and thus the toxicity of the 5-fluorouracil is explained by an impairment of the inactivation of this pyrimidine analog via DPD, which normally accounts for approximately 80% of its catabolism.

### DIAGNOSIS

Affected individuals excrete high amounts of uracil and thymine in urine. Elevations of uracil and thymine in plasma and cerebrospinal fluid are also observed. The enzyme defect can be demonstrated in the subject's fibroblasts, liver, and blood cells, with the exception of erythrocytes. The diagnosis can be confirmed by DNA sequencing of the *DPYD* gene.

### TREATMENT AND PROGNOSIS

No treatment is available. Symptoms usually remain the same, but death in early infancy of a more severely affected child has been reported. The pyrimidine analog uridine triacetate has been recently FDA approved for treatment of fluorouracil overdose or severe toxicity. Uridine triacetate, a prodrug, is deacetylated to uridine after oral administration. Excess circulating uridine is converted into uridine triphosphate, which inhibits the cytotoxic activity of 5-fluorouridine triphosphate, a fluorouracil metabolite, by competing with it for incorporation into RNA.

## DIHYDROPYRIMIDINASE DEFICIENCY

Dihydropyrimidinase (DHP) catalyzes the cleavage of dihydrouracil and dihydrothymine into β-ureidopropionate and β-ureidoisobutyrate, respectively (see Fig. 163-2). DHP deficiency is an autosomal recessive neurologic disease with similar symptoms to DPD deficiency. DHP deficiency (MIM no. 222748) results in accumulation of dihydrouracil and dihydrothymine and depletion of the end products β-alanine and β-aminoisobutyrate. Similar to DPD deficiency, the mechanism of the neurologic symptoms in DHP deficiency remains unknown; however, the reduction of β-alanine may play a role.

### CLINICAL PRESENTATION

While fewer cases have been described, as with DPD deficiency, the clinical picture is very variable, with some individuals being asymptomatic. Symptomatic children can present with psychomotor delay, hypotonia, epilepsy, growth retardation, microcephaly, and white matter abnormalities. Nearly half of the affected individuals present with gastrointestinal problems such as feeding difficulties, cyclic vomiting, gastroesophageal reflux, and malabsorption. Similar to DHP, increased sensitivity to 5-fluorouracil, leading to severe toxicity, has also been reported in DPD carriers. This is also explained by the role of DPD in the catabolism of 5-fluorouracil.

### DIAGNOSIS

Urinary dihydrouracil and dihydrothymine are very high. Moderate elevations of uracil and thymine are also found in the urine. Enzyme assay requires a liver biopsy, since more accessible tissues do not possess DHP activity. The molecular diagnosis can be achieved by DNA sequencing of the *DPYS* gene.

### TREATMENT AND PROGNOSIS

There is no therapy, and prognosis appears unpredictable. Some affected individuals were reported to improve with time, whereas others may display a progressive neurodegenerative clinical course. Similar to DPD carriers, uridine triacetate can be used for 5-fluorouracil toxicity in DHP carriers.

## UREIDOPROPIONASE DEFICIENCY

Ureidopropionase catalyzes the conversion of β-ureidopropionate and β-ureidoisobutyrate into β-alanine and β-aminoisobutyrate, respectively (see Fig. 163-2). Ureidopropionase deficiency (MIM no. 613161) is an autosomal recessive disease that results in elevations of β-ureidopropionate and β-ureidoisobutyrate and depletion of β-alanine and β-aminoisobutyrate. It has been suggested that β-ureidopropionate may act as a neurotoxin by inhibiting mitochondrial energy metabolism. As in DPD and DHP deficiency, a reduction of the concentration of β-alanine may play a role in the manifestations of ureidopropionase deficiency. This disease is relatively common in Japan due to a founder mutation p.R326Q, with prevalence of 1 in 6000.

### CLINICAL PRESENTATION

Symptoms of the disorder are widely variable, and it can be asymptomatic. Clinical manifestations can include psychomotor delay, hypotonia, epilepsy, dystonia, microcephaly, optic atrophy, pigmentary retinopathy, cerebellar hypoplasia, delayed myelination, and brain atrophy.

### DIAGNOSIS

β-Ureidopropionate (*N*-carbamyl-β-alanine) and β-ureidoisobutyrate (*N*-carbamyl-β-aminoisobutyric) are elevated in urine, plasma, and CSF. Dihydrouracil and dihydrothymine are also elevated. Assay of ureidopropionase activity in liver confirms the diagnosis. Molecular diagnosis is established by DNA sequencing of the *UPB1D* gene encoding ureidopropionase.

### TREATMENT AND PROGNOSIS

Treatment is symptomatic, and no effective therapy is available.

### SUGGESTED READINGS


Balasubramaniam S, Duley JA, Christodoulou J. Inborn errors of purine metabolism: clinical update and therapies. *J Inherit Metab Dis*. 2014;37:669-686.

Chanprasert S, Wang J, Weng SW, et al. Molecular and clinical characterization of the myopathic form of mitochondrial DNA depletion syndrome caused by mutations in the thymidine kinase (TK2) gene. *Mol Genet Metab*. 2013;110:153-161.

El-Hattab AW, Scaglia F. Mitochondrial DNA depletion syndromes: review and updates of genetic basis, manifestations, and therapeutic options. *Neurotherapeutics*. 2013;10:186-198.

Hirano M. Mitochondrial neurogastrointestinal encephalopathy disease. 2014. In: Pagon RA, Adam MP, Ardinger HH, et al, eds. *GeneReviews®* [Internet]. Seattle, WA: University of Washington, Seattle; 1993-2016.

Jurecka A, Zikanova M, Kmoch S, Tylki-Szymańska A. Adenylosuccinate lyase deficiency. *J Inherit Metab Dis*. 2015;38:231-242.

Kelley RE, Andersson HC. Disorders of purines and pyrimidines. *Handb Clin Neurol*. 2014;120:827-838.

Mechler K, Mountford WK, Hoffmann GF, Ries M. Ultra-orphan diseases: a quantitative analysis of the natural history of molybdenum cofactor deficiency. *Genet Med*. 2015;17:965-970.

Micheli V, Camici M, Tozzi MG, Ipata PL, Sestini S, Bertelli M, Pompucci G. Neurological disorders of purine and pyrimidine metabolism. *Curr Top Med Chem*. 2011:923-947.

Nakajima Y, Meijer J, Dobritzsch D, et al. Clinical, biochemical and molecular analysis of 13 Japanese patients with β-ureidopropionase deficiency demonstrates high prevalence of the c.977G > A (p.R326Q) mutation. *J Inherit Metab Dis*. 2014;37:801-812.

Nyhan WL, O'Neill JP, Jinnah HA, et al. Lesch-Nyhan syndrome. In: Pagon RA, Adam MP, Ardinger HH, et al, eds. *GeneReviews®* [Internet]. Seattle, WA: University of Washington, Seattle; 2014.

Rainger J, Bengani H, Campbell L, et al. Miller (Genee-Wiedemann) syndrome represents a clinically and biochemically distinct subgroup of postaxial acrofacial dysostosis associated with partial deficiency of DHODH. *Hum Mol Genet*. 2012;21:3969-3983.

van Kuilenburg AB, Dobritzsch D, Meijer J, et al. Dihydropyrimidinase deficiency: phenotype, genotype and structural consequences in 17 patients. *Biochim Biophys Acta*. 2010;1802:639-648.



# 164 Disorders of Metal Metabolism

Stephen G. Kaler and Tracey A. Rouault

## INTRODUCTION

Metals are indispensable elements of cell biology. They function as cofactors in many specific proteins and are involved in all major metabolic pathways. Their metabolism and implications in inborn errors of metabolism are still not fully known, but the number of inherited metabolic disorders involving the absorption, transport, or metabolism of metals is rapidly growing. Clinical presentations are very diverse and can involve all organs and systems, including the liver and the central nervous system. Deficiency in metals results in metabolic abnormalities due mostly to loss of function of metal-dependent proteins. On the other hand, excess of metals can result in the unregulated oxidation of proteins, lipids, and other cellular components, causing subsequent tissue injury. Some inherited metal disorders are treatable by chelating drugs or by daily supplementation of the missing metal at pharmacologic doses. Advances in viral gene therapy augur well for improved management of certain disorders of metal metabolism.

## IRON METABOLISM AND ASSOCIATED PEDIATRIC GENETIC DISEASES

Iron is an important cofactor for heme and for hundreds of mammalian proteins that use iron and iron sulfur clusters as cofactors. Accordingly, iron is an indispensable nutrient, and iron deficiency is one of the most common diseases in the world. In most cases, iron deficiency can be treated with oral iron supplementation. However, there are numerous iron deficiency and iron overload diseases that are caused by genetic defects in proteins involved in regulation of normal systemic iron homeostasis and normal iron cofactor assembly. The latter are less amenable to simple remedies.

To understand genetic syndromes of iron deficiency and overload, it is important to review how iron is absorbed from the diet, how it is transported through the body, and how it is distributed to various tissues to ensure that cells acquire sufficient iron, while not incurring damage from excess iron deposition, which results in generation of harmful free radicals.

Iron is taken up from the duodenal lumen by the iron transporter DMT1, which is aided by DCYTB, a reductase that reduces ferric (3+) iron to ferrous (2+) iron, the substrate for transport by DMT1. Iron transits across the polarized basolateral membrane of mucosal cells, where ferroportin, the sole known iron exporter, exports ferrous iron to the circulation, aided by ferroxidase activity provided by membrane-bound hephaestin or circulating ceruloplasmin to generate ferric iron. Transferrin binds ferric iron and transports iron to tissues throughout the body. Cells that need iron express transferrin receptors (TFRC) on their plasma membrane. Upon binding ferric transferrin (TF), the TF-TFRC complex undergoes endosomal internalization and acidification. Iron is released from TF, oxidized by STEAP3, and exported into the cytosol by DMT1. In the cytosol, iron can be incorporated into numerous iron proteins, transported into mitochondria by mitoferrin (MFRN), or sequestered by the multimeric iron storage protein, ferritin.

The interaction of 2 proteins, hepcidin, a soluble peptide hormone synthesized by hepatocytes, and ferroportin, a membrane-bound iron exporter, governs the regulation of systemic iron homeostasis. Many proteins collaborate to regulate hepcidin synthesis so that it quantitatively reflects systemic iron status. These proteins are mainly located on the surface membrane of the hepatocyte, and they communicate signals derived from circulating iron levels into pathways that regulate hepcidin transcription. Mutations of proteins in this hepatocytic sensing pathway, including HFE, hemojuvelin (HJV), HAMP (hepcidin), transferrin receptor 2 (TFR2), TMPRSS6, and erythroferrone (ERFE), interfere with appropriate regulation of hepcidin transcription, causing abnormally low or high hepcidin levels. Hepcidin binds to an extracellular loop of ferroportin and causes internalization, ubiquitination, and degradation of the hepcidin-ferroportin complex. By causing ferroportin degradation, high hepcidin levels interfere with dietary iron uptake and release of iron from macrophages, which store iron that they acquire when they phagocytose senescent red cells and metabolize heme. Erythropoiesis uses about two-thirds of total bodily iron (Fig. 164-1).

Important genetic diseases of iron metabolism include iron overload in hemochromatosis and iron deficiency diseases. Hemochromatosis is a systemic iron overload disease that can be caused by mutations in HFE, HJV, HAMP, and TFR2. Mutations of HJV, the cause of hemochromatosis type 2a (HFE2A; Mendelian Inheritance in Man [MIM] no. 602390), and HAMP, the cause of hemochromatosis type 2b (HFE2B; MIM no. 235200), cause severe iron overload, whereas mutations of HFE, the cause of hemochromatosis type 1 (HFE1; MIM no. 235200), or TFR2, the cause of hemochromatosis

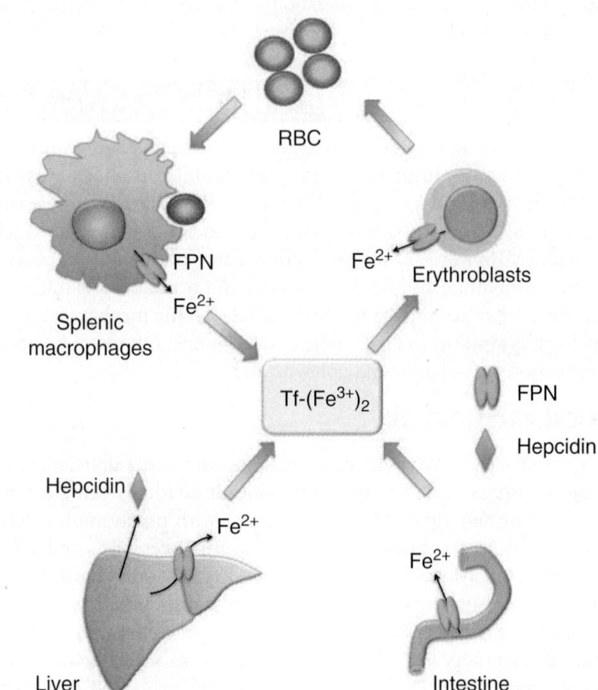


**FIGURE 164-1** An overview of systemic iron homeostasis. Iron is absorbed through the intestine, binds to serum transferrin, is taken up by multiple cells including erythroblasts, and is exported by ferroportin mainly from the duodenal mucosa and macrophages. Hepcidin is secreted by hepatocytes, and it binds to surface ferroportin, leading to ferroportin degradation.

type 3; (HFE3; MIM no. 604250) cause mild iron overload that may not be detected until adulthood. Mutations in ferroportin (*SLC40A1*; MIM no. 606069) can cause iron overload; autosomal dominant hemochromatosis type 4 (HFE4), when they cause resistance to hepcidin-mediated degradation; or iron deficiency when they interfere with the transport activity of ferroportin, leading to diminished iron uptake and release of iron from macrophages. Mutations of TMPRSS6, a matriptase that cleaves HJV, cause high hepcidin levels, which leads to refractory iron deficiency, a condition known as iron-refractory iron deficiency anemia (IRIDA; MIM no. 206200).

Hemochromatosis caused by mutations of HFE can be treated by removing excess iron through monthly phlebotomies. Treatment of IRIDA and FPN-mediated iron deficiency can include red cell infusions, but pharmacologic therapies that act as hepcidin agonists or antagonists are being developed for conditions in which hepcidin levels are abnormal.

Neuronal brain iron accumulation (NBIA) diseases are a group of rare diseases characterized by development of psychomotor symptoms during childhood. In some patients, prominent abnormal iron deposition has been repeatedly detected in the basal ganglia. There are no known treatments, but patients can be diagnosed through sequencing of candidate disease genes.

Numerous rare childhood diseases are caused by mutations in genes that encode proteins involved in synthesis of iron-sulfur clusters, specialized prosthetic groups that are very important in electron transfer in respiratory chain complexes of mitochondria, in numerous DNA repair proteins, and proteins crucial for function of numerous other metabolic pathways such as the citric acid cycle. Many of these patients present with neonatal lactic acidosis and leukoencephalopathy.

## COPPER

Copper is readily available in the diet. After absorption through the stomach and duodenum, it is rapidly removed from the portal circulation by hepatocytes (Fig. 164-2). Biliary excretion is the major

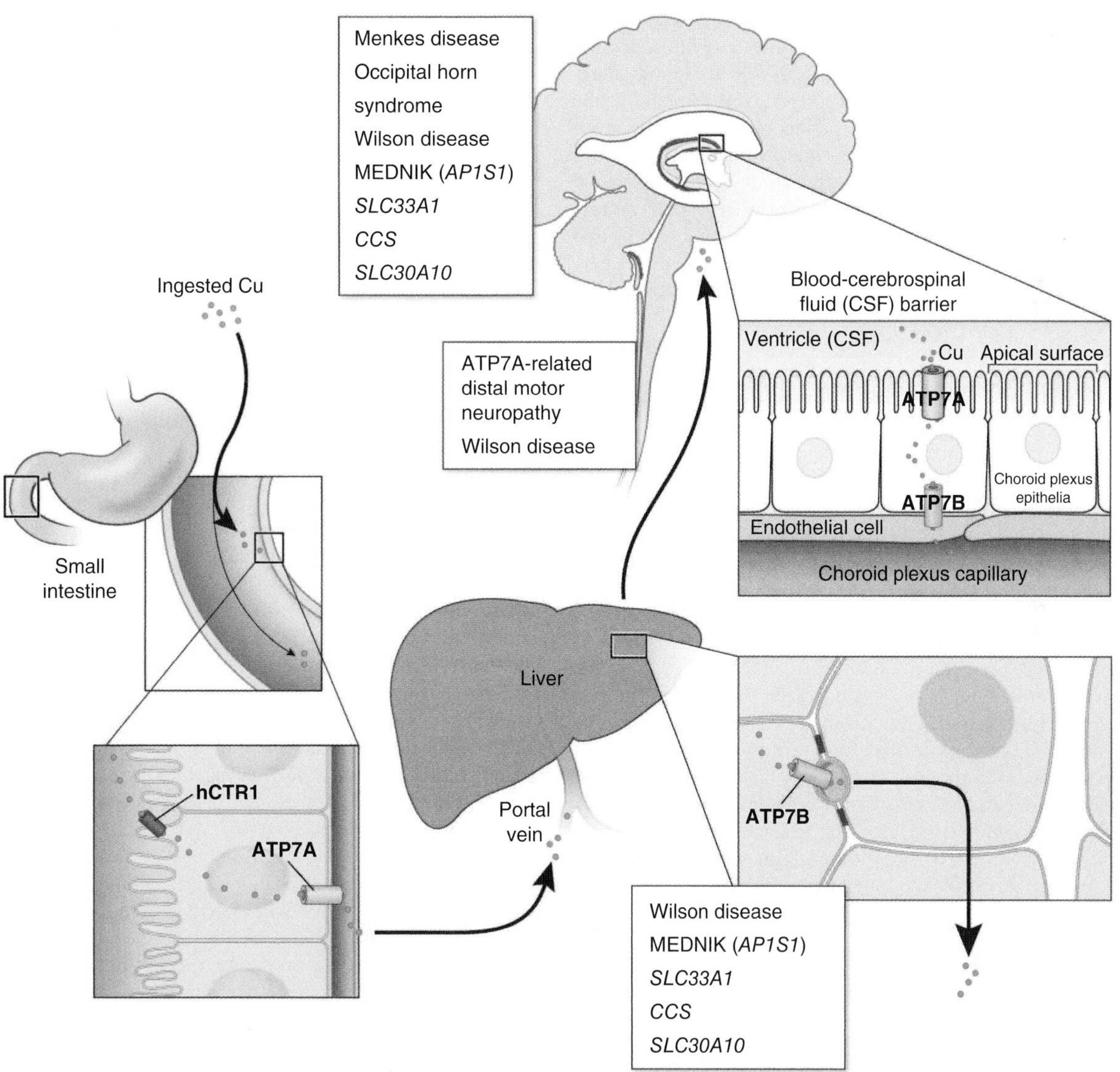


**FIGURE 164-2** Normal copper metabolism and molecular mechanisms of copper transport disease. Copper absorption occurs in the small intestine with passage into the blood mediated by ATP7A at the basolateral aspect of duodenal epithelia. Copper is conveyed to the liver via the portal circulation and excess removed by excretion into the bile at the apical aspect of hepatocytes, a process impaired by mutations in *ATP7B*. Copper diseases of the liver also involve the *AP1S1* gene implicated in MEDNIK syndrome; an acetyl-CoA transporter, *SLC33A1*; and a cytosolic copper chaperone, *CCS*. See text for details. Mutations in a manganese transporter, *SLC30A10*, produce hepatic cirrhosis that can mimic Wilson disease. ATP7A and ATP7B are believed to mediate copper entry and exodus, respectively, at the blood-CSF (cerebrospinal fluid) barrier of choroid plexus epithelia. Brain copper deficiency (Menkes disease) or excess (Wilson disease) results from mutations in these essential copper transporters. The brain is also affected by alterations of *AP1S1*, *SLC33A1*, *SLC30A10*, and *CCS*. Isolated motor neuron degeneration occurs in association with unique *ATP7A* missense mutations affecting axonal trafficking, and sensory peripheral neuropathy can be a component of Wilson disease.

physiologic mechanism of copper elimination, and at steady state, the amount of copper excreted into the bile is equivalent to that absorbed from the intestine. Human Ctr1 (hCTR1) is a plasma membrane protein essential for early embryonic development, intestinal copper uptake, and transportation from the serum into the brain. Ninety percent of serum copper is bound to ceruloplasmin. Intracellular copper metabolism is dependent on the copper-transporting ATPases, ATP7A and ATP7B. Intracellular trafficking also requires proteins termed metallochaperones (Atox1, CCS, Cox 17, Sco1, and Sco2), which direct copper to specific intracellular destinations.

## COPPER METABOLISM AND ASSOCIATED INHERITED PEDIATRIC DISEASES

Menkes disease is an X-linked recessive disorder of copper transport caused by diverse mutations in a copper-transporting ATPase, ATP7A (MIM no. 309400). As early as 1937, Australian veterinary scientists recognized the critical role of copper in mammalian neurodevelopment through the association of copper deficiency with demyelinating disease in ataxic lambs. Fifty years after Kinnear's description of Wilson disease, Menkes and colleagues described 5 male infants in a family of English-Irish heritage who were affected with a distinctive syndrome of neurologic degeneration, peculiar hair, and failure to thrive. These boys appeared normal at birth and throughout the first several months of life, but then experienced seizures and developmental regression and ultimately passed away between the ages of 7 months and 3.5 years. The pedigree of the family strongly suggested that the condition was an X-linked genetic disease. In 1972, it was recognized that the unusual hair of infants with Menkes disease appeared similar in texture to the brittle wool of sheep raised on copper-deficient soil in Australia, and very low serum copper was observed in 7 Menkes disease patients.

Menkes disease typically presents in males at 2 to 3 months of age with loss of previously obtained developmental milestones and the onset of hypotonia, seizures, and failure to thrive. Characteristic physical changes of the hair and facies in conjunction with typical neurologic findings often suggest the diagnosis. The less distinctive appearance of very young affected infants before the onset of symptoms is discussed separately below.

Scalp hair in classically affected infants is short, sparse, coarse, and twisted. Light microscopy of the hair will illustrate pathognomonic pili torti (180° twisting of the hair shaft) and often other abnormalities, including trichoclasis (transverse fracture of the hair shaft) and trichoptilosis (longitudinal splitting of the shaft). The hair tends to be lightly pigmented and may show unusual colors such as white, silver, or gray, but in some cases, it is normally pigmented. The face is jowly with sagging cheeks and ears that often appear large. The palate tends to be high-arched and tooth eruption delayed. Pectus excavatum is a common thoracic finding. Umbilical and/or inguinal herniae may be present. The skin often appears loose and redundant, particularly at the nape of the neck, the axillae, and on the trunk. Neurologically, profound truncal hypotonia with poor head control is invariably present. Appendicular tone may be increased with thumbs held in an adducted, cortical posture. Deep tendon reflexes are often hyperactive.

Certain clinical diagnostic tests are characteristic. White matter abnormalities reflecting impaired myelination, diffuse atrophy, ventriculomegaly, and tortuosity of cerebral blood vessels are typical findings on brain magnetic resonance imaging (MRI). Subdural hematomas are common in infants, and cerebrovascular accidents can occur in patients who survive longer. The "corkscrew" appearance of cerebral vessels is well visualized by magnetic resonance angiography, a noninvasive method for study of the vasculature. Dysplastic coronary vessels may be detectable by echocardiography. Electroencephalograms (EEGs) are usually moderately to severely abnormal including high rates of status epilepticus and infantile spasms. Normal tracings may be recorded in some classically affected individuals; however, 3 prior surveys indicated clinical seizures and EEG abnormalities in a combined 27 (93%) of 29 symptomatic Menkes disease patients diagnosed at 2 months of age or older.

Pelvic ultrasonography reveals diverticula of the urinary bladder in nearly all patients. Radiographs often disclose abnormalities of bone formation in the skull (wormian bones), long bones (metaphyseal spurring), and ribs (anterior flaring, multiple fractures). Connective tissue problems in Menkes disease that have been identified more recently include neck masses due to dilation of internal jugular veins, aneurysms of the brachial arteries, and gastrointestinal polyps.

Classical Menkes disease often escapes attention in the newborn period due to its very subtle manifestations in neonates and the fact that healthy newborns have low serum copper levels that overlap those in affected infants. However, several nonspecific physical and metabolic findings are commonly cited when birth histories of these infants are reviewed. These include premature labor and delivery, large cephalohematomas, hypothermia, hypoglycemia, and jaundice. Occasionally, unusual hair pigmentation may suggest the diagnosis in newborns. Often, however, the appearance of the hair is unremarkable, and the pili torti found on microscopic examination of hair from older Menkes patients is not evident in the hair of affected newborns. Neurologically, newborns with Menkes disease generally appear normal. Since the success of treatment with subcutaneous copper histidinate injections in this disorder depends heavily on early diagnosis and treatment, newborn screening for Menkes disease based on neurochemical levels from dried blood spots or via high-throughput molecular assays is highly desirable.

The biochemical phenotype in Menkes disease involves (1) low levels of copper in plasma, liver, and brain due to impaired intestinal absorption; (2) reduced activities of copper-dependent enzymes; and (3) paradoxical accumulation of copper in certain tissues (duodenum, kidney, spleen, pancreas, skeletal muscle, placenta). The copper retention phenotype is also evident in cultured fibroblasts and lymphoblasts, in which reduced egress of radiolabeled copper is demonstrable in pulse-chase experiments. Certain clinical features of Menkes disease are related to deficient activity of specific copper-requiring enzymes. Partial deficiency of dopamine-β-hydroxylase (DBH), a critical enzyme in the catecholamine biosynthetic pathway, is responsible for a distinctively abnormal plasma and cerebrospinal fluid (CSF) neurochemical pattern in Menkes patients.

Peptidylglycine-α-amidating monooxygenase (PAM) is required for removal of the carboxy-terminal glycine residue characteristic of numerous neuroendocrine peptide precursors (eg, gastrin, cholecystokinin, vasoactive intestinal peptide, corticotropin-releasing hormone, thyrotropin-releasing hormone, calcitonin, vasopressin). Failure to amidate these precursors results in 100- to 1000-fold reduction of bioactivity compared to the mature, amidated forms. Deficiency of tyrosinase, a copper enzyme needed for melanin biosynthesis, is considered responsible for reduced hair and skin pigmentation in patients with Menkes disease. Deficient cytochrome c oxidase (CCO) activity is likely a major factor in the neuropathology of Menkes disease; the brain findings (marked neuronal cell loss in the cerebral cortex and cerebellum, severe demyelination, dystrophic Purkinje cells, mitochondrial proliferation) are partly similar to those in individuals with Leigh disease (subacute necrotizing encephalomyelopathy) in whom, among other causes, CCO deficiency is caused by defects in complex IV of the respiratory chain. Deficiency of copper/zinc superoxide dismutase (Cu/Zn SOD) may lower protection against oxygen free radicals and theoretically have cytotoxic effects.

In the natural history of classical Menkes disease, death usually occurs by 3 years. Survival and outcomes are clearly improved through early diagnosis and early copper replacement treatment. The effective rescue of a lethal mouse model of severe Menkes disease using brain-directed viral gene therapy indicates considerable hope for curative remedies of this difficult illness in humans.

The occipital horn syndrome is a milder allelic variant of Menkes disease, so named in reference to the pathognomonic wedge-shaped calcifications that form within the trapezius and sternocleidomastoid muscles at their attachment to the occipital bone in affected individuals. This protuberance can be palpated in some patients and is demonstrable radiographically on lateral and Towne's view skull x-rays or appropriate sagittal computed tomography (CT) or MRI images. Occipital horn syndrome shares the hair and connective tissue abnormalities of classical Menkes disease. Because the neurologic phenotype in this variant is mild (slight generalized muscle weakness and dysautonomia including syncope, orthostatic hypotension, and chronic diarrhea), affected individuals often escape detection until mid-childhood or later. Patients with occipital horn syndrome have low-normal levels of serum copper and ceruloplasmin and abnormal levels of catecholamines in plasma and CSF. The neurochemical abnormalities are distinctive, although of lower magnitude than in classic Menkes disease. The molecular basis for typical occipital horn syndrome most often involves exon skipping with reduction of correct mRNA processing compared to normal.

The natural history of patients with occipital horn syndrome is not well known due to the scarcity of patients for whom long-term follow-up has been reported. Potential vascular complications could be anticipated for these patients in terms of their connective tissue problems, although there are no reports of catastrophic vascular rupture, stroke, or cardiac events in patients with this phenotype.

A third ATP7A phenotype, distal motor neuropathy without overt abnormalities of copper metabolism, was recently found in association with mutations in the ATP7A copper transporter. Distal hereditary motor neuropathies (HMNs) comprise a clinically and genetically heterogeneous group of disorders predominantly affecting motor neurons in the peripheral nervous system. Distal HMNs have been classified into 7 subgroups based on mode of inheritance, age of onset, distribution of muscle weakness, and clinical progression. Fifteen genetic loci for distal HMN have been mapped, with 14 genes identified to date. These encode a functionally diverse array of gene products including a transfer RNA synthetase, 2 heat shock proteins, and a microtubule motor protein involved in axonal transport.

The ATP7A allelic variant involves progressive distal motor neuropathy with minimal or no sensory symptoms. Signs include weakness of distal muscles with curled fingers, pes cavus foot deformities, and diminished deep tendon reflexes. Neurophysiologic studies indicate reduced compound motor amplitudes with normal conduction velocities. Affected patients do not manifest the severe infantile central neurologic deficits observed in Menkes disease, the signs of autonomic dysfunction seen in occipital horn syndrome, the hair and connective tissue abnormalities found in both conditions, or any of the typical biochemical features of those well-characterized phenotypes. These facts highlight the distinction between this isolated distal motor neuropathy and syndromes previously associated with ATP7A mutations. The phenomenon of late-onset, often adult-onset, distal muscular atrophy implies that the ATP7A missense mutations causing this phenotype are unique and have attenuated effects that require decades to provoke pathologic consequences.

Three other autosomal recessive disorders of copper metabolism have recently been described: (1) MEDNIK syndrome, which revealed that mutations in the sigma 1A subunit (σ1A) of adaptor protein complex 1 (AP-1) have detrimental effects on trafficking of ATP7A and ATP7B; (2) Huppke-Brendel syndrome caused by mutations in an acetyl-coenzyme A (CoA) transporter SLC33A1 needed for acetylation of 1 or more copper proteins; and (3) copper chaperone for SOD (CCS) deficiency caused by a variant in a copper chaperone to SOD.

MEDNIK represents an acronym for the syndromic constellation of mental retardation, enteropathy, deafness, neuropathy, ichthyosis, and keratodermia. This condition is known to be caused by mutations in *AP1S1*, encoding σ1A, the small subunit of the adaptor protein 1 complex. This subunit plays a crucial role in clathrin coat assembly and mediates transmembrane protein trafficking between the trans-Golgi network, endosomes, and the plasma membrane. MEDNIK syndrome (MIM no. 609313) was first reported in French-Canadian families sharing common ancestors, presenting a complex neurocutaneous phenotype, but its pathogenesis was not completely understood. A Sephardic-Jewish patient, carrying a new *AP1S1* homozygous mutation, showed severe perturbations of copper metabolism with hypocupremia, hypoceruloplasminemia, and liver copper accumulation along with intrahepatic cholestasis. Zinc acetate treatment strikingly improved the clinical condition, as well as liver copper and bile acid overload. Subsequent evaluation of copper-related metabolites and liver function in the original French-Canadian patients suggested disturbed intracellular copper metabolism and hepatopathy in those MEDNIK patients. Thus, this multisystem disease is characterized, at least in part, by a phenotype that combines clinical and biochemical signs of Wilson and Menkes diseases, presumably related to adverse effects on ATP7B and ATP7A trafficking, respectively.

Huppke-Brendel syndrome (MIM no. 614482) was described in 5 patients from 4 unrelated families with low serum copper and ceruloplasmin who presented with a lethal autosomal recessive syndrome of congenital cataracts, hearing loss, and severe developmental delay. Cerebral MRI showed pronounced cerebellar hypoplasia and hypomyelination. Homozygosity mapping was performed and displayed a region of commonality among 3 families at chromosome 3q25. Deep and conventional sequencing disclosed homozygous or compound heterozygous mutations for all affected subjects in *SLC33A1*, which encodes a highly conserved acetyl-CoA transporter (AT-1) required for acetylation of multiple gangliosides and glycoproteins. The mutations were found to cause reduced or absent AT-1 expression and abnormal intracellular localization of the AT-1 protein. AT-1 knockdown in HepG2 cells led to reduced ceruloplasmin secretion, suggesting that posttranslational acetylation of ceruloplasmin is necessary for the normal procession of this glycoprotein in the secretory pathway. The severity of the clinical phenotype implies an essential role of AT-1 in the proper posttranslational modification of numerous proteins, without which normal lens and brain development is interrupted. AT-1 defects are a new and important differential diagnosis in patients with low copper and ceruloplasmin in serum.

In 1 of the consanguineous patients with inherited homozygous mutations in *SLC33A1*, concurrent mutations in *CCS*, the gene encoding a copper chaperone, were also identified. This patient's clinical and biochemical phenotype was more severe than found in the other 4 affected subjects in terms of neurologic and hepatic disease. The homozygous CCS variant, p.Arg163Trp, predicts substitution of a highly conserved arginine residue at position 163, with tryptophan in domain II of CCS, which interacts directly with the copper enzyme superoxide dismutase 1 (SOD1). Biochemical analyses of the patient's fibroblasts, mammalian cell transfections, immunoprecipitation assays, and Lys7Δ (CCS homolog) yeast complementation support the pathogenicity of the *CCS* mutation. Expression of CCS was reduced, and binding of CCS to SOD1 was impaired. The mutation reduces SOD1 activity and may impair other mechanisms important for normal copper homeostasis. CCS-Arg163Trp represents the primary example of a human mutation in a gene coding for a copper chaperone.

Wilson disease or hepatolenticular degeneration is due to mutations in the *ATP7B* gene (MIM no. 277900) and is an autosomal recessive disorder of copper metabolism with an incidence of approximately 1 in 30,000 live births. Affected individuals accumulate abnormal levels of copper in the liver and (later) in the brain. This gene was identified in 1993 and encodes a copper-transporting ATPase, ATP7B, expressed primarily in the liver, where its major function is excretion of hepatic copper into the biliary tract.

Presenting clinical features of Wilson disease include nonspecific liver disease, neurologic abnormalities, psychiatric illness, hemolytic anemia, renal tubular Fanconi syndrome, and various skeletal abnormalities. Age influences the specific presentation in Wilson disease. Nearly all individuals who present with liver disease are less than 30 years of age, whereas those presenting with neurologic or psychiatric signs may range in age from the first to the fifth decade. This reflects the sequence of events in the pathogenesis of this disease. However, regardless of clinical presentation, some degree of liver disease is invariably present. In a series of 400 adult patients with Wilson disease, approximately 50% presented with neurologic and psychiatric symptoms, 20% with neurologic and hepatic symptoms, and 20% with purely hepatic symptoms. In patients with neurologic presentations, abnormalities include speech difficulty (dysarthria), dystonia, rigidity, tremor, or choreiform movements, abnormal gait, and uncoordinated handwriting. Wilson disease may properly be classified as a movement disorder. The neurologic signs and symptoms reflect the predilection for basal ganglia (eg, caudate, putamen) involvement in the brain of these individuals. Parkinson disease or other movement disorders may be mistakenly diagnosed. In psychiatric presentations, changes in personality (irritability, anger, poor self-control), depression, and anxiety are common symptoms. Typically, patients presenting in this fashion are in their late teens or early twenties, a period during which substance abuse is also a diagnostic consideration. Wilson disease should be formally excluded in all teenagers and young adults with new-onset psychiatric signs.

With hepatic presentations, signs and symptoms include jaundice, hepatomegaly, edema, or ascites. Secondary endocrine effects of liver disease may include delayed puberty or amenorrhea. Viral hepatitis and cirrhosis are often initial diagnostic considerations in individuals who, in fact, have Wilson disease.

In addition to the brain and liver, the eye is a primary site of copper deposition in Wilson disease, producing a pathognomonic sign, the Kayser-Fleischer ring. The Kayser-Fleischer ring is a golden to greenish-brown annular deposition of copper in the periphery of the cornea. This important diagnostic sign first appears as a superior crescent, then develops inferiorly and ultimately becomes circumferential. Slit-lamp examinations are required to detect rings in their early stage of formation. Copper can also accumulate in the lens and produce "sunflower" cataracts. Approximately 95% of patients with neurologic signs manifest the Kayser-Fleischer ring compared to approximately 65% of those with hepatic presentations. Copper chelation therapy causes fading and eventual disappearance of corneal copper.

Renal tubular dysfunction in Wilson disease leads to abnormal losses of amino acids, electrolytes, calcium, phosphorus, and glucose. Presumably these are related to copper toxicity. High copper levels have been noted previously in the kidneys of patients with Wilson disease. Treatment with copper chelation often improves the renal disturbances.

There can also be skeletal effects of Wilson disease, including osteoporosis and rickets, and these may be attributable to renal losses of calcium and phosphorus. Osteoarthritis primarily affecting the knees and wrists also occurs in Wilson disease patients and may involve excess copper deposition in the bone and cartilage. Hemolytic anemia due to the direct toxic effects of copper on the red blood cells has been observed and is usually associated with release of massive quantities of hepatic copper into the circulation, a phenomenon that can be sudden and catastrophic.

Laboratory findings that support the diagnosis of Wilson disease include low levels of serum copper and serum ceruloplasmin, elevated hepatic transaminase levels, aminoaciduria, and hemolytic anemia. Incorporation of radiolabeled copper-64 into serum ceruloplasmin, measured as the appearance of copper in the serum after an oral load is a highly specific diagnostic test; patients with Wilson disease incorporate very little copper-64 into ceruloplasmin.

Aceruloplasminemia (MIM no. 604290), a different autosomal recessive disease caused by mutations in the ceruloplasmin gene (*CP*), may be confused with Wilson disease due to very low or absent serum ceruloplasmin level. This rare disorder of iron metabolism involves the triad of diabetes, retinal degeneration, and progressive degeneration of basal ganglia with clinical symptoms including dysarthria, dystonia, and dementia. Since ceruloplasmin is required for oxidation of ferrous iron ($Fe^{2+}$) to ferric iron ($Fe^{3+}$), ferrous iron accumulates in pancreas, retina, and brain of aceruloplasmic patients. MRI reveals distinctive iron deposition in the basal ganglia, which is not seen in Wilson disease. Of note, given the pediatric focus of this text, aceruloplasminemia has an average age of onset of 50 years and only 1 non-adult case (age 16 years) has been reported.

Increased urinary excretion of copper (> 100 µg per 24 hours) is easily demonstrated and important in the diagnosis of Wilson disease. Acid-washed (copper-free) collection containers should be used. A variation involving serial measurements of urinary copper is the penicillamine "challenge" in which 500 mg of penicillamine is administered orally after collecting a baseline 24-hour urine. The penicillamine dose is repeated after 12 hours, the midpoint of the second 24-hour urine collection. A several-fold increase in copper excretion in the second collection is suggestive of the diagnosis. Percutaneous liver biopsy for measurement of hepatic copper remains a gold standard, although invasive, technique for Wilson disease diagnosis. Hepatic copper values > 200 µg per gram of dry weight (normal 20–50) are characteristic of Wilson disease. Atomic absorption spectrometry is the preferred method; histochemical staining for copper in a liver biopsy specimen is unreliable. For families in which the mutant alleles have been determined, molecular diagnosis is highly reliable.

The era of successful treatment of Wilson disease began in 1956 with Walshe's use of penicillamine, a free thiol that binds (chelates) copper. This drug does not formally correct the basic defect of impaired copper excretion in the bile. However, it greatly enhances urinary excretion of copper and thereby corrects and prevents copper overload and its effects. Pyridoxine (vitamin $B_6$) is usually prescribed concomitantly to counter the tendency for deficiency of this vitamin to develop during chronic penicillamine administration. Certain individuals are intolerant of penicillamine, however, encountering significant side effects that include nephrotoxicity, hematologic abnormalities, and a distinctive rash, *elastosis perforans serpiginosa* (usually involving the neck and axillae). Furthermore, in some patients with neurologic presentation, penicillamine treatment induces paradoxical worsening of the clinical picture. Triethylenetetramine dihydrochloride (Trien) is a suitable alternative chelating agent with a somewhat lower side effect profile.

Oral zinc acetate also has proven highly effective in Wilson disease. The mechanism involves induction of metallothionein synthesis in intestinal epithelial cells; increased metallothionein synthesis results in greater binding of dietary copper and thus decreased absorption. Zinc therapy has particular value in (1) young, presymptomatic patients; (2) patients who are pregnant given the possible fetal teratogenic effects of other compounds; and (3) as maintenance therapy for patients after their initial "de-coppering" is accomplished. Zinc acetate has minimal side effects. The only drawback to its use is the relatively long time (4–6 months) needed for restoration of proper copper balance when used as monotherapy in the initial stages of treatment.

Tetrathiomolybdate forms stable tripartite complexes between protein, copper, and itself. This drug functions both to decrease copper absorption and to reduce circulating free copper. It is very fast acting and can restore normal copper balance within weeks compared to the months required with other copper chelators or with zinc.

Liver transplantation is a rare consideration in Wilson disease since the condition is typically responsive to medical therapy. This is generally necessary only in cases where a delay in diagnosis or poor compliance results in irreversible hepatic damage.

The prognosis in Wilson disease is generally favorable; current therapeutic approaches can prevent or reverse most of the significant clinical signs and symptoms, including the Kayser-Fleisher rings. However, if treatment is stopped, irreversible and potentially fatal liver damage will inevitably occur.

## ZINC METABOLISM AND ASSOCIATED INHERITED PEDIATRIC DISEASES

Zinc is a cofactor for more than 100 enzymes and, as such, is involved in all major metabolic pathways. It is also essential for nucleic acid metabolism and protein synthesis and their regulation through zinc-finger proteins. In humans, about 1% of the total body zinc content is replenished daily by the diet. This is accomplished principally by tight control of 2 systems: absorption from the intestine and endogenous loss via pancreatic and other intestinal secretions. Zinc transporter proteins lower intracellular zinc by mediating zinc efflux from cells or influx into intracellular vesicles. *SLC30A2* mutations are responsible for zinc deficiency in breastfed babies, while *SLC39A4* mutations are responsible for autosomal recessive acrodermatitis enteropathica. In the latter condition (MIM no. 201100), breastfed infants typically present around the time of weaning, whereas those receiving infant formula may become symptomatic within the first month of life. This difference is due to the greater bioavailability of zinc in human milk as compared with formula. The symptoms of acrodermatitis enteropathica are similar to those seen in other forms of zinc deficiency and may include acral skin lesions, alopecia, dermatitis, diarrhea, irritability, and failure to thrive. The diagnosis is made on the basis of a low serum zinc level (< 60 μg/dL), although symptomatic infants with normal or only slightly decreased serum zinc levels have been reported. Therefore, treatment should not be based solely on the zinc level.

Oral therapy with 10 mg/kg/d of zinc sulfate or zinc gluconate results in rapid reversal of symptoms and clearing of the skin lesions within several weeks. Following normalization of serum zinc levels, lifelong maintenance therapy at 1 to 2 mg/kg/d is required.

An early-onset form of acrodermatitis enteropathica occurs in breastfed infants whose mothers have decreased levels of zinc in breast milk due to mutations in the *SLC30A2* gene that encodes the zinc transporter ZNT2 in the epithelial cells of the mammary gland (MIM no. 608118). This disorder shows autosomal dominant inheritance with incomplete penetrance and can be diagnosed by measurement of the zinc content of the mother's milk. Zinc deficiency and all symptoms can be eliminated by the use of donor breast milk, formula, or zinc supplementation.

Spondylocheirodysplastic Ehlers-Danlos syndrome (SCD-EDS; MIM no. 612350) is an autosomal recessive disorder with features similar to those in Ehlers-Danlos type VI (EDS VI) that results from mutations in the gene for ZIP13 (*SLC39A13*), an intracellular zinc transporter localized to the Golgi apparatus. Clinical features of SCD-EDS include thin, hyperelastic skin with easy bruising, hypermobility of the small joints, blue sclerae, atrophy of the thenar muscles of the hand, osteopenia, and moderate short stature. Accumulation of excess zinc in the Golgi and endoplasmic reticulum is associated with reduced activity of both lysl and prolyl hydroxylases, and reduced formation of crosslinks in types 1 and 2 collagen. The serum level of zinc is normal, but urinary excretion of hydroxylated and crosslinked collagen metabolites (lysyl pyridinoline/hydroxylysyl pyridinoline) is reduced, which can be used for diagnosis. However, confirmation by molecular analysis is essential to differentiate from EDS VI, which results from mutations in lysyl hydroxylase and has similar clinical and biochemical features. Studies in a mouse model of SCD-EDS demonstrated reduced bone morphogenetic protein (BMP)/transforming growth factor (TGF)-β signaling, which is believed to be the cause of the short stature, a feature not seen in EDS VI.

Zinc deficiency, either hereditary or acquired, has major detrimental effects, whereas high serum zinc has few, probably because of its binding to albumin or $\alpha_2$-macroglobulin.

## MANGANESE METABOLISM AND HUMAN DISEASE

Manganese homeostasis remains poorly understood, but it seems certain that concentrations in subcellular compartments are closely controlled despite quite large variations in dietary manganese intake (eg, it is higher in vegetarians). Manganese plays an important role in many biologic processes as a cofactor for various enzymes in the cytoplasm, Golgi apparatus, and mitochondria. High cytoplasmic concentrations of manganese are cytotoxic. Two $Ca^{2+}$-ATPases are known to also be involved in $Mn^{2+}$ transport: the Golgi-associated secretory pathway (SPCA) and the sarco-/endoplasmic reticulum $Ca^{2+}$ ATPases (SERCA).

Several investigators have reported patients with what appear to be typical features of Wilson disease, including liver dysfunction and a movement disorder, that result from mutations in a manganese (Mn) transporter encoded by the *SLC30A10* gene (MIM no. 613280). Pathologic findings of this autosomal recessive disorder include hepatic cirrhosis, hypertrophic cardiomyopathy, basal ganglia injury, diffuse reactive gliosis of the white matter, and axonal loss in the corticospinal tracts of the spinal cord. This condition has been described by some authors as the "new Wilson disease." Patients with this disorder typically develop generalized dystonia in childhood and adolescence (2–14 years) or asymmetrical parkinsonism and early postural instability in adulthood (47 and 57 years for the 2 cases reported with this presentation so far). Typical laboratory findings include polycythemia, depleted iron stores with low ferritin, high total iron binding capacity, increased serum Mn concentrations, and basal ganglia hyperintensities on T1-weighted brain MRI. The treatment of choice for these patients is repeated intravenous $Na^2Ca$-EDTA infusions, leading to a large increase in urinary Mn excretion. Both parkinsonian and dystonic features can greatly improve after such infusions, but successful treatment response may depend on early diagnosis and initiation of treatment.

Recently, homozygous loss-of-function mutations in a different gene, *SLC39A14*, were identified in a cohort of children with hypermanganesemia and progressive parkinsonism-dystonia (MIM no. 617013). The findings demonstrated that SLC39A14 functions as a primary Mn transporter and that mutations in *SLC39A14* impair Mn uptake, without affecting zinc, iron, and cadmium blood levels. $Na^2Ca$-EDTA treatment effectively chelates Mn and increases urinary Mn excretion in affected individuals. Commenced early in the disease course, chelation therapy can lead to significant improvement of clinical symptoms and, potentially, prevention of disease progression.

## MOLYBDENUM METABOLISM AND ASSOCIATED INHERITED PEDIATRIC DISEASES

Molybdenum is an essential trace element with a recommended daily allowance ranging from 3 μg/d in infants to 45 μg/d in adults. It is well absorbed in the gut, and dietary deficiency is very rare. Molybdenum is required for the activity of at least 4 enzymes, sulfite oxidase (SUOX), xanthine dehydrogenase (XDH), aldehyde oxidase (AOX), and the mitochondrial amidoxime-reducing component (MARC1). The functionally active form of molybdenum is called the molybdenum cofactor, which consists of a molybdenum atom bound to a modified pterin (molybdopterin). Biosynthesis of the molybdenum cofactor occurs in 5 steps. The first 4 steps generate the molybdopterin, and the final step is the addition of molybdenum to the pterin ring. Studies of patient fibroblasts have identified 3 complementation groups. Complementation group A patients are unable to convert guanosine triphosphate (GTP) to precursor Z due to mutations in the *MOCSI* gene (molybdenum cofactor synthesis-1; MIM no. 252150). Group B patients have mutations in the *MOCS2* gene (MIM no. 252160) and cannot convert precursor Z to molybdopterin. Group C patients are unable to form the molybdenum cofactor from molybdopterin due to mutations in the gene that encodes gephyrin (*GPHNI*; MIM no. 615501), which catalyzes the insertion of molybdenum into molybdopterin. Both *MOCS1* and *MOCS2* encode 2 proteins (MOCS1A and MOCS1B, MOCS2A and MOCS2B, respectively), which are all required for molybdenum cofactor synthesis. A fourth gene required for synthesis of molybdenum cofactor is *MOCS3*, which encodes an enzyme required for activation of the MOCS2A protein. Mutations affecting the genes required for molybdenum cofactor biosynthesis all result in a similar clinical phenotype called molybdenum cofactor deficiency. The most common presentation of molybdenum cofactor deficiency involves severe neonatal seizures. Infants appear normal at birth but subsequently develop feeding problems, seizures, and abnormalities of muscle tone. The seizures typically are generalized and resistant to therapy. Many patients die in the neonatal period, but those who survive have severe developmental problems and rarely live beyond the third year of life. In neonates, diffusion-weighted MRI shows diffuse cytotoxic edema similar to what is observed following hypoxic-ischemic injury. Over time, there is progression to cystic encephalomalacia in the basal ganglia and other regions as well as generalized atrophy. A characteristic pattern of encephalomalacia with sparing of superficial cortex termed *ulegyria* has been observed in both molybdenum cofactor deficiency and isolated sulfite oxidase deficiency. Cystic changes have also been observed in neonates, suggesting prenatal onset of brain injury in some patients. Pathologic studies demonstrate severe neuronal loss and astrogliosis in the cortex and cystic lesions consistent with changes seen by MRI. The pathophysiology of these changes is uncertain, but they may be due to a direct excitotoxic effect of the sulfite- and sulfur-containing amino acids that accumulate as a result of the lack of sulfite oxidase activity.

Dysmorphic facial features are often seen, including hypertelorism, a small nose, puffy cheeks and lips, a long philtrum, and progressive microcephaly. Lens dislocation is seen in approximately 50% of patients but may be absent in neonates. The loss of xanthine dehydrogenase activity results in elevated renal excretion of xanthine and a risk for stones. Although most patients present as neonates, milder forms with a later onset have been reported and may be misdiagnosed as cerebral palsy.

Isolated deficiency of sulfite oxidase (MIM no. 272300) results in a clinical phenotype very similar to the severe form of molybdenum cofactor deficiency. It results from mutations in the *SUOX* gene, which has no effect on molybdenum cofactor synthesis or the activity of xanthine dehydrogenase and aldehyde oxidase, suggesting that most of the symptoms seen in molybdenum cofactor deficiency, especially the brain injury, are due to the loss of sulfite oxidase activity. Sulfite oxidase functions in the cysteine degradation pathway, and loss of activity leads to the accumulation of taurine, sulfite, thiosulfite, and *S*-sulfocysteine. Cysteine levels are decreased secondary to reaction with sulfite and formation of *S*-sulfocysteine. Total serum homocysteine is also very low in patients lacking sulfite oxidase activity. Elevated levels of sulfite in urine can be detected by a sulfite dipstick, but fresh urine must be used to avoid loss through oxidation to sulfate and a false-negative result. A more stable marker in the urine is *S*-sulfocysteine, which is the preferred metabolite for diagnosis. Urinary thiosulfite also can be measured but has a high rate of false-positive results due to cross-reaction of commonly used antibiotics.

Xanthine dehydrogenase functions in purine degradation, catalyzing the conversion of hypoxanthine to xanthine, and xanthine to uric acid. Loss of enzymatic activity leads to markedly decreased levels of both serum and urinary uric acid. Consequently, the determination of serum uric acid level is an excellent screening test in infants with neonatal seizures of unknown etiology. However, in some affected infants, particularly those with later onset or milder symptoms, the level of uric acid may be within the low-normal range and result in a false-negative test. There is also a significant elevation of xanthine and a more modest increase in hypoxanthine, which can be detected by measuring oxypurines in either urine or blood. Determination of oxypurines and uric acid allows differentiation between molybdenum cofactor deficiency and isolated sulfite oxidase deficiency. Based on the results of biochemical testing, a definitive diagnosis can be made by either enzymatic studies in cultured fibroblasts or DNA testing. This is important not only for diagnosis but also for genetic counseling. Both molybdenum cofactor deficiency and sulfite oxidase deficiency are inherited as autosomal recessive disorders and thus have a 25% recurrence risk. A prenatal diagnosis can be made by DNA testing or measurement of sulfite oxidase activity in cultured amniocytes or tissue obtained by chorionic villus sampling. The seizures associated with molybdenum cofactor deficiency are difficult to control, and no specific therapies are readily available. Direct administration of molybdenum cofactor is not practical due to its instability, but several trials with precursor Z (cyclic pyranopterin monophosphate), an intermediate in molybdenum cofactor synthesis, have been reported. The results of these trials indicate some neurologic benefit when treatment is started very early, but further study is required. This treatment is limited to patients in complementation group A, who specifically lack the ability to make precursor Z. Use of a diet with reduced levels of sulfur-containing amino acids (eg, cysteine and methionine) has been successful in 2 patients with a mild form of sulfite oxidase deficiency, resulting in a decrease in urinary thiosulphate and *S*-sulphocysteine. Both patients grew normally with no signs of neurologic deterioration. Based on the hypothesis that *S*-sulfocysteine may cause excitotoxicity via activation of *N*-methyl-D-aspartate (NMDA) receptors, 1 patient was treated with dextromethorphan (12.5 mg/kg/d), an NMDA receptor inhibitor, resulting in decreased seizures and improvement in the electroencephalogram. Dextromethorphan has also been used in isolated sulfite oxidase deficiency, but its efficacy is uncertain. Overall, the therapeutic options in molybdenum cofactor deficiency are very limited, and as a result, the outcome is usually poor.

## SUGGESTED READINGS


Bandmann O, Weiss KH, Kaler SG. Neurological effects of Wilson disease and other copper metabolism disorders. *Lancet Neurol.* 2015;14:103-113.

Drakesmith H, Nemeth E, Ganz T. Ironing out ferroportin. *Cell Metab.* 2015;22:777-787.

Kaler SG. The neurology of ATP7A copper transporter disease: emerging concepts and future trends. *Nat Rev Neurol.* 2011;7:15-29.

Koeller DM, Kaler SG. Disorders of mineral metabolism (iron, copper, zinc, and molybdenum). In: Sarafoglou K, Georg F, Hoffmann GF, Roth KS, eds. *Pediatric Endocrinology and Inborn Errors of Metabolism.* 2nd ed. New York, NY: McGraw-Hill; 2016.

Poli M, Asperti M, Ruzzenenti P, Regoni M, Arosio P. Hepcidin antagonists for potential treatments of disorders with hepcidin excess. *Front Pharmacol.* 2014;5:86.

Rouault TA. Iron metabolism in the CNS: implications for neurodegenerative diseases. *Nat Rev Neurosci.* 2013;14:551-564.

Rouault TA. Mammalian iron-sulphur proteins: novel insights into biogenesis and function. *Nat Rev Mol Cell Biol.* 2015;16:45-55.

Tuschl K, Meyer E, Valdivia LE, et al. Mutations in SLC39A14 disrupt manganese homeostasis and cause childhood-onset parkinsonism-dystonia. *Nat Commun.* 2016;7:11601.

Zhao N, Zhang AS, Enns CA. Iron regulation by hepcidin. *J Clin Invest.* 2013;123:2337-2343.

# 165 Principles for the Practice of Clinical Genetics

Tanya N. Eble and Sandesh C. S. Nagamani

## INTRODUCTION

Few specialties of medicine, if any, can match the unprecedented advances that have occurred in the field of human and medical genetics during the last 2 decades. Since completion of the sequencing of the human genome in 2003, our understanding of the genetic bases of rare single-gene disorders as well as common multifactorial disorders has increased tremendously. Molecular cytogenetic and sequencing techniques are not only being widely used for diagnosis of many disorders but also to help guide management and therapy, particularly cancer therapy. This chapter outlines the key principles of genetics that are relevant for the practice of medicine.

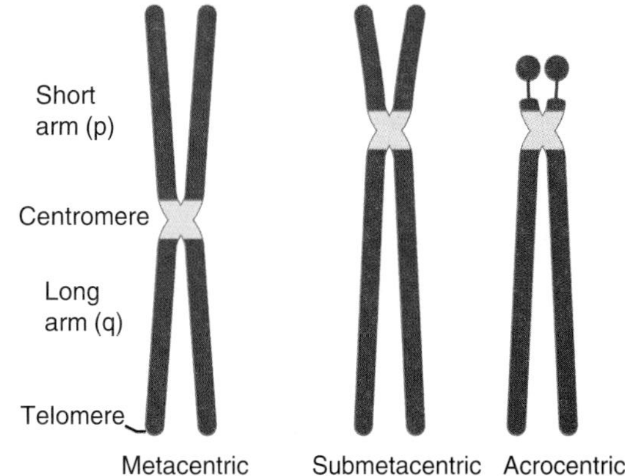


**FIGURE 165-1** Types of human chromosomes. During metaphase, each chromosome is made up of 2 chromatids. Metacentric chromosomes have a central centromere and arms of approximately equal length. Submetacentric chromosomes have an off-center centromere and arms of different lengths. Acrocentric chromosomes (13, 14, 15, 21, and 22) have a centromere toward the end of the chromosome.

## THE HUMAN GENOME

Deoxyribonucleic acid (DNA) contains within its sequence a remarkable amount of information that is essential for all developmental and physiologic processes. DNA is composed of purine (adenine and guanine) and pyrimidine (thymine and cytosine) bases bound to deoxyribose sugar moieties that are covalently linked by phosphodiester bonds. The double helix of DNA consists of 2 complementary strands coiled around a common axis in an antiparallel fashion (the 3′ end of one strand is paired with the 5′ end of the second strand). The pairing of bases between the 2 strands is highly specific; adenine is paired with thymine and guanine with cytosine. The double-stranded structure and complementarity afforded by Watson-Crick base pairing not only permit faithful replication and passing of genetic information during meiosis and mitosis, but also allow for flow of information from DNA to ribonucleic acid (RNA) to protein.

DNA associates with numerous proteins including histones to form higher order structures called chromatin that facilitates packaging of long DNA molecules within the nucleus of the cell. The basic unit of chromatin is the nucleosome, which consists of a segment of DNA wound around 8 histone proteins. The organization of chromatin is complex and involves dynamic interactions between various segments of the DNA. Topologically associating domains (TADs) are regions of DNA that preferentially interact resulting in discrete 3-dimensional chromatin structures that can affect the regulatory architecture of the region. The human genetic material or *genome* is organized into 23 pairs of chromosomes: 22 pairs of autosomes (numbered 1 to 22 from largest to smallest) and 1 pair of sex chromosomes (XX in females and XY in males). Each chromosome consists of a single, continuous, double-stranded DNA molecule, and thus, the *nuclear genome* is essentially composed of 46 linear DNA strands. Almost all cells are diploid (2n), meaning they contain homologous pairs of each chromosome; however, germ cells are haploid (n) and contain only 1 copy of each chromosome. Human chromosomes can be visualized under light microscopy and distinguished based on their size and characteristic staining patterns (e.g., G-banding with Giemsa stain). During metaphase, each chromosome consists of 2 chromatids that have a short (p for petit) and a long arm (q) connected by a centromere. The position of the centromere can be used to classify chromosomes as metacentric, submetacentric, and acrocentric (Fig. 165-1).

The haploid human genome consists of approximately 3 billion base pairs (bp), and thus, each diploid cell contains 6 billion bp. About two-thirds of the human genome is made up of *repetitive elements*, which are stretches of DNA sequences present in multiple copies in the genome. Repetitive elements show significant variations in size, number, and distribution. They can be broadly classified into tandem repeats and interspersed repeats.

Tandem repeats are short nucleotide sequences that are repeated in a head-to-tail orientation and account for approximately 4% of the human genome. Alpha satellites forming the centromeres, telomeric repeats (TTAGGG), microsatellites (typically 2–5 bp), minisatellites, and macrosatelites are tandem repeats. The interspersed repeats are derived from transposable DNA elements. A fascinating feature of the transposable DNA elements is the ability to change their position in the genome. The interspersed repeats comprising DNA transposons, long terminal repeat (LTR) retrotransposons, and non-LTR retrotransposons (short interspersed elements [SINEs] and long interspersed elements [LINEs]) account for 40% of the reference haploid human genome.

The unique sequence DNA constitutes less than half of the genome, and only a small percentage (about 1.5%) of these unique sequences code for proteins. Examples of unique sequence DNA are conserved regulatory sequences, protein coding genes, sequences that encode noncoding RNA including small nucleolar RNAs, long noncoding RNAs (lncRNAs), and microRNAs. The number of protein coding genes is estimated to be between 20,000 and 25,000.

In addition to the nucleus, each mitochondrion in the cell contains multiple copies of DNA. The human mitochondrial DNA (mtDNA) is a small circular molecule of approximately 16,500 bp in length that encodes for 2 ribosomal RNAs, 22 transfer RNAs, and 13 polypeptides that function in the mitochondria. In contrast to the nuclear genome inherited from both parents, all of the *mitochondrial genome* is maternally inherited.

A DNA segment occupying a particular position or location on the chromosome is termed a *locus*. Alternative versions of DNA at a locus are called *alleles*. A *gene* is defined as a set of DNA segments that contains the information necessary to produce a functional product, which could be a functional RNA molecule or a protein. Genes contain exons (segments that code for functional product), introns (intervening sequences that are spliced out), and regulatory sequences including promoters, enhancers, and insulators that control expression of genes (Fig. 165-2).

## GENETIC VARIATION IN HUMANS

Many collaborative efforts including the Human Genome Diversity Project, the ENCODE Project, and the 1000 Genomes Project, among others, have uncovered the remarkable extent of variations in the human genome (Table 165-1). Whereas some genetic variations are common in the general population, others may be rare and limited

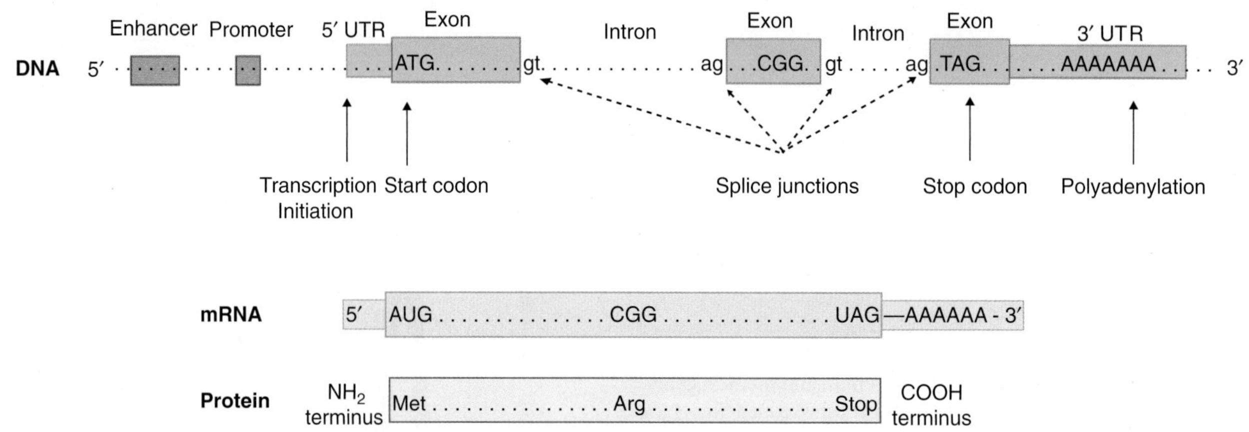


**FIGURE 165-2** Structure of a gene. The flow of information from DNA to RNA to protein is depicted. A gene consists of exons (*green boxes*), introns, and regulatory elements (*red boxes*). The exon-intron boundaries have splice junctions that allow for the removal of the intronic sequences to generate a mature messenger RNA. The RNA molecule serves as the template for translation into a peptide. The 5′ region of a gene corresponds to the amino terminus of the peptide. The untranslated regions (UTRs) in the 5′ and 3′ ends are transcribed but not translated.

**TABLE 165-1 E-RESOURCES**

| Resource | Description | URL |
|---|---|---|
| **UCSC Browser** | A collection of vertebrate and model organism genome assemblies and annotations with tools for accessing and analyzing data | https://genome.ucsc.edu/ |
| **Ensembl Browser** | Genome interface for annotated vertebrate genomes | www.ensembl.org |
| **Human Genome Diversity Project** | Genotype data at more than 650,000 single nucleotide polymorphism loci from 1000+ individuals from around the world | http://www.hagsc.org/hgdp/ |
| **ENCODE Project** | Database of the functional elements in the human genome generated from the ENCODE project | https://www.genome.gov/10005107/encode-project/ |
| **1000 Genomes Project** | Database of utility in identifying human genetic variation | http://www.1000genomes.org/ |
| **DECIPHER** | Database for the medical community to share and compare phenotypic and genotypic data | https://decipher.sanger.ac.uk/ |
| **ExAC** | Exome sequencing data from many large-scale sequencing projects | http://exac.broadinstitute.org/ |
| **Online Mendelian Inheritance in Man (OMIM)** | Compilation of detailed summaries of genes and phenotypes | http://www.ncbi.nlm.nih.gov/omim |
| **Genetic Testing Registry** | Information about genes and genetic conditions with an emphasis on clinical and research genetic testing | http://www.ncbi.nlm.nih.gov/gtr/ |
| **GeneReviews** | Clinically relevant summaries of inherited conditions | http://www.ncbi.nlm.nih.gov/books/NBK1116/ |
| **Genetics Home Reference** | Concise summaries of genetic conditions for healthcare providers and public | https://ghr.nlm.nih.gov/ |

to few individuals. Genetic variations that have a frequency of 1% or more in the population are called *polymorphisms*. The genetic variations in humans are predominantly due to single nucleotide variants (SNVs), insertions/deletions (indels), and copy number variants (CNVs) (Fig. 165-3).

SNVs represent the simplest form of variation that results from a base substitution at a locus during DNA replication. SNVs with a frequency of greater than 1% in the population are termed *single nucleotide polymorphisms* (SNPs). On average, SNPs are observed once every 300 bp in an individual genome. The vast majority of SNPs are inherited and represent changes that have accumulated over many human generations. Whereas most SNPs map outside of the coding regions, about 20,000 SNPs occur within the coding sequences; these have been referred to as cSNPs. SNPs that do not change the encoded amino acid are termed *synonymous*, while those that change the amino acids in the peptides are *nonsynonymous*. SNPs in the noncoding regions of the genome can also have functional consequences if they modify transcription factor binding sites or gene regulatory elements, change the sequence of noncoding RNAs, or generate alternate splice sites in genes.

Indels, or insertion/deletion of nucleotides, can generate multiple alleles at a particular locus. To date, several million small indels have been described in humans. Indels in the coding regions that are not in multiples of 3 alter the reading frame (ie, frameshift alleles), resulting in downstream change in the amino acid sequence that can lead to a nonfunctional protein. For example, indels in *BRCA1* (185delAG and 5382insC) and *BRCA2* (6174delT) commonly found in individuals of Ashkenazi Jewish ancestry are associated with significantly increased risk for breast and ovarian cancer.

Deletions, duplications, triplications, translocations, and complex rearrangements of the genome can result in deviation from the normal diploid state at a particular locus. Such variations, termed CNVs, are now recognized as a major contributor to genetic variation. CNVs are enriched in genomic regions with low copy repeats (DNA fragments longer than 1000 bp with sequence identity of greater than 90%). The number, size, and the population distribution of CNV are yet to be elucidated; however, it is estimated that, on average, each individual harbors 1000 CNVs of size between 500 bp and 1.2 Mb. It has been shown that an individual personal genome differs from the reference genome at more bases in total due to CNV than to all SNV combined. Whereas CNVs can be present without observable consequences, they can be responsible for Mendelian diseases, genomic disorders, and can increase the susceptibility to complex traits. CNVs can result in disease by altering the dosage-sensitive genes (e.g., extra copy of a gene with duplication of a segment), causing gene fusions or interruptions, or by a position effect, in which the rearrangement has effects on expression or regulation of a gene.

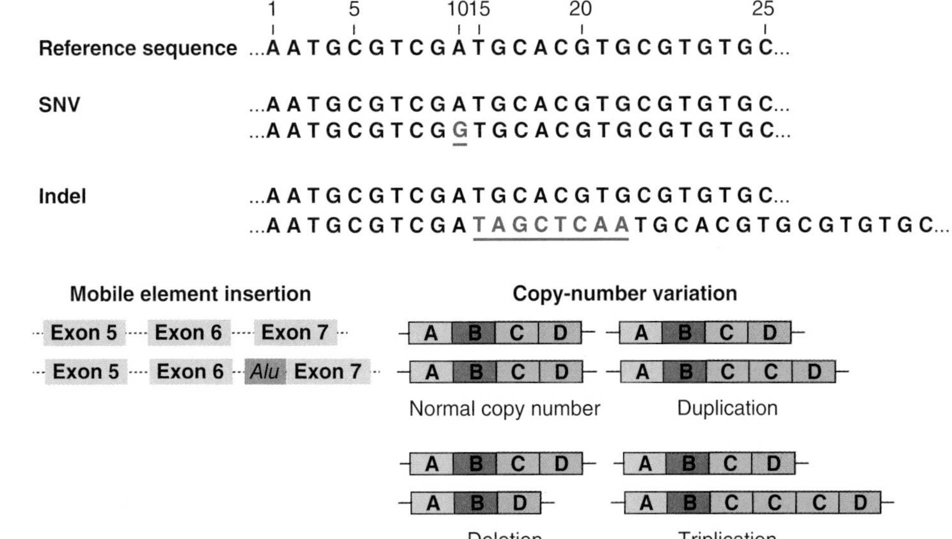


**FIGURE 165-3** Genetic variations in humans. Change in a nucleotide on one allele (G replacing A at position 10), or an indel with addition of insertion of eight bases at position 11, or insertion of *Alu*, a short interspersed element, generates two different alleles at the same locus. Deviation from the normal diploid copy at a locus results in copy number variations (deletion, duplication, and triplication are shown in the figure). These contribute to the significant variations observed in the human genome.

## COMMON TERMINOLOGY USED TO DESCRIBE GENETIC DISORDERS

*Genotype* refers to the genetic constitution, whereas *phenotype* is the expression of a physical, cellular, or biochemical trait. Alternative versions of a gene (or DNA sequence at a locus) are called *alleles*. When a locus has two identical alleles, the genotype (or the individual with the alleles) is *homozygous*; if the alleles are different, and one of them is the wild-type (normal) allele, the genotype is *heterozygous*. *Compound heterozygous* describes a genotype in which two different *mutant* alleles are present at a locus. Because males have only one X chromosome, they are *hemizygous* for most alleles on the X chromosome. *Mutation* is defined as a permanent change in the nucleotide sequence. A mutation that results in disease susceptibility is termed a pathogenic variant. A *missense* variant is one that changes the encoded amino acid; a nonsense variant changes the codon for an amino acid to a termination (stop) codons. A *splice site variant* alters the splicing of introns. *Dynamic mutations* are simple nucleotide repeat sequences that can undergo expansion during gametogenesis (e.g., CGG trinucleotide repeats in *FMR1* in fragile X syndrome). *Allelic heterogeneity* refers to the fact that various different mutations in the same genetic locus cause a similar phenotype (e.g., numerous pathogenic variants in *CFTR* lead to the classic phenotype of cystic fibrosis). *Allelic affinity* refers to different pathogenic variants in the same gene causing different diseases (e.g., pathogenic variants in *MPZ* lead to various neuropathies including early-onset congenital hypomyelinating neuropathy, Dejerine-Sottas neuropathy, and adult-onset Charcot-Marie-Tooth disease type 1B). The distinction between the two terms is that allelic heterogeneity results in different expression of the same disease, whereas allelic affinity results in distinct diagnoses that may have overlapping phenotypes. *Locus heterogeneity* is where mutations in different genetic loci lead to a similar disease phenotype (e.g., Noonan syndrome is caused by pathogenic variants in *PTPN11, SOS1, RAF1, RIT1, KRAS, BRAF, NRAF*, and *MAP2K1*). *Pleiotropy* refers to more than one phenotype caused by mutations in a single gene. For example, pathogenic variants in *FBN1* cause Marfan syndrome, a condition that can present with aortic disease, dislocation of the lens, retinal detachment skeletal abnormalities, and pneumothorax. *Penetrance* is the proportion of individuals with a genotype that expresses the phenotype. When all individuals with a genotype present with phenotype, the condition is completely penetrant. Many phenotypes can have an age-dependent penetrance. *Variable expressivity* refers to differing severity of expression of phenotype among individuals with the same genotype. *Phenocopy* is the presence of a phenotype due to environmental factors that mimics a phenotype associated with a particular genotype. For example, patients with X-linked recessive chondrodysplasia punctate have aberrant bone mineralization, distal phalangeal hypoplasia, and underdevelopment of nasal cartilage. A nearly indistinguishable phenotype can be observed with warfarin embryopathy, a condition that occurs due to teratogenic exposure to coumarin derivatives. A *proband* is an individual with a phenotype through whom the family is ascertained.

## GENETIC BASIS OF DISEASE

Almost every known human disease is influenced by genetic factors. Genetic disorders can be broadly classified into chromosomal disorders, single-gene disorders, and multifactorial disorders.

### CHROMOSOMAL DISORDERS

The normal chromosome constitution in humans is 46,XX in females and 46,XY in males. Chromosomal disorders are caused by numerical or structural aberrations in the chromosomes. Even the smallest autosome, chromosome 21, is estimated to contain 300 genes, and thus, it is not surprising that the aberrations in the number or structure of chromosomes can have significant consequences on gene expression and physiologic processes. Chromosomal abnormalities are relatively common and are a major cause of fetal loss, intellectual disability, and birth defects. Numerical aberrations include the following: polyploidy, where the number of chromosomes is in multiple of the haploid set of 23 chromosomes (e.g., 69,XXX, 92,XXYY); aneuploidy, where there is an abnormal number of chromosomes (e.g., trisomy 21 [47,XY,+21]; monosomy X [45,X]; supernumerary or marker chromosomes [47,XY,+mar(15)]). Structural abnormalities of chromosomes include deletions, duplications, triplications, translocations, inversions, complex genomic rearrangements, and ring chromosomes. Chromosomal basis of disease is detailed in Chapter 166.

### SINGLE-GENE DISORDERS

Single-gene disorders are also called Mendelian disorders because their mode of transmission obeys the principles originally outlined by Gregor Mendel in 1856. Based on the pattern of inheritance, single-gene disorders can be classified into autosomal dominant, autosomal recessive, and X-linked disorders.

More than half of the known Mendelian disorders are inherited in an autosomal dominant (AD) manner. A classical pedigree (a graphical representation of the family tree) in a family with an AD disorder typically shows appearance of the phenotype in multiple generations and transmission of the disorder from both males and females to offspring of either sex (Fig. 165-4A). Each affected individual has a 50% chance of transmitting the mutant allele to his or her offspring, and children of unaffected individuals do not develop the phenotype. Incomplete or age-dependent penetrance, variable expressivity, de novo mutations, and phenocopies have to be considered while interpreting the pedigree. An individual with an AD disorder may appear to have both parents who do not have the disease phenotype. This could be because of a de novo pathogenic variant in the proband, incomplete penetrance where a parent with the mutant allele does not manifest any phenotype, variable expressivity where the phenotype in the parent is mild enough to miss detection, somatic mosaicism in a parent, or nonpaternity. There is an association between advanced paternal age and *de novo* mutations that cause some AD disorders; achondroplasia, thanatophoric dysplasia, Crouzon syndrome, Apert syndrome, and multiple endocrine neoplasia type 2B are examples of such disorders. Rarely, two or more children can be affected by an AD disorder when their parents are clearly unaffected and do not show evidence for the mutant allele in the blood. Such a scenario is likely due to *gonadal mosaicism*, where one parent harbors the pathogenic variant only in the germ cells.

The mechanisms by which pathogenic variants cause AD disorders include haploinsufficiency (decreased amount of the encoded protein; e.g., nonsense variants in *COL1A1* in osteogenesis imperfecta type I); dominant-negative or antimorphic effect (mutant protein interferes with the activity of normal product; e.g., glycine substitution missense variants in *COL1A1* in osteogenesis imperfecta type III); increased activity of the encoded protein (e.g., *FGFR3* missense variant in

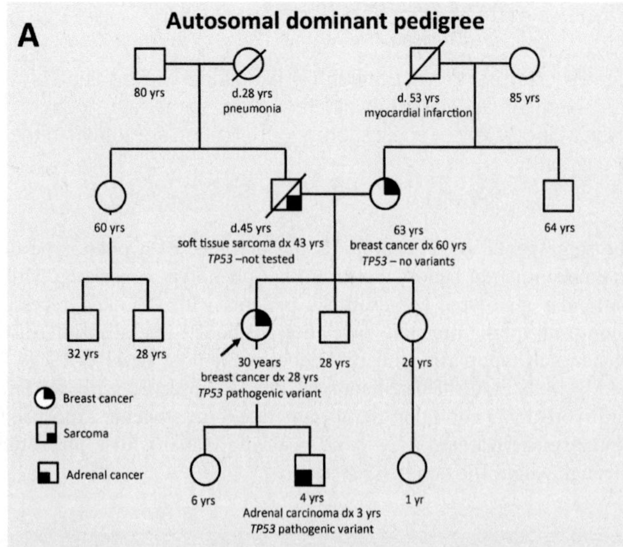


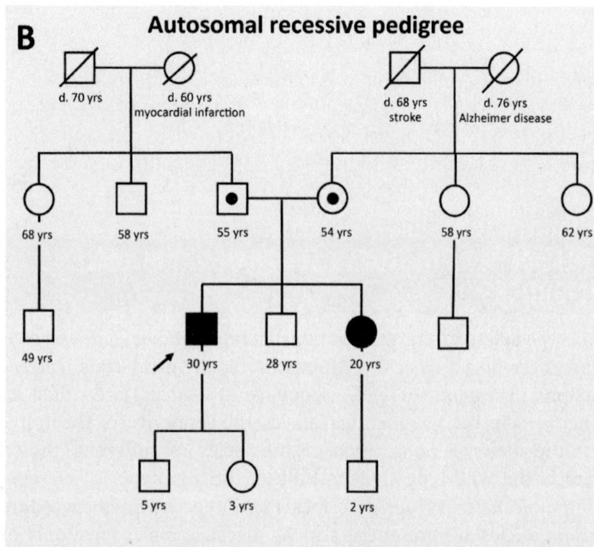


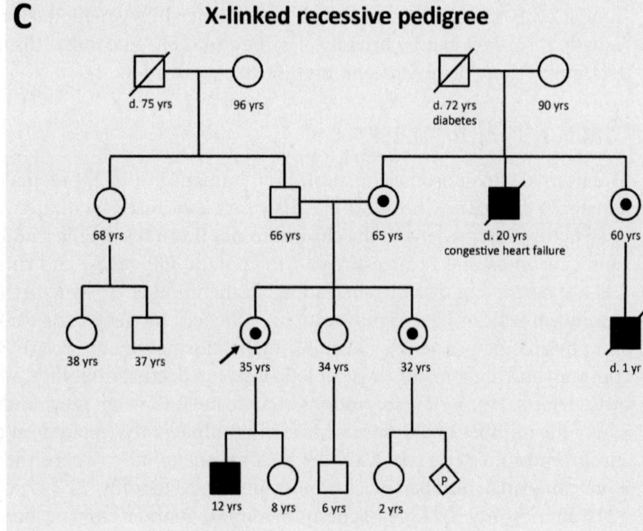


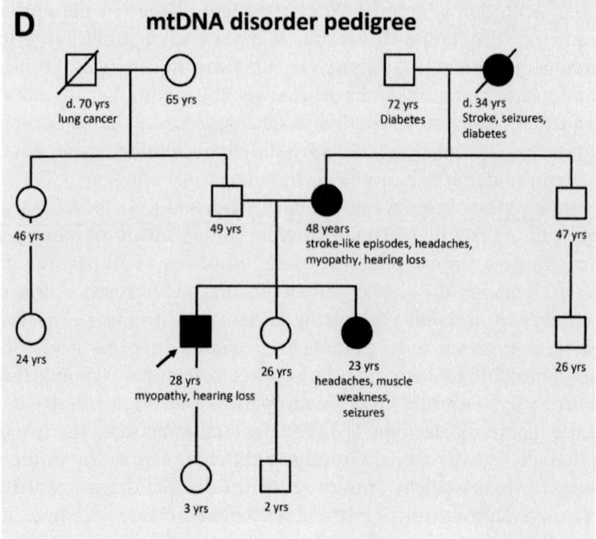


**FIGURE 165-4** Patterns of inheritance. **A.** A family with Li-Fraumeni syndrome an autosomal dominant hereditary cancer disorder caused by pathogenic variants in *TP53*. In the pedigree, circles depict females and squares depict males. The proband is marked by an arrow. Note the vertical transmission of the phenotype in multiple generations. The different types of cancer within the same family and the varying ages at which cancer developed illustrate pleiotropy and variable expressivity, respectively. The breast cancer in the mother of the probands who does not have a pathogenic variant in *TP53* illustrates the phenomenon of phenocopy. **B.** Family with Stargardt disease, an autosomal recessive (AR) form of juvenile macular degeneration caused by biallelic pathogenic variants in *ABCA4*. Note that the phenotype in AR disorders is observed within a sibship and most other family members are unaffected. The parents of the affected individuals are obligate carriers for a pathogenic variant. **C.** Pedigree of a family with Duchenne muscular dystrophy (DMD), an X-linked disorder. Mildly affected or asymptomatic females with a pathogenic variant in *DMD* have a 50% chance of passing on this condition to their male offspring. **D.** mtDNA is maternally inherited. Pedigree of a family with mitochondrial encephalomyopathy, lactic acidosis, and stroke-like episodes syndrome (MELAS) caused by mutations in *MTTL1*. Due to different proportions of mutant mitochondria in various tissues (heteroplasmy), the organ system involvement and severity are variable.

achondroplasia); and neomorphic effect (mutant protein acquires a new function; e.g., CAG trinucleotide repeat expansion in *HTT* in Huntington disease). Irrespective of the type of the variation, a hallmark of AD disorders is that one pathogenic variant is sufficient to cause disease.

### Autosomal Recessive Disorders

Autosomal recessive (AR) disorders occur only when both alleles at a locus are mutated. Individuals with AR disorders may be homozygous or compound heterozygous for a specific locus. A pedigree in a family with an AR disorder typically demonstrates phenotype in the sibship of the affected proband, equal likelihood for both males and females to be affected, and absence of phenotype in the parents and other relatives (Fig. 165-4B). Whereas consanguinity, especially between closely related individuals, increases the risk for AR phenotypes, many disorders occur in the absence of consanguinity.

Some populations have a greater risk for specific AR conditions than other groups of people. Some factors that may affect carrier frequency include *founder effect* and *heterozygous advantage*. Founder effect is the loss of genetic variation that occurs when a new population is established by a very small number of individuals—a population bottleneck. If one or more of these founder individuals harbored a pathogenic variant, the frequency of the variant in their descendants is high. For example, individuals of Ashkenazi Jewish descent have a higher likelihood of being carriers for Tay-Sachs disease, a devastating neurodegenerative condition. A heterozygous advantage is one where the heterozygote genotype has a higher relative fitness than either the homozygote dominant (wild-type alleles) or homozygote recessive genotypes. A classic example of this is the variant in the beta-globin chain of hemoglobin that results in abnormal hemoglobin (HbS). Individuals who are heterozygotes for the HbS allele exhibit increased resistance to malaria, whereas homozygous individuals develop significant anemia.

Parents of individuals affected by autosomal recessive disorders are *carriers*, which means that they each have one mutant allele and one wild-type allele at the locus. A couple with a child with an AR disorder have, with each pregnancy, a probability of 0.25 of having another child with the disorder, 0.5 probability of having a child who is a carrier, and 0.25 probability of having a child with two wild-type alleles at the locus.

The mutant alleles responsible for AR disorders lead to a reduction or abolition of protein product. Heterozygotes are generally asymptomatic because the wild-type allele is able to compensate for the loss of function of the mutant allele.

### X-Linked Disorders

In contrast to the genes on the autosomes, genes located on the X and Y chromosomes are not distributed equally between males and females. Males have only one X chromosome and have a single copy of most of the genes, except a small number of genes mapping to the pseudoautosomal region of the X chromosome that is homologous to a region on the Y chromosome. Females have two copies of every gene on the X chromosome. Dosage compensation in females is achieved by the transcriptional silencing of genes on one copy of the X chromosome in somatic cells. Early during embryonic development in females, genes on one of the X chromosomes are "turned off." Once the pattern of X chromosome inactivation has been established (paternal vs maternal chromosome inactivation), the same X chromosome will be inactivated in all cells derived from the lineage. All females thus exhibit somatic *mosaicism*, as they have two different types of cell lines—cells containing an active maternally derived X chromosome and cells with an active paternally derived X chromosome. The X-inactivation process is controlled by a gene located on the long arm of the X chromosome called *XIST* (X inactive specific transcript [non–protein coding]). The X chromosome contains approximately 1000 genes, but not all are subject to inactivation. It is estimated that 15% of genes may be expressed to some extent. The process is generally random, and there is equal probability that that the paternally and maternally inherited X chromosome will undergo inactivation. However, nonrandom X inactivation can occur and can lead to the expression of an X-linked recessive disease in a female. A cause of nonrandom X chromosome inactivation is a structural abnormality involving the X chromosome. When there are structural aberrations involving one X chromosome, the abnormal X chromosome is inactivated. In contrast, when there is a balanced translocation of an X chromosome and an autosome, the normal X chromosome is usually inactivated. This prevents silencing of the translocated autosome. In aneuploidy of X chromosomes (eg, 47,XXY, 47,XXX), X inactivation leads to transcriptional silencing of all but one X chromosome.

The inheritance pattern of X-linked conditions is distinct from autosomal disorders (Fig. 165-4C). The incidence of disease in X-linked recessive disorders is significantly greater in males than females. Because males do not contribute X chromosomes to their male offspring, male-to-male transmission is not observed. All daughters of a male with an X-linked disorder are carriers for the condition. Male offspring of female carriers with X-linked disease have a 50% chance of developing the disorder. Female carriers may be asymptomatic or exhibit a milder form of the disorder. A classic example is Duchenne muscular dystrophy (DMD), a progressive muscle disease leading to weakness, cardiomyopathy, and early mortality, caused by pathogenic variants in *DMD* on the X chromosome. Female carriers of this condition typically do not have the significant skeletal muscle weakness observed in males but can have elevated levels of creatinine kinase and develop cardiomyopathy during adulthood. Females can have a severe phenotype in X-linked recessive conditions if there is skewed or nonrandom inactivation of X chromosome or absence of a second sex chromosome (Turner syndrome, 45,X).

An X-linked disorder can be described as X-linked dominant if the phenotype is regularly expressed in heterozygotes. Examples for such disorders include focal dermal hypoplasia, X-linked Charcot-Marie-Tooth neuropathy, and X-linked hypophosphatemia. Both male and female offspring of an affected mother have a 50% chance of inheriting the pathogenic variant and developing a phenotype; however, the phenotype in the females is typically milder. However, similar to X-linked recessive inheritance, there is no male-to-male transmission. Some X-linked dominant conditions may be seen predominantly in females, as male fetuses with the condition may not be viable.

### Dynamic Mutations

In the modes of inheritance outlined earlier, the term *pathogenic variant* or *mutation* has been used in the context of a sequence change that is not altered when passed between generations. In contrast, dynamic mutations are simple nucleotide repeat sequences such as CAG, CTG, or ATTCT within genes that can undergo significant expansion between generations. Huntington disease, fragile X syndrome, Friedreich ataxia, myotonic dystrophy, and spinocerebellar ataxia are examples of disorders caused by dynamic mutations or unstable repeat expansions. The wild-type alleles of genes associated with these disorders contain a certain number of repeats; however, expansion beyond a specific limit results in disease. With increasing number of repeats with successive generations, earlier-onset disease and increased phenotypic severity are observed. This phenomenon is called *anticipation*. The disorders conveyed by dynamic mutations can be transmitted in an AD (e.g., Huntington disease), AR (e.g., Friedreich ataxia), or X-linked (e.g., fragile X syndrome) manner.

## NONMENDELIAN INHERITANCE

Many disorders, although clearly genetic, do not follow inheritance patterns in which traits segregate in accordance with Mendel's laws. Some commonly encountered disorders with non-Mendelian inheritance will be outlined in this section.

### Mitochondrial DNA-Related Disorders

The mtDNA codes for 13 subunits of enzymes involved in oxidative phosphorylation, as well as ribosomal and transfer RNA, which are required for the synthesis of mitochondria-encoded peptides. Pathogenic variants in mtDNA cause defects in energy metabolism that can present with involvement of multiple organ systems including muscle, heart, eyes, and brain. The unique characteristics of inheritance of mtDNA-related mitochondrial disorders are maternal inheritance, replicative segregation, and homoplasmy, and heteroplasmy.

Because all mitochondria in the zygote are derived from the ovum, all mtDNA is maternally inherited. Offspring of a female with an mtDNA-related disorder will inherit the mutations, while mtDNA mutations are not passed from a male to his offspring (Fig. 165-4D). The replication of mtDNA and segregation of mitochondria during cell division are rather random, and hence, different tissues contain varying proportions of mutant and normal mtDNA. This phenomenon of replicative segregation can lead to daughter cells with both mutant and normal mtDNA (*heteroplasmy*) or with a pure population of mitochondria with either wild-type or mutant mtDNA (*homoplasmy*). The proportion of mutant mitochondria in different tissues can vary significantly, and thus, pleiotropy and variable expressivity are typical features in mtDNA-related disorders. In rapidly dividing cells like the white blood cells, cells with a large proportion of normal mitochondria typically survive. Genetic tests to assess mtDNA mutations in blood cells may be unrevealing in such scenarios, and testing of other tissues like skin fibroblasts or muscle may be required to confirm the diagnosis. It is to be noted that many mitochondrial disorders are a result of pathogenic variants in the autosomal genes, and these disorders follow the non-Mendelian principles.

### Disorders of Genomic Imprinting

Most autosomal genes are expressed irrespective of whether they are inherited from the mother or the father. However, certain genes are expressed in a parent-of-origin-specific manner. This phenomenon is called *genomic imprinting*. If the allele inherited from the mother is imprinted, that particular allele is silenced and only the allele from the father is expressed and vice versa. Imprinting is an epigenetic process that results in alteration in gene expression without any changes in the nucleotide sequence. Imprinting is associated with non-Mendelian inheritance as the phenotype is dependent on the gender of the parent from whom the pathogenic variant is inherited. For example, hereditary paraganglioma-pheochromocytoma syndrome (PGL/PCC) is a condition characterized by the development of tumors in the autonomic ganglia and the adrenal medulla. A subset of PGL/PCC is caused by pathogenic variants in *SDHD*, a gene that is maternally imprinted. If a pathogenic variant that caused a loss of function of the protein were to be located on the maternal chromosome, it would not have any functional consequences, as that gene would not be expressed. However, if a pathogenic variant were to be on the paternal chromosome, the expressed protein product would be nonfunctional and hence result in the phenotype. Hence this disorder can only be transmitted from an affected father to his offspring. An affected mother can transmit the pathogenic variant but typically not the phenotype to her offspring.

### Uniparental Disomy

Rarely, both copies of a homologous pair of chromosomes may be inherited from a single parent. This distortion from biparental inheritance is termed *uniparental disomy* (UPD). The most common mechanism responsible for UPD is trisomy rescue. During the early development, if an embryo is trisomic and one chromosome is lost to restore disomy, both copies in the homologous pair could be from a single parent, thus leading to UPD. UPD can lead to disease when a uniparental chromosome contains a recessive mutation or an imprinted gene.

### Digenic Inheritance

Non-Mendelian inheritance can also be seen with digenic inheritance where pathogenic variants in two different genes are required to manifest phenotype. For example, heterozygous pathogenic variants in *CDH23* and *PCDH15*, when present together, result in Usher syndrome, type 1D/F. In some individuals with Bardet-Biedl syndrome and cortisone reductase deficiency, three abnormal alleles in two different genes have been identified, representing digenic triallelic inheritance.

### Multifactorial Inheritance

The risk for many congenital anomalies like cleft lip and palate and neural tube defects as well as adult-onset disorders like diabetes, hypertension, and cancer are increased in individuals with family history of these disorders. However, their mode of transmission is not Mendelian. Disorders that occur as a result of interactions between many genetic and environmental factors follow a complex or multifactorial inhertiance pattern.

## COMMON TESTING MODALITIES IN CLINICAL GENETICS

Laboratory testing of genetic disorders and diagnostic algorithms of clinical relevance have been outlined in Chapters 167 and 169, respectively. This section will provide a brief overview of available testing modalities.

Large aberrations of chromosomes such as translocations, deletions, or duplications greater than 5 Mb in size can be diagnosed by G-banded karyotype analysis. Genome-wide screening assays such as array-based comparative genomic hybridization (aCGH) are typically used to assess submicroscopic rearrangements like microduplications and microdeletions. Next-generation sequencing (NGS) technologies that enable simultaneous and massively parallel sequencing of DNA have made it possible to develop “gene panel tests” and whole-exome sequencing (WES). Whereas the panel tests can interrogate multiple genes implicated in particular phenotypes, WES involves sequencing of the exons or coding regions of thousands of genes. These technologies have revolutionized molecular diagnosis in clinical genetics. Currently, the diagnostic yield from the utilization of WES as a clinical test is around 25%. NGS technologies have also made it possible to amplify cell-free DNA from maternal serum for prenatal screening of trisomies of chromosomes 13, 18, or 21. With decreasing costs of sequencing and the continuous improvements in molecular technologies and interpretation of data, the diagnostic yield and the impact of genetic testing can only improve in the future.

## ETHICAL ISSUES IN GENETIC TESTING OF MINORS

While the unprecedented advances in genetic testing have undoubtedly led to improved molecular diagnosis and care of individuals with genetic disorders, such testing can have ethical, social, and legal implications. Appropriate counseling about genetic testing and its implications, obtaining informed consent for testing, and active involvement of patients and their parent(s), or legal guardian(s) in the decision making are cornerstones of the practice of clinical genetics.

Parents or legal guardians are typically entrusted with medical decision-making power with regard to minors. However, involving minors in the decision-making process fosters development of autonomy and builds trust between the patient and the healthcare provider. Obtaining assent from minors during the informed consent process with their parents should be pursued. Communicating complicated genetic information to minors who are old enough to provide assent can be challenging and is best done by clinical geneticists, genetic counselors, or other trained professionals.

The ethical issues regarding genetic testing for adult-onset disorders in asymptomatic minors have generated much discussion. Most geneticists and bioethicists agree that for disorders that clearly have manifestations only in adults and do not affect children, and for which earlier testing does not lead to any intervention, genetic testing is best deferred until adulthood. The recommendation against the testing of asymptomatic minors is meant to protect autonomy until a time when the individual can make an informed decision. However, with the use of tests that can assay genetic variants on a genome-wide level, application of this principle can be complicated. WES is fast becoming a widely used clinical test for diagnosis of birth defects and a wide range of pediatric age–onset disorders. WES involves sequencing of the entire exome and thus can uncover incidental findings that are unrelated to the phenotype being investigated. Most laboratories report not only on genes related to the phenotype, but also on medically actionable variants. It has been argued that the potential benefit of medically actionable incidental findings to the health of the child outweighs the ethical concerns of providing this information.

Genetic testing performed in an appropriate and responsible manner has the ability to significantly improve the molecular diagnosis and management of many disorders and provide risk assessment for additional family members. It is the responsibility of healthcare providers to consider and address the ethical issues associated with such testing.

## SUGGESTED READINGS


Lupski JR, Belmont JW, Boerwinkle E, Gibbs RA. Clan genomics and the complex architecture of human disease. *Cell*. 2011;147:32-43.

Pope BD, Ryba T, Dileep V, et al. Topologically associating domains are stable units of replication-timing regulation. *Nature*. 2014;515: 402-405.

Trivellin G, Daly AF, Faucz FR, et al. Gigantism and acromegaly due to Xq26 microduplications and *GPR101* mutation. *N Engl J Med*. 2014;371:2363-2374.

Wu N, Ming X, Xiao J, et al. *TBX6* null variants and a common hypomorphic allele in congenital scoliosis. *N Engl J Med*. 2015;372:341-350.

Yang Y, Muzny DM, Xia F, et al. Molecular findings among patients referred for clinical whole-exome sequencing. *JAMA*. 2014;312(18):1870-1879.


# 166 Chromosomal and Genomic Disorders

Tamar Harel, James R. Lupski, and Seema R. Lalani

## INTRODUCTION

Chromosomal disorders can be classified into numerical and structural abnormalities of the chromosomes and are frequently encountered in clinical practice. They account for the majority of spontaneous abortions in the first trimester of pregnancy and are a major cause of congenital malformations, intellectual disability, and neurodevelopmental disorders.

**Aneuploidy** is defined as the presence of an abnormal number of chromosomes in a cell, resulting from errors in chromosome segregation during meiosis and, less frequently, in mitosis. Most cases of aneuploidy of the autosomes are incompatible with life and lead to early pregnancy loss. The viable autosomal trisomies involve some of the smaller chromosomes, namely 21, 18, and 13. Aneuploidy of the sex chromosomes is tolerated more than aneuploidy of the autosomes. It is estimated that about 1 in 400 newborns has an abnormality of one of the sex chromosomes.

**Genomic disorders** involve structural abnormalities of the chromosomes and have become increasingly recognized with advanced technologies, enabling recognition of submicroscopic losses and gains of genetic material; ie, DNA deletion and duplication rearrangements. The phenotype in these disorders can result from abnormal gene dosage of 1 or more of the genes in the deleted or duplicated interval or from interruption of a gene at a breakpoint junction. Many of the disorders have a specific constellation of physical findings and congenital malformations, which can be recognized clinically.

Evaluation of chromosome number and structure should be considered in any child with multiple major and/or minor anomalies. For suspected aneuploidy such as proportionate short stature or primary amenorrhea in females (Turner syndrome) and small testes or significant gynecomastia in adolescent males (Klinefelter syndrome), an evaluation by G-banded karyotype study is warranted. Many clinicians recommend chromosomal microarray analysis (CMA), for assessment of children with intellectual disability and/or multiple congenital anomalies including congenital heart defects (CHD) (22q11.2 microdeletion syndrome). Other clinical indications for cytogenetic analysis include evaluation of stillbirths, as well as abortuses in recurrent cases, potentially due to a familial translocation.

## MECHANISMS OF ANEUPLOIDY AND GENOMIC IMBALANCE

**Nondisjunction**, the failure of homologous chromosomes or sister chromatids to separate properly during cell division, results in gametes with abnormal chromosome numbers (Fig. 166-1). Fertilization of such gametes results in either monosomy (eg, Turner syndrome, 45,X) or trisomy (eg, Down syndrome). Advanced maternal age is associated with an increasing risk of meiotic nondisjunction, most likely due to the prolonged meiotic arrest of human oocytes. Occasionally, a fertilized ovum containing 3 copies of a chromosome resulting from a meiotic error loses 1 of the chromosomes in a process known as **trisomy rescue**. If the 2 retained chromosomes originate from the same parent, **uniparental disomy** results. Uniparental disomy (UPD) can cause disease by the copy number neutral genetic mechanisms of: (1) imprinting, an epigenetic mechanism dependent on the parent-of-origin of the mutation, and (2) reduction to homozygosity of recessive disease alleles present in 1 parental carrier on the chromosome associated with UPD.

A carrier of a balanced **chromosomal translocation** can have offspring with unbalanced genomic material, with either extra or missing regions of chromosomes. **Robertsonian translocations** involve fusion of the long arms of 2 acrocentric chromosomes (13, 14, 15, 21, and 22) with loss of the p arms. The unaffected parent carrying a Robertsonian translocation has 45 chromosomes and is at an increased risk of having progeny with an unbalanced rearrangement.

The mechanisms leading to terminal deletion syndromes (where the distal portion of either a long or short arm of a chromosome is deleted, eg, cri du chat syndrome due to 5p deletion) are not yet well-defined for several chromosomal regions. These deletion syndromes

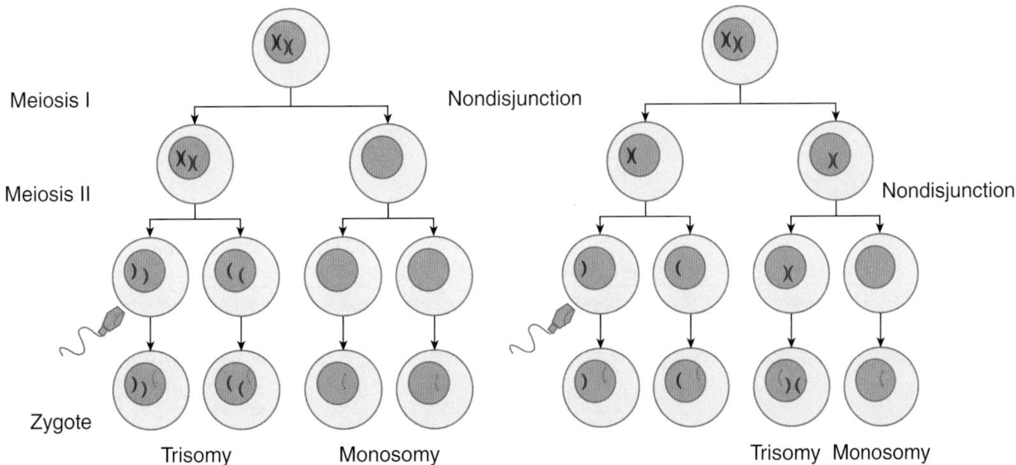


**FIGURE 166-1** Nondisjunction leads to trisomy or monosomy. Nondisjunction during meiosis I (*left*) or meiosis II (*right*) leads to gametes with an extra or missing chromosome. Fertilization of such gametes results in trisomy or monosomy.

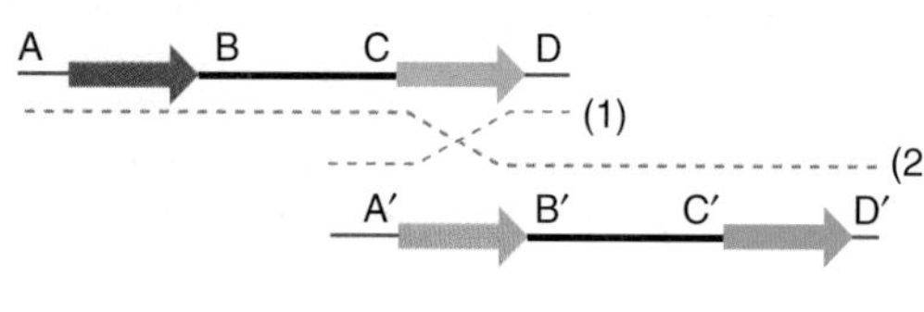


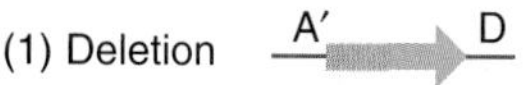


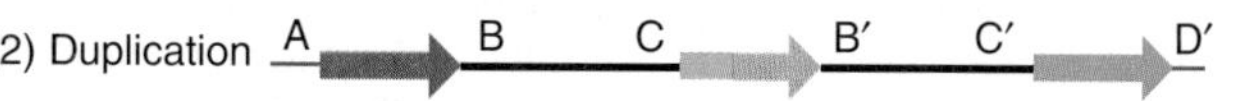


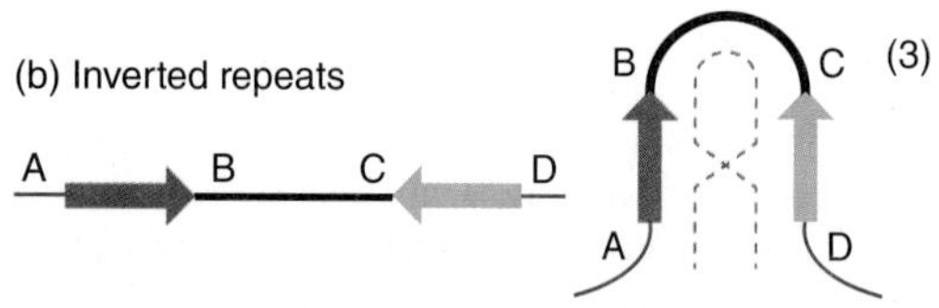


(3) Inversion A C B D

**FIGURE 166-2** Mechanism of genomic rearrangements. **A.** Recombination between direct repeats can lead to either deletion (1) or duplication (2). **B.** Recombination between inverted repeats leads to an inversion (3). *Thick arrows* represent repeated sequences, and the *thick black line* represents the genomic segment prone to rearrangement. Letters flanking the thick arrows represent unique sequences, and primed letters represent the unique sequence on the homologous chromosome. (Modified with permission from Lupksi JR. Genomic disorders: structural features of the genome can lead to DNA rearrangements and human disease traits, *Trends Genet.* 1998 Oct;14(10):417-422.)

often have variable breakpoints, with consequent wide phenotypic variability. In contrast to the terminal deletions, interstitial deletions and duplications are often recurrent, ie, occur at the same breakpoints. **Segmental duplications**, or low-copy repeats, are defined as DNA sequences of about > 1 kb in size with high (>90%) sequence identity, which occur at more than 1 site within the haploid genome. Nearly identical sequences (>97% sequence identity), typically longer than 10 kb, can predispose to ectopic synapsis and homologous recombination between nonallelic copies (ie, nonallelic homologous recombination [NAHR]) and can give rise to deletions, duplications, and inversions (Fig. 166-2).

An understanding of the mechanisms underlying chromosomal aneuploidy and genomic abnormalities is essential to the understanding of recurrence risks for these disorders.

## COMMON TRISOMY SYNDROMES

The 3 most common autosomal trisomies in live-born newborns are trisomies 21, 18, and 13 (Table 166-1). Trisomies of other chromosomes have been described, mostly in the mosaic state. The importance of appropriate counseling for the families, including an explanation of medical management, recurrence risk, and information regarding parent support groups, cannot be understated.

### TRISOMY 21: DOWN SYNDROME

Down syndrome is caused by an extra copy of chromosome 21 and is the most common cause of intellectual disability. It has an overall incidence estimated at 1 in 650 to 850 newborns. Full trisomy 21 resulting from nondisjunction of the chromosome 21 pair during meiosis is observed in about 95% of cases, while mosaic trisomy 21 and Robertsonian translocations involving chromosome 21 (usually 14/21 and 21/21) account for the remainder of cases. The majority are due to errors in maternal meiosis, which increase with maternal age; thus, the risk for having a child with trisomy 21 increases with maternal age, especially after age 30 years, and approaches 1 in 10 births in the oldest maternal age group (45–50 years). However, the birth rate in younger mothers is much higher, and therefore, the majority of babies with Down syndrome are born to mothers younger than 35 years. The paternal age appears to have no influence on the trisomy risk.

Down syndrome can often be recognized at birth, if not ascertained prenatally, by hypotonia and distinctive facial features (Fig. 166-3). Characteristic features are summarized in Table 166-2 and include brachycephaly with a flat occiput, epicanthal folds, upslanting palpebral fissures, speckling of the iris (Brushfield spots), a flat nasal bridge, protruding tongue, and small ears. The neck is short with loose folds of skin on the back of the neck, and the hands are short and broad and often have a single transverse palmar crease and incurved fifth digits (clinodactyly). A wide gap between the first and second toes is sometimes present and referred to as a "sandal gap."

Additional features include CHD, found in approximately 50% of children with Down syndrome. Atrioventricular canal defect is the most common heart defect, followed by ventricular septal defect (VSD). Echocardiogram is recommended as a screening measure in all children with Down syndrome. Common obstructive gastrointestinal malformations include duodenal atresia and Hirschsprung disease. Hematologic abnormalities include transient myeloproliferative disorder during the neonatal period and early infancy and an increased risk of leukemia later in life, specifically a 20-fold increased risk of acute lymphoblastic leukemia and a 500-fold increased risk of acute megakaryoblastic leukemia (AMKL), a subtype of acute myeloid leukemia. Children with Down syndrome have a significant risk of recurrent otitis media, hearing loss, obstructive sleep apnea, and pulmonary hypertension. Eye disease includes cataracts and refractive errors.

**TABLE 166-1 COMMON AUTOSOMAL TRISOMIES**

| Trisomy | Incidence | Key Findings on Exam | Associated Malformations and Disorders | Life Expectancy |
|---|---|---|---|---|
| Trisomy 21 (Down syndrome) | ~1/650–1/850 | Hypotonia, excess nuchal folds, flat facial profile, single transverse palmar crease | CHD, duodenal atresia, Hirschsprung disease, hypothyroidism, risk for leukemia | > 50 years |
| Trisomy 18 (Edward syndrome) | ~1/5000–1/6000 | Hypertonia, clenched fists with overlapping fingers | CHD, omphalocele, gut malrotation | >90% die within first year |
| Trisomy 13 (Patau syndrome) | ~1/10,000–1/15,000 | Microcephaly, polydactyly, ocular abnormalities, cleft lip and palate | Severe CNS malformations (holoprosencephaly), CHD | >90% die within first year |

CHD, congenital heart disease; CNS, central nervous system.

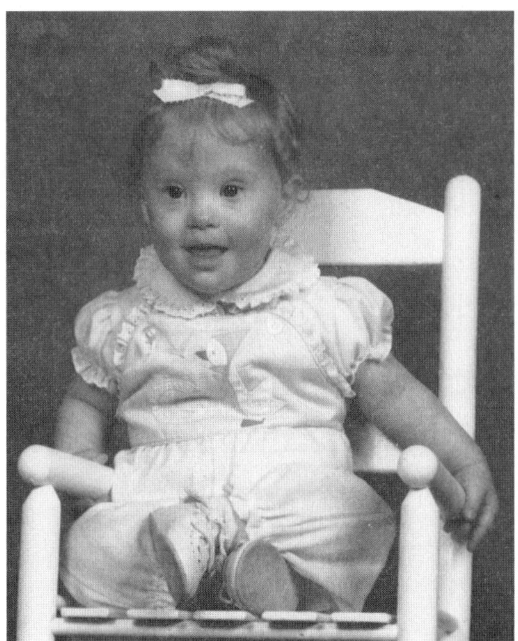

FIGURE 166-3 Child with Down syndrome. Note the upslanting palpebral fissures, epicanthal folds, and flat facial profile. (Reproduced with permission from Jorde LB, Carey JC, Bamshad MJ, White RL: *Medical Genetics*, St. Louis, Mosby, 2000.)

Orthopedic complications include hip dislocations and atlantoaxial instability with or without subluxation, requiring careful consideration during anesthetic airway management and risk assessment of certain sports. Endocrine disorders with higher incidence include type 1 diabetes mellitus and hypothyroidism. The risk of Graves disease is also increased in individuals with Down syndrome. Specific recommendations regarding surveillance in children with Down syndrome have been published by the American Academy of Pediatrics Committee on Genetics and are summarized as Table 166-3.

Intellectual disability in children with Down syndrome is variable, usually mild to moderate. Development usually progresses steadily, albeit at a slower pace, with no evidence of regression. Children learn to walk and develop communication skills and often function more effectively in social situations than would be predicted on the basis of cognitive assessment alone. Early intervention, proper medical management, and educational and vocational training can significantly affect the level of functioning in children and adolescents with Down syndrome and facilitate their transition into adulthood.

**TABLE 166-2 TYPICAL FEATURES IN DOWN SYNDROME**

| | |
|---|---|
| Head shape | Brachycephaly, flat occiput |
| Face | Flat facial profile |
| Eyes | Epicanthal folds, upslanting palpebral fissures, Brushfield spots on iris |
| Nose | Flat nasal bridge, small nose |
| Mouth | Small mouth, protruding tongue |
| Ears | Small, dysplastic auricles |
| Neck | Excessive skin on back of neck |
| Stomach | Diastasis recti |
| Extremities | Shortened |
| Hands | Single transverse palmar crease |
| Fingers | Short fifth finger due to short middle phalanx, clinodactyly |
| Toes | Wide space between first and second toes, often with plantar groove |
| Joints | Hyperextensibility or hyperflexibility |
| Skin | Dry skin |
| Tone | Hypotonia |

**TABLE 166-3 EVALUATION AND SURVEILLANCE OF NEWBORNS WITH DOWN SYNDROME, BASED ON RECOMMENDATIONS BY AMERICAN ACADEMY OF PEDIATRICS (2011)**

| Evaluate for | Recommended Evaluation | Age at Evaluation and Frequency |
|---|---|---|
| Diagnosis and determination of recurrence risk | Karyotype analysis | Newborn |
| Heart defect | Echocardiogram | Newborn |
| Cataracts | Red reflex (if abnormal, refer to ophthalmologist) | Newborn; annually until age 5 years; then space out follow-up visits |
| Hearing loss | Audiology testing (BAER or OAE) | Newborn, 6 months; then evaluate hearing every 6 months |
| TMD, polycythemia, leukemia | CBC | Newborn; Hb annually thereafter |
| Hypothyroidism | Thyroid function studies | Newborn, 6 and 12 months; annually thereafter |
| Duodenal atresia or anorectal atresia/stenosis | | Newborn |
| Apnea, bradycardia, oxygen desaturation | Car safety seat for infants at risk | Newborn |
| Obstructive sleep apnea | Sleep study | By age 4 years |
| Aspirations, feeding difficulties | Radiographic swallowing assessment | If symptomatic |
| Atlantoaxial instability | Neutral position spine films; if normal, obtain flexion and extension films | If neurologic signs and symptoms |
| Constipation (due to restricted diet, limited fluid intake, hypotonia, GI malformation) | | As indicated |
| GERD | | As indicated |
| Tracheal anomalies | | As indicated |
| Celiac disease | | As indicated |

BAER, brain stem auditory evoked response; CBC, complete blood count; GERD, gastroesophageal reflux disease; GI, gastrointestinal; Hb, hemoglobin; OAE, otoacoustic emissions; TMD, transient myeloproliferative disorder.

Life expectancy has increased dramatically in recent decades, to 50 to 55 years in the developed countries with proper health care. Neuropathologic hallmarks of Alzheimer disease (senile plaques, neurofibrillary tangles) are present in brains of nearly all individuals with Down syndrome by age 40 years. This is presumed to be secondary to the extra dosage of the amyloid precursor protein gene (*APP*) on chromosome 21; indeed, *APP* duplication has been reported in families with autosomal dominant Alzheimer disease. Premature dementia is found in about one-third of the Down syndrome population by age 60, with an estimated lifetime prevalence of 90% for all people with Down syndrome.

While the specific dosage-sensitive genes that cause the features of Down syndrome in individuals with trisomy 21 have not been fully elucidated, extra copies of *DYRK1A*, *SIM2*, *DSCAM*, and *RCAN1* have been implicated in the neurologic phenotype. Interestingly, somatic mutations in the *GATA1* gene, localized on chromosome X, have been associated with transient myeloproliferative disorder and AMKL in Down syndrome.

Therapeutic trials in mouse models and in cell lines have targeted specific transmitters and signaling pathways in the brain, which are affected by the extra dosage of genes on chromosome 21. Other trials have employed neuroprotective agents, and yet other therapies aim to normalize expression of proteins encoded by triplicated genes. A recent study showed the ability to inactivate the entire third copy of chromosome 21 in Down syndrome pluripotent stem cells via a mechanism similar to the inactivation of X chromosome in females. Due to the critical window of organ development, prenatal therapies likely have potential for the greatest impact.

Overall, the recurrence risk of trisomy 21 is estimated at approximately 1% for mothers younger than 30 years after having a child with trisomy 21 and approximates the age-related risk in older mothers. Trisomy 21, associated with Down syndrome, can be detected prenatally by karyotype analysis, chromosomal microarray, or genome-wide analyses by next-generation DNA sequencing. To address the recurrence risk for families, G-banded karyotype analysis is recommended as the study of choice. The recurrence risk for translocation carriers is higher and depends on the chromosomes involved in the translocation and the sex of the parent carrying the rearrangement.

## TRISOMY 18: EDWARDS SYNDROME

Trisomy 18, or Edwards syndrome, is the second most common autosomal trisomy and occurs in approximately 1 in 5000 to 6000 live-born infants (see Table 166-1). Around 80% of affected live-born individuals are females. Trisomy 18 is a common cause of stillbirth. Both neonatal and infant mortality are increased, with 50% of newborns succumbing to the disorder in the first week of life. Only 10% survive beyond the first birthday, even with optimal management.

The recognizable pattern of abnormalities (Fig. 166-4) includes growth deficiency of prenatal onset and a distinctive face, with prominent occiput, narrow bifrontal diameter, short palpebral fissures, small mouth, micrognathia, and low-set, malformed ears. Other features include a short sternum and a clenched hand with overlapping of index finger and fifth finger over the third and the fourth, respectively. Nail hypoplasia and a small pelvis with limited hip abduction can be observed. CHDs are frequent and most often include polyvalvular disease and VSD. Infants may have apneic episodes in the neonatal period and demonstrate poor feeding requiring nasogastric tube feeding. Children who survive beyond the first year have severe intellectual disability.

The vast majority of children with Edwards syndrome have full trisomy 18, and the risk increases with maternal age, similar to other trisomies. About 5% of infants have mosaicism for trisomy 18 or partial trisomy of the long arm of chromosome 18. Recurrence risk is approximately 1% for mothers under age 35 years and approximates the age-related risk for older females.

## TRISOMY 13: PATAU SYNDROME

The third most common viable trisomy in humans is trisomy 13, or Patau syndrome, which occurs in approximately 1 in 10,000 to 15,000 live births (see Table 166-1). Characteristic features include cleft lip and/or palate, microphthalmia, scalp defects (cutis aplasia), and postaxial polydactyly of the hands and at times, feet (Fig. 166-5).

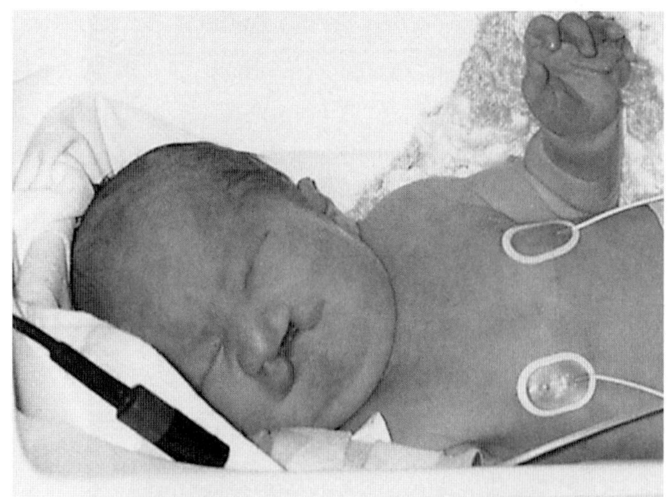

A

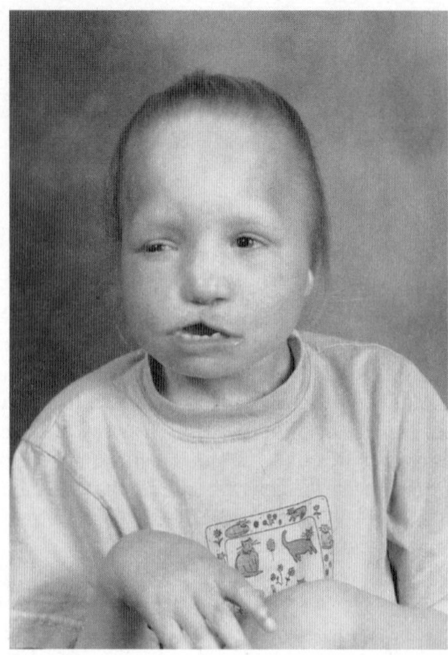

B

**FIGURE 166-5** Infant with Trisomy 13. **A.** Newborn showing typical features of trisomy 13 (Patau syndrome), including bilateral cleft lip and broad nasal bridge and postaxial polydactyly of the left hand. **B.** An older child with trisomy 13. Note the repaired cleft lip. (Reproduced with permission from Jorde LB, Carey JC, Bamshad MJ, White RL: *Medical Genetics*, St. Louis, Mosby, 2000.)

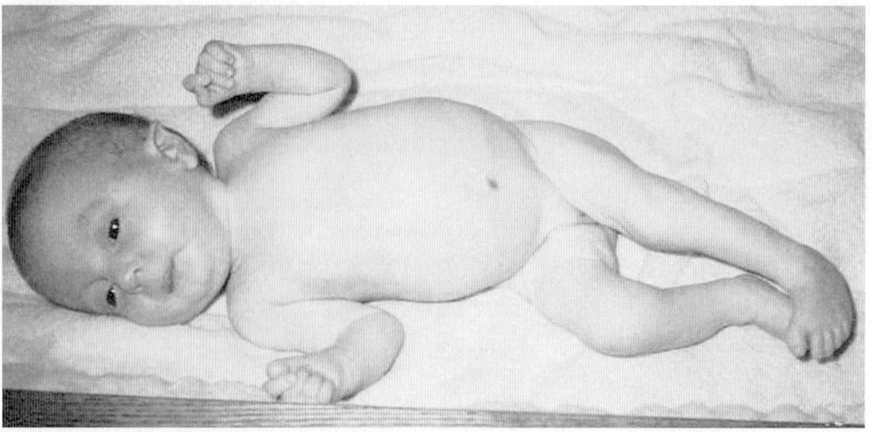

**FIGURE 166-4** Infant with trisomy 18. A newborn girl with trisomy 18 (Edwards syndrome), showing the short sternum, typical clenched fist with overlapping fingers, and left-sided clubfoot. (Reproduced with permission from Jorde LB, Carey JC, Bamshad MJ, White RL: *Medical Genetics*, St. Louis, Mosby, 2000.)

Holoprosencephaly-type defects with varying degrees of incomplete development of the forebrain and olfactory and optic nerves are common. CHDs are found in approximately 80% of patients, including VSD, patent ductus arteriosus (PDA), and atrial septal defect (ASD). Apneic spells are common in early infancy. The median survival is 1 week. Over 90% of patients die within the first year of life. Infants who survive have severe intellectual disability, seizures, and failure to thrive.

The majority of children with trisomy 13 have 3 complete copies of chromosome 13. A small number of infants with Patau syndrome have an extra copy of the long arm of chromosome 13 caused by an unbalanced Robertsonian translocation (ie, 2 long arms fused at a centromere). Infants mosaic for trisomy 13 are usually less severe and have variable presentations.

## GENOMIC DISORDERS

### CHROMOSOMAL DELETION SYNDROMES

Chromosomal deletions at the distal ends of either arm of a chromosome typically give rise to developmental delay, intellectual disability, and a chromosome-specific constellation of dysmorphic features and birth defects. Deletions at the ends of chromosomes can often be visualized on karyotype by standard G-banded chromosome analysis. These can arise de novo or result from a balanced rearrangement in a parent. Such deletions usually have variable breakpoints, such that the phenotype varies in severity depending on which genes are deleted. Overall, cytogenetically visible autosomal deletions occur with an estimated incidence of 1 in 7000 live births. Some are observed in only a few individuals, while others are sufficiently common to allow for delineation of a clinically recognizable syndrome.

Wolf-Hirschhorn syndrome, or 4p deletion syndrome, is estimated to occur in 1 in 50,000 births with female predominance. It is characterized by marked growth deficiency of prenatal onset, microcephaly, developmental delay, and a typical facial appearance described as a "Greek warrior helmet" facies, consisting of a high forehead, prominent glabella, hypertelorism, and a broad nasal bridge. CHDs are found in about 50% of the affected individuals. Seizures are frequent in infancy and childhood, but usually cease by age 10 years.

Cri du chat syndrome, with an estimated incidence of 1 in 15,000 births, is caused by a deletion of the short arm of chromosome 5 (5p). It derives its name from a distinctive cry in infancy, caused by an anatomic alteration of the larynx. The facial characteristics include a round face, hypertelorism, and epicanthal folds, and can include preauricular tags. Feeding problems and respiratory difficulties are common in the first year. Approximately 30% have a heart defect; other major malformations are rare. The degree of intellectual disability correlates with the size of the deletion, although studies suggest that particular regions within 5p14-5p15 may contribute disproportionately to severe intellectual disability.

Other well-characterized terminal deletion syndromes that are large enough to be identifiable on routine karyotype include deletions of 9p, 13q, and 18q and are summarized in Table 166-4.

### MICRODELETION SYNDROMES

A common terminal deletion syndrome, which was characterized after the introduction of molecular cytogenetics with the use of subtelomeric fluorescence in situ hybridization (FISH) technique, is the 1p36 microdeletion syndrome. At an incidence of approximately 1 in 5000, it is estimated to be the second most common deletion syndrome in humans. The breakpoints are variable and probably reflect a range of different mutational mechanisms. Phenotypic features include intellectual disability, severely delayed speech, behavioral difficulties, postnatal onset of growth deficiency, hypotonia, microcephaly, a late-closing anterior fontanel, and a characteristic facies with straight eyebrows and low-set, posteriorly rotated ears with thickened ear helices. Seizures and brain malformations are frequent. Structural heart defects can be found in approximately 70% of individuals; left ventricular noncompaction has been reported in up to approximately 20% of individuals.

**TABLE 166-4 COMMON TERMINAL DELETION SYNDROMES IDENTIFIABLE ON ROUTINE CHROMOSOME ANALYSIS**

| Deletion Syndrome | Characteristic Features | Phenotype |
|---|---|---|
| 4p (Wolf-Hirschhorn syndrome) | Microcephaly, hypertelorism, distinctive appearance of nose, short philtrum, micrognathia, simple ears | Growth deficiency of prenatal onset, severe feeding difficulties, seizures that tend to cease by age 10 years, visual and hearing problems, severe DD |
| 5p (cri du chat syndrome) | Round face, hypertelorism, epicanthal folds, downslanting palpebral fissures | Growth deficiency of prenatal onset, mewing cry in infancy, CHD, DD |
| 9p | Prominent forehead with metopic ridge, trigonocephaly | Mild to severe ID, behavioral problems |
| 13q | Microcephaly, trigonocephaly, hypertelorism, ptosis, short big toe | Growth deficiency of prenatal onset, susceptibility to retinoblastoma if 13q14 deleted, brain malformations, distal limb anomalies, GI malformations |
| 18q | Midface hypoplasia, deep-set eyes, prominent antihelix, long hands with tapering fingers | Hearing loss associated with narrow or atretic external canal, ureteral reflux, recurrent urinary tract infection, intellectual disability, growth deficiency of postnatal onset, disproportionate short stature, behavioral problems |

DD, developmental delay; GI, gastrointestinal; ID, intellectual disability.

Contiguous gene syndromes result from deletions or duplications of multiple well-characterized disease-associated genes. In such cases, an amalgamation of multiple clinical features can be observed, specific to the phenotype linked to each disease-associated gene within the deleted interval. For example, WAGR (predisposition to Wilms tumor, aniridia, genitourinary anomalies, and retardation) results from a deletion on chromosome 11p13, which encompasses *WT1*, encoding Wilms tumor 1, and *PAX6*, a gene important for ocular development. Similarly, deletion of chromosome 16p encompassing *TSC2* and *PKD1* causes tuberous sclerosis and polycystic kidney disease, respectively. Yet another example is a duplication on chromosome 17p11.2p12, encompassing both *PMP22* and *RAI1*, respectively, associated with Charcot-Marie-Tooth disease type 1A and Potocki-Lupski syndrome.

#### Reciprocal Microdeletion and Microduplication Syndromes

Recurrent deletions, wherein unrelated individuals share deletion breakpoints in precisely the same regions, arise by nonallelic homologous recombination between segmental duplications or low copy repeats (LCRs). These are often associated with clinically and molecularly recognizable reciprocal duplication syndromes. Chromosomal regions with a high concentration of LCRs are particularly prone to rearrangements, including deletions, duplications, and inversions (see Fig. 166-2). Examples of microdeletion and duplication syndromes, including several reciprocal deletions and duplications, are summarized in Table 166-5.

The 22q11.2 microdeletion syndrome is the most common autosomal microdeletion syndrome and has been associated with various alternate designations, including DiGeorge syndrome, velocardiofacial syndrome, and Shprintzen syndrome. Typical features are conotruncal

**TABLE 166-5 MICRODELETION AND DUPLICATION SYNDROMES**

| Microdeletion/Duplication | OMIM No. | Dosage-Sensitive Gene[a] | Phenotype |
|---|---|---|---|
| 1p36 deletion | 607872 | *RERE* | ID, speech delay, behavioral difficulties, growth deficiency, hypotonia, characteristic facies, seizures, brain malformations, CHD |
| 5q35 deletion[b] | — | *NSD1* | Sotos phenotype, cleft palate, language delay, ID, macrocephaly |
| 5q35 duplication[b] | — | *NSD1* | Microcephaly, short stature, DD, delayed bone maturation |
| 7q11.23 deletion[b] (Williams syndrome) | 194050 | *ELN*, others | Periorbital fullness, long philtrum, large mouth, stellate iris pattern, supravalvular aortic stenosis, ID, gregarious personality |
| 7q11.23 duplication[b] | 609757 | — | Speech delay, mild craniofacial anomalies, DD, autism, aortopathy |
| 8p23 deletion | — | *GATA4* | CHD |
| 9q34 deletion (Kleefstra syndrome) | 610253 | *EHMT1* | ID, speech, delay, hypotonia, seizures, characteristic facies, CNS abnormalities, CHD |
| 11q deletion syndrome (Jacobsen syndrome) | 147791 | *ETS1, FLI1* | ID, growth deficiency, characteristic facies, thrombocytopenia, CHD |
| 15q11-q13 deletion (Prader-Willi syndrome; paternal)[b] | 176270 | *SNRPN* | ID, hypotonia, feeding difficulties (infancy) followed by hyperphagia, obesity, hypogonadotropic hypogonadism, small hands and feet |
| 15q11-q13 deletion (Angelman syndrome; maternal)[b] | 105830 | *UBE3A* | Severe ID, significant language impairment, gait ataxia, microcephaly, seizures |
| 15q11-q13 duplication (maternal)[b] | 608636 | — | ID, autism |
| 16p11.2 deletion[b] | 611913 | — | ID, autism spectrum disorder, epilepsy, macrocephaly, Chiari malformation, cerebellar tonsillar extopia, vertebral anomalies |
| 16p11.2 duplication[b] | 614671 | — | ID, autism, schizophrenia, microcephaly, CNS abnormalities |
| 17p11.2 deletion[b] (Smith-Magenis syndrome) | 182290 | *RAI1* | ID, behavioral problems, self-injury, disturbed sleep pattern, congenital anomalies |
| 17p11.2 duplication[b] (Potocki-Lupski syndrome) | 610883 | *RAI1* | ID, autism, hypotonia, FTT, congenital anomalies |
| 17p11.2 deletion[b] (HNPP) | 600361 | *PMP22* | Hereditary neuropathy with liability to pressure palsy |
| 17p11.2 duplication[b] (CMT1A) | 601098 | *PMP22* | Charcot-Marie-Tooth disease, type 1A |
| 17q11.2 deletion[b] | 613675 | *NF1* | Neurofibromatosis, DD, ID, facial dysmorphism |
| 17q11.2 duplication[b] | — | — | DD, ID, seizures |
| 17q21.31 deletion[b] (Koolen-De Vries syndrome) | 610443 | *KANSL1* | DD, ID, hypotonia, friendly demeanor, characteristic facies, CHD, genitourinary anomalies, seizures |
| 17q21.31 duplication[b] | 613533 | — | DD, ID, autism |
| 22q11.2 deletion[b] (Di George/velocardiofacial syndrome) | 192430 | *TBX1*, others | Cardiac abnormalities, cleft palate, T cell dysfunction, learning difficulties, psychiatric issues |
| 22q11.2 duplication[b] | 608363 | — | DD, ID, growth retardation, hypotonia |
| Xq28 deletion[b] (Rett syndrome) | — | *MECP2* | Stereotypic behavior, ataxia, DD, autism, epilepsy, spastic paraparesis |
| Xq28 duplication[b] (*MECP2* duplication syndrome) | 300815 | *MECP2* | (Males): DD, severe ID, hypotonia, seizures, progressive spasticity |

CHD, congenital heart disease; CMT1A, Charcot-Marie-Tooth disease type 1A; CNS, central nervous system; DD, developmental delay; FTT, failure to thrive; HNPP, hereditary neuropathy with liability to pressure palsy; ID, intellectual disability.

[a]Dosage-sensitive gene is provided if a single gene has been associated with most of the phenotypic features of the syndrome. Many microdeletion and microduplication syndromes are contiguous gene syndromes, with more than 1 dosage-sensitive gene involved.

[b]Reciprocal microduplication or deletion.



heart malformations (including interrupted aortic arch, type B), cleft palate (may be submucosal), velopharyngeal incompetence, and absence or hypoplasia of the thymus and parathyroid glands, with associated T cell dysfunction and hypocalcemia (Fig. 166-6). Seizures may be encountered in infancy as a result of neonatal hypocalcemia. Learning problems are common, and approximately 10% to 20% of individuals develop psychiatric disorders by adulthood. Haploinsufficiency for *TBX1*, encoding a T-box transcription factor with an important role in early vertebrate development, has been implicated in much of the phenotype.

## SEX CHROMOSOME ABNORMALITIES

Sex chromosome abnormalities are among the most common genetic conditions, with an incidence of approximately 1 in 400 live-born infants. Monosomy X (Turner syndrome) is the most common chromosome anomaly reported in spontaneous abortions. Trisomic aneuploidies of the sex chromosomes (XXY, XXX, and XYY) are frequent in live-born infants, with the incidence of Klinefelter syndrome (XXY) estimated to be as high as 1 in 600 male births. Typical features of the sex chromosome aneuploidies are summarized in Table 166-6.

### TURNER SYNDROME (45,X)

Turner syndrome is caused by complete or partial loss of an X chromosome. Almost 99% of all monosomy X conceptions die in utero, commonly with massive hydrops and cystic hygroma. The most consistent clinical features in children are proportionate short stature and gonadal dysgenesis, with lack of secondary sexual characteristics. Many have cardiac defects (bicuspid aortic valve and coarctation of the aorta) and congenital lymphedema, with swelling of the dorsum of the hands and feet. Other physical features include a short webbed neck, broad chest with widely spaced nipples, and cubitus valgus. Mean IQ is approximately 90. Poor coordination and neuropsychological defects are common. Approximately 6% of females with Turner syndrome have 45,X/46,XY mosaicism; these children are at increased risk for gonadoblastoma, and an exploratory laparotomy for removal of residual gonadal tissue should be considered.

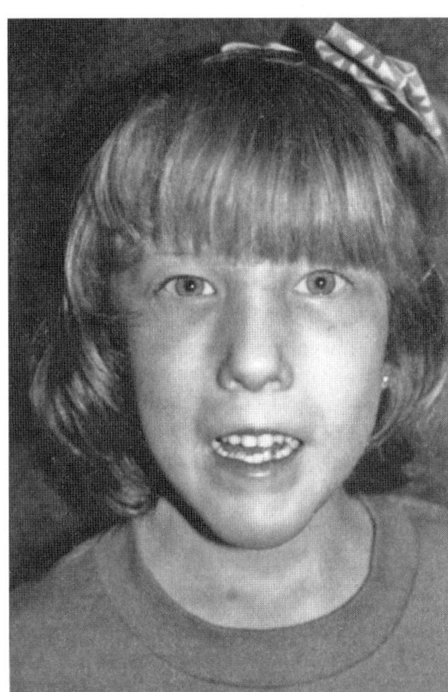

FIGURE 166-6 Child with DiGeorge syndrome. Note the tall nasal root and bridge with a bulbous nasal tip and small mouth. (Reproduced with permission from Jorde LB, Carey JC, Bamshad MJ, White RL: *Medical Genetics*, St. Louis, Mosby, 2000.)

### KLINEFELTER SYNDROME (47,XXY)

Klinefelter syndrome (47,XXY) is the most common single cause of hypogonadism and male infertility and often presents with oligospermia or azoospermia. Physical features include long limbs, gynecomastia, and relatively small penis and testes. Verbal comprehension, auditory processing abilities, and memory may be reduced. Behavior problems are frequent and reported as immaturity, shyness, and poor psychosocial adjustment. There is an increased risk for male breast cancer and extragonadal germ cell tumors.

## CHROMOSOME INSTABILITY SYNDROMES

Chromosome instability syndromes are autosomal recessive conditions characterized by increased susceptibility to chromosome breakage under specific laboratory conditions. The chromosome instability results from specific defects in DNA repair and cell cycle regulation and predisposes to malignancy. The chromosome instability syndromes include ataxia-telangiectasia, Bloom syndrome, Fanconi anemia, xeroderma pigmentosum, and Roberts syndrome (Table 166-7). These syndromes differ in mechanism from Fragile X syndrome, in that the "fragile site" in the latter is localized to a single, specific locus. Fragile X, one of the most common forms of inherited intellectual disability, is caused by expansion of the CGG trinucleotide repeat in the 5' untranslated region of the *FMR1* gene on chromosome X. It is associated with intellectual disability, an elongated face with prominent jaw and large ears, and macroorchidism in males.

**TABLE 166-6 SEX CHROMOSOME ABNORMALITIES**

| Disorder | Karyotype | Typical Features |
|---|---|---|
| Klinefelter syndrome | 47,XXY (other variants and mosaics) | Tall male, long limbs, gynecomastia, hypogonadism, infertility, reduced verbal IQ to low-normal range |
| XYY syndrome | 47,XYY | Tall, reduced verbal IQ, language delay, reading difficulties, subset with behavioral problems |
| XX testicular disorders of sex development | 46,XX | Phenotypically male |
| Turner syndrome | 45,X (other variants and mosaics) | Short stature, webbed neck, lymphedema, cardiac defects |
| Trisomy X | 47,XXX (48,XXXX and 49,XXXXX) | Hypotonia, developmental delay (severity correlated with number of extra X chromosomes), tend to be taller, reduced social skills |
| XY gonadal dysgenesis | 46,XY | Phenotypically female |

**TABLE 166-7 CHROMOSOME INSTABILITY SYNDROMES**

| Syndrome | Laboratory Abnormalities | Typical Features |
|---|---|---|
| Ataxia telangiectasia | Increased chromosome breakage, elevated alpha-fetoprotein | Cerebellar degeneration, oculocutaneous telangiectasias, immunodeficiency, radiosensitivity, cancer predisposition |
| Bloom syndrome | Increased sister chromatid exchange and increased chromosome breakage | Short stature, malar hypoplasia, telangiectatic erythema of face, immunodeficiency, cancer predisposition |
| Fanconi anemia | Spontaneous chromosome breakage | Congenital anomalies, bone marrow failure, cancer predisposition, microcephaly |
| ICF syndrome | Multiradial chromosomes | Immunodeficiency, centromere instability, and facial anomalies |
| Nijmegen breakage syndrome | Chromosome instability with rearrangements of chromosomes 7 and 14 | Progressive microcephaly, growth retardation, recurrent sinopulmonary infections, cancer predisposition |
| Roberts syndrome | Premature centromere separation | Hypomelia, midfacial defect, severe growth deficiency |
| Xeroderma-pigmentosum | Defective nucleotide excision repair | Sun sensitivity, ocular involvement, increased risk of cutaneous neoplasms |

## SUPPORT GROUPS AND INFORMATION FOR FAMILIES

Several Web sites with helpful information for families and physicians regarding aneuploidies and/or genomic disorders are listed in Table 166-8.

**TABLE 166-8 WEBSITES WITH HELPFUL INFORMATION FOR FAMILIES AND PHYSICIANS**

| URL | Web site |
|---|---|
| www.rarechromo.org | Unique, The Rare Chromosome Disorder Support Group |
| www.rarediseases.org | National Organization for Rare Disorders (NORD) |
| www.ghr.nlm.nih.gov | Genetics Home Reference |
| www.trisomy.org | Support Organization for Trisomy (SOFT) |
| www.omim.org | OMIM, Online Mendelian Inheritance in Man |
| https://decipher.sanger.ac.uk | DECIPHER, Database of Chromosomal Imbalance and Phenotype in Humans Using Ensembl Resources |

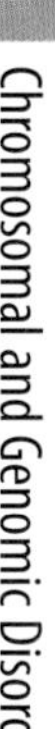

Adams DJ, Clark DA. Common genetic and epigenetic syndromes. *Pediatr Clin North Am*. 2015;62(2):411-426.

Bull MJ. Committee on Genetics. Clinical report—health supervision for children with Down syndrome. *Pediatrics*. 2011;128:393-406.

Carvalho CM, Lupski JR. Mechanisms underlying structural variant formation in genomic disorders. *Nat Rev Genet*. 2016;17(4):224-238.

Cereda A, Carey JC. The trisomy 18 syndrome. *Orphanet J Rare Dis*. 2012;7:81.

Emanuel BS, Saitta SC. From microscopes to microarrays: dissecting recurrent chromosomal rearrangements. *Nat Rev Genet*. 2007;8(11):869-883.

Levitsky LL, Luria AH, Hayes FJ, Lin AE. Turner syndrome: update on biology and management across the life span. *Curr Opin Endocrinol Diabetes Obes*. 2015;22(1):65-72.

Martin CL, Warburton D. Detection of chromosomal aberrations in clinical practice: from karyotype to genome sequence. *Annu Rev Genomics Hum Genet*. 2015;16:309-326.

Nevado J, Mergener R, Palomares-Bralo M, et al. New microdeletion and microduplication syndromes: a comprehensive review. *Genet Mol Biol*. 2014;37(1 Suppl):210-219.

Nussbaun RL, McInnes RR, Willard HF. The chromosomal and genomic basis of disease: disorders of the autosomes and sex chromosomes. In: Nussbaun RL, McInnes RR, Willard HF, eds. *Thompson & Thompson Genetics in Medicine*. 8th ed. Philadelphia, PA: Elsevier; 2016:75-105.

Schmickel RD. Contiguous gene syndromes: a component of recognizable syndromes. *J Pediatr*. 1986;109(2):231-241.

Spence JE, Perciaccante RG, Greig GM, et al. Uniparental disomy as a mechanism for human genetic disease. *Am J Hum Genet*. 1988;42(2):217-226.

Trivellin G, Daly AF, Faucz FR, et al. Gigantism and acromegaly due to Xq26 microduplications and *GPR101* mutation. *N Engl J Med*. 2014;371(25):2363-2374.



# 167 Laboratory Analysis of Copy Number and Single Nucleotide Variants

Tamar Harel, James R. Lupski, and Pengfei Liu

## INTRODUCTION

Cytogenetics is a field of genetics involved with the study of chromosomes. Clinical cytogenetics aims to delineate the gross chromosomal abnormalities, both in number and structure, associated with certain malformation syndromes. Approximately 1% of live-born babies have a cytogenetic abnormality, making this field particularly relevant in the pediatric population and the clinical practice of pediatrics. Cytogenetics includes routine analysis of G (Giemsa)-banded chromosomes, fluorescence in situ hybridization (FISH), and whole-genome array comparative genomic hybridization (aCGH) and single nucleotide polymorphism (SNP) arrays. Whole-genome sequencing (WGS), which has been viewed traditionally as a molecular technique targeting single nucleotide variants (SNVs), is gradually being introduced into the cytogenetics field because of its potential to analyze copy number variants (CNVs) as well as structural variants (SVs). WGS can be implemented postnatally as well as prenatally, from fetal DNA in maternal blood. Whole-exome sequencing (WES) focuses on the coding sequences of all genes in the human genome (~1% of the human genome). It detects small changes in DNA including SNVs and indels (insertions and deletions <50–100 bp). WES has been particularly useful clinically for elucidating the etiologic molecular diagnosis in pediatric patients whose phenotype remained a diagnostic dilemma and for finding dual molecular diagnoses in patients with blended phenotypes.

Numerical abnormalities of chromosomes, such as trisomy 21 (Down syndrome), Turner syndrome (monosomy X), and Klinefelter syndrome (47,XXY), can be detected by analysis of chromosomes under a light microscope and preparation of a **karyotype**, a standardized photomicrograph of chromosome pairs ordered from largest to smallest (with the exception of chromosome 21, which is smaller than chromosome 22). The karyotype allows for visualization of large (generally involving >5 megabases [Mb] of DNA) structural abnormalities of chromosomes, such as reciprocal translocations, Robertsonian translocations, and ring chromosomes. In addition, large terminal deletions at either end of a chromosome (eg, 5p deletion or cri du chat syndrome) and large interstitial deletions within the arms of a chromosome (eg, del(17)p11.2 associated with Smith-Magenis syndrome) can also be visualized on routine karyotype. However, smaller deletion and duplication CNVs require higher resolution techniques that can be either targeted to a specific region, as with FISH technology, or multiple loci based, as with microarrays and next-generation sequencing technologies.

Indications for use of cytogenetics in a pediatric population include recognizable syndromes, multiple congenital malformations, developmental delay, short stature and primary amenorrhea in girls, and intellectual disability. Cytogenetics is also widely used in oncology to help with diagnosis, a treatment plan, and prognosis.

## CHROMOSOME ANALYSIS

Abnormalities of chromosome number and structure can result during either type of cell division, mitosis or meiosis. **Mitosis** is the ordinary somatic cell division by which the body grows, differentiates, and renews tissues. Mitotic division results in 2 diploid daughter cells that are genetically identical to the parent cell. To prepare for mitotic division, genomic DNA is duplicated during **interphase**, in the S (synthesis) phase of the cell cycle. The duplication results in 2 **sister chromatids** held together at the **centromere.** Mitosis then ensues, with its 4 stages: prophase, metaphase, anaphase, and telophase. **Prophase** is marked by gradual condensation of the chromosomes and formation of the mitotic spindles and centrosomes. The nuclear membrane is dissolved in prometaphase. In **metaphase**, the chromosomes are maximally compacted and align at the equatorial plane of the cell. At this stage, they are clearly visible as distinct structures and are connected by spindle fibers that extend from the centromere of each chromosome to the centrosome at either pole of the cell. **Anaphase** is the stage when the chromosomes separate at the centromeres, and the sister chromatids of each chromosome become independent and migrate to opposite poles of the cell. **Telophase** is the final mitotic phase, in which chromosomes decondense, a new nuclear membrane re-forms around each of the 2 daughter nuclei, and the cytoplasm cleaves to form 2 daughter cells.

**Meiosis** is the process specific to gametogenesis, by which diploid cells (2n, or 46 chromosomes: 46,XX female or 46,XY male karyotype) give rise to haploid cells (n, or 23 chromosomes). Two successive rounds of cell division occur. The first division, meiosis I, is also known as the **reduction division**, as the chromosome number is reduced from 46 to 23 in this division. During prophase of meiosis I, homologous chromosomes pair in **synapsis,** and **genetic recombination** occurs. This process involves shuffling of genetic material, or **crossing over**, between 2 DNA strands. It ensures that the genetic content of each gamete will be unique and diversified. Errors in homologous recombination, due to unequal crossing over, can result in structural chromosomal abnormalities (eg, deletions and duplications). During metaphase I, the paired chromosomes align at the equatorial plane. At this stage, each chromosome typically contains alternating DNA segments of paternal and maternal origin. Anaphase I differs from mitotic anaphase, in that homologous chromosomes move apart rather than sister chromatids. Failure of homologous chromosomes to separate, or **nondisjunction**, results in an abnormal number of chromosomes in the progeny derived from that gamete, known as aneuploidy. Telophase I ends with 2 cells, each with 23 chromosomes. Each chromosome still has 2 sister chromatids at the end of meiosis I. These are separated during meiosis II, which is similar to mitotic division.

Spermatogenesis and oogenesis follow the same successive stages of meiosis; however, the timing of the stages is very different. In males, spermatogenesis is initiated continuously throughout adult life. In females, meiosis is initiated in a limited number of cells during fetal life and is completed years to decades later. Of several million oocytes at the time of birth, most degenerate and others remain arrested in prophase I (dictyotene, or prolonged diplotene, stage) for decades. Just before ovulation, the oocyte rapidly completes meiosis I. Meiosis II begins promptly and progresses to the metaphase stage during ovulation, where it arrests again, only to be completed if fertilization occurs. The division of the cytoplasm is asymmetric in oogenesis: meiosis I results in a large cell that will become the egg and a small cell that is the first polar body. Meiosis II, completed if fertilization occurs, results in a fertilized egg and the second polar body. These differences in gametogenesis may account for the higher incidence of nondisjunction in female gametes, which are arrested for years or decades, and for the higher incidence of de novo variants in male gametes, which are exposed to more mitotic divisions and thus more potential replicative errors.

## THE KARYOTYPE

A human karyotype is a photomicrograph of the 46 chromosomes in a particular cell, arranged from largest to smallest chromosome. The sex chromosomes are placed last (XX in female and XY in male). Karyotypes can be prepared from a variety of cell types but are most often obtained from peripheral blood lymphocytes. Fetal cells extracted from amniotic fluid or obtained by chorionic villus biopsy are used in prenatal diagnosis, and cells derived from bone marrow are used in oncology. In order to prepare a karyotype, cells are cultured, and then artificially arrested in mitosis during metaphase or prometaphase, when the chromosomes are most condensed and thus most visible under light microscopy. The cells are placed in a hypotonic solution to trigger disruption of the nuclear cell membrane, followed by fixation, banding, and staining. **G-banding** (Giemsa staining) is the most commonly used staining method. Each chromosome pair stains in a characteristic pattern of alternating dark and light bands (Fig. 167-1). The chromosome spread is then analyzed by a cytogeneticist, in terms of chromosome number and gross structure. A typical metaphase chromosome spread includes about 450 to 550 bands (ie, ~5–6 Mb of DNA per band given the $3 \times 10^9$ bp haploid human genome). Prophase and prometaphase chromosomes are less condensed and can show 550 to 850 bands, enabling higher resolution analysis. Other types of banding and staining that highlight specific portions of the chromosome (eg, R-banding, Q-banding, C-banding) are available clinically but are much less commonly used.

Chromosomes are distinguished one from another based on length and banding pattern. The position of the centromere also varies between chromosomes. The centromere divides the chromosome into a short arm, designated as the **p arm** (p for "petite"), and a long arm, designated as the **q arm** (q for the letter following p). Acrocentric chromosomes have a centromere located close to 1 end of the chromosome. In a Robertsonian translocation, the long arms of 2 acrocentric chromosomes join at the centromere and the short arms are lost. Carriers of a balanced Robertsonian translocation have 45 chromosomes, since 2 chromosomes have fused, and are phenotypically normal. However, offspring of carriers of a balanced Robertsonian translocation are at risk of aneuploidy, often manifested by resultant recurrent miscarriages. Carriers of isochromosome 21, t(21;21), have a 100% recurrence risk for Down syndrome among their live offspring, since the alternate gamete gives rise to monosomy 21, which is not viable (Fig. 167-2A). The recurrence risk for Down syndrome among carriers of the common Robertsonian translocation between chromosomes 14 and 21 (Fig. 167-2B) depends on the parental sex. Females carrying a Robertsonian translocation have a 10% to 15% risk for a child with Down syndrome, while males carrying a Robertsonian translocation have an approximately 1% risk for a child with Down syndrome.

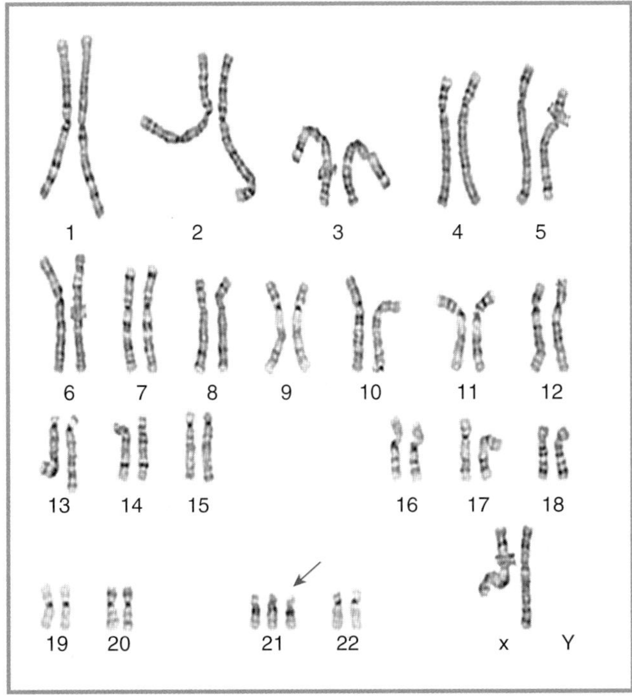


47, XX, +21

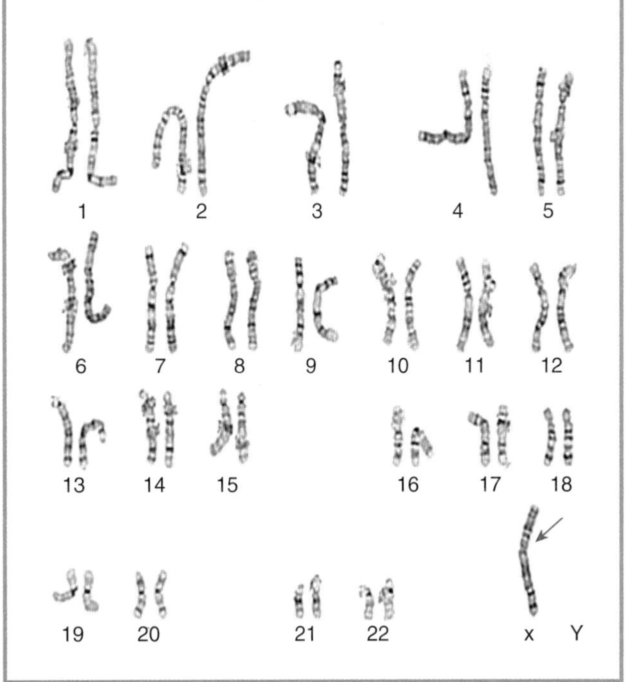


45, X

**FIGURE 167-1** Chromosome analysis. The karyotype on the left shows a total of 47 chromosomes, including 2 X chromosomes and 3 copies of chromosome 21, indicating a female with Down syndrome. The karyotype on the right shows a total of 45 chromosomes, with a single X chromosome and no Y chromosome, indicating a female with Turner syndrome. (Used with permission from Dr. Amy Breman).

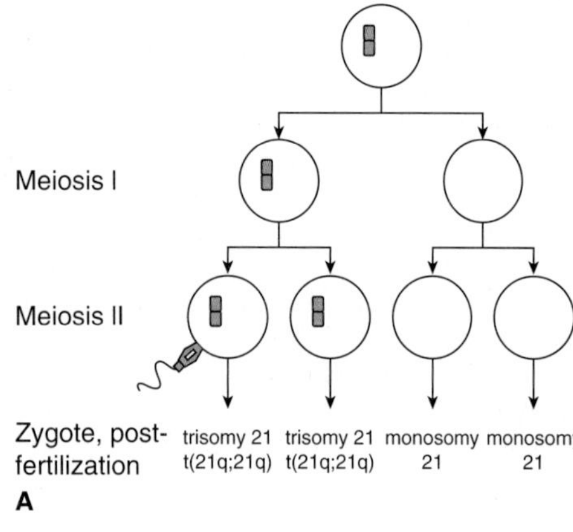


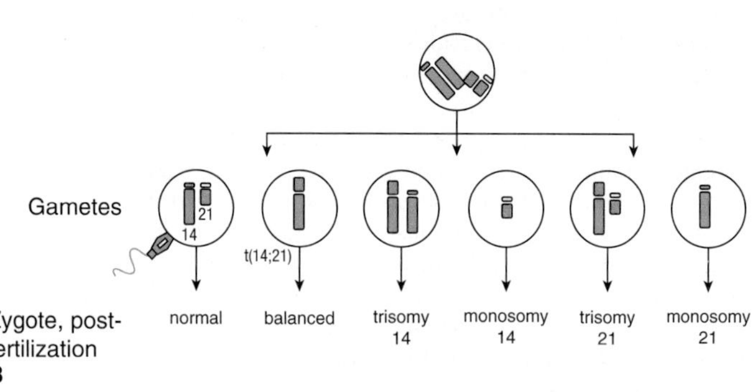


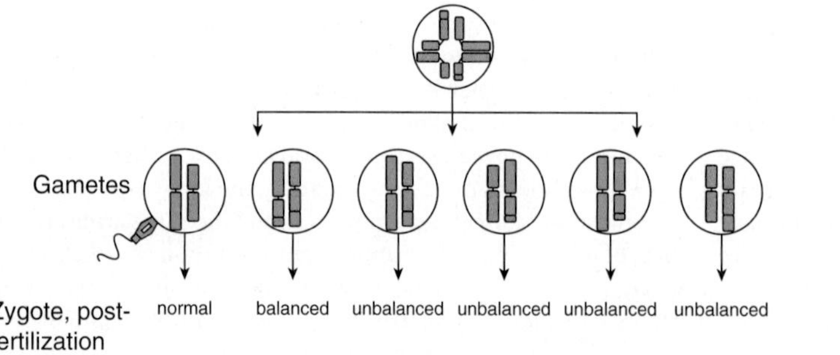


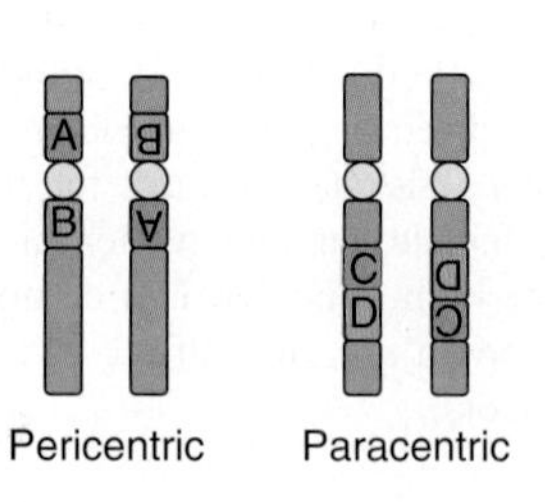


**FIGURE 167-2** Translocations and inversions. **A:** Meiotic segregation of isochromosome 21. Gametes receive either the isochromosome (indicated by the joining of the blue and orange copies of chromosome 21) or no copy of chromosome 21. After fertilization, zygotes have either 3 copies or 1 copy of chromosome 21. Since monosomy 21 is not viable, the observed recurrence risk for Down syndrome in live-born offspring is 100%. **B:** Segregation of a Robertsonian translocation between chromosomes 14 and 21 is depicted, with possible outcomes. Most cases of aneuploidy result in spontaneous miscarriage; thus, the empirical recurrence risk for Down syndrome in live offspring is much lower than the predicted recurrence risk. **C:** Segregation of a balanced translocation between 2 chromosomes can lead to normal, balanced, or unbalanced karyotypes in offspring. **D:** Pericentric inversions involve breakpoints on either side of the centromere, whereas paracentric inversions involve breakpoints on the same arm.

## NOMENCLATURE

A nomenclature has been developed by the International System for Human Cytogenetic Nomenclature (ISCN) to standardize the identification of chromosomes and the naming of chromosome bands with specific designations for abnormalities; eg, t(11;22)(q23q11.2) representing a recurrent translocation that occurs between palindromic AT rich repeat sequences (PATRRs) on the long arms of these chromosomes. Several examples are provided in Table 167-1.

## NUMERICAL AND STRUCTURAL ABNORMALITIES OF CHROMOSOMES

Chromosome abnormalities can be classified into numerical abnormalities (ie, Down syndrome, Klinefelter syndrome, Turner syndrome) and structural abnormalities. Numerical abnormalities are readily detected on routine karyotype. In addition, large structural abnormalities such as translocations (exchange of genomic material between 2 chromosomes), isochromosomes (homologous chromosomes fused at the centromere), ring chromosomes, and large inversions can also be detected on karyotype.

Approximately 1 in 500 newborns carries a balanced translocation, ie, 1 in 200 to 300 couples, and about 1 in 600 newborns has an unbalanced translocation. Carriers of balanced translocations are often phenotypically normal; however, they may be affected if the breakpoint disrupts a gene or a regulatory element. Offspring of carriers of balanced translocation are at risk of chromosomal or genomic disorders. In fact, the majority of unbalanced translocations arise from unbalanced segregation of a balanced translocation (Fig. 167-2C). Balanced translocations are frequently encountered in oncology, as acquired translocations in somatic cells that

**TABLE 167-1 EXAMPLES OF CYTOGENETIC NOMENCLATURE**

| Category | Cytogenetic Result | Interpretation |
|---|---|---|
| Normal | 46,XX | Normal female |
| Normal | 46,XY | Normal male |
| Trisomy | 47,XX,+21 | Trisomy 21 (female with gain of chromosome 21) |
| Trisomy | 47,XXY | Klinefelter syndrome (male with 2 X chromosomes and 1 Y chromosome) |
| Monosomy | 45,X | Monosomy X (Turner syndrome) |
| Mosaicism | mos 45,X[12]/46,XX[38] | Mosaic Turner syndrome (50 cells were analyzed; of these, 12 cells were 45,X and 38 cells were 46,XX) |
| Translocation | 46,XY,t(11;22)(q23;q11) | Balanced translocation between chromosomes 11 and 22, with breakpoints at bands 11q23 and 22q11 |
| Translocation | 45,XX,rob(14;21)(q10;q10) | Balanced Robertsonian translocation; long arms of chromosomes 14 and 21 were fused |
| Deletion | 46,XY,del(5)(q13) | Terminal deletion of chromosome 5 distal to band 5q13 |
| Duplication | 46,XX,dup(6)(q21q22) | Interstitial duplication of chromosome 6, bands q21 and q22 |
| Inversion | 46,XY,inv(9)(p11q13) | Pericentric inversion of chromosome 9 |
| Marker chromosome | 47,XX,+mar | Female with extra, unidentified chromosome |

drive specific forms of cancer. Examples include t(8;14) in Burkitt lymphoma and the Philadelphia chromosome t(9;22) in chronic myelogenous leukemia (CML). The latter translocation results in a chimeric oncogene encoding a constitutively active tyrosine kinase (BCR-ABL). Tyrosine kinase inhibitors have been developed to specifically target BCR-ABL and are considered first-line treatment of Philadelphia chromosome–positive CML.

Inversions within a particular chromosome can either be **pericentric** and involve the centromere, or **paracentric**, localized to 1 arm of the chromosome (Fig. 167-2D). An inversion can be relatively benign, such as the common pericentric inversion of chromosome 9, inv(9)(p11q13), estimated to occur in 1% to 3% of the population. Alternatively, it can disrupt a gene or regulatory element and lead to a phenotype, depending on the particular breakpoints involved; eg, a specific inversion that disrupts the factor VIII gene is responsible for over 45% of severe hemophilia. Carriers of pericentric inversions are at risk of having a child with duplications or deletions of the terminal ends of the chromosome involved in the inversion. The actual risk for a carrier of a balanced inversion (ie, with no loss of genomic material) to have viable offspring with an unbalanced karyotype (ie, with loss or gain of genomic material) depends on the size and content of the inversion and is estimated at 5% to 10%. Carriers of paracentric inversions have a much lower risk of having children with an unbalanced karyotype, since the unbalanced karyotypes that result from paracentric inversions are typically not viable.

## FLUORESCENCE IN SITU HYBRIDIZATION

**Fluorescence in situ hybridization (FISH)** is a molecular cytogenetic technique that utilizes a fluorescently labeled DNA probe to hybridize to a specific genomic sequence via complementary Watson-Crick base pairing of DNA (Fig. 167-3). It enables detection of subtle structural abnormalities below the resolution of conventional chromosome analysis and also serves as a method of confirmation for abnormalities such as small deletions and duplications identified by other techniques (ie, chromosomal microarrays). However, this technology is limited in that the underlying cytogenetic abnormality must be clinically suspected; the basic technique does not allow for unbiased analysis of the entire genome. Thus, it has been widely used for well-known, clinically recognizable syndromes, including Prader-Willi syndrome, Angelman syndrome, 22q11 deletion syndrome, and cri du chat syndrome.

**Spectral karyotyping** involves simultaneous "painting" of all the chromosomes, each in a different fluorescent color. This FISH-based technology can be useful to detect translocations or other structural abnormalities. **Telomere FISH** allows for simultaneous investigation of the ends of all chromosomes for rearrangements. It enabled discovery of many microdeletion and microduplication syndromes, such as the well-characterized 1p36 microdeletion syndrome. These technologies have been often replaced with the clinical availability of genome-wide arrays.

## CHROMOSOMAL MICROARRAYS

**Chromosomal microarray analysis (CMA)** is a genome-wide approach for detecting **copy number variants** (CNVs, deletions and duplications) at a high resolution (Table 167-2). The standard G-banded karyotype allows for detection of deletions and duplications of >5 to 10 million base pairs, and high-resolution chromosome analysis (at 850 bands) can detect deletions >2 to 3 million base pairs. By comparison, FISH analysis can detect CNVs as small as 50 to 250 kb but is limited in genome-wide applications. The human genome resolution for CMA is conceptually similar to FISH, with the advantage of simultaneous interrogation of the entire genome.

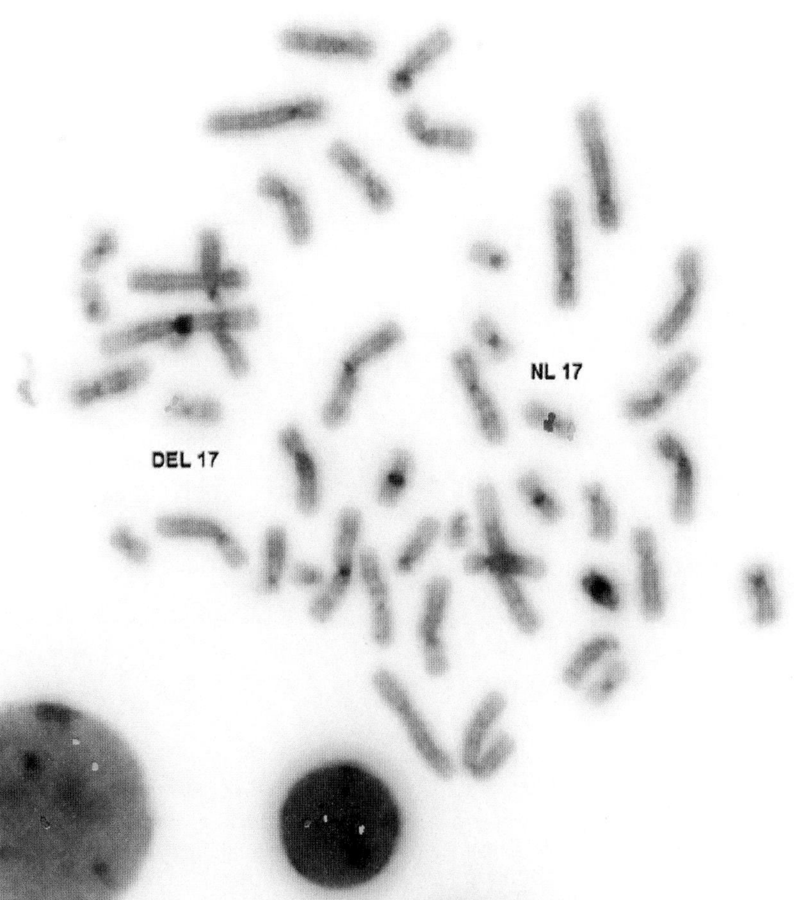


**FIGURE 167-3** Fluorescence in situ hybridization (FISH). Abnormal FISH analysis showing a deletion in the neurofibromatosis 1 region on chromosome 17, ish del(17)(q11.2q11.2)(NF1–). The red probe hybridizes to the *NF1*-specific genomic region, whereas the green probe hybridizes to a control region on chromosome 17. (Used with permission from Dr. Amy Breman).

**TABLE 167-2 COMPARISON OF METHODS FOR ASSESSING GENOMIC AND GENETIC VARIATION**

| Technology | Resolution | Limitations |
|---|---|---|
| Chromosome analysis (up to 550 G-bands) | 5–15 Mb | Low resolution |
| High-resolution chromosome analysis (up to 850 G-bands) | 2–3 Mb | Time consuming; technically difficult |
| FISH | 50–250 kb | Targeted region must be known |
| CMA | 50–250 kb | Balanced translocations give normal result |
| WES | Single base pair | Assess variation only in exome or coding region (1% of entire genome) |
| WGS | Single base pair | Costly; difficult to interpret clinical consequence of variation |

CMA, chromosomal microarray; FISH, fluorescence in situ hybridization; WES, whole-exome sequencing; WGS, whole-genome sequencing.

High-resolution CMA can readily detect CNVs of exon or sub-exon size. CMA technologies include **comparative genome hybridization (CGH)** and **single nucleotide polymorphism (SNP)** arrays.

Array CGH (aCGH) compares the amount of DNA in a patient sample to the amount of DNA in a control sample at each locus interrogated by the genome-arrayed oligonucleotide probes. Patient DNA is labeled by one dye, and control DNA is labeled by another dye. The fluorescently labeled DNA samples are then hybridized to a microarray grid of spotted DNA probes that represent different regions across the entire genome. By comparing the ratio of fluorescence of patient to control samples at each point on the microarray, CNVs can be detected (Fig. 167-4).

An alternative approach uses SNPs that are highly variable among healthy individuals. Several million SNPs are found in the human genome. By investigating the relative representation and intensity of alleles in different regions of the genome, one can detect CNVs as well as absence of homozygosity (AOH). AOH can indicate consanguinity or uniparental disomy. Many commercial arrays currently available combine aCGH and SNP array technologies. Results of abnormal microarrays (ie, CNVs) can be confirmed by FISH. Small CNVs without well-known clinical consequences are often challenging to interpret and often require parental investigations to determine whether the CNV occurred de novo (a change that is found in the child but not the parents). Changes that are inherited from a phenotypically normal parent are more readily interpreted as benign. A major limitation of CMA technologies is that they cannot detect balanced translocations or other structural abnormalities that do not lead to a loss or gain of genomic material.

## HIGH-THROUGHPUT SEQUENCING TECHNOLOGIES

The Human Genome Project, which commenced in 1990 and published the first draft of the human genome in 2001, marked a turning point for human genetics. Technical developments during the project and thereafter enabled massively parallel next-generation sequencing (NGS) of individual genomes and paved the way to personalized or precision medicine. Genetics has extended much beyond the field of rare Mendelian disorders and has pervaded every field of medicine, perhaps currently most striking in oncology, pediatrics, obstetrics and

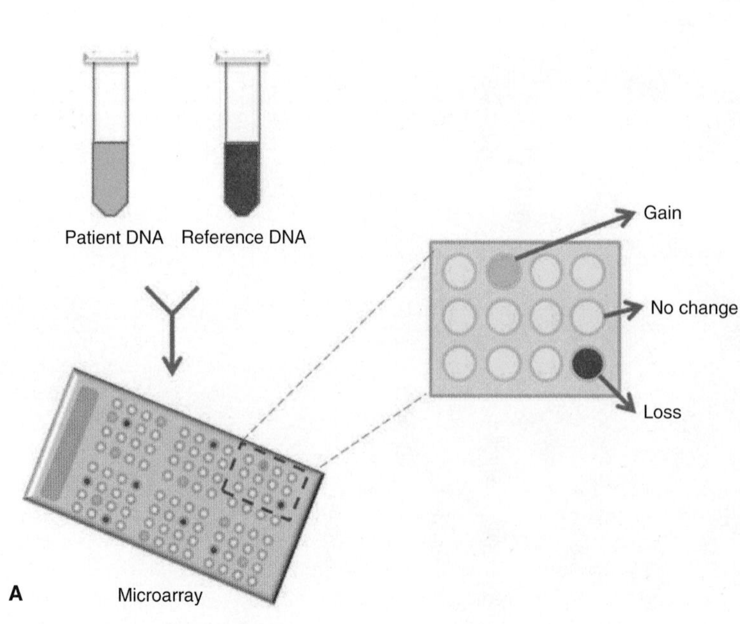


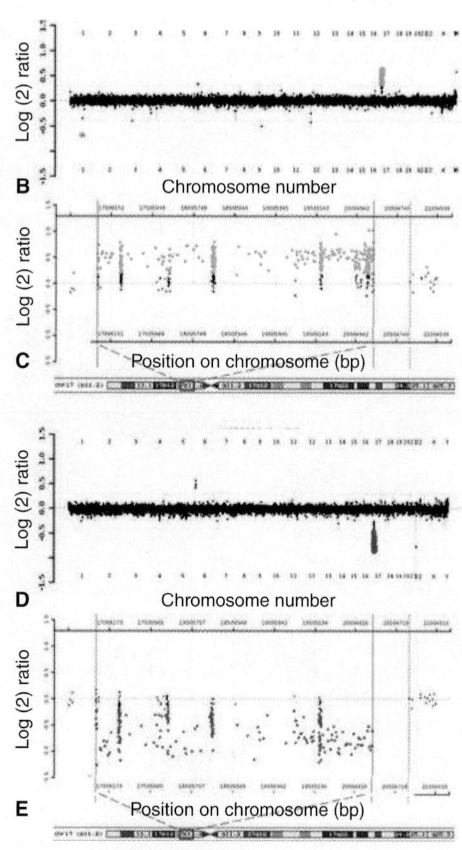


**FIGURE 167-4** Chromosomal microarray. **A:** Schematic depiction of an array based on comparative genomic hybridization (CGH). The affected individual's DNA and the reference DNA are labeled with dyes of different color. The samples are then mixed and hybridized to the array. Relative intensities of the fluorescence are measured. Yellow fluorescence indicates equal dosage of patient and reference DNA. Green fluorescence indicates a relative gain of genomic material, and red indicates a relative loss of genomic material. **B:** Array CGH result for an individual with a gain on chromosome 17. The log(2) ratio of the fluorescence ratios are plotted along the genome. **C:** Zoomed-in view of the duplication on chromosome 17p11.2, indicative of Potocki-Lupski syndrome. **D:** Array CGH result for an individual with a loss on chromosome 17. **E:** Zoomed-in view of the deletion on chromosome 17p11.2, indicative of Smith-Magenis syndrome. (Panels B-E, Used with permission from Dr. Amy Breman).

gynecology, and neurology. It has implications for diagnosis, intervention, management, recurrence risk counseling, and preventative medicine.

## WHOLE-GENOME SEQUENCING

**Whole-genome sequencing** determines the sequence of the entire genome and thus allows for the most comprehensive and highest resolution approach for detection of genetic and genomic alterations potentially contributing to disease phenotypes. It has been largely used as a research tool; however, as the ability to interpret the vast amount of data improves, as costs of genome analyses continue to decrease, and as clinical utility is continually realized, it will likely become more widely available and utilized in clinical medicine. Several techniques are available to sequence the approximately 6 billion base pairs in a human diploid genome, and bioinformatic analysis of the generated data allows for identification of both CNVs and single nucleotide variants (SNVs).

The challenge for genome-wide analyses remains to identify the disease-causing or susceptibility-conferring mutations from among the tremendous amount of benign variation, which makes each of us unique individuals, in a personal genome. A typical human genome is estimated to contain approximately 5 to 10 million single nucleotide polymorphisms (SNPs) as compared to the reference genome; 175 to 500 rare nonsynonymous SNPs that change the amino acid sequence of the encoded protein; and 70 to 80 de novo SNVs not detected in parental genomes (of these, an average of 1 nonsynonymous variant).

## WHOLE-EXOME SEQUENCING

**Whole-exome sequencing (WES)** focuses on the expressed genes, or coding region, in a genome (ie, the exome). The exome approximates 1% of the entire genome. Humans have approximately 20,000 genes, with an average of 8 to 9 exons per gene. Technical steps of WES include "capture" of genomic regions of interest from an individual patient (ie, exons) followed by amplification, or enrichment, of the target regions, and finally sequencing of the fragments.

WES is useful in diagnosis of rare Mendelian disorders, as it is the most efficient way to screen for genetic variants potentially contributing to a clinical phenotype and to establish an etiologic molecular diagnosis. It is often ordered clinically as part of an evaluation for individuals with intellectual disability (ID) and developmental delay (DD), regardless of whether additional phenotypic features are present. In sporadic DD/ID, trio exomes (proband plus parents) can be particularly useful for detecting the responsible new mutation. However, when there is a high suspicion for a specific genetic disorder based on clinical findings, targeted testing of a single gene or a gene panel by either Sanger sequencing or next-generation sequencing may be indicated. Examples include testing for well-characterized disorders such as Marfan syndrome.

Both CNVs and SNVs in the exome can be detected with WES, although traditionally, it has been used in clinical practice mainly for SNVs. Variants of interest are often confirmed by an orthogonal approach, such as Sanger sequencing for SNVs. One limitation of WES is that it does not assess variation in the remaining 99% of the human genome, which may be particularly important in complex, heterogeneous, or more subtle phenotypes. Another consequence of WES is the potential for recognition of incidental, or secondary, findings unrelated to the clinical phenotype that triggered ordering of WES. The American College of Medical Genetics and Genomics (ACMGG) has published recommendations about responsible management of incidental findings. These are often related to cancer susceptibility (eg, hereditary breast and ovarian cancer, *BRCA1* and *BRCA2*; Li-Fraumeni syndrome, *TP53*; Lynch syndrome, *MLH1, MSH2, MSH6, PMS2*) or cardiac disease (eg, genes associated with aortic aneurysms and dissections, cardiomyopathy, or arrhythmia). Finally, pharmacogenetic variants, carrier status, and extent of AOH also become readily available with WES. Ethical considerations for sharing of WES data unrelated to the indication for testing have been a wide subject of debate and merit consideration.



## SUGGESTED READINGS


Campbell IM, Shaw CA, Stankiewicz P, Lupski JR. Somatic mosaicism: implications for disease and transmission genetics. *Trends Genet.* 2015;31(7):382-392.

Carvalho CMB, Lupski JR. Mechanisms underlying structural variant formation in genomic disorders. *Nat Rev Genet.* 2016;17:224-238.

Gonzaga-Jauregui C, Lupski JR, Gibbs RA. Human genome sequencing in health and disease. *Annu Rev Med.* 2012;63:35-61.

Green RC, Berg JS, Grody WW, et al. ACMG recommendations for reporting of incidental findings in clinical exome and genome sequencing. *Genet Med.* 2013;15:565-574.

Lupski JR. Clinical genomics: from a truly personal genome viewpoint. *Hum Genet.* 2016;135(6):591-601.

Nussbaun RL, McInnes RR, Willard HF. Principles of clinical cytogenetics and genome analysis. In: Nussbaun RL, McInnes RR, Willard HF, eds. *Thompson & Thompson Genetics in Medicine.* 8th ed. Philadelphia, PA: Elsevier; 2016:57-74.

Posey JE, Harel T, Liu P, et al. Multiple molecular diagnoses unravel blended phenotypes. *N Engl J Med.* 2017;376(1):21-31.

Stankiewicz P, Lupski JR. Structural variation in the human genome and its role in disease. *Annu Rev Med.* 2010;61:437-455.

Wiszniewska J, Bi W, Shaw C, et al. Combined array CGH plus SNP genome analyses in a single assay for optimized clinical testing. *Eur J Hum Genet.* 2014;22(1):79-87.

Wu N, Ming X, Xiao J, et al. *TBX6* null variants and a common hypomorphic allele in congenital scoliosis. *N Engl J Med.* 2015; 372(4):431-350.

Yang Y, Muzny DM, Xia F, et al. Molecular findings among patients referred for clinical whole-exome sequencing. *JAMA.* 2014;312:1870-1879.




# 168 Online Resources for Genetic Disorders

Pilar L. Magoulas, Jennifer E. Posey, and Lorraine Potocki

*"We are all now connected by the Internet, like neurons in a giant brain."*
—Stephen Hawking

*"We don't heal in isolation, but in community."*
—S. Kelley Harrell

## INTRODUCTION

The Internet has the power to connect families with rare diseases to one another; to serve as a bridge across oceans when families may feel as isolated as an island surrounded by a sea of uncertainty. The support organizations and resources available online provide a sense of hope, community, and togetherness that is often lacking for families when initially faced with a rare disorder diagnosis. The speed with which new gene-syndrome associations are discovered is only matched by the speed in which a new support organization for that condition is formed. Therefore, this chapter will review some of the available Internet resources for genetic syndromes available today, with the caveat that these resources are a mere glimpse of what is currently available.

## HISTORY OF GENETIC SUPPORT AND ADVOCACY GROUPS

In the late 1970s and early 1980s, patients and families living with rare diseases felt alone and forgotten. Little was being done to study these diseases or develop treatments. Leaders of several rare disease patient organizations formed an ad hoc coalition to focus attention on this problem. That coalition became the National Organization for Rare Disorders (NORD) and was instrumental in the Orphan Drug Act of 1983, which created financial incentives for the development of treatments for rare diseases (NORD Web site: www.rarediseases.org).

By the mid-to-late 1980s and 1990s, disorder-specific and general advocacy groups were becoming key components of the genetics network. These organizations engendered partnerships among patients, families, and healthcare providers that facilitated communication and enabled more rapid dissemination of information and pathways to research. These groups continue to provide powerful resources that pediatricians can offer to their patients while still providing the foundation for which they receive their primary care. Joan Weiss, founder of the Alliance for Genetic Support Groups, believed that "those working within the walls of the pediatric clinic are in a crucial place to address the comprehensive needs of families with genetic disorders and to identify the role of the genetic support group in a treatment plan."

The growth of genetic support groups and resources for genetic conditions prospered with the parallel growth of the Internet in the late 1990s and 2000s. One example of the benefit of this unexpected union was the launch, partly in response to advocacy from NORD and others in the patient community, of a new Web site by the National Institutes of Health (NIH) that provided an overview of current clinical research trials available to patients with various genetic and rare disorders (www.clinicaltrials.gov). This repository and the information gleaned from it often serve as a beacon of hope for families affected by rare disorders where disease management and treatment, in the typical sense of the word, may not be as readily available as it may be for other chronic illnesses.

## SOCIAL MEDIA AND GENETIC SUPPORT AND ADVOCACY ORGANIZATIONS

The advent and exponential rise of social media from the late 2000s to the present signify a crucial and revolutionary shift in the way families affected by genetic disorders connect with one another. This marked one of the first times that families, and later, researchers, could share information and unite under the auspices of common goals and interests nearly instantaneously, traversing cultures, countries, and continents with the use of an Internet-abled device.

Internet resources used by parents of children with medical illnesses include social networking sites, discussion forums, blogs, wikis, video-sharing sites, and microblogs. It is not uncommon for families to receive a genetic diagnosis and to find one or more corresponding Facebook groups or pages targeted at that specific syndrome shortly thereafter. Patients have also commented on the benefits of social media in providing support and information when faced with a medical diagnosis. In addition, with the increased utility of whole-exome sequencing identifying new gene-disease associations at an increasingly common rate, families may turn to social media to seek out others with a specific gene or genetic variant that may not currently have a large cohort and slowly begin to grow their patient population.

Jacobs and colleagues performed a cross-sectional analysis and user survey to define characteristics and needs of Facebook users in relation to congenital anomalies (anorectal malformation, congenital diaphragmatic hernia, and hypospadias/epispadias). They concluded that Facebook groups or pages related to congenital anomalies are highly populated and active and stressed a need for healthcare providers and policymakers to better understand and participate in social media to support families and improve patient care.

In 2016, Cacioppo and colleagues conducted a focus group study to determine the attitudes and experiences toward Internet support groups for parents of children diagnosed with Cornelia de Lange syndrome in order to better understand the impact on emotional support and their child's medical care. In their cohort, a majority of respondents (over 70%) reported that Internet support groups have been helpful in finding emotional support, with the most common areas impacted being behavior toward their children and family dynamic. Regarding medical care, most respondents (over 60%) reported that the online support groups have been helpful in finding medical information and support, with the most commonly impacted areas of their child's care including day-to-day management, diet, therapy interventions, and healthcare providers. For provider and researchers, social networking sites may also serve as a means of research participant recruitment and source of data collection. However, families should be cautioned about information posted on social media sites such as Facebook, Twitter, Reddit, and others because the information posted on these sites is not vetted by healthcare providers or peer reviewed.

## ONLINE RESOURCES FOR GENETIC DISORDERS

The list of resources below includes online educational resources for providers as well as support resources for patients and families. Syndrome-specific resources are not listed individually because there are literally hundreds of genetic syndromes that each have one or more support group Web sites. However, a simple search of a particular syndrome in a common search engine will bring up the most relevant support group information and resources for that particular condition.

The Web sites listed below are general resources from which to gain basic information regarding genetic disorders and genetic syndrome support organizations. They also provide tools that will enable the clinician to search for a particular syndrome or groups of conditions, depending on their specific needs and interests. It is important to note that there are many different types of services and resources available within a syndrome-specific support group. For example, some organizations are primarily focused on research and fundraising endeavors, whereas others emphasize emotional support, education, and outreach. This may seem like a minor distinction, but it is one that should be underscored when providing resources to patients because the mission of the organization should be in alignment with the specific needs of the family.

**Centers for Disease Control and Prevention (CDC)**
www.cdc.gov
The CDC is our nation's health protection agency. The goal and aim of the CDC is to protect America from health, safety, and security threats, both foreign and in the United States, by fighting disease and supporting communities to do the same. They conduct science and provide health information on many health conditions, including dozens of birth defects, in the form of fact sheets, videos, and online resources that are available to the public as well as providers. They also maintain health-related and medical statistics for the United States.

**Chromosome Disorder Outreach**
www.chromodisorder.org
Chromosome Disorder Outreach is a nonprofit organization that was founded in 1992 by a group of seven parents raising children born with rare chromosome disorders. Their mission is to provide support and information to anyone diagnosed with a rare chromosome change, rearrangement, or disorder. Additionally, they actively promote research and community understanding of all chromosome disorders. They also offer an extensive library of up-to-date articles and maintain a detailed database registry.

**GeneReviews**
www.genereviews.org
GeneReviews is an international point-of-care resource for clinicians that provides clinically relevant and medically actionable information for inherited conditions in a standardized journal-style format, covering diagnosis, management, and genetic counseling for patients and their families. Each chapter is written by one or more experts on the specific condition or disease and goes through a rigorous editing and peer-review process before being published online.

**GeneTests**
www.genetests.org
GeneTests is a medical genetics information resource developed for physicians, genetic counselors, other healthcare providers and

researchers. It has two main components, a laboratory directory of over 600 international laboratories that offer molecular genetic, biochemical, and cytogenetic testing, and a clinic directory of over 1000 international genetics clinics.

**Genetic Alliance**
www.geneticalliance.org
Genetic Alliance is a nonprofit health advocacy organization. Their network includes more than 1200 disease-specific advocacy organizations and thousands of universities, private companies, government agencies, and public policy organizations. Originally founded as an alliance for support groups, their work now tries to apply solutions in health and disease, in practice and prevention, on the local and global level.

**Genetic and Rare Conditions Site**
http://www.kumc.edu/gec/support/index.html
The University of Kansas Genetic Center's Genetic and Rare Conditions Site is an online repository of information regarding lay advocacy and support groups and information on genetic conditions and birth defects for professionals, educators, and individuals.

**Genetic and Rare Disease Information Center**
http://rarediseases.info.nih.gov/gard
The Genetic and Rare Diseases (GARD) Information Center provides the public with access to current, reliable, and easy-to-understand information about rare or genetic diseases in English or Spanish. GARD also has a list of specific syndromes and birth defects with their respective Web sites and support organizations (https://rarediseases.info.nih.gov/files/GARD_Resources_Report_06012015.pdf).

**Genetics Home Reference**
https://ghr.nlm.nih.gov/
Genetics Home Reference provides consumer-friendly information about the effects of genetic variation on human health. It provides syndrome-specific information as well as general educational information about the basics of genetics and heredity.

**Genetic Testing Registry**
www.ncbi.nlm.nih.gov/gtr
The Genetic Testing Registry (GTR) provides a central location for voluntary submission of genetic test information by providers. The scope includes the test's purpose, methodology, and validity; evidence of the test's usefulness; and laboratory contacts and credentials. The overarching goal of the GTR is to advance the public health and research into the genetic basis of health and disease.

**Global Genes**
www.globalgenes.org
Global Genes is a rare disease patient advocacy organization that promotes the needs of the rare disease community under a unifying symbol of hope. They have relationships and collaboration with over 500 global organizations. Their mission is to eliminate the challenges of rare disease by building awareness, educating the global community, and providing connections and resources that equip advocates to become activists for their disease.

**March of Dimes**
www.marchofdimes.org
The mission of the March of Dimes, started initially at the request of Franklin D. Roosevelt in response to polio research, is to improve the health of babies by preventing birth defects, premature birth, and infant mortality. They provide many resources for providers and patients, as well as fact sheets on various pregnancy-related healthcare items, birth defects, and management.

**National Organization of Rare Disorders (NORD)**
http://www.rarediseases.org
NORD provides services for patients and their families, rare disease patient organizations, medical professionals, and those seeking to develop new diagnostics and treatments. NORD also works with policymakers to help inform policies that are reflective of the needs of rare disease patients. NORD works closely with 250 member organizations, which are listed on their Web site with corresponding links.



**Online Mendelian Inheritance in Man (OMIM)**
http://www.ncbi.nlm.nih.gov/omim
OMIM is a comprehensive and searchable database of human genes and genetic phenotypes for clinicians and researchers that is freely available and updated daily. It is authored and edited at the McKusick-Nathans Institute of Genetic Medicine, Johns Hopkins University School of Medicine. It is a helpful tool for reviewing a known genetic condition or for when a syndrome diagnosis may be suspected, yet is not recognized. By entering the phenotypic features of an individual (eg, microcephaly, hypertelorism), a list of syndromes that contain those search terms will be generated for further review and assessment.

**Orphanet**
www.orpha.net
Orphanet is the reference portal for information on rare diseases and orphan drugs, for all audiences. Orphanet's aim is to help improve the diagnosis, care, and treatment of patients with rare diseases. It provides an inventory and encyclopedia of rare diseases in multiple languages as well as other resources on clinics, medical laboratories, and research protocols.

**Rare Diseases Clinical Research Network (RDCRN)**
https://www.rarediseasesnetwork.org/
The RDCRN is made up of 22 research groups (consortia) and a Data Management and Coordinating Center that are working together to improve availability of rare disease information, treatment, clinical studies, and general awareness for both patients and the medical community. The RDCRN provides up-to-date information for patients and assists in connecting patients with advocacy groups, expert doctors, and clinical research opportunities.

**The Arc**
www.thearc.org
The Arc is the largest national community-based organization advocating for and serving people with intellectual and developmental disabilities and their families. It encompasses all ages and more than 100 different diagnoses including autism, Down syndrome, fragile X syndrome, and various other developmental disabilities with nearly 700 state and local chapters nationwide. The Arc tries to ensure that people with intellectual and developmental disabilities and their families have the support and services they need to be fully engaged in their communities.

**Unique**
www.rarechromo.org
Unique is an international support organization for individuals with rare chromosome abnormalities. It maintains an extensive, searchable database of members with various chromosome abnormalities. It provides comprehensive literature and educational materials on the basics of chromosomes and chromosome abnormalities as well as family-friendly medical information and management guidebooks for dozens of specific, rare chromosome abnormalities.

## ADDITIONAL RESOURCES

There are many additional resources that clinicians, and some families, may find useful. As the field of genetics and our understanding of the relationship between genetic variation and disease continue to evolve, online databases of human genome variation such as DECIPHER (https://decipher.sanger.ac.uk/) and ClinVar (http://www.ncbi.nlm.nih.gov/clinvar/) are important resources for interpretation of rare genetic variants. For conditions and genetic variants that are quite rare, various matchmaking sites allow clinicians, researchers, and families to search for other cases with the same condition and/or candidate gene in order to identify new disease genes and variants, clarify the expected clinical presentation and course of a rare condition, and/or identify specialists who study the condition. Examples of these matching tools include GeneMatcher (https://genematcher.org/), DECIPHER, PhenomeCentral (https://phenomecentral.org/), and MyGene2 (https://www.mygene2.org/MyGene2/), which are now connected through a central exchange, the Matchmaker Exchange (MME; http://matchmakerexchange.org), allowing matching to occur across a large network of clinicians and researchers. The Centers for Mendelian Genomics (CMG; www.mendelian.org) form a research program designed to support novel disease gene and variant discovery. Physicians and/or families can reach out to the CMGs regarding participation through the CMG Web site.

## CONCLUSION

The availability of Internet resources for genetic disorders has grown exponentially in the past few decades since the inception of genetic syndrome support groups in the 1980s. The reasons for this expansion are multifaceted yet serve the common goal for connectivity and community among individuals affected by rare conditions. These support and advocacy organizations provide reliable and accurate information about genetic disorders that can be readily accessed by healthcare providers and distributed to families. Given the increased utility of social media and Internet resources and often lack of regulation regarding its content, careful vetting of the accuracy and reliability of the online materials and references should be performed before distributing the information to patients. Importantly, provision of this information is only one aspect of care needed for the child and family affected by a genetic condition. Referral to a pediatric geneticist or pediatric genetic counselor will assure that the family's subsequent questions and concerns will be addressed and will facilitate an enhanced multidisciplinary approach for medical, psychosocial, and psychological wellness.

## SUGGESTED READINGS


Baas M, Huisman S, van Heukelingen J, Koekkoek G, Laan HW, Hennekam R. Building treasures for rare disorders. *Eur J Med Genet.* 2014;58:11-13.

Cacioppo CN, Conway LJ, Mehta D, Krantz ID, Noon SE. Attitudes about the use of Internet support groups and the impact among parents of children with Cornelia de Lange syndrome. *Am J Med Genet Part C Semin Med Genet.* 2016;172C:229-236.

Greene A. Patient commentary: social media provides patients with support, information, and friendship. *BMJ.* 2015;350:h256.

Greene J, Choudry N, Kilabuk E, Shrank W. Online social networking by patients with diabetes: a qualitative evaluation of communication with Facebook. *J Gen Intern Med.* 2010;26:287-292.

Griffith GM, Hastings RP, Oliver C, et al. Psychological well-being in parents of children with Angelman, Cornelia de Lange and Cri du Chat syndromes. *J Intellect Disabil Res.* 2011;55:397-410.

Jacobs R, Boyd L, Brennan K, Sinha CK, Giuliana S. The importance of social media for patients and families affected by congenital anomalies: a Facebook cross-sectional analysis and user survey. *J Pediatr Surg.* 2016;51:1766-1771.

Kirk S, Milnes L. An exploration of how young people and parents use online support in the context of living with cystic fibrosis. *Health Expect.* 2016;19:309-321.

Koteyko N, Hunt D, Gunter B. Expectations in the field of the Internet and health: an analysis of claims about social networking sites in clinical literature. *Sociol Health Illn.* 2015;37:468-484.

Merolli M, Gray K, Martin-Sanchez F, Lopez-Campos G. Patient-reported outcomes and therapeutic affordance of social media: findings from a global online survey of people with chronic pain. *J Med Internet Res.* 2015;17:e20.

Reaves AC, Bianchi DW. The role of social networking sites in medical genetics research. *Am J Med Genet A.* 2013;161A:951-957.

Weiss JO. Genetic support groups: a continuum of genetic services. *Women Health.* 1989;15:37-53.

Weiss JO. Support groups for patients with genetic disorders and their families. *Pediatr Clin North Am.* 1992;39:13-23.


# 169 Diagnostic Algorithms

Juanita Neira Fresneda, Keren Machol, and V. Reid Sutton

## INTRODUCTION

This chapter introduces clinical algorithms for the genetic causes and evaluation of relatively common pediatric conditions such as disorders of growth and development, seizures, hearing loss, and other diagnoses where genetic causes account for a significant proportion of the etiology of the condition. These algorithms are primarily focused on genetic causes of the phenotypes, and so when indicated, nongenetic causes should also be considered. These are intended as general guidelines and the approach should be tailored to the specific individual being evaluated, rather than inflexibly applied universally in the evaluation of the specific phenotype.

Diagnostic algorithms:

- Algorithm 169-1: Intellectual disability
- Algorithm 169-2: Autism spectrum disorder
- Algorithm 169-3: Failure to thrive
- Algorithm 169-4: Neonatal hypotonia
- Algorithm 169-5: Neonatal seizures
- Algorithm 169-6: Overgrowth
- Algorithm 169-7: Short stature
- Algorithm 169-8: Microcephaly
- Algorithm 169-9: Cardiomyopathy
- Algorithm 169-10: Rhabdomyolysis
- Algorithm 169.11: Hearing loss

## INTELLECTUAL DISABILITY (Table 169-1, Fig. 169-1)

There is a significant overlap between the algorithms for genetic evaluation of autism spectrum disorder (ASD) and intellectual disability (ID). Neurodevelopmental abnormalities in multiple syndromes can include ASD or ID and sometimes both. In the "Conditions to Consider" tables, we include syndromes in which the more common presentation will be either ASD or ID, but these are not mutually exclusive.

**TABLE 169-1 INTELLECTUAL DISABILITY: CONDITIONS TO CONSIDER**

| Disorder | Additional Clinical Characteristics | Specific/Genetic Testing |
|---|---|---|
| Fragile X | Intellectual disability, distinct dysmorphic features (large head, long face, prominent forehead and chin, protruding ears), large testes after puberty, family history may include tremor/ataxia and primary ovarian insufficiency | *FMR1* gene testing (trinucleotide repeat expansion) |
| Klinefelter syndrome | Males with mild to moderate intellectual disability, hypogonadism, tall stature, gynecomastia | Routine chromosome analysis |
| Prader-Willi syndrome | History of hypotonia and feeding difficulties in early infancy, followed in later infancy by excessive eating. Developmental delay, intellectual disability, and obesity | For definite diagnosis, do methylation analysis of chromosome region 15q11-q13 (abnormal in 100% of patients)<br>For further characterization of the genetic abnormality consider FISH or CMA (deletion will be found in 70% of the patients)<br>IC sequencing (abnormal in 5%) |
| Rett syndrome | Females with initial normal development followed by rapid developmental regression, intellectual disability, stereotypic hand movements | *MECP2* gene analysis |
| Atypical Rett syndrome | Intellectual disability with spasticity or tremor, mild learning disability, autism | *MECP2* gene analysis |
| Williams syndrome (7q11.2 deletion syndrome) | Cardiovascular disease (elastin arteriopathy, peripheral pulmonary stenosis), distinctive facial characteristics, connective tissue abnormalities, hypercalcemia | FISH or CMA |
| Smith-Magenis syndrome | Distinct dysmorphic features, behavioral problems, sleep disturbance, intellectual disability, early-onset obesity | Initial workup includes FISH or CMA for 17p11.2 deletions (in up to 95% of the patients)<br>*RAI1* DNA sequencing if no deletion was detected |
| Coffin-Siris syndrome | Coarse facial features, aplasia or hypoplasia of the distal phalanx or nail of the fifth digits (not universal), developmental delay, hypotonia, hypertrichosis, sparse scalp hair | Gene panel including *ARID1B, SMARCA4, SMARCB1, ARID1A, PHF6, SMARCE1, SOX11, SMARCA2* |
| Metabolic disorders | Developmental regression, failure to thrive, episodes of metabolic decompensation, +/− seizures | Obtain specific genetic testing according to clinical findings<br>Referral to metabolic specialist should be considered |
| Mitochondrial disorders | Constitutional symptoms (eg, fatigue, weight loss), reduced stress endurance, hypotonia, developmental regressions, multiple organ dysfunctions | Mitochondrial DNA testing<br>Referral to metabolic specialist should be considered |

CMA, chromosomal microarray; FISH, fluorescence in situ hybridization; IC, imprinting center.

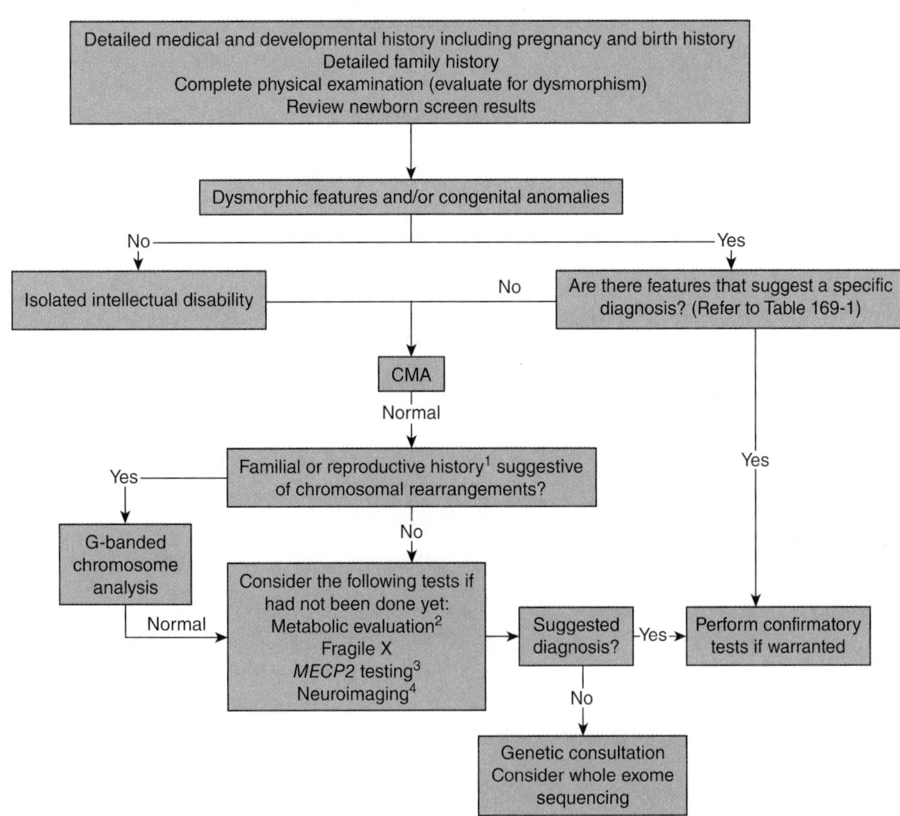


**FIGURE 169-1** Diagnostic algorithm for intellectual disability. (1) Consider familial chromosomal rearrangement with history of 3 or more miscarriages. (2) Metabolic evaluation: Initial metabolic evaluation may include blood PH, plasma lactate, ammonia, plasma amino acids profile, and urine organic acid profile. More specific metabolic testing should be obtained depending clinical picture. (3) *MECP2* duplication in males should also be considered. (4) Consider brain imaging when there is a clinical suspicion for brain structural abnormality or demyelinating disorder. Brain magnetic resonance imaging (MRI) is the preferred imaging modality. CMA, chromosomal microarray.

**TABLE 169-2 AUTISM SPECTRUM DISORDER: CONDITIONS TO CONSIDER**

| Disorder | Additional Clinical Characteristics | Specific/Genetic Testing |
|---|---|---|
| Fragile X | Intellectual disability, distinct dysmorphic features (large head, long face, prominent forehead and chin, protruding ears), large testes after puberty, family history may include tremor/ataxia and primary ovarian insufficiency | *FMR1* gene testing (trinucleotide repeat expansion) |
| Turner syndrome | Short stature, webbed neck, infantile edema of hands and feet | Routine chromosome analysis |
| PTEN-related syndromes | Macrocephaly, high risk for benign and malignant tumors | *PTEN* gene analysis |
| 16p11.2 deletion/duplication | Articulation abnormalities, seizures, hypotonia, sacral dimple, macrocephaly (deletion)/microcephaly (duplication) | CMA |
| Metabolic disorders | Developmental regression, failure to thrive, episodes of metabolic decompensation, +/– seizures | Obtain specific genetic testing according to clinical findings<br>Referral to metabolic specialist should be considered |
| Mitochondrial disorders | Constitutional symptoms (eg, fatigue, weight loss), reduced stress endurance, hypotonia, developmental regressions, multiple organ dysfunctions | Mitochondrial DNA testing<br>Referral to metabolic specialist should be considered |

CMA, chromosomal microarray.

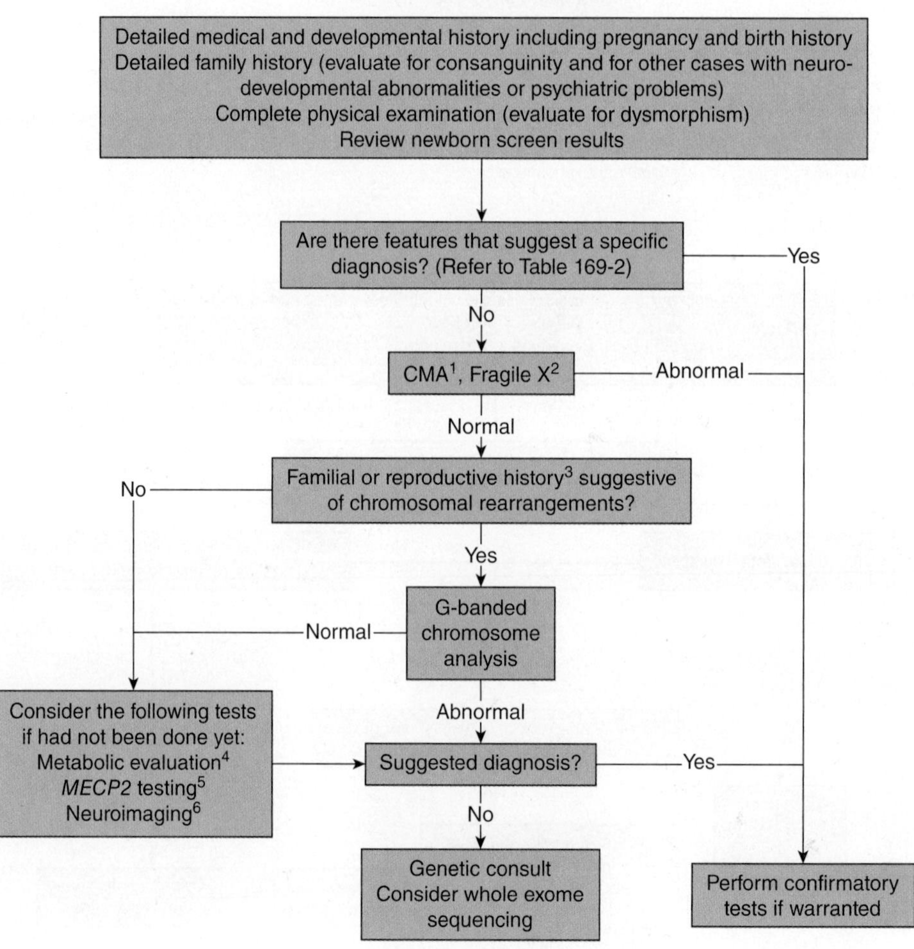


**FIGURE 169-2** Diagnostic algorithm for autism spectrum disorder (ASD). (1) Frequency of causative copy number variants in ASD cases is estimated to be 8% to 21%. The diagnostic yield of CMA increases to 30% in cases of "complex ASD" (ASD with additional findings). (2) Approximately 20% of boys with fragile X syndrome meet diagnostic criteria for ASDs. (3) Consider familial chromosomal rearrangement with history of 3 or more miscarriages. (4) Metabolic evaluation: Initial metabolic evaluation may include blood PH, plasma lactate, ammonia, plasma amino acids profile, and urine organic acids profile. More specific metabolic testing should be obtained depending on the clinical picture. (5) *MECP2* pathogenic variants were reported in nonsyndromic ASDs; *MECP2* duplication in males should also be considered. (6) Brain magnetic resonance imaging (MRI) is the preferred imaging modality. CMA, chromosomal microarray.

**TABLE 169-3 FAILURE TO THRIVE: CONDITIONS TO CONSIDER**

| Disorder | Additional Clinical Characteristics | Specific/Genetic Testing |
|---|---|---|
| **Chromosomal disorders** | | |
| Trisomy 13, 18, 21 | Distinct dysmorphic features, cardiac abnormalities | Routine chromosome analysis |
| Turner syndrome | Webbed neck, infantile edema of hands and feet | Routine chromosome analysis |
| **Microdeletion/duplication syndromes** | | |
| 22q11 deletion | Distinct dysmorphic features, palatal abnormalities, cardiac abnormalities, learning difficulties, immune deficiency, hypocalcemia | CMA or FISH |
| Williams syndrome (7q11.2 deletion syndrome) | Cardiovascular disease (elastin arteriopathy, peripheral pulmonary stenosis), distinctive facial characteristics, connective tissue abnormalities, intellectual disability, hypercalcemia | FISH or CMA |
| Potocki-Lupski syndrome (17p11.2 duplication ) | Hypotonia, oropharyngeal dysphagia with failure to thrive, cardiac abnormalities, developmental delay | CMA |
| **UPD/methylation abnormalities** | | |
| Russell-Silver syndrome | Intrauterine growth retardation, postnatal growth deficiency (2 or more SDs below the mean), normal head circumference, triangular facies, hemihypotrophy | Methylation test of imprinting center 1 (H19-IGF2 IC1) of chromosome 11p15.5 (abnormal in up to 50% of cases)<br>Maternal uniparental disomy for chromosome 7 (in 10% of cases) |
| Prader-Willi syndrome | Congenital hypotonia, feeding difficulties in the neonatal period, intellectual disability, characteristic facial features, undescended testis | For definite diagnosis, do methylation analysis of chromosome region 15q11-q13 (abnormal in 100% of patients)<br>For further characterization of the genetic abnormality, consider FISH or CMA (deletion will be found in 70% of the patients)<br>IC sequencing (abnormal in 5%) |
| **Single-gene abnormalities** | | |
| Rasopathies (Noonan syndrome) | Distinct dysmorphic features (hypertelorism, low-set posteriorly rotated ears, epicanthal folds, ptosis), broad or webbed neck, unusual chest shape, congenital heart defect, developmental delay | Rasopathies gene panel including *PTPN11, BRAF, KRAS, NRAS, RIT1, RAF1, SOS1, MAP2K1* |
| Cornelia de Lange (CDL) syndrome | Distinctive facial features (synophrys, highly arched thin eyebrows, long eyelashes), growth retardation, IUGR, hirsutism, upper limb defects | *NIPBL* sequencing (abnormal in 60% of patients) other genes associated with CDL (in ~5% of patients): *SMC1A, HDAC8, RAD21,* and *SMC* |
| 3M syndrome | Distinctive facial features (including hypoplastic midface, full eyebrows, and fleshy nose tip), severe prenatal and postnatal growth retardation, normal intelligence, hypogonadism in males | Pathogenic variants in *CUL7* will be found in up to 75% of the patients can be caused also by *OBSL1* or *CCDC8* pathogenic variants |

CMA, chromosomal microarray; FISH, fluorescence in situ hybridization; IC, imprinting center; IUGR, intrauterine growth restriction; SD, standard deviation.

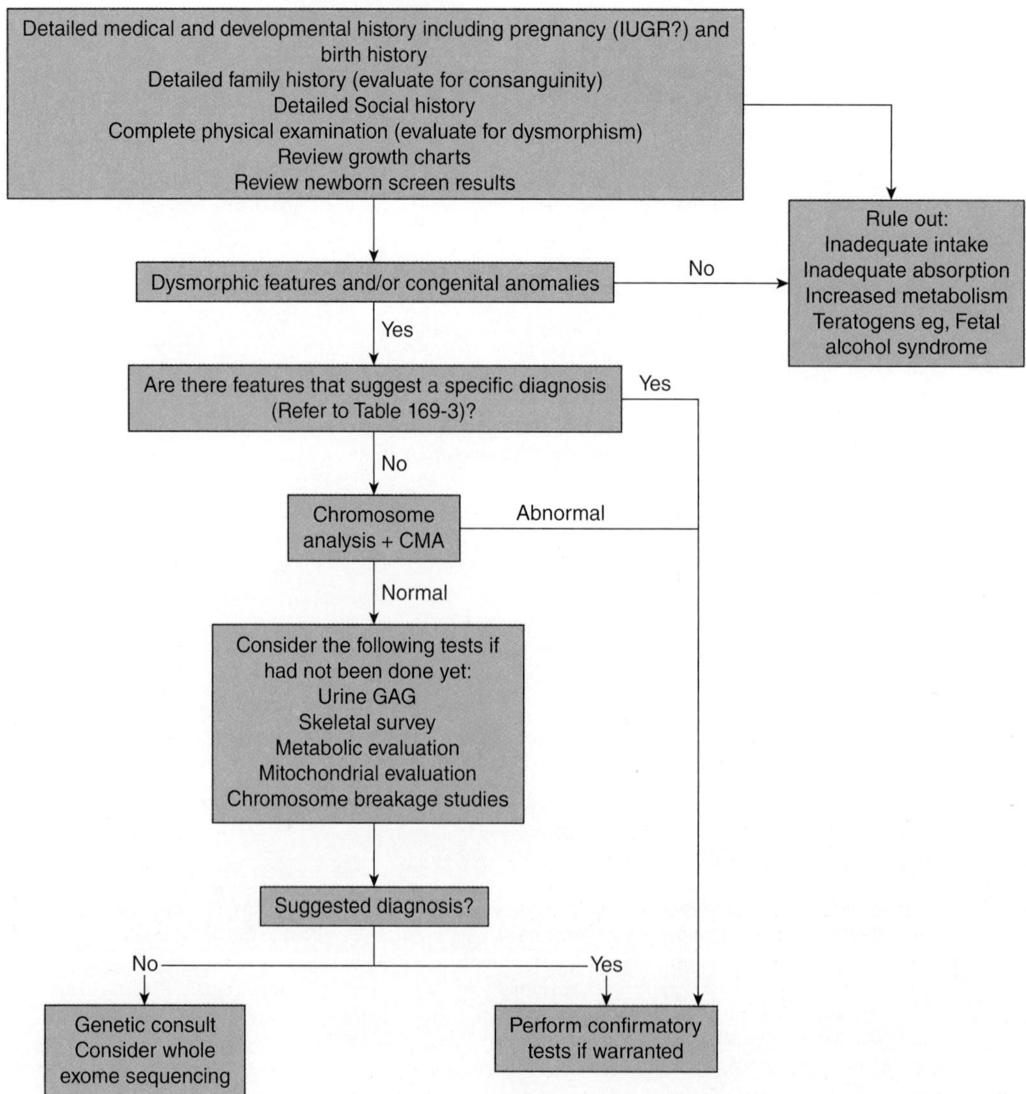


**FIGURE 169-3** Diagnostic algorithm for failure to thrive. CMA, chromosomal microarray; GAG, glycosaminoglycans; IUGR, intrauterine growth restriction.

**TABLE 169-4 NEONATAL HYPOTONIA: CONDITIONS TO CONSIDER**

| Disorder | Additional Clinical Characteristics | Specific/Genetic Testing |
|---|---|---|
| **Central Hypotonia** | | |
| Prader-Willi syndrome | Congenital hypotonia, feeding difficulties in the neonatal period, intellectual disability, characteristic facial features, undescended testis | For definite diagnosis, do methylation analysis of chromosome region 15q11-q13 (abnormal in 100% of patients)<br>For further characterization of the genetic abnormality, consider FISH or CMA (deletion will be found in 70% of the patients)<br>IC sequencing (abnormal in 5%) |
| Peroxisome biogenesis disorders (Zellweger syndrome spectrum) | Feeding difficulties, distinctive facies, seizures, liver cysts, hepatic dysfunction | Definite diagnosis can be done by biochemical assays (serum very-long-chain fatty acids and phytanic acid)<br>*PEX* genes analysis |
| Congenital disorders of glycosylation | Inverted nipples, abnormal fat distribution, cerebellar hypoplasia | Transferrin isoelectric focusing/*N*-glycan analysis/*O*-glycan analysis |
| Smith-Lemli-Opitz syndrome | Prenatal and postnatal growth retardation, microcephaly, intellectual disability, distinctive facial features, cleft palate, cardiac defects, underdeveloped external genitalia in males, polydactyly, Y-shaped 2–3 toe syndactyly | Elevated serum concentration of 7-dehydrocholesterol (DHCR) and low or low-normal plasma cholesterol |
| Glycine encephalopathy (nonketotic hyperglycinemia) | Developmental delay, seizures (myoclonic jerks) | Plasma and CSF AA: increase in CSF glycine and increased CSF-to-plasma glycine ratio |
| **Peripheral Hypotonia** | | |
| Spinal muscular atrophy | Progressive muscle weakness, fasciculation of the tongue, absence of tendon reflexes, preserved sensory, alert appearance, normal intelligence | *SMN1/SMN2* targeted mutation analysis/deletion/duplication analysis |
| Glycogen storage disease type II (Pompe disease), infantile onset | Hypertrophic cardiomyopathy, feeding difficulties, failure to thrive, respiratory distress, hearing loss | Acid alpha-glucosidase (GAA) enzyme activity in blood |

AA, amino acids; CMA, chromosomal microarray; CSF, cerebrospinal fluid; FISH, fluorescence in situ hybridization; IC, imprinting center.

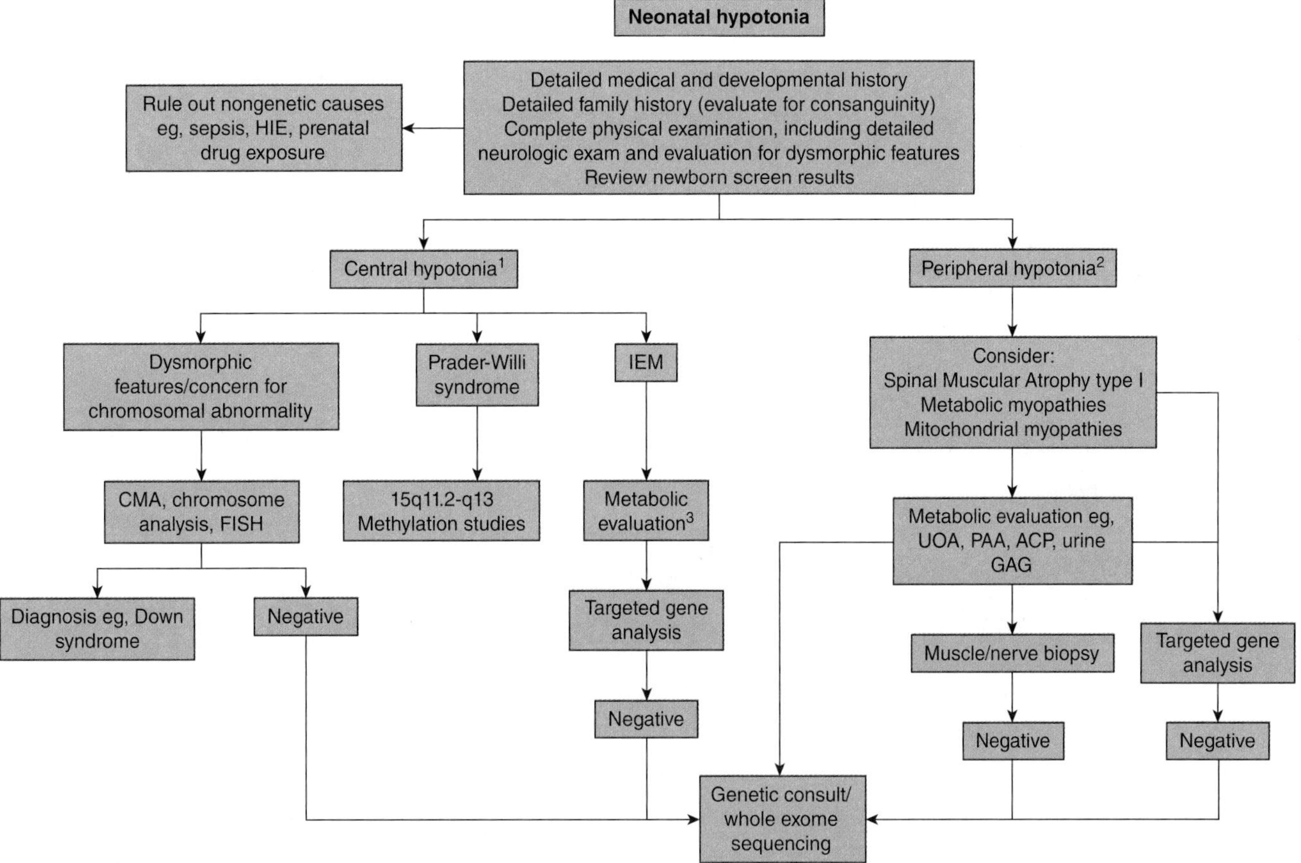


**FIGURE 169-4** Diagnostic algorithm for neonatal hypotonia. (1) Consider brain imaging to evaluate for brain structural abnormalities. (2) Consider muscle and nerve investigations (electromyography [EMG], nerve conduction velocity [NCV]). (3) Full metabolic evaluation includes ammonia, lactate, plasma amino acids, urine organic acids, very-long-chain fatty acids, carnitine/acyl carnitine profile, 7-dehydrocholesterol, transferrin isoelectric focusing, *N*- and *O*-glycan analysis, and galactose-1-phosphate. ACP, acyl carnitine profile; FISH, fluorescence in situ hybridization; GAG, glycosaminoglycans; HIE, hypoxic ischemic encephalopathy; IEM, inborn errors of metabolism; PAA, plasma amino acids; UOA, urine organic acids.

**TABLE 169-5 NEONATAL SEIZURES: CONDITIONS TO CONSIDER**

| Disorder | Additional Characteristics | Specific/Genetic Testing |
|---|---|---|
| Brain anomalies | Lissencephaly, polymicrogyra | Consider lissencephaly/brain malformation gene panel; if specific diagnosis is suspected, consider targeted gene analysis |
| **Metabolic**[a] | | |
| Pyridoxine responsive seizures | Epileptic encephalopathy presenting on day 1–2 of life (up to day ~28). Seizures respond to daily doses of pyridoxine and should be started once this condition is suspected | Pyridoxine plasma panel, *ALDH7A1* gene analysis |
| GLUT1 deficiency syndrome | Epileptic encephalopathy in infancy (70%), microcephaly, involuntary rapid eye movements | CSF glucose/blood glucose ratio <0.45; if abnormal proceed with *SLC2A1* gene analysis |
| Glycine encephalopathy | Severe epileptic encephalopathy, lethargy, hypotonia | Plasma and CSF AA: elevated glycine, increased glycine CSF/plasma ratio (>0.08) |
| Creatine metabolism | Guanidinoactetate methyltransferase: ID, seizures, behavioral disorders | Plasma and urine guanidinoacetate and creatine, urine creatine/creatinine ratio |
| | Transporter deficiency: ID, speech delay, behavioral problems | |
| Sulfite oxidase deficiency | Infantile epileptic encephalopathy, microcephaly | Urine *S*-sulfocysteine |
| Pyruvate metabolism disorders | Congenital lactic acidosis, seizures, hypotonia, progressive encephalopathy | Lactate, pyruvate, PAA |
| | Pyruvate carboxylase deficiency | *PC* gene analysis |
| | Pyruvate dehydrogenase deficiency | Multiple genes involved. *PDHA1* is the most common |
| Multiple carboxylase deficiency | Metabolic acidosis, hypotonia, ataxia, seizures, ID, skin rashes | Lactate, ammonia, plasma AA, UOA; *BTD* or *HLCS* gene analysis |
| Other single-gene disorders | Early infantile epileptic encephalopathies | Gene panel or whole-exome sequencing |

AA, amino acids; CSF, cerebrospinal fluid; ID, intellectual disability; PAA, plasma amino acids; UOA, urine organic acids.

[a]Warrant a genetics referral.



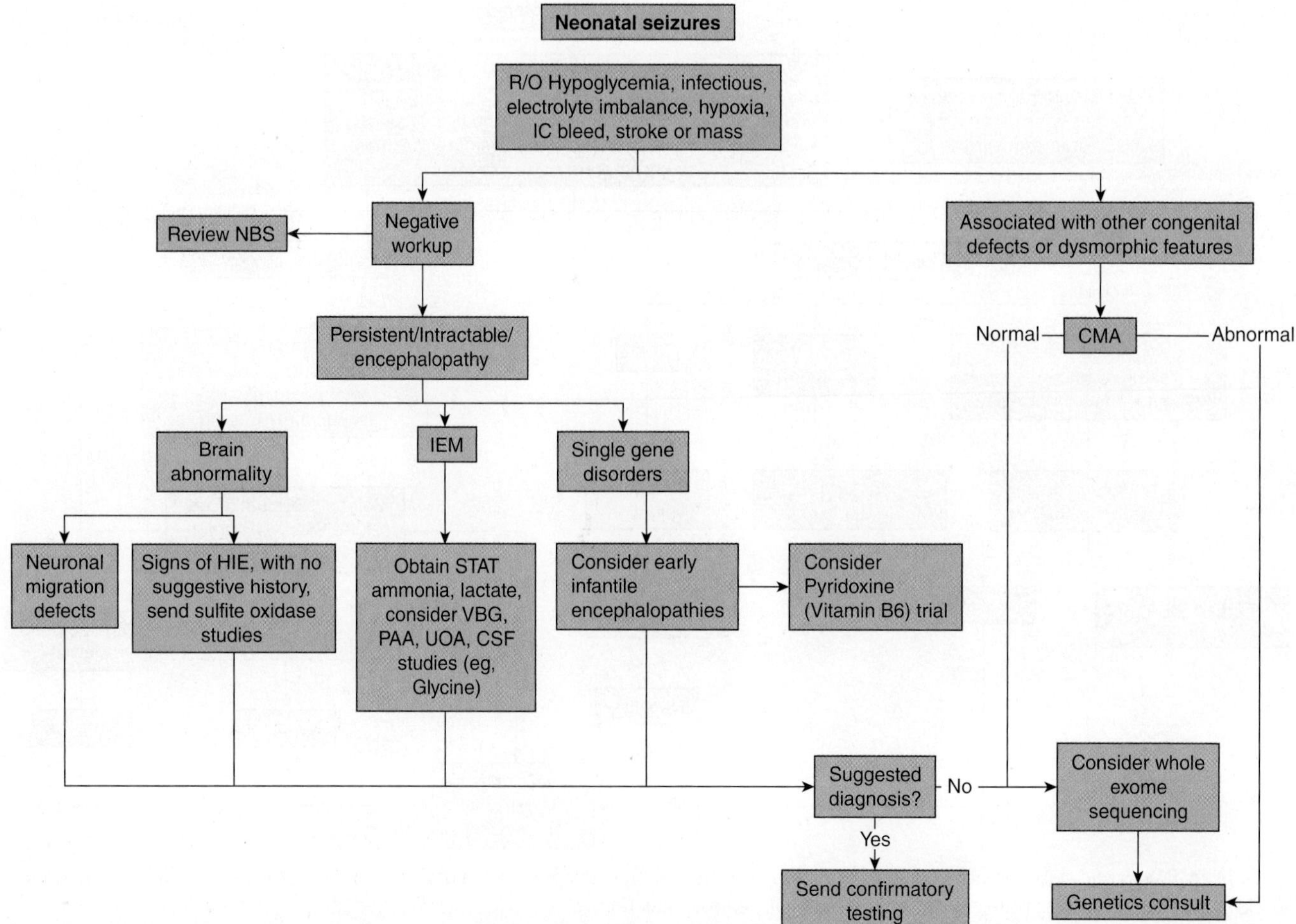


**FIGURE 169-5** Diagnostic algorithm for neonatal seizures. CMA, chromosomal microarray; CSF, cerebrospinal fluid; HIE, hypoxic ischemic encephalopathy; IC, intracranial; IEM, inborn error of metabolism; NBS, newborn screen; PAA, plasma amino acids; R/O, rule out; UOA, urine organic acids; VBG, venous blood gas; WES, whole-exome sequencing.

## OVERGROWTH (Table 169-6, Fig. 169-6)

**TABLE 169-6 OVERGROWTH: CONDITIONS TO CONSIDER**

| Disorder | Additional Characteristics | Specific/Genetic Testing |
|---|---|---|
| **Macrocephaly** | | |
| *PTEN* hamartoma tumor syndromes | **Bannayan-Riley-Ruvalcaba syndrome:** Congenital macrocephaly, hamartomas, lipomas, and pigmented macules of the glans penis<br>**Cowden syndrome:** Macrocephaly, trichilemmomas, and papillomatous papules. Presents in late 20s. High risk for thyroid, breast, and endometrium tumors | *PTEN* gene analysis |
| Achondroplasia | Disproportionate small stature, rhizomelic (proximal) shortening of the arms and legs with redundant skin folds, large head, frontal bossing, midface hypoplasia, hypotonia in infancy | *FGFR3* gene analysis |
| Neurofibromatosis type 1 | Café-au-lait spots, axillary and inguinal freckling, cutaneous neurofibromas, Lisch nodules | *NF1* gene analysis |
| **Overgrowth syndromes** | | |
| Sotos syndrome | Broad prominent forehead, sparse frontotemporal hair, downslanting palpebral fissures, long and narrow face, long chin, learning disability and overgrowth | *NSD1* gene analysis |
| Gorlin syndrome | Frontal bossing, coarse facial features, and facial milia. Development of multiple jaw keratocysts and/or basal cell carcinomas. Plantar and palmar pits | *PTCH1* or *SUFU* gene analysis |
| Weaver syndrome | Tall stature, broad forehead, hypertelorism, low-set ears, long philtrum, camptodactyly, broad thumbs, deep-set nails, advanced bone age | *EZH2* gene analysis |
| Simpson-Golabi-Behmel syndrome (SGBS) | Hypertelorism, broad nose, macrostomia, macroglossia, thickened lips, and palate anomalies. Coarse facial features. Supernumerary nipples and abdominal wall defects | *GPC3* gene analysis |
| **Visceromegaly/asymmetric overgrowth** | | |
| Beckwith-Wiedemann syndrome (BWS) | Neonatal hypoglycemia, macrosomia, ear creases/pits, macroglossia, hemihyperplasia, omphalocele, embryonal tumors (eg, Wilms tumor), renal abnormalities (eg, nephrocalcinosis) | Methylation studies for 11p15.5, IC1, and IC2<br>*CDKN1C* gene analysis if familial BWS is suspected |
| Proteus | Asymmetric, segmental overgrowth (mosaic distribution of lesions) vascular and lymphatic malformations, cerebriform connective tissue nevus, splenomegaly, kyphoscoliosis, skeletal overgrowth | Clinical criteria<br>Mosaic somatic mutation in *AKT1* |
| *PIK3CA*-related segmental overgrowth | **CLOVES syndrome:** congenital lipomatous asymmetric overgrowth of the trunk, lymphatic, capillary, venous, and combined-type vascular malformations, epidermal nevi, skeletal and spinal anomalies<br>**Fibroadipose hyperplasia:** progressive segmental overgrowth of visceral, subcutaneous, muscular, fibroadipose, and skeletal tissues, and may involve the trunk or extremities | *PIK3CA* gene analysis on affected tissue |
| **Acromegaly**[a] | | |
| Xq26.3 duplication syndrome (X-linked acrogigantism) | Early-onset gigantism (increased weight and height velocity), usually beginning during the first year of life caused by growth hormone hypersecretion. Large hands and feet | CMA<br>If suspected and negative CMA, test for *GRP101* gene |
| Pituitary adenoma, growth hormone-secreting (PAGH) | **PAGH1:** usually presents close to the second decade, menstrual irregularities and galactorrhea<br>**PAGH2:** excessive growth starts before 4 years of age. More common in females; frequently associated with hyperprolactinemia | *AIP* gene<br>*GRP101* gene analysis |
| McCune-Albright syndrome | Café-au-lait macules (usually the first manifestation). Fibrous dysplasia, can involve any part of the craniofacial, axial, and/or appendicular skeleton with isolated lesions to a severe, disabling polyostotic disease. Endocrine manifestations include hyperthyroidism, hyperparathyroidism and precocious puberty | Somatic activating mutation of *GNAS* (affected tissue) |
| Multiple endocrine neoplasia type I (MEN1) | Combinations of tumors of parathyroid, pancreatic islets, duodenal endocrine cells, and the anterior pituitary | *MEN1* gene analysis |

CMA, chromosomal microarray; IC, imprinting center.

[a]Acromegaly is characterized by coarse facial features, protruding jaw, and enlarged extremities.

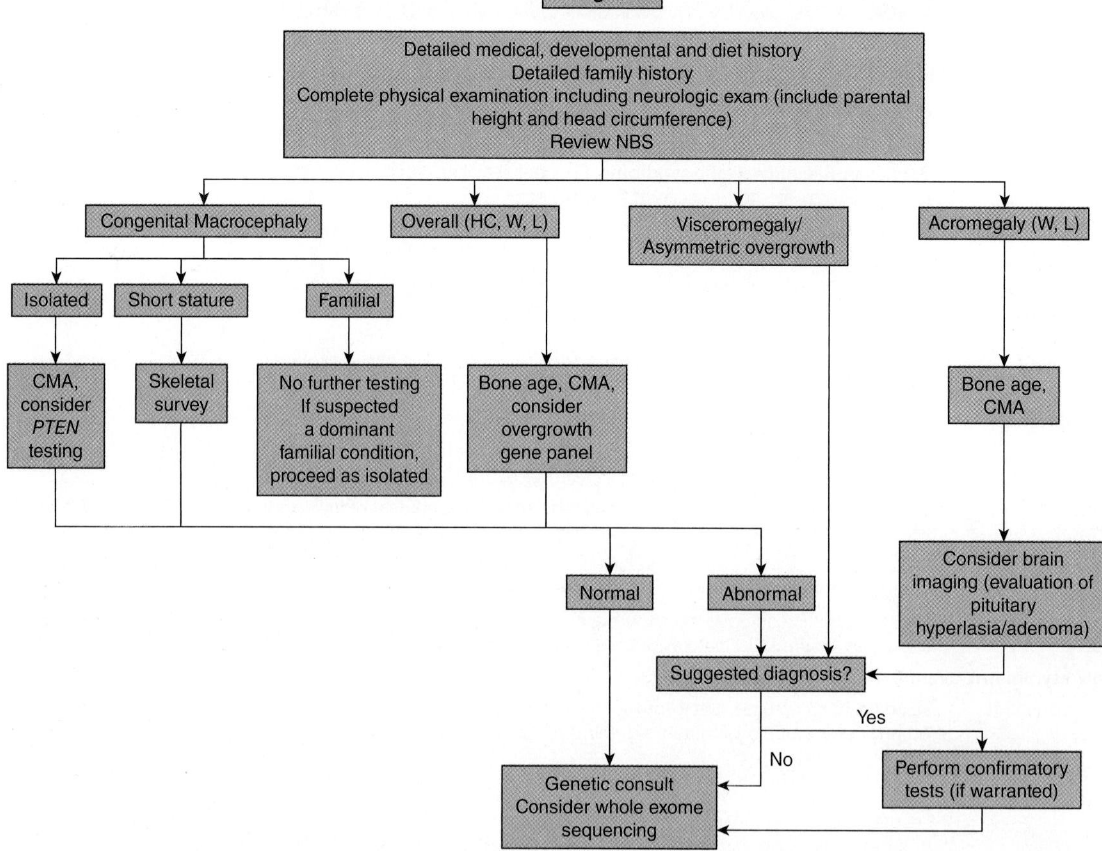


**FIGURE 169-6** Diagnostic algorithm for overgrowth. CMA, chromosomal microarray; HC, head circumference; L, length; NBS, newborn screen; W, weight.



## SHORT STATURE (Table 169-7, Fig. 169-7)

**TABLE 169-7 SHORT STATURE: CONDITIONS TO CONSIDER**

| Disorder | Additional Clinical Characteristics | Specific/Genetic Testing |
|---|---|---|
| Turner syndrome | Webbed neck, infantile edema of hands and feet | Routine chromosome analysis |
| Noonan syndrome | Distinct dysmorphic features (hypertelorism, low-set posteriorly rotated ears, epicanthal folds, ptosis), broad or webbed neck, unusual chest shape, congenital heart defect, developmental delay | Rasopathies gene panel including *PTPN11, BRAF, KRAS, NRAS, RIT1, RAF1, SOS1, MAP2K1* |
| Prader-Willi syndrome | History of hypotonia and feeding difficulties in early infancy, followed in later infancy by excessive eating. Developmental delay, intellectual disability | For definite diagnosis, do methylation analysis of chromosome region 15q11-q13 (abnormal in 100% of patients)<br>For further characterization of the genetic abnormality consider, FISH or CMA (deletion will be found in 70% of the patients)<br>IC sequencing (abnormal in 5%) |
| Russell-Silver syndrome | Intrauterine growth restriction, postnatal growth deficiency (2 or more standard deviations below the mean), normal head circumference, triangular facies, hemihypotrophy | Methylation test of imprinting center 1 (H19-IGF2 IC1) of chromosome 11p15.5 (abnormal in up to 50% of cases)<br>Maternal uniparental disomy for chromosome 7 (in 10% of cases) |
| Mucopolysaccharidoses | Coarse facial features, inguinal or umbilical hernia, hepatosplenomegaly, skeletal and joint findings, ocular findings | Urinary glycosaminoglycans<br>Measuring specific lysosomal enzyme activity |
| SHOX-related short stature | Phenotypic spectrum: Leri-Weill dyschondrosteosis (short stature, mesomelia, and Madelung deformity) to isolated short stature | *SHOX* gene analysis |
| Achondroplasia | Disproportionate short stature, rhizomelic (proximal) shortening of the arms and legs with redundant skin folds, large head, frontal bossing, midface hypoplasia, hypotonia in infancy | *FGFR3* gene analysis |
| Hypochondroplasia | Short stature, disproportionately short arms and legs, broad, short hands and feet, macrocephaly. Symptoms become prominent with age. Usually present as toddlers/early school age | *FGFR3* gene analysis |
| Pseudoachondroplasia | Disproportionate short stature that develops around the age of 2 years, waddling gait, short limbs, mild joint laxity, normocephaly, degenerative joint disease | *COMP* gene analysis |

CMA, chromosomal microarray; FISH, fluorescence in situ hybridization; IC, imprinting center.

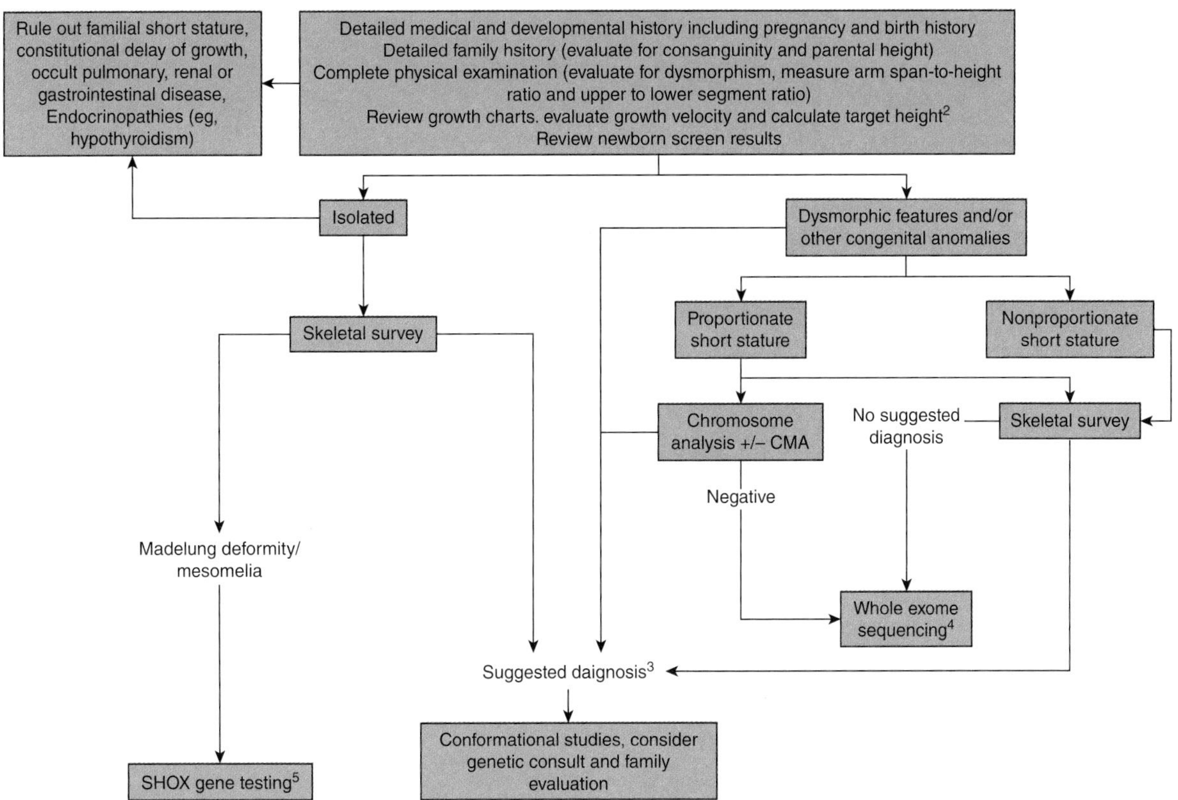


**FIGURE 169-7** Diagnostic algorithm for short stature. (1) Short stature is defined as height less than third percentile. (2) Target height for boys = [(Maternal height in cm + Paternal height in cm) + 13]/2; and target height for girls = [(Maternal height in cm + Paternal height in cm) – 13]/2. (3) See Table 169-7 for possible causes for short stature. (4) Referral to genetic counseling is recommended. (5) If *SHOX* testing is negative, consider testing for *PAR1* (pseudoautosomal region 1) deletion, which results in loss of *SHOX* enhancer. Bone age can give indication for skeletal maturity, although it is nonspecific. (Modified with permission from Seaver LH, Irons M, American College of Medical Genetics (ACMG) Professional Practice and Guidelines Committee: ACMG practice guideline: genetic evaluation of short stature. *Genet Med*. 2009 Jun;11(6):465-470.)

## MICROCEPHALY (Table 169-8, Fig. 169-8)

**TABLE 169-8 MICROCEPHALY: CONDITIONS TO CONSIDER**

| Disorder | Additional Characteristics | Specific/Genetic Testing |
|---|---|---|
| Deletion 5p syndrome (cri-du-chat) | Low birth weight, hypotonia, cat-like cry, hypertelorism, downslanting palpebral fissures | CMA |
| 1q21.1 deletion syndrome | Mild to moderate developmental delay/ID, mild dysmorphic features, prominent forehead, deep-set eyes, cardiac abnormalities, and broad thumbs and halluces. Reports of schizophrenia | CMA |
| 16p11.2 duplication syndrome | Low BMI, ASD, attention-deficit/hyperactivity, increased risk for mental health problems, eg, schizophrenia, anxiety, depression | CMA |
| Trisomy 18 | Prominent occiput, bitemporal narrowing, short palpebral fissures, micrognathia, clenched hands, structural cardiac defects | Routine chromosome analysis |
| Trisomy 13 | Sloping forehead, microphthalmia, cleft lip, cleft palate, single palmar crease, polydactyly, posterior prominence of heel, and structural cardiac defects | Routine chromosome analysis |
| Cornelia de Lange (CDL) syndrome | Distinctive facial features (synophrys, highly arched thin eyebrows, long eyelashes), growth retardation, IUGR, hirsutism, upper limb defects | *NIPBL* (abnormal in 60% of patients)<br>Other genes associated with CDL (in ~5% of patients): *SMC1A*, *HDAC8*, *RAD21*, and *SMC* |
| Williams syndrome (7q11.2 deletion syndrome) | Cardiovascular disease (elastin arteriopathy, peripheral pulmonary stenosis), distinctive facies, connective tissue abnormalities, intellectual disability and hypercalcemia | FISH or CMA |
| Smith-Lemil-Opitz syndrome | Prenatal and postnatal growth retardation, microcephaly, intellectual disability, distinctive facial features, cleft palate, cardiac defects, underdeveloped external genitalia in males, polydactyly, Y-shaped 2–3 toe syndactyly | Elevated serum concentration of 7-dehydrocholesterol (DHCR) and low or low normal plasma cholesterol |

ASD, autism spectrum disorder; BMI, body mass index; CMA, chromosomal microarray; FISH, fluorescence in situ hybridization; ID, intellectual disability; IUGR, intrauterine growth restriction.

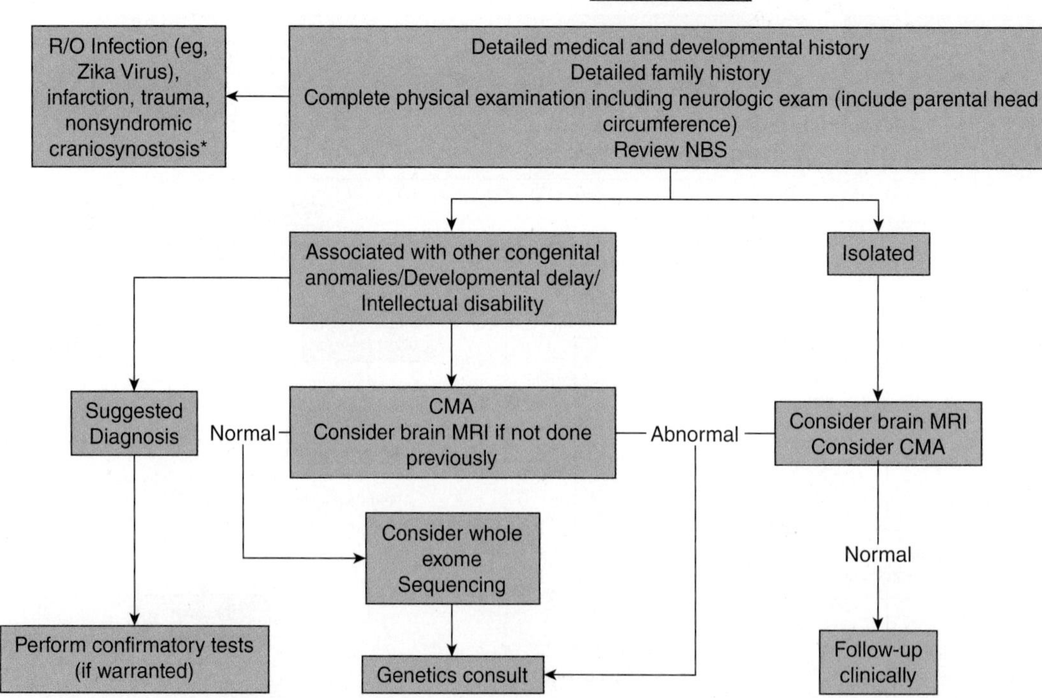


**FIGURE 169-8** Diagnostic algorithm for microcephaly. *There are multiple causes of syndromic craniosynostosis. CMA, chromosomal microarray; MRI, magnetic resonance imaging; NBS, newborn screen; R/O, rule out.

## CARDIOMYOPATHY (Table 169-9, Fig. 169-9)

**TABLE 169-9 CARDIOMYOPATHY: CONDITIONS TO CONSIDER**

| Disorder | Additional Clinical Characteristics | Specific/Genetic Testing |
|---|---|---|
| Duchenne muscular dystrophy | Delayed milestones, including delays in sitting and standing independently. Proximal weakness causes a waddling gait and difficulty climbing with calf hypertrophy. Rapidly progressive | *DMD* gene analysis |
| Becker dystrophy | Later-onset skeletal muscle weakness with calf hypertrophy; some individuals remain ambulatory into their 20s | *DMD* gene analysis |
| Fatty acid oxidation: very-long-chain acyl-CoA dehydrogenase deficiency (VLCAD) | Early onset: first months of life, pericardial effusion, arrhythmia, hypotonia, hepatomegaly, intermittent hypoglycemia | Acylcarnitine profile |
| Mitochondrial disease | Multiorgan involvement, including myopathy. Lactic acidosis | —[a] |
| Glycogen storage disease | | |
| II | Presents in first months of life with hypotonia, muscle weakness, cardiomegaly, feeding difficulties, failure to thrive, respiratory distress, hearing loss. Shortened PR interval with a broad, wide QRS complex | Acid alpha-glucosidase (GAA) enzyme activity in blood |
| IIIa | Ketotic hypoglycemia, hepatomegaly, hyperlipidemia, elevated transaminases. Cardiomyopathy usually appears during childhood | *AGL* gene analysis |
| IV | Various subtypes. Hypotonia, hepatomegaly, liver dysfunction, early death | Demonstration of glycogen branching enzyme (GBE) deficiency in liver, muscle, or skin fibroblasts<br>*GBE1* gene analysis |

[a]Warrants a genetics referral.

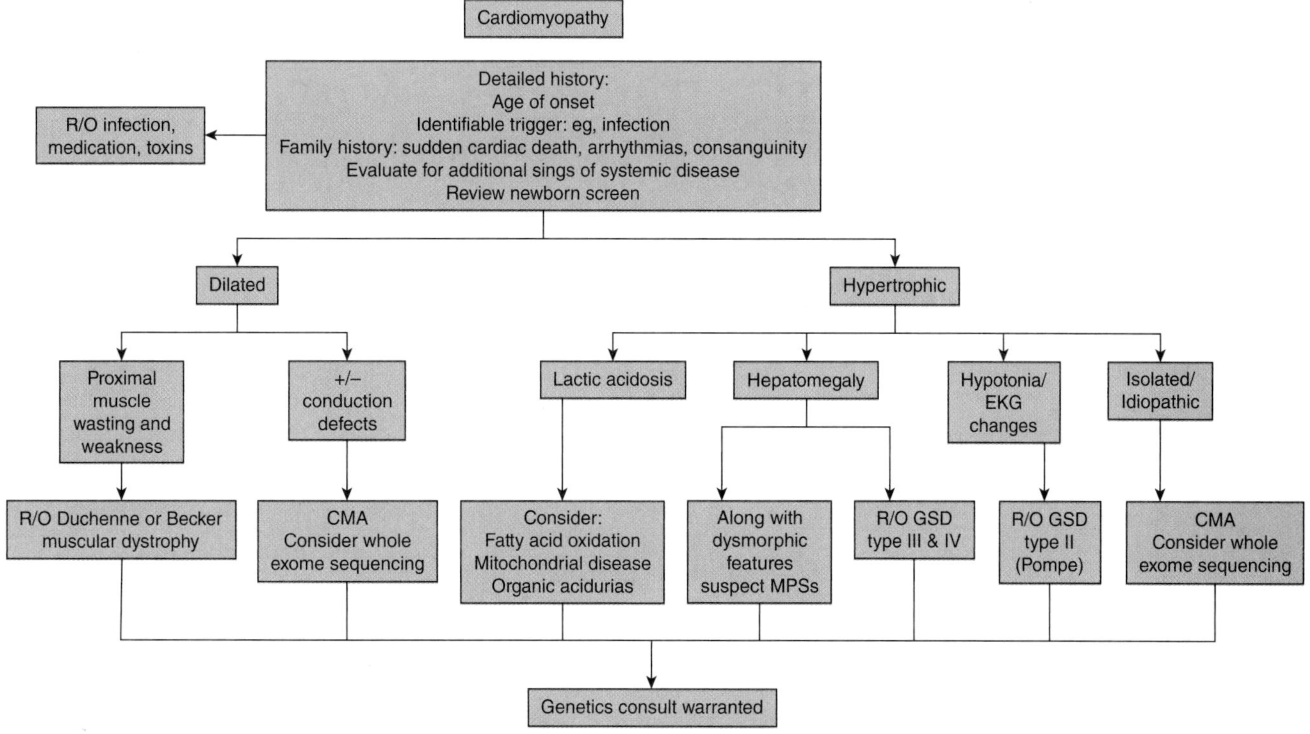


**FIGURE 169-9** Diagnostic algorithm for cardiomyopathy. CMA, chromosomal microarray; EKG, electrocardiogram; GSD, glycogen storage disease; MPS, mucopolysaccharidosis; R/O, rule out.

## RHABDOMYOLYSIS (Table 169-10, Fig. 169-10)

**TABLE 169-10 RHABDOMYOLYSIS: CONDITIONS TO CONSIDER**

| Disorder[a] | Additional Characteristics | Specific/Genetic Testing |
|---|---|---|
| Inborn error of glycogenolysis | **McArdle disease (GSD V):** Exercise intolerance, rapid fatigue, myalgia, cramps. Normal lactate. Second wind phenomenon | *PYGM* gene analysis |
| Fatty acid oxidation defects: CPT2, VLCAD, MCAD, CACTD | During stress or fasting<br>During rest or prolonged low-intensity exercise | Acylcarnitine profile |
| Carnitine palmitoyltransferase II deficiency (CPT2) | **Myopathic form**<br>Exercise-induced muscle pain and weakness, +/– myoglobinuria<br>Onset first to sixth decade<br>*Most frequent cause of hereditary myoglobinuria* | Acylcarnitine profile: elevated C12 to C18, notably **C16 and C18:1** |
| Oxidative phosphorylation | Defects in the respiratory chain. Mitochondrial myopathies | —[a] |
| MECRCN | Episodic rhabdomyolysis, intellectual disability, hypoglycemia, susceptibility to cardiac tachyarrhythmias, progressive neurodegeneration | *TANGO2* sequencing and del/dup analysis. If normal, consider CMA |
| Others | Susceptibility to malignant hyperthermia (*RYR1*)<br>Myoadenylate deaminase deficiency (*AMPD1*)<br>Muscular dystrophies<br>Acute recurrent myoglobinuria (*LPIN1*) | —[a] |

CMA, chromosomal microarray; del, deletion; dup, duplication; MECRCN, metabolic encephalomyopathic crises, recurrent, with rhabdomyolysis, cardiac arrhythmias, and neurodegeneration.

[a]Metabolic disorders warrant a genetics referral.

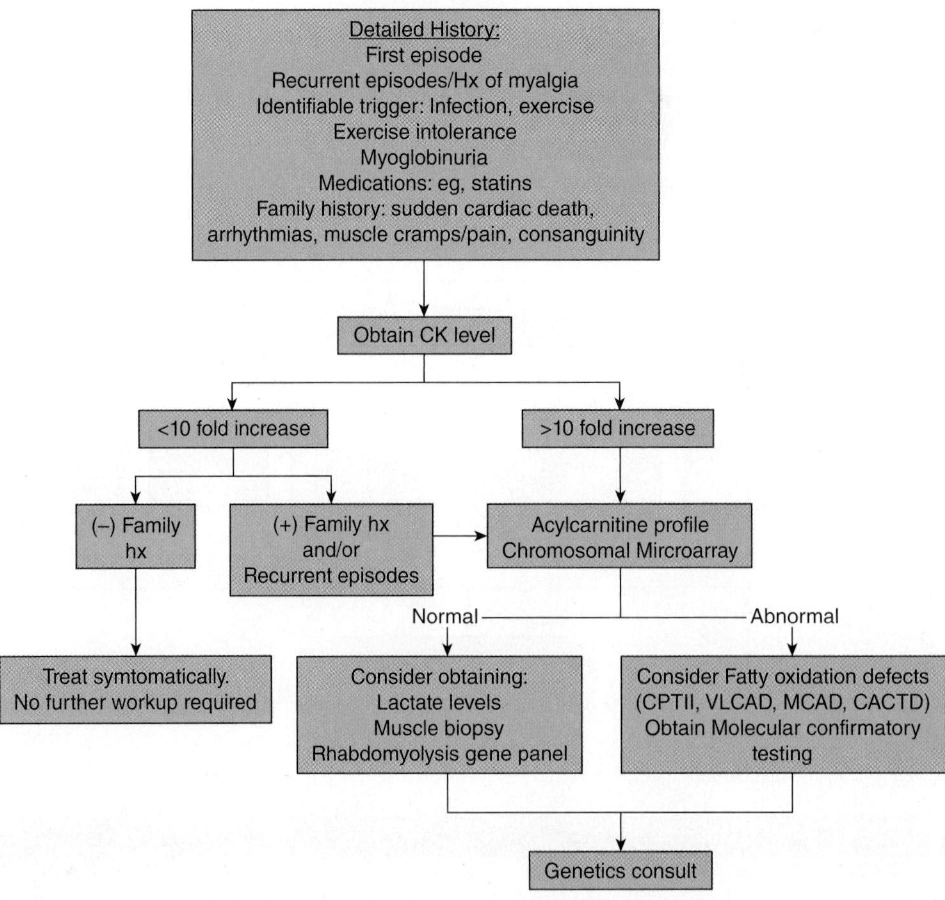


**FIGURE 169-10** Diagnostic algorithm for rhabdomyolysis. CK, creatine kinase; Hx, history.



## HEARING LOSS (Table 169-11, Fig. 169-11)

**TABLE 169-11 HEARING LOSS: CONDITIONS TO CONSIDER**

| Disorder | Additional Clinical Characteristics | Specific/Genetic Testing |
|---|---|---|
| Nonsyndromic hearing loss (NSHL) | Inheritance pattern can be autosomal dominant, autosomal recessive, or X-linked | *GJB2* and *GJB6* analysis (when autosomal recessive inheritance is suspected)<br>Multigene panel for NSHL |
| Waardenburg syndrome (WS) | Sensorineural hearing loss, pigmentary abnormalities of the skin, hair (white forelock), and eyes (heterochromia iridis) | Start with *PAX3* sequencing if WS type I is suspected<br>Multigene panel (including *MITF*, *EDNRB*, *EDN3*, and *SOX10*) is recommended if *PAX3* testing is negative or if type is not clear |
| Stickler syndrome | Progressive sensorineural hearing loss, cleft palate, spondyloepiphyseal dysplasia resulting in osteoarthritis | *COL2A1* (type I, most common), *COL11A1* (type 2, up to 20% of the cases), *COL11A2* (type 3, rare). Rare pathogenic variants had been also found in *COL9A1*, *COL9A2*, and *COL9A3* |
| Neurofibromatosis type 2 | Hearing loss secondary to bilateral vestibular schwannomas | *NF2* gene analysis |
| Biotinidase deficiency | Neurologic features (seizures, hypertonia, developmental delay, ataxia), visual problems, skin rash, alopecia, conjunctivitis | Deficient biotinidase enzyme activity in serum/plasma<br>*BTD* gene analysis |
| Alport syndrome | Progressive sensorineural hearing loss, glomerulonephritis, ophthalmologic findings | Type 4 collagen genes:<br>Start with single-gene testing based on family history (*COL4A5* for X-linked pattern, *COL4A3* for autosomal recessive/dominant pattern)<br>Multigene panel is available (including *COL4A3*, *COL4A4*, and *COL4A5*) |
| Mitochondrial DNA pathogenic variants | Neuromuscular abnormalities (Kearns-Sayre syndrome), diabetes mellitus (3243 A-to-G transition in MTTL1)<br>MELAS<br>MERRF<br>NARF | Mitochondrial deletions/pathogenic variants |
| Pendred syndrome | Enlarged/dilated vestibular aqueduct or Mondini dysplasia | *SLC26A4* gene analysis |

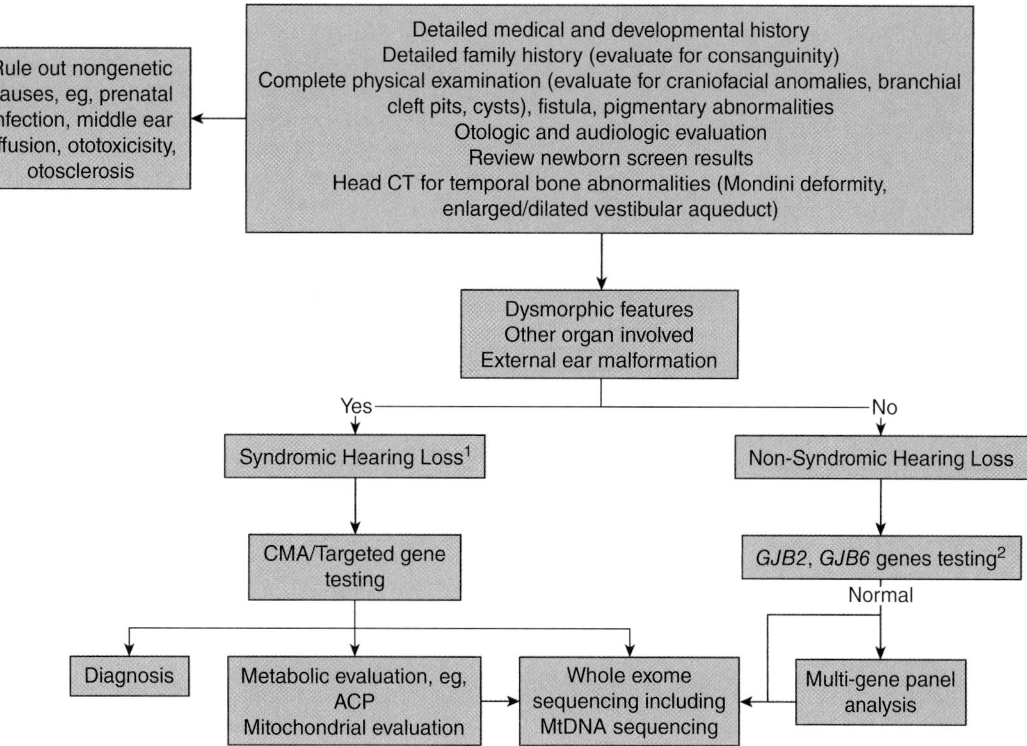


**FIGURE 169-11** Diagnostic algorithm for hearing loss. (1) Approximately 80% of nonsyndromic hearing loss is autosomal recessive, and approximately 30% of all genetic hearing loss is syndromic in nature. (2) As much as 50% of autosomal recessive nonsyndromic hearing loss is caused by *GJB2* or *GJB6* genes abnormalities. Gene panels are clinically useful when multiple genes are involved in a particular disorder or when there is extensive phenotypic overlap between different disorders. ACP, acylcarnitine profile; CMA, chromosomal microarray; CT, computed tomography; MtDNA, mitochondrial DNA.

## SUGGESTED READINGS


Benito-Sanz S, Royo JL, Barroso E, et al. Identification of the first recurrent PAR1 deletion in Leri-Weill dyschondrosteosis and idiopathic short stature reveals the presence of a novel? SHOX enhancer. *J Med Genet*. 2012;49:442-450.

Dumas LJ, O'Bleness MS, Davis JM, et al. DUF1220-domain copy number implicated in human brain-size pathology and evolution. *Am J Human Genet*. 2012;91(3):444-454.

Iacovazzo D, Caswell R, Bunce B, et al. Germline or somatic GPR-101duplication leads to X-linked acrogigantism: a clinico-pathological and genetic study. *Acta Neuropathol Commun*. 2016;4:56.

Lalani SR, Liu P, Rosenfeld JA, et al. Recurrent muscle weakness with rhabdomyolysis, metabolic crises, and cardiac arrhythmia due to biallelic *TANGO2* mutations. *Am J Human Genet*. 2016;98(2):347-357.

Lupski JR. Cognitive phenotypes and genomic copy number variations. *JAMA*. 2015;313(20):2029-2030.

Männik K, Mägi R, Macé A, et al. Copy number variations and cognitive phenotypes in unselected populations. *JAMA*. 2015; 313(20):2044-2054.

Ramocki MB, Peters SU, Tavyev YJ, et al. Autism and other neuropsychiatric symptoms are prevalent in individuals with *MECP2* duplication syndrome. *Ann Neurol*. 2009;66:771-782.

Steinman KJ, Spence SJ, Ramocki MB, et al. 16p11.2 deletion and duplication: characterizing neurologic phenotypes in a large clinically ascertained cohort. *Am J Med Genet Part A*. 2016;9999A:1-13.

Trivellin G, Daly AF, Faucz FR, et al. Gigantism and acromegaly due to Xq26 microduplications and *GPR101* mutation. *N Engl J Med*. 2014;371(25):2363-2374.


# 170 Approach to a Newborn with Birth Defects

Mohammed Almannai and Seema R. Lalani

## INTRODUCTION

Congenital anomalies occur frequently and are estimated to be present in about 13% of all admissions to neonatal intensive care units in the developed countries. Data from large studies indicate that the burden of genetic diseases in neonates with congenital anomalies in intensive care settings is approximately 5% to 7%. Congenital anomalies are a leading cause of infant mortality in the United States, accounting for about 20% of all infant deaths. There are over 4500 Mendelian disorders that have a known genetic etiology at present, and a significant fraction of these present in the neonatal period. With the rapid advancement in diagnostic technologies and our increasing ability to decipher the genetic basis of birth defects, a substantial influence of genetic perturbation is recognized in infants with birth defects. Recognition of chromosomal syndromes, genomic disorders, and single-gene Mendelian diseases, as well as imprinting diseases presenting in the newborns, is paramount in this age of rapidly advancing diagnostic and treatment alternatives. While trisomy 21 (Down syndrome) remains the most common genetic condition associated with birth defects, with an estimated incidence of 1 in 700 live births, other genetic disorders play a correspondingly significant role and should be recognized by astute clinicians. Teratogens, such as warfarin, alcohol, maternal phenylketonuria, retinoic acid, and Zika virus have an important role in causing birth anomalies and should be distinguished from inherited genetic determinants. Approaching a newborn with birth defects not only requires a comprehensive evaluation to identify the underlying cause, but also involves elucidating the genetic variants in at-risk families to prevent recurrence of often serious and life-threatening congenital anomalies.

## DEFINITIONS

Understanding different terminologies relevant to birth defects is important to determine the etiology of causation, whether genetic or environmental.

**Malformations** result from an intrinsic abnormal development during organogenesis. Etiology includes both genetic and environmental factors. Malformations typically develop early, often in the first 8 weeks of gestation. Depending on the underlying cause, malformation could involve a single organ or multiple systems in the body. Malformations can be further divided into **major malformations**, such as congenital heart disease (CHD) and meningomyelocele, and minor **malformations,** which are generally of minimal significance, particularly if seen as an isolated finding.

A **syndrome** is defined as a pattern of malformations, whether major or minor, that occurs as a predictable constellation of features due to a single underlying etiology. The basis of a syndrome could be chromosomal, genomic structural change (eg, deletion or duplication also known as copy number variant [CNV]), monogenic, epigenetic, or teratogenic exposure. Some examples of syndromes include Down syndrome, DiGeorge/velocardiofacial syndrome (DGS/VCFS) due to 22q11.2 deletion, and Beckwith-Wiedemann syndrome (BWS).

An **association** is defined by the combination of several birth defects that occur more frequently together than would be expected by chance. VACTERL/VATER association (vertebral defects, anal atresia, cardiovascular anomalies, tracheoesophageal fistula with esophageal atresia, and radial/renal abnormalities) is a good example, occurring as a sporadic defect with at least 3 of these congenital malformations in an individual. The causation has not yet been defined in the majority of the affected individuals.

**Disruptions** result from factors that disrupt normal development of an embryonic structure after its early formation. A classic example is amniotic band disruption. Amniotic bands, which are considered to result from an early injury to the amniotic sac, could cause a range of defects that include constriction rings and limb and/or digital amputations.

A **sequence** is a term used to describe conditions in which multiple defects occur secondary to an initial triggering event. A classic example is Pierre-Robin sequence (PRS), where small mandible prompts posterior displacement of the tongue, which eventually prevents the palatal shelves to fuse. This sequence is recognized in a newborn with micrognathia, glossoptosis, and cleft palate. A sequence can occur in isolation or as a part of an underlying genetic diagnosis. For example, a subset of newborns with PRS have Stickler syndrome. Other syndromes to consider with PRS include DGS/VCFS, Marshall syndrome, Treacher Collins syndrome, and Nager syndrome.

**Deformations** result from extrinsic factors causing physical restraints on fetal development. An example is oligohydramnios, where regardless of the underlying cause, the fetus is physically compressed by the uterus, resulting in Potter sequence. In comparison to malformations, deformations usually occur later in pregnancy.

# APPROACH TO A NEWBORN WITH BIRTH DEFECTS

## HISTORY

Procuring an extensive medical history is a crucial element in the diagnostic process. When evaluating a newborn with birth defects, there are elements in history that require special consideration. Some of these are highlighted below.

### Obstetric History

Inquiring about parental ages at the time of conception is particularly relevant in the evaluation process of a newborn with a birth defect. While advanced maternal age is a known risk factor for aneuploidies such as trisomies 21 (Down syndrome), 18 (Edward syndrome), and 13 (Patau syndrome), advanced paternal age at the time of conception has been linked to *de novo* mutations causing autosomal dominant disorders (syndromes such as achondroplasia and CHARGE). Exposure during pregnancy to smoking, alcohol, or drugs should be explored in detail. Travel history, household pets, and consideration for potential viral exposure/infection is relevant. Maternal pregestational diabetes mellitus is a well-known risk factor for embryopathy including CHD, renal anomalies, and caudal regression. Conotruncal malformations are known teratogenic effects of isotretinoin-exposed pregnancies. Any results available from prenatal genetic testing, including noninvasive prenatal testing (NIPT), chorionic villous sampling, or amniocentesis, should be reviewed.

### Family History

Comprehensive family history is a cornerstone of genetic evaluation and should be assessed with a pedigree drawn for at least 3 generations, using international standards. Parental relatedness, ie, consanguinity, should be addressed to potentially recognize increased risk for autosomal recessive disorders in the newborn. History of recurrent first-trimester miscarriages is important to ascertain, often suggestive of the presence of a balanced chromosomal rearrangement in a parent.

## PHYSICAL EXAM

Physical exam begins with overall observation of the newborn including facial gestalt, somatic growth, behavior (cry pattern), feeding abilities, muscle tone, and general alertness.

Abnormal growth including overgrowth or growth restriction at birth is important to elucidate. Large for gestational age infants with birth defects such as omphalocele, macroglossia, and hypoglycemia would need to be evaluated for BWS. On the other hand, significant growth restriction in the presence of multiple congenital anomalies can be an indication of trisomy 18, particularly in the presence of polyvalvular heart disease. Other chromosomal disorders should also be considered. Some of the recognizable single-gene disorders that are characterized by significant intrauterine growth retardation (IUGR) in the neonatal period include Cornelia de Lange and Smith-Lemli-Optiz syndrome. Neonatal hypotonia with prolonged requirement for nasogastric tube feedings is an important consideration and may indicate disorders such as Prader-Willi syndrome (PWS).

Dysmorphology exam focuses on recognizing major and minor malformations that collectively signify a pattern indicative of a specific diagnosis, or identify a specific group of disorders for further evaluation (eg, RASopathies including Noonan, Costello, and cardiofaciocutaneous syndromes). Several dysmorphic features are illustrated with specific measurements that are compared to the normal range for age and gender. The Human Phenotype Ontology (HPO) (http://human-phenotype-ontology.github.io/) provides over 11,000 terms that describe phenotypic abnormalities seen in different diseases. Using standardized terms is extremely helpful in clinical diagnosis. "Elements of Morphology" is another good source in which an international group of clinicians working in the field of dysmorphology has initiated standard terms to describe anomalies. Finally, what is thought to be a dysmorphic feature on exam might be a familial trait. Evaluation of other first-degree family members by brief exam or, in some cases, review of photographs may be needed for thorough evaluation.

A comprehensive dysmorphology exam requires a detailed head-to-toe evaluation. The craniofacial exam often provides invaluable clues for the underlying genetic diagnosis in a newborn, and it is not uncommon to make, or strongly suspect, a diagnosis with good exam. Head circumference and shape should be evaluated (eg, brachycephaly is seen in Down syndrome; microcephaly at birth can be indicative of a syndromic condition). Ophthalmologic evaluation includes eye position, size, and slant of palpebral fissures, color of sclerae, irides, and fundal exam. Colobomas, both iris and retinal, can be seen in newborns with CHARGE syndrome. Upslanting palpebral fissures are characteristic feature of Down syndrome. Evaluation of the size of the nose, nasal root, tip, columella, and alae nasi is important. Similarly, ears should be evaluated for size, shape, rotation, and position. Ear tags, pits, and creases can be part of several syndromes. Exam of mouth and surrounding structures includes philtrum (eg, smooth philtrum in fetal alcohol syndrome), lips, gums (eg, accessory gingival frenulae in oral-facial-digital syndrome), tongue (eg, macroglossia in BWS), palate (cleft palate in DGS/VCFS), and chin (eg, micrognathia in PRS). Neck should be evaluated for redundant skin (eg, webbed neck is common in females with Turner syndrome). Chest shape and size should be documented, as well as appearance and position of the nipples (eg, widely set nipples in Turner syndrome). Extremity evaluation involves determining distal and proximal proportions of limbs (eg, rhizomelic shortening in achondroplasia) and symmetry between left and right sides (eg, hemihyperplasia in overgrowth syndromes). Assessment of hands and feet includes hand position (eg, clenched hands in trisomy 18), creasing pattern (eg, single transverse palmar crease in Down syndrome), shape (eg, puffiness in Turner syndrome), nails and digits (eg, postaxial polydactyly in trisomy 13, 2–3 toe syndactyly in Smith-Lemli-Optiz syndrome, and broad thumbs and great toes in Rubinstein-Taybi syndrome). Cardiac exam is essential, including auscultation for heart murmurs (CHD can be part of several genetic disorders). Abdominal exam for abdominal wall defects (umbilical hernia, omphalocele) and visceromegaly should be completed. Anal atresia can be seen in VACTERL association or other genetic disorders such as cat eye syndrome. Dysmorphology exam should also include detailed exam of the genitourinary system (eg, ambiguous genitalia relevant in disorders of sexual differentiation), skin (eg, hypomelanotic macules in tuberous sclerosis), and hair (eg, hirsutism in Cornelia de Lange syndrome). Back should be evaluated for any deformities or sacral dimple. Neurologic exam includes ascertainment of tone (hypotonia observed in Down syndrome, PWS, congenital myotonic dystrophy, and other monogenic disorders) and assessment of deep tendon reflexes (absent deep tendon reflexes are characteristic of spinal muscular atrophy [SMA]).

## PUTTING EVERYTHING TOGETHER: "GENERATING A PHENOTYPE"

Based on the information gathered from history and physical exam, a phenotype is generated (Fig. 170-1). In some situations, the phenotype is distinguishing enough that a clinical diagnosis could be made with a

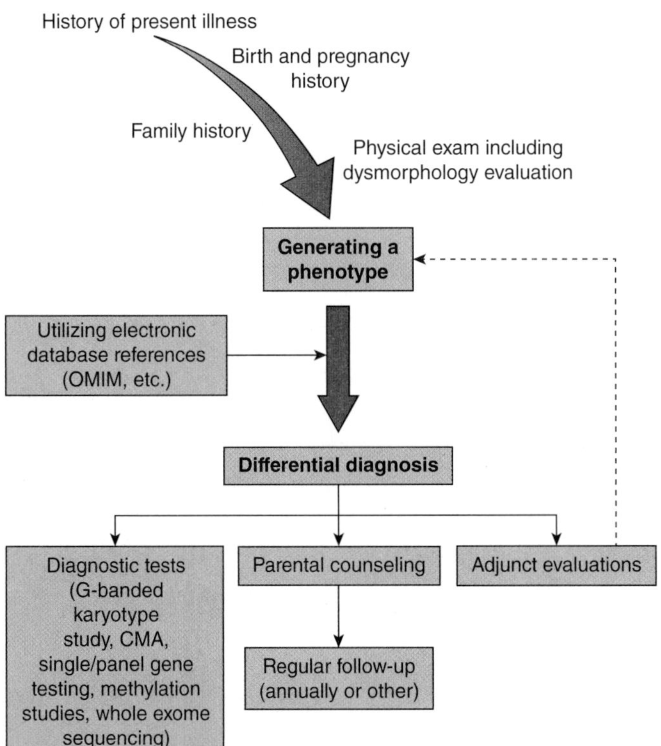


**FIGURE 170-1** Approach to a newborn with birth defects. Details gathered from history and physical exam are put together to generate a phenotype that will direct further workup, including diagnostic tests and adjunct evaluations. CMA, chromosomal microarray analysis; OMIM, Online Mendelian Inheritance in Man.

high degree of certainty before confirmatory testing is sent (Table 170-1). For example, the presence of atrioventricular septal defect (AVSD) in a newborn with hypotonia, upslanting palpebral fissures, bilateral epicanthal folds, and small ears would be characteristic of Down syndrome. On the other hand, feeding difficulties and hypotonia in a term newborn with otherwise no major malformations could be an indication of PWS. Absence of deep tendon reflexes in an alert, hypotonic infant may indicate SMA. Conotruncal heart defects, hypocalcemia, cleft palate, with feeding problems are common concerns in neonates with DGS/VCFS. A newborn with cleft lip and palate, eye anomalies (microphthalmia, anophthalmia), scalp defects, holoprosencephaly, and postaxial polydactyly would likewise need to be evaluated for trisomy 13. In other situations, the ascertained phenotype will help generate a limited list of possible diagnostic considerations that require a focused workup. However, there are several instances in which the genetic diagnosis remains uncertain, and a broad differential diagnosis is generated. In these situations, more comprehensive testing might be warranted. There are several available electronic databases that could be used as helpful tools in the diagnostic process. Based on the phenotypic characteristics entered into these databases, a summary of possible diagnoses is formulated. Examples of such databases are the Online Mendelian Inheritance in Man (OMIM) (http://www.omim.org/) and London Dysmorphology Database (https://suite.face2gene.com/lmd-library-london-medical-database-dysmorphology/; subscription is required). DECIPHER database (https://decipher.sanger.ac.uk/browser) is another resource used frequently for discerning associated phenotypes related to genomic findings in the evaluation of neonates with birth defects.

## CHOOSING THE APPROPRIATE WORKUP

### Diagnostic Tests

Based on the differential diagnosis determined, specific genetic testing is requested. In the past decade, the increasing use of chromosomal microarray analysis (CMA) has uncovered several genomic disorders that cause birth defects in infants. The escalating use of whole-exome sequencing in intensive care units for the evaluation of critically ill newborns promises to further increase the diagnostic yield from genetic testing for enhanced patient care. There are some important points to consider when selecting diagnostic tests for a newborn with birth defect(s):

- G-banded karyotype analysis remains the test of choice for evaluation of Down syndrome and other aneuploidies such as trisomy 18, trisomy 13, and Turner syndrome (45,X). This is true because chromosome studies are essential to identify the underlying molecular mechanisms for aneuploidies (ie, nondisjunction vs translocation), with very different recurrence risks for families.
- Fluorescence in situ hybridization (FISH) has the advantage of rapid turnaround time of 24 to 48 hours for evaluation of aneuploidies. It is often employed, particularly for newborns with significant cardiopulmonary disease suspected to have trisomy 18 or 13.
- CMA is the first-tier test for evaluating a newborn with multiple congenital anomalies. DGS/VCFS is a relatively common diagnosis made in the neonatal intensive care unit. While some institutions continue to use FISH for ascertaining 22q11.2 deletion, others employ CMA for a more comprehensive evaluation.
- There are several other genetic tests that could be requested in neonates based on the suspected diagnosis and the underlying molecular mechanisms, including methylation studies for Prader-Willi/Angelman and BWS, single-gene testing for infantile SMA or myotonic dystrophy, and gene panels for disorders such as Stickler syndrome, Rubinstein-Taybi syndrome, and craniosynostosis syndromes.
- Whole-exome sequencing (WES) should be considered in select cases, although consultation with a geneticist is recommended to aid in the process of informed consent and interpretation of the results. Trio WES (proband plus both parents) can be particularly useful for ascertaining potential *de novo* mutations as the underlying cause of congenital anomalies in infants.

### Adjunct Evaluations

Besides diagnostic tests, other studies are often requested for appropriate clinical management of infants with birth defects. For instance,

**TABLE 170-1 SOME EXAMPLES OF GENETIC DISORDERS DIAGNOSED IN THE NEONATAL PERIOD**

| Disorder | Features Recognized in the Newborn | Recommended Genetic Testing |
| --- | --- | --- |
| Down syndrome | • Dysmorphic features (brachycephaly, flat facial profile, small ears, upslanting palpebral fissures, epicanthal folds, single transverse palmar creases, sandal gap deformity)<br>• Hypotonia<br>• CHD (AVSD) | • Karyotype<br>• FISH (for rapid diagnosis if indicated) |
| Trisomy 18[a] | • IUGR<br>• Dysmorphic features (prominent occiput, small mouth, micrognathia)<br>• Short sternum<br>• Hypertonia<br>• CHD<br>• Clenched hands with overlapping fingers<br>• Rocker bottom feet | • Karyotype<br>• FISH (for rapid diagnosis if indicated) |
| Trisomy 13[a] | • Holoprosencephaly<br>• Microphthalmia<br>• Scalp defects (cutis aplasia)<br>• Cleft lip/palate<br>• CHD<br>• Omphalocele<br>• Postaxial polydactyly | • Karyotype<br>• FISH (for rapid diagnosis if indicated) |
| Turner syndrome | • Webbed neck/cystic hygroma<br>• CHD (coarctation of the aorta)<br>• Renal anomalies (horseshoe kidneys)<br>• Puffy hands and feet | • Karyotype<br>• FISH (for rapid diagnosis if indicated) |
| DiGeorge/velocardiofacial syndrome, 22q11.2 deletion | • Dysmorphic features (hooded eyelids, cupped ears, bulbous nasal tip)<br>• CHD (conotruncal defects)<br>• Absent thymus<br>• Cleft palate<br>• Hypocalcemia<br>• Immune deficiency | • CMA<br>• Targeted FISH |
| Prader-Willi syndrome | • Poor feeding<br>• Hypotonia | • Methylation analysis of Prader-Willi/Angelman region (15q11-q13) |
| CHARGE syndrome | • Choanal atresia/stenosis<br>• Coloboma<br>• Ear malformations (including external, middle, and inner ear)<br>• Cranial nerve dysfunction<br>• Sensorineural hearing loss<br>• CHD<br>• Cleft lip/palate<br>• Tracheoesophageal fistula<br>• Renal malformations | • *CHD7* gene sequencing and deletion/duplication analysis |
| Stickler syndrome | • Pierre-Robin sequence (micrognathia, glossoptosis, cleft palate)<br>• Myopia<br>• Flat facial profile | • NGS panel (*COL2A1, COL11A1, COL11A2, COL9A1, COL9A2, COL9A3* genes) |
| Noonan syndrome | • Dysmorphic features (hypertelorism, downslanting palpebral fissures, low-set and posteriorly rotated ears, short neck with excess nuchal skin)<br>• CHD (pulmonary valve stenosis, HCM)<br>• Widely set nipples<br>• Cryptorchidism<br>• Lymphedema | • NGS panel (*PTPN11, RAF1, SOS1, NRAS, BRAF, MAP2K1* genes) |
| Spinal muscular atrophy | • Hypotonia<br>• Absent deep tendon reflexes<br>• Tongue fasciculations | • *SMN1* gene deletion analysis |
| Congenital myotonic dystrophy | • Hypotonia<br>• Muscle weakness<br>• Respiratory compromise<br>• Lack of facial expression | • CTG trinucleotide repeat expansion analysis of *DMPK* |

(*Continued*)

**TABLE 170-1 SOME EXAMPLES OF GENETIC DISORDERS DIAGNOSED IN THE NEONATAL PERIOD (CONTINUED)**

| Disorder | Features Recognized in the Newborn | Recommended Genetic Testing |
|---|---|---|
| Beckwith-Wiedemann syndrome | • Overgrowth/hemihyperplasia<br>• Macroglossia<br>• Omphalocele<br>• Ear lobe creases<br>• Hypoglycemia | • Methylation analysis; *CDKN1C* gene sequence analysis |
| Osteogenesis imperfecta | • Fractures<br>• Bone deformities<br>• Blue/gray sclera | • *COL1A1* and *COL1A2* gene sequencing and deletion/duplication analysis |
| VACTERL/VATER association | • Vertebral defects<br>• Anal atresia<br>• CHD<br>• Tracheoesophageal fistula<br>• Renal malformations<br>• Limb defects | • No specific testing (sporadic condition)<br>• May consider CMA and chromosome breakage studies |
| Cornelia de Lange syndrome | • Dysmorphic features (synophrys, arched eyebrows, long and thick eyelashes, micrognathia)<br>• Growth restriction<br>• Hirsutism<br>• Limb anomalies (mainly upper extremities) | • NGS panel (*NIPBL, RAD21, SMC3, HDAC8*, or *SMC1A* genes) |
| Rubinstein-Taybi syndrome | • Dysmorphic features (downslanting palpebral fissures, maxillary hypoplasia, prominent nose with short columella, arched eyebrows)<br>• Broad thumbs and great toes<br>• Cryptorchidism and renal anomalies | • *EP300* and *CREBBP* gene sequencing and deletion/duplication analysis |
| Tuberous sclerosis complex | • Cerebral lesions (subependymal nodules, cortical dysplasia)<br>• Cardiac rhabdomyomas<br>• Skin lesions (hypomelanotic macules) | • *TSC1* and *TSC2* gene sequencing and deletion/duplication analysis |
| Cat eye syndrome | • Iris coloboma<br>• Preauricular pits and tags<br>• Anal atresia<br>• CHD (TAPVR)<br>• Renal malformation<br>• Biliary atresia | • CMA<br>• Karyotype |

[a]FISH study has rapid turnaround time of 24 to 48 hours. It is often indicted in infants suspected to have trisomy 18 or 13, who usually have significant cardiopulmonary disease, and a timely diagnosis is essential to determine further management.

AVSD, atrioventricular septal defect; CHD, congenital heart disease; CMA, chromosomal microarray analysis; FISH, fluorescence in situ hybridization; HCM, hypertrophic cardiomyopathy; IUGR, intrauterine growth restriction; NGS, next-generation sequencing; TAPVR, total anomalous pulmonary venous return.

echocardiogram should be obtained in neonates suspected to have Down syndrome, Turner syndrome, and DGS/VCFS, preferably before discharge from the hospital. Heart defects are present in about 50% of babies with Down syndrome. Coarctation of the aorta can be a serious consideration in females with Turner syndrome. Significant cardiac compromise due to interrupted aortic arch and other conotruncal defects in DGS/VCFS is also a concern. Other tests or evaluations that might be useful include renal ultrasound, brain imaging, newborn hearing screen, ophthalmologic exam, and skeletal survey. These studies are often valuable in making a clinical diagnosis, thereby helping in selecting the most appropriate confirmatory test.

## APPROACHING THE FAMILY

The emotional and psychological impact on families with newborns having birth defects can be overwhelming. Many parents go through the typical stages of grief, depending on the severity of the congenital anomalies. Anxiety, fear, stress, depression, and self-blame are some of the parental reactions after learning that their baby has a significant birth defect. Siblings are often affected by the diagnosis of a genetic disorder in this setting. Helping the caregivers deal with these reactions is essential. While discussing the diagnostic considerations with parents, it is important to be empathetic and compassionate, explaining the underlying genetic basis in an unassuming manner. Genetic counseling is an important aspect of evaluation of a newborn with a genetic diagnosis and should be undertaken by trained personnel, not only for addressing the medical concerns related to the birth defect, but also for discussing the risk of recurrence in future pregnancies and preventative measures that could be taken to reduce that risk. The complexity of genetic diagnosis generally necessitate serial follow-up evaluations in specialized clinics beyond the neonatal period for most infants with genetic disorders.

## SUGGESTED READINGS

Elements of Morphology: Human Malformation Terminology. https://elementsofmorphology.nih.gov/. Accessed May 10, 2017.

Firth HV, Richards SM, Bevan AP, et al. DECIPHER: database of chromosomal imbalance and phenotype in humans using Ensembl resources. *Am J Hum Genet*. 2009;84:524-533.

Gripp KW, Slavotinek AM, Hall JG, Allanson JE. *Handbook of Physical Measurements*. 3rd ed. New York, NY: Oxford University Press; 2013.

Groza T, Köhler S, Moldenhauer D, et al. The human phenotype ontology: semantic unification of common and rare disease. *Am J Hum Genet*. 2015;97:111-124.

Mazer P, Gischler SJ, Koot HM, Tibboel D, van Dijk M, Duivenvoorden HJ. Impact of a child with congenital anomalies on parents (ICCAP) questionnaire; a psychometric analysis. *Health Qual Life Outcomes*. 2008;6:102.

McKusick VA. Mendelian Inheritance in Man and its online version, OMIM. *Am J Hum Genet.* 2007;80:588-594.

Nussbaum RL, McInnes RR, Willard HF. Developmental genetics and birth defects. In: Nussbaum RL, McInnes RR, Willard HF, eds. *Thompson & Thompson Genetics in Medicine.* 8th ed. Philadelphia, PA: Elsevier; 2016:283-308.

Schaaf CP, Zschocke J, Potocki L. The diagnostic approach for a child with multiple anomalies or dysmorphic features. In: Schaaf CP, Zschocke J, Potocki L, eds. *Human Genetics: From Molecules to Medicine.* Philadelphia, PA: Lippincott Williams & Wilkins; 2012:113-121.

Slavotinek A, Ali M. Recognizable syndromes in the newborn period. *Clin Perinatol.* 2015;42:263-280.

# 171 Birth Defects, Malformations, and Syndromes

Bret L. Bostwick and Carlos A. Bacino

## INTRODUCTION

Birth defects are relatively common, with major anomalies occurring in approximately 3% to 4% of live births. More than 20% of infant deaths in the United States are directly attributable to birth defects. In addition to mortality, birth defects also cause long-term morbidity, including intellectual disability and physical dysfunction, that can limit the productivity of individuals. These long-term disabilities can have significant impact on individuals, families, healthcare systems, and communities.

The term *dysmorphology* was first used in the 1960s to refer to the study of abnormal physical features. This term is used today to encompass both the normal variation of physical traits as well as the abnormal physical features resulting from an aberrant developmental process. Experts in dysmorphology, called dysmorphologists, are trained to describe the appearance of anomalies (ie, the trait manifestations) and establish an etiologic hypothesis based on their pattern or characteristics.

The pathogenesis and clinical classification of birth defects are reviewed here. Using the knowledge of normal embryology and development, an experienced clinician is able to analyze the characteristics and patterns of birth defects to hypothesize a pathogenetic mechanism, ultimately leading to improved diagnosis and treatment as well as informed recurrence risk and natural history counseling.

## PATHOGENESIS AND EPIDEMIOLOGY

Birth defects are structural abnormalities that are present at birth (often called *congenital anomalies*) and caused by either intrinsic or extrinsic factors during intrauterine life. Birth defects are the result of genetic factors, nongenetic factors, or a combination of both. Developmental genetics, including embryology, and knowledge of molecular pathways responsible for normal human development are essential background for a physician tasked with diagnosing a newborn with congenital anomalies.

## BRIEF REVIEW OF EMBRYOLOGY AND DEVELOPMENTAL GENETICS

**Development** is a highly regulated, precise, and efficient process by which a fertilized ovum becomes a mature organism capable of reproduction. The information required for development is transmitted from parent to offspring via genes that encode signaling molecules, cellular receptors, transcription factors, enzymes, transport systems, and other proteins tasked to ensure a highly regulated series of events that can be replicated with high fidelity. Each genetic program is expressed in a spatially and temporally overlapping pattern such that it can be used repetitively to control different developmental processes. The same gene program is reused in different tissues and at different times during development, increasing efficiency and decreasing the overall amount of genetic instruction passed from one generation to the next. Mutations in the genes mediating development are a common cause of birth defects.

### Pattern Determination

**Pattern formation** is the process by which cells acquire different identities based on their relative spatial position within an embryo. The animal body plan is laid down during embryogenesis resulting in the formation of semi-autonomous regions, each of which undergo subsequent pattern formation to form organs and appendages. The hierarchical order of steps includes: (1) definition of cells in a region, (2) formation of a signaling center that provides positional information, and (3) differentiation of cells within the region in response to signaling cues.

The first major pattern formation during embryogenesis, termed **gastrulation**, occurs between days 14 and 28 of gestation and is hallmarked by the transformation of a bilaminar disk into a trilaminar embryo composed of the 3 germ layers: ectoderm, mesoderm, and endoderm.

**Ectoderm** The dorsal mesoderm and the overlying ectoderm then interact to form a hollow neural tube in an event called **neurulation**. Neurulation is a critical developmental step, initiating organogenesis and dividing the ectoderm into 3 cell populations: (1) the neural tube, fated to become the brain and spinal cord; (2) the epidermis of the skin; and (3) the neural crest cells, fated to become sensory neurons, melanocytes, and neurons for smooth muscle and bowel.

**Mesoderm** After gastrulation, the tissue sandwiched between the endoderm and ectoderm is differentiated into mesoderm. The mesoderm can then be subdivided into 5 components termed the notochord; the dorsal, intermediate, and lateral mesoderms; and the head mesenchyme. The notochord is responsible for the induction of the overlying ectoderm into the neural tube and body axis. The dorsal mesoderm produces the sclerotomes (axial and appendicular skeleton), myotomes (skeletal muscle), and dermatomes (connective tissue of the skin). Intermediate mesoderm forms the kidneys and genitourinary system. Lateral plate mesoderm becomes the heart and contributes to the viscera as well as the amnion and chorion. Finally, head mesoderm produces the muscles of the head, including periorbital muscles.

**Endoderm** The final germ layer, the endoderm, forms the linings of the gastrointestinal tract and the respiratory system. The pancreas, gallbladder, and liver are also derived from specialized outgrowths of the endoderm. The endoderm also contributes to the pharyngeal pouches, which eventually give rise to the middle ear, thymus, parathyroids, and thyroids.

### Axis Specification

The **primitive streak** defines the anterior/posterior axis of the developing mammalian embryo. The patterning of the axis is controlled by *HOX* genes that encode transcription factors that each contain a DNA-binding domain of 60 amino acids called the homeodomain. The dorsal/ventral axis is formed by concentration-dependent factors that are termed either dorsalizing or ventralizing based on the target tissue's response to the signal. Molecules that can promote tissue differentiation of undifferentiated cells as a function of concentration are termed **morphogens**.

### Formation of Organs and Appendages

After axis specification, formation of the organs and limbs occurs in a process called organogenesis. Many of the same proteins used earlier in pattern formation are now used again in the patterning and growth of the limbs. Some genes that were previously transcriptionally silent now become active to trigger organ formation. Most of the genes that are known to cause human birth defects have critical roles during this period of development. It is thought that mutations in genes that disrupt earlier developmental events, including gastrulation, germ layer formation, and axis specification, tend to be lethal.

**Development of the Limb** Tetrapod limb development is well elucidated, and many of the transcriptional control elements are shared with model organisms. The signal that first initiates induction of the forelimbs and hindlimbs arises in the intermediate mesoderm and triggers elements of the lateral and somatic mesoderms to form the bones and soft tissue components of the limb, respectively. After initiation, proximal to distal growth of the limb is orchestrated by a region of ectoderm known as the apical ectodermal ridge (AER), which extends along the dorsal/ventral boundary of the limb bud. The AER later on interacts with the zone polarizing activity (ZPA) for limb development. The longitudinal growth is mediated by fibroblast growth factors (*FGF2*, *FGF4*, and *FGF8*), while the dorsal/ventral patterning of the central nervous system (CNS) and the embryonic left/right axis is mediated in part by sonic hedgehog (*SHH*). Secreted signaling molecules of the Wnt family have important functions in limb bud initiation, limb outgrowth, and limb morphogenesis events.

**Organ Formation** The processes of organ formation are coordinated simultaneously with reciprocal induction of the mesenchyme on the epithelium and vice versa. The differentiation of many organs relies on epithelial-mesenchymal interactions, including cutaneous structures (hair cells, sweat glands, breasts), parenchymal organs (liver, pancreas, etc.), lungs, thyroid, kidneys, and teeth. Once specialized cells are terminally differentiated, transcriptional activation produces the proteins required for the cells' fated function.

## GENETIC CAUSES OF BIRTH DEFECTS

A diverse set of molecular mechanisms can lead to various birth defects. Single-gene defects, chromosomal aneuploidies, and chromosomal copy number variants (CNVs; deletions or duplications) are well-known genetic causes. Approximately 40% of all major malformations have no identifiable cause, but some are seen at a higher than expected frequency but without a specific pattern of mendelian inheritance. These groups of disorders are known as multifactorial, including polygenic inheritance or complex gene-environment interactions. Some of the most common major malformations fall within this category, including congenital heart defects, orofacial clefts in general including cleft lip with or without cleft palate, and neural tube defects.

## ENVIRONMENTAL AND INTRAUTERINE CAUSES OF BIRTH DEFECTS

Environmental or intrauterine factors can modify developmental processes and patterning, resulting in phenotypes that are often similar to those seen in primary genetic causes of birth defects. Some of these other etiologies include maternal illnesses (such as maternal phenylketonuria or maternal diabetes), pregnancy infections (Zika and microcephaly), environmental factors, physical maternal exposures (radiation, heat), drugs, twinning, and chemical agents. Teratology, a term used to describe birth defects as a result of environmental or drug/chemical exposure, is discussed separately in Chapter 172.

## CLINICAL CLASSIFICATION OF BIRTH DEFECTS

Since our knowledge of the underlying mechanisms of many birth defects is limited, all classification schemes for birth defects are somewhat arbitrary and many, thus far, are uninformed by molecular mechanism. Although classification schemes by organ system or body part may seem rational, it becomes inadequate once specific information is required regarding the etiology, natural history, or recurrence risk of the anomaly. Additionally, most diagnoses are not made by mere assignment of the anomaly to an organ system, but rather by examination of the constellation of anomalies across multiple systems, ultimately pointing to a specific syndromic diagnosis or known association.

Here, we will present the most useful classification systems and terminology for generating a hypothesis about the causative pathogenetic mechanisms. These systems typically aim to identify an underlying pathway. Although a single birth defect can result from perturbation of more than 1 pathway, which can occasionally make it difficult to identify the primary defect from classification alone, the overall categorization still proves useful to provide a background for understanding future observations.

We will present 3 different classification systems, with the first focused on the presumed etiology of the individual anomaly, the second highlighting the overall pattern of multiple anomalies, and the third concentrated on the medical significance of the anomalies.

There are 4 categories within the etiologic classification: **malformations, deformations, disruptions**, and **dysplasias**. A separate set of terms is used to describe the different patterns of anomalies: **association, sequence, developmental field defect**, and **syndrome.** The final classification simply distinguishes the medical significance of the birth defect, termed **major anomaly** or **minor anomaly**. All 3 systems are useful in characterizing the findings, and indeed, they are often used concurrently.

## ETIOLOGIC CLASSIFICATION OF BIRTH ANOMALIES

### Malformation

A malformation is a structural defect in an organ or body part that results from *intrinsic* abnormalities in early development. Etiologically, malformations are the result of perturbation in 1 or more of the genetic programs that trigger and coordinate essential developmental processes. As a result, structures are either not formed, are partially formed, or are formed in an abnormal fashion. The majority of malformations occur prior to the 8th week postconception, including those involving the heart, upper limb, lower limb, lip, and palate. However, some malformations can occur after this time, most notably those of the central nervous system, external genitalia, and teeth.

Since malformations arise from intrinsic perturbation of genetic programs that are often used redundantly in different parts of the embryo or during different stages of development, a malformation in one body part is often, but not always, associated with malformations elsewhere. Thus, when multiple congenital malformations are found in an individual, they could be caused by either a common single pathway or multiple pathways.

### Deformation

In contrast to malformations, deformations result from *extrinsic* mechanical factors that physically impinge on a fetus, ultimately modifying a previously normally formed structure. Thus, a deformation is an alteration of the form, shape, or position of a body part by mechanical forces. The most common mechanical forces include decreased amniotic fluid, uterine tumors or growths, and uterine shape abnormalities, all of which can lead to fetal compression. Early pelvic engagement of the fetal head, aberrant fetal positions, and multifetal gestations can also lead to fetal deformations.

Oligohydramnios is the most common cause of fetal deformations and can result in mechanical constraints on joint mobility (clubfoot), congenital dysplasia of the hip, or plagiocephaly. Even pulmonary hypoplasia could be considered a deformation caused by oligohydramnios. Most skeletal deformations (clubfoot, hip dysplasia, or plagiocephaly) can be corrected with physical therapy, serial casting, or the use of a specialized helmet. Since deformations are not intrinsic to the infant, they are not expected to recur.

### Disruption

A disruption occurs when there is abnormal *external* interference with an originally normal developmental process that results in destruction of irreplaceable normal fetal tissue. Although both disruptions and deformations are secondary to extrinsic sources, deformations are merely a change in the shape or form of a body part, while disruptions uniquely result in the irreversible loss of the fetal tissue. Tissue destruction most commonly occurs from vascular or mechanical processes that lead to compression, strangulation, hemorrhage, ischemia, or thrombosis. Most disruptions are a single event in time, are commonly sporadic, and have a low chance of recurrence. An example of a disruption is amniotic band–related limb injury, where a loose strand of amnion entangles or fuses with fetal tissue, resulting in absence of all or part of a limb's structures.

### Dysplasia

A dysplasia occurs when the *intrinsic* cellular architecture of a tissue is not normally maintained throughout growth and development. The abnormal cellular organization is usually specific to a single tissue type. An example of a skeletal dysplasia is achondroplasia, where fibroblast growth factor receptor 3 gene mutations lead to abnormal endochondral ossification resulting in shortened long bones, skull defects, and other generalized bone abnormalities.

#### Etiologic Classifications May Overlap and Are Not Mutually Exclusive

The pathophysiologic terms malformations, deformation, disruptions, and dysplasias are useful clinically and aid in recognition of a diagnosis or treatment; however, the terms are not mutually exclusive for a particular anomaly. What often appears to be the same birth defect can have different etiologies in different individuals. For example, a transverse limb defect could be caused by amniotic banding (a disruption) or could be a malformation of a single-gene disorder (eg, Goltz syndrome, Adams-Oliver syndrome).

In a patient with multiple anomalies, the classifications can overlap. For example, a renal malformation could lead to oligohydramnios causing a clubfoot deformation. Alternatively, a vascular malformation in the limb could lead to disruption of distal limb tissue. Thus, multiple birth defects in a single individual often represent a combination of malformations, deformations, disruptions, and dysplasias.

Malformations and dysplasia are primary disturbances of embryogenesis or histogenesis, respectively, whereas deformations and disruptions are secondary to other primary extrinsic forces. Primary disturbances can lead to secondary disturbances, but not vice versa. Thus, a malformation may lead to a deformation; however, a deformation will not give rise to a malformation.

## CLASSIFICATION BY PATTERN OF BIRTH ANOMALIES

Although detailed characterization of a single anomaly is critical to arriving at the correct diagnosis, often it is the constellation of multiple anomalies that ultimately leads to a syndromic diagnosis or known association. Classification by pattern aims to use our understanding of the typical spatial arrangements of differentiated cells to help determine if a single underlying trigger for perturbation exists.

#### Syndrome

A syndrome is defined as a well-characterized pattern of anomalies that are known to occur together in a predictable fashion and are pathogenetically related by a single underlying etiology. In a syndrome, the primary causative agent produces multiple abnormalities in parallel. Syndromes can be caused by monogenic, genomic, chromosomal, mitochondrial, or teratogenic etiologies.

An example of a well-characterized syndrome is Down syndrome, where overrepresentation of material from chromosome 21 is known to account for many predictable major and minor anomalies. This understanding has enabled a recognizable phenotype, where Down syndrome can be diagnosed clinically even when only a small subset of the physical features are present in a particular individual.

Note that the term *syndrome* is sometimes used more broadly in other fields of medicine to refer to a constellation of symptoms without a single clear etiology (ie, nephrotic syndrome); however, the more specific definition above proves more useful when diagnosing or managing an individual with multiple birth defects.

#### Sequence

A sequence is a group of related anomalies where an initial primary defect then triggers a secondary cascade of structural anomalies. The primary defect precedes the structural defects; thus, the anomalies are not formed in parallel. Most sequences are primary malformations that cause subsequent deformations or disruptions.

Potter sequence is a constellation of physical findings in a newborn, including a flattened abnormal face, depressed nasal tip, abnormal ear folding with large ears, wrinkled skin, deformations of the hands and feet, and poor pulmonary development. The primary defect is often a renal malformation, a urogenital obstruction, or some other cause of decreased urine output or severe oligohydramnios. The structural changes are all secondary to the oligohydramnios and do not occur in parallel with the primary defect.

Prune belly sequence occurs mostly in male fetuses when urethral malformations or obstruction leads to a distended bladder. The distension interferes with timely closure of the abdominal wall muscles, secondarily resulting in a flaccid and wrinkled abdomen. The cause of prune belly sequence is often unknown, although recent evidence suggests at least some cases may result from mutations in smooth muscle genes.

Robin sequence is due to a primary restriction of mandibular growth that causes secondary posterior displacement of the tongue and interference with palatal shelf closure, resulting in a classic U-shaped cleft palate. Palatal clefting is often U-shaped and is secondary to mandibular restriction and interference of palatal closure by malposition of the tongue, whereas primary failure of palatal closure is classically described as V-shaped. Robin sequence can be from an unknown cause or could be a feature of a syndrome, such as Stickler syndrome, where a type II collagenopathy results in an abnormally small mandible, as well as defects in the joints, stature, and eyes.

#### Association

An association is 2 or more anomalies that are not pathogenetically related but occur together more frequently than expected by chance alone. The etiology of most associations is not well defined, and it is possible that some associations are actually developmental field defects or syndromes.

An example of this pattern is the VATER or VACTERL association. These are acronyms to describe a series of associated structural abnormalities. VACTERL includes vertebral anomalies, anal atresia, cardiac defects, tracheoesophageal fistula, renal defects, and limb defects. Since these anomalies tend to occur more frequently together than by chance alone, the finding of one abnormality should prompt clinical evaluation for related anomalies. For example, a newborn with an imperforate anus and limb abnormality should receive additional clinical evaluation for vertebral, renal, cardiac, or esophageal anomalies.

#### Developmental Field Defect

The term *developmental field defect* is used to refer to a pattern of anomalies caused by a disturbance of a physical contiguous region of the embryo. The contiguous region is known as a developmental field. In practice, this term is not usually used rigorously and sometimes overlaps with known sequences. For example, some clinicians consider Robin sequence to be a developmental field defect, where the mandible, tongue, and palate define the contiguous developmental field.

Holoprosencephaly is a classic example of a developmental field defect where a failure of induction by the prechordal mesoderm on the forebrain results in abnormal cleavage of the embryonic forebrain that occurs at approximately 21 days of gestation and that results in a wide phenotypic spectrum ranging from an almost completely absent forebrain in severe cases to a single central incisor in mild cases. Since the embryonic forebrain influences the mesodermal processes in the midface, defining the craniofacial structures, the spectrum of contiguous abnormalities is within the developmental field of the initial forebrain.

## CLASSIFICATION BY THE MEDICAL SIGNIFICANCE OF BIRTH DEFECTS

Birth anomalies can also be classified as major or minor, where major anomalies have a significant medical or social implication while minor anomalies are not generally considered medically or socially relevant.

#### Major Anomalies

A major anomaly is a structural birth defect that has a significant medical and/or social implication. Major anomalies often require surgical repair or other medical interventions. Examples of major anomalies include orofacial clefting, omphalocele, or polydactyly.

#### Minor Anomalies

Minor anomalies, by definition, are not medically significant by themselves but, when identified, can provide important diagnostic clues. Minor anomalies often merely represent the normal morphologic variation in the general population and rarely require surgical intervention. They often have only cosmetic significance. Examples of minor anomalies include single transverse palmar creases, ear tags, frontal bossing, clinodactyly (incurving of the fifth fingers), or epicanthal folds.

Approximately 15% of newborns have a single minor anomaly, whereas 2 and 3 or more minor anomalies occur in 0.8% and 0.5% of newborns, respectively. Half of all minor anomalies are located in the head or neck. Infants with 3 or more minor anomalies are at increased risk of having a major anomaly or a syndrome; thus, the presence of multiple minor anomalies may prompt further evaluation. Many major and minor anomalies are detectable on physical exam (Table 171-1).

**TABLE 171-1 EXAMPLES OF MAJOR AND MINOR ANOMALIES DETECTABLE ON EXAM**

| System | Major Anomalies | Minor Anomalies |
|---|---|---|
| Skull | Anencephaly | Abnormal hair whorls |
| | Encephalocele | Frontal bossing |
| | Holoprosencephaly | Plagiocephaly |
| | Hydrocephaly | Flat occiput |
| | | Metopic fontanel |
| Eyes | Microphthalmia, | Epicanthal folds |
| | Anophthalmia | Hypo-/hypertelorism |
| | Colobomas | Ptosis |
| | | Synophrys |
| | | Short palpebral fissures |
| Ears | Severe microtia | Ear lobes (attached, creased, bifid) |
| | | Shapes (cupped, protruding, lop ear) |
| | | Ear tags |
| | | Preauricular sinuses |
| Nose | Arrhinia | Flat nasal bridge |
| | Congenital nasal pyriform aperture stenosis | Anteverted nostrils |
| | | Philtrum (long, short, flat) |
| Mouth | Cleft lip/palate | Micro-/macrostomia |
| | Micrognathia | Bifid uvula |
| | Macro-/microglossia | Multiple frenula |
| | | Neonatal tooth |
| Neck | Cystic hygroma | Short neck |
| | | Webbed neck |
| | | Branchial sinuses |
| Chest | Pectus excavatum | Tertiary nipples |
| | Absent or hypoplastic clavicles | |
| Back | Meningomyelocele | Sacral dimple or pit |
| | Spina bifida | Winged scapulae |
| Abdomen | Omphalocele | Diastasis recti |
| | Gastroschisis | |
| Genitalia | Hypospadias | Shawl scrotum |
| | Cryptorchidism | Vaginal tags |
| | Microphallus | |
| | Penoscrotal transposition | |
| | Ambiguous genitalia | |
| Arms/legs | Absent long bones | Cubitus valgus |
| | Transverse limb defect | Dimples over joints |
| | Limb hemi-hypertrophy | |
| Hands/feet/digits | Polydactyly | Fifth finger clinodactyly |
| | Syndactyly | Transverse palmar creases |
| | Oligodactyly | Nail hypoplasia |
| | Ectrodactyly | Persistent fetal fingerpads |
| | | Overlapping digits |
| Skin | | Nevi |
| | | Hypopigmented macules |
| | | Hyperpigmented macules |
| | | Hemangiomas |

## SUGGESTED READINGS



Carlson BM. *Human Embryology and Developmental Biology*. 5th ed. Philadelphia, PA: WB Saunders; 2014.

Dye FJ. *Dictionary of Developmental Biology and Embryology*. 2nd ed. New York, NY: Wiley-Blackwell; 2012.

Erickson RP, Wynshaw-Borris AJ. *Epstein's Inborn Errors of Development*. 3rd ed. New York, NY: Oxford University Press; 2016.

Gilbert SF. *Developmental Biology*. 10th ed. Sunderland, MA: Sinauer Associates; 2013.

Graham JM, Sanchez-Lara PA. *Smith's Recognizable Patterns of Human Deformation*. 4th ed. Philadelphia, PA: Elsevier; 2016.

Stevenson RE, Hall JG, Everman DB, Solomon BD. *Human Malformations and Related Anomalies (Oxford Monographs on Medical Genetics)*. 3rd ed. New York, NY: Oxford University Press; 2016.

Wangler M, Gonzaga-Jauregui C, Gambin T, et al. Heterozygous de novo and inherited mutations in the smooth muscle actin (ACTG2) Gene underlie megacystis-microcolon-intestinal hypoperistalsis syndrome. *PLoS Genet*. 2014;10:1-11.

Wolpert L, Tickle C. *Principles of Development*. 4th ed. New York, NY: Oxford Press; 2011.

# 172 Environmental Exposures and Health

Melissa A. Suter and Kjersti M. Aagaard



## INTRODUCTION

### EPIGENETICS 101: THE BASICS

From the moment of conception, orchestrated epigenomic changes allow for proper development of the embryo, as well as establishment of the fetal germline (and hence the subsequent generation). The organization of the sperm and egg genomes undergo rapid epigenetic remodeling, primarily in waves of methylation and demethylation, in order to assure zygote viability (Fig. 172-1). As the cell readies for its first division, these early epigenomic modifications help to ensure proper condensation of the DNA, its packaging into chromatin, and proper division of the chromosomes between subsequent cells.

The first differentiation event in human development occurs when embryonic stem cells (ESCs) differentiate to become trophoblast stem cells. These cells form the trophectoderm of the blastocyst. This differentiation event is essential, as the trophectoderm gives rise to the extraembryonic tissues required to support the pregnancy, including the placenta. However, the ESCs and the trophectoderm all have the same genetic information. This begs the question, what drives transcriptional activation and silencing along distinct lines in these 2 cells types? As development proceeds, how can cells that have the exact same genetic material eventually become hepatocytes or neurons, expressing vastly different proteins and having completely different functions?

The answer lies in the understanding of gene regulation, which inherently incorporates epigenomics (Fig. 172-2). Epigenetic modifications function to repress or activate genes, organize chromatin structure, and repair damaged DNA. These modifications enable maintenance of cellular memory of previous gene activation events and ensure genome stability. Similar to the underlying DNA backbone, epigenetic modifications are "heritable" during the cell cycle. Throughout the process of DNA replication, the DNA becomes accessible to the replication machinery. Following behind the replication machinery, chromatin remodeling enzymes are at play, reestablishing

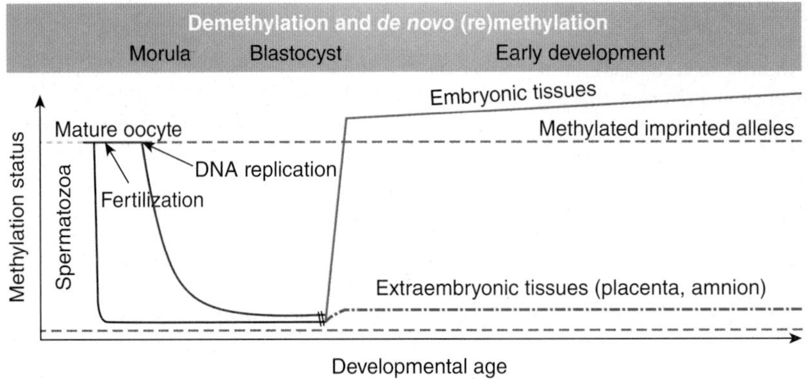


**FIGURE 172-1** The embryonic methylome is erased and reestablished in utero. Upon fertilization, the paternal genome goes through a rapid round of active demethylation. The maternal genome is also demethylated, but in a passive process involving DNA replication without rounds of active re-methylation. As the fetus develops, DNA methylation patterns are reestablished in the embryonic tissues. The extraembryonic tissues, including the placenta, remain largely hypomethylated.

the chromatin structure to its previous state. When the cell divides, the chromatin state of each cell is seemingly identical.

While mechanisms enable genomic DNA heritability with limited nucleotide variation across many generations, the mechanisms regulating heritability of the epigenome are an area of intense investigation. In essence, the epigenome must allow for generation-to-generation stability, yet enable dynamic plasticity and responsiveness to a varying intrauterine environment. As described throughout this chapter, there are environmental exposures that are associated with phenotypic outcomes in the offspring and are believed to be mediated largely via stable epigenomic modifications. In a classical experimental example of these stable modifications, Stockard demonstrated in 1913 that offspring of healthy female rats mated with male rats who had been chronically treated with alcohol had an increased risk of perinatal mortality. This phenotype persisted through a second generation. This occurrence cannot be tied to changes in the offspring nuclear genome as the phenotype is lost after 2 generations. It is hypothesized that epigenetic alterations are a major contributing factor to the transgenerational propagation of this phenotype. These and other experimental observations of heritable phenotypes have led to the hypothesis that epigenetic alterations are responsible for the "molecular memory" of distinct in utero exposure.

What constitutes epigenomic modifications? As schematically shown in Figure 172-2, histone modifications, noncoding RNA-driven suppression, and methylome events are the primary epigenomic constituents that are environmentally influenced during development. Below we give a brief overview of chromatin organization as well as background on 3 main epigenetic modifiers that have major roles in regulating chromatin structure and gene transcription.

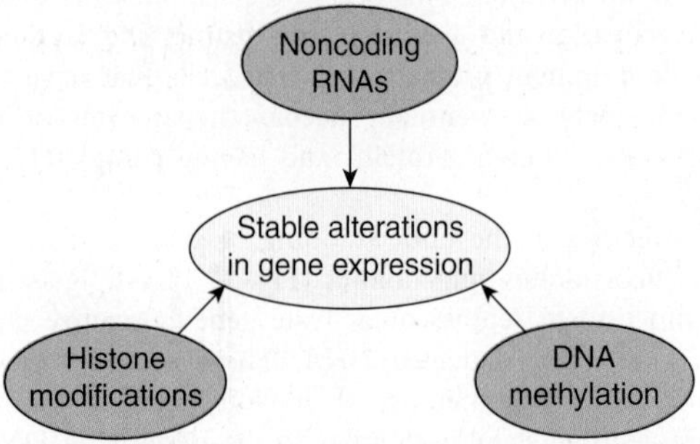


**FIGURE 172-2** Epigenetics: heritable information beyond the DNA sequence. Epigenetic modifiers aid in stable alterations of gene expression. Such modifiers include changes in DNA methylation, posttranslational histone modifications, and noncoding RNAs.

### Chromatin Organization

Chromatin structural organization is fluid, as is seen throughout the cell cycle. Regions of the chromatin can flux between a repressed and an active state depending on the necessity of transcription of the gene. The availability of substrates that contribute to these epigenomic modifiers (eg, dietary intake of folic acid) can have a profound effect on the epigenome with no effect on the underlying DNA sequence.

The approximately 6 billion base pairs of DNA, which are assembled into 46 chromosomes to make up the human genome, require intricate organization. This is achieved, at the most basic level, through the organization of the nucleosome. In all eukaryotic cells, DNA is organized at the primary level as "beads on a string," where 147 base pairs of DNA wrap around an octamer of histone proteins. Two copies each of 4 histone proteins (H2A, H2B, H3, and H4) form the histone octamer, which is the nucleosome core. These histone proteins each have an N-terminal region, termed the "histone tail," which extrudes from the nucleosome surface, making this region of the protein accessible for the addition and removal of varying modifications.

Distinct regions of the genome require tight packaging of the chromatin to inhibit genomic rearrangements that would lead to genome instability. The ends of each chromosome, called telomeres, and long stretches of repeat DNA found throughout the genome are 2 of these regions. All 3 epigenetic modifiers come into play in the telomeric and repeat regions in order to maintain this tightly packed heterochromatin. However, some regions of the DNA need to be accessible to the gene transcription machinery. Again, all 3 epigenetic modifiers contribute to the chromatin alterations that make the DNA accessible and also maintain a memory of transcription.

### DNA Methylation

With regard to the study of environmental exposures and epigenetic alterations, a great deal of work has been done exploring changes in DNA methylation. While modifiable, it is thought to be a relatively stable modification of the DNA. Methyl groups are added directly to the DNA base pairs by specialized DNA methyltransferase enzymes. The telomeric heterochromatic regions of the genome are hypermethylated, which helps maintain silencing. The majority of studies investigate methylation specifically within the context of CpG dinucleotides, where a cytosine base is immediately followed by a guanine base in the DNA sequence. However, non-CpG methylation occurs throughout the genome as well. Of note, DNA methylation is essential for proper establishment and maintenance of imprinting, which leads to parent-of-origin expression of these imprinted genes. Imprinting disorders are covered in other chapters.

### Noncoding RNAs (ncRNAs)

Large-scale sequencing studies have brought to light the importance of ncRNAs, which are more abundant than RNAs, which code for proteins. Of relevance to this chapter, microRNAs (miRNAs) are between 20 and 23 nucleotides long and are processed by Drosha and Dicer proteins from longer RNA strands. These miRNAs are involved in silencing genes through the interaction with a silencing complex consisting of proteins in the Argonaute family. The miRNA sequence aids the targeting of specific protein-coding RNAs (mRNA) for silencing. These mRNAs are then processed through an exonuclease complex, thus inhibiting translation.

Long ncRNAs (lncRNAs) are transcribed by RNA polymerase II and are over 200 nucleotides in length. They do not code for functional proteins. Instead, they help to epigenetically regulate the activation or repression of gene transcription through various mechanisms. In *trans*, lncRNAs can physically interact with DNA methyltransferases and direct DNA methylation to specific regions of the genome. They can also interact with chromatin-modifying complexes, such as polycomb repressive complex 2 (PRC2), which can then target repressive histone modifications to distinct regions of the genome that require transcriptional silencing. In *cis*, transcription of lncRNAs aids in the transcriptional activation of flanking genes through the recruitment of chromatin-modifying enzymes, which add activating histone modifications.

#### Histone Modifications

As described previously, 4 histone proteins form an octameric structure around which the DNA is wrapped to form the nucleosome. Each histone has an N-terminal region that extrudes from the nucleosome surface (the histone tail) that can be posttranslationally modified through the addition of functional groups to specific amino acid residues in the histone tail. Many studies have revealed that patterns of acetylation, methylation, and phosphorylation of the histone tails can act as a "histone code" to orchestrate chromatin-templated events.

Changes in the local histone code can aid in gene transcription, heterochromatin formation, and repair of DNA. During embryonic development, bivalent histone domains are present in the ESCs. These domains contain activating and repressive histone marks and are essential in maintaining an undifferentiated state. For differentiation to occur, specific posttranslational modifications to the histone tail can be readily removed or added. A plethora of kinases, which phosphorylate the histone tails, as well as phosphatases, which are able to remove the phosphorylation "marks," abound. Similarly, there are acetyl transferases, which add an acetyl group, and histone deacetylase enzymes (HDACs), which can remove it.

### THE EPIGENOME IS MODIFIABLE DURING FETAL DEVELOPMENT

So why are investigations of environmental exposures during pregnancy important for our lifelong health? Because the epigenome is modifiable and is especially susceptible to changes in the early stages of embryonic and fetal development, these early changes are continuously propagated in the cellular memory during that individual's lifetime. In the remaining sections of this chapter, we describe different exposures that can occur during fetal development that have been associated in human and animal studies not only with adverse neonatal and childhood outcomes but also with epigenetic changes. We focus on hazardous air pollutants (HAPs), modifiable exposures throughout pregnancy, and in utero exposure to different maternal dietary constraints (Table 172-1). This is by no means meant to be a comprehensive list of likely important environmental exposures, but rather provides contemporaneous examples with a potential high prevalence or that may be possibly modifiable.



**TABLE 172-1 PRENATAL EXPOSURES AND ASSOCIATED EPIGENETIC CHANGES**

| Exposure | Epigenetic Changes |
|---|---|
| Cadmium | • Cord blood DNA methylation levels associated with maternal exposure |
| | • Sex dimorphism in cord blood DNA methylation |
| | • Hypermethylation and increased gene expression of glucocorticoid receptor (rat) |
| Polycyclic aromatic hydrocarbons | • Genomic hypomethylation in cord blood white blood cells (human) |
| | • Association between exposure, DNA methylation levels, and developmental delays at age 3 |
| | • Hypermethylation of ACSL3 in cord blood |
| | • Changes in DNA methylation in the cortex (mouse) |
| Tobacco | • CpG-specific changes in placental DNA methylation associated with changes in gene expression |
| | • DNA methylation alterations in buccal cells in kindergarten-aged children |
| Nicotine | • Histone modifications and altered HDAC activity in offspring lung and brain (rat) |
| | • Global DNA methylation changes in ovaries and testes (rat) |
| Alcohol | • DNA methylation changes in the agouti yellow viable allele (mouse) |
| | • Decreased fetal methylase activity and decreased global DNA methylation (mouse) |
| | • Decreased DNA methylation in sperm of exposed males (mice) |
| Famine/starvation | • Changes in peripheral blood DNA methylation 50 years after exposure |
| Low-protein diet | • Changes in DNA methylation in skeletal muscle, liver, adrenal gland, and pancreas (rat) |
| High-fat diet | • Increase in histone H3 lysine 14 acetylation |
| | • Promoter-specific changes in histone acetylation and methylation associated with alterations in the fetal circadian rhythm and thyroid hormone axis |



## HAZARDOUS AIR POLLUTANTS

### BACKGROUND

The US Clean Air Act Extension was signed into federal law in 1970 and was among the first legislative acts implicating a link between environmental exposures and human health and disease. As statute, it required the Environmental Protection Agency (EPA) to develop and enforce regulations to protect the general public from exposure to ambient (outdoor) airborne contaminants that are known to be hazardous to human health. However, it was not until passage of the 1990 Clean Air Act Amendment that a Commission on Risk Assessment and Risk Management was created in order to actually establish a framework for environmental health risk assessment, management, and the development of federal air quality minimal standards. This amendment was written with the stated goal "that instead of evaluating risks singly and in isolation from each other, they are evaluated in the context of the risk management decision to be made and in the context of public health" (http://www.epa.gov/air/caa/peg/).

As an initial attempt to better study exposures and monitor air quality, the Clean Air Act Amendment defined 2 classes of pollutants: criteria pollutants and HAP. The 6 criteria pollutants (lead, nitrogen oxides, sulfur dioxide, particulate matter, ozone, and carbon monoxide) are strictly regulated by EPA-based standards that govern their permissible ambient levels and are monitored via national networks that ascertain compliance with primary and secondary standards. As a result of this established extensive network, reliable estimates on health effects and ambient concentrations of the criteria pollutants are relatively abundant. In contrast, the HAPs are comprised of 189 specific pollutants or chemical groups that are known to cause or are suspected of causing cancer, birth defects, reproductive issues, and other serious morbidity or mortality. HAPs are numerous and vary with respect to biochemical properties (half-life and toxicity), heterogeneity of distribution, magnitude of concentration, and emission source (stationary vs mobile). As such, the EPA created an air toxic component of the Cumulative Exposure Project in order to provide estimates of ambient concentration for a large portion (148 of 189) of the HAPs along the 60,803 US population census tracts. In an effort to identify air toxics of greatest potential contribution to population risk, the EPA refined its exposure project in 2002 with the development of the National Air Toxics Assessment (NATA). NATA provides a tool to inform both national and regional efforts and collect information on air toxicants, characterize emissions, and help prioritize pollutants/geographic areas of interest for more refined data collection (http://www.epa.gov/ttn/atw/natamain/index.html).

NATA risk assessment results are estimated at the census tract level and employ a computer simulation model (Assessment System for Population Exposure Nationwide [ASPEN]). This model is based on the EPA's Industrial Source Complex Long Term model (ISCLT), which simulates the behavior of the pollutants after they are emitted into the atmosphere based on toxic air pollutant emissions and meteorologic data from National Weather Service stations. As part of NATA activities, the EPA conducted a national-scale assessment of 32 of the HAPs and diesel particulate matter, which compiled 1996 data post hoc in 4 steps across the contiguous United States: (1) compilation of a national emissions inventory of the 33 pollutants from ambient sources, (2) estimation of ambient concentrations, (3) estimation of population exposures, and (4) characterization of potential public health risk (cancer and noncancer) due to inhalation of air toxics. All aspects of the development and implementation of NATA and ASPEN have been subjected to scientific peer review by both the EPA and an external panel and have been further validated and employed in other studies.

As of 2006, 80% (224 million) of the estimated 280 million Americans reside in metropolitan areas. Approximately 180 million Americans were living in areas where monitored air failed to meet the 1997 National Ambient Air Quality Standards for at least 1 of the 6 criteria air pollutants and the vast majority of HAPs. In the face of such exposure prevalence and despite advances in data attainment and modeling, it is of noted concern that in the 4 decades since passage of the Clean Air Act of 1970, ambient (outdoor) air quality as it relates to public health concerns surrounding pregnancy remains largely poorly understood and understudied. Specifically, while scientific understanding of the health effects of air pollution on child and adult respiratory and cardiovascular morbidity and mortality has increased in past decades, pregnancy-related exposure analyses are primarily limited to studies on teratogenesis and reproductive toxicology. Indeed, only in recent years has literature emerged that addresses the possibility that environmental contaminants may influence the rate and prevalence of common adverse pregnancy outcomes such as preterm birth, delivery of a small for gestational age (SGA) infant, preeclampsia, and pregnancy loss. Similarly, these HAPs are associated with asthma and neurologic problems, including learning disabilities and hyperactivity in children.

## IN UTERO EXPOSURES TO HAP AND ADVERSE OUTCOMES

There are many HAPs that have been implicated in adverse outcomes with in utero exposures (Fig. 172-3). Benzene, which is a prevalent HAP in urban areas, is associated with cancer in adults and is among the top 20 chemicals produced in the United States. It is formed during combustion of natural gas, is a by- product of gasoline combustion, and is also found in tobacco smoke. Epidemiologic studies have shown that mothers living in urban areas with the highest levels of benzene have a higher risk for having a child with spina bifida compared with those living in areas with the lowest benzene levels. In utero exposures to benzene have also been associated with an increased risk of childhood leukemia. While benzene exposures are associated with epigenetic changes in adults, no studies are available that delineate epigenetic changes associated with in utero exposures. This is a gap in the literature and reveals that more important work remains to be done.

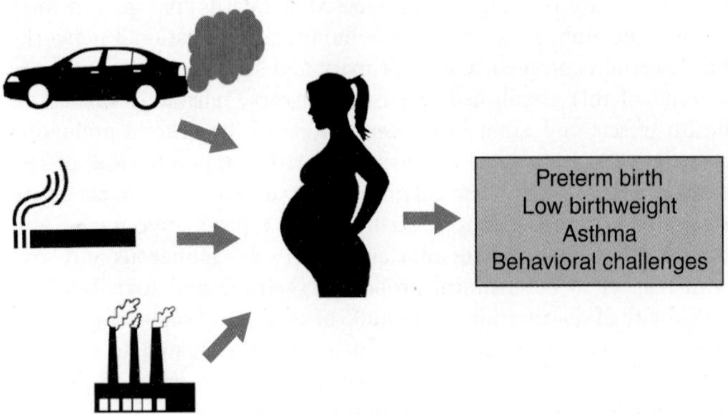


**FIGURE 172-3** Prenatal exposure to hazardous air pollutants leads to adverse neonatal and childhood outcomes. Hazardous air pollutants found in exhaust, second-hand tobacco smoke, and ambient air including benzene, polycyclic aromatic hydrocarbons, and cadmium are known to lead to adverse outcomes in the exposed offspring. Such outcomes include, but are not limited to, preterm birth, low-birthweight babies, childhood asthma, and behavioral problems in childhood and adolescence.

## EVIDENCE OF EPIGENETIC CHANGES WITH PRENATAL HAP EXPOSURE

### Cadmium

Cadmium (Cd) exposure can occur through air pollution, cigarette smoke, water, and food. While in nonpregnant individuals Cd targets the kidneys, during pregnancy, Cd has been shown to accumulate in the placenta in hamsters, rats, mice, and humans. Cd is a well-established placental toxin, causing placental necrosis and stromal edema while inhibiting trophoblast proliferation. Chronic occupational exposure to Cd is associated with recurrent pregnancy loss due to evident placental damage. High levels of placental Cd are associated with low-birthweight babies.

Evidence from epidemiologic studies as well as animal models reveals evidence of adverse outcomes with prenatal Cd exposure. Studies measuring the extent of Cd exposure through maternal urine and cord blood concentrations reveal an association with exposure and low birthweight as well as smaller head circumference. Rodent models of prenatal Cd exposure show that exposed offspring suffer from alterations in immune cell development and function. Further studies in mice yield insight into the potential for Cd to act as an endocrine-disrupting chemical (EDC) during fetal development, and offspring exposed in utero have reduced reproductive capacity.

As evidence increases that the effects of early life exposures to Cd persist throughout the lifetime of the individual, epigenetic studies that interrogate changes associated with in utero Cd exposure are becoming increasingly prevalent. However, the results are difficult to interpret. Epidemiologic studies have been conducted to examine differences in DNA methylation in cord blood with Cd exposure. In one study, global levels of DNA methylation were studied through analysis of long interspersed nuclear elements (LINE-1), which are repetitive regions located throughout the human genome, and found that with increasing amounts of Cd exposure there was hypomethylation of LINE-1 in the cord blood. Tight control of LINE-1 methylation is important for the maintenance of genome stability, as methylation of these transposable elements prevents genomic rearrangements that may lead to cancer. Another study of 127 mother-child pairs from Bangladesh correlated levels of CpG methylation with Cd levels as measured from maternal blood. Using the Illumina 450K array, which measures the methylation status of over 450,000 individual CpG dinucleotides throughout the genome, they reported a marked sex dimorphism with prenatal Cd exposure. They observed positive correlations between maternal Cd levels and site-specific CpG methylation changes in boys and negative correlations with the majority of the altered CpG sites in girls.

In light of such epidemiologic evidence, it is important to utilize animal models to get a better understanding of the nature of these changes. Studies in chick embryos have determined that there is a distinct window in early development where Cd exposure is associated with epigenetic changes. Studies in rats, where Cd is administered by addition to the drinking water, also show a sex dimorphism, revealing that males have hypermethylation and decreased gene expression of the glucocorticoid receptor, while in females they found hypomethylation and increased gene expression. The sex dimorphism of Cd exposure needs to be further explored with regard to health in adolescence and adulthood, in light of the noted epigenetic alterations that occur in utero.

### Polycyclic Aromatic Hydrocarbons

Polycyclic aromatic hydrocarbons (PAHs) are a classification of hundreds of chemicals that include 2 or more fused aromatic rings. They are formed through the incomplete combustion of fossil fuels and coal and are found in first- and second-hand tobacco smoke. Exposure to PAHs is associated with asthma and cancer, and PAHs can act as an immunosuppressant. Exposure can occur through ambient (air) exposures, as well as through water contamination and food, particularly charbroiled meat.

The Agency for Toxic Substances and Disease Registry (ATSDR) has listed PAHs as ninth in the national priority list of hazardous substances. The specific PAHs benzo(a)pyrene (BaP) and benzo(b) fluoranthene (BbF) hold numbers 8 and 10, respectively, on this priority list. PAHs are ubiquitous and can be deposited and persist in bed sediment as a sink in the aquatic system. Over time, these toxins can be released into the water, threaten the aquatic ecosystem, and bioaccumulate in food chains.

Studies reveal that prenatal PAH exposure is associated with adverse pregnancy outcomes, including preterm birth. Exposure has been shown to reduce birthweight and increase the risk for SGA infants. There is an association between PAH exposures and the cephalization index (the ratio of head size to birth weight), which is serving as a surrogate measurement of brain maturity. Upper limits of prenatal PAH exposure have also been associated with cognitive dysfunction and lower cognitive test scores in children. At age 3, children who were exposed in utero have increased recurrent wheeze and number of wheezing days. In animal models, in utero exposure to PAHs is associated with an increase in adverse birth outcomes including exacerbation of bronchopulmonary dysplasia, a disorder associated with early preterm birth. These studies reveal the need for an improved understanding of the mechanisms underlying prenatal PAH exposure and its harmful effects.

Because PAHs are ubiquitous and can cross the placenta as well as the fetal blood-brain barrier and because their exposure is associated with learning disabilities and lifelong risk of cancer, studies of epigenetic changes are essential to our understandings of the likely etiology of these risk factors. PAHs form distinct bulky DNA adducts that can be measured in blood and tissue, yielding insight into the extent of the exposure. Both cord blood and placenta can be used to measure PAH-induced adducts to quantify prenatal PAH exposures.

A major cohort study from the Columbia Center for Children's Environmental Health in New York City has interrogated the associations between prenatal PAH exposure, adverse outcomes, and epigenetic changes. They have reported that PAH exposure was associated with genomic hypermethylation in umbilical cord white blood cells in a cohort of 159 children. Levels of global DNA methylation were associated with levels of PAH adducts in the cord blood white blood cells. In a follow-up study of these subjects, they found an association between DNA methylation levels in cord blood and neurodevelopmental delay at age 3, indicating that the "footprint" of this in utero exposure persisted. In fact, further analysis of a subset of this cohort (n = 56) revealed that hypermethylation of a specific gene, *ACSL3*, was significantly associated with increased maternal PAH exposures and a higher incidence of asthma before age 5.

Animal models are also utilized to further understand the epigenetic changes associated with in utero PAH exposures. Through these models, the amount, duration, and gestational windows of exposure can be controlled. In a mouse model where the PAHs were administered through aerosol spray throughout gestation, the prenatal exposure was associated with changes in behavior that revealed increased anxiety levels in the mouse. In these same offspring, the behavioral changes were accompanied by gene expression changes in the cortex in adulthood as well as promoter-specific alterations in DNA methylation in the brain.

## MODIFIABLE EXPOSURES

### EVIDENCE OF EPIGENETIC CHANGES WITH MODIFIABLE EXPOSURES

#### Tobacco

Although public health warnings have been shown to be effective in reducing the smoking rate nationally, as many as 14% to 20% of women smoke during pregnancy. Decades of research have shown that smoking in pregnancy is associated with preterm birth, premature rupture of membranes, placental abruption, and placenta previa. Similarly, many studies have reported an association between maternal tobacco smoke exposure (MTSE) and restricted fetal growth and low-birthweight babies. However, it has also been noted that not all babies exposed in utero to MTSE are born growth restricted. Genetic studies reveal associations between polymorphisms in genes that metabolize xenobiotics, which may contribute to the altered susceptibility of the growth-restricted phenotype in neonates from smokers. However, studies of epigenetic changes may also be important in illuminating a better understanding of these observed differences in outcomes. Among the environmental exposures, tobacco smoke is unique in its understanding of the interplay between the exposure and genomic-epigenomic interactions rendering risk for adverse outcomes.

Epigenetic changes associated with MTSE have been reported in the placenta, cord blood, buccal cells, and peripheral blood of exposed offspring. In fact, in one study, cord blood levels of cotinine (a metabolite of nicotine and an indicator of nicotine exposure) were inversely correlated with DNA methylation from cord blood. Studies of the placenta from smoking and nonsmoking mothers also reveal that tobacco smoke leaves an epigenetic footprint and that these epigenetic changes are likely contributing to changes in gene expression levels. Using a genome-wide CpG methylation array side by side with a gene expression array, it was reported that 438 genes showed a significant correlation between CpG methylation and gene expression in the placenta from mothers who smoke. These correlations were not observed in the nonsmoking cohort.

Studies interrogating individuals who were exposed to tobacco smoke in utero potentially have lasting changes to their epigenomes. Studies of DNA methylation from children in kindergarten and first grade showed differential methylation of a repeat region of the genome (*Alu*Yb8) as well as gene-specific changes (*AXL*) between those exposed in utero and those who were not. DNA methylation from peripheral blood granulocytes is altered in a repeat region of the genome (Sat2) in adults who were exposed in the womb compared with those who were not.

How these epigenetic changes are manifested throughout the lifetime of the individual is unknown. However, reports that these epigenetic changes are observed at birth (placenta and cord blood), during childhood (buccal cells), and into adulthood (peripheral blood) indicate that this modifiable in utero exposure likely has lifelong consequences to the offspring.

#### Nicotine

There is an alarming trend of increased use of electronic cigarettes (e-cigarettes) and other electronic nicotine delivery systems in adolescents and women of reproductive age. While studies investigating pregnancy and neonatal outcomes due to in utero exposures to electronic cigarettes are not yet available, this is likely to become a highly investigated public health issue. In this emerging area of concern, some of the potentially best clues pertaining to what we anticipate seeing in human studies have arisen from animal models detailing the adverse effects of nicotine exposures in utero.

Tobacco smoke has over 4000 chemicals, including PAHs, benzene, and nicotine. In the previous section, we detailed PAH exposure risks, which are unique to combustible tobacco but are not found in e-cigarettes. However, while electronic cigarettes do not have nearly as many chemicals with a proven impact on the epigenome, what they do contain is not benign to the developing fetus or the young adult or adult user. Specifically, most electronic cigarettes available on the market today contain varying concentrations of nicotine, which is an addictive substance with well-delineated and well-established associations with both adverse pregnancy and infant outcomes, as well as risk of aberrant neurodevelopment.

Nicotine readily crosses the placenta and is able to bind nicotinic acetylcholine receptors in the brain and lung. From rodent and primate animal models, we know that in utero nicotine exposure is associated with decreased lung volume and weight, elevated blood pressure, increased weight and adipose accumulation, and changes in dopamine and serotonin levels in the offspring. In a rat model, an asthma-like phenotype has even been shown to persist throughout 2 generations. In this model, prenatal administration of nicotine was associated with asthma not only in the offspring, but also in the "grandchildren" as well, even though this second generation was never exposed to nicotine. Studies of multigenerational inheritance beg the question, are there epigenetic associations that could help potentiate these phenotypes in the absence of the exposure?

In addition to lung and brain tissue modifications, animal models have been used to document epigenetic changes in the fetal ovaries and testes with in utero exposures to nicotine. Specifically, global DNA methylation is altered in ovary and testes, which may contribute to the multigenerational phenotype. In the lung and brain, alterations of specific histone markers have been reported. Alterations to histones H3 and H4 acetylation are observed in these organs, which may provide a molecular memory of these exposures. In adult mice, chronic nicotine administration has been found to reduce histone deacetylase (HDAC) activity in the brain and increase the animal's behavioral response to cocaine. These observations co-occur in association with increased histone H3 and H4 acetylation in the brain. The potential for in utero exposures of nicotine to enhance the offspring's behavior for cocaine needs to be examined.

One recent study in mice uncovered a potential mechanism to explain the lasting changes in behavior and cognition that are associated with nicotine exposure in utero. They observed changes in neuronal plasticity within the cortex, by studying dendritic branching and spine density. This was associated with persistent expression changes of a gene important for the methylation of histones (*Ash2l*). Elegant studies in these offspring revealed *Ash2l* is altered with prenatal nicotine exposure and is responsible for the observed epigenetic and structural changes observed.

### Marijuana

The reported rates of marijuana use are estimated between 2% and 11% of pregnant women, making it one of the most commonly used dependent substances during pregnancy. Due to the recent changes in legislature regarding the legality of marijuana use, there has been an increase in reporting of its use in pregnancy, potentially due to a decline in perceived risk of harm. The major psychotropic ingredient in marijuana, delta-9-tetrahydrocannabinol (THC) is able to cross the placenta. Studies have shown that marijuana use is associated with lower birthweight babies and a decreased growth trajectory throughout pregnancy. Studies of neurologic function have shown that in utero marijuana exposure has a detectable impact on the social and cognitive development of school-age children. In one current study, the risk of co-use of marijuana and cigarettes suggested a synergism with higher risk of harm than either substance in isolation. The cannabinoids in marijuana have been shown experimentally to be immunosuppressive; however, it is unknown whether prenatal exposure has adverse effects on the developing immune system of the fetus.

To date, no data exist on whether or not epigenetic changes occur with in utero exposure to marijuana either alone or in combination with other exposures. However, in experimental nonhuman primate and mouse models, as well as in vitro cell culture systems, there is evidence for the associated occurrence of epigenetic changes with chronic marijuana use in adolescents and adults. Cannabinoid exposure is associated with alterations in miRNA, DNA methylation, and histone modifications in animal models and in vitro systems. For example, in a mouse model, THC administration upregulates myeloid-derived suppressor cells (MDSCs). This induction is dependent on changes in the miRNA expression profile within the MDSCs. Because prenatal exposure appears to have long-term neurologic consequences on the offspring, it is possible that epigenetic mechanisms are at play. Further investigations are warranted to understand the nature of these changes to determine mechanisms that contribute to these adverse outcomes.

### Alcohol

One of the great public health campaigns of the past century resulted in a near-complete abrogation of alcohol consumption during pregnancy. While there are genetic variables that contribute to the discrepancy in neonatal outcomes with fetal alcohol syndrome, including polymorphisms in the genes that metabolize alcohol, epigenetic factors are believed to be primary contributors.

Insight into the potential for epigenetic mechanisms to be involved in alcohol susceptibility dates back to 1913, where studies involving rats revealed that chronic exposure of the father to alcohol was associated with increased perinatal mortality, even though the mother was naive to alcohol. It was (much) later reported that the DNA methyltransferase (DNMT1) expression is altered in sperm from male rats after chronic alcohol exposure. Preconceptional alcohol consumption by females, in a mouse model, was associated with transcriptional silencing of a specific gene, the agouti yellow viable allele ($A^{vy}$), even in the absence of alcohol consumption during the pregnancy.

As early as 1991, studies in mice were being conducted to determine epigenetic effects of prenatal alcohol consumption on the fetus. In these offspring, there was decreased methylase activity in the fetuses as well as lower levels of DNA methylation. Reported changes in DNA methylation using mouse models of prenatal alcohol exposures include decreased DNA methylation in the sperm of males and gene-specific changes, including within the promoters of *Igf2*.

### Bisphenol A

Bisphenol A (BPA) is a ubiquitous chemical found in polycarbonate plastics. Bottled water, plastic food storage containers, and infant bottles are known sources of BPA. In fact, BPA is so ubiquitous that a study from the Centers for Disease Control and Prevention (CDC) in 2004 reported that 93% of participants had detectable levels of BPA in their urine. Such ubiquitous exposure is of concern, especially during development, because BPA can act as an EDC. EDCs are chemicals that mimic or disrupt the action of endogenous hormones. In the case of BPA, it can act as a weak environmental estrogen. We have included it under modifiable exposures because it is possible to limit BPA exposure through proactive measures including choosing BPA-free plastic bottles and containers as well as abstaining from heating food in BPA-containing containers.

BPA has been detected in placenta samples, cord blood, and breast milk. Much of our understanding of prenatal BPA exposure, especially concerning epigenetic changes, has been determined using rodent models. Such models have shown that BPA exposure in utero disrupts development of the male and female reproductive tracts, changes the sexual differentiation of the brain, and accelerates fetal neuronal development. The offspring undergo accelerated puberty and are at higher-risk for cancerous lesions in the mammary tissue and prostate. Behavioral changes have been noted in rodent models including increased anxiety, altered social interactions, and learning and memory impairments.

Recent studies in humans have reported a propensity for obesity with prenatal exposure as well as sex-specific changes in behavior. These studies are from the Columbia Center for Children's Environmental Health where maternal BPA levels were measured in the third trimester of pregnancy. BPA was further measured in the children at 3 and 5 years of age. From this cohort, they found that prenatal BPA levels positively correlated with the fat mass index of the children at age 7 years. In girls, but not boys, prenatal BPA also positively correlated with waist circumference. Childhood levels of BPA did not correlate with any measures of obesity, indicating that the prenatal period is an important window of exposure for these outcomes. Two studies from this cohort also found that high levels of prenatal BPA exposures were associated with increased anxiety and aggressive behaviors in boys age 7 to 9 years, and a follow-up revealed increased signs of anxiety and depression in boys age 10 to 12. No such differences were reported in the girls exposed to BPA.

Prenatal BPA exposure also induces epigenetic changes, as described in rodent models. In a mouse model, BPA exposure in utero was associated with hypomethylation of the agouti yellow locus, which ultimately altered the offspring coat color from brown to yellow. Another study in mice revealed persistent changes in DNA methylation and gene expression in the uterus of the exposed offspring. These studies also showed that the changes in DNA methylation coincided with estrogen receptor alpha (ERα)-activated genes and that the ERα protein itself had altered expression in the uterus by virtue of BPA exposure. In the mammary gland, which is susceptible to cancerous lesions in the BPA-exposed mice, site-specific CpG methylation changes were found at 4, 21, and 50 days postnatally. In male mice, neonatal BPA exposure is associated with changes in DNA methylation in the prostate. DNA methylation changes have also been reported in the offspring brain. Specifically, methylation of the ERα promoter was altered, and changes in expression of the DNA methyltransferase genes *DNMT1* and *DNMT3* were observed. In sum, epigenetic alterations have been found in the uterus, prostate, mammary tissue, and brain in rodent models. While no epigenetic changes associated with prenatal BPA exposure have been reported in humans, given the increased incidences of obesity and behavioral changes that are observed in children, such investigations are certainly warranted.

## MATERNAL DIET

### BACKGROUND

Large-scale epidemiologic studies of individuals born during the Dutch famine have greatly increased our understanding of how maternal diet constraints can have a long-lasting impact. Unlike traditional famines, the Dutch famine occurred during a defined time period during World War II. During the famine, the average Dutch citizen had a food ration of approximately 500 calories per day. Remarkably, during this time, meticulous medical records were kept, allowing researchers to know at what time point during gestation individuals were subjected to maternal starvation in utero. When the famine ended, the average citizen's daily calorie ration went from 500 to 2000 calories per day fairly rapidly.

As the individuals who were exposed to starvation across gestation grew into adulthood, a startling phenotype began to be observed. These individuals had a much higher incidence of developing cardiovascular disease than their unexposed siblings. Over time, epidemiologists studying this cohort realized that low birthweight was a strong determinant of metabolic fitness in adulthood. Furthermore, individuals who were exposed to starvation early in gestation and did not have a decreased birthweight still had a higher incidence of heart disease in later life.

Although the in utero exposure occurred early in gestation, the phenotype can take decades to emerge. How is the memory of that exposure maintained? Through comprehensive epidemiologic studies as well as using animal models, epigenetic reprogramming that occurs by virtue of exposure to varying maternal diet constraints (calorie restriction, protein restriction, overnutrition/high-fat diet) has begun to be elucidated.

### EVIDENCE OF EPIGENETIC CHANGES WITH MATERNAL DIET

Because of the long-lasting memory of the Dutch famine exposure, studies of DNA methylation levels in peripheral blood samples from these individuals were performed. Those who were exposed in utero to the Dutch famine have site-specific changes compared with unexposed siblings. Hypomethylation within the insulin-like growth factor 2 receptor (IGF2), as well as changes in DNA methylation in the promoters of six other genes, has been reported. However, these studies only begin to uncover the reprogramming that likely occurred in utero.

#### Low-Protein Diet

Perhaps the most well-characterized animal model of maternal malnutrition is maternal protein restriction (PR), which has been extensively studied in rat and mouse models. The offspring from PR dams are growth restricted in utero and experience a postnatal catch-up phase. In these models, the exposed offspring are at increased risk for type 2 diabetes, hypertension, and markers of cardiac disease (such as an increase in ventricular interstitial fibrosis). These animal models are ideal to study epigenetic reprogramming due to diet exposure as different tissues can be studied postnatally to determine what changes occur, where they occur, and how long they persist.

Such changes have been reported in the offspring liver, skeletal muscle, adrenal gland, and pancreas. Alterations in DNA methylation are observed in the promoter of the *PPARα* gene in the liver. PPARα is essential for proper lipid and carbohydrate storage. Methylation changes in the glucocorticoid receptor, which is a gene that helps to regulate blood pressure, have also been reported in these offspring. Epigenetic changes in this model also include misexpression of miRNAs in the pancreas and changes in promoter-specific histone acetylation patterns in the skeletal muscle.

It should be noted that there are reports of transgenerational inheritance of phenotypes in this model. In a mouse model, the F3 generation experiences low beta-cell mass in the pancreas in early life. Transcriptional changes in the liver in the third generation after exposure to maternal PR have been reported, while others have shown insulin resistance in the F2 generation.

#### High-Fat Diet

The latest report from the CDC informs that one-third of all Americans are obese and that susceptibility to obesity is associated with race and ethnicity as well as socioeconomic status. A map of the United States showing prevalence by state shows distinct regions within the United States with a higher prevalence of obesity than others. Many theories exist as to what factors have most strongly contributed to this prevalence of obesity and overweight, including lifestyle choices, food abundance, and caloric density as well as genetic factors. With regard to pregnancy, it is documented that obese women give birth to large for gestational age (LGA) babies and that these LGA babies are then at risk later in life for metabolic disease. Is it possible that fetal programming is underlying the current persistence of obesity?

Studies in a nonhuman primate model of maternal obesity and chronic caloric excess indeed indicate that epigenetic changes are associated with these in utero exposures. In this model, Japanese macaques are fed either a control diet or a high-fat diet (HFD) and are bred annually. Over time, the dams on the HFD become overweight and progress to obesity. The offspring have been studied, and the outcomes are profound. As early as the beginning of the third trimester, the fetuses have evidence of nonalcoholic fatty liver disease, and this pathology persists postnatally. Neurologic and behavioral changes are seen in these offspring including perturbations in the dopaminergic and serotonergic systems, increased intake of high-sugar and high-fat food, and increased levels of anxiety-like behavior.

In this model, the fetuses exposed to the maternal HFD have an altered thyroid axis, and their $T_4$ levels are significantly decreased compared with those from control diet animals. Genes involved in thyroid homeostasis are disrupted. A major transcription factor required for thyroid hormone–dependent gene expression, THRB, is epigenetically altered in these offspring. Epigenetic alterations are also observed in the fetal liver. A site-specific histone modification, acetylation of lysine 14 of histone H3, is increased with maternal HFD exposure. This modification is differentially enriched in the promoter of Npas2, a transcription factor that drives proper gene expression of genes necessary for maintaining the circadian rhythm. Altered promoter occupancy of histone modifications is observed in the postnatal liver with maternal HFD exposure.

## FUTURE DIRECTIONS

For decades, physicians, epidemiologists, and scientists have understood that there are adverse consequences for fetuses exposed in utero to various exposures. While some are modifiable, such as maternal tobacco use and alcohol consumption, other exposures are ambient and therefore difficult for a pregnant woman to avoid. Regardless, we are just beginning to understand the long-term consequences of these exposures not only for the offspring, but also for subsequent generations to come.

The findings outlined in this chapter from both animal models and epidemiologic studies describe many epigenomic changes arising from distinct exposures, looking at specific epigenetic changes at defined time points during fetal and postnatal life. Long-term studies, following the individual from birth into adulthood to monitor for stability of these changes, will help in an understanding of the potential permanence and explore the longevity of these "epigenetic memories."

## SUGGESTED READINGS


Chabarria KC, Racusin DA, Antony KM, et al. Marijuana use and its effects in pregnancy. *Am J Obstet Gynecol.* 2016;215(4):506.e1-e7.

Geraghty AA, Lindsay KL, Alberdi G, McAuliffe FM, Gibney ER. Nutrition during pregnancy impacts offspring's epigenetic status-evidence from human and animal studies. *Nutr Metab Insights.* 2015;8(Suppl 1):41-47.

Jung Y, Hsieh LS, Lee AM, et al. An epigenetic mechanism mediates developmental nicotine effects on neuronal structure and behavior. *Nat Neurosci.* 2016;19(7):905-914.

Kobor MS, Weinberg J. Focus on: epigenetics and fetal alcohol spectrum disorders. *Alcohol Res Health.* 2011;34(1):29-37.

Perera F, Herbstman J. Prenatal environmental exposures, epigenetics, and disease. *Reprod Toxicol.* 2011;31(3):363-373.

Suter MA, Mastrobattista J, Sachs M, Aagaard K. Is there evidence for potential harm of electronic cigarette use in pregnancy? *Birth Defects Res A Clin Mol Teratol.* 2015;103(3):186-195.

Vilahur N, Vahter M, Broberg K. The epigenetic effects of prenatal cadmium exposure. *Curr Environ Health Rep.* 2015;2(2):195-203.

Zumbrun EE, Sido JM, Nagarkatti PS, Nagarkatti M. Epigenetic regulation of immunological alterations following prenatal exposure to marijuana cannabinoids and its long term consequences in offspring. *J Neuroimmune Pharmacol.* 2015;10(2):245-254.




# 173 Genetic Evaluation of Intellectual Disability and Autism

Christian P. Schaaf

## INTRODUCTION

The American Association of Intellectual and Developmental Disabilities defines intellectual disability as "a disability characterized by significant limitations in both intellectual functioning and in adaptive behavior, which covers many everyday social and practical skills." Intellectual disability originates before the age of 18.

Autism spectrum disorder is a group of developmental disabilities that are characterized by significant impairments in social communication and social interaction, and affected individuals manifest restricted and repetitive behaviors, interests, or activities.

Intellectual disability and autism spectrum disorder frequently co-occur. Approximately 10% to 15% of all children with intellectual disability have autism spectrum disorder or autistic traits. On the other hand, up to 40% of all children with autism spectrum disorder have intellectual disability.

Both intellectual disability and autism spectrum disorder are extensively heterogeneous from a genetic viewpoint. Several hundred genes and chromosomal loci have been identified, mutations of which cause or predispose to the respective disorders. Some genetic syndromes manifesting intellectual disability and/or autism spectrum disorder are clinically so distinct and easily recognizable that a given set of symptoms and features will suggest the diagnosis and determine a very targeted diagnostic approach. However, most individuals with intellectual disability or autism spectrum disorder are nondysmorphic, and the overall clinical presentation is nonspecific, rendering them "idiopathic."

The genetic diagnostic approach to intellectual disability and autism spectrum disorder has changed dramatically during recent years because of the availability of genome-wide methodologies, such as chromosome microarray analysis and whole-exome sequencing.

## PATHOGENESIS AND EPIDEMIOLOGY FOR INTELLECTUAL DISABILITY

There are many possible causes of intellectual disability, including prenatal infections, teratogenic exposures, perinatal complications, as well as postnatal brain infections, traumatic brain injury, or toxic exposure. However, especially in developed countries, the majority of cases of intellectual disability (approximately 80%) have an underlying genetic cause. Using the currently available technology, that cause can be identified in up to 60% of all patients who present for diagnostic evaluation.

The prevalence of intellectual disability in the United States ranges from 0.7% to 1.4%. While males and females are equally represented among individuals with mild intellectual disability, there is an overrepresentation of males among individuals with moderate and severe intellectual disability (male-to-female ratio 1.4:1). This has mostly been attributed to genetic factors, especially X-linked forms of intellectual disability.

## PATHOGENESIS AND EPIDEMIOLOGY FOR AUTISM SPECTRUM DISORDER

The etiologic causes of autism spectrum disorder are not as well understood as those of intellectual disability. Based on twin studies, the heritability of autism spectrum disorder has been estimated to be between 60% and 90%. Nongenetic risk factors for autism spectrum disorder include prematurity and low birth weight, gestational diabetes, maternal infections during pregnancy, and prenatal drug exposure (eg, valproate, selective serotonin reuptake inhibitors). Genetic causes of autism spectrum disorder can be identified in 20% to 40% of cases referred for evaluation. The likelihood of identifying a specific genetic cause is greater in the lower functioning cases of autism spectrum disorder, as well as medically complex (syndromic) forms of autism spectrum disorder.

The prevalence of autism spectrum disorder in the United States was estimated by the Centers for Disease Control and Prevention in 2014. This study identified 1 in 68 children as having autism spectrum disorder. Boys are approximately 4 times more likely to be affected than girls (1 in 42 boys vs 1 in 189 girls). Mutations of X-linked genes seem to account for only part of that gender difference. A "female protective model" for autism spectrum disorder has been proposed, suggesting that females can tolerate a greater burden of genetic variation and mutation without clinically manifesting autism spectrum disorder.

## CLINICAL MANIFESTATIONS OF INTELLECTUAL DISABILITY

The 10th revision of the International Statistical Classification of Diseases (ICD-10) defines intellectual disability as "a condition of arrested or incomplete development of the mind, which is especially characterized by impairment of skills that contribute to the overall level of intelligence, ie, cognitive, language, motor, and social abilities." Degrees of intellectual disability are conventionally estimated by standardized intelligence tests. Based on the results of these tests, intellectual disability is defined as an intelligence quotient (IQ) of less than 70. The Diagnostic and Statistical Manual of Mental Disorders (DSM-V) states that impairments are typically recognized in 3 domains of functioning: (1) The conceptual domain, which includes skills in language, reading, writing, math, reasoning, knowledge, and memory; (2) the social domain, which refers to empathy, social judgment, interpersonal communication skills, and the ability to make and retain friendships; and (3) the practical domain, which centers on self-management in areas such as personal care, job responsibilities, money management, recreating, and organizing school and work tasks.

In most cases, individuals with intellectual disability have a history of global developmental delay (delayed acquisition of developmental

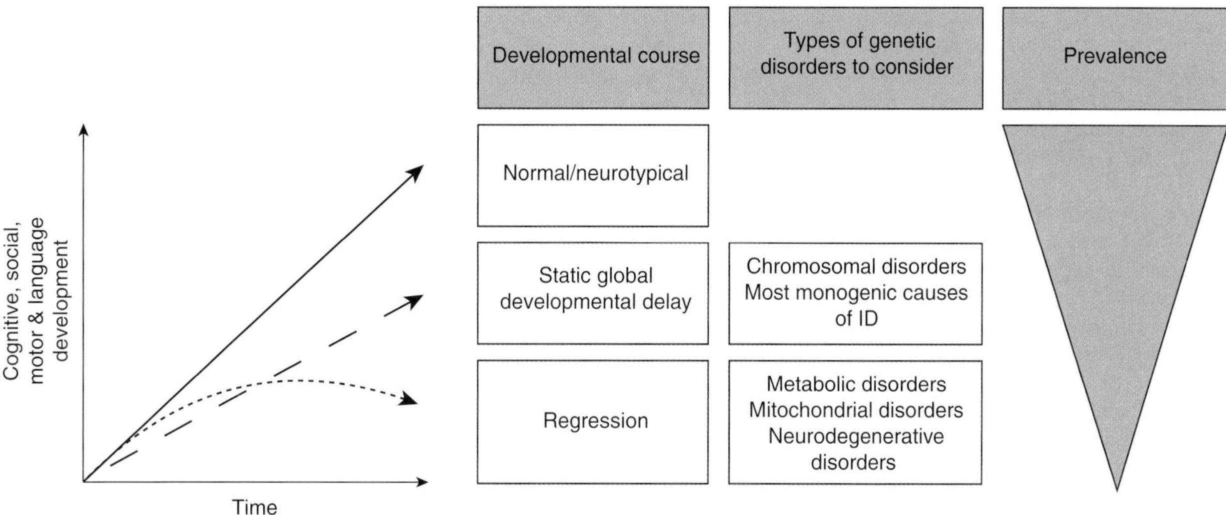


**FIGURE 173-1** Groups of genetic disorders and their typical developmental trajectories. ID, intellectual disability.

milestones). In common clinical practice, the term "developmental delay" is used for children younger than 5 years, whereas "intellectual disability" is used for children 5 years and older.

Mild intellectual disability (IQ 50–69) accounts for 80% to 85% of all cases of intellectual disability. Moderate (IQ 35–49), severe (IQ 20–34), and profound intellectual disability (IQ < 20) are much less frequently encountered.

The typical course of intellectual disability is that of a static encephalopathy, such that affected individuals show delays in cognitive development that are manifest in infancy or early childhood, and continue to be present throughout life (Fig. 173-1). Developmental regression, with a (seemingly) normal phase of early cognitive development, followed by marked loss of previously acquired developmental milestones, is rare, and requires special evaluation and investigations, as it may be seen in the context of inborn errors of metabolism or neurodegenerative disorders (see Fig. 173-1).

## CLINICAL MANIFESTATIONS OF AUTISM SPECTRUM DISORDER

Autism spectrum disorder manifests in the early developmental period. It is characterized by persistent deficits in social communication and social interaction, as well as restricted, repetitive patterns of behaviors, interests, or activities (DSM-V). The symptoms must cause clinically significant impairment in social, occupational, or other important areas of functioning, and not be better explained by intellectual disability or global developmental delay alone. In other words, to make the diagnosis of autism spectrum disorder, the level of impairment in social functioning and restricted/repetitive behaviors should be out of proportion to that which would be expected based on the overall level of functioning.

Autism spectrum disorder and intellectual disability frequently co-occur. In addition, there is a high comorbidity of other neurobehavioral and neuropsychiatric disorders with autism spectrum disorder, eg, epilepsy, anxiety, attention-deficit/hyperactivity disorder, bipolar disorder, or obsessive-compulsive disorder. Regression is reported in up to 30% of cases of autism spectrum disorder, but typically only refers to loss of communication skills and previously acquired words. As is the case for intellectual disability, regression deserves clinical attention whenever it is more pronounced and dramatic, and the differential diagnosis should then include metabolic disorders and neurodegenerative conditions.

## GENERAL APPROACH TO DIAGNOSIS AND FIRST-TIER TESTING

The diagnostic evaluation of all children with intellectual disability and/or autism spectrum disorder should include a complete neurologic and dysmorphologic examination (Fig. 173-2). The majority of cases of intellectual disability and/or autism spectrum disorder are nondysmorphic and without any major congenital malformations. The clinical appearance of the affected individuals does not suggest a specific molecular diagnosis. They would therefore be considered as having "idiopathic" nonsyndromic developmental delay/intellectual disability. The diagnostic workup of individuals with idiopathic developmental delay/intellectual disability and individuals with idiopathic autism spectrum disorder has been the subject of recommendations and practice guidelines by some of the major professional societies, such as the American College of Medical Genetics and the American Academy of Pediatrics. In both cases, chromosome microarray should

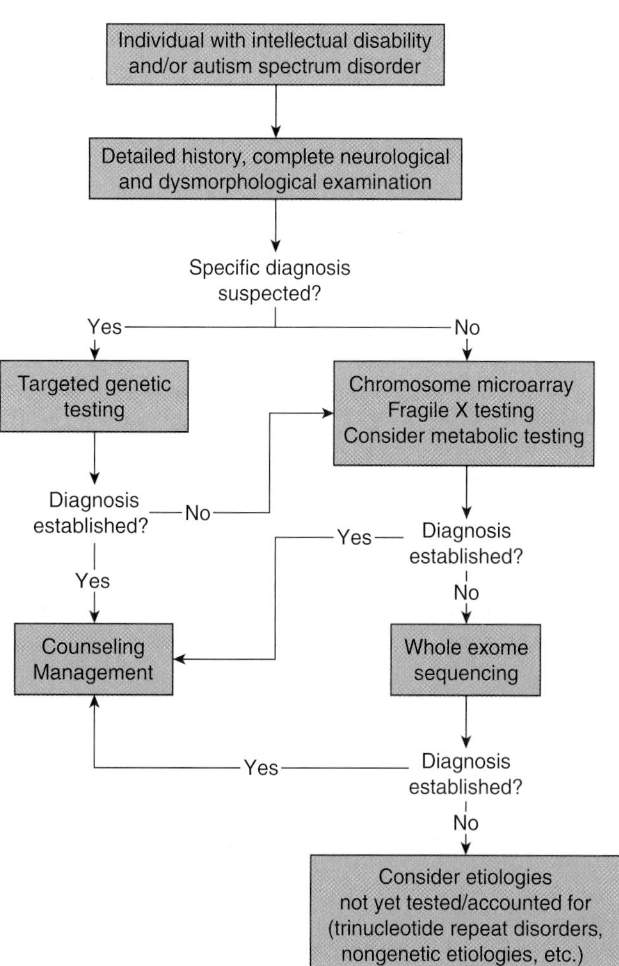


**FIGURE 173-2** Diagnostic algorithm for intellectual disability and/or autism spectrum disorder.

be ordered as a first-tier diagnostic test. Importantly, chromosome microarray testing replaces the standard karyotype analysis and fluorescent in situ hybridization (FISH) subtelomere tests, due to its greater sensitivity and therefore greater diagnostic yield. In addition, DNA testing for fragile X syndrome should be performed routinely on all male individuals with intellectual disability and/or autism spectrum disorder.

A diagnostic workup for inborn errors of metabolism may not be necessary or cost-efficient in all patients with intellectual disability, especially given the large number of conditions that would be identified by expanded newborn screening. However, certain clinical symptoms should always prompt diagnostic testing for metabolic or mitochondrial disorders. These include acid-base or electrolyte disturbances, anemia with elevated mean corpuscular volume, cyclic vomiting, developmental regression (especially when in the context of illness or fever), hypotonia/dystonia, lactic acidosis, lethargy, multisystem involvement (especially cardiac, hepatic or renal), poor growth, microcephaly, or seizures. A metabolic screening evaluation would typically include a complete blood count, a serum metabolic profile, serum amino acid analysis, urine organic acid analysis, and urine screening for glycosaminoglycans. When in doubt, a referral to a metabolic genetic specialist should be considered.

## SPECIFIC DIAGNOSES

Whenever specific clinical findings exist, then those should be considered in an attempt to establish a specific differential diagnosis.

Down syndrome is the single most common genetic cause of intellectual disability. In the presence of the typical clinical features, eg, hypotonia, cardiac defects (present in 45% of cases), dysmorphic facial features (brachycephaly, flat facial profile, upslanting palpebral fissures, epicanthal folds, small mouth), or single palmar crease, targeted diagnostic testing should be attempted. For Down syndrome, the best diagnostic test would be standard chromosome analysis (karyotype).

Fragile X syndrome represents one of the most common monogenic causes of intellectual disability and autism spectrum disorder. It is caused by trinucleotide (CGG) repeat expansion in the 5′ untranslated region of the *FMR1* gene on the X chromosome. Clinical features that can help distinguish fragile X syndrome from other forms of intellectual disability or autism spectrum disorder include relative macrocephaly, typical craniofacial symptoms, such as a long face with prominent forehead, prognathism (large jaw), and large ears. Macroorchidism is typically present in boys with fragile X syndrome, starting at the beginning of puberty.

Rett syndrome should be considered in girls with acquired microcephaly, developmental regression, and loss of purposeful hand movements (which typically occurs between age 6 months and 2.5 years). The latter are replaced by stereotypical hand movements that have been described as washing and kneading. Rett syndrome is an X-linked disorder caused by mutations in the *MECP2* gene (point mutations or deletions). The human brain is quite sensitive to *MECP2* dosage, and duplications involving the *MECP2* gene in males cause *MECP2* duplication syndrome, a severe neurodevelopmental disorder characterized by infantile hypotonia, developmental delay/intellectual disability, progressive spasticity, seizures, and recurrent respiratory infections.

Genetic testing for mutations in the *PTEN* gene should be considered among individuals with autism spectrum disorder and head circumferences greater than 2.5 standard deviations above the mean.

Tuberous sclerosis can be the cause of intellectual disability and/or autism spectrum disorder. Affected individuals most commonly manifest refractory epilepsy. Typical skin changes (hypopigmented ash-leaf spots, facial angiofibromas, subungual or periungual fibromas) can be the key to making the diagnosis. Tuberous sclerosis is caused by mutations affecting the *TSC1* or *TSC2* genes.

Angelman syndrome is a severe neurodevelopmental disorder that manifests global developmental delay/intellectual disability. Many affected individuals meet criteria for autism spectrum disorder. Absent speech, epilepsy, ataxia in combination with truncal hypotonia, microcephaly, obsession with water, and a happy demeanor with seemingly inappropriate laughter may suggest this specific diagnosis. Angelman syndrome is caused by lack of a maternally inherited normal copy of the *UBE3A* gene. While 70% of cases are caused by microdeletion of this region on chromosome 15q12, and would be detected by chromosome microarray analysis, cases caused by paternal uniparental disomy or point mutations in *UBE3A* would not be detected by array comparative genomic hybridization (the most commonly used type of chromosome microarray), and require methylation analysis and *UBE3A* sequence analysis.

Other chromosome microdeletion and microduplication syndromes commonly identified by chromosome microarray analysis in the context of intellectual disability and/or autism spectrum disorder are 16p11.2 deletion syndrome, 1q21.1 duplication, Smith-Magenis syndrome (17p11.2 deletion) and its reciprocal duplication (Potocki-Lupski syndrome), and Williams syndrome (7q11.23 deletion) and its reciprocal duplication (7q11.23 duplication syndrome). The latter provide one of the rare examples in which deletion and duplication of a given chromosome locus have opposite effects on social behavior. Individuals with Williams syndrome are unusually friendly and sociable, whereas individuals with duplication of the same locus manifest a high prevalence of autism spectrum disorder.

Whenever a unique combination of clinical features exists but does not suggest a specific diagnosis to the examiner, then online tools and software programs may be used to help establish a differential diagnosis (see Chapter 168). The Online Mendelian Inheritance in Man (OMIM) is one of those databases, as it allows searching for genetic conditions by symptoms/features and combinations thereof (www.omim.org). The more unusual and the more rare a specific clinical symptom, the more powerful it is in narrowing down the potential differential diagnoses.

## SECOND-TIER TESTING

When intellectual disability and/or autism spectrum disorder is idiopathic, and first-tier testing does not establish a diagnosis, then second-tier testing should be attempted. The test with the greatest diagnostic yield is whole-exome sequencing (see Chapter 167), ideally carried out as trio whole-exome sequencing, ie, whole-exome sequencing of the proband/patient and both biological parents. This approach allows filtering all sequence variants by their inheritance status (de novo vs inherited). The diagnostic yield of trio whole-exome sequencing in mixed patient populations of neurodevelopmental disorders is approximately 25% to 50%.

A diagnostic approach and algorithm to the patient presenting with intellectual disability and/or autism spectrum disorder is presented in Figure 173-2. In several syndromes and conditions (eg, fragile X syndrome, Prader-Willi syndrome, Angelman syndrome), the recognizable physical and behavioral phenotype evolves over time ("the patient *grows into* the phenotype"). Serial evaluations, follow-up visits, and reassessments therefore represent an important approach to the patient with intellectual disability. They may help confirm diagnostic suspicions, restructure the differential diagnosis, or eliminate certain diagnoses previously considered. In addition to clinical reassessments, the molecular diagnostic laboratories are encouraged to reanalyze whole-exome sequencing data periodically, to incorporate newly discovered human disease genes and genotype-phenotype correlations. Eventually, this leads to a definitive molecular diagnosis in a subset of patients, even without additional molecular genetic testing.

## TREATMENT

For both developmental delay/intellectual disability and autism spectrum disorder, early recognition and initiation of early intervention treatment services are key to improving the affected child's development. A referral for assessment of eligibility of early intervention services should be made for every child who is at risk and every child suspected to manifest developmental delay and/or autism spectrum disorder. This referral does not require a definitive, let alone molecular diagnosis, but initiates the formal evaluation process and access to resources when needed. Based on the deficits identified in the individual child, a therapeutic intervention plan is devised, which may include physical therapy, occupational therapy, speech therapy, and others.

## AUTISM SPECTRUM DISORDER

In the context of autism spectrum disorder, behavior and communication approaches that provide structure, direction, and organization for the affected child and that encourage family participation have proven beneficial. One of the most popular and successful treatment approaches is applied behavior analysis (ABA). ABA encourages positive behaviors and discourages negative behaviors in order to improve a variety of skills. Another therapy that has been applied widely is the Developmental, Individual Differences, Relationship-Based Approach (DIR, also called "Floortime"), which focuses on emotional and relational development (feelings, relationships with caregivers). It also addresses how the child deals with visual, auditory, and olfactory stimuli. There are currently no US Food and Drug Administration–approved drugs that treat the core symptoms of autism spectrum disorder (communication deficits, social deficits, restricted and repetitive behaviors). The only 2 medications currently approved with an indication of autism spectrum disorder are risperidone and aripiprazole. They have been approved for autism-related irritability.

## SPECIFIC TREATMENTS BASED ON THE MOLECULAR DIAGNOSIS

Only a few disorders associated with intellectual disability or autism spectrum disorder can be treated with well-established treatment regimens. Examples of such disorders include congenital hypothyroidism and phenylketonuria, both of which are detected by newborn screening. Disorders of creatine metabolism, ie, guanidinoacetate methyltransferase (GAMT) deficiency and arginine:glycine amidinotransferase (AGAT) deficiency, are at least partially treatable with high oral doses of creatine supplementation, with improved developmental outcomes, especially when treatment is started early. Other examples, especially in the area of inborn errors of metabolism, do exist.

## BENEFITS

Even when specific treatments are not available, the power of a molecular diagnosis should not be underappreciated. Identifying the exact molecular cause of intellectual disability and/or autism spectrum disorder can end "diagnostic odysseys" and prevent the patient from having additional, unnecessary tests and interventions. It can help the family with coping. It empowers them and the medical provider by allowing them to focus their effort and interest on a more specific disease entity. Understanding the natural course of the disease and obtaining some anticipatory guidance based on published literature may be important. For example, deletions of chromosome 16p11.2 are one of the more commonly identified causes of intellectual disability and autistic features. Due to an increased prevalence of cardiac malformations among individuals with 16p11.2 deletion, an echocardiogram is recommended whenever that deletion is identified. Also, individuals with 16p11.2 are at significantly increased risk for being overweight and having obesity. This typically only develops during adolescence and becomes a major challenge during adulthood. Therefore, healthy eating habits and an active lifestyle are encouraged from a young age.

Beyond medical management, a specific diagnosis allows patients and their families to connect with others affected with the same disorder, eg, via family support groups or social media. Lastly, it helps families understand the chances of recurrence for their future children and the offspring of their already existing healthy and affected children.

## PREVENTION

Generally speaking, most cases of intellectual disability and/or autism spectrum disorder cannot be prevented. There are a few exceptions to the rule, eg, fetal alcohol syndrome or maternal phenylketonuria. Also, expanded newborn screening allows the identification of a few dozen inborn errors of metabolism, many of which will compromise cognitive and social development when left untreated. Phenylketonuria is a classic example; when recognized early and treated appropriately (by phenylalanine-restricted diet and supplementation of essential amino acids and trace elements), patients will have normal development and intelligence, but when left untreated, it causes severe to profound intellectual disability, seizure disorder, and spasticity.

Once the genetic cause of intellectual disability or autism spectrum disorder has been identified in a given patient, the family should receive genetic counseling regarding the chance of recurrence in future children to the patient's biological parents, potential future children of the patient, and other family members. Depending on the genetic cause and the associated inheritance pattern, prenatal genetic testing and/or preimplantation genetic diagnosis may be an option. These technologies, and the associated ethical implications, can be discussed by a genetic counselor with the respective couple, ideally prior to conception.

## SUGGESTED READINGS


Bhat S, Acharya UR, Adeli H, Bairy GM, Adeli A. Autism: cause factors, early diagnosis and therapies. *Rev Neurosci.* 2014;25:841-850.

Lupski JR. Cognitive phenotypes and genomic copy number variations. *JAMA.* 2015;313:2029-2030.

Michelson DJ, Shevell MI, Sherr EH, et al. Evidence report: genetic and metabolic testing on children with global developmental delay: report of the Quality Standards Subcommittee of the American Academy of Neurology and the Practice Committee of the Child Neurology Society. *Neurology.* 2011;77:1629-1635.

Miles JH. Autism spectrum disorders: a genetics review. *Genet Med.* 2011;13:278-294.

Miller DT, Adam MP, Aradhya S, et al. Consensus statement: chromosomal microarray is a first-tier clinical diagnostic test for individuals with developmental disabilities or congenital anomalies. *Am J Hum Genet.* 2010;86:749-764.

Moeschler JB, Shevell M. Committee on Genetics. Comprehensive evaluation of the child with intellectual disability or global developmental delays. *Pediatrics.* 2014;134:e903-e918.

South ST, Lee C, Lamb AN, et al. ACMG Standards and Guidelines for constitutional cytogenomic microarray analysis, including postnatal and prenatal applications: revision 2013. *Genet Med.* 2013;15:901-909.

Tarailo-Graovac M, Shyr C, Ross CJ, et al. Exome sequencing and the management of neurometabolic disorders. *N Engl J Med.* 2016;374:2246-2255.

Yang Y, Muzny DM, Reid JG, et al. Clinical whole-exome sequencing for the diagnosis of mendelian disorders. *N Engl J Med.* 2013;369:1502-1511.


# 174 Hearing Loss

Bryan Liming, Iram Ahmad, and Richard J.H. Smith

## INTRODUCTION

Hearing is the perception and interpretation of biologically relevant acoustic information. The external, middle, and inner parts of the ear are responsible for sound detection and transduction into electrical signals. These signals are transmitted to the brain by the auditory nerve for central auditory processing. Hearing impairment can be associated with a variety of factors including genetics, age, trauma, drugs, and infections. In children, hearing loss is of particular clinical interest because it significantly impacts language acquisition and has lifelong implications that affect the cognitive, behavioral, and social development of a child. While its diagnosis and treatment are challenging in resource-constrained areas, childhood hearing loss remains a serious global health issue.

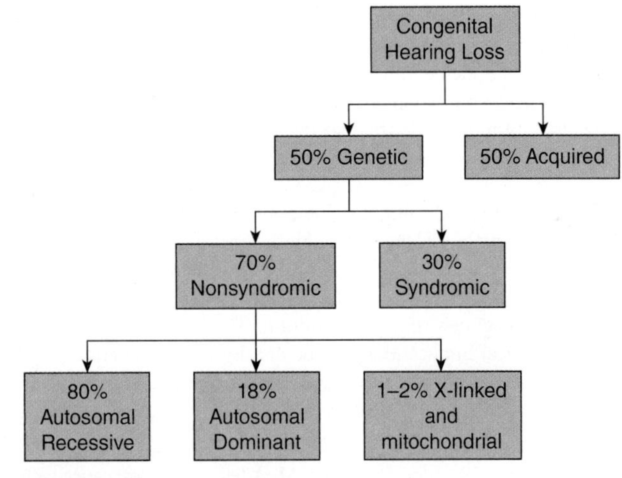


**FIGURE 174-1** Etiology of congenital hearing loss.

## EPIDEMIOLOGY

Hearing loss is the most prevalent sensory impairment in children. Worldwide, its prevalence at the severe-to-profound level is 4 in every 10,000 infants, although the number of infants with hearing loss detected by universal newborn screening programs is higher in developed countries, likely reflecting increased access to early screening. Children with moderate-to-profound degrees of hearing loss can be identified by early screening and targeted for appropriate intervention.

About 50% of newborns with hearing loss have a genetic basis for their loss, although in developed countries, this percentage rises to approximately 70%; in the remainder, the hearing loss is attributed to environmental factors (Fig. 174-1). Hearing loss, once diagnosed, is described as syndromic or nonsyndromic, depending on whether the loss occurs in isolation or is associated with concurrent clinical findings. Of genetic hearing loss, 70% is nonsyndromic and 30% is syndromic. By severity, hearing loss is graded as mild, moderate, severe, or profound, a classification based on a quantitative assessment of sound intensity measured in decibels and recorded as an audiogram (Table 174-1).

## PATHOGENESIS AND MECHANISMS OF AUDITORY PERCEPTION

Auditory perception is a complex process whereby acoustic signals from the environment are transduced by the auditory system into electrical signals that are interpreted by the brain and allow humans to interact with the acoustic environment. Acoustic energy enters the external auditory canal and vibrates the tympanic membrane where it is converted to mechanical energy. The mechanical energy is transferred from the tympanic membrane through the ossicular chain (malleus, incus, and stapes) to the inner ear. Vibration of the stapedial footplate at the oval window displaces fluid in the cochlea, leading to hair cell stimulation and depolarization. An electrical signal is transmitted from inner ear hair cells to the dendrites of the neurons that have cell bodies in the central portion of the cochlea. These cell bodies unite to form the cochlear nerve (cranial nerve VIII), which transmits this signal to the brain stem and then to central processing centers.

## TYPES OF HEARING LOSS

Hearing loss is categorized by time of onset, location of auditory pathway dysfunction, and type of loss. In principle, the 2 primary types of hearing loss are conductive hearing loss and sensorineural hearing loss; however, a third type, auditory neuropathy spectrum disorder, is of interest in at-risk children.

**TABLE 174-1 LEVELS OF HEARING LOSS**

| Severity | Hearing Loss |
|---|---|
| Mild | 20–40 dB |
| Moderate | 40–55 dB |
| Severe | 70–90 dB |
| Profound | > 90 dB |

**TABLE 174-2 CLASSIFICATION OF HEARING LOSS**

| Variable | Classification | |
|---|---|---|
| Time of onset | Congenital | Late onset |
| Language acquisition/age | Prelingual | Postlingual |
| Laterality | Unilateral | Bilateral |
| Severity of loss | Mild, moderate, severe, profound | |
| Type of loss | Conductive | Sensorineural |
| Genetics | Syndromic | Nonsyndromic |
| Inheritance | Recessive | Dominant |
| Etiology | Environmental | Genetic |
| Anatomic | External, middle, inner ear anomaly | |

### Temporal Classification of Hearing Loss

Prelingual hearing loss is present at birth or is detected shortly thereafter, before a child has acquired speech and language skills. It can be acquired or genetic. Postlingual hearing loss, in comparison, occurs after acquisition of language.

### Conductive Hearing Loss

Conductive hearing loss (CHL) occurs when pathology of the external ear, external auditory canal, tympanic membrane, middle ear, or ossicles prevents sound transmission to the cochlea. In a systematic fashion, one can assess conductive hearing loss by evaluating each of the points along the auditory pathway. For example, a congenital external ear deformity, mass in the external ear canal, cerumen impaction, or congenital atresia of the canal blocks sound transmission to the tympanic membrane, while a perforation of the tympanic membrane reduces vibration and the transmission of mechanical energy to the inner ear. The most common cause of CHL is fluid in the middle ear cavity (otitis media) (Table 174-2).

### Sensorineural Hearing Loss

Sensorineural hearing loss (SNHL) refers to dysfunction in components of hearing required for transduction of signal in the cochlea to central auditory processing centers in the brain. Hair cell dysfunction, cochlear malformations, eighth nerve malformations, and higher levels of auditory dysfunction are common causes of SNHL. See also Chapter 364 for a physiologic consideration of the ear and hearing.

### Congenital Hearing Loss

Congenital hearing loss is prelingual by definition and is either acquired or inherited. Inherited hearing loss is subclassified as nonsyndromic hearing loss (NSHL; 70%) or syndromic hearing loss (SHL; 30%), and then further subclassified based on inheritance pattern. Most congenital NSHL segregates as an autosomal recessive trait (ARNSHL), although autosomal dominant NSHL (ADNSHL) and X-linked and mitochondrial forms of hearing loss also occur (see Fig. 174-1).

### Environmental/Acquired Hearing Loss

Environmental factors that cause hearing loss vary from infections to toxins. Intrauterine infections account for about 8% of congenital hearing loss. The infections denoted by the TORCHES acronym include toxoplasmosis, rubella, cytomegalovirus (CMV), herpes simplex virus (HSV), and syphilis. Several additional infections are implicated in congenital hearing loss such as HIV, enteroviruses, Lyme disease, and Zika virus.

The most common infectious cause of congenital hearing loss is congenital CMV. Congenital CMV is transmitted from mother to infant in utero and affects 1 in 150 infants born in the United States. If the mother is asymptomatic, detection of congenitally acquired CMV is challenging. Symptomatic CMV, however, presents with the classic symptoms of hepatosplenomegaly, thrombocytopenia, petechial rash, and hypotonia and is diagnosed in about 1 in 1500 births. The remaining CMV-affected infants have so-called asymptomatic CMV; 5% to 15% of these infants will go on to develop some neurologic sequelae, which may include SNHL and/or neurocognitive impairments. It has been estimated that CMV causes up to 25% of all hearing loss present at age 4.

Perinatal or postnatal meningitis also causes hearing loss. Bacterial meningitis results in inflammation of the cochlea and SNHL in about 10% of children.

Exposure to ototoxic medications is another cause of acquired hearing loss. Aminoglycosides are frequently used in the neonatal intensive care unit population and are known to be ototoxic. Gentamicin, for example, is a widely available aminoglycoside antibiotic with strong activity against multidrug-resistant organisms. It is inexpensive and internationally available, and its use is endorsed by a World Health Organization subcommittee report when a definite indication is identified and drug levels are monitored. Babies who have inherited the mitochondrial 12S rRNA A1555G mutation are genetically predisposed to aminoglycoside-induced ototoxicity.

#### Auditory Neuropathy Spectrum Disorder

Auditory neuropathy spectrum disorder (ANSD) deserves special consideration due to challenges in its diagnosis and management. ANSD occurs when outer hair cell function is intact but the auditory brain stem response is abnormal. Like SNHL, ANSD can be genetic or acquired. Genetic cases are further subdivided into syndromic or nonsyndromic ANSD. The most common cause of nonsyndromic ANSD is mutations in the *OTOF* (DFNB9) gene. Syndromic forms of ANSD include Friedreich ataxia and Charcot-Marie-Tooth (CMT) disease. CMT deserves special mention as it is a genetically and phenotypically variable disease with over 50 known associated genes. A disease of peripheral nerve structure and function, some forms of CMT may have hearing loss as a prominent feature. Recognition of the hearing loss component may facilitate early diagnosis.

Acquired ANSD is associated with prematurity, hypoxia, and hyperbilirubinemia, and may be transient or permanent, and stable or progressive. Hearing levels often fluctuate over time, and thus as a whole, ANSD behaves differently from one child to the next.

## CLINICAL MANIFESTATIONS OF HEARING LOSS

#### Syndromic Hearing Loss

When a child presents with hearing loss and a constellation of other clinical findings, a syndromic form of hearing loss is likely. Syndromic hearing loss makes up approximately one-third of hereditary hearing loss (see Fig. 174-1). Syndromic hearing loss is subclassified by inheritance pattern. The more common types of syndromic hearing loss are described.

**Autosomal Dominant Syndromes** Waardenburg syndrome is one of the most common types of autosomal dominant syndromic hearing loss (ADSHL). Of the 4 types of Waardenburg syndrome that are recognized, the most common is Waardenburg syndrome type 1. Caused by mutations in the *PAX3* gene, it is characterized by heterochromia irides, dystopia canthorum, a white forelock, synophrys, and unilateral or bilateral SNHL. Waardenburg syndrome type 2 is also common. It is caused by mutations in the *MITF* gene and, with the exception of the dystopia canthorum, is phenotypically similar to Waardenburg syndrome type 1. Waardenburg syndrome type 3 and type 4 are rare.

Branchio-oto-renal (BOR) syndrome is a second very common type of ADSHL. Clinical findings include ear pits, cervical fistulae, and renal anomalies (agenesis to dysplasia). The hearing loss can be sensorineural (20%), conductive (30%), or mixed (50%). The most commonly implicated gene is *EYA1*.

Distinctive facial features that reflect underdevelopment of the first and second branchial arches characterize Treacher-Collins syndrome, a third example of ADSHL. The result is midface and mandibular hypoplasia, lower eyelid colobomas, and downslanting palpebral fissures. The hearing loss is most frequently conductive due to anomalous development of the ossicular chain.

The final common example of ADSHL is Stickler syndrome. Affected children have cleft palate, myopia, and a Marfanoid habitus. Their hearing loss is sensorineural or mixed. Midface and mandibular hypoplasia is also common. Of the 3 types of Stickler syndrome, the most common, Stickler syndrome type 1, is caused by mutations of *COL2A1*.



**Autosomal Recessive Syndromes** Usher syndrome, the most common autosomal recessive syndromic hearing loss (ARSHL), affects 50% of the deaf and blind population in the United States. Three types of Usher syndrome are recognized—type 1, type 2, and type 3—differentiated from each other by the degree of hearing loss, the presence or absence of vestibular dysfunction, and the age of onset of retinitis pigmentosa (RP). In general, Usher syndrome type 1 is associated with severe-to-profound hearing loss, vestibular areflexia (and delayed developmental milestones), and the onset of RP in the early teenage years. In Usher syndrome type 2, vestibular function is normal, the hearing loss is moderate to severe, and the RP tends to develop later. Usher syndrome type 3 is characterized by progressive hearing loss and is the most common cause of the deaf-blindness in Finland.

A second common type of ARSHL is Pendred syndrome, which includes profound bilateral SNHL and thyroid goiter. The syndrome arises from a defect in pendrin, a protein that is transcribed from the *SLC26A4* gene and functions as an ion symporter. Defective transport of bicarbonate in the inner ear and of iodine in the thyroid gland leads to the hearing loss and thyroid dysfunction. On temporal bone computed tomography, specific inner ear findings such as Mondini dysplasia (incomplete partitioning and reduced number of turns of the cochlea) or dilated vestibular aqueduct are seen. The euthyroid goiter is often clinically evident in the early teenage years.

**X-Linked Syndromes** Alport syndrome, caused by mutations in the *COL4A5* gene, is 1 form of X-linked syndromic hearing loss. Although autosomal recessive and dominant forms of this syndrome exist, greater than 80% are X-linked. *COL4A5* (and *COL4A3* and *COL4A4*) encodes type IV collagen and the phenotypic dysfunction in Alport syndrome is related to defective glomerular filtration in the kidneys, abnormal retinal structure, and degeneration of structures within the cochlea (stria vascularis and spiral ligament). Hearing loss often does not manifest until the second decade of life and is then progressive in nature. End-stage renal disease occurs in many patients.



#### Nonsyndromic Hearing Loss

Children with NSHL do not have additional physical findings that co-segregate with the hearing loss. The majority (75–80%) of NSHL is recessive, with mutations in connexin 26 (*GJB2*) accounting for about half of all autosomal recessive NSHL that is severe to profound in degree. Determining the genetic cause of hearing loss is critical to the comprehensive diagnosis and treatment of a child with hearing impairment. With the advent of new sequencing strategies, targeted genomic enrichment with massive parallel sequencing has become the most cost-effective test after an audiogram to obtain in the evaluation of deafness. At this time, 134 deafness loci have been identified.

#### Other Clinical Manifestations of Hearing Loss

External ear malformations are associated with hearing loss and, in 30% of cases, imply the presence of a syndrome. Anomalies can involve the shape, size, orientation, and projection of the pinna. Complete absence of an external ear is known as anotia, whereas partial loss is referred to as microtia. Other external ear malformations include accessory tragus, ear tags, and pits.

Middle ear anomalies include fusion, malformation, or disease of the ossicles. The middle ear space can also be poorly aerated, and the oval and/or round windows can be absent. Understanding the anomaly in exquisite detail is required if surgical correction of the hearing loss is offered to these children.

Inner ear malformations typically reflect anomalies in early embryogenesis. Abnormal cochlea, semicircular canals, aplasia of the cochlear nerve, and hypoplasia of the cochlear nerve have been described. Identification of the specific malformation is required for development of the appropriate treatment plan for the child.

#### Late-Onset Hearing Loss

The Federal Government mandates newborn hearing screening (NBHS), and NBHS is now offered in some form in all 50 states. Requirements and coverage vary, but overall, it is estimated that greater than 90% of infants born in the United States receive some form of NBHS. Because hearing loss can develop later, follow-up programs are essential. For example, CMV-associated hearing loss can be progressive and may not be apparent until preschool age or later, and chronic otitis media, which can significantly impact hearing, is a disease of early childhood.

Parents are often the initial persons to express concern about childhood hearing loss. These concerns must be evaluated with a full otologic exam and audiometry. Cues to possible hearing loss include delayed or missed developmental milestones especially in the speech and language category, academic difficulties, behavioral problems, and perceived inattentiveness. Older children may self-report hearing loss, especially if it is relatively rapid in onset.

## DIAGNOSIS

#### Newborn Hearing Screening

Newborn screening protocols are derived from consensus recommendations published by the Joint Committee on Infant Hearing; however, protocols vary between institutions and states. Infants categorized as "high risk for congenital hearing loss" are at a higher risk for ANSD and should be screened with both otoacoustic emissions (OAEs) and automated auditory brain stem response (ABR) testing to evaluate both outer hair cell and inner hair cell function. Factors that place an infant in this category include congenital infections (ie, TORCHES infections), birthweight less than 1500 g, hyperbilirubinemia requiring exchange transfusion, exposure to ototoxic medications (eg, aminoglycoside antibiotics), bacterial meningitis, mechanical ventilation > 5 days, head trauma, neurodegenerative disorders, neonatal intensive care unit stay greater than 5 days, and family history of hearing loss (Table 174-3).

Infants not in the high-risk category can be screened with a 2-stage procedure that utilizes OAEs alone as the initial screening test, with an automated ABR if the OAE response is absent or subthreshold. A child who fails screening protocols should undergo a confirmatory diagnostic ABR performed by an experienced audiologist. Since newborn hearing screening protocols are designed to detect hearing losses in the moderate to profound range (< 40 dB HL), mild hearing loss (20–40 dB HL) may go undetected.

#### History and Physical Examination

As with any diagnostic endeavor, the first step is a thorough and focused history. History should focus on the aforementioned risk factors as well as any family history of hearing loss. In the older child, a history must include an assessment of developmental milestones—especially related to speech and language acquisition. A noise exposure history may also be relevant, especially in a child presenting in adolescence.

The physical examination is an important part of the evaluation of suspected or identified hearing loss. The physical examination may reveal signs consistent with syndromic hearing loss (branchial cleft abnormalities, craniofacial dysmorphisms, syndromic features, or ocular abnormalities). Additionally, the entire auditory apparatus should be examined for abnormalities of the pinna, external auditory canal, tympanic membrane, and middle ear structures. Finally, a thorough examination should address vestibular function, as the majority of children with profound SNHL will have an element of vestibular dysfunction.

**TABLE 174-3 RISK FACTORS FOR CONGENITAL HEARING LOSS**

- TORCHES infections
- Birth weight < 1500 g
- Hyperbilirubinemia requiring exchange transfusion
- Ototoxic medications > 5 days
- Bacterial meningitis
- Mechanical ventilation > 5 days
- Head trauma
- Neurodegenerative disorders
- Neonatal intensive care unit stay > 5 days
- Family history of hearing loss

#### Evaluation of Older Children With Hearing Loss

Older children with suspected hearing loss should undergo a full diagnostic audiologic evaluation that includes threshold sensitivity of pure tones for both air and bone conduction, speech reception thresholds, speech discrimination testing, and acoustic immittance testing. For children, some aspects of the full battery may be truncated or skipped based on the child's ability to cooperate and participate.

When measuring pure tone thresholds, ear-specific information may be difficult to obtain in younger children. Soundfield data provide information regarding the "better hearing" ear. For example, visual reinforcement audiometry (VRA) can be performed in children as young as 6 months. In this technique, a sound is presented in a sound field or through insert phones and the child's response is reinforced by a visual stimulus. For slightly older children, conditioned play audiometry (CPA) is used. In this technique, a child is "conditioned" to perform a play task in response to a sound. When adequate conditioning is not possible, a diagnostic ABR should be done.

Speech threshold and discrimination testing provide a better assessment of a child's ability to understand speech. Speech threshold testing measures a child's ability to hear words as opposed to pure tone sounds, while speech discrimination testing assesses the ability to hear *and* identify words. These tests are important if ANSD is being considered as speech perception may be impaired to a greater degree than pure tone thresholds.

Acoustic immittance testing is also part of the test battery and includes tympanometry and acoustic reflex testing. The former is an impedance test to measure ear canal volume and tympanic membrane compliance. Tympanic membrane compliance is reduced with otitis media, which also typically causes a CHL. Acoustic reflex testing measures the response of the stapedius muscle to high-intensity sounds and is absent or diminished in ANSD, thus providing another clue to this diagnosis.

#### Genetic Testing and Imaging

A child with bilateral SNHL should receive comprehensive genetic testing, as this type of evaluation provides the highest diagnostic rate of any test in the evaluation of hearing loss. A genetic cause of hearing loss can be identified in up to 60% of children (dependent on ethnic background and the specific gene panel). This information is prognostically useful. For example, if a child with moderate hearing loss is found to have mutations in the *STRC* gene, it becomes possible to prognosticate progression of hearing loss for this family by looking at data compiled on all persons with *STRC*-associated hearing loss that graphs average hearing thresholds per decade on a single audiogram. This process is called "audioprofiling." Another example is the child with severe to profound hearing loss caused by mutations in *GJB2*. Studies have shown that these children perform exceptionally well with cochlear implants. As the field of genomic medicine advances, habilitation options for hearing loss will be guided by genetic diagnoses.

When testing reveals ANSD, the child should also be offered comprehensive genetic testing as approximately 50% of ANSD is genetic. Temporal bone imaging is optional, although up to two-thirds of children with ANSD will have imaging abnormalities like cochlear nerve deficiency, brain abnormalities, or cochlear dysplasias.

If a comprehensive genetic test using NSHL gene panels is negative, whole-exome sequencing (WES) may be considered; furthermore, physical findings may prompt a genetic referral and consideration for directed genetic testing. If the genetic consultation is negative or if there are no additional physical findings, consideration should be given to CMV. Testing for congenital CMV is not currently standardized. CMV can be reliably detected in saliva or urine by polymerase chain reaction during the first 3 weeks of life. Thereafter, blood spot CMV testing can be considered if the neonatal blood spots are available.

When a child with unilateral sensorineural hearing loss is identified, comprehensive genetic testing is not indicated, as the diagnostic rate is extremely low. Temporal bone imaging should be considered to rule out a unilateral abnormality of the bony labyrinth or the cochlear nerve. In cases of severe-to-profound unilateral loss, imaging identifies cochlear nerve abnormalities in nearly half of patients.

Temporal bone imaging is not indicated for the diagnosis of bilateral SNHL, although it is optional if genetic testing is negative. In general, imaging via high-resolution computed tomography (HRCT) or magnetic resonance imaging (MRI) has a diagnostic yield of 25% to 30%. It is also optional in the workup of children with unilateral hearing loss or ANSD. Imaging is indicated in cochlear implant candidates to evaluate for cochleovestibular anomalies, which may affect candidacy for implantation as well as surgical planning. The choice of MRI versus HRCT varies among implant surgeons.

## TREATMENT

### Early Intervention

Regardless of the cause or the severity of hearing loss, all children with hearing loss should be followed closely by a team of childhood communication specialists to ensure that appropriate habilitation is provided and that any progression is discovered. Services should include, at a minimum, an audiologist, pediatric otolaryngologist, speech-language pathologist, early intervention specialists, social workers, community support interventionalists, and teachers trained to work with deaf and hard-of-hearing individuals. Early intervention (EI) services are federally mandated through the Individuals with Disabilities Act. The team may be institutionally based and co-located or may be fragmented, with some individuals in the regional healthcare system, local school system, or community support agency.

### Amplification

The diagnostic and interventional time lines targeted by the National Institutes of Health Consensus Conference and the Joint Committee on Infant Hearing are 3 months for diagnosis and 6 months for appropriate intervention. Initial intervention, in addition to EI services, often includes fitting of hearing aids. Amplification should be mandatory in children with moderate-to-severe bilateral hearing loss (conductive or sensorineural) and in children with unilateral hearing loss, mild hearing loss, and ANSD. In children with at least moderate hearing loss, the benefits of hearing aids are clear. "Behind-the-ear" hearing aids are the style of choice as the ear is rapidly growing and this style allows for frequent adjustments of the ear mold. Behavioral interventions may be necessary to encourage consistent wear, and firm, persistent encouragement from parents improves compliance. For example, young children may have a difficult time adjusting to an unfamiliar object, and school-aged children may wrestle with the social stigma of hearing aids, especially if the degree of hearing loss is mild to moderate.

The benefits of amplification in children with unilateral or minimal to mild bilateral sensorineural hearing loss are unclear. While binaural hearing is important for sound localization and understanding speech in settings of high background noise, there is limited evidence that amplification of unilateral hearing loss or minimal to mild hearing loss improves outcomes. These children are at a high risk for speech-language and academic delays, cognitive deficits, and decreased quality of life relative to normal-hearing children. In addition, a child with unilateral or minimal to mild hearing loss may be more reluctant to comply with amplification given the lack of perception of a deficit. Private payer coverage for hearing aids in the setting of unilateral hearing loss is not universal, and thus, there may be a large financial barrier. Further complicating the matter is that in some locations, unilateral hearing loss does not qualify for EI programs. Options for rehabilitation of unilateral hearing loss include digital amplification and contralateral routing of signal (CROS) systems. In the CROS system, the sound signal is picked up from a microphone on one side of the head and then transmitted to the contralateral ear either wirelessly or electrically.



As mentioned, NBHS protocols are designed to detect moderate levels of hearing loss and thus may not detect children with mild hearing loss. These children are often identified later by school screening programs. Regardless of whether amplification is provided, these children must be closely monitored for evidence of speech language delay and academic impairment. In the classroom setting, preferential seating should be provided to all children with any degree of hearing loss to maximize the amount of information perceived. Frequency-modulated (FM) devices can be used, connected to a microphone worn by the teacher, to improve gain in the classroom setting.

With respect to ANSD, benefit from amplification is highly variable. Response to cochlear implantation may also be difficult to predict but should be an option.

### Treatment of Mixed or Conductive Loss

The child with mixed hearing loss or CHL must be treated expeditiously to ensure that any underlying SNHL is diagnosed and habilitated. A child older than 3 months with a CHL and middle ear effusion should undergo myringotomy and tympanostomy tube placement with sedated ABR to assess sensorineural hearing. A child under 3 months with an effusion should be reexamined in 3 months if the hearing loss is purely conductive and at 4 to 6 weeks if the loss is mixed. A persistent effusion mandates myringotomy and tympanostomy tube placement. SNHL should be evaluated as described earlier. Children with CHL related to congenital aural atresia or other anatomic abnormalities may benefit from bone-anchored osseointegrated hearing aids or CROS/biCROS aids.

### Cochlear Implantation

Referral for cochlear implant evaluation should be considered in children with profound, bilateral, sensorineural hearing loss (> 90 db HL). Although current US Food and Drug Administration–approved indications are for implantation at 12 months or older, many centers are performing implantation at ages less than 12 months with excellent results. If a child is thought to be a potential candidate for cochlear implantation, referral for evaluation should occur as soon as possible so that surgery can be scheduled as soon as implant criteria are met. Candidates usually undergo a trial period with a hearing aid, which should begin as per all recommended habilitation. In addition, specific developmental assessments may be used to determine candidacy.

In older children, cochlear implantation should be considered if hearing loss progresses to profound or if conventional amplification is not providing the needed benefit. Implantation should be considered in the child noted to have increasing difficulties in school and social situations with hearing aids tuned for maximum gain. If a child is known to have a genetic defect that will likely lead to a profound hearing loss, implantation may be performed prior to progression to this level.

It is important to remember that children with cochlear implants are at a higher risk for meningitis caused by *Streptococcus pneumoniae*. Thus all children with cochlear implants or preparing for implantation should receive the pneumococcal conjugate vaccine (PCV13) as per the recommended schedule. In addition, children older than 2 should receive 1 dose of the pneumococcal polysaccharide vaccine (PPSV23). In addition, careful attention should be given to ensure that all vaccinations are up to date in the cochlear implant candidate.

## TREATMENT OF CMV-ASSOCIATED HEARING LOSS

Treatment of CMV-associated hearing loss is an area of controversy. In infants with symptomatic CMV (defined by multisystem manifestations that include central nervous system, visual system, and auditory system), there is a clear benefit with regard to hearing and neurodevelopmental outcomes in treating with 6 months of valganciclovir. Some investigators have suggested that treatment for congenital CMV in which hearing loss is the only manifestation is also indicated; however, no randomized controlled trials support intervention in this circumstance.

Genomic medicine will lead to exciting new treatments for genetic causes of hearing loss. In the future, gene therapy may be used to regenerate functional hair cells within the cochlear epithelium, leading to restoration of natural hearing. Preclinical animal studies are under way, and human trials will likely begin in the next decade. Genetic treatments will revolutionize the treatment of congenital hearing loss.

## SUGGESTED READINGS

American Academy of Pediatrics: Year 2007 Position Statement: principles and guidelines for early hearing detection and intervention programs. *Pediatrics*. 2007;120(4):898-921.

Carvalho GM, Ramos P, Arthur C. Performance of cochlear implants in pediatric patients with auditory neuropathy spectrum disorder. *J Int Adv Otol*. 2016;12(1):8-15.

Cushing SL, Papsin BC. Taking the history and performing the physical examination in a child with hearing loss. *Otolaryngol Clin North Am*. 2015;48(6):903-912.

Goderis J, De Leenheer ED, Smets K. Hearing loss and congenital CMV infection: a systematic review. *Pediatrics*. 2014;134(5):972-982.

Jayawardena AD, Shearer AE, Smith RJH. Sensorineural hearing loss: a changing paradigm for its evaluation. *Otolaryng Head Neck Surg*. 2015;153(5):843-850.

Miranda-Filho Dde B, Martelli CM, Zimenes RA, et al. Initial description of the presumed congenital Zika syndrome. *Am J Public Health*. 2016;106(4):598-600.

Norrix LW, Velenovsky DS. Auditory neuropathy spectrum disorder: a review. *J Speech Language Hearing Res*. 2014;57(4):1564-1576.

Shearer AE, Black-Ziegelbein EA, Hildebrand MS, et al. Advancing genetic testing for deafness with genomic technology. *J Med Genet*. 2013;50:627-634.

Shearer AE, Smith RJH. Massively parallel sequencing for genetic diagnosis of hearing loss: the new standard of care. *Otolaryngol Head Neck Surg*. 2015;153(2):175-182.

Sloan Heggen CM, Bierer AO, Shearer AE, et al. Comprehensive genetic testing in the clinical evaluation of 1119 patients with hearing loss. *Hum Genet*. 2016;135(4):441-450.

Taylor KR, Booth KT, Azaiez H, et al. Audioprofile surfaces: the 21st century audiogram. *Ann Otol Rhinol Laryngol*. 2016;125(5):361-368.



# 175 Congenital Hypotonia

Davut Pehlivan and Fernando Scaglia

## INTRODUCTION

Congenital hypotonia is a relatively common, well-recognized entity that causes a diagnostic challenge for pediatricians due to a wide differential. Identification of the cause is crucial for determining the prognosis and possible early interventional options. Since the etiology is heterogeneous, a systematic approach to infants with hypotonia is necessary. In this chapter, we aim to give a general perspective of diseases that cause hypotonia and establish a diagnostic algorithm for infants who present with hypotonia.

## PATHOGENESIS AND EPIDEMIOLOGY

Tone is the amount of resistance/tension to stretch in a relaxed muscle, and hypotonia is the condition of low muscle tone leading to decreased postural control and movement against gravity. Thus, hypotonic infants present with poor control of movement and delayed motor skills later in life. It is important to distinguish hypotonia from weakness. Weakness is decreased maximum strength that can be generated by a muscle. Weakness is always associated with hypotonia, but hypotonia may exist without weakness.

The maintenance of normal muscle tone requires intact coordination of the brain, spinal cord, nerves, neuromuscular junction, and muscles. The spindle apparatus is the cytoskeletal structure that senses the stretch and sends impulses through the sensory nerve to the anterior horn of spinal cord. This information is transferred to the alpha motor neuron and then to the muscle under the control of the central nervous system. Disruption at any level of this pathway can cause hypotonia (Table 175-1). If the hypotonia is caused by cerebral reasons (brain and spinal cord lesion before synapse at the anterior horn cells), the term "central hypotonia" is used. Damage between the spinal cord anterior horn and muscle is called "peripheral hypotonia." A detailed neurologic exam can differentiate whether the hypotonia is of central origin, and thus localized to brain or spinal cord, versus that of peripheral origin and thus localized to spinal anterior horn disease, neuromuscular junction, and muscle.

Several studies have shown that central causes of hypotonia are far more common (60–80%) than peripheral causes (20–30%).

## CLINICAL MANIFESTATIONS

The first step in evaluating an infant with hypotonia is to obtain a detailed prenatal and birth history along with family history. The essential information regarding pregnancy history consists of fetal movements, presence of polyhydramnios/oligohydramnios, abnormal ultrasound findings, fetal position, maternal exposure to infections and maternal drug, alcohol, and medication use. Maternal exposure to infections, drugs, alcohol, and medications suggest a central cause, whereas decreased fetal movements and polyhydramnios elicit a potential underlying neuromuscular etiology.

Perinatal history should include fetal presentation at delivery, type of delivery, any birth trauma during delivery, Apgar scores, requirement for respiratory support, and feeding difficulty. Detailed birth history is usually important to rule out hypoxic ischemic encephalopathy (HIE) or exposure to medications and foods. A common reversible cause of hypotonia is due to magnesium administered for a preeclampsia delivery. If an otherwise normal full-term infant develops hypotonia after first feedings, an inborn error of metabolism should be considered.

The essential information regarding family history includes parental consanguinity, other family member(s) with hypotonia, neuromuscular disease, developmental delay/intellectual disability (DD/ID), seizure disorder, or any other neurologic or genetic disorders. Family history is paramount in making the diagnosis and for prognostication and counseling for future risks. For example, benign congenital hypotonia, which can be elucidated by family history, has a much more reassuring prognosis compared to Walker-Warburg syndrome. Of note, it is important to mention that examination of the mother for subtle clinical features can lead to the diagnosis, eg, presence of myopathic face and/or difficulty in relaxing the grip during a handshake in the mother can contribute to making the diagnosis of myotonic dystrophy.

The next step in establishing the etiologic diagnosis is a careful systemic examination. The physical examination will determine whether the hypotonia is part of a syndrome or an apparently isolated neurologic condition. Presence of dysmorphic features may lead to diagnosis in some cases, eg, presence of upslanting palpebral fissures, epicanthal folds, microbrachycephaly, and short nose can be features of trisomy 21, which is the most common, easily recognizable chromosomal abnormality. Abnormal fat pads in the buttocks and inverted nipples are diagnostic clues for a congenital disorder of glycosylation (CDG). The presence of cardiomegaly or hepatosplenomegaly can point to glycogen storage and lysosomal storage disorders, respectively. The existence of marked feeding difficulty along with central hypotonia should prompt the clinician to consider investigating for Prader-Willi syndrome (PWS), which requires specific testing such as DNA methylation assay for diagnosis.

The clinician should also document if hypotonia is static or progressive in nature, which is critical to differentiate neurodegenerative conditions from static disorders.

**TABLE 175-1 DIFFERENTIAL DIAGNOSIS OF CONGENITAL HYPOTONIA**

- Central hypotonia
  - a. Cerebral
    - i. Benign congenital hypotonia
    - ii. Static encephalopathies due to injuries pre-/perinatal
      1. Hypoxic ischemic encephalopathy (HIE)
      2. Intracranial hemorrhage
      3. Congenital infections
    - iii. Neurogenetic disorders
      1. Chromosomal disorders
      2. Single-gene disorders causing brain anomalies
      3. Neurometabolic disorders (eg, mitochondrial disorders, Zellweger syndrome, phenylketonuria, galactosemia, propionic acidemia)
      4. Methylation anomalies (Prader-Willi and Angelman syndromes)
    - iv. Maternal drug effect
  - b. Spinal cord
    - i. Spinal cord injuries (birth trauma)
    - ii. Spinal cord anomalies (syringomyelia, neural tube defects)
- Peripheral hypotonia
  - a. Anterior horn cell disorder (spinal muscular atrophy [SMA])
  - b. Neuromuscular junction disorders
    - i. Congenital myasthenic syndrome (CMS 1A-12)
    - ii. Transient acquired neonatal myasthenia
    - iii. Infantile botulism
    - iv. Drug toxicity (magnesium and aminoglycosides)
  - c. Peripheral neuropathies
    - i. Congenital hypomyelinating neuropathy
    - ii. Dejerine-Sottas syndrome
    - iii. Giant axonal neuropathy
  - d. Muscle disorders
    - i. Congenital muscular dystrophies (CMD)
      1. Extracellular matrix protein abnormalities
         - a. Merosin-deficient congenital muscular dystrophy (MDC1A)
         - b. Collagen VI–deficient CMD
      2. Collagen VI–deficient congenital muscular dystrophies
         - a. Ullrich CMD
         - b. Bethlem myopathy
      3. Defects of glycosylation
         - a. Dystroglycanopathies
         - b. Fukuyama CMD
         - c. Muscle-eye-brain disease
         - d. Walker-Warburg syndrome
         - e. Merosin-deficient CMD type 1C
         - f. Merosin-deficient CMD type 1D
      4. Defects of proteins of the endoplasmic reticulum
         - a. *SEPN1*-related myopathy
      5. Defects of nuclear envelope proteins
         - a. *LMNA*-related CMD
    - ii. Congenital myopathies
      1. Congenital myopathies with protein accumulation
         - a. Nemaline myopathy (NEM 1-7)
         - b. Cap disease
         - c. Reducing body myopathy
         - d. Myosin storage myopathy (hyaline body myopathy)
      2. Congenital myopathies with cores
         - a. Central core disease
         - b. Central core disease with rods and malignant hyperthermia
         - c. Multiminicore disease
      3. Congenital myopathies with central nuclei
         - a. Centronuclear myopathy
      4. Congenital myopathies with fiber side variation
         - a. Congenital fiber–type disproportion (CFTD 1–5)

After examining the other systems of the infant, a detailed neurologic examination should be conducted. Hypotonia evaluation starts with careful inspection. Infants with hypotonia look similar when they are in supine position regardless of the underlying etiology. In general, spontaneous movements are decreased, and their extremities are abducted and extended. Older infants may have hair loss at the back of their head with a misshapen occiput that is flat unilaterally or bilaterally (plagiocephaly and brachycephaly, respectively) due to a prolonged position of the head in the same place. Infants who are hypotonic in utero may be born with hip dislocation and/or joint contractures (arthrogryposis) due to intrauterine lack of mobility. Three techniques on exam are important in evaluating the hypotonia: (1) The first is traction response maneuver where infants with hypotonia will have obvious head lag and no apparent movements in arms and legs while pulling by both hands from lying position to sitting position. Term infants with normal tone will lift the head with minimal head lag while body is rising from the table with associated flexions in elbows, knees, and ankles. It is important to note that the traction response develops after the 32nd week of gestation. The second technique is the vertical suspension maneuver: infants with hypotonia will "slip through" the examiner's hands while the infant is held under axillae vertically without getting support from chest. Infants with normal tone will suspend without slipping through the hands and will have a flexed posture at the knee and hip joints. The third technique is the horizontal suspension maneuver: infants with hypotonia drape over the examiner's hand with the head and hip flexed, making a U-shape while the infant is held from the chest/abdomen horizontally. Healthy infants in horizontal position will make intermittent efforts to lift the head, straighten the back, and flex the limbs.

Although there is some overlap between hypotonia originating from central versus peripheral causes, certain features on exam can help to differentiate and avoid unnecessary testing such as muscle biopsy in a central hypotonia patient. Common differences are outlined in Table 175-2. In general, an infant who has predominantly axial hypotonia, appears lethargic or encephalopathic, and has other associated system anomalies points to a central etiology. If the infant appears alert, responds to surroundings appropriately, and has profound weakness, hypotonia, and severely depressed reflexes, then the hypotonia is likely caused by a peripheral etiology. It is important to mention that some infants have both central and peripheral origin of hypotonia such as those with muscle-eye-brain disease.

Due to a wide range of disease etiologies, identifying the underlying cause of hypotonia in infants remains difficult, except in widely recognized common conditions such as Down syndrome or the presence of an obvious etiology such as hypoxemia at birth. Tables 175-3 and 175-4 summarize clinical/laboratory clues for different diseases that cause hypotonia. Although the workup can be initiated by a pediatrician, a referral to a subspecialist such as neurologist or geneticist is typically warranted.

## DIAGNOSIS

Since there are a wide variety of conditions that can cause hypotonia, and each condition requires specific test(s)/procedure(s), the diagnostic evaluation should be performed after differential diagnosis is tailored according to the history and physical examination. Genetic diagnosis is crucial in counseling these families regarding future risks of having similar babies and risks of other family members. Furthermore, genetic diagnosis will help to counsel the patient and family on disease prognosis since life expectancy and potential health risk factors vary significantly between different diseases.

An infant with hypotonia during the newborn period should undergo infectious workup, including complete blood count, urinalysis, and blood/urine/cerebrospinal fluid cultures in addition to evaluation for an inborn error of metabolism. Basic metabolic workup includes blood gas and chemistries including glucose and bicarbonate for metabolic acidosis, ammonia and plasma amino acid for urea cycle defects, urine organic acid analysis and acyl carnitine profile for fatty acid oxidation defects and organic acidemias, and lactate and pyruvate for disorders of pyruvate metabolism and mitochondrial disorders.

**TABLE 175-2 LOCALIZATION AND CLINICAL FEATURES OF DISEASES CAUSING HYPOTONIA**

| | Central | Peripheral | | | |
|---|---|---|---|---|---|
| **Clinical Feature** | **CNS** | **Anterior Horn Cells** | **Peripheral Nerve** | **NMJ** | **Muscle** |
| Strength (weakness) | Mild | Moderate to severe | Moderate to severe | Moderate to severe | Moderate to severe |
| DTRs | Normal to increased | Decreased | Decreased | Decreased | Decreased |
| Babinski sign | Present | Absent | Absent | Absent | Absent |
| Infantile reflexes | Persistent | Absent | Absent | Absent | Absent |
| Fasciculation | Absent | Present | Absent | Absent | Absent |
| Muscle bulk | Normal | Atrophy | Distal atrophy | Normal to atrophy | Proximal atrophy |
| Sensation | Normal | Normal | Decreased | Normal | Normal |
| Tone | Decreased then increased | Decreased | Decreased | Normal to decreased | Decreased |

CNS, central nervous system; DTR, deep tendon reflex; NMJ, neuromuscular junction.

There are also some more specific biochemical tests that could be considered such as carbohydrate-deficient transferrin analysis for congenital disorders of glycosylation or very long chain fatty acids and plasmalogens for peroxisomal defects. We recommend consultation with a neurogeneticist/biochemical geneticist if basic metabolic studies are inconclusive.

If there is a history of hypoxia during the perinatal period or difficult delivery/abnormal presentation, eg, breech presentation, brain and/or spine magnetic resonance imaging (MRI) is warranted to see the potential extent of hypoxemia and spinal cord trauma, respectively. Brain MRI is also of great importance in central hypotonia patients since it can delineate several disorders such as structural brain malformations, abnormal signals in basal ganglia (mitochondrial abnormalities and iron accumulation disorders), brain stem defects (pontocerebellar hypoplasia, Joubert syndrome), white matter disorders (neurodegenerative conditions and peroxisomal disorders), and corpus callosum abnormalities (both anterior and posterior brain malformations). Magnetic resonance spectroscopy is an important noninvasive diagnostic tool in certain neurometabolic conditions such as Canavan disease.

To evaluate causes of peripheral hypotonia, muscle enzymes should be measured (ie, creatine phosphokinase, aldolase, and alanine aminotransferase/aspartate aminotransferase levels). Nerve conduction study/electromyogram (NCS/EMG) will be helpful in differentiating peripheral neuropathy, neuromuscular junction disorders, and myopathies. Normal NCS/EMG findings mostly suggest a central hypotonia with the exception of a few myopathies that involve both the central and peripheral nervous system, eg, Fukuyama congenital muscular dystrophy. Muscle MRI is considered in myopathic patients. Muscle biopsy was commonly used in neuromuscular disorders in the past, and sometimes it is the only test that can differentiate some myopathy subtypes. However, given the invasiveness of the biopsy procedure and availability of genome-wide genetic testing options, muscle biopsy can be used as a last resort.

The clinician must also be vigilant regarding other potential nongenetic causes such as a toxic dose of magnesium intake at birth, aminoglycoside use during pregnancy, or honey consumption during the infantile period. Simple blood level tests might be enough and will be a much more cost-effective approach in these populations.

Infants with dysmorphic features or involvement of other systems in addition to hypotonia should undergo genetic testing. The general clinician can order specific genetic testing such as a chromosome analysis in suspected Down syndrome; however, broader screening tools should be performed in patients with unknown etiologies of hypotonia. With emerging new genomic technologies, there has been a tremendous increase in understanding the etiology of neurogenetic disorders including hypotonia. Chromosome microarray analysis (CMA), including genome-wide array comparative genomic

**TABLE 175-3 CLINICAL AND LABORATORY CLUES OF DISEASES THAT CAUSE CENTRAL HYPOTONIA AND RECOMMENDED STUDY FOR DIAGNOSIS**

| Disease | Key Clinical Feature in History and Physical Exam | Recommended Study |
|---|---|---|
| HIE | Preterm birth, difficult delivery | None |
| ICH | Difficult delivery, bleeding diathesis in family | None |
| Congenital infections | Prenatal infection history | TORCH testing |
| Chromosomal disorders | Abnormal prenatal US findings, dysmorphism on exam | CMA |
| Maternal drug effect | Prenatal/birth history | Drug level |
| Single-gene disorders | Abnormal US findings, dysmorphic features on exam | WES, DNA methylation test, mitochondrial DNA NGS |
| Spinal cord anomaly/injury | Natal history, abnormal spine in prenatal US findings | Spinal MRI |

CMA, chromosomal microarray; HIE, hypoxic ischemic encephalopathy; ICH, intracranial hemorrhage; MRI, magnetic resonance imaging; NGS, next-generation sequencing; US, ultrasound; WES, whole-exome sequencing.

**TABLE 175-4 CLINICAL AND LABORATORY CLUES OF DISEASES THAT CAUSE PERIPHERAL HYPOTONIA AND RECOMMENDED STUDY FOR DIAGNOSIS**

| Disease | Key Clinical Features in History and Physical Exam | Recommended Study |
|---|---|---|
| SMA | Severe weakness, absent/diminished DTR, muscle fasciculation | *SMN* gene testing, EMG |
| NMJ disorder | | |
| Myasthenia gravis | Easy fatigability, bulbar symptoms (feeding difficulty, aspiration) | EMG/NCS, anticholinesterase response test |
| Infantile botulism | Facial weakness and pupillary defects | Toxin detection in food |
| Drug toxicity | Magnesium and/or aminoglycoside (drug exposure in history) | Drug levels |
| Peripheral nerve | Severe weakness, diminished DTR, distal muscle atrophy | Single gene testing or WES |
| Muscle | | |
| CMD | Severe weakness, diminished DTR, positive family history | Muscle enzymes/MRI, muscle biopsy, EMG/NCS, mother's neurologic exam, genetic testing including single-gene testing, WES, triple expansion disorder testing |
| Congenital myopathies | Severe weakness, diminished DTR, positive family history | Muscle enzymes/MRI, muscle biopsy, EMG/NCS, genetic testing including single gene testing, WES |

CMD, congenital muscular dystrophy; DTR, deep tendon reflex; EMG/NCS, electromyography/nerve conduction study; MRI, magnetic resonance imaging; NMJ, neuromuscular junction; SMA, spinal muscular atrophy; WES, whole-exome sequencing.

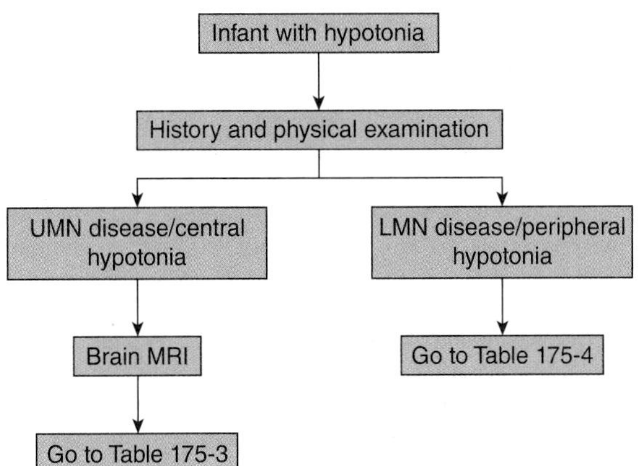


**FIGURE 175-1** A suggested approach to a patient with congenital hypotonia. Since the workup and key findings in history and physical exam are detailed in Table 175-3, please refer to Table 175-3 for central hypotonia and Table 175-4 for peripheral hypotonia. LMN, lower motor neuron; MRI, magnetic resonance imaging; UMN, upper motor neuron.

hybridization (array CGH) and single nucleotide polymorphism (SNP) arrays, is used instead of chromosome analysis for copy number variant (ie, deletions and duplications) detection, and targeted single-gene Sanger sequencing has been replaced with clinical whole-exome sequencing (WES). However, clinicians must be aware of the restrictions of diagnostic utilities of these tests; for example, these tests cannot detect triplet expansion disorders (eg, myotonic dystrophy or fragile X) or methylation abnormalities such as those that can be found causative for Prader-Willi and Angelman syndromes.

In summary, the differential diagnosis of congenital hypotonia can be extensive and is a challenge that requires a stepwise and multidisciplinary team approach including pediatricians, geneticists, and neurologists. We propose a diagnostic algorithm based on medical/family history and physical examination, which provides crucial information that differentiates each condition, thus minimizing potential unnecessary testing (Fig. 175-1).

## TREATMENT

In accordance with advances in genetics, there have been promising therapeutic options in many conditions causing hypotonia including neurometabolic disorders, spinal muscular atrophy, peripheral neuropathies, muscular dystrophies, myopathies, and myotonic dystrophies. However, most are currently undergoing different stages of clinical trials.

Besides developing disease-specific therapies, symptomatic and supportive therapies still remain the mainstay of the treatment. Regular physical and occupational therapies can improve the patient's strength and tone in mildly affected patients and delay development of contractures in severely hypotonic patients. These patients require special attention compared to the general population, and a multidisciplinary team approach is usually necessary for management and care. Hypotonic patients are prone to joint subluxations, broken bones, and scoliosis due to prolonged deconditioning. Thus, annual orthopedic evaluation should be performed in severely affected patients. Nutritional intake might be a problem especially for patients with neuromuscular disorders. Close monitoring of calorie count and weight gain is necessary for potential interventions such as G-tube placement to maintain ideal body weight. Management of anesthesia has to be more carefully considered, particularly in patients with muscle disorders, since there is a potential risk for life-threatening conditions such as malignant hyperthermia.

Other important aspects of managing patients with neurogenetic condition are the ethical/social issues. Counseling on potential future risks for respiratory failure, cardiac arrest, necessity of tracheostomy tube and gastric tube placements, and decisions on do not resuscitate/do not intubate (DNR/DNI) orders and hospice/palliative care should be discussed in a sensitive manner with the family.

# CONDITIONS CAUSING HYPOTONIA

## BENIGN CONGENITAL HYPOTONIA

Benign congenital hypotonia is a diagnosis of exclusion. The clinician has to rule out diseases that cause hypotonia before making the diagnosis of benign congenital hypotonia. Patients with benign congenital hypotonia are typically hypotonic at birth and early infantile period and later on improve to normal tone. There may be a positive family history. The neurologic exam is reassuring with the exception of tone. Diagnostic studies should not reveal any abnormality. Overall, the prognosis is good; however, some of these children may develop some delays in developmental milestones and learning disabilities in the future even if they recover from hypotonia.

## STATIC ENCEPHALOPATHIES

Static encephalopathy develops due to an insult to the brain of the fetus or baby during pregnancy or delivery, respectively. A careful pregnancy and delivery history usually unveils the etiology. Hypotonia is a common feature of prematurity and mostly correlates with the severity of prematurity. If a newborn, especially premature infant develops sudden-onset hypotonia, the development of intracranial hemorrhage should be considered. HIE is the most common cause of static encephalopathy and usually occurs due to a brain insult during birth. The clinician should obtain a detailed prenatal and perinatal history. Congenital infections remain an important cause of congenital hypotonia and severe brain injury, especially in developing countries. Recently, Zika virus became a threat to global health since it is rapidly spreading in developed countries and causing congenital infection including severe microcephaly in the developing fetus. Since mothers generally do not feel sick or may only have vague flu-like symptoms during the infection period, the prenatal history may not reveal the etiology. Furthermore, despite the fact that many babies have obvious clinical features of congenital infection at birth including microcephaly, hydrocephalus, hearing deficit, and congenital heart defects, some babies may be born with silent congenital infection and exhibit disabilities months to years later. Physical examination usually reveals hypotonia, absent/diminished deep tendon reflexes, and mild weakness around the time of insult. Features of cerebral palsy including hypertonia (scissoring of legs, constant fisting of fingers), increased deep tendon reflexes, a positive Babinski sign, and persistence of infantile reflexes develop later in life. Brain imaging is warranted in all patients who have concern for central hypotonia. Brain MRI is superior to brain computed tomography (CT) and head ultrasound (US) due to its high tissue resolution, which maximizes the attainment of a diagnosis. Brain MRI can show signs of prematurity (germinal matrix hemorrhage, delayed myelination, or rarely periventricular leukomalacia; however, the latter mostly develops later in the life) and features of hypoxic ischemia (restrictions on diffusion-weighted images, edema, and hemorrhage). Brain CT is the most sensitive test to show intracranial hemorrhage and calcifications and does not require sedation since scanning time is shorter. However, it requires high-dose radiation and has low tissue resolution. Head US is a quick, noninvasive, harmless technique that is especially useful to evaluate and monitor infants with hydrocephaly and intracranial hemorrhage. It is important to mention that a normal imaging study does not rule out sequelae of prematurity, HIE, or congenital infections. The TORCH panel and Zika virus polymerase chain reaction should be sent in infants if there is concern for congenital infections. Prognosis depends on the underlying etiology.

## NEUROGENETIC DISORDERS

Neurogenetic disorders are a heterogeneous group of neurologic disorders that occur due to a mutation that disrupts gene(s) function through various mutational mechanisms. Although mutation in any gene that has a function in the neuromuscular system, from the central nervous system to muscle, can cause hypotonia, we will specifically discuss neurogenetic disorders causing central hypotonia.

### Chromosomal Disorders

Chromosomal disorders are a group of neurogenetic disorders that occur by monosomy (a missing chromosome copy) or trisomy (an extra copy) of an entire chromosome or segment of a chromosome. There is a wide variety of chromosomal disorders, from well-known conditions such as Down syndrome and Turner syndrome to specific deletions or duplications of certain segments of chromosomes. Common features in addition to profound hypotonia include facial dysmorphism, extremity abnormalities, and organ malformations including brain, heart, and kidneys. A patient who has a chromosomal abnormality should be screened for other subclinical system abnormalities such as unilateral kidney agenesis or congenital heart disease, among others. CMA is the test that needs to be performed in this patient population. Treatment is supportive. Prognosis depends on the underlying chromosomal abnormality, and can range from normal life expectancy to death at birth or even stillborn/miscarriages.

### Single-Gene Disorders

Single-gene disorders are caused by Watson-Crick nucleotide base pair (bp) changes such as missense/nonsense single nucleotide variants (SNVs) or small-size (< 50 bp) insertions and deletions (known as indels) that are not detectable by CMA (see Chapter 167). Disorders involving genes that play a role in central nervous system development and function may present with central hypotonia. A classical example of this kind of disorder is lissencephaly (ie, "smooth brain"), a structural brain disorder characterized by the absence of normal gyrus formation of the cerebral cortex and microcephaly, caused by mutations in the *PAFAH1B1* gene. Another example for this group of disorders is pontocerebellar hypoplasia, which is caused by mutations in genes that have a role in RNA synthesis/splicing. Treatment is symptomatic. This group of disorders is usually nonprogressive. With the launch of WES in clinical practice, there has been an enormous increase in the discovery of genes that cause hypotonia, DD/ID, and/or cerebral malformations. Since the brain is not formed properly, these patients tend to have microcephaly, epilepsy, intellectual disability, and other system anomalies based on the underlying genetic defect. Brain MRI is warranted in this patient population. However, a normal brain MRI does not exclude subtle cortical malformations and neuronal migration disorders. WES is necessary since there is a substantial percentage of genetic heterogeneity.



### Neurometabolic Disorders

Neurometabolic disorders refer to a group of disorders that are characterized by a lack or dysfunction of an enzyme or vitamin necessary for a specific chemical reaction in the body. Malfunction of a chemical pathway can cause either a deficiency of an essential metabolite or accumulation of materials that may become toxic for the body. The lack of essential metabolites or accumulation of toxic metabolites can have a detrimental effect on the developing brain and lead to loss of nerve cells and breakdown of brain white and gray matter. The presenting symptoms for neurometabolic disorders vary significantly in accordance with the underlying enzyme deficiency. One of the key features of neurometabolic disorders is the progression of symptoms over time. Some patients with neurometabolic disorders have an abnormal brain even before birth, such as those with Zellweger syndrome; some become symptomatic just after birth or with the introduction of food; and some become symptomatic during infancy or early/late childhood, with symptoms mostly including hypotonia/developmental delay, seizures, lethargy, visual disturbance, vomiting, poor feeding, and respiratory abnormalities. Yet others become symptomatic during adulthood, which mostly includes psychiatric diseases, mood/behavioral disorders, or subtle neurologic symptoms.

Mitochondrial disorders are a subgroup of neurometabolic disorders that are caused by mutations in either mitochondrial DNA or genomic DNA that has a role in mitochondria function. Since mitochondria are the major source of energy for the body, diseases of the mitochondria manifest mostly in high-energy-demanding organs and tissues such as the brain, heart, liver, eye muscles, and skeletal muscles. However, mitochondrial disorders may present with any system involvement. Depending on which cells are affected, symptoms may include hypotonia, developmental delay, muscle weakness and pain, seizures, stroke-like episodes, visual problems, gastrointestinal disorders and swallowing difficulties, poor growth, cardiac disease (including left ventricular noncompaction and other cardiomyopathies), liver disease, diabetes, respiratory complications, lactic acidosis, and susceptibility to infections. Diagnostic workup should start with screening basic chemistries, complete blood count, ammonia, lactate, pyruvate, creatine phosphokinase (CPK), liver enzymes, plasma amino acids analysis, plasma acyl carnitine profile, and urine organic acid analysis and advance gradually to WES and mitochondrial next-generation sequencing (NGS). To confirm a variant of unknown significance, invasive tests such as muscle biopsy or a less invasive test such as a skin biopsy could be considered for enzymatic studies. Prognosis is variable from fatal at birth to mildly symptomatic throughout life.

### Other Genetic Mechanisms (ie, DNA Methylation Abnormality and Uniparental Disomy)

It is important to discuss these diseases separately since these disorders cannot be detected by routine genetic tests including CMA and WES. The prototypical example of these disorders is PWS. Patients with PWS typically have profound hypotonia and feeding difficulty during infancy. Infants with hypotonia and feeding difficulty should be tested for PWS, unless exam and laboratory findings suggest another disorder. Patients mostly have decreased fetal movement during pregnancy. As they become older, patients have distinctive dysmorphic features including bifrontal narrowing, almond-shaped eyes, small hands and feet, obesity, and genital hypoplasia in males.

## MATERNAL DRUG EFFECT

Drug use during pregnancy including alcohol can cause several different anomalies including facial dysmorphism, hypotonia, DD/ID, microcephaly, cardiac defects, and others. The condition is nonprogressive. Physical exam can vary from nonspecific findings to distinctive features as in fetal alcohol syndrome. There is no specific test to measure the drug level.

## SPINAL CORD INJURIES

Spinal cord injuries are part of the differential diagnosis of hypotonia only during the newborn period. Almost all cervical spine injuries occur during vaginal delivery, specifically with breech presentation. The extent of injury can vary from mild edema to complete disconnection of the spinal cord. Depending on the severity and the level of the pathology, the patients may present with hypotonia/weakness, loss of sensory modalities, absent reflexes, bowel and bladder dysfunction, and/or abnormal breathing. Screening of the spinal cord with an MRI is important if there is a concern for spinal cord injury. Treatment is supportive in these patients.

## SPINAL CORD ANOMALIES

Syringomyelia is the longitudinal formation of fluid-filled cysts within the spinal cord that may be present congenitally or later in life. Spina bifida is the incomplete closure of bones and other structures around the spinal cord. It may happen in any segment of spine; however, the most common location is the lumbar area. Spinal cord anomalies may be physically visible or occult with subtle signs on exam such as swelling, a patch or tuft of hair, dark spot, and/or dimple at the site of anomaly. Physical exam findings, diagnostic studies, and treatment are similar to other spinal cord injuries.

## SPINAL MUSCULAR ATROPHY

Spinal muscular atrophy is an autosomal recessive neurodegenerative disease of the anterior horn cells in the spinal cord that occurs due to mutation, mostly deletion of exons 7 and 8, in the *SMN1* gene. Depending on the level of the normal SMN protein, the disease may be symptomatic even before birth (decreased fetal movement) to adulthood, which also correlates with the mortality. There are 4 different types, from the most severe SMA1 to the mildest phenotype

SMA4. The distinctive finding on physical exam is the presence of fasciculations in addition to other exam findings including hypotonia, moderate to severe weakness, decreased reflexes and decreased muscle bulk. Since anterior horn cells are solely involved, sensation is intact in SMA. NCS/EMG can be diagnostic; however, the test of choice is screening for deletions in the *SMN1* gene. Serum CPK is normal or mildly increased. Recently, FDA approved the intrathecal use of Nusinersen, an antisense oligonucleotide which increases the level of SMN protein in the CNS by modulating splicing of the SMN2 gene and promoting inclusion of exon 7. In general, prognosis varies with the SMA type; however, patients deteriorate over time due to its neurodegenerative nature.

## CONGENITAL MYASTHENIC SYNDROME

Congenital myasthenic syndrome is a rare group of genetic disorders of the neuromuscular junction. Clinical features include weakness that worsens with exertion, diminished reflexes, normal to decreased muscle bulk and tone, and a normal sensation. Patients may have arthrogryposis, respiratory insufficiency, and feeding difficulty at birth. Although facial and skeletal muscles are weak, extraocular muscles are usually intact. Clinical findings vary between individuals and type of mutation. Diagnosis is based on clinical findings, a decremental response on EMG, and genetic testing. There have been about 20 genes described so far, all of which play a role in neuromuscular junction structure or function. Acetylcholine receptor (AChR) and muscle-specific kinase (MuSK) antibodies are negative. Edrophonium challenge test usually helps to establish the diagnosis. Reversible acetylcholinesterase inhibitors prevent myasthenic crisis. Prognosis varies significantly depending on the involved gene; eg, mutations in *CHRNG* cause Escobar syndrome, which may be lethal prenatally or cause severe multiple pterygium at birth. However, in general, patients may require mechanical ventilation or feeding support at birth. Mostly within weeks, infants become stronger and can be weaned from mechanical ventilation though; patients may have episodes of weakness and life-threatening apnea throughout their life with a decreasing frequency and severity.

## TRANSIENT NEONATAL MYASTHENIA

Transient myasthenia symptoms occur in 10% to 20% of babies who were born to mothers with myasthenia gravis. Passive transfer of AChR and MuSK antibodies is the underlying cause of myasthenic symptoms. Of note, severity is generally not correlated with maternal disease, and even in some cases, the mother may be asymptomatic. Onset is usually within the first few hours of life. Difficulty feeding and hypotonia are the cardinal features. Infants are eager to feed, but the ability to suck weakens quickly. Other clinical features are weak cry, facial muscle weakness, and rarely respiratory insufficiency. Diagnosis is based on detection of antibodies in the newborn, and sometimes, an edrophonium response test may be necessary. Treatment is reversible acetylcholinesterase inhibitors in milder cases. Patients may require plasma exchange in severe cases such as generalized weakness and respiratory distress. The mean duration of symptoms is 2 to 3 weeks, and recovery is almost always complete. There is no risk of developing myasthenia gravis later in life.

## INFANTILE BOTULISM

Botulism results from ingestion of preformed *Clostridium botulinum* exotoxin, which blocks the release of acetylcholine at the neuromuscular junction. A significant percentage (>90%) of cases occur in infants younger than 6 months. Honey is a well-known dietary reservoir of *C botulinum*, but it accounts for only approximately 20% of cases. In most cases, the source is not defined. Typical symptoms of infantile botulism vary from asymptomatic carrier, mild hypotonia, and constipation to severe weakness, failure to thrive, descending flaccid paralysis, and sudden infant death. Diagnosis is based on the isolation of the organism from the stool. EMG has a specific pattern and can be helpful for diagnosis. Treatment is antitoxin immune globulin along with supportive care. Infantile botulism is a self-limited condition that usually resolves within 2 to 6 weeks. Recovery is complete in most cases, but there is a small chance of relapse.

## PERIPHERAL NEUROPATHIES

Peripheral neuropathies are a very rare cause of congenital hypotonia. A typical representative disease is congenital hypomyelinating neuropathy. Clinical features are quite similar to spinal muscular atrophy, except sensation is decreased and fasciculations are absent. Treatment is mainly supportive, and prognosis is usually poor, resulting in death secondary to respiratory insufficiency during infancy.

## DRUG TOXICITY (MAGNESIUM AND AMINOGLYCOSIDES)

Magnesium is usually used to treat eclampsia and preterm labor. Infants, who were exposed to high-dose magnesium will manifest the signs of hypermagnesemia including hypotonia, hyporeflexia, poor sucking, respiratory depression, intraventricular hemorrhage, periventricular leukomalacia, cerebral palsy, DD/ID, necrotizing enterocolitis, blindness, and deafness.

Aminoglycosides are commonly used in neonates worldwide since they are recommended by the World Health Organization as the first-line antibiotics in neonates with possible serious bacterial infection. The primary toxicities of aminoglycosides are nephrotoxicity, ototoxicity, and rarely, neuromuscular blockade causing hypotonia.

In general, checking the serum and urine levels of the newborn is recommended in drug toxicity. However, clinicians should be aware that the levels do not necessarily correlate with the clinical picture and may be of little diagnostic value. Treatment for drug toxicities is supportive, and symptoms usually improve over time if there are no sequelae from the toxicity.

## CONGENITAL MUSCULAR DYSTROPHIES

Congenital muscular dystrophies (CMD) are a clinically and genetically heterogeneous group of muscle disorders with variable clinical presentation even within the family. Onset is usually at birth or early infancy, which is mainly characterized by hypotonia, progressive weakness, and atrophy of the proximal muscles. There are some syndromic forms that involve other organs including eye, brain, heart, and lungs. CPK level is usually high, but there are some forms which have normal CPK. Due to increasing knowledge in underlying genetic causes, classification frequently requires update. Current, widely accepted classification is according to genetic etiology of the affected protein. Diagnosis usually requires CPK level, NCS/EMG, brain MRI, muscle biopsy, and genetic testing. The most common CMDs in decreasing frequency are collagen VI–related disorders (eg, Ullrich CMD and Bethlem myopathy), α-dystroglycanopathy CMD (eg, Fukuyama CMD, Walker-Warburg syndrome), and merosin-deficient CMD. There is population bias; for example, Fukuyama CMD composes approximately half of the cases in Japan. It is important to examine the mother of suspected myotonic dystrophy infants since she is likely to exhibit clues of the disease such as myopathic face or difficulty in relaxing the hand grip. Treatment is usually supportive.

## CONGENITAL MYOPATHIES

Congenital myopathies are genetic disorders of the skeletal muscle characterized mainly by congenital hypotonia, muscle weakness/atrophy, and normal to slightly elevated CK levels. Onset is usually in the early infantile period, but some patients may present late in childhood or adulthood. Clinical presentation is similar to CMDs with congenital hypotonia, muscle weakness including facial muscles, predominantly lower face, and bulbar and respiratory symptoms. Other system involvements are rare and are usually nonprogressive or very slowly progressive compared to muscular dystrophies. Diagnosis mainly depends on muscle biopsy, with other tests including CPK level and NCS/EMG. The most well-known myopathies are nemaline myopathy, central-core disease, and multiminicore disease. Ryanodine receptor gene mutations can cause multiminicore disease, central core disease, central core disease with rods, and malignant hyperthermia. Mutations in this gene in combination with general anesthesia convey a high risk for malignant hyperthermia, especially during surgery. For congenital myopathies, the classification is primarily based on immunohistochemical features on biopsy. Treatment is mainly supportive.

## SUGGESTED READINGS


Douglas-Escobar M, Weiss MD. Hypoxic-ischemic encephalopathy: a review for the clinician. *JAMA Pediatr.* 2015;169(4):397-403.

Iannaccone ST, Castro D. Congenital muscular dystrophies and congenital myopathies. *Continuum (MinneapMinn).* 2013;19:1509-1534.

Karaca E, Harel T, Pehlivan D, et al. Genes that affect brain structure and function identified by rare variant analyses of mendelian neurologic disease. *Neuron.* 2015;88(3):499-513.

North KN, Wang CH, Clarke N, et al. Approach to the diagnosis of congenital myopathies. *Neuromuscul Disord.* 2014;24(2):97-116.

Paro-Panjan D, Neubauer D. Congenital hypotonia: is there an algorithm? *J Child Neurol.* 2004;19:439-443.

Peredo DE, Hannibal MC. The floppy infant: evaluation of hypotonia. *Pediatr Rev.* 2009;30(9):e66-e76.

Pina-Garza JE. *Fenichel's Clinical Pediatric Neurology: A Signs and Symptoms Approach.* 7th ed. New York, NY: Elsevier Saunders; 2013:147-169.

Prasad AN, Prasad C. Genetic evaluation of the floppy infant. *Semin Fetal Neonatal Med.* 2011;16(2):99-108.

Sparks SE. Neonatal hypotonia. *Clin Perinatol.* 2015;42(2):363-371.

Wang CH, Dowling JJ, North K, et al. Consensus statement on standard of care for congenital myopathies. *J Child Neurol.* 2012 Mar; 27(3):363-382.




# 176 Neurocutaneous Disorders

Surya Rednam and Michael Wangler

## INTRODUCTION

Neurocutaneous disorders are a heterogeneous group of genetic conditions affecting both the central and peripheral nerves that can result in brain, spine, skin, and skeletal manifestations. This chapter discusses select neurocutaneous disorders, or phakomatoses, in which seizures are not a typical component. Neurocutaneous disorders with prominent neurologic features, particularly seizures, are discussed separately (see Chapter 567). A comprehensive table of neurocutaneous disorders (Table 176-1) and selected more commonly observed conditions are described below.

**TABLE 176-1 NEUROCUTANEOUS DISORDERS**

| |
|---|
| Ataxia-telangiectasia |
| Encephalocraniocutaneous lipomatosis |
| Epidermal nevus syndrome (linear sebaceous nevus, linear epidermal nevus) |
| Nevoid basal cell carcinoma syndrome (Gorlin syndrome) |
| Hypomelanosis of Ito |
| Incontinentia pigmenti |
| Neurocutaneous melanosis |
| Neurofibromatosis type 1 |
| Neurofibromatosis type 2 |
| Schwannomatosis |
| Sturge-Weber syndrome |
| Tuberous sclerosis complex |
| Von Hippel-Lindau disease |

## NEUROFIBROMATOSIS TYPE 1

### CLINICAL MANIFESTATIONS

Neurofibromatosis type 1 (NF1, Online Mendelian Inheritance in Man [OMIM] no. 162200) is the most common neurocutaneous disorder, and one of the most common autosomal dominant disorders affecting approximately 1 in 3000 people worldwide. The hallmark features of NF1, café-au-lait macules and benign cutaneous neurofibromas, typically arise in early childhood and adolescence, respectively. Approximately two-thirds of individuals with NF1 have manifestations that generally do not require clinical intervention, whereas the remaining one-third display a myriad of medical complications that are unpredictable, both in timing and severity.

Even though NF1 has been recognized as von Recklinghausen disease by the medical community since the 19th century, both its variability and the age-dependent penetrance of its clinical manifestations made it essential to develop a well-accepted set of clinical criteria to establish the diagnosis (Table 176-2). The typical clinical manifestations allow the diagnosis to be established in children by 8 years according to a set of clinical criteria known as the National Institutes of Health (NIH) consensus criteria for NF1. By virtue of full penetrance in the adult population, diagnosis of NF1 is more straightforward in familial cases because it requires only 1 physical manifestation in addition to an affected first-degree relative. In sporadic cases, features associated with NF1 that are not part of the diagnostic criteria sometimes appear prior to the development of a second diagnostic sign, for example, characteristic T2 hyperintensities on brain magnetic resonance imaging (MRI).

The typical pattern of clinical presentation in NF1 is subject to age-dependent penetrance. Usually, multiple café-au-lait (CAL) spots are identified in the first 2 years of life (Fig. 176-1). The observation of more than 5 CAL spots that are greater than 0.5 cm in diameter and on the thoracic or abdominal skin in toddlers is a classic presentation. A number of other conditions include multiple CAL macules (eg, McCune-Albright syndrome, Noonan syndrome, Bloom syndrome), although other signs and symptoms generally make exclusion of other diagnoses fairly straightforward. The presence of familial multiple CAL spots without other signs of NF1 is a relatively rare overlapping condition, Legius syndrome, and it is caused by mutations in the *SPRED1* gene.

Axillary or inguinal freckling, which usually involves the axillae and groin (see Fig. 176-1), occurs in approximately 90% of individuals with NF1, and this sign develops by late childhood. Lisch nodules, of hamartomas of the irises, can be identified by slit lamp examination of the eyes in over 75% of preadolescents.

Neurofibromas are benign tumors that are a collection of Schwann cells, fibroblasts, mast cells, and extracellular matrix. Cutaneous neurofibromas tend to appear at the time of puberty and progress in number throughout life. They can be difficult to detect at their outset, and they are often most easily palpated along the flanks and lower abdomen as slight depressions rather than protruding bumps. Cutaneous neurofibromas may occasionally itch but are not painful and never lead to malignancy. Plexiform neurofibromas are distinct from cutaneous neurofibromas and arise in the peripheral nerve sheath.

**TABLE 176-2 NATIONAL INSTITUTES OF HEALTH CONSENSUS DIAGNOSTIC CRITERIA FOR NEUROFIBROMATOSIS 1 (NF1)**

| |
|---|
| 6 or more café-au-lait spots > 5 mm in greatest diameter in prepubertal individuals or > 15 mm in greatest diameter in postpubertal individuals |
| 2 or more neurofibromas of any type or 1 plexiform neurofibroma |
| Axillary or inguinal freckling |
| Optic pathway glioma |
| 2 or more Lisch nodules (iris hamartomas) |
| A distinctive osseous lesion such as sphenoid dysplasia or tibial pseudoarthrosis |
| A first-degree relative (parent, sibling, or child) with NF1 by the above criteria |

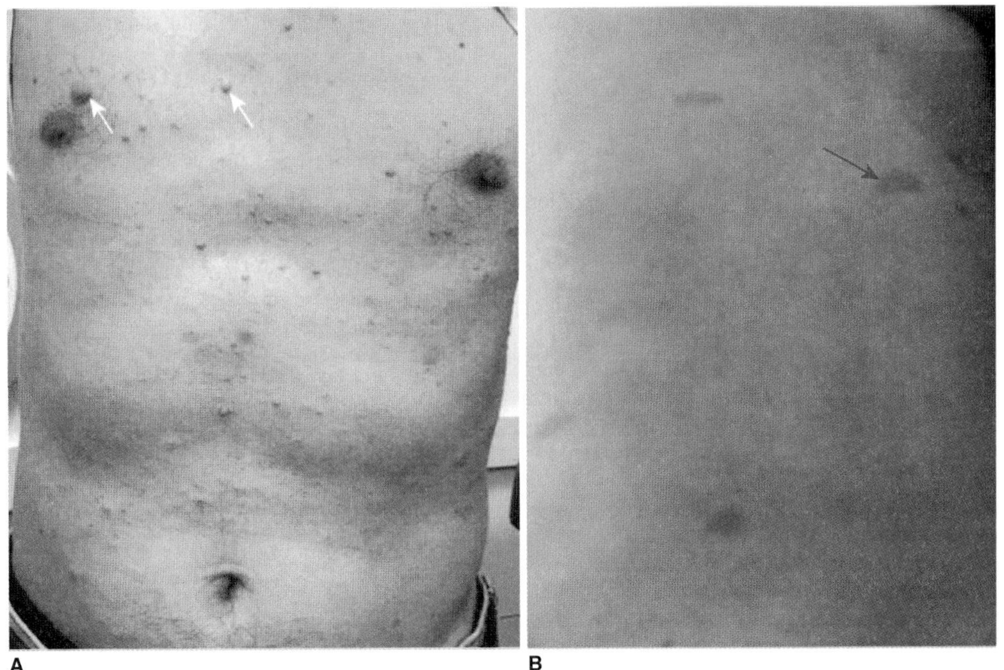


**FIGURE 176-1** **A:** Adult individual affected with neurofibromatosis type 1 (NF1) displaying neurofibromas (*white arrows*) and café-au-lait (CAL) macules affecting the torso. **B:** Child with NF1 with multiple CAL macules (*red solid arrow*) on the back.

They affect about one-half of the NF1 population, although many are not apparent on exam. Plexiform neurofibromas are typically present from birth or develop in infancy. Actively growing plexiform neurofibromas, which usually occur in young children, require close medical attention, as these tumors are diffuse and may extensively entwine with or compress internal organs and structures. Plexiform neurofibromas are at risk for transformation to malignant peripheral nerve sheath tumors (MPNST), but this is rare in the pediatric population.

Optic pathway gliomas (OPGs) are pilocytic astrocytomas (low-grade gliomas) along the length of the optic nerves or optic tracts that affect approximately 15% to 20% of individuals with NF1, but only about one-third of these become symptomatic. Symptomatic tumors tend to arise in the toddler or early childhood years and rarely develop after puberty. Screening for symptomatic tumors is critical to prevent severe visual impairment. Serial eye exams (at least annually) performed by a pediatric ophthalmologist can detect optic nerve pallor or visual symptoms and are strongly recommended by consensus opinion. Other surveillance techniques like MRI of the brain are more controversial; newer techniques are currently being developed and investigated. Pilocytic astrocytomas can occur in other locations in the brain of children with NF1 (basal ganglia, cerebellum, and brain stem). These tumors tend to behave indolently and rarely require intervention, in contrast to the behavior of the same low-grade gliomas outside of the context of NF1.

The skeletal features of NF1 are also age dependent and include sphenoid wing dysplasia, long-bone bowing (ie, tibial dysplasia with or without pseudoarthrosis) in infancy to early childhood, and dystrophic scoliosis in middle to late childhood. The pathophysiology of the various skeletal features is not understood, and it challenges the paradigm of NF1 being a disorder of neural crest origin. Both dystrophic scoliosis and pseudoarthrosis of long bones are primary defects that require significant orthopedic management and do not usually arise in the context of either plexiform or paraspinal neurofibromas.

Individuals with NF1 are prone to a number of medical complications that are quite varied. Approximately 40% to 50% have speech and language delays as preschoolers and/or learning problems in school. Early recognition and treatment within the educational environment can improve NF1-related learning problems and is 1 reason to provide a provisional diagnosis of NF1 in sporadic cases who only have multiple CAL spots. Short stature, macrocephaly, hypertension, constipation, and chronic headaches are other NF1-related features.

Approximately 1 in 10 individuals with NF1 exhibit features of Noonan syndrome, an autosomal dominant disorder most frequently due to pathogenic variants in *PTPN11*. These "Noonan/NF1" (OMIM no. 601321) individuals share features of CAL macules and freckling along with the facial features (downslanting palpebral fissures, relative macrocephaly, low-set ears, and webbing of the neck) of Noonan syndrome. These individuals almost invariably have pathogenic variants in the *NF1* gene (rather than *PTPN11*).

## MOLECULAR ASPECTS

The *NF1* gene spans approximately 350 kilobases of genomic DNA and is ubiquitously expressed. It encodes neurofibromin, a GTPase activating protein that downregulates ras signaling through the mitogen-activated protein kinase (MAPK) pathway. *NF1* mutations are generally inactivating, and double inactivation of both alleles in NF1-related tissues classifies this gene as a tumor suppressor.

Approximately half of individuals with NF1 are sporadic cases, which indicates that the gene is highly mutable. The high germline *NF1* mutation rate likely carries over to somatic mutations, which supports the tumor suppressor model for NF1 and provides one explanation for the variable and progressive nature of some clinical features. Random acquisition of somatic mutations that inactivate the normal *NF1* allele (second hit) in tissue showing abnormal growth could explain the age-related clinical presentation of many NF1 features, that is, neurofibromas, optic nerve pathway tumors, and plexiform neurofibromas. Leukemia cells, neurofibromas, malignant peripheral nerve sheath tumors, and pheochromocytomas have all demonstrated biallelic inactivation of *NF1*. The molecular diagnostic testing is able to detect pathogenic variants in > 99% of individuals who meet the NIH consensus criteria. However, the specific mutation is often of limited utility in predicting the clinical outcomes. To date, there are few genotype–phenotype correlations. Patients with a large, whole-gene deletion (~5% of all NF1 patients) tend to have a more severe phenotype with an unusually large number of cutaneous neurofibromas that present at an earlier age, distinctive facial features, and significant intellectual impairment. A relatively mild phenotype occurs in those with a specific 3-base pair deletion in exon 17 who generally have multiple CAL spots without other serious clinical manifestations. Finally, a high incidence of pulmonic stenosis and the Noonan/NF1 phenotype has been associated with missense mutations affecting Arg1809.

Counseling issues surrounding NF1 relate to its heritability, pleiotropy, variable expressivity, and age-dependent penetrance of the myriad clinical features. Even though there is a high sporadic incidence, once it is established within a family, it behaves as any other autosomal dominant condition, with a 50% risk for recurrence in each child conceived. However, unlike many other dominant conditions, the lack of genotype–phenotype correlation means that affected family members who have the same *NF1* mutation may have markedly different manifestations. This is one reason clinical mutation analysis on a routine basis is generally required.

Management decisions for tumor-related complications in NF1 can be challenging. Cutaneous neurofibromas are not at risk to undergo malignant transformation, and so observation is usually warranted. Surgical resection is reserved for lesions that are causing significant pain or irritation such as neurofibromas on the scalp or along the waistline that produce shooting sensations each time they are disturbed. Enlarging plexiform neurofibromas may also require intervention either because of the symptoms they are causing (substantial pain or functional impairment) or problems related to their impact on local structures (nerves, blood vessels, proximate tissue, and/or organs). These tumors can be controlled with complete resection; however, this is often impossible due to their entanglements. Early-phase clinical studies of therapies targeting the Ras-MAPK pathway have been in progress. Initial results with MEK inhibition have been promising. MPNST transformation may be signaled by rapid enlargement in the size of a plexiform neurofibroma and/or a worsening with the associated pattern of pain (eg, intensity, persistence). If suspicious for the possibility of an MPNST, prompt evaluation with imaging and potentially biopsy should be conducted because a complete resection is the most important prognostic factor in curing these highly aggressive cancers.

Symptomatic OPGs should be treated to prevent progressive vision loss. Various chemotherapy regimens may be effective in stabilizing these tumors (eg, carboplatin-based treatments) until the growth of these tumors spontaneously ceases with older age. MEK inhibitors may have a role in controlling OPGs as well. Radiation therapy is usually contraindicated for managing NF1-related brain tumors due to the heightened risk for secondary malignancies and the possibility of inducing or exacerbating cerebral vasculopathy.

Anticipatory guidance for NF1 includes the recognition of the age-dependent occurrence of most manifestations, some of which are uncommon and are not included in the diagnostic criteria. Issues that should be addressed on a regular basis are psychosocial adaption, development, school performance, tumors, bone abnormalities, and the consequences of NF1-related vasculopathy such as hypertension. Annual clinical assessments using a multidisciplinary approach are important to determine appropriate evaluation and management on an individualized basis.

## NEUROFIBROMATOSIS TYPE 2

### CLINICAL MANIFESTATIONS

Neurofibromatosis 2 (NF2; OMIM no. 101000) is an autosomal dominant condition characterized by the presence of bilateral vestibular schwannomas (or acoustic neuromas). The incidence of this condition is estimated at approximately 1 in 40,000. NF2 is a neurocutaneous condition with variable clinical expressivity; however, there is almost complete penetrance in adults, although the type of mutation can influence the age of onset. Diagnostic criteria have been established as shown in Table 176-3. Even though the mean age of onset of symptoms is in the third decade, clinical presentation in childhood is not rare.

In adults, the presenting symptoms of this disorder are most often related to the vestibular schwannomas; they include hearing loss, tinnitus, and imbalance. Vestibular schwannomas are found in virtually all older individuals with NF2, and they are bilateral in 90%. Approximately 20% of individuals with NF2 who are younger than age 15 have clinical features; however, only one-third of these cases have manifestations of vestibular schwannoma. Other central nervous system (CNS) tumors also occur in NF2, and they include intracranial meningiomas, schwannomas involving other cranial nerves (the fifth being most common) or peripheral nerves, and spinal cord tumors (schwannomas and ependymomas). Posterior subcapsular lenticular opacities or cataracts occur in 50% to 75% of individuals with NF2, and they serve as an early clinical sign of the disorder, and so should trigger a genetic evaluation if noted in children.

**TABLE 176-3 DIAGNOSTIC CRITERIA FOR NEUROFIBROMATOSIS 2 (NF2)**

| |
|---|
| Bilateral vestibular schwannomas |
| A first-degree relative (parent, sibling, or child) with NF2 |
| AND |
| EITHER a unilateral vestibular schwannoma OR |
| Any 2 of: meningioma, schwannoma, glioma, neurofibroma, posterior subcapsular lenticular opacities |
| Unilateral vestibular schwannoma |
| AND |
| Any 2 of: meningioma, schwannoma, glioma, neurofibroma, posterior subcapsular lenticular opacities |
| Multiple meningiomas |
| AND |
| EITHER a unilateral vestibular schwannoma OR |
| Any 2 of: schwannoma, glioma, neurofibroma, posterior subcapsular lenticular opacities |

Cutaneous manifestations of NF2 may include CAL spots, although relatively few, and skin tumors. These tumors are either characteristic plaque-like lesions or subcutaneous nodules that are pathologically diagnosed as schwannomas. Schwann cell tumors are found in both NF1 (neurofibromas) and NF2 (schwannomas); however, these 2 conditions are distinct entities and have minimal clinical overlap. Schwannomatosis (OMIM no. 162091, 615670) is an adult-onset syndrome with predisposition to schwannomas in various areas of the body. It is distinguished from NF2 by the relative lack of vestibular involvement and by the involved loci, which include the *SMARCB1* and *LZTR1* genes.

### MOLECULAR ASPECTS

NF2 genetically maps to chromosome 22q12.2 and is a 110-kb gene encoding a 595-amino acid cytoplasmic protein that has been named merlin and that shares homology with a family of cytoskeletal-associated proteins called the ERM family involved in communication between the extracellular milieu and the intracellular cytoskeleton. The *NF2* gene product is unusual because as a structural protein, it still has tumor suppressor properties. Interfamilial variability is greater than intrafamilial phenotypic differences, resulting in stronger genotype–phenotype correlations than those observed for NF1. Therefore, mutation detection in NF2 is helpful in predicting clinical severity and outcomes. Somatic mutation also plays a significant role in the pathology of this condition; loss of the normal allele in NF2-related tumors supports the hypothesis that *NF2* is a bona fide tumor suppressor gene.

### MANAGEMENT

Individuals suspected of having NF2 should undergo a thorough genetics evaluation. For affected individuals, a comprehensive initial investigation should be performed to identify CNS tumors, skin manifestations, and eye findings. Referral to a center experienced in managing NF2 is essential to ensuring all aspects of multidisciplinary care are addressed. Depending on the center, primary responsibility for NF2 care coordination may be assumed by geneticists, oncologists, neurologists, or surgeons. The availability of audiology and radiology (particularly neuroradiology) services is critical for tumor surveillance: annual audiology evaluations and MRI of the CNS with particular focus on the internal auditory canals where vestibular schwannomas arise (starting around 10–12 years of age). Management of manifestations may require the involvement and collaboration of multiple specialties including otolaryngology, neurosurgery, oncology, and ophthalmology. Early intervention for progressive tumors that are causing or are at risk for causing significant problems (severe symptoms, functional impairment, and reduced quality of life) may eliminate or reduce the severity of these issues or slow their progression.

Treatment of symptomatic and/or progressive vestibular schwannomas is the most common reason for intervention in patients with NF2. Historically, surgery or stereotactic radiosurgery has been performed to preserve hearing and achieve tumor control; however, frequent tumor regrowth and injury to the facial nerve are concerns. Alternatively, radiation has been used with the goals of stabilizing hearing and halting tumor growth; however, treatment failures are again common. More recently, treatment with bevacizumab, a monoclonal antibody directed against vascular endothelial growth factor (VEGF), has demonstrated hearing improvement in approximately half of patients. A substantial proportion of centers have started using this as an initial therapy with some advocating for indefinite treatment as long as the response is maintained and the side effects are tolerable/manageable. A spectrum of hearing assistance devices may also allow for different options for patients with hearing loss including hearing aids, cochlear implants, and auditory brain stem implants. In addition to auditory symptoms, patients with NF2 can have vestibular disorders that are severe and require lifestyle modifications. For NF2-related tumors other than vestibular schwannomas, surgery remains the mainstay of management, with the decision on whether to operate based on a deliberate consideration of the potential benefits of intervention against the possible morbidity.

## VON HIPPEL-LINDAU SYNDROME

### CLINICAL MANIFESTATIONS

Von Hippel-Lindau syndrome (VHL; OMIM no. 193300) is an autosomal dominant condition characterized by a predisposition to developing tumors in the CNS, eye, kidney, adrenal gland, pancreas, and endolymphatic sac. Diagnostic criteria based on this spectrum of tumors have been well established (Table 176-4). The prevalence has been estimated to be about 1 in 50,000 people. Like other neurocutaneous conditions, VHL demonstrates marked variability of clinical expression and near-complete penetrance in the adult population.

Most VHL-related tumors occur in young adults. However, retinal hemangioblastomas (or angiomas) and pheochromocytomas can occur in early childhood; the risk of CNS hemangioblastomas starts to rise in the teenage years. The symptoms of CNS and retinal hemangioblastomas associated with VHL differ from sporadic forms of this tumor. While the associated symptoms are similar, VHL-related hemangioblastoma usually presents earlier in life with multiple tumors developing. CNS hemangioblastomas most commonly arise in the cerebellum, and the symptoms they produce are similar to other posterior fossa tumors (ataxia, headaches, vomiting). Retinal angiomas occur in approximately 70% of patients with VHL, and about one-third of affected individuals have bilateral lesions. Without screening and treatment, these retinal tumors become symptomatic in the second and third decades of life with hemorrhage, retinal detachment, and visual loss. Pheochromocytomas develop in up to one-fourth of patients with VHL. Classic signs and symptoms may include headache, sweating, tachycardia, and elevated blood pressure, as severe as malignant hypertension. Endolymphatic sac tumors (ELSTs) and epididymal or broad ligament cystadenomas occasionally affect older children with VHL. ELSTs may cause hearing loss or repeated ear infections, while the cystadenomas are usually asymptomatic. Renal cell carcinomas can also be found in the majority of individuals with VHL, occurring predominantly in affected adults.

**TABLE 176-4 DIAGNOSTIC CRITERIA FOR VON HIPPEL-LINDAU (VHL) SYNDROME**

Multiple hemangioblastomas of the central nervous system/retina OR

Two or more of the following features:

- Family history of VHL
- One hemangioblastoma of the central nervous system/retina
- Renal cell carcinoma or cysts
- Pheochromocytoma
- Endolymphatic sac tumor
- Pancreatic neuroendocrine tumor or cysts
- Epididymal or broad ligament cystadenoma

### MOLECULAR ASPECTS

VHL genetically maps to chromosome 3p25 and is a relatively small gene (10 kb); the disease-causing gene is composed of 3 exons that encode a protein of 213 amino acids. The gene is ubiquitously expressed, and the unique VHL protein (pVHL) is present both in the nucleus and cytoplasm of cells; pVHL plays a pivotal role in regulating expression of hypoxia-response genes. The most characterized function of pVHL is its role in transcription elongation. Inactivation of pVHL by mutation of the gene leads to unregulated elongation of transcription of oncogenes and results in tumor growth. The identification of "second hits" in the *VHL* gene in tumor tissue from individuals with VHL demonstrates that it is a classic tumor suppressor.

The *VHL* gene is relatively small and test sensitivity for mutation detection is virtually 100%. Mutations are predictive of a group of distinct VHL disease phenotypes. VHL type 1 is characterized by retinal angioma, hemangioblastomas of the CNS, and renal cell carcinoma. Type 1 has low risk for pheochromocytoma and is associated with specific missense alleles in *VHL* that usually grossly disrupt folding of the protein. VHL type 2 has a high risk for pheochromocytoma, and the *VHL* mutations are usually missense mutations. In families with multiple affected members, VHL type 2 can be subdivided into 2A with low risk of renal cell carcinoma; 2B with high risk for renal cell carcinoma; and 2C with a risk for pheochromocytoma only. Complete deletion of the *VHL* gene leads to lower risk for both pheochromocytoma and renal cell carcinoma. Almost all individuals with a *VHL* mutation will demonstrate disease-related symptoms by age 65 consistent with nearly complete penetrance of the condition.

### MANAGEMENT

Medical professionals with expertise in VHL have worked with the VHL Alliance to develop extensive surveillance guidelines based on the tumor risks and the variable ages at which risk for these tumors typically emerge. These surveillance methods incorporate a combination of subspecialist exams, biochemical tests, and imaging. The regimen consists of screening for retinal angiomas with annual ophthalmology exams starting at 1 year of age, for pheochromocytomas with annual testing for fractionated metanephrines (plasma or 24-hour urine collection) starting at 5 years and annual abdominal ultrasounds starting at 8 years, for ELST with biennial audiology evaluations starting at 5 years, and for CNS hemangioblastomas and all potential abdominal tumors with biennial MRI starting at 16 years. Adjustments to this regimen may be made based on the VHL phenotype predicted by the genotype and the family history. Once diagnosed, a multidisciplinary team approach is needed to fully address anticipated clinical manifestations. In particular, the management of pheochromocytomas requires multiple subspecialties working closely in concert, including renal, surgery, anesthesia, critical care, endocrine, and oncology.

## NEVOID BASAL CELL CARCINOMA SYNDROME (GORLIN SYNDROME)

### CLINICAL MANIFESTATIONS

Nevoid basal cell carcinoma syndrome (NBCCS; OMIM no. 109400) is an autosomal dominant condition characterized by basal cell nevi, multiple jaw keratocysts, and a number of other systemic features such as calcification of the falx and palmar/plantar pits. While basal cell nevi can occur in early childhood, basal cell carcinomas (BCCs) typically start to develop later in life (teens/young adults) from these nevi or spontaneously, continuing to increase in number with age (about 10% of individuals with NBCCS do not develop them).

Medulloblastoma, the most common malignant brain tumor in childhood, develops in about 5% of individuals with NBCCS. In affected children with NBCCS, these tumors mostly arise before 3 years of age, with the oldest occurrence at 7 years. Pathology has been reported as 1 of 3 variants: desmoplastic, desmoplastic nodular, or medulloblastoma with extensive nodularity. These children rarely die from their medulloblastoma, with long-term progression-free survival exceeding 90%.

Individuals with NBCCS are also at risk of developing several benign tumors. Cardiac fibromas (2%) or infrequently rhabdomyomas, either cardiac or at other sites, may be congenital or develop in infancy. Affected females, typically young adults, may also develop ovarian fibromas with an estimated risk level of 20%. Keratocysts of the jaw, which usually appear as painless enlargements, affect most individuals with NBCCS and may arise in young children with most occurring in teenagers.

## MOLECULAR ASPECTS

NBCCS is due to heterozygous germline pathogenic variants in 1 of 2 genes, *PTCH1* or *SUFU*. The majority of individuals with NBCCS inherit the disorder from an affected parent. Point mutations in the *PTCH1* gene are seen in the majority of individuals, but gene deletions of *PTCH1* or point mutations or deletions of *SUFU* account for a smaller proportion, while approximately a quarter of patients are not molecularly diagnosed despite a clinical diagnosis. *PTCH1* maps to 9q22.32 and encodes a membrane protein that binds the secreted factor sonic hedgehog. NBCCS-associated *PTCH1* mutations lead to loss of function. The *SUFU* gene encodes a suppressor of the hedgehog pathway.

## MANAGEMENT

Consensus cancer surveillance guidelines in NBCCS do not exist. However, there is a clear role for complete unclothed skin exams performed at least annually starting from diagnosis to allow for early intervention. When concerning nevi or early BCCs are found, they are amenable to excision. Supplemental treatment with cryotherapy, laser treatment, or photodynamic therapy may also be used.

A heightened awareness of risk of medulloblastoma and the associated signs and symptoms in families and providers caring for children with NBCCS is essential. Whether imaging surveillance with serial MRI is beneficial is not straightforward. Again, survival rates from medulloblastoma in NBCCS are high. The medulloblastoma risk appears to diverge substantially depending on the causative gene; the risk of medulloblastoma for children with germline *PTCH1* mutations is less than 2%, while the risk conferred by germline *SUFU* mutations can be as much as 20-fold greater. However, consideration should be given to performing MRI of the brain every 3 to 6 months during the first 3 years of life, possibly limited to those with mutations of the *SUFU* gene. In general, medulloblastoma requires multimodality therapy for cure. For children older than 3 years of age, this includes maximal achievable tumor resection, followed by radiation to the CNS, and then chemotherapy. Radiation is often avoided or delayed in children under 3 years of age due to high risk of severe neurocognitive impairment. In children with NBCCS, radiation therapy may lead to a greatly increased incidence of BCCs of the skin encompassed within the radiation field. This risk should be strongly weighed in cases when radiation is being considered for inclusion in the treatment plan for NBCCS-related medulloblastoma.

Additional surveillance evaluations may be beneficial for assessing benign lesions. An echocardiogram at diagnosis should be performed to assess for clinically significant cardiac fibromas or rhabdomyomas. Annual panorex films initiated at about 8 years of age can reveal early jaw keratocysts, which can be excised with much less morbidity when small than when they are much larger and discovered by visual inspection.



## SUGGESTED READINGS


Aufforth RD, Ramakant P, Sadowski SM, et al. Pheochromocytoma screening initiation and frequency in von Hippel-Lindau syndrome. *J Clin Endocrinol Metab.* 2015;100:4498-4504.

Bree AF, Shah MR. BCNS Colloquium Group. Consensus statement from the first international colloquium on basal cell nevus syndrome (BCNS). *Am J Med Genet A.* 2011;155A:2091-2097.

Evans DG, Baser ME, O'Reilly B, et al. Management of the patient and family with neurofibromatosis 2: a consensus conference statement. *Br J Neurosurg.* 2005;19:5-12.

Gorlin RJ. Nevoid basal cell carcinoma (Gorlin) syndrome. *Genet Med.* 2004;6:530-539.

Hersh JH. American Academy of Pediatrics Committee on Genetics. Health supervision for children with neurofibromatosis. *Pediatrics.* 2008;121:633-642.

Hirbe AC, Gutmann DH. Neurofibromatosis type 1: a multidisciplinary approach to care. *Lancet Neurol.* 2014;13:834-843.

Listernick R, Ferner RE, Liu GT, Gutmann DH. Optic pathway glioma in neurofibromatosis-1: controversies and recommendations. *Ann Neurol.* 2007;61:189-198.

Lonser RR, Glenn GM, Walther M, et al. von Hippel-Lindau disease. *Lancet.* 2003;361:2059-2067.

Matsuo M, Ohno K, Ohtsuka F. Characterization of early onset neurofibromatosis type 2. *Brain Dev.* 2014;36:148-152.

Nguyen R, Dombi E, Widemann BC, et al. Growth dynamics of plexiform neurofibromas: a retrospective cohort study of 201 patients with neurofibromatosis 1. *Orphanet J Rare Dis.* 2012;7:75.

Plotkin SR, Stemmer-Rachamimov AO, Barker FG 2nd, et al. Hearing improvement after bevacizumab in patients with neurofibromatosis type 2. *N Engl J Med.* 2009;361:358-367.

Schwetye KE, Gutmann DH. Cognitive and behavioral problems in children with neurofibromatosis type 1: challenges and future directions. *Expert Rev Neurother.* 2014;14:1139-1152.


# 177 Craniosynostosis

Lindsay C. Burrage and V. Reid Sutton

## INTRODUCTION

Craniosynostosis (also called craniostensosis) results from a premature fusion of the cranial sutures, which consist of fibrous connective tissue that connects the bones of the cranium. Craniosynostosis may occur as an isolated birth defect or as part of a syndrome. The major cranial sutures are the coronal sutures, which separate the frontal and parietal bones; the sagittal suture, which separates the parietal bones; the metopic suture, which separates the frontal bones; and the lambdoid sutures, which separate the parietal and occipital bones. The main functions of these sutures is to facilitate deformation of the skull during passage through the birth canal and to facilitate growth of the cranium to accommodate rapid brain growth during early childhood. Typically, cranial sutures close in early adulthood with the exception of the metopic suture, which closes in early childhood. Craniosynostosis may affect 1 or more of these sutures, and premature fusion of these sutures can have a host of consequences including increased risk for raised intracranial pressure, abnormal cranial shape, and distortion of craniofacial structures, which may affect breathing patterns, vision, and hearing. Moreover, syndromic forms of craniosynostosis may be characterized by other skeletal abnormalities and involvement of other organ systems.

## PATHOGENESIS AND EPIDEMIOLOGY

Craniosynostosis affects approximately 1 in 2000 to 1 in 2500 live births, and the sagittal suture is the most common suture involved. Craniosynostosis may occur in isolation ("nonsyndromic forms") or within the context of a genetic syndrome ("syndromic form"). Nonsyndromic forms account for about 75% of cases, and these nonsyndromic forms may have genetic and/or environmental causes. Known environmental risk factors include teratogens (eg, valproic acid or methotrexate) and factors that constrain the growth of the developing fetus (eg, multiparity and macrosomia). In the nonsyndromic forms, genetic factors are more likely to contribute to isolated bilateral or unilateral coronal craniosynostosis as compared to other sutures. A recent study has implicated a 2-locus model (eg, variants in *SMAD6* and *BMP2*) to explain a subset of nonsyndromic midline craniosynostosis. Approximately 15% of craniosynostosis occurs in the setting of 1 of more than 150 recognizable genetic syndromes. Pathogenic variants in over 50 genes have been associated with either nonsyndromic or syndromic forms of craniosynostosis. The most common syndromic forms are caused by pathogenic variants in *FGFR1*, *FGFR2*, *FGFR3*, and *TWIST*. Although autosomal dominant inheritance is the most common pattern observed in genetic forms of craniosynostosis (eg, *FGFR1*, *FGFR2*, *FGFR3*), autosomal recessive and X-linked forms (eg, *EFNB1*) exist. When inherited, many of these syndromic forms of craniosynostosis are associated with reduced penetrance and/or variable expressivity within families.

## CLINICAL MANIFESTATIONS

Craniosynostosis results in a failure of growth in the plane perpendicular to the prematurely fused suture, and to accommodate, excessive growth occurs in the plane parallel to the prematurely fused suture. This abnormal growth leads to recognizable patterns of skull growth that allows for identification of the suture involved (Fig. 177-1). For instance, craniosynostosis involving the bilateral coronal sutures results in brachycephaly or a skull that is wide from side-to-side but short in the anterior-posterior dimension. Alternatively, premature fusion of the sagittal suture results in a skull that is long and narrow (scaphocephaly). When the metopic suture is fused prematurely, the skull has a triangular shape (trigonocephaly). Unilateral lambdoid suture craniosynostosis leads to flattening of the ipsilateral occipital portion of the skull (plagiocephaly) with posterior displacement of the ipsilateral ear and forehead and contralateral frontal bossing, and from above, the resulting skull shape resembles a trapezoid. The most severe form of craniosynostosis involves multiple sutures, and the resulting skull shape is similar to a cloverleaf. This cloverleaf skull shape is also known as kleeblattschädel.

For the general pediatrician, positional plagiocephaly results from flattening of 1 side of the occipital region that occurs when an infant is placed on the back to sleep; this must be distinguished from craniosynostosis. Positional plagiocephaly (or molding) causes flattening of the ipsilateral occipital bone with ipsilateral frontal bossing and anterior displacement of the ipsilateral ear, and from above, the resulting shape of the skull resembles a parallelogram. The differentiation of plagiocephaly resulting from occipital craniosynostosis versus positional plagiocephaly has important treatment implications.

The most worrisome complication of craniosynostosis is increased intracranial pressure, and thus, the clinical evaluation of individuals with craniosynostosis should include an evaluation of the fundus for papilledema and evaluation for other signs of increased intracranial pressure that would require immediate intervention. In addition, syndromic or nonsyndromic forms of craniosynostosis may show similar complications including vision or hearing abnormalities, decreased blood flow to the brain, and developmental delays.

In syndromic forms of craniosynostosis, clinical manifestations may include other skeletal manifestations and involvement of various organ systems. These additional clinical manifestations may provide clues to the underlying genetic syndrome. Several of the most common syndromic causes of craniosynostosis are outlined in the next sections and in Table 177-1.

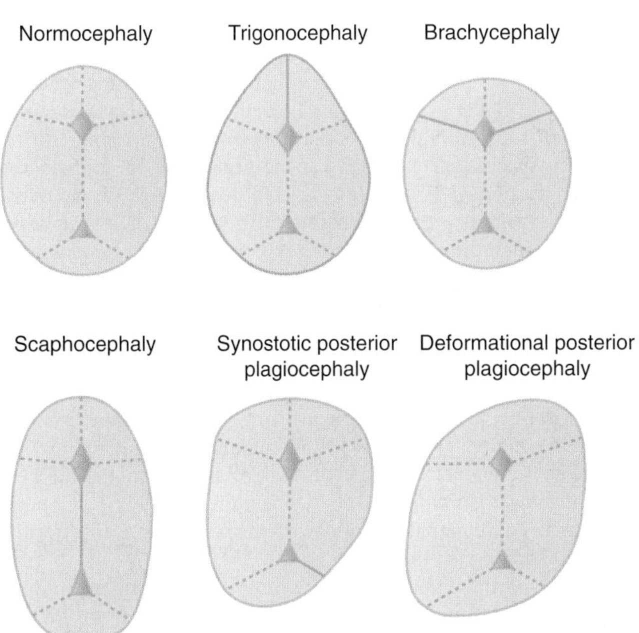


**FIGURE 177-1** Fusion of suture(s) in craniosynostosis results in excess head growth in the plane parallel to the fused suture and a characteristic shape of the head. Normocephaly and positional plagiocephaly are provided for comparison. Dotted lines indicate open sutures, and solid lines indicate prematurely fused sutures.

## CRANIOSYNOSTOSIS SYNDROMES

### Crouzon Syndrome

Crouzon syndrome is typically associated with coronal synostosis without the extremity abnormalities that may be observed in other related syndromes. However, other sutures may also be involved. Individuals with Crouzon syndrome typically have maxillary hypoplasia with the appearance of mandibular prognathism and shallow orbits causing the eyes to appear proptotic. Intellectual development in Crouzon syndrome is typically normal. A sacrococcygeal tail may be observed in some. Crouzon syndrome is typically associated with heterozygous pathogenic variants in *FGFR2*, and these variants may be inherited from affected family members in an autosomal dominant pattern or may arise de novo as a new mutation in the proband. A small subset (~5%) with Crouzon syndrome develop acanthosis nigricans early in childhood or later in life. This subset of Crouzon syndrome, called Crouzon syndrome with acanthosis nigricans, is classically associated with a specific pathogenic variant (heterozygous p.Ala391Glu) in *FGFR3*.

### Apert Syndrome

Like Crouzon syndrome, Apert syndrome is also characterized by coronal synostosis, but other sutures may also be involved. Individuals with Apert syndrome may have similar facial features to Crouzon syndrome. The distinctive features of Apert syndrome are the limb abnormalities, which typically include syndactyly of the hands and feet, giving the hands and feet a "mitten-glove" appearance. In addition, some individuals with Apert syndrome have developmental delay or intellectual disability (~50%), and a subset may also have cleft palate, rhizomelic shortening, and involvement of other organs. Typically, Apert syndrome is associated with a heterozygous pathogenic variant in *FGFR2* that is de novo or that is inherited in an autosomal dominant pattern in families.

### Pfeiffer Syndrome

Three forms of Pfeiffer syndrome have been described. All forms of Pfeiffer syndrome involve craniosynostosis of the coronal suture(s), but other sutures may also be involved. In addition, the extremities have a distinctive appearance with a broad shape and medial deviation of the first digits of the upper and lower extremities. Pfeiffer syndrome

**TABLE 177-1 COMMON SYNDROMIC CAUSES OF CRANIOSYNOSTOSIS**

| Disorder | Gene(s) | Inheritance Pattern | Thumbs | Hands | Great Toe | Feet |
|---|---|---|---|---|---|---|
| Crouzon | *FGFR2* | AD | Normal | Normal | Normal | Normal |
| Crouzon with acanthosis nigricans | *FGFR3* | AD | Normal | Normal | Normal | Normal |
| Apert[a] | *FGFR2* | AD | +/– Fused fingers | Soft tissue +/– bone syndactyly | +/– Fused toes | Soft tissue +/– bone syndactyly |
| Pfeiffer[a] | *FGFR1/FGFR2* | AD | Broad, medial deviation | Variable brachydactyly | Broad, medial deviation | Variable brachydactyly |
| Muenke | *FGFR3* | AD | Normal | +/– Carpal fusion | +/– Broad | +/– Tarsal fusion |
| Jackson-Weiss | *FGFR2* | AD | Normal | Variable | Broad, medial deviation | Abnormal tarsals |
| Saethre-Chotzen | *TWIST* | AD | Normal | +/– Syndactyly of second and third digits | +/– Broad or bifid | Normal |

[a]Intellectual disability observed frequently.

AD, autosomal dominant.

type 2 is the most severe type, with craniosynostosis affecting all sutures, which results in a cloverleaf shape to the skull. In addition, individuals with Pfeiffer syndrome type 2 have marked proptosis that may interfere with closure of the eyelids, cognitive involvement, and elbow and/or knee ankylosis. Given the severity of the abnormalities and the associated sequelae, individuals with Pfeiffer syndrome type 2 are at increased risk for premature death in early childhood. Pfeiffer syndrome type 3 is similar to type 2 except that individuals with Pfeiffer syndrome type 3 typically do not have the cloverleaf shape to the skull but rather have turribrachycephaly or a high and tall forehead, giving the skull a "tower shape." Individuals with all forms of Pfeiffer syndrome typically have a heterozygous pathogenic variant in *FGFR2*, although a small fraction (~5%) with type 1 may have a heterozygous pathogenic variant in *FGFR1*.

#### Muenke Syndrome

Muenke syndrome, the most common of the syndromic forms of craniosynostosis, is characterized by unilateral or bilateral coronal synostosis, broad toes, and fusions of the carpal bones or calcaneus. In addition, other cranial sutures may be involved, and individuals may have hearing abnormalities, vision abnormalities, or developmental delay. This developmental delay does not appear to be the consequence of the craniosynostosis itself as individuals who have Muenke syndrome but no craniosynostosis may also have developmental delays. Interestingly, all individuals with Muenke syndrome have the same heterozygous pathogenic variant (p.Pro250Arg) in *FGFR3*. This pathogenic variant may be inherited or de novo, but as with many of the pathogenic variants in the FGFRs, the de novo variants typically arise on the paternal allele. Interestingly, some individuals inherit the pathogenic variant from a parent who was thought to be unaffected, but on careful examination, the parent may have mild manifestations of the disorder as a result of variable expressivity or possibly somatic mosaicism.

#### Saethre-Chotzen Syndrome

Like the previously described syndromes, Saethre-Chotzen syndrome typically involves coronal synostosis, although other sutures may be involved. Characteristic physical exam findings may include asymmetric facial features, ptosis, strabismus, and characteristic ears that have a small pinnae and a prominent crus. First digits of the lower extremity may be broad or bifid, and syndactyly involving the second and third digits of the hands may be present. Other features that have been observed in some individuals include short stature, parietal foramina, vertebral fusions, radioulnar synostosis, cleft palate, hypertelorism, and congenital cardiac malformations. Cognitive outcome is typically normal except in those who have large chromosomal deletions associated with the phenotype. The genetic abnormality in Saethre-Chotzen syndrome is typically a heterozygous pathogenic variant in *TWIST* that is either inherited or de novo. The pathogenic variants associated with Saethre-Chotzen have been found to be distributed throughout exon 1, the only coding exon of this gene. Moreover, some individuals have contiguous gene deletions involving *TWIST* and other neighboring genes.

#### Jackson-Weiss Syndrome

Jackson-Weiss syndrome is similar to Pfeiffer syndrome in that craniosynostosis is associated with broad and medially deviated first digit of the lower extremity. However, the 2 syndromes can be distinguished because individuals with Jackson-Weiss syndrome typically do not have broad thumbs. Other phenotypic features of Jackson-Weiss syndrome include partial syndactyly of the second and third toes and short and broad metatarsals. Radiographs of the feet demonstrate calcaneocuboid fusion, short first metatarsals, and broad proximal phalanges. Individuals with Jackson-Weiss syndrome typically have normal cognitive development. Jackson-Weiss syndrome has been associated with heterozygous pathogenic variants in *FGFR2*.

## DIAGNOSIS

Early recognition of the physical examination findings of craniosynostosis is important because untreated craniosynostosis can lead to a host of complications including increased intracranial pressure, decreased blood flow to the brain, or vision and hearing deficits. The first step for diagnosing craniosynostosis is a detailed history including prenatal history (eg, teratogen exposure) and family history and a careful physical examination to determine whether an individual has a syndromic or nonsyndromic form of craniosynostosis. If an individual has features of a recognizable clinical syndrome, specific gene testing can be performed to confirm the suspected diagnosis. Typically, targeted sequencing of recurrent pathogenic variants is pursued before full gene sequencing. In addition, panels including various genes associated with craniosynostosis are also available. If a person appears to have a more complex phenotype with features that are not typical of a known syndrome, a genome-wide test such as chromosome microarray (array comparative genomic hybridization or genome-wide single nucleotide polymerphism array) is indicated to search for chromosomal deletions or duplications, which might be causing the phenotype. Whole-exome sequencing (WES) or whole-genome sequencing (WGS) might also be considered. The identification of the genetic cause for the craniosynostosis will not only confirm the underlying diagnosis but will also guide management decisions and facilitate appropriate genetic counseling for the family.

For nonsyndromic forms of craniosynostosis involving the midline sutures, genetic testing of *SMAD6* may be considered, but the yield is variable depending on the suture involved, with the highest frequency for metopic plus sagittal (37.5%), a moderate frequency for metopic alone (10%), and low frequency for sagittal alone (< 3%). On the other hand, genetic testing should be considered for unilateral or bilateral nonsyndromic coronal synostosis as pathogenic variants in *FGFR3*, *FGFR1*, *FGFR2*, and *TWIST* have been observed in up to 24% of these individuals. Identification of a pathogenic variant in individuals with nonsyndromic coronal synostosis may yield important prognostic information. Comprehensive genetic counseling should be provided to families when genetic testing is performed so that families understand the limitations of testing and so that appropriate recurrence risks can be provided. Moreover, families should be made aware that a normal genetic test result does not necessarily rule out a genetic cause for the phenotype.

## TREATMENT

The management of individuals with craniosynostosis should involve a team approach, and many hospitals have multidisciplinary clinics designed for those with craniofacial abnormalities such as craniosynostosis. These clinics typically include various surgical subspecialties, medical geneticists or genetic counselors, developmental specialists, audiologists, speech therapists, and social workers, and such clinics provide multidisciplinary care for individuals with craniosynostosis. In the absence of a need for emergent interventions for increased intracranial pressure, the timing of surgical repair may vary depending on the type of craniosynostosis but is typically in the first year of life (in some cases, as early as 3–6 months), and surgical repair may be a staged approach with multiple procedures planned. Because of the craniofacial abnormalities, these patients may be at risk for various respiratory complications such as sleep apnea and choanal stenosis, and thus, respiratory status should be monitored, and careful planning for anesthesia and sedation is recommended. Regular funduscopic exams (preoperatively and postoperatively) are indicated to monitor for papilledema, which may be a sign of increased intracranial pressure, and routine ophthalmologic evaluations are recommended to monitor for ophthalmologic complications. Given risk for chronic otitis media and hearing loss, audiology evaluations should be part of the routine management of individuals with craniosynostosis. Developmental evaluations and early childhood intervention are also recommended given risks for developmental delays and intellectual disabilities. Genetic counseling is recommended so that patients and families understand the prognosis and recurrence risks associated with their diagnosis.

## SUGGESTED READINGS


Agochukwu NB, Solomon BD, Muenke M. Impact of genetics on the diagnosis and clinical management of syndromic craniosynostoses. *Childs Nerv Syst*. 2012;28:1447-1463.

Goriely A, Wilkie AOM. Paternal age effect mutations and selfish spermatogonial selection: causes and consequences for human disease. *Am J Hum Genet*. 2012;90:175-200.

Greenwood J, Flodman P, Osann K, et al. Familial incidence and associated symptoms in a population of individuals with nonsyndromic craniosynostosis. *Genet Med*. 2014;16:302-310.

Kruszka P, Addissie YA, Yarnell CMP, et al. Muenke syndrome: an international multicenter natural history study. *Am J Med Genet Part A*. 2016;170A:918-929.

Robin NH, Falk MJ, Haldeman-Englert CR. FGFR-related craniosynostosis. In: Pagon RA, Adam MP, Ardinger HH, et al, eds. *GeneReviews*. Seattle, WA: University of Washington; 1993-2016.

Roscioli T, Elakis G, Cox T, et al. Genotype and clinical care correlations in craniosynostosis: findings from a cohort of 630 Australian and New Zealand patients. *Am J Med Genet Part C Semin Med Genet*. 2013;163C:259-270.

Speltz ML, Collett BR, Wallace ER, et al. Intellectual and academic functioning of school-age children with single-suture craniosynostosis. *Pediatrics*. 2015;135:e615-e623.

Timberlake AT, Choi J, Zaidi S, et al. Two locus inheritance of nonsyndromic midline craniosynostosis via rare *SMAD6* and common *BMP2* alleles. *Elife*. 2016;5:e20125.

Twigg SRF, Wilkie AOM. A genetic-pathophysiological framework for craniosynostosis. *Am J Hum Genet*. 2015;97:359-377.




# 178 Cleft Lip and Palate

Ariadne Letra, Brett Chiquet, and Haley Streff

## INTRODUCTION

Oral-facial clefts, including cleft lip and/or cleft palate, are the most common craniofacial birth defects, affecting approximately 135,000 newborns worldwide each year. The costs of caring for a child with an oral-facial cleft are more than $100,000 and creates significant financial and healthcare burdens for these families. Infants born with an oral-facial cleft may have feeding, swallowing, breathing, speech, and hearing complications. Therefore, a multidisciplinary team, including surgical, dental, speech, genetic, and nutrition experts, is typically involved in patient care. This chapter will discuss the pathogenesis, epidemiology, clinical manifestations, diagnosis, treatment, and prevention of oral-facial clefts.

## PATHOGENESIS OF ORAL-FACIAL CLEFTS

Development of the lip and palate results from the growth and fusion of facial prominences and involves cell migration, proliferation, differentiation, and apoptosis. At approximately the fourth week of embryonic development in humans, the medial nasal processes that originate from the frontonasal process merge with each other and with the bilateral maxillary processes to form the upper lip and the primary palate. Later, around the sixth week, the bilateral maxillary processes project downward along the sides of the tongue; then as the tongue descends into the oral cavity, the processes elevate above the tongue and fuse to form the secondary palate, separating the oral and nasal cavities. Disruptions at any stage of these developmental processes can lead to an oral-facial cleft.

## EPIDEMIOLOGY OF ORAL-FACIAL CLEFTS

The prevalence of oral-facial clefts varies according to geographic location and ethnic background. In general, Native American and Asian populations present the highest reported birth prevalence rates of ~2 to 3 per 1000 live births, whereas Caucasians present a prevalence of ~1 per 1000 births, and African populations present the lowest prevalence of 0.3 per 1000 births.

Oral-facial clefts have been categorized as syndromic or nonsyndromic based on the presence of additional structural abnormalities. Up to 44% to 64% of all cleft cases present with associated anomalies, and to date, over 500 syndromes including chromosomal abnormalities have been reported in association with an oral cleft. Relatively common syndromic forms of oral-facial clefts include Stickler syndrome, 22q11.2 deletion syndrome, Van der Woude syndrome, and ectodermal dysplasia ectrodactyly and clefting (EEC) syndrome, most of which are associated with cleft palate rather than cleft lip and palate (Table 178-1). The most common anomalies associated with cleft palate are congenital heart defects, hydrocephaly, urinary tract defects, and polydactyly. Midline (median) clefts are commonly associated with syndromic forms of clefts (eg, frontonasal dysplasia, holoprosencephaly, or other disruptions in frontonasal development). For these reasons, children with midline clefts of the lip require careful examination that should include computed tomography (CT) or magnetic resonance imaging (MRI) of the central nervous system. The majority of cleft lip and palate cases (approximately 70–75%) are isolated, also referred to as nonsyndromic, while approximately 50% of cleft palate cases are isolated.

## CLINICAL MANIFESTATIONS

The expressivity of oral-facial clefts may vary, ranging from cleft lip only (CL), cleft lip with or without cleft palate (CL/P), or cleft palate only (CPO) (Fig. 178-1). Historically, CL/P and CPO have been described as separate entities due to embryologic differences in the structural origins of the primary and secondary palates; also CL/P and CPO do not usually segregate in the same family (although a few exceptions have been reported). The frequency of CL/P varies by gender and laterality, with

**TABLE 178-1 SELECTED SYNDROMES INVOLVING CLEFT LIP AND/OR CLEFT PALATE**

| Syndrome | OMIM No. | Inheritance | Gene/Loci | Phenotype(s) |
|---|---|---|---|---|
| DiGeorge syndrome (22q11 deletion syndrome, velocardiofacial syndrome) | 188400 (*602054, 192430) | AD | Microdeletion of 22q11.2 (typical 1.5–3.0 Mb deletion including *TBX1*) | CL/P, congenital heart defect, developmental delay/intellectual disability, immune deficiency, hypocalcemia, renal anomalies, psychiatric illness |
| Van der Woude syndrome | 119300 | AD | *IRF6* | CL/P or SMCP, congenital lip pits |
| Popliteal pterygium syndrome | 119500 | AD | *IRF6* | CL/P, lower lip fistula, syndactyly of fingers and/or toes, pyramidal fold of skin over the nail of the hallux, popliteal pterygia, abnormal external genitalia |
| Pierre Robin sequence | 261800 | Multifactorial | — | Micrognathia, glossoptosis, cleft palate |
| Stickler syndrome types I, II, III | 108300, 604841, 184840 | AD | *COL2A1, COL11A1, COL11A2* | CL/P, Pierre Robin sequence, vitreous changes, retinal detachment, high-frequency sensorineural hearing loss, skeletal anomalies |
| CHARGE syndrome | 214800 | AD | *CHD7* | Coloboma, cranial nerve dysfunction, abnormal external ears, developmental delay, cardiovascular malformations, growth deficiencies, CL/P, choanal atresia, hypogonadotropic hypogonadism |
| Kabuki syndrome | 147920 | AD | *KMT2D, KDM6A* | Elongated palpebral fissures, eversion of lateral lower eyelid, arched/broad eyebrows, skeletal anomalies, persistent fetal fingertip pads, intellectual disability, postnatal growth deficiency, congenital heart defect, CL/P, genitourinary anomalies |
| Nager syndrome (acrofacial dysostosis 1) | 154400 | AD | *SF3B4* | Pierre Robin sequence, CL/P, absent/hypoplastic thumbs, phocomelia of upper limbs, downslanting palpebral fissures, abnormal external ears |
| Treacher Collins syndrome | 154500 | AD | *TCOF1, POLR1C, POLR1D* | Zygomatic bones and mandibular hypoplasia, micrognathia, retrognathia, external ear abnormalities, lower eyelid coloboma, ophthalmologic defects, CL/P |
| Beckwith-Wiedemann syndrome | 130650 | Paternally imprinted | Methylation defect of 11p15.5; *CDKN1C* | Macrosomia, macroglossia, visceromegaly, embryonal tumors, omphalocele, neonatal hypoglycemia, ear creases/pits, renal abnormalities, CPO, hemihyperplasia, organomegaly |
| Waardenburg syndrome type I | 193500 | AD | *PAX3* | Sensorineural hearing loss, white forlock, segmental or complete heterochromia, dystopia canthorum, skin hypopigmentation, CL/P |
| Craniofacial microsomia (hemifacial microsomia, oculo-auriculo-vertebral spectrum, Goldenhar syndrome, otomandibular dysostosis, facio-auriculo-vertebral syndrome, lateral facial dysplasia) | 164210 | Multifactorial | — | First and second brachial arch defects; facial asymmetry, maxillary/mandibular hypoplasia, facial tags, ear malformations, CL/P, vertebral defects, limb anomalies |
| Oral-facial-digital syndrome, type I | 311200 | X-linked dominant | *OFD1* | CL/P, dental anomalies, brachydactyly, syndactyly, clinodactyly, structural brain abnormalities, intellectual disability, renal cysts |
| Nevoid basal cell carcinoma syndrome (basal cell nevus syndrome, Gorlin syndrome) | 109400 | AD | *PTCH1, PTCH2, SUFU* | Multiple basal cell carcinomas, jaw keratocysts, palmar/plantar pits, macrocephaly, skeletal anomalies, ectopic calcification of the falx, CL/P, medulloblastoma |
| Smith-Lemli-Opitz syndrome | 270400 | AR | *DHCR7* | Microcephaly, prenatal and postnatal growth deficiency, intellectual disability, CPO, congenital heart defect, underdeveloped external genitalia, 2–3 syndactyly of toes |
| TP63-related syndromes (ankyloblepharon ectodermal dysplasia and clefting syndrome, acro-dermo-ungual-lacrimal-tooth syndrome, ectrodactyly, ectodermal dysplasia, cleft lip/palate syndrome 3, split-hand/foot malformation 4) | *603273 (106260, 103285, 604292, 605289) | AD | *TP63* | Varying combinations of ectodermal dysplasia, CL/P, split-hand/foot malformation, syndactyly, lacrimal duct obstruction, hypopigmentation, various craniofacial abnormalities |
| Ectrodactyly, ectodermal dysplasia, and cleft lip/palate syndrome | 129900 | Multifactorial | 7q11.2-q21.3 | Ectrodactyly of hands and/or feet, ectodermal dysplasia, CL/P |
| Miller syndrome (postaxial acrofacial dysostosis) | 263750 | AR | *DHODH* | Postaxial limb hypoplasia, syndactyly, absence of postaxial digits, ulnar hypoplasia, malar hypoplasia, CPO, coloboma, ectropion of lower eyelids |
| Opitz oculo-genital-laryngeal syndrome | 300000 | X-linked dominant | *MID1* | CL/P, genitourinary abnormalities, developmental delay/intellectual disability, laryngotracheoesophageal defect, heart defect, imperforate anus, midline brain defect |

Note. Not all phenotypic features listed will necessarily be present in every case.

AD, autosomal dominant; AR, autosomal recessive; CL, cleft lip; CL/P, cleft lip and palate; CPO, cleft palate; OMIM, Online Mendelian Inheritance in Man; SMCP, submucous cleft palate.

Data from Online Mendelian Inheritance in Man, OMIM. McKusick-Nathans Institute of Genetic Medicine, Johns Hopkins University (Baltimore, MD), and National Library of Medicine.

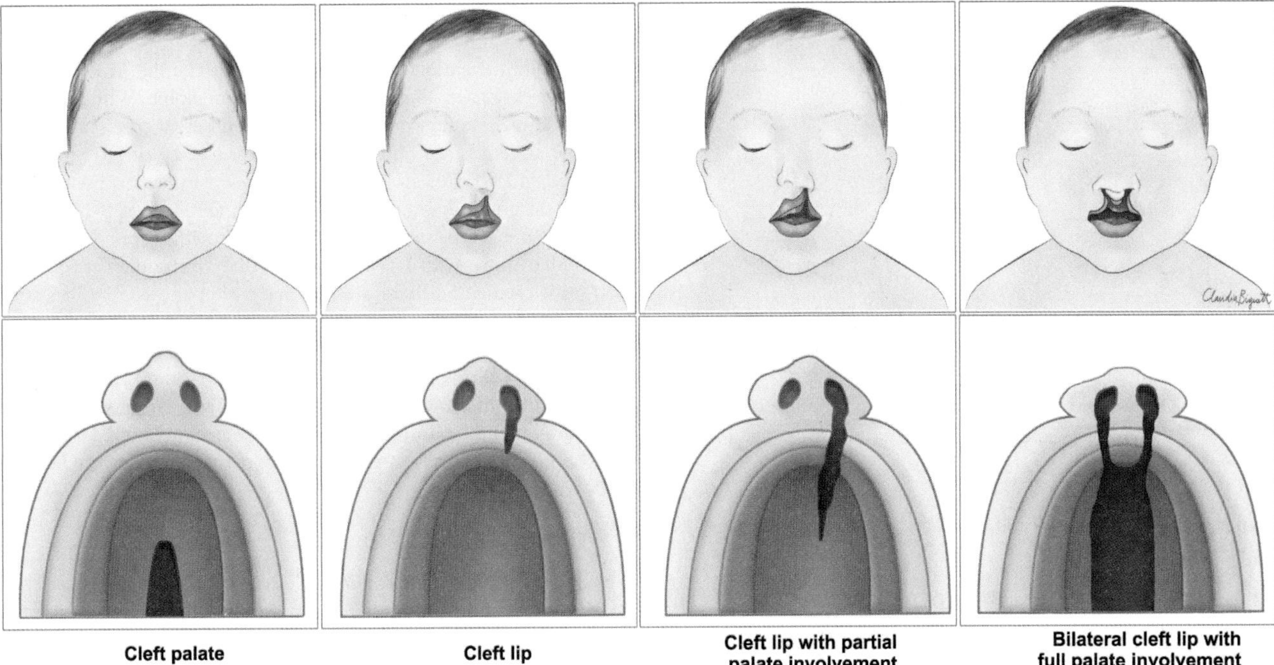


FIGURE 178-1 Clinical manifestations of oral-facial clefts. Cleft palate (CPO), cleft lip (CL), and cleft lip and palate (CL/P). CL and CL/P may be unilateral or bilateral and present with partial or full palate involvement (affecting the primary palate or the primary and secondary palates, respectively).



males being more frequently affected by CL/P than females at a 2:1 ratio, and females being more frequently affected by CPO at a 3:2 ratio. It is estimated that approximately two-thirds of all clefts are unilateral and affect the left side. Both unilateral left-sided CL/P and right-side CL/P occur more frequently than bilateral CL/P at a 6:3:1 ratio.

Observations of additional clinical features in individuals with nonsyndromic CL/P have prompted the suggestion that a broader phenotypic spectrum of oral-facial clefts exists in addition to the traditional CL, CL/P, and CPO categories. Cleft lip microforms, submucous cleft palate, defects in the orbicularis oris muscle, dental anomalies, lip whorls, velopharyngeal insufficiency, and variations in brain morphology have been reported to occur more frequently in individuals with isolated or nonsyndromic CL/P and their families in comparison to families with no history of CL/P. This observation has led to an increase in the number of affected family members for some patients, shedding light on genetic influences and possible inheritance patterns. In both nonsyndromic and syndromic CL/P, the diagnostic criteria have been rewritten to include newly recognized associated features that were not initially considered and subclinical forms that were not originally diagnosed.

## ASSESSING FOR CL/P AND CPO

The detection of CL/P during pregnancy has increased significantly as ultrasound technology has improved; typically, CL/P can be observed on an anatomy scan at 20 weeks of gestation or later. CPO is more difficult to detect with ultrasound alone and is more commonly identified after delivery. Upon discovery, referral to a cleft lip and palate multidisciplinary clinic is most appropriate. Prenatally, comprehensive ultrasounds are required to evaluate for other congenital anomalies. Postnatally, a comprehensive physical exam is always necessary to ensure that mild or microforms of clefts are not left undiagnosed. For example, a cleft of the submucous palate results in an intact soft palate with abnormal musculature and has a birth prevalence of 1/1200 to 1/2000 live births with an almost equal male-to-female ratio. Cardinal signs of a submucous cleft palate include bifid uvula, palatal muscle diastasis or furrow along the midline of the soft palate, and notch in the posterior margin of the hard palate. While 44% of patients are asymptomatic, others may exhibit speech hypernasality, translucency of the soft palate, or a short palate.

Imaging studies and specialty consultations should be considered to address symptoms related to the cleft. In all cases, comprehensive counseling and development of a care plan from all specialists need to be reviewed with the family.

## ETIOLOGY OF CL/P

### Syndromic CL/P

The number of syndromes associated with oral-facial clefts underscores the importance of a careful physical examination and the need for multidisciplinary team management. When assessing for a syndromic presentation of CL/P, comprehensive physical exam, 3-generation family history, review of pregnancy history including teratogenic exposures, and examination of past medical history including a thorough developmental assessment are necessary. CL only is the least likely to be syndromic, especially in the absence of other congenital anomalies. Conversely, Pierre Robin sequence (PRS) has the highest rate of syndromic associations, with 70% to 80% of cases considered to be syndromic. Therefore, a comprehensive evaluation to rule out other congenital malformations is necessary for any child with PRS. The most common genetic syndromes associated with CL/P are outlined in Table 178-1. There can be significant phenotypic overlap between syndromes, so genetic testing should be completed to confirm a diagnosis whenever possible.

### Nonsyndromic CL/P

The majority of instances of CL/P are sporadic and isolated events, with approximately 70% to 75% of CL/P and 45% to 60% of CPO cases being nonsyndromic. The etiology of nonsyndromic CL/P is multifactorial and includes multiple genetic and environmental factors. A variety of research approaches including linkage analysis of multiplex families, association studies and/or mutational analysis of candidate genes, and more recently, genome-wide association studies (GWAS) and whole-exome sequencing (WES), have identified candidate genes/loci for nonsyndromic CL/P. Of note, the reported associations between nonsyndromic CL/P and the interferon-regulatory factor 6 gene (*IRF6*), genes belonging to the WNT and FGF families, and loci mapping to chromosome bands 1q32, 8q24, 10q25.3 and 17q22 have been replicated in multiple populations and appear to explain ~55% of the clefting cases. However, little is known about

**TABLE 178-2 TREATMENT TIMELINE**

| Age[a] | Therapy |
|---|---|
| 0–12 months | Palatal obturator[b] |
| 0–5 months | Presurgical molding[b] |
| 3–5 months | Cheiloplasty |
| 6–12 months | Tympanostomy tube (s) |
| 9–12 months | Palate repair |
| 3–6 years | Speech therapy |
| 5–8 years | Phase I orthodontics[b] |
| 7–9 years | Alveolar bone graft |
| 9+ years | Comprehensive orthodontics |
| 15+ years | Cosmetic surgical corrections[b] |

[a]Exact age of intervention may differ between treatment protocols.

[b]Indicates therapy may not be necessary.

the functional role of these candidate genes/loci in the pathogenesis of the condition.

## TREATMENT

Management of CL/P patients is typically completed by a multidisciplinary craniofacial team, including (1) surgeons to repair the defect, (2) speech therapists to assess and treat articulation and resonance problems that exist secondary to the altered oral anatomy, (3) genetic healthcare professionals to distinguish between syndromic and nonsyndromic forms of clefting, as well as to counsel the family on recurrence risks for future pregnancies and natural histories, (4) physicians to address health complications, including airway and hearing concerns, and (5) dentists to address a number of dental-related problems, including tooth agenesis at the cleft site, supernumerary teeth, dental crowding, hypoplastic enamel, caries, and orthodontic therapies.

Treatment is an ongoing process during the first 20 years of life (Table 178-2). Prior to surgical repair, feeding complications, including poor suction, longer feedings with reduced intake, nasal regurgitation, and difficulty creating both positive and negative pressure required for normal sucking, are addressed. Feeding aids (Fig. 178-2) with specialized bottles and nipple attachments are often required, and positioning of the child in an upright position may decrease some of the feeding complications. Additionally, presurgical infant orthopedics (PSIOs), including maxillary plates, a Lantham device, lip taping, lip adhesion, and nasoalveolar molding, may be used prior to surgical intervention (Fig. 178-3). PSIOs may serve 1 or more of the following purposes: (1) obturator to separate the oral and nasal cavities, (2) facilitate feeding, or (3) molding device that uses the plasticity of the cartilage in newborns to reduce the size of the alveolar cleft and/or better approximate the lip segments at rest. While the concept of PSIOs has been around since the 1680s, the use by different craniofacial teams remains controversial as no systematic studies or evidence-based reviews for patient management exist.

Surgical intervention may begin after criteria of the "rule of 10s" are met: 10 weeks of age, 10 pounds, and 10 g hemoglobin. While the timing of surgical intervention may differ between different craniofacial teams, multiple surgeries are required, including cheiloplasty at 3 to 5 months of age (see Fig. 178-3), palatoplasty at ~1 year of age, alveolar bone grafting prior to the eruption of the maxillary permanent canines (~7–9 years of age), and surgical revisions completed after growth is complete.

Children born with CL/P are susceptible to middle ear infections and otitis media and therefore may have tympanostomy tubes surgically placed as needed. Syndromic forms of clefting, including PRS, may exhibit micrognathia, which can create an upper-airway obstruction. Intervention may be required and can range from manually repositioning the mandible, tracheostomy, and surgical techniques, including mandibular distraction osteogenesis, which lengthens a short bone by surgically separating 2 segments and allowing bony file between the segments.

## PREVENTION

Recurrence of CL/P and CPO can never be entirely prevented. The majority of CL/P is sporadic, and although empiric risks for future pregnancies will always remain, risk-reducing recommendations are in place. Genetic counseling and risk communication to family members is of utmost importance to help alleviate the associated stress and fear of recurrence of CL/P or CPO in a family.

## RECURRENCE RISKS AND GENETIC COUNSELING

It is widely accepted that nonsyndromic CL/P and CPO result from multifactorial inheritance. Genetic components and various environmental risk factors have independent and interactive effects contributing to the development of CL/P. CL only is the least likely to be syndromic, with only up to 10% being syndromic; the majority of syndromic cases have 22q microdeletion syndrome (DiGeorge/velocardiofacial syndrome) and can present with multiple other anomalies. Conversely, PRS has the highest rate of syndromic associations, with 70% to 80% of cases considered to be syndromic. Therefore, a comprehensive workup to rule out other congenital malformations is necessary for any child with PRS.

Despite an accepted hereditary component, recurrence risk for nonsyndromic clefting is based on empiric data. Current clinical genetic testing is unable to define all potentially contributing genes and account for environmental risks in an affected family. However, even when a patient appears to have isolated CL/P, various clinical genetic tests (typically a chromosomal microarray or single gene testing) are often still completed to rule out the most common syndromic forms of CL/P or CPO including genomic microdeletions and microduplications and common single-gene disorders (see Table 178-1).

The majority of syndromic forms of CL/P and CPO follow an autosomal dominant pattern of inheritance. However, many syndromes

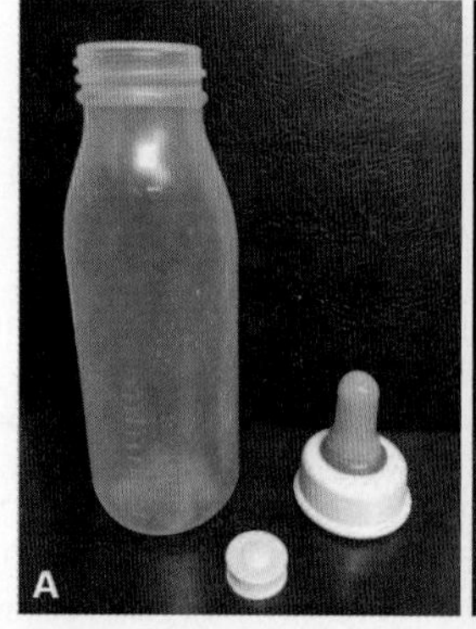

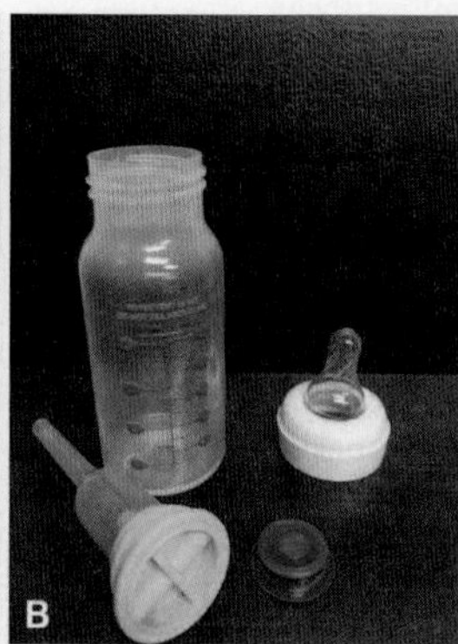

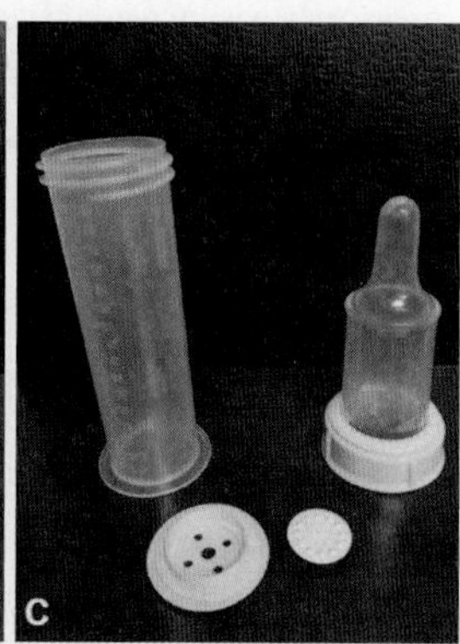


**FIGURE 178-2** Cleft feeding aids. Options for specialized bottles that assist with feeding include, but are not limited to, **A:** the Pigeon Bottle by Respironics, **B:** Dr. Brown's Specialty Feeding System, and **C:** the Special Needs Bottle by Medela (previously called the Haberman Feeder). Each family may have a preference for a particular feeding aid, including cost and ability to use with a presurgical infant orthopedic appliance.

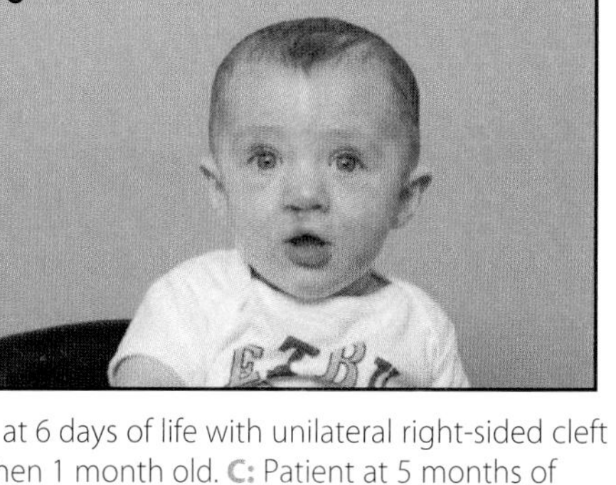
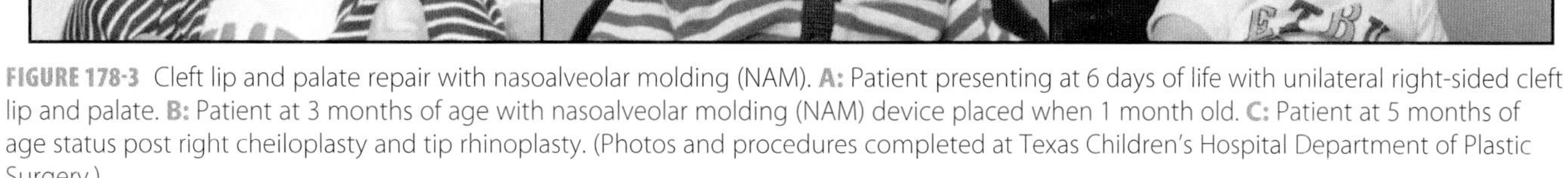

FIGURE 178-3 Cleft lip and palate repair with nasoalveolar molding (NAM). A: Patient presenting at 6 days of life with unilateral right-sided cleft lip and palate. B: Patient at 3 months of age with nasoalveolar molding (NAM) device placed when 1 month old. C: Patient at 5 months of age status post right cheiloplasty and tip rhinoplasty. (Photos and procedures completed at Texas Children's Hospital Department of Plastic Surgery.)

demonstrate variable expressivity, and there is no way to predict severity of symptoms in an affected individual. Genetic counseling for families affected by syndromic clefting with a known, mendelian inheritance pattern should include discussion of preimplantation genetic diagnosis (PGD) and prenatal diagnosis. PGD is able to use in vitro fertilization (IVF) to selectively implant unaffected embryos. Although up to 98% accurate, the known mutation(s) in the family must be identified, the process can be expensive and time-consuming, and risks should not be disregarded.

Recurrence risks in nonsyndromic CL/P and CPO are dependent on the laterality of the cleft, sex, ethnicity, family history, and environmental exposures. Family history includes first- and second-degree relatives of the affected individual (parents, siblings, grandparents, aunts/uncles); other more distantly related family members (eg, cousins) do not alter or contribute to the empiric recurrence risks. Additionally, because CPO and CL/P have different developmental etiologies, the recurrence risk for each must be considered individually. Approximate recurrence risks are detailed in Tables 178-3 and 178-4. Often the risk for a couple to have another child with an isolated cleft is not significantly above the risk for any pregnancy in the United States to have an isolated birth defect (~3%). However, if more than 1 family member is affected with an oral-facial cleft, the recurrence risk is considerably higher, and thorough examination of family history and contributing risk factors needs to be reviewed.

## TERATOGENS

A variety of teratogens have been linked to an increased risk for CL/P and CPO. These agents should be avoided during pregnancy to reduce risk of clefting as well as other birth defects. Antiepileptic medications carry the highest relative risk for CL/P during pregnancy; however, discontinuation of antiepileptic medications (folate antagonists such as carbamazepine, valproic acid, phenytoin, phenobarbital, trimethadione, and some corticosteroids) should be discussed at length with specialists as the benefits of discontinuation of medication may be determined to not outweigh other risks to the pregnancy. Sometimes medication regimens are altered to reduce risks; this discussion should occur prior to conception whenever possible. Additional known teratogens associated with an increased risk of CL/P or CPO are alcohol consumption, tobacco use, and some recreational drugs, including methamphetamine and cocaine.

## FOLATE

There is no prevention for a sporadic CL/P. However, evidence from epidemiologic studies and clinical trials has demonstrated a protective effect of folate supplementation before and during pregnancy. Typical multivitamin/folate regimens for women who are pregnant recommend 0.4 mg of folic acid every day, and it is widely recommended that "at-risk" women consume an increased dose (10 times) of folic acid during pregnancy and whenever trying to conceive a pregnancy. Therefore, for women at risk for a child with a cleft, preconceptual supplementation and supplementation during pregnancy with 4.0 mg of folate are daily recommended in many cases.

## LIFE SPAN

Children born with oral clefts have been shown to have a shorter life span, especially in the presence of other birth defects. A 15 times higher risk of mortality was reported in CPO patients when compared to the general population, and a 10 times greater risk of mortality was reported when compared to other types of clefts. A longitudinal study of Dutch patients found an infant mortality rate of ~2.5% for CPO cases, with the most common cause of death being congenital malformations of the heart. Epidemiologic studies have also assessed the relationship between cancer and oral-facial clefts, although no direct correlation has been established.

## SUMMARY

Oral-facial clefts are common birth defects caused by multiple genetic and environmental factors and require life-long multidisciplinary treatment. Corrective therapies start soon after birth and can persist through the teenage years. Most of the oral-facial cleft cases are nonsyndromic, making identification of the causative gene(s) challenging. Current research efforts aim to identify genetic and molecular networks crucial for craniofacial development and elucidate their potential roles in the developmental biology and etiology of CL/P and CPO, in order to provide valuable insights allowing the further development of management and preventive strategies in the near future. While research on the pathogenesis of CL/P and CPO continues, affected individuals and family members need to be aware of recurrence risks and preventative measures to reduce risks of oral-facial clefts in the future. Combined understanding of the etiology and best treatment

**TABLE 178-3 RECURRENCE RISKS FOR FIRST-DEGREE RELATIVES OF PATIENTS WITH NONSYNDROMIC CLEFT LIP AND PALATE (CL/P)**

| | Risk to Future Full Siblings of Proband or Children of Proband[a] | | |
|---|---|---|---|
| Cleft Type | Only Proband Affected | Proband + 1 Affected Family Member | Proband + 2 Affected Family Members |
| Unilateral CL/P | 2–3% | 3–5% | 5–7% |
| Bilateral CL/P | 3–5% | 5–7% | 7–10% |
| Cleft palate only | 2–5% | 3–5% | 7–10% |

[a]Affected family members must be within 2 degrees of relation to proband.

**TABLE 178-4 RECURRENCE RISKS FOR NONSYNDROMIC CLEFT LIP AND PALATE (CL/P) AND CLEFT PALATE ONLY (CPO)**

| | Recurrence Risk | |
|---|---|---|
| Relationship to Proband | CL/P (%) | CPO (%) |
| Sibling (overall risk) | 4.0 | 1.8 |
| Sibling (no other affected members) | 2.2 | — |
| Sibling (2 affected sibs) | 10 | 8.0 |
| Sibling and affected parent | 10 | — |
| Children of proband | 4.3 | 3.0 |
| Second-degree relatives | 0.6 | — |
| Third-degree relatives | 0.3 | — |

—, no increased recurrence risk.

practices for oral-facial clefts continues to improve toward the goal of offering all patients the best care possible.

## SUGGESTED READINGS


Burg ML, Chai Y, Yao CA, Magee W, Figueiredo JC. Epidemiology, etiology, and treatment of isolated cleft palate. *Front Physiol.* 2016;7:67.

Dixon MJ, Marazita ML, Beaty TH, Murray JC. Cleft lip and palate: understanding genetic and environmental influences. *Nat Rev Genet.* 2011;12:167-178.

Harper, Peter S. *Practical Genetic Counseling.* 7th ed. Boca Raton, FL: CRC Press; 2010.

Hennekam R, Krantz I, Allanson JE. *Gorlin's Syndromes of the Head and Neck.* 5th ed. New York, NY: Oxford University Press; 2010.

Kousa YA, Schutte BC. Toward an orofacial gene regulatory network. *Dev Dyn.* 2016;245:220-232.

Maarse W, Rozendaal AM, Pajkrt E, Vermeij-Keers C, Mink van der Molen AB, van den Boogaard MJ. A systematic review of associated structural and chromosomal defects in oral-facial clefts: when is prenatal genetic analysis indicated? *J Med Genet.* 2012;49:490-498.

Marazita ML. The evolution of human genetic studies of cleft lip and cleft palate. *Annu Rev Genomics Hum Genet.* 2012;13:263-283.

Mossey PA, Little J, Munger RG, Dixon MJ, Shaw WC. Cleft lip and palate. *Lancet* 2009;374:1773-1785.

Reiter R, Brosch S, Lüdeke M, et al. Do orofacial clefts represent different genetic entities? *Cleft Palate Craniofac J.* 2015;52:115-120.

Watkins SE, Meyer RE, Strauss RP, Aylsworth AS. Classification, epidemiology, and genetics of orofacial clefts. *Clin Plast Surg.* 2014;41:149-163.

Wehby GL, Félix T, Goco N, et al. High dosage folic acid supplementation, oral cleft recurrence and fetal growth. *Int J Environ Res Public Health.* 2013;10:590-605.

Wehby GL, Goco N, Moretti-Ferreira D, et al. Oral cleft prevention program (OCPP). *BMC Pediatr.* 2012;12:184.


# 179 Skeletal Disorders

Mahim Jain and V. Reid Sutton

## INTRODUCTION

Skeletal dysplasias represent a complex set of disorders that affect bone and/or cartilage, and typical clinical manifestations include short stature and orthopedic complications. Skeletal manifestations are common among this group of disorders; however, findings in other tissues may also be clinically relevant and can help establish the underlying diagnosis. Skeletal features can be diverse but are generally divided into the osteodysplasias (eg, osteogenesis imperfecta), chondrodysplasias (eg, achondroplasia), or dysostoses (eg, spondylocostal dysostosis). Determining the genetic basis of skeletal dysplasias is not only important for counseling and defining recurrence risk, but also for guiding pharmacologic and surgical management. In this chapter, we will review the pathogenesis and epidemiology of this set of disorders and describe clinically relevant skeletal dysplasias in which treatments or medical interventions are available.

## PATHOGENESIS AND EPIDEMIOLOGY

With the advent of novel genetic testing strategies, such as whole-exome sequencing (WES), the underlying etiologies of skeletal dysplasias are increasingly being identified. There are currently over 400 disorders in the Online Mendelian Inheritance in Man (OMIM) database (www.omim.org) with skeletal features and greater than 500 genes implicated in the pathogenesis of these disorders. Although each disorder itself is rare, together they are estimated to be present in roughly 1 in 4000 live births.

The human skeleton consists of 206 bones, and although important functions include mechanical support and protection, the skeleton is also involved in linear growth, endocrine regulation, mineral release, sound conductance, and blood cell development. During intrauterine development, skeletal elements are patterned from mesenchymal cells that differentiate into chondrocytes with subsequent mineralization of cartilage. Later, there is an invasion of vascular elements and inclusion of osteoprogenitor cells. The primary ossification center is formed, typically in the midshaft of the developing bone, and creates the cortex. At the end of the developing bone, a second ossification center forms and results in the cartilaginous growth plate between the 2 ossification centers.

A number of naming conventions exist for skeletal dysplasias; most rely on the location and radiologic findings of implicated skeletal elements. Dysostoses result in malformations from abnormal embryologic bone development and patterning. They can include the formation of abnormal bones, such as polydactyly, or the lack of bone formation, such as skeletal truncation defects. Primary abnormalities of bone or bone metabolism typically result in disorders of bone density. Chondrodysplasias involve defects in both cartilage and the resulting bone and are characterized by short stature. In addition, the naming of disorders is often based on specific skeletal features. For example, spondylometaphyseal dysplasias are characterized by the involvement of both the spine (spondylo) and long-bone metaphyses. Other naming conventions rely on classifying skeletal dysplasias by specific genes and pathways that are affected, for example, the *COL2A1*-related disorders, which have overlapping features that range in severity from the perinatal lethal disorder achondrogenesis type II to Stickler syndrome at the mildest end of the spectrum of disorders caused by variants in this gene.

## CLINICAL APPROACH TO SKELETAL DYSPLASIAS

Although the clinical manifestations can be heterogeneous among skeletal dysplasias, the evaluation involves ascertainment of historical and physical findings to group features in order to diagnose the underlying disorder. Skeletal disorders present at a variety of pediatric ages, and this can include the neonatal setting where a small trunk may result in respiratory insufficiency or the presence of skeletal malformations. In addition, disproportionate short stature or the presence of an abnormality in bone density should trigger an evaluation for an underlying skeletal dysplasia.

The clinical history should include evaluation of growth parameters, including anthropomorphic measurements at birth, and the history of longitudinal growth over time. In addition, a history that includes a review of any nonskeletal manifestations may help to classify the specific dysplasia. When a history of fracture exists, specific details about the reported cause should be elicited in order to help determine if the nature of the fracture correlates with the reported force. If the fracture history and reported cause are inconsistent, then a potential consideration should be diminished bone density or poor bone quality as a susceptibility factor. A detailed family history should be completed to evaluate for history of short stature, skeletal malformation or fracture, and, when possible, direct measurement of parental height, and evaluation for disproportion indicated by the exam on the child should be completed on both parents. A detailed pregnancy history may reveal in utero concern for poor growth or specific skeletal features that were detected by prenatal ultrasound or magnetic resonance imaging (MRI).

The physical examination should include detailed physical measurements, not only including height, weight, and fronto-occipital circumference (FOC), which are typically collected, but also arm span/height and upper/lower body segment ratios. These ratios help quantify the degree of disproportion of the limbs to the trunk if present. When possible, the arm span should be measured with the patient standing with outstretched arms flat against the wall. Normative data indicate that the arm span is typically less than the height until early adolescence, equal to height during adolescence, and then greater than height in adulthood. When evaluating short stature, if the arm span is markedly reduced compared to the height, then this indicates short upper extremities in relation to the trunk, and if the arm span is increased compared to height, this indicates a shortened trunk. The lower segment is measured from the symphysis pubis to the heel, and the upper segment is calculated from subtracting the lower segment from the height. The upper/lower body ratio is typically 1.7 at birth and decreases to 1.0 by 7 years of age. An increased upper/lower body ratio indicates short lower extremities in relation to the trunk, and a diminished ratio indicates a short trunk in relation to the lower extremities. When short limbs are indicated, further measurements should also be completed for limb segments to further classify the nature of the disproportion. Shortening of the proximal extremity is termed *rhizomelia* (humerus and femur), the intermediate extremity is *mesomelia* (ulna, radius, tibia, and fibula), the distal extremity is *acromelia* (hands and feet), and symmetric shortening of the extremity is termed *micromelia*. In addition, the physical examination should include evaluation for brachydactyly, bowing of the extremities, scoliosis, exostoses, skeletal malformations, and other dysmorphic features. Given the relation of the skeleton with joints, the evaluation should include examination for the presence of hypermobility or joint restriction.

Laboratory and radiologic studies should be considered during the initial evaluation to help classify specific findings that can lead to a diagnosis. When a skeletal dysplasia is suspected, typically a complete skeletal survey is completed and reviewed by an expert radiologist. A skeletal survey should include, from the axial skeleton, frontal and lateral skull, anteroposterior (AP) and lateral views of the spine to include views of the entire thorax, and AP of the pelvis and, from the appendicular skeleton, images of humerus, femur, forearm, lower leg, hands, and feet. Laboratory studies that can be considered include evaluation of bone metabolism and should include calcium, phosphorus, vitamin D, parathyroid hormone, and measures of bone turnover, such as alkaline phosphatase and either urinary N-telopeptide or serum C-telopeptide. Often, skeletal dysplasias have characteristic findings on radiologic and laboratory studies to identify a diagnosis (eg, delayed ossification of the pubic symphysis and calvaria and hypoplastic clavicles in cleidocranial dysplasia). For disorders with overlapping features, these studies can limit further evaluation to a subset of disorders for further diagnostic workup. To establish a diagnosis, further testing is often required. If there is a high suspicion for a single gene as the etiology, targeted testing can be completed (eg, *FGFR3* recurrent missense variant that causes achondroplasia). Often, a class of disorders can be identified and panel testing can be considered (eg, osteogenesis imperfecta and testing of both *COL1A1* and *COL1A2*). If a genetic cause is strongly suspected but the clinical presentation is not clear, WES should be considered. Furthermore, in osteogenesis imperfecta, evaluation of collagen by performing studies in fibroblasts can be used to establish a diagnosis if a genetic variant is not identified, yet there is a suspicion of the disorder. Although not routinely performed, histologic studies from a bone biopsy or postmortem sample can be undertaken to establish a diagnosis (eg, osteogenesis imperfecta type VI, thanatophoric dysplasia).

Establishing a definitive diagnosis for skeletal dysplasias is necessary for many reasons. First, identification of a molecular diagnosis will inform a plan for health supervision, which may include evaluation of hematologic, cardiac, dental, or audiologic abnormalities that can potentially identify a known complication and prompt early intervention. Second, although there is rarely a cure, there are emerging medical therapies for a subset of skeletal dysplasias, which can include enzyme replacement therapy (eg, hypophosphatasia and Morquio A disease), small-molecule therapy (eg, achondroplasia), and antibody therapy (eg, osteogenesis imperfecta). Further, molecularly confirming specific skeletal dysplasias can lead to recommendations for, or against, surgical interventions (eg, Steel syndrome). Third, a mode of inheritance can be identified to inform family planning decisions.

Table 179-1 lists a selected subset of skeletal dysplasias with clinical and radiologic features as well as the major underlying genetic etiology. Furthermore, we review osteogenesis imperfecta, hypophosphatasia, achondroplasia, cleidocranial dysplasia, and cartilage hair hypoplasia in more detail with a goal of describing a diverse set of pathologic causes of skeletal dysplasias and emerging therapies for these conditions.

## OSTEOGENESIS IMPERFECTA

Osteogenesis imperfecta (OI) is a primary bone dysplasia, and although there are 19 types currently described, the majority of cases (> 90%) are caused by autosomal dominant variants in 2 genes that form type I collagen, *COL1A1* and *COL1A2*. Type I collagen is formed by 2 COL1A1 and 1 COL1A2 proteins to create a structurally strong triple helix. These large structural proteins contain a helical domain with glycine-X-Y repeats, where X is primarily proline and Y is primarily hydroxyproline. Variants that cause a quantitative reduction in type I collagen (nonsense, frameshift, or deletions) typically result in type I OI (the mildest form), and those that are missense, specifically glycine substitutions, and thus lead to a qualitative defect of type I collagen, are more severe. Rare forms of OI have been described and are generally autosomal recessive where the implicated genes are involved in type I collagen processing. OI types I through IV are caused by variants in *COL1A1* and *COL1A2*.

OI type I is the mildest form of OI and has a prevalence of roughly 1 in 20,000 births, with most cases being familial. Classically, it is defined as nondeforming OI with blue-gray sclera. Unlike other forms of OI, there are rarely fractures or limb bowing present in utero or at birth. Associated features include deep blue-gray sclera, which does not resolve with age, and hearing loss. Further, individuals with type I OI may have findings associated with connective tissue disturbances, and this includes thin skin with prominent blood vessels, easy bruising, and hypermobility. Dentinogenesis imperfecta is uncommon. Height may be within the normal range but is generally less than expected based on calculations of midparental height. Fractures typically present with ambulation and falls in childhood; however, after puberty, there is generally a reduction in the risk of fractures. The risk again increases in late adulthood, particularly in postmenopausal women. Vertebral fractures and scoliosis are a risk in childhood and may require therapeutic intervention. Radiographic features that suggest a diagnosis of type I OI include the presence of Wormian bones in the skull and the finding of generalized osteopenia. The diagnosis of type I OI can be made by performing sequence and deletion/duplication evaluation of *COL1A1* and *COL1A2* or by collagen studies on fibroblasts.

OI type II is a perinatal lethal form of OI, typically caused by de novo glycine substitutions in *COL1A1* or *COL1A2*. There is severe fragility of the skeleton with consistent findings including the presence of in utero fracture, short and severely bowed extremities, enlarged fontanelles, and diminished birth length and weight for gestational age. There is deep blue-gray sclera. Radiographic findings include a severely bowed and/or structurally abnormal appearance of long bones and the presence of a beaded appearance on the ribs because of multiple rib fractures. Death is typically in the first week and caused by respiratory insufficiency as a result of the narrow chest, rib fractures,

**TABLE 179-1 SKELETAL DYSPLASIAS**

| Disorder (OMIM No.) | Clinical Manifestations | Radiologic and Laboratory Findings | Inheritance | Major Gene(s) |
|---|---|---|---|---|
| **Disorders of Transmembrane Receptors** | | | | |
| Achondroplasia (100800) | Macrocephaly, frontal bossing with depressed nasal bridge, limb shortening (primarily rhizomelic), trident posturing of hands | Rounded ilia, horizontal acetabula, narrow sciatic notch, narrow lumbar vertebral interpedicular distance | AD | *FGFR3* |
| Thanatophoric dysplasia type I (187600) | Macrocephaly, narrow chest, rhizomelic shortening | Platyspondyly, short ilia, bowed femur | AD | *FGFR3* |
| Thanatophoric dysplasia type II (187601) | Macrocephaly, cloverleaf skull | Platyspondyly, straight femur | AD | *FGFR3* |
| Hypochondroplasia (146000) | Macrocephaly, mild rhizomelic shortening | Narrow lumbar vertebral interpedicular distance, squared/shortened ilia | AD | *FGFR3* |
| **Disorders of Matrix Proteins and Collagen** | | | | |
| Osteogenesis imperfecta (166200, 166210, 166220, 259420) | Fractures, bone deformity, dentinogenesis imperfecta, blue/gray sclera | Wormian bones, platyspondyly, thin ribs/gracile bones | AD | *COL1A1* *COL1A2* |
| Stickler syndrome (108300) | Flat midface, myopia, cleft palate, joint degeneration | Mild epiphyseal dysplasia | AD | *COL2A1* |
| Achondrogenesis type II (200610) | Flat nose, limb shortening | Short tubular bones, poor vertebral ossification | AD | *COL2A1* |
| Steel syndrome (615155) | Bilateral hip and radial head dislocations, mild short stature, prominent forehead, hypertelorism, scoliosis | Dislocations, carpal coalition, vertebral anomalies | AR | *COL27A1* |
| Pseudoachondroplasia (177170) | Long trunk, short limbs, leg joints | Platyspondyly, epiphyseal dysplasia | AD | *COMP* |
| Multiple epiphyseal dysplasia 1 (600969) | Mildly short limbs | Epiphyseal changes | AD | *COMP* |
| **Disorders of Transmembrane Sulfate Transporter** | | | | |
| Diastrophic dysplasia (222600) | Cleft palate, hitchhiker thumb, cauliflower ear | Short long bones, scoliosis, broad metaphyses | AR | *DTDST* |
| Achondrogenesis type I (600972) | Flat nose, short limbs | Short tubular bones, poor vertebral ossification | AR | *DTDST* |
| **Disorders of DNA Transcription Factors** | | | | |
| Cleidocranial dysplasia (119600) | Delayed fontanel closure, brachycephaly, ability to approximate shoulders anteriorly, supernumerary teeth | Clavicular hypoplasia, delayed ossification of calvaria and pubic bone | AD | *RUNX2* |
| Campomelic dysplasia (114290) | Flat nose, clubfeet, dimples over tibia | Bowing of femur and tibia; narrowed ilia; hypoplastic scapulae | AD | *SOX9* |
| Spondylocostal dysostosis 5 (122600) | Congenital scoliosis | Cervical, thoracic, or lumbar hemivertebrae, butterfly vertebrae | AD/AR | *TBX6* |
| **Disorders of Bone Density** | | | | |
| Hypophosphatasia (241500, 241510, 146300) | Soft skull, short/bowed limbs, premature tooth loss | Osteopenia, bowed long bones, reduced alkaline phosphatase | AR and AD | *ALPL* |
| **Disorders of Ribosome Function** | | | | |
| Shwachman-Diamond syndrome (260400) | Narrow thorax, pelvic coxa vara, fat malabsorption | Ovoid and posteriorly wedged vertebral bodies, metaphyseal changes | AR | *SBDS* |
| Cartilage hair hypoplasia (250250) | Femoral bowing, short legs and hands, flaring of ribcage, sparse or slow-growing hair | Metaphyseal changes, cone-shaped epiphyses in the hands | AR | *RMRP* |
| **Disorders of Ciliary Function** | | | | |
| Ellis-van Creveld syndrome (225500) | Postaxial polydactyly, narrow chest, natal teeth, oligodontia, nail dysplasia | Short tubular bones, large proximal ulna and distal radius | AR | *EVC, EVC2* |
| Short rib thoracic dysplasia 2 (611263) | Postaxial polydactyly, narrow chest, brachydactyly | Short ribs, short ilia, rhizomelic or mesomelic shortening | AR | *IFT80* |

Note. For full gene names, see Online Mendelian Inheritance in Man (OMIM) at www.omim.org.

AD, autosomal dominant; AR, autosomal recessive.



and potentially the presence of a flail chest. The recurrence risk has been reported to be 6% for de novo changes in OI, given the presence of paternal gonadal mosaicism.

OI type III is a severe nonlethal form, termed *progressively deforming type*, and can present with multiple in utero or at-birth fractures and extremity bowing. This type is usually caused by missense variants in *COL1A1* or *COL1A2*. While length may be within the normal range at birth, typically there is reduction to below the normal range by 1 to 2 years. In infancy, fractures occur frequently from minimal trauma or manipulation. The presence of dentinogenesis imperfecta and scleral color are variable. Radiographic findings include long bone and vertebral anomalies from infancy. Many patients with this subtype are not able to bear weight or ambulate on their own. Orthopedic management, medical management with bisphosphonates, and physical therapy/rehabilitation care are all required to manage this form of OI. Basilar invagination, caused by compression of the skull on the cervical spine, is common and may progress to brain stem compression, obstructive hydrocephalus, or syringomyelia.

OI type IV is the moderately severe form and is highly variable in clinical presentation. Infants may present with in utero or neonatal fracture or, similar to type I OI, with fracture after ambulation. Patients typically have bowing of tibias and have moderate short stature. Dentinogenesis imperfecta and scleral color are variable. Individuals with OI type IV also benefit from close orthopedic, medical, and physical therapy management, with most being able to ambulate. This form of OI is also typically caused by single nucleotide variants in *COL1A1* and *COL1A2*.

The medical and surgical management for OI is aimed at maintaining and maximizing physical function. This includes the use of braces, orthotics, and physical therapy regimens starting at a young age with benefit seen by maintaining physical conditioning with activities such as swimming. Contact sports should be avoided. For severe forms of OI, orthopedic intervention by use of an intermedullary rod may lead to improvement in long bone deformities. Formal audiologic assessment should be completed at the time of diagnosis, and a computed tomography (CT) or MRI scan should be considered in individuals with severe OI to evaluate for basilar invagination. Twice yearly dental evaluations should be completed starting at age 3. Serum vitamin D should be measured and supplemented if low. The use of bisphosphonates in OI has been demonstrated to increase bone density and decrease bone pain, although studies have not clearly shown a reduction in fracture risk (although the studies have significant limitations). Criteria for starting intravenous (IV) bisphosphonate therapy in OI include multiple fractures within a 1-year period, the presence of bowing, or the presence of vertebral compression fractures. IV bisphosphonate therapy has also shown benefit in treating bone pain. Although, bisphosphonates improve bone density, it is unclear if they improve bone quality; thus, bisphosphonates should be used cautiously, and the presence of side effects should be closely monitored. Emerging therapies include teriparatide, an anabolic agent, which was demonstrated to improve density in OI type I, and preclinical antibody therapies against transforming growth factor-β (TGF-β), which has been demonstrated to be upregulated in OI, and an anti-sclerostin antibody. The Osteogenesis Imperfecta Foundation provides up-to-date educational resources for individuals and families with OI and clinicians (http://www.oif.org/).

## STEEL SYNDROME

Steel syndrome is a rare autosomal recessive osteochondrodysplasia that has been primarily reported in individuals with Puerto Rican ancestry. The constellation of findings includes congenital hip dislocations, radial head dislocations, short stature, carpal coalition, scoliosis with the presence of vertebral anomalies, and characteristic facial features that include hypertelorism, broad forehead, and a long ovoid face. Although congenital hip dislocation is typically treated with a surgical reduction, this should be avoided in Steel syndrome. Retrospective analysis has demonstrated that of those treated with surgical techniques, the majority of hips remain dislocated, and when not dislocated, the hips have acetabular dysplasia with significant pain. Outcomes of pain and limitation in daily activities are worse for those who have had an attempted surgical correction compared to those who have not.

Recent evidence suggests that a homozygous glycine substitution variant in *COL27A1* causes Steel syndrome and is present as a founder variant in the Puerto Rican population. Given that surgical intervention leads to worse outcomes in this condition, it is necessary to confirm the diagnosis with molecular testing, when considering patients with a presentation of hip dysplasia, because it has significant management implications. The pathogenic variant is very rare in studied human populations, seen only once in public databases, and this presumably explains the increased frequency of this rare disorder in individuals of Puerto Rican descent. This variant presumably arose in an ancestral lineage for individuals of Puerto Rican descent and has continued at a low allele frequency in the population by genetic drift. This skeletal dysplasia exemplifies the importance of not only evaluating for close consanguinity clinically, but also defining the ethnicity of parental lineages given the presence of variants that are present in subpopulations. Rare variants specific to subpopulations can further be used to understand human migration and history. This concept has been demonstrated for another rare skeletal dysplasia that is inherited in an autosomal recessive fashion, Smith-McCort dysplasia 1 (OMIM no. 607326). An identical pathogenic splicing variant has been identified in 2 families of ancestry from Guam, 1 patient of Argentinian/Chilean ancestry, and 1 patient of Spanish ancestry. Haplotype reconstruction was completed by evaluation of neighboring single nucleotide variants, and this demonstrated that the pathogenic variant was on a shared haplotype. This finding reveals the presence of shared ancestry among these geographically distinct populations. Thus, further identification of Steel syndrome in other populations and an increased understanding of rare variants in individuals of Puerto Rican descent may inform us of human migration.

## HYPOPHOSPHATASIA

Hypophosphatasia is a metabolic bone disorder, caused by variants in *ALPL*, which encodes tissue nonspecific alkaline phosphatase. Severe forms of hypophosphatasia can present with clinical overlap with severe neonatal forms of OI, including bowed extremities, fracture, poor bone mineralization, and respiratory insufficiency. However, there are distinct radiologic, clinical, and laboratory features. *ALPL* functions as a membrane-bound phosphatase in bone and cleaves inorganic pyrophosphate into 2 phosphates, which are implicated in bone formation and signaling. The disorder can either be inherited in an autosomal recessive fashion, which is typical of either severe or mild forms, or in an autosomal dominant fashion, which is typical of mild forms.

The spectrum of presentations is broad and subcategorized into 6 clinical subtypes. Perinatal severe hypophosphatasia can be identified prenatally with affected infants presenting with under-mineralization of bone; a narrow thorax, which can result in respiratory insufficiency; and hypercalcemia. The perinatal benign form of the disorder can be identified by prenatal ultrasound; however, findings are consistent with slightly diminished skeletal mineralization, and postnatally, the skeletal findings slowly resolve. Infantile hypophosphatasia presents in the first months of life and resembles rickets. There are significant risks of respiratory insufficiency and hypercalcemia, and although initially there is under-mineralization of the calvaria, there is a risk for premature fontanel closure. Juvenile hypophosphatasia can present with a clinical picture of rickets or with recurrent fracture, and there can be premature loss of teeth. Adult hypophosphatasia includes findings of premature loss of teeth and the presence of stress fractures in adulthood. Odontohypophosphatasia is classified as the presence of dental findings (early loss of primary teeth) without other skeletal features. Laboratory testing can be completed when the disorder is suspected; low serum alkaline phosphatase, elevated urine phosphoethanolamine, and elevated pyridoxal 5′-phosphate are characteristic of hypophosphatasia.

The management of nonlethal forms of the disorder includes a skeletal dysplasia expert to optimize skeletal metabolic factors, orthopedic intervention, physical therapy, and dental care. Recently, pharmacologic therapy has become available, with the development of enzyme replacement therapy of tissue-nonspecific alkaline phosphatase. A striking finding is the improvement in mortality in those with perinatal severe or infantile forms of the disorder, where previously there was 5% survival for those who required respiratory intervention; however, for those receiving enzyme replacement, there is 81% survival at an average of 3 years of age. Further studies are needed to determine if there are benefits in other forms of hypophosphatasia.

## ACHONDROPLASIA

Achondroplasia has an incidence of roughly 1 in 20,000 births and is the most common cause of disproportionate short stature. It is almost uniformly caused by 2 recurrent variants in *FGFR3* that result in a glycine change to arginine at position 380. The variant is either inherited in an autosomal dominant manner or found to be de novo if there is no family history. The causative variant results in constitutive activation of *FGFR3*, which results in decreased cartilage growth and, thus, diminished bone length. The diagnosis may be made in utero but is often made at birth.

In addition to short stature, characteristic features of achondroplasia include rhizomelic shortening with limitation of elbow extension, macrocephaly, and facial findings that include frontal bossing, a depressed nasal bridge, and midface hypoplasia. There is brachydactyly with broad fingers and a trident posturing of the hands. In infancy, there is thoracolumbar kyphosis that typically resolves and lumbar lordosis that develops with ambulation. Radiographic features include rounded ilia and horizontal acetabulum, proximal femoral radiolucency, a narrow sacrosciatic notch, narrowing of the interpedicular distances in the distal spine, and generalized metaphyseal changes. Final adult height is, on average, 131 cm for males and 124 cm for females. Growth curves are available for height and FOC.

The natural history of achondroplasia has been well studied, and there are a number of complications in the pediatric age group. In infancy, stenosis of the foramen magnum is a potentially life-threatening complication, where compression can contribute to quadriparesis, central sleep apnea, or hydrocephalus. Thus, infants and young children should be monitored closely, which may include imaging studies, for clinical signs and symptoms of compression. Neurosurgical evaluation and decompression may be required depending on imaging and clinical findings. In adolescence and adulthood, there is a risk of spinal stenosis, particularly in the lower spine. There is usually a mild gross motor delay that is attributed to macrocephaly and low muscle tone. In addition, there is an increased risk of recurrent otitis media that may affect hearing. Obstructive sleep apnea (OSA) is nearly universal, and so frequent clinical assessment and a sleep study are indicated. When present, OSA may be treated with tonsillectomy and adenoidectomy, nasal steroid spray, or continuous positive airway pressure (CPAP).

Poor socialization or psychologic maladjustments may be present. The Little People of America (www.lpaonline.org) is an informative source for patients with short stature and has peer-support and advocacy programs. Limb-lengthening procedures have been attempted with an overall increase in final adult height; however, these procedures are controversial, and in general, it is recommended that the procedure be delayed until adolescence so the child with achondroplasia can provide assent. Pharmacologic therapy with growth hormone has been studied in clinical trials, but there is only a small effect on final adult height. A new class of pharmacologic therapy is being studied, a C-type natriuretic peptide (CNP) analogue, which counteracts the constitutive effects of FGFR3 signaling; however, further analyses are ongoing to determine efficacy and safety.

While achondroplasia is the most common dysplasia associated with DNA variants in *FGFR3* that result in constitutive FGFR3 signaling, thanatophoric dysplasia and hypochondroplasia are also caused by variants in *FGFR3*. Thanatophoric dysplasia is a lethal chondrodysplasia; lethality is attributable to either severe pulmonary restriction leading to respiratory insufficiency or brain stem compression by the foramen magnum. Most cases are diagnosed prenatally. Radiographic features are similar to achondroplasia but tend to be more severe. There are 2 subtypes of thanatophoric dysplasia. Type 1 is caused by variants in the extracellular domain of *FGFR3* and has bowed femurs. Type 2 is caused by a lysine to glutamate missense variant at amino acid 650 in the intracellular domain and typically has straight femurs and the possibility of a cloverleaf skull. The variants that cause thanatophoric dysplasia are typically de novo, and thus, there is a low recurrence risk. Roughly 70% of cases of hypochondroplasia are caused by missense variants in *FGFR3*. Clinically, individuals with hypochondroplasia present with mild short stature and radiographic features that are similar to achondroplasia but less severe. Complications that are associated with achondroplasia (such as foramen magnum stenosis or OSA) are rare in individuals with hypochondroplasia.

## CLEIDOCRANIAL DYSPLASIA

Cleidocranial dysplasia is an autosomal dominant skeletal dysplasia with features of short stature compared to unaffected family members and dental anomalies. It is caused by variants in *RUNX2*, a transcription factor, with implicated roles in osteoblast differentiation, cartilage hypertrophy, and vascular development in bone. Causative variants have been demonstrated to be haploinsufficient, affecting RUNX2 transcriptional target expression. Features of cleidocranial dysplasia are based both on bones that are derived from intramembranous ossification (calvaria and clavicle) as well as effects from endochondral ossification.

The clinical presentation can be in the neonatal period, with abnormally large fontanels at birth that may remain open into adulthood. In addition to poor ossification in the calvaria, there is also delayed ossification of the pubic bone. Clavicular hypoplasia or aplasia is also a characteristic feature, and shoulders can be brought together at the midline on exam. Facial features include midface hypoplasia, and fingers typically have abnormalities such as brachydactyly, broad thumbs, and tapered fingers. In childhood, there is an increased frequency of recurrent otitis media and sinus infections. Short stature, when compared to unaffected family members, is present, and the average male adult height is 165 cm and the average female adult height is 156 cm. There is an increased risk of having low bone density, scoliosis, and genu valgus deformity. Dental features include retention of primary teeth, noneruption of permanent teeth, and the presence of extra teeth. The management of dental features typically involves aggressive removal of primary and supernumerary teeth, thus allowing permanent dentition to erupt.

## *TBX6*-RELATED CONGENITAL SCOLIOSIS

Congenital scoliosis, which is defined as greater than 10 degrees of spinal curvature (Cobb angle), is relatively common, with a prevalence of 1 in 2000 births. Congenital malformation or fusion of vertebral bodies underlies congenital scoliosis. When scoliosis is noted on physical examination, completion of plain radiograph evaluation of the spine is indicated to identify vertebral body malformations (such as hemivertebrae) or vertebral body segmentation defects that cause fusion. Once scoliosis is identified, progression should be monitored, with a goal of having a Cobb angle of less than 40 degrees at skeletal maturity, because curvature of this degree has a low chance of progressing. Orthopedic treatment options include bracing or surgical intervention.

Recent evidence has implicated *TBX6*, a putative transcription factor, as a cause of congenital scoliosis due to vertebral segmentation abnormalities. *TBX6* is crucial for mesoderm patterning of the vertebrae. The pathogenic variants that underlie the condition include evidence from one family where heterozygous loss of a stop codon leads to an extended protein product with diminished function. Further, a study of unrelated individuals with congenital scoliosis identified an autosomal recessive mechanism, where one allele is a loss-of-function (either frameshift, nonsense, or 16p11.2 deletion variants) and the second allele is a common shared haplotype, which is demonstrated to have reduced activity. *TBX6* is located within a recurrent 16p11.2 microdeletion region, and this microdeletion has been associated with a variable phenotype, including vertebral anomalies.

## CARTILAGE HAIR HYPOPLASIA

Cartilage hair hypoplasia (CHH), also known as metaphyseal chondrodysplasia McKusick type, is an autosomal recessive skeletal dysplasia with a number of nonskeletal manifestations. The disorder is caused by recessive variants in *RMRP*. Although rare overall, it is present at higher frequencies in certain genetic isolates, such as in individuals of Finnish or Amish ancestry. *RMRP* encodes an untranslated RNA subunit of a ribosomal processing complex, RNase MRP. Functional studies have demonstrated decreased ribosomal cleavage when examining variants that cause CHH, thus suggesting that the inability to process ribosomal RNA is implicated in human skeletal development.

The skeletal features of CHH include short-limb short stature with bowing of the femurs and tibia. There is also significant brachydactyly. Other skeletal findings can include limited extension at the elbow and lumbar lordosis. There is a broad range of reported adult height, from roughly 100 to 150 cm. Radiographic assessment demonstrates bullet-shaped metacarpals, cone-shaped epiphyses, and metaphyseal dysplasia of tubular bones. Although skeletal features may be identified in utero or in the neonatal period, other findings in CHH may be less apparent. Additional features include fine and sparse or slow-growing hair and joint hypermobility. Individuals with this disorder are at risk of having immunodeficiency with variable impairment of T-lymphocyte proliferation, although cases of severe combined immunodeficiency have been reported. Other hematologic findings can include macrocytic anemia and susceptibility to lymphoma and leukemia. Intestinal features have been described and include malabsorption and gastrointestinal motility problems, such as Hirschsprung disease.

## SUGGESTED READINGS


Dwan K, Phillipi CA, Steiner RD, Basel D. Bisphosphonate therapy for osteogenesis imperfecta. *Cochrane Database Syst Rev*. 2014;7:CD005088.

Gonzaga-Jauregui C, Gamble CN, Yuan B, et al. Mutations in COL27A1 cause Steel syndrome and suggest a founder mutation effect in the Puerto Rican population. *Eur J Hum Genet*. 2015;23(3):342-346.

Grafe I, Yang T, Alexander S, et al. Excessive transforming growth factor-β signaling is a common mechanism in osteogenesis imperfecta. *Nat Med*. 2014;20(6):670-675.

Lorget F, Kaci N, Peng J, et al. Evaluation of the therapeutic potential of a CNP analog in a Fgfr3 mouse model recapitulating achondroplasia. *Am J Hum Genet*. 2012;91(6):1108-1114.

Orwoll ES, Shapiro J, Veith S, et al. Evaluation of teriparatide treatment in adults with osteogenesis imperfecta. *J Clin Invest*. 2014;124(2):491-498.

Patel RM, Nagamani SC, Cuthbertson D, et al. A cross-sectional multicenter study of osteogenesis imperfecta in North America: results from the linked clinical research centers. *Clin Genet*. 2015;87(2):133-140.

Pogue R, Ehtesham N, Repetto GM, et al. Probable identity-by-descent for a mutation in the Dyggve-Melchior-Clausen/Smith-McCort dysplasia (Dymeclin) gene among patients from Guam, Chile, Argentina, and Spain. *Am J Med Genet A*. 2005;138(1):75-78.

Sinder BP, Eddy MM, Ominsky MS, Caird MS, Marini JC, Kozloff KM. Sclerostin antibody improves skeletal parameters in a Brtl/+ mouse model of osteogenesis imperfecta. *J Bone Miner Res*. 2013;28(1):73-80.

Warman ML, Cormier-Daire V, Hall C, et al. Nosology and classification of genetic skeletal disorders: 2010 revision. *Am J Med Genet A*. 2011;155A:943-968.

Whyte MP, Rockman-Greenberg C, Ozono K, et al. Asfotase alfa treatment improves survival for perinatal and infantile hypophosphatasia. *J Clin Endocrinol Metab*. 2016;101:334-342

Wu N, Ming X, Xiao J, et al. TBX6 null variants and a common hypomorphic allele in congenital scoliosis. *N Engl J Med*. 2015;372(4):341-350.


# 180 Connective Tissue Disorders


Shweta U. Dhar and Melissa Russo


## INTRODUCTION

Connective tissue provides form, strength, and support to different parts of the body. It also serves as a medium for cellular transport as well as storage and exchange of nutrients. It is made up of dozens of proteins constituting either the extracellular fibers, amorphous matrix called ground substance, or the cellular network. The most abundant extracellular fibers are composed of the protein collagen, which is also the most abundant protein found in the human body. Pathogenic variants in genes encoding the collagen proteins cause diseases such as Ehlers-Danlos syndrome, Stickler syndrome, and osteogenesis imperfecta. Other extracellular fibers consist of an amorphous protein called elastin, which is ensheathed in strong microfibrils composed of the protein fibrillin. Pathogenic variants in the gene encoding fibrillin-1 are associated with Marfan syndrome.

Connective tissue disorders are a group of disorders that affect the proteins that make up the connective tissue matrix such as collagens, proteoglycans, elastins, fibrillins, and laminins. Several hundred different heritable disorders of connective tissue have been described. Most of these recognizable disorders are caused by pathogenic variants in single genes and segregate as an autosomal dominant, autosomal recessive, or X-linked trait. Diagnosis of these disorders can be clinically challenging because of overlapping symptoms and the broad spectrum of physical findings. Identification of key clinical features will help guide diagnosis toward a specific disorder. It is imperative for a pediatrician to be cognizant of the signs and symptoms of connective tissue disorders. Management of many of these conditions needs to be initiated in early years of life as some of the main complications from these disorders are progressive and early management can lead to a better prognosis. Well-known connective tissue disorders such as Ehlers-Danlos syndrome (EDS), Marfan syndrome, Loeys-Dietz syndrome, and Stickler syndrome will be presented in this chapter.

## PATHOGENESIS

### Collagenopathies

There are numerous connective tissue disorders related to defects in collagen and its other extracellular matrix proteins such as elastin, proteoglycans, and macromolecular proteins. There are different types of collagen, and these proteins are multimeric, occurring as trimers with a central triple helical orientation. All types of collagen are synthesized first as precursor molecules of procollagen, which are then modified by specific proteases to form the subunits of extracellular fibrils. Collagenopathies result from alterations in the structure and function of collagens I, II, III, IV, V, VI, VII, IX, X, XI, and XVII and the enzymes lysyl hydroxylase and type I procollagen N-proteinase involved in the posttranslational modification of collagens. EDS is a molecularly heterogeneous disorder, as defects in different types of collagen, particularly types I, III, and V, and several extracellular matrix proteins, such as tenascin and lysyl hydroxylase, have been implicated in its pathogenesis and form the basis of the 1997 Villefranche classification of EDS (Table 180-1). Procollagen genes *COL2A1* and *COL11A1/A2* are expressed in the eye and cartilage, and defects in these genes are associated with Stickler syndrome.

### Fibrillinopathies

Marfan and Loeys-Dietz syndromes result from dysregulation of the transforming growth factor (TGF)-β pathway (Fig. 180-1). Fibrillin-1 is a large extracellular matrix protein that forms polymers called microfibrils, which closely associate with elastin fibers and sequester bioavailable TGF-β. With loss of function of fibrillin-1 in Marfan syndrome, there is decreased TGF-β sequestration and a resultant increase in TGF-β–dependent signaling, and this leads to downstream effects of aortic root dilation and pulmonary emphysema through noncanonical ERK activation. Pathogenic variants in *TGFBR1* and *TGFBR2* additionally alter and upregulate TGF-β–dependent signaling.

## CLINICAL DIAGNOSIS AND MANAGEMENT OF DIFFERENT CONNECTIVE TISSUE DISORDERS

## EHLERS-DANLOS SYNDROME

The Ehlers-Danlos syndromes (EDS) are recognized as the most common heritable connective tissue disorders. In 1997, a group of experts met at Villefranche, France, and categorized EDS into 6 major types, namely classic, hypermobility, vascular, kyphoscoliotic, arthrochalasia, and dermatopraxis types. Table 180-1 lists the different types of EDS, the genes involved, and the predominant symptoms. A recent consortium of international experts published guidelines for diagnosis of EDS using evidence-based criteria. The 2017 International Classification for EDS includes 13 sub-types, some of them associated with pathogenic variants in an array of new genes that have been identified with the advent of next-generation sequencing technologies. All of these subtypes share a varying combination of skin fragility, joint hypermobility, and easy bruisability. While there is significant overlap between the types of EDS, they are clinically diagnosed by their predominant clinical manifestations. Each type has a set of major and minor diagnostic

**TABLE 180-1 TYPES OF EDS (VILLEFRANCHE CLASSIFICATION)**

| Type of EDS | Previous Nomenclature | Major Criteria | Minor Criteria | Pattern of Inheritance | Gene |
|---|---|---|---|---|---|
| Classic | Type I (gravis) and type II (mitis) | Skin<br>Wide scars<br>Joint hypermobility | Smooth skin<br>Easy bruising<br>Molluscoid pseudotumors<br>Subcutaneous spheroids<br>Post-op hernia<br>Hypotonia | AD | *COL5A1*<br>*COL5A2* |
| Hypermobility | Type III | Generalized joint hypermobility<br>Chronic musculoskeletal pain | Recurring joint dislocations<br>Soft tissue rheumatism<br>Skin abnormalities such as striae, hyperextensibility, thin skin<br>Varicose veins<br>Organ prolapse<br>Dysautonomia and/or POTS | AD | Unknown |
| Vascular | Type IV | Excessive bruising<br>Thin, translucent skin<br>Arterial/hollow organ rupture<br>Characteristic facies | Acrogeria<br>Hypermobility of small joints<br>Varicose veins<br>Tendon and muscle rupture<br>Pneumothorax | AD | *COL3A1* |
| Kyphoscoliotic | Type VI | Severe muscular hypotonia at birth<br>Progressive scoliosis<br>Generalized joint laxity<br>Scleral fragility and rupture of the globe | Tissue fragility<br>Easy bruising<br>Arterial rupture<br>Marfanoid habitus<br>Microcornea<br>Low bone density | AR | *PLOD1* |
| Arthrochalasia | Types VII A,B | Congenital bilateral hip dislocation<br>Severe generalized joint hypermobility<br>Recurrent subluxations | Skin hyperextensibility<br>Tissue fragility including atrophic scarring<br>Easy bruising<br>Kyphoscoliosis<br>Mildly decreased bone density<br>Muscle hypotonia | AD | *COL1A1*<br>*COL1A2* |
| Dermatosparaxis | Type VIIC | Severe skin fragility<br>Sagging, redundant skin<br>Excessive bruising | Soft, doughy skin<br>Large hernias<br>Premature rupture of membranes | AR | *ADAMTS-2* |

AD, autosomal dominant; AR, autosomal recessive; EDS, Ehlers-Danlos syndrome; POTS, postural orthostatic tachycardia syndrome.



criteria that are used to make a clinical diagnosis. Diagnosis can then be confirmed by molecular testing except for hypermobile EDS (hEDS), for which the molecular etiology is not yet known.

## CLASSICAL EDS (cEDS)

Formerly known as type I EDS (EDS gravis)/type II EDS (EDS mitis), cEDS is characterized by excessive skin hyperextensibility and widened atrophic scarring. Additional features include joint hypermobility, subcutaneous spheroids, molluscoid pseudotumors, piezogenic papules (small herniations of subcutaneous fat), easy bruising, abnormal/delayed wound healing, and hernias. Hyperextensibility of skin is defined as skin that extends easily and snaps back upon release and is best tested in areas of skin not subjected to mechanical forces or scarring such as the volar surface of the forearm. It is difficult to appreciate this in younger children because of the abundance of subcutaneous fat. This subtype is classically associated with heterozygous pathogenic variants in genes coding for type V collagen such as *COL5A1* and *COL5A2*. A majority of patients with cEDS will have a pathogenic variant in one of these 2 genes. Electron microscopy of a skin biopsy may demonstrate disturbed collagen fibrillogenesis (cauliflower deformity of collagen fibrils).

## HYPERMOBILE EDS (hEDS)

This is the most common type of EDS, and its prevalence is estimated at 1 in 5000, although it is known to be underdiagnosed, and hence, some studies quote that prevalence may even be as high as 1 in 2500. This subtype is categorized by excessive joint hypermobility in association with a wide array of symptoms thought to arise either randomly or as a direct complication of the joint hypermobility. Complications of joint hypermobility include recurrent subluxations and dislocations occurring spontaneously or with minimal mechanical force, degenerative joint disease, early-onset arthritis, and chronic disabling and debilitating musculoskeletal pain. Beighton score (Fig. 180-2) is used to measure the degree of joint hypermobility. A score of 6/9 or greater in pre-pubertal individuals, 5/9 or greater in post-pubertal individuals, and 4/9 or greater in those over 50 years of age, is evidence of joint hypermobility. Other well-known associated features include dysautonomia. Patients complain of dizziness/light-headedness on changes of position, temperature intolerance, transient abdominal pain of unclear etiology, sleep disturbances, and feeling of being unwell with changes in barometric pressure and are frequently diagnosed with postural orthostatic tachycardia syndrome (POTS) and Raynaud disease. While these systemic manifestations are not part of the diagnostic criteria, their presence favors a clinical diagnosis of hEDS over other sub-types of EDS. The molecular etiology of hEDS is unknown, and hence, this remains largely a clinical diagnosis. It is believed that this subtype may be genetically heterogenous. There are currently no confirmatory biochemical or genetic tests that can confirm or rule out a diagnosis of hEDS.

## VASCULAR EDS (vEDS)

Previously known as type IV EDS, this disorder is characterized by easy bruising and skin fragility, translucent skin with visible vasculature,

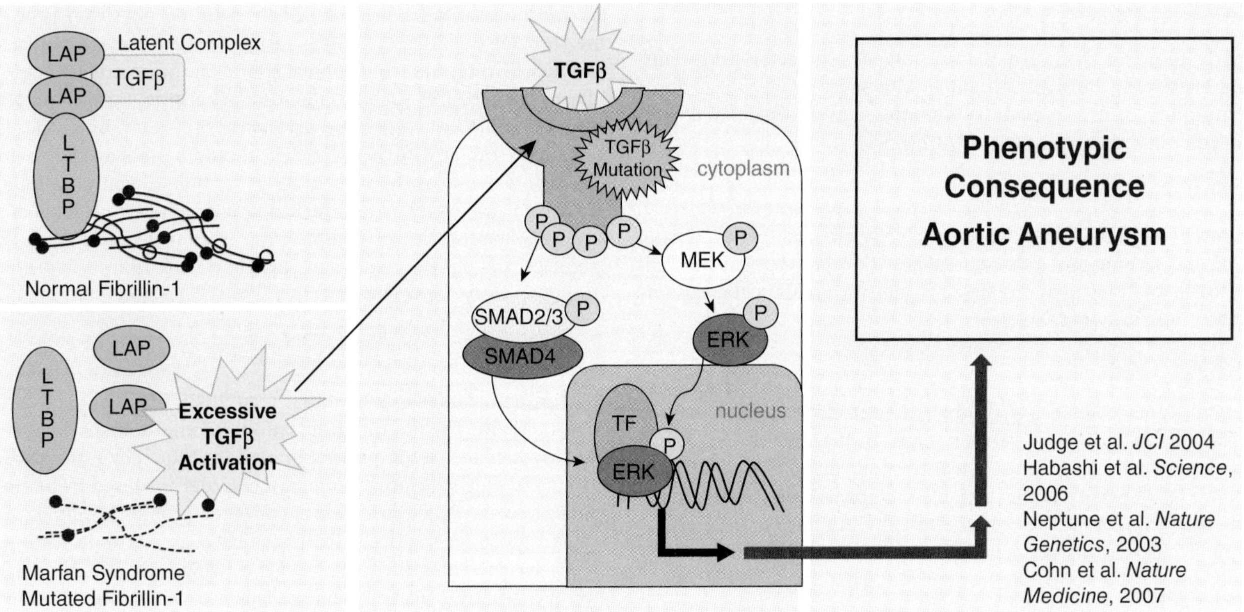


**FIGURE 180-1** Pathogenesis of aortic aneurysm in Marfan syndrome (MFS) and Loeys-Dietz syndrome (LDS). Excessive transforming growth factor (TGF)-β signaling through noncanonical ERK activation leads to phenotypic consequences.

characteristic facial appearance (Fig. 180-3), hollow organ rupture, and spontaneous dissection of aortic and other arterial vessels. The prevalence of this disorder is estimated to be 1 per 100,000. It is an autosomal dominant disorder secondary to pathogenic variants in the *COL3A1* gene, encoding type 3 procollagen. The diagnosis of vEDS is based on clinical findings and family history and confirmed by molecular testing.

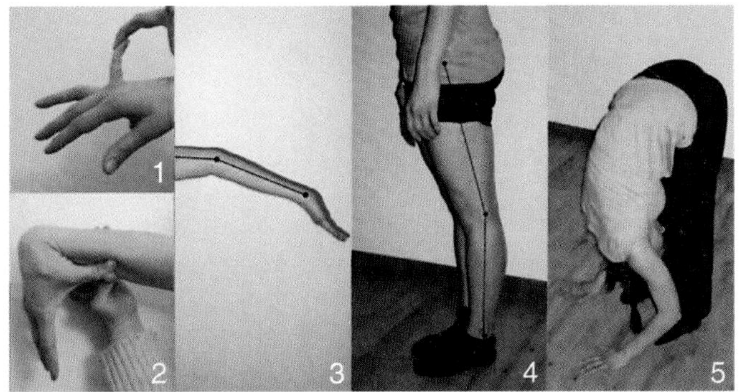


| No. | Criterion | Points |
|---|---|---|
| 1 | Passive dorsiflexion of the 5th finger >90° | 2 (bilateral) |
| 2 | Passive apposition of thumb to volar surface of forearm | 2 (bilateral) |
| 3 | Hyperextension of elbow >10° | 2 (bilateral) |
| 4 | Hyperextension of knee >10° | 2 (bilateral) |
| 5 | Ability to place the palms on the floor with knees fully extended | 1 |

**FIGURE 180-2** Beighton score: A score of 5/9 is considered an objective measure of hypermobility.

## KYPHOSCOLIOTIC EDS (kEDS)

Previously known as EDS type VI, kEDS is characterized by kyphoscoliosis, joint laxity, severe muscular hypotonia at birth, friable and hyperextensible skin with a propensity for thin scars and easy bruising, and scleral fragility with increased risk of rupture of the globe. Its prevalence is unknown but has been estimated at 1:100,000. It is caused by deficient activity of the enzyme procollagen-lysin, 2-oxoglutarate 5-dioxygenase 1 (PLOD1 or lysyl hydroxylase 1) and is distinguished from other subtypes of EDS by its autosomal recessive pattern of inheritance. The diagnosis is made based on the clinical features and confirmed by demonstrating an increased ratio of urinary deoxypyridinoline to pyridinilone crosslinks (measured by high-performance liquid chromatography). Pathogenic variants are found in the *PLOD1* gene.

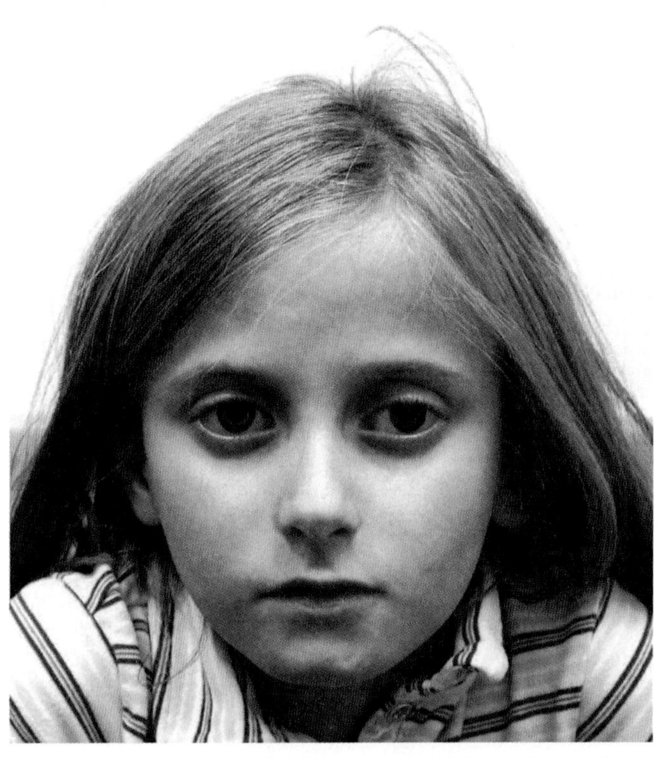

**FIGURE 180-3** Characteristic facial appearance of child with vascular Ehlers-Danlos syndrome. This child has prominence of her eyes with enophthalmos, smaller alae nasi, thin upper lip, and smaller chin.

## ARTHROCHALASIA EDS (aEDS)

Formerly known as type VIIA-B, this subtype is characterized by congenital bilateral hip dislocation along with severe generalized joint hypermobility and recurrent subluxations. It is associated with pathogenic variants in the *COL1A1/A2* genes.

## DERMATOSPARAXIS EDS (dEDS)

Previously type VIIC, this EDS type is characterized by severe skin fragility and sagging and redundant skin with excessive bruising. It is inherited in an autosomal recessive manner with pathogenic variants identified in the *ADAMTS-2* gene.

## OTHER SUB-TYPES

Other sub-types of EDS based on the newer classification include classical-like EDS, cardiac-valvular type, brittle cornea syndrome, spondylodysplastic EDS, musculocontractual, myopathic, and periodontal EDS. Owing to the variable but overlapping phenotypes among the various sub-types and the vast amount of genetic heterogeneity, molecular testing is essential to confirm the diagnosis.

## MANAGEMENT

Medical management of individuals with EDS is based on the associated complications and is essentially symptomatic. While there is no cure for EDS, most individuals benefit from knowing the diagnosis and focusing the care on symptomatic management and preventative measures. Complications from chronic joint laxity can be treated or prevented by physiotherapy aimed at global muscle strengthening and conditioning and avoidance of injurious activities or activities that cause hyperextension of joints. These individuals benefit from regular intervention from a pain management specialist. Other nonpharmacologic measures such as bracing, splinting, or taping of joints and use of ergonomic devices can help with the excessive joint mobility and to prevent further injury. Wound management requires special consideration so that the surgeon closes the skin and underlying tissues without tension with sutures applied to both surface and deeper tissues to avoid gaping of wounds. Cutaneous sutures should be left in place for twice the amount of time because individuals with EDS have a tendency for delayed wound healing. Vitamin C (ascorbic acid) is a cofactor for cross-linking of collagen fibrils and thus plays an important role in collagen formation and strengthening of ligaments, tendons, and capillary blood vessels. High-dose ascorbic acid supplementation has been recommended for improved wound healing and scarring and can be beneficial in individuals with EDS–kyphoscoliotic type, as this type of EDS is caused by a deficiency of lysyl hydroxylase and vitamin C is a known co-factor of lysyl hydroxylase. Up to 2 g can be given to patients with classic EDS to reduce easy bruising. In patients with hypermobility EDS, supplementation with up to 500 mg may improve some of the manifestations, but this has not been adequately studied. Screening for aortic aneurysms is recommended periodically in all types of EDS with echocardiography or other modalities of cardiac imaging. POTS symptoms can be controlled by β-blockers and increasing intake of salt and fluids. Periodic screening with bone densitometry (dual-energy x-ray absorptiometry [DXA]) scans and vitamin D are recommended to monitor bone health.

The management of vascular subtype of EDS demands special consideration because of the risk of catastrophic vascular and organ rupture. Arterial complications are rare in childhood; however, they occur in 25% of affected individuals by age 20 years and in greater than 80% of individuals by age 40 years with a median age of death at 48 years. The benefit of surveillance of the arterial vasculature is to attempt to identify dilation and aneurysm prior to dissection, and serial imaging is recommended on a yearly basis with echocardiograms and computed tomography and/or magnetic resonance angiography. Medical treatment with β-blockers is recommended to reduce arterial wall stress. Because of the catastrophic complications of bowel rupture, individuals with vascular EDS should be counseled to seek immediate medical attention for sudden, unexplained pain. Timely surgical intervention for bowel rupture is essential, and surgical interventions are more likely to be successful if the treating physician is aware of the vascular EDS diagnosis. It is recommended that individuals with vascular EDS refrain from contact sports and isometric exercises, and invasive procedures such as colonoscopy, arteriography, and elective surgery should be avoided and performed only if absolutely necessary. Pregnant women with vascular EDS should be managed as high-risk obstetric patients as they are more susceptible to complications such as uterine and vascular rupture during the high-volume state of pregnancy. Since the risk of complication is considered greatest during labor, during delivery, and immediately postpartum, it is prudent to decide on early delivery via elective cesarean section.

# MARFAN SYNDROME

Marfan syndrome is a hereditary, multisystem, connective tissue disorder with cardinal manifestations in the ocular, skeletal, and cardiovascular systems and a population frequency estimated to be 1 in 5000. This autosomal dominant disorder is caused by pathogenic variants in the *FBN1* gene that encodes the protein fibrillin-1 located on chromosome 15q21.1. There have been greater than 1300 pathogenic variants identified in this gene, which are highly penetrant; however, there is a great degree of phenotypic variability with this disorder. A majority of affected individuals (75%) have an affected parent, whereas the rest (25%) are de novo.

Marfan syndrome can be diagnosed clinically using the revised Ghent diagnostic criteria, which incorporate physical examination findings, cardiovascular imaging, personal medical history, and family history (Table 180-2). The clinical findings of aortic root aneurysm

**TABLE 180-2 GHENT DIAGNOSTIC CRITERIA FOR MARFAN SYNDROME AND SYSTEMIC SCORING SYSTEM**

**Diagnosis of definitive Marfan syndrome (MFS; any combination of the following)**

- Aortic root ≥ 2 z-score and ectopia lentis
- Aortic root ≥ 2 z-score and *FBN1* pathogenic variant
- Aortic root ≥ 2 z-score and systemic score of ≥ 7
- Ectopia lentis and *FBN1* pathogenic variant
- Positive family history of MFS and ectopia lentis
- Positive family history of MFS and systemic score of ≥ 7
- Positive family history of MFS and aortic root ≥ 3 z-score in those < 20 years of age or aortic root ≥ 2 z-score in those > 20 years of age

**Diagnosis of potential Marfan syndrome**

- *FBN1* mutation with aortic root < 3 z-score in those < 20 years of age

**Systemic Scoring System for the Revised Ghent Diagnostic Criteria for Marfan Syndrome**

| Feature | Value |
|---|---|
| Wrist and thumb sign | 3 |
| Wrist or thumb sign | 1 |
| Pectus carinatum | 2 |
| Pectus excavatum or chest asymmetry | 1 |
| Hindfoot deformity (valgus) | 2 |
| Pes planus | 1 |
| Pneumothorax | 2 |
| Dural ectasia | 2 |
| Protrusio acetabulae | 2 |
| Reduced upper to lower segment ratio and increased arm span to height ratio | 1 |
| Scoliosis or thoracolumbar kyphosis | 1 |
| Reduced elbow extension | 1 |
| Craniofacial features; any 3 of the following: dolichocephaly, downward-slanting palpebral fissures, enophthalmos, retrognathia, malar hypoplasia | 1 |
| Skin striae | 1 |
| Myopia | 1 |
| Mitral valve prolapse | 1 |

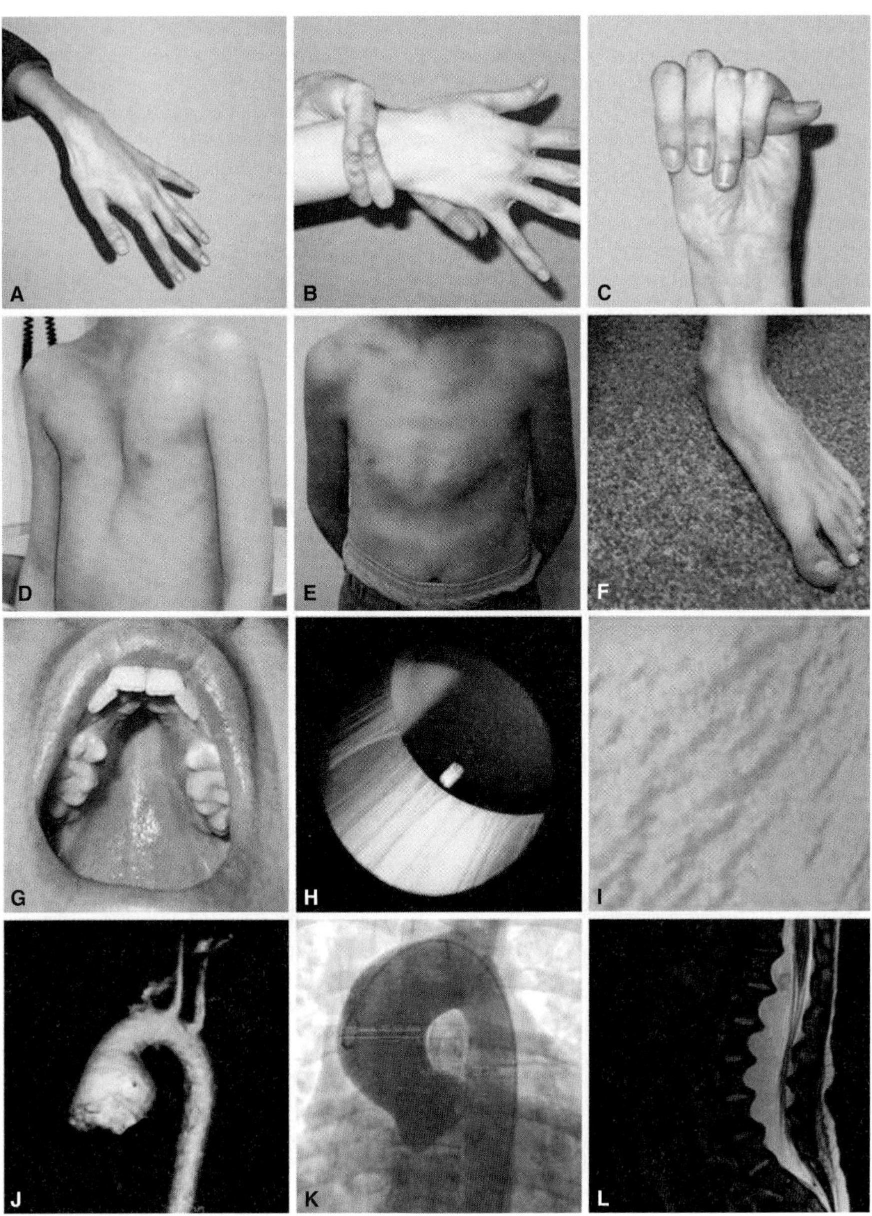


FIGURE 180-4 Clinical features of Marfan syndrome: (A) arachnodactyly, (B) Walker-Murdoch "wrist" sign, (C) Steinberg "thumb" sign, (D) pectus deformity of excavatum, (E) pectus deformity of pectus carinatum, (F) pes planus with hindfoot deformity, (G) high arched, narrow palate, (H) ectopic lentis, (I) striae of skin, (J) significant dilation of the aortic root via 3-dimensional reconstruction from magnetic resonance, (K) aortic root dilation with angiography, and (L) dural ectasia



and ectopia lentis (displacement of the lens from the center of the pupil) are particularly important diagnostic criteria because of their specificity and clinical significance. Clinical features of Marfan syndrome are outlined below, and characteristic findings are pictured in Fig. 180-4. Once a clinical diagnosis is suspected, genetic testing for *FBN1* can be initiated to confirm the diagnosis.

## CLINICAL FEATURES

**Ocular Manifestations** Myopia is the most common ocular finding in Marfan syndrome and is often progressive in children. Ectopia lentis is a hallmark feature of this disorder; however, only 60% of individuals with Marfan syndrome have this finding. It is most reliably diagnosed by slit-lamp examination with pupillary dilation. Individuals with Marfan syndrome are also at increased risk for retinal detachment, glaucoma, and early cataracts.

**Skeletal Features** Excessive bone growth is typically noted in Marfan syndrome, particularly in the long, tubular bones of the extremities, leading to disproportionally long extremities compared to the trunk (known as dolichostenomelia). This alters the arm span to height and upper to lower segment ratios. The lower segment is measured from the pubic symphysis to the floor, and the upper segment is calculated by subtracting the lower segment from the height. An increased arm span to height ratio (> 1.05) and a reduced upper to lower segment ratio (< 0.85) are considered positive findings. The fingers are also disproportionately long, which is described as arachnodactyly. The thumb and wrist signs (see Fig. 180-4B and 4C), also known as the Walker-Murdoch and Steinberg signs, highlight this disproportionality. There can be overgrowth of the ribs that can push the sternum inward, known as pectus excavatum, or outward, known as pectus carinatum, which is seen in approximately two-thirds of individuals with Marfan syndrome. Other skeletal features include progressive scoliosis or thoracic kyphosis and abnormally deep acetabulum of the hip known as protrusio acetabuli (which can be associated with pelvic or upper leg pain). Flat feet (pes planus) as well as a hindfoot deformity defined as medial rotation of the medial malleolus may also be observed in individuals with Marfan syndrome.

**Cardiovascular Manifestations** The major sources of morbidity and mortality from this disorder are the complications noted in the cardiovascular system, namely dilation of the aorta, aortic valve insufficiency, aortic aneurysm and dissection, mitral valve prolapse, tricuspid prolapse, and enlargement of the proximal pulmonary artery. The aortic dilation is seen mainly at the level of the sinuses of Valsalva but can be seen in other parts of the aorta as well. The aortic root measurements are interpreted on the basis of normal values for age and body surface area (*z*-score). Aortic dilatation is progressive over time and, if left uncorrected, increases the risk for dissection in these individuals; however, the onset and rate of progression are highly variable, and hence, close surveillance is warranted by a cardiologist familiar with Marfan syndrome.

**Skin Findings** The main skin findings in Marfan syndrome are stretch marks or striae across the back, shoulders, and inguinal and axillary regions. These individuals can also have widened scars. Individuals with Marfan syndrome are at risk for hernias, and primary hernia repairs should use synthetic mesh to minimize the risk of recurrence. These findings are not necessarily specific for this disorder.

**Central Nervous System and Dural Manifestations** The dural sac in the lumbosacral region in individuals with Marfan syndrome can stretch and result in dural ectasia. A majority of patients with this finding are asymptomatic; however, some individuals have pain, weakness, and numbness. This dural abnormality is identified by magnetic resonance imaging or computed tomography. Cognitive deficits are not known to be part of the spectrum of Marfan syndrome.

**Pulmonary Features** The pulmonary features of Marfan syndrome include spontaneous pneumothorax from lung bullae, reduced pulmonary reserve from pectus deformity or severe scoliosis, obstructive sleep apnea, and emphysematous lung disease.

**Craniofacial Features** The craniofacial features of Marfan syndrome are notable for a long narrow face with deep set eyes, enophthalmos, downward slanting palpebral fissures, malar hypoplasia, micrognathia, high arched palate, and dental crowding. The facial features are highly variable and not specific to this disorder. However, these individuals can have difficulty with anesthesia and intubation secondary to their craniofacial features.

### MANAGEMENT

Management of Marfan syndrome requires a multidisciplinary approach with involvement of different specialists. Yearly ophthalmologic exams are recommended and should be performed by a physician who is familiar with Marfan syndrome. Most eye problems are controlled with corrective lenses, but some may require surgery. In patients with pectus deformities that interfere with cardiac or pulmonary functioning, a surgical intervention is required. Yearly evaluations for scoliosis and kyphosis are recommended, and it is important to have an orthopedic surgeon involved in the care of these patients.

Important advances have been made in the cardiovascular management of patients with Marfan syndrome. Management recommendations include serial cardiac imaging, medications to decrease progressive aortic root dilation, and prophylactic aortic root replacement. Generally, yearly cardiac imaging evaluations with echocardiograms alternating with computed tomography angiography (CTA) or magnetic resonance angiography (MRA) are preferred. Due to the fragility of the aorta, contact sports and isometric exercise are prohibited in individuals with aortic root dilation. Current medical therapies that have been approved to decrease the rate of progressive aortic root dilation include β-blockers and angiotensin II type 1 receptor blockers. A large, prospective, randomized trial by the Pediatric Heart Network of losartan versus atenolol in pediatric patients did not show a significant difference in the rates of aortic root dilation, aortic root surgery, or death between the groups over a 3-year period. Surgical guidelines for aortic root repair in young children with Marfan syndrome are determined by (1) the rate of increase of the aortic root diameter (> 1 cm per year), (2) progressive and severe aortic regurgitation, and (3) size of the maximal aortic root (if it exceeds 5 cm). If possible, a valve-sparing procedure is preferred to avoid chronic anticoagulation therapy. However, valvular dysfunction can be seen, which leads to volume overload with resultant heart failure. The leading cause of morbidity and mortality in young children with Marfan syndrome is mitral valve prolapse, leading to congestive heart failure. It should be noted that children are at high risk for repeat cardiac operations.

## LOEYS-DIETZ SYNDROME

Loeys-Dietz syndrome (LDS) is a heritable connective tissue disorder that has cardiovascular, skeletal, and craniofacial features. It is an autosomal dominant condition that is caused by heterozygous pathogenic variants in the *TGFBR1* and *TGFBR2* genes that encode the TGF-β receptor 1 and 2 proteins. There is debate about the classification of the different types of this disorder and whether classification should be based on gene variants versus severity of craniofacial/cutaneous features. De novo pathogenic variants are present in 75% of individuals, and 25% of cases are inherited from a parent. The clinical features of LDS are highly variable, as described below.

### CLINICAL FEATURES

**Cardiovascular Manifestations** Individuals with LDS usually have earlier and more aggressive aortic and arterial disease compared to individuals with Marfan syndrome. Vascular aneurysms and dissections are not limited to the aorta and can occur anywhere along the arterial tree. Arterial tortuosity that commonly involves vertebral and carotid arteries of the head and neck as seen on magnetic resonance angiography or computed tomography with 3-dimensional reconstruction is a hallmark feature of patients with LDS. Quantitative measures of arterial tortuosity, such as the vertebral tortuosity index (VTI), have been developed, and increased tortuosity has been associated with earlier and more severe adverse cardiovascular events. Congenital heart diseases such as bicuspid aortic valve, atrial septal defects, and patent ductus arteriosus are seen more frequently in individuals with LDS.

**Skeletal Features** The skeletal features of LDS have some degree of overlap with those of Marfan syndrome, namely joint hypermobility, arachnodactyly, pectus deformities, pes planus, hindfoot deformity, high arched palate, dental crowding, and scoliosis. In contrast to Marfan syndrome, individuals with LDS are more often of normal stature. In addition, there is also evidence of joint contractures of the feet, leading to talipes equinovarus, and contracture of the fingers, leading to camptodactyly. These individuals also can have cervical spine instability and spondylolisthesis; thus, x-rays to determine the presence of these findings are important, especially prior to surgery.

**Craniofacial Features** The craniofacial features associated with LDS are variable in severity and include hypertelorism, cleft palate, and bifid uvula (Fig. 180-5). The uvular deformities can range from broad uvula, uvula with a raphe, to a clearly split/bifid uvula. Individuals with LDS can have craniosynostosis, micro-/retrognathia, blue sclera, and strabismus. Studies have shown that there is an association of more rapidly progressive aortic aneurysmal disease in individuals with the more severe craniofacial phenotype.

**Skin Findings** The skin findings of LDS overlap with vascular EDS and include soft, velvety, translucent skin that is fragile with easily bruising. Wound healing may be delayed, and scars can be dystrophic.

**Gastrointestinal Features** There is a higher percentage of eosinophilic gastrointestinal disease and inflammatory bowel disease in people with LDS. Infants and children with LDS frequently present with failure to thrive and constipation.

**Immune Dysregulation and Allergy** Allergic and immune conditions, such as asthma, food allergies, eczema, and allergic rhinitis, along with immunoglobulin E dysregulation, occur at higher prevalence in children with LDS.

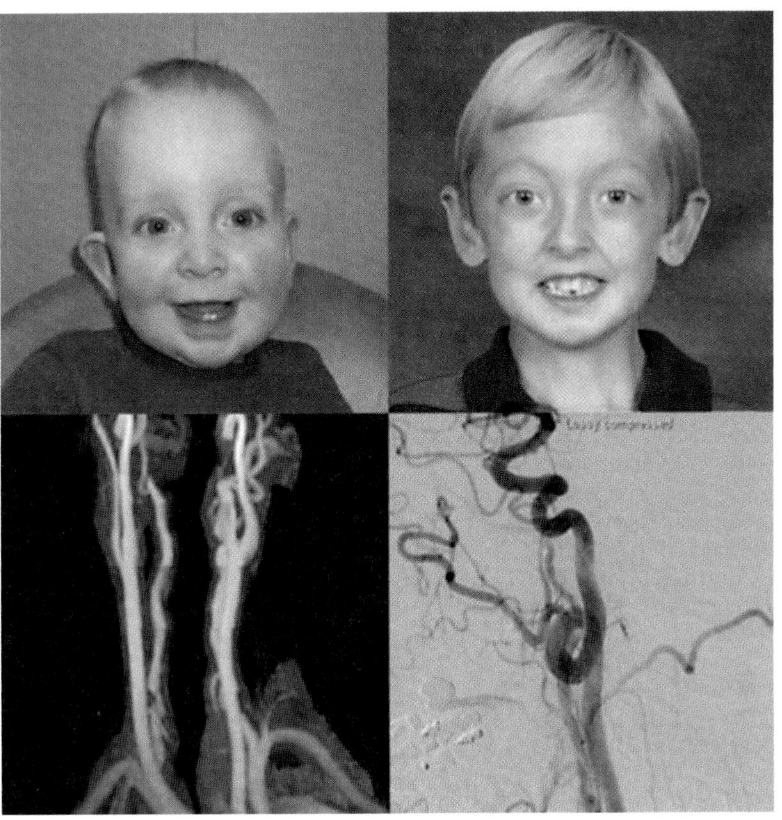

FIGURE 180-5 Clinical features of Loeys-Dietz syndrome. The craniofacial features of hypertelorism, thin upper lip, and small chin are demonstrated in the top 2 images, and the arterial tortuosity of the carotid and vertebral arteries are demonstrated on magnetic resonance angiography and computed tomography angiography in the bottom images.

## MANAGEMENT

Due to the increased risk of aortic and arterial aneurysm and dissection, the management of LDS includes serial cardiac imaging, treatment with β-blockers or angiotensin II receptor blockers to slow aortic root growth, and elective aortic root replacement. Echocardiogram and computed tomography versus magnetic resonance angiography to evaluate the whole arterial system are recommended every 6 to 12 months. In children, prophylactic aortic root replacement is recommended at a z-score of > 3 or 4 cm, depending on severe versus mild craniofacial features or rapidly expanding aortic root dilation (> 0.5 cm per year). Moreover, it is important for children to have serial evaluations with orthopedic surgeons who are familiar with LDS.

# STICKLER SYNDROME

Stickler syndrome, also known as hereditary arthro-ophthalmopathy, is a common connective tissue disorder with a population frequency estimated at 1 in 10,000. It is a clinically variable and genetically heterogenous disorder characterized by ocular, auditory, orofacial, and skeletal manifestations. Classical features of this condition include very high myopia, retinal detachment, profound hearing loss, and Pierre Robin sequence. Clinical diagnosis is challenging due to lack of minimal consensus diagnostic criteria. This is compounded by intrafamilial and interfamilial variability. This may explain why this condition remains underdiagnosed. However, consideration of the diagnosis can be made if 2 of the 4 systems are affected by typical manifestations. A diagnostic point system has been developed for type I Stickler syndrome. Table 180-3 lists the different types of Stickler syndrome based on predominant features.

## CLINICAL FEATURES

**Ocular Findings** Abnormalities of vitreous gel architecture are a pathognomonic feature and are usually associated with congenital high myopia (3 diopters in the neonatal period). There is a substantial

**TABLE 180-3 CLASSIFICATION OF STICKLER SYNDROME**

| Type of Stickler Syndrome | Clinical Features | Pattern of Inheritance | Gene |
|---|---|---|---|
| STL1; Stickler syndrome type I | Predominantly ocular (membranous vitreous form): high myopia, retinal tears<br>Normal to mild hearing loss | AD | *COL2A1* |
| STL2; Stickler syndrome type II | Beaded vitreous type: high myopia, retinal tears<br>Pierre Robin sequence<br>Cleft palate<br>Bifid uvula<br>Profound and progressive hearing loss | AD | *COL11A1* |
| STL3; Stickler syndrome type III | Nonocular form<br>Mild hearing loss<br>Pierre Robin sequence<br>Cleft palate | AD | *COL11A2* |
| STL4; Stickler syndrome type IV | Moderate to high myopia with vitreoretinopathy<br>Moderate to severe sensorineural hearing loss | AR | *COL9A1* |
| STL5; Stickler syndrome type V | High myopia with vitreoretinal degeneration; retinal detachment<br>Mild to moderate sensorineural hearing loss<br>Short stature in childhood | AR | *COL9A2* |

AD, autosomal dominant; AR, autosomal recessive.

risk for retinal abnormalities including predisposition to retinal lattice formation, holes, tears, and/or retinal detachments (onset as early as age 4–6 years) and premature cataracts. Retinal detachment leading to blindness is the most severe ocular complication of Stickler syndrome, affecting almost 50% of cases.

**Audiologic Manifestations** High-frequency sensorineural hearing loss progressive with age and hypermobile tympanic membranes are seen in patients with Stickler syndrome. There is considerable variability in the degree of hearing loss. Conductive loss can also occur secondary to middle ear disease in association with craniofacial anomalies such as cleft palate, narrow internal auditory canals, or small midface.

**Orofacial Abnormalities** Typical craniofacial features include a midface hypoplasia resulting in a flat facial profile, low nasal bridge, anteverted nares, micrognathia, and cleft palate (Fig. 180-6). Stickler syndrome is one of the most common syndromes associated with the Pierre Robin sequence, which is comprised of mandibular hypoplasia, cleft palate, and glossoptosis, leading to life-threatening obstructive apnea and feeding difficulties in neonates. While isolated Pierre Robin sequence is most prevalent (53%), as many as 30% to 50% of patients with Pierre Robin sequence actually have Stickler syndrome. Stickler syndrome should also be considered in patients with cleft lip/palate, which has an incidence of 1 per 650 live newborns.

**Skeletal Features** Musculoskeletal and joint problems are found in over 80% of individuals with Stickler syndrome. These include mild spondyloepiphyseal dysplasia with delayed ossification of the vertebrae, femoral heads, pubis, and calcanei. Young children frequently report ligamentous laxity and joint hypermobility of fingers, hips, and ankles. Osteoarthritis may begin as early as the teenage years in these individuals. The combination of slender bones, disproportionately long limbs, and joint hypermobility gives many patients a Marfanoid habitus, although some having short stature are also reported.

## MANAGEMENT

Diagnosis of Stickler syndrome should be considered in patients with skeletal dysplasias such as Kniest dysplasia, which is characterized by disproportionate short stature, numerous radiographic abnormalities, and cleft palate with or without the Pierre Robin sequence; Marshall syndrome, which is characterized by a more pronounced facial appearance that persists beyond childhood and dermatologic involvement such as hypotrichosis and hypohidrosis; and Weissenbacher-Zweymuller syndrome, which is associated with rhizomelic shortening and vertebral clefting. A point-scoring system can be used for the diagnosis of type I Stickler syndrome (Table 180-4)

Individuals suspected of having Stickler syndrome should undergo baseline evaluations by ophthalmology and audiology as well as genetics to establish the diagnosis and extent of disease. Single-gene testing for the specific type of Stickler syndrome can be undertaken. If a specific type of Stickler syndrome cannot be classified clinically, panel-based genetic testing can be ordered, which would include all the known Stickler-related genes. Treatment is based on severity of symptoms. Refractive errors should be corrected with prescription lenses, and individuals should be advised of symptoms of retinal detachment, cataracts, glaucoma, and progressive retinal disease. Infants with Pierre Robin sequence may require specialized feeding systems and tracheostomy or mandibular advancement to protect the airway from obstruction. Periodic hearing evaluations are recommended, and hearing aids may be necessary for those with hearing loss. Mild skeletal manifestations may not require special interventions, but evaluation by physical therapy and orthopedics should be considered to manage correctable deformities. Treatment for osteoarthritis needs to be initiated if it is a significant problem.

Advances in genetics and genomics have transformed the field of clinical genetics. Next-generation sequencing (NGS) technologies have now made it possible to analyze a panel of genes known to be related to a specific phenotype or the whole exome/genome if a specific diagnosis is not clinically identified. Since heritable connective tissue disorders have such overlapping phenotypes, NGS allows

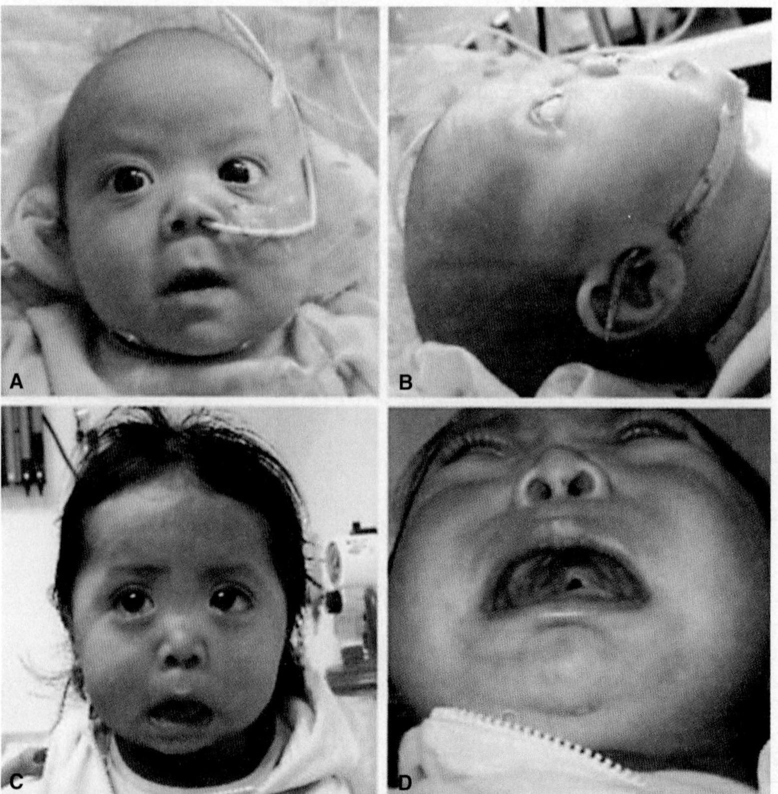


**FIGURE 180-6** Characteristic orofacial features of infants and children with Stickler syndrome. (**A, B**) Infant with flat facial profile with mandibular hypoplasia, telecanthus, low nasal bridge, upturned nasal tip, and Pierre Robin sequence. (**C**) Toddler with very similar facial features. (**D**) Cleft palate.

| TABLE 180-4 DIAGNOSTIC CRITERIA FOR TYPE I STICKLER SYNDROME (5 OR MORE POINTS WITH AT LEAST 1 MAJOR 2-POINT MANIFESTATION AND ABSENCE OF FEATURES SUGGESTIVE OF A MORE SEVERE SKELETAL DYSPLASIA OR OTHER SYNDROME) | |
|---|---|
| **Feature** | **Points** |
| Orofacial abnormalities | |
| • Cleft palate | 2 |
| • Characteristic facies | 1 |
| Ocular abnormalities | |
| • Characteristic vitreous change or retinal abnormalities | 2 |
| Auditory abnormalities | |
| • High-frequency sensorineural hearing loss | 2 |
| • Hypermobile tympanic membranes | 1 |
| Skeletal abnormalities | |
| • Femoral head failure (slipped epiphysis or Legg-Perthes–like disease) | 1 |
| • Osteoarthritis < age 40 y | 1 |
| • Scoliosis, spondylolisthesis, or kyphotic deformity | 1 |
| Family history/molecular data | |
| • Independently affected first-degree relative in an autosomal dominant pattern of inheritance or presence of pathogenic variants in *COL2A1*, *COL11A1*, or *COL11A2* | 1 |

identification of specific disorders, thus enabling understanding of the phenotypic spectrum and natural history of these disorders in more detail. A better understanding of the pathogenesis and mechanisms of disease holds promise for development of targeted molecular therapies in the future.

## SUGGESTED READINGS


Antunes RB, Alonso N, Paula RG. Importance of early diagnosis of Stickler syndrome in newborns. *J Plast Reconstr Aesthet Surg.* 2012;65:1029-1034.

Beighton P, De Paepe A, Steinmann B, Tsipouras P, Wenstrup RJ. Ehlers Danlos syndromes: revised nosology, Villefranche, 1997, for the Ehlers-Danlos National Foundation (USA) and Ehlers-Danlos Support Group (UK). *Am J Med Genet.* 1998;77:31-37.

Dietz HC. Marfan syndrome. GeneReviews. 2001 Apr 18 (updated 2014 Jun 12). Available at: www.ncbi.nlm.nih.gov/books/NBK1335/. Accessed January 17, 2017.

EDS Special ISSUE. *Am J Med Genet Part C.* 2015;169C:1-129.

Lacro RV, Dietz HC, Sleeper LA, et al. Atenolol versus losartan in children and young adults with Marfan's syndrome. *N Engl J Med.* 2014;371(22):2061-2071.

Loeys BL, Dietz HC. Loeys-Dietz syndrome. GeneReviews. 2008 Feb 28 (updated 2013 Jul 11). Available at: www.ncbi.nlm.nih.gov/books/NBK1133/. Accessed January 17, 2017.

Loeys BL, Dietz HC, Braverman AC, et al. The revised Ghent nosology for the Marfan syndrome. *J Med Genet.* 2010;47:476-485.

Mantle D, Wilkins RM, Preedy V. A novel therapeutic strategy for Ehlers-Danlos syndrome based on nutritional supplements. *Med Hypotheses.* 2005;64:279-283.

Naing BT, Watanabe A, Tanigaki S, Ono M, Iwashita M, Shimada T. Presymptomatic genetic analysis during pregnancy for vascular type Ehlers-Danlos syndrome. *Int Med Case Rep J.* 2014;7:99-102.

Robin NH, Moran RT, Ala-Kokko L. Stickler syndrome. GeneReviews 2000 Jun 9 (updated 2016 Jan 7). Available at: www.ncbi.nlm.nih.gov/books/NBK1302/. Accessed January 17, 2017.

Rose PS, Levy H, Liberfarb R, Davis J, Francomano C. Stickler syndrome: clinical characteristics and diagnostic criteria. *Am J Med Genet.* 2005;138A:199-207.

Tinkle BT, Saal H. Health supervision for children with Marfan syndrome. *Pediatrics.* 2013;132:e1059-e1072.




# 181 Genetics of Congenital Heart Disease

Seema R. Lalani and Stephanie Ware



## INTRODUCTION

Congenital heart disease (CHD) is one of the most prevalent causes of mortality among US born infants and a significant source of global economic burden, affecting almost 1% of all live-born infants. The estimate of CHD in aborted fetuses is even higher, reaching up to 10%. The underlying causes of CHD are varied and can include cytogenetic abnormalities, single-gene disorders, epigenetic alterations, environmental etiologies, or most commonly, multifactorial etiologies. Large-scale epidemiologic studies suggest that a genetic or environmental cause for CHD is identifiable in approximately 20% to 30% of cases. Infants with CHD are considered to have syndromic conditions based on the findings of multiple congenital anomalies or neurodevelopmental delays. The distinction between syndromic and nonsyndromic, or isolated, CHD can be subtle, leading to lack of recognition of syndromic cases. In addition, as genetic diagnostic modalities have become more sophisticated, the spectrum of genetic syndromic conditions has expanded, and therefore, previous assessments of syndromic cases may represent an underestimate.

High heritability provides evidence for an important genetic role in isolated CHD. Specific types of CHD show strong familial clustering in first-degree relatives, ranging from 3-fold to 80-fold compared to the prevalence in the population. Not all families show evidence of similar types of CHD, and familial clustering of discordant CHD has also been documented. Because CHD is so common, the majority of cases occur in individuals without a family history of cardiovascular malformations despite a high heritability. The prevalence of familial CHD will likely increase as more patients with CHD survive into adulthood. Securing a genetic diagnosis is important, as a definitive diagnosis not only alerts the clinician to the likelihood of noncardiac concerns that require intervention, but could also alter management considerations of CHD if a syndrome with significantly reduced life expectancy is uncovered, as observed for trisomy 18 and 13.

## PATHOGENESIS

Cardiac development is a complex, multistep process of morphogenesis that is under genetic regulation. Multiple developmental pathways act independently or in combination to affect proper cardiac lineage specification, differentiation, and subsequent patterning and organogenesis. Because of this complexity, there are multiple potential mechanisms by which genetic variations can impact both fetal cardiac development and latent cardiac disease. Systems biology approaches illustrate the functional convergence of causative CHD gene pathways and support the hypothesis that some CHD phenotypes may result from additive effects of multiple low-effect susceptibility alleles. The resulting web of developmental interactions is a highly complex milieu in which individual or multiple risk factors can act to disrupt normal heart morphogenesis. Clinical genetic testing is increasingly available for a number of genes important during cardiac development. Both monogenic and chromosomal abnormalities account for a substantial proportion of CHD, particularly when coupled with extracardiac defects.

## CHD AND CHROMOSOMAL DISORDERS

In large studies, the frequency of chromosomal abnormality in infants with CHD is estimated to be about 12%, including aneuploidies (trisomy 21, 18, or 13; monosomy X) and 22q11.2 deletion (DiGeorge/velocardiofacial syndrome). Within this group, trisomy 21 (Down syndrome) is the most common disorder, accounting for about half of all cases. Turner syndrome and other sex chromosome abnormalities are observed in about 3% of all cytogenetic aberrations uncovered in CHD. Defects in single genes are estimated to account for 3% to

5% of all cases. This is certainly an underestimate, highlighted by the pervasive use of rapidly advancing molecular diagnostic technologies in CHD.

### Down Syndrome

Down syndrome (DS; OMIM no. 190685) is the most common cause of intellectual disability and syndromic CHD, diagnosed in about 1 in 700 live births. The syndrome is easily recognized in the presence of characteristic facial features such as upslanting palpebral fissures, bilateral epicanthal folds, flat nasal bridge, small ears, and hypotonia. The prevalence of CHD in DS is approximately 50%, of which atrioventricular septal defect (AVSD) is the most common defect, observed in 30% to 40% of infants (Table 181-1). Ventricular septal defect (VSD), atrial septal defect (ASD), tetralogy of Fallot (TOF), and pulmonary valve stenosis (PS) are also seen. Coarctation of the aorta (CoA), vascular ring, and defects of single-ventricle physiology are observed less frequently. Children with DS are at greater risk of pulmonary arterial hypertension than the general population. The comorbid occurrence of upper airway obstruction contributes to the development of increased pulmonary vascular resistance in DS, leading to potentially irreversible pulmonary vascular disease. Echocardiogram in the newborn period is strongly recommended with a definitive or a suspected diagnosis, accompanied by cardiology consultation as needed. Extracardiac abnormalities include duodenal atresia, Hirschsprung disease, hypothyroidism, and risk of leukemia, which require comprehensive assessment.

### Trisomy 18

Trisomy 18, also known as Edwards syndrome, is a serious genetic disorder and is associated with CHD in about 80% to 100% of infants. The mortality is high, with about 50% of infants succumbing to the disease in the first month of life and only 5% to 10% surviving beyond the first year of life. The cause of death includes central apnea, hypoventilation, and cardiac causes. Infants are typically born with intrauterine growth retardation, clenched hands, short sternum, rocker bottom feet, and major congenital abnormalities. Polyvalvular disease is common. VSD, ASD, and patent ductus arteriosus (PDA) are also frequently reported. Endocardial cushion defects, left-sided lesions, and double outlet right ventricle (DORV) are present in about one-tenth of the affected infants.

### Trisomy 13

Trisomy 13, or Patau syndrome, is another genetic condition associated with poor survival. The median life expectancy of infants with trisomy 13 is 7 to 10 days, and over 90% of infants die in the first year of life. Clinical features of cleft lip/palate, ophthalmologic abnormalities, scalp defect, and postaxial polydactyly, in the presence of significant cardiac and brain abnormalities (eg, holoprosencephaly, absence of corpus callosum), should prompt evaluation for this aneuploidy. Typically, rapid testing by fluorescence in situ hybridization (FISH) is employed along with confirmatory karyotype study. The frequency of CHD ranges from 56% to 86%. Septal defects are the most common abnormalities. DORV, TOF, and CoA are also reported.

### Turner Syndrome

Turner syndrome (TS) is the most commonly encountered sex chromosome abnormality in females, characterized by short stature, gonadal dysgenesis, and increased risk of cardiovascular abnormalities. CHDs are present in about a third of the affected females, contributing to the high morbidity and mortality of the syndrome. Bicuspid aortic valve (BAV) is reported in approximately 30% of individuals with TS, in comparison to the 1.3% prevalence observed in healthy adults. CoA is diagnosed in up to 12% to 17% of females, and hypoplastic left heart syndrome (HLHS) is seen in about 2% of the children. The management of infants with TS and HLHS remains challenging and generally is associated with poor survival. As adults, progressive dilation of the ascending aorta is observed in 20% to 25% of patients, with the risk of dissection reported to be 6 times more common compared with healthy females. The aortopathy in TS is considered to be due to an intrinsic aortic wall abnormality and is highest for the affected females with BAV. The growing evidence of aortic disease in TS and the high risk of acquired heart disease requires close cardiac follow-up well into adulthood even in the absence of significant CHD.

### Wolf-Hirschhorn Syndrome

Wolf-Hirschhorn syndrome (WHS; OMIM no. 194190) is caused by terminal deletion of part of the short arm of chromosome 4.

**TABLE 181-1 SOME EXAMPLES OF CYTOGENETICALLY VISIBLE CHROMOSOMAL DISORDERS ASSOCIATED WITH CHD**

| Syndrome | Clinical Features | CHD | Frequency of CHD (%) |
|---|---|---|---|
| Trisomy 21 (Down syndrome) | Upslanting palpebral fissures, epicanthal folds, small ears, hypotonia, duodenal atresia, Hirschsprung disease, hypothyroidism, risk of leukemia, intellectual disability | AVSD, VSD, ASD, TOF | ~50 |
| Trisomy 18 (Edwards syndrome) | Short palpebral fissures, micrognathia, intrauterine growth retardation, overriding fingers, horseshoe kidney | Polyvalvular disease, VSD, ASD, PDA, left-sided lesions, DORV, endocardial cushion defects | 80–100 |
| Trisomy 13 (Patau syndrome) | Cleft lip/palate, microphthalmia, cutis aplasia, postaxial polydactyly, holoprosencephaly | ASD, VSD, PDA, DORV, TOF, CoA | 80 |
| 45,X (Turner syndrome) | Cystic hygroma, webbed neck, short stature, gonadal dysgenesis, renal anomalies | BAV, CoA, HLHS | ~30 |
| 4p16.3 deletion (Wolf-Hirschhorn syndrome) | Hypertelorism arched eyebrows, short philtrum, seizures, microcephaly, feeding difficulties, structural brain anomalies, intellectual disability | ASD, VSD, PS, TOF, PDA | ~50 |
| 5p minus (Cri-du-chat syndrome) | High-pitched cat-like cry, microcephaly, round facies, hypertelorism, downslanting palpebral fissures, preauricular tags, intellectual disability | PDA, VSD, ASD, TOF, pulmonary atresia | 30 |
| 11q deletion (Jacobsen syndrome) | Hypertelorism, ptosis, coloboma, downslanting palpebral fissures, V-shaped mouth, small ears, abnormal platelet function, thrombocytopenia, malrotation of the gut, pyloric stenosis, anal atresia/stenosis, growth retardation, intellectual disability | VSD, BAV, AS, HLHS, MS, CoA, Shone complex | ~50 |
| 22 inverted duplication (Cat eye syndrome) | Iris coloboma, preauricular tags or pits, imperforate anus, malrotation of the gut, biliary atresia, renal malformations | TAPVR, TOF | 50–67 |

AS, aortic valve stenosis; ASD, atrial septal defect; AVSD, atrioventricular septal defect; CHD, congenital heart disease; CoA, coarctation of the aorta; BAV, bicuspid aortic valve; DORV, double outlet right ventricle; HLHS, hypoplastic left heart syndrome; MS, mitral stenosis; PDA, patent ductus arteriosus; PS, pulmonic stenosis; TAPVR, total anomalous pulmonary venous return; TOF, tetralogy of Fallot; VSD, ventricular septal defect.

Approximately half of the affected individuals have CHDs observed as ASD, PS, VSD, and PDA. Individuals with WHS have characteristic "Greek warrior helmet" craniofacial dysmorphism, including prominent glabella, ocular hypertelorism, highly arched eyebrows, microcephaly, short philtrum, downturned corners of the mouth, feeding difficulties, seizures, urinary tract malformations, and structural brain anomalies (corpus callosum hypoplasia, enlargement of the lateral ventricles, brain atrophy). Feeding difficulties, seizures, and developmental disabilities are significant concerns.

#### Cri-du-Chat Syndrome

Cri-du-chat syndrome, also known as 5p minus syndrome (OMIM no. 123450), is characterized by a high-pitched, cat-like cry, growth retardation, and distinct craniofacial features including microcephaly, round facies, hypertelorism, epicanthal folds, downslanting palpebral fissures, preauricular tags, and downturned corners of the mouth. About 30% of the affected infants have CHDs including ASD, VSD, and PDA. Right ventricular outflow tract obstructive anomalies including TOF and pulmonary atresia have also been reported. The deletion of the short arm of chromosome 5 occurs as a de novo event in the majority of cases; however, about 10% to 15% of cases result from an unbalanced chromosomal translocation. It is recommended that parental studies be completed for the majority of families to address the risk of recurrence in future pregnancy.

#### Cat Eye Syndrome

Cat eye syndrome (CES; OMIM no. 115470) is a rare chromosomal disorder associated with CHD in over two-thirds of diagnosed patients. The majority of the affected individuals carry an extra small marker chromosome derived from the proximal part of chromosome 22 (with 4 copies instead of 2 of proximal 22q11), often present in the mosaic form. CHD, particularly total anomalous pulmonary venous return (TAPVR) and TOF, is a characteristic defect. Abnormalities such as PS, tricuspid atresia, HLHS, and single ventricle are reported in rare instances. The craniofacial phenotype in infants with CES can be subtle, with no significant dysmorphism except for preauricular pits and/or tags, downslanting palpebral fissures, and/or iris coloboma. Concomitant diagnosis of anal atresia with fistula, biliary atresia, malrotation of the gut, and/or renal malformations should alert the physician to this diagnosis. The variability in clinical features in CES is enormous, ranging from minimally affected individuals with normal cognition to those with full pattern of malformations. Both G-banded karyotype study and chromosomal microarray analysis (CMA) would be the tests to consider to establish this diagnosis. It is important to note that pertinent features of CES such as coloboma and TAPVR have also been reported in interstitial duplications of the 22q11.2 region (ie, 3 copies instead of 4).

#### Jacobsen Syndrome

Jacobsen syndrome (OMIM no. 147791), caused by partial deletion of the long arm of chromosome 11, is associated with CHD in about 56% of cases. HLHS occurs in about 5% to 10% of all patients. Other lesions include VSD, abnormalities of aortic or mitral valves, CoA, and Shone complex. Extracardiac abnormalities include craniofacial dysmorphism and thrombocytopenia or pancytopenia that are usually present at birth.

## CHD AND MICRODELETION/MICRODUPLICATION SYNDROMES

Disorders resulting from microdeletion or microduplication of the genome are an important cause of CHD, accounting for 10% to 20% of CHD, mostly in individuals presenting with extracardiac defects. These submicroscopic events, also termed *copy number variations* (CNVs), have been catalogued extensively with the ubiquitous use of CMA. Several genomic disorders are now recognized that are associated with CHD (Table 181-2).

#### 22q11.2 Deletion Syndrome (DiGeorge/Velocardiofacial Syndrome)

The most common genomic disorder linked to CHD is the DiGeorge (DGS)/velocardiofacial syndrome (VCFS) due to 22q11.2 deletion, with a prevalence of 1 in 4000 live births. CHD is reported in almost 75% of the affected individuals, typically observed as conotruncal and aortic arch defects. The conotruncal defects include TOF, truncus arteriosus, interrupted aortic arch type B, and DORV. An aberrant subclavian artery may present with feeding difficulties or respiratory symptoms. About 15% of all TOF cases are attributed to this syndrome. Extracardiac problems include characteristic features (small palpebral fissures, small dysplastic ears, bulbous nose, long digits), velopharyngeal insufficiency with or without cleft palate, hypocalcemia due to hypoparathyroidism, immunodeficiency secondary to thymic hypoplasia, renal problems, and learning disabilities. The diagnosis is confirmed either by FISH for 22q11.2 deletion or CMA.

#### Williams-Beuren Syndrome

Williams-Beuren syndrome (OMIM no. 194050) resulting from recurrent deletion of 7q11.23 is frequently characterized by cardiac defects. The characteristic facial features include periorbital fullness, a stellate pattern of the irides, flattened nasal bridge, full cheeks, an upturned nose, long philtrum, wide mouth, and full lips. Hypercalcemia is reported in about half of all patients. The classic cardiac lesion observed in WBS is supravalvular aortic stenosis (SVAS), seen in approximately 75% of children. Peripheral pulmonary artery stenosis is also encountered at a higher frequency (~60%). Arteriopathy leading to stenoses of medium and large arteries is due to loss of the elastin gene (*ELN*) within the common deleted interval.

#### 1p36 Deletion Syndrome

Terminal deletions of chromosome 1p36 (OMIM no. 607872) are associated with cardiac abnormalities in up to 70% of cases. The CHDs include PDA, valvular abnormalities, CoA, and TOF. Cardiomyopathy, largely observed as left ventricular noncompaction cardiomyopathy, is observed in about 23% to 27% of patients. Other features include deep-set eyes, straight eyebrows, late-closing anterior fontanel, microcephaly, hearing loss, seizures, brain abnormalities, and intellectual disability.

#### Smith-Magenis Syndrome and Potocki-Lupski Syndrome

Smith-Magenis syndrome (SMS; OMIM no. 182290) caused by interstitial deletion of 17p11.2 is a well-recognized genomic disorder characterized by significant behavior disorder, sleep disturbance, craniofacial dysmorphism, and short stature. About one-third of individuals with SMS have CHD, observed as septal defects, and TOF. Pulmonary atresia, PS, and TAPVR have also been described. Cardiovascular abnormalities occur in about 40% of individuals with Potocki-Lupski syndrome (PTLS), resulting from reciprocal duplication of the SMS region. Aortopathy with dilated aortic root, septal defects, patent foramen ovale, conduction abnormalities, BAV, and HLHS have been described. The extracardiac problems in PTLS include hypotonia, failure to thrive, developmental delay, intellectual disability, and sleep-disordered breathing.

#### 8p23.1 Deletion

Recurrent deletions of 8p23.1 encompassing *GATA4* are frequently associated with CHD. Congenital diaphragmatic hernia has been reported in some individuals with 8p23.1 deletion. Cardiac malformations associated with *GATA4* deletion include AVSD, ASD, PS, and TOF.

#### Kleefstra Syndrome

Kleefstra syndrome (OMIM no. 610253) is associated with CHD in about 40% of patients. The disorder is caused either by a submicroscopic deletion in the terminal region of chromosomal region 9q34.3 or a point mutation of *EHMT1*. The disorder is recognized by distinctive facial features including brachycephaly, synophrys, cupid bowed upper lip, prominent jaw, epilepsy, hypotonia, and intellectual disability. The cardiac anomalies include septal defects, PS, BAV, and PDA. Cardiac arrhythmias, including atrial flutter, have also been described.

## CHD AND SINGLE-GENE DISORDERS

With the development of next-generation sequencing approaches that have significantly increased the throughput and decreased the cost of genetic analysis, large gene sequencing panels have become

**TABLE 181-2 SOME EXAMPLES OF MICRODELETION AND MICRODUPLICATION SYNDROMES ASSOCIATED WITH CHD**

| Syndrome | Clinical Features | CHD | Frequency of CHD (%) |
|---|---|---|---|
| 1p36 deletion | Deep-set eyes, straight eyebrows, malar hypoplasia, microbrachycephaly, hearing loss, seizures, brain abnormalities, intellectual disability | Septal defects, PDA, CoA, TOF, LV noncompaction | 70 |
| 1q21.1 deletion | Microcephaly, developmental delay | CoA, IAA-A, IAA-B, BAV, aortopathy, VSD, TA, TGA, CoA, PDA | 10–25 |
| 1q21.1 duplication | Macrocephaly, developmental delay | TOF | 20 |
| 7q11.23 deletion (Williams-Beuren syndrome) | Broad forehead, periorbital fullness, stellate pattern of iris, short nose, long philtrum, full cheeks, failure to thrive in infancy, hypercalcemia, social personality, intellectual disability | SVAS, PPS | 75 |
| 8p23.1 deletion | Congenital diaphragmatic hernia | AVSD, ASD, TOF | 75–94 |
| 9q34.3 deletion (Kleefstra syndrome) | Hypertelorism, midface hypoplasia, prominent eyebrows, tented upper lip and everted lower lip, hypotonia, seizures, intellectual disability | Septal defects, PS, BAV, PDA | 40 |
| 15q26-qter deletion | Growth retardation, intellectual disability, congenital diaphragmatic hernia | VSD, ASD, CoA, HLHS, AS | ~66 |
| 17p13.3 deletion (Miller-Dieker syndrome) | Lissencephaly, corpus callosum dysgenesis/agenesis, high and prominent forehead, bitemporal hollowing, short nose with upturned nares, seizures, intellectual disability | Septal defects, TOF, PDA | 20 |
| 17p11.2 deletion (Smith-Magenis syndrome) | Brachycephaly, broad forehead, short upturned nose, tent-shaped upper lip, sleep disturbance, self-injurious behavior, intellectual disability | Septal defects, TOF, PS, PA | ~30 |
| 17p11.2 duplication (Potocki-Lupski syndrome) | Infantile hypotonia, failure to thrive, intellectual disability, autism spectrum disorder | Dilated aortic root, septal defects, conduction abnormalities, BAV, HLHS | 40 |
| 17q21.31 deletion | Upslanting palpebral fissures, large prominent ears, bulbous nose, pleasant disposition, epilepsy, urogenital abnormalities, intellectual disability | Septal defects, PS, BAV | ~40 |
| 22q11.2 deletion (DiGeorge syndrome) | Small palpebral fissures, hooded upper lids, small dysplastic ears, bulbous nasal tip, cleft palate, velopharyngeal incompetence, hypocalcemia, immunodeficiency, renal anomalies, learning difficulties | TOF, IAA-B, TrA, aortic arch anomalies | ~75 |

AS, aortic valve stenosis; ASD, atrial septal defect; AVSD, atrioventricular septal defect; BAV, bicuspid aortic valve; CHD, congenital heart disease; CoA, coarctation of the aorta; HLHS, hypoplastic left heart syndrome; IAA-A/IAA-B, interrupted aortic arch type A/B; LV, left ventricular; PA, pulmonary atresia; PDA, patent ductus arteriosus; PPS, peripheral pulmonary stenosis; PS, pulmonic stenosis; SVAS, supravalvular aortic stenosis; TA, tricuspid atresia; TGA, transposition of the great arteries; TOF, tetralogy of Fallot; TrA, truncus arteriosus VSD, ventricular septal defect.



increasingly available, as have smaller gene panels for single-gene disorders that cause genetic syndromes.

### Noonan Syndrome and RASopathies

The RAS/mitogen-activated protein kinase (MAPK) pathway is important for control of cell proliferation and differentiation. Dysregulation of this pathway results in a spectrum of disorders known as *RASopathies*, including Noonan syndrome (OMIM no. 163950 NS1), Costello syndrome, cardiofaciocutaneous syndrome, Legius syndrome, and neurofibromatosis type 1 (NF1; Table 181-3). The former syndromes are associated with a high rate of cardiac involvement, whereas cardiac abnormalities are infrequent in Legius syndrome and NF1. Noonan syndrome is a well-recognized genetic syndrome with a prevalence of approximately 1 in 2500 live births. It is inherited in an autosomal dominant pattern, although new cases are common because the *de novo* mutation rate is high. The classic manifestations of Noonan syndrome include short stature, pulmonic stenosis and/or hypertrophic cardiomyopathy, dysmorphic features including hypertelorism, downslanting palpebral fissures, low-set posteriorly rotated ears, and webbing of the neck. Pectus excavatum or mixed pectus carinatum superiorly with pectus excavatum inferiorly is common. A variety of lymphatic abnormalities have been associated with Noonan syndrome. Genitourinary abnormalities are also common, especially cryptorchidism in males. Developmental delay of variable severity occurs in approximately 25% of patients. Patients may also have a coagulopathy, and this is important to evaluate and manage appropriately prior to any surgical or invasive procedure. Finally, there is a 3-fold increased risk of malignancy in Noonan syndrome. The frequency of cardiac disease is estimated at 50% to 80% in patients with Noonan syndrome. Pulmonary valve stenosis, often with dysplasia, is the most common cardiovascular malformation, occurring in 25% to 50% of patients. Patients with Noonan syndrome need lifetime cardiac follow-up because left-sided obstructive lesions may develop in adulthood, and hypertrophic cardiomyopathy can develop at any age.

Currently, clinical testing is available for 15 genes causing Noonan syndrome and related disorders with a diagnostic yield between 70% and 85%.

### Marfan Syndrome and Related Disorders

Marfan syndrome (OMIM no. 154700) is an autosomal dominant connective tissue disorder with a high degree of clinical variability and a prevalence of 1 in 5000 to 10,000. The cardinal features of Marfan syndrome involve the ocular, skeletal, and cardiovascular systems. Up to 90% of individuals with a clinical diagnosis of Marfan syndrome have mutations in *FBN1*, a gene that codes for fibrillin-1, a structural component of microfibrils that provides mechanical stability and elastic properties to connective tissues. The primary pathology is related to alterations in transforming growth factor-β (TGFβ) signaling due to failure of sequestration of TGFβ in the extracellular matrix triggered by loss of fibrillin-1. The increase in active TGFβ signaling has been shown to cause aortic root dilation, lung bullae, and impaired muscle regeneration. Mutations in additional genes involved in TGFβ signaling are increasingly identified in individuals with thoracic aortic aneurysms (TAA) and Marfan-like features. For example, mutations in *TGFBR1* and *TGFBR2* cause the related connective tissue disorder Loeys-Dietz syndrome. Cardiovascular manifestations in Marfan syndrome include dilatation of the aorta at the level of the sinuses of Valsalva, a propensity for aortic tear and rupture, mitral valve

**TABLE 181-3 SINGLE GENES ASSOCIATED WITH CHD**

| Gene | Associated Syndrome | Features |
|---|---|---|
| *CHD7* | CHARGE | Coloboma, choanal atresia, growth retardation, genital and ear anomalies, cleft lip/palate, cranial nerve anomalies; conotruncal defects, ASD, VSD |
| *CITED2* | Isolated CHD | ASD, VSD |
| *CREBBP, EP300* | Rubinstein-Taybi syndrome | Short stature, broad thumbs and great toes, downslanting palpebral fissures, hypoplastic maxilla, GU and renal anomalies, intellectual disability; PDA, VSD, ASD, CoA, PS, BAV |
| *CRELD1* | Isolated CHD | AVSD |
| *DCHS1* | Isolated CHD | MVP |
| *ELN* | Isolated CHD | SVAS |
| *EVC1, EVC2* | Ellis-van Creveld syndrome; Weyers acrofacial dystosis | Short limbs, short ribs, postaxial polydactyly, hypoplastic nails, dental anomalies; ASD, AVSD |
| *FBN1* | Marfan syndrome | Lens dislocation, systemic features including skeletal (pes planus, hindfoot deformity, scoliosis, pectus deformity, etc.), skin, facial, spontaneous pneumothorax; dilated aorta, BAV, MVP, MPA dilation |
| *GATA4* | Isolated CHD | ASD, VSD, AVSD, TOF |
| *GATA5* | Isolated CHD | AVSD |
| *GATA6* | Isolated CHD | ASD, AVSD, PTA, TOF |
| *JAG1, NOTCH2* | Alagille syndrome | Bile duct paucity, cholestasis, broad forehead, pointed chin; posterior embryotoxon, and skeletal anomalies; PBS, PPS, TOF, pulmonary artery hypoplasia, other arterial anomalies |
| *KMT2D, KDM6A* | Kabuki syndrome | Elongated palpebral fissures with eversion of the lateral third of the lower eyelid, ptosis, arched and broad eyebrows, large, prominent, or cupped ears, persistence of fetal fingertip pads, mild to moderate intellectual disability, postnatal growth deficiency, microcephaly; ASD, VSD, LVOTO |
| *MED12-* | FG syndrome type 1; Lujan-Fryns syndrome | Typical facial features (differ by syndrome); intellectual disability, hypotonia, abnormalities of corpus callosum; ASD, VSD, AVSD, HLHS, MVP, dilated aorta |
| *MED13L* | Isolated CHD | TGA |
| *MID1* | Opitz G/BBB | Hypertelorism/telecanthus, hypospadias, laryngeal cleft, cleft lip/palate, imperforate anus, midline CNS defects, intellectual disability; VSD, PDA, LSVC |
| *MYH6* | Isolated CHD | ASD, VSD |
| *NIPBL, SMC1L1* | Cornelia de Lange syndrome | Pre-/postnatal growth retardation, low anterior hair line, synophrys, long philtrum, upper limb defects, intellectual disability; ASD, VSD, PS |
| *NKX2-5* | Isolated CHD | ASD with conduction abnormalities; VSD; TOF |
| *NKX2-6* | Isolated CHD | Conotruncal defects, PTA |
| *NOTCH1* | Isolated CHD | AS, BAV |
| *PTPN11, SOS1, RAF1, KRAS, HRAS, BRAF, MAP2K1 (MEK1), MAP2K2 (MEK2), SHOC2, NRAS, CBL, RIT1, SPRED1, ACTB, ACTG1* | Noonan, Noonan-like, cardiofaciocutaneous, Costello syndrome | Short stature, hypertelorism, epicanthal folds, webbed neck, pectus deformity, cryptorchidism, bleeding diathesis, intellectual disability; PS, HCM, PPS, ASD, VSD, PDA, AS, TOF, CoA |
| *SALL1* | Townes-Brocks syndrome | Imperforate anus, dysplastic ears, hearing impairment, thumb malformations, renal and GU anomalies; ASD, VSD, TOF, truncus arteriosus, PDA |
| *TBX1* | Isolated CHD | Conotruncal defects |
| *TBX5* | Holt-Oram syndrome | Radial ray anomalies; ASD, VSD, AVSD |
| *TBX20* | Isolated CHD | Septal defects |
| *TFAP2B* | Char syndrome | Low-set ears, ptosis, fifth finger clinodactyly, supernumerary nipples; PDA |
| *TGFBR1, TGFBR2* | Loeys-Dietz syndrome; isolated CHD | Hypertelorism, bifid uvula, vessel tortuosity, dilated aorta |
| *ZEB2* | Mowat-Wilson syndrome | Short stature, microcephaly, hypotonia, agenesis of the corpus callosum, sparse hair, Hirschsprung disease, GU anomalies, moderate/severe mental intellectual disability; PDA, ASD, VSD, TOF, PA, CoA, AS, BAV |
| *ZFPM2* | Isolated CHD | TOF |
| *ZIC3* | Heterotaxy syndrome; VACTERL | Right or left isomerism, biliary atresia, intestinal malrotation, spleen and renal anomalies, cleft lip/palate, midline CNS defects; dextrocardia, D- or L-transposition, PS, PA, DORV, AVSD, TAPVR, LSVC, interrupted IVC |

AS, aortic valve stenosis; ASD, atrial septal defect; AVSD, atrioventricular septal defect; BAV, bicuspid aortic valve; CHD, congenital heart disease; CNS, central nervous system; CoA, coarctation of the aorta; DORV, double outlet right ventricle; GU, genitourinary; HCM, hypertrophic cardiomyopathy; HLHS, hypoplastic left heart syndrome; IVC, inferior vena cava; LSVC, left superior vena cava; LVOTO, left ventricular outflow tract obstruction; MPA, main pulmonary artery; MVP, mitral valve prolapse; PA, pulmonary atresia; PDA, patent ductus arteriosus; PPS, peripheral pulmonary stenosis; PS, pulmonic stenosis; PTA, persistent truncus arteriosus; SVAS, supravalvular aortic stenosis; TAPVR, total anomalous pulmonary venous return; TGA, transposition of the great arteries; TOF, tetralogy of Fallot; VSD, ventricular septal defect; PBS, pulmonary branch stenosis.

prolapse with or without regurgitation, tricuspid valve prolapse, and enlargement of the proximal pulmonary artery. Marfan syndrome accounts for approximately 5% of all TAAs. Recent guidelines for surgical management of TAA stratify risk based on the specific gene causing the disease, indicating the importance of precisely identifying the genetic cause.

### Alagille Syndrome

Alagille syndrome (OMIM no. 118450) is a multisystem disorder with heart, skeletal, liver, eye, and facial features. It is classically characterized by paucity of bile ducts on liver biopsy, cholestasis, and/or conjugated hyperbilirubinemia. Other findings include skeletal abnormalities such as butterfly vertebrae, eye anomalies such as posterior embryotoxon, and right-sided heart defects, the latter of which occur in 75%. Peripheral and branch pulmonic stenoses are the most common findings. TOF is seen in approximately 15% of patients. Mutations in *JAG1* account for the majority of cases, occurring in approximately 89% of patients who fulfill clinical criteria. Microdeletions containing *JAG1* on chromosome 20p12 account for up to 7% of cases. *JAG1* encodes a ligand in the Notch signaling pathway. A second gene, *NOTCH2*, has been shown to cause less than 1% of cases. The clinical features are highly variable, even within families. Sequence variants in *JAG1* have also been identified in a small number of apparently isolated cases of TOF or PS.

#### CHARGE Syndrome

CHARGE (OMIM no. 214800) is an acronym for ocular coloboma, congenital heart defects, choanal atresia, retardation of growth and development, genital hypoplasia, and ear anomalies associated with deafness. Cardiovascular malformations are found in 75% to 85% of patients. The most characteristic defects include conotruncal anomalies. Atrioventricular canal defects, vascular ring, and aberrant subclavian artery are also described frequently. The phenotype is highly variable, and the spectrum of anomalies has been further expanded since the identification of *CHD7* as the causative gene in 2004. CHD7 is a chromatin remodeling ATPase that is important for epigenetic regulation of gene expression. Clinical testing for *CHD7* identifies mutations in the majority of patients with typical features of CHARGE syndrome. The remaining patients are diagnosed based on clinical findings and temporal bone imaging indicative of inner ear abnormalities.

#### Holt-Oram Syndrome

Holt-Oram syndrome (OMIM no. 142900) is a highly penetrant but variably expressed autosomal dominant disorder characterized by upper limb deformities (preaxial radial ray malformations) often accompanied by CHD. The incidence is approximately 1 in 100,000 live births with a high *de novo* mutation rate. CHD is present in 75% of patients, typically secundum ASD, muscular VSD, and/or progressive atrioventricular conduction delay. Holt-Oram syndrome is caused by mutations in the T-box transcription factor gene *TBX5*, which is expressed in the developing heart and upper limb. Approximately 75% of individuals meeting criteria for Holt-Oram syndrome have *TBX5* coding region changes, mostly nonsense or frameshift mutations predicted to result in haploinsufficiency.

### NONSYNDROMIC CHD

The majority of nonsyndromic cases of CHD are thought to result from multifactorial causes and behave as a complex trait. Like other conditions inherited as a complex trait, isolated CHD may show familial clustering with reduced penetrance. Nevertheless, Mendelian inheritance does occur, albeit less frequently, and *de novo* mutations are another important cause. Drawing a distinct boundary between syndromic and nonsyndromic causes may be an overly simplistic model given that variants in genes known to cause syndromic CHD are now identified in nonsyndromic cases.

Understanding the genetic basis of syndromic CHD can identify important genes for nonsyndromic CHD. For example, mutations in the elastin gene (*ELN*) that is deleted in Williams-Beuren syndrome are known to cause nonsyndromic familial SVAS without other features of Williams-Beuren. Recent studies have documented the utility of next-generation sequencing panels for diagnostic evaluation of CHD in nonsyndromic multiplex families. Yields range from 30% to 50% in these multiplex families, but a yield is not yet known for nonfamilial cases. Not surprisingly, genes known to be critical for cardiac development such as *NOTCH1*, *TBX5*, and *MYH6* were identified as causative (Table 181-3). The finding of a *TBX5* mutation in a family not suspected to have Holt-Oram syndrome highlights the need for careful phenotyping and ongoing data collection to determine the degree of phenotypic variability or phenotypic nonpenetrance.

CNVs are another important genetic contributor to isolated CHD. Pathogenic CNVs are reported to occur in 3% to 10% of patients with isolated heart defects. For example, a CNV at chromosome 1q21.1 has been found in 1% of nonsyndromic sporadic TOF cases.

### RECURRENCE RISK

Advances in surgical intervention and medical care have increased survival and led to an increase in CHD prevalence among patients of reproductive age such that there has been a nearly 60% increase in CHD prevalence among adult patients since the year 2000. This has clear implications for heritability. In general, recurrence estimates are more precise for syndromic than for isolated CHDs, as inheritance patterns for many CHD-associated genetic conditions are already well characterized. For dominantly inherited conditions, such as Noonan or Holt-Oram syndromes, individual recurrence risk is 50%, but not all patients with a particular syndrome will present with associated heart defects and the proportion that do can vary considerably depending on the specific diagnosis. The presence or severity of CHD in a parent is not predictive of the risk for offspring. The prevalence of CHDs in a population caused by a particular syndrome ultimately depends on the likelihood of affected individuals reaching reproductive age and the new mutation rate.

Recurrence risks for isolated CHD can be difficult to assign. The sibling or offspring recurrence risk across all types of CHDs is estimated at 1% to 4%. These estimates represent an average of different risks across the population and include individuals with higher recurrence risks due to Mendelian inheritance as well as individuals with lower risks due to a *de novo* event in the affected individual or a teratogenic etiology. Recurrence risks for specific types of CHD, such as left ventricular outflow tract obstructive defects, are higher (Table 181-4). Females with CHD have a higher recurrence risk for their offspring than males.

**TABLE 181-4 RECURRENCE RISKS FOR ISOLATED (NONSYNDROMIC) CONGENITAL HEART DISEASES (%)**

<table>
<tr><th>Defect</th><th>Father Affected</th><th>Mother Affected</th><th>1 Sibling Affected</th><th>2 Siblings Affected</th></tr>
<tr><td>ASD</td><td>1.5–3.5</td><td>4–6</td><td>2.5–3</td><td>8</td></tr>
<tr><td>AVSD</td><td>1–4.5</td><td>11.5–14</td><td>3–4</td><td>10</td></tr>
<tr><td>VSD</td><td>2–3.5</td><td>6–10</td><td>3</td><td>10</td></tr>
<tr><td>AS</td><td>3–4</td><td>8–18</td><td>2</td><td>6</td></tr>
<tr><td>PS</td><td>2–3.5</td><td>4–6.5</td><td>2</td><td>6</td></tr>
<tr><td>TOF</td><td>1.5</td><td>2–2.5</td><td>2.5–3</td><td>8</td></tr>
<tr><td>CoA</td><td>2–3</td><td>4–6.5</td><td>2</td><td>6</td></tr>
<tr><td>PDA</td><td>2–2.5</td><td>3.5–4</td><td>3</td><td>10</td></tr>
<tr><td>HLHS</td><td colspan="2">21</td><td>2</td><td>6</td></tr>
<tr><td>TGA</td><td colspan="2">2</td><td>1.5</td><td>5</td></tr>
<tr><td>L-TGA</td><td colspan="2">3–5</td><td>5–6</td><td>NR</td></tr>
</table>

Note. Merged cells indicate recurrence when one parent is affected, irrespective of gender, and are used in the absence of gender-stratified risks.

AS, aortic stenosis; ASD, atrial septal defect; AVSD, atrioventricular septal defect; CoA, coarctation of the aorta; HLHS, hypoplastic left heart syndrome; L-TGA, congenitally corrected transposition of the great arteries; NR, not reported/insufficient data; PDA, patent ductus arteriosus; PS, pulmonary stenosis; TGA, transposition of the great arteries; TOF, tetralogy of Fallot; VSD, ventricular septal defect.

Information about recurrence risk needs to take into account the specific type of cardiac malformation as well as information obtained from a detailed family history. Family history of CHD is one of the most consistently identified risk factors for identifying a CHD prenatally.

## SUGGESTED READINGS


Cowan JR, Ware SM. Genetics and genetic testing in congenital heart disease. *Clin Perinatol.* 2015;42(2):373-393.

Edwards JJ, Gelb BD. Genetics of congenital heart disease. *Curr Opin Cardiol.* 2016;31(3):235-241.

Homsy J, Zaidi S, Shen Y, et al. De novo mutations in congenital heart disease with neurodevelopmental and other congenital anomalies. *Science.* 2015;350(6265):1262-1266.

Lalani SR, Belmont JW. Genetic basis of congenital cardiovascular malformations. *Eur J Med Genet.* 2014;57(8):402-413.

McDonald-McGinn DM, Emanuel BS, Zackai EH. 22q11.2 deletion syndrome (February 2013) in GeneReviews at GeneTests: Medical Genetics Information Resource [database online]. Copyright, University of Washington, Seattle, 1997-2010. Available at: http://www.genetests.org. Accessed January 12, 2017.

Muenke M, Belmont JW, Kruszka PS, Sable CA. *Congenital Heart Disease: Molecular Genetics, Principles of Diagnosis and Treatment.* Basel, Switzerland: Karger; 2015.

Øyen N, Poulsen G, Boyd HA, Wohlfahrt J, Jensen PK, Melbye M. Recurrence of congenital heart defects in families. *Circulation.* 2009;120(4):295-301.

Roberts AE, Allanson JE, Tartaglia M, Gelb BD. Noonan syndrome. *Lancet.* 2013;381(9863):333-342.

Sifrim A, Hitz MP, Wilsdon A, et al. Distinct genetic architectures for syndromic and nonsyndromic congenital heart defects identified by exome sequencing. *Nat Genet.* 2016;48(9):1060-1065.

Yuan S, Zaidi S, Brueckner M. Congenital heart disease: emerging themes linking genetics and development. *Curr Opin Genet Dev.* 2013;23(3):352-359.

# 182 Overview of the Immune System

Kathleen E. Sullivan

## INTRODUCTION

Our immune system has evolved to provide protection from the pathogens that inhabit the natural world, and a critical aspect of immunologic function is the distinction between self tissues and non-self tissues. Self tissues must not become a target for immune responses, and training to protect self tissues is the essence of tolerance. Our host defense includes barrier functions, and we now know that the barrier interacts dynamically with the cells of the immune system as part of this defense. In this overview, we will describe the elements of the immune system, the development of different functional arms of the immune system, and the beautiful choreography that is intrinsic to an immune response.

Lymphocytes, neutrophils, monocytes, and various other myeloid cells can be detected in the blood through simple microscopy. Immunologists identify subsets of these cells through the use of flow cytometry. The cells usually are categorized by the expression of certain cell surface molecules, which are referred to as a cluster of differentiation (CD) molecules. A convenient table for reference relevant to clinical immunology and immunologic disorders is given in Table 182-1.

## ONTOGENY OF LYMPHOID CELLS AND ORGANS

The first progenitor cells of the immune system are found in the yolk sac at approximately 3 weeks of gestational age. These pluripotent stem cells migrate to the liver at 5 weeks of gestation, and clear elements of blood cells can be noted at 6 weeks of gestation. Hematopoiesis then moves to the bone marrow at 12 weeks of gestation. Certain tissue elements such as peripheral tissue macrophages and microglial cells are seeded directly from the yolk sac. Most of the immunologic cells of the bloodstream are continuously populated from bone marrow progenitors. The hematopoietic stem cell persists throughout adulthood and serves as the source for the continuous production of peripheral blood immune cells (Fig. 182-1).

In addition to the hematopoietic stem cell and its progeny, lymphoid organs also develop in early fetal life. The thymus is formed from the third and fourth branchial arches, and lymph nodes arise in response to local stimuli. These lymphoid organs become apparent at approximately 10 to 12 weeks of gestation, and shortly thereafter, mature lymphocytes can be detected in the fetal bloodstream. In fact, it is possible to sample the fetal immune system as early as 14 weeks of gestation as a strategy for diagnosis.

Myeloid cells and the innate immune system mature relatively early in fetal development. Neutrophils can be seen as early as 12 weeks of gestation. Innate responses to viruses are thought to be present even earlier, and these responses are found in a broad range of cell types and do not depend on the development of the peripheral immune system.

The distinction between the adaptive immune system and the innate immune system is important conceptually. Operationally, the *adaptive immune system* refers to T and B cells. The *innate immune system* comprises myeloid cells, innate antiviral defenses, natural killer cells, and innate lymphoid cells.

## DEVELOPMENT OF IMMUNOLOGIC FUNCTION

Infants are not born with a fully functional immune system, although they do have the capacity to defend against many infections. The immature responses to a range of pathogens result in frequent infections, particularly with encapsulated bacteria such as *Streptococcus pneumoniae* and *Haemophilus influenzae*. Recognizing the susceptibility has driven the efforts to vaccinate infants. Responses to these vaccines have demonstrated that immunity often wanes around 6 to 9 months after vaccination, and numerous boosters are required to sustain immune responses and maintain immunologic memory in young infants. In contrast, an adult would have an adequate response after a single vaccine. In utero and early in life, infants are highly dependent on their innate immune system for protection from infections. Toll-like receptor expression and responses to pathogens by neutrophils and monocytes are largely intact; however, cytokine secretion is somewhat diminished compared to adults. In addition, complement produced by reticuloendothelial cells and the liver exhibits lower levels in infants compared to adults. These aspects of the developing infant immune system are thought to contribute to susceptibility to infection.

The adaptive immune system is characterized by low numbers of memory cells in early infancy. Memory and memory-effector B cells and T cells respond rapidly to threats, and the lack of these in

**TABLE 182-1 CLUSTER OF DIFFERENTIATION (CD) CLASSIFICATION AND FUNCTION OF SELECTED MOLECULES**

| CD Number | Distribution | Function |
|---|---|---|
| CD1 | B, Mφ, DC, T | "Nonclassical" MHC |
| CD2 | T, NK | Binds CD58 (LFA-3); costimulation |
| CD3 | T | Associated with TCR; signal transduction |
| CD4 | T | Binds HLA class II; coreceptor |
| CD8 | T, NK | Binds HLA class II; coreceptor |
| CD11a | T, B, NK | CD11a/CD18 (LFA-1) binds ICAM 1–3 adhesion |
| CD11b | Activated T, M, G, Mφ, NK | CD11b/CD18 (Mac-1) receptor for iC3b and ICAM 1–3 |
| CD11c | M, G, Mφ, NK | CD11c/CD18 receptor for ICAM 1, iC3b; adhesion |
| CD16 | NK, M, G | Receptor for IgG Fc (FcγRIII); ADCC, activation |
| CD18 | T, B, NK, M, G, Mφ | $CD11_{a,b,c}$/CD18 as above; adhesion |
| CD19 | B | Forms complex with CD21, Leu-13; regulates signaling |
| CD20 | B | Calcium channel; mediates activation |
| CD21 | B | C3d/EBV receptor, associates with CD19 as above |
| CD23 | B | Low-affinity Fc IgE receptor |
| CD25 | Regulatory T, activated T | α-Chain, low-affinity IL-2 receptor |
| CD28 | T | Binds CD80 (B7-1) and CD86 (B7-2); costimulation |
| CD32 | B, M, G, P | Receptor for Fc IgG (FcγRII) |
| CD34 | SC, precursors | Adhesion |
| CD40 | B | Activation and differentiation |
| CD40L | Activated T | Ligand for CD40 |
| CD45 | All leukocytes | Many isoforms, phosphatase in signal transduction. In T cells, CD45RA is a marker for naïve T cells and CD45RO is a marker for a memory T cells |
| CD56 | NK | Mediates homophilic adhesion (NCAM) |
| CD80 | B*, Mφ, DC | Binds CD28 and CD152 on T cells; costimulation |
| CD86 | B*, M, DC | Binds CD28 and CD152 on T cells; costimulation |

B, B cell; B*, activated B cell; DC, dendritic cell; G, granulocyte; Mφ, macrophage; N, neutrophil; NK, natural killer cell; P, platelet; SC, stem cell; T, T cell.

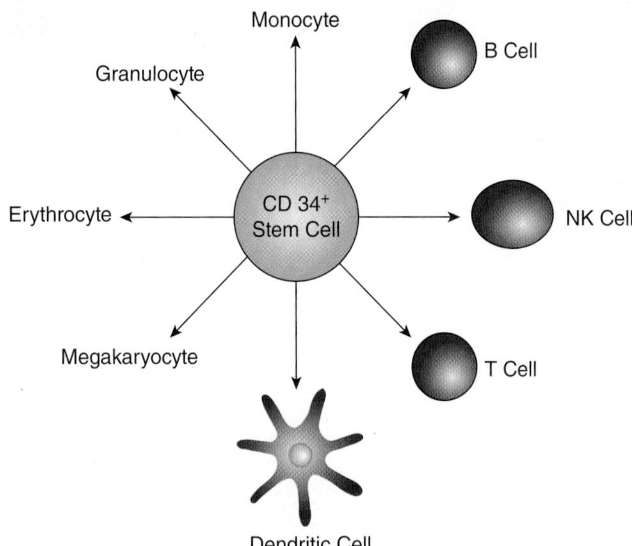


**FIGURE 182-1** Production of immune-competent cells. Hematopoiesis begins in the yolk sac and fetal liver before moving to the bone marrow. The hematopoietic stem cell gives rise to both myeloid and lymphoid cell types as well as erythrocytes and megakaryocytes. NK, natural killer.

early infancy leads to slower responses. Infant B cells are enriched in transitional B cells, and these cells are less functional than are the predominant naïve B cells seen in later childhood and adulthood. Similarly, infants are able to mount T-cell responses; however, CD4 T-cell responses develop more slowly in part because of their naïve phenotype and in part because T cells appear to be skewed toward an anti-inflammatory cytokine profile. In fetal life, regulatory T cells dominate, as is required to prevent reactions against maternal antigens. The transition from a regulatory T cell–dominated profile to one more focused on host defense leads to a period in early infancy during which T-cell function is suboptimal for the defense against viruses. In addition, T cells qualitatively are skewed more toward a Th2 response, which favors responses to helminths, as opposed to a Th1 phenotype, which favors responses to pathogens.

In addition to the cell-intrinsic deficits, lymphoid organs are also less mature in early infancy. Germinal center formation is poor until 4 months of age in humans. Although primary responses to vaccines can be elicited and are protective, the persistence of protective antibody is poor, and, therefore, the booster vaccines are required. Some of this lack of persistence no doubt reflects on the immature phenotype of germinal centers and lymphoid organs; however, it is likely that there are cell-intrinsic contributions to this deficit as well.

The development of the immune system can be affected in several ways in early life. Undernutrition leads to a smaller thymus and affects the development of T cells in an infant. It can have secondary consequences of compromised responses to vaccines. Infection, stress, and endogenous and exogenous corticosteroids also adversely affect the size of the thymus. Other studies have indicated that co-infection can compromise vaccine responses and that early responses to pathogens may distract the immune system from other types of responses. In fetal life, infections can compromise immunologic development directly. In utero infections with human immunodeficiency virus (HIV) and rubella virus have been demonstrated to impact on subsequent B-cell maturation. Maternal infections with malaria and cytomegalovirus have also been demonstrated to compromise immunoglobulin function. Thus, many variables contribute to the susceptibility to infection in early infancy. In industrialized countries, this susceptibility is mitigated by vaccine programs; nonetheless, 4 million children die each year, largely due to infection. In the United States, hospitalization of infected infants costs $690 million dollars, with nearly 50,000 deaths per year. Thus, infections in infancy represent the end result of immunologic immaturity coupled with diminished barrier function and other variables.

## INNATE IMMUNITY

Innate defense mechanisms are not confined to the classic cells of the immune system. Innate defenses include mechanical barriers as well as structural features that facilitate the host defense. In addition, most cells in the human body are able to respond to viral infections by producing type I interferons. These interferons represent the first stage of antiviral defenses and are critical for containment of the virus until the adaptive immune system can fully eradicate an infection. Innate antiviral responses are widely distributed throughout most cell types, and a variety of receptors recognize patterns intrinsic to viruses. Figure 182-2 demonstrates many of the receptors involved in innate responses to pathogens. Of note, in this figure, the majority of the responses to bacteria lead to activation of a transcription factor referred to as nuclear factor-κB (NF-κB). Antiviral responses typically induce activation of a class of transcription factors called *interferon response factors* (IRFs). The cascade of events culminating in transcription-factor activation is responsible for the cytokine secretion that recruits and activates additional cells.

Tissue macrophages represent a similar sentinel system for bacterial infections. Tissue macrophages recognize pathogen-associated molecular patterns (PAMPs) and produce cytokines that facilitate the recruitment of other cells to participate in the clearance of bacteria. Many of these PAMPs are recognized by toll-like receptors (TLR), and engagement of these receptors leads to the secretion of tumor necrosis factor (TNF), interleukin (IL)-6, and IL-12. These cytokines are central in recruiting neutrophils, activating lymphocytes, and further activating macrophages for intracellular killing.

The most critical cell responsible for the clearance of conventional bacterial infections is the neutrophil. Neutrophils are initially recruited from the bloodstream when vascular endothelial cells express adhesion molecules in response to TNF and other inflammatory mediators. These adhesion molecules engage the neutrophil and slow down the rolling. Subsequent activation of additional adhesion molecules facilitates the transmigration of the neutrophil into the tissues (Fig. 182-3). Once there, the neutrophil migrates up a chemotactic gradient until it reaches the bacteria, at which point it will engulf and kill the bacteria. The primary endogenous chemotactic signal is a complement cleavage product, C5a. Neutrophils also have receptors for a formylated peptide, f-Met-Leu-Phe, which is a pattern seen only in bacteria. The neutrophil migrates up the gradient of chemotactic molecules and finally arrives at the site of the bacteria. Here, ingestion occurs. This, too, is a highly regulated process. Neutrophils have receptors that recognize oligosaccharides typical of bacteria and can directly ingest bacteria via those receptors. Ingestion is much more efficient if the bacteria are coated with antibodies (from a previous infection) or the complement protein C3b. Once ingested, the bacterium is assaulted by reactive oxygen species produced by the NADPH complex on the membrane of the phagosome and the release of toxic granule contents into the phagosome. The combined effects are nearly uniformly fatal to bacteria. Neutrophils play little role in defense against viruses but do contribute to the clearance of bacteria, fungi, mycobacteria, and certain parasites.

Macrophages and monocytes are related by lineage. By convention, the word *monocyte* refers to the cell in the bloodstream, and the word *macrophage* refers to the cell in the tissue. There are functional differences that accompany the transformation from monocyte to macrophage, but the simplest distinction to be made is location of the cell. Tissue macrophages represent one of the main sentinel cells in the body; others are mast cells and dendritic cells. These cell types all are characterized by high expressions of receptors for pathogens discussed earlier (see Fig. 182-2). When the sentinel cells bind to a pathogen, TNF, IL-12, and IL-6 are released within a few hours. When the pathogen is a virus, a different program is followed, leading to production of type I interferons (the α and β interferons). For bacteria, the cytokines drive increased expression of adhesion molecules on the vascular

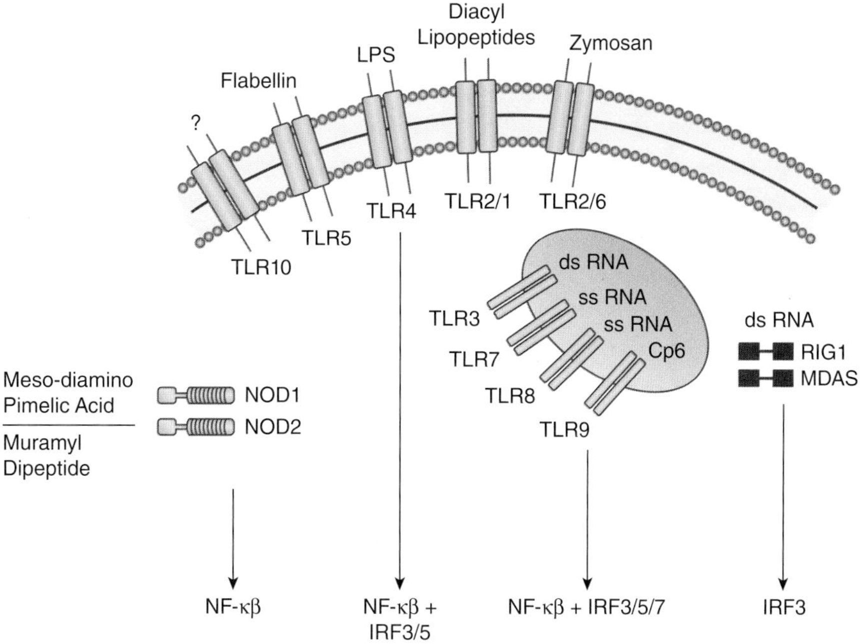


**FIGURE 182-2** Receptors involved in innate recognition of pathogens. The innate immune system utilizes a variety of hard-wired receptors to recognize pathogens. Often a given pathogen may be recognized by more than 1 receptor, which provides extra security to the system. Receptors whose primary target is bacteria are located primarily on the plasma membrane as it is most likely that they will encounter extracellular pathogens. However, there are 2 intracellular receptors for bacterial recognition, NOD1 and NOD2. They may be important for recognition of intracellular bacteria, bacterial products leaked from the phagosome, or digested bacterial products from the lysosome. Toll-like receptors whose primary target is viral patterns are located primarily in endosomes, as viruses are intracellular pathogens. Two receptors for viral patterns are located in the cytosol, RIG-I and MDA-5. These 2 receptors recognize viral nucleic acids and transmit signals that will drive type I interferon production. The bacterial receptors drive an NF-κB response, which will induce IL-6, IL-12, and TNF, all cytokines that will facilitate bacterial defenses. IL, interleukin; IRFs, interferon regulatory factors; MDA-5, melanoma differentiation-associated protein 5; NF-κB, nuclear factor-kappa light-chain enhancer of activated B cells; NOD, nucleotide-binding oligomerization domain; RIG 1, retinoid-inducible gene 1; TLR, toll-like receptor; TNF, tumor necrosis factor. (Used with permission from Kathleen E. Sullivan.)

endothelium to recruit neutrophils and enhance phagocytosis. Certain pathogens, such as mycobacteria and fungi, are resistant to neutrophil killing. They are killed by activated macrophages. Although macrophages have limited ability to kill pathogens in their resting state, activation by γ-interferon and TNF dramatically improves intracellular killing (Fig. 182-4). Macrophages can become further activated, in a poorly understood process, and then aggregate and form granulomas.

Natural killer (NK) cells are a subset of lymphocytes distinguished by their large size, granular cytoplasm, and expression of distinct surface molecules. They selectively identify and kill virally infected cells and tumor cells, using cytotoxic mechanisms to lyse target cells. Following contact with a target cell, organelles are oriented toward the target by a calcium-dependent mechanism. This event is followed by a release of granules containing granzyme A and perforin. NK cells are

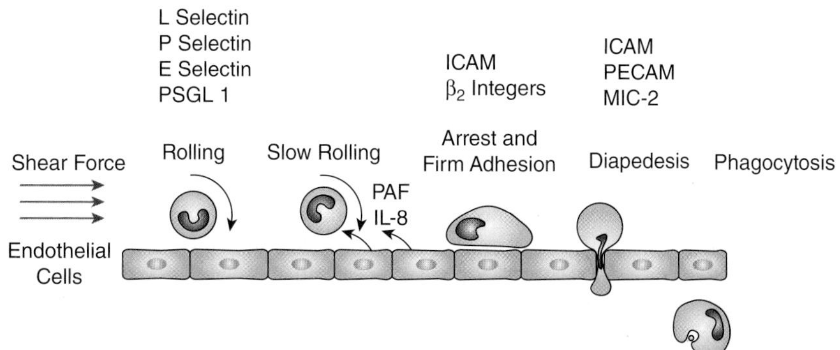


**FIGURE 182-3** Neutrophil attachment and diapedesis. Neutrophils initially engage endothelial cells via glycosylated ligands on the neutrophil such as PSGL1. These ligands interact with the selectin family only under the influence of shear stress. The selectin family of proteins is upregulated on the endothelial surface under the influence of inflammatory mediators. Endothelial production of platelet-activating factor (PAF) and interleukin (IL)-8 induces structural changes in the neutrophil $\beta_2$ integrin family after contact. The $\beta_2$ integrin molecules interact with ICAM to arrest the neutrophil movement. Diapedesis across the endothelium and into the tissue space can occur between cells, as shown, or occasionally through the cell. Additional molecules guide the cell through the endothelial barrier. Once in the tissue space, the neutrophil migrates up the chemotactic gradient toward the bacteria. Engagement of mannose receptors, scavenger receptors, Fc receptors, and complement receptors can all participate in cueing phagocytosis. Once engulfed, the bacteria are subjected to a plethora of antimicrobial substances. Finally, the neutrophil dies after phagocytosis to ensure the process is not unduly prolonged. ICAM, intercellular adhesion molecule; IL-8, interleukin 8; MIC-2, macrophage inhibitory cytokine-2; PAF, platelet activating factor; PECAM, platelet/endothelial cell adhesion molecule 1; PSGL-1, p-selectin glycoprotein binding ligand-1. (Used with permission from Kathleen E. Sullivan.)

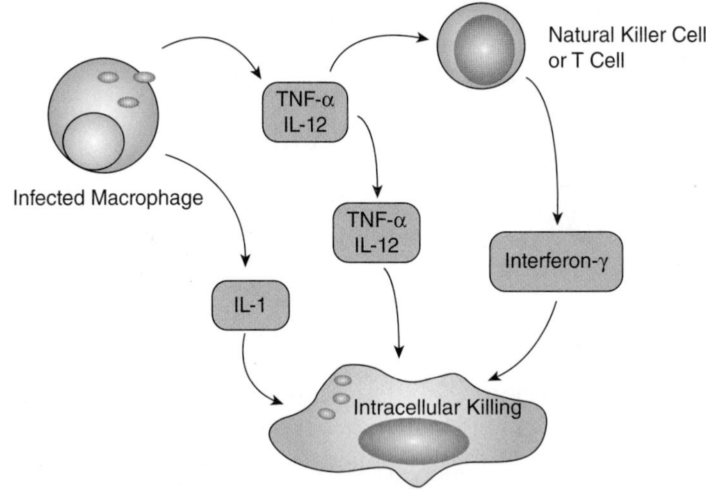


**FIGURE 182-4** Macrophage killing of intracellular organisms. Certain organisms are resistant to neutrophil killing, and macrophages are the primary defense against mycobacteria and certain other intracellular pathogens. Macrophages do not contain the same microbicidal products as neutrophils and must activate a killing program. Macrophage activation and intracellular killing require both γ-interferon and tumor necrosis factor (TNF). The source of TNF may come from an adjacent infected cell or even the same infected cell as the pattern-recognition receptors drive an NF-κB response, leading to production of TNF. The γ-interferon typically comes from a natural killer cell or a cytotoxic T cell, both of which are recruited to the location of the infection. In this setting, the role of interleukin (IL)-12 (and the closely related IL-23) is to stimulate γ-interferon production from the lymphocytes. In a typical granuloma, the activated macrophage would comprise the structure of the granuloma, and the surrounding T cells would provide the cytokines to maintain macrophage activation. Diseases such as human immunodeficiency virus, in which the T-cell component is affected, or drugs such as TNF inhibitors, in which the cytokine circuit is disrupted, all lead to increased susceptibility to mycobacteria. (Used with permission from Kathleen E. Sullivan.)

identified by their expression of CD16 (FcγRIII) and CD56 (NCAM-1) on the cell surface and comprise approximately 10% of circulating lymphocytes. Mature NK cells can be found in the spleen, lungs, and liver. During the first trimester of pregnancy, they are abundant in the placental decidua. NK cells use an array of stimulatory and inhibitory receptors to modulate their cytolytic functions. In addition to their effector functions, NK cells also have an important role in attenuating inflammatory responses. Genetically determined and acquired NK cell defects are associated with a severe autoinflammatory condition termed *hemophagocytic lymphohistiocytosis* (see Chapter 184).

The complement system is covered in detail in another chapter; however, here we will emphasize its development and interactions with other components of the immune system. Complement components are produced largely in the liver, although C1q is produced by myeloid cells. Hepatic production starts in fetal development at approximately 14 weeks of gestation, with C1q produced in the spleen by approximately 18 weeks of gestation. Complement is critical for efficient uptake of bacteria by neutrophils by serving as an opsonin, as described earlier. Complement component C3 is also critical for B-cell costimulation. Several components play a role in waste clearance, specifically the uptake of cholesterol and apoptotic cells. Direct microbicidal activity is mediated by formation of a pore, nucleated by C5, C6, C7, and C8 and stabilized by C9.

## ADAPTIVE IMMUNITY

Adaptive immune responses are broadly divided into cellular and humoral immune responses, mediated mainly by T and B lymphocytes, respectively. The adaptive responses exhibit a memory effect, where subsequent exposures elicit greater and more durable responses. The other key feature of the adaptive immune system is that T and B cells undergo education that is required to prevent self-reactivity.

### T CELLS

T cells recognize antigens through a dimeric T-cell receptor. In 95% of thymocytes, the T-cell receptor consists of 1 α chain and 1 β chain, and in approximately 5%, it is comprised of 1 γ chain and 1 δ chain. Each chain has both constant and variable gene segments. It is estimated that there are $10^{16}$ different T-cell antigen receptors. It stands to reason that with so many different receptors, some of them could potentially bind self-proteins rather than infectious agents. Education of T cells to support tolerance to self-antigens occurs mainly in the thymus.

Thymocytes commit to the T-cell lineage and undergo, in succession, rearrangement of the genes that will eventually form their respective T-cell receptors. These recombinational events are dependent on functional recombinase-associated genes, without which T-cell development is arrested or severely impaired. Maturation of T cells continues in the thymic cortex through a series of developmental stages (Fig. 182-5). Double-negative cells undergo positive selection in the cortex whereby the T cells that express T-cell receptors that recognize self are selected for further development. The thymocytes migrate to the medulla, where they become positive for CD4 and CD8 and undergo negative selection to eradicate those cells with high-affinity self-reactivity. Self-antigen expression in the thymus is controlled at least partly by the *AIRE* gene. Finally, single positive cells exit to the periphery.

T-cell receptors recognize antigen displayed by antigen-presenting cells such as dendritic cells. Macrophages and B cells represent alternative antigen-presenting cells. The antigen-presenting cells display the processed antigen to the T cell using major histocompatibility complex (MHC) molecules. When the T cell's antigen-specific receptor is engaged by a specific peptide bound to an MHC molecule expressed on the surface of the antigen-presenting cell, an "immunologic synapse" is initiated, involving intracellular signal transduction and reorganization of signaling molecules in the membrane. Activation of naïve T cells requires a second signal other than that provided through the T-cell receptor. The best-characterized costimulatory molecule on the surface of naïve T cells is CD28. CD28 binds to CD80 and CD81 on the surface of antigen-presenting cells. Upon activation, T cells that are CD4+ may further differentiate and acquire specialized effector functions, including characteristic cytokine secretion profiles. These T-cell subsets include Th1, Th2, Th17, Tfh, and Treg cells, each with a specific immune function (Fig. 182-6). Imbalances in T-cell subsets have been associated with various human diseases. Most T cells generated by a primary immune response undergo apoptotic cell death.

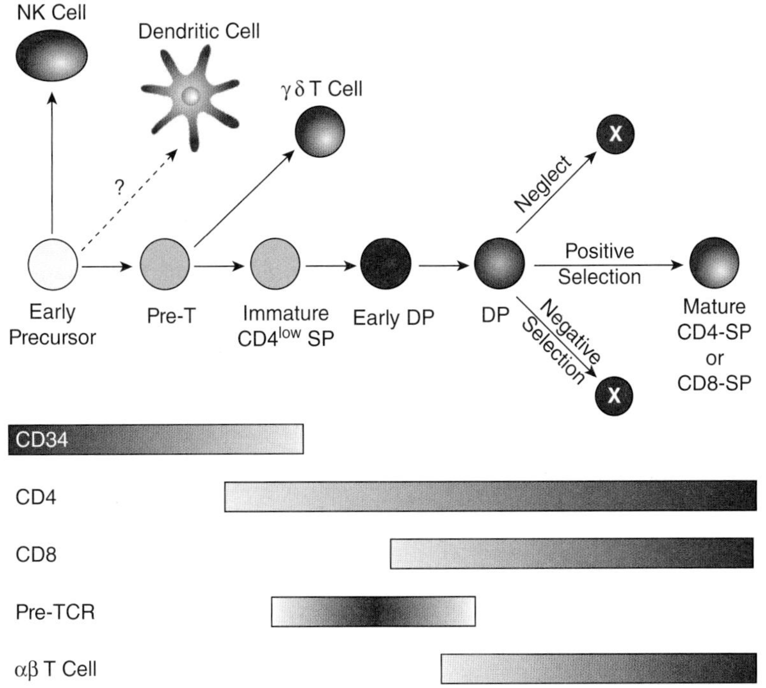


**FIGURE 182-5** The development of mature T and B cells. Both lineages arise from a common lymphoid progenitor and have comparable development. Both undergo a staged, heavy-chain rearrangement followed by the light-chain rearrangement. After the heavy chain rearranges, it is expressed on the surface with a nonrearranged light chain to test the integrity of the heavy chain. These receptors are referred to as the pre-BCR and pre-TCR. Subsequent rearrangement of the light chain leads to a functional BCR and TCR being expressed on each cell type. At this stage, negative selection of autoreactive cells occurs. Finally, immature B cells exit the bone marrow, and CD4- and CD8-positive T cells exit the thymus. BCR, B-cell receptor; TCR, T-cell receptor.

However, a small number of cells, proportional to the initial antigenic load and clonal burst size, survive and differentiate into memory cells. In general, memory cells allow a more rapid, more potent, and more enduring secondary response. Among T cells in the peripheral blood, the memory phenotype (CD45RO) increases with age.

## ANTIGEN-PRESENTING CELLS

Antigen-presenting cells are essential for T-cell function. Dendritic cells are hematopoietically derived and distributed throughout the body. Initially, they function as antigen-capturing cells, sampling their surroundings by different mechanisms, including phagocytosis, micropinocytosis, and an array of specialized receptors that recognize immunoglobulin (Ig) G, IgE, or mannose residues on the surface of pathogens. After antigen is internalized, dendritic cells are activated, leading to migration to the draining lymph nodes where they present antigen to T cells. Dendritic cells also greatly influence the nature of the ensuing T-cell response. Dendritic cells can produce cytokines with antiviral properties, such as interferons α and β, or cytokines that direct T cells toward a respective Th1, Th2, or Th17 cell phenotype. Thus, dendritic cells have a central role in initiating and controlling immune responses.

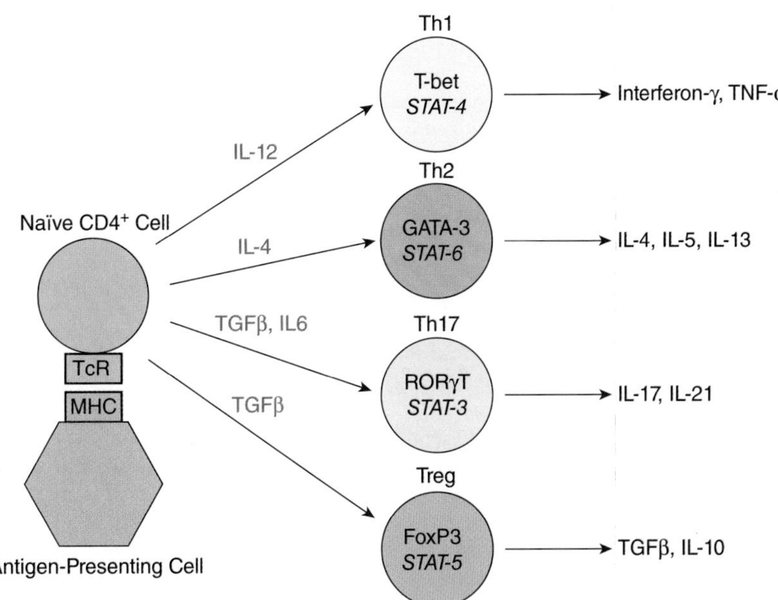


**FIGURE 182-6** T-cell lineage commitment. Naïve CD4+ T cells are stimulated by peptide presented on an antigen-presenting cell in the context of a class II HLA (major histocompatibility complex [MHC]) molecule. Cytokines direct intracellular expression of lineage-specific transcription factors, resulting in acquisition of different T-helper cell phenotypes.

Macrophages are less potent antigen-presenting cells but exhibit the same characteristics as do dendritic cells. B cells operate according to a different conceptual paradigm as they internalize antigen largely though their B-cell receptors. Thus, they present cognate antigen to T cells.

## B CELLS

B cells are the progenitors of antibody-secreting plasma cells. B-cell development involves a complex antigen-independent program that can be divided into stages, as shown in Figure 182-5. In the early pro–B-cell stage, lymphoid progenitor cells commit to the B-cell lineage, but Ig gene rearrangement has not yet occurred. Subsequently, pro-B cells undergo genetic recombinational events, partly dependent on recombinase-associated genes and terminal deoxynucleotidyltransferase, leading to generation of Ig μ heavy chain protein.

The μ chain is subsequently expressed on the cell surface together with surrogate light chains, which are invariant and are formed in the absence of DNA rearrangement, forming the pre–B-cell receptor. Expression of the pre–B-cell receptor promotes B-cell differentiation toward the pre–B-cell stage. As was true for T cells, B cells require education to eliminate self-reactive cells. Negative selection occurs at the immature B-cell stage by 2 mechanisms. Some cells with autoreactive B-cell receptors are deleted in the bone marrow by apoptosis. Alternatively, the specificity of autoreactive cells can be modified by further gene rearrangement, a process termed *receptor editing*. Surviving immature B cells are exported as transitional B cells to the spleen and other lymphoid organs.

Initially, all mature B cells express IgM and IgD on their cell surface. However, upon exposure to antigen, and under the influence of cytokines and interactions with TFH cells, B cells can undergo isotype switching. By this process, B cells bearing surface IgG, IgA, and IgE surface receptors are generated, and antigen receptor specificity is preserved. IgM, the first Ig to be generated in a primary immune response, is secreted as a pentamer. IgG is the most abundant Ig in human serum, comprising 80% of the total Ig. IgG is divided into 4 subclasses, based on structural differences. IgA comprises 10% to 15% of serum Ig and contains 2 subclasses, IgA1 and IgA2. Secreted IgA2 is the major Ig at mucosal surfaces, where it exists as a complex comprising 2 IgA monomers, a joining chain, and a secretory component. IgE plays a role in immunity to parasites and mediates allergic reactions. Antibody exerts its effects in several ways: activation of complement, engagement of Fc receptors, and direct opsonization.

## PATHOLOGIC HOST IMMUNE RESPONSES

Pathologic host immune responses often are classified into 4 categories, although it is important to remember that these processes are part of a complex pathogen defense strategy as well.

Immediate or type I hypersensitivity is the typical allergic response discussed in Section 14. Preexisting IgE directed against an antigen is bound to mast cells. Engagement of IgE by the antigen leads to immediate degranulation of mast cells with release of histamine as well as a variety of cytokines. Examples include anaphylaxis and seasonal allergies.

Type II hypersensitivity refers specifically to autoantibody-mediated tissue damage. The membrane-attack complex of the complement cascade primarily harms cells such as erythrocytes, which have no ability to repair membrane damage. Autoantibodies can also lead to tissue damage by facilitating uptake by the reticuloendothelial system. Examples include acute hemolytic anemia and myasthenia gravis.

Immune complex disease or type III hypersensitivity is best exemplified by serum sickness. Antibodies produced to antigen form a high-molecular-weight complex that deposits in organs and causes damage via Fc receptors.

Delayed or type IV hypersensitivity is familiar to clinicians as the basis of the purified protein derivative (PPD) test for tuberculosis. Here, T cells are responsible for the tissue damage.

Autoimmunity refers specifically to adaptive immune responses directed at self-antigens. The implication is that central or peripheral tolerance has failed. Breaking tolerance is complex, with a strong stochastic contribution. A cytokine's milieu can facilitate breaks in tolerance, and recurrent infections seem to be associated with a high risk of breaking tolerance. Autoinflammation represents another type of pathologic response; however, it is not mediated by lymphocytes, and there is no antigen driving the process. Autoinflammation is a result of improper control of innate responses and is associated high levels of inflammatory cytokines.

## SUGGESTED READINGS

Hannet I, Erkeller-Yuksel F, Lydyard P, Deneys V, DeBruyere M. Developmental and maturational changes in human blood lymphocyte subpopulations. *Immunol Today*. 1992;13:215-218.

Holt PG, Jones CA. The development of the immune system during pregnancy and early life. *Allergy*. 2000;55:688-697.

Levy O. Innate immunity of the newborn: Basic mechanisms and clinical correlates. *Nat Rev Immunol*. 2007;7:379-390

Simon AK, Hollander GA, McMichael A. Evolution of the immune system in humans from infancy to old age. *Proc Royal Soc B*. 2015;282:20143085.

# 183 Increased Susceptibility to Infections

Javier Chinen

## INTRODUCTION

Many children are evaluated by their physicians because of recurrent infections, a relatively common complaint in early childhood. These children are considered to have an increased susceptibility to infections as compared with children of similar age. Both extrinsic and host factors can increase the risk of developing infections, and may be found in most such cases (Table 183-1). Identification and management of these underlying conditions would result in a reduction in frequency of infectons. Examples of extrinsic factors include human immunodeficiency virus infection, use of immunosuppressor drugs, high exposure to infectious agents in a daycare setting, presence of foreign bodies, or exposure to parental smoking. Host factors that increase risks of developing infections include genetic deficiencies of the immune response and several other conditions: respiratory allergies, abnormal anatomy, and diseases affecting barriers or epithelia such as cystic fibrosis.

## ASSESSMENT OF THE CHILD WITH INCREASED SUSCEPTIBILITY TO INFECTIONS

As with other clinical conditions, a detailed history is most helpful to obtain clues and to suggest laboratory testing leading to specific diagnosis. The threshold to define high frequency of infections might not be the same for every child because of additional considerations of

**TABLE 183-1 EXAMPLES OF FACTORS CONTRIBUTING TO INCREASED FREQUENCY OF INFECTIONS**

| External Factors | Host Factors |
|---|---|
| Exposure to infectious agents | Barrier compromise (skin, mucosa) |
| Exposure to pollution or other irritants | Allergic inflammation |
| Use of immunosuppressor drugs | Genetic immunodeficiencies |
| Human immunodeficiency virus infection | Anatomic abnormalities |
| Foreign bodies | Malabsorption |

**TABLE 183-2 GENETIC DEFECTS ASSOCIATED WITH SUSCEPTIBILITY TO SPECIFIC PATHOGENS**

| Gene Defect | Pathogen |
|---|---|
| *CD40LG, CD40* | *Pneumocystis jiroveci, Cryptosporidium, Toxoplasma,* parvovirus |
| *IL12B, IL12RB1, IFNGR1/2, STAT1, IKBKG* | Mycobacteria |
| *MYD88, IRAK4* | Pyogenic and encapsulated organisms |
| *SH2D1A (SAP), XIAP* | Epstein-Barr virus |
| *TLR3, UNC93B1* | Herpes simplex virus encephalitis |
| *C5-9* | *Neisseria* species |
| *EVER1/2, CXCR4* | Human papilloma virus |

**TABLE 183-3 TESTING FOR THE EVALUATION OF THE IMMUNE RESPONSE**

| General Tests | Tests Specific for Immune Deficiencies |
|---|---|
| Complete blood count with differential | Serum levels of IgG, IgM, IgA, IgE |
| Inflammatory markers (eg, CRP, ESR) | Specific antibody titers after vaccine |
| HIV serology or viral load | Lymphocyte phenotyping by flow cytometry: T cells, B cells, NK cells |
| Chest x-ray (for thymus shadow) | T cell proliferation assays to mitogens and antigens |
| | Neutrophils oxidative burst test |
| | Total hemolytic activity (CH50) |
| | Serum levels of complement components |
| | Gene sequencing analysis |
| | Testing for specific protein expression or function. (eg, CD40 ligand expression, STAT6 phosphorylation) |

CRP, C-reactive protein; ESR, erythrocyte sedimentation rate; HIV, human immunodeficiency virus; NK, natural killer.

external factors as mentioned above. However, guidelines have been suggested: 2 or more systemic bacterial infections at any time (such as sepsis, deep-seated abscesses, or meningitis), 3 or more bacterial infections, or 6 to 8 or more upper respiratory tract infections in 1 year.

Respiratory tract infections are common in children. Two examples of host factors favoring infections are allergy conditions and cystic fibrosis. Allergic disease should be investigated because of its increasing prevalence and its role in causing respiratory airway and skin inflammation. Supporting evidence may come from family history of allergic diseases, frequent itching and sneezing, and findings on physical exam of allergic signs such as allergic shiners, clear nasal discharge, eczema, or wheezing. Diagnostic tests include allergen skin testing and serum IgE levels. Patients with cystic fibrosis are particularly susceptible to respiratory infections with *Pseudomonas aeruginosa, Burkholderia* species, and *Staphylococcus aureus.* Cystic fibrosis usually is confirmed with a sweat chloride test.

A high frequency of infections, their severity, or the nature of the infectious organism should prompt an evaluation for deficiencies of the immune response. Hospitalization or surgical intervention (eg, abscess drainage) for infections, prolonged antibiotic courses, and shortened intervals between infectious episodes are indicators of an unusual severity of infections. Other significant history associated with immunodeficiencies include weight loss, failure to thrive, presence of autoimmunity, lymphoreticular malignancy, and family history of recurrent infections.

Particular defects in the adaptive and innate immune response may lead to increased susceptibilities to specific infections (Table 183-2). Cellular immunity defects are associated with recurrent and disseminated viral, atypical mycobacterial, and fungal infections. Humoral immunodeficiency is associated with respiratory infections and/or chronic diarrhea with pathogens such as *Giardia lamblia.* Infections by encapsulated bacteria suggest both antibody deficiencies and complement deficiency, as both immunity components are involved in clearance of these bacteria. Phagocytic cell defects, such as chronic granulomatous disease (CGD), typically present with recurrent pyogenic and fungal infections. A predilection toward infections with *Neisseria* species is seen in patients with deficiencies of terminal complement components. Mutations in the IL-12/IL-23 receptor/interferon-γ receptor/STAT1 axis give rise to susceptibility to mycobacterial infections. Deficiencies of the adaptor protein MYD88 and the downstream kinase interleukin-1 receptor–associated kinase 4, both coupled to several Toll-like receptors (TLRs), are associated with invasive infections with pyogenic and encapsulated organisms. Deficiencies of the MYD88-independent TLR 3 and of the endoplasmic reticulum resident membrane protein UNC93 have been found in patients with susceptibility to herpes simplex encephalitis.

## EVALUATION OF THE IMMUNE RESPONSE

The evaluation for immunodeficiency is guided by the clinical presentation, age of onset, and type and frequency of infections. Secondary immunodeficiencies such as human immunodeficiency virus (HIV) infection might also present with frequent infections and should be investigated. A family history of severe or fatal infections suggests genetic immunodeficiencies. Opportunistic infections, such as pneumonia caused by *Pneumocystis jiroveci,* are highly suggestive of T cell immunodeficiency.

Findings in the physical exam may provide additional information suggesting impaired immunity: absent tonsil development in an infant might indicate decreased B cells, severe oral candidiasis suggests severe T cell deficiency, characteristic facial features and cardiac malformations may indicate DiGeorge syndrome, and dwarfism may point to immunodeficiency associated with the cartilage-hair hypoplasia syndrome.

Investigations useful in the child with susceptibility to infection are shown in Table 183-3 and are described in more detail in Chapter 184. A complete blood count with differential is useful to rule out immunodeficiencies associated with lymphopenia or neutropenia. Flow cytometry of lymphocyte subsets diagnoses deficits of particular cell populations characteristic of specific conditions, such as the absence of B cells in X-linked agammaglobulinemia. Quantitation of total immunoglobulin levels, considering that normal ranges vary with age, is useful to rule out hypogammaglobulinemia. Functional antibody responses can be assessed in the immunized individual by measuring specific antibody titers to tetanus toxoid and to pneumococcal serotypes present in the polyvalent pneumococcal vaccine. The integrity of the classic pathway of complement activation can be assessed by measuring the total hemolytic activity in the blood (CH50). Cellular immunity can be assessed by delayed-type hypersensitivity mitogen stimulation assays and by flow cytometric analysis of T-lymphocyte markers.

Dihydrorhodamine (DHR) assay has now replaced the nitroblue tetrazolium test to confirm deficiency of neutrophil oxidative burst, characteristic of CGD. The total hemolytic complement activity CH50, as well as serum levels of specific complement components, should be measured when infections with encapsulated organisms are frequent.

Genetic testing is currently available for a number of primary immunodeficiencies, and when gene defects are not readily identified, whole-genome sequencing approaches might be considered.

## MANAGEMENT OF A CHILD WITH RECURRENT INFECTIONS

The management of patients with recurrent infections depends on the underlying disorder. For example, the control of allergic inflammation often leads to a decreased frequency of infection in children with severe allergic disease. Antibiotic prophylaxis might be an alternative to reduce the frequency of infections for children in whom the underlying disorder is not found or could not be effectively treated, such as in cystic fibrosis, transient hypogammaglobulinemia of infancy, drug-induced immunosuppression, and phagocytic cell dysfunction. For primary immunodeficient patients, management is determined by the type and severity of the immune defect. Due to the complexity of their management, coordination of care between primary pediatricians and clinical immunologists is necessary. Frequent follow-up (eg, every 6 months) is recommended to diagnose and treat infections or other known complications early. Immunoglobulin replacement therapy is the definitive therapy for hypogammaglobulinemia and agammaglobulinemia. The use of interferon-γ has reduced infections in patients with CGD. Bone marrow transplantation and gene therapy are reserved for the most severe immunodeficiency diseases, such as severe combined immunodeficiency. Immunizations have an important role in children with recurrent infections. Booster doses might be considered if a child does not present with antibody titers at protective levels. Immunodeficient patients should not receive live vaccines or blood product transfusions without an immunologic evaluation, because these vaccines can potentially cause disease and nonirradiated blood products might induce graft-versus-host disease. Every attempt should be made to keep the immunodeficient child within his or her age-compatible social environment, and isolation procedures should be recommended only after evidence of a profound defect of immunity is found.

## SUGGESTED READINGS


Aguilar C, Malphettes M, Donadieu J, et al. Prevention of infections during primary immunodeficiency. *Clin Infect Dis.* 2014;59:1462-1470.

Arkwright PD, Gennery AR. Ten warning signs of primary immunodeficiency: a new paradigm is needed for the 21st century. *Ann N Y Acad Sci.* 2011;1238:7-14.

Bonilla FA, Khan DA, Ballas ZK, et al. Practice parameter for the diagnosis and management of primary immunodeficiency. *J Allergy Clin Immunol.* 2015;136:1186-1205.e1-78.

Cicalese MP, Aiuti A. Clinical applications of gene therapy for primary immunodeficiencies. *Hum Gene Ther.* 2015;26:210-219.

Jolles S, Orange JS, Gardulf A, Stein MR, Shapiro R, Borte M, Berger M. Current treatment options with immunoglobulin G for the individualization of care in patients with primary immunodeficiency disease. *Clin Exp Immunol.* 2015;179:146-160.

Kang E, Gennery A. Hematopoietic stem cell transplantation for primary immunodeficiencies. *Hematol Oncol Clin North Am.* 2014; 28:1157-1170.

Lanternier F, Cypowyj S, Picard C, Bustamante J, Lortholary O, Casanova JL, Puel A. Primary immunodeficiencies underlying fungal infections. *Curr Opin Pediatr.* 2013;25:736-747.

Locke BA, Dasu T, Verbsky JW. Laboratory diagnosis of primary immunodeficiencies. *Clin Rev Allergy Immunol.* 2014;46:154-168.

Maglione PJ, Simchoni N, Cunningham-Rundles C. Toll-like receptor signaling in primary immune deficiencies. *Ann N Y Acad Sci.* 2015; 1356:1-21.

Platts-Mills TA. The allergy epidemics: 1870-2010. *J Allergy Clin Immunol.* 2015;136(1):3-13.

Verhagen LM, de Groot R. Recurrent, protracted and persistent lower respiratory tract infection: a neglected clinical entity. *J Infect.* 2015;71(Suppl 1):S106-S111.


# 184 Primary Immunodeficiency Diseases

Ivan K. Chinn

## INTRODUCTION

Primary immunodeficiency diseases (PIDs) encompass a spectrum of conditions that result from more than 300 congenital defects of the immune system. These intrinsic molecular changes alter the development or function of the immune system, leading to increased susceptibility to infections, neoplasia, autoinflammation, and autoimmunity. PIDs occur more commonly than often perceived, existing at an estimated prevalence of 1 in every 1200 individuals in the United States. Higher incidence and prevalence can be expected in parts of the world with genetically homogenous populations or consanguinity. The different PIDs are established by the International Union of Immunological Societies (IUIS) and comprise 8 categories, plus an additional category for PID phenocopies, covering essentially all aspects of immune cell biology and immune function. This chapter will review distinguishing features of 7 of the 8 categories, leaving complement deficiencies for discussion in a separate chapter.

## COMBINED CELLULAR AND HUMORAL IMMUNODEFICIENCIES

Combined cellular and humoral immunodeficiencies are characterized primarily by decreased function of T cells, B cells, and sometimes natural killer (NK) cells (Table 184-1). In many cases, the T cell deficiency leads or contributes to loss of B-cell function. Within this classification scheme, severe combined immunodeficiency disease (SCID) carries distinction from other combined immunodeficiencies (CIDs).

### SEVERE COMBINED IMMUNODEFICIENCY DISEASE

Children with SCID are born with marked susceptibility to pathogens that typically results in death by 1 to 2 years of age in the absence of treatment. The diagnosis represents a true pediatric emergency. SCID is defined by specific criteria: absence or very low number of T cells (< 300 CD3+ T cells/μL) and no or very low T cell function (<10% of lower limit of normal) as measured by response to phytohemagglutinin (PHA) or presence of T cells of maternal origin. At least 16 molecular defects are recognized as causes of SCID (Table 184-1) and can often be distinguished by absence or presence of B cells or NK cells.

B-positive, NK-negative SCID typically results from defects that impair development of T and NK cells while permitting B-cell survival. The most common cause is a defect in *IL2RG*, located at Xq13, which encodes the gamma component (γc) shared in common among the receptors for interleukin (IL)-2, IL-4, IL-7, IL-9, IL-15, and IL-21. IL-7 receptor signaling is essential for T cell development, and IL-15 signaling is necessary for production of NK cells. In this form of X-linked SCID, B cells are present but do not produce protective antibodies due to failure of IL-4 signaling. B-positive, NK-negative SCID also arises from biallelic mutations in *JAK3*, which encodes Janus kinase 3, a signaling cascade molecule that is phosphorylated upon activation of γc.

B-negative, NK-positive SCID is observed in children who have defects in proteins needed for formation of lymphocyte antigen receptors. Unlike NK cells, T and B cells rearrange germline DNA to express such receptors during development. The recombination process begins when recombinase activating genes 1 (*RAG1*) and 2 (*RAG2*) cleave genomic DNA at sites of receptor V, D, or J segments. After the segments are rearranged, the DNA breaks must be repaired in a process that involves the proteins Ku 70, Ku 80, $PK_{CS}$, artemis, DNA ligase IV, XRCC4, and cernunnos. Defects in *RAG1*, *RAG2*, *DCLRE1C* (artemis), *PRKDC* ($PK_{CS}$), *LIG4* (DNA ligase IV), and *NHEJ1* (cernunnos) have all been confirmed to cause B-negative, NK-positive SCID in humans. Because artemis, $PK_{CS}$, DNA ligase IV, and cernunnos play vital DNA repair roles in other cell types, individuals with deficiencies of these proteins have radiosensitivity in addition to SCID. This additional feature must be recognized to minimize exposures to DNA-damaging processes, such as gamma radiation and alkylating agents, which are associated with poor growth, abnormal dental development, and late endocrinopathies in affected children.

B-positive, NK-positive SCID is caused by defects in molecules selective for T cell production. IL7Rα deficiency represents the most common cause of this SCID phenotype. Other examples include defects in components of the CD3 complex needed for T cell receptor signaling, such as CD3δ, CD3ε, and CD3ζ. In addition, deficiencies

**TABLE 184-1 EXAMPLES OF COMBINED CELLULAR AND HUMORAL IMMUNODEFICIENCIES**

| | Features | Associated Gene Defect(s) | Mode of Inheritance |
|---|---|---|---|
| **Severe Combined Immunodeficiency Disease (SCID)** | | | |
| T⁻B⁺NK⁻ | | *IL2RG* | XR |
| | | *JAK3* | AR |
| T⁻B⁻NK⁺ | | *RAG1* | AR |
| | | *RAG2* | AR |
| | Radiosensitivity | *DCLRE1C* | AR |
| | Radiosensitivity | *PRKDC* | AR |
| | Radiosensitivity, microcephaly | *LIG4* | AR |
| | Radiosensitivity, microcephaly | *NHEJ1* | AR |
| T⁻B⁺NK⁺ | | *IL7R* | AR |
| | | *CD3D* | AR |
| | | *CD3E* | AR |
| | | *CD247* | AR |
| | | *PTPRC* | AR |
| | Thymic shadow present | *CORO1A* | AR |
| T⁻B⁻NK⁻ | | *ADA* | AR |
| | Neutropenia, deafness | *AK2* | AR |
| **Combined Immunodeficiencies** | | | |
| Distinctive clinical features absent | | | |
| | MHC[a] class I deficiency | *TAP1, TAP2, TAPBP, B2M* | AR |
| | Other CD8+ T cell deficiency | *ZAP70* | AR |
| | MHC class II deficiency | *CIITA, RFX5, RFXANK, RFXAP* | AR |
| | Other CD4+ T cell deficiency | *MAGT1, LCK, UNC119* | XR (*MAGT1*), AR (*LCK*), AD (*UNC119*) |
| | Others | *CD3G, DOCK2, CARD11, MAP3K14, IKBKB, MALT1, BCL10* | AR |
| Distinctive clinical features present | | | |
| | Neutropenia | *CD40LG* | XR |
| | Atopic disease, cutaneous viral infections | *DOCK8* | AR |
| | Autoimmunity, inflammatory bowel disease | *LRBA* | AR |
| | Autoimmunity | *ICOS* | AR |
| | Autoimmunity, congenital heart disease | *STK4* | AR |
| | Kaposi sarcoma | *TNFRSF4* | AR |
| | Others | *ITK, CD27, CTPS1, TRAC, RHOH, IL21, IL21R* | AR |

[a]Major histocompatibility complex.

AD, autosomal dominant; AR, autosomal recessive; XR, X-linked recessive.

of CD45 and coronin 1A can lead to B-positive, NK-positive SCID. CD45 is a protein tyrosine phosphatase critical for regulation of T cell receptor signaling. Coronin 1A is necessary for T cell actin organization and egress from the thymus.

B-negative, NK-negative SCID is produced by molecular defects that impair overall lymphocyte survival. Adenosine deaminase (ADA) and adenylate kinase 2 (AK2) deficiencies provide key examples. ADA deficiency leads to failure to degrade purine metabolites in cells that are rapidly metabolizing and synthesizing DNA, such as lymphocytes. Accumulation of these metabolites causes induction of apoptosis and direct toxicity in these cells. Mitochondrial AK2, on the other hand, regulates transfer of phosphate groups between adenine nucleotides. Biallelic mutations in *AK2* result in reticular dysgenesis, a severe form of B-negative, NK-negative SCID that is accompanied by neutropenia and deafness.





Because of the severe absence of adaptive immune function in children with SCID, they must be recognized quickly to allow for prompt treatment. Before the advent of newborn screening for SCID, most affected children presented with a history of failure to thrive, recurrent infections, opportunistic infections by pathogens such as *Pneumocystis jirovecii*, or known family history. Other classic signs include lymphopenia, absence of a thymic shadow in chest radiographs (except in coronin 1A deficiency), lack of tonsils and other lymphatic tissues, and hypogammaglobulinemia. Newborn screening programs now use an assay based on quantification of DNA episomes formed during T cell receptor recombination to identify infants prior to onset of infectious complications. This process of early detection has become critical for permitting hematopoietic stem cell transplantation or gene therapy prior to 3.5 months of age and onset of active infections, both of which are known to be associated with increased mortality rates.

### COMBINED IMMUNODEFICIENCIES

CIDs are marked by decreased T- and B-cell function but fail to meet criteria for SCID. Thus, affected children may present at older ages with varying susceptibilities to certain infections. Broadly, these PIDs are distinguished by absence or presence of distinctive clinical features (see Table 184-1).

Various molecular defects are known to produce the CIDs that lack distinctive clinical features. Affected individuals carry susceptibilities to recurrent or opportunistic bacterial, viral, and fungal infections. Examples include *ZAP70* deficiency, which is characterized by low numbers of CD8+ T cells, and major histocompatibility complex (MHC) class I or class II deficiencies, which can cause lack of CD8+ or CD4+ T cells, respectively. These features often cannot be ascertained clinically but become discernible with immunologic testing.

At least 14 different molecular defects produce CIDs that are associated with recognizable clinical features and are listed in Table 184-1. For example, boys with mutations in *CD40L* classically demonstrate neutropenia and susceptibility to *P jirovecii* together with recurrent bacterial infections of the sinopulmonary tract. Some develop chronic diarrhea, failure to thrive, septicemia, meningitis, and other invasive infections. Affected patients often but not always have elevated serum IgM levels, conveying the disease nomenclature, *X-linked hyper-IgM syndrome*. Although the condition was once considered to be a humoral immunodeficiency, it is better recognized within this current category because the immunoglobulin class-switch defect results from defective CD40 ligand expression in T cells. Significant causes of long-term mortality include invasive infections, liver failure, and malignancy. Hepatic complications include sclerosing cholangitis, cirrhosis, and hepatocellular carcinoma and are associated with *Cryptosporidium parvum* infection from water parks or tap water. As another example within this category, individuals with deficiencies in dedicator of cytokinesis 8 (DOCK8) often have constellations of atopic disease, including elevated serum IgE levels and eosinophilia, along with susceptibility to herpesviral family, candidal, and staphylococcal infections. Affected persons also have increased risk for developing autoimmunity and malignancies, particularly squamous cell carcinomas or lymphomas.

## CID WITH SYNDROMIC OR OTHER ASSOCIATED FEATURES

A separate category exists for syndromic CIDs, which are generally associated with T cell defects (Table 184-2). These conditions underscore the fact that some children with PIDs may initially come to medical attention and be evaluated by providers in other subspecialties for issues other than recurrent infections. The CIDs are further subdivided into several groups based on associated features.

**TABLE 184-2 EXAMPLES OF COMBINED IMMUNODEFICIENCIES WITH SYNDROMIC OR OTHER ASSOCIATED FEATURES**

| | | Associated Gene Defect(s) | Mode of Inheritance |
|---|---|---|---|
| DNA repair defects | | *ATM, NBN, BLM, DNMT3B, ZBTB24, PMS2, RNF168, MCM4* | AR |
| Congenital thrombocytopenia | | *WAS, WIPF1* | XR (*WAS*), AR (*WIPF1*) |
| Thymic defects | DiGeorge anomaly | 22q11.2 deletion, others or none | |
| | Others | *FOXN1, CHD7, SEMA3E* | AR (*FOXN1*), AD (*CHD7, SEMA3E*) |
| Hyper-IgE syndromes | | *STAT3, SPINK5, PGM3* | AD (*STAT3*), AR (*SPINK5, PGM3*) |
| Immuno-osseous dysplasias | | *RMRP, SMARCAL1* | AR |
| Bone marrow failure syndromes | | *DKC1, TERC, TINF2, RTEL1, TERT, ACD, PARN, NOLA2, NOLA3, DCLRE1B* | XR (*DKC1*), AD (*TERC, TINF2*), AR (*NOLA2, NOLA3, DCLRE1B*), AD or AR (*RTEL1, TERT, ACD, PARN*) |
| Ectodermal dysplasias | | *IKBKG, IKBA* GOF, *ORAI1, STIM1* | XR (*IKBKG*), AD (*IKBA*), AR (*ORAI1, STIM1*) |
| Others | | *PNP, EPG5, CCBE1, SP110, RBCK1, TTC7A, POLE, STAT5B, TCN2, SLC46A1, MTHFD1* | AR |

AD, autosomal dominant; AR, autosomal recessive; GOF, gain of function; XR, X-linked recessive.

The first group consists of children with CIDs caused by defects in DNA repair. Associated features include radiation sensitivity, increased risk for developing a malignancy, facial dysmorphism or microcephaly, and neurologic disease. Ataxia-telangiectasia represents a classic example of PID that falls into this category. Affected children typically present with progressive cerebellar ataxia at around 2 years of age. Telangiectasias of the bulbar conjunctiva appear later, when patients are older. In most children with this condition, serum α-fetoprotein levels are elevated, providing a useful laboratory test for evaluation.

The next group includes children with congenital thrombocytopenia, for which Wiskott-Aldrich syndrome (WAS) serves as the archetypal example. The condition classically presents with the triad of recurrent infections, eczema, and thrombocytopenia, although only a minority of affected children exhibit all 3 features. Almost all individuals with WAS have microthrombocytopenia, which is nearly pathognomic for the diagnosis. Many exhibit poor or absent antibody responses to polysaccharide antigens. The disease is caused by highly deleterious mutations in *WAS*, which is encoded on the X chromosome. Hypomorphic mutations in *WAS* can result in X-linked thrombocytopenia, whereas *WAS* gain-of-function mutations are associated with X-linked neutropenia. Female carriers with severe lyonization of the X chromosome have been known to manifest characteristics of the disease. WAS also conveys increased risk for development of autoimmunity and malignancy, often before 10 years of age.

Thymic defects constitute an important third group within this category of PIDs, and DiGeorge anomaly offers the most well-recognized condition within this classification scheme. DiGeorge anomaly is characterized by variable defects of the heart, parathyroid glands, and thymus. The diagnosis is established clinically and not genetically, as fewer than 60% of affected individuals have 22q11.2 hemizygosity. The vast majority of infants are born with thymic hypoplasia to varying degrees and not aplasia, resulting in a spectrum of immunodeficiencies. Thus, children with DiGeorge anomaly merit immunologic evaluation to characterize their immune function and susceptibility to infectious agents, such as live viral immunizations. In as many as 2% of cases, full athymia is present, resulting in absent T- and B-cell function. These infants display the phenotype of SCID and carry the associated risk of early life mortality. Individuals with DiGeorge anomaly also typically have neurocognitive deficiencies and increased risk for autoimmunity.

The fourth group consists of the hyper-IgE syndromes (HIES), which (unlike atopic diseases) are characterized by recurrent skin abscesses or bacterial or fungal respiratory tract infections in addition to elevated serum IgE levels. The most prevalent known cause of HIES results from autosomal dominant deleterious mutations in *STAT3*. Other classic features of deficiency in signal transducer and activator of transcription 3 (STAT3) include broad nasal bridge, delayed shedding of the primary teeth, hyperextensible joints, and osteoporosis. Affected individuals exhibit significant susceptibility to *Staphylococcus aureus*. They tend to form pneumatoceles after pulmonary infections and have chronic mucocutaneous candidiasis (CMC) due to absence of $T_H17$ cells, which is nearly pathognomic for the diagnosis.

Other groups fall into the category of CID with syndromic or other associated features. Immuno-osseous dysplasias are characterized by short stature and skeletal abnormalities in addition to immune deficiency. The dyskeratosis congenita PIDs share the feature of bone marrow failure and pancytopenia. Additional traits may be present, depending on the molecular defect. Finally, a number of other less common syndromic CIDs are listed in Table 184-2. Deficiency of nuclear factor κ-B essential modulator (NEMO) is included in this list and classically presents with ectodermal dysplasia, recurrent pyogenic and mycobacterial infections, humoral immunodeficiency, and elevated serum IgM levels. Colitis also may develop. Some patients do not have ectodermal dysplasia or high IgM levels, so absence of these features cannot be used to exclude the diagnosis. The disease is caused by mutations in *IKBKG*, located on the X chromosome. Most mutations in this gene are lethal for male fetuses, and female carriers of *IKBKG* mutations can have incontinentia pigmenti. Because *IKBKG* is difficult to sequence, functional tests often are required to establish the diagnosis.

## DEFECTS PREDOMINANTLY IN B CELL FUNCTION OR NUMBER

Several PIDs are caused by defective B-cell function or regulation (Table 184-3). B-cell function is required for production of specific antibodies to pathogens. Thus, affected individuals are notably susceptible to bacterial infections, particularly of the sinopulmonary tract. Several of the more common PIDs within this category deserve further discussion.

Boys with X-linked agammaglobulinemia (XLA) are often healthy after birth due to the presence of transplacentally acquired maternal IgG. As maternal antibodies diminish, chronic or recurrent infections develop. The most common findings include recurrent otitis media, sinusitis, pneumonia, and diarrhea, but infections are not limited to mucosal surfaces. Bacteremia, meningitis, and osteomyelitis also may occur. *Mycoplasma* species infections have been implicated as a cause of a subacute, destructive arthritis, and gastrointestinal infections may be caused by *Salmonella, Shigella, Campylobacter,* or rotavirus. Chronic giardiasis with intestinal malabsorption has been observed. Affected individuals also importantly demonstrate increased risk for development of enteroviral meningoencephalitis. The defective gene (*BTK*) maps to the X chromosome and encodes a protein (Bruton's tyrosine kinase) that is a signal transduction molecule necessary for B-cell survival during maturation. Thus, XLA is marked by the absence of circulating B cells.

Common variable immunodeficiency disease (CVID) constitutes a heterogenous group of disorders that present with antibody deficiency. CVID is strictly defined using diagnostic criteria established by the European Society for Immunodeficiencies (Table 184-4). Two peaks for diagnosis have been observed: one during childhood and

**TABLE 184-3 DEFECTS PREDOMINANTLY IN B-CELL FUNCTION OR NUMBER**

| | Associated Gene Defect(s) | Mode of Inheritance |
|---|---|---|
| Absent B cells | *BTK* | XR |
| | *IGHM, CD79A, CD79B, BLNK, IGLL1, PIK3R1, GATA2* | AR |
| | *TCF7L1* | AD |
| Common variable immunodeficiency disorders | *TNFRSF13C, CD19, MS4A1, CR2, CD81* | AR |
| | *TNFRSF13B, TNFSF12, NFKB2* | AD |
| Autosomal recessive hyper-IgM syndromes | *AICDA, UNG* | AR |
| Congenital B-cell lymphocytosis | *CARD11* | AR |
| Others | *TRNT1, TTC37, MOGS, INO80, MSH6, IGKC* | AR |
| | *PIK3CD* GOF, *PIK3R1* GOF | AD |
| Selective IgA deficiency | None | |
| Transient hypogammaglobulinemia of infancy | None | |
| Specific antibody deficiency | None | |

AD, autosomal dominant; AR, autosomal recessive; GOF, gain of function; XR, X-linked recessive.

another between 30 and 40 years of age. In addition to recurrent bacterial infections of the sinopulmonary tract, noninfectious complications can arise over time. Affected individuals have increased risk for developing enteropathy or inflammatory bowel disease, autoimmunity, lymphoproliferative disease, and granulomatous disease. The latter 2 complications can manifest as lymphoid interstitial pneumonia, nodular lymphoid hyperplasia, splenomegaly, or lymphadenopathy. Numerous genetic defects have been associated with CVID (see Table 184-3).

IgA deficiency represents the most common PID. Among the Caucasian population, it appears at a frequency of 1 in 300 to 1 in 1200 persons. The vast majority of individuals with IgA deficiency are clinically asymptomatic, but some affected persons can develop recurrent infections of the respiratory tract or gastrointestinal tract.

**TABLE 184-4 COMMON VARIABLE IMMUNODEFICIENCY DISEASE DIAGNOSTIC CRITERIA**

At least 1 of the following:

- Increased susceptibility to infection
- Autoimmune manifestations
- Granulomatous disease
- Unexplained polyclonal lymphoproliferation
- Affected family member with antibody deficiency

AND marked decrease of IgG and marked decrease of IgA with or without low IgM levels (measured at least twice; less than 2 standard deviations below the normal levels for age)

AND at least 1 of the following:

- Poor antibody response to vaccines (and/or absent isohemagglutinins)
- Low switched memory B cells (<70% of the age-related normal value)

AND secondary causes of hypogammaglobulinemia have been excluded

AND diagnosis is established after the fourth year of life (although symptoms may present before that age)

AND no evidence of severe T cell deficiency, defined as 2 out of the following:

- CD4+ cells/μL: 2–6 years old < 300, 6–12 years old < 250, older than 12 years < 200
- Naive CD4+ %: 2–6 years old < 25, 6–16 years old < 20, older than 16 years < 10
- Significantly decreased T cell proliferation to stimulation

The condition is also associated with increased risk for autoimmunity. IgA deficiency is defined as the presence of serum IgA levels less than 7 mg/dL with normal IgG and IgM levels in individuals 4 years of age or older. More than 20% of children between 4 and 10 years of age who meet criteria for a diagnosis of IgA deficiency no longer have serum IgA levels below 7 mg/dL when they become adolescents. Thus, the diagnosis should be conferred with caution in the pediatric population. In terms of etiology, the pathogenesis of IgA deficiency has not been determined. Some individuals with selective IgA deficiency subsequently develop CVID, and variations in *TNFRSF13B* and *ICOS* genes have been found in families with members that have either of these conditions. IgG replacement therapy is not indicated for the treatment of patients with selective IgA deficiency. Patients with IgA-deficiency carry a small risk for development of IgE-mediated anaphylaxis if sensitized to IgA and given an IgA-containing blood product that is estimated to range between 1 in 20,000 and 1 in 47,000 transfusions. Thus, broad and routine restriction of Patients with IgA-deficiency against receiving IgA-containing blood products is not recommended.

Infants with transient hypogammaglobulinemia of infancy (THI) may come to medical attention because of recurrent respiratory tract infections and serum immunoglobulin levels below laboratory normal ranges. Septicemia, meningitis, skin infections, and other invasive infections very rarely occur. THI is caused by delayed physiologic maturation of immunoglobulin synthesis, resulting in prolongation of the relative hypogammaglobulinemia ("physiologic nadir") observed in most normal infants at 3 to 6 months of age as maternal IgG leaves the circulation. No well-established molecular etiology has been identified. Patients with THI are able to produce protective, specific, antibody responses, and more than 80% of children with THI recover to normal immunoglobulin levels by 3 years of age. Thus, because THI is self-limited and specific antibody production is normal, IgG replacement therapy is not indicated.

## DISEASES OF IMMUNE DYSREGULATION

This category includes hemophagocytic lymphohistiocytosis (HLH), other lymphoproliferative diseases, syndromes with prominent autoimmune features, colitides, and type 1 interferonopathies (Table 184-5). Because the immune dysregulation in these conditions may not necessarily lead to recurrent infections, PID should not be excluded as a potential diagnosis in children who have these disorders yet lack a history of frequent episodes of infection.

HLH is defined by criteria that specify either the identification of a genetic defect or the presence of certain clinical features (Table 184-6). Thus, absence of an identified genetic defect should not exclude the diagnosis if an affected individual meets the necessary clinical criteria. Key pathogenic mechanisms include impaired lymphocyte cytotoxicity and dysregulated production of inflammatory cytokine. Poor prognosis is associated with delayed diagnosis, age younger than 6 months, development of neurologic disease or hepatomegaly, and very high serum ferritin levels or failure of ferritin levels to decline rapidly during treatment.

Epstein-Barr virus (EBV)-associated lymphoproliferative diseases represent defects in control of EBV infection and can be associated with development of HLH. The most well-characterized PID within this category is X-linked lymphoproliferative syndrome (XLP), which is caused by mutations in *SH2D1A*. Affected boys have significant risk for development of severe or fulminant infectious mononucleosis and B-cell lymphoma. Absence of the invariant NKT-cell subset serves as a useful screening test for this disease.

PIDs that result in immune dysregulation can lead to autoimmunity with and without lymphoproliferation. Autoimmune lymphoproliferative syndrome (ALPS) is characterized by lymphadenopathy, splenomegaly, autoimmune cytopenias, and increased risk for developing B-cell lymphomas. The condition usually is caused by defects in *FAS* or *FASLG*, leading to defective lymphocyte apoptosis. Several other ALPS-related disorders have been described that exhibit other extraproliferative manifestations. Somatic activating mutations in *TNFRSF6*, *NRAS*, and *KRAS* can produce phenocopies of ALPS.

**TABLE 184-5 DISEASES OF IMMUNE DYSREGULATION**

| | | Associated Gene Defect(s) | Mode of Inheritance |
|---|---|---|---|
| Hemophagocytic lymphohistiocytosis | | *PRF1, UNC13D, STXBP2, STX11, LYST, RAB27A, AP3B1, BLOC1S6* | AR |
| Other lymphoproliferative diseases | | *SH2D1A, XIAP* | XR |
| Syndromes with prominent autoimmune features | Autoimmune lymphoproliferative syndrome | *FAS, FASLG, CASP10, CTLA4* | AD |
| | | *CASP8, FADD* | AR |
| | Others | *AIRE, IL2RA, ITCH, TPP2* | AR |
| | | *FOXP3* | XR |
| | | *STAT3* GOF | AD |
| Colitides | | *IL10, IL10RA, IL10RB* | AR |
| | | *NFAT5* | AD |
| Type 1 interferonopathies | Aicardi-Goutieres | *TREX1, RNASEH2A, RNASEH2B, RNASEH2C, SAMHD1, ADAR, IFIH1* | AD or AR (*TREX1*), AD (*IFIH1*), AR (the rest) |
| | | *ACP5, CECR1* | AR |
| | | *TMEM173* | AD |

AD, autosomal dominant; AR, autosomal recessive; GOF, gain of function; XR, X-linked recessive.

Individuals with ALPS are known to have high percentages of αβ T cells in the circulation that express neither CD4 nor CD8, elevated levels of IL-10 in the blood, and increased serum levels of vitamin $B_{12}$. Examples of immune dysregulation without lymphoproliferation include *AIRE* and *FOXP3* deficiencies. *AIRE* encodes the autoimmune regulator protein, which is necessary for proper negative selection of T cells in the thymus. Biallelic mutations in *AIRE* lead to autoimmune polyendocrinopathy-candidiasis-ectodermal dystrophy (APECED), a PID characterized by CMC, hypoparathyroidism, and Addison disease. Mutations in *FOXP3* on the X chromosome, on the other hand, produce immune dysregulation-polyendocrinopathy-enteropathy X-linked syndrome (IPEX). The disease results from failure to generate regulatory T cells. Key manifestations include enteropathy, type 1 diabetes, autoimmune cytopenias, thyroid disease, eczema, food allergies, and recurrent infections.

**TABLE 184-6 HEMOPHAGOCYTIC LYMPHOHISTIOCYTOSIS (HLH) DIAGNOSTIC CRITERIA**

Molecular diagnosis consistent with HLH

OR 5 of the following criteria:

- Fever ≥ 38°C
- Splenomegaly
- Cytopenias affecting at least 2 of 3 lineages:
  - Hemoglobin < 90 g/L (< 100 g/L in infants under 4 weeks of age)
  - Platelets < 100 × $10^9$/L
  - Neutrophils < 1.0 × $10^9$/L
- Hypertriglyceridemia and/or hypofibrinogenemia:
  - Fasting triglycerides ≥ 265 mg/dL
  - Fibrinogen ≤ 1.5 g/L
- Hemophagocytosis in bone marrow, spleen, or lymph nodes
- Low or absent NK cell activity
- Ferritin ≥ 500 μg/L
- Soluble CD25 ≥ 2400 U/mL

Immune dysregulation with colitis is exemplified by defects in the IL-10 signaling pathway. IL-10 is a key anti-inflammatory cytokine that inhibits many immunologic processes. Mutations in *IL10, IL10RA*, and *IL10RB* lead to early-onset inflammatory bowel disease that tends to be resistant to most forms of immunosuppression. Affected individuals can develop severe perianal disease and fistulas. The condition can be treated successfully with hematopoietic stem cell transplantation, emphasizing the need to establish the diagnosis in children who have early-onset inflammatory bowel disease.

## PHAGOCYTIC CELL DEFECTS

This category consists of PIDs caused by congenital defects in phagocyte number or function (Table 184-7). Congenital neutropenia can occur with or without syndromic features and includes the severe congenital neutropenia diseases and cyclic neutropenia. Severe congenital neutropenia is characterized by arrest of granulocyte maturation, markedly decreased numbers of circulating granulocytes, and severe infection. Cyclic neutropenia is an autosomal dominant defect of myelopoiesis in which periodic disappearance of granulocytes from the circulation occurs. The condition can result from mutations in *ELANE*. Periods of neutropenia usually last 5 to 7 days and occur at 14- to 35-day intervals, and the length of the cycle generally remains constant for any given person. Fever and malaise are often observed during periods of neutropenia. Affected individuals also demonstrate more frequent episodes of aphthous stomatitis, pneumonia, abscesses, sepsis, cellulitis, and peritonitis. Certain mutations in *ELANE* appear to predispose to development of myelodysplasia or acute myeloid leukemia. Defects of phagocytic function include chronic granulomatous disease (CGD) and leukocyte adhesion deficiency (LAD), both of which warrant further discussion.

CGD is caused by mutations in genes that encode components of the nicotinamide adenine dinucleotide phosphate oxidase (NADPH oxidase) complex system. The most common defect occurs in $gp91^{phox}$, which is encoded by *CYBB* on the X chromosome and accounts for almost two-thirds of cases of CGD. Mutations in genes responsible for the other components produce autosomal recessive CGD. $p47^{phox}$ deficiency accounts for 25% of cases of CGD. Defective NADPH oxidase function leads to failure to generate the respiratory burst needed for killing of phagocytized organisms, particularly catalase-positive microbes. Classic pathogens include *S aureus, Burkholderia cepacia, Serratia marcescens, Klebsiella pneumoniae, Nocardia*, and *Aspergillus* species. Of note, affected individuals do not harbor candidal susceptibility. Inappropriate production of reactive oxygen species is also thought to contribute toward dysregulated inflammation,

**TABLE 184-7 PHAGOCYTIC CELL DEFECTS**

| | | Associated Gene Defect(s) | Mode of Inheritance |
|---|---|---|---|
| Neutropenia | Nonsyndromic | *ELANE* | AD |
| | | *HAX1, JAGN1, CSF3R* | AR |
| | | *WAS* | XR |
| | Syndromic | *SBDS, G6PC3, VPS45, SLC37A4, VPS13B, C16ORF57, LAMTOR2, CLPB* | AR |
| | | *TAZ* | XR |
| Functional defects | Chronic granulomatous disease | *CYBB* | XR |
| | | *NCF1, NCF2, NCF4, CYBA* | AR |
| | Leukocyte adhesion deficiency | *ITGB2, SLC35C1, FERMT3* | AR |
| | Others | *CTSC, CEBPE* | AR |
| | | *RAC2, FPR1, ACTB* | AD |
| | | *CSF2RA* | XR |

AD, autosomal dominant; AR, autosomal recessive; XR, X-linked recessive.

resulting in noninfectious complications. Children with CGD most often present with infections of the lungs, skin, lymph nodes, and liver. Affected individuals also exhibit susceptibility to soft tissue abscesses, perirectal abscesses, central nervous system infections, and osteomyelitis. Many infections are caused by unusual (often unidentifiable) organisms, which can be pathognomonic for the diagnosis. Poor wound healing can be observed, and granulomatous obstructive lesions of the urinary and gastrointestinal tracts occur. More than 40% of patients with X-linked CGD develop an inflammatory bowel disease that mimics Crohn disease. Hepatic dysfunction can lead to portal hypertension, splenomegaly, and splenic sequestration. A small percentage of boys with X-linked CGD also have the McLeod blood phenotype, characterized by absence of the Kell antigen in red blood cells as a consequence of a contiguous gene deletion, which results in difficult cross-matching for blood transfusion and the potential for hemolytic transfusion reactions. Female carriers of a *CYBB* mutation can develop inflammatory or autoimmune clinical features, such as photosensitivity, autoimmune arthritis, discoid lupus erythematosus, aphthous stomatitis, Raynaud phenomenon, inflammatory colitis, and chorioretinitis. In terms of diagnosis, the nitroblue tetrazolium (NBT) test has been replaced by the flow cytometry–based dihydrorhodamine (DHR) assay. Falsely abnormal DHR test results can be observed in individuals who have myeloperoxidase deficiency, SAPHO (synovitis, acne, pustulosis, hyperostosis, and osteitis) syndrome, G6PD deficiency, or neutrophils that are highly activated due to significant infection. In terms of other laboratory testing, elevated erythrocyte sedimentation rates and C-reactive protein levels should warrant concern for infection. Serum galactomannan and 1,3-β-D-glucan levels may not be useful for assessing fungal infections. Prognosis remains variable and depends on the level of residual superoxide production.

Three types of LAD have been reported, caused by mutations in *ITGB2*, *SLC35C1*, and *FERMT3*. These defects lead to impaired leukocyte adherence, chemotaxis, and phagocytosis. Affected individuals develop severe and recurrent bacterial infections of the skin and soft tissues, mucosal surfaces, and gastrointestinal tract, often beginning during early infancy. A classic early presentation includes delayed separation of the umbilical cord that is associated with omphalitis. Later cutaneous infections manifest as non purulent, inflamed tissues that often become necrotic, resembling ecthyma gangrenosum or pyoderma gangrenosum. Absence of purulence is a hallmark feature of the disease. Poor wound healing, severe gingivitis, and periodontitis with progressive alveolar bone loss also occur. Affected individuals classically demonstrate marked leukocytosis. Circulating neutrophil counts may range between 15,000/μL and 75,000/μL, even in the absence of infection; and counts of 100,000/μL or greater can be observed during infections.

## OTHER INNATE AND INTRINSIC IMMUNITY DEFECTS

This PID category includes molecular defects that affect other elements of innate or intrinsic immune function (Table 184-8). Many are characterized by classic susceptibility to certain organisms and highlight defects in key mechanisms of immune function.

**TABLE 184-8 OTHER INNATE AND INTRINSIC IMMUNITY DEFECTS**

| | | Associated Gene Defect(s) | Mode of Inheritance |
|---|---|---|---|
| Susceptibilities to invasive pyogenic bacteria | | *IRAK4, MYD88, RPSA* | AR (*IRAK4, MYD88*), AD (*RPSA*) |
| Viral susceptibilities | Herpes simplex encephalitis | *UNC93B1, TLR3, TICAM1* | AR |
| | | *TLR3, TICAM1, TRAF3, TBK1* | AD |
| | Human papillomavirus | *CXCR4* GOF, *TMC6, TMC8* | AD (*CXCR4*), AR (*TMC6, TMC8*) |
| | Influenza | *IRF7* | AR |
| | Others | *STAT1* LOF, *STAT2, FCGR3A* | AR |
| Susceptibility to trypanosomes | | *APOL1* | AD |
| Fungal susceptibilities | Chronic mucocutaneous candidiasis | *STAT1* GOF, *IL17F* | AD |
| | | *IL17RA, IL17RC* | AR |
| | Others | *CARD9, TRAF3IP2* | AR |
| Susceptibility to mycobacteria | MSMD | *IFNGR1* | AD |
| | | *IFNGR1, IFNGR2, IL12B, IL12RB1, ISG15, TYK2* | AR |
| | Others | *IRF8, RORC* | AD and AR (*IRF8*), AR (*RORC*) |

AD, autosomal dominant; AR, autosomal recessive; GOF, gain of function; LOF, loss of function; MSMD, Mendelian susceptibility to mycobacterial disease; XR, X-linked recessive.

Children with defects in interleukin-1 receptor-associated kinase 4 (IRAK-4) and myeloid differentiation primary response protein 88 (MyD88) are characterized by invasive infections by pyogenic bacteria, classically unaccompanied by fever. These 2 adaptor molecules mediate signaling downstream from all Toll-like receptors (TLRs) except TLR3 and partially TLR4. Infections are most commonly caused by *S aureus*, *S pneumoniae*, and gram-negative bacteria. IRAK-4 and MyD88 deficiencies do not lead to increased susceptibility to mycobacteria, viruses, fungi, or *Pneumocystis*. These PIDs lead to high mortality rates in infants and children, but the rate of infections decreases markedly over time in survivors for reasons that remain unclear.

Several PIDs within this category result in susceptibilities to specific viruses. Numerous genetic defects are associated with development of herpes simplex encephalitis (see Table 184-8), which all have in common the ability to produce interferon-λ from the innate immune system. Autosomal dominant gain-of-function mutations in *CXCR4* result in warts, hypogammaglobulinemia, infections, and myelokathexis (WHIM) syndrome. This condition is characterized by neutropenia, B-cell lymphopenia, and low serum levels of IgG or IgM or both, leading to recurrent sinopulmonary, urinary tract, cutaneous, and invasive bacterial infections. In individuals with WHIM syndrome, human papillomavirus (HPV) infections can progress to malignancy. Disseminated cutaneous HPV infection can also develop in persons with biallelic mutations in *TMC6* or *TMC8*.

Autosomal dominant gain-of-function mutations in *STAT1* fall within this category of innate immunity defects. Hyperactive STAT1 function can produce a broad phenotype, including CMC, which is almost universally present. Affected individuals also demonstrate increased susceptibility to staphylococcal and herpesviral family infections. The condition is associated with higher risk for autoimmunity, and IPEX-like disease has been reported. On the other hand, patients have been described who exhibit solely a CVID-like phenotype. In a small percentage of affected individuals, cerebral aneurysms and malignancies can develop and portend a poor prognosis.

Although a significant number of PIDs confer impaired clearance of mycobacterial organisms within their phenotypic spectra, the molecular defects that cause Mendelian susceptibility to mycobacterial disease (MSMD) constitute a specific set of disorders that provide key insights into important immune mechanisms. Affected individuals classically present with disseminated or unusual infections from weakly virulent strains of mycobacterial organisms, such as bacillus Calmette-Guérin vaccine and atypical mycobacteria. In the normal immune response, these microbes are phagocytized by macrophages, which elicits production of IL-12. The cytokine binds to IL-12 receptors on T and NK cells, which results in production of interferon (IFN)-γ. IFN-γ then activates receptors on the macrophages, prompting killing of the internalized organisms. In homologous and autologous manners, the IFN-γ also binds to IFN-γ receptors on nearby T and NK cells and on the IFN-γ–secreting cells themselves to amplify the immune response. MSMD has been shown to be caused by genetic defects that impair production of IL-12 by macrophages, IL-12 receptor function in T and NK cells, and IFN-γ receptor function in all 3 cell types. The specific molecular defect must be identified in affected cases, as IL-12 and IL-12 receptor deficiencies can be treated with IFN-γ supplementation whereas individuals with IFN-γ receptor deficiencies do not respond to this therapy.

## AUTOINFLAMMATORY DISEASES

Autoinflammatory diseases include the periodic fevers syndromes, systemic inflammatory diseases with urticaria, sterile inflammation syndromes, and others (Table 184-9). This category possesses a remarkable number of autosomal dominant genetic defects. Many of these disorders are caused by defective inflammasome activity. The periodic fevers syndromes are characterized by recurrent fevers that appear for a given duration of time at distinct intervals, each according to the molecular defect. Autosomal dominant mutations in *NLRP3*, *NLRP12*, and *PLCG2* are responsible for the systemic inflammatory disorders with urticaria. Several diseases fall into the group of sterile inflammation syndromes, including Majeed syndrome, Blau syndrome, deficiency of IL-1 receptor antagonist (DIRA), and pyogenic arthritis-pyoderma gangrenosum-acne (PAPA). Others include CANDLE syndrome, *NLRC4* deficiency, and *COPA* deficiency.

**TABLE 184-9 AUTOINFLAMMATORY DISEASES**

| | | Associated Gene Defect(s) | Mode of Inheritance |
|---|---|---|---|
| Periodic fevers syndromes | Familial Mediterranean fever | *MEFV* | AD and AR |
| | Hyper-IgD syndrome | *MVK* | AR |
| | TNF receptor associated periodic syndrome (TRAPS) | *TNFRSF1A* | AD |
| Systemic inflammatory diseases with urticaria | Familial cold auto-inflammatory syndrome | *NLRP3, NLRP12* | AD |
| | Muckle-Wells syndrome | *NLRP3* | AD |
| | Neonatal-onset multisystem inflammatory disease (NOMID/CINCA) | *NLRP3* | AD |
| | PLCG2-associated antibody deficiency and immune dysregulation (PLAID) | *PLCG2* | AD |
| | Autoinflammation and PLAID (APLAID) | *PLCG2* | AD |
| Sterile inflammation syndromes | Blau syndrome | *NOD2* | AD |
| | Majeed syndrome | *LPIN2* | AR |
| | Deficiency of IL-1 receptor antagonist (DIRA) | *IL1RN* | AR |
| | Deficiency of IL-36 receptor antagonist (DITRA) | *IL36RN* | AR |
| | Pyogenic arthritis-pyoderma gangrenosum-acne (PAPA) | *PSTPIP1* | AD |
| | CARD14-mediated pustular psoriasis (CAMPS) | *CARD14* | AD |
| | Others | *ADAM17* | AR |
| Others | Chronic atypical neutrophilic dermatosis with lipodystrophy and elevated temperature (CANDLE) | *PSMB8* | AR |
| | COPA syndrome | *COPA* | AD |
| | Others | *NLRC4* | AD |

AD, autosomal dominant; AR, autosomal recessive; TNF, tumor necrosis factor; XR, X-linked recessive.

*COPA* deficiency particularly represents a relatively novel PID that is characterized by dysregulated inflammatory responses, leading to the constellation of renal disease, pulmonary hemorrhage, interstitial lung disease, and arthritis. The condition is caused by autosomal dominant mutations in *COPA* that can present with variable penetrance. Affected individuals develop autoantibodies, such as elevated antinuclear antibody (ANA), cytoplasmic anti-neutrophil cytoplasmic antibody (c-ANCA), and perinuclear ANCA (p-ANCA) titers. CD4+ T cells are skewed toward the $T_H17$ cell phenotype. Pathogenesis involves defective retrograde transport of vesicles from the Golgi to the endoplasmic reticulum, which results in endoplasmic reticulum stress and autophagy. This syndrome demonstrates the potential for future discoveries of additional PIDs associated with defects in cellular transport processes.

## EVALUATION AND TESTING OF CHILDREN WITH SUSPECTED PID

A comprehensive medical history remains essential for identifying children with a defective immune response. Many PIDs are characterized by a history of frequent or severe infections. An infection by an unusual organism or an unusual infectious course may also suggest the presence of an underlying PID. As noted in different parts of this chapter, specific organisms themselves can lead to infections that are associated with certain PIDs.

A variety of laboratory tests are widely available for screening for the presence of a PID and include complete blood count with differential, serum immunoglobulin levels, and specific antibody titers to different immunizations. These tests must be interpreted according to age-defined ranges, because many immunologic parameters change over time, especially in children. Specialized tests, such as lymphocyte phenotyping and proliferation assays, are also available from a number of clinical immunology laboratories.

Genetic testing is being used more routinely for diagnosis of PIDs. Targeted sequencing of specific genes can be pursued if a focused number of defects are suspected. Otherwise, because the primary features of many PIDs overlap and can sometimes result from any one of dozens of genetic defects, whole-exome sequencing (WES) provides an excellent diagnostic option for many individuals. WES has been shown to not only enhance diagnosis of PIDs but also favorably impact treatment. Interpretation of all genetic testing results remains a challenge, and testing of unaffected family members remains key for demonstrating whether autosomal-dominant variants have *arisen de novo or* compound heterozygous variants are truly biallelic. For almost all PIDs, identification of a specific gene defect can help to determine prognosis and therapeutic options. Securing a genetic diagnosis is also necessary for genetic counseling purposes. Presently, this testing can be achieved clinically by the targeted sequence analysis of individual suspected genes (direct Sanger sequencing), panels of immunologically relevant/related genes (next-generation sequencing), or WES. The decision of which sequencing modality to choose should depend on the likelihood of any 1 approach achieving the answer in light of the pretest probability for the condition(s) balanced with the time to receive the result and cost to the patient all within the context of the particular clinical diagnostic urgency.

## THERAPY

A variety of therapeutic options are available for treatment of PIDs, many of which exist beyond the scope of this chapter. Some affected individuals require only immunoglobulin replacement, whereas hematopoietic stem cell transplantation serves as the treatment of choice for many other PIDs. Allogeneic thymus transplantation provides an excellent option for treatment of congenital athymia, such as present in complete DiGeorge anomaly. Finally, gene therapy carries enormous potential for definitive treatment of PIDs in the future.

## SUMMARY

PIDs are becoming better recognized and are no longer considered rare diseases. The list of known genetic defects that cause these conditions continues to expand and evolve. Thus, awareness of the broad spectrum of phenotypic presentations associated with these disorders remains critical for optimal diagnosis and management of pediatric patients.

## SUGGESTED READINGS


Bonilla FA, Barlan I, Chapel H, et al. International Consensus Document (ICON): common variable immunodeficiency disorders. *J Allerg Clin Immunol Pract.* 2016;4(1):38-59.

Bonilla FA, Khan DA, Ballas ZK, et al. Practice parameter for the diagnosis and management of primary immunodeficiency. *J Allerg Clin Immunol.* 2015;136(5):1186-1205.

Booth C, Gaspar HB, Thrasher AJ. Treating immunodeficiency through HSC gene therapy. *Trends Mol Med.* 2016;22(4):317-327.

Bousfiha A, Jeddane L, Al-Herz W, et al. The 2015 IUIS phenotypic classification for primary immunodeficiencies. *J Clin Immunol.* 2015;35:727-738.

Chinn IK, Shearer WT. Severe combined immunodeficiency disorders. *Immunol Allergy Clin North Am.* 2015;35(4):671-694.

Kwan A, Abraham RS, Currier R, et al. Newborn screening for severe combined immunodeficiency in 11 screening programs in the United States. *JAMA.* 2014;312(7):729-738.

Lehman H, Hernandez-Trujillo V, Ballow M. Diagnosing primary immunodeficiency: a practical approach for the non-immunologist. *Curr Med Res Opin.* 2015;31(4):697-706.

Pai S-Y, Cowan MJ. Stem cell transplantation for primary immunodeficiency diseases: the North American experience. *Curr Opin Allergy Clin Immunol.* 2014;14(6):521-526.

Pai S-Y, Logan BR, Griffith LM, et al. Transplantation outcomes for severe combined immunodeficiency, 2000–2009. *N Engl J Med.* 2014;371(5):434-446.

Routes J, Abinun M, Al-Herz W, et al. ICON: the early diagnosis of congenital immunodeficiencies. *J Clin Immunol.* 2014;34(4):398-424.

Stray-Pedersen A, Sorte HS, Gambin T, et al. Primary immunodeficiency diseases: genomic approaches delineate heterogenous Mendelian disorders. *J Allergy Clin Immunol.* 2017;139(1):232-245.


# 185 Hematopoietic Stem Cell Transplantation for Primary Immune Deficiencies

Luigi D. Notarangelo

## INTRODUCTION

Primary immune deficiencies (PIDs) comprise more than 250 distinct disorders that affect the immune system's development, function, and/or homeostasis. Inability to control infections represents a major challenge in several forms of PID, leading to increased incidences of mortality early in life. Furthermore, *immune dysregulation*, defined as disorders of immune homeostasis presenting with autoimmunity or inflammatory disease, is increasingly being recognized as an important manifestation of various forms of PID and may also affect quality and duration of life. In the majority of cases, PIDs result from genetic defects that are intrinsic to the hematopoietic system. When associated with a poor prognosis, such forms of PID can be treated and cured with allogeneic hematopoietic stem cell transplantation (HCT). However, despite continuous advances in donor selection, development of less toxic chemotherapy preparatory regimens, supportive care, and prevention of transplant-related complications, mortality and late effects continue to affect the outcomes of patients with PIDs treated with HCT. In this chapter, we will review the current status of HCT for PIDs and discuss possible developments in the field.

## HEMATOPOIETIC CELL TRANSPLANTATION

### GENERAL PRINCIPLES

#### Stem Cell Sources, Donor Type, and Cell Manipulation

Transplantable hematopoietic stem cells (HSCs) can be retrieved from bone marrow, peripheral blood, or umbilical cord blood (UCB). Bone marrow HSCs are obtained by aspiration along the iliac crests, with the patient under general anesthesia. If the donor and the recipient are mismatched for AB0 blood type, red blood cell depletion of the bone marrow product must be performed prior to intravenous infusion through a central line. Otherwise, no further manipulation is required when the donor and the recipient are matched for human leukocyte antigen (HLA). By contrast, in the case of donor/recipient HLA mismatching (such as when one of the parents serves as a donor), the bone marrow is typically manipulated by depleting ex vivo the mature T cells contained in the graft (which would otherwise cause severe graft-versus-host disease [GVHD]) or by positive selection of CD34+ HSCs. Modern methods of T-cell depletion include use of monoclonal antibodies (mAb) directed against the αβ form of the T-cell receptor (TCRαβ). Often, in addition to TCRαβ T-cell depletion, B cells are depleted from the graft using anti-CD19 mAb. B-cell depletion decreases the risk of development of Epstein-Barr virus (EBV) lymphoproliferative disease after transplantation. As an alternative to ex vivo T-cell depletion, posttransplant administration of cyclophosphamide has been used recently to achieve selective depletion of alloreactive T cells in vivo following T-replete haploidentical HCT.

HSCs can be also obtained from peripheral blood by apheresis upon in vivo treatment of the donor with granulocyte-colony stimulating factor (G-CSF) and/or plerixafor, an antagonist of the chemokine receptor CXCR4, which serves as a retention signal for HSCs in the bone marrow niche.

Finally, UCB is relatively rich in HSCs. Approximately 75 mL of UCB can be collected at birth and cryopreserved. When donated to public UCB banks, UCB becomes a source of HSCs for recipients with an acceptable degree of HLA matching. Furthermore, collection of UCB at birth is recommended for families in which a previous child has been diagnosed with a severe PID that is amenable to HCT. As compared to bone marrow and peripheral blood HCT, transplantation of UCB has some distinctive features: the amount of HSCs contained in a single unit of UCB is generally insufficient to transplant to an adult or an adolescent; besides HSCs, UCB contains many other cell types, including mature T cells. There is evidence that in comparison to mature T cells contained in the bone marrow of adult donors, mature UCB T cells are less capable of mounting GFH reactions when transplanted into a partially matched recipient. On the other hand, UCB T cells are virtually exclusively naïve, and, hence, are minimally efficient in controlling ongoing infections in the recipient. By contrast, the mature T cells contained in the bone marrow of HLA-matched related or unrelated adult donors also contain antigen-specific T cells, which can expand and provide a first line of defense, before HSCs contained in the graft give rise to newly generated T lymphocytes.

Volunteer adult unrelated donors (URDs) represent an importance source of HSCs for transplantation. As of October 2016, more than 28 million URDs were included in the Bone Marrow Donors Worldwide (BMDW) registry, which also includes data on more than 700,000 units of UCB. This large database can be screened for possible HLA matching with recipients in need of HCT. The process of identifying a potentially suitable URD takes only a few weeks. Furthermore, improvements in the fine typing of HLA alleles (at the genotypic level) permits selection of the best URD available, thereby reducing the risks of development of GVHD. However, the probability of finding a suitable donor is lower for certain ethnic or racial groups that are poorly represented in the donor registry.

### Conditioning Regimens

Conditioning regimens targeting a recipient's cells may facilitate engraftment of donor cells. Depending on the nature and dosage, different intensities of conditioning regimens have been defined. Myeloablative conditioning (MAC) has the scope to oblate the recipient's bone marrow, and thus to allow more robust and durable engraftment of donor HSCs. An obvious consequence of the use of MAC regimens is the very profound pancytopenia that follows, which can last 2 to 3 weeks after HCT. Busulfan is typically used as a component of MAC regimens, most often in association with fludarabine, a nonalkylating agent with immunosuppressive properties. Fractionated total-body irradiation (TBI) also has myeloablative properties, but because of its toxicity, it is not used in patients with PID, who are typically infants and young children.

Reduced-intensity conditioning (RIC) regimens do not completely ablate the recipient's bone marrow and have less toxic effects than do MAC regimens. For this reason, RIC regimens are preferred in patients with organ damage. In addition to MAC regimens, busulfan can also be used as part of RIC regimens. The distinction between busulfan-based MAC and RIC regimens lies in the targeted level of blood busulfan concentration, which is lower for RIC regimens. Treosulfan is emerging as an alternative to busulfan in RIC regimens in Europe. The combination of fludarabine and melphalan is also frequently used in RIC regimens.

Serotherapy, based on the use of antithymocyte globulin (ATG) or alemtuzumab (anti-CD52 mAb), is frequently included in the preparation of the recipient prior to HCT. The scope of serotherapy may be 2-fold: (1) to deplete the host's lymphocytes, thereby reducing the risk of graft rejection; and (2) to provide immunosuppression and reduce the risk of developing GVHD. Especially in the case of alemtuzumab, the timing of immunosuppression with respect to the infusion of HSCs determines which effect prevails. Occasionally, serotherapy or low-dose (≤ 2 Gy) TBI is used in the absence of other chemotherapeutic agents in minimal-intensity conditioning (MIC) regimens.

Finally, for patients with severe combined immunodeficiency (SCID) who have a matched related donor, typically no conditioning regimen is used. A similar approach is also used by many centers in the case of a T-cell–depleted haploidentical HCT. In these cases, there is minimal or no engraftment of donor-derived HSCs. However, donor-derived common lymphoid progenitors that engraft demonstrate a strong selective advantage over autologous cells for T-cell differentiation, so that reconstitution of T-cell immunity is typically achieved.

In all other cases, the choice of which conditioning regimen (MAC, RIC, or MIC) to use is dictated by various factors: nature of the underlying disease, degree of matching between donor and recipient, and clinical status of the recipient at the time of transplantation. A general trend has emerged in recent years to use less intense (and, hence, also less toxic) conditioning regimens. HCT from a URD and from unrelated UCB typically requires use of a conditioning regimen, even when there is full HLA matching between the donor and the recipient and even in the case of babies with SCID. These types of transplants also require immunosuppression to prevent development of GVHD.

## COMPLICATIONS OF HCT

Several complications may affect the outcome of HCT and impact on survival and quality of life of the recipient. Some of these complications are the direct consequence of the nature and intensity of the conditioning regimen used and include posttransplant cytopenias, organ-specific toxicities, infections, and late effects on growth, development, and fertility. Furthermore, HLA mismatching between the donor and recipient can lead to rejection of the graft by the host immune system or, alternatively, to GVHD, caused by alloreactivity of donor-derived lymphocytes to the recipient's cells. The frequency and severity of these complications depend on the type of transplant, nature of the drugs used during conditioning, specific considerations related to the underlying disorder, and clinical status of the recipient at the time of HCT.

### Drug-Related Toxicities

MAC regimens cause severe pancytopenia requiring red blood cell and platelet transfusions for the first weeks after HCT. These adverse effects are also present, but less pronounced, in RIC regimens. Drug-related toxicities associated with the use of conditioning regimens are not restricted to the hematopoietic system but may also affect other organs, depending on the nature of the chemotherapeutic agent used. In particular, busulfan may damage the liver vascular endothelium and cause veno-occlusive disease (VOD), characterized by hepatomegaly, jaundice, ascites, fluid retention, and weight gain. VOD may ultimately lead to multiorgan failure (MOF) and death. Busulfan can also cause seizures and lung damage. Cyclophosphamide is a cause of hemorrhagic cystitis and of inappropriate antidiuretic hormone secretion. Conditioning regimens with busulfan and cyclophosphamide can cause delayed puberty and sterility. Other developmental problems associated with use of chemotherapy and/or radiotherapy include delayed or incomplete tooth eruption, short stature, hypothyroidism, and long-term effects on neurocognitive development. Patients with some forms of SCID due to defects of DNA repair are particularly at risk for these complications.

### Infections

The neutropenia and lymphopenia that patients experience after undergoing conditioning regimens may cause serious infections. Although filtering of blood derivatives is very important to remove leukocytes and reduce the risk of developing infections, adenovirus, cytomegalovirus (CMV), parainfluenza type III virus, and EBV infections are particularly challenging in the transplanted patient. In particular, CMV infection can cause interstitial pneumonia, enteritis, hepatitis, and encephalitis. EBV is a common cause of lymphoproliferative disease. Patients undergoing HCT should be monitored weekly for CMV and EBV viremia. Pre-emptive treatment with antiviral drugs (ganciclovir, foscarnet) or with anti-CD20 mAb is often effective in preventing dissemination of CMV and EBV infection, respectively. Parainfluenzae virus type 3 may cause severe interstitial pneumonia. Adenovirus infection may cause severe damage to the liver, lungs, and gastrointestinal tract. Cidofovir has been used with limited success in patients with adenovirus infection. Adoptive transfer of third-party, virus-specific, cytotoxic T lymphocytes (CTLs) has emerged as an important tool in the treatment of severe viral infections.

Until T-cell reconstitution is achieved, transplanted patients are at risk for development of *Pneumocystis jiroveci* pneumonia. Treatment is based on intravenous cotrimoxazole (20 mg/kg/d).

Neutropenia may facilitate development of fungal and bacterial infections. Reactivation of *Aspergillus* may occur in patients with chronic granulomatous disease (CGD). Occurrence of fever after HCT requires careful assessment, including cultures. Prompt identification of pathogens is essential to initiate specific antimicrobial treatment. Patients with SCID who have received immunization with bacillus Calmette-Guerin (BCG) at birth to prevent tuberculosis are at risk of developing local and systemic immune reconstitution inflammatory syndrome (IRIS) that becomes manifest at the time of engraftment and often requires use of immunosuppressive agents, along with administration of multiple antimycobacterial medications.

### Graft Rejection

Graft rejection may be observed when host lymphocytes specifically recognize non–self-antigens expressed by donor stem cells. Although this phenomenon is distinct from graft failure (which indicates the inability of the transplanted cells to engraft, as when the number of stem cells infused is too low), in practice, this distinction is often problematic, unless engraftment has been clearly demonstrated at an early time point after the HCT. The degree of immunocompetence of the host is important in determining the risk of graft rejection, and one of the scopes of serotherapy (and of immunosuppressive drugs contained in conditioning regimens) is indeed to reduce the risk of graft rejection. Because of the profound T-cell immunodeficiency, babies with SCID are less at risk of experiencing graft rejection. However, T lymphocytes are not the only lymphocyte population that can mediate graft rejection, as NK lymphocytes may also play an important role.

#### GVHD

Acute GVHD (aGVHD) is an inflammatory response caused by alloreactivity of donor T lymphocytes that recognize non–self-antigens on the surface of recipient's cells. Typically, it occurs during the first 100 days after the HCT, but clinical manifestations of aGVHD may also occur later. The severity of aGVHD is quantified with a grading system. Clinical manifestations of aGVHD include skin rash of variable severity (up to generalized exfoliative dermatitis), diarrhea, hepatomegaly, elevation of liver enzymes, and increased levels of direct bilirubin. Generalized edema may occur due to accumulation of fluids in interstitial tissues. Hypocellularity of the bone marrow may also be observed. During aGVHD, reactivation of latent viral infections (especially caused by CMV, EBV, and other herpesviruses) is common.

Transplantation from HLA-mismatched donors and from URDs is associated with a higher risk of developing aGVHD. In the case of HCT from haploidentical donors, rigorous T-cell depletion is the best method to prevent aGVHD. In case of T cell-replete HCT from a URD or UCB, addition of serotherapy during the preparatory regimen prior to HCT and use of immunosuppressive agents (eg, cyclosporine A, mycophenolate mofetil, tacrolimus, methotrexate) after HCT are important to reduce the risk of development of aGVHD.

Treatment of aGVHD is based on immunosuppression. Systemic steroids are the mainstay of therapy; more severe forms often require the use of second-line immunosuppressive drugs (cyclosporine A, tacrolimus, mycophenolate mofetil). Immunotherapy with anti-CD25 mAb (daclizumab) has also been used. However, grade 4 aGVHD has a severe prognosis and is associated with an increased risk of death and of chronic GVHD (cGVHD).

cGVHD typically occurs after 100 days from HCT. Fibrosis of target tissues is the hallmark of cGVHD and may manifest with cutaneous scleroderma-like lesions, sicca syndrome, fibrosis of the liver or the lungs, and limitations of joint motility. Furthermore, cGVHD compromises immune responses, with increased risk of development of infections on one hand and immune dysregulation and autoimmune manifestations on the other. Patients who have developed aGVHD are at higher risk of developing cGVHD; however, the latter may occur also without previous aGVHD. Compared to bone marrow transplantation, peripheral blood HSC transplantation has been associated with a higher risk of developing cGVHD. Whereas serotherapy and immunosuppression are efficacious in reducing the incidence of aGVHD, their efficacy in preventing cGVHD is less obvious. Immunosuppression also has limited efficacy in the treatment of this complications. Topical steroids and calcineurin inhibitors may improve skin and mucosal symptoms. Contrariwise, systemic steroids add to the increased risk of developing infections that characterizes cGVHD. Photopheresis may be used to induce tolerance, but its efficacy is often modest and delayed. Ursodeoxycholic acid may be beneficial in patients with liver disease.

## HCT FOR PRIMARY IMMUNE DEFICIENCIES: INDICATIONS AND OUTCOME

### SEVERE COMBINED IMMUNODEFICIENCY

SCID comprises a heterogenous group of genetic disorders characterized by severe impairment of T-cell development and function. Depending on the nature of the gene defect, B-cell development may or may not be affected (B-negative vs B-positive SCID), but antibody production is invariably defective, in light of the T-cell deficiency. Some forms of SCID are also characterized by lack of natural killer (NK) lymphocytes. Criteria to distinguish typical SCID from atypical forms of disease (including Omenn syndrome) have been recently developed by the Primary Immune Deficiency Treatment Consortium (PIDTC), with important implications for the appropriate approach to HCT.

If untreated, SCID is uniformly fatal within the first years of life, because affected infants succumb to overwhelming infections. Allogeneic HCT represents the mainstay of therapy; in some cases, gene therapy or enzyme replacement therapy may also be beneficial. Excellent outcomes have been reported with uses of HCT from an HLA-matched related donor (MSD), with greater than 90% long-term survival. In such cases, because of the striking advantage of donor-derived cells to differentiate to mature T lymphocytes, no conditioning regimen is needed to facilitate engraftment. Furthermore, lack of or autologous T lymphocytes renders the occurrence of graft rejection very unlikely; hence, no serotherapy is needed.

By contrast, controversy exists whether conditioning should be used for haploidentical HCT. Although most patients may attain successful T-cell reconstitution after undergoing T-cell–depleted haploidentical transplantation, poor engraftment, persistence of defective B-cell function, and waning of T-cell immunity have been reported in several cases. Use of a conditioning regimen may facilitate HSC engraftment and robust long-term T- and B-cell reconstitution in patients with SCID who receive haploidentical HCT and is typically required for URD HCT, but does carry the risk of drug-related toxicity. However, pretransplant conditioning is required to allow donor stem cell engraftment in patients with reticular dysgenesis, a form of SCID with extreme lymphopenia associated with neutropenia and sensorineural deafness.

In a recent study of outcomes of HCT in 240 consecutive patients with SCID who received HCT in North America between 2000 and 2009, the overall 5-year survival rate was 74%. Survival rate was highest among recipients of HCT from matched sibling donors (97%). Survival rate after unconditioned HCT from mismatched, related donors was 79%, which compared favorably to 66% survival after conditioned transplantation from the same donor group. Finally, the survival rates after URD and UCB transplantation were 74% and 58%, respectively. Overall, these data compare favorably to those reported in previous decades. This improved outcome reflects not only advances in transplantation, but even more importantly, improvement of supportive care and prevention and management of infections and GVHD.

The clinical status of the patient at the time of transplantation has emerged as a critical factor in determining outcome. In the North American study, among 68 infants who were treated before 3.5 months of life, 64 (94%) were reported to be alive at the time of the study. Because a similarly high survival rate has been observed also among infants older than 3.5 months with no history of infections or whose infections had resolved prior their undergoing to HCT (90% and 84% 5-year survival rates, respectively), these data clearly indicate the importance of early identification and aggressive management of babies with SCID before they undergo HCT. In this regard, a major advance is represented by the availability of newborn screening for SCID based on enumeration of T-cell receptor excision circles (TRECs), a by-product of T-cell rearrangement during thymopoiesis. Universal newborn screening for SCID has become common practice in most states in the United States and is rapidly expanding to other countries worldwide. Another important conclusion that emerged from the North American study of 240 babies with SCID treated with HCT is that for infants lacking a matched sibling donor and with an active infection, unconditioned haploidentical HCT offers better chances of survival as compared to conditioned haploidentical transplantation or HCT from a URD.

Besides donor type and the patient's clinical status at the time of HCT, the SCID phenotype and genotype may also affect the outcome. In a large European study of 699 patients, 10-year survival was higher for babies with B-positive SCID than for those with B-negative SCID (70% vs 51%, respectively). Among various factors that may contribute to this phenomenon, B-negative SCID also includes some forms of SCID with defective DNA repair, which expose these patients to a higher risk of drug-related toxicities. Furthermore, NK lymphocytes are absent in the most common variant of B-positive SCID (X-linked SCID), but they are present in B-negative SCID due to *RAG* or

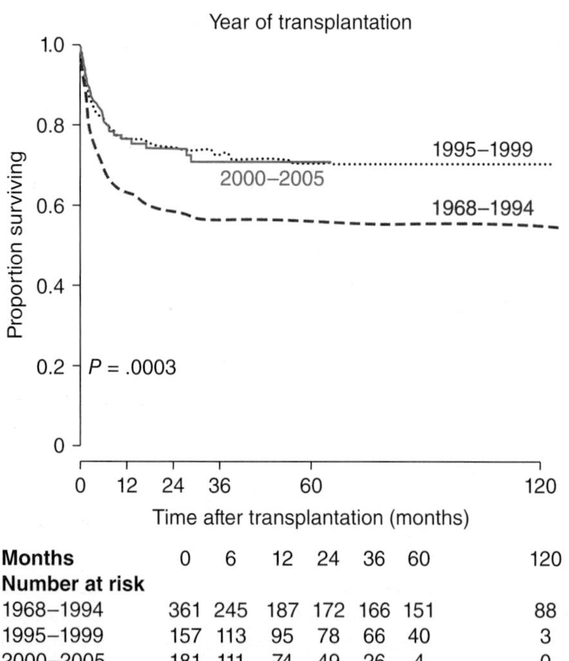


| Months | 0 | 6 | 12 | 24 | 36 | 60 | 120 |
|---|---|---|---|---|---|---|---|
| Number at risk | | | | | | | |
| 1968–1994 | 361 | 245 | 187 | 172 | 166 | 151 | 88 |
| 1995–1999 | 157 | 113 | 95 | 78 | 66 | 40 | 3 |
| 2000–2005 | 181 | 111 | 74 | 49 | 26 | 4 | 0 |

**FIGURE 185-1** Cumulative probability of survival in patients with severe combined immunodeficiency according to year of transplantation. (Reproduced with permission from Gennery AR, Slatter MA, Grandin L, et al. Transplantation of hematopoietic stem cells and long-term survival for primary immunodeficiencies in Europe: entering a new century, do we do better? *J Allergy Clin Immunol.* 2010 Sep;126(3): 602-610.)

*ARTEMIS* defects and may contribute to an increased rate of graft failure or of incomplete T-cell reconstitution. Consistent with this finding, in a series of 77 infants with SCID who received HCT in the United Kingdom, survival rate was higher among patients with NK-negative SCID than among those with NK-positive SCID

Finally, adenosine deaminase deficiency (ADA-SCID) is another genetic variant of SCID in which unconditioned haploidentical HCT is associated with a high risk of graft failure.

Notwithstanding the significant improvement in outcomes of HCT for SCID that has been achieved in recent years (Fig. 185-1), until immune reconstitution is achieved, these patients remain at high risk for development of infections. In the North American series of 240 patients with SCID who were transplanted between 2000 and 2009, infections accounted for 24 of 62 deaths. Patients who receive T-cell–depleted haploidentical HCT are at particularly high risk, because in this group of patients, T-cell reconstitution may take 4 to 6 months after transplantation. This time frame corresponds to the time required for HSCs to differentiate into mature naïve T cells that are exported from the thymus to the periphery, irrespective of the donor type and source of HSCs. However, patients who receive unmanipulated bone marrow from matched sibling donors are provided with mature T cells contained in the graft that expand and may mediate immune responses. The same is true for patients who receive bone marrow transplants from URDs; in these cases, however, chemotherapy and immunosuppression are typically used and may affect the ability of the T cells contained in the graft to expand and to participate in immune responses.

Infants with X-linked SCID or JAK3 deficiency are at higher risk of developing warts after HCT. This complication may manifest also several months or even years HCT. Although lower NK cell counts have been reported at long-term follow-up in patients with IL2RG and JAK3 deficiency, it appears that the unique susceptibility of these patients to papillomavirus infection reflects a defect in cytokine-mediated signaling that is intrinsic to keratinocytes.

Counts of total CD4+ cells and of naïve CD4+ cells at 1 year after HCT have been identified as biomarkers predictive of long-term immune reconstitution. Poor engraftment and incomplete immune reconstitution after HCT for SCID have been associated also with a higher risk of development of infections and autoimmune complications (cytopenias, hypothyroidism), and need for nutritional support. In such cases, boost infusions of HSCs are helpful only if performed early after transplantation but second transplants may be needed in patients who show late decline of immune function. Progressive waning of immunity has been reported especially among patients with SCID who received unconditioned T-cell–depleted HCT. Promising results have been reported recently with a new gene therapy protocol (that includes low-dose chemotherapy) in patients with X-linked SCID who had shown significant decline of T-cell immunity.

Although most patients with SCID attain good T-cell number and function after undergoing HCT, reconstitution of B-cell immunity is more variable. In particular, some forms of SCID involve gene defects that affect B-cell development or function in a cell autonomous manner. For example, *IL2RG* and *JAK3* mutations do not impair B-cell development, but they compromise the ability of mature naïve B cells to differentiate to plasmablasts in response to interleukin (IL)-21. *RAG* and *ARTEMIS* mutations, on the other hand, affect B-cell development, and ADA deficiency impairs both development and function of B cells. In these conditions, reconstitution of B-cell function after HCT requires robust levels of B-cell engraftment, which typically coincides with persistent HSC engraftment. Inclusion of a conditioning regimen may facilitate this. By contrast, other forms of SCID (IL7R, CD3 deficiencies) are due to genetic defects that do not directly affect B-cell function. In these patients, split lymphoid chimerism (with donor-derived T cells and autologous B lymphocytes) is typically sufficient to reconstitute antibody production, rendering use of conditioning less critical. Persistent impairment of B-cell function after HCT for SCID is associated with a higher rate of development of respiratory and intestinal infections and requires regular administration of immunoglobulins.

GVHD is another major complication after HCT for patients with SCID. In the series of 240 patients with SCID who received HCT in North America between 2000 and 2009, the cumulative incidence of grade 2 aGVHD was 20%, with no significant impact of donor type. This figure is lower than in previous reports. By contrast, the incidence of cGVHD appears to be stable at near 15%. Finally, patients with ARTEMIS deficiency are at higher risk of experiencing growth retardation, defects of tooth development, and nutritional problems.

## OMENN SYNDROME, ATYPICAL SCID, AND PROFOUND T-CELL IMMUNODEFICIENCIES

Patients with typical SCID have absent or extremely low T-cell counts, and the absence of T cells allows these patients to receive HCT without conditioning, because the chance of graft rejection is very low. By contrast, hypomorphic mutations in SCID-causing genes may allow development of a variable number of T cells, which typically are oligoclonal and have an activated phenotype. In the most extreme case (Omenn syndrome), the autologous T cells may infiltrate target tissues and create organ damage. Finally, a number of other gene defects (*ZAP70, ITK, CORO1A, STIM1, ORAI1, IKBKB, DOCK8, DOCK2, PNP*, and major histocompatibility complex [MHC] class I and MHC class II deficiencies) affect T-cell development and function without causing the severe T-cell lymphopenia that characterizes SCID. These conditions also have been defined as profound combined immunodeficiency (P-CID). In patients with atypical SCID, Omenn syndrome, and P-CID treated with HCT, some conditioning usually is required to permit T-cell engraftment. Although only limited data are available on survival and long-term outcomes of these patients after HCT, results appear to be inferior to those observed in patients with typical SCID. With the exception of Omenn syndrome (which is typically diagnosed in the first months of life), inferior outcomes in patients with these atypical forms of SCID as compared to those with typical SCID may also reflect delay in diagnosis and treatment. In a European series of 326 patients with T-cell immunodeficiencies who were treated with HCT between 1968 and 2005, 10-year survival rate was only 47%, and outcomes were poor, especially in patients with Omenn syndrome and MHC

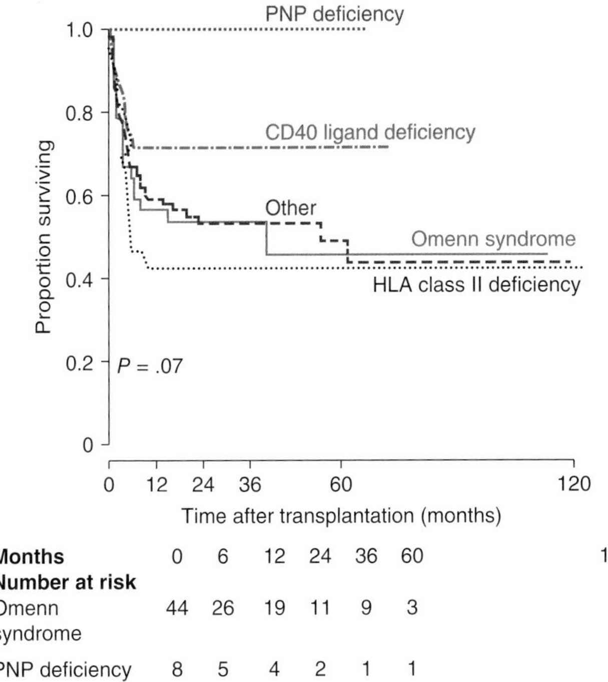


| Months | 0 | 6 | 12 | 24 | 36 | 60 | 120 |
|---|---|---|---|---|---|---|---|
| **Number at risk** | | | | | | | |
| Omenn syndrome | 44 | 26 | 19 | 11 | 9 | 3 | 0 |
| PNP deficiency | 8 | 5 | 4 | 2 | 1 | 1 | 0 |
| HLA class II deficiency | 26 | 11 | 10 | 8 | 4 | 1 | 1 |
| CD40 ligand deficiency donor | 35 | 21 | 17 | 11 | 4 | 3 | 0 |
| Other | 111 | 60 | 45 | 28 | 24 | 10 | 0 |

**FIGURE 185-2** Cumulative probability of survival in patients with various forms of combined immune deficiency who received hematopoietic cell transplantation between 1995 and 2005. (Reproduced with permission from Gennery AR, Slatter MA, Grandin L, et al. Transplantation of hematopoietic stem cells and long-term survival for primary immunodeficiencies in Europe: entering a new century, do we do better? *J Allergy Clin Immunol*. 2010 Sep;126(3):602-610.)

class II deficiency (Fig. 185-2). However, among 51 patients with P-CID who were recruited in a prospective study between 2011 and 2014, 19 underwent HCT, and only 2 of them have died, suggesting that recent improvements in HCT and in supportive care may lead to improved outcomes also in this group of patients. Finally, DOCK8 deficiency is a combined immunodeficiency characterized by atopy, sinopulmonary infections, and severe viral infections and a median survival rate at 20 years of only 47%. Excellent results have been obtained with matched related and unrelated HCT, and also with haploidentical HCT with posttransplant cyclophosphamide. Successful outcomes have also been reported after HCT in patients with DOCK2 deficiency, another combined immune deficiency with broad susceptibility to infections.

## OTHER COMBINED IMMUNODEFICIENCIES

Some forms of PID do not affect T-cell development and survival but impair immune responses. CD40 ligand (CD40LG) is a molecule that is expressed predominantly on the surface of activated CD4+ cells, and by interacting with CD40 (constitutively expressed by B cells), it plays an important role in promoting class switch recombination and generation of memory B-cells. Furthermore, interaction between CD40LG+ CD4+ cells and CD40+ dendritic cells induces production of IL-12 and initiation of Th1 responses. Patients with CD40LG deficiency are at risk of developing bacterial and opportunistic (*Pneumocystis jiroveci*, *Cryptosporidium parvum*, CMV) infections. Liver and biliary tract disease (sclerosing cholangitis) is often associated with *C parvum* and CMV infections and with tumors of the gastrointestinal tract, contributing to higher mortality rates in children and young adults. HCT may cure the disease. In a recent series of 67 patients who had been transplanted between 1964 and 2013, overall survival was 85%. Although this rate was not statistically different from that of survival with medical management only (80%), quality of life was better in transplanted patients. Liver/biliary tract disease was identified as a risk factor for mortality. Successful outcome has been also reported after HCT for CD40 deficiency.

Common variable immune deficiency (CVID) is usually managed with immunoglobulin replacement therapy and immunomodulatory drugs, when appropriate. However, a subgroup of patients with CVID experience serious complications and are at high risk of mortality. A recent study has analyzed outcomes of 25 patients with CVID who underwent HCT at 8 to 50 years of age. Severe immune dysregulation was the most common indication to transplant. Overall survival rate was only 48% and was higher (83%) for those who received HCT because they had developed lymphoma. However, the vast majority of survivors showed resolution of their major complications, and 50% of them were able to stop immunoglobulin replacement therapy.

Hypomorphic mutations of the *IKBKG* (*NEMO*) gene and heterozygous gain-of-function mutations of the *IKBA* gene impair nuclear factor-κB (NF-κB) signaling and cause combined immunodeficiency with ectodermal dystrophy. These patients are at risk for developing a wide range of infections (including mycobacterial disease). Furthermore, patients with *NEMO* deficiency often suffer from inflammatory bowel disease. HCT may cure the immunodeficiency, but graft failure has been reported when using RIC regimens. Furthermore, persistence of the colitis after transplantation has been reported in several patients with NEMO deficiency.

Wiskott-Aldrich syndrome (WAS) is characterized by immunodeficiency, eczema, and thrombocytopenia. The immunodeficiency of WAS may manifest with infections caused by a broad range of pathogens, autoimmunity, and increased risk of malignancies. The thrombocytopenia often is severe and may lead to fatal hemorrhages. HCT from matched related or unrelated donors is the mainstay of treatment in patients with severe clinical history or who lack WAS protein expression. In a multicenter study of 194 patients with WAS treated by HCT, the overall survival rate was 84%, and results were even better if the transplant was performed in children younger than 5 years of age. Pre-existing autoimmunity and recurrent/severe infections are negative risk factors. Poor myeloid chimerism may lead to persistence of thrombocytopenia, indicating that myeloablative conditioning may be helpful. For patients lacking HLA-matched donors, gene therapy may represent an alternative treatment (see below), but improved outcomes following haploidentical transplantations also have been reported recently.

## DISORDERS OF CELL-MEDIATED CYTOTOXICITY

Primary hemophagocytic lymphohistiocytosis (HLH) includes a heterogeneous groups of genetic diseases with impaired T- and NK-cell–mediated cytotoxicity. Patients with HLH develop severe clinical manifestations especially after viral infections, with cytopenias, coagulopathy, liver disease, and in some cases central nervous system involvement. Multiorgan failure often leads to death early in life. HCT is the only definitive cure for HLH. Transplantation during acute disease is associated with poor outcome, especially if myeloablative regimens are used. However, when performed during remission, transplantation from matched related or unrelated donors with use of RIC often leads to stable mixed chimerism that is sufficient to cure the disease. During the search for possible matched related donors, appropriate genetic and functional tests must be performed to avoid transplanting from a genetically affected, yet clinically asymptomatic subject.

X-linked lymphoproliferative disease type 1 (XLP1) is characterized by severe clinical manifestations (fulminant hepatitis, HLH, bone marrow aplasia, lymphoma) after infection with EBV, with high mortality rates in children and young adults. Use of RIC in preparation of matched related or unrelated HCT may cure the disease in 70% to 80% of patients.

Mutations of the X-linked inhibitor of apoptosis (*XIAP*) gene cause XLP type 2 (XLP2), which may manifest with XLP, HLH, and severe colitis. Similarly to what has been observed for HLH, HCT with MAC regimens is associated with elevated transplant-related mortality rates, but excellent results (86% survival) have been reported when HCT is performed during remission using RIC regimens.

HCT can also be used to treat some defects of cell-mediated cytotoxicity associated with defects of pigmentation. In particular, it may cure the hematologic and immune abnormalities of Chédiak-Higashi syndrome (CHS). Results are superior when the transplant is performed during remission. However, HCT does not prevent the neurologic deterioration that often accompanies the disease. Similar considerations apply to HCT for Griscelli syndrome type 2.

## DISORDERS OF IMMUNE DYSREGULATION

Immunodysregulation is being increasingly recognized as an important component of several forms of PID. Immune dysregulation, polyendocrinopathy, enteropathy, X-linked (IPEX) syndrome is due to *FOXP3* mutations that affect regulatory T ($T_{Reg}$) cell development and function. IPEX is characterized by autoimmune manifestations (enteropathy, type I diabetes, hepatitis, hypothyroidism), skin rash, and lymphoid proliferation, often leading to death early in life. HCT is curative, and selective advantage for donor-derived $T_{Reg}$ cells has been reported in patients with mixed chimerism.

Mutations of the *IL2RA* gene, encoding the α chain of the IL-2 receptor, compromise the function of both $T_{Reg}$ and effector T cells. Clinical manifestations resemble IPEX, but these patients are also at increased risk of developing severe infections. HCT can cure the disease.

CTLA4 haploinsufficiency and LRBA deficiency are characterized by autoimmunity, lymphoproliferative disease, and hypogammaglobulinemia. The LRBA protein binds to CTLA4 and permits endosomal recycling of this molecule, which plays an important role in $T_{Reg}$ function and serves as an inhibitory receptor in conventional activated T cells. In the absence of LRBA, the CTLA protein is targeted for lysosomal degradation, thereby resulting in reduced surface expression of CTLA4. Administration of a CTLA4-Ig construct (abatacept) and use of other immunosuppressive agents (sirolimus) may be beneficial, but only HCT can provide definitive cure. In a recent series of 8 patients with CTLA4 deficiency who received HCT, 6 were reported to be alive, with significant clinical improvement. However, the high degree of inflammation in which patients entered HCT may have contributed to the GVHD manifested by 4 of these patients, despite use of serotherapy and availability of well-matched donors.

*STAT1* gain-of-function mutations cause an immunodeficiency characterized by chronic mucocutaneous candidiasis; increase risk of bacterial, viral, and invasive fungal infections, frequently associated with autoimmune manifestations; aneurysms; and cancer. Patients with a complicated clinical course have poor outcomes, with fewer than 60% surviving at 40 years. Treatment is based on antimicrobials and immunosuppressive agents, and JAK inhibitors may also help. HCT has been attempted in 5 patients with severe infections, but 3 of them have died, indicating that control of the underlying disease is important to improve outcome of transplantation.

## DEFECTS OF PHAGOCYTES

Regular administration of G-CSF is the mainstay of therapy for patients with severe congenital neutropenia (SCN); however, a proportion of these patients fail to respond to treatment or develop serious complications, including acute myelogenous leukemia. In these cases, allogeneic HCT may be curative, especially if performed in patients younger than 10 years old, and with transplants from matched donors. Among 136 patients with SCN who received HCT between 1990 and 2012, the 3-year survival rate was 82%.

Chronic granulomatous disease (CGD) is the prototype of defects of phagocyte function. Despite regular prophylaxis with antibiotics and antifungals and possible use of interferon-γ, patients with CGD and absent oxidase activity remain at high risk for development of serious infections, inflammatory disease, and death. Recently, dramatic improvement in the outcome of HCT for CGD has been reported with the use of RIC-based regimens. In a series of 56 patients with CGD who received HCT from matched related (n = 21) or unrelated (n = 35) donors, after a conditioning regimen based on targeted busulfan levels, fludarabine, and serotherapy, 2-year overall survival and event-free survival rates were 96% and 91%, respectively (Fig. 185-3), and low rates of grade 3 and 4 aGVHD (4%) and cGVHD (7%) were reported. Stable and robust myeloid chimerism was observed in 93% of survivors. Similarly, excellent rates of survival (91.4%) and cure of the disease (81.4%) were observed in another study reporting outcome of 70 high-risk patients with CGD who received HCT between 2006 and 2015 using a treosulfan-based RIC.

Patients with the complete form of leukocyte adhesion deficiency type 1 (LAD-1) often die in infancy or early childhood because of severe infections. A multicenter study of 36 patients with LAD-1 who received HCT between 1993 and 2007 showed an overall survival rate of 75%. Use of haploidentical donors was associated with inferior outcome.

Mendelian susceptibility to mycobacterial disease (MSMD) includes a heterogeneous group of genetic disorders, most of which reflect defects along the IL-12/interferon (IFN)-γ pathway. Patients who lack expression of the IFN-γ receptor 1 are especially at high risk of developing infection and dying early in life. HCT represents

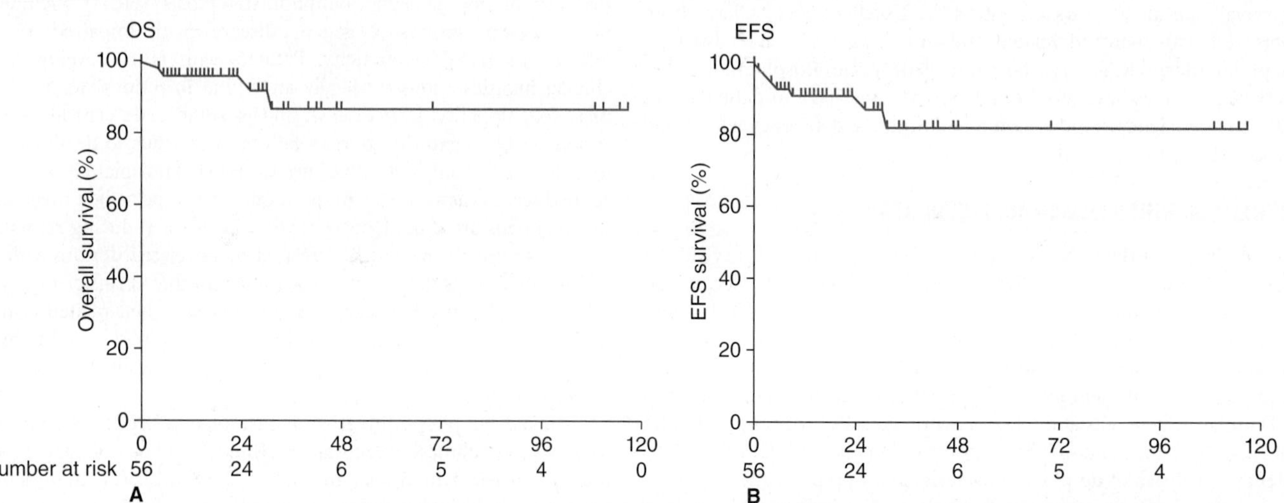


**FIGURE 185-3** Overall survival (**A**) and event-free survival (**B**) in patients with chronic granulomatous disease after hematopoietic cell transplantation with reduced-intensity conditioning. (Reproduced with permission from Güngör T, Teira P, Slatter M, et al. Reduced-intensity conditioning and HLAmatched haemopoietic stem-cell transplantation in patients with chronic granulomatous disease: a prospective multicentre study, *Lancet*. 2014 Feb 1;383(9915):436-448.)

the only curative option in these cases; however, in an international study of 8 patients who received HCT, only 2 were reported to be alive and in remission 5 years after transplantation. This unsatisfactory outcome has been attributed to the high levels of circulating IFN-γ, which would inhibit the engraftment of donor HSCs. However, a more critical factor may be represented by poor control of infections at the time of transplant.

## SUGGESTED READINGS


Gennery AR, Slatter MA, Grandin L, et al. Transplantation of hematopoietic stem cells and long-term survival for primary immunodeficiencies in Europe: entering a new century, do we do better? *J Allergy Clin Immunol.* 2010;126:602-610.

Güngör T, Teira P, Slatter M, et al. Reduced-intensity conditioning and HLA-matched haemopoietic stem-cell transplantation in patients with chronic granulomatous disease: a prospective multicentre study. *Lancet.* 2014;383:436-448.

Marsh RA, Vaughn G, Kim MO, et al. Reduced-intensity conditioning significantly improves survival of patients with hemophagocytic lymphohistiocytosis undergoing allogeneic hematopoietic cell transplantation. *Blood.* 2010;116:5824-5831.

Moratto D, Giliani S, Bonfim C, et al. Long-term outcome and lineage-specific chimerism in 194 patients with Wiskott-Aldrich syndrome treated by hematopoietic cell transplantation in the period 1980-2009: an international collaborative study. *Blood.* 2011;118:1675-1684.

Pai SY, Logan BR, Griffith LM, et al. Transplantation outcomes for severe combined immunodeficiency, 2000-2009. *N Engl J Med.* 2014;371:434-446.


# 186 Gene Therapy for Primary Immune Deficiencies


Luigi D. Notarangelo


## INTRODUCTION

Identification of the molecular basis of the disease and development of more effective strategies of gene transfer into hematopoietic stem cells (HSCs) have opened the way to innovative forms of gene therapy for primary immunodeficiency (PID). In these approaches, a normal copy of the gene of interest is introduced into the genome of autologous HSCs that are then re-infused into the patient. Gene therapy also holds the potential for gene editing, which is actually the removal and correction of an aberration in an individual PID-causing gene. In this chapter, we will review the current status of gene therapy (including gene editing) for PIDs and discuss possible developments in the field.

## GENE THERAPY

Despite improved outcomes of hematopoietic cell transplantations (HCTs) for PID, treatment-related morbidity and mortality (in particular those caused by drug toxicity, graft rejection/graft failure, graft-versus-host disease [GVHD], and incomplete immune reconstitution and immune dysregulation) remain major problems. Furthermore, HCT from human leukocyte antigen (HLA)-matched related donors is available to only approximately 15% of patients with PID, and suitable unrelated donors are not available for a significant number of patients. The identification of the genetic bases of PIDs has opened the perspective of novel therapeutic approaches based on gene therapy. With this strategy, a normal copy of the disease-related gene is delivered to the patient's own HSCs and is stably integrated in the genomic DNA, so that at each cell division, it is maintained into the genome of progeny cells (Fig. 186-1). As compared to HCT, gene therapy has the advantage that it should avoid the immunologic complications of allogeneic HSCT (graft rejection and GVHD in particular). However, current approaches of gene therapy also have important limitations. In particular, integration of the transgene into the host genome happens randomly or quasi-randomly; if the integration occurs within or near an oncogene, there is a potential for oncogene transactivation and tumor development. Furthermore, in most cases, expression of the therapeutic transgene is controlled by heterologous regulatory elements (promoters), potentially leading to dysregulated expression of the gene. These promises, but also these risks, have been confirmed in clinical trials.

## ADENOSINE DEAMINASE DEFICIENCY

Because of the strong selective advantage for genetically intact progenitor cells to differentiate into T lymphocytes (even with no or little conditioning), severe combined immunodeficiency (SCID) represents an ideal group of disorders to be treated by gene therapy. Indeed, adenosine deaminase (ADA) deficiency was the first disorder in which clinical trials of gene therapy were attempted. Initial attempts were based on use of retroviral vectors that were used to transfer ex vivo a normal copy of the ADA cDNA into either mature T lymphocytes (that had developed upon treatment with PEG-ADA) or bone marrow or umbilical cord blood autologous CD34+ HSCs, without use of any conditioning regimen. However, these attempts failed to provide clinical benefit. A major breakthrough came with the demonstration from the group at the San Raffaele Telethon Institute for Gene Therapy in Milan, Italy, that pretreatment of the patient with a low dose of busulfan made "space" in the bone marrow and facilitated long-term engraftment of gene-modified HSCs. Furthermore, in order to maximize the selective advantage for gene-corrected cells, enzyme replacement therapy was discontinued prior to initiating gene therapy. All 18 patients who received this treatment have survived (median follow-up, 6.9 years). Three patients had to resume enzyme replacement therapy due to insufficient immune reconstitution after gene therapy. In all others, multilineage gene marking was associated with metabolic detoxification, significant improvement of T-cell count, evidence of thymopoiesis, and normalization of T-cell proliferation. B-cell function was also improved, with reduced need for immunoglobulin replacement therapy and evidence of specific antibody production after immunization. There was a significant decrease in the rate of severe infections. Beneficial results of gene therapy for ADA deficiency have also been reported in other similar clinical trials at University College London/Great Ormond Street Hospital in London, Children's Hospital Los Angeles/University of California, Los Angeles, and the National Human Genome Research Institute, National Institutes of Health. Altogether, of at least 40 patients with ADA-SCID treated with gene therapy using retroviral vectors and nonmyeloablative conditioning, all are alive, and approximately 75% have gained sufficient immune reconstitution. Importantly, no adverse events related to genotoxicity (eg, leukemia due to insertional mutagenesis) have been observed.

## X-LINKED SEVERE COMBINED IMMUNODEFICIENCY

In X-linked SCID (X-SCID), mutations of the common cytokine receptor γ chain (γc) impair interleukin-7 signaling and, therefore, affect thymopoiesis. The observation that somatic reversion of an *IL2RG* mutation in a lymphoid progenitor of a patient with X-SCID allowed spontaneous recovery of T-cell number and function in the absence of other interventions has lent strong support to the idea that gene therapy could be beneficial in this disease, with no need for conditioning. Based on these premises, investigators at the Hospital Necker Enfants-Malades in Paris, France, instituted a clinical trial of gene therapy for X-SCID based on retrovirus-mediated transduction of autologous HSCs without chemotherapy. Of 10 patients treated, 9 developed normal numbers of T lymphocytes within 5 months after treatment. These patients remained initially in good health, with no

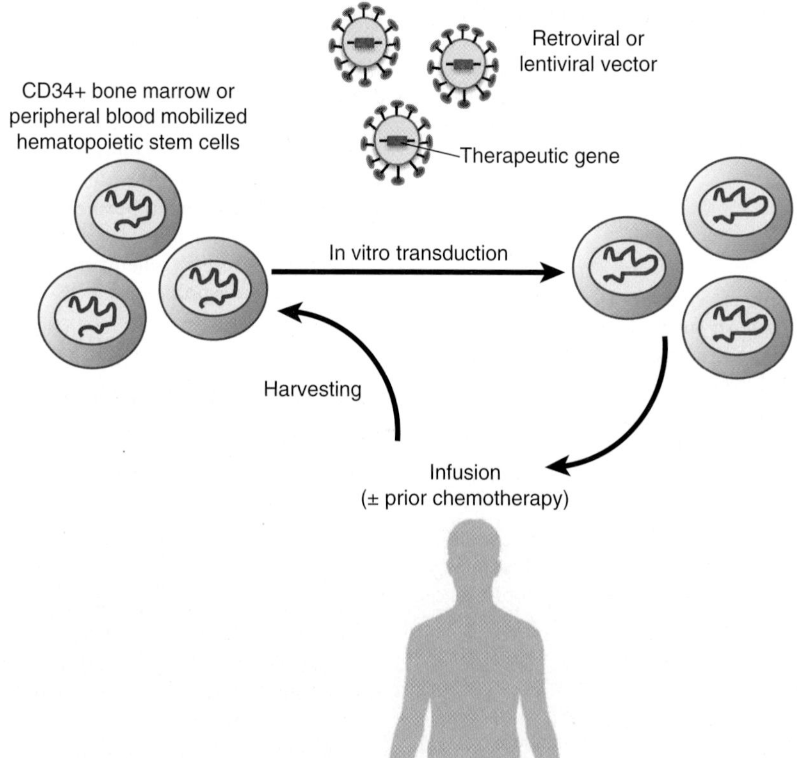


**FIGURE 186-1** Schematic representation of gene therapy. CD34+ hematopoietic stem cells (HSCs) are collected and isolated from bone marrow or upon mobilization into peripheral blood and are then subjected to in vitro transduction with viral vectors containing the therapeutic gene of interest (indicated in *red*). This allows stable integration of the transgene into the DNA of the CD34+ HSCs, which are then re-infused into the patient. Chemotherapy may be used to displace the endogenous, uncorrected HSCs, and facilitate long-term engraftment of gene-modified HSCs.

significant infections. Promising results were obtained in 10 additional patients treated with a similar approach at the Institute of Child Health, University College London, London, England. However, after a period of 2.5 to 5 years after gene therapy, 5 of the 20 patients treated in Paris and London developed leukemia. Four of them were treated successfully, but 1 of them died of this complication. Molecular investigations showed that the leukemias were the result of insertional mutagenesis, such that integration of the retrovirus within or near oncogenes had driven transactivation of the oncogene by the strong transcriptional elements contained in the long-terminal repeat (LTR) elements of the retrovirus.

These serious adverse events prompted the investigators to reconfigure the vector's design. In particular, a new retroviral vector lacking the viral LTRs has been produced, in which expression of the therapeutic *IL2RG* cDNA is driven by a weak cellular promoter. At least in theory, this new configuration should significantly reduce the risk of inducing transactivation of cellular oncogenes. Such a "self-inactivating" (SIN) retroviral vector is currently being used in another multicenter trial of gene therapy for X-SCID that is being conducted at 5 centers (Paris, London, Boston, Cincinnati, and Los Angeles). The results published so far have shown that 7 of 8 evaluable patients treated with this vector have attained T-cell immune reconstitution. Importantly, although the SIN configuration of the retroviral vector does not change the integration profile, no clonal expansions have been observed at 12 to 39 months after administration of gene therapy.

Although these results suggest that SIN retroviral vectors have a superior safety profile as compared to first-generation gamma-retroviral vectors, the propensity to integrate near transcription activation sites remains a matter of concern. For this reason, investigators have turned their attention to the development of lentiviral (LV) vectors, which should show a more neutral integration profile as compared to retroviral vectors. Furthermore, it has been shown that in the absence of chemotherapy, most patients with X-SCID who had received gene therapy in previous trials had shown lack of significant gene marking in blood cells other than T lymphocytes. In particular, lack of γc expression and function in their B lymphocytes was associated with inability to mount specific antibody responses, and, consequently, most of these patients continue to require intravenous immunoglobulins. To circumvent this problem, the group led by Harry Malech at the National Institutes of Health has used a SIN-LV vector and low-dose busulfan (6 mg/kg) to treat older patients with X-SCID who had experienced waning of immunity after HCT and presented with significant clinical problems (recurrent or chronic infections, diarrhea). Preliminary results indicate that this approach allows multilineage gene marking, restores both T- and B-cell function, and allows significant clinical improvement. These results are particularly interesting because it was thought that it would not be possible to restore thymopoiesis in older patients with X-SCID, as had been suggested by negative results that had been previously obtained in a few older patients with X-SCID who had received gene therapy without chemotherapy. Finally, none of the patients treated so far in this LV-based trial have developed clonal expansions, although the follow-up is still brief.

## WISKOTT-ALDRICH SYNDROME

A first trial of gene therapy for Wiskott-Aldrich syndrome (WAS) has been performed in Hannover, Germany, using a first-generation retroviral vector and chemotherapy. Multilineage gene marking and restoration of WAS protein (WASP) expression were achieved in 9 of 10 patients treated and associated with significant clinical improvement, increased platelet count, and restoration of immune function. However, 7 of these patients developed leukemia due to insertional mutagenesis. A SIN-LV vector in which expression of the *WAS* cDNA is driven by the autologous promoter has been used recently in 2 trials: a single-center trial at San Raffaele Telethon Institute for Gene Therapy in Milan, Italy, and a multicenter trial in Paris, London, and Boston. In both trials, patients received submyeloablative chemotherapy. In both trials, patients have experienced clinical benefit, especially in terms of infections and autoimmunity, and no leukemic events have been recorded to date. However, most patients have had only a moderate increase of the platelet count, possibly reflecting lower levels of gene marking in the myeloid compartment and suboptimal levels of expression of WASP induced by this vector.

## X-LINKED CHRONIC GRANULOMATOUS DISEASE

Initial trials of gene therapy for X-linked chronic granulomatous disease (X-CGD) were conducted in the late 1990s by targeting mobilized peripheral blood CD34+ cells with Moloney leukemia virus (MLV)-based retroviral vectors without cytoreductive chemotherapy. This approach resulted in transient reconstitution of NADPH oxidase function in a very low proportion of neutrophils, without long-lasting clinical benefit.

Subsequently, another trial was conducted in Germany using a retroviral vector derived from the murine spleen focus forming virus (SFFV), which contains strong LTR elements. Two patients were enrolled in this trial, which included cytoreductive chemotherapy with 8 mg/kg of busulfan. This approach resulted in appearance of a significant proportion (up to 60%) of functional neutrophils and resolution or significant improvement of active infections. However, both patients developed myelodysplasia, and 1 of them died of a gastrointestinal infection at a time when oxidase activity was no longer detectable in his neutrophils.

Once again, these results prompted development of a novel, hopefully safer, and more efficacious vector. In particular, a multicenter trial is being currently conducted in Europe and the United States with a LV vector in which expression of the CYBB cDNA is driven by a chimeric promoter that is particularly active in mature myeloid cells but is supposed to have reduced potential to transform stem and progenitor cells.

## FUTURE PERSPECTIVES FOR GENE THERAPY USING INTEGRATING VIRAL VECTORS IN PRIMARY IMMUNE DEFICIENCIES

Several groups are working on the development of gene therapy protocols for other forms of PID, including various forms of SCID (RAG1 and RAG2 deficiency, ARTEMIS deficiency, IL7R deficiency), leukocyte adhesion deficiency-1, hemophagocytic lymphohistiocytosis, X-linked lymphoproliferative disease type 1, IPEX (immune dysfunction, polyendocrinopathy, enteropathy, X-linked), and X-linked agammaglobulinemia. In many cases, promising results have been obtained in preclinical animal models, signaling that human clinical trials may be started in the near future.

Furthermore, attention is being paid to use of new viral vectors (such as foamy viruses and alpha-retroviruses) and to the inclusion of "insulator" sequences in the vector that should shield cellular genes from viral transcriptional elements and thereby reduce the risk of insertional mutagenesis.

## GENE EDITING

So far, all clinical trials of gene therapy for PIDs have been based on the stable integration of an additional, normal copy of the gene of interest into the patient's cells, using viral vectors. However, with this approach, the gene is integrated randomly (or semi-randomly) into the DNA, with the potential risk of insertional mutagenesis, as discussed above. Furthermore, in most cases, expression of the therapeutic gene is driven by heterologous promoters, so that physiologic control of gene expression may not be maintained. As opposed to these strategies of *gene addition*, a novel interesting approach to gene therapy is represented by *gene editing*, for which the goal is to achieve true correction of the mutation. To this purpose, a donor DNA template containing the correct DNA sequence is delivered to the cell. Upon homologous recombination (HR), the donor template is incorporated into the DNA, replacing the DNA fragment containing the mutation. If successful, this approach would avoid the risk of insertional mutagenesis and maintain physiologic regulation of gene expression intact. Unfortunately, HR occurs at extremely low frequency, even more so if the cells are not actively replicating. However, the frequency of HR can be significantly increased by introducing DNA double-strand breaks in the region of the DNA that contains the mutation. Various types of nuclei are now available that can be used to introduce targeted DNA double-strand breaks. They include zinc-finger nuclei, meganuclei TALENs, and CRISPR/Cas9. Each of these can be designed to recognize specifically the DNA sequence close to the mutation, thereby permitting introduction of targeted DNA double-strand breaks. Upon delivery of the DNA donor template with the correct sequence, the mutation can be repaired in a proportion of cells. Although efficiency of HR in HSCs remains too low at present to permit immediate application of this attractive therapy, significant progress has been made in the expression and delivery of the nuclease components and of the donor template. Hence, one may anticipate that this kind of personalized gene therapy approach for PIDs may enter clinical trials in the next few years. One problem is represented by the heterogeneity of mutations that may cause any given form of PID, which might require development of a myriad of nuclease/donor template pairs. To circumvent this problem, one approach is to target introduction of a wild-type copy of the cDNA at the translation initiation site. One alternative approach is based on the integration of the therapeutic DNA sequence in a "safe harbor," that is, in a region of the DNA that is not supposed to lead to serious adverse events when the object of targeted DNA integration. One such "safe harbor" is the AAVS1 site. Furthermore, while successful targeting of HSCs may permit permanent correction of the disease, in some cases, it may be convenient to target more mature cell types, such as T lymphocytes, in which a higher frequency of HR can be more easily achieved. Such an approach could be used, for instance, to correct CD40LG deficiency, for which gene editing of the *CD40LG* locus in circulating CD4+ cells might provide the patient with an immediate source of cells capable of fighting severe ongoing infections due to pathogens such as *Cryptosporidium*. Indeed, brilliant preliminary results, with a high rate of HR-mediated gene corrections in patients' T cells, have been recently reported in vitro. Finally, the classical approach to gene therapy, based on gene addition, would not be applicable to cure conditions due to heterozygous gain-of-function or dominant-negative mutations. In such cases, gene editing may represent a better strategy, and true correction may not even be needed, as long as the nuclease is capable of mediating selective disruption of the mutant allele, while leaving the wild-type allele intact.

## SUGGESTED READINGS


Aiuti A, Biasco L, Scaramuzza S, et al. Lentiviral hematopoietic stem cell gene therapy in patients with Wiskott-Aldrich syndrome. *Science*. 2013;341:1233151.

De Ravin SS, Wu X, Moir S, et al. Lentiviral hematopoietic stem cell gene therapy for X-linked severe combined immunodeficiency. *Sci Transl Med*. 2016;8:335ra57.

Fischer A, Hacein-Bey Abina S, Touzot F, Cavazzana M. Gene therapy for primary immunodeficiencies. *Clin Genet*. 2015;88:507-515.

# 187 Allergic Disease and Atopy

Carla M. Davis and Talal A. Chatila

## INTRODUCTION

A precipitous increase in incidence and prevalence of allergic diseases in the last 50 years has led to the current pandemic proportions. In some subpopulations, as many as 1 in 4 children suffers from asthma, and up to 1 in 12 has a food allergy. One explanation for this dramatic increase in allergic diseases is the "hygiene hypothesis," which posits that a decrease in the exposure to microbes due to improved hygiene, smaller families, less breastfeeding, more immunizations, and lack of serious childhood infections results in altered immunoregulation and deviation toward an allergic disease-promoting T-helper cell 2 (TH2) response. Microbial exposure promotes the production of regulatory T cells involved in maintaining tolerance to allergens. Lack of sufficient microbial exposure may result in weakened tolerance and, in the setting of other factors such as genetic predisposition and environmental exposures, result in the promotion of allergic diseases. The important environmental exposures that can directly decrease microbial diversity, causing increased expression of atopy, include urbanization, industrialization, climate change and rising temperatures with prolonged pollen seasons, increased viability of mold, and increased aeroallergen exposure. The increased prevalence of allergic disease is directly related to these factors.

Allergic diseases are immunologic diseases in that their genesis and manifestations result from the functioning of several components of the immune system. Disease pathogenesis is mediated by both innate immune responses, involving mast cells, basophils, eosinophils, and dendritic cells, and acquired immune responses involving T, natural killer (NK) T, and B lymphocytes. Orchestrating the allergic response is the TH2 CD4+ T-helper-cell lineage, which is now appreciated to play a central role in the pathogenesis of allergic diseases. TH2 cells recruit other components of the innate and acquired immune response by virtue of their production of a set of proatopic cytokines, including interleukin (IL)-4, IL-5, and IL-13. They promote the production of immunoglobulin (Ig) E, a key trigger of immediate hypersensitivity reactions, and help sustain chronic allergic inflammation in such diseases as asthma and eczema. Increased knowledge of allergic diseases and their pathogenesis has stimulated the development of new therapeutic approaches, including desensitization therapy with defined allergen preparations or pharmacologic interventions aimed at depleting IgE or targeting the action of mediators such as leukotrienes.

## IMMUNOLOGIC BASIS OF ATOPY

Allergic disorders develop when individuals with a genetic predisposition are exposed to environmental triggers. A unifying attribute of these disorders is *atopy*, defined as a genetically determined predisposition (and, hence, tending to be familial) to generate IgE antibodies on exposure to environmental antigens. Subsequent exposure to the offending antigen, or allergen, triggers an immediate hypersensitivity reaction. It is an IgE-mediated tissue response that is characterized by increased vascular permeability, vasodilatation, smooth muscle contraction, and local cellular inflammation. The atopic (or allergic) trait integrates pathways of the acquired immune response, including specialized T-helper cells, NKT cells, and IgE-producing B cells, as well as components of the innate immune response, including mast cells, eosinophils, basophils, and neutrophils. These pathways are critical to pathogenesis in allergic diseases. In contrast, many adverse reactions to foods, such as milk intolerance and diarrhea from lactase deficiency, are not allergic in nature in that they proceed independently of the immune system.

## TH2 CELLS

IgE production is one feature of a more fundamental specific immune response orchestrated by the TH2 subset of CD4+ T-helper cells. TH2 cells are critical for promoting acute hypersensitivity responses and maintaining the state of chronic and relapsing eosinophil-predominant inflammation that is characteristic of chronic allergic inflammation. TH2 cells represent a separate lineage of T-helper cells that arises from an uncommitted, pluripotent TH0 state. TH0 cells may differentiate toward either the TH1 state, involved in fighting intracellular pathogens, the proallergic TH2 lineage, the proinflammatory TH17 lineage, or the induced or adaptive regulatory T-cell state, which promotes immune tolerance. These different T-cell types are distinguished by their profile of cytokine production. For example, TH2 cells produce a distinct set of cytokines necessary for the allergic response, including IL-4 and IL-13, which promote IgE production, and IL-5 and granulocyte-macrophage colony-stimulating factor, which promote eosinophil production in the bone marrow. In contrast, TH2 cells do not produce IL-2 and interferon-γ, characteristic of TH1 cells, which reciprocally do not produce TH2-type cytokines. Whereas allergic diseases exhibit dominance of TH2 cytokines, TH1 and TH17 cytokines may also contribute to the pathogenesis of some allergic diseases such as atopic dermatitis.

## ROLE OF ALLERGENS AND THE CELLULAR MILIEU

Allergens enter the body through skin, respiratory, gastrointestinal, and conjunctival routes. Normal responses result in the development of tolerance. In response to inflammatory stimuli, thymic stromal lymphopoietin (TSLP), IL-33, and/or IL-25 produced by keratinocytes can upregulate OX40L on antigen-presenting cells (APCs) to promote TH2 differentiation. Induction of an allergic immune response requires uptake and processing by APCs, which then present peptide fragments to specific T cells. Among the most efficient APCs are dendritic cells and tissue-based skin and mucosal Langerhans cells. The quantity and phenotype of dendritic cells appear altered in atopic individuals in a way that promotes TH2 responses. Neighboring cells can influence the outcome of TH-cell differentiation. In particular, mast cells, basophils, and NKT cells can polarize the local cytokine milieu in ways that favor TH2 responses by virtue of their production of IL-4. Type 2 innate lymphoid cells (ILC2s) produce IL-5 and IL-13, and preexisting allergen-specific IgE may favor the induction of TH2 responses, by activating mast cells and basophils to produce IL-4 and IL-13.

## ALLERGENS

People are typically exposed to very low levels of allergens, small- to medium-sized proteins that are highly soluble and are carried on desiccated particles such as pollen. On contact with the mucosa, they are eluted from their carrier particles. A protein that is too large may not easily pass through mucosal surfaces, and proteins that are too small may not be able to cross-link IgE on mast cells. Allergens can be very complex, such as pollen, house dust mites, or foods, or simple, such as single-molecule chemicals or drugs. Glycans, chains of simple sugars, when coupled to a protein or lipid carrier, can interact with B cells, causing T-cell responses. Cross-reactive carbohydrate determinant in plant foods and α-gal (galactose-α-1,3-galatose) in animal meats are examples of proteotypic glycans with IgE-binding activity. Allergens are frequently enzymatically active. In particular, proteases feature prominently among allergens such as Der p I, the major allergen of the house dust mite *Dermatophagoides pteronyssinus,* a cysteine protease. Another industrial allergen is subtilisin, a protease that was frequently used in some laundry detergents.

## REGULATION OF IgE PRODUCTION

A critical component of the atopic phenotype and response is IgE. Its production results from the interaction of antigen-presenting B cells with antigen-specific T-helper cells. At least 2 signals are required to shift immunoglobulin production in B cells from IgM to IgE, a process called *class-switch recombination*. The first signal is provided by the TH2 cytokines IL-4 or IL-13, made by T cells, NKT cells, mast cells, and basophils, which are the only cytokines that can support IgE production through activation of the signal transducer and activator of transcription (STAT) 6 in cultured B cells. A second signal is delivered by the interaction of a B-cell protein termed CD40 with its protein ligand CD40L, which is expressed on the surface of activated T-helper cells. TH2 cells provide both signals necessary for IgE production. CD4+ TH2 cells are present in respiratory mucosa and regional lymphoid tissues of atopic individuals, where they promote IgE production by interacting with naïve B cells presenting allergen-derived peptide antigens. TH2 cells are critical to the maintenance of the allergic inflammation in atopic diseases such as asthma, and they can mediate the passive transfer of allergic airway responses.

## IgE RECEPTORS

IgE mediates 2 distinct functions in the host: initiation of the immediate hypersensitivity reaction and promotion of antigen presentation leading to augmented immune responses. These functions are mediated by dedicated receptors expressed on immune cells. The first is the high-affinity IgE receptor, or FcεRI, a multimeric protein expressed on a variety of cells, including mast cells, basophils, dendritic cells, Langerhans cells, eosinophils, platelets, and monocytes. FcεRI binds IgE with high affinity, which exceeds by 2 to 4 logs the binding affinities of other immunoglobulin Fc receptors, and with 1:1 stoichiometry. An important consequence of the high-affinity binding of FcεRI to IgE is that in atopic individuals with high IgE levels, virtually all FcεRI molecules are constitutively bound by IgE. Once attached, IgE remains permanently bound until internalized. IgE is important in regulating the density of FcεRI on the cell surface.

Cross-linking by multivalent allergenic proteins of IgE bound to FcεRI on mast cells, basophils, and activated eosinophils initiates a signal transduction cascade that results in the exocytosis of stored granules, the release of the contents, and gene transcription. This results in the de novo synthesis by these cells of cytokines IL-4, tumor necrosis factor (TNF), and IL-6 and inflammatory mediators like prostaglandins and cysteinyl leukotrienes. Because of the very high affinity of allergen–IgE and IgE–FcεRI interactions, FcεRI isoforms expressed on antigen-presenting cells, including dendritic, Langerhans, and activated monocytic cells, allow efficient antigen presentations at very low levels of antigen. The antigen-presenting function of FcεRI is important for potentiation and long-term maintenance of IgE-driven allergic and inflammatory responses. This role is especially important in chronic allergic inflammatory diseases such as eczema and asthma.

A second IgE receptor, FcεRII or CD23, is expressed on B cells, monocytes, dendritic cells, Langerhans cell, eosinophils, and gastrointestinal and respiratory epithelial cells. Its affinity for IgE, although lower than that of FcεRI, is substantial. CD23 mediates the transport of food antigens across the epithelial gut barrier, facilitates antigen presentation to T cells, and mediates transfer of antigens to dendritic cells through B cell exosomes. Soluble CD23, but not transmembrane CD23, enhances IgE production.

## IMMEDIATE- AND LATE-PHASE HYPERSENSITIVITY REACTIONS

Cross-linking of IgE bound to FcεRI on tissue mast cells or on circulating basophils triggers the release of granules containing preformed mediators, including histamine, TNF-α, proteoglycans, and neutral proteases, including tryptase, chymase, and carboxypeptidase. It also results in the rapid de novo synthesis of lipid-derived mediators, including prostaglandin $D_2$, the chief prostaglandin product of mast cells, as well as platelet-activating factor and leukotrienes $B_4$, $C_4$, $D_4$, and $E_4$. The release of these mediators induces an immediate hypersensitivity reaction, characterized by vasodilation, edema, and smooth muscle contraction. In an atopic individual, an example of this response is seen as a "wheal and flare" skin reaction on scratching of the skin with an allergenic substance. A similar reaction pattern is seen in other tissues such as bronchial airways, where mediator release on allergen inhalation rapidly induces mucosal edema, mucus production, smooth muscle constriction, and reduced airflow. This immediate hypersensitivity reaction is reversible with treatment and usually subsides within 2 hours of its initiation.

IgE-induced immediate hypersensitivity reaction often is followed by a late-phase or delayed reaction, a second wave of hypersensitivity responses occurring several hours after the acute reaction has subsided. The late-phase reaction may manifest as decreased airflow in asthmatics, gastrointestinal symptoms, skin inflammation, anaphylaxis, or recurrence of sneezing and rhinorrhea in patients with allergic rhinitis 4 to 24 hours after the initial allergen contact. The late-phase reaction arises from the recruitment to the allergen challenge site of an inflammatory cellular infiltrate that includes neutrophils, T lymphocytes, basophils, monocytes, and eosinophils.

## IgE-INDEPENDENT ALLERGIC INFLAMMATION

Despite the pivotal functions of IgE in immediate hypersensitivity reactions, there are situations in which mast cell degranulation may proceed by IgE-independent mechanisms. For example, the syndrome of active anaphylaxis, with mast cell degranulation and mediator release, can be induced in humans by repeated infusion of IgA-containing, blood-derived product (blood, plasma, or immunoglobulin preparations) in individuals who are IgA-deficient. Such infusions result in the development by these individuals of IgG (rarely IgE) anti-IgA antibodies. On rechallenge with the offending product, IgG/anti-IgA immune complexes are formed that precipitate mast cell degranulation and anaphylaxis by interaction with low-affinity Fc receptors for IgG on mast cells.

An important example of chronic allergic inflammation proceeding by IgE-independent mechanisms involves patients with so-called intrinsic allergic diseases, including asthma and eczema. In contrast to the majority of children and many adults with asthma and eczema in whom evidence of pathogenic immediate hypersensitivity can be demonstrated by skin testing, individuals with intrinsic disease forms lack evidence of IgE-mediated reactions. However, these patients exhibit a pattern of allergic inflammation and TH2 cytokine expression that is very similar to that found in patients with the extrinsic or allergic disease form.

## CELLULAR MEDIATORS OF ALLERGIC INFLAMMATION

Although IgE is a central mediator and critical component of allergic inflammation, many cells contribute to chronic inflammation in atopic conditions such as allergic rhinitis, asthma, atopic dermatitis, and eosinophilic esophagitis. TH2 cells have a central role in the propagation of allergic responses, and TH17 cells, which promote the recruitment of neutrophils through the production of IL-17, are increased in asthmatics. Type 2 innate lymphoid cells produce pro-inflammatory cytokines such as IL-5 and IL-13 after stimulation by intestinal epithelium-derived IL-25. IL-5 stimulates the production of eosinophils, which can produce immunoregulatory cytokines and soluble mediators. NKT cells produce IL-4 and IL-13. Eosinophils infiltrate the skin in atopic dermatitis and eosinophilic esophagitis. Eosinophils, when activated, deposit granule proteins in the skin, causing inflammation and priming B cells for antibody production, acting as antigen-presenting cells. Myeloid dendritic cells initiate and sustain allergic inflammation when surface histamine receptors are activated. Basophils contain secretory granules with histamine, leukotrienes, and major basic protein, which propagate atopic symptoms. All of these cells contribute to allergic responses, but on the contrary, cellular regulation of the allergic response occurs through T and B regulatory cells and the induction of inhibitory cytokines IL-10 and transforming growth factor (TGF)-β. Risk for the development of allergic diseases is associated with regulatory T-cell deficiency.

## TISSUE-SPECIFIC GENETIC FACTORS IN ALLERGIC DISEASES

The contribution of non-IgE- and non-immune-dependent mechanisms in the genesis of allergic inflammation is now recognized for diseases such as atopic dermatitis, for which defects in the skin barrier function seem to play an important role in disease evolution. Mutations that compromise the skin-barrier function, including filaggrin

(*FLG* loss of function), are associated with the development of allergic skin inflammation and ichthyosis vulgaris, which is commonly associated with atopic dermatitis. In particular, the incidence of common heterozygous mutations in filaggrin, present in as many as 10% of people of European ancestry, rises to as many as 40% in patients with atopic dermatitis of the same heritage. Filaggrin mutations are associated with allergy-associated atopic dermatitis, allergic sensitization, peanut allergy, total serum IgE levels, and asthma in those patients, suggesting that they are involved in primary development of allergic sensitization. Homozygosity of a TSLP risk allele correlates with increased basophil response in eosinophilic esophagitis patients. It regulates dendritic cell and T-cell interactions. Other tissue-expressed genes that have also been implicated in the pathogenesis of asthma include the disintegrin and metalloprotease ADAM33, which plays an important role in airway remodeling. These and other findings indicate a broad role for tissue-expressed gene products in the initiation and propagation of allergic disorders.

## TARGETING THE IMMUNOLOGIC PATHWAYS OF ATOPY

The allergic response can be attenuated or even abrogated by measures aimed at modifying its underlying immune mechanisms. Foremost is scrupulous allergen avoidance, which can result not only in symptomatic relief but, if persistent long term, also in hyposensitization. Immunotherapy with allergenic extracts also is effective in hyposensitizing the allergic response.

Several therapies target specific components of the allergic response. Antihistamines target the vasoactive effects of the mast cell. They are useful in immediate hypersensitivity reactions but ineffective for the late-phase reaction or chronic allergic inflammation, which is better managed by steroids. Steroid therapies decrease T-helper cell cytokine production, which contributes to inflammation. Leukotriene receptor antagonists combat the effects of persistent leukotriene production by eosinophils and other inflammatory cells in chronic allergic inflammation. Epinephrine counteracts anaphylaxis by dilating smooth muscle and causing cutaneous vasoconstriction.

Novel therapies being used are aimed at interrupting key pathways in atopic response. Interruption of signals delivered by IL-5, IL-4, and IL-13 by using soluble cytokine receptors is also showing promise in allergic diseases such as asthma. Anti-IL-5 is used in hypereosinophilic syndrome and severe eosinophilic asthma. Anti-IgE monoclonal antibodies that block binding of IgE to FcεRI without inducing immediate hypersensitivity reaction or anaphylaxis reduce IgE levels in humans by binding to IgE and removing it by immune complex formation. These antibodies attenuate both the early and late-phase responses to inhaled allergens and reduce the associated increase in eosinophils in sputum.

## SUGGESTED READINGS


Cabanillas B, Novak N. Atopic dermatitis and filaggrin. *Curr Opin Immunol.* 2016;42:1-8.

Campbell DE, Mehr S. Fifty years of allergy: 1965-2015. *J Paediatr Child Health.* 2015;51:91-93.

Chinthrajah RS, Hernandez JD, Boyd SD, Galli SJ, Nadeau KC. Molecular and cellular mechanisms of food allergy and food tolerance. *J Allergy Clin Immunol.* 2016;137:984-997.

Gould HJ, Sutton BJ. IgE in allergy and asthma today. *Nat Rev Immunol.* 2008;8:205-217.

Kaplan AP, Giménez-Arnau AM, Saini SS. Mechanisms of action that contribute to efficacy of omalizumab in chronic spontaneous urticaria. *Allergy.* 2016 Nov 15. doi: 10.1111/all.13083. [Epub ahead of print]

Martino DJ, Prescott SL. Progress in understanding the epigenetic basis for immune development, immune function, and the rising incidence of allergic disease. *Curr Allergy Asthma Rep.* 2013;13:85-92.

Oettgen HC. Fifty years later: Emerging functions of IgE antibodies in host defense, immune regulation, and allergic diseases. *J Allergy Clin Immunol.* 2016;137:1631-1645.

Ozdemir C, Akdis M, Akdis CA. T-cell response to allergens. *Chem Immunol Allergy.* 2010;95:22-44.

Pali-Schöll I, Jensen-Jarolim E. The concept of allergen-associated molecular patterns (AAMP). *Curr Opin Immunol.* 2016;42:113-118.

Tan HT, Sugita K, Akdis CA. novel biologicals for the treatment of allergic diseases and asthma. *Curr Allergy Asthma Rep.* 2016; 16(10):70.

Werfel T, Allam JP, Biedermann T, et al. Cellular and molecular immunologic mechanisms in patients with atopic dermatitis. *J Allergy Clin Immunol.* 2016;138:336-349.

Zellweger F, Eggel A. IgE-associated allergic disorders: recent advances in etiology, diagnosis and treatment. *Allergy.* 2016;71:1652-1661.




# 188 Clinical Aspects of Allergic Diseases

Sara Anvari and Maria Garcia-Lloret

## INTRODUCTION

Allergic rhinoconjunctivitis, asthma, and food allergy are some of the prototypical allergic diseases. Whereas allergies may develop at any age, allergic sensitization occurs predominantly early in life. *Atopy* is the inherited tendency to produce allergen-specific immunoglobulin (Ig) E antibodies. Food-specific IgE antibodies may appear in the very young child to herald an early presentation of clinical food allergies. Environmental allergen-specific IgE antibodies develop mostly after the age of 2, often leading to allergic rhinitis and/or allergic asthma in preschool or school-aged children. Although not all allergic diseases invariably develop in the same patient, in a sizeable number of children, the progressive sensitization to multiple antigens will result in sequential and often cumulative manifestations of atopy, a continuum that is known as the *allergic march*. It follows that allergic sensitization in childhood can have long-lasting effects throughout the life of the individual and implies a considerable burden to society as a whole.

## IMMUNOPATHOGENESIS

The fundamental role of the immune system is to protect the host against microbial pathogens while maintaining tolerance to "self" and to harmless exogenous antigens. This task is accomplished through a series of interactions among elements of the innate and the adaptive immune systems and involves numerous pathways of recognition, activation, response, and memory. Deficient immune responses to pathogens can lead to increased susceptibility to infection, whereas a failure in the mechanisms of tolerance results in allergy or autoimmunity. On the other hand, an uncontrolled inflammatory response during the course of an infection can increase the risk of morbidity and mortality, and augmented tolerance can hamper tumor rejection.

At the cellular level, dendritic cells and T lymphocytes are central to the regulation of immune homeostasis (Fig. 188-1). Specific interactions between these 2 key players lead to the differentiation of naïve T cells into 1 of 3 T-helper (TH) subtypes (TH1, TH2, and TH17). These effector T cells are kept in check by another set of T cells, the regulatory T cells, of which there are several subtypes that presumably represent distinct lineages.

TH1 cells express the transcription factor *T-bet* and produce the principle cytokine interferon gamma (IFN-γ), which is serves a critical role in immunity against intracellular microbes. In addition to IFN-γ, TH1 cells produce tumor necrosis factor (TNF) and other chemokines that facilitate the recruitment of leukocytes and promote inflammation. TH2 cells, which play an essential role in host defenses against helminthic infections, are defined by the expression of the transcription factor GATA-3. They produce IL-4 and IL-13, which are essential for production of IgE by B cells. Both cytokines also act to program

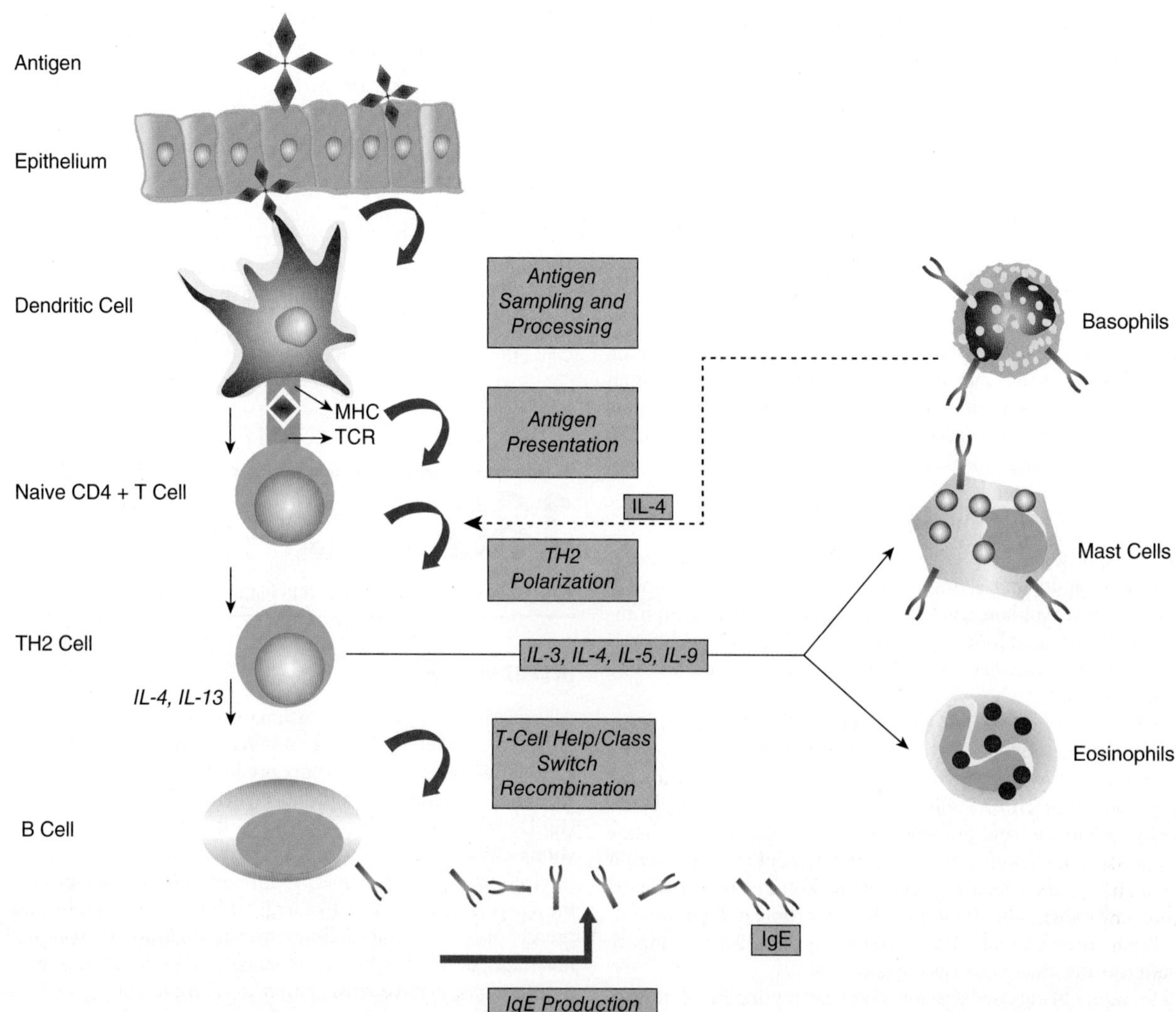


**FIGURE 188-1** TH2 differentiation and allergen sensitization. Allergens are sampled directly by dendritic cells at the mucosal surfaces or access the submucosal dendritic cells through the epithelium. Activated dendritic cells mature and process the allergen and then present it to naïve T cells in the context of major histocompatibility complex (MHC) class II molecules. Differentiation of naïve T cells toward the TH2 phenotype is favored by the availability of interleukin-4 (IL-4) in the microenvironment. Cellular sources of this early IL-4 include basophils, mast cells, T cells, and eosinophils. TH2 cells produce IL-4 and IL-13 cytokines that promote immunoglobulin (Ig) class-switch recombination and IgE production by B cells. IgE diffuses locally and then is distributed systemically, where it can bind to high-affinity receptors present on mast cells and basophils, "sensitizing" them to respond when the host is reexposed to the allergen. While sensitization is the hallmark of allergy, it does not necessarily result in clinical symptoms. Other TH2-derived cytokines (ie, IL-3, IL-9, and IL-5) promote the development and function of mast cells, basophils, and eosinophils, cellular elements that play a fundamental role in allergic inflammation.

cellular elements of the innate immune response, including macrophages and airway epithelial cells and others, to produce proallergic inflammatory products. TH2 cells also produce other cytokines such as IL-5, which is a key factor for eosinophil development and survival. The more recently discovered TH17 cells are defined by their expression of the transcription factor retinoic acid orphan receptor gamma-T. TH17 cells express signature cytokines such as IL-17, which plays a critical role in mobilizing neutrophilic inflammation and is essential to successful host defenses against certain pathogens such as fungi (especially *Candida* species).

Since the 1980s, the allergic phenotype has been understood in terms of an imbalance between TH1 and TH2 responses. This concept provided an operational mechanism behind the "hygiene hypothesis," which states that the lack of exposure to certain types of microbes early in life as a result of modern hygienic and medical practices fails to elicit robust TH1 responses and, by doing so, removes the restraint on TH2 responses that then become predominant. As a result of the TH2 skewing, there is a functional enhancement of the cellular responses to the TH2 cytokines, which predominantly target the mechanisms involved in hypersensitivity reactions such as production of IgE, mast cell maturation and survival, and development and migration of eosinophils (Fig. 188-2). In addition to a TH2 skewing, in allergy, there is a breakdown in the normal mechanisms of tolerance. This is well illustrated by the observation that patients with immune dysregulation polyendocrinopathy enteropathy X-linked (IPEX) syndrome, who have defective expression of the FoxP3 transcription factor and lack functional regulatory T cells, exhibit a phenotype characterized by severe allergies and autoimmunity. Conversely, subcutaneous allergen-specific immunotherapy induces the expansion of regulatory T cells in the periphery, and it has been shown that children who outgrow their milk allergy have more milk-specific regulatory T cells than those who remain clinically reactive.

## CLINICAL ASPECTS

Allergen-specific IgE bound to the high-affinity FcεR1 on mast cells is crucial in the initiation of the cascade of events that characterizes allergic inflammation. IgE cross-linking by its cognate antigen results in mast cell degranulation and release of biologically active products, including autacoids, prostaglandins, leukotrienes,

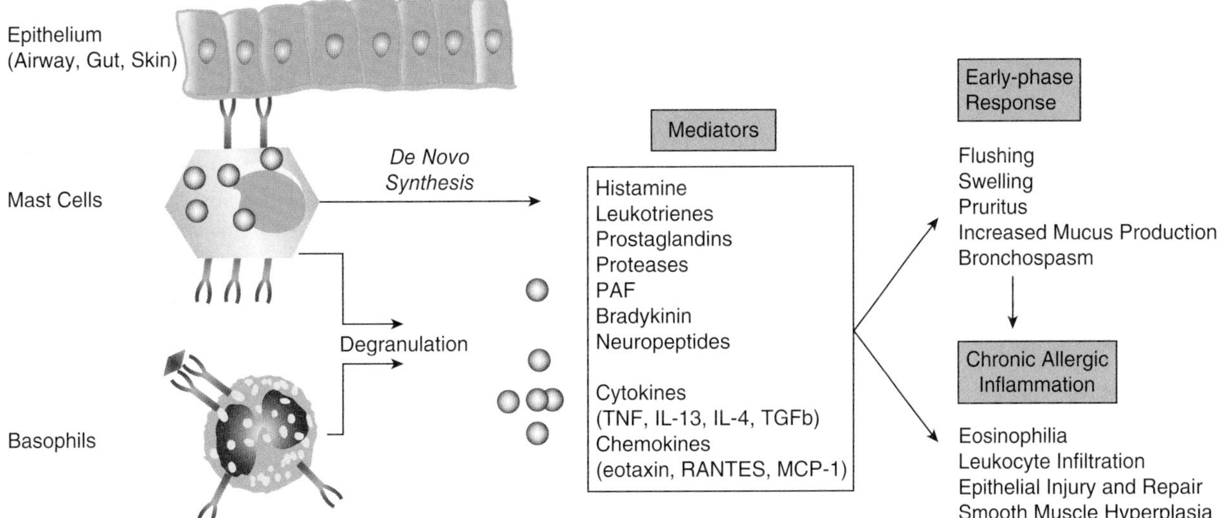


**FIGURE 188-2** Clinical and molecular aspects of the allergic response. Upon reexposure to an allergen, cross-linking of IgE molecules bound to the FcεRI expressed on tissue-resident mast cells (or on blood-borne basophils) activates these cells to secrete a host of preformed mediators that are responsible for many of the clinical manifestations of the early phase of the allergic response. This reaction is followed by synthesis of a variety of cytokines and chemokines promoting the influx of inflammatory cells at the affected sites (eg, the airway), which in turn amplifies and perpetuates the allergic response and may result in chronic inflammatory changes and tissue remodeling.

histamine, proteases, chemokines, and growth factors. The release of these mediators occurs within minutes of exposure to an allergen and contributes to the clinical manifestations associated with early-phase allergic reactions that in general depend on the target organ involved (eg, skin, gastrointestinal tract, or airway). Pruritus, sneezing, and coughing are triggered by the stimulation of sensory nerves in the airway or the skin. Some mediators promote erythema, vasodilation, and increased vascular permeability. In the skin, the result is the characteristic wheal and flare reaction, typical of the urticarial rash. Other mast cell products favor the contraction of the smooth muscles, which can lead to wheezing or to abdominal cramping and diarrhea, if the antigen encounter occurs in the gut. Whereas most allergic reactions are primarily local, systemic release of these mediators into the circulation can lead to anaphylaxis.

In some patients, the early phase is followed by a late-phase reaction, also orchestrated by the mast cell products in conjunction with T-cell–derived cytokines and chemokines. Late-phase reactions occur within 6 to 8 hours of exposure to an allergen and result from the accumulation and activation of inflammatory cells at the affected sites. Chemokines promote the infiltration of the mucosa with eosinophils, neutrophils, basophils, T lymphocytes, and macrophages. These cells become activated and release inflammatory mediators, which in turn can reactivate many of the proinflammatory reactions of the early-phase response.

Whereas the acute signs and symptoms of an allergic reaction usually subside with no sequelae, continuous or repetitive exposure to allergen can spawn a series of structural changes in the affected tissues that can have more permanent consequences for the individual. In the airway, chronic allergic inflammation can lead to epithelial injury and tissue remodeling, factors that play a central role in the pathogenesis of asthma. In the gut, continuous exposure results in mucosal damage and malabsorption, and in the skin, dysregulated epithelial repair underlies the features of chronic eczema, such as hyperkeratosis and lichenification.

In addition to increasing the risk of developing infection, the disruption of the epithelial barrier is thought to lead to further sensitizations. About one-third of infants with atopic eczema present with high levels of IgE against food allergens even before having any known oral exposure to these foods. Although exposure through breast milk cannot be ruled out, an alternative hypothesis is that encounter with allergenic foodstuffs through nonoral routes (eg, through a broken skin) favors sensitization, whereas exposure through the natural oral route results in tolerance. This hypothesis was supported in a previous study linking the rise in the prevalence of peanut allergy in Great Britain to the use of peanut-containing emollients in infants with atopic dermatitis. In turn, allergic sensitization perpetuates TH2-type responses in the skin that lead to chronic allergic inflammation and worsening of the eczema following repeated exposures to the allergen, whether through the oral or the nonoral route. This hypothesis could explain why, in some children, excluding the offending food from the diet results in improvement, if not complete resolution, of the symptoms of atopic dermatitis.

Successive sensitization to environmental allergens during childhood and early adolescence is a well-documented phenomenon and is directly linked to the progression of the atopic march. Atopic children (ie, those presumably genetically predisposed to mount IgE responses) first become sensitized to the predominant aeroallergens present in the home, such as dust mites, pet dander, and certain molds. Allergic inflammation with a local TH2 bias can alter the physiology of the nasal epithelium and favor further sensitization, this time to outdoor aeroallergens such as plant pollens. From a clinical standpoint, these children initially present with the classical symptoms of allergic rhinoconjunctivitis. Because the lower airway responds to mediators similar to those in the nasal mucosa, in the context of chronic allergic inflammation, many of these children go on to develop symptoms of allergic asthma that persist well into adulthood.

## DIAGNOSIS AND DIFFERENTIAL DIAGNOSIS

Symptoms associated with respiratory allergies (nasal congestion, cough, wheezing) are among the most common complaints encountered by pediatricians. Accordingly, the clinical history is key to establishing the correct diagnosis of allergies. Signs and symptoms will vary not only depending on the target organ and on the immunopathogenesis of the specific disorder but also on the age of the patient and the duration of the disease. The characteristic temporal association between exposure to an allergen and manifestation of clinical symptoms is not always evident and only becomes apparent after a guided questionnaire is completed. In other cases, the type of exposure is completely unknown, but the symptoms are characteristic enough to warrant further investigations.

In respiratory allergies, the age of the patient is an important consideration. In the infant or the young toddler, nasal congestion or wheezing are rarely manifestations of allergy. In this age range, common respiratory infections are the main cause of these symptoms. After the age of 3, viral infections continue to be prevalent, but allergy to indoor allergens can also play a role, especially in the presence of chronic nasal symptoms or associated ocular manifestations. Seasonal allergies (eg, "hay fever") usually present when the child is close to school age, as sensitization to pollen allergens in general occurs later in life.

Recurrent emesis and/or bloody diarrhea in a bottle-fed young infant is suggestive of a cow's milk allergy. In the older child, the typical symptoms of an IgE-mediated food-allergic reaction are flushing, urticaria, and angioedema, with or without gastrointestinal and/or respiratory manifestations, whereas heartburn, recurrent emesis, and dysphagia, even in the absence of skin manifestations, hint at the presence of eosinophilic esophagitis, an increasingly common disorder in which food allergies may play a role.

Allergies have also been implicated in the pathogenesis of several conditions such as recurrent otitis media, chronic sinusitis, and nasal polyposis. The pathogenesis of these illnesses may involve chronic allergic inflammation of the upper airway. In contrast, there is no evidence to substantiate the belief that childhood allergies are a common cause of isolated constitutional symptoms such as poor appetite, fatigue, chronic pain, or behavioral problems such as learning difficulties. A notable exception may be the child with severe, perennial allergic rhinosinusitis leading to significant nasal obstruction with or without sleep apnea. These children do benefit from medical treatment and often display significant improvement in their school performance when their allergies are under control.

When the clinical history and the presenting symptoms are suggestive of an IgE-mediated allergic condition, laboratory tests can be useful for determining the presence of specific IgE against the presumed allergen(s). Pediatricians can easily request a serum determination of allergen-specific IgE (formerly known as RAST, or radioallergoabsorbent test, but now mostly performed by other comparable technologies). To aid in the selection of tested allergens, many laboratories offer panels that include the most common allergens implicated in a particular condition (eg, food allergy panel, animal dander, molds) and, in the case of aeroallergens, a sampling of pollens relevant to the patient's environment. One has to bear in mind that sensitization (ie, IgE production) does not always correlate with clinical allergy, and, therefore, these tests should be regarded as confirmatory only in the context of a documented or highly probable reaction following exposure. The same can be said of the skin-prick tests, which are in-office tests performed routinely by pediatric allergists. They are highly sensitive and specific, and results can be obtained within minutes. Yet, in a way, they are far more useful for ruling out a particular allergen as the trigger for an allergic reaction than ruling it in because the positive predictive value of these tests has been estimated to be about 40% and the negative predictive value approaches 90% or more.

## MANAGEMENT OF ALLERGIC DISEASES

With the exception of subcutaneous immunotherapy (SCIT) and sublingual immunotherapy (SLIT), which have a proven record of success in the treatment of allergic rhinoconjunctivitis, presumably by inducing a long-lasting tolerance, most therapeutic modalities for allergic diseases are geared toward ameliorating the symptoms of the affected patients and, at the same time, preventing possible complications or involvement of other organs. This is not to say that the available therapies are not effective, and compliance with these treatments can certainly improve the quality of life of these patients.

The proper management of the allergic child requires a multipronged approach that includes minimizing the exposure to the allergic trigger(s), as well as using a cohort of medications that can revert or control an established allergic reaction (eg, antihistamines, epinephrine) or limit its development (eg, glucocorticoids, leukotriene inhibitors, and others).

### Allergen Avoidance

Exclusion of the allergenic food from a child's diet clearly reduces the likelihood of developing an allergic reaction to this food and should always be recommended. Although there have been isolated reports of nondietary exposures to food allergens (eg, through the skin or inhalation) resulting in systemic reactions, these are rare occurrences. Minimizing the exposure to allergens that act primarily on the respiratory tract has been shown to decrease symptoms and improve control in children with respiratory allergies and asthma. Environmental control measures directed at decreasing the levels of indoor allergens such as dust mites, mold, and pet dander usually result in a tangible relief in allergic symptoms, particularly in children with perennial allergic rhinoconjunctivitis and/or asthma. Removal of the pet from the home should be recommended but is not always an acceptable option for the family. In those cases, limiting the access of the animal to the child's bedroom and placing an air purifier (especially useful for cat allergens) can be helpful. Measures to prevent exposure to pollens are largely ineffective because the distribution of these allergens is widespread and they can travel airborne over large distances.

### Pharmacologic Agents

**Corticosteroids** Corticosteroids are pleiotropic, anti-inflammatory drugs with proven efficacy in the management of various aspects of the allergic inflammation. The development of highly effective topical preparations (intranasal, inhaled, or dermatologic creams) with minimal systemic effects has revolutionized the therapy of common disorders such as allergic rhinitis, allergic asthma, and atopic dermatitis. Inhaled corticosteroids are the first line of treatment for patients with persistent asthma. As monotherapy, intranasal corticosteroids are more efficacious than either leukotriene receptor antagonists or antihistamines, or their combination, in the management of both the nasal and ocular symptoms of allergic rhinoconjunctivitis. When used at the recommended doses, most intranasal corticosteroid preparations are not generally associated with clinically significant effects on the hypothalamic–pituitary–adrenal axis, ocular pressure or cataract formation, or bone density.

**Antihistamines** Histamine is a primary amine produced by mast cells and basophils that orchestrates many aspects of the allergic response by binding to specific receptors present on the surface of its target cells. So far, 4 types of histamine receptors belonging to the G protein–coupled receptor family have been identified: $H_1$, $H_2$, $H_3$, and $H_4$. Signals transduced via the $H_1$ (and to a lesser extent $H_2$) receptor mediate many of the acute symptoms and signs of allergic disease in the skin, airway, and gastrointestinal tract, whereas $H_3$ and $H_4$ appear to promote the accumulation of inflammatory cells at sites of allergic inflammation.

Histamine receptor antagonists are widely prescribed for the treatment of allergic disorders. Pretreatment with an oral $H_1$ antihistamine reduces early responses to an allergen in the conjunctiva, nose, lower airway, and skin, and administering the drug during the course of an allergic response curbs the symptoms triggered by acute allergic inflammation. Onset of action occurs within 1 to 3 hours. Newer $H_1$-antihistamines have a prolonged half-life and need to be administered only once or twice daily, whereas others have to be administered several times a day to maintain efficacy. Tolerance to doses that achieve clinical efficacy does not develop, but symptom relief may be insufficient when other mediators (leukotrienes, neuropeptides, etc.) are involved. This tolerance is often the case in the pruritus of atopic dermatitis, which, by and large, is resistant to antihistamines.

There are more than 40 $H_1$ antagonists available worldwide. These agents, which have diverse chemical structures, are in general effective and safe to use in infants and children. However, they are not interchangeable, and the safety profile varies from agent to agent. First-generation $H_1$ blockers (eg, brompheniramine, cyproheptadine, chlorpheniramine, hydroxyzine, and promethazine) are lipophilic and penetrate the central nervous system (CNS) readily, causing sedation or, in some patients, paradoxical excitation. These drugs are excreted in breast milk and have been reported to induce drowsiness or respiratory depression in nursing infants. Thus, unless sedation is a primary goal, second-generation $H_1$ antihistamines (eg, loratadine, cetirizine, and fexofenadine), which penetrate the CNS poorly, are preferable.

**Leukotriene Receptor Antagonists** Leukotrienes are products of the 5-lipoxygenase pathway synthesized by white cells in response to a variety of inflammatory stimuli. Within this family, the cysteinyl leukotrienes ($LTC_4$, $LTD_4$, and $LTE_4$) account for the biologic activity known as *slow-reacting substance of anaphylaxis*. Leukotriene receptors (BLT1 and BLT2, CysLT1 and CysLT2) are expressed in several tissues, including hemopoietic cells, smooth muscle cells, and epithelia, where they mediate a myriad of biologic functions. Pertinent to allergic disease, leukotrienes induce the migration and activation of virtually all white cells involved in allergic inflammation as well as smooth muscle and asthma.

Several studies have demonstrated the efficacy of leukotriene receptor antagonists (LTRAs) in the treatment of asthma. The best studied in this group is montelukast, which is now approved for the treatment of asthma in children age 12 months and older and for relief of symptoms of perennial allergic rhinitis in infants from 6 months on. As single drugs, LTRAs are less effective than is nasal or inhaled corticosteroids in the treatment of allergic rhinitis or asthma. Furthermore, the clinical response to LTRAs is somewhat unpredictable, which may be due in part to genetic factors. Yet, the safety profile of LTRAs renders them a suitable alternative for patients who cannot receive steroids or who are wary of their side effects. The efficacy of LTRAs in other allergic disorders such as atopic dermatitis and urticaria has been suggested but not demonstrated.

**Mast Cell Stabilizers** Mast cell stabilizers can been used in the prevention of acute and late-phase reactions associated with episodic allergen exposure in patients with allergic rhinoconjunctivitis. Mast cell stabilizers inhibit the release of histamine and other inflammatory mediators from mast cells by inhibiting the intermediate conductance chloride channel pathways of mast cells, eosinophils, epithelial and endothelial cells, fibroblasts, and sensory neurons. Although safe, their use is limited because they are not as effective as other available agents and they require frequent dosing.

**Omalizumab** Omalizumab is a recombinant humanized monoclonal antibody that has been approved for the treatment of allergic asthma in children older than 6 years of age and has also been approved for treatment of refractory chronic idiopathic urticaria in children age 12 years and older. Omalizumab inhibits IgE binding to mast cells and basophils, thereby decreasing release of a mediator. It also reduces levels of free IgE and subsequently downregulates IgE receptors.

**Allergen-Specific Immunotherapy** Allergen-specific SCIT has been practiced since the late 1950s and has proven to be clearly effective therapy for allergic airway diseases and insect venom allergy. SCIT can potentially modify the course of allergic rhinoconjunctivitis by redirecting the immune response toward a tolerant state, and its clinical benefits may be sustained years after discontinuation of treatment. Allergen immunotherapy for allergic rhinitis diminishes the risk of developing new allergen sensitizations in monosensitized children and has reduced the risk of asthma in children with allergic rhinitis.

While the cost of SCIT is comparable to that of pharmacotherapy, it is a time- and resource-consuming therapy that requires long-term (minimum of 3 years) commitment on the part of the patient. In children, who are usually fearful of shots, there is the added drawback that it implies subcutaneous injections.

The noninjection routes (sublingual immunotherapy) have been in use for years in Europe and are effective in the treatment of allergic rhinoconjunctivitis in children and adults. SLIT was recently approved for the treatment of allergic rhinoconjunctivitis due to grass or ragweed sensitivity. Immunomodulatory effects have also been observed with SLIT. Patients must demonstrate sensitivity to grass or ragweed pollens, as well as have a clinical history. SLIT is safe and effective in children as young as 3 years of age. Doses are administered daily and taken sublingually. Currently, SLIT is not available in the United States for the treatment of dust mite or tree pollen allergy.

## SUGGESTED READINGS


Abbas AK, Lichtman AH, Pillai S. *Cellular and Molecular Immunology*. 8th ed. Philadelphia, PA: Elsevier Saunders; 2015.

Jáuregui I, Mullol J, Dávila I, et al. Allergic rhinitis and school performance. *J Invest Allergol Clin Immunol*. 2009;19(Suppl 1):32-39.

Jutel M, Agache I, Bonini S, et al. International consensus on allergy immunotherapy. *J Allergy Clin Immunol*. 2015;136:556-568.

Lack G, Fox D, Northstone K, et al. Factors associated with the development of peanut allergy in childhood. *N Engl J Med*. 2003;348: 977-985.

Portnoy J, Kennedy K, Sublett J. Environmental assessment and exposure control: a practice parameter-furry animals. *Ann Allergy Asthma Immunol*. 2012;108:223.e1-e15.

Portnoy J, Miller JD, Williams PB, et al. Environmental assessment and exposure control of dust mites: a practice parameter. *Ann Allergy Asthma Immunol*. 2013;111:465-507.

Sakaguchi S, Vignali DA, Rudensky AY, Niec RE, Waldmann H. The plasticity and stability of regulatory T cells. *Nat Rev Immunol*. 2013;13:461-467.

Sampson HA, Aceves S, Bock SA, et al. Food allergy: a practice parameter update-2014. *J Allergy Clin Immunol*. 2014;134:1016-1025.

Seidman MD, Gurgel RK, Lin SY, et al. Clinical practice guideline: allergic rhinitis. *Otolaryngol Head Neck Surg*. 2015;152:S1-S43

Shreffler WG, Wanich N, Moloney M, Nowak-Wegrzyn A, Sampson HA. Association of allergen-specific regulatory T cells with the onset of clinical tolerance to milk protein. *J Allergy Clin Immunol*. 2009;123: 43-52.

Spergel JM. From atopic dermatitis to asthma: the atopic march. *Ann Allergy Asthma Immunol*. 2010;105:99-106.

Wu LC, Zarrin AA. The production and regulation of IgE by the immune system. *Nat Rev Immunol*. 2014;14:247-260.






# 189 Allergic Rhinitis and Conjunctivitis

Sara Anvari and Maria Garcia-Lloret

## INTRODUCTION

Allergic rhinitis is a chronic inflammatory disease of the upper airways caused by immunoglobulin E (IgE) sensitization to airborne allergens in genetically susceptible individuals. The clinical presentation is characteristically associated with frequent sneezing, nasal congestion, and nasal discharge. As many as 60% of patients with allergic rhinitis complain or display ocular symptoms (ie, itchy/watery eyes); thus it is termed *allergic rhinoconjunctivitis* (ARC), the term by which it is better known. Allergic rhinitis is subdivided into seasonal and perennial types based on time of occurrence and duration of symptoms. Allergic rhinitis can affect a child's quality of life and can be associated with conditions such as sleep disturbances and learning difficulties. This chapter will provide an overview of the epidemiology, pathogenesis, diagnosis, and management of allergic rhinoconjunctivitis.

## EPIDEMIOLOGY

There is a wide variation in the prevalence of ARC worldwide. In the United States, symptoms of ARC can occur in 10% to 30% of adults and as many as 40% of children. In the pediatric group, the numbers range from 0.8% to 14.9% in 6- to 7-year-olds and from 1.4% to 39.7% in 13- to 14-year-olds. The reasons behind these disparities are not completely understood, but both environmental and genetic factors are likely to play a role. Like other allergic diseases, the prevalence of ARC seems to be on the rise, particularly in industrialized countries. Risk factors for developing allergic rhinitis include family history of atopy, higher socioeconomic class, having a serum IgE > 100 IU/mL before 6 years of age, and evidence of sensitization.

Aeroallergen sensitization can occur between 6 months and 2 years of life, especially in children with a family history of atopy;

however, it is uncommon for sensitization to occur before 6 months of age. The classical symptoms of seasonal allergic rhinitis do not typically develop until the child reaches 2 to 7 years of age. In childhood, allergic rhinitis occurs more frequently in boys, but in adults, occurs more frequently in women. The prevalence of seasonal allergic rhinitis is higher in children and adolescents, whereas perennial allergic rhinitis has a higher prevalence in adults.

## PATHOGENESIS

The pathogenesis of ARC responds to the same immune mechanisms as do other allergic disorders. In this case, exposure to airborne allergens, in a genetically susceptible individual, initiates the series of events that lead to the local activation of allergen-specific T cells with a Th2 bias that directs the production of inflammatory cytokines, chemokines, and allergen-specific IgE. Upon reexposure to the same allergen, allergen-specific IgE bound to the Fcε receptors on mast cells cross-link and trigger the release of preformed mediators. Histamine released by mast cells is largely responsible for the immediate symptoms associated with ARC such as sneezing, itching, and rhinorrhea. Late responses are characterized by the recruitment of inflammatory cells to the nasal mucosa. These cells, which include eosinophils, basophils, lymphocyte, monocytes, and neutrophils, become attracted to the cytokines and chemokines released by mast cells during the immediate response. Skin-prick testing of the appropriate allergens gives a positive result, and results from nasal swabs and lavages or biopsy of the mucosa reveals eosinophils, but neutrophils are usually also present.

## DIAGNOSIS

### History

A detailed clinical and environmental history is instrumental in determining whether allergies are the cause of the patient's complaints. Questions should address not only the type and frequency of symptoms and any identified triggers but also the temporal relationship between perceived exposure and the development of symptoms consistent with an allergic reaction. In the patient with classical hay fever or cat allergies, this connection may be clear-cut, but in the child with perennial nasal congestion and complaints of cough and/or malaise, this relationship may not be readily apparent, and the diagnosis of ARC may be missed. Noisy breathing and snoring are common complaints referred by the parents of young children with ARC, and in this age range, poor appetite may also be a manifestation of ARC. In the older child, headaches may be prominent; behavioral problems or poor school performance may be the result of sleep disturbances secondary to untreated respiratory allergies. Coexisting or past atopic conditions such as atopic dermatitis, food allergies, or asthma can be suggestive of an allergic etiology, as is a history of respiratory allergies in first-degree relatives. In contrast, a lack of response to conventional antiallergy medications usually points to nonallergic causes.

### Physical Exam

Atopic children do not have any particular habitus, and for those with seasonal ARC, the physical exam may be completely normal outside of the pollen season. Examination of the nose, oropharynx, tympanic membranes, and eyes is necessary to identify features that may be consistent with ARC. Classical signs of respiratory allergies include the allergic shiners (infraorbital edema and darkening), allergic salute (transverse nasal crease), and Dennie-Morgan lines (transverse folds below the lower eyelids). Although these signs are often observed in atopic children, their presence neither confirms nor excludes the existence of allergies. The exam of the nasal cavity may be helpful in distinguishing allergic from nonallergic etiologies: pale, enlarged turbinates and clear rhinorrhea are usually a sign of ARC, whereas an erythematous mucosa with crusty secretions suggests other causes. Nasal polyps, if present, should prompt the search for a different diagnosis, such as cystic fibrosis or, in the older child, aspirin sensitivity. Ocular itch, conjunctival redness or swelling, and tearing are common symptoms of allergic conjunctivitis as part of ARC. In children, findings of dental malocclusion, a high-arched palate, and elevation of the upper lip may suggest early-onset and/or longstanding disease. A cobblestone-like appearance of the posterior pharynx is usually found in patients with ARC.

## DIAGNOSTIC TESTING

Determination of specific IgE is indicated to (1) provide additional evidence of an allergic basis for the patient's symptoms, (2) confirm suspected causes of the patient's symptoms, or (3) assess the sensitivity to a specific allergen for avoidance measures and/or allergen immunotherapy. Percutaneous skin-prick testing, when properly performed, is considered to be the most convenient and least expensive method for detecting the presence of allergen-specific IgE in most patients. The number of skin tests and the allergens selected for skin testing should be determined on the basis of the patient's age, history, and environmental exposures. Comparable results can be obtained through the determination of levels of specific IgE in serum, when skin testing is not available. However, this can be a costly approach if multiple allergens are measured. When correctly performed, both techniques display a high degree of sensitivity and specificity for the detection of allergic sensitization to aeroallergens. However, the findings should be interpreted in the context of the clinical history, because allergic sensitization does not always correlate with clinical allergy. In certain cases, radiologic exams could be indicated in order to exclude other causes of nasal congestion, such as adenoid hypertrophy or sinusitis. A polysomnographic test may be necessary to confirm the diagnosis of obstructive sleep apnea.

## DIFFERENTIAL DIAGNOSIS

Even if the coexistence of chronic or recurrent nasal and eye symptoms strongly suggests an allergic etiology, the differential diagnosis of chronic rhinitis is vast and depends on the age of the patient. Irritants or toxins can directly influence the nasal mucosa through non–IgE-dependent mechanisms and induce nasal symptoms that are similar to allergic rhinitis and occur after exposure. Other examples of nonallergic rhinitis are infectious rhinitis (usually virally induced and responsible for more than 90% of cases in infants and toddlers), vasomotor rhinitis, and the nonallergic rhinitis with eosinophilia syndrome (NARES). This syndrome is characterized by rhinitis in the absence of atopy shown by allergy skin testing and > 20% eosinophils on nasal cytology. Nasal congestion and discharge that occur after ingestion of foods or alcoholic products are vagally mediated and usually not a manifestation of food allergy. Chronic nasal congestion can present in patients who take angiotensin-converting enzyme inhibitors, nonsteroidal anti-inflammatory drugs, and other medications, and hormonal rhinitis should be considered in female adolescents. Aside from rhinitis, other conditions may mimic ARC, include nasal polyps and adenoidal hypertrophy, as well as anatomic abnormalities of the nasal or facial structures that may result in the narrowing of the upper airway.

## MANAGEMENT

Optimal management of ARC in children requires preventive measures to minimize exposure to allergens, together with the judicious use of pharmacologic agents to curtail symptoms, improve the quality of life of the child, and, ideally, prevent the development of long-term complications. Because ARC is a chronic disease, patient education is a key element in promoting adherence and optimizing treatment outcome.

## ENVIRONMENTAL CONTROL

While allergen avoidance is effective in the control of ARC, complete avoidance may not be possible or even practical. Exposure to dust mites can be reduced through implementing effective avoidance measures, which include physical barriers on the mattress, pillows, and upholstered furniture, as well as reducing dust mite colonies by controlling humidity in the home. When pet dander is the trigger, removal of the pet from the home is the safest option; however, patients should be aware that several weeks may be required before the allergen concentration reaches levels found in the animal-free home. Alternatively, considering frequent home cleaning, frequent pet bathing, and confining the pet to an uncarpeted room with high-efficiency particulate air (HEPA) filtration may reduce airborne allergen dissemination to the rest of the house.

## MEDICAL THERAPY

Intranasal corticosteroids (INCs) are the quintessential anti-inflammatory drugs used for treating ARC. As monotherapy, INCs are more efficacious than are antihistamines, leukotriene receptor antagonists, or their combination in the management of the major symptoms of ARC. INCs provide substantial relief even when used on an as-needed schedule. Local side effects (burning or stinging) are usually mild. When used at the recommended doses, INCs are not generally associated with clinically significant effects on the hypothalamic–pituitary–adrenal axis, ocular pressure or cataract formation, or bone density.

Second-generation oral antihistamines (eg, loratadine, desloratadine, fexofenadine, cetirizine, levocetirizine, and others) are preferred over first-generation medications for the treatment of ARC because of their reduced tendency to cause sedation and/or anticholinergic effects. These drugs are particularly effective in the management of the ocular and nasal symptoms associated with seasonal allergies. Because of their fast onset of action, they can be used on an as-needed basis, although maximal benefit has been reported with long-term use. In addition to the oral form, ocular and nasal preparations for antihistamines have also been demonstrated to be effective in the temporary management of ARC.

The effectiveness of leukotriene receptor antagonists in the treatment of ARC is comparable to that of oral antihistamines. As single agents, they are less effective than are INCs for the treatment of ARC, but they should be considered in patients with concomitant asthma or in those in whom corticosteroids are contraindicated. Combination of a leukotriene receptor antagonist and an antihistamine does not provide added benefit and, in general, should not be recommended.

Isotonic and hypertonic saline solutions, when used as adjunctive agents, are of benefit for reducing symptoms in patients with ARC or rhinosinusitis. Cromolyn, a mast cell stabilizer, is a safe treatment available over-the-counter and can be used to relieve nasal itch, rhinorrhea, and sneezing. However, it is less effective than are treatments and requires frequent dosing. The topical decongestants that work by constricting the blood vessels lining the nose (eg, oxymetazoline, phenylephrine, xylometazoline, and naphazoline nasal sprays) may provide temporary relief, but their longer-term use is discouraged due to the risk of rebound nasal congestion (rhinitis medicamentosa) that sets in within 5 to 7 days of repeated use. Oral decongestants are also not recommended in children due to their well-recognized cardiovascular and central nervous system side effects.

Allergen-specific subcutaneous immunotherapy is a clearly effective therapy for allergic rhinitis, particularly in patients with pollinosis and/or allergy to house dust mites. Subcutaneous immunotherapy modifies the course of ARC by redirecting the immune response toward a tolerant state, and its clinical benefits may be sustained years after discontinuation of treatment. Allergen immunotherapy for allergic rhinitis may prevent the development of new allergen sensitization and has been shown to reduce the risk of development of asthma in children and adolescents with allergic rhinitis.

Sublingual immunotherapy (SLIT) was recently approved for the treatment of ARC caused by grass or ragweed sensitivity. Immunomodulatory effects have also been observed with SLIT. Patients must demonstrate sensitivity to grass or ragweed pollens, as well as have a clinical history. SLIT is safe and effective in children as young as 3 years of age. The dose is administered under the tongue and taken once daily. The first dose should be administered under medical supervision; however, subsequent doses are administered at home. Currently SLIT is not available in the United States for the treatment of allergies to dust mites or tree pollen.

## SUGGESTED READINGS


Berger WE, Meltzer EO. Intranasal spray medications for maintenance therapy of allergic rhinitis. *Am J Rhinol Allergy*. 2015;29:273-282.

Jessen M. Malm L. Definition, prevalence and development of nasal obstruction. *Allergy*. 1997;52:3-6.

Jutel M, Agache I, Bonini S, et al. International consensus on allergy immunotherapy. *J Allergy Clin Immunol*. 2015;136:556-568.

Kulig M, Klettke U, Wahn V, et al. Development of seasonal allergic rhinitis during the first 7 years of life. *J Allergy Clin Immunol*. 2000;106:832-839.

LeMasters GK, Wilson K, Levin L, et al. High prevalence of aeroallergen sensitization among infants of atopic parents. *J Pediatr*. 2006; 149:505-511.

Muraro A, Lemanske RF Jr, Hellings PW, et al. Precision medicine in patients with allergic diseases: Airway diseases and atopic dermatitis-PRACTALL document of the European Academy of Allergy and Clinical Immunology and the American Academy of Allergy, Asthma and Immunology. *J Allergy Clin Immunol*. 2016;137:1347-1358.

Salo PM, Calatroni A, Gergen PJ, et al. Allergy-related outcomes in relation to serum IgE: results from the National Health and Nutrition Examination Survey 2005-2006. *J Allergy Clin Immunol*. 2011;127:1226-1235.

Settipane RJ, Hagy GW, Settipane GA. Long-term risk factors for developing asthma and allergic rhinitis: a 23-year follow-up study of college students. *Allergy Proc*. 1994;15:21-25.

Singh K, Axelrod S, Bielory L. The epidemiology of ocular and nasal allergy in the United States, 1988-1994. *J Allergy Clin Immunol*. 2010;126:778-783.

Skoner DP, Berger WE, Gawchik SM, Akbary A, Qiu C. Intranasal triamcinolone and growth velocity. *Pediatrics*. 2015;135:e348-e356.

Wallace DV, Dykewicz MS, Bernstein DI, et al. The diagnosis and management of rhinitis: an updated practice parameter. *J Allergy Clin Immunol*. 2008;122(2 Suppl):S1-84.

Wheatley LM, Togias A. Allergic rhinitis. *N Engl J Med*. 2015;372: 456-463.


# 190 Anaphylaxis, Urticaria, and Angioedema

Marc A. Riedl

## INTRODUCTION

Anaphylaxis, urticaria, and angioedema frequently share a common pathophysiology in that these conditions most commonly result from immunoglobulin E (IgE)-mediated mast cell activation, resulting in the release of histamine, leukotrienes, and other mast cell mediators. Urticaria and angioedema are isolated to mucocutaneous symptoms, whereas anaphylaxis is an acute systemic reaction that may rapidly lead to cardiopulmonary collapse.

## ANAPHYLAXIS

### PATHOGENESIS AND EPIDEMIOLOGY

Anaphylaxis is an acute, life-threatening, systemic syndrome mediated by sudden release of histamine, leukotrienes, and other mast cell– and basophil-derived mediators. It most often is caused by IgE-mediated hypersensitivity reactions to exposures to allergens. The estimated overall lifetime prevalence of anaphylaxis from all causes is 0.5% to 2%, and 0.7% to 2% of anaphylactic reactions are fatal. Rapid recognition, diagnosis, and therapy of anaphylaxis are imperative to prevent morbidity and mortality.

Although anaphylaxis can occur at any age, adolescents and young adults are most at risk for experiencing serious anaphylaxis. Preexisting asthma is a primary risk factor for fatal anaphylaxis, and delay in administering epinephrine therapy has been strongly associated with anaphylaxis-caused mortality. Additional risk factors for poor outcomes with anaphylaxis include concomitant therapy with β-adrenergic or α-adrenergic antagonists, which blunts the effectiveness of epinephrine treatment, and angiotensin-converting enzyme inhibitors, which interfere with physiologic compensatory mechanisms, thereby leading to severe or protracted anaphylaxis.

Risk factors for anaphylaxis include exposure to parenteral antigens (ie, intravenous [IV] medications) and repeated, interrupted exposure to antigens (ie, medication or food ingestion). The most common causes of anaphylaxis include foods, medications, stinging insects, latex, and blood products. Of these causes, foods and medications account for the majority of serious anaphylactic reactions resulting in emergency room visits or causing anaphylaxis mortality. Among foods, peanuts, tree nuts, cow's milk, egg, and seafood (crustaceans, mollusks, fish) most commonly cause anaphylaxis. Rarely, the temporal combination of ingestion of food and exercise may trigger anaphylaxis. This food-dependent, exercise-induced anaphylaxis is best evaluated by an allergy specialist. The most commonly implicated causative medications are β-lactam antibiotics (penicillins and cephalosporins), other antibiotics, radiocontrast agents (through direct mast-cell stimulation), and neuromuscular blocking agents. Other uncommon causes of anaphylaxis include physical factors such as exposure to cold, heat, or ultraviolet light. Finally, idiopathic anaphylaxis occurs when no inciting allergen can be identified through the clinical history or by diagnostic testing.

In the pediatric population, anaphylactic reactions to vaccines are a concern. True IgE-mediated anaphylaxis reaction to immunizations is rare and more commonly involves activation of IgE in response to vaccine components rather than the immunizing antigen itself. Gelatin, added to vaccines as a stabilizing agent, has been implicated in anaphylactic reactions to measles, mumps, and rubella (MMR), varicella, influenza, and Japanese encephalitis vaccines. Children with a history of allergy to egg should be seen by an allergy specialist prior to receiving influenza and yellow fever vaccines, as egg protein used in these vaccines has been implicated in anaphylactic reactions to these immunizations. IgE-mediated reaction to the specific vaccine antigen is exceedingly rare, but has been reported for diphtheria and tetanus.

Generally, previous exposure to an antigen is necessary for IgE sensitization to occur in any given individual. On subsequent exposure, the triggering antigen cross-links antigen-specific IgE bound to mast cells and basophils through high-affinity IgE (FcεRI) receptors. Activated mast cells and basophils release preformed mediators, including histamine, tryptase, chymase, and heparin. In addition, lipid-derived mediators such as cysteinyl leukotrienes (LTC4, LTD4, LTE4), prostaglandins, and platelet-activating factor are generated by activated mast cells and basophils. This sudden release of mediators into the circulation and tissues of the gastrointestinal and respiratory tract results in the multisystem syndrome of anaphylaxis.

Less commonly, non-IgE mechanisms may lead to activation of mast cells and development of symptoms of anaphylaxis. Such non-IgE reactions are sometimes called *anaphylactoid reactions*, as though they are clinically indistinguishable from IgE-mediated anaphylactic reactions. Direct mast-cell stimulation is likely a primary mechanism responsible for immediate systemic reactions to radiocontrast media. Other non-IgE alternative mechanisms leading to anaphylactic symptoms include immune complex–mediated complement activation, as occurs with blood products.

## CLINICAL MANIFESTATIONS

Anaphylaxis generally presents with a constellation of signs and symptoms, as well as a clinical history suggestive of allergen exposure. Symptoms of anaphylaxis typically appear within minutes of exposure to the allergen, though occasionally onset of symptoms may be delayed for several hours after oral ingestions. In severe cases, symptoms progress rapidly and lead to fatal shock within 60 minutes of exposure. Most anaphylactic reactions are uniphasic, although as many as 20% show a biphasic course with recurrent symptoms approximately occurring 8 to 12 hours after the exposure, or even occur as late as 72 hours after the initial anaphylactic phase. The mechanism of this clinical observation has not been established, although it has historically been attributed to mast cell cytokine production resulting in recruitment of eosinophils, basophils, macrophages, and lymphocytes into tissues, producing a second phase of inflammation.

The most common symptoms of anaphylaxis are cutaneous, respiratory, gastrointestinal, and cardiovascular. Skin symptoms may include urticaria, angioedema, erythema, pruritus, and diaphoresis. Respiratory symptoms of rhinitis, nasal congestion, wheezing, cough, chest tightness, and dyspnea are common. Laryngeal edema may also occur, causing stridor and airway compromise. Gastrointestinal symptoms including cramping, abdominal pain, nausea, vomiting, and diarrhea are frequently associated with anaphylaxis. Cardiovascular features are less common in children than adults. In the most severe or advanced stages, hypotension occurs with reflex tachycardia. Syncope and shock may result from the profound hypotension associated with severe anaphylaxis. Respiratory arrest and/or cardiovascular collapse due to hypotension are the common causes of death from anaphylaxis. Neurologic symptoms of anaphylaxis generally are less prominent but may include anxiety, a sense of impending doom, or confusion; young children may have behavioral changes such as clinging or irritability. Rarely, uterine cramping can occur during anaphylaxis.

## DIAGNOSIS

Anaphylaxis is a clinical diagnosis based on the history and constellation of presenting signs and symptoms listed above. Three diagnostic criteria for anaphylaxis have been proposed by expert opinion: (1) skin or mucosal symptoms AND involvement of respiratory compromise or hypotension *or* (2) two or more systems (skin, respiratory, cardiovascular, gastrointestinal) with allergic symptoms within a few hours following a likely exposure to a known allergen *or* (3) hypotension within a few hours following exposure to a known allergen for the patient. These criteria are helpful but do not replace clinical judgment by the health care professional. Treatment should not await laboratory confirmation, but confirmatory testing with serum tryptase levels is sometimes useful to confirm systemic mast cell activation. Histamine is detectable in plasma for only 15 to 30 minutes after the anaphylactic event, rendering appropriate collection difficult. Tryptase, a protease specific to mast cells, reaches a serum peak 30 to 120 minutes after the event and remains elevated for approximately 6 hours, rendering it more helpful to confirm systemic mast cell activation. Thus, an elevated serum tryptase level is useful to confirm systemic mast-cell activation. A normal serum tryptase level does not necessarily exclude anaphylaxis, particularly with food-induced events, which are rarely associated with elevated serum tryptase. Twenty-four-hour urine collection measurements for histamine metabolites following the event may also be helpful but are often impractical to collect. After treatment of the acute anaphylactic episode, additional diagnostic testing should include testing for allergen-specific IgE to confirm the causative antigen. It can be performed by allergy skin testing or serum-specific IgE testing to suspected allergens. Allergen skin testing should be performed at least 6 weeks after an anaphylactic event to avoid false-negative results. Evaluation by an allergy-immunology specialist is appropriate.

A number of common conditions may be confused with anaphylaxis. The differential diagnosis includes vasovagal reactions, acute urticaria and/or angioedema, acute asthma exacerbations, vocal cord dysfunction, acute anxiety disorders, and epiglottitis or foreign body aspirations resulting in respiratory distress. In addition to these common conditions, rare disorders such as mastocytosis or basophilic leukemia may present with systemic histamine-mediated symptoms.

## TREATMENT

The approach to treating anaphylaxis should focus first on maintaining the airway, breathing, and circulation. Mortality from anaphylaxis results from asphyxiation due to upper airway angioedema, respiratory failure from severe bronchial obstruction, or cardiovascular collapse. The most important initial medical therapy is epinephrine, which is most effective when administered intramuscularly (IM) within 30 minutes of onset of symptoms. There are no absolute contraindications to epinephrine use in the setting of anaphylaxis, and anaphylaxis-caused mortality is strongly correlated with delays in epinephrine therapy. Most patients respond to a single dose of IM initiating epinephrine; but, dosing may be repeated at 5- to 15-minute intervals for inadequate response, or sooner if clinically indicated. Intravenous epinephrine is rarely necessary and should be avoided whenever possible.

Any ongoing exposure to the suspected antigen should be discontinued (ie, medication infusion). Hypotension requires aggressive large-volume fluid resuscitation and, if persistent, vasopressor therapy. Supplemental oxygen is recommended, and in the presence of respiratory compromise or bronchospasm, inhaled bronchodilators such as albuterol should be administered. Intubation and mechanical ventilation may be necessary. $H_1$- and $H_2$-receptor antagonists are adjunctive medications that should be given to reduce pruritus and urticaria, although antihistamines without epinephrine are insufficient to adequately treat anaphylaxis. Corticosteroids are frequently given to attenuate the potential late-phase inflammatory response and thereby prevent recurrence of symptoms 8 to 12 hours after the initial onset; however, corticosteroids are not effective for the initial acute phase.

Anaphylactic reactions that occur in patients taking β-adrenergic antagonists may be particularly refractory to epinephrine. In this setting, glucagon or atropine administration should be considered. Whenever possible, patients should be observed for 8 to 12 hours after an anaphylactic reaction due to the possibility of recurrent symptoms from the late-phase response occurring several hours after the initial event.

## PREVENTION

All patients should be discharged with self-injectable epinephrine for home use, assuring that they receive appropriate instruction about the use of the device. Subsequent to treatment of the acute episode, identification of the triggering antigen or exposure should be pursued through diagnostic allergy skin testing or serum IgE testing whenever possible. Patients should strongly consider wearing medical alert identification detailing their specific allergies if known.

# URTICARIA AND ANGIOEDEMA

## PATHOGENESIS AND EPIDEMIOLOGY

Urticaria and angioedema are common conditions that affect as many as 20% of the population at some point during their lifespan. More than two-thirds of urticaria/angioedema cases are acute, self-limited episodes resolving in less than 6 weeks. Approximately one-third will persist with daily or near-daily symptoms for more than 6 weeks and are classified as chronic urticaria. The vast majority of urticaria and angioedema are mast-cell–mediated conditions responsive to antihistamines and corticosteroids. In contrast, angioedema in the absence of urticaria may suggest a bradykinin-related condition. Such angioedema is much less common but is important to recognize due to differences in therapy. Hereditary angioedema is a representative bradykinin-mediated angioedema with a prevalence of 1:10,000 to 1:100,000, affecting males and females equally.

Acute urticaria and angioedema are most often the result of activation of mast cells, with resultant release of histamine, leukotrienes, and other mediators into the superficial dermis (urticaria) and deep dermis (angioedema). These inflammatory mediators cause dilatation and increased permeability of capillaries and venules, leading to extravasation of fluid into tissues (angioedema). Activation of mast cells, may be the result of specific IgE cross-linking from exposure to allergens (foods, drugs, latex, insect venom, aeroallergens, parasitic infections, blood products), non-IgE activation (radiocontrast media, narcotics, vancomycin, muscle relaxants used in anesthesia), physical stimulation (pressure, cold, vibration), autoimmune activation, or immune complex formation with complement activation, as occurs in infection.

Angioedema in the absence of urticaria may be caused by mediators other than histamine. In particular, hereditary angioedema and angioedema caused by angiotensin-converting enzyme inhibitors are classified as kinin-related angioedemas, with bradykinin recognized as the most important mediator in these conditions. Hereditary angioedema is caused by mutations in the C1-inhibitor (*C1INH*) gene, resulting in low levels and/or activity of the C1INH protein. The inheritance is autosomal dominant, and most affected individuals carry 1 abnormal allele. As C1INH is a primary inhibitory protein for steps leading to bradykinin production, C1INH deficiency leads to increased tissue bradykinin, which interacts with vascular bradykinin 2 receptors, resulting in vasodilation, increased vascular permeability, and angioedema. Acquired angioedema, rarely seen in the pediatric population, is associated with malignancy or autoimmune conditions and also involves dysfunctional C1INH function. Angiotensin-converting enzyme inhibitor–associated angioedema is caused by increased bradykinin levels resulting from the inhibition of angiotensin-converting enzyme, which functions as a primary metabolizing enzyme for bradykinin.

Other mechanisms may be responsible for urticaria and angioedema caused by aspirin or nonsteroidal anti-inflammatory drugs. The pharmacologic properties of these drugs include inhibition of cyclooxygenase and reduced generation of prostaglandins from arachidonic acid, resulting in increased formation of cysteinyl leukotrienes.

## CLINICAL MANIFESTATIONS

Urticaria and angioedema are characterized by localized swelling of the skin and/or mucous membranes. Urticaria, commonly called *hives*, involves extravasation of fluid in the superficial dermis. It is characterized by well-circumscribed, pruritic, raised erythematous skin wheals, often with central pallor and blanching with applied pressure. Individual urticarial lesions typically disappear within 24 hours without any residual skin changes, unless from excoriation. Angioedema results from similar vasopermeability in the deeper layers of the dermis and subcutaneous tissue. Angioedema may appear associated with urticaria, but it occasionally presents as an isolated symptom. Angioedema typically involves the periorbital tissues, lips, tongue, posterior oropharynx, larynx, hands, feet, or genitals. Less commonly, angioedema may involve the gastrointestinal tract, resulting in abdominal pain, nausea, vomiting, and diarrhea. Edematous swelling of angioedema may take 24 to 72 hours or, in some instances, longer to fully resolve.

## DIAGNOSIS

Urticaria and angioedema are typically recognizable based on the clinical history, physical examination, and/or photographic documentation of the episodic clinical features described above. The differential diagnosis of urticaria includes viral exanthems, Sweet syndrome, atopic dermatitis, contact dermatitis, drug eruptions, insect bites, urticarial vasculitis, and erythema multiforme. The differential diagnosis for cutaneous angioedema may include edema caused by cardiac, renal, or liver dysfunction, contact dermatitis, cellulitis, lymphedema, and granulomatous disorders such as Melkersson-Rosenthal syndrome. The differential diagnosis for laryngeal or gastrointestinal angioedema is extensive but should include other potential causes for recurrent airway obstruction or abdominal pain. In accruing the patient's clinical history, important inquiries include food and medication ingestion, travel history, infections, atopy, and other systemic symptoms or conditions.

In children, common viral or bacterial infections may account for 80% of cases of acute urticaria. Food allergens frequently cause acute urticaria, with reactions generally occurring within 30 minutes of ingestion. Milk, egg, peanuts, tree nuts, soy, and wheat are the most frequently implicated foods causing urticaria in children. Among medication causes of urticaria, antibiotics (particularly β-lactams and sulfonamides) are most frequently implicated. Aeroallergen exposure is a rare cause of acute urticaria. It is important to note that in most cases of urticaria and angioedema, no external cause can be identified. Therefore, it is often reasonable to defer diagnostic testing for acute urticaria and focus on symptomatic treatment, unless there is strong clinical suspicion of an allergic trigger or a systemic medical condition. Specific IgE testing for foods, medications, or insect venom may be useful if these exposures are identified. Controlled, provocative testing may reproduce a number of physical urticarias, including those caused by pressure, cold, heat, or vibration.



Urticaria or angioedema with near daily symptoms lasting more than 6 weeks is deemed chronic, and a more thorough diagnostic evaluation may be indicated, although in most cases, no systemic underlying cause is identified. Evaluation for thyroid autoantibodies, autoimmune conditions, mastocytosis, and chronic viral infections may be considered, depending on the clinical presentation. Thirty to 50% of patients with chronic urticaria demonstrate mast-cell–stimulating autoantibodies, suggesting an autoimmune mechanism for some cases of chronic idiopathic urticaria.

Approximately 90% of mast-cell–mediated angioedema is associated with urticaria and/or pruritus, so absence of these concomitant symptoms suggests a different underlying pathway. Thus, the evaluation of isolated angioedema (ie, angioedema occurring in the absence of urticaria) should include consideration of kinin-related angioedemas such as hereditary or angiotensin-converting enzyme-inhibitor, associated angioedema. Hereditary angioedema (HAE) or C1INH deficiency often presents during the first or second decade of life, with recurrent angioedema episodes affecting the face, throat, extremities, genitals, or gastrointestinal tract. Seventy-five percent of patients with HAE experience their first attack by the age of 15.

Triggers for HAE attacks may include tissue trauma, infections, dental procedures, or emotional stress, although frequently, angioedema occurs spontaneously without an identifiable trigger. Angioedema episodes typically last for 48 to 72 hours before slow spontaneous resolution occurs. Twenty-five percent of new HAE diagnoses are attributed to de novo mutations in the *C1INH* gene, as no family history of HAE exists. Frequently, patients with HAE have been previously diagnosed with "recurrent allergic reactions," and surgical and/or gastrointestinal consultations have been obtained for recurrent, unexplained, episodic abdominal pain occurring in the absence of visible cutaneous angioedema.

Screening for hereditary angioedema is performed by testing the serum C4 level, which is typically low due to complement consumption. More comprehensive testing with quantitative and functional C1INH levels is recommended if serum C4 is low. Both quantitative and functional C1INH assays are required, as approximately 15% of HAE cases occur due to abnormal protein function (HAE type II) rather than reduced quantitative C1INH levels (HAE type I). In children younger than 1 year of age, C1INH levels are 30% to 50% lower than adult levels, and C4 levels are variable, rendering interpretation of lab results difficult. In these cases, testing should be repeated after the child reaches 1 year of age, or alternatively, genetic testing for HAE may be pursued, although it is complicated by the nearly 300 described *C1INH* gene mutations associated with HAE.

## TREATMENT

Treatment of acute urticaria and angioedema should focus on (1) identification and discontinuation of any triggering underlying process and (2) symptom suppression until resolution of the acute episode occurs. If an allergic trigger or physical urticaria is identified, avoidance of the allergen or physical stimulation is vital in terminating the reaction and preventing future episodes of urticaria. Symptom suppression can often be achieved with the administration of $H_1$-receptor antagonists, which are most effective at relieving pruritus associated with urticaria but may also reduce visible skin wheals. The use of first-generation $H_1$-receptor antagonists (ie, diphenhydramine, hydroxyzine) is limited by their sedating and anticholinergic side effects, but these agents may be particularly useful for nocturnal urticarial symptoms that interfere with sleep. Regular use of longer-acting, nonsedating antihistamines (ie, cetirizine, fexofenadine, loratadine) is generally preferred for controlling urticarial symptoms that persist for more than a few days.

$H_2$-receptor antagonists are useful adjuvant medications, but it is most efficient to maximize the $H_1$-receptor antagonist therapy prior to adding additional medications. Likewise, leukotriene inhibitors (eg, montelukast, zafirlukast, zileuton) may benefit some patients with chronic urticaria, particularly those with the autoimmune form of the condition. Short courses of oral corticosteroids can be used to control severe urticaria that is refractory to high-dose antihistamines. Long-term systemic corticosteroid use for chronic urticaria is associated with significant adverse side effects. In rare patients with severe chronic urticaria requiring frequent corticosteroids, a variety of "steroid-sparing" medications have been employed. They include omalizumab, cyclosporine, dapsone, hydroxychloroquine, and sulfasalazine.

Treatment of kinin-related angioedema is distinct because these conditions do not respond to antihistamines and corticosteroids. Angiotensin-converting enzyme-inhibitor–associated angioedema is treated primarily by withdrawing the offending drug. Generally, symptoms resolve within 48 to 72 hours of drug discontinuation. HAE symptoms are treated with plasma-derived or recombinant C1INH concentrate, ecallantide, or icatibant, all of which have been demonstrated to be effective in terminating HAE attacks. Plasma-derived C1INH is currently approved for children and adolescents, with variability in age-specific labeling for the other agents. If these proven drugs are not available, acute episodes of angioedema from HAE are managed with supportive care. Epinephrine may be useful as a temporizing measure for laryngeal attacks with airway obstruction; however, epinephrine does not effectively stop bradykinin-mediated angioedema progression and is not a substitute for the effective HAE medications listed above or for proper airway management. Intubation is sometimes necessary for significant laryngeal edema associated with HAE. The use of fresh frozen plasma, which provides a level of C1INH replacement, is complicated by rare reports of it worsening HAE attacks due to the additional substrate proteins contained in the product and the risk of transmissible blood-borne pathogens. Thus, any use of fresh frozen plasma in the therapy of HAE attacks should be undertaken with great caution.

Preventative therapy for HAE attacks should be considered in patients experiencing frequent or severe angioedema attacks. Plasma-derived C1INH has been shown to be effective for long-term prophylaxis and is the preferred preventative therapy for children affected by HAE. The attenuated androgens (ie, danazol) are effective prophylactic medications; however, their use in the pediatric population is complicated by concern for side effects, including epiphyseal closure and decreased growth. Antifibrinolytic agents such as tranexamic acid and aminocaproic acid are less effective at preventing HAE attacks but may be useful in the pediatric population when other preventative treatments are contraindicated. Specialist consultation is advised for children affected by HAE.

## SUGGESTED READINGS


Ertoy Karagol HI, Yilmaz O, Bakirtas A, et al. Angioedema without urticarial in childhood. *Pediatr Allergy Immunol.* 2013;24:685-690.

Joint Task Force on Practice Parameters. The diagnosis and management of urticaria: a practice parameter part I: acute urticaria/angioedema; part II: chronic urticarial/angioedema. *Ann Allergy Asthma Immunol.* 2000;85(Suppl 6 pt 2):525.

Kemp SF, Lockey RF, Simons FE, et al. Epinephrine: the drug of choice for anaphylaxis. A statement of the World Allergy Organization. *Allergy.* 2008;63:1061-1070.

Lieberman P, Nicklas RA, Randolph C, et al. Anaphylaxis: a practice parameter update 2015. *Ann Allergy Asthma Immunol.* 2015;115:341.

MacGinnitie AJ. Pediatric hereditary angioedema. *Pediatr Allergy Immunol.* 2014;25:420.

Novembre E, Cianferoni A, Mori F, et al. Urticaria and urticaria related skin condition/disease in children. *Eur Ann Allergy Clin Immunol.* 2008;40:5-13.

Sampson HA, Munoz-Furlong A, Campbell RL, et al. Second symposium on the definition and management of anaphylaxis: summary report–Second National Institute of Allergy and Infectious Disease/Food Allergy and Anaphylaxis Network symposium. *J Allergy Clin Immunol.* 2006;117:391.

Simons FE, Ardusso LR, Bilo MB, et al. World Allergy Organization anaphylaxis guidelines; summary. *J Allergy Clin Immunol.* 2011;127:587-593.

Wahn V, Aberer W, Eberl W, et al. Hereditary angioedema (HAE) in children and adolescents: a consensus on therapeutic strategies. *Eur J Pediatr.* 2012;171:1339-1348.

Wood RA, Camargo CA JR, Lieberman P, et al. Anaphylaxis in America: the prevalence and characteristics of anaphylaxis in the United States. *J Allergy Clin Immunol.* 2014;133:461.

Zuberbier T. A summary of the new international EAACI/GA(2)LEN/EDF/WAO guidelines in urticaria. *World Allergy Organ J.* 2012;5:S1.

# 191 Food Allergy

Carla M. Davis and Maria Garcia-Lloret

## INTRODUCTION

Food allergies, defined as adverse immune responses to food proteins, are an increasingly common concern in pediatrics. Food allergy is very distinct from food intolerance, which is defined as a nonimmune reaction that includes metabolic, toxic, pharmacologic, and undefined mechanisms. Food allergy is not one disease but a spectrum of clinicopathologic disorders. As such, manifestations of food allergies differ significantly, depending on the immune mechanism involved and the affected target organ, and range from the prototypical symptoms of acute urticaria/angioedema to chronic conditions such as eczema or eosinophilic gastrointestinal disease. The severity of a food allergic reaction may vary with similar exposures and even in the same individual. As a whole, fatalities are rare, but they do occur. Teenagers are particularly vulnerable because they are risk takers and, therefore, may ignore warning signs of an impending severe reaction.

Because a diagnosis of food allergy causes a considerable nutritional and social burden for affected children and their families, all efforts should be geared to ensure that a true food allergy is the reason for a patient's symptoms. This identification is not an easy task, given the protean clinical manifestations of these disorders and the recognized pitfalls of the routine laboratory tests. In some instances, a double-blind, placebo-controlled food challenge (DBPCFC) may be necessary. This time-consuming procedure is at present the only gold standard test for the diagnosis of food allergy.

Whereas many children will outgrow their food allergies, for others, it will remain a lifelong concern. The natural history of disease depends on the food, the patient's age, the pathophysiology of the allergy and, for many foods, is not well defined. Typically, children outgrow milk, egg, wheat, and soy allergies, but allergies to nuts, shellfish, and fish are persistent. Some allergens are heat-labile, and others are heat-resistant. For instance, most children with milk and egg allergies can tolerate extensively baked foods containing the allergen, but peanut allergenicity is not altered by baking. For the vast majority of food allergies, there are no curative treatments. Current management of these conditions relies on careful avoidance of the offending food(s) and initiating therapy to treat symptoms after accidental exposures. There have been recent clinical trials of allergen-specific immunotherapy in the treatment of food allergies and discovery of introductory feeding practices that influence the development of food allergies. These prevention and treatment strategies may be important in future management of children at risk for food-allergy reactions.



## EPIDEMIOLOGY

Food allergies are prevalent globally, but the rates vary widely in different countries. Estimates of the burden of food allergies depend on the method of diagnosis, with self-report overestimating the true prevalence. As many as one-fourth of the general population may report food-allergic disease, but true food allergy occurs in 1% to 10% of children. In the United States, the overall prevalence of food allergies has been estimated in 3% of the general population, with roughly 3 times as many children as adults afflicted by these disorders. Like other allergic diseases, the prevalence of food allergies appears to be on the rise. The prevalence of peanut allergy in the United States, for instance, has more than doubled from 1999 to 2009, and the majority of countries worldwide report an increasing prevalence.



Food allergies have a strong genetic component. Male children are more likely than are females to have food allergies. Ethnic and racial background influence the expression of food allergies, which is increased in Asian and non-Hispanic black children. Studies in twins show that 7% of dizygotic and 64% of monozygotic twins share a peanut allergy, and siblings of a peanut-allergic child are 7 times more likely to develop this condition. Susceptibility to peanut allergy has also been linked to human leukocyte antigen (HLA) class II polymorphisms and genetic defects such as the loss-of-function mutation in filaggrin, a skin barrier protein. Severe eczema and egg allergy are linked to the presence of immunoglobulin E (IgE) reaction to peanut. A family history of atopy is associated with food allergy, and asthma is a risk factor for severe food-induced life-threatening anaphylaxis.

Dietary customs may influence sensitization to food allergens, with increasing evidence that early introduction of particular foods, such as peanut, into an infant's diet may offer protection from development of allergy. Significant differences in the prevalence of peanut allergy have been reported in countries with early versus later introduction of peanuts in infants, such as in Israel and Great Britain (0.04% and 5%, respectively). In addition, geographical variations in the cooking or processing of foods can affect the food's allergenic properties. For example, roasting peanuts (customary in the United States) tends to increase allergenicity, and boiling or frying decreases it. Dietary changes, such as reduced consumption of antioxidants and omega-3-polyunsaturated fatty acids, as well as vitamin D insufficiency, are also risk factors for development of food allergies.

Environmental and lifestyle factors also affect the development of food allergies. The "hygiene hypothesis" links the paucity of infections and exposure to microbes during childhood in the developed world to an increased risk of development of allergies. Conversely, the higher number of infections and/or microbial exposures in children from rural communities seems to protect against the development of atopic diseases, including food allergies. In addition, increasing birth order is protective, potentially reflecting an increased exposure to infections from siblings.

Prevention of food allergy may be possible through early introduction of allergenic foods in infants at risk for allergic disease. Recent studies have suggested delayed introduction of peanuts may promote the development of peanut allergy in infants with eczema and egg allergy. Therefore, current guidelines on prevention of food allergies recommend the introduction of allergenic foods at 6 months of age and avoidance of delayed introduction.

## IMMUNOPATHOGENESIS

Food allergy can be viewed as a failure in the body's normal tolerance state to innocuous food antigens. The fetus and the young infant may be influenced shortly after birth to either develop or be protected against allergic disease, driven in part by the bacterial colonization of the gut and the skin as well as by exposure to nutrients and other immune regulatory elements in maternal milk. Infants who develop atopic disease show early evidence of allergic immune responses, often in the first year of life, before allergies manifest.

The tolerance to food antigens is maintained by the innate and adaptive compartments of the intestinal immune system. Food proteins are ingested and digested, and the antigens are processed by the intestinal epithelial cells, which interact with immune cells in the lamina propria. The epithelial barrier, phagocytic innate immune cells, tolerogenic antigen-presenting cells, and regulatory T cells all maintain tolerance to food. Typically, these immune mechanisms are defective in food-allergic disease. The disruption of tolerance occurs due to defects in the intestinal barrier function, decreased regulatory T-cell function, and the development of antigen-presenting cells, which stimulate CD4+ T-helper cell production of cytokines interleukin (IL)-4, IL-5, and IL-13, promoters of allergic responses. B cells are activated to produce antigen-specific IgE, which binds to mast cells and basophils. Upon reexposure to the food, IgE cross-linking triggers degranulation of these innate immune cells, releasing the preformed mediators histamine and platelet-activating factor. These mechanisms cause food-allergy symptoms.

In addition, commensal gut bacteria help establish intestinal homeostasis, which favors the tolerance to orally ingested food proteins. The microbiome has gut microflora, which promote the barrier function of the epithelium through interaction with dendritic cells, macrophages, and innate lymphoid cells. Defensins are produced by crosstalk between intestinal epithelium and gut microbes, which help maintain the intestinal barrier function. Commensal microflora promote the neutralization of allergic responses through uptake by dendritic cells, which signal CD4+ T cells to produce cytokines such as IL-10 and transforming growth factor-β which promote tolerance through signaling B cells to make food antigen–specific IgA and IgG4. Dysbiosis at critical times in the infant's development can disrupt these homeostatic mechanisms. Diet, mode of delivery, antibiotic treatment, and exposure to pets or other environmental allergens can influence the establishment of the gut microbiome, causing dysbiosis and increased susceptibility of food allergic disease.

## CLINICAL MANIFESTATIONS

Food allergies can be grouped into 2 general categories: IgE-mediated and non–IgE-mediated (Table 191-1). IgE-mediated reactions are typically of rapid onset with clinical symptoms usually developing within minutes to a few hours of ingestion of the offending food. These reactions exhibit a characteristic pattern of a type I hypersensitivity reaction, mediated by mast cell and basophil degranulation. Skin manifestations (ie, flushing, urticaria, and/or angioedema) occur in more than two-thirds of affected children, but some may present with respiratory or gastrointestinal manifestations exclusively (Table 191-2). Progression to full-blown anaphylaxis with cardiovascular collapse may occur.

An IgE-triggered reaction in the oral mucosa underlies oral allergy syndrome, in which subjects complain of pruritus of the mouth and/or throat when they eat raw vegetables and fruits. This syndrome develops exclusively in the older child or teenager with prior pollen sensitization and is due to heat-labile, cross-reactive antigens present in plant and food antigens. Usually, these foods are well tolerated when cooked.

Delayed reactions to mammalian meat 3 to 6 hours after ingestion are caused by an IgE-mediated reaction to the carbohydrate antigen galactose-α-1,3-galactose (also known as "alpha-gal"), a sugar moiety lining the surface of nonprimate mammalian tissue. Allergic reactions to beef, lamb, and pork are caused by reaction of IgE to alpha-gal. The production of the alpha-gal–IgE can be triggered by tick bites, so many patients with delayed reactions to mammalian meat have a prior history of tick bites.

In non–IgE-mediated food hypersensitivity reactions, T-cell–mediated mechanisms provide the predominant pathogenic stimulus that drives the clinical manifestations. In some individuals, there may be findings of concomitant sensitization (ie, detection of food-specific IgE), but symptoms of a type I hypersensitivity reaction as such are usually absent. T-cell–mediated, delayed hypersensitivity (T-helper cell 2 responses) has been suggested to delay onset of inflammation in patients with atopic dermatitis and eosinophilic esophagitis.

Food allergies contribute to the development of atopic dermatitis in the pediatric age group. Allergies exacerbate atopic dermatitis in about one-third of cases. Infants and young children may exhibit worsening symptoms when exposed to particular foods, either directly or through breast milk. Onset of atopic dermatitis occurs most frequently at 3 to 6 months of age, and food-specific IgE are highest in infants who develop eczema within the levels of first 3 months of age. Flare-ups of atopic dermatitis can occur within hours or days of exposure to foods in susceptible patients. The rash usually improves following an elimination of known food allergens. However, there is little evidence that use of exclusion diet in unselected individuals with atopic eczema is useful.

The clinical phenotypes of allergic gastrointestinal disorders are discussed further in Chapter 406. Food protein–induced enterocolitis (FPIES) is a disease of infancy, typically triggered by the ingestion of whole cow's-milk–based formulas, although it can also be triggered by soy and solid food proteins. FPIES affects both the small bowel and the colon, with diffuse inflammation of the gastrointestinal tract, mild villous atrophy, and crypt abscesses. Clinically, it is characterized by profuse vomiting and diarrhea that develop within a few hours of ingestion of the allergenic food and may progress to dehydration and shock in 20% of patients.

In contrast to FPIES, which is a severe disorder that requires prompt diagnosis management, infants with dietary protein proctocolitis usually look well and thrive but have presenting symptoms of the passage of frequent mucousy and sometimes overtly bloody stools. Some infants with allergic proctocolitis are breast-fed and become sensitized as a result of maternally ingested proteins excreted in breast milk. Cow's milk and soy products are the most commonly implicated allergens, and elimination of these foods from the child's or the maternal diet usually results in the resolution of the symptoms.

Eosinophilic esophagitis (EoE) is typically a disease of an atopic male, with a male-to-female ratio of 3:1, and it can occur at any age. Complaints of failure to thrive, vomiting, and prolonged mealtimes are common symptoms in infants and toddlers; recurrent vomiting, regurgitation, and abdominal pain are common manifestations in children. Coughing and choking can also be found in the initial stages, progressing to overt dysphagia and, in the most severe cases, food impaction secondary to strictures and a narrow-caliber esophagus. Adolescents most commonly experience these symptoms of late-stage disease. Many children with EoE have concomitant symptoms of environmental allergies.

**TABLE 191-1 FOOD HYPERSENSITIVITY DISORDERS**

| Acute Onset (IgE mediated) | Delayed Onset (IgE and/or cellular mediated) |
|---|---|
| Urticaria/angioedema | Atopic dermatitis |
| Anaphylaxis | Eosinophilic esophagitis and other eosinophilic gastroenteropathies |
| Oral allergy syndrome | |
| Food-associated, exercise-induced anaphylaxis | Food protein-induced enterocolitis syndrome |
| Alpha-gal mammalian meat allergy | Allergic proctocolitis |
| | Contact dermatitis |

## DIAGNOSIS

The importance of a thorough clinical history in the diagnosis of a food allergy cannot be overstated. Children may present with a variety of complaints that mimic other common pediatric disorders, and the diagnosis of a food allergy can be either overlooked or given hastily without proper evaluation. Patients or caretakers may see food as a causal factor in situations for which the likelihood of a true food allergy is very low. Non–immune-mediated adverse food reactions (eg, digestive enzyme deficiencies, gastrointestinal infections, food aversions) are common occurences in the pediatric age group and often can be excluded on the basis of the clinical history alone.

A complete history and physical exam are necessary because consideration of the symptoms characteristic of various food-associated

**TABLE 191-2 CLINICAL MANIFESTATIONS OF FOOD HYPERSENSITIVITY**

| Cutaneous | Respiratory | Gastrointestinal | Cardiovascular | Neurologic/Other |
|---|---|---|---|---|
| Urticaria | Rhinorrhea | Abdominal pain | Loss of consciousness | Lethargy |
| Flushing | Swelling of lips, tongue, and/or throat | Dysphagia | Hypotension | Headache |
| Angioedema | Cough | Emesis | Shock | Anxiety |
| Atopic dermatitis | Wheeze or stridor | Diarrhea | Tachycardia or bradycardia | Confusion |
| Contact dermatitis | Shortness of breath | Hematochezia | | Lightheadedness |
| Pruritus | Pain with swallowing | Malabsorption | | Loss of bladder control |
| | Hoarseness | Failure to thrive | | Pelvic pain |



diseases and the epidemiology of the allergic triggers are important for establishing an accurate diagnosis. Foods that have been eaten on numerous occasions are less likely to be triggers compared to foods ingested rarely. Breastfeeding history is important to consider. Factors such as the amount of food ingested as well as the time to the development of the symptoms also need to be taken into consideration. A detailed food diary may help clarify these factors and provide an assessment of potential nutritional deficiencies.

The history alone is not sensitive or specific enough to diagnose a food allergy, so the diagnostic workup of a suspected IgE-mediated food allergy includes a skin-prick test and/or the measurement of serum food-specific IgE antibodies. Both modalities have similar sensitivity, estimated to be better than 85%. Specificity, however, falls below 40%, mostly due to the fact that allergic sensitization may or may not correlate with clinical allergy. True clinical food allergy can be assessed only by means of an oral challenge, which continues to be the gold standard for diagnosis. These tests are routinely performed safely in an allergist's office. Serologic tests also provide a reproducible quantitative assessment of allergic sensitization. For some common food allergens, cut-off values have been established for serum food-specific IgE antibodies that can predict the likelihood of developing systemic allergic reactions in any particular patient.

Whereas immediate-type clinical reactions to food can quite easily be identified by the patient's history or measurement of specific IgE in combination with positive oral-food challenges, non-IgE and or delayed reactions still present diagnostic difficulties. In vitro determinations of allergen-specific T-cell responses, while scientifically sound, are still at the investigational level. The atopy patch test with foods represents another potential avenue, but its use is still nonstandarized and is not routinely performed in most centers. Diets with elimination of food followed by reintroduction over days to weeks are recommended to clarify triggering foods in non–IgE-mediated delayed food allergies.

## THERAPY

Current management of food allergies relies on the careful elimination of the offending food from the diet and, in IgE-mediated disease, the prompt institution of therapeutic measures to treat severe reactions in cases of accidental exposure. The latter treatment measures are not required in non–IgE-mediated reactions because these delayed chronic conditions rarely evolve into acute life-threatening reactions. Follow-up with a physician is required after a severe food allergic reaction for observation for 4 to 6 hours to monitor for biphasic reactions such as anaphylaxis, which can occur in up to 6% of cases.

Elimination of offending foods from the diet sounds like a trivial exercise, but due to often surprising uses of various food products in industrial food preparation processes, and problems of cross-contamination in food-processing facilities, it can be very challenging. Instruction about the fastidious avoidance of specific allergens by reading labels (note that the components of commercial food products often change without notice) often requires education of the parents by a dietitian or other provider with specific expertise in appropriate counseling of families. In children, elimination diets carry a risk of inducing malnutrition with poor growth due to the elimination of essential nutrients. In cases of multiple food allergies, monitoring by an experienced pediatric dietitian to assure adequate nutrient intake is useful.

All patients with a history of a systemic allergic reaction to food should be prescribed self-injectable epinephrine with a formulation appropriate for the patient's age and instructed on its use. A written plan outlining the symptoms requiring epinephrine use can facilitate appropriate treatment. This drug should be employed promptly in the case of an impending anaphylactic reaction. Patients should carry 2 doses at all times because biphasic reactions can occur and 1 epinephrine dose may not halt the progression of symptoms. A second dose should be given if the reaction is progressive. Milder reactions, defined as those involving exclusively the skin or the gastrointestinal system, can be managed with oral $H_1$ and $H_2$ antihistamines. Albuterol and glucocorticoids can be used as second-line agents.

The use of oral, sublingual, and epicutaneous immunotherapy for desensitization to food allergens is currently an area of intense investigation. All 3 routes of immunotherapy cause some degree of desensitization, with oral being the most effective. However, the risk of development of systemic reactions and gastrointestinal symptoms are highest with oral immunotherapy. So, although promising, the risk of reactions occurring during treatment compared to the therapeutic benefit for food oral immunotherapy has yet to be established as favorable in infants and children. In the future, lessons learned from these studies are likely to result in improved treatment of food allergies.

## SUGGESTED READINGS

Boyce JA, Assa'ad A, Burks AW, et al. Guidelines for the diagnosis and management of food allergy in the United States: report of the NIAID-sponsored expert panel. *J Allergy Clin Immunol.* 2010;126:S1-S58.

Du Toit G, Sayre PH, Roberts G, et al. Effect of avoidance on peanut allergy after early peanut consumption. *N Engl J Med.* 2016;374:1435-1443.

Iweala OI, Burks AW. Food allergy: our evolving understanding of its pathogenesis, prevention, and treatment. *Curr Allergy Asthma Rep.* 2016;16:37.

Lake AM. Food-induced eosinophilic proctocolitis. *J Pediatr Gastroenterol Nutr.* 2000;30(Suppl):S58-S60.

Nowak-Wegrzyn A, Assa'ad AH, Bahna SL, et al. Work Group report: oral food challenge testing. *J Allergy Clin Immunol.* 2009;123(6 Suppl):S365.

Prescott SL1, Pawankar R, Allen KJ, et al. A global survey of changing patterns of food allergy burden in children. *World Allergy Organ J.* 2013;6:21.

Rachid R, Chatila TA. The role of the gut microbiota in food allergy. *Curr Opin Pediatr.* 2016;28:748-753.

Sampson HA, Aceves S, Bock SA, et al. Food allergy: a practice parameter update-2014. *J Allergy Clin Immunol.* 2014;134:1016-25.e43.

Sicherer SH, Sampson HA. Food allergy. *J Allergy Clin Immunol.* 2010;125:S116-S125.

Sicherer SH, Sampson HA. Food allergy: epidemiology, pathogenesis, diagnosis, and treatment. *J Allergy Clin Immunol.* 2014;133:291-307.

Wood RA. Food allergen immunotherapy: current status and prospects for the future. *J Allergy Clin Immunol.* 2016;137:973-982.

# 192 Insect Sting Allergy

David B. K. Golden and Maria Garcia-Lloret

## INTRODUCTION

Allergic reactions to insect stings range in pattern and severity from relatively harmless to fatal. A detailed history and appropriate diagnostic tests can identify those who need the protection of venom immunotherapy to prevent life-threatening reactions to future stings. Providing the best guidance to patients requires a knowledge of the patterns of reaction, the natural history of the disease, and the utility and interpretation of diagnostic tests. Insect bites cause toxic rather than anaphylactic reactions and are discussed further in Chapter 190.



## EPIDEMIOLOGY

Systemic reactions (including anaphylaxis) to insect stings occur in 3% of adults and 0.5% to 1% of children. Fatal reactions are rare and may occur on the first reaction, but most of these deaths can be avoided with appropriate treatment, including venom immunotherapy. The frequency of allergic reactions to insect stings is related to the frequency of exposure, occurring more often in beekeepers and in rural areas.

The different families of Hymenoptera have different behaviors and degrees of aggressiveness. Honeybees (*Apis mellifera*) are minimally aggressive and will sting only in defense, such as being accidentally grabbed or stepped on. Africanized honeybees (*Apis mellifera scutellata*), which are indistinguishable from ordinary honeybees and do not have more potent venom, are much more aggressive and often sting in swarms. In contrast, yellow jackets and hornets (*Vespula, Dolichovespula,* and *Vespa* species) are more aggressive and will sting with less provocation. The paper wasps (*Polistes*) are less aggressive than are the vespids but tend to build their nests near buildings and under eaves, rendering them more likely to encounter people and contribute to a large number of stings. Imported fire ants (*Solenopsis*) are present throughout the Gulf coast and southeastern United States, and as many as 50% of people living in infested areas get stung each year. This danger is particularly true for children when they play outside.

## CLINICAL PRESENTATION

Hymenoptera stings normally cause swelling, redness, and pain at the site of the sting, with a rapid onset within minutes and resolution within hours. This reaction is expected and does not require medical treatment but may be relieved with ice, antihistamines, and analgesics. Unusual nonallergic reactions to stings include serum sickness-like reactions, neurologic reactions (peripheral and central neuropathy, seizure), or toxic reactions (constitutional). They can be caused by a single sting, but toxic reactions usually are related to a large number of stings. Anyone who has sustained more than 50 stings should be monitored for the complications of Hymenoptera venom overdose, which includes rhabdomyolysis, renal failure, and myocardial infarction.

Large local reactions occur in 5% to 10% of people who are stung. They represent immunoglobulin (Ig) E-mediated reactions and cause prolonged swelling contiguous with the sting site, with delayed onset 6 to 12 hours after the sting, increasing for 24 to 48 hours, and resolving over the course of 5 to 10 days. Large local reactions frequently are confused with cellulitis, but infections rarely occur from insect stings, and antibiotic treatment is not recommended. Systemic allergic reactions usually begin within minutes after a sting and may be cutaneous (generalized pruritus, urticaria, flushing, angioedema) or anaphylactic (airway edema, dyspnea, hypoxemia, dizziness, hypotension, loss of consciousness, diarrhea, vomiting, cardiac arrhythmia, acute coronary syndrome).

## DIAGNOSIS

Allergic reactions to insect stings (large local and systemic) are mediated by venom-specific IgE antibodies. These specific IgE antibodies can be demonstrated by standardized intradermal venom skin tests or by measurement of serum IgE to venoms. These 2 tests correlate closely but not perfectly, and the 2 test methods can be complimentary. The strength of the tests does not accurately predict the severity of sting reactions. The basal serum tryptase does predict the severity of allergic reactions.

Sensitization can occur after any sting and is found in more than 30% of adults who have been stung recently, but disappears spontaneously in most people. Those with persistent IgE to venom proteins (but no abnormal reactions to stings) have approximately 10% chance of having a systemic reaction to a future sting. Those with a history of large local reactions to stings and positive venom IgE tests have approximately 5% chance of having a systemic reaction to a future sting, and those with a history of systemic reactions and positive tests have a 20% to 70% chance of having a systemic reaction (depending on the severity of the previous reaction).

## TREATMENT

Most children (60%) with systemic reactions to stings have symptoms limited to the skin, whereas 80% of adults also have respiratory or circulatory involvement. Systemic reactions to Hymenoptera stings should be managed as are other causes of anaphylaxis, with early use of epinephrine, intravenous fluids, oxygen, and airway management. There is no immediate benefit from corticosteroids or antihistamines, but they may be administered after the basic treatment modalities. Patients with anaphylaxis should be monitored for at least 4 hours after the sting in case of persistent, recurrent, or biphasic reactions and should be discharged with a prescription for epinephrine autoinjectors (and instruction on proper use) and a referral to an allergist for evaluation, counseling, and possible immunotherapy.

Perhaps because of the relatively low rate of referrals to allergists for sting allergy, venom immunotherapy (VIT) is an underutilized therapy. Protection from systemic reactions to stings can be achieved in 8 weeks in 80% to 98% of patients (standard schedule). Rush (accelerated) immunotherapy regimens are equally safe and can achieve this protection in 2 to 7 days. Thereafter, maintenance doses are given every 1 to 2 months for at least 5 years. Therapy can be discontinued after 5 years in most people, after which treated individuals have a 10% chance of having a mild systemic reaction to a sting. Some patients should continue VIT indefinitely because of high-risk factors such as very severe (near-fatal) sting reactions, elevated basal serum tryptase, or systemic reactions during VIT. There is a relatively low frequency of adverse effects with VIT. This risk is slightly increased in patients taking angiotensin-converting enzyme inhibitors or β-blockers, but it is not a contraindication to VIT because the risk of not treating the patient exceeds the risk of treatment.

Although all patients with systemic reactions may be offered venom immunotherapy, those with only cutaneous manifestations may not require treatment because the chance of a more severe (anaphylactic) reaction occurring after a future sting is less than 3%. The same is true for those with large local reactions, although those with frequent unavoidable stings can reduce the size and duration of large local reactions with VIT. In some "low-risk" cases, impaired quality of life may justify VIT to provide security and normalize activities.

## PREVENTION

Allergic reactions to insect stings can be prevented by avoidance, prompt treatment, and most of all, VIT. However, VIT cannot be administered until after the patient has had 1 allergic reaction and a confirmed diagnosis of insect sting allergy. There is no screening test that predicts the first reaction. Patients who have had an allergic reaction should be advised about the relative risk of having future reactions to stings, the appropriate use of an epinephrine autoinjector, and the potential benefit of VIT.

## SUGGESTED READINGS

Bilò BM, Bonifazi F. Epidemiology of insect venom anaphylaxis. *Curr Opin Allergy Clin Immunol.* 2008;8:330-337.

Golden DBK, Kagey-Sobotka A, Norman PS, et al. Outcomes of allergy to insect stings in children, with and without venom immunotherapy. *N Engl J Med*. 2004;351:668-674.

Golden DBK, Moffitt J, Nicklas RA, et al. Stinging insect hypersensitivity: a practice parameter update 2011. *J Allergy Clin Immunol*. 2011;127:852-854.

Simons FER, Gu X, Silver NA, Simons KJ. EpiPen Jr versus EpiPen in young children weighing 15 to 30 kg at risk for anaphylaxis. *J Allergy Clin Immunol*. 2002;109:171-175.

Steigelman DA, Freeman TM. Imported fire ant allergy: case presentation and review of incidence, prevalence, diagnosis and current treatment. *Ann Allergy Asthma Immunol*. 2013;111:242-245.

Valentine MD, Schuberth KC, Kagey-Sobotka A, et al. The value of immunotherapy with venom in children with allergy to insect stings. *N Engl J Med*. 1990;323:1601-1603.

Yavuz ST, Sackesen C, Sahiner UM, et al. Importance of serum basal tryptase levels in children with insect venom allergy. *Allergy*. 2012;68:386-391.

# 193 Latex Allergy

Sara Anvari and Marc A. Riedl

## INTRODUCTION

The major source of natural rubber is derived from the latex, or milky sap, of the tree *Hevea brasiliensis*. Latex is a ubiquitous natural resource found in a variety of occupational and domestic commercial products. Latex hypersensitivity has become a significant medical concern in the last several decades among patients and healthcare providers. The apparent increased prevalence of latex allergy during the last few decades is due in part to the widespread use of latex gloves to prevent transmission of bloodborne pathogens such as human immunodeficiency virus (HIV). The frequent use of latex-containing materials within the healthcare system generates concern and anxiety in individuals with adverse reactions to latex. True latex allergy can cause serious complications, including death. This chapter will provide an overview of the epidemiology, pathogenesis, clinical manifestations, diagnosis, treatment, and prevention of latex of allergy.

## EPIDEMIOLOGY AND PATHOPHYSIOLOGY

IgE-mediated allergic reactions to latex, while not common in the general population, are a leading cause of anaphylaxis in children, particularly during hospitalization. Life-threatening allergic reactions may be the presenting symptom in as many as 30% of latex-allergic children. The majority of latex-allergic individuals are highly atopic, with histories of allergic conditions such as rhinitis or asthma. Those at highest risk of having a latex hypersensitivity include healthcare workers, children with spina bifida and genitourinary abnormalities, and individuals with occupational exposure to latex. Latex allergy has been reported to be one of the top causes of perioperative anaphylaxis.

The prevalence of clinical latex allergy in the general population has not been established. In a study evaluating latex specific IgE in volunteers who were not clinically symptomatic to latex, the rate of sensitization to natural rubber latex was between 3% and 9.5% in the mid-1990s, but the prevalence of latex sensitization fell to less than 1% by 2006. Approximately 10% to 17% of healthcare workers are sensitized to latex. Children with spina bifida have the highest prevalence of latex sensitization, with reports ranging from 18% to 73%. Although these prevalence rates indicate the presence of latex-specific IgE by diagnostic testing rather than clinical allergic reactions, the high rate of sensitization and potential severity of reactions suggest that all patients with spina bifida should be evaluated for latex allergy prior to undergoing surgical procedures, to minimize complications as much as possible.



Most allergic reactions to latex occur with exposure to latex "dipped" products such as gloves or balloons. These products made from liquid latex rubber have a large number of soluble proteins capable of binding IgE. Currently, 15 principle latex allergens have been well characterized and are known to cause the IgE-mediated allergic reactions. The International Nomenclature Committee of Allergens in the International Union of Immunological Societies (IUIS) has labeled them Hev b 1-15. Specifically, latex allergens Hev b 1 and Hev b 3 are known to cause sensitization to natural rubber latex from direct mucosal exposure during surgery. Healthcare workers sensitized to natural rubber latex from direct contact or inhalation have sensitivity to the major allergens Hev b 5 and Hev b 6.01/6.02.



Latex allergy has been associated with allergy to several fruits and vegetables, including avocado, kiwi, banana, potato, tomato, chestnut, and papaya. Termed the *latex-fruit syndrome*, this clinical observation has been traced to homology between major latex allergen proteins (Hev b 5, Hev b 6, Hev b 7) and various proteins found in these foods. Approximately 50% of latex-allergic individuals show laboratory or clinical symptoms of allergy to 1 or more fruits cross-reactive with latex.

Reactions to latex can manifest as an immediate (type I) hypersensitivity reaction or delayed (type IV) hypersensitivity reaction. A type 1 reaction to latex is mediated by antigen-specific IgE, which triggers mast cell activation with latex exposure. Atopic individuals generate latex-specific IgE after an initial exposure to latex antigen. This sensitizing exposure usually is mucosal, cutaneous (as with latex gloves or balloons), or intraoperative, as latex antigens are leached from rubber products by moisture. Latex antigen may also be adsorbed onto cornstarch powder inside gloves, thereby facilitating respiratory exposure from airborne particles. With subsequent latex exposure, latex-specific IgE bound to mast cells and basophils is cross-linked by the antigen, and activation of mast cells occurs via high-affinity IgE receptor signaling. Activated mast cells release preformed histamine, tryptase, chymase, and heparin, as well as generate other inflammatory mediators, such as cysteinyl leukotrienes, prostaglandins, and inflammatory cytokines. This release of mediators into tissues and circulation leads to localized or generalized urticaria, rhinitis, conjunctivitis, bronchospasm, and/or anaphylaxis, which can be observed within minutes following exposure.

Reactions to latex can also manifest as a delayed (type IV) hypersensitivity reaction. A type IV reaction is a T-cell–mediated reaction that typically presents 48 to 72 hours after exposure to the offending allergen. It is important to determine if the offending allergen is latex because type IV reactions are typically due to chemicals added during the manufacturing of a latex-containing item and not the latex. Allergic contact dermatitis, appearing days after cutaneous exposure, is a type IV inflammatory cutaneous reaction caused by specific T cell activation.

## DIAGNOSIS

Investigation of a latex allergy begins with a clinical diagnosis made by a healthcare provider. The diagnosis of a latex allergy begins by obtaining a detailed history of adverse reactions to exposures to latex products. IgE-mediated latex allergy may cause various symptoms consistent with a mast cell–mediated reaction. They may include urticaria, angioedema, acute rhinitis or conjunctivitis, bronchospasm, and anaphylaxis. As is typical of IgE-mediated reactions, symptoms generally occur up to 2 hours following exposure. Contact urticaria is the most common early manifestation of latex allergy. Generally, such symptoms result from physical contact with latex products either in the home setting (balloons, household rubber products) or the healthcare setting (gloves, blood pressure cuffs). Less commonly, symptoms of rhinitis and asthma may result from respiratory exposure to aerosolized latex particles adsorbed by cornstarch particles in powdered gloves. Latex-induced anaphylaxis usually is encountered during medical procedures such as bladder catheter placement, barium enemas, and surgical procedures. Latex allergy should always be considered in the differential diagnosis of causes for intraoperative anaphylaxis, as it is one of the most common causes.

When IgE-mediated latex allergy is suspected based on the clinical history and symptoms, diagnostic testing for latex-specific IgE should be pursued. Such confirmatory testing is important in order to avoid misdiagnosing patients as being latex-allergic. Inappropriately classifying patients leads to a great deal of anxiety, difficulty, and cost in navigating the healthcare system due to unnecessary avoidance measures. Specific IgE testing for latex can be accomplished by allergy skin testing or serum fluorescence enzyme-linked immunosorbent assays (ELISA). Currently in the United States, there is no commercially available standardized latex reagent for skin testing, rendering latex-allergy skin testing a challenging endeavor.

Historically, some specialists have performed skin testing using solutions extracted from latex rubber gloves. These methods are not recommended, due to be variability in the concentrations of specific latex allergens, the lack of established specificity and sensitivity of such testing, and the uncertainty in the amount of allergen being delivered increases the risk of a serious reaction from exposure to high doses of allergen. Serum testing for latex-specific IgE is commercially available with immunoassays licensed by the US Food and Drug Administration (FDA). While some variability exists in the sensitivity and specificity of these assays, a reasonable expectation is a sensitivity of 70% and a specificity of >95% from the FDA-licensed tests. False-positive results occur in 10% to 25% of individuals undergoing serologic testing for antilatex IgE antibody.

IgE-mediated latex allergy should be distinguished from dermatitis that occurs with exposure to synthetic rubber products such as synthetic elastomers, polymers of 2-chlorobutadiene, and copolymers of butadiene and acrylonitrile. Latex rubber products can induce both irritant and allergic contact dermatitis. Allergic contact dermatitis, a type IV immunologic reaction, may be caused by a variety of chemical accelerators and antioxidants added to the rubber mixture during production of the gloves. Thus, while this form of dermatitis may be a risk factor for IgE sensitization to latex, presumably due to compromised skin-barrier function, this delayed dermatitis is not generally due to latex IgE sensitization. Therefore, it does not confer the potential associated risks of acute, immediate life-threatening reactions with latex exposure. In the setting of rubber-induced dermatitis, it is important to distinguish latex allergy from sensitization to low-molecular-weight chemicals in synthetic or natural rubber products. Allergy patch testing to these compounds may be helpful in establishing a diagnosis.

## TREATMENT

Acute allergic reactions to latex are managed in the same manner as are other IgE-mediated reactions based on specific symptoms. The patient should be removed from the source of the latex exposure to prevent further allergic reactions. Symptoms should be treated with the appropriate emergency medications. Epinephrine (1:1000) 0.01 mg/kg should be first-line treatment for anaphylaxis. Following epinephrine, additional supportive medications to help treat anaphylaxis include $H_1$ and $H_2$ receptor antagonists, corticosteroids, intravenous fluids, and bronchodilators.

## PREVENTION

Once a diagnosis of latex allergy has been established and documented, the long-term management of such patients requires strict avoidance of latex and patient education. Minimization of exposure to dipped rubber products such as gloves, balloons, and condoms is of primary importance. Patients should inform all healthcare providers of their latex allergy and consider obtaining medical alert identification. Even though the healthcare system is often equipped with appropriate alternative rubber-free products, it is advisable for patients to have a personal supply of nonlatex gloves for use when medical or dental care is required. Latex-allergic patients should carry self-injectable epinephrine.

Medical procedures on latex-allergic patients should be conducted in a latex-free environment where nonlatex gloves are worn by medical providers and no latex accessories come in direct contact with the patient. Anecdotal reports have described latex-allergic patients developing reactions from the injection of medications through latex ports in intravenous tubing. However, the dry rubber products in such closures generally have low levels of extractable protein compared to dipped products (eg. gloves) made from liquid latex. Thus, the need to eliminate latex in IV tubing and medication vial closures is controversial. Patients diagnosed with latex allergy should also be asked about allergic signs or symptoms with ingestion of foods included in the latex-fruit syndrome. If patients tolerate these foods without symptoms, there is no compelling reason to avoid them; however, latex-allergic individuals should be cautious when eating these foods for the first time.

## SUGGESTED READINGS


Ahmed DD, Sobczak SC, Yunginger JW. Occupational allergies caused by latex. *Immunol Allergy Clin North Am.* 2003;23(2):205-219.

Bernardini R, Catania P, Caffarelli C, et al. Perioperative latex allergy. *Int J Immunopathol Pharmacol.* 2011;24(3 Suppl):S55-S60.

Caffarelli C, Stringari G, Miraglia Del Giudice M, Crisafulli G, Cardinale F, Peroni DG. Prevention of allergic reactions in anesthetized patients. *Int J Immunopathol Pharmacol.* 2011;24(3 Suppl): S91-S99.

Dong SW, Mertes PM, Petitpain N, Hasdenteufel F, Malinovsky JM. Hypersensitivity reactions during anesthesia. Results from the ninth French survey (2005-2007). *Minerva Anesthesiol.* 2012;78:868-878.

Kelly KJ, Pearson ML, Kurup VP, et al. A cluster of anaphylactic reactions in children with spina bifida during general anesthesia: epidemiologic features, risk factors, and latex hypersensitivity. *J Allergy Clin Immunol.* 1994;94:53-61.

Kurup VP, Kelly T, Elms N, et al. Cross-reactivity of food allergens in latex allergy. *Allergy Proc.* 1994;15:211-216.

Mari A, Scala E, A'mbrosio C, Breiteneder H, Wagner S. Latex allergy within a cohort of not-at-risk subjects with respiratory symptoms: prevalence of latex sensitization and assessment of diagnostic tools. *Int Arch Allergy Immunol.* 2007;143:135-143.

Reinheimer G, Ownby DR. Prevalence of latex-specific IgE antibodies in patients being evaluated for allergy. *Ann Allergy Asthma Immunol.* 1995;74:184-187.

Seyfarth F, Schliemann S, Wiegand C, Hipler UC, Elsner P. Diagnostic value of the ISAC allergy chip in detecting latex sensitizations. *Int Arch Occup Environ Health.* 2014;87:775-781.

Sussman GL, Tarlo S, Dolovich J. The spectrum of IgE-mediated responses to latex. *JAMA.* 1991;265:2844-2847.

Turjanmaa K, Alenius H, Reunala T, Palosuo T. Recent developments in latex allergy. *Curr Opin Allergy Clin Immunol.* 2002;2(5):407-412.

Yeang HY, Cheong KF, Sunderasan E, et al. The 14.6 kd rubber elongation factor (Hev b 1) and 24 kd (Hev b 3) rubber particle proteins are recognized by IgE from patients with spina bifida and latex allergy. *J Allergy Clin Immunol.* 1996;98:628-639.


# 194 Drug and Vaccine Allergy

John M. Kelso

## INTRODUCTION

Any adverse event occurring around the time a child takes a medication or receives a vaccine may be labeled as "allergy." The patient or caregivers typically are told to avoid the suspected and/or similar medications in the future. However, unnecessary avoidance of medication carries a risk because alternative medications may be less effective, more expensive, or have more side effects. In the case of vaccines, withholding future doses leaves children susceptible to serious vaccine-preventable diseases. True allergic reactions are immunologically mediated, and immunologic memory poses a risk for recurrence. In such cases, avoidance of the medication in the future may be appropriate. However, many such adverse events are coincidental or not immunologically mediated and, hence, the medication does not need to be avoided. Therefore, it is important to conduct an appropriate investigation of drug or vaccine allergy before labeling children as "allergic."

## PATHOGENESIS AND EPIDEMIOLOGY

Allergic reactions involve immunologic hypersensitivity in patients who have been sensitized by prior exposure. Such reactions can include not only type I, immunoglobulin (Ig) E-mediated, immediate-type hypersensitivity but also types II (cytotoxic), III (immune complex), and IV (delayed-type, cell-mediated) hypersensitivity of the Gell and Coombs classification scheme. The vast majority of allergens provoking IgE-mediated reactions are proteins. Some drugs and vaccines have protein constituents that may be allergenic, such as the gelatin component of some live viral vaccines. Most drugs are small molecules and, as such, would seem unlikely to be potential allergens. However, metabolism of these drugs leads to hapten molecules, which can attach to endogenous proteins to form complete hapten-carrier protein complexes. These complexes can react with IgE antibodies on mast cells and basophils to produce mild urticarial or more severe anaphylactic reactions. These IgE-mediated reactions are potentially life-threatening. Most late-onset reactions are presumed to involve types II, III, or IV hypersensitivity. Most such reactions including maculopapular rashes and serum sickness are not life-threatening, with the notable exceptions of Stevens-Johnson syndrome (SJS)/toxic epidermal necrolysis (TEN) and occasionally drug reaction with eosinophilia and systemic symptoms (DRESS).

## CLINICAL MANIFESTATIONS

Most suspected drug reactions involve a rash, often urticarial. Urticarial lesions are red, raised, pruritic, and most characteristically fleeting, with individual lesions typically not persisting for more than a few hours or a day and leaving no residual skin changes. Nonurticarial rashes are most often maculopapular, variably pruritic, and most characteristically persistent, lasting for days or weeks. These rashes often result in residual skin changes, including scaling, peeling, or bruising as they resolve. SJS and TEN involve extensive exfoliation or sloughing of the skin as well as mucosal lesions involving the eyes, nose, mouth, and/or genitalia.

Systemic symptoms suggestive of anaphylaxis include naso-ocular (stuffy or runny nose; sneezing; red, itchy, watery eyes), oropharyngeal (swelling of tongue or throat leading to difficulty speaking, breathing, or swallowing), lower respiratory (cough, wheeze, shortness of breath, chest tightness), gastrointestinal (nausea, vomiting, cramps, diarrhea), and cardiovascular (palpitations, lightheadedness, loss of consciousness). Respiratory symptoms, cardiovascular changes, and a combination of systems involved in the reaction are most characteristic of an anaphylactic reaction. The systemic symptoms of DRESS, which typically begin after the patient has been on the medication for 2 to 6 weeks, include fever, lymphadenopathy, and evidence of liver involvement.

## DIAGNOSIS

The first step in establishing the diagnosis of possible drug or vaccine allergy is to obtain additional information about the child's apparent reaction, which almost always involves a rash. The key elements of this history are the nature and timing of the rash. The rash should be categorized as urticarial or nonurticarial. The timing of the rash is also important; it should be determined when the rash appeared in relation to taking the medication, for example, within minutes of the first dose, the following day, or several days into or after the course. Urticarial reactions that began after the first dose or 2 of medication would be typical of IgE-mediated allergy, whereas a maculopapular rash that appeared after several days would be typical of a delayed-type hypersensitivity reaction. However, typical nature and timing do not always go together; for example, in some cases, the child can develop an urticarial rash several days into a course of medication. Another important element of the history is prior exposure to the suspect medication or similar medications. If the rash appeared with the child's first exposure to a medication, this dramatically decreases the likelihood that the rash represents any sort of immune reaction, as such reactions require prior sensitization through prior exposure.

The nature and timing of the rash also are important to determine what type of testing is appropriate to evaluate the reaction. Immediate-type hypersensitivity skin testing is appropriate to evaluate urticarial or potentially anaphylactic reactions that may have been IgE-mediated. Nonirritating skin test concentrations have been established for many drugs and vaccines. Although in vitro assays for specific IgE antibodies are useful for evaluating reactions to aeroallergens and food allergens, they are not useful for evaluating medication reactions due to lack of both sensitivity and specificity. Immediate-type skin testing, however, would shed no light on a late-onset, maculopapular rash, which, by its very nature and timing, could not have been IgE-mediated. Although patch tests and delayed reading of intradermal tests have been investigated to evaluate late-onset reactions that may represent cell-mediated immunity, their lack of standardization limits their clinical utility.

The primary differential diagnosis for drug allergy is coincidence. When a child develops a rash while taking a medication, it does not necessarily mean that the medication caused the rash. It is very common for underlying infections, for example, to cause both urticarial and maculopapular rashes. The other important differential diagnosis is side effect, a known adverse effect of the medication that occurs in some proportion of patients who take it, usually due to a known pharmacologic property.

## TREATMENT

The first step in treatment of a suspected allergic reaction to a medication is to discontinue the medication, including immediately stopping an intravenous infusion or not taking additional oral doses.

The treatment of urticaria without symptoms of anaphylaxis is initiation of antihistamine therapy. Both diphenhydramine (5 mg/kg/d divided in 4 doses every 6 hours) and cetirizine (once daily; age 6–23 months, 2.5 mg; 2–5 years, 2.5 or 5 mg; 6 years or older, 5 or 10 mg) have a rapid onset of action, with the latter also having the advantage of being less sedating and longer lasting. Once urticarial lesions appear, they often are recurrent. As mentioned earlier, individual urticarial lesions typically last only hours, but an episode of urticaria with new lesions appearing as old ones resolve can go on for days or weeks. If the hives were due to an IgE-mediated reaction to medication, recurrent hives may be due to residual medication in the body. However, once triggered, mast cells can stay activated and may continue to release histamine, causing hives long after the triggering medication is completely metabolized or excreted. If the hives recur as each dose of antihistamine wears off, it is best to treat continuously with scheduled antihistamines to suppress the hives for a few days before attempting to wean the antihistamine.

The first and most important treatment of anaphylaxis is epinephrine, which not only reverses the 2 most life-threatening symptoms of this condition, namely bronchospasm and hypotension, but also helps to stabilize mast cells to prevent further release of histamine and other preformed mediators. Thus it is essential that epinephrine (1:1000) be used early in the reaction course. The dose is 0.01 mg/kg up to 0.3 mg. The appropriate dose can be measured in a syringe from vials containing a 1-mg/mL concentration. Epinephrine also is available in the autoinjectors containing 0.15 mg, which can be given to children weighing between 10 and 24 kg, and 0.3 mg, which can be given to children weighing 25 kg or more. The dose can be repeated at 5- to 10-minute intervals if life-threatening symptoms persist. Additional early treatment includes intravenous access for fluid resuscitation with normal saline to replace volume lost to third spacing, recumbant positioning, oxygen by nasal cannula or face mask, and albuterol by nebulizer if there is any wheezing. Antihistamines also can be administered as above, but only in addition to, not instead of, epinephrine.

Treatment of SJS/TEN is supportive and often includes care in a burn unit. The use of intravenous immunoglobulin in treatment of TEN has been reported but is controversial. Treatment of DRESS also is supportive.

### PREVENTION

The main prevention strategy for medication allergy is to avoid administration to children who would be at risk of having serious reactions. Although immediate-type hypersensitivity reactions involve IgE antibodies, children with other atopic diseases such as atopic dermatitis, allergic rhinitis, asthma, and food allergy, which often involve IgE antibodies, are not at increased risk for having a drug allergy. Similarly drug allergies do not run in families so, for example, a child with a parent or sibling with penicillin allergy is not at increased risk for this allergy.

The major risk factor for an allergic reaction to medication is a prior history of such a reaction. However, given the risk of unnecessarily withholding a medication to which a child is not allergic, it is important to base such a decision on the history and a detailed investigation with appropriate testing, not history alone.



## SPECIFIC DRUGS AND VACCINES

### PENICILLIN

Most penicillin-allergic patients have developed IgE antibodies directed against the central β-lactam portion of the molecule and may react to a number of different penicillins. However, a small subset of patients develop IgE antibodies directed against a side chain and react only to penicillins with that specific side chain. Amoxicillin is the penicillin most often associated with these side-chain reactions. The vast majority of penicillin-allergic patients tolerate cephalosporins uneventfully. Those who do not tolerate both classes of drug may be reacting to side chains common to the specific penicillin and cephalosporin medications. For example, amoxicillin shares an identical side chain with cefadroxil, cefprozil, and cefatrizine.

Recent studies have demonstrated that patients who are labeled penicillin-allergic have longer, more expensive hospital stays and are more prone to having adverse reactions such as *Clostridium difficile*/antibiotic–associated pseudomembranous colitis. If a child is truly allergic, it is appropriate for penicillin-class antibiotics to be avoided because the risk of a serious allergic reaction outweighs the risks associated with use of other antibiotics. However, if the child is not truly allergic, being "mislabeled" is not benign, but rather leads to increased morbidity and healthcare costs.

Six percent of all children are labeled as penicillin-allergic, yet only 4% to 9% of these children are truly allergic, (ie, most are mislabeled). Many of these children may have developed coincidental rashes while taking penicillin. A common example is a maculopapular rash occurring after amoxicillin administration during an Epstein-Barr virus infection. Others may have been allergic to penicillin in the past, but this allergy tends to wane with the passage of time. It is appropriate to determine which children labeled as being allergic to penicillin are truly allergic so that they can continue to avoid it but also, just as importantly, to determine which children labeled as being allergic to penicillin are not so that they can receive it.

Thus, children labeled as being allergic to penicillin should be evaluated by an allergist. The current standard of care is for both prick and intradermal skin tests to be performed using penicillin itself as well as its major metabolite (the penicilloyl determinant) and appropriate controls. If these tests are negative, the child undergoes an oral challenge under observation with amoxicillin. The vast majority of these evaluations will be negative, and the child can be "delabeled" and able to receive penicillin and other β-lactam biotics in the future.

### INFLUENZA VACCINE IN EGG-ALLERGIC CHILDREN

The most common specific clinical question relative to vaccines is actually related to food allergy rather than a vaccine reaction. The majority of influenza vaccines are grown in egg cells and contain residual egg protein measured as ovalbumin. Thus, egg allergy was previously thought to be a contraindication to influenza vaccination. However, numerous studies have demonstrated that children with egg allergy, even those with a history of anaphylactic reactions to the ingestion of egg, tolerate both the injectable inactivated influenza vaccine (IIV) and the intranasally administered live attenuated influenza vaccine (LAIV) with no greater rates of adverse reactions than children without egg allergy. Thus, children with egg allergy of any severity should be vaccinated annually against influenza using any age-approved vaccine administered in the usual manner. Urticarial or anaphylactic reactions can occur on rare occasion after the administration of any vaccine to any patient, so vaccine providers should be prepared to recognize and treat such reactions. Children who have had an apparent allergic reaction with influenza vaccination or any other vaccine should be evaluated by an allergist prior to receiving future doses.

### SUGGESTED READINGS


Committee on Infectious Diseases, American Academy of Pediatrics. Recommendations for prevention and control of influenza in children, 2015-2016. *Pediatrics.* 2015;136:792-808.

Joint Task Force on Practice Parameters. Drug allergy: an updated practice parameter. *Ann Allergy Asthma Immunol.* 2010;105:259-273.

Kelso JM. Drug and vaccine allergy. *Immunol Allergy Clin North Am.* 2015;35:221-230.

Kelso JM, Greenhawt MJ, Li JT. Update on influenza vaccination of egg allergic patients. *Ann Allergy Asthma Immunol.* 2013;111:301-302.

Kelso JM, Greenhawt MJ, Li JT, et al. Adverse reactions to vaccines practice parameter 2012 update. *J Allergy Clin Immunol.* 2012;130:25-43.

Macy E, Contreras R. Health care use and serious infection prevalence associated with penicillin "allergy" in hospitalized patients: a cohort study. *J Allergy Clin Immunol.* 2014;133:790-796.

Macy E, Ngor EW. Safely diagnosing clinically significant penicillin allergy using only penicilloyl-poly-lysine, penicillin, and oral amoxicillin. *J Allergy Clin Immunol Pract.* 2013;1:258-263.

Turner PJ, Southern J, Andrews NJ, et al. Safety of live attenuated influenza vaccine in young people with egg allergy: multicentre prospective cohort study. *BMJ.* 2015;351:h6291.

# 195 Pathogenesis of Inflammatory and Autoimmune Disorders

Kathleen E. Sullivan

## INTRODUCTION

An overview of the immune system is provided in Chapter 182. This chapter is focused upon those aspects of inflammation, tolerance, and genetics that are particularly relevant to autoimmune disorders.

The immune system may be broadly divided into the innate immune system and the adaptive immune system. The *innate immune system* is distinguished by hard-wired programs to recognize patterns characteristic of pathogens, also known as pathogen-associated molecular patterns (PAMPs). The *adaptive immune system* consists of T-cell and B-cell functions. T cells and B cells adapt to the environment and undergo a training process to learn to distinguish foreign antigens from self-proteins. As the training process will be distinct for each individual, there is opportunity for errors. Autoimmunity arises from errors in the process of establishing self-tolerance. In contrast, defects in the regulation of innate responses lead to autoinflammatory disorders. These concepts are useful in understanding the underlying pathogenesis of autoimmune disorders, but inflammation can drive breaks in tolerance, and most such conditions are accompanied by inflammation. Thus, the clinical picture in a patient can often reflect both inflammation and autoimmunity.

## INNATE IMMUNE SYSTEM

Neutrophilic infiltrates accompany many autoimmune diseases of childhood. Many of the vasculitides and nearly all types of arthritis are accompanied by a neutrophilic infiltrate. These cells may be extremely destructive. Housed within granules are a multitude of proteolytic enzymes, antimicrobial peptides, and proteins, all of which typically are released into the phagosome holding the bacteria. Neutrophils also have a strategy to entrap larger pathogens in a NET (neutrophil extracellular trap). This killing pathway is favored for large pathogens and in the setting of type I interferon excess. Neutrophil NETs represent extruded granule contents enmeshed in a DNA-histone matrix. NETs have significant potential for tissue damage. Because of their destructive enzymes and reactive oxygen species, neutrophils in tissues are associated with end-organ injury, regardless of whether they were recruited for pathogen defense or as part of an inflammatory process.

Tissue macrophages represent one of the main sentinel cells in the body; others are mast cells and dendritic cells. Certain pathogens, such as mycobacteria and fungi, are resistant to neutrophil killing. In some autoimmune and autoinflammatory diseases, characterized by high levels of tumor necrosis factor (TNF), macrophages can become activated in a poorly understood process, then aggregate and form granulomas. All granulomas are comprised of activated macrophages, called *epithelioid cells*, but not all activated macrophages are found in granulomas. Because macrophages are dependent on γ-interferon and TNF, TNF inhibitors can effectively treat granulomatous diseases.

Natural killer (NK) cells were originally defined by their ability to kill tumor cells in vitro. NK cells kill their targets by forming a synapse and releasing cytotoxic granules into the synaptic cleft. The granules contain granzyme B, which activates apoptosis in the target cell, and perforin, which is thought to act as a pore to facilitate entry of granzyme B. The role of the NK cell is poorly understood in autoimmune disease, but murine models of arthritis suggest that NK cells can down-modulate inflammation, possibly because NK cells kill antigen-presenting cells as part of the homeostatic process. NK cells and the closely related cytotoxic CD8 T cells participate in macrophage activation syndrome by secreting inflammatory cytokines without being able to downregulate the pathway.

The complement proteins are a set of evolutionarily ancient molecules involved in innate recognition of bacteria and other pathogens (see Chapter 182). Patients with early classical pathway component deficiencies not only suffer from recurrent infections because of the loss of opsonic activity, but also are prone to developing lupus. This observation led to the demonstration of an important role for complement in the clearance of apoptotic cells and the establishment of tolerance. The complement cascade often is involved in antibody-mediated destructive processes such as autoimmune hemolytic anemia.

## REGULATION OF INNATE RESPONSES

The autoinflammatory diseases are characterized by dysregulation of myeloid cells. Their pathophysiology will be discussed in detail in Chapter 206, but it is useful to describe the concept here as an example of dysregulation. Innate responses do not exhibit classic memory, and after each episode of activation, the cells largely return to baseline. Neutrophils and macrophages often apoptose, and termination of a typical neutrophil response involves death of the responding cell. NK cells and macrophages are potent cytokine producers, and mechanisms exist to restore the cells to the resting state after cytokine production. Autoinflammatory disorders primarily represent defects in control of innate responses.

The unique monogenic autoinflammatory diseases, including familial Mediterranean fever, TNF receptor–associated periodic fever syndrome, mevalonate kinase deficiency, and CIAS1 autoinflammatory disorders, have been helpful in shedding light on the less understood polygenic disorders. All of these single-gene disorders have a dysregulated inflammatory pathway involving interleukin (IL)-1β and IL-18 expression (Fig. 195-1). As a consequence, they are also associated with a compromise in apoptosis, a major regulatory mechanism responsible for reestablishing homeostasis following immune activation. Neutrophils survive in peripheral blood for only 18 to 24 hours. To prevent undesirable perpetuation of inflammation, neutrophil apoptosis accelerates after phagocytosis of bacteria. Most known autoinflammatory diseases have delayed apoptosis, which prolongs the inflammatory process. In the case of the NALP3/CIAS1-associated syndromes, defects in cryopyrin appear to lead to increased cell death. However, the death is not the immunologically cold form seen in apoptosis, but a distinct type accompanied by cytokine overexpression, a process that enhances inflammation.

These disorders demonstrate clearly the critical balance between proinflammatory pathways needed for effective host defense and control mechanisms necessary for limiting damage. Both downregulation of cytokine production and downregulation of the cells themselves are critical, and defects disrupting these processes usually are detrimental.

## ADAPTIVE IMMUNE SYSTEM

B cells develop in the bone marrow, mature in secondary lymphoid organs, and circulate back to the bone marrow when they become plasma cells. Almost every developmental step is accompanied by checkpoints to ensure that autoreactive B cells do not persist and cause damage. The numerous strategies that B cells have evolved to prevent development of autoreactivity are critical because the recombination events that lead to immunoglobulin molecule generation are random, as likely to lead to autoreactivity as pathogen reactivity. Despite these strategies, a significant number of autoreactive cells exit into the periphery. These cells must compete for T-cell help, and B cells that do not receive T-cell help survive only briefly. Generally, the help that B cells require is cognate (ie, the B cell and T cell recognize the same antigen), although this requirement for help from cognate T cells is not absolute. It is thought that during infections, T cells may rescue autoreactive B cells nonspecifically and cytokines such as IL-6, IL-10, and type I interferons can facilitate survival of B cells that would

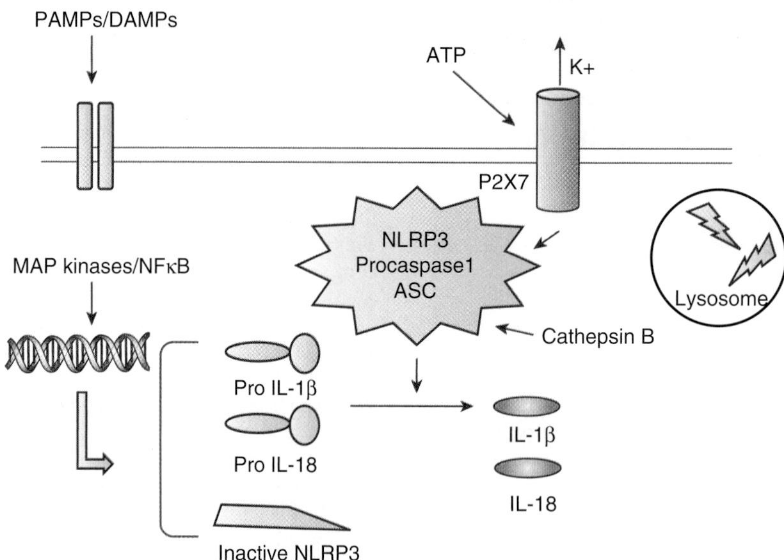


**FIGURE 195-1** The inflammasome is a complex of intracellular proteins that integrate a variety of signals. Production of inflammasome components can be induced by pathogen-associated molecular patterns (PAMPs) and damage-associated molecular patterns (DAMPs). The inflammasome can be activated by such diverse agents as uric acid, bacterial toxins, bacterial cell wall products, and some viruses. The classic inflammasome is composed of NLRP3/CIAS1 (nucleotide binding domain, leucine-rich-containing family, pyrin domain-containing 3), ASC (apoptosis-associated speck-like protein containing a CARD), and procaspase 1. Activation and association of this complex lead to cleavage of procaspase 1 into active caspase 1 and the downstream production of interleukin (IL)-1β and IL-18. Pyrin, the protein defective in familial Mediterranean fever, forms a similar inflammasome with similar functions. Defects in NLRP3, also known as CIAS1, are associated with neonatal-onset multisystem inflammatory disease (NOMID), Muckle-Wells syndrome, and familial cold urticaria. The mutations in these cases are activating mutations that drive chronic production of IL-1β and IL-18.



otherwise be deleted. Some of the autoinflammatory disorders are associated with autoantibody development on this basis.

T cells also must undergo an education process to prevent the development of autoreactivity. T-cell progenitors enter the thymus and can develop into T cells bearing either the γδ or the αβ T-cell receptor. Much less is known about γδ T-cell development than αβ T-cell development. The αβ T cells develop in the thymus, responding to chemokine signals. They proliferate vigorously in the subcapsular zone as double-negative (DN) T cells, named because they lack both CD4 and CD8. At this point, the T cells undergo rearrangement of their T-cell receptor genes. There is an interaction of T cells and thymic stromal cells that is required to develop the corticomedullary structure, suggesting that signals travel both *from* the thymic epithelium and *to* the thymic epithelium. Once a successful rearrangement has occurred, the T cells begin to express both CD4 and CD8, and these T cells are termed *double-positive (DP) T cells.* It is these cells that undergo the rigorous selection process. Initially, the highly motile DP T cells interact with stromal cells. T-cell receptors capable of interacting with self-major histocompatibility complex (MHC) receive a survival signal, whereas T cells with no ability to recognize self die of neglect.

The DP T cells that survive this first screening migrate to the thymic medulla, where they test their receptor against a variety of tissue-specific antigens. The thymus becomes a "mirror of self," and, thus, negative selection of self-reactive T cells can occur. Regulatory T cells also develop in the medulla. Further development in the medulla additionally leads to the expression of either CD4 or CD8, in such a way that the cells become single-positive T cells. The single-positive T cells exit the thymus into the periphery, where they recirculate via lymphatics. T cells only recognize antigen in the context of MHC. CD4 T cells recognize antigen in the context of MHC class II; CD8 T cells recognize antigen in the context of MHC class I. The antigen-presenting cell is more than a passive repository of antigen; it must also deliver a second signal to instruct the T cell as to whether it should treat the antigen as a threat. Dendritic cells, macrophages, and B cells are the main antigen-presenting cells. Each of them can upregulate costimulatory molecules, which provide the second signal for T cells. The signal for upregulation of the costimulatory molecules is the pathogen itself, recognized by a toll-like receptor (TLR), or, alternatively, it is inflammatory cytokines. Antigen plus a costimulatory signal drives the T cell to proliferate and ultimately to execute its effector function, including production of cytokines, providing help for B cells, and killing infected targets. In addition, T cells provide critically important regulatory functions for other T cells and immunologically competent cells. Antigen in the absence of a costimulatory signal drives the T cell to become anergic and unable to proliferate. In the absence of a perceived threat, the T cell presumes the antigen is self and ignores it. In infections in which the danger signal is not spatially limited, bystander T cells may be coincidentally activated, potentially leading to a break in tolerance.

## MECHANISMS OF TISSUE DAMAGE

Pathologic host immune responses classically are divided into 4 categories. Immediate or type I hypersensitivity refers to the typical allergic response. Preexisting immunoglobulin (Ig) E directed against an antigen is bound to mast cells. Engagement of IgE by the antigen leads to immediate degranulation of mast cells with release of histamine as well as a variety of cytokines. IgE-mediated tissue damage seldom is relevant in autoimmune conditions, but recent data have implicated IgE autoantibodies in systemic lupus erythematosus.

Type II hypersensitivity refers specifically to autoantibody-mediated tissue damage. The membrane attack complex of the complement cascade primarily harms cells such as erythrocytes, which have no ability to repair membrane damage. Autoantibodies can also lead to tissue damage by facilitating uptake by the reticuloendothelial system, as in idiopathic thrombocytopenia purpura. In other cases, autoantibodies serve as an opsonin for self-tissue and lead to the recruitment of neutrophils and macrophages, which then induce tissue damage. This type of autoantibody-mediated damage occurs in rheumatic fever, in which antibodies to *Streptococcus* cross-react with myocardial antigens, leading to inflammation and symptoms. Autoantibodies may also induce harm by acting as agonist/antagonists for a receptor or interfering with receptor function, as is in myasthenia gravis.

Immune complex disease, or type III hypersensitivity, is best exemplified by serum sickness. Originally described in the course of passive immunization with horse diphtheria toxin antiserum, it now most often occurs secondary to drug use. Typically, 7 to 10 days after beginning a medication, as antibody production begins, the patient develops fever, arthritis, and proteinuria. A vasculitic rash may be seen. Skin, joints, and kidneys are characterized by small arterial beds with high oncotic pressure, the anatomic region most likely to be involved during serum sickness. This high oncotic pressure leads to deposition of immune complexes in involved areas, in turn activating Fc receptors. This activation then drives the production of inflammatory cytokines and recruitment of neutrophils and other inflammatory cells. Some manifestations of systemic lupus erythematosus may be mediated through this process.

Delayed or type IV hypersensitivity is familiar to clinicians as the basis of the purified protein derivative (PPD) test for tuberculosis. Here, T cells are responsible for the tissue damage. Although a break in T-cell tolerance is hypothesized to underlie many autoimmune diseases, there are few disorders in which the main mechanism of tissue damage is thought to be driven by T cells. Despite the association of many autoimmune diseases with MHC haplotypes, dramatic infiltrates of T cells are seen in relatively few diseases of childhood. Examples include multiple sclerosis and diabetes mellitus. In juvenile idiopathic arthritis, the synovial fluid often contains high numbers of neutrophils, a testament to the role of the innate immune system in the signs and symptoms of the disease. In the synovial membrane, however, the infiltrating cells are largely macrophages and T cells. In some cases, infiltrating cells adopt a lymph node-like architecture, including a germinal center. This lymphoid aggregate is thought to require a T-cell contribution, but the exact role of the T cell in this complex process is not known. One theory is that the recognition of antigen by T cells may drive cytokine production, thereby leading to many of the downstream effects.

## INFLAMMATION

### Microcirculation Changes

Clinicians identify inflammation on the basis of very obvious manifestations: erythema, tenderness, induration, warmth, and often loss of function. These features arise owing to changes in microcirculation. In the setting of autoimmune or autoinflammatory disorders, effects of inflammation seem largely pathologic. When viewed as a response to infection, however, these changes can be seen as physiologic.

Regardless of the cause of inflammation, damaged capillaries activate Hageman factor, also known as *factor XII*, of the coagulation pathway. Hageman factor activates factor XI and initiates coagulation at the site of tissue damage. This process stems bleeding but also traps platelets and slows the flow of blood to the site. This, in turn, facilitates neutrophil adhesion. Hageman factor also activates the kallikrein pathway, leading to production of bradykinin. Bradykinin is responsible for the vascular leak that leads to induration and swelling, and for local hyperalgesia and pain. It is also one of the mediators of vascular dilatation, causing the characteristic redness seen in inflammation. The kallikrein pathway can also directly cleave complement protein C5, a potent chemotactic factor that attracts neutrophils to the site. These microcirculatory changes provide the optimal setting for the recruitment of neutrophils.

Bacteria interact with TLRs on the surface of sentinel cells, leading to the production of TNF. This cytokine increases P-selectin and E-selectin expression by the adjacent vascular endothelium. These selectins bind P-selectin glycoprotein ligand-1 (PSGL1) and other glycoproteins to initiate the rolling phase of neutrophil adhesion. Inflammatory cytokines, platelet-activating factor, and chemokines can activate the β2 integrins, which mediate the firm adhesion of the neutrophil to the vascular endothelium. This process is aided by the slowed flow of blood in the inflamed site. The arrested neutrophil can undergo diapedesis across the vascular endothelium and chemotax toward the bacteria. Vascular leak allows complement and antibody to escape from the blood and join neutrophils in the tissue, facilitating opsonization and ingestion of bacteria. Thus, each of the pathologic changes in inflammation has a clear physiologic benefit.

## TOLERANCE

*Tolerance* is the term used for the process whereby T cells and B cells are instructed to avoid self-responses. In a perfect world, there would be no self-reactive T cells and B cells and no autoimmunity. Understanding tolerance induction is important as a foundation for understanding autoimmunity.

### B-Cell Development and Tolerance

B cells develop in the bone marrow, and the B-cell receptor, or surface immunoglobulin, is generated via a series of recombination events. The events lead to random generation of receptors, only a few of which will be useful in host defense. The heavy chain initially undergoes rearrangement at the pro–B-cell stage. This heavy chain is expressed with surrogate light chains, and at this stage, the ability of the heavy chain to pair appropriately with a light chain is tested. An effective pairing stimulates rearrangement of the light chain, which is completed at the pre–B-cell stage in the bone marrow. A functional B-cell receptor exists at this phase of B-cell development, and it becomes fully expressed on the cell surface at the immature B-cell stage. The B-cell receptor is expressed with 2 proteins, Igα and Igβ, which transmit signals to the interior of the cell. At the immature B-cell stage, strong engagement of the B-cell receptor leads to apoptosis. Complement proteins appear to play a role in this important process because complement-deficient mice have impaired B-cell tolerance and complement-deficient humans (C1, C2, C4) are more prone to development of lupus. B-cell signaling defects interfere with deletion and are associated with a high rate of autoimmunity.

This developmental sequence serves to prevent autoreactive B cells from reaching the periphery, but it is not particularly efficient, perhaps because relatively few self-antigens are expressed in the bone marrow environment. Another option for deleting autoreactive B cells, known as *receptor editing*, also takes place at the pre–B- to immature B-cell stage. Approximately 25% of peripheral B cells appear to have undergone receptor editing, which consists of an additional round of light-chain recombination that eliminates autoreactive B-cell receptors. Studies have shown that 55% to 75% of all early immature B cells express autoreactive receptors. The processes of clonal deletion and receptor editing reduce the frequency to approximately 40%, meaning that a large number of autoreactive cells still manage to leave the bone marrow.

There is a further checkpoint in B-cell development through which the number of autoreactive mature B cells is further diminished to 20%. It is thought to be the result of competition for niches in the secondary lymphoid organ follicles and the effects of regulatory T cells. Even though these checkpoints eliminate 80% of autoreactive B cells, a relatively large number of potentially pathologic B cells remain. In addition, patients with rheumatoid arthritis and lupus have been shown to have defective checkpoints such that even larger numbers of cells escape deletion.

In general, the autoreactive B cells do not cause harm as long as they do not receive T-cell help. This process can be short-circuited by infection, explaining why autoimmune diseases may be precipitated or exacerbated by infections. Marginal zone B cells appear to be particularly prone to activation by bacterial products via TLRs. Conversely, viral infections may activate autoreactive B cells via the production of type I interferons, which stimulate B-cell proliferation and antibody production.

### T-Cell Development and Tolerance

As described in Chapter 182, T cells develop in the thymus. Similar to B cells, they initially generate a heavy chain, which is expressed with a surrogate alpha chain protein. It occurs in the DN T-cell stage. The alpha chain subsequently undergoes rearrangement, and the cells progress to become DP T cells. Positive selection for cells that have some capacity for self-recognition occurs in the cortex. This initial screening process ensures that the receptor will engage self-MHC. Unlike B cells, T cells continue to undergo rearrangements until they receive a positive signal. Recombination here too leads to random receptor specificities, and the majority of T cells fail to produce a

T-cell receptor that can positively interact with self-MHC. Consequently, most T cells die at this stage.

Medullary epithelial cells express organ-specific antigens. A transcription factor termed *AIRE* induces the expression of approximately 500 to 1200 genes in the thymus. Each of these genes encodes proteins whose expression would otherwise be limited to a distant tissue. In this way, the DP T cell can survey a set of antigens it is likely to encounter in the periphery. Autoreactive T cells undergo apoptosis. As was true for B cells, T-cell signaling defects are associated with high rates of autoimmunity due to inefficient elimination of autoreactive cells. Defects in the *AIRE* gene are associated with the progressive accumulation of autoimmune processes, a disorder called *autoimmune polyendocrinopathy, candidiasis, ectodermal dysplasia* (APECED). This condition vividly demonstrates the importance of negative selection in the thymus.

Antigens are presented to T cells in the context of an MHC molecule. An unstable MHC provides a poor platform for antigen presentation; markedly diminished expression of MHC can lead to both poor positive selection and poor negative selection. Thus, patients with an inherited immune deficiency that causes diminished MHC class I expression (the bare lymphocyte syndrome) typically have very few CD8 T cells, because CD8 T cells are positively selected though MHC class I. They also have a high frequency of autoimmune diseases. Similarly, patients with markedly diminished MHC class II expression have few CD4 T cells and also have a relatively high frequency of autoimmune disease. As one would expect, stem cell transplantation is not particularly effective in these conditions unless the graft can provide some antigen-presenting cells to populate the thymus.

Another type of αβ T cell is the regulatory T cell. These cells have particularly high affinity for self and enter a separate developmental pathway dependent on the transcription factor *FoxP3*. Regulatory development of T cells can also be compromised by T-cell signaling defects, as is demonstrated by the rare patients who have mutations in the critical transcription factor *FoxP3*. They develop immune deficiency, polyendocrinopathy, enteropathy, X-linked syndrome (IPEX), which is manifested by a T-cell infiltrate in the small bowel and accumulation of other autoimmune organ involvement. The process usually is fatal in the absence of a stem cell transplant. The role and potential manipulation of regulatory T cells in human diseases is now an active area of investigation.

The balance of antigen presentation, thymic selection, and development of cells destined to provide a safety net in the periphery (regulatory T cells) interact to prevent autoimmune disease. As is the case for B cells, environmental factors appear to affect the process, but they are not well understood.

## GENETIC FACTORS CONTRIBUTING TO AUTOIMMUNITY

A break in tolerance is thought to initiate synovitis, although the ultimate joint damage is due to the collaborative effects of many downstream pathways (Fig. 195-2). The cellular interactions defined in joint inflammation may be partially extrapolated to other types of autoimmunity. Still, there are significant differences among various types of autoimmune pathology, and there is much to learn about the subtle differences that can mold a particular disease phenotype.

## PATHOGENIC MECHANISMS IN COMPLEX POLYGENIC DISORDERS

Juvenile idiopathic arthritis (JIA) is the most common pediatric rheumatologic disorder. However, little is understood concerning its genetics. The relative risk in siblings, a rough estimate of the genetic contribution to a disease, is approximately 15, similar to that of multiple sclerosis and insulin-dependent diabetes mellitus. The concordance among twins is approximately 25%, which suggests the interplay of both genetic and environmental factors. Significant racial

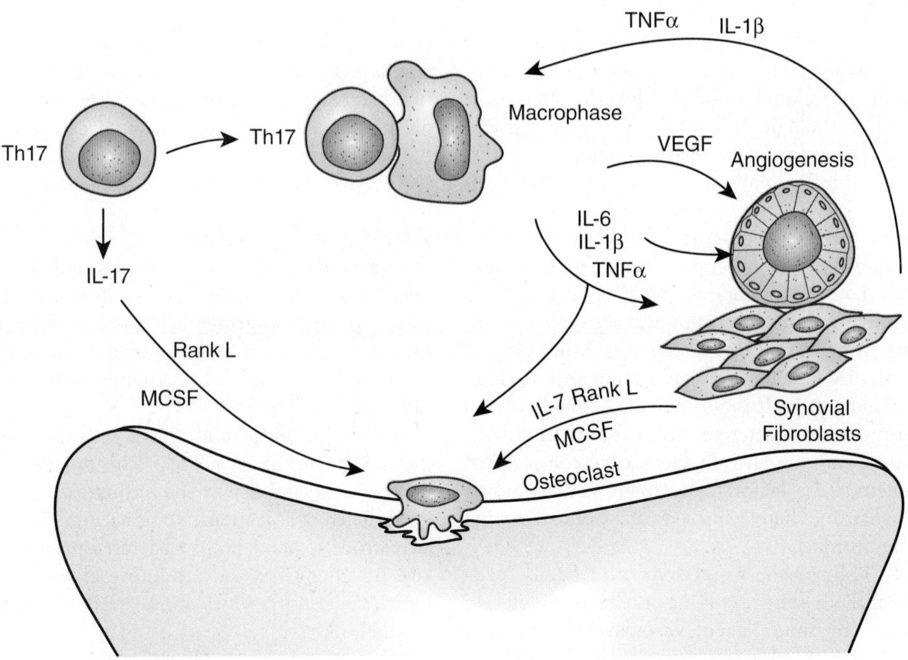


**FIGURE 195-2** Major inflammatory pathways in the joint. Bone destruction, seen in a minority of patients with juvenile idiopathic arthritis (JIA), is mediated predominantly by osteoclasts. These cells are related to macrophages but are part of normal bone homeostasis. With increased interleukin (IL)-17, macrophage colony-stimulating factor (MSCF), and receptor activator of nuclear factor-κB ligand (RANKL), the osteoclasts become disproportionately activated compared with bone development, leading to erosions. The inciting antigen is not known, but IL-17–producing T cells (Th17 cell) migrate into the joint and are present in the synovium. There is a complex interplay of the Th17 cells and synovial macrophages that is contact dependent and leads to macrophage expression of tumor necrosis factor (TNF), IL-6, and IL-1β. These cytokines contribute to osteoclast activation but also very importantly stimulate synovial fibroblast proliferation and activation. These cells form the structure of the synovial hypertrophy, often seen in JIA. Activated synovial cells produce MCSF and RANKL, which contribute to osteoclast activation, as well as TNF and IL-1β, which further activate the synovial macrophages. Finally, angiogenesis, which is required to support the metabolism associated with growth and activation, is aided by activated macrophage production of vascular endothelial growth factor (VEGF).

and ethnic differences in the incidence of arthritis may reflect either environmental or genetic contributions, including the human leukocyte antigen (HLA) variations between different human populations.

Epidemiologic studies in JIA similarly suggest a genetic component, and the same is true for pediatric lupus and dermatomyositis. In the case of lupus, the sibling relative risk is 20, and the twin concordance rate is 24% to 65%. Genome-wide association studies have identified numerous loci that appear to confer risk and protection in pediatric rheumatologic conditions. In nearly every case, the MHC is the strongest genetic risk factor.

The association of various pediatric rheumatologic conditions with MHC polymorphisms has 2 important implications. First, antigen is presented to T cells in the context of MHC, suggesting that autoreactive T cells are driving much of the pathologic autoimmunity. Supporting this idea is the fact that T cells are found in the synovium of JIA patients and in the muscle of patients with dermatomyositis. Nonetheless, T-cell–targeted interventions have not been particularly effective for treating pediatric rheumatologic conditions, possibly be due to the very strong linkage disequilibrium of the MCH region: the association of disease with an MHC type may in fact be the result of linkage with another gene in the region.

The second implication of the finding that most pediatric rheumatologic conditions are associated with MHC genes relates to the fact that there are numerous genes that contribute to overall genetic risk. In most cases, the relative risk associated with inheritance of any individual MHC allele is approximately 2 to 3; other genes thus must contribute to the overall genetic risk. Perhaps best studied in murine models of lupus, individual loci appear to contribute 1 of a series of steps that together lead to the development of lupus. Inheritance of 1 locus confers increased B-cell activation, and inheritance of another leads to increased antigen presentation. The implication is that effects of individual risk factors are cumulative.

An aspect related to genetics, but which is not inherited, is called *epigenetics*. It refers to features of the genome regulating transcription that are not encoded by the DNA, but rather are modified by environmental factors. Operationally, it refers to DNA methylation or histone modifications that alter DNA packaging into active or inactive regions. Histone modifications can also serve as a scaffold for transcription factor binding and other regulatory proteins. The sequence of the DNA may be the same in twins, but the expression of individual genes may differ significantly between the 2 because of epigenetic factors. It is not a simple issue of semantics; deliberate alteration of epigenetic characteristics has led to the development of lupus in 2 distinct models.

## EVIDENCE SUPPORTING AN ENVIRONMENTAL CONTRIBUTION

Potential environmental factors involved in the etiopathogenesis of JIA include high income, no siblings, and urban living. In general, JIA does not have seasonal clustering, although in some studies, systemic JIA was found to occur more often during colder months. The most strongly seasonal pediatric rheumatologic disease is Kawasaki syndrome, for which many studies in different geographic regions demonstrate a strong winter-spring seasonality. Studies also demonstrate temporal clustering, a finding similarly consistent with an infectious etiology. Although many researchers have attempted to identify a single infectious agent responsible for this condition, results to date have failed to confirm such a cause. As with other pediatric vasculitides such as polyarteritis nodosa and IgA vasculitis (IgAV) (Henoch-Schönlein purpura), perhaps many different infectious triggers may lead to the pattern of inflammation known as Kawasaki disease.

One of the more intriguing findings in lupus is the fact that pediatric patients are more likely to have been infected with Epstein-Barr virus (EBV) than have controls. Strong data demonstrating that type I interferons drive B-cell development and the recognition that type I interferons are produced preferentially after viral infections may provide an explanation for flares after common infections, and perhaps an explanation for the initial insult itself. On the other hand, EBV infection is ubiquitous in virtually all populations, yet lupus develops in fewer than 10 children per 100,000. Further, lupus tends to evolve over a 5- to 10-year period. Thus, whereas infection may contribute to initiation of the disease, there must be other mechanisms that propel the process. Estrogen, medications, and exposure to sun have been implicated as environmental cofactors, but how the disease evolves is not well understood.



A further aspect to environmental contributions involves the microbiome. The universe of bacteria and viruses that cohabitate our bodies clearly impacts immunologic function and can alter responses to antigens. Changes in the microbiome have been identified in several autoimmune disorders, but the implications for cause and effect are not yet clear and represent a fertile area for current investigations.

## ENVIRONMENT-GENE-IMMUNITY INTERACTIONS

One explanation for the development of most types of disease, including autoimmunity, is to hypothesize that patients inherit a genetic predisposition. This predisposition, whether strong or weak, interacts with environmental and stochastic events and eventually leads to pathology. In the case of autoimmune diseases, the intermediate event is amplification of an autoreactive B-cell or T-cell clone. This clone, in turn, is regulated by a more-or-less robust homeostatic process that may or may not keep it under control. If control is breached, the clone continues to expand and disease ensues. The disease manifests itself after recruitment of varied inflammatory cells. Some autoimmune phenomena are naturally self-limited, suggesting that a mistake need not become a chronic disease. Examples of short-lived autoimmune phenomena include idiopathic thrombocytopenia purpura, some vasculitides such as IgAV, and autoimmune hemolytic anemia. In many cases, however, the process does become chronic, and the processes that perpetuate the disease need not be the same as those that precipitate it. The infiltrate that contributes to end organ damage may be composed of mixed lymphocytes and phagocytic cells that were recruited long after the inciting event. As understanding of these factors advances, it is clear that the earlier in the process of disease evolution medical intervention begins, the better off the patient will be.

## SUGGESTED READINGS

Gilbert M, Punaro M. Blood gene expression profiling in pediatric systemic lupus erythematosus and systemic juvenile idiopathic arthritis: from bench to bedside. *Pediatr Rheum*. 2014;12:16.

Huttonlocher A, Smith JA. Neutrophils in pediatric autoimmune disease. *Curr Opin Rheum*. 2015;27:500-504.

Kochi Y. Genetics of autoimmune diseases: perspectives from genome-wide association studies. *Int Immunol*. 2016;28:155-161.

Strietesky GL, Jameson SC, Hogquist KA. Selection of self-reactive T cells in the thymus. *Ann Rev Immunol*. 2012;30:95-114.

Yokota S, Kikuchi M, Nozawa T, et al. Pathogenesis if systemic inflammatory diseases in childhood. *Mod Rheum*. 2015;25:1-10.

# 196 History and Physical Examination in Rheumatology

Robert P. Sundel

## INTRODUCTION

Extremity complaints are common in children; they are estimated to account for as many as 10% of non–well-child visits to pediatricians' offices. Conversely, rheumatologic conditions are rare, affecting fewer than 200,000 children in the United States. Thus, clinicians caring for children need an efficient and effective means of distinguishing arthritis, lupus, and other autoimmune conditions from injuries, infections, tumors, and noninflammatory causes of extremity complaints. This chapter will discuss the key components of a focused history and physical examination, the basic tools for evaluating a child with musculoskeletal symptoms. The next chapter discusses laboratory and imaging studies that may be used to confirm or refute the caregiver's clinical suspicions.

## EPIDEMIOLOGY

The reported incidence and prevalence of musculoskeletal diseases in children worldwide vary significantly. For example, among more than 30 epidemiologic studies of juvenile arthritis, new cases are reported to arise at a rate of 0.008 to 0.226 per 1000 children, yielding a reported prevalence of 0.07 to 4.01 per 1000 children. Although geographic, genetic, and environmental factors result in true variations in the incidence of rheumatologic conditions, several additional factors also contribute to reported differences. First among them is that most pediatric rheumatologic conditions are diagnosed on the basis of clinical criteria rather than definitive laboratory, imaging, or histopathologic findings. New signs may develop over time, leading to reclassification of conditions. Thus, children treated for ankylosing spondylitis may later develop colitis, resulting in a new diagnosis of Crohn disease–related arthritis. Arthritis that remits after several months and does not recur may be called *monocyclic juvenile idiopathic arthritis* by one caregiver and *postinfectious arthritis* by another. Despite these imprecisions inherent in a field based on clinical diagnoses, outcomes in virtually all autoimmune conditions are optimized by expeditious diagnosis and early initiation of effective therapy. Thus, classifying a child's rheumatologic condition as accurately as possible is essential.



## PATHOPHYSIOLOGY

The presenting symptoms of musculoskeletal conditions are more dependent on the location of the abnormality than on the specific diagnosis. Thus, fractures, tumors, and osteomyelitis all present with pain that may awaken the patient from sleep because of the constant stimulation of sensory nerves by lesions within bone. Conversely, for unknown reasons, children with arthritis seldom complain of pain. One study of more than 400 children presenting to a pediatric rheumatology clinic found that 90% of those with joint or extremity pain did not have arthritis, and more than 90% of those with arthritis did not complain of pain. Inflammatory arthritis may cause children to limp because their joints are stiff, but pain generally is absent (distinct from adults in whom arthritis is universally described as painful). Thus, differences in the location, timing, and characteristics of a child's symptoms enable a pediatrician to rapidly narrow the potential causes of musculoskeletal complaints. Confirmation of the suspected diagnosis may then be obtained from findings on physical exam, often without need for further investigations.

When a child presents with a musculoskeletal complaint, it is helpful to categorize the symptoms according to the nature of onset (acute vs chronic), the number of sites involved, and whether there is evidence of systemic or extra-articular involvement. It is also important to remember that most normally active children will have a history of trauma during the preceding 24 hours. Unless the trauma is significant (typically a football injury, automobile accident, or bicycle fall), however, it is more likely to have unmasked preexisting pathology than to have caused damage to the resilient tissues of a child's musculoskeletal system. Thus, 10% to 20% of osteogenic sarcomas present after trauma, but the symptoms reflect the underlying pathology rather than an actual traumatic injury.

## GENETICS

Although there is a strong genetic component to most rheumatologic and inflammatory disorders, susceptibility typically is generated by numerous interacting alleles (see Chapter 165). Many of the genes affect immune responses (Chapter 184), resulting in a predilection for responding to self rather than preordaining development of a particular syndrome. Thus, a family history of psoriasis or inflammatory bowel disease may indicate that the next generation is more likely to develop arthritis or lupus. In most cases, however, having a parent with a particular autoimmune condition, such as rheumatoid arthritis, does not further identify children as being at risk for developing the same disease.

## CLINICAL FEATURES

### History

Key elements of the history that help identify the cause of symptoms include the complaints' timing, character, and nature. Thus, knowing whether pain is dull, sharp, radiating, or burning may suggest whether the source is bone, soft tissue, or nerve. Alleviating and exacerbating factors, particularly response to activity, help distinguish rheumatologic from orthopedic conditions. Questions may have to be posed in a variety of ways in order to extract useful information, and interrogation of several different people may reveal subtle nuances of critical importance. Further, in younger or nonverbal children who are not able to articulate the specifics of their symptoms, observations of the parents and other caregivers may have to substitute for the patient's description. Nonetheless, the time spent obtaining a thorough and precise history is invariably repaid many times in the information it yields (Table 196-1).

#### Inflammatory Conditions

The single most characteristic feature of discomfort related to inflammatory processes is the classic *morning stiffness* of arthritis. Difficulties also often are exacerbated after naps or other periods of prolonged inactivity such as long car rides, movie watching, or sitting in classes at school (the "theater sign"). It is thought to be the result of decreased levels of hyaluronic acid in inflamed synovial fluid. The protein-rich fluid can more readily gel at higher temperatures, leading to decreased lubrication of the joints at physiologic temperatures. Thus, children with arthritis typically feel better after a warm bath or several minutes of activity. These activities help to raise the temperature within the joint, allowing the synovial fluid to return to the liquid state in which it lubricates most efficiently. Accordingly, a child with arthritis may suffer joint stiffness in the morning, yet be quite comfortable exercising strenuously later in the day. It is decidedly atypical for inflammatory arthritis to awaken children from sleep. Cold, damp weather or swimming in cool water tends to be more difficult for children with arthritis, whereas warm weather generally relieves symptoms. An atypical symptom profile—especially nighttime pain or discomfort with activity—should raise suspicion of an alternative diagnosis, even in the setting of what appears clinically to be an arthritic joint.

#### Mechanical Pain

The timing of mechanical pain is essentially the mirror image of the pattern of inflammatory pain. Children typically feel well in the morning, but the more active they are, the more uncomfortable they are. *Chondromalacia patella* is called "runner's knee" because of the timing of the pain. Like inflammation, however, mechanical pain does not generally awaken children from sleep. Rest and ice tend to alleviate mechanical symptoms, as opposed to the activity and heat that typically are salubrious in arthritis. Once the broad category causing a child's symptoms is determined, the precise type of overuse syndrome or injury can generally be determined from a careful history and physical examination. Demographic information also is helpful:

**TABLE 196-1 CATEGORIES OF MUSCULOSKELETAL PAIN BASED ON TIMING OF SYMPTOMS**

| | AM | PM | Night | Effect of Activity on Symptoms |
|---|---|---|---|---|
| Inflammatory (eg, arthritis) | +++ | + | – | Improves |
| Mechanical (eg, overuse syndromes) | ± | ++ | ± | Worsens |
| Bony (eg, tumors) | ++ | ++ | ++ | No consistent change |
| Neuropathic (eg, radiculopathy) | + | ++ | +++ | No consistent change |
| Functional | +++ | +++ | +++ | No physiologic pattern |

An adolescent boy experiencing knee pain while playing basketball is more likely to have Osgood-Schlatter syndrome, whereas aching knees in a 12-year-old girl on the cross-country team are more likely to result from iliotibial band syndrome. Even if the precise cause of discomfort is not apparent, at the very least, the caregiver may be confident that consultation with an orthopedist is likely to be more useful than referral to a rheumatologist when pain has the characteristics of a mechanical problem.

#### Bony Pain

Pain originating in the osseous compartment tends to be constant and does not change significantly with activity. Bone pain raises concerns for infection, trauma, and tumor. Although inflammatory and mechanical pains seldom awaken children at night, bony pain may do so, particularly when related to leukemia or other tumors. Consequently, when a history of nighttime awakening is elicited, special consideration must be given to possible oncologic etiologies. Cytopenias usually are seen with leukemia, although a normal complete blood count (CBC) does not preclude the possibility of a malignancy. Other tumors, such as sarcomas or metastatic neuroblastoma, are far less common, but they, too, must be considered in children with pain suggesting a bone source.

#### Neuropathic Pain

Nerve pain tends to be worst at bedtime, when the usual focus on daily activities no longer distracts the child from her discomfort. In children old enough to describe the sensation, neuropathic pain typically has a burning or lancinating character. It is also commonly associated with allodynia, hypersensitivity of overlying normal soft tissues. Although joints may be involved, neuropathic pain generally encompasses extra-articular areas as well, and it may follow a dermatomal distribution. Activity does not have a significant effect on neuropathic pain. The complaints associated with chronic pain syndromes also are most characteristic of neuropathic pain. Thus, if pain is sharp or radiating but is not associated with identifiable trauma, tumors, neuropathy, or vasculitis, then a pain syndrome such as fibromyalgia or reflex sympathetic dystrophy should be considered.

Although pain syndromes traditionally have been regarded as diagnoses of exclusion, this approach is both an inefficient and an undesirable way to arrive at such a conclusion. First, having numerous tests and studies tends to confirm families' suspicions that symptoms are caused by a medical condition that is evading the clinician's notice. Second, prolonged searches for organic etiologies tend to lead to consideration of increasingly obscure or unlikely possibilities. Rather, when pain that does not fit any apparent temporal or anatomic pattern is accompanied by significant dysfunction, particularly excessive school absences, pain syndromes should rise to the top of the list of diagnostic possibilities. Further support for such a diagnosis is provided by a family history of dysfunctional responses to pain (eg, prolonged disability after apparently minimal trauma or severe cases of fibromyalgia or irritable bowel syndrome). More evidence need not be required for a pain syndrome to be seriously considered (see Chapter 204).

## PHYSICAL EXAMINATION

Assessment of a child with musculoskeletal complaints must include both a general examination and a complete assessment of the musculoskeletal system. It is facilitated by the results of the history: If a child has complaints suggestive of an inflammatory condition involving multiple joints, then signs of systemic conditions such as inflammatory bowel disease and systemic lupus erythematosus should be sought. Conversely, monoarticular pain could point toward mechanical, infectious, or proliferative conditions.

#### Observation

It is often useful to begin by having the child run in the examining room or down the hall. This activity is unexpected and enjoyable for most children, and, therefore, helps alleviate anxiety. Further, most children find it difficult to focus on running while consciously altering their movements, so true pathology is likely to be revealed. Conversely, children often are self-conscious when asked to walk, potentially altering their movements and misleading the examiner. Absolute refusal to run, especially in an older child, might also yield important clues of a volitional or functional component to the complaints.

When observing a child who is running, it is important to remember that a normal gait is the most efficient and stable means for a bipedal creature such as a human to ambulate. In order to cause a child to dramatically alter his gait, strong factors must be at work. They usually are anatomic disruptions (eg, broken bone, loss of balance) or attempts to avoid pain, with the latter being the most common cause of a limp in children.

Different types of pathology result in predictable alterations in a child's movement. Lower extremity involvement is most common in rheumatologic conditions, and assessment of gait is, therefore, a particularly useful tool. Although formal gait analysis is not necessary, recognizing specific abnormalities will facilitate localization and identification of specific conditions. For example, abnormalities in the pelvis, hip, or upper femur cause a child to favor the involved area, usually resulting in leaning to the involved side and substituting support using the bones of the pelvis and upper leg for the midline weight-bearing. The result is hip circumduction and/or a Trendelenburg gait. Conversely, such a gait can be caused only by pathology involving the proximal femur or the pelvis. Involvement of the knee, on the other hand, causes loss of full flexion and extension of the knee, resulting in a gait with a characteristic 30° knee flexion (the most comfortable, neutral position for that joint). Similar considerations for additional sites of pathology are listed in Table 196-2.

Once the child's gait has been observed, a complete and systematic examination should be performed. Observation is the most sensitive tool for detecting abnormalities, as they are likely to be evident as subtle asymmetries between the right and left sides (Fig. 196-1). Further assessment should then focus on the areas of asymmetry. As long as the examiner is familiar with a joints' normal appearance and range, evaluation of either passive or active range of motion will yield the necessary information. Pathology typically first becomes evident at the extremes of range of motion: cervical arthritis, for example, leads to loss of full extension at the neck, whereas arthritis in the elbow renders full flexion unbearable. In both cases, the final degrees of motion are lost first, so assessment of joints only at the midranges of movement is not adequate.

#### Palpation

The next component of the exam is palpation. Examiners are understandably reluctant to cause undue discomfort in a child, but overly gentle palpation is useless. If a child does not complain of pain at any stage of the exam, it is impossible to know whether it represents an absence of pathology or simply a failure to reach the threshold for

**TABLE 196-2 SITE-SPECIFIC ALTERATIONS IN GAIT IN RHEUMATOLOGIC CONDITIONS**

| Location | Example | Alteration in Gait | Description | Mechanism |
|---|---|---|---|---|
| Pelvis | Psoas abscess | Trendelenburg gait | Pelvis tilts away from affected side | Minimize use of painful muscle |
| Hip | Septic arthritis | Refuses to walk | Hip flexed, externally rotated | Joint effusion distends joint capsule, causing pain with movement in any plane |
| Knee | Unequal leg lengths | Vaulting gait | Leg fails to clear ground in extension | "Vaults" over knee that does not provide adequate clearance |
| Ankle | Achilles tendinitis | Steppage (equinus) gait | Minimizes ankle dorsiflexion | Pain in Achilles with dorsiflexion |
| Foot | Metatarsal stress | Favors involved foot | Everts foot to redistribute weight | Pain in involved toe fracture |

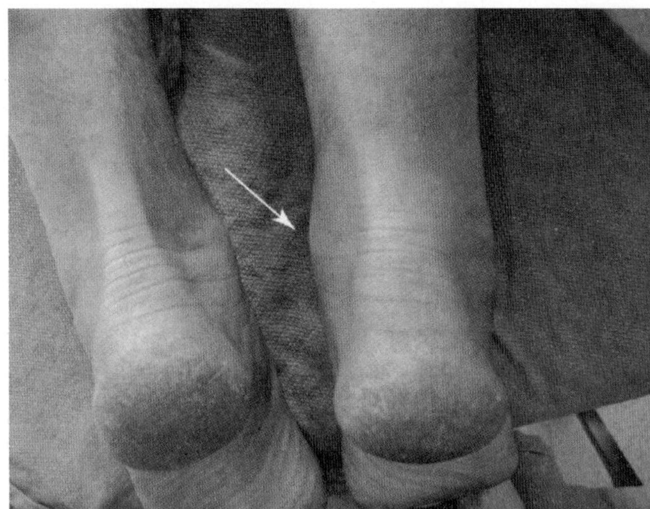

FIGURE 196-1 Asymmetry of ankles, with subtle fullness adjacent to right medial malleolus identifying abnormal joint.



pain. Thus, at least 1 area must be palpated forcefully enough to evoke an "Ouch!" from the child. The amount of pressure used may then be compared to palpation at other sites in order to provide a means of differentiating normal from affected areas. The knee may exhibit a ballotable effusion, meaning that applying pressure directly to the patella forces it downward, displacing synovial fluid and causing the patella to bounce against the femur. The characteristic springiness is not noted when fluid does not intervene between patella and femur, as in healthy children. The joint may also be swollen from synovial proliferation, which has a boggier consistency than does the free fluid of a joint effusion.

Signs of inflammation are the hallmark of arthritis. Warmth and swelling are most characteristic, whereas overlying erythema is more characteristic of septic arthritis. The child with a chronic inflammatory arthritis may report that she is uncomfortable, but the sensation is more commonly described as stiffness than as pain. In fact, at least 20% of children with juvenile arthritis never complain of pain.

Careful examination of an inflamed joint also may allow estimation of the duration of the arthritis. Synovitis is characterized by increased blood flow, typically more pronounced in the portion of the joint compartment subjected to the maximum force. In the knee, it is the medial femoral condyle, where hyperemia leads to increased delivery of nutrients and accelerated growth. Initially, it may be seen as prominence of the medial aspect of the knee, later as genu valgus. Ultimately, the leg with the inflamed knee grows more rapidly and a discrepancy in the lengths of the legs develops. The lower leg may bow in order to compensate for the greater length. At the same time, the knee loses extension and develops a flexion contracture, with resultant atrophy of the vastus medialis muscle. In contrast, significant inflammation in the hip or temporomandibular joint often damages the growth plate and leads to foreshortening of the involved side. Because minimal longitudinal growth occurs at the distal tibia, ankle arthritis causes little, if any, discrepancy in leg lengths.

## DIFFERENTIAL DIAGNOSIS

### Pattern of Joint Involvement

In addition to categorizing the type of pain a child is experiencing, it is critical to determine how many joints are affected. The potential causes of a monoarticular process differ significantly from those of polyarticular conditions, so careful examination of all joints is mandatory even when the complaint involves only a single location. It is also important to determine the type of onset (sudden or gradual), duration of symptoms, and any associated systemic features such as fever or rash. Distinct differential diagnoses must be considered for monoarticular and polyarticular processes, as well as for joint complaints associated with fever or other extra-articular signs and symptoms (Table 196-3).

**TABLE 196-3 COMMON CAUSES OF ARTHRITIS**

| |
|---|
| **Monoarticular** |
| *Acute Onset* |
| Septic arthritis |
| Reactive arthritis |
| Trauma |
| Hemophilia |
| Lyme disease |
| *Chronic* |
| Juvenile idiopathic arthritis |
| Lyme disease |
| Tuberculosis (rare without pulmonary disease) |
| Tumor (eg, pigmented villonodular synovitis) (rare) |
| **Polyarticular** |
| Juvenile rheumatoid arthritis |
| Spondyloarthropathies |
| Systemic autoimmune diseases |
| Systemic lupus erythematosus |
| Vasculitis |
| Sarcoidosis |
| Arthritis associated with inflammatory bowel disease |
| Viral arthritis |
| Reactive arthritis |
| Serum sickness |
| Rheumatic fever (migratory arthritis) |
| Malignancies |
| Periodic fever syndromes |

When generating a list of possible diagnoses, it is important to consider which presenting features are being considered. Because children usually do not have comorbid conditions as adults do, pediatricians typically assume that several symptoms share a common cause. This assumption narrows the list of possibilities and hastens arrival at a working diagnosis. Thus, if a child has an excruciatingly painful hip and a fever of 38.9°C, it is reasonable to worry about septic arthritis of the hip. If it turns out that the child fell off a ladder and broke his femoral neck, however, but was afraid to tell anyone, then other scenarios are more likely, and arthrocentesis of the hip might not be such a good diagnosis after all.

### Monoarthritis

The potential etiologies of a monoarticular process may be narrowed down by consideration of the nature of onset and duration of symptoms.

### Acute Onset

Rapid development of pain and swelling of a single joint necessitates consideration of a bacterial infection. Unlike most types of inflammatory arthritis, for which delaying the diagnosis by several days is unlikely to have long-term implications, treatment of septic arthritis must not be postponed. In fact, a history of fever associated with a single red, swollen, painful, or hot joint necessitates arthrocentesis for cell count and culture. Conversely, in an afebrile child, traumatic injury is a more likely explanation for acute joint symptoms. Documentation of an antecedent trauma is helpful, but confirmation of such may be difficult to elicit from young children who are unable to verbalize specifics of the history.

Once these possibilities are excluded, postinfectious or "reactive arthritis" must be considered in the case of an acutely symptomatic joint. This process may involve 1 or many joints, but it characteristically causes less inflammation than does an acute infection. Thus, postinfectious arthritis usually does not cause erythema overlying the joint, and although it may be uncomfortable, excruciating pain is less common. Reactive arthritis generally responds well to nonsteroidal anti-inflammatory agents and usually is transient. Lyme disease also may be difficult to distinguish clinically from septic arthritis, although generally, it causes more indolent symptoms.

#### Subacute Onset

Diagnostic considerations of an isolated, chronically swollen joint differ from those in the case of an acute arthritis. Bacterial infections are far less likely, whereas lower grade infections, especially Lyme disease in endemic areas, must be excluded. Chronic monoarthritis also may be caused by *Mycobacterium tuberculosis*, particularly in immunocompromised children. Also within this category are chronic forms of synovitis, especially pauciarticular juvenile arthritis and psoriatic arthritis. Rarer inflammatory arthropathies, such as arthritis caused by sarcoidosis, also may cause monoarthritis. Primary tumors of the cartilage and synovium, although extremely rare, also are most likely to present as discomfort in a single joint. The most common of these tumors, pigmented villonodular synovitis (PVNS), typically causes a chronically painful and swollen knee. A nontraumatic arthrocentesis that yields bloody fluid is suggestive of an articular tumor.

#### Polyarthritis

When several joints are involved, rheumatologic conditions rise to the top of the differential diagnosis. Most common among these conditions is polyarticular juvenile arthritis, although other autoimmune diseases such as systemic lupus erythematosus and vasculitis typically also involve several joints. Infections are instead progressively less likely as more joints are involved, with the exceptions of gonococcal arthritis in sexually active or abused children and *Salmonella* arthritis in immunocompromised patients. Arthritis associated with systemic conditions, such as inflammatory bowel disease or cystic fibrosis, also must be considered. Usually, extra-articular involvement (such as a new murmur in rheumatic fever or hives in serum sickness) offers a clue to multiorgan conditions. The pattern of joint involvement also may be suggestive: rheumatic fever, vasculitis, and serum sickness characteristically cause a migratory polyarthritis, whereas most other conditions cause additive or fixed involvement of several joints. In general, children with polyarthritis are most likely to benefit from consultation with a pediatric rheumatologist.

### PROGNOSIS AND OUTCOMES

Rheumatologic conditions typically take long periods of time to be diagnosed. The average delay in diagnosis of arthritis varies from a few weeks in children with systemic-onset juvenile arthritis (likely due to its acute, dramatic presentation with hectic fever, rash, and arthritis) to more than 6 months in dermatomyositis (with the more indolent and subtle loss of physical ability). Current treatment protocols stress the importance of early, aggressive therapy because chronic joint damage may start becoming evident within 6 months of the onset of synovitis. Thus, the most important thing that caregivers can do for children with suspected rheumatologic disorders is to expeditiously and efficiently diagnose their condition. Overlooking key points in the history and physical exam and referring to the wrong specialist are among the most common causes of delays in establishing diagnoses; focusing on mechanical or infectious causes of joint complaints and obtaining imaging studies or performing arthrocenteses in a child with morning stiffness will only delay the initiation of treatment for arthritis. By remembering that most rheumatologic conditions in children are clinical diagnoses established on the basis of history and physical exam, caregivers can avoid delays and optimize outcomes. Only after a short list of possibilities is generated are laboratory studies and imaging likely to be useful. On the other hand, no matter what diagnostic test is performed, if you don't know what you are looking for, you probably won't find it.

### CONCLUSION

Pediatric rheumatology is one of the few specialties in which laboratory and imaging studies have not gained outsized importance in the diagnostic process. History and physical exam remain the most effective and efficient tools that a clinician has. Hence, one must be particularly thorough and systematic as one questions and examines the child. Every patient represents a riddle, and no clinic visit is routine. The corollary, however, is that when one embraces this challenge and accurately confirms a clinical diagnosis with a magnetic resonance image or a blood test, then one has reinforced a skill that will make one just a bit better the next time.

### SUGGESTED READINGS


Bergl P, Farnan JM, Chan E. Moving toward cost-effectiveness in physical examination. *Am J Med.* 2015;128:109-110.

Herrle SR, Corgett EC Jr, Fagan MJ, et al. Bayes' theorem and the physical examination: probability assessment and diagnostic decision-making. *Acad Med.* 2011;86:618-627.

Hersh AO, Prahalad S. Immunogenetics of juvenile idiopathic arthritis: a comprehensive review. *J Autoimmun.* 2015;30:113-124.

Hinze C, Gohar F, Foell D. Management of juvenile idiopathic arthritis: hitting the target. *Nat Rev Rheumatol.* 2015;11:290-300.

Li YR, Li J, Zhao SD, et al. Meta-analysis of shared genetic architecture across ten pediatric autoimmune diseases. *Nat Med.* 2015;21: 1018-1027.

McGhee JL, Burks FN, Sheckels JL, Jarvis JN. Identifying children with chronic arthritis based on chief complaints: absence of predictive value for musculoskeletal pain as an indicator of rheumatic disease in children. *Pediatrics.* 2002;110(2 part 1):354-359.

Prakken B, Albani S, Martini A. Juvenile idiopathic arthritis. *Lancet.* 2011;377:2138-2149.

Robert I, Clear G. Evaluation of the limping child. *Pediatr Child Health.* 2009;20:195-200.

Thierry S, Fautrel B, Lemelle I, Guillemin F. Prevalence and incidence of juvenile idiopathic arthritis: a systematic review. *Joint Bone Spine.* 2014;31:112-117.

Trueworthy RC, Templeton KJ. Malignant bone tumors presenting as musculoskeletal pain. *Pediatr Ann.* 2002;31:355-359.

Vostrejs M, Hollister JR. Muscle atrophy and leg length discrepancies in pauciarticular juvenile rheumatoid arthritis. *Am J Dis Child.* 1988;142:343-345.

Willis AA, Widmann RF, Flynn JM, Green DW, Onel KB. Lyme arthritis presenting as acute septic arthritis in children. *J Pediatr Orthop.* 2003;23:114-118.




# 197 Diagnostic Testing in Rheumatology

Peter A. Nigrovic

### INTRODUCTION

Laboratory and imaging studies rarely establish a definitive diagnosis of rheumatologic diseases in children. The prevalence of rheumatic diseases in childhood is low, and even very specific tests generate high false-positive rates unless there is a well-founded clinical suspicion for a particular illness based on an informed differential diagnosis guided by the history and physical exam. Further, the utility of an assay will vary with the nature and stage of the illness. Nonetheless, diagnostic testing can provide information that is essential for the evaluation and treatment of children with rheumatic diseases.

## LABORATORY STUDIES

### MARKERS OF INFLAMMATION

Most rheumatologic diseases arise from aberrant immune attacks on normal cells and tissues. In many cases, these immune activities are reflected in indices of systemic inflammation. Two principal markers are the erythrocyte sedimentation rate (ESR) and the C-reactive protein (CRP), but other tests also may be useful. It is important to remember that localized inflammation, such as glomerulonephritis in systemic lupus erythematosus (SLE) or synovitis in pauciarticular juvenile idiopathic arthritis (JIA), may not be reflected in these indices.

#### Erythrocyte Sedimentation Rate

The ESR measures the speed with which red blood cells precipitate from suspension in a sample of anticoagulated blood and are quantitated at millimeters per hour. In the patient with inflammation, hepatic synthesis of positively charged, acute-phase reactants such as fibrinogen enables negatively charged erythrocytes to overcome electrostatic repulsion and stack together in columns (rouleaux), which fall from suspension in the blood more swiftly. The ESR thus serves as an indirect measure of the hepatic acute-phase response, in turn reflecting the presence of circulating proinflammatory cytokines such as interleukin (IL)-1, tumor necrosis factor (TNF), and, especially, IL-6. Changes in the ESR follow a time course commensurate with hepatic protein synthesis and the degradation and clearance of the relevant proteins, rising and falling gradually over the course of days.

The advantages of the ESR are its technical simplicity and low cost and its long track record of use. Whereas mild elevations of ESR (eg, <40 mm/h) arise in the course of many routine illnesses, more substantial increases warrant scrutiny for a worrisome underlying cause such as infection, malignancy, or rheumatologic disease, depending on the clinical situation. In rheumatologic patients who manifest an elevated ESR, this lab value may help track the response to therapy.

Although it is a robust and useful tool, the ESR has limitations intrinsic to the assay. Processes that alter red cell properties or the plasma protein milieu may alter the ESR. ESR decreases with elevated hematocrit, aberrant red cell shape (eg, sickle cell disease and spherocytosis), and disseminated intravascular coagulation (DIC) caused by consumption of circulating fibrinogen. ESR rises with anemia, pregnancy, nephrotic syndrome, and hypergammaglobulinemia, for which positively charged immunoglobulins promote rouleaux formation that can markedly elevate ESR in the absence of systemic inflammation.

#### C-Reactive Protein

CRP is an innate antibacterial compound of the pentraxin class that is produced as part of the hepatic acute-phase response. It was identified originally as a protein that bound the C polysaccharide of pneumococcus but is capable of recognizing numerous other bacterial ligands as well as surface lipids on dying human cells, where it may assist with the noninflammatory clearance of apoptotic debris. Present at low to undetectable levels in healthy individuals, the CRP rises briskly within hours of the onset of inflammation, and once an inflammatory stimulus ceases, the CRP level falls with a half-life of 19 hours. Accordingly, the CRP reflects hepatic acute-phase protein synthesis more tightly and directly than does the ESR, and it is not influenced by the factors that confound the ESR, such as sickle cell disease. However, certain conditions, including SLE manifest with CRP values lower than might be expected. Of course, this rapid responsiveness precludes inferring information about the duration and cumulative intensity of an inflammatory process from the CRP (as is possible with the ESR). In practice, both CRP and ESR shed light on the global inflammatory state but vary in their reliability from patient to patient. Often, interpreting the 2 together provides the most useful information.

#### Other Inflammatory Markers

Beyond the ESR and CRP, other blood indices that can reflect systemic inflammation include the white blood cell count, the platelet count, ferritin, the von Willebrand factor antigen, and total immunoglobulin level. The importance of each of these as a disease marker varies with the condition in question. The white blood cell count rises with inflammation of many causes, including rheumatic diseases. The platelet count also rises with inflammation, mediated in part by the IL-6–stimulated production of thrombopoietin by hepatocytes. Such elevation occurs slowly, over the course of days, and therefore implies a degree of chronicity. Conversely, a platelet count that is lower than expected for the degree and duration of inflammation suggests peripheral consumption (eg, DIC) or marrow dysfunction, such as may be seen in myelophthisis in acute leukemia. Ferritin is a hepatic acute-phase reactant as well as a measure of body's iron stores. Ferritin levels elevated out of proportion to other inflammatory markers are commonly seen in systemic JIA, whereas extreme elevation (often > 10,000 ng/mL) suggests a hemophagocytic complication of this condition called *macrophage activation syndrome* (see Chapters 459 and 184). The von Willebrand factor antigen is released by endothelial cells and can suggest endothelial injury, but levels can also rise nonspecifically with inflammation. Measurement of von Willebrand factor antigen is particularly useful in some patients with small-vessel vasculitides and microangiopathic conditions such as juvenile dermatomyositis, for which it can help track disease activity. The total immunoglobulin G (IgG) level may also rise with prolonged immune activation. Elevation in the IgG level is especially characteristic of SLE and related disorders as well as certain viral infections (eg, Epstein-Barr virus and human immunodeficiency virus) that are marked by prominent B-cell activation.

## AUTOANTIBODIES IN THE RHEUMATIC DISEASES

The production of antibodies to self-antigens is a hallmark of many rheumatologic diseases (Table 197-1). The presence of these antibodies indicates a defect in normal mechanisms of immune tolerance. Many of these antibodies serve simply as diagnostic markers, whereas others may participate directly in disease pathogenesis. Because autoantibody titers generally do not correlate with disease activity, in most cases, serial monitoring of autoantibody levels contributes little to disease management.

**TABLE 197-1 IMPORTANT AUTOANTIBODIES IN THE RHEUMATOLOGIC DISEASES**

| Autoantibody | Disease Association |
|---|---|
| Antinuclear antibodies (ANA) | Healthy normals (low titer), SLE, drug-induced SLE, SS, SSc, JIA, JDM, MCTD, Raynaud, autoimmune thyroiditis, autoimmune hepatitis |
| Anticentromere pattern | Limited SSc (CREST) |
| dsDNA | SLE (renal disease) |
| Ro/SS-A | SLE, SS, neonatal SLE |
| La/SS-B | SLE, SS, neonatal SLE |
| Ribonucleoprotein (RNP) | SLE, MCTD |
| Smith | SLE |
| Scl70 | SLE, SSc |
| Histone | SLE, drug-induced SLE |
| Jo-1 | Lung disease in JDM |
| Ribosomal P | SLE (possibly neuropsychiatric SLE) |
| Antineutrophil cytoplasmic antibody (ANCA) | |
| c-ANCA (cytoplasmic, antiproteinase 3) | AAV (especially granulomatosis with polyangiitis) |
| p-ANCA (perinuclear, antimyeloperoxidase) | AAV (especially microscopic polyarteritis) |
| Rheumatoid factor (RF) | Rheumatoid arthritis and RF-positive polyarticular JIA |
| | SS |
| | Cryoglobulinemia, usually related to hepatitis C |
| | Mixed connective tissue disease and other "overlap" syndromes |
| | Chronic bacterial infection |
| Cyclic citrullinated peptide (CCP) | Rheumatoid arthritis and RF-positive polyarticular JIA |

AAV, ANCA-associated vasculitis; CREST, calcinosis, Raynaud's phenomenon, esophageal dysmotility, sclerodactyly, and telangiectasia; JDM, juvenile dermatomyositis; JIA, juvenile idiopathic arthritis; MCTD, mixed connective tissue disease; SLE, systemic lupus erythematosus; SS, Sjögren syndrome; SSc, systemic sclerosis (scleroderma).

#### Rheumatoid Factor

Rheumatoid factor (RF) is the general term given to antibodies that recognize the Fc portion of IgG. Generally of the IgM class, RF of IgA, IgG, or even IgE isotypes may be seen; they occur somewhat more commonly with RF-associated arthritis, but the additional diagnostic value of isotype determination is limited.

RF may be observed in many states of immune activation, including multiple autoimmune diseases, hepatitis C, cryoglobulinemia, and chronic bacterial infection (see Table 197-1). The prevalence of a positive RF in normal children is not well established but is likely less than 3%, and then typically in low titer. Among the childhood rheumatic diseases, the presence of RF defines a subset of polyarticular JIA and is associated with a chronic, aggressive course with little likelihood of long-term disease remission apart from medications (see Chapter 198). This form of JIA typically begins in preadolescence or the teenage years. It appears to represent the earliest cases of adult rheumatoid arthritis (RA), with which it shares essentially identical clinical features and genetic associations. RF is also observed in Sjögren syndrome, often at high titer. Unlike most non–arthritis-associated RFs, the RFs seen in RA have typically undergone somatic hypermutation in germinal centers to increase their binding affinity for IgG. The significance of this observation is not clear, however, because no pathogenic role for RF has been identified.

Despite these disease associations, the diagnostic role for RF testing in pediatrics is limited. Although the presence of RF in the setting of an active polyarthritis helps to classify and prognosticate, JIA remains a clinical diagnosis. Since RF is rarely meaningfully positive in arthritis occurring in younger children (eg, before age 8), it is not routinely warranted as part of the evaluation of arthritis below this age. The optimal evaluation for a child noted to have a high-titer RF in the absence of evident clinical disease remains undefined. RF is known to predate the onset of arthritis in a substantial fraction of adult patients who go on to have RA.

#### Anti-Cyclic Citrullinated Peptide Antibodies

The identification of antibodies against citrullinated peptides represents a major advance in the understanding of the pathogenesis of some forms of arthritis. Citrulline is an amino acid that results from the enzymatic deimination of arginine. Citrullination occurs in some proteins as part of routine posttranslational modification, whereas in others, it develops in the setting of tissue injury and inflammation. The presence of autoantibodies against citrullinated peptides is highly specific for adult RA and its juvenile counterpart, RF-positive polyarticular JIA, and is generally assessed as reactivity to a synthetic cyclic citrullinated peptide (CCP). CCP-positive arthritis overlaps substantially with RF-positive arthritis, with the advantage of fewer false-positive results than are seen with RF. Like RF, CCP positivity is associated with more aggressive arthritis unlikely to enter spontaneous remission. In the context of a documented inflammatory arthritis, a positive CCP provides strong support for classification and prognosis.

#### Antinuclear Antibodies

The most common autoantibodies detected in children with rheumatic disease are the antinuclear antibodies (ANAs). ANA is assessed by layering the patient's serum over cells fixed to a surface, counterstaining with a fluorescent anti-human immunoglobulin, and visually assessing the lowest serum dilution at which fluorescence remains detectable. Normal is less than 1:40 in most laboratories. Enzyme-linked immunosorbent assays (ELISAs) are also available. The significance of a positive test rises with antibody titer. Further specificity is provided by testing for antibodies against defined targets, sometimes termed *extractable nuclear antigens* (ENAs), by ELISA. The immunofluorescence pattern of staining (eg, homogenous, speckled, rim, nucleolar) is of limited utility now that specific antigen testing is available. The single exception is the anticentromere pattern associated with limited systemic sclerosis (see Chapter 203).

ANAs are found in a wide range of immune disorders in children. They include SLE and related conditions, JIA, autoimmune thyroid disease, and autoimmune hepatitis. ANAs are also found at low titer in many normal children, ranging from 1.6% to 15% in healthy children tested at a serum dilution of 1:10. Given the low prevalence of ANA-associated disorders, the ANA has a poor positive predictive value in the absence of compelling historical, examination, or laboratory features of a specific rheumatic illness. In particular, SLE is highly unlikely in children with an ANA titer of 1:160 or less. By contrast, the presence of an ANA at any titer in a patient with JIA is relevant as a predictor of elevated risk of the presence of uveitis (see Chapter 198). Follow-up of patients referred to a pediatric rheumatology clinic with a positive ANA but no clinical rheumatic disease at presentation has established that subsequent development of an ANA-related disease is rare, although the positive ANA itself may persist for years. In patients with Raynaud phenomenon, a positive ANA is associated with an increased risk of subsequent development of an associated autoimmune process, yet most patients remain well.

The clinical significance of a positive ANA may be defined further by testing for specific, disease-associated targets of the autoantibodies. These specific antibodies are rare findings in ANA-positive healthy children and those with JIA, but they are usually positive in patients with SLE and related disorders (see Table 197-1). Most patients with SLE have at least 1 of these autoantibodies; dsDNA and Sm are relatively specific for this diagnosis. Within SLE, the presence of dsDNA correlates with an increased risk for nephritis, and the titer tends to rise and fall with disease activity. Ro and La are found in SLE but are prominent in Sjögren syndrome. Maternal Ro and La antibodies are associated with a risk for development of neonatal SLE in the newborn, in particular congenital heart block, because of cross-reactivity with antigens expressed in the fetal myocardium. RNP is common in SLE generally but is found in high titer in mixed connective tissue disease (MCTD), an overlap syndrome with features of SLE, scleroderma, and dermatomyositis. Scl70 is associated with SLE and scleroderma. Antihistone antibodies are common occurrences in patients with SLE, but they are a hallmark of SLE induced by exposure to drugs such as hydralazine and procainamide when found in the absence of antibodies against other ENAs. However, SLE induced by other drugs, including minocycline, usually is negative for antihistone antibodies, so a negative test does not definitively rule out the possibility of drug-induced SLE. Jo-1 positivity correlates with increased risk of interstitial lung disease in patients with dermatomyositis. Antiribosomal P antibody has been associated with central nervous system manifestations of SLE but is of limited sensitivity and specificity.

#### Antiphospholipid Antibodies

The term *antiphospholipid antibodies* (aPLs) refers broadly to a group of autoantibodies associated with increased risk of clotting in some patients. Many of these antibodies target phospholipid-associated proteins rather than membrane phospholipids themselves. They are thought to promote coagulation by interference with normal anticoagulant mechanisms and by the direct promotion of inflammation. In practice, only a small proportion of patients with measurable antiphospholipid antibodies ever experience clinical hypercoagulability, reflecting differential pathogenicity of specific antibodies as well as variation in predisposing genetic and environmental factors.

The most commonly measured aPLs are anticardiolipin antibodies and the lupus anticoagulant. Anticardiolipin antibodies are measured by ELISA. By contrast, the presence of a lupus anticoagulant is assessed functionally: (1) The patient's serum is induced to clot; (2) if clotting fails to occur, coagulation factor deficiency is excluded by admixture of control serum; (3) if the clotting defect fails to correct, excess phospholipid is added to adsorb aPL antibodies, and a lupus anticoagulant is said to be present if the clotting defect corrects. Testing can also be performed to look for antibodies against specific phospholipid-associated proteins, including beta-2 glycoprotein 1 (β2GP1) and prothrombin.

The clinical significance of a positive test for aPL antibodies changes dramatically with context. Transient aPLs appear to be rather common after viral infections and some other triggers. In past years, they were usually uncovered during routine testing for syphilis (the VDRL [Venereal Disease Research Laboratory] test employs cardiolipin as antigen) and during preoperative testing of the partial thromboplastin time (PTT), which is prolonged by a lupus anticoagulant. Follow-up of such patients has generally been reassuring, with a low risk of pathologic thrombosis. Patients with SLE commonly express aPL antibodies, which may be somewhat more predictive of thrombosis than in healthy subjects, though the area remains controversial. By contrast, an aPL identified in a patient with a history of clot is likely of pathogenic importance and can help to explain the index event.

There is no role for aPL testing as a screen of asymptomatic patients. In patients with SLE, testing for anticardiolipin and lupus anticoagulant may help define the risk of developing a thrombosis. By contrast, in a patient with unexplained thrombosis, testing for anticardiolipin, lupus anticoagulant, and often anti-β2GP1 is critical to define the clotting diathesis; even more refined testing may be appropriate if the clinical suspicion warrants. The role of antibody titer monitoring to assess future risk in patients who have experienced aPL-related thrombosis is controversial. Even if antibody levels fall below the limit of detection, the pathogenic plasma cell clones remain susceptible to reactivation and renewed aPL secretion by a viral illness or other unpredictable event. Thus, these patients may indefinitely to be at increased risk of developing a pathologic thrombosis.



### Antineutrophil Cytoplasmic Antibodies

Antineutrophil cytoplasmic antibodies (ANCAs) were originally identified in patients with granulomatosis with polyangiitis (GPA, formerly termed *Wegener granulomatosis*) as an antibody-mediated reactivity to the cytoplasm of fixed neutrophils. Subsequently two staining patterns were identified: a uniform cytoplasmic stain (c-ANCA) and a stain clustered around the borders of the nucleus (perinuclear or p-ANCA). In patients with ANCA-associated vasculitis (AAV), these patterns correspond to antibody reactivity against specific antigens: proteinase 3 (PR3) for c-ANCA and myeloperoxidase (MPO) for p-ANCA. The presence of anti-PR3 and anti-MPO antibodies is often assessed by ELISA during ANCA testing, avoiding the subjectivity inherent to immunofluorescence microscopy while providing a quantitative antibody titer. These ELISAs offer the further important advantage of specificity: Beyond PR3 and MPO, other antigenic targets can mimic the ANCA immunofluorescence pattern. ELISA is particularly important for p-ANCA because 200 this staining pattern is relatively nonspecific and remains strongly associated with vasculitis only when specific for MPO.

ANCA positivity defines a class of life-threatening, small-vessel vasculitides affecting the renal and pulmonary vessels, among others (see Chapter 200). PR3-ANCA (c-ANCA) occurs most often in GPA, a granulomatous vasculitis affecting the sinuses, airway, lungs, and kidneys. MPO-ANCA (p-ANCA) associates more tightly with microscopic polyangiitis (MPA), a vasculitis associated with pulmonary hemorrhage and less prominent renal disease. However, GPA and MPA disease manifestations overlap, and the association of staining pattern (and antigen reactivity) with clinical disease is variable. ANCA positivity also may be seen in Churg-Strauss vasculitis, but the association in this condition is less consistent, and many patients have no detectable ANCA. In the proper clinical setting, the specificity of a positive ANCA assay is very high, in some cases obviating the need for tissue biopsy. However, in situations in which the clinical picture diverges from typical findings in a small-vessel vasculitis, false positives may be observed, especially for p-ANCA. Conversely, cases of so-called "limited GPA" (sinus and upper respiratory disease sparing kidney and lung parenchyma) are often ANCA-negative. As with other autoantibodies, only certain isotypes and specificities of ANCA appear to play a pathogenic role.

## OTHER TESTS IN RHEUMATOLOGY

### Joint Fluid Examination

Inflamed joint tissues produce an excess of synovial fluid that can be sampled clinically by joint aspiration. Normal joint fluid is straw-colored, relatively viscous, and contains no more than a few hundred white blood cells per milliliter, including few if any neutrophils. Joint inflammation of any cause results in the influx of inflammatory cells, most commonly neutrophils. In children, the major purpose of joint aspiration is to exclude bacterial infection; examination of joint fluid under polarized light microscopy is also the method of choice to evaluate for crystal-induced synovitis (gout, pseudogout). An elevated white blood cell count (eg, >50,000/mL) with a neutrophil predominance in the joint fluid is usual in bacterial infections, but this degree of pleocytosis also may be seen in other joint processes, such as JIA or Lyme disease. Thus, infection cannot be confirmed without consistent findings on Gram stain and culture. When bacterial infection is not suspected, the characterization of joint fluid contributes minimally to the diagnostic evaluation of pediatric arthritis. The presence of grossly bloody or rust-colored joint fluid is observed with intra-articular trauma, hemophilia-associated arthropathy, and, more rarely, synovial neoplasms such as pigmented villonodular synovitis (PVNS) and synovial sarcoma. Joint fluid may also be tested for *Borrelia burgdorferi* DNA by polymerase chain reaction (PCR), but this test is imperfectly sensitive, especially after treatment with antibiotics. Assays for other joint-fluid parameters such as viscosity, glucose, or lactate dehydrogenase are rarely helpful.

### HLA Typing

The human leukocyte antigen (HLA) locus on chromosome 6 encodes the critical antigen-presenting molecules major histocompatibility complex (MHC) I and II. These receptors are variable across the human population and help determine the antigens to which an individual may develop an immune response. Many autoimmune diseases exhibit strong genetic associations with particular HLA alleles. Among the strongest are the association of the MHC I molecule HLA-B27 with ankylosing spondylitis (relative risk ~20) and of specific HLA-DR alleles (MHC II) with arthritis exhibiting RF and/or anti-CCP antibodies (relative risk ~5–11). While these associations are pathophysiologically significant, the value of clinical testing for HLA type is limited. The alleles in question are much more prevalent than after their associated diseases, whereas not all patients with the disease bear the relevant allele. The result is that both positive and negative predictive values for individual patients are limited. For example, approximately 7% to 10% of the Caucasian population expresses HLA-B27, whereas ankylosing spondylitis has a population prevalence of less than 1% (of whom 10% do not have HLA-B27). Further, appropriate management of these HLA-linked diseases rests on assessment of disease activity, something that patient genotype cannot answer. The major clinical utility of HLA-B27 status is in cases for which a diagnosis of spondyloarthropathy remains uncertain after clinical and imaging evaluations have been performed.

### Complement

The complement system is discussed in Chapter 182. In clinical practice, quantitation of the integrity and activity of the complement system can provide important diagnostic information. Most commonly measured are the levels of C3 and C4. Low levels of these proteins usually reflect complement consumption by an inflammatory process, although increased hepatic synthesis of both these acute-phase reactants may mask activation of the complement system. (Alternative measures of complement turnover, such as the complement fragment C5a, are too unstable to be practical markers in the clinical setting.) Levels of both C3 and C4 are typically low in patients with active SLE, although they do not invariably normalize with successful treatment. A correlation between decreased complement levels and the activity of renal or hematologic disease in SLE has been noted. C3 may be low in patients with poststreptococcal glomerulonephritis, whereas C4 is typically depressed (sometimes with C3 also) in cryoglobulinemia.

### Cryoglobulins

Cryoglobulins are antibody–antibody or antibody–antigen complexes that remain soluble at physiologic temperatures but precipitate in the cold. They are associated with superficial and, less commonly, deep small-vessel vasculitis resulting in features such as cutaneous ulcers and mononeuritis multiplex (see Chapter 200). Cryoglobulins may be monoclonal (type I), arising as part of a clonal B-cell dyscrasia, or polyclonal, involving numerous different antibodies. Polyclonal (mixed) cryoglobulins are far more common and are sometimes divided into subtypes (type II and type III) depending on whether the associated anti-antibody (rheumatoid factor) activity is monoclonal or polyclonal, a distinction of little practical importance. All types of cryoglobulins are rare findings in children.

The measurement of cryoglobulins requires that the blood sample remain warm until the serum can be removed, to prevent loss of the cryoprecipitate in the cellular pellet. Blood should be drawn into a warmed, anticoagulant-free tube, kept warm in transport, and spun down in a warmed centrifuge, after which the serum is placed in a refrigerator for several days to observe for precipitate formation. The degree of cryoglobulinemia is quantitated as a fraction of serum volume taken up by the precipitate (cryocrit) and can be followed to assess response to therapy. The leading cause of mixed cryoglobulinemia is chronic hepatitis C infection, so an anti–hepatitis C antibody level should be checked when cryoglobulinemic vasculitis is a strong consideration. Rarely, the hepatitis C antibody may be completely bound up in the cryoglobulins and will be falsely negative, although a hepatitis C RNA assay will still be positive.

## IMAGING STUDIES

### INTRODUCTION

Imaging is an important adjunct to clinical and laboratory evaluation in the rheumatic diseases. Broadly speaking, plain radiography and ultrasound have low risk and cost but limited sensitivity. Computed tomography (CT) provides excellent spatial resolution of bony structures but limited soft tissue characterization at the expense of increased irradiation. Magnetic resonance imaging (MRI) offers the greatest visualization of soft tissue structures, especially cartilage and synovium, benefits that must be balanced against high cost and the need for sedation in younger children. The choice of imaging modality depends on the clinical scenario, and, in all cases, one must remember that radiographic studies are seldom diagnostic, but rather are useful for confirming or refuting the clinical impression.

#### Diseases of the Joints

Many of the hallmark rheumatic diseases primarily affect the musculoskeletal system. Imaging can help define the extent of joint inflammation or injury. In arthritis, the synovial lining hypertrophies and generates an abundance of inflammatory joint fluid. Over time, this process erodes cartilage and bone, damages ligaments and tendons, and induces regional osteopenia through inflammation and disuse. In skeletally immature children, inflammation also impacts surrounding growth centers and can affect bone growth and morphology. These processes can be assessed and followed by imaging.

In the acutely inflamed joint, plain films can document the presence of thickened soft tissue and effusion (Fig. 197-1). Radiographs can assist with the initial evaluation if the differential diagnosis includes such entities as trauma, tumor, or chronic nonbacterial osteomyelitis; otherwise, clinical examination without imaging is typically sufficient. In deeper joints that cannot be palpated directly, particularly the hip, ultrasound can identify swelling and guide aspiration if necessary. If the joint examination for active synovitis is equivocal, MRI can generally provide a definitive answer. MRI reliably detects even small effusions, and intravenous contrast with gadolinium highlights the inflamed synovial lining (Fig. 197-2). It is of particular utility for joints that are difficult to examine, such as the sacroiliac joints, wherein not only joint effusion but also adjacent bone marrow edema represent important diagnostic clues (Fig. 197-3). MRI can identify early erosions of cartilage and bone that remain undetected by plain film (Fig. 197-4). Beyond inflammatory processes, MRI can define mechanical causes for joint pain, such as injury to the menisci or ligaments of the knee.

Plain radiographs help in the assessment of structural integrity in chronically inflamed joints. Substantial cartilage thinning may be visualized as the loss of radiographic joint space, often with reactive bony sclerosis (Fig. 197-5). However, clinically important cartilage degradation may go undetected in this technique. When precise assessment of the extent of active synovitis and cartilage injury is required, MRI again remains the superior tool, although skilled clinical assessment is usually adequate. In adults with joint pain, the pattern of bony changes can suggest specific causes of arthritis, such as osteoarthritis, crystal disease (gout, pseudogout), or spondyloarthritic variants. In children with chronic joint swelling, however, the radiograph infrequently narrows the differential diagnosis in a therapeutically meaningful way.

The role of ultrasound in the evaluation of inflammatory arthritis in children is evolving. Increasingly, some clinicians are employing

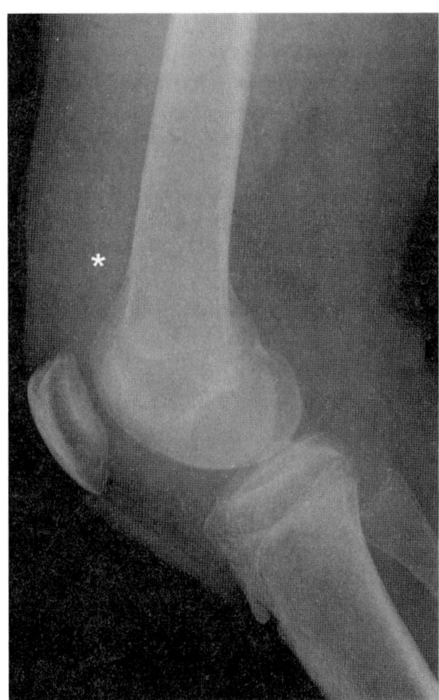


**FIGURE 197-1** Knee effusion. Plain radiograph of the right knee of a 15-year-old boy with Lyme disease, showing the large suprapatellar effusion (*). A similar effusion could result from infection, trauma, or any of the idiopathic inflammatory arthritis diseases.

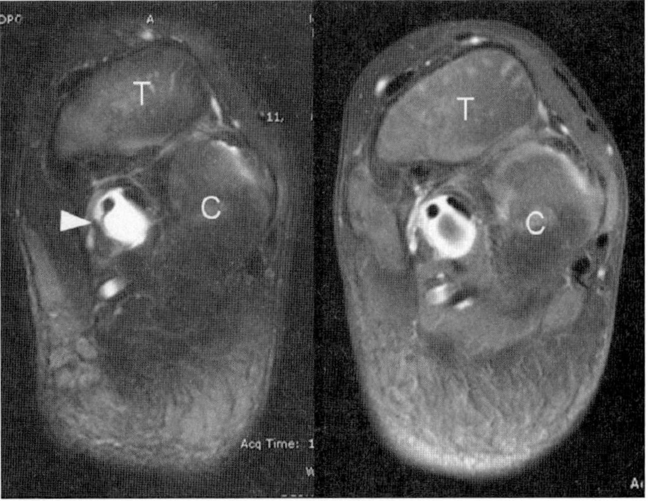


**FIGURE 197-2** Synovial enhancement with gadolinium. Shown are axial magnetic resonance images of the left ankle in a 4-year-old girl with psoriatic arthritis. **A:** Intense T2-bright signal (corresponding to fluid) surrounding the flexor digitorum tendon (*arrowhead*). **B:** The same region imaged following administration of gadolinium, enabling distinction between the enhancing synovial tendon sheath (bright) and the nonenhancing synovial fluid (dark).

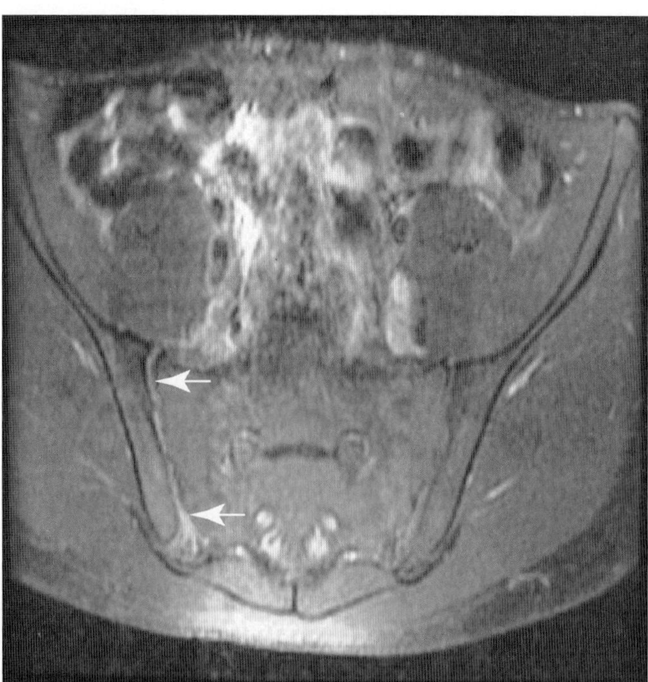

**FIGURE 197-3** Sacroiliac joint inflammation by magnetic resonance imaging (MRI). The patient is an adolescent boy who developed lower-back pain accompanied by morning stiffness. In this T2-weighted pelvic MRI, inflammation in the right sacroiliac joint may be seen as bright signal, reflecting local edema and effusion (*arrows*).

bedside ultrasound as an adjunct to the clinical examination, including detection of abnormally elevated blood flow in the synovium. Ultrasound can assist especially with the evaluation of "deep" joints such as hip and shoulder and with providing guidance for diagnostic and therapeutic arthrocentesis. However, ultrasound remains highly user-dependent, and the wide range of normal findings across the pediatric age spectrum often limits the ability to render definitive findings.

The role of CT scan in musculoskeletal imaging is generally restricted to complex 3-dimensional spaces where bone cortex detail, lost in MRI, is required. The main examples include the bones of the skull, cervical spine, and ankle.

#### Diseases Affecting Soft Tissues

Imaging contributes also to the assessment of rheumatologic processes affecting the soft tissues, including blood vessels, muscles, lungs, and brain.

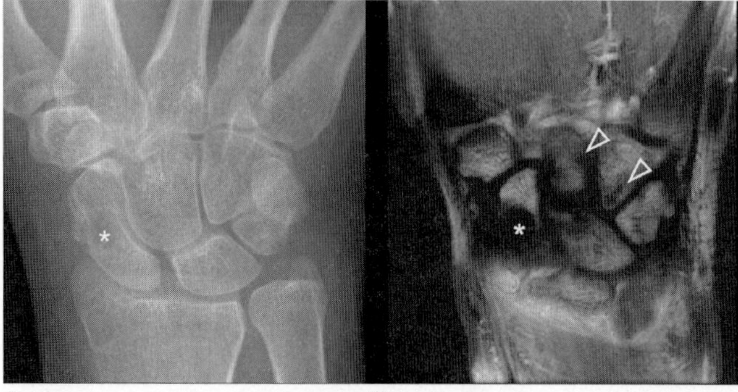


**FIGURE 197-4** Superior resolution of erosions by magnetic resonance imaging (MRI). Shown are paired images of the right wrist from a young woman, age 18, with psoriatic arthritis of juvenile onset. **A:** The plain radiograph demonstrates a large scaphoid erosion (*) but no other bony changes. **B:** An MRI obtained several weeks later shows the scaphoid erosion (*) but also shows multiple smaller erosions affecting other carpal bones (examples marked by *arrowheads*).

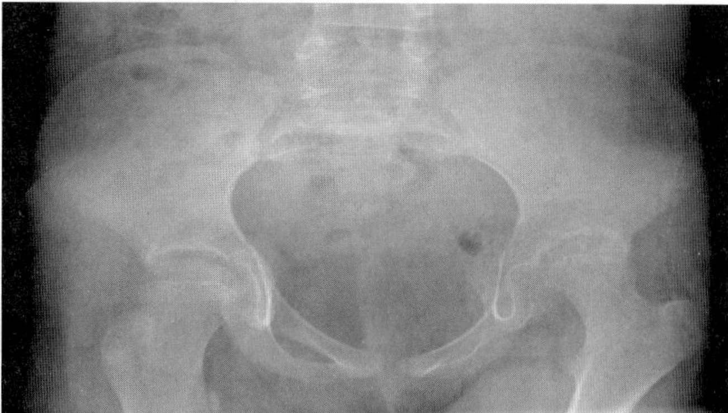

**FIGURE 197-5** Chronic joint injury detected by plain radiographs. The pelvis film from a 10-year-old girl with systemic juvenile idiopathic arthritis shows joint space loss and reactive bony sclerosis of both hips, left greater than right.

- *Vasculitis.* Although vasculitis affecting small blood vessels is commonly diagnosed with the aid of laboratory tests, such as cryoglobulins or ANCA, medium- and large-vessel vasculitides lack specific laboratory hallmarks. For these diseases, including Takayasu arteritis, polyarteritis nodosa, and Kawasaki disease, the diagnosis is anatomic—via tissue histology or, more commonly, imaging. The optimal tool for identifying inflammatory injury to blood vessels depends on the site of inflammation and the caliber of vessels involved. Conventional contrast angiography represents the historical gold standard, especially for a disease that affects smaller arteries. However, angiography is invasive and cannot be repeated regularly to monitor response to therapy. Ultrasound may be employed to image certain vessels, such as the coronary arteries in Kawasaki disease. CT angiography provides excellent cross-sectional images but with considerable exposure to radiation and iodinated contrast. MRI and contrast-enhanced magnetic resonance angiography require no exposure to radiation and have the potential to image edema/inflammation in the vessel wall and perivascular tissues, but smaller arteries cannot be reliably assessed. Thus, although numerous modalities are available for the imaging of vasculitis, the optimal study for a particular patient remains highly context-dependent.
- *Muscles.* Inflammatory disease of muscle may be imaged best by MRI, revealing edema in the inflamed muscle tissue. This finding can help to define an optimal location for biopsy or, in the right clinical setting, obviate the need for a biopsy altogether. Because myositis in children generally favors the proximal musculature, MRI evaluation commonly focuses on the muscles in the gluteal region and proximal thigh, revealing edema on fat-suppressed imaging sequences (Fig. 197-6). Alternate MRI findings are seen in degenerative and metabolic myopathies.
- *Lungs.* The chest radiograph remains the first step in lung imaging, but it is of limited sensitivity in the identification of rheumatologic processes affecting the lung, including vasculitis and interstitial fibrosis. These processes are better defined through high-resolution CT scanning (Fig. 197-7). Vasculitis and alveolar hemorrhage produce "ground-glass" opacities from alveolar filling. Interstitial fibrosis results in reticular densities, nodules, traction changes, and, at end stage, a "honeycomb" appearance reflecting the replacement of normal alveolar architecture with fibrous cysts. It is important to note that these imaging studies are complemented by pulmonary function studies, in particular the diffusion capacity for carbon monoxide ($DL_{CO}$), which is decreased by fibrotic thickening of diffusing surfaces and increased by intra-alveolar blood.
- *Brain.* The principal rheumatologic processes affecting the brain in children include vasculitis, autoimmune encephalitides, and central nervous system (CNS) lupus. Vasculitis and encephalitis often, but not invariably, may be seen as focal changes on MRI or as regional infarction on CT. CNS lupus is a heterogeneous disorder

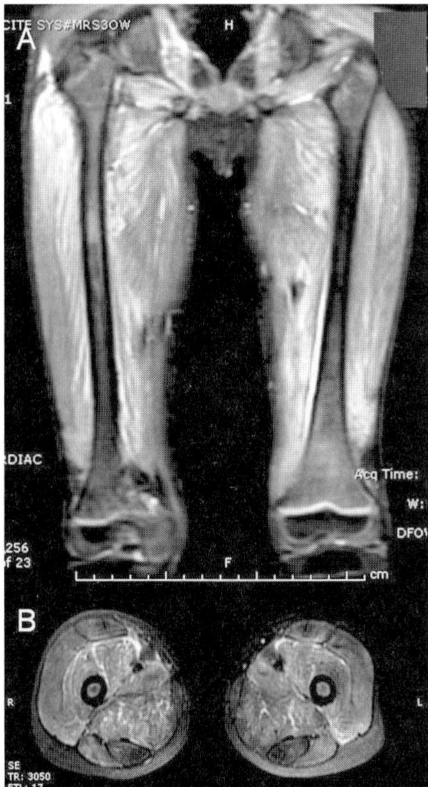


**FIGURE 197-6** Magnetic resonance image of active juvenile dermatomyositis. These T2-weighted, fat-suppressed images demonstrate extensive edema affecting the gluteal and thigh muscles of this 7-year-old boy with juvenile dermatomyositis. **A:** A coronal image of the pelvis and thighs. **B:** An axial section at midthigh. Both images show regional variation in the intensity of inflammation, with relative sparing of the anterolateral and posterior musculature.

that can result from vascular injury, but in fact more often arises through poorly understood pathophysiologic processes that do not compromise regional blood flow or cause local edema. Therefore, CT and MRI images may be normal. Further, nonspecific abnormalities are common among patients with SLE, rendering interpretation of imaging difficult. Where available, functional and metabolic scanning (eg, single photon emission CT [SPECT]) may identify regional variation of nutrient utilization. Such changes can suggest CNS lupus, although they are nonspecific.

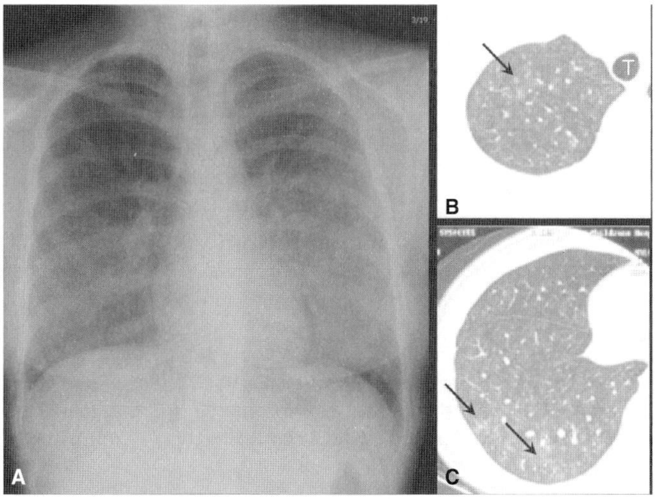

**FIGURE 197-7** Enhanced sensitivity of chest computed tomography (CT) for vasculitis. This patient presented at age 13 with hemoptysis, hematuria, and an extremely elevated erythrocyte sedimentation rate. A plain chest radiograph was normal (**A**), but high-resolution CT scanning showed patchy ground-glass opacities in all lung fields (*arrows* in **B**, mid-left lung). P-ANCA was positive with specific reactivity to myeloperoxidase, and a renal biopsy showed crescentic glomerulonephritis, consistent with the diagnosis of microscopic polyangiitis.

## SUGGESTED READINGS


Arbuckle MR, McClain MT, Rubertone MV, et al. Development of autoantibodies before the clinical onset of systemic lupus erythematosus. *N Engl J Med.* 2003;349:1526.

Chauvin NA, Khwaja A. Imaging of inflammatory arthritis in children: status and perspectives on the use of ultrasound, radiographs, and magnetic resonance imaging. *Rheum Dis Clin North Am.* 2016;42(4):587-606.

Deane PM, Liard G, Siegel DM, Baum J. The outcome of children referred to a pediatric rheumatology clinic with a positive antinuclear antibody test but without an autoimmune disease. *Pediatrics.* 1995;95(6):892-895.

England BR, Thiele GM, Mikuls TR. Anticitrullinated protein antibodies: origin and role in the pathogenesis of rheumatoid arthritis. *Curr Opin Rheumatol.* 2017;29(1):57-64.

Ferucci ED, Majka DS, Parrish LA, et al. Antibodies against cyclic citrullinated peptide are associated with HLA-DR4 in simplex and multiplex polyarticular-onset juvenile rheumatoid arthritis. *Arthritis Rheum.* 2005;52(1):239.

Gabay C, Kushner I. Acute-phase proteins and other systemic responses to inflammation. *N Engl J Med.* 1999;340(6):448.

Jones OY, Spencer CH, Bowyer SL, Dent PB, Gottlieb BS, Rabinovich CE. A multicenter case-control study on predictive factors distinguishing childhood leukemia from juvenile rheumatoid arthritis. *Pediatrics.* 2006;117(5):e840-e844.

McGhee JL, Kickingbird LM, Jarvis JN. Clinical utility of antinuclear antibody tests in children. *BMC Pediatr.* 2004;4:13.

Murray KJ, Moroldo MB, Donnelly P, et al. Age-specific effects of juvenile rheumatoid arthritis-associated HLA alleles. *Arthritis Rheum.* 1999;42(9):1843-1853.

Stone JH, Talor M, Stebbing J, et al. Test characteristics of immunofluorescence and ELISA tests in 856 consecutive patients with possible ANCA-associated conditions. *Arthritis Care Res.* 2000;13(6):424.

Tan EM, Feltkamp TE, Smolen JS, et al. Range of antinuclear antibodies in "healthy" individuals. *Arthritis Rheum.* 1997;40(9):1601-16111.


# 198 Juvenile Idiopathic Arthritis

Marietta M. de Guzman, Carol A. Wallace, David A. Cabral, and Robert P. Sundel

## INTRODUCTION

*Arthritis* is a clinical finding of persistent joint swelling or painful restriction of joint movement. *Arthralgia* is pain in a joint, with or without inflammation. Thus, a patient with arthralgia will not necessarily have arthritis, nor does a patient with arthritis always have arthralgia. There are many causes of arthritis and arthralgia in children, and this section will be limited to the chronic arthritides of childhood that have no known cause.

The heterogeneous nature of childhood arthritis continues to impose challenges as to the most descriptive terminology. At least 3 different classification schemes have been developed: juvenile rheumatoid arthritis (JRA) by the American College of Rheumatology (ACR), juvenile chronic arthritis (JCA) by the European League of Rheumatology (EULAR), and juvenile idiopathic arthritis (JIA) by the International

**TABLE 198-1 COMPARISON OF CLASSIFICATION SYSTEM NOMENCLATURE OF CHRONIC ARTHRITIS IN CHILDREN**

| ACR | EULAR | ILAR |
|---|---|---|
| Juvenile Rheumatoid Arthritis | Juvenile Chronic Arthritis | Juvenile Idiopathic Arthritis |
| • Systemic onset | • Systemic onset | • Systemic arthritis |
| • Polyarticular onset | • Polyarticular onset | • Persistent oligoarthritis |
| • Pauciarticular onset | • Oligoarticular onset | • Extended oligoarthritis |
| | • Juvenile rheumatoid arthritis | • RF-negative polyarthritis |
| | | • RF-positive polyarthritis |
| | • Juvenile psoriatic arthritis | • Psoriatic arthritis |
| | | • Enthesitis-related arthritis |
| | • Juvenile ankylosing spondylitis | • Undifferentiated arthritis |

NOTE. Terminologies apply to children less than age 16 years.

ACR, American College of Rheumatology; EULAR, European League against Rheumatism; ILAR, International League of Associations for Rheumatology; RF, rheumatoid factor.



League of Associations for Rheumatology (ILAR) (Table 198-1). These classifications share some common features: disease onset before age 16 years; minimum period of duration of arthritis (6 weeks for ACR and ILAR and 6 months for EULAR); and use of terms to describe the pattern of disease during the first 6 months from onset, with *oligoarticular* (or pauciarticular) arthritis occurring in 4 or fewer joints and *polyarticular* arthritis occurring in 5 or more joints. *Systemic* in all schemes refers to arthritis in association with characteristic fever and other extra-articular features, including rash, lymphadenopathy, hepatosplenomegaly, or serositis. The presence of rheumatoid factor has also been recognized as a defining feature for subclassification, and in the EULAR system, patients with rheumatoid factor are classified as having JRA, whereas in the ILAR system, these patients are classified as having rheumatoid factor–positive polyarthritis.

A major deficiency of the ACR, EULAR, and current ILAR classification systems is in how they deal with childhood spondyloarthropathies. They are respectively not included, incompletely included, or inadequately described in the context of adult disease. These deficiencies are further discussed in the section on enthesitis-related arthritis and the spondyloarthropathies (see Chapter 199).

The ILAR classification system has gained a great deal of international acceptance to replace the 2 previous parallel systems, and although at times it is complicated to use and is decidedly imperfect, it has been the preferred system for most of the world, giving it a cache lacking in the previous systems. As studies have enrolled patients according to the ILAR criteria, the transition in nomenclature has been made, and it is hoped that the next modification in terminology will be based firmly on genetic and pathogenic data.

Clinicians, however, need to be reminded that there is a wealth of literature on JRA and JCA that cannot be ignored and that must be applied to patients within the new ILAR classifications.

Juvenile arthritis lasting for at least 6 weeks, with onset before age 16, and not the result of infections, neoplasms, orthopedic disorders, other chronic inflammatory or autoimmune conditions, or metabolic inherited and endocrine diseases, will be referred to as *juvenile idiopathic arthritis* (JIA) in this chapter. Details of the definitions and subcategories within this system are shown in Table 198-2.

## EPIDEMIOLOGY

In the United States, the prevalence of JIA is 1 in 1000 and the incidence is 1.4 in 10,000. JIA is subdivided into 7 categories based on the number of joints involved and other identified features present within the first 6 months of disease onset. Consequently, etiologic and prognostic differences among the oligoarticular, polyarticular, and psoriatic categories are not striking. As fundamental genetic and pathogenic information about these disorders increases, the manner in which we describe, categorize, understand, and treat childhood arthritis will likely undergo significant modification, if not dramatic changes.

## PATHOPHYSIOLOGY AND GENETICS

A disease of persistent inflammation of the synovium, JIA has long been considered a manifestation of autoimmunity; however, intense investigation has failed to identify autoantibodies or target antigens. The contribution of human leukocyte antigen (HLA) alleles in persistent oligoarticular JIA (DRB1*1301, 0801) and polyarticular JIA (DPB1*0301) is indeed important, possibly through their effects on T-lymphocyte receptor function. Recent thinking led to the understanding that these heterogeneous categories of JIA as autoinflammatory, rather than autoimmune, diseases. It is postulated that persistence of microbial antigens initiates synovial inflammation through the action of antibodies against microbial antigens that cross-react with self (molecular mimicry). Another line of investigation presents evidence that an infection promotes the presentation of self-HLA peptides to T cells.

Evidence for an infectious initiation of synovial inflammation includes the persistent arthritis seen after a variety of infections, including rubella and parvovirus. The clinical features (abrupt onset, high-spiking fever, rash, hepatosplenomegaly, lymphadenopathy, and serositis) and a clustering of cases in the autumn also suggest infection as an inflammatory trigger. Further, polymerase chain reaction has allowed identification of microbes and their antigens in synovial tissue in some arthritides not previously thought to be due to infection.

The immunologic cascade involved in JIA appears to be initiated by presentation of antigen(s) to T lymphocytes by antigen-presenting cells (macrophages, B cells, dendritic cells, fibroblasts, and endothelial cells). Subsequent activation of T-cells, development of specific subsets of CD4+ lymphocytes (including the recently described Th17 lineage), and production of IL-17 stimulate cell activation and release of cytokines such as TNF-α, IL-1, and IL-6. Cytokines then trigger polyclonal T-cell expansion and production of a variety of additional inflammatory mediators including prostaglandins, complement proteins, kinins, proteases, matrix metalloproteases, and lysosomal enzymes. The result is migration of additional inflammatory cells into the synovial tissue and fluid, increased vascular permeability, and damage to cartilage and bone (see Chapter 195).

The histology of the inflamed synovium in all categories of JIA is identical to that of adult rheumatoid arthritis, with characteristic lymphocytic and plasma cell infiltration, and later villous hypertrophy and hyperplasia of the synovial lining. This process is accompanied by prominent vascular endothelial cell hyperplasia and angiogenesis, resulting in the secretion of large amounts of protein-rich synovial fluid and the migration of neutrophils, lymphocytes, and macrophages into the joint. Synovial-fluid white cell counts usually range from 2000 to 30,000/mL. However, even counts exceeding 100,000/mL may be seen in patients with systemic JIA.

An exuberant inflammatory process leads to aggressive expansion of the synovium onto the articular cartilage, resulting in the so-called *pannus formation*. Lysosomal hydrolyses that break down proteoglycans and collagen facilitate invasion of the avascular cartilage by the pannus. Prolonged synovial inflammation causes irreparable damage to the cartilage, as well as erosion and destruction of subchondral bone. Formation of synovial-lined bony cysts can occur. New investigations have documented migration of activated macrophages into subchondral bone, with activation of osteoclasts, further contributing to chronic erosive changes.

Small areas of bone at the margins of articular cartilage (bare areas) are exposed directly to the inflamed synovium; erosions at these sites provide an early radiographic clue to bony destruction in inflammatory arthritis.

## CLINICAL PRESENTATIONS

The patient's history and physical examination assume critical importance in establishing the diagnosis of JIA. A cardinal feature of inflammatory synovitis is morning stiffness of at least 30 minutes, with improvement over time or following movement and warming of the joint. Parents and other caregivers may observe changes in walking, running, climbing stairs, or eagerness to play. Children may need help

**TABLE 198-2 INTERNATIONAL LEAGUE OF ASSOCIATIONS FOR RHEUMATOLOGY CLASSIFICATION SYSTEM FOR JUVENILE IDIOPATHIC ARTHRITIS (JIA)**

JIA is arthritis of unknown etiology that begins before the 16th birthday and persists for at least 6 weeks; other known conditions including infections, neoplasms, orthopedic disorders, chronic inflammatory or autoimmune conditions, or metabolic inherited and endocrine diseases.

**Systemic Arthritis**

Arthritis in 1 or more joints with or preceded by fever of at least 2 weeks in duration that is documented to be daily ("quotidian") for at least 3 days, and accompanied by 1 or more of the following:

1. Evanescent (nonfixed) erythematous rash
2. Generalized lymph node enlargement
3. Hepatomegaly and/or splenomegaly
4. Serositis

*Exclusions:* a, b, c, d

**Oligoarthritis**

Arthritis affecting 1–4 joints during the first 6 months of disease. Two subcategories are recognized:

1. Persistent oligoarthritis: Affecting not more than 4 joints throughout the disease course
2. Extended oligoarthritis: Affecting a total of more than 4 joints after the first 6 months of disease

*Exclusions:* a, b, c, d, e

**Polyarthritis (Rheumatoid Factor [RF] Negative)**

Arthritis affecting 5 or more joints during the first 6 months of disease; a test for RF is negative.

*Exclusions:* a, b, c, d, e

**Polyarthritis (RF Positive)**

Arthritis affecting 5 or more joints during the first 6 months of disease; 2 or more tests for RF at least 3 months apart during the first 6 months of disease are positive.

*Exclusions:* a, b, c, e

**Psoriatic Arthritis**

Arthritis and psoriasis, or arthritis and at least 2 of the following:

1. Dactylitis
2. Nail pitting or onycholysis
3. Psoriasis in a first-degree relative

*Exclusions:* b, c, d, e

**Enthesitis-Related Arthritis**

Arthritis and enthesitis, or arthritis or enthesitis with at least 2 of the following:

1. The presence of or a history of sacroiliac joint tenderness and/or inflammatory lumbosacral pain
2. The presence of HLA-B27 antigen
3. Onset of arthritis in a male over 6 years of age
4. Acute (symptomatic) anterior uveitis
5. History of ankylosing spondylitis, enthesitis-related arthritis, sacroiliitis with inflammatory bowel disease, Reiter syndrome, or acute anterior uveitis in a first-degree relative

*Exclusions:* a, d, e

**Undifferentiated Arthritis**

Arthritis that fulfills criteria in no category or in 2 or more of the above categories.

**Exclusions:** (a) Psoriasis or a history of psoriasis in the patient or first-degree relative. (b) Arthritis in an HLA-B27–positive male beginning after the 6th birthday. (c) Ankylosing spondylitis, enthesitis-related arthritis, sacroiliitis with inflammatory bowel disease, Reiter syndrome, or acute anterior uveitis, or a history of one of these disorders in a first-degree relative. (d) The presence of IgM rheumatoid factor on at least 2 occasions at least 3 months apart. (e) The presence of systemic JIA in the patient.

**Definitions of Terms:** *Dactylitis:* Swelling of 1 or more digits, usually in an asymmetric distribution, which extends beyond the joint margin. *Enthesitis:* Tenderness at the insertion of a tendon, ligament, joint capsule, or fascia to bone. *Inflammatory lumbosacral pain:* Lumbosacral spinal pain at rest with morning stiffness that improves on movement. *Nail pitting:* A minimum of 2 pits on 1 or more nails at any time. *Positive test for RF:* At least 2 positive results (as routinely defined in an accredited laboratory), at least 3 months apart, during the first 6 months of disease. *Quotidian fever:* Fever that rises to ≥ 39°C once a day and returns to ≤ 37°C between fever peaks. *Serositis:* Pericarditis and/or pleuritis and/or peritonitis. *Sacroiliac joint arthritis:* Presence of tenderness on direct compression over the sacroiliac joints. *Spondyloarthropathy:* Inflammation of entheses and joints of the lumbosacral spine. *Uveitis:* Chronic anterior uveitis as diagnosed by an ophthalmologist.

Data from Petty RE, Southwood TR, Manners P, et al: International League of Associations for Rheumatology classification of juvenile idiopathic arthritis: second revision, Edmonton, 2001, *J Rheumatol.* 2004 Feb;31(2):390-392.



with dressing, eating, bathing, toileting, and other activities that were previously performed independently. Enuresis may recur in a recently toilet-trained child, and developmental milestones may be lost. Children not old enough to describe stiffness or pain may be cranky or irritable in the morning or after a nap or have generally decreased activity.

On physical examination, all joints must be thoroughly assessed for swelling, tenderness, pain, motion, and bony enlargement. Muscles should be examined for strength and possible atrophy. In addition, extra-articular signs of juvenile arthritis, including abnormal pupils, rash, lymphadenopathy, organomegaly, and pericardial and pleural rubs, should be sought. Occasionally, synovitis may be painless, but the diagnosis requires the physical finding of swelling resulting from inflammation. Loss or decreased motion with pain of the affected joints indicates chronicity of the joint inflammation and is indirect evidence of synovitis in those joints where swelling cannot be visualized (ie, spine, hip, and shoulder). Observing how the child walks and runs or moves about in the exam room can be as important as direct examination, which may be difficult in an uncooperative, frightened toddler or infant.

## OLIGOARTICULAR JIA

*Oligoarticular JIA*, defined as arthritis in 4 or fewer joints over the first 6 months of symptoms, occurs in approximately 40% of children with JIA. The ratio of males to females is 1:6.5; the usual age of onset is 1 to 3 years. Typically, the arthritis has an insidious onset and is minimally symptomatic. Many of these children will report no pain and come to medical attention after joint swelling is found incidentally. The knee is most frequently involved, followed by the ankle and then the small joints of the hand or the wrist; almost any joint, however, may be affected. Isolated hip or neck arthritis occurs rarely, although it may also portend evolution into enthesitis-related arthritis, ankylosing spondylitis, or psoriatic arthritis. Involvement of only the temporomandibular joints has been described. Children with oligoarticular JIA are systemically well otherwise.

Asymptomatic uveitis (inflammation of the uveal tract—iris, ciliary body, and choroid) develops in approximately 20% of children with oligoarticular JIA, and 80% of these children will have a positive antinuclear antibody (ANA) test. Prompt diagnosis and treatment of uveitis are critical to prevent later cataracts and glaucoma and potential loss of vision. Consequently, ophthalmologic screening by slit-lamp examination every 3 to 4 months is essential for these high-risk children. Persistent or difficult-to-treat uveitis becomes the most prominent chronic feature in a subset of children with JIA. Less frequent screening is adequate in other forms of arthritis that carry a lower risk of developing uveitis. Guidelines for ophthalmologic screening for children with different JRA subtypes are shown in Table 198-3.

Over time, approximately 80% of children with oligoarthritis will continue to have episodes of arthritis with 4 or fewer joints involved (*persistent oligoarthritis*), whereas 20% will have extension of synovitis into additional joints will be labeled as having *extended oligoarthritis*.

Seventy percent of children with oligoarticular JIA are ANA-positive, usually in low titer (≤ 1:320). Mild elevation of erythrocyte sedimentation rate (ESR) or C-reactive protein (CRP) and mild thrombocytosis with a slight decrease in hemoglobin may be found, but these tests are usually normal, as are other laboratory tests. The rheumatoid factor test is rarely positive, but if it is, it often portends conversion to a polyarticular course. Fever, rash, night pain, weight loss, thrombocytopenia, and leukopenia are not seen in this disease and should prompt further investigations for alternative diagnoses.

## POLYARTICULAR JIA

*Polyarticular JIA*, defined as involvement of at least 5 joints during the first 6 months of illness, is found in approximately 25% of children with JIA. This group is further subclassified into the categories of rheumatoid facto (RF)-negative and RF-positive disease. Those children who are considered to be RF-positive must have this test confirmed with repeat testing at least 3 months from the initial test. Females predominate, with 2 peak ages of onset: 1 to 3 years, and again during early adolescence. Both large and small joints may be affected; presentations vary from scattered joint involvement to symmetric synovitis of nearly all joints in the body. Involvement of the cervical spine, hips, shoulders, and temporomandibular joints (TMJ) is common finding. In most patients, the onset is insidious and accompanied by fatigue. Additionally, some patients have low-grade fever, weight loss, hepatosplenomegaly, lymphadenopathy, pleuritis, pericarditis, and pneumonitis. These patients are more likely to have elevated acute-phase reactants, including ESR, CRP, and platelet counts, and often may have mild anemia of chronic disease. White blood cell counts typically are normal.

The disease of children with a positive RF closely resembles adult rheumatoid arthritis, including occasional development of rheumatoid nodules, vasculitis, and Felty syndrome (splenomegaly and leukopenia). Antibodies to cyclic citrullinated peptide (anti-CCP) are found in many of the same patients, although they may develop earlier than the RF and may be a more sensitive marker of severe disease. Other serologic markers generally are negative; approximately 30% of patients with polyarticular JIA have positive ANA test results. Five percent of patients with polyarticular JIA develop asymptomatic chronic uveitis, but in general, children with more than 5 involved joints are at less risk to do so than are children with oligoarticular disease.

## SYSTEMIC JIA

Approximately 10% of children with JIA have a systemic onset. This subgroup of patients with JIA present with high-spiking daily fevers and arthritis in 1 or more joints and often with other systemic findings. Males and females are affected equally. The age of onset peaks at 5 to 10 years but spans infancy through adulthood. The characteristic finding is daily fever, which, although erratic, usually spikes once or twice a day, rising above 39.3°C (103°F) and then spontaneously falling to or below normal (so-called quotidian fever). The peak of the fever curve is often in the evening and may be accompanied by intense arthralgia and myalgia. When the temperature is normal, the child may feel quite well only to appear ill again when the fever spikes. Often the fever and other systemic features will precede the development of arthritis, so in general, systemic-onset JIA is a diagnosis of exclusion. Such patients must have an extensive or most reasonable evaluation to rule out other sources of fever, especially infections and malignancies.

Patients with systemic JIA may have a wide variety of systemic manifestations. Among them is a macular, evanescent, salmon-colored rash (Fig. 198-1). It typically exhibits discrete borders with or without central clearing and is often best seen during the fever. The rash may be raised, is usually nonpruritic, and is migratory, appearing anywhere, but most commonly over the trunk, thighs, and axillae. It may be induced by mild trauma (Koebner phenomenon). Other common systemic manifestations include pericarditis, myocarditis, pleuritis, lymphadenopathy, hepatosplenomegaly, abdominal pain, fatigue, anorexia, weight loss, and, rarely, asymptomatic iritis. With time, a few or many inflamed joints will appear. They tend to be markedly swollen and more painful than the arthritis of other subgroups. Nighttime pain and awakening are not unusual, but they nonetheless should prompt investigation for underlying malignancy or infection.

The child with typical fever and rash but without arthritis may be treated empirically for probable systemic JIA after other diagnoses are exhaustively excluded. The diagnosis is not firm until synovitis

**TABLE 198-3 GUIDELINES FOR OPHTHALMOLOGIC EXAMINATIONS**

| | Arthritis Onset ≤ Age 6 | | | Arthritis Onset > Age 6 | |
|---|---|---|---|---|---|
| JRA Subtype at Onset | First 4 years after onset, exam every: | Next 3 years after onset, exam every: | After 7 years from onset, exam every: | First 4 years after onset, exam every: | After 4 years from onset, exam every: |
| Pauci-ANA + | 3 mo | 6 mo | 12 mo | 6 mo | 12 mo |
| Pauci-ANA – | 6 mo | 6 mo | 12 mo | 6 mo | 12 mo |
| Poly-ANA + | 3 mo | 6 mo | 12 mo | 6 mo | 12 mo |
| Poly-ANA – | 6 mo | 6 mo | 12 mo | 6 mo | 12 mo |
| Systemic | 12 mo | 12 mo | 12 mo | 12 mo | 12 mo |

ANA, antinuclear antibodies; JRA, juvenile rheumatoid arthritis.

Data from American Academy of Pediatrics Section on Rheumatology and Section on Ophthalmology: Guidelines for ophthalmologic examinations in children with juvenile rheumatoid arthritis, *Pediatrics*. 1993 Aug;92(2):295-296; Cassidy J, Kivlin J, Lindsley C, et al: Ophthalmologic examinations in children with juvenile rheumatoid arthritis, *Pediatrics*. 2006 May;117(5):1843-1845.

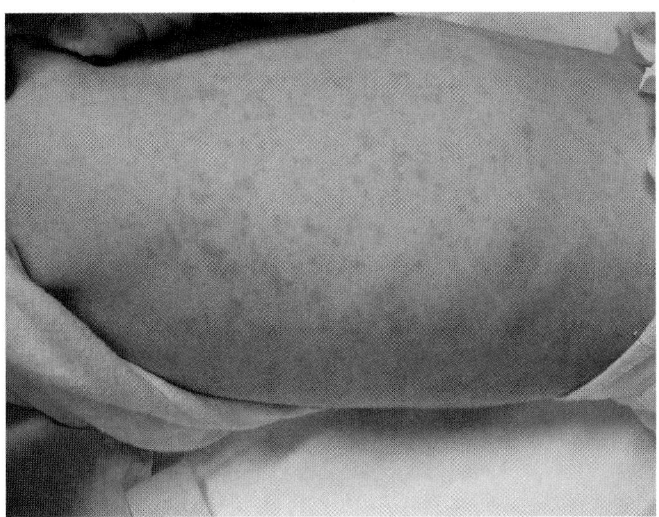

**FIGURE 198-1** Salmon-pink rash in systemic-onset juvenile idiopathic arthritis.

appears and other potential causes of the child's symptoms have been duly considered. Many of these children will require bone marrow aspiration and/or lymph node biopsy to exclude malignant diseases. Laboratory abnormalities of systemic JIA are often dramatic, including significant leukocytosis (> 40,000), thrombocytosis (> 1 million), and elevated inflammatory markers (eg, CRP > 20 mg/dL and ESR > 100 mm/h). Elevated transaminases, anemia, and low serum albumin levels are found frequently, but urinalysis is normal and RF and DNA are rarely positive. During the acute phase of disease, some children become severely ill, with development of leukopenia, thrombocytopenia, profound anemia, and hypofibrinogenemia, and an acute decrease in the sedimentation rate. In addition, D-dimer and ferritin levels may rise dramatically, and prothrombin time and partial thromboplastin time become prolonged, consistent with disseminated intravascular coagulation. This crisis is called *macrophage activation syndrome* (MAS), and it appears to be related to hereditary lymphohistiocytosis. As it progresses, serum transaminases may abruptly increase to greater than 1000 U/L, the bone marrow may exhibit hemophagocytosis, and further sequelae of disseminated intravascular coagulation and cytokine storm may develop. With delayed or inappropriate management, MAS carries a 10% to 20% mortality rate. However, severe sequelae largely may be avoided with prompt recognition and treatment with pulse intravenous (IV) methylprednisone and further immunosuppression (eg, with interleukin blockade with anakinra, or IV cyclosporine).

## DIAGNOSIS OF JIA

### Laboratory Evaluation

As described for each category of JIA, there is no test or combination of tests that can differentiate JIA from other diseases. JIA remains a clinical diagnosis dependent on the finding of unexplained synovitis. The major role of laboratory tests is to exclude other potential diagnoses, particularly infection and/or malignancy, and to stratify patients' risk of developing disease sequelae. In cases of systemic JIA, laboratory tests additionally help define severity of systemic inflammation.

### Imaging in JIA

In general, imaging studies demonstrate joint inflammation, but they do not distinguish JIA from infectious or proliferative conditions. Although conventional radiographs may rule out diseases that mimic JIA, such as leukemia, tumors, or chronic recurrent multifocal osteomyelitis, they have a limited role in the assessment of JIA. The earliest changes are soft tissue swelling and periarticular osteopenia, although this latter finding is only visible on plain radiographs when 50% of the bone mineral content has been lost because of inflammation. The intense inflammation of the tendon sheath, joint, and tendon attachments can stimulate periosteal new bone formation in the tubular bones of the phalanges, metacarpals, and metatarsals, and, occasionally, long bones. A characteristic radiographic finding in children with JIA involving a finger is widening of the mid-portion of a phalange from periosteal new bone formation. Plain radiographs are also useful for monitoring chronic joint changes and effectiveness of treatment, but ultrasound, computed tomography (CT), and magnetic resonance imaging (MRI) evaluations are more sensitive.

In young children, joint space widening can initially be seen because of increased intra-articular fluid or synovial hypertrophy. The hypervascularity of involved joints may stimulate adjacent growth plates and result in bony enlargement (eg, knee or ankle) or epiphyseal advancement or closure (often seen in the wrist or hip).

Bone scans may be normal or reveal increased uptake on both sides of an affected joint during the flow phase, indicative of increased synovial vascularity. Increased uptake on just one side of a joint would suggest another diagnosis. Ultrasonography can identify synovial expansion, increased synovial fluid, and bony erosions. Ultrasound provides an inexpensive, easily available imaging technique that can assist clinicians in demonstrating subclinical synovitis and enthesitis as an adjunct to clinical examination and assessment, especially on the hips, shoulders, wrists, and ankles. MRI with IV gadolinium contrast provides the most complete imaging analysis, can assess the extent of synovitis and bone marrow edema, and can reliably show early erosive changes. CT is most useful for identifying bony abnormalities and erosions.

Joint space narrowing on plain radiographs and CT scanning is detectable only after a significant amount of cartilage has been destroyed. This detection typically takes longer in children than in adults because of the relative thickness of cartilage during growth and may first become manifest in the TMJ. The TMJ is at particular risk for destruction because the epiphysis is as immediately adjacent to a thin fibrocartilage, which is not as robust as is true articular cartilage. When the epiphysis is destroyed, micrognathia due to lack of mandibular growth becomes evident. Coronal CT of the TMJ currently provides the best images for evaluation of joint damage in the TMJ, whereas MRI with IV gadolinium can detect active synovitis.

As arthritis progresses, further erosions become evident radiographically when inflamed synovium and activated osteoclasts and macrophages destroy cartilage and bone. Cysts can be formed when the inflamed synovium invades subchondral bone. In late stages, these cysts may collapse, leading to marked joint irregularity. Fibrous ankylosis and bony fusion can occur and are not uncommon in JIA, particularly in the wrist, cervical spine, and tarsal areas. Erosion of the odontoid process can lead to subluxation of C1 on C2. Children with JIA involving the neck should be followed with flexion and extension lateral radiographs of the cervical spine to assess the stability of C1 and C2 movement. Repeat films should be obtained before general anesthesia and if children are involved in gymnastics and contact sports.

Of note, the gap in knowledge regarding the spectrum of normal appearance in healthy growing musculoskeletal system provides challenges in the interpretation of all the imaging modalities used in JIA. Thus, a continued research for more information and a validated scoring system are needed.

## DIFFERENTIAL DIAGNOSIS

The importance of a thorough and diligent evaluation to exclude other processes such as infection and malignancy must be emphasized. The diagnoses of oligoarticular, polyarticular, or systemic JIA require swollen joints or evidence of synovitis (see Table 198-1). A well child with joint pain but no swelling may have an orthopedic condition (avascular necrosis, slipped femoral epiphysis, benign joint tumor, Osgood-Schlatter disease), so-called growing pains (benign nocturnal limb pains of childhood), hypermobility, or a pain syndrome. An ill child may have infection (of joints, bone, or generalized), postinfectious arthritis, a metastatic tumor, leukemia, lymphoma, or multifocal osteomyelitis or other rheumatologic disorders. Thus, a thorough workup is mandatory, more so in a child presenting with systemic disease.

## TREATMENT

Early diagnosis of JIA is the cornerstone of most effective therapy. Goals of treatment are to minimize or resolve symptoms, prevent joint destruction, maintain normal growth and development, and achieve inactive disease. *Inactive disease* is defined as no joints with active arthritis; no systemic features such as fever, rash, serositis, splenomegaly, or generalized lymphadenopathy attributable to JIA; no uveitis; normalization of inflammatory markers such as ESR or CRP; and normal physician's global evaluation. The pillars of treatment are patient/family education, early aggressive medical management, and physical and occupational therapy.

### Education

Educating the patient and family is a critical component of treatment, with children and their caregivers included as active partners in the treatment plan. Knowledge about the disease, understanding of the goals of treatment, and realistic expectations regarding the medications used are necessary to promote adherence to therapeutic regimens. Patients and families must be provided with careful, detailed explanations about joint functioning, the effects of untreated inflammation on growing joints, the need for early aggressive therapy, the goals of therapy, and potential adverse effects of treatments. These topics need to be reviewed repeatedly during the treatment course to make sure that the family's goals remain congruent with those of the caregiving team. The emotional impact of this chronic, often painful, and disabling disease on the child, siblings, and parents should not be underestimated. The unpredictable course of JIA, including the potential for exacerbations of disease after a long period of remission, is particularly stressful for most patients and families. Most children and parents do not need long-term counseling, but many benefit from short-term family or individual treatment.

The Arthritis Foundation is an excellent source for additional information and peer support. Other online educational resources are provided by the American College of Rheumatology.

### Medications

Timely use and correct choice of currently available medications to achieve sustained remission with as few side or adverse effects as possible remain the most challenging issues in the treatment of JIA.

Our current understanding of how quickly synovitis can cause joint destruction and the traditionally poor long-term outcome of JIA have led to earlier and more aggressive treatments over the past decade and a half. In 2011, the ACR provided a treatment guideline for oligoarticular, polyarticular, and systemic JIA, and in 2013, modification was further done for systemic-onset JIA.

Nonsteroidal anti-inflammatory drugs (NSAIDs) are no longer the mainstay of treatment for arthritis, but they continue to be useful in the initial treatment for reduction of pain and as mild anti-inflammatory agents. Intra-articular injections of triamcinolone acetonide or triamcinolone hexacetonide, in place of or in addition to systemic therapies, can be particularly effective in quickly suppressing inflammation in a limited number of joints. Depending on the age of the child and the number and location of joints to be injected, brief general anesthesia may be necessary for the injections. Repeat injections (up to 3 per joint) can be an important treatment strategy. The administration (orally or intravenously) of systemic corticosteroids is mainly restricted to the management of the extra-articular features of systemic JIA (eg, fever, anemia, pericarditis). A short course of low-dose prednisone may be considered for severe polyarthritis refractory to other therapies or while awaiting the effect of the recently initiated second-line or biologic therapy. Adult data indicate that this treatment strategy may persistently decrease the likelihood of joint damage when begun early in the course of the disease. Although there is concern for potential side effects from the use of corticosteroids, the benefits of better disease control and improved physical activity may be tremendous. Weight gain is temporary, and many patients on 0.15 mg/kg/d or less grow normally and have normal bone density studies.

Methotrexate remains the most widely used initial disease-modifying therapy in JIA because of its efficacy at achieving disease control and acceptable adverse effects. Methotrexate can be given either orally or as a subcutaneous injection, with the latter having greater bioavailability at higher doses. For patients with polyarthritis or persistent or extended oligoarthritis, methotrexate should be started as early as possible. Folic or folinic acid supplementation may help prevent some of the adverse effects of methotrexate, in particular oral sores and ulcerations, nausea, and hematologic and liver enzyme abnormalities. Leflunomide may have efficacy and safety similar to those of methotrexate and is a reasonable alternative in a child with intolerance to methotrexate.

During the past decade and a half, there has been quite a remarkable evolution in biologic therapy for adult and childhood arthritis. More focused anticytokine agents have been introduced and, to date, have been shown to be effective in better controlling arthritis and preventing joint damage, especially when administered earlier in the disease process. Etanercept was the first anti–tumor necrosis factor (TNF) therapy that was approved in the treatment of JIA; others with similar pharmacologic activity include infliximab, adalimumab, and golimumab. Co-stimulatory blocking agents (abatacept) provided another therapeutic option for those without good control with an anti-TNF agent. Anti-IL-1 (anakinra, rilonacept, canakinumab) and anti-IL-6 (tocilizumab) agents have shown efficacy and tolerability for the treatment of systemic JIA. In 2011, the (ACR) published recommendation for the treatment and safety monitoring for JIA. The first update on these recommendations was provided in 2013 addressing treatment for systemic JIA. The ACR emphasized, however, that these recommendations are for the "purpose of providing guidelines for particular patterns of practice and not to dictate care for a particular patient."

All of the medications mentioned here (including NSAIDs) have potential side effects and require ongoing laboratory monitoring. Cytopenias and liver function abnormalities are seen most commonly. For patients on methotrexate, complete blood count (CBC), aspartate aminotransferase (AST), blood urea nitrogen (BUN), and creatinine are recommended after 1 month of treatment and then every 2 to 4 months. For NSAID use, the same monitoring (with a urinalysis) should be done 1 month after starting the medication and then every 4 months thereafter. Similar monitoring is recommended for most biologic agents. Tuberculosis screening should be done prior to initiation of any biologic treatment, and repeat surveillance should be performed annually while on anti-TNF agents.

Clinical follow-up of children with active JIA should occur every 1 to 3 months to allow for thorough evaluations and medication adjustments, with the goal of achieving disease remission. Meticulous surveillance for medication-related adverse effects is of prime importance, especially with the use of biologic agents. After inactive disease is achieved, medications are kept stable for 6 months to several years before they are gradually tapered and discontinued. Evolving management strategies may be similar to cancer protocols, with induction regimens using many medications together early in the disease course followed by milder maintenance regimens aimed at maintaining remission.

### Physical Therapy

Physical and occupational therapies are important components of the care and treatment of children with JIA. Goals include improving range of motion, strength, and function and preventing further deterioration. Because loss of age-appropriate developmental skills can occur, functional skills should be monitored by a therapist experienced in working with children with arthritis. Frequency of therapy visits varies considerably, but all therapy is based on a daily home program done by the child and parent. With severe ongoing disease, long-term cooperation with physical and occupational therapy can be difficult but is enhanced if the therapist tailors the home program to take into account age, extent and severity of disease, school activities, sports, hobbies, and family dynamics. An active lifestyle is important for maintaining bone and joint health; low-impact exercises such as swimming are preferable when disease is active.

Nighttime splinting of the wrist, hand, knee, elbow, or ankle may decrease morning stiffness and help to prevent flexion contractures during active disease. Loss of extension can often be improved after corticosteroid injection followed by serial casting of a knee, ankle, wrist, finger, or elbow. Ice, heat, ultrasound, or a combination of these modalities may help restore motion and decrease pain caused by muscle spasm. When a difference in leg-length is present, a shoe lift for the shorter limb will help to prevent contralateral knee or hip flexion contractures. Children with arthritis of the tarsal and metatarsal joints may ambulate more easily with shoe splints (soft orthotics).

School can present a particular challenge for children with arthritis. Morning stiffness may render a timely arrival difficult, and stiffness from prolonged sitting may render moving between classes problematic. Daytime stiffness can be ameliorated by allowing the child to get up and move about the classroom, and some children may need extra time to pass from class to class. Upper-extremity involvement may render writing, drawing, working on the blackboard, and participating in class difficult. An extra set of books at home greatly lessens the load that needs to be carried to and from home. Physical education and sports can be a challenge when arthritis is active; most children do well when allowed to participate as much as they are able. Exercise and nonimpact sports will not damage joints or worsen arthritis if bony destruction is not present. Rarely, a child may need a shortened school day, but home tutoring is almost never indicated.

In the United States, Public Law 94-142 (the Education for All Handicapped Children Act of 1975) mandates that public schools provide transportation to and from school and therapy for those individuals with disabilities that affect their education. This law applies to many children with JIA who have limitations of range, strength, and coordination that alter their functioning at school. Physical and occupational therapists are available in the school to treat severely involved children whose disease precludes them from meeting their educational goals in a timely fashion. All therapists, whether at home, in school, or at a hospital, can be the most helpful when they work in conjunction with the other members of the patient's rheumatology team.

## OUTCOME

The outcome of juvenile rheumatoid arthritis is variable for all categories. Some patients may experience a single episode of disease lasting 6 to 12 months, whereas others are afflicted with continuous chronic inflammation, progressive joint destruction, and chronic disability. Outcomes can be measured by functional ability, persistence of synovitis, or radiographic findings. Most long-term outcome studies report cross-sectional information on patients at defined time points in the disease course rather than characterizing the longitudinal course of patients. One investigation described the entire course of each of 437 patients followed 4 to 22 years with respect to time spent with active or inactive disease and time on or off medications. This investigation revealed that although the majority of patients with oligoarticular JIA spent nearly 60% of their disease course with inactive disease, 64% of patients with RF-negative polyarticular JIA and 84% of children with RF-positive polyarticular JIA spent 60% or more of the time with active disease. Although, overall, 44% of patients achieved clinical remission off medications, only 18% remained in that state for more than 2 years and only 4% for 5 years. Thus, many patients begin their adult life with ongoing joint inflammation, and they remain at risk for all of the potential complications that it can cause.

Radiographic changes are yet another measure of the severity and outcome of arthritis. All patients with JIA are at risk for experiencing joint damage; it is common and can occur early in disease. Twenty-eight percent of patients with pauciarticular-onset develop radiologic evidence of joint damage at a median time of 5 years, whereas half of those with polyarticular and systemic-onset JIA develop joint damage within 2 years of onset of disease.

Despite these challenges, mortality from JIA in North America is rare and largely confined to children with systemic-onset disease. It is calculated at 0.29% of all patients with JIA; although a low number, this rate greatly exceeds overall mortality rates for American children.

## SUGGESTED READINGS


Beukelman T, Patkar NM, Saag KG, et al. American College of Rheumatology recommendations for the treatment of juvenile idiopathic arthritis: initiation and safety monitoring of therapeutic agents for the treatment of arthritis and systemic features. *Arthritis Care Res (Hoboken)*. 2011;63:465-482.

Chauvin NA, Khwaja A. Imaging of inflammatory arthritis in children: Status and perspective on the use of ultrasound, radiograph and magnetic resonance imaging. *Rheum Dis Clin N Am*. 2016;42:587-606.

Grom AA, Horne AC, De Benetti F. Macrophage activation syndrome in the era of biologic therapy. *Nat Rev Rheumatol*. 2016;12:259-268.

Lovell DJ, Giannini EH, Reiff A, et al. Etanercept in children with polyarticular juvenile rheumatoid arthritis. *N Engl J Med*. 2000;342:763-769.

Petty RE, Southwood TR, Manners P, et al. International League of Associations for Rheumatology classification of juvenile idiopathic arthritis: second revision, Edmonton, 2001. *J Rheumatol*. 2004;31: 390-392.

Padeh S, Passwell JH. Intra-articular corticosteroid injection in the management of children with chronic arthritis. *Arthritis Rheumatol*. 1998;41:1210-1214.

Ringold S, Weiss PF, Beukelman T, et al. 2013 update of the 2011 American College of Rheumatology recommendations for the treatment of juvenile idiopathic arthritis: recommendations for the medical therapy of children with systemic juvenile idiopathic arthritis and tuberculosis screening among children receiving biologic agents. *Arthritis Rheum*. 2013;65:2499-2512.

Wallace CA. Use of methotrexate in childhood rheumatic diseases. *Arthritis Rheumatol*. 1998;41:381-391.

Wallace CA, Giannini EH, Spalding SJ, et al. Clinically inactive disease in a cohort of children with new-onset polyarticular juvenile idiopathic arthritis treated with early aggressive therapy: time to achievement, total duration, and predictors. *J Rheumatol*. 2014;41:1163-1170.

Wallace CA, Huang B, Bandeira M, Ravelli A, Giannini EH. Patterns of clinical remission in select categories of juvenile idiopathic arthritis. *Arthritis Rheum*. 2005;2:3354-3562.


# 199 Spondyloarthropathies

David A. Cabral and Lori B. Tucker

## INTRODUCTION

The word *spondyloarthropathy* (referring to arthritis of the spine and sacroiliac joints) evolved in the adult population to distinguish a group of chronic arthritides that differ from rheumatoid arthritis. These conditions are distinct in that they involve axial joints, are associated with the HLA-B27 haplotype, have a frequent family history of these diseases, and are rheumatoid factor-negative. Traditionally, the specifically named spondyloarthropathies included ankylosing spondylitis, psoriatic arthritis, the arthropathy of inflammatory bowel disease (IBD), and reactive arthritis (previously referred to as Reiter disease).

This characterization has not been entirely satisfactory because many patients do not comfortably fit into 1 of these explicitly defined categories. The efficacy of current pharmacotherapy for ankylosing spondylitis has driven the development of clinical algorithms (judiciously using magnetic resonance imaging [MRI]) to identify early disease with a view to initiating appropriate therapy before the development of irreversible damage.

A major deficiency of the earlier classification systems for pediatric chronic arthritis was the failure to adequately distinguish children with arthritis who have, or who might ultimately develop, a

**TABLE 199-1 COMPARISON OF PSORIATIC ARTHRITIS, OLIGOARTHRITIS, ENTHESITIS-RELATED ARTHRITIS, AND JUVENILE ANKYLOSING ARTHRITIS**

| | Enthesitis-Related Arthritis | Juvenile Ankylosing Spondylitis | Psoriatic Arthritis | Oligoarthritis |
|---|---|---|---|---|
| **Mean onset age (years)** | 10–13 | > 10 | 6 | 3 |
| **Male-to-female ratio** | 4:1 | 7:1 | 1:2 | 1:4 |
| **Family history** | Frequent for HLA-B27–associated disease | Frequent for HLA-B27–associated disease | Frequent for psoriasis | Rare |
| **Enthesitis** | Common | Very common | Unknown | Very uncommon |
| **Uveitis** | Symptomatic | Symptomatic | Asymptomatic | Asymptomatic |
| **ANA positive** | < 10% | < 10% | 50% | 80% |
| **HLA-B27 positive** | 75% | 90% | 15% | 10% |

ANA, antinuclear antibody.



spondyloarthropathy, from those with juvenile rheumatoid arthritis. Although the European League Against Rheumatism (EULAR) classification included juvenile ankylosing spondylitis (JAS) and juvenile psoriatic arthritis, these conditions were defined according to adult criteria that require the presence of radiologically identified sacroiliitis or psoriasis, respectively. Children who ultimately develop AS, however, will generally not present with back pain or sacroiliitis (the primary requisites for diagnosing AS in adults). Rather, they typically have peripheral arthritis and a constellation of other features including enthesitis, onset in late childhood, a family history of AS or related diseases, and presence of HLA-B27 antigen. To address these deficiencies, such patients have been variously described as having the syndrome of seronegative enthesopathy and arthropathy (SEA syndrome), pauciarticular-onset juvenile rheumatoid arthritis (JRA) type II, late-onset pauciarticular juvenile chronic arthritis (LOPA), and HLA-B27–associated arthropathy and enthesopathy syndrome. Patients with these various syndromes could also be characterized as having "early" or "undifferentiated" spondyloarthropathy.

The current nomenclature for classification of pediatric chronic arthritis according to the International League of Associations for Rheumatology (ILAR) has encapsulated all of these syndromes in the juvenile idiopathic arthritis (JIA) subcategory of enthesitis-related arthritis (ERA) (see Chapter 198). *Enthesitis,* the most common defining clinical feature of these syndromes, refers to inflammation (pain, tenderness, and swelling) of the enthesis, the site of attachment of tendon, ligament, or fascia to bone. Thus, children with JAS also fulfill criteria for ERA. As will be discussed under the section "Juvenile Psoriatic Arthritis," children with arthritis and either psoriasis or psoriatic features probably do not represent a homogeneous subset of children with childhood arthritis despite their current classification within spondyloarthropathies (Table 199-1). Children with IBD associated arthritis or reactive arthritis may or may not develop axial arthritis, and these conditions will also be discussed below.

## ENTHESITIS-RELATED ARTHRITIS

ERA should be distinguished from other forms of chronic childhood arthritis for etiologic, genetic, prognostic, and therapeutic reasons. ERA by ILAR criteria is a subcategory of JIA and is defined as arthritis *plus* enthesitis of greater than 6 weeks in duration in a child younger than 16 years, or arthritis *or* enthesitis *plus* at least 2 of the following: sacroiliac tenderness or inflammatory lumbosacral pain, presence of HLA-B27, onset of arthritis in a boy older than 6 years, acute anterior uveitis associated with pain, redness or photophobia, and a family history of HLA- B27–associated disease (AS, ERA, sacroiliitis with IBD, reactive arthritis, acute anterior uveitis) in a first-degree relative (see Table 199-1). In addition to these disease-defining features, peripheral arthritis that tends to asymmetrically involve the lower limbs is also more typical of ERA than other categories of JIA. The prevalence of ERA is likely to be approximately 20 per 100,000 children, which is approximately half as common as is oligoarthritis and 3 to 4 times as common as is psoriatic arthritis. These numbers may vary considerably in different communities depending on factors such as the prevalence of HLA-B27.

### ETIOLOGY

As with other forms of JIA, the cause of ERA is unknown; however, the strong familial tendency and the high frequency of HLA-B27 may suggest a genetic predisposition. The similarity of ERA to *reactive arthritis* in epidemiology and gut histology additionally implicates bacterial antigens in the process. There may also be hormonal influences on the expression of the disease.

### CLINICAL PRESENTATIONS

Although often insidious and episodic, the onset of ERA also may be acute and may resemble septic arthritis when presenting as a monoarthritic process (see also "Reactive Arthritis" below). Children with ERA usually present with morning pain and stiffness, predominantly in joints of the lower extremities but often in the low back and buttocks, that are relieved by activity. They may also complain of pain at the entheses, commonly around their heels, feet, and knees. Pain felt in the buttocks when sitting on hard surfaces may represent enthesitis over the ischial tuberosities. Examination may reveal evidence of oligoarthritis asymmetrically involving the knees or ankles, and sometimes the hips or small joints of the feet. (Hip joint involvement at disease onset is uncommon in other types of JIA.) Early involvement of the midfoot (tarsitis, enthesitis, and tenosynovitis) with pain, tenderness, and swelling is less common but, if present, is very characteristic of ERA. Exquisite tenderness may be elicited by palpation of the entheses, particularly at the calcaneal insertions of the Achilles tendon and the plantar fascia; beneath the metatarsal heads and the base of the fifth metatarsal; the tibial tuberosities; the 2, 6, and 10 o'clock positions of the patella; over the greater trochanters of the hips, across the iliac crests; and in the ischial tuberosities (Fig. 199-1). Pelvic compression and distraction or direct palpation may elicit sacroiliac joint pain.

Axial involvement should be determined by history and by examining the back for range of movement and flattening of the lower back on forward flexion. Costovertebral motion can be monitored by serial measurements of maximum chest expansion. Cervical disease is not common at presentation and usually develops after lumbar involvement; however, atlantoaxial instability has been reported in early disease.

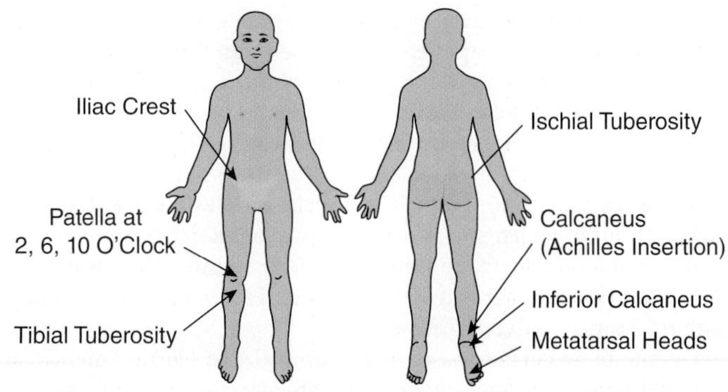


**FIGURE 199-1** Common sites of enthesitis in children with enthesis-related arthritis.

High fever with constitutional symptoms of anorexia, fever, and weight loss may occur in 5% to 10% of children with ERA; however, these findings should also alert the physician to the possibility of IBD, particularly if there is growth delay. Subclinical ileocolonoscopic evidence of gut inflammation is reported to occur in as many as 80% of patients and may be predictive of development of AS; it also may have etiologic significance. Acute symptomatic uveitis, commonly unilateral, may occur in 5% to 10% of children with ERA. Aortic valve insufficiency is a rare complication. Restrictive lung disease, which has been reported in adults with spondyloarthropathy, probably does not occur in children.

## DIAGNOSIS

The diagnosis of chronic arthritis and enthesitis is based on clinical findings and history. Pain and tenderness at the entheses can also be caused by mechanical factors related to physical activities, flat feet, or poor posture. Osteochondroses of the tibial tuberosity (Osgood-Schlatter disease), inferior pole of the patella (Sinding-Larsen-Johansson syndrome), or calcaneal apophysis (Sever disease) should also be differentiated from enthesitis. Tenderness also may be elicited at these sites (in addition to other soft tissue sites) in patients with pain amplification. In the absence of arthritis, care should be taken in making a diagnosis of ERA simply on the basis of mild tenderness at fewer than 3 entheses. Laboratory investigations are not diagnostic. Patients may have nonspecific inflammatory changes with a normocytic normochromic anemia, mild leukocytosis, thrombocytosis, and a high erythrocyte sedimentation rate (ESR); however, many patients may have normal inflammatory markers even in the face of active arthritis and enthesitis on examination. Immunoglobulins, and specifically immunoglobulin A, may be elevated. HLA-B27 is frequently present and with other criteria may help with classification.

## IMAGING

Peripheral joint-space narrowing, erosions, and radiographically evident sacroiliitis are often a late findings in children with ERA. Radiographically evident joint damage is a poor prognostic feature used in the new American College of Rheumatology (ACR) Treatment Recommendations for JIA to guide the choice of therapeutic agents. Contrast-enhanced magnetic resonance imaging (MRI) is more effective than are conventional radiographs at early detection and monitoring of disease activity in peripheral and axial joints and entheses in patients with ERA through demonstration of synovitis, joint fluid, bone marrow edema, and peri-entheseal soft tissue swelling and edema. Whole-body MRI is used by some clinicians to detect the extent of active disease and provide a method for monitoring therapeutic response. Ultrasonography with power Doppler can be highly effective at distinguishing inflammatory enthesitis from other types of entheseal conditions, but equipment and specific expertise may not be universally available.

## TREATMENT

As for all forms of JIA, the child with spondyloarthritis is best served by treatment in a multidisciplinary setting by professionals specifically trained in the treatment of childhood rheumatic diseases, including pediatric rheumatologists, nurses, and pediatric physiotherapists and occupational therapists.

The first line of pharmacotherapy for all children with ERA is regular doses of nonsteroidal anti-inflammatory drugs (NSAIDs) such as naproxen, ibuprofen, or indomethacin. Optimal effect from these medications requires at least a month of continuing treatment. While such continuous use of NSAIDs, as distinct from sporadic "symptomatic" use, is the standard of care for peripheral arthritis, evidence in adults with AS suggests that continuous use also reduces the rate of radiologic progression of axial disease. Intra-articular injection of triamcinolone hexacetonide (1 mg/kg per joint) is valuable if there are a few peripheral joints that are responding poorly to NSAID therapy.

The pain of enthesitis is often difficult to treat; local injection of corticosteroids generally is unsuccessful, and patients often require use of low-dose oral prednisone. For patients with moderate disease activity, when NSAID therapy provides inadequate disease control, sulfasalazine and methotrexate are safe and effective second-line therapies. Patients taking these medications require regular monitoring of blood count and hepatic transaminases. Although these 2 medications have been shown not to be effective in the treatment of axial disease in adult AS, it is not known whether early aggressive use of these medications in juvenile spondyloarthropathy prevents or delays progression of axial arthritis. Anti–tumor necrosis factor (TNF) therapy has been shown to be effective in the treatment of peripheral arthritis and axial arthritis and is the treatment choice for patients with peripheral arthritis who fail standard therapy with sulfasalazine or methotrexate. It may be that early use of anti-TNF therapy should be initiated once axial involvement becomes apparent.

In 2011, treatment guidelines for JIA were published by a pediatric rheumatology consensus group of the ACR. Recommended treatment pathways were determined by disease activity (assessed by a combination of raised inflammatory markers and physician/parent-rated disease activity) and presence of poor prognostic factors (presence of radiographic damage). Thus, children with spondyloarthropathy who have high disease activity and poor prognostic features should be treated with a TNF inhibitor if there is lack of adequate response to a 1- to 2-month trial of NSAIDs.

Treatment of mechanical factors affecting symptoms is also important. Many children with ERA benefit from custom-made hard orthotics to redistribute the weight from sites of painful enthesitis; heel cups in the shoes can alleviate stress in the retrocalcaneal area and the knee. Physiotherapy is an important component of treatment for all children with ERA. Treatment should be aimed at promoting general physical fitness, maintaining a healthy body weight, and restoring muscle strength and range of movement of affected joints and surrounding structures. Special attention should be paid to preserving range of movement of the back and chest.

## PROGNOSIS

Disease course is highly variable. Some patients have a short duration of illness, with oligoarthritis and/or enthesitis that resolves completely within 3 to 6 months. This pattern resembles *reactive arthritis,* although an inciting pathogen with preceding gastrointestinal or genitourinary symptoms may not be identifiable. More common, however, is a course with episodic flares that lasts for years. A recent Canadian cohort study demonstrated a 40% risk of a significant disease flare within 2 years of achieving a period of inactive disease for children with ERA. Within approximately 10 years, a majority of patients with a more chronic course have a high likelihood of developing symptomatic and radiologically confirmed sacroiliitis with spondylitis and of fulfilling classic criteria for AS. They may have an intermittent or slowly progressive course with loss of lumbosacral flexion and decreasing chest expansion. In the most severe cases, involvement progresses to a symmetric erosive and ankylosing polyarthritis by the time they reach adulthood, predominantly in the lower limbs, together with ankylosing disease of the back and sacroiliac joints and restrictive lung disease. A study of the long-term outcomes (median 15-year follow-up) of a group of children with ERA from Norway showed that these children had poorer physical functioning and health and more pain than a control group of patients who had oligoarticular or polyarticular JIA. Sacroiliitis developed in 35% of the patients with ERA, and predictors of poor outcome included a family history of AS, early hip or ankle disease, and a high number of affected joints during the first 6 months of having the disease.

# JUVENILE ANKYLOSING SPONDYLITIS

Although juvenile ankylosing spondylitis (JAS) is the archetypal spondyloarthropathy in children, it is relatively rare, occurring in fewer than one-third of children who present with spondyloarthropathy. Several criteria have evolved to define AS in adults and include the Rome Criteria (1963), New York Criteria (1968), and the more recent Modified New York Criteria. In general, AS is distinguished by the presence of persistent low back pain, limitation of motion of the lumbar spine and decreased chest expansion, and sacroiliitis. Although these criteria have been used in children to classify JAS, they are inherently difficult to apply. Presumably because the disease process affects a developing musculoskeletal system differently, disease manifestations in childhood AS differ from those in adult-onset AS. Thus, in children, back symptoms are uncommon manifestations. Approximately 10% of children with AS present with spinal or sacroiliac disease, compared with 80% of adults. Direct comparison of juvenile and adult-onset disease is further hampered by the limited data for normal lumbar spine motion and chest expansion in pediatric patients and difficulty standardizing and interpreting radiographs of growing sacroiliac joints. Conversely, 90% of children with AS have peripheral arthritis, compared with approximately 37% of adults. There is a particularly high frequency of tarsitis (78%) and enthesitis (64%), rates that are 2 to 3 times higher than in adults. In follow-up, the cumulative frequencies of peripheral arthritis, tarsitis, and enthesitis in pediatric-onset patients are approximately double those of patients with adult-onset disease.

Children with back pain are often referred to the pediatric rheumatology clinic with a presumptive diagnosis of arthritis or AS. Although children with chronic synovitis may develop inflammatory back pain, generally it would be an uncommon finding at disease presentation. The differential diagnosis of back pain in a child must include consideration of orthopedic, traumatic, infectious, and malignant disorders, many of which are more likely causes of back pain than is arthritis in children. For example, preschool-age children virtually never develop back arthritis, and malignancy (eg, neuroblastoma), discitis, or bone infections should be the primary considerations. In older children, problems such as Scheuermann disease, spondylolisthesis, scoliosis, or trauma must be considered. If night pain, fever, or other constitutional symptoms are present, infection or malignancy must be considered (see Chapter 229). The presence of HLA-B27 is not diagnostic for ankylosing spondylitis, as it is present in 2% to 10% of the general population (higher in frequency in Native American and Scandinavian communities), of whom 80% to 90% never develop arthritis. As with all forms of juvenile arthritis, the diagnosis of AS requires supportive clinical evidence of inflammatory joint disease.

Once a diagnosis of AS has been made, treatment strategies should be undertaken as outlined under the section "Enthesitis-Related Arthritis," above. Because the outcomes of children and youth with JAS who receive conventional therapy with NSAIDs and methotrexate are likely to be poor, an aggressive approach to treatment, including early consideration of TNF inhibitors, is warranted.

## ARTHRITIS OF INFLAMMATORY BOWEL DISEASE

Inflammatory arthritis occurs in 7% to 20% of patients with IBD, either Crohn disease or ulcerative colitis. Arthralgia is fairly common, likely occurring in 30% of children and adolescents with IBD (see Chapter 405). Musculoskeletal pain in children with IBD may arise from causes other than inflammatory arthritis, including nonspecific myalgia and mechanical and orthopedic issues such as pes planus, deconditioning secondary to illness, glucocorticoid-induced osteopenia, or hypertrophic osteoarthropathy. Joint disease may occur at the onset of IBD, and on occasion, it may precede the diagnosis of IBD by months to years. For all children with arthritis, systemic complaints such as prominent fatigue, weight loss, unexplained growth failure (height more delayed than weight), and fevers should suggest the diagnosis of IBD. In addition, gastrointestinal complaints, including oral ulcers; abdominal pain or tenderness; diarrhea or hematochezia; and extraintestinal manifestations such as erythema nodosum, pyoderma gangrenosum, or clubbing, suggest underlying intestinal inflammation. Suspicion is heightened by a family history of IBD and by evidence of chronic inflammation on laboratory studies (marked anemia, hypoalbuminemia, markedly elevated ESR). Definitive confirmation of a diagnosis of IBD requires gastrointestinal endoscopy and biopsy with histologic evidence of colitis or enteritis. More recently, measurement of serum and/or fecal calprotectin is being used as a less invasive test for making a diagnosis of IBD.

In patients with IBD, peripheral arthritis (usually involving the large weight-bearing joints) is twice as common as is axial arthritis, occurs more frequently in girls, is not associated with HLA-B27, and usually occurs in association with flares of gut inflammation. Active arthritis associated with active gut disease may be relatively transient and generally will resolve as the gut inflammation is treated and resolves. Patients with IBD are also at increased risk of developing axial joint involvement, although initially a peripheral arthritis and/or enthesitis consistent with ERA is most characteristic. These patients are predominantly males with HLA-B27. When such patients ultimately develop axial joint inflammation, its course resembles that of JAS, typically persistent and independent of bowel inflammation.

Peripheral arthritis in association with a flare of bowel inflammation often responds to aggressive treatment of the enterocolitis with corticosteroids, sulfasalazine, or other second-line agents. NSAIDs are generally beneficial, but there is some concern that they may exacerbate the bowel disease. Otherwise, treatment of the arthritis does not differ significantly from that of ERA: Intra-articular glucocorticoid injections may be indicated for persistent joint disease, and anti-TNF agents (notably infliximab and adalimumab) are effective for treating both the IBD and the peripheral and axial arthritis.

## REACTIVE ARTHRITIS

In the context of the "spondyloarthropathies," reactive arthritis describes a disease occurring 1 to 4 weeks following gastrointestinal (commonly *Yersinia enterocolitica, Yersinia tuberculosis, Shigella flexneri, Salmonella typhimurium, Campylobacter jejuni*) or genitourinary (*Chlamydia trachomatis* and *Ureaplasma urealyticum*) infection. Less commonly, respiratory infection with *Mycoplasma pneumoniae* or *Chlamydia pneumoniae* and enteric infections with *Clostridium difficile* or the protozoans *Giardia lamblia* or *Cryptosporidium* may precede manifestation of the arthritis. Reactive arthritis can be accompanied by extra-articular manifestations of conjunctivitis and urethritis, although they rarely occur in children. Other forms of reactive arthritis (eg, poststreptococcal, postgonococcal) differ in pattern of involvement, course, and prognosis; they are traditionally not considered among the spondyloarthropathies but should be considered in the differential diagnosis, as should viral arthritis and Lyme disease.

The frequency of reactive arthritis in any community reflects genetic factors as well as the prevalence of arthritogenic infections in the population. Although arthritis can occur in both HLA-B27–positive and HLA-B27–negative individuals, HLA-B27–positive individuals may be more susceptible to the infection and also are more likely to develop persistent arthritis following infection.

Reactive arthritis commonly presents as florid inflammation of 1 or 2 of the large weight-bearing joints and may have associated fever, fatigue, polyarthralgia, and muscle pains. Asymmetric involvement of small and large joints with dactylitis, as well as enthesitis, tenosynovitis, and bursitis, also may occur. The joints may be very hot, red, tender, and painful, and laboratory investigation may show markedly elevated inflammatory indices. A history in the patient of recent infection, infectious contact, or travel should alert to the possibility of reactive arthritis. In the case of monoarthritis, the possibility of septic arthritis may necessitate treatment with intravenous antibiotics while awaiting the results of arthrocentesis and joint fluid culture. In the presence of relatively normal "inflammatory" blood tests, several other acutely presenting conditions may have to be excluded. Acute orthopedic conditions of the hips such as slipped capital femoral epiphysis or Legg-Calve-Perthes should be distinguishable radiographically. Reflex sympathetic dystrophy (RSD) may present with an acutely painful, swollen joint that may be difficult to distinguish from reactive arthritis despite the presence of the characteristic "la belle indifference." A nuclear bone scan may be diagnostically helpful, with inflammatory processes demonstrating increased perfusion, but RSD characterized by decreased blood flow in the involved area. Support for the diagnosis of reactive arthritis is also provided by intestinal, urethral, and conjunctival cultures revealing 1 of the organisms known to incite reactive arthritis. However, although suggestive, it is no more definitive in proving the existence of reactive arthritis than the absence of organisms is for excluding the possibility. Fortunately, reactive arthritis is most often transient, lasting only days to weeks, so a diagnosis may be assumed in retrospect, following a severe, self-limited arthritis. In some cases, the arthritis may persist for months, sometimes with remissions and exacerbations, and in 1% to 3% of cases, patients (especially those with positive HLA-B27) develop chronic synovitis following an arthritogenic infection.

When the course of reactive arthritis is transient or self-limited, treatment with NSAIDs may be effective and sufficient in the short term. Sometimes the degree of discomfort and inflammation requires short-term use of glucocorticoids given orally as prednisone, or by intra-articular injection for resistant synovitis. Uncommonly, a patient may develop a persistent arthritis that is indistinguishable from ERA. It should be treated like ERA, and in the long term, such patients risk development of back pain or sacroiliitis and evolution into full-blown ankylosing spondylitis.

## JUVENILE PSORIATIC ARTHRITIS

The association of arthritis and psoriasis has been described in the adult literature for more than a century, with both conditions occurring in approximately 3% of the population. Among cohorts of children with JIA, approximately 7% are classified as having psoriatic arthritis. Classifying psoriatic arthritis will remain difficult until the biologic basis of the association between psoriasis and arthritis is understood; it remains unclear whether psoriatic arthritis is a unique entity or whether coincidental psoriasis simply modifies the expression of arthritis. There are well-characterized psoriatic phenotypes described in adults: asymmetric oligoarthritis, symmetric rheumatoid-like arthritis, predominant distal interphalangeal joint disease, arthritis mutilans, and spondylitis. At least 2 similar subtypes have been described in children. Psoriatic arthritis traditionally has been classified as a seronegative spondyloarthropathy, even though sacroiliitis or spondylitis at most occurs in only 40% of these patients. Overall, it seems likely that psoriatic arthritis represents a heterogeneous group of diseases that probably should not be lumped together as a spondyloarthropathy.

The association of psoriasis and arthritis in children versus adults was recognized much later, in part because most affected children develop psoriasis months to years after they develop arthritis. In 1980, the "Vancouver criteria" recognized psoriasis-specific clinical features (in the absence of psoriatic rash) that would facilitate early recognition and diagnosis of this subcategory of chronic childhood arthritis. These features are currently incorporated into the current ILAR criteria for subcategorizing JIA. Thus, psoriatic arthritis is defined as arthritis *plus* psoriasis, or arthritis *plus* at least 2 of the following: dactylitis, psoriatic nail abnormalities (pitting or onycholysis), and a family history of psoriasis in a first-degree relative (see Table 199-1).

Psoriatic arthritis is seen more frequently in girls than in boys and has a bimodal onset, in early childhood and in middle-late childhood. All of the adult psoriatic arthritis phenotypes described earlier, except arthritis mutilans, may occur in children; however, the most common pattern of joint disease at onset is asymmetric involvement of both large and small joints. Over time, many patients develop polyarthritis. Like young children with JIA, those with psoriatic arthritis are at risk of developing asymptomatic chronic anterior uveitis, particularly in the presence of a positive test for antinuclear antigen (ANA). Only approximately 10% to 30% of children with psoriatic arthritis develop sacroiliitis, primarily among those positive for the HLA-B27 haplotype and those with later onset disease. Overall, therefore, it seems even less relevant than in adults to classify the whole group of children with psoriatic arthritis as having a spondyloarthropathy (see Table 199-1).

Long-term outcome studies are limited, although they seem to confirm ongoing disease activity. At 8 to 10 years of follow-up, approximately one-half of children diagnosed with psoriatic arthritis had persisting synovitis, 8% to 10% had severe functional impairment, and approximately half of these had had joint replacements. Thus, principles of treatment are similar to those for children with other forms of arthritis, with an accent on early, aggressive management aimed at preventing chronic joint changes and disability. Treatment guidelines for polyarticular course JIA are generally applied to children with psoriatic arthritis. Further, it is important to remember that children with psoriatic arthritis require monitoring for asymptomatic uveitis with slit-lamp examinations performed every 3 to 6 months.

### SUGGESTED READINGS


Aquino MR, Tse SML, Gupta S, Rachlis AAC, Stimec J. Whole-body MRI of juvenile spondyloarthritis: protocols and pictorial review of characteristic patterns. *Pediatr Radiol.* 2015;45:754-762.

Burgos-Vargas R, Vazquez-Mellado J. The early clinical recognition of juvenile-onset ankylosing spondylitis and its differentiation from juvenile rheumatoid arthritis. *Arthritis Rheum.* 1995;38(6):835-844.

Flato B, Hoffmann-Vold AM, Reiff A, Forre O, Lien G, Vinje O. Long-term outcome and prognostic factors in enthesitis-related arthritis: a case-control study. *Arthritis Rheum.* 2006;54:3573-3582.

Herregods N, Delhoorne J, Pattyn E, et al. Diagnostic value of pelvic enthesitis on MRI of the sacroiliac joints in enthesitis related arthritis. *Pediatr Rheumatol.* 2015;13:46.

Katsicas MM, Russo R. Biologic agents in juvenile spondyloarthropathies. *Pediatr Rheumatol.* 2016;14:17.

Lin C, MacKenzie JD, Courtier JL, Gu JT, Milojevic D. Magnetic resonance imaging findings in juvenile spondyloarthropathy and effects of treatment observed on subsequent imaging. *Pediatr Rheumatol Online J.* 2014;12:25.

Passo MH, Fitzgerald JF, Brandt KD. Arthritis associated with inflammatory bowel disease in children: relationship of joint disease to activity and severity of bowel lesion. *Dig Dis Sci.* 1986;31:492-497.

Roberton DM, Cabral DA, Malleson P, Petty RE. Juvenile psoriatic arthritis: follow-up and evaluation of diagnostic criteria. *J Rheumatol.* 1996;23:166-170.

Stoll ML, Zurakowski D, Nigrovic LE, et al. Patients with juvenile psoriatic arthritis comprise two distinct populations. *Arthritis Rheum.* 2006;54:3564-3572.

Tse SML, Laxer RM. New advances in juvenile spondyloarthritis. *Nat Rev Rheumatol.* 2012;8:269-279.

Weiss PF. Evaluation and treatment of enthesitis-related arthritis. *Curr Med Lit Rheumatol.* 2013;32:33-41.

Weiss PF, Xiao R, Biko DM, Chauvin NA. Assessment of sacroiliitis at diagnosis of juvenile spondyloarthritis by radiography, magnetic resonance imaging and clinical examination. *Arthritis Care Res.* 2016;68(2):187-194.


# 200 Vasculitides

Karyl S. Barron

### INTRODUCTION

Vasculitis, defined as inflammation of blood vessels, is a feature of many rheumatic and nonrheumatic diseases of childhood. This chapter addresses only those diseases in which vasculitis plays a central role in both pathogenesis and clinical presentation. Criteria used for establishing a diagnosis of vasculitis in adults are often problematic when applied to children. Recently, a consensus was reached on a new classification of vasculitis, and these criteria will be used in this chapter. Classification of vasculitis is based on the size of the blood vessels involved or the pathology of the lesions (Table 200-1). This chapter will be limited to the more commonly seen vasculitides of childhood.

**TABLE 200-1 CLASSIFICATION OF VASCULITIS ACCEPTED IN THE 2012 INTERNATIONAL CHAPEL HILL CONSENSUS CONFERENCE**

| |
|---|
| **Large-vessel vasculitides** |
| Takayasu arteritis |
| Giant cell arteritis |
| **Medium-vessel vasculitides** |
| Polyarteritis nodosa |
| Kawasaki disease |
| **Small-vessel vasculitides** |
| Antineutrophilic cytoplasmic antibody (ANCA)–related vasculitides |
| Microscopic polyangiitis |
| Granulomatous polyangiitis (Wegener) |
| Eosinophilic granulomatous polyangiitis (Churg-Strauss) |
| Immune complex–related small-vessel vasculitides |
| Antiglomerular basal membrane disease |
| Cryoglobulinemic vasculitis |
| IgA vasculitis (Henoch-Schönlein purpura) |
| Hypocomplementemic urticarial vasculitis (anti-C1q vasculitis) |
| **Vasculitides involving vessels with variable size** |
| Behçet disease |
| Cogan syndrome |
| **Single-organ vasculitides** |
| Cutaneous leukocytoclastic vasculitis |
| Cutaneous arteritis |
| Primary central nervous system vasculitides |
| Isolated aortitis |
| **Vasculitides related with systemic diseases** |
| Lupus vasculitis |
| Rheumatoid vasculitis |
| Sarcoid vasculitis |
| **Vasculitides with known etiology** |
| Hepatitis C virus–related cryoglobulinemic vasculitis |
| Hepatitis B virus–related vasculitis |
| Syphilis-related aortitis |
| Drug-induced immune complex vasculitis |
| Drug-induced ANCA associated vasculitis |
| Deficiency of adenosine deaminase 2[a] |

[a]Recognized after the consensus conference.

## HENOCH-SCHÖNLEIN PURPURA (IGA VASCULITIS)

Henoch-Schönlein purpura (HSP), recently renamed *IgA vasculitis*, is an acute leukocytoclastic vasculitis, affecting mainly the small vessels of the skin, joints, gastrointestinal tract, and kidneys. HSP is the most common form of systemic vasculitis in childhood, with an incidence of about 10 cases per 100,000 per year. The main features of the disease include nonthrombocytopenic palpable purpura (present in 100% of affected children), arthritis or arthralgias (75–85%), colicky abdominal pain with or without gastrointestinal hemorrhage (60–85%), and renal involvement (10–50%). The diagnostic criteria are shown in Table 200-2. Although it can occur at any age, HSP is overwhelmingly a disease of childhood. The mean age of patients is 6 years; 75% of patients are younger than age 8, and 90% are younger than 10 years of age. The clinical features of HSP may be atypical at the extremes of age, typically presenting with milder manifestations in infants younger than 2 years of age and a more severe course in adults. The disease occurs more frequently in males, although sex differences are not seen in patients older than age 16 years. HSP has a seasonal pattern, with peaks in winter and spring. It is an IgA-mediated, leukocytoclastic vasculitis characterized by neutrophil infiltration and fibrinoid necrosis in the walls of arterioles, capillaries, and postcapillary venules, with deposition of IgG, IgA, and C3.

**TABLE 200-2 DIAGNOSTIC CRITERIA FOR HENOCH-SCHÖNLEIN PURPURA**

Purpura or petechiae (mandatory) more extensive in the lower extremities and 1 of the following 4 criteria:

- Abdominal pain
- Histopathology (IgA deposition on biopsy)
- Arthritis or arthralgia
- Renal involvement

### ETIOLOGY

The etiology of the disease is unknown. HSP often follows a respiratory infection. A wide variety of pathogens and other environmental exposures that have been associated with HSP include bacterial infections (group A β-hemolytic streptococci, *Legionella, Yersinia, Mycoplasma*), viral infections (Epstein-Barr virus, varicella-zoster virus, cytomegalovirus, parvovirus, hepatitis B virus), drugs (penicillin and other β-lactam antibiotics, chlorpromazine, quinidine, thiazide diuretics), vaccines (measles, yellow fever, cholera), food additives, and insect bites. Of all the pathogens linked to HSP, group A β-hemolytic *Streptococcus* has been studied the most. Positive throat cultures have been reported in 10% to 30% of patients, and titers to antistreptolysin O are raised in 20% to 50% of patients. Thus, a substantial minority of patients have a current or recent streptococcal infection, but most cases have no direct link to this organism.

### CLINICAL FEATURES

The onset of HSP may be acute or subacute, with clinical features of the disease most commonly developing in an additive manner over a short time span. Overall, HSP is a self-limited disease that usually lasts 1 to 2 weeks. It has a tendency to recur within the initial 6-week period, but exacerbations may occur as late as 2 years after onset. Overall, the prognosis of HSP is excellent; morbidity is determined in most cases by gastrointestinal complications during the acute phase and by renal involvement in the long term.

Skin lesions, present in all patients because the diagnosis depends on a recognizable rash, are the initial manifestation in about 50% of patients. The typical rash begins as small wheals or erythematous maculopapules that evolve into petechial or purpuric lesions, more prominent on dependent and pressure-bearing areas (Fig. 200-1). Although usually located over the lower extremities or buttocks, the rash may involve the upper extremities, trunk, and face. In young children, HSP might present as edema and purpura involving the face and ears. Skin lesions tend to occur in crops and last from 5 days to 4 weeks. Angioedema of the scalp, perineal area, and extremities may precede the onset of the rash.

Arthritis is the second most common feature of HSP, occurring in roughly 75% of patients and most often affecting knees and ankles. In about 25% of patients, arthritis/arthralgias of large joints is the initial symptom of HSP, often preceding the appearance of a skin rash by 24 to 48 hours. Because joint swelling is often periarticular, there may be no true joint effusion despite significant pain on motion. Joint symptoms typically resolve spontaneously after a few days without residual deformity but may recur with exacerbations or recurrences of HSP.

Gastrointestinal (GI) involvement occurs in 50% to 75% of patients. The most common complaint is colicky abdominal pain, frequently associated with vomiting. Pain may be severe enough to mimic an acute abdomen and may precede the onset of rash in as many as 10% to 15% of patients, again confusing the clinical picture. GI bleeding is usually occult, but 30% of patients have grossly bloody or melanotic stools. Upper GI series show nonspecific changes such as thickening of the bowel wall, "thumb printing," and filling defects. Ultrasound studies are abnormal in as many as 80% of patients with GI involvement and reveal increased echogenicity and thickening of the wall of the second portion of the duodenum and/or hydrops of the gallbladder. Endoscopy may reveal lesions with similar appearance to the palpable purpura seen in the skin. These findings are not present in patients

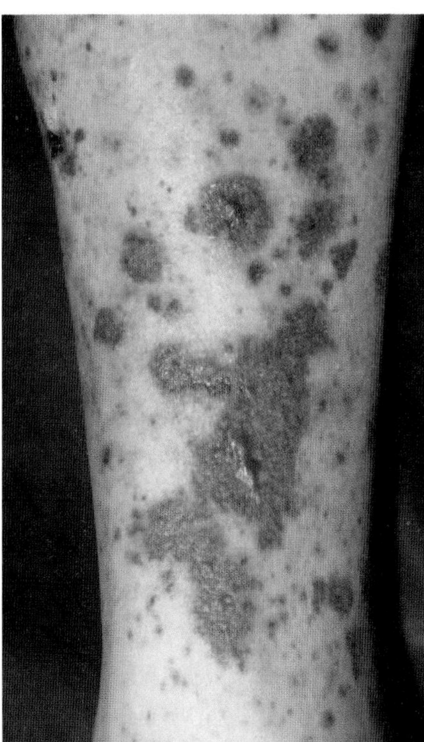

**FIGURE 200-1** Classical palpable purpura on the lower legs of a patient with Henoch-Schönlein purpura. (Reproduced with permission from Wolff K, Johnson RA. *Fitzpatrick's Color Atlas & Synopsis of Clinical Dermatology*, 6th ed. New York: McGraw-Hill; 2009.)

with HSP without GI complaints. Intussusception has been reported in 1% to 5% of patients; other uncommon GI complications may include perforation or bowel infarct.

Renal involvement occurs in 40% to 50% of patients with HSP and is most commonly limited to transient urinary abnormalities such as microscopic hematuria or hematuria plus mild proteinuria. Unlike arthritis and GI involvement, nephritis rarely, if ever, precedes the onset of purpura. About 75% to 90% of patients with nephritis develop urinary abnormalities within 4 weeks, but they may occur up to 3 months after the onset of symptoms. Urinalysis should be done each week while the disease is active, then monthly for the next 3 months. If all analyses are normal, nephritis is unlikely to occur. If at any time there is evidence of nephritis, long-term monitoring of urinalyses, protein excretion, renal function, and blood pressure is warranted until the urinary abnormalities resolve. Renal histopathology shows lesions indistinguishable from those of IgA nephropathy (Berger disease). Prognosis for those patients with renal involvement is excellent: Only 1% to 2% with severe renal involvement will have residual nephropathy, with fewer less than 1% progressing to end-stage renal disease. An age of more than 7 years at onset, persistent purpura for more than 1 month, and decreased factor XIII are significant risk factors for progression of renal involvement.

Less common manifestations of HSP include acute scrotal swelling or hemorrhage of the scrotal vessels, pancreatitis, pulmonary hemorrhage, encephalopathy, anterior uveitis, myositis, hemiparesis, and convulsions.

### DIAGNOSIS

The diagnosis of HSP is made on clinical grounds because laboratory tests are not diagnostic. Elevations of acute-phase reactants and white blood cell count are frequent findings. Platelet count and coagulation studies are normal. Serum levels of IgA frequently are elevated. Hemoglobin may be depressed in the context of severe bleeding. Elements of arthritis, acute abdominal pain, or renal involvement may confuse the picture if they precede the appearance of the characteristic rash. Patients with severe abdominal pain frequently require hospital admission. Ultrasonography is the preferred imaging technique to rule out intussusception because barium enema may miss an ileoileal intussusception, which is common in HSP.

### TREATMENT

Treatment is largely supportive. Most children may be managed as outpatients with appropriate analgesia and hydration. Development of GI and renal complications may be monitored by assessing stool guaiac tests, blood pressure, and urine dipsticks as an outpatient, unless severe intestinal or renal involvement necessitates hospital admission. Nonsteroidal anti-inflammatory drugs (NSAIDs) may be used to manage severe joint pain, although they should be avoided in the setting of significant renal disease. Prednisone in a dosage of 1 to 2 mg/kg/d is helpful in the management of painful edema, scrotal swelling, and severe, disabling arthritis. Steroids also may be used in children with severe abdominal pain, although its efficacy has not been proven. Treatment of HSP nephritis remains controversial. Therapies of severe renal disease, particularly chronic changes such as crescent formation, include intravenous pulses of methylprednisolone, cyclophosphamide, and azathioprine, alone or in different combinations.

## KAWASAKI DISEASE

Kawasaki disease (KD) is an acute febrile childhood vasculitis that involves mainly the coronary arteries and is the primary cause of acquired heart disease in children in the United States and Japan. The diagnostic criteria are listed in Table 200-3. The course of the disease is divided into 3 three phases. The *acute phase* encompasses a febrile period of 1 to 2 weeks and is characterized by fever to 104°C or higher; injection of the bulbar conjunctiva with sparing of the limbus; mouth and lip changes without oral ulcerations or exudates; rash; reddening of the palms and soles and/or swelling of the hands and feet; and cervical lymphadenopathy. During this phase, as many as 30% of patients develop arthralgias or arthritis, usually polyarticular, involving knees, ankles, and hands. Arthritis is self-limited, generally resolving within 3 weeks, although it may persist for as long as 3 months. The *subacute phase* typically begins 10 to 25 days after the onset of fever and lasts until all signs of disease activity subside. The most significant clinical manifestation of the subacute phase is cardiovascular involvement, which may lead to severe morbidity or mortality. Coronary arteries may be dilated and may form actual aneurysms. During the second to third week of illness, patients can develop a self-limited pauciarthritis involving the hips, knees, or ankles. The *convalescent phase* begins during the third or fourth week of illness, when clinical signs disappear, and continues until all parameters of inflammation normalize, usually 6 to 8 weeks after onset. Intravenous immunoglobulin is the standard treatment for KD, decreasing the risk of coronary artery aneurysms by more than 70%. KD is discussed in detail in Chapter 482.

## POLYARTERITIS NODOSA

Polyarteritis nodosa (PAN) is a necrotizing vasculitis associated with aneurysmal nodules along the walls of medium-sized arteries. The diagnostic criteria are listed in Table 200-4. The disease is rare in

**TABLE 200-3 DIAGNOSTIC CRITERIA FOR KAWASAKI DISEASE**

Fever (mandatory) in addition to 4 of the following 5 criteria:

- Nonpurulent conjunctivitis
- Mucosal changes
- Cervical lymphadenopathy
- Polymorphous rash on the trunk
- Extremity changes

**TABLE 200-4 DIAGNOSTIC CRITERIA FOR CHILDHOOD POLYARTERITIS NODOSA**

A systemic illness characterized by the presence of either a biopsy showing small and midsize artery necrotizing vasculitis OR angiographic abnormalities[a] (aneurysm or occlusion) (mandatory criteria), plus at least 2 of the following:

- Cutaneous involvement (livedo reticularis, tender subcutaneous nodules, other vasculitis lesions)
- Myalgia or muscle tenderness
- Systemic hypertension, relative to childhood normative data
- Peripheral neuropathy
- Renal involvement (abnormal urine analysis and/or impaired renal function)[b]
- Testicular pain or tenderness
- Signs or symptoms in any other major organ system (gastrointestinal, cardiac, pulmonary, or central nervous system)

[a]Should include conventional angiography if magnetic resonance angiography is negative.

[b]Glomerular filtration rate of less than 50% normal for age.



childhood. Mean age of presentation recorded in most series is 9 years. When the disease occurs in childhood, there is a male predominance (1.6–2.5:1). The exact cause and pathogenesis of PAN in children are unknown. In general, vasculitis is thought to occur when a susceptible host encounters an environmental trigger, typically an infection that cannot be handled appropriately. An association with hepatitis B virus (HBV) infection has been described in adults and occasionally in children; streptococcal infection has also been associated with juvenile PAN. Certain mutations in the Mediterranean fever (*MEFV*) gene increase the risk of developing PAN.

### CLINICAL FEATURES

The main features of PAN are constitutional symptoms (fever, malaise, anorexia, and fatigue), which are present in almost 100% of affected children, together with skin rash, abdominal pain, and musculoskeletal involvement, which is reported in as many as 80% of patients. Cutaneous manifestations include erythematous rashes, maculopapular purpuric lesions (similar to those of HSP), painful skin nodules, livedo reticularis, cutaneous ulcers, and, rarely, digital infarction or gangrene. Arthralgia, arthritis, myalgia, and myositis are common manifestations as well. Renal involvement manifesting as hematuria, proteinuria, hypertension, or rapidly progressive glomerulonephritis may be present in as many as 60% of patients. Gastrointestinal disease (bleeding, ulcerations) and neurologic involvement (mononeuritis multiplex, peripheral neuropathy, hemiparesis, encephalopathy, and stroke) are less frequent occurrences. Orchitis is a classical symptom of PAN, although it is seen less frequently in patients without concomitant HBV infection.

A subset of the disease is cutaneous PAN, characterized by crops of painful skin nodules and livedo reticularis, and sometimes nonspecific musculoskeletal findings such as myalgia and arthralgia. There is often a history of preceding upper respiratory infection, particularly *Streptococcus*. Constitutional symptoms are not present, and acute phase reactants are often normal. Skin biopsy reveals necrotizing vasculitis. The condition is treated with oral corticosteroids and has a favorable prognosis; however, relapses often occur. Every child with a diagnosis of cutaneous PAN should be followed closely for systemic symptoms. Constitutional symptoms should prompt consideration of immunosuppressive treatment. Penicillin prophylaxis may be needed to prevent recurrences when streptococcal infections are implicated.

### LABORATORY DIAGNOSIS

Establishing a diagnosis of PAN is often difficult because of the variability of presenting complaints. There are no specific laboratory tests. Acute-phase reactants are elevated, and anemia, polymorphonuclear leukocytosis, and thrombocytosis are common findings. Other laboratory abnormalities depend on specific organ involvement. The diagnosis is based primarily on the presence of either a biopsy showing necrotizing vasculitis of small and midsize arteries, or angiographic abnormalities in addition to skin, muscle, and/or renal involvement, hypertension, neuropathy, testicular pain or tenderness, or signs or symptoms suggesting vasculitis of any other major organ system (see Table 200-4).

### TREATMENT

In severe cases, treatment consists of corticosteroids, antiplatelet agents, and a cytotoxic agent, typically cyclophosphamide. Cyclophosphamide is usually administered orally for 2 to 3 months at 2 mg/kg/d to induce remission. Pulsed intravenous cyclophosphamide may have an advantage over the oral route in reducing the total cumulative dose and potential side effects, but it may not be as effective as the daily oral regimen for preventing relapses in aggressive disease. Maintenance therapy is usually with oral azathioprine at a dose of 2 mg/kg/d, with low-dose, alternate-day prednisone and antiplatelet agents. If remission with this regimen is not maintained, then cyclosporine or mycophenolate mofetil may prove useful, although the published evidence for use of these agents in this context is lacking.

Relapses occur in as many as 20% of patients. The overall prognosis of this disease has improved during the past decades primarily because of earlier diagnosis and rapid initiation of more effective treatments.

## DEFICIENCY OF ADENOSINE DEAMINASE 2

Deficiency of adenosine deaminase 2 (DADA2) is a disorder characterized by recurrent fevers, a spectrum of vascular pathologic features, and mild immunodeficiency. The most common clinical presentation includes early onset of recurrent strokes, childhood PAN, fever, livedo racemosa, hepatosplenomegaly accompanied by portal hypertension, and humoral immune deficiency. Magnetic resonance imaging (MRI) of the brain may reveal evidence of acute or chronic subcortical infarcts involving the deep-brain nuclei and brain stem, which is consistent with small-vessel occlusions (lacunar stokes). Magnetic resonance angiography (MRA) usually is negative. The disorder is associated with recessively inherited mutations in *CECR1* (cat eye syndrome chromosome region, candidate 1), which encodes adenosine deaminase 2 (ADA2). Patients have a marked reduction in the levels of ADA2 and ADA2-specific enzyme activity in blood. Skin, liver, and brain biopsies reveal vasculopathic changes characterized by compromised endothelial integrity, endothelial cell activation, and inflammation. Early studies have shown that treatment with anti–tumor necrosis factor (TNF) agents prevents the occurrence of subsequent strokes. Avoidance of antiplatelet agents is recommended, as treatment with these medications has been associated with subsequent hemorrhagic strokes. DADA2 should be considered in children with recurrent strokes, especially if there is a family history of early-onset strokes, cutaneous PAN, and/or recurrent fevers.

## MICROSCOPIC POLYANGIITIS

Microscopic polyangiitis (MPA) is a necrotizing pauci-immune vasculitis affecting predominantly small vessels. Rapidly progressive necrotizing glomerulonephritis is very common. Pulmonary capillaritis with resultant pulmonary hemorrhage often occurs, in the absence of granulomatous lesions of the respiratory tract. MPA is a rare finding in children. Patients frequently have perinuclear-staining antineutrophil cytoplasmic antibodies (p-ANCA) targeting myeloperoxidase (MPO). The disease has a worse prognosis than does PAN, with a 5-year survival rate of 60% to 65%. Patients require aggressive therapy with corticosteroids, immunosuppressive drugs, and possibly plasmapheresis. Relapses are common occurrences.

## GRANULOMATOSIS WITH POLYANGIITIS (WEGENER GRANULOMATOSIS)

Granulomatosis with polyangiitis (GPA; formerly Wegener granulomatosis) is a necrotizing granulomatous vasculitis of small to medium-sized vessels characterized by the triad of paranasal sinus involvement, pulmonary infiltration, and pauci-immune glomerulonephritis (Table 200-5). The disease is an uncommon occurrence in children. Prior to adulthood, GPA usually presents during adolescence and affects females more often than males. The indolent nature of the disease may delay the diagnosis for months, although some patients present acutely with life-threatening manifestations such as pulmonary hemorrhage or acute renal failure.

### CLINICAL FEATURES

At onset, clinical features are similar to those seen in polyarteritis nodosa (fever, rash, weight loss, and arthralgia). There are, however, particular features that might point to the diagnosis, including upper airway illness such as persistent cough, nasal stuffiness, mucosal ulceration, sinusitis, epistaxis, hoarseness, or earache. Localized disease, such as saddle nose deformity owing to damage to the nasal cartilage and subglottic stenosis (SGS) from granulomatous involvement of the trachea, is seen more frequently in children than in adults. A high proportion of patients with SGS require surgical intervention to maintain airway patency. Overall, nasal, sinus, tracheal (including tracheal stenosis), and ear abnormalities are seen in 91% of patients with childhood-onset disease. Lung disease occurs in 74% of children. Lower respiratory tract symptoms include cough, dyspnea, and hemoptysis. Nodular pulmonary infiltrates are often visible on radiographs at presentation and may masquerade as infection. Renal involvement is uncommon at presentation, although as many as 70% of children develop pauci-immune glomerulonephritis during the evolution of the disease. The renal disease may take the form of an aggressive crescentic glomerulonephritis and is discussed in more detail in Chapter 468. Ocular abnormalities, including conjunctivitis, dacryocystitis, scleritis, episcleritis, and proptosis, may be present in 10% to 15% of children at disease onset. Other manifestations of GPA include arthritis, present in one-third of children at presentation and two-thirds at follow-up; cutaneous disease including palpable purpura, skin ulceration, and subcutaneous nodules; pericarditis; and neurologic involvement.

### DIAGNOSIS

The diagnosis of GPA has been greatly facilitated by its association with the presence of cytoplasmic staining of antineutrophil cytoplasmic antibodies (c-ANCA). The target of these antibodies is the cytoplasmic protein proteinase 3 (PR3). Chest computed tomography (CT) may reveal multifocal infiltrates with or without small peripheral nodules. Urinalysis characteristically demonstrates proteinuria, microscopic hematuria, and red blood cell casts in as many as 50% of patients, although a normal urine sediment does not rule out renal involvement. Gross hematuria is an uncommon finding. Confirmation of the disease is established by the detection of granulomatous inflammation on biopsy of the upper airway, lung, kidney, or skin.

### TREATMENT

The disease was uniformly fatal in children before the use of a combination of glucocorticoids and cytotoxic agents. Treatment with steroids in combination with cyclophosphamide induces remission in 90% of patients. Cyclophosphamide (2 mg/kg/d) with prednisone at a dose of 1 mg/kg/d for 4 weeks and then tapered to an alternate-day regimen is recommended to induce remission. The median time to remission using this regimen is 3 months, whereas steroids can usually be discontinued after 6 to 8 months. When remission is achieved, the cyclophosphamide is switched to methotrexate or azathioprine maintenance therapy, which is continued for at least 2 years in an attempt to limit relapses. Nonetheless, relapses of disease requiring retreatment occur in a majority of patients with GPA. In adults, rituximab has been shown to provide a noninferior alternative to cyclophosphamide for remission induction, and use as maintenance therapy significantly decreases the risk of disease relapses. No therapeutic trials have been published involving children. For non–life-threatening disease, therapy may be initiated with glucocorticoids and methotrexate. For patients with pulmonary hemorrhage, intensive care management may be required. Plasmapheresis is commonly used in grave situations in an attempt to stabilize the patient, although data demonstrating its efficacy are lacking.

## TAKAYASU ARTERITIS

Takayasu arteritis (TA), also known as *pulseless disease*, is characterized by granulomatous vasculitis of large vessels leading to stenosis and aneurysms. It is a rare occurrence in children younger than age 16 years. The underlying pathology is a segmental arteritis of the aorta and its major branches, which can cause weak or absent pulses in the upper extremities. It occurs most frequently in young women, particularly those of Japanese origin. Hypertension is the most common reason for coming to medical attention, followed by headache. However, fever, back pain, claudication, or visual complaints may also be presenting manifestations. TA may present as chest pain due to coarctation of the aorta or congestive heart failure in association with features of systemic vasculitis such as fever and constitutional symptoms. Ischemic manifestations such as visual disturbances, neurologic deficits, or claudication are frequently present in adults, but uncommon in children. A triphasic pattern of disease has been described. *Phase I* is the pre-pulseless period with nonspecific systemic complaints such as fever, night sweats, anorexia, arthralgia/arthritis, and weight loss. In *phase II*, vessel inflammation occurs. The *final phase* is the fibrotic state during which bruits and significant ischemia become prominent. Not all patients go through all phases, and some may present with a mixture of symptoms. Criteria to aid the diagnosis of TA are listed in Table 200-6.

There is an association between TA and *Mycobacterium tuberculosis* in some geographical areas. Laboratory abnormalities are nonspecific, including anemia and elevation of acute phase reactants, but patients, especially children, may have active inflammatory vasculitis with normal acute-phase reactants. Other autoantibodies associated with vasculopathies, including antinuclear antibodies (ANA) and ANCA, are seldom detectable. Chest radiographs may demonstrate cardiomegaly or an irregular contour of the aortic arch and descending aorta. There may be areas of vascular calcification or widening associated with prestenotic dilatation. Arteriography may reveal multiple

**TABLE 200-5 DIAGNOSTIC CRITERIA FOR GRANULOMATOUS POLYANGIITIS (WEGENER GRANULOMATOSIS)**

Three of the following 6 features should be present:

- Histopathology (granulomatous inflammation)
- Upper respiratory tract involvement
- Laryngotracheobronchial obstruction
- Lung involvement
- Antineutrophil cytoplasmic antibodies positivity
- Renal involvement

**TABLE 200-6 DIAGNOSTIC CRITERIA FOR TAKAYASU ARTERITIS**

Aneurysm or dilatation in the aorta or its main branches and pulmonary artery shown by angiography (mandatory) plus 1 of the following 5 criteria:

- Decreased peripheral artery pulse(s) or claudication
- Blood pressure differences in 4 extremities
- Bruits over aorta and/or its major branches
- Hypertension (related to childhood normative data)
- Increased acute phase response

sites of segmental involvement of the aorta and major branches. MRA, CT, and ultrasonography may document early inflammatory changes occurring before the development of obstructive lesions.

There are no controlled treatment trials of TA in children. High-dose glucocorticoids (1–2 mg/kg/d) often constitute the initial treatment, although as many as 40% to 50% of patients require the addition of a disease-modifying agent, such as methotrexate, a TNF inhibitor, or, in refractory cases, cyclophosphamide. Antiplatelet agents can be added to the therapy in patients with transient neurologic deficits. Aggressive treatment of hypertension is critical. Operative management may benefit stenotic lesions that do not regress after medical therapy, but recurrence rates are very high if vascular inflammation is not completely controlled prior to surgery.

## BEHÇET DISEASE

Behçet disease (BD) is a vasculitis affecting arteries and venules that is characterized by the clinical triad of painful recurrent oral and genital ulcers and inflammatory eye disease. The disease is an uncommon occurrence in children, with most cases reported from the eastern Mediterranean or the Far East. The cause of BD is unknown.

### CLINICAL FEATURES

The most common clinical feature of BD is recurrent oral ulceration, which usually occurs at onset of the disease and may persist for much of the course of the disease. The ulcers occur in painful crops on the lips, tongue, palate, and elsewhere in the gastrointestinal tract (Fig. 200-2). They may persist for 3 to 10 days and often heal without scarring. Skin lesions may be in the form of erythema nodosum, papulopustular (acneiform) lesions, folliculitis, pustules, ulcers, or purpura. Pathergy, noted by the appearance of a pustule or papule surrounded by erythema 24 to 48 hours after a needle prick, is highly characteristic but not pathognomonic of the syndrome. Genital ulcers usually occur after the onset of oral ulcers and more commonly may scar with healing. The spectrum of eye lesions includes posterior uveitis, papilledema, and optic atrophy. Hypopyon may occur, and severe uveitis may lead to blindness. Four neurologic syndromes are recognized in patients with BD: encephalomyelitis, aseptic meningitis, benign intracranial hypertension, and organic psychiatric disturbances. Arthritis commonly affects the knees, ankles, wrists, and elbows and does not usually result in erosions or joint destruction. Arthralgia is also a common finding. Less prevalent manifestations of the disease include venous or arterial thrombosis or gastrointestinal involvement. Vascular complications may occur in the form of arterial aneurysms or thrombosis of veins or arteries.

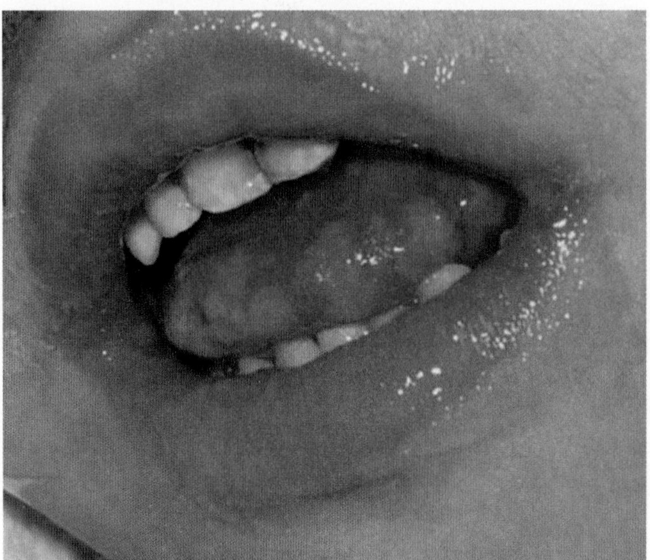

**FIGURE 200-2** Behçet disease. Extensive aphthae involving the lips and tongue. (Reproduced with permission from Wolff K, Johnson RA. *Fitzpatrick's Color Atlas & Synopsis of Clinical Dermatology*, 6th ed. New York: McGraw-Hill; 2009.)

### DIAGNOSIS AND TREATMENT

The diagnosis of BD is based on the criteria of the International Study Group for BD, which requires recurrent oral ulceration and at least 2 of the following: recurrent genital ulceration, eye lesions, skin lesions, and positive pathergy test. There is often a delay in making the diagnosis; therefore, children who satisfy only some of the criteria should be followed closely. Boys and girls are affected with equal frequency, in contrast to adults, in which men are affected almost twice as often as women.

There are no controlled studies evaluating treatment of BD in children. Recommendations are based on adult experience. For oral and genital ulcers, mouth washes with sucralfate suspension or topical and/or oral corticosteroids may be helpful. During the acute stage of ulceration, a short course of oral prednisone often provides rapid relief of the symptoms. Long-term colchicine is effective in controlling the frequency and severity of oral and genital ulceration. For severe lesions, thalidomide may be useful, but the risk of peripheral neuropathy and its contraindication during pregnancy limit its usefulness.

For erythema nodosum and arthralgia or arthritis, nonsteroidal anti-inflammatory drugs and colchicine are usually sufficient. Eye disease should be followed by an experienced ophthalmologist. For central nervous system (CNS) disease and vasculitis, corticosteroids and immunosuppressive agents such as cyclophosphamide are indicated in regimens such as those used for other vasculitides. Sulfasalazine has been reported to be of benefit in gastrointestinal disease. BD tends to run a very long and relapsing course. Young age of onset and male sex are both indicators of a prolonged disease course. Mortality because of the disease is 3%, usually secondary to CNS involvement, large-vessel thrombosis, or GI perforation.

## CENTRAL NERVOUS SYSTEM VASCULITIS

Isolated CNS vasculitis is an inflammatory brain disease characterized by an angiocentric inflammation of the vascular wall of cerebral blood vessels and/or the perivascular space. Isolated or primary blood vessel inflammation of the brain and/or spinal cord is the hallmark of primary CNS vasculitis or angiitis (PACNS). In the pediatric age group, primary CNS angiitis is considered one of the most common inflammatory brain diseases. Criteria to aid the diagnosis of PACNS are listed in Table 200-7. Childhood PACNS is divided into 3 subtypes based on the primary vessel size affected and characteristic disease course: angiography-positive, medium-large vessel progressive (PcPACNS); angiography-positive, medium-large vessel nonprogressive (NPcPACNS); and angiography-negative, biopsy positive, small-vessel CNS vasculitis (SVcPACNS). The cause of primary CNS vasculitis remains to be determined. Genetic factors have not been studied systematically.

### CLINICAL MANIFESTATIONS

Children with CNS vasculitis can present with a wide spectrum of symptoms, including headache, neck stiffness, focal neurologic deficits, brain stem or spinal cord symptoms, seizures, and encephalopathy. Children may manifest diffuse deficits including psychiatric symptoms, with behavioral, mood, or concentration problems, and constitutional symptoms, including fever, nausea, and fatigue. In

**TABLE 200-7 DIAGNOSTIC CRITERIA FOR PRIMARY VASCULITIS OF THE CENTRAL NERVOUS SYSTEM (CNS)**

- Acquired neurologic or psychiatric finding that cannot be explained by another cause
- Histopathologic or angiographic changes indicating vasculitis in the CNS
- Absence of systemic vasculitis or any disease that could cause these pathologic changes in the CNS

SECTION 15 Rheumatology

general, children with angiography-positive PACNS present with newly acquired focal deficits such as hemiparesis, hemisensory loss, and/or facial droop. The perforator arteries are most commonly affected. These vessels branch from the proximal middle cerebral artery segment and feed the basal ganglia. Children with progressive angiography-positive PACNS commonly present with both focal and diffuse neurologic deficits. In this subtype, vessel wall inflammation can affect proximal and distal vascular segments, the latter causing brain irritation, manifesting as loss of higher executive function, behavior change, and memory loss. Seizures are the most common presenting symptom of childhood small-vessel PACNS.

### DIAGNOSIS

The first step in the diagnostic evaluation of children with suspected CNS vasculitis includes ruling out systemic illnesses and nonvasculitis inflammatory disorders, which generally includes blood and cerebrospinal fluid analysis. Inflammatory markers may be seen in PACNS, but they are not consistently present. von Willebrand factor (vWF) antigen is an endothelial cell–derived protein, which is elevated in 60% to 70% of children with confirmed PACNS, most commonly in those with small-vessel disease. Cerebrospinal fluid analysis should include cell count and differential, cytospin for malignancies, protein and glucose levels, infectious evaluation, oligoclonal banding, opening pressure, and testing for neural antibodies. MRI is useful to detect inflammatory and ischemic brain lesions. Brain biopsy may be indicated in children with suspected PACNS and negative angiography findings. The characteristic finding of childhood PACNS is an angiocentric transmural and/or perivascular infiltrate and reactive endothelial cells. Associated features may include perivascular demyelination and glial cell reactions. In childhood PACNS, a predominantly lymphocytic infiltrate is seen.

### TREATMENT

Treatment of CNS vasculitis aims to control the active intramural inflammation, prevent secondary ischemic events, improve vessel remodeling, control CNS symptoms such as seizures and psychiatric manifestations, and prevent disease- and treatment-related adverse events. Children with nonprogressive PACNS are thought to have a monophasic inflammatory disease and are often treated with intravenous daily pulsed methylprednisone for 3 to 4 days, followed by tapering doses of oral prednisone over several months. Antithrombotic therapy is often added. Children with progressive PACNS and small-vessel PACNS require immunosuppression beyond corticosteroids.

### SUGGESTED READINGS


Barut K, Sahin S, Kasapcopur O. Pediatric vasculitis. *Curr Opin Rheumatol.* 2016;28:29-38.

Bohm M, Fernandez MIG, Ozen S, et al. Clinical features of childhood granulomatosis with polyangiitis (Wegener granulomatosis). *Pediatr Rheumatol.* 2014;12:18-22.

Elkan PN, Pierce SB, Segel R, et al. Mutant adenosine deaminase 2 in a polyarteritis nodosa vasculopathy. *N Engl J Med.* 2014;370:921-931.

Jennette JC, Falk RJ, Bacon PA, et al. 2012 revised international Chapel Hill consensus conference nomenclature of vasculitides. *Arthritis Rheum.* 2013;65:1-11.

Morishita K, Brown K, Cabral D. Pediatric vasculitis: advances in treatment. *Curr Opin Rheumatol.* 2015;27:493-499.

Soliman M, Laxer R, Manson D, et al. Imaging of systemic vasculitis in childhood. *Pediatr Radiol.* 2015;45:1110-1125.

Ting TV. Diagnosis and management of cutaneous vasculitis in children. *Pediatr Clin N Am.* 2014;61:321-346.

Twilit M, Benseler SM. Central nervous system vasculitis in adults and children. *Handb Clin Neurol.* 2016;133:283-300.

Zhou Q, Yang D, Ombrello A, et al. Early-onset stroke and vasculopathy associated with mutations in ADA2. *N Engl J Med.* 2015; 370:911-920.




# 201 Systemic Lupus Erythematosus, Overlap Connective Tissue Diseases, and Mixed Connective Tissue Disease

Linda Tayeko Hiraki and Earl Dean Silverman

## SYSTEMIC LUPUS ERYTHEMATOSUS

Systemic lupus erythematosus (SLE) represents the prototype of autoimmune disease, with the presence of autoantibodies as its hallmark. The incidence of SLE diagnosed in patients younger than age 16 is approximately 0.25 to 11 new cases per 100,000 annually, with an overall prevalence of 1.89 to 63.1 per 100,000 depending on ascertainment and ethnicity of the population. The prevalence and incidence rates are higher in the 12- to 18-year age group. Both the incidence and prevalence rates are 2.4 to 4.9 times higher in African Americans, Native Americans, Asians, Southeast Asians, and Hispanics compared with white children. The female predominance (4–5:1) in pediatric patients is lower than that in adults (9:1), although some but not all studies suggest that the female-to-male ratio may vary in different ethnic populations. The mean age at diagnosis is approximately 12 to 13 years, but presentation of patients as young as age 5 years is routinely reported, and the age of onset varies by ethnicity, with nonwhite populations tending to have onset of disease at younger ages. Presentation prior to age 3 to 5 years is frequently associated with a genetic defect. Despite significant improvements in the outcome of childhood-onset SLE (cSLE), mortality rates remain substantial, with a United Kingdom study reporting standardized mortality ratios (compared to national statistics in the general population) as high as 18.3 for all cSLE and 87 for those with SLE onset at <10 years of age (however, the confidence intervals were wide).

Neonatal lupus erythematosus (NLE) must not be mistaken for early-onset SLE. NLE is a disease caused by the transplacental passage of maternal autoantibodies, and the fetus/neonate has a normal immune system that is not actively producing autoantibodies. A minority of these children develop true SLE many years later. In contrast, cSLE is a disease in which the child produces autoantibodies and the immune abnormalities are intrinsic to the child's immune system.

### ETIOLOGY

SLE, similar to most autoimmune diseases, is the result of a combination of genetic and environmental factors leading to the clinical and laboratory phenotype. The reported environmental risk factors include viral infections, estrogens, cigarette smoke, pesticides, and sunlight. The mechanism leading to the production of autoantibodies, the hallmark of SLE, is the break of tolerance of self-antigens. It is theorized that increased/abnormal apoptosis, necrosis, autophagy, or netosis leads to the decreased clearance of self- or viral dsDNA and ssRNA. This clearance, in turn, stimulates autoreactive T and B cells, leading to the production of autoantibodies and proinflammatory cytokines, resulting in tissue damage. The autoantibodies usually are directed against histone, nonhistone, RNA-binding, cytoplasmic, and nuclear proteins. However, more than 100 different autoantigens have been described to date. Antinuclear antibodies (ANAs) occur in most patients, but ANA-negative SLE does occur. ANA-negative SLE usually is seen in patients having only anti-Ro antibodies and is an artefact of the immunofluorescent testing for ANA. Anti-DNA antibodies are present in approximately 50% to 60% of patients, whereas antibodies directed against the small nuclear ribonuclear proteins (anti-Sm and anti-70-kDa RNP antibodies) occur in 40% to 50% of patients. Antibodies directed against small cytoplasmic ribonuclear proteins (anti-Ro and/or anti-La antibodies) occur in 30% to 40% of patients, anticardiolipin antibodies in 40% to 50% of patients, and rheumatoid factor in 15% to 20% of patients. Antiribosomal P antibodies are present in approximately 25% to 30% of patients and may be associated with psychosis and depression.

In 1997, the American College of Rheumatology (ACR) revised the 1982 criteria for classification of SLE (Table 201-1). These criteria were not designed to be used for diagnosis, but rather for classifying patients with a known autoimmune disease in order to facilitate comparison of those with SLE to those with another autoimmune disease. Patients are classified as having definite SLE if they meet 4 of 11 criteria, but some series report 5% to 15% of patients who have only 3 criteria. In 2012, the Systemic Lupus International Collaborating Clinics (SLICC) classification criteria were proposed, which had a higher sensitivity but lower specificity than those of the revised 1982 criteria (Table 201-2). A study from 1994 showed that the ACR 1982 criteria had good sensitivity and specificity for cSLE. In 2014, a multicenter study showed that the SLICC criteria were more sensitive and led to fewer misclassifications but were less specific than were the ACR criteria for cSLE. It is currently recommended that the SLICC criteria be used.

Arthritis, skin involvement, and nephritis are the most common manifestations, but any organ may be affected (Table 201-3). Systemic symptoms reflecting a generalized inflammatory process (fever, malaise, weight loss, and lethargy) are very common findings. In 80% to 90% of patients, a disease manifestation either occurs within the first year of diagnosis or it fails to arise. The exception is central nervous system (CNS) disease, in which as many as 25% of patients will have the first episode of CNS involvement more than 1 year after diagnosis. Clinical features seen in flares of SLE tend to mimic the clinical features seen at presentation, but generally there is less systemic inflammation in patients who are followed closely.

**TABLE 201-1 1982 REVISED CRITERIA FOR CLASSIFICATION OF SYSTEMIC LUPUS ERYTHEMATOSUS**

| Criterion | Definition |
|---|---|
| Malar rash | Fixed erythema, flat or raised, over the malar eminences, tending to spare the nasolabial folds |
| Discoid rash | Erythematous raised patches with adherent keratotic scaling and follicular plugging; atrophic scarring may occur in older lesions |
| Photosensitivity | Skin rash as a result of unusual reaction to sunlight, by patient history or physician observation |
| Oral ulcers | Oral or nasopharyngeal ulceration, usually painless, observed by physician |
| Arthritis | Nonerosive arthritis involving 2 or more peripheral joints, characterized by tenderness, swelling, or effusion |
| Serositis | Pleuritis—convincing history of pleuritic pain or rubbing heard by a physician or evidence of pleural effusion or pericarditis—documented by electrocardiogram or rub or evidence of pericardial effusion |
| Renal disorder | Persistent proteinuria > 0.5 g/d (or > 3+ if quantitation not performed) or cellular casts; may be red cell, hemoglobin, granular, tubular, or mixed |
| Neurologic disorder | Seizures in the absence of offending drugs or known metabolic derangements (eg, uremia, ketoacidosis, or electrolyte imbalance) or psychosis in the absence of offending drugs or known metabolic derangements (eg, uremia, ketoacidosis, or electrolyte imbalance) |
| Hematologic disorder | Hemolytic anemia with reticulocytosis or leukopenia < 4000/μL total on 2 or more occasions, or lymphopenia < 1500/μL on 2 or more occasions, or thrombocytopenia < 100,000/μL in the absence of offending drugs |
| Immunologic disorder | Anti-DNA antibody to native DNA in abnormal titer, or presence of anti-Sm nuclear antigen, or positive finding of antiphospholipid antibodies based on (1) an abnormal serum level of IgG or IgM anticardiolipin antibodies, (2) a positive test result for lupus anticoagulant using a standard method, or (3) a false-positive serologic test for syphilis known to be positive for at least 6 months and confirmed by *Treponema pallidum* immobilization or fluorescent treponemal antibody absorption test. |
| Antinuclear antibody | An abnormal titer of antinuclear antibody by immunofluorescence or an equivalent assay at any point in time and in the absence of drugs known to be associated with drug-induced lupus syndrome |

The proposed classification is based on 11 criteria. For the purpose of identifying patients in clinical studies, a person shall be said to have SLE if any 4 or more of the 11 criteria are present, serially or simultaneously, during any interval of observation.

Reproduced with permission from Tan EM, Cohen AS, Fries JF, et al: The 1982 revised criteria for the classification of systemic lupus erythematosus, *Arthritis Rheum.* 1982 Nov;25(11):1271-1277.

### Renal Disease

The incidence of renal involvement varies between 48% and 90% of patients, although most estimates are around 50% to 60%. An extensive discussion of the diagnosis and management of renal complications of SLE is provided in Chapter 468.

### Central Nervous System

CNS disease, or neuropsychiatric SLE (NP-SLE), occurs in 20% to 40% of patients and is associated with significant morbidity and mortality rates. Both the CNS and/or the peripheral nervous systems may be involved with multiple syndromes and presentations. The wide range of reported frequency of CNS involvement is in part due to studies' variations in defining CNS involvement. The ACR criteria list only seizures and psychosis, and the SLICC criteria additionally include mononeuritis multiplex, myelitis, peripheral or cranial neuropathy, and acute confusional state. To make it even more complicated, in 1999, the ACR developed a nomenclature and case definition for NP-SLE (Table 201-4). The 1999 ACR neuropsychiatric case definitions are preferred as they include the full range of possible manifestations seen in SLE patients, rather than identifying a feature as a manifestation of neuropsychiatric involvement in SLE based on its sensitivity and specificity.

Psychiatric illnesses range from mood disorders such as depression to organic brain syndrome. Neurocognitive testing detects impairments in cognitive function or learning difficulties in a high percentage of patients, but the true incidence of clinically important cognitive dysfunction is unknown.

Depression or anxiety as a manifestation of active disease must be differentiated from a secondary depression arising from environmental factors or from medication side effects. One cross-sectional study using a validated depression and anxiety screening instrument found that 45% of cSLE patients had moderate to severe depression and 20% had anxiety. Overt psychosis or organic brain syndrome occurs in approximately 10% of all patients with SLE and is consistently associated with significant cognitive impairment. Visual distortions with preservation of insight are characteristic of NP-SLE early in the illness. In patients with psychosis and organic brain syndrome, secondary causes including metabolic imbalance, infection, and medications (such as steroids and hydroxychloroquine) must be ruled out. In most patients with psychosis or organic brain syndrome, a lumbar puncture is indicated to rule out infection.

Seizures, seen in approximately 10% to 20% of patients, may be the presenting sign of more significant organic brain disease, the result of an infarction, or the sole manifestation of CNS involvement. Movement disorders encompass cerebellar ataxia, hemiballismus, tremor, parkinsonian-like movements, and chorea. SLE, or antiphospholipid antibody syndrome, is currently the most common cause of chorea in developed countries.

Cranial nerve involvement occurs more frequently than does peripheral neuropathy. Rarely, hemiparesis or transverse myelitis may occur. Although not studied in children, the incidence of autonomic dysfunction in adults is 40% to 50%. It usually is mild and, among other symptoms, may lead to changes in heart rate.

Headache occurs in 25% to 50% of patients with SLE. The typical headache responds to mild analgesia. However, a severe, unremitting headache, sometimes referred to as a *lupus headache,* usually reflects active disease or CNS vasculitis, or it may represent cerebral vein thrombosis. In all cases of unremitting headache, appropriate investigations must be performed to rule out cerebral vein thrombosis or infection. Migraine-like headaches likely reflect active NP-SLE, in particular when they were not present prior to the diagnosis of SLE and in the absence of a family history of migraines. A more benign cause of

**TABLE 201-2 CLINICAL AND IMMUNOLOGIC CRITERIA USED IN THE SLICC CLASSIFICATION SYSTEM[a]**

*Clinical criteria*

1. **Acute cutaneous lupus, including:**
   Lupus malar rash (do not count if malar discoid)
   Bullous lupus
   Toxic epidermal necrolysis variant of SLE
   Maculopapular lupus rash
   Photosensitive lupus rash
   *in the absence of dermatomyositis*
   OR subacute cutaneous lupus (nonindurated psoriaform and/or annular polycyclic lesions that resolve without scarring, although occasionally with postinflammatory dyspigmentation or telangiectasias)
2. **Chronic cutaneous lupus, including:**
   Classic discoid rash
   Localized (above the neck)
   Generalized (above and below the neck)
   Hypertrophic (verrucous) lupus
   Lupus panniculitis (profundus)
   Mucosal lupus
   Lupus erythematosus tumidus
   Chilblains lupus
   Discoid lupus/lichen planus overlap
3. **Oral ulcers**
   Palate
   Buccal
   Tongue
   OR Nasal ulcers
   *in the absence of other causes, such as vasculitis, Behcet disease, infection (herpesvirus), inflammatory bowel disease, reactive arthritis, and acidic foods*
4. **Nonscarring alopecia** (diffuse thinning or hair fragility with visible broken hairs)
   *in the absence of other causes such as alopecia areata, drugs, iron deficiency, and androgenic alopecia*
5. **Synovitis involving 2 or more joints,** characterized by swelling or effusion
   OR tenderness in 2 or more joints and at least 30 minutes of morning stiffness
6. **Serositis**
   Typical pleurisy for more than 1 day
   OR pleural effusions
   OR pleural rub
   Typical pericardial pain (pain with recumbency improved by sitting forward) for more than 1 day
   OR pericardial effusion
   OR pericardial rub
   OR pericarditis by electrocardiography
   *in the absence of other causes, such as infection, uremia, and Dressler pericarditis*
7. **Renal**
   Urine protein-to-creatinine ratio (or 24-hour urine protein) representing 500 mg protein/24 hours OR red blood cell casts
8. **Neurologic**
   Seizures
   Psychosis
   Mononeuritis multiplex
   *in the absence of other known causes such as primary vasculitis*
   Myelitis
   Peripheral or cranial neuropathy
   *in the absence of other known causes such as primary vasculitis, infection, and diabetes mellitus*
   Acute confusional state
   *in the absence of other causes, including toxic/metabolic, uremia, drugs*
9. **Hemolytic anemia**
10. **Leukopenia** (≤ 4000/μL at least once)
    *in the absence of other known causes such as Felty syndrome, drugs, and portal hypertension*
    **OR**
    **Lymphopenia** (≤ 1000/μL at least once)
    *in the absence of other known causes such as corticosteroids, drugs, and infection*
11. **Thrombocytopenia** (≤ 100,000/μL) at least once
    *in the absence of other known causes such as drugs, portal hypertension, and thrombotic thrombocytopenic purpura*

*Immunologic criteria*

1. **ANA** level above laboratory reference range
2. **Anti-dsDNA antibody** level above laboratory reference range (or 2-fold the reference range if tested by ELISA)
3. **Anti-Sm:** presence of antibody to Sm nuclear antigen
4. **Antiphospholipid antibody positivity** as determined by any of the following:
   Positive test result for lupus anticoagulant
   False-positive test result for rapid plasma reagin
   Medium- or high-titer anticardiolipin antibody level (IgA, IgG, or IgM)
   Positive test result for anti–2-glycoprotein I (IgA, IgG, or IgM)
5. **Low complement**
   Low C3
   Low C4
   Low CH50
6. **Direct Coombs test** *in the absence of hemolytic anemia*

[a]Criteria are cumulative and need not be present concurrently.

ANA, antinuclear antibody; anti-dsDNA, anti–double-stranded DNA; ELISA, enzyme-linked immunosorbent assay; SLE, systemic lupus erythematosus; SLICC, Systemic Lupus International Collaborating Clinics.

Reproduced with permission from Petri M, Orbai AM, Alarcon GS, et al. Derivation and validation of the Systemic Lupus International Collaborating Clinics classification criteria for systemic lupus erythematosus, *Arthritis Rheum.* 2012 Aug;64(8):2677-2686.

headache is pseudotumor cerebri, ascribable either to the underlying disease or to steroid medication.

Examination and culture of cerebrospinal fluid (CSF) are performed to rule out the possibility of CSF infection or hemorrhage. An elevated CSF protein and/or CSF white blood cell count in the absence of infection is suggestive of lupus cerebritis. Neuroradiologic investigation of the CNS (computed tomography [CT] or magnetic resonance imaging [MRI] scan) may demonstrate specific structural lesions such as infarction, embolus, cerebral vein thrombosis, and subdural or intracranial hemorrhage, but these modalities are generally not helpful in measuring overall CNS disease activity. MRI with magnetic resonance angiography and venography (indicated for investigation of possible cerebral vein thrombosis) is the imaging modality of choice in patients suspected of having CNS involvement. Levels of complement proteins and anti-DNA antibodies, which may correlate with disease activity at other sites, may be normal with CNS involvement.

The therapy of CNS disease varies with the manifestation. Most clinicians do not treat isolated cognitive impairment. Active psychosis and/or organic brain syndrome are potentially life-threatening complications and should be treated aggressively with an immunosuppressive regimen that includes high-dose corticosteroids and azathioprine,

**TABLE 201-3 FREQUENCIES OF CLINICAL FEATURES OF SYSTEMIC LUPUS ERYTHEMATOSUS IN CHILDREN AND ADOLESCENTS**

| Clinical Features (n = 321) | Within First Year of Diagnosis | At Any Time During Disease |
|---|---|---|
| Generalized symptoms | | |
| Fever | 58% | 86% |
| Lymphadenopathy | 38% | 41% |
| Hepatosplenomegaly | 32% | 32% |
| Organ disease | | |
| Arthritis | 80% | 82% |
| Any skin rash | 80% | 88% |
| Malar rash | 40% | 42% |
| Nephritis | 49% | 66% |
| Neuropsychiatric disease | 25% | 33% |
| Cardiovascular disease | 20% | 22% |
| Pulmonary disease | 22% | 28% |
| Gastrointestinal disease | 14% | 16% |

Data from a multiethnic cohort of patients followed at The Hospital for Sick Children in a combined rheumatology/nephrology clinic.

mycophenolate mofetil (MMF), or cyclophosphamide. Psychotropic drugs serve as adjunctive, but not primary, therapy.

### Dermatologic Disease

Skin involvement manifesting as malar rash, discoid rash, or photosensitivity occurs in 50% to 90% of patients with SLE. A rash in the malar area involving cheeks and sparing the nasolabial folds is quite specific for SLE; dermatomyositis is the only other disease in the differential diagnosis for malar rash (Figs. 201-1 and 201-2). A discoid rash is rarer than a malar rash. Although isolated discoid lupus is commonly seen in adults, all pediatric patients with a discoid rash must be followed for the development of true SLE: only 29% of 40 patients who presented with childhood-onset discoid rash still had isolated discoid rash after a median follow-up period of 5 years. Discoid rashes are more prevalent in nonwhite than in white patients.

Many, but not all, patients with a rash exhibit photosensitivity, and sun exposure may lead to a flare of skin and/or systemic disease.

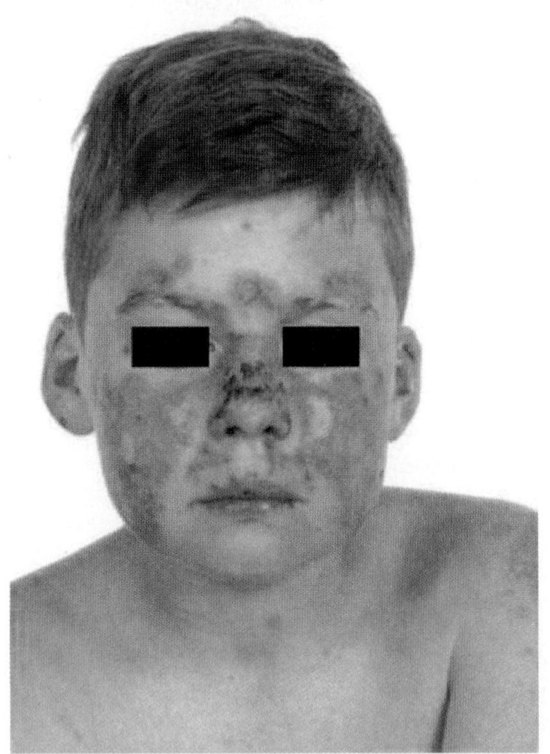

**FIGURE 201-1** Photosensitive malar rash with sparing of the nasolabial folds in systemic lupus erythematosus. Note increased rash over lips, chin, and forehead.

**TABLE 201-4 NEUROPSYCHIATRIC MANIFESTATIONS OBSERVED IN CHILDHOOD-ONSET SYSTEMIC LUPUS ERYTHEMATOSUS (SLE)**

| 1999 ACR Nomenclature and Case Definitions for Neuropsychiatric SLE | Toronto Series (n = 70) | Other Literature |
|---|---|---|
| Central nervous system | 93% | 70–97% |
| Aseptic meningitis | 3% | Not reported |
| Cerebrovascular disease | 24% | 12–30% |
| Demyelinating syndrome | 1% | 4–10% |
| Headache | 70% | 22–95% |
| Isolated headache | 24% | Not reported |
| Movement disorder | 10% | 3–15% |
| Myelopathy | 1% | 1–8% |
| Seizure disorder | 20% | 10–42% |
| Acute confusional state | 17% | 20–40% |
| Anxiety disorder | 15% | 10–28% |
| Cognitive dysfunction | 30% | 20–57% |
| Mood disorder/depression | 32% | 28–57% |
| Psychosis | 36% | 12–50% |
| Peripheral nervous system | 7% | 3–30% |
| Guillain-Barré syndrome | 0% | Not reported |
| Autonomic disorder | 0% | Not reported |
| Mononeuropathy | 3% | Not reported |
| Cranial neuropathy | 1% | Not reported |
| Myasthenia-like syndrome | 0% | Not reported |
| Plexopathy | 0% | Not reported |
| Peripheral neuropathy | 3% | Not reported |

Many patients have more than 1 neuropsychiatric manifestation.

Data from a multiethnic cohort of patients followed at The Hospital for Sick Children in a combined rheumatology/nephrology clinic.

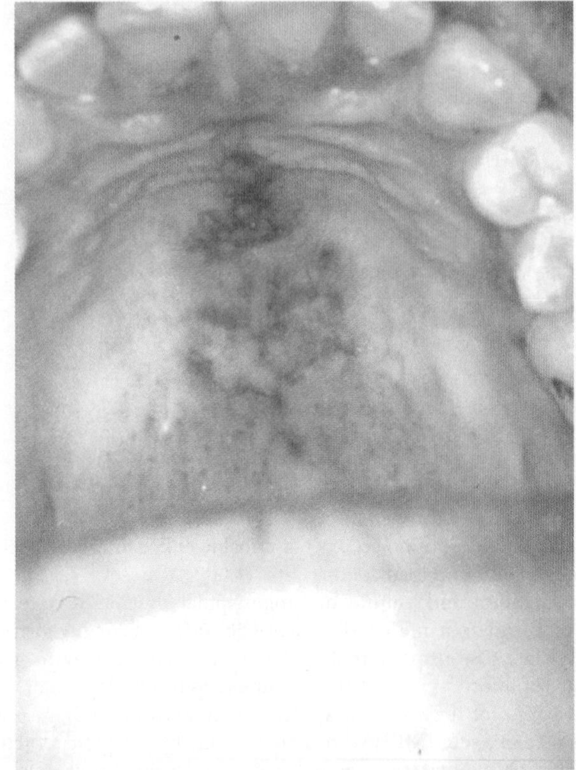

**FIGURE 201-2** Multiple oral ulcers on hard palate. The ulcers were asymptomatic.

Sun-exposed areas should be protected with light clothing and a sunscreen with a high ultraviolet (UV) light protection rating against both UVA and UVB. The rash of subacute cutaneous SLE appears as an annular rash with a raised border and central sparing; it, too, has a photosensitive component and often is associated with anti-Ro and anti-La antibodies. Alopecia occurs in 25% to 35% of patients and may be diffuse or patchy. In pediatric patients, alopecia in the presence of a systemic autoimmune disease is quite specific for SLE. A vasculitic rash consisting of oral/nasal erythema or erosions or ulcers on the arms, legs, or ears may occur in as many as 25% of patients and often is associated with systemic involvement (see Fig. 201-1). Table 201-3 lists the rashes that are manifestations of SLE.

#### Musculoskeletal Involvement

As many as 90% of patients exhibit joint involvement, typically a polyarticular arthritis that affects both large and small joints; severe pain and significant morning stiffness occur in half the patients, whereas in the other 50%, polyarthritis may produce few symptoms. Control of extra-articular sites of disease activity is frequently sufficient to treat the arthritis. An arthritic flare may herald a more generalized flare. Most patients with active arthritis without major organ involvement have normal serum complement levels. Septic arthritis and osteomyelitis must always also be considered if a fever is present. Therapy with nonsteroidal anti-inflammatory agents and antimalarial agents may control arthritis as an isolated symptom, but low-dose corticosteroid therapy is frequently required.

Patients with SLE are at a high risk for the development of avascular necrosis (AVN) of many bones; this complication is likely secondary to a combination of the disease process, antiphospholipid antibodies, and/or the use of corticosteroids. AVN occurs in 5% to 10% of patients who present with acute pain, joint tenderness, and effusion. The other major musculoskeletal complication of cSLE is osteopenia and osteoporosis with fracture. Adolescence is a time of rapid bone mass accrual, and peak bone mass usually is reached in early adulthood. Recent studies have shown that most patients with cSLE have low bone mineral density and bone mass, with an increased fracture rate as a result of the combination of chronic inflammation and the use of corticosteroids. Unfortunately, longitudinal studies have suggested that even when both disease activity and corticosteroid doses are low, patients only infrequently recover bone mass.

#### Hematologic Involvement

Anemia, thrombocytopenia, and leukopenia occur in 50% to 75% of patients. Only a Coombs-positive hemolytic anemia satisfies the ACR classification criteria (SLICC criteria do not require hemolysis), but both normochromic, normocytic anemia and microcytic, hypochromic anemia are common findings in SLE. The Coombs test is positive in approximately 30% to 40% of patients, but fewer than 10% of patients have overt hemolysis. Thrombocytopenia is present in 30% to 45% and may precede the diagnosis of SLE. SLE should be considered in anyone with chronic thrombocytopenia, although a higher percentage of adults with chronic thrombocytopenia have SLE, whereas children are more likely to have a postinfectious drop in platelets. Leukopenia occurs in 20% to 40% of cases (lymphopenia and/or granulocytopenia). The total white blood cell count usually is ≥ 2500/μL with a lymphocyte count usually > 1000/μL. Pancytopenia may occur, and when present, one must also consider macrophage activation syndrome or a concomitant herpes-family viral infection.

Antiphospholipid and anticardiolipin antibodies are detected in approximately 50% of patients. Anticardiolipin antibodies are the most common antiphospholipid antibody seen in cSLE, followed by anti-beta$_2$ glycoprotein I antibodies and then lupus anticoagulant (LAC). LAC is an antibody that reacts with phospholipids in the reagent used in the partial thromboplastin time (PTT) determination. LAC is seen in approximately 20% of cases of cSLE; as many as 50% of patients with LAC will present with or develop evidence of a thromboembolic event. Presence of LAC is also a risk factor for development of chorea. LAC often is seen in conjunction with anticardiolipin antibodies. Patients with LAC do not bleed; instead, they have an increased incidence of deep vein thrombosis, thromboemboli, or, less commonly, arterial thrombosis. Antiphospholipid antibodies are associated with multiple neurologic manifestations including stroke, seizures, chorea, and other movement disorders, pseudotumor cerebri, and migraine headaches. Antiphospholipid antibodies also may predispose to nonneurologic disorders such as thrombocytopenia and recurrent miscarriage. Most pediatric patients with evidence of venous thromboembolic disease will have evidence of LAC. LAC-negative patients with venous thromboembolic disease will frequently have a different primary or secondary thrombophilic defect.

Although 20% to 30% of patients have splenomegaly on physical examination, of more importance is the presence of functional asplenia, which may increase the incidence of bacterial sepsis, in particular, with encapsulated organisms.

#### Cardiac Involvement

Although cardiac tamponade is rare, symptomatic pericarditis occurs in approximately 20% to 25% of patients and often is associated with pleurisy. In contrast, clinically important myocarditis or endocarditis is uncommon (< 10% of patients). Longer survival times and the use of corticosteroid therapy have led to an increase in the incidence of atherosclerotic heart disease and myocardial infarction. Other factors predisposing to atherosclerotic heart disease in those with SLE include hypertension, hyperlipidemia, antiphospholipid antibodies, and coronary vasculitis, which may lead to acute myocardial infarction. Cardiac valve involvement, particularly Libman-Sacks endocarditis, frequently is seen in autopsy studies but rarely is clinically significant.

#### Pulmonary Disease

The reported incidence of pulmonary involvement varies between 25% and 75% of all patients with SLE. There are protean pulmonary manifestations ranging from severe life-threatening pulmonary hemorrhage or infection, to chronic interstitial lung disease, to asymptomatic abnormalities on pulmonary function tests. Decreased diffusion capacity is the most common abnormality. Abnormalities of pulmonary function tests account for the 75% incidence of lung disease. In the acutely ill patient with severe lung disease, the differential diagnosis includes acute lupus pneumonitis, pulmonary hemorrhage, or pulmonary infection; the last may be present even prior to steroid or immunosuppressive treatment. Pleural involvement occurs in as many as 30% of cases, frequently is seen in association with pericarditis, and usually is easy to treat with either nonsteroidal anti-inflammatory drugs or, when more severe, corticosteroids.

#### Gastrointestinal and Hepatic Disease

Gastrointestinal (GI) involvement occurs in 20% to 40% of patients with cSLE. Abdominal pain is the most common GI symptom and can be the result of peritoneal inflammation (serositis), vasculitis, pancreatitis, and/or direct bowel wall involvement (enteritis). Peritoneal inflammation of underlying SLE must be differentiated from an infective peritonitis. Pancreatitis is a rare cause of abdominal pain in pediatric SLE. Azathioprine may cause drug-induced pancreatitis, but the majority of cases of pancreatitis in patients with SLE are idiopathic, typically occurring in the setting of active disease.

Hepatomegaly occurs in 40% to 50% of patients. Abnormalities on liver function tests are seen in as many as 25% of patients but usually are mild and transient. When jaundice is a prominent feature in a patient with SLE, then a second disease, such as obstruction, hemolysis, or viral hepatitis, is the likely cause. Patients with SLE are at an increased risk of developing drug hepatotoxicity.

Liver involvement and autoimmune hepatitis require specific mention because the literature often uses the terms lupoid hepatitis, liver involvement in lupus, and autoimmune hepatitis with SLE interchangeably. The major problem arises from the definition of autoimmune hepatitis, which includes many features of SLE. However, the distinction is important because, in contrast to autoimmune hepatitis, which requires prolonged immunosuppression to prevent permanent liver damage, SLE with liver involvement usually is a benign entity that resolves without hepatic injury. We suggest that in the absence of anti-LKM or high-titer anti-smooth muscle antibodies and the presence of clinical/laboratory features of SLE (in particular autoantibodies associated with SLE), these patients should be considered to have liver involvement secondary to SLE, rather than an overlap autoimmune syndrome with autoimmune hepatitis.

#### Endocrine Involvement

The thyroid is the most common endocrine organ involved in SLE, with antithyroid antibodies present in 40% to 50% of patients and clinical hypothyroidism present in 10% to 20%. Graves disease is much less common than is hypothyroidism. Steroid-induced diabetes mellitus occurs in as many as 10% of patients, but a lower percentage require insulin treatment. Rare cases of hypoparathyroidism and growth hormone deficiency have been reported in patients with SLE.

### TREATMENT AND COMPLICATIONS

Although corticosteroids are the mainstay of therapy in patients with severe disease, side effects frequently occur and include avascular necrosis (described above), osteoporosis with fracture or vertebral body collapse, growth failure, cataracts, glaucoma, steroid-induced diabetes mellitus, hyperlipidemia, hypertension, and premature atherosclerosis. Unfortunately, patients with pediatric-onset SLE generally require steroids more frequently and at higher doses than do adults. Therefore, although steroids can be lifesaving in SLE, every attempt should be made to avoid their use or to use the minimal dose required.

The rational use of cytotoxic agents is limited by the lack of good clinical studies; their use should be reserved for severe and/or life-threatening disease. Azathioprine has a good safety profile, but leukopenia and increased susceptibility to infection must be considered in all patients using this medication. In addition to all the side effects of azathioprine, long-term use of cyclophosphamide also is associated with an increased risk of malignancy and infertility. MMF has been used successfully in large trials of adults with proliferative lupus nephritis. The outcomes of these patients are equal or superior to those of patients treated with cyclophosphamide with similar toxicity. Smaller pediatric case series have shown similarly good results with MMF, although evidence of efficacy in acute, life-threatening SLE or NP-SLE at any age is inadequate to recommend its use in these situations. Many pediatric rheumatologists will treat almost all patients with hydroxychloroquine (5–6 mg/kg/d) because studies suggest that its use is associated with fewer disease flares and an improved lipid profile. Because the major toxicity is ophthalmologic, patients require retinal examinations every 6 to 12 months.

## OVERLAP SYNDROMES AND MIXED CONNECTIVE TISSUE DISEASE

By definition, patients with overlap syndromes have features of more than 1 identifiable connective tissue disease. There are no true definitions and no estimates of how frequently they occur in pediatric patients. The diagnosis may be confounded by the acceptance of atypical features within the definitions of defined connective tissue diseases. Examples of this phenomenon include the presence of myositis in patients with SLE and arthritis in patients with dermatomyositis. In addition, patients with overlap syndromes should be differentiated from patients with diseases in evolution that do not yet meet the criteria for a defined connective tissue disease. Two recognized overlap syndromes are mixed connective tissue disease (MCTD) and a scleroderma/polymyositis overlap. These patients with the latter have features of definite scleroderma and significant myositis. They frequently have the specific autoantibody anti-PM/Scl (polymyositis/scleroderma).

MCTD, one of the most controversial of the rheumatic illnesses, is the prototype of an overlap syndrome. The controversy centers on its definition and its existence as a unique, separate condition. It has been suggested that a defined overlap syndrome must include a distinct constellation of clinical signs and/or serologic features. The main reason for defining MCTD as a separate entity is its association with antibodies against the U1 70Kd small nuclear ribonucleoprotein (RNP), which is part of what is referred to as the *extractable nuclear antigens* (ENAs). MCTD is also characterized by features of more than 1 connective tissue disease, in particular features of SLE, polymyositis/dermatomyositis, scleroderma (SSc), and rheumatoid arthritis or, in children, juvenile idiopathic arthritis (JIA).

In 1972, Sharp described a series of adult patients with MCTD and very high levels of anti-U1RNP antibodies. The common features included arthritis, swollen fingers, tight skin, abnormal esophageal motility, Raynaud phenomenon, and myositis. In contrast to SLE, anti-DNA antibodies were not detected in these patients, and they were corticosteroid-responsive and free of renal disease. Although high-titer circulating antibodies were thought to be specific for the U1RNP autoantigen, these antibodies are found in 30% to 40% of patients with SLE. Because SLE is significantly more common in a pediatric population, the vast majority of patients with even high-titer anti-U1RNP antibodies will have SLE. In patients with SLE, these antibodies are frequently but not exclusively found in the presence of other specific autoantibodies. Currently, there are 4 classification criteria of MCTD in adults, of which 3 are most commonly used: (1) Sharp, (2) Kasukawa, and (3) Alarcon-Segovia. In pediatric MCTD, only Kasukawa and Alarcon-Segovia criteria are used (Table 201-5). One adult study using the Alarcon-Segovia criteria showed that 92% also met the Kasukawa criteria, but only 70% met the Sharp criteria. The most recent study to examine MCTD criteria suggested that Kasukawa's criteria were the most sensitive of the 3 schemes for classifying MCTD in the long-term. Similar studies have not been performed in the pediatric age group.

Another controversy relates to whether MCTD is a distinct disease over time or simply a disease in transition that will differentiate into another defined illness. Even advocates for the existence of the disease acknowledge that patients may differentiate into SLE, SSc, or myositis 5 to 10 years after receiving a diagnosis of MCTD. Regardless, defining a consistent population by using established disease criteria will be the only way to ultimately resolve this issue.

The pediatric literature is even more confusing than the adult literature. The first reports of MCTD in the pediatric age group (pMCTD) were from Singsen and colleagues in 1977 and Fraga and colleagues in 1978. They described children with significant cardiac and renal involvement and thrombocytopenia in the presence of high-titer speckled ANA and anti-RNP antibodies. In this regard, the clinical and laboratory features of pediatric patients more closely resembled those of a subgroup of SLE with anti-RNP antibodies, although some patients had myositis. Some of the case reports in the literature also had anti-Sm and/or anti-DNA antibodies, which most authors consider to be specific for SLE within a group of patients with an autoimmune disease. Indeed, many pediatric patients who have been described will meet criteria for the diagnosis of definite SLE or scleroderma. A 2016 French, multicenter study of 19 patients with pMCTD observed that 47% had anti-Sm antibodies and 21% had anti-dsDNA at presentation. Many pediatric rheumatologists would have said that these patients had SLE based on the presence of either one of these antibodies; therefore, controversy remains about the definition of pMCTD. However, a subgroup of patients with only high-titer anti-U1RNP antibodies have a disease that meets the criteria for MCTD. This group is not to be confused with patients with overlap symptoms without anti-U1RNP antibodies, as fewer than 50% of children with overlap symptoms have these autoantibodies. Conversely, most pediatric patients with anti-U1RNP antibodies do not have clinical features consistent with MCTD, but instead have clinical features that meet the classification criteria for SLE. It is important to make these distinctions if we are to understand the long-term prognosis and optimal treatment for patients with pMCTD.

### EPIDEMIOLOGY

A nationwide retrospective study from Norway found a point prevalence of MCTD of 3.8 per 100,000 adults, an incidence of 2.1 per million per year over a 20-year period with a 77% female predominance. Because the definition of the disease has varied and not all studies used

**TABLE 201-5 DIAGNOSTIC CRITERIA FOR MIXED CONNECTIVE TISSUE DISORDERS**

**I. Kasukawa Criteria**

Diagnosis requires A, B, and C

A. Presence of either:
   1. Raynaud phenomenon
   2. Swollen fingers or hands

B. Positive snRNP antibody

C. Positive in 1 or more findings in 2 of the 3 disease categories listed below:
   1. SLE-like symptoms
      a. Polyarthritis
      b. Lymphadenopathy
      c. Facial erythema
      d. Pericarditis or pleuritis
      e. Leukothrombocytopenia
   2. SSc-like findings
      a. Sclerodactyly
      b. Pulmonary fibrosis, restrictive changes of lung, or reduced diffusion capacity
      c. Hypomotility or dilatation of esophagus
   3. PM-like findings
      a. Muscle weakness
      b. Elevated serum levels of muscle enzymes (CPK)
      c. Myogenic pattern on EMG

**II. Alarcon-Segovia Criteria**

Anti-RNP at a hemagglutination titer of ≥ 1600 and at least 3 of the following:

A. Edema in the hands
B. Synovitis
C. Myositis
D. Raynaud phenomenon
E. Acrosclerosis

**III. Sharp Criteria**

Definite diagnosis requires 4 major criteria with positive anti-U RNP > 1:4000 and a negative anti-Sm Ab.

Possible diagnosis requires 3 major criteria without serologic evidence of disease, or if anti-U1RNP is greater than 1:1000, 2 major criteria or 1 major and 3 minor criteria.

A. Major
   1. Severe myositis
   2. Lung involvement: Diffusion capacity < 70% normal and/or pulmonary hypertension and/or proliferative vascular lesion on lung biopsy
   3. Raynaud phenomenon or esophageal hypomotility
   4. Swollen hands or sclerodactyly
   5. Anti-ENA ≥ 10,000 and anti-U1RNP positive and anti-Sm negative

B. Minor
   1. Alopecia
   2. Leukopenia
   3. Anemia
   4. Pleuritis
   5. Pericarditis
   6. Arthritis
   7. Trigeminal neuropathy
   8. Malar rash
   9. Thrombocytopenia
   10. Mild myositis
   11. History of swollen hands

CPK, creatine phosphokinase; EMG, electromyography; PM, polymyositis; SLE, systemic lupus erythematosus.

Adapted with permission from Alarcon-Segovia, D. and Cardiel MH: Comparison between 3 diagnostic criteria for mixed connective tissue disease. Study of 593 patients, *J Rheumatol.* 1989; Mar;16(3):328-334.

defined criteria, the true incidence of pMCTD is difficult to ascertain. The youngest reported patient with MCTD was age 5, and the number of patients increases with increasing age. It has been estimated that fewer than 1% of patients followed in pediatric rheumatology clinics have MCTD.

## CLINICAL FEATURES AND DIAGNOSIS

The most common features of pMCTD are Raynaud phenomenon, fever, arthritis, skin rashes, edema of the hands with or without sclerodermatous-like skin changes, and myositis (Table 201-6). Although originally described as a relatively benign disorder, subsequent reports have found involvement of multiple internal organs. CNS manifestations are rare, but aseptic meningitis may be seen, particularly after the use of nonsteroidal anti-inflammatory medications. Clinically significant eye involvement is very rare. Acute pericarditis and/or pericardial effusion and mitral valve prolapse are the most common cardiac features, whereas myocarditis and cardiomyopathy (uncommon manifestations) tend to be severe, progressive, and life-threatening. Pulmonary and GI involvement requires special consideration.

MCTD commonly involves the lungs, and pulmonary function tests frequently show small airway obstruction early in the disease course, with a progressive impairment of alveolar gas exchange. Restrictive airway disease may be seen in more than 50% of patients, and pulmonary hypertension, when present, tends to be severe. The largest long-term outcome study in pMCTD, a nationwide survey in Norway, showed that 46% of patients had evidence of interstitial lung disease, including reduced diffusion or vital capacity, and pulmonary fibrosis on CT scan in 28%. These manifestations, characteristic of changes in SSc that may lead to pulmonary hypertension, are similar to the findings in adult MCTD patients. The corresponding pathologic finding is intimal proliferation and hypertrophy of the pulmonary arterioles with sparing of the interstitial areas.

GI abnormalities similar to those found in patients with SLE, myositis, or SSc are frequent. Any area of the GI tract may be affected,

**TABLE 201-6 CLINICAL FEATURES OF PEDIATRIC MIXED CONNECTIVE TISSUE DISEASE**

| | Clinical Feature | Percentage |
|---|---|---|
| **SLE-like** | Raynaud phenomenon[a] | 93–100% |
| | Arthralgia | 94% |
| | Arthritis | 78–97% |
| | Lymphadenopathy | 14–43% |
| | Alopecia | 7–18% |
| | Mucosal ulcers | 13–18% |
| | Pericarditis | 3–28% |
| | Pleuritis | 10–21% |
| **Scleroderma-like** | Swollen fingers/hands | 68–91% |
| | Sclerodactyly | 26–86% |
| | Restrictive lung disease | 24–64% |
| | Decreased carbon monoxide diffusion | 15–42% |
| | Gastroesophageal reflux | 24–44% |
| | Esophageal dysmotility | 7–21% |
| | Finger pitting/ulcers | 27%[a] |
| | Telangiectasias | 18[a] |
| **Myositis-like** | Muscle weakness | 29–70% |
| | Gottron papules | 9–24% |
| | Heliotrope | 0–15% |
| **Other** | Fatigue | 88%[b] |
| | Headache | 34–44% |
| | Aseptic meningitis | 4%[a] |

[a]May also be considered as scleroderma feature.

[b]Results are from only 1 series.

SLE, systemic lupus erythematosus.

**TABLE 201-7 LABORATORY FEATURES OF PEDIATRIC MIXED CONNECTIVE TISSUE DISEASE**

| Laboratory Feature | % of Patients |
|---|---|
| Anti-U1RNP antibodies | 100% |
| Antinuclear antibodies | 100% |
| Rheumatoid factor | 14–81% |
| Anti-dsDNA antibodies[a] | 21–44% |
| Anti-Sm antibodies[a] | 0–17% |
| Muscle enzyme elevations | 24–68% |
| White blood cell count < 4000/μL | 21–36% |
| Platelets < 100,000/μL | 6–21% |

[a]This is considered by many pediatric rheumatologists to be an exclusion from classification as mixed connective tissue disease and diagnostic of systemic lupus erythematosus.

but the esophagus is the most common location. The incidence of esophageal symptoms is as high as 85% and includes heartburn and dysphagia, and/or abnormal esophageal function as demonstrated by manometric abnormalities. Liver disease is an infrequent finding. GI abnormalities are not related to disease duration or to the presence of Raynaud phenomenon. Renal involvement is seen in 45% to 50% of pediatric patients and only 3% to 5% of adults. Thrombotic microangiopathy affects 25% of patients, whereas the remainder have mesangial proliferative (class II) glomerular nephritis on pathologic specimens.

Arthritis is a common occurrence, and deforming arthritis and/or loss in joint function may be seen in as many as one-third of cases, whereas erosive arthritis rarely is seen. Vasculitis may present with splenic vasculitis and oral, digital, GI, or genital ulceration. Over time, other autoimmune diseases, including Hashimoto thyroiditis, myasthenia gravis, and cold agglutinin syndrome, may develop.

All patients have a positive, speckled ANA at high titer with high-titer anti-U1RNP antibodies. Patients usually have a positive rheumatoid factor and hypergammaglobulinemia (Table 201-7). Other laboratory abnormalities may include elevated muscle enzymes, thrombocytopenia, lymphopenia, mild anemia, elevated erythrocyte sedimentation rate, and hypocomplementemia.

## TREATMENT

As originally described, MCTD was thought to be a corticosteroid-responsive illness with a good prognosis. However, more recent reports suggest that only a subgroup of patients respond to corticosteroids alone, and some of them may require high-dose intravenous methylprednisolone. Optimal therapy and long-term prognosis are determined by the disease into which the patient's condition differentiates. The outcomes in patients who develop SLE are similar to those of most patients with SLE, as is the therapy. The same is true for the patients who develop systemic scleroderma. These patients usually are unresponsive to therapy, although there have been reports of improvement with immunosuppression in patients with MCTD with predominantly SSc features. The largest long-term study in pMCTD suggests that the majority of patients require treatment with prednisone and an additional immunosuppressive agent. Commonly used agents include methotrexate, MMF, azathioprine, and, rarely, cyclophosphamide or cyclosporine. Of note, in adults, esophageal dysfunction has been reported to improve with corticosteroid therapy. Overall, given the wide variety of manifestations, therapy must be individualized, targeting first and foremost the patient's predominant vital organ involvement.

## PROGNOSIS

Follow-up studies have indicated that the majority of pediatric patients develop either severe disease or differentiate into definite SSc or SLE. A large review of pediatric patients initially diagnosed with MCTD demonstrated worse 5-year prognosis than those initially diagnosed with SLE. Large prospective and retrospective studies of adult patients with high-titer anti-RNP antibodies in the absence of anti-Sm and anti-DNA antibodies reported that only 25% to 50% of patients followed for 7 years or more still had features of an overlap, rather than another defined rheumatic disease. The transformation occurred after a mean of 2 to 3 years, but there was a large standard deviation (3 years or more). In contrast, a review at 5 large pediatric rheumatology centers in England and the United States found only a minority of patients still carrying the diagnosis pMCTD after follow-up of more than 5 years. The nationwide Norwegian follow-up showed that pMCTD most frequently evolved into a sclerodermatous phenotype, followed by SLE-like disease. After a mean follow-up of 16 years, fully 67% still had active disease.

Mortality rates in adults have been reported to be as high as 25%, with the worst prognosis associated with severe Raynaud phenomenon and clinical features of scleroderma at presentation. Infection is the leading cause of death, followed by cardiac complications or pulmonary hypertension and renal failure. The only pediatric study to examine this issue showed a much lower mortality rate of 5.1% at mean follow-up of 16 years.

## SUGGESTED READINGS


Ambrose N, Morgan TA, Galloway J, et al. Differences in disease phenotype and severity in SLE across age groups. *Lupus*. 2016;25(14):1542-1550.

Barsalou J, Bradley TJ, Tyrrell PN, et al. Impact of disease duration on vascular surrogates of early atherosclerosis in childhood-onset systemic lupus erythematosus. *Arthritis Rheumatol*. 2016;68(1):237-246.

Chiewchengchol D, Murphy R, Edwards SW, Beresford MW. Mucocutaneous manifestations in juvenile-onset systemic lupus erythematosus: a review of literature. *Pediatr Rheumatol Online J*. 2015;13(1):1.

Fonseca AR, Gaspar-Elsas MI, Land MG, de Oliveira SK. Comparison between three systems of classification criteria in juvenile systemic lupus erythematous. *Rheumatology (Oxford)*. 2015;54(2):241-247.

Gunnarsson R, Hetlevik S, Lilleby V, Molberg Ø. Mixed connective tissue disease. *Best Pract Res Clin Rheumatol*. 2016;30(1):95-111.

Hetlevik SO, Flato B, Rygg M, et al. Long-term outcome in juvenile-onset mixed connective tissue disease: a nationwide Norwegian study. *Ann Rheum Dis*. 2017;76(1):159-165.

Hiraki LT, Benseler SM, Tyrrell PN, Harvey E, Hebert D, Silverman ED. Ethnic differences in pediatric systemic lupus erythematosus. *J Rheumatol*. 2009;36(11):2539-2546.

Olsen NJ, Karp DR. Autoantibodies and SLE—the threshold for disease. *Nat Rev Rheumatol*. 2014;10(3):181-186.

Petri M, Orbai AM, Alarcon GS, et al. Derivation and validation of the Systemic Lupus International Collaborating Clinics classification criteria for systemic lupus erythematosus. *Arthritis Rheum*. 2012;64(8):2677-2686.

Pineles D, Valente A, Warren B, Peterson MG, Lehman TJ, Moorthy LN. Worldwide incidence and prevalence of pediatric onset systemic lupus erythematosus. *Lupus*. 2011;20(11):1187-1192.

Tellier S, Bader-Meunier B, Quartier P, et al. Initial presentation and outcome of pediatric-onset mixed connective tissue disease: a French multicenter retrospective study. *Joint Bone Spine*. 2016;83(3):369-371.

Thorbinson C, Oni L, Smith E, Midgley A, Beresford MW. Pharmacological management of childhood-onset systemic lupus erythematosus. *Paediatr Drugs*. 2016;18(3):181-195.

# 202 Juvenile Dermatomyositis

Lisa G. Rider

## INTRODUCTION

*Juvenile dermatomyositis* (JDM), a systemic autoimmune disease with onset in childhood, is characterized by chronic skeletal muscle and cutaneous inflammation of unknown cause. JDM is relatively responsive to immunosuppressive therapy, and rapid diagnosis and adequate therapy improve outcomes.

JDM is the most common clinical subset of a larger family of disorders known as the *idiopathic inflammatory myopathies* (IIMs) (Table 202-1). Juvenile polymyositis (JPM), which constitutes 4% to 8% of childhood myositis cases, has similar features without the characteristic cutaneous manifestations, but patients with JPM often have more severe and distal weakness. Overlap myositis, which constitutes 6% to 12% of childhood IIM, occurs when JDM or JPM is associated with another autoimmune disease, such as systemic lupus erythematosus, scleroderma, juvenile idiopathic arthritis, systemic vasculitis, or type 1 diabetes mellitus. JDM and JPM also have been reported in combination with primary immunodeficiencies, such as Wiskott-Aldrich syndrome and common variable immunodeficiency, without apparent infectious triggers. Other clinical forms of IIMs rarely have been described in children and include clinically amyopathic dermatomyositis (DM), as well as focal, orbital, cancer-associated, eosinophilic, granulomatous myositis and immune-mediated necrotizing myopathy (see Table 202-1).

The juvenile IIMs are also classified based on certain autoantibodies that are present specifically in myositis patients (myositis-specific autoantibodies) as well as other autoantibodies that are present in myositis patients and patients with other autoimmune diseases (myositis-associated autoantibodies). These autoantibodies help to define patients with similar clinical and demographic features, to predict responses to therapy, and to determine prognosis (Table 202-2). The most common of these autoantibodies in juvenile IIMs include anti-p155/140 (transcriptional intermediary factor-1 [TIF-1]), anti-MJ, and anti-melanoma-differentiation-associated gene 5 (MDA5) autoantibodies. The myositis autoantibodies have been increasingly recognized, with as many as 75% of patients with juvenile IIM currently having a defined specificity. New specificities continue to be identified.

## EPIDEMIOLOGY

In various countries around the world, the annual incidence of JDM and JPM ranges from 1.5 to 5 cases per 1 million children. In the United States, an estimate from a national registry of new-onset JDM cases was 3.2 cases per million children per year. JDM and JPM are 3.5- to 5-fold less common than are adult DM and polymyositis. JDM has a median age at onset at approximately 7 years, with a bimodal age distribution peaking first at 3 to 7 years and second during the early teenage years. Girls are affected 2 to 4 times more frequently than are boys. The incidence is similar in different racial groups, with the overall racial distribution similar to that of the general population.

**TABLE 202-1 CLINICAL CLASSIFICATION OF THE JUVENILE IDIOPATHIC INFLAMMATORY MYOPATHIES (IIMs)**

| Subgroup | Important Features |
|---|---|
| Juvenile dermatomyositis (JDM) | Characteristic skin rashes of Gottron papules on extensor surfaces or heliotrope rash over eyelids, with chronic, progressive, proximal, and axial weakness. CD4+ T cells and plasmacytoid dendritic cells in muscle in perivascular distribution with resultant type I interferon signature. Calcinosis is present in 25–40%, cutaneous or gastrointestinal ulceration in up to 25%, and lipodystrophy in 10% of patients; may have systemic manifestations. Accounts for 85% of juvenile IIM. |
| Myositis associated with another autoimmune disease (overlap myositis) | Patients meet criteria for myositis and another autoimmune disease. Overlap with scleroderma, systemic lupus erythematosus, or juvenile idiopathic arthritis is most common in children. Raynaud phenomenon, interstitial lung disease, arthritis, and calcinosis are more frequent in this subgroup. Higher mortality, related to lung disease. Seen in 6–12% of juvenile IIM. |
| Polymyositis | Characteristic skin rashes are absent. May have severe weakness, including distal weakness, falling episodes, higher serum creatine kinase level, myalgia, more frequent cardiac involvement. Pathogenesis involves CD8+ muscle endomysial inflammation. Seen in 4–8% of juvenile IIM. |
| Clinically amyopathic dermatomyositis | Typical JDM skin rashes without muscle involvement for at least 2 years, or with subclinical muscle involvement detected by additional testing (elevated serum muscle enzymes, abnormal electromyogram, magnetic resonance imaging, or muscle biopsy). Calcinosis, cutaneous ulcerations, and interstitial lung disease are lower in frequency, and associated malignancy has not been reported, in contrast to adults where these features are more frequent. Seen in 1% of juvenile IIM. |
| Focal myositis | Most often presents as an enlarged mass within the affected muscle, which is usually painful or tender to palpation. The most common sites of involvement are the thighs and calves, followed by neck. Seen in 1–2% of juvenile IIM. |
| Orbital myositis | A form of focal myositis involving the extraocular muscles. Presents with orbital pain worsened by eye movement. Diplopia, proptosis, conjunctival injection, periorbital edema, and globe retraction with narrowing of the palpebral fissure, in the presence of normal visual acuity, are common symptoms. Seen in 1–2% of juvenile IIM. |
| Immune-mediated necrotizing myopathy | Polymyositis or dermatomyositis in which the muscle biopsy demonstrates prominent muscle necrosis, myophagocytosis, and little inflammation. Thought to be mediated by autoantibodies, including anti–signal recognition particle or anti-3-hydroxy-3-methylglutaryl-coenzyme A reductase autoantibodies. Seen in approximately 1% of juvenile IIM. |
| Cancer-associated myositis | Myositis develops within 2 years of a diagnosis of cancer. Solid organ tumors, lymphoma, and leukemia reported. Only a few case reports in children, mainly with atypical cases of JDM. Screening for malignancy is not performed routinely in the evaluation of children with myositis. Prominent adenopathy, hepatosplenomegaly, palpable masses, and atypical rashes suggest possible malignancy. Seen in less than 1% of juvenile IIM. |
| Granulomatous myositis | Granulomas prominent in muscle, often with distal weakness. Primarily idiopathic or associated with Wegener granulomatosis, sarcoidosis, or tuberculosis in pediatric cases. Case reports in juvenile IIM. |
| Macrophagic myofasciitis | Myositis of the deltoids or quadriceps that is predominantly macrophagic. Childhood cases may also present with hypotonia, developmental delay, and failure to thrive. Intramuscular injection of aluminum-adjuvant vaccines predates diagnosis and may be responsible. Seen in < 1% of juvenile IIM. |
| Eosinophilic myositis | Prominent eosinophilic infiltrates on muscle biopsy, associated with peripheral eosinophilia. Generally requires treatment with corticosteroids. It is important to exclude muscular dystrophies, including calpainopathy, Becker dystrophy, and gamma-sarcoglycanopathy, which can present with eosinophilic myositis. Case reports in juvenile IIM. |

Data from Rider LG, Katz JD, Jones OY. Developments in the classification and treatment of the juvenile idiopathic inflammatory myopathies, *Rheum Dis Clin North Am*. 2013 Nov; 39(4):877-904.

**TABLE 202-2 MYOSITIS-SPECIFIC AND MYOSITIS-ASSOCIATED AUTOANTIBODIES IN JUVENILE IDIOPATHIC INFLAMMATORY MYOPATHIES**

| Myositis-Specific Autoantibodies | Associated Clinical Features |
|---|---|
| Anti-p155/140 (TIF-1) | Patients often have extensive photosensitive skin rashes, including characteristic rashes of juvenile dermatomyositis (JDM), but also malar rash, V- and shawl sign rashes, linear extensor erythema, and periungual capillary changes. Cutaneous ulceration, edema, and generalized lipodystrophy are also more frequent. Most frequently have a chronic illness course. Present in 23–30% of patients with JDM, can also be seen in overlap dermatomyositis, and is associated with cancer in adult dermatomyositis, but not in children. |
| Anti-MJ (NXP-2) | Associated with frequent muscle cramps, joint contractures, muscle atrophy, and dysphonia. Patients tend to be weaker and have lower physical function, with some reports of increased frequency of calcinosis. Characteristic Gottron papules and heliotrope and malar rashes are present, but truncal rashes are absent. More frequent hospitalizations, less frequent remission, and associated gastrointestinal ulceration. Associated primarily with dermatomyositis, but also polymyositis or overlap myositis, present in 20–25% of juvenile myositis patients. |
| Anti-MDA5 | Associated with JDM or clinically amyopathic JDM. Seen in 8% of American/British patients and 33% of Japanese patients. Frequent interstitial lung disease, which may be chronic or rapidly progressive, with the latter associated with higher mortality. Mild muscle disease, frequent arthritis, and oral and cutaneous ulcerations. |
| Anti-synthetase autoantibodies | Moderate to severe dermatomyositis or polymyositis frequently associated with arthritis, interstitial lung disease, fevers, Raynaud phenomenon, and mechanic's hands. Anti-Jo-1 is the most common anti-synthetase autoantibody. Present in up to 5–10% of juvenile myositis patients with dermatomyositis, polymyositis, or overlap myositis. Associated with higher mortality. |
| Anti-signal recognition particle | Very severe polymyositis or immune-mediated necrotizing myopathy with proximal and distal weakness, frequent falling episodes, wheelchair use, cardiac involvement, Raynaud phenomenon, and very high creatine kinase levels. Refractory to multiple immunosuppressive therapies. Patients uniformly have a chronic illness course. Seen in 1% of juvenile myositis patients. |
| Anti-Mi-2 | Typical dermatomyositis features, with mild to moderate disease, more severe muscle biopsy features. Usually responsive to therapy. Present in as many as 5% of cases of JDM or overlap myositis with dermatomyositis; more common in Hispanic patients. |
| **Myositis-Associated Autoantibodies** | **Associated Clinical Features** |
| Anti-PM-Scl | Associated with myositis-scleroderma overlap. Myositis is usually mild, and there is a high frequency of arthritis, Raynaud phenomenon, calcinosis, and interstitial lung disease. |
| Anti-URNP | Seen in 12–27% of patients with juvenile polymyositis or overlap myositis. Associated with arthritis, Raynaud phenomenon, and sclerodactyly. |
| Anti-Ro | Seen in myositis overlap syndromes as well as JDM and polymyositis, in 5–15% of patients. Little known about clinical associations. |
| Anti-Ku | Associated with myositis-scleroderma overlap syndrome (2% of patients), with frequent Raynaud phenomenon, arthralgia, and gastroesophageal reflux. |

Data from Rider LG, Katz JD, Jones OY. Developments in the classification and treatment of the juvenile idiopathic inflammatory myopathies. *Rheum Dis Clin North Am.* 2013;39:877-904. Rider LG, Nistala K. The juvenile idiopathic inflammatory myopathies: pathogenesis, clinical and autoantibody phenotypes, and outcomes. *J Internal Med.* 2016;280(1): 24-38.

## GENETICS AND PATHOPHYSIOLOGY

Evidence for genetic risk factors includes increased prevalence of other autoimmune diseases in relatives of patients with IIM. In white patients, the 8.1 ancestral haplotype of the major histocompatibility complex (MHC) locus DRB1*03:01 _ DQB1*02:01 _ B*08:01 _ DPB1*01:01 _ C*02:02 is the major risk factor for JDM, with DRB1*03:01 the strongest risk factor allele for JDM in the 8.1 complex. Patients with autoantibodies have different human leukocyte antigen (HLA) risk factor alleles, with the anti-p155/140 (TIF-1) autoantibody associated with DQA1*03:01. A genome-wide association study found that other single-nucleotide polymorphisms outside the MHC region that are risk factors for other autoimmune diseases are also risk factors for JDM. These single-nucleotide polymorphisms include phospholipase C-like 1, B lymphoid tyrosine kinase, and chemokine (C-C motif) ligand 21.

JDM is a polygenic disorder, and other polymorphic loci appear to be risk factors in white patients with JDM. These loci include the tumor necrosis factor-α (TNF-α) polymorphism TNFα-308A, which is associated with an increase in stimulated peripheral blood mononuclear cell production of TNF-α. This allele has been found to be a severity factor that is associated with the development of calcinosis and a chronic illness course. Several interleukin-1 (IL-1) polymorphisms have also been associated with calcinosis. Other loci are currently being investigated as possible risk factors.

Evidence supporting a role for environmental triggers in the pathogenesis of juvenile IIMs includes an association with ultraviolet light exposure in the month before onset of illness, based on residential location, in patients with JDM and with the anti-p155/140 (TIF-1) myositis autoantibody. A case-controlled epidemiologic study from Brazil has suggested maternal smoking and secondhand smoke during pregnancy, maternal occupational exposure to school chalk dust or gasoline vapor, and inhalation exposure to carbon monoxide during late pregnancy as risk factors for development of JDM. Subgroups of patients with JDM, including Hispanic patients, those with the HLA-DRB1*03:01 risk-factor allele, or those with the anti-p155/140 (TIF-1) autoantibody, have seasonal birth distributions that differ from patients without those features, suggesting a role for perinatal factors in the development of JDM. In addition, most children with JDM report an antecedent respiratory or gastrointestinal infection within 3 months before onset of symptoms, further supporting the suggestion that environmental factors potentially affect the development of JDM. Group A β-hemolytic *Streptococcus* has been associated as a risk factor in a case-control study, and other organisms, including coxsackievirus B, influenza, parvovirus, and *Toxoplasma*, have been variably associated with onset of JDM and inconsistently detected in affected muscle by polymerase chain reaction.

Pathologically, affected muscle and cutaneous tissues demonstrate chronic perivascular and perimysial inflammation, with a predominance of plasmacytoid dendritic cells, CD4+ T cells, and macrophages. Gene expression profiling studies reveal an upregulation of the type I interferon pathway in the muscle, skin, and peripheral blood of patients with JDM and a correlation between type I interferon-inducible genes and disease activity in JDM and other inflammatory myopathies. In JDM, there is also prominent upregulation of T-helper type 17 cells and associated pathway cytokines, such as IL-6. There is also oligoclonal expansion of CD8+ T cells and restricted T-cell receptor V gene usage. TNF-α, IL-1α and IL-1β, IL-8, and transforming growth factor-β, as well as a number of other pro- and anti-inflammatory cytokines, are also variably produced by affected muscle. The role of myositis autoantibodies in the disease's pathogenesis is unresolved. However, the target autoantigens are upregulated on the cell surface of regenerating myoblasts, and some of the myositis autoantibodies promote type I interferon activation or chemokine production. An upregulation of MHC class I on muscle cells from patients with IIM also leads to activation of the endoplasmic reticulum stress response and ongoing inflammation and muscle damage.

Several promoters and inhibitors of angiogenesis as well as genes promoting endothelial differentiation and activation are overexpressed in the affected muscle tissue of patients with IIMs. In JDM, angiostatic chemokines have elevated expression and correlate with the degree of capillary loss and mononuclear cell infiltration. Upregulation of leukocyte adhesion molecules on the muscle arterioles and venules, particularly intercellular adhesion molecule-1, results in the infiltration of B and CD4+ T lymphocytes, dendritic cells, and macrophages. Proinflammatory cytokines result in damage and further infiltration of cells.

## CLINICAL FEATURES AND COMPLICATIONS

JDM is a systemic disease, with involvement of a number of organ systems (Table 202-3). Symptoms commonly develop over a period of weeks to months, although the disease occasionally presents acutely.

Patients with JDM most often present initially with rash followed by muscle weakness. Characteristic rashes of JDM include the heliotrope rash (Fig. 202-1) and Gottron papules. The heliotrope rash is a faint lilac to erythematous discoloration over the eyelids that may be accompanied by periorbital edema. Gottron papules are erythematous plaques on the extensor surfaces, particularly overlying the small joints of the hands (Fig. 202-2) but also frequently over the elbows, knees (Fig. 202-3), and ankles. One of those characteristic rashes is present in virtually all children with JDM. Periungual capillary changes, including dilatation, dropout, and tortuosity, are seen in more than 90% of patients. This sign might reflect vasculopathy and active disease in other organs, particularly in the skin (Fig. 202-4). Overgrowth of the cuticle onto the nailbed also may be seen. Malar rash, facial erythema, V-sign and shawl sign rashes over the anterior neck and upper back involving the shoulders, and other erythematous rashes involving both sun-exposed and covered areas are also common manifestations. Cutaneous ulceration resulting from vasculopathy of dermal vessels is a serious complication associated with more severe illness, but it is seen in fewer than 25% of patients.

Muscle weakness is characteristically progressive and chronic and involves the proximal limb and axial muscles, although distal muscle weakness is evident in more severely affected children. The first muscular symptoms of JDM may be fatigue, decreased endurance, or muscle pain. A subtle decrease in activity and inability to keep up with peers in sports and play activities is followed by progressive inability to perform daily life activities involving the proximal and axial muscles, such as climbing stairs, combing or shampooing the hair, bathing, and dressing. If those symptoms remain untreated, after weeks or months, the child may become unable to rise from a chair or bed. Many children exhibit the Gower sign, that is, difficulty rising from the floor due to hip extensor weakness, and they use their hands to climb up the legs as an aid. Weakness progresses at a variable and unpredictable pace in different children, and not all patients progress to the most severe stages, described below.

Dystrophic calcification of the skin, subcutaneous tissue, or muscle, often at pressure-point sites, is seen in 15% to 45% of patients with JDM (Fig. 202-5). Its development is associated with a delay in diagnosis and treatment, more severe disease, a chronic or polycyclic illness course with more longstanding active disease, and cardiopulmonary involvement. Calcinosis typically becomes evident 1 to 3 years after onset of the illness. Cellulitis, skin breakdown, joint contractures, or ulceration can develop at the deposit sites. Calcinosis can resolve over an unpredictable time frame; progression of calcifications, however, generally is indicative of ongoing active disease.

Involvement of the striated and smooth muscle of the gastrointestinal tract resulting in dysphagia or difficulty handling secretions is a sign of severe disease requiring aggressive treatment and may be present in as many as 40% of patients. Such patients are at risk for developing aspiration pneumonia. Subclinical abnormalities on modified barium swallow examination may be seen in as many as 80% of patients with JDM. Vasculitis of the gastrointestinal tract, observed in fewer than 10% of patients with JDM, may result in severe abdominal pain, gastrointestinal bleeding, or perforation. Abdominal pain that is persistent, progressive, or severe should be evaluated carefully, and stool should be tested for occult blood. Children not at imminent risk of perforation can undergo barium examination or contrast-enhanced computed tomography, which might demonstrate dilation or thickening of the bowel wall, intraluminal air, or evidence of bowel necrosis. Lower gastrointestinal tract dysmotility, resulting in constipation, abdominal pain, or bloating, also occurs as a result of smooth muscle involvement.

Palatal involvement leading to hoarseness and dysphonia is seen in as many as 30% of patients. Respiratory muscle weakness with dyspnea on exertion and restrictive lung disease is seen frequently;

**TABLE 202-3 SIGNS AND SYMPTOMS ASSOCIATED WITH JUVENILE DERMATOMYOSITIS**

| Sign or Symptom | Frequency in JDM (%) |
|---|---|
| **Musculoskeletal** | |
| Progressive proximal muscle weakness | 100 |
| Muscle pain or tenderness | 25–83 |
| Myalgia/arthralgia | 25–73 |
| Arthritis | 10–65 |
| Joint contractures | 9–55 |
| Falling episodes | 40 |
| **Cutaneous** | |
| Heliotrope rash | 66–100 |
| Gottron papules | 57–100 |
| Periungual nailfold capillary changes | 35–91 |
| Malar/facial rash | 42–73 |
| Photosensitive rashes | 5–51 |
| Limb edema | 11–34 |
| Calcinosis | 5–34 |
| Skin ulcers | 5–30 |
| Gingivitis | 6–30 |
| V- or shawl sign rash | 19–29 |
| Raynaud phenomenon | 9–28 |
| Lipodystrophy | 4–14 |
| Alopecia | 10 |
| Sclerodactyly/mechanic's hands | 4–7 |
| **Constitutional** | |
| Fatigue | 80–100 |
| Lymphadenopathy | 8–75 |
| Fever | 16–65 |
| Weight loss | 33–36 |
| Anorexia | 18 |
| **Gastrointestinal, Pulmonary, Cardiac** | |
| Dysphagia or dysphonia | 15–44 |
| Dyspnea | 7–43 |
| Gastrointestinal symptoms (nausea, abdominal pain, constipation, gastroesophageal reflux) | 5–38 |
| Cardiac involvement | 2–13 |
| Interstitial lung disease | 5–8 |
| Gastrointestinal bleeding or ulceration | 3–4 |

Data from Shah M, Mamyrova G, Targoff IN, et al. The clinical phenotypes of the juvenile idiopathic inflammatory myopathies. *Medicine (Baltimore)*. 2013;92(1):25-41; Ramanan AV, Feldman BM. Clinical features and outcomes of juvenile dermatomyositis and other childhood onset myositis syndromes. *Rheum Dis Clin North Am*. 2002;28:833-858; McCann LJ, Juggins AD, Maillard SM, et al. The Juvenile Dermatomyositis National Registry and Repository (UK and Ireland)—clinical characteristics of children recruited within the first 5 yr. *Rheumatology (Oxford)*. 2006;45(10):1255-60.

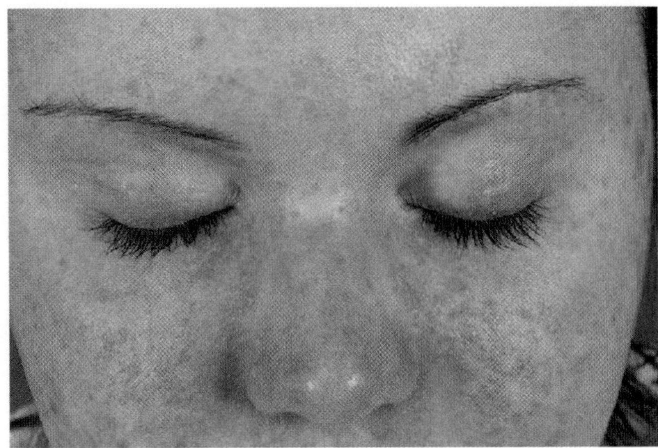

**FIGURE 202-1** Heliotrope rash, a purplish discoloration over the eyelids with associated periorbital edema, which is characteristic of dermatomyositis. This child also has a malar rash.



however, interstitial lung disease is relatively infrequent in juvenile IIM, occurring most frequently in patients with overlap myositis or in those with anti-synthetase or anti-MDA5 autoantibodies. Arthritis is present in two-thirds of patients and typically involves the knees, wrists, elbows, or interphalangeal joints. Contractures of large joints often accompany severe, persistent muscle weakness or may be seen in isolation. Tenosynovitis also may be present. Constitutional symptoms, including fatigue, fever, Raynaud phenomenon, and lymphadenopathy, may be noted, particularly at the onset of the illness.

Growth failure and osteoporosis are common manifestations, resulting from either active disease or prolonged treatment with glucocorticoids. Insulin resistance and hyperlipidemia, in isolation or in conjunction with partial or total lipodystrophy (Fig. 202-6), increasingly have been recognized in association with long-standing, active JDM.

Numerous other manifestations of JDM have been reported infrequently. They include cardiac disease with arrhythmias, pericarditis, or myocarditis; pulmonary involvement with pneumomediastinum or pneumothorax; hypoalbuminemia resulting in diffuse edema; gastrointestinal complications, including hepatitis and cholestasis; hematologic sequelae, such as hemolytic anemia, thrombocytopenia, and myelofibrosis; neurologic manifestations, including central nervous system vasculitis, peripheral neuropathy, and retinopathy; and genitourinary involvement with reports of myoglobinuria, testicular inflammation, and ureteral necrosis of the middle segment of the renal pelvis.

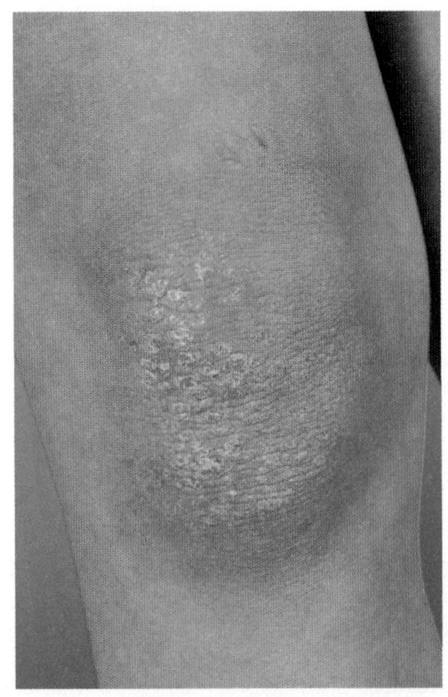

**FIGURE 202-3** Gottron papule overlying the knee.

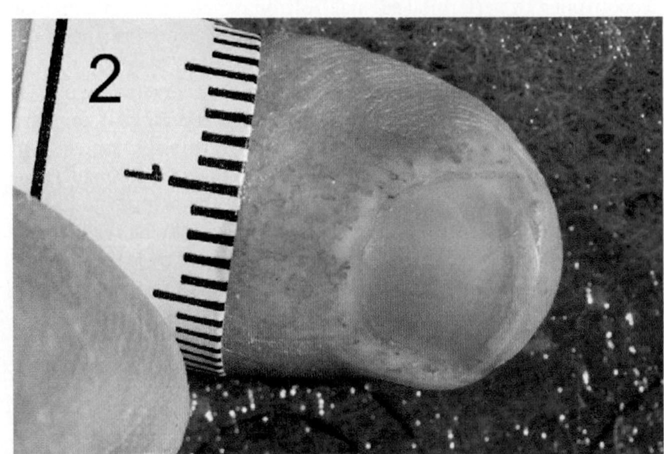


**FIGURE 202-4** Dilation, dropout, and tortuosity of periungual nailfold capillaries and bushy loop formation, which are some of the frequent nailfold vessel changes present in patients with juvenile dermatomyositis.

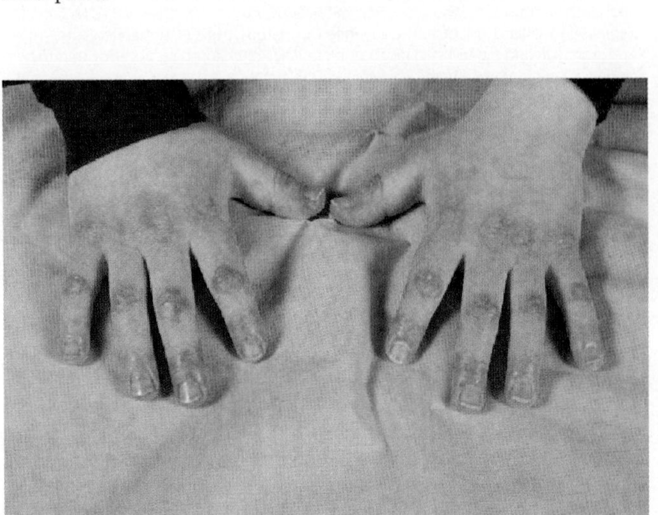

**FIGURE 202-2** Gottron papules. Raised erythematous plaques over joint extensor surfaces, here over the finger joints, which are generally symmetric and characteristic of dermatomyositis.

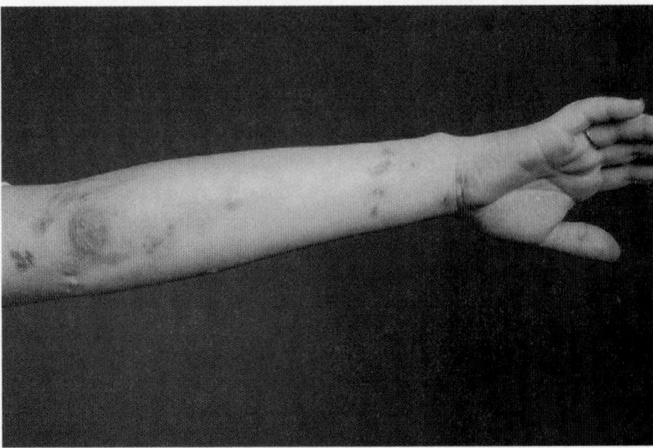

**FIGURE 202-5** Calcinosis, here seen as superficial nodules along the arm and wrist in a girl with juvenile dermatomyositis. Some lesions have depressed scars at sites of previous lesions that have extruded through the skin. Note the Gottron papule over the elbow joint.

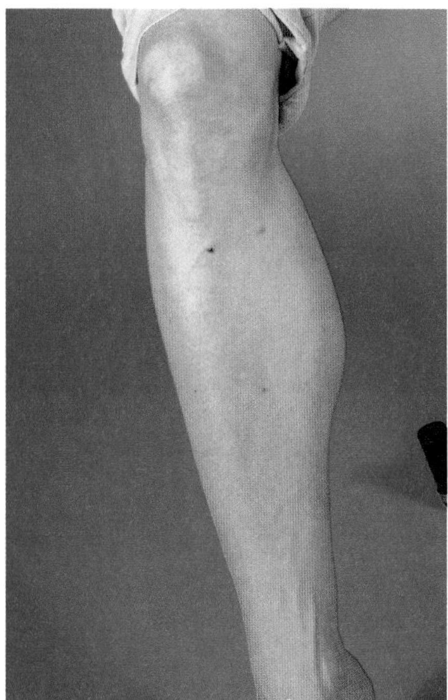

**FIGURE 202-6** Partial lipodystrophy, with subcutaneous loss of fat in the calf and thigh, and an impression of calf hypertrophy, in a young woman with juvenile dermatomyositis.

**TABLE 202-4 CRITERIA FOR THE DIAGNOSIS OF DERMATOMYOSITIS AND POLYMYOSITIS**

Definite disease: for dermatomyositis, inclusion of the rash and presence of 3 other criteria; for polymyositis, exclusion of rash and presence of the other 4 criteria.

Probable disease: for dermatomyositis, inclusion of the rash and presence of 2 other criteria; for polymyositis, exclusion of rash and presence of 3 other criteria.

1. Symmetric, often progressive proximal and axial weakness
2. Characteristic rashes of dermatomyositis (required)
   a. Scaly, erythematous papules over the metacarpophalangeal or interphalangeal joints, elbows, knees, or medial malleoli (Gottron papules) OR
   b. Purplish or erythematous discoloration of the eyelids (heliotrope rash)
3. Elevation of serum levels of muscle-associated enzymes, including creatine kinase, aldolase, lactate dehydrogenase, transaminases
4. Characteristic electromyographic changes in a triad, including:
   a. Short-duration, small, low-amplitude polyphasic potentials
   b. Fibrillation potentials, positive sharp waves, and insertional irritability, present even at rest
   c. Bizarre high-frequency repetitive discharges
5. Evidence of chronic inflammation on muscle biopsy, including the presence of necrosis of type I and type II muscle fibers, degeneration and regeneration of myofibers with variation in myofiber size, perivascular and interstitial infiltration of mononuclear cells, and perifascicular atrophy

These criteria require exclusion of all other forms of myopathies.

Data from Bohan A, Peter JB. Polymyositis and dermatomyositis (first of two parts). *N Engl J Med.* 1975;292:344-347. Bohan A, Peter JB. Polymyositis and dermatomyositis (second of two parts). *N Engl J Med.* 1975;292:403-407.

Laboratory abnormalities include elevated serum levels of muscle enzymes, including creatine kinase, transaminases, lactate dehydrogenase, and aldolase. Serum creatine kinase is elevated in two-thirds of patients with JDM and often returns to normal early in the illness, so the other serum muscle enzymes need to be followed in order to monitor the disease's activity later in its course. Two international collaborative study groups have standardized and validated measures of disease activity and disease damage.

## DIAGNOSIS

The diagnosis of JDM often is made using the classification criteria of Bohan and Peter, which require the presence of the characteristic skin findings of heliotrope rash or Gottron papules. An additional 2 of the other 4 criteria are necessary to classify a patient as having "probable" JDM, and 3 are necessary to qualify as having "definite" JDM (Table 202-4). Other forms of myopathy must be excluded to confirm a diagnosis. Only 30% to 55% of pediatric rheumatologists use electromyography, and only 50% to 60% perform a muscle biopsy to diagnose JDM, suggesting that many diagnoses of JDM can only be called "probable" by the Bohan and Peter criteria. Muscle edema on magnetic resonance imaging (MRI) is used by most North American pediatric rheumatologists to confirm a diagnosis of myositis. New classification criteria for myositis have been developed. A diagnosis of "probable" JPM requires the presence of 3 criteria, and "definite" JPM requires 4 criteria. JPM is characterized by muscle weakness without the characteristic rashes of JDM, rendering differentiation from other myopathies more difficult. Thus, it is recommended that patients suspected of having JPM undergo a muscle biopsy.

MRI of the thigh muscles is useful to confirm a diagnosis, to select a site for a directed muscle biopsy, and to assess disease activity when the extent of myositis is unclear. During active phases of illness, edema in the muscles, myofascia, subcutaneous tissue, or skin may be evident on the short tau inversion recovery (STIR) or fat-suppressed T2 images (Fig. 202-7A), whereas T1-weighted images can demonstrate muscle atrophy and fatty infiltration (Fig. 202-7B). The presence of muscle edema is not specific for myositis and can also be seen in muscular dystrophies and other inflammatory myopathies.

More than 70% of patients with JDM have a positive antinuclear antibody. The presence of a myositis-specific autoantibody can help confirm a diagnosis in the approximately 75% of patients with juvenile IIM who demonstrate these markers. The myositis-specific autoantibodies are directed against cellular translational proteins and transcription factors that are found only in patients meeting diagnostic criteria for an IIM. Tests for myositis-specific and myositis-associated autoantibodies using immunoprecipitation and immunoblotting methods are reliable but are available only in a few laboratories. The epidemiologic and clinical features, as well as therapeutic responses and outcomes for each autoantibody subset, appear to be distinct and have many similarities with corresponding subsets of adult IIM patients (see Table 202-2). Juvenile and adult patients with IIM and anti-synthetase autoantibodies, for example, have severe muscle weakness frequently in association with arthritis, fever, interstitial lung disease, Raynaud phenomenon, and mechanic's hands. In these patients, myositis often flares when glucocorticoids are reduced, and they often require cytotoxic therapies and have a chronic illness course. Juvenile and adult patients with polymyositis and antisignal recognition particle autoantibodies have severe proximal and distal weakness and extremely elevated serum creatine kinase levels. They often have a chronic illness course and require multiple cytotoxic therapies because they respond poorly to most treatments.

Recently, a myositis-specific autoantibody, anti-p155/140 (TIF-1), has been detected by protein immunoprecipitation and immunoblotting in 23% to 30% of patients with JDM, 20% of adult patients with DM, and in most adult patients with cancer-associated DM. Patients with this autoantibody have typical features of DM with prominent photosensitive rashes. Pediatric patients tend to have more extensive cutaneous involvement, including a higher frequency of cutaneous ulcerations, subcutaneous edema, and lipodystrophy, and most often have a chronic illness course. Another common myositis autoantibody in patients with juvenile IIM is anti-MJ, seen in 20% to 25% of patients, which is associated with more severe weakness, muscle cramps, muscle atrophy, joint contractures, an absence of truncal rashes, and possibly an increased frequency of calcinosis. Anti-MDA5 autoantibody, the third most common of the myositis-specific autoantibodies in children, is seen in as many as 8% of North American and European patients with JDM or clinically amyopathic JDM. This autoantibody is associated with mild muscle disease, frequent arthritis, interstitial lung disease, and cutaneous ulcerations. These

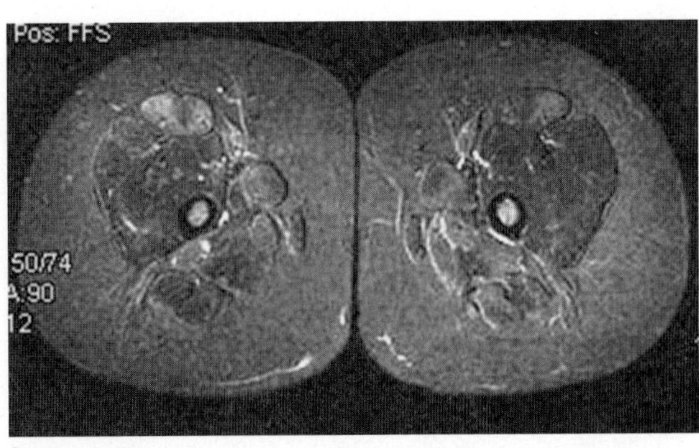


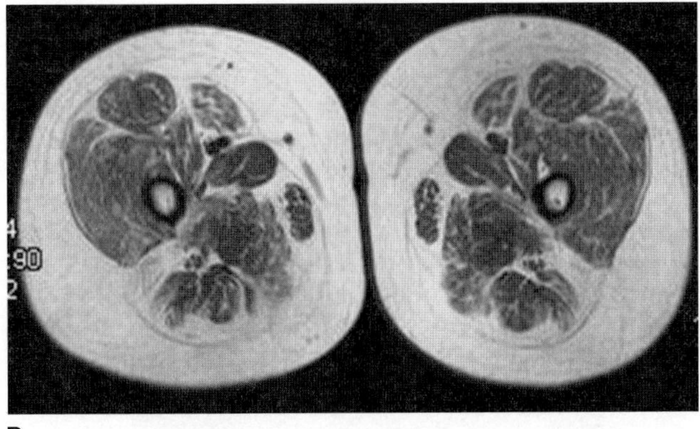


A B

**FIGURE 202-7** **A:** Short tau inversion recovery (STIR) magnetic resonance image of the thighs demonstrating patchy edema in the quadriceps, gluteus medius, and hamstrings in a girl with juvenile dermatomyositis. The edema appears bright or white, in contrast to a dull or gray appearance of normal muscle. **B:** T1 magnetic resonance image of the thighs demonstrating moderate to severe fatty infiltration and muscle atrophy in a girl with juvenile dermatomyositis.



myositis-specific autoantibodies could become important as diagnostic tests when clinical assays become available.

Other tests can also help confirm a diagnosis of IIM and include nailfold capillaroscopy. Although periungual capillary changes are present in as many as 90% of patients with JDM, the abnormalities are not specific to JDM and may be seen in other systemic connective tissue diseases, especially scleroderma and mixed connective tissue disease. A skin biopsy can be used to confirm a diagnosis, demonstrating interface dermatitis, although that condition is not specific for JDM and is seen in systemic lupus erythematosus.

## DIFFERENTIAL DIAGNOSIS

In the differential diagnosis, other conditions must be eliminated, including those with isolated weakness, those in which weakness is associated with cutaneous and even systemic manifestations, and isolated skin conditions that are often confused with the characteristic JDM findings of Gottron papules and heliotrope rash (Table 202-5). Children presenting with signs of a myopathy without cutaneous involvement should have other inflammatory and noninflammatory myopathies excluded prior to establishing a diagnosis of JPM. Noninflammatory myopathies that can mimic JPM include muscular dystrophies, metabolic myopathies, mitochondrial myopathies, and endocrinopathies. Neurologic illnesses, as well as drug-induced myopathies, also should be excluded (see Table 202-3).

Several helpful clues in the history, physical examination, and laboratory results aid in discriminating the IIMs from other myopathies. Patients with an IIM often have a family history of autoimmunity, which is not typical of patients with other myopathies. Patients with JDM and other IIMs generally have symmetric, chronic, proximal, and axial weakness, which contrasts with other myopathies in which the weakness is related to activity or fasting or involves different muscle groups, such as facial or scapular muscles. Patients with myositis develop muscle atrophy after chronic symptoms, whereas patients with other myopathies develop early muscle atrophy or even muscle hypertrophy. Patients with other myopathies may develop cramping, fasciculations, or an associated neuropathy, but those symptoms are rarely present in patients with IIMs. Patients with IIMs often have signs of systemic connective tissue diseases, including fevers, arthritis, periungual capillary nailfold changes, and photosensitive skin rashes. In patients with myositis, serum levels of the enzymes listed above tend to be mildly to moderately elevated, but rarely are they all normal or elevated, as in other myopathies. As many as 70% of patients with juvenile IIM patients have a positive antinuclear antibody. Patients with overlapping systemic sclerosis often have extractable nuclear antibodies. Finally, children with IIMs typically respond to corticosteroids and other immunosuppressive agents, whereas patients with noninflammatory myopathies respond poorly or not at all.

Benign acute childhood myositis is a self-limited illness presenting acutely after a prodromal infectious illness in which myalgia, distal lower extremity weakness, elevated serum muscle enzymes, myoglobinuria, and leukopenia are seen. It is associated with infectious agents, such as influenza, coxsackievirus, varicella, adenovirus, herpesviruses, and *Mycoplasma*. Pyomyositis resulting from *Staphylococcus aureus* and group A *Streptococcus pyogenes* is a localized infection that frequently involves thigh or hip muscles and is associated with fever, muscle pain, and tenderness. Infectious myositis from hepatitis B, human T-lymphotropic virus type 1, and parasitic infections may present with symptoms and biopsy findings identical to those of JPM.

Steroid myopathy should be considered in patients with IIM treated for prolonged periods with high-dose glucocorticoids, particularly in patients experiencing an insidious progression of proximal muscle weakness of the pelvic girdle muscles who have normal serum muscle enzymes and other associated corticosteroid toxicities. Characteristic changes on MRI may help distinguish active muscle inflammation or edema from steroid myopathy, in which muscle edema is absent and hip girdle muscle atrophy and fatty infiltration are prominent.

## TREATMENT

A general treatment algorithm for JDM is provided in Figure 202-8. The goals of treatment include eliminating inflammation of the muscle, skin, and other involved organs; treating and preventing acute life-threatening complications; restoring muscle strength and function; and preventing complications, such as calcinosis and osteoporosis. Therapy must be tailored to each patient according to the disease's severity, prognostic factors, and the likelihood of adverse events developing from medications. Risk factors for poor prognosis include severe and/or chronic disease activity, ulceration, calcification, severe dysphagia, interstitial lung disease, cardiac involvement, certain myositis-specific autoantibodies, muscle biopsy features, delayed treatment, and persistent skin disease activity.

Daily corticosteroid therapy is the foundation of treatment for JDM. It has contributed to a significantly improved prognosis, including a decrease in mortality from 40% in the presteroid era to the current rate of less than 1%. Prednisone is commonly started in the range of 1 to 2 mg/kg daily, often in 2 or 3 divided doses, then consolidated and slowly reduced over months as serum muscle enzymes return to normal and strength improves. Corticosteroids can be continued for 18 months or longer if the illness remains active, although a group of North American pediatric rheumatologists recommends discontinuation within 12 months for many patients. Premature reduction of dose or termination often results in flares of myositis and calcinosis.

Many pediatric rheumatologists also use methotrexate (15 mg/m$^2$ or 1 mg/kg/wk), initiating this medication at diagnosis. A recent therapeutic trial for new-onset JDM indicates that patients benefit

**TABLE 202-5 DIFFERENTIAL DIAGNOSIS OF JUVENILE IDIOPATHIC INFLAMMATORY MYOPATHIES**

| | |
|---|---|
| **Weakness Alone** | |
| Inherited muscle structural protein defects (muscular dystrophies) | Dysferlinopathies, Emery-Dreifuss muscular dystrophy, calpain-3, sarcoglycanopathies, and other limb girdle dystrophies |
| | Facioscapulohumeral dystrophy |
| | Duchenne and Becker dystrophies |
| | Myotonic dystrophies |
| | Other dystrophies |
| Inherited metabolic myopathies | Glycogenoses: phosphorylase deficiency (McArdle disease), acid maltase deficiency, phosphofructokinase deficiency |
| | Lipid storage disorders: carnitine deficiency, palmitoyltransferase deficiency |
| | Myoadenylate deaminase deficiency |
| | Familial periodic paralysis; sodium, potassium, calcium, chloride ion channel disorders |
| Mitochondrial myopathies | Mitochondrial encephalomyopathy, lactic acidosis, stroke (MELAS) |
| | Myoclonic epilepsy, ragged red fibers (MERRF) |
| | Kearns-Sayre syndrome |
| Endocrine myopathies | Hypothyroidism, hyperthyroidism |
| | Cushing syndrome/exogenous steroid myopathy |
| | Diabetes mellitus |
| Drug-induced myopathy | Statins and fibrates, interferon-α, glucocorticoids, hydroxychloroquine, diuretics, -caine anesthetics, growth hormone, cimetidine, cyclosporine, colchicine, D-penicillamine |
| Neurologic disorders | Myasthenia gravis |
| | Guillain-Barre syndrome |
| | Multiple sclerosis |
| **Weakness with or Without Rash** | |
| Infectious myopathies | |
| Viral | Enterovirus, coxsackievirus, echovirus, influenza, parvovirus, poliovirus, hepatitis, human T-cell lymphotropic virus 1, benign acute myositis |
| Bacterial | Group A *Streptococcus*, *Staphylococcus aureus*, pyomyositis, Lyme disease |
| Parasitic | Trichinosis, toxoplasmosis, filariasis, *Trypanosoma*, cysticercosis |
| Systemic autoimmune diseases | Systemic lupus erythematosus (SLE), systemic sclerosis, juvenile idiopathic arthritis (including systemic onset), mixed connective tissue disease, polyarteritis nodosa, and other vasculitides |
| Autoinflammatory diseases | Chronic atypical neutrophilic dermatosis with lipodystrophy and elevated temperature (CANDLE) syndrome, tumor necrosis factor (TNF) receptor–associated periodic syndrome (TRAPS), STING-associated vasculopathy with onset in infancy (SAVI) |
| Other autoimmune diseases | Celiac disease, Crohn disease, ulcerative colitis |
| **Rash Without Weakness** | |
| Hypersensitivity conditions | Seborrheic dermatitis, eczema/atopic dermatitis, allergies, hypersensitivity reaction, contact dermatitis |
| Immune-mediated conditions | Psoriasis, hypereosinophilic syndrome |
| Infections | Verrucae vulgaris, scabies, impetigo |

This is a partial list of conditions in the differential diagnosis of juvenile idiopathic inflammatory myopathies. Muscle biopsy should be strongly considered in the absence of typical juvenile dermatomyositis rashes in order to confirm a diagnosis. For further information, see Feldman BM, Rider LG, Reed AM, Pachman LM. Juvenile dermatomyositis and other idiopathic inflammatory myopathies of childhood. *Lancet*. 2008;371(9631):2201-12; and Pestronk A. Neuromuscular Disease Center, Washington University, St. Louis, MO. Available at: http://neuromuscular.wustl.edu/.

from the combination of methotrexate with prednisone therapy at diagnosis, including greater improvement in disease activity, shorter time to remission, and shorter time to discontinuation of prednison, albeit with increased risk of infection, in patients treated with the combination as compared to prednisone alone. Several retrospective and uncontrolled prospective studies also found that early introduction of methotrexate resulted in a lower likelihood of developing calcinosis and a chronic disease course. Patients who received methotrexate from the start of the illness were able to reduce their dose of corticosteroid more quickly and, therefore, were less likely to experience corticosteroid-related side effects, such as cataracts, weight gain, and impaired height velocity. Benefits of treatment are apparent within 4 to 8 weeks, and methotrexate may be effective for treating cutaneous disease. Intravenous pulse methylprednisolone often is used to obtain rapid control of symptoms and to reduce toxicity from long-term, high-dose daily oral corticosteroids. Parenteral administration can improve bioavailability compared to oral preparations, the absorption of which can be diminished in patients with JDM due to gastrointestinal vasculopathy. Most patients with JDM respond at least partially to first-line therapies.

From the consensus of North American pediatric rheumatologists, additional therapy as part of the initial treatment may also include intravenous pulse doses of methylprednisolone (30 mg/kg) in 3 doses with an option to continue weekly and/or monthly intravenous immunoglobulin (IVIG), particularly in patients with moderately active or severe disease. Additional first-line therapies for managing JDM include photoprotective measures, such as sunscreen and avoidance of exposure to the sun, use of topical steroids and hydroxychloroquine for cutaneous manifestations, and supplemental calcium and vitamin D for patients with inadequate dietary intake. Physical therapy is an integral part of first-line management to improve and prevent joint contractures and to maintain and restore muscle strength and endurance. During active myositis, passive range-of-motion exercises and pool therapy are used. Once the disease is stabilized, isometric strengthening exercises, later followed by isotonic strengthening and aerobic endurance-building exercises, are suggested. Graded exercise therapy does not appear to induce disease flares.

Second-line therapies should be considered in refractory patients, patients with unacceptable corticosteroid toxicity, patients with more severe manifestations, or patients with risk factors for a poor prognosis.

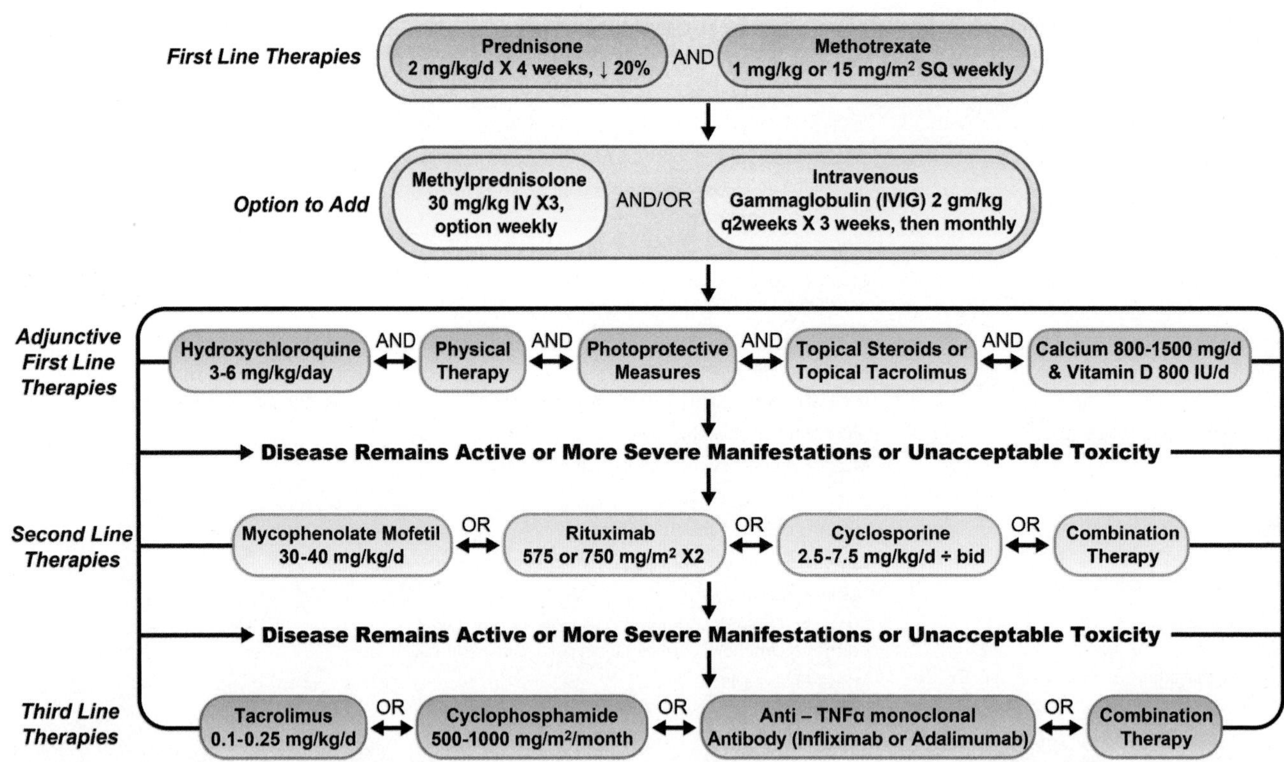


**FIGURE 202-8** Therapeutic algorithm for juvenile dermatomyositis. First-line therapies are based on the consensus treatment protocols for moderately active juvenile dermatomyositis. (See Huber AM, Giannini EH, Bowyer SL, et al. Protocols for the initial treatment of moderately severe juvenile dermatomyositis: results of a Children's Arthritis and Rheumatology Research Alliance Consensus Conference. *Arthritis Care Res (Hoboken)*. 2010;62(2):219-225.) bid, twice daily; d, day; IV, intravenous; IVIG, intravenous immunoglobulin; IU, international units; q, every; SQ, subcutaneous; TNFα, tumor necrosis factor-α.

IVIG is particularly useful in acute settings for patients who are seriously ill or at high risk for development of infection. IVIG may be useful as a short-term agent in JDM, particularly for treating severe cutaneous disease or for treating certain patients with infectious triggers. IVIG has been found to be efficacious in a randomized, placebo-controlled trial in adult DM at a dose of 1 g/kg on each of 2 days each month. A randomized trial of rituximab found it useful in treatment-refractory JDM patients, resulting in clinical improvement and decreased corticosteroid dosage in most patients. Response was greatest in patients with certain myositis autoantibodies associated with higher interferon-chemokine scores and was evident a median of 12 weeks after administration of the infusion. Recent case series support the use of mycophenolate mofetil (20–40 mg/kg/d). Treatment-refractory patients showed improved muscle strength and skin activity and reduced corticosteroid dose. Cyclosporine (2.5–7.5 mg/kg/d) is useful as a steroid-sparing agent, including as a treatment for JDM rashes. It is effective in controlling the activity of JDM but is associated with more adverse events.

For patients with extremely recalcitrant disease, it might be necessary to use combinations of second- and/or third-line therapies. Anecdotal reports and small case series support the use of oral tacrolimus and intravenous cyclophosphamide for patients with severe, refractory disease. Responses to anti-TNF-α agents have been mixed and include reports of disease development or flares after anti-TNF-α therapy. Open-label studies of infliximab report improvement in muscle strength and function, skin rashes, activity of the JDM disease, and calcinosis in the majority of treatment-refractory patients, but an open-label study of etanercept in patients with JDM showed no benefit. Newly available biologic therapies that have been used successfully to treat other autoimmune-mediated diseases have not yet been tested in patients with JDM. Open-label studies in adult patients with myositis and case reports of abatacept (CTLA4-Ig), anakinra (IL-1 receptor antagonist), tocilizumab (IL-6R), sifalimumab (anti–interferon-α monoclonal antibody), and drugs that inhibit Janus kinases suggest that they might benefit treatment-refractory patients. Stem-cell transplantation has been tried in a few patients with myositis but is associated with relatively high mortality rates. Consequently, its use currently is suggested only as a last resort for severe unremitting disease.

Patients with acute, life-threatening complications, such as severe dysphagia, gastrointestinal ulceration associated with bleeding or perforation, myocarditis, or severe, early interstitial lung disease might benefit from repeated pulses of high-dose intravenous methylprednisolone, IVIG, and/or cyclophosphamide. Patients with dysphagia, who have a high risk for developing aspiration pneumonia, often require dietary modifications, including pureed foods, eating upright, or nasojejunal feedings.

Amelioration of underlying myositis disease activity is important to prevent calcinosis and might also improve calcinosis associated with active inflammation. Colchicine has been effective in reducing the acute inflammation associated with dystrophic calcification. No controlled studies have been conducted for treating calcinosis, but anecdotal reports suggest improvement with diltiazem, bisphosphonate therapy, and sodium thiosulfate. In severe circumstances, surgical removal can be attempted once the myositis is quiescent. Progression of calcinosis is de facto evidence of active disease.

## PROGNOSIS AND OUTCOME

Although data on long-term outcomes are limited, prompt diagnosis and treatment have dramatically reduced mortality rates to <3%. Approximately 37% to 60% of patients with JDM recover from the illness within 2 years without clinical relapse, 11% to 37% develop a relapsing-remitting (polycyclic) illness course, and 9% to 52% have continuously active disease longer than 2 years. Calcinosis of varying severity, from minimal to severely debilitating, occurs in 16% to 43% of patients with JDM. As many as 30% of patients have residual weakness or functional disability, and 17% to 40% have ongoing rashes, weakness, and need for medications at more than 3 years of follow-up. A large percentage of patients with clinically inactive disease have reduced tolerance for aerobic exercise. As work on disease biomarkers, genomics, pathogenesis, and new therapies progresses, it is hoped that the outcomes of children with inflammatory myopathies will continue to improve.

## SUGGESTED READINGS


Feldman BM, Rider LG, Reed AM, Pachman LM. Juvenile dermatomyositis and other idiopathic inflammatory myopathies of childhood. *Lancet*. 2008;371:2201-2212.

Huber AM, Giannini EH, Bowyer SL, et al. Protocols for the initial treatment of moderately severe juvenile dermatomyositis: results of a Children's Arthritis and Rheumatology Research Alliance Consensus Conference. *Arthritis Care Res (Hoboken)*. 2010;62(2):219-225.

Khanna S, Reed AM. Immunopathogenesis of juvenile dermatomyositis. *Muscle Nerve*. 2010;41(5):581-592.

Martin N, Li CK, Wedderburn LR. Juvenile dermatomyositis: new insights and new treatment strategies. *Ther Adv Musculoskelet Dis*. 2012;4(1):41-50.

Oddis CV, Reed AM, Aggarwal R, et al. Rituximab in the treatment of refractory adult and juvenile dermatomyositis and adult polymyositis: a randomized, placebo-phase trial. *Arthritis Rheum*. 2013;65(2):314-324.

Pestronk A. Neuromuscular Disease Center, Washington University, St. Louis, MO. http://neuromuscular.wustl.edu/. Accessed July 24, 2016.

Ravelli A, Trail L, Ferrari C, et al. Long-term outcome and prognostic factors of juvenile dermatomyositis: a multinational, multicenter study of 490 patients. *Arthritis Care Res (Hoboken)*. 2010;62(1):63-72.

Rider LG, Katz JD, Jones OY. Developments in the classification and treatment of the juvenile idiopathic inflammatory myopathies. *Rheum Dis Clin North Am*. 2013;39:877-904.

Rider LG, Nistala K. The juvenile idiopathic inflammatory myopathies: pathogenesis, clinical and autoantibody phenotypes, and outcomes. *J Intern Med*. 2016;280(1):24-38.

Robinson AB, Hoeltzel MF, Wahezi DM, et al. Clinical characteristics of children with juvenile dermatomyositis: the Childhood Arthritis and Rheumatology Research Alliance Registry. *Arthritis Care Res (Hoboken)*. 2014;66(3):404-410.

Ruperto N, Pistorio A, Oliveira S, et al. Prednisone versus prednisone plus cyclosporin versus prednisone plus methotrexate in new-onset juvenile dermatomyositis: a randomised trial. *Lancet*. 2016;387(10019):671-678.

Shah M, Mamyrova G, Targoff IN, et al. The clinical phenotypes of the juvenile idiopathic inflammatory myopathies. *Medicine (Baltimore)*. 2013;92(1):25-41.


# 203 Juvenile Scleroderma

Francesco Zulian

## INTRODUCTION

Juvenile scleroderma syndromes are multisystem autoimmune rheumatic diseases for which the unifying characteristic is the development of hard skin before age 16. They can be separated into 2 main categories: 1) juvenile systemic sclerosis (JSSc), characterized by diffuse skin sclerosis involving many sites of the body together with internal organ involvement, and 2) juvenile localized scleroderma (JLS), characterized by circumscribed skin induration but no vascular or internal organ involvement.

## JUVENILE SYSTEMIC SCLEROSIS

JSSc is a chronic multisystem connective tissue disease characterized by the symmetrical thickening and hardening of the skin, associated with fibrous changes in such internal organs as the esophagus, intestinal tract, heart, lungs, and kidneys, plus arthritis and myositis.

**TABLE 203-1 PRELIMINARY CLASSIFICATION CRITERIA FOR JUVENILE SYSTEMIC SCLEROSIS**

| **Major Criterion** | |
|---|---|
| Proximal sclerosis/induration of the skin | |
| **Minor Criteria** | |
| Skin | Sclerodactyly |
| Vascular | Raynaud phenomenon |
| | Nailfold capillary abnormalities |
| | Digital tip ulcers |
| Gastrointestinal | Dysphagia |
| | Gastroesophageal reflux |
| Renal | Renal crisis |
| | New onset arterial hypertension |
| Cardiac | Arrhythmias |
| | Heart failure |
| Respiratory | Pulmonary fibrosis (high-resolution computed tomography/x-ray) |
| | Reduced diffusion capacity for carbon monoxide ($DL_{CO}$) |
| | Pulmonary hypertension |
| Musculoskeletal | Tendon friction rubs |
| | Arthritis |
| | Myositis |
| Neurologic | Neuropathy |
| | Carpal tunnel syndrome |
| Serology | Antinuclear antibodies |
| | SSc selective autoantibodies (anticentromere, antitopoisomerase I, antifibrillarin, anti-PM-Scl, antifibrillin, or antiRNA polymerase I or III) |

Note. A patient, younger than 16 years old, shall be classified as having juvenile systemic sclerosis if a major and at least 2 of the 20 minor criteria are present. This set of classification criteria has 90% sensitivity, 96% specificity, and a κ statistic value of 0.86.

Reproduced with permission from Zulian F, Woo P, Athreya BH, et al. The Pediatric Rheumatology European Society/American College of Rheumatology/European League against Rheumatism provisional classification criteria for juvenile systemic sclerosis, *Arthritis Rheum*. 2007 Mar 15;57(2):203-12.

A Committee on Classification Criteria for JSSc, including pediatricians, rheumatologists, and dermatologists, recently proposed new classification criteria (Table 203-1).

## EPIDEMIOLOGY AND PATHOGENESIS

Systemic sclerosis is a rare condition in any age group. Onset in childhood is particularly uncommon: the estimated incidence is approximately 0.27 cases per million children per year. Children younger than age 16 years account for fewer than 5% of all cases, and fewer than 10% develop systemic sclerosis before reaching age 20. JSSc develops at a mean age of 8.1 years, with a peak incidence between ages 10 and 16. The disease is almost four fold more prevalent in females, but there is no recognized racial predilection.

The cause of systemic sclerosis is unknown, and the pathogenesis appears to be complex. The process involves 3 components: immune activation, endothelial (vascular) damage, and excessive synthesis of extracellular matrix with increased deposition of structurally normal collagen. Genetic factors appear to increase susceptibility to development of systemic sclerosis.

## CLINICAL MANIFESTATIONS

Children developing scleroderma typically present with Raynaud phenomenon and skin changes (Fig. 203-1). Raynaud phenomenon is the first sign of the disease in 70% of patients, and in 10%, it is complicated by digital infarcts (Fig. 203-2). It may precede other manifestations by years. The classical Raynaud attack consists of 3 phases: the first phase reflects vasoconstriction, during which the fingers turn white; this phase is followed by a second phase of bluish discoloration; the third and final phase is reddish discoloration resulting from reperfusion. Raynaud phenomenon mostly occurs distal to the proximal

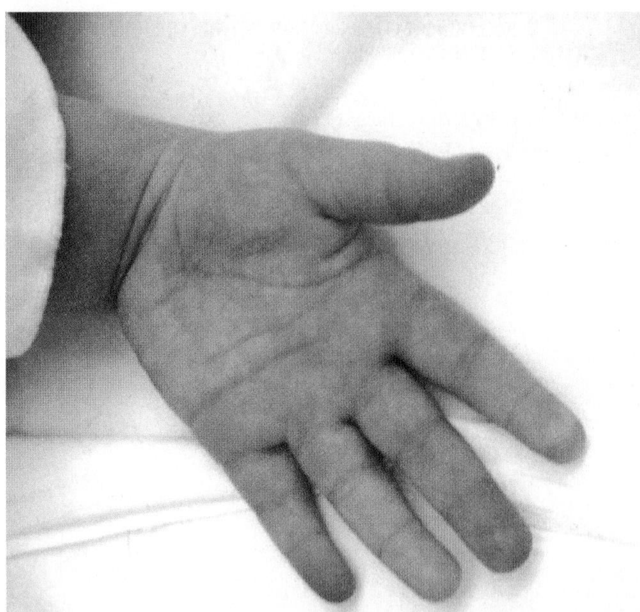

**FIGURE 203-1** Classic Raynaud phenomenon in a 4-year-old girl. Note the ischemic changes (blanching phase) of the second and fourth fingers and the cyanosis (bluish phase) of the fifth finger.



interphalangeal joint of the fingers, and usually the thumbs are spared. Vasospasm is seen more frequently in the fingers but may be observed in other acral regions including the toes, ears, lips, tongue, and tip of the nose.

Proximal skin induration usually develops somewhat later and is the second most common complaint, present in 41% of patients at onset of the disease. Cutaneous changes characteristically evolve in a sequence beginning with edema, followed by induration, and eventually resulting in marked skin tightening and joint contractures. The skin becomes waxy in texture, tight, hard, and bound to subcutaneous structures. It is particularly noticeable in skin of the digits and face, where the characteristic expressionless appearance of the skin may be the first clue to the diagnosis (Fig. 203-3).

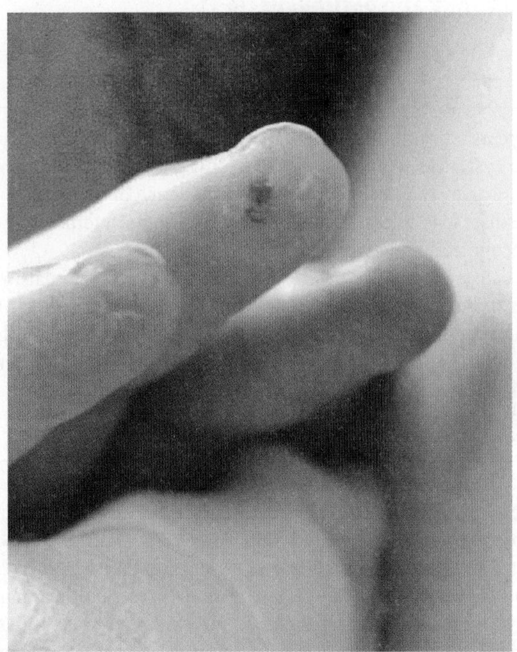

**FIGURE 203-2** Pitting of the fingertips. Note a small ulceration of the tip of the right third finger and shiny, tightly stretched skin over the fingertips.

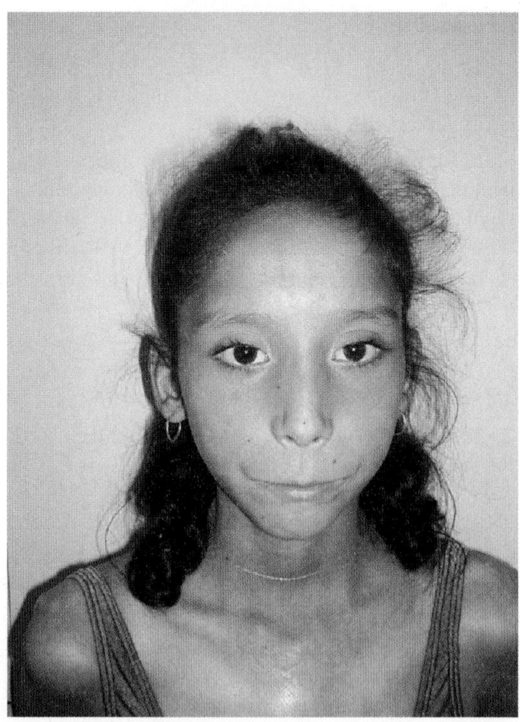

**FIGURE 203-3** Classical expressionless appearance of a 10-year-old girl with systemic sclerosis. Note also the waxy, translucent appearance of the skin in the upper trunk.

Other presenting complaints include arthralgias, arthritis, and, less frequently, muscle weakness, dyspnea, and calcinosis. Unlike adult disease, telangiectasis is rarely present in children with JSSc. Examination of the periungual nailfolds with an ophthalmoscope may demonstrate capillary dropout, tortuous dilated loops, and, occasionally, distorted capillary architecture. As with other manifestations of the disease, changes in the nail bed capillary tend to evolve over time.

In children with JSSc, visceral organ involvement may be widespread; when it occurs, it is associated with significant morbidity. The gastrointestinal and cardiopulmonary systems are most commonly involved, but effects on the kidneys, peripheral nerves, and musculoskeletal system also can lead to significant discomfort and disability. Cardiorespiratory complications are the leading cause of death in children with JSSc.

Gastrointestinal involvement occurs in 30% to 70% of children with JSSc. Most affected patients have esophageal dysfunction, resulting in gastroesophageal reflux and dysphagia (GERD). Aspiration of regurgitated acidic gastric contents may exacerbate to pulmonary disease. Manometry, esophageal scintigraphy, and intraesophageal 24-hour pH monitoring provide more sensitive indicators of diminished lower esophageal sphincter tone and gastroesophageal reflux. Large bowel involvement occurs less frequently and presents as alternating complaints of constipation and diarrhea, bloating, or abdominal discomfort. Lactulose breath test to evaluate bacterial overgrowth, fecal calprotectin, endoscopy, and colon scintigraphy are useful tools to evaluate this portion of the intestinal tract.

Pulmonary involvement, although frequently asymptomatic, may present as a dry, hacking cough or as dyspnea on exertion. Other abnormalities associated with JSSc may include pleuritis, abnormal diffusion capacity for carbon monoxide ($DL_{CO}$) (which may be the earliest manifestation of interstitial fibrosis), or pulmonary arterial hypertension. Unlike adult scleroderma, JSSc is infrequently complicated by pulmonary interstitial fibrosis. The classic radiographic features of interstitial lung disease consist of symmetric, reticulonodular shadowing, most pronounced at the lung bases. High-resolution computed tomography (HRCT) may reveal pulmonary disease, even in the presence of a normal chest radiograph. In children, HRCT findings include ground-glass opacification, subpleural micronodules, linear opacities, and honeycombing. Pulmonary hypertension occurs rarely in pediatric scleroderma. When it develops, it may be either a result of angiopathy of the pulmonary vascular bed or secondary to pulmonary fibrosis. Thus, regular screening with echocardiography is an important tool for detecting early pulmonary hypertension, while regular pulmonary function tests including $DL_{CO}$ and spirometry are sensitive means of detecting early involvement of the respiratory tract.

Cardiac involvement is present in approximately one-fifth of pediatric patients with scleroderma and represents a primary cause of morbidity among children with JSSc. Pericardial effusions are not common findings and when present are usually of no hemodynamic significance. Pulmonary hypertension caused by pulmonary vascular disease can lead to myocardial damage and right-sided heart failure. Severe cardiomyopathy, although rare, requires prompt and aggressive immunosuppressive therapy and represents one of the most common causes of early death, especially in children.

There are limited data on the prevalence of renal involvement in children with JSSc. One case series found that approximately 10% of children with systemic sclerosis had some kind of renal involvement including either increased urinary protein excretion or an elevated serum creatinine level. Although renal involvement in children appears to be less severe or frequent than in adults, the abrupt onset of accelerated hypertension with acute renal failure (scleroderma renal crisis) remains one of the most severe and dangerous complications of JSSc.

## LABORATORY AND DISEASE MONITORING

Approximately one-fourth of JSSc patients have anemia of chronic disease, or less commonly, macrocytic anemia due to malabsorption of vitamin $B_{12}$ or folate. Patients with myositis have elevated levels of a variety of muscle enzymes, including aldolase, lactose dehydrogenase (LDH), and creatine kinase.

High titers of antinuclear antibodies (ANA) are found in as many as 80% of children with JSSc. The prevalence of both antitoposomerase I (Scl-70) and anticentromere antibodies (ACA), quite specific for this condition, is lower in children as compared to adults. Thus, 34% of children with JSSc test positive for anti-Scl-70 and 7% for ACA, compared to as many as 70% and 55% of adult patients, respectively.

Objective assessment is necessary for organ-based complications, such as pulmonary fibrosis, pulmonary hypertension, or renal involvement. To provide a more global index of severity, a multidimensional severity score, the Juvenile Systemic Sclerosis Severity Score (J4S), has been developed. This instrument includes 9 organ-related categories, weighting involvement of different end-organs on the basis of clinical importance. Pulmonary function tests such as forced vital capacity (FVC) and $DL_{CO}$ should be performed regularly. If results are abnormal, pulmonary artery systolic pressure (sPAP) by Doppler echocardiography and HRCT of the chest should be performed. To exclude cardiac involvement, electrocardiogram (ECG) and echocardiogram should be performed, and in the presence of arrhythmias, Holter ECG and cardiac magnetic resonance imaging (MRI) are indicated.

## TREATMENT

No controlled trials and very few reports of any sort are available to help guide the treatment of JSSc. Nonpharmacologic measures for alleviating symptoms in JSSc begin with avoiding cold and trauma, which can exacerbate vasospasm and tissue damage. In addition, physiotherapy can help maintain functional ability, muscle strength, and joint movement while preventing flexion contractures. Corrective splints, especially while patients sleep, are also useful for treating or preventing joint and muscle contractures.

Pharmacologic management of patients with JSSc is particularly challenging: No medication has been shown to be of unequivocal benefit in either children or adults with systemic sclerosis. Calcium channel blockers, usually oral nifedipine or nicardipine, are used as first-line therapy for Raynaud phenomenon. Iloprost or other available parenteral prostanoids are used to treat more severe systemic sclerosis–related peripheral vasospasm and digital ulcers. Steroids may be used with care for treating myositis or arthritis, but they may precipitate scleroderma renal crisis. Pulmonary involvement accompanied by inflammation may be treated with cyclophosphamide, although when interstitial lung disease is purely fibrotic, no therapies are known to be effective.

Low-dose methotrexate has been shown to benefit sclerodermatous skin changes in adults, and, therefore, it is the treatment of choice for skin manifestations in children, especially during the early phase of the disease.

Angiotensin-converting enzyme (ACE) inhibitors (eg, captopril, losartan) are effective for the long-term control of blood pressure and are life-saving in cases of scleroderma renal crisis. It is not clear whether or not they have a role in preventing this condition.

Proton pump inhibitors (PPIs) such as omeprazole and lansoprazole are indicated for the prevention of gastroesophageal reflux disease and esophageal ulcers. Prokinetic drugs such as domperidone may be beneficial in the management of symptomatic motility disturbances. Rotating antibiotics, such as metronidazole and doxycycline, are indicated to treat malabsorption owing to bacterial overgrowth.

Among the evolving treatments for adults with systemic sclerosis are mycophenolate mofetil (MMF) for early diffuse scleroderma and lung disease and autologous hemopoietic stem cell transplantation (HSCT) for refractory cases. The rationale for this latter therapy is the ablation of self-reactive lymphocytic clones, which are responsible for the disease process. Patients early in the disease course who have not yet developed irreversible organ damage also might benefit from such an immune resetting, although reports of such an approach are minimal. In addition, limited experience suggests that rituximab, a monoclonal chimeric antibody directed against the CD20 antigen on B lymphocytes, might stabilize and/or improvement sclerodermatous lung disease for as long as 2 years after treatment. There is insufficient experience at present to estimate the risks and benefits of these treatments in children, but so far, a few case reports and the direct experience of the author are promising.

## PROGNOSIS

Generally, the prognosis of JSSc is poor. Skin tightness and joint contractures inevitably lead to severe disability, despite the fact that the skin may eventually soften years after onset of the disease. The most common causes of death in children are related to involvement of the cardiac, renal, and pulmonary systems. Interstitial lung disease and renal failure or acute hypertensive encephalopathy supervene as a potentially fatal outcome in a few children and seem more likely to occur early in the disease course. Survivorship has not been determined in any large series of children because of the rarity of this disease and paucity of longitudinal data. The overall mortality rate at 5 years is approximately 6% to 15% and is better than that for adults. The causes of death in JSSc include cardiac failure (67%), end-stage renal failure (13%), respiratory failure (10%), infections (7%), and hypertensive encephalopathy (3%).

# JUVENILE LOCALIZED SCLERODERMA

JLS, known as *morphea*, comprises a group of conditions with involvement essentially limited to the skin and subcutaneous tissues. They have various features and range from very small plaques to extensive fibrotic lesions that may cause significant functional and cosmetic deformity.

Although JLS is relatively uncommon, it is far more common than systemic sclerosis in childhood, by a ratio of at least 10:1. There is a mild female predilection, with girls developing the condition approximately 2.4 times as frequently as boys. Onset is usually during late infancy, although a few cases with onset at birth have been described.

## CLINICAL MANIFESTATIONS

JLS can be classified into 5 subtypes: circumscribed morphea, linear scleroderma, generalized morphea, pansclerotic morphea, and a mixed subtype in which a combination of 2 or more of the previous subtypes is present (Table 203-2).

*Circumscribed morphea (CM)* is characterized by oval or round circumscribed areas of induration surrounded by a violaceous halo.

**TABLE 203-2 CLASSIFICATION CRITERIA OF JUVENILE LOCALIZED SCLERODERMA**

| Main Group | Subtype | Description |
|---|---|---|
| Circumscribed morphea | Superficial | Oval or round circumscribed areas of induration limited to epidermis and dermis, often with altered pigmentation and a violaceous, erythematous halo (lilac ring). They can be single or multiple. |
| | Deep | Oval or round circumscribed deep induration of the skin involving subcutaneous tissue extending to fascia and potentially involving underlying muscle. The lesions can be single or multiple. |
| | | Sometimes the primary site of involvement is in the subcutaneous tissue without involvement of the skin. |
| Linear scleroderma | Trunk/limbs | Linear induration involving dermis, subcutaneous tissue, and, sometimes, muscle and underlying bone and affecting the limbs and/or the trunk. |
| | Head | *En coup de sabre* (ECDS). Linear induration that affects the face and/or the scalp and sometimes involves muscle and underlying bone. |
| | | Parry-Romberg syndrome or progressive hemifacial atrophy. Loss of tissue on one side of the face that may involve dermis, subcutaneous tissue, muscle, and bone. The skin is mobile. |
| Generalized morphea | | Indurations of the skin starting as individual plaques (4 or more and larger than 3 cm) that become confluent and involve at least two anatomic sites |
| Pansclerotic morphea | | Circumferential involvement of limb(s) affecting the skin, subcutaneous tissue, muscle, and bone. The lesion may also involve other areas of the body without internal organ involvement. |
| Mixed morphea | | Combination of 2 or more of the previous subtypes. The order of the concomitant subtypes, specified in brackets, will follow their predominant representation in the individual patient [ie, mixed (linear-circumscribed)]. |

Data from Consensus conference, Padua, Italy, 2004.

It is confined to the dermis with only occasional involvement of the superficial panniculus. Sometimes, as in deep morphea, the entire skin feels thickened, taut, and bound down. By convention, morphea characterized by 4 or more discrete or coalescent plaques larger than 3 cm is known as generalized morphea (GM) (Fig. 203-4).

*Linear scleroderma*, the most common subtype of morphea in children and adolescents, is characterized by 1 or more linear streaks that can extend through the dermis, subcutaneous tissue, and muscle to the underlying bone, potentially causing significant deformities (Fig. 203-5). The extremities are typically affected, but the face or scalp also may be involved. In such cases, the condition is known as the *en coup de sabre* variety (ECDS), so called because the lesion looks like the depression caused by a sword strike (Fig. 203-6). When deeper structures are involved, ECDS may be complicated by abnormalities of the teeth, eyes, or central nervous system, including calcifications, vasculitis, seizures, or simply nonspecific MRI changes.

*Pansclerotic morphea*, an extremely rare but severe subtype, is characterized by generalized full-thickness involvement of the skin of the trunk, extremities, face, and scalp with sparing of the fingertips and toes.

Children with JLS may present with extracutaneous involvement, such as arthritis (19%), neurologic abnormalities (4%), autoimmune conditions (eg, thyroiditis) (3%), Raynaud phenomenon or deep vein thrombosis (2%), or ocular and gastrointestinal abnormalities (2%). The most frequent neurologic complications are seizures and headaches, although behavioral changes and learning disabilities have also been described.

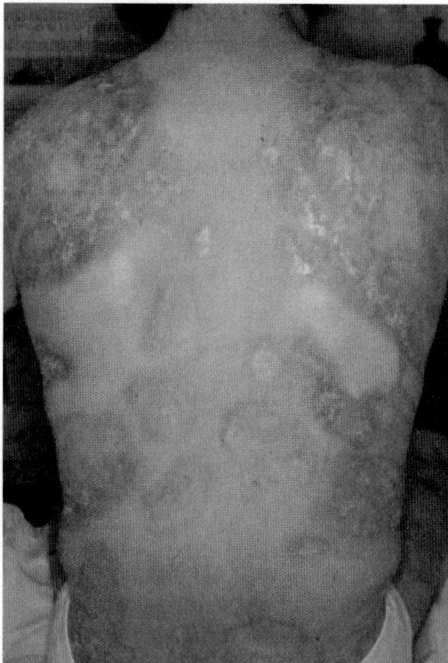

**FIGURE 203-4** Generalized morphea in a 15-year-old: indurated plaques that become confluent and involve the trunk symmetrically.

## LABORATORY AND DISEASE MONITORING

The diagnosis of JLS is not dependent on laboratory testing. Routine studies, such as complete blood count, blood chemistries, and urinalysis, are normal.

In a large cohort of patients, ANAs were found in 42%, rheumatoid factor in 16%, and antiphospholipid antibody in 13% of patients, but there is no correlation between their presence and a particular subtype or disease course (Table 203-3). Antitopoisomerase I antibodies (anti-Scl-70) and ACAs, specific markers of systemic sclerosis, were found to be positive in 2% to 3% of children with JLS. Whether these antibodies merely reflect the immunologic effects of the disease process or also have prognostic significance is unclear. Low-titer rheumatoid factor, detected in 1 in 6 patients with JLS, correlates significantly with the presence of arthritis.

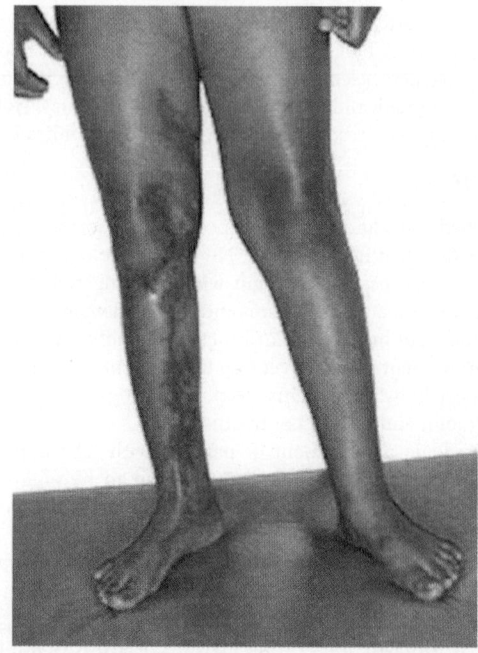

**FIGURE 203-5** Linear scleroderma involving the whole right lower limb and resulting in undergrowth of the foot and hyperpigmented skin.

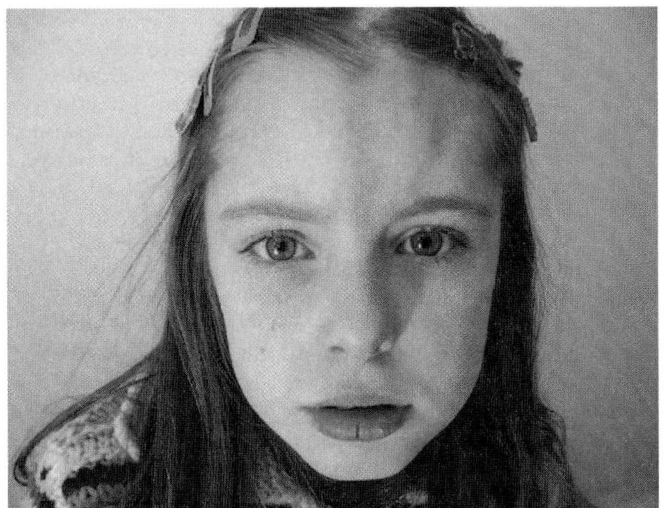

**FIGURE 203-6** Linear scleroderma *en coup de sabre* affecting the left forehead and resulting in 2 lines of induration, hyperpigmentation, and depression of the scalp.

Monitoring the progression or response to therapy of JLS includes clinical scoring methods, such as the Localized Scleroderma Severity Index (LoSSI), and noninvasive technology, such as thermography, ultrasonography, and MRI in selected patients. Infrared thermography (IRT) has been shown to be of value in the detection of active lesions. MRI is also an important tool when central nervous system or eye involvement is suspected. In other forms involving the limbs, MRI is able to demonstrate the extent and depth of soft tissue lesions, particularly in linear scleroderma and pansclerotic morphea.

## TREATMENT

Over the years, many treatments have been tried for JLS. Unfortunately, the rarity of this disease and the difficulty of reproducibly assessing outcomes have limited the interpretation of most of these studies. Circumscribed morphea generally is of cosmetic concern only, and lesions usually remit with residual pigmentation as the only abnormality. Therefore, treatment should emphasize topical therapies such as moisturizing agents and topical glucocorticoids. Phototherapy with ultraviolet wavelengths represents another possible therapeutic choice, but the increased risk for premature aging of the skin or carcinogenesis limits its use in pediatric patients.

Systemic treatment is recommended when there is a significant risk for disability, such as in deep pansclerotic morphea, progressive linear scleroderma crossing joint lines or involving the face (*en coup de sabre*), or generalized morphea. In these cases, the drug of choice is methotrexate, given as a weekly single oral or subcutaneous dose for at least 1 year. During the first 3 months of therapy, a course of glucocorticoids may be used as adjunctive bridge therapy. Patients who do not respond to this treatment approach may be treated with mycophenolate mofetil.

Surgical reconstruction, especially for face and limbs, may be required if the disease has caused significant damage to subcutaneous or musculoskeletal structures. Surgery should be performed only after the active phase of the disease has abated and when the child's growth is complete.

**TABLE 203-3 SERUM AUTOANTIBODIES IN JUVENILE LOCALIZED SCLERODERMA**

| Serum Autoantibody | Patients | Healthy Controls |
|---|---|---|
| Antinuclear antibody | 42.3% | 0–3% |
| Antitopoisomerase I | 3.2% | 0% |
| Anticentromere | 1.7% | 0% |
| Anti–double-stranded DNA | 4.2% | 0% |
| Rheumatoid factor | 16% | 0–4% |
| Antiphospholipid antibody | 12.6% | 1.5–9.4% |

## SUGGESTED READINGS


Herrick AL, Ennis H, Bhushan M, et al. Incidence of childhood linear scleroderma and systemic sclerosis in the UK and Ireland. *Arthritis Care Res*. 2010;62:213-218.

La Torre F, Martini G, Russo R, et al. A preliminary disease severity score for juvenile systemic sclerosis. *Arthritis Rheum*. 2012;64:4143-4150.

Martini G, Foeldvari I, Russo R, et al. Systemic sclerosis in childhood: clinical and immunological features of 153 patients in an international database. *Arthritis Rheum*. 2006;54:3971-3978.

Martini G, Ramanan AV, Falcini F, et al. Successful treatment of severe or methotrexate-resistant juvenile localized scleroderma with mycophenolate mofetil. *Rheumatology*. 2009;48:1410-1413.

Martini G, Vittadello F, Kasapçopur Ö, et al. Factors affecting survival in juvenile systemic sclerosis. *Rheumatology*. 2008;48:119-122.

Schanz S, Fierlbeck G, Ulmer A, et al. Localized scleroderma: MR findings and clinical features. *Radiology*. 2011;260:817.

Zulian F, Athreya BH, Laxer RM, et al. Juvenile localized scleroderma: clinical and epidemiological features in 750 children. An international study. *Rheumatology*. 2006;45:614-620.

Zulian F, Cuffaro G, Sperotto F. Scleroderma in children: an update. *Curr Opin Rheumatol*. 2013;25:643-650.

Zulian F, Martini G, Vallongo C, et al. Methotrexate treatment in juvenile localized scleroderma: a randomized, double-blind, placebo-controlled trial. *Arthritis Rheum*. 2011;63:1998-2006.

Zulian F, Vallongo C, de Oliveira SKF, et al. Congenital localized scleroderma. *J Pediatr*. 2006;149:248-251.

Zulian F, Vallongo C, Woo P, et al. Localized scleroderma in childhood is not just a skin disease. *Arthritis Rheum*. 2005;52:2873-2881.

Zulian F, Woo P, Athreya BH, et al. The PRES/ACR/EULAR provisional classification criteria for juvenile systemic sclerosis. *Arthritis Rheum*. 2007;57:203-212.




# 204 Musculoskeletal Pain Syndromes

William Bernal and Yukiko Kimura

## INTRODUCTION

With a prevalence as high as 15%, chronic pain is increasingly being recognized as a common problem in children and adolescents but one that remains poorly understood. This chapter describes evolving concepts of several syndromes in which musculoskeletal pain is a prominent feature. Interestingly, these pain syndromes frequently have overlapping features. However, most children can be readily diagnosed by the typical pattern of somatic complaints and the salient physical findings specific to each syndrome.

## GROWING PAINS

### PATHOGENESIS AND EPIDEMIOLOGY

*Growing pains* are the most common cause of recurrent limb pain in children, and references to it can be found in the medical literature dating back more than 150 years. Growing pains occur in children between the ages of 3 and 12 and are characterized by intermittent nighttime nonarticular aching or pain most commonly in the legs. Recent prevalence estimates vary from less than 3% to as high as 36.9% in 4- to 6-year-olds in Australia. An extension of the syndrome in adolescents and adults may include restless legs syndrome. In a recent population study, the prevalence of restless legs syndrome was found to be 1.9% in 8- to 11-year-olds and 2% in 12- to 17-year-olds; a history of growing pains and sleep disturbances was more common in the study population. Interestingly, restless legs syndrome also is reported to be common in patients with fibromyalgia, another pain syndrome that is described later in this chapter. The pathogenesis of growing pains is unknown. Despite the name, it is almost certainly not due to growing. Perhaps this term is used because the condition occurs in children (who are always growing) and does not occur in adulthood (after cessation of growth). Theories have abounded about the etiology and have included overuse, anatomic abnormalities, perfusion problems, and emotional issues, but most have not been supported by subsequent research. Recently, investigators have shown that children with growing pains may have increased pain sensitivity and decreased bone strength as measured by quantitative ultrasound.

### CLINICAL MANIFESTATIONS

Growing pains typically are bilateral, usually occurring in the evening or at night, and not associated with limping or limited mobility. There is no history of trauma or infection, and objective findings are lacking on physical examination. The areas most frequently involved include the thighs, calves, and, occasionally, the forearms and trunk. In contrast to patients with juvenile idiopathic arthritis (JIA), who usually have more pain and stiffness when first arising in the morning, these children usually are asymptomatic in the morning.

Parents of children with growing pains report no swelling, color changes, or warmth of the affected limb. The physical examination is unrevealing. X-rays and laboratory tests may be necessary to alleviate parental concern, but if the clinical picture is typical, they are not necessary. If testing is done, it typically includes the erythrocyte sedimentation rate, complete blood count, and muscle enzyme determination, all of which should be normal.

### DIAGNOSIS

If the child has a limp, is complaining of pain in or around the joint, or has an abnormal musculoskeletal exam, growing pains is probably not the correct diagnosis. A thorough investigation for known causes of joint pain, such as infection, inflammatory arthritis, and neoplasm, as well as orthopedic and endocrine disorders, should be pursued. A frequent mistake is to use *growing pains* as a convenient diagnosis for any vague musculoskeletal complaint, rather than reserving the term for a child whose symptoms truly fit the clinical picture as outlined above.

### TREATMENT

Treatment for this condition is symptomatic. Heat, massage, and analgesics (typically nonsteroidal anti-inflammatory agents or acetaminophen) generally ameliorate the pain, but none has been tested in a prospective fashion. Regardless of the treatment used, children tend to outgrow their pain by middle school, with no long-term sequelae. It is important to reassure patients and their parents that growing pains do not reflect a serious organic disease and will not progress to arthritis or other damaging conditions.

## HYPERMOBILITY SYNDROMES

### PATHOGENESIS AND EPIDEMIOLOGY

*Hypermobility* is quite prevalent in children and adolescents and may be responsible for a wide variety of musculoskeletal complaints including benign joint hypermobility syndrome (BJHS), patellar subluxation, articular dislocation, premature osteoarthritis, and increased susceptibility to ligamentous injury. In addition to causing joint-specific problems, BJHS is also now known to be associated with chronic pain, fatigue, and possibly dysautonomia in adults. Additional hereditary diseases that must be considered in the differential diagnosis of joint laxity include: (1) Ehlers-Danlos syndrome, (2) Marfan syndrome, (3) marfanoid hypermobility syndrome, (4) osteogenesis imperfecta, (5) Williams syndrome, and (6) inborn errors of metabolism such as homocystinuria and hyperlysinemia.

The reported prevalence of joint hypermobility in the general population varies widely, with studies citing incidences from as low as 2% to as high as 30%. Hypermobility appears to be more common in younger children and females. Children affected by BJHS usually are school-aged and adolescents, although patients younger than age 5 years have been described. There may be racial and ethnic differences as well, with hypermobility apparently occurring more frequently in persons of African, Asian, and Middle Eastern descent, although studies are somewhat conflicting. The prevalence of pain in adults with BJHS varies between 5% and 45% depending on the group studied. Not all hypermobile patients have pain: one recent study found that only approximately 5% of hypermobile adults had symptomatic BJHS. On the other hand, a study of a rheumatology clinic population found that as many as 45% had BJHS if patients were systematically examined. Segregation of joint hypermobility within families has also been noted, with parents often reporting that they were loose-jointed as youngsters. Many patients consider themselves "double-jointed" and participate in activities for which hypermobility may be advantageous, such as ballet or gymnastics.

### CLINICAL MANIFESTATIONS

The symptoms attributed to BJHS include joint and muscle pain, transient joint swelling, and subjective stiffness; they usually are worse with increased physical activity. The joints most commonly involved are the lower extremity joints, but the back also may be affected. If joint swelling is present, consideration must be given to an inflammatory arthropathy such as JIA. A high frequency of hypermobility was found in a group of children with recurrent episodes of joint pain that was called *juvenile episodic arthritis/arthralgia*. These children most likely simply have hypermobility syndrome, with the swelling likely due to edema from strain and sprain injuries rather than true joint effusions.

Congenital abnormalities of the hips including actual developmental dysplasia have also been associated with hypermobility. Anterior knee pain syndrome, a frequent diagnosis in preadolescent and adolescent patients, may be due in some individuals to hypermobility of the patellae and genu recurvatum or genu valgus. Pes planus, which becomes apparent on weight bearing, is also common in hypermobility and may cause musculoskeletal pain that tends to improve with the use of orthotics. Chronic nonspecific back pain may also be secondary to hypermobility, which can also predispose to injuries such as spondylolysis and spondylolisthesis.

Growing evidence suggests that hypermobility is not just a "benign" problem limited to the joints. One recent study of 15 children with BHJS found that these children had increased laxity of other tissues compared to asymptomatic prepubertal children. Furthermore, children and adults with BJHS tend toward osteopenia, and there appears to be overlap of hypermobility with chronic pain, fatigue, and dysautonomia, as well as with fibromyalgia.

A recent study of 125 children with BJHS found that 48% had "clumsiness," poor coordination, developmental motor delay, major physical limitations, and school absences because of symptoms. Up to 20% had recurrent joint sprains and 10% had actual subluxation/dislocation of a joint, among many other features that overlapped with collagen abnormalities such as Ehlers-Danlos and Marfan syndromes. Another study by Pacey and colleagues (see Suggested Readings) identified 5 subtypes of joint hypermobility syndrome using factor analysis of history and exam findings: joint affected, athletic, systemic, soft tissue, and high body mass index. Identification of these subtypes may enhance detection of clinically significant joint hypermobility and thus improve patient outcomes and quality of life.

### DIAGNOSIS

The 1998 Revised Brighton Criteria are the most recently published criteria for hypermobility. They include both the Beighton score, which quantifies the extent of joint hypermobility, and other manifestations of connective tissue laxity often seen in BJHS. The 5 simple Beighton maneuvers are: (1) extension of the wrist and fifth metacarpophalangeal joint so that the fifth digit is parallel to the dorsum of the forearm; (2) passive apposition of the thumb to the flexor aspect of the forearm; (3) hyperextension of the elbows 10 degrees or more; (4) hyperextension of the knees 10 degrees or more; and (5) flexion of the trunk with the knees fully extended so the palms

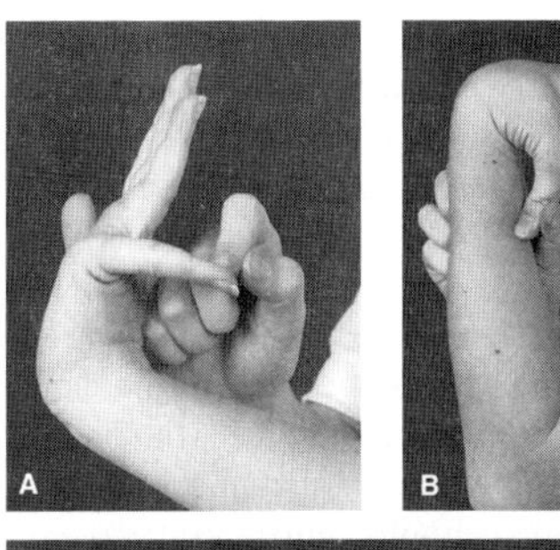

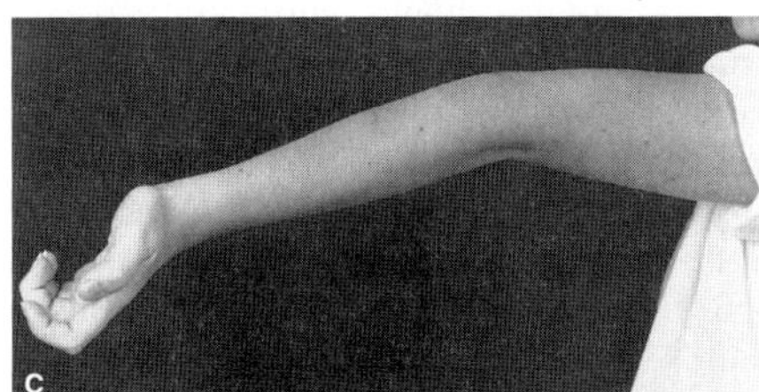

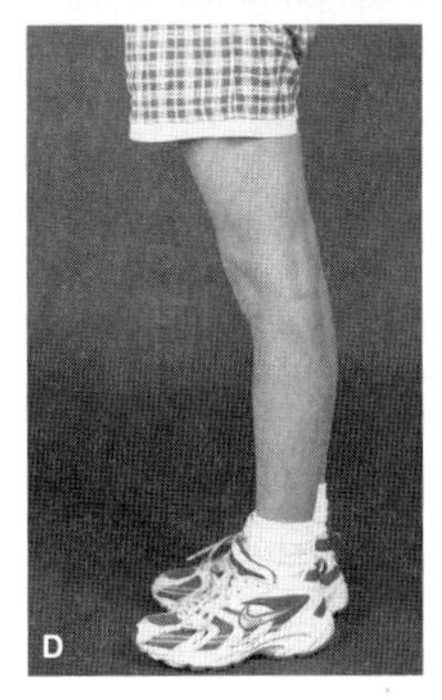

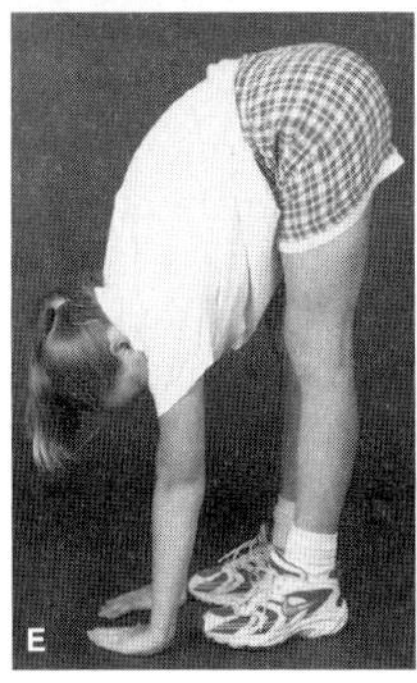

**FIGURE 204-1** Demonstrations of Beighton score components. **A:** Extension of the wrist and metacarpophalangeal joints so that the fingers are parallel to the dorsum of the forearm. **B:** Passive apposition of the thumb to the flexor aspect of the forearm. **C:** Hyperextension of the elbows 10 degrees or more. **D:** Hyperextension of the knees 10 degrees or more. **E:** Flexion of the trunk with the knees fully extended so the palms rest on the floor.

rest on the floor (Fig. 204-1). Patients are scored on a 9-point scale, with 1 point awarded for each hypermobile site. A Beighton score of 4 or more points fulfills criteria for hypermobility. However, the use of the Beighton score to diagnose hypermobility in children may not be optimal: since children are more hypermobile than adults, it may identify as many as 50% of children as being "abnormal" in terms of excessive hypermobility.

Whether or not the Beighton hypermobility score is used, the other criteria for the diagnosis of BJHS are shown in Table 204-1. The

**TABLE 204-1 1998 REVISED BRIGHTON CRITERIA FOR BENIGN JOINT HYPERMOBILITY SYNDROME**

**Major Criteria**

1. A Beighton score of 4 out of 9 or greater (either currently or historically)
2. Arthralgia for longer than 3 months in 4 or more joints

**Minor Criteria**

1. A Beighton score of 1, 2, or 3 out of 9
2. Arthralgia (≥ 3 months) in 1–3 joints or back pain (≥ 3 months), spondylosis, spondylolysis/spondylolisthesis
3. Dislocation/subluxation in > 1 joint, or in 1 joint on > 1 occasion
4. Soft tissue rheumatism, at least 3 lesions (eg, epicondylitis, tenosynovitis, bursitis)
5. Marfanoid habitus (tall, slim, span/height ratio < 1.03, upper-to-lower segment ratio < 0.89, arachnodactyly (positive Steinberg/wrist signs)
6. Abnormal skin: striae, hyperextensibility, thin skin, papyraceous scarring
7. Eye signs: drooping eyelids or myopia or antimongoloid slant
8. Varicose veins or hernia or uterine/rectal prolapse

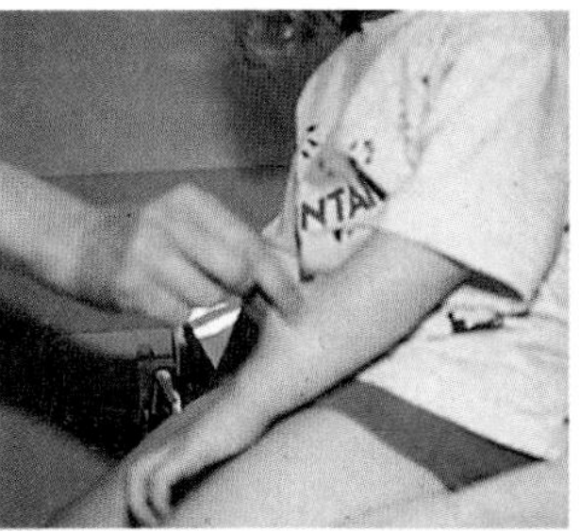

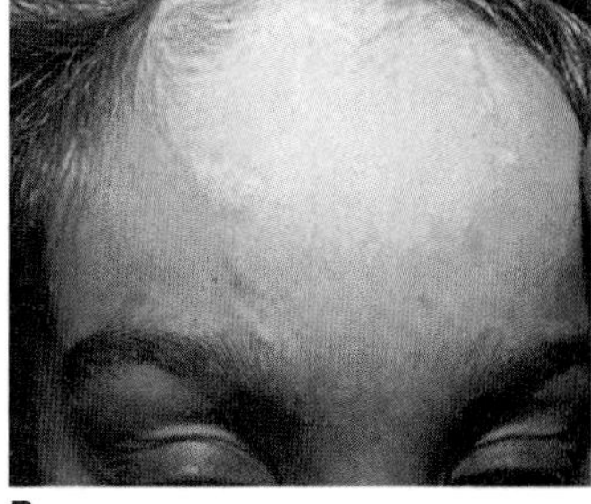

**FIGURE 204-2** Dermatologic features of Ehlers-Danlos syndrome. **A:** Increased skin elasticity. **B:** Papyraceous scars.

examiner should also look for stigmata of heritable connective tissue diseases such as Marfan syndrome (Marfanoid habitus, arachnodactyly, high-arched palate, ocular abnormalities such as drooping eyelids and dislocated lens) and Ehlers-Danlos syndrome, including increased elasticity of the skin, abnormal "papyraceous" scars, and a velvety texture of the skin (Fig. 204-2).

Basic laboratory investigations, such as a complete blood count, erythrocyte sedimentation rate, serum chemistries, thyroid function tests, and urinalysis, are usually negative unless there is a coexisting inflammatory or endocrinologic condition. A Lyme titer may be done if a joint effusion is present and the child has spent time in an endemic area. Joint radiographs show no evidence of joint space narrowing, osteopenia, or erosive changes. Invasive studies, such as arthrocentesis, arthroscopy, or biopsy, are not necessary. If an arthrocentesis is done for some reason, the synovial fluid is typically noninflammatory, with less than 200 leukocytes (in contrast to that in inflammatory arthritis, which contains at least several thousand [and sometimes many more] leukocytes).

## TREATMENT

The treatment of benign joint hypermobility syndrome includes (1) explanation of joint laxity and the mechanism of pain; (2) reassurance that an underlying arthritis does not exist; (3) analgesics; (4) a physical therapy program to improve periarticular muscle strength; and (5) avoidance of activities that aggravate the musculoskeletal pain. When overpronation and pes planus are present, the use of an orthotic to correct pronation and support the arch may be helpful in normalizing the gait and deceasing lower extremity joint symptoms. The intermittent use of nonsteroidal anti-inflammatory drugs (NSAIDs) or application of warmth or cold may help relieve pain or stiffness in some patients. Swimming is an excellent sport to improve strength and cardiovascular endurance without excessive impact loading and strain on the supportive tissues, especially because exercise tolerance in children with BJHS is reduced. The rehabilitation program should address both the physical and emotional needs of the child, and in severe cases, the child will benefit from a multidisciplinary approach involving physical and occupational therapy, psychology, and podiatry. The prognosis is thought to be good in most cases if BJHS is identified early and interventions are begun prior to the development of a chronic pain syndrome.

# COMPLEX REGIONAL PAIN SYNDROME

*Complex regional pain syndrome (CRPS)* is characterized by pain, swelling, and disuse of an extremity associated with signs of vasomotor instability. This syndrome has had many names, including reflex sympathetic dystrophy (RSD), Sudeck atrophy, causalgia, reflex neurovascular dystrophy, and hysterical edema.

## PATHOGENESIS AND EPIDEMIOLOGY

The pathogenesis of CRPS has yet to be elucidated. Disorders precipitating CRPS in adult patients include infection, fracture, surgery, peripheral neuropathy, and trauma (mild to severe), but such conditions

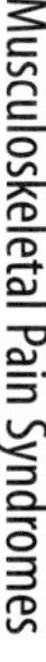

rarely antedate pediatric CRPS. Instead, the antecedent injury usually is relatively minor in relation to the severity of the pain. In one of the first series of pediatric CRPS, Bernstein reported that only 11 (46%) of 24 of his cases in children had an antecedent illness or trauma.

Although findings on physical exam would suggest that CRPS is a local phenomenon, current evidence suggests multisystem dysfunction, both neurologic and immunologic. Adult patients with CRPS have been shown to have changes in the motor and sensory cortexes, some of which have been shown to respond to treatment. The autonomic system is involved to varying degrees in CRPS as well, both locally in the region of pain and diffusely in the form of lightheadedness and dizziness. Changes in peripheral innervation have been documented in patients with CRPS, although the significance of these changes has not been established. Lastly, neurogenic inflammation may play a role in the early stages of CRPS, although it has not been well characterized in pediatric CRPS. The extent to which each of these factors plays a role in CRPS is not yet known, and questions remain as to whether they are causal to, or a result of, CRPS.

The incidence of CRPS in children is not known, but the usual age of onset is between 9 and 15 years, and it is much more common in girls than boys. CRPS occurs more frequently in white children. Risk factors for pediatric CRPS have not been well characterized, but characteristic psychological features have been suggested. Several authors have reported that children with CRPS tend to demonstrate psychosocial stress or psychopathological trends, including a tendency to somaticize. Therefore, psychotherapy is considered to be an important component of the therapeutic regimen in many patients.



### CLINICAL FEATURES AND DIAGNOSIS

The patient with CRPS often complains of a continuous burning sensation. Typically, even gentle stroking of the skin causes marked discomfort and withdrawal of the limb, a phenomenon referred to as *allodynia*. The limb usually is held in a spastic posture, and the patient refuses to bear weight on it or move it actively or passively because of pain. There is often diffuse swelling of the distal extremity as well as vasomotor changes, including coolness or warmth, pallor or erythema, and accompanying hyperhidrosis. If the CRPS has been present for an extended period of time, the patient may develop trophic skin changes, with alterations in the nails, hair, and pigmentation. The International Association for the Study of Pain has established ("Budapest") criteria for adult CRPS, which require continuing pain out of proportion to initial injury, as well as reported symptoms and physical exam findings involving the following domains: sensory (allodynia, hyperesthesia), vasomotor (skin temperature or color asymmetry), sudomotor (asymmetry of sweating or edema), and motor/trophic (spasticity, dystonia, or hair/nail changes). Although the Budapest criteria were not developed for use in pediatric CRPS, in clinical practice, many of the criteria apply to children. Typically, children with CRPS report worsening pain during rest and immobilization after a minor injury. In contrast to adults, in whom upper extremity CRPS predominates, children more often have involvement of the feet and legs.

As in other pain syndromes, laboratory studies are negative in this syndrome. Bone radiographs in the adult patient characteristically reveal a patchy osteoporosis, but children do not uniformly have demineralization, and when it occurs, it is usually diffuse but mild. Arterial Doppler ultrasonography may show decreased flow on the affected side. Bone scintigraphy using $^{99m}$Tc-labeled phosphate or polyphosphates may be abnormal, showing diffusely increased (and sometimes decreased) uptake in the juxta-articular tissues of the affected distal extremity. Magnetic resonance imaging may show edema in the bones and/or marrow. These imaging abnormalities are not specific, and, therefore, they are not necessary to diagnose a patient with the typical signs and symptoms of CRPS.

### TREATMENT

Numerous treatment modalities have been suggested to break the pain cycle and to reduce increased sympathetic tone, but it is clear that early mobilization is the single most critical intervention. Therefore, the mainstay of treatment is physical therapy to encourage the child to use the affected limb. Graded motor imagery, which includes mirror therapy, is a form of rehabilitative therapy that has been shown to be effective in adult CRPS and to treat other types of pediatric pain, although its efficacy in pediatric CRPS remains to be studied. Immobilization is contraindicated and only aggravates the pain and edema. The family should be taught range-of-motion exercises that are done frequently throughout the day. The regimen should include desensitization techniques, which include contrast baths with cold and heat application and rubbing or massaging. Patients and their families should understand that although these maneuvers will be painful initially, perseverance with a regular exercise routine will ultimately be rewarded with relief. With aggressive therapy, many children with early CRPS are quickly able to resume weight bearing.

Given the difficulties in rehabilitating the affected limb, many patients benefit from psychotherapy to learn healthy coping strategies that minimize distress. Psychotherapy, biofeedback, and cognitive-behavioral therapy (CBT) may be efficacious in children who do not have rapid resolution with physical therapy, analgesics, and desensitization techniques. One study of 28 children with CRPS showed that CBT was more important than the frequency of physical therapy in the treatment of CRPS. Other treatments studied include continuous peripheral nerve blocks and regional anesthetic and surgical approaches (including sympathetic or somatic nerve blocks, spinal cord stimulation, and surgical sympathectomy). However, such techniques are rarely necessary in children: in most case reports and series, pediatric patients generally achieve complete resolution of their pain and disability with active physical therapy with or without CBT.

As in patients with other forms of amplified pain syndromes, patients with CRPS who do not respond to outpatient therapy may benefit from intensive interdisciplinary pain rehabilitation programs. The prognosis in children usually is good, although relapses may occur at times of stress or following repeat trauma to the limb. Vitamin C supplementation has been shown to decrease the occurrence of CRPS in areas of physical injury or surgical intervention in adult women. Given its benign nature, pediatric pain specialists often recommend vitamin C supplementation prior to planned surgeries or soon after injuries to prevent occurrence of CRPS. Vitamin C supplementation should be continued until the affected area has healed. Vitamin C has not been shown to be efficacious for treating active CRPS, however.

## JUVENILE PRIMARY FIBROMYALGIA SYNDROME

*Fibromyalgia* is a common but poorly understood chronic pain condition characterized by widespread musculoskeletal aching, fatigue, and sleep disturbance. The prevailing theory of pathogenesis is that it is a dysregulation of pain pathways that leads to central pain sensitization, which is marked by neurohormonal, neurotransmitter, and sleep dysregulation. Fibromyalgia is often unrecognized or misdiagnosed in adults, but the situation is even worse for children, who may have symptoms for years before the diagnosis is made. In addition, skepticism and controversy over the existence of fibromyalgia continue because of the paucity of objective abnormalities in patients diagnosed with the condition. Despite the absence of characteristic physical, laboratory, radiographic, and pathologic findings, growing evidence supports the consensus that fibromyalgia is not a psychosomatic condition.

### PATHOGENESIS AND EPIDEMIOLOGY

Although it is classified as a "central sensitization" disorder, the precise etiology and pathophysiology of fibromyalgia remain unclear. Patients with fibromyalgia have dysregulated pain perception associated with neuroendocrinologic changes in the central and peripheral nervous systems. Heightened pain perception and hypersensitivity occur as a result. There appears to be some genetic predisposition, suggested by a significantly increased incidence of the disorder in first-degree relatives with fibromyalgia. In addition, physical or emotional factors are also thought to act as possible triggers.

Fibromyalgia is diagnosed most frequently in women from ages 20 to 50 and is reported to occur in as many as 2% of the general population. In children, it is most prevalent in 13- to 15-year-old girls but can occur in younger children; it has been reported in children as young as 5 years old. This pain syndrome was estimated to account for 7.5% of new-patient referrals to the US pediatric rheumatology disease registry, reported in 1998. In large population-based studies, fibromyalgia or diffuse musculoskeletal pain similar to fibromyalgia is seen in 1.2% to 7.5% of children.

## CLINICAL FEATURES AND DIAGNOSIS

The diagnosis of this syndrome is based on the presence of diffuse aching, pain and stiffness, associated clinical features, and the demonstration of *multiple* tender points in the absence of other physical findings. The presence of true joint swelling or other physical abnormalities militates against this diagnosis and should prompt further evaluation for an underlying inflammatory, infectious, or traumatic disorder. Similarly, laboratory studies to exclude other conditions typically include complete blood count, erythrocyte sedimentation rate, rheumatoid factor, antinuclear antibody, muscle enzyme, and thyroid function tests. Fibromyalgia does not cause identifiable abnormalities in imaging studies either. Nonetheless, it is important to remember that fibromyalgia and rheumatic diseases often coexist in a single patient.

Diagnostic criteria for adult fibromyalgia were updated by the American College of Rheumatology (ACR) in 2010. The new preliminary criteria use a combination of widespread pain and symptom severity, with numerical values for each, to determine the diagnosis. Unlike the 1990 ACR diagnostic criteria for fibromyalgia, the 2010 criteria no longer include the tender point exam as a factor. Instead, widespread pain, defined as pain present in the last week, is assessed for 19 areas of the body. Two components compose the symptom severity scale: 3 core symptoms (fatigue, waking unrefreshed, cognitive difficulties) and the extent of somatic symptoms in general. The clinician scores each of the 3 core symptoms on a scale from 0 to 3, and the extent of somatic symptoms overall on a scale from 0 to 3. The metric for diagnosis of fibromyalgia is the sum of scores of the widespread pain and symptom severity scales. Depending on the level of symptom severity, a pain score as low as 3 is sufficient for a diagnosis of fibromyalgia.

In juvenile fibromyalgia, diagnostic criteria were developed by Yunus and Masi in 1985. Since the publication of the 2010 ACR preliminary criteria for adult fibromyalgia, pediatric researchers have begun developing similar criteria for children and adolescents. An initial study concluded that it can be done successfully but recommended that modifications be made to adult criteria. As such, formal diagnostic criteria for juvenile fibromyalgia are still in development.

Patients variously describe the pain as sharp, dull, constant, intermittent, burning, heavy, or numb. Patients typically complain of stiffness, especially in the morning, which when coupled with complaints of joint pain, may cause confusion with arthritis. Patients may also report a subjective feeling of joint fullness, usually a diffuse transient puffiness in the hands and fingers, but objective joint swelling is not present. Nonrestorative sleep (not feeling refreshed when first arising in the morning, even after adequate sleep) is a hallmark of this disorder. Sleep disturbances are common, especially difficulty falling and remaining asleep, but some patients may not recognize their sleep alterations. Instead, the parents or roommate might have noticed frequent "tossing and turning" and awakening during the night. Interestingly, fibromyalgia appears to be associated with restless legs syndrome. Some patients complain that pain keeps them up at night. Studies show that adults with fibromyalgia have a significant disturbance of alpha wave activity in stage 4 non-rapid eye movement (NREM) sleep. A study of children with fibromyalgia confirmed that they also have sleep disturbances.

Further associations include irritable bowel syndrome, migraine or tension headaches, paresthesias, Raynaud phenomenon, and dizziness attributed to postural orthostatic tachycardia syndrome (POTS) or neurocardiogenic orthostatic hypotension. Patients also tend to share certain personality traits and behavior patterns, such as anxiety and depression, compulsion, overwork, and perfectionism. Mood disturbances, especially depression, are common findings. Familial aggregation of fibromyalgia is common in adults as well as among children. One study found an 8-fold increase in the chances of having a first-degree relative with fibromyalgia among children with fibromyalgia compared with controls. Specific genetic polymorphisms in genes controlling serotonin, catecholamines, dopamine, and other monoamines have been reported to modify the risk of developing fibromyalgia. Additionally, certain psychosocial, environmental, and family factors appear to affect the development of fibromyalgia in children.

Long-term outcomes in juvenile fibromyalgia reveal the detrimental effects this condition can have in early adulthood. Kashikar-Zuck and colleagues studied pain levels, as well as physical and psychological functioning, in a group of 94 young adults with a past diagnosis of juvenile fibromyalgia. More than 80% of patients continued to report chronic pain, and more than 50% met adult criteria currently for fibromyalgia. Among patients with a history of juvenile fibromyalgia, 60% had moderate or severe anxiety, and more than 25% had moderate or severe depression. Whether these findings reflect underlying mental health issues that predispose to juvenile fibromyalgia or result from having to deal up with chronic pain, most children with juvenile fibromyalgia clearly warrant psychosocial support.

## TREATMENT

The physician should establish a supportive and understanding relationship with the patient in order to promote his or her active role in managing the pain and disability of fibromyalgia. The management of fibromyalgia involves multidisciplinary approaches to relieving pain, including moderate but regular aerobic activities, salutary sleep hygiene, returning to normal activities as much as possible, and emotional support. The first priority is to establish the diagnosis and to reassure the patient and family that symptoms are not caused by arthritis or another mysterious and/or life-threatening disorder. A positive diagnosis, detailed explanation, and establishment of a trusting therapeutic relationship provide the foundation for treatment of fibromyalgia. Just knowing the diagnosis is often a great relief to the patient and the family, who typically have been evaluated by several doctors who minimized or dismissed the myriad symptoms. An important point is that these patients must come to understand that the aim of treatment is to reduce pain, and most importantly, to allow the return to normal or near-normal activities. Complete elimination of pain and discomfort associated with fibromyalgia, however, may not be possible.

Various nonmedical approaches to treatment have had variable success. Two approaches that have been studied in detail in adults and have been shown to be efficacious in children are exercise and CBT. CBT typically involves 8 to 10 weekly sessions, which can include distraction, relaxation, coping and stress-reducing techniques, as well as activity pacing, biofeedback, and self-hypnosis. Not only does CBT appear to be effective in the short term during the sessions, but benefits also appear to be maintained for months afterward. In terms of exercise, a regular physical therapy program should be recommended for muscle stretching and strengthening, and a gradually escalating aerobic exercise program, which may include bicycling, walking, or swimming, should be incorporated to recondition the patient. Moreover, aerobic exercise has been demonstrated in patients with fibromyalgia to be efficacious in reducing pain. Despite a gradual approach to increasing demands in physical therapy, patients are expected to work through the pain and not be limited by it, which is an important distinction from traditional rehabilitative therapy. For patients disabled by fibromyalgia who have not responded to outpatient therapy, consideration of an intensive interdisciplinary rehabilitation program is warranted. Such intensive approaches have a combination of psychotherapy, physical therapy, and occupational therapy, usually in a day hospital or inpatient setting. Programs such as these have been shown to promote both short- and long-term gains in physical functioning, psychological health, and pain reduction.

Most reviews of existing studies agree that the combination of nonpharmacologic and pharmacologic interventions is most helpful in fibromyalgia in both adults and children. In terms of pharmacologic treatments, conventional analgesics such as nonsteroidal anti-inflammatory agents and acetaminophen often are prescribed but rarely are effective. Likewise, other analgesics, including narcotic analgesics, are not beneficial and should not be prescribed, except for possibly tramadol, for which there is some evidence of efficacy.

Treatment with medications that alter neurotransmitter balance, such as antidepressants, has been found to be helpful for some patients. Low doses of a tricyclic antidepressant (TCA) such as amitriptyline at bedtime have been found to be useful, but the morning drowsiness and increased daytime fatigue that are sometimes a side effect of these medications may limit their usefulness. Other classes of antidepressants, for example, specific selective serotonin reuptake inhibitors (SSRIs) such as fluoxetine and the more "balanced" serotonin-norepinephrine reuptake inhibitors (SNRIs) such as duloxetine, have proven to be modestly effective in trials of adults with fibromyalgia. One study in adults evaluated the use of a combination of a TCA (amitriptyline) and an SSRI (fluoxetine) and found it to be effective. It is important that children and adolescents using SSRIs and SNRIs be monitored carefully because of the possible development of increased depression and suicidality in some patients taking these medications. Gabapentin (a γ-aminobutyric acid [GABA] analogue) and pregabalin (a GABA agonist), which are used to treat neuropathic pain, have been modestly effective in clinical trials in adults. Studies of pregabalin for the treatment of juvenile fibromyalgia are ongoing.



## SUGGESTED READINGS


Kashikar-Zuck S, Cunningham N, Sil S, et al. Long-term outcomes of adolescents with juvenile-onset fibromyalgia in early adulthood. *Pediatrics.* 2014;133:e592-e600.

Kashikar-Zuck S, Parkins IS, Graham TB, et al. Anxiety, mood, and behavioral disorders among pediatric patients with juvenile fibromyalgia syndrome. *Clin J Pain.* 2008;24:620-626.

Kashikar-Zuck S, Ting TV, Arnold LM, et al. Cognitive behavioral therapy for the treatment of juvenile fibromyalgia: a multisite, single-blind, randomized, controlled clinical trial. *Arthritis Rheum.* 2012;64:297-305.

Logan DE, Carpino EA, Chiang G, et al. A day-hospital approach to treatment of pediatric complex regional pain syndrome: initial functional outcomes. *Clin J Pain.* 2012;28:766-774.

Murray KJ. Hypermobility disorders in children and adolescents. *Best Prac Res Clin Rheumatol.* 2005;20(2):329-351.

Pacey V, Adams RD, Tofts L, et al. Joint hypermobility syndrome subclassification in paediatrics: a factor analytic approach. *Arch Dis Child.* 2015;100:8-13.

Pavone, V, Lionetti E, Gargano V, et al. Growing pains: a study of 30 cases and a review of the literature. *J Pediatr Orthopaed.* 2011;31:606-609.

Sherry DD, Brake L, Tress JL, et al. The treatment of juvenile fibromyalgia with an intensive physical and psychosocial program. *J Pediatr.* 2015;167:731-737.

Ting TV, Barnett K, Lynch-Jordan A, et al. 2010 American College of Rheumatology adult fibromyalgia criteria for use in an adolescent female population with juvenile fibromyalgia. *J Pediatr.* 2016;169:181-187.

Wolfe F, Clauw DJ, Fitzcharles MA, et al. The American College of Rheumatology preliminary diagnostic criteria for fibromyalgia and measurement of symptom severity. *Arthritis Care Res.* 2010;62:600-610.


# 205 Chronic Fatigue Syndrome

David S. Leslie and Monica L. Marcus

## INTRODUCTION

Generalized fatigue is a frequent complaint during many common pediatric infectious illnesses. Additionally, chronic diseases of childhood often are characterized by associated fatigue. The symptoms experienced by children with these conditions typically resolve with treatment of the acute illness or of the underlying chronic disease. In contrast, *chronic fatigue syndrome* (CFS) is distinguished by prolonged fatigue and associated constitutional symptoms that persist after improvement in the triggering disorder. CFS may be a debilitating illness that significantly impacts activities of daily living and family dynamics. A systematic approach directed at first ruling out identifiable causes of profound fatigue and associated symptoms is essential before arriving at the diagnosis of CFS. Through a careful history and physical exam and narrowly focused laboratory testing based on clinical presentation, underlying diseases responsible for fatigue may be eliminated. Attention then switches to maximizing the ability to function and initiating an appropriate treatment plan. Although the specific cause of this illness remains to be elucidated and appropriate treatment strategies continue to be controversial, a multidisciplinary, holistic, symptom-based approach can provide the best tools for managing CFS and achieving full recovery.

## EPIDEMIOLOGY

The symptoms of CFS-like illnesses were described in adults for many years, even prior to the acceptance of specific diagnostic and research criteria. However, the recognition that this illness affects children is a relatively recent phenomenon. Bell and colleagues initially described a cluster of pediatric patients who presented during the late 1980s with symptoms consistent with CFS and further defined the incidence in a rural community through a retrospective review. During the past several years, several published reports have demonstrated that prolonged fatigue states and CFS do indeed occur in the pediatric population, and in fact, they may not be rare. Although the etiology of CFS remains unknown, reports of clusters of cases imply that environmental triggers, such as infection, may play a role.

Children of all ages may present with CFS, but evidence suggests that it is more common in the adolescent population than in younger children. The incidence and prevalence of CFS in children are somewhat difficult to assess given the absence of specific pediatric criteria, geographical variations, and other variables. Nonetheless, a few key studies in the 1990s were performed: one indicated that Australian children reported an overall prevalence of 37 per 100,000, whereas another retrospective study done by Bell in the United States reported an estimated prevalence of 23 per 100,000. Most recently, the Centers for Disease Control and Prevention (CDC) estimated that between 0.2% and 2.3% of children or adolescents suffer from CFS. As is the case in adults, pediatric CFS seems to be more common in girls, with an overall female-to-male ratio of 2:1, although some studies have failed to demonstrate such a female predominance. In addition, children in higher socioeconomic groups appear be affected more frequently.

## PATHOPHYSIOLOGY

As in adults, the specific mechanisms through which children develop CFS remain unknown. Many theories have been proposed regarding the etiology of CFS. They include immune dysfunction, dysregulation of the hypophyseal-pituitary axis, chronic infection, and alterations in the autonomic nervous system. In addition, new research involving human metabolomics has implicated metabolic derangement, in the form of a highly concerted hypometabolic response to environmental stress, as a potential mechanism for CFS. However, to date, there is no convincing evidence for a single genetic, metabolic, or environmental cause. Most specialists agree that the manifestations of CFS are likely multifactorial, with both physiologic and psychological factors playing roles in development of the condition. Similarly, specific genetic influences on the development of CFS remain unknown, although the observation that CFS and related disorders appear to be more common within certain families suggests a possible heritable factor. The development of more sophisticated methods of genetic analysis may provide insight into the influence of inheritance on CFS.

## CLINICAL FEATURES AND DIFFERENTIAL DIAGNOSIS

Several case definitions have been used to diagnose CFS in adults. Most researchers use the adult diagnostic criteria established by the CDC in 1988 and modified in 1994. A Canadian case definition was established in 2003 incorporating a change in nomenclature to *myalgic encephalomyelitis/chronic fatigue syndrome* (ME/CFS) and indicated more specific inclusion criteria. More recently, the 2011 International Consensus Criteria for Myalgic Encephalomyelitis were established. These case definitions originally served as a framework upon which to establish a likely diagnosis in children. However, in 2006, the International Association of Chronic Fatigue Syndrome Pediatric Case Definition Working Group developed a case definition specifically for children and adolescents with ME/CFS. Although the currently accepted CDC diagnostic criteria for adults require fatigue for a duration greater than 6 months for the diagnosis of CFS, the pediatric literature suggests that this diagnosis may be more appropriately made after 3 months in children.

Following a careful exclusion of identifiable causes, the diagnosis of ME/CFS for children is made based on the following criteria:

I. Clinically evaluated, unexplained, persistent, or relapsing chronic fatigue over the past 3 months that:
   A. Is not the result of ongoing exertion
   B. Is not substantially alleviated by rest
   C. Results in substantial reduction in previous levels of educational, social, and personal activities
   D. Must persist or reoccur for at least 3 months
II. The concurrent occurrence of the following classic ME/CFS symptoms, which must have persisted or recurred during the past 3 months of illness (symptoms may predate the reported onset of fatigue):
   A. Postexertional malaise and/or postexertional fatigue
   B. Unrefreshing sleep or disturbance of sleep quantity or rhythm
   C. Pain (or discomfort) that is often widespread and migratory in nature
   D. Two or more neurocognitive manifestations: Impaired memory, difficulty focusing, difficulty finding the right word, frequently forgetting what wanted to say, absent mindedness, slowness of thought, difficulty recalling information, need to focus on 1 thing at a time, trouble expressing thought, difficulty comprehending information, frequently losing train of thought, new trouble with math or other educational subjects
   E. At least 1 symptom from 2 of the following 3 categories:
      a. Autonomic manifestations: Neurally mediated hypotension, postural orthostatic tachycardia, delayed postural hypotension, palpitations with or without cardiac arrhythmias, dizziness, feeling unsteady on the feet/disturbed balance, shortness of breath
      b. Neuroendocrine manifestations: Recurrent feelings of feverishness and cold extremities, subnormal body temperature and marked diurnal fluctuations, sweating episodes, intolerance of extremes of heat and cold, marked weight change/loss of appetite or abnormal appetite, worsening of symptoms with stress
      c. Immune manifestations: Recurrent flu-like symptoms, non-exudative sore or scratchy throat, repeated fevers and sweats, lymph nodes tender to palpitation/generally minimal swelling noted, new sensitivities to food, odors, or chemicals

These clinical criteria for identifying patients with possible CFS represent common pediatric symptoms that may be seen in a broad swath of childhood illnesses. For example, sore throat and tender lymph nodes may be present during acute viral infection or in the setting of streptococcal pharyngitis. Myalgias and arthralgias may be suggestive of acute infection, primary muscle disease, benign hypermobility syndrome, or chronic inflammatory diseases. Headaches and alteration in memory may occur secondary to infections, inflammatory diseases, mass lesions, or new-onset headache disorder. Additionally, the primary symptom of prolonged fatigue may be present secondary to altered sleep as a result of obstructive sleep apnea, or due to chronic diseases including anemia, rheumatologic conditions, malignancy, chronic infection, and hypothyroidism. Given these considerations, the potential differential diagnosis for a child presenting with fatigue and associated constitutional symptoms is broad. In addition to carefully reviewing the medical condition of a child with suspected CFS, a thoughtful psychosocial assessment is essential for ruling out psychiatric illness, social factors such as disruption of family dynamics, or other stressors that may present with somatic symptoms.

## DIAGNOSTIC EVALUATION

Because many pediatric diseases can manifest with symptoms similar to those of CFS, this illness remains a diagnosis of exclusion. The first step in evaluating a pediatric patient for possible CFS is to obtain a detailed history (both medical and psychosocial) directed at diagnosing recognizable diseases that require a specific treatment plan. Additionally, performing laboratory studies in order to evaluate basic parameters, as well as focused laboratory testing based on information gathered via history and physical exam, is prudent. The CDC has recommended that adults undergoing consideration for possible CFS have basic laboratory testing as summarized in Table 205-1. These tests should also be considered in children presenting with possible CFS. Further laboratory testing, imaging, or other studies should be conducted in a focused manner based on the history and physical exam. A general algorithm for assessment of children with possible CFS is presented in Figure 205-1.

## TREATMENT

The treatment of children with CFS should be directed toward relief of the specific primary symptoms manifested by the individual patient. Therapy should be multidisciplinary, focused on maintaining ability to function in activities such as school, sports, and social interactions. Medical therapy primarily consists of appropriate analgesics such as acetaminophen or nonsteroidal anti-inflammatory medications to treat musculoskeletal pain or symptoms such as headache. Evidence suggests that some patients with CFS also are affected by the postural orthostatic tachycardia syndrome (POTS). Patients with primary symptoms such as lightheadedness or dizziness with change

| TABLE 205-1 BASIC SCREENING LABORATORY STUDIES TO ASSESS FOR UNDERLYING DISEASE |
|---|
| Alanine aminotransferase (ALT) |
| Albumin |
| Alkaline phosphatase |
| Complete blood count |
| Blood urea nitrogen (BUN) |
| Calcium |
| Electrolytes, glucose |
| Erythrocyte sedimentation rate |
| Thyroid-stimulating hormone |
| Urinalysis |
| Total protein |
| Other tests as indicated by clinical presentation |

Data from Fukuda K, Straus SE, Hickie I, et al: The chronic fatigue syndrome: a comprehensive approach to its definition and study. International Chronic Fatigue Syndrome Study Group, *Ann Intern Med.* 1994 Dec 15;121(12):953-959.

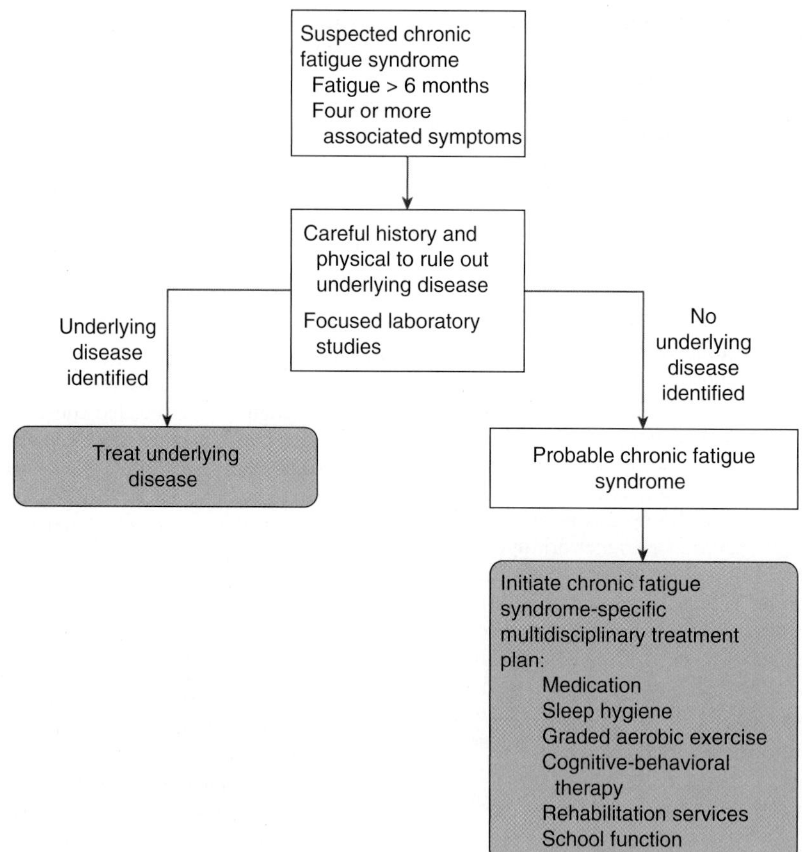


**FIGURE 205-1** Algorithm for the evaluation and treatment of suspected chronic fatigue syndrome.

in body position may feel better with medications such as fludrocortisone, α-agonists, or β-blockers, and these medications are also often helpful in children with POTS-like symptoms complicating CFS.

A significant percentage of children with significant prolonged fatigue may experience comorbid depression, anxiety, or other psychiatric illnesses, either as a preexisting condition or as a reaction to illness. Antidepressants, anxiolytics, or other psychotropic medications may be indicated in these individuals at least in the short term to potentiate other interventions. Additionally, among the complex components of CFS, there is often a significant psychosocial contribution. Not surprisingly, therefore, cognitive behavioral therapy (CBT) typically has a salubrious effect. In a study of adults, CBT was more effective in restoring psychological well-being and tolerance of exercise than was either a conventional medical therapy or a program of education and support. Studies in adolescents with CFS also have suggested that CBT is an important component of treatment promoting improved ability to function and long-term outcome.

The specific recommendations for physical exercise in children with CFS remain controversial. Additionally, studies in adults have been somewhat conflicting in determining whether aerobic capacity is impaired in patients with CFS. Nonetheless, a program of graded aerobic exercise consisting of a 1:3 ratio of exercise time to rest is currently recommended by the CDC. Overly vigorous exercise may lead to increased postexertional malaise with recurrent cycles of relapse (the so-called *overtraining syndrome*). It presents a particular problem in the management of the child and adolescent with CFS because it is often difficult for children to self-regulate their activities. Conversely, children with CFS often feel worse in the short term after exercising, so in order to avoid either excessive or inadequate exertion, careful oversight of exercise programs is important. Regular aerobic exercise may also help children adjust the disrupted sleep patterns that typify CFS. Therapeutic goals should include restoring normal sleep–wake cycles through appropriate sleep hygiene characterized by consistent bedtime and elimination of napping.

Because symptoms of CFS may persist for prolonged periods of time, it is essential to also focus on maintaining the ability of the child to function, particularly in the school environment. The practitioner should advocate for appropriate educational accommodations while promoting the affected child's school attendance. An individualized educational plan often facilitates active school participation, which can be augmented by supportive services such as tutoring as needed. In a study by Lim et al, adolescents with CFS were treated using a 4-week in-patient program incorporating gradual reintroduction of physical activity, psychological therapy, and reintroduction into the school environment. Although 66% of patients were not attending school prior to the program, 78% were able to attend school full time at long-term follow-up. No control group was reported, but these data still support the idea that multidisciplinary treatment may be effective in promoting the ability of individuals to cope with symptoms of CFS.

## OUTCOMES

The prognosis for children and adolescents with CFS appears to be more favorable than that of adults. Krilov et al reported that on long-term follow-up, approximately 95% of patients were somewhat improved, whereas 43% noted complete resolution of symptoms. Additionally, in a 13-year follow-up of the patient population originally described by Bell et al, approximately 80% of patients reported improvement, with 37% reporting that the illness had completely resolved. This is not to say that the condition may be taken lightly or that good outcomes may be assumed without expert management. As with many pediatric conditions, however, the combination of early aggressive therapy with a child's natural resilience does allow caregivers to be optimistic when explaining expectations for children with CFS.

## SUGGESTED READINGS


Bell KM, Cookfair D, Bell DS, Reese P, Cooper L. Risk factors associated with chronic fatigue syndrome in a cluster of pediatric cases. *Rev Infect Dis.* 1991;13(suppl 1):S32-S38.

Bell DS, Jordan K, Robinson M. Thirteen-year follow-up of children and adolescents with chronic fatigue syndrome. *Pediatrics.* 2001;107(5):994-998.

Fang H, Xie Q, Boneva R, Fostel J, Perkins R, Tong W. Gene expression profile exploration of a large dataset on chronic fatigue syndrome. *Pharmacogenomics.* 2006;7(3):429-440.

Fukuda K, Straus SE, Hickie I, Sharpe MC, Dobbins JG, Komaroff A. The chronic fatigue syndrome: a comprehensive approach to its definition and study. International Chronic Fatigue Syndrome Study Group. *Ann Intern Med.* 1994;121(12):953-959.

Jason LA, Jordan K, Miike T, et al. A pediatric case definition for myalgic encephalomyelitis and chronic fatigue syndrome. *J Chronic Fatigue Syndr.* 2006;13(2-3):1-44.

Jordan KM, Landis DA, Downey MC, Osterman SL, Thurm AE, Jason LA. Chronic fatigue syndrome in children and adolescents: a review. *J Adolesc Health.* 1998;22(1):4-18.

Knoop H, Stulemeijer M, de Jong LW, Fiselier TJ, Bleijenberg G. Efficacy of cognitive behavioral therapy for adolescents with chronic fatigue syndrome: long-term follow-up of a randomized, controlled trial. *Pediatrics.* 2008;121(3):e619-e625.

Krilov LR, Fisher M, Friedman SB, Reitman D, Mandel FS. Course and outcome of chronic fatigue in children and adolescents. *Pediatrics.* 1998;102(2 Pt 1):360-366.

Lloyd AR, Hickie I, Boughton CR, Spencer O, Wakefield D. Prevalence of chronic fatigue syndrome in an Australian population. *Med J Aust.* 1990;153(9):522-528.

Naviaux RK, Naviaux JC, Li K, et al. Metabolic features of chronic fatigue syndrome. *Proc Natl Acad Sci U S A.* 2016;113(37):E5472-E5480.

Stewart JM, Gewitz MH, Weldon A, Arlievsky N, Li K, Munoz J. Orthostatic intolerance in adolescent chronic fatigue syndrome. *Pediatrics.* 1999;103(1):116-121.

Van Den Eede F, Moorkens G, Van Houdenhove B, Cosyns P, Claes SJ. Hypothalamic-pituitary-adrenal axis function in chronic fatigue syndrome. *Neuropsychobiology.* 2007;55(2):112-120.


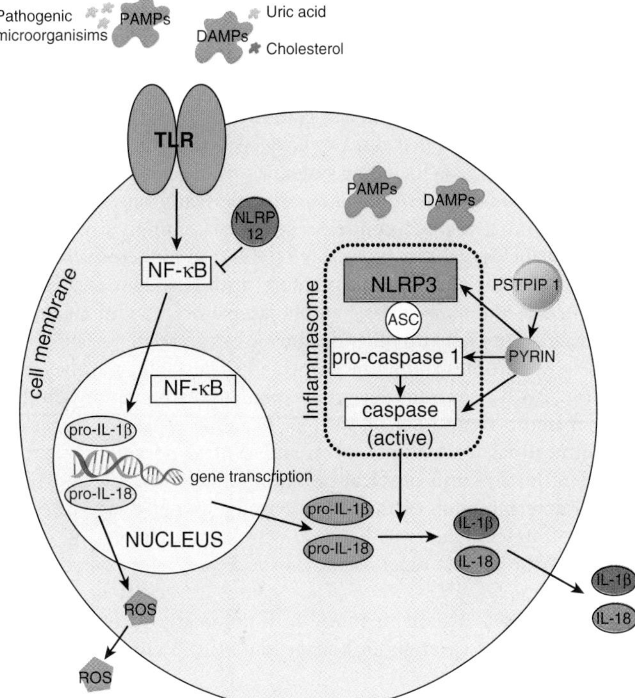


**FIGURE 206-1** Schema of selected innate immune inflammatory pathways related to the autoinflammatory syndromes. The schema demonstrates the effect of external stimuli on the development of inflammation and the relationship of several regulatory proteins (pyrin, NLRP3, NLRP12, PSTPIP1) that when mutated result in the development of autoinflammatory diseases. DAMP, damage-associated molecular patterns; IL, interleukin; NLR, nod-like receptors; NLRPs, NLRs with pyrin domain–containing proteins; PAMP, pathogen-associated molecular patterns; PSTPIP, proline-serine-threonine phosphatase-interacting protein; TLR, toll-like receptors.

# 206 Autoinflammatory Disorders

Philip J. Hashkes

## INTRODUCTION

Autoinflammatory syndromes, formerly known as *periodic fever syndromes*, are defined as recurrent attacks of often unprovoked systemic inflammation that are related to a lack of adequate regulation of the innate immune system. Unlike autoimmune diseases, these conditions are not generally marked by autoantibodies or autoreactive T cells. Many of these syndromes have a genetic etiology (Table 206-1). The pathogenesis of a large proportion of the major syndromes involves the excessive production and activity of interleukin (IL)-1β (Fig. 206-1). However, other immune mechanisms are also implicated in the pathogenesis of these diseases. The conditions are no longer known as periodic fever syndromes because most are not truly periodic and fever is not a necessary feature.

**TABLE 206-1 GENETIC CHARACTERISTICS OF THE MAJOR[a] INHERITED AUTOINFLAMMATORY SYNDROMES**

| Disease | Inheritance | Gene Defect | Protein Product | Common Mutations |
|---|---|---|---|---|
| Familial Mediterranean fever (FMF) | Recessive[b] | *MEFV* | Pyrin | M694V, M694I, M680I, V726A, E148Q |
| Mevalonate kinase deficiency (MKD)/hyperimmunoglobulin D syndrome (HIDS) | Recessive | *MVK* | Mevalonate kinase | V377I, I268T |
| Tumor necrosis factor (TNF) receptor–associated periodic syndrome (TRAPS) | Dominant | *TNFRSF1A* | 55 kDa TNF receptor | T50M, C52Y, R92Q, P46L |
| Familial cold autoinflammatory syndrome (FCAS) | Dominant | *NLRP3* | Cryopyrin | R260W |
| Muckle-Wells syndrome (MWS) | Dominant | *NLRP3* | Cryopyrin | L264V, D303N |
| Neonatal-onset multisystem inflammatory disease (NOMID) | Dominant[c] | *NLRP3* | Cryopyrin | L264F, H, D303H, V351M, L |
| Pyogenic sterile arthritis, pyoderma gangrenosum, acne (PAPA) syndrome | Dominant | *PSTPIP1* | CD2 antigen binding | A230T, E250Q,K |
| Deficiency of interleukin (IL)-1 receptor antagonist (DIRA) | Recessive | *IL1RN* | IL-1 receptor antagonist | E77X, Q54X, 175-kb deletion |
| Deficiency of adenosine deaminase 2 (DADA2) | Recessive | *CERC1* | Adenosine deaminase 2 | G47R, A |
| Chronic atypical neutrophilic dermatosis with lipodystrophy and elevated temperature (CANDLE) syndrome | Recessive | *PSMB8* | Proteasome subunit β type 8 | T75M |

[a]Readers are referred to more detailed reviews on very rare monogenic autoinflammatory syndromes

[b]Dominant transmission has been reported; many patients have only 1 mutation.

[c]Cases without germ-line mutations (many have somatic mosaic mutations) are common

As understanding of the pathogenesis of autoinflammatory syndromes increases, so does the spectrum of conditions that may be included within this category. The field of autoinflammatory disorders is probably the most rapidly changing discipline in pediatric rheumatology, and since the last edition was published, numerous new monogenic and other diseases have been added to the list. Thus, inflammatory diseases including systemic juvenile idiopathic arthritis, genetic inflammatory granulomatous diseases (early-onset sarcoidosis and Blau syndrome), Behçet disease, and even common diseases such as gout, diabetes mellitus (especially type II), and atherosclerosis are now considered to be autoinflammatory disorders. This chapter will be limited to the major/classic autoinflammatory conditions and to those that do not fall into other diagnostic categories.

These syndromes should be suspected in patients, mainly young children, with recurrent fever unexplained by infections and/or with episodic symptoms in various systems, especially the skin, gastrointestinal tract, joints, eyes, and central nervous system. A complete history and physical examination are crucial, and often careful determination of the organ systems involved, age of onset, length of attacks, intervals between attacks, and triggering events will allow the correct diagnosis to be suspected before genetic tests are performed (Tables 206-2, 206-3, and 206-4). It is useful to examine patients during an attack or, if not possible, to ask parents to record attacks carefully in a diary and send pictures of relevant physical findings.

The role of genetic testing is often used more for prognostic information than for diagnosis, as the diagnosis of most syndromes is based on clinical criteria. Genetic test results need to be interpreted by experts due to frequent false-positive and false-negative results as well as genetic variants/polymorphisms with unclear clinical significance. Algorithms and guidelines for the performance and interpretation of genetic testing for the autoinflammatory disorders have been published.

Autoinflammatory syndromes also should be considered in patients with unexplained elevations of acute-phase reactants, even in the absence of symptoms. It is also useful to measure markers of inflammation during and between attacks, because in some syndromes attacks are only the "tip of the inflammatory iceberg" and patients consistently have increased inflammatory indices. These patients are at higher risk of developing amyloid A (AA) amyloidosis, the major adverse outcome of some of the autoinflammatory syndromes (Table 206-5). A family history often reveals relatives with similar symptoms, including unexplained cases of renal failure, hearing loss, or amyloidosis. Specific autoinflammatory syndromes often show a predilection for certain ethnic groups.

## FAMILIAL MEDITERRANEAN FEVER

Familial Mediterranean fever (FMF), first described in 1945, is the most common inherited autoinflammatory syndrome. It is an autosomal recessive disorder that results in recurrent attacks of fever, serositis, arthritis, and rash. Late complications of untreated FMF include the development of renal AA amyloidosis leading to the nephrotic syndrome and renal failure. The highest prevalence of FMF is in Sephardic Jews, Armenians, Arabs, and Turks. Because of the availability of genetic diagnosis, FMF is now recognized more frequently among Ashkenazi Jews, Greeks, and Italians as well. A national study in Turkey found a prevalence of 0.093%. The prevalence of FMF varies from 1:100 to 1:2000 (carrier rate of 1:5 to 1:45) among Sephardic Jews and 1:87 to 1:1000 (carrier rate of 1:7 to 1:32) among Armenians. Recently, FMF has also been found in Far East populations, particularly in Japan. There are an estimated 100,000 to 120,000 patients worldwide.

### PATHOPHYSIOLOGY AND GENETICS

The FMF gene (*MEFV*) has been localized to the short arm of chromosome 16. The product of this gene is a 781-amino acid protein termed *pyrin* (*marenostrin* in Europe). There may be a phenotype–genotype correlation, with more severe disease and amyloidosis occurring in patients with the M694V, M694I, and M680I mutations. However, not all patients have homozygous or compound heterozygous pyrin mutations. In various series, between 30% and 70% of patients diagnosed with definitive FMF by clinical criteria lack 1 or even both mutations,

**TABLE 206-2 CHARACTERISTICS OF THE MAIN AUTOINFLAMMATORY SYNDROMES**

| Disease | Onset Age | Typical Ethnicity | Common Triggers | Episode Duration | Interval Between Episodes |
|---|---|---|---|---|---|
| Familial Mediterranean fever (FMF) | Mostly first decade (~80%) | Sephardic Jewish, Armenian, Arab Moslem, Turks, Italian | None known, exercise, stress, menstrual period | Hours to 3 days | Variable |
| Mevalonate kinase deficiency (MKD)/hyperimmunoglobulin D syndrome (HIDS) | First year of life | Dutch, western Europe | Vaccines, infections | 3–7 days | 3–6 weeks |
| Tumor necrosis factor (TNF) receptor–associated periodic syndrome (TRAPS) | Mostly first decade<br>Can start in adults (~25%) | Any, mainly Scottish, Irish (Hibernian) | Exercise, stress, minor trauma | Days to 6–8 weeks | Variable, usually > 8 weeks |
| Familial cold autoinflammatory syndrome (FCAS) | First year of life | United States | Cold | < 24 hours | Variable |
| Muckle-Wells syndrome (MWS) | Any age | Western Europe | None known | 1–3 days | Variable |
| Neonatal-onset multisystem inflammatory disorder (NOMID) | Birth, infancy | Any | None known | Continuous | None |
| Pyogenic sterile arthritis, pyoderma gangrenosum, acne (PAPA) syndrome | Mostly first decade | Western Europe | Minor trauma | Variable | Variable |
| Periodic fever, aphthous stomatitis, pharyngitis, adenitis (PFAPA) | Toddler (1–5 years) | Any | None known | 5–7 days | 3–4 weeks, truly periodic |
| Deficiency of interleukin-1 receptor antagonist (DIRA) | Birth, infancy | Puerto Rico, Lebanon, Newfoundland, Netherlands | None known | Continuous | None |
| Deficiency of adenosine deaminase 2 (DADA2) | First year of life, adolescence | Georgian Jewish | None known | Unclear, often episodic | Years |
| Chronic atypical neutrophilic dermatosis with lipodystrophy and elevated temperature (CANDLE) syndrome | Early childhood | Any | None known | Continuous | None |

**TABLE 206-3 SYSTEM INVOLVEMENT OF THE MAIN AUTOINFLAMMATORY SYNDROMES**

| Disease | Serositis | Skin | Musculoskeletal | Eyes | Mucous Membranes | Reticuloendothelial | Neurologic |
|---|---|---|---|---|---|---|---|
| Familial Mediterranean fever (FMF) | Peritonitis, pleuritis pericarditis, scrotum swelling | Erysipelas-like, vasculitis | Acute monoarthritis, 5–10% chronic arthritis, exercise-related myalgia, prolonged febrile myalgia | No | No | Splenomegaly, adenopathy | Headaches |
| Mevalonate kinase deficiency (MKD)/hyperimmunoglobulin D syndrome (HIDS) | Abdominal pain, vomiting, diarrhea | Maculopapular, morbilliform, erythema multiforme | Arthralgia, polyarthritis | No | Aphthous, vaginal sores | Cervical adenopathy | No |
| Tumor necrosis factor (TNF) receptor–associated periodic syndrome (TRAPS) | Peritonitis, pleuritis, pericarditis | Painful, migratory erythema, vasculitis | Myalgia, fasciitis, arthralgia, arthritis | Periorbital edema | Aphthous (R92Q mutation) | Splenomegaly, adenopathy | Focal neuropathy |
| Familial cold autoinflammatory syndrome (FCAS) | No | Urticaria-like | Arthralgia | Conjunctivitis | No | No | Headaches |
| Muckle-Wells syndrome (MWS) | No | Urticaria-like | Arthralgia, arthritis | Conjunctivitis, episcleritis, uveitis | No | No | Hearing loss, headaches |
| Neonatal-onset multisystem inflammatory disorder (NOMID) | No | Urticaria-like | Epiphyseal overgrowth with deformities, cartilage defect, arthritis | Conjunctivitis, uveitis, papillitis | No | Adenopathy | Chronic meningitis, hearing loss, mental retardation, headaches |
| Pyogenic sterile arthritis, pyoderma gangrenosum, acne (PAPA) syndrome | No | Pyoderma gangrenosum, acne | Destructive "pyogenic" large-joint arthritis | No | No | No | No |
| Periodic fever, aphthous stomatitis, pharyngitis, adenitis (PFAPA) | No | No | Arthralgia | No | Aphthous, pharyngitis | Cervical | No lymphadenopathy |
| Deficiency of interleukin-1 receptor antagonist (DIRA) | No | Pustular rash | Bone lytic lesions, bone overgrowth | No | No | No | No |
| Deficiency of adenosine deaminase 2 (DADA2) | No | Vasculitis, nodular | Arthralgia, arthritis, myalgia | No | No | No | Stroke (often early onset) |
| Chronic atypical neutrophilic dermatosis with lipodystrophy and elevated temperature (CANDLE) syndrome | No | Panniculitis, pernio-like | Arthritis, joint deformities (mainly hands) | No | No | Splenomegaly | No |

especially patients from western Europe or the United States. In some families, transmission of the condition appears to be autosomal dominant. Mutations or polymorphisms in genes other than pyrin may impact the development of FMF or the severity of the disease, including the development of amyloidosis.

**TABLE 206-4 IMPORTANT HISTORICAL POINTS TO CONSIDER DURING INVESTIGATIONS OF AUTOINFLAMMATORY SYNDROMES**

| |
|---|
| Age of onset |
| Ethnicity (eg, Mediterranean) |
| Consanguinity |
| Family history |
| Triggers for attack (eg, infection, cold, vaccines, stress, exercise) |
| Duration of attacks |
| Frequency of attacks (including periodicity) |
| Clinical features (eg, fever, rash, serositis, gastrointestinal, chest, musculoskeletal, eye, neurologic) |
| Response to therapy (colchicine, corticosteroids, tumor necrosis factor and interleukin-1 inhibitors) |

The pyrin protein consists of 3 main domains, the N-terminal 92-amino acid pyrin domain, the B-box, and the C-terminal B30.2 domain. Most mutations occur in exon 10 of the *MEFV* gene encoding the B30.2 domain. The pyrin protein plays a role in apoptosis and regulation of the innate immune response, mainly via the pyrin domain. Pyrin directly interacts with and binds to caspase 1 and inhibits the conversion of pro-IL-1β to IL-1β. Mutations in the B30.2 region of pyrin, particularly those mutations considered more severe (positions 680 and 694), interfere in this binding process, thus contributing to increased levels of IL-1β and inflammation. Increased levels of IL-1β and inflammation with and without stimulation by exogenous stimuli have been demonstrated in mouse models and in people with pyrin mutations, including gain of function in mice with only 1 mutation. Recently, a researcher found that *MEFV* mutations decrease the binding of the anti-inflammatory protein 14-3-3 to phosphorylated pyrin.

## CLINICAL FEATURES

Clinical signs of FMF develop by age 10 in 80% of patients and by age 20 in 90%. A typical attack of FMF results in a 12- to 72-hour attack of fever, serositis, and monoarthritis of the knee or ankle,

**TABLE 206-5 THE RISK OF AMYLOIDOSIS IN UNTREATED AUTOINFLAMMATORY SYNDROMES**

| Disease | Risk of Amyloidosis | Risk Factors |
|---|---|---|
| Familial Mediterranean fever (FMF) | Yes (up to 25%) | 680, 694 mutations |
| | | Ethnicity (increased in Armenians, Sephardic Jewish, Arab Moslems) |
| | | Geography of patients (decreased in United States, western Europe) |
| | | Family history |
| | | Increased in males |
| | | Serum amyloid A genotype |
| Mevalonate kinase deficiency (MKD)/hyperimmunoglobulin D syndrome (HIDS) | Rare (0–5%) | |
| Tumor necrosis factor (TNF) receptor associated periodic syndrome (TRAPS) | Yes (14–25%) | Cysteine mutations |
| Familial cold autoinflammatory syndrome (FCAS) | Rare | |
| Muckle-Wells syndrome (MWS) | Yes (25–33%) | Unknown |
| Neonatal-onset multisystem inflammatory disorder (NOMID) | Yes, in survivors | Unknown |
| Pyogenic sterile arthritis, pyoderma gangrenosum, acne (PAPA) syndrome | Unknown | |
| Periodic fever, aphthous stomatitis, pharyngitis, adenitis (PFAPA) | No | |



often accompanied by an erysipelas-like rash over the involved joint. Severe abdominal pain that may mimic peritonitis or appendicitis accompanies fever in nearly 90% of patients. Other symptoms related to serositis include pleuritis (30–45% of patients), pericarditis, and scrotal swelling. Acute arthritis is seen in 50% to 75% of patients and is characterized by massive neutrophilic effusions. It usually resolves within 1 week, although in 5% to 10% of cases, the arthritis takes a chronic course, especially in the hip and sacroiliac joints.

Since the discovery of the genetic cause of FMF, additional presentations of the condition have been recognized. They include recurrent abdominal pain of childhood, recurrent arthritis without fever, prolonged febrile myalgia, and exercise-induced myalgia. Less commonly, vasculitis, especially leukocytoclastic vasculitis (similar to Henoch-Schonlein purpura without deposition of immunoglobulin [Ig] A), or polyarteritis nodosa, may be a manifestation of an *MEFV* mutation. For unclear reasons, the course of polyarteritis nodosa related to FMF is usually more benign than that of the idiopathic form and is characterized by perirenal hematoma. Children with frequent attacks and a chronic increase of inflammatory indices often have growth abnormalities and short stature. Splenomegaly is also a frequent finding.

## AMYLOIDOSIS

Prior to the discovery of colchicine as an effective therapy for FMF by Goldfinger in 1972, amyloidosis was the major cause of morbidity and mortality. Amyloidosis usually presents with proteinuria and progresses to the nephrotic syndrome and renal failure within 3 to 5 years. Rarely, FMF can present with amyloidosis ("type II phenotype"), although when analyzed retrospectively, most patients reported clinical symptoms prior to development of amyloidosis. Later manifestations include signs of gastrointestinal involvement such as abdominal pain, diarrhea, malabsorption, and weight loss, as well as cardiomyopathy, macroglossia, joint stiffness, bleeding disorders, and peripheral neuropathies.

Risk factors for the development of amyloidosis include the particular genotype (especially patients homozygous for 694 and 680 mutations), family history of amyloidosis, geography of the patient (less amyloidosis in the United States), male gender, serum amyloid A genotype (there is an odds ratio of 7 for patients with an α/α genotype), and poor compliance with colchicine therapy.

Amyloidosis should be suspected when regular screening urinalysis demonstrates proteinuria. Renal biopsy then confirms the diagnosis, although less invasive diagnostic methods such as subcutaneous abdominal fat aspiration, rectal biopsy, and nuclear $^{123}$I-labeled scan for serum amyloid P component may be considered. The last method can also be used to monitor the total body load of amyloid. Treatment once amyloidosis has developed is generally limited to minimizing its progression by controlling inflammation. An agent to decrease or inhibit fibril formation by blocking polymerization of serum amyloid A, eprodisate disodium, has been shown to slow the decrease in creatinine clearance, although few patients actually have a marked improvement in their amyloidosis.

## DIAGNOSIS

Diagnostic criteria for FMF were described for adults in 1997 and in children in 2009 based on the clinical pattern, ethnicity, family history, and response to colchicine. Recently, evidence-based classification criteria have been published based on patient ethnicity and the presence and absence of clinical features. Laboratory tests are nonspecific and reflect elevated acute-phase reactants. Elevations in the erythrocyte sedimentation rate, C-reactive protein, leukocyte count, fibrinogen, and serum amyloid A are usually present during attacks and frequently also between attacks. Serum amyloid A levels may be useful in monitoring treatment efficacy. Recently, an evidence-based score to determine disease severity and the potential need to escalate therapy has been published.

The diagnosis should not rely only on genetic testing because at least 30% of patients with FMF are either heterozygote for the *MEFV* gene or do not show any mutations when tested in commercial laboratories. Questions regarding the testing of relatives of patients with genetically proven FMF and concerning the management of asymptomatic patients with homozygote genetic mutations remain controversial, although recommendations on some of these topics have been issued.

## TREATMENT

Treatment with colchicine (1–2 mg/d) is effective in preventing development of amyloidosis in nearly all patients and in preventing attacks in 60% to 70% of patients. However, 20% to 30% of patients are only partially responsive to maximal tolerated doses of colchicine, whereas 5% of patients are totally unresponsive and continue to have frequent attacks. Unresponsive patients may include those with more severe genetic mutations or patients with modifying genes that may inhibit the activity of colchicine, such as polymorphisms in MDR-1 P-glycoprotein pump transporter genes that result in lower intracellular concentration of colchicine. Good adherence to therapy is crucial and is likely the most common reason for "unresponsiveness"; in some patients, missing even one dose of colchicine can precipitate an attack. Recently, a composite score to establish the effectiveness of treatments has been published and may serve as a base to determine "unresponsiveness."

Colchicine generally is well tolerated. The most common adverse effects include abdominal pain and diarrhea, especially in those receiving higher doses of colchicine and in patients with lactose intolerance. These effects are usually transient and respond to gradual dose changes, dividing the daily dose, lactose avoidance, and antidiarrheal and antibloating agents. Liver enzyme abnormalities may occur but are rarely of clinical significance. Other rare adverse effects include myalgia/myositis, peripheral neuropathy, and bone marrow suppression, particularly in patients with renal disease. Colchicine does not affect growth or development and is safe to continue during pregnancy.

Based on the pathogenesis of FMF, many case series, open studies, and recently a controlled study have shown that IL-1 inhibitors (canakinumab, rilonacept, anakinra) are very effective and safe alternatives for those who fail or do not tolerate colchicine. Corticosteroids are effective only for prolonged febrile myalgia and FMF-related vasculitis.

## MEVALONATE KINASE DEFICIENCY/HYPERIMMUNOGLOBULINEMIA D WITH PERIODIC FEVER SYNDROME

Mevalonate kinase deficiency (MKD)/hyperimmunoglobulinemia D with periodic fever syndrome (HIDS), an autosomal recessive disease, was first described in 1984 in 6 Dutch patients. The mean age of onset is 6 months, with greater than 70% of patients having the first episode prior to reaching 12 months of age. The disease is seen mainly in the Netherlands and western Europe.

### PATHOPHYSIOLOGY AND GENETICS

MKD/HIDS is actually a metabolic disease caused by mutations in the *MVK* gene on the long arm of chromosome 12, encoding mevalonate kinase. The vast majority of patients have mutations in the V377I (founder gene) and I268T positions. Mutations result in an unstable enzyme that is less active than is the wild type, particularly when patients are febrile. Hence, attacks are often precipitated by infection and by vaccines that are pyrogenic. The cause of the fever and other symptoms is related to the deficiency of geranylgeranyl and other isoprenoid substrates, rather than excessive mevalonate. This deficiency affects IL-1β processing by the pyrin inflammasome through effects on the anti-inflammatory RhoA-type GTPase, dependent on prenylation. Total absence of *MVK* results in mevalonic aciduria, a syndrome characterized by severe neurologic sequelae in addition to febrile episodes.

### CLINICAL FEATURES

Attacks typically occur every 3 to 6 weeks and last for 3 to 7 days. Besides fever, patients develop a maculopapular, often morbilliform, rash; abdominal pain with vomiting and diarrhea; cervical lymphadenopathy, arthralgia or arthritis; and oral and genital ulceration (Fig. 206-2A). Amyloidosis is a rare complication of HIDS (< 3%).

### DIAGNOSIS AND TREATMENT

Acute-phase reactants are elevated during attacks. IgD levels are usually elevated above 100 IU/mL, and IgA is elevated in 80% to 90% of patients. Mevalonate kinase activity is decreased, and urinary mevalonic acid is elevated, mainly during attacks. Homozygous genetic mutations are present in 75% of patients. However, HIDS may be seen in patients without genetic mutations when tested commercially (termed *variant HIDS*). If clinical suspicion is high, serum IgD and either *MVK* genetic testing or urinary mevalonic acid should be obtained. False-positive causes of increased IgD levels (usually not to the degree in HIDS) include other autoinflammatory diseases, human immunodeficiency virus (HIV), diabetes mellitus, smoking, and pregnancy. Normal IgD levels may represent a false-negative test, especially in patients younger than 3 years of age. Recently, evidence-based classification criteria have been published based the presence and absence of clinical features.

Nonsteroidal anti-inflammatory drugs (NSAIDs) and corticosteroids have some symptomatic benefit. Colchicine is ineffective. Simvastatin may reduce the number of febrile days but has no effect on the frequency of attacks. Case reports and series also suggest occasional benefit from etanercept and anakinra, with the latter likely more effective. Anakinra can occasionally be used in patients with infrequent attacks on demand at the start of an attack. Tocilizumab, an anti-IL-6 receptor antibody, may be beneficial in patients not responsive to anti-IL-1 therapy. A recent controlled study showed the benefit of the IL-1β antibody canakinumab. Regardless of treatment, attacks usually decrease in severity and frequency over time.

## TUMOR NECROSIS FACTOR RECEPTOR–ASSOCIATED PERIODIC SYNDROME

First described in 1982 as *familial Hibernian fever*, the gene mutation for the autosomal dominant disorder tumor necrosis factor (TNF) receptor–associated periodic syndrome (TRAPS) was discovered in 1999. TRAPS is the most common autosomal dominant autoinflammatory disorder. Although initially described in patients of Irish or Scottish descent, TRAPS is found in all ethnic groups. TRAPS presents in 75% of cases during the first decade of life (median age, 3 years), but it can present at any age. There is a slight male predominance (3:2).

### PATHOPHYSIOLOGY AND GENETICS

The TRAPS gene (*TNFRSF1A*) has been localized to the short arm of chromosome 12. The product of this gene is the 55-kDa TNF cell membrane receptor. There is a phenotype-genotype correlation with more severe disease and amyloidosis occurring in patients with cysteine residue mutations that alter the structure of the protein. Milder mutations of low penetrance, including R92Q and P46L, are frequently seen in normal controls (up to 9% of the population). These mutations

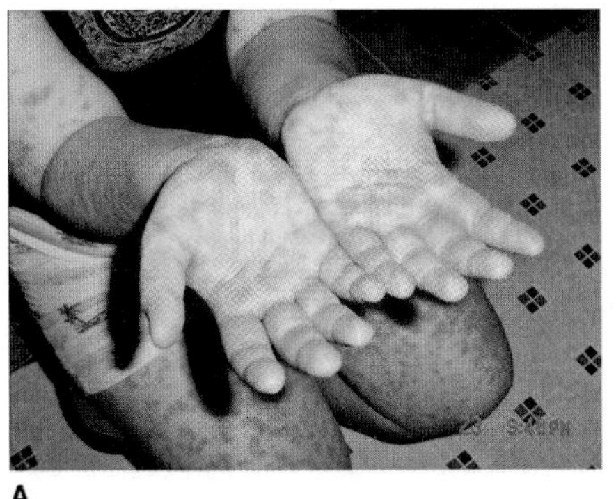
A

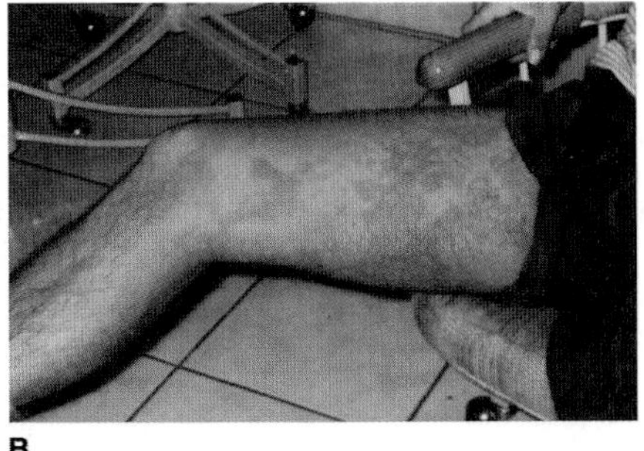
B

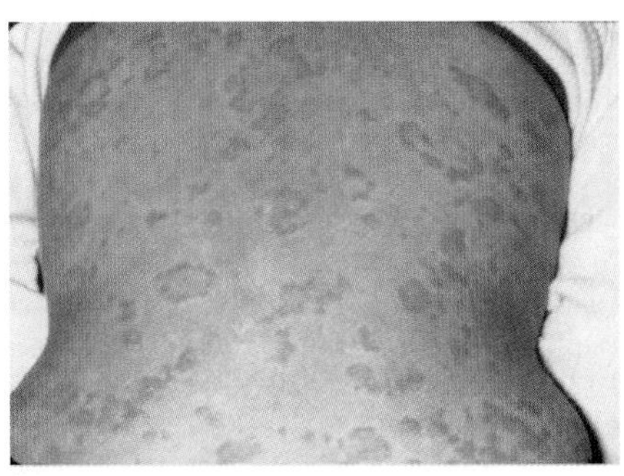
C

**FIGURE 206-2 A:** Erythematous macular and papular rash distributed over the arms and hands during an attack of mevalonate kinase deficiency (MKD)/hyperimmunoglobulinemia D syndrome (HIDS). The rash is almost morbilliform. **B:** Migratory erythematous rash of a patient with tumor necrosis factor–associated periodic syndrome (TRAPS). The rash is typically painful and migrates distally. **C:** Urticaria-like skin rash in a patient with cryopyrin-related periodic syndrome (CAPS). Unlike most urticarial rashes, the cellular infiltrate is predominately polymorphonuclear. (Panel A: Reproduced with permission from Takada K, Aksentijevich I, Mahadevan V, et al. Favorable preliminary experience with etanercept in two patients with the hyperimmunoglobulinemia D and periodic fever syndrome, *Arthritis Rheum.* 2003 Sep;48(9):2645-2651. Panels B and C: Reproduced with permission from Wolff K, Lowell A, Goldsmith A, et al. *Fitzpatrick's Dermatology in General Medicine.* New York: McGraw-Hill; 2008.)

may not be pathogenic by themselves but may contribute to other still unclear causes of increased inflammation. Decreased shedding of mutated membrane-bound TNF receptors was thought to explain the unopposed serum TNF effects observed in TRAPS. However, it is clear that not all mutations result in defective shedding. The pathogenesis of TRAPS may involve defects in TNF-induced apoptosis, protein misfolding, and abnormal intracellular trafficking, leading to stimulation of intracellular inflammatory pathways, including formation of reactive oxygen species, which also may result in a decrease in the concentration of surface receptors.

### CLINICAL FEATURES

Attacks typically last 1 to 6 weeks and occur 2 to 6 times per year, commonly triggered by exercise. They are marked by fever as well as serositis (abdominal, chest, and testicular pain), conjunctivitis, arthralgia, and myalgia. Two unique features are periorbital edema and a painful, distally migrating, erythematous rash (Fig. 206-2B). This rash represents a mononuclear perivascular infiltrate of the subcutaneous fascia and occasionally panniculitis. Patients with certain mutations, particularly R92Q and P46L, may develop a shorter and milder attack, with involvement of the pharynx and oral ulcerations. Less common manifestations include recurrent pericarditis and central and focal neurologic abnormalities. Amyloidosis develops in 14% to 25% of patients, particularly those with cysteine mutations and a family history of amyloid.

### DIAGNOSIS AND TREATMENT

Unlike other autoinflammatory diseases in which genetic abnormalities are only supportive of the diagnosis, the identification of TRAPS is based on finding a genetic mutation in the *TNFRSF1A* gene. However, evidence-based classification criteria have been published based on the presence and absence of clinical features.

NSAIDs may be effective for mild attacks. Corticosteroids are often beneficial for severe attacks, but escalating doses are often required as the efficacy tends to decrease over time. Colchicine is not effective.

In view of the role of defective shedding of the TNF receptor in the pathogenesis of TRAPS, researchers hypothesized that etanercept, a soluble TNF fusion protein receptor developed for the treatment of inflammatory arthritis, would be beneficial. Initial case reports supported this hypothesis. However, follow-up indicates that etanercept is not effective in all patients, and in others it loses effectiveness over time. IL-1 inhibitors are effective in most patients. A controlled study showed the effectiveness of canakinumab. In general, aggressive therapy with etanercept or IL-1 inhibitors should be reserved for patients with severe disease or those at increased risk of developing amyloidosis.

## THE CRYOPYRIN-ASSOCIATED PERIODIC SYNDROMES

Three autosomal dominant syndromes constitute the cryopyrin-associated periodic syndromes (CAPS). All are caused by single-base mutations on the *NLRP3* gene located on the long arm of chromosome 1 encoding the protein cryopyrin. Some mutations are specific to 1 of the syndromes, and some mutations overlap among all 3 syndromes (see Table 206-1). Often, especially in patients with neonatal-onset, multisystem inflammatory disease, no germ cell mutations are found. However, using advanced genetic techniques, somatic mutations are often found in some cells. Thus, as with other autoinflammatory syndromes, it is clear that other factors influence the development and severity of CAPS.

The cryopyrin protein contains an N-terminal pyrin domain and has an important role in regulation of the assembly of the inflammasome (see Fig. 206-1). This group of proteins, once assembled, activates caspase-1, leading to cleavage of pro-IL-1β to active IL-1β. Mutations of cryopyrin protein probably increase the rate of spontaneous assembling of inflammasomes. Cryopyrin is present mainly in neutrophils and chondrocytes, explaining the target organs of these diseases.

The 3 diseases that compose CAPS are considered variants of the same process, varying by severity of symptoms, systems involved, and outcome. Recently, evidence-based classification criteria have been published based on the presence and absence of clinical features. All 3 diseases respond dramatically to IL-1 inhibition.

### FAMILIAL COLD AUTOINFLAMMATORY SYNDROME

Familial cold autoinflammatory syndrome (FCAS), the mildest of the CAPS, was first described in 1940 as *familial cold urticaria*. The genetic mutation was discovered in 2001. Most patients with FCAS are located in the United States. Almost all patients have a genetic mutation in the *NLRP3* gene. FCAS often starts at birth and is apparent in 95% of patients by 6 months of age.

Typically, the attack starts 2 to 3 hours after general exposure to cold (as opposed to the direct contact that triggers cold-induced urticaria). Patients develop a urticarial-like rash that starts on the extremities and spreads to the trunk (Fig. 206-2C), low-grade fever, arthralgia, conjunctivitis, nausea, extreme thirst, sweating, and headaches. The attack peaks at 6 to 8 hours and lasts up to 24 hours. The frequency of attacks is variable, but they may occur with debilitating regularity. The rash is not true urticaria (mast cells); rather there is a perivascular polymorphonuclear cellular infiltrate in the dermis. Amyloidosis is a rare complication of FCAS (2–4%).

NSAIDs and antihistamine therapies are not effective. Corticosteroids may alleviate symptoms, but the magnitude and frequency of effective doses may result in significant adverse effects. IL-1 inhibition is very effective in alleviating symptoms. Rilonacept and canakinumab have been shown to be effective in controlled trials and also during long-term follow-up.

### MUCKLE-WELLS SYNDROME

Muckle-Wells syndrome (MWS), the CAPS of intermediate severity, was described in 1962, and the genetic mutation was found together with that of FCAS in 2001. MWS starts later in life than does FCAS and can appear at any age. Most cases are in Europe. Germ cell genetic mutations in the *NLRP3* gene are found in 65% to 75% of patients.

Attacks are usually not triggered by exposure to cold. A typical attack includes fever, rash, arthralgia, arthritis, myalgia, headaches, conjunctivitis, episcleritis, and uveitis. Attacks are more persistent than those of FCAS, lasting up to 3 days. Fifty to 70% of patients develop sensorineural hearing loss that typically starts in adolescence with loss of high-frequency sounds. Amyloidosis develops in 25% of patients with MWS. MWS also responds dramatically to IL-1 inhibition. However, hearing loss is reversible (usually partially) in only 20% to 33% of patients.

### NEONATAL-ONSET MULTISYSTEM INFLAMMATORY DISEASE

Neonatal-onset multisystem inflammatory disease (NOMID), which in Europe is called *chronic infantile neurologic, cutaneous, articular syndrome* (CINCA), is the most severe of the CAPS. It was first described in 1981, and the association with the *NLRP3* gene was reported in 2002. However, only approximately 50% to 60% of patients have germline mutations in this gene, whereas somatic mosaic mutations are found by new genetic technologies in the majority of other patients.

The onset of NOMID is at or within several weeks of birth. As many as half of affected infants are born prematurely. Patients present with a urticarial-like rash and fever, often occurring daily. They also have symptoms related to chronic aseptic meningitis such as headaches, irritability, and vomiting. Late neurologic complications include hydrocephalus, developmental delay, mental retardation, and hearing loss. Ocular findings include conjunctivitis, uveitis, and papillitis of the optic nerve, resulting in visual loss. By approximately 2 years of age, around 50% of patients have developed a severe arthropathy, consisting mainly of cartilage growth abnormalities leading to severe pain, metaphyseal and epiphyseal overgrowth, ossification irregularities, deformities, and disabilities. There is little synovial inflammation in NOMID. Patients have typical morphologic changes including short stature, frontal bossing, macrocephaly, saddle nose, short and thick extremities with clubbing of fingers, and wrinkled skin. Without treatment, approximately 20% of patient die by age 20, and others develop amyloidosis.

NSAIDs, antihistamines, corticosteroids, colchicine, methotrexate, and other immunosuppressive medications are marginally effective and do not change the disease course. Anakinra, a recombinant IL-1 receptor antagonist, is dramatically effective in treating the rash, fever, and meningitis of NOMID, with normalization of acute-phase reactants and a steroid-sparing effect. However, existing joint/bone damage and mental retardation are not reversible. Canakinumab is less effective in treating central nervous system disease. Early recognition and treatment are crucial in preventing long-term damage and disability.

## PYOGENIC STERILE ARTHRITIS, PYODERMA GANGRENOSUM, ACNE SYNDROME

Pyogenic sterile arthritis, pyoderma gangrenosum, acne (PAPA) syndrome was first described in 1997. PAPA syndrome usually presents in the first decade of life but can become manifest at any age. It is the result of mutations on the long arm of chromosome 15 in the *PSTPIP1* gene encoding the CD2 antigen-binding protein. This cytoskeleton protein also binds to pyrin, thereby enabling its function. Similar to FMF, mutations in *PSTPIP1* may affect IL-1 activity. The protein also inhibits apoptosis.

### CLINICAL MANIFESTATIONS

Attacks are often triggered by minor trauma, resulting in fever and massive neutrophilic joint effusion primarily affecting large joints. Patients also may develop pyoderma gangrenosum, severe acne (mainly during adolescence), and diabetes mellitus.

### TREATMENT AND OUTCOME

Intra-articular corticosteroid injections and surgical drainage do not affect outcome. Case reports suggest that anti-TNF and IL-1 agents may be effective in some patients.

If incompletely controlled, PAPA syndrome results in progressive destructive arthritis, skin scarring from acne, and significant depression from the severe sequelae of the disease. Longevity often depends on whether diabetes develops.

## DEFICIENCIES IN CYTOKINE RECEPTOR ANTAGONISTS

Receptor antagonists often function as natural protein inhibitors of inflammatory processes by competing with proinflammatory cytokines for membrane or intracellular receptors. At least 2 autoinflammatory syndromes related to mutations in genes that encode receptor antagonists have been described.

### DEFICIENCY OF THE IL-1 RECEPTOR ANTAGONIST

Deficiency of the IL-1 receptor antagonist (DIRA) is an autosomal recessive disease caused by a mutation (or deletion) in the *IL1RN* gene on the long arm of chromosome 2, which encodes the IL-1 receptor antagonist. DIRA has been described in families from Newfoundland, Puerto Rico, Lebanon, and southern Netherlands.

DIRA presents at birth or shortly after with multifocal osteomyelitis/lytic bone lesions, a sterile pustular rash, nail pits, oral ulcers, and respiratory distress with pneumonitis. Prior to the discovery of effective treatment, patients developed severe skeletal deformities and failure to thrive and often succumbed to the disease. Treatment with anakinra, an IL-1 receptor antagonist, is remarkably effective.

### DEFICIENCY OF THE IL-36 RECEPTOR ANTAGONIST

Deficiency of the IL-36 receptor antagonist (DITRA) is a rare autosomal recessive disease caused by a mutation in the *IL36RN* gene at the long arm of chromosome 3, near the *IL1RN* gene, that encodes the IL-36 receptor antagonist. DITRA has been described in Tunisian families and sporadically in Europe.

DITRA can start any time from infancy to mid-adulthood. Pregnancy has been a trigger in several patients. Patients develop flares of high fever lasting 1 to 3 days and a generalized pustular psoriatic rash lasting days to weeks. Approximately 30% develop arthritis and a chronic course of psoriasis vulgaris. Treatment includes use of oral retinoids, immunosuppressive medications, and IL-1 and TNF inhibitors. The mortality rate is high, and death occurs mainly from sepsis related to loss of the skin barrier during acute attacks.

## INTERFERONOPATHIES

The pathogenesis of these diseases is related to upregulation of type I interferon intracellular signaling and gene expression (mainly α and β) causing autoinflammation, which can overlap with features of autoimmunity. Recently, 4 monogenic diseases have been described. These diseases are not responsive to conventional anti-inflammatory therapies, including IL-1 inhibition, but may respond to inhibition of the interferon signaling pathways by Janus kinase inhibitors or to retroviral inhibitors.

### PROTEASOME-ASSOCIATED AUTOINFLAMMATORY SYNDROME

Proteasomes are large intracellular complexes that degrade unnecessary or abnormal proteins. The *PSMB8* gene located on the short arm of chromosome 6 encodes a ring subunit in the proteasome. Mutations in *PSMB8* cause an autosomal recessive autoinflammatory disease related to cellular stress, leading to stimulation of interferon pathways. Three conditions that probably represent 1 disorder have been described. The *Nakajo-Nishimura syndrome* was described in Japan. The *joint contractures, muscular atrophy, microcytic anemia, and panniculitis-induced lipodystrophy* (JMP) syndrome was described in Spain. However, the most commonly used term for this disease is *chronic atypical neutrophilic dermatosis with lipodystrophy and elevated temperature* (CANDLE) syndrome. These syndromes are characterized by early onset (usually in the first year of life) of recurrent fevers. Classic skin manifestations include purpuric rash and erythematous/violaceous plaques representing panniculitis primarily on the upper limbs, face, and eyelids and progressive lipodystrophy. Other features include arthralgia/arthritis with joint deformities (particularly in the fingers), hepatomegaly, failure to thrive with anemia, and increased acute-phase reactants. Patients may also develop hypertrichosis, acanthosis nigricans, alopecia areata, scleritis, interstitial lung disease, and aseptic meningitis.

### STIMULATOR OF INTERFERON GENES (STING)–ASSOCIATED VASCULOPATHY WITH ONSET IN INFANCY

This rare autosomal dominant disease is caused by gain-of-function mutations in the *TMEM173* gene, encoding STING, located on the long arm of chromosome 5. Soon after birth, patients develop a systemic inflammatory disease with capillary vasculopathy/vasculitis characterized by a violaceous pustular scaly rash on the digits, nose, cheeks, and ears with telangiectasia, worsened by exposure to cold. The vasculopathy may progress to acral necrosis and gangrene. Most patients develop interstitial lung disease and have episodes of low-grade fever and failure to thrive. Acute-phase reactants are markedly elevated. Most patients succumb to pulmonary disease or infection.

### OTULOPENIA

Autosomal recessive loss-of-function mutations in *OTULIN* encoding a deubiquitinase was described in a Pakistani and 2 Turkish families with 4 affected patients. Patients presented with neonatal-onset fever, neutrophilic dermatitis/panniculitis, and failure to thrive, but without obvious primary immunodeficiency. Evidence was found in the nuclear factor-κB pathway, as accumulated linear ubiquitin aggregates induced increases in the interferon pathway.

## DEFICIENCY OF ADENOSINE DEAMINASE 2

This autosomal recessive disease results from mutations in the *CERC1* gene on the long arm of chromosome 1, encoding the protein adenosine deaminase 2. Unlike deficiency of adenosine deaminase 1, which is associated with severe combined immunodeficiency, adenosine deaminase 2 is mostly an extracellular protein acting mainly as a factor important to vascular growth and cell differentiation, particularly monocytes. Therefore, deficiency of adenosine deaminase 2 (DADA2) is less associated with severe immunodeficiency. Rather, as demonstrated in a Zebra fish model, DADA2 may affect the integrity of blood vessels, particularly the endothelial barrier. DADA2 has been shown to decrease the differentiation of monocytes into anti-inflammatory, tissue-repairing M2 monocytes.

There are several phenotypes of DADA2. The *first*, primarily seen in patients of Georgian Jewish origin, is that of polyarteritis nodosa (PAN). The disease can vary in severity from mild cutaneous PAN, most commonly presenting with a livedoid rash with or without skin ulcerations, to severe life-threatening gastrointestinal and central nervous system disease. There may be long periods (years) of inactive disease between flares. The *second* phenotype combines early-onset stroke, most commonly thalamic and often hemorrhagic with fever, livedoid rash, and inflammatory markers. Many patients have low-grade immunodeficiency with recurrent infections, and some have low immunoglobulin levels, especially low IgM. Patients may have low B-cell counts, B-cell switching, and natural killer cells. *Other phenotypes* include early-onset pure red blood cell aplasia and hepatic disease with nodular hyperplasia and portal hypertension.

TNF inhibitors are extremely effective in treating DADA2, even in severe cases not responsive to cyclophosphamide and corticosteroids, although the reason for the effectiveness is still unclear. Anticoagulation is contraindicated, and aspirin should be used with caution for concern of developing brain hemorrhage. Severe cases have been treated with bone marrow transplantation.

## PERIODIC FEVER, APHTHOUS STOMATITIS, PHARYNGITIS, ADENITIS

Periodic fever, aphthous stomatitis, pharyngitis, adenitis (PFAPA) syndrome is probably the most common periodic fever syndrome in childhood and was initially described in 1987. The etiology is unknown. Although no specific genetic mutations have been found, familial cases of PFAPA are common occurences (> 10%), and many Middle Eastern patients have heterozygous *MEFV* mutations.

### CLINICAL FEATURES

The onset of PFAPA is usually in early childhood (< 5 years). It is the only autoinflammatory syndrome that is truly periodic (especially at onset), with attacks occurring usually every 21 to 28 days and fever lasting 3 to 7 days. Patients usually report an aura of feeling unwell several hours before the onset of an attack. Pharyngitis and cervical adenopathy are present in 80% to 100% of patients and aphthous stomatitis in 60% to 70%. Patients also frequently have abdominal pain, nausea/vomiting, arthralgias, and headaches.

### DIAGNOSIS AND TREATMENT

Diagnostic criteria have been defined for children with typical clinical features. In addition, patients must be completely asymptomatic between attacks, exhibit normal growth and development, and not have cyclic neutropenia. Other autoinflammatory syndromes, particularly TRAPS or MKD/HIDS, need to be considered in patients with atypical features or in those who are not completely well between attacks. Patients have increased acute-phase reactants during attacks, which normalize between attacks. Some patients have a mild increase in IgD, and some have heterozygous mutations of other autoinflammatory genes, especially *MEFV*.

A single dose of prednisone (0.6–2 mg/kg) at the onset of symptoms usually aborts that attack, although it may also decrease the intervals between attacks. Colchicine is effective as a prophylactic agent in approximately 50% of patients, especially those with *MEFV* mutations, and cimetidine is effective in approximately 33% of patients (40 mg/kg/d in 2 divided doses). Two controlled studies, large series, and a Cochrane review suggest that tonsillectomy (± adenoidectomy) is curative in the vast majority of patients, although the indication and timing of performing surgery are still unclear. On-demand anakinra at the onset of symptoms may shorten attacks.

The natural course of PFAPA in untreated patients is benign. The frequency and severity of attacks diminish over time, and PFAPA usually, but not always, resolves fully during the second decade of life. Amyloidosis is not a complication of PFAPA.

## CHRONIC RECURRENT MULTIFOCAL OSTEOMYELITIS

Chronic recurrent multifocal osteomyelitis (CRMO) was first described in 1972. The term *chronic nonbacterial osteomyelitis* may be more accurate, as this disease is often not recurrent or multifocal. The disease is usually sporadic, and the etiology is unknown. The median age of onset of isolated CRMO is 10 years. Several related autoinflammatory bone disorders have been found to have a genetic etiology. A rare autosomal recessive disorder of CRMO with congenital dyserythropoietic anemia (Majeed syndrome) is associated with mutations in the *LPIN2* gene. Cherubism, an autosomal dominant chronic inflammatory disease of excessive bone degradation of the upper and lower jaws followed by development of fibrous tissue masses, is associated with mutations in the *SH3BP2* and possibly *PTPN11* genes. A mouse model of CRMO with mutations in the *PISPIP2* gene has been described. Lytic inflammatory bone lesions are found in patients with DIRA (see earlier section).

Patients with classic CRMO develop recurrent episodes of bone pain and fever. Bone lesions include osteolytic lesions surrounded by sclerotic bone, especially in the metaphysis of long bone. Any bone may be involved, particularly the clavicle, ribs, and vertebrae. Asymptomatic lesions may be demonstrable on technetium bone scan and magnetic resonance imaging (MRI). Whole-body MRI is now considered the imaging modality of choice in following these patients. Bacterial cultures of biopsies are negative for usual bacteria. Other associated clinical findings may include synovitis, acne, pustulosis, hyperostosis, and osteitis (SAPHO syndrome), isolated palmoplantar pustulosis, psoriasis, sacroiliitis, inflammatory bowel disease, and pyoderma gangrenosum. A diagnostic score based on clinical, laboratory, and imaging features has been developed, although a biopsy is necessary in the majority of cases to exclude other causes of bone lytic lesions, particularly malignancies.

The natural history of CRMO is waxing and waning symptoms, often with spontaneous remissions and healing of lesions followed by relapses. In the past, patients were thought to have a good long-term prognosis, but recent studies have found chronic disease in approximately 50% of patients. Without treatment, chronic bone deformities, leg-length inequality, and disability are common, especially in males.

Antibiotics usually are not effective. NSAIDs are the first line of treatment. Other patients may benefit from corticosteroids, methotrexate, sulfasalazine, azithromycin, interferon, infliximab, or bisphosphonates, especially pamidronate. Pamidronate and infliximab should be used in severe disease, particularly disease affecting the vertebrae.

## SCHNITZLER SYNDROME

Schnitzler syndrome, first described in 1972, is characterized by a chronic urticarial eruption with a monoclonal IgM gammopathy. Other findings include intermittent fever, joint and/or bone pain with radiologic evidence of osteosclerosis, lymphadenopathy, hepatosplenomegaly, and elevated acute-phase reactants. The etiology is still unknown, but IL-1 plays an important role in the pathogenesis. Some patients were found to have somatic mosaic mutations in the

*NLRP3* gene associated with CAPS. The disease pursues a chronic course, without remission. Traditional NSAID, colchicine, dapsone, and antihistamine therapy usually is not effective. Late evolution to a lymphoproliferative malignancy, often Waldenström macroglobulinemia, occurs in at least 15% of patients. Amyloidosis has been reported in some cases. IL-1 inhibition is remarkably effective.

## THE CONTRIBUTION OF AUTOINFLAMMATORY GENE MUTATIONS TO OTHER DISEASES

Autoinflammatory gene mutations also may play a role in the severity and clinical presentations of other diseases including Behçet disease, inflammatory bowel disease, juvenile idiopathic arthritis, rheumatic fever, pericarditis, and palindromic arthritis. Recently, a monogenic, gain-of-function, autosomal dominant disorder causing a Behcet disease–like syndrome was described with a mutation in the NF-κB inhibitory protein A20. Reports have suggested that these gene mutations may affect the outcome of septic shock and may increase the risk of the development of secondary amyloidosis and atherosclerotic plaque.

### SUGGESTED READINGS


Crow YJ. Type I interferonopathies: Mendelian type I interferon up-regulation. *Curr Opin Immunol.* 2015;32C:7-12.

Federici S, Gattorno M. A practical approach to the diagnosis of autoinflammatory diseases in childhood. *Best Pract Res Clin Rheumatol.* 2014;28:263-276.

Federici S, Sormani MP, Ozen S, et al. Evidence-based provisional clinical classification criteria for autoinflammatory periodic fevers. *Ann Rheum Dis.* 2015;74:799-805.

Giancane G, Ter Haar NM, Wulffraat N, et al. Evidence-based recommendations for genetic diagnosis of familial Mediterranean fever. *Ann Rheum Dis.* 2015;74:635-641.

Hashkes PJ, Laxer RM. The cryopyrin-associated periodic syndromes: CAPS is underrecognized, undiagnosed and undertreated. *Rheumatologist.* 2014;9:18-22.

Hedrich CM, Hofmann SR, Pablik J, Morbach H, Girschick HJ. Autoinflammatory bone disorders with special focus on chronic recurrent multifocal osteomyelitis (CRMO). *Pediatr Rheumatol Online J.* 2013;11:47.

Hentgen V, Grateau G, Kone-Paut I, et al. Evidence-based recommendations for the practical management of familial Mediterranean fever. *Semin Arthritis Rheum.* 2013;43:387-391.

Hofer M, Pillet P, Cochard MM, et al. International periodic fever, aphthous stomatitis, pharyngitis, cervical adenitis syndrome cohort: description of distinct phenotypes in 301 patients. *Rheumatology (Oxford).* 2014;53:1125-1129.

International Society for Systemic AutoInflammatory Diseases. Infevers. http://fmf.igh.cnrs.fr/ISSAID/infevers/. Accessed May 19, 2016.

Lachmann HJ, Papa R, Gerhold K, et al. The phenotype of TNF receptor-associated autoinflammatory syndrome (TRAPS) at presentation: a series of 158 cases from the Eurofever/EUROTRAPS international registry. *Ann Rheum Dis.* 2014;73:2160-2167.

Shinar Y, Obici L, Aksentijevich I, et al. Guidelines for the genetic diagnosis of hereditary recurrent fevers. *Ann Rheum Dis.* 2012;71:1599-1605.

ter Haar NM, Oswald M, Jeyaratnam J, et al. Recommendations for the management of autoinflammatory diseases. *Ann Rheum Dis.* 2015;74:1636-1644.

# 207 Growth and Development

Indranil Kushare and John G. Birch

## INTRODUCTION

Growth and development of the musculoskeletal system, in tandem with gross and fine motor development, are overshadowed perhaps only by intellectual development in terms of magnitude, complexity, and sophistication from conception to skeletal maturity. The pathway delineated by postnatal development defines infancy, childhood, and adolescence. In the simplest terms, the growth plates (or *physes*) of long bones are the "motors" of skeletal development. Their physical characteristics and function help separate the "child" from the "adult," orthopedically speaking. In this chapter, we will briefly review musculoskeletal embryology, postnatal musculoskeletal development, and the structure and function of the growth plate and their clinical implications.

## MUSCULOSKELETAL EMBRYOLOGY

Embryologically, the musculoskeletal system develops from the dorsal (somatic) mesoderm. Approximately 26 days after fertilization, the upper limb "bud" appears on the ventrolateral body wall, consisting of mesenchymal cell swelling covered by ectoderm. The lower limb bud appears about 2 days after the upper; this slight delay relative to the upper limb in appearance, organization, and maturation continues throughout the limbs' development. With continued growth and development, a chondrogenic core forms, beginning proximally and progressing distally (characteristic of both upper and lower limb formation). This chondrogenic core evolves to the point that the upper limb skeletal elements, except for the distal phalanges, are present by the seventh week (eighth for the lower limb). Subsequent to the development of the chondrogenic skeletal structure, invasion of nerves of the limb occurs, followed quickly by formation of skeletal muscle tissue. Joints form by programmed chondrogenic cell death (apoptosis) producing clefts within the chondrogenic skeleton. Further healthy joint development is dependent on movement, which in turn is dependent on the development and maturation of innervated skeletal muscle. By the eighth week, differentiation of major tissues in the limbs is complete, and the majority of the remaining fetal period is dedicated to growth.

## BONE DEVELOPMENT AND POSTNATAL GROWTH

Bone is a composite tissue, consisting of an organic component (osteoid) and inorganic matrix (primarily hydroxyapatite) that give bone its hardness.

Bone is formed by 1 of 2 pathways: intramembranous and enchondral ossification. *Intramembranous ossification* is characterized by direct ossification of fibrous primitive connective tissue; the clavicle and bones of the skull form intramembranously. During intramembranous ossification, dense nodules of mesenchymal cells convert to capillaries and osteoblasts. These osteoblasts secrete osteoid that subsequently becomes mineralized. All other appendicular and axial bones form by *enchondral ossification*—that is, by gradual ossification of a cartilaginous anlage. Instead of converting directly into osteoblasts, condensations of mesenchymal cells transform into cartilage matrix-secreting chondroblasts.

Long bones are anatomically characterized by a central shaft (*diaphysis*) flaring to a broader *metaphysis* at either end, and they terminate in a typically bulbous, articular cartilage-capped, *epiphysis* (Fig. 207-1). In the central region of each cartilage anlage, capillary invasion results in the replacement of chondroblasts by osteoblasts and the formation of *primary centers of ossification*. Ossification of

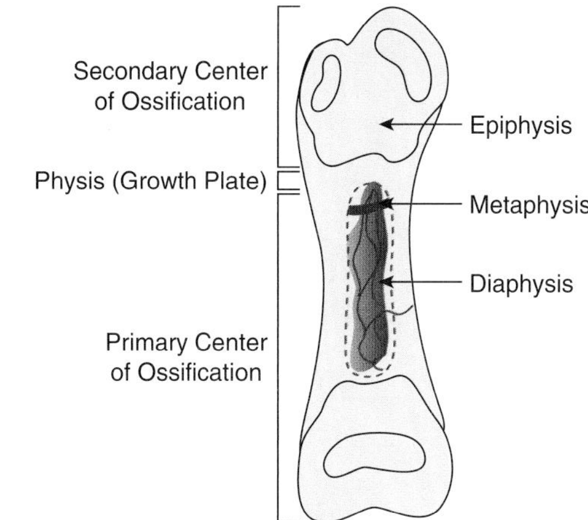


FIGURE 207-1 Scheme of anatomic regions of long bones.

the cartilaginous anlage then continues centrifugally. The epiphyses at various stages of development, particular to the individual bone, experience vascular invasion as well, resulting in the formation of *secondary centers of ossification*. Once the secondary centers of ossification have appeared, the cartilaginous growth plate (*physis*) can be "visualized" radiographically as the radiolucent disk between the bony metaphysis and epiphysis. The appearance of the various secondary centers of ossification typically occurs within a relatively narrow age range, so that their absence or appearance may be used to estimate the age of the fetus and infant (Fig. 207-2). Similarly, the physes will disappear ("close") at skeletal maturity; the timing of physeal closure is specific to the individual physes and is location- and gender-dependent (Fig. 207-3). At a more sophisticated level during later stages of growth, careful analysis of the maturation of the distal radial and ulnar epiphyses, carpals, metacarpals, and phalanges forms the basis for the calculation of skeletal (or "bone") age. These estimations may be used to identify inhibition of hormonal growth and allow a calculation of growth remaining in long bones and, to a lesser extent, the spine.

The central shaft (diaphysis) flares to the metaphyses, which are capped by the usually bulbous, joint-forming ends (epiphyses). In skeletally immature children, the physis or growth plate is sandwiched between the epiphysis and metaphysis. Earliest ossification is characterized by vascular invasion of the diaphysis and ossification of the "primary center of ossification." Later, secondary centers of ossification form within the epiphyses by a similar process. After the appearance of the secondary centers of ossification, the physis is identifiable as the radiolucent zone between the metaphyseal and epiphyseal bone.

The process of enchondral ossification continues throughout skeletal growth in the epiphyses and particularly in the physes of long bones. The physis is a highly organized disk of replicating and subsequently ossifying cartilage located between the epiphysis and metaphysis. The physes are the primary source of longitudinal skeletal growth. Each long-bone physis will elongate a typical and known amount per year of skeletal growth. The major long bones of the upper and lower limbs have a physis at either end, whereas the metacarpals, metatarsals, and phalanges usually have only 1. The "globular bones" (carpals and tarsals) are more "jelly bean"–like in their cartilaginous-bony structure, with a central ossific nucleus embedded in an ever-thinning rind of growing cartilage. The physes are highly complex cartilaginous structures microscopically divided into 4 layers or "zones" (Fig. 207-4): germinal (or "resting"), proliferative, hypertrophic, and zone of provisional calcification. The germinal layer, adjacent to the secondary ossific nucleus once the latter has appeared, is characterized by a relatively large amount of extracellular matrix with apparently randomly located chondroblasts. The

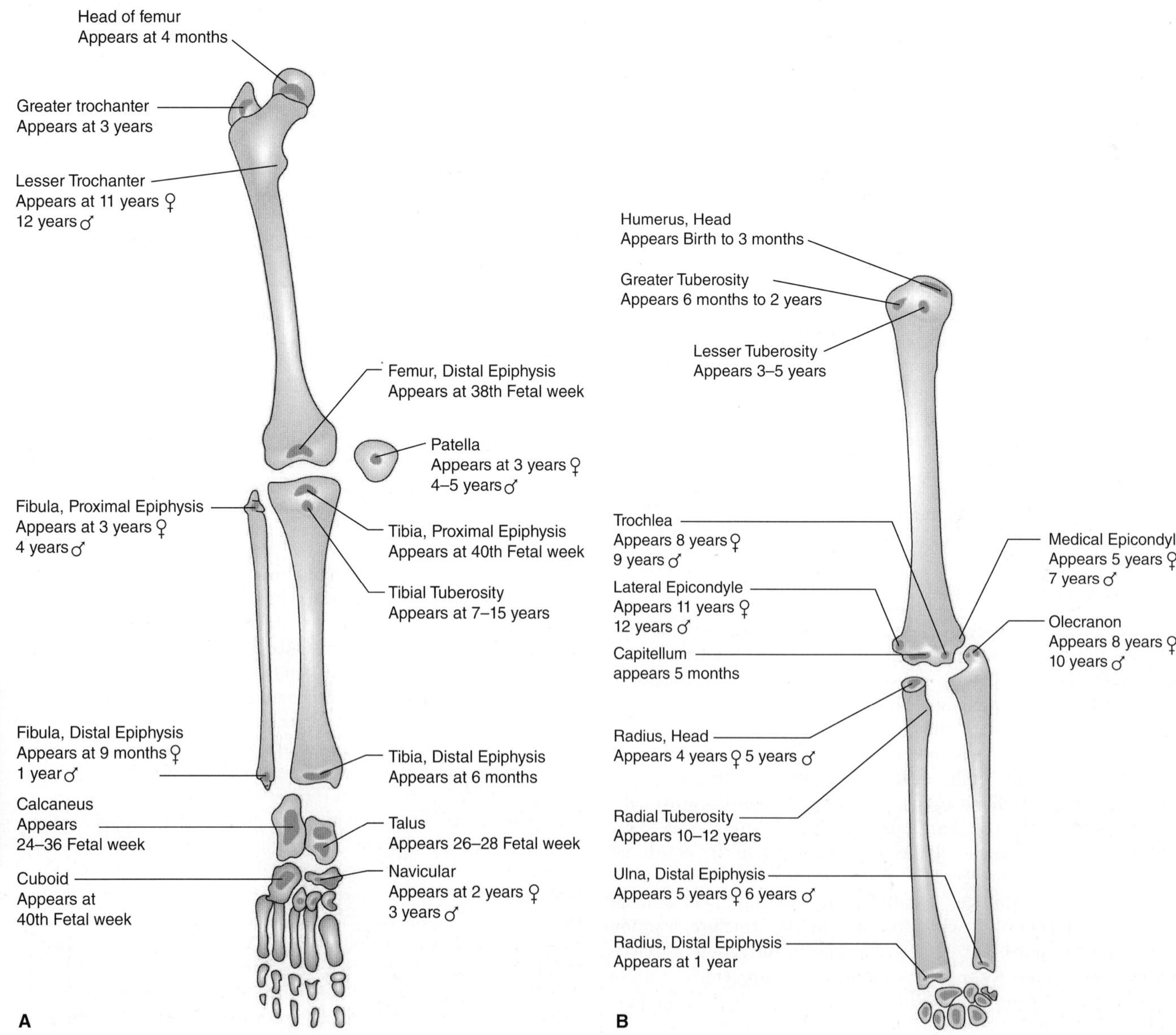


**FIGURE 207-2** Age of radiographic appearance of the secondary ossific centers of long-bone epiphyses: (**A**) upper extremity and (**B**) lower extremity. These appearances can be used to estimate a child's skeletal age and identify skeletal growth abnormalities and need to be differentiated from fractures.

proliferative layer has proportionately more cells and less extracellular matrix. The chondroblasts are strikingly arranged into longitudinal columns. Toward the metaphyseal region, these cells become larger in size, with even less extracellular matrix between them. This extracellular matrix becomes calcified, with chondroblast apoptosis, in the zone of provisional calcification. The zones of hypertrophy and provisional calcification are the structurally weakest layers, and it is here that fractures of the physes are most typically propagated. At the metaphyseal base of the zone of provisional calcification, vascular invasion and early ossification of the matrix occur (see Fig. 207-4).

The modulation of growth through the physis is subject to many hormonal and mechanical influences that are not thoroughly understood. Insulin-like growth factors, growth hormone, thyroid hormone, and the estrogens all influence physeal activity during prenatal, postnatal, and preadolescent growth. The absence of certain vitamins and minerals (most notably vitamin D, vitamin C, and calcium) also adversely affects physeal growth and ossification in the provisional calcification zone of the physis (see Fig. 207-4). In addition, the physis responds favorably and unfavorably, respectively, to physiologic and nonphysiologic loading, referred to as *the Hueter-Volkmann principle.* In general, excessive compressive forces decelerate normal physeal growth, whereas modest traction or distraction forces may result in accelerated physeal growth.

It is important to recognize that even in long bones, growth does not occur exclusively at the physes. Appositional growth of the diaphysis and metaphysis occurs, primarily under the periosteum, by intramembranous ossification. The epiphyses expand in a centrifugal manner, resulting in enlargement of the ends of long bones and contributing to the overall increase in the total length of a long bone. Simultaneous with growth at all of these locations, reshaping (or "remodeling") occurs, under both genetic and physical influences. The metaphyses tapers and condenses into the diaphysis, and the overall long bone remodels.

Each physis contributes a known amount to a long bone's length during each year of skeletal maturation, both in percentage and actual amounts. The average growth of specific physes of upper and lower extremities is presented in Table 207-1.

Thus, injury, inadvertent or deliberate via surgery, can have a calculable effect on the ultimate length of a limb. This information is important because physeal injuries occur frequently in children. Physes can be damaged physically by direct trauma, infection, or encroachment by both benign and malignant tumors. Physeal growth

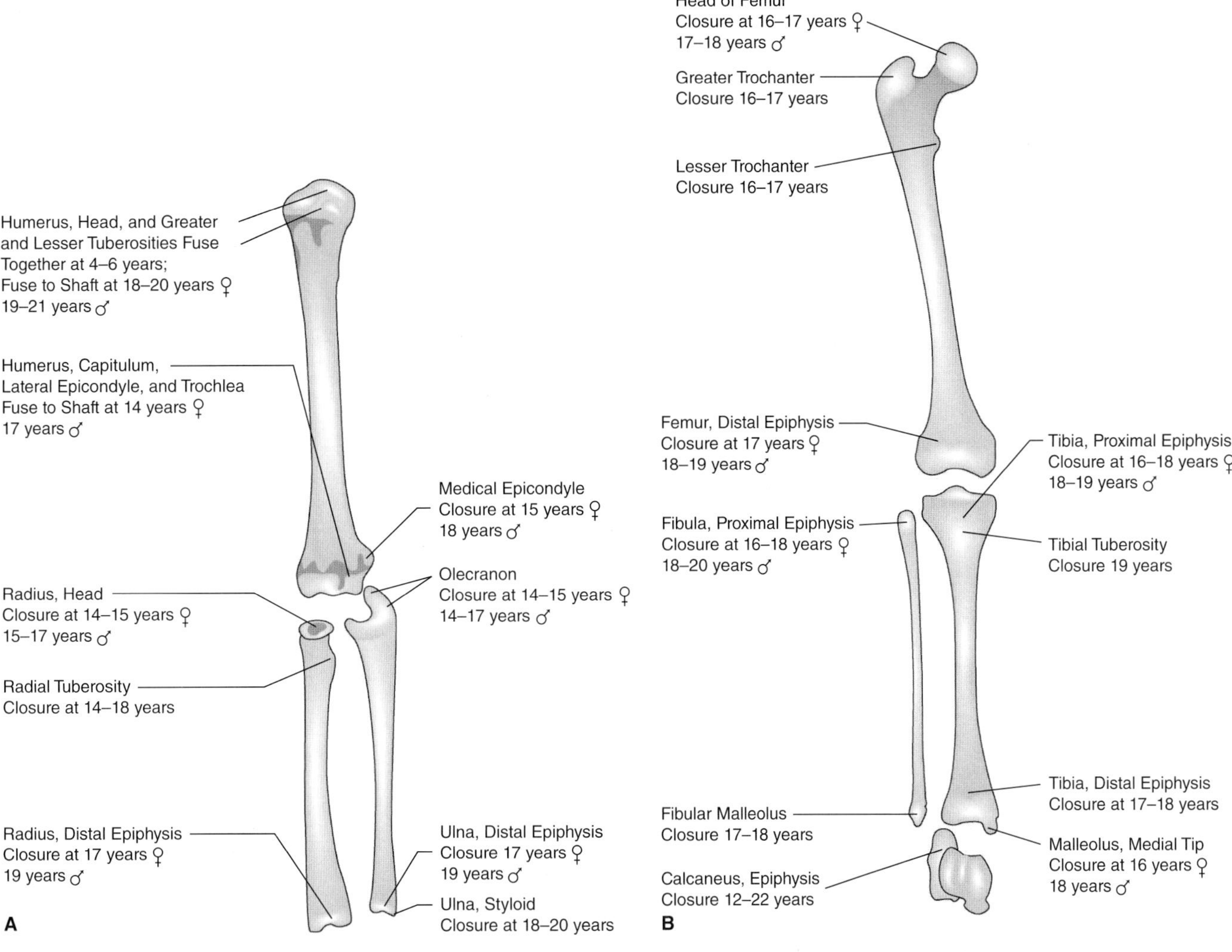


**FIGURE 207-3** Age of physeal (growth plate) closure: (**A**) upper extremity and (**B**) lower extremity for males and females.



disturbances are, fortunately, not common, but significant deformities may result when they occur, and extensive orthopedic reconstruction treatment may be required. Similarly, pathologic angular deformities or inequality in the length of the limbs may be corrected by harnessing physeal growth using appropriately timed surgical growth-modulation procedures (Fig. 207-5).

Lower-limb growth is characterized by 4 different periods: antenatal growth (exponential); birth to 5 years (rapid growth); 5 years to puberty (stable growth); and puberty, which is the final growth spurt characterized by a rapid acceleration phase lasting 1 year followed by a more gradual deceleration phase lasting 1.5 years.

Secondary Center of Ossification
Resting (Germinal) Zone
Proliferative Zone
Hypertrophic Zone
Zone of Provisional Calcification

**FIGURE 207-4** Scheme of the microscopic organization of the physis or growth plate. Traditionally, the physis is separated into 4 contiguous layers from epiphysis to metaphysis: resting (or germinal), proliferative, hypertrophic, and zone of provisional calcification.

## GROSS MOTOR DEVELOPMENT

Maturation of the neurologic system after birth, particularly the peripheral nervous system, is integral to musculoskeletal growth. Gross motor milestones cannot be met without a complex interaction of central and peripheral nervous system development, as well as musculoskeletal growth and maturation. The average age and range of achievement of gross and fine motor milestones (discussed in Chapters 82, 84, and 88) should be well understood by all physicians and allied healthcare workers involved in the care of children. The major gross motor milestones and their average age of attainment are summarized in Table 207-2.

**TABLE 207-1 AVERAGE GROWTH PER YEAR AT VARIOUS PHYSES**

| Location of the Physis | Estimated Average Growth per Year |
|---|---|
| Proximal humerus | 7 mm |
| Distal humerus | 2 mm |
| Proximal femur | 3.5 mm |
| Distal femur | 9 mm |
| Proximal tibia | 6 mm |
| Distal tibia | 5 mm |

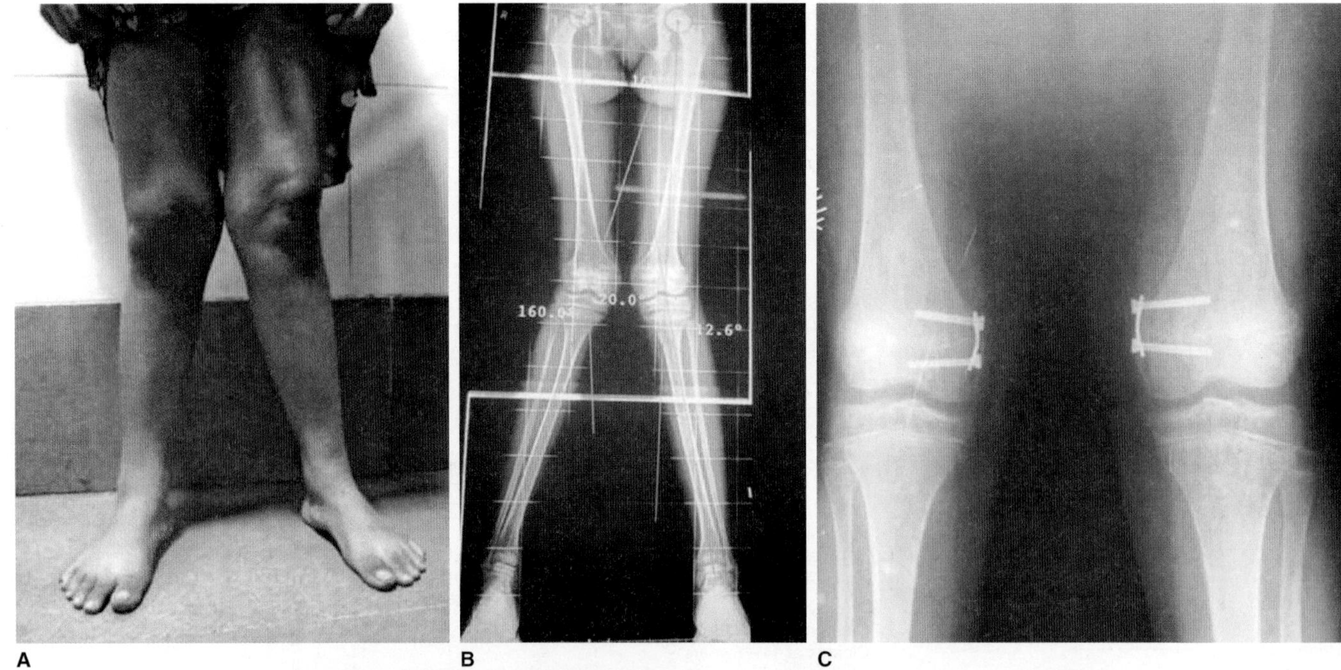


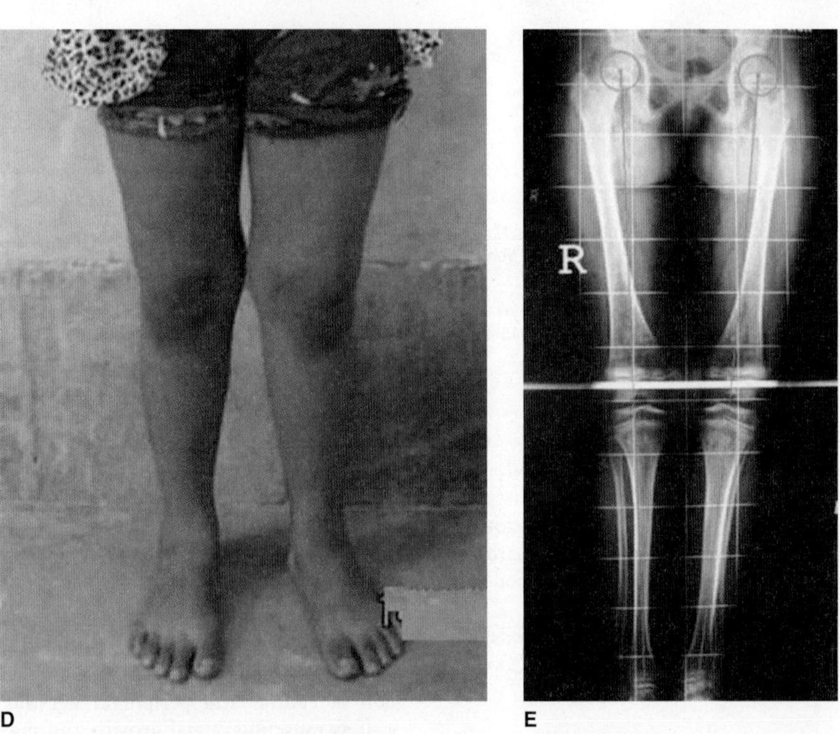


**FIGURE 207-5** Longitudinal growth can be "harnessed" by surgical procedures to correct deformity in growing children. **A:** A patient with bilateral idiopathic genu valgum. **B:** Preoperative radiograph. **C:** Surgical implantation of 8 plates straddling the medial distal femur for growth modulation (temporary epiphysiostasis). **D:** Correction of the knock knee deformity; by tethering of the medial with continued lateral, distal femoral physeal growth has occurred. **E:** Postcorrection radiograph.

**TABLE 207-2 AGE OF APPEARANCE OF CERTAIN GROSS MOTOR MILESTONES[a]**

| Milestone | Age (Months, Average) |
|---|---|
| Rolls over (front to back) | 5 |
| Rolls over (back to front) | 6 |
| Sits independently | 7 |
| Crawls | 8 |
| Pulls to stand | 9 |
| Cruises (walks holding on) | 11 |
| Walks independently | 12 |
| Runs well | 24 |

[a]Note that achievement of these milestones requires development of the neurologic and musculoskeletal systems.

## SUGGESTED READINGS

Ballock RT, O'Keefe RJ. Physiology and pathophysiology of the growth plate. *Birth Defects Res C Embryo Today*. 2003;69(2):123-143.

Colnot C. Cellular and molecular interactions regulating skeletogenesis. *J Cell Biochem*. 2005;95(4):688-697.

Dietz FR, Morcuende JA. Embryology and development of the musculoskeletal system. In: Morrissey RT, Weinstein SL, eds. *Lovell and Winter's Pediatric Orthopaedics*. 6th ed. Philadelphia, PA: Lippincott Williams & Wilkins; 2005:1-34.

Forriol F, Shapiro F. Bone development: interaction of molecular components and biophysical forces. *Clin Orthop Relat Res*. 2005;432:14-33.

Ghanem I, Widmann RF. Surgical epiphysiodesis indications and techniques: update. *Curr Opin Pediatr.* 2011;23(1):53-59.

Illingworth RS. *The Development of the Infant and Young Child: Normal and Abnormal.* 9th ed. New York, NY: Churchill Livingstone; 1987.

Mackie EJ, Tatarczuch L, Mirams M. The skeleton: a multi-functional complex organ: the growth plate chondrocyte and endochondral ossification. *J Endocrinol.* 2011;211(2):109-121.

# 208 The Limping Child

Aharon Z. Gladstein and Lawson A.B. Copley

## INTRODUCTION

Among the causes of gait abnormality in children, those that should be kept in mind in acute settings include infection, trauma, and malignancy. Children who develop a limp acutely should be evaluated carefully with a detailed history and physical examination, appropriate radiographs and laboratory studies, and timely subspecialty evaluation in order to exclude these potentially worrisome causes. When infection is suspected, the workup should be conducted in either an observation or inpatient status until the diagnosis is confirmed or excluded. An age-based approach to diagnosis can help the clinician focus his or her approach.

## HISTORY

A thorough history will point the clinician toward the correct diagnosis in most cases. Factors to note are the onset and duration of symptoms, the presence and location of pain, the presence of fever or malaise, or any history of witnessed injury. Although trauma is far more common in children than is infection or malignancy, it is less commonly the source of an unexplained limp. The history is consistent with injury, without suggestion of fever or malaise. The clinician must maintain a high index of suspicion for nonaccidental injury when objective findings point toward trauma but the history is inconsistent. Physical findings often demonstrate bruising or swelling without erythema. Trauma may be reported as an antecedent event in approximately 35% of children with infection. In these circumstances, the physician should be mindful of subtle details in the history and physical examination. One should ask about the timing of the injury with respect to the onset of symptoms, the mechanism of injury, and the presence of fever.

## PHYSICAL EXAMINATION

Gait should be observed by having the child walk and run while distracted. Antalgic gait is characterized by shortening the stance phase to minimize weight bearing on a painful limb. Limp with a nonantalgic gait pattern is less likely the result of an infectious or traumatic etiology.

The lower extremities should be observed for symmetry, noting any areas of swelling or deformity. Range of motion of the hips, knees, and ankles should be assessed. Keep in mind that hip disorders may present with knee pain, but movement of the hip may exacerbate the pain. Affected areas should be palpated for swelling or tenderness. Sites that are painful with range of motion or tender to palpation may warrant radiographic evaluation.

## DIAGNOSTIC MANEUVERS

### Leg Lengths

Discrepancy in the length of the legs should be assessed with the patient standing and the examiner's hands on the iliac crests. Discrepancy can be further evaluated by observing the heights of the knees with the patient supine and the hips and knees flexed (Galeazzi sign), followed by prone observation of length of the lower leg.

### Trendelenburg Test

The child stands on 1 leg with the other raised off the ground. The test is positive if the pelvis tilts away from the planted leg. A positive test indicates weakness in the hip abductor.

### Flexion and External Rotation

A child with a painful hip due to intra-articular pathology will keep it flexed and externally rotated to avoid tightening the joint capsule. A helpful maneuver in a young child is to have the patient's caregiver hold him or her under the arms. The irritable hip will be kept in a flexed and externally rotated position compared to the unaffected hip.

## LABORATORY TESTS

Whenever infection is suspected, laboratory studies should be obtained to assess for a systemic response to the infection. They should include a complete blood count (CBC) with differential, C-reactive protein (CRP), and the erythrocyte sedimentation rate (ESR). Among these studies, the most sensitive test for identifying the inflammation associated with acute musculoskeletal infection is the CRP. Abnormalities of the infectious indices should raise the level of concern and motivate the physician to perform more dedicated imaging to help define the nature and extent of the problem.

## IMAGING

### X-Ray

Areas of tenderness or deformity, including the joints above and below the area of concern, should be examined with biplanar radiography. Any suspected hip pathology should be evaluated with anteroposterior (AP) pelvis and bilateral frog-leg lateral views. These views allows side-to-side comparison for the detection of subtle abnormalities.

### Ultrasound

Suspected hip joint effusion can be confirmed with ultrasound (Fig. 208-1). The absence of effusion in the setting of suspected hip infection may warrant magnetic resonance imaging (MRI) evaluation to rule out osteomyelitis or soft tissue infection.

### MRI

MRI is a sensitive and specific test for both soft tissue infection and trauma. Its use in the acute setting is reserved for assessing areas of

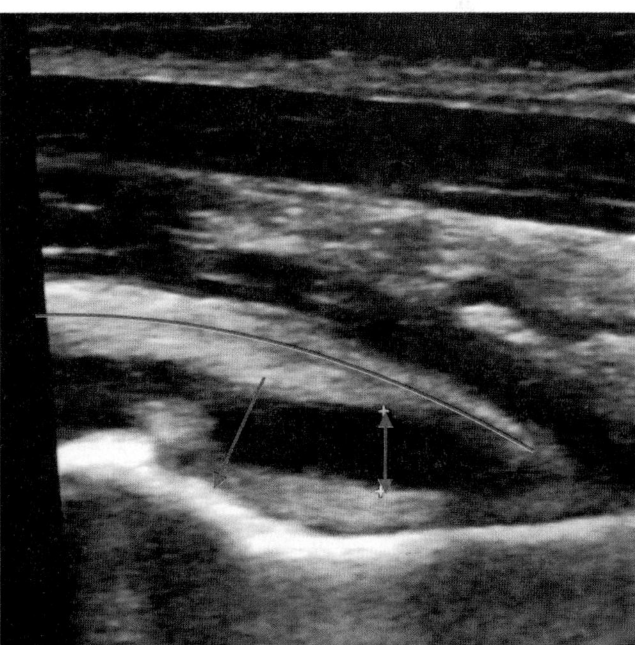

**FIGURE 208-1** Ultrasound of the hip shows a joint effusion with elevation of the capsule off of the proximal femur. *Double arrowed-line:* effusion; *single-arrowed line:* proximal femur; *curved line:* hip joint capsule.

suspected infection for which an obvious intra-articular source is not readily apparent. If a precise location can be determined from physical examination, then MRI with and without intravenous contrast is the most sensitive and specific study to evaluate for infection, even if the onset has been within 24 hours. Findings from the MRI will be useful to guide surgical decision-making, if indicated, as the spatial extent and involvement of various tissue types can be identified. If infection is suspected, but the location is uncertain, then bone scintigraphy is preferable.

## AGE-BASED DIFFERENTIAL DIAGNOSIS

### 0 to 3 Years

**Septic Arthritis or Osteomyelitis** Septic arthritis of the hip causes pain at rest that is exacerbated by motion. Subspecialty consultation is warranted, and consideration should be given for image-guided aspiration and possible surgical drainage.

**Developmental Dysplasia of the Hip** Unilateral *developmental dysplasia of the hip* (DDH) may present with a painless limp due to a shortening of the affected extremity. It also may lead to a Trendelenburg gait due to shortening of the hip abductor lever arm. Bilateral DDH may lead to a waddling gait but may be difficult to diagnose as limb lengths may be equal. The diagnosis can be confirmed with x-ray examination of the hips (Fig. 208-2). X-rays should include an AP pelvis and bilateral frog-leg lateral views.

**Fracture or Soft Tissue Injury** Trauma is a more unusual cause of unexplained limp, as in most cases the antecedent traumatic event is witnessed. Toddlers' fractures (eg, spiral fracture of the distal tibial metaphysis), however, may be the result of a low-energy trauma that does not arouse concern until the onset of pain. Radiographs are indicated to evaluate for fracture, dislocation, or physeal injury. These radiographs should include at least 2 views of the area of injury and should span the regions including the joint above and below the area of involvement.

When radiographs do not demonstrate obvious skeletal injury, the soft tissues should be inspected to look for other signs of injury, such as joint effusion, ligament avulsions, or soft tissue swelling. Clinical findings of tenderness directly over a growth plate, despite negative radiographs, may suggest a possible growth plate injury that should be protected as a fracture, as this is a far more common injury than a sprain in childhood.

Fractures in children below walking age should arouse suspicion of nonaccidental trauma.

### 4 to 10 Years

**Transient Synovitis** *Transient synovitis,* or irritable hip, is a benign, self-limited condition that affects children in this age group. Differentiating it from septic arthritis of the hip can be very challenging. Clinical-prediction algorithms have been proposed, but their clinical value is the subject of debate.

**Septic Arthritis of the Hip** If septic arthritis is suspected, subspecialty consultation should be obtained. Ultrasound-guided aspiration may be warranted for diagnosis, followed by urgent surgical decompression.

**Legg-Calvé-Perthes Disease** *Legg-Calvé-Perthes disease* is a rare, idiopathic cause of hip pain in this age group. Patients may present with unilateral hip pain and limp. Initial x-rays may be normal, but follow-up films will show abnormality of the proximal femoral epiphysis (Fig. 208-3).

**Fracture or Soft Tissue Injury** Again, fracture is an unusual cause of unexplained limp in this age group as patients will report an antecedent event.

### 11 to 15 Years

**Slipped Capital Femoral Epiphysis** An important condition to keep in mind in the discussion of a traumatically related limp is *slipped capital femoral epiphysis* (SCFE; see also Chapter 212).

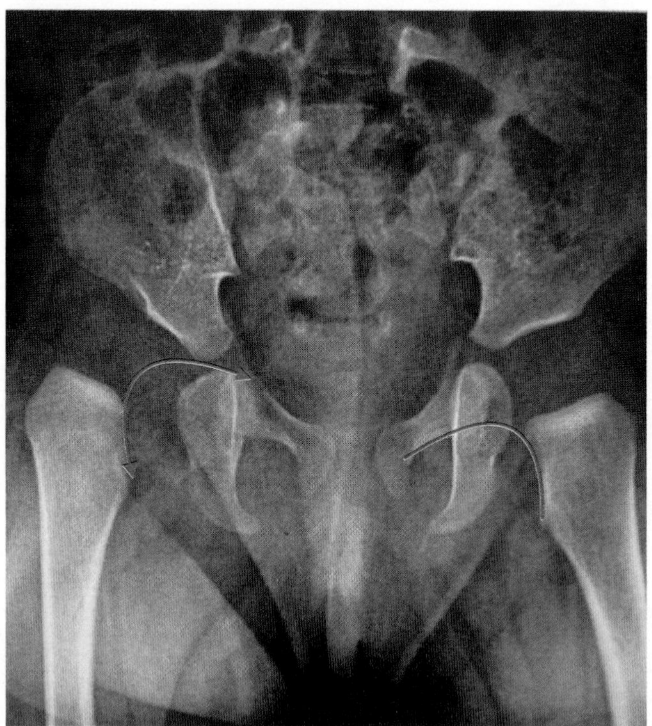

A

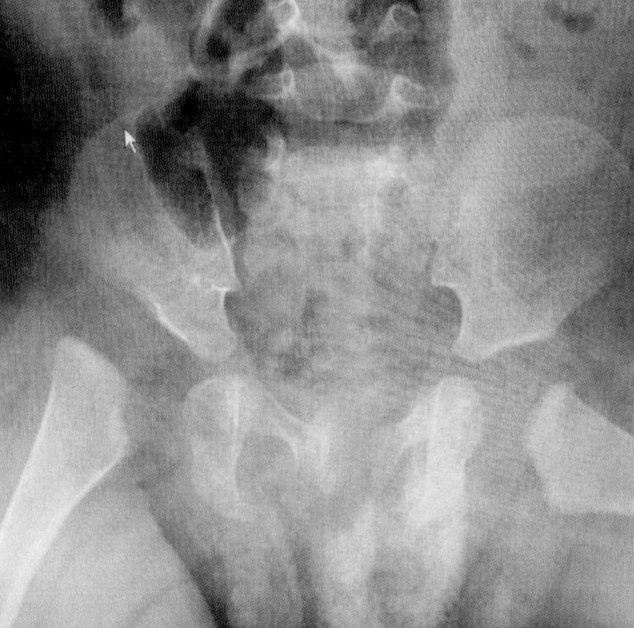

B

**FIGURE 208-2 A and B:** Anteroposterior pelvis and bilateral frog-leg lateral views show developmental dislocation of the right hip. *Double arrowed line:* broken Shenton's arc; *nonarrowed line:* intact Shenton's arc.

Children and adolescents from approximately age 9 to 14 years are at risk for developing this condition if they are overweight or have underlying endocrine abnormalities. If a limp is present with associated pain in the thigh or knee in an individual in this age group, it is important to obtain AP and lateral radiographs of both hips to evaluate for this condition (Fig. 208-4, A and B). Physical examination of the affected hip will show obligate external rotation with hip flexion (Fig 208-5). If SCFE is suspected, consultation with a subspecialist

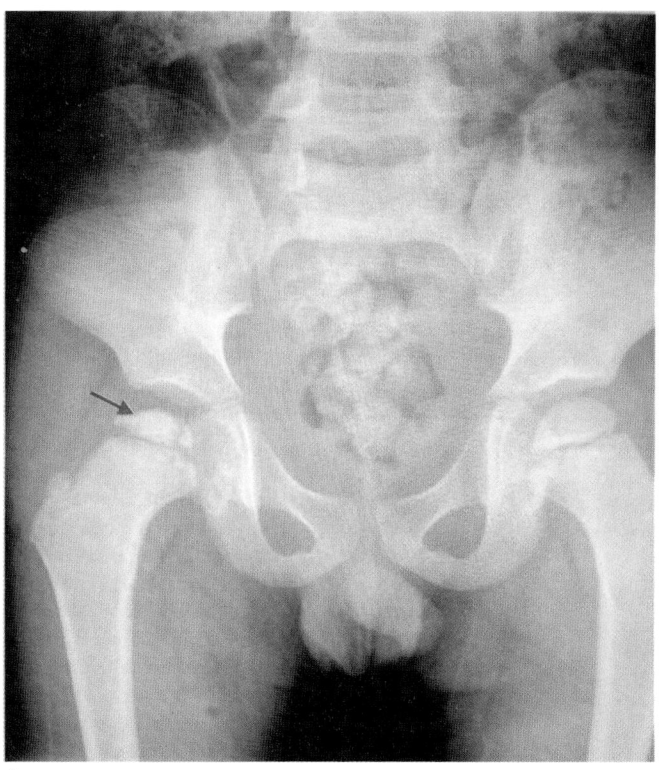

A

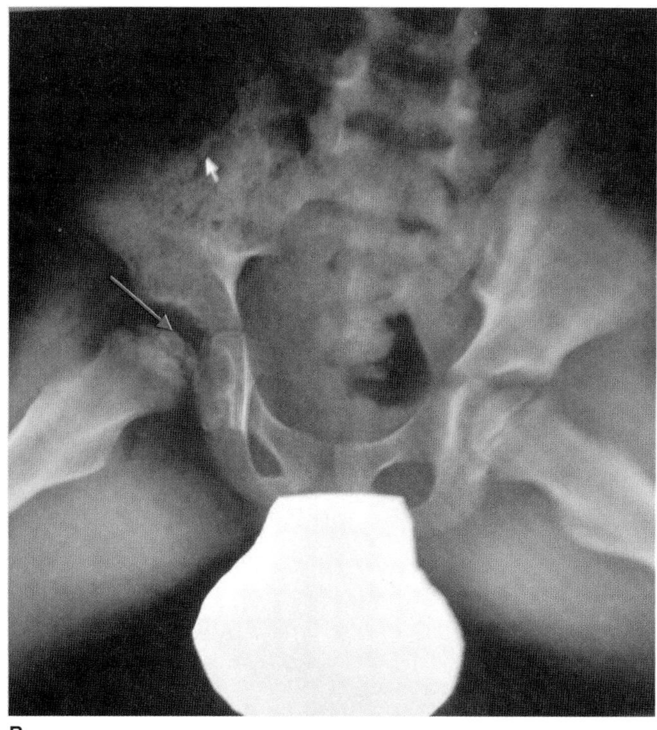

B

**FIGURE 208-3 A and B:** Anteroposterior pelvis and bilateral frog-leg lateral views show Legg-Calvé-Perthes disease of the right hip. Note sclerosis and fragmentation of the proximal femoral epiphysis. *Arrow:* proximal femoral epiphysis.



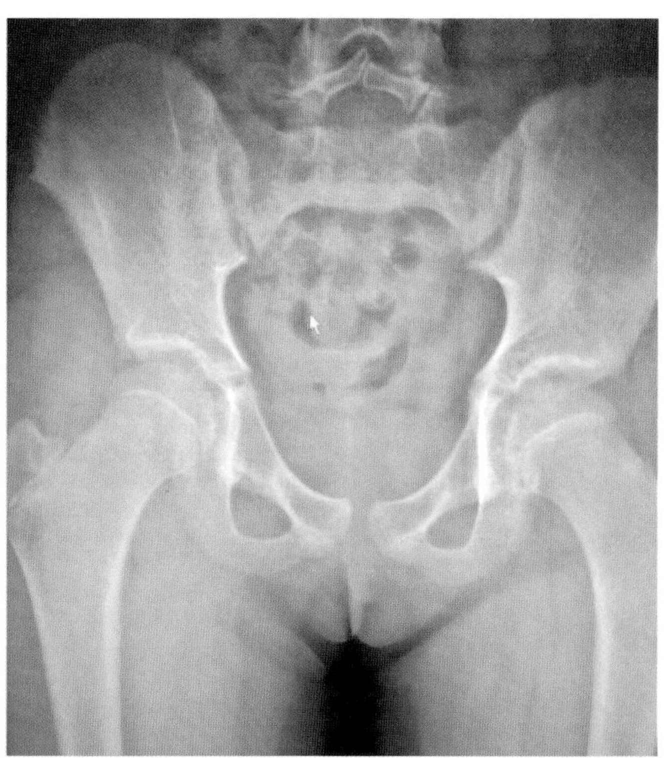

A

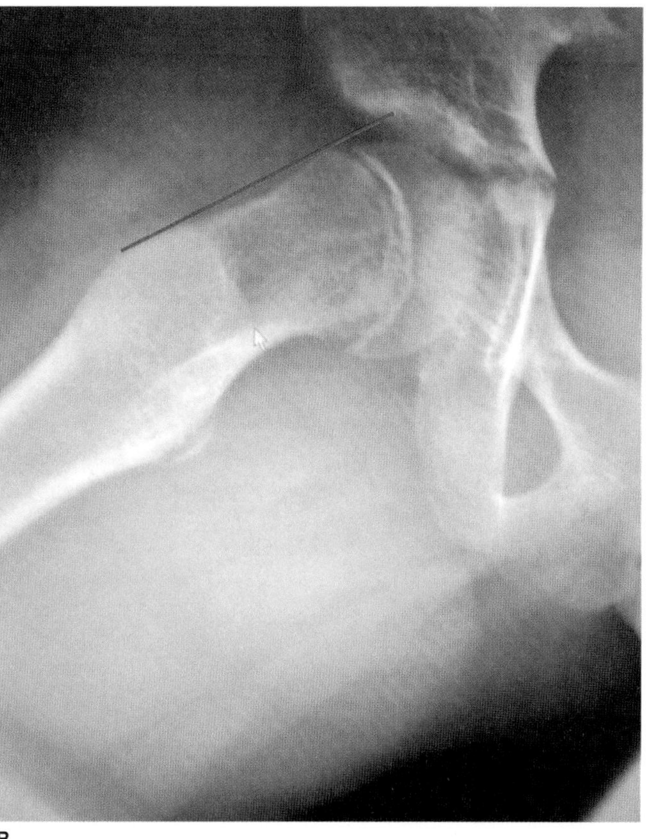

B

**FIGURE 208-4 A and B:** Anteroposterior pelvis and frog-leg lateral views of the right hip show a slipped capital femoral epiphysis, best demonstrated on the lateral view. It was missed on initial evaluation.

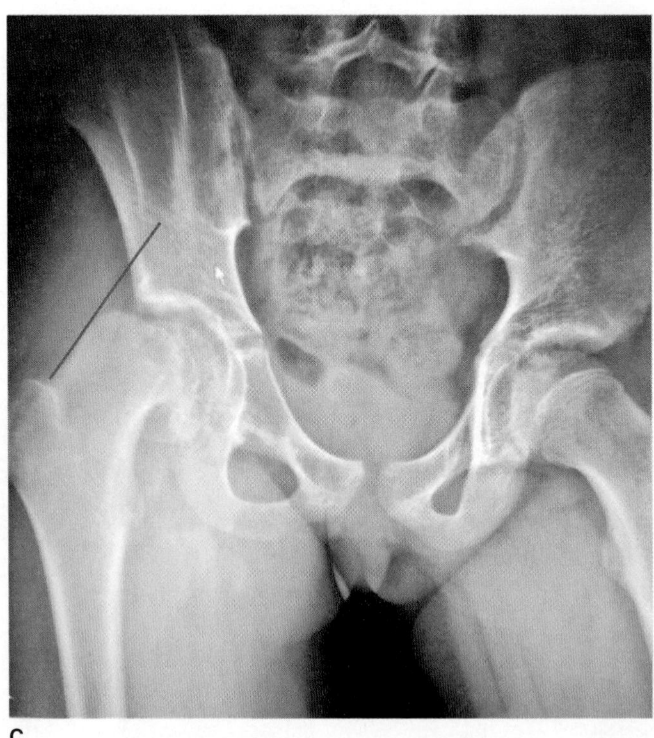

C

**FIGURE 208-4** (*Continued*) **C:** Progression of the slip 6 weeks after the initial x-rays. Line: Klein's line projected along femoral neck, should intersect the epiphysis of the proximal femur.



should be obtained immediately to determine the treatment plan. Children with suspected SCFE are admitted to the hospital to prevent inadvertent progression of the slip and undergo surgical stabilization at the time of availability of the surgical team (Fig. 208-4C).

### Any Age

**Malignancy** Although extremely rare as a cause of limp in childhood, malignancy should be considered whenever a clearly identifiable cause is not determined. Radiographs of the region of concern should be inspected for permeative changes, periosteal elevations, and marrow replacement or lucencies. Laboratory studies should be reviewed for subtle elevations of the inflammatory indices or alterations of the hematopoietic elements to include red cells, white cells, and platelets. An automated white blood cell differential should not be trusted under circumstances of increased clinical suspicion, as blast cells may be mistakenly identified as atypical lymphocytes. Rather, a manual differential should be requested.

*Acute lymphoblastic leukemia* (ALL) (Chapter 445) is the most common childhood malignancy, with a peak incidence at age 4 years (range 3–9 years). Other forms of malignancy that may be seen in childhood or adolescence include Ewing sarcoma and osteogenic sarcoma (Chapters 449 and 450). ALL tends to present with diffuse bone pain, whereas osteosarcoma and Ewing sarcoma present with a localized area of swelling or discomfort. When clinical suspicion exists of these diagnoses, subspecialty referral should be made. Typically, a biopsy would be performed to obtain histopathologic confirmation of the diagnosis. See Table 208-1 for age-based differential diagnosis.

## SUMMARY

There are many causes of gait abnormality in childhood. The most worrisome causes, including trauma, infection, and malignancy, should be excluded by a diligent, timely workup including a careful history and physical examination, appropriate radiographic and laboratory studies, and prompt subspecialty referral when necessary.

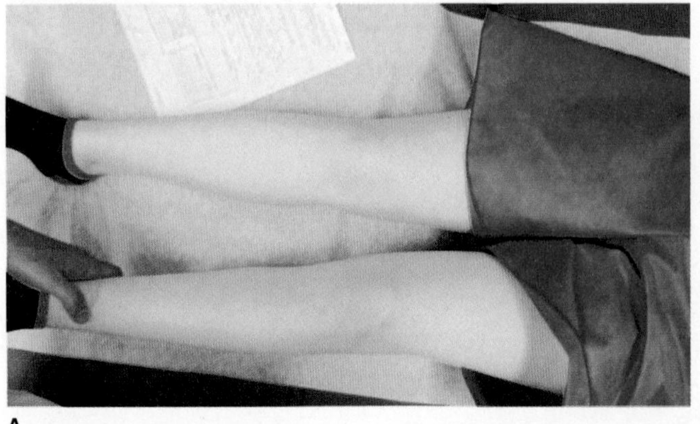

A

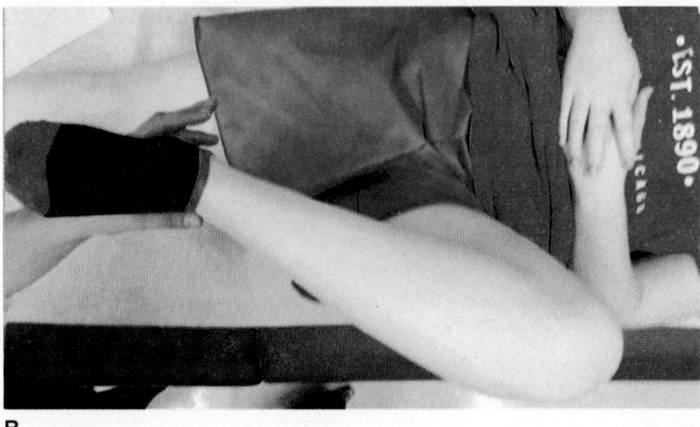


B

**FIGURE 208-5 A and B:** Clinical photos of a patient with healed left slipped capital femoral epiphysis show obligate external rotation of the hip with flexion.

**TABLE 208-1 AGE-BASED DIFFERENTIAL DIAGNOSIS**

| Age (years) | Differential Diagnosis of Limp |
|---|---|
| 0–3 | Septic arthritis |
| | Osteomyelitis |
| | Developmental dysplasia of the hip |
| | Fracture or soft tissue injury |
| | Nonaccidental trauma |
| 4–10 | Septic arthritis |
| | Osteomyelitis |
| | Transient synovitis |
| | Legg-Calvé-Perthes disease |
| | Fracture or soft tissue injury |
| 11–15 | Slipped capital femoral epiphysis |
| | Septic arthritis |
| | Osteomyelitis |
| | Legg-Calvé-Perthes disease |
| | Fracture or soft tissue injury |
| Any age | Malignancy (acute lymphoblastic leukemia, osteosarcoma, Ewing sarcoma) |
| | Leg length discrepancy |

## SUGGESTED READINGS

Copley LA, Kinsler MA, Gheen T, Shar A, Sun D, Browne R. The impact of evidence-based clinical practice guidelines applied by a multidisciplinary team for the care of children with osteomyelitis. *J Bone Joint Surg Am.* 2013;95(8):686-693.

Herman MJ, Martinek M. The limping child. *Pediatr Rev.* 2015;36: 184-195.

Hosseinzadeh P, Iwinski HJ, Salava J, Oeffinger D. Delay in the diagnosis of stable slipped capital femoral epiphysis. *J Pediatr Orthop.* 2016;170:250-254.

Jonsson OG, Sartain P, Ducore JM, et al. Bone pain as an initial symptom of childhood acute lymphoblastic leukemia: association with nearly normal hematologic indexes. *J Pediatr.* 1990;117(pt 1): 233-237.

Kocher MS, Bishop JA, Weed B, et al. Delay in diagnosis of slipped capital femoral epiphysis. *Pediatrics.* 2004;113(4):e322-e325.

Kocher MS, Mandiga R, Zurakowski D, Barnewolt C, Kasser JR. Validation of a clinical prediction rule for the differentiation between septic arthritis and transient synovitis of the hip in children. *J Bone Joint Surg.* 2004;86:1629-1635.

Luhmann SJ, Jones A, Schootman M, Gordon JE, Schoenecker PL, Luhmann JD. Differentiation between septic arthritis and transient synovitis of the hip in children with clinical prediction algorithms. *J Bone Joint Surg.* 2004;86:956-962.

Mueller AJ, Kwon JK, Steiner JW, et al. Improved magnetic resonance imaging utilization for children with musculoskeletal infection. *J Bone Joint Surg Am.* 2015;97(22):1869-1876.

Perry D, Harper A, Bruce C. A limping child. *Br Med J.* 2011;342: d3565-d3565.

van der Have N, Nath SV, Story C, et al. Differential diagnosis of paediatric bone pain: acute lymphoblastic leukemia. *Leuk Res.* 2012;36(4):521-523.



# 209 Torsional and Angular Deformities

Howard R. Epps and Karl E. Rathjen

## INTRODUCTION

Rotational and angular deformities of the lower extremities are among the most common orthopedic complaints to primary care providers. Fortunately, most patients have nothing more than normal physiologic variance, and the majority may be treated with education and observation. However, there are a variety of uncommon, but significant, orthopedic and neuromuscular conditions that may present as rotational or angular deformity. Thus, an understanding of both anatomy and potential pathologies is important. Recognition of normal variations in normal growth and development can reduce the number of unnecessary referrals for specialist evaluation.

## ROTATIONAL ABNORMALITIES

Although the vast majority of parental concerns regarding rotational difference will represent nothing more than developmental norms, it is paramount to remember that rotational differences may be the presenting complaint in patients with mild neuromuscular differences; thus, a careful history and physical exam focusing on neuromuscular development should be incorporated with every patient who presents for evaluation of in- or out-toeing.

### IN-TOEING

*In-toeing* is perhaps the most common gait deviation that presents for medical assessment. Assessment should begin with observation of the gait to determine the foot progression angle, namely the angle described by the intersection of the axis of the foot with the axis of progression. Although the torsional alignment of the lower extremities changes during skeletal development, most parents are unaware of this fact and will consider any deviation from the normal adult value of 10 to 20 degrees external as pathologic (Fig. 209-1). If an internal foot progression angle is identified, careful examination of the lower extremities can identify the anatomic location responsible for the inward deviation. Fortunately, because of normal physiologic variance, usually a strong correlation exists between the age of the patient and the anatomic location producing the inward deviation.

#### Metatarsus Adductus

*Metatarsus adductus* is the most frequent reason for in-toeing in the first year of life and is the most common congenital foot deformity, affecting approximately 3% of all births. Metatarsus adductus occurs when there is inward torsion of the mid- or forefoot with the hindfoot in normal position or slight valgus. It is bilateral in 60% of children. It is important to distinguish metatarsus adductus from more significant foot pathology—namely, talipes equinovarus (clubfoot). This distinction may be accomplished by assessing the position of the hindfoot or heel. In clubfoot, the heel will be in equinus (plantar flexion) and varus, and the foot will not achieve neutral dorsiflexion. The severity of metatarsus adductus is determined by the amount of flexibility of the forefoot and is graded 1 to 3, with 3 being the most severe. A foot that neutralizes itself spontaneously with tickling of the lateral border is termed mild or grade 1. A moderate, or grade 2, foot is passively correctable but does not actively correct itself to neutral. A severe, or grade 3, foot cannot be completely corrected with stretching. Because developmental dysplasia of the hip has been identified in as many as 10% of the children with metatarsus adductus, a careful hip exam is paramount in these children.

There are no well-defined treatment indications for metatarsus adductus. Infants younger than 3 months of age with moderate to

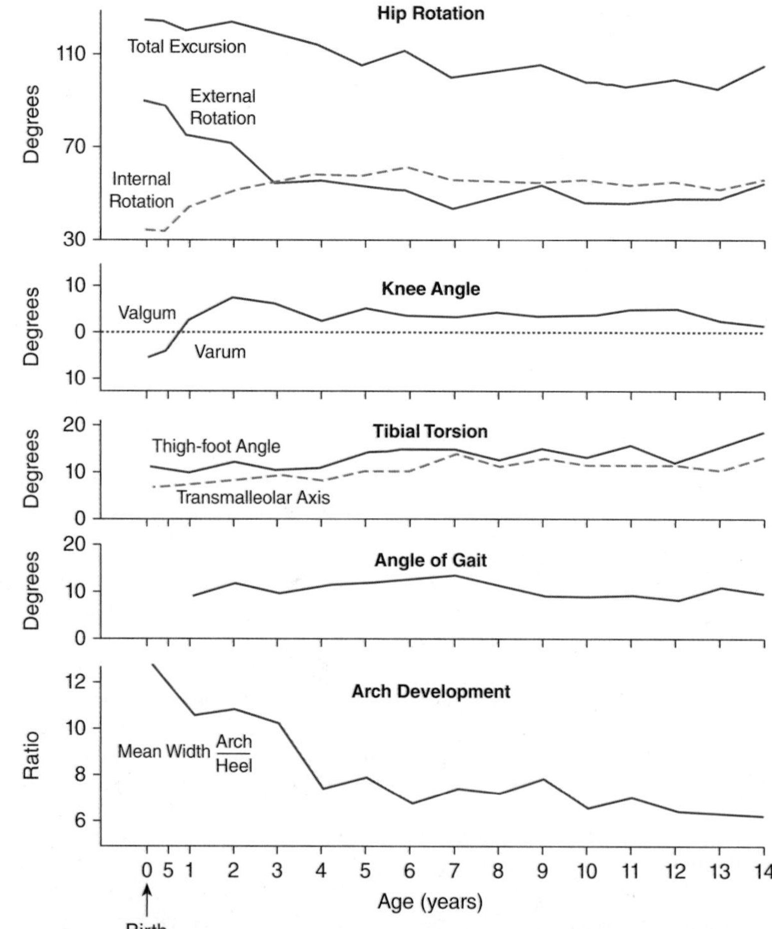


**FIGURE 209-1** The normal evolution of hip rotation, knee angle (ie, mechanical axis), tibial torsion, angle of gait (ie, foot progression angle), and arch development in children between 0 and 14 years of age. (Reproduced with permission from Engel, G.M. and L.T. Staheli, The natural history of torsion and other factors influencing gait in childhood. A study of the angle of gait, tibial torsion, knee angle, hip rotation, and development of the arch in normal children, *Clin Orthop Relat Res* 1974; Mar-Apr;(99):12-17.)

severe, rigid metatarsus adductus may be treated with serial casting; children between 3 and 12 months can be treated with *straight* or *reverse last shoes*. The natural history of metatarsus adductus, however, is usually quite benign. Parents can be assured that it is seldom, if ever, a functional problem, and improvement can be seen into adolescence. Surgery is reserved for older patients with severe residual adductus that interferes with function or wearing shoes.

#### Internal Tibial Torsion

*Internal tibial torsion* is the most common cause of in-toeing in children between the ages of 12 and 36 months. Parents of patients with significant internal tibial torsion may note bowed legs as well as in-toeing, as it is often difficult to differentiate between the 2 in this age group. Internal tibial torsion can be identified by assessing the thigh–foot angle in the prone position (Fig. 209-2). As with all lower extremity rotational parameters, the thigh-foot angle varies with age (see Fig. 209-1). Internal tibial torsion usually spontaneously improves throughout skeletal growth, and treatment seldom is required. Historically, special shoes connected to a bar (*Denis Browne splint*) were a popular treatment for internal tibial torsion; however, there has never been any scientific validation that these splints are efficacious.

#### Excessive Femoral Anteversion

Excessive femoral anteversion is the most common etiology of in-toeing in children older than 4 years of age. Parents of these children often report a preference for sitting in the "W" position. These children sit in this position because it is comfortable for them, and there is no evidence that doing so causes the abnormality. Femoral anteversion is associated with increased internal rotation of the hip, which is best assessed with the patient in the prone position (Fig. 209-3). As with other lower extremity rotational characteristics, hip rotation is dynamic and changes throughout growth (see Fig. 209-1).

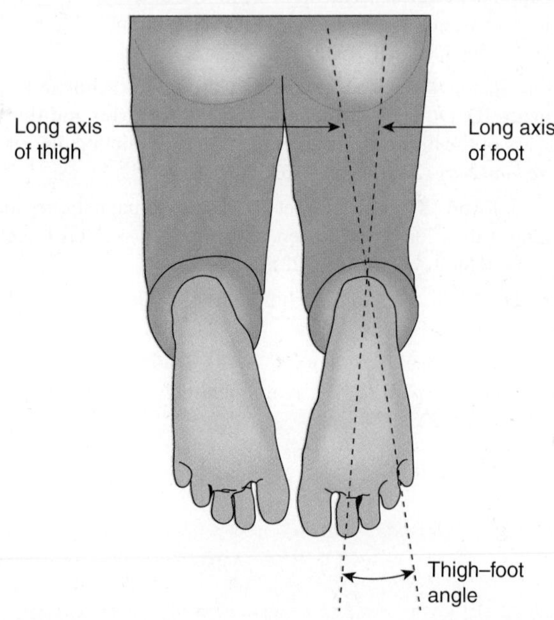


**FIGURE 209-2** Determination of the thigh–foot angle in the prone position.

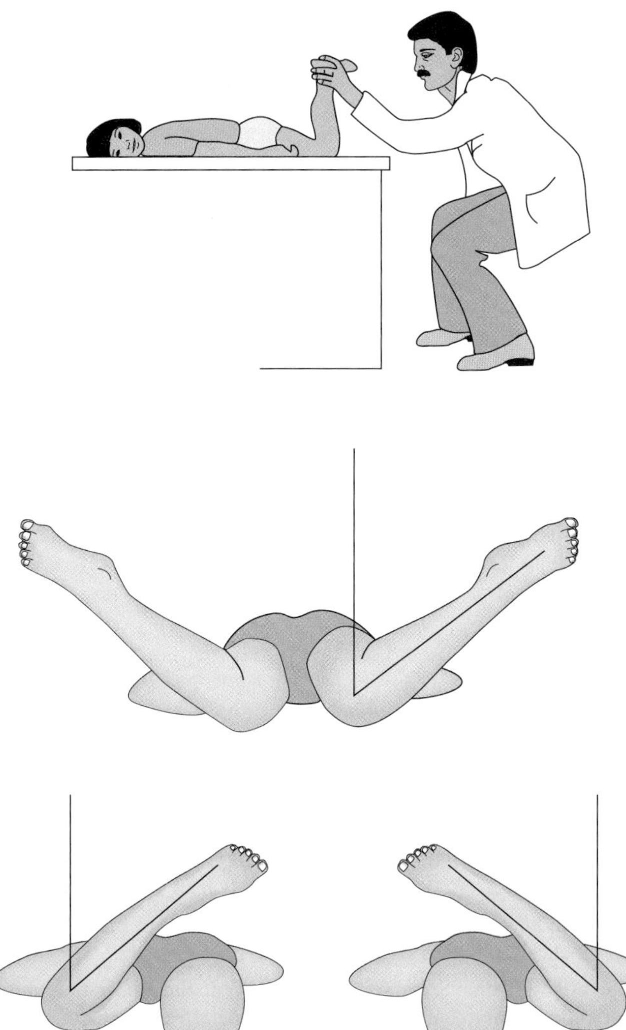

FIGURE 209-3 Determination of hip rotation (and, subsequently, femoral anteversion) in the prone position.

Although some authors suggested a correlation exists between excessive femoral anteversion and osteoarthritis of the hip, the vast majority of literature indicates that the natural history of increased femoral anteversion is completely benign without functional or degenerative impact. Orthotic management of increased femoral anteversion has not been shown to be efficacious.

Correction of both internal tibial torsion and excessive femoral anteversion can be accomplished surgically through rotational osteotomy. However, because of the benign natural history of these conditions, it is important to recognize that such treatment is essentially for the rare patient approaching skeletal maturity with residual deformity and functional difficulties. Cosmesis and physical appearance should not be a priority in surgical decision-making. It is important that parents and patients be fully apprised of the risks and benefits before surgical procedures are entertained.

### OUT-TOEING

Complaints of out-toeing are less common than those of intoeing, and these patients rarely have more than normal physiologic variance. As with in-toeing, it is important to remember that patients with out-toeing may have subtle occult neuromuscular pathology; thus, a careful developmental history and neurologic assessment are of paramount importance. Adolescents with slipped capital femoral epiphyses may develop new-onset out-toeing, which may be asymmetrical. Surgical treatment rarely is necessary and is performed for patients close to skeletal maturity with residual external femoral or tibial torsion and functional limitations.

## ANGULAR DEFORMITIES

Angular deformities of the lower extremities include pure coronal plane deformities (genu varum or bowed legs and genu valgum or knock knees) as well as less common multiplane deformities, such as anterior lateral and posterior medial bowing of the tibia. As with rotational alignment, the coronal plane alignment of the lower extremities changes during the first 7 years of life (see Fig. 209-1). Thus, a pediatric practitioner must understand coronal plane evolution during growth to be able to determine when patients have alignment that falls outside the realm of normal. As demonstrated in Figure 209-1, children are at their maximum varus or bowlegged deformity as infants, and it slowly corrects to a maximal valgus or knocked knee deformity sometime between 2 and 4 years of life. An adult angular profile usually is achieved by 8 years of age.

### GENU VARUM

*Genu varum* may present in children of any age. The differential diagnosis includes normal physiologic variance, Blount disease, metabolic bone disease, and skeletal dysplasias. Despite the fact that genu varum is most severe at birth, it is uncommon for parents to consult with providers before walking age. Parents, however, frequently express concern about the "bowleggedness" of their toddlers. As previously mentioned, increased tibial torsion often is responsible for the appearance of genu varum in toddlers with normal physiologic varus (Fig. 209-4). If evaluation of the lower extremities reveals symmetrical alignment with internal tibial torsion as would be expected at this age, patients simply need observation, and the parents should be reassured. However, in older patients (older than 2 years of age) with significant deformity or asymmetry in the limbs, or a positive family history of metabolic bone disease, short stature, or risk factors for nutritional rickets, a standing anterior to posterior radiograph of both lower extremities should be obtained.

### BLOUNT DISEASE

*Idiopathic genu varum,* frequently referred to as *Blount disease,* can present at any age, particularly when the child has an elevated body mass index (BMI). One hypothesis is that the increased compressive

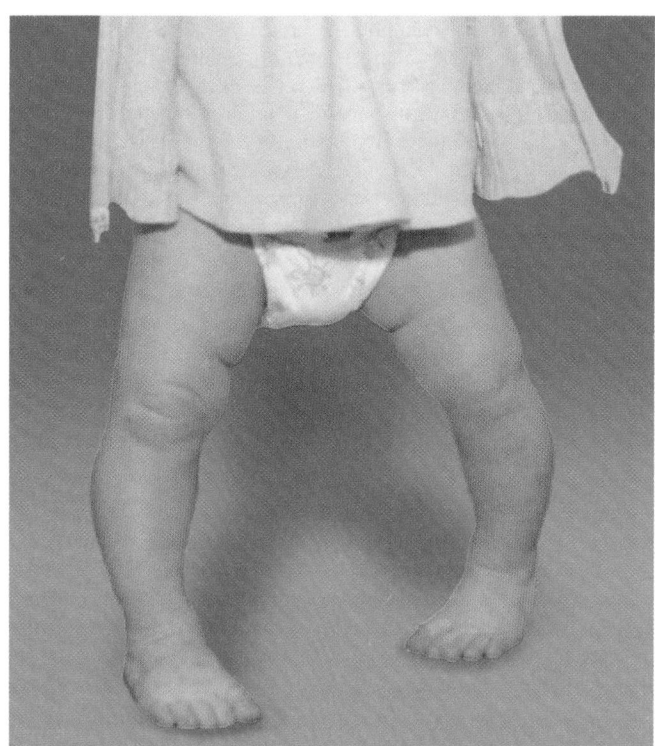

FIGURE 209-4 Two-year-old with internal tibial torsion. Note the knee is directly anterior, but the foot progression angle is medial. Note how the torsion of the distal tibia produces a "bowed-leg" appearance.

forces from obesity cause a growth disturbance at the knee, affecting primarily the tibia but sometimes the femur as well. Children with *infantile Blount disease,* the term used when the child presents before 4 years of age, have significantly higher BMIs compared to children with physiologic bowing. Risk factors for infantile Blount disease include early walking age and obesity. The classic radiographic finding is calcification in the medial aspect of the proximal tibial epiphysis. Bracing has been shown to be effective in treating children with infantile Blount disease, particularly those with unilateral disease. If bracing fails to resolve the deformity, patients are usually treated with hemiepiphysiodesis or tibial osteotomy. If the deformity is not corrected before the child reaches 4 years of age, permanent growth disturbance may develop, resulting in progressive deformity and discrepancy in lengths of the legs. Bracing has no role in children older than 4 years of age. Adolescent *Blount disease* is the entity when the age of onset is older than 10 years. The hallmark radiographic finding is widening of the medial aspect of the proximal tibial physis. Patients with significant deformity are treated with growth modulation or tibial osteotomy.

## RICKETS

*Rickets* refers to a variety of metabolic conditions that produce a disturbance in calcium homeostasis, which leads to abnormalities in areas of rapid calcium turnover, most notably the physis. Nutritional rickets is the result of inadequate vitamin D intake. Although less common in the developed world, nutritional rickets still occurs, particularly in children with dark skin who are breastfed past 12 months of age. Other causes of rickets include hypophosphatemia, renal tubular acidosis, and end-stage renal disease. The radiographic hallmark of rickets is widening of the physis and associated "cupping" of the metaphysis. Angular deformity in patients with rickets may spontaneously correct through normal remodeling after optimization of their metabolic condition. Those with persistent deformity despite optimal medical treatment may require hemiepiphysiodesis or corrective osteotomy.

## SKELETAL DYSPLASIAS

Genu varum in patients with short stature should raise the suspicion of a skeletal dysplasia. *Skeletal dysplasias* are a heterogenous group of conditions that are inherited in Mendelian fashion, although spontaneous mutations are common. The diagnosis of skeletal dysplasias usually requires a skeletal survey and consultation with a pediatric musculoskeletal radiologist or geneticist. The list of causative genetic etiologies is growing and encompasses a number of distinct biological mechanisms. Because there are no effective nonoperative treatments in the majority of patients, children with skeletal dysplasias and symptomatic genu varum require surgical correction.

## GENU VALGUM

*Genu valgum* or "knock knee" is less common than is genu varum and is less likely to represent pathology. As discussed earlier, coronal plane alignment of the legs evolves during growth, and genu valgum becomes most noticeable between 4 and 6 years of age (see Fig. 209-1). During this stage of development, genu valgum is best treated with observation. Occasionally, adolescents will present with persistent genu valgum. A thorough history should be obtained to assess for the possibility of subtle growth arrest from trauma or infection, particularly if the limbs are asymmetrical. Most commonly, genu valgum in adolescents is predominately a cosmetic complaint, although valgus at the knee may cause difficulty running or knee pain or predispose to dislocation of the patella. There is no effective nonoperative treatment for genu valgum. Surgical treatment of idiopathic genu valgum, however, is occasionally indicated and best accomplished in adolescents with growth modulation techniques.

## ANTERIOR LATERAL BOWING OF THE TIBIA

*Anterior lateral bowing of the tibia* is a rare condition that is usually a precursor to congenital pseudarthrosis of the tibia. *Congenital pseudarthrosis of the tibia* is a poorly understood bone dysplasia that produces angular deformity and fracture of the tibia that can be challenging to treat. Fifty percent of patients with this diagnosis will have neurofibromatosis. Usually, children with anterior lateral bowing of the tibia are managed in a brace until deformity progresses and pain interferes with function, at which time surgical attempts to achieve union of the congenital pseudarthrosis are indicated. Treatment frequently fails or is complicated by recurrence with growth. Occasionally, patients with severe disease eventually require a below-knee amputation.

## POSTERIOR MEDIAL BOWING OF THE TIBIA

*Posterior medial bowing of the tibia* is a benign congenital deformity of unknown etiology. It is present at birth and can be quite dramatic, with the dorsum of the foot pressed back onto the anterior aspect of the tibia. The differential diagnosis includes a severe calcaneus valgus foot deformity.

Unlike anterior lateral bowing of the tibia, the natural history of posterior medial bowing is favorable, and the deformity usually spontaneously corrects in the first 2 years of life. However, patients should be followed until they attain skeletal maturity, as they are likely to develop limb length inequalities that may require surgical treatment with epiphysiodesis or lengthening.

## SUGGESTED READINGS

Carli A, Saran N, Kruijt J, Alam N, Hamdy R. Physiological referrals for paediatric musculoskeletal complaints: a costly problem that needs to be addressed. *Paediatr Child Health.* 2012;17:e93-e97.

Davids J, Davis R, Jameson L, Westberry D, Hardin J. Surgical management of persistent intoeing gait due to increased internal tibial torsion in children. *J Pediatr Orthop.* 2014;34:467-473.

Engel G, Staheli L. The natural history of torsion and other factors influencing gait in childhood. A study of the angle of gait, tibial torsion, knee angle, hip rotation, and development of the arch in normal children. *Clin Orthop Relat Res.* 1974;99:12-17.

Farsetti P, Weinstein S, Ponseti I. The long-term functional and radiographic outcomes of untreated and nonoperatively treated metatarsus adductus. *J Bone Joint Surg Am.* 1994;76:257-265.

Mooney J. Lower extremity rotational and angular issues in children. *Pediatr Clin North Am.* 2014;61:1175-1183.

Richards B, Katz D, Sims J. Effectiveness of brace treatment in early Blount's disease. *J Pediatr Orthop.* 1998;18:374-380.

Sabharwal S. Blount disease: an update. *Orthop Clin North Am.* 2015;46:37-47.

Schoenecker P, Rich M, Gordon J. The lower extremity. In: Weinstein S, Flynn J, eds. *Lovell and Winter's Pediatric Orthopaedics.* Vol 2. 7th ed. Philadelphia, PA: Wolters Kluwer; 2014:1261-1340.

Stevens P. Guided growth for angular correction: a preliminary series using a tension band plate. *J Pediatr Orthop.* 2007;27:253-259.

Uden H, Kumar S. Non-surgical management of a pediatric "intoed" gait pattern: a systematic review of the current best evidence. *J Multidiscip Healthc.* 2012;2:27-35.

# 210 Disorders of the Foot

Jaclyn F. Hill and Charles E. Johnston

## INTRODUCTION

A common reason for referral to a pediatric orthopedist is for foot deformities that may or may not be symptomatic. Conditions range from benign, self-resolving, perceived abnormalities involving the forefoot and toes, to more severe congenital and neuropathic deformities including clubfoot, congenital vertical talus, and cavus foot. Frequently, differentiation between a benign, resolving condition and a more severe pathologic deformity can be made by clinical examination and level of suspicion. A review of the common disorders, both benign and pathologic, will be presented to assist in the clinical evaluation of pediatric foot conditions.

## CONGENITAL POSITIONAL FOOT DEFORMITIES

### METATARSUS ADDUCTUS

*Metatarsus adductus* is the medial deviation of the forefoot on the hindfoot (Fig. 210-1). It is thought to be secondary to intrauterine positioning, with the foot medially rotated across the fetal torso. The deformity is classified as either flexible or stiff. When viewed from the plantar surface, the lateral border of the foot is curved and appears "bean shaped" (Fig. 210-1B). The degree of severity is classified using the heel-bisector line. In this method, a line is drawn through the center of the heel and extended up through the toes. In a normal foot, the line extends to the interspace between the second and third toes (Fig. 210-2). Treatment of metatarsus adductus varies from observation to casting in more severe presentations. If the forefoot can be passively manipulated into a corrected position, then the parents can be instructed in passive stretching, and the "deformity" can be observed. Full resolution can be expected in most cases by the time the child reaches 3 years of age. If the forefoot is stiff, serial long-leg casting or a short period of casting may be warranted. Surgical correction is reserved for the rare patient with a fixed adductus and is controversial. Orthopedic consensus is that, even with moderately fixed residual adductus, adult function is still normal.

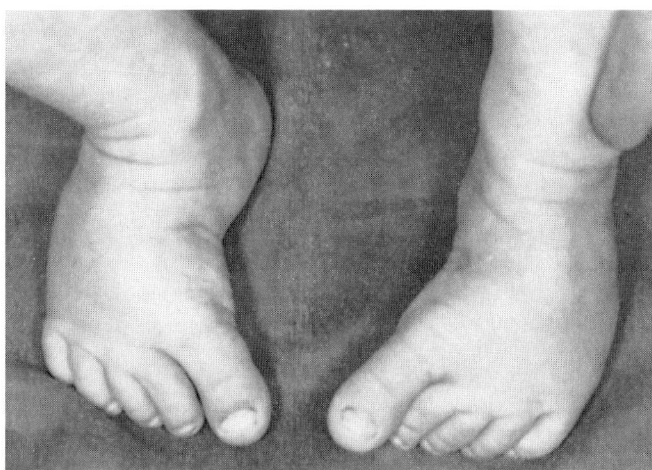

A

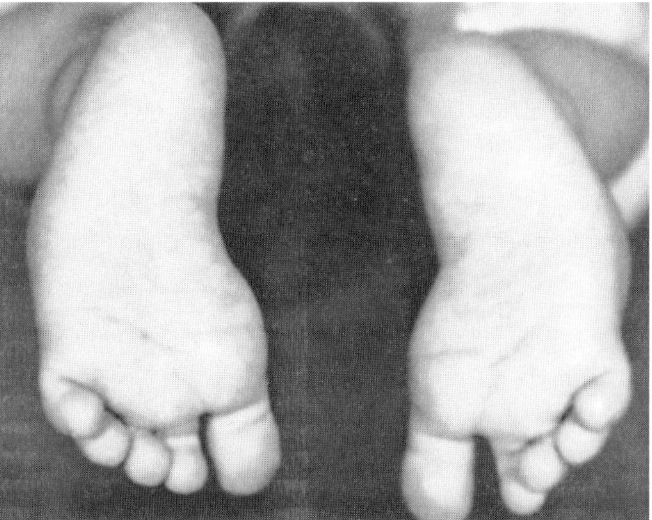

B

**FIGURE 210-1 A:** Dorsal view of bilateral metatarsus adductus. Note the medial deviation of all toes. **B:** Plantar view. The lateral border of the foot is curved and "bean shaped." (Reproduced with permission from Herring JA: *Tachdjian's Pediatric Orthopaedics*, 4th ed. Philadelphia: Elsevier; 2007.)



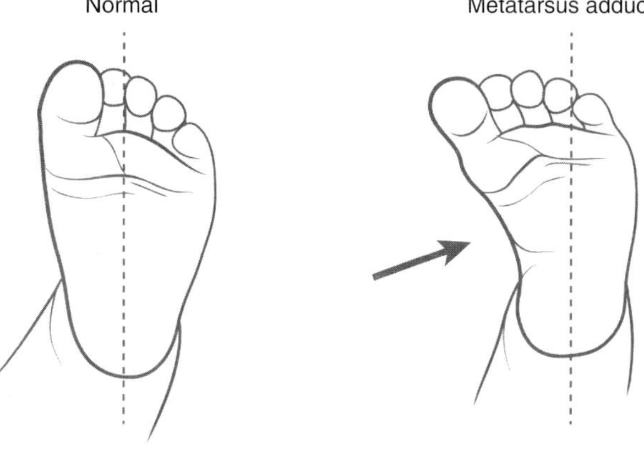


**FIGURE 210-2** Illustration of heel-bisector line in normal foot and in metatarsus adductus. (Printed with permission from Texas Children's Hospital.)

### CALCANEOVALGUS FOOT

Calcaneovalgus foot is a postural deformity of infancy characterized by a sometimes dramatic hyperdorsiflexion position, in which the dorsum of the foot is plastered to the anterior surface of the tibia (Fig. 210-3). Plantarflexion is limited, and the foot may also be deviated laterally, the "valgus" portion of the deformity. This benign deformity needs to be differentiated from congenital vertical talus. The 2 conditions can be differentiated by the position of the heel and the appearance of a "rocker-bottom" foot in congenital vertical talus. Calcaneovalgus foot can also be associated with a posteromedial bow of the tibia, which requires some orthopedic intervention due to discrepancy in the leg's length (Fig. 210-4).

The hyperdorsiflexed foot can be treated by gentle manipulation and stretching by pushing the foot into plantarflexion (see Fig. 210-3). Such stretching exercises can be taught to the parents, although it may not affect the rate of deformity's correction. Typical calcaneovalgus foot will resolve spontaneously in a period of 3 to 6 months. Parents should be educated as to the benign nature of this deformity, but they should also be warned that there may be a flatfoot appearance when ambulation begins.

## CONGENITAL STRUCTURAL FOOT DEFORMITIES

### CLUBFOOT (TALIPES EQUINOVARUS)

*Clubfoot* is a structural deformity with the heel in marked equinus and the foot severely inverted on the end of the tibia (Fig. 210-5). The foot may approach a position of being upside down in relation to the normal position. Lack of correctability of the inversion and the equinus of the heel separates the true clubfoot from a more mild postural deformity. It represents congenital dysplasia of all musculoskeletal tissues distal to the knee and is present in 1 to 2 per 1000 live births. At the time a newborn infant with a clubfoot is evaluated, other associated syndromes or conditions, such as Down syndrome, arthrogryposis (Fig. 210-6), skeletal dysplasias, spina bifida or spinal dysraphism, or other trisomy and dysmorphic conditions, should be considered. Although concomitant hip dysplasia is reported to occur in fewer than 1% of patients with idiopathic clubfeet, a screening hip examination should always be done.

Nonoperative treatment has become the mainstay because of the unsatisfactory long-term results obtained with surgery. Many studies have demonstrated that surgically treated feet are stiffer and weaker,

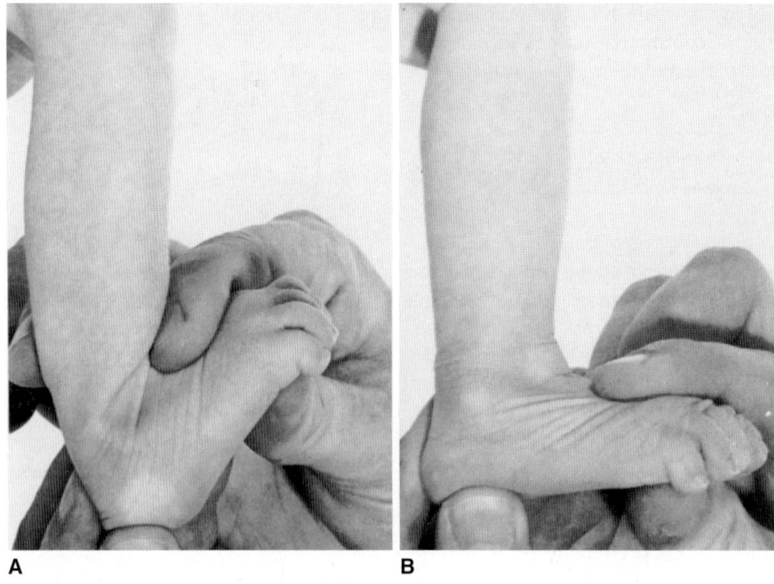


**FIGURE 210-3 A, B:** Manipulation of a calcaneovalgus foot into plantar flexion, stretching the contracted anterior ankle structures. Note the upward movement of the heel as the forefoot is plantarflexed. (Reproduced with permission from Herring JA: *Tachdjian's Pediatric Orthopaedics*, 4th ed. Philadelphia: Elsevier; 2007.)



due to scarring and muscle atrophy. The most common method of nonoperative treatment is serial casting, described and popularized by Dr. Ponseti. This method involves weekly manipulation and application of a cast, followed by a percutaneous heel-cord release done prior to applying the final cast to bring the foot out of equinus (Fig. 210-7). Following removal of the last cast, an equally important period begins of bracing the foot in the corrected position by the use of a *Denis Browne bar* attached to shoes, which maintains the feet in 50 to 70 degrees of external rotation (Fig. 210-8). The orthosis is worn full time for a period of 3 months, and then part time for up to 4 years to maintain the correction. The outcome of treatment depends significantly on the severity of the deformity at presentation, the timeliness and competence of the nonoperative treatment, and the compliance of the family in maintaining the corrected foot in an appropriate orthosis until walking age. Limited surgery for residual deformity or recurrence following the initial nonoperative method of infancy may be recommended.

## CONGENITAL VERTICAL TALUS

*Congenital vertical talus* (CVT) is a rare foot anomaly that is differentiated from clubfoot by the appearance of the foot resembling a rocker-bottom deformity (Fig. 210-9A). The pathology in CVT is a teratologic dorsolateral dislocation of the navicular on the talus, in which the midfoot and subtalar joints are dislocated dorsally and laterally while the heel is still fixed in equinus (Fig. 210-9B). The talus is vertically aligned with the tibia (Fig. 210-9C). CVT often presents in association with arthrogryposis or myelomeningocele and various trisomy syndromes.

Treatment of the congenital vertical talus includes early casting in a method reverse of Ponseti casting (Dobbs casting). Casting attempts to stretch the contracted dorsolateral structures and reduce the navicular on the talus, followed by operative open reduction of the talonavicular joint and release of the hindfoot equinus. Long-term functional outcome of CVT is uncertain because most patients with

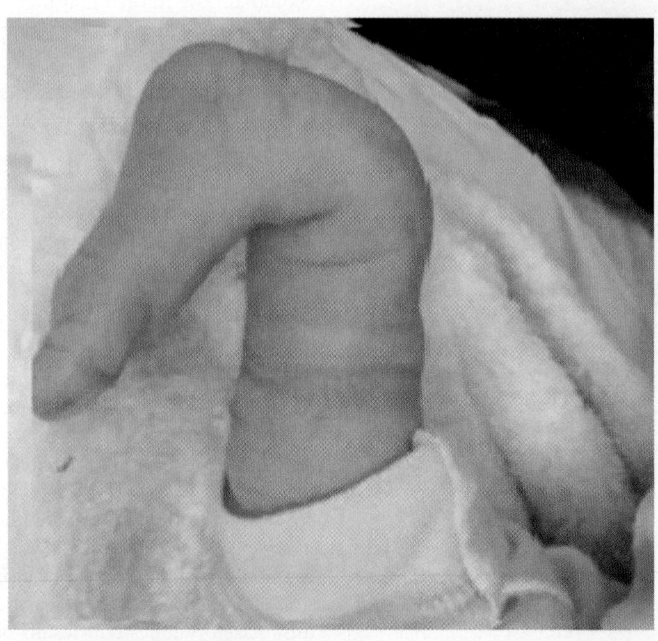

**FIGURE 210-4** Clinical photo of posteromedial bow with calcaneovalgus foot.

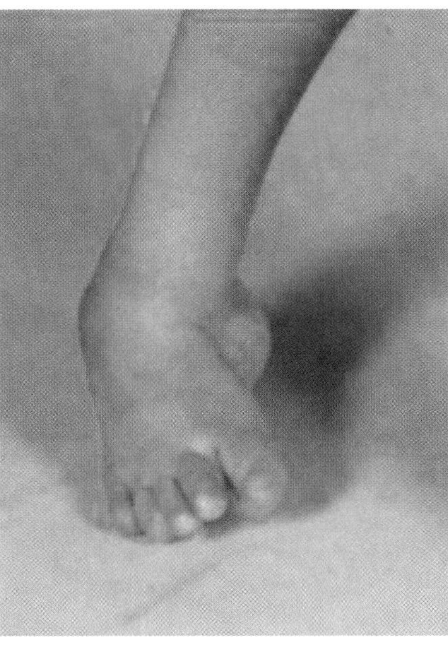

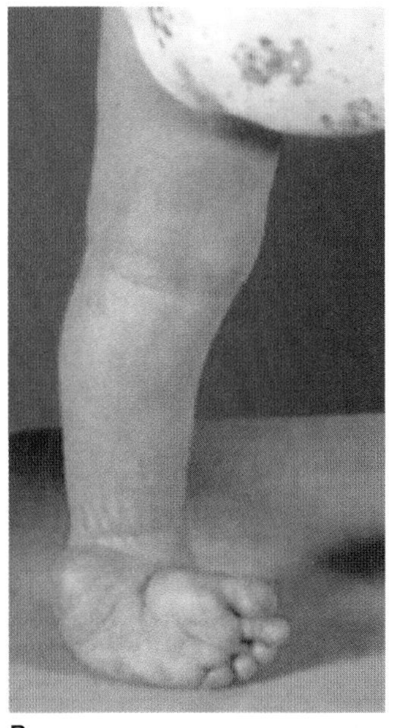

A B

FIGURE 210-5 A: Dorsal view of untreated clubfoot, showing equinus, cavus, heel, and forefoot varus. B: Posterior view. Due to severe inversion/varus, the patient bears weight on the dorsum of the lateral side of the foot. (Reproduced with permission from Herring JA: *Tachdjian's Pediatric Orthopaedics*, 4th ed. Philadelphia: Elsevier; 2007.)

CVT have various disabilities and low functional demands due to comorbidities associated with their underlying syndrome or chromosomal abnormality.

## OTHER FOOT AND ANKLE DEFORMITIES

### FLEXIBLE FLATFOOT (PES PLANOVALGUS)

*Flatfoot* is probably the most common "deformity" evaluated by pediatric orthopedists. Whether it constitutes an actual deformity is, in fact, questionable. In general, the weight of the child's body in the presence of lax ligaments in the foot flattens the normal arch. In the infant and pretoddler child, a "fat" foot should not be mistaken for a flatfoot, as the arches of infants and young children are often obscured by subcutaneous fat. This appearance usually does not improve until the child reaches the age of 8 years, and even after this age, a lower arch is a normal variant in approximately 20% of the population.

The appearance of a flatfoot is well known—the heel is everted with a loss of height, and the talar head and navicular appear to rest on the floor medially (Fig. 210-10A). When viewed from behind, the examiner may note that all 5 toes are visible to the lateral side of the tibia (called "too many toes" sign) (Fig. 210-10B). However, while observing the child from behind, the examiner may request that the child go up on tiptoes, at which time in the flexible flatfoot, the longitudinal arch will reconstitute, and the heels will invert (Fig. 210-10C). This simple maneuver rules out any significant foot pathology. Similarly, when examining the foot with the child seated and the foot dangling, the flexible flatfoot will demonstrate good subtalar motion and reconstitution of the longitudinal arch.

Treatment of flexible pes planovalgus depends on the presence or absence of symptoms. Asymptomatic flatfeet require no treatment, with education and reassurance being given to the parents. There is no evidence that prophylactic treatment of flexible pes planovalgus, such as orthotics or inserts, prevents either the development of symptoms or the progression of a deformity. Symptomatic patients almost all have a heel-cord contracture and should be instructed in stretching exercises (Fig. 210-11). Occasionally, older adolescents, who have pain despite stretching exercises and shoe and orthotic prescriptions, are candidates for surgical management.

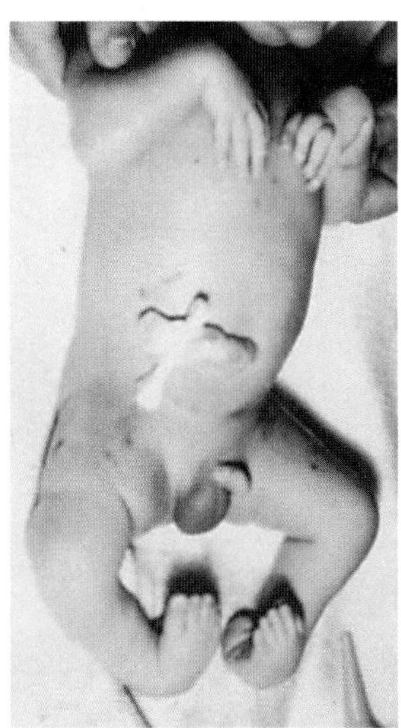

FIGURE 210-6 Clinical photograph of severe clubfeet in a neonate with arthrogryposis.

### TARSAL COALITIONS

Tarsal coalitions usually presents as a painful, stiff flatfoot. By definition, there is an abnormal lack of segmentation between 2 or more bones of the foot, which accounts for the rigidity and pain that bring the patient for evaluation. Because of the rigidity and appearance of the foot, the condition is also known as *peroneal spastic flatfoot*. Patients typically present between the ages of 12 and 16 years with activity-related pain. The predominant physical finding is decreased range of motion at the subtalar joint. Patients often are unable to stand on tiptoes without discomfort, and there is a noticeable lack of inversion of the heel when the tiptoe position is requested. Plain radiographs and computed tomography (CT) scan are used to make the diagnosis (Fig. 210-12). Treatment of tarsal coalition is conservative initially, including the use of orthoses

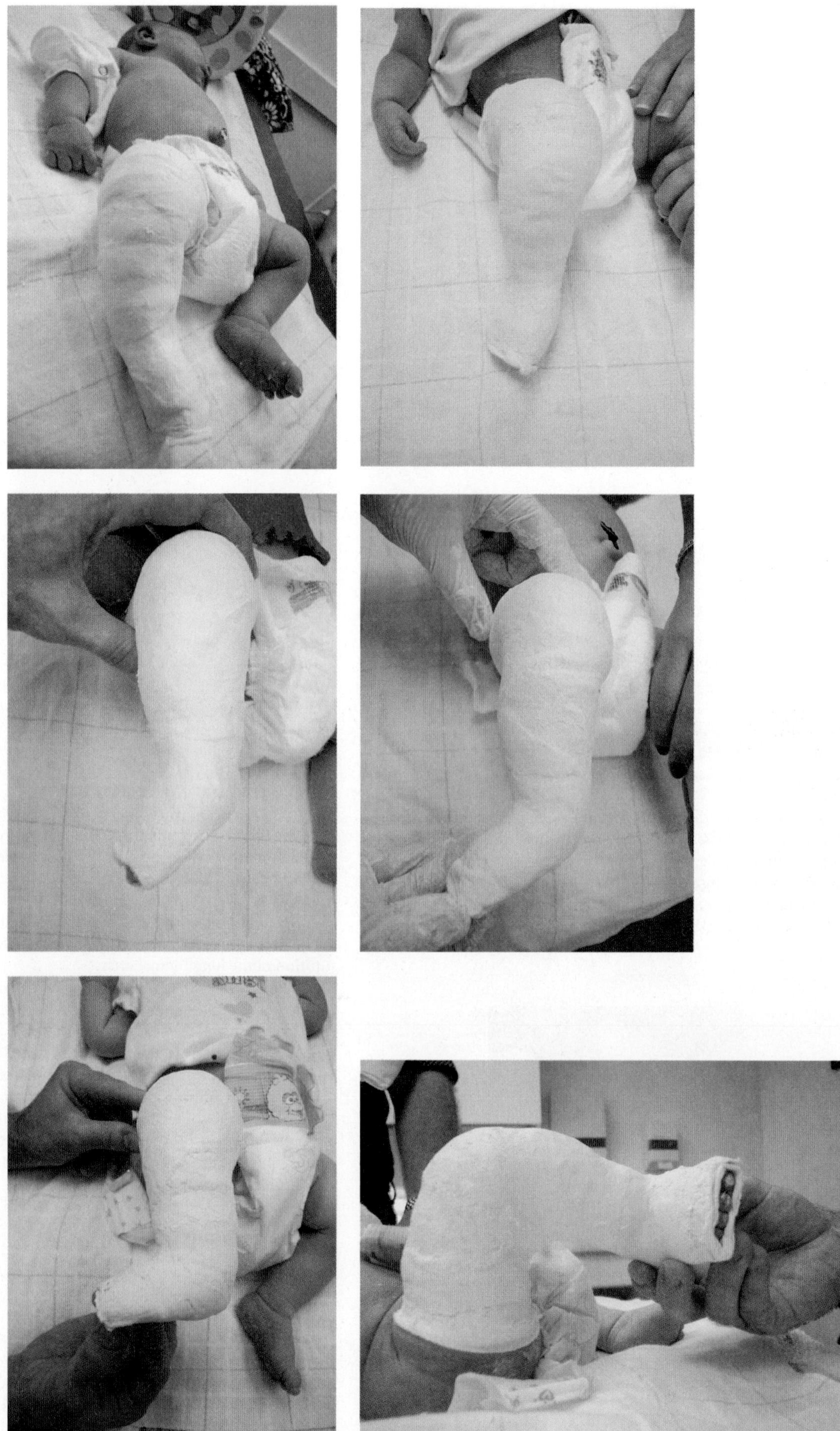

**FIGURE 210-7** Progression of clubfoot correction with serial casting. The final cast is applied after percutaneous heel-cord lengthening to bring the foot out of equinus. (Reproduced with permission from Herring JA: *Tachdjian's Pediatric Orthopaedics*, 4th ed. Philadelphia: Elsevier; 2007.)

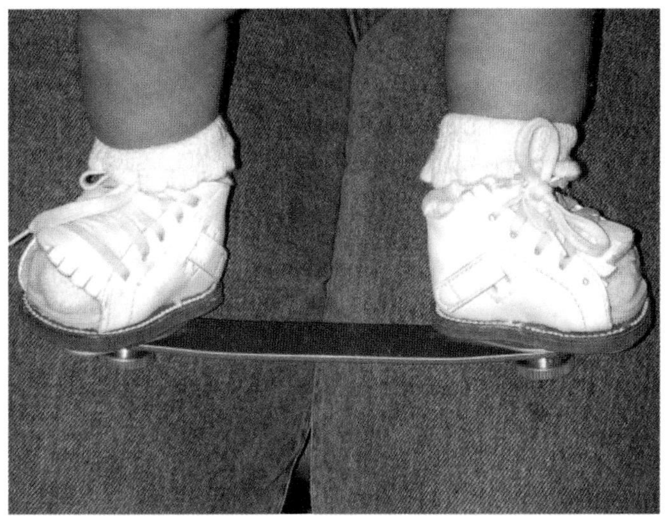

FIGURE 210-8 The Denis Browne/Ponseti brace. (Reproduced with permission from Herring JA: *Tachdjian's Pediatric Orthopaedics*, 4th ed. Philadelphia: Elsevier; 2007.)

and a short period of casting. Patients who fail conservative treatment with documented coalitions are then candidates for either resection of the coalition or subtalar midfoot arthrodesis.

### CAVUS FOOT (PES CAVUS)

The *cavus foot* is defined by an abnormal elevation of the longitudinal arch. The etiology often is neurologic, with the most common underlying diagnoses being peripheral neuropathies such as Charcot Marie Tooth disease and tethered spinal cord. Other diagnoses include cerebral palsy, poliomyelitis, Friedrich ataxia, and myelomeningocele. Idiopathic pes cavus exists but must be made as a diagnosis of exclusion. The clinical features of a cavus foot include plantarflexion of the forefoot with a high arch, with some degree of varus of the hindfoot and pronation of the first metatarsal (Fig. 210-13). Patients typically present because of pain under the lateral aspect of the foot caused by excessive weight bearing, as well as complaints of frequent lateral ankle sprains caused by the forced inversion in association with whatever muscle imbalance or weakness is present from the neuropathic etiology. Secondary changes, due to the progression of neuropathic changes, include cock-up and clawing deformities of the toes (Fig. 210-14).

Determining the underlying etiology of a cavus foot is the first priority because of possible treatment of conditions involving the spinal cord (including tumors) or the underlying neurologic condition. Conservative measures to relieve the abnormal weight bearing and ankle instability include orthoses to balance the weight-bearing surface of the foot or ankle-foot orthoses (AFOs) to stabilize the ankle and, in the case of a muscle weakness etiology, assist with dorsiflexion. The foot deformity frequently progresses to require surgical stabilization. The surgical goal is to provide stable, plantigrade feet that do not require bracing unless the patient also has a foot drop due to weakness of the tibialis anterior muscle.

## TOE DEFORMITIES AND MALFORMATIONS

### HALLUX VALGUS

*Hallux valgus* in a pediatric orthopedic practice is usually seen in adolescent females who are concerned about cosmesis as well as pain. A positive family history is present in as many as three-quarters of the patients, and the concern becomes more significant as the child enters adolescence. The deformity consists of lateral deviation of the great toe, with the apex at the first metatarsophalangeal joint (Fig. 210-15). The prominence of the head of the first metatarsal usually is responsible for the discomfort, but the lateral deviation with under- or overlapping of the second toe produces the cosmetic concern. Patients with hallux valgus usually have a rather wide forefoot, rendering narrow "fashionable" shoes difficult, if not impossible, to don.

Pediatric patients with hallux valgus should initially be strongly encouraged to avoid surgical treatment. Surgical procedures to

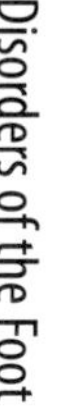


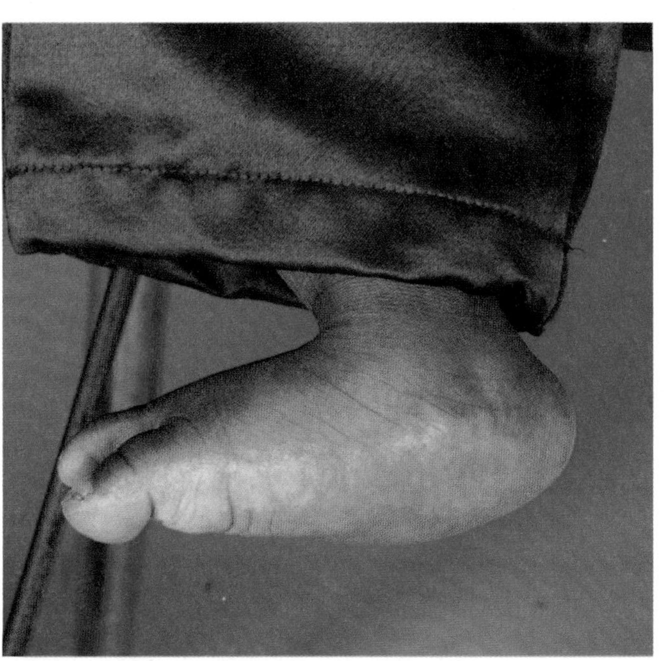
A

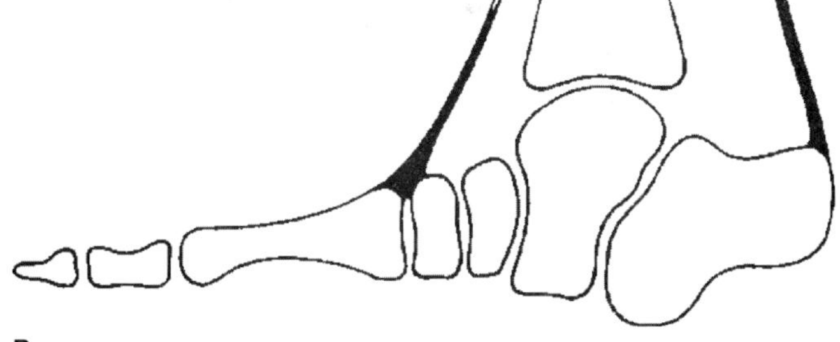
B

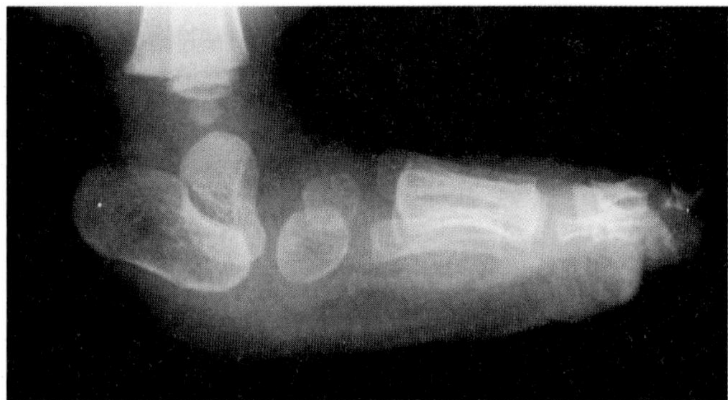
C

FIGURE 210-9 A: Congenital vertical talus with "rocker-bottom" appearance. B: Dorsal dislocation of talonavicular joint combined with heel equinus. C: Lateral radiograph of a congenital vertical talus. The calcaneus is in equinus (plantar flexion) and the talus appears to be vertical, parallel to the long axis of the tibia and fibula. (Reproduced with permission from Herring JA: *Tachdjian's Pediatric Orthopaedics*, 4th ed. Philadelphia: Elsevier; 2007.)

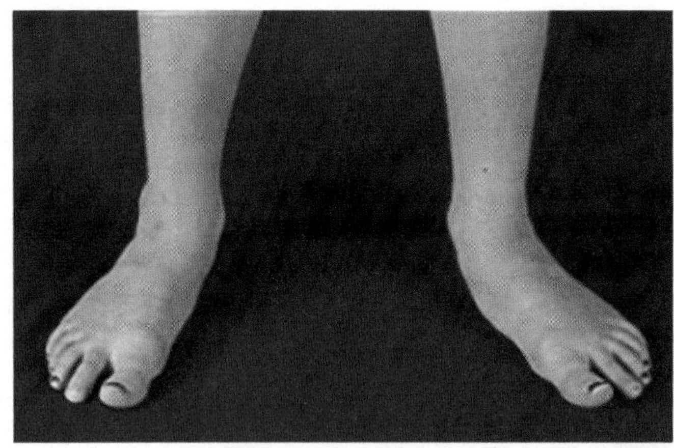

A

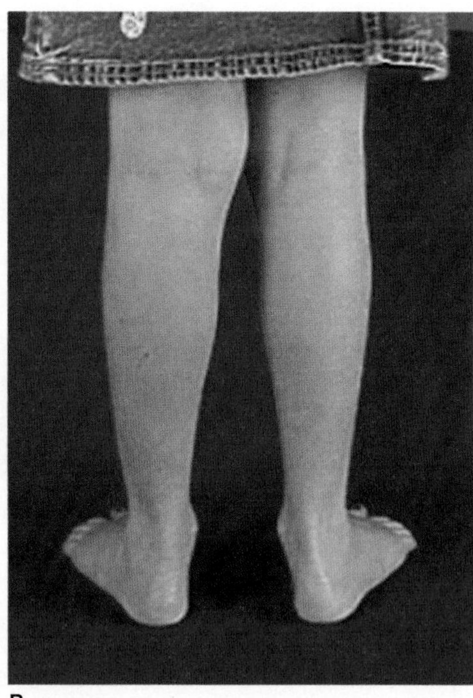

B

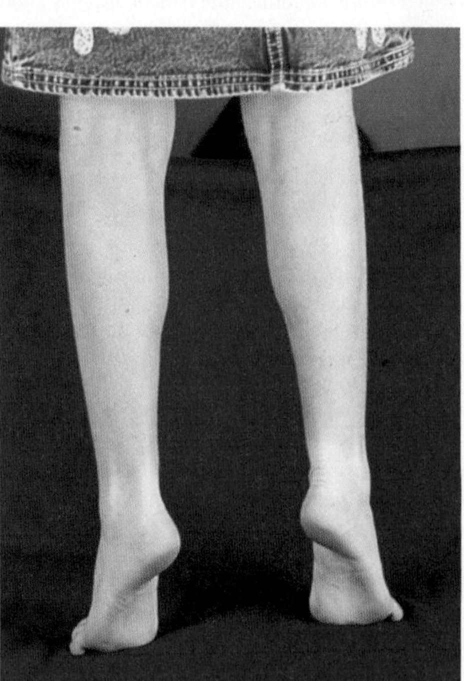

C

**FIGURE 210-10** **A, B:** Front and back views of pes planovalgus, "flatfeet," showing weight bearing on the medial column of the everted foot and "too many toes" visible when viewed from behind. **C:** On tiptoes, the heel inverts and the arch is reconstituted. (Reproduced with permission from Herring JA: *Tachdjian's Pediatric Orthopaedics*, 4th ed. Philadelphia: Elsevier; 2007.)

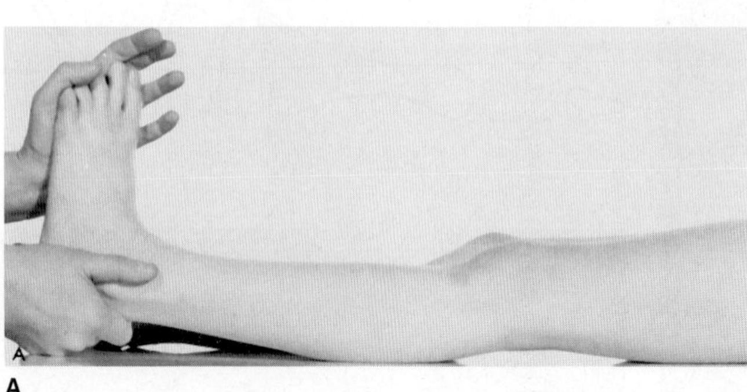

A

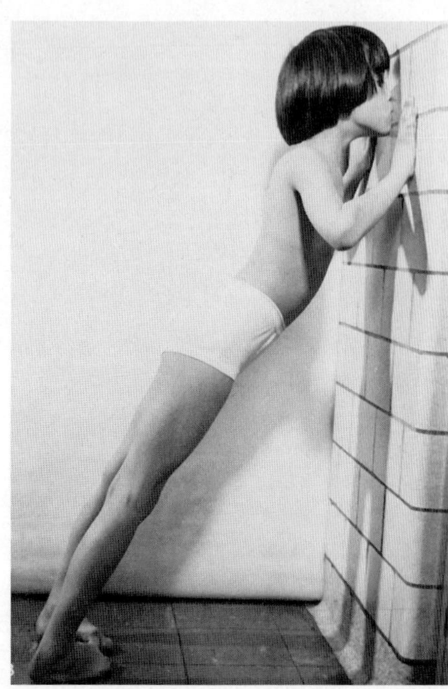

B

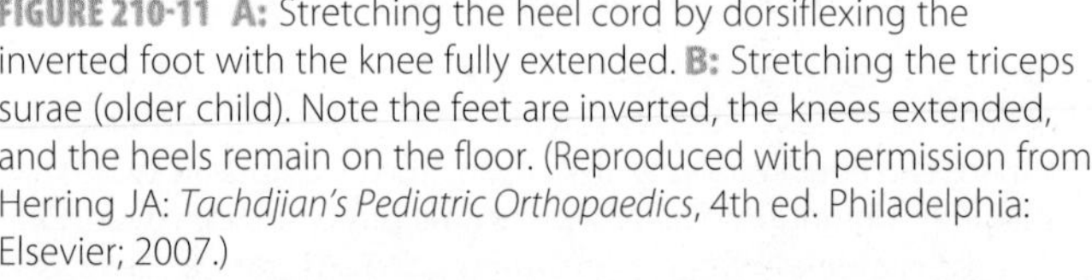

**FIGURE 210-11** **A:** Stretching the heel cord by dorsiflexing the inverted foot with the knee fully extended. **B:** Stretching the triceps surae (older child). Note the feet are inverted, the knees extended, and the heels remain on the floor. (Reproduced with permission from Herring JA: *Tachdjian's Pediatric Orthopaedics*, 4th ed. Philadelphia: Elsevier; 2007.)

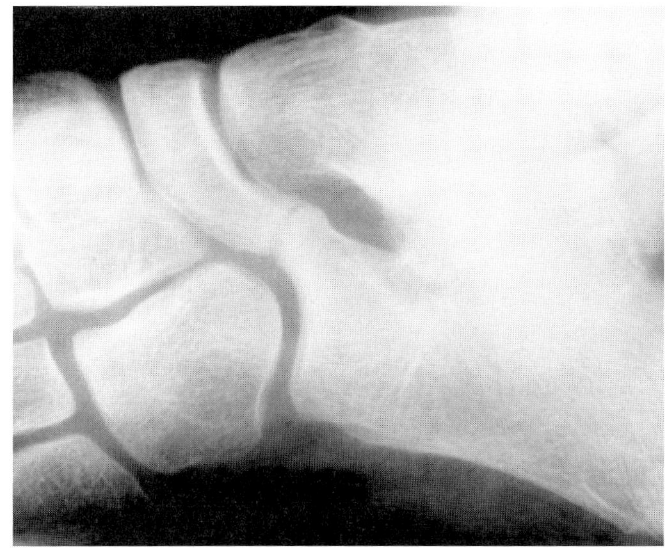

A

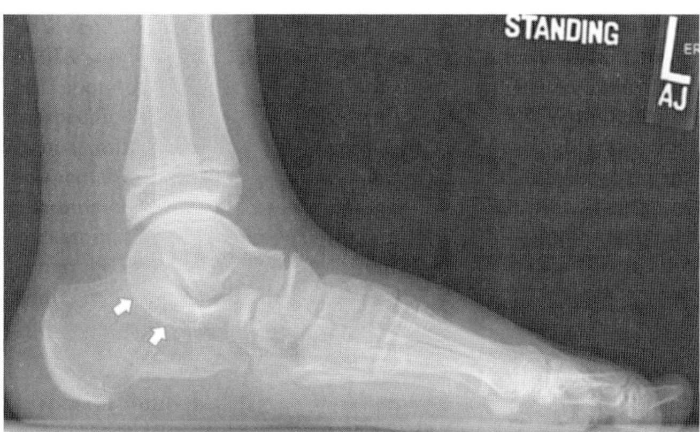


B

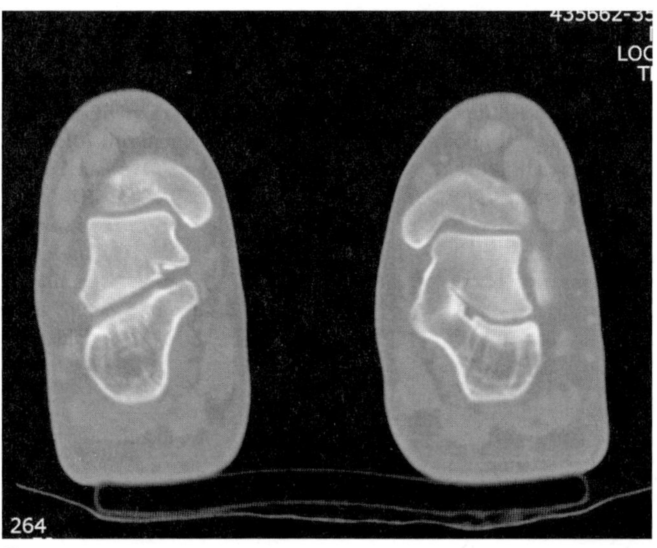


C

**FIGURE 210-12** **A:** The bony bridge connecting the calcaneus and navicular on an oblique radiograph of the foot. **B:** Lateral x-ray of talocalcaneal coalition. Note the "C" sign (*arrows*) outlining the edge of the medial facet coalition. **C:** Computed tomography scan of complete medial facet coalition on right (left normal).

straighten the deformity are fraught with untoward effects and complications, including a high rate of recurrence if the patient is skeletally immature or has a significant flexible flatfoot. Surgical treatment for the mature adolescent is similar to the treatment for the adult, in that a combination of osteotomies, soft tissue releases, and capsular imbrication are usually used.

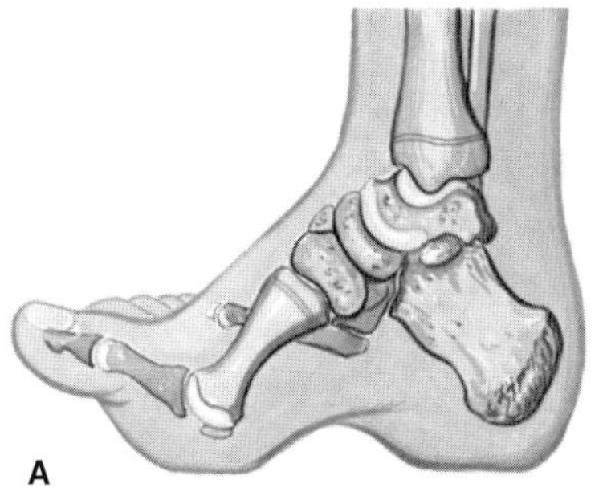

A

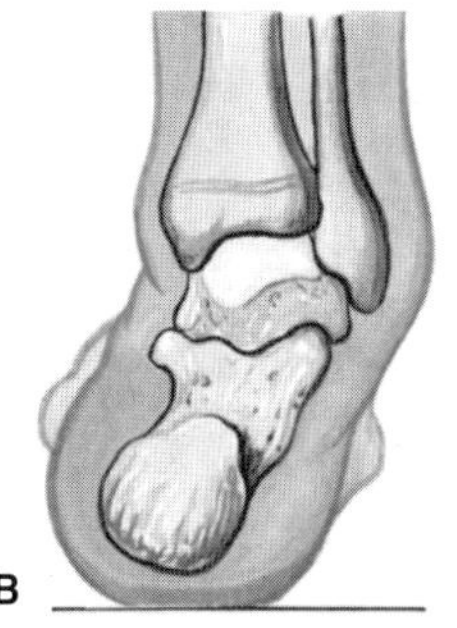

B

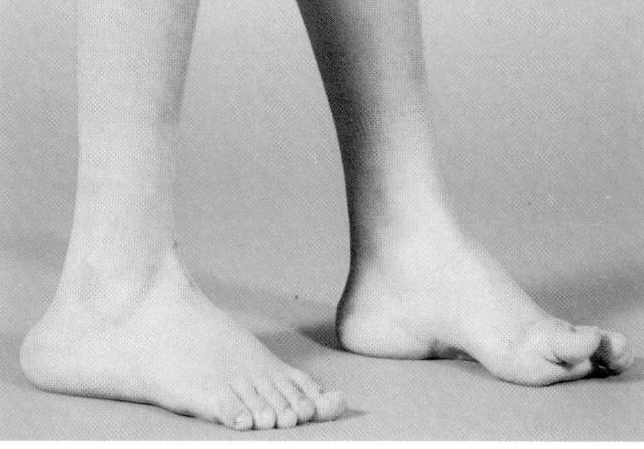

C

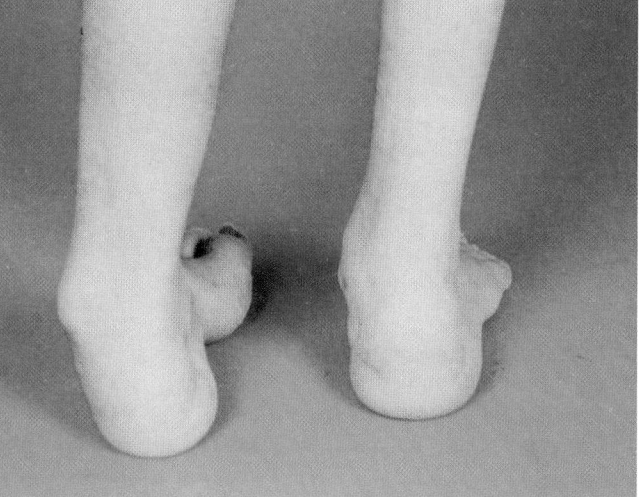

D

**FIGURE 210-13** **A, B:** Illustration of cavus foot with plantarflexed metatarsals and heel in varus position. **C, D:** Clinical photographs of forefoot cavus and supination and heel inversion.

## POLYDACTYLY

Extra toes are probably the most common congenital toe deformities noted, with an incidence of almost 2 per 1000 live births. A positive family history is present in one-third of the patients, with the fifth toe being the most frequently duplicated (postaxial polydactyly) (Fig. 210-16). Preaxial polydactyly (duplication of the great toe) is less common (Fig. 210-16C) and is seen in association with syndromes including trisomy 13, tibial hemimelia, and Down syndrome. The widened foot can cause an issue with wearing of shoes, and most parents request removal of the extra toe for this and cosmetic reasons.

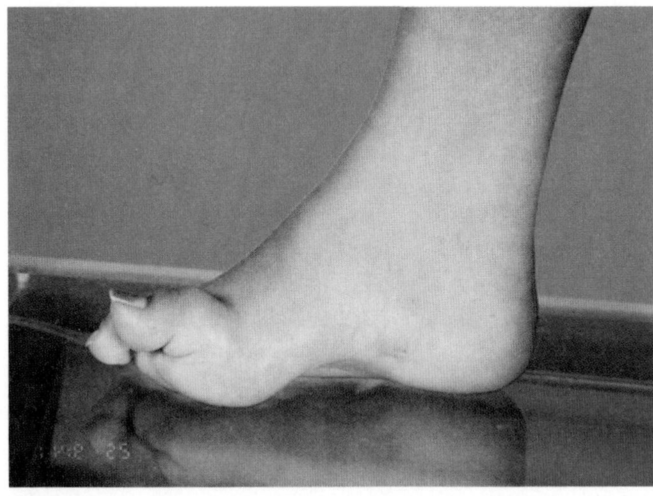

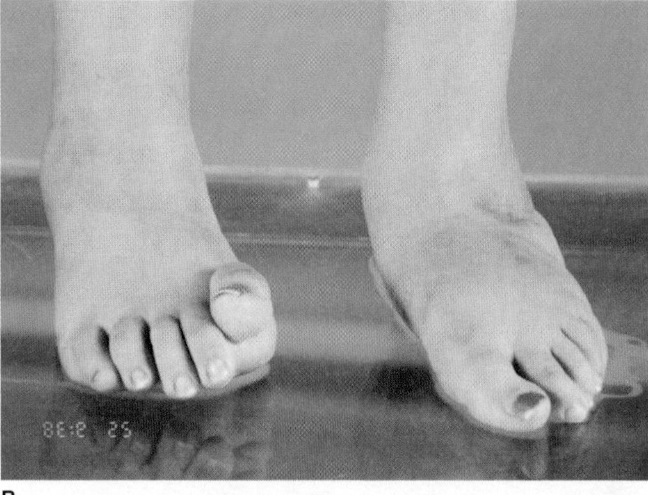

**FIGURE 210-14** "Cock-up" deformity of great toe on right secondary to muscle imbalance (substitution of toe extensors for a weak tibialis anterior in a patient with Charcot-Marie-Tooth disease). (Reproduced with permission from Herring JA: *Tachdjian's Pediatric Orthopaedics*, 4th ed. Philadelphia: Elsevier; 2007.)

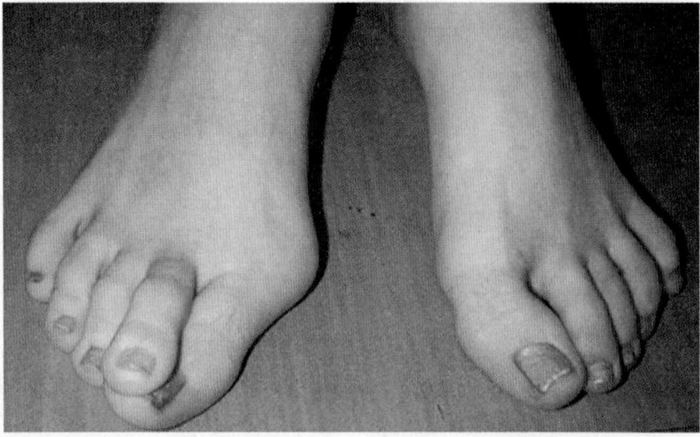

**FIGURE 210-15** Bilateral hallux valgus, "bunions," more severe on the right, in a 16-year-old female. The increased width of the right forefoot is noted. (Reproduced with permission from Herring JA: *Tachdjian's Pediatric Orthopaedics*, 4th ed. Philadelphia: Elsevier; 2007.)

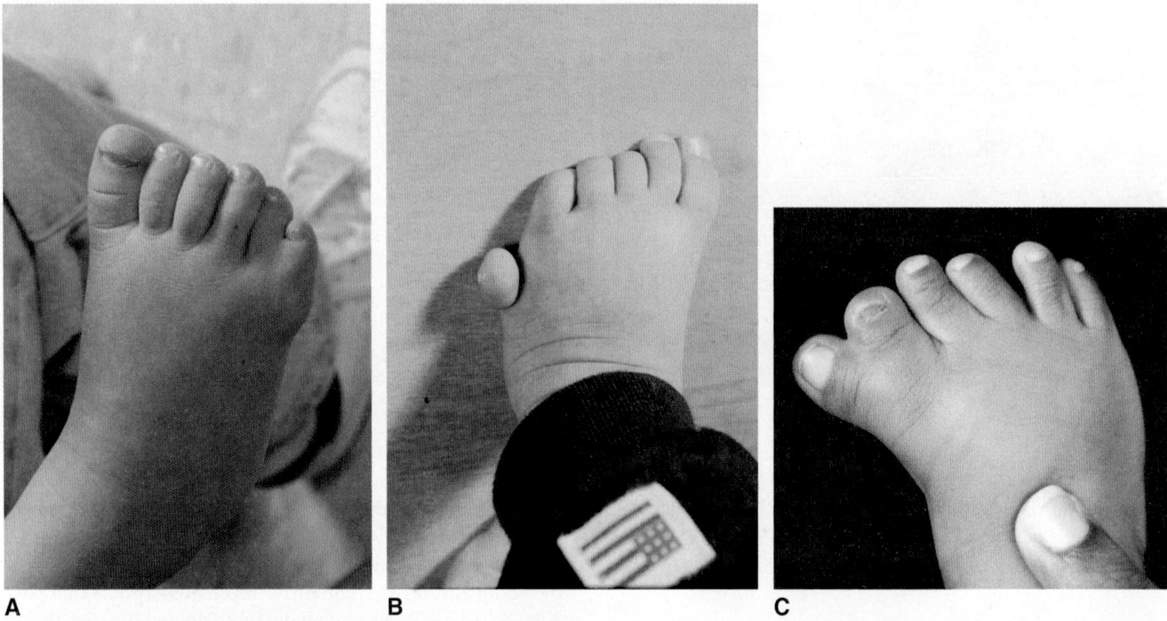

**FIGURE 210-16** **A:** Postaxial polydactyly involving a complete extra sixth ray (metatarsal and phalanges). **B:** Rudimentary sixth toe with no function or skeletal attachment to the rest of the foot. **C:** Preaxial polydactyly with hallux varus. Excision and realignment of the first toe are indicated due to the deformity. (Reproduced with permission from Herring JA: *Tachdjian's Pediatric Orthopaedics*, 4th ed. Philadelphia: Elsevier; 2007.)

Removal can be accomplished at essentially any time, but is probably best done around walking age. It allows the toes to enlarge to a point such that the surgery is technically simple due to ample skin and soft tissue for coverage and decreases the risk of anesthesia.

## SUGGESTED READINGS


Bauer K, Mosca VS, Zionts LE. What's new in pediatric flatfoot? *J Pediatr Orthop*. 2016;36(8):865-869.

Chell J, Dhar S. Pediatric hallux valgus. *Foot Ankle Clin*. 2014; 19(2):235-243.

Lee H-S, Lee W-C. Congenital lesser toe abnormalities. *Foot Ankle Clin*. 2011;16(4):659-678.

Mahan ST, Spencer SA, Vezeridis PS, Kasser JR. Patient-reported outcomes of tarsal coalitions treated with surgical excision. *J Pediatr Orthop*. 2015;35(6):583-588.

Miller M, Dobbs MB. Congenital vertical talus: etiology and management. *J Am Acad Orthop Surg*. 2015;23(10):604-611.

Mosca VS. Subtalar coalition in pediatrics. *Foot Ankle Clin*. 2015; 20(2):265-281.

Sullivan JA. Pediatric flatfoot: evaluation and management. *J Am Acad Orthop Surg*. 1999;7(1):44-53.

Zionts LE. What's new in idiopathic clubfoot? *J Pediatr Orthop*. 2015;35(6):547-550.


# 211 Disorders of the Knee

Scott D. McKay and John A. Herring

## KNEE INJURIES

Knee injuries present frequently in virtually all age groups within a pediatric practice. The age and mechanism of injury are guidelines to a correct diagnosis. A swollen, painful knee in an infant should raise the suspicion of child abuse or infection. In the young child, significant ligament or meniscal injuries are rare, but epiphyseal separations and fractures are more frequent. In the adolescent, internal injuries to menisci and ligaments are frequent findings and most often result from sports activities, with or without contact. Patellar dislocations are also more common in adolescents.

The examiner should note bruising, swelling about the knee, the presence or absence of an effusion, and the ability to walk or bear weight. Most significant injuries are accompanied by an effusion or hemarthrosis, and the swollen knee is difficult to examine due to pain and limited motion. After the initial swelling has resolved, specific findings of an internal derangement can be elicited. The torn anterior cruciate is indicated by a positive Lachman test, in which the tibia can be translated anteriorly with the knee flexed 20°. Meniscal tears often produce pain when the knee is fully flexed and extended with medial or lateral rotational stress. Medial collateral and lateral collateral ligament injuries allow the joint to open either medially or laterally with stress in a 20° flexed position.

Radiographs should be evaluated and will show effusion in the case of internal derangement such as ligamentous injury or injury to the articular cartilage or meniscus. Widening of the distal femoral growth plate suggests a separation injury of the growth plate (Salter-Harris 1). Elevation of the tibial spine indicates an injury in which the anterior cruciate pulls a fragment of bone from the tibial articular surface. Other avulsion fractures about the knee are commonly detected on radiographs.

Initial treatment usually consists of splinting with compression using a prefabricated knee immobilizer and flexible elastic bandage (ie, ACE[t] brand). Aspiration of the knee is not necessary. Reevaluation at 2 weeks allows for a better physical exam for significant injury. Minor injuries will usually be recovering by then, and significant injuries will show persistent physical findings by that time. A magnetic resonance imaging (MRI) examination will help to define internal injuries that will require orthopedic consultation.

## DISCOID MENISCUS

A *discoid meniscus* is an abnormally shaped lateral meniscus found in children of all ages (Fig. 211-1). The spectrum of abnormalities ranges from a minor excess of central tissue in an otherwise normal meniscus, to a grossly malformed unstable mass of meniscoid tissue with few tibial or capsular attachments. It may slip in and out of the joint, causing the patient to feel something pop over the lateral aspect of the knee joint. It may be somewhat painful. The examiner can feel something pop along the lateral joint line as the knee is flexed and extended. Over time, it may become more painful, and the "popping" may begin to limit function.

An anteroposterior radiograph of the knee may show widening of the lateral joint space, and an MRI examination provides a definitive diagnosis. Arthroscopic reconstruction of the meniscus is the treatment of choice for those with significant symptoms. The natural history depends on the severity of malformation and the extent of the resection. Knees having little functional meniscus predictably go on to development of premature arthritis.

## PATELLOFEMORAL PAIN SYNDROME

Adolescents with vague anterior knee pain are seen frequently in a primary care office. The complaint is pain around the patella, aggravated by physical activities. The knee often is painful when the person sits in a car or theater where it is difficult to extend the knee. Straightening the knee gives immediate relief. This condition has been called *chondromalacia patella,* yet there is little evidence of damage to the cartilage of the patella. It has also been associated with malalignment, as many patients have excessive femoral anteversion with patellae that face toward one another as the patient walks.

Radiographs will show no abnormalities, and the treatment is aimed at relieving symptoms. Nonsteroidal anti-inflammatory drugs (NSAIDs) are helpful. A well-planned physiotherapy program that emphasizes strengthening of the quadriceps and hamstrings as well as the hip abductors and external rotators will help most patients recover.

## PATELLAR INSTABILITY AND DISLOCATION

In patellar instability and dislocation, there is a baseline anatomic malalignment of the patella and quadriceps complex that results in recurrent lateral subluxation or dislocation of the patella. The dislocations may reduce spontaneously or may require sedation and closed reduction. The subluxations are annoying and painful to the patient but do not require reduction. This condition usually is seen in adolescents rather than young children. It is common in Down syndrome and difficult to treat.

The examination will show that the patella tends to move laterally as the knee approaches full, active extension. As the knee begins to flex, the patella moves medially into its normal position in the femoral notch, a physical finding called the *"J" sign.* With the patient relaxed and the knee in full extension, the examiner can push the patella laterally and begin to flex the knee. The patient with this condition will quickly react to prevent this action, and this is termed *the apprehension sign.*

Treatment begins with quadriceps strengthening and rehabilitation as described for patellofemoral pain syndrome. Patellar stabilization braces can also be helpful. The patient with recurrent dislocation often requires surgical correction in which the medial restraints to patellar motion are reconstructed and/or the extensor mechanism is realigned.

Rarely, the patella will never be located in its proper position in the trochlea, a condition called *congenital patellar dislocation.* It should be suspected in cases of congenital knee flexion contracture and valgus alignment. Because the patella is hard to feel in the newborn and radiolucent, diagnosis may require ultrasound or MRI.

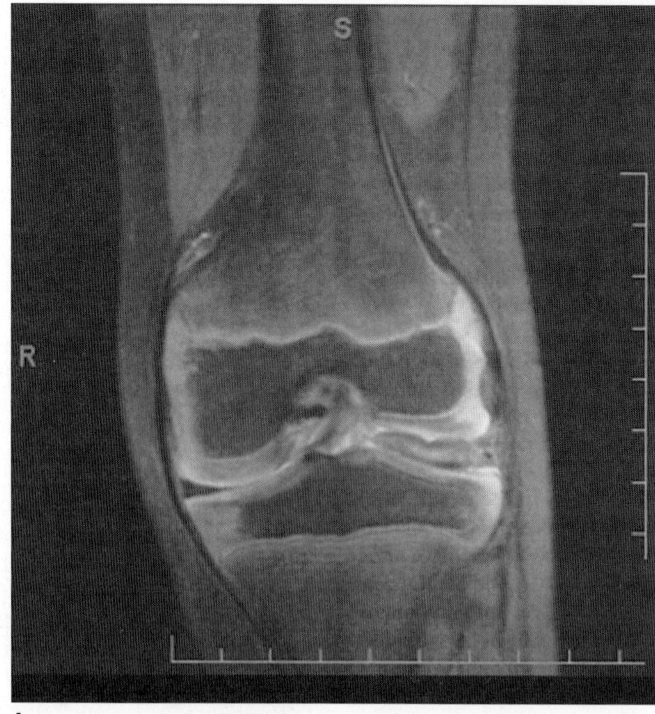


A



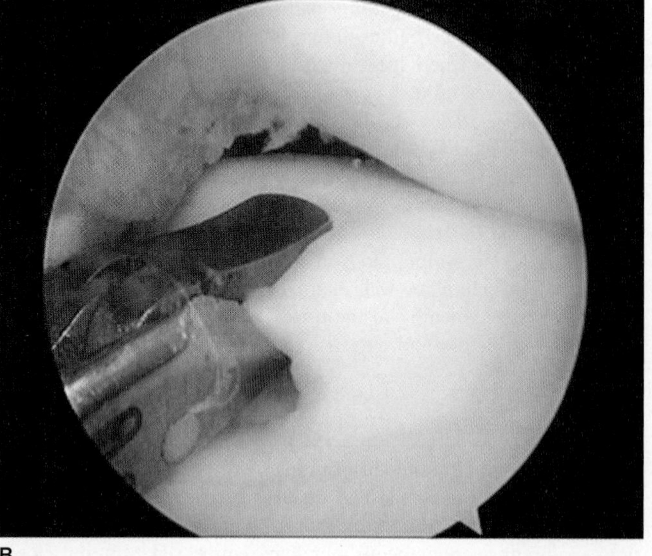

B

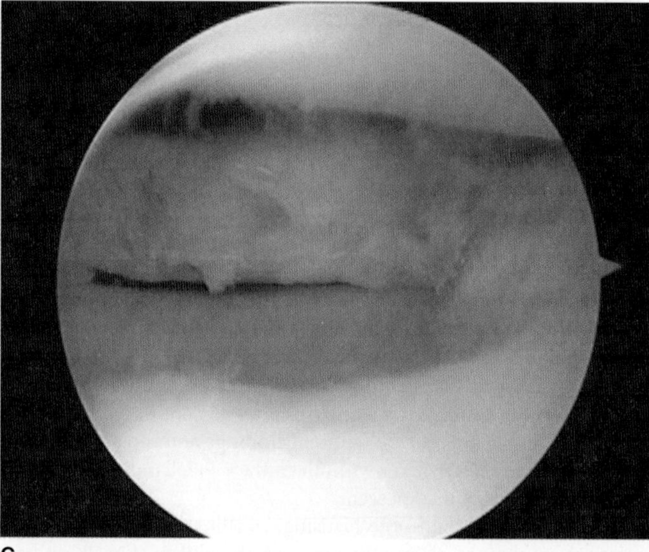

C

**FIGURE 211-1** **A:** Coronal magnetic resonance imaging of a 7-year-old patient with painful left knee popping due to large, unstable discoid meniscus. **B:** Intraoperative photo with instrument grasping the discoid meniscus. **C:** Intraoperative photo after reshaping and repair of the discoid meniscus

## OSTEOCHONDRITIS DISSECANS

An *osteochondritis dissecans lesion* is an idiopathic disease of subchondral bone that can lead to softening, fissuring, or even frank separation of the corresponding articular surface. These lesions vary in size from a few millimeters to several centimeters in diameter. In the early stages, the lesion is painful but not mobile. Later, the fragment becomes mobile and leads to an intra-articular loose body, leaving a large divot in the articular surface. Histology shows bone necrosis without inflammation. The etiology likely includes repetitive microtrauma and decreased blood supply.

The patient complains of soreness on the affected side of the knee with activity and occasionally swelling, popping, or crepitance. The physical findings are nonspecific unless there is tenderness next to the patella, or palpable crepitance or effusion. Radiographs show a lucent area on the femoral condyle, especially seen on a tunnel view with the knee partially flexed. Initial treatment is conservative, followed by arthroscopic evaluation and treatment when the condition persists (Fig. 211-2).

## OSGOOD-SCHLATTER DISEASE

In *Osgood-Schlatter disease,* there is tenderness and enlargement of the tibial tubercle in a growing child, usually in early adolescence. It is aggravated by activity, especially stair climbing and running. It represents a stress reaction of the growth cartilage into which the patellar tendon inserts. The enlargement often creates concern for a possible tumor. Radiographs will show variable fragmentation of the tibial tubercle, which are normal findings in the involved age group. Treatment is symptomatic, with reduction of activities to tolerance. If the child can continue sports without limping during the activity, he or she should be allowed to continue. The symptoms usually resolve

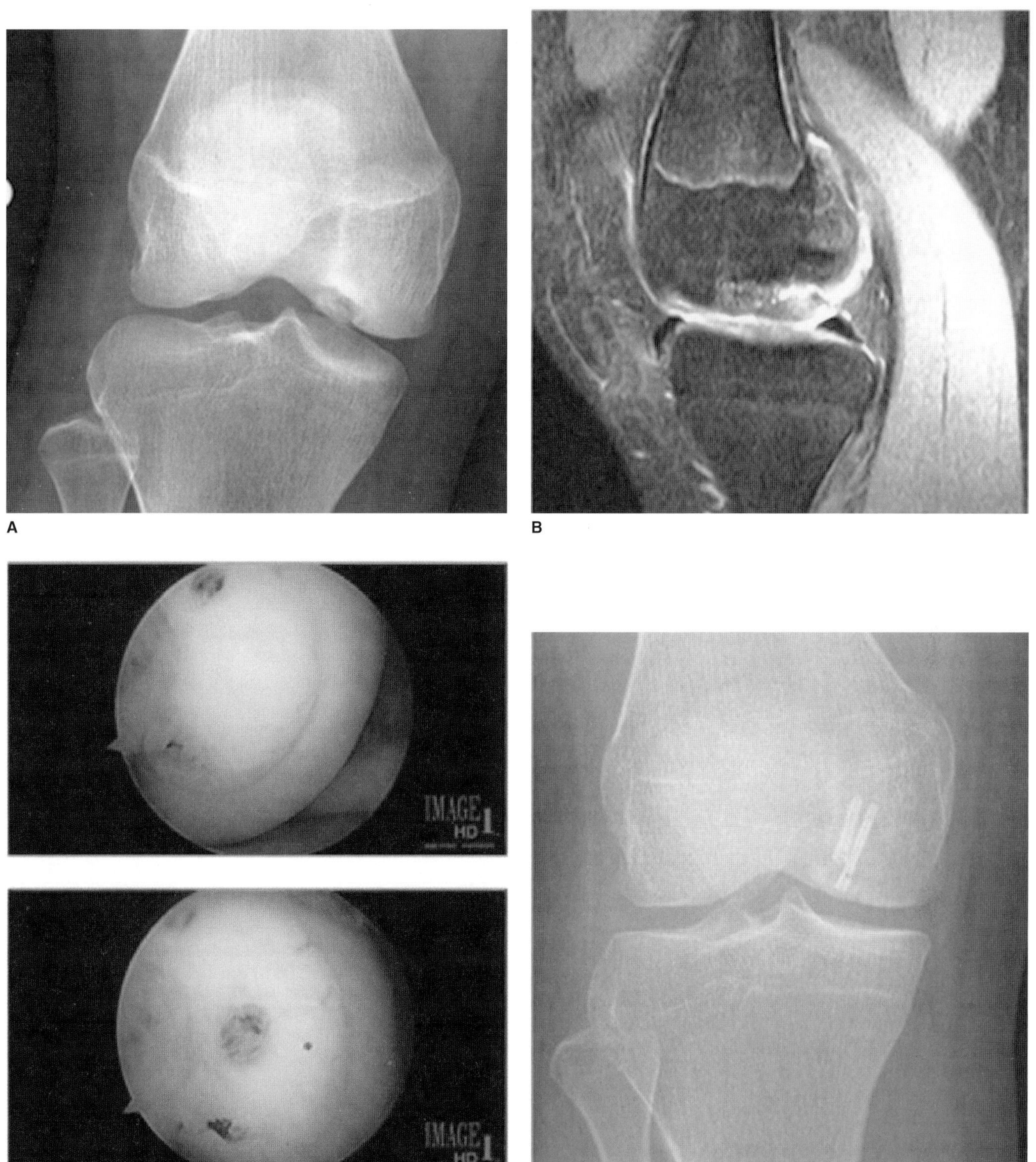


FIGURE 211-2 **A:** Anteroposterior (AP) radiograph of a 16-year-old patient with activity-related medial knee pain showing osteochondritis dissecans of the medial femoral condyle. **B:** Sagittal magnetic resonance imaging showing fragment instability. **C:** Intraoperative photo showing in situ fixation of the lesion. **D:** Follow-up AP radiograph showing healed osteochondritis dissecans fragment.



with skeletal maturity, with only an occasional person having a symptomatic nodule at the tubercle as an adult.

## SINDING-LARSEN JOHANSSON DISEASE

*Sinding-Larsen Johansson disease* is similar to Osgood-Schlatter disease in which there is a stress reaction at the distal pole of the patella. The patient typically complains of pain and tenderness at the lower pole of the patella, and the symptoms are aggravated by activities that load the knee. The patient may complain of generalized knee pain, but the exam should reveal exquisite tenderness at the inferior patellar pole. Radiographs will show fragmentation of the bone at the distal pole of the patella. Treatment is symptomatic, directed toward reducing loading activities such as jumping, running the stairs, and deep knee bends. Children will outgrow this condition without any residual problems.

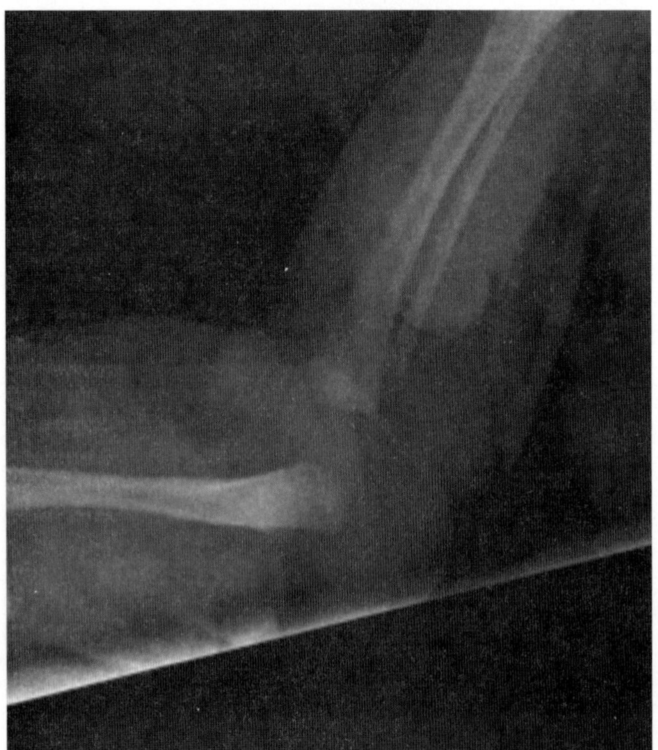

**FIGURE 211-3** Lateral radiograph of left knee in a newborn showing hyperextension and anterior tibial subluxation. This child has congenital dislocation of the knee.



## CONGENITAL DISLOCATION OF THE KNEE

When a baby is born with the knees markedly hyperextended, with the feet under the chin, parents and medical personnel alike are usually very distressed (Fig. 211-3). Fortunately, this is a condition that usually responds very well to treatment and generally has a good outcome. This condition, frequently associated with breech position, is divided into 3 categories. *Hyperextension* of the knee implies that the tibia and femur are in alignment, *subluxation* indicates that the tibia is in contact with the femur but is anterior to it, and *dislocation* means that the tibia is all the way anteriorly displaced relative to the femur.

The first 2 degrees of deformity usually respond to serial cast manipulation and have a benign prognosis with fully normal function. True dislocation of the knee, often associated with other syndromes, such as Larsen syndrome, may require surgical correction and may have some lasting disability.

## POPLITEAL (BAKER) CYST

Children with Baker cyst present with a mass in the popliteal fossa that may or may not be painful. It arises spontaneously and is not usually related to trauma or activity. The cyst, which is filled with a congealed, jelly-like condensation of joint fluid, arises as an extension of the synovium of the joint. In adults, they are usually associated with an internal derangement of the knee, but in children, the knee is usually normal.

The examiner finds a firm mass in the popliteal fossa, best appreciated with the patient prone and the knee fully extended. With the knee flexed, there is some mobility to the mass, but it remains firm. In a dark room, the mass will transilluminate. Radiographs show no abnormalities. Ultrasound can typically distinguish between a benign cystic lesion and a more solid tumor. If there is suspicion of a tumor, an MRI will be extremely helpful in resolving the issue.

Treatment is observation and reassurance. The mass will usually resolve gradually but may occasionally enlarge for a time. Excision is often complicated with recurrence and is generally discouraged.

## SUGGESTED READINGS


Abbasi D, May MM, Wall EJ, Chan G, Parikh SN. MRI findings in adolescent patients with acute traumatic knee hemarthrosis. *J Pediatr Orthop*. 2012;32(8):760-764.

Abdelaziz TH, Samir S. Congenital dislocation of the knee: a protocol for management based on degree of knee flexion. *J Child Orthop*. 2011;5(2):143-149.

Akagi R, Saisu T, Segawa Y, et al. Natural history of popliteal cysts in the pediatric population. *J Pediatr Orthop*. 2013;33(3):262-268.

Edmonds EW, Polousky J. A review of knowledge in osteochondritis dissecans: 123 years of minimal evolution from König to the ROCK study group. *Clin Orthop Relat Res*. 2013;471(4):1118-1126.

Kushare I, Klingele K, Samora W. Discoid meniscus: diagnosis and management. *Orthop Clin North Am*. 2015;46(4):533-540.

McKay SD, Chen C, Rosenfeld S. Orthopedic perspective on selected pediatric and adolescent knee conditions. *Pediatr Radiol*. 2013;43(Suppl 1):S99-S106.

2016 Patellofemoral pain consensus statement from the 4th International Patellofemoral Pain Research Retreat, Manchester. Part 1: Terminology, definitions, clinical examination, natural history, patellofemoral osteoarthritis and patient-reported outcome measures. *Br J Sports Med*. 2016;50(14):839-843. doi:10.1136/bjsports-2016-096384.

2016 Patellofemoral pain consensus statement from the 4th International Patellofemoral Pain Research Retreat, Manchester. Part 2: recommended physical interventions (exercise, taping, bracing, foot orthoses and combined interventions). *Br J Sports Med*. 2016;50(14):844-852.

Weber AE, Nathani A, Dines JS, et al. An algorithmic approach to the management of recurrent lateral patellar dislocation. *J Bone Joint Surg Am*. 2016;98(5):417-427.

Yen Y-M. Assessment and treatment of knee pain in the child and adolescent athlete. *Pediatr Clin North Am*. 2014;61(6):1155-1173. doi:10.1016/j.pcl.2014.08.003.


# 212 Developmental Conditions of the Hip

Scott B. Rosenfeld and David A. Podeszwa

## INTRODUCTION

*Developmental dysplasia of the hip* (DDH) is a spectrum of disorders of the developing hip ranging from a slightly shallow acetabulum (hip socket) with a well-located femoral head to a moderately shallow socket with joint subluxation to a severely shallow socket with complete dislocation of the joint. DDH evolves over time and may present in different forms at different ages. DDH may not be detectable at birth, and hence, the preferred term is *developmental* and not *congenital*. The American Academy of Pediatrics (AAP) defines DDH as a condition in which the femoral head has an abnormal relationship to the acetabulum, specifically, the acetabulum does not completely cover the femoral head. It can result in hip joint instability. *Dislocation* is defined as complete displacement of a joint, with no contact between the original articular surfaces. *Subluxation* is defined as displacement of a joint with some contact remaining between the articular surfaces. *Dysplasia* refers to abnormal or deficient development of the acetabulum. A teratologic dislocation is a distinct condition that occurs before birth, is generally nonreducible on physical exam, and causes the hip to be stiff. Teratologic dislocations often are associated with other syndromes and conditions, particularly arthrogryposis and myelodysplasia, and treatment depends on the underlying condition.

The incidence of DDH varies based on the criteria for diagnosis, method of diagnosis (clinical exam vs radiologic exam), race, age of the patients, and geography. Clinical instability and ultrasound abnormalities are quite common findings in newborns, with rates of 2.3 cases per 100 live births and 8 cases per 100 live births, respectively. However, the majority of these cases in newborns resolve spontaneously. As such, the overall incidence of DDH with instability or dislocation that requires treatment is approximately 1 to 1.5 per 1000 live births. Bilateral DDH occurs in 20% of all patients with this disorder.

The natural history of untreated DDH depends on the age at diagnosis and severity of dysplasia. Most neonatal hip dysplasia and instability will resolve spontaneously by the time the infant is 2 to 3 months of age. Patients with persistent hip dysplasia typically have few problems in the first decade of life. DDH generally does not affect the patient's ability to reach normal developmental milestones such as crawling and walking. However, a patient with persistent hip dysplasia is at risk of developing problems, including pain, leg length differences, and ultimately hip arthritis, in adolescence and young adulthood.

## ETIOLOGY

The etiology of DDH is multifactorial, but numerous predisposing factors have been identified. The classic risk factors for DDH include breech positioning, family history of DDH, first born, female sex, and a history of oligohydramnios. Breech positioning is considered a "packaging" issue (intrauterine crowding) predisposing to DDH. The footling breech presentation (both hips flexed) is associated with a 2% risk of DDH, and the frank breech position (1 or both knees extended) is associated with a 20% risk of developing DDH. Gestational age does not appear to have a protective effect on the incidence of DDH as there is a similar incidence in breech preterm infants as in breech term infants. Torticollis, metatarsus adductus, and oligohydramnios are other packaging-related conditions strongly associated with DDH. A child with torticollis has a 14% to 20% risk of also having DDH. Although clubfoot has not been strongly associated with DDH, as many as 10% of children with metatarsus adductus will also have DDH. DDH is more common in females and first-born children and most frequently affects the left hip. Family history also strongly influences the risk of having DDH. The risk of a subsequent child having DDH is 6% if there are healthy parents and an affected child, 12% with an affected parent, and 35% with an affected parent and an affected child. Other factors include ligamentous laxity and postnatal positioning. The maternal relaxin hormone, which allows the maternal pelvis to expand, crosses the placenta and can induce laxity in the child, an effect known to be stronger in females than in males. It can lead to instability in an immature or dysplastic hip joint. Newborn babies wrapped in a hip-extended position (papoose boarding), common in the Native American culture, also have a higher incidence of developing DDH. Healthy-hip swaddling with the hips positioned in flexion and abduction, however, does not increase the risk of DDH but instead is a healthy position allowing for normal hip development. Despite the increased incidence in patients with these well-known factors, most patients with DDH have no risk factors, emphasizing the importance of physical examination of the hip in all young children.

## CLINICAL FEATURES

The clinical evaluation and diagnosis of DDH can be difficult and can change over time. Thus, close follow-up and documentation of the physical exam are critical. The AAP recommends a hip exam at birth, 2 weeks, and every subsequent well-child visit until walking age. The physical exam findings will vary depending on the age of the child and the severity of the condition. The stability of the hip in the neonate is clinically diagnosed by performing the Barlow and Ortolani maneuvers. In the neonatal period, these maneuvers are generally the only physical exam finding suggestive of DDH. These maneuvers are best performed with the child placed supine on a warm, firm surface. The child and examiner must be as relaxed as possible. Dimming the room lights or feeding the child a bottle will often help. If the child is fussy or the examiner is impatient, the exam will be inaccurate.

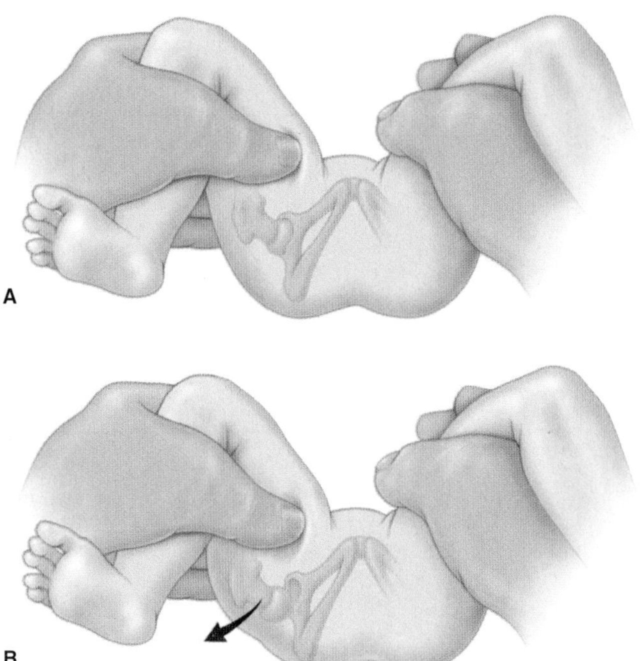


**FIGURE 212-1** The Barlow test for developmental dislocation of the hip in a neonate. **A:** With the infant supine, the examiner holds both of the child's knees and gently adducts 1 hip and pushes posteriorly. **B:** When the examination is positive, the examiner will feel the femoral head slide (*arrow*) out of the acetabulum (Barlow's sign). When the pressure is released, the head is felt to slip back into place. (Reproduced with permission from Herring JA: *Tachdjian's Pediatric Orthopaedics*, 4th ed. Philadelphia: Elsevier; 2007.)

The examiner holds the child's knees, 1 in each hand, with the fingers of the examiner over the greater trochanter and the thumb placed along the inner thigh. The hips are examined 1 at a time. The Barlow test (Fig. 212-1) is an attempt to dislocate the femoral head from within the acetabulum. With the hip flexed 90° with neutral rotation, the hip is adducted and pressure is applied in a posterior direction in an attempt to slide the hip posteriorly out of the acetabulum. With a positive Barlow test, the hip, which resides in the reduced position, will slide posteriorly out of the acetabulum and will be felt to slip back as the posterior pressure is relaxed. The Ortolani test (Fig. 212-2) is an attempt to reduce a dislocated femoral head back into the acetabulum (the opposite of the Barlow maneuver). With the hip flexed 90° and in neutral rotation, the hip is abducted while simultaneously the ring and small fingers are used to gently lift the greater trochanter. With a positive Ortolani test, the hip, which resides in the dislocated position, will slide back into the acetabulum with a palpable "clunk" of reduction and will be felt to slip back out of the acetabulum when pressure is released. In the absence of an obviously positive test, both of these maneuvers should be repeated multiple times as a smooth arc of motion before proceeding to the opposite hip.

In the infant (> 3 months of age), more specific physical exam findings of the dislocated hip, such as limited hip abduction and a more proximal location of the greater trochanter, will appear. The Galeazzi sign, highly suggestive of developmental dysplasia of the hip, is a relative shortening of the thigh when comparing the height of the knees with both hips flexed 90° (Fig. 212-3). With a unilateral dislocation, the thigh will be foreshortened, resulting in additional thigh folds on the affected side (Figure 212-4). However, extra thigh folds are commonly a normal variant and do not necessarily indicate a hip dislocation when found in isolation. Limitation of abduction, the most reliable sign of a dislocated hip, is best appreciated by abducting both hips simultaneously with the child on a firm surface. The dislocated side will have a distinct decrease in abduction as compared to the healthy side (Fig. 212-5).

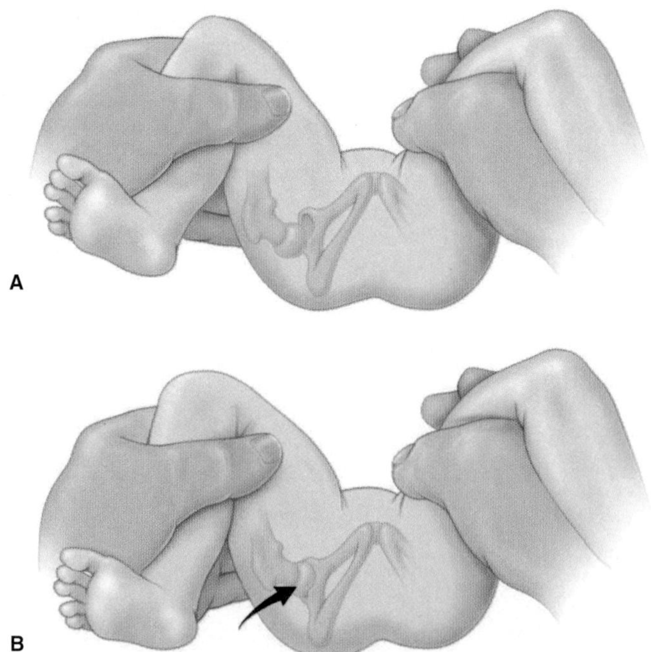


FIGURE 212-2 The Ortolani test for developmental dislocation of the hip in a neonate. **A:** The examiner holds the infant's knees and gently abducts the hip while lifting up on the greater trochanter with 2 fingers. **B:** When the test is positive, the dislocated femoral head will fall back into the acetabulum (*arrow*) with a palpable (but not audible) "clunk" as the hip is abducted (Ortolani's sign). When the hip is adducted, the examiner will feel the head redislocate posteriorly. (Reproduced with permission from Herring JA: *Tachdjian's Pediatric Orthopaedics*, 4th ed. Philadelphia: Elsevier; 2007.)

The evaluation of the infant with bilateral hip dislocations can be difficult. There may be symmetric abduction (although symmetrically decreased) and similar thigh lengths with the Galeazzi test. The Klisic test is a helpful examination maneuver in this situation. It is performed by placing the middle finger on the greater trochanter and the thumb on the anterior-superior iliac spine. Normally, an imaginary line drawn between the 2 fingers will point at or above the umbilicus. If the hip is dislocated, the line will point below the umbilicus (Fig. 212-6).

The physical findings in a child of walking age with a unilateral dislocated hip may include decreased abduction of the affected hip,

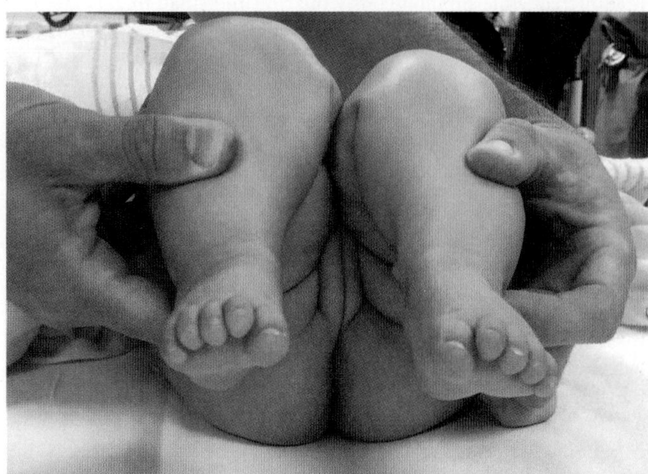

FIGURE 212-3 The Galeazzi test for developmental dislocation of the hip in an infant. The examiner holds the infant's hips and knees flexed with the pelvis on a level surface. The left knee is lower than the right, demonstrating a positive Galeazzi sign.

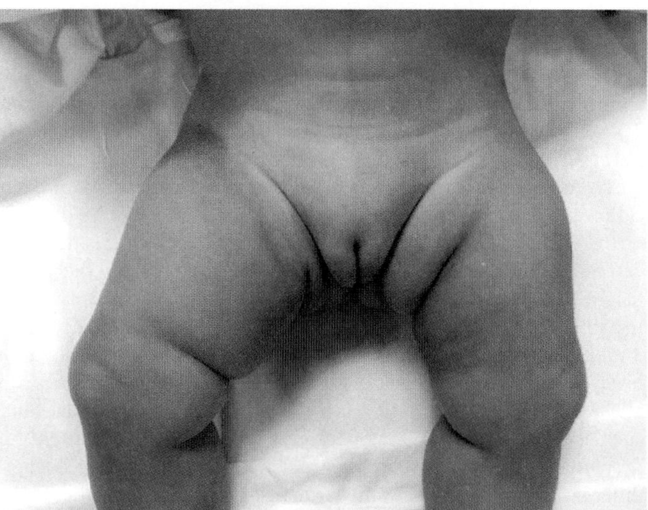

FIGURE 212-4 Asymmetric thigh folds in developmental dislocation of the hip in an infant. The left leg appears foreshortened, resulting in additional thigh folds, suggesting a left hip dislocation.

a positive Klisic test, a positive Galeazzi sign, a limp, and a leg-length discrepancy. A walking patient with bilateral hip dislocations often presents with only a complaint of increased lumbar lordosis (sway back) secondary to bilateral hip flexion contractures but may also have a waddling gait on both sides.

Imaging in DDH depends on the age of the child. The neonate's femoral head and acetabulum are primarily cartilaginous, rendering conventional radiographs difficult to interpret in this age group. Ultrasonography visualizes the cartilage and soft tissue structures of the hip and the relationship of the femoral head and acetabulum very well. The AAP recommends ultrasonography for female infants either carried breech or with a positive family history for DDH. An infant with a positive Ortolani or Barlow sign does not require an immediate ultrasound but should be referred to a pediatric orthopedic surgeon for evaluation and possible treatment. At 3 to 6 months of age, the femoral head begins to ossify and, by 6 months of age, plain radiographs replace ultrasound as the imaging study of choice for DDH.

## TREATMENT

Treatment of DDH depends on the child's age and the location of the hip. The Pavlik harness (Fig. 212-7) is the first choice of treatment for patients younger than 6 months old with a dysplastic, unstable, or dislocated hip. The harness should hold the hip in 100° of flexion. If the hip cannot be placed into this position, the treatment will fail. The hip, however, does not have to be reducible at the time of the examination to be successfully treated with the harness. The child should be evaluated within 3 weeks with clinical and ultrasound examination to document the reduction of the femoral head. If the femoral head is not reduced within 3 to 4 weeks, the harness is abandoned.

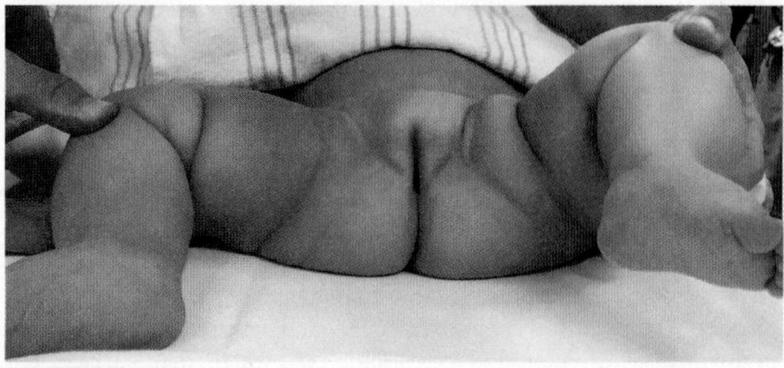

FIGURE 212-5 Asymmetric hip abduction in developmental dislocation of the hip in an infant. The left hip exhibits decreased abduction as compared to the right suggesting a left hip dislocation.

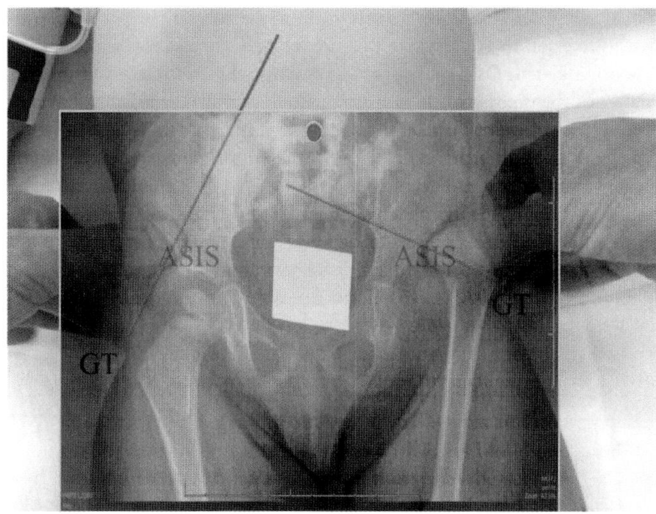


FIGURE 212-6 The Klisic sign in developmental dislocation of the hip in an infant. In the patient's normal right hip, a line drawn between the finger on the greater trochanter (GT) and the thumb on the anterior-superior iliac spine (ASIS) points above the umbilicus (red oval). In the patient's dislocated left hip, that line points below the umbilicus.

If the hip successfully reduces, use of the harness is continued for an additional 6 to 12 weeks until the ultrasound is normal. Treatment with a Pavlik harness has success rates of 85% to 95% and a very low complication rate. The most severe reported complication of Pavlik harness use is iatrogenic avascular necrosis (AVN) of the hip with an incidence of approximately 1%. AVN usually is associated with inappropriate positioning of the hip in the Pavlik harness. For this reason,

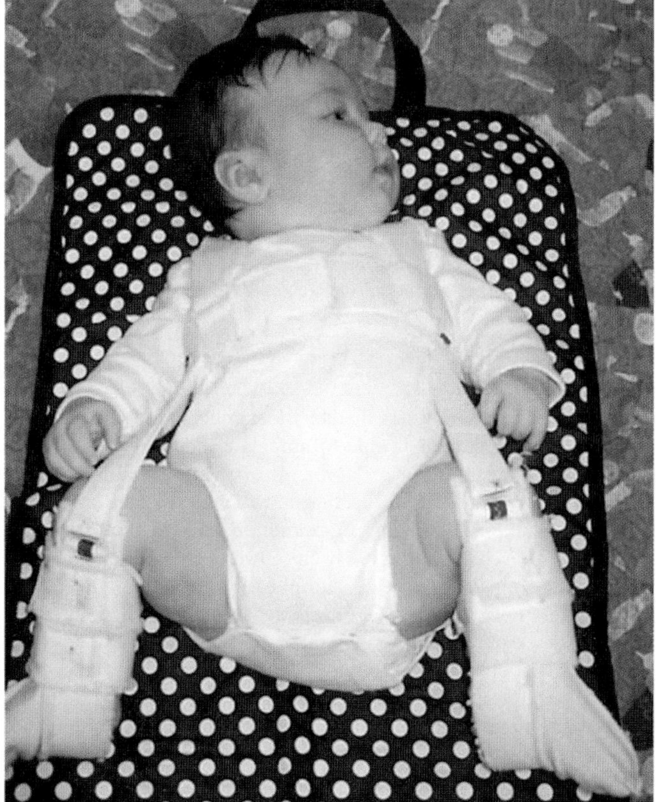

FIGURE 212-7 The Pavlik harness. The transverse chest strap should be placed just below the nipple line. The hips should be flexed to 100°, and the posterior straps should not produce forced abduction. (Reproduced with permission from Herring JA: *Tachdjian's Pediatric Orthopaedics*, 4th ed. Philadelphia: Elsevier; 2007.)

it is recommended that treatment with a Pavlik harness be performed by a physician experienced in its use. If treatment with a Pavlik harness fails to reduce a dislocated hip by 3 to 4 weeks, a rigid abduction orthosis such as a Rhino brace may be considered for an additional 3 to 4 weeks.

For the child between 6 months and 2 years of age who presents with a dislocated hip or who has failed initial harness treatment, the goal of treatment is to obtain and maintain a concentric reduction of the hip without damaging the femoral head. It can be performed with either a closed or open reduction. Both procedures are performed in the operating room with the patient under general anesthesia. In a closed reduction, the hip is reduced by manipulating the femoral head into the acetabulum utilizing an Ortolani maneuver. Often this procedure is combined with lengthening of the contracted adductor tendon and an arthrogram to confirm reduction. Once the hip is reduced, the patient is placed into a spica cast in the "human position" for 3 to 4 months. An open reduction involves surgically opening the hip joint and placing the femoral head back in the socket. The child who is older than 2 years of age and presents with a dislocated hip usually requires an open reduction in combination with a femoral shortening osteotomy and a pelvic osteotomy to correct the persistent femoral and acetabular bony deformities. Follow-up with regular radiographs until skeletal maturity is essential as persistent acetabular dysplasia may be present despite the perfect execution of prior treatments at any age. The incidence of residual or recurrent dysplasia after successful treatment is estimated to be between 10% and 20%. AVN of the femoral head is the most significant complication associated with the treatment of developmental dysplasia of the hip and can occur with any nonoperative or operative treatments.

## LEGG-CALVÉ-PERTHES DISEASE

*Legg-Calvé-Perthes disease* (LCPD) is idiopathic AVN of the femoral head. In this condition, the vascular supply to part or all of the femoral head is disrupted, leading to the cessation of growth of the femoral head and increased bone density in the femoral head. Once the blood supply returns, the dense bone is resorbed and replaced by new bone. However, during this process, the femoral head bone becomes weakened, typically resulting in fragmentation and flattening of the femoral head.

### ETIOLOGY

Despite being recognized as a distinct entity a century ago, the exact etiology of LCPD is still unknown and is probably multifactorial. Factors that have been associated with the etiology of LCPD include coagulopathy, trauma, hereditary influences, hyperactivity or attention-deficit disorder, and environmental factors, including exposure to cigarette smoke. These factors may work in combination in a "predisposed child" with certain growth and developmental abnormalities such as low birth weight, short stature for age, and delayed bone age relative to chronologic age. However, how these findings relate to the pathogenesis of the disease is still uncertain.

LCPD can be diagnosed at any time between 18 months of age and skeletal maturity but is most prevalent in children between 4 and 12 years of age. The disease is 4 to 5 times more likely to develop in boys than girls, more common in whites and those of Asian descent, and rare in African Americans and Native Americans. African Americans presenting with clinical and radiographic signs of LCPD should undergo evaluation for an underlying hemoglobinopathy. Bilateral disease occurs in 10% to 12% of patients but usually is not symmetric or concurrent. A patient with bilateral, symmetric AVN should be evaluated for other systemic conditions such as hypothyroidism, an epiphyseal dysplasia, Gaucher disease, sickle cell disease, and use of steroid medications.

### CLINICAL FEATURES

The most common presenting symptom is a painless limp, frequently first noticed by a parent. The limp often is exacerbated by physical activity and alleviated with rest. Pain is the second most common presenting symptom and may be located in the groin, anterior hip region, or laterally around the greater trochanter. It is important to recognize that pain may be referred to the knee, which, if unrecognized as coming from the hip, can lead to a delay in establishing the diagnosis. The patient or parent may note an isolated traumatic event (fall or twisting injury) prior to the onset of the symptoms. These initial symptoms may completely resolve after a few days, followed by the waxing and waning of symptoms for some time.

Upon physical examination, the patient will have a limp in addition to limitations of hip abduction and internal rotation. During the early phase of the disorder, reduction of hip motion commonly occurs as a result of muscle spasm and synovitis within the hip joint. A hip flexion contracture also may be present, as may varying degrees of atrophy of the gluteus, quadriceps, and hamstring muscles.

Initial radiographic imaging should include a standing anteroposterior (AP) and a frog-lateral radiograph of both hips. Significant radiographic changes will be evident for 18 to 24 months as the femoral head goes through fragmentation and healing followed by remodeling of the femoral head and acetabulum that will last until skeletal maturity occurs. The extent of radiographic changes is quite variable from patient to patient, and the radiographic appearance may not correlate with the patient's symptoms or function. Perfusion magnetic resonance imaging (MRI), a recently developed imaging technique, has been shown to be useful early in the disease process for both diagnosis and prognosis of LCPD disease by calculating the percentage of the femoral head that is hypoperfused.

In the absence of radiographic changes, the differential diagnosis of a child with limp, hip pain, and decreased range of motion should include trauma and infection. In the presence of radiographic changes, the differential diagnosis should include other causes of AVN such as sickle cell disease (and other hemoglobinopathies), thalassemia, use of steroid medications, the sequela of a traumatic hip dislocation, or a complication of treatment of DDH. In addition, epiphyseal dysplasias, such as multiple epiphyseal dysplasia, spondyloepiphyseal dysplasia, mucopolysaccharidoses, and hypothyroidism, should be ruled out, especially in the case of bilateral disease.

The severity of the disease can range from very mild (minimal pain and limp) to severe (marked activity limitation). Most children experience moderate symptoms for 12 to 18 months followed by complete resolution of their symptoms and a return to normal physical activities. The patient's age at onset of symptoms has been found to be the most consistent factor affecting the course and outcome of the disease. The natural history of LCPD is affected by the age of onset, which is related to the remodeling ability of the growing hip. Patients with early onset (before 6 years of age) have more growth and remodeling capability and, therefore, tend to have the best outcomes. Conversely, those with onset after reaching 11 years of age tend to have the worst outcomes. Outcomes are also affected by the duration from the onset of the disease to complete resolution: the shorter the duration, the better the final results. The most important predictor of long-term outcomes of LCPD is the shape of the healed femoral head and its congruency with the acetabulum at maturity. A patient with a femoral head that heals with a round shape that matches the shape of the acetabulum will generally do very well with few long-term consequences. However, a patient with a femoral head that heals out of round with poor congruency with the acetabulum is at increased risk of developing hip arthritis in the future.

### TREATMENT

The goal of treatment is to allow the femoral head to heal with a round shape and to prevent permanent deformity of the femoral head. Treatment is indicated for patients with pain, limitation of motion, early hip subluxation (femoral head uncovering), and severe femoral head deformity. The initial treatment for all symptomatic patients should include elimination of hip joint irritability (rest, crutches, and/or nonsteroidal anti-inflammatory medications) and the maintenance or restoration of a normal range of hip motion, especially abduction. Maintaining range of motion can be achieved by teaching the family exercises to stretch the adductor muscles. However, in some cases, physical therapy may be required. Short periods of bed rest with or without traction for major episodes of pain or loss of joint motion may be needed. Other nonoperative treatment methods used in early stages of the disease to prevent deformity and hip subluxation include abduction casts (Petrie casts) and abduction bracing.

Surgical treatment for LCPD is controversial because there are few large, long-term, prospective studies describing outcomes. Surgical options include muscle-tendon lengthening and osteotomies of the femur and/or pelvis. A proximal femoral varus osteotomy and/or a pelvic osteotomy (Salter or Shelf osteotomy) may be recommended for patients between the ages of 6 and 11 years at the onset of symptoms and in the early radiographic stage of disease. Recent studies have shown that for certain patients between the ages of 8 and 11 years at the onset of symptoms, these osteotomies are likely to prevent deformity of the femoral head and improve outcome.

## SLIPPED CAPITAL FEMORAL EPIPHYSIS

*Slipped capital femoral epiphysis* (SCFE) is a displacement of the femoral epiphysis from the proximal femoral metaphysis (femoral neck). The femoral epiphysis actually maintains its normal relationship within the acetabulum, and it is the femoral neck and shaft that displace relative to the femoral epiphysis, most commonly slipping anteriorly and externally rotating.

The incidence of SCFE is estimated to be approximately 2 per 100,000, but this figure varies according to race, sex, and geographic location. SCFE typically occurs during adolescence (boys 13 to 15 years of age, girls 11 to 13 years of age), a period of maximal skeletal growth. African American males and adolescents residing in the eastern states appear to be at greatest risk. When SCFE occurs in a juvenile (10 years of age or younger) or in a patient older than 16 years of age, careful assessment for an underlying endocrinopathy should be considered.

### ETIOLOGY

The exact etiology of a SCFE is still unclear, but mechanical and endocrine factors are thought to play a role. The mechanical factors that contribute to an SCFE include thinning of the perichondral ring complex (a fibrous band that encircles the physis at the cartilage-bone junction), relative or absolute retroversion of the femoral neck, and an increased obliquity of the adolescent proximal femoral physis relative to the femoral neck and shaft. The most common endocrine disorders associated with SCFE are hypothyroidism, growth hormone deficiency (SCFE will occur during hormone replacement), and chronic renal failure (due to uncontrolled secondary hyperparathyroidism).

### CLINICAL FEATURES

SCFE is most commonly classified by the stability of the slip. An SCFE is "stable" if the patient is able to ambulate independently or with crutches. An "unstable" SCFE is when the patient is unable to ambulate at all. The difference is likely due to increased pain associated with an unstable SCFE having more motion, similar to a fracture, at the physis. This classification has been shown to be predictive of AVN, which is the most devastating complication of SCFE. The rate of AVN is very low in stable SCFE, whereas in unstable SCFE, the rate of AVN has been reported to be as high as 58%.

Bilateral involvement of the hips either on initial presentation or subsequently occurs in approximately 20% to 25% of patients. Of those with bilateral SCFE, 50% will present initially with both hips involved simultaneously. In more than 80% of patients who present with unilateral involvement and subsequently develop a contralateral SCFE, the contralateral SCFE will develop within 18 months of presentation for treatment of the first hip. Younger patients and those with endocrine or metabolic abnormalities are at much higher risk for having bilateral involvement.

The most common clinical presentation is that of a chronic, stable SCFE. The adolescent is commonly an obese male with a few months

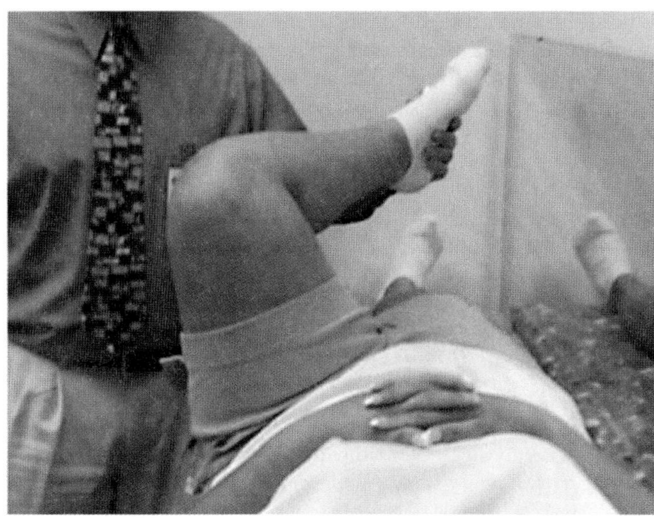

**FIGURE 212-8** Clinical examination of a patient with stable slipped capital femoral epiphysis. Hip flexion and external rotation are limited. With flexion of the affected hip, the limb rotates externally. (Reproduced with permission from Herring JA: *Tachdjian's Pediatric Orthopaedics*, 4th ed. Philadelphia: Elsevier; 2007.)

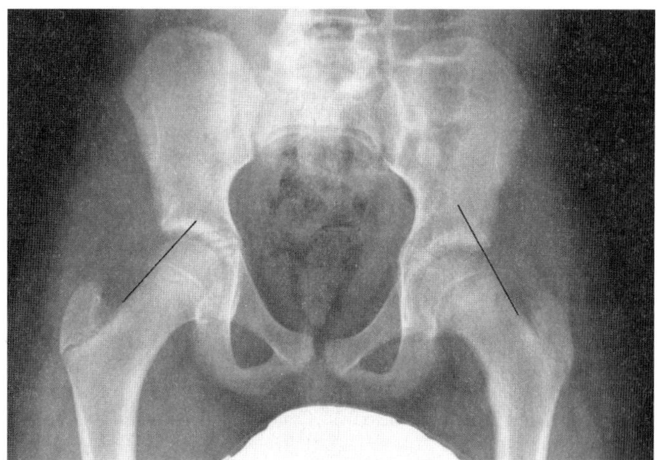

**FIGURE 212-9** Klein's line for slipped capital femoral epiphysis (SCFE) on an anteroposterior pelvis radiograph. Klein's line is drawn tangential to the superior femoral neck. In the normal hip on the right, Klein's line intersects the femoral head. In the left hip, Klein's line does not intersect the femoral head, indicating a SCFE.

of gradual-onset groin pain, thigh pain, knee pain, or a limp. Pain referred to the knee may be the only presenting symptom; therefore, any adolescent (especially if obese) who presents with pain between the umbilicus and the knee must have the hips evaluated radiographically to rule out an SCFE. Clinically, patients with an SCFE have a shortened lower extremity with increased external rotation at rest and an obligate abduction and external rotation of the hip with passive or active hip flexion (Fig. 212-8). An acute, unstable SCFE, one that occurs in a patient with minor prior symptoms, often presents as a sudden, fracture-like episode with severe pain and an inability to bear weight after relatively trivial trauma. Most patients who present with unstable SCFE report having pain and limp for months prior to their sudden onset of severe pain. This pain is likely the result of a chronic, stable SCFE suddenly converting to an unstable SCFE, underscoring the importance of early diagnosis of chronic stable SCFE.

AP and frog-lateral plain radiographs of both hips are the primary and often the only imaging studies needed to diagnose an SCFE. The earliest radiographic sign is widening and irregularity of the physis, and displacement may not be evident. In the normal hip, a line drawn tangential to the superior femoral neck (Klein's line) on the AP radiograph should intersect a portion of the femoral head. With posterior displacement of the typical SCFE, this line will not intersect the head. The frog-lateral radiograph is the most helpful view for identifying the slip because the posteriorly slipped head is easily seen (Fig. 212-9).

## TREATMENT

A patient with an acute, unstable SCFE presents with a sudden onset of severe, fracture-like pain in the affected hip, usually the result of a minor fall or twisting injury. An acute, unstable SCFE usually is treated urgently because these patients are at significant risk for developing AVN. The patient is unable to bear weight and will seek immediate medical attention. These patients should be immobilized on a stretcher and provided appropriate analgesics. Any attempt at ambulation or transportation by wheelchair will cause severe pain and risk further slippage of the capital epiphysis.

Once the diagnosis of a chronic, stable SCFE is confirmed, the patient should be made non–weight bearing and transported by wheelchair or stretcher. The patient should be admitted to the hospital and placed on bed rest until prompt, definitive surgical treatment is undertaken. Conversion to an unstable SCFE with acute displacement of the epiphysis after diagnosis of a mild, chronic slip has been well documented and can dramatically alter the patient's prognosis. For this reason, patients with a diagnosis of SCFE should not be sent home and advised to follow-up with an orthopedic surgeon. Instead, the SCFE should be evaluated and treated urgently.

The primary goal of definitive treatment for SCFE is to stabilize the capital femoral epiphysis to the femoral neck to prevent further slipping. Most orthopedic centers treat stable SCFE by single in situ percutaneous screw fixation with no attempt at reducing the deformity. Postoperatively, patients will generally remain crutch-assisted, foot-flat weight bearing for 4 to 6 weeks followed by full weight bearing with restricted running and jumping activities for an additional 6 weeks. Unstable SCFE is usually treated with 2 screws. Alternatively, some centers may treat unstable SCFE with a larger, more extensive reconstructive surgery aimed at correcting the deformity (surgical hip dislocation with modified Dunn osteotomy). This treatment method is controversial because it is a relatively novel procedure without large studies reporting long-term follow-up comparing the results with in situ fixation.

Diligent follow-up is required for these patients after treatment because they have approximately a 20% risk of having a slipped epiphysis of the contralateral hip. In skeletally immature patients, particularly in those with open triradiate cartilage, this risk may be even greater. In addition, patients with unstable SCFE must be followed for the development of AVN of the femoral head, the most severe complication associated with SCFE, which most often manifests within 6 to 12 months following treatment. Patients with AVN will present with increasing hip pain, decreased range of motion, and radiographic changes that may include increased femoral head density, fragmentation, and collapse. Before and after treatment, families must be reminded that in situ screw fixation will not change the deformity of the proximal femur and, thus, will not change the range of motion of the hip, the externally rotated position of the lower extremity, or the patient's limp. If correction of the proximal femoral deformity is desired, reconstructive surgery, including osteochondroplasty of the femoral head-neck junction and proximal femoral flexion, and internal rotation osteotomy may be performed after healing of the SCFE. Unequal lengths of the legs is also a common finding with longer-term follow-up as a result of shortening secondary to the slippage as well as early closure of the growth plate. In addition, early arthrosis of the hip joint secondary to residual SCFE deformity or AVN is a leading cause of degenerative hip joint disease in adults.

# TRANSIENT SYNOVITIS OF THE HIP

*Transient (toxic) synovitis of the hip joint* is one of the most common causes of lower extremity pain and limping due to an irritable joint. The condition is most commonly seen in children between 3 and

8 years of age who present with a history of acute-onset hip pain, limited hip range of motion, and limping (or an inability to walk in more severe cases). Frequently, they have a history of a recent viral illness.

### ETIOLOGY

The etiology of transient synovitis of the hip is unclear. Associations have been made with minor trauma, allergies, and recent illness. Frequently, there is a history of recent viral upper respiratory illness.

### CLINICAL FEATURES

Clinically, at presentation, transient synovitis mimics septic arthritis with hip pain and irritability along with limp or even inability to walk (see Chapter 199). However, patients with transient synovitis usually have a temperature below 38°C, no evidence of systemic illness, white blood cell count (WBC) < 12,000 cells/mL, C-reactive protein level (CRP) < 2.0 mg/dL, and erythrocyte sedimentation rate (ESR) < 20 mm/h (although mild elevations are possible). Radiographs may show widening of the hip joint space, and an ultrasound of the affected hip will show an effusion. Aspiration of the joint may be necessary to rule out septic arthritis. The joint aspirate will usually show a WBC count between 5000 and 15,000 cells/mL.

### TREATMENT

Treatment is aimed at eliminating the underlying inflammatory synovitis. A brief period of bed rest, progressive weight bearing with crutches if needed, and around-the-clock nonsteroidal anti-inflammatory medications for 3 to 5 days are usually all that are required. Clinical symptoms usually resolve gradually and completely over a period of several days to weeks (the average duration is 10 days). However, it is common for the patient to have symptoms that wax and wane for months. The long-term outcome usually is favorable without long-term consequences.

### SUGGESTED READINGS


American Academy of Orthopaedic Surgeons. Detection and nonoperative management of pediatric developmental dysplasia of the hip in infants up to six months of age. Evidence-based clinical practice guideline. September 2014. Available at http://www.aaos.org/research/guidelines/DDHGuidelineFINAL.pdf.

American Academy of Orthopaedic Surgeons Advisory Statement. *"CDH" Should Be "DDH."* Park Ridge, IL: American Academy of Orthopaedic Surgeons; 1991.

Bialik V, Bialik GM, Blazer S, et al. Developmental dysplasia of the hip: a new approach to incidence. *Pediatrics.* 1999;103:93-99.

Barlow TG. Early diagnosis and treatment of congenital dislocation of the hip. *Proc R Soc Med.* 1963;56:804-810.

Carroll KL, Schiffern AN, Murray KA, et al. The occurrence of occult acetabular dysplasia in relatives of individuals with developmental dysplasia of the hip. *J Pediatr Orthop.* 2016;36:96-100.

Choudry Q, Goyal R, Paton RW. Is limitation of hip abduction a useful clinical sign in the diagnosis of developmental dysplasia of the hip? *Arch Dis Child.* 2013;98:862-866.

Committee on Quality Improvement, Subcommittee on Developmental Dysplasia of the Hip. American Academy of Pediatrics. Clinical practice guideline: early detection of developmental dysplasia of the hip. *Pediatrics.* 2000;105:896-905.

Daniel AB, Joseph B. Epidemiology, pathogenesis, and treatment of Legg-Calvé-Perthes disease: current concepts. *Curr Orthop Pract.* 2013;24:28-33.

Gans I, Flynn JM, Sankar WN. Abduction bracing for residual acetabular dysplasia in infantile DDH. *J Pediatr Orthop.* 2013;33:714-718.

Hailer YD, Haag AC, Nilsson O, et al. Legg-Calvé-Perthes disease: quality of life, physical activity, and behavior pattern. *J Pediatr Orthop.* 2014;34:514-521.

Harcke HT, Karatas AF, Cummings S, Bowen JR. Sonographic assessment of hip swaddling techniques in infants with and without DDH. *J Pediatr Orthop.* 2016;36:232-235.

Herring JA. Legg-Calvé-Perthes disease at 100: a review of evidence-based treatment. *J Pediatr Orthop.* 2011;31:S137-S140.

Herring JA, Kim HT, Browne R. Legg-Calve-Perthes disease. Part II: prospective multicenter study of the effect of treatment on outcome. *J Bone Joint Surg Am.* 2004;86-A(10):2121-2134.

Holman J, Carroll KL, Murray KA, et al. Long-term follow-up of open reduction surgery for developmental dislocation of the hip. *J Pediatr Orthop.* 2012;32:121-126.

Joseph B. Natural history of early onset and late-onset Legg-Calve-Perthes disease. *J Pediatr Orthop.* 2011;31:S152-S155.

Kim HKW, Wiesman KD, Kulkarni V, et al. Perfusion MRI in early stage of Legg-Calve-Perthes disease to predict lateral pillar involvement: a preliminary study. *J Bone Joint Surg.* 2014;96:1152-1160.

Ortiz-Neira CL, Paolucci EO, Donnon T. A meta-analysis of common risk factors associated with the diagnosis of developmental dysplasia of the hip in newborns. *Eur J Radiol.* 2012;81:e344.

Price CT, Schwend RM. Improper swaddling a risk factor for developmental dysplasia of the hip. *AAP News.* 2011;32:11. Available at http://aapnews.aappublications.org/content/32/9/11.1.full.

Sarkissian EJ, Sankar WN, Zhu X, et al. Radiographic follow-up of DDH in infants: are X-rays necessary after a normalized ultrasound? *J Pediatr Orthop.* 2015;35:551-555.

Terjesen T. Residual hip dysplasia as a risk factor for osteoarthritis in 45 years follow-up of late-detected hip dislocation. *J Child Orthop.* 2011;5:425-430.

Terjesen T, Wiig O, Svenningsen S. Varus femoral osteotomy improves sphericity of the femoral head in older children with severe form of Legg-Calvé-Perthes disease. *Clin Orthop Relat Res.* 2012;470:2394-2401.

Weinstein SL. Natural history of congenital hip dislocation (CDH) and hip dysplasia. *Clin Orthop Relat Res.* 1987;225:62-76.

Zaltz I, Baca G, Clohisy JC. Unstable SCFE: review of treatment modalities and prevalence of osteonecrosis. *Clin Orthop Relat Res.* 2013;471:2192-2198.


# 213 Disorders of the Neck and Spine

William A. Phillips, Lee S. Haruno, and Daniel J. Sucato

## CONGENITAL MUSCULAR TORTICOLLIS

*Torticollis* (wryneck) is a head position whereby the ear is tilted to 1 shoulder and the chin is rotated to the opposite shoulder. The most common form of torticollis is known as *congenital muscular torticollis* and is due to overpull of the sternocleidomastoid (SCM) muscle. This deformity is typically noted within the first 2 to 4 weeks of life and almost always by 6 months of age. The incidence of congenital muscular torticollis is reported to be approximately 3 to 5 per 1000 births. Although its etiology is not completely understood, the condition has been previously linked to breech presentation, increased infant size, difficult forceps delivery, and first-born children. Orthopedic disorders associated with torticollis include hip dysplasia, clubfoot, and metatarsus adductus.

Clinical presentation of congenital muscular torticollis ranges from a benign postural preference without range of motion limitation to severely restricted mobility with a very tight SCM. In some cases of congenital muscular torticollis, the SCM may have a palpable, painless, olive-like swelling in its mid-substance (fibromatosis colli). Physical examination demonstrates a tilt of the head to 1 side with rotation to the opposite side. For example, a left-sided SCM muscle contracture

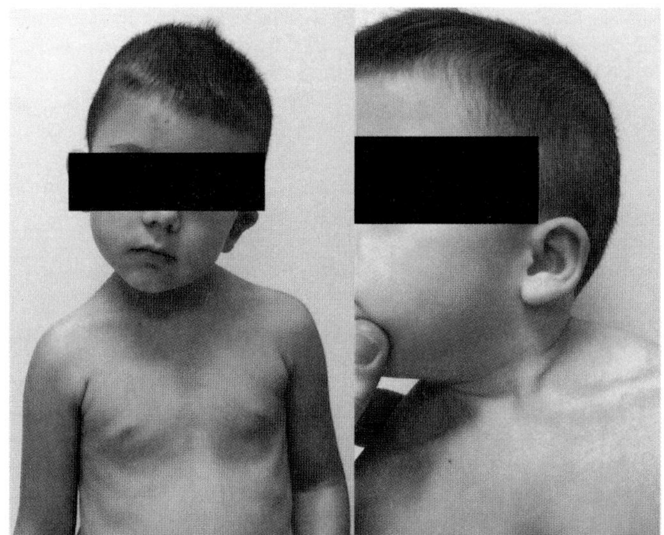

FIGURE 213-1 Congenital muscular torticollis in a young boy. The tight left sternocleidomastoid causes the left head tilt and chin rotation to the right. The tight left sternocleidomastoid muscle is evident.

would result in head tilt to the left and rotation of the chin to the right (Fig. 213-1). It should be noted that chin rotation toward a tight SCM is atypical for congenital muscular torticollis and should prompt further evaluation of other nonmuscular causes. Although rare, head tilt may be absent with involvement of both SCMs. Craniofacial asymmetry is noted in as many as 90% of patients with congenital muscular torticollis at initial presentation.

Due to the persistence of abnormal head positioning, particularly for prolonged periods in the supine position, skull abnormalities including plagiocephaly can result. In general, plagiocephaly will improve over time with the correction of torticollis as the asymmetric pressure is alleviated. There is some evidence that use of an orthotic helmet can improve plagiocephaly when compared with traditional repositioning techniques.

The differential diagnosis of congenital muscular torticollis includes vertebral anomalies, atlantoaxial rotatory displacement, central nervous system (CNS) tumors of the posterior fossa or cervical spinal cord, and visual abnormalities (eg, strabismus). Diagnosis is based on characteristic clinical findings including head positioning and asymmetry, tightness of the SCM, and restricted neck range of motion. Routine imaging is not recommended, although neurologic and visual examination can help to narrow the differential.

Treatment for congenital muscular torticollis consists of stretching exercises to reverse the direction of the deformity (ie, rotating the infant's chin and tilting the head toward the opposite shoulder). These exercises should be performed several times throughout the day and usually result in correction of the deformity over a 6- to 12-month period of time. Strategic positioning of the child in the crib and other surfaces such as a changing table can encourage them to overcome their restricted motion to look at people and objects. For instance, if the chin points to the right shoulder, the infant should be positioned so he or she has to look to the left. Prone positioning ("tummy time") should also be encouraged to allow active stretching of the SCM. If appropriate physical therapy is begun early, surgical treatment for congenital muscular torticollis is rarely needed, and excellent outcomes including restoration of mobility and resolution of head tilt and craniofacial asymmetry are usually achieved. Operative intervention for refractory cases entails releasing or lengthening 1 or both ends of the SCM muscle. It is rarely indicated in the first few years of life.

## KLIPPEL-FEIL SYNDROME

*Klippel-Feil syndrome* is a spectrum of abnormalities resulting from congenital fusion of the cervical vertebrae secondary to failed segmentation. It is important to recognize Klippel-Feil syndrome because neck

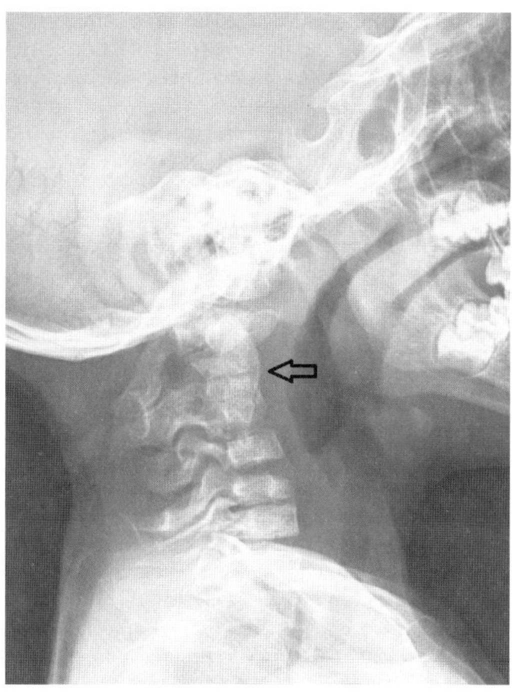

FIGURE 213-2 Lateral radiograph of a patient demonstrating congenital fusion of the cervical spine (Klippel-Feil syndrome).

mobility is limited and may predispose the child to a cervical spine injury with a traumatic event from participation in collision sports.

The classic triad of a short, webbed neck, low posterior hairline, and limited mobility of the cervical spine is seen in 40% to 50% of patients. A neurologic examination to assess for upper motor neuron signs should be performed. Variable degrees of restricted motion are observed because both a mild single-level fusion and an almost complete fusion of the cervical spine meet diagnostic criteria. Klippel-Feil syndrome can be associated with an elevated scapula (Sprengel deformity) in approximately 30% of patients, and congenital scoliosis may be present in as many as 60% of patients. Additional evaluation should include an echocardiogram to screen for cardiac abnormalities (primarily ventricular septal defect), audiologic evaluation for possible hearing impairment, magnetic resonance imaging (MRI) for neural axis abnormalities (eg, Chiari malformations or tethered cord), and a screening renal ultrasound to look for urologic anomalies.

Radiographs demonstrate fusion of single or multiple levels of the cervical spine (Fig. 213-2). There may be numerous blocks of fused vertebrae separated by open motion segments. Flexion and extension lateral radiographs are used to assess for possible instability. Fusions involving the upper cervical spine are sometimes better appreciated on a lateral radiograph of the skull rather than one of the cervical spine. The remainder of the spine should be inspected for possible deformity. Further investigation with MRI is necessary for patients who demonstrate neurologic abnormalities.

Patients with Klippel-Feil syndrome and their families require education about refraining from contact sports, which may lead to cervical spine injuries. Surgical intervention may be necessary when neurologic deficits are present or with progression of the deformity or instability.

## SCOLIOSIS

### INTRODUCTION

*Scoliosis* is a lateral curvature of the spine with rotational deformity. Scoliosis is a descriptor of any abnormal curvature of the spine and not a diagnosis. Small curves measuring less than 10° by the Cobb method are common and should be classified as spinal asymmetry and not as scoliosis. They do not require any further imaging or orthopedic follow-up.

Scoliosis has numerous etiologies. The most common etiology is idiopathic, accounting for approximately 85% of cases. Neuromuscular scoliosis is seen in children with conditions such as cerebral palsy, myelomeningocele, dystrophinopathies, and spinal cord injury in childhood. Congenital malformations of the vertebrae (failures of formation and/or segmentation) can result in scoliosis from asymmetric growth of the spine. Other conditions associated with scoliosis include neurofibromatosis and connective tissue disorders such as Marfan syndrome and osteogenesis imperfecta. The following sections will provide a brief overview of the common types of scoliosis.

## IDIOPATHIC SCOLIOSIS

*Idiopathic scoliosis* is the most common diagnosis in pediatric patients and represents more than 80% of cases. Epidemiologic studies estimate that scoliosis may affect as many as 2% to 3% of children; however, only a small fraction of them (approximately 10%) will require treatment. Idiopathic scoliosis can be subdivided by age at presentation into infantile (0–3 years), juvenile (4–9 years), and adolescent (≥ 10 years). Some authors classify infantile and juvenile idiopathic scoliosis to be "early onset" and adolescent idiopathic scoliosis as "late onset." Adolescent idiopathic scoliosis (AIS) is by far the most common type of scoliosis. Females are more frequently affected and have a substantially higher risk of curve progression. There is a genetic component to AIS, but the exact inheritance pattern has not yet been determined. There is no definitive study to confirm the diagnosis of AIS, so it is a diagnosis of exclusion.

The deformity may be first noticed by family members, by school nurses performing screening, during sports physicals, or by a primary care practitioner on a routine visit. School screening is variably performed and may have a high false-positive rate.

The assessment of a child with scoliosis has 3 purposes: first, to determine the type of scoliosis; second, to assess for problems the child may have from the scoliosis; and third, to determine the child's degree of skeletal maturity and remaining growth. A thorough history should include age at onset, presence of pain and if present its effect on the child, neurologic or respiratory problems, and assessment of remaining growth. In females, the age at menarche (if started) should be noted. Neurologic symptoms or complaints of severe pain are not typical of AIS and suggest an alternative diagnosis.

Physical examination should include evaluation of the gait as well as strength, sensation, and deep tendon reflexes of the lower extremities. Intrinsic wasting of the hands and an asymmetric abdominal reflex are suggestive of a nonidiopathic etiology. The child's spine should be examined from behind with the back uncovered. Any asymmetry in the level of the shoulders, waist spaces, or skin creases should be noted (Fig. 213-3). The iliac crests can be palpated to screen for a limb-length discrepancy, which can cause a compensatory nonstructural scoliosis. The skin should be inspected for any dimples, hairy patches, or birthmarks such as café-au-lait spots, which can suggest a nonidiopathic cause.

Because scoliosis includes rotation of the spine as well as lateral deviation, affected children will not have a level back. The spine and attached ribs on the convexity of the curve rotate up, whereas those on the concavity of the curve rotate down. In the Adams bending test, the child bends forward to touch his or her toes, and asymmetry at any level of the back should be noted (Fig. 213-4). A level known as a *scoliometer* can be used to quantify the slope, otherwise known as the angle of trunk rotation (ATR). There is a fair correlation between the ATR and the degree of curvature seen on radiographs. An ATR of 7° corresponds roughly with a scoliosis curve measuring approximately 20° Cobb and is commonly regarded as a curve warranting orthopedic referral.

Most children with AIS will have curves with the convexity to the right in the thoracic spine and/or curves with the convexity to the left in the lumbar spine, resulting in elevation of the right ribs and/or left paraspinal muscles. Left thoracic curves with elevation of the left side ribs are uncommon, and many physicians recommend a screening MRI for such patients. In addition, while the child is bending forward, the spine should be inspected from the side to look for reduced or increased thoracic kyphosis. Children with thoracic AIS commonly have decreased thoracic kyphosis. Normal or increased thoracic kyphosis is suggestive of other etiologies and may warrant a screening MRI.

Radiographs should be taken with the child standing upright to load the spine and more accurately depict the degree of deformity. Ideally, the entire spine should be captured on a single image, although not all facilities have the equipment to do so. A posteroanterior (PA) radiograph allows adequate visualization of the spine and reduces the radiation dose to the breast and thyroid tissues. The image should be inspected for bony abnormalities including defects in formation or segmentation. Widening of the pedicles may be a sign of an intraspinal lesion.

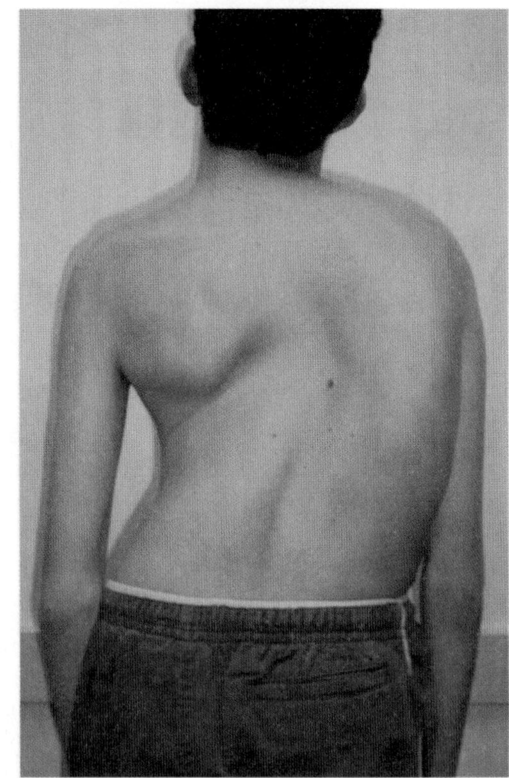

**FIGURE 213-3** Male patient with adolescent idiopathic scoliosis resulting in a trunk shift to the right and waistline asymmetry.

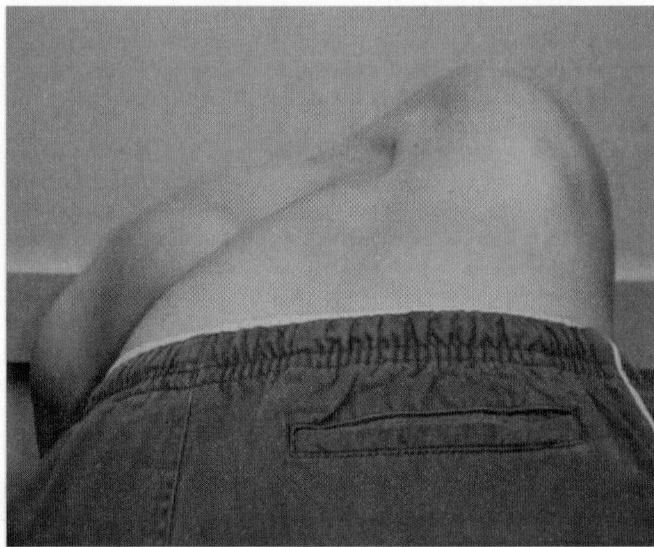

**FIGURE 213-4** The Adams forward bend test is used to visualize the axial plane deformity seen in idiopathic scoliosis.

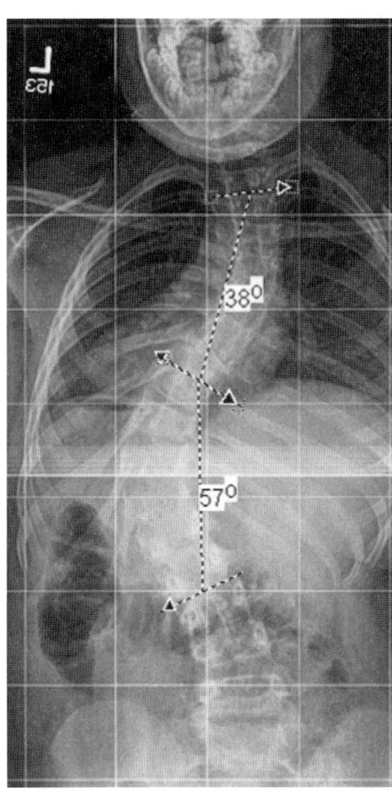


FIGURE 213-5 Posteroanterior radiograph demonstrating measurement of the deformity in a patient with scoliosis using the Cobb method.

The magnitude of the curve usually is determined by the Cobb method. The vertebrae most tilted from horizontal at the top and bottom of each curve are selected. A line is drawn along the upper endplate of the topmost vertebra in the curve. A second line is drawn along the lower endplate of the bottommost vertebra in the curve. The angle between these 2 lines determines the degree of curvature for a scoliosis (Fig. 213-5). For practical reasons, perpendiculars drawn to each of these lines may also be used to determine the Cobb angle. Most digital imaging systems have software to calculate the Cobb angle once the endplates are selected. On the lateral radiograph, the degree of thoracic kyphosis and lumbar lordosis can be measured in a similar manner. The lateral radiograph should also be inspected for structural problems at the lumbosacral junction such as spondylolysis or spondylolisthesis.

Advanced imaging studies such as computed tomography (CT) or MRI are usually not necessary in the initial evaluation of a child with scoliosis. CT may be used to determine the bony anatomy in difficult cases but carries the risk of substantial radiation exposure. An absolute indication for MRI is the patient with scoliosis who presents with an abnormality on neurologic examination. Children with early-onset (infantile or juvenile) idiopathic scoliosis are more likely to have abnormalities in the central nervous system such as syringomyelia, Arnold-Chiari malformation, or tethered spinal cord. A screening MRI of the spine is similarly recommended. Other relative indications for MRI include rapid progression, severe back pain, and "atypical" curves, although none of them is well defined in the literature.

Few children with AIS present with a curve so large that surgery is immediately recommended. The risk of curve progression is related to the size of the curve at presentation and the amount of remaining growth. The larger the curve and the younger the child, the greater is the risk of progression. As menarche occurs after peak height velocity, the risk of progression for a postmenarchal patient is much lower than for one with the same size curve who has not yet started her menstrual cycles.

Radiographic determinants of remaining growth include bone age of the hands and the Risser sign. The Risser sign grades the ossification of the iliac apophysis on a scale of 0 to 5, with 0 being no ossification and 5 being complete ossification. Risser grades 1 through 4 represent 25%, 50%, 75%, and 100% ossification, respectively. The triradiate cartilage of the acetabulum closes prior to any ossification of the iliac crest. Children with open triradiate cartilages on presentation have extremely high risks for progression.

The primary care objective for a child with AIS is to prevent progression. There are 3 management options for AIS: observation, orthosis (bracing), or operation. Initial management should include a thorough evaluation, as outlined earlier, to rule out other types of scoliosis. Children are observed at 6-month intervals with examination of the spine and neurologic system. At follow-up visits for AIS, only PA radiographs are routinely required; repeated lateral radiographs are not necessary in most cases. No restrictions on activity, including contact sports and backpack wearing, are needed. Children with scoliosis should be observed until skeletal maturity as determined radiographically (Risser grade 5 or appropriate bone age for sex) and clinically (2 years after menarche for girls and daily shaving for boys) is achieved.

Curves under 25° Cobb can be observed with no active intervention needed. Evidence supporting the efficacy of exercise, physical therapy, or chiropractic manipulation in preventing curve progression is very limited.

Bracing is a consideration for children with substantial growth remaining (Risser grade 2 or less) with curves between 25° and 45° Cobb. Bracing is designed to prevent progression and not to correct the curve. The family needs to understand that a successful outcome of bracing is prevention of curve progression, not necessarily correction. The brace needs to be worn at least 13 hours a day, and there appears to be a dose-response relationship with greater daily brace wear time further reducing the risk of progression.

A recent large, multicenter, randomized prospective study demonstrated that use of a thoraco-lumbar-sacral orthosis (TLSO) can reduce the risk of curve progression in AIS. In this study, 25% of the children who were compliant with bracing (13+ hours per day) still progressed to the point that surgery was recommended. Children with similar curves who did not wear a brace or were noncompliant progressed to the point that surgery was recommended 60% of the time. These results suggest that for some children the extent of progression is independent of brace usage. Unfortunately, at present, there is no way to identify these patients in advance.

Children undergoing brace treatment can remove the brace for physical education and athletic activities, including contact sports. They should be observed with serial in-brace PA radiographs every 6 months until maturity. Continued progression of the curve in the brace warrants careful questioning and inspection to ensure compliance and proper fit.

Skeletally mature patients with a curve less than 40° are unlikely to progress and do not require regular follow-up. Conversely, patients with a larger curve at maturity should be evaluated on an individual basis to weigh the benefits of surgery and risk for progression in adulthood. Curves greater than 50° Cobb are considered to be at high risk for continued progression after skeletal maturity, and surgery should be discussed with the family. Curves greater than 80° Cobb may impair pulmonary function. The goal of operative management of scoliosis is to prevent further curve progression while safely correcting, at least partially, the spinal deformity.

Surgical correction of scoliosis consists of an instrumented spinal fusion, which results in a permanent loss of motion of the affected segment (Fig. 213-6). Preoperative bending radiographs assist the surgeon in planning the extent of the fusion. The decreased spinal motion is generally well accommodated; however, the long-term health of the spine may be somewhat compromised because the remaining motion segments, particularly those below the fusion, bear increased load. In general, surgery for AIS results in a 50% to 70% curve correction.

The risks of surgery include infection and the possible need for blood transfusions. Although very rare, the most feared complication is spinal cord injury, which could result in paraplegia. Later problems such as pseudarthrosis (failure of the bone to fuse) with implant breakage or loosening have been reported. Overall, surgical treatment

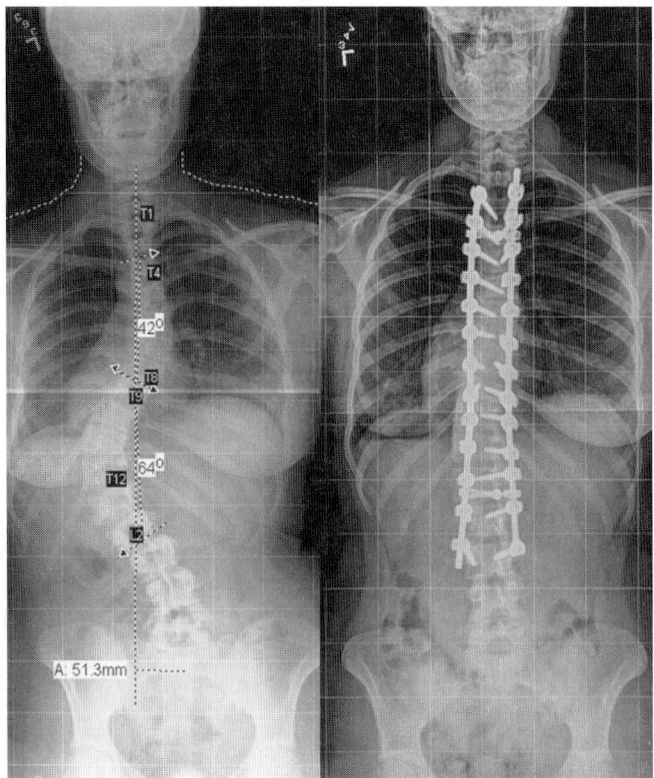


FIGURE 213-6 Posterior spinal fusion in a patient with adolescent idiopathic scoliosis. The preoperative (*left*) and the postoperative (*right*) radiographs.

for idiopathic scoliosis has a high success rate, with cosmesis being one of the most consistently reported positive outcomes in patient surveys. The overall complication rate for spine surgery in a patient with AIS is not insignificant (between 4% and 5%), although the incidence of neurologic deficit is less than 1%. Following surgical correction and a recovery period of 4 to 12 months, patients may return to their usual activities, including athletic competition, with caution regarding high-impact or collision sports.

## EARLY-ONSET SCOLIOSIS

The goal of management is to prevent progression while allowing as much growth of the spine as possible. In children younger than 5 years of age, serial casting (Mehta technique) can buy time and even completely correct the scoliosis in some cases. Older children may benefit from bracing. New techniques and implants allow surgery to control the deformity while allowing for growth but have high morbidity.

## CONGENITAL SCOLIOSIS

*Congenital scoliosis* is caused by abnormal development of the vertebrae. Spinal development occurs between the fourth and eighth week of gestation. At this same time, the renal and cardiac systems also form, and concurrent anomalies of these systems are often seen in children with congenital scoliosis. Congenital scoliosis may result from complete or partial failure of vertebral formation, a failure of vertebral segmentation, or some combination of both (Fig. 213-7). For example, a hemivertebra (Fig. 213-8) is a failure of formation, whereas a congenital bar or fusion is a failure of segmentation. Abnormalities in the thoracic spine may also result in rib and chest wall abnormalities. Management ranges from observation to aggressive and early operation, depending on the curve configuration and progression. In contrast to idiopathic scoliosis, bracing has a limited role in management. Documented progression with substantial growth remaining usually requires operative intervention, regardless of age. Preoperative evaluation of the spinal cord with MRI is necessary because of a high likelihood of neural axis abnormalities.

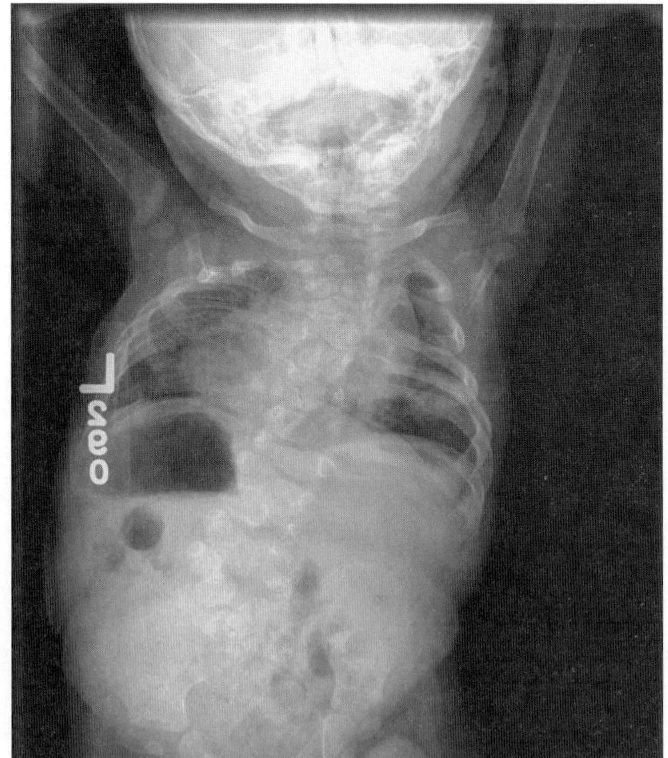

FIGURE 213-7 A radiograph of an infant with severe congenital scoliosis with multiple vertebral body anomalies present.

Some patterns of congenital scoliosis are known to have a high risk of progression, such as a hemivertebra with a contralateral unsegmented bar.

## NEUROMUSCULAR SCOLIOSIS

Children with a variety of neuromuscular disorders, such as cerebral palsy, myelomeningocele, or Duchenne muscular dystrophy, are more likely to develop scoliosis secondary to muscle imbalance or weakness, particularly those who are wheelchair ambulators. Neuromuscular scoliosis can develop at any age and may progress rapidly during the adolescent growth spurt. In contrast to idiopathic scoliosis, curves seen in neuromuscular scoliosis are usually long, sweeping, and C-shaped, often spanning almost the entire thoracolumbar spine

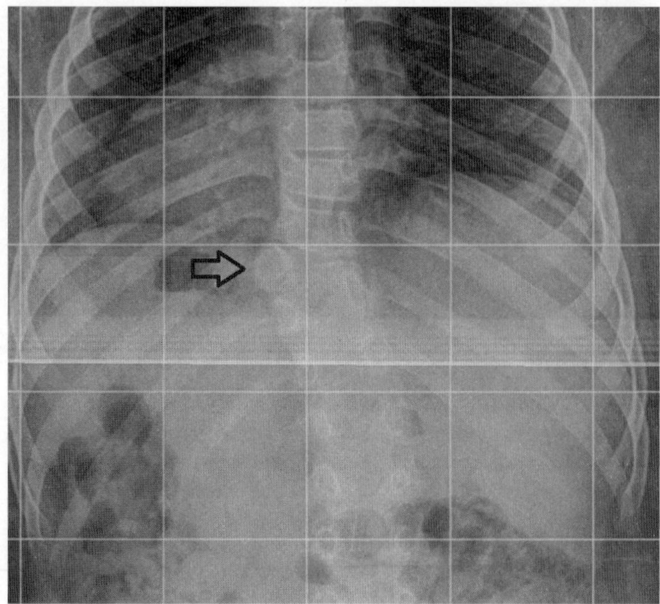

FIGURE 213-8 A radiograph demonstrating a left T10 hemivertebra that has resulted in scoliosis.

and pelvis. This pelvic obliquity may present challenges with sitting comfortably. Wheelchair modifications can improve sitting balance and posture but are rarely effective in preventing progression. Bracing usually is ineffective and difficult, as many of these children will not tolerate use due to restrictions in pulmonary function from the brace. Surgery for neuromuscular scoliosis has a much higher complication rate, and a thorough preoperative assessment of nutrition, pulmonary function, and other medical issues is warranted.

### SYNDROMIC SCOLIOSIS

Scoliosis may also be a feature of a variety of syndromes. Connective tissue disorders associated with spinal deformity include Ehlers-Danlos syndrome, Marfan syndrome, and osteogenesis imperfecta. Scoliosis has also been linked to metabolic deficits such as homocystinuria and the cohort of mucopolysaccharidoses. Neurofibromatosis (von Recklinghausen disease) has been recognized as an important syndromic cause of scoliosis. In addition to the classic clinical manifestations of café-au-lait spots, Lisch nodules, and neurofibromas, spinal deformities may be present in up to 50% of patients. It is not unheard of for a child with Marfan syndrome or neurofibromatosis to first present with scoliosis. Management of syndromic scoliosis is similar to AIS, although the success rate of bracing has not been well documented and the surgery can be more challenging due to increased complexity of the child's spinal anatomy.

## KYPHOSIS

Although the spine in the coronal plane is normally straight, the spine in the sagittal plane is normally curved. The cervical and lumbar spines are in lordosis, with the convexity pointing forward, and the thoracic spine is in kyphosis, with the convexity pointing backward. Alterations in these normal curves can be problematic.

Cervical kyphosis can result from congenital abnormalities such as Klippel-Feil syndrome as well as conditions such as Larsen syndrome, diastrophic dysplasia, camptomelic dysplasia, and neurofibromatosis. The assistance of an experienced radiologist and geneticist can be invaluable in determining the exact diagnosis and prognosis. Iatrogenic kyphosis can result from previous removal of the posterior vertebral elements to gain access to the neural structures for treatment of tumors, infection, or syringomyelia. Cervical kyphosis may cause pressure on the spinal cord and subsequent neurologic deficits. Operative intervention is indicated for progressive deformity or when neurologic deficits occur.

Normal thoracic kyphosis measures between 20° and 45° Cobb from T5 to T12. Increased thoracic kyphosis can present as a roundback deformity. This deformity may be either postural, in which the spine is flexible, or more rigid, a condition known as *Scheuermann kyphosis*. Distinction between the 2 is based on both clinical and radiographic examinations. A patient with roundback that self-corrects on hyperextension while standing or lying is considered to have postural hyperkyphosis and usually does not need treatment, although hyperextension exercises may be recommended in some cases. A child with marked stiffness in the spine and a rigid kyphosis requires further evaluation. In Scheuermann kyphosis, a lateral radiograph will demonstrate at least 3 consecutive vertebrae with ≥ 5° of anterior wedging. This finding is associated with decreased disk spaces, irregular endplates, and Schmorl nodes (slight disruptions or cavitations in the endplates of the vertebrae). Scheuermann kyphosis has an estimated prevalence of 2% to 3%.

Patients with Scheuermann kyphosis often complain of pain over the apex of the curve or pain in the lumbar spine secondary to the compensatory lumbar hyperlordosis. Like idiopathic scoliosis, curve exacerbation is seen in periods of rapid spinal growth. Neurologic deficits from Scheuermann kyphosis are rare. Nonoperative treatment of Scheuermann kyphosis includes physical therapy, core strengthening, and bracing. Surgical treatment for Scheuermann kyphosis usually is reserved for patients who have demonstrated continued progression of the kyphosis despite skeletal maturity or prolonged pain refractory to conservative treatment. Typically, symptoms do not begin until curves are greater than 70°. Surgical intervention resembles treatment for scoliosis in that implants are used to correct the kyphosis while fusion occurs. Surgical complications are similar to those in scoliosis operations; however, a slightly greater neurologic risk is seen.

## BACK PAIN

### INTRODUCTION

Whereas at one time back pain was considered an infrequent occurrence in children and adolescents, later studies have found it to be almost as common as in adults and equally as challenging to assess and manage. The musculoskeletal differential for pediatric back pain is broad, and a definitive cause often is difficult to determine. When a specific etiology is not identified, the back pain can be termed *mechanical low back pain* and possibly results from spasms as the paraspinal muscles fatigue during or following activities. It usually occurs at the end of a very active day. Pain is localized to the low back without radiation into the lower extremities, improves with rest, and is not associated with bowel or bladder symptoms.

Mechanical low back pain is the most common etiology of back pain in children and adolescents. Additional differential considerations include trauma and vertebral body injury, spinal deformity such as scoliosis or kyphosis, intervertebral disk disease, infectious processes such as osteomyelitis, inflammatory or rheumatologic conditions, and primary or metastatic neoplasms. Several of the more common specific causes of pediatric back pain will be discussed in further detail below.

Initial evaluation of back pain should include a thorough history and physical examination. Attempts to characterize any localizing or radiating pain symptoms are useful. The exam should include inspection, palpation, range-of-motion testing, a general examination of the pelvis, abdomen, and extremities, and a thorough neurologic assessment. Concerning "red flags" include night pain (pain that awakens the child from sleep), neurologic symptoms, or constitutional symptoms including fevers, night sweats, or loss of weight, and age younger than 4 years old.

The need for further workup with laboratory or radiologic evaluation should be based on the presence or absence of "red flag" findings. If there is no suspicion of concerning pathology, conservative management is warranted. Plain radiographs (anteroposterior and lateral) are the only indicated imaging. Of note is that many children and adolescents will have normal imaging studies, and the presence of an abnormal radiographic finding must be correlated with findings from the history and physical examination. MRI scan is indicated for an abnormal neurologic exam or concern for malignancy and should not be ordered for nonspecific back pain. In the past, a radionuclide bone scan was often recommended to assess children with back pain; however, its use has largely been supplanted by MRI. Helpful lab studies include a complete blood count (CBC) and inflammatory markers including the erythrocyte sedimentation rate (ESR) and C-reactive protein (CRP).

### SPONDYLOLYSIS AND SPONDYLOLISTHESIS

*Spondylolysis* is a stress fracture of the pars interarticularis. It usually occurs in the lower lumbar spine (L5 is most common level, followed by L4). Spondylolysis may be asymptomatic initially, and it is often impossible to determine when the fracture occurred. It can present as an incidental finding on radiographs, for example, during evaluation for scoliosis. Whereas at one time oblique radiographs of the lumbar spine were recommended to assess for spondylolysis, more recent studies have shown that the defect can be identified on routine PA and lateral radiographs (Fig. 213-9). Children typically describe an insidious onset of pain that is sometimes exacerbated by extension of the spine. Buttock and thigh pain are common complaints, although true radicular pain radiating below the knee is not. Spondylolysis is seen more frequently in athletes who perform activities resulting in repeated hyperextension of the lumbar spine such as gymnasts and football linemen, although it can also be seen in sedentary

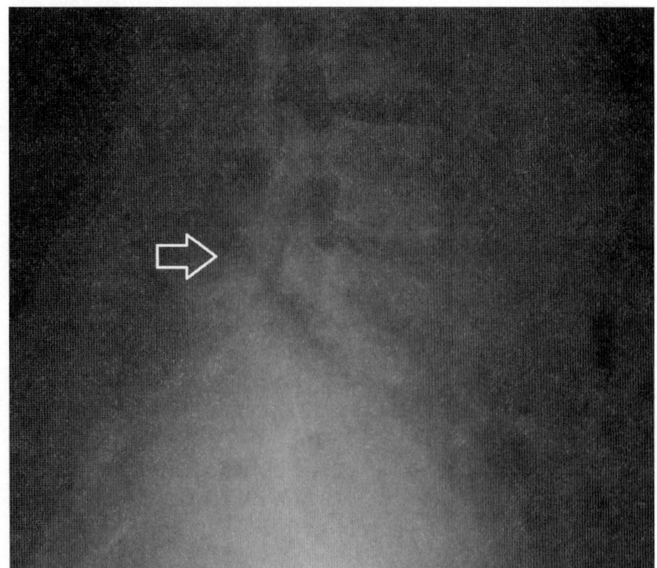

**FIGURE 213-9** A lateral radiograph demonstrating spondylolysis at the L5 level, resulting in a low-grade spondylolisthesis at L5-S1.

children, occurring in as many as 5% of the general population. Most patients with spondylolysis respond to conservative management with physical therapy and activity restrictions. The goal of treatment is to reduce pain and allow a return to regular activities, including athletics. Attempts to repair the defect are not necessary as there is poor correlation between the appearance of the defect (healed or not) and the presence or absence of pain. Surgical treatment is rarely indicated and reserved for prolonged failure to respond to nonoperative interventions.

*Spondylolisthesis* is a forward slippage of a vertebra on the one below. The most common level is L5 on S1. Spondylolisthesis may be classified based on etiology (dysplastic, elongation of the pars, lytic, or microfracture of the posterior elements) and degree of slippage (percentage of anterior translation). High degrees of slippage (> 50%) may be associated with severe hamstring tightness and neurologic deficits (Fig. 213-10). The hamstring tightness can result in an unusual gait with marked alternating lateral rotation of the pelvis. Lower-grade slips can be observed or managed with physical therapy. High-grade slips may benefit from surgical stabilization. Complete reduction is not necessary and may increase the risk of L5 nerve root injury.

## DISK HERNIATION

Herniated disks, or a *herniated nucleus pulposus* (HNP), are extremely uncommon in children and adolescents. Risk factors include obesity, trauma, family history, or participation in certain athletic activities (eg, collision sports, weight lifting, and gymnastics). The HNP may impinge on a nerve root and cause pain that radiates down the leg below the knee. The disks between the L4-L5 and L5-S1 levels are most commonly involved (Fig. 213-11).

In a child with an HNP, the leg pain often is more severe than is the back pain. True radicular pain radiates below the knee, and the nerve compression by the disk can result in diminished sensation and weakness in the distribution of the affected nerve roots. The child may complain of increased pain with coughing, sneezing, or straining to defecate, as these actions all increase intra-abdominal pressure, placing more pressure on the disk.

Physical examination may demonstrate pain with passive straight leg raising in the supine position ("the straight leg raise test") and other nerve-root tension signs. MRI confirms an HNP, but mild bulging of disks is a common finding of asymptomatic individuals who have had MRIs for other reasons. Generally, conservative management, including over-the-counter pain medication and core-strengthening exercises, is helpful. Surgical excision can be considered with failure of conservative treatment or unremitting pain.

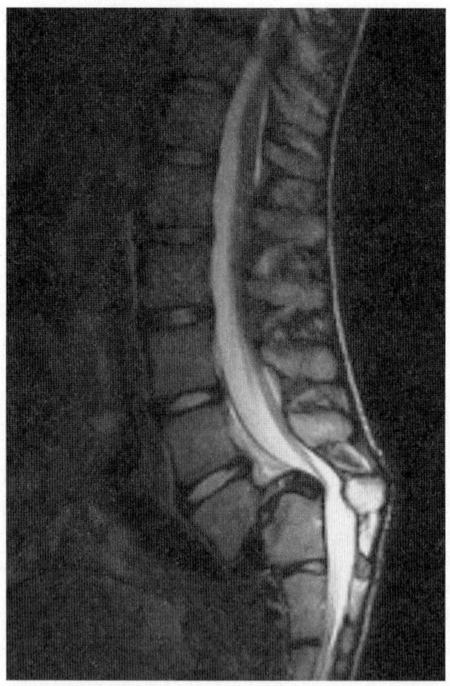

**FIGURE 213-10** A high-grade spondylolisthesis seen on magnetic resonance imaging at the L5-S1 level resulting in compression of the thecal sac and narrowing of the spinal canal at S1. There is marked sclerosis and deformity of the posterior inferior endplate of L5 and the anterior superior endplate of S1.

## TUMORS OF THE SPINAL COLUMN

Central nervous system (CNS) tumors are the second most frequent type of neoplasm in children. Lesions affecting the spinal column are relatively rare, accounting for fewer than 10% of CNS tumors.

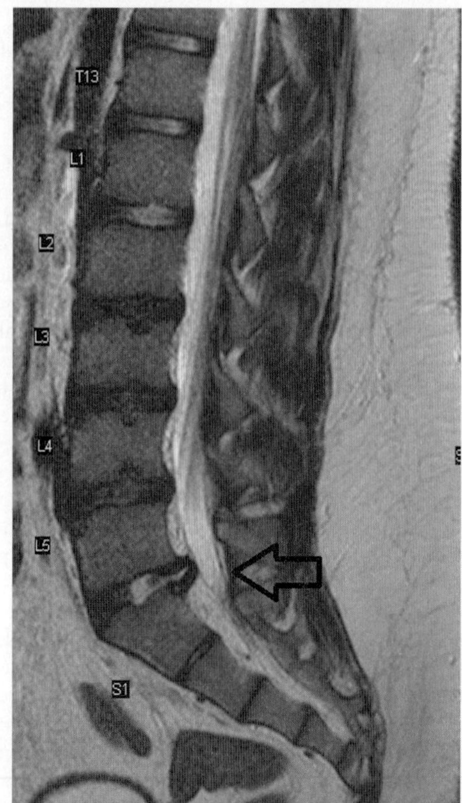


**FIGURE 213-11** A centrally herniated L5-S1 disk, as seen on magnetic resonance imaging, that comes into contact with the S1 nerve root.

Patients will typically note persistent pain, neurologic symptoms, or progressive gait abnormalities. The most common tumors of the spinal cord are neurodevelopmental, namely dermoid and epidermoid growths and teratomas, all of which are generally benign. Astrocytomas and neuroblastomas are also prevalent in the spine. Developmental tumors occur most often in the lumbosacral region, whereas neuroblastomas occur predominantly in the thoracic region.

The bones of the spinal column develop different neoplasms. Eosinophilic granulomas, giant cell tumors, and osteosarcomas have a predilection for the anterior vertebral body, whereas osteoid osteoma, osteoblastomas, and Ewing sarcoma tend to occur more frequently in the posterior elements. An observable spinal deformity such as scoliosis, kyphosis, or lordosis is noted in as many as 25% of patients and results from osseous invasion and destruction. Constitutional symptoms such as fever, night sweats, and weight loss may be indications of hematologic neoplasms involving the spine. Physical examination may demonstrate tenderness to palpation of the spine, both upper and lower motor neuron signs, bowel or bladder dysfunction, and inability to bear weight without pain.

Osteochondromas are the most common bone tumors seen in children and adolescents. The lesion may be solitary or occur as a result of multiple hereditary exostoses (MHE). Osteochondromas occur primarily in the cervical spine. Due to the cartilaginous nature of the tumor, advanced imaging with CT or MRI is useful in diagnosis and often will demonstrate a characteristic pedunculated or sessile mass with a cartilaginous cap. Surgical excision for relief of symptoms usually is curative, and although the risk of recurrence is low, there are previously described cases of malignant transformation to osteosarcoma.

The most common anterior vertebral neoplasm is eosinophilic granuloma, which is a benign but destructive osteolytic lesion. It can result in vertebra plana, a deformity in which the vertebral body (normally rectangular) becomes flattened. This tumor usually occurs in the cervical and thoracic spine. It usually is a self-resolving condition, but other lesions should be searched for as this may obviate the need for vertebral biopsy or at least allow biopsy of a more accessible lesion.

Osteoid osteomas are benign bone tumors associated with pain that typically occurs at night and is relieved with nonsteroidal anti-inflammatory medications. A CT scan demonstrates the characteristic nidus (a central bony spicule) surrounded by reactive bone that usually is less than 2 cm in size. Osteoid osteomas do tend to resolve over time; however, symptoms can persist for many years, causing enough discomfort for patients that surgical excision should be explored. Osteoblastomas are also generally benign but are more locally aggressive and tend to be larger (> 2 cm) and more vascular than are osteoid osteomas. Instances of malignant transformation of osteoblastoma to osteosarcoma have been reported. Due to increased size and disruption of the local environment, patients with osteoblastomas are more likely to have neurologic symptoms or pain refractive to nonsteroidal anti-inflammatory drugs. Both osteoid osteoma and osteoblastoma tend to affect the lumbosacral spine. Surgical excision is warranted after failed conservative management; however, both osteoid osteoma and osteoblastoma have a risk of recurrence of approximately 10%, related at least in part to inadequate initial resection.

Aneurysmal bone cysts occur in the posterior elements, usually in the lumbar spine, which may cause neurologic problems or pathologic fractures. Although generally benign, aneurysmal bone cysts are locally aggressive and can be very challenging to treat. Plain radiographs demonstrate a significant radiolucent lesion whereas advanced imaging will show fluid levels within cortical bone. The blood supply to these lesions is robust and can result in significant bleeding at the time of surgery. An angiogram often is performed prior to surgery in order to identify the blood supply, and a preoperative embolization to limit blood loss during surgery may also be considered.

Ewing sarcoma is the most common primary malignant pediatric spine tumor. It usually occurs in children between the age of 5 and 15 years. The classic imaging findings of a "moth-eaten" lesion with periosteal "onion-skin" reaction seen in Ewing sarcoma of the extremities are not as readily observed in spinal locations. MRI will usually show a soft tissue mass. As many as 25% of patients may present with evidence of metastatic disease (most commonly involving the lungs). Depending on the nature of the disease at diagnosis, management options include surgical resection and both radiotherapy and chemotherapy.

Osteosarcoma is the most common primary malignant bone tumor and occasionally occurs in the lumbar and thoracic regions. Advanced imaging may reveal a destructive lesion or soft tissue mass with invasion into the neural elements. Unfortunately, even after adequate surgical resection and chemotherapy, the median overall survival of patients with osteosarcoma of the spine remains less than 3 years.

## DISK INFECTION

*Diskitis* is a rare inflammatory condition of the intervertebral disk or vertebral endplate (spondylodiskitis) and should be considered in patients who present with back pain and refusal to bear weight. Patients are usually younger than 10 years of age and demonstrate restricted range of motion, abnormal gait, and possibly referred pain to the abdomen, hip, or knee; systemic symptoms are less common. Diskitis predominately affects the lumbar region of the spine, although cases of cervical and thoracic diskitis have been described (Fig. 213-12).

The examination is nonspecific. Affected children will walk gingerly to minimize jarring of the spine, and younger children may refuse to walk or even sit up due to pain. Blood cultures and white blood cell count are typically normal; however, inflammatory indices including ESR and CRP will usually be elevated. Radiographs often are unremarkable initially but eventually demonstrate a narrow or irregular disk space within a few weeks. MRI can be used to confirm the diagnosis and differentiate from vertebral osteomyelitis or oncologic lesions.

Routine biopsy of the affected disk is not needed if the findings are classic. *Staphylococcus aureus* is the most commonly identified bacteria implicated in diskitis, and empiric antibiotic treatment should target both *S aureus* and *Kingella kingae*. Because the disk space is still highly vascular in younger children, the infection may improve with only rest and supportive care. This condition usually resolves and does not require surgical treatment.

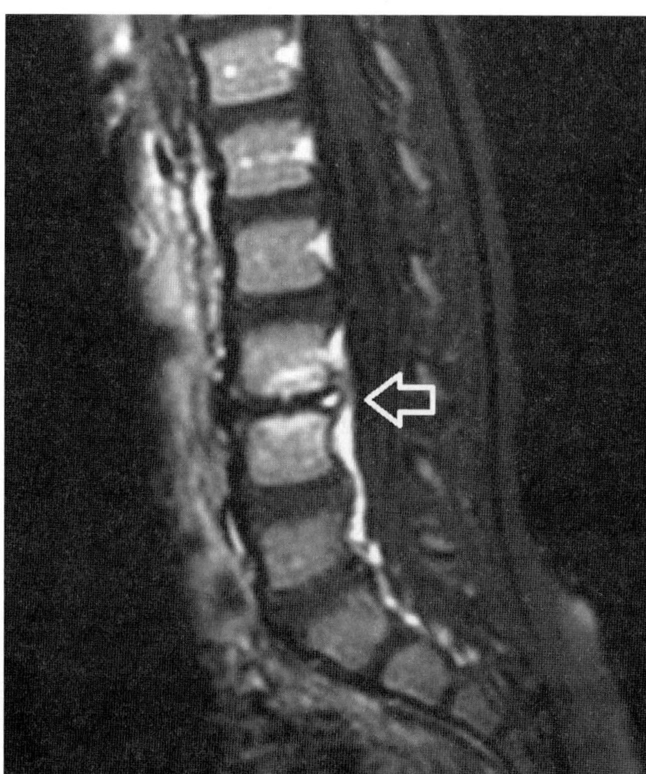

**FIGURE 213-12** L3-L4 diskitis and vertebral body osteomyelitis as seen on magnetic resonance imaging.

Garg S, Dormans JP. Tumors and tumor-like conditions of the spine in children. *J Am Acad Orthop Surg*. 2005;13:372-381.

Hresko MT. Idiopathic scoliosis in adolescents. *N Engl J Med*. 2013; 368:834-841.

Hresko MT, Talwalkar V, Schwend R. Early detection of idiopathic scoliosis in adolescents. *J Bone Joint Surg Am*. 2016;98:e67(1-4).

Kuo AA, Tritasavit S, Graham JM. Congenital muscular torticollis and positional plagiocephaly. *Pediatr Rev*. 2014;35:79-87.

Mo F, Cunningham ME. Pediatric scoliosis. *Curr Rev Musculoskelet Med*. 2011;4:175-182.

Ravindra VM, Eli IM, Schmidt MH, Brockmeyer DL. Primary osseous tumors of the pediatric spinal column: review of pathology and surgical decision making. *Neurosurg Focus*. 2016;41(2):E3.

Shah SA, Saller J. Evaluation and diagnosis of back pain in children and adolescents. *J Am Acad Orthop Surg*. 2016;24:37-45.

Spencer SJ, Wilson NI. Childhood discitis in a regional children's hospital. *J Pediatr Orthop B*. 2012;21:264-268.

Weinstein SL, Dolan LA, Wright JG, Dobbs MB. Effects of bracing in adolescents with idiopathic scoliosis. *N Engl J Med*. 2013;369: 1512-1521.

# 214 Disorders of the Upper Extremity

Bryce Bell, Scott Oishi, and Marybeth Ezaki



## INTRODUCTION

Certain upper extremity conditions are commonly seen or are important for timely diagnoses and treatment or referral. This section is not meant to be comprehensive or inclusive of all upper extremity conditions that may be seen, but rather is a brief overview of those that every pediatric resident and practicing pediatrician should know about. A "triage" list is provided at the end.

## EMERGENCY CONDITIONS

### TRAUMA

Physical examination of the hand injured by trauma is critical to determine if tendons or nerves have been damage. The active range of motion of the fingers distal to the injury should be assessed, and the depths of the wound should be inspected directly for partial or complete injuries to tendons. Sensation in all fingers and function of the intrinsic muscles in the hand should be assessed while inspecting the wound fro evidence of nerve injury. The presence of arterial injury renders the possibility of nerve injury much higher. If an injury is confirmed or suspected, refer the patient to a hand surgeon.

All open wounds should be gently cleansed and assessed for nerve, vessel, and tendon injury. If bleeding cannot be adequately controlled by direct pressure or if the distal circulation has been compromised, the patient should be referred to an emergency department for further evaluation. Open wounds should never be clamped to control bleeding. If sensation is normal in all fingers, and tendon function is intact, the wound can be closed and the entire forearm and hand splinted to allow the wound to heal. If there are deficits in tendon or nerve function, follow-up evaluation and definitive treatment by a hand surgeon should be arranged within the next 5 to 7 days.

An important note is that some fingertip amputations do not have to go to the emergency department when they occur. If no bone is exposed, the finger wound can be gently cleansed and then covered with a nonadherent dressing (Telfa, Adaptic, Xeroform gauze, petrolatum gauze, etc). Fluffed gauze can then be put between all the fingers and then over the injured finger, which can then be wrapped with cast padding, followed by a short or long arm cast, and examined subsequently by a hand surgeon for further care. If a child is younger than 5 years, a long arm cast with the elbow bent to 90° is preferred. For a child older than age 5 years, a short arm cast is appropriate. The wound will heal by secondary intention, and after approximately 3 weeks in a cast, most of these minor injuries will be healed and pain free. If bone is exposed or if the nail plate has been pulled out of the eponychial fold (otherwise known as an open Seymour physeal fracture), the patient should be referred to an emergency department for urgent care.

### BITE WOUNDS

Superficial dog and cat bites from domestic animals should be cleansed and dressed and appropriate antibiotics administered. The most common organisms that can cause an infection from a bite are staphylococcal and streptococcal species, but for cat bites, coverage for *Eikenella corrodens* should be added. Snake bites with envenomation require emergency evaluation in the emergency department and may require antivenom or surgical debridement. Spider bites rarely are life-threatening, but local reaction may require individualized treatment. Human bites that penetrate fascial and synovial spaces in the hand require surgical debridement and aggressive antibiotic care.

### PAINT GUN AND INJECTION INJURIES

High-pressure injection injuries from paint guns or water pressure nozzles are surgical emergencies. The injected substance travels along tissue planes and, depending on the material injected, can result in chemical necrosis, tissue destruction, and proximal spread of infective material. Compartment syndrome is possible. These types of injuries require emergent surgical evaluation, even if the initial wound is small or appears benign.

### FRACTURES

An acutely displaced fracture is not difficult to diagnose and requires urgent care. The nondisplaced, closed fracture without neurologic or vascular deficit or excessive swelling can be splinted, elevated, and referred in the next 24 to 48 hours to the orthopedist for semi-urgent evaluation and definitive care. Open fractures constitute an emergency and require surgical debridement and definitive fracture care.

A compartment syndrome is a true emergency. Any condition that leads to an increase in the pressure within a fascial compartment that exceeds the tissue perfusion pressure results in ischemia and impending tissue death. Emergent medical care should be arranged. Common causes for compartment syndrome include direct vessel injury, kinking or spasm of a vessel due to fracture, bleeding into the compartment and resultant swelling from blunt or open trauma, bleeding associated with a coagulopathy, and prolonged entrapment of the hand or forearm in a tight space. Clinical findings should be recognized by all physicians and include pain out of proportion to the associated condition, increased pain on stretch of the muscles involved (usually the finger flexors), and fullness or hardness of the muscle compartment. If the compartment syndrome is unrelieved, loss of sensation and paralysis of muscles occur because of nerve ischemia.

A rare but devastating variant of compartment syndrome occurs in the neonate. It develops during the immediate antepartum period, but the exact etiology is unknown. Intrinsic thrombophilic mechanisms as well as extrinsic compression have both been implicated. The neonate presents in the delivery room with a swollen, paralyzed, dysvascular limb. There is typically a sentinel bullous or open lesion on the forearm (Fig. 214-1).

Unrelieved ischemia resulting from compartment syndrome results in muscle necrosis, cellular breakdown, hemoglobinuria, and permanent functional loss of the limb. The only treatment that may salvage some function is emergency surgical fasciotomy. For additional details on injuries and fractures please refer to the other chapters within Section 16.

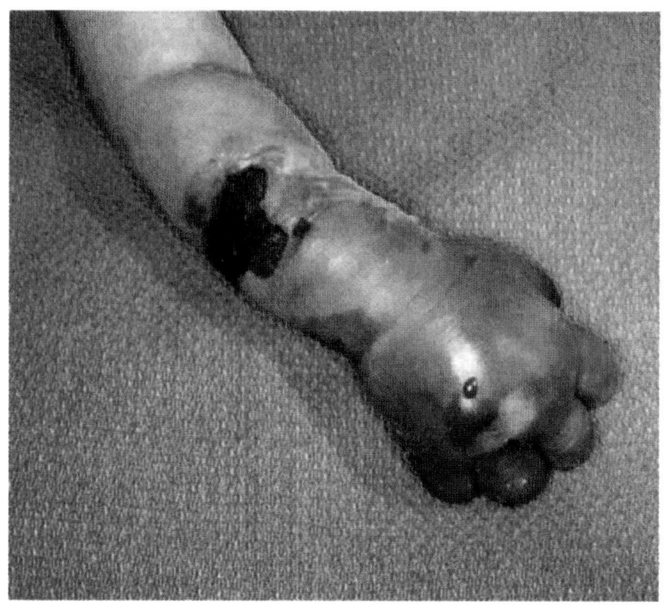

FIGURE 214-1 The appearance of the forearm with a neonatal compartment syndrome. Note the sentinel lesion and the discoloration.

### INFECTION

Early diagnosis and appropriate treatment of children's hand infections should be part of primary care practice. The most common infections are bacterial and result from direct inoculation by a puncture wound or minor trauma. A *paronychia* is an infection of the paronychium, or the cuticle and delicate superficial tissue around the base of the fingernail. Warm soaks, elevation, and gently pushing the cuticle back will often resolve these minor infections. Oral antibiotics may hasten the resolution of a paronychia. A *felon* by contrast is an infection in the closed space of the pulp of the fingertip and usually requires surgical drainage. Deep infections that involve synovial-lined spaces, bones, or joints require emergency surgical care. Any child with a swollen tender hand, fever, and systemic signs of sepsis such as blood pressure instability or a rapid heart or respiratory rate should be referred emergently to a hand surgeon or hospital.

*Herpetic whitlow* is a relatively common infection in children, especially a child who sucks a thumb or finger. This infection is recognized by the absence of swelling but either vesicles or pustules on a red base. Oral lesions are often present. Treatment is symptomatic and time-limited, although a primary infection may benefit from use of acyclovir.

Chronic swelling of joints or tendon sheaths may be indicative of unusual infectious or inflammatory conditions. The differential diagnosis should include atypical mycobacterial infections, juvenile chronic arthritis, and psoriatic arthritis. Obtaining tissue for culture and pathology may be necessary to diagnose or rule out the cause of the chronic condition.

## SUBACUTE OR SEMIURGENT CONDITIONS

### NEONATAL BRACHIAL PLEXUS PALSY

Stretch injury to the brachial plexus in a newborn is a common condition following the birth of a large baby. The diagnostic findings are diminished or asymmetric motion of the involved upper extremity in the neonate. Initial treatment is to protect the limb and support for comfort. Most of these birth palsies will recover spontaneously in the first several weeks. Treatment of these injuries is evolving, and there is not yet consensus as to the optimal timing or nature of treatment. If recovery is not complete by age 2 months, the infant should be referred to a team of specialists who can manage early physical therapy, neurologic evaluation, musculoskeletal care, and decision making regarding appropriateness of direct surgical intervention in the brachial plexus. Decisions about appropriate treatment are made after a period of observation.

### AMNION DISRUPTION SEQUENCE WITH IMPENDING TISSUE LOSS

*Amnion disruption sequence* (amniotic band syndrome, constriction band syndrome) typically presents with fenestrated syndactyly, finger amputations and tissue loss, distal edema, and constriction bands. Rarely, a band may entwine a finger or limb and cause increasing edema and impending tissue loss in the early newborn period. Immediate surgical release of the encircling bands may salvage the endangered part.

## CHRONIC OR ELECTIVE CONDITIONS

### CONGENITAL ANOMALIES

In general, there is rarely an indication for early surgery if congenital anomalies of the upper extremity are noted at birth, even though they can be quite distressing to the parents, who want immediate answers and reassurance about their infant. Most care for congenital conditions is nonoperative, and reconstructive procedures are postponed until anesthetic risk is lessened after approximately 1 year of age. Larger size and maturation of airway and critical organ systems render surgical care more predictable.

Certain conditions necessitate a search for related conditions. They include, in particular, the spectrum of "radial dysplasia." Recognition of a small thumb or other elements of radial dysplasia requires evaluation of the cardiac, spinal, renal, and hematologic systems. The hand anomaly may be the presenting finding in VACTERRL association, Fanconi anemia, thrombocytopenia absent radius (TAR) syndrome, and other conditions (see Chapter 171).

Other congenital conditions such as syndactyly, polydactyly with broad connection to the hand, and major morphologic limb malformation can be referred to a hand surgeon when the child reaches 3 to 6 months of age. The postaxial polydactyly with a small, pedunculated base can be tied off or ligaclipped by the primary pediatrician. If the base is too wide, surgical care is best delayed until the child is 1 year of age.

Trigger thumbs and fingers are mislabeled as truly being congenital because most occur in infancy and early childhood, and some will resolve spontaneously. A trigger thumb appears as a flexed distal joint of the thumb, usually locked in flexion. There is a characteristic nodule at the flexor aspect of the metacarpophalangeal joint. There is no need for radiographs or other imaging with this condition. Treatment is by surgical release if the deformity is bothersome and still present by age 3 years. Trigger fingers are more complicated than are trigger thumbs and require surgical care as well. Corticosteroid injection has no place in the treatment of trigger thumbs or trigger fingers.

Congenital contractures and angled digits should be referred for diagnosis, splinting, and treatment. The hand deformity may be the presenting complaint in a number of conditions, including the myriad forms of arthrogryposis.

Oligodactyly, or too few fingers, and missing parts of fingers are common congenital upper limb malformations. *Few* of these are related to amnion disruption sequence, and this diagnosis should not be given if there is any uncertainty. The most common diagnosis is symbrachydactyly, which has a broad spectrum of presentation and is thought to be related to insufficient mesoderm during early limb formation. Other diagnoses include ulnar dysplasia and clefting syndromes (Fig. 214-2). Referral for diagnosis and treatment can be delayed until after the child reaches 3 to 6 months of age.

Infants with enlarged parts of their hand or arm should be referred early for evaluation and diagnosis. The differential diagnosis includes tumorous conditions, malformations, lymphedema, and hamartomas, as well as the various forms of gigantism and hemihypertrophy. Hemihypertrophy has been reported to be associated with Wilms tumor. Although it is rare, the potential for early diagnosis should initiate ultrasonographic screening of the perinephric area.

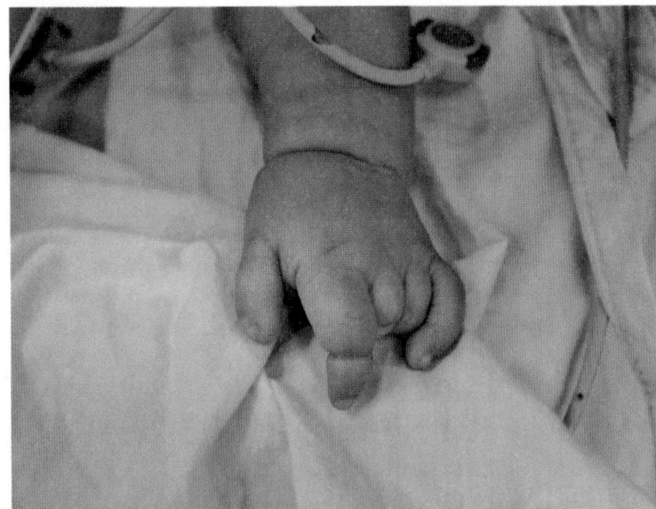

A

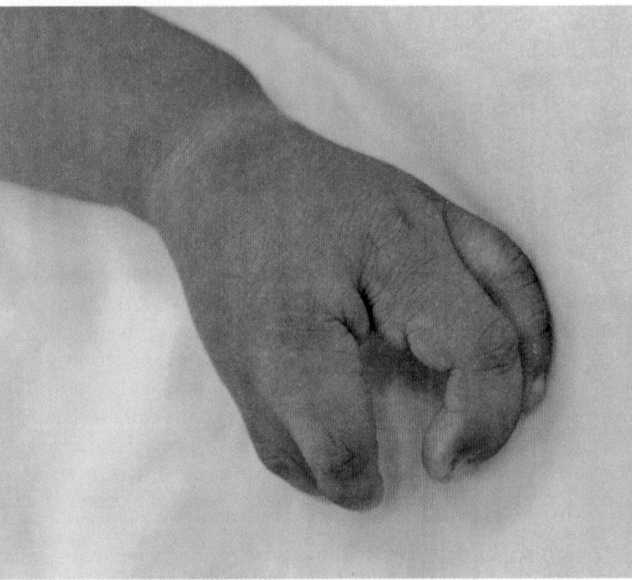

B

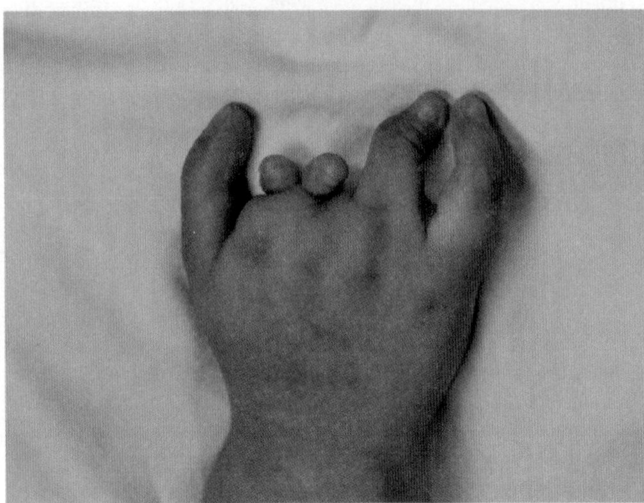

C

FIGURE 214-2 A comparison of causes of oligodactyly. A: Note the circumferential indentation around the index finger and the lack of fingernail in the truncated digits in the patient with constriction bands. B: The cleft hand typically has a V-shaped cleft and absence of digits starting with the middle ray. C: In symbrachydactyly, the digits are shortened but will still have a rudimentary fingernail.



TABLE 214-1 TRIAGE CLASSIFICATION OF UPPER EXTREMITY EMERGENCIES

| Emergencies Requiring Immediate Evaluation and Care by Hand Surgeon |
|---|
| Compartment syndrome |
| Bone, joint, or deep soft tissue infection |
| Paint gun injection injury |
| Open fracture including Seymour fracture |
| Fractures with displacement or angulation |
| Penetrating injuries with nerve, vessel, or tendon injury |
| Deep bites |
| Amnion disruption sequence with impending tissue loss |
| **Minor Emergencies That Should Be Treated in the Primary Care Setting** |
| Most fingertip injuries |
| Paronychiae and minor infections |
| **Semiurgent Referral** |
| Nondisplaced fractures |
| Lacerations with potential nerve or tendon injury |
| **Nonurgent, Elective Referral** |
| Congenital conditions |
| Trigger digits |
| Developmental conditions |

## MASSES

*Ganglion cysts* are common benign masses found in children and teenagers on flexor sheaths and in the wrist area. This type of synovial cyst must be differentiated from a solid tumor. An otoscope can be used to transilluminate the mass. If there is transillumination, then the mass likely is a cyst. If transillumination is equivocal, ultrasonography is the preferred imaging modality to confirm the diagnosis. Treatment seldom is needed. There is a very high spontaneous resolution rate with observation and a very high recurrence rate if these cysts are surgically excised. Surgery is rarely indicated. If the mass is solid, painful, or of great concern to the parents, referral to the hand surgeon is appropriate.

## INFLAMMATORY CONDITIONS

Juvenile chronic arthritis and other inflammatory and collagen vascular conditions can occur in young children (see Chapters 198 and 201). Psoriasis in particular can mimic chronic infection. A pediatric rheumatologist should be involved in management of children with these conditions.

## DEVELOPMENTAL

*Madelung deformity* is a progressive deformity of the wrist due to abnormal growth of the ulnar and volar part of the distal radius. It typically presents in adolescence and is more common in girls. Recognition and surgical intervention before skeletal maturity may prevent worsening of this deformity. Corrective procedures can restore alignment in severe cases.

*Kirner deformity* is a rare progressive hooking of the small fingernail. It is sometimes painful and can be treated surgically if severe (Table 214-1).

## SUGGESTED READINGS


Abzug JM, Kozin SH. Evaluation and management of brachial plexus birth palsy. *Orthop Clin North Am.* 2014;45(2):225-232.

Gellman H. Fingertip-nail bed injuries in children: current concepts and controversies of treatment. *J Craniofac Surg.* 2009;20(4):1033-1035.

Goldfarb CA, Sathienkijkanchai A, Robin NH. Amniotic constriction band: a multidisciplinary assessment of etiology and clinical presentation. *J Bone Joint Surg Am.* 2009;91(Suppl 4):68-75.

Kanj WW, Gunderson MA, Carrigan RB, Sankar WN. Acute compartment syndrome of the upper extremity in children: diagnosis, management, and outcomes. *J Child Orthop.* 2013;7(3):225-233.

Kozin SH, Zlotolow DA. Common pediatric congenital conditions of the hand. *Plast Reconstr Surg*. 2015;136(2):241e-257e.

Osterman M, Draeger R, Stern P. Acute hand infections. *J Hand Surg Am*. 2014;39(8):1628-1635; quiz 1635.

Plancq MC, Buisson P, Deroussen F, Krim G, Collet LM, Gouron R. Successful early surgical treatment in neonatal compartment syndrome: case report. *J Hand Surg Am*. 2013;38(6):1185-1188.

Williams AA, Lochner HV. Pediatric hand and wrist injuries. *Curr Rev Musculoskelet Med*. 2013;6(1):18-25.

# 215 Injuries

Philip Wilson and Vinitha Shenava

## INTRODUCTION

Injury to the growing skeleton is common as an isolated event and is also seen in the child with multiple injuries. Nearly 1 of 3 children will have at least 1 fracture during childhood. Pediatricians, primary care physicians, orthopedic surgeons, and emergency room personnel often will need to evaluate and treat fractures and other musculoskeletal trauma in children and, therefore, need an understanding of the basic diagnostic and treatment principles. The patterns and incidence depend on a number of variables including sex, age, climate, and time of year. From birth to 16 years of age, 42% of boys and 27% of girls suffer a fracture. Upper extremity fractures account for two-thirds of childhood fractures, with the forearm being the most common location. The vast majority of these injuries are treated in an outpatient setting.

## INJURY EVALUATION

Most orthopedic injuries present with obvious pain and swelling. At times, decreased use of an extremity or limp may be the only presenting signs. Despite challenges in communications with younger children, methodical and directed palpation will often localize the injury. Screening for symmetry during an exam with a focus on range of motion, pain, swelling, and warmth allows the identification of injuries even in the uncooperative or nonverbal patient. When no reasonable history of injury is present, nonaccidental trauma or musculoskeletal infection also should be considered with the presenting signs of pain and swelling.

## FRACTURES

### OCCULT FRACTURES

Radiographs in at least 2 planes (typically anterior/posterior and lateral) should be obtained in cases with significant signs of injury or duration of symptoms. When bony abnormalities are not readily apparent, a close examination of radiographic soft tissue swelling may help to localize an injury and redirect examination. In younger children, occult fractures are common findings. Common occult fracture locations are the lateral malleolus, evidenced by lateral ankle swelling, and the elbow, in which fat pad signs demonstrate a joint effusion (Fig. 215-1A–C). Three weeks of splint or cast immobilization is appropriate treatment for suspected occult fractures. In older children and adolescents, RICE (rest, ice, compression, and elevation) is appropriate for most soft tissue injuries.

### INCOMPLETE FRACTURES

#### Buckle (Torus) Fractures

*Buckle fractures*, also called *torus fractures* because of a shape similar to the base of a decorative column, are characterized by a buckling of 1 side of the bone while the other cortex remains intact (Fig. 215-2). The presence of an intact cortex accounts for the stable nature of these fractures. Cast or splint treatment for 3 to 4 weeks allows symptomatic relief while rapid healing occurs.

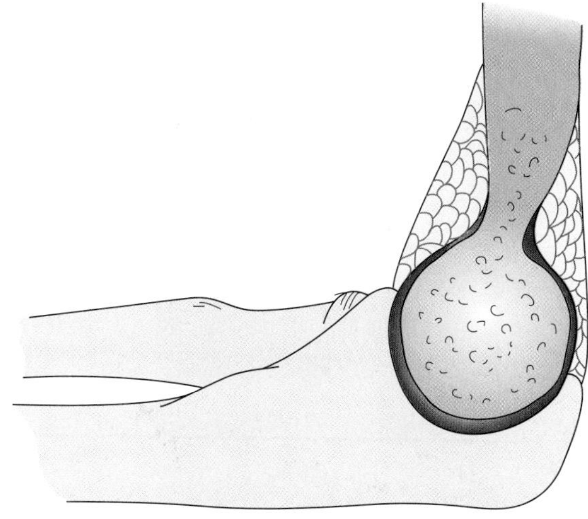

A

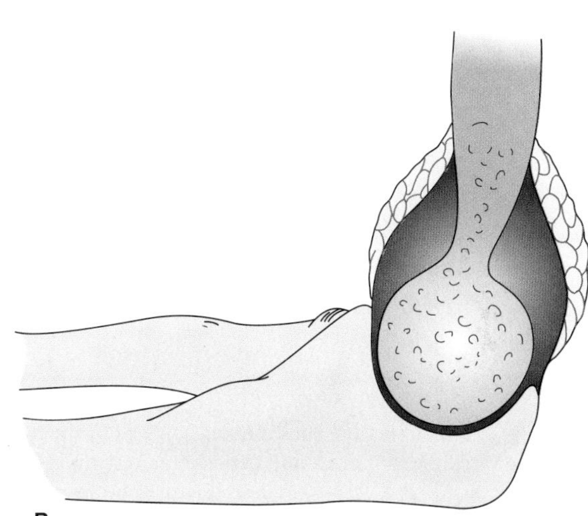

B

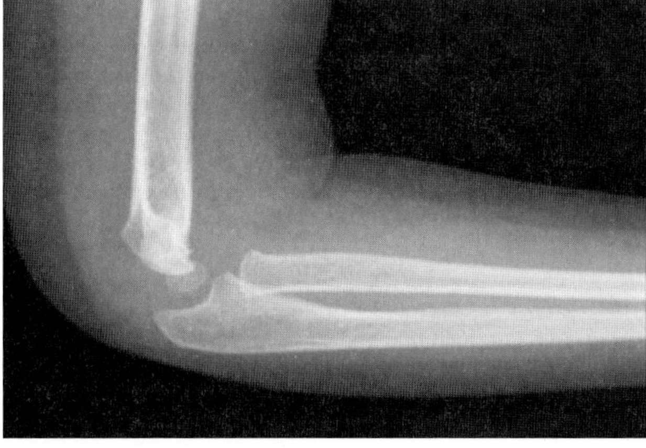

C

FIGURE 215-1 A: Anterior and posterior fat pad positions in a normal elbow. B: Elevation of fat pads secondary to elbow effusion as seen in occult fractures. C: Radiograph with anterior and posterior fat pad signs.

#### Greenstick

*Greenstick fractures* may occur in children due to the combination of the plastic quality of immature bone and the thick periosteum present.

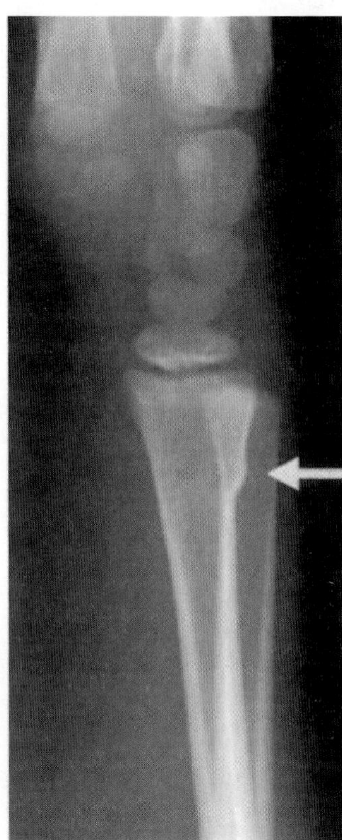

FIGURE 215-2 Buckle fracture of the distal radius. Note that there is no break or deformity of the bone opposite the buckle.

As in breaking a "green" immature stick, the tension side of the bone fractures completely while the cortex and periosteum in compression remain intact but bend (Fig. 215-3). These fractures often require manipulative reduction of gross deformity and are unstable injuries compared to buckle fractures.

## PHYSEAL FRACTURES

In addition to deformity and instability that may be seen in other fracture patterns, *growth plate fractures* may also result in permanent alteration of normal growth that can result in a discrepancy in the lengths of the limbs or angular deformity of the limb that progresses with growth. Arrest of growth generally occurs in fewer than 10% of all physeal fractures and may be seen most frequently at the distal femur. While early reduction of the fracture prior to onset of callus formation and minimizing the number of attempts at manipulation are thought to be protective of physeal arrest, the literature suggests that the quality of an anatomic reduction may be the most important factor for reducing the risk of growth arrest. The Salter-Harris classification is the most common system used to describe patterns of growth plate fractures and is useful when communicating regarding orthopedic care (Fig. 215-4). As a general rule, displaced physeal fractures should be treated within 7 days because treatment after that time results in additional trauma to the growth plate and increases the likelihood that permanent injury will occur. Physeal fractures also require longer follow-up to monitor for physeal injury as it is desirable to recognize and address the physeal arrest early in order to minimize any deformity that will progress with further growth.

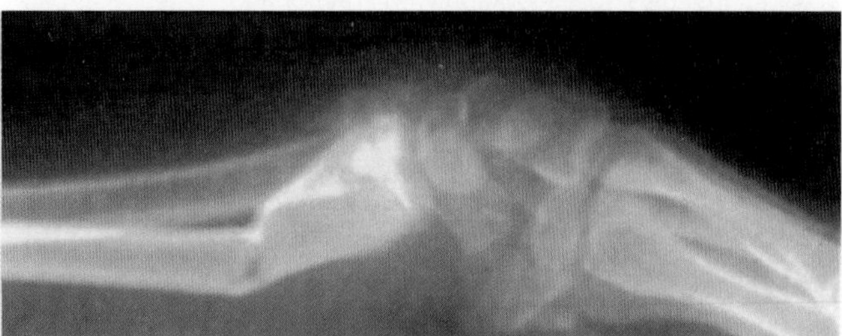

FIGURE 215-3 Greenstick fracture. Note that there is deformity of both sides of the bone, but some bone remains intact.

## COMMON FRACTURES

### Distal Radius and Ulna

Fractures of the distal radius and ulna are the most common childhood fractures and usually occur from a routine fall. Buckle fractures can be treated in short arm casts or volar splints for 4 weeks of immobilization. Deformity or physeal involvement is best treated within 1 to 2 days following injury. Displaced fractures may be reduced with traction, splinted, and referral for orthopedic office evaluation and treatment.

### Elbow

Elbow fractures occur commonly from a fall on an outstretched hand. Common mechanisms of injury include a fall on a trampoline or a fall from playground monkey bars. Displaced fractures with significant deformity and swelling should be referred for prompt evaluation and orthopedic treatment. Even though relatively uncommon, neurovascular injury from deformity or swelling can occur. Occult fractures are common and may be diagnosed by focal pain to palpation and fat pad signs on radiographs. Nondisplaced supracondylar, radial neck, and olecranon fractures are common and may be seen only later as they heal or by magnetic resonance imaging (MRI). Treatment for an occult elbow fracture is 3 weeks of casting with subsequent return to activity once the patient is pain free and full range of motion is achieved.

### Nursemaid's Elbow

Although not a fracture, nursemaid's elbow may be a common presentation of elbow pain and decreased use of the arm. This injury classically results from traction on the extended arm in a child younger than 5 years of age (Fig. 215-5). At this age, the shape of the immature radial head allows subluxation of the annular ligament over the margin of this structure and into the radiocapitellar articulation. In this situation, the child presents with pain and decreased use of the affected limb. The elbow is held slightly flexed and pronated (palm down), and the child may complain of pain in the wrist or elbow.

Radiographs in this condition are negative, and the diagnosis is typically made based on the mechanism of the injury. A reduction maneuver is best performed upon suspicion of the diagnosis and does not require anesthetic or sedating medications. Flexing the elbow to 90° and rapidly and firmly rotating the forearm into full supination (palm up) will allow reduction of the annular ligament and radial head. The child should begin to use the arm within minutes. Immobilization is not necessary following reduction. Parents should be counseled regarding the potential risk of recurrence in children younger than 5 years of age. With further growth, the proximal radial shape enlarges, preventing annular ligament subluxation.

### Toddler's Fracture

A *toddler's fracture* is a nondisplaced or occult spiral tibia fracture that occurs during the first 2 to 3 years of ambulation. Three to 4 weeks in a long-leg, weight-bearing cast will provide relief from the pain and allow union of the fracture. Occult fractures may be diagnosed by diffuse new periosteal bone formation, which is evident 3 weeks following the injury.

### Finger Fractures

Finger fractures may occur from a twisting injury or from an axial load while attempting to catch a ball. When joint swelling is present beyond 2 days, anteroposterior (AP) and true lateral radiographs of the finger are important to evaluate for a periarticular fracture. Quality finger x-rays are obtained by using the fingernail as a visual guide for appropriate positioning for x-rays. Angulated phalangeal

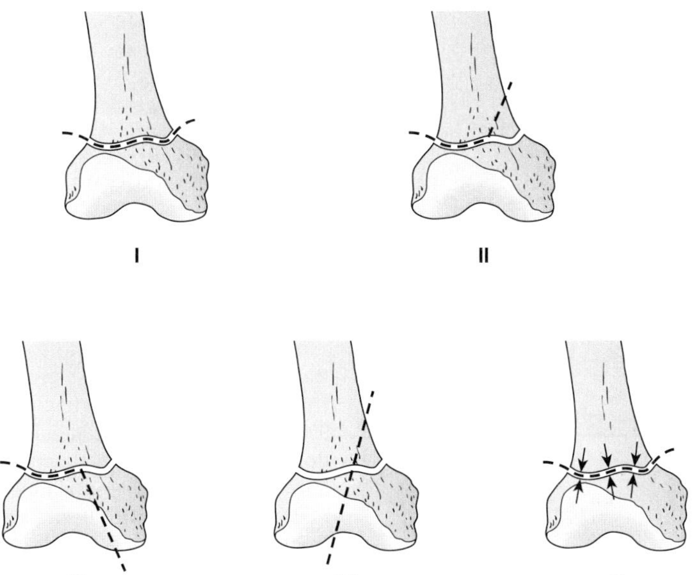


**FIGURE 215-4** Salter classification of fractures. I. Shearing separation of epiphysis from metaphysis. II. Fracture line passing through the physis involving small segment of metaphysis attached to epiphysis. III. Intra-articular fracture of the epiphysis that also passes through the physis. IV. Vertical fracture through metaphysis, epiphyseal plate, and epiphysis. V. Crush injury of physeal plate.

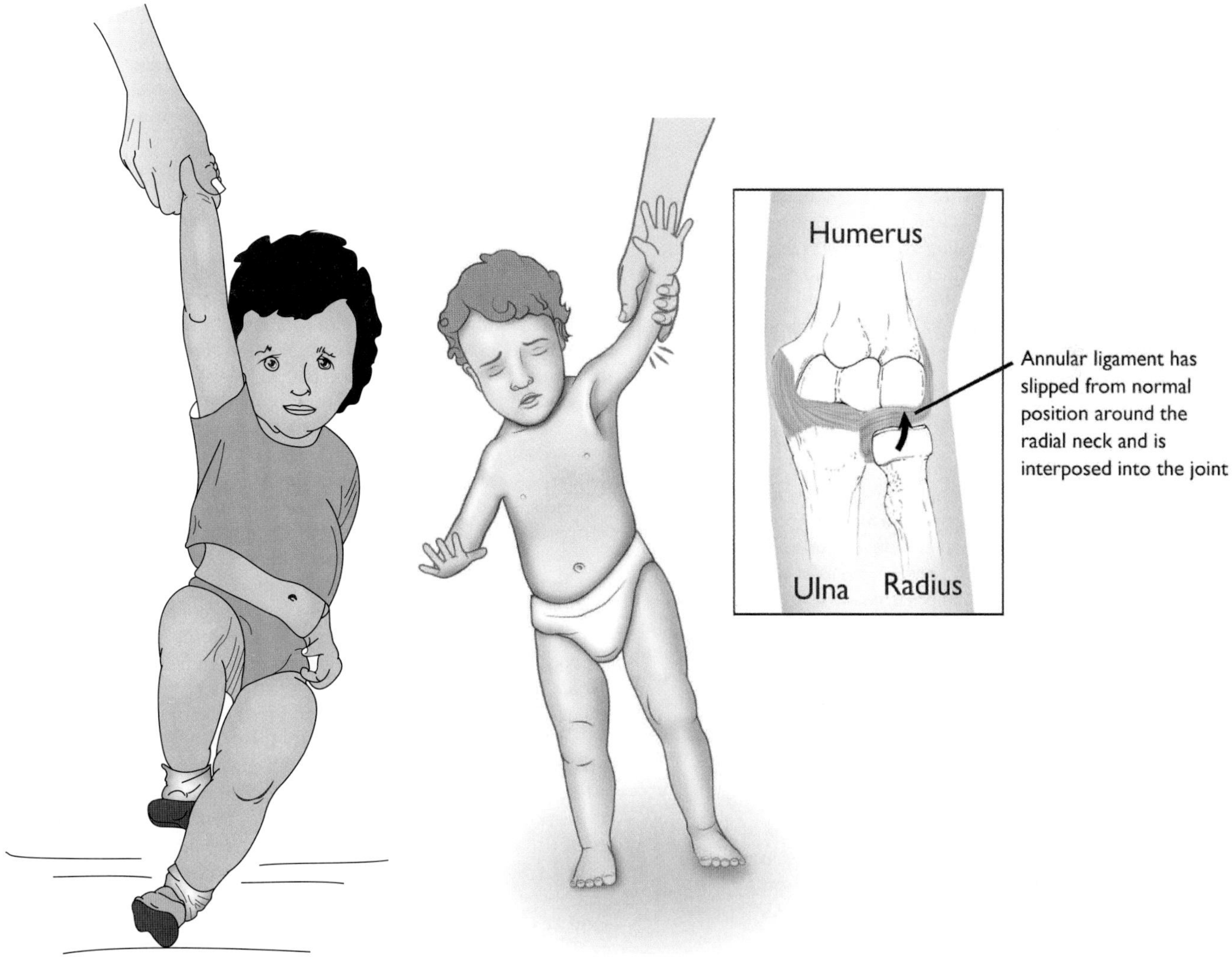

**FIGURE 215-5** Longitudinal traction on the arm of a young child may result in nursemaid's elbow. Inset figure reveals radial head subluxing below annular ligament.

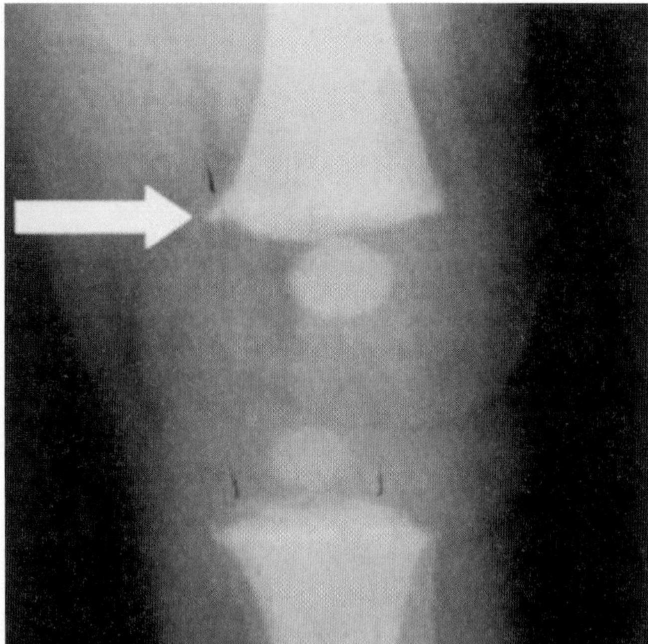

**FIGURE 215-6** Corner fracture of the distal femur is highly specific for child abuse in children < 1 year old.

shaft and periarticular fractures require orthopedic evaluation and treatment.

## CHILD ABUSE

There are few actual "pathognomonic" signs of abuse, and fractures in children younger than 1 year of age should be evaluated carefully for history or other indications of nonaccidental trauma. Metaphyseal corner fractures (Fig. 215-6), posterior rib fractures, and several fractures in varied stages of healing are highly correlated with abuse. Femur fractures and elbow fractures in children younger than 12 months of age should also be evaluated with a high index of suspicion for abuse or neglect. A skeletal survey should be obtained when nonaccidental trauma is a consideration.

## GENERAL FRACTURE CARE

Many fractures in children can be treated with casting. Pain, swelling, and neurovascular status are important factors in the initial evaluation of a fracture. Management with a cast or splint is appropriate when neurovascular examination is normal and pain and swelling are reasonably controlled. With more severe injuries, splinting, which allows for increased volume with swelling, is a safer alternative than is casting. Follow-up is important to prevent cast-related complications. Poorly controlled pain or ongoing narcotic requirement, swelling unresponsive to elevation, or changes in neurovascular exam should prompt immediate treatment. Removal of the cast and thorough evaluation for pressure sores or swelling leading to compartment syndrome should be undertaken in this setting.

As a general rule, fractures of the metaphysis (the bony flare by the growth plate) in children most often heal in 4 to 5 weeks. Shaft fractures typically require 6 to 8 weeks of treatment. In children younger than 3 years old, the cast or splint should be placed on the entire extremity (above the elbow or knee with the joint flexed) to avoid slippage and decrease the risk of skin pressure complications.

## REMODELING

Remodeling is the reshaping of a bone that may occur with growth following a fracture (Fig. 215-7A–D). The determinants that increase remodeling capability are younger age, proximity of the fracture to the physis, and deformity that exists in the same plane as the primary motion of the nearest joint. The potential for remodeling is significantly decreased following adolescence and occurs very little around the elbow at any age following infancy.

## SPORTS AND OVERUSE INJURIES

The assessment of a patient for an injury either during a game or practice or with regard to checking the status of an old injury begins with a focused sports-oriented history and physical exam. The basic features of a sports examination involve joint range of motion, muscle strength screening, and palpation for discomfort. Cervical spine motion can be evaluated by asking the patient to face the examiner and look at the ceiling, the floor, and over the shoulders, and touch ears to shoulders. Shoulder screening involves trapezius muscle strength screening by shrugging shoulders against resistance, and deltoid testing by resisted abduction of shoulders at 90°. Standing and supine shoulder external rotation at 90° of abduction can screen for motion asymmetry or patient apprehension that may indicate shoulder instability. Evaluate elbows for tenderness or motion asymmetry with flexion and extension, and forearm rotation (symmetric palm up and palm down) with the elbows held against the torso in 90° of flexion. Pain-free loss of elbow extension may often be the first sign of an intra-articular or ligamentous injury. Resisted thumbs-up, finger spreading, and clinched-fist testing can be used for peripheral-nerve-function screening and finger-motion deficits or deformity. Lower extremity screening for gross strength and motion deficits may be accomplished by "duck walking" 4 steps away from examiner, standing from squatting position, and rising up first on heels and then toes. The examiner evaluates for symmetry in motion and muscle bulk. With the patient in a supine position, the hips are flexed and rotated to evaluate for symmetry. The quadriceps are compared in contraction, and the knees are examined for symmetric flexion and extension, ligamentous laxity (anterior/posterior drawer testing and varus/valgus testing), and the presence of an effusion (as evidenced by a mobile fluid wave at the medial and lateral patellar margins). The ankles are evaluated for symmetric flexion and extension, pain or laxity with rotation and inversion, and the presence of an effusion (as evidenced by mobile fluid at the anterior ankle joint crease).

In addition to fractures and dislocations, children active in sports may incur injuries to ligaments and cartilage, epiphysitis, or stress fractures. Most commonly a result of rotational or bending forces around a joint, the term *sprain* is used to describe some degree of injury to ligament fibers. Sprains result in pain and swelling of soft tissue along joint margins. A sprain is often a common diagnosis of exclusion when the exam reveals soft-tissue tenderness to a greater degree than bony tenderness, and radiographs are normal. If soft-tissue swelling and tenderness are concentrated at the bony physis, a clinical diagnosis of a nondisplaced physeal fracture should be made, and immobilization is appropriate. With a history of a twisting injury and exam findings of swelling of soft tissue and pain along the ligament, a diagnosis of a sprain may be appropriate. By convention, sprains are classified into 3 clinical grades. *Type I sprains* involve pain along a ligament, but no laxity in comparison to the contralateral corresponding joint. *Type II sprains* involve some detectible degree of asymmetry in laxity testing. *Grade III sprains* describe injuries to a ligament that result in greater than 10 mm of laxity in comparison to the contralateral joint. Most sprains are grade I or grade II injuries with minimal fiber injury and are appropriately treated by the RICE protocol. In addition to the RICE protocol during the initial 72 hours, low-grade sprains benefit from early range of motion and weight bearing as tolerated. Slow return to activity is allowed as pain and swelling resolve over 3 to 4 weeks. Suspected grade III sprains and lower-grade sprains that fail to improve following the initial 3 weeks should be referred to a musculoskeletal specialist for further evaluation.

The ankle is often injured in sporting activities with inversion and rotational mechanisms resulting in bone and soft tissue injuries. Any bony tenderness or significant swelling of soft tissue around the malleoli or joint should prompt radiographic examination centered on the ankle joint. Obvious fractures or widening of the soft tissue shadow overlying the bony physes are indications for immobilization and

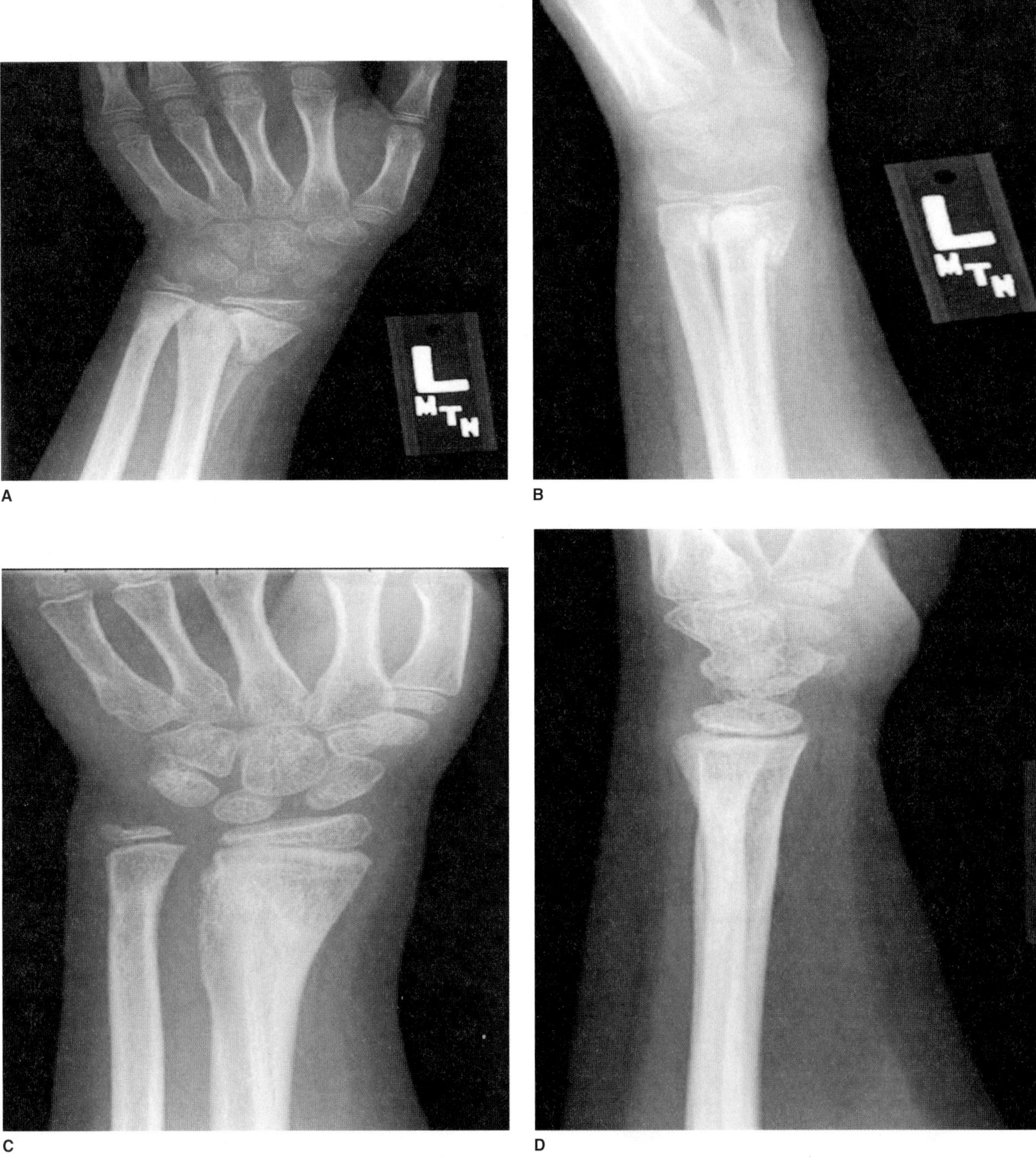


FIGURE 215-7 **A, B:** Distal radius and ulna fracture with early union in a displaced position with deformity present. **C, D:** Remodeling of the fracture with growth from the physis and comparison to the contralateral side.



orthopedic referral. Comparison radiographs of the uninjured side may be useful for identifying more subtle findings. The anterior lateral ankle is a common site of sprains, as described earlier. A sprain of the anterior talofibular ligament may occur following an inversion of the foot and hyperplantarflexion, or rotation through the ankle. A patient with an anterior lateral ankle sprain presents with pain and swelling anterior to the lateral malleolus and limited ankle range of motion. As described earlier, the RICE protocol with slow return to activity is appropriate when this clinical diagnosis is made in the setting of normal radiographs.

Contusions and fractures are common injuries around the knee, and a posttraumatic knee effusion (Fig. 215-8) should also prompt evaluation for injury to ligaments or cartilage. Tibial spine fractures (Fig. 215-9), patellar dislocations, anterior cruciate ligament tears, and meniscal tears are possible causes of a knee effusion in children regardless of skeletal maturity. In addition to routine examination and radiographs, history of the knee giving way or shifting may assist with diagnosis of patellar dislocation or anterior cruciate ligament tear. The patient's apprehension with a lateral patellar translation maneuver is seen following patellar dislocation, and asymmetry with Lachman or

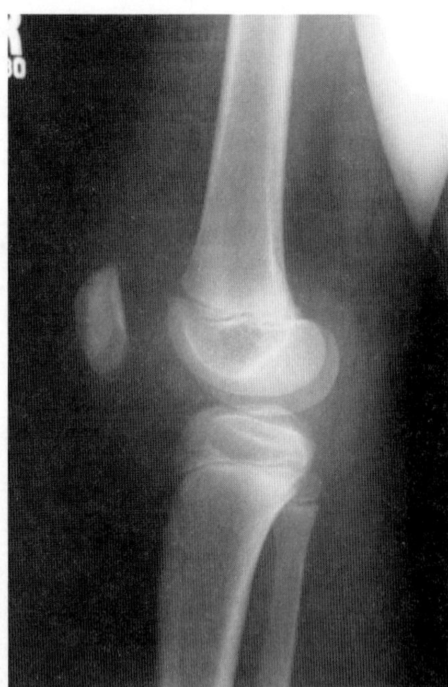

FIGURE 215-8 An x-ray without visible fracture demonstrating a post-traumatic knee effusion.



anterior drawer testing is seen with anterior cruciate ligament injury. A persistent effusion should prompt further examination and imaging when the diagnosis remains uncertain.

A high volume of repetitive activity can result in stress to tissues that overcomes the mechanisms of repair. In children, it can occur in the growth plate as well as in bone and soft tissues. *Epiphysitis* is bone edema and physeal widening that occurs at the growth plate as a result of repetitive stress. It can be seen most commonly at the proximal humerus (Fig. 215-10) or medial epicondyle of the elbow, secondary to pitching in baseball. Forced rest and count limits for little league pitches are important for treatment and prevention of injury. Stress fractures can occur at the distal femur or proximal tibia following rapid increases or high volumes of running activity. Diagnosis is made by history of a high level of activity, or increased training, and activity-related pain, corresponding with characteristic radiographic changes of nondisplaced linear fracture or increased radiodensity. Bone scan or MRI may assist with early diagnosis. As with all injuries related to overuse, treatment is forced rest, with immobilization when indicated, and activity modification.

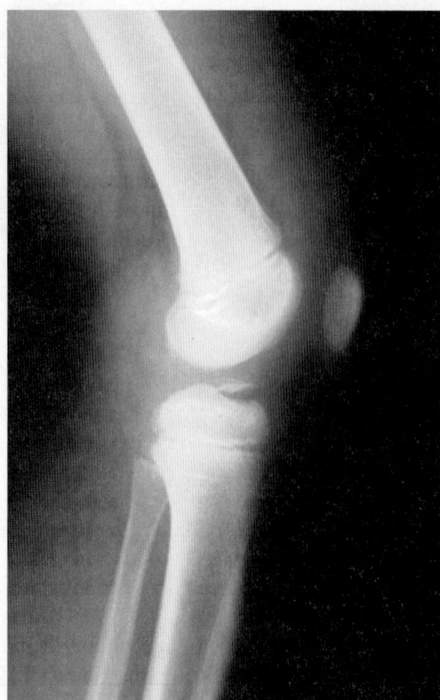

FIGURE 215-9 Lateral knee x-ray demonstrating a displaced tibial spine fracture—the bony insertion point of the anterior cruciate ligament.

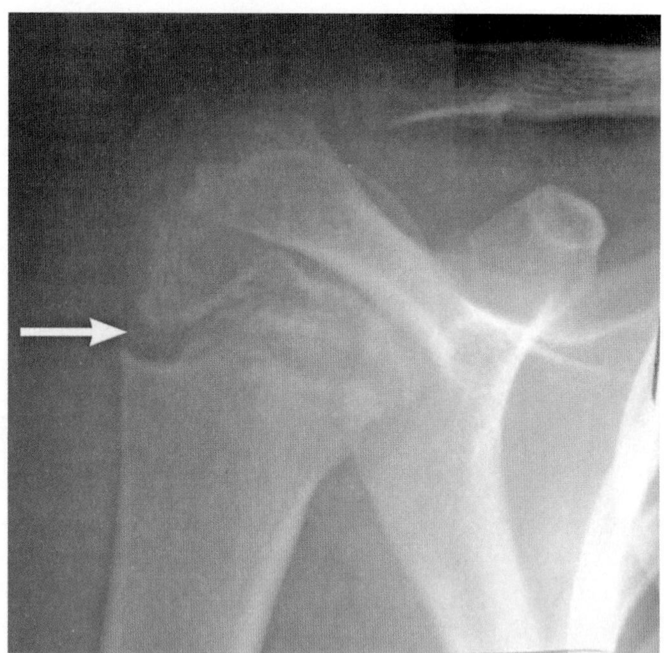

A

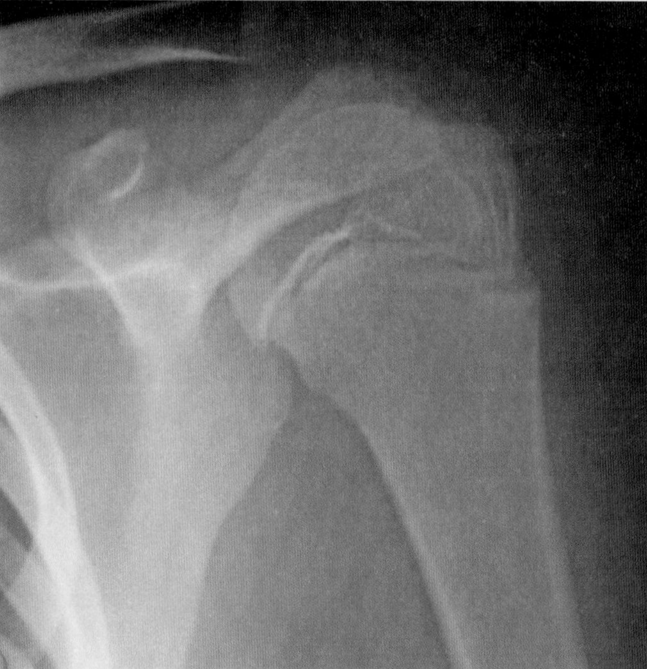

B

FIGURE 215-10 Epiphysitis of the proximal humerus with radiographic widening of the proximal humeral physis (*arrow*).

## SUGGESTED READINGS


Danseco ER, Miller TR, Spicer RS. Incidence and costs of 1987-1994 childhood injuries: demographic breakdowns. *Pediatrics*. 2000; 105(2):E27.

Flaherty EG, Perez-Rosselio JM, Levine MA, et al. Evaluating children with fractures for child physical abuse. *Pediatrics*. 2014;133(2): e477-e489.

Flynn JM, Bashyal RK, Yeger-McKeever M, Garner MR, Launay F, Dponseller PD. Acute traumatic compartment syndrome of the leg in children: diagnosis and outcome. *J Bone Joint Surg Am.* 2011;93(10):937-941.

Goldflam K. Evaluation and treatment of the elbow and forearm injuries in the emergency department. *Emerg Med Clin North Am.* 2015;33:409-421.

LaBella CR. Common acute sports-related lower extremity injuries in children and adolescents. *Clin Pediatr Emerg Med.* 2007;8:31-42.

Pandya NK, Upsani VV, Kulkarni VA. The pediatric polytrauma patient: current concepts. *J Am Acad Orthop Surg.* 2013;21(3):170-179.

Thornton MD, Della-Giustina K, Aronson PL. Emergency department evaluation and treatment of pediatric orthopaedic injuries. *Emerg Med Clin North Am.* 2015;33:423-449.

# 216 Tumors

Nicole Montgomery and Richards B. Stephens

## SOLITARY OSTEOCHONDROMA

Osteochondroma, a cartilage-capped bony projection protruding from the surface of a bone, is the most common benign bone tumor. It reportedly accounts for 36% to 41% of all bone tumors. More than 50% of solitary osteochondromas occur in the metaphyseal area of the knee (distal femur and proximal tibia) and shoulder (proximal humerus).

Its cause is related to a localized herniation of a portion of the growth plate, which results in the formation of a cartilage-capped eccentric small bone. Unlike the more extensive hereditary (autosomal-dominant) multiple exostoses, solitary osteochondromas do not appear to be genetically transmitted.

Osteochondromas may be sessile (broad based) or pedunculated (narrow based). The surface usually is lobular, with multiple bluish-gray cartilaginous caps covering the irregular bony mass. The cartilaginous cap usually is 1 to 3 mm thick, but in the younger patient, it may be noticeably thicker. The thickness of the cartilaginous cap may be much greater if the tumor has undergone sarcomatous change.

In the majority of patients, the osteochondroma becomes evident when the patient is between the ages of 10 and 20 years, with a slight male preponderance. An osteochondroma may be discovered as an incidental radiographic finding, or it may be detected by the patient who feels a protruding bump. Other factors that often draw attention to the osteochondroma include localized pain, growth disturbance, limited joint motion, or abnormal cosmetic appearance.

On the radiograph, the cortex and cancellous bone of the osteochondroma blend with the cortex and cancellous bone of the normal bone. This is the main radiographic finding, and any deviation from this feature should raise suspicion of a more serious lesion. Steady growth of the cartilaginous cap is acceptable during childhood and early adolescence, but growth should cease when skeletal maturity is reached. If the cartilaginous cap continues to grow after skeletal maturity, malignant transformation should be considered and the appropriate follow-up studies undertaken.

### TREATMENT

Because a solitary osteochondroma is a benign tumor, it does not need to be surgically excised if it is asymptomatic. Excision usually is reserved for those lesions that cause pain or symptomatic impingement on neurovascular structures or that interfere with joint function. Pain usually becomes an issue when an osteochondroma is repeatedly bumped on its prominence. Sometimes the osteochondroma is considered cosmetically unacceptable, and the adolescent will ask to have it removed, preferring a scar to a bump. Malignant degeneration of a peripheral solitary osteochondroma can lead to chondrosarcoma in adulthood. However, malignant degeneration of solitary osteochondromas is a rare occurrence, found in fewer than 0.25% of lesions. The prognosis following excision of a chondrosarcoma is excellent.



## HEREDITARY MULTIPLE EXOSTOSES

Hereditary multiple exostoses, or multiple osteochondromatosis, is considered an autosomal-dominant condition affecting numerous areas of the skeleton. Its overall prevalence approaches 1 in 50,000 persons. The median age at the time of diagnosis is approximately 3 years. Hereditary multiple exostoses have a penetrance of 50% by age 3 years. By the end of the first decade of life, 80% of affected persons will have exostoses. By 12 years of age, nearly all affected individuals have evidence of exostoses, as penetrance of the disorder has been found to reach 96% to 100%.

Numerous genetic studies have found anomalies on chromosomes 8, 11, and 19, rendering this a genetically heterogeneous disorder. Specifically, the 3 loci include 8q24.1 (*EXT1*), 11p11–12 (*EXT2*), and 19p (*EXT3*). Mutations of *EXT1* and *EXT2* genes lead to an absence of heparan sulfate, which plays a critical role in growth plate signaling and remodeling essential in normal endochondral ossification.

The gross pathologic and microscopic features of hereditary multiple exostoses are similar to those described for solitary osteochondromas. Numerous sites can be involved. On presentation, several exostoses typically may be found, involving both the upper and lower extremities. Seventy percent will have involvement of the distal femur (Fig. 216-1A), 70% the proximal tibia, and 30% the proximal fibula. The likelihood of involvement near the knee in at least one of these three locations is approximately 94%. Functionally, involvement of the forearm and subsequent radial head dislocation are the most devastating manifestations of the disease (Fig. 216-1B).

### TREATMENT

The only treatment for hereditary multiple exostoses is surgery. However, the mere presence of an osteochondroma is not an indication for surgery. Reasonable indications include: (1) pain from external trauma or irritation of surrounding soft tissues; (2) growth disturbance leading to angular deformity or limb-length discrepancy; (3) joint motion compromised by juxta-articular lesions; (4) soft tissue impingement or tethering of the soft tissue (tendon, nerve, or vessel) (5) compression of the spinal cord; (6) false aneurysm produced by an osteochondroma; (7) formation of painful bursa; (8) obvious cosmetic deformity; and (9) a rapid increase in the size of a lesion. Life expectancy is average unless malignant degeneration of an osteochondroma has occurred and metastases have developed.

Transformation of a lesion in hereditary multiple exostoses to chondrosarcoma during childhood is exceedingly rare. In general, transformation in adulthood remains uncommon, with current reports indicating the risk to be 0.9% to 5%. The most frequent sign of sarcomatous change is a painful, enlarging mass after a long period of quiescence.

## ENCHONDROMA AND MULTIPLE ENCHONDROMATOSIS

Solitary enchondromas are found at the average age of 35. However, multiple enchondromatosis as seen in patients with Ollier disease or Maffucci syndrome can manifest in childhood. They are characterized by islands of cartilage in metaphyseal and diaphyseal bone. Proximity to the growth plate may lead to growth disturbance and angular deformity or limb-length discrepancy. Maffucci syndrome is a condition of enchondromatosis associated with multiple hemangiomas involving soft tissue.

Histologically, enchondromas are proliferating nests of cartilage cells that lack obvious atypia. Foci of calcification are present, and lamellar bone surrounds the cartilage. In multiple enchondromatosis, the lesions may be more cellular, with ominous nuclei mimicking a low-grade chondrosarcoma. The rate of eventual malignant transformation is 20% to 33% in Ollier disease and described as 100% in Maffucci syndrome. Hematopoietic malignant diseases

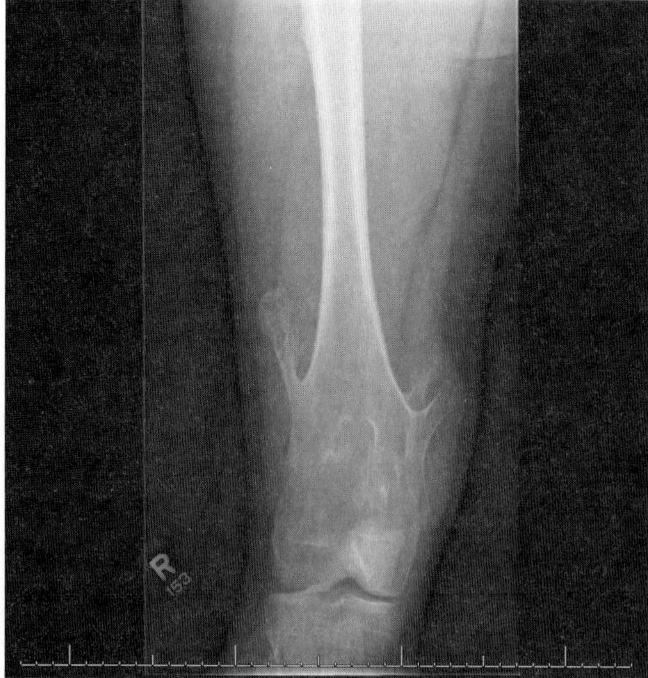

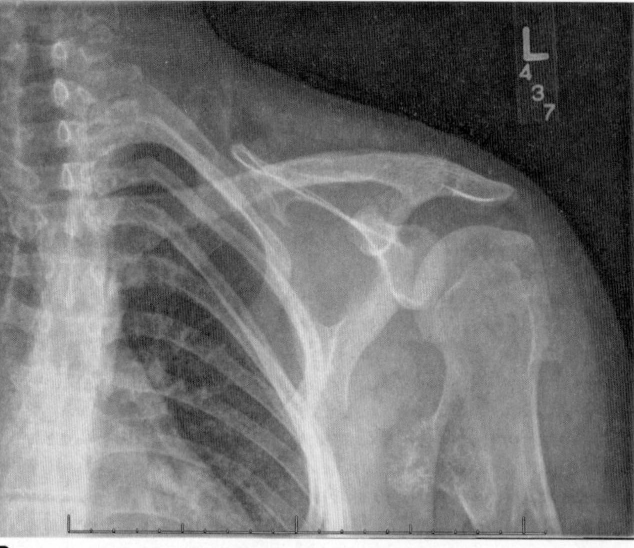


**FIGURE 216-1** **A:** Anteroposterior radiograph of the right distal femur demonstrating multiple osteochondromas. **B:** Radiograph of the left shoulder of the same patient demonstrating multiple osteochondromas.

(acute lymphoid leukemia and chronic myeloid leukemia) have been described in both Ollier disease and Maffucci syndrome.

Radiographically in long bones, enchondromatosis is recognized as radiolucent longitudinal streaks that involve the metaphysis and extend into the diaphysis. The cortex is thin, and calcification within the lesion is common. In Maffucci syndrome, superficial calcifications representing phleboliths in the hemangiomas may be seen. Computed tomography (CT) imaging may be useful to better classify the lesion and demonstrate cortical scalloping suggestive of malignant transformation.

### TREATMENT

Multiple enchondromatosis cannot be cured by curettage and bone grafting. Potentially malignant lesions are treated with wide excision. Treatment is largely aimed at correcting limb angular deformities and limb length inequalities with corrective procedures such as growth manipulation, osteotomies, and distraction osteogenesis.

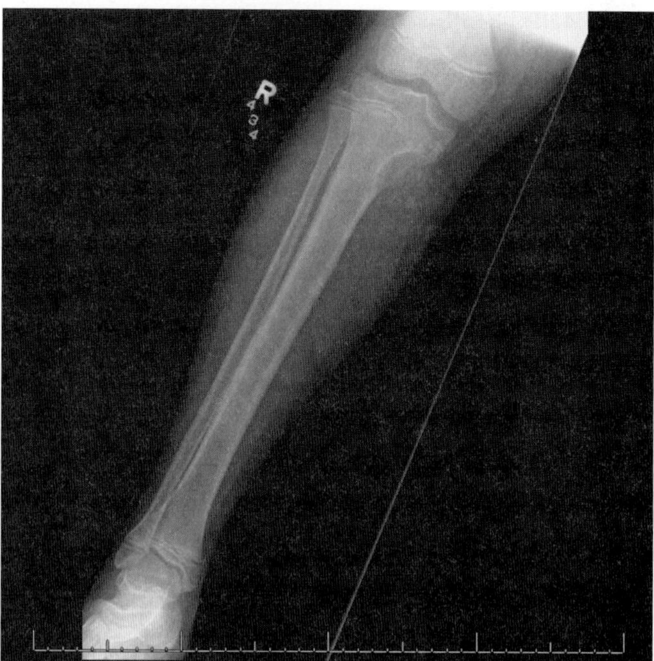

**FIGURE 216-2** Nonossifying fibroma of the left proximal tibia with typical features: eccentric, radiolucent lesion with well-defined sclerotic margins.

## NONOSSIFYING FIBROMA AND FIBROUS CORTICAL DEFECT

Fibrous defects in bone are common lesions in children. They are found in the metaphyseal regions of the long bones, particularly the femur and the tibia. These lesions contain fibrous tissue, thus leading to the terms *fibrous cortical defect* and *nonossifying fibroma.* These fibrous lesions appear to be developmental defects due to a localized disturbance of bone growth and may not be representative of true neoplasms. Most are asymptomatic, picked up as an incidental finding during radiographs taken for other reasons, and eventually resolve during remodeling at the metaphyseal (growing) end of the bone. As many as 30% of people may have a fibrous cortical defect present in the first two decades of life.

On radiographs, these lesions are sharply delineated, radiolucent, multiloculated, eccentric, and outlined by a sclerotic border (Fig. 216-2). These findings are usually so characteristic that further radiologic studies are unnecessary. Commonly, the lesion regresses spontaneously, becoming smaller and less distinct and eventually disappearing.

### TREATMENT

Fibrous cortical defects do not require treatment because they usually regress over time. Larger, nonossifying fibromas can be monitored without surgical intervention, and if fractures do occur, they can be successfully managed nonoperatively. Occasionally, discomfort or repeated fractures may require intralesional excision by curettage down to normal bone, with the defect filled with bone graft.

## SIMPLE BONE CYSTS (SOLITARY BONE CYST, UNICAMERAL BONE CYST)

Simple or unicameral bone cysts are benign, fluid-filled cavities that can expand and weaken bone but are not true neoplasms. Simple bone cysts represent approximately 3% of all biopsied primary bone tumors and nearly always occur during the first 2 decades of life, most often between 3 and 14 years of age. They occur more commonly in boys than girls (2:1). Most of cysts occur in the metaphyseal region of the proximal humerus or femur, with approximately 50% of cases involving the humerus and 18% to 27% affecting the femur. Its cause remains uncertain.

Rarely does more than 1 cyst occur in an individual, thus the term *solitary bone cyst.* The term *unicameral bone cyst* implies that 1 chamber exists. These bone cysts tend to expand by eroding the cortex, resulting in a localized bulge of the bone. Where the cortical tissue is thinnest, the wall can actually be fluctuant and a bluish tinge from the underlying fluid can be seen. The fluid found within is straw-colored, or serosanguineous, a feature distinguishing simple bone cysts from aneurysmal bone cysts. Cysts can be asymptomatic and may be discovered incidentally when radiographs are obtained for other reasons. More often, though, the cysts are diagnosed because of pain. The pain may be mild and reflective of a microscopic pathologic fracture. More abrupt discomfort occurs when a pathologic fracture occurs following relatively minor trauma, such as a fall. These fractures occur in as many as 90% of patients and heal readily, although the cysts do not.

There are several characteristic radiographic features of simple bone cysts. The cyst is metaphyseal and usually extends to, but not across, the growth plate (physis). Typically, the cyst is symmetrically expansile and radiolucent, with a thin cortical rim surrounding it. Magnetic resonance imaging (MRI) demonstrates high signal intensity on T2-weighted imaging and low signal intensity on T1-weighted imaging (Fig. 216-3).

### TREATMENT

A common misconception in the treatment of simple bone cysts in children is that once the pathologic fracture heals, the cyst also has an excellent chance of healing spontaneously. However, most investigators examining this phenomenon have found that the likelihood of spontaneous healing of the cyst following pathologic fracture is very low, probably less than 5%. In mature individuals, if the cyst has a sufficiently thick cortex and is located in the upper extremity, periodic observation may be all that is needed. If the patient is asymptomatic, it may not be necessary to restrict activities.

The treatment approach is more aggressive for all simple bone cysts in younger children. Plans should be made for definitive treatment of the cyst in order to prevent future fractures and possible associated complications (eg, shortening due to growth arrest and deformity). The diagnosis is usually confirmed at surgery, when straw-colored fluid is aspirated through a large-bore needle introduced into the cystic cavity. Treatment modalities include injection of corticosteroids into the cyst, injection of autologous bone marrow, injection of calcium phosphate paste that later hardens, several drillings and drainage of the cavity, and decompression of the cavity and curettage of the membranous wall followed by bone grafting. A relatively high recurrence rate has been associated historically with treatment of simple bone cysts, but more modern percutaneous techniques combining curettage, decompression, and grafting have been described, with excellent results. Older forms of treatment, such as subtotal resection with or without bone grafting and total resection, have been associated with increased cyst recurrence and are rarely, if ever, used today.

## ANEURYSMAL BONE CYST

An aneurysmal bone cyst is a solitary, expansile, radiolucent lesion generally located in the metaphyseal region of the long bones. They are much less common than are simple bone cysts and represent 1% of all biopsied primary bone tumors. Nearly 70% of affected patients are between 5 and 20 years of age, with approximately half of cases occurring in the second decade of life.

The most common sites are the femur, tibia, spine, humerus, pelvis, and fibula, with approximately half of reported cases occurring in the long bones of the extremities. Although they usually involve the metaphyseal region, aneurysmal cysts may on occasion cross the growth plate into the epiphysis or may extend into the diaphysis. Approximately 20% of aneurysmal bone cysts involve the spine. They may cause cord compression or spinal deformity. Within the vertebra,

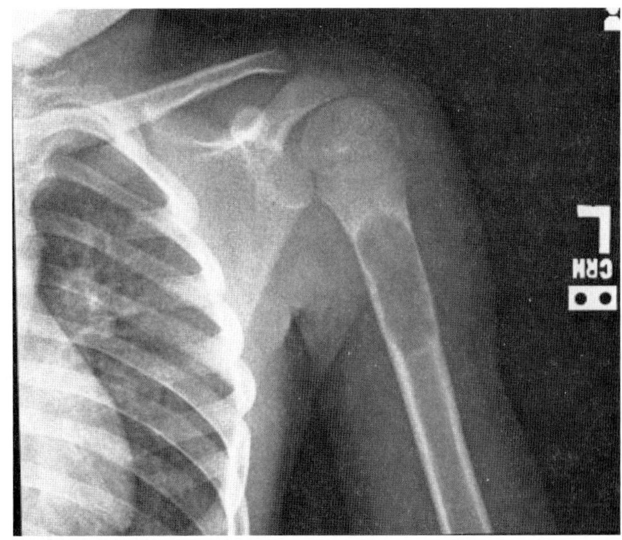


A

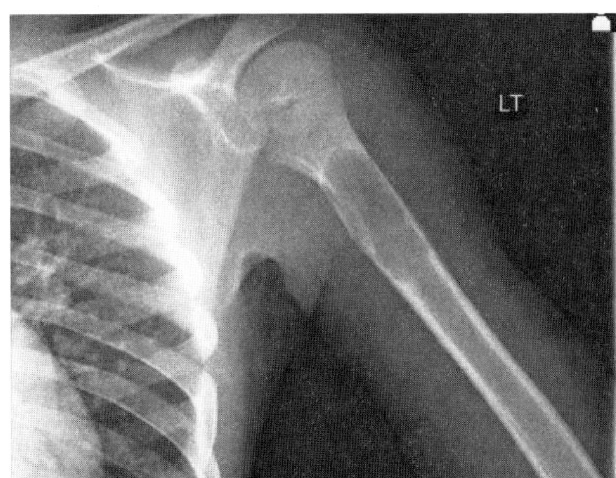


B

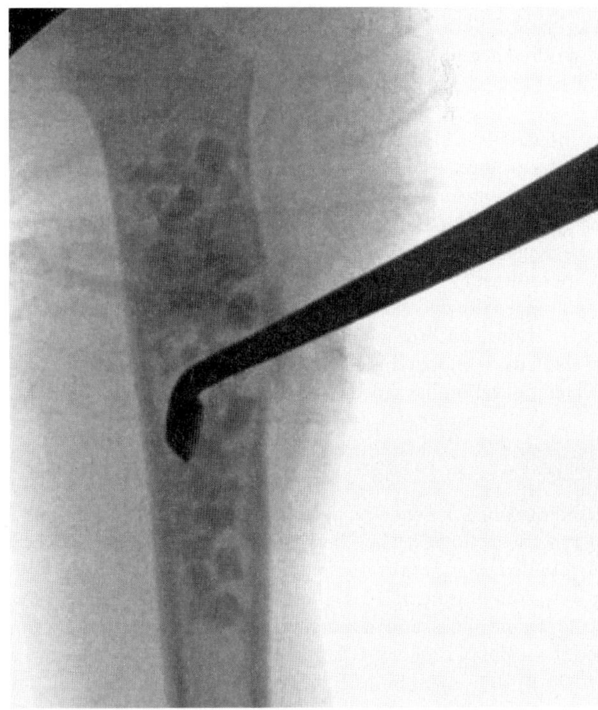

C

**FIGURE 216-3 A and B:** Unicameral bone cyst of the left humerus associated with pain and multiple pathologic fractures. **C:** Intraoperative image of the left humerus after the cyst was curettaged, decompressed, and packed with graft.

the cyst may be found in the body, pedicles, lamina, and spinous process.

Aneurysmal bone cysts represent either a primary neoplastic condition or a secondary response (arteriovenous malformation) to the destructive effects of an underlying primary tumor, such as nonossifying fibromas, fibromyxomas, fibrous dysplasia, chondroblastomas, giant cell tumors, simple bone cysts, telangiectatic osteosarcomas, chondrosarcomas, and metastatic disease. A reported 65% of aneurysmal bone cysts are thought to be primary, with 35% thought to be secondary to other lesions.

The clinical presentation includes localized pain of several weeks or months in duration, tenderness, and, if the aneurysmal bone cyst occurs in an extremity, swelling. When the cyst involves the spine, progressive enlargement may compress the spinal cord or nerve roots, resulting in neurologic deficits such as motor weakness, sensory disturbance, and loss of bowel or bladder control.

The classic radiographic feature of an aneurysmal bone cyst is a ballooned-out lesion outlined by a thin shell of subperiosteal new bone formation. In about 80% of cases, the cyst involves the metaphyseal region of the long bones and, unlike simple bone cysts, is eccentric in its location. Once a lesion is identified on radiographs, the tumor can be better clarified with CT, particularly if it is located in the spine. The extent of involvement of the vertebra and any encroachment of the spinal canal will be readily evident. CT will also demonstrate the characteristic fluid–fluid levels if the patient is able to lie still long enough for the serosanguineous fluid to separate from the blood within the chambers of the cyst that do not have active circulation. Fluid-fluid levels are easily identified on magnetic resonance images (MRIs). The differential diagnosis with regard to malignant conditions includes atypical osteosarcoma and telangiectatic osteosarcoma.



### TREATMENT

Although spontaneous healing of aneurysmal bone cysts has been reported, it is uncommon. Thus, expectant management should be considered only when the diagnosis has been made with confidence and the lesion is in a location and at a stage that do not entail any risk of fracture or further destruction. More often, when the diagnosis of aneurysmal bone cyst is made, active treatment is recommended.

Curettage followed by bone grafting of aneurysmal cysts has been the standard treatment for many years. Unfortunately, this tumor has a high incidence of local recurrence (14–59%) after curettage. Adjunctive therapy, such as cementation, cryotherapy, or embolization, should be considered along with curettage, as it can significantly reduce recurrence. Embolization is useful as a primary treatment of aneurysmal cysts located in areas of limited access, such as the spine and pelvis. Radiation therapy has been used for some aneurysmal bone cysts, especially those that are recurrent, inoperable, or located in areas that are difficult to gain access to, such as the spine. The dose should be minimized to decrease the risk of radiation-induced sarcoma. Because of this concern, radiation therapy should be limited to cases of cysts that are inoperable or have become inoperable and cases in which embolization has failed.

## OSTEOID OSTEOMA

Osteoid osteomas are solitary, benign, painful lesions of the bone and have unknown etiology. They have a nidus, 1.5 to 2.0 cm in size, which is surrounded by an area of reactive, dense bone. Osteoid osteomas are relatively common benign bone lesions, exceeded in incidence only by osteochondromas and nonossifying fibromas. Osteoid osteomas account for approximately 10% to 11% of benign bone tumors and 2% to 3% of all primary biopsied bone neoplasms. They are characteristically seen in children and adolescents.

Patients with osteoid osteoma typically present with a history of dull, aching pain in the region overlying the affected long bone. The pain may have been present for several months before presentation, tends to be worse at night, and is relieved significantly by nonsteroidal anti-inflammatory drugs (NSAIDs). The most commonly involved sites are the femur and tibia. A limp often is noted during evaluation of the patient's gait. Muscle atrophy may be apparent if the lesion has been present for several months. However, direct tenderness, erythema, or swelling is uncommon.

On radiographs, most of the tumors are intracortical, with the nidus appearing as a radiolucent lesion. This nidus rarely exceeds 1 cm in diameter but may be as large as 2 cm. The dense surrounding reactive sclerotic bone may extend for several centimeters away from the nidus. Cross-sectional imaging with CT will best demonstrate the well-circumscribed area representing the nidus.

Over the long term, these lesions are described as self-limiting and may mature spontaneously. The nidus may gradually calcify, then ossify, and finally blend into the sclerotic surrounding bone. However, few patients are willing to continue with conservative management long term because of the intensity of the pain and the favorable outcomes that are achieved with surgery.

### TREATMENT

NSAIDs are effective in relieving symptoms of pain associated with osteoid osteoma. If the symptoms are moderate and controlled by this treatment program, observation alone is sufficient. Most patients recognize persistent pain and elect to undergo more aggressive treatment. Surgical excision has proven extremely effective. Relief from the pain usually is immediate, dramatic, and permanent unless the nidus has been incompletely excised. CT-guided radiofrequency ablation also is very effective in carefully chosen anatomic sites.

## FIBROUS DYSPLASIA

Fibrous dysplasia is characterized by the presence of expanding intramedullary fibro-osseous tissue in 1 or more bones. Its incidence is not known. Although most lesions probably are present in early childhood, they usually do not become evident before late childhood to adolescence (Fig. 216-4).

In general, fibrous dysplasia can be classified into 1 of 3 categories: involving 1 bone only (monostotic), involving multiple bones (polyostotic), and polyostotic form with endocrine abnormalities. Precocious puberty, premature skeletal maturation, hyperthyroidism, hyperparathyroidism, acromegaly, and Cushing syndrome can occur in these patients.

The outer surface of expanded bone usually is smooth and covered by reactive periosteal bone. The underlying dysplastic tissue is grayish white, and the fibrous tissue may feel gritty when palpated, almost like sandpaper. Histologically, the bony spicules are described as looking like the letters C, J, or Y, or as resembling Chinese characters.

The clinical manifestations usually are mild in monostotic fibrous dysplasia. Pain and a limp may be evident when the femur is involved. Local swelling may be seen when the lesion is in a superficial bone, such as the mandible, skull, or tibia. The skeletal changes usually are more severe in the polyostotic form and may result in pain, swelling, deformity, and limb length discrepancies.

The most common nonskeletal manifestation associated with fibrous dysplasia is abnormal cutaneous pigmentation, or café au lait spots. They have irregular borders, are not raised from the surrounding skin, and may be extensive, involving large areas of the trunk, face, or limbs. The pigmentation changes usually are not present in the monostotic fibrous dysplasia.

### TREATMENT

The mere presence of fibrous dysplasia in bone is not, in itself, an indication for surgery, and surgical overtreatment should be avoided. Surgery is indicated when the lesions (1) are complicated by fractures, (2) cause significant or progressive deformity that jeopardizes the integrity of the long bone or that results in unacceptable disfigurement, or (3) are symptomatic and cause the patient pain.

In children, restoring dysplastic bone to normal bone after surgery is nearly impossible. Thus, if the rare biopsy is needed to

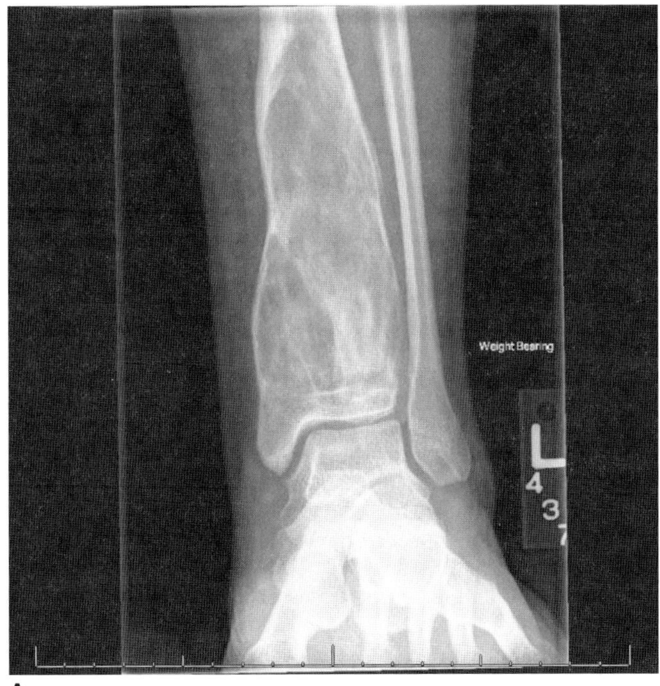

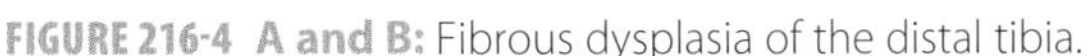
A

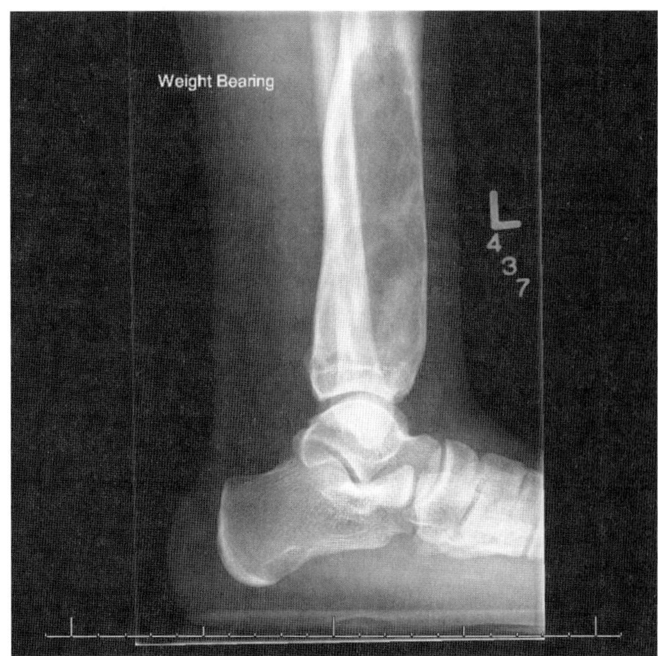

B

**FIGURE 216-4 A and B:** Fibrous dysplasia of the distal tibia.

confirm the diagnosis of a monostotic lesion, surgical intervention probably should not be undertaken unless there is a fracture or painful deformity. Operative intervention is needed when repeated pathologic fractures have occurred, deformity increases, or associated pain becomes persistent. These pathologic fractures can occur following mild trauma, are often minimally displaced, and heal at a normal rate.

## HISTIOCYTOSIS X (LANGERHANS CELL HISTIOCYTOSIS)

Histiocytosis X has frequently been referred to as *eosinophilic granuloma*, a term introduced in 1940 to describe solitary bone destruction by large histiocytic cells intermingled with eosinophilic leukocytes. Approximately 80% of cases of histiocytosis X are solitary eosinophilic granulomas, 6% are multiple eosinophilic granulomas, 9% are Hand-Schüller-Christian disease, and 1.2% are Letterer-Siwe disease.

The etiology is poorly understood. There is speculation that immunologic stimulation of a normal presenting cell, the Langerhans cell, continues in an uncontrolled manner, resulting in the proliferation and accumulation of these cells. It may not truly represent a neoplasm but, instead, a proliferative lesion that may be secondary to a defect in immunoregulation. No hereditary pattern has been described.

Langerhans cell histiocytosis can present at any age, from birth to old age. The incidence in children has been estimated at 3 to 4 per million, with a 2:1 male-to-female ratio. The mildest, most favorable form of histiocytosis X is an eosinophilic granuloma that is confined to a single bone, or occasionally to several bones, without extraskeletal involvement. The lesion is a benign process.

The first symptom is localizing pain, occasionally accompanied by swelling and low-grade fever. The skull is the most common site of involvement, followed by the femur. About 40% of solitary eosinophilic granulomas are found at 1 of these 2 sites. In the case of multiple lesions, the skull and femur again are most commonly affected. Other sites of involvement include the pelvis, ribs, and spine.

Radiographically, a rapidly destructive lytic process occurs in the bone, producing a "punched-out" appearance on radiographs. In the early phases, the lesion may be poorly delineated and show a "moth-eaten" erosive pattern of the bone. It may mimic osteomyelitis or Ewing sarcoma, and, therefore, a biopsy often is necessary to rule out a malignant process. Approximately 10% of patients who initially present with a solitary eosinophilic granuloma develop multifocal lesions with extraskeletal involvement such as diabetes insipidus and exophthalmos (Hand-Schüller-Christian disease). Nearly any bone other than those in the hands and feet may be affected. Histiocytic disorders are discussed in Chapter 459.

### TREATMENT

Patients with solitary eosinophilic granulomas generally have a benign clinical course. They have a good chance of experiencing spontaneous remission and a favorable outcome over a period of months to years. The single bony lesion usually does not require treatment other than a biopsy to confirm the diagnosis.

## MALIGNANT TUMORS

Osteosarcoma is discussed in Chapter 449, Ewing sarcoma in Chapter 450, and histiocytic disorders in Chapter 459.

### SUGGESTED READINGS

Betsey M, Kupersmith LM, Springfield DS. Metaphyseal fibrous defects. *J Am Acad Orthop Surg*. 2004;12(2):89-95.

Biermann JS. Common benign lesion of bone in children and adolescents. *J Pediatr Orthop*. 2002;22(2):268-273.

Cottalorda J, Bourelle S. Current treatments of primary aneurysmal bone cysts. *J Pediatr Orthop B*. 2006;15(3):155-167.

Darilek S, Wicklund C, Novy D, et al. Hereditary multiple exostosis and pain. *J Pediatr Orthop*. 2005;25(3):369-376.

Krych A, Odland A, Rose P, et al. Oncologic conditions that stimulate common sports injuries. *J Am Acad Orthop Surg*. 2014;22(4):223-234.

Pretell-Mazzini J, Murphy RF, Kushare I, Dormans JP. Unicameral bone cysts: Characteristics and management controversies. *J Am Acad Orthop Surg*. 2014;22:295-303.

Santiago FR, Del Mar Castellano Gaercia M, Montes JL, Garcia MR, Fernandez JM. Treatment of bone tumours by radiofrequency thermal ablation. *Curr Rev Musculoskeleta Med*. 2009;2(1):43-50.

# 217 Neuromuscular Disorders

Jeffrey S. Shilt, Lee S. Haruno, and Lori A. Karol

## INTRODUCTION

Neuromuscular disorders are conditions that impair the skeletal or voluntary muscle system. Strictly speaking, these afflictions are primary defects of muscle and the peripheral nervous system. Conditions resulting in impaired central control of muscles, however, are commonly considered secondary neuromuscular disorders with regard to treatment or research.

The spectrum of primary neuromuscular and secondary nervous system disorders is expansive and can be found in Table 217-1. This chapter first focuses on basic orthopedic interventions, both operative and nonoperative, that are commonly applied in the course of management for neuromuscular disorders. This topic is followed by a review of selected neuromuscular disorders that require orthopedic attention and has been expanded to include arthrogryposis, as the general treatment principles are similar and not covered in other textbook sections. Where appropriate, the disease process and medical management are cross-referenced to chapters that provide greater details of specific entities.

## OVERVIEW OF MANAGEMENT

### NONOPERATIVE: ORTHOTICS AND BRACING

The general purpose of orthoses is to help patients achieve stability in standing or walking and control the position of the extremities. They serve a purpose in both correction and prevention of deformities and may act as a compensatory mechanism for deficient muscle strength or activity. Orthoses may be considered positional (comparatively more rigid) or functional (adaptive to movement). The following paragraphs provide a brief introduction to common orthotic devices.

#### Spinal Orthoses

Neuromuscular scoliosis can result from a variety of neuropathic or muscular conditions including cerebral palsy, myelodysplasia, and muscular dystrophy. Orthoses and bracing are commonly used in the early management of spinal disorders in pediatric patients, particularly to facilitate sitting, but generally are viewed as a temporary measure until the timing of surgical intervention is ideal. Unlike in idiopathic scoliosis, bracing does little to prevent progression of the curve. The most commonly used brace is the thoracolumbosacral orthosis (TLSO).

#### Extremity Orthoses

Upper and lower extremity orthoses are used in the management of neuromuscular disorders to address a lack of strength and range of motion and to facilitate gait and function. The nomenclature of the devices typically denotes the joints they cross. For example, hip-knee-ankle-foot orthoses (HKAFO) provide stabilization and support for the entire lower extremity, whereas ankle-foot orthoses (AFO) cross only the ankle joint.

#### Mobility Aids

Assistive devices such as walkers, crutches, and wheelchairs can improve the mobility and independence of patients with neuromuscular disorders. In nonambulatory patients, for example those with thoracic-level myelodysplasia or severe cerebral palsy, wheelchair modifications to accommodate preferred posture and the specific needs of the patients are warranted. Mobility devices often are used in conjunction with the previously described extremity orthoses and bracing to maximize individual ability and function.

### SURGICAL INTERVENTION

Despite the widespread use of nonoperative measures in children with neuromuscular disorders, many patients will eventually require operative management to improve deformity, comfort, and/or function. This section provides a brief overview of surgical techniques and principles.

#### Soft Tissue Surgery

Tendon transfers commonly are performed in patients with neuromuscular conditions to correct deformity and improve function. The tendon is surgically released from its insertion site and rerouted through the soft tissue to a different insertion point. This procedure alters the mechanical purpose of the tendon and associated muscle to replace or supplement a previously deficient motor function.

Tendon lengthening serves to correct joint contractures or deformities in patients with neuromuscular disorders. Lengthening typically is accomplished by 2 general techniques: by surgically cutting the tendon in a z-like fashion or by release of the fascia over the musculotendinous junction, both of which effectively reduce tension across a

**TABLE 217-1 OVERVIEW OF SELECTED NEUROMUSCULAR AND RELATED DISORDERS**

| Primary Neuromuscular Disorders: Muscle and Peripheral Nerve Defects | | | |
|---|---|---|---|
| **Peripheral Nerve Disease** | **Muscular Dystrophies** | **Metabolic Diseases** | **Myopathies** |
| • Charcot-Marie-Tooth<br>• Chronic inflammatory demyelinating polyneuropathy<br>• Guillain-Barré syndrome<br>• Friedreich ataxia | • Duchenne<br>• Becker<br>• Congenital<br>• Distal<br>• Emery-Dreifuss<br>• Fascioscapulohumeral<br>• Limb-Girdle<br>• Myotonic<br>• Oculopharyngeal | • Acid maltase deficiency<br>• Carnitine deficiency<br>• Carnitine palmityl transferase deficiency<br>• Debrancher enzyme deficiency<br>• Lactate dehydrogenase deficiency<br>• Mitochondrial myopathy<br>• Myoadenylate deaminase deficiency<br>• Phosphorylase deficiency<br>• Phosphofructokinase deficiency<br>• Phosphoglycerate kinase deficiency | • Central core disease<br>• Hyperthyroid myopathy<br>• Congenital myotonia<br>• Myotubular myopathy<br>• Nemaline myopathy<br>• Congenital paramyotonia<br>• Periodic paralysis |
| **Neuromuscular Junction Disorders** | | | **Inflammatory Myopathies** |
| • Lambert-Eaton syndrome<br>• Congenital and adult myasthenia gravis<br>• Botulism | | | • Dermatomyositis<br>• Calcinosis cutis<br>• Polymyositis<br>• Inclusion body myositis |
| **Secondary Neuromuscular Disorders: Defects in the Brain and Spinal Cord** | | | |
| **Motor Neuron Diseases** | **Diseases of Brain and Spinal Cord** | | **Miscellaneous** |
| • Amyotrophic lateral sclerosis (ALS)<br>• Spinal muscular atrophy | • Cerebral palsy<br>• Neural tube defects/myelodysplasia<br>• Dejerine-Sottas syndrome | | • Arthrogryposis |

given joint by increasing the length of the muscle tendon. Tenotomies, transverse incisions across the tendon releasing the ends from one another, are also used to reduce musculotendinous tightness. The intervening space between the 2 tendon ends commonly fills in with scar tissue, which typically is weaker than the repair in the lengthening methods mentioned earlier.

The approach to lengthening of the tendon may be percutaneous for superficial structures or through a larger incision (open lengthening) for more extensive procedures. The cut tendon heals in its newly lengthened state, achieving ultimate strength between 6 and 12 months after the procedure. Typically, orthoses are used to protect the tendon from overlengthening until the healing process is complete. However, braces may be used beyond the protective postoperative period as well.

#### Bone and Joint Surgery

Reduction of dislocated joints often is important in the management of children with neuromuscular disorders to reduce pain or improve biomechanics. Joint subluxation or dislocation is common in neuromuscular disorders. For example, the incidence of hip displacement in patients with cerebral palsy is approximately 35%. Correction usually is achieved by osteotomy, which involves cutting and reorienting the bones on either side of the joint. Redirectional osteotomies are performed in the pelvis to increase the femoral head coverage by the acetabulum. Rotational osteotomies realign segments of bone to allow for a more functional position. For example, patients with an intoeing deformity resulting from excessive anteversion may undergo a "derotational" femoral osteotomy to realign the foot in an improved forward position rather than an internally rotated position.

Arthrodesis or surgical fusion of a joint may be required for severe pain, instability, or deformity. Triple arthrodesis of the foot (specifically the talocalcaneal, talonavicular, and calcaneocuboid joints) is performed on rare occasion in individuals with cerebral palsy or Charcot-Marie-Tooth disease. Fusion typically is achieved with placement of internal fixation hardware and bone graft to encourage bony union.

## SPECIFIC CONDITIONS

### MYELODYSPLASIA

Myelodysplasia, a congenital condition, is discussed in Chapter 213. Briefly, myelodysplasia is a broad spectrum of abnormalities resulting from incomplete closure of the neural tubes during the fourth week of embryogenesis. Although myelodysplasia remains the most common neural-tube defect, its incidence has decreased over the last 2 decades due to recommendations for folic acid supplementation and prenatal screening. Myelodysplasia is associated with a variety of congenital spinal deformities and acquired musculoskeletal deformities including scoliosis, kyphosis, clubfoot, and hip dislocations. The presence of potentially complex medical comorbidities, including hydrocephalus, renal anomalies, and syringomyelia, necessitates a multidisciplinary approach to care. Depending on the level in which the vertebral defect occurs, patients present with a spectrum of both motor and sensory issues ranging from weakness to paralysis and bowel/bladder incontinence.

The level of myelodysplasia is defined by the most caudal functioning nerve root. Patients with lesions in the thoracic region have absent quadriceps function and require orthoses for positioning and a wheelchair for mobility. Some individuals with high lumbar lesions may have limited ambulation with extensive orthoses but usually rely on wheelchairs for mobility as well. Patients with involvement of the low lumbar levels retain function of their quadriceps but lack strength in the gluteus musculature. A majority maintain a reasonable degree of ambulation. An individual with a lesion in the sacral region has the most favorable prognosis of achieving a sustainable gait, although the lack of distal motor innervation and protective plantar sensation may lead to foot deformity and problematic ulcerations.

Treatment of patients with myelodysplasia begins with neurosurgical closure of the defect in the perinatal period. Orthopedic intervention should be considered when the child is ready to begin weight bearing. Almost all patients with spina bifida above the sacral level will require some form of orthoses for ambulatory assistance. HKAFOs or reciprocating gait orthoses (RGOs) are frequently used in patients with thoracic or lumbar level lesions. Knee-ankle-foot orthoses (KAFOs) may be used in patients with mid-lumbar lesions who require knee-extension support due to weak or absent quadriceps muscle function. AFOs may be of benefit for individuals with low lumbosacral spina bifida who have comparatively better lower extremity strength and function but lack ankle dorsiflexion and/or plantarflexion function.

Hip dislocations are commonly seen in this population; however, there remains a debate regarding management and the approach to reduction. Recent studies have highlighted the importance of emphasizing functionality when considering treatment, and surgical reduction has not conclusively been shown to correlate with improved ambulation.

Spinal deformity is common in patients with myelodysplasia. Scoliosis can result from congenital malformations of the vertebrae in young children but more commonly occurs in later childhood or adolescence as a result of neuromuscular weakness. The latter presents as a long sweeping curve with pelvic obliquity and is more common in patients with proximal-level spinal lesions. Bracing may be useful in young children with flexible curves to maintain posture as a temporary measure, but anterior and posterior spinal fusion with instrumentation is the treatment of choice for larger curves.

Kyphosis may be present in very young children with thoracic-level spina bifida. Sharp angular kyphosis can interfere with the ability to sit comfortably in a wheelchair and may lead to chronic skin breakdown over the spine, with subsequent infection. Surgical treatment, typically kyphectomy, is technically challenging. See Chapter 213 for further discussion.

### CEREBRAL PALSY

Cerebral palsy (CP) is the most common neuromuscular disorder seen in children. It is defined as a nonprogressive (static) encephalopathy resulting from injury, ischemia, or infection of the brain in the perinatal period until 2 years of life. Cerebral palsy is discussed in detail in Chapter 547. It is important to note that whereas the neurologic damage is considered static, the condition may be progressive from an orthopedic standpoint as the pediatric musculoskeletal system develops. As with most neuromuscular conditions, a multidisciplinary approach to care is essential. CP often is accompanied by medical comorbidities such as intellectual disability, seizures, visual impairment, autonomic dysfunction, or bladder incontinence.

CP can be classified by the movement disorder present or by the severity of involvement of an affected area of the body. The functional status of the patient can be qualified by the Gross Motor Function Classification System (GMFCS), as described in Table 217-2. Spasticity is the most common single movement disorder in patients with cerebral palsy, although a mixed motor deficit usually is present.

**TABLE 217-2 GROSS MOTOR FUNCTION CLASSIFICATION SYSTEM (GMFCS) FOR CEREBRAL PALSY**

| | |
|---|---|
| Level I | Ambulatory patients who walk without restrictions, but may have issues with advanced motor skills, balance, and coordination. |
| Level II | Ambulatory patients who may have difficulty walking in outdoors and likely experience limitations with advanced gross motor tasks. May use orthoses for stability and support. |
| Level III | Patients who use assistive devices for mobility such as crutches or a walker and have limitations walking outdoors and in the community. |
| Level IV | Patients who rely on wheelchairs, powered mobility, or physical assistance in most settings. Self-mobility is limited to short distances. |
| Level V | Patients who are completely dependent on others for care and mobility, even with the use of assistive technology. |

Spasticity is defined as increased tone that is exacerbated by increasing the velocity of movement of a given limb. The muscle imbalance results in limited range of motion in the extremities and can lead to contractures. Dystonia, increased muscle tone that is not velocity dependent, may also be seen in this population, whereas ataxia is relatively rare.

The geographic classification of CP describes the area of the body affected. *Spastic hemiplegia* is defined as ipsilateral upper and lower extremity involvement, with the upper limb typically more severely involved. A patient with *spastic diplegia* has bilateral lower extremity involvement, with abnormalities seen to a lesser extent in the upper extremities. *Spastic quadriplegia* describes a patient who has upper and lower extremity involvement. Patients with spastic quadriplegia often have poor trunk and head control.

The cognitive level of the child is not always related to the severity of spasticity or geographic classification and must be kept in mind when considering treatment. Function for an intellectually normal individual with spastic quadriplegia is equally important to that of an individual with spastic diplagia, although achieved in a different fashion.

Orthopedic treatment in the ambulatory child typically begins with early physical therapy and the prescription of orthoses. The use of intramuscular botulinum toxin can be an effective therapeutic intervention for young children with CP. The toxin causes selective and reversible chemodenervation at the neuromuscular junction, which can subsequently improve ambulatory status, range of motion, and tone. It is used frequently in the treatment of ankle equinus due to gastroc-soleus spasticity in young children who walk on their toes. As the patient's skeletal system grows, the imbalanced muscle forces acting across the growth plates and joints cause an increased incidence of contractures and joint deformities.

Baclofen, a γ-aminobutyric acid (GABA) agonist, is another important pharmacologic agent in the management of CP, particularly for patients with impaired gait and significant spasticity limiting function. Because of the short half-life, the drug is administered through an intrathecal catheter via an implanted pump that can be electronically modulated for proper dosing. This therapy has been shown to effectively reduce tone and spasticity.

Surgery is considered a salvage procedure for the child with musculoskeletal deformities and contractures that interfere with functional activities or positioning. Common surgeries performed in patients with CP include Achilles tendon or gastrocnemius fascial lengthening for ankle equinus, hamstring lengthening for excessive knee flexion, and hip flexor lengthening or adductor release. Rotational osteotomies are considered in children to improve alignment, by repositioning the foot in the same direction as the patient is walking (foot-progression angle). Foot surgery may be useful in providing a stable plantigrade walking surface and is composed of both tendon transfers, osteotomies, and on rare occasions, arthrodesis. Gait analysis may aid in guiding proper surgical management for ambulatory children but is not available in all centers providing care.

Hip subluxation and dislocation are frequently seen in patients with extensive neurologic impairment who are nonambulatory, with an approximated incidence of 90% for children who are classified as GMFCS level V. Treatment may consist of both nonoperative (analgesia, antispasticity medications) and operative measures including adductor tendon release and femoral or pelvic osteotomy, all in an effort to remedy pain, restore range of motion, or reduce instability. Bilateral surgery often is performed in cases of contralateral subluxation. Recurrent hip subluxation is not infrequent in the years following surgical treatment, particularly in patients who do not have adequate control of their spasticity.

Scoliosis is another important consideration in patients with CP, with the overall incidence estimated at 25% and approaching 75% in individuals with near total-body involvement and poor trunk control. Bracing typically is ineffective in preventing progression of the curve in CP, likely secondary to the combination of spasticity preventing comfortable brace wear and the residual muscular imbalance. In young, skeletally immature patients with adequate spasticity control, bracing may be considered as a temporary measure. Wheelchair modifications are frequently employed to provide an improved sitting position. When surgery is required, fusion of the entire spine from the second thoracic vertebra to the pelvis is most effective in obtaining correction of sitting balance. Medical complications are encountered frequently following both hip and spine surgery in this high-risk population. Please see Chapter 213 for further discussion.

## MUSCULAR DYSTROPHY

A variety of different myopathies and muscular dystrophies are discussed in more detail in Chapters 563. Duchenne muscular dystrophy (DMD) is an X-linked recessive condition that arises from a mutation in the dystrophin gene and will serve as the index condition for general treatment guidelines across the other dystrophies.

Patients with DMD typically present with complaints of weakness, abnormal gait, toe-walking, or clumsiness. The age at which DMD patients begin to walk is only slightly delayed. Symptoms are rarely apparent until age 3 to 5 years, but, unfortunately are progressive and eventually lead to the loss of ambulation and ultimately death.

Physical examination reveals proximal muscle weakness, classically exhibited by the Gower maneuver in which the child is unable to rise from a seated position on the floor without the assistance of their arms to "walk up" the legs and achieve extension of the hips. Pseudohypertrophy of the gastroc-soleus complex can be seen and represents replacement of normal muscle with fibrofatty tissue. Limited ankle dorsiflexion frequently is present.

Serum creatine phosphokinase (CPK) is markedly elevated in patients with DMD. Diagnosis by DNA analysis for mutations in the dystrophin gene is confirmatory in approximately 80% of individuals. Muscle biopsy with dystrophin analysis may be pursued for patients in whom mutations are not identified or to rule out other forms of muscular dystrophy.

Orthopedic interventions include both nonoperative bracing and surgical management of the contractures that develop due to DMD. Commonly, operative lengthening of the Achilles tendon and release or tendon transfer of the posterior tibialis to maintain a shoeable foot are performed. Correction of hip and knee contractures is indicated in a small subset of patients to aid or prolong ambulatory function. Historically, most patients ultimately lost walking ability between 10 and 12 years old, necessitating transition to a wheelchair or other ambulatory device. However, the use of glucocorticoids from the time of diagnosis has considerably prolonged ambulation ability in patients.

Scoliosis is a common problem in this disorder, developing in as many as 90% of individuals who do not receive steroid treatment. Early spinal fusion when the curve reaches 30 degrees often is considered to avoid pulmonary complications with disease progression and enable the patient to sit comfortably. Studies have demonstrated promising results with glucocorticoid treatment in delaying motor regression and substantially reducing the incidence of scoliosis. It is important to be aware of increased fracture frequency in patients following long-term therapy.

## ARTHROGRYPOSIS

Congenital contractures are divided into those that affect only 1 joint (isolated) versus those that are present in 2 or more body parts. Arthrogryposis describes the latter and is a term used to indicate the presence of multiple contractures in multiple areas of the body. It is not a specific diagnosis but rather a clinical finding characteristic of more than 300 different disorders. Arthrogryposis is further classified based on the presence or absence of neurologic abnormalities or by anomalies aside from those in the musculoskeletal system.

Many patients with arthrogryposis have a history of decreased fetal movement or restricted intrauterine space that alters the development of joints and results in abnormal connective tissue deposition. Maternal comorbidities such a diabetes, multiple sclerosis, myotonic dystrophy, or myasthenia gravis may also contribute to arthrogryposis. An underlying neurologic etiology is implicated in approximately 70% to 80% of all patients, and approximately 50% of infants who have central nervous system dysfunction along with the joint contractures do not survive beyond their first year. Patients with other causes of arthrogryposis can have a normal life span.

Common subtypes of arthrogryposis include amyoplasia (most common), distal arthrogryposis, and syndromic or neuropathic arthrogryposis. Clinical findings vary and are dependent on the subtype. Amyoplasia is classically characterized by symmetrical upper and lower extremity deformities including internal rotation of the shoulders, flexed wrists, hip dislocations, and clubfoot anomalies. A characteristic midfacial hemangioma often is described, and the extremities appear thin and tapered due to lack of muscle development. Distal arthrogryposes by definition involve the distal extremities (ie, hands and feet) and present without underlying neurologic pathology. A spectrum of deformities of the hand or contractures of the foot may be observed. In the neuropathic form of arthrogryposis, failure of anterior horn cell development in the spinal cord leads to a lack of normal musculature. The extremities do not move due to the resulting weakness and fibrosis of the joints that occurs. Scoliosis accompanies 10% to 30% of cases.

Nonsurgical treatment of musculoskeletal deformities typically is limited in patients with arthrogryposis, although both bracing and physical therapy play a role in individual circumstances. Surgical intervention for lower extremity contractures should be explored if the patient has eventual potential for ambulation, for instance, knee contractures in patients who are able to demonstrate quadriceps muscle activity. Early operative reduction of hip dislocations and correction of clubfoot at standing age are recommended.

Treatment of the upper extremity contractures is guided by the functional needs of the child. Release of elbow extension contractures or triceps tendon transfers can assist the child in self-feeding. In addition, wrist carpectomy or fusion can place the hand in a more functional orientation. Intensive orthopedic efforts, both operative and nonoperative, that optimize joint mobility, strength, and positioning are of great potential benefit for patients, with as many as 85% of affected individuals able to ambulate or perform their activities of daily living following care.

## SUGGESTED READINGS


Bamshad M, Van Heest AE, Pleasure D. Arthrogryposis: a review and update. *J Bone Joint Surg Am*. 2009;91(suppl 4):40-46.

Bushby K, Finkel R, Birnkrant D, et al. Diagnosis and management of Duchenne muscular dystrophy, part 1: diagnosis, and pharmacological and psychosocial management. *Lancet Neurol.* 2010;9:77-93.

Bushby K, Finkel R, Birnkrant D, et al. Diagnosis and management of Duchenne muscular dystrophy, part 2: implementation of multidisciplinary care. *Lancet Neurol.* 2010;9:177-189.

Chambers HG. Update of neuromuscular disorders in pediatric orthopaedics: Duchenne muscular dystrophy, myelomeningocele, and cerebral palsy. *J Pediatr Orthop*. 2014;34:S44-S48.

Ferguson J, Wainwright A. Arthrogryposis. *Orthopaed Trauma*. 2013;27(3): 171-180.

Koman LA, Smith BP, Shilt JS. Cerebral palsy. *Lancet*. 2004;363: 1619-1631.

Liptak GS, Dosa NP. Myelomeningocele. *Pediatr Rev*. 2010;31(11): 443-450.

Palisano R, Rosenbaum P, Walter S, Russell D, Wood E, Galuppi B. Development and reliability of a system to classify gross motor function in children with cerebral palsy. *Dev Med Child Neurol.* 1997;39:214-223.

Swaroop VT, Dias L. Orthopaedic management of spina bifida—part II: foot and ankle deformities. *J Child Orthop*. 2011;5:403-414.

Swaroop VT, Dias L. Orthopedic management of spina bifida—part I: hip, knee, and rotational deformities. *J Child Orthop*. 2009;3:441-449.




# 218 Common Orthopedic Misses

Dorothy Y. Harris and John A. Herring

## INTRODUCTION

This chapter is designed to alert the pediatric practitioner to common conditions that are frequently missed in primary care practice. These conditions are those in which an early diagnosis can prevent long-term future problems. Although they are mentioned elsewhere in this text, an awareness of the diagnostic features of these conditions gives primary care persons the ability to prevent the complications that occur as the disorders progress. Thus, they are specifically considered in this chapter.

## LOWER EXTREMITY "MISSES"

### Slipped Capital Femoral Epiphysis

Slipped capital femoral epiphysis should be suspected when an obese teenager with an outturned foot limps into the office complaining of knee pain. Although hip and groin pain may be present, knee pain is quite common. Anteroposterior (AP) and frog-lateral radiographs of the pelvis show characteristic changes (Fig. 218-1A and B). The patient should be made weight-bearing immediately to avoid sudden, drastic slipping of the femoral head and referred urgently for surgical stabilization.

### Developmental Dislocation of the Hip

The diagnosis of developmental dislocation of the hip is sometimes missed in pediatric practice. The examiner must try to feel the hip move in and out of the joint with delicate pressure over the knee and greater trochanter. Sometimes it is easy to feel it, and at other times, the finding is missed or not there at all. The exam is hard to teach because the babies with this finding are few. Consequently, the examiner must have a high index of suspicion based on the presence of known risk factors. Ultrasound examination and orthopedic referral are appropriate for babies with breech presentation, especially females, for those with a positive family history, for firstborn girls, and for any infant with abnormal exam findings. For further information, see Chapter 212.

### Adolescent Septic Knee

Septic arthritis of the knee in adolescence can be subacute with subtle physical findings and grave consequences. Patients may present with mild pain and swelling, low-grade fever, and history of recent infection treated with antibiotics. Aspiration of joint fluid may show only moderate leukocytosis, and cultures may be negative, especially if antibiotics have been given. Joint lavage or drainage and appropriate antibiotic treatment, beginning with intravenous dosage and transitioning to oral medications after clinical response, are the treatments of choice. Failure to treat may result in serious loss of joint function. For further information, see Chapter 211.

### Cozen Fracture

The Cozen fracture is a proximal tibia fracture with minimal displacement in a young child (Fig. 218-2A). As the fracture heals, the leg grows fairly rapidly into a valgus or knock-knee alignment (Fig. 218-2B). The parent returns alarmed 3 or 4 months after the cast is removed, wondering what happened. Fortunately, most of these alignments correct spontaneously, and if the family is forewarned at the time of injury, there is much less distress for all concerned.

### Tumors

Bone tumors are rare. They usually present with persistent pain and often produce night pain and enlargement of the extremity. Radiographic examination for unusually persistent complaints of knee pain or thigh pain enables an earlier diagnosis. Bilateral leg pain at night is typical of growing pains, whatever that entity is, and usually

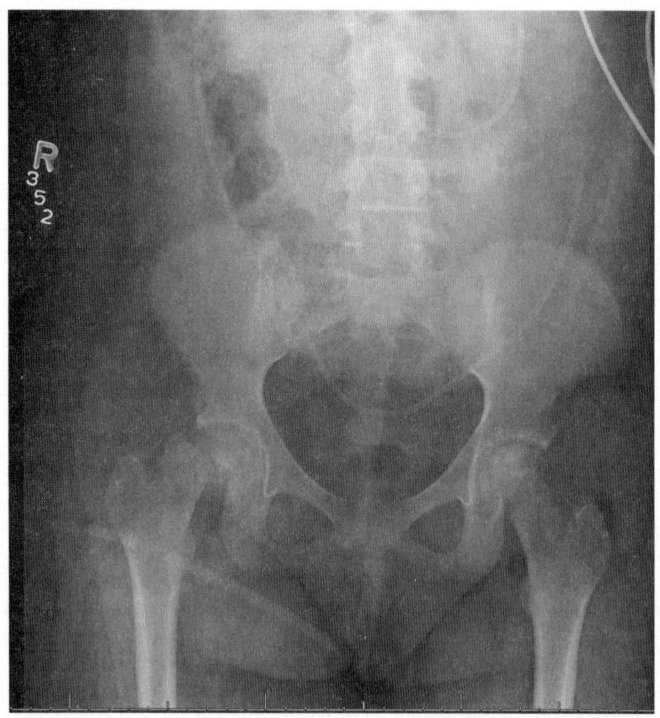


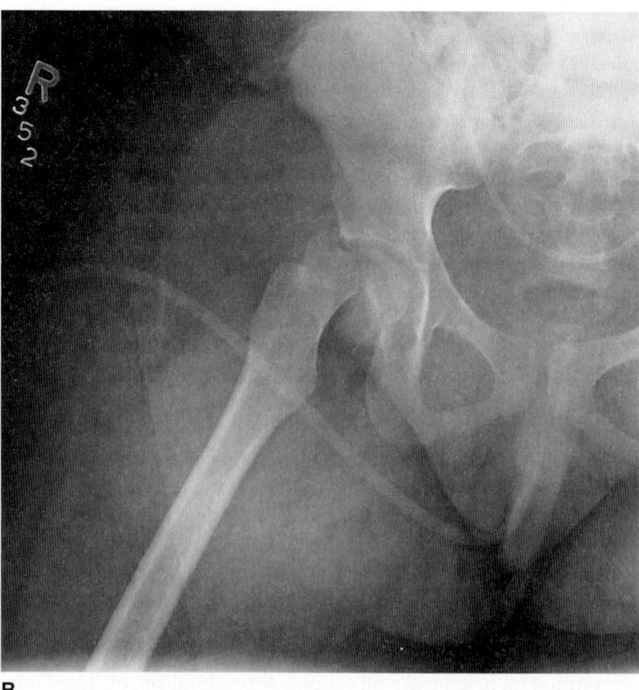


A B

**FIGURE 218-1** **A and B:** Right slipped capital femoral epiphysis. Note the malposition of the femoral head on the metaphysis.



does not require radiographs or referral. For further information, see Chapter 216.

## UPPER EXTREMITY "MISSES"

### Missed Monteggia Fracture

The Monteggia fracture is a fracture or even a deformation of the ulna, which results in dislocation of the radial head at the elbow (Fig. 218-3). At times, the ulnar fracture is not severely displaced, and it is easy to overlook the finding of a radial head that does not line up with the capitellum. The diagnosis is made by making certain that a line along the radius intersects the capitellum on all views of the elbow. Acutely, it is easily treated, but late presentation may require major surgery and the outcome may be compromised.

### Missed Lateral Condyle Fracture of the Elbow

The lateral condyle fracture is easily missed at the elbow. It appears as a tiny crescent of bone slightly displaced from the distal humerus

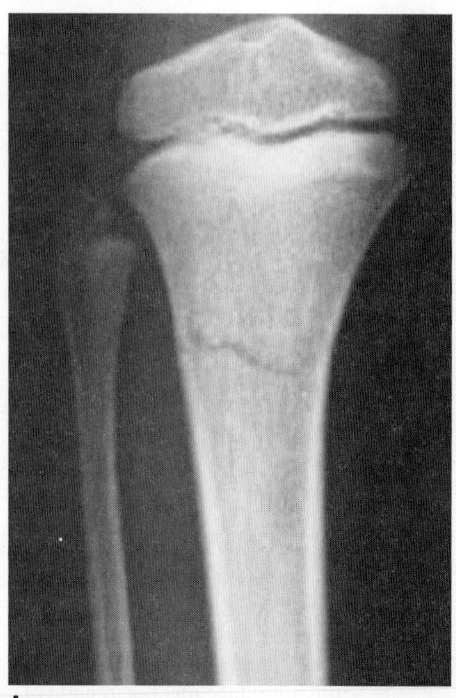

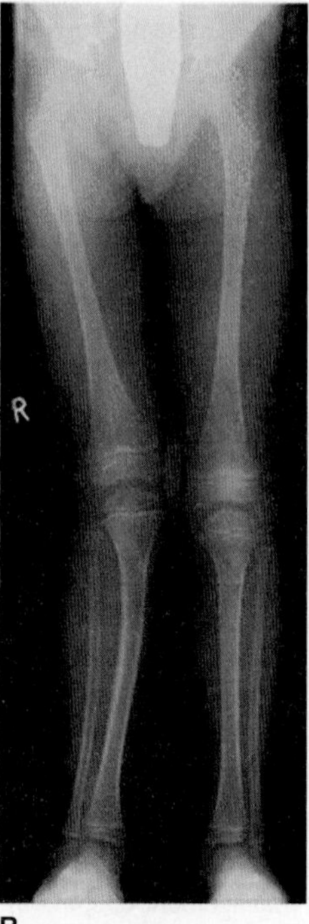


A B

**FIGURE 218-2** Cozen fracture. **A:** There is a minimally displaced fracture of the proximal tibia on the right. **B:** The fracture has healed, and the tibia has grown into a marked valgus alignment. It will usually self-correct but requires orthopedic attention.

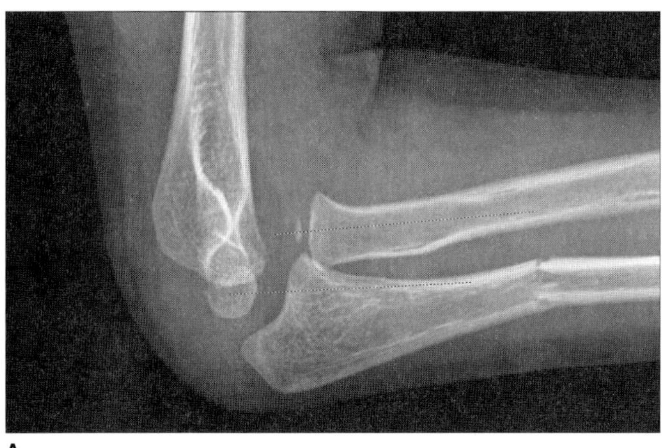

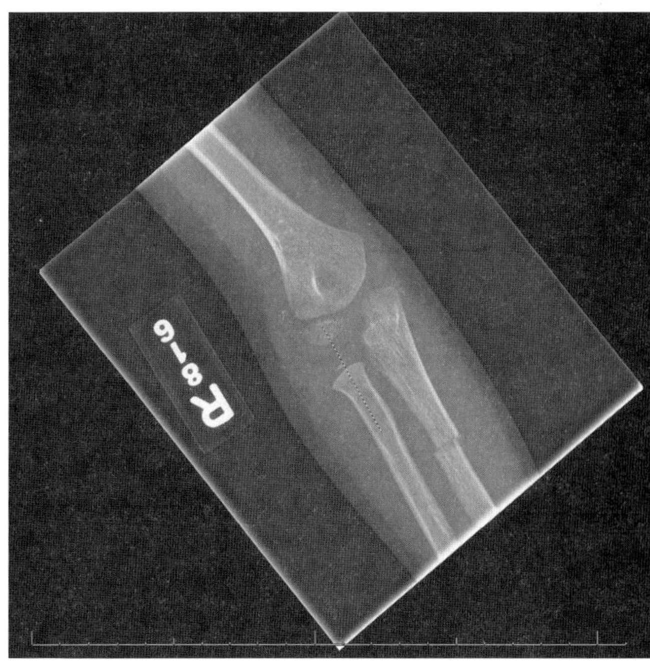


A B

FIGURE 218-3 A: Lateral view of right elbow showing mildly angulated fracture of the ulna and anterior radial head subluxation with disruption of radiocapitellar line. B: Anteroposterior view of right elbow showing ulna fracture and minimal disruption of radiocapitellar line.

in the young child (Fig. 218-4). The elbow will be swollen and tender laterally. This injury requires surgical stabilization to prevent later displacement and deformity.

## SPINE "MISSES"

### Screening for Scoliosis

Screening for scoliosis, a seemingly simple procedure, is fraught with pitfalls. Patients with slight shoulder asymmetry, mild discrepancy in length of legs, and tiny curves need no treatment and are subjected to unnecessary anxiety by the referral process. Heavy patients may show mild asymmetry and hide fairly large curves that do require treatment. Because scoliosis progresses with growth, mild curves in postmenarchal girls and mature boys have little potential to progress, but mild curves in young children have significant potential to do so. For further information, see Chapter 213.

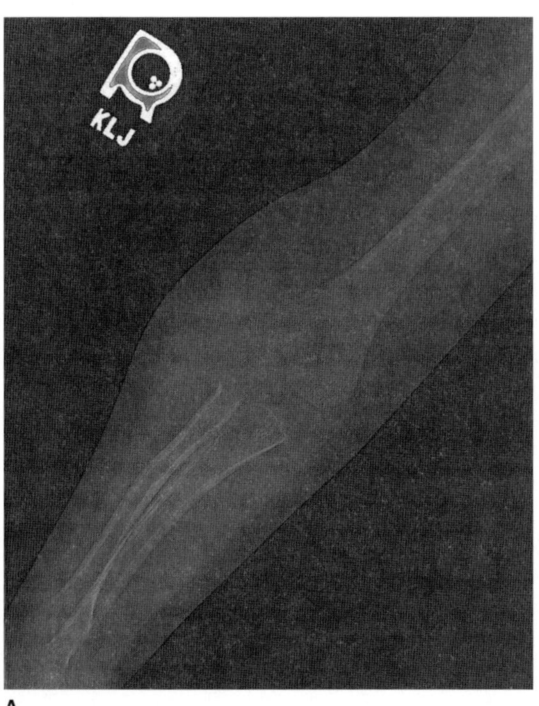


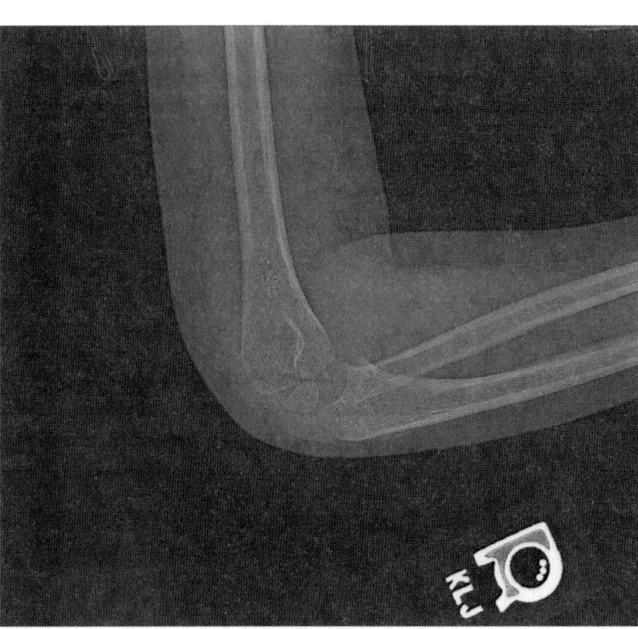


A B

FIGURE 218-4 A: Anteroposterior view of right elbow with fracture of the lateral condyle; note small crescent fragment. B: Oblique view of right elbow with improved visualization of lateral condyle fracture.

Georgiadis AG, Zaltz I. Slipped capital femoral epiphysis: how to evaluate with a review and update of treatment. *Pediatr Clin North Am*. 2014;61(6):1119-1135.

Herring JA, ed. *Tachdjian's Pediatric Orthopaedics*. Vol. 5. Philadelphia, PA: Saunders/Elsevier; 2014

Mooney JE, Hennrikus WL. Fractures of the shaft of the tibia and fibula. In: Flynn JM, Skaggs DL, Waters PM, eds. *Rockwood and Wilkins' Fractures in Children*. 8th ed. Philadelphia, PA: Wolters Kluwer Health; 2015:1137-1172.

Mulpuri K, Song KM, Goldberg MJ, et al. Detection and nonoperative management of pediatric developmental dysplasia of the hip in infants up to six months of age. *J Am Acad Orthop Surg*. 2015;23(3):202-205.

Tejwani N, Phillips D, Goldstein RY. Management of lateral humeral condyle fractures in children. *J Am Acad Orthop Surg*. 2011;19(6):350-358.

Tuten HR, Keeler KA, Gabos PG, Zionts LE, Mackenzie WG. Post-traumatic tibia valga in children; a long-term follow-up note. *J Bone Joint Surg*. 1999;81:799-810.

# PART 1 PRINCIPLES OF INFECTIOUS DISEASE

## 219 Bacteremia, Sepsis, and Septic Shock

Stephanie H. Stovall and Michelle A. Hoffman

### INTRODUCTION

Definitions of sepsis over the last 2 decades have changed multiple times as they relate to adult critical care. The definition of sepsis and sepsis syndromes in pediatric patients has been less well defined. The most recent published consensus definitions of sepsis in pediatric patients were published in 2005. These definitions were modeled after the adult definition and consensus guidelines published first in 1991 and then revised in 2001, 2008, 2012, and, most recently, 2016. The biggest change in adult consensus definitions occurred in the 2016 publication, which discarded systemic inflammatory response syndrome (SIRS) and severe sepsis; however, pediatric definitions continue to use these terms.

Based on the 2005 guidelines for pediatrics, SIRS requires both abnormal temperature and abnormal leukocyte count or 1 of those plus either tachypnea (> 2 standard deviations [SDs] above the mean for age) or abnormal heart rate (> 2 SDs above the mean for age or under the 10th percentile for age for those < 1 year old) without other explanation. Sepsis is defined as SIRS plus proven or suspected infection (bacteria, virus, fungus, or rickettsia). Severe sepsis is defined as sepsis plus dysfunction of at least 2 organs, acute respiratory distress syndrome, or cardiovascular dysfunction. Septic shock is sepsis plus cardiovascular dysfunction. The most recent adult definitions include sepsis, as defined previously with introduction of the use of sepsis-related organ failure assessment (SOFA) score, and septic shock requiring vasopressors despite appropriate fluid resuscitation and elevated lactate. It is likely that the definitions of pediatric sepsis will be reevaluated in light of the recent changes in adult practice.

### PATHOGENESIS AND EPIDEMIOLOGY

The development of SIRS, sepsis, severe sepsis, and septic shock in the pediatric patient depends on a complex series of interrelated factors that include: host factors such as age, immunologic competence including vaccination status, comorbid conditions (including the presence of foreign material such as a central vascular, urinary, peritoneal, or intraventricular catheter), exposures (such as travel or day care), host response, site of entry of the infectious agent, and invading organism factors (including inoculum, virulence factors, and toxin production).

Central to the definition of sepsis is organ dysfunction as a result of infection. A variety of barriers, such as the skin and mucous membranes, serve as the first line that is breached at the beginning of the continuum of sepsis. After that breach, a series of events, first triggered by the innate immune response recognizing pathogen-associated molecular patterns (PAMPs) on the surface of invading organisms, starts the sepsis cascade by triggering release of cytokines and also awakening of the adaptive immune response, which is relatively slow because the adaptive immune response requires maturation and proliferation. This release triggers a systemic reaction to even a localized invasion, which ultimately results in loss of vascular integrity, apoptosis of immune cells, and reduced perfusion of vital organs. Clinically, this is evidenced by low blood pressure, cyanosis, delayed capillary refill, reduced urine output, and alterations in mental status.

Bacteremia may or may not be associated with a specific focus of infection. It may result from the extension of an infection originating elsewhere (eg, genitourinary, gastrointestinal, upper or lower respiratory tracts, or skin and soft tissue), or it may result in infection at other sites (eg, endocarditis, meningitis, facial cellulitis, osteomyelitis, pyelonephritis, or peritonitis). Recurrent or persistent bacteremia may result from established infectious foci (eg, endocarditis, abscess, or foreign body).

The epidemiology of pediatric sepsis is not well described globally and varies significantly between geographic regions in part due to environmental conditions, poor nutrition and vaccine use, and limited access to care. Globally, however, it is a significant cause of infant and child mortality. In the United States, it is a less common occurrence and cause of death. The most recently available National Vital Statistics report, from the year 2014, showed that sepsis was the seventh leading cause of death in the first year of life and the tenth leading cause of death in children age 1 to 19 years (this does not include sepsis deaths that were coded for other diagnoses such as deaths caused by influenza and pneumonia, which was the sixth leading cause of death in the first year of life and the seventh leading cause of death in children age 1–19 years).

The prevalence of sepsis in hospitalized patients increased significantly in the past 20 years, attributable mainly to an increase in the prevalence of sepsis in neonates, particularly those with a very low birth weight (VLBW; < 1500 g); in some studies, the diagnosis of sepsis accounted for more than 25% of admissions to high-acuity units, with an associated mortality approaching 10%. A review of severe sepsis in 43 US children's hospitals between 2004 and 2012 found an increasing prevalence of severe sepsis of 7.7% overall and an associated mortality rate of 14.4% with a significant reduction in mortality from 18.9% in 2004 to 12% in 2012.

In term newborns, culture-proven early-onset sepsis (EOS; < 7 days old) occurs in approximately 0.77 to 1 neonate per 1000 live births, with a case fatality rate of 10.9%. Overall, among preterm infants, the highest rates of EOS were found in black preterm infants, at 5.14 per 1000 live births with a case fatality rate of 24.4%. VLBW premature infants have an increased incidence of EOS; for those weighing < 1000 g, the incidence is estimated to be 26 per 1000 live births. In EOS, bacteremia typically results from colonization and subsequent invasion by organisms acquired from the maternal genital tract.

The most common bacterial agents of neonatal sepsis are *Streptococcus agalactiae* (group B *Streptococcus* [GBS]) and *Escherichia coli*; the 2 bacteria combined account for approximately 70% of infections. Additional organisms include viridans group streptococci, *Staphylococcus aureus, Haemophilus influenzae* (typically nontypeable since the introduction of the *H influenzae* type b [Hib] conjugate vaccine), *Enterococcus* species, *Listeria monocytogenes,* and other gram-negative enteric bacilli. Nonbacterial causes of neonatal sepsis include herpes simplex viruses, which affect between 12 and 60 per 100,000 live births; and enteroviruses or parechoviruses, which infect about 13% of babies < 29 days of age, nearly 20% of whom are readmitted.

Once beyond the newborn period, *Streptococcus pneumoniae, Neisseria meningitidis, S aureus, Streptococcus pyogenes* (group A streptococcus [GAS]), and *Salmonella* species are the most common bacteria causing community-acquired sepsis in the normal infant and child. Immunocompetent children with bacteremia must be evaluated for a source of the bacteremia. Such sources may include pneumonia (*S pneumoniae, S aureus,* GAS), gastroenteritis (*Salmonella* species), pyelonephritis (*E coli, Klebsiella pneumoniae*), salpingitis (*Neisseria gonorrhoeae*), and cutaneous or osteoarticular infections (*S aureus,* GAS).

In immunocompromised children without foreign bodies, endogenous sources, such as the gastrointestinal tract, become important causes of bloodstream infections commonly caused by Enterobacteriaceae, *Enterococcus* species, and *Candida* species. Different immunodeficiencies predispose patients to different pathogens causing sepsis: children with agammaglobulinemia are at higher risk of pneumococcal and Hib sepsis; children with neutropenia are at higher risk for infections due to *Pseudomonas* species; children with (functional) asplenia have higher rates of pneumococcal and meningococcal disease; and children with terminal complement deficiency are prone to *Neisseria* infections.

Indwelling vascular lines, urinary catheters, and endotracheal tubes, as well as other foreign material, predispose newborns and children to nosocomial infections due to *S aureus*, coagulase-negative staphylococci (most commonly, *Staphylococcus epidermidis*), Enterobacteriaceae, *Enterococcus* species, fungi, and other less common opportunistic infections.

## CLINICAL FEATURES

Signs and symptoms of sepsis are highly variable in children, depending on many factors including the age of the patient, comorbid conditions, duration of illness, etiology, and host response to the infection. Because of the ability of the young, healthy heart to maintain significant tachycardia for sustained periods, children can increase their cardiac output to compensate for sepsis and maintain a normal blood pressure more easily than adults with sepsis. For this reason, children frequently do not exhibit the classic sign of hypotension until late in the course of sepsis. Physical exam findings of lethargy or agitation, cyanosis, delayed capillary refill, and reduced pulses are often found in children with sepsis; reduced urinary output and temperature dysregulation are also common. Cutaneous findings, such as petechiae and purpura, may be present in children with sepsis.

In the pediatric patient, specific attention must focus on evaluating the possibility of a localized site of infection. As an example, osteoarticular infections in children are common and can be difficult to recognize in young children. History from family members focusing on the use of extremities can be helpful in recognizing osteomyelitis or a septic joint. In infants, osteomyelitis may present with pseudoparalysis of a limb. In older children, the family may report that the child had a recent injury to a limb. Often, osteomyelitis in a septic child can be recognized by erythema, swelling, or tenderness over a long bone near the epiphysis. Likewise, in young children, the urinary tract can be a source of infection that leads to sepsis. Children who are not normally continent may not have typical signs of urinary tract infection, like dysuria or back pain. Past history of urinary tract infections can be a clue, and caregivers may report malodorous or discolored urine in the diaper. Another common source of infection that can precede sepsis in children is a recent viral respiratory tract infection. Children with secondary bacterial pneumonia after viral respiratory infection may present with splinting with respirations and lack of breath sounds on exam.

## DIAGNOSIS

Much effort has been expended to more rapidly recognize and treat sepsis. Studies have shown that rapid treatment of sepsis reduces morbidity and mortality. Scoring algorithms have been developed to characterize early sepsis. These are largely dependent on vital signs, which, of course, vary with the age of the child. In adult medicine, the abbreviated form of the SOFA score, called the quick SOFA, utilizes mental status, respiratory rate, and systolic blood pressure. This score is not easily transferrable to pediatrics due to differences in baseline mental status at various ages and the relative delay in hypotension as a clinical sign.

Laboratory methods to support or refute the diagnosis of sepsis are varied. Laboratory features may include hypoxemia, acidosis, renal insufficiency, leukopenia or leukocytosis, thrombocytopenia, and/or disseminated intravascular coagulopathy (DIC). Classically, certain inflammatory markers, such as C-reactive protein and erythrocyte sedimentation rate, have been utilized, but these have limitations due to their inherent lack of specificity in regard to infection, as both can be elevated in noninfectious illnesses such as burns, trauma, and ischemia-reperfusion injury. In 2012, the Surviving Sepsis Campaign identified serum lactate as an important biological marker of sepsis that could also be used to monitor response to therapy. Unfortunately, this marker is less reliable in children as many children with sepsis have normal lactate levels. Instead, utilizing vital signs, capillary refill, urine output, and cardiac index as markers for pediatric patients is recommended. Over 100 other markers have been considered, although none have become standard practice for diagnosis of sepsis due to their lack of availability and reliability. Some of these include proinflammatory proteins such as procalcitonin, endothelial proteins such as angiopoietins, cell surface markers like CD64, and cytokines such as interleukin-6 and -10. Certain immunomodulatory effects of sepsis, such as depletion of dendritic cells and upregulation of T regulatory lymphocytes, could also be evaluated, although cutoff values are not well established and measuring is not readily available in many institutions.

The gold standard for the diagnosis of bacterial sepsis is blood culture, although in some patients with sepsis, the offending organism may not be detected in blood. Evaluation of cerebrospinal fluid, urine, or other body fluids/sites should be performed as appropriate (eg, examination of the peripheral blood smear for evidence of splenic dysfunction [Howell-Jolly bodies] or DIC [fragmented red blood cells]). Prior administration of antibiotics to the patient (or the mother prior to birth of the neonate), the concentration of bacteria in the blood, and the amount of blood drawn can all affect the ability to isolate an organism from routine blood cultures. Inherent in the process of obtaining cultures are the delays associated with current culture systems. Even automated blood culture identification and susceptibility systems often require 24 hours at a minimum. Because of these issues, much effort has focused on utilizing molecular mechanisms to improve both the likelihood of determining the causative agent and the time to actionable diagnosis. Over the past few years, molecular-based platforms have been developed that utilize specific antimicrobial markers for identification in combination with specific known resistance markers (such as the *mecA* gene in methicillin-resistant *S aureus* [MRSA]). Newer methodologies, such as DNA microarray-based methods, are also being studied as alternatives to culture. In many instances, viral infections can also be diagnosed rapidly by molecular testing through detection of viral nucleic acids.

## TREATMENT

### Supportive Care

Supportive management of sepsis, severe sepsis, and septic shock is directed toward restoration of adequate tissue perfusion and maintenance of efficient respiratory function. In the Surviving Sepsis Campaign of 2012, recommendations for treatment of pediatric sepsis are delineated. The initial resuscitation phase requires providing oxygen and fluids and recognizing that young infants have poor functional residual capacity and may require early intubation, but also that they are at risk for worsening shock if volume-depleted when reduced venous return occurs after increased intrathoracic pressure from mechanical ventilation. Noninvasive ventilation is offered as an alternative when it is adequate for oxygenation and ventilation. The American College of Critical Care Medicine Pediatric Advanced Life Support guidelines should be followed including initial fluid resuscitation of up to 60 mL/kg (or beyond) of isotonic saline or colloid until improvement in perfusion or signs of fluid overload develop (eg, hepatomegaly or auscultation of rales in the lungs). Fluid-refractory shock requires administration of inotropic support rapidly, as delay in use of inotropic support has been associated with increased mortality. Hydrocortisone to treat adrenal insufficiency in the case of catecholamine-resistant shock should be considered early. During the initial resuscitation phase, glycemic stability should also be evaluated and corrected as needed. Hyperglycemia is defined as > 180 mg/dL. Extracorporeal membrane oxygenation (ECMO) should be considered in the pediatric patient with refractory shock or refractory respiratory failure and sepsis, as about 40% of pediatric patients (and 70% of newborns) with sepsis requiring ECMO for respiratory failure survive. Other measures such as mechanical ventilation with lung protective strategies, diuretics, and renal replacement therapy may also be considered to support the pediatric patient with sepsis.

#### Antimicrobial Therapy

Delayed delivery of appropriate antimicrobial therapy has been associated with increased mortality. Diagnostic cultures should be obtained as rapidly as possible, although antimicrobial therapy should not be delayed in order to obtain these cultures. The initial selection of empiric antimicrobial therapy for a child with bacteremia, sepsis, severe sepsis, or septic shock is dependent on many factors including the age of the patient, the patient's underlying immunologic and vaccination status, the patient's risk for nosocomial infection, the site of infection, likely pathogens, and local antibiotic resistance patterns.

In newborns with EOS, the combination of ampicillin plus gentamicin in standard dosages for gestational age has been the mainstay of therapy for infants with sepsis in the first week of life. With an increase in extended-spectrum β-lactamase (ESBL)-producing Enterobacteriaceae, monitoring of local antibiogram data is important as empiric therapies may need to be altered regionally. Currently in the United States, most neonatal *E coli* infections are susceptible to gentamicin. Addition of cefotaxime in the neonate with EOS and meningitis is encouraged. After the first week of life (late-onset sepsis), vancomycin should be considered in neonates with indwelling devices such as central venous catheters. In neonates with severe necrotizing enterocolitis, additional gram-negative coverage should be considered (as should anaerobic coverage) based on regional antibiogram data. In the infant 1 to 3 months of age, the age-specific pathogens include those found in neonates, as well as those found in older children. A third-generation cephalosporin is appropriate presumptive antibiotic coverage in these patients; if there are significant risk factors for *Listeria monocytogenes* or *Enterococcus* species (eg, complicated or recurrent urinary tract infection), ampicillin should be added, as should vancomycin in the case of meningitis.

In immunocompetent children older than 3 months, third-generation cephalosporins (cefotaxime or ceftriaxone) are standard empiric antibiotic regimens. With drug resistance now identified as a common problem in many areas, the use of vancomycin, plus cefotaxime or ceftriaxone, is standard therapy for life-threatening sepsis, sepsis with meningitis, patients predisposed to invasive pneumococcal disease, and any patient with a concurrent or recent soft tissue or osteoarticular focus or other cause of suspicion of MRSA infection. Once a bacterial etiology is confirmed and susceptibility results are available, targeted antimicrobial therapy should be used.

Immunocompromised children with neutropenia (eg, those receiving chemotherapy) should receive agents to cover the typical causes of sepsis for their age as well as targeting *Pseudomonas aeruginosa*. This can be accomplished with a third (ceftazidime) or fourth (cefepime) generation cephalosporin or a carbapenem (meropenem); if resistant gram-negative organisms are suspected, addition of an aminoglycoside should be considered. An intravascular catheter, other indwelling foreign material, skin and soft tissue infection, or mucositis should prompt additional coverage with vancomycin for gram-positive organisms such as *S aureus*, coagulase-negative staphylococci, α-hemolytic streptococci, or enterococci. In immunocompromised patients not responding to broad-spectrum antibacterial therapy, presumptive antifungal therapy should be considered. Indwelling devices (eg, intravascular catheters) should be removed if at all possible if they are the source of infection.

### SOURCE CONTROL AND ADJUNCTIVE THERAPIES

Sources of infection such as abscesses should be debrided and indwelling devices removed to decrease the microbial load. Patients should be evaluated carefully for discrete sites of infection, such as bones, joints, and pleural cavity.

The use of intravenous immunoglobulin (IVIG) for the prevention or treatment of sepsis has been controversial. At this time, there are no definitive data to support the use of IVIG in pediatric sepsis. Routine administration of IVIG for neonatal sepsis has not been shown to be beneficial and is not recommended. It is recommended that use of IVIG be considered for sepsis associated with toxic shock syndrome with refractory hypotension. The addition of clindamycin to β-lactam therapy in treatment of toxic shock syndrome has been shown to improve mortality due to its effect on decreasing toxin production by the bacteria.

Corticosteroid administration during sepsis has been studied extensively. Critical illness-related corticosteroid insufficiency (CIRCI) should be considered in the pediatric patient (as should classical adrenal insufficiency); however, routine administration of corticosteroids for pediatric sepsis is not recommended. Current recommendations include consideration of corticosteroid administration in pediatric patients with catecholamine-resistant septic shock and evidence of adrenal insufficiency.

The failure of other adjunctive therapies, directed at single mediators of the sepsis cascade (eg, antibodies directed against tumor necrosis factor), reiterates both the complex and multifactorial nature of sepsis. Further, such therapies are less well examined in the pediatric population.

Hemofiltration through continuous renal replacement therapy (CRRT) is not recommended in adult or pediatric sepsis guidelines. Plasmapheresis may play a role in certain situations; it has shown promising results in reversing DIC associated with sepsis in adults and in thrombocytopenia-associated multiorgan failure.

### PREVENTION

Although there are many preventive methods that are not specific for a particular microorganism (eg, simple hand washing), agents causing sepsis can be targeted individually to decrease the incidence of disease. This is true especially for vaccination against bacteria such as Hib, which is quite rare in immunized populations in developed countries. Likewise, after the widespread use of the pneumococcal conjugate vaccine, a significant decline in invasive pneumococcal disease has been noted. It is recommended that young children with sickle cell disease also receive daily penicillin prophylaxis as an additional protection against pneumococcal disease. Meningococcal disease is targeted with vaccination of high-risk groups including teenagers, (functionally) asplenic individuals, and those with terminal complement deficiency. Patients with agammaglobulinemia receive passive immunization via repeated infusions of IgG.

### SUGGESTED READINGS

Balamuth F, Weiss SL, Neuman MI, et al. Pediatric severe sepsis in US children's hospitals. *Pediatr Crit Care Med.* 2014;15:798-805.

Biron BM, Ayala A, Lomas-Neira JL. Biomarkers for sepsis: what is and what might be? *Biomark Insights.* 2015;10:7-17.

Bizzarro MJ, Shabanova V, Baltimore RS, Dembry LM, Ehrenkranz RA, Gallagher PG. Neonatal sepsis 2004-2013: the rise and fall of coagulase negative staphylococci. *J Pediatr.* 2015;166:1193-1199.

Dellinger RP, Levy MM, Rhodes A, et al. Surviving sepsis campaign: international guidelines for management of severe sepsis and septic shock, 2012. *Intensive Care Med.* 2013;39:165-228.

Hanna W, Wong HR. Pediatric sepsis: challenges and adjunctive therapies. *Crit Care Clin.* 2013;29:203-222.

Hartman ME, Linde-Zwirble WT, Angus DC, Watson RS. Trends in the epidemiology of pediatric severe sepsis. *Pediatr Crit Care Med.* 2013;14:686-693.

Randolph AG, McCulloh RJ. Pediatric sepsis: Important considerations for diagnosing and managing severe infections in infants, children and adolescents. *Virulence.* 2014;5:172-182.

Ruth A, McCracken CE, Fortenberrry JD, Hall M, Simon HK, Hebbar KB. Pediatric severe sepsis: current trends and outcomes from the pediatric health information systems database. *Pediatr Crit Care Med.* 2014;15:828-838.

Simonsen KA, Anderson-Berry AL, Delair SF, Davies HD. Early-onset neonatal sepsis. *Clin Micro Rev*. 2014;27:21-47.

Singer M, Deutschman CS, Seymour CW, et al. The third international concensus definitions for sepsis and septic shock. *JAMA*. 2016;315:801-810.



# 220 Infection Control and Prevention

Judith R. Campbell

## INTRODUCTION

Hospital infection control and prevention programs protect patients and healthcare providers from acquiring or transmitting infectious diseases. Through surveillance and reporting, healthcare-associated infections are identified, and policies and best practices are implemented to limit such infections. The Joint Commission and the Joint Commission International inspect hospitals and other healthcare delivery systems to ensure that appropriate infection control and prevention practices are being followed. Infection control is a major patient safety effort that involves all members of the healthcare team.

General principles of infection control and prevention should also be applied in outpatient settings. Although less is written about outpatient clinics, offices, and outpatient procedure and surgical centers, the practice of infection control remains an integral part of patient care in these settings. The goal is the same as for inpatients: protection of patients and healthcare personnel from acquiring and transmitting infectious diseases.

On a national level, the Occupational Safety and Health Administration (OSHA) is responsible for promoting a safe work environment. The OSHA bloodborne standards apply to hospitals and all other healthcare facilities. Another important federal agency is the National Institute for Occupational Safety and Health (NIOSH), which is responsible for conducting research and making recommendations for the prevention of work-related injury and illness.

## TRANSMISSION OF INFECTIOUS AGENTS

To practice effective infection control and prevention, one must understand the routes of transmission of infectious agents. The most common route of transmission is by contact with contaminated hands, body sites, or objects. Organisms are carried from the hands of one person to another and are frequently implicated in the transmission of bacteria, fungi, parasites, and viruses. Adequate hand hygiene removes most organisms transiently carried on the hands and thus is central to all infection prevention programs.

Some pathogens are aerosolized in small or large droplets. Small droplets can be carried by air currents, remain suspended, and infect persons at longer distances than large droplets, which require relatively close contact (within a few feet) in order for the droplet to move from one person to the next. Body fluids, such as oral and nasal secretions, vomitus, feces, or urine, may be common modes for transmission of microorganisms, both among children and between children and healthcare workers. Direct contact between children and caregivers transmits skin organisms such as bacteria, fungi, and mites.

A variety of fomites can be involved in the transmission of infectious agents. Stethoscopes, equipment, and toys have been cultured and shown to harbor pathogens. These pathogens then can be spread from the fomites to the hands of healthcare providers or body surfaces of patients. Most of the time, this does not result in disease; however, these fomites serve as potential reservoirs of pathogens.

Transmission of pathogens by food or water is rare in the healthcare setting; however, outbreaks related to contaminated foods, products, or medications have been reported. Intrinsic or extrinsic contamination of intravenous fluids, oral or tube feedings, and medications is an occasional cause of healthcare-associated infection. Vector-borne agents are rarely transmitted in the healthcare setting.

Surgical and medical procedures are associated with varying risk of infection depending on the disruption of cutaneous or mucosal barriers, thus allowing for inoculation of pathogens into body spaces. In general, the longer the surgical procedure, the greater is the risk for infection. Patients who require intensive care are at higher risk for infection because they stay in the hospital longer, are exposed to more invasive devices, and undergo more procedures. Infection rates vary from 1 to 3 per 100 discharges in those receiving care in non–intensive care unit settings, and from 30 to 50 per 100 discharges in newborn intensive care units.

Bloodborne pathogens are transmitted by transfusion of blood products or by inadvertent inoculation of blood from an infected person to an uninfected person. Organs that are transplanted may carry pathogens, usually viruses of the herpes family, particularly cytomegalovirus and Epstein-Barr virus. Tissues are used in a variety of procedures and are potential sources of bloodborne viruses such as hepatitis B, hepatitis C, human immunodeficiency virus, and human T-lymphotropic viruses.

Immunocompromised hosts are at risk for healthcare-associated infection, most often due to their own flora, which is altered after antibiotic exposure, increasing the risk for infection with resistant bacteria and fungi. The intestinal tract serves as a reservoir for pathogens including Enterobacteriaceae, *Clostridium difficile*, and *Candida* species.

The site and frequency of transmission will depend on the host and the pathogens in the environment. Hospitalized children may be exposed to other ill children in the hospital room, surgical or diagnostic imaging suites, hallways, and playrooms.

Infection rates in outpatients have not been extensively studied. In general, children who visit doctors' offices have had better outcomes and fewer infections than those who do not receive regular care. Nonetheless, the opportunity to acquire infection exists in the outpatient setting. The healthy child who comes for a routine office visit may be exposed to infectious agents while in the waiting room, during play with other patients, in the examination room, and during procedures.

## COMMON ETIOLOGIES AND MANIFESTATIONS

The most common cause of infection in the hospitalized child is viral illness, which is acquired from other patients, visitors, or hospital staff. Healthcare-associated respiratory infections are most common during the winter and are due to seasonal viruses such as influenza and respiratory syncytial virus. Patients who require respiratory support are at risk for bacterial pneumonia (see Chapter 235). Endotracheal and tracheostomy tubes bypass the normal body defenses. Tubes can occlude the orifices of the sinus ostia and eustachian tubes, increasing the risk for hospital-acquired sinusitis and otitis media. Certain medications may impair natural immune function.

Gastrointestinal infections acquired in healthcare settings typically occur after transfer of viruses or bacterial pathogens on hands or instruments or by ingestion of contaminated foods or medicines. Outbreaks of colitis due to *C difficile* and transmission of vancomycin-resistant *Enterococcus* have been traced to medical devices such as electronic thermometers. In these cases, the thermometer box becomes contaminated during use and allows spread of the pathogen from patient to patient. Children with rotavirus or norovirus infection may be asymptomatic; thus, any children hospitalized or visiting offices during the winter and spring may be shedding rotavirus or norovirus. These viruses are transmitted from child to child by the fecal-oral route and by the contaminated hands of caregivers.

Bacteremia is usually a complication of intravenous catheters and associated therapy; the site, duration of catheterization, and underlying condition of the patient are important factors determining the frequency of bacteremia (see Chapter 219). The convenience of intravascular catheters carries with it the concomitant risk of infection; in contrast to adults, in whom peripheral venous catheters are changed every 3 to 4 days, infants' limited vascular access often prevents routine rotation of sites. The risk of infection of peripheral or central venous catheters can be minimized by adhering to strict aseptic technique during catheter insertion and manipulation of the catheter. Entry into the system should be minimized. The most common pathogens are those colonizing the skin of the patient or caregiver: *Staphylococcus epidermidis* and other coagulase-negative staphylococci and *Staphylococcus aureus.* The skin of the groin and damaged skin (burns or eczema) are colonized by gram-negative rods such as *Escherichia coli, Klebsiella* species, and *Pseudomonas* species, increasing the risk of such infections when these sites are used.

Healthcare-associated urinary tract infections occur in patients who are catheterized and in those with obstruction to urine flow. Catheterization to obtain urine for analysis or culture carries with it a 1% risk of subsequent infection. Indwelling urinary catheterization is complicated by infection at a rate of 3% to 5% per day, and all long-term indwelling urinary catheters become colonized with bacteria. Infection of the lower urinary tract can be complicated by spread to the kidneys and bloodstream. Common causes of infection in the urinary tract include those organisms colonizing the perineum: Enterobacteriaceae (eg, *E coli, Klebsiella* species), enterococci, and *Candida* species.

Indwelling devices placed for the management of trauma, neurosurgical processes, or monitoring can lead to infection of the central nervous system. Ventricular shunts, ventricular reservoirs, and lumbar drains are all susceptible to infection; manipulation increases the risk. Once infected, foreign bodies in the central nervous system typically cannot be sterilized simply with the use of antibiotics; thus, they must be removed as soon as medically feasible.

Hospital-acquired skin infections are generally a complication of surgery and burns. Rarely, common bacterial or fungal infections, such as impetigo or ringworm, are transmitted by direct contact of one child's skin with another or by the contaminated hands of a caregiver. Musculoskeletal infections acquired in a healthcare setting are uncommon; the highest risk patients are neonates and those in intensive care who suffer bacteremia, which may seed the bones or joints. These also may occur in patients with postoperative infections of internal orthopedic devices (eg, spinal rod instrumentation). Direct inoculation of muscles, bones, and joints is rare.

## PREVENTION

General guidelines, as well as guidelines to prevent specific infections published by multidisciplinary groups of experts, are found in several resources (Table 220-1). There are additional guidelines designed to protect healthcare workers, specifically through immunizations and postexposure care. The Healthcare Infection Control Practices Advisory Committee (HICPAC) of the Centers for Disease Control and Prevention (CDC) and the Committee on Infectious Diseases of the American Academy of Pediatrics (AAP) publish guidelines and policies to decrease the incidence of infection. These policies address infection in the inpatient and outpatient settings. The policies are updated on a regular basis, generally every 3 to 5 years. CDC recommendations are published in the *Morbidity and Mortality Weekly Report,* whereas AAP recommendations appear in *Pediatrics.*

### Hand Hygiene

Hand hygiene is central to infection control and prevention. Alcohol-based hand rubs are preferred for use in direct patient care; however, these rubs are not effective in the presence of dirt or large amounts of proteinaceous material. Hands should be washed with soap and water whenever visibly contaminated with dirt or proteinaceous material, including blood and body fluids. Hand washing also is preferred for caregivers of patients with *C difficile* colonization or disease; alcohol does not kill spores, and the friction of hand washing is more effective in removing spores. Patients and parents should be encouraged to clean their hands and to request hand hygiene of all caregivers. Staffing levels should be appropriate for the number of patients and level of care; outbreaks in nurseries and critical care areas have coincided with overcrowding and understaffing.

**TABLE 220-1 SOURCES FOR GUIDELINES ON PREVENTION OF HEALTHCARE-ASSOCIATED INFECTIONS**

| |
|---|
| **Healthcare Infection Control Practices Advisory Committee (HICPAC)** provides advice and guidance regarding the practice of infection control and strategies for surveillance, prevention, and control of healthcare-associated infections, antimicrobial resistance, and related events in US healthcare settings. |
| www.cdc.gov/hicpac/ |
| **The Division of Healthcare Quality Promotion (DHQP) of the Centers for Disease Control and Prevention (CDC)** seeks to protect patients; protect healthcare personnel; and promote safety, quality, and value in both national and international healthcare delivery systems. |
| www.cdc.gov/ncezid/dhqp/index.html |
| **Guideline for Isolation Precautions: Preventing Transmission of Infectious Agents in Healthcare Settings, 2007** |
| www.ajicjournal.org/article/S0196-6553(07)00740-7/pdf |
| **World Health Organization Guideline on Hand Hygiene in Health Care** |
| http://apps.who.int/iris/bitstream/10665/70126/1/WHO_IER_PSP_2009.07_eng.pdf?ua=1 |
| **Guidelines for the Prevention of Intravascular Catheter-Related Infections** |
| www.cdc.gov/hicpac/pdf/guidelines/bsi-guidelines-2011.pdf |
| **Management of Multidrug-Resistant Organisms in Healthcare Settings** |
| www.cdc.gov/hicpac/pdf/MDRO/MDROGuideline2006.pdf |
| **Guideline for the Prevention of Surgical Site Infection** |
| www.cdc.gov/ncidod/dhqp/gl_surgicalsite.html [*Infect Control Hosp Epidemiol.* 1999;20:247-280] |
| **Occupational Safety and Health Administration (OSHA)** |
| www.osha.gov |
| **Influenza Vaccination of Healthcare Personnel** |
| www.cdc.gov/flu/healthcareworkers.htm |
| **Immunization of Healthcare Workers** |
| Recommendations of the Advisory Committee on Immunization Practices (ACIP) and the Hospital Infection Control Practices Advisory Committee (HICPAC) |
| www.cdc.gov/mmwr/pdf/rr/rr6007.pdf |
| **Guidelines for Environmental Infection Control in Healthcare Facilities** |
| Recommendations of CDC and the HICPAC |
| *MMWR Recomm Rep.* 2003;52(RR-10):1-42. |
| **Professional Organizations with Additional Guidelines** |
| The Society for Healthcare Epidemiology of America (www.shea-online.org) |
| Association for Professionals in Infection Control and Epidemiology (www.apic.org) |
| Committee on Infectious Diseases, American Academy of Pediatrics (www.aap.org) |

### Procedures and Devices

Preparation of the skin prior to injections can be accomplished with alcohol wipes. Standardized practices for insertion and maintenance of medical devices are recognized as an effective method to reduce healthcare-associated infections. Aseptic technique is essential whenever skin or mucous membranes are breeched. Skin preparation for suturing lacerations, incising skin, or obtaining blood for culture requires the use of tincture of iodine, povidone-iodine, or chlorhexidine. Preparation for long-term catheter placement should be similar to that used for surgery. Chlorhexidine preparation and use of chlorhexidine-impregnated dressings have been shown to decrease the incidence of bacteremia associated with indwelling central catheters. Catheter care must be meticulous whether the catheter is in the bloodstream or bladder. In general, manipulation increases the risk for contamination and infection. Medical necessity of all catheters should be assessed daily and they should be removed as soon as medically feasible. There is conflicting evidence regarding the efficacy of antibiotic- and antiseptic-coated catheters in decreasing the incidence of infection; in adult studies, the consensus is that antibiotic-coated catheters are effective; little evidence is available in pediatric patients.

### Environmental Controls

Environmental controls are important in preventing infection. Airflow for inpatient and outpatient areas can contribute to spread of airborne pathogens. Water sources must be free of potential pathogens. Disinfection and cleaning are important in keeping the environment free of pathogens. Furniture and floors must be cleaned regularly; the type of furnishings and equipment are selected with consideration of cleaning and durability. Toys in the healthcare environment must be cleaned regularly as well. Linens and patient clothing must be handled and processed in ways that prevent transmission of pathogens to healthcare personnel and patients. Disinfection and sterilization are necessary for instruments or materials that bypass the skin or mucous membranes. Medical waste must be identified and handled appropriately.

### Isolation Precautions

Isolation procedures for hospitalized children involve use of standard precautions for all patients and additional transmission-based precautions for those infected with agents transmitted by the airborne, droplet, and contact routes, as well as those colonized or infected with multidrug-resistant bacteria. Standard precautions are appropriate in all healthcare settings. The basis of standard precautions is the assumption that every person is potentially infected or colonized with an organism that could be transmitted. Hand hygiene should be performed before and after all patient contacts. Gloves should be worn when touching blood, body fluids, secretions, excretions, and items contaminated with any of these fluids. Masks, eye protection, and face shields should be worn whenever it is likely that splashes or sprays of body fluids will be generated. Gowns are used when appropriate to protect the skin and clothing. Every effort should be made to prevent injuries caused by needles, scalpels, and other sharp items used in patient care. Needles must be disposed of properly: they should not be recapped; instead, used needles should be deposited in puncture-proof containers. Mouthpieces, resuscitation bags, and other ventilation devices should be available in all patient care areas so that mouth-to-mouth resuscitation is not necessary. Every healthcare area must have environmental controls with procedures for routine care, cleaning, and disinfection of environmental surfaces.

Transmission-based isolation is used for hospitalized children with contagious infections; these are in addition to standard precautions. *Airborne precautions* are used to prevent airborne pathogens such as *Mycobacterium tuberculosis,* measles virus, and varicella-zoster virus. Airborne precautions require a single room with negative airflow (ie, the air comes from the hallway into the room and exits to the outdoors or to a high-efficiency particulate air filtration system). Use of N95 or N100 respirators that have been fitted for the provider is necessary for caregivers of patients with active tuberculosis who are contagious. *Droplet precautions* are used for care of children with illness transmitted by droplets, such as influenza, pertussis, or adenovirus. Patients are placed in a single room or patients with the same infection are cohorted; masks are worn when entering the room to provide care. *Contact precautions* (gloves and gowns) are used for patients with infections transmitted by contact and for those infected or colonized with multidrug-resistant bacteria.

Policies for outpatient care of children colonized with multidrug-resistant bacteria have not been standardized. Some experts recommend strict isolation of these patients in offices and outpatient clinics, whereas others believe that this is necessary only during hospitalization. Whenever possible, children colonized with multidrug-resistant bacteria should be placed in an examination area as soon as feasible, thus minimizing time in the waiting area and direct contact with other patients. Other multidrug-resistant bacteria, such as *Streptococcus pneumoniae,* may be frequent colonizers of the nasopharynx of otherwise well children; devising isolation procedures for these children is impractical.

Respiratory hygiene has been recommended to decrease the transmission of droplet and airborne pathogens. Patients with respiratory infections should be identified; if possible, they should not spend time in the waiting areas. Use of masks should be considered. Tissues should be available in waiting areas for use by children and families. Alcohol-based hand rub solutions for disinfecting hands should be present in all patient care settings. If feasible, these solutions should be available in waiting areas.

### Antimicrobial Prophylaxis

Judicious use of antimicrobial agents is important to prevent the emergence and spread of multidrug-resistant organisms. Antimicrobial stewardship is a term applied to programs used to help physicians use antibiotics appropriately. Multidisciplinary teams of infectious disease specialists, microbiologists, infection control practitioners, and pharmacists work together to help the physician make the best choice of antimicrobials for their patients. Guidelines for management of multidrug-resistant organisms in healthcare settings have been developed; surveillance, screening, isolation, and judicious antibiotic use are important procedures to follow.

Prophylactic antibiotics have been used in an attempt to prevent infections related to surgery or other invasive procedures. The timing of surgical prophylaxis is important; the antibiotic should be in the tissues at the time of skin incision. There is no evidence that continuing antibiotic prophylaxis beyond the surgical procedure is useful; in fact, this increases the risk for adverse effects of the antibiotics and alteration of normal bacterial flora. Surgical prophylaxis should be limited to cases where the risk of infection justifies the use of an antibiotic. In general, if bowel is entered or mucous membranes are crossed, prophylaxis is indicated. The choice of antibiotic is based on the expected pathogens and the susceptibilities of these organisms. Antibiotic prophylaxis has been used in an attempt to prevent infection following vascular or urinary bladder procedures; generally, these are effective for short periods. Prolonged therapy increases the emergence of multidrug-resistant flora. If surgery involves infected tissues, then the antibiotics are therapeutic rather than prophylactic.

### Healthcare Personnel

Because healthcare workers are capable of transmitting disease, each healthcare facility should have written policies regarding restriction of staff members with contagious illnesses (Table 220-2). Respiratory symptoms in the absence of fever are not usually a reason for exclusion with the exception of during influenza season. Emphasis should be placed on hand hygiene and use of tissues to prevent transmission of respiratory viruses to patients and other staff members.

Skin testing or interferon-gamma release assay for tuberculosis is recommended at the time of employment for hospital personnel; it should also be considered for outpatient areas where the employees are at risk for tuberculosis or where the background rate of infection is high. Yearly influenza vaccination of all healthcare workers should be mandatory. Hepatitis B vaccination is recommended for healthcare personnel who perform tasks that may involve exposure to blood or body fluids. Measles, mumps, rubella (MMR) vaccination is recommended for healthcare personnel born in or after 1957. All healthcare workers should be immune to varicella, tetanus, and diphtheria, and appropriately immunized against pertussis.

## SURVEILLANCE

Surveillance is important to detect clusters or outbreaks of infection in healthcare settings. Most surveillance is performed within hospitals; however, surveillance may be appropriate in outpatient and home care settings for high-risk patients. Clusters of healthcare-associated infections due to the same organism may warrant a detailed investigation to identify potential sources and interventions to interrupt further transmission and cases. In addition to hospital epidemiology, molecular techniques add to our ability to determine when healthcare-associated infections are due to identical strains. Infection control and prevention managers for healthcare systems should work closely with local and regional health agencies during seasons of community outbreaks

**TABLE 220-2 WORK RESTRICTIONS FOR ILLNESS IN HEALTHCARE PERSONNEL**

| Condition | Work Restriction | Length of Restriction |
|---|---|---|
| Conjunctivitis | Restrict from direct patient care | Until discharge resolved |
| Common cold (afebrile) | Stress hand washing and use of tissues for nasal discharge | |
| Cytomegalovirus | None | |
| Gastroenteritis | Restrict from direct patient care and food preparation | Until symptoms resolve or person deemed noncontagious |
| Hepatitis A | Restrict from direct patient care | Until 1 week after onset of jaundice |
| Hepatitis B | None unless performing procedures with a high risk of transmission of blood from provider to patient | |
| Herpes simplex, orofacial | Restrict from direct care of newborn infants | Until lesions dry |
| Human immunodeficiency virus (HIV) | None unless performing procedures considered to be at risk for transmission of blood from provider to patient | |
| Measles | Exclude from office or hospital | Until 7 days after onset of rash |
| Mumps | Exclude from office or hospital | Until 9 days after onset of parotitis |
| Pediculosis | Restrict from direct patient contact | Until treated |
| Pertussis | Exclude from office or hospital | Until treated for 5 days |
| Rubella | Exclude from office or hospital | Until 5 days after onset of rash |
| Scabies | Restrict from direct patient care | Until treated |
| Staphylococcal skin infection | Restrict from direct patient care | Until treated for 24 hours |
| Streptococcal infection, group A | Restrict from direct patient care | Until treated for 24 hours |
| Tuberculosis, active | Exclude from office or hospital | Until proven noncontagious |
| Varicella-zoster | Exclude from office or hospital. If zoster lesions covered, restrict from care of immunocompromised patients; if lesions cannot be covered, restrict from all patient care | Until lesions crust |

(eg, influenza) and report patients with reportable conditions (eg, pertussis, tuberculosis). Furthermore, this partnership is essential to address concerns for emerging infectious diseases or conditions with significant public health implications (eg, Ebola).

## SUGGESTED READINGS


American Academy of Pediatrics. Infection control for hospitalized children. In: Kimberlin DW, Brady MT, Jackson MA, Long SS, eds. *Red Book: 2015 Report of the Committee on Infectious Diseases.* 30th ed. Elk Grove Village, IL: American Academy of Pediatrics; 2015:161-176.

Bizzarro MJ. Health care-associated infections in the neonatal intensive care unit: barriers to continued success. *Semin Perinatol.* 2012;36:437-444.

Committee on Infectious Diseases, American Academy of Pediatrics. Infection prevention and control in pediatric ambulatory settings. *Pediatrics.* 2007;120:650-665.

Huskins WC. Quality improvement interventions to prevent health-care-associated infections in neonates and children. *Curr Opin Pediatr.* 2012;24:103-112.

Klompas M, Branson R, Eichenwald EC, et al; Society for Healthcare Epidemiology of America (SHEA). Strategies to prevent ventilator-associated pneumonia in acute care hospitals: 2014 update. *Infect Control Hosp Epidemiol.* 2014;35:915-993.

Miller MR, Niedner MF, Huskins C, et al. Reducing PICU central line-associated bloodstream infections: 3-year results. *Pediatrics.* 2011;128:e1077-e1083.

Patrick SW, Kawai AT, Kleinman K, et al. Health care-associated infections among critically ill children in the US, 2007-2012. *Pediatrics.* 2014;134:705-712.

Rutledge-Taylor K, Matlow A, Gravel D, et al. A point prevalence survey of health care-associated infections in Canadian pediatric inpatients. *Am J Infect Control.* 2012;40:491-496.

Saint S, Greene MT, Krein SL, et al. A program to prevent catheter-associated urinary tract infection in acute care. *N Engl J Med.* 2016;374:2111-2119.


# 221 Diagnostic Approaches for Infectious Diseases

Elizabeth L. Palavecino

## INTRODUCTION

Although not all infectious diseases require diagnostic laboratory testing, clinicians often rely on laboratory tests to help identify a causative agent, select an appropriate antimicrobial agent, and/or assess response to therapy. Children are more susceptible than adults to certain infections such as viral respiratory infections, streptococcal pharyngitis, and otitis media. The variety of potential pathogens and difficulties in collection of specimens create diagnostic challenges that are specific to children. Ordering the right test at the right time is paramount for laboratory diagnosis of infectious diseases and for preventing false-positive and false-negative results. Therefore, it is important that clinicians have a basic understanding of diagnostic microbiology so that they collect the optimal specimen and order the most appropriate test for diagnosing and selecting the most appropriate therapy for the infectious process.

## BACTERIA

### COLLECTING AND PROCESSING BACTERIAL CULTURES

No test methodology or degree of laboratory expertise can correct the error of inappropriately collected and transported specimens. The proper collection and handling of clinical specimens is as important as selecting the correct medication for treatment. Common problems with clinical specimen collection and handling include insufficient quantity, contamination, inappropriate transport conditions, and delay in transport to the laboratory. Swabs, although commonly used, are less likely to yield reliable results, and their use for obtaining bacterial cultures should be discouraged, except when submitted for throat culture (or for rapid antigen tests, which include swabs as part of the test kit). Submission of sterile body fluid, scrapings, biopsy, or tissue

**TABLE 221-1 KEY RECOMMENDATIONS FROM THE MICROBIOLOGY LABORATORY**

| Specimen or Culture Type or Test | Recommendations |
|---|---|
| All specimens | Obtain all specimens for culture before initiating antimicrobial therapy.<br>Inform the lab if unusual organisms are possible (such as *Brucella*, *Bartonella*, etc). |
| Cerebrospinal fluid (CSF) | CSF samples submitted for bacterial culture should not be refrigerated. Samples submitted for molecular tests, preferred for detection of herpes simplex virus 1 and 2, enterovirus, and *Mycobacterium tuberculosis*, should be stored and transported at 4°C. |
| Blood culture | Collect the appropriate volume per bottle. Volume of blood collected is the most important factor in successful isolation of the causative organism. |
| Synovial fluid | Inoculate fluid into an aerobic blood culture bottle, preferably at the bedside, in addition to submitting fluid in a sterile container for Gram stain. |
| Abscess | Submit tissue, fluid, or aspirate. Swab is not the specimen of choice. |
| Stool samples | Ova and parasite exam are of low yield; do not order routinely. |
| Urine culture | Urine should not sit at room temperature for more than 30 minutes. Hold at refrigerator temperature if delay is expected. |
| Skin and soft tissue | Submit tissue of the advancing margin of the lesion. Pus swab and surface swab are inadequate specimens. |
| *Clostridium difficile* toxin | Do not order in children younger than 12 months. |
| Antimicrobial susceptibility testing | Minimal inhibitory concentration (MIC) values vary, depending on the antibiotic and organism being tested. A lower MIC value for one agent does not necessarily represent a more active agent than another with a higher MIC. |

samples increases the chance of recovery of pathogens and reduces the isolation of contaminants that may mislead or result in misdiagnosis. Table 221-1 provides important and useful tips for collection of specific specimens.

Transport media are necessary to maximize pathogen survival. They are designed to prevent drying, provide minimal nutrients, and maintain a balanced physiochemical environment that prevents the oxidation and enzymatic destruction of the pathogen. When specimens cannot be transported or processed immediately, appropriate alternatives are available. Holding conditions are specimen- or pathogen-specific. Urine can be refrigerated at 2°C to 8°C for up to 24 hours. Inoculated blood culture bottles can be held at room temperature for up to 24 hours. Ideally, specimens for bacterial culture should not be stored longer than 24 hours before processing. Blood culture bottles should be inoculated by the bedside with the required volume of blood. Synovial joint and peritoneal fluids can also be inoculated into blood culture bottles to enhance yield. Specimens from infected sites where anaerobic bacteria may be causative agents, such as brain or lung abscesses, require a special anaerobic transport media. Transporting the fluid in a syringe to the laboratory for an anaerobic culture is not adequate. Sterile screw-cap containers can be used to transport urine, feces, cerebrospinal fluid (CSF), and other body fluids. Frequently, transport kits are assembled and supplied by local laboratories to ensure the optimal recovery of microorganisms. For rapid antigen tests (eg, group A *Streptococcus* [GAS, *Streptococcus pyogenes*], influenza virus, or respiratory syncytial virus [RSV]), the appropriate swab included in the test kit and supplied by the microbiology laboratory should be used.

Various types of culture media are used within the clinical microbiology laboratory. Enriched media support the growth of fastidious bacteria and are commonly used for culture of normally sterile sites. Selective media permit the selective growth of certain groups of bacteria, while suppressing others. These selective media are commonly used for isolation and detection of pathogens from specimens that contain normal flora. Differential media assist in distinguishing among similar groups of bacteria. MacConkey agar is both selective (permitting the growth of aerobic gram-negative bacteria only) and differential (distinguishing gram-negative bacilli by their ability to ferment lactose). The use of these special media increases the recovery of certain fastidious organisms and hastens the time to identification and availability of susceptibility data.

The Gram stain is used routinely by clinical microbiology laboratories to classify organisms on the basis of their Gram stain reaction, which provides invaluable information for the presumptive diagnosis of infectious agents. The Gram stain not only provides information about staining characteristics and the size, shape, and morphology of the organism, but also allows examination of the quality of the clinical specimen and evaluation of the presence of particular host cell types indicating the type of inflammation present.

The acid-fast stain is used to identify mycobacteria and other bacteria such as *Nocardia* and *Rhodococcus* that have mycolic acid in the cell wall. These organisms resist decolorization by acid-alcohol; hence the name "acid-fast." Most clinical laboratories use the auramine-rhodamine fluorescent stain, which is the recommended stain for specimen examination because of its increased sensitivity for detecting mycobacteria.

## SPECIMEN-SPECIFIC ISOLATION METHODS

### Blood

Blood cultures contaminated with skin flora during collection should not exceed 3% of blood cultures submitted. Contaminated blood cultures are very costly for the healthcare system and provide misleading results to the clinical team. Therefore, meticulous care should be taken in skin preparation prior to venipuncture. Peripheral venipuncture is the preferred technique for obtaining blood for culture instead of collecting the sample through an intravascular catheter or other device.

Venipuncture sites are cleansed with 70% isopropyl alcohol, followed by disinfection with iodine tincture, chlorine peroxide, or chlorhexidine gluconate, as these skin disinfectants have shown better performance than that of povidone-iodine. It is important to note that chlorhexidine gluconate is *not* recommended for use in infants less than 2 months of age. The manufacturer's recommendations should be strictly followed when using prepackaged kits for disinfection of the venipuncture site for collection of blood culture as the required application time for effective activity may vary by disinfectant type.

Current blood culture systems were developed to increase yield, reduce the time to recovery of bacteria, and standardize interpretation of results. Newer systems also maximize the recovery of fastidious organisms. Commonly used systems in today's microbiology laboratories include the VersaTREK (Thermo Scientific), the BacT/Alert (bioMérieux), and the BACTEC system (BD Diagnostics). The VersaTREK system detects microbial growth by measuring the headspace gas pressure within the blood culture bottle, whereas the BacT/Alert and BACTEC systems monitor increase in carbon dioxide ($CO_2$), which is detected by colorimetric or fluorometric dyes. A variety of media formulations are available for use with each system. The BacT/Alert and the BACTEC systems offer pediatric-specific blood culture bottles, while the VersaTREK system does not.

The lysis centrifugation system (Isolator; Du Pont) refers to a blood culture method in which red and white blood cells in the blood specimen are lysed, leading to the release of microorganisms that are then separated by centrifugation. The lysate is removed and inoculated directly onto agar medium, which is incubated and examined daily for growth. Media can be selected to maximize the recovery of suspected pathogens. Unfortunately, contamination has been a problem with this system, and for this reason, use of the Isolator system has been limited to specific situations, such as when infection with intracellular bacteria (eg, *Brucella* species, *Bartonella* species) or fungal infection (eg, *Histoplasma capsulatum*) is suspected.

The BacT/Alert and the BACTEC systems require a minimum of 0.5 mL of blood per pediatric-specific blood culture bottle. The VersaTREK system requires a minimum of 0.1 mL for their standard blood culture bottle. However, the most important factor that influences the recovery of pathogens from blood cultures is the volume of blood inoculated into each blood culture bottle. Numerous studies in adults and some in children have clearly shown that the recovery yield increases significantly with each additional milliliter of blood collected. Depending on the patient's precise weight, it is recommended that for patients weighing 12.7 kg or less, for each blood culture set (may consist of 1 aerobic and 1 anaerobic bottle), a total volume of 2 to 6 mL be collected, and for patients weighing more than 12.7 kg, 20 mL for each blood culture set should be collected.

Pediatric blood culture bottles were introduced into the market to allow the use of a low volume of blood per bottle while supporting the recovery of fastidious organisms such as *Streptococcus pneumoniae*, *Haemophilus influenzae*, and *Neisseria meningitidis*. However, use of conjugated vaccines has resulted in a reduction of infections caused by these pathogens, and for this reason, many hospitals have discontinued the use of pediatric-specific bottles as these offer only a very slight advantage over standard bottles for detecting bacteremia when a low volume of blood is obtained.

It is important to be aware that pediatric blood culture bottles do not support the growth of strict anaerobes, but the prevalence of bacteremia caused by anaerobes is low in pediatric patients, except in those with head, neck, and intra-abdominal infections. In these cases, separate adult anaerobic bottles can be submitted to the laboratory.

The standard incubation time when using continuously monitored blood culture systems is 5 days. Most bacterial pathogens are detected within 48 hours. Unfortunately, contaminants such as coagulase-negative staphylococci (CONS) may also grow within this time frame, and careful evaluation of the clinical aspects is important for differentiation of contamination versus infection.

In the era of automated blood culture systems, there is no need for prolonged incubation for fastidious organisms, including the HACEK group of microorganisms (*Haemophilus*, *Aggregatibacter*, *Cardiobacterium*, *Eikenella*, and *Kingella*), which are rare causes of bacteremia and endocarditis, because these organisms will grow within the routine 5-day incubation period used by automated blood culture systems. Prolonged incubation (14–21 days) may be necessary for isolation of *Bartonella* and *Brucella* species.

### Urine

Although clean-voided midstream urine is an acceptable specimen for culture in older children and adults, this technique is difficult in young children. The collection of urine by a bag fixed to the perineum is a poor substitute (because of contamination), especially when antibiotic therapy will be initiated after collection. In young infants, urine obtained by bladder catheterization or by suprapubic aspiration is preferred. Urine culture is the gold standard for diagnosis of urinary tract infection (UTI). Rapid techniques to predict UTI include urine dipstick tests for leukocyte esterase and nitrites, various forms of urinalysis, and Gram stain of unspun urine. Studies have shown that all these approaches may have false positives and false negatives. Urine dipstick, showing the presence of leukocyte esterase or nitrates or both, may be a practical approach in outpatient settings. However, urine culture is recommended to detect cases of UTI that are not detected by dipstick or urinalysis. Urine samples should be tested within 2 hours of collection, but refrigeration or chemical preservation may be used if processing within a 2-hour window is not possible.

A quantitative culture is required to differentiate significant isolates from contaminants because the distal urethra is normally colonized with bacteria. Detection of ≥ 100,000 colony-forming units (CFUs) per milliliter of a single bacterial species from a clean-voided midstream urine specimen (≥ 50,000 CFUs/mL from a specimen obtained by catheter) indicates a probable UTI. Any bacterial growth from urine obtained by suprapubic aspiration is considered clinically relevant.

### Cerebrospinal Fluid

Identification of the infecting pathogen in meningitis is one of the most important functions of the microbiology laboratory. CSF must be transported to the laboratory immediately because the fluid is hypotonic and cells can lyse, thereby affecting the cell count and also contributing to a falsely abnormal biochemical analysis (low glucose). Refrigeration can render fastidious bacteria such as *Neisseria* species nonviable. If a delay is expected, samples should be stored at room temperature or incubated at 37°C. The minimal volume acceptable for culture of fungi and mycobacteria is 2 mL; a volume of 10 to 15 mL is preferred. It is important to be aware that mycobacterial culture from CSF has a very low sensitivity, and the current recommendation is to order nucleic acid amplification test (NAAT) for detection of *Mycobacterium* species in CSF samples.

CSF may contain very few microorganisms per milliliter of fluid, and therefore, concentration of the specimen is recommended. Centrifugation by cytospinning (2000 rpm; 350 *g*) maximizes pellet formation of bacteria, producing a yield on direct examination of CSF by Gram stain superior to that of unconcentrated samples. Bacterial antigen detection in CSF is no longer recommended as it is not useful in the diagnosis and management of meningitis. The multiplex molecular panel for laboratory detection of pathogens causing meningitis is described later in this chapter.

### Respiratory Tract Specimens

**Throat Culture** Pharyngitis, or sore throat, remains a common reason for consult in pediatric clinics. Although GAS is the most common bacterial cause of pharyngitis, many viral pathogens can also cause pharyngitis. The signs and symptoms of GAS pharyngitis are often indistinguishable from viral or other causes of sore throat. Therefore, a laboratory diagnosis is essential to identify and limit treatment to those with confirmed GAS infection. Proper collection of the sample by swabbing a tonsillar surface, the posterior pharyngeal wall, and the opposite tonsillar surface, while avoiding the tongue and saliva, increases the yield of the culture.

Routine culture requires 24 to 48 hours to detect GAS and may result in a delay in therapy for some patients. Rapid antigen diagnostic tests (RADTs) have increasingly been used for diagnosis of GAS pharyngitis because of the availability of results while the patient is still present, and because they are easy to perform and many of them are approved for point-of-care testing, they can be performed in physicians' offices. However, although the specificity is very high, meaning that there are few false-positive results, the sensitivity of these tests varies by manufacturer and has been reported to range from 30% to 85%. For that reason, the current guidelines from the Infectious Diseases Society of America (IDSA), American Heart Association (AHA), and American Academy of Pediatrics (AAP) recommend a culture also be performed for children with a negative RADT. In recent years, rapid molecular assays have been developed. The reported sensitivity and specificity of these molecular tests are greater than 95%, eliminating the need for back-up culture, and they are becoming a good alternative for the laboratory diagnosis of GAS pharyngitis in patients for whom testing is clinically indicated.

**Nasopharyngeal Specimens** The routine use of nasopharyngeal (NP) swabs for bacterial culture is not recommended and should be submitted primarily to diagnose *Bordetella pertussis* infection. Culture is best done from NP swabs collected during the first 2 weeks of cough transported using a special transport media such as Regan-Lowe or the organism will not be viable for culture. Isolation of *B pertussis* requires immediate inoculation on special agar media, which may not be readily available in local microbiology laboratories, and the results may not be available for several days. For these reasons, polymerase chain reaction (PCR) and other NAAT methods have been developed and are increasingly being used for the laboratory diagnosis of *B pertussis* infection. PCR has excellent sensitivity, but specificity varies among the different PCR tests and false positives may occur. The Centers for Disease Control and Prevention (CDC) recommends separating the area where *B pertussis* vaccines are prepared and administered from the area where specimens are collected so that the opportunity for cross-contamination is reduced.

**Other Respiratory Specimens** Tympanocentesis and sinus aspiration for culture are extremely useful in special situations (eg, immunocompromised patients, patients with suppurative complications, and those who fail to respond to antimicrobial therapy). Data are conflicting regarding the validity of culture of the NP in predicting the pathogens of sinusitis and otitis media, and their routine use is not indicated.

Collection of sputum from children with lower respiratory tract infection is technically difficult. Aspiration of deep pharyngeal/tracheal secretions (with a Lukens trap) is used by many. In older children, sputum can be a valuable specimen. The presence of 10 or more squamous epithelial cells per low-power field is highly suggestive of oropharyngeal contamination, and the specimen should not be processed. Conversely, the presence of more than 25 white blood cells per low-power field denotes an adequate specimen.

Transtracheal aspirates are technically difficult to obtain in young children and are seldom performed. Bronchoscopy, especially a quantitative bronchoalveolar lavage (BAL) specimen or protected brush, is extremely useful in the diagnosis of *Pneumocystis jirovecii* and mycobacterial, fungal, and bacterial infections.

Induced sputum can be obtained in children as young as 1 month, and 1 well-collected, induced sputum has been found to have a similar yield for isolation of *Mycobacterium tuberculosis* to that from 3 gastric aspirates. Induced sputum and gastric aspirates should arrive in the laboratory soon after collection to prevent overgrowth of contaminant bacteria, which can decrease the yield of mycobacterial culture. If transport is delayed more than 1 hour, the specimen should be refrigerated at 4°C. Most laboratories use solid and liquid media for isolation of mycobacteria from respiratory specimens. Automated liquid mycobacteria culture systems such as the BD Bactec MGIT system or BACT/Alert HB monitor for mycobacterial growth continuously and have shown improved recovery of mycobacteria compared to solid media. More recently a molecular test—the Xpert MTB/RIF (Cepheid)—has been approved by the US Food and Drug Administration (FDA) for detection of *M tuberculosis* directly from sputum samples. Studies have shown that the molecular test is about 40% more sensitive than direct microscopy for sputum and gastric aspirates.

### Stool

**Bacterial Enteric Pathogens** Most children with diarrhea have an uncomplicated course that resolves within days without antimicrobial therapy. These children rarely require laboratory testing. Infants and children with fever and/or bloody diarrhea may require specific antibacterial therapy or need close monitoring for complications such as hemolytic-uremic syndrome (HUS). Stool specimens are then submitted routinely to laboratories for isolation of *Salmonella, Shigella, Campylobacter*, and *Escherichia coli* O157:H7. When clinically and epidemiologically indicated, the isolation of other bacterial causes such as *Plesiomonas, Aeromonas*, and *Yersinia* can be attempted.

The yield of stool cultures (and examinations for ova and parasites [O&P]) in persons with onset of diarrhea more than 3 days after hospitalization is extremely low (< 1%). In these patients, nosocomial pathogens such as rotavirus and norovirus are more likely. Institutions should educate clinicians not to order "routine" stool cultures on these patients, or the laboratory should implement rejection criteria where the test would not be performed if ordered.

**Shiga Toxin** Shiga toxin–producing *E coli* (STEC) serotype O157:H7 has been responsible for many outbreaks of gastrointestinal illness in the United States, although some regions are reporting outbreaks related to non-O157 STEC. To detect STEC O157:H7, stool culture is performed using a MacConkey sorbitol plate. Serotype O157:H7 is sorbitol-negative (clear colonies) and can be differentiated from other *E coli* strains (pink colonies) present in the sample. Because culture does not identify STEC serotypes other than O157:H7, CDC guidelines for clinical laboratories recommend that all stools submitted for diagnosis of acute community-acquired diarrhea should be simultaneously cultured and tested for Shiga toxin by using enzyme immunoassay (EIA) or NAAT.

***Clostridium difficile*** Diagnostic tests and recommendations for *C difficile* testing have changed drastically in the last few years. EIAs for detecting *C difficile* toxins A and B are no longer recommended due to poor sensitivity. As a result, molecular tests have been implemented as stand-alone tests, but because molecular tests detect the toxin genes rather than the toxins, it is unclear whether a positive PCR result reflects clinical disease. More recently, laboratories have adopted a 2-step algorithm for toxin detection. Stool is simultaneously screened for *C difficile* glutamate dehydrogenase antigen and *C difficile* toxins. If both tests are negative or if both tests are positive, no further testing is merited. When the antigen is positive and the toxin is negative and other common causes of diarrhea have been ruled out, NAAT testing can be performed. The diagnosis of *C difficile* infection in young children is very challenging due to the high rate of colonization in this population. The AAP guidelines published in 2013 recommend testing only in patients with diarrhea (3 or more loose stools in a 24-hour period) and no testing in children less than 1 year of age unless there are specific gut motility disorders. In children up to 3 years of age, testing should be considered only if other causes, such as viral infection or noninfectious causes, have been investigated. In children older than 3 years of age, a positive *C difficile* test indicates probable *C difficile* infection if clinical signs and risk factors are present.

### Synovial and Peritoneal Fluid

Inoculation of synovial fluid and peritoneal fluid into blood culture bottles at the bedside results in a higher bacteria recovery rate than inoculation onto conventional media in the microbiology laboratory. In one study, *Kingella kingae*, a cause of septic arthritis in children less than 4 years old, was exclusively detected in specimens inoculated into blood culture bottles. Pediatric bottles were inferior to standard bottles for recovery of *K kingae* at low bacterial concentrations. In patients with bacterial peritonitis, inoculation of peritoneal fluid into blood culture bottles more than doubled the recovery of gram-negative bacteria compared to those inoculated onto conventional media. Further, although none of the peritoneal fluids inoculated onto conventional media yielded streptococci or enterococci, 33% of those inoculated into blood culture bottles grew these organisms. Similar findings have been demonstrated in patients with peritonitis complicating continuous ambulatory peritoneal dialysis.

## ANTIGEN TESTS

Bacterial antigen detection assays were developed for the rapid diagnosis of bacterial meningitis. Unfortunately, these tests have suffered from poor sensitivity and specificity, and therefore, their use is no longer recommended.

Two urinary antigen tests are commercially available—one for diagnosis of *S pneumoniae* infection and the other for detection of *Legionella pneumophila* serogroup 1. Although the *S pneumoniae* urine antigen test has a high sensitivity and specificity in adult patients, particularly in cases of bacteremic pneumococcal pneumonia, studies have reported a 21% to 54% false-positive rate in children with NP carriage and no evidence of pneumonia. For this reason, general use of *S pneumoniae* urine antigen in febrile infants and children is not recommended at this time.

*Legionella* species are a potential cause of pediatric pneumonia and are particularly important because infection can be especially severe in immunocompromised children. The immunochromatographic urinary antigen assay (BinaxNOW; Binax, Inc.) for *L pneumophila* serogroup 1 has shown high sensitivity, and the antigen may be detectable in the urine as early as 3 days after onset of symptoms. A negative result for *L pneumophila* serogroup 1 antigen in urine suggests no recent or current infection with that serogroup, but infection with other serogroups of *L pneumophila* or with *Legionella* species other than *L pneumophila* cannot be ruled out. The antigen test can be positive for an extended period; therefore, patient history must be considered when evaluating results.

## IDENTIFICATION OF MICROORGANISMS

### Matrix-Assisted Laser Desorption Ionization–Time of Flight Mass Spectrometry

Traditionally, clinical microbiology laboratories have performed identification of bacteria using a series of biochemical reactions by either manual or automated methods. The traditional methodology is time consuming, and it can take 1 to 3 days for the final identification to become available. In the last few years, clinical laboratories have started to implement a new methodology for identification of bacteria and fungi: matrix-assisted laser desorption ionization–time of flight mass spectrometry (MALDI-TOF MS), which represents a revolutionary change in the way microorganisms are identified. This technology analyzes the protein profile of the microorganism and has evolved into a rapid and highly reliable and specific method for the characterization of bacteria and fungi commonly isolated in clinical laboratories. In MALDI-TOF, a bacterial or fungal colony is applied directly onto a MALDI-TOF plate and subsequently loaded into the MALDI-TOF MS instrument. The ionized microbial molecules are separated from each other on the basis of their mass-to-charge ratio and then measured using a time-of-flight (TOF) mass analyzer to determine the time required to travel the length of the flight tube. A mass spectrum is generated, and the pattern is analyzed by the instrument software, allowing the identification of each organism. The entire process takes only a few minutes. In the past year, 2 systems, the VITEK MS (bioMérieux) and the MALDI Biotyper CA system (Bruker Daltonics, Inc.), have been approved by the FDA for identification of cultured bacteria and yeasts. Compared to traditional methodology, MALDI-TOF has shortened the time required for identification by at least 24 hours for bacterial and by weeks for mycobacteria and fungal isolates.

## ANTIMICROBIAL SUSCEPTIBILITY TESTING

In vitro antimicrobial susceptibility testing (AST) is one of the most important functions of clinical microbiology laboratories worldwide. AST results have enormous implications for the entire healthcare system, influencing decisions on the selection of antimicrobials for patients, development of antibiotic formularies, recommendations for treatment of infectious syndromes, and implementation of infection prevention policies.

### Indications

The role of in vitro AST is to estimate the effectiveness of the antimicrobial therapy against a specific organism. However, laboratory testing is performed under standardized conditions using constant bacterial growth and drug exposure, while in vivo none of these conditions are standardized and the organisms are exposed to fluctuating concentrations of drug and bacterial growth parameters. As a result, in vitro susceptibility does not ensure clinical efficacy. Discrepancies between in vitro susceptibility test results and clinical outcomes occur as a result of a variety of factors that are intrinsic to the antimicrobial agent used, the host, and the pathogen causing the infection. For example, the antimicrobial agent's route of administration, protein binding, and accessibility to the site of infection; the immune status of the host; the inoculum size at the site of infection; virulence factors produced by the organism; and the presence of an abscess requiring drainage may influence response to antimicrobial treatment.

Organisms warrant testing if the susceptibility profile cannot be reliably predicted. Therefore, AST is most often indicated when the causative organism is thought to commonly exhibit resistance to often used antibiotics. Susceptibility testing of GAS is seldom necessary because of its predictable susceptibility pattern, whereas testing for *Pseudomonas aeruginosa* is always indicated. The selection of the most appropriate antimicrobial agents to test and to report is a decision made by each laboratory in consultation with the different stakeholders within the healthcare system, particularly pharmacists and infectious disease practitioners.

Despite the standardization of susceptibility testing methods for common pathogens by the Clinical and Laboratory Standards Institute (CLSI) and other professional organizations, there are many organisms that can cause serious infections in which methods are still not standardized and interpretive guidelines are not available. The choice of antimicrobial therapy for these infections is based on clinical experience including that published in the medical literature, rather than in vitro susceptibility testing.

Routine susceptibility testing of anaerobic bacteria is not recommended. Testing should be limited to laboratories with special qualifications. CLSI publishes an annual report, and a local laboratory may also publish its own cumulative report, with the susceptibility rates for different anaerobic organisms to provide guidance for therapy selection.

### Laboratory Methods

Disk diffusion, or the Kirby-Bauer test, is a standardized technique for testing rapidly growing pathogens. An inoculum is prepared by direct suspension of colonies to yield a standardized inoculum that is swabbed onto the surface of a Mueller-Hinton agar plate. Reproducibility depends on the log-growth phase of organisms; therefore, fresh subcultures are always required. Filter paper disks, each impregnated with a standardized concentration of an antimicrobial agent, are placed on the surface, and the size of the zone of inhibition around the disk is measured after overnight incubation. Classification of zone diameters into susceptible, intermediate, or resistant categories is accomplished by following CLSI interpretive guideline tables.

Another commonly employed susceptibility method is broth microdilution (BMIC). This method allows a quantitative measurement of in vitro activity by determining the minimal inhibitory concentration (MIC). Usually, 5 to 8 concentrations representing therapeutically achievable ranges are tested against each organism to determine activity at the breakpoint MIC. One must be careful with the interpretation of these values because they apply to a specific organism, the concentration of the organism at the site of infection, and the type of antimicrobial agent being used.

The gradient method or E-test is a method that integrates disk diffusion to determine an actual MIC value and that provides accurate, reproducible results. An impervious inert strip carries a marked, continuous concentration gradient of a predefined antibiotic consisting of more than 15 two-fold dilutions. After incubation on seeded agar, the MIC is read at the edge of the zone of inhibition as it intersects the strip (Fig. 221-1). The E-test methodology is especially useful for testing organisms isolated from sterile sites when an exact MIC may be needed for optimization of drug dosage.

### Automated Systems

Automated AST can provide results in 2 to 18 hours depending on the system and the organism. Systems commonly used in the United States are the VITEK2 system (bioMérieux), the MicroScan WalkAway (Beckman Coulter), and the BD Phoenix automated microbiology system (BD Diagnostics). The VITEK2 system uses plastic reagent cards containing small wells or microcuvettes that allow simultaneous testing for many different antimicrobial agents. Growth is detected by means of a densitometer. It uses turbidimetrically determined kinetic measurements of growth to compute MIC values by regression analysis. The MicroScan WalkAway system utilizes microdilution panels of 96 wells containing several dilutions of different antimicrobial agents. Panels are monitored and read using turbidimetric end points. The Phoenix system uses microdilution panels, and a redox indicator measures bacterial growth.

Advantages of automated systems are that they can be connected to the laboratory computer system, provide rapid test results, allow intra- and interlaboratory standardization, are less labor intensive, and have software that can apply interpretation rules before reporting and offer flexibility for data review. Automated systems can be too restrictive for some laboratories, as panels and cards are formatted by the manufacturer with predetermined antimicrobial agents and these may not match the hospital pharmacy formulary. Automated systems are not appropriate for all organisms, and therefore, laboratories frequently use more than 1 method for susceptibility testing to cover all the organisms that require testing.

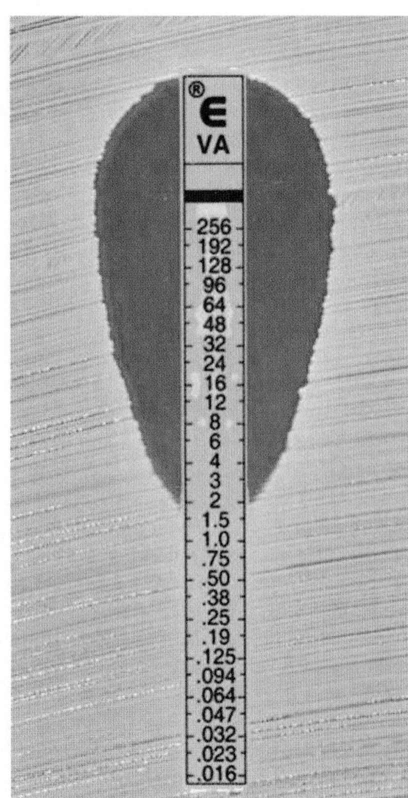


**FIGURE 221-1** A *Staphylococcus* isolate tested by the E-test gradient diffusion method. The minimal inhibitory concentration (MIC) of vancomycin is determined by reading the value where the inhibition ellipse intersects the strip. In this case, the vancomycin MIC is 2 µg/mL.

### Special Antimicrobial Testing Methods

**Gram-Positive Cocci** Resistance to oxacillin in staphylococci is mostly mediated by the *mec*A gene, which encodes the supplemental penicillin-binding protein, PBP2a. Therefore, tests for the *mec*A gene or PBP2a are the most accurate methods for prediction of oxacillin (methicillin) resistance. Staphylococci that test positive for *mec*A or PBP2a are reported as oxacillin-resistant. Resistance to oxacillin in most staphylococci is expressed heterogeneously, making it difficult to detect by routine AST because only a fraction of the cells within a population are expressing resistance. For this reason, special test conditions are used to improve the detection of oxacillin resistance in staphylococci, such as incubation at lower temperatures (33–35°C) and incubation for a full 24 hours before reporting if susceptible.

Vancomycin resistance in *Staphylococcus aureus* is still rare. In the United States, since 2002, *S aureus* strains with vancomycin MICs in the resistant range (MICs ≥ 32 µg/mL) have been detected, although infrequently. *S aureus* with vancomycin MICs of ≥ 8 µg/mL can be reliably detected by broth microdilution, agar screen test, and automated susceptibility systems, but standard broth microdilution using a full 24-hour incubation is the recommended method for detection of staphylococci with vancomycin MICs in the intermediate range (MIC of 4 µg/mL).

Macrolide-resistant isolates of *S aureus*, CONS, *S pneumoniae*, and β-hemolytic streptococci may express constitutive or inducible resistance to clindamycin. In the case of constitutive resistance, routine AST shows the organism to be resistant to both clindamycin and erythromycin. When routine AST shows the organism to be susceptible to clindamycin but resistant to erythromycin, the recommended disk diffusion test for evaluation of inducible macrolide-clindamycin phenotypes consists of an erythromycin disk in close proximity to a clindamycin disk. Organisms that cause flattening of the clindamycin zone of inhibition adjacent to the erythromycin disk, and thus a "D-shaped" zone around the clindamycin disk (D-test positive), have inducible resistance and should be considered clindamycin-resistant. Organisms that do not show flattening of the clindamycin zone should be reported as clindamycin-susceptible. More recently, broth microdilution methods have been standardized to detect inducible clindamycin resistance for all staphylococci, *S pneumoniae*, and β-hemolytic streptococci in a single well test.

**Gram-Negative Bacilli** The major mechanism of resistance to β-lactam antimicrobial agents by gram-negative bacilli (GNB) is production of β-lactamase enzymes. Many different types of these enzymes have been reported in GNB. β-Lactamase enzymes inactivate β-lactam antimicrobial agents at different rates, and combined resistance mechanisms carried by the organism may also affect different groups of β-lactam agents. Extended-spectrum β-lactamases (ESBLs) hydrolyze expanded-spectrum cephalosporins and monobactams; these ESBLs may be inhibited by β-lactamase inhibitors.

Carbapenemases represent the most versatile family of β-lactamases as they hydrolyze almost all β-lactam agents including the carbapenems. In the last decade, identification of plasmid-encoded carbapenemases, such as *Klebsiella pneumoniae* carbapenemases (KPC) and New Delhi metallo-β-lactamases (NDM-1), has changed the patterns of dissemination of these carbapenemases, and laboratories are now isolating GNB that are resistant to most antimicrobial agents currently used for treatment of antimicrobial-resistant organisms. Outbreaks due to infection caused by carbapenem-resistant Enterobacteriaceae (CRE) have been reported in the United States and other countries, and these infections are associated with a high mortality.

### Interpretation of Antimicrobial Susceptibility Results

The laboratory must interpret the susceptibility results prior to releasing the report to clinicians. MIC values and disk diffusion zone diameters must be interpreted based on proven efficacy of each antibiotic for the various species and, in some situations, according to the specimen type or site of infection because the MIC breakpoints can be different for the same bacteria at different body sites. Pharmacokinetics (PK) refers to drug concentration at the site of infection, while pharmacodynamics (PD) refers to the effect of the drug over time at a particular site of infection. The effectiveness of treatment depends on the relationship between the MIC of the organism and the exposure of the organism to the agent at the site of infection. Based on this, in recent years, PK/PD parameters have been used to set up breakpoints for specific sites of infections. For example, the susceptible breakpoint for penicillin and *S pneumoniae* is ≤ 0.12 µg/mL for meningitis and ≤ 0.5 µg/mL for nonmeningitis infections.

### Interpretive Criteria

The recommended interpretive categories for various MIC and zone diameter values are included in the tables for each organism published every year by CLSI. The CLSI definitions for each interpretive category are described below:

Susceptible: The susceptible category implies that isolates are inhibited by the achievable concentrations of antimicrobial agent using the recommended dosage for that type and site of infection and that the patient should respond to therapy.

Intermediate: The intermediate category implies that the isolate falls into a range of susceptibility with an MIC that approaches usually achievable blood and tissue levels, and for which clinical response is likely to be less than with a susceptible isolate. The antimicrobial agent can be used if it is physiologically concentrated in a body fluid such as urine (eg, quinolones and β-lactams) or if higher than normal dosages of the antimicrobial agent can be safely used.

Resistant: The resistant category implies that the isolate is not inhibited by the concentration of the antimicrobial agent achieved with the dosages normally used, and/or the MIC value or zone diameter fall in the range seen with organisms that carry mechanisms of resistance (eg, β-lactamases).

Susceptible-dose dependent (SDD): This category implies that susceptibility of an isolate is dependent on the dosing regimen that is used in the patient. For organisms with an MIC or zone diameter interpretation of SDD, it is necessary to use a dosing regimen that results in higher drug exposure than that used for susceptible isolates.

**TABLE 221-2 ANTIMICROBIALS TO WHICH BACTERIA MAY APPEAR SUSCEPTIBLE BY IN VITRO TESTING BUT ARE NOT CLINICALLY USEFUL**

| Organism | Antimicrobials That Should Not Be Reported as Susceptible | Comments |
|---|---|---|
| *Enterococcus* species | Aminoglycosides, cephalosporins, clindamycin, and trimethoprim-sulfamethoxazole | Only high-level concentrations should be reported for aminoglycosides. |
| Methicillin-resistant *Staphylococcus* species | All penicillins, cephalosporins, β-lactam/β-lactamase inhibitor combinations, and carbapenems | This rule does not apply to the cephalosporins with anti-MRSA activity such as ceftaroline and ceftobiprole. |
| *Salmonella* species, *Shigella* species | First- and second-generation cephalosporins and aminoglycosides | A third-generation cephalosporin should be reported for *Salmonella* species isolated from extraintestinal sources. |

MRSA, methicillin-resistant *Staphylococcus aureus*.

When interpreting MIC results, lower MIC values for a specific antimicrobial agent do not imply that that agent is more active than another agent with a higher value when both are considered susceptible for that organism. Thus, such comparisons warrant caution.

#### Expert Rules

Expert rules are used by clinical microbiology laboratories to assist in the interpretation of AST results, provide accurate information, facilitate selection of the appropriate antibiotic for that particular infection, and contribute to quality assurance by highlighting unusual results. For example, some antimicrobial agents may appear susceptible in vitro, but they are not effective in vivo or there are no data about correlation with clinical efficacy (Table 221-2). Some antimicrobial agents should not be reported for certain sites of infection (Table 221-3), and others should only be reported for organisms isolated from urine samples.

Organisms can have intrinsic resistance that may be a characteristic of all or almost all isolates of the bacterial species. AST testing is unnecessary in these cases, and the organisms should be considered resistant to the antimicrobial agent even if the MIC is within the susceptible range. For additional information about expert rules and examples of organisms with intrinsic resistance, please refer to the article by Leclercq et al in the Suggested Readings.

It is important for laboratories to use the most current breakpoint tables and expert rules as these are updated in view of new microbiologic or clinical information. For example, for Enterobacteriaceae, in 2010 CLSI lowered the MIC breakpoints for cephalosporins and in 2013 for carbapenems. The breakpoints were revised due to the emergence of new mechanisms of resistance against these agents, changes in bacterial population distributions, new PK/PD data, and adoption of newer treatment practices by clinicians. The revised breakpoints provide improved information for direct patient care since the MIC of an organism correlates better with clinical outcome than do known mechanisms of resistance carried by the organism, and for that reason, laboratories should use these updated breakpoints when reporting susceptibility test results.

**TABLE 221-3 ANTIMICROBIALS THAT SHOULD NOT BE REPORTED FOR CERTAIN SPECIMEN TYPES**

| Specimen Type | Antimicrobials | Comments |
|---|---|---|
| Cerebrospinal fluid (CSF) | Agents that can be administered by the oral route only, first- and second-generation cephalosporins, clindamycin, macrolides, tetracyclines, and fluoroquinolones | These agents are not drugs of choice and may not be effective for treating CSF infections. |
| Urine | Clindamycin, macrolides, chloramphenicol | These agents should not be routinely reported for organisms isolated from the urinary tract. |
| All specimen types, except urine | Fosfomycin, nitrofurantoin | These agents should be reported only for organisms isolated from urine samples and when treatment with these agents is approved by the US Food and Drug Administration. |

## FUNGI

### SPECIMEN COLLECTION AND PROCESSING

There are several challenges associated with fungal cultures: clinical specimens have a lower concentration of organisms compared to those with bacterial infection and therefore a larger volume may be needed for culture, and they require a long incubation period (4–6 weeks) and different incubation temperature settings (30°C vs 37°C) for optimal growth. Tissue is the preferred specimen for culture, whereas BAL may be adequate for lung infections. Specimens such as nail scrapings or hair clippings are submitted for dermatophyte culture. Swabs should not be submitted for fungal culture. Blood samples, as indicated above, should be inoculated directly into blood culture bottles designed for isolation of fungal pathogens. A recent study evaluated the use of the pediatric Isolator system over a 10-year period and found that this system only rarely provided useful clinical information for the diagnosis of fungemia in children, with the exception of *Malassezia furfur* and possibly endemic mycoses caused by dimorphic fungi such as *H capsulatum* and *Coccidioides immitis/posadasii*, which are isolated very rarely.

Specimens submitted for fungal culture are inoculated onto primary isolation media as soon as possible to ensure a high yield of recovery. If delay is anticipated, the specimens can be stored in the refrigerator at 4°C to 8°C for up to 8 hours, except blood and CSF specimens, which should be stored at room temperature. It is important to prevent desiccation of tissue specimens by adding a small amount of sterile 0.85% saline.

All samples are examined by fluorescent microscopy with 0.1% Calcofluor white, a substance that binds to the chitin and cellulose of cell walls and causes bright fluorescence. Giemsa and Wright stains are used for examination of blood or bone marrow specimens and can reveal intracellular yeast forms such as *H capsulatum*.

### ISOLATION AND IDENTIFICATION

No single culture medium is appropriate for all specimens. Sabouraud dextrose (SAB) with and without antimicrobial agents is the fungal medium most commonly used to isolate most fungal pathogens.

Fungi are classified as either yeasts or molds. Yeasts are single cells that typically form a smooth, creamy bacteria-like colony and grow in 24 hours (*Candida* species) or in 48 hours (*Cryptococcus* species). Most molds, as opposed to yeasts, have a fuzzy or woolly appearance that is due to the mycelium, which is made up of many tube-like structures called hyphae. Some species in the Mucorales family can grow within 24 hours, whereas *Aspergillus* species may take 3 to 14 days. *Fusarium* species and dermatophytes can take several weeks. After isolation, molds are frequently identified by the morphologic characteristics of spores and structures. To determine dimorphism, the organism is incubated at 30°C and 37°C to detect the presence of mold and yeast forms, respectively. Dimorphic fungi include *Blastomyces dermatitidis, H capsulatum, C immitis, Paracoccidioides, Sporothrix schenckii*, and *Penicillium marnefii*. Identification of yeasts is based primarily on biochemical differences. MALDI-TOF is increasingly being used for identification of yeasts growing in solid media because of the speed and accuracy of this new methodology.

## ANTIGEN TESTS

Fungal antigen tests include the antigen detection latex agglutination test for *Cryptococcus neoformans*, which is commercially available and has been a highly useful clinical tool for detecting *Cryptococcus* in blood and CSF.

Immunoassays performed on blood, CSF, BAL fluid, and urine can detect *H capsulatum* and *B dermatitidis* antigens. Caution in interpreting results is merited because cross-reactivity between fungi does occur.

*Aspergillus* galactomannan antigen can be detected in blood and BAL specimens from immunosuppressed patients with invasive aspergillosis by using an EIA method. A single positive test result should be followed by testing a second sample because many agents (eg, antibiotics, food) may cross-react with the test.

Another antigen test used for the diagnosis of invasive fungal infections is the Fungitell assay, which detects 1,3-β-d-glucan, a component of the cell wall of many medically important fungi, such as *Candida* species, *Aspergillus* species, *Fusarium* species, *P jirovecii*, *C immitis*, *H capsulatum*, and *B dermatitidis*. False positives have been reported due to the presence of glucans in body fluids containing albumin, immunoglobulin, coagulation factors, or plasma proteins. *Cryptococcus* and the *Zygomycetes* species produce little or none of this substance, and therefore, the 1,3-β-d-glucan results would likely be negative in these infections.

## HISTOPATHOLOGY EXAMINATION

In some fungal infections, particularly those causing chronic diseases, the histopathology examination may provide the first diagnostic evidence of a fungal infection, but the identification of the fungal pathogen should be confirmed by culture.

The most commonly used stains for the diagnosis of fungal infections from tissue specimens include the hematoxylin-eosin (H&E), the Grocott-Gomori methenamine silver (GMS), and the periodic-acid shift (PAS) stains. H&E is the stain of choice for examining the morphologic appearance of yeasts and fungi and for assessing the pattern of inflammation, which, in conjunction with the clinical information, is key in formulating a possible diagnosis. The H&E stain can also help to determine whether the fungus is hyaline (colorless) or dematiaceous (naturally pigmented) and whether the hyphae are septate or nonseptate (Fig. 221-2). GMS stains the fungal walls brown to black and provides high contrast with minimal background staining, so their sparse, isolated fungal elements are detected easily. With the PAS stain, fungi appear pinkish-red. The pathology report usually includes description of the morphologic characteristics of the yeast (size, presence of capsule and budding characteristics) and the fungal hyphae (eg, septate or nonseptate hyphae, colorless or dark hyphae) for the presumptive identification of the causative pathogen, but culture is needed for confirmation of identification.

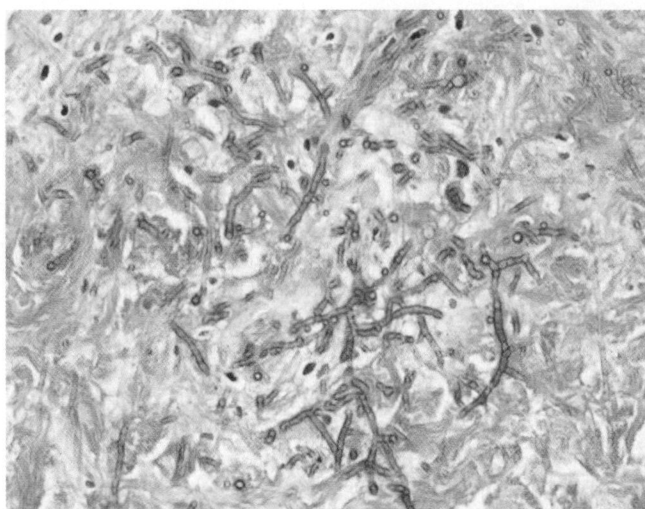

**FIGURE 221-2** Section of skin tissue showing branching, septate hyphae. The most likely diagnosis is aspergillosis, but hyphae of other fungi, particularly *Fusarium* and *Scedosporium* species, have a similar appearance. Fungal culture is required for identification (hematoxylin-eosin stain, original magnification ×60).

## ANTIFUNGAL SUSCEPTIBILITY TESTING

Susceptibility testing methods and interpretive criteria have been standardized for the main *Candida* species with MIC breakpoints developed for 6 antifungal agents. In contrast to yeast susceptibility, the relationship between susceptibility testing for filamentous fungi and clinical response to therapy is unclear and seems to be related to the high rate of intrinsic resistance present in these fungi.

Routine antifungal susceptibility testing is not recommended. There are specific situations in which antifungal susceptibility testing should be considered: *Candida glabrata* isolated from blood or deep sites should be tested for susceptibility to fluconazole, voriconazole, and an echinocandin; and invasive disease that is unresponsive to the initial antifungal regimen, especially if caused by species with significant rates of acquired resistance.

Many fungal species have predictable antifungal susceptibility patterns. For example, *Candida krusei* strains have high rates of intrinsic resistance, and antifungal susceptibility testing is not necessary. Rather, empiric therapy with agents known to have activity against the species should be used.

# PARASITES

## COLLECTION AND PROCESSING OF STOOL

Proper collection and handling of stool specimens are critical for the detection of parasites. Stool should be collected in a clean, wide-mouthed container with a tightly fitting lid. The specimen should not be contaminated with urine or water from the toilet. If transportation to the laboratory is not prompt, the specimen should be stored in the refrigerator. Dry samples are not acceptable. To ensure the recovery of parasitic organisms that are passed intermittently, a minimum of 3 samples over a period of 7 to 10 days is highly recommended.

Liquid stool should be examined or preserved within 30 minutes of collection, soft or semi-formed stool within 1 hour, and formed stool the same day. Specimens that cannot be examined within the recommended time must be transferred to an appropriate preservative such as polyvinyl alcohol (PVA) or formalin.

Stools are examined grossly for consistency, the presence of mucus and blood, and the presence of adult worms or proglottids. Trophic amebae and flagellates are encountered more commonly in liquid and soft specimens. However, testing must be performed quickly because these organisms disintegrate rapidly at room temperature.

*Cryptosporidium* species are not usually seen with routine permanent stains and require the use of special stains such as modified Kinyoun or Ziehl-Neelsen. Such stains can also be used to detect *Isospora belli* and *Cyclospora*.

A simple way of obtaining larvae and adult worms of *Enterobius vermicularis* (pinworms) for examination is the cellulose tape method. Tape reversed on a tongue depressor is pressed against the anus in the early morning. The tape is then placed over a slide and sent to the laboratory for examination.

## ANTIGEN TESTS

There are several commercial products (direct and indirect fluorescent antibodies, EIA, and rapid immunochromatographic assays) available in the United States for the detection of protozoa antigens in stool samples that provide increased sensitivity over modified acid-fast staining techniques. Several kits combine tests for detection of either *Cryptosporidium* and *Giardia* or *Cryptosporidium*, *Giardia*, and *Entamoeba histolytica*.

Laboratories should have specific protocols or algorithms for ordering parasitology tests in stool samples for patients with diarrhea. For example, for patients with watery diarrhea who are ≤ 5 years old (or their contacts) or who are involved in daycare, resort, or community outbreaks, *Cryptosporidium* and *Giardia* antigen testing is recommended. Traditional O&P examination is reserved only for patients who are residents of or visitors to developing countries or areas of North America where infections caused by worms are reported with some frequency.

Multiplex molecular tests are replacing the traditional O&P examination. Gastrointestinal molecular panels are discussed later in this chapter.

### BLOOD PARASITES

Examining thin- and thick-film smears stained with Giemsa or Wright stain is still one of the most reliable and efficient ways of diagnosing bloodstream parasitic infections caused by *Plasmodium, Babesia, Trypanosoma,* and *Leishmania.* Unfortunately, because most of these parasites are infrequently observed in laboratories in developed countries, maintaining a sufficient level of expertise is difficult. A single blood sample is not sufficient to exclude a diagnosis of these parasitic diseases. Blood samples should be submitted every 6 to 12 hours until a diagnosis is made or infection is no longer suspected (usually 2–3 days). Blood obtained by fingerstick is preferred for examination when malaria is suspected. Blood should be inoculated into anticoagulated tubes (with ethylenediaminetetraacetic acid [EDTA]), but smears should be made within 1 hour of collection for reliable staining.

Newer technology such as the BinaxNOW malaria antigen assay compares favorably with microscopic smear examination in the diagnosis of malaria of moderate-to-high parasitemia. The use of the malaria antigen does not eliminate the need for malaria microscopy, as microscopy is necessary to determine the species of *Plasmodium* that was detected by the rapid antigen test, as well as to quantify the proportion of red blood cells that are infected (parasitemia), which is an important prognostic indicator.

### OTHER SITES AND ORGANISMS

*Trichomonas vaginalis* can be observed on direct saline wet mounts from vaginal secretions, first-voided urine, or other fluids such as respiratory secretions from neonates.

*P jirovecii* pneumonia can be diagnosed by demonstrating morphologically consistent organisms from respiratory specimens by a variety of methods, including Giemsa or Giemsa-like rapid stains (eg, Diff-Quik), Gomori methenamine silver stain, toluidine blue O stain, and fluorescein-conjugated monoclonal antibody (direct fluorescent antibody [DFA]) stain.

Tissue obtained by biopsy is the preferred specimen for certain severe parasitic infections. Parasites in tissue samples can be observed with H&E stain. This stain allows detection of most parasites and eggs. PAS stain helps to distinguish intracellular yeast of *H capsulatum* (PAS-positive) from *Leishmania* species (PAS-negative).

## VIRUSES

The laboratory diagnosis of viral infections is based on several different methodologies, including culture, antigen assays, molecular methods, histology, and serology. The development of molecular diagnostic testing with PCR and reverse transcriptase PCR has allowed the clinician a better understanding of the epidemiology and clinical presentations of many viral agents, provided an assessment of viral load for monitoring effectiveness of antiviral therapeutic regimens, and defined the natural course and outcomes after therapy for many viral diseases. Currently, there are numerous different molecular assays and platforms for qualitative and quantitative detection of a variety of viruses, which are now being used in most clinical laboratories. PCR assays including multiplex PCR assays are discussed later in this chapter.

### SPECIMEN COLLECTION AND PROCESSING

In general, specimens for virus identification should be collected within 4 days after onset of illness, as virus shedding decreases rapidly after that time. All specimens for viral culture should be placed in viral transport medium (VTM) and submitted at 4°C. If collecting a sample from a vesicular lesion, sample only fresh vesicles and, using a swab, collect fluid and cellular material by vigorously sampling the base of the lesion. For collection of NP samples, pass a flexible, fine-shafted swab into the NP and allow secretions to absorb before removing the swab.

### CULTURE

Traditional culture and shell vial culture are the 2 methodologies used for isolation of respiratory viruses (eg, influenza, RSV, parainfluenza, adenovirus), cytomegalovirus (CMV), enterovirus, herpes simplex virus (HSV), and varicella-zoster virus (VZV). The cell lines used for culture are available commercially and consist of a monolayer of cells adherent to the side of a glass (traditional culture) or to the surface of a cover slip contained inside a shell vial. The time of incubation varies depending on the virus—from 3 to 5 days for the shell vial method and from 3 days to 3 weeks for traditional culture. In many centers, viral culture has been replaced by molecular assays, particularly for laboratory diagnosis of HSV infection in the neonate.

### ANTIGEN TESTS

Rapid antigen tests are frequently used for respiratory viruses such as RSV and influenza. It is important that clinicians be aware that the predictive values of the rapid diagnostic influenza tests vary significantly year-to-year and during a single season with higher positive predictive values (PPVs) during the peak of the influenza season and low PPVs in times of low prevalence. False negatives are common, especially when influenza activity is high, and false positives occur when influenza activity is low. Many of the antigen influenza tests are point-of-care tests and can be performed by nonlaboratory personnel. The performance of the test is based on the specimen source, how the specimen was obtained, and the transport conditions, so it is of the utmost importance to strictly follow the manufacturer's instructions for the specific assay in use.

### SEROLOGY

Although acute and convalescent serologic testing has high sensitivity and specificity, it has limited utility for management of viral infections. Clinicians should be careful when ordering IgM antibodies, as specific IgM assays, particularly those for measles, mumps, and rubella, may be associated with false-positive results.

For the last 2 decades, the standard algorithm used by clinical laboratories in the United States for serologic diagnosis of (nonacute) human immunodeficiency virus (HIV) infection beyond infancy has been a 2-step process involving a screening immunoassay followed by a confirmatory Western blot. The current algorithm consists of screening with a fourth-generation assay, which detects a combination of p24 antigen and HIV-1 and HIV-2 antibodies, and recommends follow-up of any reactive screening results with an HIV-1/HIV-2 differentiation assay for confirmation of HIV-1 and/or HIV-2 antibodies. Specimens with a reactive screen followed by negative or indeterminate results by the differential assay are followed up with nucleic acid testing to identify acute HIV infection.

## MOLECULAR ASSAYS

### QUALITATIVE AMPLIFICATION ASSAYS

These are PCR tests designed to detect a particular pathogen in the appropriate clinical specimen. There are numerous FDA-approved molecular assays as well as laboratory-developed tests for detection of bacteria and viruses from different clinical specimens. For example, qualitative molecular assays are available for detection of methicillin-resistant *S aureus* (MRSA), *B pertussis*, influenza, and RSV in NP swabs; HSV and enterovirus in CSF; group B *Streptococcus* in vaginal/rectal swabs of pregnant women; HSV in skin and genital specimens; VZV in skin; *N gonorrhoeae* and *Chlamydia trachomatis* in genital and urine samples; and adenovirus in blood and stool. A variety of different platforms and fully automated systems are available for laboratories to choose from depending on the needs of their patient population.

Newly FDA-approved assays for use as waived tests (ie, easy to perform and interpret so they can be performed by nonlaboratory personnel) will increase the availability of molecular assays in point-of-care settings.

### QUANTITATIVE AMPLIFICATION ASSAYS

These assays give clinicians the ability to assess baseline levels and to monitor virologic response to antiviral therapies or adjustments in an antirejection regimen. There are different commercial platforms and assays currently available for quantitative detection (viral load) for HIV, CMV, hepatitis B and C viruses, BK virus, and Epstein-Barr virus (EBV). Specific discussion of the utilization of PCR for diagnosis and therapy is found in the chapters focusing on each viral pathogen.

### MULTIPLEX PCR ASSAYS

The ability to use a single sample to detect multiple targets is especially important when clinical samples are difficult to collect or can only be collected in limited volumes (eg, CSF), or when multiple different pathogens can cause the same clinical presentation, making it difficult for clinicians to unambiguously identify the causative pathogen based on clinical findings.

One of the drawbacks of multiplex assays is that offering a preset panel with multiple targets compels physicians to order a test with targets that may not be needed for a particular patient. On the other hand, the causative pathogen may not have been in the physician's differential diagnosis but can be detected by the panel.

The multiplex PCR assays that are currently commercially available and approved by the FDA in the United States for the diagnosis of infectious diseases are briefly described below.

#### Blood Culture Panel

To date, there are 2 molecular blood culture panels that are FDA-approved for detection of microorganisms directly from positive blood cultures: the FilmArray blood culture identification panel (Biofire Diagnostics) and the Verigene blood culture test (Nanosphere).

Evaluation of both of these panels has shown that these tests accurately identify most leading causes of bloodstream infections and provide results significantly faster than traditional methodologies, allowing the clinicians to prescribe appropriate therapy much earlier, shortening hospital stay and reducing costs, and at the same time improving patient outcomes.

#### Meningitis Panel

At the time of this writing, there is 1 FDA-approved panel for the diagnosis of central nervous system infections. The FilmArray meningitis/encephalitis (ME) panel identifies the most common viral, bacterial, and yeast pathogens that cause infections in the central nervous system. Because the laboratory usually receives a small volume of CSF, use of multiplex PCR is very advantageous as many different pathogens can be tested using 1 sample. The meningitis panel detects most but not all organisms responsible for meningitis and encephalitis, and therefore, culture and other traditional laboratory studies are still necessary.

#### Respiratory Viral Panel

Clinicians are becoming more aware that viral respiratory infections other than influenza can be very severe, driving interest in a rapid and comprehensive multiplex PCR test that can detect the most common viral respiratory pathogens. At the time of this writing, there are 4 FDA-approved multiplex molecular respiratory viral panels (RVPs). Sensitivity varies by assay and by target, but all show high specificity for all targets included in the panels. The different multiplex PCR tests for the diagnosis of respiratory infections have been evaluated in various clinical settings and found to be important tools in the management of hospitalized children.

#### Gastrointestinal Panel

Infectious diarrhea can be caused by bacterial, viral, and parasitic pathogens. Because the pathogen cannot be ascertained by clinical presentation, clinicians often order a bacterial culture and also an O&P exam of stool samples from patients with diarrhea. This approach may not be clinically helpful because it can take 2 to 4 days for results of bacterial culture to be available and the O&P exam lacks sensitivity. The current gastrointestinal panels available commercially detect very rapidly and accurately most common pathogens causing diarrhea. Clinicians should be cautious and correlate the results with the clinical findings to differentiate colonization from infection.

## ANTIMICROBIAL STEWARDSHIP PROGRAMS

Antibiotics are prescribed in more than half of all hospitalizations for children, often unnecessarily. The problem of overuse of antibiotics is even more prevalent in pediatric outpatient settings. Since 2007 when IDSA published the guidelines for developing antimicrobial stewardship programs (ASPs), the number of institutions with stewardship programs in children's hospitals has been growing. Studies from single pediatric centers show that formalized ASPs in children's hospitals are effective in reducing antibiotic prescribing compared to hospitals without ASPs.

### ACKNOWLEDGMENT

I thank Carlos A. Fasola for helpful editorial suggestions.

### SUGGESTED READINGS

Baron EJ, Miller JM, Weinstein MP, et al. A guide to utilization of the microbiology laboratory for diagnosis of infectious diseases: 2013 recommendations by the Infectious Diseases Society of America (IDSA) and the American Society for Microbiology (ASM). *Clin Infect Dis.* 2013;57:e22-e121.

Clinical and Laboratory Standards Institute (CLSI). *Performance Standards for Antimicrobial Susceptibility Testing.* 26th ed. CLSI Supplement M100S. Wayne, PA: Clinical and Laboratory Standards Institute; 2016.

Dien Bard J, McElvania TeKippe E. Diagnosis of bloodstream infections in children. *J Clin Microbiol.* 2016;54:1418-1424.

Dingle TC, Butler-Wu SM. MALDI-TOF mass spectrometry for microorganism identification. *Clin Lab Med.* 2013;33:589-609.

Dudley MN, Ambrose PG, Bhavnani SM, Craig WA, Ferraro MJ, Jones RN. Antimicrobial susceptibility testing subcommittee of the Clinical and Laboratory Standards Institute. Background and rationale for revised Clinical and Laboratory Standards Institute interpretive criteria (Breakpoints) for *Enterobacteriaceae* and *Pseudomonas aeruginosa*: I. Cephalosporins and aztreonam. *Clin Infect Dis.* 2013;56:1301-1309.

Guarner J, Brandt ME. Histopathologic diagnosis of fungal infections in the 21st century. *Clin Microbiol Rev.* 2011;24:247-280.

Leclercq R, Cantón R, Brown DFJ, et al. EUCAST expert rules in antimicrobial susceptibility testing. *Clin Microbiol Infect.* 2013;19:141-160.

Palavecino EL. Clinical, epidemiologic, and laboratory aspects of methicillin-resistant *Staphylococcus aureus* infections. *Methods Mol Biol.* 2014;1085:1-24.

Schutze GE, Willoughby RE; Committee on Infectious Diseases; American Academy of Pediatrics. *Clostridium difficile* infection in infants and children. *Pediatrics.* 2013;131:196-200.

Society for Healthcare Epidemiology of America; Infectious Diseases Society of America; Pediatric Infectious Diseases Society. Policy statement on antimicrobial stewardship by the Society for Healthcare Epidemiology of America (SHEA), the Infectious Diseases Society of America (IDSA), and the Pediatric Infectious Diseases Society (PIDS). *Infect Control Hosp Epidemiol.* 2012;33:322-327.

Yagupsky P. *Kingella kingae*: carriage, transmission, and disease. *Clin Microbiol Rev.* 2015;28:54-79.

# 222 Acute Fever Without a Focus

Elizabeth P. Schlaudecker and Steven Black

## INTRODUCTION

Fever is one of the most common causes for sick child visits to healthcare providers (HCPs). Fever, as distinct from hyperthermia, is defined as a regulated rise in core body temperature. Most clinicians define fever as an oral or rectal temperature of 38°C (100.4°F) or higher. In the pediatric age group, infection due to a virus (most likely) or bacteria (eg, urinary tract infection) is the most common cause of fever, and the HCP must always be alert to serious etiologies. The tendency to seek medical attention for fever is very much age-dependent, with younger children brought to care most often. Although part of the tendency to seek medical attention for fever rests with parental anxiety, part rests appropriately with the increased risk of serious infection associated with fever in the youngest children (especially neonates), as well as in special high-risk groups.

## CLINICAL MANIFESTATIONS

Fever is not a diagnosis per se. Fever is a nonspecific response to many adverse stimuli, including inflammation, infection, and malignancy, among others. As noted, the challenge to the HCP is to separate serious causes of fever from more minor or self-limited illnesses. The most useful tool in the diagnosis of the etiology of fever is the clinical examination. One key goal of training and experience is to hone the HCP's ability to identify the truly sick or "toxic" child. Perhaps no clinical skill is more important for an HCP, who is often dealing with young children who are not able to communicate directly. Often the signs of serious infection are subtle, and the child just "does not look right." Listlessness, poor feeding, weakness, rapid pulse, and lethargy are all clues, as is the more sinister presence of poor perfusion of the extremities, shock, cyanosis, or purpura.

## DIAGNOSIS

Once the child is identified as being potentially seriously ill, then, following appropriate resuscitation, laboratory evaluation should be undertaken including peripheral white blood cell (WBC) count with differential, electrolytes, and urinalysis, as well as cultures, often including urine, blood, and cerebrospinal fluid (CSF). The CSF may also be sent for other studies as appropriate (eg, polymerase chain reaction [PCR] for herpes simplex virus [HSV] or enterovirus). Some clinicians also use erythrocyte sedimentation rate (ESR), C-reactive protein (CRP), or procalcitonin testing to evaluate febrile children, because these are often elevated in children with bacterial infection. For the truly toxic child and especially for younger children, age-appropriate antimicrobials that include treatment of sepsis and possibly meningitis should be started after obtaining appropriate studies. In most areas of the world, this must now include coverage against resistant gram-positive organisms through the inclusion of vancomycin.

For the child who is less seriously ill, a more measured evaluation is warranted. Such an evaluation should include a thorough history and physical examination to delineate the patient's symptoms and clinical course. Knowledge of the most common infectious etiologies in a given age group is also important. Upper respiratory infection, pharyngitis, otitis media, gastroenteritis, and bronchiolitis are all common causes of fever and can often be diagnosed by history and physical examination alone. Similarly, roseola and scarlet fever, as well as Kawasaki disease, can often be diagnosed on the basis of physical examination. For other entities, it may not be possible to identify a specific infection. For children without an identifiable likely cause, the most common etiology is a self-limited viral illness. Another common cause of fever in infants and children is urinary tract infection. Urinary tract infection is discussed further in Chapter 233. Prolonged fever of unknown origin is a separate entity and is discussed in Chapter 223, and fever in the immunocompromised child is discussed in Chapter 224. An algorithm summarizing the evaluation and management of febrile infants and children is shown in Fig. 222-1.

Fever patterns can occasionally be useful in the diagnosis of specific conditions such as malaria. Dissociation between the pulse rate and the peak of temperature (high temperature, lower pulse than normally expected) can be seen in typhoid fever and brucellosis, but not in all cases. In most situations, the patterns tend to be nonspecific. Neoplasia is often associated with fever, especially with leukemia or lymphoma. Other noninfectious causes of fever include drug fever, hyperthyroidism, adrenal insufficiency, and autoimmune disorders such as lupus and juvenile idiopathic arthritis. Rarely, factitious fever can be seen in the young child. However, the most common cause of acute fever in children is infection, with most children having experienced at least 1 such febrile episode in the first year of life.

## FEVER IN A YOUNG CHILD

Occult bacteremia is usually defined as bacteremia occurring without the expected associated symptoms of toxicity, cardiorespiratory changes, or evidence of focal infection. Prior to the introduction and routine use of the pneumococcal conjugate vaccine in infancy, occult bacteremia due to pneumococcus was a relatively common cause of fever in young children, accounting for 90% or more of positive blood cultures in children younger than 3 years of age in the United States. About 8% of children with fever and an absolute neutrophil count (ANC) > 10,000/μL had a positive blood culture for *Streptococcus pneumoniae,* and children with such an ANC and a fever of > 41°C had about a 20% risk of bacteremia. Of children with pneumococcal bacteremia, the majority recovered spontaneously, but about 3% to 5% developed meningitis, and another 5% developed another focal infection, most commonly pneumonia.

Following introduction of conjugate vaccines against pneumococcus and *Haemophilus influenzae* type b, the remaining pathogens causing occult bacteremia are meningococcus and *Salmonella. Salmonella* is more common in the developing world. Meningococcus is the most feared of the 2, with as many as 50% of such children developing meningitis and others developing sepsis. However, occult meningococcal bacteremia is rare, occurring in less than 1% of febrile young children. Because of the severity of meningococcal infection, any association of petechiae or purpura with fever should instigate rapid clinical assessment and institution of appropriate therapy. In a survey of practicing pediatricians and emergency physicians, it was found that febrile infants (< 1 year of age) with petechiae received intensive evaluations, whereas older children did not. This may reflect the higher incidence of meningococcal disease in infancy, but it should be realized that children of all ages are susceptible to meningococcal disease and that cautious evaluation is warranted in all children who present with fever and petechiae of unknown cause. Although almost all children who present with meningococcal disease present with fever, only 62% present with a petechial or purpuric rash. At some centers, rapid diagnosis of meningococcal infection is undertaken using PCR. However, given the potential for this disease to rapidly evolve, therapy should not be withheld pending test results for suspected cases.

## FEVER IN THE NEONATE

Fever in the neonatal period (0–60 days of age) warrants special consideration. The neonate's ability to respond to infection is not fully developed. Neutrophils exhibit decreased chemotaxis, adherence, and ability to kill bacteria. The germinal centers in lymph nodes are not fully developed until about 8 weeks of age. There is also decreased ability to kill viruses such as HSV and varicella-zoster virus (VZV) in this age group. Immunoglobin G and complement levels are lower than those of older children. These developmental deficiencies make the infant more susceptible to serious infections and infections by organisms that are much less common in older children or adults. Group B streptococcus, *Escherichia coli, Listeria monocytogenes, Enterococcus, Staphylococcus aureus*, and HSV can cause sepsis in the first 2 months of life. Identification of sepsis in the neonate is more challenging than in older children. The febrile response is less developed such that a

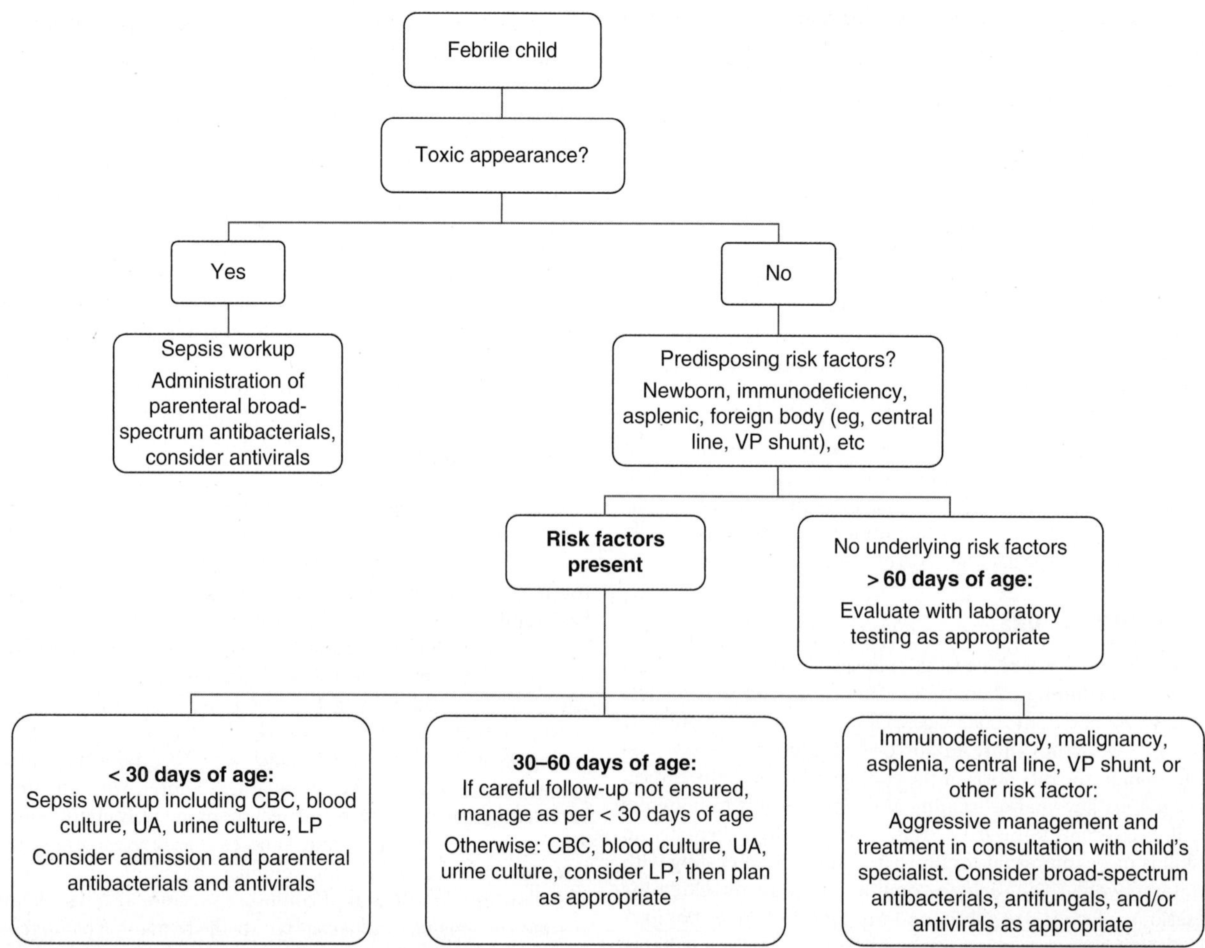


**FIGURE 222-1** Summary algorithm for evaluation of the febrile child. CBC, complete blood count; LP, lumbar puncture; UA, urinalysis; VP, ventriculoperitoneal.

seriously ill infant may not develop fever. Behavioral changes are more difficult to identify because the range of behaviors in this age group is limited. Although lethargy or changes in feeding habits, sleep pattern, or stool pattern can occur, their presence does not always indicate serious infection.

Because of the difficulty in identifying sepsis in the neonate and because such infections can progress so rapidly, special precautions should be taken in the evaluation and treatment of febrile neonates. In the first month of life, most experts believe that a "full septic workup" should be performed, including blood and urine cultures as well as a lumbar puncture. Admission to the hospital is warranted in this age group, with parenteral antibacterials given pending results. If there is no obvious bacterial cause after initial evaluation, many experts also recommend the addition of parenteral acyclovir (for HSV) in this age group. For children 31 to 60 days of age, there is less consensus regarding management. Some HCPs will evaluate and treat these children the same as children 0 to 30 days of age. Other HCPs will perform the same assessment; however, if the CBC, urinalysis, and CSF are normal and the child is feeding well and appears otherwise normal, children who have reliable parents are often cautiously observed at home with frequent visits to their HCP. This approach requires the willingness of the HCP to stay in contact with the parents as well as confidence in the parents' ability to reassess the child. Several scales have been developed to facilitate assessment of potentially ill young infants, but the specificity of these varies.

## THE FEBRILE CHILD IN A RESOURCE-LIMITED COUNTRY

Children who live in or have traveled to a resourced-limited country are subject to all of the conditions mentioned earlier, but also are at risk of other diseases including malaria, *Ascaris* or other parasitic infections, *Shigella,* typhoid fever, and other *Salmonella* infections. In malaria-endemic areas, appropriate testing for malaria should be included in the first round of testing. Typhoid fever and other *Salmonella* infections are common causes of fever in many tropical countries. Infected children may not present with gastroenteritis, but with fever only. *Ascaris* infection is often associated with abdominal distention and irritability. In addition, dengue and other arbovirus infections must be considered in areas where they occur.

## PREDISPOSING CONDITIONS

Several underlying conditions predispose children to bacterial infections. Children with asplenia or sickle cell disease are especially susceptible to overwhelming pneumococcal infections and infections due to *Salmonella, E coli,* and other gram-negative organisms. Even if the child has received pneumococcal vaccine, the risk of pneumococcal infection due to serotypes not in the vaccine remains. Febrile young children with asplenia or sickle cell disease should receive prompt assessment and antibacterial treatment. Similarly, immunosuppressed or human immunodeficiency virus (HIV)-infected children often present with severe infection. An approach to diagnosis and treatment of patients with HIV/acquired immunodeficiency syndrome (AIDS) can be found in Chapter 310. Fever in the immunocompromised child is discussed in Chapter 224. Children with foreign bodies such as central venous catheters, ventriculoperitoneal shunts, or implanted cardiac valves are all at increased risk of bacteremia and, when febrile, require early evaluation with cultures obtained and antimicrobial treatment as appropriate.

## TREATMENT

The primary decision facing the HCP in the evaluation of the febrile child is whether the child's condition warrants presumptive antimicrobial therapy and whether such therapy should be given on an outpatient or inpatient basis. As discussed previously, for neonates, immunosuppressed or HIV-infected children, and children with asplenia, sickle cell disease, or other predisposing conditions, the decision is relatively straightforward, with aggressive diagnostic measures and antimicrobial therapy often being required. For children without a history of underlying conditions, consideration must be given to the child's age (with children younger than 2 years with fever and without an obvious focus warranting laboratory evaluation, especially including a urinalysis), as well as the reliability of the parents and home situation. For the HCP who knows the child and family, it is often easier to rely on clinical judgment and careful follow-up. For the emergency room doctor, this approach may be more difficult. In all cases, one of the most important components of the evaluation and therapy of febrile infants and children is careful follow-up of the child.

## SUGGESTED READINGS


Arora R, Mahajan P. Evaluation of child with fever without source: review of the literature and update. *Pediatr Clin North Am.* 2013;60:1049-1062.

Colvin JM, Muenzer JT, Jaffe DM, et al. Detection of viruses in young children with fever without an apparent source. *Pediatrics.* 2012;130:e1455-e1462.

Iroh Tam PY, Obaro SK, Storch G. Challenges in the etiology and diagnosis of acute febrile illness in children in low- and middle-income countries. *J Pediatr Infect Dis Soc.* 2016;5:190-205.

Mekitarian Filho E, Carvalho WB. Current management of occult bacteremia in infants. *J Pediatr.* 2015;91:S61-S66.

Rudinsky SL, Carstairs KL, Reardon JM, Simon LV, Riffenburgh RH, Tanen DA. Serious bacterial infections in febrile infants in the post-pneumococcal conjugate vaccine era. *Acad Emerg Med.* 2009;16:585-590.

Watt K, Waddle E, Jhaveri R. Changing epidemiology of serious bacterial infections in febrile infants without localizing signs. *PLoS One.* 2010;5:e12448.


# 223 Fever of Unknown Origin

Russell W. Steele

## INTRODUCTION

The definition of fever of unknown origin (FUO) in an immunologically normal host requires an oral or rectal temperature ≥ 38.0°C (100.4°F) at least twice a week for more than 3 weeks and a noncontributory history and physical examination. FUO should not be confused with fevers of shorter duration variously termed "fever without localizing signs" (< 7 days) and "fever without source" (FWS) (7–14 days). Management of patients with comorbidity factors such as acquired or congenital immunodeficiency, neutropenia, and occurrence of fever during prolonged hospital stays is not considered in the following discussion since the differential diagnosis and evaluation of these patients vary considerably.

Because of the ready availability of more sensitive polymerase chain reaction (PCR) and serologic antibody assays and more precise radiographic scanning procedures, the assigned etiologies of FUO in children, as well as in adults, have changed over the past 3 decades, and more causes of fever are diagnosed earlier in the course of illness by primary care physicians.

Three pathogens now account for most identified infectious disease causes of FUO: Epstein-Barr virus, *Bartonella henselae* (cat scratch disease), and *Escherichia coli* urinary tract infections (Table 223-1). All can be confirmed with serologic assays or cultures for the respective pathogens. Cat scratch disease can also be confirmed with compatible liver lesions documented by abdominal sonogram or computed tomography (CT) scan.

**TABLE 223-1 ETIOLOGY OF FEVER OF UNKNOWN ORIGIN IN CHILDREN**

| Disease Category | 1970–1980 | 1980–1990 | 1990–1996 | 1991–2015 |
|---|---|---|---|---|
| Infectious | 38% | 22% | 44% | 21% |
| Epstein-Barr virus | 2% | 8% | 15% | 4% |
| Cat-scratch disease | 0% | 2% | 5% | 2% |
| Urinary tract infection | 5% | 4% | 4% | 2% |
| Osteomyelitis | 1% | 1% | 10% | 1% |
| Tuberculosis | 2% | 0% | 0% | 1% |
| Others | 28% | 7% | 10% | 11% |
| Autoimmune | 17% | 6% | 8% | 6% |
| Juvenile idiopathic arthritis | | 3% | 3% | 4% |
| Systemic lupus erythematosus | | 1% | 2% | 1% |
| Others | | 2% | 2% | 1% |
| Malignancy | 9% | 2% | 3% | 4% |
| Leukemia | | 1% | 1% | 1% |
| Lymphoma | | 1% | 1% | 1% |
| Others | | 0% | 1% | 2% |
| Others | 18% | 3% | 2% | 8% |
| No diagnosis | 18% | 67% | 43% | 61% |

Over 60% of children who now present with FUO resolve their fever without determination of a cause, in contrast to only 10% to 20% in series published 20 to 30 years ago. In addition, a higher percentage of children with malignancies are now definitively diagnosed earlier in the course of illness, and such cases lead to an overall reduction in total cases of FUO. A greater percentage of the remainder likely have viral illnesses that are more difficult to diagnose but more likely to resolve without intervention.

## CLINICAL EVALUATION

An oral or rectal temperature ≥ 38°C (100.4°F) is 2 standard deviations above the average for normal children and most appropriately defines fever. Rectal recordings are preferred for younger children. Tympanic and temporal artery temperatures are so unreliable that they cannot be used to monitor febrile patients. Many parents believe that any temperature above the average—that is, ≥ 37°C (98.6°F)—is abnormal and seek consultation for these observations. Unless there are other clinical findings, either historically or during physical examination, reassurance is the only intervention warranted for temperatures < 38°C (100.4°F).

For "subjective" fevers, usually meaning that the child feels warm to the parent or another caregiver, a diary recording of morning and afternoon rectal temperature measurements for at least 1 week should be obtained before initiating diagnostic evaluation. Children often feel warm, particularly when environmental temperatures are high enough to induce flushing or perspiration. Despite widespread public perceptions, few parents (or grandparents) can determine low-grade temperature elevations by simply touching their child's forehead. However, core temperatures > 39.4°C (103°F) consistently produce skin temperature changes that can be recognized by most caregivers.

The number of documented febrile recordings during a 21-day observation period considered abnormal is suggested as 2 per week. However, cases should be individualized. Well-defined events such as otitis media or limited viral illnesses can account for some febrile periods. Conversely, antipyretic therapy might mask significant temperature spikes. Rarely, an observation period in the hospital is the only way to verify fever in children whose parents insist that fever exists, but in whom the observation cannot be confirmed. In cases of factitious fever (Munchausen syndrome by proxy), potential underlying family psychopathology should be assessed and managed with appropriate professional evaluation and counseling.

Although there is a natural tendency to consider unusual or exotic diseases when confronted with prolonged fever in children, common viral or bacterial pathogens that present atypically are much more frequent than exotic or unusual diseases. Therefore, epidemiologic information and history of exposure prior to illness are major components of the initial evaluation. Diagnoses quite common in one area of the United States might not even be considered in other locations. Examples include Lyme disease (Northeast and certain areas of the Midwest), tularemia (Midwest and far West), coccidioidomycosis (Southwest), and tuberculosis (urban).

Patient history should be more detailed than that obtained for acute illnesses, carefully examining family history, previous illnesses, recent symptoms, current medications, travel, and exposure to pets or humans with potential communicable pathogens. Weight loss, failure to thrive, and decreased activity during afebrile periods are more ominous systemic signs that will usually require a more rapid diagnostic evaluation. Prolonged fever and bone pain may be the only manifestations of bone tumors, leukemia, osteomyelitis, syphilis, cat scratch disease, tuberculosis, or Langerhans cell histiocytosis. In the presence of documented fever and constitutional symptoms, a history of abdominal pain necessitates evaluation for autoimmune diseases, pyelonephritis, Crohn disease, tuberculosis, and hepatitis, as well as abdominal abscesses and tumors.

Of all symptoms, the presence of pain is the single finding that is likely to suggest specific laboratory studies. Therefore, pain should be completely characterized by its severity, location, periodicity, precipitating factors, and response to attempted therapy.

Age is the next critical factor. Leukemia peaks in early childhood, whereas lymphomas are unusual before age 8 years. Human immunodeficiency virus (HIV) infection presenting as FUO is more prevalent during the first year of life or during adolescence. Most autoimmune disease is seen in school-age children and adolescents, so screening tests for this category would usually be limited to this older age group.

Physical examination occasionally provides the first diagnostic clue, especially when directed toward areas where abscesses or solid tumors are less apparent. Thorough abdominal and rectal exams are essential because the abdomen and pelvis represent the largest areas for such masses. Bones and joints can be adequately evaluated if the child is cooperative. Transillumination of sinuses is only useful in the older child and adolescent; younger children require selective CT scans to diagnose sinusitis.

## LABORATORY AND RADIOGRAPHIC EVALUATION

Diagnostic evaluation should begin with basic studies done during outpatient observation, as summarized in Table 223-2. The complete blood count with a manual differential accomplishes 3 goals: (1) it is a screen for leukemia, anemia, and neutropenia; (2) it identifies some acute phase reactant changes by quantitating polymorphonuclear leukocytes, immature granulocytes, and platelets; and (3) it helps eliminate some specific, although unusual, diagnostic considerations, such as eosinophilia (present in some parasitic diseases), Howell-Jolly bodies (congenital or functional asplenia), or pathogens on blood smear (malaria, relapsing fever). Additional screening for leukemia is achieved with a serum lactate dehydrogenase and uric acid. Urinalysis and urine culture should be obtained because urinary tract infection is the second most commonly identified infectious cause of FUO, remembering that fever is second only to abdominal pain as a symptom of pyelonephritis. Chest roentgenograms may identify an unexpected pneumonia, but they are also important in screening for tumors, particularly lymphomas, and for tuberculosis. An interferon-γ release assay (IGRA) is now preferred to the tuberculin skin test (TST) to rule out tuberculosis in older children. Also in older children, an antinuclear antibody (ANA) determination is beneficial in screening for autoimmune diseases such as systemic lupus erythematosus, although no single test consistently identifies autoimmune processes. Patients with systemic juvenile idiopathic arthritis (JIA) are most likely to present with fever alone, but JIA is rarely associated with a positive ANA response. Both a C-reactive protein (CRP) and procalcitonin should be considered since the CRP is elevated in all inflammatory conditions, whereas the procalcitonin is usually not elevated during viral infection and autoimmune diseases.

The greatest clinical concern in evaluating FUO is identifying patients whose fever has a serious or life-threatening etiology for whom a delay in diagnosis could jeopardize successful intervention. However, the majority of children with prolonged FUO resolve their illness without a diagnosis and do not exhibit long-lasting effects. Therefore, it appears appropriate for most children to delay extensive diagnostic evaluation until the child has remained febrile for at least 6 weeks. The initial outpatient evaluation (see Table 223-2) generally requires 1 week for completion of laboratory testing and for reporting of final results. After this time, the physician must decide whether continued observation or progressive laboratory investigation is more appropriate. Decisions are based primarily on the clinical status of the child and the results of the initial evaluation. If a decision is made to pursue testing beyond the initial screen, selection of subsequent studies is guided primarily by knowledge of the more common etiologies. This approach takes into consideration patient age, epidemiologic and geographic information, and any positive findings from a detailed history and physical examination. In addition, testing for some less common etiologies should be included for diseases known to progress in severity if diagnosis and treatment are delayed. Examples of the latter category include abdominal tumors, Lyme disease, and Crohn disease.

Table 223-3 summarizes a practical approach to a stepwise, yet systematic, evaluation. Earlier studies can be accomplished during continued outpatient evaluation, although hospitalization is required for those more invasive (and costly) procedures suggested during later phases of investigation. The rationale for each test should be apparent. Individual circumstances will certainly modify selection of tests to the extent that any 2 patients are unlikely to have the same studies ordered. More invasive and expensive testing is not recommended unless there is a clear clinical indication. Such tests might include bone marrow examination, sonograms, CT, whole-body magnetic resonance imaging or fluorine-18 fluorodeoxyglucose positron emission tomography ($^{18}$F-FDG-PET). Other nuclear medicine tests such as indium or gallium scanning have fallen out of favor due to the relatively high dose of radiation the patient receives and the need to wait for several days until these studies are completed.

Finally, patience on the part of the physician is required. The best tests to arrive at a final etiologic diagnosis remain repeated careful clinical assessment with interim histories and physical examinations. Even under these conditions, fever will usually resolve before a specific cause has been delineated.

| TABLE 223-2 INITIAL OUTPATIENT EVALUATION FOR A PEDIATRIC PATIENT WITH FEVER OF UNKNOWN ORIGIN |
|---|
| History and physical examination (all causes) |
| Complete blood cell count with manual differential (leukemia and infection) |
| Lactate dehydrogenase and uric acid (leukemia and lymphoma) |
| Urinalysis and culture (urinary tract infection) |
| Chest roentgenogram (infection and malignancy) |
| Interferon-γ release assay (tuberculosis) |
| Antinuclear antibody titer—older children (autoimmune disease) |
| Procalcitonin and C-reactive protein (all causes) |

**TABLE 223-3 ADVANCED EVALUATION FOR A PEDIATRIC PATIENT WITH FEVER OF UNKNOWN ORIGIN**

| |
|---|
| **Phase 1: Outpatient 3–6 weeks of fever** |
| Complete blood cell count with manual differential (repeat) |
| C-reactive protein and procalcitonin (repeat) |
| Urinalysis and culture (repeat) |
| Epstein-Barr virus serology (VCA-IgG, VCA-IgM, EA, and EBNA) |
| *Bartonella henselae* serology IgG and IgM (if history of cat exposure) |
| Chest roentgenogram (review if already obtained) |
| 2 Blood cultures |
| Antistreptolysin O (ASO) titer |
| Human immunodeficiency virus (HIV) antibody if there are risk factors |
| Twice-daily temperature recordings (by parents at home) |
| **Phase 2: Inpatient (if clinically ill after 6 weeks of fever)** |
| Observation |
| Lumbar puncture for routine studies |
| Repeat blood cultures |
| Sinus radiographs |
| Ophthalmologic examination for iridocyclitis |
| Liver enzymes |
| Serologic screens (IgG and IgM) |
| Cytomegalovirus |
| *Toxoplasma gondii* |
| Hepatitis A, B, and C (if liver enzymes elevated) |
| Tularemia (agglutination titer) |
| Leptospira (microscopic agglutination test) |
| **Phase 3: Inpatient (after 6 weeks of fever if condition worsens)** |
| Abdominal ultrasonography |
| Abdominal computed tomography scan |
| Upper and lower gastrointestinal endoscopy (older child with any abdominal symptoms or suspicion for Crohn disease, eg, mouth ulcers) |
| Bone marrow (including aspirate, biopsy, and culture) |
| Technetium bone scan |
| Whole-body magnetic resonance imaging |
| Fluorine-18 fluorodeoxyglucose positron emission tomography |

## SUGGESTED READINGS


Antoon JW, Knudson-Johnson M, Lister WM. Diagnostic approach to fever of unknown origin. *Clin Pediatr (Phila)*. 2012;51(11): 1091-1094.

Damasio MB, Magnaguagno F, Stagnaro G. Whole body MRI: non-oncological applications in paediatrics. *Radiol Med*. 2016;121: 454-461.

Lachmann HJ. Autoinflammatory syndromes as causes of fever of unknown origin. *Clin Med*. 2015;15:295-298.

Marshall GS. Prolonged and recurrent fevers in children. *J Infect*. 2014;68(suppl 1):S83-S93.

Oostenbrink R. Implementation of procalcitonin in the management of febrile children. *Pediatr Infect Dis J*. 2012;31(7):792-793.

Seashore CJ, Lohr JA. Fever of unknown origin in children. *Pediatr Ann*. 2011;40(1):26-30.

Shammas A, Charron M. Pediatric nuclear medicine in acute care. *Semin Nucl Med*. 2013;43:139-156.

Statler VA, Marshall GS. Characteristics of patients referred to a pediatric infectious diseases clinic with unexplained fever. *J Pediatr Infect Dis Soc*. 2016;5(3):249-256.

Tolan RW Jr. Fever of unknown origin: a diagnostic approach to this vexing problem. *Clin Pediatr*. 2010;49:207-213.


# 224 Fever and Infection in the Immunocompromised Patient

Christopher C. Dvorak and Jeffery J. Auletta



## INTRODUCTION

A key element in the effective care of immunocompromised patients with fever is hypervigilance. Not only are these patients at increased risk for a diverse range of microorganisms, but also infections caused by these organisms can present in subtle or atypical ways and often progress to difficult-to-treat chronic disease states or rapid clinical decompensation. Therefore, empiric anti-infective therapy is justified for new-onset fever in immunocompromised patients while a thorough investigation into the source of fever is performed. Because antimicrobial therapies often have adverse side effects, an accurate evaluation to guide definitive antimicrobial therapy becomes crucial.

General features of a thoughtful diagnostic approach to fever in immunocompetent patients remain valid for immunocompromised patients, including consideration for noninfectious diagnoses (see Chapter 223). Likewise, exposure history remains essential and must be expanded to include microorganisms traditionally considered to be "environmental" or of "low virulence." Published guidelines for the use of antimicrobial agents in immunocompromised children outline contemporary standards of care and can provide useful algorithms to help improve patient outcomes. One key principle is the importance of frequent reevaluations of immunocompromised patients' course and care. Furthermore, optimal care may require input from an infectious diseases physician with expertise in treating immunocompromised patients infected with microorganisms that are often difficult to diagnose or treat like fungi or mycobacteria.

## EPIDEMIOLOGY AND PATHOGENESIS

In developed countries, immunodeficiency is commonly acquired. Severe connective tissue disease, hematopoietic cell transplantation (HCT), and solid organ transplantation (SOT) inherently cause immune suppression, which is often worsened by immunosuppressive drugs used to prevent deleterious auto- and allo-immunity. In developing countries, acquired conditions such as human immunodeficiency virus (HIV)/acquired immunodeficiency syndrome (AIDS) and severe malnutrition cause significant immunodeficiency.

Patients with primary immunodeficiency often cannot eradicate infection until immune function is restored through allogeneic HCT, enzyme replacement therapy (for patients with adenosine deaminase deficiency), or gene therapy. Similarly, immune function in patients with acquired immunodeficiencies like HIV or immunosuppressive therapy can sometimes be clinically improved via immunomodulatory therapies that suppress viral load (eg, antiretroviral therapy [ART]) or stimulate neutrophil production (eg, granulocyte colony-stimulating factor [GCSF]), which work in combination with antimicrobial therapy to eradicate infection.

Defects in immunologic functions (see Chapters 183 and 184) correlate with increased patient risk for infection (Table 224-1). For example, T-cell–mediated immunity is particularly important for defense against fungal and viral infections. The reticuloendothelial function of the spleen is necessary to clear encapsulated bacteria from the blood, and terminal complement components lyse opsonized bacteria such as *Neisseria meningitidis*. Neutrophil oxidative bursts kill catalase-positive bacteria and fungi within neutrophils, and antitoxin antibodies prevent toxic shock induced by the toxic shock syndrome toxin (TSST)-1 superantigen as well as directly kill bacterial pathogens. Therefore, immune defect–specific risks offer basic insights into the diagnostic workup and the use of prophylactic and empiric antimicrobials for immunocompromised children. Conversely, certain infectious disease presentations provide clues to trigger and guide an

**TABLE 224-1 IMMUNOLOGIC FUNCTIONAL DEFECTS AND SUSCEPTIBILITY TO INFECTIONS**

| Immune Defect | Underlying Etiology | Increased Infection Susceptibility |
|---|---|---|
| **Barriers/Clearance** | | |
| Skin barrier defects | Burns, mucositis, intravenous catheters, urinary catheters | Gram-negative rods (especially *Pseudomonas*); gram-positive cocci (staphylococci, streptococci); fungi (especially *Candida* and *Aspergillus*) |
| Respiratory clearance defects | Ciliary motility defects, cystic fibrosis | Respiratory tract pathogens, including *Streptococcus pneumoniae, Staphylococcus aureus, Pseudomonas, Klebsiella, Stenotrophomonas, Burkholderia cepacia*, fast-growing atypical mycobacteria (eg, *Mycobacterium abscessus*) |
| Asplenia | Sickle cell anemia, splenic trauma or surgery, splenic developmental defects | Encapsulated bacteria (*S pneumoniae, Neisseria meningitidis, Haemophilus influenzae*), *Salmonella* |
| **Neutrophils** | | |
| Neutropenia | Cytotoxic chemotherapy for neoplasia, bone marrow transplantation, severe congenital neutropenia | Gram-negative rods (especially *Pseudomonas, Escherichia, Klebsiella*); gram-positive cocci (staphylococci, streptococci, enterococci); *Corynebacterium*; fungi (especially *Candida* and *Aspergillus*) |
| Neutrophil oxidative burst defect | Chronic granulomatous disease | Catalase-positive bacteria such as staphylococci, Enterobacteriaceae (eg, *Escherichia coli, Klebsiella, Serratia*), *Aspergillus, Candida, Nocardia* |
| Neutrophil adhesion or migration defects | Intracellular adhesion molecule or cytoskeletal molecular defects | Periodontal disease, omphalitis, skin infections (staphylococci, streptococci, *Pseudomonas, Klebsiella, Enterobacter, Candida*), pneumonia |
| **Lymphocytes** | | |
| Combined T- and B-cell defects | Severe combined immunodeficiency, combined immunodeficiency | Herpes viruses (HSV, CMV, VZV, EBV); respiratory and enteric viruses (parainfluenza, rotavirus, norovirus), fungi (*Candida, Pneumocystis jirovecii*), atypical *Mycobacteria* |
| CD4 T-cell deficiency | HIV infection, Bare lymphocyte syndrome | Bacteria (*S pneumoniae* and other encapsulated organisms, *Salmonella*, enteric organisms, *Mycobacterium tuberculosis*, atypical mycobacteria); herpes viruses (HSV, CMV, VZV, EBV); fungi (*Candida, Aspergillus, P jirovecii*) |
| T-cell development defect | Athymia, as in DiGeorge syndrome | Similar to patterns seen in HIV infection |
| T-cell proliferation defect | T-cell immunosuppressive medications[a] | Fungi (eg, *Aspergillus, Candida, Cryptococcus*, molds, *Mucormycosis*), latent herpes viruses (HSV, CMV, VZV, EBV), polyomaviruses (BK, JC), adenovirus, hepatitis viruses, *P jirovecii, Listeria, Nocardia, Toxoplasma* |
| B-cell dysfunction | X-linked agammaglobulinemia | Overwhelming EBV infections |
| | Hyper-IgE syndrome | Recurrent skin abscesses (especially *S aureus*) |
| | Wiskott-Aldrich syndrome | Encapsulated organisms, herpes viruses |
| Antibody class-switching defect | CD40/CD40 ligand defects | Encapsulated organisms, herpes viruses, *Cryptosporidium, Cryptococcus, Candida, Histoplasma, Bartonella, P jirovecii* |
| Absence of specific antibody titers | Host variation in neutralizing antibody response | TSS (toxic shock syndrome) toxin-1 |
| Natural killer cell defects | *RTEL1, GATA2*, or *MCM4* deficiency | Herpes viruses, HPV |
| **Innate Immunity** | | |
| TNF-α blockade | Anti–TNF-α therapy | Mycobacteria, including *M tuberculosis*; fungi, including histoplasmosis |
| Terminal complement component deficiency | Defects in complement genes for C5 through C9 | *N meningitidis* |

[a]T-cell immunosuppressant medications include antithymocyte globulin, calcineurin inhibitors, tacrolimus/sirolimus, corticosteroids, and azathioprine.

CMV, cytomegalovirus; EBV, Epstein-Barr virus; HPV, human papilloma virus; HSV, herpes simplex virus; TNF, tumor necrosis factor; VZV, varicella-zoster virus.

evaluation into specific immune defects in children, many of which are primary or genetic in nature.

From a clinical perspective, the pathophysiology of infections in immunocompromised hosts often reflects a combination of immune defects (see Table 224-1). For example, following cytotoxic chemotherapy for cancer, patients are predisposed to sepsis due to acquired neutropenia, mucosal breakdown, foreign bodies like intravascular catheters, and broad-spectrum antimicrobials that eliminate commensal bacteria, select for drug-resistant microbial flora, and increase fungal infection risk. Similarly, patients with genetic immune defects in T-cell development can also have defective B-cell function, producing combined immunodeficiency.

## CLINICAL MANIFESTATIONS

Infections in immunocompromised children vary in their clinical presentation depending on the underlying immune functional defect (see Table 224-1). The most common clinical presentations are fever in patients with neutropenia (F&N), resulting from genetic, autoimmune, and iatrogenic causes, and fever in patients receiving immunosuppressive therapies for rheumatologic diseases, HCT, or SOT. In patients with F&N, many of the clinical signs of a localized infection such as erythema or pus may be absent given the lack of functionally competent neutrophils and other white blood cells. In patients receiving immunosuppression, certain therapies, especially corticosteroids, can attenuate the fever response, even in the context of serious infection.

### Febrile Neutropenia

Following antineoplastic therapy, neutropenia has traditionally been defined as an absolute neutrophil count (ANC) < 500 cells/μL or as an ANC < 1000 cells/μL with a predicted decrease to < 500 cells/μL. Distinct from prolonged fever duration required for classic fever of unknown origin (FUO), fever in the context of neutropenia is defined as a single oral temperature ≥ 38.3°C (101°F) or ≥ 38.0°C (100.4°F) sustained for 1 hour. The depth and duration of neutropenia determine the risk for microbiologically documented infection, particularly invasive fungal infection. For example, nearly 50% of febrile neutropenic patients may ultimately prove to have infections, and 1 in 5 patients with fever and profound neutropenia (ANC < 100 cells/μL) will have bacteremia (see Table 224-1). Profound and prolonged neutropenia, particularly among patients who have received broad-spectrum antibacterial therapy, predisposes to severe fungal infections, most commonly *Candida* and *Aspergillus* species.

### Transplant Recipients

Febrile transplant recipients have contrasting presentations and infections versus patients with F&N. Transplant patients have

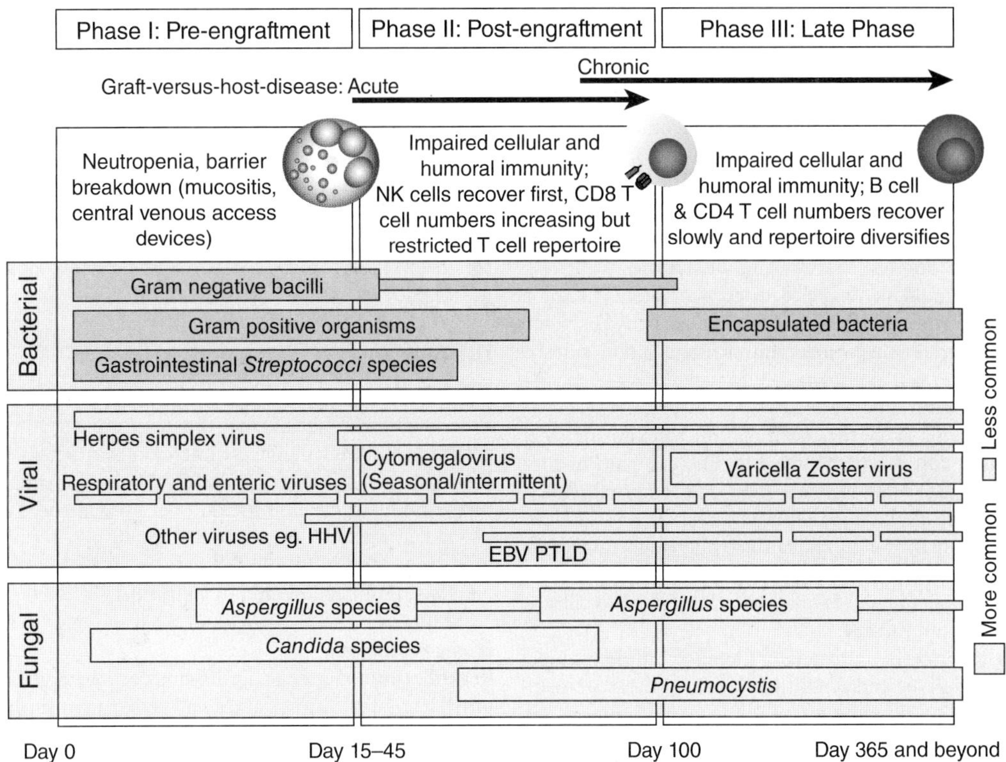


**FIGURE 224-1** Phases of risk for opportunistic infections in allogeneic hematopoietic cell transplantation (HCT) recipients over time based on type of immunocompromise. EBV PTLD, Epstein-Barr virus–associated posttransplant lymphoproliferative disorder; HHV, human herpes virus. (Reproduced with permission from Tomblyn M, Chiller T, Einsele H, et al. Guidelines for preventing infectious complications among hematopoietic cell transplantation recipients: a global perspective, *Biol Blood Marrow Transplant.* 2009 Oct;15(10):1143-1238.)

compromised lymphocyte function, which increases susceptibility to different infections over time. Early after HCT (< 1 month), organisms associated with breaks in mucosal or skin barriers and neutropenia predominate (Fig. 224-1). Early after SOT (< 1 month), nosocomial infections predominate, including aspiration pneumonia and catheter, wound, or anastomotic leak infections. Recipient-derived infections are most common, which reflect host microbial colonization with *Aspergillus*, *Pseudomonas*, or resistant species like methicillin-resistant *Staphylococcus aureus*, vancomycin-resistant *Enterococcus*, and *Candida* non-*albicans* species.

In the intermediate post-HCT period (1–6 months), immunosuppression is often at its most intense. During this time, there are notably high risks for pneumocystis pneumonia and infections due to herpes simplex viruses (HSV), varicella-zoster virus (VZV), cytomegalovirus (CMV), and Epstein-Barr virus (EBV), risks that can be partially attenuated by prophylaxis with trimethoprim-sulfamethoxazole and antivirals, respectively. Other opportunistic infections classically seen during this stage include *Listeria*, *Nocardia*, *Toxoplasma*, *Mycobacterium tuberculosis*, hepatitis B and C viruses, adenovirus, influenza, BK polyomavirus, and endemic fungi such as coccidiomycosis or histoplasmosis. In relevant geographic contexts, *Strongyloides*, *Leishmania*, and *Trypanosoma cruzi* infections can also occur. Lastly, EBV-associated posttransplant lymphoproliferative disorder (EBV-PTLD) is most common in the intermediate post-HCT period, reflecting incomplete donor-derived immune recovery. SOT patients in the intermediate posttransplant period (1–6 months) are predisposed to similar opportunistic infections, as are HCT patients.

In the late post-HCT period (> 6 months), immunosuppressive medications are typically tapered and discontinued, and immunity is restored unless the patient develops graft-versus-host disease (GVHD). In addition to requiring ongoing immunosuppression, GVHD itself adversely affects secondary lymphoid organ and bone marrow function, resulting in functional asplenia and peripheral pancytopenia, respectively. In the late post-SOT period (> 6 months), immunosuppressive medications are traditionally decreased, but host susceptibility remains significantly increased for *Listeria*, *Nocardia*, and invasive fungal infections. Likewise, late viral infections with CMV, HSV, and JC polyomavirus can occur. Finally, EBV-PTLD and late allograft rejection can also present with fever during the late SOT period, often more than 2 years after transplant.

Analogous to the level of neutropenia predisposing to infection, the degree of immunosuppression in HCT and SOT patients influences infection risk. However, clinical biomarkers for quantifying the level of immunosuppression are less robust than quantitative measurements like ANC in patients with neutropenia or absolute CD4 count for patients with HIV. Immune recovery after HCT is measured by levels in quantitative T- and B-cell subtypes, quantitative immunoglobulins, and lymphocyte proliferative response assays. Serum levels of immunosuppressive drugs and clinical concern for GVHD (for HCT patients), allograft rejection (for SOT patients), or host infection are used to titrate immunosuppressive therapies.

## DIAGNOSIS

Immunocompromised patients often lack classic signs and symptoms of inflammation, such that severe infections can exhibit remarkably occult clinical presentations. Furthermore, lack of classic inflammation on physical exam can still result in rapid clinical decompensation in immunocompromised patients. Indeed, a fundamental challenge in caring for these patients is that they can initially present in extremis from overwhelming infection. Accordingly, vigilant attention to signs of shock, hypoxia, or deep-organ infections is essential.

Physical examination should seek even subtle signs of infection, such as pain in anatomic sites, including the eyes, periodontium, pharynx, esophagus, lung, perineum, skin and nails, and near vascular access sites. A thorough examination is critical. In particular, localized signs of pain or discomfort should result in diagnostic investigation directed at defining an underlying etiology.

The evaluation of febrile immunocompromised patients should always include attempts to identify the responsible pathogens as well as to define the pathogen's susceptibility to antimicrobials, as unrecognized and untreated infections can be lethal. Blood cultures, including those drawn from all lumens of central venous lines (CVLs), are a cornerstone of diagnostic evaluation to detect bacteremia or fungemia. Quantitative cultures, drawn concomitantly from CVL lumens and peripheral blood, and assessing time to positivity (TTP) can help establish if the CVL is the nidus of infection. To increase diagnostic yield, at least 2 sets of blood cultures are suggested. Furthermore, pediatric blood culture sensitivity decreases with low-volume blood samples. Therefore, blood cultures using less than 1 mL of blood should be recorded to appropriately discount their value for negative prediction. To improve sensitivity, particularly for recovery of certain mycobacteria and fungi, blood culture methods in immunocompromised hosts should include use of special media and prolonged culture incubation.

CVL infection is more likely for particular microorganisms (eg, *Staphylococcus* species) and can be heralded by line site pain or discharge (ie, tunnel infection) or by systemic symptoms temporally associated with line infusions. Rapid microbiologic stains of any exudates, biopsy specimens, or positive cultures can provide important early insights to direct antimicrobial therapy. Importantly, evidence of deep infections on imaging often necessitates direct biopsy and culture for definitive diagnosis and therapy.

Additional diagnostic tests traditionally include complete blood count with differential, liver and renal function, and measurement of electrolytes. Other blood tests that can aid in the diagnosis of opportunistic infections include galactomannan (GMN) assay for the polysaccharide cell wall component of *Aspergillus* species, as well as quantitative polymerase chain reaction (PCR) for double-stranded DNA viruses (eg, CMV, EBV, adenovirus, BK virus, human herpes virus [HHV]-6). Indeed, PCR-based diagnostic assays are particularly important for diagnosing and guiding appropriate antiviral drug therapy against CMV infections, which can manifest as direct invasive disease or can be associated with indirect immunomodulatory effects, such as GVHD, allograft rejection, or co-viral infection.

Use of nonspecific tests of inflammation, such as the C-reactive protein (CRP) or interleukin-6 (IL-6) levels, has not been widely adopted given problems with either sensitivity or specificity. Depending on symptoms, other potentially useful tests include urinalysis and culture, stool studies for enteric pathogens (eg, *Clostridium difficile*, rotavirus, norovirus, *Cryptosporidium*), nasopharyngeal swabs for respiratory virus antigen or PCR testing, bronchoalveolar lavage (BAL), and cerebrospinal fluid (CSF) evaluation for total protein, glucose, cell counts, viral PCR, and stains and cultures. In the near future, next-generation sequencing for nonhuman DNA may prove to be a more powerful technique to identify unusual infections in immunocompromised hosts.

Imaging studies should include a chest radiograph for patients with any respiratory signs or symptoms or for those who will be managed as outpatients. However, computed tomography (CT) or magnetic resonance imaging (MRI) of the chest, abdomen, pelvis, sinuses, or other sites may also be recommended based on relevant symptoms or previous history of infection at these sites.

The astute clinician must also remain cognizant that not all fevers in immunocompromised hosts ultimately prove to be infectious in nature. Many primary immunodeficiencies have a propensity to develop hemophagocytic lymphohistiocytosis (HLH), a syndrome of dysregulated cytokine storm that can mimic infection and even sepsis. Patients with malignancies can occasionally develop noninfectious fevers during relapse of the primary disease, and allograft rejection in SOT patients can also manifest with fevers. Finally, fevers may be due to medications, either commonly (eg, with antithymocyte globulin, some monoclonal antibodies) or as a diagnosis of drug fever by exclusion.

Complications from infections in immunocompromised hosts often relate to 3 core issues: (1) missed initial diagnosis secondary to altered features of disease presentation as compared to those observed in immunocompetent hosts; (2) traditionally "nonpathogenic" organisms in immunocompetent patients can cause severe disease in immunocompromised hosts; and (3) antimicrobial agents may not adequately prevent infectious disease progression in the context of immune defects. These concerns reiterate the importance of maintaining a broad differential diagnosis for possible infections, in which almost any microorganism isolated from a normally sterile body site should be considered a potential pathogen. Prognosis is improved with enhanced patient and physician awareness and rapid response to infection risk and diligence in diagnosing infection in order to provide timely antimicrobial therapy. In the event of an immunocompromised patient's death, autopsy findings may offer meaningful infectious disease insights, particularly for the benefit of future patients.

## TREATMENT

A common clinical scenario for patients undergoing chemotherapy, or following HCT or SOT, is the development of fever. Especially for patients with implantable central venous catheters, standard management involves a prompt clinical evaluation, obtainment of blood cultures, and typically administration of a broad-spectrum antibiotic with a long half-life, such as ceftriaxone. In the absence of neutropenia, risk prediction models to identify patients at high risk for having actual bloodstream infection are not yet robust.

### Febrile Neutropenia

Regardless of the absence of findings on physical examination and in initial laboratory investigations, all F&N patients, whether after myelosuppressive chemotherapy or following HCT, should receive empiric antimicrobial therapy directed at the microorganisms most commonly identified in this setting. In children receiving chemotherapy, whereas gram-negative rods (particularly *Escherichia coli, Klebsiella* species, and *Pseudomonas* species) were formerly the most commonly isolated, recent trends have shown that gram-positive organisms now account for more than 50% of blood culture pathogens. Coagulase-negative staphylococci (CoNS), which are the most commonly isolated organisms, typically are associated with a relatively indolent clinical effect in patients. However, some gram-positive bacteria, such as *S aureus* and the viridans group *Streptococcus*, can be associated with rapidly progressive shock, noncardiogenic pulmonary edema, and multiorgan failure, which have been more traditionally associated with gram-negative sepsis.

Current practice guidelines suggest that there are 2 major risk groups in F&N patients: (1) low-risk patients (ie, patients with anticipated neutropenia ≤ 7 days and clinically stable with no major medical comorbidities); and (2) high-risk patients (ie, all other F&N patients; Fig. 224-2). Some centers have adopted guidelines that allow outpatient management of selected low-risk children with F&N after a single dose of parenteral antibiotics is administered and if reliable follow-up is ensured. For example, after thorough history and physical examination are completed, laboratory evaluation including a complete blood count and blood cultures is obtained. The child is then given a dose of a parenteral antibiotic such as ceftazidime and discharged on oral antibiotics, such as ciprofloxacin and amoxicillin/clavulanate, with follow-up arranged. Such initial outpatient management is not acceptable for patients with hemodynamic instability or severe mucositis or for patients receiving induction chemotherapy or who have received HCT.

For patients admitted, empiric parenteral antimicrobial therapy should reflect contemporary local patterns of infection and antimicrobial resistance. As a general rule, a regimen should provide broad coverage for gram-negative organisms, including *Pseudomonas*, and provide some coverage for *S aureus*. US Food and Drug Administration–approved single-agent regimens meeting these criteria include ceftazidime, cefepime, and carbapenems (eg, meropenem or imipenem). Carbapenems are preferred if local rates of extended-spectrum β-lactamase (ESBL)–positive strains are high or if *Klebsiella* infection is suspected. To date, studies have not demonstrated marked differences in outcomes between patients receiving empiric monotherapy and combination antimicrobial therapy. Therefore, current recommendations are only to administer combination therapy in the setting of complications such as hypotension or other clinical instability.

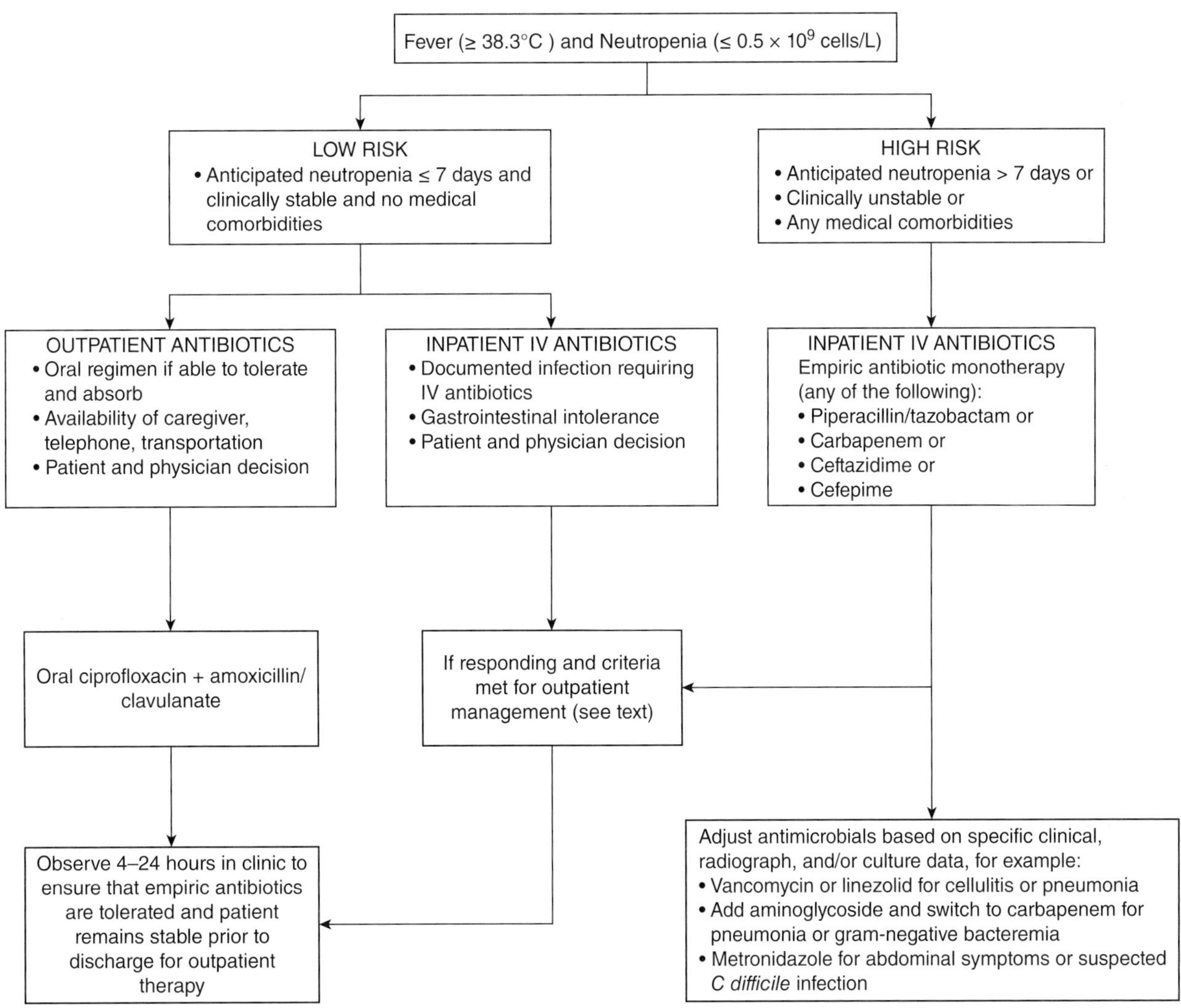


**FIGURE 224-2** Initial management of fever and neutropenia by risk category. (Modified with permission from Freifeld AG, Bow EJ, Sepkowitz KA, et al: Clinical practice guideline for the use of antimicrobial agents in neutropenic patients with cancer: 2010 update by the infectious diseases society of america, *Clin Infect Dis*. 2011 Feb 15;52(4):e56-e93.)

The decision of whether to include vancomycin as initial empiric therapy deserves particular attention. Unwarranted use of vancomycin has significant potential negative effects, including selection for vancomycin-resistant *Enterococcus* (VRE). The recommendation from the Infectious Diseases Society of America (IDSA) states that vancomycin should only be added to empiric therapy if the patient has an obvious catheter-related infection, severe mucositis, hypotension or other signs of sepsis, or known colonization with methicillin-resistant *S aureus* (MRSA). In general, vancomycin therapy should be discontinued after 48 hours if the clinical course is stable, no gram-positive organisms are isolated, and no skin or soft tissue infection is found.

After approximately 2 to 4 days of empiric antimicrobial therapy, the condition of the patient primarily determines the need for further therapy (Fig. 224-3). Patients with no signs of sepsis on admission, no evident source of current infection, resolution of fever, continued clinical stability, negative cultures after 48 hours, and an ANC > 100/μL may be considered for de-escalation to an appropriate oral antibiotic. Alternately, such patients may be discharged from the hospital to continue parenteral antibiotics at home. Either approach requires a reliable social situation and the ability to provide close follow-up. These antibiotics would continue until the ANC is > 500/μL, although some centers consider an earlier marker of bone marrow recovery (ANC ≥ 200/μL and increasing). Patients in whom the ANC is ≤ 100/μL or who have ongoing mucositis or other factors predisposing to recurrent infection should continue parenteral antibiotics as an outpatient, even if they become afebrile.

The median time to defervescence in adequately treated patients is approximately 4 days. Accordingly, if a patient remains febrile but is otherwise clinically stable and if a definitive pathogen is not identified by culture, the clinician may wait up to 4 days prior to considering making changes in the antimicrobial regimen. Among neutropenic patients whose fevers continue for more than 4 days, the following should be considered: (1) a nonbacterial infection, such as fungus; (2) a drug-resistant organism (particularly if blood cultures are persistently positive); (3) an infection site poorly accessible to antibiotics (eg, an abscess or catheter-associated infection); (4) inadequate antimicrobial administration (dose, frequency); or (5) a noninfectious source of fever. To assess these possibilities, patients should be examined thoroughly for a previously unidentified focus of infection. Blood cultures, including fungal cultures, should be repeated. Relevant drug serum levels should also be obtained. Finally, CT of the chest, abdomen, pelvis, or sinuses should be considered.

Depending on the condition of the patient, 3 treatment options are available for continued F&N after 4 days of initial empiric antimicrobial therapy (Fig. 224-4): (1) to continue antimicrobials without change with ongoing close observation, as long as the patient is clinically stable, particularly if neutropenia is expected to resolve in the near future; (2) to change or add antibacterial agents, including broadening gram-negative coverage and adding vancomycin; or (3) to add empiric antifungal therapy, including amphotericin B, a triazole (eg, voriconazole, posaconazole, isavuconazole), or an echinocandin (eg, caspofungin, micafungin).

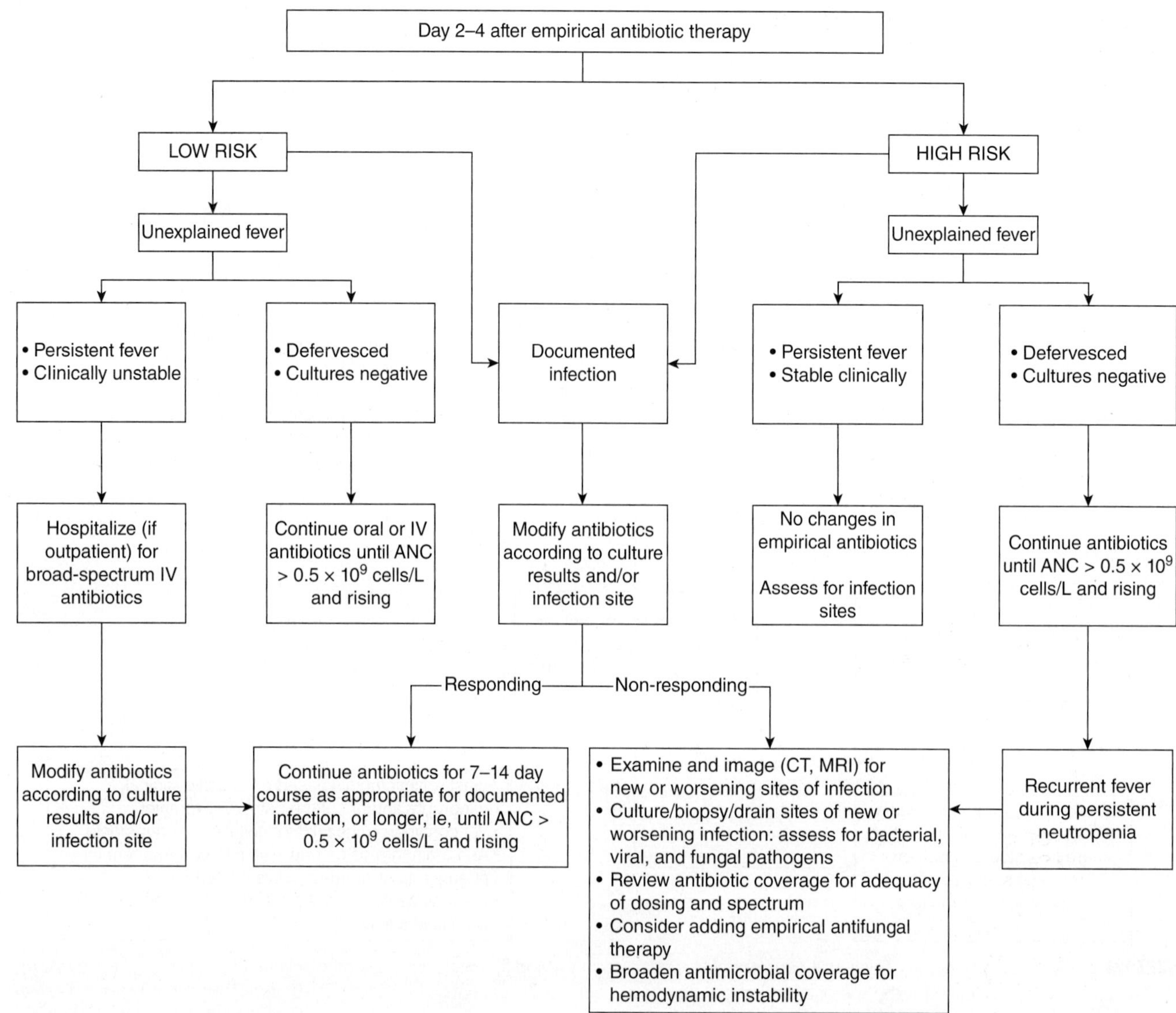


**FIGURE 224-3** Management of patients after 2 to 4 days of empiric therapy. ANC, absolute neutrophil count; CT, computed tomography; IV, intravenous; MRI, magnetic resonance imaging. (Modified with permission from Freifeld AG, Bow EJ, Sepkowitz KA, et al: Clinical practice guideline for the use of antimicrobial agents in neutropenic patients with cancer: 2010 update by the infectious diseases society of america, *Clin Infect Dis.* 2011 Feb 15;52(4):e56-e93.)

Despite neutropenia being a key predictor of risk for infection, neither granulocyte infusions nor GCSF is recommended as routine treatment in patients with F&N. Although it can shorten the duration of neutropenia, GCSF has not decreased mortality or shortened duration of fever. Accordingly, GCSF is used primarily in severely neutropenic patients with documented infections who do not respond to appropriate therapy or when prolonged delay in marrow recovery is anticipated.

#### Pathogen-Specific Immunity

An important theme in treating both viral and fungal infections in immunocompromised patients, including those post-HCT or post-SOT, is that antimicrobials alone are often insufficient to eradicate infection, and often, immune restoration is needed. In patients with primary immunodeficiencies, this may require that the patient undergo corrective allogeneic HCT while actively infected, while patients receiving immunosuppressive medications may need their immunosuppression tapered, as in the context of EBV-PTLD following HCT or SOT. In recent years, a large amount of research has demonstrated that antiviral third-party T cells directed against CMV, EBV, adenovirus, HHV-6, and BK can be safely administered to patients and help with control of disease. Use of these cells currently remains investigational and limited to certain centers but may provide a novel method to help control viral infections in immunocompromised hosts in the future.

## PREVENTION

To decrease the likelihood of infection in immunocompromised children, preventive strategies include attempts to minimize exposure to known infectious disease risks through the use of environmental "isolation" restrictions and use of prophylactic antimicrobials, passive immunity via administration of immunoglobulin (IG), and vaccination.

#### Isolation

Attempts to minimize exposures to known infectious disease risks remain fundamentally important. Immunocompromised patients should be educated on avoiding potential environmental sources of pathogens, including unpasteurized dairy products; well and lake water and even previously treated water in standing collections; soil (eg, building sites, caves, gardening, or agricultural work); contact with feces or secretions; exposure to animals of notable zoonotic risk (eg, birds, reptiles, rodents, cats); and undercooked meats or unwashed produce. Feasible application of these exposure control recommendations varies. In some cases (eg, histoplasmosis),

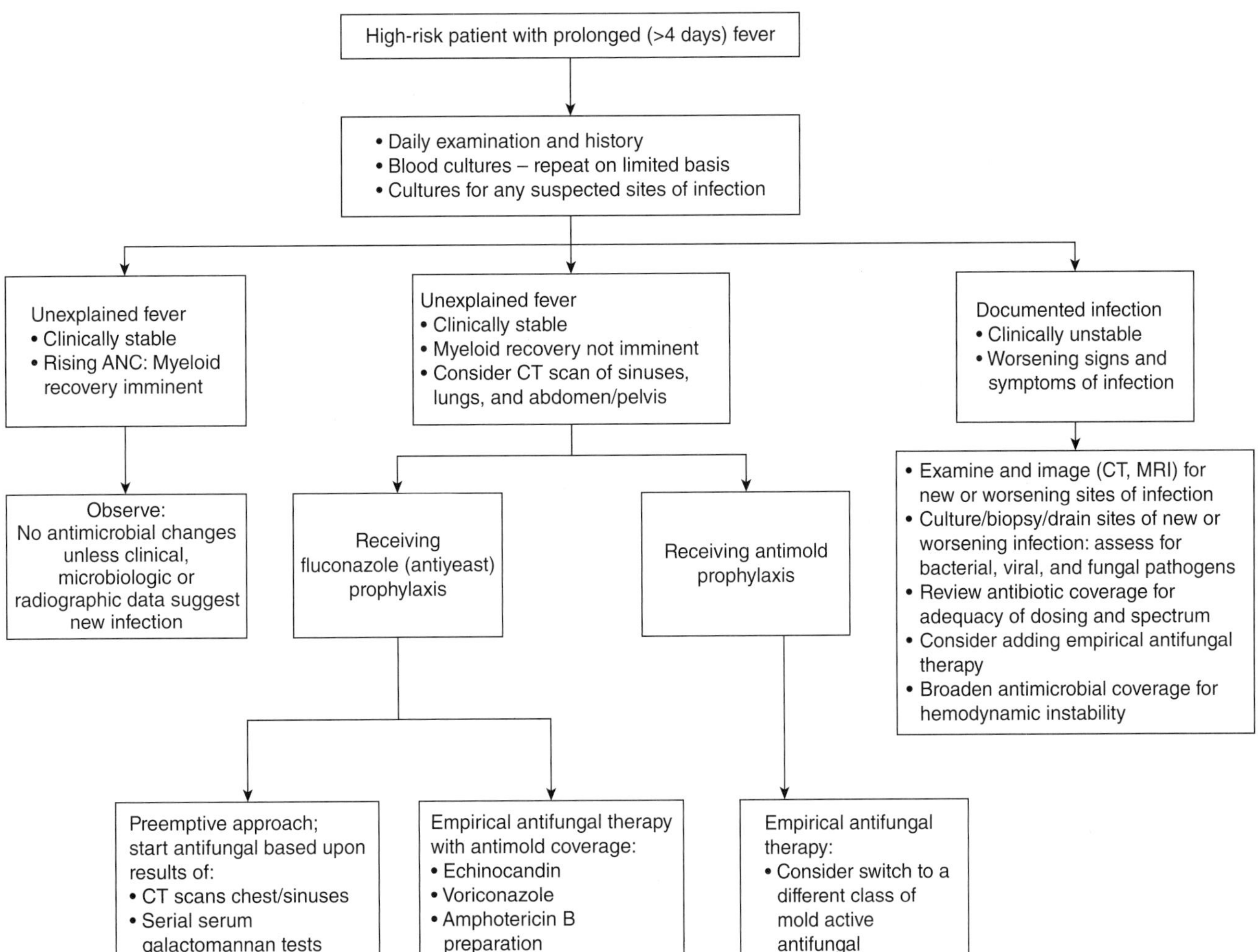


**FIGURE 224-4** Management of high-risk patients with persistent fevers. ANC, absolute neutrophil count; CT, computed tomography; MRI, magnetic resonance imaging. (Modified with permission from Freifeld AG, Bow EJ, Sepkowitz KA, et al: Clinical practice guideline for the use of antimicrobial agents in neutropenic patients with cancer: 2010 update by the infectious diseases society of america, *Clin Infect Dis.* 2011 Feb 15;52(4):e56-e93.)

inoculum size appears most relevant to disease risk, and thus avoiding exposure to high-inoculum microorganisms may be possible without significant restriction in activities of daily life. However, for hospitalized HCT patients, even small breaches of isolation measures have been associated with catastrophic infections, including nosocomial mold and viral infections. Due to its inherent difficulties and negative psychosocial sequelae, the isolation strategy is primarily practiced for short durations while awaiting definitive correction in the immune defect. The classic example would be a patient with severe combined immunodeficiency (SCID) who is kept isolated until his or her T-cell compartment has numerically and functionally developed following successful allogeneic HCT.

Other additional environmental considerations include fastidious central line care and restriction in the use of broad-spectrum antimicrobials without a clear indication, as inappropriate broad antimicrobial use is a known risk factor for subsequent serious infections with invasive fungi and highly resistant bacteria. Furthermore, an expanding body of research is demonstrating the critical interplay between the normal flora of the body, termed the microbiome, and the immune system. This interaction has been most clearly demonstrated in the allogeneic HCT setting, where limited intestinal bacterial diversity due to broad-spectrum antimicrobial therapy is associated with development of severe GVHD and increases transplant-related mortality. As a result, trials are now evaluating whether restoration of normal flora through probiotics or fecal transplant from healthy "donors" can attenuate GVHD severity and treat nosocomial *Clostridium difficile*–associated diarrhea (CDAD), respectively.

#### Prophylactic Antimicrobials and Immunoglobulins

Use of prophylactic antimicrobials is indicated in some well-studied contexts. Trimethoprim-sulfamethoxazole (TMP-SMX) prophylaxis significantly decreases risk of both *Pneumocystis jirovecii* pneumonia and *Toxoplasma* in patients with primary T-cell immunodeficiencies or acquired compromised T-cell immunity following chemotherapy or transplantation and in patients with advanced HIV infection. TMP-SMX is sometimes used as prophylaxis for patients with chronic granulomatous disease (CGD), primarily to prevent *Nocardia* infections. Routine antibiotic prophylaxis (typically with a fluoroquinolone) has been studied in adults with neutropenia from chemotherapy or HCT, where it has shown some efficacy in decreasing bacteremia and all-cause mortality. However, data for the efficacy and safety of this approach in children are not yet available, so it is currently not recommended.

Antifungal prophylaxis in severely immunocompromised patients has historically utilized fluconazole, as several studies have demonstrated its protective benefit and good safety profile in this patient population. Yet an expanded armamentarium of antifungal drug options is now available, and several trials evaluating efficacy and safety profiles of echinocandins and mold-active triazoles in adult immunocompromised patients have demonstrated their benefit. For example, posaconazole prophylaxis has been shown to decrease invasive fungal infections and improve mortality in adults with neutropenia or GVHD. Antiviral drugs against herpesviruses are often used in transplant patients, either as universal prophylaxis or preemptive therapy to decrease CMV and HSV risk.

Passive immunization with intravenous (IV) or subcutaneous (SC) IG preparations may be indicated in 2 main contexts: (1) patients for whom profoundly depressed levels of immunoglobulin cause their immunocompromised state and polyvalent immunoglobulin is essential as a replacement factor (eg, Bruton agammaglobulinemia); and (2) when pathogen-specific immunoglobulins may prevent or abrogate disease progression (eg, the use of varicella hyperimmune globulin administration to highly immunocompromised, varicella-susceptible hosts soon after putative virus exposure; or CMV hyperimmune globulin for transplant patients with CMV pneumonia).

#### Vaccination

Vaccination recommendations for immunocompromised hosts are regularly updated by the Centers for Disease Control and Prevention and the IDSA. Key recommendations include the following:

1. Live viral vaccines (eg, measles-mumps-rubella [MMR], varicella, rotavirus, intranasal influenza) are typically withheld from children with immunodeficiency, especially those with T-cell defects. However, live vaccines are considered as net benefit in certain circumstances and might be considered in consultation with infectious disease specialists. Transplant patients with restored immunity may also receive live virus vaccines.
2. Patients with an inability to make specific immunoglobulins in response to exposures and who are receiving passive immunoglobulin preparations may still benefit from T-cell response to certain vaccines.
3. Annual killed influenza vaccination is recommended for immunocompromised patients in general.
4. Vaccination against pneumococcus using both the conjugated 13-valent vaccine and the polysaccharide 23-valent vaccine is recommended for immunocompromised patients and may be especially beneficial for patents with asplenia or splenic dysfunction. Patients with asplenia, splenic dysfunction, or complement deficiency should also be vaccinated against meningococcus with administration relatively early in childhood.

### SUGGESTED READINGS


Chellapandian D, Lehrnbecher T, Phillips B, et al. Bronchoalveolar lavage and lung biopsy in patients with cancer and hematopoietic stem-cell transplantation recipients: a systematic review and meta-analysis. *J Clin Oncol.* 2015;33:501-509.

Freifeld AG, Bow EJ, Sepkowitz KA, et al. Clinical practice guideline for the use of antimicrobial agents in neutropenic patients with cancer: 2010 Update by the Infectious Diseases Society of America. *Clin Infect Dis.* 2011;52:427-433.

Lehrnbecher T, Phillips R, Alexander S, et al. Guideline for the management of fever and neutropenia in children with cancer and/or undergoing hematopoietic stem-cell transplantation. *J Clin Oncol.* 2012;30:4427-4438.

Naik S, Nicholas SK, Martinez CA, et al. Adoptive immunotherapy for primary immunodeficiency disorders with virus-specific T lymphocytes. *J Allergy Clin Immunol.* 2016;137:1498-1505.

Rubin LG, Levin MJ, Ljungman P, et al. 2013 IDSA clinical practice guideline for vaccination of the immunocompromised host. *Clin Infect Dis.* 2014;58:309-318.

Taur Y, Jenq RR, Perales MA, et al. The effects of intestinal tract bacterial diversity on mortality following allogeneic hematopoietic stem cell transplantation. *Blood.* 2014;124:1174-1182.

Tomblyn M, Chiller T, Einsele H, et al. Guidelines for preventing infectious complications among hematopoietic cell transplantation recipients: a global perspective. *Biol Blood Marrow Transplant.* 2009;15:1143-1238.

Wilson MR, Naccache SN, Samayoa E, et al. Actionable diagnosis of neuroleptospirosis by next-generation sequencing. *N Engl J Med.* 2014;370:2408-2417.


# 225 Therapy for Perinatal and Neonatal Infections

Debra L. Palazzi, C. Mary Healy, and David W. Kimberlin

### INTRODUCTION

Limitations in the immunologic response predispose the infant to certain viral and bacterial infections acquired during the prenatal, perinatal, and immediate postpartum periods. The development of the immune system and the mechanisms of response to both bacterial and viral infections are discussed in Chapter 182. Common viral and bacterial infections of neonates are discussed in this chapter.

### NEONATAL VIRAL PATHOGENS

Viral pathogens can infect the fetus or neonate in utero via transplacental or ascending transmission of microorganisms; in the peripartum period at delivery by passage through an infected birth canal; or in the postpartum period by acquisition within the first several weeks of life. Human cytomegalovirus (CMV) and rubella virus can cause significant sequelae when acquired in utero, whereas herpes simplex virus types 1 and 2 (HSV-1 and HSV-2) and enteroviruses can cause life-threatening disease when acquired in the peripartum and postpartum periods.

The usual timing of transmission, clinical presentation, diagnosis, treatment, and prevention of common neonatal viral infections are discussed in the following sections and summarized in Table 225-1.

## HERPES SIMPLEX VIRUS

### PATHOGENESIS AND EPIDEMIOLOGY

HSV infections can be acquired in utero (5%) or in the peripartum (85%) or postpartum (10%) periods. Peripartum or postpartum disease can be classified as disseminated disease involving multiple visceral organs, including lung, liver, adrenal glands, skin, and eye, with or without brain involvement; central nervous system (CNS) disease, with or without skin involvement; and disease limited to the skin, eyes, and/or mouth (SEM disease). This classification system is predictive of both morbidity and mortality. Patients with disseminated or SEM disease generally present to medical attention at 10 to 12 days of life, and patients with CNS disease present on average somewhat later, at 16 to 19 days of life.

Historically, disseminated HSV infections have accounted for approximately one-half to two-thirds of all children with neonatal HSV disease. However, this figure has been reduced to about 25% since the development and utilization of antiviral therapy, likely the consequence of recognizing and treating SEM infection before its progression to more severe disseminated disease. CNS involvement is a common component of this category of infection, occurring in 60% to 75% of infants with disseminated disease. Although the presence of a vesicular rash can greatly facilitate the diagnosis of HSV infection, over 20% of neonates with disseminated HSV disease will not develop cutaneous vesicles during the course of their illness. Patients with disseminated HSV infection commonly present with viral sepsis, including respiratory collapse, liver failure, and disseminated intravascular coagulation (DIC). Death from disseminated neonatal HSV infection is usually the result of the pulmonary involvement, liver dysfunction, or severe coagulopathy.

### CLINICAL MANIFESTATIONS

Almost one-third of all neonates with HSV infection are categorized as having CNS disease (with or without SEM involvement). Clinical manifestations of CNS disease include seizures (focal or generalized), lethargy, irritability, tremors, poor feeding, temperature instability, and bulging fontanel. Between 60% and 70% of babies classified as

**TABLE 225-1 NEONATAL VIRAL PATHOGENS AND TREATMENT**

| Organism | Usual Time of Transmission | Clinical Manifestations | Diagnosis | Antiviral Treatment | Prevention |
|---|---|---|---|---|---|
| Herpes simplex virus (HSV) | Perinatal, postnatal | Hepatitis, disseminated intravascular coagulation (DIC), pneumonitis, seizures (focal or generalized), lethargy, irritability, tremors, poor feeding, temperature instability, bulging fontanel, skin vesicles | Culture of lesions, surface sites; polymerase chain reaction (PCR) from CSF and whole blood; ALT | Acyclovir (IV) | Cesarean delivery, Suppressive acyclovir in the pregnant woman may be useful |
| Enterovirus | Perinatal, postnatal | Fever, irritability, anorexia, lethargy, rash, emesis, diarrhea, abdominal distention, jaundice, hepatomegaly, seizures, apnea, bulging anterior fontanel | Culture or PCR of CSF, blood, culture of surface sites | Consider intravenous immune globulin (IVIG); pleconaril is an experimental therapy | Hand washing |
| Cytomegalovirus (CMV) | Prenatal | Petechiae, jaundice, hepatosplenomegaly, purpura, microcephaly, periventricular calcifications, lethargy, hypotonia, poor suck, seizures, intrauterine growth restriction, hearing impairment | Shell vial or tissue culture or PCR of urine, saliva | Valganciclovir (PO) or ganciclovir (IV) for infants born with symptomatic congenital CMV disease | Unproven, experimental therapies include CMV hyperimmune globulin and a vaccine now in development |
| Rubella | Prenatal | Dermal erythropoiesis ("blueberry muffin" rash), chronic rash, thrombocytopenic purpura, hemolytic anemia, generalized lymphadenopathy, interstitial pneumonitis, hepatitis, hepatosplenomegaly, nephritis, myositis, myocarditis, bone radiolucencies, meningoencephalitis, structural defects of the cardiovascular system, cataracts, retinopathy, microphthalmia, deafness | Culture of blood, urine, CSF, saliva, rubella-specific IgM in neonatal serum | None | Vaccination |

ALT, alanine aminotransferase; CSF, cerebrospinal fluid; IgM, immunoglobulin M; IV, intravenous; PO, oral.

having CNS disease have associated skin vesicles at some point in the disease course. In the absence of skin lesions and frank CNS signs, the initial presentation can be indistinguishable from other viral and bacterial infections that lead clinicians to suspect possible sepsis in neonates. With CNS neonatal HSV disease, mortality is usually the product of devastating brain destruction, with resulting acute neurologic and autonomic dysfunction. Neonatal HSV can involve any and often multiple parts of the brain, in contrast with the typical temporal lobe involvement seen with HSV encephalitis with onset beyond the neonatal period.

Infection localized to the skin, eyes, and/or mouth (SEM disease) historically accounted for approximately 20% of all cases of neonatal HSV disease. With the introduction of early antiviral therapy, this has increased to approximately 45%. By definition, babies with SEM disease have limited infection, and 80% to 85% have associated vesicular lesions apparent on physical examination.

A number of other conditions, both infectious and noninfectious, can mimic neonatal HSV infection. These include hyaline membrane disease, intraventricular hemorrhage, and necrotizing enterocolitis. Bacterial pathogens of newborns with systemic and/or cutaneous manifestations that can be confused with neonatal HSV disease include group B *Streptococcus* (GBS), *Staphylococcus aureus*, *Listeria monocytogenes*, and gram-negative bacteria. Exanthemous viral agents that can be confused with neonatal HSV infection include varicella-zoster virus, adenovirus, enteroviruses, and disseminated CMV infection. Other infectious pathogens in the differential diagnosis include toxoplasmosis, rubella, and syphilis. Noninfectious cutaneous disorders should also be considered, including erythema toxicum, neonatal melanosis, acrodermatitis, and incontinentia pigmenti. See Chapter 304 for further discussion of methods of laboratory diagnosis for HSV infection.

## TREATMENT

Neonatal HSV disease is treated with parenteral acyclovir administered at 60 mg/kg/d in 3 divided doses. Duration of therapy is 21 days for babies with disseminated and CNS disease and 14 days for babies with SEM disease. All babies with CNS involvement should have a repeat lumbar puncture near the end of intravenous therapy to document polymerase chain reaction (PCR) negativity prior to stopping parenteral therapy; in the unlikely event that the PCR remains positive near the end of the 21-day treatment course, intravenous acyclovir should be administered for another week, with repeat cerebrospinal fluid (CSF) PCR assay performed near the end of the extended treatment period and another week of parenteral therapy if it remains positive. Consultation with an infectious diseases specialist is warranted in these cases. Oral acyclovir suppressive therapy (300 mg/m$^2$/dose administered 3 times per day) should be administered to all babies following completion of parenteral therapy and continued for 6 months; patients with CNS disease benefit from suppressive therapy in terms of neurodevelopmental outcomes, while all disease classifications of neonatal HSV benefit in terms of preventing cutaneous recurrences.

In the pre-antiviral era, 85% of those with disseminated HSV disease died by 1 year of age, as did 50% of those with CNS disease. With current antiviral therapy, 12-month mortality has been reduced to 29% for disseminated disease and to 4% for CNS disease. At initial presentation, lethargy and severe hepatitis are associated with increased mortality among patients with disseminated disease, and prematurity and seizures are associated with increased mortality in patients with CNS disease.

Until recently, improvements in morbidity rates with antiviral therapies were not as dramatic as with mortality. The proportion of survivors of disseminated HSV disease who have normal neurologic development has increased from 50% in the pre-antiviral era to 83% today. In the case of CNS disease, though, it was only the recent utilization of oral acyclovir suppressive therapy that improved the proportion of patients with normal neurologic developmental outcomes, from 30% without antiviral suppression to 70% with antiviral suppression. Seizures at or before the time of initiation of antiviral therapy are associated with increased risk of morbidity both in patients with CNS disease and in patients with disseminated infection.

In contrast to disseminated or CNS disease, morbidity following SEM disease has dramatically improved during the antiviral era due in large part to prevention of SEM disease progressing to disseminated disease. Prior to the development of vidarabine or acyclovir, 38% of SEM patients experienced developmental difficulties at 12 months of age. Today, fewer than 2% of acyclovir recipients have developmental delays following recovery from SEM disease.

## PREVENTION

A number of approaches are employed by obstetricians to try to prevent neonatal HSV disease. Cesarean delivery in a woman with active genital lesions can reduce the infant's risk of acquiring HSV and is recommended when genital HSV lesions or prodromal symptoms are present at the time of delivery. Physicians caring for neonates delivered by cesarean section should be aware that neonatal HSV infections have occurred despite cesarean delivery performed prior to the rupture of membranes.

An increasingly common practice among obstetricians is the use of oral antiviral suppressive therapy near the end of pregnancy to prevent genital HSV recurrences at delivery. Several small studies suggest that suppressive acyclovir or valacyclovir therapy during the last weeks of pregnancy decreases the occurrence of clinically apparent genital HSV disease at the time of delivery, with an associated decrease in cesarean section rates for the indication of genital HSV. However, because viral shedding still occurs (albeit with reduced frequency), the potential for neonatal infection likely is not completely avoided. Cases of neonatal HSV disease have occurred among babies born to women who were on suppressive antiviral therapy at the end of pregnancy, and pediatricians should not assume that the risk of neonatal HSV is completely eliminated by a woman receiving suppressive oral antiviral therapy at the time of delivery.

Currently, an HSV glycoprotein vaccine is under investigation. Even if efficacious for genital HSV infection, its impact on neonatal herpes will remain to be established. See Chapter 304 for further discussion of HSV infection including methods of laboratory diagnosis, and Chapter 240 expanded discussion of recommended antiviral treatment.

## ENTEROVIRUSES

### PATHOGENESIS AND EPIDEMIOLOGY

Enteroviral infection is a serious and important health problem in the newborn infant. Prospective studies have documented that nonpolio enteroviruses are the most commonly identified cause of fever without an apparent focus among infants under 1 month of age who present for emergent care. During the summer and fall months, enteroviruses account for at least 53% to 63% of these cases. Fever is often the sole finding among babies with postnatally acquired enteroviral disease, although some infants will present with other nonspecific findings such as irritability, lethargy, poor feeding, vomiting, diarrhea, exanthem, and signs of upper respiratory tract infection. Approximately half of all enterovirus-infected infants younger than 3 months of age who undergo lumbar puncture for fever are diagnosed with meningitis, although there are no clinical features that distinguish those with meningitis from those without meningitis. The most consequential outcome of enteroviral infection, neonatal enteroviral sepsis, occurs following perinatal transmission from a mother shedding enterovirus at the time of delivery.

Approximately 60% to 70% of infants diagnosed with enteroviral disease within the first 10 days of life acquire their infection by transmission from the mother at the time of delivery. Infected mothers usually report a febrile gastrointestinal or respiratory illness in the 2-week period preceding delivery of the infant. Congenital infection is rare but often fatal. Importantly, postnatal transmission of enteroviral infection in newborn nurseries also has been implicated as an important route of spread of disease. During periods of high prevalence of enterovirus infection in the community, there are many other potential sources of infection both during the stay and after discharge from the nursery, including the mother and other family members.

### CLINICAL MANIFESTATIONS

Babies with neonatal enteroviral sepsis syndrome usually present in the first 2 weeks of life with any number of symptoms including fever, irritability, lethargy, rash, anorexia, emesis, diarrhea, or abdominal distention. Other symptoms and signs relate to specific organ infection and include jaundice, hepatomegaly, seizures, apnea, and bulging anterior fontanel. Common laboratory abnormalities include CSF pleocytosis, peripheral leukocytosis, thrombocytopenia, hyperbilirubinemia, transaminase elevation, and infiltrates on chest radiographs.

Echoviruses and parechoviruses are isolated most frequently in cases of neonatal enteroviral sepsis syndrome, with coxsackievirus group B occurring less often.

Severe hepatitis can result from neonatal echovirus infection or may occur along with myocarditis and other manifestations of neonatal coxsackievirus B disease. Although severe hepatitis is usually the consequence of echovirus 11 infection, neonatal disease caused by echovirus serotypes 6, 7, 9, 14, 17, 19, and 21 can also demonstrate dramatic hepatic involvement. Extensive hepatic necrosis and overwhelming liver failure can result. Severe hepatitis syndrome has been defined as a serum transaminase level of greater than 3 times the upper limit of normal; a prothrombin time or partial thromboplastin time greater than twice the control value; or evidence of hepatic necrosis or extensive hemorrhage at postmortem examination. Postmortem examination of neonates who die of echovirus disease usually reveals inflammatory changes limited to the liver. Survivors may have residual hepatic dysfunction. Neonatal myocarditis is most frequently caused by group B coxsackievirus serotypes 2 through 5. Such infants frequently demonstrate concomitant meningoencephalitis, pneumonia, hepatitis, pancreatitis, or adrenalitis.

### DIAGNOSIS

The diagnosis of enterovirus infection has traditionally been based on isolating virus in cell culture from specimens obtained during the acute illness. The most common sites of virus isolation are blood, CSF, throat, urine, and feces. The echoviruses and group B coxsackieviruses are isolated readily in cell lines used by most clinical virology laboratories. A combination of human fibroblasts, primary monkey kidney cells, and human rhabdomyosarcoma cells are optimal for cell culture isolation of a broad range of enteroviruses. Echoviruses and group B coxsackieviruses can be recovered from infants with severe myocarditis or hepatitis from multiple sites, including blood, CSF, respiratory secretions, feces, and urine. However, the utility of diagnosis of enteroviral infections by viral culture is limited by a sensitivity of only 65% to 75%. PCR detection of enteroviral RNA, on the other hand, has been shown to be an effective alternative to viral culture in the diagnosis of enteroviral meningitis using CSF specimens, and in the diagnosis of neonatal enteroviral infections with serum and urine specimens. Sensitivity and specificity, respectively, of PCR for the detection of enteroviral RNA have been reported as 100% and 97% (CSF); 92% and 98% (serum or plasma); 95% and 88% (throat); and 77% and 95% (urine). However, routine enteroviral PCR testing will not detect parechoviruses. Parechovirus PCR testing of CSF is available through commercial laboratories.

### TREATMENT

Management of neonates who present with possible enteroviral sepsis syndrome is directed toward the symptom complex. Cultures and PCR of body fluids for bacterial and viral pathogens are performed and broad-spectrum antibacterial therapy initiated until the results of bacterial cultures are available. Acyclovir is frequently administered as well until HSV disease is excluded. Supportive care has been the rule in the management of severe enteroviral disease. Intravenous gamma-globulin has been used in case reports and small clinical trials, but definitive proof of efficacy has not been established. No enteroviral-specific antiviral medication is currently available for the management of these gravely ill neonates, although use of the experimental drug pleconaril may be discussed with the US Food and Drug Administration.

Approximately 75% of cases of neonatal enteroviral disease carry a benign outcome, with diagnosis and symptomatic treatment in nonintensive care unit settings. For the remainder of patients, more serious consequences can result from systemic enteroviral infection, including meningoencephalitis, cardiovascular collapse, myocarditis, or hepatitis. These last 2 organ-specific complications carry high mortality rates. More than 80% of babies with enteroviral sepsis syndrome involving the liver will die within 1 to 3 weeks of onset of symptoms, and mortality among infants with myocarditis alone is generally reported to be 30% to 50%.

## PREVENTION

Given the ubiquity of enteroviruses in the environment during the summer and fall, specific measures designed to diminish transmission of virus to neonates are lacking. Careful hand washing likely can have an impact on viral transmission to young babies and remains the best preventative method. For further discussion of enteroviruses, see Chapter 301.

# CYTOMEGALOVIRUS

## PATHOGENESIS AND EPIDEMIOLOGY

CMV is a ubiquitous virus, and humans are its only reservoir. In populations with higher socioeconomic conditions, approximately 40% of adolescents are seropositive, with another 1% seroconverting annually thereafter. Approximately 70% of adults from higher socioeconomic strata and 90% from lower socioeconomic strata eventually become infected with CMV.

Transmission of CMV occurs by contact with infected secretions via direct (including sexual) contact or indirect contact. Sources of virus include tears, oropharyngeal secretions, cervical and vaginal secretions, breast milk, semen, urine, blood, and transplanted organs. Intrauterine transmission of CMV is especially important. Spread among children in group childcare facilities is the result of horizontal transmission from child to child through saliva on hands and toys. This mode of viral transmission is so efficient that it is not unusual to find excretion rates as high as 20% to 40% in young toddlers attending group childcare. Young children acquiring primary CMV infection at childcare facilities are at risk of transmitting CMV to their seronegative parents, which in turn can lead to intrauterine transmission should a mother be pregnant at the time. Seronegative caretakers working in daycare centers are also at increased risk for acquisition of CMV infection.

Intrauterine infection follows maternal viremia and associated placental infection. CMV is the most common congenital infection in humans, with approximately 0.5% of all live births in the United States being infected with CMV (~20,000–25,000 babies per year). CMV can be acquired in utero during any trimester of pregnancy. Congenital CMV infection is the most frequent known viral cause of mental retardation and is the leading nongenetic cause of neurosensory hearing loss in many countries including the United States. Of infected fetuses, approximately 10% will be symptomatic at birth, and approximately 20% of those will die in the neonatal period; of the survivors, 90% will have significant neurologic sequelae, including hearing deficits in 30% to 65%.

Children born with congenital CMV infection but without overt symptoms may nevertheless develop sequelae on follow-up, particularly sensorineural hearing loss. A systematic review of prospective studies published worldwide reported that 13.5% of all babies with congenital CMV infection develop sensorineural hearing loss on follow-up. Approximately one-quarter of sensorineural hearing loss in the early childhood years is due to congenital CMV infection.

## CLINICAL MANIFESTATIONS

Approximately 10% of neonates infected in utero with CMV will be born with "classic" symptoms. These include being small for gestational age, microcephaly, hepatosplenomegaly, jaundice, and petechiae over the body (blueberry muffin appearance). Laboratory examination will reveal thrombocytopenia, elevated liver function test, and periventricular calcifications on a cranial ultrasound. The majority of these babies will have other complications show up over their lifetime, including vision loss, progressive deafness, and learning disabilities. Even though the majority of infants congenitally infected with CMV are asymptomatic at birth, another 10% to 20% may also have vision and hearing deficits develop.

## DIAGNOSIS

Detection of CMV by culture or PCR from urine or saliva within the first 3 weeks of life is diagnostic for congenital infection. Human fibroblasts are routinely used to support CMV replication in vitro. Cultures are observed at least twice weekly for the typical focal cytopathic effect (CPE) of CMV. Occasionally, urine samples from cases of congenital infection produce widespread CPE within 24 to 48 hours, which resembles that of HSV. More usually, the CPE evolves slowly, typically becoming apparent at 14 to 16 days, so that cultures must be maintained for a minimum of 21 days before being reported as negative. To facilitate more rapid finalization of culture results, the shell vial assay utilizes monoclonal antibody for detection of CMV antigens early in the culture process to confirm infection in a specimen. More recently, as with the diagnosis of HSV, the application of PCR from saliva or urine is supplanting tissue culture confirmation of CMV.

## TREATMENT

Either parenteral ganciclovir or oral valganciclovir is used for the treatment of babies born with symptomatic congenital CMV disease to improve audiologic and neurodevelopmental outcomes. The initial controlled study of antiviral therapy for symptomatic congenital CMV assessed 6 weeks of intravenous ganciclovir therapy (6 mg/kg/dose administered intravenously every 12 hours), the results of which documented that antiviral therapy reduces the progression of hearing loss. The availability of a liquid formulation of oral valganciclovir allowed for assessment of longer treatment, and a recent randomized controlled trial comparing 6 weeks versus 6 months of valganciclovir oral solution (16 mg/kg/dose administered orally twice daily) for the treatment of symptomatic congenital CMV disease found that children who received 6 months of antiviral therapy had further improvement in hearing outcomes at 2 years of age. Further, neurodevelopmental outcomes were also better in the group receiving 6 months of therapy compared with the 6-week group. Given the toxicities of ganciclovir and valganciclovir, treatment to improve audiologic and developmental outcomes at this time is limited to infants with symptomatic disease at birth; the preferred treatment duration is 6 months. Antiviral therapy is not routinely recommended for infants with mild symptomatic congenital CMV infection, including isolated sensorineural hearing loss.

Two-thirds of babies receiving intravenous ganciclovir and one-fifth of babies receiving oral valganciclovir for the treatment of symptomatic congenital CMV disease develop significant neutropenia. When it occurs, the neutropenia usually develops during the first 6 weeks of treatment. It usually can be managed with serial observations or withholding the antiviral medication for 1 to 7 days until the neutrophil count recovers. Discontinuation of treatment may be necessary in cases where neutropenia recurs upon reinstitution of antiviral therapy.

In some animal models, ganciclovir (and therefore valganciclovir) is carcinogenic and gonadotoxic. To date, such serious toxicities have not been seen in humans. There are no data on antiviral treatment of babies with asymptomatic congenital CMV infection. Given the toxicities, antiviral therapy in this larger population cannot be recommended at this time.

As noted, approximately 20% of babies with symptomatic congenital CMV disease will die in the neonatal period. Of the survivors, 90% will have significant neurologic sequelae, including hearing deficits in 30% to 65% of patients. In at least 30% of untreated babies, their CMV-induced hearing loss will not be static but will progress over time. Even with antiviral treatment, progression of hearing loss can occur, albeit at a lower frequency. Thus, the majority of symptomatically infected babies will have sensorineural hearing loss, mental retardation, microcephaly, seizures, and/or paresis/paralysis. These impairments frequently result in spastic quadriplegia requiring lifelong dependence on a wheelchair, along with cognitive and speech impairments that dramatically limit their ability to interact with and function in the world. Patients with this degree of neurologic impairment generally have a life expectancy of less than 10 to 15 years.

## PREVENTION

In 1999, the Institute of Medicine assessed the need for a CMV vaccine as the highest of all priorities. A glycoprotein B CMV vaccine demonstrated promise in phase II trials in adolescent girls and women of childbearing age, with approximately 50% efficacy in the prevention of CMV infection in the women. CMV hyperimmune globulin administered to pregnant women with primary CMV infection was shown in one study to protect against in utero transmission of CMV to the fetus. However, methodologic difficulties with the selection of subjects in this trial make it difficult to know the extent, if any, to which such an intervention is beneficial, and a subsequent well-controlled study did not demonstrate any benefit of such a therapeutic approach.

## RUBELLA

### PATHOGENESIS AND EPIDEMIOLOGY

Rubella is a highly contagious disease, and the incidence of rubella infection during an epidemic cycle approaches 100% of susceptible hosts in closed populations (eg, military recruits and household contacts). At least half of all serologically confirmed childhood primary rubella infections result in clinically apparent illness. Reinfection with rubella virus can occur following natural infection or vaccination but is usually asymptomatic. Up to 80% of persons previously vaccinated against rubella will be infected during an epidemic. Rubella reinfection during pregnancy can result in congenital rubella syndrome, although this is a rare event.

Fetal infection can occur throughout pregnancy, with the risk being greatest during the first trimester, decreasing during the second trimester, and then rising again as the fetus approaches term. The risk of congenital anomalies in live-borne children following fetal infection also varies according to the month of pregnancy in which maternal infection occurs, with over 85% of infants born to women infected with rubella virus during the first 8 weeks of pregnancy having anomalies detected during the first 4 years of life. This risk declines to 50% of infants born to mothers infected at 9 to 12 weeks of gestation, 15% of infants born to women infected at 13 to 20 weeks of gestation, and close to 0% of infants born to mothers infected beyond 20 weeks of gestation.

### CLINICAL MANIFESTATIONS

The clinical manifestations of congenitally acquired rubella usually are severe. The classic triad of congenital rubella consists of cataracts, cardiac abnormalities, and deafness. The consequences of in utero rubella infection can be considered broadly as belonging to 1 of 3 categories: signs and symptoms that are transiently apparent in affected infants; permanent manifestations that are noted within the first year of life; and manifestations that are delayed in onset until later in life (2 years of age to adulthood). Transient findings include dermal erythropoiesis ("blueberry muffin" rash), chronic rash, thrombocytopenic purpura, hemolytic anemia, generalized lymphadenopathy, interstitial pneumonitis, hepatitis, hepatosplenomegaly, nephritis, myositis, myocarditis, bone radiolucencies, and meningoencephalitis. Among the more common of these findings are rash (petechial or blueberry muffin rash), hepatosplenomegaly, jaundice, pulmonary involvement, meningoencephalitis, and radiographic abnormalities. The majority of such infants are intrauterine growth restricted at delivery. Sensorineural hearing loss is the most common permanent manifestation of congenital rubella, with cardiovascular anomalies, ophthalmologic findings, and neurologic impairment also occurring commonly.

### DIAGNOSIS

Rubella infection is definitively diagnosed by isolation of rubella virus in tissue culture, using one of several cell lines and primary cell strains. Viral interference in African green monkey kidney cells is one common culture technique by which the presence of rubella virus is demonstrated. Infection in African green monkey kidney tissue culture by rubella virus is suggested by failure of the typical enteroviral CPE to occur after challenge with echovirus 11 or other enteroviruses. The presence of rubella virus is then confirmed by an additional technique, such as neutralization or fluorescence with specific antirubella serum. In rubella acquired horizontally, virus can be readily isolated from throat swabs for 6 days before and after the onset of rash. Virus also can be isolated from specimens from the nasopharynx, conjunctivae, urine, blood buffy coat, and CSF of patients with congenital rubella. In utero infection with rubella can be demonstrated by nucleic acid hybridization or by virus-specific antigen detection in specimens from the chorionic villus or the fetus. PCR assays have also been developed.

Despite the definitive results afforded by direct viral isolation in tissue culture, the majority of rubella cases are diagnosed serologically. A 4-fold rise in rubella-specific immunoglobulin (Ig) G between acute and convalescent serum specimens confirms the diagnosis of horizontally acquired rubella. Commercially available rubella virus IgG avidity assays are of variable sensitivity. Demonstration of rubella-specific IgM is also diagnostic for recent infection with rubella virus. Rarely, rubella-specific IgM can be detected with reinfection. Serologic diagnosis of congenital rubella can be demonstrated by the presence of rubella-specific IgM in neonatal serum. Confirmation of congenital rubella based solely on the presence of IgG is difficult. In such cases, it is necessary to test sequential sera from the infant for rubella-specific IgG. In most cases, the IgG titer will decrease over several months if it is solely of maternal origin, whereas it will rise if congenital infection has occurred and the infant is producing rubella-specific IgG.

### TREATMENT

Interferon and amantadine have been used in individual cases of congenital rubella syndrome. Patients with congenital rubella require supportive care not only in the neonatal period but throughout life for such permanent impairments as deafness and heart defects. Prompt identification of such afflictions is of the utmost importance so that they can be managed with adjunct interventions.

Permanent sequelae from infancy onward include sensorineural hearing loss in 80% of congenitally infected patients, as well as cardiovascular anomalies, ophthalmologic findings, and neurologic impairment. Structural defects of the cardiovascular system occur in the majority of infants whose mothers acquired rubella during the first 2 months of gestation. Patent ductus arteriosus (PDA) is the most common of these cardiovascular sequelae, followed by pulmonary artery stenosis and pulmonary valvular stenosis. Two-thirds of patients with PDAs will have other cardiovascular lesions present. Ophthalmologic findings include cataracts (bilateral or unilateral), retinopathy, and microphthalmia. The retinopathy results from pigmentary defects in the retina and usually does not interfere with vision. In contrast, a small number of patients have congenital glaucoma that, if undetected, can result in visual impairment. Permanent neurologic impairment can result from the active replication in the CNS of rubella virus both in utero and following delivery. Indeed, such neurologic sequelae as mental retardation and motor disabilities correlate with the severity and persistence of the acute meningoencephalitis that is present at delivery in 10% to 20% of infants with congenital rubella syndrome. Movement and behavioral disorders can also be seen in surviving patients.

Sequelae of congenital rubella that develop in childhood or adulthood but are not present in infancy include endocrinopathies, deafness, ocular damage, vascular effects, and progressive rubella panencephalitis. Of these, the development of insulin-dependent diabetes mellitus (IDDM) occurs most frequently, with approximately 20% of patients being diagnosed with IDDM by the time they reach adulthood. Autoimmune-mediated thyroid dysfunction can also be seen.

### PREVENTION

Rubella and congenital rubella syndrome prevention are among the hallmark successes of the vaccination programs of the United States. By 2005, endemic transmission of rubella was eliminated in the United States, and cases of rubella and of congenital rubella syndrome in the United States in 2007 were 99.9% and 99.3% lower, respectively, compared to the prevaccine era. Fewer than 10 rubella cases have been reported each year in the United States since its elimination was declared, and only 7 cases of congenital rubella syndrome were reported from 2005 through 2013. Rubella vaccination coverage is at least 95% among school-aged children. An estimated 91% of the US population is immune to rubella. The remarkable success in decreasing the incidence of rubella in this country and others has led scientists and international organizations to consider the goal of rubella eradication. Further information on rubella is provided in Chapter 315.

Since 1979, the RA27/3 rubella vaccine has been the only rubella vaccine used in the United States. Vaccination results in IgG antibody production in more than 98% of vaccine recipients, and a single dose confers long-term (probably lifelong) immunity against clinical and asymptomatic infection in more than 90% of vaccinees. Subcutaneous administration of vaccine induces production of IgM antibodies that peak at 1 month postvaccination. Additionally, the generation of secretory IgA following subcutaneous vaccination may provide protection against reinfection by wild-type virus by blocking mucosal replication of virus. Postpubertal females who are not known to be immune to rubella should be immunized. Based on data from the Centers for Disease Control and Prevention, the maximal theoretical risk for the occurrence of congenital rubella syndrome following administration of the RA27/3 vaccine during the first trimester of pregnancy is 1.6%. Although asymptomatic rubella infection has been reported in 2% of such infants, no cases of congenital rubella syndrome resulting from live virus vaccination of pregnant women have been reported. Persistence of fetal infection following inadvertent rubella vaccination during early pregnancy has been documented, but with no apparent adverse clinical sequelae. Finally, prenatal or antepartum serologic screening for rubella immunity should be routinely performed. Women who are found to be rubella-susceptible should receive rubella vaccine in the immediate postpartum period prior to discharge. Breastfeeding is not a contraindication to such immunization.

Exposure to rubella virus during pregnancy can be especially anguishing. If a woman with such an exposure is known to be rubella-immune from a previous pregnancy, she can be reassured with no further evaluation required. If, on the other hand, she is not immune to rubella or her rubella status is unknown, serologic testing should be performed immediately. If such testing performed around the time of the exposure demonstrates the presence of rubella antibody, it can be assumed that she is immune and thus not at risk. However, if no rubella-specific antibody is detected, she should have a second serum sample obtained 2 to 3 weeks after the exposure, and it should be tested for antibody simultaneously with the first specimen; seroconversion suggests that infection occurred with the exposure. If the second test is also negative, a final serologic analysis should be performed on a serum sample obtained 6 weeks following the initial exposure and also tested concurrently with the first specimen; a negative test result in both specimens indicates that infection has not occurred. A positive test in the 6-week sample but not the first (seroconversion) indicates recent infection.

For counseling purposes, determination of the risk of congenital defects after confirmed maternal infection can be calculated by multiplying the rates of fetal infection by the rates of defects in infected infants. As such, the risks of congenital defects are 90% for maternal infection before the 11th week of gestation; 33% for infection occurring during weeks 11 and 12; 11% for infection from weeks 13 to 14; and 24% for infection between weeks 15 and 16.

## NEONATAL BACTERIAL INFECTIONS

Intrauterine bacterial infection can result from overt or subclinical maternal infection, and sequelae depend on the infectious agent and timing of the infection in gestation. Congenital bacterial infection can cause spontaneous abortion, stillbirth, premature birth, and symptomatic neonatal infection. Intrapartum infection commonly is caused by bacteria that colonize the maternal genitourinary and gastrointestinal tracts; postpartum infection can occur by direct maternal contact or through exposure to organisms and other persons in the environment.

## NEONATAL SEPSIS

Neonatal sepsis is a clinical syndrome characterized by systemic signs of infection in the first month of life. Neonatal systemic bacterial infections occur in 1 to 5 per 1000 live births. Over the past 20 years, the mortality rate due to neonatal bacterial infections has declined from 30–40% to 2–15%, in part due to enhanced awareness of maternal and infant risk factors and to earlier treatment. *Early-onset* and *late-onset sepsis* are 2 patterns of illness that characterize systemic bacterial infections during the first month of life (Table 225-2).

Neonates with early-onset disease have symptoms before 7 days of life, but the majority present with fulminant, systemic illness within 24 hours of birth. Infants who develop early-onset disease usually have a history of 1 or more risk factors associated with pregnancy and delivery such as premature or prolonged rupture of maternal membranes, preterm onset of labor, preterm delivery, low birth weight, chorioamnionitis, peripartum maternal fever, septic or traumatic delivery, lack of prenatal care, and maternal urinary tract infection. Bacteria responsible for early-onset disease are acquired from the maternal genital tract. The typical clinical presentation often is of nonspecific signs and respiratory distress. The mortality rate is generally from 3% to 15%, but can be as high as 40%, depending on the infecting organism (eg, gram-negative pathogens) and the patient's gestational age.

Late-onset disease is variably defined as occurring after 72 hours in hospitalized infants to after 6 days in neonates in the community, up through 89 days of age. Patients with late-onset infections may have a history of obstetric complications, but these are less characteristic than in early-onset sepsis. The bacteria causing late-onset infection can be from the maternal genital tract, the hospital environment, or the community. The mortality rate usually is lower than that in early-onset sepsis, generally between 2% and 10%, but can be up to 60% for gram-negative pathogens in very low birth weight (VLBW, < 1500 g) infants. The clinical presentation for late-onset disease also varies but often is focal and may manifest as pneumonia, meningitis, soft tissue infection, or other focal illness. With increasing survival of VLBW and extremely low birth weight (ELBW, < 1000 g) infants over the last decades, a third category of neonatal sepsis, late late-onset disease (≥ 90 days), has emerged. These infants, because of their ongoing

**TABLE 225-2 FEATURES OF EARLY-ONSET VERSUS LATE-ONSET BACTERIAL INFECTIONS IN NEONATES**

| Feature | Early Onset | Late Onset | Late Late Onset |
|---|---|---|---|
| Day of life at onset of illness | 0–6 | 7–89 | ≥ 90 |
| Maternal complications of labor or delivery | Common | Less common | Common |
| Prematurity | 25% | Less common | All |
| Organism source | Maternal genital tract | Maternal genital tract, postnatal environment, hospital | Postnatal environment, hospital |
| Clinical presentation | Multisystem, pneumonia common | Focal, meningitis frequent | Focal, meningitis frequent |
| Case fatality rate | 3–15% | 2–10% | 5–60% |

Adapted with permission from Long SS, Pickering LK, Prober CG: *Principles and Practice of Pediatric Infectious Diseases.* 4th ed. Philadelphia: Elsevier Saunders; 2012.

**TABLE 225-3 PATHOGENS CAUSING NEONATAL SEPTICEMIA**

| | Importance | |
|---|---|---|
| **Bacteria** | **Early Onset** | **Late Onset** |
| **Gram positive** | | |
| Group B *Streptococcus* | +++ | + |
| *Enterococcus* spp | + | ++ |
| *Listeria monocytogenes* | + | + |
| *Viridans* streptococci | + | + |
| *Streptococcus pneumoniae* | – | + |
| Coagulase-negative staphylococci | – | +++ |
| *Staphylococcus aureus* | + | +++ |
| **Gram negative** | | |
| *Escherichia coli* | +++ | ++ |
| *Klebsiella* spp | + | ++ |
| *Enterobacter* spp | + | ++ |
| *Citrobacter* spp | – | + |
| *Pseudomonas* spp | – | + |
| *Serratia marcescens* | – | + |
| *Haemophilus influenzae* | + | – |
| *Neisseria meningitidis* | – | + |
| Other enteric bacilli | + | + |
| **Anaerobic** | | |
| *Bacteroides* spp | + | + |
| Others | – | + |

+++, classically associated; ++, often associated; +, occasionally associated; –, rarely associated.

Reproduced with permission from Long SS, Pickering LK, Prober CG: *Principles and Practice of Pediatric Infectious Diseases*. 4th ed. Philadelphia: Elsevier Saunders; 2012.

hospitalization and corrected gestational age of less than 38 weeks, are considered to have an extended period of time during which they are classified as neonates.

The most common pathogens causing early-onset bacterial infection are GBS and *Escherichia coli* as well as other gram-negative bacilli (Table 225-3). These organisms account for two-thirds of all cases of early-onset disease and remain common as causes of late-onset sepsis. Other pathogens that cause early-onset sepsis include streptococci such as *Enterococcus*, α-hemolytic streptococci, and, rarely, *Streptococcus pneumoniae, Haemophilus influenzae* (nontypeable and type b), and other flora of the maternal genital tract.

Late-onset infection can be caused by the organisms listed above, but gram-negative pathogens also include those acquired in the healthcare setting that are potentially multidrug resistant, such as *Serratia marcescens, Klebsiella* species, *Pseudomonas aeruginosa, Citrobacter* species, and *Enterobacter* species.

## CLINICAL MANIFESTATIONS

Clinical signs of bacterial sepsis in the neonate may be subtle and do not distinguish among organisms in most cases. Fever or hypothermia can be the sole finding, although they are absent in approximately half of infants with sepsis. Sustained fever for more than 1 hour generally indicates infection. Many infants will present with nonspecific findings such as irritability, lethargy, poor feeding, abdominal distention, vomiting, diarrhea, or exanthem. One-third to one-half of neonates with bacterial infection will have signs of respiratory distress, such as apnea, cyanosis, or bradycardia. In infants from birth to 8 weeks of age, the most reliable clinical signs of sepsis can include changes in affect, peripheral perfusion, and respiratory status. Alterations in feeding pattern, level of alertness, level of activity, and muscle tone, although often present, may be less sensitive indicators. Jaundice (direct hyperbilirubinemia) can indicate infection, especially when it occurs within the first 24 hours of life without Rh or ABO blood group incompatibility. Infants with bacterial meningitis can present with seizures, bulging fontanel, or nuchal rigidity in addition to manifesting the same nonspecific signs as those with septicemia.

In VLBW infants, the nonspecific and subtle nature of the signs of neonatal sepsis makes recognizing infection even more problematic. The clinical signs of late-onset sepsis in these infants can include increasing apnea and bradycardia episodes (55%), increasing oxygen requirement (48%), feeding intolerance, abdominal distention, or guaiac-positive stools (46%), lethargy and hypotonia (37%), and temperature instability (10%). Unexplained metabolic acidosis and hypoglycemia can be present and are laboratory indicators of the metabolic derangement accompanying sepsis. In infants with nonfocal and nonspecific signs of illness, the differential diagnosis includes noninfectious etiologies such as congenital heart disease, birth asphyxia, hyaline membrane disease, metabolic disorders, and intraventricular hemorrhage.

Infants with sepsis can present with focal infection of any organ. However, excluding pneumonia and meningitis, focal infection in neonates occurs more often with late- rather than early-onset disease. Evaluation of infants with suspected septicemia should include a careful search for primary or secondary foci such as meningitis, pneumonia, urinary tract infection, peritonitis, otitis media, conjunctivitis, septic arthritis, osteomyelitis, or soft tissue infection.

# COMMON BACTERIAL PATHOGENS IN THE NEONATE

## GROUP B *STREPTOCOCCUS*

*Streptococcus agalactiae*, or Lancefield group B *Streptococcus*, has been the most frequent organism causing invasive disease in neonates for the past 4 decades. GBS is classified immunochemically into serotypes on the basis of its capsular polysaccharides. Ten capsular types, Ia, Ib, II, III, IV, V, VI, VII, VIII, and IX, have been characterized. Types Ia, Ib, II, III, and V account for nearly all cases of early-onset disease, and type III strains predominate among late-onset infections, especially those accompanied by meningitis.

GBS frequently is found in the lower genital and gastrointestinal tracts of up to 30% of healthy adult women and men and in the upper respiratory tracts and lower gastrointestinal tracts of neonates. The organism also has been isolated from various body fluids and sites including blood, pleural or peritoneal fluids, CSF, stool, urine, cervix, vagina, throat, skin, joints, bones, and wounds.

Early-onset disease caused by GBS presents as a multiorgan system illness, frequently characterized by severe respiratory distress, with rapid onset usually during the first day or two of life. The mortality rate is estimated at 3% but was as high as 50% in the 1970s. Late-onset neonatal sepsis frequently is accompanied by meningitis and usually is more insidious in clinical presentation than early-onset disease. Many of these infants are products of normal-term pregnancies and deliveries. In addition to sepsis and meningitis, other manifestations of neonatal disease caused by GBS include pneumonia, empyema, facial cellulitis, adenitis, ethmoiditis, orbital cellulitis, conjunctivitis, necrotizing fasciitis, osteomyelitis, suppurative arthritis, and impetigo. Bacteremia without systemic or focal signs of sepsis can occur.

## GROUP A *STREPTOCOCCUS*

Streptococcal puerperal sepsis and obstetric infections have been recognized for centuries as causes of morbidity and mortality among parturient women and their newborns. Group A *Streptococcus* (GAS) now is an infrequent cause of neonatal sepsis but can occur rarely including in nursery outbreaks. Maternal GAS disease can affect the fetus or newborn in 3 ways: in utero infection resulting in fetal loss or stillbirth can result from maternal bacteremia during pregnancy; GAS toxins from maternal infection can be transmitted transplacentally to the fetus and can cause intrauterine demise, premature delivery, and systemic illness; or GAS can be acquired from the maternal genital tract and can result in early-onset neonatal sepsis similar to early-onset GBS disease. Focal infections such as cellulitis, omphalitis, pneumonia, and osteomyelitis also have been reported.

## NON-GROUP A OR B STREPTOCOCCI

Group C streptococci have caused puerperal sepsis but rarely neonatal sepsis or meningitis. Similarly, group G streptococci uncommonly cause neonatal sepsis and pneumonia. Group D streptococci such as *Streptococcus mitis* and *Streptococcus bovis* also rarely cause neonatal disease. The clinical signs of sepsis in neonates with streptococcal infection are indistinguishable from signs of sepsis caused by other etiologies.

Viridans streptococci are normal flora of the respiratory and gastrointestinal tracts and are a heterogeneous group of streptococci with both alpha and nonhemolytic growth characteristics. Neonatal sepsis caused by viridans streptococci is uncommon but has been reported. As is the case in other immunocompromised patient populations, growth of viridans streptococci in the blood culture of a neonate suspected to have sepsis should not be considered a contaminant.

## ENTEROCOCCI

Enterococci may cause sepsis in neonates, with *Enterococcus faecalis* being the most common cause and a smaller number of cases caused by *Enterococcus faecium*. In most cases, the clinical presentation of enterococcal sepsis in neonates is similar to that of early-onset sepsis of any etiology. Prominent respiratory distress can be accompanied by a chest radiograph demonstrating the hyaline membrane–appearing pattern of other etiologies such as GBS. Septicemia may manifest as apnea, bradycardia, shock, respiratory failure, or other signs of illness. Meningitis and urinary tract infection also can occur. Nursery outbreaks have been reported. Recently, vancomycin-resistant enterococci have emerged as significant pathogens in hospitalized, usually premature neonates.

## STAPHYLOCOCCI

Staphylococci have been an important cause of late-onset infections in neonates for 100 years. For most of the last century, methicillin-susceptible *Staphylococcus aureus* (MSSA) was the organism causing endemic and sporadic disease, in addition to staphylococcal epidemics occurring in 20- to 30-year cycles. In adults, healthcare-associated methicillin-resistant *S aureus* (MRSA) infections emerged in the 1980s. Strains of virulent, community-associated MRSA (CA-MRSA), which are distinct from the typical healthcare-associated MRSA, have been reported since the late 1990s. Over the past decade, MRSA has emerged as a significant pathogen in neonatal intensive care units as a cause of late-onset sepsis. Infants with late-onset infection due to *S aureus* can present with septic shock characterized most often by respiratory distress, temperature instability, and poor perfusion. Staphylococcal syndromes, such as toxic shock and toxic epidermal necrolysis, also have been reported. A distinctive feature of *S aureus* infection in the neonate is its ability to frequently and rapidly result in focal pyogenic complications in skin, soft tissues, lungs, bones, and joints. Prolonged bacteremia despite appropriate antimicrobial therapy can occur and suggests foci of infection, such as endocarditis. Focal infection without bacteremia is less likely to cause fulminant disease but can cause cervical adenitis, impetigo, furunculosis, soft tissue abscesses, pneumonia, and pleural empyema. Outbreaks of MRSA skin infection among otherwise healthy, full-term newborns less than 30 days of age have been reported.

With the increased survival of VLBW and ELBW premature infants, coagulase-negative staphylococci (CoNS) have emerged as significant pathogens causing late-onset sepsis. Premature infants are at risk for infection with this commensal organism due to their developmentally immature immune systems and invasive procedures, such as placement of vascular access devices that further compromise their already poor skin integrity. Other risk factors for CoNS infection include mechanical ventilation, intravenous intralipid use, and duration of total parenteral nutrition. Although CoNS is present on the skin and is usually considered a contaminant in immunocompetent individuals, in the premature infant or in those with vascular catheters, isolation of this organism from the bloodstream may be indicative of infection. Clinical signs and features of late- and late late-onset sepsis caused by CoNS can include apnea, bradycardia, hypoxia, hypotension, temperature instability, serum glucose alterations, and other findings. The mortality rate from CoNS infection is approximately 5%.

## *LISTERIA MONOCYTOGENES*

*Listeria monocytogenes* is a ubiquitous organism and is an important cause of zoonoses. Listeriosis primarily is foodborne and can be found in animal products, including unpasteurized milk and soft cheeses, hot dogs, deli meat, pâté, and undercooked poultry, as well as on unwashed fresh fruits and vegetables. Most people exposed to *Listeria* do not develop illness, but maternal infection can result in miscarriage or stillbirth, and neonates can develop early- or late-onset sepsis and meningitis. Infection in pregnant women occurs most frequently in the third trimester and is associated with an influenza-like illness accompanied by fever, headache, malaise, myalgias, and gastrointestinal tract symptoms in two-thirds of infected women. Perinatal listeriosis results in stillbirth or neonatal death in approximately 22% of cases.

Both early- and late-onset listeriosis are uncommon. In infants with early-onset listeriosis, prematurity, pneumonia, and septicemia are common. Chorioamnionitis and brown-staining amniotic fluid can occur. Mothers can be asymptomatic. Granulomatosis infantiseptticum, a diffuse erythematous nodular rash characterized by granulomas on histopathology, can occur in neonates with severe listerial disease. The lesions also commonly occur in the liver and placenta but also can be found in the brain, lungs, adrenal glands, kidney, spleen, and gastrointestinal tract. Late-onset disease caused by *Listeria* is even less common than the early-onset form, but it usually occurs in the perinatal period in term infants and results in meningitis. Frequently, there is no history of pregnancy complications. Neonatal septicemia or meningitis caused by *Listeria* cannot be distinguished clinically from other infectious causes of sepsis.

## *ESCHERICHIA COLI*

Most infants are colonized with enteric bacilli in the lower gastrointestinal or respiratory tract during or just before delivery. *E coli* has a complex antigenic structure with more than 145 different somatic (O), approximately 50 flagellar (H), and 80 capsular (K) antigens. Despite this genetic diversity of human commensal isolates, a limited number of clones cause neonatal pathology.

*E coli* strains with the K1 capsular polysaccharide antigen are associated with 40% of cases of septicemia and 80% of cases of neonatal meningitis. The presence, amount, and persistence of K1 antigen in CSF have been related to a more severe outcome in infants with meningitis.

Neonatal septicemia or meningitis caused by *E coli* and other gram-negative bacilli cannot be distinguished clinically from other infectious causes of sepsis. Signs of sepsis can include apnea, bradycardia, cyanosis, fever or temperature instability, poor perfusion, lethargy, irritability, poor feeding, vomiting, abdominal distension, diarrhea, jaundice, organomegaly, bulging fontanel, seizure, or other nonspecific clinical findings.

## HOSPITAL-ASSOCIATED GRAM-NEGATIVE PATHOGENS

Both *Klebsiella* and *Enterobacter* species inhabit the gastrointestinal tracts of hospitalized infants and have emerged as significant hospital-associated neonatal pathogens. These pathogens more commonly cause late-onset rather than early-onset sepsis. Infections of the bloodstream, CNS, lung, urinary tract, skin, and soft tissues can occur. *Klebsiella* species may account for up to 20% to 30% of late-onset sepsis, and the mortality rate can approach 30%. *Enterobacter* species, especially *Enterobacter sakazakii*, have been associated with a severe form of necrotizing meningitis with a high mortality rate (50%). Risk factors for infection include prematurity, low birth weight, prolonged rupture of maternal membranes, and instrument or cesarean section delivery, as well as the presence of indwelling devices. Routine extended-spectrum cephalosporin usage in some nurseries has resulted in the emergence of multidrug resistance, in the form of extended-spectrum β-lactamase production by isolates of *Enterobacter* and *Klebsiella* species. Infections with these organisms are associated with increased morbidity and mortality.

*Citrobacter* and *Serratia* species, also occasional inhabitants of the gastrointestinal tracts of hospitalized infants, can cause sporadic and epidemic clusters of neonatal late-onset sepsis and meningitis. Clinical features can include septicemia, pneumonia, empyema, meningitis, urinary tract infection, skin and soft tissue infection, and bone infection. Like *E sakazakii, Citrobacter koseri* and *Serratia marcescens* are associated with necrotizing meningitis and the formation of brain abscesses. The mortality rate following meningitis due to either *Citrobacter* or *Serratia* species is estimated at 30%, and most survivors suffer significant neurodevelopmental morbidity. Risk factors for infection include prematurity, low birth weight, mechanical ventilation, indwelling vascular device, prior receipt of antibiotics, intraventricular hemorrhage, and necrotizing enterocolitis. Outbreaks of multidrug-resistant *S marcescens* infections in neonates have been reported.

*Pseudomonas aeruginosa* is a cause of late-onset neonatal sepsis, and infants are infected from their environment or their endogenous flora. The clinical presentation can be identical to other bacterial causes of neonatal infection, although infants with *Pseudomonas* sepsis frequently present with clinically fulminant disease. With rapid disease progression, mortality is approximately 50%. Risk factors for pseudomonas sepsis include prematurity, low birth weight, feeding intolerance, prolonged parenteral hyperalimentation, conjunctivitis, and necrotizing enterocolitis.

### RARE BACTERIAL ETIOLOGIES

Although non-typhi *Salmonella* is an uncommon cause of sepsis and meningitis in neonates, a significant number of cases of *Salmonella* meningitis occur in young infants. Meningitis can be complicated by subdural empyema and communicating hydrocephalus and can result in death.

Another uncommon cause of invasive bacterial infection in neonates is *Neisseria meningitidis*. This organism can colonize the maternal genital tract and infect the infant at the time of delivery, or intrauterine infection can occur as a result of maternal meningococcemia. Meningococcus can cause early- and late-onset sepsis in neonates. The clinical presentation can include septicemia, meningitis, and conjunctivitis. Purpura are rare. Serogroups B, C, and Y and nongroupable isolates have been reported.

*Haemophilus influenzae* type b disease in infants in the United States is rare since the introduction of *H influenzae* type b conjugate vaccines in 1989. In addition, invasive infections caused by nontypeable *H influenzae* in neonates remain uncommon. The clinical presentation of neonatal *H influenzae* disease can include septicemia, meningitis, pneumonia, soft tissue or joint infection, otitis media, and mastoiditis. Clinical and epidemiologic characteristics are similar to those of GBS disease, including early- and late-onset presentations.

Pneumococci are not usually isolated from cultures of the cervix or vagina of pregnant and nonpregnant women. However, *S pneumoniae* rarely can present as early-onset neonatal sepsis with clinical features similar to those of early-onset GBS infection. The illness can be associated with respiratory distress, abnormal chest roentgenogram, poor peripheral perfusion, hypotension, leukopenia, and rapid clinical decline. Late-onset infection accompanied by meningitis, though rare, also can occur.

Anaerobes have been isolated from the external genitalia or vagina of pregnant and nonpregnant women, and newborns are colonized with these organisms at the time of birth. Anaerobes are thought to cause fewer than 5% of the cases of neonatal sepsis, but the true incidence is uncertain. The clinical presentation is indistinguishable from other bacterial causes of sepsis, but predisposing factors include premature rupture of membranes, maternal amnionitis, preterm delivery, and neonatal postoperative complications and necrotizing enterocolitis. Intrauterine infection can cause septic abortion. *Bacteroides* and *Clostridium* species are the most frequent pathogens isolated from neonates with anaerobic sepsis, and the mortality rate is estimated at 26%. Neonatal bacteremia caused by *Clostridium perfringens* can present with the characteristics seen in adults such as active hemolysis, hyperbilirubinemia, and hemoglobinuria. In addition to causing sepsis and meningitis, *Clostridium* species can cause localized infection, such as omphalitis, cellulitis, and necrotizing fasciitis.

## MISCELLANEOUS SYNDROMIC INFECTIONS

### PATHOGENS CAUSING CONJUNCTIVITIS

Eyelid edema, hyperemia of the conjunctivae, and purulent discharge are common manifestations of infectious conjunctivitis in neonates. The most common pathogen in infants is *Chlamydia trachomatis*. Various organisms including gram-negative (eg, *Haemophilus* species, *Neisseria gonorrhoeae*) and gram-positive (eg, *S aureus*, enterococci, and *S pneumoniae*) organisms also can cause disease. In hospitalized and premature infants, bacteremia and meningitis can occur in association with conjunctivitis caused by *P aeruginosa*.

### PATHOGENS CAUSING OTITIS MEDIA

Infants with acute otitis media in the newborn period generally are not systemically ill. Signs of upper respiratory tract infection are common, but fever often is absent. The most common pathogens are the same as those found in older infants and children, such as *S pneumoniae, Moraxella catarrhalis*, and *H influenzae*. Tympanic aspiration reveals that approximately 40% of middle ear aspirates in this age group do not yield a pathogen. In hospitalized and premature infants with otitis media, systemic signs of illness such as fever, poor feeding, vomiting, diarrhea, and abdominal distention are more common than signs of upper respiratory tract infection. The same pathogens causing late-onset sepsis, including staphylococci and enteric bacilli, are common.

### DIAGNOSTIC EVALUATION FOR BACTERIAL PATHOGENS

The diagnosis of systemic infection in the newborn infant cannot be reliably established on the basis of clinical findings alone. A history of risk factors for neonatal sepsis often is associated with early-onset infection, but up to 20% of infants who develop early-onset disease are born without pregnancy or delivery complications. The development of late-onset sepsis in the term infant often is accompanied by only subtle signs of infection.

The isolation of a pathogenic bacteria from the blood is the "gold standard" and is the only definitive method of establishing the diagnosis of neonatal septicemia. The optimal volume of blood to obtain for culture is unknown, but an amount of 1.0 to 2.0 mL, depending on the patient's weight and gestational age, generally is recommended and yields the pathogenic organism in greater than 90% of cases. Multiple blood cultures generally are not necessary. In those cases in which a pathogen cannot be cultivated, sepsis sometimes may be presumed from the clinical course.

A lumbar puncture for CSF studies is recommended to evaluate for meningitis. A negative blood culture occurs in approximately 15% to 38% of neonates with meningitis. In the neonate whose unstable condition precludes the performance of a lumbar puncture when sepsis is initially suspected, CSF should be obtained as soon as the infant's condition permits and parameters evaluated for partially treated meningitis.

Urine cultures generally are not useful in the evaluation of the neonate with early-onset sepsis but should be obtained by catheter or suprapubic aspiration when infants are evaluated for sepsis beyond the first few days of life. The yield is 7% to 10% for late-onset disease.

Cultures and Gram stain of foci of suspected infection are recommended, except in select clinical circumstances, such as brain abscess not amenable to surgery or lung abscess at high risk of fistula formation, where obtaining cultures can be associated with excessive morbidity or even mortality. In general, cultures from surface sites or mucous membranes reveal colonizing microorganisms and correlate poorly with invasive disease. Gastric aspirate and placental cultures provide information about exposure to possible pathogens and may be helpful in guiding empirical therapy in an infant with signs of or risk factors for sepsis.

Screening tests for neonatal sepsis (eg, total white blood cell count, percentage of neutrophils and/or immature forms, platelet count, C-reactive protein, serum procalcitonin, and cytokine levels) are of variable utility in the evaluation of those with clinical signs of illness. No one screening test or combination of tests is sufficiently sensitive or specific to affect the necessity of performing blood, CSF, or other appropriate studies, such as chest roentgenogram, in infants with signs of or risk factors for infection. Normal screening test results should not deter a clinician from fully evaluating an infant for sepsis; however, screening tests, clinical signs of illness, and risk factors for infection should be considered together. A concern in any area should prompt immediate evaluation of the infant and initiation of appropriate antimicrobial therapy.

## TREATMENT

Table 225-4 lists common antibacterial agents used for the treatment of neonatal infections. The choice of empirical antimicrobial therapy for the treatment of suspected sepsis is influenced by factors such as the prevalent organisms responsible for neonatal sepsis by age of onset and other risk factors, patterns of antimicrobial susceptibility of isolates in a community or hospital, penetration of an antimicrobial agent into the CNS or other site, and potential toxicity of an agent in neonates in general or in a particular neonate. For infants who develop clinical signs of illness during the first few days of life, initial therapy must include agents active against GBS, other streptococci, other gram-positive cocci, *L monocytogenes*, and gram-negative enteric bacilli. Treatment of the infant with suspected late-onset sepsis who remains in the nursery also must include therapy for hospital-associated and commensal pathogens, such as *S aureus*, CoNS (especially in infants with intravascular catheters or CSF shunts), and potentially multidrug-resistant gram-negative bacilli. These infants also remain at risk for sepsis due to maternally acquired etiologic agents.

Empirical antimicrobial therapy for early-onset sepsis consists of ampicillin and gentamicin in order to provide bactericidal activity against GBS and other streptococci, enterococci, *Listeria*, *E coli*, and other gram-negative bacilli. If CSF parameters are concerning for meningitis, cefotaxime is added because of its ability to achieve bactericidal concentrations in the CSF. Gentamicin serum concentrations are not necessary unless therapy is continued beyond 72 hours, renal dysfunction is present, or the neonate is a VLBW infant.

As an initial choice of empirical antimicrobial therapy in infants with presumed early-onset septicemia, an aminoglycoside is recommended over a third-generation cephalosporin for the following reasons: third-generation cephalosporins are not active against *Listeria* and enterococci; superior efficacy with third-generation cephalosporins has not been demonstrated; routine empirical use of third-generation cephalosporins for neonatal septicemia has been associated with sepsis due to multidrug-resistant organisms; and empirical cephalosporin use for treating early-onset neonatal sepsis has independently been shown to be associated with a higher case fatality rate. Use of cefotaxime should be restricted to those with initial evidence of gram-negative sepsis or meningitis. Ceftazidime should be used if *Pseudomonas* sepsis is suspected. Continued cephalosporin therapy should be limited to those infants with gram-negative meningitis caused by susceptible organisms or those with ampicillin-resistant infections. Unless it is the only agent effective against the pathogen causing disease, ceftriaxone is not recommended for use in neonates because it can displace bilirubin from serum albumin. The typical duration of therapy for early- or late-onset septicemia is 10 to 14 days with the most effective, least toxic, and preferentially most narrow-spectrum antimicrobial agent based on culture and susceptibility results.

**TABLE 225-4 INITIAL ANTIBACTERIAL THERAPY FOR NEONATAL BACTERIAL INFECTIONS**

| Clinical Presentation | Antibiotics | Potential Adverse Effects with Ongoing Therapy | Expected Duration (days) |
|---|---|---|---|
| **Septicemia or pneumonia** | | | |
| Early onset; term or preterm infant | Ampicillin | Neutropenia, bone marrow suppression, renal impairment, interstitial nephritis | 10 |
| | Gentamicin | Renal impairment, hearing deficit | |
| Late-onset; term infant, readmitted | Ampicillin | See above | 10 |
| | Gentamicin | | |
| Late-onset; hospitalized infant | Vancomycin | Renal impairment, neutropenia | 10–14 |
| | Gentamicin or amikacin | Hearing deficit, renal impairment | |
| **Meningitis** | | | |
| Early onset | Ampicillin | See above | 14–21 |
| | Gentamicin | See above | |
| | Cefotaxime | Neutropenia, bone marrow suppression, renal impairment | |
| Late onset | Ampicillin | See above | 14–21 |
| | Gentamicin or amikacin | See above | |
| | Cefotaxime | See above | |
| **Gastrointestinal infection** | Include clindamycin | Elevated transaminases | 10–21 |
| | or | | |
| | Piperacillin-tazobactam | Neutropenia, renal impairment, elevated transaminases | |
| **Bone or joint infection** | Nafcillin | Neutropenia, phlebitis, interstitial nephritis, renal impairment, elevated transaminases | 3–6 weeks |
| | or | | |
| | Vancomycin | See above | |
| | Gentamicin | See above | |

Adapted with permission from Long SS, Pickering LK, Prober CG: *Principles and Practice of Pediatric Infectious Diseases*. 4th ed. Philadelphia: Elsevier Saunders; 2012.

For neonates with early-onset meningitis, a third-generation cephalosporin should be administered in addition to ampicillin and gentamicin or in place of gentamicin because it provides concentrations of drug in the CSF that greatly exceed the minimum inhibitory concentrations of susceptible pathogens and there is no dose-related toxicity. In patients with gram-negative meningitis, combination therapy with a cephalosporin and an aminoglycoside may be used until drug susceptibility results are known and the CSF is sterile. Most experts recommend treating meningitis caused by enteric bacilli for a minimum of 21 days and 14 days for most other bacteria.

For suspected late-onset sepsis in the nursery or for sepsis associated with skin, soft tissue, bone, or joint infection, initial antimicrobial therapy should provide coverage against MRSA, commensal species such as CoNS, and other nonstaphylococcal gram-positive organisms as well as gram-negative pathogens. β-Lactamase production is present in most species of CoNS, and they also are resistant to methicillin and cephalosporins. In addition, ampicillin has no activity against *S aureus*. In such cases, vancomycin is substituted for ampicillin and is administered with an aminoglycoside pending further culture data. Except in cases of neurosurgery, indwelling CNS devices, or intraventricular hemorrhage, staphylococci are rare causes of meningitis. For empirical therapy of hospital-associated meningitis, a third-generation cephalosporin should be added to vancomycin and an aminoglycoside.

For infants in whom infection caused by anaerobic organisms is suspected, such as those with signs of omphalitis, peritonitis, or necrotizing enterocolitis, initiating therapy that includes an agent such as clindamycin, metronidazole, or piperacillin-tazobactam is indicated. Penicillin G is not considered adequate anaerobic coverage for most neonatal infections because *B fragilis* is usually resistant.

Virtually all infants with neonatal sepsis died before the advent of antibiotics. In the present day, if the evaluation for bacterial sepsis and the initiation of antibacterial therapy are prompt, infants are less likely to experience death or long-term health problems associated with neonatal bacterial infection. However, if appropriate therapy is delayed because early signs are subtle or missed, the mortality rate increases. Cases of fulminant early-onset sepsis are associated with a high mortality rate of 14% to 20% to as much as 70%.

In the 1960s, mortality from neonatal sepsis was approximately 50% but decreased to 10% to 20% in the 1970s and 1980s. The mortality rate for premature infants is higher than for term infants. A more recent report indicated that in preterm infants with GBS sepsis, the mortality rate was 23% and 9% for early-onset and late-onset cases, respectively. In comparison, among term infants, 4% with early-onset disease and no infants with late-onset disease died during the same time period. Outcomes in neonates with meningitis are discussed in Chapter 226.

## PREVENTION

Improvements in the health of pregnant women with increased use of prenatal care facilities, improvements in diagnostics and therapeutics, the development of neonatal intensive care expertise and dedicated units, and adherence to proper hand hygiene and disinfection of materials involved in the care of neonates have improved infant outcomes. Improved care of the mother and infant contributes to a decreased incidence of neonatal infection. The use of antimicrobials to prevent neonatal infection can be valuable when a specific pathogen-directed approach is employed for a limited period of time. An example is the application of antimicrobials to the eye or intramuscular administration of ceftriaxone to prevent neonatal gonococcal ophthalmia. Intrapartum chemoprophylaxis of pregnant women with rectovaginal colonization of GBS has been shown to be a highly effective method of preventing early-onset neonatal GBS disease. Consensus guidelines developed for intrapartum chemoprophylaxis were modified in 2010 and provide recommendations based on maternal screening cultures (and risk factors). The guidelines also state that routine administration of antibiotics to newborn infants who are born to mothers who have received intrapartum chemoprophylaxis is not recommended.

The neonatal immune system is quantitatively and functionally immature. It is characterized by decreased antibody levels against common bacterial pathogens; inadequate neutrophil production, mobilization, and function; decreased complement activity, especially in the alternative pathway; and inadequate T lymphocyte cytokine production to many antigens, as well as other defects.

Breastfeeding has been recognized for many years to provide neonates a degree of protection against viral and bacterial pathogens. Breastfeeding can protect infants against neonatal sepsis and meningitis, urinary tract infection, respiratory illness, gastroenteritis, otitis media, and other infections. Uncommonly, breastfeeding can be the source of neonatal bacterial infection.

Infants are somewhat protected from bacterial infection by placental transfer of maternal IgG. Immunization of pregnant women against pathogens causing severe infection in neonates has been studied and is recommended on a limited basis. The immunization of pregnant women with tetanus toxoid is widely practiced and, in resource-limited countries, has markedly decreased the incidence of neonatal tetanus. In the United States, administration of a dose of Tdap (tetanus, diphtheria, and pertussis) with every pregnancy is recommended to provide transplacental antibody to the fetus and protect it during the critical first months of life, especially from pertussis. New candidate polysaccharide-protein conjugate vaccines against GBS for use in pregnant women have been or are being tested in phase I and II trials; however, no licensed vaccine is yet available.

Numerous studies have explored whether the use of intravenous immune globulin or granulocyte colony-stimulating factor, especially in preterm infants, can reduce the incidence of sepsis. Analysis of these studies and others reveals that there currently is insufficient evidence to support the routine use of intravenous immune globulin or granulocyte colony-stimulating factor to prevent systemic bacterial infection in high-risk neonates.

## SUGGESTED READINGS


Abzug MJ, Michaels M, Wald E, et al. A randomized, double-blind, placebo-controlled trial of pleconaril for the treatment of neonates with enterovirus sepsis. *J Pediatr Infect Dis Soc.* 2016;5:53-62.

Camacho-Gonzalez A, Spearman PW, Stoll BJ. Neonatal infectious diseases: evaluation of neonatal sepsis. *Pediatr Clin North Am.* 2013;60:367-389.

Centers for Disease Control and Prevention. Perinatal group B streptococcal disease. *Morb Mortal Wkly Rep.* 2010;59:1-32.

Chu HY, Englund JA. Maternal immunization. *Clin Infect Dis.* 2014;59:560-568.

Kimberlin DW, Jester PM, Sánchez PJ, et al. Valganciclovir for symptomatic congenital cytomegalovirus disease. *N Engl J Med.* 2015;372:933-943.

Kimberlin DW, Whitley RJ, Wan W, et al. Oral acyclovir suppression and neurodevelopment after neonatal herpes. *N Engl J Med.* 2011;365:1284-1292.

Nizet V, Klein JO. Bacterial sepsis and meningitis. In: Remington JS, Klein JO, Wilson CB, et al, eds. *Infectious Diseases of the Fetus and Newborn Infant.* 7th ed. Philadelphia, PA: Elsevier Saunders; 2011:222-275.

# 226 Bacterial Infections of the Central Nervous System

Thomas S. Murray and Robert S. Baltimore

## BACTERIAL MENINGITIS

Meningitis, an infection of the subarachnoid space and leptomeninges caused by a variety of pathogenic organisms, continues to be an important source of mortality and morbidity. Despite the introduction of new vaccines that prevent the most severe causes, bacterial or purulent meningitis remains the most important form of meningitis in the United States in terms of incidence, sequelae, and ultimate loss of productive life. Aseptic meningitis, usually caused by viruses, especially enteroviruses, is more common; however, significant sequelae are uncommon, and the disease is usually self-limited. Granulomatous meningitis, caused either by *Mycobacterium tuberculosis* or fungi, is a major cause of neurologic injury and death in the developing world.

### PATHOGENESIS AND EPIDEMIOLOGY

The most common progression of infection in children with bacterial meningitis is hematogenous spread from the nasopharynx followed by bacterial entry into the subarachnoid space where the cerebrospinal fluid (CSF) contains few fixed or circulating scavenger cells to remove bacteria. Different bacteria cross the blood-brain barrier using a variety of cell surface receptors. There is poor opsonic and bactericidal capability in the CSF, so there is not a rapid cellular or humoral immune response, and bacteria can grow to the level of $10^6$ to $10^7$ organisms per milliliter of CSF. Meningitis may also occur as a direct extension from a contiguous focus or as a result of congenital, traumatic, or surgical disruption of normal anatomic barriers. Examples of such disruption include congenital dermal sinuses along the craniospinal axis, basilar skull fractures, and placement of CSF shunts.

Many of the neurologic sequelae of bacterial meningitis are a consequence of altered physiology due to the host's inflammatory response to the infecting organism (Fig. 226-1). In the subarachnoid space, components of the surface of the multiplying bacteria (lipopolysaccharide, lipo-oligosaccharide, teichoic acid) stimulate generation of proinflammatory cytokines (tumor necrosis factor [TNF]-α, interleukin [IL]-1β, IL-6, platelet activating factor [PAF], and others). These, in turn, increase adhesion of leukocytes to cerebral vascular endothelium, promoting increased blood-brain barrier permeability and migration of leukocytes into the subarachnoid space. White blood cell (WBC) and endothelium-derived reactive oxygen species, and perhaps nitric oxide, then participate in altering cerebrovascular reactivity. Cerebral edema associated with meningitis represents a combination of vasogenic, cytotoxic, and interstitial edema. Cerebral perfusion is reduced in meningitis in approximately 30% of children in whom brain blood-flow studies have been performed. Cerebral edema not only contributes to reduced cerebral perfusion, but may also cause cerebral herniation due to increased intracranial pressure.

Direct cytotoxic neuronal injury, frequently found in postmortem studies, is likely caused by reactive oxygen and nitrogen species (oxygen radical, nitric oxide, peroxynitrite, hydroxyl radical), excitatory amino acids, caspases, and matrix metalloproteinases (MMPs). Experimental animal studies demonstrate improved neuronal survival when specific inhibitors of these compounds are used. Abnormalities of brain metabolism include hypoglycorrhachia and CSF lactic acidosis. Low CSF glucose levels occur by impaired glucose transport across the blood-brain barrier and possibly by increased cerebral glucose utilization. CSF lactic acidosis indicates anaerobic glucose utilization within the central nervous system.

Pathologic changes in meningitis reflect the inflammatory mass in the subarachnoid space, cerebral vasculitis, cerebral edema, and cellular injury. The inflammatory mass usually begins in the basilar cisterns, spreads around the cerebellum, and then spreads over the cerebral convexities. The cranial nerves that traverse the subarachnoid space are particularly prone to injury in meningitis, perhaps due to the surrounding inflammation. Vasculitis of both arteries and veins occurs, particularly in meningitis caused by *Streptococcus pneumoniae*, resulting in tissue ischemia and arterial and venous infarcts. Direct cellular injury, as a result of bacterial toxins, host factors, or ischemia, is frequently noted in postmortem studies.

The first month after birth represents the period of highest attack rate for meningitis, with likely pathogens including *Streptococcus agalactiae* (group B *Streptococcus*), *Escherichia coli*, other gram-negative enteric organisms, and less commonly, *Listeria monocytogenes* (Table 226-1). Beyond the neonatal period, the most important pathogens are *S pneumoniae* and *Neisseria meningitidis*. In the past, *Haemophilus influenzae* type B (Hib) was the most common pathogen causing meningitis in toddlers and children, but the incidence has been reduced dramatically by immunization with conjugate vaccines in developed countries. Recent studies of conjugate pneumococcal vaccine, introduced in the United States in 2000, demonstrate that it is effective in preventing pneumococcal meningitis. Similarly, the meningococcal conjugate vaccine first introduced in 2005 as part of

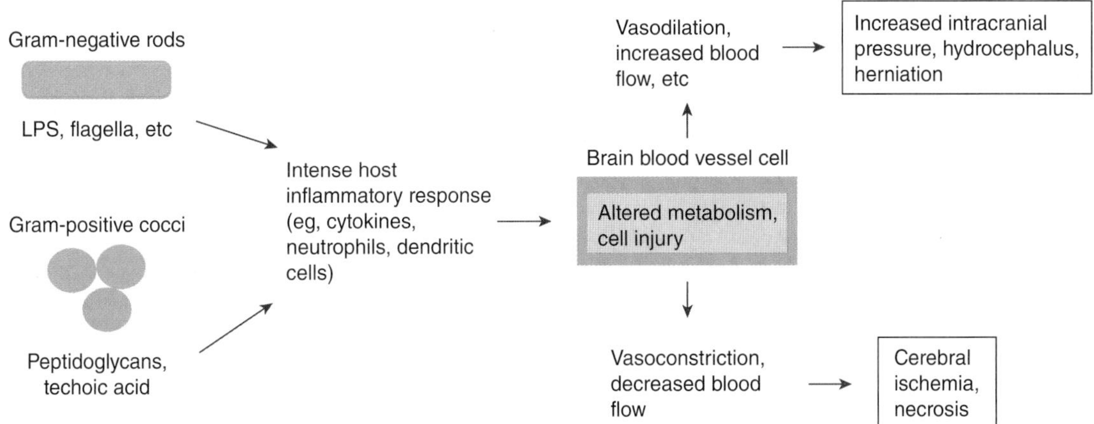


**FIGURE 226-1** Pathophysiologic changes that occur in the brain in response to invasion by bacteria in meningitis. Note that different regions of the brain may be hyperperfused or hypoperfused. LPS, lipopolysaccharide; TNF, tumor necrosis factor.

**TABLE 226-1 BACTERIAL CAUSES OF MENINGITIS**

| Relative Frequency | 0–1 Month | > 1 Month |
|---|---|---|
| Common | *Streptococcus agalactiae* | *Streptococcus pneumoniae* |
| | *Escherichia coli* | *Neisseria meningitidis* |
| | *Listeria monocytogenes* | |
| | *Klebsiella* species | |
| | *Enterobacter* species | |
| Uncommon | *Staphylococcus aureus*[a] | *Streptococcus pyogenes* |
| | Coagulase-negative staphylococci[a] | Gram-negative bacilli |
| | | *Haemophilus influenzae* type b[b] |
| | Enterococcal species | |
| | *Pseudomonas aeruginosa* | |
| Rare | *S pneumoniae* | *L monocytogenes* |
| | *Streptococcus pyogenes* | *S aureus*[a] |
| | *Citrobacter diversus* | Coagulase-negative staphylococci[a] |
| | *H influenzae* non–type b | |
| | *Salmonella* species | |

[a]Usually associated with neurosurgical procedures.

[b]Common where *Haemophilus influenzae* type b vaccine is unavailable.

the routine vaccination schedule for US adolescents has been effective in reducing meningococcal meningitis due to serogroups A, C, Y, and W135. More recently a vaccine has been approved for serogroup B *N meningitidis* for at-risk children. Thus, the incidence of infection and prevailing predominant causative organisms vary depending on both the age and the immunization status of the population.

Bacterial meningitis is reported with increased frequency among African Americans, Native Americans, and individuals in rural areas. It is unclear whether environmental or genetic factors are responsible for enhanced susceptibility. Seasonal patterns of disease have been noted to occur, with meningitis caused by *N meningitidis* and *S pneumoniae* peaking in the winter months, Hib showing a biphasic distribution with peaks in the early winter and spring, and *L monocytogenes* occurring most frequently in the summer months. In the "meningitis belt" of sub-Saharan Africa, the shift from the wet to the dry season is associated with an increase in meningitis. These patterns are likely due to the modes for acquiring the organisms, with *N meningitidis, S pneumoniae*, and Hib spread by the respiratory route in months with increased incidence of common respiratory diseases, and *L monocytogenes* acquired from contaminated food or contact with farm animals.

Host factors such as asplenia and lack of opsonizing antibody predispose to increased susceptibility to encapsulated organisms such as *S pneumoniae* and increase the risk of meningitis. *Neisseria* infections including *N meningitidis* occur with increased frequency in persons with terminal complement deficiencies. Polymorphisms in toll-like receptor proteins and other adaptor molecules that are integral parts of the innate immune response have also been associated with increased risk for invasive disease caused by *N meningitidis*.

The emergence of bacteria resistant to commonly prescribed antibiotics has changed empiric treatment of presumed bacterial meningitis. In the past decade, *S pneumoniae* with reduced susceptibility to penicillins and cephalosporins has been identified in virtually all parts of the world and, in some areas, may compromise the utility of those drugs for empiric therapy. The 13-valent pneumococcal conjugate vaccine (PCV) currently available in the United States is directed at several strains associated with increased antibiotic resistance. According to the Centers for Disease Control and Prevention, in 2013, 30% of invasive infections due to *S pneumoniae* were caused by pneumococci that were not susceptible to at least 1 drug used for therapy with increased resistance to older β-lactam antibiotics and macrolides. Of children who received the pneumococcal conjugate vaccine, 18.4% of those with invasive pneumococcal disease had strains intermediately susceptible to penicillin, and 19.1% had strains with high-level resistance to penicillin. A serotype (19A) that was not included in the initial 7-valent PCV and was resistant to multiple antibiotics that caused invasive disease has been incorporated in the currently available PCV. Increased antibiotic resistance has also been seen with gram-negative enteric species such as *E coli*. However, *S agalactiae* and *N meningitidis* have remained susceptible to penicillin and third-generation cephalosporins. The clinician must be aware of emerging patterns of antibiotic resistance within the local community and in the hospital setting for patients who develop symptoms suspicious for invasive bacterial disease, including meningitis.

## CLINICAL MANIFESTATIONS

The classic triad of symptoms in meningitis includes fever, headache, and stiff neck. However, in children under 2 years of age, and especially in young infants, stiff neck or other signs of meningeal irritation may be absent. Alteration of level of consciousness is usual, occurring in up to 90% of patients. The majority present with irritability, lethargy, or confusion, and 10% to 15% present in coma, a very poor prognostic sign. Physical examination of older children may reveal typical signs of meningeal irritation—stiff neck and positive Kernig and Brudzinski signs. Infants often have a bulging fontanel. Cranial nerve abnormalities, particularly of the sixth cranial nerve, may be the consequence of increased intracranial pressure or of inflammation in the subarachnoid space. Focal neurologic abnormalities are uncommon early in the disease but, when present, may be indicators of cerebral infarct.

Systemic signs may also be present in children with meningitis. The most common occur in the setting of meningococcal disease. The rash in meningococcal sepsis evolves from a transient erythematous, macular eruption to the presence of petechiae, ecchymoses, and purpura. These may lead to frank tissue ischemia and tissue death. Approximately 50% of these patients will have concurrent meningitis. Meningitis due to *N meningitidis* and gram-negative rods frequently results in hypotension due to the systemic effects of endotoxin. Most other causes of meningitis, including those due to *S pneumoniae*, Hib, and *L monocytogenes*, are usually not accompanied by endotoxic shock. Hypotension in the setting of disease caused by these other organisms is most commonly the result of volume depletion or purpura fulminans. Purpura fulminans is a condition associated with overwhelming infections and includes rapidly evolving disseminated intravascular coagulation (DIC), fever, chills, and ecchymotic skin lesions that may ulcerate and progress to peripheral gangrene, shock, and death.

## DIAGNOSIS

Once the diagnosis of meningitis is suspected, immediate examination of the CSF is indicated unless there is a strong suspicion of an intracranial mass lesion. Such a mass may be the cause of herniation of the brain through the foramen magnum during the lumbar puncture. Worrisome findings include papilledema or a history of an indolent process with focal neurologic findings. In those instances, lumbar puncture can be delayed until a mass is excluded by cranial computed tomography (CT) or magnetic resonance imaging (MRI) of the brain. CSF abnormalities in bacterial meningitis include elevated numbers of WBCs, elevated protein concentration, hypoglycorrhachia, elevated opening pressure, and bacteria observed on Gram stain. Pleocytosis is typical in bacterial meningitis, with CSF WBC concentrations in the range of 100 to 10,000 cells/μL, although occasionally early in the disease, the WBC concentration may be normal or slightly elevated. In bacterial meningitis, polymorphonuclear cells predominate and usually account for more than 90% of the total. Very high WBC concentrations (> 50,000/μL) raise the possibility of an intracranial abscess that has ruptured into the ventricles.

Hypoglycorrhachia is commonly found in bacterial meningitis, with CSF glucose usually less than 50% of simultaneous serum glucose. Other causes of hypoglycorrhachia include tuberculous and fungal meningitis, subarachnoid hemorrhage, and carcinomatous meningitis. CSF protein concentration is usually elevated, in the range of 100 to 500 mg/dL, but because elevated protein reflects an alteration in the blood-brain barrier, it is not, by itself, diagnostic of bacterial infection.

In contrast to bacterial meningitis, CSF from patients with aseptic (including viral) meningitis is typically characterized by lower WBC counts and a glucose concentration near or within the normal range. Although the percentage of neutrophils may be variable, it is usually much lower in aseptic meningitis where lymphocyte predominance is more common. CSF protein concentration may be normal or elevated in patients with meningitis caused by enterovirus or *M tuberculosis*.

The Gram stain is positive in more than 90%, and the CSF culture is positive in 70% to 90% of patients with untreated hematogenous bacterial meningitis. The Gram stain must be interpreted by an experienced microbiologist, as errors in interpretation are common. Pneumococci, when overdecolorized, may resemble meningococci, Hib may be thought to be gram-negative enteric organisms or vice versa, and debris may resemble gram-positive cocci. *L monocytogenes* is frequently difficult to identify on direct smear.

Prior treatment with oral antibiotics substantially reduces the yield of CSF bacterial cultures. More recently, molecular diagnostic methods, including polymerase chain reaction (PCR) of a portion of the bacterial gene encoding the 16S ribosome, have been successful in the early diagnosis and speciation of bacterial meningitis. Novel diagnostic platforms that detect nucleic acid from bacteria, viruses, and fungi that cause meningitis and encephalitis are available, with US Food and Drug Administration (FDA) approval having occurred in 2015 for a platform that detects 14 of the most common central nervous system (CNS) pathogens.

In addition to culture and Gram stain of the CSF, blood culture may be useful in specific etiologic diagnosis. Blood cultures are positive in 40% to 75% of cases of bacterial meningitis, depending on the pathogen, and should be performed routinely.

Studies other than those aimed at making an etiologic diagnosis are indicated as well. Peripheral blood WBC and differential are useful in assessing the likelihood of a serious bacterial infection, and leukopenia may be a poor prognostic sign, indicating failure of the inflammatory response, particularly in the settings of overwhelming meningococcal or pneumococcal disease. Other inflammatory markers such as C-reactive protein and procalcitonin may also be helpful, as high levels correlate with the likelihood of serious bacterial infection, including meningitis, when patients present with symptoms consistent with meningitis. Prolongation of blood coagulation studies in conjunction with thrombocytopenia may indicate DIC, which is often present with serious gram-negative infection. Serum and urine electrolytes and osmolality should be measured routinely to look for the syndrome of inappropriate antidiuretic hormone (SIADH) secretion, marked by hyponatremia in association with increased urine osmolality and increased urine concentration of sodium. Radiologic studies are rarely needed in the diagnosis of meningitis; however, they may be useful in identifying coexisting complicating factors. Cranial CT may indicate cerebral edema early in the infection and later may show subdural effusion or subdural empyema.

## TREATMENT

### Antimicrobial Therapy

Effective treatment of meningitis depends on early aggressive supportive therapy and selection of empiric antimicrobials appropriate for the likely pathogens. The principles of antimicrobial therapy of meningitis include selection of an antibiotic that is bactericidal against the suspected pathogens and that achieves a concentration in CSF at least 10 times the minimal bactericidal concentration (MBC) for the organism, as this is the concentration that has been shown in animal studies to correlate with most effective sterilization of CSF. Suggested choices for empiric therapy are listed in Table 226-2 and should be based on the likely pathogens for the age group, known exposures, and any unusual risk factors for the patient. Resistance to third-generation cephalosporins is increasing, so empiric therapy with vancomycin as well as ceftriaxone or cefotaxime is warranted when pneumococcal meningitis is suspected. An exception may be in a country or region where monitoring for pneumococcal resistance has shown resistance to be absent.

**TABLE 226-2 EMPIRIC ANTIMICROBIAL THERAPY FOR PRESUMED BACTERIAL MENINGITIS**

| Age | Drug of Choice[a] | Alternative Drug[a] |
|---|---|---|
| Newborns (0–1 month) | Ampicillin plus gentamicin | Ampicillin plus cefotaxime or meropenem[c] |
| Infants and toddlers (1 month to 4 years) | Ceftriaxone[b] or cefotaxime plus vancomycin | Meropenem[c] or ampicillin[a] plus chloramphenicol[d] |
| Children and adolescents (5–13 years) and adults | Ceftriaxone or cefotaxime plus vancomycin | Meropenem[c] or ampicillin[a] plus chloramphenicol[d] |

[a]Consider vancomycin in areas with substantial pneumococcal penicillin resistance.

[b]Not for newborns younger than 1 week with hyperbilirubinemia because of the possibility of bilirubin displacement from albumin.

[c]Meropenem is preferred therapy for gram-negative species if the organism expresses an extended-spectrum β-lactamase.

[d]Used in resource-limited countries.

Definitive antibiotic therapy depends on the antibiotic susceptibility of the causative organism. *N meningitidis* remains susceptible to penicillin, but ceftriaxone or cefotaxime also can be used. For patients who must avoid all β-lactam antibiotics, meropenem or chloramphenicol would be appropriate. Chloramphenicol is not used in the United States, but in the developing world, it is available, is low cost, can be used intravenously or intramuscularly, can be given orally to complete a course of therapy, and is effective for older children with meningitis due to susceptible organisms. For *S pneumoniae* strains susceptible to penicillin, penicillin, ceftriaxone, or cefotaxime would be appropriate. If the isolate is nonsusceptible to penicillin but susceptible to ceftriaxone or cefotaxime, 1 of these 2 drugs is recommended, and vancomycin should be discontinued. If the isolate is also nonsusceptible to ceftriaxone or cefotaxime, then vancomycin and ceftriaxone or cefotaxime should be continued for the full course of treatment. In this instance, under selected circumstances, rifampin also may be added if the isolate is susceptible. Hib is uniformly susceptible to ceftriaxone or cefotaxime, but the majority of isolates are susceptible to ampicillin, which is the drug of choice if the isolate is susceptible. Doses of antibiotics used to treat the more common causes of bacterial meningitis in children are shown in Table 226-3.

**TABLE 226-3 SUGGESTED DOSAGES FOR BACTERIAL MENINGITIS TREATMENT IN PERSONS WITH NORMAL RENAL FUNCTION**

| Drug | Dosage | Maximum Daily Dose |
|---|---|---|
| Amikacin | 22.5 mg/kg/d divided q8–12h IV | 1.5 g |
| Ampicillin | 200–400 mg/kg/d divided q4–6h IV | 12 g |
| Cefotaxime | 200–300 mg/kg/d divided q6–8h IV | 12 g |
| Ceftriaxone | 100 mg/kg/d divided q12h IV or IM or 80 mg/kg/d given q24h IV or IM | 3–4 g |
| Chloramphenicol | 100 mg/kg/d divided q6h IV | 4 g |
| Trimethoprim-sulfamethoxazole | 15 mg/kg/d (as trimethoprim) divided q8h IV | 1.2 g (as trimethoprim) |
| Gentamicin | 7.5 mg/kg/d divided q8h IV | 7.5 mg/kg |
| Meropenem | 120 mg/kg/d divided q8h IV | 6 g |
| Nafcillin | 150–200 mg/kg/d divided q6h IV | 12 g |
| Oxacillin | 150–200 mg/kg/d divided q6h IV | 12 g |
| Penicillin G | 250,000–500,000 U/kg/d divided q4–6h IV | 20–24 MU |
| Rifampin | 20 mg/kg/d divided q12h IV | 600 mg |
| Tobramycin | 7.5 mg/kg/d divided q8h IV | 7.5 mg/kg |
| Vancomycin | 45–60 mg/kg/d divided q6h IV | 2 g |

IM, intramuscular; IV, intravenous.

Duration of antibiotic therapy is 14 to 21 days for neonatal meningitis caused by group B streptococci, and a minimum of 21 days for gram-negative enteric organisms. For meningitis in older infants or children, treatment should be 7 days for *N meningitidis*, 7 to 10 days for Hib, and 10 to 14 days for *S pneumoniae*.

#### Supportive and Adjunctive Therapies

Regarding the possible benefits of adjunctive early corticosteroid treatment, despite numerous studies, there have been inconsistent results in children with bacterial meningitis not caused by Hib. Dexamethasone, 0.15 mg/kg per dose, administered prior to or concurrently with the start of antibiotic treatment and continued every 6 hours for 2 to 4 days is the regimen used in published studies. Some data suggest steroid administration improves mortality in adults with pneumococcal meningitis and improves morbidity and mortality in neonates, but there is insufficient literature to support this as a blanket recommendation for children.

There are supportive measures that address the consequences of serious intracranial pathology. Patients who are comatose or who have impaired gag reflex should have their stomach contents emptied, and intubation should be considered to protect the airway. Hypoxia should be treated with supplemental oxygen. Hypoventilation is particularly worrisome in these patients because elevated $Paco_2$ may cause cerebral vasodilatation and potentiate increased intracranial pressure. Hypercarbia should be considered another indication for intubation and assisted ventilation.

Fluid management is critically important in patients with meningitis. SIADH occurs in approximately 30% of patients with bacterial meningitis and warrants fluid restriction after restoration of normal blood volume. However, a clinical study has documented the importance of maintaining an adequate cerebral perfusion pressure in this disease. Inappropriate fluid restriction may result in volume depletion, leading to inadequate circulating volume if carried to extremes. If SIADH is present, fluids should be limited to replacement of insensible losses plus urine output (generally, approximately two-thirds of maintenance requirement) until ADH excess resolves. If SIADH is not present, fluids should be administered in an amount appropriate to maintenance requirements plus intercurrent losses, and electrolytes should be carefully monitored.

Therapy of increased intracranial pressure must be directed at maintaining an adequate degree of cerebral perfusion pressure as in other conditions complicated by intracranial hypertension. Available modalities may include elevation of the head of the bed, hyperventilation, withdrawal of CSF through an intraventricular catheter, or possibly the careful use of osmotic diuretic agents.

Mortality rates in bacterial meningitis vary considerably depending on the age of the patient, the pathogen, and the degree of illness at the time of initial evaluation. Individuals with meningococcal meningitis without overwhelming meningococcemia have a fatality rate of 12%, whereas newborns with gram-negative meningitis succumb up to 70% of the time. Death rates from Hib and *S pneumoniae* are approximately 3% and 6%, respectively, at children's hospitals in developed countries.

Morbid sequelae occur in approximately 30% of survivors, but there is also an age and pathogen predilection, with the greatest incidence of sequelae occurring among the very young and in those infected with either gram-negative bacteria or *S pneumoniae*. Although many patients with meningitis have good neurologic outcomes with standard supportive measures and antibiotics, patients with more profound CNS disturbance require more intensive treatment to reduce intracranial pressure in conjunction with supportive care and antimicrobial therapy. In addition to depressed mental status at the time of presentation, other poor prognostic factors include the presence of comorbid conditions, leukopenia, and severe hypoglycorrhachia. The most common neurologic sequelae include deafness in 3% to 25% of patients; cranial nerve palsies in 2% to 7%; and severe injury, such as hemiparesis or global brain injury, in 1% to 2% of patients. More than 50% of patients with neurologic sequelae at discharge from the hospital will improve with time, and recent advances in cochlear implant therapy may provide hope for the child with permanent hearing loss.

### PREVENTION

Prevention of meningitis currently takes 2 forms: chemoprophylaxis for susceptible individuals known to be exposed to an index patient and active immunization. Chemoprophylaxis is currently indicated for preventing secondary cases of meningitis due to Hib and *N meningitidis*. Active immunization with conjugate vaccine against Hib has resulted in a dramatic reduction in invasive disease, with a > 95% reduction in meningitis caused by that organism. Universal infant Hib vaccination is recommended in the United States. The introduction of the conjugate pneumococcal vaccine has also reduced rates of invasive pneumococcal disease such as meningitis, including in high-risk communities, such as Native American communities. Initially, a multivalent polysaccharide vaccine was approved but was not immunogenic for children under 2 years old. This was followed by the first conjugated pneumococcal vaccine, which conferred immunity in infants to the 7 most common pneumococcal serotypes causing invasive disease. This has since been superseded by a conjugated vaccine containing 13 pneumococcal serotypes in the United States as part of the universal infant vaccination.

A quadrivalent conjugate meningococcal vaccine has become available against *N meningitidis* groups A, C, Y, and W-135. It is administered to all adolescents and to children over 2 years of age who are considered to be at increased risk of meningococcal infection in the United States. The Centers for Disease Control and Prevention's Advisory Committee on Immunization Practices (ACIP) has not recommended the recently licensed group B vaccine for universal immunization but rather for "certain persons aged ≥ 10 years who are at increased risk for meningococcal disease. These persons include persons with persistent complement component deficiencies, persons with anatomic or functional asplenia, microbiologists routinely exposed to isolates of *N meningitidis*, and persons identified as at increased risk because of a serogroup B meningococcal disease outbreak."

### FUTURE DIRECTIONS

The increasing availability of rapid molecular testing for the early diagnosis of bacterial and viral etiologies of meningitis and encephalitis will potentially have several benefits: (1) early diagnosis of viral disease can reduce the use of empiric antimicrobials that might contribute to increasing microbial resistance; (2) early identification of a bacterial pathogen can direct and narrow antibiotic choices and ensure early appropriate therapy with potential for improved clinical outcomes; and (3) in cases where the Gram stain and culture are negative due to previous antibiotic administration, the rapid identification of a pathogen can help direct therapy.

While much work has gone into adjuvant therapies to improve clinical outcomes for bacterial meningitis, a groundbreaking intervention has proven elusive. While steroids given early may have some clinical benefit, when recommended, it is only in high-income countries and this is not uniformly endorsed. Hypothermia for bacterial meningitis resulted in improved outcomes in animal studies. However, a human trial found it caused more harm than benefit. The use of the antidepressant fluoxetine has had favorable results in animals preventing hippocampal damage during bacterial meningitis, but more data are required to determine if this is a viable therapeutic option. Ongoing studies are examining glycerol as an adjuvant to antibiotic therapy, but results to date have been mixed.

## BRAIN ABSCESS

Brain abscess is relatively uncommon yet remains a serious disease. Early diagnosis with neuroradiologic imaging, rapid neurosurgical intervention (including stereotactic brain biopsy and aspiration), and the initiation of broad-spectrum antimicrobial therapy, to cover both anaerobic and aerobic bacteria, provide the best opportunity for a favorable outcome. Nevertheless, because there are no prospective controlled or comparative trials, management relies largely on retrospective studies and clinical experience.

## PATHOGENESIS AND EPIDEMIOLOGY

Most abscesses start at the gray-white matter junction. Encapsulation proceeds more rapidly and profusely on the cortical side than on the side facing the white matter. With abscesses in paraventricular sites, rupture into the ventricle may occur at any time, an event that carries a very high mortality.

Investigations of experimental abscesses and correlation of CT scans with both experimental and operative histologic findings have led to a definition of stages in the course of abscess formation. These stages include early and late cerebritis followed by early and late capsule formation. The findings from CT and MRI differ according to the stage of abscess formation. In early cerebritis, there is only patchy enhancement and an ill-defined area of low density or attenuation. As the abscess matures to late cerebritis and early capsule formation, a large enhancing ring is identified. This occurs during the formation of a collagen capsule, and the central portion of the abscess begins to necrose. In the final late capsular stage, there is a well-defined collagen capsule and necrotic center. Contrast images at this stage reveal only a faint thin rim of enhancement.

Brain abscess can arise in association with infection elsewhere in the body or can be caused by penetrating injury or a neurosurgical procedure. Extension and spread of infection via the bloodstream through venous channels to the brain from paranasal, mastoid, or inner ear sites has been reported as the most common cause of brain abscess in many series. However, the incidence of infection from otorhinologic sources has fallen markedly since the introduction of antibiotics. Metastatic abscesses usually originate in either the heart or the lungs, although osteomyelitis, renal infections, and skin abscess (including the scalp) can be the primary source. Anatomic anomalies that predispose children to brain infections include congenital dermoids or dermal sinus tracts. Although treatment of the brain abscess is the primary responsibility, detection and treatment of the infective source must proceed simultaneously. A history of inadequate treatment of an initial source infection, usually with a broad-spectrum antibiotic of insufficient potency, is frequently elicited when patients present with brain abscess. In approximately 6% of patients, the primary source of infection is undetectable.

Material from abscess cavities must be cultured immediately, both aerobically and anaerobically. Anaerobic bacteria, including *Bacteroides fragilis*, play a prominent role in brain abscess formation, accounting for almost 80% of nontraumatic brain abscesses in some series. Another common isolate is *Streptococcus* with a predominance of *Streptococcus milleri* species in the *viridans* group. Abscesses resulting from trauma most commonly are due to *Staphylococcus aureus*. Other causative organisms are other *Bacteroides* species, hemolytic streptococci, *Proteus* species, *H influenzae, E coli*, and, rarely, *Cryptococcus, Nocardia, Aspergillus*, or *Corynebacterium* species. Still, more than 10% of cultures will be sterile, using the best contemporary culture techniques.

The bacterial spectrum in neonates with brain abscesses differs from that in older infants and children. Brain abscesses in infants less than 3 months of age are often due to gram-negative organisms, such as *E coli, Citrobacter* species, *Proteus* species, *Chronobacter*, or *Salmonella* species, almost half of the time. The incidence of brain abscess is difficult to evaluate but is probably 2 to 3 per 10,000 general hospital admissions. A preponderance of male patients has been noted in most large series. Nearly one-third of all brain abscesses occur in the pediatric age group. The low incidence of brain abscesses in infants is related to their lack of well-formed frontal or mastoid sinuses.

One risk factor for the development of brain abscesses is cyanosis, caused either by congenital heart disease or by pulmonary arteriovenous shunting. Postmortem studies have indicated that brain abscesses are found in 0.4% of patients dying from all causes, whereas in patients with congenital heart disease, the incidence may be as high as 6%. The incidence of brain abscess in all children with congenital cyanotic heart disease is 2% to 3%. Children with right-to-left intracardiac shunting are deprived of the phagocytic filtering action of the pulmonary capillary bed, and in these children, the cerebral circulation is subject to recurrent bacteremia. These children are also likely to have focal encephalomalacia resulting from hypoxia and decreased cerebral blood flow caused by increased viscosity because of polycythemia. The coincidence of an area of recent infarction and bacteremia will predispose to abscess formation. A relationship has been shown between the severity of hypoxemia and the development of and prognosis for brain abscess in these patients.

Immunosuppressed children are also at risk for brain abscess. This category includes children receiving chemotherapy or radiation therapy for malignancy, a small group who have had transplants, and a smaller group with acquired immunodeficiency syndrome (AIDS). The increased risk in these groups of children is related to their generally high risk for opportunistic infection, rather than to specific CNS factors. The children are usually debilitated, and the abscesses are more likely to be multiple and to contain multiple species, including fungi.

## CLINICAL MANIFESTATIONS

The initial symptoms of brain abscess are more likely to be related to its intracranial mass effect than to the infectious nature of the illness. Lethargy, anorexia, and vomiting are noted, and older children will complain of headache. Focal or grand mal seizures may be the first indication of cerebral involvement and may lead to discovery of previously unnoticed neurologic deficits that are due to the abscess. Fever may be low-grade; almost half of children are afebrile on hospital admission, even though there is a history of recent febrile illness. Brain abscesses are usually rapidly progressive; the duration of symptoms is often less than a week and seldom more than a month. Specific neurologic deficits will depend on the area of involvement and may include hemiparesis, sensory impairment, and visual field abnormalities. Posterior fossa abscess will cause ataxia, dysmetria, and cranial nerve palsies.

## DIAGNOSIS

Both CT scanning and MRI are useful to diagnose and follow intracranial abscess (Fig. 226-2). MRI will often provide better resolution of the abscess and surrounding edema when compared with CT, but CT imaging is usually more rapidly available in the emergency department. CT and MRI scans should be performed with and without contrast enhancement. Following contrast injection, scans performed both immediately and after delay of 30 to 60 minutes will allow for more precise staging of the abscess. Multiple lesions, which cause high mortality among patients with brain abscesses, are easily diagnosed. Dosages of steroids, antibiotics, and even mannitol may be adjusted according to the changes observed over time.

In patients who receive adjunctive anti-inflammatory therapy, steroids may reduce the contrast enhancement of abscesses, especially during the cerebritis stages. This effect of steroids should not shorten the duration of antibiotic therapy or decrease consideration of surgery if symptoms progress. The results of routine laboratory studies may be normal or may reveal moderate leukocytosis and an elevated erythrocyte sedimentation rate. Skull films may indicate a chronic otorhinologic infection, and rarely, there is evidence of mass effect or increased intracranial pressure.

Many reports have stressed the danger of lumbar puncture in the presence of abscess. If there are indications of increased intracranial pressure or shifting of intracranial structures, lumbar puncture is contraindicated. The information obtained from the CSF in patients with brain abscess is usually nonspecific; often the causative organisms cannot be demonstrated, and lumbar puncture may introduce a potentially fatal risk.

## TREATMENT

The initiation of appropriate therapy requires a rapid assessment of the patient's clinical status and the expertise of an experienced neurosurgeon. An intracerebral abscess can act as a rapidly expanding intracranial mass because of both the purulent collection and the surrounding cerebral edema. Secondary brain stem compression can

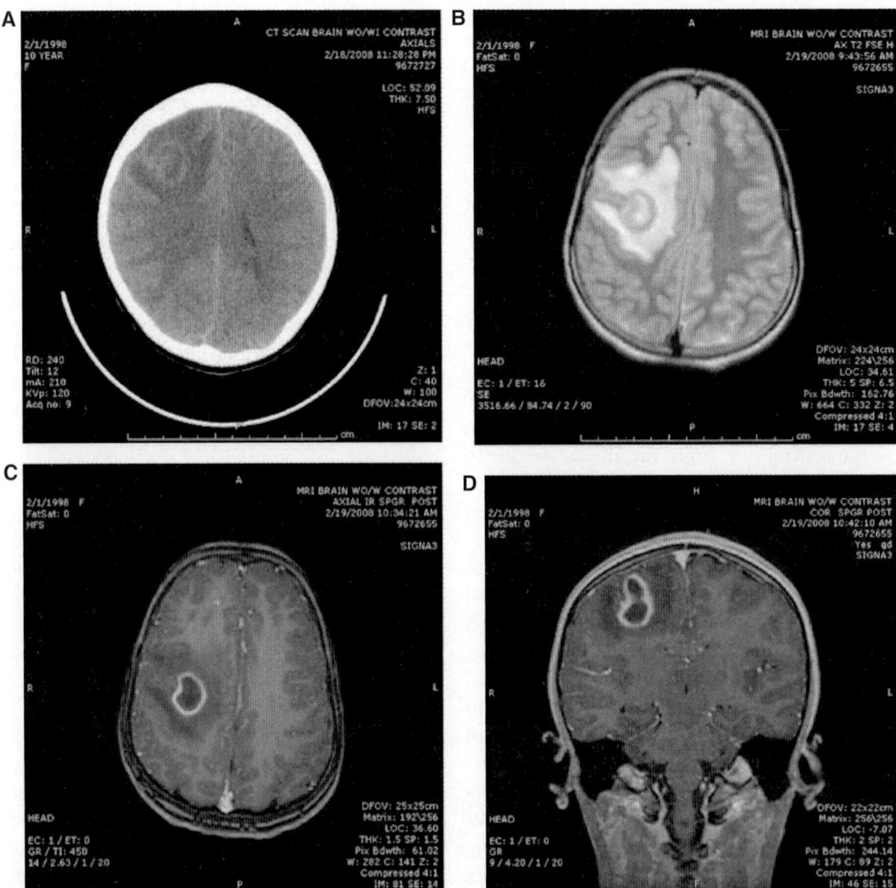


**FIGURE 226-2** Computed tomography (CT) and magnetic resonance imaging (MRI) scans of a 10-year-old patient with a brain abscess in the posterior aspect of the right frontal lobe, due to *Streptococcus milleri*. **A:** Axial noncontrast CT showing an indistinct rim surrounding a mass. **B:** Axial T2-weighted MRI showing low signal capsule and surrounding vasogenic edema. **C and D:** Axial and coronal SPGR (spoiled gradient echo T1) MRIs of bright rim-enhancing lesion.

lead to coma and death in a very short time. Uncal herniation causing midbrain compression is almost uniformly found in fatal brain abscess. For patients who display clinical or radiographic evidence of increased intracranial pressure, initial therapy is aimed at decreasing the intracerebral pressure and mass effect and includes steroids. Peri-abscess edema derives from both the local mass and the stasis effect and inflammation response that causes a diffuse increase in brain water. Steroids in large doses decrease the endothelial permeability of vessels in the inflammatory area and reduce the excessive edema. Although the restorative effect of steroids on the blood-brain barrier may reduce antibiotic activity in the infected region, this effect is usually of lesser concern than the need to reduce increased intracranial pressure. Patients who do not have evidence of increased intracranial pressure or mass effect may not require steroids or immediate neurosurgical intervention but must have frequent neurologic exams to check for changes in the patient's status.

### Antimicrobial Therapy

Appropriate initial empiric antibiotic therapy for brain abscess is broad to cover the most likely pathogens while awaiting culture data. During the stage of cerebritis, antibiotics with appropriate protein and lipid-binding characteristics can readily diffuse into the area of inflammatory response. Contrast studies have shown that once an abscess has formed, bacteria may still be isolated from the abscess, despite measurable levels of appropriate antibiotics within the abscess. It has been postulated that the intensely acidic environment associated with the necrotic debris may decrease antimicrobial action. This mechanism may explain reported treatment failure despite appropriate antibiotic therapy.

Gram-negative anaerobic organisms (eg, *Bacteroides* species) often associated with otogenic brain abscesses are susceptible to metronidazole. Metronidazole is bactericidal for most anaerobes; it penetrates into brain abscesses well and is not degraded in purulent debris. Gram-positive cocci such as streptococci usually respond to one of the β-lactam antibiotics or to vancomycin. Vancomycin is increasingly required as the incidence of methicillin-resistant *S aureus* (MRSA) increases. First-line therapy for gram-negative aerobic bacilli includes the third-generation cephalosporins (cefotaxime, ceftazidime, and ceftriaxone). Bactrim and ciprofloxacin are alternative choices in patients who are unable to tolerate cephalosporins. Thus, empiric therapy might include vancomycin, a third-generation cephalosporin, and metronidazole. Intravenous antibiotic therapy is required intraoperatively and for at least several weeks thereafter. Antimicrobial therapy can be altered as soon as susceptibility testing has been performed on organisms recovered from the purulent material obtained at operation.

### Surgical Intervention and Adjunct Therapy

Timing of surgical intervention will depend on the general condition of the child, the location and stage of the abscess, knowledge of the infecting organism, and the response to medical therapy. Patients who have multiple small abscesses are usually best treated medically. Even large areas of cerebritis and early encapsulation may be treated with steroids and appropriate antibiotics if these patients are followed carefully by both clinical observation and serial scanning. However, the process of waiting for abscess stabilization and encapsulation places the patient at risk for abrupt brain herniation or rupture of the abscess. Early aspiration of an abscess in a paraventricular locus is warranted.

Several techniques have been devised for operative treatment of abscesses, and selection of the appropriate procedure will depend on the condition of the patient, abscess location, and degree of abscess encapsulation. The patient's clinical condition at the time of operation is more important in determining the result than is the choice of operative procedure. Decompression of the mass effect is the primary goal of surgery. Management of children with a brain abscess should be cooperative between experts in infectious diseases and neurosurgery.

Aspiration of the abscess through a burr hole is preferable for severely ill children, as well as for known multiple abscesses and instances where the abscess has a thin or poorly developed wall. CT- and/or MRI-assisted stereotactic equipment is available in most centers. These devices allow for the safe aspiration of even deep abscesses. Abscesses may require 2 or 3 further aspirations in the postoperative period. Total excision can be attempted if the abscess is single, well encapsulated, and away from critically functional cortex. Excision has the advantage of immediately decompressing the mass and decreasing the risk of recurrence from remaining infected material. Excision may be delayed until aspiration and a period of antibiotic and steroid therapy allow stabilization of the cavity and formation of a thick capsule, facilitating total excision. Mortality is highest in children with cyanotic heart disease, and aggressive surgical intervention has been recommended for these patients.

Anticonvulsants should be given to all patients with supratentorial purulent lesions for at least 2 years after surgery. Seizures are frequently present during the preoperative period, and the incidence of seizures after surgery is almost 50%. The choice of operative procedure does not appear to alter the incidence of seizures.

High mortality rates from brain abscess in previous decades have been related to 2 major factors: late diagnosis and the presence of multiple lesions. If diagnosis is delayed until children are obtunded or comatose, the mortality is 65% to 90%. Mortality rates as high as 80% were reported for children with multiple abscesses. With current diagnostic and therapeutic options, a recent case series of 96 patients including both children and adults reported a mortality rate of 6% with an additional 34% of patients suffering moderate to severe sequelae.

## SPINAL ABSCESS

Spinal abscesses are rare in children. Infection can occur in any of the intraspinal planes, but most infections occur in the epidural space. Subdural empyema and intramedullary spinal abscesses are even rarer and, when seen, are often associated with a congenital dermal sinus tract or dermoid tumor.

### PATHOGENESIS

Spinal epidural abscesses are usually the result of hematogenous seeding. They may be metastatic, from another focus by the veins of the Batson plexus. A minority occur by direct extension, from spondylitis, or from lung or perinephric infections. In adults, there frequently are preexisting systemic illnesses, but children are usually previously normal. If a distant source is identified, it is often a cutaneous furuncle. Local trauma can result in a hematoma, which can provide a nidus for infection. The most common organism is *S aureus* including MRSA. In *S aureus* spinal epidural infections, sometimes there is a history of a preceding skin infection, but cases with no risk factors have also been reported. Rarely, spinal epidural abscesses have cultured coagulase-negative staphylococci, gram-negative rods, anaerobes, fungi, and other organisms. Spinal abscesses are most frequent in the midthoracic and lumbar regions.

### CLINICAL MANIFESTATIONS

The initial complaint is usually backache, with well-defined localization of tenderness. Initially fever may not be present but usually appears as the condition progresses. As the purulence expands, there is sharp unilateral or bilateral pain at the level of the abscess. As the pain intensifies, the child may refuse to sit or walk. Sensory deficits appear, and weakness of the legs is noted. If untreated, gait difficulty, sphincteric loss, and finally paraplegia follow in rapid order. The chance of recovery after total loss of leg, bladder, and bowel functions is small; therefore, early diagnosis and surgical decompression are of great importance. Surgical consultation should be obtained immediately if an epidural abscess is suspected. Spinal infections in children are generally more acute than are those in adults, and the symptoms may progress rapidly. Infections have been reported in which only several hours have elapsed between the onset of symptoms and the paraplegic state. Differential considerations include spinal and paraspinal tumors such as neuroblastoma or sarcomas, transverse myelitis, discitis, spontaneous hematoma, and Guillain-Barré syndrome.

### DIAGNOSIS

Laboratory examination will usually reveal leukocytosis and an elevated erythrocyte sedimentation rate and C-reactive protein. Spine radiographs may show local spondylitis, fracture, or a paraspinal soft tissue mass. Lumbar puncture studies will demonstrate pleocytosis, elevated protein concentration, and decreased glucose concentration. However, it is important to note that lumbar punctures may be contraindicated if a lumbar epidural abscess is suspected because of the potential of seeding the infection into the sterile CSF if the needle traverses the abscess. Therefore, it is best if the diagnosis is made on the basis of history, physical examination, and MRI. Scanning by CT or MRI may diagnose the disorder, and currently, MRI is the imaging study of choice.

### TREATMENT

Surgical drainage combined with antibiotics is usually the treatment of choice. Vancomycin is a reasonable empiric choice in communities where MRSA is prevalent. There have been reports of patients treated medically alone with good results when they are a poor operative risk or have a small abscess and lack of neurologic progression. However, there can be no blanket recommendation for medical therapy alone because of the paucity of data. Oral antibiotic treatment (following parenteral) is not advised unless the infecting organism is determined either by a positive blood culture or aspirate. Generally, if an epidural or subdural collection is demonstrated, surgery should be performed immediately. Decompressive laminectomy, removal of the purulent material, and copious irrigation should be done. Antibiotic irrigation has been recommended, but systemically administered antibiotics enter the spinal epidural space easily. In general, the degree of recovery is directly related to the neurologic function at the time of surgery.

## INTERVERTEBRAL DISC INFECTION

Discitis is an inflammation of the intervertebral disc or vertebral endplates. It primarily affects children, often in the first 5 years of life, but is also rarely encountered in adults. Although it is considered to be an infectious disease, cultures are often sterile.

### PATHOGENESIS

In the young age group, the developing spinal disc has a rich blood supply coming from the vertebrae. It is believed that these vessels provide a pathway to the disc space during bacteremia. In adolescence and into the third decade of life, the disc becomes avascular, and infection in the disc space is secondary to osteomyelitis. Discitis usually affects the lumbar spine, particularly the L3–4 and L4–5 spaces.

Cultures from blood or disc-space material have been positive in less than 50%, leading some to postulate an inflammatory cause rather than an infectious cause in a portion of these children. When cultures are positive, *S aureus* is usually the cause. Less commonly, *Pseudomonas aeruginosa*, streptococci, and other gram-negative bacilli have been recovered. Biopsy specimens typically show acute or chronic inflammation.

### CLINICAL MANIFESTATIONS

Children usually present with fever and back pain that may be localized. Children may limp or may refuse to stand or walk or may be unable to do so. Severe spinal muscle spasms may lead to splinting, giving the appearance of scoliosis or lordosis, and the physical exam may reveal localized tenderness over the spine and decreased spinal motion. A smaller group of children present with abdominal pain alone, or just irritability, and discitis has been reported to be found in children with prolonged fever of unknown origin. Vertebral osteomyelitis usually occurs in older children, who are more likely to have fever and specific complaints of pain. The differential also includes fracture, epidural abscess, spinal tumors, perinephric or renal infections, transverse myelitis, hematoma, and Guillain-Barré syndrome.

## DIAGNOSIS

Discitis is most frequently diagnosed on the basis of diagnostic imaging, although there may be a lag between the radiologic findings and the onset of symptoms. The intervertebral space becomes narrowed, and there is demineralization of adjacent vertebral body margins. CT or MRI scanning is more accurate than plain radiograph in this condition, and the MRI scan usually is the test of choice. A radionuclide scan, with technetium or gallium, is usually positive. The most consistent laboratory finding is an elevation in the erythrocyte sedimentation rate. Culture of the blood may grow a pathogen, and direct aspirates from the disc or vertebral endplate may yield the infecting organism. These cultures are more likely to be positive in vertebral osteomyelitis. In the appropriate clinical setting, biopsy or disc space cultures are not mandatory.

## TREATMENT

Treatment is started and usually consists of intravenous administration of antibiotics, usually with antistaphylococcal antibiotics, and immobilization by a brace or body cast. If initial antimicrobial therapy does not include activity against MRSA, failure to respond to therapy may be due to the presence of MRSA, and this would be an indication for obtaining a culture of the involved tissue. If discitis may be associated with MRSA or if MRSA is highly prevalent in the community, it may be necessary to commence empiric therapy with an agent such as vancomycin. Continuation of therapy is best guided by isolation of a pathogen from the blood or disc culture. In the absence of an isolate, there is no one accepted protocol. Four to 6 total weeks of antibiotics with a combination of 2 weeks of intravenous antibiotics followed by a month of oral antibiotics is a common regimen. Failure of the treatment plan to relieve the pain and/or fevers should prompt consideration of needle aspiration or biopsy of the disc space, if this has not already been performed. Open surgery is rarely required, and bracing usually continues until resolution of the symptoms, typically 3 to 4 months. Overall, the outcome for discitis is excellent.

## SUGGESTED READINGS


Bonfield CM, Sharma J, Dobson S. Pediatric intracranial abscesses. *J Infect*. 2015;71:S42-S46.

Brouwer MC, McIntyre P, Prasad K, van de Beek D. Corticosteroids for acute bacterial meningitis. *Cochrane Database Syst Rev*. 2015;9: CD004405. doi:10.1002/14651858.CD004405.pub5.

Kim KS. Acute bacterial meningitis in infants and children. *Lancet Infect Dis*. 2010;10:32-42.

Thigpen MC, Whitney CG, Messonnier NE, et al. Bacterial meningitis in the United States, 1998–2007. *N Engl J Med*. 2011;364: 2016-2025.

Wooten SH, Aguilera E, Salazar L, et al. Enhancing pathogen identification in patients with meningitis and a negative Gram stain using the BioFire FilmArray Meningitis/Encephalitis panel. *Ann Clin Microbiol Antimicrob*. 2016;15:26-30.

Yildirim I, Shea KM, Pelton SI. Pneumococcal disease in the era of pneumococcal conjugate vaccine. *Infect Dis Clin North Am*. 2015;29:679-697.


# 227 Viral Infections of the Central Nervous System

Kristen A. Wendorf and Carol Glaser

## INTRODUCTION

Viral infections of the central nervous system (CNS) may be variously categorized by type of onset (eg, acute, subacute, chronic, or recurrent), by the level of the CNS involved (eg, brain, brain stem, or spinal cord), and by the viral agent causing disease. The approach to diagnosis and management of CNS viral infection depends greatly on the age, immunization history, and immune status of the patient, and also the epidemiologic setting including season, location, and exposure to viruses that are circulating in the community or transmitted by arthropod vectors. Molecular testing techniques continue to evolve to improve identification of viral agents causing CNS diseases.

## VIRAL MENINGITIS

### ACUTE VIRAL MENINGITIS

Community-acquired viruses and arthropod-borne viruses are the major causes of the acute "aseptic meningitis" syndrome that, by definition, is accompanied by symptoms and signs of meningeal inflammation in the absence of acute bacterial or fungal meningitis. Although meningitis may occur in the course of infection with many viruses (Table 227-1), the human enteroviruses (EVs) have been shown to be responsible for the majority of cases of viral meningitis, most prominently the nonpolio EVs. Other well-known causes of viral meningitis include herpesviruses (herpes simplex virus [HSV], Epstein-Barr virus [EBV], cytomegalovirus [CMV], human herpesvirus [HHV]-6, and varicella-zoster virus [VZV]), mumps virus, lymphocytic choriomeningitis virus (LCMV), influenza virus, and the arthropod-borne viruses (including West Nile virus [WNV],

**TABLE 227-1 IMPORTANT CAUSES OF VIRAL MENINGITIS AND ENCEPHALITIS IN NORTH AMERICA**

| | Meningitis | Encephalitis |
|---|---|---|
| Enteroviruses | ++++ | ++ |
| Parechoviruses | + | ++ |
| Herpes simplex virus | | |
| Type 1 | | ++/+++ |
| Type 2 | + | |
| Arthropod-borne viruses | ++ | ++ |
| Flaviviruses | | |
| West Nile virus | | |
| St. Louis encephalitis virus | | |
| Bunyaviruses | | |
| California encephalitis virus | | |
| La Crosse virus | | |
| Togaviruses | | |
| Eastern equine encephalitis virus | | |
| Western equine encephalitis virus | | |
| Lymphocytic choriomeningitis virus | + | + |
| Mumps virus | + | + |
| Human immunodeficiency virus | + | + |
| Rabies virus | | + |
| Influenza virus (H1N1) | + | + |

++++, causes > 50% of cases of known etiology; +++, causes 10% to 50% of cases of known etiology; ++, causes 1% to 10% of cases of known etiology; +, causes < 1% of cases of known etiology.

St. Louis encephalitis virus, La Crosse [LAC] virus, and eastern equine encephalitis virus).

Because EVs cause more than 90% of cases, even during periods of peak arbovirus transmission, the epidemiology of viral meningitis usually reflects the trends of EV infection in the population, including seasonal peaks in late summer and fall and a strong inverse correlation between age and observed rates of disease. Overall rates of EV infection are several-fold higher for infants under 12 months of age than older children. The observed rates of meningitis among children with documented EV infection are highest under 4 months of age when approximately 50% of infants undergoing lumbar puncture in the course of an evaluation for fever will have laboratory evidence of meningitis.

Viral meningitis syndrome due to HSV occurs mainly in adolescents and young adults with primary HSV-2 genital infections, but it is also reported in young children (see Chapter 304).

Mumps virus infection, once a common cause of viral meningitis, is now primarily seen in locations where mumps virus circulation is not controlled by immunization (see Chapter 313). However, mumps meningitis has been identified along with or in the absence of clinical mumps infection in the context of outbreaks and is more likely to occur in young adults several years after vaccination. Signs of meningeal irritation occur in approximately 5% of patients identified in mumps outbreaks.

Children acquire LCMV infection from exposure to household environments contaminated by rodent urine. Common house mice are most often implicated; an estimated 5% of these rodents asymptomatically carry LCMV and can transmit the infection throughout their lifetimes. LCMV infection is more common during winter months.

### CLINICAL MANIFESTATIONS

The clinical manifestations of EV meningitis vary with age. For young infants, fever and other nonspecific symptoms might be the only manifestations. Older children might first experience a brief prodrome of fever and sore throat followed by headache that is often severe. Signs of meningeal irritation are variable. Children with LCMV infection usually present with an influenza-like systemic illness in addition to headache and signs of meningeal irritation. Complications such as complex seizures, lethargy, coma, and movement disorders that are reported in 5% to 10% of patients with viral meningitis suggest a more precise diagnosis of meningoencephalitis.

### DIAGNOSIS

Although the diagnosis of viral meningitis can be suspected based on clinical findings, examination of cerebrospinal fluid (CSF) is necessary when bacterial meningitis must be excluded. The CSF white blood cell (WBC) count typically ranges from 0 to 1000 WBC/mL, but levels > 1000 are also reported in proven cases of viral meningitis. There might be a predominance of neutrophils during the first 1 to 2 days of illness with an inevitable shift to a lymphocyte predominance later. In most cases, the CSF glucose concentration is normal, but values slightly lower than normal are reported in 18% to 33% of cases, and the CSF protein concentration is normal or mildly elevated. Notably, LCMV and mumps infections can be associated with low CSF glucose concentrations. A proportion of children have peripheral leukocytosis, some with a left shift. Confirmation of the diagnosis of EV infection depends on detection of virus in the CSF by polymerase chain reaction (PCR) or by virus isolation. For LCMV, diagnosis usually depends on documentation of seroconversion in paired serum samples. CSF samples from those with HSV infection might reveal lymphocytosis along with an increased number of red blood cells.

### TREATMENT

Patients with viral meningitis are given analgesics for headache and are often hospitalized in order to receive intravenous antibiotics until bacterial disease can be ruled out with confidence. Identification of specific agents with available medical therapies should be treated accordingly, including use of acyclovir or valacyclovir for HSV, antiretrovirals for human immunodeficiency virus (HIV) infection, and neuraminidase inhibitors for influenza. However, most viral agents have no specific treatment. The symptoms of acute viral meningitis can be more severe and persist longer in adults compared with young children.

### PROGNOSIS

Subtle disturbances of motor function such as limitation of passive motion, muscle spasms, and poor coordination might persist for weeks after resolution of the acute illness but slowly resolve. Despite concern raised by early studies, viral meningitis does not lead to long-term neurologic or cognitive sequelae.

## RECURRENT ASEPTIC MENINGITIS

Recurrent aseptic meningitis (Mollaret syndrome) is a rare disease characterized by 3 or more distinct episodes of lymphocytic meningitis of 2 to 5 days in duration, each of which is separated by weeks to years. HSV-2 has been strongly associated with recurrent meningitis by identification of virus in CSF by PCR, but many patients do not have evidence of genital lesions at the time of presentation. A small number of cases are reported to be caused by HSV-1 and EBV, and many have no established etiology. Prophylactic treatment with acyclovir or another anti-HSV drug might suppress recurrent episodes.

## ACUTE ENCEPHALITIS

The terms *encephalitis*, *meningoencephalitis*, and *encephalomyelitis* are generally used interchangeably to denote inflammation of the brain, brain stem, and/or spinal cord. The International Encephalitis Consortium defines encephalitis as altered mental status (decreased or altered level of consciousness, lethargy, or personality change) lasting ≥ 24 hours with no alternative cause identified. Additionally, patients must have at least 2 of the following: fever, seizure, focal neurologic findings, CSF pleocytosis, abnormality of brain parenchyma on neuroimaging suggestive of acute encephalitis, or abnormality on electroencephalography (EEG) that is consistent with encephalitis.

Encephalitis causes an estimated 19,000 hospitalizations a year in the United States, with a case fatality rate > 5%. It is a general presumption that most acute encephalitis cases are caused by viral infections, although active surveillance studies are able to identify a specific viral etiology for only 9% to 22% of cases, and the cause of approximately 60% of cases cannot be determined. Important nonviral causes of encephalitis include infections such as bacteria, fungus, and *Mycobacterium tuberculosis*. Noninfectious causes include autoimmune etiologies such as anti-*N*-methyl-D-aspartate receptor (NMDAR) and limbic encephalitis, which might present with more psychiatric symptoms than viral causes, but symptom overlap occurs. The list of viruses proven or suspected to cause acute encephalitis is extensive and is prominently represented by herpesviruses, EVs, flaviviruses, togaviruses, bunyaviruses, adenoviruses, mumps virus, LCMV, HIV, and rabies virus that all replicate in neural cells causing neuronal destruction and inflammation, primarily in gray matter (see Table 227-1).

The terms postinfectious encephalitis and acute demyelinating encephalomyelitis (ADEM) are interchangeably applied to acute CNS disease that rarely complicates infection with some common viruses, including measles virus, rubella virus, influenza viruses, and other respiratory viruses. Evidence for CNS viral replication is generally lacking, and immunopathologic mechanisms are considered to be responsible for the characteristic perivascular inflammation and demyelination associated with postinfectious encephalitis.

Overall, children with normal neuroimaging and higher Glasgow Coma Score on presentation have been found to be more likely to recover from acute encephalitis. Neurologic sequelae are associated with younger age at time of illness and presentation with seizure. In particular, children who present with seizures, require more antiepileptic medications for seizure control, and have an abnormal EEG are more likely to develop epilepsy following encephalitis.

## HERPES SIMPLEX VIRUS ENCEPHALITIS

HSV causes only 8% to 12% of encephalitis cases of known etiology, but deserves special consideration because HSV is identified in population-based studies as the most common cause of viral encephalitis. The virus affects males and females equally, as well as people of all ages, and has no seasonal variation. Unlike other viral infections, the outcome of HSV encephalitis can be improved with prompt and safe antiviral therapy. HSV-1 and HSV-2 are closely related alpha herpesviruses that share a tropism for mucocutaneous sites and are able to establish latency in neural tissues and reactivate repeatedly, causing recurrent disease. HSV encephalitis is characterized by inflammation with perivascular lymphocytic cuffing, edema, and hemorrhagic necrosis of affected areas of the CNS.

### CLINICAL MANIFESTATIONS

#### Neonates

In neonates, HSV encephalitis can occur as isolated CNS disease or develop in the course of disseminated HSV disease; altogether, about half of infants with neonatal HSV infection develop encephalitis. Viremia probably represents the major route of transmission to the CNS during disseminated neonatal HSV infection, resulting in diffuse, patchy CNS involvement. In contrast, transport to the brain is likely to occur via peripheral sensory neurons in neonates who present with localized CNS disease. In either case, the absence of preexisting immunity and immature T-cell responses permits a high level of virus replication and spread within the immature brain. Both HSV-1 and HSV-2 can be transmitted to the newborn in the perinatal period, but encephalitis occurs more commonly and severely with HSV-2 infection. Infants who survive infection with HSV-2 are likely to have long-term neurologic sequelae. As many as 35% of infants with HSV encephalitis have no skin findings. Overall, infants less than 4 weeks of age are at risk, although disseminated HSV infection typically begins within the first 10 days of life, and infants with disease limited to the CNS are more likely to have onset of disease in the second or third week of life. Neonates with HSV encephalitis typically present with lethargy, poor feeding, and focal and/or generalized seizures. Motor abnormalities in the form of tremors, paresis, and hypo- or hyperreflexia might be noted on exam.

#### Infants and Children

About one-third of HSV encephalitis cases beyond the newborn period occur in children and adolescents, with an approximate annual incidence of 2 to 4 per 1,000,000. Virtually all are a consequence of sporadic HSV-1 disease that occurs as either a primary or recurrent infection. The hallmark of HSV encephalitis is focal neurologic disease that can affect any part of the brain, brain stem, or spinal cord, but most commonly involves 1 or both temporal lobes. More than 90% of patients present with fever and altered consciousness, and more than two-thirds exhibit headache, personality change, dysphagia, and focal or generalized seizure activity. Other common early findings are memory loss, hemiparesis, ataxia, and cranial nerve palsies. Among children < 4 years of age, presenting symptoms often include febrile seizure.

### DIAGNOSIS

The initial evaluation of suspected HSV encephalitis includes brain imaging, EEG, and CSF examination. Diffusion-weighted magnetic resonance imaging (MRI) is reported to be most sensitive, more than standard MRI or computed tomography (CT) for detection of focal brain lesions. The periodic lateralized epileptiform discharges (PLEDs) demonstrated by EEG represent sensitive but relatively nonspecific evidence of HSV encephalitis. At least 90% of patients at presentation will have an abnormal CSF examination with an elevated CSF WBC count and elevated protein concentration.

Confirmation of HSV encephalitis depends on detection of HSV virus in CSF or CNS tissue. PCR detection of viral DNA in CSF is highly sensitive and specific when compared with virus isolation from brain biopsy specimens. Viral culture of the CSF has low sensitivity (< 10%) for HSV, whereas PCR testing is reported to have ≥ 94% sensitivity and ≥ 98% specificity. PCR can be positive as early as 24 hours after symptom onset; however, testing early in the course of HSV encephalitis might produce a false-negative PCR. Repeat testing in cases with an initial false-negative PCR will often reveal a positive PCR by day 4 or later after symptom onset. Despite treatment, HSV DNA has been shown to persist in CSF in virtually all patients who have repeat lumbar punctures up to 7 days after symptom onset. Infectious virus can also be isolated when brain biopsy is performed 4 or more days after the start of antiviral therapy.

### TREATMENT

Untreated HSV encephalitis is fatal in more than two-thirds of cases, and only about 10% of survivors recover with normal neurologic function. Intravenous acyclovir given at a dose of 10 mg/kg every 8 hours for 10 days reduces mortality and improves the prognosis for survivors. A higher acyclovir dose of 20 mg/kg every 8 hours for 21 days improves survival for neonates and reduces the risk of poor neurologic outcomes. For those with CNS disease, CSF should again be tested for DNA by PCR near the completion of the parenteral acyclovir course, and if DNA remains present, parenteral acyclovir should be continued for another week, with repeat of this weekly process until DNA is not detected. Continued oral treatment with acyclovir for 6 months following completion of parenteral therapy can improve neurodevelopmental outcomes in those with CNS disease and is recommended for all neonates with HSV disease (CNS or other type). See also the chapter on therapy for perinatal and neonatal infections (Chapter 225).

### PROGNOSIS

Delayed initiation of therapy has been associated with poorer outcomes in children. Despite treatment, > 60% of children have neurologic sequelae, particularly seizures or developmental delays. Relapse of CNS disease with recurrent fever, focal neurologic symptoms, and CSF pleocytosis is reported in 10% to 25% of patients with acute HSV encephalitis. Relapse occurs within days to months of discontinuation of antiviral therapy and is associated with similar signs and symptoms compared with the initial episode. Although HSV can be recovered from some cases of recurrent disease, the inability to demonstrate the presence of HSV by virus isolation or PCR in many others suggests a second mechanism that may be immunologically mediated. Relapse with HSV should be distinguished from autoimmune encephalitis since anti-NMDAR encephalitis can be triggered by HSV encephalitis, presumably by triggering an antineuronal autoimmune response.

## ENCEPHALITIS CAUSED BY OTHER HERPESVIRUSES

Although HSV is the most common herpes viral agent to cause encephalitis, other herpesviruses have been implicated. Epstein-Barr virus is an important cause of encephalitis, especially among adolescents. Both HHV-6 and HHV-7 have been shown to cause encephalitis in children, although the majority of cases occur among younger or immunocompromised children. Varicella-zoster virus is more likely to cause encephalitis in adults, although cases in children typically present either concurrently with varicella disease or in a postinfectious form. Cytomegalovirus has also been reported to cause encephalitis, particularly in severely immunocompromised children.

## ENTEROVIRUS AND PARECHOVIRUS ENCEPHALITIS

Encephalitis is a rare complication of EV infection, but because these infections are ubiquitous, they are a leading cause of encephalitis in children and are responsible for 10% to 15% of encephalitis cases for which an etiology is identified. Children with EV encephalitis tend to be younger and might have a less severe clinical presentation than children with encephalitis caused by other viruses. Additionally, human parechoviruses (HPeV) are an important cause of encephalitis in children younger than 2 years. At least 16 HPeV serotypes have been described to date; many have been associated with encephalitis. For diagnostic workup of suspected EV/HPeV encephalitis, molecular testing of CSF is important. It is important to also test for EV/HPeV in non-CNS sites (throat, stool, and serum) to increase the likelihood of detection.

## ARTHROPOD-BORNE ENCEPHALITIS

Several viruses cause acute encephalitis in humans and other mammals following the bite of an infected mosquito or tick, including certain flaviviruses, togaviruses, and bunyaviruses. These taxonomically distinct viruses are often collectively referred to as "arboviruses" due to the common requirement for an arthropod vector, and all exist within diverse ecologic systems that include animal reservoirs in nature. More than 20 arboviruses cause acute encephalitis worldwide; among the most prevalent are Japanese encephalitis virus, responsible for widespread disease throughout East and Southeast Asia, and WNV, the predominant cause of arthropod-borne encephalitis in North America during the past decade. In general, serologic testing with acute and convalescent titers is preferable to molecular testing for arboviruses because viremia precedes symptoms. Molecular testing following symptom onset is often insensitive and fails to detect virus.

### JAPANESE ENCEPHALITIS VIRUS

Japanese encephalitis virus, a flavivirus, is the leading cause of vaccine-preventable encephalitis in Asia and the Western Pacific and is responsible for thousands of human encephalitis cases in the region. Culex mosquitoes breed in marshy environments including rice patties, leading to human transmission that primarily occurs in agricultural areas. The ratio of symptomatic to asymptomatic infections is approximately 1:250, and most illness is mild and self-limited. Cases can occur among susceptible people of any age, but in endemic areas, encephalitis primarily occurs among children younger than 15 years. Individuals who develop encephalitis have an estimated mortality of 25%, and 30% to 50% will experience significant neurologic and cognitive sequelae. The spectrum of CNS manifestations includes meningismus, altered consciousness, seizures, extrapyramidal signs, and acute motor neuron disease.

The laboratory diagnosis of Japanese encephalitis virus infection is based on demonstration of specific antibodies in the CSF or serum, which can usually be detected by 4 to 7 days after onset of symptoms. There is no available specific antiviral therapy.

Although the risk of Japanese encephalitis is low for most travelers to endemic areas, immunization is recommended when there is a high risk of exposure, such as travel to rural areas during the rainy season when mosquito activity is high. Vaccines are available in the United States and are approved for children 2 months and older prior to high-risk travel.

### WEST NILE VIRUS

WNV is a member of the same flavivirus complex as Japanese encephalitis virus and St. Louis encephalitis virus. Human infections with WNV occur widely in Africa, Europe, South Asia, and Australia, but were unknown in the Americas until 1999 when an outbreak occurred in the New York City metropolitan area caused by a virus with close genetic identity to WNV circulating in Israel and elsewhere in the Middle East. The virus has since spread across the North American continent, causing hundreds to thousands of cases each year. In most locations, human disease coincides with a summer–fall sylvatic cycle that includes viral amplification in birds and transmission via multiple mosquito species. Person-to-person spread might occur via transfusion of blood and blood products, organ transplantation, or rarely from mother to baby during pregnancy, delivery, or while breastfeeding.

Seventy to 80% of people infected by WNV have no symptoms. Approximately 20% of infected persons develop illness that in the majority of patients is limited to fever, malaise, arthralgias, and rash that last for 3 to 10 days. Neurologic disease occurs in a smaller proportion of laboratory-confirmed infections (< 1%) but in a higher percentage of reported cases due to the propensity to test and report cases with serious disease. Overall case fatality rate is 10% for individuals with neurologic disease, although many more deaths occur among individuals with encephalitis compared to meningitis. Children are at lower risk of developing CNS disease than adults, and risk is increased among persons with chronic disease and immunodeficiency, including patients with solid organ transplants and hematologic malignancies. WNV encephalitis can coincide with a number of manifestations indicating different levels of CNS involvement, including seizures, movement disorders (tremor, myoclonus, parkinsonism), cerebellar ataxia, acute motor neuron disease, optic neuritis, chorioretinitis, cranial nerve palsy, radiculopathy, Guillain-Barré syndrome, and demyelinating peripheral neuropathy.

A specific laboratory diagnosis depends on demonstration of WNV IgM antibodies detectable 3 to 8 days after onset, which can persist for several weeks or even months after exposure. Plaque-reduction neutralization tests can help differentiate between flaviviruses and can confirm acute infection when a ≥ 4-fold increase is noted between acute and convalescent samples. Viral RNA can be identified in serum or CSF early in the course of disease but should not be used as the sole test due to insensitivity. There are no specific antiviral therapies for WNV infection, and no vaccine is yet available. Full recovery from WNV neuroinvasive disease occurs in less than half of survivors. Long-term sequelae include fatigue, dizziness, alterations in cognition, inability to concentrate, and residual muscle weakness.

### OTHER NORTH AMERICAN ARTHROPOD-BORNE VIRUS DISEASES

La Crosse virus (LAC), eastern equine encephalitis (EEE) virus, western equine encephalitis (WEE) virus, and St. Louis encephalitis (SLE) virus are mosquito-borne viruses that are also important causes of CNS infection. Each of these viruses has a distinct sylvatic cycle, geographic distribution, and spectrum of disease. Each is associated with a high ratio of subclinical infections compared with clinical disease. LAC, EEE, and WEE have higher clinical attack rates among children, and SLE virus, like its close relative WNV, is more often observed in adults.

LAC is the second most common cause of arboviral infections in the United States (after WNV) and the most common cause of neuroinvasive arboviral disease in children. The LAC virus is a bunyavirus transmitted from small mammals by mosquitoes and is endemic in Midwest states. LAC causes approximately 75 cases of encephalitis per year in the United States. In contrast, EEE and WEE viruses are members of the *Alphavirus* genus (family: Togaviridae) that cause sporadic and unpredictable regional outbreaks of human encephalitis when conditions are optimal for breeding of mosquitoes that maintain these viruses in a natural cycle that includes migratory birds. Compared with other causes of arthropod-borne encephalitis, disease due to LAC virus is relatively mild, and most children recover from infection with minimal or no neurologic sequelae. Disease caused by EEE or WEE viruses is more severe in children, with high rates of death and disability among survivors. EEE has the highest case fatality rate of up to 35%. As of this printing, no human cases of WEE have been reported to the Centers for Disease Control and Prevention (CDC) since 1994.

Virus-specific IgM antibody is present in the serum and CSF at the time of presentation for most arthropod-borne virus encephalitis cases. Serologic testing for regionally prevalent arthropod-borne virus diseases is generally available in state and some local public health laboratories in the United States and Canada. Treatment is limited to supportive measures because no antiviral therapy is available.

## OTHER VIRAL CAUSES OF ENCEPHALITIS

Less frequent, but important, viral causes of encephalitis include rabies virus and LCMV.

Although rare in the United States, rabies should always be considered in patients with rapidly progressive encephalitis. Rabies is a lyssavirus that spreads from infected animals primarily through bites. Only 1 or 2 cases are generally seen in the United States annually, but worldwide, there are approximately 24,000 to 60,000 deaths each year, with the majority of deaths occurring in Africa and Asia. Paresthesia at the site of a bite is a distinctive feature of rabies and is a relatively common finding, but not uniformly described. Most patients with rabies present with agitation, hydrophobia, delirium, and seizures ("furious form"). A minority of patients present with ascending paralysis, followed by confusion and then coma ("paralytic form"). Fatality is generally 100%, with only a handful of survivors.

### LYMPHOCYTIC CHORIOMENINGITIS VIRUS

LCMV is an arenavirus that is acquired from infected house mice, guinea pigs, and hamsters. Humans become infected when saliva, urine, or feces from LCMV-infected rodents is ingested or inhaled. The incidence of LCMV is unknown, but it is likely that infection goes undiagnosed in many instances. Infections occur more frequently in winter months, when rodents are more likely to migrate indoors. Emerging zoonotic viruses associated with encephalitis include Nipah virus, Hendra virus, and Bornavirus.

## POSTINFECTIOUS ENCEPHALITIS

Postinfectious encephalitis, or ADEM, is an acute, inflammatory brain disease that is associated with an antecedent or concomitant (often viral) infection. It has also been observed following administration of several vaccines, including smallpox, measles, diphtheria-tetanus-polio, and Japanese B encephalitis. The pathologic features of postinfectious encephalitis are accurately replicated in the experimental allergic encephalomyelitis animal model in which an immune-mediated reaction against myelin protein can be demonstrated. Antimyelin basic protein antibodies can be demonstrated in some patients with postinfectious encephalitis, but evidence of viral replication within the CNS is virtually never demonstrated.

Postinfectious encephalitis is estimated to represent about 10% to 15% of acute encephalitis cases in the United States. Disease is much more common in children than adults, and there is a slightly higher burden of cases in males and during the winter and spring seasons. The current incidence is probably lower than in the past when smallpox vaccines were universally administered. Abrupt onset of fever, altered mental status, seizures, or focal neurologic signs may occur before, during, or, more commonly, within 3 weeks after a respiratory, gastrointestinal, or rash illness, although preceding illness is only reported in about two-thirds of children. The inflammatory changes in the CSF do not distinguish postinfectious encephalitis from other causes of acute encephalitis, but contrast-enhanced MRI examination often reveals characteristic abnormalities on T2 and fluid-attenuated inversion recovery (FLAIR) images in white matter, cerebellum, basal ganglia, and brain stem. Treatments typically include corticosteroids as first-line treatment, with intravenous immunoglobulin or plasma exchange for those who do not respond to corticosteroids. However, the natural course of postinfectious encephalitis is spontaneous resolution, so it is difficult to be certain of the benefits of these treatments. Recovery may be very slow, however. Patients who develop recurrent episodes might ultimately receive a diagnosis of multiple sclerosis.

## ACUTE HEMORRHAGIC LEUKOENCEPHALITIS

Acute hemorrhagic leukoencephalitis is a rare form of acute encephalitis of unknown etiology characterized by abrupt onset, a rapid course, and often a fatal outcome. The pathologic changes reflect those of postinfectious encephalitis with edema, demyelination, and perivascular inflammation but also include extensive hemorrhagic lesions within white matter. Compared with postinfectious encephalitis, the CSF findings in acute hemorrhagic encephalitis include elevated opening pressure, relatively high WBC count, predominance of polymorphic leukocytes, and the characteristic presence of red blood cells. Because patients with acute hemorrhagic encephalitis are usually treated with high-dose steroid therapy based on anecdotal experience, it is important to rule out HSV encephalitis that has many similar clinical features.

## ACUTE CEREBELLAR ATAXIA

Acute cerebellar ataxia is a common, distinct clinical entity of young children usually caused by acute cerebellitis without evidence of other serious CNS disease. Both direct infection and postinfectious, immunopathologic mechanisms are postulated to occur. Patients typically report recent viral illness. Reported coincident infections include VZV, EV, measles, mumps, rubella, parvovirus, mycoplasma, and EBV. It is also described following vaccinations.

The typical patient is a toddler or young child who develops a truncal ataxia and a wobbly gait 5 to 10 days after onset of the inciting infectious episode, which may have resolved. More severe cases might be accompanied by nausea, vomiting, nystagmus, dysarthria, or dysmetria, but fever and other signs of CNS disease are rare. Disability is often maximal at onset. Even though symptoms resolve slowly over days to weeks, most children recover completely without residual deficits. The most important task of the pediatrician is to rule out a more serious cause for ataxia.

## BRAIN STEM ENCEPHALITIS

Enterovirus 71 possesses a unique ability to invade the cerebellum, ventral brain stem, and spinal cord, producing a spectrum of serious neuromotor syndromes including acute flaccid paralysis of 1 or more extremities, cranial nerve paresis, tremors, myoclonus, or ataxia. The majority of cases occur among infants and young children, particularly during outbreaks in Southeast Asia; many children demonstrate rash consistent with hand, foot, and mouth disease prior to the onset of neurologic disease. Although many children recover without deficits, a subset of children develop a devastating, often fatal syndrome of acute neurogenic pulmonary edema and hemorrhage that may result from destruction of medullary vasomotor and respiratory centers. There is some evidence that treatment of pulmonary edema with milrinone improves mortality. Pulmonary hemorrhage often develops rapidly, with most fatalities occurring within 24 hours of admission.

## MYELITIS

Acute viral infection of the spinal cord occurs in 2 different forms: segmental (or "transverse") myelitis of a section of the cord producing motor and sensory dysfunction at a level below the involved segment; and disease limited to gray matter producing acute motor neuron disease.

Acute transverse myelitis (ATM) is a focal inflammatory disorder of the spinal cord, resulting in motor, sensory, and autonomic dysfunction. It occurs at any age, and approximately 20% of cases in the United States occur during childhood. Most children report mild illness during the few weeks prior to neurologic symptoms. Initially, many children report pain later followed by lower extremity weakness (often bilateral), loss of sensation below the level of the lesion, and loss of bladder and bowel control. Transverse myelitis most frequently occurs in the thoracic spinal cord and involves the entire width of the cord within a limited number of segments. Pediatric cases are most often associated with herpesvirus infection, although evidence for infection with other viruses has been presented, and some cases might be caused by immunopathologic mechanisms. Direct infection with HSV1, HSV2, VZV, CMV, and EBV has been demonstrated by detection of virus in CSF by virus isolation or by PCR. HSV is the most common cause of acute transverse myelitis in children, and VZV myelitis is more common in patients who are immunosuppressed. CSF pleocytosis is present in most cases. The presence of oligoclonal immunoglobulin bands on CSF protein electrophoresis in a minority of patients might suggest a diagnosis of multiple sclerosis. Contrast-enhanced MRI is a sensitive and specific technique for demonstrating the inflammatory changes and swelling of the involved cord segments. Anti-herpesvirus drugs and steroids are often administered without clear evidence of benefit or harm. Recovery is slow and often incomplete. Only 30% to 50% of children make a full recovery, while many children experience some permanent disability.

The prototype of acute motor neuron disease is poliomyelitis caused by 1 of 3 poliovirus serotypes. However, other viruses cause acute paralysis by the same pathophysiologic mechanism, including other EVs and flaviviruses. HHV-7 has been detected in immunocompromised individuals, and recent evidence has associated several EVs, including EV71 and EV68, with acute flaccid myelitis. Acute myelitis has also been observed to occur in association with infections due to hepatitis A virus, hepatitis B virus, LCMV, measles virus, mumps virus, rubella virus, and adenovirus. Illness in children often follows a biphasic course over 5 to 12 days with initial nonspecific symptoms including fever, headache, and (for EVs) sore throat followed by a brief period of improvement. The second phase is heralded by onset of intense myalgia, headache, and meningismus, followed by motor weakness that progresses over 1 to 3 days. Paresis ranges from mild weakness to complete flaccid paralysis and characteristically involves 1 or more extremities in an asymmetric manner. Deep tendon reflexes are diminished in the affected extremities, but sensation remains intact. Lumbar puncture reveals a moderate CSF pleocytosis. MRI of the spinal cord demonstrates evidence of acute inflammation in the anterior horns, especially in the regions innervating the arms and legs. Acute motor neuron disease must be differentiated from Guillain-Barré syndrome, which causes symmetrical paralysis and sensory abnormalities in the absence of fever and meningitis.

Most recently, cases of a polio-like syndrome were described in California and then later in other areas of the United States. Many of the affected individuals were children with fever and respiratory or gastrointestinal symptoms prior to onset of neurologic symptoms. Patients had radiologic and neurophysiologic findings of acute motor neuron involvement. This illness is called acute flaccid myelitis (AFM). Preliminary data suggest that at least some of the cases might be associated with EVD68. This apparent increase in AFM cases coincided with a nationwide outbreak of EVD68 respiratory illness.

## SUGGESTED READINGS


Bennetto L, Scolding N. Inflammatory/post-infectious encephalomyelitis. *J Neurol Neurosurg Psychiatry*. 2004;75(suppl 1):i22-i28.

Bloch KC, Glaser CA. Encephalitis srveillance through the Emerging Infections Program, 1997-2010. *Emerg Infect Dis*. 2015;21:1562-1567.

DuBray K, Anglemyer A, LaBeaud AD, et al. Epidemiology, outcomes and predictors of recovery in childhood encephalitis: a hospital-based study. *Pediatr Infect Dis J*. 2013;32:839-844.

Fowlkes AL, Honarmand S, Glaser C, et al. Enterovirus-associated encephalitis in the California Encephalitis Project, 1998-2005. *J Infect Dis*. 2008;198(11):1685-1691.

Glaser CA, Gilliam S, Schnurr D, et al. In search of encephalitis etiologies: diagnostic challenges in the California Encephalitis Project, 1998-2000. *Clin Infect Dis*. 2003;36(6):731-742.

Rismanchi N, Gold JJ, Sattar S, et al. Neurological outcomes after presumed childhood encephalitis. *Pediatr Neurol*. 2015;53:200-206.

Sabah M, Mulcahy J, Zeman A. Herpes simplex encephalitis. *BMJ*. 2012;344:e3166.

Teoh HL, Mohammad SS, Britton PN, et al. Clinical characteristics and functional motor outcomes of enterovirus 71 neurological disease in children. *JAMA Neurol*. 2016;73:300-307.

Van Haren K, Ayscue P, Waubant E, et al. Acute flaccid myelitis of unknown etiology in California, 2012-2015. *JAMA*. 2015;314:2663-2671.

Venkatesan A, Tunkel AR, Bloch KC, et al. Case definitions, diagnostic algorithms, and priorities in encephalitis: consensus statement of the International Encephalitis Consortium. *Clin Infect Dis*. 2013;57:1114-1128.

Wolf VL, Lupo PJ, Lotze TE. Pediatric acute transverse myelitis overview and differential diagnosis. *J Child Neurol*. 2012;27:1426-1436.


# 228 Sexually Transmitted Infections

Loris Y. Hwang and Anna-Barbara Moscicki

## INTRODUCTION

Sexual activity is common among adolescents. A large ongoing national survey of US high school students reported that 24% of adolescents have had sexual intercourse by ninth grade and 58.1% by 12th grade, based on data collected in 2014 to 2015. Although rates of sexual activity have slowly decreased during 1991 to 2015, the adolescent age group continues to be at the highest risk for common sexually transmitted infections (STIs) compared to other age groups.

This chapter provides an overview of STIs including the common clinical presentations, screening guidelines, and treatment for bacterial, fungal, protozoal, and viral infections. For the most up-to-date clinical guidelines on treatment regimens, readers are strongly advised to refer to the Centers for Disease Control and Prevention (CDC) Web site since the optimal treatment regimens are frequently updated based on antibiotic resistance patterns and logistical availability of specific medications in the United States. Table 228-1 summarizes the major points about chlamydia, gonorrhea, human papillomavirus (HPV), *Trichomonas*, and *Candida*. Detailed discussions of syphilis, human immunodeficiency virus (HIV), and herpes simplex virus (HSV) infections are found in Chapters 283, 310, and 304, respectively.

## EPIDEMIOLOGY

Adolescents and young adults 15 to 24 years of age represent one-quarter of the sexually active population, but they acquire nearly half of the 20 million new STIs each year in the United States. These STIs place our youth at risk for substantial morbidity and mortality, including pelvic inflammatory disease (PID) and its associated sequelae of ectopic pregnancy, infertility, and chronic pelvic pain; HPV-associated genital dysplasia; and HIV-associated immunosuppression and life-threatening complications.

Annual epidemiologic data are published by the CDC, based on state and local STI case reports made from private and public sources. Chlamydia, gonorrhea, and syphilis are reportable infections, whereas other STIs such as HPV, HSV, and *Trichomonas* are not routinely reported to the public health authorities. In 2014, among women, the highest reported rates of chlamydia infection were found in those age 15 to 24 years (3309.4 cases per 100,000 females), compared to other age groups. The gonorrhea rate is similarly highest in women age 15 to 24 years (484 cases per 100,000 females), and the syphilis rate is highest in women age 20 to 24 years (4.5 cases per 100,000 females). HPV is not a reportable infection, but data from large surveillance studies show that 34% of women age 14 to 24 years have genital HPV, which is roughly 7.5 million females with HPV. Among the men, the highest chlamydia and gonorrhea rates are in those age 20 to 24 years (1368.3 cases per 100,000 males and 485.6 cases per 100,000 males, respectively). Syphilis rates are highest in men age 25 to 29 years (34 cases per 100,000 males), although syphilis rates in men age 20 to 24 years are similarly concerning (31.1 cases per 100,000 males).

The higher STI rates observed in adolescents and young adults are associated with several risk factors. For example, gender is an important factor, as STIs are disproportionately more common among females compared to males, as evidenced from the gender-specific rates discussed above. Among adolescents, those with higher rates of

**TABLE 228-1 COMMON SEXUALLY TRANSMITTED INFECTIONS (STIs) AND VAGINITIS IN ADOLESCENTS**

| STI | Clinical Presentations | Screening/Diagnosis | Recommended Treatment[a] | Alternative Treatment[a] | Comments |
|---|---|---|---|---|---|
| *Chlamydia trachomatis* (chlamydia) | *Females:*<br>Endocervicitis<br>Pelvic inflammatory disease<br>*Males:*<br>Epididymitis<br>*Both females and males:*<br>Urethritis<br>Pharyngitis<br>Proctitis<br>Conjunctivitis | *Females:*<br>NAATs: self-collected or clinician-collected vaginal specimen preferred, endocervical site acceptable, urine is less sensitive<br>*Males:*<br>NAATs: urine preferred, urethral specimen acceptable<br>*Extragenital sites:*<br>NAATS: rectal, oropharyngeal, if validated according to CLIA regulations<br>*Suspected sexual abuse cases in younger children:*<br>Culture (better specificity than NAAT in younger children), recommend referral to clinic for specialized medicolegal evaluation | *Uncomplicated Chlamydia:*<br>Azithromycin 1 g orally single dose<br>OR<br>Doxycycline 100 mg orally 2 times a day for 7 days | *Uncomplicated Chlamydia:*<br>Erythromycin base 500 mg orally 4 times a day for 7 days<br>OR<br>Erythromycin ethylsuccinate 800 mg orally 4 times a day for 7 days<br>OR<br>Levofloxacin 500 mg orally once daily for 7 days<br>OR<br>Ofloxacin 300 mg orally 2 times a day for 7 days | Abstain from sex at least 7 days after single-dose treatment or after 7-day antibiotic course and until all partners treated; recommend prompt evaluation and treatment of all partners from past 60 days; offer testing for other STIs; encourage consistent condom use; retest in 3 months to monitor for reinfection |
| *Neisseria gonorrhoeae* (gonorrhea) | *Females:*<br>Endocervicitis<br>Pelvic inflammatory disease<br>*Males:*<br>Epididymitis<br>*Both females and males:*<br>Urethritis<br>Pharyngitis<br>Proctitis<br>Conjunctivitis<br>Disseminated gonococcal infection | *Females:*<br>NAATs: self-collected or clinician-collected vaginal specimen preferred, endocervical site acceptable, urine is less sensitive<br>*Males:*<br>NAATs: urine preferred, urethral specimen acceptable<br>*Extragenital sites:*<br>NAATS: rectal, oropharyngeal, if validated according to CLIA regulations<br>*Suspected persistent infection (persistent symptoms 3–5 days after treatment):*<br>Culture with antimicrobial resistance testing; work with public health and CDC for further evaluation<br>*Suspected sexual abuse cases in younger children:*<br>Culture, recommend referral to clinic for specialized medicolegal evaluation | *Uncomplicated gonorrhea of cervix, urethra, rectum, pharynx:*<br>Ceftriaxone 250 mg IM single dose<br>PLUS<br>Azithromycin 1 g orally single dose<br>*Disseminated gonococcal infection (DGI)[c] including arthritis and arthritis-dermatitis syndrome:*<br>Ceftriaxone 1 g IM or IV every 24 hours<br>PLUS<br>Azithromycin 1 g orally single dose<br>Switch to oral agent 24–48 hours after substantial clinical improvement, for total treatment course of at least 7 days<br>*DGI[c] with meningitis and/or endocarditis:*<br>Ceftriaxone 1–2 g IV every 12–24 hours<br>PLUS<br>Azithromycin 1 g orally single dose, 10–14 days for meningitis, 4 weeks for endocarditis | *Uncomplicated gonorrhea of cervix, urethra, rectum, pharynx:*<br>*If ceftriaxone is not available:*<br>Cefixime 400 mg orally single dose<br>PLUS<br>Azithromycin 1 g orally single dose<br>*If azithromycin allergy:*<br>Ceftriaxone 250 mg IM single dose<br>PLUS<br>Doxycycline 100 mg orally twice per day for 7 days<br>*DGI[c] including arthritis and arthritis-dermatitis syndrome:*<br>Cefotaxime 1 g IV every 8 hours<br>OR<br>Ceftizoxime 1 g IV every 8 hours<br>PLUS<br>Azithromycin 1 g orally single dose<br>Switch to oral agent 24–48 hours after substantial clinical improvement, for total treatment course of at least 7 days | Abstain from sex at least 7 days after single-dose treatment or after 7-day antibiotic course and until all partners treated; recommend prompt evaluation and treatment of all partners from past 60 days; offer testing for other STIs; encourage consistent condom use; retest in 3 months to monitor for reinfection |

| | | | | | |
|---|---|---|---|---|---|
| *Trichomonas vaginalis* | *Females:*<br>Vaginitis<br>cervicitis<br>*Both females and males:*<br>Urethritis | *Females:*<br>NAATs preferred: self-collected or clinician-collected vaginal, endocervical, or urine<br>Point-of-care OSOM Rapid Test (immunochromatographic capillary-flow enzyme immunoassay dipstick): vaginal<br>Point-of-care Affirm VP III (DNA hybridization probe) vaginal<br>Wet mount microscopy: vaginal<br>Culture: vaginal<br>*Males:*<br>NAATs: urine or urethral, if validated according to CLIA regulations<br>Culture: urethral | Metronidazole 2 g orally single dose<br>OR<br>Tinidazole 2 g orally single dose | Metronidazole 500 mg orally twice a day for 7 days | Counsel patient about disulfiram-like reaction, abstain from alcohol until at least 24 hours after completion of metronidazole or 72 hours after completion of tinidazole.<br>Abstain from sex until patient and all partners treated; recommend prompt evaluation and treatment of all partners from past 60 days; offer testing for other STIs; encourage consistent condom use; retest in 3 months to monitor for reinfection |
| *Candida albicans* | *Females:*<br>Vulvovaginitis<br>*Males:*<br>Balanitis | *Females:*<br>Signs and symptoms<br>AND<br>Either:<br>wet mount microscopy that shows budding yeast forms or hyphae (pH usually < 4.5)<br>OR<br>culture that shows yeast species | *Uncomplicated:*<br>Fluconazole 150 mg orally single dose<br>OR<br>Over-the-counter intravaginal antifungals<br>OR<br>Prescription intravaginal antifungals<br>*Recurrent VVC:*<br>Initial therapy fluconazole 100-, 150-, or 200-mg dose on days 1, 4, and 7 for 3 total doses, followed by maintenance therapy fluconazole once weekly for 6 months<br>*Severe VVC:*<br>Fluconazole 150 mg on days 1 and 4 for 2 total doses<br>*Non-albicans VVC:*<br>Consider non-fluconazole azole for 7–14 days; for recurrence, consider boric acid vaginal capsule once daily for 2 weeks<br>OR<br>Refer to specialist | | Self-treatment using over-the-counter antifungals is common. Unnecessary or inappropriate self-treatment can delay clinical evaluation for other causes of genitourinary symptoms. |
| Bacterial vaginosis | *Females:*<br>Vaginitis | *Females:*<br>Wet mount microscopy using Amsel's criteria<br>Gram stain using Nugent's criteria<br>Point-of-care Affirm VP III (DNA hybridization probe for *G vaginalis*)<br>Point-of-care OSOM BV Blue test (detects vaginal fluid sialidase activity) | Metronidazole 500 mg orally twice daily for 7 days<br>OR<br>Metronidazole gel 0.75% (5 g) intravaginally once a day for 5 days<br>OR<br>Clindamycin cream 2% 1 full applicator (5 g) intravaginally at bedtime for 7 days | Tinidazole 2 g orally daily for 2 days<br>OR<br>Tinidazole 1 g orally daily for 5 days<br>OR<br>Clindamycin 300 mg orally twice a day for 7 days<br>OR<br>Clindamycin ovules 100 mg intravaginally once at bedtime for 3 days | Clindamycin cream may weaken latex condoms.<br>Counsel patient about disulfiram-like reaction. Abstain from alcohol until at least 24 hours after completion of metronidazole or 72 hours after completion of tinidazole. |

(Continued)

**TABLE 228-1 COMMON SEXUALLY TRANSMITTED INFECTIONS (STIs) AND VAGINITIS IN ADOLESCENTS (CONTINUED)**

| STI | Clinical Presentations | Screening/Diagnosis | Recommended Treatment[a] | Alternative Treatment[a] | Comments |
|---|---|---|---|---|---|
| Human papillomavirus (HPV) | *Females*:<br>Abnormal cervical cytology: LSIL, HSIL<br>Invasive cancer<br>*Females and males:*<br>Condyloma acuminatum (genital skin wart) | *Females:*<br>Cervical cytology[c]<br>Colposcopy (cervical, vaginal, vulvar lesions visible using 3–5% acetic acid wash and iodine; areas appear dense, white with neovascular changes)<br>HPV DNA detection (only FDA-approved methods should be used for testing of high-risk types)<br>*Females and males:*<br>Visible inspection of genital skin for warts | Based on lesion type, location, extent<br>*LSIL or HSIL:*<br>LSIL can be followed with cytology; HSIL should be referred to colposcopy specialist for evaluation<br>*Condyloma acuminatum, self-applied therapies:*<br>Imiquimod 3.75% or 5% cream<br>OR<br>Podofilox 0.5% solution or gel<br>OR<br>Ableinecatechins 15% ointment<br>*Condyloma acuminatum, clinician applied*: Cryotherapy with liquid nitrogen or cryoprobe<br>OR<br>Trichloroacetic acid (TCA) or bichloroacetic acid (BCA) 80–90% solution<br>OR<br>Surgical removal | | Liquid nitrogen: pain on application<br>TCA: safe with mucosa and pregnancy, local sensitivity |

[a]Adapted from Workowski KA, Bolan GA. Sexually transmitted diseases treatment guidelines, 2015. *MMWR Recomm Rep.* 2015;64(Rr-03):1-137. Check https://www.cdc.gov/std/tg2015/ for the most current updates to the treatment guidelines.

[b]Guidelines for the management of abnormal cytology are found in Massad LS, Einstein MH, Huh WK, et al. 2012 updated consensus guidelines for the management of abnormal cervical cancer screening tests and cancer precursors. *Obstet Gynecol.* 2013;121(4):829-846.

[c]Consultation with an infectious disease specialist and/or the CDC is also advised, as the optimal treatment regimen (antibiotic selection and duration of therapy) for an individual case may vary, depending on the specific clinical presentation, antimicrobial susceptibility results, and clinical response to treatment.

CDC, Centers for Disease Control and Prevention; CLIA, Clinical Laboratory Improvement Amendments; FDA, US Food and Drug Administration; HSIL, high-grade squamous intraepithelial lesion; IV, intravenous; LSIL, low-grade squamous intraepithelial lesion; NAATs, nucleic acid amplification tests; VVC, vulvovaginal candidiasis.

STIs report a younger age of their first sexual encounter, have multiple concurrent sex partners, multiple sequential sex partners, inconsistent use of condoms, or use of injection drugs. Higher risk is also found in certain populations, such as young men who have sex with men (MSM), adolescents evaluated in STI clinics and some adolescent clinics, and those in detention facilities. Race and ethnicity are another important factor to consider for all age groups overall, given the correlation of race and ethnicity to other critical determinants of health, including socioeconomic status, differential educational attainment, and access to quality health care. One challenge in data collection is the missing data on race and ethnicity, since many case reports to public health are submitted without the race and ethnicity information, but population-based studies and national surveys provide clearly confirmatory evidence of the substantial burden of STIs on certain racial and ethnic groups. In 2014, the CDC reported that the overall ratios of chlamydia for African American, Native American, Native Hawaiian/Pacific Islanders, Hispanic, and whites were 6:4:6:2:1. The ratios for gonorrhea were 11:4:3:2:1, and the ratios for primary and secondary syphilis were 5:2:2:2:1. In considering the substantial risk associated with race and ethnicity, it is important to recognize that individuals who reside in geographic areas of high STI prevalence face a greater challenge to reduce their own personal risk for STI exposure. Public health interventions must address not only individual-level risk factors but also community-level risk factors involving social and cultural conditions that impact STI risk.

### SCREENING RECOMMENDATIONS

The overall screening recommendations for adolescents and young adults are listed below:

- Sexually active females age < 25 years: Routine annual screening for chlamydia and gonorrhea is recommended, and HIV screening should be offered. The frequency of HIV screening should be based on risk factors. Cervical cancer screening by cervical cytology is recommended to start at age 21 years. Routine screening for other infections (syphilis, HSV, trichomonas, bacterial vaginosis) is not generally recommended in asymptomatic females.
- Sexually active males age < 25 years: Evidence is not sufficient for a broad recommendation for routine screening for all males for chlamydia and gonorrhea, but screening for chlamydia and gonorrhea in high-prevalence settings or men with risk factors should be strongly considered. HIV screening should be offered. The frequency of HIV screening should be based on risk factors.
- Men who have sex with men (MSM): Routine annual screening for HIV and syphilis serology is recommended. For MSM who have had insertive anal intercourse in the preceding year, routine annual screening for urethral chlamydia and gonorrhea is recommended. For MSM who have had receptive anal intercourse in the preceding year, routine annual screening for rectal chlamydia and gonorrhea is recommended. For MSM who have had receptive oral intercourse in the preceding year, routine annual screening for pharyngeal gonorrhea is recommended.

## BACTERIAL INFECTIONS

## CHLAMYDIA

*Chlamydia trachomatis* is the most common reported bacterial STI in the United States. Chlamydiae are obligate intracellular bacteria, and disease appears to result from both the destruction of cells during the growth cycle and the body's immune response to the infection producing inflammation.

### CLINICAL MANIFESTATIONS

Uncomplicated endocervicitis is the most common clinical manifestation of chlamydial infection in sexually active female adolescents. However, the majority of chlamydial lower genital infections in women are asymptomatic, thus underscoring the importance of routine screening. When symptomatic, clinical findings may include abnormal vaginal discharge or bleeding, especially after intercourse. Another possible finding is mucopurulent cervicitis (MPC), which presents with a yellow endocervical discharge or by identification of increased polymorphonuclear cells on a Gram stain from the discharge (> 10–30 white blood cells per high-power field). However, MPC is not a sensitive diagnostic indicator of infection because most infected women do not have MPC. The most serious complication of endocervical infection is PID, including a subclinical upper tract infection that can lead to infertility. Routine annual screening for chlamydia has been shown to decrease PID rates in female populations. Patients with multiple risk factors or concern for possible exposures may warrant more frequent screening.

Urethritis is the most common clinical manifestation of chlamydial infection in sexually active male adolescents and occurs commonly in women as well. In men, chlamydia is the most common cause of nongonococcal urethritis (NGU), responsible for 15% to 40% of cases. Chlamydial urethritis is typically identified through testing of symptomatic men (presenting with discharge and dysuria), contact tracing from a chlamydia-positive partner, or routine screening of asymptomatic men. Additionally, 20% to 50% of those with gonococcal urethritis are co-infected with chlamydia.

Extragenital sites represent another clinical presentation, especially in MSM, and most are asymptomatic. In a 2003 study of 6434 MSM seen at an STI clinic, chlamydia prevalence was 7.9% rectal, 5.2% urethral, and 1.4% pharyngeal.

### DIAGNOSIS

Diagnosis of chlamydia by direct detection is recommended using US Food and Drug Administration (FDA)–approved nucleic acid amplification tests (NAATs) for both women and men, with or without symptoms. NAATs have demonstrated superior sensitivity and specificity compared to other testing technologies; thus, the older approaches including culture, enzyme immunoassays, nucleic acid probe tests, genetic transformation tests, and serology are not recommended. The exception is the preferred use of culture in cases of suspected sexual abuse in younger children because of the high specificity of culture. Clinicians are advised to refer cases of suspected sexual abuse to centers that are equipped to address the complex medicolegal aspects of these scenarios.

For women, NAATs are available for vaginal, cervical, and urine specimens, with the vagina being the preferred site of collection. Self-collected and clinician-collected vaginal swabs are equivalent in assay performance, and many adolescent women appreciate the convenient option of a self-collected vaginal swab when a pelvic exam is not otherwise indicated, for example in asymptomatic women. In the setting of a pelvic exam, vaginal specimens are still appropriate, but cervical samples are also acceptable. Although a first-catch urine specimen is acceptable in women, urine is less preferred due to lower sensitivity compared to vaginal and cervical specimens.

For men, the preferred detection method is the NAATs using the first-catch urine specimen, which demonstrate equivalent performance to urethral swabs and much higher acceptability from the patient perspective. For MSM, the CDC recommends routine annual screening of extragenital sites (rectal and/or oropharyngeal as indicated by the patient's history of sexual behaviors) using NAATs, due to superior sensitivity and specificity compared to culture. Since NAATS are not FDA-approved for extragenital sites, rectal and oropharyngeal NAAT testing must be performed by laboratories that meet Clinical Laboratory Improvement Amendments (CLIAs) regulations for assay performance specifications.

### TREATMENT

The recommended and alternative treatment regimens are found in Table 228-1. The goals of prompt treatment are to relieve symptoms and to prevent reproductive sequelae and further transmission to partners and neonates. Single-dose azithromycin offers the opportunity for direct administration and observation by clinical staff to ensure adherence. Patient counseling should include advice to abstain from sexual activity for at least 7 days after the single-dose azithromycin or until the other options of 7-day antibiotic courses are completed. Patients should further abstain until all sexual partners are treated. All partners in the past 60 days should ideally receive presumptive treatment and a full STI evaluation. If the patient reports no partners in the past 60 days, then the most recent partner beyond the 60 days should be offered treatment and services. If partners might not be able to access care, expedited partner treatment (EPT) should be offered as an alternative where allowed by state laws. EPT consists of prescription of antibiotic treatment and written counseling, which are delivered by the infected patient to the partner(s). EPT has been shown to decrease rates of recurrent or persistent chlamydia and is endorsed by several national medical societies and public health organizations. Of note, EPT is not ideal for MSM infected with chlamydia because of concern for co-existing STIs in the partners and thus the need for full evaluation in person. All patients diagnosed with chlamydia should also be offered testing for other STIs if not already performed and counseled about consistent condom use for STI prevention. Test-of-cure within a few weeks after treatment is not routinely recommended except in cases of questionable adherence to treatment, persistent symptoms, or repeat exposure to chlamydia. However, it is important to note that a positive result from an NAAT can persist up to 3 weeks after successful treatment due to nonviable chlamydia organisms that cause false-positive results. Rather than conducting routine tests-of-cure, retesting at 3 months after treatment is advised in order to detect reinfection from repeated exposure to an infected partner.

## GONORRHEA

*Neisseria gonorrhoeae* is the second most commonly reported bacterial STI in the United States. *N gonorrhoeae* is a gram-negative bacterium that has the unique genetic ability to change the antigenic expression of its surface-exposed proteins, making development of a vaccine challenging. Gonorrhea prevalence varies by geographic communities, and clinicians are encouraged to be familiar with public health recommendations for screening in their areas. Additional discussion of *N gonorrhoeae* can be found in Chapter 269.

### CLINICAL MANIFESTATIONS

The majority of gonorrhea infections in men and women are asymptomatic and found on routine screening. Endocervicitis is the most common clinical manifestation of gonorrhea in women, as most gonococcal infections in women affect the lower genital tract with a particular predilection for the columnar cells of the endocervix. When symptomatic, gonorrhea in women leads to vaginal discharge, bleeding, pelvic discomfort, and/or PID. Urethritis is another clinical presentation in women but is often associated with endocervicitis. In men, urethritis is the most common clinical manifestation of gonorrhea. Symptomatic men report dysuria and/or discharge, appearing as soon as 2 to 4 days after urethral exposure. The discharge may be scant, or mucus may be present as a profuse purulent discharge. Approximately 10% of cases progress to acute epididymitis and urethral strictures. Additionally, 5% to 30% of men and 25% to 50% of women with *N gonorrhoeae* infection have concurrent *C trachomatis* infection.

Of particular note is the serious condition of disseminated gonococcal infection (DGI), a bloodborne infection that has been classically described as a triad of petechial or pustular skin lesions, polyarthralgia, and tenosynovitis but may also manifest as septic arthritis alone (culture-positive joint fluid in approximately 50% of cases only), which occurs in 2% to 5% of gonorrhea-infected individuals, or involvement of joint and skin alone, known as the arthritis-dermatitis syndrome. Complications of DGI include meningitis and endocarditis, which are very rare. DGI is more common in African Americans than in other race/ethnicity groups. When considering the typical STI risk factors during an evaluation for gonorrhea, clinicians should also inquire about travel history and patients' sexual exposures outside the United States, given the antimicrobial resistance patterns observed across international geographic regions for gonorrhea in particular.

### DIAGNOSIS

Direct diagnosis of gonorrhea by NAATs is the preferred method because NAAT sensitivity is superior to culture but varies by the type of NAAT. FDA-approved NAATs are available for vaginal, endocervical, and urine testing for women, and urine and urethral testing for men. Similar to chlamydia, the vaginal site is recommended for gonorrhea screening for women and the urine for men. As noted, NAATs are not FDA-approved for rectal and oropharyngeal sites but can be used by laboratories that meet CLIA regulations for assay performance specifications. However, culture retains an important role in gonorrhea management due to antimicrobial resistance issues. The US Gonococcal Isolate Surveillance Project (GISP) is a national sentinel surveillance system in place since 1986. Fluoroquinolone-resistant gonorrhea became apparent in 2007, and ongoing concerns for cephalosporin resistance are being monitored in several countries. When treatment failure is suspected, it becomes essential to perform culture and antimicrobial susceptibility testing. Furthermore, similar to chlamydia, culture is preferred in cases of suspected sexual abuse in younger children. Any gonorrhea isolates should be retained for additional testing.

Another diagnostic tool for use only in symptomatic men is the Gram stain of urethral secretions, which is considered diagnostic when polymorphonuclear leukocytes with intracellular gram-negative diplococci are observed. Gram stain is not recommended in asymptomatic men or for endocervical, pharyngeal, or rectal specimens because of low sensitivity in these scenarios.

### TREATMENT

The recommended and alternative treatment regimens for uncomplicated gonorrhea of the cervix, urethra, rectum, and pharynx are found in Table 228-1. After fluoroquinolone-resistant gonorrhea emerged in 2007, cephalosporins became the only antibiotics sufficiently effective for gonorrhea treatment. Current guidelines recommend dual therapy using a cephalosporin plus either azithromycin or doxycycline for gonorrhea treatment, regardless of chlamydia test results. Furthermore, rising resistance to cefixime and other oral cephalosporins in several countries as well as concerns about tetracycline resistance have led to the preferred recommended regimen of ceftriaxone and azithromycin as dual treatment administered simultaneously and with direct observation by clinical staff. Of note, the older regimen of azithromycin 2 g orally as monotherapy is no longer recommended in light of concerns for macrolide resistance. In situations of azithromycin allergy, doxycycline may serve as an alternative second antibiotic agent in place of azithromycin. For patients with persistent symptoms 3 to 5 days after treatment, treatment failure should be suspected, and the clinician should perform culture and antimicrobial susceptibility testing, report the case to public health, and work with the CDC to provide isolates for further testing.

The treatment of DGI is not as well-established as is the treatment of uncomplicated cases. The CDC has made recommendations for treatment of DGI cases involving arthritis, arthritis-dermatitis syndrome, meningitis, and endocarditis, as listed in Table 228-1. However, the CDC concurrently advises consultation with an infectious disease specialist and/or the CDC to discuss individual cases, as the optimal treatment regimen for an individual patient may vary. The antibiotic selection and duration of treatment in a particular case are influenced by the specific clinical presentation, antimicrobial susceptibility results, and clinical response to treatment.

Similar to the management of chlamydia, gonorrhea-infected patients should receive counseling about partner treatment, EPT if indicated (cefixime 400 mg and azithromycin 1 g), abstaining from sex until all partners are treated, consistent condom use for future STI prevention, testing for other STIs, and retesting in 3 months to monitor for reinfection.

Treatment for DGI requires hospitalization for parenteral therapy and further evaluation for possible meningitis or endocarditis.

# PROTOZOAN AND FUNGAL INFECTIONS

## TRICHOMONAS

*Trichomonas* is the most common nonviral STI in the United States (Fig. 228-1). These organisms are sexually transmitted flagellated protozoans that attach to epithelial cells and can survive for up to 1.5 hours on a wet sponge and 24 hours on a wet cloth. *Trichomonas* is not reportable to public health authorities, but a US national survey reported an overall prevalence of 3.1%, with the highest prevalence of 13.3% found in non-Hispanic African American women. Similar to other STIs, higher prevalence is observed in populations such as patients with multiple partners, inconsistent condom use, racial/ethnic minorities, those seen in STI clinics, and those in detention facilities, but it is notable that the epidemiology of *Trichomonas* differs from chlamydia and gonorrhea in that older women also bear the burden of higher prevalence, and lower prevalence is found in MSM.

### CLINICAL MANIFESTATIONS

The majority of infected patients are asymptomatic or have minimal symptoms. Untreated infections can persist for months to years. In women, *Trichomonas* can cause vaginitis, cervicitis, and urethritis. Symptoms include pruritus, vaginal discharge, dyspareunia, postcoital bleeding, lower abdominal pain, dysuria, and frequency. The vulva may appear erythematous, and the vaginal walls may appear granular. The "classical" frothy yellow-green vaginal discharge occurs in only 12% and can be found with other infections. The "strawberry cervix" consisting of punctate hemorrhages on the ectocervix occurs in only 2% and is not pathognomonic for *Trichomonas* cervicitis. Important implications of *Trichomonas* infection include the 2- to 3-fold increased risk for HIV acquisition and adverse pregnancy outcomes (eg, preterm birth). In HIV-infected women, *Trichomonas* carries a higher risk for PID, and thus annual screening is advised in this population. In men, the infection is usually self-limited, and most men are asymptomatic or present with features of nongonococcal urethritis. Infrequently, epididymitis or proctitis may develop.

### DIAGNOSIS

In the last several years, new diagnostic assays for *Trichomonas* have become available. Currently, the most sensitive tests are the FDA-approved NAATs. The APTIMA NAAT (Hologic Gen-Probe, San Diego, CA) can be used for vaginal, endocervical, or urine specimens from women, with both sensitivity and specificity of 95% to 100%. Laboratories fulfilling CLIA regulations can use APTIMA for urine or urethral specimens from men. The BD Probe Tec Q$^x$ Amplified DNA Assay (Becton Dickinson, Franklin Lakes, NJ) is another NAAT available for vaginal, endocervical, or urine specimens from women. Point-of-care assays are also available and FDA-approved for women only. The OSOM Rapid Test (Sekisui Diagnostic, Framingham, MA) is an immunochromatographic capillary flow enzyme immunoassay dipstick that can be used for vaginal specimens, with sensitivity of 82% to 95%, specificity of 97% to 100%, and results in 10 minutes. The Affirm VP III (Becton Dickinson) is a DNA hybridization probe used for vaginal specimens with a sensitivity of 63%, a specificity of 99.9%, and results in 45 minutes.

These newer assays are becoming more widely available, but the traditional wet mount microscopy continues to be commonly used because of convenience, low cost, and immediate results, although sensitivity is only 51% to 65% for vaginal specimens and even lower for specimens from men. Wet mount also requires prompt evaluation for the motile organisms as *Trichomonas* motility decreases quickly with time. Some clinicians may adopt the option of wet mount first and then NAAT if the wet mount is negative. Culture was traditionally considered the gold standard because of the specificity close to 100%, but it offers sensitivity of only 75% to 96% and is not commonly used currently. Pap cytology sometimes identifies an incidental *Trichomonas* infection but should not be used for routine testing because of false negatives and false positives.

### TREATMENT

The recommended and alternative treatment regimens are found in Table 228-1. For metronidazole and tinidazole, the consumption of alcohol can cause a disulfiram-like reaction. Thus, patients should avoid alcohol-containing drinks until at least 24 hours after metronidazole use or 72 hours after tinidazole use. Metronidazole gel is not recommended because of subtherapeutic levels and insufficient efficacy for the urethra and perivaginal glands.

## VULVOVAGINAL CANDIDIASIS

Vulvovaginal candidiasis (VVC) is estimated to occur at least once in 75% of women, and 2 or more episodes are estimated to occur in 40% to 45%. The majority are caused by *Candida albicans*, but other *Candida* species are possible. Risk factors include immunocompromise, genetic host factors, medication use, and behavioral factors such as douching. Although sexual transmission of *C albicans* may occur, the role of such transmission in promoting infection among sexually active women is unclear.

### CLINICAL MANIFESTATIONS

Uncomplicated VVC typically presents with nonspecific symptoms of vaginal pruritus, discomfort, or discharge; vulvar edema, fissures, or excoriations; dyspareunia; or dysuria. Approximately 10% to 20%

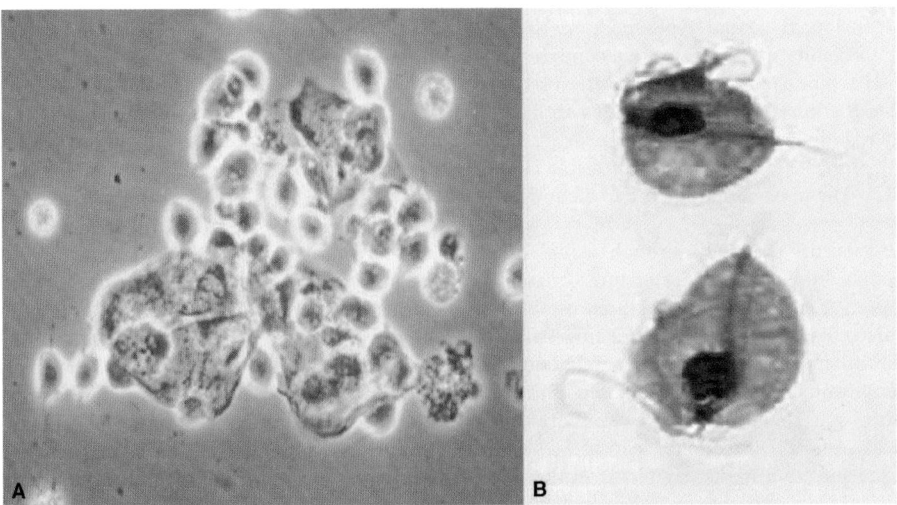


**FIGURE 228-1** *Trichomonas vaginalis.* **A:** Wet mount microscopy. **B:** Giemsa stained.

of cases are classified as complicated VVC, including recurrent VVC, severe VVC, or non-albicans species VVC. Recurrent VVC is defined as 4 or more episodes of symptomatic VVC in 1 year. Many of these patients do not have any clear risk factors, and non-albicans species VVC is found in 10% to 20% of recurrent VVC cases. Severe VVC involves extensive vulvar erythema, edema, excoriations, and fissures.

### DIAGNOSIS AND TREATMENT

One diagnostic challenge is distinguishing pathogenic infection from nonpathogenic colonization. Accordingly, diagnosis is typically made when a woman has signs and symptoms of vaginitis and either wet mount microscopy that shows budding yeast forms or hyphae (pH is usually < 4.5) or culture that shows yeast species. For patients with signs or symptoms but negative wet mount microscopy, empiric treatment is an option. However, positive culture without signs or symptoms may simply indicate normal colonization because 10% to 20% of women have yeast in the vagina and would not warrant treatment. Treatment regimens are found in Table 228-1.

## VIRAL INFECTIONS

## HUMAN PAPILLOMAVIRUS

HPV is a member of the papillomavirus family capable of infecting humans. It is a closed, circular, double-stranded DNA virus of approximately 8000 base pairs. The viral genome is enclosed in an icosahedral capsule composed of 2 protein capsomeres (referred to as late [L] 1 and 2 proteins) and lacks the lipid-containing envelope common to many other viruses such as HSV. Unlike other human STIs such as HSV, HPV growth in traditional cell culture has been difficult because its replication is dependent on epithelial cell differentiation and maturation requiring the use of cell raft systems.

### PATHOGENESIS AND EPIDEMIOLOGY

For infection, HPV requires access to basal epithelial cells through a wound or inflammation. Sites most vulnerable to infection are those where basal cells are actively dividing including the active squamous metaplasia of the transformation zone of the female cervix and areas of wound healing in the genital area. Although perinatal transmission has been shown to occur, the infections are usually only found in the respiratory tract of the infant. Rarely, genital warts occur in infants from perinatal transmission. Common clinical presentations of HPV include genital warts or condyloma acuminatum. In addition, HPV is the cause of precancerous and cancerous lesions of the genitals, including vulvar, vaginal, cervical, anal, and penile cancers. Genital HPV types are also associated with oropharyngeal cancers. Subclassification of HPV into over 100 types has been based on differences in degree of DNA homology. Of the > 100 types, approximately 40 are considered genital types because they are found predominantly in the genital area only. Genital condyloma are usually associated with HPV type 6 or 11. These types are considered to be low-risk HPV types because they are rarely seen in cancers. Twelve types are considered high risk (HR; 16, 18, 31, 33, 35, 39, 45, 51, 52, 56, 58, and 59), 1 probable HR (68b), and 7 possible HR (66, 26, 53, 67, 70, 73, and 82), The most common type in all anogenital cancers is HPV-16.

Genital HPV infection occurs primarily through sexual behavior and may include genital-to-genital contact or intercourse. The role of hands or sex toys in transmission has not been established, but HPV DNA can be detected on hands and under fingernails. In adolescents and young women, infections are extremely common, with over 50% of young women acquiring the infection within 2 to 4 years after initiating sex. The infections, however, are mostly transient, with 70% to 90% of HPV infections clearing within 1 to 2 years. Persistence of the infection is the key factor in the development of anogenital precancers and cancers. The length of time of persistence required for cancer development is not known. Because HPV is acquired commonly through sexual intercourse during adolescence and cancer is not seen until 2 or 3 decades later, it is thought that years of persistence are required for most individuals before cancer develops. Viral–host protein interactions result in the loss of cell cycle control and are considered crucial steps in the development of the cancers. The roles of other cofactors are less compelling. Those thought to play important roles include cigarette use and immune suppression. More specifically, HIV-infected persons and organ transplant patients are at higher risk for cervical and anal cancers. Other factors with conflicting data include prolonged use of hormonal oral contraceptives, increased parity, and infection with *C trachomatis*.

### CLINICAL MANIFESTATIONS

HPV can cause multicentric disease, including much of the anogenital area, including the vulvar labia minora and majora, clitoris, vaginal introitus, vagina, cervix, urethra, anus, and perineum in women, and the penis (including the prepuce, frenulum, corona, glans, urethra, and shaft), scrotum, and anus in men. The common genital warts, condyloma acuminatum, seen on the skin surfaces present as polypoid masses with fissured and irregular surfaces. They are often multiple and polymorphic and commonly coalesce into large masses. Genital HPV types also often appear as flat, smooth, or pedunculated papules, specifically on mucosal surfaces. These lesions can also occur on conjunctival, nasal, oral, respiratory, gastrointestinal, and bladder mucosa.

Infections with HPV can result in the development of lesions in the anogenital area referred to as low-grade squamous intraepithelial lesions (LSIL) and high-grade squamous intraepithelial lesions (HSIL). The term *low grade* refers to benign changes caused by the virus described in cell morphology. These lesions will usually clear spontaneously and require no intervention. *High grade* refers to changes that are considered truly precancerous (ie, the chance of progression is high and regression less).

### DIAGNOSIS

Screening for HPV infections in adolescents and young adult women is currently limited to visual inspection for external genital warts, and for women 21 years and older, cervical cancer screening using cytology is recommended for intraepithelial lesions and invasive cancers. No routine screening recommendations are made for vulvar, anal, and penile precancerous lesions in adolescents and young adults (defined as < 25 years of age) including MSM. This includes immunocompromised individuals.

Diagnosis of genital warts by visual inspection is considered adequate, and HPV testing plays little to no role in confirming the diagnosis unless the diagnosis is questioned. In this case, biopsy is the best confirmation. The differential diagnosis includes bowenoid papulosis, vulvar intraepithelial neoplasia, Bowen disease, condylomata, skin tags, nevocellular nevus, benign tumors, sebaceous glands, seborrheic keratosis, pearly penile papules, molluscum contagiosum, squamous cell carcinoma, vulva papillomatosis, and vestibular papillae.

### TREATMENT

Treatment (see Table 228-1) for genital warts includes self-administered and provider-administered options. Provider-administered therapies are primarily ablative including application of trichloroacetic acid (TCA) or bichloroacetic acid (BCA) (85–90%) to the wart. Cryotherapy with liquid nitrogen is also quite effective. Treatments are usually applied weekly for 4 to 6 weeks. If there is no improvement, therapy should be switched, or the diagnosis should be questioned. The current role of podophyllin resin in therapy is questioned because its potency is unpredictable, and it is contraindicated on mucosal surfaces and in pregnancy. Other therapies include cidofovir, intralesion interferon, or 5-fluorouracil/epinephrine gel implant or laser therapy. Surgical removal by experienced clinicians is also an alternative using tangential scissor excision, tangential shave excision, curettage, or electrosurgery. Urethral meatus and vaginal wart treatments include liquid nitrogen or surgical removal. Cervical and intra-anal warts should be treated with cryotherapy with liquid nitrogen, surgical removal, or TCA/BCA. Referral to a trained specialist is recommended for both cervical and anal warts. Cervical warts require biopsy prior to treatment to rule out HSIL.

There are now several options for self-applied therapies. Podofilox is applied directly to the warts twice daily for 3 consecutive days and repeated weekly up to 4 to 6 weeks. Imiquimod (5%), which is a cytokine-inducing agent, is applied directly once daily at bedtime 3 times a week (alternating days) for up to 16 weeks. Sinecatechins is used 3 times daily topically for up to 16 weeks. Disadvantages to all therapies include irritation, inflammation, and ulceration from local applications.

Despite known limitations in sensitivity, cytology remains the primary screening tool for squamous intraepithelial lesions (SIL) and invasive cancers in women age 21 years and older. Although HPV testing assists in triage of borderline abnormal cytology (atypical squamous cells of undetermined significance [ASCUS]) and SIL screening in older women, its role appears less specific in adolescents because of the high rates of HPV infections and LSIL and low rates of HSIL and invasive cancer in this age group. HPV DNA testing in adolescents is not currently recommended under any circumstance. Because HPV is often acquired early after the onset of sexual activity and is likely to be transient, cytology screening is not recommended under 21 years of age unless the patient is immunocompromised. Screening with cytology is then recommended every 3 years. At 25 years of age, primary screening with HPV DNA using the FDA-approved assays is allowed. Immunocompromised adolescent females should be screened within 1 year after the onset of sexual activity.

The cellular changes associated with these lesions can be identified on cytology (cervical cancer screening) and histology. The lesions can usually be visualized with the aid of colposcopy. Typical appearances on colposcopy associated with LSIL, HSIL, and invasive cancers assist in directing biopsy. Final diagnosis is dependent on histologic interpretation of the biopsy, not colposcopic appearance or cytologic diagnosis, specifically in adolescents. HPV DNA detection can be common in women with normal cytology, specifically in young women. Whether these women truly have no lesion remains controversial because cytology alone is an insensitive test to detect SIL. However, most of these infections in women with normal cytology appear transient, as in LSIL, and therefore, detection of HPV DNA in adolescents and young women is not cost-effective as a clinical tool and, as noted, should not be used. There are no treatments available or indicated for HPV DNA detection without abnormal cytology or histology.

### PREVENTION

Prevention of HPV types 6, 11, 16, 18 31, 33, 45, 52, and 58 can now be achieved with vaccination prior to exposure. In the United States, the nonavalent (HPV9) vaccine is currently recommended for all females and males age 11 to 12 years. It is also recommended for males and females up to age 26 years, particularly targeting those who are not yet sexually active. In the United States, the HPV vaccine is a 2-dose regimen for those starting the vaccine before their 15th birthday, and a 3-dose regimen for those starting the vaccine after their 15th birthday. The vaccine is not therapeutic and has no effect on women already infected with the HPV types included in the vaccine. A bivalent vaccine for HPV-16 and -18 is also approved for females only. The vaccine can be given starting at 9 years of age. If there is a history of sexual abuse, it is recommended to vaccinate starting at the age of 9 years. Readers should refer to vaccine guidelines frequently updated from the CDC Advisory Committee on Immunization Practices (ACIP).

## SYNDROMES

A constellation of symptoms and signs is characteristic of specific STI syndromes. Common lower genital tract syndromes in women include those characterized by vaginal discharge, which include bacterial vaginosis, *Trichomonas vaginalis*, and candidiasis, as well as endocervicitis and urethritis. In men, urethritis is the most common STI syndrome, but epididymitis also occurs. Proctitis occurs in both females and males.

## BACTERIAL VAGINOSIS

The dominant organism (> 95% of organisms) in the normal flora of healthy women is hydrogen peroxide–producing *Lactobacillus* species. Bacterial vaginosis (BV) results from the replacement of vaginal hydrogen peroxide–producing *Lactobacillus* species with high concentrations of anaerobic bacteria, including *Bacteroides* species, *Mobiluncus* and *Prevotella* species, and other bacteria such as *Gardnerella vaginalis* and *Mycoplasma hominis*. Reported prevalence varies widely from 10% to 50%, depending on the population sampled.

### CLINICAL MANIFESTATIONS

BV is the most common cause of abnormal vaginal discharge, although half the women who meet the clinical criteria for the diagnosis have no symptoms. BV is rarely found in non–sexually active women and is associated with multiple sexual partners and lack of condom use as well as douching. However, the cause of the microbial alterations remains unknown. BV has been associated with premature labor, as well as increased risk of acquiring HIV, gonorrhea, chlamydia, HSV, and HPV. Symptoms include pruritus, irritation, and a thin white vaginal discharge with a "fishy" odor.

### DIAGNOSIS

Various criteria have been used to diagnose BV. Amsel's clinical criteria are based on presence of 3 of the following 4 factors: (1) homogenous, thin white discharge that coats the vaginal walls; (2) > 20% of squamous cells with a clue cell appearance (vaginal epithelial cells studded with adherent coccobacilli); (3) pH of vaginal fluid > 4.5; and (4) fishy odor before or after addition of 10% KOH (whiff test). Nugent's gram stain criteria are used to quantify the absence of lactobacilli, and abundance of gram negative and variable rods and cocci and curved gram negative rods, which are seen in BV. The Nugent score is calculated and categorized as follows: 0 to 3 (normal), 4 to 6 (intermediate abnormal), and 7 to 10 (BV). Newer tests include the Affirm VP III (Becton Dickinson), which detects high concentrations of *G vaginalis*, and the OSOM BV Blue Test (Sekisui Diagnostics), which detects sialidase activity. Cervical Pap tests should not be used because they have low sensitivity and specificity.

### TREATMENT

Treatment of nonpregnant women is linked only to relief of symptoms; male partners of infected women are almost always asymptomatic, and treating men does not affect the woman's disease course. Treatment may lower risk of other STIs including HIV. Treatment regimens are found in Table 228-1. Additionally, treatment of symptomatic pregnant women is recommended using oral or vaginal treatments as recommended for nonpregnant women. Evidence is insufficient to recommend routine screening and treatment in asymptomatic pregnant women for the prevention of preterm birth.

## PELVIC INFLAMMATORY DISEASE

PID is used to describe a variety of inflammatory disorders of the upper female genital tract including endometritis, salpingitis, tubo-ovarian abscess, and peritonitis. PID is thought to reflect ascending infections initiated in the vagina or endocervix. STIs, in particular, *C trachomatis* and *N gonorrhoeae*, are often identified, but other vaginal organisms have also been implicated (eg, anaerobes, *G vaginalis*, *Haemophilus influenzae*, enteric gram-negative rods, *Streptococcus agalactiae*, *M hominis*, *Ureaplasma urealyticum*, and possibly *Mycoplasma genitalium*). The notable sequelae of PID include ectopic pregnancy and infertility. Risk factors that may predispose young women to develop acute PID include young age, history of an STI,

**TABLE 228-2 DIAGNOSTIC CRITERIA FOR PELVIC INFLAMMATORY DISEASE (PID)**

| Diagnostic Criteria |
|---|
| *Treat empirically if any are present and no other illness can be identified as causal:* |
| Cervical motion tenderness |
| OR uterine tenderness |
| OR adnexal tenderness |
| **Additional Criteria to Enhance and Support Diagnosis** |
| Oral temperature > 38.3°C |
| Abnormal cervical mucopurulent discharge or cervical friability |
| Elevated erythrocyte sedimentation rate or C-reactive protein |
| Laboratory-documented *Neisseria gonorrhoeae* or *Chlamydia trachomatis* cervical infection |
| Abundant white blood cells on saline wet prep |
| **Definitive Criteria (Selected Cases)** |
| Evidence of endometritis on biopsy |
| Thickened or fluid-filled tubes with or without free pelvic fluid or tubo-ovarian mass on transvaginal ultrasound |
| Laparoscopic findings of PID |

Data from Workowski KA, Bolan GA: Sexually transmitted diseases treatment guidelines, 2015, *MMWR Recomm Rep.* 2015 Jun 5;64(RR-03):1-137. Check https://www.cdc.gov/std/tg2015/ for the most current updates to the treatment guidelines.

previous PID diagnosis, greater number of sexual partners, and recent gynecologic interventions (eg, therapeutic abortion or endometrial biopsy). Although the relationship of oral contraceptives to acute PID has been controversial, most current research supports a protective role of oral contraceptives in the development of PID.

## DIAGNOSIS

PID is challenging to diagnose because there is no single historical, physical, or laboratory finding that is definitively diagnostic. The clinical diagnosis for PID is imprecise and requires the consideration of multiple possible findings. Although laparoscopy is thought to offer a definitive diagnosis, endometritis and subtle fallopian tube inflammation will be missed. In addition, laparoscopy is frequently unavailable. Since most episodes go undiagnosed because of mild symptoms such as dyspareunia or abnormal vaginal bleeding, it is recommended to have a low threshold for diagnosis. Symptoms and signs of acute PID include lower abdominal pain, vaginal discharge, cervical motion tenderness, and uterine and adnexal tenderness (Table 228-2). The differential diagnosis to be considered in a young woman presenting with acute lower abdominal pain, in addition to PID, includes acute appendicitis, acute cholecystitis, mesenteric lymphadenitis, acute cystitis, acute pyelonephritis, ectopic pregnancy, intrauterine pregnancy, septic abortion, endometriosis, ovarian cyst with or without torsion, hemorrhagic ovarian cyst, ovarian tumor, severe constipation, and trauma.

Principles to remember in the clinical approach to PID include the following: rule out other causes including pregnancy; when in doubt, err on the side of "overdiagnosis" of PID to prevent sequelae, especially in view of the possibility of subclinical infections, while pursuing further workup for other causes; treat with broad-spectrum antibiotics to cover *C trachomatis, N gonorrhoeae*, and other pathogens discussed earlier and begin the course promptly; and, finally, follow up with clinical evaluations (within 24–48 hours) to confirm the original clinical diagnosis and reevaluate the treatment regimen.

## TREATMENT

Treatment regimens are outlined in Table 228-3. Criteria for hospitalization include uncertain diagnosis or the need to rule out surgical emergencies; presence of a pelvic or tubo-ovarian abscess; pregnancy; severe illness, nausea, and vomiting; inability to take oral medications; failure of outpatient therapy within 48 hours; and inability to arrange

**TABLE 228-3 TREATMENT REGIMENS FOR ACUTE PELVIC INFLAMMATORY DISEASE (PID)**

| Recommended Inpatient Regimens |
|---|
| Parenteral regimen A |
| Cefotetan 2 g IV q12h or cefoxitin 2 g IV q6h, plus doxycycline 100 mg IV q12h. Use IV for minimum of 24 hours after patient improves. After hospital discharge, continue doxycycline 100 mg PO twice daily to complete 14-day course |
| or |
| Parenteral regimen B |
| Clindamycin 900 mg IV q8h, plus gentamicin 2 mg/kg IV or IM in 1 loading dose followed by a maintenance dose of 1.5 mg/kg IV q8h in patients with normal renal function. |
| Transition to oral outpatient therapy can be initiated 24–48 hours after clinical improvement. For those on cefotetan or cefoxitin, continue doxycycline 100 mg orally twice daily to complete 14-day total; for those on clindamycin/gentamicin regimen, continue clindamycin 450 mg orally 4 times daily or doxycycline 100 mg twice daily to complete 14-day course therapy. If tubo-ovarian abscess is present, clindamycin or metronidazole, 500 mg twice daily, should be used to complete the 14 days of therapy with doxycycline. Alternative regimens can be found at CDC website. |
| **Recommended Outpatient Regimens** |
| Ceftriaxone 250 mg IM |
| or |
| Cefoxitin 2 g IM and probenecid 1 g PO given concurrently in a single dose |
| or |
| Other third-generation cephalosporin (ceftizoxime or cefotaxime) |
| PLUS |
| Doxycycline 100 mg PO twice daily for 14 days |
| with or without |
| Metronidazole 500 mg PO twice daily for 14 days |
| Patients should demonstrate substantial clinical improvement within 3 days of start of treatment. For a diagnosis of chlamydial or gonococcal PID, patients should be retested 3 months after treatment. |
| **Management of Sex Partners** |
| Partners with sexual contact within 60 days prior should be evaluated and treated empirically for *Neisseria gonorrhoeae* and *Chlamydia trachomatis* infection. If a woman's last intercourse was > 60 days ago, then her most recent sexual partner should be evaluated and treated. |

CDC, Centers for Disease Control and Prevention; IM, intramuscular; IV, intravenous; PO, orally; q, every.

Data from Workowski KA, Bolan GA. Sexually transmitted diseases treatment guidelines, 2015, *MMWR Recomm Rep.* 2015 Jun 5;64(RR-03):1-137.

follow-up within 72 hours of starting antibiotics. Some recommend inpatient treatment for HIV-infected women because of greater sequelae. A serious complication of acute PID is the development of a tubo-ovarian abscess. Although most abscesses can be managed medically, occasional surgical intervention is necessary when medications fail. Screening and treatment of the sexual partner(s) are important parts of PID management, as with any STI. Intrauterine devices (IUDs) do not need to be routinely removed. If no improvement is noted after 48 to 72 hours of treatment, IUD removal should be considered.

# FITZ-HUGH-CURTIS SYNDROME

Fitz-Hugh-Curtis (FHC) syndrome results from ascending pelvic infection and inflammation of the liver capsule and/or diaphragm. It presents in females with right upper quadrant pain that can occur without other signs of PID. Bacteria that are typically associated with PID spread from the pelvis along the paracolic gutters to the liver capsule. *N gonorrhoeae* was the most common cause, but now *C trachomatis* is causative in about 80% of cases.

The disorder initially presents with acute pain that is similar to cholecystitis and may be referred to the right shoulder. It can then become chronic with persistent, but not severe, right upper quadrant pain.

Physical findings are otherwise not specific except for an occasional finding of a friction rub over the right upper quadrant. Diagnosis is most often inferred based on the symptoms and a finding of a positive cervical culture for gonorrhea or chlamydia. Liver function tests are usually normal. Imaging studies may be normal, although ultrasonography or abdominal computed tomography scan may identify perihepatic adhesions. Diagnostic laparoscopy demonstrates the pathognomonic finding of "violin-string" adhesions from the anterior abdominal wall to the liver capsule. Treatment is the same as for PID.

## EPIDIDYMITIS

Epididymitis is a clinical syndrome of inflammation of the epididymis caused by infection or trauma. Acute epididymitis is defined as pain and swelling of the epididymis for less than 6 weeks; chronic epididymitis is defined as discomfort in the scrotum, testicle, or epididymis for more than 6 weeks. The patient's age and sexual history are important in determining the causative agent. *C trachomatis* and *N gonorrhoeae* are the most common organisms in sexually active adolescents, being responsible for approximately two-thirds of infections. Enteric organisms such as *Escherichia coli* must be considered in youth who have engaged in insertive anal intercourse.

### CLINICAL MANIFESTATIONS

The patient typically presents with acute onset of unilateral testicular and/or scrotal pain and swelling (hydrocele), often accompanied by asymptomatic urethritis. Urinary frequency, dysuria, and urethral discharge may also occur. Upon examination, the epididymis is swollen and tender. Early in the course of the infection, the epididymis is easily discernible from the testicle, but with progression, the testis becomes involved, producing epididymo-orchitis, thereby making it difficult on examination to differentiate the epididymis from a swollen and tender testicle. The cremasteric reflex may be absent. Fever is a sign of systemic infection.

### DIAGNOSIS

Proper STI evaluation is similar to that for urethritis. Epididymitis is often difficult to differentiate from torsion of the spermatic cord. If the diagnosis is unclear, evidence for urethritis is not found, or the pain is very sudden and severe, urgent referral to a urologist should be made since testicular viability is at risk. Diagnosis should include evaluation by 1 of the following point-of-care tests: > 2 white blood cells (WBCs) per oil immersion field on Gram, methylene blue, or gentian violet stain of urethral secretions (this test also allows for the diagnosis of gonococcal infection showing intracellular gram-negative or purple diplococci); positive leukocyte esterase test on first-void urine; or > 10 WBCs per high-power field from a spun first void urine sediment.

Radionucleotide scanning is currently the most accurate method to diagnosis epididymitis. Ultrasound is often unable to distinguish between spermatic cord torsion and epididymitis. Scrotal masses are discussed in other sections. Hospitalization for presumptive acute epididymitis is typically not necessary but should be considered in cases of severe pain when further workup is indicated, when there is fever or concern for systemic disease, or when there is inability to adhere to treatment.

### TREATMENT

If chlamydial or gonococcal epididymitis is suspected, empiric treatment should start promptly. The recommended regimen is ceftriaxone 250 mg intramuscularly (IM), plus a 10-day course of doxycycline 100 mg twice daily. For infection likely caused by sexually transmitted chlamydia, gonorrhea, and enteric organisms (men who practice insertive anal intercourse), suggested treatment includes ceftriaxone 250 mg IM plus levofloxacin 500 mg orally once a day for 10 days or ofloxacin 300 mg orally twice a day for 10 days. For infection most likely caused by enteric organisms, suggested treatment is levofloxacin 500 mg orally once a day for 10 days or ofloxacin 300 mg orally twice a day for 10 days. All sexual partners within the prior 60 days should be contacted for evaluation and treatment. If last intercourse was > 60 days, the most recent partner should be evaluated. Additional therapy should include bed rest, scrotal elevation, and analgesics. If there is no improvement within the first 3 days of treatment, the diagnosis and treatment plan should be reconsidered. Other diagnostic possibilities include abscess, tuberculosis, fungal epididymitis, infarction, or tumor. Full resolution of discomfort may take weeks after treatment.

Epididymitis usually resolves without sequelae if treatment is administered promptly. However, there are some indications that oligo- or azoospermia may result, particularly if *C trachomatis* was the etiologic agent. Other sequelae include atrophy, infarct, or abscess formation.

## PROCTITIS, PROCTOCOLITIS, AND ENTERITIS

Proctitis is defined as inflammation of the distal 10 to 12 cm of the rectal mucosa and is associated with anorectal pain, mucus or blood in stools, tenesmus, or rectal discharge. Many infections involve the anus as well and are therefore considered "anorectal" infections. Although STI-related rectal infections are frequently associated with anal intercourse among MSM, they may also occur in heterosexual men and women. Such infections in women are less well defined and, with gonorrhea, are often asymptomatic and associated with endocervical gonorrhea. The most common sexually transmitted anorectal infections among sexually active adolescents include *N gonorrhoeae, C trachomatis* (including lymphogranuloma venereum [LGV] strains), HSV, and *Treponema pallidum* (syphilis). HIV-infected persons may also have severe herpes proctitis. Proctocolitis is proctitis with inflammatory extension to the colonic mucosa (> 12 cm above the anus) and is associated with diarrhea or abdominal cramps. Sexually transmitted enteric organisms, most commonly associated with anal intercourse or oral-anal sex, include *Entamoeba histolytica, Campylobacter* species, *Shigella* species, and LGV serovars of *C trachomatis.* Enteritis can present with or without proctitis or proctocolitis and commonly presents with diarrhea and abdominal cramping. It is most commonly associated with oral-anal sex practices. *Giardia lamblia* is the most common pathogen. Among HIV-infected persons, enteritis may be associated with organisms generally not sexually transmitted, including cytomegalovirus, *Mycobacterium avium-intracellulare, Cryptosporidium, Microsporidium, Isospora,* and others.

### DIAGNOSIS

Diagnostic evaluation for acute proctitis includes a careful sexual history to determine risk (eg, oral-anal sex, anal intercourse); examination including anoscopy; Gram stain of an anal sample; rectal sample tests (NAAT or culture) for *N gonorrhoeae, C trachomatis,* and HSV (or polymerase chain reaction [PCR]); and *T pallidum* (and darkfield, if available) serologic testing. If *C trachomatis* is identified, a molecular PCR test for LGV should be done.

### TREATMENT

Empiric treatment is indicated if the examination reveals anorectal exudates or if a Gram stain smear of an anorectal sample reveals polymorphonuclear leukocytes. Ceftriaxone 125 mg IM plus doxycycline 100 mg orally twice daily for 7 days are given while awaiting other test results. Presumptive treatment for HSV in addition to ceftriaxone and doxycycline is indicated for painful perianal or mucosal ulcers found on examination. If symptoms of proctocolitis and enteritis are found in association with oral-anal or anal intercourse, tests for enteric pathogens can be obtained. In the absence of this typical history and findings, other causes of proctitis need to be considered such as non-STI infectious colitis or inflammatory bowel disease (see Chapter 405). Partners of patients with STI-associated (eg, gonorrhea, chlamydia, including LGV) proctitis who had sexual contact within the prior 60 days should be evaluated and treated presumptively.

## CHANCROID

The majority of genital ulcers in sexually active youth in the United States are caused by HSV. Syphilis and chancroid are less common. Rates of chancroid have declined in the United States, and chancroid is associated with sporadic outbreaks. Patients infected with chancroid also have a high prevalence of HIV, HSV, and syphilis. Typical signs include painful genital ulcer and tender suppurative inguinal adenopathy.

### DIAGNOSIS

Presumptive diagnosis is made when all of the following criteria are present:

1. One or more painful genital ulcers
2. Negative darkfield examination of the ulcer exudate or negative syphilis serology within 7 days
3. Regional inguinal adenopathy
4. Negative HSV test from ulcer exudates

A definitive diagnosis of chancroid requires special culture media that is not widely available in many labs. Currently, there is no FDA-cleared PCR test for *Haemophilus ducreyi* (the causative agent), but some labs have developed in-house assays.

### TREATMENT

Four treatment options are currently recommended: azithromycin 1 g orally once; ceftriaxone 250 mg IM once; ciprofloxacin 500 mg orally twice daily for 3 days; or erythromycin base 500 mg orally 3 times daily for 7 days. Repeat examination should occur within 3 to 7 days of starting treatment in order to confirm improvement. Suppurative inguinal adenopathy may require needle aspiration or incision and drainage if no improvement is seen. Complete healing of larger ulcers may require more than 2 weeks. Patients who are uncircumcised or infected with HIV tend to demonstrate slower healing. All patients infected with chancroid should routinely be tested for HIV and receive repeat testing for syphilis and HIV 3 months later if initial tests were negative. Sex partners should be evaluated and treated if they had sexual contact within 10 days prior to the onset of symptoms.

### SUGGESTED READINGS


Centers for Disease Control and Prevention. Recommendations for the laboratory-based detection of *Chlamydia trachomatis* and *Neisseria gonorrhoeae*–2014. *MMWR Recomm Rep*. 2014;63:1-19.

Centers for Disease Control and Prevention. *Sexually Transmitted Disease Surveillance, 2014*. Atlanta, Georgia: U.S. Department of Health and Human Services; November 2015.

Kann L, McManus T, Harris WA, et al. Youth risk behavior surveillance–United States, 2015. *MMWR Surveill Summ*. 2016;65:1-174.

Markowitz LE, Dunne EF, Saraiya M, et al. Human papillomavirus vaccination: recommendations of the Advisory Committee on Immunization Practices (ACIP). *MMWR Recomm Rep*. 2014;63:1-30.

Massad LS, Einstein MH, Huh WK, et al. 2012 updated consensus guidelines for the management of abnormal cervical cancer screening tests and cancer precursors. *Obstet Gynecol*. 2013;121:829-846.

Petrosky E, Bocchini JA Jr, Hariri S, et al. Use of 9-valent human papillomavirus (HPV) vaccine: updated HPV vaccination recommendations of the Advisory Committee on Immunization Practices. *MMWR Morb Mortal Wkly Rep*. 2015;64:300-304.

Saslow D, Solomon D, Lawson HW, et al. American Cancer Society, American Society for Colposcopy and Cervical Pathology, and American Society for Clinical Pathology screening guidelines for the prevention and early detection of cervical cancer. *Am J Clin Pathol*. 2012;137:516-542.

Trojian TH, Lishnak TS, Heiman D. Epididymitis and orchitis: an overview. *Am Fam Physician*. 2009;79:583-587.

Wiesenfeld HC, Hillier SL, Meyn LA, Amortegui AJ, Sweet RL. Subclinical pelvic inflammatory disease and infertility. *Obstet Gynecol*. 2012;120:37-43.

Workowski KA, Bolan GA. Sexually transmitted diseases treatment guidelines, 2015. *MMWR Recomm Rep*. 2015;64:1-137.


# 229 Bone, Joint, and Soft Tissue Infections

Robin B. Churchill and Blanca E. Gonzalez

### INTRODUCTION

Bone and joint infections may occur at any age but are more common in children than adults. Optimal management requires early diagnosis and aggressive initial treatment to prevent disabling sequelae. This is best achieved with care provided by a multidisciplinary team of pediatricians and orthopedic surgeons experienced in the specific issues encountered in care of growing children. Soft tissue infections in children, generally less difficult to diagnose and treat than skeletal infections, remain important because of their greater frequency of occurrence and the need for antibiotic therapy, occasionally in conjunction with hospitalization and surgery.

## ACUTE HEMATOGENOUS OSTEOMYELITIS

### PATHOGENESIS AND EPIDEMIOLOGY

The majority of bone infections in children are of hematogenous origin. The vascular anatomy of long bones in children underlies the predilection for localization of blood-borne bacteria. In children, unlike young infants, the blood supply of the epiphysis is separate from the metaphysis. The nutrient artery to the metaphysis empties into a system of venous sinusoids in which sluggish flow presumably facilitates deposition of bacteria. During the *cellulitic phase* of acute osteomyelitis, infection originates on the venous side of the system and then spreads to the nutrient artery, causing thrombosis of the nutrient artery. The resultant ischemia prevents host defense mechanisms from reaching the area and allows bacterial proliferation. Formation of an abscess can then occur, which can rupture into the subperiosteal space with subsequent elevation of the periosteum, which is loosely adherent in children. If infection is uncontrolled, purulent material may extend up and down the diaphysis and circumferentially around the bone (Fig. 229-1). In areas in which the metaphysis is intra-articular, such as the hip and shoulder, the intraosseous abscess may rupture into the joint, resulting in septic arthritis. In young infants, blood vessels connect the metaphysis and epiphysis, and rupture of pus into the adjacent joint space is more common.

Thrombosis of blood vessels and elevation of the periosteum deprive the bone of its blood supply, resulting in necrosis, which can be extensive without early surgical drainage. Left untreated, granulation tissue forms around the dead bone, which separates from live bone and becomes a *sequestrum*. New bone growing around the dead bone is called an *involucrum*. Sinus tract formation occurs in the involucrum allowing pus to escape and eventually form sinus tracts through the skin. The involucrum is mechanically weak and may become the site of pathologic fractures.

Acute hematogenous osteomyelitis (AHO) is one of the most common and important invasive bacterial infections affecting children. The incidence ranges from 2 to 13 per 100,000 in developed countries, but is considerably higher (up to 200/100,000) in developing countries. Historically, the highest incidence occurred in young children, usually less than 5 years of age. More recent studies, including a large meta-analysis, show the mean age to be 6 to 9 years and the majority of children in multiple series to be in the school-age range, with only

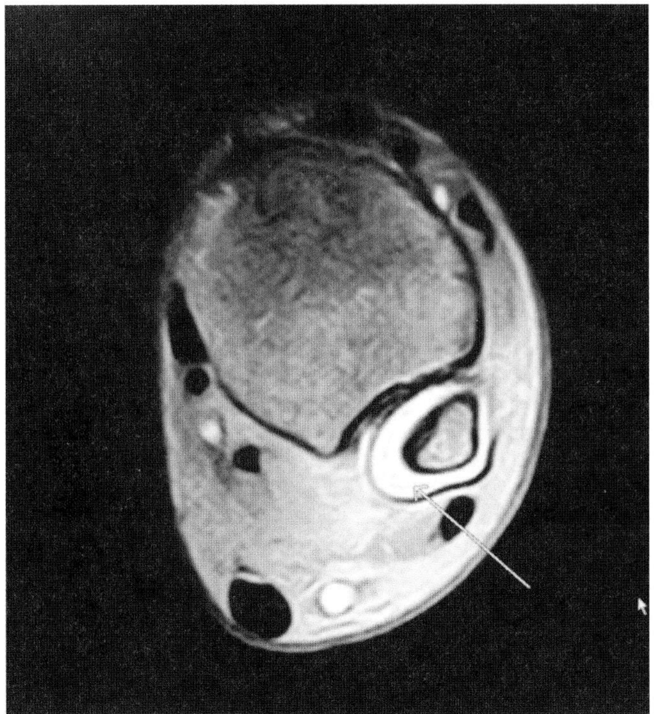

**FIGURE 229-1** Magnetic resonance imaging scan axial view demonstrating an extensive subperiosteal abscess (*arrow*) surrounding the cortex of the fibula secondary to *Staphylococcus aureus*.

40% being preschool age. There is a consistent male predilection, with males outnumbering females approximately 2:1 in published series. There is frequently a history of some type of minor blunt trauma or illness such as an upper respiratory tract infection. Other risk factors for AHO include immunodeficiency states, sickle cell anemia, and indwelling vascular catheters.

## ETIOLOGIC AGENTS

The predominant etiologic organism in AHO in all age groups is *Staphylococcus aureus*, accounting for 50% to 90% of cases. While methicillin-sensitive *S aureus* (MSSA) continues to cause the majority of infections, community-acquired methicillin-resistant *S aureus* (CA-MRSA) has also become a significant pathogen in AHO in particular geographic areas since its emergence in the late 1990s. The majority of strains circulating in the community harbor the genes encoding for the exotoxin panton valentine leukocidin (PVL). This important virulence factor has been associated with severe musculoskeletal infections in children. Studies have shown that osteomyelitis caused by PVL-positive *S aureus* strains (MSSA or MRSA) are of greater severity and are characterized by more frequent presence of subperiosteal and intraosseous abscesses as well as complications such as multifocal disease and deep venous thrombosis. This may account for the more severe disease seen in patients in certain geographic areas and should be taken into consideration in patient management.

*Streptococcus pyogenes* osteomyelitis accounts for approximately 10% of cases of AHO and is more prevalent in preschool and early school-aged children. *Streptococcus pneumoniae* is a less frequent cause of AHO, accounting for 1% to 10% of cases primarily in children less than 3 years of age and immunocompromised patients. Widespread usage of the conjugated pneumococcal vaccine may have resulted in a decline in incidence as it has with other invasive pneumococcal infections.

*Kingella kingae*, a fastidious gram-negative coccobacillus that colonizes the respiratory tract, has been increasingly recognized as an important pathogen in osteoarticular infections in children younger than 4 years of age. This organism has been reported in more than one series to cause > 50% of cases of AHO. This organism is difficult to recover and requires bone aspirates be inoculated into blood culture bottles, which then need to be incubated longer than many laboratories routinely do or sent for polymerase chain reaction (PCR) for diagnosis. *K kingae* infections tend to be associated with a less aggressive clinical course than those seen with other bacteria, causing fewer symptoms and less bone destruction.

*Streptococcus agalactiae* (group B *Streptococcus* [GBS]) and enteric gram-negative organisms occur almost exclusively in neonates. *Salmonella* is most commonly isolated in patients with AHO who have sickle cell anemia, although it can occasionally occur in normal hosts. *Haemophilus influenzae* type b, an important pathogen in older series, is now rarely seen in countries that routinely use the *H influenzae* type b conjugate vaccine. Less common organisms causing osteomyelitis include *Bartonella henselae* (the cause of cat scratch disease), *Brucella*, and *Mycobacterium tuberculosis*.

Causes of nonhematogenous osteomyelitis in children include *Pseudomonas* osteochondritis, usually resulting from puncture wounds to the feet through sneakers, and anaerobic, gram-negative, and polymicrobial infections that occur after puncture wounds or open fractures.

## CLINICAL MANIFESTATIONS

Early signs of skeletal infection may be subtle, especially in the neonate who may not appear ill. The earliest signs of osteomyelitis in infants may be failure to move the affected extremity (pseudoparalysis), pain on passive movement, or both. Older children typically present with fever, pain at the site of infection, and refusal to use the affected extremity, which usually translates to limping or refusal to bear weight because lower extremity bones are affected more frequently. Nonspecific constitutional symptoms can occur, but are not prominent. There can be intense tenderness over the metaphysis of the bone on palpation, and muscles of the adjacent joint are frequently in spasm. The joint is held in a position of comfort, usually mild flexion, but to a lesser degree than with septic arthritis. Soft tissue changes of swelling, erythema, and heat are generally late findings in osteomyelitis. After several days, a sympathetic sterile effusion may form in a nearby joint, presenting a problem in differentiation from septic arthritis. It is imperative for the evaluating physician to remember that any infant or child with fever and failure to bear weight or use an extremity needs to be carefully evaluated for potential musculoskeletal infection.

Although essentially any bone can be involved, long bones are most often involved in AHO in children. As noted, the majority of infections occur in the lower extremities, and the most common sites of involvement are the distal femoral and proximal tibial metaphyses. Next in frequency are the proximal femoral metaphysis and distal metaphyses of the radius and humerus. Infection in flat bones occurs most often in the pelvis and calcaneus, both of which can present challenges in diagnosis.

The differential diagnosis of osteomyelitis includes cellulitis, septic arthritis, pyomyositis, malignancy, collagen vascular disease, and trauma. In differentiating cellulitis from bone infection, tenderness disproportionate to physical findings suggests osteomyelitis. Septic arthritis may be differentiated from osteomyelitis by its more discrete joint findings and its greater degree of joint immobility, in addition to a lack of metaphyseal tenderness. History, physical examination, clinical scenario, and radiologic studies are helpful in differentiating skeletal infection from other diagnoses. Recovery of the causative organism is best obtained by biopsy or aspiration, which not only establishes the diagnosis but also facilitates susceptibility testing and rules out other pathologic processes.

## SPECIAL CLINICAL SITUATIONS

### Neonatal Osteomyelitis

Diagnosis of osteomyelitis in an infant who is less than 3 months of age requires a high index of suspicion. Young infants with bone infections often lack fever and other systemic signs of illness. Symptoms may be confined to failure to move an extremity and fussiness or poor feeding. Predisposing factors include a history of any of the following: prematurity, infection, bacteremia, exchange transfusion, or intravascular catheter. GBS, *S aureus*, and enteric gram-negative bacteria are the most common etiologic agents. *Candida* must also be considered, especially in the premature infant who has had previous antibiotic therapy or intravascular catheters. As noted, neonates are more likely to have decompression of pus into the adjacent joint, resulting in an associated septic arthritis, and they are also more likely to have multifocal disease.

### Pelvic Osteomyelitis

Pelvic osteomyelitis often presents a diagnostic dilemma. Most patients present with fever, limp, or refusal to bear weight. Pain may seem to be localized to the hip, groin, or buttocks, but evaluation of these areas may not reveal the site of infection. Initial diagnostic impressions often include intra-abdominal pathology, other intrapelvic problems, and septic arthritis of the hip joint. In these cases, imaging studies such as computed tomography (CT) or magnetic resonance imaging (MRI) are usually necessary to establish the diagnosis.

### Osteomyelitis in Children with Sickle Cell Disease

Aseptic bone infarcts are common in children with sickle cell disease. The signs, symptoms, and radiographic changes may mimic those of acute osteomyelitis, making differentiation between the diagnoses difficult. Neither bone scan nor MRI reliably discriminates between the 2 conditions. Ultrasonography (US) has been reported as a method assisting in differentiation between infarction and infection. A recent case-control study looking at the utility of US in distinguishing between osteomyelitis and vaso-occlusive crisis in sickle cell patients detected periosteal elevation/fluid in 84% of the osteomyelitis patients, whereas in vaso-occlusive crisis, this finding was absent in 91% on initial US and all patients on repeat US. Diagnostic aspiration of the site should be performed in an attempt to recover the organism and confirm the diagnosis. *Salmonella* species and *S aureus* are the most frequent causes of bone infection in sickle cell patients depending on the series. A recent meta-analysis showed no evidence favoring one over the other. Aggressive surgery and prolongation of parenteral therapy may be necessary for successful treatment of osteomyelitis in the child with sickle cell disease.

### Vertebral Osteomyelitis /Discitis

Vertebral osteomyelitis and discitis are 2 entities that may present similarly, with patients complaining of back pain, limp, or refusal to bear weight. Vertebral osteomyelitis accounts for 1% to 4% of osteomyelitis in children. It is seen in older children and adolescents who are usually febrile on presentation and may have had symptoms for several weeks or months. The lumbosacral area is most commonly involved. *S aureus* is the predominant organism isolated. Discitis is seen more frequently in children less than 5 years of age when blood supply to intervertebral discs is rich. These patients are seldom ill appearing, and fever is uncommon.

Plain radiographs may show narrowing of the intervertebral space with destruction of vertebral endplates in discitis. Destruction of the vertebrae is seen in vertebral osteomyelitis, but findings may not appear until later in the disease course. MRI has become the modality of choice to differentiate one entity from the other.

## DIAGNOSIS

Figure 229-2 outlines an approach to the diagnosis and management of a patient with suspected AHO. No specific laboratory test for the diagnosis of osteomyelitis exists with the exception of isolation of a pathogen from bone.

### Bone Aspiration and Biopsy

Bone cultures are positive in 38% to 91% of cases and confirm the diagnosis. Blood cultures are also very useful, demonstrating the organism in 30% to 76% of cases. The highest diagnostic yield occurs when both blood and bone specimens are submitted for culture. Recovery of organisms is enhanced by inoculating bone aspirates into blood culture bottles. This is particularly important when fastidious organisms (eg, *Kingella*) are suspected, which may require up to

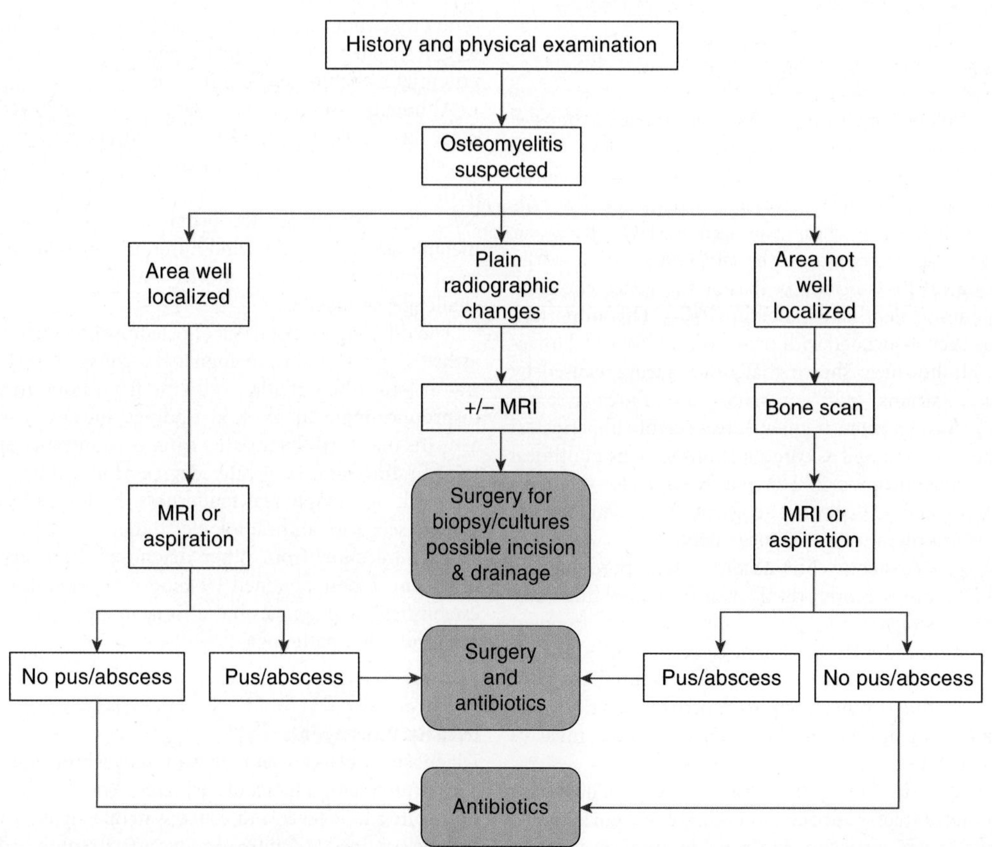


**FIGURE 229-2** An algorithmic approach to the management of suspected acute hematogenous osteomyelitis. MRI, magnetic resonance imaging. (Adapted with permission from Churchill JA, Mazur JM: Ankle Pain in Children: Diagnostic Evaluation and Clinical Decision Making, *J Am Acad Orthop Surg*. 1995 Jul;3(4):183-193.)

a week of incubation before growth is evident. Alternatively, bone aspirates can be submitted for PCR testing when trying to establish a diagnosis in culture-negative osteomyelitis. In multiple studies, PCR testing has been shown to be particularly useful for the diagnosis of *Kingella* AHO, but when available, can also be used to identify other organisms in cases where conventional cultures are negative.

The ability to recover an organism from blood or bone cultures decreases significantly with prior antimicrobial therapy. Therefore, if the patient is stable, and blood and bone cultures can be done in a timely fashion, it is preferable to delay the initiation of antibiotics until cultures are obtained.

#### Other Laboratory Studies

Peripheral white blood cell count (WBC) and differential may or may not be abnormal. The erythrocyte sedimentation rate (ESR) rises slowly and initially may be normal or minimally elevated. ESR usually peaks 3 to 5 days after the initiation of therapy and returns to normal in 3 to 6 weeks. Many experts find C-reactive protein (CRP) to be more useful because it rises earlier, peaks within 48 hours of onset of symptoms, and may return to normal after approximately 1 week of effective therapy. Surgical intervention itself increases inflammatory markers; therefore, baseline ESR and CRP values used for monitoring disease progression should be repeated after surgical intervention if such are necessary.

#### Plain Radiographs

Plain films begin to show destructive changes approximately 7 to 14 days after the onset of bone infection. Subtle osteopenic changes may sometimes be discerned after 5 days. Plain films may be helpful acutely in demonstrating changes in the deep soft tissue adjacent to the affected bone, or joint effusion, as well as excluding other pathology such as fractures. To detect alterations of the soft tissue, identical views of the contralateral limb are recommended.

#### Radionuclide Scanning

When a bone scan is indicated, radiophosphate bone scintigraphy using technetium ($^{99}$Tc) is most commonly used. Isotope accumulates to a greater degree in areas of increased vascularity and rapid bone turnover, resulting in a *hot spot* reflected on the scan. Conversely, infected areas may have associated compromise of the vascular supply, causing the area to appear *cold* or normal, resulting in a false-negative interpretation. Although bone scans have a high degree of sensitivity, they do not make the diagnosis of skeletal infection. Bone scans indicate abnormal areas of bone without revealing whether the abnormality is due to infection, tumor, injury, or other causes. Although the ready availability of MRI in many areas has largely replaced bone scanning, there is still a role in selected cases. Bone scans are particularly helpful in cases where the site of infection is not readily apparent by physical examination or when multiple sites of involvement are suspected. If the site of infection can be localized by physical examination, a bone scan is not necessary. It has been shown experimentally that aspiration of bone (or joint) does not compromise results of subsequent bone scans.

Gallium scans or indium-labeled leukocyte scans are less commonly used techniques in the diagnosis of skeletal infection. Indium-labeled leukocyte scans, which reflect migration of WBCs into areas of inflammation, are useful in the diagnosis of osteomyelitis associated with trauma, recent surgery, or prosthetic devices.

#### Magnetic Resonance Imaging

MRI has become the most commonly used imaging study for the diagnosis of osteomyelitis. It is an effective modality for imaging bone and is quite sensitive and specific in diagnosis of musculoskeletal infections. It is not recommended as a screening study but is very useful when there is an indication of where the pathology is localized, either from physical examination or radionuclide scanning. It can be especially helpful in cases in which the spine or the pelvis is the site of infection, or conflicting clinical data exist, or in planning surgical intervention. Many orthopedic surgeons request a preoperative MRI because the spatial resolution of MRI is far superior to other modalities. Additionally, conditions requiring surgical intervention such as bone abscesses, subperiosteal abscesses, joint effusions, and pyomyositis are readily determined by MRI.

### TREATMENT

Initial antibiotic therapy for osteomyelitis should be based on Gram-stained specimens obtained from bone aspiration, when possible. The importance of obtaining the exact bacteriologic diagnosis by blood or bone culture cannot be overemphasized. In the absence of such data, initial therapy is empiric and must be directed at likely pathogens based on the age of child, considering underlying medical conditions and the clinical presentation of the patient (see Fig. 229-2).

Because *S aureus* is the major pathogen of AHO, empiric therapy for all age groups should include an appropriate antistaphylococcal agent. Nafcillin, oxacillin, or a first-generation cephalosporin remain the antibiotics of choice for coverage of MSSA and are also effective against *K kingae* and *S pyogenes*. However, it is important to know the rates of infection caused by CA-MRSA locally prior to choosing empiric treatment regimens. Multiple studies have proven the effectiveness of clindamycin in the treatment of osteomyelitis. However, *S aureus* (MSSA or MRSA) may be resistant to this drug, either inherently or induced during treatment. In cases where initial studies show *S aureus* to be susceptible to clindamycin but resistant to erythromycin, the presence of inducible resistance should be evaluated in vitro with a D-test. When the inherent or inducible resistance rates in the community are greater than 10% to 15%, some experts recommend clindamycin alone not be used for initial treatment. Use of vancomycin, particularly in combination with a β-lactam, can be considered in the critically ill patient or in areas with high rates of MRSA and clindamycin resistance. It is important to recognize that *Kingella* isolates tend to be resistant to both clindamycin and vancomycin.

In the young infant, GBS and *S aureus* are the major pathogens, but coverage for enteric gram-negatives must be included. An appropriate initial therapeutic regimen includes an antistaphylococcal agent plus a third-generation cephalosporin, such as cefotaxime.

In children less than 4 years of age, a regimen providing coverage for *S aureus, S pyogenes, S pneumoniae*, and *Kingella* should be used. An antistaphylococcal agent plus a third-generation cephalosporin may provide appropriate coverage.

In immunocompromised children or those with underlying medical conditions, broader-spectrum coverage may be appropriate. If *Pseudomonas* is a consideration, an antipseudomonal agent may be part of the regimen.

Once an organism is identified, therapy should be guided by susceptibilities. If MSSA is identified, nafcillin, oxacillin, or a first-generation cephalosporin is the agent of choice. Cefazolin and other cephalosporins have been shown to reach adequate concentrations in bone tissue, provide convenient dosing schedules, and generally be better tolerated.

Newer antimicrobials have been shown to be acceptable alternatives for the treatment of MRSA osteomyelitis. Linezolid can be used in selected situations. It achieves excellent levels in bone and has equivalent intravenous and oral bioavailability. It has been shown to be effective in step-down therapy of AHO caused by gram-positive organisms but has several disadvantages. It remains expensive, and long-term therapy (> 2 weeks) has been associated with anemia and thrombocytopenia, and thus, weekly blood counts are required when using it. It can also have other serious adverse effects including optic neuritis, peripheral neuropathy, and serotonin syndrome when used in combination with selective serotonin reuptake inhibitors (SSRIs) and sympathomimetic drugs. Daptomycin is another alternative that can be considered in selected situations, but has no oral equivalent and is not approved by the US Food and Drug Administration (FDA) for treatment of osteomyelitis in children. Daptomycin has FDA approval for treatment of pediatric skin and soft tissue infections.

If possible, initiating treatment with a single agent is preferred. If cultures remain sterile, treatment should be continued based on the most common organism for the age group, usually *S aureus*. If there is no response to treatment, less common organisms may be suspected, although there may be other causes as well (eg, the common etiologic agent is resistant to the chosen antibiotic regimen or there are complications of the infection). In children under 4 years of age with negative cultures, *K kingae* should strongly be considered.

There are several options for delivery of antibiotic therapy in the treatment of osteomyelitis. Therapy may be completed parenterally through a central venous catheter or a peripherally inserted central catheter (PICC); however, this is much less common today than it was in the past. The most commonly used option currently is to initiate therapy parenterally, followed by orally administered drugs after any necessary surgical procedures have been performed and the clinical condition has stabilized. Oral therapy instituted after an initial course of parenteral therapy is equally effective compared to continued parenteral therapy when the responsible organism and its susceptibilities are defined, although parenteral treatment is associated with more adverse events related to the catheter. The selected option depends on a patient's particular situation considering factors such as location, extent, and severity of disease, as well as the patient's ability to tolerate oral therapy and the likelihood of compliance. It is important to recognize that the length of parenteral therapy is dependent on the patient's response to therapy and may need to be extended in severe disease or in immunocompromised patients. Evidence that a patient can safely be transitioned to oral therapy per some experts has been a combination of subjective and objective clinical findings such as defervescence, increased use of the affected extremity, and a decrease in CRP.

When sequential parenteral/oral therapy is implemented, the oral drug chosen should be active against the identified pathogen, or if the pathogen has not been isolated, when possible, it should be identical in spectrum of activity to the parenteral drug to which the patient has shown clinical response. Contraindications to oral therapy include the inability to swallow or retain medication, lack of an effective oral agent, and failure to demonstrate adequate clinical response to parenteral antibiotics. In older literature, failure to demonstrate the etiologic agent and an inability to monitor the degree of drug absorption were considered contraindications to oral therapy; however, that edict is no longer followed. Especially in young children, palatability of oral suspensions is an important feature. In general, cephalosporins are more palatable than antistaphylococcal penicillins, which are seldom used. Clindamycin is an excellent drug for staphylococcal osteomyelitis in older children, but many young children may not tolerate the taste of the oral solution.

Dosages of oral antibiotics required in sequential intravenous-oral regimens are 2 to 3 times those used for minor infections. It is optimal to monitor absorption of oral antibiotics and compliance by measurement of serum bactericidal levels against the isolated organism or measurement of antibiotic serum levels; however, in practice, these are almost never done.

The minimum or optimum duration of antimicrobial therapy for acute osteomyelitis is unknown. The usual recommended duration is 4 to 6 weeks, but depends on the cause and extent of infection as well as clinical and laboratory response. Older literature suggested that courses of 3 weeks or less were associated with a greater likelihood of relapse or recurrence. However, some newer studies have shown successful outcomes with 3 weeks of therapy. Each patient must be evaluated individually, taking into account the speed of clinical response, whether surgical debridement was done, normalization of CRP or ESR, and radiologic findings.

The need for open surgery in osteomyelitis depends on the extent of the pathologic process in individual patients and likely somewhat on the virulence of the specific pathogen. In children who present early in the "cellulitic phase," antibiotic therapy alone is usually sufficient for treatment. If pus is encountered during diagnostic aspiration, if a subperiosteal or intramedullary abscess is detected by ultrasound or MRI, or if a bone lesion is evident on plain films, surgical intervention may be warranted. Patients initiated on medical therapy who do not promptly improve should also be evaluated for surgical intervention. Surgical drainage and debridement removes inflammatory products more rapidly than do host defense mechanisms, providing a more effective environment for antibiotic penetration and preventing further bone necrosis. Drainage of an abscess also reduces the inoculum of bacteria present. Any patient with a lytic lesion on plain films should have, in addition to cultures, the bone biopsy sent to pathology for histology and special stains to rule out other pathologic processes such as malignancy and to evaluate for unusual organisms such as fungi or acid-fast bacilli.

It is well accepted that *Pseudomonas* osteochondritis of the foot following a nail penetrating the foot through a sneaker is mainly a surgical disease. When thorough curettage and debridement are achieved, 10 days of antipseudomonal therapy are usually sufficient.

### COMPLICATIONS AND OUTCOMES

#### Chronic Osteomyelitis

The most common complication of AHO is chronic or recurrent osteomyelitis, which occurs in fewer than 5% of cases. Symptoms may include chronic or recurrent pain, swelling, erythema, or purulent discharge, and in some cases, sinus tract formation. Development of chronic osteomyelitis is more common following nonhematogenous osteomyelitis (eg, following penetrating trauma). The hallmark of chronic osteomyelitis is bone necrosis. Therapy is primarily surgical with adjunctive long-term antibiotics. A bone biopsy should be obtained in chronic osteomyelitis for culture and for histopathology to exclude Langerhans cell histiocytosis, malignancy, and other causes.

With the increase in PVL-positive *S aureus* strains, especially in CA-MRSA, there has been an increase in cases of severe sepsis in adolescents with the involvement of multiple sites of osteomyelitis and septic arthritis. Deep venous thromboses have also been encountered more frequently in patients with CA-MRSA osteomyelitis but can also occur in patients infected with PVL-positive strains of MSSA. The thrombosis is usually in a vein adjacent to the infected bone site. Septic emboli have been seen in such patients leading to severe respiratory compromise. Patients who have evidence of septic emboli or persistent bacteremia should be evaluated for deep venous thrombosis by Doppler ultrasonography. Those with persistent bacteremia should also be evaluated for other causes such as endocarditis.

#### Other Complications and Outcomes

Pathologic fractures can occur but are rare. If the bone growth plate is involved, there is a risk of abnormal length of the affected bone. In general, the outcome of well-managed cases of acute osteomyelitis in pediatric patients is favorable.

## SEPTIC ARTHRITIS

### PATHOGENESIS AND EPIDEMIOLOGY

The anatomy of the synovial joint provides an environment conducive to bacterial infection. The synovial tissue lining the joint lacks a basement membrane and therefore secretes a transudate of serum. The rest of the joint surface is composed of avascular cartilage. Bacteria enter the joint by hematogenous seeding, direct extension from an adjacent focus, or direct inoculation during a joint aspiration, arthrotomy, or trauma. Initially, after bacterial invasion occurs, the synovial membrane swells and produces increased amounts of fluid, distending the joint. If infection persists without treatment, pus accumulates in the area and destruction of cartilage follows. Subluxation or dislocation of the joint may result from increased intra-articular pressure occurring when the joint capsule is distended by purulent fluid. This increased pressure may compromise blood supply in certain areas. In the hip, this may lead to avascular necrosis of the femoral head.

Delayed or inadequate treatment of a septic joint can result in permanent joint damage with subsequent disability. Septic arthritis is most common in children less than 3 years of age. In most cases, a single, large joint is involved, usually in the lower extremity. As with osteomyelitis, males are affected more frequently. There may be a history of trauma or recent infection of the skin or upper respiratory tract. Predisposing factors for the development of septic arthritis vary with age. For example, in neonates, the presence of indwelling catheters including those in the umbilical vessels increases the risk, whereas in older children, risk factors include underlying medical conditions such as immunodeficiencies, diabetes, juvenile idiopathic arthritis (JIA), and hemoglobinopathies.

## ETIOLOGIC AGENTS

As in osteomyelitis, etiologic agents of septic arthritis vary by age. *S aureus* (MSSA and MRSA) is the leading organism in all age groups. In neonates, GBS and enteric gram-negative organisms are also important to consider and may be isolated from an affected joint as a consequence of an adjacent osteomyelitis. *S aureus, S pyogenes, K kingae*, and *S pneumoniae* are the most prominent causative pathogens in children less than 4 years of age. *H influenzae* type b, the most common organism in this age group in the past, is rarely seen now in countries that routinely vaccinate against this agent. In children older than 4 years, *S aureus* and *S pyogenes* are the chief pathogens.

Other bacteria reported to cause septic arthritis in children include *Neisseria meningitidis, Pseudomonas* (eg, following a nail injury through a sneaker), and enteric gram-negative organisms, including *Salmonella* (eg, sickle cell patients). *Neisseria gonorrhoeae* is a consideration in neonates and sexually active adolescents. Rat bite fever, an uncommon zoonotic disease caused by *Streptobacillus moniliformis* usually presents with the triad of fever, rash, and polyarthritis, and may be seen in children with exposure to rats as pets or otherwise.

Fungal septic arthritis is rare but occasionally encountered, especially in the immunocompromised host. Neonates, especially premature infants, who often have indwelling catheters and are exposed to broad-spectrum antibiotics, may develop septic arthritis caused by *Candida* species. Certain endemic mycoses such as coccidiomycosis, blastomycosis, and histoplasmosis may cause extrapulmonary manifestations in which bones and joints may be involved. The most common joint affected in patients with extrapulmonary blastomycosis is the knee followed by the ankle and elbow joints.

## CLINICAL MANIFESTATIONS

Children generally present acutely with a painful, erythematous, warm joint, and refusal to move or bear weight on the affected extremity. Fever, toxicity, and irritability are often accompanying features. The joint is held in the position of most comfort, usually mild flexion. When the hip is involved, erythema or joint swelling is generally not obvious, but the affected hip is held in a position of flexion, abduction, and external rotation. Young children may exhibit the phenomenon of "referred pain," in which symptoms from an infected hip joint are referred to the ipsilateral knee. The differential diagnosis of septic arthritis includes cellulitis, bursitis, osteomyelitis (including patellar) with or without a sympathetic effusion, reactive arthritis, transient synovitis, arthritis associated with systemic disease such as JIA, or malignancy.

## DIAGNOSIS

Because of the risk of long-term orthopedic complications, septic arthritis is an orthopedic emergency. Joint aspiration is the most important component of the diagnostic evaluation. Other laboratory tests and radiologic studies are generally nonspecific, but findings may be useful to direct the evaluation (Fig. 229-3).

### Joint Aspiration

For patients in whom the diagnosis of septic arthritis is suspected, aspirating the affected joint can be both diagnostic and in many cases therapeutic. Synovial fluid should be sent for Gram stain, aerobic cultures, and cell count with a leukocyte differential. Anaerobic, fungal, and acid-fast bacilli (AFB) cultures may be considered in some instances (eg, immunocompromised patients, penetrating injuries to the joint, postprocedure septic arthritis). Joint fluid cultures are positive in 30% to 60% of cases. Inoculation of joint fluid into blood culture bottles increases the yield of cultures, particularly when the etiologic agent is fastidious such as in the case of *K kingae*. Leukocyte counts greater than 50,000 cells/μL, with a predominance of segmented neutrophils, are suggestive of bacterial arthritis, even in the absence of a positive culture. However, it should be recognized that WBCs in infected joint fluid can vary widely, ranging from 2000 to 300,000/μL. Synovial fluid glucose and protein may be measured but are nonspecific.

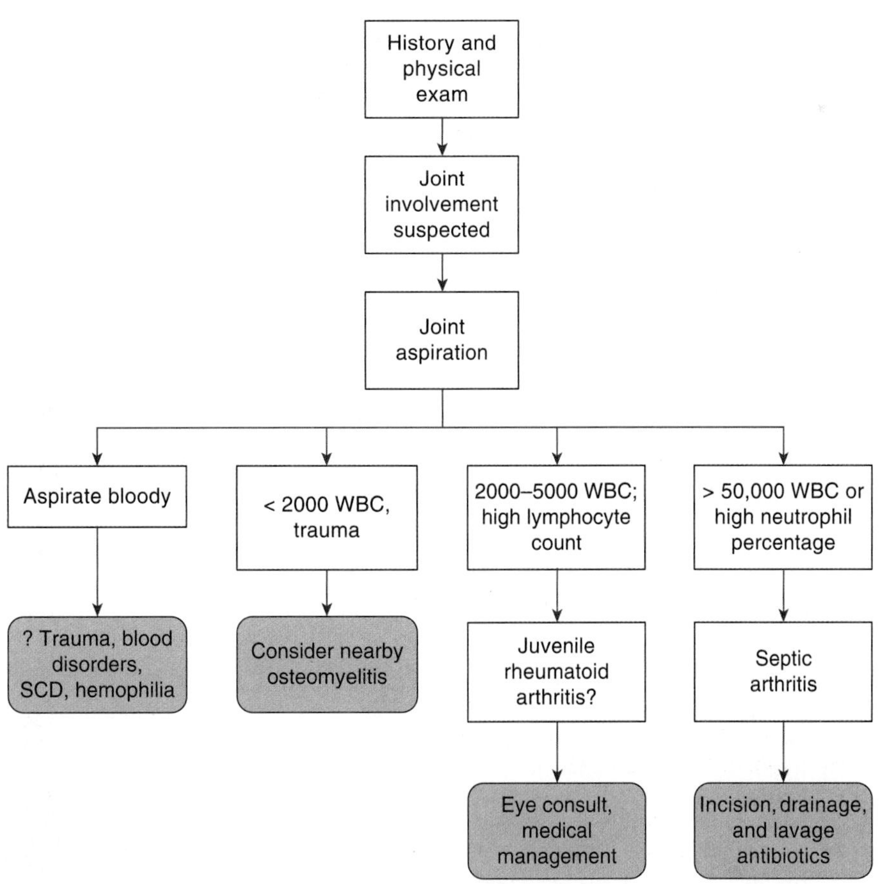


**FIGURE 229-3** An algorithmic approach to the management of suspected septic arthritis. SCD, sickle cell disease.

### Other Laboratory Tests

In addition to cultures of joint fluid, it is important to obtain blood cultures, which are positive 30% to 40% of the time. The combination of blood and joint fluid cultures reveals an etiologic agent in approximately 70% of cases. As in osteomyelitis, peripheral WBC, ESR, and CRP may be useful in the workup of the patient with suspected joint infection but are nonspecific. Although frequently abnormal, they do not confirm or exclude the diagnosis. CRP and ESR are valuable adjuncts in gauging response to therapy.

Molecular techniques have improved the diagnosis of culture-negative septic arthritis. PCR techniques are being more frequently utilized, especially when fastidious organisms such as *Kingella* species are suspected or in patients pretreated with antimicrobial agents. These techniques are currently available only in specialized laboratories, are costly, and may have long turnaround times, limiting their widespread use at this time.

### Radiologic Studies

Plain films may demonstrate evidence of soft tissue swelling or widening of the joint space. In the hip, lateral displacement or subluxation of the femoral head may be evident. Normal plain films do not eliminate the possibility of pyogenic arthritis of a joint. Ultrasonography is a reliable method of detecting joint fluid, especially in the hip. It has the advantage of being noninvasive, usually does not require sedation, and generally is more readily available than MRI. MRI is also a sensitive method for detecting joint fluid and may demonstrate abnormalities in adjacent bone or soft tissues. The need for MRI should be discussed with the consulting orthopedic surgeon.

## TREATMENT

Figure 229-3 illustrates an approach to the diagnosis and management of septic arthritis. An orthopedic surgeon experienced in the treatment of children should be involved in the management of the child with septic arthritis. The goals of therapy are as follows: decompression of the joint space and removal of inflammatory debris by adequate drainage; sterilization of the joint through the use of appropriate antimicrobial agents; relief of pain; and prevention of joint deformity.

Drainage of the infected joint may require repeated aspiration, arthroscopic lavage, or open drainage with lavage. Repeated aspiration may be appropriate in a setting where no surgeon is readily available to perform arthroscopic or open drainage, but drainage with lavage, either via an arthroscopic or an open procedure, is superior because it allows thorough cleansing and removal of inflammatory debris that cannot be evacuated by aspiration. Arthrotomy may not be necessary for infection of all joints, but is indicated for patients who fail to respond to repeated joint aspirations and in those with infections of the hip (and perhaps the shoulder). Recently, arthroscopic techniques have become more popular and cause less morbidity with similar results.

Antimicrobial therapy should be instituted immediately after blood cultures and joint fluid samples are obtained. Empiric, initial antibiotic choice is based on the likely pathogens at various ages, the results of Gram stain of the joint aspirate, and any special considerations dictated by the patient's underlying medical problems or clinical situation.

Empiric choice of antimicrobials is similar to that recommended for osteomyelitis, and regimens for all age groups should include an antistaphylococcal agent with coverage for MRSA as dictated by local prevalence. If *N gonorrhoeae* is a consideration, ceftriaxone or cefotaxime should be used. Parenteral antibiotics are used initially and continued until there is no further need for surgical intervention and the child is afebrile with clinical improvement and improvement of laboratory parameters. Exact length of therapy is dependent on the clinical situation, the patient's response, and the particular organism. Traditionally, therapy is continued for at least 2 weeks after the patient is afebrile, joint fluid accumulation has resolved, and laboratory parameters have normalized. A prospective, randomized study in Finland showed that shorter courses (3–4 days of intravenous therapy followed by oral therapy to complete 10–14 days) may suffice for MSSA septic arthritis. Clindamycin and oral cephalosporins at high doses were used in the study. In immunocompromised individuals, neonates, and other special populations, therapy should be individualized.

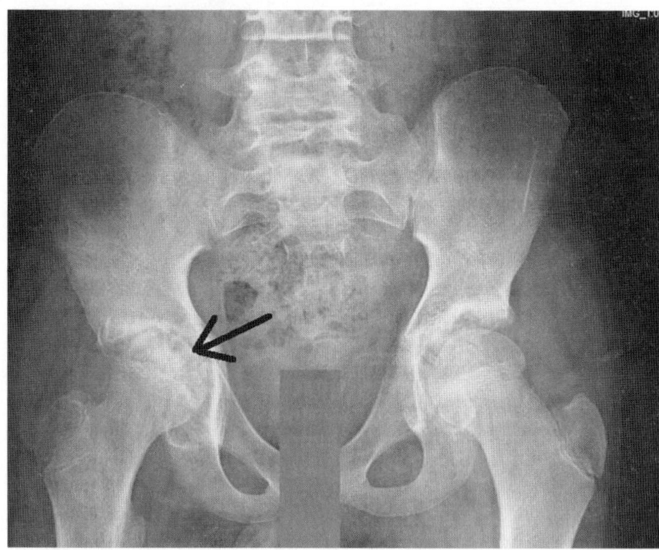

**FIGURE 229-4** Anteroposterior pelvis x-ray showing chondrolysis as evidenced by narrowing of the joint space and mottling of the femoral head of the right hip suggestive of early avascular necrosis (*arrow*) in an adolescent patient with *Staphylococcus aureus* septic arthritis in whom the diagnosis was delayed.

## PROGNOSIS AND OUTCOMES

Sequelae of septic arthritis include joint deformity and residual dysfunction, abnormal bone growth, and in the hip, avascular necrosis of the femoral head (Fig. 229-4). Risk factors for subsequent complications include delay in drainage, age < 1 year, involvement of the hip or shoulder, adjacent osteomyelitis, and infection with *S aureus*.

# SKIN AND SOFT TISSUE INFECTIONS

In many areas of the United States, the emergence of CA-MRSA has been accompanied by a marked increase in the incidence of skin and soft tissue infections, which are one of the most common manifestations of this pathogen.

It is important to differentiate uncomplicated cellulitis from other more serious disorders that require more aggressive therapy. For example, it is often difficult to determine if there may be underlying pyomyositis, osteomyelitis, or septic arthritis. Tenderness disproportionate to the soft tissue findings suggests involvement of deeper structures. It is also very important to differentiate uncomplicated cellulitis from the more serious condition of necrotizing fasciitis due to *S pyogenes*. Single or multiple skin abscesses often develop in conjunction with cellulitis caused by *S aureus*. In 2014, the Infectious Disease Society of America (IDSA) updated the Practice Guidelines for the Diagnosis and Management of Skin and Soft Tissue Infections, which are available at www.idsociety.org.

## CELLULITIS, ERYSIPELAS, AND ABSCESSES

Cellulitis is an acute localized infection of the skin involving the subcutaneous tissues. Infection usually develops as a result of a breach in skin integrity or an associated skin lesion. The term has been used interchangeably with "erysipelas," although for some, the latter refers to an infection limited to the superficial layers of the skin, whereas cellulitis involves deeper structures. Gram-positive organisms, primarily *S aureus* (including MRSA) and *S pyogenes*, account for the majority of infections. Other organisms may occasionally be involved, particularly in neonates, in the immunocompromised host, or after trauma. Extremities are frequent sites of infection because they are more subject to minor trauma that may go unnoticed. Cellulitis in certain locations may be associated with an underlying process. Some examples include cellulitis over the buccal area associated with an odontogenic infection or cellulitis behind the ear, which is a common feature of mastoiditis.

The presence of cellulitis is usually easily recognized clinically by findings of erythema, warmth, and edema of an area. Isolating the etiologic agent in the absence of an associated abscess or purulent skin lesion is frequently difficult. Blood cultures are positive in a minority of cases, usually only those with systemic symptoms. If there is an abscess or purulent skin lesion present, material for Gram stain and culture should be obtained during drainage, which should be performed. Some literature discusses skin aspiration of cellulitis; however, in practice this is seldom performed because the yield of these cultures is low. Cultures of the skin via aspiration or punch biopsy is important in patients with malignancies, in patients who develop cellulitis after penetrating trauma, and in immunocompromised patients, as less common organisms may be isolated. Purulent collections within the skin are abscesses, and the most common etiology in children is *S aureus*.

Therapy in the immunocompetent child should be aimed at *S aureus* and *S pyogenes* and based on local susceptibility patterns for them. Incision and drainage constitute the primary therapy for purulent skin and soft tissue infections. Failure to perform incision and drainage has been associated with a lack of clinical response in patients with *S aureus* skin and soft tissue infections in a recent series. In the afebrile, nontoxic child, drainage alone is sometimes sufficient treatment. Oral therapy for cellulitis alone or as an adjunct to the incision and drainage of abscesses should include agents with coverage for MSSA, MRSA, and *S pyogenes*. First-generation cephalosporins provide excellent coverage if MRSA is not suspected. Clindamycin is a reasonable choice in areas where most MRSA and *S pyogenes* are susceptible. Doxycycline is an alternative for older children but may not provide adequate coverage for *S pyogenes* strains. Trimethoprim/sulfamethoxazole is also an option if *S pyogenes* is unlikely based on Gram stain results. Parenteral therapy should be used in the febrile patient if progression is rapid or if associated lymphangitis or lymphadenitis is present. Again, initial Gram stain results, if available, can be used to guide selection of therapy. Five to 10 days of therapy are usually sufficient for uncomplicated cellulitis if the infection has improved after 5 days. In more severe infections, treatment can be achieved by sequential parenteral-oral therapy as the patient's condition warrants.

## NECROTIZING SOFT TISSUE INFECTIONS

Some of the most feared skin and soft tissue infections are the necrotizing group: necrotizing fasciitis (NF), gas gangrene, and Fournier necrosis. These infections are life threatening and require a prompt and multidisciplinary approach between the pediatrician, surgeon, and infectious diseases physician. NF is a rare but rapidly progressive condition in which infection spreads to the fascia and subcutaneous tissues causing tissue necrosis. This condition was classically described in patients with varicella complicated by *S pyogenes* superinfection and subsequent development of NF. Other organisms that have been associated with the development of NF are *Pseudomonas* species, *Aeromonas hydrophila*, *Vibrio vulnificus*, *S aureus*, and anaerobic streptococci. Initially, NF may be indistinguishable from cellulitis, but usually the patients are toxic and experience pain that is out of proportion to the physical findings. As the disease progresses, bullous lesions, gas in the soft tissues (crepitation), and skin necrosis may become evident. Even though CT and MRI may help establish the diagnosis, the diagnosis is mainly clinical, and obtaining additional imaging may delay prompt initiation of appropriate treatment, which is surgical. It is common for patients to go to the operating room repeatedly until no further debridement is needed. Cultures obtained at the time of surgical intervention usually establish the infecting agent. Initial antibiotic therapy should be broad and should cover *S pyogenes, S aureus*, and anaerobic organisms. Frequently used antimicrobials include vancomycin or linezolid combined with either piperacillin/tazobactam, a carbapenem, or ceftriaxone plus metronidazole. Once an organism has been identified, then the antimicrobial spectrum should be narrowed. IDSA guidelines recommend continuation of therapy until no further surgical debridement is required, there is clinical improvement, and fever is absent for 48 to 72 hours.

Fournier necrosis is a clinical condition very similar to NF, but is localized to the perineum and external genitalia. It is a rare occurrence in pediatrics; however, cases have been described, especially in premature infants and immunocompromised children. Contrary to adults, the outcome is not as often fatal but necessitates the same aggressive therapy as NF.

Gas gangrene, also known as clostridial myonecrosis, is a rapidly progressive infection of the muscles caused by *Clostridium* species. When the infection stems from trauma, the usual organism is *Clostridium perfringens*, whereas when it is a result of seeding from a gastrointestinal source, *Clostridium septicum* is the most common organism. In the case of trauma, pain ensues 24 hours after the injury, progressing rapidly to necrosis with changes in skin color and the appearance of bullous lesions. Crepitation is a later finding. These patients are very ill, progressing rapidly to multiorgan system failure. In the nontrauma form, it is mainly seen in neutropenic patients (including patients with congenital or cyclic neutropenia) and presents with abrupt onset of severe pain accompanied by fever. The involved extremity may become edematous and change color to a purplish hue. Bacteremia precedes the infection, and therefore, blood cultures are useful. Similar to NF, combination therapy to cover *Clostridium* species in addition to *S aureus*, streptococci, and anaerobes is recommended; however, surgery is the mainstay of treatment.

## PYOMYOSITIS

Also known as tropical pyomyositis, pyomyositis is an infection of the skeletal muscle characterized by phlegmon or abscess formation within the muscle tissue. Usually nonpenetrating trauma and vigorous activity seem to be predisposing factors in children. The most common symptoms include fever, swelling, and pain over the affected area and limp depending on the involved area. The most common involved sites are the proximal thigh and the hip. *S aureus* is the most common isolated organism (75%) followed by *S pyogenes, S pneumoniae*, and occasionally enteric gram-negatives. Laboratory studies usually reveal an elevated WBC, CRP, and ESR, but the creatinine kinase may be normal in the cases of hematogenous spread. The diagnosis is usually established by MRI. Occasionally, pyomyositis is associated with osteomyelitis. The treatment will vary depending whether a drainable abscess is present, in which case incision and drainage should be performed promptly. In patients in whom only a phlegmon is found, prolonged antibiotic therapy should be curative. The length of therapy for pyomyositis is usually 3 to 4 weeks using sequential parenteral-oral therapy.

## SUGGESTED READINGS

Arnold JC, Bradley JS. Osteoarticular infections in children. *Infect Dis Clin North Am*. 2015;29:557-574.

Dartnell J, Ramachandran M, Katchburian M. Haematogenous acute and subacute paediatric osteomyelitis. A systematic review of the literature. *J Bone Joint Surg Br*. 2012;94-B:584-585.

Ilharredorbe B. Sequelae of pediatric osteoarticular infection. *Orthop Traumatol Surg Res*. 2015;101:S129-S137.

Keren R, Shah S, Srivastava R, et al. Comparative effectiveness of intravenous vs oral antibiotics for postdischarge treatment of acute osteomyelitis in children. *JAMA Pediatr*. 2015;169:120-128.

Liu C, Bayer A, Cosgrove S, et al. Clinical practice guidelines by the infectious diseases society of america for the treatment of methicillin-resistant *Staphylococcus aureus* infections in adults and children. *Clin Infect Dis*. 2011;52:1-38.

Pannaraj P, Hulten KG, Gonzalez BE, et al. Infective pyomyositis and myositis in children in the era of community-acquired, methicillin-resistant *Staphylococcus aureus* infection. *Clin Infect Dis.* 2006;43:953-960.

Peltola H, Paakkonen M, Kallio P, et al. Short- versus long-term antimicrobial treatment for acute hematogenous osteomyelitis of childhood: prospective, randomized trial of 131 culture-positive cases. *Pediatr Infect Dis J.* 2010;29:1123-1127.

Peltola H, Paakkonen M, Kallio P, et al. Prospective, randomized trial of 10 days versus 30 days of antimicrobial treatment, including a short-term course of parenteral therapy, for childhood septic arthritis. *Clin Infect Dis.* 2009;48:1201-1210.

Sukswai P, Kovitvanitcha D, Thumkunanon V, et al. Acute hematogenous osteomyelitis and septic arthritis in children: clinical characteristics and outcome study. *J Med Assoc Thai.* 2011;94:S209-S216.

Tanwar YS, Jaiswal A, Singh S, Arya RK, Lal H. Acute pediatric septic arthritis: a systematic review of literature and current controversies. *Pol Orthop Traumatol.* 2014;79:23-29.

# 230 Cardiac Infections

Joseph R. Block and Rodney E. Willoughby

## ENDOCARDITIS

### INTRODUCTION

Infective endocarditis (IE) in pediatric patients is rare (5–12 per 100,000 pediatric admissions) and often associated with an underlying congenital heart defect or, increasingly, central indwelling intravascular catheters. However, structurally normal hearts may also be infected. Premature infants now account for 10% of pediatric IE. Endovascular infections outside the heart and infected thrombi are close cognates of IE.

### PATHOGENESIS AND EPIDEMIOLOGY

Establishment of IE results from the interaction of several host and microbial factors. Experimental animal models have demonstrated that damage to the endocardium (as with a plastic catheter or a high-velocity jet of blood) leads to formation of a nonbacterial thrombotic lesion. Following endocardial damage, bacterial access to the bloodstream from elsewhere and subsequent adherence to endocardial surfaces are required for the establishment of IE. It is now thought that the great majority of IE develops as the result of transient bacteremia related to activities of daily life, but not all bacteria are capable of initiating this process. The endocardium appears to be a preferential site of microbial adherence and may have some specificity for binding with certain bacteria. The presence of several factors, including bacterial adhesins, endothelial binding proteins, and agglutinating antibodies that clump bacteria, promotes adherence of organisms to damaged endocardial surfaces. The Venturi effect (the reduction in fluid pressure that results when blood flows through a constricted area) deposits bacterial colonies immediately beyond the orifice that separates high- and low-pressure areas.

Bacteremia in patients with established endocarditis is generally low grade and continuous. As many as 10% of cases of IE yield consistently negative blood cultures, most often as a result of prior antibiotic therapy or organisms that are difficult to culture. Bacteria infecting right-sided heart lesions may be filtered by pulmonary phagocytes, significantly reducing the number of bacteria in a peripheral blood sample.

Classically, viridans streptococci have been the most common cause of IE, progressing along a subacute course in patients with preexisting cardiac lesions in which fever, fatigue, and immune complex–mediated clinical manifestations develop slowly over weeks or months. Enterococci behave in a fashion similar to the viridans streptococci. IE caused by *Staphylococcus aureus* has historically followed an acute course with rapid progression and poor outcome, including death, often in patients with normal hearts. Prosthetic heart valves within 2 months after implantation are prone to infection with coagulase-negative staphylococci and *S aureus*, as are neonates who require intensive care and intracardiac central lines. Gram-negative infections of the heart, although infrequent, are increasing in frequency and are most often associated with intravenous drug use, prosthetic or otherwise abnormal valves, invasive procedures, or nosocomial acquisition.

HACEK is an acronym for a group of small, fastidious gram-negative coccobacilli (***H****aemophilus aphrophilus,* ***A****ggregatibacter actinomycetemcomitans,* ***C****ardiobacterium hominis,* ***E****ikenella corrodens,* and ***K****ingella kingae*). These organisms that normally inhabit the upper respiratory tract are often associated with IE when recovered from the bloodstream. Anaerobic and microaerophilic bacteria as well as polymicrobial infections are responsible for a minority of cases of IE. In adults, these infections occur mostly among intravenous drug users or originate from oropharyngeal, gastrointestinal, or genitourinary sites. *Candida* IE occurs occasionally, often associated with indwelling catheters. *Aspergillus* IE has been reported in children following open heart surgery; the blood is always culture-negative. *Streptococcus pneumoniae* accounts for a small minority of cases of childhood IE in both structurally normal and abnormal hearts. Infections at additional sites (eg, meningitis and pneumonia) often accompany *S pneumoniae* IE, and despite antibiotic therapy, intracardiac complications are frequent. Culture-negative endocarditis includes infections suppressed by prior courses of antimicrobials as well as poorly cultivable pathogens such as *Bartonella, Coxiella, Tropheryma,* and *Brucella* species that are diagnosed serologically or by nucleic acid amplification tests (NAATs). Non–culture-based methods have also identified rare or previously unrecognized organisms in IE of uncertain pathogenicity and significance; consultation with an expert in infectious diseases is advised in this circumstance.

### CLINICAL MANIFESTATIONS

The "incubation period" of IE, that is, the time from initial bacteremia to onset of symptoms, is generally less than 2 weeks, although diagnosis may be delayed for weeks or months. Early manifestations may be mild or nonspecific, and patients may not seek medical attention promptly. Improper use of short courses of antibiotics for nonspecific complaints may contribute to delays in diagnosis. Fever (88%), fatigue (60%), gastrointestinal complaints (47%), and weight loss (43%) are common manifestations of IE in children. In a child with underlying congenital heart disease (CHD) and fever, fatigue, or worsening cardiac function, the diagnosis of IE requires a high index of suspicion. Patients with cyanotic CHD with artificial systemic-pulmonary shunts may show declining systemic oxygen saturation due to obstruction of flow. Splenomegaly (48%) is common, while new or changing murmurs are infrequent (24%). Among all pediatric series, extracardiac manifestations of IE are infrequent (all < 4%), including Roth spots (small hemorrhagic retinal lesions with pale centers), Osler nodes (small, tender, reddish-purple nodules typically found on the digital pads), Janeway lesions (painless hemorrhagic macules on the palms or soles), and splinter hemorrhages (linear streaks in the nail beds). Many of the classic manifestations of IE are immunologically mediated. In IE patients with arthralgia and arthritis, splenomegaly, Roth spots, glomerulonephritis, and thrombocytopenia, circulating immune complex levels are significantly higher than in IE patients without these manifestations. Levels of immune complexes decline as these physical manifestations resolve.

Common laboratory findings include anemia (37%) and elevated erythrocyte sedimentation rate (ESR; 75%). The presence of rheumatoid factor (19%) is dependent on the duration of infection. Hematuria and associated hypocomplementemia reflecting immune complex–mediated nephritis occur in 35% of patients, and aseptic meningitis has been reported in a minority of children with IE. Many neonates have neurologic signs (apnea, seizures, and paresis). Some presentations of IE are fulminant, with high fever, rapidly evolving sepsis, metastatic disease, and heart failure. Fulminant IE requires urgent intervention.

## DIAGNOSIS

Proper diagnosis is key given the severity of IE and burden of treatment. In evaluating patients for IE, continuous bacteremia is typical; therefore, it is preferable to obtain at least 3 separate blood cultures over a 24- to 48-hour period while antibiotics are withheld if the patient is not acutely ill. Blood should not be drawn through indwelling vascular catheters because contamination may be misleading. If only 1 of several blood cultures of adequate volume is positive, IE is less likely. The blood culture bottles should be filled with their maximal volume using both aerobic and anaerobic bottles. If these are negative, the director of the microbiology laboratory should be alerted and 2 more cultures should be drawn before antibiotic therapy is instituted. Fungal blood cultures are rarely indicated. Commercial NAATs of blood are insensitive and do not detect HACEK organisms. Culture of explanted surgical specimens is poorly specific and should be complemented by NAATs in replicates of the explants and blood cultures.

The subtlety of clinical and laboratory findings in IE necessitates use of complex diagnostic criteria—the modified Duke criteria. In 1994, the Duke University Endocarditis Service developed new diagnostic criteria for IE based on pathologic evidence or on a combination of clinical findings, and these were modified in 2000. According to the Duke criteria, definite IE must meet 2 major criteria, or 1 major and 3 minor criteria, or 5 minor criteria. Major criteria are (1) multiple positive blood cultures for typical IE organisms and (2) evidence of endocardial involvement, either by echocardiography or by the development of a new regurgitant murmur. Minor criteria are a predisposition to IE (eg, CHD), fever, vascular phenomena, immunologic phenomena, and microbiologic or serologic evidence that does not meet major criteria. Each of the major and minor criteria has qualifying details. Modified Duke criteria may be less specific in children than adults.

Echocardiography aids in the diagnosis of IE. Transthoracic echocardiogram (TTE) should be the first-line diagnostic tool. TTE has sensitivities for diagnosis of IE from 59% to 82% in children. Transesophageal echocardiography (TEE) may improve the sensitivity for visualizing prosthetic valves and the aortic outflow tract, but it has more associated risks than TTE in children. Use of TEE should be considered when TTE acoustic window views are inadequate, when suspicion remains high despite negative TTE, when aortic lesions are suspected, for optimal evaluation of prosthetic valves, or for patients > 60 kg.

## TREATMENT

Prior to the availability of antibiotics, IE was uniformly fatal. With timely and appropriate medical therapy, IE can be cured and complications minimized. As noted, when patients are clinically stable, specificity of the diagnosis is improved by multiple blood cultures of generous volume collected over a period of 24 to 48 hours before antibiotic therapy is initiated. In patients with severe toxicity, heart failure, or arrhythmias highly suggestive of acute IE, collection of multiple blood cultures over 1 to 2 hours is appropriate, followed by initiation of empiric antibiotic therapy. Following identification of an infecting organism, selection of antibiotics should be based on results of susceptibility testing.

Some basic considerations apply in determining therapy for IE. High doses of parenteral antibiotics are required to exceed the minimum bactericidal concentration for the infecting organism, and synergistic combinations are recommended in some situations (eg, enterococci) to improve effectiveness or to shorten duration of treatment. Oral antibiotics are insufficient unless bioavailability approaches 100%. Antibiotics used should be bactericidal rather than bacteriostatic, because the relatively avascular vegetations of IE offer little access to host defenses. Pediatric and adult guidelines for therapy of specific pathogens, based on susceptibility testing and the presence or absence of prosthetic material, were published by the American Heart Association (AHA) in 2015. Beta-lactams (including penicillins and cephalosporins) and vancomycin are used most frequently. Gentamicin is commonly added for a period of time to achieve synergy with a β-lactam or vancomycin, especially when enterococci or *S aureus* is the causative organism. Rifampin is useful as an adjunct when *S aureus* infects prosthetic valves.

Surgical intervention, in addition to medical therapy, is generally indicated in fungal IE, when bacteremia persists despite appropriate antibiotic therapy, when congestive heart failure is uncontrolled by medical therapy, or in the presence of any of the following: abscess of the valve annulus or the myocardium, systemic embolic events, rupture of a valve leaflet or chordae, or acute valvar insufficiency with cardiac failure. Prosthetic valve endocarditis per se is not an indication for surgery, but early surgical intervention may improve the outcome

The most frequent complications of IE are congestive heart failure and arterial embolization. Intracardiac lesions that may lead to congestive heart failure include valvar insufficiency caused directly by vegetations or by chordal rupture, abscesses of the myocardium or valvar annulus, myocardial infarction, and conduction defects. Arterial emboli occur most frequently when large (> 10 mm) mobile vegetations develop on valves, particularly the anterior leaflet of the mitral valve. Although vegetations slowly regress with effective therapy, sudden disappearance of a vegetation should raise the possibility of embolization.

Emboli originating from left-sided vegetations can affect vascular beds in the systemic or cerebral circulation, whereas right-sided lesions produce pulmonary emboli. Cerebral emboli occur in 30% of left-sided IE and are mostly clinically silent. Head magnetic resonance imaging (MRI) is often considered for detection. Mycotic aneurysms most commonly occur at vessel bifurcations and can involve any artery. Intracranial mycotic aneurysms often require surgery.

Pericarditis may result from bacteremic spread or direct extension of infection. It is usually associated with IE due to *S aureus*.

## PREVENTION

The AHA's most recent recommendations for prevention of bacterial endocarditis recognize the lack of evidence to support widespread use of antibiotic prophylaxis. Only patients with cardiac conditions with the very highest risk of adverse outcomes from IE should receive prophylaxis for dental procedures (Table 230-1). The importance of good oral hygiene and routine dental care (personal and professional) should be emphasized to all cardiac patients. Table 230-2 provides

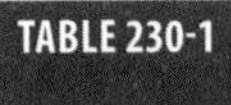

**TABLE 230-1 CARDIAC CONDITIONS WITH THE HIGHEST RISK OF ADVERSE OUTCOMES FROM BACTERIAL ENDOCARDITIS FOR WHICH ANTIMICROBIAL PROPHYLAXIS WITH DENTAL PROCEDURES IS RECOMMENDED[a]**

| Cardiac conditions |
| --- |
| Prosthetic cardiac valve or prosthetic material used for cardiac valve repair |
| Previous infective endocarditis |
| Unrepaired cyanotic congenital heart disease, including palliative shunts and conduits |
| Completely repaired congenital heart defect with prosthetic material or device, whether placed by surgery or by catheter intervention, during the first 6 months after the procedure[b] |
| Repaired congenital heart disease with residual defects at the site or adjacent to the site of a prosthetic patch or prosthetic device (which inhibit endothelialization) |
| Cardiac transplantation recipients who develop cardiac valvulopathy |

[a]Except for the conditions listed, antibiotic prophylaxis is no longer recommended for any other form of congenital heart disease.

[b]Prophylaxis is recommended because endothelialization of prosthetic material occurs within 6 months after the procedure.

Modified with permission from Wilson W, Taubert KA, Gewitz M, et al: Prevention of infective endocarditis: guidelines from the American Heart Association: a guideline from the American Heart Association Rheumatic Fever, Endocarditis, and Kawasaki Disease Committee, Council on Cardiovascular Disease in the Young, and the Council on Clinical Cardiology, Council on Cardiovascular Surgery and Anesthesia, and the Quality of Care and Outcomes Research Interdisciplinary Working Group, *Circulation*. 2007 Oct 9; 116(15):1736-1754.

TABLE 230-2 REGIMENS FOR ALL DENTAL PROCEDURES THAT INVOLVE MANIPULATION OF GINGIVAL TISSUE OR THE PERIAPICAL REGION OF TEETH OR PERFORATION OF THE ORAL MUCOSA[a]

| | | Regimen: Single Dose 30–60 Minutes Before Procedure | |
|---|---|---|---|
| Situation | Agent | Adult | Children |
| Oral | Amoxicillin | 2 g | 50 mg/kg |
| Unable to take oral medication | Ampicillin | 2 g IM or IV | 50 mg/kg IM or IV |
| | OR | | |
| | Cefazolin or ceftriaxone | 1 g IM or IV | 50 mg/kg IM or IV |
| Allergic to penicillins or ampicillin—oral | Cephalexin[b,c] | 2 g | 50 mg/kg |
| | OR | | |
| | Clindamycin | 600 mg | 20 mg/kg |
| | OR | | |
| | Azithromycin or clarithromycin | 500 mg | 15 mg/kg |
| Allergic to penicillins or ampicillin and unable to take oral medication | Cefazolin or ceftriaxone[c] | 1 g IM or IV | 50 mg/kg IM or IV |
| | OR | | |
| | Clindamycin | 600 mg IM or IV | 20 mg/kg IM or IV |

[a]The following procedures and events do not need prophylaxis: routine anesthetic injections through noninfected tissue, taking dental radiographs, placement of removable prosthodontic or orthodontic appliances, adjustment of orthodontic appliances, placement of orthodontic brackets, shedding of deciduous teeth, and bleeding from trauma to the lips or oral mucosa.

[b]Or other first- or second-generation oral cephalosporin in equivalent adult or pediatric dosage.

[c]Cephalosporins should not be used in an individual with a history of anaphylaxis, angioedema, or urticaria with oral or respiratory symptoms following exposure to penicillins or ampicillin.

IM, intramuscular; IV, intravenous.

Modified with permission from Wilson W, Taubert KA, Gewitz M, et al: Prevention of infective endocarditis: guidelines from the American Heart Association: a guideline from the American Heart Association Rheumatic Fever, Endocarditis, and Kawasaki Disease Committee, Council on Cardiovascular Disease in the Young, and the Council on Clinical Cardiology, Council on Cardiovascular Surgery and Anesthesia, and the Quality of Care and Outcomes Research Interdisciplinary Working Group, *Circulation*. 2007 Oct 9;116(15):1736-1754.

the AHA's definition of dental procedures for which prophylactic antibiotics are and are not indicated and antibiotic recommendations for the limited group of qualified patients. Because normal oral flora are altered in patients already taking antibiotic prophylaxis (eg, penicillin for rheumatic fever prophylaxis), a different class of drugs (eg, clindamycin, azithromycin, or clarithromycin) may provide more protection against the patient's own oral microbes in that circumstance. When patients with cardiac lesions at highest risk of adverse outcomes from endocarditis (see Table 230-1) have established gastrointestinal or genitourinary infections or receive antibiotics for wound or sepsis prophylaxis during a gastrointestinal or genitourinary procedure, their antibiotic regimen should include enterococcal coverage.

## ACUTE RHEUMATIC FEVER

### INTRODUCTION

Acute rheumatic fever (ARF) is a nonsuppurative sequela of pharyngeal infection with group A *Streptococcus* (GAS). Target organs of the resultant autoimmune process include the heart, joints, central nervous system, and subcutaneous tissues. Permanent cardiac damage is the most important consequence of this disease.

### PATHOGENESIS AND EPIDEMIOLOGY

Antigenic differences among GAS serotypes are related to the bacterial M protein, found within its cell wall. Recent data demonstrated a shift in prevalence from "rheumatogenic" to "nonrheumatogenic" M types in the United States over the past 40 years that parallels the decrease in the incidence of ARF over this period. The 10 days to 3 weeks period between streptococcal pharyngitis and ARF is consistent with a cellular and humoral immune response. Cross-reactivity of streptococcal antigens and human cardiac, synovial, and brain antigens also supports an immune mechanism of ARF.

Pathologic changes are found throughout the body in connective tissue and around small blood vessels. The pathognomonic lesion of rheumatic fever is the Aschoff body, a painless nodular connective tissue lesion consisting of fibrinoid changes and a collection of lymphocytes, plasma cells, and histiocytes. Within the heart, the endocardium and myocardium are most often affected; the pericardium may also be involved by extension or as serositis. Active valvulitis results in variable degrees of valve insufficiency, with chronic changes possibly leading to valvar stenosis. The mitral and aortic valves are affected most commonly, the tricuspid less frequently, and the pulmonary valve rarely.

Pathologic changes in the joints consist of joint effusion, exudation with edema of synovial membranes, focal necrosis in the joint capsule, and edema and inflammation in periarticular tissue. These changes are completely reversible. Subcutaneous nodules seen during the acute phase of the disease histologically resemble Aschoff bodies. "Rheumatic pneumonia" consists of exudative and inflammatory changes without Aschoff bodies. Pathologic changes in patients with chorea are not consistent, and little postmortem information is available because patients with active chorea rarely die.

ARF occurs most often in the winter and spring seasons and in children ages 5 to 15 years. Much less commonly, it has been reported in the preschool age group. There is familial susceptibility to ARF. Asian/Pacific Islander children have recently been identified as a group with possible increased genetic susceptibility. Patients with ARF have a high likelihood of recurrence when reinfected with GAS; this tendency declines with age and with increased time since the last episode. Environmental factors such as nutrition, crowding, and age all appear to influence the incidence of ARF, probably because the same factors influence the incidence of streptococcal pharyngitis.

### CLINICAL MANIFESTATIONS

Many of the clinical manifestations of ARF occur in other infectious and inflammatory disorders, and so ARF must meet complex diagnostic criteria. The revised Jones criteria vary for areas of high and low ARF endemicity. Diagnosis requires that an individual have either 2 major criteria or 1 major criterion plus 2 minor criteria along with evidence of streptococcal infection. Exceptions are chorea or indolent carditis, which each may by itself indicate rheumatic fever. The diagnostic criteria are listed in Table 230-3.

Classic ARF presents with acute migratory polyarthritis associated with fever. The joints are red, hot, swollen, exquisitely tender, and painful if moved. In general, the larger joints of the extremities are affected, but arthritis rarely may occur in the spine and other joints such as the temporomandibular and sternoclavicular joints; arthritis of fingers and toes is more common in older than younger patients. Usually, pain and effusion subside in 1 joint as another becomes involved, but several joints may be involved simultaneously. Polyarthritis is the most common of the major criteria and lasts less than 4 to 6 weeks when untreated. Characteristic is a dramatic response to salicylates and nonsteroidal anti-inflammatory drugs (NSAIDs); early use in febrile children may confound diagnosis.

Rheumatic carditis may be asymptomatic. Echocardiography diagnoses 17% more cases of carditis than auscultation. Carditis may affect the endocardium (valves), myocardium, or pericardium. Endocarditis manifested by pathologic murmurs is the hallmark of ARF carditis. The most frequent murmur is an apical regurgitant systolic murmur of mitral regurgitation. With severe mitral regurgitation, the third heart sound may be followed or replaced by a low-pitched mid-diastolic rumble. The early diastolic murmur of aortic regurgitation is the second most common murmur in ARF and generally occurs only in patients who also have mitral regurgitation.

Myocarditis may be manifested by tachycardia disproportionate to the fever, a gallop rhythm, or arrhythmias. Cardiomegaly may be

**TABLE 230-3 CRITERIA FOR THE DIAGNOSIS OF ACUTE RHEUMATIC FEVER WITH EVIDENCE OF STREPTOCOCCAL INFECTION**

| | |
|---|---|
| A. For all patient populations with evidence of preceding GAS infection | |
| Diagnosis: initial ARF | 2 Major manifestations or 1 major plus 2 minor manifestations |
| Diagnosis: recurrent ARF | 2 Major or 1 major and 2 minor or 3 minor |
| B. Major criteria | |
| Low-risks populations[a] | Moderate and high-risk populations |
| Carditis[b] | Carditis |
| • Clinical and/or subclinical | • Clinical and/or subclinical |
| Arthritis | Arthritis |
| • Polyarthritis only | • Monoarthritis or polyarthritis |
| | • Polyarthralgia[c] |
| Chorea | Chorea |
| Erythema marginatum | Erythema marginatum |
| Subcutaneous nodules | Subcutaneous nodules |
| C. Minor criteria | |
| Low-risks populations[a] | Moderate and high-risk populations |
| Polyarthralgia | Monoarthralgia |
| Fever (≥ 38.5°C) | Fever (≥ 38°C) |
| ESR ≥ 60 mm in the first hour and/or CRP ≥ 3.0 mg/dl[d] | ESR ≥ 30 mm/h and/or CRP ≥ 3.0 mg/dl[d] |
| Prolonged PR interval, after accounting for age variability (unless carditis is a major criterion) | Prolonged PR interval, after accounting for age variability (unless carditis is a major criterion) |

[a]Low-risk populations are those with ARF incidence ≤ 2 per 100,000 school-aged children or all-age rheumatic heart disease prevalence of ≤ 1 per 1000 population per year.

[b]Subclinical carditis indicates echocardiographic valvulitis.

[c]See section on polyarthralgia, which should only be considered as a major manifestation in moderate- to high-risk populations after exclusion of other causes. As in past versions of the criteria, erythema marginatum and subcutaneous modules are rarely "stand-alone" major criteria. Additionally, joint manifestations can only be considered in either the major or minor categories but not both in the same patient.

[d]CRP value must be greater than upper limit of normal for laboratory. Also, because ESR may evolve during the course of ARF, peak FSR values should be used.

ARF indicates acute rheumatic fever; CRP, C-reactive protein; ESR, erythrocyte sedimentation rate; and GAS, group A streptococcal infection.

Reproduced with permission from Gewitz MH, Baltimore RS, Tani LY, et al. Revision of the Jones Criteria for the diagnosis of acute rheumatic fever in the era of Doppler echocardiography: a scientific statement from the American Heart Association, *Circulation*. 2015 May 19;131(20):1806-1818.

evident on radiograph. Severe myocarditis may result in congestive heart failure with signs including jugular-venous distention, hepatomegaly, and pulmonary edema with rales. Prolongation of the P-R demonstrated on an electrocardiogram interval is common but does not indicate carditis.

Pericarditis may appear suddenly and may be associated with precordial pain and a friction rub. More often, however, patients with pericarditis are asymptomatic. Pericarditis seldom appears without endocarditis and myocarditis, the combination being termed pancarditis. Death may occur during the acute phase of carditis; permanent cardiac damage may result in long-term disability, usually because of mitral or aortic valvar insufficiency and/or stenosis.

Sydenham chorea is characterized by sudden, aimless, irregular movements of the extremities frequently associated with emotional instability and muscle weakness. Whereas carditis and arthritis develop within weeks after an inciting streptococcal infection, chorea presents after several months and is not often associated with other features of ARF except perhaps mild carditis. The onset may be gradual, with complaints that the child is nervous. The child may become clumsy and stumble, fall, or drop objects. Often there are complaints of poor attention and deteriorating handwriting and school performance. Facial grimacing and various speech disorders occur. As chorea becomes more severe, irregular jerking movements can be sufficiently violent to cause injuries. Muscle weakness may be profound. The choreiform movements subside during sleep and are exaggerated

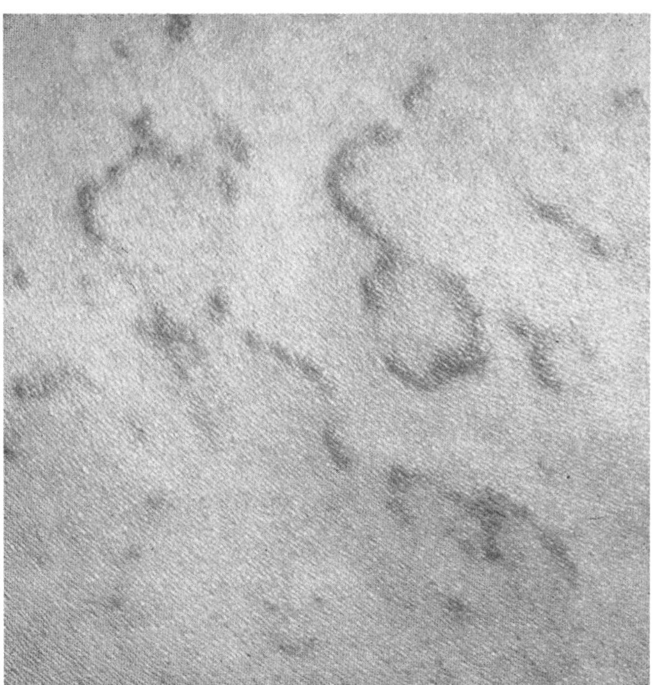

**FIGURE 230-1** Erythema marginatum of rheumatic fever. Enlarging and shifting transient annular and polycyclic lesions. (Reproduced with permission from Wolff K, Goldsmith L, Katz S, et al: *Fitzpatrick's Dermatology in General Medicine*, 7th ed. New York: McGraw-Hill; 2008.)

by emotion. Characteristically, when the patient is asked to extend the arms, hands, and fingers, flexion of the wrists and hyperextension of the metacarpophalangeal joints ("silver forking") are observed. The pronator sign may be elicited: after the arms are raised above the head, there is gradual pronation of the hands (apposition of the dorsal aspects of the hands). Other signs are an inability to hold the tongue still when it is protruded and spasmodic contractions of the hands when the patient intentionally grips objects or the examiner's hand (milkmaid's grip). Chorea can also be caused by diseases other than ARF, such as systemic lupus erythematosus (SLE) or Wilson disease, and patients who present with chorea as the only manifestation of ARF should undergo a full evaluation.

Subcutaneous nodules are rare and manifest as painless small (0.5–1 cm) swellings over bony prominences, primarily over the extensor tendons of the hands, feet, elbows, scalp, scapulae, and vertebrae. Nodules tend to occur in crops and may persist for days to months after the onset of ARF, generally with severe carditis. Subcutaneous nodules are not specific for ARF and may occur in rheumatoid arthritis as well as SLE.

Erythema marginatum occurs in less than 10% of ARF patients; it may be seen more frequently in children less than 5 years old. The characteristic rash consists of an evanescent, pink, erythematous macule, with a clear center and serpiginous outline (Fig. 230-1). The rash is transient, migratory, and not pruritic; it blanches with pressure, is exacerbated by warmth, and is found primarily on the trunk and proximal extremities, sparing the face.

## DIAGNOSIS

Proof of previous streptococcal infection is required in addition to combinations of major and minor criteria. Paired, increasing serum antistreptococcal antibody titers are probably the most specific and reliable proof of previous streptococcal infection. A rising antibody titer to specific streptococcal antigens is more specific than a single elevated value. However, if the patient presents with chorea more than 3 months after the acute streptococcal infection, then antibody titers may be declining or low. The most widely used serologic test is antibody formation against streptolysin O. Titers of at least 333 U in children and 250 U in adults are usually considered elevated. Other available antibody tests are antideoxyribonuclease B, antihyaluronidase, antistreptokinase, and antinicotinamide-adenine-dinucleotidase. A 4-fold rise in titer to 1 or more of the above antigens can be demonstrated in virtually all cases of acute or recurrent rheumatic fever if serum samples are obtained within 2 to 3 months of the streptococcal infection. Titers may remain high for up to a year. Patients who present with fever, rash, arthritis, or carditis should also have studies to exclude SLE and rheumatoid arthritis. These include antinuclear antibodies, anti-deoxyribonucleic acid (DNA) titers, and rheumatoid factor.

Demonstration of GAS by rapid antigen detection, NAATs, or culture of the throat of a patient suspected of having ARF provides strong evidence for the diagnosis. Because of lower sensitivity, negative rapid antigen tests should be followed by culture. Caution is needed, however, as most ARF patients clear their streptococcal pharyngitis without antibiotic therapy, and many children are chronic pharyngeal carriers of GAS unrelated to ARF. Failure to demonstrate GAS in the throat of patients with ARF may be related to prior antibiotic therapy, small numbers of organisms, or improper testing technique, but most often reflects spontaneous clearance.

The 2015 revised Jones criteria recommend use of echocardiography for suspected or confirmed ARF and consideration of serial use in such patients. This should be done even in the absence of auscultatory findings.

Absence of ESR > 60 mm/h and C-reactive protein (CRP) > 3.0 mg/dL argues against ARF. Leukopenia and abnormal urinalysis probably do not occur in rheumatic fever, and if found in a patient with joint and cardiac abnormalities, they are more suggestive of SLE

## TREATMENT

A full course of oral or intramuscular penicillin as given for GAS pharyngitis should be administered to all patients with ARF even if testing for GAS is negative. An oral cephalosporin is an acceptable alternative; macrolide antibiotics, such as erythromycin, clarithromycin, or azithromycin, should be limited to penicillin-allergic patients. Tetracyclines and sulfonamide drugs are not appropriate for treatment of the streptococcal infection.

If a child with ARF is free of clinical carditis, normal activity can be resumed once the pain and fever resolve. If there is mild carditis, a period of 1 to 2 weeks resting at home is reasonable. The murmur may persist indefinitely, and its disappearance is not a requisite for return to activity. The ESR may remain high for weeks, showing gradual decline. Patients with severe carditis, as evidenced by marked cardiomegaly or congestive heart failure, should remain at bed rest for several weeks, until the heart size returns to normal or is at least stable.

Salicylates, NSAIDs, and steroids are beneficial in controlling the acute clinical manifestations of ARF. Arthritis and fever respond dramatically to salicylate therapy, often within hours of initiation. Acetylsalicylic acid is usually used in relatively high doses (50–70 mg/kg/d) for a duration related to the course and severity of the disease; the minimum period is usually 6 weeks. Prior to discontinuation, the dose should be reduced gradually over 2 to 4 weeks. If rebound of rheumatic activity occurs, full therapy may have to be reinstituted for an additional 4 to 6 weeks.

In patients with moderate to severe carditis, neither salicylates nor steroids demonstrate superiority over the other drug in modifying the duration of acute disease or lessening the residual heart damage. However, steroids are indicated in patients who develop congestive heart failure. Current understanding suggests unlikely benefit from digoxin, with the exception of associated arrhythmias. Occasionally, severe incompetence of aortic and/or mitral valves leads to refractory heart failure, which requires surgical implantation of a prosthetic valve.

Specific treatment for chorea is not available. Physical and mental stress should be minimized, and protective measures to prevent injury during severe episodes should be instituted. In very severe cases, steroids, phenobarbital, and valproic acid have been helpful.

Prophylaxis against recurrent ARF should be instituted immediately following acute therapy. The most effective prophylaxis consists of benzathine penicillin G intramuscular injections every 4 weeks; the injection can be painful and may lead to reactions. Alternative therapy consists of either oral penicillin V twice daily or oral sulfisoxazole once daily. Patients without rheumatic heart disease are at lower risk of recurrence than are patients with carditis or valvar disease. In pediatric ARF patients without carditis, prophylaxis should continue for at least 5 years or until age 21, whichever is longer. When ARF includes carditis but no clinical or echocardiographic evidence of residual valvar disease, the duration of prophylaxis should be extended to at least 10 years or well into adulthood, whichever is longer. Patients with persistent valvar disease following ARF with carditis should continue prophylaxis for at least 10 years and until at least age 40. Lifelong prophylaxis should also be considered in this group.

Approximately 75% of patients with ARF are well after 6 weeks. By 6 months, fewer than 5% remain symptomatic with chorea or intractable carditis. Up to 70% of patients who develop carditis during the initial episode of ARF recover without any residual heart disease. Whereas 70% of ARF patients with congestive heart failure and pericarditis develop permanent heart disease, only 20% of patients with mild carditis are permanently affected. When more than 8 weeks have elapsed after stopping treatment, ARF does not recur in the absence of recurrent streptococcal infection. In individual patients, the clinical features of recurrent episodes of ARF tend to be similar to that of the initial episode. The likelihood of permanent residual heart damage following carditis increases with each recurrence. Patients who have had chorea without apparent carditis may present years later with mitral stenosis.

## PREVENTION

Most acute pharyngitis is caused by viruses and, less commonly, other bacteria. Only GAS pharyngitis leads to ARF, and ARF is rare in the United States. Well under 3% of confirmed streptococcal pharyngitis infections cause ARF in the United States, while carriers of GAS (with minimal risk of ARF) approximate 10% to 15% of children. The emphasis is therefore on the specificity of diagnosing acute streptococcal pharyngitis to minimize inappropriate therapy and attendant medical risks. The clinical syndrome of streptococcal pharyngitis is variable (abrupt sore throat, cervical adenopathy, fever, headache, often abdominal pain and rash) and not specific; laboratory testing is necessary. Gold standard laboratory testing is by culture. As noted, rapid antigen testing is usually less sensitive than culture, although NAATs approximate culture sensitivity and specificity. The epidemiologic peak of GAS pharyngitis and the risk for developing ARF are between 5 and 15 years of age. Protocols for testing for acute GAS pharyngitis in adults account for the lower GAS prevalence and risk for ARF beyond 15 years of age and are not to be used in children.

Children with compatible clinical presentation, the absence of signs of viral disease (conjunctivitis, coryza, cough, diarrhea, or characteristic viral exanthems or enanthems), and rapid antigen testing, NAAT, or culture detecting GAS in the throat should be treated to prevent ARF (Table 230-4). Preferred regimens include oral penicillin V 2 to 3 times daily or a single daily dose of amoxicillin for 10 days. Parenteral benzathine penicillin is generally reserved for patients with poor compliance. Penicillin-allergic patients should receive a first-generation cephalosporin, clindamycin, or a macrolide. Macrolide resistance by GAS varies geographically. Testing for cure is not generally indicated.

# MYOCARDITIS AND PERICARDITIS

## INTRODUCTION

The myocardium is specialized muscle and a conduction system that is isolated from the bloodstream by the endocardium; it is perfused by the coronary arteries. The pericardium is made up of 2 layers, which form a sac around the heart, anchored at the origins of the great vessels. The visceral layer is a single layer of mesothelial cells adherent to the myocardium. The parietal layer lies against the mediastinal and pleural spaces and is made up of collagen and elastin fibers. The pericardium is relatively avascular but well innervated.

**TABLE 230-4 PRIMARY PREVENTION OF RHEUMATIC FEVER (TREATMENT OF STREPTOCOCCAL TONSILLOPHARYNGITIS)[a]**

| Agent | Dose | Mode | Duration | Rating |
|---|---|---|---|---|
| Penicillins | | | | |
| Penicillin V (phenoxymethyl penicillin) | Children: 250 mg 2–3 times daily for ≤ 27 kg (60 lb); children > 27 kg (60 lb), adolescents, and adults: 500 mg 2–3 times daily | Oral | 10 days | IB |
| | or | | | |
| Amoxicillin | 50 mg/kg once daily (maximum 1 g) | Oral | 10 days | IB |
| | or | | | |
| Benzathine penicillin G | 600,000 U per patients ≤ 27 kg (60 lb); 1,200,000 U for patients > 27 kg (60 lb) | Intramuscular | Once | IB |
| For individuals allergic to penicillin | | | | |
| Narrow-spectrum cephalosporin[b] (cephalexin, cefadroxil) | Variable | Oral | 10 days | IB |
| | or | | | |
| Clindamycin | 20 mg/kg per day divided in 3 doses (maximum 1.8 g/d) | Oral | 10 days | IIaB |
| | or | | | |
| Azithromycin | 12 mg/kg once daily (maximum 500 mg) | Oral | 5 days | IIaB |
| | or | | | |
| Clarithromycin | 15 mg/kg per day divided BID (maximum 250 mg BID) | Oral | 10 days | IIaB |

Rating indicates classification of recommendation and LOE (eg, IB indicates class I, LOE B); BID, twice per day.

[a]For other acceptable alternatives, see text. The following are not acceptable: sulfonamides, trimethoprim, tetracyclines, and fluoroquinolones.

[b]To be avoided in those with immediate (type I) hypersensitivity to a penicillin.

Reproduced with permission from Gerber MA, Baltimore RS, Eaton CB, et al: Prevention of rheumatic fever and diagnosis and treatment of acute Streptococcal pharyngitis: a scientific statement from the American Heart Association Rheumatic Fever, Endocarditis, and Kawasaki Disease Committee of the Council on Cardiovascular Disease in the Young, the Interdisciplinary Council on Functional Genomics and Translational Biology, and the Interdisciplinary Council on Quality of Care and Outcomes Research: endorsed by the American Academy of Pediatrics, *Circulation*. 2009 Mar 24;119(11):1541-1551.

## ACUTE MYOCARDITIS

### PATHOGENESIS AND EPIDEMIOLOGY

Acute myocarditis is an acute, patchy inflammation of the heart muscle that accounts for 2% of cases of heart failure. Most pediatric heart failure is due to genetic cardiomyopathies (14%) or is associated with severe CHD (69%) or arrhythmias (15%). In developing countries, nutritional deficiencies and ARF (see above) also contribute to heart failure.

In developed countries, acute myocarditis can be associated with viral infections. Respiratory symptoms are common (56%). The virus infection is usually cleared and then followed by an autoimmune attack and the presence of sarcolemmal antibodies. The myocardium may recover fully from the infection and autoinflammation. If damage is extensive, the heart may dilate chronically. The myocardium is not well innervated, so acute myocarditis often manifests as exertional fatigue, difficulty feeding and abdominal pain, peripheral edema, and palpitations.

The most common organisms infecting the myocardium are enteroviruses (including coxsackieviruses). Adenovirus, Epstein-Barr virus (EBV), herpes simplex virus (HSV), human herpesviruses (HHVs) 6 and 7, cytomegalovirus (CMV), and human immunodeficiency virus (HIV). Many of these are endemic human infections that reactivate commonly. Human parvovirus B19 may be detected for up to a year after primary infection. Genomic material from these persistent or prolonged infections may persist for months to years in tissues. Distinguishing true infection of the myocardium by viruses other than enteroviruses is challenging and best accomplished in population studies that include healthy controls. Acute bacterial myocarditis is rare and most often caused by *Mycoplasma pneumoniae*, *Coxiella burnetii*, or *Borrelia* species. Sepsis, notably pneumococcal, meningococcal, and rickettsial, may lead to severe myocardial dysfunction. Cardiac "stunning" associated with high neurogenic peripheral vascular resistance is a hallmark of enterovirus-71 infection.

### CLINICAL MANIFESTATIONS

Acute myocarditis is characterized by reduced ejection fraction of the heart, usually affecting both pulmonary and systemic circulations. In most pediatric patients, the presentation is acute heart failure following a viral prodrome. In infancy, this may manifest by sweating, pallor, tachycardia disproportionate to fever, tachypnea, gastroesophageal reflux and difficulty feeding with consequent growth failure. In older children, there is fatigue (17%), dyspnea, orthopnea, exercise intolerance, cough, nausea, vomiting, and abdominal pain, pericarditis/chest pain (7%), or syncope (5%). Fever, regurgitant murmurs, gallops, jugular venous distension, and peripheral edema or ascites are variable. There may be associated findings of a respiratory or systemic infection, autoinflammatory or autoimmune disorder, or endocrinopathy.

### DIAGNOSIS

Echocardiography should be prioritized because it is highly sensitive and specific for acute or fulminant myocarditis. An echocardiogram commonly demonstrates wall motion abnormalities and ventricular dysfunction proportionately less than dilation when compared to myocarditis with dilated cardiomyopathy. Cardiac magnetic resonance (CMR) imaging can provide additional and often superior information to echocardiography. CMR can further assess tissue characteristics such as edema, hyperemia, and fibrosis/scarring of the myocardium. It also can show patchy areas of inflammation and may delineate adjacent pathology in the lung, pleural space, and mediastinum. Chest x-ray is insensitive but may show an enlarged heart. Electrocardiogram is not specific but often abnormal. Electrolytes and renal and hepatic function may be altered. Blood levels of CRP, B-type natriuretic peptides (BNP) or N-terminal (NT)-proBNP, troponin, and creatine kinase-MB concentrations are often elevated. *Borrelia* and rabies infections are often also associated with progressive heart block. Blood NAAT is highly sensitive for enteroviruses during systemic infection; enteroviruses persist for weeks in respiratory and fecal samples, which may mislead the clinician. NAAT of blood for adenovirus, EBV, HSV, CMV, HHV-6 and -7, and human parvovirus B19 are difficult to interpret. The gold standard for diagnosis and staging of myocarditis (infectious, autoimmune, and chronic forms) is endomyocardial biopsy (EMB). The patchy nature of the disease (evident by CMR), thinner right hearts, and lack of evidence for benefit of standard therapies in children often lead to individualized decisions regarding EMB. Gene panels and metabolic tests for cardiomyopathies are recommended.

### TREATMENT

Treatment is mainly supportive and symptomatic care. Therapy involves cardiac monitoring in hospitals capable of electrophysiologic and mechanical circulatory support, diuretics, and inotropes. Use of corticosteroids and intravenous immune globulin (IVIG) is not supported by meta-analyses or large registries. Broad-spectrum antivirals under development (eg, favipiravir) may be useful in the near future. Outcome is generally good, with 66% recovering fully. Paradoxically, patients with the worst ejection fraction acutely often recover the best. Damage in 24% of cases may result in cardiac transplantation or death.

Acute myocarditis may be associated with chest pain and pericarditis (perimyocarditis) and is treated as myocarditis. Pericarditis may be associated with mild myocarditis (myopericarditis) and is treated as pericarditis.



## ACUTE PERICARDITIS

### PATHOGENESIS AND EPIDEMIOLOGY

Acute pericarditis is an acute inflammation of the pericardial layers. It is most common in early adolescence, particularly in males. Pericarditis in developing countries is usually tuberculous but is viral or idiopathic in industrialized regions. Viral pericarditis often follows a respiratory infection. Enteroviruses, especially the Coxsackie B viruses, are well known to affect the pericardium, with or without associated myocarditis. Sometimes the causative agent can be identified in pericardial fluid by antigen detection tests, NAAT, or viral culture, or may be demonstrated in blood. Detection of viruses from nasopharyngeal or rectal sites often does not correlate with results from pericardial fluid or tissue.

Purulent pericarditis occurs either by hematogenous spread or extension from a septic focus in the lung (pneumonia or empyema), liver abscess, or, rarely, after cardiac surgery. The most common organisms are staphylococci, pneumococci, streptococci, meningococci, and *Haemophilus influenzae* type B (the latter is much less common in countries with universal childhood vaccination against this pathogen); these organisms can usually be isolated from blood, pleural or pericardial fluid, or other metastatic sites. Fungal pericarditis generally occurs in immunocompromised hosts.

### CLINICAL MANIFESTATIONS

Acute pericarditis is most often manifested by pain (85%), irritability, anorexia, and sometimes fever. The pain is precordial or referred to the epigastrium, neck, shoulder, or left arm; it may be relieved by leaning forward and made worse by deep inspiration or coughing. A friction rub (in < 33%) may be heard along the left sternal border as a high-pitched grating sound, similar to the sound of sandpaper rubbing on wood. It is always in phase with the heart sounds, but may vary by respiration or posture and disappears with an enlarging effusion. Tamponade and constrictive pericarditis are rare. Recovery occurs spontaneously in 2 to 4 weeks.

Purulent pericarditis has an acute onset, with high spiking fever, marked blood polymorphonuclear leukocytosis, and severe toxicity. Symptoms may be modified if the patient has received antibiotics.

### DIAGNOSIS

There is usually a polymorphonuclear leukocytosis. The electrocardiogram (in < 60%) initially shows elevation of the S-T segments in most leads; after about 1 week, the S-T segments return to normal and are associated with T-wave flattening and then inversion in the same leads. These changes may persist for months after the acute lesion resolves. Echocardiography reveals an effusion (in < 60%) that is usually mild and excludes cardiac tamponade (present in 2%). CMR and computed tomography provide superior visualization of associated chest abnormalities, pericardial thickening, and evidence of inflammation. CRP is recommended in patients with effusion.

ARF, juvenile inflammatory arthritis, SLE, uremia, Kawasaki disease, dissecting aneurysm, hypothyroidism, neoplasm, sarcoidosis, acute myocardial infarction, and acute pancreatitis are rare causes of pericardial disease. Pericardial effusions are also seen with fetal hydrops.

### TREATMENT

Treatment for isolated pericarditis is NSAIDs, aspirin, low-dose colchicine, or combinations when response is poor. Corticosteroids may lead to more recurrences and are reserved for specific diseases causing pericarditis (eg, leukemia, tuberculosis, SLE). Risk factors for poor prognosis include fever > 38.0°C, subacute course, large pericardial effusion, and failure to respond within 7 days to NSAIDs.

Specific antibiotic treatment of purulent pericarditis depends on the bacteria identified, but initial empiric antibiotic therapy should include coverage of the usual organisms. Antibiotic therapy should be continued for 3 to 4 weeks. Close observation for tamponade is essential. Surgical drainage of the pericardial cavity is recommended to reduce high mortality and the 25% risk of constrictive pericarditis, which may follow cure; extended follow-up is necessary.

### SUGGESTED READINGS


Adler Y, Charron P, Imazio M, et al. 2015 ESC Guidelines for the diagnosis and management of pericardial diseases: the Task Force for the Diagnosis and Management of Pericardial Diseases of the European Society of Cardiology (ESC) endorsed by: the European Association for Cardio-Thoracic Surgery (EACTS). *Eur Heart J.* 2015;36:2921-2964.

Baddour LM, Wilson WR, Bayer AS, et al. Infective endocarditis in adults: diagnosis, antimicrobial therapy, and management of complications: a scientific statement for healthcare professionals from the American Heart Association. *Circulation.* 2015;132: 1435-1486.

Baltimore RS, Gewitz M, Baddour LM, et al. Infective endocarditis in childhood: 2015 update: a scientific statement from the American Heart Association. *Circulation.* 2015;132:1487-1515.

Gerber MA, Baltimore RS, Eaton CB, et al. Prevention of rheumatic fever and diagnosis and treatment of acute streptococcal pharyngitis: a scientific statement from the American Heart Association Rheumatic Fever, Endocarditis, and Kawasaki Disease Committee of the Council on Cardiovascular Disease in the Young, the Interdisciplinary Council on Functional Genomics and Translational Biology, and the Interdisciplinary Council on Quality of Care and Outcomes Research: endorsed by the American Academy of Pediatrics. *Circulation.* 2009;119:1541-1551.

Gewitz MH, Baltimore RS, Tani LY, et al. Revision of the Jones Criteria for the diagnosis of acute rheumatic fever in the era of Doppler echocardiography: a scientific statement from the American Heart Association. *Circulation.* 2015;131:1806-1818.

Kantor PF, Lougheed J, Dancea A, et al. Presentation, diagnosis, and medical management of heart failure in children: Canadian Cardiovascular Society guidelines. *Can J Cardiol.* 2013;29:1535-1552.

Shakti D, Hehn R, Gauvreau K, Sundel RP, Newburger JW. Idiopathic pericarditis and pericardial effusion in children: contemporary epidemiology and management. *J Am Heart Assoc.* 2014;3:e001483.

Shulman ST, Bisno AL, Clegg HW, et al. Clinical practice guideline for the diagnosis and management of group A streptococcal pharyngitis: 2012 update by the Infectious Diseases Society of America. *Clin Infect Dis.* 2012;55:1279-1282.

Wilson W, Taubert KA, Gewitz M, et al. Prevention of infective endocarditis: guidelines from the American Heart Association: a guideline from the American Heart Association Rheumatic Fever, Endocarditis, and Kawasaki Disease Committee, Council on Cardiovascular Disease in the Young, and the Council on Clinical Cardiology, Council on Cardiovascular Surgery and Anesthesia, and the Quality of Care and Outcomes Research Interdisciplinary Working Group. *Circulation.* 2007;116:1736-1754.

# 231 Gastrointestinal Infections

Monica I. Ardura and Ivor D. Hill

## INTRODUCTION

Diarrheal disease due to infectious enteritis remains a significant global health burden, accounting for 1 in 9 child deaths worldwide, and is the second leading cause of mortality in children less than 5 years of age in resource-poor countries. In the United States, it is estimated that young children have 1 to 3 episodes of diarrhea each year, with the highest rates reported in those attending childcare centers. This chapter will focus on common enteric pathogens causing acute diarrhea in children.

## PATHOGENESIS AND EPIDEMIOLOGY

Many enteric pathogens cause gastrointestinal (GI) infections in children, especially in those less than 5 years of age (Table 231-1). These pathogens are acquired via the fecal-oral route directly from another person or indirectly following ingestion of food or water contaminated with feces. Person-to-person transmission generally requires only a low-dose inoculum to produce infection and has a short incubation period.

Enteric pathogens cause diarrhea by altering the balance between secretion and absorption of fluids and electrolytes in the GI tract. This can occur by means of a direct effect on enterocyte ion transport and the tight junction barrier or indirectly through virulence factors that cause inflammation. Based on pathophysiology, infectious diarrhea can be categorized as secretory, osmotic, or inflammatory. Secretory diarrhea is the result of active water loss into the GI tract with minimal inflammation, as is classically described with infections such as *Vibrio cholerae*. Osmotic diarrhea occurs when there is failure to absorb solutes, which then retain water within the GI tract (eg, consuming undiluted concentrated formula). Damage to enterocytes can result in transient lactase deficiency, which in turn results in lactose malabsorption. Inflammatory diarrhea occurs when pathogens, or their enterotoxins, damage enterocytes, leading to villous destruction and impaired water absorption. Infections caused by *Salmonella* and *Clostridium difficile* primarily cause inflammatory diarrhea and are characterized by detection of polymorphonuclear white cells in stool.

In cases of suspected infectious enteritis, epidemiologic risk factors may allow consideration of a specific pathogen. Exposures to animals (eg, reptiles), contaminated water, travel to endemic areas, recent receipt of antibiotics, or attendance at a childcare center are important risk factors. For example, *Giardia* and *Cryptosporidium* are the most common gastrointestinal infections reported with waterborne outbreaks. Outbreaks of enteric infections in children attending childcare centers have included bacteria (*Shigella, Escherichia coli* including O157:H7), viruses (adenovirus, astrovirus, norovirus, and rotavirus), and parasites (*Cryptosporidium parvum* and *Giardia lamblia*). National outbreaks of infectious bacterial enteritis have followed ingestion of undercooked ground beef, chicken, or pork (*E coli* O157:H7 and other Shiga-toxin producing *E coli* [STEC], *Salmonella* species), raw fish (*Salmonella* species), milk products (*Listeria monocytogenes*), nuts (*E coli* O157:H7, *Salmonella* species), and raw fruits or vegetables (*E coli* O157:H7, *L monocytogenes, Salmonella* species).

In developed countries, viral agents are the most frequent cause of infectious diarrhea in children. In the United States, rotavirus was the most common cause of gastroenteritis before the introduction of routine rotavirus vaccination in 2006. Currently, human caliciviruses such as norovirus are the most frequent cause of infectious enteritis in children < 5 years of age. The most commonly isolated bacteria causing acute infectious enteritis are *Campylobacter* and *Salmonella* species, followed by *Shigella* and *E coli* O157:H7 and other STEC. An increasing incidence of antimicrobial-associated *C difficile*–associated diarrhea (CDAD) in hospitalized children has been reported.

**TABLE 231-1 COMMON AGENTS CAUSING GASTROINTESTINAL INFECTIONS IN CHILDREN**

| Bacteria | Viruses | Parasites |
|---|---|---|
| *Aeromonas* species | Adenovirus | *Cryptosporidium parvum* |
| *Bacillus cereus* | Astrovirus | *Cyclospora cayetanensis* |
| *Campylobacter* species | Enterovirus | *Entamoeba histolytica* |
| *Clostridium difficile* | Norovirus | *Giardia lamblia* |
| *Clostridium perfringens* | Rotavirus | *Isospora belli* |
| *Escherichia coli*[a] | Sapovirus | Microsporidia |
| *Plesiomonas shigelloides* | | |
| *Salmonella* species | | |
| *Shigella* species | | |
| *Staphylococcus aureus* | | |
| *Vibrio* species | | |
| *Yersinia enterocolitica* | | |

[a]Diarrheagenic *E coli* pathogens including Enteroaggregative, Enterohemorrhagic, Enteroinvasive, Enteropathogenic, Enterotoxigenic, and Shiga-toxin producing *E coli*.

## CLINICAL MANIFESTATIONS

Most GI infections present with acute diarrhea, defined as 3 or more loose stools per day and generally lasting less than 7 to 14 days. In breastfed and young infants who normally have 3 to 10 stools per day, diarrhea can be defined as an increase in stool frequency to twice the usual number per day. Diarrhea may be accompanied by other signs of enteric involvement including vomiting, abdominal pain or distension, bloody stools, or fever. In children with acute viral gastroenteritis, nausea and vomiting may be the predominant symptoms early in the illness. Enteric fluid losses can lead to dehydration and electrolyte imbalance. In severe cases, children may present with hypovolemic shock with hypotension and altered mental status.

In general, the effects of enteric infections are confined to the intestinal mucosa. Extraintestinal manifestations result from spread of the enteric infection beyond the GI tract or from immune-mediated mechanisms. Young infants and immunocompromised children are at higher risk for extraintestinal invasive disease. *Salmonella* species can lead to bacteremia or focal infections in susceptible hosts. In the United States, the incidence of invasive *Salmonella* infections is highest among infants < 3 months of age and can present with bacteremia and/or meningitis. Additional extraintestinal manifestations include osteomyelitis, suppurative arthritis, peritonitis, hepatitis, pneumonia, and endovascular conditions (eg, endocarditis, arteritis, thrombophlebitis). Immune-mediated extraintestinal manifestations tend to occur after the bacterial enteritis has resolved and include reactive arthritis, Guillain-Barré syndrome, hemolytic anemia, erythema nodosum, and renal complications including glomerulonephritis, IgA nephropathy, or hemolytic-uremic syndrome.

## DIAGNOSIS

Most cases of infectious enteritis in otherwise healthy children are self-limiting and, as such, do not require diagnostic testing. Clinical practice guidelines recommend diagnostic testing of stool in cases of dysentery (characterized by the presence of frequent, small-volume diarrheal stools that contain mucus or visible blood), moderate to severe disease, patients with prolonged symptoms (lasting > 7–14 days), and those at high risk for complications. Testing is also recommended when there is an outbreak in communities or childcare centers. The combination of fever and bloody stools is highly indicative of a bacterial enteric pathogen such as *Campylobacter, Salmonella, Shigella,* and *E coli* 0157:H7 or other STEC. The presence of fecal leukocytes is associated with inflammatory enteroinvasive infections, such *Shigella, Salmonella,* enteroinvasive *E coli,* and amoeba, but not with toxin-producing bacteria such as *V cholerae* or enterotoxigenic *E coli.* Fecal leukocyte detection by microscopy is approximately 90% specific in differentiating bacterial from nonbacterial causes of diarrhea, but leukocytes can also be identified in noninfectious inflammatory bowel diseases such as Crohn disease or ulcerative colitis. Additional fecal markers of intestinal inflammation include lactoferrin, which has a high sensitivity (95%) but low specificity for infectious enteritis, and fecal calprotectin, which is reported to be 93% sensitive and 88% specific for detection of bacterial infection. In general, use of fecal biomarkers is considered insufficiently reliable for detecting infectious causes of diarrhea, and pathogen-directed diagnostic methods remain the standard of care.

Identification of specific enteric pathogens in some cases may be labor intensive, costly, and time consuming, and require a combination of culture, antigen assay, and nucleic acid detection by polymerase chain reaction (PCR). Recent application of culture-independent methods using broad-range multiplexed molecular assays has allowed for simultaneous testing for multiple pathogens. These syndromic panels detect multiple bacterial, viral, and parasitic pathogens that have been associated with infectious diarrhea, and they offer improved sensitivity over culture. While these assays provide a more rapid means of identifying bacterial enteric pathogens, they may lack specificity for the cause of the current illness and do not detect all potential pathogens. For these reasons, bacterial culture remains an important means of identifying a specific pathogen and performing antibiotic susceptibility testing.

## TREATMENT

Because children have greater insensible water loss and limited renal compensation compared with adults, they are at greater risk for fluid depletion and dehydration during an episode of acute diarrhea. As such, they should be assessed for signs of dehydration and hypovolemia on clinical examination and have therapy directed at fluid and electrolyte replacement. In those with severe dehydration and hypovolemic shock, intravenous fluids with isotonic crystalloid should be initiated and continued until circulating blood volume is restored while monitoring the patient's vital signs and urine output. Electrolyte derangements may occur and require correction in patients with severe diarrhea.

Oral rehydration therapy (ORT) is recommended by the American Academy of Pediatrics and the World Health Organization (WHO) as the preferred treatment for fluid and electrolyte losses in children with mild to moderate dehydration. Commercial ORT solutions are recommended. Fruit juices, sports drinks, and sodas are contraindicated and may aggravate fluid losses in the acute phase due to their high osmolar concentration. Following rehydration, children should be offered an unrestricted age-appropriate diet together with additional oral fluids to replace ongoing stool losses.

Empirical antimicrobials are not recommended for children with suspected infectious gastroenteritis. An exception may be made for children with suspected traveler's diarrhea as bacterial causes are more frequent than parasitic or viral causes and occur most commonly in the first 2 weeks of travel. Antibiotics effectively shorten the duration of moderate to severe traveler's diarrhea in adults. Because there are no good data for children in this regard, recommendations are derived from adult studies. Ciprofloxacin and azithromycin as single doses or 3-day therapy regimens are generally the preferred agents, with azithromycin favored in younger children. Nalidixic acid has also been used to treat traveler's diarrhea in children. The choice of agent also depends on the geographic destination; for example, a high rate of fluoroquinolone resistance in Southeast Asia makes azithromycin a more prudent choice if traveling to these areas. Use of antimotility agents is not recommended for the treatment of acute diarrhea in children.

Antimicrobial therapy may be indicated when certain bacterial and parasitic pathogens are detected in patients with moderate to severe disease, but the benefits and risks of antimicrobial therapy should be carefully considered. Targeted antibiotic therapy is effective in shortening the duration of dysentery and reducing the shedding of *Campylobacter* and *Shigella* species in stool. Antimicrobial therapy has proven efficacy against CDAD and most parasitic causes of infectious enteritis, including *Giardia* and *Cryptosporidium*. Conversely, antibiotics should be avoided in patients with enterohemorrhagic *E coli* and STEC because there is some evidence that their use increases the risk for hemolytic-uremic syndrome. Antibiotics are also not indicated in uncomplicated gastroenteritis caused by *Salmonella* species in otherwise healthy patients as this can lead to prolonged shedding or a chronic carrier state. Antimicrobial therapy against *Salmonella* species is recommended for children at risk for invasive or complicated disease, including children less than 3 months of age and those with underlying chronic GI tract disease, malignancies, hemoglobinopathies, or other known immunosuppressive illnesses or therapies.

A single dose of ondansetron has been shown to reduce the frequency of vomiting and allow successful rehydration with ORT. The role of other adjunctive therapies such as probiotics for the treatment of infectious enteritis is less clear and requires additional controlled data.

## PREVENTION

Because enteric pathogens are acquired via the fecal-oral route, strict hand washing, observing safe food preparation including washing of raw products and thorough cooking of eggs and other foods of animal origin, and access to clean drinking water are imperative to prevent spread of infection. In areas where clean water is not available, use of alcohol-based hand sanitizers containing at least 60% alcohol may be considered, although when hands are heavily soiled, sanitizers may be less effective than handwashing with soap and water for infections caused by *C difficile*, *Cryptosporidium*, or norovirus.

Certain bacterial infections (*Campylobacter, Cryptosporidium, E coli* O157:H7 and other STEC, *Shigella, Salmonella, Vibrio* species) are reportable to local and state US public health departments given concern for potential epidemic spread. In general, children are considered contagious for as long as the diarrhea is present. However, the risk of transmission of infection persists for as long as an infected person excretes the organism. For example, in children < 5 years of age with nontyphoidal *Salmonella* species GI infections, 45% will continue to excrete organisms 12 weeks after infection, long after symptoms have resolved.

Since the introduction of routine rotavirus vaccination in the United States in 2006, rates of healthcare utilization and hospitalization for rotavirus gastroenteritis have significantly decreased. As such, the WHO recommended inclusion of rotavirus vaccination in all national immunization programs globally in 2009, with expectations to lower the global burden caused by rotavirus diarrhea. Typhoid vaccine, both as oral live-attenuated and intramuscular polysaccharide formulations, is available for use in patients ≥ 6 years of age and ≥ 2 years of age, respectively. Overall efficacy of these vaccines ranges from 50% to 80%. They do not provide complete protection against *Salmonella typhi* serovars, do not provide reliable protection against *Salmonella paratyphi*, and have a variable duration of protection. Use of the oral typhoid vaccine is contraindicated in immunocompromised patients. Currently, recommended indications for typhoid vaccination include travelers to the Indian subcontinent, South and Southeast Asia, Latin America and the Caribbean, the Middle East, and the African continent who will have prolonged exposure to contaminated food and drink and intimate exposure to a household contact known to be a carrier. Typhoid vaccine is not a substitute for careful hand hygiene and safe food and water practices. A live cholera vaccine was recently approved by the US Food and Drug Administration for the prevention of *V cholerae* caused by serogroup 01 in otherwise healthy patients ≥ 18 years of age traveling to cholera-endemic countries. The single-dose, oral cholera vaccine should be taken at least 10 days before travel and may be shed in the stool of recipients for at least 7 days.

## SUGGESTED READINGS

Cortes JE, Curns AT, Tate JE, et al. Rotavirus vaccine and health care utilization for diarrhea in U.S. children. *N Engl J Med.* 2011;365:1108-1117.

Desai R, Curns AT, Steiner CA, Tate JE, Patel MM, Parashar UD. All-cause gastroenteritis and rotavirus-coded hospitalizations among US children, 2000-2009. *Clin Infect Dis.* 2012;55:e28-e34.

Freedman SB, Ali S, Oleszczuk M, Gouin S, Hartling L. Treatment of acute gastroenteritis in children: an overview of systematic reviews of interventions commonly used in developed countries. *Evid Based Child Health*. 2013;8:1123-1137.

Goldenberg JZ, Lytvyn L, Steurich J, Parkin P, Mahant S, Johnston BC. Probiotics for the prevention of pediatric antibiotic-associated diarrhea. *Cochrane Database Syst Rev*. 2015;12:CD004827.

Guarino A, Ashkenazi S, Gendrel D, Lo Vecchio A, Shamir R, Szajewska H. European Society for Pediatric Gastroenterology, Hepatology, and Nutrition/European Society for Pediatric Infectious Diseases evidence-based guidelines for the management of acute gastroenteritis in children in Europe: update 2014. *J Pediatr Gastroenterol Nutr*. 2014;59:132-152.

Humphries RM, Linscott AJ. Laboratory diagnosis of bacterial gastroenteritis. *Clin Microbiol Rev*. 2015;28:3-31.

Khare R, Espy MJ, Cebelinski E, et al. Comparative evaluation of two commercial multiplex panels for detection of gastrointestinal pathogens by use of clinical stool specimens. *J Clin Microbiol*. 2014;52:3667-3673.

Steffen R, Hill DR, DuPont HL. Traveler's diarrhea: a clinical review. *JAMA*. 2015;313:71-80.

# 232 Infections of the Liver

Grzegorz Telega

## INTRODUCTION

Patients with infections of the liver generally present with nonspecific symptoms such as fever, fatigue, abdominal pain, or weight loss. The abdominal pain may be diffuse, be confined to the right upper quadrant, or radiate to the shoulder or back. Other symptoms may include headache, arthralgias, and adenopathy. The initial history should focus on geographic location or travel, unprotected sex or drug use, use of hemodialysis or blood products, other recent exposures, vaccination/immune status, chronicity of symptoms, anatomical anomalies or surgery that may affect the biliary tracts, and family history of hepatitis. Physical exam is often normal; some patients will have right upper quadrant or diffuse abdominal tenderness and hepatomegaly. Jaundice or stigmata of chronic liver disease is infrequent. For additional details regarding viral hepatitis, please refer to Table 232-1 and Chapter 303.

Laboratory findings of liver infection often consist of leukocytosis, elevated erythrocyte sedimentation rate (ESR), and variable elevation of bilirubin, aminotransferases (alanine aminotransferase [ALT], aspartate aminotransferase [AST]), alkaline phosphatase, and γ-glutamyl transferase (GGT). Liver ultrasound is useful in initial evaluation of suspected liver infection because it can screen for liver abscess or bile duct anomalies.

## BACTERIAL CHOLANGITIS

Cholangitis is an infection of the biliary tracts and is seen most commonly in patients with abnormal biliary tracts such as post-Kasai (portoenterostomy) for biliary atresia. After portoenterostomy, nearly 60% of patients have 1 or more episodes of cholangitis, with decreasing frequency over time. Other conditions that cause functional or mechanical obstruction of the bile ducts such as gallstones, congenital hepatic fibrosis, Caroli syndrome, choledochal cysts, and primary sclerosing cholangitis (PSC) also increase the risk of cholangitis. When these patients present with fever and no other obvious source of infection, they should be evaluated for possible cholangitis. Cholangitis classically presents with fever, jaundice, and right upper quadrant pain (Charcot triad); however, in children, not all symptoms may be present. In patients post-Kasai, fever is seen in nearly 100% of patients with cholangitis, usually with increased bilirubin or acholic stools and laboratory values showing either leukocytosis or leukopenia. Evaluation of cholangitis should include ALT, AST, alkaline phosphatase, GGT, and blood and urine cultures, although blood cultures will be positive in less than 50% of cases. Imaging should also be undertaken by either ultrasound or computed tomography (CT) scan to rule out the presence of abscess, calculi, ductal dilatation, or other anatomic lesions. If concern persists regarding the presence of a stone, a magnetic resonance cholangiogram may be helpful in delineating the location. Liver biopsy can be used to support the diagnosis; however, the diagnostic value of the biopsy should be balanced with the risk of the procedure.

Therapy for cholangitis begins with ensuring that the patient is hemodynamically stable with fluid resuscitation as needed. The patient may require nasogastric suction if an ileus is present. Antibiotics are given parenterally and should cover the most likely pathogens considering local antibiotic sensitivities and have adequate biliary penetration. Cholangitis is most commonly caused by enteric pathogens such as *Escherichia coli*, *Klebsiella*, *Enterobacter*, and *Enterococcus*; thus, antibiotic coverage often involves a third-generation cephalosporin or broad-spectrum penicillin such as ampicillin-sulbactam in addition to an aminoglycoside. At times, coverage should be expanded to include anaerobic bacteria, with a drug such as metronidazole. If the patient remains febrile, with evidence of obstruction, bile duct decompression is necessary. Available options include endoscopic retrograde cholangiopancreatography (ERCP), percutaneous drainage, or open surgical intervention. The type of intervention depends on clinical stability, anatomy of the lesion, and available procedural expertise. Following therapeutic measures, patients should demonstrate response with defervescence and corresponding decrease in bilirubin, aminotransferases, and white blood cell count. Treatment should continue for 14 to 21 days.

## LIVER ABSCESS

Liver abscesses are usually classified as pyogenic or amoebic based on etiology. The distinction is important because treatment varies substantially. Important aspects of the patient's history that suggest amoebic rather than pyogenic abscess include bloody diarrhea or travel to tropical areas preceding the illness.

### Pyogenic Liver Abscess

Pyogenic abscesses may be associated with trauma to the biliary tract or hematogenous spread through the portal vein in conditions such as appendicitis or inflammatory bowel disease. Other risk factors include pelvic inflammatory disease and altered immune status such as chronic granulomatous disease or leukemia. Signs and symptoms are usually nonspecific but commonly include fever, weight loss, abdominal pain, right upper quadrant tenderness, and hepatomegaly. A more fulminant presentation associated with septic shock may occur when multiple abscesses or a ruptured abscess occurs. Laboratory findings often demonstrate leukocytosis and an elevated ESR, but aminotransferases, alkaline phosphatase, and bilirubin may be normal or only mildly elevated. Diagnosis requires a high degree of suspicion and appropriate imaging.

Ultrasound may identify focal hypodense lesions and suggest presence of liver abscess. Abdominal CT or magnetic resonance imaging (MRI) scans are used to further define lesions. They may demonstrate abscesses as small as 1 cm. Abscesses appear as areas of hypoattenuation, with surrounding edema. These findings are enhanced through the use of intravenous contrast. A solid appearance should suggest tumor. Pyogenic abscesses are frequently multifocal. Amoebic abscesses, on the other hand, are usually single, most often in the right lobe, near the diaphragm; these findings, however, do not reliably distinguish between pyogenic abscess and amoebic abscess.

Abscess fluid should be obtained by either needle aspiration or placement of a drainage catheter. Indications for open surgery are noted in Figure 232-1. Specimens should be sent for Gram stain and culture. Gram-positive bacteria are most common in children, although gram-negative bacteria and anaerobes are frequently involved, and the specimen may grow more than 1 pathogen. Antibiotic therapy is aimed at covering the most likely pathogens and is then refined based on culture results and susceptibilities. Treatment parenterally for 4 to 6 weeks is generally recommended.

**TABLE 232-1 COMMON VIRAL INFECTIONS OF THE LIVER AND PRESENTATION**

| | Acute Hepatitis | Chronic Hepatitis | Acute Liver Failure | Comments |
|---|---|---|---|---|
| **Hepatotrophic** | | | | |
| HAV | ++ | – | + | More common in developing countries; children may be asymptomatic |
| HBV | + | +++ | + | Children may be asymptomatic |
| HCV | + | +++ | – | |
| HDV | + | +++ | – | Only affects HBV(+) patients, worsens outcome |
| HEV | ++ | – | + | More common in developing countries |
| **DNA** | | | | |
| CMV | + | + | – | Affects infants/children more than adolescents/adults |
| EBV | ++ | + | – | Lymphadenopathy; PTLD in immunosuppressed patients |
| HSV-1, -2 | ++ | – | + | Occurs in setting of overwhelming viremia/sepsis |
| Adenovirus | ++ | – | + | |
| VZV | ++ | – | + | Most often affects immunocompromised patients |
| HHV 6, 7 | ++ | – | + | |
| Parvovirus | + | – | + | Often causes aplastic anemia simultaneously |
| **RNA** | | | | |
| HIV | ++ | ++ | – | Symptoms often due to coinfection |
| Enterovirus | ++ | – | + | |
| Measles | + | – | + | |
| Rubella | + | – | – | |
| TTV | + | – | – | |
| Reovirus | – | + | – | Possible association with EHBA, cholangiopathy |
| Parechovirus | + | – | + | |
| Coronavirus | + | – | – | |

(–) unlikely; (+) infrequent to (+++) most likely form of liver involvement for each pathogen.

CMV, cytomegalovirus; DNA, deoxyribonucleic acid; EBV, Epstein-Barr virus; EHBA, extrahepatic biliary atresia; HAV, hepatitis A virus; HBV, hepatitis B virus; HCV, hepatitis C virus; HDV, hepatitis D virus; HEV, hepatitis E virus; HHV, human herpesvirus; HIV, human immunodeficiency virus; HSV, herpes simplex virus; PTLD, posttransplant lymphoproliferative disorder; RNA, ribonucleic acid; TTV, transfusion-transmitted virus; VZV, varicella-zoster virus.

### Amoebic Liver Abscess

Amoebic abscess presents similarly to pyogenic liver abscess but is caused by *Entamoeba histolytica*, which is reported to cause hepatic abscesses in up to 7% of invasive cases (see Chapter 336). Younger children and those living in or traveling from tropical regions such as Southeast Asia or Central or South America are most commonly affected. Jaundice is infrequently seen, and diarrhea may be seen in less than half of patients at the time of presentation; however, a history of dysentery should raise suspicion for this disease.

As with pyogenic liver abscess, the leukocyte count and ESR are usually elevated, and ALT and AST, bilirubin, and alkaline phosphatase are normal to mildly elevated. Imaging studies should include ultrasound or CT of the abdomen. Additional studies include evaluation of the stool for ova and parasites looking for trophozoites or cysts and testing the stool for *E histolytica* antigen; note that stool tests may be negative in the case of extraintestinal amebiasis and that routine ova and parasite examination does not permit differentiation of *E histolytica* from nonpathogenic *Entamoeba*. Serologic testing of the blood is positive in > 90% of patients. Many patients from endemic areas, however, will already have antibodies from previous exposure; the tests can also be falsely negative for the first 7 days of infection. Aspiration of the abscess may also be used to distinguish between pyogenic and amoebic liver abscess. In amoebic liver abscess, the fluid is classically sterile and reddish-brown in color; amoebic organisms will be seen in less than one-third of cases.

Treatment most often begins with metronidazole (50 mg/kg/d divided into 3 doses) for 10 days, with alternatives of tinidazole, ornidazole, and nitazoxanide, which can be given for shorter periods of time. This should then be followed by a luminal amoebicide such as paromomycin or iodoquinol for 10 or 20 days, respectively. This combination is effective at eradication in > 90% of patients. Surgery or invasive therapy usually is not needed. Aspiration may be indicated when fever and abdominal pain persist after 4 to 5 days of treatment and in large abscesses with imminent risk of rupture. In these patients, repeated aspiration may be helpful in improving symptoms and speeding symptom resolution. Complications are generally related to delay in diagnosis or rupture of the abscess, which can cause peritonitis, as well as pulmonary or even cardiac involvement. Mortality is directly related to these findings.

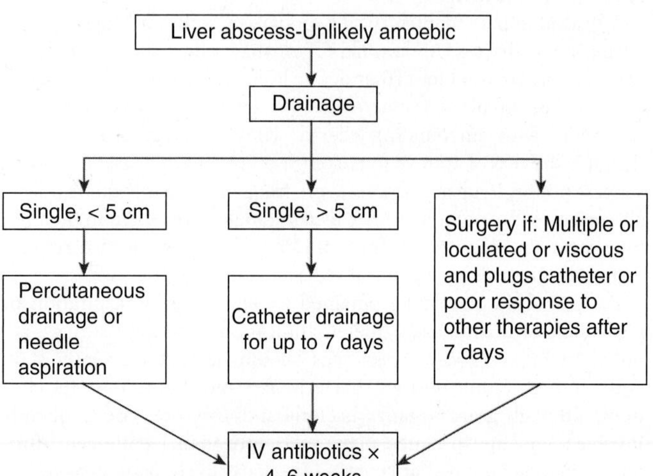


**FIGURE 232-1** Surgical management of pyogenic liver abscess.

## OTHER INFECTIONS OF THE LIVER

A list of nonviral liver pathogens is provided in Table 232-2. Bacterial infections can also result in liver involvement as part of the systemic manifestations. Cat scratch disease (CSD), caused by *Bartonella henselae*, is most often found in warm, humid climates and, in addition to

**TABLE 232-2 COMMON NONVIRAL INFECTIONS OF THE LIVER AND TYPES OF LIVER INVOLVEMENT**

| | Parenchymal | | | | |
|---|---|---|---|---|---|
| | Abscess | Diffuse | Cholangitis | Immunocompromised | Comments |
| **Bacteria** | | | | | |
| **Gram positive** | | | | | |
| *Actinomyces israelii* | + | – | – | – | Sulfur granules on Gram stain are diagnostic |
| *Enterococcus* | + | – | +++ | ++ | |
| *Listeria monocytogenes* | – | + | – | ++ | Granulomas |
| *Staphylococcus aureus* | +++ | + | + | + | Diffuse involvement in toxic shock syndrome |
| *Streptococcus* species | + | ++ | + | + | Diffuse involvement in toxic shock syndrome |
| **Gram negative** | | | | | |
| *Bacteroides* species | + | – | + | + | |
| *Bartonella henselae* | ++ | + | – | + | Multiple abscesses |
| *Brucella* species | + | ++ | – | + | Granulomas |
| *Coxiella burnetii* | – | + | – | + | Q fever |
| *Ehrlichia chaffeensis* | – | ++ | + | + | |
| *Escherichia coli* | +++ | + | +++ | ++ | Hyperbilirubinemia with sepsis/urinary tract infections |
| *Francisella tularensis* | + | + | – | – | Tularemia |
| *Klebsiella* | +++ | + | +++ | + | |
| *Neisseria gonorrhoeae* | – | – | – | – | Adhesions, white plaques; perihepatitis (Fitz-Hugh–Curtis) |
| *Pseudomonas* species | – | – | + | + | |
| *Rickettsia rickettsii* | – | + | – | + | Rocky Mountain spotted fever |
| *Salmonella* species | + | ++ | + | + | "Typhoid nodules," rare granulomas |
| **Other** | | | | | |
| *Mycobacterium avium intracellulare* | – | – | – | ++ | |
| *Mycobacterium tuberculosis* | + | + | + | ++ | Caseating granulomas in portal areas |
| *Borrelia burgdorferi* | – | + | – | – | Lyme disease |
| *Chlamydia trachomatis* | – | – | – | – | Adhesions, white plaques; perihepatitis (Fitz-Hugh–Curtis) |
| *Leptospira interrogans* | – | + | – | + | 5–10% with icterohemorrhagic presentation |
| *Treponema pallidum* | + | ++ | + | + | Jaundice in newborns |
| **Parasites**[a] | | | | | |
| *Ascaris lumbricoides* | – | – | ++ | + | |
| *Clonorchis sinensis* | – | – | ++ | + | May lead to secondary abscess with *E coli* |
| *Cryptosporidium* | – | – | ++ | +++ | |
| *Echinococcus* species | – | – | + | + | Cyst formation |
| *Entamoeba histolytica* | ++ | + | – | + | |
| *Fasciola hepatica* | – | ++ | ++ | + | |
| *Leishmania donovani* | – | ++ | – | + | Possible granulomas |
| *Plasmodium* species | – | + | – | + | |
| *Schistosoma* species | – | + | – | + | "Pipestem fibrosis" on liver biopsy |
| *Toxocara canis* | – | – | – | + | Granulomas |
| **Fungi** | | | | | |
| *Aspergillus* species | + | + | – | + | |
| *Candida* species | ++ | ++ | – | +++ | |
| *Coccidioides immitis* | – | + | – | + | Disseminated in immunocompromised patients |
| *Cryptococcus neoformans* | – | + | + | + | |
| *Histoplasma capsulatum* | – | + | – | + | |
| *Penicillium marneffei* | ++ | + | – | ++ | |

(–) unlikely; (+) infrequent to (+++) most likely form of liver involvement for each pathogen.

[a]Parasites are all more likely in developing countries.

lymphadenitis, can cause hepatitis, granulomatous hepatitis, hepatosplenomegaly, and hepatic or splenic abscesses. Symptoms are often nonspecific (eg, fever) but may be similar to other liver infections previously discussed; in addition, patients often present with chronic adenopathy. The evaluation, therefore, should focus on a history of cat exposure, adenopathy, and seeking an inoculation site. Imaging studies may show multiple small lesions in both spleen and liver parenchyma, and antibody titers are typically elevated. Antibiotics may not be needed unless the patient is immunosuppressed; complete recovery is expected.

Fitz-Hugh–Curtis syndrome is the common name for perihepatitis in association with salpingitis most often seen in young females.

Among adolescents with salpingitis, rates of Fitz-Hugh–Curtis syndrome range from 4% to 12% in most reports, but have been described in up to 27%. Signs and symptoms generally include severe right upper quadrant pain at the lower costal margin with occasional radiation to the back or shoulder that increases with inspiration or deep palpation, in addition to a friction rub over the anterior costal margin. Laboratory values are not typically as helpful as is the clinical picture taken in context. The most common organisms are those that cause pelvic inflammatory disease (*Neisseria gonorrhoeae* and *Chlamydia trachomatis*), which can be identified in urine or cervical or rectal swabs. Treatment should cover the most likely bacteria; recommendations for treatment are updated periodically and are available on the Centers for Disease Control and Prevention (CDC) website.

### LIVER INFECTIONS IN THE IMMUNOCOMPROMISED

Fungal liver infections are a serious and a significant cause of morbidity and mortality most often seen in immunocompromised patients, especially neutropenic patients undergoing chemotherapy or post-transplant patients. Because the symptoms are nonspecific, this condition should be suspected when a neutropenic patient remains febrile on broad-spectrum antibiotics and blood cultures have shown no growth. Fever, hepatomegaly, and splenomegaly are frequently seen with elevated alkaline phosphatase more often than elevated bilirubin or liver enzymes. Ultrasound appears to be less sensitive than CT in the diagnosis of fungal liver infection. Different etiologies are listed in Table 232-2. Pertinent geographic clues include living or traveling in the southwestern United States or Mexico (*Coccidioides*) or living or traveling through the Ohio or Mississippi River Valleys in the United States (histoplasmosis).

In the immunocompromised patient, special attention should be given to opportunistic pathogens causing cholangiopathy, a condition with similar clinical and radiologic appearance as PSC. Cholangiopathy is seen in patients with deficient cell-mediated immunity such as those who have acquired immunodeficiency syndrome (AIDS), severe combined immunodeficiency (SCID), common variable immunodeficiency (CVID), Wiskott-Aldrich syndrome, major histocompatibility complex class II deficiency, interferon-γ deficiency, DiGeorge syndrome, or hyper-IgM syndromes. Signs and symptoms are similar to acute cholangitis with abdominal pain and fever, but jaundice is less common. Other findings may include hepatomegaly and diarrhea. Laboratory values often demonstrate an elevated alkaline phosphatase with only mild elevation of bilirubin and mild to no change in liver enzymes. Mild hypoalbuminemia, anemia, or leukopenia may also be noted. Abdominal ultrasound may demonstrate mild dilation of the bile ducts, an enlarged gallbladder, and abnormal liver texture with possible splenomegaly. Detailed evaluation of the bile ducts may require magnetic resonance cholangiogram or ERCP. The most common pathogens include cryptosporidium and cytomegalovirus, but microsporidia and mycobacteria can also cause cholangiopathy. Efforts are more often aimed at prevention rather than treatment of the disease, as cholangiopathy often reflects an advanced disease stage and carries a poor prognosis. Therefore, in patients with AIDS, antiretroviral therapy remains the best option; with the introduction of highly active antiretroviral therapy and subsequent improved immune status, cholangiopathy is seen less frequently in human immunodeficiency virus (HIV)-infected patients. Patients with congenital immunodeficiencies may require bone marrow transplantation.

### SUGGESTED READINGS

Belvisi V, Tieghi T, Grenga PL, et al. *Bartonella henselae* infection presenting with ocular and hepatosplenic manifestations in a immunocompetent child. *Pediatr Infect Dis J*. 2012;31:882-883.

Decharun K, Leys CM, West KW, Finnell SM. Prophylactic antibiotics for prevention of cholangitis in patients with biliary atresia status post-Kasai portoenterostomy: a systematic review. *Clin Pediatr*. 2016;55:66-72.

Hsu YL, Lin HC, Yen TY, Hsieh TH, Wei HM, Hwang KP. Pyogenic liver abscess among children in a medical center in Central Taiwan. *J Microbiol Immunol Infect*. 2015;48:302-305.

Law ST, Kong Li MK. Is there a difference in pyogenic liver abscess caused by *Streptococcus milleri* and *Klebsiella* spp? Retrospective analysis over a 10-year period in a regional hospital. *J Microbiol Immunol Infect*. 2013;46:11-18.

Ng KF, Tan KK, Ngui R, et al. Fatal case of amoebic liver abscess in a child. *Asian Pac J Trop Med*. 2015;8:878-880.

# 233 Urinary Tract Infection

Ruthie R. Su and Ellen R. Wald

### INTRODUCTION

Since the introduction of routine immunization against *Haemophilus influenzae* type b and *Streptococcus pneumoniae*, urinary tract infections (UTIs) have replaced bacteremia and meningitis as the most common serious bacterial infection in children. Identification and treatment of UTIs are important in managing signs and symptoms such as fever and dysuria, and also for preventing and minimizing the morbidity associated with pyelonephritis and sepsis. The site of infection may be the bladder (cystitis), ureters (ureteritis), pelvis (pyelitis), and/or renal parenchyma (pyelonephritis).

### PATHOGENESIS AND EPIDEMIOLOGY

The pathogenesis of UTI depends on a complex interaction between bacterial and host factors. The urinary tract is normally a sterile environment with nearby bacterial reservoirs in the distal urethra, periurethral region, perianal region, perineum, and vagina. With normal hydration and spontaneous voiding, the urinary flow through the distal urethra helps to prevent bacterial ascension into the bladder. Maintenance of normal flora prevents more virulent strains from colonizing the gut and the periurethral area; an individual's microbiome may be influenced by age, hormones, recent antibiotic use, hygiene, or spermicides.

The majority of UTIs are initiated by bacteria that ascend the urethra and adhere to the mucosal lining of the bladder; a hematogenous source that seeds the urinary tract is much less common but is also possible. The most studied model of bacterial adhesion in the urinary tract is the "P" fimbriae expressed on the surface of uropathogenic *Escherichia coli*. These bacterial proteins enable adherence of uropathogenic *E coli* to the bladder. They are referred to as P fimbriae because they can recognize and agglutinate erythrocytes of the P1 blood group. The P blood group antigen is also present on human uroepithelial cells.

Following adhesion, the bacteria may invade across the mucosal barrier and trigger an inflammatory host reaction. White blood cells (WBCs) are then recruited to respond to the bacterial invasion, resulting in leukocytes appearing in the urine (pyuria). The inflammatory response results in the typical symptoms of cystitis including dysuria, urinary frequency, and urgency.

Understanding the pathogenesis of UTI clarifies how certain factors can increase the risk of UTI. For example, bacterial ascension via adherence to the urethra and bladder may be facilitated by infrequent or dysfunctional voiding. Dysfunctional voiding refers to the lack of coordination between 2 processes that are essential for normal voiding to occur—relaxation of the urethral sphincter and contraction of the detrusor muscle of the bladder. The failure of the voluntary sphincter to relax causes an obstruction to the urine outflow during voiding. Coordinated bladder-sphincter control and efficient elimination of urine with a brisk urine outflow across the urethra is a natural defense mechanism against bacterial ascension and adherence. Toilet training is a period during which the risk for UTI rises as the child may inappropriately tighten and relax the sphincter to be socially continent. Children being evaluated for recurrent UTIs will often exhibit dysfunctional voiding on their urologic workup. They will also often have constipation whereby the distended rectum pushes up against the bladder outlet and obstructs the urine flow.

There can be mechanical, anatomic, or structural risk factors that promote UTIs. Indwelling catheters breach the separation between urinary tract and colonized body surface. Congenital genitourinary anomalies indicated by dilation anywhere along the urinary tract often present with UTI because there has been obstruction to normal antegrade urine flow. On the other hand, if during gestational development there was abnormal migration of the Wolffian ducts resulting in laterally displaced ureters, the ureterovesical valve may be faulty, resulting in vesicoureteral reflux (VUR). VUR increases the risk of pyelonephritis by promoting bacterial ascension to the kidneys.

*E coli* is the most common uropathogen and causes about 80% of all UTIs; other common gram-negative uropathogens include *Klebsiella*, *Proteus*, *Enterobacter*, and *Citrobacter*. Common gram-positive uropathogens include *Staphylococcus saprophyticus*, *Enterococcus*, and rarely, *Staphylococcus aureus*. According to the American Academy of Pediatrics 2011 guidelines, *Lactobacillus* species, other coagulase-negative staphylococci, and *Corynebacterium* species are not considered clinically relevant urine isolates. Factors that affect the incidence of UTIs include gender, age, race, circumcision status, and general health. Throughout childhood, adolescence, and adulthood, females are at higher risk for UTI than males. In contrast, during the early part of the first year of life, boys have a higher incidence of UTI than girls (2.7% vs 0.7%). After the first year of life, the incidence of UTI in males drops to 0.03% to 2% and rises in females to 1% to 3%. Caucasians are at higher risk for UTI than blacks. Uncircumcised boys have up to 12 times the risk of UTI than circumcised boys. Factors such as dysfunctional voiding, constipation, sexual activity, and bladder catheterization increase the risk of UTI.

## CLINICAL MANIFESTATIONS

Cystitis is the most common clinical manifestation of infection of the urinary tract. Classic symptoms include urgency, frequency, or dysuria. Children may also have a history of difficulty in initiating the urinary stream. Occasionally, children may complain of abdominal or suprapubic pain. If fever is present, it is usually low grade. The urine may be foul smelling and cloudy.

The clinical presentation of acute pyelonephritis (APN) is more severe; those who have APN have chills, spiking fevers, and complaints of back pain. They may have associated gastrointestinal complaints of diarrhea and especially vomiting. Lower urinary tract symptoms, such as frequency, urgency, dysuria, and suprapubic discomfort, may or may not be present. Other findings vary, such as irritability, poor feeding, vomiting, decreased urinary output, and clinical evidence of dehydration. Infants with APN usually have high fever without other localizing features; since their clinical presentation of UTI tends to be nonspecific, diagnosis relies heavily on laboratory studies outlined below.

Features of the physical examination that should be emphasized include (1) an accurate measurement of blood pressure (hypertension may be present in patients who have chronic renal disease), (2) general growth and development (failure to thrive may be a sign of chronic or recurrent UTI), and (3) a careful abdominal examination (which might reveal tenderness or a mass caused by either an enlarged bladder or an obstructed urinary tract). An effort should be made to elicit the finding of costovertebral angle tenderness in children of all ages. The perineum should be inspected carefully to search for signs of irritation, scars, tears, signs of trauma, labial adhesions, or evidence of vulvovaginitis. A rectal examination should be considered to detect masses or poor sphincter tone, which might be associated with a neurogenic bladder. The lower back should be observed for any lipoma, sinus, pigmentation, or tuft of hair that may be evidence of an occult myelodysplasia.

## DIAGNOSIS



In infants or children who are not toilet trained, a sample of urine should be obtained for urinalysis and urine culture via catheterization or suprapubic aspiration (SPA). SPA yields a specimen of urine that completely avoids any contamination from the perineal flora. When urine is obtained via catheterization, the first few drops of urine should not be collected in the sterile container as they may be contaminated by the bacteria in the distal urethra. If the first attempt at catheterization is not successful, a new catheter is required for the next attempt. Urine collected with a bag affixed to the perineum results in a high false-positive rate due to contamination from colonization of the perineum, the vagina in girls, and the prepuce in uncircumcised boys. Bagged specimens are only helpful when the results are negative; if the results from a bagged specimen suggest infection (urine dipstick is positive for leukocyte esterase [LE] or nitrites or microscopic analysis is positive for WBCs or bacteria), then another specimen should be obtained via catheterization or SPA before initiating treatment. In the child who is toilet trained, a freshly voided midstream clean catch urine specimen may be obtained. If the urine is kept at room temperature, it should be analyzed within 1 hour; otherwise the urine should be refrigerated and analyzed within 4 hours.

A diagnosis of UTI requires that there is pyuria ($\geq$ 3 WBCs per high-power field [hpf] or $\geq$ 10 WBCs/μL or $\geq$ trace LE on dipstick) and at least 50,000 colony-forming units (CFUs) of a single bacterial species per milliliter of urine when obtained by clean catch or catheter. The presence of pyuria helps to distinguish asymptomatic bacteriuria from true UTI. Asymptomatic bacteriuria occurs in 0.8% of preschool girls and 1% to 2% of school-age girls. Results from the urinalysis will likely be available before the preliminary urine culture, which requires at least 24 hours. In a febrile infant or a child with symptoms suggestive of UTI, a urinalysis suspicious for UTI may include the presence of bacteria or WBCs on microscopy or the presence of LE or nitrites on dipstick (Table 233-1). Nitrites result from the conversion of dietary nitrates to nitrites by gram-negative enteric bacteria such as *E coli* and require about 4 hours in the bladder. A false-negative nitrite on a dipstick may be due to insufficient bladder time in young children who frequently empty their bladders in less than 4 hours or due to infection with bacteria that do not convert dietary nitrates to nitrites (eg, *Enterococcus*, *Pseudomonas*, *Acinetobacter*, and *S saprophyticus*). LE is an enzyme found in WBCs and is a surrogate marker for WBCs in the urine. LE has a specificity of about 78%; accordingly, false-positive results may be observed. The presence of bacteria on a Gram stain of a sample of fresh, uncentrifuged urine correlates with $10^5$ CFUs/mL but requires more equipment and expertise than dipsticks.

It should be noted that the definition or threshold of what constitutes a positive urine culture varies according to different guidelines. In general, the varying thresholds take into account the risk of contamination from the distal urethra and periurethral region with a higher threshold used for clean catch specimens and a lower threshold used for urines obtained by catheterization or SPA. The $10^5$ cutoff is based on morning-voided urine samples from adult women with pyelonephritis and applies to clean catch specimens. With the added stipulation that there must be evidence of pyuria, a lower cutoff of

**TABLE 233-1 SENSITIVITY AND SPECIFICITY OF URINALYSIS COMPONENTS**

| Positive Test | Sensitivity (%) | Specificity (%) |
|---|---|---|
| Leukocyte esterase (LE) | 83 | 78 |
| Nitrite | 53 | 98 |
| LE or nitrite | 93 | 72 |
| Microscopy, white blood cells | 73 | 81 |
| Microscopy, bacteria | 81 | 83 |

Adapted with permission from Subcommittee on Urinary Tract Infection, Steering Committee on Quality Improvement and Management, Roberts KB: Urinary tract infection: clinical practice guideline for the diagnosis and management of the initial UTI in febrile infants and children 2 to 24 months, *Pediatrics* 2011 Sep;128(3):595-610.

50,000 CFUs/mL is acceptable and is also the general standard for specimens obtained by catheter. Any growth in urine collected by SPA should be considered a positive culture; however, most samples have high colony counts.

## TREATMENT

For febrile UTI, the length of treatment should be 7 to 14 days. In an otherwise healthy child with suspected afebrile acute cystitis and without a history of recurrent UTI, a shorter course may be sufficient.

Oral and parenteral antibiotics are equally efficacious treatment for a UTI; the latter is indicated if the patient is either toxic or vomiting or if there are no oral options available (Tables 233-2 and 233-3). Empiric treatment should be based on the local antibiogram, if possible, due to the community variability in resistance and then, if necessary, adjusted according to the antimicrobial susceptibility profile of the uropathogen isolated. Initial oral antibiotic options include cephalosporins, amoxicillin-clavulanate, or trimethoprim-sulfamethoxazole. Sulfonamides should be avoided in premature infants or newborns younger than 4 weeks given the risk of hyperbilirubinemia, jaundice, and kernicterus. Nitrofurantoin does not reach adequate concentrations in tissue, so it is not a good option if pyelonephritis is suspected. Nitrofurantoin should also be avoided in neonates and those with renal insufficiency, liver dysfunction, and glucose-6-phosphate dehydrogenase deficiency.

Infection with *Enterococcus* is more common during early infancy; accordingly, antibiotic coverage for neonates should include intravenous ampicillin. Broader coverage should also be considered for patients with recent antibiotic exposure, recent hospitalization, or history of genitourinary anomaly because they are at risk for infection with a drug-resistant bacterial species. Increased coverage includes antipseudomonal penicillins, β-lactam/β-lactamase inhibitor combinations, fluoroquinolones, second-, third-, or fourth-generation cephalosporins, and carbapenems. Fluoroquinolones are not a first-line consideration but are an effective choice when *Pseudomonas aeruginosa* is suspected or proven to be the cause of infection.

The risk of recurrent UTI is highest 3 to 6 months after the index infection. Parents should be educated regarding this possibility and encouraged to seek prompt treatment if a fever or symptomatic UTI develops again. Besides a recent UTI, risk factors for recurrent UTI include bladder and bowel dysfunction (voiding dysfunction and constipation) and congenital anomalies.

A renal and bladder ultrasound is indicated following a first febrile UTI for patients 3 months to 2 years of age; if the ultrasound shows hydronephrosis, a dilated ureter, other evidence of obstructive uropathy, or another significant abnormality, then a voiding cystourethrogram (VCUG) is recommended. A VCUG can also be considered depending on the presence of a family history of VUR; the child's age, sex, and race; the severity and course of the initial infection; bladder and bowel dysfunction; and importance that parents place on preventing recurrences. The incidence of reflux in girls evaluated after a first UTI is 25% to 40%. If VUR is detected, antibiotic prophylaxis may be considered. A recent large, randomized, placebo-controlled trial (the RIVUR study) showed that antibiotic prophylaxis with trimethoprim-sulfamethoxazole approximately halves the risk of recurrent UTI. The rate of recurrent febrile or symptomatic UTI in these patients with VUR was 24% in the placebo group and 13% in the trimethoprim-sulfamethoxazole group over 2 years. These data can be discussed with parents during shared decision making regarding the use of prophylactic antimicrobials.

**TABLE 233-2 EMPIRIC PARENTERAL ANTIBIOTIC OPTIONS**

| Agent | Dosage |
|---|---|
| Ceftriaxone | 75 mg/kg/d |
| Cefotaxime | 150 mg/kg/d, divided every 6–8 hours |
| Ceftazidime | 100–150 mg/d, divided every 8 hours |
| Gentamicin | 7.5 mg/kg/d, divided every 8 hours |
| Tobramycin | 5 mg/kg/d, divided every 8 hours |
| Piperacillin | 300 mg/kg/d, divided every 6–8 hours |

Adapted with permission from Subcommittee on Urinary Tract Infection, Steering Committee on Quality Improvement and Management, Roberts KB: Urinary tract infection: clinical practice guideline for the diagnosis and management of the initial UTI in febrile infants and children 2 to 24 months, *Pediatrics* 2011 Sep;128(3):595-610.

**TABLE 233-3 EMPIRIC ORAL ANTIBIOTIC OPTIONS**

| Agent | Dosage |
|---|---|
| Amoxicillin-clavulanate | 20–40 mg/kg/d, divided in 3 doses |
| Trimethoprim-sulfamethoxazole | 6–12 mg/kg trimethoprim and 30–60 mg/kg sulfamethoxazole/d, divided in 2 doses |
| Sulfisoxazole | 120–150 mg/kg/d, divided in 4 doses |
| Cefixime (third generation) | 8 mg/kg/d |
| Cefpodoxime (third generation) | 10 mg/kg/d, divided in 2 doses |
| Cefprozil (second generation) | 30 mg/kg/d, divided in 2 doses |
| Cefuroxime (second generation) | 20–30 mg/kg/d, divided in 2 doses |
| Cephalexin (first generation) | 50–100 mg/kg/d, divided in 4 doses |
| Nitrofurantoin | 5–7 mg/kg/d, divided in 4 doses |

Adapted with permission from Subcommittee on Urinary Tract Infection, Steering Committee on Quality Improvement and Management, Roberts KB: Urinary tract infection: clinical practice guideline for the diagnosis and management of the initial UTI in febrile infants and children 2 to 24 months, *Pediatrics* 2011 Sep;128(3):595-610.

## PREVENTION

The use of prophylactic antimicrobial agents in order to prevent recurrences of UTIs in patients with VUR is controversial. The RIVUR study showed that although prophylaxis does not prevent renal scarring, it does reduce the risk of recurrence by 50%. Many support the use of prophylactic antimicrobial therapy in patients with grade III to V VUR with the understanding that eventual antimicrobial resistance to the prophylactic agent is likely to develop.

Among preschool and school-age children, bladder and bowel dysfunction are common. A history of dysfunctional voiding can be elicited by inquiring about voiding postponement, urinary incontinence, and constipation. First-line therapy is behavioral modification with more frequent, timed voiding every 2 to 3 hours, increased water intake (1 L/d) in addition to all other fluids consumed, correction of constipation, and improved perineal hygiene if possible. Children who exhibit persistent inability to relax their sphincters may require training that involves relaxation techniques reinforced with biofeedback. Referral to a pediatric urologist may be necessary in some instances.

## SUGGESTED READINGS


Cooper CS, Storm DW. Infection and inflammation of the pediatric genitourinary tract. In: Wein AJ, Kavoussi LR, Partin AW, Peters CA, eds. *Campbell-Walsh Urology*. 11th ed. Philadelphia, PA: Elsevier Saunders; 2016:2926-2948.

Mathews R, Mattoo TK. The role of antimicrobial prophylaxis in the management of children with vesicoureteral reflux—the RIVUR study outcomes. *Adv Chronic Kidney Dis*. 2015;22:325-330.

RIVUR Trial Investigators, Hoberman A, Greenfield SP, et al. Antimicrobial prophylaxis for children with vesicoureteral reflux. *N Engl J Med*. 2014;370:2367-2376.

Roberts KB, Downs SM, Finnell SME, et al. Reaffirmation of AAP clinical practice guideline. The diagnosis and management of the initial urinary tract infection in febrile infants and young children 2 to 24 months of age. *Pediatrics*. 2016;138(6):e20163026.

Wald ER. Cystitis and pyelonephritis. In: Cherry JD, Harrison GJ, Kaplan SL, Steinbach WJ, Hotez PJ, eds. *Feigin and Cherry's Textbook of Pediatric Infectious Diseases*. 7th ed. Philadelphia, PA: Elsevier Saunders; 2014:535-553.

# 234 Catheter-Associated Bloodstream Infections

Candace Johnson and Marc Foca

## INTRODUCTION

Intravascular catheters are used for a wide range of therapies in pediatric patients, such as administering total parenteral nutrition and chemotherapy, providing reliable access for hemodynamic monitoring, blood drawing, and performing interventions such as hemodialysis. No longer limited to the acute care setting, intravascular catheters are also used in outpatient settings. For the purposes of discussing management, complication risks, and preventive strategies, these catheters can be subdivided into short-term, intermediate-term, and long-term devices based on planned duration of use. While there is overlap between catheter types used for given planned durations, it is generally accepted that nontunneled central venous catheters are used for short-term access, peripherally inserted central catheters (PICCs) are often used as intermediate-term catheters, and long-term catheters include tunneled catheters and implantable ports.

## PATHOGENESIS AND EPIDEMIOLOGY

Catheter-related bloodstream infections (CR-BSIs) are one of the more common types of healthcare-associated infections and result in increased healthcare costs, increased use of antimicrobials, prolonged hospital stays, morbidity, and death. The pathogenesis of CR-BSI varies. Different types include migration of potential pathogens from the skin at the exit site along the external surface of the catheter to the catheter tip; intraluminal migration of organisms from the catheter hub; contaminated infusates; and rarely, seeding of the catheter hematogenously from a distant focus. Current evidence suggests that migration of pathogens along the external surface of the catheter is more common in CR-BSIs associated with short- and intermediate-term, nontunneled catheters, with a higher rate of extraluminal source of infection in the first 1 to 2 weeks after placement of the central line. In contrast, intraluminal migration of organisms is more commonly seen in CR-BSIs associated with long-term, tunneled catheters. This differential is due in part to mechanical differences in the lines with the presence of a cuff on tunneled catheters acting as a fibrotic dam to migration of organisms along the external lumen. That said, external migration of organisms is possible in tunneled catheters and is associated with tunnel infections. Hematogenous seeding is one proposed mechanism of CR-BSIs in children with dysfunctional bowel; however, the true incidence of bowel translocation of microorganisms with subsequent seeding of the catheter is unknown.

The most commonly reported organisms implicated in CR-BSIs include skin flora such as coagulase-negative *Staphylococcus* and *Staphylococcus aureus*, *Enterococcus* species, enteric gram-negative organisms (particularly in patients with gastrointestinal dysfunction), and *Candida* species. Of concern is the growing number of CR-BSIs due to multidrug-resistant organisms.

Risk factors for CR-BSIs include prolonged use of systemic antimicrobials, catheter location (short- and intermediate-term lines placed in the femoral vein compared to other sites are more prone to infection in some pediatric studies), infusion of hyperalimentation with lipids, prolonged duration of catheterization (associated with increased formation of pathogenic biofilm), age < 2 years (especially premature infants with immature skin integrity), burn patients, immunocompromised patients, and those with intestinal integrity issues.

## CLINICAL MANIFESTATIONS

The clinical manifestations of catheter-related infections are variable and related to the type of infection. Fever is classically associated with CR-BSIs, while erythema, tenderness, and purulent drainage can be seen with exit site, tunnel, and pocket infections. The definitions of different types of catheter-associated infections are presented in Table 234-1.

**TABLE 234-1 DEFINITIONS OF CATHETER-ASSOCIATED INFECTIONS**

| Infection | Definition |
|---|---|
| Catheter-related bloodstream infection (CR-BSI) | Patient has a pathogen cultured from 1 or more blood cultures and the organism is not related to infection at another site *or* the patient has at least 1 of the following signs or symptoms: fever (> 38°C), chills, or hypotension, and signs and symptoms and positive laboratory results are not related to infection at another site, while a commensal is grown from ≥ 2 blood cultures drawn on separate occassions[a] |
| Colonized catheter | Growth of ≥ 15 (semiquantitative) or > $10^3$ (quantitative) colony-forming units from a proximal or distal catheter segment without accompanying signs or symptoms of infection |
| Exit site infection | Erythema, tenderness, induration, or purulence within 2 cm proximal to the exit site of the catheter |
| Tunnel infection | Erythema, tenderness, induration in the tissues overlying the catheter and > 2 cm proximal to the exit site |
| Pocket infection | Erythema and necrosis of the skin over the reservoir of a totally implantable device or purulent exudate in the pocket containing the device reservoir |
| Infusate-related bloodstream infection | Isolation of the same organism from the infusate and from a peripheral blood culture with no other identifiable source of infection |

[a]Additional diagnostic criteria include at least 1 of the following: (1) a positive catheter tip culture, either semiquantitative (≥ 15 colony-forming units/catheter tip segment) or quantitative (≥ 1000 colony-forming units/catheter tip segment), and the same microorganism (species and antibiogram) isolated from the peripheral blood; (2) simultaneous quantitative blood cultures with a ≥ 3:1 ratio (central venous catheter:peripheral); (3) differential time to positivity of ≥ 2 hours between the central venous catheter blood culture (positive first) and the peripheral blood culture; or (4) pus from the catheter exit site, growing the same microorganism as peripheral blood.

## DIAGNOSIS

Any discussion of the diagnosis of catheter-associated infections should differentiate between CR-BSIs and central line–associated bloodstream infections (CLABSIs), another term frequently encountered in the catheter-associated infection literature. The diagnosis of a CR-BSI requires that more stringent diagnostic criteria be met, which include detection of the same pathogen on peripheral blood and central venous catheter cultures in the absence of an alternative source (see Table 234-1). CLABSI is defined as a bloodstream infection identified in a patient with a central line either at the time of or within the previous 48 hours of detection of a positive culture regardless of whether the bloodstream infection is secondary to infection at another site; this is the definition typically used for surveillance purposes.

Our ability to accurately diagnose CR-BSIs has evolved over time but remains imperfect. Typically, blood cultures are drawn from patients with intravascular catheters when they develop fever. In the past, nontunneled lines were removed immediately if a blood culture became positive. The line tip was then cultured and, if there were ≥ 15 colony-forming units/catheter tip segment of the same organism as in the blood, a CR-BSI was diagnosed. Although this method is accurate and meets the more stringent CR-BSI definition, it requires removal of the catheter. With the advent of tunneled and totally implanted catheters, a diagnostic strategy that does not require removal of the catheter has been sought. Ideally, in lieu of catheter removal, when a CLABSI is suspected, blood cultures would be drawn from the catheter and a peripheral vein. If both cultures grow the same organism, a CLABSI can be diagnosed. For a more accurate diagnosis (ie, to diagnose CR-BSI), strategies using either quantitative cultures or differential time to positivity (DTP) of blood cultures have been suggested. The diagnostic use of quantitative cultures is based on the idea that, if an infection is truly line-related, the largest burden of organisms would be at the catheter tip. As organisms are shed into the bloodstream, they are filtered through the lungs and, as a result, are present in lower concentrations in the peripheral blood. By definition, to diagnose a CR-BSI, the colony count of organisms in blood obtained via the catheter should be at least 3 times higher than an equal-volume culture obtained from the peripheral blood. This method is sensitive and specific but is not widely used because of its labor intensiveness and expense. It may have its greatest utility in specific patient populations, such as those with bowel dysfunction, where one might expect a greater incidence of bacterial translocation. With the advent of blood culture analyzers that are capable of storing time of entry and time to positivity in the computer, it is possible to calculate the DTP. This method involves drawing blood cultures peripherally and from the catheter at the same time. Growth occurring in the culture obtained from the catheter at least 2 hours before growth from the peripheral culture is indicative of a CR-BSI. The current Infectious Diseases Society of America (IDSA) guidelines also allow for diagnosis of a CR-BSI by use of cultures drawn from 2 different lumens of a central catheter if a peripheral culture cannot be obtained. If quantitative cultures demonstrate at least 3-fold greater colony counts of an organism on the culture from one lumen compared to the other lumen, a CR-BSI is likely.

Controversy remains as to the optimal combination of central and peripheral blood cultures to obtain in pediatric patients. Studies looking at the sensitivity, specificity, and positive and negative predictive values (PPV and NPV, respectively) of central versus peripheral blood cultures have been performed predominantly in adults. The simultaneous acquisition of equal volumes of blood from a peripheral vein and from a potentially infected catheter provides the best combination of sensitivity, specificity, PPV, and NPV. In children, especially infants and toddlers, equal blood volume is not always guaranteed (nor is successful obtainment of any blood) from a peripheral vein. As a result, because the volume of blood has been shown to predict culture positivity, with a greater volume associated with higher likelihood of positivity in the setting of bloodstream infection, inadequate peripheral blood volume could lead to a high false-negative rate compared to a central culture, where blood volume is not an issue. Consequently, it has become more common in children to draw blood cultures only from the catheter. Utilization of the optimal combination of central and peripheral blood cultures must take into consideration the age and clinical status of the child; the type of catheter, number of catheter lumens, and ability to draw from each lumen; and the type of blood culture vial (pediatric blood culture vials have an optimal liquid medium-to-blood ratio for smaller volumes of blood). Unless clearly prohibitive, every effort should be made to obtain adequate peripheral and central blood cultures before antimicrobials are initiated as per current guidelines. As always, clinical judgment is paramount in interpreting results and deciding on appropriate management strategy.

The diagnosis of nonbloodstream catheter-related infections such as exit site, tunnel, or pocket infection is clinical, based on compatible signs and/or symptoms of infection (see Table 234-1). These infections are not always associated with concurrent bloodstream infection.

## TREATMENT

A proposed algorithm for the general management of short- and intermediate-term catheters suggests: (1) removal of catheters when they are no longer needed for patient care and (2) replacement over a guidewire if clinically indicated (ie, a line that is still needed but has mechanical difficulty or suspected but not yet documented infection). Replacement by guidewire exchange has been shown to reduce insertional complications. However, if a line is exchanged because of presumed infection, the old line should be cultured and, if positive, the new line should be removed and a new catheter placed in a different body site. Similarly, whenever a catheter is removed because of a documented infection, then the new line should be placed in a different location. When possible, placement of a new line should await documentation of negative blood cultures.

Short- or intermediate-term catheters ideally should be removed when a catheter-associated infection is documented. Removal of a long-term catheter may not be practical in some clinical situations, as when it may risk the loss of life-sustaining vascular access. It is now generally routine practice to attempt to treat an infection in a long-term catheter without removal of the catheter. Guidance on decisions regarding immediate versus delayed removal of catheters is provided in Table 234-2.

**TABLE 234-2 IMMEDIATE VERSUS DELAYED REMOVAL OF SHORT-TERM AND LONG-TERM CATHETERS**

| | Short-Term Catheters | Long-Term Catheters |
|---|---|---|
| **Immediate removal** | CLABSI associated with signs of sepsis | CR-BSI associated with septic shock |
| | Exit site infection with bacteremia | Continued BSI after > 72 hours of appropriate antimicrobial therapy |
| | Infection with *S aureus*, gram-negative bacilli, fungi, mycobacteria | Endocarditis |
| | Metastatic infection | Infection with *S aureus*, *Pseudomonas aeruginosa*, *Bacillus* spp, *Micrococcus* spp, Propionobacteria, fungi, mycobacteria |
| | Tunnel infection | Tunnel infection |
| **Consideration of delayed removal** | CLABSI without signs of sepsis | Exit site infection |
| | Exit site infection without bacteremia | Uncomplicated bacteremia |

BSI, bloodstream infection; CLABSI, central line–associated bloodstream infection; CR-BSI, catheter-related bloodstream infection

Whether or not to remove a long-term line secondary to recrudescence of infection after completion of antimicrobial therapy is more problematic and should be based on the pathogenicity of the offending organism, the status of the patient, and the need to maintain appropriate access; however, most experts would recommend line removal in such situations.

Major complications of central line infections include sepsis, septic emboli, endocarditis, endovascular infection, abscess formation, and death. The true incidence of these complications is unknown in the pediatric population. Certain organisms, including *S aureus*, *Pseudomonas* species and other gram-negative bacilli, *Candida* species and other fungi, and mycobacteria, are more difficult to clear and have greater metastatic potential; thus, early consideration should be given to removing central lines when these pathogens are present. Studies analyzing the outcomes of central line–related infections have shown increased length of stay with associated increases in medical costs, and morbidity and mortality rates as high as 10% to 20%. Complications in immunocompromised patients would be expected to be greater and to carry a greater morbidity and mortality burden, although this has yet to be confirmed in pediatric studies.

### Treatment of Cathe-ter-Related Bloodstream Infections

There are a large variety of acceptable regimens for treatment of CR-BSIs depending on the likely organism(s) and the patient's status. In general, empirical therapy for suspected CR-BSI should include coverage for gram-positive organisms, including drug-resistant gram-positive organisms such as methicillin-resistant *S aureus* (depending on local prevalence). Those also requiring coverage for gram-negative organisms include seriously ill patients, patients with neutropenia, and patients with a femoral line. Additionally, for neutropenic patients, severely septic patients, and patients known to be colonized with multidrug-resistant organisms, gram-negative coverage should be combination therapy, initiated with agents that work by different mechanisms (eg, a β-lactam agent and an aminoglycoside or a quinolone and an aminoglycoside). When catheter-related candidemia is suspected, initiation of an echinocandin is typically recommended; fluconazole is an acceptable alternative for patients who have not received fluconazole in the prior 3 months and who are in a facility for which risk of infection due to *Candida krusei* or *Candida glabrata* is very low. As with all empirically treated infections, once an organism is identified and susceptibilities known, antimicrobial therapy should be de-escalated and tailored as appropriate.

Duration of antimicrobial therapy depends on several factors including the clinical status of the patient, type of catheter-related infection, offending pathogen, duration of bloodstream infection, and status of involved line (retained vs removed). In general, infection with a less virulent organism (eg, coagulase-negative *Staphylococcus*), short duration of bacteremia, and removal of the catheter are all factors amenable to a shorter course of therapy. It should be noted that the duration of therapy for bloodstream infections is counted starting from the day of the first negative blood culture. A workup for bacterial dissemination to other sites (eg, to the heart resulting in endocarditis, the bone resulting in osteomyelitis) should be initiated for all patients who fail to clear their peripheral blood culture despite line removal or who remain persistently symptomatic despite negative blood cultures. If this workup is negative at the end of a standard 2-week course of antimicrobial therapy and the bloodstream infection and symptoms have resolved, then it is reasonable to discontinue treatment. In addition, bloodstream infection with *Candida* species should prompt a search for additional foci of infection, especially in neutropenic patients; this search should include an ophthalmologic exam, echocardiogram, and imaging of the chest and abdomen (as well as the head if shunting of blood may occur across the heart).

#### Adjunctive Treatment Strategies for Catheter-Related Bloodstream Infections

Antibiotic and ethanol locks have been used as adjuncts in the treatment of catheter-related infections. Antibiotic lock therapy—instilling an antibiotic solution into the lumen of the involved catheter and allowing it to dwell for a set amount of time, typically hours—is currently a recommended strategy in the IDSA guidelines for management of CR-BSI in the setting of a retained catheter. Ethanol lock therapy, although not currently recommended, has shown some promise for the treatment of CR-BSI in this setting as well. The major complication of ethanol lock therapy is catheter occlusion, presumably from biofilm destruction. This often necessitates the use of catheter thrombolysis procedures but rarely requires catheter removal.

#### Treatment of Exit Site/Tunnel Infections

The treatment of more localized exit site/tunnel infections depends on the catheter type in use. For short-term catheters, an exit site infection associated with bacteremia should prompt catheter removal and the initiation of systemic as well as topical antimicrobials. If the exit site infection is not associated with bacteremia, then an attempt can be made to treat the infection with topical agents alone. The treatment of long-term catheter exit site infections is essentially the same, except that unlike short-term catheters, long-term catheters can be salvaged, even in the face of bacteremia, if the infection responds to appropriate antimicrobial therapy with sterilization of the blood and resolution of the local infection. In contrast, tunnel tract infections require systemic antimicrobial therapy and usually necessitate catheter removal. Pocket infections require catheter removal for eradication of the offending organism.

## PREVENTION

Preventive strategies should be employed at all points of catheter management—from insertion, to catheter access, to dressing changes. Maximal barrier precautions during insertion, including the use of masks, sterile gowns and gloves, and large sterile fields, have been shown to significantly reduce the incidence of catheter infection. Additionally, antisepsis with chlorhexidine should be used before insertion of a catheter. Prior to any later manipulation of the catheter, hand hygiene and hub antisepsis are mandatory to reduce the incidence of catheter contamination. Sterile gauze, a transparent dressing, or a chlorhexidine patch can be used to cover the exit site. Preference is usually given to use of a transparent dressing (which may be coated with chlorhexidine) because it is easier to evaluate the exit site while maintaining the barrier integrity provided by the dressing. Frequency of dressing changes is determined by type of dressing, with gauze dressings typically changed every 2 days and transparent dressings changed every 7 days. Additionally, dressings should be changed when they are loose, soiled, or damp. With dressing changes, the exit site should be cleansed with chlorhexidine in 70% alcohol, although povidone iodine is still used, typically in children who have displayed allergy/sensitivity to chlorhexidine. Use of topical antibiotic ointments or creams is discouraged due to concern for the development of antimicrobial resistance and promotion of fungal growth. To further reduce infections, some catheters have been coated with either external chlorhexidine-silver sulfadiazine or internal and external minocycline/rifampin. Both types of catheters have proven effective in reducing the incidence of catheter-related infections in prospective randomized trials in adults when compared to catheters without coating, with minocycline/rifampin-coated catheters found in some studies to be superior in this respect. There remains a need for further studies in children.

The use of antibiotic lock therapy has also emerged as a potential preventive strategy. Studies have shown that vancomycin instilled into the catheter lumen and allowed to dwell for a period of time is effective in reducing the number of gram-positive infections in long-term lines. The use of ethanol lock therapy is also being explored as a means to prevent CR-BSIs.

## SUGGESTED READINGS


Mermel LA. What is the predominant source of intravascular catheter infections? *Clin Infect Dis.* 2011;52:211-212.

Mermel LA, Allon M, Bouza E, et al. Clinical practice guidelines for the diagnosis and management of intravascular catheter-related infection: 2009 Update by the Infectious Diseases Society of America. *Clin Infect Dis.* 2009;49:1-45.

O'Grady NP, Alexander M, Burns LA, et al. Guidelines for the prevention of intravascular catheter-related infections. *Clin Infect Dis.* 2011;52:e162-e193.

Tan M, Lau J, Guglielmo BJ. Ethanol locks in prevention and treatment of catheter-related bloodstream infections. *Ann Pharmacother.* 2014;48:607-615.

Ullman AJ, Marsh N, Mihala G, Cooke M, Rickard CM. Complications of central venous access devices: a systematic review. *Pediatrics.* 2015;136:e1331-e1344.

Wolf J, Curtis N, Worth LJ, Flynn PM. Central line-associated bloodstream infection in children: An update on treatment. *Pediatr Infect Dis J.* 2013;32:905-910.

Zacharioudakis IM, Zervou FN, Arvanitis M, Ziakas DZ, Mermel LA, Mylonakis E. Antimicrobial lock solutions as a method to prevent central line-associated bloodstream infections: a meta-analysis of randomized controlled trials. *Clin Infect Dis.* 2014;59:1741-1749.

# 235 Community-Acquired Pneumonia in Children

Stephen I. Pelton

## INTRODUCTION

Worldwide, community-acquired pneumonia (CAP) is a leading cause of infectious morbidity and mortality in children. A major clinical challenge persists—determining the role of viral and bacterial pathogens in pediatric pneumonia. Studies that employ blood and respiratory cultures, serology, and molecular detection suggest a small role for bacterial pathogens, while those that rely on pneumococcal conjugate vaccines (PCVs) as a probe to determine the proportion of disease due to *Streptococcus pneumoniae* suggest that pneumococcus is the major pathogen. Evolving insight from epidemiologic, molecular detection, and vaccine probe studies suggests that viral-bacterial interactions have a substantial role in the pathogenesis of pediatric pneumonia. In addition, the importance of comorbid illness as a risk factor for both increased incidence and poorer outcomes of pneumonia has emerged from recent studies.

## EPIDEMIOLOGY

CAP is most frequent in infants and toddlers and remains the most common cause of hospitalization in children. During the period from 2010 to 2012, following the introduction of the 13-valent PCV (PCV13) in the United States, the incidence of CAP requiring hospitalization was 15.7 per 100,000 in those < 18 years of age, with the highest rate among those less than 2 years of age (62 per 100,000). Mortality due to CAP in high-income countries is low, at < 1 per 1000 patient-years in children less than 5 years of age. Males are affected almost twice as commonly as females. Differences in incidence are also reported by socioeconomic status and ethnicity. Rates of pneumococcal pneumonia are higher in native Alaskan children than in nonnatives, as well as in children of African American, Hispanic, and Asian ethnicity compared to Caucasian children. These differences have narrowed, but have not been completely eliminated, in the era of universal immunization with PCVs. The incidence of CAP also varies by season; studies in the United States and Israel report greater frequency in the winter and spring months and in association with annual peaks of respiratory syncytial virus (RSV), influenza A, and, in older children, *Mycoplasma pneumoniae*. Comorbid illness has been recognized as both predisposing to pneumonia and as being associated with increased severity and morbidity. Children with congenital and acquired immune deficiencies represent a well-known high-risk group, but excess risk and morbidity are also found in children with chronic cardiac and pulmonary disease (including severe asthma), diabetes mellitus, neuromuscular disorders, prematurity, and specific genetic disorders (ie, trisomy 21).

Lower respiratory tract infections (RTIs) are both more frequent and associated with increased mortality in low-income countries. The incidence among children less than 5 years old in 10 low-income countries is estimated to range from 0.2 to 8.1 new episodes per 100 child-weeks. Mortality from pneumonia has become uncommon in high-income countries as noted, yet it remains a major cause of death in low-income countries. The countries with the highest incidence of pneumonia in children are located in Africa and Southeast Asia; case fatality rates for pneumococcal pneumonia are estimated to be 5% globally, with 10 countries accounting for most of the deaths (India, China, Nigeria, Pakistan, Bangladesh, Indonesia, Ethiopia, Democratic Republic of the Congo, Kenya, and the Philippines).

## MICROBIAL ETIOLOGY

### COMMUNITY-ACQUIRED PNEUMONIA

A large spectrum of pathogens have the capacity to cause CAP in children. In recent studies using routine and molecular methods, potential pathogens are detected in 65% to 80% of cases. Figure 235-1 details the distribution of viral pathogens, bacterial pathogens, neither, and both isolated from hospitalized, radiograph-confirmed cases of pneumonia, and Figure 235-2 details the frequency of various pathogens recovered from these cases. However, in studies comparing pediatric pneumonia cases with asymptomatic controls, only RSV, influenza viruses, and human metapneumovirus (HMPV) were found more frequently and with greater density in the nasopharynx of pneumonia cases, whereas coronavirus and parainfluenza viruses were found more frequently, and rhinoviruses and others were found no more frequently, cautioning the conclusion that recovery from the nasopharynx implies causation of pneumonia.

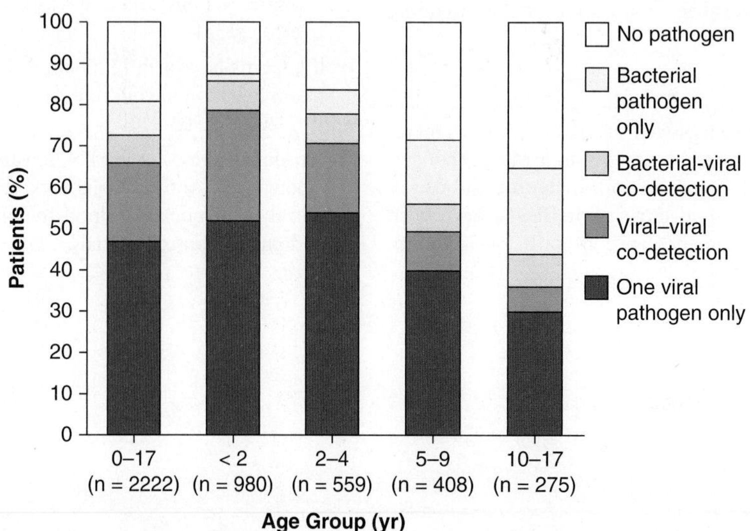


**FIGURE 235-1** Proportion of pathogens detected in 2222 hospitalized cases of radiograph–confirmed pneumonia in children by age. (Reproduced with permission from Jain S, Williams DJ, Arnold SR, et al. Community-acquired pneumonia requiring hospitalization among U.S. children, *N Engl J Med*. 2015 Feb 26;372(9):835-845.)

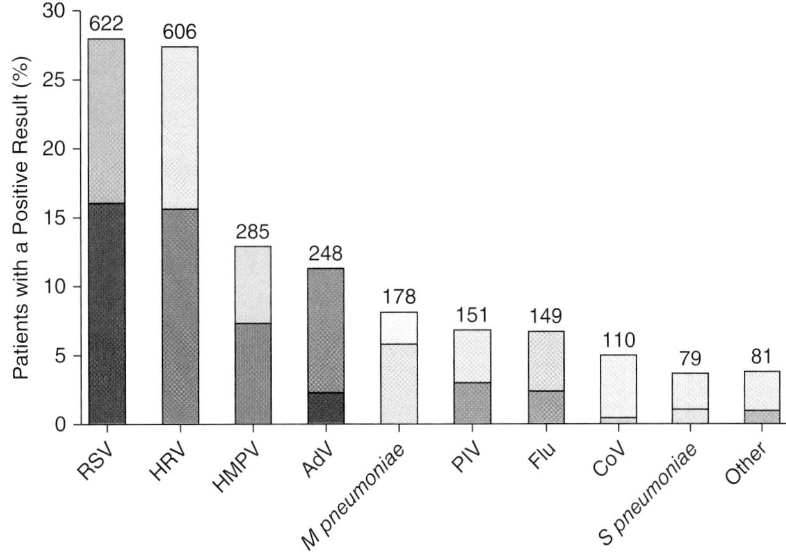


**FIGURE 235-2** Frequency of detection of specific pathogens among 2222 hospitalized children with radiograph–confirmed pneumonia. Darker shading indicates that only a single pathogen was detected; lighter shading indicates the pathogen was detected in combination with at least one other pathogen. AdV, adenovirus; CoV, coronavirus; Flu, influenza virus; HMPV, human metapneumovirus; HRV, human rhinovirus; PIV, parainfluenza virus; RSV, respiratory syncytial virus. (Reproduced with permission from Jain S, Williams DJ, Arnold SR, et al. Community-acquired pneumonia requiring hospitalization among U.S. children, *N Engl J Med.* 2015 Feb 26;372(9):835-845.)

Studies of vaccine efficacy suggest that the pneumococcus may have a larger role in CAP than revealed through blood or respiratory specimen testing including molecular diagnostics. Such studies report declines of approximately 40% in ambulatory pneumonia and 50% in hospitalization for pneumonia in US children less than 2 years old following universal immunization of infants with the 7-valent PCV (PCV7) and additional declines of approximately 25% following the introduction of PCV13. Black and colleagues have reported a decline of 35% in pneumonia characterized by an abnormal chest radiograph in children immunized with PCV7 compared to unvaccinated controls. Klugman and colleagues observed an approximate 40% decline in children hospitalized for pneumonia associated with influenza, RSV, and HMPV in South African children immunized with 9-valent PCV compared to controls, providing further support for viral-bacterial interaction (specifically *S pneumoniae*) in the pathogenesis of a large proportion of cases of pneumonia in children. Such interactions are further supported by epidemiologic studies demonstrating an increase in bacteremic pneumococcal pneumonia during the RSV season. These data support a role for *S pneumoniae* in the etiology of pneumonia beyond those identified by concurrent bacteremia and beyond those with empyema or consolidated lobar pneumonia to include as many as one-third of young children with acutely abnormal chest radiographs and clinical symptoms or signs of RTIs.

Additional bacterial pathogens are also important causes of pneumonia in children. *Streptococcus pyogenes* is associated with rapid onset of large pleural effusions, significant toxicity, and prolonged fever. *Haemophilus influenzae* type b (Hib), prior to the introduction of the Hib conjugate vaccine and in countries where Hib vaccination has not been incorporated into national immunization programs, and possibly nontypeable *H influenzae* (NTHi) strains appear to be associated with prolonged symptoms and are disproportionately found in children with respiratory comorbid illnesses. A substantial role for NTHi is supported by results of lung aspirate studies from Gambia and Papua New Guinea, where NTHi strains are recovered from 25% to 53% of children with *Haemophilus* pneumonia (Table 235-1). In addition, NTHi has been reported as a major pathogen in children with recurrent CAP undergoing bronchoalveolar lavage (BAL). Most recently, *Staphylococcus aureus*, specifically community-acquired (CA) methicillin-resistant *S aureus* (MRSA), has emerged as an important cause of complicated pneumonia. On autopsy, these cases frequently demonstrate microabscesses and hemorrhage. Cavitation, pleural empyema, pneumatocele, bronchopleural fistula, and/or pyopneumothorax also can complicate staphylococcal pneumonia. Karen and colleagues reported *S aureus* as the most common cause of pleural empyema in children in the decade between 1993 and 2002. However, following the introduction of PCV7, an increase in pneumococcal empyema due to nonvaccine serotypes (those not contained within PCV7) was observed. Following introduction of PCV13, such cases have declined.

The atypical/intracellular pathogens *M pneumoniae* and *Chlamydophila pneumoniae* are recognized as important pathogens causing CAP in children. Both are difficult to culture; therefore, most studies rely on nonstandardized serologic tests or molecular detection from the respiratory tract/nasopharynx. Studies of children with ambulatory pneumonia identify *M pneumoniae* infection in 26.5% to 29.5% of cases and *C pneumoniae* in 15.0% to 28.5% of cases. These pathogens are found most commonly in children age > 5 years; however, they also occur in younger children. Data from 2222 hospitalized children with radiograph–confirmed pneumonia showed *Mycoplasma* recovered from 8% of cases overall (see Fig. 235-2), accounting for 19% of the total cases over 5 years old and only 3% of those under the age of 5 years. *Mycoplasma* should be suspected in children with pneumonia who have headache and wheezing in the setting of a family cluster of lower RTI. Perinatally acquired *Chlamydia trachomatis* pneumonia, a once common etiology of pneumonia in the first 2 months of life in the United States, has been largely eliminated in

**TABLE 235-1 SEROTYPES OF *HAEMOPHILUS INFLUENZAE* RECOVERED FROM CHILDREN WITH PNEUMONIA**

| Lung Aspiration | Children (No.) | *Haemophilus* (Total No.) | Type b, No. (%) | Type a, c, d, e, f, No. (%) | Nontypeable, No. (%) |
|---|---|---|---|---|---|
| Papua New Guinea | 83 | 34 | 7 (21) | 9 (26) | 18 (53) |
| Gambia | 51 | 9 | 3 (33) | 2 (22) | 4 (44) |
| Gambia | 94 | 8 | 5 (63) | 1 (12) | 2 (25) |
| TOTAL | 228 | 51 | 15 (39) | 12 (20) | 24 (41) |

Modified with permission from Shann F: Haemophilus influenzae pneumonia: type b or non-type b? *Lancet.* 1999 Oct 30;354(9189):1488-1490.

high-income countries through the systematic screening and treatment of pregnant women.

### Complicated Pneumonia

In children, the microbiology of patients with complicated pneumonia (eg, those with large pleural effusion, empyema, necrotic lung parenchyma, lung abscess, or pneumatocele) differs somewhat from ambulatory patients. In children with complicated bacterial pneumonia with necrosis and/or empyema, *S pneumoniae* (often serotype 3) and both methicillin-sensitive *S aureus* (MSSA) and MRSA are dominant. Other less common bacterial pathogens recovered from hospitalized children with pneumonia include group A β-hemolytic streptococci, Hib, and *Moraxella catarrhalis*. Pneumonia with Group A β-hemolytic streptococci is often rapidly progressive, severe, and associated with sepsis syndrome. Infection with Hib has been virtually eliminated wherever Hib conjugate vaccine has been introduced; however, Hib may still be a significant pathogen in countries where Hib conjugate vaccine has not, as yet, had high penetration in the infant population. *Mycobacterium tuberculosis* may also present as acute pneumonia with fever, respiratory signs, and alveolar infiltrate with or without pleural effusion. Tuberculosis should be considered in children who recently immigrated to the United States, those returning from travel to countries with endemic tuberculosis, those with human immunodeficiency virus (HIV), and those who have had contact with recently diagnosed individuals. Skin testing for tuberculosis should be a routine part of evaluation of children with pneumonia.

## CLINICAL MANIFESTATIONS

Clinical signs and symptoms of bacterial pneumonia overlap with many aspects of viral pneumonia, preventing clear discrimination between the 2. Fever, frequently greater than 102°F (38.9°C), ill appearance, and respiratory and/or abdominal signs are found in the majority of patients with pneumonia due to pneumococcus or RSV (Table 235-2). Tachypnea and rales/crackles are reported in 40% to 50% of such patients. Focal chest pain is uncommon with pneumonia, but when present should strongly suggest bacterial pneumonia. Bacteremic pneumonia is more frequently associated with greater severity of clinical signs and symptoms such as higher fever.

## DIAGNOSIS

Determining the etiology of pneumonia in children is challenging because bacteremia is uncommon even in those thought to have bacterial pneumonia; pleural effusion is present in only a small percentage of children, and antimicrobial therapy has often been administered prior to collection of body fluids for culture; nasopharyngeal cultures are not necessarily representative of lower respiratory tract secretions; and the vast majority of children do not produce sputum. More aggressive procedures, such as lung puncture and BAL, may be diagnostic but are generally reserved for hospitalized patients with significant respiratory distress and, therefore, only inform us about a select population of children with pneumonia.

**TABLE 235-2 COMPARISON OF SIGNS AND SYMPTOMS IN CHILDREN WITH RESPIRATORY SYNCYTIAL VIRUS VERSUS PNEUMOCOCCAL PNEUMONIA**

| Clinical Signs/ Symptoms | RSV Pneumonia (%) | Pneumococcal Pneumonia (all)[a] (%) | Bacteremic Pneumococcal Pneumonia (%) |
|---|---|---|---|
| Fever | | | |
| > 37.5°C | 92 | 100 | 100 |
| > 39°C | 60 | 84 | 93 |
| Ill appearance | 54 | 50 | 79 |
| Cough | 89 | 71 | 55 |
| Rhinorrhea | 58 | 45 | 49 |
| Dyspnea | 62 | 24 | 11 |
| Lethargy | 27 | 29 | 39 |
| Vomiting | 31 | 32 | 32 |
| Abdominal pain | 4 | 8 | 14 |
| Chest pain | 0 | 21 | 8 |
| Acute otitis media | 58 | 13 | 12 |

[a]Diagnosis by either positive blood culture or serology.

Data from Juvén T, Mertsola J, Waris M, et al: Etiology of community-acquired pneumonia in 254 hospitalized children, *Pediatr Infect Dis J*. 2000 Apr;19(4):293-298.

## LABORATORY TESTING

Acute-phase reactants such as total and differential white blood cell count, erythrocyte sedimentation rate, C-reactive protein, and procalcitonin have been evaluated for their usefulness in discriminating between viral and bacterial etiologies. In general, these markers of inflammation demonstrate a correlation with bacterial etiology but have limited sensitivity and specificity. Serologic tests have been evaluated for diagnosis of pneumonia due to *S pneumoniae, M pneumoniae,* and *C pneumoniae*. Using a number of different techniques, these tests detect immunoglobulin (IgM or IgG) against antigens specific for each of these pathogens. In general, many of the tests are moderately specific, have wide variation in sensitivity, lack reproducibility, and have not been standardized. In addition, serologic tests may provide only retrospective diagnosis because they often require comparison of acute and convalescent serum specimens.

Detection of bacterial antigens in urine and detection of bacterial DNA in nasopharyngeal secretions, sputum, BAL specimens, or blood have been pursued as possible strategies for identifying the etiology of pneumonia. Pneumococcal capsular polysaccharide antigens have been detected in children with pneumococcal pneumonia; however, children with dense nasopharyngeal colonization have also had antigen detected in urine, suggesting the specificity of such assays is limited. Molecular strategies for detection of pneumococcus in blood or nasopharyngeal specimens have received increasing attention. Potentially, DNA from *S pneumoniae, M pneumoniae,* and *C pneumoniae* can be detected in clinical samples from children with acute pneumonia. Molecular detection of pneumococcus has proven to be successful in children with culture-negative empyema.

## IMAGING

A chest radiograph is often used to confirm the presence of pulmonary infiltrates/consolidation in patients with suspected pneumonia. Lobar consolidation has a high correlation with bacterial pneumonia, while mild interstitial and perihilar changes are considered to be due to viral infection or possibly underlying asthma. While the association of lobar consolidation with pneumococcal disease is well accepted, the role of pneumococcus in cases with interstitial or mixed findings is less certain. Several studies suggest that the presence of alveolar infiltrates is an insensitive but reasonably specific indicator of bacterial infection. In a Finnish study of hospitalized children with pneumonia (n = 254), 71% of those with alveolar infiltrates had bacterial infection. More recent studies (Table 235-3) found no significant correlation between the radiologic picture and the etiologic agent—ie, it was not possible from the chest radiograph alone to predict whether the child had viral infection, bacterial infection, or mixed infection—but rather there was a correlation between age and radiographic findings.

Vaccine probe studies demonstrate that PCV efficacy is greatest in cases with alveolar infiltrates confirming an important role for pneumococcus in such cases. However, efficacy is also demonstrated in children, with interstitial infiltrates and recovery of virus from the nasopharynx strongly suggesting that the pneumococcus, at least in low-income settings, has a significant role in such cases (Table 235-4). Whether its role is direct tissue invasion or to enhance the severity of the viral infection remains uncertain.

## SPECIAL POPULATIONS

Despite widespread use of PCVs and an overall decline in rates of all-cause pneumonia and pneumococcal pneumonia in children with high-risk conditions (eg, immunodeficiency, nephrotic syndrome, functional or anatomic asplenia, HIV), the incidence of pneumonia remains disproportionately high compared to otherwise healthy children. Children with chronic heart or lung disease or diabetes mellitus demonstrate a 2- to 3-fold increase in the incidence of pneumonia. Children with comorbid conditions are also at increased risk for treatment failure and

**TABLE 235-3 RADIOGRAPHIC FINDINGS[a] RELATED TO ETIOLOGY IN CHILDREN BY AGE**

| | Interstitial | Alveolar | Mixed | Hyperinflation |
|---|---|---|---|---|
| **A. 0–1 years (n = 166)** | | | | |
| Bacterial and viral co-infection | 21% | 31% | 14% | 21% |
| Bacterial infection only | 11% | 15% | 11% | 12% |
| Viral infection only | 40% | 35% | 32% | 41% |
| No evidence for viral or bacterial infection | 28% | 19% | 43% | 26% |
| **B. 2–5 years (n = 119)** | | | | |
| Bacterial and viral co-infection | 20% | 15% | 14% | 27% |
| Bacterial infection only | 22% | 25% | 10% | 20% |
| Viral infection only | 29% | 39% | 38% | 31% |
| No evidence for viral or bacterial infection | 29% | 21% | 38% | 22% |
| **C. 6 years and older (n = 61)** | | | | |
| Bacterial and viral co-infection | 14% | 8% | 25% | 20% |
| Bacterial infection only | 43% | 45% | 25% | 40% |
| Viral infection only | 14% | 12% | 25% | 10% |
| No evidence for viral or bacterial infection | 29% | 20% | — | 30% |
| *Mycoplasma* only | 7% | 15% | 25% | — |

[a]Parenchymal infiltrates are described as interstitial, alveolar, or mixed interstitial and alveolar. The presence of general hyperinflation is noted separately and is found together with, as well as without, infiltrates.

poor outcome, making prevention a high priority and requiring additional strategies beyond pneumococcal immunization.

### Children with Asthma

A link between RTIs and asthma in children is well established. Recent studies find that those with more severe asthma are at greater risk for all-cause and pneumococcal pneumonia compared to those with mild disease. It has been suggested that asthma exacerbations in children are associated with viral or atypical/intracellular pathogens such as *C pneumoniae* and *M pneumoniae.* Both of these agents have also been detected more frequently in children with wheezing than in control subjects (for *C pneumoniae*, 11.0% vs 4.9%, respectively). In addition, 9 (75%) of 12 children with wheezing and evidence of *C pneumoniae* infection showed clinical and laboratory improvement of their reactive airways disease after eradication of chlamydial infection with erythromycin or clarithromycin. Furthermore, a history of recurrent wheezing is more common in children with *C pneumoniae* or *M pneumoniae* infections than in those without either infection. Some investigators estimate that these organisms may trigger 5% to 30% of wheezing episodes and asthma exacerbations. A recent observation suggested that certain children with recurrent asthma may benefit from azithromycin prophylaxis with a subsequent reduced frequency of exacerbations. Further confirmation is required before this can be widely recommended.

### Children with Sickle Cell Disease

The prevalence of pneumonia in children with sickle cell disease (SCD) is significantly higher than in healthy controls. By age 4, children with SCD have a 4 times greater risk of bacterial pneumonia compared with age- and sex-matched controls with normal hemoglobin genotype. Pneumonia in children with SCD also has a more serious clinical course compared to otherwise healthy children. *M pneumoniae* has been associated with severe pneumonia, including pleural effusion and multilobar infiltrates in children with SCD. Acute chest syndrome (ACS) is a common cause of hospitalization in patients with SCD and is associated with substantial morbidity and mortality (see also Chapter 430). Recent reports indicate that pneumonia may be a common cause of ACS in children with SCD. The report from a 30-center study demonstrated that infection—especially CAP—is a common cause of ACS. In this study, 27 different infectious pathogens as well as pulmonary fat embolism were identified as causes; *C pneumoniae* and *M pneumoniae* were the most prevalent infectious agents. Infection was considered a contributing factor in 56% of deaths. Other potential bacterial pathogens include *S pneumoniae, S aureus,* and *H influenzae.*

**TABLE 235-4 REDUCTION IN HOSPITALIZED CASES OF "VIRAL" PNEUMONIA IN SOUTH AFRICAN CHILDREN IMMUNIZED WITH PCV9**

| | All Children[e] | | | | HIV-Uninfected Children[f] | | | |
|---|---|---|---|---|---|---|---|---|
| Clinical Diagnosis | Vaccine n = 18,245 | Placebo n = 18,268 | Efficacy (95% CI) | *P* value | Vaccine n = 17,065 | Placebo n = 17,086 | Efficacy (95% CI) | *P* value |
| Total number of pneumonia cases[a] | 544 | 679 | 20 (10, 28) | 0.00009 | 348 | 452 | 23 (11, 33) | 0.0002 |
| Pneumonia with alveolar consolidation[b] | 251 | 303 | 17 (2, 30) | 0.03 | 119 | 158 | 25 (4, 40) | 0.02 |
| Pneumonia without identified virus[c] | 419 | 486 | 14 (2, 24) | 0.03 | 252 | 299 | 16 (0, 29) | 0.05 |
| Any identified virus-associated pneumonia[d] | 160 | 231 | 31 (15, 43) | 0.0004 | 111 | 167 | 33 (15, 48) | 0.0008 |
| Influenza A | 31 | 56 | 45 (14, 64) | 0.01 | 21 | 32 | 34 (–14, 62) | 0.1 |
| RSV | 90 | 115 | 22 (–3, 41) | 0.08 | 64 | 94 | 32 (6, 50) | 0.02 |
| PIV types 1-3 | 24 | 43 | 44 (8, 66) | 0.02 | 15 | 27 | 41 (–10, 68) | 0.09 |
| Adenovirus | 14 | 15 | 7 (–94, 55) | 0.9 | 9 | 13 | 31 (–62, 70) | 0.4 |

[a]First episodes are shown; thus, a child with episodes of pneumonia associated both with and without a virus are counted in that category for each first episode, but only once in the total number of pneumonia cases.

[b]Alveolar consolidation (WHO-AC)[5].

[c]Includes episodes of pneumonia that tested negative for all of the respiratory viruses examined.

[d]Includes the first episode of any identified virus-associated pneumonia including influenza B.

[e]Includes children whose HIV status was unknown.

[f]Although the number of children receiving vaccine or placebo are known, the denominator of HIV-uninfected children is estimated at 93.53%.

HIV, human immunodeficiency virus; PCV, pneumococcal conjugate vaccine; PIV, parainfluenza; RSV, respiratory syncytial virus.

Data from Madhi SA, Klugman KP; Vaccine Trialist Group: A role for *Streptococcus pneumoniae* in virus-associated pneumonia, *Nat Med.* 2004 Aug;10(8):811-813.

The data above support the selection of antibiotics that include activity against atypical/intracellular pathogens when selecting suitable antibacterial coverage for patients with ACS.

### Recurrent Community-Acquired Pneumonia

Children with recurrent CAP can be categorized as those with recurrent pneumonia in the same location (on chest radiograph) and those in whom the episodes of pneumonia occur at different locations. In the former situation, anatomical abnormality, foreign body, recurrent aspiration (especially with upper lobe pneumonia), and tracheoesophageal fistula should be considered. In those in whom the pulmonary infiltrate varies in location with each episode, immune deficiency (including cilia dysfunction syndrome) is more likely.

## TREATMENT

In 2011, the Pediatric Infectious Diseases Society, in collaboration with the Infectious Diseases Society of America, developed and published guidelines for the management of pneumonia in children. The guidelines address a spectrum of challenges in managing children with pneumonia, including the following: criteria for admission to the hospital or intensive care unit; appropriate diagnostic testing; anti-infectives indicated for ambulatory and inpatient CAP; appropriate duration of therapy; expected response to treatment; management of parapneumonic effusions; management of CAP failing to respond to initial therapy; and prevention of CAP. The guidelines address whether all children with pneumonia require antimicrobial therapy or whether therapy should be limited to those with moderate or severe clinical symptoms and signs. Because a microbiologic diagnosis is not commonly established and the selection of initial antibacterial therapy is primarily empirical, there are no absolutes about which children with CAP require antimicrobial therapy. In addition, the new insights about bacterial-viral interaction in the pathogenesis of CAP and the reduction in hospitalization for "viral" pneumonia in children immunized with PCVs blur the picture.

Most children with CAP can be treated with oral antimicrobial agents. The treatment choice is based on age, clinical severity, and epidemiologic factors. When therapy for CAP is indicated, antibiotics targeting *S pneumoniae,* the most common bacterial pathogen, should be prescribed. The British Thoracic Society has proposed guidelines for treatment that support withholding antimicrobial therapy in young children presenting with mild symptoms of lower RTIs but do not specifically address whether to treat all children diagnosed with pneumonia. Amoxicillin is the first choice for oral antibiotic therapy in children less than 5 years old. Because β-lactam antibiotics are not active against atypical pathogens, macrolides are often recommended for children age > 5 years or whenever infection with atypical/intracellular pathogens is suspected, such as when headache and wheezing are present. The British Thoracic Society guidelines recommend management in the hospital for children with evidence of more severe disease (Table 235-5). In children hospitalized with severe CAP, initial therapy must include coverage for *S pneumoniae,* including multidrug-resistant strains in the community and community-acquired MRSA, especially when complicated pneumonia is present (see Chapter 279). The highlights of the Pediatric Infectious Diseases Society guidelines are summarized in Table 235-6.

**TABLE 235-5 ASSESSMENT OF SEVERITY OF COMMUNITY-ACQUIRED PNEUMONIA IN CHILDREN**

| | Mild | Severe |
|---|---|---|
| Infants | Temp < 38.5°C | Temperature > 38.5°C |
| | RR < 50 breaths/min | RR > 70 breaths/min |
| | Feeding well | Poor feeding |
| | | Intermittent apnea |
| | | Nasal flaring, cyanosis, grunting |
| Older children | Temp < 38.5°C | Temp > 38.5°C |
| | RR < 50 breaths/min | RR > 50 breaths/min |
| | Mild breathlessness | Severe difficulty breathing |
| | No vomiting | Dehydration |
| | | Nasal flaring, cyanosis, grunting |

RR, respiratory rate.

Reproduced with permission from Harris M, Clark J, Coote N, et al: British Thoracic Society guidelines for the management of community acquired pneumonia in children: update 2011, *Thorax.* 2011 Oct;66 Suppl 2:ii1-ii23.

**TABLE 235-6 HIGHLIGHTS FROM THE PEDIATRIC INFECTIOUS DISEASES SOCIETY GUIDELINES FOR THE MANAGEMENT OF COMMUNITY-ACQUIRED PNEUMONIA IN CHILDREN**

| |
|---|
| Most children > 6 months of age can be managed as outpatients; children with moderate to severe CAP defined as respiratory distress and/or hypoxemia are best managed as inpatients. |
| Testing for viral pathogens (specifically RSV and influenza viruses) is valuable because a positive test may decrease the need for additional diagnostic studies and antimicrobial therapy and allows for the appropriate use of antiviral agents. |
| Testing for *Mycoplasma pneumoniae* may be of value in selected children with CAP (headache and wheezing; family members with lower respiratory tract illness). |
| Routine chest radiograph is not necessary in children with clinically suspected CAP who are well enough to be treated as outpatients but is recommended for those requiring inpatient management. |
| Antimicrobial therapy is not routinely required in preschool children (as viral illness is more common) with mild disease. |
| Amoxicillin should be first-line treatment in children with mild to moderate CAP suspected to be of bacterial origin. |
| Macrolide antibiotics should be prescribed for children with signs and symptoms compatible with atypical pathogens (predominantly school age and adolescents). |
| For inpatients, ampicillin is first-line therapy for fully immunized children when local epidemiology reports a low incidence of high-level penicillin resistance among pneumococcal isolates. |
| Third-generation cephalosporins should be prescribed for hospitalized children where local epidemiology documents high-level penicillin resistance, those with sepsis accompanying CAP, and those with empyema or complex pneumonia. |
| Empiric macrolide therapy should be initiated when *M pneumoniae* is of significant concern. |
| Vancomycin or clindamycin (dependent on local antimicrobial resistance patterns) should be added if clinical, laboratory, or radiographic findings are suggestive of disease due to *Staphylococcus aureus.* |
| Clinical and laboratory signs of improvement should be observed within 48 to 72 hours. |
| Repeat chest radiograph is not routinely of value. |
| If pleural effusion is present, the size of the effusion and the degree of respiratory distress are important in determining management. |
| Moderate pleural effusion associated with respiratory distress should be drained. |
| Both chest tube drainage with fibrinolytic agents and VATS are effective. |
| Children not responding to initial treatment should have repeat clinical and laboratory evaluation, imaging as needed, and consideration for BAL for Gram stain and culture in those who are on mechanical ventilation. |
| The guidelines apply to otherwise healthy children; special consideration should be given to high-risk children such as those with sickle cell disease, immunodeficiency, or trisomy 21. |
| Influenza vaccine, PCV, and Hib conjugate vaccines are valuable for prevention of CAP and should be routinely administered to all children without specific contraindications as per published recommendations. |

BAL, bronchoalveolar lavage; CAP, community-acquired pneumonia; Hib, *Haemophilus influenzae* type B; PCV, pneumococcal conjugate vaccine; RSV, respiratory syncytial virus; VATS, video-assisted thoroscopy.

### Impact of Antimicrobial Resistance

As can be seen in Table 235-6, antibacterial resistance has an important influence on the selection of antibacterial therapy for childhood CAP. Multidrug-resistant *S pneumoniae* has been reported in children with pneumococcal pneumonia. The minimal inhibitory concentration (MIC) for some of these pneumococcal isolates for amoxicillin, amoxicillin clavulanate, azithromycin, and trimethoprim-sulfamethoxazole exceed the pharmacokinetic and pharmacodynamic parameters than can be achieved within the lung with oral administration. Resistance to ceftriaxone (MIC ≥ 4.0 μg/mL) is, however, uncommon among current isolates. Susceptibility to vancomycin and levofloxacin persists among almost all pneumococci isolated from children. Vancomycin or levofloxacin should be considered in children with type I allergy to cephalosporins; however, in 2016, the US Food and Drug Administration (FDA) added a black box warning for adverse events from fluoroquinolones affecting tendons, muscles, nerves, and the central nervous system. The FDA recommended that systemic fluoroquinolones be used only in patients with bacterial sinusitis, chronic bronchitis, and uncomplicated urinary tract infection in the absence other treatment options.

## SUGGESTED READINGS


Agnello L, Bellia C, Di Gangi M, et al. Utility of serum procalcitonin and C-reactive protein in severity assessment of community-acquired pneumonia in children. *Clin Biochem*. 2016;49:47-50.

Das A, Patgiri SJ, Saikia L, Dowerah P, Nath R. Bacterial pathogens associated with community-acquired pneumonia in children aged below five years. *Indian Pediatr*. 2016;53:225-227.

Griffin MR, Mitchel E, Moore MR, Whitney CG, Grijalva CG. Declines in pneumonia hospitalizations of children aged < 2 years associated with the use of pneumococcal conjugate vaccines: Tennessee, 1998-2012. *Morb Mortal Wkly Rep*. 2014;63:995-998.

Jain S, Finelli L. Community-acquired pneumonia among U.S. children. *N Engl J Med*. 2015;372:2167-2168.

Medjo B, Atanaskovic-Markovic M, Radic S, Nikolic D, Lukac M, Djukic S. *Mycoplasma pneumoniae* as a causative agent of community-acquired pneumonia in children: clinical features and laboratory diagnosis. *Ital J Pediatr*. 2014;40:104.

Millman AJ, Finelli L, Bramley AM, et al. Community-acquired pneumonia hospitalization among children with neurologic disorders. *J Pediatr*. 2016;173:188-195.

Picot VS, Bénet T, Messaoudi M, et al. Multicenter case-control study protocol of pneumonia etiology in children: Global Approach to Biological Research, Infectious diseases and Epidemics in Low-income countries (GABRIEL network). *BMC Infect Dis*. 2014;14:635.

Ross RK, Hersh AL, Kronman MP, et al. Impact of Infectious Diseases Society of America/Pediatric Infectious Diseases Society guidelines on treatment of community-acquired pneumonia in hospitalized children. *Clin Infect Dis*. 2014;58:834-838.

Self WH, Williams DJ, Zhu Y, et al. Respiratory viral detection in children and adults: comparing asymptomatic controls and patients with community-acquired pneumonia. *J Infect Dis*. 2016;213:584-591.


# 236 Viral Respiratory Infections Including Influenza

Claudia P. Vicetti Miguel and Asuncion Mejias

## INTRODUCTION

Respiratory viral infections are a major cause of morbidity in children around the world. Healthy infants and preschool children experience between 6 and 10 respiratory illnesses per year, and school-age children and adolescents experience 3 to 5 illnesses annually. Respiratory viral infections are classified into (1) upper respiratory tract infections (URIs), also known as the common cold, rhinitis, pharyngitis, otitis media, and conjunctivitis; and (2) lower respiratory tract infections (LRTIs), namely croup, laryngitis, tracheobronchitis, bronchiolitis, and pneumonia. With molecular techniques becoming the new gold standard for the detection of respiratory viruses, important changes have occurred in our understanding of the role of these viruses in respiratory illnesses in children, particularly in LRTIs. Newly discovered viruses have been identified in the last decade (eg, human bocaviruses, human coronaviruses) that have been associated with respiratory illnesses. In addition, areas that require further research have been uncovered such as the causality between newly discovered viruses and clinical disease, the significance of viral co-detections, and the role of viral quantitation and its correlation with disease severity. Despite these changes, epidemiologic studies have demonstrated that the major associations established by traditional techniques (eg, viral culture, antigen detection, and serology) remain valid. Despite the major advances observed with the development of diagnostic tools, there has been a paucity of major changes in the availability of specific antivirals and vaccines, although many are currently under investigation with the potential to become available in the next few years.

## RESPIRATORY SYNCYTIAL VIRUS

Respiratory syncytial virus (RSV) is the leading cause of viral lower respiratory tract disease in infants and toddlers. It accounts for approximately 60% of all LRTIs in preschool-aged children worldwide. In the developing world, RSV is second only to malaria as a cause of death during the first year of life. Severe disease is generally associated with primary infection, although LRTI can also occur upon reinfection. Bronchiolitis, which refers to inflammation of smaller intrapulmonary airways, is the single most distinctive clinical syndrome of RSV infection.

### PATHOGENESIS AND EPIDEMIOLOGY

RSV belongs to the genus *Pneumovirus* within the Paramyxoviridae family. It is an enveloped, single-stranded, negative-sense RNA virus with a diameter spanning 100 to 350 nm. The viral envelope is studded with spike-like projections that include the fusion (F) and attachment (G) surface glycoproteins, but unlike most paramyxoviruses, RSV surface proteins lack both hemagglutinin (HA) and neuraminidase (NA) activity. The G protein initiates the infection, while the F glycoprotein mediates viral penetration by fusing viral and cellular membranes, contributing to syncytia formation. These 2 proteins carry the antigenic determinants that elicit the production of neutralizing antibodies by the host. Nevertheless, the F protein represents the major target for antiviral drug development, especially in its prefusion form (preF), which has been shown to be highly superior at inducing neutralizing antibodies compared to its postfusion (postF) form. Human RSV exists as 2 antigenic subgroups, A and B, which can co-circulate during the same season and exhibit genome-wide sequence divergence.

RSV infection is first established in the upper respiratory tract by infecting the ciliated cells of the nasopharynx, paranasal sinuses, or eustachian tubes of the inner ear. One to 3 days later, 30% of infants who experience their first infection will demonstrate involvement of the lower respiratory tract. In the lower respiratory tract, RSV infects the small bronchial epithelium, spreading to the type 1 and type 2 alveolar pneumocytes. RSV infection is restricted to the respiratory epithelium and rarely spreads outside the respiratory tract. Disseminated disease has been documented in patients with T-cell deficiency.

Infants are more likely to develop severe distal airway disease, because of an immature immune system, the lack of full protection from maternal antibodies, and also the smaller bronchiolar lumen of infants compared with older children and adults. In addition, in infants, collateral ventilation in alveolar regions is not well developed; thus, the impact of obstruction resulting from infection and inflammation is greater.

Histopathologically, airway plugging with mucus, necrosis of the bronchial and bronchiolar epithelium, and peribronchial inflammation with mononuclear cell predominance has been noted. The peribronchial infiltrate may extend into the adjacent pulmonary interstitium. Cytoplasmic inclusion bodies have been described, but syncytia formation is uncommon. Neutrophils are found between small airways and vascular structures and represent the predominant cell type in the bronchoalveolar lavage of RSV-infected infants.

During RSV infection, a number of cytokines and chemokines (eg, interleukin [IL]-8, IL-6, interferon-γ) are released and appear to play a role in the pathogenesis of the disease. Recent data suggest that host innate immune responses are actually inadequately activated or even suppressed in infants with severe RSV disease. With regard to adaptive immunity, the immune response to RSV is neither complete nor long lasting, and reinfections are the rule. Protection against reinfection is greater with homologous than heterologous RSV subtypes. Cellular immunity is not well understood in humans. Nevertheless, the role of CD8+ T cells in viral clearance is highlighted by the fact that patients with profound T-cell deficiency (eg, bone marrow transplantation, severe combined immunodeficiency) often have prolonged viral shedding and develop fatal disease. Regarding humoral immunity, as noted, it appears that antibody responses are important in ameliorating the severity of the disease rather than completely preventing the infection. In addition, passively acquired maternal antibody is not adequate to ensure complete protection from RSV infection and disease. However, children with high titers of maternally derived neutralizing antibody usually have milder symptoms, and the infection is restricted to the upper respiratory tract. These observations have led to use of passive immunoprophylaxis with antibodies as a method for protecting children at highest risk of severe RSV disease.

RSV has a worldwide distribution. In temperate climates, RSV annual midwinter epidemics occur predictably; in the United States, epidemics usually begin in November or December and last until March or April. In the tropics or subtropical areas, RSV activity is present all year long (eg, Florida).

RSV is the single leading cause of infant hospitalization, causing approximately 150,000 hospital admissions per year in children under 2 years of age in the United States. Globally, it is estimated that RSV causes about 34 million episodes of acute LRTIs in children under 5 years of age, resulting in approximately 3.4 million hospitalizations per year. The burden of RSV, however, is significantly larger in the outpatient setting, accounting for 18% of emergency department visits in children less than 5 years of age. In addition, RSV is also a major pathogen in immunocompromised and elderly individuals.

Disease in the immediate neonatal period is uncommon; however, by their first birthday, nearly one-half to two-thirds of infants have been infected with RSV. Seropositivity approaches 100% by 2 years of age. Reinfection with RSV occurs throughout life and may occur even during the same winter season. The annual risk of reinfection falls from between 33% and 75% in the preschool years to approximately 20% among school-age children. The risk of severe LRTI from reinfections also falls with increasing age and number of exposures, likely from the presence of partially neutralizing antibodies following previous infection.

Besides young age (< 6 months) at the start of the RSV season, epidemiologic studies have identified select groups of infants at high risk for severe disease and mortality including premature birth, compromised cardiopulmonary function (chronic lung disease or congenital heart disease [CHD]), trisomy 21, or immunocompromise). Males with severe RSV LRTI outnumber females by 1.6 to 1. Risk factors such as low socioeconomic status and modifiable risk factors such as exposure to secondhand smoke or out-of-home daycare attendance have also been associated with an increased risk for more severe RSV disease.

Humans are the only known reservoir for RSV. Studies of transmission dynamics suggest that infection of infants often follows infection of older siblings. The incubation period ranges from 2 to 8 days, most commonly 4 to 6 days. In infants hospitalized with primary RSV infection, continuous viral shedding for 10 or 11 days detected by polymerase chain reaction (PCR) is commonly observed; young infants and immunocompromised children may shed the virus for 3 to 4 weeks.

Transmission primarily occurs by inoculation of nasopharyngeal or ocular mucous membranes after direct contact with contaminated secretions or fomites. RSV can persist for 30 minutes or more on hands and for several hours on environmental surfaces. Close adherence to infection control policies is critical to limit healthcare-associated transmission. Nosocomial outbreaks of RSV infection in hematopoietic stem cell transplant units and neonatal units have been reported and carry significant morbidity and mortality. Therefore, strict handwashing and contact precautions using gown and gloves for the duration of the RSV-associated illness must be practiced routinely.

## CLINICAL MANIFESTATIONS

The vast majority of infants with RSV infection develop a mild illness with upper respiratory tract symptoms; however, 20% to 30% will develop lower respiratory tract disease (eg, bronchiolitis and/or pneumonia) with the first infection. Of those, 2% to 3% will require hospitalization.

RSV infection is heralded by initial symptoms indistinguishable from those of the common cold. The infant may show rhinitis and cough, and there may be fever. Within 1 to 2 days, the cough becomes more prominent and tachypnea may develop. With increasing respiratory effort, substernal and intercostal retractions are noted along with nasal flaring and abdominal breathing. Grunting can be present in more severe cases. The expiratory phase is prolonged, and the chest is hyperexpanded and hyperresonant, providing further evidence of generalized expiratory airflow obstruction. Crackles or rales with or without diffuse expiratory wheezing are usually heard. In children requiring hospitalization, hypoxemia is typical, reflecting ventilation-perfusion mismatch. Chest radiographs reveal hyperinflation, increased peribronchial markings, and frequently, areas of atelectasis or infiltrate. Densities on chest radiographs are predominantly areas of atelectasis, and although these patients may be labeled as having RSV pneumonia rather than bronchiolitis, this distinction is often arbitrary.

Apnea can be an early manifestation of RSV infection in young infants, particularly infants < 8 weeks old or those with a history of premature birth or apnea of prematurity. Apnea can occur associated with respiratory tract symptoms or may be the only sign at presentation.

Severe bacterial infections, namely bacteremia or meningitis, are extremely rare in infants with RSV bronchiolitis, while urinary tract infections have been documented in approximately 5% of patients. Acute otitis media during or after RSV bronchiolitis occurs in approximately 60% of children. RSV-related fatality rates for hospitalized children in developed countries are < 1%. Although children with underlying conditions such as prematurity or cardiopulmonary disease are at increased risk of death, most fatalities occur in previously healthy infants. The average duration of hospitalization for previously healthy infants without complications is approximately 2 to 3 days. Full recovery may take 2 to 3 weeks. Approximately 50% of infants who develop RSV LRTI will develop recurrent wheezing during childhood. The highest risk for wheezing occurs in the first 6 years of life. It is still unclear whether RSV infection plays a causal role in this pulmonary sequela or whether it is simply a sign of individuals predisposed to asthma. The agent is nevertheless an important precipitant of wheezing in children with reactive airway disease.

## DIAGNOSIS

Bronchiolitis is a clinical diagnosis; however, other respiratory viruses also cause bronchiolitis in young children, and clinical features are insufficient to reliably distinguish RSV from these other viral infections. Specific viral diagnosis may be helpful in certain scenarios: when the diagnosis is uncertain; to reduce unnecessary use of antibiotics; or in hospitalized children at risk for severe disease or for infection control purposes. Detection of RSV from nasopharyngeal specimens may be achieved by rapid antigen tests including fluorescence-based methods such as direct fluorescent antibody (DFA: sensitivity 90–95%, specificity 92–97%) or immunoassays such as enzyme immunoassay (EIA: sensitivity 80%, specificity 75–100%). Molecular-based methods such as real-time reverse transcriptase (rt) polymerase chain reaction (PCR) also may be used to detect RSV. The sensitivity of rapid antigen tests may be lower in older children and is poor in adults, because they shed low concentrations of RSV. Detection by viral culture or by serology is not clinically practical for early diagnosis of acute RSV infection. Serology also is challenging to interpret in young infants because of the presence of maternal antibodies.

In cell culture, RSV growth is detected within 5 to 7 days by the typical plaque morphology with syncytium formation. Cell culture was traditionally the gold standard for diagnosis, but this technique has been replaced by the more rapid and sensitive rt-PCR assays, although many outpatient settings still rely on rapid antigen detection by DFA or EIA due to operational challenges and costs. rt-PCR is the most sensitive method for RSV detection and allows the differentiation between A and B subgroups (which is useful for surveillance purposes in cases of respiratory disease outbreaks). Multiplex PCR assays allow the simultaneous detection of several respiratory viruses, including RSV. Recently, an automated real-time molecular station was developed (FilmArray, Biomerieux, Marcy-l'Étoile, France) that performs nucleic acid extraction, then reverse transcription, followed by PCR identification of as many as 20 respiratory pathogens within 1 hour. Using these assays, studies have shown that approximately 30% of children hospitalized with RSV bronchiolitis may be co-infected with another respiratory virus. Whether children with RSV bronchiolitis who are co-infected with another respiratory virus develop more severe disease is still unclear.

## TREATMENT

Currently, the primary treatment for RSV infection is supportive and includes nasal suctioning, hydration, and, in hospitalized patients, close cardiorespiratory monitoring and measurement of oxygen saturation. Nasal suctioning may provide relief of upper airway obstruction, but deep suctioning of the nasopharynx is not recommended. Nasogastric or intravenous fluids may be used to maintain hydration or when severe tachypnea is present. Although infants with bronchiolitis are at risk of developing subsegmental atelectasis, chest physiotherapy has not been shown to be of clinical benefit. Humidified oxygen is frequently required when managing hospitalized infants since hypoxemia is common (oxygen saturation < 90%) in more severe illness. The complications associated with hypoxemia and carbon dioxide ($CO_2$) retention generally begin when the respiratory rate surpasses 60 breaths per minute. Admission to pediatric intensive care units and use of noninvasive or invasive ventilatory support because of severe respiratory distress, hypoxemia, or apnea are required in 10% to 20% of children hospitalized with RSV bronchiolitis.

Inhaled bronchodilators, such as albuterol or racemic epinephrine, or inhaled or systemic corticosteroids are not recommended for the management of children with RSV bronchiolitis. Nebulized hypertonic saline has been shown to increase mucociliary clearance and may be beneficial in infants who are expected to have prolonged hospitalizations (> 72 hours). Last, except for acute otitis media, bacterial infections of the lower respiratory tract are rarely associated with RSV infection; thus, antibiotic treatment is usually not indicated for LRTI.

Ribavirin is a broad-spectrum virostatic antiviral agent with activity against RSV and other RNA viruses. Early on, small, double-blinded, placebo-controlled studies showed a beneficial effect in infants treated with aerosolized ribavirin soon after onset of disease. The required aerosol route of administration, concerns about potential toxic effects among exposed healthcare personnel, possible teratogenicity in pregnant women, conflicting results of efficacy trials, and high cost have led to infrequent use of ribavirin. The American Academy of Pediatrics (AAP) does not recommend its routine use in children but notes that it may be considered for use in selected patients with, or at risk for, life-threatening RSV infection (Table 236-1). It is also important to note that in immunocompromised children at high risk for severe disease, treatment with ribavirin is most helpful during the stage of URI before LRTI has developed. Uncontrolled studies in hematopoietic stem cell transplant recipients using combination therapy with ribavirin and intravenous polyclonal immunoglobulin or monoclonal antibodies (palivizumab) or in lung transplant recipients using ribavirin and intravenous immunoglobulin or corticosteroids have been performed demonstrating potential benefit. There are a number of promising antiviral drugs currently under development, including new monoclonal antibodies with extended half-life, fusion inhibitors, nucleoside analogs, and small molecules. These newer antivirals have the potential to impact both the prevention and treatment of RSV disease in the main target populations. In hospitalized patients, standard and contact precautions are recommended for the duration of the RSV illness, including patients receiving antivirals. Children with RSV should be cared for in single rooms or cohorted with other RSV-infected children.

## PREVENTION

Preventive strategies against RSV infection are available. Education of parents and other caregivers on ways to decrease the infant's exposure not only to RSV but also to factors that may contribute to the severity of the infection must form the basis of any RSV prophylaxis program. Hand hygiene is crucial in all settings. High-risk infants and children should not be exposed to individuals with respiratory infections, and if at all possible, they should not be in settings (eg, childcare centers) where such exposures are likely. Exposure to tobacco smoke must be eliminated since it has been associated with more severe RSV disease. These measures will have the added benefit of decreasing transmission of other respiratory pathogens.

Passive immunoprophylaxis to prevent RSV infection in infants and children at increased risk for severe disease is available in the form of a monoclonal anti-RSV antibody. Palivizumab targets the F surface glycoprotein of RSV, which is highly conserved among RSV isolates. In the original randomized clinical trials, safety and efficacy were established in infants with a history of premature birth (≤ 35 weeks of gestational age), children with chronic lung disease of prematurity (CLD), and children with hemodynamically significant CHD. Mainly because of costs, the AAP has updated the guidance on palivizumab prophylaxis on different occasions. For the specific updated recommendations, see the current edition of the AAP Report of the Committee on Infectious Diseases. The following recommendations are based on the committee's 2015 report. Palivizumab prophylaxis should be considered at the start of the RSV season for: (1) infants or children with CLD of prematurity born at < 32 weeks of gestation who are younger than 12 months, or younger than 24 months and require medical therapy for their CLD within 6 months before the RSV season; (2) infants born before 29 weeks of gestation who are younger than 12 months at the start of the RSV season; and (3) infants younger than 12 months of age with acyanotic CHD with congestive heart failure and possibly cyanotic CHD. Others to consider palivizumab prophylaxis include children during the first year of life with neuromuscular disorders or pulmonary abnormalities that impair their ability to clear secretions from the lower airway and hematopoietic stem cell transplant patients who are profoundly immunosuppressed during the RSV season.

Palivizumab has a half-life of 28 days, and thus, it is administered once a month during the RSV season intramuscularly. It should be initiated immediately before the RSV season and continued monthly until the end. Although there is significant regional and year-to-year variability in the season onset and offset in the United States, administration of 5 monthly doses starting in November will usually ensure adequate serum concentrations throughout the season. Practitioners outside the United States or in regions with different RSV seasonality should contact their health departments or diagnostic virology laboratories to determine the optimal time to initiate prophylaxis.

Epidemiologic and clinical studies suggest that there are different target populations that will benefit from active immunization with RSV vaccines and that they might require different approaches: young RSV-naïve infants (< 6 months), children > 6 months, pregnant women, and the elderly. Although a safe and effective RSV vaccine has not yet been developed, there are many vaccine candidates currently undergoing testing in preclinical and phase I, II, and III clinical trials.

## HUMAN METAPNEUMOVIRUS

First described in 2001, human metapneumovirus (hMPV) is now recognized as a globally distributed respiratory pathogen affecting children and adults. hMPV is one of the causes of bronchiolitis in

**TABLE 236-1 ANTIVIRALS FOR RESPIRATORY VIRUSES**

| Virus | Clinical Situation | Agent of Choice | Alternative/Comment |
|---|---|---|---|
| Respiratory syncytial virus (RSV) | Treatment | Ribavirin aerosols:<br>Continuously as 6 g over 18 hours per day<br>Alternatively, 2 g/dose over 2–3 hours 3 times daily (only in patients who are not mechanically ventilated) | Ribavirin treatment of RSV is controversial and should be limited to patients with severe disease or at high risk for severe disease. |
| | Prophylaxis | Palivizumab 15 mg/kg IM monthly<br>Duration: RSV season | |
| Human metapneumovirus | Treatment | None | Ribavirin (as above) |
| | Prophylaxis | None | None |
| Parainfluenza virus | Treatment | None | Ribavirin (as above) |
| | Prophylaxis | None | None |
| Influenza A[a] | Treatment | Oseltamivir:<br>Age < 1 year: 3 mg/kg/dose twice daily<br>Age > 1 year weight based:<br>– weight ≤ 15 kg: 30 mg PO twice daily<br>– weight 15–23 kg: 45 mg PO twice daily<br>– weight 23–40 kg: 60 mg PO twice daily<br>– weight > 40 kg: 75 mg PO twice daily<br>Duration: 5 days<br>Zanamivir:<br>Age ≥ 7 years: 2 inhalations (one 5-mg blister per inhalation, for total 10 mg per dose) twice daily<br>Duration: 5 days<br>Peramivir:<br>Age > 18 years: 600 mg via intravenous infusion for 15–30 minutes<br>Duration: 1 day | Amantadine and rimantadine currently not recommended for treatment or prophylaxis in the United States because of high rates of resistance. |
| | Prophylaxis | Oseltamivir:<br>Age 3 months to 1 year: 3 mg/kg once daily<br>Age > 1 year weight based: same dose as for treatment but once daily<br>Duration: 7 days | Zanamivir:<br>Age ≥ 5 years: 2 inhalations (one 5-mg blister per inhalation, for total of 10 mg per dose) once daily<br>Duration: 7 days |
| Influenza B[a] | Treatment | Oseltamivir or zanamivir as for influenza A | None |
| | Prophylaxis | Oseltamivir as for influenza A | Zanamivir as for influenza A |
| Influenza C | Treatment | None | None |
| | Prophylaxis | None | None |
| Adenovirus | Treatment | None | Cidofovir 5 mg/kg once weekly or 1 mg/kg 3 times a week |
| | Prophylaxis | None | None |

[a]See the Centers for Disease Control and Prevention Web site, http://www.cdc.gov/flu, for updated influenza antiviral therapy recommendations.

IM, intramuscularly; PO, orally.

infants and is also associated with different presentations of URIs and LRTIs in children.

## PATHOGENESIS AND EPIDEMIOLOGY

hMPV is an enveloped, single-stranded, negative-sense RNA virus that belongs to the Paramyxoviridae family. Like RSV, which is of the genus *Pneumovirus*, hMPV has projecting F and G envelope glycoproteins and lacks HA activity. However, differences in its genomic sequence and structure result in its placement in the separate genus *Metapneumovirus*. There are 2 major groups of hMPV, A and B, which are further divided into 4 clades: A1, A2, B1, and B2. These different subgroups co-circulate each year in different proportions.

The pathogenesis of hMPV is based on limited studies in children, but it appears that the virus causes inflammatory changes of the lower airways once infection has become established. The interaction of hMPV and the immune system is poorly understood. Although humans mount a very robust antibody response to hMPV, immunity wanes over time and provides limited cross-protectivity between genotypes of the virus.

hMPV causes respiratory infections across the globe. Although discovered in 2001, archived sera from the 1950s contain antibodies against this agent, suggesting that this virus has been circulating for at least 60 years. In temperate regions, the virus is present year-round but peaks in late winter and early spring, later than the usual peak of RSV infection. In subtropical areas, hMPV circulation is most prevalent during the spring and summer. It may account for approximately 10% of LRTIs and 3% of URIs in young children. Almost all children are infected at least once by age 5. LRTIs from hMPV are usually associated with primary infection, and the peak age for severe disease and need for hospitalization is older than for RSV, often between 6 and 12 months of age. Studies have demonstrated symptomatic subsequent infections with hMPV from different hMPV subgroups in young children, although most reinfections are generally limited to the upper respiratory tract, which suggests partial immune protection and cross-protection against other hMPV subgroups following natural infection. Limited data suggest that co-circulation of related viruses, such as RSV or parainfluenza virus (PIV), may reduce the incidence of hMPV infections due to the presence of partial cross-protective immunity. Waning immunity is suggested by the fact that hMPV can cause severe respiratory infections in older adults including pneumonia requiring hospitalization. Asymptomatic infections are rare but may be seen in healthy young adults. Humans are the only reservoir, and like RSV, hMPV is thought to be transmitted through direct contact or contact with contaminated secretions. The incubation period is 3 to 5 days, and viral shedding in otherwise immunocompetent infants may last up to 2 weeks. Healthcare-associated infections have been reported.

## CLINICAL MANIFESTATIONS

Children infected with hMPV cannot be distinguished clinically from those infected by other respiratory viruses such as RSV or PIVs. URIs with rhinorrhea, cough, or fever are common and can be present in 50% to 90% of cases. Pharyngitis and croup have been described in 40% and 18% of cases, respectively. Acute otitis media is a common complication, occurring in 25% to 50% of children with hMPV infection. Between 5% and 10% of children may also develop a rash during the infection. The most common lower respiratory tract syndromes include bronchiolitis (59%), asthma exacerbation (14%), and pneumonia (8%). When compared to RSV, more children with hMPV are diagnosed with pneumonia versus bronchiolitis, with a higher incidence of radiologic findings such as alveolar disease, focal infiltrates, bronchopneumonic changes, and pleural effusions. Like RSV, prematurity, cardiopulmonary disease, and immunosuppression are associated with more severe infection and higher hospitalization rates.

## DIAGNOSIS

In the clinical setting, rt-PCR of respiratory specimens is the most sensitive technique and the gold standard for diagnosis of hMPV. In many clinical laboratories, hMPV is included in the multiplex diagnostic PCR assays, allowing for simultaneous detection of other respiratory pathogens, with a rapid turnaround time. Antigen detection by immunofluorescence using monoclonal antibodies is quite specific, but sensitivity is typically reported as < 75% with these assays. hMPV growth is fastidious in cell culture, with cytopathic effect often not apparent until after 10 to 14 days of incubation, which is not clinically useful. Shell vial culture with immunofluorescence staining improves speed and sensitivity over traditional viral culture but does not reach that of PCR. Serology is useful for epidemiology purposes. A definitive serologic diagnosis requires seroconversion or at least a 4-fold increase in convalescent samples.

## TREATMENT

Care for children infected with hMPV is supportive and includes fever control, hydration, and close monitoring of respiratory status and oxygen saturation. Ribavirin is effective against hMPV in vitro and in animal models. In humans, there are a few small studies as well as anecdotal data with conflicting results regarding its benefit. There are also case reports of successful treatment of severe hMPV infection in immunocompromised patients with combined intravenous immunoglobulin and ribavirin. Antibiotics are not indicated for the treatment of hMPV bronchiolitis or pneumonia unless there is evidence of a concurrent bacterial infection.

## PREVENTION

In hospitalized patients, standard and contact precautions are warranted for the duration of illness.

# PARAINFLUENZA VIRUSES

PIVs are common causes of acute respiratory infections in young children. Croup is the most distinctive clinical syndrome caused by these agents, although bronchiolitis and pneumonia also occur. The initial infection usually occurs in the first few years of life, and reinfections are common.

## PATHOGENESIS AND EPIDEMIOLOGY

PIVs are negative-sense, single-stranded, enveloped RNA viruses belonging to the genus *Paramyxovirus* in the Paramyxoviridae family, which also includes RSV and hMPV. The 4 PIVs have been separated into 2 genera, *Respirovirus* (serotypes PIV-1 and PIV-3) and *Rubulavirus* (PIV-2 and PIV-4 with 2 PIV-4 serotypes A and B). The large viral envelope (150–200 nm) is covered with spike-like projections containing 2 glycoproteins, the hemagglutinin-neuraminidase (HN) and fusion (F) proteins. These proteins are important for viral attachment and fusion with host cell membranes and are the major targets for neutralizing antibodies. The serotypes can be distinguished by type-specific antigens, but the viruses also share common antigens, such that infection with one PIV can lead to heterotypic serologic responses to the other serotypes. PIV-3 is the most prevalent serotype, with 90% to 100% of children demonstrating antibody by age 5.

Pathologic studies of children reveal that inflammation as evidenced by necrosis of the epithelium occurs throughout the respiratory tract with primary infection. In croup, the subglottic tissues appear particularly involved, but with primary infection, the airways at all levels, including the alveoli, can be involved. Most children with bronchopneumonia due to PIVs will have cellular necrosis and destruction of bronchial columnar epithelium in addition to diffuse alveolar damage. Infection with PIVs induces initial innate immune responses, serum and mucosal antibody responses, and cellular immune responses (both CD4+ and CD8+). Immunity to reinfections with PIVs is at best incomplete. Naturally acquired serum immunoglobulin (Ig) G provides the most durable protection against reinfection and may protect against LRTIs. However, infection of adult volunteers reveals that mucosal IgA was better correlated with protection from reinfection than serum IgG. After repeated infections, antibodies may develop that cross-neutralize different PIV strains, mostly noted within the genera (PIV-1 and PIV-3, or PIV-2 and PIV-4). Studies of hospital epidemics indicate a high attack rate and implicate shedding of virus before symptom onset.

Although all PIV serotypes are distributed globally and are capable of causing the full spectrum of respiratory illnesses, they tend to occur in distinct epidemiologic and clinical patterns. Humans are the only source of infection. PIV-1 causes the largest, most defined outbreaks of croup. In the United States, these have occurred for several decades during the fall of odd years. PIV-2 produces smaller, less severe epidemics of croup also in the fall months. PIV-1 and PIV-2 infections occasionally result in bronchiolitis or pneumonia. PIV-3 is the most frequently recovered PIV, is endemic, and circulates throughout the year with annual outbreaks typically extending from late spring through summer. It regularly causes bronchiolitis, pneumonia, or croup. The seasonal pattern of PIV-4 has been increasingly recognized with the use of molecular diagnostic tools. PIV-4 has been mainly associated with upper respiratory disease. A large retrospective study conducted in the United States from 2009 to 2012 showed that PIV-4 had year-round prevalence with biennial peaks during the fall of odd-numbered years. PIV infections are associated with substantial morbidity and mortality in immunocompromised hosts. Most PIV outbreaks in transplant units coincide with the peak incidence of these infections in the community.

Most children are infected with all PIV serotypes by age 5. Infection with PIV-1 usually occurs between year 1 and 5, whereas PIV-3 occurs earlier, with up to two-thirds of infants infected before age 1. Acquisition of PIV-4 also occurs during preschool years following the pattern observed with PIV-1 and PIV-2. Reinfection occurs in children and adults with all serotypes and is usually confined to the upper respiratory tract. Person-to-person transmission of PIV occurs via direct contact with large-droplet aerosols or fomites, and illness follows an incubation period of 2 to 6 days. Depending on the serotype, viral shedding can last up to 3 weeks after symptoms resolve.

## CLINICAL MANIFESTATIONS

PIVs cause a variety of URIs and LRTIs that may vary based on age and serotype. Most primary infections are symptomatic, and disease prevalence is greater in the outpatient setting. In healthy children, most illnesses involve the upper respiratory tract, and up to 35% are complicated with otitis media. In a subset of children, the infection progresses to the lower respiratory tract causing croup (acute laryngotracheobronchitis), bronchiolitis, or pneumonia. As noted, in general, PIV-1 and PIV-2 are associated with croup, and PIV-4 is associated with mild URI in both children and adults, whereas PIV-3 causes bronchiolitis and pneumonia. Overall, croup is the most common PIV-associated diagnosis. Croup begins with a URI of several days in duration, followed by hoarseness and a "barking seal" croupy cough. Inspiratory stridor and marked retractions are evident in more severe infections. Fever is usually mild. Most children recover after 48 to 72 hours, but some children progress to severe airway obstruction. When croup occurs in children younger than 6 months of age or is prolonged or recurrent, underlying anatomic pathology should be suspected. However, recurrent "spasmodic" (noninfectious) croup can occur in children with normal airway anatomy. The differential diagnosis for severe stridor includes bacterial tracheitis, which may be seen as a secondary bacterial infection following viral croup and is most commonly caused by *Staphylococcus aureus*, or epiglottitis, which is a life-threatening infection that was usually caused by *Haemophilus influenzae* type b or diphtheria. These last 2 entities are extremely rare now due to routine immunization. Bronchiolitis and pneumonia caused by PIVs are clinically indistinguishable from those associated with RSV, hMPV, or other respiratory viruses. Rare reports implicate PIVs in cases of aseptic meningitis, encephalitis, myopericarditis, Guillain-Barré syndrome, and parotitis.

## DIAGNOSIS

PIV infection should be suspected in a child with compatible symptoms during a known outbreak, but definitive diagnosis requires identification by culture, antigen detection, or PCR from nasopharyngeal or lower respiratory tract specimens. PCR assays for detection of type-specific PIV RNA have the highest sensitivity and specificity, and thus, PCR is currently the preferred method for diagnosis. All 4 PIV serotypes are also included in available multiplex PCR assays, which may allow for simultaneous detection of several other respiratory viruses. Although used less frequently now because of availability of these other tests, if viral culture is performed, as with other respiratory viruses, care must be taken to promptly place specimens in viral transport media and maintain temperature near 4°C during transport due to the lability of these viruses. Antigen detection by immunofluorescent staining or EIA allows rapid diagnosis but is less sensitive than PCR assays. Serologic diagnosis can also be performed but has limited value in patient management.

## TREATMENT

In immunocompetent children, treatment of PIV infection is supportive. For the management of croup, nebulized epinephrine and steroids (parenteral, oral, or nebulized) can be used. Close monitoring is needed for those with severe disease, and occasionally, intubation of the airway is necessary. No specific antiviral treatment is currently available for PIV infections. Ribavirin has activity against PIVs in vitro, but retrospective studies in immunocompromised patients have failed to show benefit in preventing progression to the lower respiratory tract. Novel drugs are currently being evaluated in clinical trials. DAS181 is a recombinant sialidase fusion protein with activity against PIV that is currently undergoing phase II clinical trials. DAS181 has been used with success for the treatment of PIV LRTI in lung and stem cell transplant patients, including children, resulting in reductions of viral loads and improvement in clinical symptoms. BCX2798 and BCX2855 (hemagglutinin-neuraminidase inhibitors) have demonstrated antiviral activity against PIV-3 in vitro and in murine models, but no human studies are currently available.

## PREVENTION

There is no available PIV vaccine, but many clinical trials are being conducted on vaccine efficacy in healthy infants and children. In addition to standard precautions, contact precautions are recommended for hospitalized infants and young children for the duration of illness.

# INFLUENZA VIRUSES

Influenza is an acute respiratory illness typically accompanied by fever and systemic symptoms. Annual global epidemics interspersed with occasional pandemics result in considerable morbidity and mortality in children and adults.

## PATHOGENESIS AND EPIDEMIOLOGY

The influenza viruses are members of the Orthomyxoviridae family and are separated into 3 genera: *Influenzavirus A, Influenzavirus B*, and *Influenzavirus C*. These viruses contain a negative-sense, single-stranded, segmented RNA genome. Each of the 8 RNA segments codes for 1 or 2 of 11 viral proteins. The segmented nature of the influenza genome allows for exchange of RNA segments when 2 different influenza virions infect the same cell (genetic reassortment). This property is responsible for the antigenic shifts and drifts and has great significance for the epidemiology of influenza including pandemics.

The enveloped virion is about 100 nm in diameter and studded with spike-like projections consisting of its surface glycoproteins HA and NA. Influenza A viruses are further divided into subtypes based on these 2 surface glycoproteins. Major influenza A subtypes circulating in humans have been A (H1N1) and A (H3N2) and, most recently, the pandemic A (H1N1). Protective antibodies directed against particular subtypes of HA or NA are of little or no cross-protective benefit against alternative subtypes. Although human infections with avian influenza viruses are uncommon, they may result in severe lower respiratory tract disease, acute respiratory distress syndrome (ARDS), and death. There are 18 known HA subtypes and 11 NA subtypes of avian influenza viruses, and of those, H5N1 and H7N9 have been associated with severe disease and high mortality rates in humans. Humans are also occasionally infected with swine origin influenza viruses, which usually manifest as the typical influenza-like illness. Influenza B and C have less antigenic variability and are not divided into subtypes. Type C influenza viruses cause sporadic mild influenza-like illness in children, and type C antigens are not included in influenza vaccines.

Influenza infection is initiated by virus inoculation in the upper or lower airways. If present, virus-specific IgG and IgA antibodies against the surface antigens, particularly HA, may block the infection. Neuraminidase facilitates penetration through the sialyloligosaccharide-rich respiratory mucous layer for access to the epithelial cells and later is important for release of newly packaged viruses from cells. The viral HA allows viral attachment and later membrane fusion with respiratory epithelial cells. Upon infection and replication in the respiratory epithelium, virus is shed into respiratory secretions, and local spread ensues, with eventual desquamation. The entire airway from pharynx to alveoli may be involved. Diffuse pneumonia due to alveolar infection can be life threatening. Viral infection usually remains limited to the respiratory tract, although viremia has been described with specific strains and has been associated with enhanced disease severity. Systemic symptoms are mostly due to the high levels of cytokines and chemokines released upon infection. Influenza infection results in damaged mucociliary function, reduced neutrophil function, and impairment of other immune mechanisms that are probably responsible for the increased risk of bacterial superinfections.

The virus type and subtype have an effect on the virulence of the circulating influenza strain. The HA and NA represent the major determinants of immunity. Minor mutations in these enveloped glycoproteins are referred as "antigenic drifts" and occur almost annually. Antigenic drifts are responsible for the circulation of new viral variants to which the individual may be susceptible, perpetuating the annual epidemics of variable extent and severity. At varying intervals, major changes in the HA and NA occur and are referred as "antigenic

**TABLE 236-2 GROUPS AT HIGH RISK FOR COMPLICATIONS OF INFLUENZA INFECTION**

| |
|---|
| Children < 2 years of age[a] |
| Adults ≥ 65 years of age |
| Chronic pulmonary (including asthma), cardiovascular (except hypertension), renal, hepatic, hematologic (including sickle cell disease), metabolic (including diabetes mellitus), neurologic, neuromuscular, and neurodevelopmental disorders (including disorders of the brain, spinal cord, peripheral nerve and muscle such as cerebral palsy, epilepsy, stroke, intellectual disability [mental retardation], moderate to severe developmental delay, muscular dystrophy, or spinal cord injury) |
| Immunosuppression (including immunosuppression caused by medications or by human immunodeficiency virus) |
| Women who are pregnant or postpartum (within 2 weeks after delivery) |
| Children < 19 years of age receiving long-term aspirin therapy |
| Morbidly obese (body mass index [BMI] ≥ 40 for adults or BMI > 2.33 standard deviations above the mean for children) |
| Residents of chronic care facilities or nursing homes |
| Native Americans and Alaskan Natives |

[a]All children < 5 years of age are considered to be at higher risk for complications of influenza; however, the highest risk is in those < 2 years of age, with the highest hospitalization and death rates among infants < 6 months of age.

shifts." Antigenic shifts are associated with genetic reassortment of RNA segments between human and animal viruses or adaptation of a new animal virus to humans and are responsible for pandemics of influenza A. These events, which occurred 4 times during the 20th century and once in 2009, render antibody to previously circulating influenza A viruses unprotective. Worldwide pandemics associated with considerable excess mortality ensue.

In temperate climates, seasonal influenza epidemics occur during winter months. In the United States, influenza activity usually peaks between January and March, although occasionally, it can occur as early as November or as late as May. Community outbreaks usually last 4 to 8 weeks; however, circulation of 2 or 3 influenza viruses may be associated with a prolonged influenza season of 3 or more months and bimodal peaks in activity. Rates of hospitalization and death associated with influenza vary from year to year because influenza seasons are unpredictable and fluctuate in duration and severity. The severity of the disease is related in part to the presence of preexisting immunity as a result of prior exposure or immunization with a related strain and underlying risk factors (Table 236-2). In the United States, the annual epidemics usually result in more than 200,000 hospitalizations. Hospitalization rates are similarly high for children < 2 years of age and adults age 65 years or older. The number of influenza-associated deaths, which is probably underestimated due to underreporting, can vary from 3000 to 50,000 people annually, with the majority of deaths occurring in adults age 65 years or older. During influenza season, the virus accounts for approximately 20% of outpatient visits for children and adults with acute respiratory infections and fever (influenza-like illness). Surveillance activity is updated weekly during influenza season and available from the Centers for Disease Control and Prevention (CDC).

Young children shed higher concentrations of virus for a longer duration than their older counterparts. The virus is highly contagious and is transmitted person-to-person primarily through contact with respiratory secretions (aerosolized droplets) generated by coughing or sneezing, or through contact with contaminated surfaces. Symptoms follow a 1- to 4-day incubation period, and patients may be infectious 24 hours before symptom onset. Viral shedding lasts for approximately 7 days, although virus can be shed for a longer period of time in young children or in patients with immunodeficiency. Viral shedding and fever are directly correlated.

## CLINICAL MANIFESTATIONS

In children, influenza typically presents with sudden onset of fever and respiratory symptoms, but ultimately, the clinical manifestations depend on the age of the child and his or her preexisting immunity. Fever is more prominent than with other viral respiratory infections, occurring in 95% of children, routinely reaching 39°C (102.2°F) to 40°C (104°F), and lasting 3 to 6 days in the absence of complications. In older children, the typical influenza-like illness starts with fever, often accompanied by chills or rigor, headache, myalgias, malaise, sore throat, and dry cough, followed later by a more productive cough and rhinitis. Children under age 5 usually present with a febrile URI, but some manifest severe croup, bronchiolitis, or pneumonia, while neonatal influenza may mimic bacterial sepsis. Tracheitis or tracheobronchitis may be particularly severe or complicated by bacterial superinfection (bacterial tracheitis). Asthma exacerbations are also common in children with influenza infection. The most common complication of influenza is acute otitis media, affecting approximately 10% to 50% of children, followed by pneumonia, especially in high-risk patients. Viral bronchopneumonia is more common in children < 2 years of age and is typically mild, rarely leading to severe disease or death in otherwise healthy children. Bacterial pneumonia has been reported in 2% of hospitalized children and usually manifests as recurrent fever and pulmonary symptoms after 5 to 7 days of influenza illness. The most common causative agents are *Streptococcus pneumoniae* and *Staphylococcus aureus* (including methicillin-resistant *S aureus* [MRSA]). *S aureus* pneumonia may be particularly severe and rapidly fatal and usually occurs in children with no underlying medical condition.

Other complications of influenza include Reye syndrome in association with aspirin use, toxic shock syndrome due to secondary bacterial infection, myositis or myocarditis and neurologic complications that range from febrile seizures to acute encephalitis, aseptic meningitis, Guillain-Barré syndrome, or transverse myelitis. Postinfectious encephalitis has also been reported.

## DIAGNOSIS

Influenza virus infection should be considered when clinically compatible symptoms are present irrespective of the immunization status. However, diagnostic confirmation requires viral isolation or detection of viral antigens or viral RNA in respiratory samples (nasal swab or wash), ideally within the first 3 days of symptoms as viral load decreases afterward. Influenza can be cultured from respiratory secretions upon inoculation into monkey or canine kidney cell cultures or embryonated eggs. Viral growth can be detected after 2 to 6 days by hemadsorption, hemagglutination, or, on occasion, by evidence of cell destruction. However, with the availability of specific antiviral treatment and the need to initiate therapy quickly in high-risk or hospitalized patients, culture methods are not preferred in clinical practice. Similarly, serology testing requires acute and convalescent sampling and thus is not practical for clinical decision making. Rapid antigen detection assays (by immunofluorescence or EIA) are also available, with reported sensitivities of 45% to 97% and specificities of 76% to 100% compared with PCR. Most of these assays cannot differentiate between influenza subtypes, which may be needed for choice of antiviral agents. RNA detection by rt-PCR is the most sensitive and specific diagnostic method and allows for rapid diagnosis, differentiating between influenza types and subtypes. Influenza viruses are included in the commercially available multiplex PCR assays. Diagnostic testing also is helpful because it may reduce additional testing to identify the cause of the child's influenza-like illness. Treatment should not be withheld in high-risk patients while awaiting rt-PCR test results.

## TREATMENT

In general, influenza infection in children is a self-limited condition. Supportive care includes antipyretics to reduce fever (and discomfort). Salicylates should not be used to treat influenza in children or adolescents because of the increased risk of Reye syndrome. Bed rest and maintenance of adequate fluid intake may also provide comfort.

Antiviral therapy is recommended regardless of the immunization status or whether or not symptoms have been present for more than 48 hours for any patient with confirmed or suspected influenza who is hospitalized, has severe or complicated disease, or is at high risk for complications (see Table 236-2). Clinical benefit is greater when antiviral therapy is initiated within 48 hours of symptom onset; however, treatment should be considered even if later in the disease course, especially in hospitalized patients, in whom antiviral therapy has been shown to shorten the duration of hospitalization and decrease mortality. The duration of treatment is 5 days.

Antiviral therapies are discussed in Chapter 240, and use in specific respiratory infections is outlined in Table 236-1. The CDC has a surveillance program in place to identify antiviral resistance each year and updates recommendations for influenza antiviral use accordingly. Two classes of antivirals are approved for treatment and prophylaxis of influenza infections in the United States: NA inhibitors (oseltamivir, zanamivir, and peramivir); and adamantanes (amantadine and rimantadine). NA inhibitors have activity against influenza A and B viruses and can be administered through different routes. Oral oseltamivir is the preferred antiviral and is approved for treatment in children as young as 2 weeks old. Inhaled zanamivir is an alternative, but it is difficult to administer. It is approved for treatment in children over 7 years of age and is not recommended in children with underlying airway disease because of association with bronchospasm. A parenteral form of zanamivir is currently in a phase III clinical trial for patients who cannot tolerate or absorb oseltamivir. Peramivir is another NA inhibitor approved for those over 18 years of age and is also administered intravenously. Dosages are detailed in Table 236-1. Laninamivir is a long-acting inhaled NA inhibitor available only in Japan. Amantadine and rimantadine are active against influenza A only, and levels of resistance in past seasons have been reported to be > 99%; thus, these agents are not recommended for treatment or chemoprophylaxis in the United States.

## PREVENTION

Immunoprophylaxis with trivalent and quadrivalent inactivated influenza vaccines (IIVs) or live attenuated, cold-adapted influenza vaccines (LAIVs) and chemoprophylaxis using NA inhibitors are available measures that are effective in reducing the number of influenza virus infections and the impact of influenza disease.

### Influenza Vaccines

Since the late 1940s, the vaccination each year prior to the onset of influenza season of individuals at high risk for complications has been the most effective approach for reducing the impact of influenza. Each year, influenza vaccines are modified to contain 3 or 4 antigens (2 for influenza A and 1 or 2 for influenza B) based on the influenza circulation in the Southern Hemisphere, which precedes the circulation in the Northern Hemisphere. From 2005 to 2016, the overall adjusted vaccine effectiveness has varied widely from 10% to 60%. Vaccine effectiveness is highest when the vaccine strains and circulating strains are closely related. The IIVs contain no live virus and are administered either intramuscularly or intradermally. IIVs are available in both trivalent (IIV3) formulations, including a high-dose vaccine for those at least 65 years of age, and quadrivalent (IIV4) formulations. In addition, there are 2 trivalent IIVs that have been developed without using eggs and are available for people older than 18 years with severe egg allergy: recombinant influenza vaccine (RIV3), and cell culture–based influenza vaccine (ccIIV3), which contains trace amounts of ovalbumin. Although intramuscular IIV formulations are licensed for administration in children 6 months and older, the intradermal formulation is only licensed for use in those 18 to 64 years of age.

LAIV4 is a quadrivalent formulation that is administered intranasally and is licensed for healthy children older than 2 years of age and adults less than 50 years old. It is contraindicated in children < 5 years of age with a history of asthma or wheezing in the preceding 12 months, children between 2 and 17 years of age who are receiving chronic aspirin therapy, pregnant women, immunocompromised individuals, and people who have received influenza antiviral treatment within the previous 48 hours. Since 2016, the CDC does not recommend LAIV administration in children because of low effectiveness.

LAIV and most of the IIV formulations are produced in eggs. Except for severe, life-threatening allergic reactions to any ingredient in the vaccine, egg allergy is not a contraindication to influenza vaccination. Recent studies have shown that IIV administered in a single, age-appropriate dose is well tolerated by most recipients with a history of egg allergy. If a child with mild egg allergy (eg, hives) is vaccinated, close observation for 30 minutes and availability of appropriate resuscitation equipment are required. See the CDC recommendations for further information regarding use of influenza vaccines in egg-allergic individuals. The risk of developing Guillain-Barré syndrome is rare (no more than 1–2 cases per million doses).

All children 6 months and older should receive annual influenza vaccination. Children 6 months to 8 years who have not received influenza vaccine previously require 2 doses of vaccine in their first year of influenza vaccination, administered at least 4 weeks apart to boost antibody responses. Children older than 8 years require 1 dose of influenza vaccine regardless of their previous immunization status. Special emphasis for IIV administration should be directed to patients at increased risk (see Table 236-2). Influenza vaccination should be mandatory for healthcare workers. People who care for severely immunocompromised patients (eg, in bone marrow transplant units) should not receive LAIV unless patient contact can be avoided for 7 days following administration. See http://www.cdc.gov/flu for the Public Health Service Advisory Committee on Immunization Practices (ACIP) updated recommendations on influenza vaccine target populations, dosage, administration instructions, and adverse effects. For further discussion of influenza vaccination, see Chapter 239.

### Chemoprophylaxis

Chemoprophylaxis should not be substituted for vaccination, even in high-risk patients, but can be considered for prevention of infection in children at high risk of complications during the first 2 weeks following vaccination, children who may not respond to vaccination due to immunosuppression, or children who cannot receive vaccination due to a contraindication. It can also be used during influenza outbreaks for prevention of infection among residents of institutions. Chemoprophylaxis can be administered concomitantly with IIV formulations to provide protection until antibody develops but cannot be administered with LAIV formulations, since antivirals may have activity against vaccine strains. Chemoprophylaxis can be administered before or after exposure in children at high risk for complications. Given the development of resistance to other antiviral agents, the NA inhibitor oseltamivir is now the primary agent recommended for children. It is approved for use in children age 3 months and older. Zanamivir may also be used and is approved as a prophylactic agent for children over age 5. CDC recommendations should be consulted for further information regarding prophylaxis.

### Other Preventive Measures

In hospitalized patients, strict infection prevention measures to avoid nosocomial infections should be implemented, and patients should be placed in droplet (and standard) precautions for the duration of illness. Hand washing is essential. Respiratory secretions should be considered infectious.

Other preventive measures that are key when managing children with influenza infection, especially those at increased risk of complications, include influenza vaccination of household contacts and out-of-home caregivers, general infection prevention measures, and avoidance of sick contacts.

# ADENOVIRUSES

Adenoviruses account for 5% to 10% of all febrile illnesses in children and are also important causes of ocular, gastrointestinal, and urologic infections. In addition, they are recognized as serious pathogens in immunocompromised hosts in whom fatal disseminated infection can develop following primary infection or viral reactivation.

## PATHOGENESIS AND EPIDEMIOLOGY

Adenoviruses are nonenveloped, double-stranded DNA viruses that are icosahedral in shape and measure 70 to 80 nm in diameter. They are members of the Adenoviridae family in the genus *Mastadenovirus* and are divided into 7 species (A–G) on the basis of their DNA sequence. There are 57 recognized human adenovirus serotypes. Adenoviruses 1 to 5, 7, 14, and 21 are primarily associated with respiratory tract disease, while adenoviruses 40 and 41 mainly cause gastroenteritis. Antigenically important coat proteins include hexon, penton base, and fiber. Infection with one adenovirus type confers type-specific immunity.

In most respiratory disease, the initial infection by adenovirus involves the nose, oropharynx, and conjunctiva, but the severity will vary based on the serotype. In severe pneumonia, total destruction with necrotizing bronchitis, bronchiolitis, and pneumonia has been described. Hyaline membrane and necrosis may be present, whereas cilia and goblet cells may be absent. Often epithelial cells take on a characteristic appearance with adenoviral infection.

Adenoviruses have worldwide distribution, and infections occur throughout the year. Spread is primarily via respiratory droplets, but transmission can also occur by fecal routes or via contact with contaminated fomites. Most children have serologic evidence of prior adenovirus infection by age 10. Care must be taken in associating adenovirus detection with disease entities because these viruses, especially species C, are capable of establishing persistent or latent infection in lymphoid tissues including tonsils, adenoids, and the gut of infected children, and recurrent shedding without acute symptoms can occur. Nevertheless, many epidemics of adenovirus disease including keratoconjunctivitis, pharyngoconjunctival fever, or acute respiratory disease as well as nosocomial transmission have been described. The incubation period ranges from 2 to 14 days for adenoviral respiratory tract infections and 3 to 10 days for gastroenteritis.

## CLINICAL MANIFESTATIONS

Adenoviruses are capable of causing a broad spectrum of clinical diseases due to the organ tropism of different species. Species A is primarily associated with respiratory and gastrointestinal infections; species B, C, and E with respiratory infections; species D with ocular and gastrointestinal infections; and species F and G with gastrointestinal infections. The clinical manifestations of adenoviral disease vary based on the age and the host immune status. Severe disease has been reported with types 5, 7, 14, and 21.

### Respiratory Illness

Adenoviruses are some of the most common viruses that cause febrile respiratory illnesses in children. The usual duration of illness is 5 to 7 days, although symptomatology can last up to 2 weeks. Infants and children most commonly manifest URI symptoms with conjunctivitis, otitis media, coryza, or pharyngitis, and less commonly with croup or a pertussis-like syndrome. Exudative tonsillitis may be present, and systemic symptoms such as fever, malaise, and headache may be prominent. Respiratory symptoms may be accompanied by a benign follicular conjunctivitis, febrile pharyngitis. and cervical adenitis in a condition termed pharyngoconjunctival fever (adenovirus B types 3 and 7 are the most common isolates). Outbreaks of pharyngoconjunctival fever have been documented in summer camps and in association with public swimming pools. Bronchiolitis or pneumonia occurs in a small percentage of children and can be fatal in neonates and children with underlying medical conditions. The incidence of bronchiolitis obliterans or bronchiectasis is high following adenoviral pneumonia in young children. Although most children recover without complications, some outbreaks caused by species B types 3, 7, 11, 14, and 21 have resulted in fulminate disease with significant mortality.

### Epidemic Keratoconjunctivitis

In this more serious form of ocular adenovirus infection, conjunctivitis is followed by bilateral corneal infiltrates and enlargement of preauricular nodes. It has been associated primarily with adenovirus D types 8, 19, and 37 and causes severe pain and blurry vision. Outbreaks of keratoconjunctivitis have been reported in medical facilities.

### Extrarespiratory Manifestations

The enteric adenoviruses, species F types 40 and 41 and species G type 52, are important causes of diarrheal illness that may last from 8 to 12 days. Adenoviruses (not necessarily the enteric serotypes) have been recovered from mesenteric lymph nodes of children with intussusception, suggesting a role for these viruses in the pathogenesis of the disease. Adenovirus species B types 11 and 21 are associated with acute hemorrhagic cystitis and hematuria lasting several days to 2 weeks. Adenovirus infection, especially subgroup C type 5, may cause severe hepatitis and liver failure, particularly in infants or immunocompromised patients. Viral myocarditis, meningoencephalitis, hepatitis, and rhabdomyolysis are occasionally associated with adenovirus infection. Severe disseminated adenovirus disease with or without exanthem has been reported in immunocompetent and immunocompromised children, including neonates, and is associated with high mortality.

## DIAGNOSIS

Adenoviruses can be identified by PCR in nasopharyngeal, oropharyngeal, and eye secretions, blood, cerebrospinal fluid, urine, stool, and biopsy specimens. Other means less commonly used for adenovirus isolation include traditional culture in primary or permanent cell lines, shell vial culture, and antigen detection that is generally less sensitive than culture but may provide a rapid diagnosis. Serologic evidence of increasing antibody titers could be useful to confirm recent infection.

Because virus shedding from the pharynx may persist for weeks or even recurrently following adenovirus infection, the diagnostic significance of adenovirus detection in respiratory or fecal samples is not as strong as it is with many of the other respiratory viruses. In these cases, measuring viral burden may be useful to confirm acute infection. In immunocompromised patients, quantitative PCR for adenovirus in the blood may be useful for detecting patients at risk of dissemination.

## TREATMENT

For most healthy children, treatment is symptomatic. Antiviral therapy is reserved for immunocompromised children and patients with severe disease. Although there are no available controlled trials, the nucleotide analog cidofovir has been used at different doses and intervals for the treatment of adenovirus infection in immunocompromised patients. The major limiting factor of cidofovir is nephrotoxicity. CMX001 (brincidofovir) is a lipid conjugate form of cidofovir with enhanced in vitro activity against adenoviruses, improved bioavailability when administered orally, and lower potential for nephrotoxicity and myelosuppression. Brincidofovir is currently being evaluated in phase III clinical trials, and preliminary results have indicated good safety and efficacy in treating adenoviral infections in transplant recipients. Intravenous immunoglobulin has also been used for the treatment of adenovirus disease in immunocompromised patients. Other emerging therapies include the transfusion of donor-derived adenovirus-specific T lymphocytes, which is currently being used in some centers for stem cell transplant recipients who do not respond to antiviral therapy.

## PREVENTION

An effective, live, enteric-coated oral vaccine against serotypes 4 and 7 has been used in military recruits but has not been employed in civilian populations. Hospitalized children with conjunctivitis or gastroenteritis should be placed in contact isolation, and those with respiratory tract disease in contact and droplet isolation for the duration of illness. Adenoviruses are difficult to inactivate with alcohol-based gels and can remain viable on environmental surfaces for prolonged periods; thus, strict hand hygiene and use of disposable gloves are recommended when caring for infected patients.

# RHINOVIRUSES AND RESPIRATORY ENTEROVIRUSES

Rhinoviruses have been known to cause the majority of URIs in adults and children, which are also known as the "common cold," with a generally benign, self-limited course. Currently, they are also increasingly recognized as important triggers of LRTIs and asthma exacerbations.

## PATHOGENESIS AND EPIDEMIOLOGY

Rhinoviruses and enteroviruses are small, nonenveloped, single positive-stranded RNA viruses belonging to the *Enterovirus* genus within the Picornaviridae family. They are divided into 7 species: 3 rhinovirus species (A, B, and C) and 4 non-rhinovirus enterovirus species (A, B, C, and D). There are more than 100 serotypes. Most rhinoviruses replicate optimally at low pH (< 5) and high temperature (> 34°C), the temperature of the upper respiratory tract mucosa. Cross-protection after rhinovirus infection is incomplete and short lasting.

Rhinoviruses infect and replicate in the upper respiratory tract through the intracellular adhesion molecule-1 (ICAM-1), the host receptor for most rhinoviruses. On the other hand, enteroviruses can replicate in different cells, causing clinical syndromes such as febrile illness, viral meningitis and encephalitis, and myopericarditis. Some species of enteroviruses, however, are mainly associated with respiratory tract infections (species C and D) and are clinically indistinguishable from those caused by rhinovirus.

Rhinovirus infections occur year-round, but 2 peaks have been classically reported, 1 between April and May and a second between September and October. Some studies have shown that species C has a different peak of infection, typically over the winter months. Children are the major reservoir for rhinovirus. Transmission occurs primarily by person-to-person contact through self-inoculation with contaminated secretions (hand-to-nose or hand-to-eye). Large-droplet spread is also possible. Viral shedding in respiratory secretions is greatest during the first 2 to 3 days of illness and can last from 10 to 21 days. The incubation period is 2 to 3 days.

Enteroviruses with respiratory tropism, such as species C and D, have a worldwide distribution and can cause respiratory disease with varying degrees of severity ranging from mild URI to pneumonia. Enterovirus D68 was first described in 1962 from children with bronchiolitis and pneumonia, with a few clusters of cases reported over the past decade in different parts of the world. The largest outbreak of enterovirus D68 occurred in the United States in 2014 with over 1000 cases reported in 49 states mainly affecting children with a history of asthma. In addition to its respiratory tropism, enterovirus D68 infection has been associated with neurologic disease including acute flaccid myelitis.

## CLINICAL MANIFESTATIONS

Rhinovirus infection can be asymptomatic or symptomatic. The most common manifestation of rhinovirus infection is the common cold—an illness dominated by nasal obstruction or discharge, with accompanying cough, sore throat, and mild or absent fever. It has also been linked to acute otitis media complicating approximately one-third of patients with URI. Rhinoviruses can also cause LRTI, such as bronchiolitis and pneumonia, and are well-established triggers of wheezing in children with asthma.

## DIAGNOSIS

rt-PCR is the most sensitive and the preferred test for diagnosis and is the only method available to diagnose rhinovirus C. Commercially available multiplex PCR assays include both rhinoviruses and enteroviruses. Most of these assays target a region that is conserved among both species, making their differentiation difficult. Rhinovirus can be positive by PCR in asymptomatic children, which may indicate residual viral RNA from a prior rhinovirus infection.

## TREATMENT

No specific antiviral treatment is currently available for rhinovirus infections. Over-the-counter cough and cold preparations do not provide significant benefit for children with the common cold and are not recommended. Vitamins (ascorbic acid), minerals (zinc), and herbal remedies (*Echinacea*) are frequently used for the treatment and prevention of the common cold, with limited evidence of any benefit in reducing symptoms. To date, there are no vaccines available or in clinical trials.

## PREVENTION

Hand washing and avoidance of hand contact with respiratory secretions of affected individuals reduce viral transmission. For symptomatic hospitalized children, contact and droplet precautions are recommended for the duration of illness.

# CORONAVIRUSES

The human coronaviruses are enveloped, pleomorphic, nonsegmented, single-stranded RNA viruses named after their corona or crown-like surface projections that correspond to their surface glycoproteins. Coronaviruses have long been identified as causes of the common cold in adults and children, causing 5% to 18% of childhood respiratory infections. Cases of croup, bronchiolitis, and pneumonia are increasingly recognized. Emergence of 2 highly virulent coronaviruses with zoonotic transmission causing severe LRTI has been described in the past 15 years. In 2003, the SARS coronavirus was identified as a novel virus responsible for the 2002 to 2003 global outbreak that resulted in thousands of cases and more than 700 deaths. Technologies developed during the SARS epidemic contributed to the discovery of additional coronaviruses such that 4 non-SARS coronaviruses (HCoV-229E, HCoV-NL63, HCoV-OC43, and HCoV-HKU1) are currently known to circulate in humans and have been associated with respiratory disease. Non-SARS coronavirus epidemics have also occurred. In 2012, the Middle East respiratory syndrome (MERS) coronavirus (CoV) was identified, and since then, hundreds of people have been affected in different countries. Most people affected with MERS-CoV developed acute febrile respiratory illness, and many died. The incubation period of non-SARS-CoV is approximately 3 days, for SARS-CoV approximately 4 days, and for MERS-CoV approximately 5 days. The growth of CoVs in tissue culture is limited, and rt-PCR has enhanced the ability to detect these viruses. The diagnosis of SARS-CoV or MERS-CoV should not be based on a single test and needs to be confirmed by an approved laboratory. Treatment is supportive, and no vaccines are currently available.

# BOCAVIRUSES

Human bocaviruses (HBoVs) of the family Parvoviridae are single-stranded DNA viruses that were discovered in 2005 using novel molecular techniques in children with respiratory infections. HBoVs circulate throughout the year, with peaks in winter and spring months. The virus is most frequently identified in children < 2 years of age. By age 6 years, most children have evidence of previous HBoV infection, with reinfections occurring into adulthood. Four genotypes are included in the *Bocavirus* genus (HBoV 1–4). HBoV1 is the genotype associated with respiratory disease in children, having been found in approximately 8% of young children with acute respiratory infections including otitis media, pneumonia, bronchiolitis, and wheezing. Although this virus is not commonly found in asymptomatic individuals, its causal role in childhood respiratory infections has been called into question because of the high frequency of co-detection with other respiratory viruses (as high as 80%) and the potential for asymptomatic persistence in some individuals. HBoV1 has also been detected in low levels in the stool of children with gastroenteritis; however, co-pathogens were detected in 100% of the patients, potentially reflecting ingestion of the virus without causation of disease. HBoV2, HBoV3, and HBoV4 seem to be associated with gastrointestinal symptoms, but their prevalence is low. Detection of HBoV1–3 from cerebrospinal fluid in children with encephalitis associated with seroconversion has occasionally been reported. Diagnosis is made mainly with rt-PCR, but serology is also available. Treatment is supportive.

## SUGGESTED READINGS

Broccolo F, Falcone V, Esposito S, Toniolo A. Human bocaviruses: possible etiologic role in respiratory infection. *J Clin Virol.* 2015;72:75-81.

Debiaggi M, Canducci F, Ceresola ER, Clementi M. The role of infections and coinfections with newly identified and emerging respiratory viruses in children. *Virol J*. 2012;9:247.

Jacobs SE, Lamson DM, St George K, Walsh TJ. Human rhinoviruses. *Clin Micro Rev*. 2013;26:135-162.

Mazur NI, Martinon-Torres F, Baraldi E, et al. Lower respiratory tract infection caused by respiratory syncytial virus: current management and new therapeutics. *Lancet Respir Med*. 2015;3:888-900.

Nair H, Nokes DJ, Gessner BD, et al. Global burden of acute lower respiratory tract infections due to respiratory syncytial virus in young children: a systematic review and meta-analysis. *Lancet*. 2010;375:1545-1555.

Principi N, Esposito S. Paediatric human metapneumovirus infection: epidemiology, prevention and therapy. *J Clin Virol*. 2014; 59:141-147.

Ralston SL, Lieberthal AS, Meissner HC, et al. Clinical practice guideline: the diagnosis, management, and prevention of bronchiolitis. *Pediatrics*. 2014;134:e1474-e1502.

Sandkovsky U, Vargas L, Florescu DF. Adenovirus: current epidemiology and emerging approaches to prevention and treatment. *Curr Infect Dis Rep*. 2014;16:416.

Schomacker H, Schaap-Nutt A, Collins PL, Schmidt AC. Pathogenesis of acute respiratory illness caused by human parainfluenza viruses. *Curr Opin Virol*. 2012;2:294-299.

Williams JV, Harris PA, Tollefson SJ, et al. Human metapneumovirus and lower respiratory tract disease in otherwise healthy infants and children. *N Engl J Med*. 2004;350:443-450.

# 237 Fungal Respiratory Infections

Tim Flerlage, Aditya H. Gaur, and Joshua Wolf

## INTRODUCTION

Fungi are widely distributed in the environment and are uncommon respiratory pathogens in children or adolescents. Fungi causing infection can be viewed as 2 main groups: those that cause endemic mycoses (eg, *Histoplasma* and *Blastomyces* species), which can lead to disease in both immunocompetent and immunocompromised hosts; and those considered opportunistic fungal pathogens (eg, *Aspergillus* and *Mucor* species), which primarily cause disease in immunocompromised hosts (Fig. 237-1). Although the endemic mycoses can be severe in otherwise healthy hosts, especially when exposed to a large infectious inoculum, infection is more often mild and self-limiting or even subclinical. In contrast, the endemic mycoses and opportunistic fungal pathogens can cause life-threatening pulmonary infections in patients with primary or secondary immunodeficiency. Early diagnosis of respiratory fungal infection is a challenge in both immunocompetent and immunocompromised patients. The initial clinical findings are nonspecific and are similar to other more common bacterial and viral infections. Critical to an early diagnosis is a clinician's index of suspicion, which is influenced by recognition of the host's immune status and vulnerability to fungal infections.

## THE ENDEMIC MYCOSES

The endemic mycoses are diseases caused by fungi with shared characteristics, including thermal dimorphism (mycelial form in the environment and yeast in tissue), the ability to cause clinically significant disease in otherwise well hosts, and specific geographic distributions.

### PATHOGENESIS AND EPIDEMIOLOGY





The respiratory tract serves as the most common primary site of infection and portal of systemic entry for many of the endemic mycoses, including *Histoplasma capsulatum*, *Blastomyces* species, *Coccidioides* species, and *Paracoccidioides* species. Exposure typically occurs as a result of inhalation of infectious conidia aerosolized from soil disrupted due to wind or human activity. Although *Blastomyces* species may cause primary cutaneous infection by direct inoculation in children, it most frequently causes primary pulmonary infection. Organisms within the *Sporothrix schenckii* complex predominantly cause a cutaneous infection acquired through traumatic inoculation and only rarely cause primary respiratory tract disease. The mechanism by which humans become infected with *Talaromyces marneffei* is incompletely understood, but epidemiologic studies suggest that, similar to these other organisms, inhalation of infectious conidia from disrupted soil is a likely route of acquisition.

After inhalation of conidia, intact cell-mediated immunity appears to be of critical importance for control of infection. Underlying deficiencies in cell-mediated immune function predispose to severe or disseminated disease and to reactivation of latent infection. Examples of medications and conditions that increase risk of severe disease include the acquired immunodeficiency syndrome (AIDS), anticancer chemotherapy, solid organ or hematopoietic stem cell transplantation, chemotherapy, and immunomodulatory medications (including systemic corticosteroids) used for the treatment of rheumatologic and other conditions.

Although cases are documented in patients with apparently normal immunologic function, disseminated histoplasmosis and penicilliosis are considered AIDS-defining illnesses in human immunodeficiency virus (HIV)-infected individuals. Similarly, a diagnosis of penicilliosis in a pediatric patient without a known underlying immunologic deficit may increase the suspicion for a primary or secondary immunodeficiency.

In general, the fungi that cause the endemic mycoses dwell in soil. Each has a specific geographical and environmental predilection (Table 237-1). For this reason, obtaining a careful (past) social history is necessary; it is important to ask patients about travel to endemic regions, occupational activities, and recreational endeavors. Localized outbreaks or disease clusters of endemic mycoses can occur, such as outbreaks of coccidioidomycosis following earthquakes in California.

### CLINICAL MANIFESTATIONS

The clinical manifestations of each of the endemic mycoses vary depending on factors such as inoculum burden and host immune competence. In otherwise healthy individuals, infection is commonly subclinical or mild and self-limiting, but on occasions, such as with a large inoculum exposure (eg, cleaning barns), severe clinical disease may develop.

Endemic mycoses, including histoplasmosis, blastomycosis, and coccidioidomycosis, can present with pneumonia. The associated symptoms can range from fever, cough, chest pain, and dyspnea to the acute respiratory distress syndrome. Because symptoms overlap with community-acquired bacterial and viral pneumonias, diagnosis and management of a fungal etiology can be delayed. In endemic areas, lack of clinical improvement following routine treatment of community-acquired pneumonia should raise concern for endemic mycoses.

Pulmonary histoplasmosis typically presents subacutely over the course of weeks with fever, malaise, and progressive cough or dyspnea as a result of lymphadenopathy causing compression of the tracheobronchial tree. Other presentations include mediastinal granulomatous disease, mediastinal lymphadenitis, mediastinal fibrosis, broncholithiasis, and nodular pulmonary disease. Some manifestations are asymptomatic and usually noted incidentally (eg, solitary pulmonary nodules), others produce local respiratory symptoms (eg, mediastinal lymphadenitis or mediastinal fibrosis), and others produce dysphagia, hemoptysis, or the superior vena cava (SVC) syndrome secondary to mass effect or erosion into adjacent structures (eg,

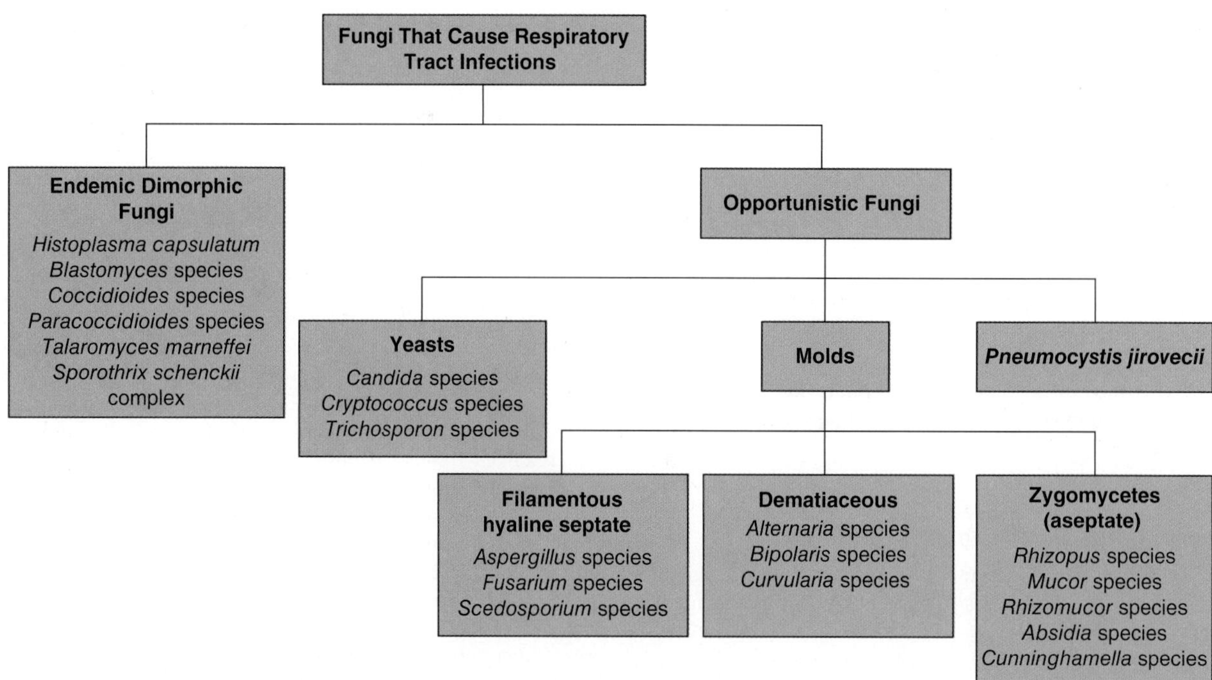


**FIGURE 237-1** Classification of fungal respiratory pathogens.

mediastinal lymphadenitis). Primary disseminated histoplasmosis, which occurs predominantly in young infants and immunocompromised hosts, can affect any organ system often without any respiratory symptoms.

Pulmonary blastomycosis commonly presents acutely with symptoms of fever, fatigue, chest pain, and cough that mimics typical bacterial pneumonia. In contrast, pulmonary coccidioidomycosis usually presents as a subacute infection with similar symptoms present for weeks to months. Arthralgias, malaise, and skin rashes may also be seen.

Chronic cavitary pulmonary disease has been described following infection with *H capsulatum* and *Coccidioides* species in adults, but these indolent forms of disease are rarely encountered in pediatric patients.

Paracoccidioidomycosis and penicilliosis are acquired via the respiratory route, but generalized systemic findings are more common than isolated pulmonary signs and symptoms in pediatric patients. The acute/subacute (or "juvenile") presentation of paracoccidioidomycosis, more often seen in children, is characterized by a generalized infection involving the reticuloendothelial system and other tissues; pulmonary symptoms are often absent. Attributed to reactivation of disease acquired earlier in life, the chronic (or "adult") type of paracoccidioidomycosis increases in incidence in early adulthood and usually presents with chronic lung disease, upper respiratory tract ulceration, and local lymphadenopathy. Penicilliosis is characterized by a progressive systemic illness with multisystem involvement that can also include respiratory symptoms in pediatric patients.

Sporotrichosis typically presents with cutaneous lesions, but a pulmonary presentation, including involvement of the nasal mucosa and lower respiratory tract, has been described.

## DIAGNOSIS

Pulmonary histoplasmosis produces hilar or mediastinal adenopathy, often with calcification, sometimes associated with diffuse or localized

**TABLE 237-1 GEOGRAPHIC LOCATIONS OF ENDEMIC DIMORPHIC FUNGI**

| Fungus (Endemic Mycosis) | Location | Soil Characteristics |
|---|---|---|
| *Histoplasma capsulatum* (histoplasmosis) | 1. North America: Ohio and Mississippi River Valleys, localized foci in other areas, most notably in mideastern states<br>2. Central/South America<br>3. Africa<br>4. Asia-Pacific regions | Soil enriched with bat or bird excrement (eg, caves, barns, and construction sites) |
| *Blastomyces* species (blastomycosis) | 1. North America: Ohio and Mississippi River Valleys, Great Lakes region, St. Lawrence River, and in the southeast<br>2. Africa, particularly southern Africa | Soil enriched with organic material, particularly in wooded areas close to bodies of water |
| *Coccidioides* species (coccidioidomycosis) | 1. North America: Texas, Arizona, New Mexico, much of central and southern California, and Mexico<br>2. Central America: Small endemic areas within Central America<br>3. South America: Brazil, Argentina, and other areas | Arid soil of desert regions |
| *Paracoccidioides* species (paracoccidioidomycosis) | Central America and South America between 25 degrees North and 35 degrees South | No particular characteristics |
| *Talaromyces marneffei* (formerly *Penicillium marneffei*) (penicilliosis) | Tropical Asia: Vietnam, Thailand, China, India, Hong Kong, and Taiwan, as well as other countries in the region | Incompletely understood; potentially associated with soil around bamboo rat burrows |
| *Sporothrix schenckii* complex (sporotrichosis) | Worldwide, especially in tropical and subtropical regions | Decaying organic material including hay, wood, and moss |

infiltrates. If the diagnosis is delayed or incidental, infiltrates may be absent. In contrast to adults, pleural effusion is rare in children. Cavitary lung lesions may occasionally be seen in chronic pulmonary histoplasmosis. Blastomycosis most frequently causes parenchymal infiltrates, often lobar; pleural effusion is noted in about one-third of cases. Pulmonary coccidioidomycosis commonly produces focal consolidation, often associated with an ipsilateral pleural effusion, with or without adenopathy. Residual findings on thoracic imaging, such as nodules or cavities, may remain following pulmonary coccidioidomycosis in a small number of patients.

Although respiratory signs and symptoms are rare in pediatric paracoccidioidomycosis, abnormal thoracic radiographic findings comparable to pulmonary tuberculosis may be seen during acute disease. Pediatric patients with penicilliosis may have parenchymal infiltrates, nodular lung disease, and pleural effusions.

Pulmonary sporotrichosis produces nonspecific thoracic imaging findings that can include upper lobe cavitary lesions, tracheobronchial lymphadenopathy, and nodular parenchymal lesions.

Histopathology, direct examination of clinical specimens, culture, serology, and antigen-based methods are available to support the diagnosis of an endemic mycosis in the appropriate clinical context (Table 237-2). For many endemic mycoses, the gold standard for diagnosis remains culture or microscopic examination of clinical tissue or body fluid samples. Serologic and antigen-based testing is available to be performed on blood or urine samples for many endemic mycoses. For each of the endemic mycoses, individual tests have their own sensitivity, specificity, advantages, and limitations (see Table 237-2). Molecular diagnostic tests (eg, polymerase chain reaction [PCR]-based tests) are in various stages of development but not currently available for routine clinical use.

**TABLE 237-2 TESTING AVAILABLE FOR THE ENDEMIC MYCOSES**

| Endemic Mycosis | Available Testing | Comments |
|---|---|---|
| Histoplasmosis | Histopathology or direct examination with fungal stains of clinical specimens demonstrating narrow-based budding yeast (eg, mediastinal lymph node or BAL fluid) | May be visualized with calcofluor (fluids), PAS (tissue), or GMS (tissue) stains |
| | Culture of tissue or body fluid (eg, sputum or BAL fluid) | Low sensitivity in patients with mild disease |
| | Serologic testing: Complement fixation (CF) using yeast and mycelial antigens. A 4-fold rise in antibody titers over 2–6 weeks confirms a diagnosis. A single titer ≥ 1:32 is suggestive. | Lower sensitivity in immunocompromised patients; specificity may be limited by cross-reaction with other fungal infections |
| | Serologic testing: Immunodiffusion (ID) detecting M and H precipitin bands. The M band is more commonly positive and persists longer than the H band. | Lower sensitivity in immunocompromised patients; use of both serologic tests (CF and ID) improves sensitivity |
| | Antigen detection in urine or serum | Higher sensitivity in patients with disseminated or severe acute disease; use of both blood and urine antigen tests improves sensitivity; specificity may be limited by cross-reaction with other fungi |
| Blastomycosis | Culture of tissue or body fluid (eg, sputum, BAL fluid, gastric aspirates) | Sensitive, but may take weeks for results |
| | Histopathology or direct examination with fungal stains of clinical specimens demonstrating characteristic large yeast with broad-based budding | May be visualized with calcofluor (fluids), PAS (tissue), or GMS (tissue) stains; direct examination of sputum has low sensitivity |
| | Several serologic tests have been developed | None has appropriate sensitivity or specificity for clinical use |
| | Antigen detection in urine or serum | High sensitivity for disseminated and pulmonary infections (urine higher than blood); specificity may be limited by cross-reaction with other fungi |
| Coccidioidomycosis | Histopathology or direct examination with fungal stains of clinical specimens demonstrating mature spherule with endospores | May be visualized with calcofluor (fluids), PAS (tissue), or GMS (tissue) stains |
| | Culture of tissue or body fluid (eg, sputum, BAL fluid, tissue biopsy) | Relatively easy to cultivate; if coccidioidomycosis is suspected, the microbiology laboratory should be notified (for laboratory staff safety) |
| | IgM by latex agglutination (LA), EIA, or ID | May be falsely negative in immunocompromised patients; EIA is more sensitive than ID, but less specific; LA is sensitive but lacks specificity |
| | IgG by EIA, ID, or CF | May be falsely negative in immunocompromised patients; EIA is more sensitive than ID, but less specific; CF provides quantitative titer |
| | Antigen detection in urine | Studied in patients with disseminated disease or immunocompromise; specificity may be limited by cross-reaction with other fungi |
| Paracoccidioidomycosis | Histopathology or direct examination with fungal stains of clinical specimens demonstrating narrow-based budding yeast cells of variable size | May be visualized with calcofluor (fluids), PAS (tissue), or GMS (tissue) stains |
| | Culture of tissue or body fluid | Establishes a definitive diagnosis, but may take weeks to cultivate |
| | Serologic testing by immunodiffusion (preferred test) | Sensitivity lower in immunocompromised patients; specificity may be limited by cross-reaction with other fungi |
| Penicilliosis | Culture from clinical specimens (eg, blood or skin biopsy) | Establishes a definitive diagnosis; yield varies depending on cultured site: bone marrow is most sensitive, sputum poorly sensitive |
| | Histopathology or direct examination with fungal stains of clinical specimens demonstrating intracellular and extracellular basophilic, elliptical yeast-like forms with a clear central septation | May be visualized with Giemsa (tissue) and GMS (tissue) stains |
| Sporotrichosis | Culture from tissue | Establishes a definitive diagnosis |
| | Histopathology demonstrating "cigar-shaped" budding | May be visualized using PAS (tissue) and GMS (tissue) stains; low sensitivity (few fungal organisms typically encountered) |
| | Serologic testing | Limited diagnostic value |

BAL, bronchoalveolar lavage; EIA, enzyme immunoassay; GMS, Gomori methenamine silver; Ig, immunoglobulin; PAS, periodic acid-Schiff.

## TREATMENT

The route, composition, and duration of antifungal treatment for respiratory tract infections caused by endemic mycoses vary with the severity and chronicity of clinical presentation, presence or absence of multisystem organ involvement, and underlying patient characteristics. Clinical practice guidelines for the treatment of histoplasmosis, blastomycosis, coccidioidomycosis, and sporotrichosis, published by the Infectious Diseases Society of America (IDSA), are available to assist management.

Some patients with self-limiting conditions or who present with postinfective symptoms require no antifungal therapy. If therapy is required, active antifungal agents include the various forms of amphotericin and drugs within the azole class. For many of the endemic mycoses, itraconazole has favorable activity and past clinical experience and is the first-line recommended azole antifungal in many cases. Newer extended-spectrum azoles, including voriconazole and posaconazole, may have activity against the fungi that cause the endemic mycoses, but evidence and clinical experience supporting their use as first-line medications are presently limited. Echinocandins (eg, micafungin) demonstrate limited activity against many of the fungi that cause the endemic mycoses, and their use is not routinely recommended.

Ketoconazole and fluconazole can be used for coccidioidomycosis. Trimethoprim-sulfamethoxazole demonstrates effectiveness in the management of paracoccidioidomycosis, although the required treatment duration may be longer than when an azole antifungal is prescribed.

Adjunctive therapy for management of symptomatic lymphadenopathy from histoplasmosis may include surgery or systemic corticosteroids to decompress the SVC or tracheobronchial tree. The role of steroids is still poorly defined, and symptoms often eventually resolve without treatment, but many clinicians prescribe anti-inflammatory doses of corticosteroids for symptomatic hilar or mediastinal lymphadenopathy. If steroids are used, antifungal therapy is often given concurrently.

## PREVENTION

Prevention efforts against endemic mycoses are largely focused on minimizing airborne exposure in patients susceptible to severe or disseminated disease. For prevention of histoplasmosis, especially in immunocompromised patients, exposure to soil and dust should be minimized. In contrast to certain adult patients, primary prophylaxis of histoplasmosis in HIV-infected children with antifungal medications is not recommended. Immunocompromised patients residing in or traveling to areas endemic for *Coccidioides* species should be counseled to avoid exposure to activities that may aerosolize spores in contaminated soil. There are no recommendations for primary antifungal prophylaxis for coccidioidomycosis in patients with AIDS, even in endemic regions. No specific control measures, regarding either exposure avoidance or primary prophylaxis, are recommended for blastomycosis, paracoccidioidomycosis, and sporotrichosis.

# THE OPPORTUNISTIC FUNGI

The opportunistic fungi, including yeasts and molds (see Fig. 237-1), lead to disease of the respiratory tract, including sinuses, lower airways, and lung parenchyma, predominantly in immunocompromised hosts. Occasionally, *Aspergillus* species and other molds cause allergic, saprophytic, or invasive infections in immunocompetent hosts.

## PATHOGENESIS AND EPIDEMIOLOGY

Opportunistic fungal infections are the result of the interplay between host susceptibility, the virulence of the pathogen, and inoculum of exposure. Clinical manifestations are related to both the pathogen and the immune response.

Inhalation of airborne fungal conidia is the main route of acquisition for many opportunistic fungal respiratory infections. Phagocytes resident in the respiratory tree provide the first line of defense against fungal pathogens. Conidia that are not contained by this initial response begin mycelial growth, which subsequently triggers a neutrophil response. Compromise of either of these host defense mechanisms allows for further germination into the hyphal form in sinus or lung tissue (in the case of molds), which leads to growth and tissue invasion. Immunologic abnormalities that make patients susceptible to fungal respiratory infections include neutropenia, especially profound neutropenia with an absolute neutrophil count (ANC) less than 100 cells/μL (eg, hematologic malignancies or anticancer chemotherapy), impaired phagocyte function (eg, chronic granulomatous disease), and disruption of cutaneous and mucosal barriers (eg, radiation, chemotherapy, or indwelling catheters).

Defects in cell-mediated immunity, such as those seen in AIDS or therapy for malignancy, also increase the risk of invasive fungal infection and are the primary contributors to the risk of *Pneumocystis jirovecii* pneumonia (PCP).

Respiratory infections caused by opportunistic fungi are generally not geographically restricted. The incidence, etiology, and presentation of respiratory tract infections secondary to opportunistic fungi can vary from center to center based on differences among centers in immunosuppressive protocols, transplant types (solid organ vs hematopoietic stem cell), and antifungal prophylaxis strategies.

## DIAGNOSIS

Persistent fever in an immunocompromised host while on broad-spectrum antibacterials, with or without focal symptoms or signs, is a common presentation of invasive fungal infection. In this setting, pain in the face or chest, mild cough, or visualization of an eschar in the nose may be the first clue to an invasive respiratory fungal infection. A thorough skin exam can also help identify deep-seated invasive fungal infections as skin lesions can be seen in disseminated candidiasis, aspergillosis, and fusariosis and are readily accessible for skin biopsy. When fever persists in a high-risk neutropenic host, computed tomography (CT) of the chest should be performed to pursue a diagnosis of pulmonary infection, even in the absence of local signs or symptoms. A negative CT may need to be repeated after several days or after neutrophil recovery as imaging changes are sometimes absent early in infection during profound neutropenia.

Consensus criteria have been published for the diagnosis of invasive fungal infections. However, many of the recommendations are based on data obtained in adults that are not necessarily directly applicable to pediatrics. As a general construct, the diagnosis requires appropriate patient characteristics (immunocompromising conditions that place the patient at risk of developing a fungal infection) in combination with suggestive radiographic findings or mycologic support (either direct or indirect). Direct mycologic support is provided by histopathology demonstrating fungal forms in association with local tissue damage or by a positive culture for a yeast or mold from a sterile site. Indirect mycologic support is provided by antigen-based testing methods (Table 237-3).

## APPROACH TO SPECIFIC ORGANISMS

### Yeasts

*Candida* species may colonize portions of the respiratory tract. As such, identification in sputum or bronchoalveolar lavage (BAL) fluid often represents colonization only. For instance, endotracheal intubation increases the likelihood of airway colonization, and *Candida* species can be isolated from intubated patients without clinical or radiographic lower respiratory tract disease. However, in immunocompromised or very young patients, *Candida* species may cause lower respiratory tract disease. Primary pulmonary candidiasis follows aspiration of *Candida* from the upper respiratory tract, may be associated with oropharyngeal or esophageal candidiasis, and is diagnosed by confirmation of parenchymal disease without candidemia or other organ involvement. The imaging findings differ from secondary pulmonary candidiasis; they consist predominantly of confluent parenchymal opacities that may be multifocal. Secondary pulmonary candidiasis is much more common and represents a component of disseminated candidiasis. Imaging typically reveals a pattern of bilateral innumerable small nodules. Although definitive

**TABLE 237-3 TESTING AVAILABLE FOR OPPORTUNISTIC FUNGAL INFECTIONS**

| Pathogen | Test | Comments |
|---|---|---|
| *Cryptococcus* species | Histopathology or direct examination of clinical specimens revealing yeast with a large capsule | May be visualized by India ink (fluid), Mayer's mucicarmine (tissue), or GMS (tissue) stains |
| | Culture from clinical specimens (eg, tissue biopsies, BAL fluid, sputum) | Positive respiratory cultures may be confounded by the potential for cryptococci to colonize the respiratory tract; consider clinical context |
| | Capsular polysaccharide antigen detection in serum. Both LA and EIA testing is available. | Sensitivity is decreased in isolated pulmonary disease; testing BAL fluid is not well studied |
| *Aspergillus* species | Galactomannan antigen by EIA in serum or BAL fluid. In serum, a positive test is an optical density index > 0.5. In BAL fluid, a positive test is an optical density index > 1.0. | Limited pediatric data in nonsurveillance contexts (serum); specificity may be limited by false-positive results (eg, cross-reaction with other fungi or poor extraction techniques) |
| Various opportunistic fungi | (1-3)-β-D-glucan testing in serum | Thresholds for positivity have not been established in pediatric patients; specificity for fungal infections may be limited by false-positive results (eg, with bacterial infections, in patients receiving hemodialysis) |
| *Pneumocystis jirovecii* | Direct examination with fungal stains or histopathologic examination of clinical specimens (eg, induced sputum or BAL fluid) demonstrating *Pneumocystis* cysts | May be visualized by calcofluor or GMS stains; sensitive and specific DFA testing available; BAL fluid is more accurate than sputum in children |
| | PCR testing on respiratory specimens (eg, induced sputum or BAL fluid) | High sensitivity; positive tests may be confounded by the potential for *P jirovecii* to colonize the lower respiratory tract; consider clinical context |
| | Serum LDH | If elevated, may increase concern, but it is not specific enough to make a diagnosis |
| | (1-3)-β-D-glucan in serum | May be elevated in PCP, but further study in pediatric patients is needed before routine use |

BAL, bronchoalveolar lavage; DFA, direct fluorescent antibody; EIA, enzyme immunoassay; GMS, Gomori methenamine silver; LA, latex agglutination; LDH, lactate dehydrogenase; PCP, *Pneumocystis jirovecii* pneumonia; PCR, polymerase chain reaction.

diagnosis requires biopsy or positive blood cultures, typical imaging and clinical findings in an immunocompromised, typically neutropenic host should lead to presumptive diagnosis and empiric treatment. Most positive cultures from the respiratory tract require no specific therapy. Treatment of confirmed primary pulmonary candidiasis usually involves amphotericin B, an echinocandin, or an azole antifungal drug, depending on organism susceptibility, and duration of therapy is shorter than for disseminated infection. Treatment for secondary pulmonary candidiasis is directed toward disseminated infection. In immunocompromised patients, an echinocandin is the treatment of choice. Azole antifungals and amphotericin may be alternatives depending on organism susceptibility and host factors.

Cryptococcosis is caused by *Cryptococcus neoformans* and *Cryptococcus gattii*, which are environmental fungi. *C neoformans* is associated with exposure to bird droppings; the niche for *C gattii* is less well understood. Humans are exposed to *Cryptococcus* species through inhalation of infectious fungal elements from the environment. Secondary dissemination from the lungs with involvement of other organ systems (eg, the central nervous system) may follow. Pulmonary cryptococcosis can present with asymptomatic pulmonary nodules in both healthy and immunocompromised patients, incidentally or as part of a workup for cryptococcal meningitis. Symptomatic pulmonary cryptococcosis presents subacutely with cough, dyspnea, chest pain, and constitutional symptoms. Imaging findings are variable and are a function of the host's immune status. Nodular, cavitary, and consolidative patterns may all be demonstrated with thoracic imaging. Immunocompromised patients are more likely to have multiple pulmonary nodules, cavitary lung disease, and pleural effusion. A diagnosis of pulmonary cryptococcosis can be made using direct examination of clinical specimens, culture, and antigen detection methods (see Table 237-3). Treatment guidelines have been published by the IDSA and vary with the clinical presentation and host immune status. Azole antifungals (including fluconazole), amphotericin, and flucytosine all have activity against *Cryptococcus*.

Trichosporonosis is caused by fungi within the *Trichosporon* genus. They are pathogenic in neonates and patients with compromised skin barriers (eg, skin burns or indwelling central venous lines) or immunologic function (eg, hematologic malignancies or transplant recipients). Infection is typically disseminated and accompanied by pulmonary infiltrates and skin lesions. Diagnosis is made by histopathology and/or culture (can be isolated from blood with disseminated infection). The most active antifungals are the azoles; amphotericin and echinocandins may have little activity.

### Molds

Suggestive signs and symptoms of a lower respiratory tract mold infection include fever, cough, dyspnea, and chest pain. Hemoptysis may also be present, especially after neutrophil recovery, and can potentially be life threatening if resulting from erosion into a large blood vessel. However, the only presenting sign of lower respiratory tract infection may be persistent fever despite the provision of broad-spectrum antibacterial agents. For this reason, thoracic imaging is recommended for high-risk neutropenic patients with fever persisting more than 4 days.

Although chest radiograph can identify abnormalities, including nodules and air space consolidation, it has a low sensitivity and specificity for the detection of pulmonary fungal infections in immunocompromised patients. Thoracic CT is more sensitive and specific and provides the advantage of further defining the location, type, and extent of pulmonary lesions to facilitate tissue sampling. Thoracic CT findings may include nodules, cavitary lesions, the "halo" sign, the "reversed halo" sign, and the "air-crescent" sign (Fig. 237-2). The halo sign, classically described in aspergillosis, is a nodule surrounded by a ground-glass opacity thought to be representative of angioinvasion. The reversed halo sign, classically described in zygomycosis, is a rounded area of ground-glass opacity surrounded by consolidation thought to appear as a result of pulmonary infarction. The air-crescent sign is a later finding that may be seen on repeat imaging, especially following neutrophil recovery, and is characterized by air surrounding a radiopaque mass within a cavitary lung lesion. These "typical" CT findings of invasive pulmonary fungal infection are much less common in children, especially those who are less than 5 years old.

Biopsy of areas suspicious for invasive mold infections on thoracic imaging, when possible, is indicated to establish a diagnosis and guide choice of antifungal treatment. Depending on the location of the pulmonary lesion and available expertise, transbronchial, percutaneous radiologically guided (commonly with CT), or open lung biopsies may provide adequate tissue for diagnostic studies. Transbronchial biopsies can be performed in small children if adequate clinical expertise is available. Percutaneous CT-guided biopsy has been demonstrated to have moderate diagnostic yield with relatively low adverse event rates, but utility may be operator-dependent. Open lung biopsy or

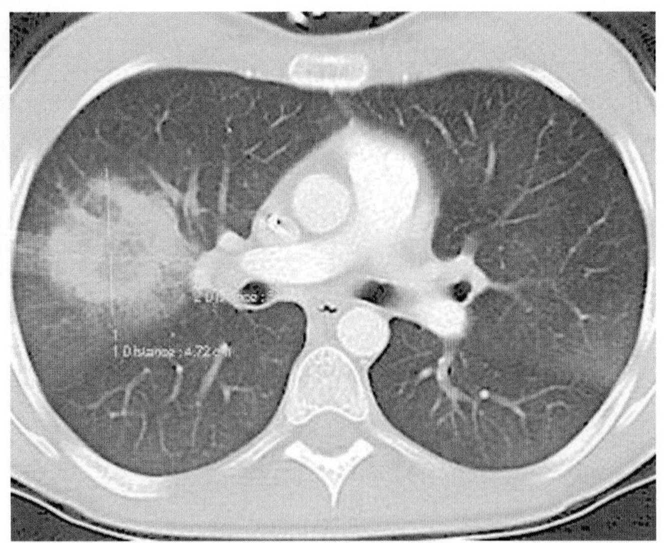

**FIGURE 237-2** An irregular and heterogeneous right mid lung mass surrounded by a poorly defined halo suggestive of an angioinvasive infection in a 14-year-old with acute myelogenous leukemia presenting with fever, neutropenia, cough, and chest pain. The patient underwent thoracotomy and mass resection, which demonstrated invasive pulmonary mucormycosis.

lobectomy provides the opportunity to sample a larger tissue volume and has the added benefit of removing infected tissue, but is associated with higher perioperative risks. Once acquired, the specimen should be sent for histopathology and culture. Histopathology will show fungal elements in association with local tissue destruction. Although stains (eg, Gomori methenamine silver [GMS] or periodic acid-Schiff [PAS]) can demonstrate characteristic morphologies of an organism (eg, presence or absence of septation and hyphal branching pattern), definitive identification of the underlying etiology is made by culture.

Bronchoscopy with BAL sent for fungal stains, culture, and antigen testing (see Table 237-3) also may provide support for a lower respiratory tract mold infection. However, the diagnostic yield of BAL in immunosuppressed patients, especially those on antifungal agents, is relatively low, so a negative BAL does not necessarily exclude a mold infection. Bronchoscopy with BAL does offer the additional advantage of establishing a diagnosis of alternative infectious processes (eg, viral, bacterial, *Pneumocystis*).

An enzyme immunoassay (EIA) for the galactomannan antigen, which is found in the cell walls of all *Aspergillus* species, is available to provide indirect mycologic support of invasive *Aspergillus* infections and can be performed on serum, plasma, BAL fluid, and cerebrospinal fluid (see Table 237-3). Galactomannan EIA testing has been more rigorously evaluated as a serial prospective surveillance tool for invasive aspergillosis in hematopoietic stem cell transplant recipients; its clinical performance outside this setting has not been as well studied. However, when positive in blood or BAL fluid in an appropriate clinical context, it can help support a diagnosis of invasive pulmonary aspergillosis.

Testing blood for the presence of (1-3)-β-D-glucan, a component of the cell wall in most fungi (excluding the zygomycetes and *Cryptococcus* species), is also available (see Table 237-3). Based on its favorable performance in adult patients, this test has been included in consensus criteria for the diagnosis of invasive fungal infections. However, performance of this test in children has been less well explored, and preliminary data suggest that the test may be less specific or require a different cutoff in the pediatric population. For this reason, its use as a diagnostic test is not recommended until further clinical data are available.

Once the diagnosis of invasive lower respiratory tract mold infection is suspected or established, antifungal medication should promptly be administered. While awaiting the results of diagnostic tests, amphotericin or voriconazole is usually the drug of choice for initial empirical management. Once identification is made, management guidelines have been published by the IDSA for several of the invasive mold infections, including invasive pulmonary aspergillosis. Long-term therapy, at least 12 weeks and until resolution of profound immunosuppression, is usually required. Adjunctive surgery to remove infected tissue may improve clinical outcomes, especially if the lesion is unifocal or close to large vessels.

#### *Pneumocystis jirovecii*

*P jirovecii* is a globally distributed fungal organism that causes pneumonia (PCP) in immunocompromised hosts. The mode of primary acquisition and habitat are unknown. Exposure to *P jirovecii* is common in early childhood. Symptomatic disease occurs in patients with compromised cell-mediated immunity (eg, after anticancer chemotherapy, AIDS, or primary immunodeficiencies), so primary prophylaxis with trimethoprim-sulfamethoxazole is recommended in these populations. Signs and symptoms of PCP include nonproductive cough, tachypnea, dyspnea, and hypoxemia. The acuity of presentation varies with the cause and degree of immune suppression and can be acute to subacute with continued progression without treatment. Similarly, the severity of clinical manifestations can be mild to severe. Except for infants less than 4 months of age, who may experience upper and lower respiratory tract disease, infection is commonly subclinical in otherwise well children.

Thoracic imaging most commonly identifies bilateral interstitial infiltrates that may be described as reticular or ground-glass opacities. In less severe disease, chest radiographs may be normal. Thoracic CT is more sensitive and specific than plain chest radiographs for diagnosing PCP.

Because *P jirovecii* cannot routinely be cultured, the diagnosis relies on identification of the organism in sputum or BAL fluid. Several cytologic stains (eg, GMS), direct fluorescent antibody (DFA) testing, and molecular testing (PCR) are available for clinical use on respiratory samples. Lactate dehydrogenase (LDH) and (1-3)-β-D-glucan may also be elevated in cases of PCP (see Table 237-3). Trimethoprim-sulfamethoxazole is the initial treatment of choice in children over 2 months of age. Alternative agents include pentamidine, atovaquone, dapsone, and clindamycin in combination with primaquine, but these may be less effective. Despite limited evidence, adjunctive corticosteroids are usually administered to patients with significant hypoxemia because response to antimicrobial therapy alone is often delayed.

#### Aspergilloma and Allergic Bronchopulmonary Aspergillosis

*Aspergillus* species may cause a noninvasive infection in preexisting pulmonary parenchymal cavities, which is termed a pulmonary aspergilloma. These are composed of fungal hyphae and cellular debris and are most commonly caused by *Aspergillus fumigatus*. Conditions leading to structural lung abnormalities, including congenital pulmonary malformations, cystic lung disease, or prior tuberculosis, predispose patients to this condition. Patients may be asymptomatic or present with hemoptysis. Characteristically, a cavity containing a rounded mass with a rim of surrounding air and local pleural thickening is seen on thoracic imaging. Aspergillomas do not uniformly necessitate treatment. Surgical resection is commonly the initial treatment of choice; bronchial artery embolization can also be used acutely for patients with life-threatening hemoptysis. No benefit is seen with systemic antifungal administration.

Allergic bronchopulmonary aspergillosis (ABPA) is caused by a hypersensitivity reaction within the respiratory tract to antigens produced by *A fumigatus* after it becomes trapped in the thick mucus of patients with asthma or cystic fibrosis (CF). The incidence of ABPA in these patient populations increases with age. Signs and symptoms may include fever, productive cough, malaise, and a decrease in pulmonary function test performance. There are diagnostic criteria available for patients with asthma and with CF. Clinical decline, demonstration of hypersensitivity to *A fumigatus* serologically and by skin testing, and imaging changes are included in the diagnostic schema. The primary treatment is with systemic corticosteroids (eg, prednisone). Azole antifungals (eg, itraconazole) can reduce fungal burden and steroid exposure.

## SINUS DISEASE

Owing to their environmental ubiquity, molds frequently colonize the paranasal sinuses. Several distinct clinical diseases, each with unique presentations, pathogenesis, and underlying host risk factors, may be caused by environmental fungi within the paranasal sinuses.

Localized collections of mucous and fungal elements, typically from *Aspergillus* species, without tissue invasion or inflammatory reaction may develop in an obstructed sinus. Terms have been variably used to describe these collections, including sinus mycetoma and sinus aspergilloma, although these names have been replaced by fungus ball, a more general term. These have not been described in young children, and cases have rarely been diagnosed in adolescence. Affected patients are not usually immunocompromised. The clinical presentation is chronic and includes symptoms of headache and facial pain. Diagnosis is made by clinical history and imaging demonstrating a thickly opacified sinus. Endoscopic sinus surgery is the treatment of choice, and there is no established role for antifungal agents in management.

Allergic fungal sinusitis is a clinical subtype of chronic rhinosinusitis that may be encountered in children and adolescents. It is thought to result from a prolonged IgE-mediated response to antigens expressed by colonizing molds (eg, *Alternaria* and *Curvularia*) in the process of noninvasive growth. The presentation is often chronic, and symptoms include nasal congestion, rhinorrhea, and facial pain. Diagnostic criteria include the appropriate clinical findings in an immunocompetent patient, nasal polyposis, suggestive findings on sinus imaging, histopathology of sinus contents demonstrating eosinophilic mucous and fungal elements without mucosal invasion, and type 1 hypersensitivity to fungal antigens. Treatment is both medical and surgical, although the role of antifungal agents in management is unclear.

The most feared form of fungal sinusitis is invasive disease in patients with compromised immune function. This can be disfiguring or fatal if not diagnosed and addressed expediently. Patient characteristics predisposing to invasive fungal sinusitis include neutropenia (eg, anticancer chemotherapy or hematologic malignancy), solid organ or hematopoietic stem cell transplantation, uncontrolled diabetes mellitus, chronic systemic glucocorticoid exposure, and primary or secondary hemochromatosis. Signs and symptoms may include fever, headache, facial pain, periorbital edema, nasal congestion, and epistaxis, although inflammatory findings may be less prominent in patients with significant immunocompromise due to the lack of an associated immune response. Infection may be complicated by invasion into contiguous structures, including the brain, orbits, and local blood vessels. Invasion can result in hemorrhage, infarction, mental status changes, facial paresthesias, proptosis, and diplopia. Molds (eg, *Aspergillus* species, dematiaceous molds, and the zygomycetes) are most commonly implicated. Suspicion of fungal sinusitis in a susceptible host should prompt immediate endoscopic sinus examination with biopsy of apparently involved nasal or sinus tissue to obtain specimens for histopathology and culture. Imaging with either CT or magnetic resonance imaging (MRI) has limited diagnostic sensitivity and specificity but can define the extent of infection and involvement of adjacent structures. Histopathology typically demonstrates locally invasive fungal hyphae associated with tissue necrosis. An identification of the causal organism may subsequently be made by culture. Surgical consultation, early and repeated debridement, and antifungal therapy are critical to management. Empiric therapy with amphotericin or posaconazole is the treatment of choice for suspected invasive fungal rhinosinusitis while awaiting pathology and culture results. Treatment is subsequently tailored to pathologic and microbiologic findings. These infections are difficult to treat, and significant morbidity often results from repeated surgical intervention or invasion into orbit, eye, or brain.

## SUGGESTED READINGS

Chapman S, Dismukes WE, Proia LA, et al. Clinical practice guidelines for the management of blastomycosis: 2008 update by the Infectious Diseases Society of America. *Clin Infect Dis*. 2008;46:1801-1812.

Cooley L, Dendle C, Wolf J, et al. Consensus guidelines for diagnosis, prophylaxis and management of *Pneumocystis jirovecii* pneumonia in patients with haematological and solid malignancies, 2014. *Int Med J*. 2014;44:1350-1363.

Groll AH, Castagnola E, Cesaro S, et al. Fourth European Conference on Infections in Leukaemia (ECIL-4): guidelines for diagnosis, prevention, and treatment of invasive fungal diseases in paediatric patients with cancer or allogeneic haematopoietic stem-cell transplantation. *Lancet Oncol*. 2014;15:e327-e340.

Kauffman CA, Bustamante B, Chapman SW, et al. Clinical practice guidelines for the management of sporotrichosis: 2007 update by the Infectious Diseases Society of America. *Clin Infect Dis*. 2007;25:1255-1265.

Lehrnhecher T, Phillips R, Alexander S, et al. Guideline for the management of fever and neutropenia in children with cancer and/or undergoing hematopoietic stem cell transplantation. *J Clin Oncol*. 2012;30:4427-4438.

Pappas PG, Kauffman CA, Andes DR, et al. Clinical practice guideline for the management of candidiasis: 2016 update by the Infectious Diseases Society of America. *Clin Infect Dis*. 2016;62:e1-e50.

Perfect JR, Dismukes WE, Dromer F, et al. Clinical practice guidelines for the management of cryptococcal disease: 2010 update by the Infectious Diseases Society of America. *Clin Infect Dis*. 2010;50:291-322.

Walsh TJ, Anaissie EJ, Denning DW, et al. Practice guidelines for the diagnosis and management of aspergillosis: 2016 update by the Infectious Diseases Society of America. *Clin Infect Dis*. 2016;doi:10.1093/cid/ciw326.

Wheat LJ, Freifeld AG, Kleiman MB, et al. Clinical practice guidelines for the management of patients with histoplasmosis: 2007 update by the Infectious Diseases Society of America. *Clin Infect Dis*. 2007;45:807-825.

# 238 Infection of the Middle Ear

Tasnee Chonmaitree

## INTRODUCTION

Infection of the middle ear, or otitis media (OM), includes acute, nonacute, and chronic types of infections. Acute otitis media (AOM) is defined as an acute illness marked by the presence of middle ear fluid and inflammation of the mucosa that lines the middle ear space. Otitis media with effusion (OME) is defined by the presence of middle ear fluid without signs of acute illness and usually follows AOM but may also occur as a result of viral upper respiratory tract infection (URTI), allergy, or barotrauma. Synonyms for OME include serous otitis, secretory otitis, and glue ear. Less common chronic variations of OM include permanent perforation of the tympanic membrane (TM) and perforation or retraction of the TM with trapped epithelium that is unable to spontaneously clear desquamated debris, forming a cholesteatoma. Both perforations and cholesteatoma may be associated with recurrent foul-smelling otorrhea, termed chronic suppurative otitis media (CSOM). CSOM occurs more commonly after repeated and untreated AOM in low- and middle-income countries. Infection may spread from the middle ear space to contiguous structures such as the inner ear, mastoid air cells, petrous bone, and intracranial structures, leading to infection of the central nervous system.

## PATHOGENESIS AND EPIDEMIOLOGY

The middle ear system includes the nasopharynx, the eustachian tube (ET), the middle ear space, and the adjacent structures, including the mastoid air cells and inner ear. The middle ear is an air-filled space between the TM and the inner ear. It has a mucosal lining of respiratory epithelium and contains 3 bony ossicles—malleus, incus, and stapes—that form a lever mechanism important for the conduction of sound. The size of the middle ear cavity and the ossicles is the same at birth as in the adult. The ET originates in the anterior middle ear space and courses anteriorly to empty into the lateral nasopharynx. The normal physiologic functions of the ET include: pressure regulation or ventilation of the middle ear, which equilibrates gas pressure in the middle ear with atmospheric pressure; protection of the middle ear by anatomic, immunologic, and mucociliary defenses; and clearance or drainage of secretions produced within the middle ear via mucociliary activity and muscular clearance. In infancy, the ET is short, wide, and in a straight position, permitting easy access of nasopharyngeal flora into the middle ear space. With increasing age, the ET elongates, narrows, and assumes an oblique position, corresponding to a decrease in the incidence of OM as age increases.

AOM usually occurs concurrently or just after URTI; more than 90% of children with AOM have concurrent URTI symptoms. The 3 most common bacterial otopathogens include *Streptococcus pneumoniae*, nontypeable *Haemophilus influenzae*, and *Moraxella catarrhalis*. These organisms colonize the infant's nasopharynx from early age and do not infect the respiratory tract or cause symptoms until viral URTI (nasopharyngitis) occurs, causing changes in the nasopharyngeal milieu. Steps in the pathogenesis of AOM are outlined in Table 238-1.

Even when there is no nasopharyngeal colonization by bacterial otopathogens, viral URTI alone may cause AOM through similar mechanisms. URTI may also lead to OME, likely through similar mechanisms, but with less degree of inflammation. In children 6 months to 4 years of age who were closely followed, 37% of viral URTI resulted in AOM, while another 24% resulted in OME. The mean duration of middle ear effusion after an episode of AOM is approximately 3 weeks, with 10% persisting after 12 weeks.

OM is a disease of infancy and early childhood. AOM is the most frequent reason that children visit healthcare facilities in the first 3 years of life and has been one of the most frequent reasons that physicians prescribe antimicrobial agents for infants and children. The peak age-specific attack rate of AOM occurs between 6 and 18 months. Children who have had little or no experience with OM by age 3 years are unlikely to have subsequent severe or recurrent disease. Previous data from the 1980s have shown that, on average, children have 1.2 and 1.1 episodes of AOM in the first and second years of life, respectively. Recent data have shown reduced incidence to 0.67 episodes in the first year. Many factors are likely to contribute to the decline in OM incidence in the past few decades. First, introduction in the United States of the 7-valent conjugate pneumococcal vaccine (PCV7) in 2000, and the 13-valent vaccine (PCV13) in 2010, and later in countries throughout the world, has reduced OM-related healthcare use and the number of episodes of vaccine-type pneumococcal AOM and decreased the incidence of severe and recurrent disease. In addition, routine influenza vaccination was recommended in 2004, 2006, and 2008 for children age 6 to 23 months, 6 months to 5 years, and then all children, respectively. Influenza vaccination has been shown to reduce AOM during yearly influenza epidemics. Second, publication of the Diagnosis and Management Guideline by the American Academy of Pediatrics (AAP) in 2004, which was updated in 2013, presented uniform criteria for diagnosis, choice of antimicrobial agents, and recommendations for use or withholding of antibiotics for children with AOM. Healthcare providers may have felt less pressure to diagnose and treat AOM knowing that observation is an acceptable option. Third, there were programs developed by Centers for Disease Control and Prevention advocacy groups to inform physicians and consumers about the appropriate use of antimicrobial agents to decrease the development of multidrug-resistant bacteria. Last, there has been a decrease in cigarette smoking and an increase in breastfeeding in the United States.

**TABLE 238-1 STEPS IN THE PATHOGENESIS OF ACUTE OTITIS MEDIA**

1. Asymptomatic nasopharyngeal bacterial colonization.
2. Viral infection of the upper respiratory tract epithelium.
3. Inflammatory responses in the nasopharynx and eustachian tube (ET), including cytokine/chemokine/inflammatory mediator generation, etc.
4. Increased bacterial colonization and adherence in the nasopharynx, partly through upregulation of host cell-surface antigens that serve as bacterial receptor sites. Bacterial and viral interactions, bacterial activation, and increased bacterial virulence.
5. Swelling of the nasopharyngeal and ET mucosa; diminished mucociliary clearance.
6. ET dysfunction/obstruction of the narrowest portion of the tube, the isthmus, resulting in negative middle ear pressure.
7. Entry of the colonized bacteria and upper respiratory tract infection viruses into the middle ear.
8. Immune and inflammatory responses in the middle ear mucosa and generation of effusion by middle ear mucosa.
9. Acute otitis media signs and symptoms.

The more severe suppurative complications are infrequent in developed countries, where access to medical care is readily available, although these complications are still a frequent cause of morbidity in developing countries. It is unclear whether early prescribing of antibiotics has been responsible for decreasing the incidence of mastoiditis in developed countries.

OME is even more common than AOM. Up to 90% of school-age children have OME at some time. In the first year of life, > 50% of children experience OME, increasing to > 60% by 2 years of age.

### Risk Factors

OM is a multifactorial disease. Risk factors include demographic, prenatal/perinatal, immunologic, anatomic, intrinsic genetic, and environmental risks. Young age at first episode of AOM is significantly associated with recurrent episodes. Males have a higher incidence of single and recurrent episodes of AOM than do females. Selected racial groups, many in developing countries or hostile environments, appear to be otitis prone. Native Americans and Alaskan and Canadian Inuit infants and children have a high incidence of severe AOM and suppurative complications. In an Apache community, a draining ear or perforation was found in 8.4% of patients of all ages. Several studies indicate that African American children have less OM than white children, but it is unclear if this is explained by underdiagnosis in the African American community due to less access to medical care or due to differences in the position of the bony ET among races.

Premature infants and those born with low serum levels of maternally derived pneumococcal antibodies are more prone to OM. Altered host defenses, such as congenital or acquired immune deficiencies, and use of immunosuppressive drugs may play a role in recurrent and severe AOM. Among the anatomic risks are cleft palate, cleft uvula, and submucous cleft. Alteration of normal physiologic defenses (patulous ET) and malignant neoplasms that may alter the anatomy of the upper respiratory tract add to OM risk. An increased incidence of AOM also occurs in children with Down syndrome.

Genetic predisposition to AOM is suggested by the aggregation of cases in families: AOM risk increases if any other member of the family had AOM. There is also a strong genetic component to the amount of time with OME and the number of AOM episodes in monozygotic twins. Severe and recurrent disease may be associated with genetically determined features, such as skull configuration, or with overt or subtle immunologic defects. A range of genes regulating innate and adaptive immunity are associated with predisposition to OM. Some of the heritable risk for OM might result from cytokine gene polymorphisms (eg, tumor necrosis factor [TNF]-α, interleukin [IL]-6), and others such as toll-like receptor (TLR)-2 polymorphisms, affecting signal transduction pathways, have been associated with increased rates of OM and disease severity.

For environmental factors, passive cigarette smoking has been shown to be responsible for structural and physiologic changes in the respiratory tree. Smoke exposure can result in goblet cell hyperplasia and mucus hypersecretion, ciliostasis, and decreased mucociliary transport in the respiratory tract. High concentrations of serum cotinine, a biochemical marker for cigarette smoke exposure, were associated with increased incidence of AOM and increased duration of middle ear effusion (MEE) after AOM. Daycare attendance is an OM risk factor; children in daycare not only have more episodes of AOM than children in home care but also have more resultant surgical procedures. The more children in the daycare group, the more exposures there are to bacterial otopathogens and respiratory viruses and the higher the risk for OM. Similarly, crowded conditions (eg, as seen with low socioeconomic status or a large number of siblings in the household) increase OM risk. On the other hand, breastfeeding of 3 to 6 months in duration has been documented to prevent nasopharyngeal bacterial colonization, as well as URTI and AOM. Among the possible reasons for the beneficial effect of breastfeeding are the presence in breast milk of various immunoglobulins, B and T cells, macrophages and neutrophils, and nonimmune factors including interferon and glycoproteins. Oligosaccharides in breast milk that correspond to the pneumococcal carbohydrate receptor suggest that breast milk may protect against OM by blocking attachment of bacterial pathogens to respiratory mucosa. Thus, lack of breastfeeding is an OM risk factor.

## MICROBIOLOGY

Our understanding of the microbiology of AOM is attributed to needle aspiration (tympanocentesis) of the MEE. Results vary depending on the methods used to detect the microorganisms. Bacteria and/or viruses are most commonly detected. AOM is often due to bacterial and viral co-infection.

When only bacterial culture was used to study the MEE, bacterial otopathogens were detected in 70% to 85% of cases. When conventional diagnostic assays including bacterial and viral cultures plus rapid antigen detection for respiratory syncytial virus (RSV) were performed, results showed: bacteria alone in 55% of cases; bacteria and viruses in 15%; viruses alone in 5%; and no pathogens in 25%. Using bacterial culture and polymerase chain reaction (PCR) assays to detect bacteria and viruses, data showed: both bacteria and viruses in 66%; bacteria alone in 27%; viruses alone in 4%; and no pathogen in 4% of cases.

### Bacterial Otopathogens

The 3 most common bacterial otopathogens are *S pneumoniae*, nontypeable *H influenzae*, and *M catarrhalis*. Less common bacteria include *Streptococcus pyogenes* (group A), which causes 2% to 10% of AOM, tends to occur in older children, and is more frequently associated with TM perforation and mastoiditis. Rare pathogens detected in the MEE include *Chlamydia*, *Mycoplasma*, *Mycobacterium tuberculosis*, and fungi.

Bacterial causes of AOM and the diversity of strains within *S pneumoniae* have been dynamic, with the major contributor to such change being the introduction of PCVs. *S pneumoniae* is the most important cause of AOM as it often produces the most severe, persistent, or refractory AOM. There are at least 90 distinct serotypes of *S pneumoniae*, although relatively few types are responsible for most AOM. Before the advent of PCVs, *S pneumoniae* was the most commonly detected bacteria in MEEs. In the first few years after widespread use of PCV7 (serotypes 4, 6B, 9V, 14, 18C, 19F, and 23F) in 2000, there were decreases in frequencies of persistent AOM and AOM associated with early treatment failure, along with an increase in *H influenzae* AOM. After several years of PCV7 use, vaccine serotypes of *S pneumoniae* disappeared, but a surge in nonvaccine, multidrug-resistant serotypes, such as 19A, emerged. The widespread use of PCV13 (with added serotypes 1, 3, 5, 6A, 7F, and 19A) since 2010 has been associated with further decline in healthcare use for OM and further decline in AOM caused by serotypes in the PCV13, especially serotypes 19A and 6A.

Nontypeable *H influenzae* accounts for approximately 45% of AOM; the disease caused by this pathogen is not clinically distinguishable from that caused by *S pneumoniae*, although AOM caused by *H influenzae* is more often bilateral than unilateral and particularly associated with older age and recurrent disease. Approximately one-third of strains of *H influenzae* recovered from MEE produce β-lactamase.

*M catarrhalis* accounts for approximately 10% of the MEE isolates from children with AOM; it is more often found in polymicrobial AOM. The relative proportion of AOM due to *M catarrhalis* has been less affected by universal immunization of infants with PCVs. More than 90% of *M catarrhalis* strains produce β-lactamase.

### Respiratory Viruses

Viral URTI is exceedingly common in infants and children and often leads to AOM. It has been suggested that certain viruses are more likely to cause AOM than others. It is likely, however, that any virus that causes URTI is able to induce AOM. A broad spectrum of respiratory viruses cause URTI; rhinoviruses and coronaviruses are the most common among them. Other common URTI viruses are adenoviruses, RSV, parainfluenza viruses, human metapneumovirus, influenza viruses, enteroviruses, and human bocavirus.

Viruses that infect the nasopharynx may enter the middle ear along with bacteria that colonize the nasopharynx. Presence of live virus in the MEE likely indicates AOM causation as it is evidence of viral replication in the middle ear. Ample evidence has shown that live viruses infect the middle ear. First, in experimental animals, virus alone without bacteria can cause AOM; furthermore, the virus interacts with bacteria to generate more severe inflammation. Second, live viruses have been detected in the MEE of children, and their presence interferes with bacteriologic responses to antibiotic. Third, viruses have been found to generate additional cytokines/inflammatory mediators in cases with combined bacterial and viral infection, compared to bacterial infection alone. The presence in MEE of viral nucleic acids alone as detected by PCR has created debate on whether finding nucleic acids suggests that the virus is the pathogen or just a bystander.

### Bacterial-Viral Interactions

Due to the wide variety of respiratory viruses and bacterial otopathogens, analyses of viral-bacterial interactions are complex. Interactions between specific viruses and bacteria are the topics of numerous studies in animal models and in vitro. Overall, synergisms between bacteria and viruses are evident and the co-infections increase the degree of inflammation, compared to bacterial infection alone. In infants and children, viral-bacterial interactions during AOM enhance the degree of middle ear inflammation and interfere with the penetration of antibiotic into the middle ear. Recent studies have shown interesting bacterial-viral interactions during URTI. The presence of otopathogens such as *S pneumoniae* and *M catarrhalis* increases URTI risk. In addition, specific URI symptoms are associated with the presence of *H influenzae* or *M catarrhalis* colonization. These data together suggest that colonizing bacteria may enhance URTI symptoms during viral infection.

# ACUTE OTITIS MEDIA

## CLINICAL MANIFESTATIONS

Symptoms of AOM are generally nonspecific, including fever, irritability, restless sleep, decreased appetite, vomiting, and diarrhea. Fever occurs in one-third to two-thirds of children with AOM, but temperatures of 40°C or more are unusual unless accompanied by invasive bacterial disease or foci elsewhere. Because AOM most often occurs during URTI, there are also symptoms such as cough, sneezing, runny nose, stuffy nose, and red/watery eyes. Purulent conjunctivitis has been associated with AOM due to nontypeable *H influenzae*.

Ear pain may manifest as ear tugging in infants. In children 6 months to 3 years of age with URTI, ear tugging does not differentiate children with URTI and AOM from those with only URTI. Earache is not universal in AOM; about one-fifth of children older than age 2 do not complain of ear pain. The ear pain is due to pressure of the increasing suppuration in the middle ear and is relieved when the pressure leads to ischemia of the central vessels in the capillary bed of the TM. Persistent ischemia leads to necrosis of the TM with rupture and discharge of the contents of the middle ear abscess and virtual elimination of the otalgia. Parents often report that a child who had cried with pain was relieved and bloody pus was observed. However, the TM is so vascular that the site of perforation may not be evident even 24 hours later, and the resealed membrane may result in reaccumulation of the purulent MEE.

Hearing loss is a frequent sign in infants. It may be expressed by verbal children or detected by a parent who sees the child not responding to spoken voice.

## DIAGNOSIS

Otologic examination should include evaluation of the position, color, and degree of translucency and mobility of the TM. The normal eardrum should be in the neutral position. Mild retraction of the TM usually indicates the presence of negative middle ear pressure, an effusion, or both. Severe retraction of the TM identifies high negative pressure associated with MEE. Fullness or bulging of the TM is caused by increased middle ear pressure or MEE.

The normal TM has a ground-glass appearance and is translucent. The otoscopist should be able to look through the TM and visualize the middle ear landmarks. A blue or yellow color identifies MEE seen through a translucent TM. A red TM may indicate inflammation but may also identify engorgement of the blood vessels of the TM caused by crying, sneezing, or nose-blowing. Adequate examination of the TM to confirm the MEE is sometimes difficult, particularly in infants and small children. Normal and abnormal findings on otoscopic examination are shown in Figure 238-1.

The diagnosis of AOM generally requires: (1) abrupt onset of symptoms; (2) presence of MEE (bulging of the TM, limited or absent mobility of the TM, or otorrhea); and (3) signs or symptoms of middle ear inflammation. As AOM develops, there is a spectrum of signs seen during the progression of TM inflammation and MEE accumulation.

The current Clinical Practice Guideline for the Diagnosis and Management of AOM was published in 2013 by the AAP. The AAP guideline requires bulging TM as evidence for middle ear inflammation. Three degrees of bulging are defined: mild, moderate, and severe. For mild bulging of the TM, intense erythema must also be present. The AAP guideline has tightened the AOM working definition, in order to differentiate AOM from OME, recognizing that the AOM definition likely results in high specificity but less sensitivity as it may exclude less severe presentations of AOM.

Pneumatic otoscopy is the most feasible and cost-effective method for diagnosis of AOM and OME. Mobility of the TM is identified by pressure applied to the rubber bulb attached to the pneumatic otoscope. The normal or air-filled middle ear is identified by a brisk movement inward with slight positive pressure and outward with slight negative pressure. MEE or high negative pressure within the middle ear dampens movement of the TM. Movement of the TM is best seen in the posterosuperior quadrant of the TM.

Tympanometry and acoustic reflectometry can supplement pneumatic otoscopy. Tympanometry involves varying the pressure in the external canal accompanied by a probe tone. A graphic presentation, the tympanogram, provides information on middle ear pressure and the presence of an air-filled or fluid-filled middle ear space. Because tympanometry and pneumatic otoscopy require a seal in the external canal for a few seconds, they may be difficult to perform in the young infant who is irritable due to ear pain. Acoustic reflectometry accompanied by spectral gradient analysis determines the probability of MEE by measuring the response of the eardrum to a frequency sweep in the audible range of 1.8 to 4.4 kHz and provides information on the probability of an air- or a fluid-filled middle ear space.

MEE can also be demonstrated by evidence of pus on the pillow or bedding of the child as a result of TM perforation, observation of fluid in the external canal, needle aspiration (tympanocentesis), or myringotomy (an incision in the TM that drains the MEE).

## TREATMENT

Treatment of AOM includes 3 main approaches: pain management and initial observation alone, or when appropriate, antibiotic therapy.

Pain may be a major symptom of AOM due to pressure within the middle ear and can be substantial in the first few days of onset of illness. Antibiotic treatment does not relieve pain within the first 24 hours. Analgesics can relieve pain associated with AOM early in the course. Therefore, the child should be assessed for pain, and if pain is present, treatment for pain should be given. Oral analgesics such as acetaminophen or ibuprofen are the mainstay of AOM pain management; they are effective for mild to moderately severe pain. Narcotic analgesics with codeine or analogs may be prescribed for severe pain; risks and benefits of using these drugs, including potential toxic effects, need to be considered. Topical agents such as benzocaine or lidocaine may offer additional brief benefit over acetaminophen in children older than 5 years.

Numerous studies of AOM, including studies of children younger than age 2 diagnosed with stringent criteria, have shown that AOM may resolve (improvement of symptoms and TM appearance) without antibiotic treatment. While ET dysfunction leads to AOM development, return to normal ET function facilitates drainage of pus from the middle ear; this may take a few to several days.

The 2013 AAP guideline on AOM management suggests the use of 4 factors in deciding whether to choose initial observation or prescribing antibiotics: age, severity of symptoms, presence of otorrhea, and laterality of AOM. Table 238-2 summarizes the recommendations for initial management of uncomplicated AOM. All infants and children with severe AOM, as defined by a toxic-appearing child, persistent otalgia for more than 48 hours, or temperature ≥ 39°C (102.2°F), should receive antibiotic therapy. AOM with otorrhea, presumably with rupture of the TM, also should receive antibiotic therapy. For those with nonsevere symptoms, initial observation is an option for children younger than 2 years of age with unilateral AOM. Children at least 2 years old with unilateral or bilateral AOM may also be observed initially. Initial observation without antibiotic prescription must be a shared decision with the child's family. If observation is offered, a mechanism must be in place to ensure follow-up and initiation of antibiotics if the child worsens or fails to improve within 72 hours of AOM onset.

The rationale for antibiotic therapy in children with AOM is based on the high rate of positive bacterial cultures of the MEE. However, it has been shown that 19% of children with *S pneumoniae* and 48% with *H influenzae* who were not treated with antibiotics had cleared the bacteria cultured from the first tympanocentesis by the time of repeat tympanocentesis 2 to 7 days later. It is estimated that 75% of children infected with *M catarrhalis* experience bacteriologic cure without antibiotic treatment. Therefore, recommended antibiotics for AOM mostly aim for elimination of *S pneumoniae* and nontypeable *H influenzae*. Further considerations for antibiotic selection include cost of the drug, taste, convenience, and adverse effects. Table 238-3 lists recommended antibiotics for (initial or delayed) treatment and for patients who have failed initial antibiotic treatment.

High-dose amoxicillin is recommended as the first-line treatment because of its effectiveness against *S pneumoniae* and *H influenzae*, as well as its safety, low cost, acceptable taste, and narrow microbiologic spectrum. In children who have taken amoxicillin in the previous 30 days, those with concurrent conjunctivitis, or those for whom coverage for β-lactamase–positive *H influenzae* and *M catarrhalis* is desired, therapy should be initiated with high-dose amoxicillin-clavulanate. Alternative initial antibiotics including cefuroxime and third-generation cephalosporins are less efficacious than the first-line drugs. For penicillin-allergic children, cefdinir, cefuroxime, cefpodoxime, or ceftriaxone may be used as they are unlikely to be associated with cross-reactivity with penicillin; the exceptions are children with severe and/or recent penicillin allergy.

Treatment with an effective antibiotic results in significant resolution of acute signs and symptoms within 48 to 72 hours. Persistent ear pain or systemic signs, including fever after 72 hours of antibiotic

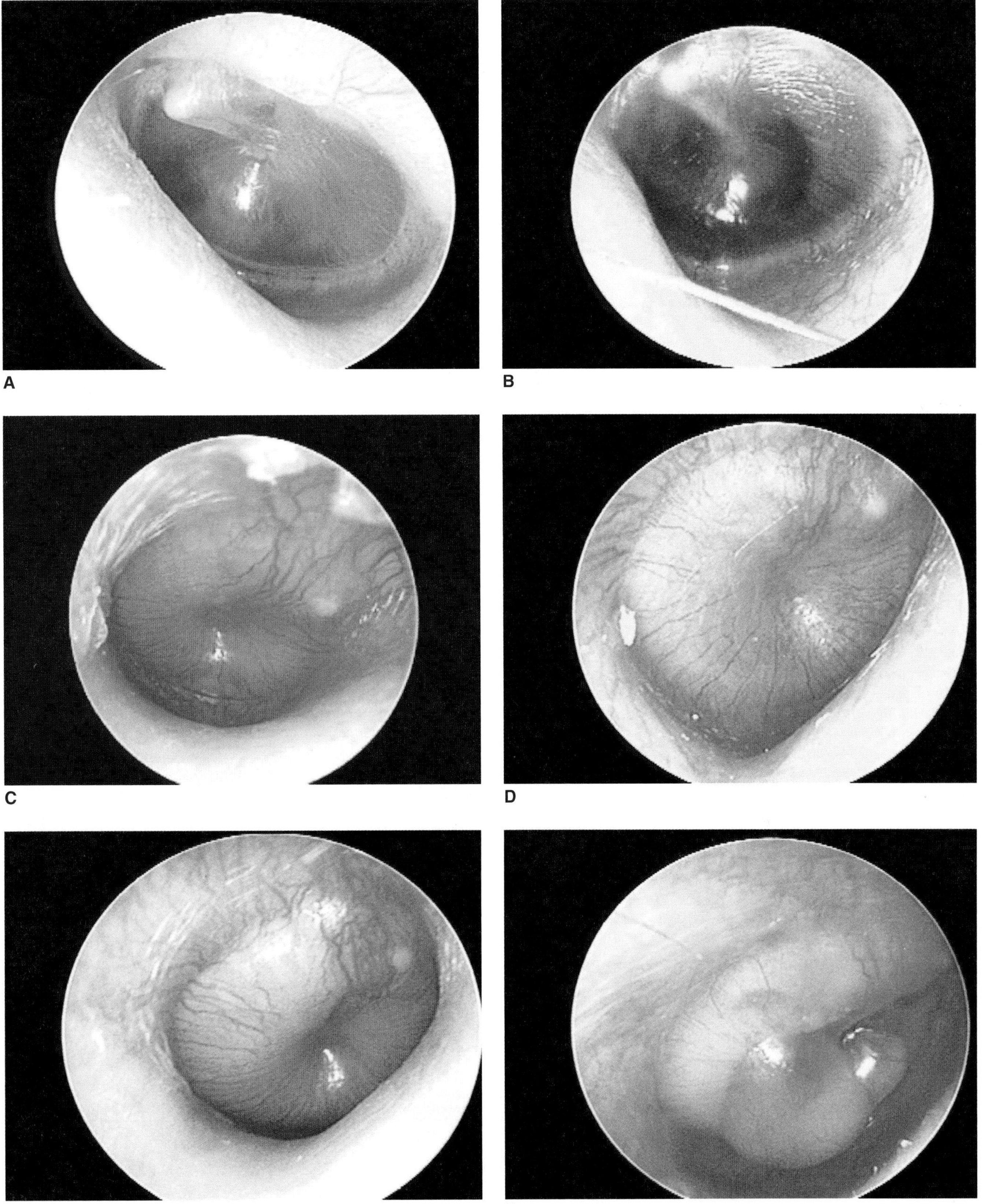


**FIGURE 238-1** **A:** Normal tympanic membrane. **B:** Otitis media with effusion; dark-colored chronic effusion. **C:** Early acute otitis media with mild bulging. **D:** Acute otitis media with moderate bulging. **E:** Acute otitis media with severe bulging. **F:** Acute otitis media with bullous myringitis. (Used with permission from David P. McCormick, MD.)

therapy, indicate a need for reevaluation for persistent AOM or foci elsewhere. If otologic findings support the diagnosis of persistent AOM, antibiotic treatment should be changed, depending on the initial drug (Table 238-3).

Surgical treatment, including tympanocentesis or myringotomy, results in immediate relief by draining the abscess and should be considered for the child who is toxic, who fails to improve on repeated antibiotic therapy, who has severe suppurative or nonsuppurative

**TABLE 238-2 GUIDELINES FOR INITIAL MANAGEMENT OF UNCOMPLICATED ACUTE OTITIS MEDIA (AOM)**

| Age | Otorrhea with AOM | Unilateral or Bilateral AOM with Severe Symptoms[a] | Bilateral AOM Without Severe Symptoms | Unilateral AOM Without Severe Symptoms |
|---|---|---|---|---|
| 6 months to 2 years | Antibiotic therapy | Antibiotic therapy | Antibiotic therapy | Antibiotic therapy or initial observation[b] |
| ≥ 2 years | Antibiotic therapy | Antibiotic therapy | Antibiotic therapy or initial observation[b] | Antibiotic therapy or initial observation[c] |

[a]A toxic-appearing child, persistent otalgia for > 48 hours, temperature ≥ 39°C (102.2°F) in the past 48 hours, or if there is uncertain access to follow-up after the visit.

[b]This plan of initial management provides an opportunity for shared decision making with the child's family for those categories appropriate for initial observation. If observation is offered, a mechanism must be in place to ensure follow-up and begin antibiotics if the child worsens or fails to improve within 72 hours of AOM onset.

Reproduced with permission from Lieberthal AS, Carroll AE, Chonmaitree T, et al. American Academy of Pediatrics-Clinical Practice Guideline: the diagnosis and management of acute otitis media, *Pediatrics*. 2013 Mar;131(3):e964-e999.

complications (eg, mastoiditis or facial nerve palsy), or who has an underlying immunodeficiency. The middle ear fluid should be cultured for bacteriologic diagnosis and susceptibility testing. Presence of multidrug-resistant bacteria in the MEE may necessitate the use of antibiotics that are not approved by the US Food and Drug Administration (FDA) for treatment of AOM, such as levofloxacin or linezolid. Levofloxacin is a quinolone antibiotic that is not approved by the FDA for use in children. Linezolid is a relatively recent and expensive antibiotic that is effective against resistant gram-positive bacteria. Consultation with a pediatric infectious disease expert may help with selection of unconventional drugs.

Duration of antibiotic treatment should be 10 days for children under age 2 years, while a 7-day course should be adequate for AOM in children age 2 to 5 years. For children age 6 years or older with nonsevere symptoms, a 5- to 7-day course is adequate.

Antihistamines have not been shown to be of any value in the management of AOM and may prolong the duration of MEE. Similarly, nasal and oral decongestants are ineffective for treatment of AOM. A 5-day course of systemic corticosteroid therapy, in addition to antibiotics, has not resulted in improvement in treatment failure rate or duration of MEE. Therefore, none of these adjunctive treatments is recommended.

#### Recurrent Otitis Media

Recurrent AOM is defined as the occurrence of ≥ 3 separate, well-documented AOM episodes in a 6-month period, or ≥ 4 episodes in a 12-month period with at least 1 episode in the preceding 6 months. Antibiotic prophylaxis has been used to prevent recurrent AOM. Studies have shown that an estimated 5 children would have to be given 1 year of antibiotic prophylaxis in order to prevent 1 AOM episode. The modest benefit afforded by a prolonged course of antibiotic prophylaxis does not have longer-lasting benefit after cessation of therapy. Because of the modest benefit and the potential adverse effects associated with prolonged antibiotic use and emergence of resistance, the AAP guideline does not recommend antibiotic prophylaxis.

The use of tympanostomy tubes is recommended for recurrent AOM. Tympanostomy tubes prevent approximately 1.5 episodes of AOM in the 6 months after surgery. The disadvantages of tube placement include the cost, surgical and anesthetic risk, and long-term sequelae such as tympanosclerosis and chronic perforation.

#### Acute Otitis Media Associated With Tympanostomy Tubes

In a child with tympanostomy tubes, AOM may still occur, presenting as ear discharge, usually without pain or fever. Although this may occur as a result of contaminated water (eg, bath water, pool water) penetrating the tympanostomy tube to enter the middle ear space, it is much more likely to occur as a result of a concurrent URTI. The most common bacterial causes of AOM in children with tympanostomy tubes are *S pneumoniae*, nontypeable *H influenzae, M catarrhalis, Staphylococcus aureus*, and *Pseudomonas aeruginosa*. Treatment with either broad-spectrum antibiotic eardrops that are nontoxic or systemic antibiotics for AOM is recommended. Recent studies have shown that antibiotic ear drops with corticosteroids are superior to systemic antibiotics. However, for antibiotic eardrops to be effective, they must penetrate the tympanostomy tube to reach the middle ear space. A proportion of children with recurrent ear discharge may have bacterial colonization of the tympanostomy tube itself, usually because of bacterial biofilm, which may be extremely resistant to bacterial eradication. In such circumstances, removal of the tympanostomy tube may be required.

## OTITIS MEDIA WITH EFFUSION

OME is defined as the presence of fluid in the middle ear without signs and symptoms of acute ear infection. The major concern is resultant hearing loss. Persistent MEE results in decreased mobility of the TM

**TABLE 238-3 RECOMMENDED ANTIBIOTICS FOR (INITIAL OR DELAYED) TREATMENT AND FOR PATIENTS WHO HAVE FAILED INITIAL ANTIBIOTIC TREATMENT**

| Initial Antibiotic Treatment at AOM Diagnosis or After Observation | | Antibiotic Treatment After 48–72 Hours of Initial Antibiotic Treatment Failure | |
|---|---|---|---|
| **Recommended First-Line Treatment** | **Alternative Treatment** | **Recommended First-Line Treatment** | **Alternative Treatment** |
| Amoxicillin (80–90 mg/kg/d)<br>OR<br>Amoxicillin-clavulanate[a] (90 mg/kg/d of amoxicillin, with 6.4 mg/kg/d of clavulanate) | Cefdinir (14 mg/kg/d in 1 or 2 doses)<br>Cefuroxime (30 mg/kg/d in 2 divided doses)<br>Cefpodoxime (10 mg/kg/d in 2 divided doses)<br>OR<br>Ceftriaxone (50 mg/kg/d IM or IV for 1–3 days) | Amoxicillin-clavulanate (90 mg/kg/d of amoxicillin, with 6.4 mg/kg/d of clavulanate)<br>OR<br>Ceftriaxone (50 mg/kg/d IM or IV for 3 days) | Ceftriaxone, 3 days, or clindamycin (30–40 mg/kg/d in 3 divided doses), with or without second- or third-generation cephalosporin<br>Clindamycin plus second- or third-generation cephalosporin<br>Tympanocentesis[b]<br>Consult specialist[b] |

[a]May be considered in patients who have received amoxicillin in the previous 30 days or who have the otitis-conjunctivitis syndrome.

[b]Perform tympanocentesis/drainage if skilled in the procedure or seek consult from an otolaryngologist for tympanocentesis/drainage. If the tympanocentesis reveals multidrug-resistant bacteria, then seek infectious disease consultation.

AOM, acute otitis media; IM, intramuscular; IV, intravenous.

Reproduced with permission from Lieberthal AS, Carroll AE, Chonmaitree T, et al. American Academy of Pediatrics-Clinical Practice Guideline: the diagnosis and management of acute otitis media, *Pediatrics*. 2013 Mar;131(3):e964-e999.

and serves as a barrier to sound conduction. OME may be silent in its presenting symptomatology and may be an incidental finding. There may be subjective symptoms such as mild balance disturbance, especially in younger children, or a change in a child's behavior. Diagnosis of OME is made by pneumatic otoscopy and/or tympanometry. Many OME episodes resolve spontaneously, but at least 25% of OME persist for ≥ 3 months, and 5% to 10% of episodes last ≥ 1 year. In addition, 30% to 40% of children have repeated OME. Children diagnosed with OME should be assessed for risk for speech, language, or learning problems from MEE because of baseline sensory, physical, cognitive, or behavioral factors.

The American Academy of Otolaryngology–Head and Neck Surgery published the Clinical Practice Guideline: Otitis Media with Effusion in 2016. The guideline recommends watchful waiting for 3 months from the date of effusion onset (if known) or 3 months from the date of diagnosis in the child with OME who is not at risk for developmental difficulties. They recommend against the use of intranasal or systemic steroids, systemic antibiotics, antihistamines, or decongestants. If OME persists for ≥ 3 months in a child or for any duration in an at-risk child, age-appropriate hearing testing should be performed. If bilateral hearing loss is documented, the family should be counseled about the potential impact on speech and language development. The child should be reevaluated for persistent OME at 3- to 6- month intervals until the MEE is no longer present, significant hearing loss is identified, or structural abnormalities of the TM are suspected.

Surgical management for OME primarily aims to restore hearing. Tympanostomy or ventilation tube placement is an option in children with documented hearing difficulties after 3 months. Adenoidectomy as a stand-alone operation or as an adjunct to tube insertion is most beneficial in children age ≥ 4 years. Therefore, surgical management for OME in children ≥ 4 years of age should include adenoidectomy and/or tympanostomy tubes, while tympanostomy tube placement alone is recommended for OME in children < 4 years old.

## COMPLICATIONS AND OUTCOMES

### Hearing Loss

Hearing loss is the most common complication of OM and can be conductive, sensorineural, or both. Some degree of conductive hearing loss is present whenever fluid fills the middle ear space. In AOM, the loss is usually between 15 and 40 dB; the average loss due to AOM or OME is 27 dB. Reversible or irreversible sensorineural hearing loss can occur during AOM or OME. Reversible sensorineural loss is due to increased tension and stiffness of the round window membrane. Permanent sensorineural hearing loss is most likely due to the spread of infection or products of inflammation through the round window membrane into the labyrinth, development of a perilymphatic fistula in the oval or round window, or suppurative complications such as labyrinthitis or meningitis. Hearing testing is recommended whenever language delay, learning problems, or a significant hearing loss is suspected. Negative pressure in the middle ear, in the absence of MEE, can also be a cause of hearing loss.

### Effect of Otitis Media on Child Development

MEE and the resulting conductive hearing loss may lead to decreased perception of language, impaired development of speech and language, lower scores on tests of cognitive abilities, and poor performance in school. Many studies have been performed relating experience with AOM and OME to developmental outcomes, but the differences in design of the studies and inconsistencies of the results limit conclusions about the effect of OM on development. While some studies reported delay in speech and language development related to hearing loss from persistent MEE, others showed that early placement of ventilating tubes in children with prolonged time spent with MEE did not measurably improve developmental outcomes at age 3 years.

### Suppurative Complications

CSOM occurs when episodes of recurrent AOM are untreated or inadequately treated; a perforation of the TM persists and there is chronic infection of the middle ear and mastoid. The hallmark of CSOM is a purulent, mucoid, or serous discharge through the persistent perforation. CSOM is a major health problem in many developing countries but is of particular concern in regions and populations with limited access to medical care, including the Inuit of Alaska, Canada, and Greenland; Australian Aborigines; and Native Americans.

Extension of infection from suppurative AOM into the mastoid air cells is frequent; the mastoid infection resolves with treatment of AOM but, in some cases, may progress to an acute periostitis or osteitis. Labyrinthitis may follow the spread of infection from the middle ear into the cochlear and vestibular organs, resulting in sensorineural hearing loss and/or vertigo.

Intracranial complications of OM include meningitis, epidural abscess, subdural empyema, brain abscess, dural sinus thrombosis, and otitic hydrocephalus. Suppurative meningitis and other intracranial complications usually follow bacteremia, but may also occur as a result of spread from the middle ear/mastoid infection through the dura. The pus can accumulate between the dura and the cranial bone (epidural abscess) or the potential space between the dura and the arachnoid (subdural empyema) or progress to the meninges to cause meningitis.

### Nonsuppurative Complications

Nonsuppurative complications of AOM include facial paralysis, avascular necrosis of the long process of the incus with an associated conductive hearing loss, atelectasis of the middle ear (with or without a retraction pocket), adhesive OM, tympanosclerosis, and cholesteatoma.

Cholesteatoma consists of keratinized squamous epithelium and may accumulate within the middle ear and expand, resulting in necrosis of surrounding tissues. Cholesteatoma may be a sequela of recurrent OM and may develop from epithelium that has migrated through a perforation of the TM or from epithelium deposited from alternating infection and healing. Cholesteatoma may be due to chronic negative middle ear pressure that retracts a portion of the TM, inhibiting the natural epithelium migration of desquamated squamous debris. This can then become wet and infected, producing foul-smelling otorrhea and/or an expansile mass lesion that can cause local bony erosions. In a patient with a history of chronic otorrhea, pneumatic otoscopy may demonstrate retraction of the TM or granulation tissue or debris within a retraction pocket. However, the diagnosis of cholesteatoma is best made with otomicroscopy using an operating microscope. Computed tomography scanning of the temporal bone may provide further information on the size of the lesion. Aside from otorrhea, symptoms may include conductive hearing loss due to ossicular erosion, sensorineural hearing loss, or disequilibrium due to vestibular involvement. Treatment is surgical.

Although the facial nerve normally travels in a bony canal in its complicated course through the middle ear, up to 55% of individuals have small areas where the bony covering is incomplete, particularly in the area of the oval window. Inflammation may cause edema of the exposed facial nerve as it passes through the middle ear, compromising its venous return within the surrounding bony canal and resulting in peripheral facial nerve palsy. Although full recovery of facial nerve function can be expected in virtually all cases, it is usually recommended that the patient have insertion of a tympanostomy tube and be started on systemic antibiotic therapy. A tympanostomy tube not only serves to drain pus, but also allows for antibiotic and steroid eardrops to be placed directly into the middle ear space.

## PREVENTION

Because of the multifactorial nature of OM, there are a variety of prevention strategies. These strategies mainly focus on reducing modifiable risk factors and vaccination against bacterial and viral infections. Chemoprophylaxis using antibiotics to prevent recurrent AOM is currently discouraged due to relative inefficacy, costs, and potential adverse effects. Surgical interventions for recurrent OM prevention are discussed in the earlier section on recurrent OM.

### Reducing Environmental Risks

During the OM peak age incidence (6–18 months), avoidance of well-known environmental risks, such as exposure to tobacco smoke, daycare attendance, and use of pacifiers, has been associated with reduction of OM. The benefit of breastfeeding in preventing OM has long been known. Breastfeeding protects against OM until 2 years of age, and protection is greater for exclusive breastfeeding. Based on current data, the AAP Clinical Practice Guideline for the Diagnosis and Management of AOM recommends avoidance of tobacco smoke exposure, and exclusive breastfeeding for at least 6 months. The guideline also discusses other lifestyle changes such as avoiding supine bottle feeding (eg, bottle propping), reducing use of pacifiers, and altering childcare center attendance patterns.

### Bacterial Vaccines

The goal of vaccines in this setting is to reduce or eliminate nasopharyngeal colonization of the 3 most common otopathogens: *S pneumoniae*, nontypeable *H influenzae*, and *M catarrhalis*. As noted, PCV7 was first available in 2000. Its use was associated with a 29% reduction in AOM caused by pneumococcal serotypes contained in the vaccines and a 6% to 7% reduction in overall AOM. However, there was subsequent replacement of vaccine serotypes of *S pneumoniae* in the nasopharynx and as AOM pathogens by nonvaccine serotypes and nontypeable *H influenzae*. PCV13, available since 2010, has been associated with further reduction of AOM, mastoiditis, and ventilating tube insertion. A 10-valent pneumococcal-nontypeable *H influenzae* protein D-conjugate vaccine (PHiD-CV) is available in Europe. While effective for pneumococcal OM, PHiD-CV may be less broadly protective for nontypeable *H influenzae* than originally reported in the earlier prototype vaccine study. Even with serotype replacement phenomenon after new PCVs, there are data suggesting that pneumococcal AOM may continue to decrease with PCV vaccination as the serotypes with greater capacity to cause AOM are replaced by less otopathogenic serotypes. More recent evidence suggests that preventing early OM episodes by PCVs may reduce progression to recurrent/chronic OM, although these conditions are not usually caused by *S pneumoniae*. However, PCVs do not prevent OM in previously unvaccinated children with a history of recurrent OM. There are no licensed vaccines against nontypeable *H influenzae* or *M catarrhalis*, but numerous vaccines are in various stages of development.

### Viral Vaccines

AOM is usually preceded by symptomatic viral URTI; therefore, prevention of viral URTI will impact AOM incidence. To date, the only available vaccines against viral respiratory infection are for influenza. Both trivalent, inactivated influenza vaccines and live attenuated influenza vaccines have been shown repeatedly to reduce AOM during influenza seasons. The vaccines work through preventing influenza infection and influenza-associated AOM, which may occur in as many as two-thirds of young children with influenza. The efficacy and effectiveness in AOM prevention vary from year to year depending on the level of influenza activity in the community and how well matched the vaccine strains are with the circulating strains. The higher the level of influenza activity and the better matched the vaccines are, the higher the efficacy/effectiveness in prevention of influenza-associated AOM. Influenza vaccines are currently recommended for all children 6 months of age and older.

Future goals to prevent OM by preventing viral URTI will need to include vaccines against other viruses that are important in AOM development. Vaccines against viruses with high antigenic diversity such as rhinovirus and adenovirus will be difficult to develop. Efforts have been made in RSV vaccine development, mostly to prevent RSV lower respiratory tract infection. Numerous RSV vaccines are in phase I and II clinical trials, some of which are targeting pregnant women to induce maternal immunity for prevention of infection in young infants.

### Nonvaccine Approaches to Prevent Viral URTI and AOM

The occurrence of AOM in the course of URTI peaks between days 2 and 5 after URTI onset. Therefore, early administration of antiviral drugs during URTI may prevent AOM development. Currently, antirespiratory viral drugs are available only for influenza. Studies have shown 43% to 85% reduction in AOM development in young children given oseltamivir within 12 to 48 hours of symptom onset. However, a recent meta-analysis of studies in adults and children concluded that neither oseltamivir nor zanamivir significantly reduced OM. Echinacea, a home remedy, immune modulator, and mild antiviral, has been shown to reduce risks of recurrent respiratory infections (including virologically confirmed cases) and OM. Xylitol, a 5-carbon naturally occurring sugar alcohol with antibacterial properties, has been shown to prevent recurrent AOM with some success. However, the successful dose regimens (eg, chewing gum or syrup given 5 times per day) are not practical, while more practical regimens (eg, 3 times per day) are not effective. Probiotics, mostly *Lactobacillus* and *Bifidobacterium*, have recently been used to reduce risks of respiratory symptoms and OM in infants and children; results have been encouraging. Further studies are required to identify the most promising probiotic strains and to elucidate the mechanisms by which these probiotics prevent infants and children from developing OM.

## SUGGESTED READINGS

Ben-Shimol S, Givon-Lavi N, Leibovitz E, Raiz S, Greenberg D, Dagan R. Impact of widespread introduction of pneumococcal conjugate vaccines on pneumococcal and nonpneumococcal otitis media. *Clin Infect Dis*. 2016;63:611-618.

Chonmaitree T, Trujillo R, Jennings K, et al. Acute otitis media and other complications of viral respiratory infection. *Pediatrics*. 2016;137:e20153555.

Hoberman A, Paradise JL, Rockette HE, et al. Treatment of acute otitis media in children under 2 years of age. *N Engl J Med*. 2011;364:105-115.

Kalu SU, Ataya RS, McCormick DP, Patel JA, Revai K, Chonmaitree T. Clinical spectrum of acute otitis media complicating upper respiratory tract viral infection. *Pediatr Infect Dis J*. 2011;30:95-99.

Carroll AE, Chonmaitree T, et al. The diagnosis and management of acute otitis media. American Academy of Pediatrics Clinical Practice Guideline [published correction appears in *Pediatrics*. 2014;133:346]. *Pediatrics*. 2013;131:e964-e999.

Marom T, Tan A, Wilkinson GS, Pierson KS, Freeman JL, Chonmaitree T. Trends in otitis media-related health care use in the United States, 2001-2011. *JAMA Pediatr*. 2014;168:68-75.

Rosenfeld RM, Shin JJ, Schwartz SR, et al. Clinical practice guideline: otitis media with effusion executive summary (update). American Academy of Otolaryngology-Head and Neck Surgery. *Otolaryngol Head Neck Surg*. 2016;154:201-214.

Ruohola A, Pettigrew MM, Lindholm L. Bacterial and viral interactions within the nasopharynx contribute to the risk of acute otitis media. *J Infect*. 2013;66:247-254.

Tähtinen PA, Laine MK, Huovinen P, Jalava J, Ruuskanen O, Ruohola A. A placebo-controlled trial of antimicrobial treatment for acute otitis media. *N Engl J Med*. 2011;364:116-126.

# 239 Immunizations

H. Cody Meissner

## INTRODUCTION

Childhood immunizations represent one of the great public health achievements of the 20th and 21st centuries. According to the World Health Organization, immunization prevented at least 2 million child deaths in 2003 alone. Less than 250 years after Edward Jenner reported that inoculation with cowpox protected against smallpox, immunization against 15 different diseases before age 2 is routinely recommended in the United States. The individual, societal, and economic benefits of disease prevention resulting from the childhood and adult immunization programs in the United States are without question. A report from the Centers for Disease Control and Prevention (CDC) describing the benefits of vaccination of the 2009 birth cohort through 18 years of age estimated that 20 million cases of vaccine-preventable disease will not occur, 42,000 early deaths related to these diseases will be avoided, and $76 billion in direct and indirect costs will be averted. This economic benefit stands in stark contrast to the comparatively small cost for vaccine purchases. The estimated vaccine purchasing cost for a similar birth cohort based on 2015 pricing is $7.8 billion based on CDC cost and $11.6 billion at private sector pricing. The benefit from the reduction in suffering because of vaccine-preventable disease avoidance cannot be quantified.

## IMMUNE RESPONSE

Many vaccines can be categorized as live or inactivated vaccines. Live vaccines contain organisms that have been attenuated or weakened so that the vaccine strain replicates in the host but rarely causes disease. The cowpox vaccine administered by Jenner in 1796 to prevent smallpox is an example of a live vaccine. In the late 19th century, Louis Pasteur and others discovered methods to attenuate both viruses and bacteria through chemical means, leading to the development of early vaccines. In the 1940s, John Enders and his colleagues perfected viral culture techniques that enabled the attenuation of viruses through serial passage in cell culture, paving the way for vaccines against polio, measles, mumps, and rubella. Some of the newest live vaccines are the products of genetic engineering. For example, one available rotavirus vaccine is produced by reassortment: the vaccine strains are derived from viral cultures co-infected with both human and bovine rotaviruses and contain genes from both "parent" viruses.

The immune response elicited by live attenuated vaccines is similar to that produced with natural infection. Live attenuated vaccines stimulate both humoral and cell-mediated immunity. Most live attenuated vaccines produce immunity in recipients after a single dose. Because a small number of recipients do not respond to the first dose of an injected live vaccine (such as measles, mumps, and rubella [MMR], or varicella), a second dose is recommended routinely to ensure a high level of immunity in the population (herd immunity). Although live attenuated vaccine strains replicate in the vaccinee, they usually do not cause disease such as may occur with the "wild" form of the organism. When a live attenuated vaccine does cause symptoms, it is usually much milder than the natural disease. At times, active immunity from a live attenuated viral vaccine may not develop because of interference from previously acquired circulating antibody to the virus. Antibody from any source (eg, transplacental, transfusion) can interfere with replication of a live attenuated vaccine strain and lead to a poor immune response. Currently available live attenuated viral vaccines include MMR, varicella, zoster, and rotavirus. Oral polio vaccine is a live viral vaccine but is no longer available in the United States, having been replaced by an inactivated polio vaccine. Licensed live attenuated bacterial vaccines include oral typhoid vaccine, oral cholera vaccine, and bacillus Calmette-Guérin (BCG), a cutaneous vaccine against tuberculosis.

In contrast to the immune response to a live vaccine, the immune response to an inactivated vaccine is mostly humoral. Inactivated vaccines cannot replicate and therefore require multiple doses to stimulate a protective immune response. In general, the first dose primes the immune response but does not produce protective immunity. A protective immune response develops after the second or third dose. Antibody titers against inactivated antigens diminish with time. As a result, some inactivated vaccines require periodic supplemental doses to maintain protective antibody titers. The immune response to inactivated antigens is less affected by circulating antibody than that of live agents, so they may be given when antibody is present in the blood. Currently available whole-cell inactivated vaccines include the whole viral vaccines (polio, hepatitis A, and rabies). Inactivated whole virus influenza vaccine and whole inactivated bacterial vaccines (pertussis, typhoid, cholera, and plague) are no longer available in the United States.

Vaccines can also be composed of fractions of bacteria or viruses. Fractional vaccines can be either protein-based or polysaccharide-based. Protein-based vaccines include toxoids (inactivated bacterial toxin) and subunit or subvirion products. Fractional subunit vaccines include hepatitis B, influenza, acellular pertussis, and human papillomavirus (HPV). A subunit vaccine for Lyme disease is no longer available in the United States.

Polysaccharide-based vaccines are composed of pure cell wall polysaccharide from bacteria. Conjugated polysaccharide vaccines contain polysaccharide that is chemically linked to a protein. In the late 1980s, it was demonstrated that the limited immunogenicity associated with polysaccharide vaccines could be overcome through conjugation. Conjugation changes the immune response from T-cell independent to T-cell dependent, leading to increased immunogenicity in infants and antibody booster response to subsequent doses of vaccine. The first conjugated polysaccharide vaccine was *Haemophilus influenzae* type b (Hib), licensed in 1989. A conjugated vaccine for pneumococcal disease was first licensed in 2000. A meningococcal conjugated vaccine was licensed in 2005. A pure polysaccharide vaccine is still available for pneumococcus, but pure polysaccharide vaccines for Hib or meningococcus are no longer available in the United States.

As noted, vaccine antigens may be produced by genetic engineering. Some are recombinant vaccines: hepatitis B and HPV vaccines are produced by insertion of a segment of the respective viral gene into the gene of a yeast cell or an insect virus that infects a susceptible cell line. The modified yeast cell or insect cell line produces pure hepatitis B surface antigen or HPV capsid protein. Live attenuated influenza vaccine has been engineered to replicate more effectively in the cooler temperature of the mucosa of the nasopharynx and less well at the core temperature in the lungs. Live typhoid vaccine (Ty21a) consists of *Salmonella typhi* bacteria that were genetically modified to not cause illness.

## VACCINE LICENSURE

Vaccines are licensed by the US Food and Drug Administration (FDA) based on results of clinical trials submitted by the manufacturer. Recommendations for use of these licensed vaccines are provided by the Advisory Committee on Immunization Practices (ACIP) of the CDC and representatives from participating committees including, the Committee on Infectious Disease (COID) of the American Academy of Pediatrics (AAP), and the American Academy of Family Physicians (AAFP). The addition of new vaccines as well as changes to the existing national immunization schedules for both children and adults are based on numerous factors such as efficacy, safety, burden of disease that may be prevented, equity, compatibility with existing vaccines, and cost. Recommendations for the immunization of children and adolescents are updated annually, including catch-up schedules for children who start their immunizations late or who fall 1 month or more behind, and can be located at the CDC Web site (http://www.cdc.gov/vaccines/schedules/downloads/child/0-18yrs-child-combined-schedule.pdf).

## VACCINE ADMINISTRATION

Recommendations from the CDC and from manufacturers regarding transport and storage, schedule, dose, route, and site of administration should be followed for each vaccine. Most routinely recommended childhood vaccines are administered intramuscularly or subcutaneously. Failure to administer a vaccine as recommended may result in decreased vaccine effectiveness or increased adverse effects.

In general, intramuscular injections are administered in the anterolateral thigh in infants and the deltoid muscle of older children and adolescents. For toddlers, either the anterolateral thigh or the deltoid may be used. The buttock should be avoided as a site of injection because of the potential for sciatic nerve damage and the presence of varied amounts of subcutaneous fat which impairs absorption. Changing needles after withdrawing a vaccine dose from a vial but before administration to a patient is not necessary, nor is pulling back on the vaccine plunger after insertion of the needle but before administration. The route of administration of injectable vaccines is determined in part by the presence of an adjuvant. Inactivated vaccines containing an adjuvant should be injected into a muscle because subcutaneous administration may cause local irritation, induration, skin discoloration, inflammation, or granuloma formation. Unlike intramuscular injections, subcutaneous injections are administered at a 45-degree angle to the skin. The preferred needle length will vary with age. Guidance for selection of proper needle length is available at http://www.immunize.org/catg.d/p3085.pdf.

When vaccines are administered according to the recommended schedule, a child may receive 3 or more injections in a single visit. The pain associated with the administration of immunizations may be a source of distress and anxiety for patients and their families. Parents can be coached to present a calm, matter-of-fact demeanor. They may be taught distraction techniques to minimize the discomfort experienced by their children. Sucrose water (12–50% or 1 packet of sugar in 10 mL of water) may decrease pain in children younger than 6 months when administered shortly before a procedure. When a child needs multiple injections at a single visit, simultaneous administration (multiple staff members injecting separate sites at the same time) is preferred to sequential administration (one after the other). Combination vaccines represent one solution to the issue of increased numbers of injections during single clinic visits and generally are preferred over separate injections of equivalent component vaccines. Combination vaccines can be administered instead of separately administered vaccines if licensed and indicated for the patient's age. Considerations should include provider assessment, patient/guardian preference, and the potential for adverse events. Different vaccines should not be mixed in the same syringe unless specifically licensed for use in this manner. Partial doses of vaccines should never be administered, as this may result in decreased immunogenicity and inadequate protection.

Topical anesthetic agents applied to the skin may help to reduce the pain of an injection by blocking transmission of pain signals. EMLA (lidocaine 2.5%/prilocaine 2.5%) is approved by the FDA for patients greater than 37 weeks of gestational age and should be applied 60 minutes in advance of the injection. Lidocaine 4% is approved by the FDA for children older than 2 years and should be applied 30 minutes before the injection. Available data indicate no known adverse effect of topical anesthetics on the immune response. Evidence does not support the routine use of oral analgesics before or at the time of vaccination. Reduced immunogenicity of some vaccines may be associated with prophylactic use of acetaminophen. An oral analgesic may be used for treatment of fever and local discomfort following immunization. Studies of children with previous febrile seizures have not demonstrated antipyretics to be effective in the prevention of febrile seizures.

The timing and spacing of vaccine doses are 2 of the most important issues in the appropriate use of vaccines. All age appropriate vaccines can be administered at the same visit, with rare exceptions. In those with functional or anatomic asplenia, the Menactra (Sanofi Pasteur) meningococcal conjugate vaccine should not be given until at least 4 weeks after all doses of pneumococcal conjugate vaccine (PCV13) have been administered. PCV13 and pneumococcal polysaccharide vaccine (PPSV23) should be separated by at least 8 weeks. Live MMR and varicella vaccines, if not administered on the same day, should be separated by at least 4 weeks. Otherwise, in order to facilitate completion of the vaccine schedule and minimize the period during which a child is susceptible to vaccine-preventable disease, all vaccines for which a child is eligible at a given visit should be administered.

There are no minimum intervals between doses of different inactivated vaccines or between administration of live parenteral or oral vaccines and any other vaccine. Likewise, there are no maximum intervals between doses of routinely recommended vaccines. When there is a lapse in the administration of sequential doses of vaccines in a given series, the series need not be restarted but may simply be continued. There is no increase in risk of an adverse event from immunizing an individual who already has had the disease.

There are minimum ages for the administration of all routinely recommended vaccines except hepatitis B vaccine. Likewise, there are minimum intervals between the doses of the same vaccine. Because vaccine administration before the recommended age or interval can result in decreased immunogenicity, doses administered more than 4 days early ("grace period") should not be considered valid doses and should be repeated at the appropriate interval.

Antibody-containing products, including whole blood, packed red blood cells, plasma, hyperimmune globulin, and intravenous immune globulin, can interfere with the immune response to some live viral vaccines. Measles and varicella vaccines must be deferred for a minimum of 3 or more months after the receipt of an antibody-containing product. The interval varies with the amount of antigen-specific antibody in the product received (Table 239-1).

## ADVERSE EVENTS

All vaccines undergo rigorous safety testing before licensure. However, no vaccine is completely risk free. The value of a given vaccine depends on the prevalence and severity of the disease targeted, the vaccine's ability to prevent or modify disease, and the incidence and severity of vaccine-related morbidity. Although most adverse events after vaccination are minor and self-limited, some vaccines have been associated with rare but serious side effects.

A vaccine adverse event refers to any medical event that occurs following vaccination. An adverse event could be a true adverse reaction or just a coincidental event, with further research needed to distinguish between them. Acute vaccine adverse reactions fall into 3 general categories: local, systemic, and allergic. The most common type of adverse reactions are local reactions, such as pain, swelling, and redness at the site of injection. Local reactions may occur with up to 80% of vaccine doses, depending on the type of vaccine. Local adverse reactions generally occur within a few hours of the injection and are usually mild and self-limited. On rare occasions, local reactions may be exaggerated or severe. Systemic adverse reactions may occur following receipt of live attenuated vaccines. Live attenuated vaccines must replicate in order to produce immunity. The adverse reactions that follow live attenuated vaccines, such as fever or rash, represent symptoms produced from viral replication and are similar to a mild form of the natural disease. Systemic adverse reactions following live vaccines occur 3 to 21 days after the vaccine is administered (ie, after an incubation period of the vaccine virus). The third type of acute vaccine adverse reactions is allergic reactions. Allergic reactions may be caused by the vaccine antigen itself or some other component of the vaccine, such as cell culture material, stabilizer, preservative, or antibiotic used to inhibit bacterial growth. Severe allergic reactions (anaphylaxis) occur at a rate of 1 case per 1–2 million doses administered.

Thimerosal is a mercury-containing organic compound used for decades in the United States and other countries as a preservative

**TABLE 239-1 SUGGESTED INTERVALS BETWEEN ADMINISTRATION OF ANTIBODY-CONTAINING PRODUCTS AND VACCINATION FOR MEASLES OR VARICELLA[a]**

| Indication and Product | Usual Dose (of mg IgG/kg administered)[a] | Recommended Interval Before Measles or Varicella Vaccination (months) |
|---|---|---|
| Monoclonal antibody (palivizumab) | 15 mg/kg intramuscularly (IM) | None |
| Tetanus IG | 250 units (10 mg IgG/kg) IM | 3 |
| Hepatitis A IG | | |
| Contact prophylaxis | 0.02 mL/kg (3.3 mg IgG/kg) IM | 3 |
| International travel | 0.06 mL/kg (10 mg IgG/kg) IM | 3 |
| Hepatitis B IG | 0.06 mL/kg (10 mg IgG/kg) IM | 3 |
| Rabies IG | 20 IU/kg (22 mg IgG/kg) IM | 4 |
| Varicella IG | 125 units/10 kg (20–40 mg IgG/kg) IM, maximum 625 units | 5 |
| Botulinum immune globulin | 1.5 mL/kg IV intravenously (IV) | 6 |
| Measles prophylaxis IG | | |
| Standard (ie, nonimmunocompromised) contact | 0.25 mL/kg (40 mg IgG/kg) IM | 5 |
| Immunocompromised contact | 0.50 mL/kg (80 mg IgG/kg) IM | 6 |
| Blood transfusion | | |
| Red blood cells (RBCs), washed | 10 mL/kg negligible IgG/kg IV | None |
| RBCs, adenine-saline added | 10 mL/kg (10 mg IgG/kg) IV | 3 |
| Packed RBCs (hematocrit 65%)[b] | 10 mL/kg (60 mg IgG/kg) IV | 6 |
| Whole blood (hematocrit 35–50%)[b] | 10 mL/kg (80–100 mg IgG/kg) IV | 6 |
| Plasma/platelet products | 10 mL/kg (160 mg IgG/kg) IV | 7 |
| Cytomegalovirus intravenous immune globulin (IGIV) | 150 mg/kg maximum | 6 |
| IGIV | | |
| Replacement therapy for immune deficiencies | 300–400 mg/kg IV | 8 |
| Varicella prophylaxis (IGIV) | 400 mg/kg | 8 |
| Immune thrombocytopenic purpura | 400 mg/kg IV | 8 |
| Immune thrombocytopenic purpura | 1000 mg/kg IV | 10 |
| Kawasaki disease | 2 g/kg IV | 11 |

[a]This table is not intended for determining the correct indications and dosages for using antibody-containing products. Unvaccinated persons might not be fully protected against measles during the entire recommended interval, and additional doses of immune globulin or measles vaccine might be indicated after measles exposure. Concentrations of measles antibody in an immune globulin preparation can vary by manufacturer's lot. Rates of antibody clearance after receipt of an immune globulin preparation might vary also. Recommended intervals are extrapolated from an estimated half-life of 30 days for passively acquired antibody and an observed interference with the immune response to measles vaccine for 5 months after a dose of 80 mg IgG/kg.

[b]Assumes a serum IgG concentration of 16 mg/mL.

in vaccines and other biologic products. Thimerosal prevents contamination of multidose vials, primarily by bacteria and fungi, during repeated entry of the vial. In humans, thimerosal is metabolized to ethyl mercury and thiosalicylate. Ethyl mercury is cleared quickly via excretion in stool without an opportunity to accumulate to harmful levels. In contrast, methyl mercury is formed in the environment when mercury metal is metabolized by bacteria. Consumption of fish is a common source of methyl mercury. Methyl mercury is not cleared from the body quickly, thereby allowing the chemical to reach neurotoxic levels. Ethyl mercury has not been associated with the neurotoxic effects seen with methyl mercury accumulation. Despite the absence of evidence of harm, in 1999, the AAP and the US Public Health Service recommended removal of thimerosal from vaccines. By 2001, thimerosal was removed or reduced to trace amounts in all vaccines routinely recommended for children 6 years of age or younger in the United States. In January 2003, the last vaccine containing thimerosal as a preservative expired. Thimerosal is present in some multidose vials of influenza vaccine.

## CONTRAINDICATIONS AND PRECAUTIONS

Contraindications and precautions to vaccination generally dictate circumstances when vaccines should not be given. Many contraindications and precautions are temporary, and the vaccine can be given at a later time. A contraindication is a condition that increases the likelihood of a serious adverse reaction to a vaccine for a patient with that condition. Administration of the vaccine could result in harm to the recipient. For instance, administering MMR vaccine to a person with a true anaphylactic allergy to gelatin could cause serious illness or death in the recipient. In general, vaccines should not be administered when a contraindication condition is present. A precaution is a condition in a recipient that might increase the chance or severity of a serious adverse reaction or that might compromise the ability of the vaccine to produce immunity (such as administering measles vaccine to a person with passive immunity to measles from a blood transfusion). The chance of injury or adverse event is less than with a contraindication. In general, vaccines are deferred when a precaution condition is present. However, situations may arise when the benefit of protection from the vaccine outweighs the risk of an adverse reaction, and a provider may decide to give the vaccine. Contraindications and precautions for routinely used vaccines are available at http://www.bhsj.org/Clinic/immz/contraindications-guide-508.pdf.

Any clinically significant adverse event that occurs after the administration of any vaccine licensed in the United States should be reported to the Vaccine Adverse Event Reporting System (VAERS). Providers should report a clinically significant adverse event even if they are unsure whether a vaccine caused the event. Questions regarding VAERS are addressed at the VAERS Web site at https://vaers.hhs.gov/index.

In the United States, the National Vaccine Injury Compensation Program (VICP) was created by the National Childhood Vaccine Injury Act (NCVIA) of 1986. A no-fault alternative to civil litigation, the VICP was created to adjudicate vaccine injury claims and compensate individuals found to be injured by certain vaccines. Claimants alleging injury from vaccines must file with the VICP before pursuing any legal action against vaccine manufacturers or healthcare providers.

They are not required to prove negligence by the manufacturer or healthcare provider in order to receive compensation. Rather, settlements are based on a Vaccine Injury Table (available at http://www.hrsa.gov/vaccinecompensation/vaccineinjurytable.pdf), which summarizes adverse events associated with vaccines. The Vaccine Injury Table is updated by a panel of experts as new research on vaccine adverse events becomes available. VICP settlements are funded by an excise tax on each covered vaccine.

The VICP has reduced legal claims against manufacturers and healthcare providers, helped ensure national vaccine supplies, and stabilized vaccine costs. Providers who administer covered vaccines in both the public and private sectors have specific responsibilities defined by the NCVIA. For example, patients and/or their parents or guardians must be informed of the risks and benefits of vaccines. A current version of the Vaccine Information Statement (VIS) for each covered vaccine must be provided each time the vaccine is administered (available at http://www.cdc.gov/vaccines/hcp/vis/current-vis.html). Providers must also document key components of the vaccination process, including the date of administration, the manufacturer, the lot number, the VIS version date, and the date the VIS was given.

## PARENTAL REFUSAL

Concerns about vaccine safety have eroded parental confidence in immunizations, leading to antivaccine movements in some countries and occasionally a resurgence of vaccine-preventable diseases due to the lack of immunization. Increasingly, pediatric healthcare providers encounter families who refuse 1 or more immunizations for their children. The AAP Committee on Bioethics has published guidance for pediatricians faced with vaccine refusal. Despite education of parents about the effectiveness of vaccines and the low chance of vaccine-associated adverse events, some parents will decline to have their children vaccinated. This often results from families misinterpreting or misunderstanding information presented by the media and on unmonitored and biased Web sites, causing substantial and often unrealistic fears. Providing parents with an opportunity to ask questions about their concerns regarding recommended childhood immunizations, attempting to understand parents' reasons for refusing 1 or more vaccines, and maintaining a supportive relationship with the family are all part of a good risk management strategy. Physicians are encouraged to explain what is known about the risks and benefits of vaccines, helping parents consider the risks of a given vaccine with the risks of remaining unimmunized.

Continued parental refusal of vaccines should be respected unless a child faces serious harm, as might be the case during an outbreak. However, communication about vaccines should continue at each subsequent healthcare visit. To facilitate the process of informed refusal, the AAP has developed a refusal waiver (https://www.aap.org/en-us/Documents/immunization_refusaltovaccinate.pdf). This "Refusal to Vaccinate" form outlines potential risks of vaccine refusal, including severe illness, death, and the transmission of disease to others. It is suggested that this information be reviewed with the parent and a signature obtained at each medical encounter. This form is not a legal document, however, and should not be presumed to provide immunity from liability if a patient develops a vaccine-preventable disease or transmits a vaccine-preventable disease to others. The AAP encourages physicians to attempt to avoid discharging families who refuse vaccines from their practice unless a "significant level of distrust develops" or there are "significant differences in the philosophy of care."

## DIPHTHERIA–TETANUS–ACELLULAR PERTUSSIS VACCINES

Routine childhood immunization has virtually eliminated once-common diseases such as diphtheria and tetanus and significantly reduced cases of pertussis. Although cases of pertussis have been on the rise for the past 2 decades, the 20,762 reported cases in 2015 reflect a significant decrease from the more than 200,000 cases reported annually in the 1930s. Pertussis is one of the few vaccine-preventable disease that is not at record low levels.

Diphtheria–tetanus–whole cell pertussis (DTwP) vaccines were introduced in the 1940s. These vaccines combined diphtheria and tetanus toxoids (toxin from *Corynebacterium diphtheriae* and *Clostridium tetani* treated with formaldehyde) with a suspension of whole cell, inactivated *Bordetella pertussis*. Although effective in reducing disease, these vaccines were associated with local and systemic reactions. Febrile seizures, for example, were observed in 6 to 9 per 100,000 vaccinees, usually on the day of immunization. Rare systemic reactions included inconsolable crying lasting 3 hours or longer (up to 3%), fever ≥ 104.9°F (0.3%), and an unusual, high-pitched cry (0.1%). Hypotonic-hyporesponsive episodes were observed in 1 in 1750 immunizations.

Since the 1990s, because of less reactogenicity than with DTwP vaccines, only diphtheria–tetanus–acellular pertussis (DTaP) vaccines have been used. They contain diphtheria and tetanus toxoids combined with 3 or more purified *B pertussis* antigens. Licensed DTaP vaccines and combination vaccines that include DTaP all contain pertussis toxin (PT), a cell wall protein that promotes attachment to respiratory epithelial cells, and filamentous hemagglutinin (FHA). Pertactin (PRN) and fimbrial proteins (FIM) are included in some DTaP vaccines. DTaP and DTaP-containing vaccine products and their pertussis antigen components are listed in Table 239-2. Two pediatric acellular pertussis vaccines are currently available for use in the United States. Both vaccines are combined with diphtheria and tetanus toxoids as DTaP and are approved for children 6 weeks through 6 years of age (until the 7th birthday).

In 2002, the FDA approved Pediarix (GlaxoSmithKline), the first pentavalent (5-component) combination vaccine licensed in the United States. Pediarix contains DTaP (Infanrix), hepatitis B (Engerix-B), and inactivated polio vaccine (IPV). Pentacel (Sanofi-Pasteur) is a combination vaccine that contains lyophilized Hib (ActHIB) vaccine and is reconstituted with a liquid DTaP-IPV solution. Pentacel is licensed by the FDA for doses 1 through 4 of the DTaP series among children 6 weeks through 4 years of age. Kinrix (GlaxoSmithKline) is a combination vaccine that contains DTaP and IPV. Kinrix is licensed only for the fifth dose of DTaP and fourth dose of IPV in children 4 through 6 years of age whose previous DTaP vaccine doses have been with Infanrix and/or Pediarix for the first 3 doses and Infanrix for the fourth dose.

Despite differences in antigen content, licensed DTaP vaccines are considered equally effective, although estimates of effectiveness vary. More than 95% of infants develop protective antibody against diphtheria after 4 doses of vaccine, and clinical effectiveness is estimated at 97%. Essentially 100% of vaccinated infants develop protective antibody against tetanus. There are no widely accepted serologic correlates of protection for pertussis, but point estimates of clinical effectiveness range from 80% to 85%.

Children ages 2 months to 6 years should receive 5 doses of DTaP vaccine. Each 0.5-mL dose is administered intramuscularly. The primary series consists of 4 doses typically given at ages 2 months, 4 months, 6 months, and 15 to 18 months, although the first dose may be given as early as age 6 weeks. The minimum interval between each of the first 3 doses is 4 weeks. The fourth dose must be given at least

**TABLE 239-2 DIPHTHERIA, TETANUS, ACELLULAR PERTUSSIS (DTaP) AND DTaP-CONTAINING VACCINES**

| Trade Name | Manufacturer | Pertussis Antigens |
|---|---|---|
| **DTaP Vaccines** | | |
| Infanrix | GlaxoSmithKline | PT, FHA, PRN |
| Daptacel | Sanofi Pasteur | PT, FHA, PRN, FIM-2, FIM-3 |
| **Combination Vaccines** | | |
| Pediarix (DTaP-IPV-Hep B) | GlaxoSmithKline | PT, FHA, PRN |
| Pentacel (DTaP-IPV/Hib) | Sanofi Pasteur | FHA, PRN, PT, FIM-2, FIM-3 |
| Kinrix (DTaP-IPV) | GlaxoSmithKline | FHA, PT, PRN |

FHA, filamentous hemagglutinin; FIM-2, FIM-3, fimbrial proteins; Hep B, hepatitis B; Hib, *Haemophilus influenzae* type B; IPV, inactivated polio vaccine; PRN, pertactin; PT, pertussis toxin;

6 months after the third, and not before age 12 months. The fifth dose of DTaP is not necessary if the fourth dose is administered at 4 years or older. When feasible, the same brand of DTaP vaccine should be used for all doses in the immunization series. If the brand of DTaP vaccine used previously is not available or is not known, any brand may be used. Adverse reactions—both mild and severe—are significantly less common with DTaP vaccines than with DTwP vaccines. Mild reactions include injection site reactions such as redness, tenderness, and swelling; fever < 101°F (2–7%); and irritability (12–30%). Swelling of an entire limb has been reported in children receiving 4 or 5 doses of DTaP vaccine. The swelling resolves without sequelae and does not preclude further doses of vaccine.

Until 2005, no pertussis-containing vaccines were licensed for use in individuals older than 7 years of age. Immunity from pediatric DTwP/DTaP vaccines wanes after approximately 5 to 10 years, leaving adolescents susceptible to infection. Although the majority of deaths from pertussis occur among babies younger than 3 months of age, they acquire the infection from contacts, often adolescents. In 2005, 2 different tetanus–diphtheria–acellular pertussis (Tdap) vaccines were licensed for use in adolescents. One product, licensed for persons 10 years and older (Boostrix [GlaxoSmithKline]) contains 3 different pertussis antigens and is similar to the infant product Infanrix but with reduced quantities of antigen. A second product (Adacel [Sanofi Pasteur]) is licensed for adolescents and adults ages 10 through 64 years and, like the infant product Daptacel, contains 5 different pertussis antigens. However, Adacel contains less diphtheria toxoid and detoxified pertussis toxin than Daptacel.

Both Tdap vaccines result in immune responses to tetanus and diphtheria similar to those observed after immunization with tetanus-diphtheria (Td) vaccine. Immunity to pertussis antigens is similar to that observed in infants following 3 doses of the respective DTaP vaccine.

A single dose of Tdap vaccine is recommended for all adolescents at age 11 to 12, replacing the previously recommended Td booster. A dose of 0.5 mL is given intramuscularly. Tdap may be administered to adolescents whether or not they completed a childhood immunization series with DTwP or DTaP. Those not immunized at age 11 or 12 may be immunized later. Adolescents who received a dose of Td at age 11 or 12 may be subsequently immunized with Tdap in order to provide protection against pertussis. Tdap can be administered regardless of the interval since the last tetanus- or diphtheria toxoid–containing vaccine. A single lifetime dose of Tdap is recommended except during pregnancy when a repeat dose is recommended during each pregnancy, as the immunity provided by Tdap vaccines is short lived. Booster vaccination of a pregnant woman and subsequent transplacental antibody may protect her infant during the first few months of life when most at risk of serious complications from pertussis including death.

Local injection site reactions may occur after Tdap vaccination. Pain at the injection site occurs in 75% of vaccinees; 20% to 30% experience some redness and swelling. Headache and fatigue are the most frequent systemic side effects. Precautions and contraindications can be found at http://www.bhsj.org/Clinic/immz/contraindications-guide-508.pdf.

## POLIO VACCINES

Polio incidence reached a peak in the United States in 1952, with more than 21,000 paralytic cases annually. Following introduction of effective vaccines, polio incidence declined rapidly. The last case of wild-virus polio acquired in the United States was in 1979. Global polio eradication possibly may be achieved within the next decade.

Both live attenuated and inactivated poliovirus vaccines (IPVs) are used worldwide. In the United States, IPV was licensed in 1955 and was used extensively from that time until the early 1960s. In 1963, trivalent live attenuated oral poliovirus vaccine (OPV) was licensed. Trivalent OPV was the vaccine of choice in the United States and most other countries after its introduction in 1963. Advantages of OPV include the stimulation of intestinal as well as systemic immunity. In addition, fecal shedding of the vaccine strains occurs for several weeks after immunization, leading to indirect immunization of contacts. Rarely, however, OPV causes paralytic disease in vaccine recipients or their contacts. Between 1980 and 1996, an average of 8 cases of vaccine-associated paralytic polio (VAPP) were reported annually in the United States. In an effort to eliminate VAPP, exclusive use of IPV vaccine in the United States was recommended in 2000. An enhanced-potency IPV was licensed in 1987. It contains formaldehyde-inactivated poliovirus types 1, 2, and 3 and 2-phenoxyethanol as a preservative. The vaccine is immunogenic, with at least 90% of vaccinees developing protective antibody after 2 doses and 99% after 3 doses. IPV is also available as part of combination vaccines.

All children in the United States should receive 4 doses of IPV. The primary series consists of 3 doses, with the first 2 doses administered at ages 2 and 4 months. The third dose is given at age 6 to 18 months. Children who receive 3 doses of IPV before their fourth birthday should receive a fourth dose at school entry (age 4–6). If the fourth dose is given before age 4, a fifth dose should be administered at 4 through 6 years and at least 6 months after the previous dose. Each 0.5-mL dose can be administered subcutaneously or intramuscularly.

Like other injectable vaccines, IPV causes minor local reactions such as pain and redness at the injection site. Allergic reactions attributed to trace amounts of streptomycin, neomycin, and polymyxin B in the vaccine have been reported. No serious adverse events have been attributed to IPV.

## HEPATITIS B VACCINES

An estimated 850,000 to 2.2 million people in the United States are chronically infected with hepatitis B virus. Before immunization of infants with hepatitis B vaccine became routine, up to 30% to 40% of chronic infections were thought to have resulted from perinatal or early childhood transmission of the virus. Infants infected perinatally have a 90% risk of chronic infection, and up to 25% die of chronic liver disease as adults. Key components of a national immunization strategy to eliminate hepatitis B transmission via infant immunization are based on prevention of mother-to-infant transmission of hepatitis B and, importantly, subsequent prevention of acquisition of hepatitis B later in life associated with high-risk activities.

Two recombinant hepatitis B vaccines (Recombivax HB [Merck] and Engerix B [GlaxoSmithKline]) are licensed in the United States. Both vaccines contain hepatitis B surface antigen (HBsAg) protein synthesized in *Saccharomyces cerevisiae* (common baker's yeast) and then purified and adsorbed onto aluminum hydroxide. Each is available in pediatric and adult formulations (Table 239-3). A combination vaccine for the prevention of hepatitis B infection in children consists of DTaP–hepatitis B–IPV (Pediarix [GlaxoSmithKline]). A combination hepatitis A–hepatitis B vaccine (Twinrix [GlaxoSmithKline]) is licensed only for use in adults age 18 or older. Hepatitis B vaccines are efficacious, inducing a protective antibody response in over 95% of infant recipients after 3 doses.

Three doses of hepatitis B vaccine are recommended for all infants. A dose of 0.5 mL is administered intramuscularly. Only monovalent hepatitis B vaccine is indicated and all newborn infants should receive the first of 3 doses within 24 hours of birth. Infants born to HBsAg-positive mothers should receive the vaccine within 12 hours of birth plus 0.5 mL of hepatitis immune globulin (HBIG) administered at a separate site. When a mother's HBsAg is unknown, infants should receive hepatitis B vaccine within 12 hours of birth and HBIG no later than age 1 week if the mother is subsequently found to be HBsAg-positive. Either monovalent vaccine or a combination hepatitis B vaccine may be used to complete the series with subsequent doses given at age 1 to 2 months and 6 to 18 months (give at 6 months for those born to HBsAg-positive mothers). Monovalent vaccine may be administered as early as at birth, but the combination vaccine containing hepatitis B (DTaP-HepB-IPV) cannot be given before age 6 weeks. Some infants will receive 4 doses of hepatitis B vaccine (birth dose and 3 subsequent doses) when combination vaccine is used to complete the vaccine series.

Infants born to HBsAg-positive mothers should be tested for HBsAg and antibody to HBsAg sometime between 9 and 18 months,

**TABLE 239-3 RECOMMENDED DOSES AND SCHEDULES OF LICENSED FORMULATIONS OF HEPATITIS B VACCINE**

**Single-Antigen Vaccines**

| | Recombivax HB | | | Engerix | | |
|---|---|---|---|---|---|---|
| **Age** | **Dose[a] (µg)** | **Volume (mL)** | **Schedule[b] (months)** | **Dose[a] (µg)** | **Volume (mL)** | **Schedule[b]** |
| Infants (< 1 year) | 5 | 0.5 | Birth, 1–4, 6–18 | 10 | 0.5 | Birth, 1–4, 6–18 |
| Children (1–10 years) | 5 | 0.5 | 0, 1, 6 | 10 | 0.5 | 0, 1, 6 |
| Adolescents | | | | | | |
| 11–15 years | 10[c] | 1.0 | 0, 4–6 | N/A | N/A | N/A |
| 11–19 years | 5 | 0.5 | 0, 1, 6 | 10 | 0.5 | 0, 1, 6 |

[a]Recombinant hepatitis B surface antigen protein dose.

[b]Infants of hepatitis B surface antigen–positive mothers dosed at birth, 1 month, and 6 months.

[c]Adult formulation administered in 2-dose schedule, with second dose 4–6 months after the first.

N/A, not applicable.

**Combination Vaccine**

| | Pediarix | | |
|---|---|---|---|
| **Age** | **Dose[a] (µg)** | **Volume (mL)** | **Schedule[b,c] (months)** |
| Infants (< 1 year) | 10 | 0.5 | 2, 4, 6 |
| Children (1–10 years) | 10 | 0.5 | 0, 2, 4[b] |
| 11–15 years | N/A | N/A | N/A |
| 11–19 years | N/A | N/A | N/A |

Pediarix also includes diphtheria, tetanus, acellular pertussis, and inactivated polio vaccine.

[a]Recombinant hepatitis B surface antigen protein dose.

[b]Infants who received a birth dose of hepatitis B vaccine will receive a total of 4 doses of hepatitis B–containing vaccine.

[c]May not be administered before 6 weeks of age or at 7 years of age or older.

or between 1 and 2 months after completion of the series if the series was delayed. HBsAg-negative infants with nonprotective levels of anti-HBs (< 10 mIU/mL) should be reimmunized with 3 doses of hepatitis B vaccine. Serologic testing is not required for infants born to HBsAg-negative mothers.

Diminished immune responses have been noted in infants weighing less than 2000 g who receive hepatitis B vaccine before age 1 month. The immunization strategy for these infants depends on the HBsAg status of the mother. When the maternal HBsAg status is positive or unknown, hepatitis B vaccine is administered within 12 hours of birth, but this dose is not counted in the 3-dose series; routine 3-dose hepatitis B immunization should begin at 1 month of age. For infants weighing less than 2000 g born to HBsAg-negative mothers, the first dose of hepatitis B vaccine is postponed until age 1 month or hospital discharge.

Hepatitis B vaccination is contraindicated for persons with a history of hypersensitivity to yeast or any other vaccine component. Despite a theoretic risk for allergic reaction to vaccination in persons with allergy to *S cerevisiae* (baker's yeast), no evidence exists to document adverse reactions after vaccination of persons with a history of yeast allergy. Persons with a history of serious adverse events (eg, anaphylaxis) after receipt of hepatitis B vaccine should not receive additional doses. As with other vaccines, vaccination of persons with moderate or severe acute illness, with or without fever, should be deferred until illness resolves.

## *HAEMOPHILUS INFLUENZAE* TYPE B CONJUGATE VACCINES

Before licensure of vaccines for the prevention of Hib infection, 1 in 200 children developed invasive Hib disease (see Chapter 258). This organism was the most common cause of childhood meningitis in the United States and a frequent cause of other invasive diseases (eg, bacteremia, pneumonia, septic arthritis, facial cellulitis, epiglottitis). With universal childhood immunization, initially with polysaccharide Hib vaccine followed by the licensure of the conjugated vaccine in 1989, cases of invasive Hib disease decreased more than 99%.

Three single-antigen conjugate Hib vaccines are available in the United States (Hiberix, GlaxoSmithKline; ActHIB, Sanofi Pasteur; PedvaxHIB, Merck). All vaccines contain Hib capsular polysaccharide (PRP) conjugated to either tetanus toxoid (PRP-T: ActHIB, Hiberix) or an outer membrane protein (PRP-OMP) from *Neisseria meningitidis* serogroup B (PedvaxHIB). Two combination vaccines are available that contain conjugated Hib polysaccharide: Pentacel with DTaP and IPV; and MenHibRix with *N meningitidis* serotypes C and Y (also conjugated).

All Hib conjugate vaccines are highly immunogenic, inducing protective antibody against Hib polysaccharide in > 95% of children after a primary series. Effectiveness against invasive disease is estimated at 95% to 100%. However, PRP-OMP is unique in its ability to elicit high levels of antibody in young children with the first dose of vaccine. Therefore, a PRP-OMP–containing vaccine (PedvaxHIB) is preferred for children at high risk of invasive Hib disease, including American Indian and Alaskan Native children. Hib vaccines do not elicit protective antibody against the carrier protein and do not protect against non–type B strains of *H influenzae*, including non-typeable strains.

The schedule for Hib vaccine differs by the product used and the age at initiation of the series. The primary series of ActHIB or Hiberix consists of 3 doses of vaccine given at ages 2 months, 4 months, and 6 months. The primary series of PedvaxHIB consists of 2 doses given at ages 2 months and 4 months. The vaccines are considered interchangeable for the primary series, but when at least 1 dose of ActHIB or Hiberix is used, 3 doses are required. The first dose of the primary series should not be given to infants younger than age 6 weeks because of the risk of inducing immunologic tolerance against subsequent doses. A booster dose of Hib vaccine is given at age 12 to 15 months. For those not immunized during the first 6 months of life, catch-up schedules can be found in the recommendations of the AAP COID as published in the Red Book.

Generally, healthy children not immunized before age 59 months do not require immunization with Hib vaccine. However, previously unvaccinated individuals older than age 59 months who are at increased risk for invasive Hib disease, including those with functional or anatomic asplenia or human immunodeficiency virus (HIV) infection, should be given 1 dose of Hib vaccine. Recipients of hematopoietic stem cell transplant require 3 doses regardless of prior vaccine history. Adverse reactions following Hib conjugate vaccines are not common. Swelling, redness, or pain has been reported in 5% to 30% of recipients and usually resolves within 12 to 24 hours. Systemic reactions such as fever and irritability are infrequent. Serious reactions are rare.

## PNEUMOCOCCAL CONJUGATE VACCINES

*Streptococcus pneumoniae* is a common cause of invasive and noninvasive infection in children worldwide. The organism colonizes the upper respiratory tract, and disease results from local spread (otitis media, sinusitis) or hematogenous dissemination (eg, bacteremia, pneumonia, meningitis). Before the licensure of a 7-valent pneumococcal conjugate vaccine (PCV7, Prevnar, Wyeth) in 2000, pneumococci accounted for 17,000 cases of invasive disease in the United States each year in children under age 5, including 500 deaths. The highest rates of disease were seen in children age 6 to 11 months and in Alaska Natives, African Americans, and specific American Indian populations. With universal immunization of young children, cases of invasive pneumococcal disease in children younger than age 5 decreased by 77%.

PCV7 contained purified capsular polysaccharide from *S pneumoniae* serotypes 4, 6B, 9V, 14, 18C, 19F, and 23F, conjugated to CRM 197 (a nontoxic mutant of diphtheria toxin) and, in prelicensure trials involving approximately 40,000 children, was 97% effective in reducing invasive pneumococcal disease due to vaccine serotypes. However, serotypes not included in the vaccine (eg, 19A) then began to increase in incidence, so in 2010, a 13-valent pneumococcal conjugate vaccine (PCV13) was licensed in the United States. PCV13 contains the 7 serotypes included in PCV7 plus serotypes 1, 3, 5, 6A, 7F, and 19A.

As with PCV7, a 4-dose series of PCV13 is recommended at ages 2, 4, 6, and 12 to 15 months of age. The 0.5-mL dose is administered intramuscularly. When initiation of the series is delayed, the total number of recommended doses depends on the age at the first dose of vaccine.

A 23-valent pneumococcal polysaccharide vaccine (PPSV23) is also licensed in the United States. This vaccine is used for those at least 2 years of age who are at high risk of invasive pneumococcal disease. When both vaccines are indicated, PCV13 should be administered first and PPSV23 should be given at least 8 weeks after the last dose of PCV13.

Local reactions (such as pain, swelling, or redness) following PCV13 occur in up to half of recipients. Approximately 8% of local reactions are considered to be severe (eg, tenderness that interferes with limb movement). Local reactions are generally more common with the fourth dose than with the first 3 doses. In clinical trials of pneumococcal conjugate vaccine, fever (> 100.4°F [38°C]) within 7 days of any dose of the primary series was reported for 24% to 35% of children. High fever was reported in less than 1% of vaccine recipients. Nonspecific symptoms such as decreased appetite or irritability were reported in up to 80% of recipients.

## MEASLES, MUMPS, AND RUBELLA VACCINES

Since the licensure of an effective vaccine against measles, mumps, and rubella (MMR) in the 1960s, the incidences of measles, mumps, rubella, and congenital rubella syndrome have decreased more than 90%. Sporadic outbreaks of disease occur mostly among unvaccinated or incompletely vaccinated populations.

MMR vaccine (MMR II [Merck]) contains 3 live attenuated viruses. Vaccine strains of measles and mumps are grown in chick embryo cell culture; rubella is grown in human diploid cell culture. A combination measles, mumps, rubella, varicella vaccine (MMRV; ProQuad [Merck]) is also available. Each vaccine contains small quantities of neomycin to prevent bacterial overgrowth.

A single dose of MMR vaccine confers protection to measles and rubella in more than 95% of vaccine recipients age 12 months or older. Individuals who do not develop serologic evidence of immunity after the first dose of vaccine (primary vaccine failure) typically respond to the second dose. The duration of protective immunity is long lasting and probably lifelong. Postlicensure studies indicate that 1 dose of mumps or MMR vaccine is approximately 78% effective against disease caused by mumps virus. Two-dose mumps vaccine effectiveness is approximately 88%.

Two doses of MMR vaccine are recommended for all children. The dose is 0.5 mL and is administered subcutaneously. The first dose is administered at age 12 to 15 months, and the second dose at age 4 to 6 years. The second dose may be administered earlier as long as 4 weeks have elapsed since the first dose. During measles outbreaks or when the risk of exposure to measles is high because of travel outside the United States, children as young as age 6 months should receive the vaccine, but doses administered before age 12 months are not counted in the 2-dose series. These children should be revaccinated with 2 additional doses of MMR with the first dose administered at age 12 through 15 months. The persistence of maternal measles antibody in young infants may modify the immune response to the vaccine. MMRV may be used instead of separate injections of MMR and varicella in healthy children ≥ 12 months to 12 years.

MMR vaccine may be administered on the same day with any other live or inactivated childhood vaccines as long as the vaccines are given in separate syringes at separate sites. Injected live virus vaccines not given on the same day as MMR vaccine should be deferred for at least 4 weeks. Measles vaccination may temporarily suppress tuberculin skin test reactivity for 4 to 6 weeks after immunization but will not interfere with the accuracy of a test placed on the same day. MMR vaccine must be deferred for 3 or more months after the receipt of an antibody-containing product (including immune globulin, whole blood, packed red blood cells, and intravenous immune globulin) because passively transferred antibody interferes with the immune response (see Table 239-1). The interval varies with the amount of antigen-specific antibody in the product received.

Redness, induration, or soreness at the injection site may occur after MMR vaccine. Local hypersensitivity consisting of wheal-and-flare reactions or urticaria is occasionally seen. Fever and rash are the most common systemic side effects, with 5% to 15% of vaccinees developing a fever ≥ 39.4°C (103°F) 6 to 12 days after immunization (among seronegative vaccinees) and 5% developing a morbilliform rash. Higher rates of fever as well as a slight increase in febrile seizures have been reported with the first dose of combination MMRV vaccine in comparison to children who receive separate injections of MMR and varicella vaccines on the same day. For children age 12 to 23 months, the rate of febrile seizures after MMR vaccine is 4 cases per 10,000 vaccinations. In contrast, the rate of febrile seizures after MMRV vaccination is 9 per 10,000 vaccinations. Neither vaccine is associated with the development of chronic seizure disorders. The above should be discussed with parents, as should the benefit of receiving only a single injection when MMRV is used. When the first dose is given at ≥ 48 months of age or for dose 2 at 15 months to 12 years, MMRV is preferred over separate MMR and varicella vaccine injections. Transient thrombocytopenia occurring within 2 months of MMR immunization has been observed in less than 1 in 30,000 vaccinees and is presumably due to the measles component of the vaccine. Because of the risk of vaccine-induced thrombocytopenia, a history of thrombocytopenia is considered a precaution to MMR immunization. It should be noted, however, that the risk of thrombocytopenia with vaccination is less than that observed with natural measles infection. Arthralgias occur in up to 25% of adult women given rubella-containing vaccines, including MMR, but joint complaints in children are much less common. Although the measles and mumps viruses are grown in chick embryo cell culture, MMR does not contain significant quantities of cross-reacting egg protein (ovalbumin) to elicit an allergic reaction, and children with egg allergy may safely be vaccinated. Skin testing for egg allergy is not predictive of adverse reactions to vaccine and is not recommended.

Live virus vaccines including MMR are generally contraindicated in individuals known or suspected to be immunodeficient. However, HIV-infected children who are not severely immunocompromised (defined by age-specific quantitation of CD4 lymphocytes) should receive MMR because the risk associated with the vaccine is much less than that associated with wild-type measles infection. MMRV vaccine should not be used in place of MMR vaccine for immunization of HIV-infected children because the MMRV vaccine contains a higher concentration of varicella vaccine virus. Other precautions and contraindications can be found at http://www.bhsj.org/Clinic/immz/contraindications-guide-508.pdf.

In 1998, a connection between receipt of MMR vaccine and autism was postulated. This theory was based on a case series of 12 children, 8 of whom developed regressive neurologic symptoms 1 to 14 days after receipt of MMR vaccine. The paper published in *The Lancet* describing this association contained methodologic flaws and has subsequently been retracted by the journal. In addition, a number of well-controlled epidemiologic studies involving thousands of children have failed to find evidence that MMR causes autism. Both the AAP and the Institute of Medicine have concluded that there is no association between MMR vaccine and autism.

MMR is contraindicated in pregnant women because of a theoretical risk to the fetus. However, because the attenuated viruses in the MMR vaccine are not transmitted from person-to-person after immunization, household contacts of either pregnant women or immunosuppressed individuals can and should be immunized to prevent introducing natural virus into the household. Breastfeeding mothers immunized with rubella-containing vaccines may occasionally transmit rubella vaccine virus to their infants via breast milk. Because transmission results only in a mild rash illness and does not interfere with response to MMR vaccine administered at age 12 months, breastfeeding is not a contraindication to receipt of rubella-containing vaccines.

## VARICELLA VACCINES

Before the licensure of varicella vaccine in 1995, approximately 4 million cases of chickenpox occurred annually in the United States. Although most infections were self-limited, secondary complications including pneumonia, encephalitis, and secondary bacterial infections (usually soft tissue infections) that occasionally were quite severe (eg, necrotizing fasciitis), resulted in more than 10,000 hospitalizations and 100 deaths each year.

Two live attenuated varicella-zoster virus–containing vaccines are available for use in children. A monovalent varicella vaccine (Varivax [Merck]) is licensed for children older than age 12 months, adolescents, and adults. A combination measles, mumps, rubella, varicella vaccine (ProQuad [Merck]) is approved for use in children ages 12 months to 12 years. Both vaccines contain live attenuated varicella-zoster virus (Oka strain), although the combination vaccine contains a higher concentration of varicella vaccine virus, with a minimum of 10,000 plaque-forming units (PFUs) compared to 1350 PFUs in the monovalent product. Both vaccines contain minute quantities of neomycin and gelatin.

A single dose of varicella vaccine is approximately 72% to 85% effective against varicella disease, with even higher protection against severe varicella disease. Because primary vaccine failure (failure to make protective antibodies) after 1 dose of varicella vaccine occurs and frequent school-based outbreaks of varicella have been observed in populations with high single-dose vaccination rates, 2 doses of varicella-containing vaccine are recommended for all children. Recipients of 2 doses of varicella vaccine are 3.3 times less likely to have breakthrough varicella compared to recipients of 1 dose (2.2% vs 7.3%; $P < .001$). Following the recommendation for 2 doses instead of 1 varicella vaccine dose, varicella cases declined 97% between 1995 and 2010 in areas of active surveillance.

The first dose is administered at age 12 to 15 months, and the second dose is generally administered at age 4 to 6 years, although it can be given as early as 3 months after the first dose (if inadvertently given between 28 days and 3 months after the first dose, the second dose need not be repeated). A dose of 0.5 mL is administered subcutaneously. Catch-up immunization is recommended for susceptible older children not previously immunized or those immunized with a single dose of vaccine.

Varicella vaccine is associated with few side effects. Approximately 20% of monovalent varicella vaccine recipients experience transient pain and tenderness at the site of injection. A mild varicelliform eruption develops at the injection site in 3% of children within 1 month of immunization, and 5% of children may develop a generalized rash. Transmission of the attenuated vaccine virus from immunocompetent individuals who develop a rash soon after vaccination to susceptible individuals has been reported but is extremely rare (1 case of transmission per 10 million doses).

Precautions and contraindications can be found at http://www.bhsj.org/Clinic/immz/contraindications-guide-508.pdf. Varicella-containing vaccines should not be administered to individuals with a history of anaphylactic reaction to neomycin or gelatin. Monovalent varicella vaccine does not contain egg protein and thus may be safely administered to individuals with egg allergy. Although the measles and mumps vaccine viruses in MMRV are grown in chicken-embryo cell culture, the amount of egg protein is not significant, and children with egg allergy may receive MMRV.

Specific recommendations have been published for immunization of individuals with altered immunity. Varicella-containing vaccines are not recommended for children receiving treatment for leukemia, lymphoma, or other malignancies affecting the bone marrow or lymphatic systems; children receiving long-term immunosuppressive therapy; or children with most congenital or acquired T-cell immunodeficiencies. Immunodeficiency should be excluded in children with a family history of hereditary immunodeficiency before a varicella-containing vaccine is administered. For individuals receiving high-dose systemic corticosteroids (≥ 2 mg/kg/d of prednisone or its equivalent or 20 mg/d of prednisone) for ≥ 14 days, immunization should be deferred with a minimum interval of 1 month between the last dose of steroids and subsequent vaccination. Monovalent varicella vaccine may be administered to children with certain humoral immune deficiencies and HIV-infected children defined by age specific CD4+ lymphocyte counts. Household contacts of immunocompromised hosts should be vaccinated to decrease the likelihood of introducing wild varicella into the household. However, those vaccinees who then develop rash should avoid contact with immunocompromised persons who are not immune to varicella for the duration of the rash.

Varicella vaccine is contraindicated in pregnant women, but children living in the same household may be vaccinated. Caution is advised when vaccinating children taking salicylates. No adverse events associated with salicylate use and varicella vaccine have been reported. However, the manufacturer recommends that salicylates be avoided for 6 weeks after vaccine administration because of the well-established relationship between Reye syndrome and use of salicylates during natural varicella infection. According to the ACIP, varicella vaccine with subsequent close monitoring should be considered for children requiring chronic salicylate therapy because the risk of aspirin-associated complications is likely to be greater with natural varicella infection.

## HEPATITIS A VACCINES

Before the implementation of a targeted hepatitis A immunization program in the United States, there were 180,000 infections reported annually, resulting in approximately 100 deaths (see Chapter 303). The highest incidence of infection occurred in children ages 5 to 14 years. Children younger than age 6 years frequently developed asymptomatic (anicteric) infection and were a source of transmission of the virus to others. Native Americans, Alaska Natives, and Hispanics were at increased risk for disease.

National recommendations for hepatitis A immunization have evolved from a targeted strategy focused on groups of individuals at increased risk for infection to one that includes universal immunization of infants. Beginning in 1996, routine hepatitis A immunization was recommended for children age 2 years or older living in communities with high rates of hepatitis A infection or periodic outbreaks, namely children living in Alaska Native villages or Native Americans. In 1999, the recommendations were expanded to include children ages 2 to 18 years living in states, counties, or communities with annual hepatitis A infection rates that were at least twice the national average or ≥ 20 cases per 100,000 population. Locales with hepatitis A infection rates of at least 10 cases per 100,000 population were encouraged to "consider" immunization of children ages 2 to 18 years.

In 2005, hepatitis A vaccine was licensed for children as young as age 12 months, and the CDC amended recommendations to include all children beginning at 1 year of age, regardless of state of residence. Two doses of hepatitis A vaccine are currently recommended for all children in the second year of life, with at least 6 months between doses. Anyone aged 2 to 18 years old and not previously immunized may be vaccinated if immunity against hepatitis A is desired. States, counties, and communities with existing programs for immunization of children ages 2 to 18 are encouraged to maintain these programs.

Two hepatitis A vaccines are currently licensed for use in children age 12 months or older (Havrix [GlaxoSmithKline] and Vaqta [Merck]). Both contain whole hepatitis A virus propagated in human fibroblasts, formalin-inactivated and adsorbed to aluminum hydroxide adjuvant. More than 95% of children and adults will have protective antibody 4 weeks after the first dose, and nearly 100% seroconvert after a second dose. A combination hepatitis A–hepatitis B vaccine (Twinrix [GlaxoSmithKline]) is licensed for use in those age 18 years or older. A dose of 0.5 mL is administered intramuscularly. Although administration of the same hepatitis A vaccine is preferable for both doses, either single-antigen hepatitis A vaccine may be used to complete the series, regardless of what product was given for the first dose. Local injection site reactions, including erythema, swelling, and tenderness, occur in approximately 20% of children immunized with hepatitis A vaccine. These reactions are generally mild and resolve within 24 hours. Decreased appetite and fatigue occur less commonly. Serious adverse events have not been associated with hepatitis A vaccine. Contraindications and precautions are found at http://www.bhsj.org/Clinic/immz/contraindications-guide-508.pdf.

## INFLUENZA VACCINES

Annual epidemics of influenza result in 50 million to 60 million infections, with the highest attack rates in school-age children. The risks for serious disease, hospitalization, and death from influenza are highest among children age 2 years and younger, adults age 65 and older, and individuals of any age with underlying medical conditions that place them at increased risk for complications from influenza (Table 239-4).

The effectiveness of influenza vaccines varies by vaccine type, the number of doses administered, the age and immune status of the vaccinee, and the match between circulating strains of influenza and those contained in the vaccine. Inactivated vaccines typically are protective in about 60% of healthy vaccinated people less than 65 years of age. The role of high dose or adjuvanted influenza vaccine in persons > 65 years of age is not yet determined.

**TABLE 239-4 GROUPS ESPECIALLY TARGETED FOR INFLUENZA VACCINATION**

- Children ages 6 months through 59 months
- All persons age 50 or older
- Individuals with chronic medical conditions, including:
  - Pulmonary disorders (including asthma)
  - Cardiovascular disease (except isolated hypertension)
  - Renal dysfunction
  - Hepatic dysfunction
  - Hemoglobinopathies (including sickle cell disease)
  - Metabolic disorders (including diabetes mellitus)
  - Immune suppression due to illness or medication
  - Neurologic disorders, especially those that compromise respiratory function or handling of respiratory secretions or increase the risk of aspiration
- Household contacts and caregivers of at-risk children and adults, especially contacts of children < 6 months of age
- Women who will be pregnant or are pregnant during the influenza season
- Persons who are morbidly obese (body mass index > 40)
- Residents of long-term care facilities
- Healthcare workers

**TABLE 239-5 SCHEDULE AND DOSING OF INACTIVATED INFLUENZA VACCINE IN CHILDREN**

| Age | Number of Doses | Dose (mL) | Route |
|---|---|---|---|
| 6–35 months | 1 or 2[a] | 0.25 | Intramuscular |
| 3–8 years | 1 or 2[a] | 0.5 | Intramuscular |
| ≥ 9 years | 1 | 0.5 | Intramuscular |

[a]Two doses separated by ≥ 4 weeks are indicated for children receiving influenza vaccine for the first time or who were vaccinated for the first time in the prior season but received only 1 dose.

Both live attenuated and inactivated influenza vaccines were used in previous years. A live attenuated influenza vaccine (LAIV) containing 2 influenza A viruses and 2 influenza B viruses previously was recommended for use in the United States. The viruses in this vaccine were reassortants that contained genes encoding for the surface proteins hemagglutinin and neuraminidase from circulating wild-type influenza viruses and genes from master influenza A and B viruses that confer cold adaption and temperature sensitivity. The vaccine strains were designed to replicate in the cooler temperature of the nasopharynx in order to simulate the route of infection by wild-type virus, but because of their temperature sensitivity, vaccine strains were designed not to replicate in the lower airway. The CDC and the AAP recommend that LAIV not be offered in any setting during the 2016 to 2017 and 2017 to 2018 seasons because of lack of effectiveness during the 3 prior influenza seasons.

The trivalent inactivated vaccine (IIV3) contains 2 inactivated influenza A viruses (types H1N1 and H3N2) and 1 influenza B virus. The quadrivalent inactivated vaccine (IIV4) contains 2 inactivated influenza A viruses and 2 influenza virus B strains representing each lineage. The composition of the vaccine changes annually based on circulating influenza types. Most vaccine strains are grown in chicken eggs and then inactivated by formaldehyde or β-propiolactone treatment. Organic solvents or detergents are then used to disrupt the viruses into viral subunits or subvirions. Other influenza vaccines are prepared using strains grown in continuous cell lines or using recombinant technology. In general, IIV vaccines are approved for use in individuals age 6 months or older, including those with underlying medical conditions. Unlike other vaccines routinely recommended for children, influenza vaccines contain thimerosal if a multidose vial is used.

Annual influenza immunization is recommended for all people 6 months of age and older (Table 239-5 lists schedules and doses). No influenza vaccine is licensed for use in children younger than 6 months; therefore, immunization of household and other close contacts is the preferred way to protect these children from influenza. Similarly, other groups at high risk of complications from influenza infection (and their close contacts) are especially targeted for influenza vaccination (see Table 239-4). Vaccination of pregnant women with IIV can protect them and their infant. Annual vaccination of healthcare workers should be mandatory. Inactivated influenza vaccines can be administered as soon as the vaccine is available in late summer or early fall.

Transient, local reactions, including tenderness, erythema, and induration at the injection site, occur in 15% to 20% of IIV3 vaccine recipients. Systemic reactions such as fever and myalgias occur in 1% or less. Hypersensitivity reactions including anaphylaxis are rare. Precautions and contraindications can be found at http://www.bhsj.org/Clinic/immz/contraindications-guide-508.pdf.

## ROTAVIRUS VACCINES

In the prevaccine era in the United States, rotavirus gastroenteritis resulted in 55,000 to 70,000 hospitalizations annually with 20 to 60 deaths (see Chapter 231). Because of the effectiveness of the rotavirus vaccines, norovirus has replaced rotavirus as the most common cause of severe gastroenteritis in this country.

The first vaccine for the prevention of rotavirus gastroenteritis was licensed in the United States in 1998. However, this live attenuated tetravalent rhesus reassortant vaccine was withdrawn from the market in 1999 because a slight increase in risk of intussusception was noted in vaccine recipients, particularly after the first dose of vaccine.

Currently, 2 oral live attenuated rotavirus vaccines are licensed in the United States. A pentavalent rotavirus vaccine (RV5, RotaTeq [Merck]) contains 5 reassortant viruses derived from human and bovine rotavirus strains. A monovalent vaccine is also available (RV1, Rotarix [GlaxoSmithKline]). RV1 contains live attenuated human rotavirus. In clinical trials, RV5 demonstrated 74% efficacy against all rotavirus gastroenteritis and 98% efficacy against severe rotavirus gastroenteritis. RV1 performs similarly.

The schedule for rotavirus immunization depends on the product used. RV5 is administered as a 3-dose series for infants at age 2 months, 4 months, and 6 months. RV1 is administered as a 2-dose series with doses given at ages 2 months and 4 months. The first dose of either vaccine can be administered as early as age 6 weeks, but not later than age 14 weeks, 6 days. The minimum interval between vaccine doses is 4 weeks, and the last dose should be administered no later than age 8 months, 0 days. All doses in the series should be completed with the same product, but immunization should not be delayed if the product used for previous doses is unknown or not available. If any dose in the series is RV5 or an unknown product, 3 total doses should be given. Redosing is not indicated when an infant spits out or vomits the vaccine, and subsequent doses should be administered at recommended intervals.

In 2010, rotavirus vaccination was temporarily suspended because DNA sequences from porcine circovirus type 1 were found in vaccine lots. Subsequently, live porcine circovirus type 1 was identified in RV1, and porcine circoviruses types 1 and 2 were identified in RV5. The FDA ultimately determined that these viruses posc no risk to humans, and at present, both vaccines are available for administration.

Precautions and contraindications for rotavirus vaccine are available at http://www.bhsj.org/Clinic/immz/contraindications-guide-508.pdf. Altered immunocompetence should be considered a precaution to vaccine administration; however, severe combined immunodeficiency is a contraindication to immunization. Postmarketing studies have identified a minimal risk of intussusception after any available rotavirus vaccine. A history of intussusception is a contraindication to vaccination. Premature infants who are at least 6 weeks of age and clinically stable are eligible for immunization and should be vaccinated using the same schedule as term infants. The vaccine should be administered at or after discharge from the hospital nursery.

## MENINGOCOCCAL VACCINES

In the United States in 2016, a total of 375 cases of invasive disease due to *N meningitidis* were reported. This is a historically low rate, and the reason for the falling rates of disease is not known. The highest rates of disease occur in children younger than age 1 year, but 62% of cases occur in individuals age 11 years or older. Rates of meningococcal disease due to serogroups A, C, W, and Y (included in the quadrivalent vaccines) among adolescents exceed those of the general population. Other individuals at increased risk of meningococcal disease include those with functional or anatomic asplenia and those with deficiencies of properdin and terminal complement components.

Two meningococcal conjugated vaccines are licensed for use in infants at increased risk of meningococcal infection: MenHibrix (GlaxoSmithKline), licensed for use at 6 weeks through 18 months of age; Menactra (Sanofi Pasteur), for 9 months through 55 years of age; and Menveo (Novartis), for 2 months through 55 years of age. These 2 meningococcal quadrivalent vaccines (MCV4s) are active against serogroups A, C, W, and Y: Menactra employs a diphtheria toxoid carrier protein, while Menveo contains a nontoxic mutant diphtheria toxin. These 2 vaccines are given intramuscularly. Like all protein conjugate vaccines, they elicit immune responses from T cells as well as B cells, resulting in some degree of immunologic memory.

Routine vaccination using MCV4 should be administered at 11 or 12 years of age with a booster dose at 16 years of age. Individuals 13 through 18 years of age who were not previously immunized should be immunized, and those receiving the first dose at 13 to 15 years of age should receive a booster dose at 16 to 18 years of age. College freshmen living in dormitories who have not previously received a dose of MCV4 should also be immunized. Those at least 2 months of age who are at increased risk for invasive meningococcal disease should be immunized with a meningococcal conjugate vaccine, but the different products are given at different schedules. Because vaccine-induced antibodies against *N meningitidis* wane over time, children initially vaccinated with MCV4 who remain at increased risk for meningococcal disease require revaccination. Local reactions, including redness, tenderness, and swelling at the injection site, are common after MCV4 administration but generally resolve within 1 to 2 days. Systemic reactions, including headache and malaise, are observed in up to 60% of vaccinees.

Two serogroup B meningococcal protein vaccines were recently licensed by the FDA. Although these vaccines are not recommended for routine use, the ACIP recommends vaccination of people age 10 years and older who are at increased risk for serogroup B meningococcal disease including: during outbreaks of serogroup B disease, those with functional or anatomic asplenia including those with sickle cell disease, those with persistent deficiencies in the complement pathway, persons receiving eculizumab, and microbiologists who routinely work with isolates of *N meningitidis*. The vaccines are administered in either a 2- or a 3-dose series. The efficacy of serogroup B meningococcal vaccines at disease prevention is unknown, as licensure was based on a serologic response using a presumed measure of immunity. Neither vaccine is expected to provide protection against all circulating serogroup B strains, and the duration of immunity is likely to be limited to a few years.

## HUMAN PAPILLOMAVIRUS VACCINES

HPV is the most common sexually transmitted disease in the United States (see Chapter 228). Seventy-four percent of the 6.2 million new infections each year occur in individuals age 15 to 24 years. Although most infections are asymptomatic and self-limited, persistent infection may cause genital warts and, more worrisome, cancers of the anogenital region and cervix. Two HPV types, 16 and 18, account for 70% of all cases of cervical cancer.

The vaccine is composed of noninfectious virus-like particles (VLPs) prepared from recombinant L1 viral capsid protein are available in the United States. Previously, 2 vaccines were FDA-approved. A bivalent vaccine (2vHPV; Cervarix [GlaxoSmithKline]) including oncogenic HPV types 16 and 18, licensed for females 9 through 25 years of age, has been shown to be highly effective in preventing cervical cancer due to the HPV types contained in the vaccine. A quadrivalent vaccine (4vHPV; Gardasil [Merck]) contains types 6 and 11, which are common causes of genital warts, is licensed for males and females 9 through 26 years of age, and has been shown to protect against genital warts in males and females, as well as vaccine type cervical cancer and anal precancers in males. Neither vaccine is available in the United States. A 9-valent HPV vaccine (9vHPV; Gardasil 9, Merck) includes types 6, 11, 16, 18, 31, 33, 45, 52, and 58 and is currently available. 9vHPV is recommended for females 9 through 26 years of age and for males 9 through 21 years of age for prevention of vulvar, vaginal, cervical, and anal cancer and anogenital warts (condyloma acuminata), as well as precancerous and dysplastic lesions caused by serotypes contained in the vaccine. Males aged 22 through 26 years also may be vaccinated with 9vHPV.

Females and males age 11 or 12 years should be vaccinated with HPV vaccine routinely, although the series may be started as early as age 9 years. Each 0.5-mL dose is administered intramuscularly. If the first dose is administered before the 15th birthday, only 2 doses are necessary with the second dose 6 to 12 months after the first dose. If the series is begun on or after the 15th birthday, 3 doses are recommended with the second dose 1 to 2 months after the first dose and the third dose at least 6 months after the first dose. The HPV vaccine should be administered before the onset of sexual activity because the vaccine has no efficacy against an established infection, and HPV infection is acquired soon after sexual activity begins.

Local injection site reactions, including pain, swelling, and erythema, are common after vaccination with HPV vaccine but are generally mild. Systemic symptoms such as headache, fatigue, and myalgias are also observed. Because syncope may occur as with adolescents administered any vaccine, vaccine recipients should be observed sitting or lying down for 15 minutes following vaccination. Precautions and contraindications are available at http://www.bhsj.org/Clinic/immz/contraindications-guide-508.pdf.

## SUGGESTED READINGS


Ahmed F, Temte JL, Campos-Outcalt D, Schünemann HJ. ACIP evidence based recommendations work group (EBRWG). Methods for developing evidence-based recommendations by the Advisory Committee on Immunization Practices of the United States Centers for Disease Control and Prevention. *Vaccine.* 2011;29:9171-9176.

American Academy of Pediatrics Committee on Infectious Diseases. Immunization. In: Kimberlin DW, Brady MT, Jackson MA, Long SS, eds. *Red Book: 2015 Report of the Committee on Infectious Diseases* (30th ed). Elk Grove Village, IL: American Academy of Pediatrics; 2015:7-107.

Centers for Disease Control and Prevention. General recommendations on immunization. Recommendations of the Advisory Committee on Immunization Practices. *Morb Mortal Wkly Rep.* 2011;60:1-61.

Centers for Disease Control and Prevention. Advisory Committee on Immunization Practices recommended immunization schedules for persons aged 0 through 18 years—United States, 2016. *Morb Mortal Wkly Rep.* 2016;65:86-87.

Hamborsky J, Kroger A, Wolfe C, eds. *Epidemiology and Prevention of Vaccine-Preventable Disease* (13th ed). Washington, DC: Public Health Foundation; 2015.

Rubin LG, Levin MJ, Ljungman P, et al. Clinical practice guidelines for vaccination of the immunocompromised host. *Clin Infect Dis.* 2014;58:e44-e100.

Smith JC, Snider DE, Pickering LK. Immunization policy development in the United States: the role of the Advisory Committee on Immunization Practices. *Ann Intern Med.* 2009;150:45-49.

Top KA, Billard MN, Gariepy MC, et al. Immunizing patients with adverse events following immunization and potential contraindications to immunization: a report from the Special Immunization Clinics Network. *Pediatr Infect Dis J.* 2016;35(12):e384-e391.

Walton LR, Orenstein WA, Pickering LK. The history of the United States Advisory Committee on Immunization Practices. *Vaccine.* 2015;33:405-414.


# 240 Antiviral Therapy


Mark R. Schleiss


## INTRODUCTION

The deployment of antiviral therapy typically requires the clinician to strike a delicate balance between targeting virally encoded functions required for production of progeny viruses and avoiding toxicity to the host cellular functions subverted by the viral replication machinery. Accordingly, as a part of the trade-off for eliciting antiviral effect, many antivirals historically have induced considerable toxicity in the host cell as well. A watershed moment in the history of antiviral drug discovery was the development of the drug acyclovir, one of a series of drugs that was developed that blocked nucleic acid synthesis only in virally infected cells without damaging the uninfected host cells (because a viral enzyme, thymidine kinase, is required to phosphorylate the compound to its active form). This discovery resulted in the awarding of a Nobel Prize to Dr. Gertrude Elion in 1988.

Today, a number of effective antivirals currently are licensed and available, and are important in the management of infections caused by herpes simplex virus (HSV), varicella-zoster virus (VZV), cytomegalovirus (CMV), hepatitis B and C viruses, influenza A and B viruses, and human immunodeficiency virus (HIV). To maximize therapeutic effectiveness, treatment should generally be initiated as early as possible in the course of infection. Under some circumstances, antivirals may be effective in prophylaxis against acquisition or reactivation of infection. The advent and increased utilization of rapid-diagnosis molecular platforms for viral infections has enabled the more timely use of antiviral therapy in many clinical settings, so a working knowledge of available antivirals in pediatric practice is essential.

Although most early experience with antivirals in pediatric practice was accrued in the inpatient setting, structural and biochemical modifications of antiviral compounds have led to the development of many agents with excellent bioavailability after oral administration. Many of these drugs are now used extensively in the outpatient setting (Table 240-1). However, severe viral infections, especially in immunocompromised hosts, still require aggressive parenteral therapy, usually in the inpatient setting (Table 240-2).

## HERPESVIRUSES

### Herpes Simplex Virus and Varicella-Zoster Virus

Acyclovir is the most useful agent for the treatment of HSV and VZV infections. Acyclovir is a synthetic purine nucleoside analog that, as noted above, has specificity for the HSV thymidine kinase, which phosphorylates the drug to the monophosphate form. The drug is then further phosphorylated by host cell thymidine kinases to the triphosphate form, which inhibits viral DNA polymerase. This initial dependence upon a viral, not a cellular, enzyme is the basis for acyclovir's selectivity and favorable safety profile. Acyclovir is most active against HSV-1 and HSV-2. It also has substantial activity against VZV but requires approximately 10-fold higher concentrations to inhibit replication of VZV compared to HSV. Typically in pediatric practice, acyclovir should be administered by parenteral or oral routes.

Acyclovir is available in oral formulations; however, less than 20% of an orally administered dose is absorbed. Therefore, oral administration is not appropriate for serious or life-threatening infections. Valacyclovir is the L-valyl ester of acyclovir, and after oral administration, it is rapidly converted to acyclovir by hepatic first-pass metabolism. Its bioavailability after oral administration exceeds 50%. Although valacyclovir has been used in adults for the treatment and suppression of genital herpes infections, there is currently no oral suspension available for children, and pediatric pharmacokinetic data are limited. Valacyclovir oral suspension (25 mg/mL or 50 mg/mL) may be prepared extemporaneously from 500-mg capsules for use in pediatric patients for whom a solid dosage form is not appropriate (Table 240-1).

Alternatives to acyclovir for HSV infections include penciclovir, a nucleoside antiviral agent, and its oral diacetyl ester prodrug, famciclovir. Both drugs have the same spectrum of activity as acyclovir. Following oral administration, famciclovir is converted by the liver into the active drug, penciclovir. Its bioavailability is approximately 70%. Famciclovir has been used in the suppression of genital herpes. Penciclovir is available for topical use and is licensed by the US Food and Drug Administration (FDA) for herpetic gingivostomatitis but should not be used in neonates or young infants with mucocutaneous herpetic infections.

Other topical antivirals are available for HSV infection. These are occasionally used to treat keratoconjunctivitis caused by HSV and include trifluorothymidine, iododeoxyuridine, and vidarabine ophthalmic drops. Parenteral vidarabine was formerly used in the treatment of HSV encephalitis, but is no longer available in an intravenous formulation.

Acyclovir is safe and generally well tolerated, although patients should be monitored for potential side effects. Neurotoxicity (paresthesias and other neurologic symptoms such as tremor, ataxia, and hallucinations) can occur in patients receiving acyclovir, particularly in the setting of renal insufficiency. Doses should be adjusted for patients with impaired creatinine clearance. Serum creatinine should be monitored in patients treated with acyclovir, especially if more

**TABLE 240-1 DOSAGES FOR ORAL (EXCEPT AS NOTED) ANTIVIRAL AGENTS COMMONLY USED FOR OUTPATIENTS**

| Drug | Indication | Age | Recommended Dosage |
|---|---|---|---|
| Acyclovir (Zovirax) | Varicella in immunocompetent host | ≥ 2 yr | 80 mg/kg/day in 4 divided doses × 5 days; maximum dose 3200 mg/day |
| | Herpes zoster in immunocompetent host | ≥ 12 yr | 4000 mg/day in 5 divided doses × 5–7 days |
| | Herpes simplex virus infection in immunocompromised host | ≥ 2 yr | 1000 mg/day in 3–5 divided doses × 7–14 days |
| | Herpes simplex virus prophylaxis in immunocompromised host | ≥ 2 yr | 600–1000 mg/day in 3–5 divided doses |
| | Suppression following neonatal herpes simplex virus infection | Following IV treatment of neonatal infection | 300 mg/m²/dose three times a day × 6 mo |
| | Genital herpes simplex virus infection (primary) | ≥ 12 yr | 1000–1200 mg/day in 3–5 divided doses × 7–10 days |
| | Genital herpes simplex virus infection (recurrent) | ≥ 12 yr | 1000–1200 mg/day in 3 divided doses × 3–5 days |
| | Chronic suppressive therapy for recurrent genital herpes simplex virus infection | ≥ 12 yr | 800–1200 mg/day in 2 divided doses for up to 1 yr |
| Adefovir (Hepsera) | Chronic hepatitis B | ≥ 12 yr | 10 mg once daily |
| | | | Not recommended in children <12 yr of age |
| Entecavir (Baraclude) | Chronic hepatitis B | ≥ 2 yr | Dosage dependent on age, weight, and prior therapy |
| Famciclovir (Famvir) | Genital herpes simplex virus infection (primary) | Adult | 750 mg/day in 3 divided doses × 7–10 days |
| | Genital herpes simplex virus infection (recurrent) | Adult | 250 mg/day in 2 divided doses × 3–5 days |
| | Chronic suppressive therapy for recurrent genital herpes simplex virus infection | Adult | 500 mg/day in 2 divided doses for up to 1 yr |
| Interferon α2b | Hepatitis B, hepatitis C | ≥ 3 yr | 3 to 6 million international units/m² 3 times weekly, subcutaneous/intramuscular; combined with oral ribavirin for chronic hepatitis C |
| Pegylated interferons α2a (Pegasys) | Hepatitis B, hepatitis C | ≥ 5 yr | 180 mcg/1.73 m² body surface area subcutaneously once weekly, to a maximum dose of 180 μg; combined with oral ribavirin for chronic hepatitis C; see Chapter 303 for further information. |
| α2b (PegIntron) | | ≥ 3 yr | 1.5 μg/kg once per week subcutaneously; no information on dosing in children <3 yr old; |
| | | | combined with oral ribavirin for chronic hepatitis C; side effects less common with pegylated formulations; see Chapter 303 for further information |
| Lamivudine (3TC; Epivir) | Chronic hepatitis B | ≥ 3 mo | For children 3 mo to 16 yr of age, 4 mg/kg, up to 150 mg per dose, twice daily |
| Oseltamivir (Tamiflu) | Influenza A and B | 1–12 yr | Treatment (× 5 days): |
| | | | < 15 kg: 30 mg twice daily |
| | | | 15–23 kg: 45 mg twice daily |
| | | | 23–40 kg: 60 mg twice daily |
| | | | > 40 kg: 75 mg twice daily |
| | | | Prophylaxis (× 7 days): |
| | | | Same doses as above but once daily |
| | | ≥ 13 yr | 75 mg twice daily for treatment (× 5 days); once daily for prophylaxis (× 7 days) |
| Ribavirin (Rebetol) | Chronic hepatitis C (with interferon therapy) | ≥ 3 yr | Dosing dependent on weight |
| Tenofovir (Viread) | Chronic hepatitis B | ≥ 12 yr | 300 mg daily |
| Telbivudine (Tyzeka) | Chronic hepatitis B | ≥ 16 yr | 600 mg daily |
| | | | Concomitant use of α interferon not recommended (increased neuropathy risk) |
| Valacyclovir (Valtrex) | Genital herpes simplex virus infection (primary) | Adolescent | 2 g/day in 2 divided doses × 10 days |
| | Genital herpes simplex virus infection (recurrent) | Adolescent | 1 g/day in 2 divided doses × 3 days |
| | Chronic suppressive therapy for recurrent genital herpes simplex virus infection | Adolescent | 500–1000 mg once daily for up to 1 yr |
| | Herpes labialis | ≥ 12 yr | 2 grams twice daily for 1 day taken 12 hours apart; therapy should be initiated at the earliest symptom (eg, tingling, itching, or burning). |
| | Varicella-zoster (chickenpox) | ≥ 2 yr | 20 mg/kg administered 3 times daily × 5 days; total dose should not exceed 1 gram 3 times daily |
| Valganciclovir (Valcyte) | Symptomatic congenital cytomegalovirus infection | Infants | 32 mg/kg/day in 2 divided doses × 6 months |
| Zanamivir (Relenza) | Influenza A and B | ≥ 7 yr (treatment) | Inhaled |
| | | ≥ 5 yr (prophylaxis) | |
| | | | 10 mg twice daily × 5 days (treatment) |
| | | | 10 mg once daily × 7 days (prophylaxis) |

**TABLE 240-2 DOSAGES FOR ANTIVIRAL AGENTS GIVEN PARENTERALLY (EXCEPT AS NOTED) FOR HOSPITALIZED PATIENTS**

| | | | |
|---|---|---|---|
| Acyclovir (Zovirax) | Neonatal herpes simplex virus infection | Birth–3 mo | 60 mg/kg/day in 3 divided doses × 14–21 days |
| | Herpes simplex virus encephalitis | ≥ 3 mo–12 yr | 60 mg/kg/day in 3 divided doses × 21 days |
| | | ≥ 12 yr | 30 mg/kg/day in 3 divided doses × 21 days |
| | Varicella in immunocompetent host | ≥ 2 yr | 30 mg/kg/day in 3 divided doses × 7–10 days |
| | Varicella in immunocompromised host | < 1 yr | 30 mg/kg/day in 3 divided doses × 7–10 days |
| | | ≥ 1 yr | 1500 mg/m²/day<br>OR<br>30 mg/kg/day in 3 divided doses × 7–10 days |
| | Herpes zoster in immunocompromised host | < 12 yr | 60 mg/kg/day in 3 divided doses × 7–10 days |
| | | ≥ 12 yr | 30 mg/kg/day in 3 divided doses × 7 days |
| | Herpes simplex virus in immunocompromised host | < 12 yr | 30 mg/kg/day in 3 divided doses × 7–14 days |
| | | ≥ 12 yr | 15 mg/kg/day in 3 divided doses × 7–14 days |
| | Herpes simplex virus prophylaxis in immunocompromised host (seropositive) | All ages | 15 mg/kg/day in 3 divided doses |
| | Genital herpes simplex virus infection (primary) | ≥ 12 yr | 15 mg/kg/day in 3 divided doses × 5–7 days |
| Cidofovir (Vistide) | Cytomegalovirus retinitis | Adult dose | 5 mg/kg once weekly × 2 doses, then 5 mg/kg once every 2 weeks |
| | Resistant herpes simplex virus | Adult dose | 5 mg/kg once weekly<br>OR<br>1 mg/kg 3 times per week<br>Concomitant therapy: 2 grams of probenecid 3 hours prior to each cidofovir dose, 1 gram at 2 hours and again at 8 hours after completion of 1 hour cidofovir infusion (total of 4 grams probenecid); ingestion of food prior to each dose of probenecid may reduce drug-related nausea and vomiting<br>Hydration: Suggested that 1 L of 0.9% (normal) saline solution be administered IV prior to each infusion of cidofovir; should administer over 1–2 hours; may administer a second liter over 1–3 hours at start of cidofovir infusion or immediately following infusion if tolerated |
| Foscarnet (Foscavir) | Cytomegalovirus retinitis | Adult dose | 180 mg/kg/day in 2 divided doses × 14–21 days, then 90–120 mg/kg once daily |
| | Resistant herpes simplex virus in immunocompromised host | Adult dose | 80–120 mg/kg/day in 2–3 divided doses |
| Ganciclovir (Cytovene) | Cytomegalovirus retinitis | Adult dose | 10 mg/kg/day in 2 divided doses × 14–21 days<br>Long-term suppression:<br>5 mg/kg/day × 7 days/wk<br>or<br>6 mg/kg/day × 5 days/wk |
| | Cytomegalovirus prophylaxis | Adult dose | 10 mg/kg/day in 2 divided doses × 1 wk, then 5 mg/kg/day daily for 100 days |
| | Symptomatic congenital cytomegalovirus infection | Neonates | 12 mg/kg/day, dosing every 12 h IV until able to complete 6 mo course with oral valganciclovir |
| Peramivir (Rapivab) | Influenza A<br>Influenza B | Adult dose | 600 mg single IV infusion over 15 to 30 minutes |
| Ribavirin (Virazole) | Respiratory syncytial virus | Pediatric dose | Standard ribavirin aerosol therapy: 6 g per 300 mL water for 18 h daily; short-duration therapy: 6 g per 100 mL water given for 2 h, 3 times per day |

than 5 to 7 days of therapy is anticipated. Acyclovir therapy can induce neutropenia, particularly in the context of long-term suppressive therapy following neonatal HSV infection, but this side effect is reversible with dose reduction or discontinuation. Acyclovir also can cause gastrointestinal symptoms, including anorexia, nausea, vomiting, and diarrhea.

The decision to treat HSV-1, HSV-2, and VZV infections depends on whether the infection is primary or recurrent; the clinical presentation; and host factors, such as age and underlying conditions. Primary infections are more often treated than recurrent infections because of the absence of viral-specific immunity. Because neonates and other immunodeficient hosts infected with HSV or VZV can experience substantial morbidity and mortality, parenteral antiviral therapy for these patients is recommended.

The diagnosis of infection caused by HSV-1 or HSV-2 in neonates is an indication for intravenous antiviral therapy. The use of high-dose intravenous acyclovir (60 mg/kg/day) is indicated for all clinical presentations of neonatal HSV infection (Chapters 225 and 304). Further, following such parenteral therapy, 6 months of oral suppressive treatment has been shown to improve outcomes. Intravenous acyclovir is also indicated for HSV encephalitis at any age and regardless of immune status. Antiviral therapy also is indicated for immunocompromised children with primary HSV-1 or HSV-2 infection. Although the risk of life-threatening dissemination is low even among severely immunocompromised patients, severe local symptoms can persist for 2 weeks or longer.

Acyclovir also can be considered for treatment of serious HSV infections in other patients in whom the indications are less well established. Examples of such patients include otherwise healthy children with severe herpetic gingivostomatitis and children with *eczema herpeticum*. If the patient is hospitalized, intravenous acyclovir may be used, but if the patient is not, oral therapy may be appropriate. Acyclovir in the oral capsule formulation is FDA-approved for treating primary and recurrent genital HSV virus infection, usually caused by HSV-2. The recommended dosage for adults and adolescents is 200 mg 5 times per day. Sexually active teenagers or sexually abused children may present with this infection and should be treated if the clinical symptoms are significant and the child is able to take capsules. Severe primary genital HSV, particularly in pregnant women, should be treated with intravenous acyclovir.

HSV isolates resistant to acyclovir, on the basis of mutations in the viral thymidine kinase or viral DNA polymerase genes, have been reported. Although these isolates have demonstrated diminished virulence in animal models, they have been associated with progressive mucosal infections in immunocompromised hosts. Alternative antiviral agents to consider for the therapy of patients infected with acyclovir-resistant isolates include foscarnet and cidofovir (Table 240-2). Foscarnet is an inorganic pyrophosphate analog that has activity against all human herpesviruses. It is only available in an intravenous formulation. Side effects of foscarnet include nephrotoxicity and electrolyte disturbances, including symptomatic derangements of both calcium and phosphate. Cidofovir is an acyclic phosphonate nucleotide analog that does not require viral thymidine kinase to convert it to its active form. Therefore, it is well suited to treat viruses that are resistant to acyclovir due to alterations in viral thymidine kinase. Cidofovir has a very long half-life because it accumulates intracellularly; it can be given once per week. Cidofovir therapy is associated with significant nephrotoxicity. Co-administration with probenecid and pre-hydration with crystalloid can ameliorate nephrotoxicity. Experience with these agents in pediatric patients is limited.

Acyclovir has good activity in vitro against VZV, but its use in acute varicella should be limited to patients at high risk for severe disease, such as children older than age 12 or immunocompromised individuals. If acyclovir is administered within 24 hours of the onset of rash, a more rapid decrease in fever and a modest reduction in the total number of lesions can be expected. Acyclovir also is effective in the treatment of reactivated VZV (herpes zoster, shingles). For immunocompromised patients with herpes zoster who have a high risk of dissemination, high-dose intravenous acyclovir should be administered. In healthy individuals with herpes zoster, treatment with oral acyclovir can decrease acute pain but may not have an impact on the development of postherpetic neuralgia. Oral valacyclovir or famciclovir is approved for the treatment of herpes zoster in adults, but no pediatric recommendations are available for this indication.

### Cytomegalovirus

Ganciclovir was the first effective antiviral agent available for the treatment of infections due to CMV. Ganciclovir is an acyclic analog of the nucleoside guanosine, which is phosphorylated by a CMV-specific viral kinase, the *UL97* gene product. It is subsequently triphosphorylated by host kinases. The triphosphate form of the drug has high affinity for CMV DNA polymerase and can inhibit viral replication. Ganciclovir has been used extensively in bone marrow and solid organ transplant recipients in prophylactic, preemptive, and treatment regimens. It also has been shown to be effective in the treatment of CMV retinitis in patients infected with HIV. In addition, ganciclovir has been demonstrated to be of benefit in newborns with symptomatic congenital CMV infection, improving both audiologic and neurodevelopmental outcomes. Ganciclovir has very poor oral bioavailability and should only be administered intravenously. Valganciclovir, the L-valine ester of ganciclovir, has excellent bioavailability after oral administration and has been used to prevent CMV disease in transplant patients, and to treat symptomatic congenital CMV infection in which 6 months of therapy has been shown to improve outcomes.

The main side effects of ganciclovir include myelosuppression (primarily neutropenia and, to a lesser extent, anemia and thrombocytopenia) and nephrotoxicity. Therefore, blood counts and serum creatinine should be monitored during treatment. Liver function tests should also be monitored in infants on long-term therapy for symptomatic congenital CMV infection. Because viral shedding in urine and oropharyngeal secretions is common in the context of CMV infection, care should be taken by the clinician to consider the goals of antiviral therapy, and not commence ganciclovir or valganciclovir therapy solely in response to a positive laboratory test for CMV. CMV isolates that are resistant to ganciclovir (most commonly because of mutations in the *UL97* phosphotransferase) have been described. Infection due to CMV isolates that are resistant to ganciclovir can be treated with either foscarnet or cidofovir.

## INFLUENZA VIRUSES

Although influenza vaccination remains the best strategy to reduce morbidity and mortality attributable to influenza virus infection, antiviral drugs are also effective for both prophylaxis and treatment. Two main classes of antivirals are available—adamantanes and neuraminidase inhibitors.

Amantadine and rimantadine are the two adamantanes that historically have been used for both prevention and treatment of influenza A virus infections. The mechanism of action of these drugs involves binding to the M2 ion channel, preventing acidification of host endosomes, a step that is essential for virus uncoating. Unfortunately, because of the high prevalence of resistance among circulating strains of influenza A virus, the use of adamantanes is no longer generally recommended.

The neuraminidase inhibitors, oseltamivir, zanamivir, and peramivir, are active against both influenza A and B viruses and act by inhibiting the release of the newly formed influenza virus from host cells. Oseltamivir or zanamivir, given to household contacts of influenza-infected individuals as prophylaxis, has been shown to reduce the incidence of proven influenza infections by 68% to 89%. Treatment with either drug, if initiated within 2 days of onset of symptoms, has been shown to shorten the duration of fever and other symptoms by 1 to 2 days. Oseltamivir may be used in children older than 2 weeks for treatment and older than 3 months as prophylaxis. Further, treatment with these drugs has been shown to improve the outcome in those severely ill (and should be given to all hospitalized for influenza) and those at risk for severe illness, which includes all children under 2 years of age. See Table 240-1 for dosing. For further recommendations for the use of these drugs for treatment or prophylaxis of high-risk people and their contacts, see the Centers for Disease Control and Prevention (CDC) Web site.

Oseltamivir is available as a suspension or tablet. Nausea and vomiting are the most common side effects. Zanamivir is administered by aerosol and its primary side effects include bronchospasm. It is approved for treatment of influenza in children 7 years and older, and for prophylaxis in children 5 years and older (Table 240-1). Peramivir is an intravenous neuraminidase inhibitor. It is not FDA-approved for use in children, but case reports have described its use in critically ill patients with influenza who have deteriorated following enterally administered oseltamivir therapy or those unable to tolerate enteral therapy. Resistant viruses have been identified, but they are not widespread.

## RESPIRATORY SYNCYTIAL VIRUS

Primary respiratory syncytial virus (RSV) infection often causes pneumonia or bronchiolitis, which can be particularly severe in children with chronic lung disease, congenital heart disease, or immunodeficiency, and in infants younger than 6 weeks. Recommendations for the use of the RSV-specific monoclonal antibody, palivizumab, for prophylaxis against RSV infection in high-risk infants are revised periodically by the American Academy of Pediatrics (AAP).

Ribavirin is a nucleoside analog that inhibits a wide spectrum of RNA and DNA viruses including RSV. It is approved by the FDA for administration as an aerosol to treat lower respiratory tract infections caused by RSV. Because the improvement associated with ribavirin use in studies has been limited to a small increase in oxygen saturation; because it must be given by aerosol, which causes concern about exposure of healthcare workers and pregnant women to ribavirin; and because of its high cost, the AAP suggests that therapy with ribavirin be considered for use in selected patients with documented, potentially life-threatening RSV infection.

### HEPATITIS B AND HEPATITIS C VIRUSES

Currently, seven antiviral agents have been approved by the FDA for treatment of adults with chronic hepatitis B infection. These agents, categorized as either interferons (IFN-α2b and pegylated interferon-α2a/α2b) or nucleoside or nucleotide analogues (eg, lamivudine, adefovir, entecavir, tenofovir, telbivudine), are used as monotherapy or in combination. Lamivudine is now considered the first-line therapy in adults, eclipsing interferon. Experience with and indications for antiviral therapy for chronic hepatitis B infection in children are limited. IFN-α, lamivudine, and adefovir were the first drugs approved for treatment of chronic hepatitis B infection in children, but success is widely variable. In September 2012, tenofovir was FDA-approved for children 12 years or older weighing over 35 kg with chronic hepatitis B infection. More recently, entecavir was approved for use in children 2 years and older with chronic hepatitis B infection and evidence of active viral replication and disease activity, and, with IFN-α, entecavir is emerging as a first-line antiviral regimen for children with chronic hepatitis B infection who are candidates for antiviral therapy.

For chronic hepatitis C infection, IFN-α therapy combined with oral ribavirin has been shown to be effective and is the only approved therapy for use in children (approved for children older than 3 years). The main adverse effects seen are an influenza-like illness, which usually resolves with continued therapy; neuropsychiatric problems, occurring in 10% to 20% of patients; and bone marrow suppression. Until recently, only IFN-α and ribavirin were approved by the FDA to treat adults and children with chronic hepatitis C infection. The recent development of novel and highly effective antivirals for hepatitis C virus has revolutionized the care of adults, but unfortunately these drugs are not yet licensed for pediatric use. Novel drugs include ledipasvir, sofosbuvir, daclatasvir, elbasvir, beclabuvir, grazoprevir, paritaprevir, ombitasvir, velpatasvir, and dasabuvir. Ledipasvir, ombitasvir, daclatasvir, elbasvir, and velpatasvir inhibit the virally encoded phosphoprotein, NS5A, which is involved in viral replication, assembly, and secretion, while sofosbuvir is metabolized to a uridine triphosphate mimic, which functions as an RNA chain terminator when incorporated into the nascent RNA by the NS5B polymerase enzyme. Dasabuvir and beclabuvir are also NS5B inhibitors. Paritaprevir and grazoprevir inhibit the nonstructural protein 3 (NS3/4) serine protease, a viral nonstructural protein that is the 70 kDa cleavage product of the hepatitis C virus polyprotein. It is hoped that these compounds will soon be licensed for pediatric use.

### SUGGESTED READINGS


Birkmann A, Zimmermann H. HSV antivirals-current and future treatment options. *Curr Opin Virol.* 2016;18:9-13.

De Clercq E, Li G. Approved antiviral drugs over the past 50 years. *Clin Microbiol Rev.* 2016;29:695-747.

Defresne F, Sokal E. Chronic hepatitis B in children: Therapeutic challenges and perspectives. *J Gastroenterol Hepatol.* 2016;doi: 10.1111/jgh.13459.

El-Guindi MA. Hepatitis C viral infection in children: Updated review. *Pediatr Gastroenterol Hepatol Nutr.* 2016;19:83-95.

Kimberlin DW, Baley J; American Academy of Pediatrics Committee on Infectious Diseases; Committee on Fetus and Newborn. Guidance on management of asymptomatic neonates born to women with active genital herpes lesions. *Pediatrics.* 2013;131:e635-e646.

Kimberlin DW, Jester PM, Sánchez PJ, et al. Valganciclovir for symptomatic congenital cytomegalovirus disease. *N Engl J Med.* 2015;372:933-943.

Mejias A, Ramilo O. New options in the treatment of respiratory syncytial virus disease. *J Infect.* 2015;71:S80-S87.

Naesens L, Stevaert A, Vanderlinden E. Antiviral therapies on the horizon for influenza. Curr Opin Pharmacol. 2016;30:106-115.

Zopf S, Kremer AE, Neurath MF, Siebler J. Advances in hepatitis C therapy: what is the current state—what comes next? *World J Hepatol.* 2016;8:139-147.


# 241 Antibacterial Therapy

Mark R. Schleiss

### INTRODUCTION

Antibacterial therapy in infants and children presents many unique challenges not faced in other clinical specialties. A major problem is the paucity of pediatric data regarding efficacy, pharmacokinetics, and optimal dosages; pediatric recommendations are therefore often extrapolated from studies in adults. Age-appropriate antibiotic dosing and toxicities must also be considered, taking into account the developmental status and physiology of children. The clinician must consider important differences among various age groups with respect to the pathogenic bacterial species responsible for pediatric infections. Specific antibiotic therapy is optimally driven by a microbiologic diagnosis, predicated on isolation of the pathogenic organism from a normally sterile body site, and supported by antimicrobial susceptibility testing. Given the inherent difficulties that can arise in collecting specimens from pediatric patients and given the increased risk of serious bacterial infection in young infants, much of pediatric infectious diseases practice is based on clinical diagnosis with empirical use of antibacterial agents before or even without eventual identification of the specific pathogen.

Several key considerations must be incorporated in decisions about the appropriate empirical use of antibacterial agents in infants and children. Recommendations for therapy often are dictated by the clinical syndrome and/or anatomic site of infection and the age of the child (Table 241-1). This information affects the choice of antimicrobial agent(s) and also the dose, dosing interval, route of administration (oral vs parenteral), and degree of urgency. The vaccination history may reflect reduced risk for some invasive infections but not necessarily elimination of risk of them. The risk of serious bacterial infection in pediatrics is also affected by the child's immunologic status, which may be compromised by immaturity (neonates), underlying disease (immunodeficiency), or treatment of underlying diseases with chemotherapy (malignancy) or immune modulators (rheumatologic disease). Infections in immunocompromised children often result from bacteria that are not considered pathogenic in immunocompetent children. The possibility of central nervous system (CNS) involvement must be considered in pediatric patients, because some bacteremic infections in childhood carry a significant risk for hematogenous spread to the CNS including *Haemophilus influenzae* type b, pneumococcus, and meningococcus.

Potential causative pathogens being empirically treated and patterns of antimicrobial resistance in the community must also be considered. Resistance to penicillins and cephalosporins (Table 241-2) is common among strains of *Streptococcus pneumoniae* and *Staphylococcus aureus* (ie, methicillin-resistant *S aureus* [MRSA]), often necessitating the use of other classes of antibiotics.

Although empirical broad-spectrum antibiotics are often employed in pediatric practice, empiricism must be balanced against the risk of potentiating selection of resistant microorganisms. Overuse of antibiotics is a major contributing factor to antimicrobial resistance, and the indiscriminate use of antibiotics alters the drug-resistance patterns of isolates not only from the individual being treated but also the community in general. Particular care should be taken not to treat viral diseases with antibiotics. Although overuse of antibiotics is often driven by the sincere desire to help patients, antibiotics do carry a significant risk, including side effects.

**TABLE 241-1 EMPIRIC DRUGS OF CHOICE BASED ON THE TYPE OF INFECTION**

| Diagnosis | Probable Pathogen(s) | Recommended Antibiotics | |
|---|---|---|---|
| | | **First-Line** | **Alternative** |
| **Ears and Sinuses** | | | |
| Acute otitis media | *Streptococcus pneumoniae*<br>*Haemophilus influenzae* (nontypeable)<br>*Moraxella catarrhalis* | Amoxicillin or amoxicillin-clavulanate | Cefdinir or azithromycin |
| Acute sinusitis | As above | Amoxicillin or amoxicillin-clavulanate | Cefdinir or cefuroxime |
| Otitis externa | *Staphylococcus aureus*<br>*Pseudomonas* | Neomycin/polymyxin B otic drops, +/– steroid drops | Ciprofloxacin or ofloxacin otic drops, +/– steroid drops |
| **Upper Airway** | | | |
| Pharyngitis | | | |
| Exudative | Group A *Streptococcus* (GAS) | Penicillin | Cephalexin or azithromycin or clindamycin |
| Membranous | *Corynebacterium diphtheriae* | Erythromycin | Penicillin |
| Epiglottitis | *H influenzae* type b | Cefotaxime or ceftriaxone | Cefuroxime or meropenem |
| **Lower Airway** | | | |
| Lobar pneumonia | *S pneumoniae* | Cefuroxime or amoxicillin-clavulanate | Clindamycin |
| Empyema | *S pneumoniae*<br>*S aureus*<br>GAS | Clindamycin + ceftriaxone<br>Vancomycin (if MRSA suspected) | |
| Interstitial and/or atypical pneumoniae | *Mycoplasma pneumoniae*<br>*Chlamydia pneumoniae*<br>*Legionella pneumophila* | Azithromycin or erythromycin | Doxycycline for children > 8 years of age |
| Pneumonia in infants | *Chlamydia trachomatis* | Azithromycin or erythromycin | Trimethoprim-sulfamethoxazole |
| **Ophthalmologic** | | | |
| Preseptal cellulitis | *S aureus*<br>GAS | Clindamycin | |
| Orbital cellulitis | *S aureus*<br>*H influenzae*<br>*S pneumoniae*, GAS, anaerobes | Meropenem<br>(+ vancomycin if MRSA suspected) | Ampicillin-sulbactam<br>(+ vancomycin if MRSA suspected) |
| Conjunctivitis | | | |
| Neonate < 5 days | *Neisseria gonorrhoeae* | Cefotaxime | |
| Neonate > 5 days | *Chlamydia trachomatis* | Azithromycin | Erythromycin |
| **Central Nervous System** | | | |
| Meningitis | | | |
| Neonate | Group B *Streptococcus*<br>*Escherichia coli*<br>*Listeria monocytogenes* | Ampicillin + cefotaxime | Meropenem |
| Infant, child, or adolescent | *S pneumoniae*<br>*Neisseria meningitidis* | Vancomycin, and cefotaxime or ceftriaxone | Vancomycin and meropenem |
| Brain abscess | | | |
| Without trauma | *S aureus*<br>Streptococci<br>Anaerobes | Vancomycin + ceftriaxone + metronidazole | Vancomycin + meropenem |
| **Abdomen** | | | |
| Peritonitis | | | |
| Primary | *S pneumoniae*<br>*E coli* | Ceftriaxone or cefotaxime | Meropenem |
| After perforation | Enterobacteriaceae<br>Anaerobes | Ampicillin + ceftriaxone + metronidazole | Meropenem, cefoxitin, cefotetan, or piperacillin-tazobactam |
| Peritoneal dialysis associated | *S aureus*<br>Coagulase-negative staphylococci<br>Enterobacteriaceae | Vancomycin + cefotaxime or ceftriaxone | Vancomycin + meropenem |
| **Renal** | | | |
| Urinary tract infection (pyelonephritis) | Enterobacteriaceae (*E coli* most frequent) | Cefotaxime or ceftriaxone | Ceftazidime or meropenem or piperacillin-tazobactam |
| Perinephric abscess | Enterobacteriaceae<br>*S aureus* | Oxacillin + cefotaxime or ceftriaxone<br>Vancomycin (if MRSA suspected) + cefotaxime or ceftriaxone | Oxacillin + gentamicin<br>Vancomycin + gentamicin (if MRSA suspected) |

(Continued)

**TABLE 241-1 EMPIRIC DRUGS OF CHOICE BASED ON THE TYPE OF INFECTION (CONTINUED)**

| | | Recommended Antibiotics | |
|---|---|---|---|
| **Diagnosis** | **Probable Pathogen(s)** | **First-Line** | **Alternative** |
| **Skin and Soft Tissue** | | | |
| Cellulitis | *S aureus*<br>GAS | Oxacillin or cefazolin or vancomycin (if MRSA suspected) | Clindamycin |
| Impetigo | GAS<br>*S aureus* | Cephalexin or dicloxacillin | Clindamycin or topical mupirocin |
| Fasciitis | GAS<br>*S aureus* | Oxacillin ± clindamycin or vancomycin ± clindamycin (if MRSA suspected) | |
| Myositis | *S aureus*<br>GAS | Oxacillin or vancomycin (if MRSA suspected) | Clindamycin |
| **Bones (Osteomyelitis)** | | | |
| Neonates | Group B *Streptococcus*<br>*S aureus*<br>Enterobacteriaceae | Oxacillin + cefotaxime or vancomycin + cefotaxime (if MRSA suspected) | |
| Acute hematogenous | *S aureus*<br>GAS | Oxacillin or cefazolin or vancomycin (if MRSA suspected) | Clindamycin |
| Children with sickle cell disease | *S aureus*<br>*Salmonella* (spp) | Oxacillin + cefotaxime or vancomycin + cefotaxime (if MRSA suspected) | |
| After puncture wound through gym shoe | *Pseudomonas aeruginosa* | Piperacillin/tazobactam | Ceftazidime |
| **Joints (Arthritis)** | | | |
| Neonates | Group B *Streptococcus*<br>*S aureus*<br>Enterobacteriaceae | Oxacillin + cefotaxime or vancomycin + cefotaxime (if MRSA suspected) | |
| Infants and children | *S aureus*<br>GAS<br>*S pneumoniae*<br>*Kingella kingae* | Oxacillin ± cefotaxime or vancomycin ± cefotaxime (if MRSA suspected) | |
| Adolescents | *S aureus*<br>GAS<br>*S pneumoniae*<br>*N gonorrhoeae* | Oxacillin or vancomycin (if MRSA suspected), and ceftriaxone (if *N gonorrhoeae* suspected) | |
| Postoperative infections | *S aureus*<br>Enterobacteriaceae | Vancomycin + cefotaxime | Vancomycin + piperacillin/tazobactam or vancomycin + meropenem |
| **Blood (Septicemia/Bacteremia)** | | | |
| Neonates | Group B *Streptococcus*<br>*E coli*<br>*L monocytogenes* | Ampicillin + cefotaxime or ampicillin + gentamicin (if meningitis excluded) | |
| Children | *S pneumoniae*<br>*S aureus*<br>GAS<br>*N meningitidis* | Ceftriaxone or cefotaxime (add vancomycin if MRSA suspected) | |
| Adolescents | *S pneumoniae*<br>*S aureus*<br>GAS<br>*N meningitidis*<br>*N gonorrhoeae* | Ceftriaxone or cefotaxime (add vancomycin if MRSA suspected) | |
| **Pericardium** | | | |
| Pericarditis | *S aureus*<br>*H influenzae*<br>*S pneumoniae* | Oxacillin ± ceftriaxone or cefotaxime; or vancomycin ± cefotaxime or ceftriaxone (if MRSA suspected) | Meropenem |

MRSA, methicillin-resistant *Staphylococcus aureus*.

## GENERAL PRINCIPALS OF ANTIBIOTIC THERAPY

### ANTIBIOTIC SELECTION

The decision to prescribe an antibiotic is generally based on proof or strong suspicion that the patient has a bacterial infection. In the febrile neonate or in the critically ill patient in whom there is some chance that bacterial infection may be a contributing factor, it is prudent to administer antibiotics effective against the most likely pathogens. If more than 1 antibiotic is active against the most likely pathogen(s), the antimicrobial agents should be chosen on the basis of relative toxicity and other factors. An important tenet of the use of antibiotic therapy is that once the pathogen is identified, the antibiotic with the narrowest spectrum of activity, lowest cost, and most convenient administration should be used.

**TABLE 241-2 MECHANISMS OF RESISTANCE TO β-LACTAM AGENTS**

- Alter target site (penicillin-binding protein)
  - A. Decrease affinity of PBP for β-lactam antibiotic
    - 1. Modify existing PBP
      - Create mosaic PBP
      - Mutate structural gene of PBP(s) (eg, ampicillin-resistant, β-lactamase–negative *Haemophilus influenzae*)
    - 2. Import new PBP (eg, mecA in methicillin-resistant *Staphylococcus aureus*)
- Destroy β-lactam antibiotic
  - A. Increase production of β-lactamase (increased transcription/translation, deregulation of expression, or modification of promoter)
  - B. Modify structure of resident β-lactamase (eg, extended-spectrum β-lactamases in *Klebsiella pneumoniae*)
  - C. Import new β-lactamase(s) with different spectrum of activity (eg, NDM-1 metallo-β-lactamase; requires zinc for function)
- Decrease concentration of β-lactam antibiotic inside cell
  - A. Restrict its entry (loss of porins)
  - B. Pump it out (efflux mechanisms)

### Age- and Risk-Specific Use of Antibiotics in Children

**Neonates** The causative pathogens of neonatal infections are typically acquired around the time of delivery from the maternal birth canal. Thus, empirical antibiotic selection must take into account the importance of these pathogens in neonates. Among the causes of neonatal sepsis in infants, group B *Streptococcus* (GBS) is the most common, although intrapartum antibiotic prophylaxis has greatly decreased the incidence of neonatal disease due to this agent. Gram-negative enteric organisms, in particular *Escherichia coli*, are other common causes of neonatal sepsis. Although rare, *Listeria monocytogenes* is also an important pathogen, insofar as it is intrinsically resistant to cephalosporin antibiotics, which are often used as empirical therapy in young children. All of these organisms can be associated with meningitis in the neonate; therefore, lumbar puncture should always be considered in the setting of bacteremic infections in this age group, and, if meningitis cannot be excluded, antibiotic management should include agents capable of crossing the blood-brain barrier.

**Older Children** Antibiotic choices in toddlers and young children were once driven by the high risk of this age group for invasive disease caused by *H influenzae* type b, but since the advent of conjugate vaccines, invasive disease due to this agent has declined dramatically. It is still appropriate to consider the use of antimicrobials that are active against this pathogen, particularly if meningitis is a consideration. The unfortunate refusal by some parents to accept immunizations in their children means that these agents must continue to be considered in the differential diagnosis of serious bacterial infections especially if vaccine compliance cannot be assured. Particularly important pathogens to be considered in this age group include *S pneumoniae, Neisseria meningitidis*, and *S aureus*. Antimicrobial resistance is commonly exhibited by *S pneumoniae* and *S aureus*. Strains of *S pneumoniae* that are resistant to penicillin and cephalosporin antibiotics are frequently encountered in clinical practice. Similarly, MRSA is highly prevalent in many regions. Resistance of *S pneumoniae* and that of MRSA is due to mutations that confer alterations in penicillin-binding proteins (PBPs), the molecular targets of penicillins and cephalosporins (see Table 241-2).

Depending on the specific clinical diagnosis, other pathogens that are commonly encountered include *Moraxella catarrhalis*, nontypeable strains of *H influenzae*, and *Mycoplasma pneumoniae*, which cause respiratory tract infections including pneumonia; group A *Streptococcus* (GAS), which causes pharyngitis, skin and soft tissue infections, osteomyelitis, septic arthritis, and, rarely, bacteremia with toxic shock syndrome; *Kingella kingae*, which causes bone and joint infections in young children; *Salmonella*, which causes enteritis, bacteremia, osteomyelitis, and septic arthritis; and viridans streptococci and *Enterococcus*, which cause endocarditis. This complexity underscores the importance of formulation of a clear clinical diagnosis, including an assessment of the severity of the infection, in concert with knowledge of local susceptibility patterns in the community.

**Immunocompromised and Hospitalized Patients** It is important to consider the risks associated with immunocompromising conditions (eg, malignancy, solid organ or hematopoietic stem cell transplantation) and the risks conferred by conditions leading to prolonged hospitalization (eg, intensive care, trauma, burns). Immunocompromised children are predisposed to develop a wide range of bacterial, viral, fungal, or parasitic infections. Prolonged hospitalization can lead to nosocomial infections, often associated with indwelling lines and catheters and commonly caused by gram-negative enteric organisms. In addition to the usual bacterial pathogens, *Pseudomonas aeruginosa* and enteric organisms, including *E coli, Klebsiella pneumoniae, Enterobacter*, and *Serratia*, are important considerations as opportunistic pathogens in these settings.

Selection of appropriate antimicrobials is challenging because of the diverse causes and scope of antimicrobial resistance exhibited by these organisms. Many strains of enteric organisms have resistance due to extended-spectrum β-lactamases (ESBLs). *P aeruginosa* encodes proteins that function as efflux pumps to eliminate multiple classes of antimicrobials from the cytoplasm or periplasmic space. In addition to these gram-negative pathogens, infections caused by *Enterococcus faecalis* and *Enterococcus faecium* are inherently difficult to treat. These organisms may cause urinary tract infection or infective endocarditis in immunocompetent children and may be responsible for a variety of syndromes in immunocompromised patients, especially in the setting of prolonged intensive care. The emergence of infections caused by vancomycin-resistant *Enterococcus* (VRE) has further complicated antimicrobial selection in high-risk patients and has necessitated the development of newer antimicrobials that target these highly resistant gram-positive infections. Although experience with many of these newer agents in the management of complex hospitalized pediatric patients is limited, they are important agents to be aware of.

A special situation affecting antibiotic use is the presence of an indwelling medical device, such as a venous catheter, ventriculoperitoneal shunt, stent, or other catheter. In these patients, in addition to *S aureus*, coagulase-negative staphylococci are also a major consideration. Coagulase-negative staphylococci seldom cause serious disease without a predisposing risk factor such as an indwelling medical device. Empirical antibiotic regimens must take this risk into consideration. In addition to appropriate antibiotic therapy, removal or replacement of the colonized prosthetic material is commonly required for cure.

## ROUTE OF ADMINISTRATION

The route chosen for the administration of antibiotics depends on a number of factors, including the severity of infection, pharmacokinetics, logistics of administration, and anticipated patient compliance. In some situations, intramuscular administration of antibiotics is appropriate. These situations include settings where parenteral administration of a long-acting agent, such as ceftriaxone, is desirable (eg, in the emergency department where a child is not ill enough to justify hospital admission).

A common practice, particularly for pediatric bone and joint infections, is to commence therapy by an intravenous route and then transition to oral therapy for completion of the treatment course. A number of prerequisites are desirable. The child should be demonstrating a positive clinical response with improvement on intravenous therapy, and a downward trend should be noted in elevated acute-phase reactants such as C-reactive protein, erythrocyte sedimentation rate, serum procalcitonin, or platelet count. Importantly, parental compliance must be assured. Oral antibiotic therapy, resulting in decreased costs and reduction of the risks attendant to maintenance of an indwelling venous catheter for long-term treatment of infections, is underused and should be considered if the above criteria can largely be met.

## DURATION OF THERAPY

With only rare exception, the duration of antibiotic administration recommended for specific infections is often based on uncontrolled experience, not on controlled trials. Guidelines concerning the duration of therapy for common pediatric infections are provided in this chapter. Clinicians should not commit patients to a rigid duration of therapy when the infection is initially identified; rather, therapy should be guided by clinical and laboratory response rather than by an arbitrary number of days.

Clinical monitoring usually involves sequential physical examinations with special reference to body temperature and the site originally infected. Fever and signs of inflammation should resolve within several days after appropriate antibiotics are initiated. Laboratory monitoring may include repeat bacterial cultures (eg, blood) to ensure sterilization, and for severe infections, it may be useful to monitor the peripheral white blood cell count and acute-phase reactants. Serial imaging studies may be valuable in some situations. An important principle to bear in mind is that the persistence of fever is not necessarily indicative of "antibiotic failure." Some infections (eg, pyelonephritis or empyema) are characterized by persistence of fever even in the setting of successful therapy. Unrelenting fever beyond that expected for the illness in question, lack of anticipated clinical improvement, a lack of sustained improvement in laboratory markers, and continued culture positivity from the focus of infection are appropriate reasons to consider changes in antibiotic therapy. In some settings, persistence of fever can indicate a focus of infection that may require surgical drainage.

## CLASSIFICATION OF ANTIBIOTICS

Antibiotics typically target unique gene products important in bacterial physiology and replication that fundamentally differ from those found in human cells. Four of the most common sites of antibacterial action that provide the molecular basis for antimicrobial therapeutics are: (1) inhibition of the synthesis of the bacterial cell wall; (2) inhibition of nucleic acid replication; (3) inhibition of protein synthesis; and (4) interference with folate metabolism (Table 241-3). The mechanism of action of an antibiotic impacts whether that agent is "bacteriostatic" (prevents the growth of the organism or maintains it in a stationary phase of growth) or "bactericidal" (kills the bacteria). Cell wall–active agents (eg, the penicillins, cephalosporins, carbapenems) are typically bactericidal, since disruption of cell wall integrity rapidly leads to lysis of the organism.

## ANTIBIOTIC RESISTANCE

The development of microbial drug resistance results from the widespread use of the growing array of antimicrobial agents, coupled with the ability of bacteria to acquire and spread resistance in addition to the capacity of humans to spread bacteria. There are, unfortunately, a large number of mechanisms by which bacteria develop resistance to antibiotics. Recent years have seen the emergence of ESBLs, β-lactamases that hydrolyze extended-spectrum cephalosporins that have an oxyimino side chain. Agents that are subject to hydrolysis include cefotaxime, ceftriaxone, and ceftazidime, as well as the oxyimino-monobactam agent aztreonam. ESBLs are frequently encoded by plasmids carrying genes encoding resistance to other drug classes, including aminoglycosides. Therefore, antibiotic options in the treatment of ESBL-producing organisms are sparse but generally include carbapenems. Another emerging class of resistant organisms in the United States demonstrates resistance mediated by the *K pneumoniae* carbapenemases (KPCs). These organisms are resistant to all β-lactam, cephalosporin, and carbapenem antibiotics, and reconsideration (and use) of agents developed many decades ago and not used for a long time until recently, such as colistin, needs to be considered in some cases.

Table 241-2 lists several of the resistance mechanisms relevant to β-lactam antibiotics. These include the production of enzymes that inactivate or modify the antibiotic, mutations that lead to decreased antibiotic uptake or an active efflux system, and alterations in molecular targets of antibiotic activity. Mechanisms differ across different species of bacteria, and this knowledge in turn impacts clinical decision making. For example, a bacterial strain that is resistant based on β-lactamase production may be treated with an antibiotic combined with a β-lactamase inhibitor, such as ampicillin-sulbactam. A bacteria that is resistant to β-lactamase based on modified PBPs (eg, *S pneumoniae*), on the other hand, will be impervious to treatment with a β-lactam/β-lactamase inhibitor combination.

**TABLE 241-3 CLASSIFICATION OF ANTIBIOTICS BY MECHANISM OF ACTION**

| | |
|---|---|
| Inhibition of cell wall synthesis | Vancomycin |
| | Penicillins |
| | Cephalosporins |
| | Aztreonam |
| | Carbapenems |
| Inhibition of nucleic acid synthesis | Rifampin |
| | Quinolones |
| | Metronidazole |
| Inhibition of protein synthesis | Aminoglycosides |
| | Tetracyclines |
| | Macrolides |
| | Clindamycin |
| | Linezolid |
| Inhibition of folate synthesis | Sulfonamides |
| | Trimethoprim |

## SPECIFIC ANTIBIOTICS

Table 241-4 provides a summary of currently licensed antibiotics in the United States that may be useful in clinical practice. For some agents, data on drug dosage in children are limited.

### PENICILLINS

Penicillin G is the "natural" or "native" penicillin; all other penicillins are semisynthetic compounds. The basic structure of penicillin consists of a 6-aminopenicillanic acid (6-APA) nucleus. A variety of side chains have been added to penicillin to produce the semisynthetic penicillins. The 6-APA nucleus has a thiazolidine ring connected to a β-lactam ring. The integrity of the β-lactam ring is necessary for antibacterial activity. Hence, organisms that produce β-lactamases, which break the ring configuration, render the drug inactive.

The penicillins are divided into 3 groups on the basis of their antibacterial spectrum as detailed in the following discussion.

#### Narrow-Spectrum, β-Lactamase–Sensitive Penicillins

The prototype of this group is penicillin G. Penicillin G is active against GAS, GBS, and many other streptococci, most *Neisseria* species, some Gram-negative anaerobes, and *Treponema pallidum*. Penicillin G is not active against most gram-negative aerobic organisms. Bacteria sensitive to penicillin generally have a minimal inhibitory concentration (MIC) less than 0.05 mg/L.

A 100,000-IU/kg dose of penicillin G (1 IU = 0.6 μg) administered intravenously results in serum concentrations in excess of 10 mg/L, 200-fold higher than the MIC of most sensitive bacteria. This antibiotic also diffuses widely, attaining therapeutic concentrations in most body tissues. For example, up to 25% of serum concentrations are attained in the cerebrospinal fluid (CSF) during the treatment of bacterial meningitis. The terminal half-life ($t_{1/2}$) of penicillin G is less than 1 hour, and penicillin G is eliminated primarily by renal tubular secretion. This secretion can be inhibited by co-administration of probenecid. Because renal dysfunction will compromise the elimination of penicillin, dosages may need to be reduced in patients with renal insufficiency. This is necessary only in the most severe renal insufficiency owing to the low toxicity of penicillin.

Penicillin V, the phenoxymethyl analog of penicillin G, is much more stable than is its parent compound and therefore better absorbed

**TABLE 241-4 COMMONLY USED PARENTERAL ANTIBACTERIAL AGENTS IN PEDIATRIC PRACTICE**

| Drug | Half-Life (hours) | Daily Dose | Side Effects |
|---|---|---|---|
| ***Antibiotics That Inhibit Cell Wall Synthesis*** | | | |
| **Penicillins** | | | |
| *Natural Penicillins* | | | |
| Penicillin G | 0.5 | 100,000–300,000 IU/kg divided every 4–6 h (maximum dose 4 million IU) | Coombs-positive hemolytic anemia, neutropenia, thrombocytopenia<br>Seizures if renal insufficiency present<br>Interstitial nephritis |
| Procaine penicillin G | 12 | 25,000–50,000 IU/kg IM × 1 | |
| Benzathine penicillin G | 2 weeks | 600,000 IU IM × 1 if < 27.5 kg<br>1.2 million IU IM × 1 if > 27.5 kg | |
| *Antistaphylococcal Penicillins* | | | |
| Nafcillin | 1 | 100–200 mg/kg divided every 6 h (maximum dose 2 g) | Neutropenia<br>Hepatitis |
| Oxacillin | 1 | 100–200 mg/kg divided every 6 h (maximum dose 2 g) | Neutropenia<br>Hepatitis |
| *Aminopenicillins* | | | |
| Ampicillin | 1.2 | 100–400 mg/kg divided every 4–6 h (maximum dose 2 g) | Rash if given with Epstein-Barr virus–related mononucleosis |
| *Antipseudomonal Penicillins* | | | |
| Piperacillin | 1 | 200–300 mg/kg divided every 4–6 h (maximum dose 4 g) | |
| *Penicillin + β-Lactamase Inhibitors* | | | |
| Ampicillin-sulbactam | 1.2 | 100–200 mg/kg divided every 6 h (maximum dose 3 g) | |
| Piperacillin-tazobactam | 1 | 240–300 mg/kg divided every 8 h (maximum dose 4 g) | Rash, eosinophilia, increased serum creatinine |
| **Cephalosporins** | | | |
| *First Generation* | | | |
| Cephalothin | 1 | 75–125 mg/kg divided every 6 h | Coombs-positive hemolytic anemia |
| Cefazolin | 2 | 50–100 mg/kg divided every 8 h (maximum dose 2 g) | |
| *Second Generation* | | | |
| Cefuroxime | 1 | 75–150 mg/kg divided every 8 h (maximum dose 1.5 g) | Serum sickness |
| Cefoxitin | 1 | 80–150 mg/kg divided every 4–6 h (maximum dose 2 g) | Coagulopathy |
| Cefotetan | 1.8–3.5 | 40–80 mg/kg divided every 12 h (maximum dose 2 g) | |
| *Third Generation* | | | |
| Ceftriaxone | 8.5 | 50–100 mg/kg divided every 12–24 h (maximum dose 2 g) | Gallbladder sludging, displacement of bilirubin from albumin binding sites |
| Cefotaxime | 1.2 | 100–150 mg/kg divided every 6–8 h (maximum dose 2 g) | |
| Ceftazidime | 1.8 | 100–150 mg/kg divided every 8 h (maximum dose 2 g) | |
| Ceftazidime-avibactam | 2 | 2.5 g (2 g ceftazidime/0.5 g avibactam) every 8 h (adults)<br>Pediatric dose not established; dosages based on ceftazidime are recommended | Diarrhea, nausea, vomiting, headache<br>Dosage adjustment necessary for patients with moderate to severe renal failure |
| *Fourth Generation* | | | |
| Cefepime | 2 | 150 mg/kg divided every 8 h (maximum dose 2 g) | |
| *Fifth Generation* | | | |
| Ceftaroline | 2.5 | 400 mg every 8 h or 600 mg every 12 h (adults)<br>12 mg/kg every 8 h (age 2–18 years)<br>8 mg/kg every 8 h (age 2 months through 2 years) | Diarrhea, nausea, headache<br>Dosage adjustment necessary for patients with moderate to severe renal failure |
| Ceftolozane-tazobactam | 2.5 | 1.5 g (1.0 g of ceftolozane and 0.5 g of tazobactam) every 8 h (adults)<br>Pediatric dose not established, but doses of 18 mg/kg of ceftolozane and 9 mg/kg of tazobactam are currently under study in children 3 months to 12 years, and 12 mg/kg of ceftolozane and 6 mg/kg of tazobactam in infants under 3 months | Nausea, headache, diarrhea, pyrexia |
| ***Glycopeptides*** | | | |
| Vancomycin | 4–6 | 40–60 mg/kg divided every 6–8 h (maximum dose 1 g) | Nephrotoxicity when used concomitantly with other potentially nephrotoxic agents<br>Histamine release (red man syndrome) during infusion |
| **Monobactams and Carbapenems** | | | |
| Aztreonam | 2 | 90–120 mg/kg divided every 6–8 h (maximum dose 2 g) | |
| Imipenem-cilastatin | 1 | 40–60 mg/kg divided every 6 h (maximum dose 1 g) | Lowers seizure threshold |
| Meropenem | 1 | 60–120 mg/kg divided every 8 h (maximum dose 1 g) | Neurotoxicity |

(Continued)

**TABLE 241-4 COMMONLY USED PARENTERAL ANTIBACTERIAL AGENTS IN PEDIATRIC PRACTICE (CONTINUED)**

| Drug | Half-Life (hours) | Daily Dose | Side Effects |
|---|---|---|---|
| ***Antibiotics That Inhibit Nucleic Acid Synthesis*** | | | |
| Ciprofloxacin | 4 | 20–30 mg/kg divided every 12 h (maximum dose 400 mg) | Cartilaginous damage in juvenile animals |
| Metronidazole | 6–14 | 30 mg/kg divided every 6 h (maximum dose 1 g) | Neutropenia, peripheral neuropathy, seizures, encephalopathy, disulfiram effect with alcohol |
| Rifampin | 1–6 | 20 mg/kg divided every 12 h (maximum dose 600 mg) | Hepatotoxicity |
| ***Antibiotics That Inhibit Protein Synthesis*** | | | |
| Aminoglycosides | | | |
| Gentamicin | 2 | 5–7.5 mg/kg divided every 8 h | Nephrotoxicity with trough > 2 μg/mL |
| | | | Irreversible vestibular ototoxicity with sustained peak > 12 μg/mL |
| | | | Neuromuscular blockade after IV push or with copious irrigation |
| Tobramycin | 2 | 5–7.5 mg/kg divided every 8 h | Nephrotoxicity with trough > 2 μg/mL |
| | | | Cochlear ototoxicity |
| Amikacin | 2 | 15 mg/kg divided every 8 h | Nephrotoxicity with trough > 10 μg/mL |
| | | | Cochlear ototoxicity |
| Others | | | |
| Azithromycin | 68 | 10 mg/kg once daily | Diarrhea, nausea, abdominal pain, loose stools |
| Clindamycin | 2.4 | 20-45 mg/kg/d divided every 6 or 8 h | Diarrhea, nausea, abdominal pain, rash |
| | | | *Clostridium difficile* infection, pseudomembranous colitis (less common in children than in adults) |
| Doxycycline | 15-24 | Adults: 100 mg administered every 12 h | Rash, photosensitivity, diarrhea, nausea, vomiting |
| | | Pediatrics: 2.2–4.4 mg/kg/d (up to 200 mg/d) divided every 12 h | Bone and tooth discoloration in children < 8 years of age, though not seen with short course |
| Colistin (colistimethate) | | 2.5–5 mg/kg divided every 6–12 h | Renal insufficiency |
| | | | Higher doses required in cystic fibrosis |
| Erythromycin | 2–4 | 15–50 mg/kg divided every 6–8 h (maximum dose 1 g) | Pyloric stenosis in neonates |
| | | | Increased transaminases |
| | | | Neuromuscular blockade |
| Linezolid | 4.5 | 30 mg/kg divided every 8 h (< age 12) | Reversible monoamine oxide inhibitor |
| | | 20 mg/kg divided every 12 h (adolescents and adults; maximum dose 600 mg) | |
| ***Antibiotics That Inhibit Folate Synthesis*** | | | |
| Trimethoprim (TMP)-sulfamethoxazole | 11 | 5–20 mg/kg TMP component divided every 6–8 h (maximum dose 320 mg TMP) | Bone marrow suppression |
| | | | Stevens-Johnson syndrome |

from the gastrointestinal tract. A 250-mg dose of this preparation results in concentrations roughly equivalent to those attained after twice the dose of orally administered penicillin G. Procaine penicillin is a commonly used intramuscular preparation that produces low (3 mg/L) concentrations of drug sustained over several days. It is best suited to the single-dose outpatient treatment of very sensitive organisms. Benzathine penicillin is another preparation given intramuscularly. Serum concentrations of less than 0.1 mg/L, sustained for as long as 3 to 4 weeks, are attained with this formulation. It is used to prevent recurrent GAS infections in patients with rheumatic fever when compliance with oral therapy may be an issue.

#### Broad-Spectrum, β-Lactamase–Sensitive Penicillins

**Aminopenicillins** Examples of aminopenicillins include (parenteral) ampicillin and (oral) amoxicillin. The activity of the aminopenicillins against most gram-positive bacteria is similar to that of penicillin. Aminopenicillins are, however, more active than penicillin against enterococci, *L monocytogenes,* and non-β-lactamase–producing *H influenzae.* They also are active against some *E coli, Shigella, Salmonella,* and indole-negative *Proteus* species. Amoxicillin is a drug of choice for the treatment of acute otitis media. It is also available in a formulation combined with the β-lactamase inhibitor clavulanate, which is also recommended for treatment of otitis media and sinusitis. Similarly, ampicillin is available in combination with the β-lactamase inhibitor sulbactam.

The serum concentration of ampicillin after a 1-g intravenous dose is approximately 40 mg/L; after a 500-mg dose taken orally, it is approximately 4 mg/L. Concentrations of amoxicillin are usually twice those of ampicillin after an equivalent oral dose. The distribution, $t_{1/2}$, and excretion characteristics of the aminopenicillins are similar to those of penicillin.

**Ureidopenicillins** Ureidopenicillins include piperacillin, azlocillin, and mezlocillin. These antibiotics have a broader spectrum of gram-negative activity than do the aminopenicillins and include activity against most strains of *P aeruginosa.* The usual MICs of *P aeruginosa* range from 12 to 25 mg/L, with piperacillin consistently being the most active agent. Maximum serum concentrations of these agents are usually in excess of 150 mg/L after a 3- to 5-g parenteral dose. These antibiotics are used almost exclusively in the treatment of urinary tract, lung, and bloodstream infections caused by ampicillin-resistant enteric gram-negative pathogens. Piperacillin is also available combined with the β-lactamase inhibitor tazobactam in a proprietary formulation to enhance activity against β-lactamase–producing bacteria.

**β-Lactamase–Resistant Penicillins**

These penicillins include parenteral agents (methicillin, nafcillin, and oxacillin) and oral agents (cloxacillin, dicloxacillin, and flucloxacillin). The principal bacteriologic advantage of this group of antibiotics is their activity against β-lactamase–producing staphylococci. Most isolates of methicillin-sensitive *S aureus* have MICs of 0.25 to 0.5 mg/L. These antibiotics are less active than penicillin G against other gram-positive bacteria, and they are inactive against gram-negative enteric organisms and anaerobes. Maximum serum concentrations after a 1-g intravenous dose of methicillin, nafcillin, or oxacillin range from 20 to 40 mg/L, whereas after a 500-mg oral dose of cloxacillin, they range from 4 to 8 mg/L. Dicloxacillin and flucloxacillin have enhanced absorption after oral administration. Thus, serum concentrations of these agents are twice those of cloxacillin after an equivalent oral dose. This group of penicillins is used almost exclusively for the treatment of mild, moderate, and severe infections caused by methicillin-sensitive *S aureus,* including cellulitis, pyomyositis, septic arthritis, osteomyelitis, pneumonia, and septicemia.

**Toxicity of Penicillins**

The adverse reactions of all penicillins are similar. In general, these agents are well tolerated; however, suspension formulations tend to have an unpleasant taste and aftertaste and, as a result, may be poorly accepted. All penicillins have a wide toxic-to-therapeutic ratio, although they can cause hypersensitivity reactions, neurotoxicity, nephrotoxicity, and hematologic toxicity.

Hypersensitivity reactions are relatively common and include rashes, serum sickness, anaphylaxis, nephritis, and drug fever. Urticarial skin reactions and anaphylaxis, which occur within 20 to 30 minutes after a dose, are termed immediate reactions. These are the most dangerous reactions and constitute absolute contraindications to future treatment with a penicillin derivative. Fortunately, the incidence of anaphylaxis is only 0.01% to 0.02% of individual courses of therapy.

Nonurticarial skin eruptions that occur several days after the initiation of a course of penicillin are relatively common. Many such eruptions represent the rash of a viral infection for which an antibiotic has been inappropriately prescribed. Patients manifesting these sorts of reactions should not be labeled "penicillin-allergic."

Convulsions and other forms of CNS irritation may occur when high doses of a penicillin have been administered, particularly to patients with compromised renal function. Such reactions are also more likely when high CSF concentrations of drug are attained, such as in patients with meningeal inflammation.

Interstitial nephritis can occur during therapy with any penicillin, although it is most frequently associated with the administration of methicillin. Hypokalemia is another side effect of high-dose penicillin therapy.

Coombs-positive hemolytic anemia may occur with any of the penicillins, as may neutropenia. Neutropenia is most common among patients receiving a β-lactamase–resistant penicillin and usually resolves when the antibiotic is stopped. Decreased platelet aggregation, which may precipitate bleeding, has been noted at high concentrations of most penicillins.

In addition to the reactions noted above, which are common to all of the penicillins, ampicillin or amoxicillin can cause a characteristic nonurticarial maculopapular rash that does not appear to have an allergic etiology. This rash usually appears 3 to 4 days after the onset of therapy and is classically described with ampicillin when given during intercurrent infectious mononucleosis.

## CEPHALOSPORINS

The cephalosporins are currently divided into 5 "generations," with original agents being referred to as first-generation cephalosporins and the most recent agents being fourth or fifth generation (Table 241-5). In general, the spectrum of activity of the cephalosporins increases with each generation (ie, enhanced activity against many gram-negative organisms). Cephalosporins should not be used to treat infections due to *L monocytogenes* or *Enterococcus.*

These agents may also be useful in patients who are intolerant to penicillins. Although cephalosporins and penicillins share the β-lactam ring structure, the true incidence of cross-reactivity to cephalosporins in skin test–confirmed penicillin-allergic patients is less than 5%. Cephalosporins should not be administered to patients with a history of immunoglobulin (Ig) E–mediated hypersensitivity reactions to penicillins, as similar reactions to cephalosporins may be observed.

**First-Generation Cephalosporins**

These cephalosporins are active against most staphylococci (excluding MRSA), pneumococci, and streptococci. MICs against sensitive gram-positive organisms are usually less than 0.5 mg/L. Their activity against aerobic gram-negative bacteria and against anaerobes is limited. Maximum serum concentrations after a 500-mg dose of oral cephalexin are approximately 20 mg/L, whereas they are 100 mg/L after 1-g intravenous doses of cefazolin. These antibiotics distribute widely throughout the body but do not penetrate well into CSF. Therefore, they must not be used to treat meningitis. Their $t_{1/2}$ ranges from 30 minutes to 1.5 hours, and they are eliminated unchanged in the urine. Doses may need adjustment in the presence of renal insufficiency, although these agents have a wide toxic-to-therapeutic ratio.

The first-generation cephalosporins are rarely drugs of first choice, although they are useful in outpatient management of skin and soft tissue infection not due to MRSA. Liquid suspensions are more palatable than those prepared for dicloxacillin or clindamycin, which has implications for compliance in young children. These antibiotics are useful in the perioperative prophylaxis of surgical procedures that carry a high risk of postoperative infections caused by staphylococcal species, such as those involving the cardiovascular system and bones.

**Second-Generation Cephalosporins**

These cephalosporins have a broader bacteriologic spectrum than do the first-generation agents. For example, cefuroxime is not only more active against gram-negative enteric bacteria but is active against both

**TABLE 241-5 REPRESENTATIVE CEPHALOSPORINS CLASSIFIED BY GENERATION**

| Route | First | Second | Third | Fourth | Fifth |
|---|---|---|---|---|---|
| Parenteral | Cephalothin | Cefotetan | Cefotaxime | Cefepime | Ceftaroline fosamil |
| | Cefazolin | Cefoxitin | Ceftazidime (also available with avibactam) | Cefpirome | Ceftobiprole |
| | | Cefuroxime | Ceftizoxime | | Ceftolozane (plus tazobactam) |
| | | | Ceftriaxone | | |
| Oral | Cephalexin | Cefaclor | Cefixime | | |
| | Cefadroxil | Cefuroxime | Cefdinir | | |
| | | Cefprozil | Cefditoren | | |
| | | | Cefpodoxime | | |
| | | | Ceftibuten | | |

β-lactamase-negative and -positive strains of *H influenzae,* generally at concentrations below 2 mg/L. The major bacteriologic advantage of the cephamycins cefoxitin and cefotetan is their activity against a broad range of anaerobic pathogens, with most anaerobes being inhibited by less than 16 mg/L. Maximum serum concentrations of cefuroxime and cefoxitin after a 1-g intravenous dose are approximately 100 mg/L. The half-lives of the second-generation agents are similar to those of the first-generation agents. Also, like the first-generation, excretion of second-generation cephalosporins is primarily renal, and they distribute widely but do not attain sufficient concentrations in CSF to warrant their use in the treatment of bacterial meningitis.

Second-generation cephalosporins, like the first-generation agents, are rarely drugs of first choice. Cefuroxime, available in intravenous and oral forms, has been actively promoted because of its activity as a good agent for the treatment of a variety of infections in children, including cellulitis, osteomyelitis, septic arthritis, and pneumonia. The most common use of cefuroxime is in respiratory tract infections and occasionally in acute otitis media and sinusitis. Cefoxitin and cefotetan are effective agents in the prevention and treatment of intra-abdominal or pelvic infections.

#### Third-Generation Cephalosporins

Third-generation cephalosporins retain much of the gram-positive activity of the first 2 generations, although their antistaphylococcal activity is reduced 5- to 10-fold. They are remarkably active against most gram-negative enteric isolates, with MICs usually less than 0.5 mg/L. Ceftazidime is also active against most isolates of *P aeruginosa.* Maximum serum concentrations of the third-generation agents range from 50 to 150 mg/L after a 1-g intravenous dose. In healthy subjects, their half-lives range from 1 hour (cefotaxime) to between 6 and 8 hours (ceftriaxone). These antibiotics diffuse well into most tissues. Cefotaxime and ceftriaxone, in particular, penetrate well into the CSF, and they are approved by the Food and Drug Administration (FDA) for the therapy of bacterial meningitis in children. Excretion of these agents is primarily renal.

Settings in which third-generation cephalosporins are recommended include empiric therapy of suspected bacterial meningitis, pyelonephritis, and suspected infections in certain immunocompromised hosts. Ceftriaxone also is the drug of choice for infections caused by *N gonorrhoeae.*

Although these antibiotics show excellent activity against a wide variety of Enterobacteriaceae, their widespread use has led to the development of antibiotic resistance. Bacteria containing plasmid-encoded ESBLs are considered resistant to all cephalosporins and have rapidly spread over the past decades, especially among strains of *E coli* and *K pneumoniae.* Although their prevalence has been low in US pediatric populations, clinicians should continue to be judicious in their use of third-generation cephalosporins. All microbiology laboratories should screen Enterobacteriaceae for the presence of ESBL.

Ceftriaxone is eliminated by both renal and biliary clearance. It can cause biliary sludging. It can precipitate if used together with calcium, leading to severe reactions. The FDA specifies that ceftriaxone should not be mixed with calcium-containing products and that ceftriaxone and calcium should not be administered in the same or different infusion lines or sites in any patient within 48 hours of each other. This can be problematic in children requiring total parenteral nutrition. Due to its high level of protein binding with subsequent displacement of bilirubin, ceftriaxone should not be used in neonates with hyperbilirubinemia, due to the theoretical risk of kernicterus.

Ceftazidime/avibactam was approved by the FDA in 2015. This antibiotic is a fixed-dose combination drug containing ceftazidime and a novel non-β-lactam β-lactamase inhibitor avibactam. Current indications include complicated intra-abdominal infections and complicated urinary tract infections. It may also be useful for the treatment of infection due to KPCs. Pediatric experience is limited.

#### Fourth-Generation Cephalosporins

This generation of cephalosporins combines the antistaphylococcal activity (excluding MRSA) of first-generation agents with enhanced gram-negative spectrum compared with third-generation cephalosporins. Currently, cefepime is the only available fourth-generation cephalosporin in the United States. Cefepime has excellent activity against multidrug-resistant gram-negative bacteria including *P aeruginosa,* as well as bacteria that produce the AmpC-inducible β-lactamase. Use might include therapy of infections suspected or proved to be caused by multidrug-resistant pathogens or in treating infections in immunocompromised hosts at risk of infections caused by *Pseudomonas* species and other multidrug-resistant gram-negative rods (eg, cystic fibrosis).

#### Fifth-Generation Cephalosporins

The first-in-class of the fifth-generation cephalosporins is ceftaroline. This agent exhibits broad-spectrum activity against gram-positive bacteria, including MRSA and more resistant strains of *S aureus,* such as vancomycin-intermediate *S aureus* (VISA), heteroresistant VISA (hVISA), and vancomycin-resistant *S aureus* (VRSA). Ceftaroline is also active against many respiratory pathogens including *S pneumoniae, H influenzae,* and *M catarrhalis.* Although pediatric experience is limited, it is indicated in complicated skin and soft tissue infections and community-acquired pneumonia. A second agent from this group, ceftobiprole, is not yet approved for use in the United States.

Another fifth-generation cephalosporin, ceftolozane, is a derivative of ceftazidime with improved activity against *Pseudomonas* species. It is not stable against most ESBLs or carbapenemases. It is marketed in combination with the β-lactam inhibitor tazobactam to improve its activity against β-lactamase–producing Enterobacteriaceae. Ceftolozane-tazobactam is approved in a dosage of 1 g/0.5 g administered every 8 hours by the intravenous (IV) route. Clinical decisions based on MIC determinations will be essential to make the best use of a specific β-lactam/β-lactamase inhibitor combination in individual patients.

#### Toxicity of Cephalosporins

Serious adverse reactions due to cephalosporins are uncommon. Allergic reactions are seen in approximately 5% of courses. As with most antibiotics, the full spectrum of hypersensitivity reactions may occur, including rash, fever, eosinophilia, serum sickness, and anaphylaxis. Adverse reactions attributable to irritation at the site of administration are common. Reactions also include local pain after intramuscular injection, phlebitis after intravenous administration, and minor gastrointestinal complaints after oral administration.

Therapy with cephalosporins leads to the development of a positive direct Coombs reaction during approximately 3% of courses. This is, however, not commonly associated with hemolytic anemia. Some of the cephalosporins are associated with dose-related nephrotoxicity, whereas others are associated with interstitial nephritis.

The third-generation drugs may cause transient elevations of liver function tests and blood urea nitrogen. These broad-spectrum cephalosporins also have a profound inhibitory effect on the vitamin K–synthesizing bacterial flora of the gastrointestinal tract.

### GLYCOPEPTIDES

#### Vancomycin

The prototypical member of this class of antibiotics is vancomycin. The primary activity of this cell wall–active antibiotic is against gram-positive bacteria. Despite its introduction several decades ago, vancomycin recently has gained widespread use. The reasons relate to the emergence and increasing prevalence of several important multidrug-resistant pathogens. Most clinical isolates of *S aureus* and coagulase-negative staphylococci, including those that are methicillin-resistant, are inhibited by less than 1.6 mg/L of this antibiotic. However, recent reports of increasing MICs of *S aureus* strains to vancomycin have been associated with treatment failure. VRE also are being reported at an increasing rate, especially with hospital-acquired infections. Vancomycin is active against multidrug-resistant pneumococci. Gram-positive bacilli, including *Clostridium* species, are very sensitive to vancomycin, but gram-negative bacteria are resistant.

Vancomycin is not absorbed from the gastrointestinal tract. Maximum serum concentrations after a 10-mg/kg intravenous dose are approximately 25 mg/L, 6-fold higher than the MICs of the usual bacteria being treated. It diffuses quite widely throughout the body and, during meningeal inflammation, attains concentrations in CSF that are approximately 10% to 20% of serum concentrations. The $t_{1/2}$ of vancomycin is approximately 4 to 6 hours in patients with normal renal function. The drug is excreted unmetabolized, almost exclusively in the urine. Doses should be reduced in patients with decreased renal function and levels monitored.

**Toxicity** Vancomycin historically has had a reputation for toxicity. Many of its original adverse reactions, including ototoxicity and nephrotoxicity, were probably due to impurities in the formulation. Now that a more purified form is available, these adverse reactions are uncommon, although nephrotoxicity may occur with concomitant administration of other potentially nephrotoxic agents (eg, aminoglycosides). One of the more common side effects is the "red man" syndrome, which occurs during the infusion. It is characterized by fever, chills, and a pruritic rash usually involving the head, neck, and chest. Although more likely to occur after rapid infusion of vancomycin, red man syndrome may also occur after slow infusions and appears to be mediated by histamine. It may be treated or prevented with the use of antihistamines. It is not a contraindication to further vancomycin therapy.

### Telavancin

Telavancin is a novel glycopeptide antibiotic recently approved by the FDA. Pediatric experience is limited. It is indicated for skin and skin structure infections caused by *S aureus* (including MRSA), GAS, and *E faecalis* (vancomycin-susceptible isolates only). It is also approved for hospital-acquired (including ventilator-associated) pneumonia caused by *S aureus*. The recommended adult dose is 10 mg/kg IV every 24 hours for 7 to 21 days. It appears to be more nephrotoxic than vancomycin. Telavancin has been associated with prolongation of the QT interval.

**Dalbavancin and Oritavancin** Dalbavancin's unique characteristic is its long half-life (150–250 hours). In adults with normal renal function, the dose is 1000 mg IV, followed 1 week later by 500 mg IV. This agent can be considered when MRSA is confirmed or strongly suggested. Dalbavancin is not active against vancomycin-resistant *S aureus*. It is approved by the FDA for bacterial skin and soft tissue infections.

Oritavancin is a vancomycin derivative with indications similar to that of dalbavancin. It has a half-life of approximately 250 hours. The dosage for adults is a single 1200-mg dose, administered IV over 3 hours. There is no pediatric experience yet with this agent.

## COLISTIN

Colistin, also known as polymyxin E, belongs to the class of polypeptide antibiotics known as polymyxins. It was developed many decades ago but fell out of favor because of its substantial nephrotoxicity. Colistin is effective against most gram-negative bacilli, including strains producing ESBL or KPCs, and so has re-emerged in recent years as a therapeutic option in critically ill patients with infections caused by these highly resistant organisms. Resistance to colistin is rare. Two forms of colistin are available commercially: colistin sulfate and colistimethate sodium. Colistimethate sodium is the formulation marketed in the United States.

## AZTREONAM

Aztreonam is the first member of a unique class of antibiotics referred to as monobactams. Although monobactams are β-lactam antibiotics, their structure is so different that cross-reactivity does not appear to be a problem; they can be prescribed for patients with penicillin or cephalosporin allergies. Aztreonam is resistant to a broad range of β-lactamases produced by gram-negative bacteria and therefore is active in vitro against many gram-negative organisms. Activity against gram-positive bacteria is minimal. In comparison with the aminoglycosides, aztreonam appears to be less nephrotoxic and ototoxic. Clinical experience in children is limited.

## CARBAPENEMS

Imipenem, meropenem, doripenem, and ertapenem are members of the carbapenem β-lactam antibiotic family. Because imipenem is rapidly metabolized by renal brush-border enzymes, it is administered with cilastatin, a substance that inhibits imipenem metabolism by the kidney. Insofar as they are more stable in vivo to inactivation by human renal dehydropeptidase, meropenem, doripenem, and ertapenem are administered without cilastatin. The carbapenems have activity against gram-negative and gram-positive aerobes and anaerobes. Carbapenems are useful in the treatment of ESBL-producing gram-negative bacteria that are resistant cephalosporins. In addition, they can be used as monotherapy for polymicrobial infections, which potentially include anaerobes such as intra-abdominal infection and necrotizing fasciitis. An important limitation of ertapenem is its lack of activity against *P aeruginosa*. Doripenem, on the other hand, has exceptional activity against *P aeruginosa*. These antibiotics diffuse widely throughout the body and have excellent penetration into CSF. Only meropenem has an FDA-approved indication for the therapy of meningitis in children. These agents are all administered by the parenteral route. They appear to have toxicity profiles similar to that of other β-lactam agents. Imipenem is epileptogenic in high doses, whereas meropenem appears to have less neurotoxicity.

## RIFAMPIN

Rifampin is active against a wide range of gram-positive and gram-negative bacteria. It also is active against the majority of *Mycobacterium tuberculosis* strains, with MICs less than 0.5 mg/L. Rifampin is given orally and is well absorbed from the gastrointestinal tract. Maximum serum concentrations of 8 mg/L are usually attained after a 600-mg dose. Rifampin penetrates well into most body tissues and fluids, including tears; saliva; bone; liver; lungs; and other fluids such as pleural, ascitic, and CSF (the latter even in the absence of inflammation). The $t_{1/2}$ of rifampin ranges from 2 to 5 hours. It is metabolized in the liver and excreted principally in the bile and, to a lesser degree, in the urine. All patients receiving this antibiotic should be advised that their bodily secretions, including tears, saliva, sweat, and urine will develop a reddish-orange discoloration. This is especially important for patients who wear soft contact lenses, which may be permanently discolored. Important drug interactions with rifampin have been recognized. For example, it enhances the metabolism of fluconazole, oral contraceptives, warfarin, propranolol, and anticonvulsants, all of which are metabolized in the liver. Doses of these concurrently administered agents may need to be increased to maintain therapeutic concentrations.

The use of rifampin as a single agent is limited by the fact that bacteria can rapidly develop resistance. It is, however, one of the first-line agents to be used as part of combination therapy for most forms of tuberculosis. It also is the antibiotic of choice for the prophylaxis of children with exposure to patients with infections caused by *H influenzae* type b and *N meningitidis*. Rifampin also has been used to eradicate upper respiratory carriage of GAS. It may also be useful in combination with antistaphylococcal agents in the management of catheter-associated infections due to these organisms.

Hypersensitivity reactions include dermatitis and a flu-like syndrome occasionally with thrombocytopenia, hemolytic anemia, and acute renal failure. Cholestatic hepatitis is another possible adverse reaction.

## QUINOLONES

The prototype of the quinolone antibiotics is nalidixic acid. This naphthyridine derivative has been used almost exclusively as a urinary antiseptic. It is as active as ampicillin against gram-negative enteric isolates, but has no useful activity against *Pseudomonas* species or gram-positive bacteria. Because nalidixic acid is only partially absorbed from the gastrointestinal tract, large doses are necessary to attain therapeutic urinary concentrations. These high doses have caused side effects, including visual disturbances. An additional problem has been the rapid development of bacterial resistance during therapy. These factors have limited the use of this antibiotic.

Research directed at modifying the chemical structure of nalidixic acid resulted in the development of the ever-growing family of fluorinated quinolone derivatives, including ciprofloxacin, ofloxacin, levofloxacin, gatifloxacin, and moxifloxacin. The spectrum of activity of these derivatives now includes gram-positive bacteria (including some strains of MRSA) and many enteric organisms. Quinolones may be given IV, and most quinolones are absorbed well after oral administration, and thus represent the first agents available for the oral treatment of systemic infections caused by multidrug-resistant gram-negative enteric isolates. Ciprofloxacin has the most activity against *Pseudomonas*, and thus, it is often useful for oral therapy of such infections. These agents are also of great value because their activity is unrelated to that of other antibiotics and resistance is not plasmid-borne. In adults, the quinolones may be preferred over alternate agents for treatment of complicated urinary tract infection, suspected bacterial gastroenteritis, osteomyelitis caused by gram-negative bacilli, and invasive external otitis.

#### Toxicity

In animal studies, the quinolones cause cartilaginous damage in young animals. This limited their use in children to recalcitrant infections for which alternatives were lacking. A body of data emerging over the past 25 years suggests that quinolones may be generally safe for administration to children. However, the American Academy of Pediatrics Committee on Infectious Diseases recommends that the use of quinolones should be limited in children because of high rates of resistance seen with overuse and the theoretical risk of joint injury. There are specific circumstances in which a quinolone may be the most appropriate antibiotic, such as in urinary tract infections due to *Pseudomonas* species or other multidrug-resistant gram-negative bacteria or if other antibiotics are contraindicated because of allergy.

## METRONIDAZOLE

The antibacterial activity of metronidazole is limited to anaerobes, with greatest activity against gram-negative anaerobic bacilli such as *Bacteroides* and *Fusobacterium,* most of which have MICs under 3.12 mg/L. Activity against gram-positive anaerobic cocci is less consistent, with about 75% of such strains being inhibited by 12.5 mg/L.

Metronidazole can be administered intravenously, orally, or rectally. Maximum serum concentrations after a 7.5-mg/kg dose administered intravenously are 20 to 25 mg/L. Concentrations after an equivalent oral dose are similar, and those after an equivalent rectal dose are about half. The drug diffuses well into all tissues; therapeutic concentrations can be attained in CSF, bile, bone, and abscesses. The $t_{1/2}$ of metronidazole is approximately 8 hours. It is metabolized to acid and hydroxy metabolites. Between 60% and 80% is eliminated by the kidneys, and 6% to 15% is eliminated in the feces. Hepatic insufficiency prolongs the $t_{1/2}$ of unchanged metronidazole, and doses usually have to be adjusted. Renal insufficiency usually does not necessitate dose adjustment.

Metronidazole therapy often is associated with a metallic taste and nausea. More serious but less frequent adverse reactions include a reversible peripheral neuropathy, seizures, encephalopathy, and neutropenia. A disulfiram-like reaction can occur when metronidazole is taken with alcohol. Several studies conducted in laboratory animals have indicated that prolonged use of high-dose metronidazole can be carcinogenic; however, there is no evidence that it is carcinogenic in humans.

Metronidazole has been shown to be effective in a wide variety of infections caused by anaerobes. The most common indications for this antibiotic are the treatment of pelvic and intra-abdominal sepsis and brain abscesses. It also is an effective treatment for pseudomembranous colitis caused by *C difficile.*

## AMINOGLYCOSIDES

The aminoglycoside group of antibiotics contains a large number of structurally related compounds. Streptomycin was the first of these agents to be discovered. Agents subsequently developed include neomycin, kanamycin, gentamicin, tobramycin, amikacin, and netilmicin. Streptomycin is primarily used to treat tuberculosis. Gentamicin, tobramycin, and amikacin are the most common aminoglycosides used; they are discussed below as a group, with only their clinically important differences emphasized.

These antibiotics are active primarily against gram-negative and limited numbers of gram-positive aerobes. They are inactive against the vast majority of anaerobes. All 3 of these aminoglycosides are active against most strains of *P aeruginosa,* with tobramycin consistently demonstrating the greatest activity. Gentamicin is consistently the most active of these agents against strains of *Serratia marcescens.* Otherwise, their relative antibacterial activities are similar, with most sensitive strains being inhibited by less than 3 to 4 mg/L.

An important aspect of aminoglycoside activity against gram-negative aerobes is the increasing resistance developed since their introduction. Resistance is most often due to antibiotic inactivation by enzymes produced by the bacteria. There are at least 12 such inactivating enzymes. Gentamicin is susceptible to the largest number of these enzymes (9 of 12), and amikacin is susceptible to the smallest number (1 of 12). When widespread bacterial resistance develops to one of the aminoglycosides being used in a particular hospital, changing to an alternate agent usually results in a return to increased sensitivity.

The pharmacokinetics of all the aminoglycosides are similar. They are poorly absorbed from the gastrointestinal tract, but well absorbed after intramuscular or intravenous administration. Maximum serum concentrations of gentamicin and tobramycin are 5 to 8 mg/L after unit doses of 1 to 2.5 mg/kg. Maximum serum concentrations of amikacin range from 15 to 30 mg/L after a unit dose of 7.5 mg/kg. The aminoglycosides are distributed in most extracellular fluids, but do not attain therapeutic concentrations in CSF. The main site of deposition of these drugs is the kidney, which accounts for approximately 40% of the total antibiotic in the body. The renal cortex accumulates approximately 85% of the kidney load, and the resulting concentrations are more than 100-fold greater than serum concentrations. The half-lives of the aminoglycosides range from 1.5 to 2.5 hours, and they are eliminated, primarily unchanged, by glomerular filtration. The doses of the aminoglycosides must be carefully monitored and adjusted in the presence of renal insufficiency. In such cases, the total daily dose is decreased by either prolonging the dosing interval or reducing the unit dose. Nomograms, based on the measured or approximated glomerular filtration rate, are available to guide these adjustments.

Aminoglycosides demonstrate concentration-dependent killing, that is, the bactericidal activity increases with increasing concentration of drug. In addition, aminoglycosides exhibit a substantial postantibiotic effect (ie, aminoglycosides will inhibit growth of bacteria even after the serum level has fallen below the MIC for that antibiotic). Because of these pharmacodynamic characteristics, aminoglycosides may be effective when administered as a single daily dose. Toxicity is not increased using this dosing strategy.

#### Indications

Aminoglycosides are indicated for treatment of endocarditis due to certain bacteria where they are used for synergy with the primary agent (eg, ampicillin and gentamicin for enterococcal endocarditis). The aminoglycosides also are useful in combination with a cell well–active agent in the empiric therapy of febrile neutropenic episodes in immunocompromised patients. Other indications include treatment of proven or suspected gram-negative infections of the blood or urinary tract. Aminoglycosides are used less frequently since the development of third-generation cephalosporins.

#### Toxicity

The most important toxicities of the aminoglycosides are ototoxicity and nephrotoxicity. These toxic effects are more common in adults than in children, who generally tolerate this class of drugs well. Ototoxicity may be primarily vestibular or cochlear. The agent most commonly associated with vestibular toxicity is gentamicin, with an estimated incidence in adults of 2%. This ranges from mild vertigo to severe Ménière syndrome. Damage is usually permanent, but symptoms may eventually be reduced by adaptation. The agents most likely to cause cochlear toxicity are amikacin and tobramycin. Although the frequency of hearing loss following treatment with these drugs is low, it may occur without any warning and may be irreversible. Risk factors that seem to predispose to ototoxicity include cumulative dosage, advanced age, and maternal history of preexisting renal compromise or hearing loss. Controlled trials in adult patients have found little difference overall in the incidence of ototoxicity following treatment with gentamicin, tobramycin, or amikacin.

Early manifestations of nephrotoxicity may include hypokalemia, glycosuria, alkalosis, hypomagnesemia, and hypocalcemia. Renal damage is dose-related and generally reversible.

Another less common but important side effect of the aminoglycosides is a competitive type of neuromuscular blockade, seen most often after intraperitoneal administration or after intravenous push. For this reason, aminoglycosides should not be administered to those with infant botulism. Hypersensitivity reactions to systemically administered aminoglycosides are uncommon.

Because of their relatively narrow toxic-to-therapeutic ratio, serum concentrations of the aminoglycosides should be monitored. When using multiple daily dosing, peak concentrations of gentamicin and tobramycin should not exceed 10 mg/L, and trough concentrations should be below 2 mg/L. Amikacin peak and trough concentrations should not exceed 30 mg/L and 10 mg/L, respectively. When using single daily dosing, levels approximately 8 hours after the start of dosing should be in the range of 2 to 5 mg/L for gentamicin and tobramycin and 10 to 15 mg/L for amikacin.

## TETRACYCLINES

The tetracyclines are not frequently prescribed for children because of age-related toxicities. The antibiotics in this category include tetracycline, doxycycline, minocycline, and the newer agent tigecycline. The tetracyclines are active against a wide range of gram-positive and gram-negative bacteria, *Mycoplasma, Rickettsia,* and *Chlamydia.* They also are active against *Treponema pallidum* and moderately active against a wide range of anaerobes. All tetracyclines are absorbed adequately, but incompletely, from the gastrointestinal tract. They are chelated by various cations and are absorbed more completely during fasting. These antibiotics distribute widely and attain concentrations in the CSF of 10% to 50% of simultaneous serum concentrations. Most of these agents are excreted primarily by renal glomerular filtration, with lesser amounts being eliminated in the bile. Doxycycline is an exception, with 90% appearing in the feces. The half-lives of the tetracyclines range from 6 hours for tetracycline to approximately 20 hours for doxycycline.

### Indications

Indications for tetracycline therapy in adults and children over 8 years of age include infections caused by *Mycoplasma pneumoniae,* Q fever, psittacosis, brucellosis, and lymphogranuloma venereum. Tetracyclines may be used in children irrespective of age in the treatment of Rocky Mountain spotted fever, ehrlichiosis, and anaplasmosis, since there are no reasonable alternative agents for these infections. Minocycline is frequently prescribed to patients with acne vulgaris. Doxycycline is an effective chemoprophylactic agent against *E coli*–induced diarrhea and anthrax.

Tigecycline, a semisynthetic derivative of minocycline, is a parenteral agent of a new class of antibiotics (glycylcyclines). It has a broader spectrum of (bacteriostatic) activity than traditional tetracyclines but retains the side effect profile of tetracyclines. Tigecycline is active against tetracycline-resistant gram-positive and gram-negative pathogens, including MRSA, and possibly VRE, but not *Pseudomonas.* It also may be useful for multidrug-resistant Enterobacteriaceae.

### Toxicity

The adverse effects of tetracyclines relate to tooth and bone deposition. Permanent binding to dental calcium can produce a dose-related, brownish, fluorescent discoloration of the teeth when administered during the period of dental calcification (5 months to 8 years). Bone deposition of tetracycline may result in temporary cessation of bone growth. This effect is reversible when the drug is discontinued. Doxycycline is one of the least offensive tetracyclines in relation to bone staining and does not appear to cause teeth staining in children < 8 years of age until the child has consumed over 5 courses of treatment.

Other adverse effects of tetracyclines that are not age-related include gastrointestinal disturbances, photosensitivity, hepatotoxicity, and neurotoxicity. Hypersensitivity reactions to the tetracyclines are rare.

Photosensitivity reactions may be caused by any of the tetracyclines but are most frequent with doxycycline. Unfortunately, doxycycline is sometimes prescribed as a prophylactic agent against diarrhea in individuals traveling to tropical, sunny climates. Hepatotoxic reactions are uncommon, but fatal liver necrosis has been described after large intravenous doses in pregnant women. The pathogenesis of this reaction is unknown.

Manifestations of neurotoxicity are observed frequently and almost exclusively with minocycline. Dizziness, weakness, vertigo, and ataxia appear within the first few days of therapy. Another neurologic side effect of these agents is benign intracranial hypertension that is self-limited and resolves when the therapy is discontinued.

## OXAZOLIDINONES

Linezolid is the first member of the recently developed oxazolidinone class of antibiotics. Linezolid binds to the bacterial 50S ribosomal subunit. It has 100% bioavailability after oral administration and has wide distribution throughout the body, including lung extracellular lining fluid and CSF. Maximum serum concentrations of 11 to 16.7 μg/mL are achieved within 1 to 2 hours of an oral dose. Linezolid is cleared primarily by nonrenal mechanisms, with only 30% of the drug eliminated by the kidneys. The $t_{1/2}$ is 1.5 to 5 hours; infants and young children clear the medication more rapidly. Linezolid has been approved for the treatment of complicated skin and skin-structure infections and nosocomial pneumonia. It demonstrates activity against gram-positive bacteria such as *Staphylococcus, Streptococcus,* and *Enterococcus,* including MRSA and VRE. It also has been used as second-line therapy for both tuberculous and nontuberculous mycobacterial infections. Recommended dosages are 600 mg orally or IV twice daily for children ≥ 12 years of age and 10 mg/kg/dose orally or IV every 8 hours for children < 12 years of age.

Tedizolid is a second-generation oxazolidinone derivative that is 4-to-16-fold more potent against staphylococci and enterococci compared to linezolid. It was approved by the FDA in 2014 for the treatment of acute bacterial skin and skin-structure infections caused by *S aureus* (including MRSA), GAS, GBS, *Streptococcus anginosus,* and *Enterococcus.* The recommended dosage in patients over 18 years of age is 200 mg once daily for 6 days; pediatric studies to date are limited.

### Toxicity

Linezolid is generally well-tolerated in children. Most adverse effects occur only with prolonged (> 2 weeks) therapy. These include reversible hepatotoxicity and bone marrow suppression. Linezolid is also a reversible monoamine oxidase inhibitor, so concurrent treatment with selective serotonin reuptake inhibitors is contraindicated as this combination has been associated with serotonin syndrome.

## LINCOSAMIDES

The prototype of the lincosamide class of antibiotics is clindamycin. Clindamycin is well absorbed from the gastrointestinal tract. An oral dose of 300 mg results in maximum serum concentrations of 4 to 5 mg/L. It may be prescribed as a capsule or suspension. Maximum serum concentrations after an intravenous dose are 2- to 3-fold higher than after an oral dose. Clindamycin distributes widely but penetrates into CSF poorly. The drug is metabolized primarily in the liver, with less than 25% excreted in the urine. Thus, hepatic insufficiency has a more profound effect on the disposition of this drug than does renal insufficiency. The $t_{1/2}$ of clindamycin is 2 to 4 hours.

Clindamycin acts at the 50S subunit of the bacterial ribosome. It is active against most gram-positive bacteria, both aerobic and anaerobic. It also is active against most gram-negative anaerobic rods, but it is inactive against most gram-negative aerobes. Sensitive organisms usually have MICs less than 0.5 mg/L.

An important role for clindamycin has emerged in the management of infections due to MRSA. Because of its outstanding penetration into body fluids (excluding the CSF) as well as tissues and bone, clindamycin can be used for therapy of serious infections caused by *S aureus* or GAS. Even when using vancomycin or a β-lactam agent for treatment, clindamycin may be co-administered for treatment of serious infection due to *S aureus* or GAS (toxic shock syndrome or necrotizing fasciitis), as its effect on ribosomes may decrease toxin production by the bacteria. There is a form of inducible clindamycin resistance exhibited by some strains of *S aureus*; therefore, consultation with the clinical microbiology laboratory or an infectious diseases specialist is necessary before treating a serious infection due to *S aureus* with clindamycin. Clindamycin is also useful in the management of anaerobic infections. Clindamycin plays an important role in the treatment of malaria and babesiosis (when each is co-administered with quinine), *Pneumocystis jirovecii* pneumonia (when co-administered with primaquine), and toxoplasmosis.

#### Toxicity

The most important adverse reactions to clindamycin are gastrointestinal disturbances. Approximately 30% of patients treated with this drug develop diarrhea. This diarrhea is usually self-limited and subsides when therapy is discontinued. It may be associated with nausea, vomiting, and abdominal cramps. A more severe gastrointestinal side effect is pseudomembranous colitis, which was first described in association with this antibiotic. It is caused by gastrointestinal overgrowth of toxin-producing *C difficile.* Almost every antibiotic has now been implicated in the pathogenesis of pseudomembranous colitis, and clindamycin is not the most frequent culprit. Furthermore, pseudomembranous colitis is much less common in children than in adults.

Minor abnormalities of liver function tests are quite common during clindamycin therapy, and cardiovascular collapse has been observed after rapid intravenous administration.

### MACROLIDES

The macrolide antibiotics most commonly used in pediatric practice include erythromycin and the newer agents clarithromycin and azithromycin. This class of antimicrobials exerts its antibiotic effect through binding to the 50S subunit of the bacterial ribosome, producing a block in elongation of bacterial polypeptides. Clarithromycin is metabolized to 14-hydroxy clarithromycin, and interestingly, this active metabolite also has potent antimicrobial activity. Azithromycin has largely replaced erythromycin for use in many infections.

The spectrum of activity of these drugs includes many gram-positive bacteria. Unfortunately, resistance to these agents among *S aureus* and GAS is fairly widespread, limiting the usefulness of macrolides for many skin and soft tissue infections and for streptococcal pharyngitis. Azithromycin and clarithromycin have demonstrated efficacy for otitis media. Although many *S pneumoniae* are becoming resistant, members of this class have an important role in the management of pediatric respiratory infections, including atypical pneumonia caused by *M pneumoniae, Chlamydia pneumoniae*, and *Legionella pneumophila*, as well as infections caused by *Bordetella pertussis.* Azithromycin is also useful for the treatment of gastrointestinal disease due to some bacteria (eg, *Salmonella*, *Shigella*, and *Campylobacter*) and is the treatment of choice for traveler's diarrhea in children.

Azithromycin is an azalide antibiotic that is structurally related to erythromycin. It may be given IV or orally, and its biochemical modifications result in excellent oral bioavailability, greatly extended serum and tissue half-lives (both exceeding 48 hours), and excellent in vivo activity against most of the organisms susceptible to erythromycin. In addition, it has excellent activity against *Chlamydia trachomatis,* with MICs between 0.03 and 0.5 mg/L. It is particularly well suited for treating genital infections caused by *Chlamydia.* A single oral dose is as effective as a 7-day course of erythromycin or doxycycline. Similarly, for other infections for which a 10- to 14-day course of other antibiotics is routinely given, a 5-day course of azithromycin may be adequate. Further, an extended-release microsphere formulation has recently been released that allows for single-dose treatment of some infections, such as community-associated pneumonia (CAP).

Clarithromycin is another macrolide antibiotic that is similar to azithromycin. A special feature of clarithromycin is its activity against selected mycobacteria; thus, it is particularly useful in the treatment of atypical mycobacteria infections, especially those caused by *Mycobacterium avium-intracellulare.*

#### Toxicity

Oral erythromycin formulations often result in gastrointestinal disturbances, including nausea, vomiting, diarrhea, and abdominal cramps. These adverse effects are likely to occur at high doses. A much more serious adverse reaction, fortunately rare among children, is cholestatic hepatitis. It occurs most commonly with the estolate preparation and is probably due to the propionyl ester linkage. Manifestations can include fever, jaundice, pruritus, rash, increased liver size, and eosinophilia. Resolution usually occurs when the antibiotic is discontinued. Oral erythromycin (and azithromycin) use in neonates has been associated with the development of pyloric stenosis. Intravenous erythromycin is frequently associated with thrombophlebitis. Ototoxicity, manifested as tinnitus and transient deafness, is a rare adverse reaction.

Drug interactions are common with erythromycin and to a lesser extent with clarithromycin. These agents can inhibit the CYP3A4 enzyme system, resulting in increased levels of certain drugs such as astemizole, cisapride, statins, pimozide, and theophylline. Itraconazole may increase macrolide levels, whereas rifampin, carbamazepine, and phenytoin may decrease macrolide levels. There are few reported adverse drug interactions with azithromycin. Clarithromycin has been associated with prolonged QT interval and auditory and visual hallucinations in some recipients of the drug.

### SULFONAMIDES AND TRIMETHOPRIM

Sulfonamides were the first group of synthetic antibacterial compounds. They originally had a wide range of activity, but this range is considerably compromised by acquired bacterial resistance. Trimethoprim and the sulfonamides are bacteriostatic agents that inhibit the bacterial folate synthesis pathway, in the process impairing both nucleic acid and protein synthesis. Sulfonamides interfere with the synthesis of dihydropteroic acid from para-aminobenzoic acid, whereas trimethoprim acts at a site further downstream, interfering with synthesis of tetrahydrofolic acid from dihydrofolic acid. The sulfonamides are available in both parenteral and oral formulations. Although there have historically been a large number of sulfonamides developed for clinical use, relatively few remain available for pediatric practice. The most important agent is the combination of trimethoprim-sulfamethoxazole (TMP-SMZ), which is commonly used for treatment of urinary tract infections. TMP-SMZ has also emerged as a commonly prescribed agent for staphylococcal skin and soft tissue infections, since this antibiotic retains activity against MRSA. TMP-SMZ should not be used when infection may be due to GAS. TMP-SMZ also plays a unique role in immunocompromised patients as a prophylactic and therapeutic agent for *P jirovecii* infection. Bacteria that are usually sensitive to sulfonamides include *Nocardia* species, many Enterobacteriaceae, *H influenzae,* and *B pertussis*, and *Chlamydia* and nonbacterial pathogens such as *Toxoplasma* and *Plasmodium falciparum* are also sensitive to the sulfonamides. Other commonly used sulfonamides include sulfisoxazole, which is useful in the management of urinary tract infections, and sulfadiazine, which is a drug of choice in the treatment of toxoplasmosis.

The sulfonamides are often classified on the basis of their half-lives, which range from 2 to 6 hours with the short-acting sulfonamides, such as sulfanilamide, sulfadiazine, and sulfisoxazole, to 150 to 200 hours with the ultralong-acting sulfonamide sulfadoxine. Most of the sulfonamides are well absorbed from the gastrointestinal tract. Serum concentrations vary somewhat among the different agents, but after the usual recommended orally administered doses, maximum concentrations are typically in the range of 50 to 100 mg/L. Concentrations are higher after intravenous administration. These drugs are distributed widely and attain therapeutic concentrations in CSF. The sulfonamides are acetylated in the liver, and some also undergo glucuronidation. Free and conjugated sulfonamides are excreted by renal glomerular filtration and secretion. The longer-acting sulfonamides undergo more complete tubular resorption than do the shorter-acting agents. Minimal amounts of the sulfonamides are excreted in the bile.

#### Toxicity

Sulfonamides may cause a variety of hypersensitivity reactions, ranging from mild rashes to life-threatening Stevens-Johnson syndrome. The latter reaction is more common with the longer-acting sulfonamides. Hematologic toxicity also may occur with sulfonamide use. Reactions include agranulocytosis, which is usually reversible on discontinuation of the drug, and hemolytic anemia in patients with deficiency of glucose-6-phosphate dehydrogenase (G6PD). Renal damage was common with the older sulfonamides, which were poorly water soluble. Patients developed crystalluria, which led to urinary obstruction and hematuria. Renal damage may also be a manifestation of a hypersensitivity reaction. Sulfonamides are contraindicated in the neonate and during the latter part of pregnancy, as they may displace bilirubin from protein-binding sites, possibly leading to jaundice and kernicterus. Neonates also seem to be more susceptible to the potential renal toxicity of these agents.

### NITROFURANTOIN

Although nitrofurantoin was approved by the FDA in 1953, its exact mechanism of action is still not known. It has a hydantoin ring with a nitro-substituted furanyl side chain that is metabolized by bacteria to activate its bactericidal activity. Nitrofurantoin has broad activity against gram-positive and gram-negative enteric bacteria.

Nitrofurantoin is well absorbed after oral administration and rapidly cleared by the kidneys. It has an extremely short half-life (~30 minutes) and a high volume of distribution, which may be due to both rapid distribution into tissue compartments and enzymatic degradation at those sites. Therefore, serum levels are not maintained, but the antibiotic concentrates in the urine, making it a useful antibiotic for urinary tract infections.

#### Indications

Because of the high concentrations of nitrofurantoin in urine and its broad spectrum of activity, it has primarily been used as therapy or prophylaxis in urinary tract infections. Some data suggest that nitrofurantoin may be more effective than other antibiotics in preventing recurrent urinary tract infections in children. However, its gastrointestinal side effects may limit its utility.

#### Toxicity

The primary side effect of nitrofurantoin is nausea and vomiting. These adverse effects are the most common reason for discontinuing therapy. Although there have been reports of acute lung injury and pulmonary fibrosis in adults on long-term nitrofurantoin therapy, similar toxicities have not been seen in children. Hemolysis can occur in patients with G6PD deficiency.

### STREPTOGRAMINS

The emergence of highly resistant gram-positive organisms, in particular VRE, has necessitated development of new classes of antibiotics. One such class that is especially useful for resistant gram-positive infections is the streptogramins. The currently licensed agent in this category is dalfopristin-quinupristin, which is available in a parenteral formulation. It is appropriate for treatment of MRSA, methicillin-resistant coagulase-negative staphylococci, and vancomycin-resistant *E faecium* but not *E faecalis*. The recommended dose for children and adults is 7.5 mg/kg by intravenous route every 8 hours. This antibiotic is a potent inhibitor of CYP3A4 and so may be associated with substantial drug-drug interactions.

### DAPTOMYCIN

Daptomycin is a novel member of the cyclic lipopeptide class of antibiotics. Its spectrum of activity includes virtually all gram-positive organisms, including *E faecalis* and *E faecium* (including VREs) and *S aureus* (including MRSA). The structure of daptomycin is a 13-member amino acid peptide linked to a 10-carbon lipophilic tail, which results in a novel mechanism of action of disruption of the bacterial membrane through the formation of transmembrane channels. These channels cause leakage of intracellular ions, leading to depolarization of the cellular membrane and inhibition of macromolecular synthesis. A theoretical advantage of daptomycin for serious infections is its bactericidal activity against MRSA and enterococci. It is administered IV. Experience in children is limited. Doses ranging from 6 to 10 mg/kg/d have been used in children. Myopathy and elevations in creatine phosphokinase have been described. Daptomycin is inactivated by surfactant and should not be used to treat pneumonia.

### SUGGESTED READINGS


Boucher HW, Talbot GH, Benjamin DK Jr, et al. 10 x '20 Progress—development of new drugs active against gram-negative bacilli: an update from the Infectious Diseases Society of America. *Clin Infect Dis.* 2013;56:1685-1694.

Bradley JS. Which antibiotic for resistant gram-positives, and why? *J Infect.* 2014;68:S63-75.

Dryden MS. Novel antibiotic treatment for skin and soft tissue infection. *Curr Opin Infect Dis.* 2014;27:116-124.

Golan Y. Empiric therapy for hospital-acquired, gram-negative complicated intra-abdominal infection and complicated urinary tract infections: a systematic literature review of current and emerging treatment options. *BMC Infect Dis.* 2015;15:313.

Long SS. Optimizing antimicrobial therapy in children. *J Infect.* 2016;72:S91-97.

McMullan BJ, Andresen D, Blyth CC, et al. Antibiotic duration and timing of the switch from intravenous to oral route for bacterial infections in children: Systematic review and guidelines. *Lancet Infect Dis.* 2016;16:e139-152.

Murphy JL, Fenn N, Pyle L, et al. Adverse events in pediatric patients receiving long-term oral and intravenous antibiotics. *Hosp Pediatr.* 2016;6:330-338.

Principi N, Esposito S. Antimicrobial stewardship in paediatrics. *BMC Infect Dis.* 2016;16:424.

Sutter DE, Milburn E, Chukwuma U, Dzialowy N, Maranich AM, Hospenthal DR. Changing susceptibility of Staphylococcus aureus in a US pediatric population. *Pediatrics.* 2016;137:e20153099.

Turk VE, Simic I, Likic R, et al. New drugs for bad bugs: what's new and what's in the pipeline? *Clin Ther.* 2016;38:e9.


# 242 Antifungal Therapy

Akinobu Kamei and Patricia M. Flynn

### INTRODUCTION

Antifungal agents are available in systemic and/or topical formulations. The choice of antifungal agent(s) and duration of therapy depend not only on the causative pathogen but also the anatomic location and severity of the infection and host immune status. For example, topical antifungal agents are less likely to cause toxicity and should, as a rule, be the first choice for treating skin and mucous membrane infections, whereas tinea capitis and onychomycosis (fungal infection of the nails) are best treated systemically (see Chapter 362). Infections that are severe, are disseminated, or involve the bloodstream should be treated with systemic therapy. In some instances, aggressive initial therapy using more potent antifungal agents with higher toxicity profiles may be warranted as initial therapy for life-threatening invasive fungal diseases in immunocompromised hosts. This aggressive initial therapy may be followed by less aggressive "step-down" therapy until immune reconstitution occurs. It is not uncommon that drug-drug interactions (eg, azole agents with anticancer chemotherapies) limit antifungal options in practice. To guarantee the maximum effectiveness and safety, therapeutic drug monitoring (TDM) is essential, especially for some of the systemic azole agents and flucytosine. In contrast to antibacterial therapy, correlation between in vitro susceptibility test results (eg, minimal inhibitory concentrations [MICs]) and clinical outcome has not been established for each antifungal-pathogen combination except for fluconazole, voriconazole, and echinocandins with *Candida* species. Organism- and disease-specific antifungal therapies are summarized in Table 242-1.

## SYSTEMIC ANTIFUNGAL THERAPY

The most commonly used systemic antifungal agents can be divided into 3 major groups based on their structure and function: polyenes, azoles, and echinocandins.

### Polyenes

The polyenes bind to sterols in the fungal cell membrane, causing increased cell membrane permeability followed by leakage of cellular contents and cell death. They have been reported to be both fungistatic and fungicidal, depending on the fungal organism as well as host factors. Currently amphotericin B, available as amphotericin B deoxycholate (AMBD) or its lipid formulations, is the only polyene agent for systemic use. Amphotericin B is active against most fungi, including yeasts such as *Candida* species, *Cryptococcus neoformans, Histoplasma capsulatum, Blastomyces dermatitidis, Coccidioides immitis,* and also a variety of molds including but not limited to *Aspergillus* species and zygomycetes (eg, *Rhizopus* species and *Mucor* species). Because of its broad antifungal spectrum, amphotericin B is often used for the empiric treatment of febrile neutropenic cancer patients. It is also indicated for visceral leishmaniasis. Of note, amphotericin B is not active against *Scedosporium* species, some isolates of *Fusarium* species, *Aspergillus terreus,* and *Candida lusitaniae.* All amphotericin B formulations have poor penetration into the cerebrospinal fluid (CSF), vitreous humor, and amniotic fluid.

AMBD is typically administered as a 1- to 6-hour (usually 2- to 4-hour) daily intravenous infusion of 0.6 to 1.5 mg/kg. The dosage is dependent on the infecting organism and the extent of infection. AMBD is highly protein bound and accumulates in tissues, especially the liver and spleen. Thus, after therapy has been established, some experts opt to administer the drug every other day or 3 times weekly. Common side effects include acute infusion-related reactions and nephrotoxicity (often reversible). Infusion-related fever and chills can be treated with meperidine, antipyretics, slowing the infusion rate, or a combination of these options. Patients who experience severe reactions can be given these agents or a hydrocortisone infusion before AMBD is administered. Neonates and children are less likely than adults to experience infusion-related toxicity. Frequency and severity of infusion-related side effects often diminish with continued treatment. Nephrotoxicity and electrolyte disturbances (hypokalemia and hypomagnesemia) are also common, but usually reversible, side effects. Volume expansion with normal saline prior to administration of AMBD has reduced nephrotoxicity in adults, but there are no comparable data for children.

Amphotericin B has been administered directly into the CSF via intraventricular/intrathecal routes in cases of meningitis; however, no data exist to suggest that this improves the outcome of candidal meningitis, and significant toxicity due to administration has been reported. It has also been used as a bladder irrigant for treating uncomplicated candidal cystitis. However, the availability of new systemic antifungal agents with better penetration into these compartments has almost eliminated the use of intraventricular/intrathecal CSF and bladder administration.

Lipid formulations of amphotericin B result in less infusion-related and renal toxicities compared to AMBD. Thus, these agents can be given at higher doses than AMBD; however, infusion-related symptoms and nephrotoxicity remain the dose-limiting toxic effects. Two lipid formulations are commercially available: liposomal amphotericin B (LAMB, AmBisome) and amphotericin B lipid complex (ABLC, Abelcet). LAMB and ABLC have lower kidney penetration but achieve higher amphotericin B concentrations in the liver and spleen compared to AMBD. LAMB achieves higher amphotericin B concentrations in the brain than the other amphotericin B formulations, whereas ABLC achieves higher amphotericin B concentrations in the lung. Recommended daily dosages are variable and depend on the infecting organism and host susceptibility. Current recommendations are 3 to 5 mg/kg for LAMB and 5 mg/kg for ABLC. In general, most experts recommend 5 mg/kg of either lipid formulation for the treatment of serious fungal infections in pediatric patients. Despite the much higher cost of the lipid formulations and the necessity for higher dosages, utilization of these agents is increasing in pediatric patients because of their improved safety profile.

### Azoles

Azoles inhibit the fungal cytochrome P450 enzyme, sterol 14-α-demethylase, thereby impairing fungal ergosterol synthesis and leading to damage in the fungal cell membrane. Azoles are fungistatic in general. The azole family contains 2 classes of drugs: the imidazoles and the triazoles. Although the 2 classes are similar in their spectrum of activity and their mechanism of action, the triazoles are more commonly prescribed, because they are more slowly metabolized (requiring less frequent dosing) and have less effect on human sterol synthesis (and thus are associated with less toxicity). The available systemic azoles include the imidazoles, miconazole and ketoconazole, and the triazoles, fluconazole, itraconazole, voriconazole, posaconazole, and isavuconazole. Isavuconazole has been recently approved by the US Food and Drug Administration (FDA) for treatment of invasive aspergillosis and mucormycosis in adults, but clinical data in the pediatric population are still very limited. The introduction of second-generation triazoles (voriconazole, posaconazole, and isavuconazole) has expanded the target organisms and use of azoles. In general, the azole family has activity against *Candida albicans*, the dimorphic fungi (eg, *H capsulatum, B dermatitidis, C immitis,* and *C neoformans*), and the dermatophytes. Itraconazole, voriconazole, posaconazole, and isavuconazole have activity against *Aspergillus* species. Voriconazole, posaconazole, and isavuconazole have even extended activities, being active against other hyaline and dematiaceous molds and against some of the fluconazole-resistant *Candida* species. Importantly, voriconazole lacks activity against zygomycetes, whereas posaconazole and isavuconazole have some activity depending on the isolate. All azole agents inhibit human cytochrome P450 enzymes to varying degrees. Therefore, possible drug-drug interactions should be carefully considered. Investigation of the pharmacokinetics of the newer azoles in neonates, children, and adolescents is ongoing. As new information emerges, recommended dosing regimens are likely to change. The recommended dosages indicated below should be verified prior to prescribing. Therapeutic drug monitoring for systemic azoles except for fluconazole or isavuconazole is recommended because of the wide inter- and intraindividual variability of serum drug levels.

Fluconazole (Diflucan) is effective for the treatment of esophageal, laryngeal, and vaginal candidiasis. It should also be considered in cases of oropharyngeal candidiasis unresponsive to topical therapy. Fluconazole can also be used for serious candidal infections in hemodynamically stable patients unless the infection is suspected to be caused by a fluconazole-resistant strain such as *Candida krusei, Candida guilliermondii,* or *Candida glabrata* (see Table 242-1). The drug has also been used for antifungal prophylaxis in adult and pediatric recipients of hematopoietic stem cell transplants or solid organ transplants and in premature infants. Fluconazole can be used as initial therapy for mild cases of cryptococcal meningitis in adults with acquired immunodeficiency syndrome (AIDS) and for long-term suppression

**TABLE 242-1 ANTIFUNGAL THERAPY**

| Organism or Condition | Disease | Therapy |
|---|---|---|
| *Aspergillus* species | Invasive, central nervous system (CNS), or sinus infection | Voriconazole is the first-line therapy. Alternate therapies include liposomal amphotericin B or isavuconazole. Some experts recommend combination therapy with voriconazole plus echinocandin. Therapy should continue for a minimum of 6–12 weeks based on clinical course and underlying host status. CNS infections may require prolonged duration of therapy. Surgical removal of involved tissue is recommended in some cases. Note that *Aspergillus terreus* may be resistant to amphotericin B. |
| | Skin | Surgical debridement or wide margin surgical resection. Antifungal therapy same as above. Following adequate debridement and recovery of immunosuppression, shorter duration of therapy may be acceptable. |
| *Blastomyces dermatitidis* | Pulmonary and disseminated | Amphotericin B deoxycholate (AMBD) or its lipid formulations. Itraconazole for mild to moderate infections (for 6–12 months) or as step-down therapy for severe infections (for a total of 12 months). Voriconazole and posaconazole may also be active, but there is limited clinical experience. |
| *Candida* species | Oropharyngeal candidiasis (thrush) | Infants: nystatin oral suspension for at least 7 days. |
| | | Children: nystatin oral suspension swish and swallow, or clotrimazole troche for 7 days. |
| | | Immunocompromised or failed topical therapy: fluconazole for 14 days. |
| | Cutaneous | Nystatin or clotrimazole or miconazole cream, lotion, or powder applied twice a day for at least 7 days. |
| | Vulvovaginitis | Topical azole or nystatin for 1–7 days or single-dose oral fluconazole (150 mg, adult dosage) for uncomplicated cases. Duration of therapy and selection of topical or systemic therapy based on clinical features. |
| | Esophagitis | Fluconazole (intravenous [IV] or oral [PO]) for 14–21 days. Alternatives, especially when fluconazole-resistant *Candida* is suspected, are: voriconazole, posaconazole, itraconazole, echinocandin, AMBD, or its lipid formulations for 14–21 days. For recurrent esophagitis, suppressive therapy with fluconazole. |
| | Cystitis | Investigate possibility of disseminated disease. Remove urinary catheter if feasible. Fluconazole (IV or PO) for 14 days. AMBD for 1–7 days for fluconazole-resistant *Candida* species. |
| | Peritonitis (peritoneal dialysis catheter) | 5-Flucytosine or fluconazole PO or intraperitoneally [IP] for 4–6 weeks. Remove catheter if no improvement in 4–7 days. |
| | Uncomplicated candidemia in nonneutropenic and neutropenic hosts | An echinocandin as initial therapy, then can be switched to fluconazole if patient is clinically stable, has negative blood cultures, and the isolate is susceptible to fluconazole (eg, *Candida albicans:* all blood isolates should be tested for azole susceptibility). Continue for total of 2 weeks after resolution of candidemia in the absence of metastatic complications. Duration of therapy may be longer in neutropenic patients. Alternatives for the initial therapy include lipid formulation amphotericin B or fluconazole (in selected cases). Voriconazole can be used when additional mold coverage is desired (eg, in neutropenic patients). |
| | Neonatal candidiasis (including CNS infection) | AMBD (lipid formulations of amphotericin B are alternatives in the absence of urinary tract infection). Fluconazole is an alternative if resistance is unlikely or ruled out. Echinocandins are not generally recommended as primary treatment. Duration of 2 weeks after resolution of candidemia in the absence of metastatic complications. |
| | Vascular catheter-related | Catheter removal. Treat as recommended above for uncomplicated candidemia. Note that *Candida tropicalis* and *Candida parapsilosis* may require treatment for up to 3–4 weeks. |
| | Chronic disseminated (hepatosplenic) candidiasis | Lipid formulation amphotericin B or echinocandins for several weeks, followed by oral fluconazole if fluconazole-resistant *Candida* infection is unlikely. Therapy should continue until lesions resolve on repeat imaging (usually takes several months). |
| *Coccidioides immitis* | Nonmeningeal | Fluconazole is recommended therapy, but the duration of therapy is not well defined; some experts suggest 12–18 months. AMBD results in similar cure rates in adults and should be considered in severely ill or immunocompromised patients. Lipid formulations of amphotericin B, itraconazole, voriconazole, or posaconazole may also be effective. Itraconazole is preferred in bone disease. Long-term suppressive antifungal therapy in patients with ongoing immune suppression or in cases of osteomyelitis. Uncomplicated pulmonary disease in normal hosts may be monitored without therapy. |
| | Meningeal | Same as above, but duration of therapy indefinite. |
| *Cryptococcus neoformans* | Pneumonia | Fluconazole for 6–12 months. Itraconazole, voriconazole, posaconazole, or lipid formulations of amphotericin B may also be effective. Patients with HIV infection require chronic suppressive therapy with fluconazole (discontinuation after CD4 count recovery following effective antiviral treatment is poorly studied in pediatric populations). |
| | Meningeal or disseminated disease | AMBD plus flucytosine for 2 weeks followed by fluconazole for 8 weeks. For AMBD-intolerant cases, lipid formulations of amphotericin B. Monitoring flucytosine levels and complete blood counts is recommended. |
| Dermatophytes: *Trichosporon* species, *Microsporum* species, *Epidermophyton* species | Tinea corporis, cruris, pedis | Topical clotrimazole or miconazole in cream, lotion, ointment, or powder applied twice daily for 2–3 weeks. For failures, consider other azole or allylamine preparation. Duration of therapy 2–3 weeks. |
| | Tinea capitis | Griseofulvin or itraconazole for 4–6 weeks. |
| | Onychomycosis | Itraconazole for 3–4 months or itraconazole pulse therapy for 2 months or terbinafine for 6 weeks for fingernail and 12 weeks for toenail disease. |

(Continued)

**TABLE 242-1 ANTIFUNGAL THERAPY (CONTINUED)**

| Organism or Condition | Disease | Therapy |
|---|---|---|
| *Malassezia furfur* | Tinea versicolor | Ketoconazole cream or shampoo applied for 2 weeks or selenium sulfide, leave on 10 minutes daily for 7 days or 3–5 times weekly for 2–4 weeks. Successful therapy in adults with ketoconazole 400 mg single dose or 200 mg daily for 7 days. |
| *Fusarium* species | Fungemia or disseminated infection | Options include voriconazole, lipid formulations of amphotericin B, or posaconazole. Duration of therapy undetermined, but 6 weeks minimum and typically until immune reconstitution. |
| *Histoplasma capsulatum* | Pulmonary | No therapy in normal host for asymptomatic or very mild pulmonary disease. Itraconazole for mild to moderate infections. For moderate to severe infections, AMBD or lipid formulations of amphotericin B for 1–2 weeks followed by itraconazole, for a total of 12 weeks. |
| | Disseminated | AMBD or lipid formulations of amphotericin B for 1–2 weeks followed by itraconazole. For severe disease, duration of therapy is usually 12 months, but some experts treat for shorter time (eg, 6 months). HIV-infected patients require indefinite suppressive therapy with itraconazole. |
| *Scedosporium* species | Fungemia or disseminated infection | Voriconazole, based on anecdotal experience. All the commercially available agents show poor in vitro activity against *Scedosporium prolificans*, for which experts recommend voriconazole, plus terbinafine or an echinocandin (or both) with surgical excision if feasible. Duration of therapy is undetermined, but 6 weeks minimum and typically until immune reconstitution. Amphotericin B is ineffective. |
| *Sporothrix schenckii* | Cutaneous or lymphocutaneous | Itraconazole for 3–6 months. |
| *Trichosporon* (species) | Fungemia or disseminated infection | Voriconazole. Central venous catheter removal if it is involved. Duration of therapy is undetermined, but 6 weeks minimum. |
| Zygomycoses: *Rhizopus* species, *Mucor* species, *Rhizomucor* species, *Cunninghamella bertholletiae* | Rhinocerebral, pulmonary, and disseminated | AMBD or lipid formulations of amphotericin B. Some experts recommend combination therapy with liposomal amphotericin B plus echinocandin for initial therapy. Isavuconazole seems as effective as amphotericin B. Posaconazole can also be considered. Discontinuation of steroids, controlling diabetes mellitus. Surgical excision of lesion if feasible. Duration of therapy is undetermined, but 6 weeks minimum and also until immune reconstitution. |
| Empiric therapy of presumed fungal infection in febrile neutropenic patients | | Echinocandin or liposomal amphotericin B until resolution of neutropenia (absolute neutrophil count > 100–500/μL) in the absence of documented or suspected invasive fungal diseases. Agents already given as prophylaxis and risk for invasive mold infections (eg, severity and duration of neutropenia) should be taken into account in antifungal choice. |

of cryptococcal infection. Its usefulness in treating patients with non-AIDS–associated cryptococcal meningitis has not been defined. Fluconazole is also effective in coccidioidal meningitis and other types of coccidioidomycosis.

Fluconazole is available as an oral suspension, a tablet, and an intravenous solution. It is well absorbed from the gastrointestinal tract, and the recommended oral and intravenous dosages are identical. For patients with moderate to severe oropharyngeal candidiasis, a dose of 100 to 200 mg daily for 7 to 14 days for adults, or a loading dose of 6 mg/kg followed by 3 mg/kg daily for 2 weeks for children is recommended. The recommended daily dosage for patients with systemic fungal infection is 400 to 800 mg for adults and approximately 6 to 12 mg/kg for children. Dosing recommendations for premature infants are based on both the gestational age and the postnatal age of the infant at drug initiation. Fluconazole has excellent penetration into the CSF and vitreous humor. Unlike the other azoles that are metabolized in the liver, fluconazole is concentrated and excreted unchanged in the urine (favorable for treating cystitis); thus, the dosage must be adjusted for patients with renal impairment. The most common side effects are gastrointestinal complaints; less frequently, hepatic enzyme activity may be elevated. Development of resistance to fluconazole, especially among *Candida* species, is reported with increasing frequency. Failure of fluconazole treatment may be attributable to resistance, especially in patients who have received chronic suppressive therapy, and to the drug's fungistatic, rather than fungicidal, effects. Similar to the other azoles, fluconazole has many potential drug interactions to consider.

Itraconazole (Sporanox) has activity similar to that of fluconazole but is also active against *Aspergillus* species and certain dematiaceous molds. It is indicated for the treatment of sporotrichosis, blastomycosis, histoplasmosis, aspergillosis, and onychomycosis. It is also effective in tinea capitis in adults and children. Itraconazole has also been used for the prophylaxis and empiric therapy of fungal infections in neutropenic cancer patients and hematopoietic stem cell transplant recipients. The oral solution of itraconazole is effective therapy for oropharyngeal and esophageal candidiasis. Currently, the agent is available as an oral solution and a capsule. The preparations are not interchangeable; the oral solution produces greater systemic drug exposure than the equivalent dose in capsule form. Bioavailability of the capsule form is affected by the acidity of the stomach, and the capsules should be taken with food. The oral solution is less affected by stomach pH and should be taken on an empty stomach. Itraconazole is highly protein bound, and very little penetrates into the CSF. It is metabolized by the liver and excreted as inactive metabolites in the feces and urine. Although neither formulation is approved by the FDA for use in children, multiple pediatric studies describe the administration of itraconazole at dosages as high as 10 mg/kg/d for severe infections and 2.5 to 5 mg/kg/d for tinea capitis and onychomycosis. Serum itraconazole concentration for the treatment of invasive fungal infections, such as histoplasmosis and blastomycosis, should be at least 1 μg/mL by high-performance liquid chromatography (HPLC) or 3 μg/mL by bioassay. The duration of therapy for onychomycosis is 3 to 4 months. However, because the drug accumulates in the nail tissues, "pulse therapy" (repeated courses of 1 week of therapy, 3–5 mg/kg/d, followed by 1–3 weeks without therapy) has been reported to be effective for onychomycosis. As with fluconazole, gastrointestinal side effects occur most frequently. Use of itraconazole with terfenadine, cisapride, or astemizole can cause a serious drug interaction that produces life-threatening cardiac arrhythmias. Itraconazole has been reported to potentiate vincristine toxicity in children undergoing concurrent chemotherapy for leukemia.

Voriconazole (Vfend), a second-generation triazole and synthetic derivative of fluconazole, is approved for use in the treatment of invasive aspergillosis, serious *Candida* infections in nonneutropenic patients (eg, candidemia, disseminated disease, and infections caused by fluconazole-resistant species), and serious infections due to *Scedosporium apiospermum* and *Fusarium* species in patients refractory to or intolerant of other therapy. Voriconazole is currently the recommended initial therapy for invasive aspergillosis as it was shown to be superior to AMBD. Published reports suggest voriconazole also demonstrates activity in a variety of less common or refractory fungal infections. However, voriconazole is not active against the zygomycetes, and clinical reports have noted emergence of these infections following prophylactic administration of voriconazole.

Voriconazole is available as an intravenous preparation, tablet, and oral suspension. The pharmacokinetics of voriconazole are nonlinear in adults but appear to be linear in children. Thus, children require higher doses of voriconazole than adults. The most recent recommendation for children age 2 to 11 years is to start with an intravenous loading dosage of 9 mg/kg every 12 hours for 2 doses followed by 8 mg/kg every 12 hours. Serum drug concentrations should be monitored because of the intrapersonal variability in metabolism of this drug (eg, CYP2C19 polymorphism). Studies show that trough levels less than 1 μg/mL were associated with poorer clinical response and trough levels above 5.5 μg/mL with higher risk for neurotoxicity; therefore, a therapeutic target for trough levels in the range of 1.5 to 4.5 μg/mL has been proposed. Voriconazole concentrations in tissue and CSF exceed those of the trough plasma level several-fold. Similar to the other azoles, voriconazole has many potential drug interactions to consider.

Visual disturbances, elevated liver transaminases, and dermatologic reactions are the most common adverse effects associated with voriconazole administration. Visual disturbances include blurred vision, photophobia, and altered or enhanced visual perception and occur in approximately 25% to 45% of recipients. These reactions typically occur within 30 minutes of drug administration and have a median duration of 30 minutes. Increased liver transaminases occur in approximately 10% to 20% of recipients. For patients with mild to moderate hepatic insufficiency (Child-Pugh class A and B, scores 5 to 9), the manufacturer recommends giving the normal loading dose but halving the maintenance dose. There are no data available on administration in patients with more severe hepatic dysfunction. Rash, including photosensitivity, occurs in less than 10%. Dose adjustments for patients with renal insufficiency are not necessary for the oral formulation. However, the intravenous formulation of voriconazole is not generally recommended for patients with moderate to severe renal impairment because of possible accumulation of the cyclodextrin vehicle used in the intravenous formulation that may lead to nephrotoxicity. Of note, unlike fluconazole, urine concentrations of voriconazole do not reach therapeutic levels; thus, this agent should not be relied on to treat urinary tract infections.

Posaconazole (Noxafil) is a second-generation triazole that is closely related to itraconazole. It has even broader coverage than voriconazole with activity against the zygomycetes. Currently, posaconazole is indicated for treatment of oropharyngeal candidiasis (including refractory cases) and for antifungal prophylaxis in patients older than 13 years undergoing hematopoietic stem cell transplant or with prolonged neutropenia. In addition, posaconazole has demonstrated efficacy as salvage therapy in a variety of fungal infections, including aspergillosis, fusariosis, and zygomycosis.

Posaconazole is available as an oral suspension, an extended-release tablet, and an intravenous solution. Bioavailability of the oral suspension is unpredictable, but its absorption is improved with divided daily dosing and high-fat meals. Delayed-release tablets demonstrate less variability in pharmacokinetic parameters related to food intake when compared with the oral suspension and thus are useful in patients who cannot eat full meals. Dosage recommendations are the same for the delayed-release tablets and the intravenous form; these dosing recommendations are not interchangeable with the oral suspension dosing recommendations. In general, the intravenous formulation of posaconazole should be restricted to patients ≥ 18 years of age who are unable to take the extended-release tablet or suspension for the treatment of invasive fungal disease and whose infections are unable to be adequately treated by other intravenous antifungal agents. The recommended dose of the delayed-release or intravenous formulation for adolescents and adults is 300 mg twice daily as a loading dose followed by 300 mg daily for prophylaxis and treatment. Using the oral suspension, the recommended dose for adults is 200 mg 3 times daily for prophylaxis or 800 mg daily (divided 2–4 times) for treatment of serious infections. The adult dose is recommended for adolescents because a small number of older children, age 8 to 17 years, have demonstrated similar serum concentrations as adults. There are limited pharmacokinetic data for posaconazole in younger children. For antifungal prophylaxis in infants and children ≥ 8 months to < 12 years, 4 mg/kg/dose of oral suspension administered thrice daily is recommended. For treatment purposes, we suggest an oral suspension dosage of 4.5 to 6 mg/kg/dose 4 times daily in children weighing less than 34 kg or the adult dosage if weight is 34 kg or more. Posaconazole is generally well tolerated; gastrointestinal symptoms, including vomiting, abdominal pain, and diarrhea, are the most commonly reported side effects. The drug is primarily eliminated in feces as an unchanged form and is not a choice for urinary tract infection. Therapeutic drug monitoring is recommended, and experts suggest a trough concentration of ≥ 0.7 μg/mL for prophylaxis and ≥ 1.0 μg/mL for treatment of severe infections.

Isavuconazole (Cresemba) was recently approved by the FDA for treatment of invasive aspergillosis and invasive mucormycosis in adults (18 years and older). It is formulated as the prodrug, isavuconazonium sulfate, and available as both intravenous (IV) and oral formulations (capsules). The oral capsule has excellent bioavailability and a longer half-life, and it is easier to achieve good serum levels compared with the other second-generation triazoles. Neither IV nor oral formulations contain cyclodextrin vehicle, a solubilizing agent used in voriconazole or posaconazole; thus, IV isavuconazole can be used in patients with renal dysfunction, another advantage of this new agent. Isavuconazole is generally safe and well tolerated but has drug-drug interactions like the other azole agents. A double-blind, randomized controlled trial has shown noninferiority of this agent compared with voriconazole as initial therapy for invasive aspergillosis. Furthermore, isavuconazole was associated with less frequent adverse events than voriconazole. A single-arm, open-label trial with a matched control from the FugiScope database suggested equivalent efficacy of isavuconazole for zygomycosis compared with amphotericin B. Clinical experience with isavuconazole in the pediatric population is still very limited.

#### Echinocandins

The echinocandins act by inhibiting the synthesis of 1,3-β-d-glucan, a major component of the fungal cell wall. Because there is no counterpart in the mammalian cell, the echinocandins are predictably much better tolerated compared to other antifungal agents. Currently, 3 echinocandins are commercially available. They are available only as IV formulations and have the same general spectrum of activity. They have long half-lives and can be dosed once daily. Echinocandins are fungicidal against *Candida* species, including azole-resistant species, and fungistatic against *Aspergillus* species. Echinocandins are not active against most of the noncandidal yeasts (eg, *Cryptococcus* species) or the majority of molds other than *Aspergillus* species.

Caspofungin (Cancidas) is approved for treatment of esophageal candidiasis, candidemia, and other candidal infections; as treatment of aspergillosis in patients who are refractory to or intolerant of other therapies; and as empiric therapy for presumed fungal infections in febrile, neutropenic patients. The agent is highly protein bound and penetrates into all major organs including the brain. However, the concentration in uninfected CSF is low, and there is a lack of clinical data to support its use in central nervous system infections. The recommended dosage for children is a loading dose of 70 mg/m$^2$ followed by daily administration of 50 mg/m$^2$ (maximum loading and daily maintenance dose of 70 mg). If concomitant inducers of hepatic cytochrome P450 enzymes are also given, the daily dose in pediatric patients should be 70 mg/m$^2$ (still with a daily maximum of 70 mg). No dose adjustment is indicated for patients who are on dialysis or have renal or mild hepatic insufficiency. Reduction in the daily dose from 50 to 35 mg is recommended for adults with moderate hepatic insufficiency (Child-Pugh class B, or score 7 to 9). There is no information on administration in patients with severe hepatic dysfunction. The most common adverse events reported with the use of caspofungin are mild increases in hepatic transaminases, gastrointestinal upset, and headache.

Micafungin (Mycamine) is similar to caspofungin and is indicated for the treatment of esophageal candidiasis and as prophylaxis in patients undergoing stem cell transplant. In addition, there are clinical studies demonstrating efficacy in disseminated candidiasis and in invasive aspergillosis in patients refractory to or intolerant of other antifungal therapy. Micafungin is highly protein bound and achieves highest tissue concentrations in the lung. Low levels can be detected in the brain, and levels are undetectable in CSF. Micafungin has been studied in children and neonates. The drug was well tolerated without dose-related toxicities. Recommended pediatric dosing for adolescents, children, or infants ≥ 4 months of age is 1 mg/kg/d (maximum dose of 50 mg daily) for prophylaxis and 2 to 3 mg/kg/d (maximum dose of 150 mg daily) for treatment. In salvage treatment studies of aspergillosis, children received doses up to 8.6 mg/kg/d safely. Premature infants less than 1000 g have a shorter half-life and more rapid clearance, and a dose of 10 mg/kg/dose once daily is recommended. For neonates > 1000 g, 7 to 10 mg/kg/dose once daily is recommended. Patients with renal insufficiency and mild or moderate hepatic dysfunction do not require dose adjustments of micafungin.

Anidulafungin (Eraxis) has a similar spectrum of activity and safety profile compared to other echinocandins. Animal data indicate a large volume of distribution, suggesting extensive tissue distribution. Tissue concentrations are highest in the lung and liver. Measurable concentrations were detected in the brain. The half-life is even longer than that of the other echinocandins, greater than 24 hours in adults. Anidulafungin is indicated for the treatment of esophageal candidiasis and candidemia and other forms of *Candida* infections (intra-abdominal abscess and peritonitis) in nonneutropenic patients. The recommended dosing for adults is a loading dose of 200 mg followed by a 100 mg daily dose for systemic *Candida* infections and a 100-mg loading dose followed by 50 mg daily for esophageal candidiasis. The pediatric equivalent is approximately 1.5 mg/kg/d and 0.75 mg/kg/d, respectively. Dose adjustment is not needed for renal insufficiency and mild, moderate, or severe hepatic insufficiency. As with the other echinocandins, anidulafungin is well tolerated, with gastrointestinal symptoms and mild increases in hepatic transaminases as the most commonly attributed events.

#### Other Systemic Antifungal Agents

Flucytosine (5-FC, Ancobon), a fluorinated pyrimidine related to fluorouracil, is indicated for treating serious infections caused by *Candida* species and *C neoformans*. It is converted to fluorouracil within fungal cells, where it interferes with ribonucleic acid (RNA) and deoxyribonucleic acid (DNA) synthesis. Flucytosine is available in capsule form and is readily absorbed from the gastrointestinal tract. Because the drug is poorly protein bound and penetrates the blood-brain barrier, it is effective as adjunctive therapy for meningitis, in combination with amphotericin B. The recommended daily dosage is 50 to 150 mg/kg, divided into 4 equal doses. The dosage must be adjusted for patients with renal impairment, and caution should be used when flucytosine is administered to patients with underlying renal dysfunction. The target serum peak concentration of 5-FC for cryptococcal infection is between 30 and 80 μg/mL, and levels above 100 μg/mL should be avoided to avert bone marrow suppression, which is the most serious toxicity. Gastrointestinal complaints, hepatitis, and jaundice are frequent adverse effects. Flucytosine should be used in combination with other antifungal agents, such as amphotericin B, because pathogens rapidly acquire resistance to flucytosine when it is used alone.

Griseofulvin (Gris-peg and Grifulvin V) is indicated for treatment of superficial fungal infections of skin, hair, and nails that are caused by various species of dermatophytes, including *Trichophyton, Microsporum*, and *Epidermophyton*. The drug inhibits fungal cell mitosis by binding to fungal microtubules. The drug also binds to human keratin and renders keratin-rich tissue resistant to fungal infection. Absorption from the gastrointestinal tract is markedly variable but is thought to be increased by fatty meals and by the use of smaller griseofulvin crystals. Currently, formulations containing microsized and ultramicrosized griseofulvin crystals are commercially available. The daily dosage for children is approximately 10 mg/kg of ultramicrosized and 15 mg/kg of microsized griseofulvin, given as 1 dose or 2 divided doses. The duration of therapy depends on the location of the fungal infection; therapy must be continued until the infected tissue is replaced by normal tissue. Tinea corporis requires 2 to 4 weeks of therapy, tinea capitis 4 to 6 weeks of therapy, and infection of toenails at least 6 to 12 months of therapy. The safety of griseofulvin treatment is not established for children younger than 2 years of age. Griseofulvin is usually well tolerated; rash and urticaria are the most common adverse effects. Headache is also common. When given with warfarin, griseofulvin may result in decreased plasma warfarin concentration; it may also reduce the effectiveness of oral contraceptives. Phenobarbital may diminish the effectiveness of griseofulvin.

Terbinafine (Lamisil) is an allylamine that acts by inhibiting fungal synthesis of ergosterol, a component of the fungal cell membrane. It is available as a topical agent and also as an oral tablet for treatment of onychomycosis. The drug has not been tested in children and should be reserved for patients with refractory disease. The recommended adult regimen is 250 mg daily for 6 weeks for fingernail disease and 12 weeks for toenail disease. Children who weigh more than 40 kg should receive the adult dosage. The dosage should be 125 mg/d for children who weigh between 20 and 40 kg and 62.5 mg/d for children who weigh less than 20 kg. Gastrointestinal toxicity is observed most frequently.

### COMBINATION SYSTEMIC ANTIFUNGAL THERAPY

As multiple classes of systemic antifungal agents are now available, there is considerable interest in combining agents for the treatment of serious invasive fungal infections. The combination of AMBD plus 5-flucytosine in cryptococcal meningitis and AMBD plus fluconazole in candidemia remained the only combinations supported by evidence from randomized clinical trials until recently. A randomized controlled trial has recently shown that combination therapy with voriconazole plus anidulafungin for invasive aspergillosis had trends for better survival compared to voriconazole monotherapy. Outside these settings, however, there are limited clinical data to support the use of combination antifungal therapy as definitive antifungal therapy. Considering the increased toxicity associated with dual therapy and some animal data suggesting antagonistic effects (eg, amphotericin B vs azoles), combination antifungal therapy (other than those currently supported by clinical trials) should be used with caution.

### TOPICAL ANTIFUNGAL AGENTS

Topical antifungal agents are available in many different preparations, including ointment, cream, solution, lotion, powder, oral and vaginal troches, and vaginal tablets. Topical agents are the treatment of choice for superficial fungal infections of the skin, mucosa, and cornea, such as dermatophytosis (tinea corporis, tinea cruris, tinea pedis), tinea versicolor, candidiasis, and fungal keratitis. Creams and lotions are generally preferable to ointments for treating diseases of the skin. Powders are used only in moist areas such as the feet, groin, or other intertriginous areas. Several of the agents used as systemic therapy are also available as topical preparations. In such cases, the mechanism of action is the same, but the efficacy of the topical agents depends on their direct interaction with the fungal organisms on the surface of the skin or mucous membranes. In selecting a topical antifungal agent, consideration should be given to the type of preparation needed and the cost. Several agents now available without prescription may be used as first-line therapy for tinea corporis, with more expensive preparations reserved for resistant infection.

#### Polyene Antifungals

Nystatin belongs to the polyene class with the mechanism of action similar to that of amphotericin B, but nystatin is active only against superficial candidiasis. The agent is available as a cream, ointment, powder, vaginal tablet, oral tablet, pastille, and suspension. Nystatin suspension is the treatment of choice for oral candidiasis and should be administered 4 times daily. Children who are able should be instructed to swish the suspension around the mouth and then swallow. Side effects include nausea and bad taste, but both are manageable. Topical nystatin is also frequently used for candidiasis in the diaper area and is available in combination with corticosteroids. Nystatin powder is effective for treating superficial candidiasis in skin folds, but care should be taken to prevent young infants from inhaling the powder when it is applied to their necks.

#### Azoles

Multiple azole antifungal agents are available as topical preparations. They are active against *Candida* species, *Trichophyton* species, *Microsporum* species, and, in some cases, *Malassezia furfur*. When used as directed, topical azoles cause few side effects. Some redness and irritation can occur.

Clotrimazole is available as an oral troche, vaginal tablet, vaginal cream, cream, and lotion. All but the oral troches are available over the counter. A clotrimazole and corticosteroid combination is also available, but it should be used with caution in children, who may absorb proportionally larger amounts of corticosteroid and thus be more susceptible to systemic toxicity. Miconazole is also available over the counter as a cream, spray, powder, lotion, and vaginal cream. These agents are readily available and inexpensive, and they should be the treatment of choice for tinea corporis (including tinea pedis and tinea cruris) and vaginal candidiasis. Topical ketoconazole, econazole, sulconazole, sertaconazole, and oxiconazole are also available. These agents should be considered second-line agents because of cost. Ketoconazole is available as a shampoo for treatment of tinea versicolor but is ineffective for tinea capitis. Terconazole, butoconazole, and tioconazole are available only as vaginal preparations.

#### Allylamines

Three topical allylamine agents—terbinafine, naftifine, and butenafine—are currently available. As a group, allylamines are active against the dermatophytes.

#### Other Topical Antifungal Agents

Tolnaftate is a synthetic thiocarbamate active against dermatophytes but ineffective for infections caused by *Candida* species and less effective than the azoles for tinea corporis. Many preparations of tolnaftate are available without prescription. Ciclopirox is a synthetic topical antifungal agent with broad-spectrum activity against the dermatophytes, including *M furfur*.

### SUGGESTED READINGS

Felton T, Troke PF, Hope WW. Tissue penetration of antifungal agents. *Clin Microbiol Rev*. 2014;27:68-88.

Maertens JA, Raad II, Marr KA, et al. Isavuconazole versus voriconazole for primary treatment of invasive mould disease caused by *Aspergillus* and other filamentous fungi (SECURE): a phase 3, randomised-controlled, non-inferiority trial. *Lancet*. 2016;387:760-769.

Marr KA, Schlamm HT, Herbrecht R, et al. Combination antifungal therapy for invasive aspergillosis: a randomized trial. *Ann Intern Med*. 2015;162:81-89.

Marty FM, Ostrosky-Zeichner L, Cornely OA, et al; VITAL and FungiScope Mucormysosis Investigators. Isavuconazole treatment for mucormycosis: a single-arm open-label trial and case-control analysis. *Lancet Infect Dis*. 2016;16:828-837.

Nucci M, Marr KA, Vehreschild MJ, et al. Improvement in the outcome of invasive fusariosis in the last decade. *Clin Microbiol Infect*. 2014;20:580-585.

Pappas PG, Kauffman CA, Andes DR, et al. Clinical practice guideline for the management of candidiasis: 2016 update by the Infectious Diseases Society of America. *Clin Infect Dis*. 2016;62:e1-e50.

Patterson TF, Thompson GR 3rd, Denning DW, et al. Practice guidelines for the diagnosis and management of aspergillosis: 2016 update by the Infectious Diseases Society of America. *Clin Infect Dis*. 2016;63:e1-e60.

# PART 5 BACTERIAL INFECTIONS

## 243 Actinomycosis

Nahed Abdel-Haq

### INTRODUCTION

Actinomycosis is a slowly progressive, suppurative infection characterized by fistula formation. A number of gram-positive, non–spore-forming bacteria from the genus *Actinomyces* are the etiologic agents. It is encountered worldwide in 3 main clinical forms: cervicofacial, thoracic, and abdominal. Metastatic lesions to other sites are also reported. With appropriate therapy, most patients with cervicofacial or abdominal infection recover completely.

### EPIDEMIOLOGY AND PATHOGENESIS

*Actinomyces* species are part of the normal flora of the human gastrointestinal tract. Actinomycosis is not considered a communicable disease. It affects both immunocompetent and immunocompromised individuals. Diabetes mellitus, malnutrition, and immunosuppression may be predisposing factors. Although uncommon in children, actinomycosis has been reported even in infancy. The disease is not related to occupation, season, or race.

With the use of 16S rRNA sequencing, at least 21 species of *Actinomyces* have been identified in humans. *A israelii*, the species that most commonly produces human disease, is part of normal oral flora. *A viscosus, A naeslundii, A odontolyticus, A meyeri*, and *Propionibacterium* (*Arachnia*) *propionica* are also established etiologic agents. *Actinomyces* species require an anaerobic or microaerophilic environment for growth and demonstrate gram-positive branching filaments, often appearing as beaded filaments. It has also been shown that *Actinomyces* species require the presence of other bacteria to multiply. Thus, actinomycosis is frequently polymicrobial in nature, and concomitant bacterial species such as *Eikenella corrodens, Aggregatibacter actinomycetemcomitans, Fusobacterium, Capnocytophaga, Staphylococcus*, microaerophilic streptococci, and Enterobacteriaceae are often isolated from actinomycotic lesions.

### CLINICAL MANIFESTATIONS

Actinomycosis may present as a chronic indolent process, as an acute rapidly progressive infection, or somewhere between these extremes. However, the most common presentation remains the chronic indolent form. The hallmark of actinomycosis is the spread of infection that fails to respect fascial or tissue planes.

#### Cervicofacial Disease

Cervicofacial disease is the most common type of infection in immunocompetent individuals, accounting for 60% of patients with actinomycosis. Predisposing factors include gingivitis, gingival trauma, dental procedures, and tooth-related infections. It presents as a slowly progressive, indurated swelling or mass, usually at the angle of the jaw (lumpy jaw), but it can occur anywhere on the cheek, mandible, or anterior neck. The duration of illness is typically several months. Pain is seldom prominent. A low-grade fever may occur in as many as 50% of patients. Most patients do not appear systemically ill. Inflammatory markers such as the erythrocyte sedimentation rate and C-reactive protein as well as the white blood cell count are often normal.

The clinical progression may be marked by episodes of suppuration that are contained by reactive fibrosis. Although the lesions may be intermittently fluctuant and appear as cold abscesses, they will eventually progress to a hard mass with a lumpy appearance. The disease spreads to adjacent tissues without regard to anatomic structures. Lymphatic spread and associated lymphadenopathy are uncommon. The skin overlying the mass may become violaceous, and sinus tract formation with spontaneous discharge often occurs. These sinus tracts have little tendency to heal and may remain chronic. There may be associated trismus. The drainage may reveal 1-mm diameter yellow friable masses termed *sulfur granules*, which are actual colonies of *Actinomyces*. The diagnosis of actinomycosis should be considered in virtually any chronic mass or recurrent abscess in the head and neck region.

Maxillary and ethmoid sinusitis may occur. Actinomycosis is an uncommon but important cause of otitis media, as untreated cases can extend into the mastoid and central nervous system and cause death. As a cause of middle ear disease, actinomycosis is characterized by numerous episodes of otitis media that transiently respond to antibiotics (conventional short-course therapy) or by resistance to myringotomy. The diagnosis can be made by microbiologic examination of cholesteatoma-like material from the middle ear.

Periostitis or osteomyelitis may develop if the infection extends to the mandibular or maxillary bones. In children presenting with osteomyelitis due to *Actinomyces*, the mandible is the most common site of involvement. More than 1 surgical debridement procedure is frequently needed. Most affected children are school-aged, and about half of them have underlying medical predisposing conditions.

Actinomycosis of the tonsils is a rare and poorly defined clinical entity. *Actinomyces* species may be isolated from tonsillar crypts of both inflamed and uninflamed tonsils. Patients with tonsillar actinomycosis may present with coughing and expectoration of particulate material or a tonsillar mass. *Actinomyces* species may have a role in tonsillar hypertrophy. Patients with tonsillar actinomycosis may require tonsillectomy, particularly if antibiotic treatment fails.

Actinomycosis of the thyroid is another rare clinical entity. Predisposing factors include the persistence of a thyroglossal duct or a pyriform sinus fistula, which facilitates communication between the oral flora and the thyroid gland. Acute thyroiditis and abscess have been reported. An affected child may present with a painless neck mass. Treatment is a combination of surgical drainage and antibiotics. Primary actinomycosis may rarely occur in the palate, tongue, larynx, hypopharynx, or trachea.

Central nervous system (CNS) involvement has been documented in 2% to 10% of cases of cervicofacial actinomycosis. Most cases of CNS actinomycosis are due to hematogenous or lymphatic spread from a distant focus such as the mouth, lungs, abdomen, or pelvis. Other mechanisms of CNS infection include direct extension from soft tissues, orbit, sinus, or auditory canal, spread through foramina, and perineural spread. Spread to the meninges may cause meningitis, meningoencephalitis, and brain abscess. Other forms of CNS involvement include tumor-like lesions called actinomycetomas as well as subdural and epidural abscesses.

### Thoracic Disease

Thoracic involvement accounts for about 15% of patients with actinomycosis. It results from inhalation of contaminated aerosol particles or aspiration of contaminated secretions from the oropharynx or upper gastrointestinal tract. Less commonly, pulmonary involvement occurs following esophageal perforation or as an extension of cervicofacial or abdominal disease. Poor oral and dental hygiene is a predisposing condition. Immunocompromised and neurologically impaired patients are at increased risk. Thoracic actinomycosis is rare in children and young adults. Most cases are due to *A israelii*.

The most common presentation is a slowly progressive disease involving the parenchyma and pleura. Fever and weight loss may be the only clinical manifestations; thus, a high index of suspicion is required for diagnosis. Hemoptysis has been reported. Tachypnea, chest pain, and productive cough are not common. As the disease progresses, the lung becomes consolidated and an abscess may form; the pleura and thoracic wall are invaded and produce empyema, rib involvement with osteolytic lesions, subcutaneous abscesses, a thoracic mass, or draining sinuses. Delayed diagnosis may result in bacteremic dissemination with increased risk of death. Pulmonary actinomycosis must be differentiated from nocardiosis, tuberculosis, fungal infection, pyogenic lung abscess, and cancer. Due to the slow progression of the disease, if bone is involved, both destruction and new bone formation occur, producing wavy periostitis in the ribs or sawtooth changes in the vertebral bodies. Mediastinal actinomycosis is uncommon.

Isolation of *Actinomyces* species in sputum cultures is unusual, due to the overgrowth of synergistic bacteria, prior use of antibiotics, and improper handling of anaerobic cultures. In addition, *Actinomyces* species are found normally in saliva samples. Transbronchial biopsy or needle aspiration biopsy may be used to confirm the diagnosis. However, surgery is frequently needed to establish the diagnosis. Other indications for surgery are recurrent or severe hemoptysis, prolonged illness, poor response to antibiotics, and suspected carcinoma.

Cardiac actinomycosis is rare and follows direct spread from pulmonary disease. Pericardial involvement is the most common form. Myocarditis and endocarditis are less frequent. The clinical presentation of pericarditis is more insidious than other causes of purulent pericarditis. The diagnosis is usually made by histopathologic identification of the typical *Actinomyces* filaments and sulfur granules in a pericardial biopsy. Esophageal actinomycosis is a rare clinical entity that mainly affects immunocompromised patients including those with cancer or human immunodeficiency virus.

### Abdominal Disease

Abdominal actinomycosis accounts for 20% of patients. Any structures in the abdomen may be involved. The majority of cases begin in the ileocecal region as a complication of appendicitis or appendectomy (65% of cases). It may also follow gastric bypass surgery. Actinomycosis may arise from a perforating gastrointestinal ulcer or after the intestinal mucosa is penetrated by a sharp object such as a knife, ingested bone, or bullet. Unrecognized perforation by a pin or needle also may lead to actinomycosis. Abdominal infections are polymicrobial; gram-negative bacilli are frequent concomitant pathogens.

The initial symptoms are insidious and include abdominal discomfort, fever, weight loss, change in bowel habits, and malaise. Abdominal tenderness and guarding in the right iliac fossa are common with perforated appendix. During the initial stage of infection, an abscess forms that is followed by extension to the peritoneum. The abscess consists of pus surrounded by a thick layer of granulation tissue. Abdominal examination often reveals a mass. Months to years may pass from the time of the inciting event to clinical recognition of this indolent infection. In advanced stages, the disease progresses to fistula formation, both internally and externally, simulating inflammatory bowel disease. Abscess rupture through the abdominal wall produces a typical draining sinus from which sulfur granules are detected.

Colonic involvement accounts for approximately 15% of abdominal actinomycosis, often presenting with obstruction or fistula. Isolation of *Actinomyces* species or identification of characteristic sulfur granules in sinus drainage material is diagnostic. However, in the absence of these findings, differentiation from appendicitis, regional enteritis, cancer, abscess, tuberculosis, amebiasis, and other intra-abdominal disorders may only be possible by biopsy. The infection may extend to involve other abdominal organs or the spine, or it may penetrate the diaphragm to produce thoracic disease.

Hepatic infection occurs in 5% of cases of abdominal actinomycosis, usually by direct extension. Most cases are unilobar. Patients present with nonspecific signs and symptoms. Ultrasound may show an abscess or a solid mass suggestive of a tumor. Most hepatic abscesses can be drained percutaneously in contrast to abscesses elsewhere in the abdomen. Rarely, actinomycosis may present secondary to hematogenous spread to the liver.

### Other Clinical Presentations

Renal involvement is rare and often occurs due to direct extension from abdominal or pelvic abscesses. Hematogenous seeding of the kidney may rarely occur. Most cases of renal actinomycosis are diagnosed following nephrectomy for renal masses. However, nephrectomy can be avoided by suspecting the diagnosis and obtaining fine-needle aspirate and biopsy.

Pelvic actinomycosis is commonly associated with the presence of any type of intrauterine contraceptive device (IUD) and appears to occur rarely unless the IUD has been in place for at least 2 years. It has been reported months after removal of an IUD, making a history of prior use important. *Actinomyces* species have been identified in 8% to 20% of women using IUDs. Although most of those colonized individuals are asymptomatic, up to 25% develop symptoms of pelvic infection. Pelvic actinomycosis may also occur as a complication of abortion, endometriosis, pelvic inflammatory disease, or tubo-ovarian abscess. Presentation is most frequently that of an indolent infection, with fever, weight loss, abnormal vaginal bleeding, and pain being common. Less frequently, patients may present more acutely if the concomitant pathogen is *Staphylococcus aureus* or β-hemolytic streptococci. Actinomycosis should be considered in women using IUDs who present with any abdominal pathology. Involvement of the bladder and ureters may cause hydroureter and hydronephrosis. Extensive disease leading to liver abscesses, intestinal obstruction, and pleural effusion has also been reported. Women frequently undergo surgery because of suspicion of ovarian cancer due to masses of pelvic actinomycosis. Because of the extensive soft tissue involvement and the lack of well-defined surgical margins, early surgical intervention in stable patients is limited to relief of obstructive symptoms or drainage of large abscesses. Surgery is also indicated in patients with no clinical or radiologic evidence of improvement on antibiotic treatment.

Rarely, actinomycotic skin and soft tissue lesions mimicking tumors are seen on extremities secondary to traumatic inoculation (including toothpick injuries). Human bites have caused localized skin infection with *Actinomyces* species. Musculoskeletal disease involving bones other than those noted thus far have also been reported. Some cases of actinomycosis have been linked to specific conditions, such as osteoradionecrosis or bisphosphonate-related osteonecrosis of the jaws, the use of anti–tumor necrosis factor-α drugs, and hereditary disorders such as hereditary hemorrhagic telangiectasia and chronic granulomatous disease.

## DIAGNOSIS

The diagnosis of actinomycosis is obvious when a draining sinus in the neck, chest, or abdomen produces sulfur granules. Microscopic examination of these granules reveals gram-positive, beaded filaments that are not acid fast. Sulfur granules are characteristic but not a universal finding of actinomycosis. Further, they can be produced by other bacteria such as *S aureus, Nocardia*, and *Actinobacillus lignieresii*, and fungi such as *Sporotrichum* and *Phialophora*.

Biopsies for histopathologic evaluation and culture are frequently needed for diagnosis of actinomycosis. Pathologic examination will reveal a central suppurative area surrounded by chronic granulation tissue and a thick fibrous capsule. Sulfur granules, if present, are found in the necrotic centers. The capsule is characteristically intensely collagenous, fibrotic, and avascular, and thus helps to maintain the anaerobic environment, limit antibiotic penetration, and allow for progression of infection.

Isolation of *Actinomyces* species in tissue samples is essential to confirm the diagnosis. Optimal isolation often requires specimens to be transported and cultured on semi-selective anaerobic media. Because these organisms are normal oral flora, isolation of the organisms is not sufficient for diagnosis in the absence of sulfur granules. The use of immunofluorescent-conjugated monoclonal antibodies (IFAs) has improved identification of *Actinomyces* species. Partial or complete 16S rRNA gene sequencing has been used for definitive molecular identification of clinical *Actinomyces* isolates that fail to be identified by routine phenotypic methods.

## TREATMENT

Prolonged and intensive penicillin therapy remains the mainstay of treatment for most cases of actinomycosis. Initially, intravenous aqueous penicillin should be given for 2 to 4 weeks for cervicofacial disease and 4 to 6 weeks for pulmonary and abdominal infection, depending on the extent of disease and response to therapy. Subsequently, patients should receive high-dose oral penicillin V for 6 to 12 months. Ampicillin/amoxicillin may be substituted for penicillin. Patients allergic to penicillin may be treated with erythromycin, clindamycin, or doxycycline (such long courses of this drug are not recommended for use in children under 8 years of age). Most patients with cervicofacial disease respond to antibiotic therapy alone.

If the duration of treatment is not extended beyond the resolution of measurable disease, relapses will occur. Successful treatment with shorter courses of antibiotics (< 6 months) has been reported; such patients typically had localized disease and underwent appropriate drainage procedures. Accessible abscesses should be incised and drained. Because extensive fibrosis may limit antibiotic penetration of abscesses, surgical excision should be considered for refractory fibrotic lesions that respond slowly to antibiotic therapy. Persistent sinus tracts should be marsupialized. Successful treatment of actinomycosis often requires surgery, which should always be accompanied by appropriate antibiotic therapy.

## SUGGESTED READINGS


Attaway A, Flynn T. *Actinomyces meyeri*: from "lumpy jaw" to empyema. *Infection*. 2013;41(5):1025-1027.

Bartlett AH, Rivera AL, Krishnamurthy R, Baker CJ. Thoracic actinomycosis in children: case report and review of the literature. *Pediatr Infect Dis J*. 2008;27(2):165-169.

Budenz CL, Tajudeen BA, Roehm PC. Actinomycosis of the temporal bone and brain: case report and review of the literature. *Ann Otol Rhinol Laryngol*. 2010;119(5):313-318.

Kononen E, Wade WG. Actinomyces and related organisms in human infections. *Clin Microbiol Rev*. 2015;28(2):419-442.

Moskowitz SM, Shailam R, Mark EJ. Case records of the Massachusetts General Hospital. Case 25-2015. An 8-year-old girl with a chest-wall mass and a pleural effusion. *N Engl J Med*. 2015;373(7):657-667.

Thacker SA, Healy CM. Pediatric cervicofacial actinomycosis: an unusual cause of head and neck masses. *J Pediatr Infect Dis Soc*. 2014;3(2):e15-e19.

Valour F, Senechal A, Dupieux C, et al. Actinomycosis: etiology, clinical features, diagnosis, treatment, and management. *Infect Drug Res*. 2014;7:183-197.

Wong VK, Turmezei TD, Weston VC. Actinomycosis. *BMJ*. 2011;343:d6099.


# 244 Anaerobic Infections

Ayesha Mirza and Mobeen H. Rathore

## INTRODUCTION

Anaerobes form the predominant bacterial components of the normal human skin and mucous membranes. They are responsible either alone or in combination with aerobes for a wide variety of infections ranging from superficial skin infections to intra-abdominal and intracranial infections.

## PATHOGENESIS AND EPIDEMIOLOGY

Anaerobic organisms are widely distributed in nature. They are present in the soil as well as the skin, mucous membranes, and gastrointestinal tracts of animals and humans. Only a few of these organisms have been identified as responsible for disease in humans (Table 244-1).

Infection with these organisms usually results secondary to disruption in the normal skin or mucous membrane barriers of the host, resulting in entry of the bacteria into deeper tissues and leading to, at times, potentially severe infections from an individual's own endogenous flora. Although some are strict anaerobes, others may be facultative anaerobes, able to survive in conditions with or without oxygen. The presence of devitalized tissues, low oxygen tension, and low pH serve to greatly contribute to the pathogenesis of anaerobic infections. Other conditions that may play a role include host defense mechanisms, virulence factors (bacterial adherence factors), production of toxins (eg, *Clostridium* species), and the presence of other bacteria in polymicrobial infections.

Due to their fastidious nature, as well as inconsistent use of adequate methods for isolation and identification, anaerobic bacteria are not easily isolated, which makes their exact frequency difficult to ascertain. Although anaerobes have been reported to account for 1% to 20% of episodes of bacteremia in adults, anaerobic organisms have rarely been isolated from blood cultures in pediatric patients. This may partly be explained by higher prevalence of chronic or debilitating conditions in adults, like malignant neoplasms, secondary immunodeficiencies, diabetes, obstetric and gynecologic surgery, and the presence of decubitus ulcers.

In recent years, increased use of advanced technology such as matrix-assisted laser desorption/ionization–time of flight mass spectrometry (MALDI-TOF MS) has greatly increased the ability to identify, speciate, and type anaerobes. Determination of in vitro antimicrobial susceptibility or resistance is also possible. This will serve to enhance early recognition as well as institution of appropriate and timely therapy in patients with severe infections.

## CLINICAL MANIFESTATIONS

Commonly encountered diseases caused by anaerobic bacteria in children are listed in Table 244-2. The principal sites of infection are deep soft tissue around the mouth and oropharynx, peritonitis and peritoneal abscesses following appendicitis or bowel rupture, and brain and lung abscesses. In females, beyond menarche, anaerobic bacteria may cause pelvic infections, such as salpingitis, tuboovarian abscesses, pelvic inflammatory disease, and bacterial vaginosis. Recently, various eye infections such as conjunctivitis and keratitis have been associated with contact lens use. Overuse of antibiotics leading to pseudomembranous colitis, which may be quite refractory to treatment, has also emerged as a significant problem, more so in adults than in children.

Clinically differentiating anaerobic from aerobic infections is often difficult. Although anaerobic infections may be more putrid, there is generally no gas formation unless *Clostridium perfringens* infection is present. Bacteremia, although rare, has been associated with a high mortality rate (15–35%) and is invariably secondary to a primary focal infection. Mortality rates vary, however, depending on the underlying condition of the host, other existing comorbidities, and the specific microorganism involved. Disease in neonates and immunocompromised children is often more severe and needs to be recognized and treated early.

**TABLE 244-1 ANAEROBIC BACTERIA COMMONLY CAUSING DISEASE IN CHILDREN**

**Gram Positive**

Cocci: *Peptococcus, Peptostreptococcus, Microaerophilic streptococcus*

Bacilli (spore-forming): *Clostridium* species

Bacilli (non–spore-forming): *Actinomyces, Propionibacterium, Lactobacillus, Eubacterium, Bifidobacterium, Arcanobacterium haemolyticum*

**Gram Negative**

Cocci: *Veillonella*

Bacilli: *Bacteroides, Prevotella, Porphyromonas, Fusobacterium*

**TABLE 244-2 ANAEROBIC BACTERIAL INFECTIONS IN CHILDREN**

**Central Nervous System**
Brain abscess
Subdural empyema

**Eye**
Conjunctivitis
Keratitis (in association with contact lens use)

**Oropharyngeal and Respiratory Tract**
Chronic sinusitis
Chronic otitis media
Mastoiditis
Periodontal infections
Gingivitis
Ludwig angina
Parapharyngeal abscess
Retropharyngeal abscess
Tonsillar abscess
Peritonsillar abscess
Cervical adenitis
Lung abscess
Pleural empyema
Lemierre syndrome[a]
Aspiration pneumonia

**Intra-abdominal and Pelvic**
Peritonitis
Peritoneal abscess
Intra-abdominal visceral abscess
Necrotizing enterocolitis
Bacterial vaginosis
Salpingitis
Pelvic inflammatory disease

**Skin and Soft Tissue**
Cellulitis
Fasciitis
Paronychia
Animal and human bite infections

**Toxin-Mediated**
Botulism
*Clostridium difficile*–associated diarrhea

**Miscellaneous**
Bacteremia associated with gastrointestinal disease
Septicemia in immunocompromised individuals
Puerperal sepsis, rarely bone and joint infections

[a]Soft tissue infection of the neck caused by *Fusobacterium*, rarely *Arcanobacterium haemolyticum*.

### Central Nervous System Infections

Although not commonly isolated, anaerobes can cause a variety of central nervous system infections including those that are relatively common (eg, brain abscess, subdural empyema) and those that are rare (eg, epidural abscess, meningitis). Chronic infections of the adjacent structures (eg, ears, mastoids, sinuses, and teeth) commonly predispose to these infections, either as a result of direct extension or less commonly due to bacteremia. Meningitis may also follow the infection of a cerebrospinal fluid shunt with skin flora such as *Propionibacterium acnes*. Anaerobes of enteric origin (eg, *Bacteroides fragilis*) may be isolated when these shunts perforate the gut. Following intracranial surgery or trauma, infections with *C perfringens* tend to be seen more commonly than infections with the other anaerobes. Respiratory and dental infections leading to brain abscess as a secondary complication are generally caused by *Prevotella, Porphyromonas, Bacteroides, Fusobacterium*, and *Peptostreptococcus*, as well as microaerophilic and other streptococci.

### Ocular Infections

Anaerobic bacteria may also play an important role in ocular infections such as conjunctivitis, keratitis, and dacrocystitis. Although anaerobes are part of the normal flora of the conjunctival sac, this does not exclude their ability to become pathogenic given the correct milieu (eg, injuries, foreign bodies, underlying diseases). Apart from this, direct contamination from other than an endogenous source is a frequent mode of transmission. In studies that employed adequate methods for isolation, anaerobes were recovered from about a third of patients with conjunctivitis, half of the time being the only isolate.

Conjunctivitis associated with anaerobic bacteria is not clinically distinguishable from inflammation caused by other bacteria, although patients who use contact lenses may be at higher risk of developing infections caused by anaerobes. Although the vast majority of cases of acute conjunctivitis are caused by viruses or aerobic bacteria (eg, *Staphylococcus aureus, Streptococcus pneumoniae, Haemophilus influenzae*), anaerobic gram-positive cocci (eg, *Peptostreptococcus*) have also been recovered in significant numbers from these patients. Other anaerobic bacteria that have been recovered include *Propionobacterium, B fragilis*, pigmented *Prevotella, Porphyromonas, Fusobacterium*, and *Bifidobacterium*. Often these are found in conjunction with aerobic bacteria. *Neisseria gonorrhoeae* infection may occur in sexually active adolescents. *Chlamydia trachomatis* may cause conjunctivitis in young infants. Corneal ulcerations may be infected by *S pneumoniae, Pseudomonas* species, and *Peptostreptococcus*.

Keratitis is a relatively serious infection that may result in corneal scarring, opacification, and blindness. Although mostly associated with a variety of aerobic gram-positive and gram-negative bacteria, it has been reported in conjunction with *C perfringens*, in which case it can result in a fulminant endophthalmitis. This has been associated with perforating ocular injuries. *Clostridium tetani* has also been associated with ocular trauma. Corneal susceptibility to infection is secondary to its continuous exposure and avascularity. Anaerobic bacteria should also be considered in cases of chronic dacryocystitis.

#### Head and Neck Infections

Anaerobes may be isolated in cases of acute as well as chronic infections involving the ears, sinuses, mastoids, and other head and neck structures. Members of the oropharyngeal flora (eg, *Prevotella, Porphyromonas, Bacteroides, Fusobacterium*, and *Peptostreptococcus*) are the predominant anaerobic flora involved in these infections. In addition, *Streptococcus salivarius* and microaerophilic streptococci may be involved in the pathogenesis of dental infections.

Anaerobes have been isolated from approximately 5% to 15% of cases of acute otitis media as well as 50% of cases of chronic suppurative otitis media, including those with the presence of a cholesteotoma. Absorption of bone may be enhanced by organic acids produced by anaerobic bacteria.

Recovery of anaerobes in up to 75% of tonsils of children with recurrent group A β-hemolytic *Streptococcus* (GABHS) as well as 40% of those with non-GABHS tonsillitis has been one of the possible explanations offered for the failure of penicillin to treat these infections. Selection of β-lactamase–producing strains of aerobic or anaerobic bacteria may render penicillin ineffective in these situations.

Other infections, such as thyroiditis, have been associated with anaerobic bacteria, including gram-negative bacteria and *Peptostreptococcus* species.

#### Lemierre Syndrome

Fusobacteria, which are normal inhabitants of the oropharynx, have become increasingly recognized as a cause of acute and chronic otitis, sinusitis, tonsillitis, peritonsillar, and retropharyngeal infections. Lemierre syndrome, or postanginal sepsis, is the most common life-threatening manifestation of infection with fusobacteria, caused mainly by *Fusobacterium necrophorum*, although other anaerobes and *Staphylococcus* have also been implicated. Lemierre syndrome begins with tonsillitis, followed by septic thrombophlebitis of the internal jugular vein, which is then followed by septicemia with septic emboli in lungs and other sites. Lemierre syndrome, although seen primarily in healthy adolescents, has also been reported in young infants and children, as well as in adult patients.

Lemierre syndrome was a relatively common entity in the preantibiotic era but seemed to virtually disappear with widespread use of antibiotics for upper respiratory tract infection. In the last several years, however, there appears to have been a rise in incidence, possibly related to a decrease in antibiotic usage for sore throat, although available data are not sufficient to support this conclusively.

Approximately 10% of published cases are associated with infectious mononucleosis, which may facilitate invasion. Lymphatic obstruction, deficient translocation of leukocytes, and impaired immunoglobulin production also may help facilitate the disease. Factors that increase the virulence of fusobacteria include the lipopolysaccharide in the bacterial cell wall and the production of a heat-stable toxin that mediates inflammation and stimulates the production of tumor necrosis factor. Additionally, activation of human platelets may lead to thrombus formation.

#### Pleuropulmonary Infections

Severe periodontal or gingival disease and aspiration of oropharyngeal secretions or gastric contents are the major risk factors associated with the development of pleuropulmonary disease, which can range from uncomplicated pneumonia to severe necrotizing pneumonia with the formation of pleural empyema or lung abscess. Like most anaerobic infections, these are generally polymicrobial in nature. The predominant anaerobes isolated in these situations include *Prevotella, Porphyromonas, Fusobacterium*, and *Peptostreptococcus*. These may be mixed with aerobic organisms such as α-hemolytic and microaerophilic streptococci and, in nosocomially acquired pneumonia, gram-negative organisms such as *Pseudomonas* species and Enterobacteriaceae. *S aureus* may be isolated as well.

#### Intra-abdominal Infections

Perforation of abdominal viscera, either traumatically or during surgery, may lead to peritonitis and the formation of intra-abdominal abscesses. Necrotizing enterocolitis is a common entity seen in preterm neonates where anaerobic organisms are most often implicated. The specific microorganisms involved here are the normal flora of the gastrointestinal tract where the anaerobic bacteria outnumber aerobes in a ratio of 1000:1 to 10,000:1. These infections often tend to be biphasic, with the initial infection being caused by Enterobacteriaceae followed by a later phase with the development of abscesses from which *B fragilis* or *Peptostreptococcus* may be isolated. Because *Bacteroides* species tend to make up 25% of the anaerobes in the gut, infections with these organisms are seen most commonly. Members of the *Clostridium* species are another common group of anaerobic organisms isolated in these situations.

#### Osteomyelitis and Septic Arthritis

These anaerobic infections also tend to be polymicrobial, with osteomyelitis after trauma and fracture most commonly involving the long bones, whereas osteomyelitis involving the spine may be seen following decubitus ulcers. Cranial and facial bones may be involved as well, particularly following trauma. Anaerobes are also associated with infected bites and cranial infections.

Anaerobic streptococci and *Bacteroides* are the most common anaerobic organisms at all sites. Pigmented *Prevotella* and *Porphyromonas* are other common organisms isolated in these infections. Clostridia may be isolated in compound fractures involving the lower extremities and pelvis.

Septic arthritis involving anaerobes may be seen following hematogenous or direct spread of infection, following trauma, and in association with prosthetic joints.

#### Infections of the Female Genital Tract Including Pelvic Inflammatory Disease

Genital tract infections mimic other infections caused by anaerobes in the sense that they are usually polymicrobial. This includes bacterial vaginosis, endometritis, salpingitis, tubo-ovarian abscesses, and intrauterine-device–associated infections. The predominant anaerobic bacteria include *Prevotella* species, *Peptostreptococcus, Porphyromonas*, and *Clostridium* species. Bacterial vaginosis occurs when the normal vaginal flora, such as *Lactobacillus* species, are replaced by other anaerobes such as *Mobiluncus curtisii, Gardnerella vaginalis*, or *Mycoplasma hominis*.

In addition to these infections, more than 1 million women in the United States are treated for pelvic inflammatory disease (PID) annually. Although *C trachomatis* (20–40%) and *N gonorrhoeae* (30–80%) are the organisms most frequently associated with PID, up to 75% of cases are neither gonococcal nor chlamydial. Anaerobic gram-negative rods are frequently involved in these infections.

The most current Centers for Disease Control and Prevention guidelines for the treatment of PID include both oral and parenteral regimens. Since these guidelines are subject to periodic updates, readers are encouraged to check for the most recent guidelines at http://www.cdc.gov/std/default.htm.

#### Neonatal Infections

In addition to infections in older children, anaerobes colonize the newborn during vaginal delivery and have been recovered from several types of newborn infections, including cellulitis, conjunctivitis, aspiration pneumonia, omphalitis, bacteremia, and infant botulism. The wide range of endogenous infections caused by anaerobes in neonates and older children is not surprising, being that they form the predominant component of the normal human skin and mucosa.

## DIAGNOSIS

Knowledge of host risk factors and the organ system involved may aid in the diagnosis of anaerobic infection. Presence of a foul odor in the clinical specimen or site from which the specimen was obtained may provide a useful clue as well.

In the diagnosis of anaerobic infections, use of optimal culture conditions for the growth of anaerobic organisms in appropriate specimens is especially important. Antimicrobial susceptibility studies for anaerobic bacteria are often not available from hospital laboratories; however, they should be requested in exceptional and life-threatening cases.

Given the overall low incidence of anaerobic infections in children, the routine use of anaerobic blood cultures in childhood illness has been debated. However, with the reemergence of anaerobic bacteremia, the evidence favors obtaining anaerobic blood cultures in the appropriate clinical setting. Diagnosis made on clinical grounds can prove difficult because the clinical features of anaerobic bacteremia are not very different from those associated with other types of bacteremias in children. Diagnosis may also be delayed due to the more fastidious growth requirements and time needed for identification of these bacteria, although with the increasing use of MALDI-TOF MS, this is likely to improve.

## TREATMENT

Because of the mortality associated with anaerobic infections, it is important to establish timely and appropriate therapy. Critically ill patients or those suspected of having infections involving anaerobic bacteria should be started on broad-spectrum antibiotics effective against both aerobic and anaerobic organisms. Site of the infection, antimicrobial resistance patterns when available, pharmacokinetics of the different drugs used, and potential side effects should all be taken into consideration when choosing an antimicrobial agent. Penicillin G remains the drug of choice against most non–β-lactamase-producing organisms, including anaerobic streptococci, *Clostridium* species other than *C difficile*, and nonsporulating anaerobic bacilli. This makes it appropriate for treatment of most oropharyngeal infections. Other than oropharyngeal infections, penicillin G has largely been replaced by antibiotic combinations with β-lactamase inhibitors (amoxicillin/clavulanic acid, ampicillin/sulbactam, and piperacillin/tazobactam), which are all preferred due to their broad-spectrum coverage and the ability to overcome β-lactamase production. Metronidazole and clindamycin also have excellent activity against anaerobes, including those producing β-lactamase (eg, *Bacteroides*). Clindamycin is superior to penicillin for serious lung infections. The second-generation cephalosporins cefotetan and cefoxitin also have good anaerobic activity, although cefoxitin is relatively inactive against most species of *Clostridium* except *C perfringens*.

The carbapenems (imipenem, meropenem, ertapenem, and doripenem) all have excellent anaerobic activity. The macrolides have moderate to good in vitro activity against anaerobic bacteria other than *B fragilis* and fusobacteria. Although the quinolone antibiotics moxifloxacin and levofloxacin have antianaerobic activity, especially against the *B fragilis* group, their use in children is limited due to the possible adverse effects on cartilage. Vancomycin has good activity against all gram-positive anaerobes including *C difficile*. For *C difficile*–associated diarrhea, metronidazole is usually the antimicrobial of choice. Recommendations for treatment of these patients depends on multiple factors (eg, the severity of disease).

In addition to antimicrobial therapy, drainage of any abscesses and debridement of necrotic tissue are important. Certain types of adjunct therapy, such as hyperbaric oxygen, although controversial, may also be considered in select circumstances.

Simple cases of conjunctivitis may be treated with topical antibiotics. Bacitracin is very effective against pigmented *Prevotella* and *Porphyromonas* as well as *Peptostreptococcus* species but is usually not effective against *B fragilis* and *Fusobacterium*. Similarly, erythromycin is active against pigmented *Prevotella* and *Porphyromonas*, microaerophilic and anaerobic streptococci, *Clostridium* species, and gram-positive non–spore-forming anaerobic bacilli but has poor activity against gram-negative anaerobic bacilli. Sulfonamides, polymyxin B, and aminoglycoside preparations may not be very effective against most anaerobes.

## SUGGESTED READINGS


Brook I. Fusobacterial head and neck infections in children. *Int J Pediatr Otorhinolaryngol*. 2015;70:953-958.

Brook I. Microbiology of chronic rhinosinusitis. *Eur J Clin Microbiol Infect Dis*. 2016;35:1059-1068.

Brook I. Ocular infections due to anaerobic bacteria in children. *J Pediatr Ophthalmol Strabismus*. 2008;45:78-84.

Brook I. Spectrum and treatment of anaerobic infections. *J Infect Chemother*. 2016;22:1-13.

Centers for Disease Control and Prevention. 2015 CDC STD treatment guidelines. http://www.cdc.gov/std/tg2015/pid.htm. Accessed August 2, 2016.

Clark AE, Kaleta EJ, Arora A, et al. Matrix-assisted laser desorption ionization-time of flight mass spectrometry: a fundamental shift in the routine practice of clinical microbiology. *Clin Microbiol Rev*. 2013;26:547-603.

Dierig A, Frei R, Egli A. The fast route to microbe identification: matrix assisted laser desorption/ionization-time of flight mass spectrometry (MALDI-TOF MS). *Pediatr Infect Dis J*. 2015;34:97-99.

Duarte R, Fuhrich D, Ross JD. A review of antibiotic therapy for pelvic inflammatory disease. *Int J Antimicrob Agents*. 2015;46:272-277.

Vena A, Muñoz P, Alcalá A, et al. Are incidence and epidemiology of anaerobic bacteremia really changing? *Eur J Clin Microbiol Infect Dis*. 2015;34:1621-1629.


# 245 Clostridial Infections

Jose J. Zayas and Mobeen H. Rathore

## *CLOSTRIDIUM DIFFICILE*

*Clostridium difficile* is a spore-forming, obligate anaerobic, gram-positive bacillus that is spread via the fecal-oral route. The most common manifestations of *C difficile*–associated disease (CDAD) are mediated by toxins A and B produced by the organism.

### PATHOGENESIS AND EPIDEMIOLOGY

Treatment with antibiotics and chemotherapeutic agents (eg, fluorouracil, methotrexate) that alter the natural gastrointestinal flora favor the emergence of *C difficile*. Risk factors for developing CDAD include recent gastrointestinal surgery, prolonged stays in healthcare facilities, immunocompromised patients, proton pump inhibitor therapy, repeated enemas, prolonged use of nasogastric tubes (or other gastrointestinal feeding devices), inflammatory bowel disease, cystic fibrosis, Hirschsprung disease, and a history of cancer. Breastfeeding, on the other hand, may offer some protective benefits. Studies report that 3% to 7% of children with *C difficile* develop a complication, such as hypotension, ileus, or toxic megacolon.

CDAD results directly from toxin-mediated effects to the large intestine. The exact incubation period is unknown, but symptoms are known to develop up to 10 weeks after discontinuation of antibiotics. Infants and children are more likely than adults to carry *C difficile* asymptomatically in the gastrointestinal tract; it is estimated that 15% to 63% of neonates, up to 33% of infants and toddlers younger than 2 years of age, and up to 8.3% of children older than 2 years of age are asymptomatic carriers. It is postulated that infants do not manifest illness because they lack the necessary toxin-binding sites in their colon. In children who have diarrhea not caused by *C difficile*, many may still carry *C difficile*. Over the past decade, more severe, sometimes fatal infections have been seen with outbreaks of *C difficile* infection caused by a virulent strain (NAP-1/027) that appears to have increased production of toxins A and B, as well as binary toxin, and fluoroquinolone resistance.

In 2011, the estimated incidence of *C difficile* infection in the United States in children < 18 years old was 24.2 cases per 100,000 population, with approximately two-thirds of cases being community-associated. With the rate of *C difficile* colonization or infection in hospitalized patients being 13 per 1000, CDAD is now the most common cause of healthcare-associated infection, with an estimated 453,000 incidents of CDAD, including 29,300 deaths, in the United States, resulting in an estimated cost of $5 billion in 2011.

## CLINICAL MANIFESTATIONS

Colonization is defined as a patient who exhibits no clinical symptoms but tests positive for the *C difficile* organism and/or its toxin. Colonization is more common than symptomatic CDAD.

The presentation of CDAD can range from mild diarrhea to life-threatening disease. Initial signs and symptoms of CDAD include watery diarrhea, fever, loss of appetite, nausea, and abdominal tenderness. Progressive signs and symptoms include bloody diarrhea, cramping, and flatulence. If pseudomembranous colitis is suspected, it requires a colonoscopy to confirm the diagnosis. More severe complications include toxic megacolon, perforation, and bacteremia with distant metastatic infection. Therefore, a high index of suspicion is critical, as is awareness of the limitations of current diagnostic tests.

## DIAGNOSIS

Asymptomatic colonization occurs frequently in neonates and young infants, and therefore, current guidelines recommend not testing children under 1 year of age.

Stool cultures that are positive for *C difficile* are not diagnostic. The diagnosis of *C difficile* colitis should only be made if toxin is found in the stool. Commercially available enzyme immunoassays (EIAs) can detect both toxins A and B. Approximately 5% to 20% of patients, however, may require more than 1 stool sample be sent to detect toxin. Molecular assays using nucleic acid amplification tests (NAATs) are approved by the US Food and Drug Administration (FDA) and are now the preferred test. NAATs combine good sensitivity and specificity, have turnaround times comparable to EIAs, and are not required to be part of a 2- or 3-step algorithm. In a recent study, the sensitivity of the real-time polymerase chain reaction (PCR) assay for toxin A/B was superior compared with EIA for toxin A/B (95% vs 35%, respectively), and the specificities were equal (100%).

The presence of symptoms compatible with CDAD and identification of the toxin in a patient over 1 year of age are considered diagnostic for CDAD. When symptoms are severe and CDAD is a consideration, endoscopic evaluation is indicated even in the absence of toxin identified by assays. There are typical findings of pseudomembranous colitis on colonoscopy, characterized by the presence of an adherent inflammatory "pseudomembrane" overlying the mucosa (Fig. 245-1).

## TREATMENT

Potentially offending antimicrobial or chemotherapeutic agents should be discontinued if possible in an attempt to restore balance to the gut flora. Supportive care addressing hydration, nutrition, and electrolyte abnormalities should be provided. In approximately 20% of immunocompetent patients, CDAD will resolve within 2 to 3 days after discontinuing the offending agent with no additional treatment necessary. Immediate initiation of antimicrobial therapy for CDAD is indicated for patients with immunodeficiency, Hirschsprung disease, inflammatory bowel disease, or severe disease, or in patients whose diarrhea persists beyond 3 days after the offending agent is discontinued.

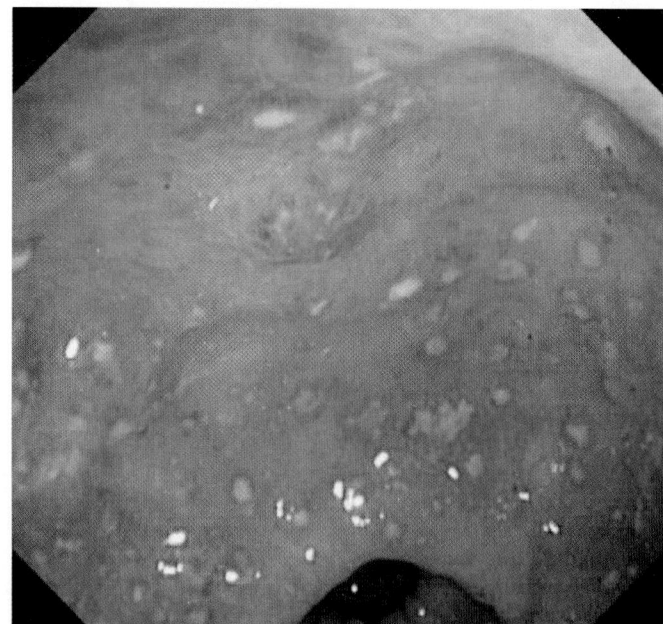

**FIGURE 245-1** Colonoscopic image of pseudomembranous colitis in a patient with the acute onset of bloody diarrhea due to *Clostridium difficile*. Note the pseudomembranes adherent to the mucosal surface. (Used with permission from Colin Rudolph.)

*C difficile* is susceptible to metronidazole and vancomycin, and both are effective for the treatment of mild CDAD. Metronidazole is the more cost-effective choice for the initial treatment of patients with CDAD. The recommended dose is 30 to 50 mg/kg/d (maximum 2 g/d) orally divided in 4 doses, and the length of therapy should be at least 10 days. Up to 40% of patients experience a relapse after discontinuing such therapy, but the infection usually responds to a second course of the same treatment. Up to 10% have a second relapse, and oral vancomycin is recommended in this case. Vancomycin is also recommended as initial therapy for CDAD with hypoalbuminemia (< 2.5 g/dL), severe manifestations, and infection suspected or proven to be due to NAP-1/027. The dose is 40 mg/kg/d (maximum 2 g/d) orally divided in 4 doses. Alternative treatments include rifaximin and nitazoxanide. Fidaxomicin is a macrolide drug that is approved for individuals with CDAD who are at least 18 years of age; however, there is limited experience in children.

On the basis that restoration of the normal fecal microbiota may be valuable for resolving infections refractory to oral metronidazole or vancomycin, fecal transplantation of donor stool has been reported to be highly successful. The exact complement of fecal bacteria that is required to restore a normal fecal microbiota is not established.

Monoclonal antibodies offer potential for improving treatment and prevention of CDAD in the future. Phase III clinical studies for bezlotoxumab (an investigational *C difficile* antitoxin) showed reduction in *C difficile* recurrence through 12 weeks compared to placebo, when used in conjunction with antibiotics for the treatment of *C difficile*.

Since the excretion of the organism and the toxin can be prolonged after clinical cure, follow-up testing for *C difficile* is discouraged. Antimotility agents should be avoided. Surgical intervention may be required in severe cases of CDAD unresponsive to medical therapy or to manage complications such as toxic megacolon or colonic perforation.

## PREVENTION

The first step in prevention of CDAD is the judicious use of antibiotics. Probiotics are both safe and moderately effective in preventing CDAD in immunocompetent children. There is very limited evidence to support the use of probiotics to prevent simple antibiotic-associated diarrhea and no evidence that it is beneficial for treatment of CDAD.

In the hospital environment, contact precautions should be implemented for patients with known or suspected CDAD to prevent nosocomial transmission of *C difficile*. Note that alcohol-based hand hygiene products (now commonly used in healthcare facilities as a substitute for soap and water) are not sporicidal and should not be relied upon to prevent person-to-person spread of *C difficile*. Hand washing with soap and water involving vigorous mechanical scrubbing and rinsing is more effective for physical removal of bacterial spores. Adherence to glove use in the care of symptomatic patients is critically important for preventing transmission of *C difficile*. There is evidence that chlorhexidine baths reduce hospital-acquired CDAD, but the optimal strategy for this application is not established. Children with CDAD should be excluded from child care for the duration of their diarrhea.

## *CLOSTRIDIUM BOTULINUM*

*Clostridium botulinum* is a gram-positive, obligate anaerobic bacillus most commonly found in the soil. *C botulinum* generates spores that survive extreme weather and temperature conditions, so unlike the toxins, which are heat labile, the spores are relatively heat resistant. Neuromuscular blockade by one of these neurotoxins produced by the organism results in a descending paralysis of varying degrees.

Classically, 3 clinical presentations of botulism are described: infant botulism, foodborne botulism, and wound botulism. An average of 110 cases of botulism are reported each year in the United States according to the Centers for Disease Control and Prevention (CDC). Approximately 72% of cases are infant botulism, 25% are foodborne botulism (vegetables being the most common source in the United States), and the remaining 3% are wound botulism. In the United States, foodborne botulism has been largely reduced by implementing safe canning and food manufacturing processes. However, improperly home-canned foods are still a cause of outbreaks. Recently, inadvertent botulism has been described as an iatrogenic disease occurring in patients treated with botulinum toxin injections for dystonia, other movement disorders, or cosmetic procedures. The increase in iatrogenic botulism underscores the importance of using botulinum toxin only for clinically established and approved indications.

In foodborne botulism, it is the preformed toxin that is directly ingested from inappropriately handled food. Wound botulism is caused by contamination of the wound with *C botulinum*.

## INFANT BOTULISM

### PATHOGENESIS AND EPIDEMIOLOGY

Infant botulism results from ingested spores of *C botulinum* that germinate in the colon and produce a neurotoxin. The neurotoxin is absorbed and carried by the circulatory system to the peripheral cholinergic synapses. The toxin binds irreversibly and produces a flaccid paralysis by producing a presynaptic blockade, preventing the release of acetylcholine. The toxin also blocks acetylcholine from parts of the autonomic system, inducing symptoms of dry mouth and reduced sweating.

Infant botulism has been the most common form of botulism reported in the United States. There is no gender predilection. Between 2006 and 2011, there has been an annual average of 96 laboratory-confirmed cases with an age range of < 1 to 60 weeks. The median age of presentation is 16 weeks. Infant botulism occurs at a significantly younger age in formula-fed infants compared to breast-fed infants. There are no clear epidemiologic risk factors for the development of infant botulism. Possible spore sources include foods, dust, and soil. A history of honey ingestion is present in a minority of cases, and honey is not recommended for children younger than 12 months of age. *C botulinum* spores have also been identified in corn syrup. In most cases, the source of the spores is unidentifiable.

### CLINICAL MANIFESTATIONS

Infant botulism displays a wide spectrum of presentations from transient mild weakness and hypotonia that may go unnoticed, to a fulminant, even fatal, illness. Choking with feeds and/or decreased tone are what often initially illicit parental concern. The infant is usually afebrile unless the course is complicated by a secondary bacterial infection (such as aspiration pneumonia).

The classic presentation of infant botulism includes decreased stool frequency (constipation) followed by poor feeding due to a weak suck, a weak cry, and progressive, symmetrical descending weakness beginning with the cranial nerves. This results in an expressionless face, ptosis, weak cry, and impaired gag or suck reflexes, which are followed by a generalized progressive hypotonia. Deep tendon reflexes are normal initially but diminish later in the course of the illness. Despite a sad, lethargic appearance and a feeble cry, the infant conveys a paradoxical sense of alertness because the toxin does not cross the blood-brain barrier. Impaired respiratory effort may evolve to respiratory failure.

### DIAGNOSIS

Botulism should be suspected in any infant who presents with poor feeding, constipation, and symmetric progressive weakness. Clinical suspicion is the cornerstone of diagnosis, and the initiation of treatment should not be delayed awaiting laboratory confirmation. Sepsis is the most common admitting diagnosis. Other frequent admission diagnoses include dehydration, viral syndrome, and failure to thrive. The differential diagnosis includes drug or heavy metal poisoning, hypothyroidism, metabolic disorders, myasthenia gravis, poliomyelitis, Guillain-Barré syndrome, Werdnig-Hoffmann disease, and Hirschsprung disease.

A stool specimen for toxin assay is the confirmatory test of choice for infant botulism. Although not always helpful, if electromyography (EMG) is used, the most prominent finding is an incremental increase of evoked muscle potentials at high-frequency nerve stimulation (20–50 Hz). Additionally, small-amplitude, overly abundant motor action potentials may be seen after stimulation of muscle, but their absence does not exclude the diagnosis.

### TREATMENT

In infant botulism, supportive care is the mainstay of therapy. In addition, the early use of botulism immune globulin-intravenous (human BIG-IV or baby BIG) is now standard. Specific treatment with BIG-IV is highly effective, shortening hospital stays from 5.5 to 2.5 weeks and reducing morbidity and mortality. It is not recommended in other forms of botulism. Treatment with BIG-IV should be instituted as soon as possible and not delayed awaiting laboratory confirmation. It is available from the California Department of Public Health (24-hour phone number: 510-231-7600). BIG-IV immediately binds and neutralizes all circulating botulinum toxin and remains present in neutralizing amounts in the circulation for up to 6 months. This allows regeneration of nerve endings to proceed and leads to full recovery. Treatment with BIG-IV within 0 to 3 days after admission shortens the hospital stay by up to 1 week or more when compared to administration 4 to 7 days after admission. Equine-derived heptavalent botulinum antitoxin has been used on a case-by-case basis to treat type F infant botulism since that antitoxin is not contained in BIG-IV, unlike the other 6 toxin serotypes (A–E and G).

Theoretically, antibiotic usage may lead to lysis of *C botulinum*, releasing further neurotoxin, which could result in prolonged or more severe illness. Therefore, antibiotics should not be routinely employed. Aminoglycosides, due to their potential for additional neuromuscular blockade, should particularly be avoided because they may exaggerate the paresis.

## OTHER FORMS OF BOTULISM

The symptoms of foodborne botulism begin several hours to days after the ingestion of a preformed toxin. Similar to infant botulism, these patients present with some degree of flaccid paralysis that manifests initially with prominent cranial nerve paralysis with descending progression and an absence of sensory nerve involvement. Early symptoms include blurred or double vision, dizziness, trouble swallowing, and difficulty speaking. Because the toxin is in the gastrointestinal tract, decreased stool frequency and increased consistency are also common features.

The neurologic manifestations of wound-associated botulism are indistinguishable from those seen in foodborne botulism; however, gastrointestinal symptoms are absent. Associated wounds are not necessarily outwardly impressive, although they are frequently deep and associated with avascular injuries. The average incubation period in cases of trauma is 7 days (range 4–21 days). This clinical entity should be kept in mind with injection drug users; recurrent wound botulism has been described in this population.

Iatrogenic botulism demonstrates the same clinical characteristics as naturally occurring botulism. Some patients develop associated autonomic nervous system effects following the toxin injections. Patients treated with toxin for cervical dystonia often experience dysphagia. This focal weakness likely results from the local spread of toxin from the injected muscles. Generalized weakness and autonomic symptoms are likely a result of circulating toxin in the blood.

### DIAGNOSIS

Routine laboratory tests are typically unremarkable. The tensilon test helps distinguish botulism from myasthenia gravis. In suspected cases, serum and stool samples should be sent for toxin confirmation. Detection of toxin in the patient's serum, stool, wound, or food is diagnostic. This testing is performed at the CDC.

### TREATMENT

Patients older than 1 year of age and adults with botulism should be treated with equine-derived heptavalent botulinum antitoxin that contains antitoxin against all 7 (A–G) botulinum toxin types. Immediate administration of antitoxin is critical, because it arrests the progression of paralysis, although it does not reverse it. Similar to infant botulism, antibiotics should not be routinely used because of concerns of lysis of *C botulinum* and further neurotoxin release. Aminoglycosides should especially be avoided in cases of botulism for the reasons previously mentioned.

Antibiotics are recommended for wound botulism after antitoxin has been administered. Penicillin G (250,000–400,000 U/kg/d, up to 24 million U/d, divided every 4 hours) provides coverage. For penicillin-allergic patients, metronidazole orally, 30 to 50 mg/kg/d divided every 8 hours (maximum 2250 mg/d), or intravenously, 22.5 to 40 mg/kg/d divided every 8 hours (maximum 1500 mg/d), is an alternative.

## *CLOSTRIDIUM PERFRINGENS*

*Clostridium perfringens* is the most common cause of clostridial myonecrosis. It is also implicated in cellulitis, necrotizing fasciitis, and food poisoning.

### PATHOGENESIS AND EPIDEMIOLOGY

*C perfringens* is readily found in soil samples, contaminated surgical and other objects, and the intestinal contents of animals and humans. It is also present in raw meat and poultry. Factors that facilitate the growth of *C perfringens* include penetration of deep tissue, extensive tissue devitalization, tissue anoxia, an anaerobic environment, polymicrobial infection, and the presence of a foreign body.

Myonecrosis may occur after trauma, postoperatively, or spontaneously in the presence of other primary pathology. Nontraumatic myonecrosis occurs occasionally from clostridia in the gastrointestinal tract of immunocompromised hosts. Food poisoning caused by *C perfringens* is usually due to the ingestion of the organism that produces enteric toxins. Symptoms may also result from ingestion of preformed toxin. Necrotizing enteritis (pigbel) is associated with β-enterotoxin produced by *C perfringens* type C following consumption of undercooked pork. It is rarely seen in the United States.

### CLINICAL MANIFESTATIONS

Clostridial myonecrosis is marked by significant, disproportionate pain that is sudden and progressive at the site of injury. It is accompanied by local, tense swelling, pallor, and a thin hemorrhagic exudate. Pallor gives way to a bronze or magenta discoloration, and hemorrhagic purplish bullae appear. Myonecrosis caused by *Clostridium* species is called gas gangrene. Crepitus from gas production is suggestive but not pathognomonic and may not be present at all. A peculiar offensive odor, sometimes described as sweet, may be noted, with a brown serosanguinous discharge. Eventually, the muscle becomes "gangrenous"—black, friable, and liquefied.

The toxins from this organism have systemic effects such as direct cardiodepressive effects. Systemic findings include tachycardia disproportionate to the degree of fever, pallor, diaphoresis, hypotension, renal failure, and changes in mental status. Untreated clostridial myonecrosis can lead to disseminated myonecrosis, suppurative visceral infection, sepsis, and death within hours. Additionally, *C perfringens* can also cause a simple localized cellulitis.

In food poisoning from *C perfringens*, the illness starts 8 to 12 hours after ingestion of contaminated products containing high numbers of organisms. Symptoms usually last under 24 hours and include nausea, severe abdominal pain, and profuse nonbloody, watery diarrhea. Fever is absent, and vomiting is uncommon.

Neonatal necrotizing enterocolitis has been associated with *C perfringens, Clostridium butyricum*, and *C difficile*. The exact role of these organisms needs further elucidation. Neutropenic enterocolitis (typhlitis) is a similar syndrome that occurs in the cecum of neutropenic patients. *Clostridium septicum* is the usual agent. Symptoms are fever, right lower quadrant abdominal pain, and diarrhea. Initial treatment is with antibiotics, but surgical resection may be necessary.

### DIAGNOSIS

Clostridial myonecrosis is a clinical diagnosis including the characteristic appearance of necrotic muscle noted at surgery. Early recognition is critical for a successful outcome. Anaerobic cultures of wound exudate and blood should be performed. Tissue specimens and aspirates (not swab specimens) are appropriate for anaerobic culture. If gram-positive bacilli are present with a consistent clinical picture, the diagnosis of clostridial myonecrosis should be assumed until proven otherwise. A radiograph of the affected site can demonstrate gas in the tissue, but this is a nonspecific finding and not always present.

In foodborne illnesses, isolation of large concentrations of *C perfringens* or demonstration of enterotoxin in the stool supports the diagnosis. For most cases of self-limited food poisoning, however, diagnostic testing is not performed.

### TREATMENT

A high index of suspicion and immediate surgical excision of necrotic tissue with removal of any foreign material are essential to the management of clostridial myonecrosis. Decompressing fascial compartments is essential to prevent further tissue anoxia. Broad-spectrum antibiotics are indicated until culture and sensitivity reports allow for appropriate antibiotic adjustments given the prevalence of polymicrobial necrotizing infections.

High-dose penicillin G (250,000–400,000 U/kg/d, up to 24 million U/d, divided every 4 hours) administered intravenously has excellent activity against *C perfringens* and should be included in the initial antibiotic regimen. Approximately 5% of clostridial species show variable degrees of resistance to penicillin. Clindamycin (40 mg/kg/d divided every 8 hours), metronidazole, meropenem, and ertapenem (not approved for individuals ≤ 18 years of age) can be considered as alternative drugs for patients with a penicillin allergy or for treatment of polymicrobial infections. The combination of penicillin G and clindamycin is considered superior to penicillin alone because of clindamycin's toxin-inhibiting action. Polyvalent clostridial myonecrosis antitoxin has no proven benefit. Hyperbaric oxygen may be beneficial when used adjunctively along with antibiotics and aggressive surgical debridement. Clostridial cellulitis can be treated with antibiotics alone and with any associated fluid collection being drained.

Treatment of food poisoning is primarily symptomatic support. Antibiotics are not indicated.

## PREVENTION

For the prevention of myonecrosis, during initial wound management, prompt and careful debridement, flushing of contaminated wounds, and removal of foreign material should always be performed. Clindamycin (20–30 mg/kg/d) may be of value for prophylaxis in patients with grossly contaminated wounds. In hospitalized cases, isolation is not necessary.

For foodborne illness, prevention is achieved by cooking foods thoroughly and maintaining food at warmer than 60°C. Meat dishes should be served hot shortly after cooking. Foods should never be held at room temperature to cool; they should be refrigerated after removal from warming devices or serving tables as soon as possible and within 2 hours of preparation. Refrigerators should keep food cooler than 7°C (45°F).

## SUGGESTED READINGS


American Academy of Pediatrics Committee on Infectious Diseases. Botulism and infant botulism. In: *Red Book: 2015 Report of the Committee on Infectious Diseases*. 30th ed. Elk Grove Village, IL: American Academy of Pediatrics; 2015:294-297.

American Academy of Pediatrics Committee on Infectious Diseases. Clostridial myonecrosis. In: *Red Book: 2015 Report of the Committee on Infectious Diseases*. 30th ed. Elk Grove Village, IL: American Academy of Pediatrics; 2015:297-298.

American Academy of Pediatrics Committee on Infectious Diseases. *Clostridium difficile*. In: *Red Book: 2015 Report of the Committee on Infectious Diseases*. 30th ed. Elk Grove Village, IL: American Academy of Pediatrics; 2015:298-301.

American Academy of Pediatrics Committee on Infectious Diseases. *Clostridium perfringens* food poisoning. In: *Red Book: 2015 Report of the Committee on Infectious Diseases*. 30th ed. Elk Grove Village, IL: American Academy of Pediatrics; 2015:301-302.

Centers for Disease Control and Prevention. Botulism. http://www.cdc.gov/botulism/. Accessed August 2, 2016.

Centers for Disease Control and Prevention. *Clostridium difficile* infection. http://www.cdc.gov/HAI/organisms/cdiff/Cdiff_infect.html. Accessed August 2, 2016.

Division of Communicable Disease Control, California Department of Health Services. Infant Botulism Treatment and Prevention Program. www.infantbotulism.org. Accessed June 1, 2016.

Goldenberg JZ, Ma SSY, Saxton JD, et al. Probiotics for the prevention of *Clostridium difficile*-associated diarrhea in adults and children (review). *Cochrane Database Syst Rev*. 2013;5:1-153.

Lessa FC, Mu Y, Bamberg WM, et al. Burden of *Clostridium difficile* infection in the United States. *N Engl J Med*. 2015;372:825-834.

Schutze GE, Willoughby RE. Committee on Infectious Diseases: American Academy of Pediatrics. *Clostridium difficile* infection in infants and children. *Pediatrics*. 2013;131:196-200.


# 246 Anthrax (*Bacillus anthracis*)

Denise Bratcher

## INTRODUCTION

Anthrax is an acute infectious disease caused by the gram-positive, encapsulated, nonmotile, spore-forming rod *Bacillus anthracis*. The incubation period is 1 to 7 days (may be longer in the inhalation form). Person-to-person transmission from cutaneous lesions rarely occurs.

## PATHOGENESIS AND EPIDEMIOLOGY

An antiphagocytic capsule and 2 exotoxins (lethal toxin, edema toxin) are responsible for the clinical illness cause by *B anthracis*. The toxins are responsible for the clinical manifestations (eg, hemorrhage, edema, necrosis) of the various clinical presentations as well as the morbidity and mortality associated with illness due to anthrax. Therefore, treatment not only requires antimicrobial therapy to kill the organism, but antitoxin therapy may also be indicated.

*B anthracis* affects domestic and wild animals throughout the world. Human infections are a result of contact with infected animals or contaminated animal products (eg, meat, skin, hair). In the United States, the most common form has been cutaneous infections among animal handlers, but more invasive cases (eg, inhalation) have been described in drum makers working with contaminated animal hides or in people participating in drumming events where spore-contaminated drum heads were being used. In 2001 in the United States, 22 cases of anthrax occurred due to purposeful contamination of the mail. Because of the potential of biological terrorism with this organism, every suspected case should be reported to the local or state health department.

## CLINICAL MANIFESTATIONS

Cutaneous anthrax occurs when *B anthracis* spores enter through an abrasion. A small, erythematous papule vesiculates to form a painless, black eschar with marked edema. Lymphadenopathy or lymphangitis may occur. Untreated, mortality is up to 20%, but with appropriate treatment, it is less than 1%.

Inhalation anthrax occurs after respiratory exposure to *B anthracis* spores. Initial symptoms are nonspecific, mimicking influenza. Symptoms become fulminant over a few days, often leading to death. Mediastinal widening and pleural effusions on chest radiograph are common. Hemorrhagic meningitis and bacteremia are often present. Even with treatment, mortality rates are 40%.

Gastrointestinal anthrax follows ingestion of contaminated, undercooked meat. It may present in 2 forms. In the intestinal form, patients present with nausea, vomiting, and malaise, progressing to bloody diarrhea, gross ascites, hemorrhagic lymphadenitis, and sepsis. The oropharyngeal form of anthrax may present with dysphagia and oropharyngeal necrotic ulcers, profound submental swelling, regional adenopathy, and sepsis. Like inhalation, mortality rates are 40%.

Injection anthrax is a rare clinical manifestation of disease and has not been reported in children but has been described primarily in heroin-injecting populations.

## DIAGNOSIS

Gram stain and culture of vesicular fluid, necrotic tissue, tissue biopsy specimens, blood, cerebrospinal fluid, respiratory specimens, or rectal swabs or stool may confirm the diagnosis of anthrax. *B anthracis* grows in ordinary nutrient broth and on blood agar, appearing as large, gram-positive, sporulating bacilli on Gram stain. Polymerase chain reaction testing may also be available. Definitive identification is available through the Laboratory Response Network (https://emergency.cdc.gov/lrn/). If possible, specimens should be obtained prior to antimicrobial therapy as antimicrobials may decrease positivity rates.

## TREATMENT

Most patients with inhalation or gastrointestinal anthrax have systemic disease, although systemic disease may follow any form, and anthrax meningitis may occur in anyone with systemic disease. Antibiotic resistance to penicillins and tetracyclines is assumed in bioterrorism cases until proven otherwise.

Empiric therapy of inhalational or gastrointestinal bioterrorism-related anthrax or any form that progresses to systemic disease without meningitis includes a bactericidal agent, preferably ciprofloxacin (alternatives include meropenem, imipenem-cilastatin, levofloxacin, or vancomycin), plus a protein synthesis inhibitor, such as clindamycin, linezolid, doxycycline, or rifampin. Penicillin or ampicillin is preferred once susceptibility is confirmed. Full recommendations for pediatric anthrax clinical management are detailed in a 2014 Clinical Report of the American Academy of Pediatrics Committee on Infectious Diseases and Disaster Preparedness Advisory Council.

For anthrax meningitis (where the mortality rate is near 100%), or disseminated infection when meningitis cannot be ruled out, treatment regimens include 2 bactericidal antimicrobial agents (ciprofloxacin plus meropenem) and 1 protein synthesis inhibitor (linezolid preferred). If meningitis is ruled out, a single bacteriostatic agent and a protein synthesis inhibitor (clindamycin preferred) should be used.

First-line therapy for cutaneous anthrax is oral ciprofloxacin. Doxycycline and clindamycin are alternatives. If cutaneous lesions involve the head and neck, if extensive edema is associated, or for any form that evolves to systemic involvement, combination intravenous regimens are recommended. Corticosteroid adjunctive therapy is considered for severe cerebral edema and for meningitis. Either anthrax immune globulin or raxibacumab (GlaxoSmithKline, Research Triangle Park, NC), a humanized monoclonal antibody, is indicated in patients with systemic disease after consultation with the Centers for Disease Control and Prevention.

As spores may persist in the respiratory tract, in bioterrorism-associated disease or disease following exposure to aerosolized spores, treatment should be continued for 60 days. Otherwise, 7 to 10 days of therapy are adequate for uncomplicated cutaneous disease, and at least 14 days are necessary for other forms. Therapy may be completed orally when clinically appropriate.

## PREVENTION

Standard barrier precautions are advised for patients with anthrax, and contact precautions should be added when cutaneous lesions are draining until 24 hours of appropriate therapy have been given. Human anthrax vaccine is recommended for those with occupational risks and is mandated for US military personnel assigned to high-risk areas. In the setting of a bioterrorism attack, vaccination of exposed persons and 60 days of antibiotic administration are recommended. No data on vaccine safety or effectiveness in children are available.

## SUGGESTED READINGS


American Academy of Pediatrics. Anthrax. In: Kimberlin DW, Brady MT, Jackson MA, Long SS, eds. *Red Book: 2015 Report of the Committee on Infectious Diseases.* 30th ed. Elk Grove Village, IL: American Academy of Pediatrics; 2015:234-240.

Bradley JS, Peacock G, Krug SE, et al. Pediatric anthrax clinical management. *Pediatrics.* 2014;133:e1411-e1436.

Conlin AM, Bukowinski AT, Gumbs GR; Department of Defense Birth and Infant Health Registry Team. Analysis of pregnancy and infant health outcomes among women in the National Smallpox Vaccine in Pregnancy Registry who received anthrax vaccine adsorbed. *Vaccine.* 2015;33:4387-4390.

Guh A, Heyman ML, Barden D, Fontana J, Hadler JL. Lessons learned from the investigation of a cluster of cutaneous anthrax cases in Connecticut. *J Public Health Manag Pract.* 2010;16:201-210.

Pillai SK, Huang E, Guarnizo JT, et al. Antimicrobial treatment for systemic anthrax: analysis of cases from 1945 to 2014 identified through a systematic literature review. *Health Secur.* 2015;13: 355-364.

Wright JG, Quinn CP, Shadomy S, Messonnier N; Centers for Disease Control and Prevention. Use of anthrax vaccine in the United States: recommendations of the Advisory Committee on Immunization Practices (ACIP), 2009. *MMWR Recomm Rep.* 2010;59:1-30.


# 247 *Arcanobacterium*

Dennis L. Murray

## INTRODUCTION

The bacterium *Arcanobacterium* was first described in 1946 as a pathogen causing pharyngitis and cutaneous infections in US service members and people in the South Pacific. *Arcanobacterium* means "secretive bacteria." *Arcanobacterium haemolyticum* is the most well-known species of *Arcanobacterium* affecting humans.

## EPIDEMIOLOGY AND PATHOGENESIS

*A haemolyticum* can be isolated from approximately 0.4% of adults in the United States presenting with pharyngitis. This pleomorphic, nonsporulating, hemolytic, catalase-negative, gram-positive (sometimes gram-variable) bacillus resembles *Corynebacterium pyogenes* and is a facultative anaerobe as well as non–acid fast. Humans are the main environmental reservoir, but *Arcanobacterium* is not part of the normal respiratory tract flora. Disease is suspected to be spread from person to person by respiratory droplet. The incubation period is unknown.

*A haemolyticum* is responsible for up to 2% to 2.5% of bacterial pharyngitis by culture in the United States as well as other countries. This bacterium appears to cause disease most commonly in those 10 to 30 years of age, with the maximum incidence occurring in those 15 to 18 years of age. There appears to be no difference in incidence between men and women or among different races.

Although the mechanism for adherence of *Arcanobacterium* to pharyngeal mucosa remains unknown, *A haemolyticum* can liberate toxins, including a dermonecrotic toxin, using a mechanism similar to the production of erythrogenic toxin by group A β-hemolytic streptococci (GABHS).

## CLINICAL MANIFESTATIONS

Presentation of disease caused by *A haemolyticum* is similar to GABHS pharyngitis, with fever, pharyngeal exudate, and lymphadenopathy, but palatal petechiae and a strawberry tongue are usually absent. A sore throat occurs in 97% to 100% and a patchy gray to white exudate in 70% of patients with *A haemolyticum* infection; however, fever and lymphadenopathy occur in only 50% of patients with pharyngitis. An exanthema, described only in patients with pharyngitis, develops 1 to 4 days after the symptoms of sore throat begin. This exanthema, which may be pruritic in up to 33% of patients, includes the extensor surfaces of the extremities and spreads centrally. The face, palms of the hands, and soles of the feet are not typically involved. Other forms of rash that occur include scarlatiniform and maculopapular. Some form of rash occurs in up to 75% of patients with *A haemolyticum* pharyngitis. Nonsuppurative sequelae have not been reported following pharyngitis caused by *A haemolyticum*.

Infections of the skin caused by *A haemolyticum*, especially chronic ulcerations, occur mainly in tropical countries. Invasive infections, including brain abscess, endocarditis, meningitis, osteomyelitis, pneumonia, pyogenic arthritis, and sepsis, have been reported. *A haemolyticum* can be a rare cause of mortality, most often associated with endocarditis. Co-infection with *Fusobacterium necrophorum* can occur in cases of Lemierre disease. Severe, invasive disease occurs most frequently among immunocompromised hosts.

## DIAGNOSIS

Adolescents with clinical findings typical for *A haemolyticum* pharyngitis and whose tests for GABHS are negative should be considered for testing for *A haemolyticum*. Isolation of *A haemolyticum* from a clinical specimen is diagnostic as the organism is rarely identified from healthy persons. While *A haemolyticum* will grow from a pharyngeal exudate culture on 5% sheep's blood agar when held at 37°C for 48 hours in 5% carbon dioxide ($CO_2$), the organism grows best on either human or rabbit blood agar or trypticase soy agar with 5% horse blood in 5% $CO_2$. At 48 hours, these bacteria produce nonpigmented 1-mm colonies with a 3- to 5-mm zone of hemolysis. Colonies often have a small dark dot in the center.

Although infrequently used in clinical laboratories, BioMérieux (Durham, NC, and St. Louis, MO) has developed an anaerobe and *Corynebacterium* identification card kit for the Vitek2 automated bacterial identification system that can identify *A haemolyticum* from clinical specimens.

In terms of differential diagnosis, the patient's age and clinical presentation, especially the occurrence of pharyngitis with delayed rash, should help narrow the possibilities. Enteroviruses, GABHS, and, perhaps, human immunodeficiency virus infection with cutaneous manifestations deserve consideration in those cases where *A haemolyticum* is suspected.

## TREATMENT

No prospective clinical trials have been performed to evaluate the efficacy of antimicrobial treatment of *A haemolyticum* pharyngitis; however, erythromycin is considered the drug of choice for this infection. Bacteriologic failure has occurred when penicillin was used to treat *A haemolyticum* pharyngitis. The organism is sensitive in vitro to erythromycin, azithromycin, clindamycin, cefuroxime, and vancomycin. *A haemolyticum* has shown some resistance (30%) to tetracycline and is typically resistant to trimethoprim-sulfamethoxazole.

Whereas pharyngitis has resolved in untreated patients with *A haemolyticum*, invasive disease caused by *Arcanobacterium* can be fatal. The use of parenteral penicillin combined with an aminoglycoside, such as gentamicin or tobramycin, should be considered empirically while awaiting antimicrobial susceptibility testing in invasive and/or disseminated infection due to *A haemolyticum*.

## PREVENTION

Judicious handwashing and avoidance of sharing food and utensils with someone infected with *A haemolyticum* may be of benefit in limiting disease transmission. For patients hospitalized with invasive *A haemolyticum* infection, standard precautions are recommended.

## SUGGESTED READINGS


American Academy of Pediatrics. Arcanobacterium haemolyticum infections. In: Kimberlin DW, Brady MT, Jackson MA, Long SS, eds. *Red Book 2015 Report of the Committee on Infectious Diseases.* 30th ed. Elk Grove Village, IL: American Academy of Pediatrics; 2015:246-247.

Carlson P, Kontiainen S, Renkonen OV. Antimicrobial susceptibility of *Arcanobacterium haemolyticum. Antimicrob Agents Chemother.* 1994;38:142-143.

Garcia-de-la-Fuente C, Campo-Esquisabel AB, Unda F, et al. Comparison of different culture media and growth conditions for recognition of *Arcanobacterium haemolyticum. Diagn Microbiol Infect Dis.* 2008;61:232-234.

Horner KL. *Arcanobacterium.* http://www.emedicine.medscape.com/article/1054547-overview. Updated January 13, 2014. Accessed March 27, 2016.

Mackenzie A, Fuite LA, Chen FT, et al. Incidence and pathogenicity of *Arcanobacterium haemolyticum* during a 2-year study in Ottawa. *Clin Infect Dis.* 1995;21:177-181.

Minarik T, Sufliarsky J, Trupl J, Krcmery V Jr. *Arcanobacterium haemolyticum* invasive infections, including meningitis in cancer patients. *J Infect.* 1997;34:91.




# 248 *Bacillus cereus*

Denise Bratcher

## INTRODUCTION

*Bacillus cereus* is a gram-positive, spore-forming, motile aerobic rod that also grows well anaerobically. It is ubiquitous in the environment, frequently isolated from plants, meat, eggs, dried cereal, and dairy products.

## PATHOGENESIS AND EPIDEMIOLOGY

*B cereus* commonly causes toxin-mediated foodborne illness due to the formation and release of an emetic and diarrheal toxins. Spores of this organism can survive pasteurizations, brief cooking, and boiling. The emetic form of disease is usually associated with the consumption of contaminated cooked rice (eg, fried rice). Unlike the diarrheal toxins, the emetic toxin is preformed in foods so the presence of living organism is not necessary to cause disease.

For infections not related to food consumption, neonates, immunocompromised hosts, intravenous drug users, patients with recent eye surgery or trauma, or those with intravascular devices or artificial prosthesis are at risk. *B cereus* does not persist in the intestine after ingestion and therefore is not spread by the fecal-oral route.

## CLINICAL MANIFESTATIONS

The 2 primary forms of infection due to *B cereus* are food poisoning and invasive disease. Further, there are 2 types of food poisoning due to *B cereus*. In both forms, the disease is due to the organism's enterotoxin. If the food is contaminated with *B cereus* spores, the diarrheal form results, manifested as abdominal cramps and profuse, watery diarrhea, and in about 25% of patients, vomiting. Following ingestion of the preformed toxin, the emetic form results, manifested as nausea, vomiting, and abdominal cramps, followed by diarrhea in up to 30% of patients. Following the ingestion of the contaminated food, the incubation of the emetic form is less than 6 hours (similar to food poisoning due to *Staphylococcus aureus*) while the incubation period of the diarrhea form is more than 6 hours (similar to food poisoning due to *Clostridium perfringens*). Either form is usually mild and self-limited, lasting 6 to 24 hours, although the diarrhea form may be more severe than the emetic form. Fulminant liver failure has been associated with the emetic form.

*B cereus* is a significant cause of virulent posttraumatic endophthalmitis, typically following a penetrating injury or intravenous drug use. Severe pain, reduced visual acuity, chemosis, swelling, and proptosis, often with systemic symptoms, are noted. Full vision recovery is rare. Postsurgical, traumatic, or burn wounds due to *B cereus* and severe deep infections such as necrotizing fasciitis and gangrene have occurred.

*B cereus* bacteremia is reported among neonates, intravenous drug users, immunocompromised patients, and those with central lines. *B cereus* endocarditis is associated with intravenous drug use or valvular disease. Pneumonia is also reported in neonates and immunosuppressed patients. Meningitis and brain abscesses due to *B cereus* may occur in neonates or in children with ventricular shunts. A cluster of necrotizing enterocolitis was linked to *B cereus* contamination of human milk fortifier in a neonatal intensive care unit.

## DIAGNOSIS

*B cereus* grows readily on nutrient agar or peptone media at 25°C to 37°C (77°F–98.6°F) and may require the addition of certain amino acids. *Bacillus* species are commonly considered contaminants when isolated from normally sterile sites; however, among the at-risk populations noted earlier, *B cereus* should be considered a potential pathogen. In foodborne outbreaks, isolation of *B cereus* from vomitus, stool, or implicated food suggests causation, and in suspected foodborne outbreaks, specimens may be obtained from multiple people.

## TREATMENT

*B cereus* food poisoning is self-limited, requiring no antimicrobial therapy. Antimicrobial therapy is indicated in invasive *B cereus* infections. Empiric therapy with vancomycin or clindamycin, with or without an aminoglycoside, is most commonly recommended. *B cereus* is resistant to β-lactam antibiotics but is usually susceptible to vancomycin, clindamycin, aminoglycosides, erythromycin, fluoroquinolones, carbapenems, and linezolid. Surgical intervention is usually necessary in ophthalmic or skin infections due to *B cereus*. In addition to parenteral therapy, intravitreal vancomycin is often employed in ophthalmic infections. Removal of prosthetic devices is essential for cure.

## PREVENTION

Foodborne *B cereus* disease is prevented by appropriate storage and preparation of food. Bacterial growth may be prevented if hot food is kept above 60°C (140°F) or rapidly cooled to less than 10°C (50°F). Careful attention to aseptic technique and handwashing is helpful in preventing *B cereus* infections among immunocompromised patients and those with indwelling devices.

## SUGGESTED READINGS


American Academy of Pediatrics. *Bacillus cereus* infections. In: Kimberlin DW, Brady MT, Jackson MA, Long SS, eds. *Red Book: 2015 Report of the Committee on Infectious Diseases*. 30th ed. Elk Grove Village, IL: American Academy of Pediatrics; 2015:255-256.

Bottone EJ. *Bacillus cereus*, a volatile human pathogen. *Clin Microbiol Rev*. 2010;23:382-398.

Centers for Disease Control and Prevention. Diagnosis and management of foodborne illness: a primer for physicians and other health care professionals. *Morb Mortal Wkly Rep*. 2004;53:1-33.

Long C, Liu B, Xu C, et al. Causative organisms of post-traumatic endophthalmitis: a 20-year study. *BMC Ophthalmol*. 2014;14:34.

Nichols M, Purcell B, Willis C, et al. Investigation of an outbreak of vomiting in nurseries in South East England, May 2012. *Epidemiol Infect*. 2016;144:582-590.

Tewari A, Abdullah S. *Bacillus cereus* food poisoning: international and Indian perspective. *J Food Sci Technol*. 2015;52:2500-2511.


# 249 Brucellosis

Avinash K. Shetty

## INTRODUCTION

Brucellosis is a zoonotic infection caused by species of the genus *Brucella*. *Brucella* are nonencapsulated, nonmotile, aerobic, gram-negative coccobacilli. Human infections are usually caused by 4 species, which are classified based on their animal reservoir: *Brucella melitensis* (goat, sheep), *Brucella abortus* (cattle), *Brucella suis* (pig), and *Brucella canis* (dog). *B melitensis* is the most common cause of human infection. Other species rarely causing human disease include *Brucella ceti* and *Brucella pinnipedialis* (marine animals). *Brucella inopinata* has been associated with infection of prosthetic implants.

## PATHOGENESIS AND EPIDEMIOLOGY

*Brucella* are facultative intracellular microorganisms with a tendency to establish latent and chronic infection. *Brucella* replicate within vacuoles of macrophages, monocytes, dendritic cells, trophoblasts, and epithelial cells. After the organisms penetrate the mucosal barriers and enter the bloodstream, *Brucella* multiply in the tissues of the reticuloendothelial system and result in granulomas. The organism evades the host immune response by using a wide repertoire of virulence factors and immunomodulatory strategies. The virulence of *Brucella* may be related to the smooth lipopolysaccharides that cover the bacterium. The development of type 1 (Th1) cellular immune response with production of proinflammatory cytokines such as interferon-γ (IFN-γ) by T cells and natural killer cells results in clearance of the organism.

Human brucellosis is a major public health problem in many areas of the globe, with an estimated 500,000 new cases reported annually. Brucellosis is endemic in Mediterranean countries, the Middle East, Central Asia, India, Mexico, and Central and South America. The disease is rare in the United States and other high-income countries due to effective eradication programs in domestic livestock. In 2013, only 8 of 99 brucellosis cases reported to the Centers for Disease Control and Prevention were in patients younger than 15 years old.

Transmission of *Brucella* to humans can occur via ingestion of contaminated animal products, inoculation of the skin or conjunctiva during direct contact with infected animals or their products (such as placenta or aborted tissues), and inhalation of contaminated aerosolized particles. Consumption of unpasteurized milk or other dairy products imported primarily from Mexico accounts for the majority of cases of childhood brucellosis in the United States.

*Brucella* infection has been reported with recreational activities such as hunting feral swine in California, Florida, and Texas. Brucellosis is an occupational hazard for laboratory personnel, abattoir workers, veterinarians, and shepherds. *Brucella* is considered a potential agent for bioterrorism given airborne transmission. Human-to-human transmission is very unusual. Mother-to-baby transmission during pregnancy and breastfeeding has been reported.

## CLINICAL MANIFESTATIONS

Brucellosis is a disease of protean manifestations and can involve any organ system. Symptoms typically develop 2 to 4 weeks after exposure and can be acute or insidious. Fever is present in almost every patient and may wax and wane over a prolonged period of time, which is how it earned the name "undulant fever." The classic triad of brucellosis consists of fever, arthralgia or arthritis, and hepatosplenomegaly. Brucellosis can present as a fever of unknown origin accompanied by nonspecific symptoms such as night sweats, malaise, anorexia, weight loss, abdominal pain, and joint pain. Physical examination may reveal hepatosplenomegaly, lymphadenopathy, and monoarticular arthritis involving the hip or knee. Laboratory abnormalities may include mild leukopenia (with relative lymphocytosis), anemia, thrombocytopenia, and elevated liver enzymes.

Compared to adults, chronic brucellosis is less common in children. Complications include endocarditis, meningitis, osteomyelitis, hepatosplenic abscess, or pneumonia. Brucellosis during pregnancy can result in spontaneous abortion, preterm labor, fetal death, and maternal/neonatal death.

The differential diagnosis includes other granulomatous infections such as tularemia, cat scratch disease, blastomycosis, coccidiomycosis, histoplasmosis, and tuberculosis. Typhoid fever and malaria can mimic brucellosis in endemic areas. Given the nonspecific symptomatology, fastidious growth on blood culture, and difficulty in serologic diagnosis, the diagnosis of brucellosis can be challenging. History of travel to an endemic area, consumption of unpasteurized milk products, and contact with livestock are important epidemiologic clues.

## DIAGNOSIS

Definite diagnosis of brucellosis requires the isolation of the organism from blood, bone marrow, body fluid, or tissue. Laboratory personnel should be notified when brucellosis is suspected because (1) the laboratory must take precautions and (2) *Brucella* grows slowly on routine media, and blood cultures must be incubated for 3 to 4 weeks to increase yield. However, modern BACTEC systems can detect the organism by 7 days. Serologic diagnosis is made using the serum agglutination test (SAT), which detects antibodies to *B melitensis*, *B suis*, and *B abortus*. SAT does not detect antibodies to *B canis*. A 4-fold or greater rise in antibody titer between acute and convalescent sera obtained at least 14 days apart confirms the diagnosis. A single titer is not diagnostic, but a titer of ≥ 1:160 is considered significant in nonendemic areas. False-positive SAT for *Brucella* is a concern since serologic cross-reactions may occur with other gram-negative pathogens (eg, *Francisella tularensis*, *Yersinia enterocolitica*, *Vibrio cholerae*). Enzyme immunoassays, although sensitive, are not standardized and are only recommended for suspected cases with negative SAT or for evaluation of patients with suspected complicated or chronic disease or reinfection. Polymerase chain reaction assays have been developed but also lack standardization.

## TREATMENT

Combination antibiotic therapy for a prolonged period is recommended for successful treatment of human brucellosis. For uncomplicated brucellosis, oral doxycycline combined with rifampin for 6 weeks is recommended for children age ≥ 8 years. For children age < 8 years, oral trimethoprim-sulfamethoxazole combined with rifampin for 6 weeks is recommended. For complicated or serious disease, a 1- to 2-week course of gentamicin should be added to the 6-week regimens above. Meningitis or endocarditis often requires 4 to 6 months of antibiotic therapy. Surgical intervention may be indicated in complicated disease (eg, hepatosplenic abscess, epidural abscess, endocarditis). Relapses are common (3–10%) in treated patients. Monotherapy and shorter duration of combination regimens are associated with higher relapse rates. Thus, relapses are not usually associated with drug resistance but are related to the intracellular persistence of the organism and lack of adherence to the prolonged antimicrobial therapy required.

## PREVENTION

No human vaccine is available. Prevention is achieved by eradication of brucellosis in animals, pasteurization of milk, and public education. Individuals should avoid the ingestion of unpasteurized animal-milk products from endemic areas. Consumption of raw milk supplied by "certified" dairies may transmit *Brucella*. Brucellosis is a reportable disease in the United States.

## SUGGESTED READINGS


Ahmetagić S, Porobić Jahić H, Koluder N, et al. Brucellosis in children in Bosnia and Herzegovina in the period 2000-2013. *Med Glas (Zenica)*. 2015;12:177-182.

American Academy of Pediatrics. Brucellosis. In: Kimberlin DW, Brady MT, Jackson MA, Long SS, eds. *Red Book: 2015 Report of the Committee on Infectious Diseases*. 30th ed. Elk Grove Village, IL: American Academy of Pediatrics; 2015:268-270.

Atluri VL, Xavier MN, de Jong MF, et al. Interactions of the human pathogenic *Brucella* species with their hosts. *Annu Rev Microbiol.* 2011;65:523-541.

Bosilkovski M, Kirova-Urosevic V, Cekovska Z, et al. Osteoarticular involvement in childhood brucellosis: experience with 133 cases in an endemic region. *Pediatr Infect Dis J*. 2013;32:815-819.

Bosilkovski M, Rodriguez-Morales AJ. Brucellosis and its particularities in children travelers. *Recent Pat Antiinfect Drug Discov.* 2014;9:164-172.

Committee on Infectious Diseases; Committee on Nutrition; American Academy of Pediatrics. Consumption of raw or unpasteurized milk and milk products by pregnant women and children. *Pediatrics*. 2014;133:175-179.

Fruchtman Y, Segev RW, Golan AA, et al. Epidemiological, diagnostic, clinical, and therapeutic aspects of *Brucella* bacteremia in children in southern Israel: a 7-year retrospective study (2005-2011). *Vector Borne Zoonotic Dis.* 2015;15:195-201.

Yagupsky P. Pediatric brucellosis: an (almost) forgotten disease. *Adv Exp Med Biol.* 2011;719:123-132.


# 250 *Pseudomonas, Burkholderia,* and *Stenotrophomonas*

Karen P. Acker and Lisa Saiman



## INTRODUCTION

*Pseudomonas*, *Burkholderia*, and *Stenotrophomonas* species are non–lactose-fermenting gram-negative bacilli that are frequently multidrug resistant and are important pathogens, particularly in healthcare-associated infections in immunocompromised patients and in individuals with cystic fibrosis (CF). Previously, *Burkholderia* and *Stenotrophomonas* species were classified as *Pseudomonas* due to their similar biochemical properties. In 1992, the genus *Burkholderia* was proposed for 7 species. There has been a rapid increase in newly identified species to > 70 species that are very similar phenotypically, thus making taxonomic classification somewhat perplexing without the use of molecular strategies. The most commonly identified species within the *Burkholderia cepacia* complex are *Burkholderia cenocepacia* and *Burkholderia multivorans. Stenotrophomonas* was initially reclassified as *Xanthomonas* in 1983 and acquired its present classification in 1993. *Stenotrophomonas maltophilia* is the only species within its genus known to cause human disease.

## EPIDEMIOLOGY AND PATHOGENESIS

*Pseudomonas*, *Burkholderia*, and *Stenotrophomonas* are ubiquitous environmental organisms found in water, soil, and plants, and are distributed worldwide. Some *Burkholderia* species are well-known causes of disease in plants. For example, *B cepacia* causes crop rot in onion fields.

*Pseudomonas aeruginosa* and *S maltophilia* are endemic in most hospital environments and can contaminate medical devices such as suction tubing, indwelling catheters, and sinks and faucets. *P aeruginosa* colonization of artificial nails worn by healthcare workers has been linked to outbreaks. *Burkholderia* species are less easily isolated from sources in the hospital environment, although *B cepacia* complex has a unique ability to grow in disinfectant solutions, which can result in nosocomial outbreaks. Similarly, intrinsic contamination of medications, including nasal sprays and bronchodilators, has been linked to human infections.

In individuals with CF, acquisition of environmental strains of *P aeruginosa* and *Burkholderia* species has been documented. There are well-documented instances of person-to-person transmission of both *P aeruginosa* and *B cepacia* complex.

One of the primary virulence mechanisms shared by these organisms is the ability to produce biofilms, which enable them to adhere to surfaces such as wounds and medical tubing, evade immune responses such as phagocytosis, and resist antimicrobial killing. Neutrophils are the most important defense against *Pseudomonas*, and thus, severe and prolonged neutropenia predisposes patients to severe infections. Similarly, patients with chronic granulomatous disease (CGD) who have impaired phagocytic killing due to defective function of NADPH oxidase are particularly susceptible to *Burkholderia* infections. Additional virulence factors include flagella and pili that aid these organisms in motility and facilitate binding to epithelial surfaces. In addition, they produce exotoxins that possess enzymatic activity and cause tissue damage. Mechanisms of antibiotic resistance that render these organisms quite difficult to treat include β-lactamase and carbapenemase production, multidrug efflux pumps, porin loss, and antibiotic modification via aminoglycoside-modifying enzymes.

## CLINICAL MANIFESTATIONS

The most clinically important *Pseudomonas* species is *P aeruginosa*. This opportunistic pathogen rarely causes disease in immunocompetent hosts. However, there are several well-described clinical syndromes that can occur in individuals with normal host immunity;

*P aeruginosa* can cause folliculitis from hot tub exposure, otitis externa or "swimmer's ear," and osteochondritis/osteomyelitis following a puncture wound of the foot through the sole of a sneaker. The association with sneakers is thought to be due to the moist inner sole, which facilitates growth of *P aeruginosa* within the sneaker.

*P aeruginosa* causes serious infections in patients with underlying conditions, such as neutropenia, immunodeficiency, prematurity, or CF, and in hospitalized patients with wounds, burns, or indwelling devices. The most common healthcare-associated infections caused by *P aeruginosa* include bacteremia, pneumonia, and urinary tract infection. Neutropenia puts patients at particularly high risk for such infections; thus, patients receiving induction chemotherapy for leukemia or lymphoma or myeloablative regimens for stem cell transplantation should be empirically covered with antipseudomonal therapy in the setting of fever and neutropenia. Burn wounds are often colonized with *Pseudomonas* species, predisposing hospitalized burn patients to sepsis and delayed wound healing. *P aeruginosa* can also cause other invasive infections including meningitis following trauma and endocarditis and osteomyelitis in intravenous drug users.

Other *Pseudomonas* species, such as *Pseudomonas fluorescens* and *Pseudomonas putida*, have also been implicated in cases of bacteremia and pseudobacteremia; the latter refers to false-positive blood cultures due to contamination of blood culture samples within the microbiology laboratory. *P fluorescens*, in particular, has been associated with bacteremia linked to contaminated transfusion products and intravenous fluids. *Pseudomonas oryzihabitans* has been increasingly identified as an agent of catheter-associated infections, and *Pseudomonas stutzeri* and *Pseudomonas luteola* are occasional causes of human infections.

The *B cepacia* complex includes the most clinically significant *Burkholderia* species and encompasses at least 17 genetically related species, causing lung infections in patients with CF and CGD. Respiratory tract infections in patients without CF are the most common manifestations of *Burkholderia*, and ventilator-associated pneumonia has been linked to contaminated respiratory equipment or medications. Outbreaks of *B cepacia* bacteremia have been reported in neonatal intensive care units and have been linked to contaminated medical solutions. A variety of other clinical manifestations such as bacteremia, urinary tract infection, and septic arthritis have been described.

Non-*cepacia* species can also cause human disease. *Burkholderia pseudomallei* is the etiologic agent of melioidosis, an infection endemic in Southeast Asia and northern Australia caused by direct contact, inhalation, or ingestion of contaminated surface water or soil. Clinical manifestations of melioidosis reflect the route of acquisition and include localized skin and soft tissue infections, pulmonary infections, bloodstream infections, and/or disseminated infections. *Burkholderia mallei* is the etiologic agent of glanders, which is rarely transmitted from infected animals to humans in Africa, Asia, the Middle East, and Central and South America. Clinical manifestations of *B mallei* are similar to those of *B pseudomallei*, including localized acute or chronic skin and soft tissue infections and abscesses. *Burkholderia gladioli* can be isolated from the lungs of individuals with CF.

*S maltophilia* is generally regarded as a low-virulence organism but has emerged as an important multidrug-resistant organism that can cause serious healthcare-associated infections in immunocompromised patients. The incidence of isolation of this organism is increasing, particularly in immunocompromised patients, although community-acquired infections have been reported as well. Clinical manifestations of *S maltophilia* include, but are not limited to, respiratory tract infections, which are the most common, followed by central line–associated bacteremia, and more rarely, urinary tract infection, eye infection, and skin and soft tissue infection. Risk factors for infection are similar to those for *Pseudomonas* and *Burkholderia* and include presence of indwelling catheters and endotracheal tubes, chronic respiratory disease, immunocompromised state, prior antibiotic exposure, and intensive care unit hospitalization.

*Pseudomonas, Burkholderia*, and *Stenotrophomonas* species are all recovered from the lungs of individuals with CF. *P aeruginosa* plays a prominent role in CF pathogenesis; chronic infection persists despite aggressive antibiotic therapy and leads to excessive lung inflammation resulting in progressive loss of lung function. *P aeruginosa* and *B cepacia* complex are well-described pathogens in CF, but the role of *S maltophilia* is less well understood. The prevalence of *P aeruginosa* in individuals with CF increases with age; approximately 20% to 25% of children under 2 years of age and approximately 50% of adolescents have *P aeruginosa* isolated from their respiratory tract. Once chronic infection with *Pseudomonas* is established, these organisms undergo mutations from a nonmucoid to a mucoid form, a transition that is associated with worsening pulmonary function and poorer prognosis. CF pulmonary infections caused by *P aeruginosa* are also complicated by multidrug resistance due to the frequent courses of antipseudomonal antibiotics used to treat pulmonary exacerbations. Approximately 3% of CF patients in the United States are infected with *B cepacia* complex species, with *B cenocepacia* and *B multivorans* being the most common. Infection with *Burkholderia* portends declined lung function and increased mortality, including after lung transplantation, and thus is a contraindication to receiving a lung transplant in many CF centers. *S maltophilia* is increasingly isolated from the CF lung, and approximately 13% of CF patients have had this organism isolated (see Chapter 507).

## DIAGNOSIS

Diagnosis of an invasive infection caused by *Pseudomonas* species, *Burkholderia* species, or *S maltophilia* is based on the isolation of these organisms from a normally sterile site using standard culture methods. However, *P aeruginosa* and other *Pseudomonas* species are increasingly identified using molecular techniques such as polymerase chain reaction (PCR) amplification of 16s rRNA genes. Identification of *Burkholderia* and *Stenotrophomonas* still relies primarily on culture methods, but molecular methods may be needed to distinguish species of *Burkholderia*. It is not uncommon for *Burkholderia* to be misidentified as other non–lactose-fermenting gram-negative bacilli such as *Achromobacter, Ralstonia, Pandoraea*, and *Cupriviavidus* species unless molecular methods are used. Although molecular methods were formerly confined to research settings, they are increasingly available in clinical microbiology laboratories or public health laboratories.

In hospitalized patients, isolation of these organisms from nonsterile body sites may represent colonization, rather than infection. This is particularly an issue for patients with endotracheal tubes or tracheostomies. Thus, it is important to review all the associated signs and symptoms including chest radiographs to ensure the judicious use of antimicrobial therapy.

## TREATMENT

*Pseudomonas, Burkholderia*, and *S maltophilia* are resistant to many antibiotics, and thus, susceptibility testing is required to determine optimal therapy. In addition, organisms can readily develop resistance after exposure to antimicrobial agents. Commonly used antimicrobial agents are shown in Table 250-1. For uncomplicated infections caused by *P aeruginosa* in a normal host, treatment with a single agent and removal of a foreign body, when appropriate, may be adequate therapy. In immunocompromised hosts or for management of a pulmonary exacerbation in CF, 2-drug combinations from different classes of antimicrobial agents are recommended.

*B cepacia* complex organisms are even more intrinsically resistant to antibiotics than *P aeruginosa* and are uniformly resistant to the aminoglycosides and polymyxin. The only drugs recommended for testing by the Clinical Laboratory Standards Institute (CLSI) are ceftazidime, minocycline, meropenem, and trimethoprim/sulfamethoxazole (TMP/SMX). Additional agents that may have activity against *B cepacia* complex are shown in Table 250-1. Due to the risk of developing resistance during therapy, repeating susceptibility testing may be warranted in the setting of clinical or microbiologic failure.

*S maltophilia* is intrinsically resistant to many antibiotics, and although TMP/SMX is recommended as first-line treatment, resistance often limits its use. CLSI interpretative criteria for susceptibility

**TABLE 250-1 ANTIMICROBIAL TREATMENT OPTIONS**

| | First-Line Therapy | Alternative Therapy and New Agents | Comments |
|---|---|---|---|
| *Pseudomonas* species | Piperacillin-tazobactam, ceftazidime, cefepime, or meropenem | Tobramycin, gentamicin, amikacin, ceftolozane/tazobactam, ceftazidime/avibactam | Aminoglycosides often recommended in combination with β-lactam agent for serious infections |
| *Burkholderia cepacia* complex | Trimethoprim/sulfamethoxazole (TMP/SMX), meropenem, or ciprofloxacin | Minocycline | Susceptibility testing generally recommended for TMP/SMX, meropenem, and minocycline |
| *Stenotrophomonas maltophilia* | TMP/SMX | Fluoroquinolones, tigecycline, polymyxin, minocycline | Higher dosing of TMP/SMX is required (15 mg/kg/d)<br>Susceptibility testing generally recommended for TMP/SMX, fluoroquinolones, and minocycline |

testing are available for minocycline, levofloxacin, and TMP/SMX, although hospital laboratories will often perform susceptibility testing for additional antibiotics if initial testing demonstrates resistance to first-line agents.

## PREVENTION

Both active and passive immunization strategies have been attempted for the prevention of *P aeruginosa* infections in high-risk populations, including patients with CF, immunocompromised patients, and following burns or major trauma. IC43, a recombinant outer membrane–based vaccine against *P aeruginosa*, is the only gram-negative vaccine that has progressed beyond phase I trials. Currently, there are no licensed vaccines or prophylactic antibiotic strategies aimed at preventing infections caused by *Pseudomonas, Burkholderia,* and *Stenotrophomonas.*

Prevention primarily employs strategies aimed at preventing healthcare-associated infections. These include strategies to prevent catheter-associated bloodstream infection, catheter-associated urinary tract infection, and ventilator-associated pneumonia. Key strategies to prevent these device-associated infections is to limit use of the devices as much as feasible and to consistently implement evidence-based strategies aimed to prevent infections. In addition, antimicrobial stewardship programs can improve appropriate use of antibiotics and reduce inappropriate use of broad-spectrum agents, which promotes resistance.

## SUGGESTED READINGS


Abbott IJ, Peleg AY. *Stenotrophomonas, Achromobacter,* and nonmelioid *Burkholderia* species: antimicrobial resistance and therapeutic strategies. *Semin Respir Crit Care Med.* 2015;36:99-110.

Brooke JS. *Stenotrophomonas maltophilia*: an emerging global opportunistic pathogen. *Clin Microbiol Rev.* 2012;25:2-41.

Hoiby N, Ciofu O, Bjarnsholt T. *Pseudomonas.* In: Jorgensen JH, Pfaller MA, eds. *Manual of Clinical Microbiology.* 11th ed. Washington, DC: ASM Press; 2015:773-787.

Lipuma JJ, Currie BJ, Peacock SJ, Vandamme PAR. *Burkholderia, Stenotrophomonas, Ralstonia, Cupriavidus, Pandoraea, Brevundimonas, Comamonas, Delftia,* and *Acidovorax.* In: Jorgensen JH, Plalier MA, eds. *Manual of Clinical Microbiology.* 10th ed. Washington, DC: ASM Press; 2013:791-812.

Saiman L, Siegel JD, LiPuma JJ, et al. Infection prevention and control guideline for cystic fibrosis: 2013. *Infect Control Hosp Epidemiol.* 2014;35:S1-S67.

Vandamme P, Dawyndt P. Classification and identification of the *Burkholderia cepacia* complex: past, present and future. *Syst Appl Microbiol.* 2011;34:87-95.

van Duin D, Bonoma RA. Ceftazidime/avibactam and ceftolozane/tazobactam: second-generation β-lactam/β-lactamase combinations. *Clin Infect Dis.* 2016;63:234-241.

Waters V, Smyth A. Cystic fibrosis microbiology: advances in antimicrobial therapy. *J Cyst Fibros.* 2015;14:551-560.

Wiersinga WJ, Currie BJ, Peacock SJ. Melioidosis. *N Engl J Med.* 2012;367:1035-1044.


# 251 *Campylobacter*

Gueorgui Dubrocq and Benjamin Hanisch

## INTRODUCTION

*Campylobacter* species are among the most common pathogens in humans and are commensal in birds, swine, and cattle. The incidence and prevalence of campylobacteriosis have increased in both developed and developing countries over the last 10 years, causing an estimated 92 to 300 million illnesses annually. Although diarrhea is the most frequent clinical manifestation, a broad clinical spectrum is associated with this infection, from asymptomatic carriage to systemic illness. Guillain-Barré syndrome (GBS), reactive arthritis, irritable bowel syndrome, and inflammatory bowel disease have been reported as postinfectious complications of or associations with campylobacteriosis.

## PATHOGENESIS AND EPIDEMIOLOGY

*Campylobacter* organisms are motile, comma-shaped, gram-negative bacilli that derive their name from the Greek words meaning "curved rod." *Campylobacter* has been recognized as a pathogen of many animal species including humans. There are 26 species of the genus *Campylobacter,* of which 17 have been isolated or detected in humans. The species most frequently associated with human infections include *C jejuni* and *C coli. C concisus, C ureolyticus, C upsaliensis,* and *C lari* are emerging *Campylobacter* species that contribute to the etiology of gastroenteritis. *C fetus* is an infrequent cause of bacteremia and meningitis in immunocompromised individuals and neonates.

Rates of *C jejuni and C coli* infection in the United States are more common during the summer months, but cases occur throughout the year. Modes of transmission of *Campylobacter* differ between economically developed and developing countries. The main vehicles of transmission have been associated with improperly cooked poultry, untreated water, and unpasteurized milk consumption. *Campylobacter* outbreaks are uncommon in the United States but have occurred in schoolchildren who drank unpasteurized milk. Person-to-person spread occurs occasionally, particularly among very young children, and the risk is greatest during the acute phase of the illness. The incubation period for *Campylobacter* infection is usually 2 to 5 days, but it can be longer. Person-to-person transmission also has occurred in neonates of infected mothers and has resulted in healthcare-associated outbreaks in nurseries. Excretion usually lasts about 2 to 3 weeks without treatment.

Among *Campylobacter* isolates reported in FoodNet (2014) with species information, 88% are *C jejuni*, 9% are *C coli*, 2% are *C upsaliensis*, and the remaining 1% are other species. *C jejuni* is found in the intestinal tract of chickens, turkeys, ducks, ostriches, sheep, cattle, pigs, and other farm animals, all of which serve as reservoirs of infection. Consumption of contaminated poultry, beef, pork, and unpasteurized milk is the leading cause of human foodborne illness. Poultry is estimated to account for 50% to 70% of human *Campylobacter* infections. Confinement of animals in farms promotes increased carriage and horizontal transmission of *Campylobacter*.

In the United States, an estimated 1.3 million cases of campylobacteriosis occur each year. It is the second most common bacterial cause of foodborne illness after salmonellosis. The overall incidence of laboratory-confirmed *Campylobacter* infection in 2015 in the United States was 12.9 cases per 100,000 population, representing a 9% increase from the 2006 to 2008 baseline. Age-specific rates of *C jejuni* isolation in patients with diarrhea differ among countries. The disease occurs in all ages, but the highest incidence is in children less than 5 years of age (21 per 100,000 persons vs 8 per 100,000 in children 5–19 years of age). Infection occurs more frequently in males than females. It is the second most common bacterial cause of hospitalization for gastroenteritis after *Salmonella* species infection, with a hospitalization rate of 15% for all *Campylobacter* species infections. Studies of the disease burden of *Campylobacter* species infection in the world have estimated that the highest rates of intestinal infection in general account for 2221 disability-adjusted life-years (DALYs) per 100,000 persons in the African region, while in the Americas region, it is lower at 1389 DALYs. The total cost annually for all gastrointestinal infections in the United States was $51 billion, with *Campylobacter* accounting for an estimated $1.5 billion each year. *Campylobacter* species infection is generally associated with mild illness and only occasionally is fatal. The mortality rate associated with symptomatic *Campylobacter* species infection has been estimated at < 1%, with only 12 deaths occurring in 2013 in the United States. In developing countries, the isolation rate in children with diarrhea ranges from 5% to 20%.

## CLINICAL MANIFESTATIONS

The most common clinical manifestation of *C jejuni* and *C coli* infection is gastroenteritis. Predominant symptoms include diarrhea with or without blood, abdominal pain often with fever, and malaise. In neonates and young infants, bloody diarrhea without fever can be the only manifestation of infection. Diarrhea caused by *C coli* is clinically undistinguishable from that caused by *C jejuni*. The onset of symptoms usually occurs 1 to 3 days following ingestion, depending on the quantity of bacteria ingested. The infectious dose is low and can be as little as 360 colony-forming units. The peak of the illness may last 1 to 2 days, and the abdominal pain may mimic appendicitis or intussusception. A study in Denmark that evaluated the consistency of stool of persons infected with *C jejuni* or *C coli* who had no co-infection and no prior gastrointestinal disease showed that 98% of persons experienced watery stools, and 24% contained blood in the stool. Most persons reporting diarrhea due to *C jejuni* or *C coli* recover in less than 14 days without treatment, but in 32% of persons, it can be prolonged. Severe or persistent infection in older children and adolescents can mimic acute inflammatory bowel disease.

Immunoreactive complications including GBS, Miller Fisher variant of GBS (ophthalmoplegia, areflexia, ataxia), pericarditis, erythema nodosum, and reactive arthritis with or without urethritis, conjunctivitis, or uveitis all have been associated with the convalescent stage of infection. *C jejuni* is the most commonly identified bacterial cause of GBS, preceding paralysis in 30% of patients with GBS. In Europe and North America, the subtype of GBS that predominates with *Campylobacter* infection includes acute inflammatory demyelinating polyneuropathy, while in the developing world of Asia and Central and South America, persons are more likely to experience the acute motor axonal neuropathy subtype. The underlying mechanism of nerve damage associated with GBS is likely due to cross-reactivity between antibodies produced in response to *C jejuni* lipooligosaccharide (LOS) and human gangliosides, such as the GM1 ganglioside.

*Campylobacter* bacteremia is one of the most common extragastrointestinal manifestations of *Campylobacter* species. It is most commonly associated with *C jejuni*, *C coli*, and *C fetus* infections, although there are at least 10 species documented, including *C lari* and *C upsaliensis*, that cause bacteremia. Most cases occur from a single gastroenteritis infection or as recurrent episodes in immunocompromised persons. Bacteremia has been estimated to occur in 2.9 cases per 100,000 persons. Other rare extragastrointestinal infections caused by *C jejuni* include cholecystitis, urinary tract infection, acute febrile illness, myocarditis, meningitis, and Bell palsy.

Perinatal infections including neonatal sepsis and meningitis have been associated with *C fetus* but rarely with *C jejuni*. *C fetus* is generally associated with abortion in pregnant women following an aggressive bowel infection that results in sepsis, with the infection eventually transmitted to the fetus. Perinatal complications include premature birth and low birth weight.

## DIAGNOSIS

The diagnosis of *Campylobacter* enteritis can be suggested clinically by the occurrence of watery diarrhea sometimes followed by blood-streaked stools and preceded or accompanied by abdominal pain, although a microbiologic diagnosis is needed to differentiate this condition from other causes of watery diarrhea or colitis. In some cases, blood cultures can also be positive. A rapid diagnosis of *Campylobacter* enteritis can be made by direct examination of fresh stool sample by identifying the characteristic comma-shaped organism with phase contrast or dark-field microscopy. *C jejuni* and *C coli* also can be detected directly via enzyme immunoassays, but false-positive results have been reported. Nucleic acid amplification tests have become available and may help distinguish between the different types of *Campylobacter* species, but accuracy data are preliminary. Isolation of *C jejuni* and *C coli* in culture requires use of selective media, microaerobic conditions, and an incubation temperature of 42°C.

## TREATMENT

Rehydration and correction of electrolyte abnormalities are the mainstays of treatment for patients with *Campylobacter* enteritis. Antimicrobial therapy should be considered for persons with severe disease who are experiencing bloody diarrhea, fever, a large number of stools, and worsening or prolonged symptoms. Therapy also should be considered for those at high risk for severe disease, such as those with immune systems severely weakened from medications or other illnesses. Azithromycin (children) and fluoroquinolones (adults) commonly are used for treatment of these infections. Ideally, the antibiotic regimen should be selected based on the antimicrobial susceptibility results. Antimotility agents should be avoided as they have been associated with prolongation of symptoms and fatalities. *Campylobacter* species, particularly *C jejuni* and *C coli,* often are resistant to penicillin, ampicillin, cephalosporins (except a few third-generation agents), and trimethoprim/sulfamethoxazole. *Campylobacter* resistance to azithromycin remains low in the United States, with less than 2% of *C jejuni* and 9% of *C coli* isolates reported as resistant. In contrast, fluoroquinolone resistance has been increasing, with 25% of *C jejuni* and 34% of *C coli* isolates resistant to ciprofloxacin. This rise in resistance coincides with the increased usage of fluoroquinolones in food production of animals to control, prevent, and treat infections. When antimicrobial therapy is indicated, treatment with azithromycin given at 10 mg/kg/d for 3 days or erythromycin given at 40 mg/kg/d for 5 days usually eradicates the organism from the stool within 2 to 3 days. When given early in the course of infection, antimicrobial therapy serves to shorten the duration of clinical symptoms and the period of stool shedding of the organism. A longer duration of therapy may be needed in immunocompromised individuals. Antibiotic therapy for bacteremia should be selected on the basis of antimicrobial susceptibility tests and commonly is given for approximately 2 weeks.

## PREVENTION

Control measures that could reduce transmission substantially include proper hand hygiene after handling raw poultry and its associated products, hand hygiene following contact with feces of dogs and cats that have diarrhea, avoidance of raw milk ingestion, and cooking poultry thoroughly. Appropriate handling, storage, and cooking of poultry should be stressed. Poultry and meat should be cooked until no longer pink in the middle (internal temperature at least 165°F). Unpasteurized milk should not be consumed. In the hospital, in addition to standard precautions, contact precautions are recommended for diapered and incontinent children for the duration of illness.

## SUGGESTED READINGS


American Academy of Pediatrics. *Campylobacter* In: Kimberlin DW, Brady MT, Jackson MA, Long SS, eds. *Red Book: 2015 Report of the Committee on Infectious Diseases.* 30th ed. Washington, DC: American Academy of Pediatrics; 2015:273-275.

Crim SM, Griffin PM, Tauxe R, et al. Preliminary incidence and trends of infection with pathogens transmitted commonly through food: Foodborne Diseases Active Surveillance Network, 10 U.S. sites, 2006-2014. Centers for Disease Control and Prevention (CDC). *Morb Mortal Wkly Rep.* 2015;64:495-499.

Epps SV, Harvey RB, Hume ME, Phillips TD, Anderson RC, Nisbet DJ. Foodborne *Campylobacter*: infections, metabolism, pathogenesis and reservoirs. *Int J Environ Res Public Health.* 2013;10:6292-6304.

Humphries RM, Schuetz AN. Antimicrobial susceptibility testing of bacteria that cause gastroenteritis. *Clin Lab Med.* 2015;35:313-331.

Kaakoush NO, Castaño-Rodríguez N, Mitchell HM, Man SM. Global epidemiology of *Campylobacter* infection. *Clin Microbiol Rev.* 2015; 28:687-720.

Keithlin J, Sargeant J, Thomas MK, Fazil A. Systematic review and meta-analysis of the proportion of *Campylobacter* cases that develop chronic sequelae. *BMC Public Health.* 2014;14:1203.

Nielsen HL, Engberg J, Ejlertsen T, Bücker R, Nielsen H. Short-term and medium-term clinical outcomes of *Campylobacter concisus* infection. *Clin Microbiol Infect.* 2012;18:e459-e465.


# 252 Cat Scratch Disease (*Bartonella henselae*)

Moshe Ephros and Michael Giladi

## INTRODUCTION

Cat scratch disease (CSD) is a ubiquitous, self-limited infection characterized by prolonged regional lymphadenitis and often an inoculation site papule, usually after a cat's (frequently a kitten's) scratch or bite, and caused primarily by *Bartonella henselae.* In 10% to 20% of cases, the lymph node will suppurate. In a minority of cases (approximately 10%), a wide range of extranodal manifestations collectively known as atypical CSD may occur, including fever of unknown origin (FUO), as well as visceral, neurologic, and ocular involvement. In immune-competent individuals, prognosis is generally good, but infection may be life-threatening and its manifestations different in the immunocompromised.

## PATHOGENESIS AND EPIDEMIOLOGY

Bartonellae are fastidious, slow-growing, pleomorphic gram-negative *Proteobacteria* related to *Brucella.* All *Bartonella* species can be cultured on cell-free media (eg, rabbit-heart infusion or chocolate agar plates). Results are optimized if media are fresh. Culture of *B henselae* may require several weeks of incubation before colonies can be detected. Routine bacterial cultures in the clinical microbiology laboratory are not likely to detect *Bartonella* growth. Although *B henselae* frequently can be isolated from infected cats, sensitivity of blood or lymph node cultures is extremely low in immunocompetent patients with CSD. Therefore, cultures are not recommended for the routine diagnosis of most CSD cases. *B bacilliformis, B quintana,* and *B henselae* are the most important human pathogens; rarely, other *Bartonella* species also cause human disease.

CSD was clinically recognized in the early 20th century and was first described in 1950 by Debré. In 1983, organisms were visualized by silver staining of CSD lymph nodes. Finally, in the 1990s, *B henselae* was proven to be the major cause of CSD—epidemiologically, serologically, by culture, and by molecular methods. The pathogenesis of CSD is poorly understood, and the reasons some patients develop typical CSD with localized infection and regional necrotizing granulomatous adenitis while others develop serious atypical disease, presumably due to bloodborne dissemination with visceral or other end-organ involvement, are not clear. Bacterial and host factors play a role. *B henselae* strains particularly associated with human disease (eg, ST1 genotype) or with only cat infection (eg, ST7 genotype) were identified. The type and severity of the host immune response to infection also modify the clinical picture. Immunocompromised individuals, especially those with cell-mediated immune deficiency, either congenital or acquired (particularly HIV-AIDS but also solid organ transplant patients), are at risk of developing severe or atypical disease. *Bartonella* infection has also been increasingly reported in patients treated with biological immune modulators such as monoclonal antibodies (eg, infliximab, tocilizumab). *B henselae,* like other Bartonellae, interacts with endothelial cells and is capable of inducing angiogenesis. *B henselae* can induce a Th1 inflammatory response, and interferon-γ and nitric oxide play important roles. Dendritic cells and humoral immunity also play a role in the host response to *B henselae.*

CSD occurs worldwide and is prevalent in warm and humid climates. In temperate zones, CSD occurs primarily during fall and winter, sometimes also during the summer, while in the tropics, it occurs throughout the year. CSD was, in the past, considered to be mainly a disease of children and adolescents, with approximately 90% of patients younger than 18 to 21 years old and with about 55% males. Newer studies, however, have reported that 45% and 43% of CSD patients are more than 18 and 20 years of age, respectively. CSD almost never occurs in children under 2 years of age but otherwise is increasingly recognized in all age groups, including the elderly. Intrafamilial clustering of CSD occurs rarely, although anti–*B henselae* seropositivity is more frequent in families with a case of CSD than in the general population, indicative of asymptomatic infection. Immune-deficient people, especially those with HIV, may become severely ill with a unique spectrum of disease. In 1993, the annual incidence of CSD in the United States was estimated at 9 to 10/100,000 with about 10% hospitalization, and most patients were younger than 21 years old. In 2000, the US annual hospitalization rate for CSD was estimated at 0.6/100,000 and 0.86/100,000 for children under 18 and under 5 years old, respectively; not surprisingly, 24% of admissions were for atypical disease, 12% for central nervous system (CNS) disease, and 7% for visceral disease. Cats, especially kittens under 1 year of age, are the major reservoir and tend to have prolonged, asymptomatic intra-erythrocytic bacteremia. They infect humans by scratch, bite, or mucous membrane (conjunctival, respiratory) inoculation. The cat flea, *Ctenocephalides felis,* is associated with increased cat infectivity and with cat-to-cat transmission of *B henselae,* although it probably does not play a major role in cat-to-human *B henselae* transmission. The observation that in temperate zones CSD incidence peaks in fall and winter while flea infestation of cats primarily occurs during spring and summer argues against the role of the cat flea in human CSD pathogenesis. Felids, dogs, monkeys, and other animals may harbor *B henselae,* and some have been anecdotally associated with CSD. Trauma associated with inanimate objects (eg, thorns, splinters, fencing) probably also causes CSD, although overall, approximately 90% of CSD is cat associated. Certain ticks, noncat fleas, and even lice may harbor Bartonellae including *B henselae,* but their role in human disease is as yet undefined. Direct human-to-human spread has not been reported; however, indirect transmission of *B henselae* by red cell transfusion may be possible.

## CLINICAL MANIFESTATIONS

Typical CSD is probably the most common cause of prolonged subacute regional lymphadenitis in children. Cutaneous inoculation of *B henselae* is 90% cat-, especially kitten-associated, 50% to 75% of which is via scratch or bite. A few days to a few weeks later, often unrecognized by the patient, a 2- to 5-mm erythematous, nonpainful papule appears at the inoculation site in up to two-thirds of patients (Fig. 252-1) and persists for a few weeks; *B henselae* can be found in these lesions. When inoculation is presumably respiratory and involves mucous membranes (especially about the head and neck), inoculation lesions are absent. The hallmark of typical CSD is chronic regional lymphadenitis in a node or nodes draining the site of inoculation. Most frequently, CSD involves a solitary lymph node or a group of nodes at a single site, while only rarely will CSD manifest as generalized adenopathy. Usually tender initially and often remaining tender, these nodes appear from 1 week to 1 to 2 months after inoculation. Size may vary from 1 to 2 cm to 5 to 10 cm, and erythema of the overlying skin may occur. Suppuration occurs in 10% to 20% of cases, and drainage of pus due to breakdown of overlying skin may persist for weeks. CSD usually involves the nodes draining the upper extremity, head, neck, and groin, but any lymph node location is possible. Epitrochlear lymphadenopathy with or without axillary adenopathy is typical though not pathognomonic of CSD. Between 30% and 50% of patients will have an elevated temperature that can be accompanied by malaise, anorexia, night sweats, headache, and other nonspecific complaints, all of which are more prominent with increasing age. Resolution is slow, usually over weeks to a few months, though rarely, recovery may be prolonged, over a year or more.

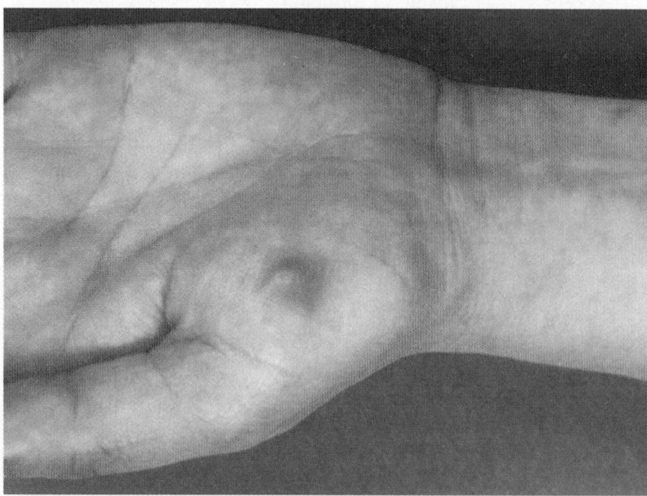

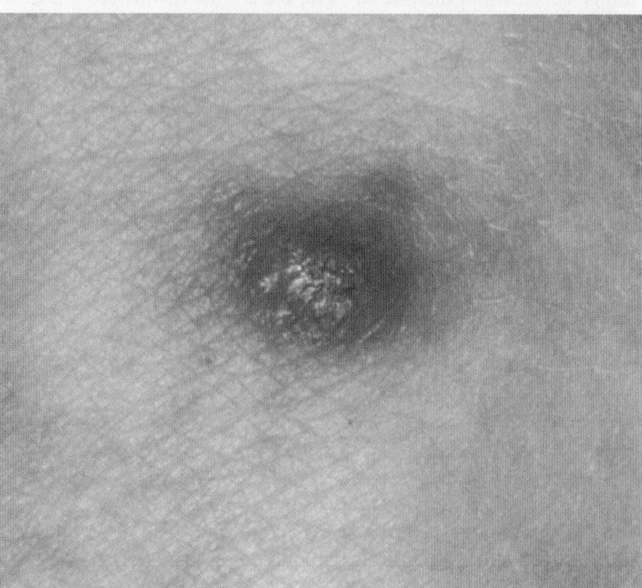

**FIGURE 252-1** Primary inoculation lesions associated with cat scratch disease.

## TYPICAL CAT SCRATCH DISEASE

The causes of regional adenopathy/adenitis with or without an inoculation lesion are numerous, with infectious etiologies leading the list. Bacterial (eg, staphylococcal, streptococcal, and other entities), viral (eg, Epstein-Barr virus or cytomegalovirus), mycobacterial (eg, nontuberculous and tuberculous), and fungal (eg, blastomycosis, histoplasmosis, and coccidioidomycosis) causes should be considered. The prolonged course of CSD lymphadenopathy, often without the stigmata of pyogenic lymphadenitis (eg, local erythema, warmth, and leukocytosis), particularly when accompanied by fever, night sweats, or weight loss, may mimic malignancy, especially lymphoma. This often is a cause of serious concern for the patient, the parents, and the treating physician. Noninfectious, nonneoplastic causes include sarcoidosis, Kawasaki disease, sinus histiocytosis with massive lymphadenopathy, congenital neck anomalies, autoimmune lymphoproliferative syndrome, histiocytic necrotizing lymphadenitis (Kikuchi disease), idiopathic facial aseptic granuloma, and drug-induced lymphadenopathy (eg, due to phenytoin). CSD rarely coexists with another pathological entity. In the few reported cases of CSD during pregnancy, neither deleterious effects nor long-term sequelae were found. One early spontaneous abortion occurred.

## COMPLICATED CAT SCRATCH DISEASE

The term *atypical CSD* is confusing and should be replaced by *extranodal CSD* or *complicated CSD*. In immune-competent children, typical CSD occurs in 85% to 90%, and complicated CSD in the remainder. Occasionally, *B henselae* disseminates to liver, spleen, eye, central nervous system (CNS), bone, and other sites. Even these manifestations are usually self-limited, and recovery without sequelae is usually the rule. The most common complicated presentation of CSD (about 50% of all atypical CSD) is Parinaud oculoglandular syndrome (Fig. 252-2), where the patient has granulomatous conjunctivitis and

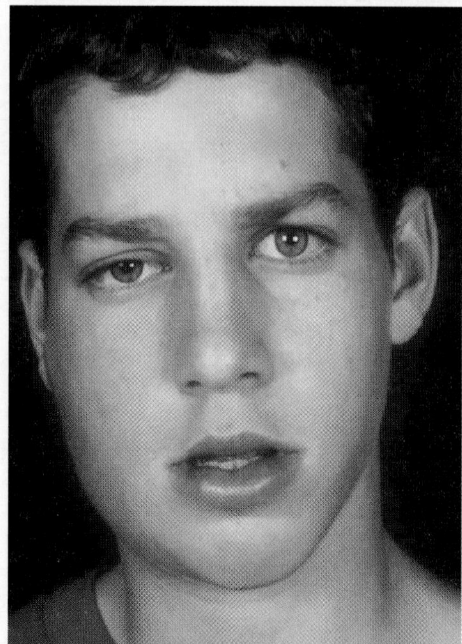

**FIGURE 252-2** Parinaud oculoglandular syndrome: This boy's right eye is partially closed due to palpebral granulomatous conjunctivitis (not shown); in addition, ipsilateral preauricular swelling due to lymphadenopathy is present.

preauricular lymphadenitis. In fact, this is actually typical CSD with conjunctival inoculation and regional adenitis. Dissemination to viscera usually involves liver or spleen, often with prolonged fever, abdominal pain, weight loss, and tender visceromegaly, sometimes abnormal hepatocellular enzymes, elevated erythrocyte sedimentation rate (ESR) or C-reactive protein (CRP), and frequently without an inoculation site or regional adenopathy. Ultrasound and computed tomography (CT) suggest microabscesses, which histologically are necrotizing granulomata of liver or spleen. CSD is a relatively common cause of FUO in children, and FUO due to CSD may occur in the context of visceral dissemination or in its absence. Eye manifestations other than conjunctivitis include neuroretinitis, papillitis, posterior uveitis, retinal vascular occlusion, optic neuritis, and focal retinochoroiditis, where most commonly the patient complains of acute, usually unilateral, visual deterioration, and occur in about 2% of CSD. Optic nerve edema with stellate macular exudates ("macular star") is seen funduscopically and can persist for months. This is associated with sequelae in some, although most recover. Neurologic complications (2–4% of CSD) include encephalopathy with or without focal or generalized seizures, transverse myelitis, Guillain-Barré syndrome, radiculitis, cerebellar ataxia, cranial nerve palsies especially of the facial nerve, and compression neuropathy (due to the enlarged lymph node's mass effect). These presentations can occur with or without typical CSD symptoms or signs. Encephalopathy, the most common neurologic complication, usually begins abruptly 1 to 4 weeks after exposure to *B henselae.* Lumbar puncture is either normal or with a mild, predominantly mononuclear pleocytosis, or mildly elevated CSF protein. Culture is negative, head CT usually is normal, and electroencephalogram is characteristically encephalopathic. Most recover within weeks to months, sequelae are rare, but CNS involvement can be fatal. CSD should be considered in any previously healthy school-aged child with new-onset status epilepticus. Other atypical manifestations of CSD consist of osteomyelitis/osteolytic granulomatous lesions including those of vertebrae and pelvis; multifocal osteomyelitis; numerous rashes including erythema nodosum, erythema multiforme, and vasculitic; deep neck space infection; arthropathy and myopathy (mostly in adults); hypercalcemia; pneumonitis; thrombocytopenic purpura; hemolytic anemia; and glomerulonephritis. *B henselae* also has been associated with Henoch-Schönlein purpura as determined in 2 small studies where the seropositivity rate for *B henselae* was found to be significantly higher than in controls. Two very important kinds of *B henselae* infection not within the scope of this chapter are bacterial endocarditis, rare in children, and infection of immunocompromised patients including vascular proliferative cutaneous and visceral lesions of bacillary angiomatosis and bacillary peliosis, with persisting or relapsing bacteremia.

## DIAGNOSIS

Maintaining a high index of suspicion and taking a detailed history, particularly that of cat contact, are important in making the correct diagnosis and thus avoiding diagnostic procedures that are often unnecessary (eg, CT scan, biopsies). Historically, diagnosis was made when a patient presented with a cat scratch or bite, a primary inoculation lesion, regional lymphadenitis and a characteristic biopsy, or sterile pus or a positive skin test with cat scratch antigen. Clinical suspicion in the appropriate epidemiologic context is still extremely important, but given the expanded spectrum of CSD, specific diagnostic tools may be required, especially when a classical history is absent. Routine laboratory tests are usually not helpful: white blood cell count, ESR, and CRP may be normal or elevated, hepatocellular enzymes may be abnormal with visceral involvement, and imaging (ultrasound, CT, magnetic resonance imaging) is also nonspecific. Culture of *B henselae* from blood or tissue is slow, cumbersome, and requires special and impractical techniques, and in the immune-competent host, negative cultures are the rule rather than the exception. Skin test (prepared from pus aspirated from affected lymph nodes of CSD patients) was deemed useful, but because it was never standardized and is potentially dangerous, its use has been discontinued, especially with current, better diagnostic tools available. Biopsy of the inoculation papule or lymph node (or deep lesions) shows a characteristic but nondiagnostic histologic picture with epithelioid granuloma and Langhans giant cells. Later, necrotizing stellate granulomata are seen, and in some nodes, microabscesses enlarge and coalesce, leading to suppuration. The inflammatory process often involves surrounding tissue (eg, the skin). When present (primarily early in the course of infection), *B henselae* may be visualized by silver staining, but a positive stain for bacteria is not specific. Immunohistochemical assays can improve specificity but are of limited availability in routine diagnostic laboratories. The most practical way to diagnose CSD is serologically. The IgG-based immunofluorescent antibody test (IFAT), such as that performed at the Centers for Disease Control and Prevention, has a sensitivity of 84% to 95% and a specificity of 94% to 98%. Results from studies performed in Europe are less satisfactory and inconsistent, perhaps due to higher background seroprevalence. Cross-reactivity with other organisms including other *Bartonella* species (eg, *B quintana*) has been reported. Enzyme immunoassay (EIA) tests are also used, but variable sensitivity is also a problem. An outer-membrane protein-based EIA has a sensitivity of 85% (when IgG and/or IgM anti-*B henselae* antibodies are positive) and a specificity of 98% and can be useful in differentiating old from acute disease. Both IFAT and EIA antibodies develop slowly; thus, seroconversion may occur only after ≥ 3 weeks of illness. Repeat serologic testing may be required to make the diagnosis. Polymerase chain reaction (PCR) of lymph node or pus aspirate, primary skin lesions, or of other tissue is a highly sensitive and specific diagnostic tool. Both broad-range and species-specific PCR assays have been developed. PCR is particularly useful when serology is negative and definitive diagnosis is urgent (eg, in those who are particularly ill, who have atypical disease or complications, whose lesions are not resolving, the immunocompromised, or when other diagnoses such as malignancy are being entertained). Fine-needle aspiration of a lymph node for PCR may suffice when the pretest probability for CSD is high. Excisional biopsy is indicated when malignancy needs to be ruled out. Particularly difficult is considering the diagnosis of CSD, particularly complicated CSD, in the absence of cat exposure or lymphadenopathy.

## TREATMENT

Few studies, mostly small, anecdotal, or retrospective, have addressed the question of therapy for CSD. In addition, in vitro susceptibility testing does not correlate with in vivo results of therapy. Possible explanations include the fact that lymph node disease may be host response driven, that most antibiotics are not bactericidal for Bartonellae, and that the intracellular location of the bacteria may be protective. A large, retrospective study showed that treating with rifampin, ciprofloxacin, gentamicin, and trimethoprim-sulfamethoxazole resulted in a shorter duration of disease when compared to no therapy or to therapy with other antimicrobials. However, it is difficult to draw conclusions from this retrospective review, especially because CSD is a self-limited disease, and cure without sequelae is the rule even without treatment. Only one small, randomized, prospective, double-blind, placebo-controlled study was performed to assess the effects of treating CSD: azithromycin reduced lymph node volume significantly during 30 days after therapy. Thereafter, there were no differences noted. Antimicrobial therapy for CSD has been reviewed critically, and some specific recommendations for therapy have been made. It is logical to conclude, due to the minimal effects of antibiotic therapy on typical CSD (a self-limited disease with a good prognosis), that many if not most nonimmunocompromised patients need not be treated. Treatment should be limited to patients with moderate to severe illness who have not begun to improve spontaneously (eg, those with severe systemic symptoms, those whose nodes are large and significantly painful). Azithromycin seems to be a reasonable choice if treatment for typical CSD is desired. Doxycycline, rifampin, ciprofloxacin, gentamicin, and trimethoprim-sulfamethoxazole may be considered as alternatives. However, despite antimicrobial treatment, CSD patients may have a prolonged course or develop lymph node suppuration or complications. Symptomatic therapy including analgesics, and locally applied warm compresses can relieve pain. Aspiration of fluctuant, suppurating nodes with a 16- to 18-gauge needle yields thick, beige, odorless, often blood-tinged pus and will relieve the associated discomfort. This may need to be repeated up to 2 to 3 times. Incision and drainage should be avoided in order to prevent sinus formation with chronic drainage. Complicated CSD (eg, hepatosplenic, bacteremic) is often treated, although no strong evidence-based recommendations can be made. Various protocols have been proposed, usually with doxycycline, rifampin, and azithromycin, alone or in combination. Rarely, a Jarisch-Herxheimer reaction occurs. Treating neuroretinitis may decrease the incidence and severity of sequelae, and a combination of doxycycline and rifampin for 4 to 6 weeks is recommended for adults, though a regimen for children younger than 8 years old has not been defined. CNS complications are often treated similarly but for shorter durations, though evidence to support this is lacking. Corticosteroids have been of benefit anecdotally, but their use should not be considered routinely. It must be emphasized that the treatment of endocarditis due to *B henselae* or of immunocompromised patients with *B henselae* infection including bacillary angiomatosis, peliosis, and bacteremia is not within the scope of this chapter.

In healthy individuals, especially in the pediatric age group, a good prognosis is the rule. Even atypical disease or complications usually resolve without sequelae. Patience is required because the infection's course often spans weeks to months. If not immunocompromised, lifelong immunity is nearly 100%, and reinfection or relapse is exceedingly rare. In the immunocompromised, infection may be life threatening, and immunity may not develop.

## PREVENTION

People play no role in transmitting infection to other people, and therefore, isolation of a CSD patient is unnecessary. Avoiding cats, especially kittens, is an excellent way to prevent CSD but is not always practical. Preventing flea infestation may indirectly diminish a cat's infectivity and theoretically also may prevent cat-to-human infection. Declawing may be partially protective. Vaccination of cats to prevent *B henselae* infection is not available. Because intrafamilial clustering is rare, removal of the cat from the household should not be necessary. When immunocompromised patients or patients with valvular heart disease are involved, older, less potentially infective cats (> 1 year old) might make safer pets than would kittens.

## SUGGESTED READINGS


Chang CC, Lee CJ, Ou LS, Wang CJ, Huang YC. Disseminated cat-scratch disease: case report and review of the literature. *Paediatr Int Child Health*. 2016;36:232-234.

Chi SL, Stinnett S, Eggenberger E, et al. Clinical characteristics in 53 patients with cat scratch optic neuropathy. *Ophthalmology*. 2012; 119:183-187.

Gandhi TN, Slater LN, Welch DF, Koehler JR. *Bartonella*, including cat-scratch disease. In: Bennet JE, Dolin R, Blaser MJ, eds. *Principles and Practice of Infectious Diseases*. 8th ed. Philadelphia, PA: Elsevier Saunders; 2015:2649-2663.

Giladi M, Ephros M, Welch DF. *Bartonella* infections, including cat-scratch disease. In: Scheld WM, Whitley RJ, Marra CM, eds. *Infections of the Central Nervous System*. 4th ed. Philadelphia, PA: Wolters Kluwer Health; 2014:434-443.

Klotz SA, Ianas V, Elliott SP. Cat-scratch disease. *Am Fam Physician*. 2011;83;152-155.

Nelson CA, Saha S, Mead PS. Cat-scratch disease in the United States, 2005-2013. *Emerg Infect Dis*. 2016;22:1741-1746.

Rostad CA, McElroy AK, Hilinski JA, et al. *Bartonella henselae*-mediated disease in solid organ transplant recipients: two pediatric cases and review of the literature. *Transpl Infect Dis*. 2012;14: e71-e81.


# 253 Chancroid (*Haemophilus ducreyi*)

Melissa Del Castillo

## INTRODUCTION

Chancroid is a sexually transmitted disease (STD) caused by the organism *Haemophilus ducreyi*. It is characterized by painful genital ulcers and tender inguinal adenopathy that may suppurate. Also known as "soft chancre," chancroid is 1 of the 3 major causes of genital ulcer disease (GUD) among young sexually active patients in the United States; the other major causes are genital herpes and syphilis.

## PATHOGENESIS AND EPIDEMIOLOGY

*H ducreyi* invades the skin after disruption of the epithelial surface following trauma. An infecting dose of as few as 30 colony-forming units is thought to be able to produce papules in the skin. Once a papule appears, the disease progresses to a pustule in the majority of patients, although as many as 30% of those infected may have spontaneous resolution of their pustule. Although the pathogenesis of this organism has been well studied, additional studies are required to clearly define the virulence factors.

The prevalence of chancroid is low in the United States. The reason for this low prevalence may be due to underdiagnosis. Most clinicians do not have clinical experience with chancroid and thus do not consider it in the differential diagnosis. Additionally, most laboratories do not have the capability of isolating *H ducreyi*. Chancroid cases peaked to a high of 5001 in the United States in 1988 and have steadily declined, with the lowest number (6 cases) in 2014, reported by the states of California, Texas, and Massachusetts. In comparison, there were 19,999 cases of primary and secondary syphilis reported in 2014.

Some data suggest that the disappearance of chancroid in the United States may be due to lack of testing and underreporting. In a survey of 405 STD clinics in 1996, only 32 (8%) tested patients for chancroid. Surveys in California from 1996 to 2003 found that less than 300 tests for chancroid were done, accounting for less than 0.1% of all tests done for STDs. However, in genital ulcer studies during the late 1990s where testing for *H ducreyi* was done, chancroid was frequently found. In a study in Brooklyn, New York, *H ducreyi* was identified in 27 (42%) of 65 cases in which a microbiologic diagnosis was established. Coinfection with syphilis was common. In New Orleans, Louisiana, similar findings were reported in 299 men with non-syphilitic GUD; 39% had *H ducreyi*, 19% had herpes simplex virus (HSV), and the culture was negative in 41%. Using the sensitive polymerase chain reaction (PCR), it appears that chancroid may be even more common than previously thought. In a PCR study in Jackson, Mississippi, in 1995, 59% of genital ulcer cases were due to *H ducreyi*. In 1998, cases of chancroid identified by PCR in Memphis and Chicago accounted for 12% to 20% of genital ulcers. In 10 patients with chancroid in Memphis, none were identified clinically. Thus, the burden of chancroid in the United States is unknown.

Chancroid was an extremely common cause of GUD in sub-Saharan Africa and in many parts of southeast Asia and Latin America. Definitive epidemiologic data are not generally available in these resource-poor countries because diagnosing chancroid is extremely problematic. However, a recent meta-analysis of available data seems to indicate that the rates of GUD due to *H ducreyi* have steadily declined around the world since 2000. This is largely due to the widespread adoption of syndromic management of GUD with antimicrobial drugs effective against syphilis and chancroid, without microbiologic confirmation. While rates of sexually transmitted *H ducreyi* appear to have declined worldwide, it is interesting to note that this bacterium has recently been identified as the causative agent of nongenital cutaneous ulcers in children in tropical regions (proportions range from 9% to 60% from 6 studies in 4 countries). Chancroid should be considered in high-risk groups such as prostitutes, drug users, and travelers to a part of the world where chancroid is endemic. As many as 10% of patients with chancroid are coinfected with syphilis or HSV.

## CLINICAL MANIFESTATIONS

The incubation period of chancroid is 3 to 10 days. The first lesion is generally a small papule that is surrounded by erythema. Within 2 to 3 days, a pustule forms that ruptures and leaves a circumscribed ulcer with ragged, undermined edges without induration (Fig. 253-1). The base of the ulcer is painful, is erythematous with a granular appearance, and usually is covered with a gray or yellow purulent exudate that bleeds when scraped. A typical chancroid ulcer is about 1 to 2 cm in diameter, but the size is variable, especially in HIV-infected patients. Often, infected persons have more than 1 ulcer. In men, the most common sites for the ulcers are on the distal prepuce, the mucosal surface of the prepuce on the frenulum, or in the coronal sulcus. In women, the majority of lesions are at the entrance to the vagina, the labia, or perianal areas. With vaginal or cervical lesions, there may be no symptoms. Unilateral painful tender inguinal adenopathy is present in as many as 50% of patients. Involved lymph nodes may become fluctuant to form painful buboes, and if untreated, these may rupture, forming inguinal ulcers. Adenopathy is less common in women. Most buboes arise 1 to 2 weeks after the appearance of the primary ulcer. As with other STDs, coinfection with HIV may result in atypical manifestations of chancroid. There may be numerous lesions, extragenital involvement, and delays in resolution after treatment.

The differential diagnosis of genital ulcer disease in sexually active persons is broad and is greatly influenced by the geographic location in which the infection was acquired. Worldwide, the main infectious causes of GUD are HSV (genital herpes), *Treponema pallidum* (syphilis), *H ducreyi* (chancroid), *Chlamydia trachomatis* (lymphogranuloma venereum), and *Klebsiella granulomatis,* formerly known as *Calymmatobacterium granulomatis* (donovanosis or granuloma inguinale). In the United States, most cases are due to HSV, followed by syphilis and chancroid. Noninfectious causes include drug eruptions and Behçet disease. In the United States, the combination of a painful ulcer with tender inguinal adenopathy is suggestive of chancroid and is almost pathognomonic when accompanied by suppurative inguinal adenopathy. However, patients with *H ducreyi* infection may have ulcers that can be confused with other causes of GUD such as HSV or syphilis; as many as 10% with chancroid may be coinfected with *T pallidum* or HSV.

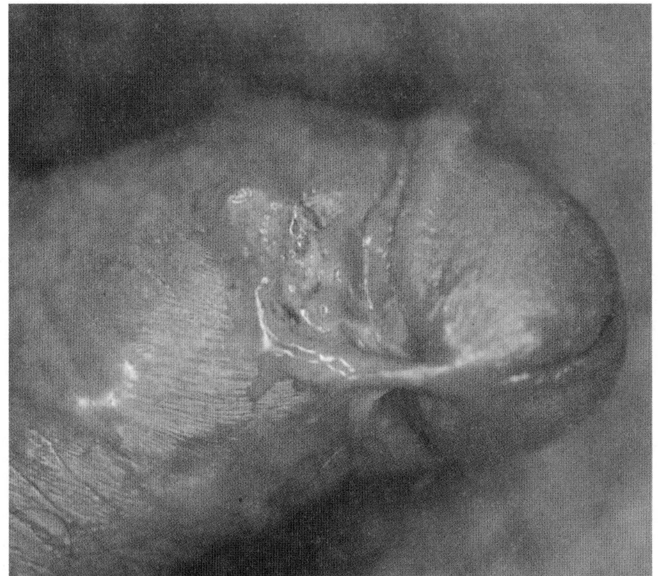

**FIGURE 253-1** Chancroid of the penis. Note the ragged edges of a soft ulcer. (Reproduced with permission from Goldsmith LA, Katz SI, Gilchrest BA et al: *Fitzpatrick's Dermatology in General Medicine*. 8th ed. New York: McGraw-Hill Companies; 2012.)

## DIAGNOSIS

Diagnosis of chancroid on clinical grounds alone is difficult because the presentation is often not classic, and many clinicians have little experience with the disease. Definitive diagnosis requires isolation of the organism from a genital ulcer or involved lymph nodes. However, the organism is fastidious and is difficult to isolate. For culture, a swab should be used to obtain material from the purulent base of an ulcer (undermined edge after removing superficial pus) and should be plated directly onto culture medium. The material should be cultured on special media (GC agar base containing 1–2% hemoglobin, 5% fetal bovine serum, and 3 μg/mL of vancomycin) that is not widely available. Sensitivity of culture is approximately 75% compared to PCR. Gram stain of purulent material may be misleading because most genital ulcers are polymicrobial; therefore, it is not recommended as a diagnostic test.

Given the low sensitivity of culture, alternative non–culture-based diagnostic tests have been evaluated. Serologic assays lack sensitivity during the acute infection and are not available commercially. Most promising are PCR-based techniques. These assays have high sensitivity and identify patients with chancroid, from whom bacterial cultures for *H ducreyi* are negative. Multiplex PCR assays that can simultaneously amplify and subsequently detect DNA from *H ducreyi, T pallidum,* and HSV from genital ulcer specimens are undergoing field trials and show promise. There is currently no FDA-approved PCR test for *H ducreyi* in the United States. However, some commercial laboratories have PCRs for *H ducreyi.* Even if chancroid is diagnosed definitively, it is recommended that patients also be tested for HIV and syphilis, and if these initial tests are negative, retesting for both syphilis and HIV should be done 3 months later.

The Centers for Disease Control and Prevention (CDC) criteria make a definite diagnosis of chancroid only with isolation of *H ducreyi* from a lesion. A probable diagnosis is made if there are clinical findings compatible with the diagnosis (painful genital ulcer and tender, suppurative, inguinal adenopathy) with a negative dark-field microscopic examination for *T pallidum,* a negative serologic test for syphilis performed at least 7 days after onset of ulcers, and a negative culture or PCR for HSV. Even with careful evaluation, the sensitivity and specificity of using clinical criteria for diagnosing chancroid are limited. Because there is a lack of rapid and reliable diagnostic tests and typically treatment consists of single-dose therapy, treatment decisions for chancroid are generally based on a clinical diagnosis.

## TREATMENT

Successful antimicrobial treatment of genital ulcers caused by *H ducreyi* cures infection, resolves clinical symptoms, and prevents transmission to others. However, in cases of extensive ulcerative disease, scarring may result despite successful antimicrobial therapy. A number of agents have been used and are recommended for the treatment of chancroid including erythromycin, ciprofloxacin, ceftriaxone, and azithromycin. The CDC currently recommends 1 of 4 antibiotic regimens for treatment of chancroid: azithromycin in a single dose; ceftriaxone in a single dose; ciprofloxacin 500 mg for 3 days; or erythromycin base for 7 days.

All 4 regimens are effective for treatment of chancroid in patients with HIV infection. Ciprofloxacin presents a possible risk to the fetus during pregnancy, with a potential for toxicity during breastfeeding, so other regimens are preferred. A successful response to therapy is usually evident within 48 to 72 hours, as evidenced by decreased ulcer tenderness and pain. Complete healing of ulcers may take up to 28 days but is often achieved in 7 to 14 days. Clinical improvement of ulcerative disease without lymphadenitis usually occurs shortly after treatment is initiated. Relief of pain is noted by most patients within 48 hours, and objective improvement in the ulcers is usually evident within 72 hours. Patients should be reexamined 3 to 7 days after beginning therapy. If no clinical improvement is evident after 7 days, the diagnosis may be incorrect or the patient could be coinfected with syphilis, HIV, or HSV. Other considerations include poor adherence with medications or that the organism may be resistant to the regimen prescribed. Globally, *H ducreyi* isolates with resistance to either ciprofloxacin or erythromycin have been reported.

Prior to effective antimicrobial therapy, failure to aspirate fluctuant buboes was associated with the development of draining fistulas or secondary ulcers at the site of the ruptured bubo. Even since the availability of antimicrobial agents for chancroid, healing of fluctuant adenopathy has been shown to be slower than that of the ulcers. Needle aspiration through adjacent intact skin or incision and drainage may be necessary for relief of pain in some cases.

Response may be delayed in some patients. In uncircumcised men, healing is slower with ulcers under the foreskin. Patients with HIV infection must be closely monitored, as they may require longer courses of treatment than the standard regimens outlined above. Treatment failures have been observed with several of these regimens, and there is some suggestion that those individuals who are most immunosuppressed are at the greatest risk for failure of standard regimens. The erythromycin 7-day regimen and azithromycin 1 g in a single dose are preferred by some experts for HIV-infected patients, provided follow-up for these patients can be ensured.

## PREVENTION

To prevent further spread of *H ducreyi* disease, it is critical to identify all sexual contacts of infected individuals. The CDC recommends that all persons who have had sexual contact with a patient with proven *H ducreyi* infection within the 10 days before onset of the patient's symptoms should be examined and treated. The examination and treatment of contacts should be administered even in the absence of symptoms. Standard precautions are recommended. Regular condom use may decrease transmission.

## SUGGESTED READINGS


Gonzalez-Beiras C, Marks M, Chen C, et al. Epidemiology of *Haemophilus ducreyi* infections. *Emerg Infect Dis.* 2016;22:1-8.

Lewis DA. Epidemiology, clinical features, diagnosis and treatment of *Haemophilus ducreyi*: a disappearing pathogen? *Expert Rev Anti Infect Ther.* 2014;12:687-696.

Lewis DA, Mitjà O. *Haemophilus ducreyi*: from sexually transmitted infection to skin ulcer pathogen. *Curr Opin Infect Dis.* 2016;29:52-57.

Marks M, Chi K, Pillay A, et al. *Haemophilus ducreyi* associated with skin ulcers among children, Solomon Islands. *Emerg Infect Dis.* 2014;20:1705-1707.

Mitja O, Lukehart S, Pokowas G, et al. *Haemophilus ducreyi* as a cause of skin ulcers in children from a yaws-endemic area of Papua New Guinea: a prospective cohort study. *Lancet Glob Health.* 2014;2:e235-e241.

Workowski KA, Bolan GA. Sexually transmitted disease treatment guidelines, 2015. *MMWR Recomm Rep.* 2015;64:26-27.


# 254 Chlamydia

Ankoor Y. Shah and Bernhard L. Wiedermann

## INTRODUCTION

Chlamydiae are nonmotile, gram-negative, obligate intracellular bacteria. These organisms cannot produce energy and thus survive by acting as a parasite using the energy mechanics of their infected host; they all have biphasic cycles of replication. The elementary body that represents the "infectious" particle enters the host cell and lives within the host's cytoplasmic inclusion particles. The organism then begins its secondary vegetative state known as the reticulate body and replicates by binary fission. Each inclusion body begins to form multiple progeny that will be extruded as new infectious elementary bodies to begin the cycle once again.

**TABLE 254-1 CHLAMYDIAL INFECTIONS IN HUMANS**

| Species | Serovars | Clinical Manifestations |
|---|---|---|
| *C trachomatis* | A, B, C | Trachoma |
| | D–K | Urethritis, epididymitis, cervicitis, pelvic inflammatory disease, inclusion conjunctivitis, infantile pneumonia |
| | L1–L3 | Lymphogranuloma venereum |
| *C psittaci* | | Psittacosis, ornithosis |
| *C pneumoniae* | | Pharyngitis, cough, pneumonia |

Some controversy exists as to whether chlamydiae should be split into 2 genera; this discussion will use the more commonly used nomenclature for the 3 recognized species that cause human disease: *Chlamydophila psittaci, Chlamydophila pneumoniae,* and *Chlamydia trachomatis* (Table 254-1). *C psittaci* is responsible for psittacosis (ornithosis). *C pneumoniae* causes pneumonia, pharyngitis, and bronchitis. *C trachomatis* has at least 15 different serotypes, known as serovars, that are associated with a spectrum of diseases. Serovars A to C are associated with trachoma, D to K with genital infections, and L1 to L3 with lymphogranuloma venereum. The most common infections of *C trachomatis* are those of the genital tract, which present as urethritis and epididymitis in the male and cervicitis and salpingitis in the female. Neonates can present with conjunctivitis and pneumonia acquired by passage through an infected mother's genital tract.

## *CHLAMYDOPHILA PSITTACI*

*C psittaci* causes psittacosis, also known as ornithosis. Psittacosis is contracted by humans from infected birds and their contaminated droppings. All birds, including pet birds (parrots, parakeets, macaws, and cockatiels) and poultry (turkeys, ducks, chickens, and other fowl), are most frequently involved in transmission to humans; however, mammals such as sheep, cattle, goats, and cats have also been shown to transmit infection to humans. The birds show a spectrum of disease that ranges from no evidence of illness to the severely ill. Birds transmit the disease to humans by the respiratory route from feces, fecal dust, or secretions of infected animals. The incidence among poultry workers, pet shop workers, and exotic bird importers can be high. Since 1996, the US Centers for Disease Control and Prevention (CDC) reports around 50 cases a year. This is likely an underestimate because *C psittaci* is difficult to diagnose and may not be considered in a differential diagnosis. Person-to-person transmission also is possible, and healthcare personnel can acquire the disease from patients. Children infrequently acquire the disease, perhaps because they are less likely to be exposed to infected animals.

### CLINICAL MANIFESTATIONS

*C psittaci* should be included in the differential diagnosis for atypical pneumonia. It is difficult to distinguish between *C psittaci* pneumonia and other causes of atypical pneumonia such as *Legionella pneumophila, Mycoplasma pneumoniae,* or *Coxiella burnetii.* The onset of symptoms of psittacosis typically present 5 to 14 days after exposure. Clinically, 2 main forms of the infection occur. The more common form presents with symptoms of fever, chills, headache, and pneumonia; less commonly, the illness may present as a severe influenza-like illness. The patient's temperature rises steadily, and there may be complaints of headache, malaise, and nausea. Mental confusion may be observed. If pneumonia is present, as it is in most patients, the cough is prominent and the sputum may be blood-streaked. Delay in diagnosis and treatment can lead to septic shock, multiorgan failure, pancreatitis, and myocarditis, which are all severe complications of the disease. *C psittaci* can be associated with significant morbidity and mortality during pregnancy in mothers exposed to infected sheep. Radiologically, the appearance is that of an extensive interstitial pneumonia, which can be confused with other atypical pneumonia etiologies. If the infection is left untreated, the disease can last several weeks and present as a nonremitting chronic cough. There is an important association between *C psittaci* and an extranodal non-Hodgkin lymphoma termed ocular adnexal mucosa-associated lymphoid tissue (MALT) lymphoma. The incidence of psittacosis has decreased since the implementation of importation controls of parrots and other exotic birds into the United States. Confirmed cases of psittacosis should be reported to the local or state health department.

### DIAGNOSIS

A diagnosis of psittacosis can be confirmed by 1 of 3 confirmatory laboratory studies combined with a history of potential exposure and a clinical history suggestive of the illness. The first laboratory method is culture from respiratory secretions yielding positive growth of *C psittaci.* The second method is using complement fixation (CF) or microimmunofluorescence (MIF) techniques to demonstrate a 4-fold or greater increase between paired acute- and convalescent-phase serum specimens collected 2 weeks apart. Antimicrobial treatment can suppress the antibody response, leading to a need of a third serum sample 4 to 6 weeks later in order to confirm the diagnosis. The third method is detection of immunoglobulin (Ig) M antibody against *C psittaci* by MIF. Elevated CF titers also may result from *C pneumoniae* and *C trachomatis* infections; therefore, MIF assays should be used to distinguish *C psittaci* infection from infection with other chlamydial species.

### TREATMENT

The treatment of choice for *C psittaci* infection is tetracycline or doxycycline given orally. Clinical improvement occurs in 48 to 72 hours, and treatment should continue for a minimum of 10 days and at least 10 to 14 days after the fever resolves to avoid relapse. In patients with severe infection, intravenous doxycycline will be needed. Erythromycin or azithromycin is recommended for children less than 8 years of age and for pregnant women. Standard precautions are appropriate for infection control.

## CHLAMYDOPHILA PNEUMONIAE

*C pneumoniae* is a common respiratory pathogen worldwide. Over the past 2 decades, with improvements in diagnostics and epidemiologic studies, *C pneumoniae* has been found to be a common and important cause of community-acquired pneumonia in children and adults. It is transmitted by aerosolized respiratory secretions from person-to-person contact. The average incubation period is 21 days.

In the United States, about 50% of adults have evidence of past infection with *C pneumoniae* by age 20. Hospital-based studies have shown that *C pneumoniae* is responsible for 2% to 10% of community-acquired pneumonia in adults. In children, studies using the MIF method show increasing *C pneumoniae* antibody prevalence rates beginning in school-age children, which reach 30% to 45% in adolescents. Small epidemics have also been described in colleges and among military recruits.

### CLINICAL MANIFESTATIONS

*C pneumoniae* can cause upper and lower respiratory tract infections; the most common clinical manifestations of *C pneumoniae* include pneumonia and bronchitis. In studies examining the etiology of pediatric community-acquired pneumonia worldwide, *C pneumoniae* was found in 3% to 14% of cases. In addition to pneumonia, acute otitis media, rhinitis, sinusitis, and pharyngitis also can be seen.

The most common symptoms include cough, rhinitis, fever, and sore throat, followed by headache, dyspnea, and earache. Clinical findings may resemble influenza. The initial rhinitis and pharyngitis are followed by the development of a chronic cough with bronchitis or pneumonia that can last for several weeks. In addition to a prominent cough, the patient may have rales, rhonchi, or wheezing. A radiograph of the chest typically shows patchy infiltrates. The overall nature of this infection is typically nonspecific and resembles other etiologic agents of atypical pneumonia such as *Legionella* or *Mycoplasma pneumoniae* (see Chapters 259 and 268).

### DIAGNOSIS

*C pneumoniae* may be identified by culture, polymerase chain reaction (PCR), antigen detection, and serologic testing; however, no reliable commercial diagnostic tests have been approved by the US Food and Drug Administration for clinical use. In the clinical setting, serology is the testing of choice. The MIF antibody test is the most sensitive and specific serologic test for acute infection. IgM antibodies appear within 2 to 3 weeks after onset of illness followed by IgG antibodies, which peak 6 to 8 weeks after onset. A confirmatory test will show an IgM titer of 1:16 or greater or a 4-fold rise in IgG titer when comparing acute to convalescent titers.

Because *C pneumoniae* is a fastidious and slow-growing organism, culture is not useful clinically. PCR has been used to detect *C pneumoniae* in the nasopharynx, sputum, blood, or tissue, but it is mainly used in research settings and is not readily available clinically. A positive PCR may reflect asymptomatic shedding of *C pneumoniae* and may not actually identify the cause of the patient's illness.

### TREATMENT

Macrolides (erythromycin, azithromycin, and clarithromycin) and doxycycline are recommended as first-line treatment options. For tetracyclines, it is important to note the association to permanent teeth staining in children under 8 years of age, but it is uncertain whether this property applies to doxycycline. Newer fluoroquinolones such as levofloxacin and moxifloxacin are alternatives. Treatment is for 10 to 14 days, except for azithromycin, which is given for 5 days. Standard precautions are appropriate for infection control.

## CHLAMYDIA TRACHOMATIS

*C trachomatis* is the leading bacterial pathogen of sexually transmitted infections (see Chapter 228) worldwide. The World Health Organization (WHO) estimated that 10.1 million new cases of *C trachomatis* infections occurred globally. In the United States in 2014, there were 1,441,789 chlamydia diagnoses reported to the CDC, with 63% in those aged 15 to 24 years. However, it is estimated that there are as many as 2.8 million new cases of *C trachomatis* infection each year because the majority of cases go undiagnosed. Most infected men and women are asymptomatic and are diagnosed from either routine screening or as a result of a known infected partner. Men usually do not have long-term complications from infection but are important in continued transmission as carriers. Women are at greater risk for complications because most infections are initially asymptomatic and unrecognized. If the infection is not diagnosed and treated, severe complications including pelvic inflammatory disease (PID), ectopic pregnancy, and infertility can occur. Therefore, *C trachomatis* infections present an enormous public health problem throughout the world. The highest age-specific rates of chlamydia were in females 20 to 24 years of age (3651 cases per 100,000 females), followed by females 15 to 19 years of age (2941 cases per 100,000 females). These higher rates compared to men reflect increased detection from higher rates of screening in women. Given the high prevalence of chlamydia in women 15 to 24 years of age, the CDC recommends annual chlamydia screening for all sexually active women who are younger than 26 years of age (Fig. 254-1). It is important for clinicians to have a high suspicion for sexual abuse when children present with a *C trachomatis* infection.

### CLINICAL MANIFESTATIONS

#### Nongonococcal Urethritis

Nongonococcal urethritis in the male is a common sexually transmitted disease caused by *C trachomatis* in 15% to 55% of cases. The presumptive diagnosis is made by examining the urethral discharge and excluding gonorrhea by smear and culture; or by rapid tests using ligase or nucleic acid amplification technique (PCR) testing of urine for *C trachomatis.* The definitive diagnosis is made by culturing chlamydia from a urethral specimen.

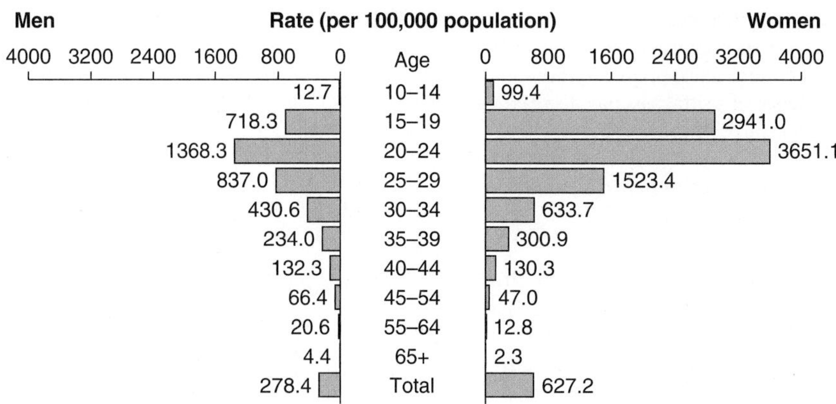


**FIGURE 254-1** Chlamydia rates of reported cases by age and sex, United States, 2014. (Reproduced with permission from Centers for Disease Control and Prevention.)

The treatment of choice for chlamydial urethritis is azithromycin in a single dose or doxycycline for 7 days. Erythromycin, ofloxacin, and levofloxacin are alternative drugs. Successful treatment requires that the sexual partners of the patient be treated as well. In one study of a closed population of adolescents receiving observed treatment for urogenital *C trachomatis* infection, the efficacy of azithromycin against doxycycline was 97% versus 100%.

#### Epididymitis

Epididymitis, an important complication of sexually transmitted urethritis in young men, may be caused by *Neisseria gonorrhoeae* or *Chlamydia trachomatis* and is treated with a 10-day course of oral doxycycline and a single dose of ceftriaxone. A 10-day course of ofloxacin or levofloxacin, in conjunction with ceftriaxone, is recommended when concern for enteric pathogens is possible, such as for men practicing insertive anal sex.

#### Female Genital Tract Infections

In most women, chlamydial infections are asymptomatic, but women with *C trachomatis* can present with endocervical erosions, a mucopurulent cervical exudate, or urethritis. In addition, chlamydial infection is a common cause of PID in sexually active adolescents and women. Diagnosis depends on demonstration of *C trachomatis* in a cervical specimen either by culture or the rapid direct slide immunofluorescence method using monoclonal antibodies. Nucleic acid amplification tests (NAATs) are widely available and are able to detect small amounts of chlamydial nucleic acid in urine or in a urethral or endocervical swab. Treatment for uncomplicated female genital tract infections in children over 8 years of age and over 45 kg includes doxycycline for 7 days or azithromycin given orally in a single dose, whereas erythromycin for 14 days is used for children less than 45 kg. Azithromycin, erythromycin, or amoxicillin is recommended for treatment in pregnant women. Sexual partners also must be treated to prevent reinfection.

As with other inflammatory sexually transmitted infections, chlamydia infection can facilitate the transmission of HIV infection. In addition, pregnant women infected with chlamydia can pass the infection to their infants during delivery, potentially resulting in neonatal ophthalmia and pneumonia.

#### Lymphogranuloma Venereum

Lymphogranuloma venereum (LGV) is a sexually transmitted chlamydial disease caused by serovars L1 to L3. The incidence of this disease has declined in the United States, but it is still quite prevalent in tropical and subtropical areas. Tender, unilateral inguinal or femoral lymphadenopathy is the most common clinical manifestation of LGV among heterosexual men. Women and homosexually active men may have proctocolitis or involvement of perirectal or perianal lymphatic tissues resulting in fistulas and strictures. The disease is rare in children and infrequently seen in adolescents.

LGV can manifest as acute or chronic disease because it is a disease of the lymphatic tissue. First, there is a primary lesion, which is transient and clinically mild, usually appears as a papule or a shallow ulcer on the penis or vaginal wall, and generally heals without scar formation. Systemic manifestations can include fever, chills, and anorexia. In the secondary stage, occurring 2 to 6 weeks after the primary lesion, there is pronounced lymphadenitis or lymphadenopathy in the inguinal area (Fig. 254-2). The nodes are large and often fluctuant, forming buboes. This stage of disease is found predominantly in males. In the tertiary stage, which is not necessarily preceded by lymphadenopathy, there is a chronic inflammatory response with fibrosis, which can result as strictures in the anal, rectal, and vaginal areas. The diagnosis is made on clinical suspicion, epidemiologic correlation, and exclusion of other possible diagnoses. The diagnosis can be supported but not confirmed by CF (titers > 1:64) or MIF (titers > 1:256) tests, using the specific antigens. The treatment of choice is doxycycline for 21 days. For children less than 8 years of age, erythromycin base for 21 days is recommended.

#### Perinatal Infections

*C trachomatis* can be transmitted to newborns and can cause purulent conjunctivitis and pneumonia. Notably, 50% to 75% of infants born to infected mothers become infected at one or more sites including the conjunctiva, nasopharynx, vagina, and rectum. The most frequent site

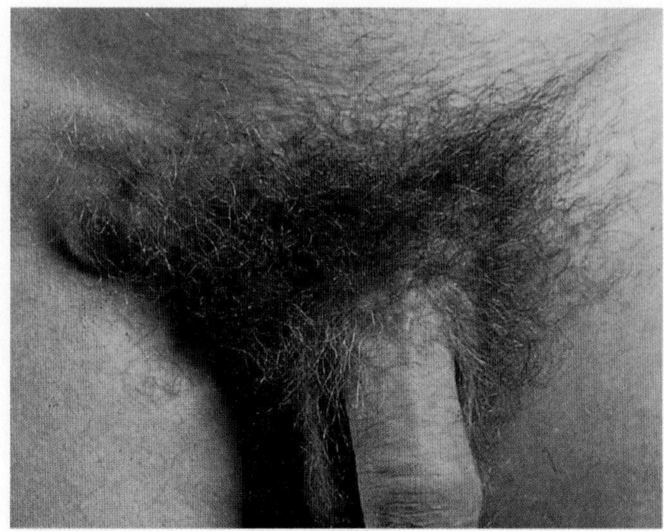

**FIGURE 254-2** Lymphogranuloma venereum (LGV): striking tender lymphadenopathy occurring at the femoral and inguinal lymph nodes, separated by a groove made by Poupart's ligament. This "sign-of-the-groove" is not considered specific for LGV; for example, lymphomas may present with this sign. (Reproduced with permission from Fauci AS, Braunwald E, Kasper DL, et al: *Harrison's Principles of Internal Medicine*, 17th ed. New York: McGraw-Hill; 2008.)

of perinatally acquired chlamydia infection in neonates is the nasopharynx with rates as high as 70% in exposed infants. Furthermore, in those with nasopharyngeal infection, chlamydia pneumonia develops in 30% of infants. However, prophylactic therapy for infants born to mothers with untreated chlamydial infection is not recommended due to lack of efficacy data.

#### Newborn Conjunctivitis

Acute purulent chlamydial conjunctivitis in the newborn has an incubation period from 5 to 12 days. There is a watery discharge from the eyes that becomes progressively more purulent, with swelling of the eyelids. Left untreated, lymphoid follicles and a membranous conjunctivitis can develop and persist for weeks or months. The conjunctivitis should be distinguished from other pyogenic bacterial infections (*N gonorrhoeae* and *Staphylococcus aureus*) and from chemical conjunctivitis resulting from silver nitrate prophylaxis. *N gonorrhoeae* conjunctivitis typically occurs in the first 2 to 5 days after birth, whereas chlamydia conjunctivitis occurs later, but it may be difficult to distinguish between the two clinically.

Conjunctival cultures on blood and chocolate agar media will identify bacterial pathogens. Examination of Giemsa-stained conjunctival scrapings for inclusion bodies of *C trachomatis* may be helpful. Because chlamydia are obligate intracellular agents, the conjunctivae must be scraped rather than swabbed to obtain an adequate specimen. The infection also can be diagnosed by culture, immunofluorescence, or enzyme-linked immunosorbent assay (ELISA). NAATs currently are not approved as a diagnostic tool for chlamydial conjunctivitis.

Optimal management is oral erythromycin 50 mg/kg/d in 4 divided doses daily for 14 days. Because treatment is not 100% effective, a second course may be needed. It is important to note the association between erythromycin and infantile hypertrophic pyloric stenosis, which can be seen in infants less than 6 weeks of age.

Topical treatment of neonatal conjunctivitis is not recommended because local eye treatment does not prevent or clear nasopharyngeal carriage and thus results in further risk of developing pneumonia or repeated episodes of conjunctivitis.

Similarly, attempts to provide prophylaxis through erythromycin or tetracycline regimens administered topically to the eyes shortly after delivery have not been highly effective because these regimens do not eliminate nasopharyngeal colonization and further increase the risk for pneumonia. Prevention can be achieved only by identifying and treating pregnant women prior to delivery.

#### Pneumonia of Infancy

*C trachomatis* pneumonia usually occurs during an infant's first 4 months of life. Chlamydial pneumonia is seen in 30% of infants with nasopharyngeal infection. The classic symptoms of chlamydial pneumonia of infancy include a staccato cough that worsens over time; nasal obstruction; and a respiratory exam showing tachypnea or rales, but no wheezing. Fever usually is absent. The infant may appear mildly to moderately ill. On chest radiologic imaging, hyperinflation with bilateral interstitial infiltrates is the classic finding. The recommended treatment is azithromycin for 3 days or erythromycin for 14 days. The diagnosis of chlamydial pneumonia (or conjunctivitis) in a neonate is clear evidence of maternal infection, and thus, the mother and her partner should be treated.

#### Trachoma

Trachoma is responsible for about 3% of blindness worldwide, with a prevalence of 1.3 million people worldwide blind from trachoma; 84 million people have active trachoma infection. Trachoma is caused by *C trachomatis* serovars A, B, and C, which spread through contact with eye discharge from the infected person (on towels, handkerchiefs, fingers, etc.) and through transmission by eye-seeking flies. It is associated with poverty and unsanitary living conditions. In hyperendemic areas, active disease is most common in preschool children, with prevalence rates as high as 60% to 90%.

Active trachoma starts as the presence of follicles on the tarsal conjunctiva. The follicles heal with necrosis and cause severe conjunctival scarring. This in turn produces lacrimal stenosis, lid distortion, and entropion and trichiasis. The chronic keratoconjunctivitis then progresses to severe scarring of the cornea and finally to blindness. The end result occurs after many years of active disease. The WHO developed a grading system including at least 2 of the following 4 criteria to diagnose trachoma: lymphoid follicles on the upper tarsal conjunctiva, typical conjunctival scarring, vascular pannus, and limbal follicles.

The diagnosis of trachoma is usually clinical but can be confirmed by examining conjunctival scrapings with a Giemsa stain or immunofluorescence demonstrating the infective particles. Chlamydia can also be cultured. Serologic tests are not very helpful, but they are important epidemiologic tools to assess prevalence.

The WHO recommends utilizing 4 prevention and treatment methods: *s*urgery for trichiasis, *a*ntibiotics, *f*ace washing, and *e*nvironmental improvement (SAFE). Antibiotic treatment is azithromycin as a single oral dose, as well as treating all household contacts. Mass antibiotic treatment with azithromycin once or twice a year can be effective to treat large populations in areas of high endemicity.

## SUGGESTED READINGS


American Academy of Pediatrics. Chlamydial infections. In: Kimberlin DW, Brady MT, Jackson MA, Long SS, eds. *Red Book: 2015 Report of the Committee on Infectious Diseases*. 30th ed. Elk Grove Village, IL: American Academy of Pediatrics; 2015:284-294.

Geisler WM. Diagnosis and management of uncomplicated *Chlamydia trachomatis* infections in adolescents and adults: summary of evidence reviewed for 2015 Centers for Disease Control and Prevention sexually transmitted disease guidelines. *Clin Infect Dis*. 2015;61:S774-S784.

Geisler WM, Uniyal A, Lee JY, et al. Azithromycin versus doxycycline for urogenital *Chlamydia trachomatis* infection. *N Engl J Med*. 2015;373:2512-2521.

Newman L, Rowley J, Vander Hoorn S, et al. Global estimates of the prevalence and incidence of four curable sexually transmitted infections in 2012 based upon systematic review and global reporting. *PLoS One*. 2015;10:e0143304.

Torrone E, Papp J, Weinstock H; Centers for Disease Control and Prevention. Prevalence of *Chlamydia trachomatis* genital infection among persons aged 14–39 years: United States, 2007-2012. *Morb Mort Wkly Rep*. 2014;63:834-838.

Workowski KA, Bolan GA; Centers for Disease Control and Prevention. Sexually transmitted diseases treatment guidelines, 2015. *MMWR Recomm Rep*. 2015;64:1-137.


# 255 Cholera

Mohammad Mhaissen and Chokechai Rongkavilit

## INTRODUCTION

Cholera is an acute life-threatening disease characterized by enormous loss of fluid and electrolytes due to profuse diarrhea and vomiting. This waterborne disease has been responsible for global scourges for centuries; it is often seen in the wake of disaster situations, both manmade and natural.

## PATHOGENESIS AND EPIDEMIOLOGY

*Vibrio cholerae* is an oxidase-positive, gram-negative, highly mobile, curved bacillus with a single polar flagellum. It is a slow lactose fermenter and also ferments glucose and sucrose. It grows easily in alkaline media in the presence of bile salts and is exquisitely sensitive to acid and to drying. The organism can be isolated on a variety of culture media, but a selective media, such as thiosulfate-citrate-bile salt sucrose (TCBS) agar, is recommended. On TCBS agar, *V cholerae* appear as 2- to 4-mm large, smooth, round, yellow colonies with opaque centers and translucent edges that contrast with the blue-green agar. Suspicious colonies can be rapidly identified by agglutination tests using specific *V cholerae* O1 and O139 antisera. Nontoxigenic strains of *V cholerae* are occasionally isolated from patients with diarrhea or sepsis.

There are at least 200 somatic serogroups based on somatic (O) antigens. The strains of only 2 serogroups, O1 and O139, have been associated with epidemic cholera. Other non-O1/O139 *V cholerae* serogroups result in sporadic diarrhea and occasionally cause a variety of severe extraintestinal infections including wound infections and sepsis, especially among patients with liver disease or immunosuppression. The *V cholerae* O1 are divided into 3 serotypes, Ogawa, Inaba, and Hikojima, based on specific antigenic determinants. The *V cholerae* O1 are further divided into 2 biotypes, classical and El Tor. *V cholerae* O139, first identified in 1993, originated from *V cholerae* O1 El Tor strain through a mutation in the O1 antigen leading to the substitution of O139 antigen.

Several genes are responsible for the virulence of *V cholerae.* Only epidemic strains of *V cholerae* O1 and *V cholerae* O139 possess the *ctxA* and *ctxB* genes that encode for enterotoxin subunits A and B. The B subunits bind to $G_{M1}$ ganglioside receptors on enterocytes, after which the A subunit enters the cell. The A subunit irreversibly activates the adenylate cyclase system in the mucosa, leaving it in the "on" position, leading to increases in the intracellular concentration of cyclic adenosine monophosphate, which results in sodium and water loss. Thus, the active secretion of sodium and chloride into the gut lumen with water following it passively results in secretion of isotonic fluid into the small intestine surpassing the absorptive capacity of the colon. This results in volume depletion and shock. Loss of bicarbonate and potassium also occurs, and this leads to metabolic acidosis and hypokalemia.

The current characterization of the ecology of cholera includes global weather patterns, aquatic reservoirs, bacteriophages, zooplankton, the collective behavior of surface-attached cells, an adaptable genome, and the deep sea, together with the bacterium and its host. Strains of *V cholerae* have been isolated from aquatic environments in areas where the disease is endemic as well as where no cholera cases occur. The organism is well adapted to warm stagnant environments with increased salinity. The ecological relationship of cholera and planktonic copepods was first described in 1983; *V cholerae* attach to live copepods in the Chesapeake Bay and around Bangladesh. This suggests that cholera is probably not an eradicable disease, because its causative organism lives naturally in riverine, brackish, and estuarine ecosystems. Outside of the host and in the aquatic phase, *V cholerae* can be found as free-swimming cells attached to plants, filamentous green algae, copepods, crustaceans, insects, and egg masses of chironomids. Biofilm formation and entry into a viable but nonculturable state in response to nutrient deprivation are thought to be important in facilitating environmental persistence during periods between epidemics. Although *V cholerae* is part of the normal estuarine flora, toxigenic strains are mostly isolated from the environment in areas where infected individuals are present.

Until the early 19th century, cholera was confined primarily to the Indian subcontinent, although seven pandemics have been described over the past 2 centuries. The most recent pandemic started in Indonesia in 1937, with spread to India in 1964, the Middle East in 1965, Africa and southern Europe in 1970, and South America in 1991. This pandemic was important because it led to the recognition of the importance of the use of oral rehydration solutions (ORS) to treat cholera. Until 1992, only the *V cholerae* O1 serogroup caused epidemic cholera. Other serogroups were identified in sporadic gastroenteritis cases. However, the 1992 cholera outbreak in India was caused by a new *V cholerae* serogroup, designated O139 or Bengal strain.

Cholera has pronounced seasonality. In Bangladesh, 2 peaks occur each year corresponding to the warm seasons before and after the monsoon season. In Peru, epidemics are strictly confined to the warm season. The seasonality seems to be related to the ability of vibrios to grow rapidly in a warm environment. Other than shellfish and plankton, there are no animal reservoirs.

Endemic cholera caused by *V cholerae* O1 primarily affects children. For instance, in Bangladesh, the infection was most prevalent among children in the 2- to 4-year age group; however, *V cholerae* O139 has been reported in infants as young as a 4-day-old newborn with diarrhea. In the United States, the average number of cholera cases during 2001 to 2005 was 4.6 cases per year, all of which were caused by *V cholerae* O1. This has increased after the recent outbreak in Haiti. In 2012, 18 cases of *V cholerae* serogroup O1 infection were reported. All but 1 were associated with travel to Haiti or other cholera-affected countries.

## CLINICAL MANIFESTATIONS

The incubation period for cholera is short, ranging from 6 hours to 5 days, with most cases occurring between 1 and 3 days. Toxigenic strains of *V cholerae* O1 and O139 produce infections ranging from asymptomatic infection to a severe fatal illness. Most infected individuals have no symptoms, and approximately 25% develop mild to moderate symptoms, while less than 5% of infected individuals develop the classic symptoms of cholera. Symptoms are generally abrupt and include watery diarrhea and vomiting. Anorexia and mild abdominal pain may precede the onset of diarrhea. Initially there is brownish fecal matter in the liquid stools. Once the diarrhea becomes copious, the stools are pale gray in color with a faint fishy smell and contain mucous flecks, giving them a classic "rice water" look. Vomiting may occur after the onset of diarrhea. The patient may be normothermic, hypothermic, or have a low-grade fever. Because of the massive amount of fluid and electrolyte loss, occasionally exceeding 1 L per hour, severe dehydration and shock may develop within a few hours. Patients at first are restless and extremely thirsty, but as shock progresses, they become apathetic and may lose consciousness. Many also show respiratory signs of metabolic acidosis with Kussmaul gasping breathing. If not treated vigorously and promptly, fluid loss may be so rapid that the patient is at risk of death within hours of the onset of symptoms.

Children also may develop seizures, hypoglycemia, and loss of consciousness. Hyponatremia and hypokalemia are more pronounced in children because of the greater loss of sodium and potassium in stools. Acute renal failure from protracted hypotension may develop if insufficient fluids are given. Many patients have hypoglycemia, which occasionally can be severe. In pregnant women, cholera can be severe, resulting in very high fetal mortality and premature labor as a complication of shock and placental hypoperfusion.

## DIAGNOSIS

Immunoassays that detect cholera toxin or *V cholerae* O1 and O139 lipopolysaccharide directly in stool are available and can be used in settings with limited laboratory capacity. The dipstick immunoassay has a 97% sensitivity and 71% to 76% specificity compared with polymerase chain reaction under field conditions for both O1 and O139 cholera. Rapid etiologic diagnosis can also be made by dark-field or phase microscopy. Actively motile *Vibrio* organisms are seen in large numbers in stool. Adding specific antisera for *V cholerae* O1 and O139 to the sample will immobilize and extinguish the characteristic "shooting star" movement of the *Vibrio*. Rectal swab or stool culture in Carry-Blair transport medium should be used for transportation of the specimen to the laboratory. The sample should then be placed onto TCBS agar. In addition, the specimen should be inoculated into alkaline peptone water, a high pH enrichment broth, which preferentially supports the growth of *Vibrio*. After 6 to 12 hours of incubation in the enrichment broth, a second TCBS plate is inoculated. The subsequent identification of the organism is established by agglutination test with O1- or O139-specific antisera. Molecular methods including polymerase chain reaction assay and DNA probes also are available but are not widely used and are not practicable in many areas where cholera is common.

**TABLE 255-1 INTERNATIONALLY AVAILABLE ORAL CHOLERA VACCINES**

| Vaccine | Composition | Primary Course | Booster Interval | Comments |
|---|---|---|---|---|
| Monovalent inactivated whole-cell *V cholerae* plus recombinant B subunit toxin vaccine (rCTB-WC, Dukoral) | *V cholerae* O1 classic Inaba<br>*V cholerae* O1 El Tor Inaba<br>*V cholerae* O1 classic Ogawa | Children 2 to 6 years: 3 doses at 1- to 6-week intervals<br>Adults and children 6 years or older: 2 doses at 1- to 6-week interval | Every 6 months[a]<br>Every 2 years[a] | Overall efficacy, 60–86%<br>Efficacy against severe disease, 82%<br>Decreasing to baseline by 2–3 years<br>Provides short-term protection against enterotoxigenic *Escherichia coli* |
| Bivalent inactivated whole-cell *V cholerae* vaccine (Shanchol, mORCVAX) | *V cholerae* O1 classic Inaba<br>*V cholerae* O1 El Tor Inaba<br>*V cholerae* O1 classic Ogawa<br>*V cholerae* O139 | Adults and children 1 year or older: 2 doses 14 days apart | Every 2 years | Overall efficacy, 50–65%[b]<br>Currently more affordable than Dukoral |

[a]If more than 2 years since last dose, primary course should be repeated.

[b]A recent study showed no decline in vaccine efficacy over 5 years, with protective efficacy of 65% (95% confidence interval, 52–74%)

## TREATMENT

Without appropriate treatment, the case-fatality rate for severe cholera can be as high as 50%. The primary therapy is replacement of fluid and electrolyte losses as outlined in Chapter 380. Antibiotic therapy is of secondary importance.

Antibiotic treatment for 2 to 3 days will shorten the clinical course from 4 to 5 days to 2 to 3 days, reduce the volume requirement for rehydration, and decrease the period of bacterial excretion. Tetracycline, 50 mg/kg/d given every 6 hours, or a single dose of doxycycline, 4 to 6 mg/kg, is the antibiotic of choice. *V cholerae* also is generally sensitive to trimethoprim-sulfamethoxazole, erythromycin, azithromycin, ciprofloxacin, furazolidone, chloramphenicol, and the aminoglycosides. The rapid global emergence of multidrug-resistant isolates is of grave concern. Therefore, during an outbreak, samples from representative patients should be tested for antibiotic susceptibility in order to select the most appropriate antibiotic on the basis of current sensitivity patterns. Antibiotics should not be given to asymptomatic contacts because that could increase the risk of development of resistance and is not cost-effective.

## PREVENTION

Sanitation, a safe water supply, and good personal hygiene are of primary importance in controlling cholera, but these measures are often difficult to implement in poor, developing countries. Vaccine programs must be integrated with other key public health interventions including safe water and sanitation, hand hygiene, and health education.

Clinical cholera confers effective and long-lasting immunity. The protection stems from the development of local vibriocidal antibodies directed against the *V cholerae* cell wall lipopolysaccharide and antitoxin antibodies directed against the cholera toxin B subunits. Either class of antibody is protective; however, together they exert synergistic protective effects. Hence, the ideal vaccine should stimulate production of both types of antibody in the intestinal mucosa.

The World Health Organization has endorsed the inclusion of an oral vaccine in cholera control programs. Currently, there are 2 inactivated whole-cell oral cholera vaccines that are licensed for commercial use in many countries except the United States (Table 255-1): the monovalent vaccine derived from *V cholerae* O1 plus recombinant B subunit of cholera toxin vaccine (rCTB-WC; Dukoral; SBL Vaccin AB, Stockholm, Sweden) and the bivalent vaccines containing killed *V cholerae* O1 and O139 serogroups without cholera toxin B subunit (Shanchol; Shantha Biotechnics-Sanofi Pasteur, Hyderabad, India; and mORCVAX; VaBiotech, Hanoi, Vietnam).

The rCTB-WC vaccine does not contain the A subunit toxin, and therefore no pathogenic toxin is present. A large randomized, double-blind, placebo-controlled trial in Peru evaluated the rCTB-WC vaccine given as 2 doses followed by a booster dose at 10 months. Protection starts 10 days after the second dose. The overall protective efficacy after 3 doses was 61%. The efficacy against severe cholera requiring hospitalization was 82%. The vaccine efficacy was 52% for children 2 to 5 years old, 46% for those 6 to 15 years old, and 72% for those older than 15 years. In a report of mass vaccination using a 2-dose regimen of rCTB-WC vaccine before cholera outbreak in Mozambique, receipt of 1 or more doses of the vaccine was associated with 78% to 84% protection. The vaccine was found to be equally effective in children younger than 5 years of age and in older persons. The rCTB-WC vaccine has been shown to confer moderate immunity up to 3 years in adults. Young children, however, develop immunity that lasts less than 1 year. Therefore, the booster interval is shorter for children. This vaccine is currently recommended for use in refugee settings at risk of cholera.

The second killed whole-cell oral cholera vaccine (Shanchol) was developed and licensed in India in 2009. It contains the same *V cholerae* O1 whole-cell strains as the rCTB-WC vaccine plus killed *V cholerae* O139 strain, but it does not have the B subunit component. In a placebo-controlled, cluster-randomized trial, the vaccine was shown to be safe and conferred 67% efficacy against cholera severe enough to require treatment in a health facility at 2 years and 66% efficacy at 3 years of follow-up. At 5 years after vaccination, the protective efficacy was maintained at 65%.

Cholera immunization is not required for travelers entering the United States from cholera-affected areas, and the World Health Organization no longer recommends immunization for travel to or from areas with cholera infection.

## SUGGESTED READINGS


Ali M, Lopez AL, You YA, et al. The global burden of cholera. *Bull World Health Org.* 2012;90:209-218A.

Bhattacharya SK, Sur D, Ali M, et al. 5 year efficacy of a bivalent killed whole-cell oral cholera vaccine in Kolkata, India: a cluster-randomised, double-blind, placebo-controlled trial. *Lancet Infect Dis.* 2013;13:1050-1056.

Dick MH, Guillerm M, Moussy F, Chaignat CL. Review of two decades of cholera diagnostics: how far have we really come? *PLoS Negl Trop Dis.* 2012;6:e1845.

Harris JB, LaRocque RC, Qadri F, Ryan ET, Calderwood SB. Cholera. *Lancet.* 2012;379:2466-2476.

Leibovici-Weissman Y, Neuberger A, Bitterman R, Sinclair D, Salam MA, Paul M. Antimicrobial drugs for treating cholera. *Cochrane Database Syst Rev.* 2014;19:CD008625.

Mutreja A, Kim DW, Thomson NR, et al. Evidence for several waves of global transmission in the seventh cholera pandemic. *Nature.* 2011;477:462-465.

Newton AE, Heiman KE, Schmitz A, et al. Cholera in United States associated with epidemic in Hispaniola. *Emerg Infect Dis.* 2011;17:2166-2168.

World Health Organization. Cholera Annual Report, 2015. *Wkly Epidemiol Recor.* 2016;38:433-440.

Tran NT, Taylor R, Antierens A, Staderini N. Cholera in pregnancy: a systematic review and meta-analysis of fetal, neonatal, and maternal mortality. *PLoS One.* 2015;10:e0132920.

# 256 Diphtheria

Andrew Abreo and Bernhard L. Wiedermann

## INTRODUCTION

Diphtheria is an acute infection caused by *Corynebacterium diphtheriae*. The incidence of diphtheria is inversely related to the percentage of immune individuals in an area, and it remains endemic in countries without effective immunization programs. The incidence of diphtheria in the United States has declined dramatically since aggressive immunization efforts were begun in 1980. Concurrently, diphtheria shifted from a disease of children to a disease of adults with waning immunity. The potential for outbreaks continues, however, if segments of a community are not immunized.

## PATHOGENESIS AND EPIDEMIOLOGY

*C diphtheriae* is an irregularly staining, non–spore-forming, nonmotile, unencapsulated, gram-positive bacillus. Metachromatic granules and a cuneiform appearance help distinguish the organism on smear. There are 4 biotypes (ie, *mitis, intermedius, gravis, belfanti*) that are differentiated by colony morphology, growth characteristics, and biochemical reactions. All biotypes are capable of producing a cytotoxic exotoxin that inhibits protein synthesis in host cells. The ability of a strain to produce the exotoxin is conferred by a lysogenic bacteriophage that carries the gene for toxin production. The toxin leads to the formation of pseudomembranes in the pharynx and respiratory tract, as well as systemic toxicity including myocarditis and polyneuropathy. *C diphtheriae* also presents as a cutaneous infection that often is associated with homelessness and tropical areas.

*C diphtheriae* inhabits mucosal epithelial cells (primarily respiratory tract) and skin of humans, the only reservoir. Transmission occurs from person-to-person by respiratory droplets and close contact with respiratory secretions or discharge from cutaneous lesions. Diphtheria occurs worldwide, and it may present at any time of the year, although it is most common during winter. Because humans are the only significant reservoir, closeness and duration of contact with an ill person or a healthy carrier are important determinants of infection spread. As a result, attack rates in households and in crowded living conditions are high.

## CLINICAL MANIFESTATIONS

The presentation of diphtheria depends on the primary site of infection. Respiratory tract diphtheria is characterized by either membranous nasopharyngitis or obstructive laryngotracheitis. Cutaneous diphtheria is associated with infected skin lesions that lack a characteristic appearance. With either presentation, toxin produced by the organism results in further symptoms.

## RESPIRATORY DISEASE

After an average incubation period of 2 to 4 days, symptoms of a sore throat with mild pharyngeal injection and low-grade fever develop. Systemic signs of illness are absent in the early stages. Within 1 to 2 days, areas of yellow or "dirty" white exudate appear, most frequently on or adjacent to the tonsils. Subsequently, these areas coalesce to form a light reflective, sharply outlined pseudomembrane. The pseudomembrane consists of necrotic epithelium embedded in an inflammatory, organized exudate at the surface. Inflammatory changes in the underlying epithelium may extend into the submucosa and induce hemorrhage. Dislodgement of the pseudomembrane exposes an edematous, bleeding submucosa. The organisms remain in the surface lesions and rarely invade deeper structures or cause bacteremia. However, the diphtheria exotoxin may be systemically absorbed from the local lesion, causing damage to distant organs and tissues.

Persons with partial antitoxin immunity may not progress beyond the exudative stage. In those lacking immunity, the pseudomembrane may spread to the mucous membranes of the uvula, soft palate, oropharynx, and nasopharynx. Cervical lymph nodes may be mildly enlarged, but the single, large, anterior cervical nodes characteristic of streptococcal infection are not found. Dysphagia and drooling may develop due to significant soft-tissue swelling and cervical lymphadenopathy caused by extensive membrane formation. After approximately 5 days, the pseudomembrane changes to a grayish color secondary to hemorrhage as it loosens and sloughs. In approximately 10% of patients, the illness has a hyperacute, grave presentation with high fever, systemic toxicity, cerebral obtundation, and rapid proliferation of the pseudomembrane associated with marked edema of the face and neck, a phenomenon referred to as "bull neck" diphtheria.

In less than 5% of patients, diphtheria of the laryngeal area occurs in the absence of tonsillopharyngeal involvement, but in about 10% of patients, there is secondary downward spread from the pharynx. Symptoms include hoarseness, stridor, and a barking cough. The severity of respiratory distress depends on the extent and thickness of the membrane in relation to the caliber of the airway. Young children are at higher risk of compromise because of small airways. Rarely, the membrane extends into the bronchial tree, resulting in a virtual cast of the airway, which is invariably fatal.

Anterior nasal diphtheria is more common in infants and young children. The nasal discharge is mucoid, profuse, and grayish in color, but may become blood-tinged once the membrane begins sloughing after a few days. This is the mildest form of diphtheria and seldom has toxic manifestations.

## SKIN AND MUCOUS MEMBRANE DISEASE

Skin lesions of diphtheria are most often superficial, have no characteristic appearance, and are not associated with pseudomembrane formation. Occasionally, ulcerating or ecthymatous lesions develop. The lesions occur in persons with preexisting antitoxic immunity, or they induce immunity because they are not associated with toxic manifestations. Individual lesions heal, but new ones may form at the sites of breaks in the integrity of skin from insect bites or trauma over a period of weeks. Rarely, the primary site of infection is the mucous membrane of the eye, vagina, or ear. An ulcerating lesion with exudate or pseudomembrane forms, but these self-limited lesions are only rarely associated with toxicity.

## EFFECTS OF TOXIN PRODUCTION

The heart, nervous system, and kidneys are susceptible to damage by diphtheria toxin. The degree of toxic damage is determined by 2 factors: (1) the extent of disease at the primary site and, hence, the amount of toxin produced and disseminated hematogenously; and (2) the amount of circulating antitoxin. The amount of antitoxin is determined by both the preexisting antitoxin resulting from prior subclinical infection or immunization and by the therapeutic amounts of antitoxin administered. Previously immunized persons may become susceptible to toxin as immunity wanes over time.

Clinical myocarditis develops in approximately 10–25% of patients with diphtheria. Myocarditis generally develops during the first week of illness; however, onset can be delayed for 1 month or longer. On histology, myocarditis is characterized by degenerative or "toxic" damage rather than by inflammation. Minute hemorrhages or accompanying round-cell infiltration may be present. Dysrhythmias are common given the frequent involvement of the electrical conduction system. Electrocardiographic changes are present in many patients without clinical evidence of myocarditis. Death occurs more often from severe dysrhythmia (including complete heart block) than from heart failure.

Nervous system involvement occurs in 5% to 10% of patients. Local paralysis of contiguous muscles in the soft palate, pharynx, and larynx can occur as early as the first week of disease, but more often develops between the second and sixth week after onset of the respiratory illness. Paralysis leads to dysphagia and increases the risk for aspiration. Cranial neuropathies develop later in the disease course and lead to oculomotor and ciliary paralysis. Polyneuropathy develops 10 days to 3 months after initial symptom onset and is characterized by a symptom complex mimicking Guillain-Barré syndrome, including motor weakness, diminished deep tendon reflexes, and paralysis of the diaphragm.

If the patient does not succumb to respiratory complications of paralysis, full recovery can be expected within a few weeks. Degenerative changes in the nervous system occur in nearly all fatal infections. In the spinal cord, changes are seen in the ganglion cells of the anterior horns and in the posterior root ganglia. The cranial nerves and their nuclei can be affected, but the cortex is spared.

Renal failure is rare, but minor injury as reflected by changes in the urinalysis (proteinuria, cylindruria, increased cells) is common. If toxic nephropathy develops, it is almost uniformly fatal. Hemolytic-uremic syndrome has been reported in diphtheria. The kidneys may exhibit cloudy swelling with swollen granular epithelial cells of the convoluted tubules. Interstitial nephritis may occur. Lesions in the adrenal cortex, similar to those present in meningococcemia, are often found in fatal infections. Hepatic function may be mildly impaired; liver cells show degenerative changes with scattered areas of focal necrosis at autopsy.

## DIAGNOSIS

The differential diagnosis for pseudomembranous tonsillitis includes many bacterial and viral pathogens, the most common being *Streptococcus pyogenes,* adenoviruses, and Epstein-Barr virus. However, in these conditions, the pseudomembrane does not otherwise extend away from the tonsil. In rare instances of laryngeal diphtheria without oropharyngeal involvement, the diagnosis is suspected if there is a history of exposure to diphtheria or when a pseudomembrane is seen at the time of laryngoscopy or bronchoscopy. Otherwise, distinguishing diphtheria from other viral causes of croup is exceedingly difficult.

When diphtheria is suspected, attempts should be made to isolate the organism from the local lesion. It is advisable to obtain specimens for culture from the nasopharynx and throat because the yield of positive result is 20% greater with 2 cultures as opposed to 1. A portion of the pseudomembrane or underlying material should be submitted for culture. Laboratory staff should be alerted if *C diphtheriae* is suspected given that special medium is needed for culture. The swab can be transported in a laboratory-recommended commercial transport medium (eg, Amies, Stuart media) or sterile container at 4°C. If transport will take longer than 24 hours, the swab should be placed in a silica gel pack. Specimens are inoculated onto recommended media (eg, cystine-tellurite blood agar or modified Tinsdale agar). Suspicious colonies may be stained with Neisser's or Loeffler's methylene blue and examined for the characteristic morphologic appearance of *C diphtheriae* (eg, metachromatic granules). If *C diphtheriae* is present, the toxigenicity of the strain is usually determined using the Elek test in reference or state laboratories. Polymerase chain reaction (PCR) identification of the gene for toxin production (dtxR) and the diphtheria toxin gene (*tox*) helps support the diagnosis.

The degree of leukocytosis in the peripheral blood generally reflects the severity of disease. In mild to moderate disease, the leukocyte count is between 10,000 and 20,000/μL. The likelihood of a fatal outcome rises sharply in patients with leukocyte counts higher than 25,000/μL. Thrombocytopenia and disseminated intravascular coagulation (DIC) are rare. Some patients develop mild anemia. Albuminuria is common, and in severe disease, there may be cells and casts in the urine.

In postdiphtheritic paralysis, protein concentrations increase in the cerebrospinal fluid (CSF), but there is no increase in the number of cells, and the glucose content is normal, as occurs in idiopathic Guillain-Barré syndrome. The protein content continues to increase during the initial weeks of neurologic symptoms and slowly returns to normal after clinical recovery.

## TREATMENT

Diphtheria antitoxin neutralizes circulating toxin but has no effect on toxin that is already bound to cells. A single dose of intravenous antitoxin (Table 256-1) should be administered as soon as the clinical diagnosis is suspected. The decision to treat is usually made before culture results are available and is based on a compatible clinical picture in a susceptible individual. Antitoxin is of dubious value for patients with cutaneous diphtheria, but some authorities recommend it because toxic manifestations have been reported. Diphtheria antitoxin is an equine serum, so tests for sensitivity are completed prior to administration. If the patient has an immediate reaction, a desensitization procedure is completed. Details of appropriate sensitivity testing and interpretations of results are provided with antitoxin available from the Centers for Disease Control and Prevention.

**TABLE 256-1 GUIDELINES FOR DIPHTHERIA ANTITOXIN THERAPY**

| Status of Disease | Dosage of Antitoxin (Units) |
|---|---|
| Pharyngeal or laryngeal of ≤ 2 days in duration | 20,000–40,000 |
| Nasopharyngeal | 40,000–60,000 |
| "Bull neck" or any disease of ≥ 3 days in duration | 80,000–120,000 |
| Skin lesions | 20,000–40,000 |

Antibiotic therapy has little or no effect on the clinical evolution of diphtheria. It is given primarily to eliminate the organism, stop toxin production, and render the patient noncontagious. Erythromycin and penicillin are recommended to treat *C diphtheriae,* although the organism is susceptible to other antibiotics in vitro. Erythromycin (40 mg/kg/d divided every 6 hours; maximum 2 g/d) is given orally or intravenously for 14 days. Alternatively, daily procaine penicillin G (300,000 units/d if < 10 kg; 600,000 units/d if > 10 kg) can be given intramuscularly for 14 days, or aqueous crystalline penicillin G (100,000–150,000 units/kg/d divided every 6 hours) can be given intramuscularly or intravenously for 14 days. Eradication of the organism should be confirmed after completion of antibiotic therapy by obtaining 2 negative cultures from the nasopharynx and throat separated by at least 24 hours. Respiratory isolation precautions are maintained until there is culture confirmation of eradication. Some patients with cutaneous diphtheria have asymptomatic respiratory tract colonization with *C diphtheriae,* and thus, throat and nasopharyngeal cultures are necessary in these patients as well. A repeat course of erythromycin therapy is given if there is persistent nasopharyngeal carriage after the first course of therapy. Treatment is otherwise supportive with an emphasis on bed rest during the acute illness. Corticosteroid therapy (to mitigate myocarditis or nephritis) is ineffective and not recommended.

A patent airway must be maintained in patients with diphtheria. Nasotracheal intubation or tracheostomy may be needed. Patients should be monitored carefully for signs or symptoms of myocarditis, nephropathy, or neuropathy. Patients should be observed closely for signs of laryngeal, pharyngeal, or diaphragmatic paralysis. Respiratory paralysis is managed by standard procedures. If difficulty with swallowing is observed, oral feedings should be withheld and parenteral nutrition provided. During the stage of sloughing of the pseudomembrane, tracheal suction may be successful in removing obstructive fragments.

The overall fatality rate is about 10%; however, the prognosis depends on type of disease, patient age, general condition of the patient, and the interval from disease onset to receipt of antitoxin therapy. More than half of patients with bull neck diphtheria die despite aggressive intensive care. The prognosis is grim if myocarditis or renal failure occurs early in the disease course. Patients managed in an intensive care facility are unlikely to die from airway obstruction unless the pseudomembrane extends into the bronchi. After recovering from the acute illness, patients remain at risk for late development of paralysis or myocarditis. There are no permanent sequelae of diphtheria unless anoxic damage has occurred.

## PREVENTION

Immunization with diphtheria toxoid is the only effective preventive measure. In fact, recovered patients should receive diphtheria toxoid since an attack of diphtheria does not provide reliable immunity to the toxin. Immunity is associated with a minimum diphtheria antitoxin level of 0.01 IU/mL. Immunization recommendations are found in Chapter 239.

Exposed household members and other close contacts of an index patient with diphtheria are at increased risk of becoming asymptomatic carriers or of developing disease. Immunization provides antitoxin immunity, but no immunity to infection with *C diphtheriae*. All exposed persons need to be examined promptly, and individuals with symptoms consistent with diphtheria should be investigated and treated appropriately. Regardless of immunization status, all exposed, asymptomatic persons should be cultured for *C diphtheriae*, kept under surveillance for 7 days, and started on prophylactic antimicrobial therapy with oral erythromycin (40 mg/kg/d; maximum 1 g/d) for 7 to 10 days or a single intramuscular injection of benzathine penicillin G (600,000 units if < 30 kg; 1.2 million units if > 30 kg). The exposed persons are considered potentially contagious until the culture results are known. Individuals who cannot be kept under surveillance should receive benzathine penicillin G.

Asymptomatic, previously immunized contacts should be given a booster dose of age-appropriate diphtheria toxoid if they have not received a booster within 5 years. In addition, individuals who are underimmunized or whose immunization status is unknown should receive an age-appropriate diphtheria toxoid-containing vaccine. Diphtheria antitoxin is not recommended for unimmunized close contacts.

## SUGGESTED READINGS

American Academy of Pediatrics. Diphtheria. In: Kimberlin DW, Brady MT, Jackson MA, Long SS, eds. *2015 Red Book: Report of the Committee on Infectious Diseases*. 30th ed. Elk Grove Village, IL: American Academy of Pediatrics; 2015:325-329.

Centers for Disease Control and Prevention. Diphtheria. In: Hamborsky J, Kroger A, Wolfe S, eds. *Epidemiology and Prevention of Vaccine-Preventable Diseases. The Pink Book: Course Textbook*. 13th ed. Washington, DC: Public Health Foundation; 2015. http://www.cdc.gov/vaccines/pubs/pinkbook/downloads/dip.pdf. Accessed January 29, 2017.

Centers for Disease Control and Prevention. General recommendations on immunization: recommendations of the Advisory Committee on Immunization Practices. *MMWR Morb Mortal Wkly Rep*. 2011;60(No. RR-02):1-60.

Tewari T, Clark T. Use of diphtheria antitoxin (DAT) for suspected diphtheria cases. Atlanta, GA: Centers for Disease Control and Prevention; 2014. https://www.cdc.gov/diphtheria/downloads/protocol.pdf. Accessed January 29, 2017.

# 257 Enterococcus

Mark S. Needles

## INTRODUCTION

Enterococci are gram-positive facultative anaerobic bacteria and are normal flora of the human gastrointestinal tract. Historically classified as group D streptococci, enterococci are now classified as a separate genus with at least 35 different species.

## PATHOGENESIS AND EPIDEMIOLOGY

Only 2 species, *Enterococcus faecalis* and *Enterococcus faecium*, account for all but a rare case of human disease. *E faecalis* is responsible for about 80% to 90% of human cases, but several studies show a rising proportion of cases due to *E faecium*. Enterococci are facultatively anaerobic catalase-negative gram-positive cocci that normally inhabit the bowel. Approximately half of newborn infants have acquired colonization with enterococci by 1 week of age. These very hardy organisms grow at temperatures of 10°C to 60°C (50–140°F) and remain viable for weeks on environmental surfaces such as bed rails, sinks, faucets, and doorknobs. Human-to-human spread is common in hospital settings.

Enterococci generally are not highly invasive pathogens and typically are classified as opportunists. They lack not only the major exotoxins and endotoxins associated with virulent streptococci and staphylococci, but also the enzymes that enable rapid tissue spread. Infections are most often associated with prolonged hospitalization, particularly in intensive care or hematology/oncology units; use of broad-spectrum antibiotics; indwelling lines; immunocompromised state; or loss of integrity of the gastrointestinal tract, urinary tract, or skin.

## CLINICAL MANIFESTATIONS

The 3 most common types of infection associated with enterococci are urinary tract infection (UTI), polymicrobial abdominal infections, and bacteremia or sepsis. Although infrequent, cases of focal organ infection, such as endocarditis, meningitis, and wound infections, may be severe. UTI caused by enterococci almost never occurs in otherwise healthy children. They are most often associated with indwelling urinary catheters and account for approximately 15% of nosocomial UTIs in children. Anatomic urinary tract anomalies, particularly vesicoureteral reflux, are more common in community-acquired enterococcal UTIs than those associated with gram-negative Enterobacteriaceae.

Enterococci may be involved in intra-abdominal polymicrobial infections following intestinal perforation such as ruptured appendix or necrotizing enterocolitis. Although there has been controversy regarding the pathogenic role of enterococci in such infections, most authorities recommend adding an antibiotic to cover for enterococci in the setting of healthcare-associated intra-abdominal infections, particularly postoperative infections. Empiric therapy also should be considered for severe sepsis of abdominal origin in immunocompromised patients or patients who recently received broad-spectrum antibiotics selecting for *Enterococcus* species. Enterococcal bacteremia or sepsis in children may not be identified with a specific focus, but common risk factors are use of broad-spectrum antibiotics or intravascular catheters in association with underlying conditions such as surgery, immunosuppression, transplants, or major organ dysfunction. Bacteremia without a focal infection may result in a self-limited illness or a severe and life-threatening illness, particularly in newborns or children with underlying disease. Bacteremia is often polymicrobial with other enteric microorganisms. Mortality occurs in up to 25% of cases but is hard to separate from the underlying health problems.

In newborns, infection may present as early-onset sepsis in the first several days of life, similar to early-onset group B streptococcal sepsis. However, most neonatal enterococcal infections are nosocomial and occur after the second week of life, typically in the setting of bacteremia attributable to line infection or necrotizing enterocolitis. The most common presenting signs are apnea, bradycardia, respiratory dysfunction, fever or hypothermia, and abdominal distention.

## DIAGNOSIS

Enterococci are easily isolated on standard bacterial culture plates or broth media. They are distinguished from nonenterococcal, catalase-negative, gram-positive cocci by the PYR reaction (hydrolysis of L-pyrrolidinyl-β-naphthylamide), the ability to hydrolyze esculin in the presence of 4% ox gall (bile), and growth in 6.5% NaCl at 10°C to 45°C.

## TREATMENT

The most important aspect of treating enterococcal infections is determination of antibiotic susceptibility. Enterococci have an intrinsic resistance to cephalosporins, monobactams, antistaphylococcal penicillins, clindamycin, and aminoglycosides. For penicillin-susceptible strains, ampicillin is considered more active than penicillin. Generally, *E faecium* are more resistant to β-lactam antibiotics than strains of *E faecalis*. Although low-grade β-lactam resistance is mediated by β-lactamase production, most β-lactam resistance is high grade and mediated by altered penicillin-binding protein.

Aminoglycoside resistance, due to decreased drug uptake, is either low or high grade (minimal inhibitory concentration ≥ 500 μg/mL for gentamicin or ≥ 1000 μg/mL for streptomycin). If susceptible, use of penicillin, ampicillin, or vancomycin improves aminoglycoside uptake and results in synergistic activity. Synergy is not possible with high-grade resistant enterococci isolates.

Resistance to the glycopeptide antibiotics vancomycin and teicoplanin is mediated by the production of novel peptidoglycan, with decreased affinity for glycopeptides. This alters the ability of vancomycin and teicoplanin to inhibit cell wall formation. Resistance is transferred by gene clusters Van A, B, C, D, F, and G, carried in transposon 1546. Although the gene clusters vary in the degree of resistance to vancomycin or teicoplanin, for practical clinical purposes, they are grouped as vancomycin-resistant enterococci (VRE).

Most enterococci are susceptible to the oxazolidinone antibiotic linezolid and/or susceptible to the lipopeptide antibiotic daptomycin. However, there are now reports in the United States and Europe of linezolid-resistant enterococci, and daptomycin resistance may arise during therapy.

Ampicillin alone is the antibiotic of choice for UTIs with susceptible enterococci (about 98% of *E faecalis* and 15% of *E faecium*). Most authorities recommend that serious infections such as meningitis and endocarditis be treated with the addition of an aminoglycoside to achieve synergistic bactericidal activity. Unfortunately, high-level aminoglycoside resistance, which precludes synergistic activity, is increasing among enterococci. The role of combination therapy for uncomplicated enterococcal bacteremia is unresolved. The risks for aminoglycoside-associated nephrotoxicity may surpass the benefits when used for this indication. For ampicillin-resistant enterococci, vancomycin is the antibiotic of choice. However, vancomycin-resistant strains of enterococci are increasing at an alarming rate. The National Nosocomial Surveillance Network Database–USA reported a vancomycin resistance rate of 35% among enterococci causing hospital-associated infections in intensive care units in 2010. This was an 18.5% increase from 1991. Several hospital outbreaks of VRE have been reported in children. Antibiotic selection for treatment of VRE must depend on laboratory susceptibility profiles because many strains are multidrug resistant. Some *E faecalis* VRE retain ampicillin susceptibility, whereas most *E faecium* VRE do not.

If linezolid resistance is confirmed in a VRE *E faecium* strain, it may be susceptible to daptomycin or to the streptogramin antibiotic quinupristin-dalfopristin. Neither daptomycin nor quinupristin-dalfopristin is approved for pediatric use. Quinupristin-dalfopristin is not active against *E faecalis.*

## PREVENTION

Prevention of further spread of VRE will depend on appropriate control measures such as active surveillance for VRE in intensive care settings, contact isolation to minimize person-to-person transmission, and restriction of the use of vancomycin and other broad-spectrum antibiotics.

## SUGGESTED READINGS

Baddour LM, Wilson WR, Bayer AS, et al. Infective endocarditis in adults: diagnosis, antimicrobial therapy, and management of complications: a scientific statement for healthcare professionals from the American Heart Association: endorsed by the Infectious Diseases Society of America. *Circulation.* 2015;132:1435-1486.

Ford CD, Lopansri BK, Gazdik MA, et al. The clinical impact of vancomycin-resistant *Enterococcus* colonization and bloodstream infection in patients undergoing autologous transplantation. *Transpl Infect Dis.* 2015;17:688-694.

Ibrahim SL, Zhang L, Brady TM, et al. Low-dose gentamicin for uncomplicated *Enterococcus faecalis* bacteremia may be nephrotoxic in children. *Clin Infect Dis.* 2015;61:1119-1124.

Lister DM, Kotsanas D, Ballard SA, et al. Outbreak of vanB vancomycin-resistant *Enterococcus faecium* colonization in a neonatal service. *Am J Infect Control.* 2015;43:1061-1065.

O'Driscoll T, Crank CW. Vancomycin-resistant enterococcal infections: epidemiology, clinical manifestations, and optimal management. *Infect Drug Resist.* 2015;8:217-230.

# 258 *Haemophilus influenzae*

Mark R. Schleiss



## INTRODUCTION

The types of infectious diseases caused by *Haemophilus influenzae* have changed considerably in recent years as a result of the widespread implementation of routine childhood immunization against type b organisms, but the organism remains an important pathogen. There are 2 major categories of disease caused by *H influenzae*: infections caused by unencapsulated strains (nontypeable [NTHi]) and disease induced by encapsulated strains (typeable). The unencapsulated strains are responsible chiefly for infections at mucosal surfaces, including conjunctivitis, otitis media, sinusitis, and bronchitis. In contrast, encapsulated strains are associated with invasive disease. Of the 6 encapsulated strains, type b in particular is associated with septicemia, meningitis, cellulitis, septic arthritis, epiglottitis, and pneumonia. Prior to the availability of an effective vaccine, *H influenzae* type b (Hib) was the most common cause of pediatric bacterial meningitis in the United States.

## PATHOGENESIS AND EPIDEMIOLOGY

*H influenzae* is a small gram-negative coccobacillus that shows considerable microscopic pleomorphism, necessitating careful and cautious interpretation of Gram stains of clinical specimens (Fig. 258-1). Biochemical identification of *H influenzae* has classically been based on the demonstration that growth on rich media (blood agar) is dependent on supplements, factors X (hemin) and V (β-nicotinamide adenine dinucleotide [NAD]), as found in chocolate agar. Although both factors are present in erythrocytes, the V factor must be released from the cell in order to sustain replication, and hence, standard blood agar is an unsatisfactory media for growth of *H influenzae*. The V factor may be exogenously provided or derived from lysed red blood cells; heated blood agar (chocolate agar) provides both factors. The growth of *H influenzae* is fastidious, and the viability of the organism is lost rapidly, necessitating expeditious handling of clinical specimens.

The polysaccharide capsule of *H influenzae* has a central role in the virulence of the organism and plays a role in the pathogenesis of invasive disease. Six antigenically and biochemically distinct capsular polysaccharide subtypes (a–f) have been identified. All isolates associated with invasive infection should be serotyped, either through slide agglutination serotyping or genotyping by polymerase chain reaction. Although type b encapsulated strains have historically been of primary clinical and immunologic importance (because of the association with invasive infection, including meningitis), the other encapsulated

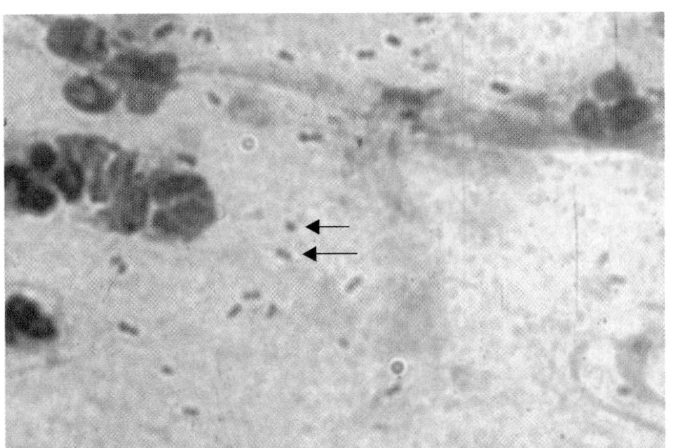

**FIGURE 258-1** Gram stain of *Haemophilus influenzae. Arrows* point to 2 small "cocco-bacillary" gram-negative rods. (Used with permission from Professor Shirley Lowe, University of California, San Francisco School of Medicine.)

strains also are capable of producing invasive disease. Lipopolysaccharide (LPS) is another important component of the *H influenzae* cell wall that contributes to pathogenesis. Although chemically different from the LPS of the Enterobacteriaceae, the biological activity of Hib LPS is similar to that of other gram-negative endotoxins. Multiple adhesins target specific cells of the airway and provide redundancy for adherence to respiratory tissues. *H influenzae* encodes 3 distinct immunoglobulin (Ig) A proteases that may play a role as virulence factors by interfering with host mucosal defenses. The molecular determinants responsible for nasopharyngeal colonization and subsequent invasiveness of *H influenzae* remain poorly understood.

Another clinically important aspect of the molecular microbiology of *H influenzae* has been the identification of genes responsible for antimicrobial resistance. Plasmid-mediated ampicillin resistance due to production of β-lactamase has become extremely common in Hib and NTHi, ranging from 5% to 50% of isolates in various parts of the world. Non-β-lactamase–mediated ampicillin resistance is increasing in the United States; thus, susceptibility testing should be performed on all isolates identified in invasive infections.

Humans are the only natural host for *H influenzae*. Maintenance of the organism in the human population depends on person-to-person transmission via respiratory tract mucosal colonization, which occurs by a hand-to-respiratory tract route. This mode of transmission was best documented during nosocomial outbreaks of NTHi pneumonia in the elderly. Nontypeable strains colonize the upper respiratory tract of as many as 75% of healthy adults. Hib strains colonize the nasopharynx of children at a rate of 3% to 5%; the effectiveness of the conjugate vaccines is related in part to their ability to diminish the incidence of nasopharyngeal colonization. Although both nontypeable and type b strains of *H influenzae* are easily spread via person-to-person transmission, only the Hib strains have historically been associated with invasive disease in children. Nasopharyngeal colonization by Hib is for the most part asymptomatic, but breakthrough bacteremia with subsequent development of invasive disease was at one time a common occurrence in the United States.

In the prevaccine era, invasive Hib disease characteristically had a striking age-related incidence, with approximately 85% of disease occurring in children younger than 5 years. The peak incidence of the most serious form of invasive disease, meningitis, occurred between 6 and 12 months of age. Hib epiglottitis was, in contrast, predominantly a disease of older children, with more than 80% of the infections occurring in children older than 2 years. In the prevaccine era, approximately 20,000 instances of invasive Hib disease occurred annually in the United States, affecting about 1 in 200 children younger than 5 years.

Chronic illnesses associated with increased risk for invasive Hib disease include sickle cell disease, asplenia, agammaglobulinemia, trisomy 21, Hodgkin disease, and complement deficiencies. Increased risk also has been associated with childcare attendance, the presence of siblings younger than 5 years, household crowding, lower socioeconomic status, and passive smoke exposure. Breastfeeding confers some protection against disease. Although invasive Hib infection is uncommon in adults, remarkably, in the post-Hib vaccine era, Hib meningitis has now become more common in adult patients than in children.

The epidemiology of invasive Hib disease has changed dramatically in recent years as a consequence of the widespread administration of conjugate vaccines. In 1987, the first Hib polysaccharide-containing vaccine (polyribosylribitol phosphate [PRP]) was licensed in the United States for administration to children 18 months of age and older. Over the next few years, some decreases in the incidence of invasive disease were seen in older children. However, because Hib meningitis had always been a more significant problem in children younger than 1 year, the most significant decline in invasive disease was not observed until late 1990, when protein-PRP conjugate vaccines were approved for use in infants, beginning at 2 months of age. In populations with high rates of vaccine coverage, the incidence of Hib disease was reduced by more than 95%. The protective efficacy of these vaccines exceeded initial expectations because of an unanticipated decrease in nasopharyngeal carriage, ultimately leading to a decreased environmental burden of Hib and a resultant protection even of unimmunized children, a manifestation of "herd immunity." The conjugate vaccines are so effective in preventing Hib infection that the finding of invasive disease in a fully immunized child should prompt further diagnostic evaluation for the possibility of an underlying immunodeficiency.

An important aspect of Hib epidemiology is the risk it poses to contacts. Although the direct contagiousness of invasive Hib infection is limited, a significant risk for secondary disease exists among household contacts of a patient with invasive Hib disease, particularly in the 30 days following exposure to an index patient. This is a consequence of spread under conditions of continuous household exposure. Colonization rates higher than 70% have been noted following exposure in closed populations, such as within families or in daycare centers. This becomes the rationale for chemoprophylaxis following exposure to an invasive case of Hib disease.

Another less common but recently recognized route of acquisition of NTHi may be vertical transmission via the birth canal causing neonatal bacteremia, pneumonia, and meningitis. These strains are genetically distinct from those colonizing the upper respiratory tract and occasionally are a cause of neonatal conjunctivitis.

Age-dependent susceptibility to Hib infections correlates with an age-dependent nature of immune response to Hib surface components, particularly the PRP component. The failure to make serum anti-PRP antibodies is typical of the natural delay in immune response of infants to polysaccharide antigens. PRP stimulates B cells but does not adequately activate macrophages and appropriate T-helper cells, and therefore, it is considered to be a T-cell–independent antigen. The characteristics of T-cell–independent antigens include limited immune responses, particularly in young infants; no booster response occurrence with repeated antigenic stimulation; and production of antibody that is of low affinity and mostly consisting of IgM. The development of an Hib vaccine that was more immunogenic and protective for young infants required conversion of PRP from a T-cell–independent antigen to a T-cell–dependent antigen, using the principles of carrier-hapten linkage.

## CLINICAL MANIFESTATIONS

Noninvasive or mucosal infections, including otitis media, sinusitis, bronchitis, and pneumonia, are much more frequent than invasive disease, particularly in the postvaccine era. NTHi seldom causes bacteremia in children beyond the neonatal period. It is therefore presumed that these infections represent extensions of *H influenzae* from the respiratory mucosa to contiguous body sites. Disease is more likely if normal clearance mechanisms or immune function are impaired, such as after viral infection, sinus obstruction, or eustachian tube dysfunction.

### Meningitis

Prior to Hib conjugate vaccines, meningitis was the most common and serious manifestation of invasive Hib disease. The differential diagnosis and clinical manifestations of meningitis are detailed in Chapter 226. The sequelae from Hib meningitis differ in some aspects from other causes of bacterial meningitis. Approximately 30% of children will have seizures at some point in the course of Hib meningitis. Like patients with meningococcal disease, children with Hib bacteremia can have a petechial rash. They can also have a secondary site of infection, such as a septic arthritis or facial cellulitis. Shock is present in approximately 20% of cases. Anemia is common, the result of a combination of accelerated red blood cell destruction and diminished erythropoiesis. Complications of *H influenzae* type b meningitis include subdural effusion or empyema, ischemic or hemorrhagic cortical infarction, cerebritis, ventriculitis, intracerebral abscess, and hydrocephalus. Intravenous antibiotics and supportive care are the mainstays of therapy, but the mortality from Hib meningitis remains approximately 5%, even with prompt diagnosis. Long-term sequelae occur in 15% to 30% of survivors and are manifest as sensorineural hearing loss, language disorders, and developmental disorders. A meta-analyses of randomized controlled clinical trials in children has shown that the incidence of severe hearing loss due to *H influenzae* was decreased by the administration of corticosteroids concomitant with antibiotics, an effect that was more evident in children in high-income countries.

### Epiglottitis

Acute upper airway obstruction caused by Hib infection of the epiglottis and supraglottic tissues is perhaps the most dramatic and rapidly progressive form of disease caused by this organism. In contrast to the peak incidence of meningitis in children younger than 1 year, epiglottitis occurs primarily in older children (2–7 years of age) and usually has an abrupt onset with high fever, dysphagia, drooling, and toxicity. Occasional cases of Hib epiglottitis are still observed in older children who were never fully immunized, and Hib is also an important cause of epiglottitis in adult patients.

Classically, the child with Hib epiglottitis will drool because of an inability to swallow oropharyngeal secretions. Progressive respiratory distress develops over a period of hours with tachypnea, stridor, cyanosis, and retractions. The patient may sit forward with the chin extended to maintain an open airway ("tripod" position). Few conditions produce such a striking constellation of symptoms and findings. A lateral neck radiograph (Fig. 258-2) is helpful if the clinical presentation is subtle, but the study should be performed cautiously and without undue delays, with a physician experienced in airway management in attendance. Diagnostic studies should not delay the need for direct inspection of the epiglottis in the operating room and insertion of an endotracheal tube (Fig. 258-3). The mortality rate is 5% to 10% and is invariably related to poor control of the airway early in illness.

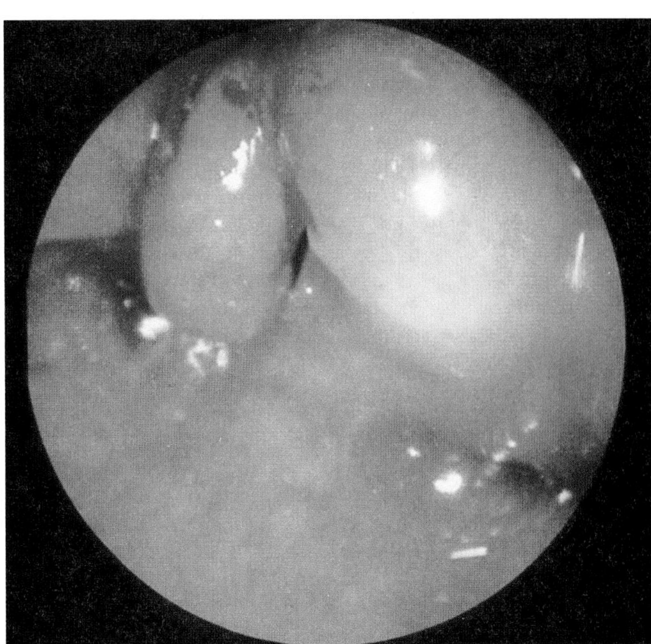

**FIGURE 258-3** Epiglottitis: Endoscopic view of almost complete airway obstruction secondary to epiglottitis. Note the slit-like opening of the airway. (Used with permission from Department of Otolaryngology, Children's Hospital Medical Center, Cincinnati, OH.)

### Septic Arthritis and Osteomyelitis

In the prevaccine era, Hib was the leading cause of septic arthritis in children younger than 2 years. Approximately 8% of *H influenzae* invasive disease presents as septic arthritis, typically affecting large joints such as knees, ankles, hips, or elbows. A contiguous osteomyelitis may be present, but isolated osteomyelitis without an adjacent septic joint is uncommon. Characteristically, there is a preceding nonspecific illness, followed by pain, swelling, and erythema of the involved joint. Clinical signs in children with a septic hip may be less prominent than for other joints, with findings limited to decreased range of motion of the joint, often with the leg abducted at the hip and externally rotated. In some cases, pain is referred from the hip to the lower leg. Septic arthritis of the hip joint requires surgical drainage; the majority of cases involving the shoulder also require open drainage. There is a strong association of septic arthritis with meningitis, necessitating lumbar puncture in these patients.

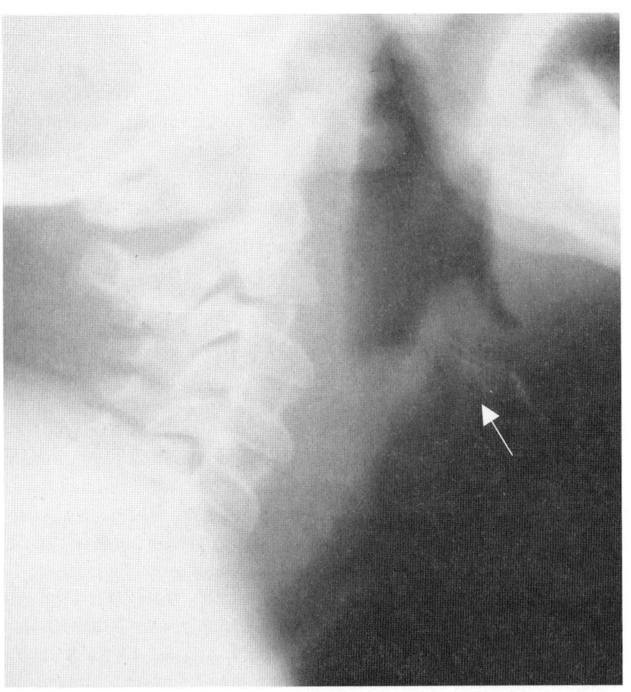

**FIGURE 258-2** Lateral soft tissue radiograph of the neck demonstrating thickening of aryepiglottic folds and thumbprint sign of epiglottis (*arrow*). (Used with permission from Richard M. Ruddy, MD.)

### Cellulitis

Hib cellulitis usually involves the face, head, or neck. The vast majority of cases occur in the first 2 years of life. Buccal cellulitis, seen almost exclusively in children during the first year of life, presents as a raised, warm, tender, and indurated area that progresses to a violaceous hue. The clinical presentation may mimic erysipelas. Periorbital (preseptal) cellulitis is similarly seen in young children and often occurs in the setting of contiguous sinus disease. It must be differentiated by appropriate imaging from the more serious orbital cellulitis. Hib cellulitis is a bacteremic disease, and concomitant meningitis must be excluded by lumbar puncture.

### Occult Bacteremia

Although the vast majority of children with Hib bacteremia present with a focus of infection, occasionally bacteremia can be the sole manifestation of disease in the febrile child. These children are usually younger than 2 years and have temperatures of 39°C (102.2°F) or higher. In the prevaccine era, Hib was the second leading cause of occult bacteremia, behind *Streptococcus pneumoniae*. However, there is an important distinction between Hib and pneumococcal bacteremia; whereas most episodes of untreated occult pneumococcal bacteremia resolve spontaneously without sequelae, 30% to 50% of children with occult Hib bacteremia will develop focal infections, including meningitis. Hence, in any child with a positive blood culture for Hib, the possibility of meningitis must be seriously considered.

### Pneumonia

Hib pneumonia is clinically indistinguishable from other bacterial pneumonias. It was estimated to cause as many as one-third of cases of documented bacterial pneumonias in the prevaccine era. Radiologically, it can appear as a segmental, subsegmental, interstitial, or lobar pattern. There is a strong association with pleural effusion; 50% of cases have evidence of pleural involvement on initial radiographic examination. The most useful diagnostic test is the blood culture, which is positive in almost 90% of cases. Complications of Hib pneumonia include pericarditis, meningitis, and pleural empyema often requiring decortication.

### Pericarditis

The classic presentation of *H influenzae* pericarditis is that of a toxic child with fever, respiratory distress, and a clear chest on examination. Associated conditions include pneumonia and meningitis. Hib pericarditis may become clinically manifest while a child is receiving antibiotic therapy and should be considered in the differential diagnosis of the child with persistent fever while receiving therapy for *H influenzae* meningitis. Although the diagnosis may be suggested after careful inspection of the cardiac silhouette and jugular veins, echocardiography is the best modality for establishing the diagnosis of pericardial effusion. Pericardiocentesis is the diagnostic procedure of choice. Early pericardiectomy, in conjunction with antibiotics, is the treatment of choice.

### Neonatal Disease

In recent years, *H influenzae* has been increasingly recognized as a cause of bacteremia and meningitis in the neonatal period. Neonatal infections are usually caused by nontypeable *H influenzae*, which can also be cultured from the maternal genital tract, the presumed source of the infection. The disease is one of early-onset sepsis, with the majority of cases occurring within the first 24 hours following delivery. Maternal-to-fetal transmission is presumed to occur in utero insofar as the infection is associated with prematurity, low birth weight, and maternal complications such as premature rupture of membranes and chorioamnionitis. Routine therapy with ampicillin and gentamicin for presumptive neonatal sepsis may not be effective if an ampicillin-resistant strain of *H influenzae* has caused the infection.

### Nontypeable Infections

Nontypeable strains of *H influenzae* frequently cause otitis media, sinusitis, conjunctivitis, and bronchitis, the latter in adults. Conjunctivitis is usually bilateral and purulent and is often associated with acute otitis media ("conjunctivitis-otitis" syndrome). Although these respiratory tract infections are common, they are rarely life threatening and are not associated with bacteremia. Prematurity, cerebrospinal fluid (CSF) leak, congenital heart disease, and immunoglobulin deficiency may predispose to invasive disease with nontypeable strains of *H influenzae*. In the absence of these predisposing conditions, nontypeable *H influenzae* systemic infection should prompt an immunologic investigation. Importantly, immunization with conjugate Hib vaccines does not confer protection against nontypeable strains: nontypeable *H influenzae* remains a major cause of otitis media in children and appears to be increasing in prevalence since the introduction of pneumococcal conjugate vaccines. Encapsulated non-Hib strains of *H influenzae* have been identified as causes of invasive disease. One unusual example is Brazilian purpuric fever (BPF), caused by nonserotypeable *H influenzae* biogroup III, which has characteristics identical to the *Haemophilus aegyptius* group and was first recognized in children in southern Brazil. Following an antecedent episode of purulent conjunctivitis, children with BPF become bacteremic and present with fever, shock, and purpura clinically similar to meningococcemia. A single case of the disease was reported in the United States, and no cases of BPF have been reported in Brazil since the 1990s.

## DIAGNOSIS

The primary criterion for the diagnosis of *H influenzae* infection is isolation of the organism from the infectious focus (eg, blood, CSF, or any other site of infection, such as joint, pericardial, or empyema fluid). Patients with epiglottitis usually have positive blood cultures; cultures from the inflamed epiglottis should be obtained only after the airway has been secured. Whenever invasive disease is encountered or meningitis is suspected on clinical grounds, lumbar puncture should be performed. Because the organism is fastidious, specimens should be processed immediately after they are acquired. Gram stain (see Fig. 258-1) should be performed on any body fluid possibly infected with *H influenzae*. Organisms are seen in about 90% of stained CSF smears in patients with meningitis, and the Gram stain appearance of CSF has important implications in the management of pediatric meningitis. Key pathogens to consider in the differential diagnosis include *S pneumoniae* and *Neisseria meningitidis* for central nervous system (CNS) infections, and *Staphylococcus aureus* and *Streptococcus pyogenes* for bone, joint, skin and soft tissue, and epiglottic infections. The appearance of gram-positive cocci in CSF suggests the possibility of pneumococcal meningitis and the possible need for empiric vancomycin therapy, whereas the appearance of organisms consistent with *H influenzae* suggests that antibiotic administration should consider local resistance patterns. The CSF of a child with Hib meningitis characteristically has a marked pleocytosis, a low glucose concentration, and an elevated protein concentration, but these findings are not specific for the diagnosis of Hib meningitis.

For noninvasive infections caused by nontypeable strains of *H influenzae*, antigen detection and blood cultures are of little diagnostic value because bacteremia is rare. The diagnosis is usually clinical, although a microbiological diagnosis can be established for pneumonia/bronchitis by culture of sputum, for otitis media by diagnostic tympanocentesis, for sinusitis by culture of sinus aspirate, and for conjunctivitis by vigorous culture of the eye exudate containing epithelial cells with adherent bacteria.

## TREATMENT

Because bacteremia is central to the pathogenesis of invasive *H influenzae* type b disease, therapy must anticipate the need for adequate CNS penetration and be of sufficient duration to sterilize the primary and any secondary foci. The emergence of antibiotic resistance further necessitates that therapy of invasive infections includes β-lactamase–stable agents. Although touted as an aid to management of otitis media, the antibiotic susceptibility of *H influenzae* isolated from the nasopharynx does not correlate well with middle ear isolates, and nasopharyngeal culturing should not be used.

Because of the emergence of ampicillin-resistant isolates of *H influenzae* in the setting of proven or suspected Hib meningitis, cefotaxime or ceftriaxone is recommended until the antibiotic susceptibility of the organism is known or an alternative diagnosis is established. Both antibiotics have bactericidal activity against Hib, including β-lactamase–producing strains, and both penetrate well into infected CSF. Ceftriaxone is approved for once-daily therapy of meningitis at a dose of 100 mg/kg/d and can be administered by daily intramuscular injections if intravenous access is difficult or used to complete a course of outpatient therapy in the patient who is clinically stable. Empiric therapy with ampicillin alone is not justified because approximately 50% of Hib isolates in the United States are resistant, although it is effective for isolates that are documented to be susceptible. Other extended-generation cephalosporins with indications for meningitis include ceftazidime and cefepime, but because of their overly broad spectrum, they are not desirable choices for therapy of documented Hib meningitis. Vancomycin should be included empirically (until culture results are available) for all cases of pediatric meningitis in those areas of the United States where levels of *S pneumoniae* resistance to penicillin are high and when *S pneumoniae* cannot be excluded.

Meropenem is an acceptable alternative to third-generation cephalosporins with a well-established track record of efficacy for pediatric meningitis, including meningitis caused by Hib. However, meropenem does not appear to have activity for strains of *S pneumoniae* with high-level resistance to penicillins, and therefore should not be used as single-agent therapy when pneumococcal meningitis is suspected.

Cefuroxime has good activity against *H influenzae* and *S aureus* and is a reasonable choice for empiric therapy of some infections when *H influenzae* is in the differential diagnosis, such as pneumonia, cellulitis, or bone and joint infections. However, caution must be taken with this agent if the diagnosis of meningitis has not been excluded because cefuroxime is associated with delayed sterilization of the CSF.

The duration of antibiotic therapy is determined by the site of infection and the clinical response. Children with uncomplicated Hib meningitis can be treated intravenously for 7 to 10 days. Patients with septic arthritis should receive at least 14 to 21 days of therapy in conjunction with appropriate surgical care. Children with pericarditis, empyema, or osteomyelitis may require longer courses of antibiotic treatment. Stepdown from intravenous to oral therapy is determined based on clinical course.

Supportive therapy is also vital in the management of children with invasive Hib disease. The recommended dose of dexamethasone for infants and children with Hib meningitis is 0.6 mg/kg/d divided every 6 hours for 4 days, with the first dose given just before or with the first antibiotic dose. Management of the child with meningitis requires anticipation of complications such as shock, inappropriate antidiuretic hormone secretion, subdural empyema, and secondary foci of infection. Prolonged fever during treatment of Hib meningitis is common and does not imply failure of the antibiotic regimen but should prompt consideration of additional foci of infection (eg, pericarditis, subdural effusion). Children treated with dexamethasone have a shorter duration of fever acutely but are still at risk to develop secondary fevers late in the course of illness.

In children with epiglottitis, the first priority is airway management. Endotracheal intubation is optimally performed in the operating room by an experienced anesthesiologist. If it can be done safely, cultures of the epiglottis may be obtained at this time, and blood cultures should be obtained once the airway is secure. Intravenous antibiotics should be provided as soon as possible.

Surgical drainage may be helpful in patients with joint infections, subdural empyema, pericarditis, or pleural empyema. Arthrocentesis is particularly important with septic arthritis of the hip joint to reduce pressure and to prevent avascular necrosis of the femoral head. Most orthopedic surgeons prefer open drainage of the hip.

Numerous orally administered antimicrobials are available to treat respiratory tract infections caused by nontypeable *H influenzae*. Generally, therapy in this setting is empiric, without specific culture confirmation of *H influenzae* as the etiology. Despite the increasing prevalence of β-lactamase–producing organisms, both among Hib strains and nontypeable *H influenzae*, amoxicillin remains the drug of choice for empiric therapy of acute otitis media and sinusitis because of its low cost and safety. In the United States, approximately 30% to 40% of *H influenzae* isolates produce β-lactamase, so agents with activity against these organisms should be used if amoxicillin therapy fails. Consideration must be given to performance of diagnostic tympanocentesis in such patients, particularly to exclude the possibility of high-level, penicillin-resistant isolates of *S pneumoniae*. Among the available alternative antimicrobials are amoxicillin-clavulanate; macrolides such as azithromycin; and second- and third-generation oral cephalosporins, such as cefuroxime axetil, cefprozil, cefixime, cefpodoxime, and cefdinir.

## PREVENTION

Two modalities are available to prevent Hib disease: chemoprophylaxis to prevent secondary disease and active immunization to prevent endemic disease. The widespread success of immunization has rendered chemoprophylaxis largely of historical interest only.

Many studies have documented the increased risk of invasive disease among household contacts in the month following onset of disease in the index case. The attack rate is a function of age, approaching 4% in children younger than 2 years. Rifampin is the most effective antibiotic for eradicating Hib from the nasopharynx, primarily because of its ability to concentrate in respiratory secretions. Current recommendations call for household contacts of an index case of invasive Hib disease only under certain circumstances. These include a household with at least one contact younger than 4 years of age who is unimmunized or incompletely immunized; a household with a child younger than 12 months of age who has not received the primary Hib vaccine series; or a household with a contact who is an immunocompromised child. For circumstances when 2 or more cases of Hib invasive disease have occurred within 60 days in a preschool or childcare center, contact prophylaxis is recommended and should be managed in consultation with the local public health department.

For individuals who are candidates for prophylaxis, rifampin at a dose of 20 mg/kg (maximum 600 mg) once daily for 4 days should be administered. The quinolones may also be effective, although they are not approved for this use in children. Prophylaxis should be instituted as soon as possible because the risk of secondary disease is greatest during the first few days after disease onset in the index patient. Prophylaxis is most effective if it can be given within 2 weeks of disease onset. Treatment of Hib disease with cefotaxime or ceftriaxone eradicates Hib colonization in the index patient, eliminating the need for prophylaxis when these antibiotics are used.

The first vaccine used in an effort to prevent Hib invasive disease was a purified type b capsular polysaccharide vaccine, introduced in the United States in 1985. After licensure, the majority of studies suggested that protection afforded by this vaccine was, at best, marginal. By 1988, this vaccine was replaced by the more immunogenic conjugate vaccines. These vaccines covalently linked PRP (the process of "conjugation") to an immunogenic carrier protein, in the process creating a semisynthetic carrier-hapten. With these vaccines, much higher levels of antibodies are induced, particularly in infants and young children; booster responses are seen with subsequent injections; and the antibody is predominantly IgG. Six Hib-conjugate vaccines have undergone extensive evaluation in humans and have been licensed for use in infants beginning at 2 months of age. All Hib-conjugate vaccines evoke protective immunity and are considered interchangeable as long as recommendations for a total of 3 doses in the first year of life are followed. Recommendations for Hib vaccination are detailed in Chapter 239.

## SUGGESTED READINGS


Cerquetti M, Giufrè M. Why we need a vaccine for non-typeable *Haemophilus influenzae*. *Hum Vaccin Immunother*. 2016;12:2329-2331.

Davis S, Feikin D, Johnson HL. The effect of *Haemophilus influenzae* type B and pneumococcal conjugate vaccines on childhood meningitis mortality: a systematic review. *BMC Public Health*. 2013; 13(suppl 3):S21.

Duell BL, Su YC, Riesbeck K. Host-pathogen interactions of nontypeable *Haemophilus influenzae*: from commensal to pathogen. *FEBS Lett*. 2016;590:3840-3853.

Gilsdorf JR. What the pediatrician should know about non-typeable *Haemophilus influenzae*. *J Infect*. 2015;71:S10-S14.

Khan MN, Ren D, Kaur R, Basha S, Zagursky R, Pichichero ME. Developing a vaccine to prevent otitis media caused by nontypeable *Haemophilus influenzae*. *Expert Rev Vaccines*. 2016;15:863-878.

Low N, Redmond SM, Rutjes AW, et al. Comparing *Haemophilus influenzae* type b conjugate vaccine schedules: a systematic review and meta-analysis of vaccine trials. *Pediatr Infect Dis J*. 2013;32:1245-1256.

Mohanty S, Gaind R, Paul P, Deb M. Bacteraemic *Haemophilus influenzae* type B pneumonia complicated with empyema: report of a case and review of literature. *J Commun Dis*. 2013;45;95-100.

Murphy TF. Vaccines for nontypeable *Haemophilus influenzae*: the future is now. *Clin Vaccine Immunol*. 2015;22:459-466.

Reilly BK, Reddy SK, Verghese ST. Acute epiglottitis in the era of post-*Haemophilus influenzae* type B (HIB) vaccine. *J Anesth*. 2013;27:316-317.


# 259 *Legionella* Pneumonia

Lorry G. Rubin

## INTRODUCTION

*Legionella pneumophila* was first recognized as the etiology of an outbreak of pneumonia among attendees at a 1976 American Legion convention. Pneumonia caused by *Legionella*, known as Legionnaires' disease or legionellosis, is a relatively common cause of community-acquired pneumonia in adults and is a cause of healthcare-associated pneumonia and pneumonia in immunocompromised adults and children. *Legionella* is also associated with Pontiac fever, an uncommon, short incubation, self-limited influenza-like illness that primarily affects adults, presenting in epidemic form with symptoms of fever, malaise, myalgia, chills, headache, and pleuritic pain.

## PATHOGENESIS AND EPIDEMIOLOGY

Although more than 50 *Legionella* species have been identified, less than one-half have been isolated from humans. *L pneumophila*, comprised of 14 serogroups, is the most virulent species, accounting for the majority of human infections. *L pneumophila* serogroup 1 causes 50% to 90% of human infections, whereas *L pneumophila* serogroup 6, other *L pneumophila* serogroups, and *Legionella longbeachae, Legionella bozemanii, Legionella dumoffi*, and *Legionella micdadei* cause most of the remainder of human infections. These bacilli are nutritionally fastidious, aerobic rods that, after recovery on artificial media, stain as gram negative. *L micdadei* is unique among *Legionella* species in that it can be visualized in specimens using a modified acid-fast stain.

Infection with *Legionella* results from inhalation of contaminated aerosols from environmental or aquatic sources, except for *L longbeachae* that is transmitted via exposure to soil. *Legionella* species are ubiquitous in natural freshwater habitats such as lakes, rivers, and groundwater. From these sources, they gain entry into water systems of buildings, including hospitals. These bacteria grow at temperatures between 30°C (86°F) and 54°C (129°F) and are killed at temperatures above 60°C (140°F). *Legionella* species are facultative intracellular pathogens, surviving and multiplying in both mammalian macrophages and monocytes and in free-living amoebae in the environment. Most cases are sporadic and presumably related to exposure to aerosols of contaminated water in the home including water heaters, particularly electric water heaters; workplace; or public places. Community outbreaks, almost all due to *L pneumophila*, have occurred and have been linked to aerosol-generating machinery such as cooling towers and evaporative condensers; however, showers, respiratory therapy devices, air conditioners, ultrasonic mist machines for vegetables, whirlpool spas, and humidifiers also have been associated with outbreaks. Healthcare-associated infections and outbreaks also occur and are most commonly traced to the water supply, particularly the hot water supply.

*Legionella* are not transmitted from person to person. Most cases of Legionnaires' disease occur in susceptible elderly or middle-age adults and are responsible for 1% to 15% of community-acquired pneumonias in adults that require hospitalization. The incubation period has been estimated to range from 2 to 14 days, with a median of 7 days. The main risk factors in adults are chronic lung disease; immunosuppression, especially associated with corticosteroid treatment, anti–tumor necrosis factor therapy, or organ transplantation; and cigarette smoking.

Legionellosis is uncommon in the pediatric age group. Only 18 (0.36%) of 4954 cases of legionellosis reported to the Centers for Disease Control and Prevention in 2013 were in persons 15 years of age or younger. In pediatric legionellosis, the risk factors for serious infection are immune compromise due to cancer therapy, corticosteroid treatment, primary immune deficiency, organ transplantation, end-stage renal disease, or underlying lung disease including healthcare-associated infection in children on ventilators. *Legionella* pneumonia is increasingly being recognized as a healthcare-associated cause of serious or fatal pneumonia in healthy full-term infants as well as premature infants and those with congenital heart disease. Cases have been related to tap water, humidifiers, and birthing pools. *Legionella* species are probably responsible for 1% to 3% of mild-to-moderately severe community-acquired pneumonias in healthy children. These infections may resolve without antibiotic therapy effective against these pathogens. Subclinical infection probably occurs, as evidenced by serosurvey data that the prevalence of anti-*Legionella* antibody titers increase with age.

The pathogenesis of Pontiac fever may involve a host response to endotoxin from lipopolysaccharide of *Legionella* or other gram-negative bacteria without multiplication of *Legionella*.

## CLINICAL MANIFESTATIONS

The most important clinical presentation of infection in both children and adults with legionellosis is acute pneumonia presenting as an acute febrile illness with cough that may be accompanied by chest pain and progressive respiratory distress. Initially patients may have symptoms not referable to the lungs, such as chills, abdominal pain, myalgias, confusion, malaise, anorexia, and watery diarrhea. However, these clinical findings are not sufficiently specific to differentiate *Legionella* pneumonia from community-acquired or nosocomial pneumonia of other etiologies. Chest radiographs more commonly show evidence of alveolar, rather than interstitial, infiltrates. Disease is usually unilateral but may progress to bilateral disease. Pulmonary nodules with or without cavitation may occur, particularly in immunocompromised hosts. The incidence of pleural effusion is not different from other bacterial pneumonias. Progressive respiratory distress, and often respiratory failure, may develop over several days. Co-pathogens are rarely recovered. *Legionella* infection is relatively common in renal or cardiac transplant patients presenting within several weeks after transplantation with fever and pulmonary nodules on chest radiograph. Alternatively, these patients may have prodromal symptoms of malaise, myalgias, and headache, followed by an abrupt onset of dyspnea, cough, and pleuritic chest pain indicating pneumonia.

In neonates, the clinical presentation is that of acute respiratory distress that often results in a need for mechanical ventilation. Because of the fulminant nature of the infection, the failure to consider this organism, and the uncommon use of empiric antimicrobial therapy active against this pathogen, the diagnosis is established in some infants only at autopsy.

Extrapulmonary infection occurs rarely, with the heart a specific site of infection. In children, extrapulmonary infection has been found in the liver, spleen, and brain. Localized extrapulmonary infection from irrigation of a postoperative wound with *Legionella*-contaminated water has been reported.

## DIAGNOSIS

Specific laboratory diagnosis is established by culture of respiratory tract secretions or tissue (the "gold standard"), by antigen or DNA detection in clinical samples, or by serology. In practice, the vast majority of cases are diagnosed using urinary antigen detection. A useful clue to the diagnosis of *Legionella* pneumonia is the presence of inflammatory cells without bacteria on a Gram-stained preparation of lower respiratory secretions; *Legionella* induce a polymorphonuclear leukocyte inflammatory response, but stain poorly with Gram stain. However, the absence of significant numbers of polymorphonuclear leukocytes does not exclude the diagnosis. *L micdadei* may stain with acid-fast stains.

*Legionella* do not grow on ordinary laboratory media and must be cultured on special medium, most commonly buffered charcoal yeast extract (BCYE) agar enriched with α-ketoglutarate and supplemented with antibiotics. To optimize growth and inhibit overgrowth of other microorganisms present in the clinical specimen that may interfere with recognition of colonies of *Legionella*, sputum may be diluted 1:10 in tryptic soy broth, decontaminated by washing with acid or heating prior to inoculation, and plated on special media. Colonies take an average of 3 days to appear.

Because of the difficulty of recovering the organism in culture, urine antigen detection is frequently used to diagnose legionellosis. Antigen detection tests detect *Legionella* lipopolysaccharide antigens in urine using an enzyme immunoassay or immunochromatographic card assay. These tests are rapid and exhibit very high specificity and sensitivities of up to 80% to 90%, particularly in patients with severe infections, and can detect antigen as early as a few days after onset of infection. These assays primarily detect antigen of *L pneumophila* serogroup 1 but are positive in urine from some patients infected with nonserogroup 1 or with other *Legionella* species. The preferential use of these tests may have resulted in the overrepresentation of *L pneumophila* type 1 in national surveillance data. Antigenuria is typically prolonged beyond resolution of clinical infection and should not be used to judge the adequacy of therapy. Detection of organisms on smears of respiratory secretions using specific antibodies by direct (or indirect) immunofluorescence using polyclonal or monoclonal antibodies is now uncommonly performed because the specificity is technician-dependent and the sensitivity is lower than culture or urine immunoassay.

Nucleic acid amplification–based assays have been developed that are sensitive and specific for detection of *L pneumophila* serogroup 1 alone, *L pneumophila*, or all *Legionella* species primarily in respiratory or blood specimens, but they are not commercially available in the United States. A commercial assay is available for polymerase chain reaction (PCR)-based amplification and detection of *Legionella* DNA in environmental specimens. Serology by indirect immunofluorescence demonstrating a 4-fold rise in antibody titer to more than 1:128 is diagnostic of a recent infection, but neither a single elevated titer nor detection of immunoglobulin (Ig) M antibodies is useful for diagnosis. Furthermore, not all patients seroconvert, and seroconversion may take 6 weeks or longer. Another drawback is that seroconversion is occasionally the result of serologic cross-reaction after infection with another organism (eg, *Pseudomonas* species, *Bacteroides fragilis*, or *Campylobacter jejuni*). Although it has been stated that infected children younger than 1 year do not seroconvert, seroconversion has been documented in several young children with legionellosis. In summary, although culture is the gold standard and has the advantage of detecting non–*L pneumophila* type 1, detection of antigen in urine is the most commonly used test to diagnose infection with *Legionella*.

## TREATMENT

Legionnaires' disease may be fatal; therefore, appropriate therapy should be instituted promptly in suspected cases. Based on extensive but uncontrolled clinical experience, the antibiotic of choice for treatment of *Legionella* infection in children is intravenously administered azithromycin. After a definite clinical response, oral azithromycin may be substituted to complete a 5- to 10-day course. For immunocompromised children and those with severe diseases, fluoroquinolone antibiotics (eg, levofloxacin) are the drug of choice. Unlike azithromycin and erythromycin, fluoroquinolone antibiotics are bactericidal for *Legionella* and may be superior to azalide/macrolide therapy, at least in adults. If levofloxacin or erythromycin is used, a 14- to 21-day course should be completed with the longer courses for patients who are immunocompromised or have severe disease. Limited experience supports the addition of rifampin to azithromycin or a fluoroquinolone and should be considered for patients with severe infections, for those who fail to respond to azithromycin, and for severely immunocompromised patients. When treating a patient with a solid organ transplant, it is important to consider that azithromycin and erythromycin inhibit the metabolism of cyclosporine, and rifampin has the opposite effect. Doxycycline has been used successfully in some patients as has trimethoprim-sulfamethoxazole, including in some patients infected with *L micdadei* or patients who failed treatment with erythromycin. Clinical experience shows that β-lactam antibiotics, clindamycin, and aminoglycosides are ineffective in treating *Legionella* pneumonia.

## PREVENTION

Hospitals with hematopoietic stem cell or solid organ transplantation programs should use sterile water for filling and terminal rinsing of nebulization devices and consider routine testing of water samples by culture for *Legionella* or detecting *Legionella* in water by PCR; nosocomial cases and outbreaks in hospitals should be similarly investigated. For emergency disinfection of the water supply, methods include hyperchlorinating ("shock chlorination") or superheating the water to 60°C (140°F) or higher with flushing of the distal sites. For longer term prevention, methods include copper-silver ionization, maintenance of a hot water temperature above 50°C (with periodic superheating and flushing), chlorination to achieve a free residual chlorine concentration of 1 to 2 mg/L, ultraviolet light, or point-of-use filtration of faucets and shower heads.

## SUGGESTED READINGS


Burdet C, Lepeule R, Duval X, et al. Quinolones versus macrolides in the treatment of legionellosis: a systematic review and meta-analysis. *J Antimicrob Chemother.* 2014;69:2354-2360.

Cunha BA, Burillo A, Bouza E. Legionnaires' disease. *Lancet.* 2016;387:376-385.

Edelstein PH, Lück C. *Legionella.* In: Jorgensen JH, Pfaller MA, Carroll KC, et al, eds. *Manual of Clinical Microbiology.* 11th ed. Washington, DC: American Society for Microbiology; 2015: 887-904.

Gamage SD, Ambrose M, Kralovic SM, Roselle GA. Water safety and *Legionella* in health care: priorities, policy, and practice. *Infect Dis Clin North Am.* 2016;30:689-712.

Lin YE, Stout JE, Yu VL. Controlling *Legionella* in hospital drinking water: an evidence-based review of disinfection methods. *Infect Control Hosp Epidemiol.* 2011;32:166-173.

Mercante JW, Winchell JM. Current and emerging *Legionella* diagnostics for laboratory and outbreak investigations. *Clin Microbiol Rev.* 2015; 28:95-133.

van Heijnsbergen E, Schalk JA, Euser SM, Brandsema PS, den Boer JW, de Roda Husman AM. Confirmed and potential sources of *Legionella* reviewed. *Environ Sci Technol.* 2015;49:4797-4815.


# 260 Leptospirosis

Madan Kumar

## INTRODUCTION

Leptospirosis is a zoonotic illness caused by spirochetes of the genus *Leptospira*. Traditional classification held 1 pathologic species (*Leptospira interrogans*) with separate strains. However, genetic classification has identified at least 19 species (13 pathogenic). Numerous synonyms for the disease were named prior to understanding of the causative agent: Weil disease (used most commonly for the severe icteric form of the disease), swineherd's disease, swamp fever, field fever (Europe), nanukayami, autumnal fever (Japan), canefield fever (Australia), and Fort Bragg fever (United States).

## PATHOGENESIS AND EPIDEMIOLOGY

Humans become infected with leptospirosis via contact with animal urine, either directly or secondarily through contaminated soil or water. *Leptospira* species are very sensitive to acid and perish in solutions of low pH in a few hours; however, in alkaline or neutral medium, they persist for weeks. Infection can be acquired through cut or abraded skin or through respiratory or conjunctival epithelium with immersion. It is more frequent in summer and early fall and has a 3:1 predominance of males. Seventy percent of infections occur in individuals between 10 and 40 years of age.

Leptospirosis is the most common zoonosis in the world and is emerging as a major public health problem. Unfortunately, clinical leptospirosis is not always recognized, and countries with a high disease burden often lack notification systems. As such, it remains an underreported disease, and there are no reliable incidence figures globally. However, in 2009, the World Health Organization established a Leptospirosis Burden Epidemiology Reference Group (LERG). Modeling exercises in their annual reports estimate there are 873,000 cases worldwide and an annual mortality rate of 48,600 individuals.

Reservoir animals for leptospirosis include rodents, cattle, swine, dogs, horses, sheep, and goats. Reservoir animals retain the spirochete in their renal tubules and shed large numbers of these organisms in the urine for months after infection. Aside from contact with these animals, a strong association is also found with the use of rainwater catchment systems, farming, camping, and fishing.

## CLINICAL MANIFESTATIONS

Clinical manifestations vary somewhat with the infecting serogroup. The majority of *Leptospira* infections are subclinical or produce very mild symptoms that would not lead an individual to seek medical attention. Clinically significant leptospirosis is a biphasic disease that develops after a median incubation period of 1 week, with a range of 2 to 30 days. The initial phase, lasting 4 to 7 days, is the septicemic stage. There is sudden onset of fever, headache, myalgia, and gastrointestinal disturbances, such as abdominal pain, nausea, and vomiting. Physical examination usually reveals an acutely ill patient, who may be confused or delirious. Conjunctivitis, uveitis, pharyngeal infection, lymphadenopathy, hepatosplenomegaly, macular exanthem, proteinuria, and icterus may be seen. Up to two-thirds of patients develop abnormal radiographic findings in the lungs. Small nodular densities predominate, but a few patients have larger areas of consolidation. The patient may remain well and comfortable for 1 to 3 days, until the start of the second phase of the disease.

In patients who have symptoms, the second phase begins with meningitis (which may be subclinical) and fever (may be of a lower grade than during the first phase). Examination of the cerebral spinal fluid (CSF) shows features characteristic of aseptic meningitis: mononuclear pleocytosis (usually not exceeding 500 cells/μL), a normal glucose, and an elevated protein concentration. During this phase, the patient no longer has leptospiremia but does have leptospiruria. Because the patient has developed antibodies to the organism by now, this phase is sometimes referred to as the immune stage.

Ten percent of patients develop a severe form of the disease, characterized by prolonged fever, jaundice, azotemia, hemorrhage, vascular collapse, and an altered state of consciousness. Severe disease is mediated by a cytokine storm characterized by high levels of interleukin (IL)-6, tumor necrosis factor-α, and IL-10. The same biphasic pattern of the disease can be seen in this severe form, but the severity of symptoms and their prolongation may last well into the second phase, obscuring the signs that mark the end of the first phase. Thrombocytopenia and renal failure can develop and appear to be correlated, although a causal relationship has not been demonstrated. Other complications include acute acalculous cholecystitis, hydrops of the gallbladder, cholangitis, pancreatitis, and peripheral gangrene.

## DIAGNOSIS

Leptospirosis must be considered in patients with aseptic meningitis, hepatitis, generalized malaise with myalgia, and fever of undetermined origin. Those who have recently returned from tropical environments and have an illness resembling hemorrhagic fever should also be suspected of having leptospirosis. Definitive diagnosis involves demonstrating spirochetes in the patient's blood or urine by culture or by inoculation of guinea pigs, hamsters, or mice, but this method is laborious and prolonged. A rapid diagnosis can be made by determining the specific IgM using the dot enzyme-linked immunosorbent assay (Dot-ELISA) method, which is accurate and inexpensive and is therefore preferable to the older, commonly used microscopic agglutination test (MAT). The Dot-ELISA method is based on a series of leptospiral antigens, may be performed in a routine laboratory, and is more sensitive and easier to perform than the older method. A sensitive polymerase chain reaction (PCR) assay for *Leptospira* species has been applied to human CSF and urine. Although not widely available, sensitivity and specificity are promising. However, PCR-based assays can only identify the infecting organism to the genus level; it cannot distinguish a serovar. For this purpose, the aforementioned MAT is the most accurate.

## TREATMENT

Most cases resolve spontaneously and require only supportive care. Although the efficacy of antimicrobial therapy had been somewhat debated, current evidence suggests it is useful in shortening the duration of illness and reducing the shedding of organisms. Doxycycline, amoxicillin, and azithromycin have been used for outpatient cases. Severe disease requiring hospitalization traditionally has been treated with penicillin G, but can also be managed with ceftriaxone or doxycycline. Immunization of humans with killed, whole-cell vaccines is restricted to individuals in high-risk occupations and in response to floods and epidemics. The limited immunity provided is moderately protective against infections only within the same serovar.

The prognosis depends on 2 principal factors: virulence of the infecting organism and the age of the patient. In anicteric leptospirosis, death is virtually unknown, but in severe disease, case fatality may be as high as 20%. Mortality tends to be higher in the oldest age group and lower in children.

## PREVENTION

Immunization of livestock and dogs can help prevent infections from serovars of the organism contained within the vaccine. Use of the vaccine, however, may not stop the shedding of leptospires in the urine, still allowing contamination of the environment. Swimming should be discouraged in potentially contaminated waters. Doxycycline (200 mg once a week) may provide effective prophylaxis against clinical disease among adults from high-risk groups (eg, swimmers, triathletes) with short-term exposure.

## SUGGESTED READINGS

Abela-Ridder B, Sikkema R, Hartskeerl RA. Estimating the burden of human leptospirosis. *Int J Antimicrob Agents*. 2010;36:S5-S7.

Costa F, Hagan JE, Calcagno J, et al. Global morbidity and mortality of leptospirosis: a systematic review. *PLoS Negl Trop Dis*. 2015; 9:e0003898.

Haake DA, Levett PN. Leptospirosis in humans. *Curr Top Microbiol Immunol*. 2015;387:65-97.

Lau C, Smythe L, Weinstein P. Leptospirosis: an emerging disease in travelers. *Travel Med Infect Dis*. 2010;8:33-39.

Signorini ML, Lottersberger J, Tarabla HD, Vanasco NB. Enzyme-linked immunosorbent assay to diagnose human leptospirosis: a meta-analysis of the published literature. *Epidemiol Infect*. 2013;141:22-32.

Taylor AJ, Paris DH, Newton PN. A systematic review of the mortality from untreated leptospirosis. *PLoS Negl Trop Dis*. 2015;9:e0003866.

World Health Organization. Report of the second meeting of the leptospirosis burden epidemiology reference group. 2011. Available at: http://apps.who.int/iris/bitstream/10665/44588/1/9789241501521_eng.pdf.

Wynwood SJ, Graham GC, Weier SL, Collet TA, McKay DB, Craig SB. Leptospirosis from water sources. *Pathog Glob Health*. 2014;108: 334-338.

# 261 Listeriosis

Andrés E. Alarcón and Barbara A. Jantausch

## INTRODUCTION

*Listeria monocytogenes* is a saprophytic organism (found in multiple environments including water, soil, and decaying vegetation) and a foodborne pathogen that causes disease primarily in pregnant women, the elderly, immunocompromised hosts, and neonates. It has a worldwide distribution and is acquired relatively frequently in developed countries due to consumption of refrigerated, contaminated, ready-to-eat food, mostly dairy products and cold cuts. Listeriosis is a zoonosis of many animal species that can directly transmit infection to humans. In humans, it causes epidemic and sometimes sporadic outbreaks of febrile gastroenteritis.

## PATHOGENESIS AND EPIDEMIOLOGY

*L monocytogenes* is a facultatively anaerobic, gram-positive, motile bacillus, often observed in clinical specimens as gram-variable. Systemic infection results from passage of the organism across the intestinal mucosal barrier by endocytosis, coupled with its ability to evade immune surveillance by cell-to-cell spread; deficiencies in T-cell immunity such as in pregnancy and immunosuppression increase the risk of listeriosis. Extraintestinal disease results from hematogenous dissemination with particular predilection for central nervous system and placental infections. The mode of acquisition in neonates is mainly by vertical transplacental transmission or through the birth canal in parturition.

In 2009 to 2011, there were 1651 reported cases of *Listeria* illness in the United States, with an annual incidence of 0.29 cases per 100,000 population and a case fatality rate of 21%. Adults over 65 years of age accounted for 58% of the cases and pregnant women for 14% of the cases. The majority of nonpregnant patients younger than 65 years of age (74%) were immunocompromised.

## CLINICAL MANIFESTATIONS

Bacteremic illness in a pregnant woman presents with a nonspecific febrile illness (eg, flulike or gastrointestinal symptoms) and may progress to amnionitis, with brown staining of amniotic fluid, preterm labor, or septic abortion in 3 to 7 days. Perinatal listeriosis results in neonatal death or stillbirth in 22% of the cases. Neonatal listeriosis has both early- and late-onset presentations. Neonates with early-onset listeriosis, typically acquired in utero through transplacental transmission, usually present at 1 to 2 days of age with sepsis. Respiratory distress, pneumonia, and, rarely, meningitis and granulomatosis infantisepticum also are described. The latter is manifested by diffuse granulomas in the liver, skin, and placenta as well as other organs in addition to a papular rash on the skin. The fatality rate for early-onset listeriosis is 14% to 56%. Late-onset listeriosis of the neonate can result from infection acquired during passage through the birth canal or through environmental sources or through healthcare-associated acquisition. Late-onset disease typically presents at 2 weeks of age (range, 8–30 days), most commonly as meningitis. The fatality rate for late-onset neonatal listeriosis is approximately 25%.

After the neonatal period, invasive listeriosis most commonly presents in an immunocompromised or elderly patient as bacteremia without a source or as meningitis (30–55% of cases), leading to neurologic sequelae in 30%. Other forms of central nervous system infection include meningoencephalitis, cerebritis, brain stem or spinal cord abscesses, and brain stem involvement (rhombencephalitis).

## DIAGNOSIS

The diagnosis of listeriosis is established by positive blood or cerebrospinal fluid (CSF) cultures. Peripheral leukocytosis is common. In meningitis, the CSF is usually purulent with polymorphonuclear cell predominance, an elevated protein level, and a low or normal glucose. Rarely, the CSF is devoid of inflammatory cells, and CSF Gram stain is positive in only 40% of cases. Concomitant blood cultures are positive in about two-thirds of patients.

## TREATMENT

Although there have been no randomized, well-controlled trials to evaluate a drug of choice or duration of therapy, expert consensus is that the drug of choice for the treatment of listeriosis is ampicillin. Gentamicin is added based on demonstration of synergy in in vitro studies and on animal data only. For patients allergic to penicillin or aminoglycosides, trimethoprim-sulfamethoxazole is the alternative of choice. Cephalosporins have poor activity against *Listeria*. The recommended treatment duration is 14 days for nonmeningitic invasive infection and 21 days for *L monocytogenes* meningitis. Longer courses of treatment are necessary for endocarditis, cerebritis, rhombencephalitis, and brain abscess.

## PREVENTION

Prevention relies on decreasing the risk of exposure. Public health measures to control and monitor contamination of ready-to-eat foods have resulted in a significant decrease in invasive listeriosis since 1996, including a 37% reduction in pregnancy-associated disease. The consumer should thoroughly cook raw food from animal sources, wash raw vegetables, avoid unpasteurized dairy products, avoid contamination of cooking utensils with uncooked foods, use careful handwashing after contact with uncooked food, and disinfect the interior of refrigerators. Leftover food in the refrigerator should be consumed within 3 to 4 days. High-risk persons should also avoid consumption of soft cheeses unless labeled as pasteurized and of hot dogs or cold cuts unless heated thoroughly. (Complete guidance is available at http://www.cdc.gov/listeria/prevention.html.)

## SUGGESTED READINGS


Centers for Disease Control and Prevention. Summary of notifiable diseases, 2014. *MMWR Morb Mort Wkly Rep*. 2016;63:18.

Centers for Disease Control and Prevention. Vital signs: *Listeria* illnesses, deaths and outbreaks: United States, 2009-2011. *MMWR Morb Mort Wkly Rep*. 2013;62:448-452.

Committee on Infectious Diseases. *Listeria monocytogenes* infections. In: Kimberlin DW, Brady MT, Jackson, MA, Long SS, eds. *Report of the Committee on Infectious Diseases: Red Book: 2015*. 30th ed. Elk Grove Village, IL: American Academy of Pediatrics; 2015:513-516.

Okike IO, Lamont RF, Heath PT. Do we really need to worry about *Listeria* in newborn infants? *Pediatr Infect Dis J*. 2013;32:405-406.


# 262 Lyme Disease

Eugene D. Shapiro

## INTRODUCTION

Lyme disease is the most commonly reported vector-borne illness in the United States. It is caused by the spirochete *Borrelia burgdorferi*, and is transmitted to humans through the bite of an *Ixodes* tick.

## PATHOGENESIS AND EPIDEMIOLOGY

*B burgdorferi* is transmitted into the skin while the tick is feeding on its host. Once in the skin, the organism does not produce toxin but is able to produce disease primarily through an immunologic host response. Lyme disease cannot be transmitted either from person-to-person or by direct contact with infected animals. There have been no documented cases of congenital Lyme disease. Transmission in breast milk has not been documented. Although *B burgdorferi* can survive in stored blood for several weeks, there also have not been any documented cases of transmission via blood transfusion.

Since it became a nationally notifiable disease in 1991, the annual number of reported cases of Lyme disease in the United States has more than doubled, with approximately 25,000 new cases reported annually in recent years. More than 90% of the cases of Lyme disease are reported from 10 states along the northeastern and mid-Atlantic seaboard and from Wisconsin. The highest incidence of Lyme disease is in children 5 to 9 years of age. The principal risk factor for acquiring Lyme disease in endemic areas is residence in suburban or rural areas that are wooded or overgrown with brush and are infested by infected vector ticks. The ticks that transmit Lyme disease (*Ixodes scapularis*, the black-legged tick or the deer tick, in the eastern and the midwestern United States, and *Ixodes pacificus*, the western black-legged tick, in the western United States) are found in wooded areas, high grasses, marshes, and gardens. *B burgdorferi* is transmitted to humans while the tick is taking a blood meal.

## CLINICAL MANIFESTATIONS

The clinical manifestations of Lyme disease depend on the stage of the illness—early, localized disease; early, disseminated disease; or late disease. The most common manifestation of early, localized Lyme disease, erythema migrans (EM), appears 3 to 30 days (but typically within 7–14 days) after and at the site of a tick bite (although most often, the bite is not recognized). EM begins as a red macule or papule and usually expands over days to weeks to form a large, annular, erythematous lesion that is at least 5 cm and as much as 70 cm in diameter (median of 15 cm). The rash most often is uniformly erythematous, but it may appear as a "bull's eye" lesion with variable degrees of central clearing (Fig. 262-1). It can vary greatly in shape and, occasionally, may have vesicular or necrotic areas in the center. EM is usually asymptomatic, but may be pruritic or painful and may be accompanied by nonspecific systemic symptoms such as fever, malaise, headache, myalgia, or arthralgia.

The most common manifestation of early, disseminated Lyme disease is multiple EM. The skin lesions, which usually occur from 3 to 5 weeks after the tick bite, are comprised of multiple annular erythematous lesions similar to, but usually smaller than, the primary lesion (Fig. 262-2). Other relatively common manifestations of early, disseminated Lyme disease are cranial nerve palsy, especially facial nerve palsy, and meningitis. Carditis, which usually is manifested by various degrees of heart block, is rare but is another manifestation of this stage of the illness. Systemic symptoms such as myalgia, arthralgia, headache, and fatigue are common at this stage.

Late Lyme disease, which occurs weeks to months after a tick bite, is characterized by arthritis, which is usually monoarticular or oligoarticular and affects the large joints, particularly the knee. Although the affected joint is typically swollen and tender, patients do not have the intense pain associated with septic arthritis. Encephalitis, encephalopathy, and polyneuropathy are also manifestations of late Lyme disease but are extremely rare, especially in children.

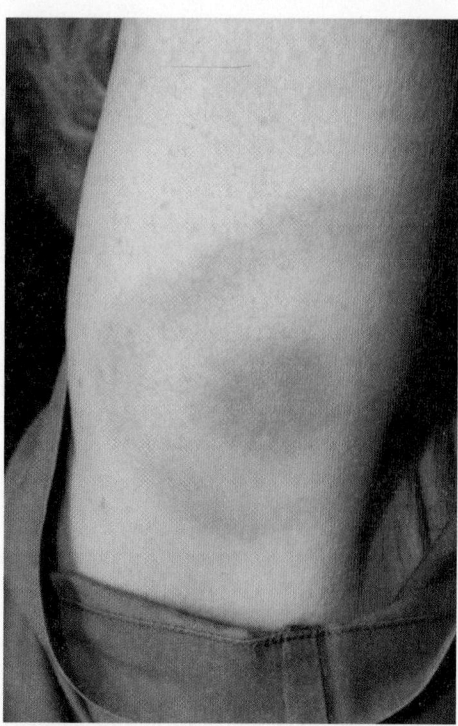

**FIGURE 262-1** Erythema migrans in a patient with Lyme disease. (Reproduced with permission from Centers for Disease Control and Prevention. http://www.cdc.gov/ncidod/dvbid/lyme/ld_LymeDiseaseRashPhotos.ht.)

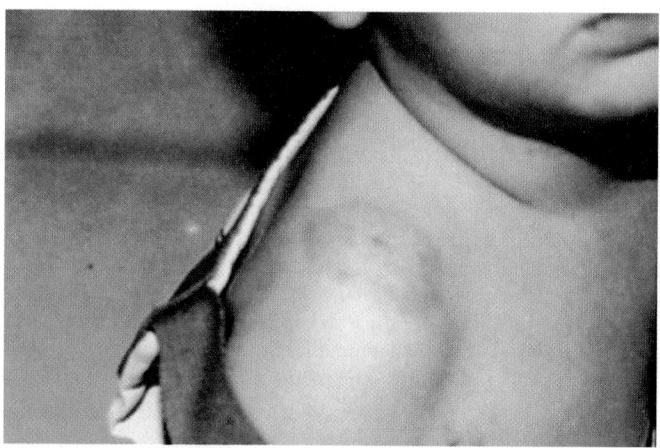

**FIGURE 262-2** Multiple erythema migrans in a patient with Lyme disease.

## DIAGNOSIS

For patients who present with an EM rash (80–90% of patients), the diagnosis should be based on the clinical presentation alone. For patients who do not have EM, the diagnosis also should be based on clinical findings, but support from laboratory tests also is usually necessary to make the diagnosis. Methods for directly detecting *B burgdorferi* in patients (eg, culture, antigen detection, histopathology) generally have poor sensitivity and often require invasive procedures (eg, skin biopsy) to obtain an appropriate specimen to test. Laboratory confirmation usually depends on serologic testing for antibodies to *B burgdorferi*.

While sensitivity and specificity of tests for antibodies may vary, by far the most important factor that determines the predictive value of a test result is the prior probability that the patient has Lyme disease. One exception to this principle is patients with EM. Because the rash usually develops before antibodies to the bacteria are detectable, antibody test results in most patients with EM will be negative. Furthermore, some patients who are treated with antimicrobial agents early in the course of their illness never develop antibodies to *B burgdorferi*. However, most patients with other manifestations of early, disseminated Lyme disease, and virtually all patients with late Lyme disease, have antibodies to *B burgdorferi*. As with other infections, once such antibodies develop, they (both immunoglobulin [Ig] G and IgM antibodies) may persist for many years despite cure of the disease. Consequently, tests for antibodies should not be used to assess the success of treatment.

The enzyme immunosorbent assay (EIA) is the most commonly used test for detection of antibodies to *B burgdorferi*. This test may give false-positive results because of cross-reactive antibodies in patients who do not have Lyme disease. Because the specificity of the EIA is relatively poor, a 2-step approach is recommended for serologic testing for Lyme disease. Sera that are positive or equivocal by a sensitive EIA should then be tested by a standardized Western immunoblot for the presence of antibodies to proteins specific for *B burgdorferi*; if the result of the EIA is negative, a Western blot should not be performed since the result is uninterpretable without a concomitant quantitative test result that is positive or equivocal.

A major problem in diagnosing Lyme disease is the widespread practice of ordering serologic tests in patients with only nonspecific symptoms (eg, fatigue, arthralgia), virtually all of whom will have a low pretest probability of having Lyme disease. Almost all positive serologic test results in such patients are false positives. Patients with Lyme disease almost always have specific signs (eg, EM, facial nerve palsy, arthritis). Although nonspecific symptoms commonly accompany these specific signs, such symptoms are extremely common in the general population and almost never will be the only clinical manifestation of Lyme disease.

## TREATMENT

Table 262-1 lists the recommended treatment for children with Lyme disease. Doxycycline is the drug of choice for treatment of early, localized disease in children 8 years of age or older, and new

**TABLE 262-1 RECOMMENDED TREATMENT OF LYME DISEASE IN CHILDREN**

| Disease Category | Drugs and Dosages |
|---|---|
| **Early, Localized Disease** | |
| All ages[a] | Doxycycline, 4 mg/kg/d in 2 divided doses (maximum, 100 mg/dose) for 10–14 days<br>Amoxicillin, 50 mg/kg/d in 3 divided doses (maximum, 500 mg/dose) for 10–14 days<br>Cefuroxime axetil 30 mg/kg/d in 2 divided doses (maximum, 500 mg/dose) for 10–14 days |
| **Early, Disseminated Disease** | |
| Multiple EM | Same as for early, localized disease for 14–21 days |
| Isolated facial nerve palsy | Same as for early, localized disease for 14–21 days |
| Facial nerve palsy with evidence of central nervous system involvement | Same as for meningitis |
| Carditis | |
| Mild | Same as for early, localized disease for 14–21 days |
| Severe | Same as for meningitis |
| Meningitis | Ceftriaxone, 50–75 mg/kg, IV or IM once daily (maximum, 2 g/d); or penicillin, 200,000–400,000 U/kg/d, IV, in divided doses every 4h (maximum, 18–24 million U/d) for 14 days |
| **Late Disease** | |
| Arthritis | Same as early, localized disease but for 28 days |
| Neurologic disease | Same as for meningitis |

[a]At the time this chapter was going to print, American Academy of Pediatrics 2018 recommendations were to allow use of doxycycline for up to a 14-day course for chlidren of all ages. Readers should consult a current version of the Red Book for definitive recommendations.

EM, erythema migrans; IM, intramuscular; IV, intravenous.

recommendations likely will allow use of doxycycline for children of all ages for up to 14 days (see Table 262-1 footnote). Precautions to avoid exposure to the sun (eg, the use of sunscreen) should be taken because a rash develops in sun-exposed areas in about 20% of persons who take doxycycline (see Table 262-1 footnote). Amoxicillin is recommended for children younger than 8 years and for those who cannot tolerate doxycycline. Cefuroxime axetil is an alternative first-line therapy for Lyme disease. Macrolide antibiotics should be reserved for patients who are unable to tolerate doxycycline, amoxicillin, and cefuroxime axetil, because of limited data that they may be less efficacious. Most experts treat persons with early, localized Lyme disease for 10 to 14 days. EM usually resolves within several days of initiating therapy. Treatment of EM almost always prevents development of later stages of Lyme disease.

Multiple EM and arthritis should be treated with orally administered antimicrobial agents. Most experts also recommend orally administered antimicrobial agents for facial nerve palsy. A lumbar puncture usually is recommended only for patients with facial nerve palsy for whom there also is a strong clinical suspicion of concomitant meningitis. There is evidence from Europe that even meningitis can be safely treated with orally administered doxycycline. For patients with recurrent or persistent arthritis, most recommend a second course of orally administered antibiotics before using a parenterally administered agent. Mild carditis is usually treated orally with doxycycline or amoxicillin. Most experts treat severe carditis with parenterally administered therapy, at least initially. The optimal duration of antimicrobial therapy for the various stages of Lyme disease is not well established, but there is no evidence that children with any manifestation of Lyme disease benefit from either prolonged (> 4 weeks) or multiple courses of either orally or parenterally administered antimicrobial agents.

There is a widespread misconception that Lyme disease is difficult to treat successfully and that persistent or recurrent disease is common. The long-term prognosis for children with either early or late stages of Lyme disease who are treated with appropriate antimicrobial therapy is excellent. The most common reason for a lack of response to appropriate antimicrobial therapy for Lyme disease is misdiagnosis (ie, the patient actually does not have Lyme disease). Approximately 10% of adults and fewer than 5% of children with Lyme arthritis develop inflammatory joint disease (usually the knee) that persists despite appropriate antimicrobial treatment. This "treatment-resistant" arthritis is unlikely to be due to failure to kill the bacteria. It may be due to an autoimmune process or simply to very slow clearance of fragments of killed bacteria. Nonsteroidal anti-inflammatory agents are often helpful in treatment of the arthritis.

It is not uncommon for children with early Lyme disease to have persistence of vague, nonspecific symptoms after completing an appropriate course of antimicrobial therapy. The persistence of such symptoms is not an indication of treatment failure. Within 6 months of completing the initial course of antimicrobial therapy, these vague, nonspecific symptoms will almost always resolve without additional antimicrobial therapy. There is no evidence that "chronic Lyme disease" exists, and there is substantial evidence that it does not.

## PREVENTION

The best currently available method for preventing Lyme disease is to avoid tick-infested areas in areas where Lyme disease is endemic. If this is not possible, a number of measures may help decrease the risk that ticks will attach and subsequently transmit infection. Frequent visual inspection of skin and clothing may help identify ticks before attachment. Transmission of *B burgdorferi* from infected ticks usually requires a prolonged (≥ 48 hours) duration of attachment. Therefore, careful inspection and prompt removal of ticks can substantially reduce the risk of Lyme disease. Use of protective clothing may interfere with attachment of ticks, and wearing light-colored clothing may facilitate the recognition of ticks. Application of repellents that contain DEET (*N,N*-diethyl-*m*-toluamide) or picaridin to the skin provides additional, though transient, protection and is safe when used according to instructions on the label of the product. Repellent sprays that contain permethrin are also effective when applied to clothing. There is evidence that a single dose of 200 mg of doxycycline, administered within 72 hours of recognition of the bite of an *I scapularis* tick, can prevent Lyme disease. However, because the risk of Lyme disease is low after a recognized tick bite, even in highly endemic areas, administration of antimicrobial prophylaxis for a tick bite is not recommended routinely, but only for high-risk bites (eg, for nymphal-stage deer ticks that have been attached for ≥ 36 hours). Serologic tests for Lyme disease either at the time of or subsequent to a recognized tick bite are also not recommended. When preventive measures have failed, morbidity can be substantially reduced by detecting and treating persons with Lyme disease in the early stages. A Lyme disease vaccine was approved in 1999 for persons 15 to 70 years of age, but it was withdrawn from the market in 2002 because of poor sales and litigation.

## SUGGESTED READINGS


Centers for Disease Control and Prevention. Lyme disease. Available at: http://www.cdc.gov/lyme/. Accessed October 16, 2016.

Sanchez E, Vannier E, Wormser GP, Hu LT. Diagnosis, treatment, and prevention of Lyme disease, human granulocytic anaplasmosis, and babesiosis: a review. *JAMA*. 2016;315:1767-1777.

Seriburi V, Ndukwe N, Chang Z, Cox ME, Wormser GP. High frequency of false positive IgM immunoblots for *Borrelia burgdorferi* in clinical practice. *Clin Microbiol Infect*. 2012;18:1236-1240.

Shapiro ED. *Borrelia burgdorferi* (Lyme disease). *Pediatr Rev*. 2014; 35:500-509.

Shapiro ED. Clinical practice: Lyme disease. *N Engl J Med.* 2014; 370:1724-1731.

Warshafsky S, Lee DH, Francois LK, Nowakowski J, Nadelman RB, Wormser GP. Efficacy of antibiotic prophylaxis for the prevention of Lyme disease: an updated systematic review and meta-analysis. *J Antimicrob Chemother.* 2010;65:1137-1144.



# 263 *Moraxella catarrhalis*

Basim I. Asmar

## INTRODUCTION

*Moraxella catarrhalis* is a gram-negative aerobic diplococcus that belongs to the Neisseriaceae family. In the past, it has been known as *Micrococcus catarrhalis, Neisseria catarrhalis,* and *Branhamella catarrhalis.* It commonly inhabits the upper respiratory tract. For many years, it was considered a nonpathogenic member of the resident flora of the nasopharynx. Over the past 30 to 35 years, it has been recognized as a genuine mucosal pathogen and is now considered an important cause of otitis media and sinusitis in healthy children and adults. It also causes lower respiratory tract infections and exacerbation of bronchitis in adults with chronic lung disease. Occasionally, it can cause a variety of severe infections, including septicemia, pneumonia, and meningitis, especially in immunocompromised hosts.

## PATHOGENESIS AND EPIDEMIOLOGY

*M catarrhalis,* an exclusively human pathogen, is an aerobic gram-negative diplococcus that has a striking resemblance to meningococcus and gonococcus, except that it is unencapsulated. After the nasopharynx is colonized, the organism appears to spread contiguously from its respiratory colonizing position to the infection site and cause mainly otitis media and sinusitis in children and less often pneumonia in adults. There is no pathognomic feature of *M catarrhalis* otitis media, sinusitis, or pneumonia. The mode of transmission of the organism is presumed to be direct contact with contaminated respiratory tract secretions and/or droplet spread.

In children, pneumonia may develop in those with intercurrent viral infection, underlying lung disease, prematurity, or immunoglobulin deficiency. Risk factors for development of bacterial tracheitis and pneumonia in children in an intensive care setting include endotracheal intubation and frequent suctioning.

The predominant bacteria associated with otitis media in children are *Streptococcus pneumoniae,* nontypeable *Haemophilus influenzae,* and *M catarrhalis.* Since 1980, there has been an increase in the isolation of *M catarrhalis* from middle ear exudates. Presently, it accounts for 15% to 20% of pathogens recovered from middle ear fluids of children with acute otitis media (AOM); however, these isolation rates might be an underestimation. In a study using polymerase chain reaction (PCR), *M catarrhalis* DNA was detected in 46.4% of 97 middle ear specimens compared to 54.6% for *H influenzae* DNA and 29.9% for *S pneumoniae* DNA. The increase in the isolation rate of *M catarrhalis* has been accompanied by the appearance of β-lactamase-producing strains, which now account for approximately 95% to 100% of the isolates. In a cohort of 306 infants followed from birth through 12 months to determine frequency and duration of nasopharyngeal colonization and risk of AOM and otitis media with effusion (OME), *M catarrhalis* was the most common bacterium isolated. Infants colonized at 3 months of age or younger were at increased risk of AOM and OME. Early colonization with *M catarrhalis* revealed the greatest risk (relative risk [RR] = 1.24), especially for OME (RR = 1.57). A strong relationship was noted between the frequency of colonization and OM ($r = 0.37$, $P < .001$) for each pathogen. *M catarrhalis* is a normal inhabitant of the upper respiratory tract. Nasopharyngeal colonization rate is highest during infancy and early childhood and lowest in adulthood. Colonization rates as high as 36% to 50% in infants and young children and 1% to 3% in adults have been reported. More recently, the widespread use of pneumococcal vaccines has altered nasopharyngeal colonization patterns and caused an increased prevalence of colonization and infection by *M catarrhalis.*

## CLINICAL MANIFESTATIONS

Otitis media is the most frequent infection caused by *M catarrhalis* in children. AOM due to *M catarrhalis* and *H influenzae* is milder than that caused by *S pneumoniae.* However, substantial overlap in clinical severity is observed such that one cannot clinically predict the etiology in an individual patient.

Sinusitis is a very common infection in early childhood, accounting for about 5% to 10% of upper respiratory tract infections. It is often underdiagnosed in children because the symptoms are nonspecific, and diagnosis is difficult without quantitative sinus cultures. In both acute and subacute sinusitis in children, *S pneumoniae, H influenzae,* and *M catarrhalis* are the most frequently isolated pathogens. *S pneumoniae* is found in 30% to 40% of patients, whereas *H influenzae* and *M catarrhalis* each account for about 20% of cases. The clinical manifestations of sinusitis caused by *M catarrhalis* are similar to those caused by *S pneumoniae* and *H influenzae.*

Although bronchopulmonary infections caused by *M catarrhalis* generally have been noted in adults with chronic lung disease, pneumonia also has been reported in children. Lower respiratory tract infections due to *M catarrhalis* appear to be relatively rare during childhood, with most infections occurring in children younger than 1 year. Expectorated sputum and tracheal aspirates are more likely to yield a clinically significant isolate than nasopharyngeal aspirates. Therefore, data concerning the role of *M catarrhalis* in lower respiratory tract infection are not conclusive. Because sputum samples usually are not available in children, most documented pneumonia cases were severe and occurred primarily in immunocompromised patients. In one report, 5 premature infants younger than 6 months with preexisting lung disease were diagnosed as having pneumonia following a 2- to 4-day prodrome of cough, tachypnea, and retractions. *M catarrhalis* was recovered from bronchial aspirations. All patients required assisted ventilation for marked hypoxia. Associated *M catarrhalis* bacteremia has been reported in other patients with pneumonia. In adults, *M catarrhalis* pneumonia is more common in patients with chronic lung disease, acquired immunodeficiency syndrome (AIDS), and malignancy.

Underlying conditions associated with increased predisposition to *M catarrhalis* infections in children include AIDS, leukemia, and immunoglobulin deficiencies. *M catarrhalis* has also been reported as a cause of bacterial tracheitis, as well as a variety of other infections including urethritis, conjunctivitis, pyogenic arthritis, peritonitis, preseptal cellulitis, bacteremia, and urinary tract infection. Meningitis caused by *M catarrhalis* occasionally results from hematogenous spread or as a complication of ventriculoperitoneal shunt infection. Endocarditis is rare, and the few reported cases were associated with a high mortality rate. Urethritis caused by *M catarrhalis* can be mistaken for gonococcal urethritis. Conjunctivitis caused by *M catarrhalis* in the newborn can mimic ophthalmia neonatorum caused by *Neisseria gonorrhoeae.*

Bacteremia caused by *M catarrhalis* is less well understood and has been reported sporadically in a variety of clinical settings, in both children and adults. The clinical severity of *M catarrhalis* bacteremia has varied from self-limited febrile illness to lethal sepsis. Some reviews indicate that a significant proportion of children with *M catarrhalis* bacteremia had an underlying immune defect (eg, malignancy, AIDS, neutropenia, low immunoglobulin G level) or a predisposing respiratory factor (eg, chronic lung disease, tracheostomy, mechanical ventilation). However, some healthy, immunocompetent patients with no predisposing factors have presented with *M catarrhalis* bacteremia. In most such patients, the source of the infection was an upper airway focus (otitis, sinusitis) or pneumonia. Children with *M catarrhalis* bacteremia may present with different clinical manifestations. Some children present with petechial or purpuric rashes resembling infection caused by *N meningitidis*. Other patients present with nonspecific symptoms and no focus of infection, similar to patients with occult pneumococcal bacteremia.

## DIAGNOSIS

*Moraxella* can be recovered by culturing specimens of bodily fluids using blood or chocolate agar. The organism grows as round, gray, opaque, nonhemolytic convex colonies that can be pushed intact over the surface of the agar (ie, hockey puck sign). Recovery can be enhanced by the use of selective media (eg, modified Thayer Martin). Newer molecular techniques such as PCR have been used to help in the diagnosis but are not yet widely available.

## TREATMENT

Presently, almost all *M catarrhalis* isolates are producers of β-lactamases (prevalence > 90%) and therefore resistant to ampicillin. The β-lactamase inhibitors clavulanic acid and sulbactam are active against the β-lactamase enzymes produced by *M catarrhalis*.

In vitro, *M catarrhalis* isolates are generally susceptible to ampicillin/sulbactam and amoxicillin/clavulanic acid, erythromycin, azithromycin, clarithromycin, trimethoprim-sulfamethoxazole, chloramphenicol, tetracycline, aminoglycosides, fluoroquinolones (eg, ciprofloxacin), and both second- and third-generation cephalosporins (cefuroxime, cefaclor, cefprozil, cefpodoxime, cefixime and cefdinir). Most β-lactamase-producing strains respond to treatment with a β-lactam/β-lactamase inhibitor combination, as well as second- and third-generation cephalosporins. Treatment of otitis media and sinusitis, the 2 most common infectious diseases caused by *M catarrhalis* in children, is generally empirical. Therefore, antimicrobial agents that are active against *S pneumoniae* and *H influenzae,* in addition to *M catarrhalis*, are usually administered. However, antimicrobial treatment should be guided by in vitro susceptibility testing, especially for invasive infections. *M catarrhalis* strains are resistant to vancomycin, oxacillin, and clindamycin.

## PREVENTION

The mode of transmission of the organism is by direct contact with contaminated respiratory tract secretions and/or droplet spread. Therefore, good handwashing technique and sterilization of instruments used in intubations and aspiration may reduce or prevent nosocomial infections caused by *M catarrhalis*. Cessation of smoking, as well as prevention of passive smoking, may reduce *M catarrhalis* infections. Presently, no vaccine is available for the prevention of *M catarrhalis* infections.

## SUGGESTED READINGS

Bernhard S, Spaniol V, Aebi C. Molecular pathogenesis of infections caused by *Moraxella catarrhalis* in children. *Swiss Med Wkly.* 2012;142:w13694.

Funaki T, Inoue E, Miyairi I. Clinical characteristics of patients with bacteremia due to *Moraxella catarrhalis* in children: a case-control study. *BMC Infect Dis.* 2016;16:73.

Hassan F. Molecular mechanisms of *Moraxella catarrhalis*-induced otitis media. *Curr Allerg Asthma Rep.* 2013;13:512-517.

Oikawa J, Ishiwada N, Takahashi Y, et al. Changes in nasopharyngeal carriage of *Streptococcus pneumoniae*, *Haemophilus influenzae* and *Moraxella catarrhalis* among health children attending a day-care centre before and after official financial support for the 7-valent pneumococcal conjugate vaccine and *H. influenza*, type b vaccine in Japan. *J Infect Chemother.* 2014;20:146-149.

Su YC, Singh B, Riesbeck K. *Moraxella catarrhalis*: from interactions with the host immune system to vaccine development. *Future Microbiol.* 2012;7:1073-1100.



# 264 Tuberculosis (*Mycobacterium tuberculosis*)

Heather Y. Highsmith and Jeffrey R. Starke

## INTRODUCTION

Despite important advances in its treatment over the past 2 decades, tuberculosis (TB) remains a major infectious disease. Approximately one-third of the world's population harbors *Mycobacterium tuberculosis* and is at risk for developing disease in the near or distant future. The incidence and prevalence of TB increased in the 1990s and 2000s partly due to the human immunodeficiency virus (HIV) epidemic and the prevalence of drug-resistant TB. The failure to control TB in both developed and developing countries represents one of our greatest public health failures.

*M tuberculosis* produces a spectrum of clinical entities that have differing diagnostic and management approaches. TB exposure occurs when one individual has been in recent contact with an individual who has a contagious form of TB disease. The exposed individual has negative tests of infection, a normal chest radiograph, and normal physical exam findings. Whereas adults in this stage usually do not get treated, children under 5 years of age are treated because progression to disease may occur rapidly, even before the tests of infection turn positive. TB infection occurs when an individual has inhaled *M tuberculosis*, has a positive test of infection, has no signs or symptoms of disease, and has a chest radiograph that is normal or only reveals granulomas or calcifications. TB disease occurs when an individual with TB infection develops signs and symptoms and/or radiographic changes characteristic of TB.

## PATHOGENESIS AND EPIDEMIOLOGY

Mycobacteria are nonmotile, non–spore-forming, pleomorphic, weakly gram-positive rods that are typically slender and slightly bent. The cell walls contain lipid and wax that make these organisms more resistant than most others to light, alkali, acid, and the bactericidal action of antibodies. Growth is slow, with a generation time of 14 to 24 hours. Acid fastness, the capacity to perform stable mycolate complexes with certain aryl methane dyes, is the hallmark of mycobacteria. Cells appear red when stained with fuchsin (Ziehl-Neelsen or Kinyoun stain; Fig. 264-1), appear purple with crystal violet, or exhibit yellow-green fluorescence under ultraviolet light (auramine and rhodamine, as in Truant stain). Truant stain is the most sensitive method for visualizing mycobacteria in a clinical specimen.

Identification of mycobacteria species depends on their staining properties and their biochemical and metabolic characteristics.

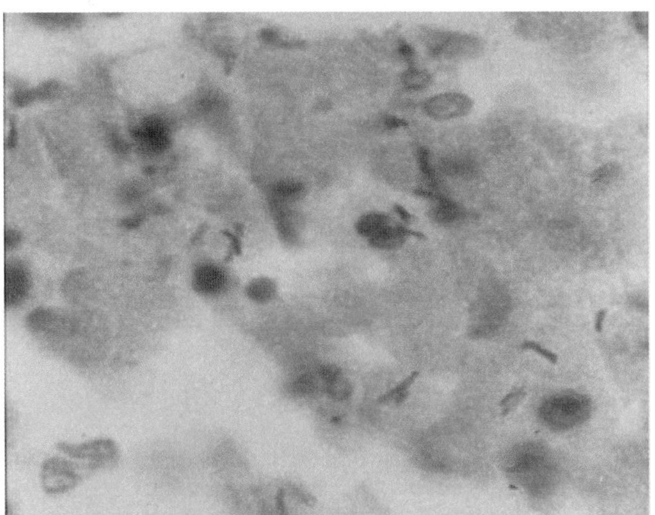

**FIGURE 264-1** *Mycobacterium tuberculosis* on a Kinyoun stain.

Isolation of these obligate aerobes on solid media often takes 3 to 6 weeks, after which the growth can be replated onto solid media with antituberculosis drugs to allow for drug susceptibility testing. Full drug susceptibility results can take up to 2 to 4 additional weeks for drug susceptibility testing. The automated methods using liquid broth allow isolation and identification from clinical specimens and identification of mycobacteria within 7 to 10 days. Other molecular methods of identification are available, including polymerase chain reaction (PCR) techniques that are discussed in the Tests for Disease section.

In more than 95% of cases, the portal of entry for *M tuberculosis* is the lung. Small particles are inhaled beyond the normal clearance mechanisms of the lungs and multiply initially within the alveoli and alveolar ducts. The initial inflammation with polymorphonuclear leukocytes is replaced by epithelioid cell proliferation and the appearance of giant cells with lymphocytic infiltration. Macrophages ingest the bacilli but are not able to kill them initially. Replication of the organisms occurs within the macrophages, which carry some of the organisms through lymphatics to the regional lymph nodes.

As the initial cycle of macrophage ingestion and replication of bacilli continues, development of cutaneous hypersensitivity and cell-mediated immunity occurs most often between 4 and 8 weeks after onset of infection. During this time, the initial focus grows larger and has not yet become encapsulated. Occasionally, this focus is visible on the chest radiograph, but the radiograph usually remains normal and the child is asymptomatic. If adequate immunity is established, the parenchymal portion of the primary complex heals completely by fibrosis and/or calcification after undergoing caseous necrosis and encapsulation.

During the creation of the parenchymal lesion and the accelerated caseation brought on by the development of hypersensitivity, the bacilli from the primary complex spread via the bloodstream and lymphatics to the apices of the lungs, liver, spleen, meninges, peritoneum, lymph nodes, bones, and joints. This dissemination can involve large numbers of bacilli, which leads to disseminated TB disease, which is commonly called miliary disease because of the late radiographic changes in the lungs. More commonly, small numbers of bacilli circulate and leave microscopic foci scattered in various tissues, including superficial and visceral lymph nodes, the meninges, the middle ear, bone and joints, and kidneys. These metastatic foci are usually clinically inapparent, but they may be the origin of either extrapulmonary TB or reactivation pulmonary TB later in life.

In most cases of TB infection in children, the infection is held in check locally and distantly. However, in some individuals, hilar or paratracheal lymph nodes become enlarged by the host inflammatory reaction to the tubercle bacilli (Fig. 264-2A). The nodes may encroach on the regional bronchus or bronchiole. Partial obstruction caused by external compression leads to hyperinflation in the distal lung segment. Inflamed, caseous nodes may attach to the bronchial wall and erode through it, leading to endobronchial TB. Air is reabsorbed beyond this obstruction, and collapse of the segment of the lung occurs. The resulting lesion is a combination of pneumonia and atelectasis, commonly referred to as a collapse-consolidation or segmental lesion. Cavitary lung lesions (Fig. 264-2B) are observed less frequently among children with pulmonary TB than among adults with the disease.

A fairly predictable timetable is apparent for events that may complicate the initial TB infection and complications. Massive lymphohematogenous dissemination leading to tuberculous meningitis and miliary or disseminated disease occur no later than 2 to 6 months after infection. Clinically significant lymph node or endobronchial TB usually appears within 3 to 9 months. Lesions of the bones and joints usually take at least a year to develop, whereas disease of the genitourinary tract may be evident 5 to 25 years after infection.

Extrapulmonary TB occurs when the quiescent disseminated foci of *M tuberculosis* become active. The most common manifestation of extrapulmonary TB is peripheral lymphadenitis, especially of the cervical lymph nodes. Rarely, cutaneous TB can occur when an individual has had infectious substances such as sputum enter through a break in the skin. In areas of the world where *Mycobacterium bovis* infects cattle, children can develop similar peripheral lymphadenitis or abdominal disease from ingesting contaminated milk or cheese. In these situations, *M bovis* forms a primary complex in the oropharynx or intestines and then disseminates to nearby lymph nodes.

Control of the initial infection with the organism requires a complex balance between the host defenses and the organism, with heavy dependence on intact cell-mediated immunity. Macrophages initially ingest the bacilli and present TB antigens to naïve CD4 T cells, which then proliferate and release several cytokines, including interferon-γ, interleukin-2 and -12, and tumor necrosis factor (TNF)-α, among others. These cytokines stimulate the macrophages to effectively contain, if not rid the body of, the infection. In cases when cell-mediated immunity is compromised, as in severe HIV infection or therapy with immunomodulating drugs such as TNF-α antagonists, TB infection can progress to disease quickly. Individuals with cell-mediated immune defects are at increased risk of disseminated and extrapulmonary disease as compared to immunocompetent individuals.

Transmission of *M tuberculosis* is virtually always by person-to-person spread via the respiratory route. Mucous droplets become airborne when the index case coughs, sneezes, laughs, or sings. Infected droplets dry and become droplet nuclei, which remain suspended in the air for hours. Environmental factors, such as poor

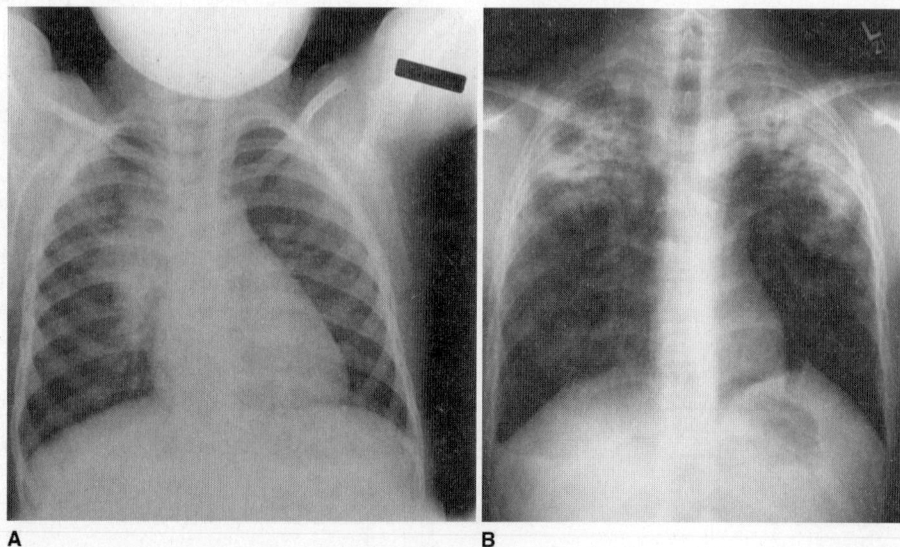


**FIGURE 264-2** **A:** A chest radiograph from a child with early pulmonary tuberculosis demonstrating hilar adenopathy and perihilar infiltrate. **B:** An adolescent with severe bilateral upper lobe tuberculosis, with cavitation on the right side.

air circulation, secondhand smoking, and indoor wood-burning stoves enhance transmission. Rarely, transmission occurs by direct contact with infected body fluids such as urine or purulent sinus tract drainage.

Of the several patient-related factors associated with transmission of *M tuberculosis*, a positive acid-fast smear of the sputum correlates most closely with infectivity. However, adults with a negative acid-fast sputum smear may still be contagious. Extensive epidemiologic studies show that most children with typical TB disease rarely, if ever, infect other children or adults. In the absence of cavitary lesions, which are extremely rare in childhood, the bacilli are relatively sparse in the endobronchial secretions of children with pulmonary TB. When children with TB cough, they rarely produce sputum and lack the tussive force necessary to suspend infectious particles in the air. However, adolescents with reactivation forms of pulmonary TB, particularly if they have pulmonary cavities or extensive infiltrates, may be infectious to others. Many experts initially place hospitalized children with pulmonary TB in respiratory isolation, especially if their parents or adult visitors have not yet been fully evaluated for TB. However, the risk of transmission from the young child with primary TB is remote.

Estimates of the incidence and prevalence of TB depend on the ability of healthcare professionals to diagnose and report cases of TB disease to public health agencies. Due to reasons discussed later in the chapter, TB is a difficult diagnosis to confirm in children, which leads to both misdiagnosis and underreporting. Estimates have improved in the 2010s due to increased age-segregated reporting and mathematical modeling studies. It is estimated that approximately 2 billion people worldwide harbor asymptomatic infection with *M tuberculosis*, including 67 million children. The World Health Organization (WHO) estimates that in 2014, 9.6 million people developed symptomatic disease, including 1 million children. In addition, 1.5 million people died from TB, including 400,000 individuals infected with HIV and 140,000 children. Furthermore, the WHO estimates that there were 480,000 total multidrug-resistant TB (MDR-TB) cases worldwide in 2014, with mathematical modeling studies estimating the number of childhood MDR-TB cases at 25,000 in 2014.

The majority of childhood TB cases occur in Asia, particularly in the Indian subcontinent, and sub-Saharan Africa (Fig. 264-3). In the United States in 2014, there were 460 cases of TB disease in children less than 15 years of age out of 9421 total US cases.

Two elements determine a child's risk for developing TB disease. The first is the likelihood of exposure to an individual with infectious TB, which is primarily determined by the individual's environment. The second is the ability of the person's immune system to control the initial infection and keep it clinically dormant. Without treatment, disease develops in 5% to 10% of immunologically normal adults with TB infection. In young children, the risk is greater; as many as 50% of those younger than 1 year with untreated TB infection develop radiographic or clinical evidence of TB disease. Methods of preventing disease in infected individuals benefit children and adolescents even more than adults.

About 60% of cases of childhood TB occur in infants and children younger than 5 years. The ages of 5 to 14 years are often called the "favored age" because children in this range may become infected, but usually have the lowest rate of TB disease. The gender ratio for TB in children is about 1:1 in contrast to adults, in whom males predominate.

Children acquire *M tuberculosis* from adults in their environment. Environmental risk factors include those characteristics that make it more likely that the child shares the air with an adult with infectious TB. Factors that increase the risk of a child being infected with *M tuberculosis* include (1) birth or travel/residence in a country in which TB is endemic; (2) early childhood environments with exposures to multiple high-risk caregivers, for example, some orphanages; or (3) contact with high-risk adults who have had previous residence in a jail, prison, or high-risk nursing home, and homelessness in some communities. Also included are use of illegal drugs, experience as a healthcare worker who cares for high-risk patients, having unscreened

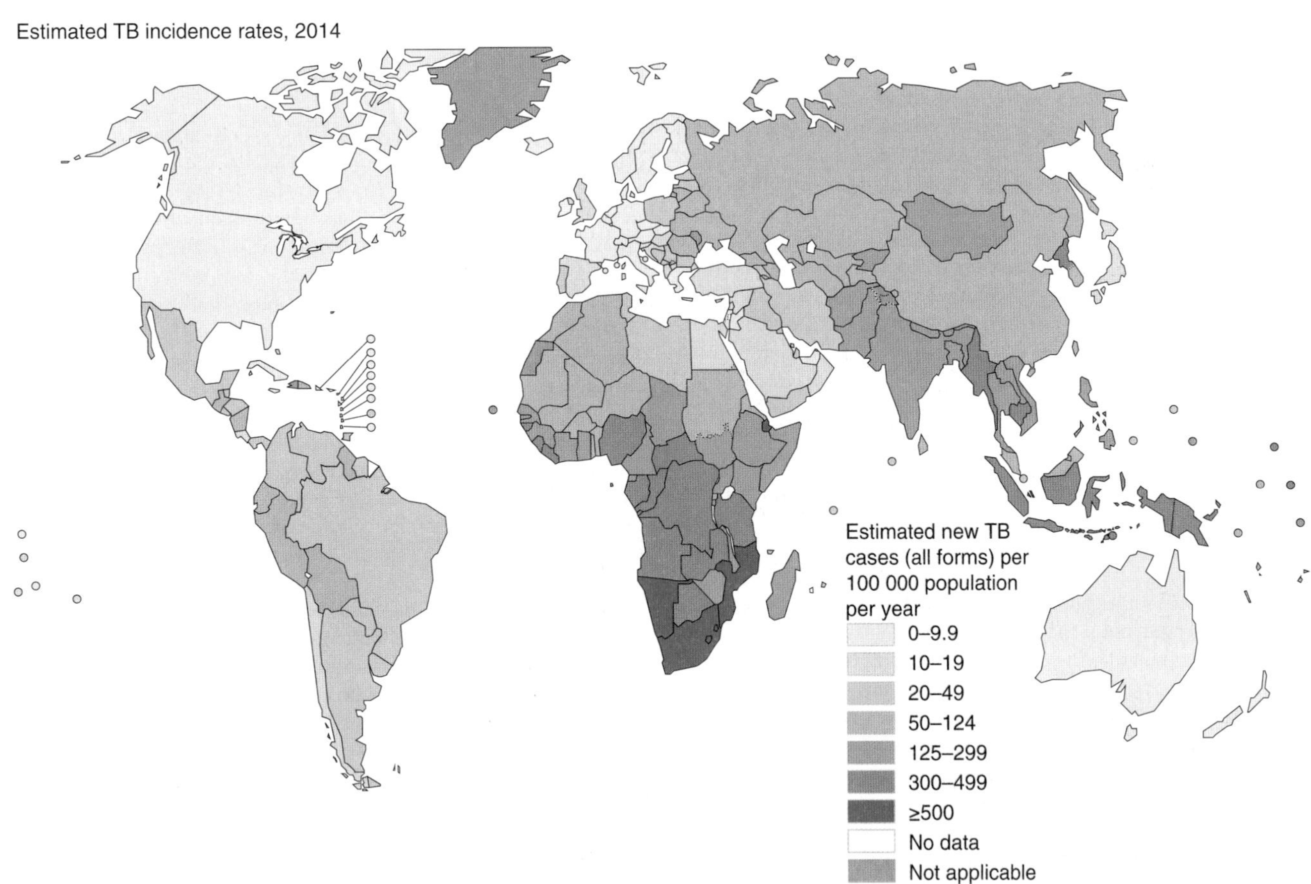


**FIGURE 264-3** Estimated global tuberculosis (TB) disease incidence rates in 2014, from the World Health Organization Global Report 2015. (Reproduced with permission from the World Health Organization Global Report 2015.)

foreign visitors stay in the home, or locally defined risk factors. Factors that increase the risk of developing disease once infected include age younger than 2 years, coinfection with HIV, other immunocompromising diseases or treatments (corticosteroids, TNF-α inhibitors), and malnutrition.

Most children in the United States are infected with *M tuberculosis* in the home, but outbreaks of childhood TB centered in elementary and high schools, nursery schools, family daycare homes, churches, school buses, and stores have occurred. Childhood TB case rates in the United States and in other developed countries are strikingly higher among ethnic and racial minority groups and among the poor. In the United States, approximately 85% of TB cases in children occur among African American, Hispanic, Asian, and Native American children.

The more recent epidemic of HIV infection has 2 major effects on the epidemiology of childhood TB. First, HIV-infected adults with TB may transmit the infection to children, some of whom will develop TB disease. Second, children with HIV infection are at increased risk of progressing to TB disease once infected. TB may be difficult to diagnose in HIV-infected children because of the similarity of its clinical presentation to other opportunistic infections and because of the difficulty in confirming the diagnosis with positive cultures. Children with TB should have HIV serotesting because the 2 infections are linked epidemiologically.

## CLINICAL MANIFESTATIONS

### Tuberculosis Infection

The vast majority of children with TB infection develop no signs or symptoms at any time. Occasionally, the initiation of infection is marked by several days of low-grade fever and mild cough. Rarely, the child experiences a clinically significant disease with high fever, cough, malaise, and flulike symptoms that resolve within a week. These children have a positive test of infection, and the purpose of treating them is to prevent them from developing reactivation TB in the future.

### Tuberculosis Disease

**Pulmonary** The symptoms and physical signs of pulmonary TB in children are surprisingly meager, considering the degree of radiographic changes often seen. The physical manifestations of disease tend to differ by the age of onset. Young infants and adolescents are more likely to have significant signs or symptoms, whereas school-age children usually have clinically silent radiographic disease. In some locales, more than 50% of infants and children with pulmonary TB have no physical findings and are discovered only via active contact tracing of an adult with TB. Infants are more likely to experience signs and symptoms because of their small airway diameters relative to the parenchymal and lymph node changes that occur. Nonproductive cough and mild dyspnea or wheezing, especially at night, are the most common symptoms. Systemic complaints such as fever, night sweats, anorexia, and decreased activity occur less often. Some infants have difficulty gaining weight or develop a true failure-to-thrive presentation that does not improve significantly until after several months of treatment.

Pulmonary signs are even less common. Some young children with bronchial obstruction have signs of air trapping, such as localized wheezing or decreased breath sounds, that may be accompanied by tachypnea or frank respiratory distress. These nonspecific symptoms and signs are sometimes alleviated by antibiotics, suggesting that bacterial superinfection distal to the focus of bronchial obstruction caused by TB has contributed to the clinical presentation of disease.

In chest radiography, the hallmark of pulmonary TB in infants and children is the relatively large size of the hilar or paratracheal lymphadenitis as compared with the less significant size of the initial parenchymal focus (see Fig. 264-2A). Hilar lymphadenopathy is almost invariably present with childhood TB, but it may not be distinct on a plain radiograph when calcification is not present. Significant atelectasis and/or pulmonary infiltrate make it impossible to discern the lymph node enlargement. A computed tomography (CT) scan of the chest may show the adenopathy, but this is rarely required to establish the correct diagnosis. As the hilar or mediastinal lymph nodes continue to enlarge, partial bronchial obstruction caused by external compression from the enlarged nodes causes air trapping, hyperinflation, and even lobar emphysema. As the lymph nodes attach to and infiltrate the bronchial wall, reabsorption of air and atelectasis occurs. The radiographic findings are similar to those caused by aspiration of a foreign body; in effect, the lymph node is acting as the foreign body. Multiple segmental lesions in different lobes may be apparent simultaneously, and segmental atelectasis and hyperinflation lesions can occur together. Children with TB may have the radiographic picture of lobar pneumonia without impressive or specific adenopathy. Rarely, bullous lesions occur in the lungs that can lead to pneumothorax. Enlargement of the subcarinal lymph nodes causes compression of the esophagus and, rarely, a bronchoesophageal fistula. A sign of subcarinal TB is horizontal splaying of the main stem bronchi.

The course of thoracic lymphadenopathy and bronchial obstruction can follow several paths if antituberculosis chemotherapy is not given. In many cases, the segment or lobe reexpands and the radiographic abnormalities resolve completely. However, these children are still at risk for developing reactivation TB later in life. In some cases, this segmental lesion resolves, but residual calcification of the parenchymal focus and regional lymph node occurs. Finally, bronchial obstruction may cause scarring and progressive contraction of the lobe or segment, which may be associated with cylindrical bronchiectasis and chronic pyogenic infection.

A rare but serious complication of TB in children occurs when the parenchymal focus enlarges and develops a large, caseous center. This progressive primary TB presents like bronchopneumonia and may be accompanied by high fever, severe cough, dullness to percussion, rales, and decreased breath sounds. Liquefaction in the center may result in formation of a thin-walled cavity. Before the advent of antituberculosis chemotherapy, the mortality rate of this form of TB was 30% to 50%. With effective treatment, the prognosis is excellent for full recovery.

Adolescents with pulmonary TB may develop segmental lesions with adenopathy typical of initial infection in young children, or apical infiltrates with or without cavitation that are typical of adult reactivation TB (see Fig. 264-2B). Regional lymphadenitis is absent in the latter type of disease. Adolescents with adult-type pulmonary TB often present with cough, fever, weight loss, fatigue, and, eventually, hemoptysis.

**Pleural** Tuberculous pleural effusions, which can be local or general, originate from the discharge of bacilli into the pleural space from a subpleural pulmonary focus or caseated subpleural lymph node. Asymptomatic local pleural effusion is so frequent in childhood pulmonary TB that it is basically a component of the primary complex. Most large and clinically significant effusions occur months to years after the initial infection. Tuberculous pleural effusion is uncommon in children younger than 6 years and rare in those younger than 2 years. Effusions are usually unilateral, but can be bilateral. They are virtually never associated with a segmental pulmonary lesion and are rare in miliary TB.

The clinical onset of tuberculous pleurisy is usually fairly sudden. It is characterized by low to high fever, shortness of breath, chest pain on deep inspiration, dullness to percussion, and diminished breath sounds on the affected side. The presentation is similar to that of pyogenic pleurisy. The fever and other symptoms may last for several weeks after the start of ultimately effective antituberculosis chemotherapy. Although corticosteroids may reduce the clinical symptoms, they have little effect on the ultimate outcome. The tuberculin skin test is positive in only 70% to 80% of cases. The prognosis is excellent, but radiographic resolution may take months. Scoliosis rarely complicates recovery of a long-standing effusion.

**Cardiac** Tuberculous pericarditis occurs in only 0.4% of infected children. It arises from hematogenous dissemination or direct invasion from caseous lymph nodes in the subcarinal area. Pericardial fluid may be serofibrinous or hemorrhagic. However, tubercle bacilli rarely are found on direct smear of the fluid. Extensive fibrosis of the pericardial sac may lead to obliteration with development, usually years later, of constrictive pericarditis. The presenting systems are usually nonspecific: low-grade fever, poor appetite, failure to gain weight, and chest pain. A pericardial friction rub may be heard, or, if a large effusion already is present, distant heart sounds, tachycardia, and narrow pulse pressure may suggest the diagnosis. In the prechemotherapy era, half the patients died; now, with appropriate drugs and use of corticosteroid therapy to diminish the size of the effusion, the prognosis is excellent.

**Disseminated (Miliary)** The lymphohematogenous spread of bacilli that accompanies the initial infection is usually asymptomatic. Patients rarely experience protracted hematogenous TB caused by the intermittent release of tubercle bacilli as a caseous focus erodes through the wall of the blood vessel in the lung. Although the clinical picture may be acute, more often, it is indolent and prolonged, with high fevers accompanying the release of organisms into the bloodstream. Early pulmonary involvement is surprisingly mild, but diffuse lung involvement becomes apparent if treatment is not given promptly. Culture confirmation can be difficult. Bone marrow or liver biopsy with appropriate stains and cultures may be necessary and should be performed if the diagnosis is considered and other tests are unrevealing.

The most common clinically significant form of disseminated TB is miliary disease, which occurs when massive numbers of bacilli are released into the bloodstream, causing disease in at least 2 organs. This form of disease usually occurs within 2 to 6 months of the primary infection. The clinical manifestations are protean, depending on the number of organisms that disseminate and the focus of infection. Lesions are usually larger and more numerous in the lungs, spleen, liver, and bone marrow than in other organs (Fig. 264-4). This form of TB is most common in infants and in malnourished or immunosuppressed patients. The onset of clinical disease is sometimes explosive, with the patient becoming gravely ill in several days. More often, the onset is insidious, with the patient not being able to pinpoint the true time of initial symptoms. The most common signs include malaise, anorexia, weight loss, and low-grade fever. Within several weeks, hepatosplenomegaly and generalized lymphadenopathy develop in about 50% of cases. About this time, the fever may become higher and more sustained, but the chest radiograph is usually normal and respiratory symptoms are few. Within several more days to weeks, the lungs become filled with tubercles, causing dyspnea, cough, rales, and wheezing. As pulmonary disease progresses, alveolar air block syndrome may result in frank respiratory distress, hypoxia, and pneumothorax or pneumomediastinum. Signs or symptoms of meningitis or peritonitis are found in 20% to 40% of patients with advanced disease. Severe headache in a patient with miliary TB usually indicates the presence of meningitis. Abdominal pain or tenderness is usually a sign of tuberculous peritonitis. Choroid tubercles occur in 13% to 87% of patients and are highly specific for miliary TB. Unfortunately, the tuberculin skin test is nonreactive in as many as 50% of patients with advanced disease.

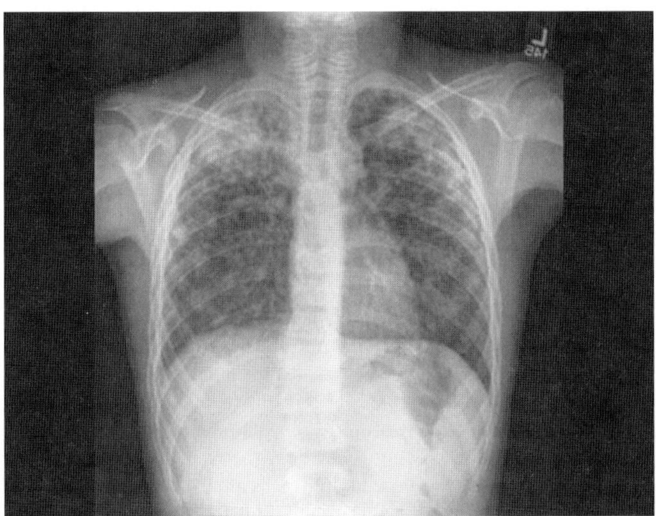

**FIGURE 264-4** A chest radiograph from a child with disseminated (miliary) disease.

**Central Nervous System** Central nervous system TB is the most serious complication in children and is fatal without effective treatment. This condition can arise from massive hematologic dissemination of organisms, but usually arises from the formation of a caseous lesion in the cerebral cortex or meninges that develops during the occult lymphohematogenous dissemination of the initial infection. This lesion, called a *Rich focus,* increases in size and discharges small numbers of tubercle bacilli into the subarachnoid space. The resulting exudate may infiltrate the cortical or meningeal blood vessels, producing inflammation, obstruction, and subsequent infarction of the cerebral cortex. This exudate also interferes with the normal flow of cerebrospinal fluid (CSF) in and out of the ventricular system at the level of the basal cisterns, leading to a communicating hydrocephalus. The combination of vasculitis, infarction, cerebral edema, and hydrocephalus results in severe damage that occurs gradually or rapidly. Abnormalities in electrolyte metabolism, especially hyponatremia caused by syndrome of inappropriate antidiuretic hormone or salt wasting, also contribute to the pathophysiology.

Tuberculous meningitis complicates about 0.3% of untreated TB infections in children. This condition is extremely rare in infants younger than 3 months because pathologic events usually need this much time to develop. It is most common in children between 6 months and 4 years of age.

The clinical progression of tuberculous meningitis may be rapid or gradual. Rapid progression occurs more frequently in infants and young children who may experience symptoms for only several days before the onset of acute hydrocephalus, seizures, and cerebral edema. More often, the signs and symptoms progress slowly over several weeks and can be divided into 3 stages. The first stage, which typically lasts 1 to 2 weeks, is characterized by nonspecific symptoms such as fever, headache, irritability, drowsiness, and malaise. Focal neurologic signs are absent, but infants may experience a stagnation or loss of developmental milestones. The second stage usually begins more abruptly. Lethargy, nuchal rigidity, Kernig and Brudzinski signs, seizures, hypertonia, vomiting, cranial nerve palsies relevant to basilar meningitis, and other focal neurologic signs are apparent. This clinical picture usually correlates with the development of hydrocephalus, increased intracranial pressure, and vasculitis. The third stage is marked by coma, hemiplegia or paraplegia, hypertension, decerebrate posturing, deterioration in vital signs, and, eventually, death. The prognosis of tuberculous meningitis correlates closely with the clinical stage of illness at the time treatment with antituberculosis chemotherapy and corticosteroids begins. The majority of patients in the first stage have an excellent outcome, whereas most patients diagnosed in the third stage who survive have permanent disabilities, including blindness, deafness, paraplegia, and mental retardation. It is imperative that antituberculosis chemotherapy be considered for any child who develops basilar meningitis and hydrocephalus or cerebral infarction with no other apparent etiology. The key to diagnosis is often identifying the adult from whom the child acquired *M tuberculosis.*

Another manifestation of central nervous system TB is the tuberculoma, which presents clinically as a brain tumor. Tuberculomas account for as many as 40% of brain tumors in children in some areas of the world, but they are rare in North America. These lesions, which occur most often in children younger than 10 years, are usually singular, but they may be multiple. In adults, lesions are usually supratentorial, but in children, they are often infratentorial, located at the base of the brain near the cerebellum. The most common symptoms are headache, fever, and seizures. The paradoxical development of tuberculomas in patients with tuberculous meningitis while receiving effective chemotherapy has been recognized since the advent of CT. The cause and nature of these tuberculomas are poorly understood, but their development does not require a change in the therapeutic regimen. Whenever a child with tuberculous meningitis deteriorates or develops focal neurologic findings while on treatment, this phenomenon should be considered. Corticosteroids may help alleviate the occasionally severe clinical signs and symptoms. These lesions may be very slow to resolve clinically, persisting radiographically for months or years.

**Lymph Node** TB of the superficial lymph nodes is the most common form of extrapulmonary TB in children. Most cases occur within 6 to 9 months of the initial infection, although some cases appear years later. The tonsillar, anterior cervical, and submandibular nodes become involved secondary to extension of a primary lesion of the upper lung fields or abdomen. In areas of the world where children ingest unpasteurized products contaminated with *M bovis*, an identical clinical entity can arise from this organism. It is important to distinguish between the 2 pathogens as *M bovis* is inherently resistant to pyrazinamide, one of the first-line antituberculosis medications. Infected nodes in the inguinal, epitrochlear, or axillary regions, which are rare in children, result from regional lymphadenitis associated with TB of the skin or skeletal system.

In the early stages of infection, the lymph nodes usually enlarge gradually. The nodes are firm but not hard, discrete, and nontender. The nodes usually feel fixed to underlying or overlying tissue. Disease is most often unilateral, but bilateral involvement may occur. As infection progresses, multiple nodes are affected, resulting in a mass of matted nodes. Systemic signs and symptoms other than low-grade fever are usually absent. The chest radiograph is usually normal, although adenopathy in the chest may be apparent. Occasionally, the illness is more acute with rapid enlargement of cervical nodes, high fever, tenderness, and fluctuance. The infection may resolve if left untreated, but more often progresses to caseation and necrosis of the lymph node. The capsule of the node breaks down, resulting in the spread of infection to adjacent nodes. The skin overlying the massive nodes becomes thin, shiny, and erythematous. Rupture results in a draining sinus tract that may require surgical removal; if the correct diagnosis is made prior to rupture, however, the process can be cured with antituberculous therapy alone.

**Skeletal** Skeletal TB results from lymphohematogenous seeding of tubercle bacilli during the initial infection. Bone infection also may originate as a result of direct extension from a regional lymph node or a neighboring infected bone. The time interval between infection and clinical disease can be as short as 1 month in cases of tuberculous dactylitis, or as long as 30 months or more for TB of the hip. The infection usually begins in the metaphysis. Granulation tissue and caseation destroy bone by direct infection and by pressure necrosis. Soft tissue abscess and extension of the infection through the epiphysis into the nearby joint often complicate the bony lesion.

Weight-bearing bones and joints are most commonly affected. The majority of cases of bone TB occur in the lower thoracic and upper lumbar vertebrae, causing TB of the spine or Pott disease. Involvement of 2 or more vertebrae is common; these vertebrae are usually contiguous, but there may be skip areas between lesions. Infection in the body of the vertebra leads to bony destruction and collapse. The infection may extend out from the bone, causing a paraspinal, psoas, or retropharyngeal abscess. The most frequent clinical signs and symptoms of tuberculous spondylitis in children are low-grade fever, irritability, and restlessness, especially at night; back pain; and abnormal positioning in gait or refusal to walk. Spinal rigidity may be caused by profound muscle spasm. Other sites of skeletal TB, in approximate order of frequency, are the knee, hip, elbow, and ankle (Fig. 264-5). The degree of involvement can range from mild joint effusion without bone destruction to frank destruction of bone and restriction of the joint caused by chronic fibrosis. The tuberculin skin test is reactive in 80% to 90% of cases, and culture of joint fluid or bone biopsy usually yields the organism.

Tuberculous dactylitis is a form of bone TB that is peculiar to infants and toddlers. Affected children develop distal endarteritis followed by painless swelling and cystic bone lesions in the hands.

**Abdominal and Gastrointestinal** TB of the oral cavity or pharynx is very unusual. TB of the larynx causes chronic hoarseness and is often accompanied by upper-lobe apical pulmonary disease and sputum production in adolescents and adults. TB of the esophagus is very rare in children and may be associated with a tracheoesophageal fistula. Tuberculous peritonitis is uncommon in adolescents and rare in young children. Whereas generalized peritonitis is caused by dissemination of organisms, most localized disease is caused by direct extension from an abdominal lymph node, intestinal focus, or tuberculous salpingitis. Initial pain and abdominal tenderness are mild. Rarely, the lymph nodes, omentum, and peritoneum become matted in children and can be palpated as a "doughy," irregular, nontender mass. Ascites and low-grade fever are common. Tuberculous enteritis is caused by hematogenous dissemination of organisms in most cases. However, ingestion of unpasteurized cow's milk laden with *M bovis* causes an identical clinical picture and is still common in many areas of the world. The jejunum and ileum near Peyer patches and the appendix are the most common sites of involvement. Mesenteric adenitis usually complicates this disease. Lymph nodes may cause intestinal obstruction or erode through the omentum to cause generalized peritonitis. This entity should be considered in any child with chronic gastrointestinal complaints and a reactive tuberculin skin test.

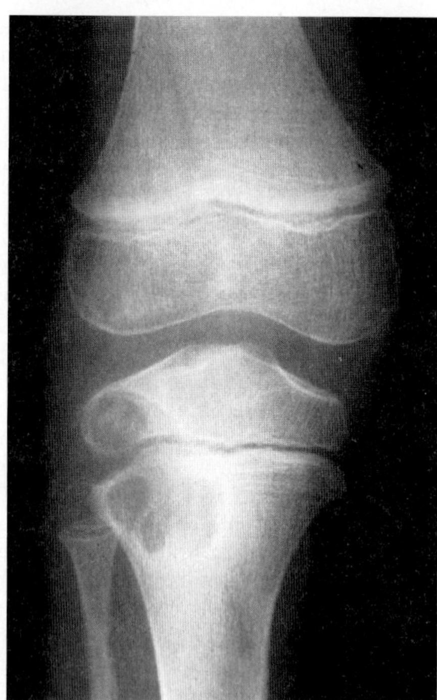

**FIGURE 264-5** Radiograph of tuberculous osteomyelitis in the proximal tibia of a 10-year-old girl. (Reproduced with permission from Skinner HB. *Current Diagnosis & Treatment in Orthopedics*, 4th ed. New York: McGraw-Hill; 2006.)

**Genitourinary** Renal TB is rare in children, and the incubation period is several years or longer. Tubercle bacilli can be isolated from the urine in cases of miliary TB, even in the absence of renal disease. In true renal TB, small caseous tubercles develop in the renal parenchyma and release *M tuberculosis* into the tubules. A mass may develop near the renal cortex that discharges large numbers of bacteria through a fistula into the renal pelvis. Infection can spread locally to the ureters, prostate, or epididymis. Renal TB is often clinically silent in the early stages. The only signs may be sterile pyuria and microscopic hematuria. As the disease progresses, dysuria, flank, or abdominal pain and gross hematuria develop. Superinfection by other bacteria is frequent and may delay recognition of the underlying TB. Hydronephrosis or ureteral stricture may complicate the disease.

TB of the genital tract is uncommon in both males and females before puberty. This condition usually originates from lymphohematogenous spread, but can complicate direct spread from the intestinal tract or bone. In adolescent girls, the fallopian tubes are most often involved, followed by the endometrium, the ovaries, and the cervix. The usual symptoms are low abdominal pain and dysmenorrhea or amenorrhea. Chronic infection usually leads to infertility. Genital TB in adolescent males is rare. Tuberculous orchitis presents as a nodular, painless swelling of the scrotum that is usually unilateral.

**Other Sites** Cutaneous TB, which was more common decades ago, arises as an extension of disease from the primary infection, from hematogenous dissemination, or from hypersensitivity to the bacilli. Skin lesions associated with the initial infection can be caused by direct inoculation of the skin through an abrasion, cut, or insect bite. Regional lymphadenitis is striking, but systemic symptoms are usually absent. The most common form of hypersensitivity lesion is erythema nodosum, which is characterized by large, painful, purple-brown, indurated nodules on the shins and forearms. Scrofuloderma occurs when a caseous lymph node ruptures to the outside and leaves an ulcer or sinus tract. Papulonecrotic tuberculids are miliary lesions of the skin that appear most frequently on the face, trunk, and upper thighs. Their characteristic "apple jelly" center is best demonstrated by placing a glass slide over the lesions. Tuberculosis verrucosa cutis is a wartlike lesion, most common on the arms or legs, caused by auto-inoculation of bacilli in a person already sensitized to the organism.

Ocular TB is very rare in children. This condition usually involves the conjunctiva or cornea and results from direct inoculation. Unilateral redness and lacrimation are often associated with enlargement of the preauricular, submandibular, or cervical lymph nodes. Iritis can also occur in conjunction with systemic TB. Frequently individuals will suffer from pain and blurry vision, with constricted or poorly reactive pupils. Typically, iritis is a unilateral process.

TB of the middle ear results from a primary focus in neonates who aspirate infected amniotic fluid or from hematogenous dissemination in older children. The most common signs and symptoms are painless otorrhea, tinnitus, decreased hearing, facial paralysis, and perforated tympanic membrane. Enlargement of local lymph nodes may accompany infection. Diagnosis can be difficult because stain and cultures of material from the ear are frequently negative, and the histology of affected tissue usually shows acute and chronic inflammation without granuloma formation.

**Congenital Tuberculosis** True congenital TB is exceedingly rare, with less than 400 cases reported. *M tuberculosis* can pass from the placenta to the fetus through the umbilical vein. The mothers of these infected infants frequently suffer from tuberculous pleural effusion, meningitis, or disseminated disease during pregnancy or soon afterward. However, the diagnosis of TB in the newborn often leads to the discovery of the mother's TB. Initial infection in the mother just before or during pregnancy is more likely to lead to congenital infection than previous infection. However, even massive involvement of the placenta with TB does not usually give rise to congenital infection. The tubercle bacilli first reach the fetal liver, where an initial focus develops with associated involvement of regional lymph nodes. Organisms then pass through the liver into the main fetal circulation, leading to foci in the lung and other tissues. The bacilli in the lung usually remain dormant until after birth, when oxygenation and pulmonary circulation increase significantly. Congenital TB also may occur by aspiration or ingestion of infected amniotic fluid if a caseous placental lesion ruptures directly into the amniotic cavity.

Symptoms of true congenital TB may be present at birth, but more commonly begin in the second or third week of life. The most common signs and symptoms, in order of frequency, are respiratory distress, fever, hepatic or splenic enlargement, poor feeding, lethargy or irritability, lymphadenopathy, abdominal distention, failure to thrive, ear drainage, and skin lesions. Many infants have an abnormal chest radiograph, most often a miliary pattern. Only one-third of affected infants have meningitis. This clinical presentation in newborns is similar to that caused by bacterial sepsis and other congenital infections. The diagnosis of neonatal TB should be suspected in an infant with signs and symptoms of bacterial or congenital infection whose response to antibiotic and supportive therapy is poor and whose mother has risk factors for developing TB.

**Tuberculosis in Adolescents** There are no global estimates of TB disease in adolescents, as the definition of the adolescent time period varies across cultures. Internationally, childhood TB is defined as TB in individuals less than 15 years of age, and TB in children older than 15 is reported in aggregate with adults. In the United States, adolescents age 13 to 17 years account for 30% of all pediatric TB cases, with the majority of cases occurring in foreign-born adolescents. Compared to younger school-age children, adolescents have an increased risk of progression from infection to disease, and for unknown reasons, the risk is higher for girls than for boys.

TB disease in adolescents typically presents as pulmonary disease or peripheral lymphadenitis, but other forms of extrapulmonary disease, including those types with long incubation periods, can also occur. Genitourinary disease, with an incubation period of 4 to 5 years, is the second most common presentation of extrapulmonary TB in adolescents. Adolescents with pulmonary TB frequently will have constitutional symptoms and cough but rarely develop night sweats and hemoptysis. Up to one-third of adolescents with pulmonary TB have cavities on chest radiograph, and these adolescents can transmit TB to others (Fig. 264-2B). Pleural effusions are fairly common in adolescents and can also occur in the presence or absence of parenchymal lung disease.

**Tuberculosis and HIV Infection** In general, the clinical presentation of TB in children with HIV infection is similar to that in children without HIV infection. However, children with HIV infection more commonly have extrapulmonary TB (especially meningitis, tuberculoma, and abdominal disease), and pulmonary TB has a more aggressive picture, more often leading to substantial infiltrates or cavitation within the lung. Establishing the diagnosis of TB in an HIV-infected child can be difficult because the skin test is often negative, microbiologic confirmation of disease is difficult to achieve in many cases, and other opportunistic conditions can mimic TB. An aggressive evaluation for TB should be undertaken for any child with known HIV infection, or risk factors for HIV infection, who develops pulmonary disease or any unusual constellation of signs and symptoms.

## DIAGNOSIS

### General Tests

There are 2 primary ways in which a child with TB can be discovered. The first is when TB is considered part of the differential diagnosis of a symptomatic child. This passive discovery is usually the only means of diagnosis in resource-poor countries, and children often have advanced disease. The second is when children with TB in developed countries are discovered through contact investigations of adults who are believed to have infectious TB. In these cases, children usually have relatively asymptomatic disease that would have either progressed or escaped detection if the contact tracing had not occurred. The importance of the epidemiologic setting of the child in establishing the diagnosis of TB cannot be overemphasized. Often, the most important maneuver in determining whether the child has TB is testing the adults in close contact with the child to determine whether any adult has or recently has had infectious pulmonary TB.

General laboratory and other tests are usually unrevealing for children with TB. Screening tests such as a complete blood count and differential, erythrocyte sedimentation rate, and blood chemistries are usually normal. When considering a diagnosis of extrapulmonary TB, analysis of appropriate tissue or fluids often leads to establishing the correct diagnosis. In cases of tuberculous meningitis, the CSF leukocyte count usually ranges from 10 to 500 cells/μL, but is occasionally higher. Polymorphonuclear leukocytes may be common initially, but in a majority of cases, lymphocytes are predominant. The CSF glucose level is typically less than 40 mg/dL, but rarely goes below 20 mg/dL. The protein level is elevated and may be markedly high (400–5000 mg/dL) secondary to hydrocephalus and spinal block. Although the lumbar CSF is grossly abnormal, ventricular CSF may have normal chemistries and cell counts because samples are obtained proximal to the site of obstruction.

In cases of pleural TB, the pleural fluid usually yields results indicative of a mild exudate: specific gravity is 1.012 to 1.025, the protein level is usually 2 to 4 g/dL, and the glucose may be low, although it is often in the low-normal range (20–40 mg/dL). There are typically several hundred to several thousand white blood cells per microliter, with an early predominance of polymorphonuclear cells followed by a high concentration of lymphocytes. Biopsy of the pleura may show evidence of granuloma formation and the organisms.

### Tests of Infection

**Tuberculin Skin Testing** A positive tuberculin skin test (TST) is the hallmark of infection with *M tuberculosis.* The definitive test is the Mantoux skin test technique, which in the United States involves intradermal injection of 0.1 mL of purified protein derivative containing 5 tuberculin units. The results are interpreted as the transverse diameter of induration present 48 to 72 hours after injection (Fig. 264-6). A variety of host-related factors—including very young age, malnutrition, immunosuppression by disease or drugs, viral infection, measles vaccination, and overwhelming TB—can depress tuberculin reactivity in a child infected with *M tuberculosis.* Approximately 10% of immunocompetent children with TB disease do not react initially to a TST; however, most become reactive after several months of treatment, suggesting that the disease contributed to this anergy. Anergy with TB may be global or specific to tuberculin, so a positive control skin test with a negative tuberculin test never rules out TB disease. False-positive reactions to a TST can be caused by cross-sensitization to antigens of nontuberculous mycobacteria or, in some cases, previous immunization with bacille Calmette-Guérin (BCG) vaccine. No reliable method distinguishes tuberculin reactions caused by a BCG vaccination from those resulting from infection with *M tuberculosis.* However, many infants who receive a BCG vaccine never develop a positive tuberculin reaction. When a reaction does occur, the induration is often less than 10 mm, and the reaction tends to wane after several years. One study of BCG cross-reaction in Native American children vaccinated at birth showed that all positive TST reactions occurred within the first 6 months after vaccination. In general, a reactive area of 10 mm or more in a BCG-vaccinated child indicates infection with *M tuberculosis* and necessitates further diagnostic evaluation and treatment. A history of prior BCG vaccination is never a contraindication to tuberculin testing.

The interpretation of the TST should be influenced by the purpose for which the test was given and the consequences of false classification. Because there is always some overlap in reactions to the TST between groups of individuals with and without infection with *M tuberculosis,* false-positive and false-negative results always occur within a population. To try to minimize false results, reaction size limits for determining a positive result are made. Patients are then stratified by risk of infection (Table 264-1). For adults and children at the highest risk of having infection progress to disease, a reactive area of at least 5 mm is classified as a positive result. For other high-risk groups, including children younger than 4 years, a reactive area of at least 10 mm is considered positive. For all other low-risk persons, the cutoff point for a positive reaction is raised to 15 mm. The key to this scheme is obtaining an adequate history of possible risk factors for acquiring infection with *M tuberculosis.* Classifying children by this scheme depends on the willingness and ability of the clinician and family to create a thorough history for the child and for the adults who are in the child's environment. In general, tuberculin skin testing of low-risk children yields few positive results, and in low-prevalence populations, the majority of these positive results will be false positive (see Table 264-1).

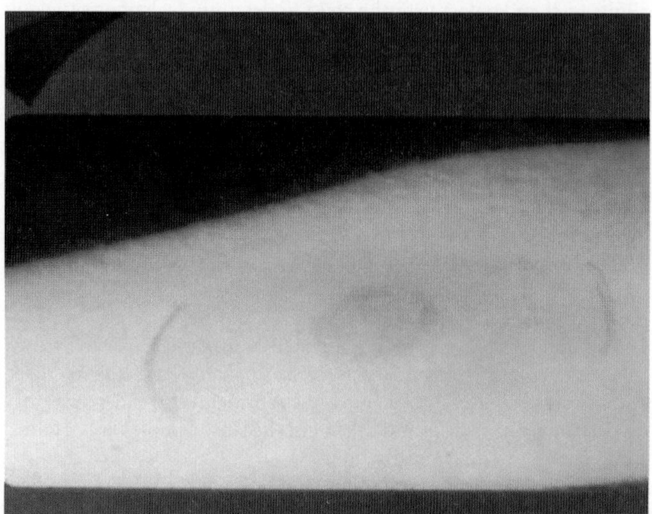

**FIGURE 264-6** An image showing a positive tuberculin skin test. The ink marks on either side denote the area of induration as opposed to the area of erythema. The area of induration is the area to be measured.

**TABLE 264-1 AMOUNT OF INDURATION THAT DEFINES A POSITIVE MANTOUX TUBERCULOSIS SKIN TEST**

| Reaction Size | Risk Factors |
|---|---|
| ≥ 5 mm | Contacts of infectious cases |
| | Abnormal chest radiograph |
| | Human immunodeficiency virus infection or other immunocompromise |
| ≥ 10 mm | Birth or previous residence in a high-prevalence country |
| | Certain medical risk factors: diabetes mellitus, silicosis, renal disease |
| | Occupation in health case field; exposure to tuberculosis patients |
| | Member of a locally defined high-risk group |
| | Close contact of a high-risk adult (except healthcare workers) |
| | Age < 4 years |
| ≥ 15 mm | No risk factors |

**Interferon-γ Release Assays** Advances in molecular biology and genomics have led to alternatives to the TST: the interferon (IFN)-γ release assays (IGRAs). The first test, QuantiFERON-TB (QFT; Cellestis, Carnegie, Australia), measures whole-blood IFN-γ production by enzyme-linked immunosorbent assay after stimulation of lymphocytes ex vivo by 3 proteins: early secreted antigen target-6 (ESAT-6), culture filtrate protein-10 (CFP-10), and TB 7.7. The second format is the enzyme-linked immunospot (ELISPOT) (T-SPOT.*TB*; Oxford Immunotec, Abindgon, United Kingdom), which detects the number of T cells that produce INF-γ after stimulation with ESAT-6 and CFP-10. The proteins used to stimulate INF-γ production are not found in BCG vaccine strains or most common nontuberculous mycobacteria, such as *Mycobacterium avium* complex. Due to this lack of cross-reactivity, these tests have higher specificity than the TST.

Both IGRAs contain negative and positive controls in addition to the *M tuberculosis*–specific antigens. These are used in test interpretation. A positive result is defined as when the difference in the amount of IFN-γ measured between the test antigen and the negative control is greater than a certain threshold: over 8 spots in T-SPOT.*TB* and greater than 0.35 IU/mL in QFT. Too much IFN-γ response to the negative control or too little response to the positive control yields indeterminate (QFT) or invalid (T-SPOT.*TB*) results. For the QFT, failure to shake the sample as per manufacturer instruction increases the likelihood of an indeterminate result. Other factors associated with indeterminate results include young age and immunocompromised status.

In many clinical situations, these tests have a higher specificity than the TST, better correlation with surrogate measures of recent exposure to *M tuberculosis* in low-incidence settings, and less cross-reactivity than the TST with previous BCG vaccination. Two clear advantages of the IGRAs are the need for only 1 patient encounter (2 with the TST) and the lack of possible boosting of the result because the patient is not exposed to any biologic material. However, the sensitivity of IGRAs is similar to the TST, which ranges from 50% to 84% in studies of culture-proven TB disease in children.

IFN release assays are being increasingly used and are recommended by the Centers for Disease Control and Prevention (CDC) and the

American Academy of Pediatrics (AAP) for BCG-vaccinated children over the age of 4 years. The AAP recommends to do *either* an IGRA or a TST if the child who already is or is about to be immunocompromised has no known risk factors for TB, but do *both* the TST and an IGRA and pursue a positive result with either test (to maximize sensitivity) if the child has at least 1 risk factor. Furthermore, there is a relative lack of data concerning the reliability of negative IGRA results in very young children; as these children are at increased risk for progression to disease, the AAP recommends against the routine use of IGRAs to detect infection in children under the age of 2 years. The AAP provides an algorithm as a guide for the appropriate use of IGRAs in children with at least 1 risk factor for TB infection (Fig. 264-7).

#### Tests for Disease

**Acid-Fast Stains and Cultures** The most important laboratory tests for the diagnosis of TB are the acid-fast stain and mycobacterial culture. The traditional culture specimen for pulmonary TB in a child has been the early-morning gastric aspirate obtained before the child has risen and before peristalsis has emptied the stomach of the pooled secretions that were swallowed overnight. In general, acquisition of these samples has required hospitalization. Unfortunately, even under optimal conditions, 3 gastric aspirates yield *M tuberculosis* in less than 50% of cases; in clinical practice, the yield is usually lower. Therefore, negative cultures never exclude the diagnosis of TB in a child. The culture yield from bronchoscopy in children with TB is usually less than the yield from properly obtained gastric samples. However, bronchoscopy can be useful to define the anatomy of the airways and helps to distinguish TB from other pulmonary diseases. Recent studies have demonstrated that the culture yield from one outpatient-induced sputum (using warm nebulized saline and a suction catheter to capture the mucus) is equal to that for several inpatient gastric aspirates in children with extensive pulmonary disease. With practice, sputum can be induced from children as young as 18 months of age.

Fortunately, the need for culture confirmation in children with TB is not always necessary. If a child has a positive test of infection, clinical or radiographic findings suggestive of TB, and known

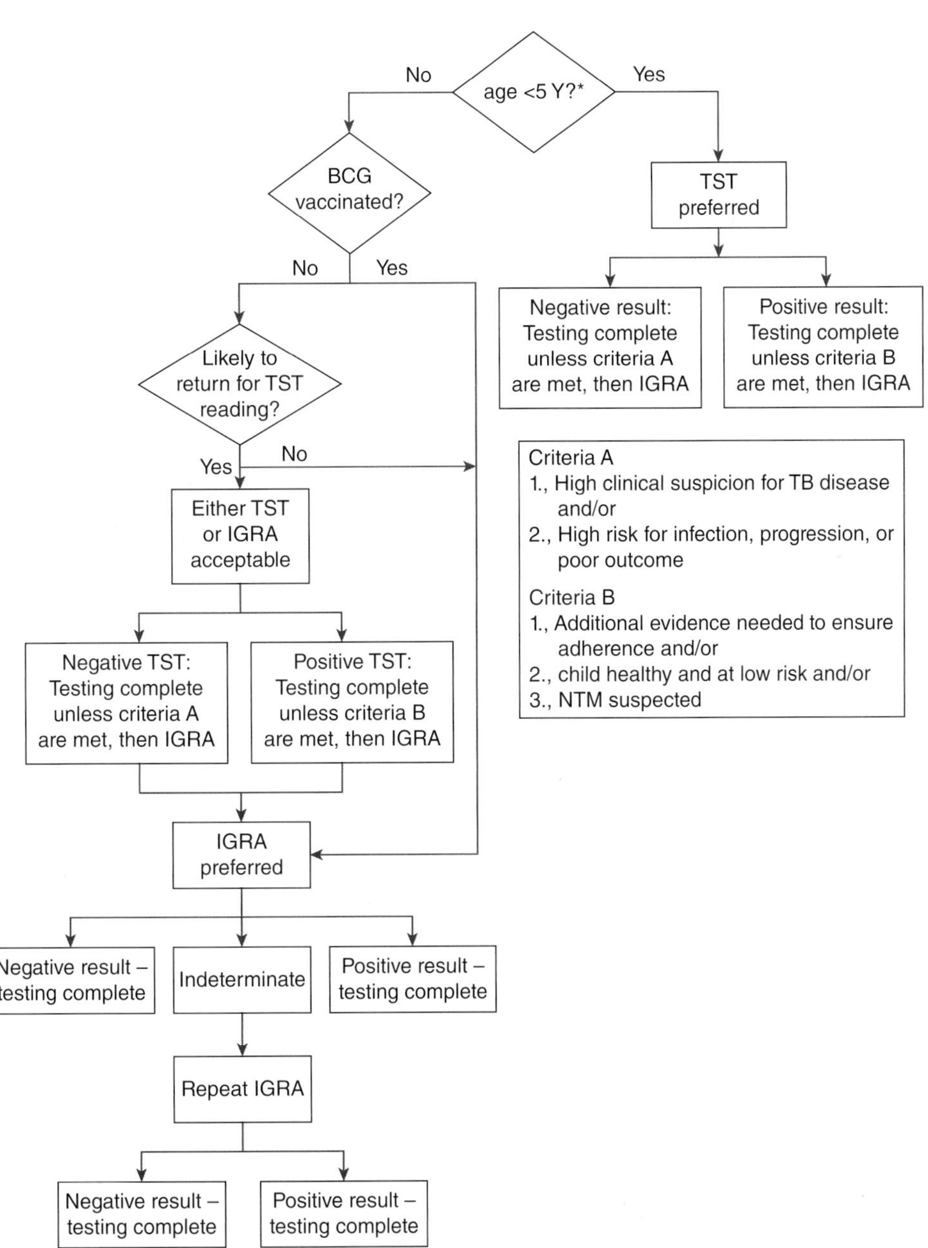


**FIGURE 264-7** An algorithm provided for the use of tuberculin skin tests (TSTs) and interferon-γ release assays (IGRAs) in children with at least 1 risk factor for tuberculosis (TB) infection. BCG, bacille Calmette-Guérin; NTM, nontuberculous *Mycobacterium*. *New data may allow lowering the age for use of IGRAs to children as young as 2 years. Readers should consult a current edition of the American Academy of Pediatrics Red Book for best advice. (Reproduced with permission from Starke JR; Committee On Infectious Diseases. *Pediatrics*: Interferon-γ release assays for diagnosis of tuberculosis infection and disease in children, 2014 Dec;134(6):e1763-e1773.)

contact with an adult case of TB, the child should be treated for TB disease. The drug susceptibility test results from the adult case can be used to determine the best therapeutic regimen for the child. Cultures always should be obtained from a child with suspected TB when the source case is not known or when the source case has a drug-resistant isolate.

Unfortunately, acid-fast stain of various fluids and tissues from children with TB disease is often unrevealing. Acid-fast stain of gastric samples is positive in less than 10% of cases, and staining and culture of other infected material is positive in less than 25% to 50% of cases.

**Nucleic Acid Amplification and GeneXpert** The main form of nucleic acid amplification studied in children with TB is the polymerase chain reaction (PCR), which uses specific DNA sequences as markers for microorganisms. Various PCR techniques have a sensitivity and specificity of more than 90% compared with sputum culture for detecting pulmonary TB in adults. However, in children, the sensitivity of traditional PCR has varied from 25% to 83%, and specificity has varied from 80% to 100% when compared to clinical diagnosis. A negative PCR result never eliminates TB as a diagnostic possibility. The major use of PCR is in evaluating children with significant pulmonary disease when the diagnosis is not established readily by clinical or epidemiologic grounds. PCR may be particularly helpful in evaluating immunocompromised children with pulmonary disease or in children with extrapulmonary disease.

The most readily available PCR-based test detects the presence of *M tuberculosis* as well as the presence of rifampin resistance. GeneXpert MTB/RIF (Xpert; Cepheid, Sunnyvale, CA) is an easy-to-use, automatic, cartridge-based platform that yields results in 2 hours. For pulmonary TB, the test has excellent specificity (98%) when compared to sputum smear and culture in adults. In a systematic review and meta-analysis of all pediatric studies, GeneXpert MTB/RIF had greater pooled sensitivity than sputum smear (62–66% vs 22–26%). However, GeneXpert is not as sensitive as routine culture techniques and should not replace culture. There are few studies determining the sensitivity and specificity of GeneXpert compared with acid-fast smear and culture in extrapulmonary TB samples, but WHO recommends its use as part of the evaluation of extrapulmonary samples, excluding blood, urine, and stool samples.

## TREATMENT

Mycobacteria replicate slowly and remain dormant in the body for prolonged periods. The treatment of TB is affected by the presence of naturally occurring drug-resistant organisms in large bacterial populations, even before chemotherapy is initiated. This drug resistance is caused by mutation at one of several chromosomal loci. The loci for resistance to one drug are not linked to the loci for resistance to other antituberculosis drugs. Although a population as a whole may be considered drug susceptible, a subpopulation of drug-resistant organisms occurs at fairly predictable frequencies within the main population. The frequency for these drug-resistant organisms varies for the various drugs: streptomycin, $10^5$; isoniazid, $10^6$; and rifampin, $10^7$. A cavity containing $10^9$ bacilli will have thousands of drug-resistant organisms, whereas a caseous lesion with a much smaller population contains few, if any, resistant organisms.

These microbiologic characteristics of *M tuberculosis* explain why single antimicrobial drugs cannot cure TB disease in adults. The major biologic determinant of the success of antituberculosis therapy is the size of the bacterial population within the host. For patients with a large population of bacilli, such as adults with cavities or extensive infiltrates, many drug-resistant organisms are present initially, and at least 2 antituberculosis drugs must be given. Conversely, for patients with infection but no disease, the bacterial population is small, drug-resistant organisms are rare or nonexistent, and a single drug, such as isoniazid, can be given. Children with pulmonary TB and patients with extrapulmonary TB have medium-size populations in which significant numbers of drug-resistant organisms may or may not be present. In general, these patients are treated with at least 2, and usually 3 or 4, drugs.

### Drugs for Tuberculosis

Table 264-2 details the first-line antituberculosis drugs used to treat TB in children.

**Isoniazid** Isoniazid (INH), a synthetically produced drug, is the most potent and valuable single drug in the treatment of TB. An oral dose attains a plasma concentration 20 to 80 times the usual level required to inhibit the growth of tubercle bacilli (0.02–0.05 μg/mL) within several hours, with high concentrations persisting for 6 to 8 hours in plasma and sputum. Isoniazid penetrates readily into the CSF, even in the absence of inflammation, and into caseous tissue. It is partially conjugated in the liver to an acetylated, inactive, nontoxic form. The rate and degree of acetylation are genetically determined.

The principal side effects of isoniazid are peripheral neuritis and hepatitis. Peripheral neuritis results from competitive inhibition of pyridoxine metabolism. This is more likely to occur at higher dosages of isoniazid (> 10 mg/kg/d) in alcoholics and people who are poorly nourished. This is rarely a problem in children, although precautions must be taken during adolescence, for breastfeeding babies, during pregnancy,

**TABLE 264-2 FIRST-LINE DRUGS USED TO TREAT TUBERCULOSIS INFECTION AND DISEASE IN CHILDREN**

| Drug | Dosage Forms | Daily Dose (mg/kg/d) | Twice-Weekly Dose (mg/kg/d) | Maximum Dose |
|---|---|---|---|---|
| Ethambutol | Tablets:<br>100 mg<br>400 mg | 15–25 | 50 | 2.5 g |
| Isoniazid[a,b] | Scored tablets:<br>100 mg<br>300 mg<br>Syrup: 10 mg/mL | 10–15 | 20–30 | Daily: 300 mg<br>Twice weekly: 900 mg |
| Pyrazinamide[b] | Scored tablets:<br>500 mg | 30–40 | 50 | 2 g |
| Rifampin[b] | Capsules:<br>150 mg<br>300 mg<br>Syrup: formulated in syrup from capsules | 10–20 | 10–20 | 600 mg |

[a]Most experts advise against the use of isoniazid syrup because of its instability and because of a high rate of gastrointestinal adverse reaction (diarrhea, cramps). When isoniazid is used in combination with rifampin, the incidence of hepatotoxicity increases when the dose exceeds 10 mg/kg/d.

[b]Rifamate is a capsule containing 150 mg of isoniazid and 300 mg of rifampin. Two capsules provide the usual adult (> 50 kg body weight) daily dose of each drug. Rifater capsules contain isoniazid, rifampin, and pyrazinamide.

or when the total daily dose of isoniazid exceeds 300 mg. Pyridoxine (10 mg for each 100 mg of isoniazid) should be given daily when indicated.

Hepatotoxicity is more common in patients older than 35 years. In children, hepatitis is rare and usually mild. Slight elevation of serum liver enzymes occurs in 1% to 5% of children taking isoniazid, but symptomatic hepatitis is very rare. Concomitant use of rifampin or phenytoin increases the likelihood of hepatitis, as do isoniazid dosage regimens in excess of 15 mg/kg/d. Children who are taking isoniazid need not have serum liver enzyme testing unless they have a previous history of liver disease, predisposition to the development of liver disease, or are taking other hepatotoxic drugs. A careful symptom review should be performed monthly, with warnings to report such symptoms as nausea, loss of appetite, or right upper-quadrant pain promptly.

Other infrequent adverse effects of isoniazid are convulsions (usually from a large and often intentional overdose), psychoses, loss of memory, allergic manifestations, and a lupus-like syndrome with arthritis and antinuclear antibodies.

**Rifampin** Rifampin is a semisynthetic drug that has wide antimicrobial activity against bacteria and mycobacteria. It is absorbed readily from the gastrointestinal tract after oral administration, with peak concentrations of 6 to 32 μg/mL (mean inhibitory concentration for *M tuberculosis*, 0.5 μg/mL) occurring in 3 hours. Rifampin readily diffuses to most tissues and body fluids; CSF levels are low but adequate for treatment. It is excreted primarily through the biliary tract and kidneys.

Rifampin is relatively nontoxic; the principal side effect is hepatitis, which occurs with a frequency of $< 1\%$. Hepatitis seems to be more common in patients who are treated with the combination of rifampin and isoniazid. Gastrointestinal disturbances, rashes, reversible leukopenia, thrombocytopenia, and elevation of blood urea nitrogen have been reported. Rifampin interacts with many drugs, including dicumarol, corticosteroids, antifungal agents, and many anti-HIV agents. Rifampin may chemically interfere with birth control pills, making them ineffective. Administration of the drug may also impart an orange-red color to feces, urine, sputum, saliva, tears, and sweat. The suggested dosage is 10 to 20 mg/kg/d (maximum, 600 mg). A liquid preparation is not commercially available, but can be prepared in community pharmacies. A newer, longer-acting rifamycin called rifapentine is now available for use in combination with longer-acting for treatment of TB infection. It is not used in treatment of TB disease in children. It has the same drug interactions and adverse effects as rifampin.

**Pyrazinamide** Pyrazinamide (PZA) is a bactericidal drug that attains a therapeutic concentration in the CSF and in macrophages. It is recommended as the third drug of a 3- or 4-drug regimen, particularly for the first 2 months of therapy. In doses of 20 to 40 mg/kg/d (adult dose, 2 g/d), it is well tolerated by children. Adverse reactions are rare in children but may include hepatitis, joint pain (caused by elevated levels of uric acid), and itching with or without a rash.

**Ethambutol** Ethambutol is an odorless water-soluble compound rapidly absorbed from the gastrointestinal tract and excreted in the urine, mainly with its form unchanged. It is bacteriostatic at the usual dose of 20 mg/kg/d. It is excreted via the kidneys and must be used with caution in patients with renal dysfunction. The only important toxic effect is a retrobulbar neuritis that infrequently results in loss of visual acuity, defects in visual fields, and inability to distinguish between red and green; the visual changes are usually reversible. This side effect should be monitored by monthly studies of visual acuity and visual fields and tests for green color vision when possible. At doses of 20 mg/kg/d, it can be safely administered to children of all ages. Ethambutol is used as the fourth drug in a multidrug regimen, and its major purpose is to prevent emergence of resistance to other drugs.

**Corticosteroids** These drugs are controversial in the management of TB. They can be used only if effective antituberculosis therapy is in place. They are useful when the host inflammatory response to *M tuberculosis* contributes to tissue damage. Generally accepted indications are for the management of tuberculous meningitis, tuberculous pleural effusion, pericarditis, and endobronchial disease. Prednisone at 2 mg/kg/d is used commonly for 4 to 6 weeks and then weaned slowly.

**Second-Line Drugs for Resistant *M tuberculosis*** The emergence of multidrug-resistant *M tuberculosis* strains means that second-line drugs must be used to treat children who have acquired these strains. Second-line drugs also can be used if children are intolerant of the first-line drugs. An expert in TB should be consulted whenever a second-line drug is being considered for a child. Second-line drugs are divided into several classes: the injectables, the fluoroquinolones, oral bacteriostatic agents, and other agents. These classes are used to determine the treatment regimens for drug-resistant TB, generally using 1 from each class to comprise 3 to 4 drugs active against the individual's isolate. First-line drugs with activity against the isolate are also used.

The fluoroquinolones, specifically levofloxacin and moxifloxacin, have bactericidal activity against *M tuberculosis*. They also penetrate the tissues and central nervous system well. Side effects include neuropsychiatric issues, joint problems, Achilles tendon inflammation and rupture (rare in children), and prolonged QT interval. Levofloxacin is available as an oral suspension for younger children, whereas moxifloxacin must be compounded into a suspension. If an isolate is resistant to one fluoroquinolone, it is likely resistant to the other.

Streptomycin, capreomycin, amikacin, and kanamycin comprise the injectable class of second-line drugs. The injectable drugs are nephrotoxic, can cause hearing loss after prolonged use, and are quite painful when administered as intramuscular injections. The WHO recommends that children with milder forms of multidrug-resistant disease can forego the injectable drugs as their risks may outweigh the benefit.

The oral bacteriostatic agent class includes cycloserine and the closely related terizidone, prothionamide and the closely related ethionamide, as well as para-aminosalicylic acid (PAS). The fifth class includes other agents: clofazimine (used often in the treatment of *Mycobacterium leprae*, the etiologic agent responsible for leprosy, or Hansen disease), meropenem, and linezolid. Two newly developed drugs, bedaquiline and delamanid, are being studied for their use in adult MDR-TB but can be used on a compassionate-release basis for children.

## TREATMENT OF EXPOSURE AND INFECTION

In the United States, children exposed to potentially infectious adults with pulmonary TB should be started on treatment with isoniazid if the child is younger than 5 years or has other risk factors for the rapid development of TB disease. Failure to do so may result in the development of severe TB even before a test of infection becomes positive; the "incubation" of disease may be shorter than that for the test. The child is treated for a minimum of 3 months after contact with the infectious case is broken. After 3 months, the test of infection is repeated. If the second test is positive, infection is documented and isoniazid should be continued for a total of 9 months; if the second test is negative, the treatment can be stopped.

Two circumstances of exposure deserve special attention. A difficult situation arises when exposed children are anergic because of HIV infection or other immunocompromise. These children are particularly vulnerable to rapid progression of TB, and it may not be possible to tell whether infection has occurred. In general, these children should be treated as if they have TB infection. The second situation is potential exposure of a newborn to a mother or other adult with possible pulmonary TB. In general, this exposure should be treated the same as for an older infant. The neonate should be started on isoniazid and continued on it until TB disease in the adult can be ruled out, or for 3 months after the person with TB is no longer contagious.

The treatment of children infected with *M tuberculosis* before they have developed disease is a mainstay of modern TB control. Many large, well-documented studies have shown that isoniazid is extremely effective in preventing the development of TB disease in infected children. Because isoniazid is so safe, any child or adolescent with TB infection and no evidence of TB disease should receive treatment.

Historically, treatment consisted of 9 months of isoniazid, but in recent years, new regimens have become available. Isoniazid is usually taken every day, but can be administered twice weekly under the direct observation of a healthcare worker in cases of high-risk infection, particularly if an adult with TB disease who is also being treated twice a week is present in the home. The optimal length of isoniazid therapy has been debated for 40 years. The summary opinion of experts is that 9 months of therapy is the optimal length of treatment for children with TB infection. The major difficulty with taking isoniazid for 9 months is completing the regimen; many studies have documented completion rates of only 50% to 80%. Rifampin taken daily for 4 months is effective, and completion rates with this regimen are much higher compared to those with 9 months of isoniazid. The rifampin regimen causes fewer adverse events, but as children typically tolerate isoniazid well, there is little difference between the 2 regimens in terms of safety.

The newest treatment for TB infection is a 12-dose, once-a-week regimen consisting of isoniazid and the long-acting rifamycin rifapentine; this regimen is referred to as 3HP. This has been studied in children 2 to 17 years of age; it is well tolerated and at least as effective as 9 months of isoniazid taken daily. Adults occasionally develop a flu-like illness, joint pains, and/or skin rash caused by the rifapentine, but these are extremely rare in children. Currently, 3HP may be limited in availability and, in many locales, is available only via directly observed therapy given by the local health department.

If a child is exposed to or infected with an isoniazid-resistant but rifampin-susceptible strain of *M tuberculosis*, rifampin should be given for 4 months. If the infecting strain is resistant to both isoniazid and rifampin, a fluoroquinolone-based treatment regimen is often used, but an expert in TB should be consulted for this situation.

## TREATMENT OF TUBERCULOSIS DISEASE

Over the past 3 decades, a large number of trials of antituberculosis therapy for children with drug-susceptible pulmonary TB have demonstrated that the optimal regimen is 6 months in duration, starting with at least 3 antituberculosis medications, usually isoniazid, rifampin, and pyrazinamide. Isoniazid and rifampin are continued for the entire 6 months, whereas pyrazinamide is used only for the first 2 months of therapy. Medications are usually given every day for the first 2 weeks to 2 months of therapy. After this time, medications can be given safely and effectively twice or thrice weekly under the direct observation of a healthcare worker. In all the reported trials for these regimens, the overall success rate for therapy was greater than 98%, and the incidence of clinically significant adverse reactions was less than 2%. If the child is at risk for being infected with isoniazid-resistant TB because of previous treatment of the adult source case or because the child has lived in an area of the world where resistance rates are high, most experts would add a fourth drug, usually ethambutol, to the initial regimen, until the exact drug susceptibility of either the child's isolate or the adult source case's isolate can be established.

Controlled clinical trials for treating various forms of extrapulmonary TB are almost nonexistent. Extrapulmonary TB is usually caused by fairly small numbers of mycobacteria. Most non–life-threatening forms of extrapulmonary TB respond well to a 6-month treatment regimen using 3 or 4 drugs in the initial phase, similar to that used for pulmonary TB. One exception is bone and joint TB, which is associated with a higher failure rate when only 6 months of chemotherapy are used, especially if surgical intervention has not been performed. Some experts recommend at least 9 to 12 months of therapy for bone and joint TB. Tuberculous meningitis has not usually been included in trials of extrapulmonary TB because of its serious nature and low incidence. Several more recent trials suggest that 6 to 9 months of therapy are effective if isoniazid, rifampin, and pyrazinamide are administered during the initial phase of treatment. The official recommendation of the American Academy of Pediatrics for tuberculous meningitis is 9 to 12 months of therapy that includes at least isoniazid and rifampin and usually 1 or 2 other drugs in the initial phase of treatment. Most experts add a fourth drug at the beginning of therapy to protect against initial drug resistance; the most commonly used fourth drugs are amikacin (intravenous) and ethionamide (oral).

In general, the treatment of TB in HIV-infected children is the same as it is in children without HIV infection. Although some experts previously recommended lengthening the duration of therapy to 9 to 12 months in HIV-infected children, many trials have shown that adults with HIV infection and TB can be treated for the same length of time as adults without HIV infection who have TB. The same principle is usually applied to HIV-infected children with TB disease.

The incidence of drug-resistant TB is increasing in many areas of the world. In the United States, approximately 10% of isolates of *M tuberculosis* are resistant to at least 1 drug. Many countries in Latin America, Eastern Europe, and Asia routinely report drug resistance rates of 20% to 30%. Rates of drug resistance are unknown in many African countries. Patterns of drug resistance among children tend to mirror those found in adults in the same population. For children in the United States, certain epidemiologic factors, such as being immigrants from high-prevalence countries, or a history of previous antituberculosis treatment in the adult source, correlate with drug resistance. Therapy for drug-resistant TB is successful only when at least 2 bactericidal drugs to which the infecting strain of *M tuberculosis* is susceptible are given. When a child has a possible drug-resistant TB disease, at least 3, and usually 4 or 5, drugs should be administered initially, until the susceptibility pattern is determined and a more specific regimen can be designed. The specific treatment plan must be individualized for each patient. The length of treatment can be as short as 9 months if the patient has not been treated with second-line drugs before and there is no evidence for resistance to second-line agents, but can extend to 18 to 24 months if these criteria are not met.

Activity does not need to be restricted in children with TB unless the child develops respiratory embarrassment or immobilization is needed for treatment, as in some cases of vertebral TB. Adequate nutrition is important, although reestablishment of weight gain may take several months. The major problem with treating TB in children and adults is nonadherence with therapy. Suspected cases of TB must be reported to the local health department so that it can compile accurate statistics, perform necessary contact investigations, and assist both patients and healthcare providers in overcoming barriers to adherence with therapy. In general, patients with TB disease should be treated with directly observed therapy, employing the help of a third party, such as a health department worker who observes the child and family during the administration of medication.

In general, children undergoing treatment for TB infection or disease should be seen every 4 to 6 weeks to monitor adherence, to observe for adverse reactions to medications, and to follow improvement in clinical course. Routine biochemical monitoring for adverse reactions is not necessary in asymptomatic children. Radiographic changes with intrathoracic TB occur slowly, and frequent chest radiographic monitoring is not necessary. A common practice for treating pulmonary TB is to obtain a chest radiograph at diagnosis and several months after the initiation of therapy to ensure that no unusual changes have occurred. Children with TB infection do not need a repeat chest radiograph.

The prognosis of TB in infants, children, and adolescents is excellent with early recognition and effective chemotherapy. In most children with pulmonary TB, the disease completely resolves and, ultimately, radiographic findings are normal. The prognosis for bone and joint TB and for tuberculous meningitis depends on the stage of disease at the time antituberculosis medications are started. With all forms of extrapulmonary TB, the major problems are usually delayed recognition of the cause of disease and delayed initiation of treatment.

## PREVENTION

The only available vaccine against TB is BCG, which employs live attenuated bacilli. The BCG vaccines are extremely safe in immunocompetent hosts. BCG vaccination given during infancy has little effect on the ultimate incidence of TB among adults in a population. However, many experts believe that BCG vaccines are more effective in preventing disseminated TB among infants and young children. Retrospective studies from Europe and Asia yielded estimates of the protective effect of BCG in young children of 60% to 80%, and the effect is particularly strong for tuberculous meningitis and severe forms of disease.

The BCG vaccines are among the safest of the childhood vaccines. Many children develop a small local ulceration, but regional suppurative lymphadenitis occurs in only 0.1% to 1% of vaccinees. These lesions usually resolve spontaneously, but occasionally require chemotherapy with either isoniazid or erythromycin. Rarely, needle aspiration or surgical incision and drainage of the suppurative draining node is necessary, but this should be avoided rather than encouraged. Systemic complaints such as fever, convulsions, and irritability are extraordinarily rare after BCG vaccination. Children with undiagnosed serious immunocompromising conditions (eg, severe combined immunodeficiency) can develop systemic and even fatal infection after neonatal BCG vaccination.

BCG vaccination works well in some situations, but poorly in others. Clearly, BCG vaccination has had little effect on the ultimate control of TB throughout the world. Any protective effect created by BCG probably wanes over time. BCG vaccination has never been adopted as part of the strategy of control of TB in the United States. Its only recommended use in the United States is for children who will invariably be exposed to adults with multidrug-resistant TB due to family and other epidemiologic factors.

## SUGGESTED READINGS


Chiang SS, Swanson DS, Starke JR. New diagnostics for childhood tuberculosis. *Infect Dis Clin North Am.* 2015;29:477-502.

Cruz AT, Ahmed A, Mandalakas AM, Starke JR. Treatment of latent tuberculosis infection in children. *J Pediatr Infect Dis Soc.* 2013;2:248-258.

Dodd PJ, Gardiner E, Coghlan R, Seddon JA. Burden of childhood tuberculosis in 22 high-burden countries: a mathematical modelling study. *Lancet Glob Health.* 2014;2:453-459.

Dodd PJ, Sismanidis C, Seddon JA. Global burden of drug-resistant tuberculosis in children: a mathematical modelling study. *Lancet Infect Dis.* 2016;16:1193-1201.

Horsburgh CR, Barry CE, Lange C. Treatment of tuberculosis. *N Engl J Med.*2015;373:2149-2160.

Jenkins HE, Tolman AW, Yuen CM, et al. Incidence of multidrug-resistant tuberculosis disease in children: systematic review and global estimates. *Lancet.* 2014;383:1572-1579.

Mandalakas AM, Kirchner HL, Lombard C, et al. Well-quantified tuberculosis exposure is a reliable surrogate measure of tuberculosis infection. *Int J Tuberc Lung Dis.* 2012;16:1033-1039.

Nahid P, Doman SE, Alipanah N, et al. Official American Thoracic Society/Centers for Disease Control and Prevention/Infectious Diseases Society of America Clinical Practice Guidelines: treatment of drug-susceptible tuberculosis. *Clin Infect Dis.* 2016;63: e147-e195.

Pinto LM, Dheda K, Theron G, et al. Development of a simple reliable radiographic scoring system to aid the diagnosis of pulmonary tuberculosis. *PLoS One.* 2013;8:e54235.

Starke JR, Committee on Infectious Diseases, American Academy of Pediatrics. Interferon gamma release assays for diagnosis of tuberculosis infection and disease in children. *Pediatrics.* 2014;134: e1763-e1773.


# 265 Nontuberculous Mycobacterial Infections

Jeffrey R. Starke

## INTRODUCTION

The nontuberculous mycobacteria (NTM) have been collectively identified by a variety of terms, including mycobacteria other than tuberculosis, atypical, nonpathogenic, unclassified, and environmental or opportunistic mycobacteria. Although grouping these organisms can be helpful, classification based on specific etiologic agent is preferable because this has implications for the predisposing factors, usual clinical course, diagnosis, and appropriate medical and surgical management of the infection.

Mycobacteria are true bacteria. They are nonmotile, non–spore-forming, weakly gram-positive slender pleomorphic rods. Their cell walls have a complex structure that includes a variety of proteins, carbohydrates, and lipids. Traditional species identification involved various biochemical tests that were time consuming and sometimes difficult to interpret. Studies using high-pressure liquid chromatography (HPLC) reveal a variable species-related distribution of mycolic acids, with each species having a distinct mycolic acid fingerprint that can be used for identification. However, genetic sequencing is used to identify species in research laboratories and is increasingly being used by reference clinical laboratories.

## PATHOGENESIS AND EPIDEMIOLOGY

More than 60 species of *Mycobacterium* have been described, of which about half are pathogenic in humans. The most commonly encountered are *Mycobacterium avium, Mycobacterium intracellulare,* and *Mycobacterium scrofulaceum,* which are classified together as the *M avium* complex (MAC). The prevalence of infections caused by the so-called rapid growers—*Mycobacterium fortuitum, Mycobacterium chelonae,* and *Mycobacterium abscessus*—appears to be increasing, especially in patients with indwelling catheters and patients with immune compromise or cystic fibrosis (CF).

Transmission of NTM to humans occurs from environmental sources, including soil, water, dust, and aerosols. NTM have been isolated from as many as 80% of soil samples, and certain strains of MAC are found in fresh and brackish waters in warmer climates. Other mycobacteria have been isolated from natural water supplies and tap water. Although mycobacteria are frequently found in animals, particularly swine and poultry, there is little evidence to suggest direct animal-to-human transmission. There is no evidence that person-to-person transmission occurs, although concern has been raised that transmission of NTM can occur between patients with CF. Clusters and isolated cases of healthcare-associated disease due to NTM are being reported with increasing frequency. Most common are outbreaks caused by the rapid growers, which are associated with injectors, continuous ambulatory peritoneal dialysis, contaminated skin marking, and injection solutions and hemodialysis.

The direct detection of NTM is similar to that for *Mycobacterium tuberculosis.* All NTM are acid fast, but they are visualized in stains of clinical fluid and tissue samples less than 50% of the time. Although even a single organism visualized on an entire slide is suspicious, false-positive results can be caused by contamination of stain solutions, tap water, distilled water, delivery tubes, or immersion oil. Direct detection of the various NTM by nucleic acid amplification is advancing, but appropriate primers and reagents are not yet commercially available for many species.

The true incidence and prevalence of NTM infections are difficult to determine because there is no mandatory reporting. Isolation of the organism does not prove infection, and distinguishing among saprophytes, colonizers, and pathogenic organisms can be difficult. A survey in the 1980s estimated the prevalence of NTM disease in the United States as 1.8 cases per 100,000 population, approximately 20%

of the prevalence of tuberculosis. Rates were highest for disease due to MAC, *Mycobacterium kansasii,* and *M fortuitum.* The age distribution of NTM disease varies by mycobacterial species and site of disease. Pulmonary disease is rare in otherwise healthy children, but occurs more often in older adults. The majority of cases of NTM lymph node infection occur in children younger than 5 years.

Clinical disease caused by NTM is common among both adults and children with untreated and advanced human immunodeficiency virus (HIV) infection and other immunosuppressing conditions, including increasingly recognized rare autosomal recessive primary immunodeficiency syndromes involving specific gene mutations that interfere with host responses to NTM. Prior to the advent of antiretroviral therapy, almost 25% of deceased patients with acquired immunodeficiency syndrome (AIDS) in the United States had autopsy evidence of widespread disease caused by MAC. In one epidemiologic survey, 7.8% of children 0 to 9 years of age with AIDS had disseminated NTM infection; MAC caused more than 90% of cases. Patients with malignancies, especially leukemia and lymphoma, appear to have a higher incidence of NTM infections than the general population in the same geographic area. NTM infections are being diagnosed more often in transplant patients, including children.

The majority of NTM that cause human disease are of low virulence. Infections in immunocompetent hosts require an unusual exposure or direct route of inoculation such as trauma. These infections are generally characterized by findings limited to the inoculation site. NTM infections do not exhibit lymphohematogenous dissemination in normal hosts. Immunocompromised hosts are at increased risk for systemic and disseminated NTM infection, but these typically occur in the setting of extreme and prolonged immunocompromise, such as in individuals with advanced HIV infection and blood CD4+ cell counts below 50/μL. Although the portal of entry for the MAC is usually the oropharynx or respiratory tract, the pattern of disseminated disease in patients with HIV infection is most consistent with an intestinal portal.

## CLINICAL MANIFESTATIONS

### Lymph Node

The most common site of clinically significant NTM infection in children is the superficial lymph nodes of the head and neck. The vast majority of cases are caused by MAC. Lymph node infection as a result of NTM is most common in young children because of their tendency to put objects contaminated with soil, dust, or standing water into their mouths. Although NTM adenitis is more common in North America than is tuberculous adenitis, clinicians should never presume NTM to be the cause of apparent mycobacterial cervical adenitis until tuberculosis has been ruled out by a thorough epidemiologic history, evaluation of the family for tuberculosis, tests of tuberculosis infection (tuberculin skin test and/or an interferon-γ release assay [IGRA]), and culture. The vast majority of children who develop NTM adenitis are immunologically normal.

Lymphadenitis caused by NTM usually involves a group of lymph nodes, most often located unilaterally, in the anterior cervical chain or submandibular region, but can also involve anterior or posterior auricular nodes. Involvement of the supraclavicular lymph nodes is unusual and suggests infection with *M tuberculosis* or malignancy.

Lymph node enlargement usually occurs over weeks to months. Systemic signs or symptoms are rare in immunocompetent children. The involved lymph nodes are usually painless and nontender, firm but not hard, and usually seem fixed to the underlying or overlying tissues. The overlying skin often has a red to purple hue (Fig. 265-1). With further progression, the lymph nodes soften, become fluctuant, and may rupture through the skin, causing drainage and formation of a sinus tract that can persist for months or years. Healing is characterized by fibrosis and scarring of the skin, which can be extensive and disfiguring.

The standard tuberculin skin test may show a reaction with any NTM lymph node infection but is more likely to cause a reaction with disease caused by *M fortuitum, M kansasii,* or MAC organisms. However, the IGRA tests are negative except for when the infection is

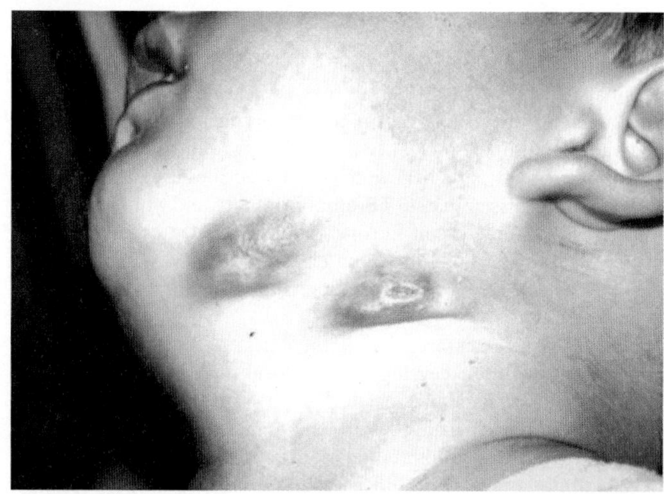

**FIGURE 265-1** *Mycobacterium avium* complex infection of cervical lymph nodes in a young child.

caused by one of several species including *M kansasii, Mycobacterium marinum,* and *Mycobacterium szulgai.* The greatest difficulty in differential diagnosis is usually distinguishing between adenitis caused by NTM and *M tuberculosis.* The most important distinguishing feature is the epidemiologic setting, which determines whether children may have been exposed to *M tuberculosis.* Lack of contact with an adult with tuberculosis, a skin test reaction of less than 10 mm or a negative IGRA result, and a poor response to standard antituberculosis chemotherapy suggest the diagnosis of NTM cervical adenitis.

**Cutaneous and Soft Tissue** In immunocompetent hosts, the most common form of cutaneous nontuberculous mycobacteria infection is the skin granuloma, frequently called swimmer's granuloma, caused by *M marinum.* These infections are associated with aquatic activities such as swimming, boating, fishing, or even care of tropical fish. Direct trauma from contact with shrimp, barnacles, coral, or fish hooks may lead to infection. This mycobacterium can be isolated from swimming pools and natural sources of freshwater and saltwater. Cases of *M marinum* infection usually are sporadic, although outbreaks of swimming pool granuloma involving hundreds of people have been reported. Typical skin lesions are nontender inflammatory nodules that progress to ulcerated granuloma or to chronic warty lesions over several weeks to months. The most commonly affected sites are areas where trauma is frequent such as the elbows, knees, feet, and hands (Fig. 265-2). The typical lesion is 1 to 2 cm in diameter and is not accompanied by regional adenopathy. Most lesions heal spontaneously within a few months, but occasionally, a nodular, sporotrichoid-like area spreads up an extremity. The clinical diagnosis is confirmed by culture of the discharge from the lesions or by biopsy. Many of these children have a highly reactive Mantoux tuberculin skin test.

In many tropical areas throughout the world, *Mycobacterium ulcerans* causes an itching nodule on the arms or legs, which then breaks down to form a shallow ulcer. This lesion is referred to as a *Buruli ulcer* (see Chapter 267). Isolation of *M ulcerans* is extremely difficult, and the diagnosis is usually made on clinical grounds. Excision of the lesion usually constitutes therapy, and treatment with several different antibiotics has led to variable success.

An increasing number of mycobacterial cutaneous infections are caused by the rapidly growing mycobacteria, particularly *M fortuitum, M abscessus,* and *M chelonae.* These localized skin or subcutaneous lesions are associated with accidental penetrating or iatrogenic trauma such as an injection or catheter site. Manifestations usually include cellulitis, a draining abscess that may be single or multiple, or tender nodules. Seropurulent drainage, poor wound healing, and development of sinus tracts after an operative procedure should suggest this diagnosis.

### Pulmonary

The most common NTM infection in adults is pulmonary disease with MAC, with or without some form of underlying chronic lung disease.

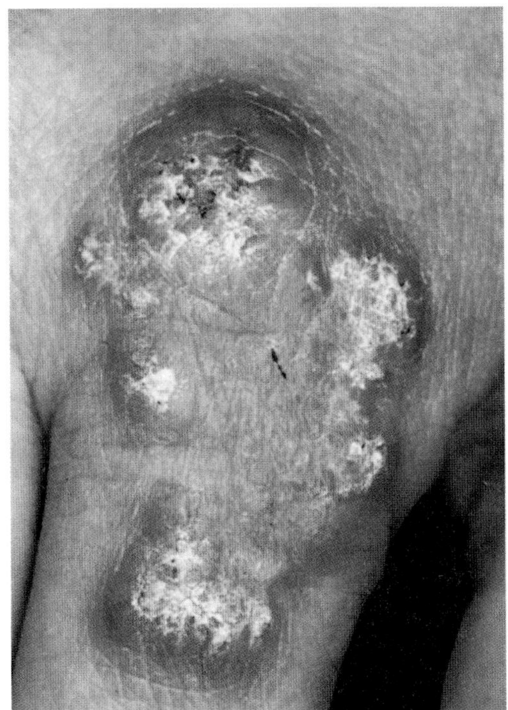

**FIGURE 265-2** *Mycobacterium marinum* lesion showing a verrucous violaceous plaque with central spontaneous clearing at the site of an abrasion on the hand sustained in a fish tank. (Reproduced with permission from Wolff K, Goldsmith LA, Katz SI, et al: *Fitzpatrick's Dermatology in General Medicine*, 7th ed. New York: McGraw-Hill; 2008.)

The clinical presentation includes cough, production of sputum, low-grade fever, and weight loss. In addition, hemoptysis, pleuritic chest pain, and night sweats may occur. Pleural effusions caused by NTM are rare. *M kansasii* is the most frequent cause of mycobacterial lung disease in the Midwestern and Southwestern United States. Some patients have underlying chronic lung disease, and the infection may resemble pulmonary tuberculosis. Dissemination beyond the lung is rare in immunocompetent patients but is common in immunosuppressed hosts.

Pulmonary infection by NTM in children is rare. Strains of MAC are the most frequent cause of pediatric NTM pulmonary infection. The majority of infected children are immunocompetent with no underlying pulmonary disease. The most common presentation is similar to the primary tuberculosis complex. Patients have mild cough and low-grade fever with few systemic signs or symptoms. Occasionally, localized wheezing is noted, and the diagnosis of an aspirated foreign body should be considered. Enlargement of hilar or mediastinal lymph nodes is common. These species can be isolated from the gastric secretions of healthy children, so diagnosis requires repeated isolation of the same mycobacterium in association with pulmonary deterioration.

Special mention should be made of the association between NTM colonization and infection and CF. Unfortunately, a standard definition of NTM disease in CF patients, using clinical, radiographic, and pulmonary function testing results, is not possible. A single isolation of an NTM in the sputum of a CF patient who is not experiencing a decline in pulmonary function probably represents colonization, and treatment is not usually necessary. However, repeated isolation of the same species of NTM in association with declining pulmonary function or worsening radiographic appearance of the lungs is more suggestive, but not diagnostic, of invasive NTM disease in the lung.

### Other Sites

Several cases of osteomyelitis caused by the MAC have been described in children. In these cases, the bony lesions are usually the only sites of infection. The most frequent findings are lytic lesions of the long bones or lesions of the small bones of the hands, feet, skull, ribs, and sternum. In most patients, the lesions persist for several years and then become inactive or resolve spontaneously.

Very few cases of NTM meningitis have been reported in children. The clinical presentation and laboratory values are generally similar to those commonly seen in patients with tuberculous meningitis. Before the HIV epidemic, disseminated NTM infection had been reported in less than 20 children. Most of these children died. Lesions of the lungs, long bones, liver, gastrointestinal tract, and bone marrow were common.

## NONTUBERCULOUS MYCOBACTERIA AND HIV INFECTION

The major risk factor for NTM infection in patients with HIV infection is the level of immune dysfunction, reflected by the concentration of CD4+ cells in the blood. The mean concentration of CD4+ cells in patients with disseminated NTM infection is less than 60/μL. The most frequent causative agent of disseminated NTM infection is MAC, but disease also results from infection with *M kansasii, M fortuitum, M chelonae, Mycobacterium xenopi, Mycobacterium haemophilum,* and other novel, unidentified mycobacteria. The incidence of NTM infection in persons with HIV infection is reduced dramatically by highly active antiretroviral therapy.

Disseminated NTM infection most commonly affects the blood, bone marrow, liver, spleen, and lymph nodes, but organisms have been recovered from virtually every organ of the body. Patients have a variety of signs and symptoms. The most common presentation is persistent fever with weight loss or failure to thrive. Gastrointestinal symptoms are common, especially chronic diarrhea, abdominal pain, and extrahepatic biliary obstruction. Radiographic imaging of the abdomen and physical examination often reveal marked hepatosplenomegaly, focal lesions in the liver or spleen, diffuse thickening of bowel walls, and enlarged mesenteric lymph nodes. Severe anemia requiring transfusion is frequent. Less commonly, cutaneous lesions, superficial lymph node enlargement, or endobronchial disease without pneumonia may occur. Many of the signs and symptoms described previously are common in patients with HIV infection and other conditions or infections; however, fever, abdominal pain, diarrhea, anemia, and weight loss are significantly associated with disseminated NTM infection. Diagnosis of disseminated NTM infection is easily established by culture of a normally sterile site. Only 1 or 2 mycobacterial blood cultures are necessary to confirm the diagnosis in most cases.

## DIAGNOSIS

The key to diagnosis of NTM infection is a high level of suspicion based on epidemiologic factors and clinical presentation. This etiology should be especially considered in patients with chronic cervical lymphadenitis or pulmonary abnormalities, in cases of chronic cutaneous ulcers or other skin lesions with poor wound healing, and in immunosuppressed hosts.

Methods used for the isolation of *M tuberculosis* from clinical samples also are useful for the isolation of NTM. All mycobacteria are obligate aerobes that grow best in the presence of 5% to 10% $CO_2$. Isolation on solid media of slow-growing NTM takes 2 to 6 weeks. Only the rapid growers form visible colonies in less than 10 days. Use of liquid media systems usually leads to isolation of any species of NTM within 14 days, with the rapid growers often being detectable in 3 to 5 days. Some NTM have specific growth requirements, such as low temperature for *M haemophilum*. Some newly recognized species of mycobacteria cannot be cultivated and can be detected only by nucleic acid amplification. Some clinical laboratories continue to use HPLC analysis to speciate these organisms.

Determining the species of NTM causing infection is crucial to directing chemotherapy. However, in most cases, there is little correlation between the in vitro susceptibility results for individual drugs and the clinical response to treatment. One exception is that susceptibility to clarithromycin among members of the MAC does predict a positive clinical response. In addition, drug susceptibility testing for the rapid-growing mycobacteria can be informative and somewhat predictive

**TABLE 265-1 FIVE CLINICAL OBSERVATIONS TO USE WHEN DETERMINING WHETHER A NONTUBERCULOUS *MYCOBACTERIUM* (NTM) SPECIES IS THE CAUSE OF DISEASE**

| |
|---|
| Repeated isolation of the same *Mycobacterium* from the same site is likely to indicate true infection. |
| Quantity of growth is usually moderate to heavy, especially in respiratory tract specimens, when disease occurs. |
| The site of origin of a positive specimen is important. The majority of NTM isolated from urine, gastric aspirates, and oropharyngeal secretions are contaminants, whereas NTM isolation from closed aspiration of lymph nodes or abscesses, as well as from deep tissue fluids, biopsy specimens, or resected tissues, usually indicates disease. |
| The species of mycobacteria is important. Isolates of NTM that rarely cause human disease should be viewed with caution. |
| Host risk factors should be considered. In the presence of predisposing conditions, the index of suspicion should be raised so that less stringent criteria are applied to the evaluation of specimens that are culture-positive for NTM. |

of clinical success. For these mycobacteria, susceptibility testing to antibiotics such as amikacin, cefoxitin, doxycycline, sulfonamides, linezolid, imipenem, tigecycline, and the macrolides may be particularly helpful. Unfortunately, many strains of *M abscessus* are resistant to most individual antibiotics.

Nonspecific laboratory tests such as blood counts, erythrocyte sedimentation rate, urinalysis, and serum chemistry tests are usually normal in children with NTM infections. Skin testing with purified protein derivative from *M tuberculosis* may be helpful in the detection of infections caused by NTM. These infections are usually associated with skin test reactions less than 10 mm in diameter, but larger areas of induration may be seen. A negative tuberculin skin test never eliminates consideration of NTM infection. Of course, similar reactions may be caused by *M tuberculosis* infection. NTM antigens for skin testing are no longer available commercially because of poor sensitivity and specificity, as well as a lack of quality control during production.

Acid-fast stains of appropriate patient samples may give an early clue to the presence of NTM infection but are frequently negative because the number of organisms in tissues and fluids is small. Histologic studies of affected tissues may be helpful if classic granulomatous changes are evident; however, NTM infection may cause only acute and chronic inflammation without distinct granulomas.

The most direct method for diagnosing NTM disease is culture of involved fluid or tissue specimens. Because of their ubiquity in the environment, isolation of NTM may represent colonization or infection without recognizable disease. Most experts suggest considering 5 clinical observations when determining whether an isolated NTM is the cause of disease (Table 265-1).

## TREATMENT

Specific treatment of NTM disease depends on the location and extent of the infected tissue, the host immune system, and the mycobacteria species involved. In general, surgery plays a more important role in the management of NTM disease than in tuberculosis because chemotherapy is often ineffective for NTM, and most NTM infections are localized and therefore amenable to surgical excision. An important initial consideration is determination that *M tuberculosis* is not the causative pathogen. Until NTM are identified by culture, treatment is usually directed at *M tuberculosis,* both for therapeutic reasons and for infection control.

To properly direct chemotherapy, it is important to determine the infecting species of NTM. In general, *M kansasii, M marinum, M xenopi, Mycobacterium gordonae, Mycobacterium malmoense, M szulgai,* and *M haemophilum* are susceptible to some or all standard antituberculosis drugs. Treatment of the rapidly growing mycobacteria and most strains of MAC requires other antibiotics, guided by the drug susceptibility profile. The macrolides, particularly clarithromycin, are a staple of treatment of many NTM infections, especially for MAC and *M abscessus.* However, monotherapy should be avoided because of the propensity of the organisms to develop drug resistance when a single agent is used.

The natural history of NTM cervical adenitis is resolution over many months, although the patient is commonly left with significant scarring and, occasionally, chronic sinus tract formation. In general, excisional biopsy remains the treatment of choice for cervical lymphadenitis caused by NTM. Incisional biopsy should not be performed because it frequently leads to development of a draining sinus tract or recurrent disease. Total excision of the inflammatory mass usually precludes persistence or recurrence. However, removal of all involved lymph nodes may be impossible due to the close proximity of vital structures. Excision is best performed early, in order to improve the cosmetic outcome before extension of disease into the subcutaneous structures occurs. Chemotherapy is not generally necessary for children with NTM lymphadenitis if surgical excision can be achieved safely. If tuberculosis cannot be reasonably excluded, an initial course of antituberculosis therapy should be considered. Many cases of cervical adenitis caused by the MAC resolve during treatment with standard antituberculosis medications, although no controlled trials have been reported. In a small percentage of cases in which complete surgical excision is not possible, recurrence of adenitis is a problem. Chemotherapy may be helpful; the purpose is to prevent extension of recurrence so that a second surgical procedure is not necessary. The most commonly used regimen is a combination of at least 2 drugs, including clarithromycin, rifampin or rifabutin, and ethambutol.

Many cases of cutaneous disease caused by *M marinum* resolve spontaneously. Acceptable chemotherapy regimens for more extensive lesions include doxycycline, or rifampin plus ethambutol, administered for a minimum of 3 months. The rate of resolution is variable, but therapy must be given for at least 3 to 4 weeks before the clinical response can be evaluated. No controlled clinical trials for treatment of cutaneous or soft tissue disease caused by rapid-growing mycobacteria have been reported. Most isolates of *M fortuitum* are susceptible to amikacin, cefoxitin, ciprofloxacin, clarithromycin, and imipenem. Drug susceptibility for *M chelonae* and *M abscessus* is more variable, and treatment must be individualized. For serious disease, intravenous therapy is recommended until clinical improvement is evident. Removal of foreign bodies is essential for resolution of infection at these sites. In cases of extensive disease, surgical excision of affected tissue may shorten the duration and morbidity of the infection.

Pulmonary infections with NTM in children are rare, and no controlled therapy trials have been reported. Most isolates of MAC are resistant to antituberculosis drugs used singly. However, combination therapy with standard antituberculosis drugs generally has been successful in the treatment of adults with pulmonary MAC infection. If standard therapy is not effective, second-line drugs with significantly more side effects and greater toxicity must be used. Resectional surgery may be necessary for localized disease. Treatment of disease caused by *M kansasii* is usually successful because it is susceptible to rifampin, ethambutol, often isoniazid, and streptomycin. The usual length of recommended combination therapy is 12 to 18 months. Patients with CF may develop pulmonary disease caused by *M abscessus*; management is often difficult and must be handled on an individual basis, based on the patient's functional status and the drug susceptibility profile. In these cases, the goal is often management rather than cure.

The most effective way to prevent or help treat disseminated mycobacterial infections in patients with HIV infection is by administration of effective antiretroviral regimens. Certain multiple-drug antimycobacterial regimens can provide symptomatic relief, prolong life, and lead to partial clearing or reduction in the level of NTM bacteremia in patients with HIV infection. However, treatment with various antimycobacterial agents may be associated with considerable toxicity. Patients with HIV infection usually have significantly higher rates of adverse reactions to most antimycobacterial drugs, just as they do to many other classes of drugs. The most commonly used drugs for patients with disseminated MAC infection are clarithromycin, azithromycin, amikacin, ciprofloxacin, ethambutol, and rifampin or rifabutin. Although many different therapeutic regiments have been studied, recommendation of any specific drug regimen or duration of therapy for disseminated MAC disease in patients with HIV infection is difficult. Most experts use the combination of clarithromycin, a rifamycin, and ethambutol as initial therapy.

## PREVENTION

Most experts recommend placing HIV patients with CD4+ counts of less than 100 cells/μL on azithromycin, clarithromycin, or rifabutin prophylactically in order to prevent disseminated MAC disease. The best method in preventing disseminated disease, however, is to maintain immune function with antiretroviral therapy. Rifabutin is less effective than azithromycin or clarithromycin and should not be used until disease from *M tuberculosis* has been excluded. Combination therapy for prophylaxis is not indicated since it has not been shown to be cost-effective while increasing rates of adverse events.

## SUGGESTED READINGS


Atkins BL, Gottlieb T. Skin and soft tissue infections caused by nontuberculous mycobacteria. *Curr Opin Infect Dis.* 2014;27:137-145.

Floto RA, Olivier KN, Saiman L, et al. US Cystic Fibrosis Foundation and European Cystic Fibrosis Society consensus recommendations for the management of non-tuberculous mycobacteria in individuals with cystic fibrosis. *Thorax.* 2016;71:1-22.

López-Varela E, García-Basteiro AL, Santiago B, Wagner D, van Ingen J, Kampmann B. Non-tuberculous mycobacteria in children: muddying the waters of tuberculosis diagnosis. *Lancet Respir Med.* 2015;3:244-256.

Perdikogianni C, Galanakis E. Non-tuberculous mycobacterial cervical lymphadenitis in the immunocompetent child: diagnostic and treatment approach. *Expert Rev Anti Infect Ther.* 2014;12:959-965.

Wu UI, Holland SM. Host susceptibility to non-tuberculous mycobacterial infections. *Lancet Infect Dis.* 2015;15:968-980.

Xu HB, Jiang Rh, Li L. Treatment outcomes for *Mycobacterium avium* complex: a systematic review and meta-analysis. *Eur J Clin Microbiol Infect Dis.* 2014;33:347-358.


# 266 Leprosy

Douglas S. Walsh, Françoise Portaels, Bouke C. de Jong, and Wayne M. Meyers

## INTRODUCTION

Leprosy is a chronic infectious disease caused by *Mycobacterium leprae*, an acid-fast bacillus (AFB) first recognized by Hansen in 1873 in Bergen, Norway, while examining smears from lepromas of Norwegian patients. Notably, the organism was the first reported bacterium causing chronic disease in humans and principally affects the cooler parts of the body, especially the skin, upper respiratory tract, testes, eyes, and superficial segments of peripheral nerves. The stigma suffered by patients with leprosy has historically been severe. Because of the stigma of leprosy, physicians must carefully consider the social implications of a diagnosis of leprosy, especially in children.

## PATHOGENESIS AND EPIDEMIOLOGY

*M leprae* is an AFB in the order Actinomycetales and the family Mycobacteriaceae. The acid fastness of *M leprae* is weaker than that of other mycobacteria, but as in other mycobacteria, the acid fastness is related to mycolic acids in the cell wall. Viable, undamaged *M leprae* organisms stain solidly, but degenerating bacilli first stain irregularly, then become granular, and eventually lose acid fastness completely. The persistence of bacillary carcasses can be verified by silver staining techniques. Staining quality, therefore, provides a rapid method for determining the effectiveness of therapy. *M leprae* still cannot be cultivated in vitro. Therefore, identification depends on criteria other than those used routinely for cultivable mycobacteria. Current criteria for *M leprae* are the following: (1) it does not grow on routine laboratory media, (2) it infects the footpads of mice in a characteristic manner, (3) acid fastness is abolished by exposure to pyridine, (4) the organism invades nerves of the host, (5) suspensions of dead bacilli produce a characteristic pattern of reactions when injected into the skin of patients (lepromin reaction) in accordance with the various clinical forms of leprosy, (6) it produces the species-specific antigen phenolic glycolipid-1 (GLP-1), and (7) it exhibits species-specific DNA sequences.

*M leprae* causes disease by its ability to survive and multiply in macrophages. If macrophages of the host digest the bacilli early, disease is not detectable, or the patient has only minimal lesions. If the macrophages are totally incapable of destroying the organisms, widely disseminated lepromatous leprosy (LL) will follow. Apoptosis of host cells occurs but is not as important in the pathogenesis of leprosy as in some other mycobacterial infections. Survival of *M leprae* in macrophages depends on the immune response of the patient.

The role of immunologic processes in damage to nerves in leprosy is poorly understood. Some observations suggest that antineural antibodies in the sera of many patients, especially those with lepromatous disease, are related to such damage. Tumor necrosis factor (TNF) is associated with macrophage infiltration of peripheral nerves in reversal reactions. Infected Schwann cells present antigens to T cells, making them targets for immune attack.

The highest prevalence of leprosy is in tropical Southeast Asia, South America, and Africa. Approximately 64% of all patients are in Southeast Asia (65% in India), 19% in the Americas, and 8% in Africa. The World Health Organization (WHO) reports annually the prevalence of leprosy, unlike other infectious diseases where incidence is reported; leprosy prevalence includes those on treatment and new case detections. In 1999, WHO reported that approximately 800,000 patients were being treated for active leprosy, with 738,000 new case detections. By 2006, the numbers had dropped to about 225,000 and 260,000 cases, respectively, and have generally remained at approximately that level through 2014. The notable drop in prevalence between 2001 and 2006 is partly because around 2001 WHO shortened the treatment regimen for disseminated (lepromatous) disease from 2 years to 1 year, effectively halving the prevalence. However, based on limited whole-population surveys in endemic areas, the total number of active patients may exceed the number reported by WHO by a significant margin. Many authorities consider that the total global prevalence of patients with active leprosy is much higher (1.5–2 million) and that, after many years of decline, new case rates are no longer rapidly declining. Indeed, that children are still developing leprosy in many locations underscores active transmission. The stigma of the disease and inefficiency in healthcare delivery systems further contribute to this disparity in statistics.

Geographic, ethnic, and socioeconomic factors may contribute to the spread of leprosy by affecting the number of untreated or ineffectively treated bacillary-positive patients and the opportunities for exposure. Lymphocyte transformation studies show that occupational contacts of leprosy patients in Ethiopia have the highest rate of sensitization (58%) to *M leprae*, followed closely by household contacts (47%). Noncontacts living in endemic areas have a lower rate of sensitization, but approximately 29% of the population is still sensitized. Nutritional status may or may not be important. Several leprosy epidemics have occurred in nutritionally debilitated populations, although there is still no convincing evidence that the prevalence of leprosy is unusually high in chronically malnourished populations. The percentage of patients who harbor large numbers of bacilli, generally those with LL, is often related to ethnic background. In some Asian populations, for example, 50% or more of those with leprosy have LL; in Africans, this figure is 5% to 10%. Improvements in housing and other living conditions may play a role in the declining prevalence of leprosy. No other set of factors satisfactorily explains the virtual disappearance of leprosy from northern Europe after the Middle Ages and from Scandinavia in the 20th century, long before any effective chemotherapy was available.

The proportion of children among all detected leprosy patients is 20% to 30%, with a gender ratio of approximately 1:1. Of the 615 known patients who were diagnosed in Louisiana between 1855 and 1970, 5% had disease onset at 0 to 9 years of age, and 19% were 10 to 19 years old. A study of 2000 children who lived in a leprosarium in the Philippines in an era when effective chemotherapy was not available found that leprosy developed in 470 (23%). Of these 470 patients, 254 were monitored closely and, in approximately 75%, the lesions healed spontaneously. Thus, active, persistent disease developed in approximately 6% of the children who were heavily exposed to leprosy. In adults, leprosy occurs more commonly in men than in women (2:1–3:1).

From 2005 to 2014, a total of 868 new cases (range, 66–103 cases per year) were reported to the Centers for Disease Control and Prevention, down from an annual high of 361 cases in 1985. Most patients are immigrants, but a few indigenous patients regularly come from Hawaii, as well as Louisiana, Texas, and several other southeastern states, with the mainland cases sometimes related to contact with wild nine-banded armadillos having naturally acquired disease, first described in the 1970s. Reports on the prevalence of naturally acquired leprosy in wild armadillos range from 3% to 53% in the southern region of the United States.

Modes of transmission of *M leprae* in nature have not been fully established. The prevailing concept has been that an individual becomes infected only after experiencing repeated exposure. This concept is now doubted, and a single exposure may be sufficient in optimal conditions. Indeed, one report describes leprosy transmission after a single exposure, from a patient to a surgeon who practiced in a leprosy nonendemic area. However, in any patient contact situation, the number of viable *M leprae* being shed by the patient and the degree of susceptibility of the contact may both vary. Thus, long periods of association may be necessary before optimal conditions for infection exist.

The frequency of a single early lesion in the skin of children that is usually covered by clothing argues against the development of such lesions at the site of contact with *M leprae*. For many years, skin-to-skin contact between the patient and healthy subjects was considered the most important means of transmission, and this concept cannot be abandoned readily. Intact skin of heavily infected patients discharges small numbers of *M leprae*, but ulcers in the skin may be a source of large numbers of bacilli. Thus, skin-to-skin contact and fomites containing *M leprae* could be sources of infection.

However, it is currently accepted that nasorespiratory transmission is most common. The nasal mucosa of lepromatous patients harbors massive numbers of *M leprae*, known since Hansen's original discovery. *M leprae* appears to bind to nasal mucosal cells by first binding fibronectin and then attaching to fibronectin receptors on mucosal cells. *M leprae* organisms ejected during sneezing remain viable under ambient conditions for as long as 1 week, and disseminated leprosy develops in immunosuppressed mice after the inhalation of aerosol that contains *M leprae*. Breast tissue and milk from lepromatous patients contain *M leprae*, and infants may acquire infection from this source.

## CLINICAL MANIFESTATIONS

The period from infection to clinical disease varies (usually 2–5 years but up to 15 years reported), and no prodromal manifestations are well established. After an incubation period, lesions of varying description appear. The nature of the lesions depends on the immune response of the patient to *M leprae*. Most clinicians today follow the classification scheme outlined by Ridley and Jopling (Table 266-1). Classification is important because it aids in establishing the treatment program and prognosis of the patient.

The cardinal signs of leprosy are hypoesthetic lesions of the skin, enlarged peripheral nerve or nerves, and AFB in skin smears. In the absence of another clear explanation, any one of these signs strongly suggests leprosy.

Virtually all patients with leprosy have peripheral neuropathy if cutaneous sensory changes are included, and approximately 25% have significant deformity, depending on the intensity of leprosy case finding and the inherent delays in detection. In experimental studies, the pathogenesis of peripheral neuritis in leprosy involves uptake of bacilli by the endothelial cells of epineural and perineural blood vessels and lymphatics. Surface proteins of *M leprae* may bind the bacillus to Schwann cells via laminin. Detailed discussions of peripheral neuropathy in leprosy may be consulted for further coverage of this important topic.

**TABLE 266-1 CLINICAL AND HISTOPATHOLOGIC RIDLEY-JOPLING CLASSIFICATION OF LEPROSY**

| Classification | Clinical Features | Histopathologic Features |
|---|---|---|
| Indeterminate (I) | Vaguely defined, hypopigmented or erythematous macule(s). | Small lymphocytic infiltrates around nerves and appendages. Rare bacilli, usually in nerves. |
| Tuberculoid (TT) | Few well-defined anesthetic macules or plaques. Neural involvement common. | Granulomas with or without giant cells. Rare bacilli. Nerves damaged. No subepidermal free zone. |
| Borderline-tuberculoid (BT) | More lesions, borders less distinct. Neural involvement common. | Similar to TT but with occasional bacilli, usually in nerves. Subepidermal free zone. |
| Mid-borderline (BB) | More lesions than BT, borders vague. Neural involvement common. | Epithelioid cells and histiocytes. Focal lymphocytes. Increased cellularity of nerves. Bacilli readily found, mostly in nerves. Subepidermal free zone. |
| Borderline-lepromatous (BL) | Numerous lesions, borders vague, sometimes central clearing. Less neural damage than in BB. | Histiocytes, few epithelioid cells, some foamy cells. Bacilli plentiful in nerves and histiocytes. Subepidermal free zone. |
| Lepromatous (LL) | Multiple macules, nodules or diffuse infiltrations, symmetrically distributed. Neural lesions develop late. | Foamy histiocytes with large numbers of bacilli. Few lymphocytes. Numerous bacilli in nerves. Minimal intraneural cellular infiltration. Subepidermal free zone. |

Ocular complications in leprosy are well known. All patients with leprosy should be evaluated by an ophthalmologist at diagnosis and periodically thereafter, especially during any reactional episodes.

### Indeterminate Leprosy

An indeterminate lesion is the first manifestation of leprosy in most patients, and may heal spontaneously, remain unchanged for months or years, or gradually progress toward tuberculoid leprosy (TT) or LL disease. Patients with indeterminate leprosy have a single or a few macules in the skin (Fig. 266-1). The macule is poorly defined and mildly hypopigmented in deeper pigmented skin and slightly erythematous in lighter skin. Skin texture, sensation, and sweating within early macules are normal or only slightly altered. Peripheral nerves are not affected, and skin smears from lesions rarely contain bacilli.

### Tuberculoid Leprosy

Patients with TT have a single or several asymmetrically distributed hypopigmented skin lesions (Fig. 266-2). Tuberculoid lesions arise de novo or evolve from indeterminate macules. The lesion may be macular or infiltrated, but the borders are always sharply demarcated from the surrounding normal skin and are frequently finely papulated. Lesions range from less than 1 cm to those that cover entire regions such as the thigh or buttock. Many TT lesions heal spontaneously. In large, active lesions, the centers are often healed and repigmented, although somewhat atrophic.

In TT lesions, there is sensory loss with impaired sweating and eventually loss of hair. On the face, because of its rich innervation, the detection of hypoesthesia in early lesions requires discriminating tests. Conversely, clinicians may mistakenly diagnose leprosy in areas

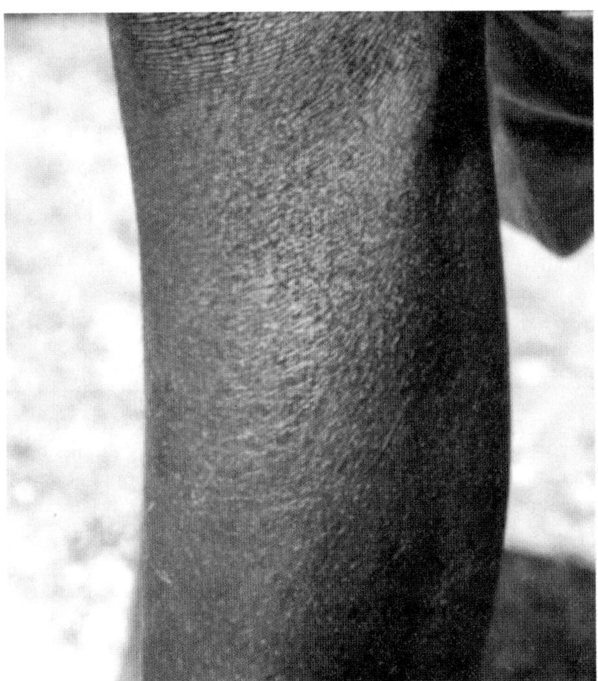

**FIGURE 266-1** Hypopigmented macule of indeterminate leprosy on the calf of an Indian child.

of the body that normally have reduced sensory acuity (eg, over the elbows or knees).

Involvement of peripheral nerves commonly develops in TT leprosy (Fig. 266-3), and cutaneous nerves can often be palpated adjacent to or within lesions. The regional nerve trunks most commonly enlarged are the ulnar nerve from the olecranon groove to midarm, the lateral popliteal nerve just distal to the head of the fibula, and the posterior tibial nerve in the medial aspect of the ankle. Enlarged or tender nerves anywhere should alert the clinician to the possibility of leprosy. Any readily palpable cutaneous nerve is probably enlarged, but evaluating the size of nerve trunks requires experience because of the wide range in normal size.

#### Borderline Leprosy

Borderline leprosy, sometimes called dimorphous or intermediate leprosy, has features of both the LL and the TT forms and represents a continuous spectrum of disease ranging from near-tuberculoid to near-lepromatous. It is an unstable form of leprosy and may evolve gradually toward TT leprosy by undergoing reversal reactions (see below) or be downgraded toward LL leprosy. Table 266-1 describes the 3 major subgroups of borderline leprosy: borderline-tuberculoid (BT), borderline (BB), and borderline-lepromatous (BL).

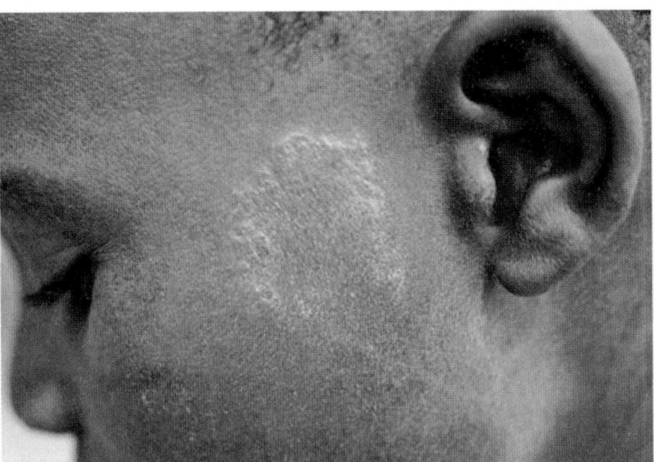

**FIGURE 266-2** Tuberculoid leprosy in a 12-year-old boy. This was the only lesion, and it had a well-defined papulated border with central healing.

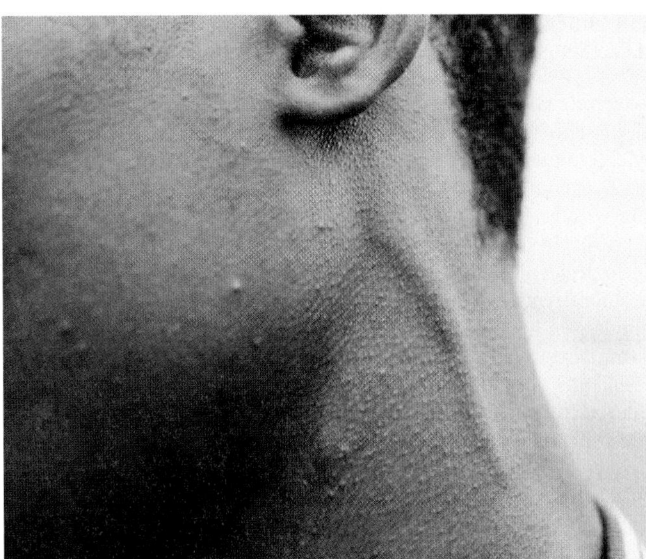

**FIGURE 266-3** Thickened great auricular nerve in an adolescent boy. A large macule of tuberculoid leprosy in the area of the angle of the mandible is now nearly inactive and barely visible.

In BT leprosy, the number of lesions is usually greater than in TT leprosy, and the borders of each lesion, macule, or plaque are defined less sharply than in TT leprosy. There may be central clearing within lesions. Small satellite lesions may develop around larger macules or plaques. BL leprosy often presents with widespread nodular infiltrations or plaques of varying size (Fig. 266-4)

Damage to nerves and the resulting deformity develop early and are often widespread. Pain in nerves or neuropathic changes (eg, sensory changes that lead to damaged hands or feet or muscular weakness such as footdrop) frequently bring the patient to the physician. Severe damage to nerves is infrequent in early childhood but can be disastrous.

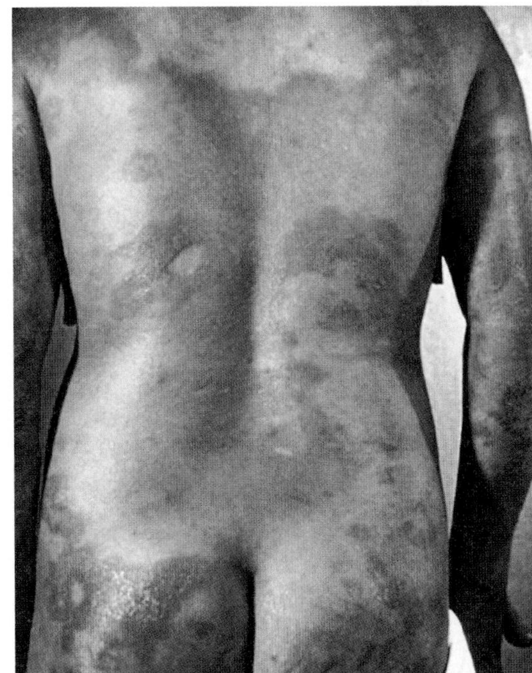

**FIGURE 266-4** Borderline lepromatous leprosy. Among many plaques, some have defined borders, and others are vague. Note central clearing in some lesions. The erythematous lesions suggest patient is undergoing a reversal reaction (type 1).

Prevention of this complication is an important goal of leprosy detection programs and of treatment of every leprosy patient.

**Lepromatous Leprosy**

In LL leprosy, the bacilli multiply freely and the disease disseminates widely, often before striking cutaneous manifestations develop, in contrast to the strict localization of lesions in TT leprosy. LL leprosy may evolve from indeterminate or BB leprosy or may be the first recognizable form.

In its earliest form, LL leprosy manifests as "juvenile leprosy," a clinical entity delineated from observations on large numbers of children in homes for children of patients with leprosy in India. This form, also called pre-lepromatous leprosy, is difficult to detect and frequently goes unrecognized until a more advanced stage develops. Skin texture may be altered slightly, but the vague macules with indistinct borders are detected only under appropriate lighting, preferably daylight. There are no changes in sensation or sweating in the macules, and frequently AFB are not detectable in smears from skin. Histopathologic sections may reveal a few bacilli to confirm the diagnosis. If leprosy is suspected, the patient should be monitored until an explanation for the mild skin changes is found. If leprosy is present but not detected and treated, advanced forms of LL leprosy will develop in many of these patients.

The hypopigmented or slightly erythematous macules of early LL leprosy, like those of juvenile leprosy, are missed easily because they are vague and have slight, if any, sensory changes. These macules are usually small but gradually may coalesce and cover large areas of skin, even nearly the entire body. A clinical diagnosis then is often missed, and over the course of a few years, advanced LL leprosy develops. If skin smears or biopsy specimens are taken in the macular stage, diagnosis is almost assured. If the disease is not diagnosed and treated in the macular stage, infiltration of the skin will increase gradually, and nodules may develop. The skin is infiltrated most heavily in the cooler portions of the body, notably the ears (pinnae) and face. By this time, nerves are usually enlarged, with early signs of sensory loss in the hands and feet. Eyebrows are thinned and eventually lost, beginning at the lateral edges. These advanced changes of LL leprosy are not common findings in young children but are well known (Fig. 266-5).

**Neuritic Leprosy**

Rarely, leprosy involves 1 or more major nerve trunks unaccompanied by cutaneous lesions. These patients have anesthesia, paresis, or wasting of muscles in the affected area. Nerve trunks are frequently painful, enlarged, and tender. Leprosy must be suspected in patients with any peripheral neuritis that has these features. Chronic neuritis with pain, enlargement, and tenderness of peripheral nerves often persists for years after the patient has completed chemotherapy for leprosy. Large leprotic nerve abscesses are rare but are exquisitely painful and may require surgical intervention for drainage. However, most clinicians prefer to treat such lesions with corticosteroids.

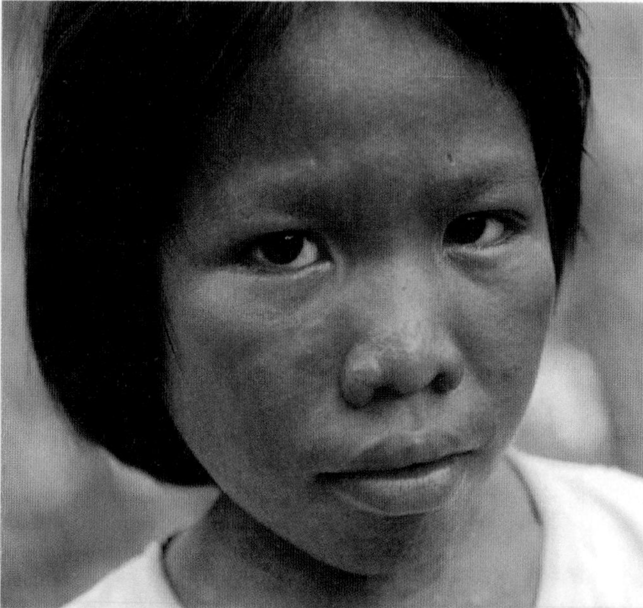

**FIGURE 266-5** Advanced lepromatous leprosy in an adolescent girl. Skin of face is diffusely thickened, especially the alae nasi. Eyebrows are thinned.

**Reactions**

The course of leprosy, treated or untreated, is often interrupted by acute immunologically based episodes called reactions, which fall into 2 general categories: reversal reactions (or type 1) and erythema nodosum leprosum (ENL) or type 2 reactions.

**Reversal Reactions** Reversal reactions complicate borderline leprosy and represent delayed hypersensitivity reactions with an upgrading of cell-mediated immunity toward TT leprosy. Existing lesions become erythematous and edematous, and neuritis is common. Patients who are lepromin positive and have immunoglobulin (Ig) M antibodies to PGL-1 are most at risk for reversal reactions. Proliferation of sensitized T lymphocytes initiates reversal reactions, releasing lymphokines that amplify the inflammatory response, calling in and activating macrophages. Immunohistopathologic evidence has shown that effective chemotherapy for both paucibacillary and multibacillary patients may activate cell-mediated immunity and provoke clinical or subclinical reversal reactions. Differentiating reversal reactions from relapsing lesions is frequently difficult and requires careful correlation of clinical and histopathologic findings.

**Erythema Nodosum Leprosum** Formerly, ENL developed in approximately 50% of LL patients after they had undergone a few months of chemotherapy; however, with the addition of clofazimine to the standard therapeutic regimen, ENL frequency is much reduced. Tender erythematous subcutaneous nodules develop rapidly (Fig. 266-6); the nodules are often accompanied by fever and occasionally by synovitis and iridocyclitis. ENL resembles the Arthus reaction and is believed to result from immune complex formation.

The differential diagnosis of leprosy is discussed only briefly here. Superficial mycoses and postinflammatory changes are commonly confused with early leprosy. Changes in pigmentation may be caused, for instance, by scars, birthmarks, and actinic dermatitis. In areas where dermal filariasis is endemic, vague macules in a dark-skinned patient may appear identical to the early macules of leprosy. Among the many infiltrated lesions of the skin that can resemble leprosy are leishmaniasis, lymphoma, granuloma annulare, granuloma multiforme (Mkar disease), lupus erythematosus, psoriasis, pityriasis rosea, sarcoidosis, and neurofibromatosis. Peripheral neuropathies that may simulate leprosy are those seen in Morvan disease, syringomyelia, lead intoxication, diabetes mellitus, primary amyloidosis of nerves, and familial hypertrophic neuropathy. Cardiolipin-based assays of sera

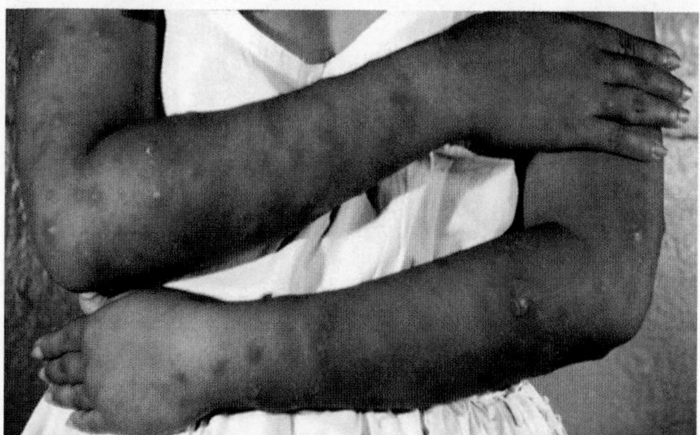

**FIGURE 266-6** Erythema nodosum leprosum in a Filipino adolescent girl with lepromatous leprosy. Papules on upper extremities are erythematous and tender.

from patients with advanced LL leprosy frequently give false-positive reactions for syphilis.

## DIAGNOSIS

An experienced observer can make a clinical diagnosis in most patients, except those with very early leprosy, with a high degree of accuracy. However, as leprosy is considered one of the "great imitators" with a substantial differential diagnosis, histopathologic evaluation, including mycobacterial stains, is strongly recommended to supplement and confirm the clinical diagnosis. History is important. Contact with patients with leprosy or residence in an endemic area raises suspicion of leprosy in a patient with a chronic lesion of the skin. Sensory loss or unexplained damage to hands or feet suggests damage to nerve trunks. Sometimes, a foot drop or claw hand will bring the patient to a physician. Occasionally, LL patients will consult an otolaryngologist first because of a chronic stuffy nose.

Globally, leprosy is the most common cause of peripheral neuropathy and must be considered in any patient with peripheral neuropathy. Clinicians must evaluate sensory changes in a lesion by testing light touch with the use of a few fibers of cotton or calibrated nylon filaments and heat-cold discrimination with the use of warm and cold water in test tubes. Much patience and repeated testing are often necessary in evaluating young children. Spontaneous sweating can be observed directly, or induced sweating can be evaluated. Hair may be completely preserved in early lesions but lost in advanced lesions. The main nerve trunks must be palpated for tenderness and enlargement. Skin in the area of discrete lesions must also be palpated gently to detect enlargement of cutaneous nerves.

Obtaining and examining smears for AFB is an important diagnostic procedure and should be controlled carefully by experienced laboratories. Briefly, smears are made from the edge of discrete macules or plaques, nodules, ear lobes, and nasal mucosa. Skin smears are made by squeezing and holding a fold of skin between the thumb and forefinger to avoid getting blood in the smear and by making a short, shallow slit in the skin with a sterile razor blade or scalpel. The instrument is then turned at a right angle to the slit, and the edges of the incision scraped. The cells and fluid thus obtained are spread on a slide, heat-fixed, and stained by the Ziehl-Neelsen method. Evaluation of smears should not be done by researchers unfamiliar with their interpretation. An occasional AFB may be, for example, a contaminant in the staining reagents, although with appropriate quality controls, such false positives can be minimized.

Biopsy specimens from well-defined lesions of leprosy should be taken from the active border and fixed in buffered 10% formalin or other suitable fixative, unless molecular studies are requested, in which case formalin should be avoided. The Fite-Faraco staining method is used because the Ziehl-Neelsen stain does not demonstrate *M leprae* optimally in tissue sections. A histopathologic diagnosis of leprosy must not be made unless the evidence is convincing. DNA probes specific for *M leprae* are available and are useful in identifying leprosy bacilli in tissue or nasal secretions. Specimens for DNA evaluation or polymerase chain reaction (PCR) amplification should be preserved in 70% ethyl alcohol.

The lepromin reaction is useless for the diagnosis of leprosy, and currently available skin tests with soluble *M leprae* antigens are unreliable for diagnosis. Enzyme-linked immunosorbent assays and gelatin particle agglutination tests for antibodies to the PGL-1 of *M leprae* are available. Although specificity for *M leprae* is high, these tests detect antibodies to PGL-1 in only approximately 50% of paucibacillary patients. PGL-1 antigen is detectable in the serum and urine of most multibacillary patients. Other serologic tests for antibodies to *M leprae*–specific epitopes on protein moieties of the bacillus are being evaluated, with the NDO-LID test commercially available in Brazil and purporting to detect notable numbers of early-stage infections.

Reliance on DNA probes and PCR technology may prove useful in the diagnosis of leprosy in tissue sections, skin smears, nasal smears, and oral mucosa. Different PCR targets were used, and the recent development of real-time PCR has improved the sensitivity and specificity of the tests. Because these methods can detect a single leprosy bacillus, interpretation of results, particularly in highly endemic areas, is difficult. Careful clinicopathologic correlation is essential when basing diagnosis on DNA findings.





## TREATMENT

Once a diagnosis of leprosy is established, chemotherapy must be initiated. Because of drug-resistant *M leprae*, combined multiple-drug treatment (MDT) regimens, such as WHO-MDT, are mandatory for the treatment of all forms of leprosy. Currently, drugs used in WHO-MDT and US-MDT are a combination of rifampicin, clofazimine, and dapsone for multibacillary leprosy, and rifampin and dapsone for paucibacillary leprosy. Rifampin, the most important antileprosy drug, is used in both types of leprosy (Table 266-2).

Appropriate measures are also begun for preventing or correcting deformity in patients with neuropathic changes. Neuropathic changes involve primarily nerves and other structures in the cooler parts of the body and are most profound in the eyes, face, hands, and feet. Damage to the hand, for example, is related to loss of normal autonomic, sensory, and motor function. Early appropriate surgical intervention can often restore motor function, and physiotherapy will maintain useful hands.

### WHO-MDT

In 1982, a WHO study group recommended MDT regimens for all forms of leprosy. For ease of use in the field, especially sites without histopathologic capability, patients were divided into paucibacillary and multibacillary groups. Paucibacillary patients (to include indeterminate, TT, and BT) were originally defined as those with negative skin smears at all sites or those who have fewer than 4 lesions and no clinical peripheral neuritis. Subsequently, paucibacillary patients were classified only as those who have 5 or fewer lesions, without reference to skin smear evaluation. All other patients are multibacillary. In the United States, recommendations of the National Hansen's Disease Program (US-MDT) differ slightly from the WHO-MDT recommendations (Table 266-2).

WHO-MDT was designed primarily for field programs, and uses, for example, pulsed supervised monthly rather than daily rifampin. WHO-MDT is well tolerated, and compliance in large-scale control programs has been satisfactory. For dapsone, given at relatively low doses, glucose-6-phosphate levels are not done. The efficacy of MDT has been promising. In 2 surveys involving approximately 112,000 multibacillary patients monitored for as long as 9 years after therapy, the cumulative risk of relapse was 0.77%. Anecdotal descriptions of

**TABLE 266-2 MULTIDRUG TREATMENT REGIMENS FOR PAUCIBACILLARY AND MULTIBACILLARY LEPROSY IN ADULTS[a]**

| | Paucibacillary (Indeterminate, Tuberculoid, Borderline-Tuberculoid) | Multibacillary (Borderline, Borderline-Lepromatous, Lepromatous) |
|---|---|---|
| WHO-MDT | Dapsone 100 mg daily, unsupervised, rifampin 600 mg monthly, supervised; both for 6 months<br>Single lesion disease: combined single dose: rifampin 600 mg + ofloxacin 400 mg + minocycline 100 mg | Dapsone 100 mg + clofazimine 50 mg, both daily, unsupervised; rifampin 600 mg + clofazimine 300 mg monthly, supervised; all ≥ 1 year |
| US-MDT[b] | Dapsone 100 mg + rifampin 600 mg, both daily, all unsupervised; both for 1 year | Dapsone 100 mg daily + rifampin 600 mg daily, for 2 years; clofazimine 50 mg daily,[c] for 2 years, all unsupervised |

[a]Pediatric dosages of multidrug therapy are given as a percentage of adult dose: less than 15 kg body weight, 25% of adult dose; 15–30 kg, 50%; 30–45 kg, 75%; and greater than 45 kg, 100% of adult dose.

[b]Because the US National Hansen's Disease Program (Baton Rouge, LA) may change their recommendation for treatment, clinicians in the United States should consult them before treating a patient (telephone: 1-800-862-7326).

[c]For patients in whom the hyperpigmentation caused by clofazimine is unacceptable, 250–375 mg of prothionamide or ethionamide daily, or minocycline 100 mg daily, may be substituted for clofazimine.

MDT, multiple-drug therapy; WHO, World Health Organization.

certain groups of highly bacilliferous patients with relapse rates of up to 20% and recurrences developing 5 years or more after therapy have been reported. These and other results suggest that therapeutic regimens for multibacillary patients should be given for at least 2 years, as was done earlier, but WHO-MDT has reduced the treatment to 1 year. Indeed, the trend since 2001 has been to reduce the duration of treatment and change the therapeutic regimens, even to the extreme of a combined single-dose regimen composed of rifampin, ofloxacin, and minocycline (coined "ROM") for single-lesion therapy. Some have observed high early relapse rates. Many of these innovations are interwoven into the WHO Elimination of Leprosy Program and have provoked critical concern by some authorities.

In most reports, relapse rates in paucibacillary patients exceed those in multibacillary patients. In our experience in evaluating histopathologic specimens, many patients classified clinically as paucibacillary are, in fact, multibacillary. The potential for relapse after multidrug therapy regimens must await long-term, large-scale, follow-up results. Peripheral neuropathy sometimes persists after completion of these therapeutic regimens.

Another alternate therapy for multibacillary leprosy, for those especially unwilling to accept the hyperpigmentation of clofazimine or for those who are noncompliant with other regimens, consists of rifampin (600 mg), ofloxacin (400 mg; if unavailable, moxifloxacin 400 mg could be considered), and minocycline (100 mg) (ROM or RMM), all of which are administered under supervision on a single day, once monthly, for at least 2 years. In India and Brazil, low-level drug resistance to ofloxacin has been observed. Other potential antileprosy drugs that are undergoing advanced clinical evaluation and may gain general use include a combination of fluoroquinolones (eg, pefloxacin, moxifloxacin), the macrolide clarithromycin, and as described, minocycline.

Once treatment is stopped, the patient should be seen every 3 to 6 months for a number of years. All apparent relapses require histopathologic examination for establishing whether the lesions represent relapses or reversal reactions. Relapsing or absconded patients must be treated again, with the latter defined as a patient who misses 3 or more supervised doses in a row. The aforementioned multidrug therapy is not used alone in patients with concurrent tuberculosis. In cases where rifampin, ofloxacin, or dapsone resistance is suspected, either in a new or a relapsed patient, molecular studies can help identify resistance-conferring mutations, such as with the commercially available GenoType LepraeDR (Hain Lifesciences).

#### Treatment of Reactions

Patients undergoing a reversal (type 1) reaction or ENL (type 2) reaction should be observed daily in the early stages and hospitalized if the symptoms are severe, so that sensory loss and deformities are minimized. By repeated reversal reactions, borderline leprosy, and even cases close to LL disease, may be gradually upgraded to TT leprosy, often with disastrous peripheral neuropathy.

Formerly, specific antileprosy therapy was stopped or the dosage reduced during reactions, but these measures are no longer recommended. Damage to eyes and neuropathic changes may ensue rapidly without immediate attention. Nerve tenderness and function must be assessed frequently during reactions. Acute inflammation of isolated lesions without damage to nerves is likely to be of little consequence except for cosmetic considerations.

Without chemotherapy, prognosis in all patients except those with limited and self-healing disease is potentially poor. Patients with borderline or advanced TT leprosy frequently become mutilated because of damage to nerves. Borderline patients can downgrade toward LL leprosy. In patients with LL leprosy, the disease is progressive and can cause death from laryngeal obstruction. Amyloidosis is a frequent late sequela. Blindness may result from lagophthalmic-related keratitis or repeated episodes of iridocyclitis. General debility and deformity eventually prevent gainful employment in many patients. Iridocyclitis requires emergency measures. Local corticosteroids must be added to systemic anti-inflammatory regimens and ophthalmologic consultation obtained.

With adequate specific chemotherapy and control of reactions, prognosis is good in nearly all patients. Leprosy patients receiving oral steroids may develop life-threatening strongyloidiasis and must receive appropriate therapy. If therapy is started early, prognosis is usually excellent, and deformity and mutilation are prevented. Even after successful chemotherapy, however, some patients continue to suffer significant neuritis and loss of peripheral nerve function. Sometimes this "silent neuropathy" goes unnoticed by both the patient and the physician. Appropriate early attention to anesthetic hands and feet and restoration of function by reconstructive surgery can prevent most mutilation.

**Reversal Reactions** For reversal reactions, analgesics are given, and the affected area is put at rest. Large daily doses of corticosteroids are started and tapered to a minimal effective dose until the reaction subsides. Conversion to alternate-day steroid regimens may be attempted when long-term treatment is necessary. Some clinicians use clofazimine for chronic reversal reactions, but it is not recommended for the initial treatment of reactions with acute neuritis. For reactions, clofazimine is probably consistently efficacious only for ENL.

**Erythema Nodosum Leprosum** Mild ENL reactions are treated with analgesics; more severe ENL is treated with thalidomide or corticosteroids. Pediatric doses of thalidomide in ENL have not been established, but the initial adult dose is 100 mg 4 times daily followed by a minimal effective dose, usually 100 mg daily. The teratogenic action of thalidomide demands that appropriate measures be taken in the treatment of fertile females. For the rare patient who does not respond to thalidomide or in fertile females, corticosteroids or clofazimine is used. Corticosteroids, if used, are administered in the usual dosage schedules, beginning with large doses and tapering to a minimal effective level. Some clinicians use an alternate-day regimen when long-term steroid therapy is necessary, thus minimizing the well-known side effects. A few studies suggest that pentoxifylline or pentoxifylline plus clofazimine may be effective for ENL. Clofazimine is effective in most patients with ENL and does not have the disadvantages of thalidomide or corticosteroids. The anti-inflammatory action of clofazimine is not manifested until after 4 to 6 weeks of continuous use. The dosage must be adjusted to the minimal effective level.

## PREVENTION

Precise recommendations for the prevention of leprosy in individuals have not been formulated. Control programs today are based on the general principles that (1) the number of contagious patients is reduced by chemotherapy and (2) the surveillance of contacts will detect early leprosy. To accomplish these goals, appropriate education of the public and medical personnel and population surveys in areas of higher prevalence must be implemented. In endemic areas, improved housing is probably a highly important preventive measure by reducing close contact of patients with healthy individuals. The most important obstacles to improving control of leprosy include persistence of *M leprae* in treated patients, loss of expertise and interest in leprosy, transmission occurring via asymptomatic infected persons, cost and toxicity of antileprotic medications, long duration of therapeutic regimens, patient compliance, and social stigma of leprosy.

Chemoprophylaxis with dapsone for close contacts has limited usefulness but is not recommended for large populations. This recommendation is based on the probability that long-term use would be irregular and dapsone-resistant *M leprae* may develop. Rifampin prophylaxis may have some value, at least in the short term, but the risk of increasing the rates of drug-resistant tuberculosis, or even leprosy, must be considered.

WHO initiated an Immunology of Leprosy Program (IMMLEP) in 1974 with 2 primary goals: (1) development of a vaccine against leprosy and (2) development of reagents for detecting subclinical leprosy. Achievement of both goals could profoundly diminish the incidence of leprosy. *M leprae*, or specific antigens thereof, for the IMMLEP studies were obtained from experimentally infected armadillos. Vaccines composed of heat-killed whole *M leprae* alone or in combination with live bacille Calmette-Guérin (BCG) have been found to be safe but induce delayed-type hypersensitivity to *M leprae* in a high percentage of lepromin-negative individuals. Several other vaccines based on cultivable mycobacteria (*Mycobacterium vaccae, Mycobacterium "w,"* and the ICRC bacillus, named for the Indian Cancer Research Centre) induce similar responses. Field trials of these vaccines for the immunoprophylaxis of leprosy have been conducted; however, because of the chronicity and low prevalence of the disease, meaningful evaluation of their efficacy will require extended follow-up observations.

Because infection-induced immunity is not observed regularly in leprosy, a reasonable doubt exists that vaccines containing only *M leprae* will be protective. Hence, combined vaccines of killed *M leprae* and live BCG have been studied. Such vaccines convert lepromin-negative contacts of leprosy patients to positive reactors and upgrade LL patients toward the tuberculoid region of the disease spectrum. WHO does not recommend BCG vaccination for the prevention of leprosy. This decision was based on the highly variable results of extensive studies in Burma, Papua New Guinea, and Uganda. Another trial in India involving 270,000 individuals confirmed that over a 12.5-year follow-up, BCG vaccination was only approximately 25% effective against leprosy.

Initial evaluations of a large-scale immunoprophylaxis trial of heat-killed *M leprae* plus BCG vaccine in humans in Venezuela showed no better protection than did BCG alone 5 years after vaccination. A randomized trial of a single BCG vaccination, repeated BCG, or BCG plus killed *M leprae* involving 121,020 individuals in Malawi gave the following results over a 5- to 9-year follow-up: a single BCG vaccination afforded 50% protection against leprosy, a second BCG vaccination added appreciably to this protection, but the addition of killed *M leprae* to BCG did not enhance protection against leprosy.

## SUGGESTED READINGS

Duthie MS, Raychaudhuri R, Tutterrow YL, et al. A rapid ELISA for the diagnosis of MB leprosy based on complementary detection of antibodies against a novel protein-glycolipid conjugate. *Diagn Microbiol Infect Dis.* 2014;79:233-239.

Gillis TP, Scollard DM, Lockwood DN. What is the evidence that the putative *Mycobacterium lepromatosis* species causes diffuse lepromatous leprosy? *Lepr Rev.* 2011;82:205-209.

Oliveira MB, Diniz LM. Leprosy among children under 15 years of age: literature review. *An Bras Dermatol.* 2016;91:196-203.

Richardus JH, Oskam L. Protecting people against leprosy: chemoprophylaxis and immunoprophylaxis. *Clin Dermatol.* 2015;33:19-25.

Roset Bahmanyar E, Smith WC, Brennan P, et al. Leprosy diagnostic test development as a prerequisite towards elimination: requirements from the user's perspective. *PLoS Negl Trop Dis.* 2016;10:e0004331.

Schreuder PA, Noto S, Richardus JH. Epidemiologic trends of leprosy for the 21st century. *Clin Dermatol.* 2016;34:24-31.

Sharma R, Singh P, Loughry WJ, et al. Zoonotic leprosy in the southeastern United States. *Emerg Infect Dis.* 2015;21:2127-2134.

Smith CS, Noordeen SK, Richardus JH, et al. A strategy to halt leprosy transmission. *Lancet Infect Dis.* 2014;14:96-98.

Truman RW, Singh P, Sharma R, et al. Probable zoonotic leprosy in the southern United States. *N Engl J Med.* 2011;364:1626-1633.

# 267 Buruli Ulcer (*Mycobacterium ulcerans* Infection)

Bouke C. de Jong, Douglas S. Walsh, Françoise Portaels, and Wayne M. Meyers

## INTRODUCTION

*Mycobacterium ulcerans* causes indolent, necrotizing cutaneous lesions known as Buruli ulcers, an appellation given by Dodge and Lunn who described the first large epidemic, located in Buruli County (now called Nakasongola), Uganda. Today, *M ulcerans* infections are recognized to present a spectrum of clinical disease: nodules, plaques, severe edemas, and massive ulcers in the skin, and osteomyelitis. Buruli ulcer, after tuberculosis and leprosy, is the third most common and perhaps least understood major mycobacterial infection. In contrast to tuberculosis and leprosy, Buruli ulcer is closely related to environmental factors.

Since 1998, the World Health Organization (WHO) has recognized Buruli ulcer as a reemerging infectious disease in West and Central Africa with an important public health impact. In endemic countries, Buruli ulcer is a major public health and psychosocial problem because of potential disabling sequelae. The disease tends to afflict children in those countries in which it is highly endemic.

## PATHOGENESIS AND EPIDEMIOLOGY

*M ulcerans* is strongly acid-fast, with an optimal growth temperature of 30°C to 32°C on routine mycobacteriologic media such as Löwenstein-Jensen medium. The organism is a slow grower, often requiring several months of incubation to achieve isolation in primary culture. Microaerophilic conditions promote the growth of *M ulcerans,* and the organism is strikingly sensitive to temperatures of 37°C or higher. After a multitude of attempts to cultivate the organism from the environment by many investigators over half a century, the first isolation of *M ulcerans* from nature was reported in 2008. The development of polymerase chain reaction (PCR) techniques specific for *M ulcerans* facilitated detection of DNA in the environment in Australia and West Africa, although the significance of environmental *M ulcerans* DNA remains unclear.

Modes of transmission to humans have not been delineated completely; however, the most plausible route is by trauma at sites of skin recently contaminated by *M ulcerans.* Many patients give a history of specific antecedent penetrating trauma at the site of the initial lesion, which may include wounds from a gunshot or land mine, thrown stones, human bite, and hypodermic injection. Nonpenetrating trauma may also provoke lesions at the site of injury. Additionally, the organism may be spread by aerosol from the surface of ponds or be carried by fomites or insects to skin surfaces.

Globally, the highest incidence of Buruli ulcer is in West and Central Africa, followed by Australia, where one endemic focus is in a tropical region (Queensland), yet a larger focus is located in a temperate climate (Victoria). The greatest number of reported patients live in West Africa (Benin, Côte d'Ivoire, and Ghana), with 2200 Buruli case notifications from 12 countries received by WHO in 2014. Other known endemic countries include Angola, Cameroon, Democratic Republic of Congo, Equatorial Guinea, French Guiana, Gabon, Kenya, Malaysia, Papua New Guinea, Peru, Suriname, Togo, and Uganda. In some West African countries, the number of Buruli ulcer patients exceeds those of leprosy and tuberculosis. Human immunodeficiency virus (HIV) co-infection rates are higher in Buruli patients than in the general population, and co-infected patients tend to have more severe disease, with larger and more edematous lesions. Rarely, patients have acquired Buruli ulcer in Asian countries, including China, Japan, and Malaysia. In South America, known countries in which Buruli ulcer is endemic include French Guyana, Suriname, and Peru. While Mexico is the only North American country in which it is endemic, travelers to endemic areas occasionally present to European, American, and Canadian medical centers.

Individuals of all ages are affected, but children 15 years of age or younger constitute about 75% of all cases. Approximately 80% of the lesions are located on the limbs, with highest frequencies involving the lower extremities. The sexes are affected equally, and racial predilection is unknown. Anecdotal observations of children in families of multiple parentage have suggested a possible genetic predisposition. This possibility is supported by molecular studies. Seasonal changes in climate affect incidence in some foci. Focal prevalence within countries varies greatly and must be assessed at the community level of geopolitical subdivisions.

Buruli ulcer infection is rarely, if ever, contagious. The distribution of patients, even in highly endemic foci, is random, suggesting that each patient is exposed to environmental sources such as swamps

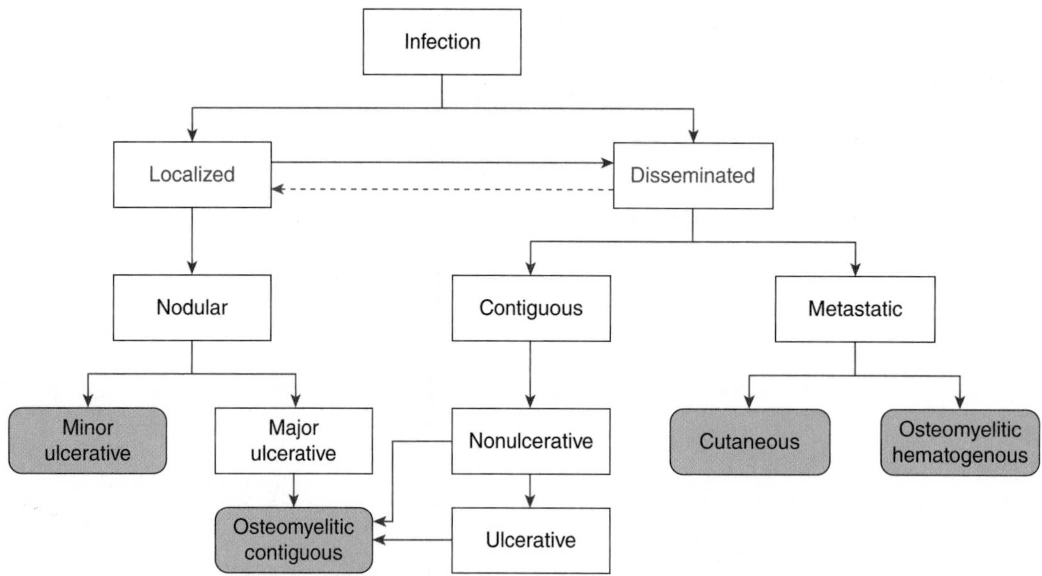


**FIGURE 267-1** A proposed classification of clinical forms of active *Mycobacterium ulcerans* disease and possible pathways of development if the disease is not treated.

where villagers work their gardens and obtain water for domestic use and where children play. The following additional risk factors have been determined in African populations: use of unprotected water for domestic purposes, swimming and wading in rivers, low level of schooling, and HIV infection.

## CLINICAL MANIFESTATIONS

A proposed classification of most of the clinical forms of *M ulcerans* is provided (Fig. 267-1). Besides suggesting categories based on the extent of the lesion(s), the WHO designations of the various forms of lesions of *M ulcerans* infection include: (1) *papules* that are painless, elevated, measure up to 1 cm in diameter, and ulcerate early (seen only in Australia); (2) *nodules* that are primarily subcutaneous and firm, measure approximately 2 cm in diameter, and are painless, although often pruritic (a nodule is the initial stage in most African patients; Fig. 267-2); (3) plaques that are firm, elevated, painless, well-defined lesions more than 2 cm in the largest dimension with skin over the lesion that is reddened or discolored (these lesions may ulcerate late, producing stellate ulcers without extensive undermining; Fig. 267-3); (4) *edematous* lesions that do not begin in the nodular stage but spread rapidly from the initial nidus of infection and often cover wide areas like entire limbs or major portions of the face or trunk; and (5) *ulcerative* lesions that are more or less symmetric, have undermined edges surrounded by a zone of induration, and often have desquamation of the surrounding epidermis. These are classified as minor and major lesions. In the base of the ulcerated area, a whitish necrotic slough and, sometimes, eschar develop. Microscopically, the active ulcer shows extensive coagulation necrosis of the subcutaneous tissue down to and often including the fascia. Marked edema is present, and fat cells are enlarged and dead, leaving only their cellular ghost outlines.

Bone involvement is due to both contiguous or metastatic osteomyelitis in about 10% of all patients, although 20% of patients with osteomyelitis may not have an apparent portal of entry. Reactive osteitis occasionally develops beneath destroyed overlying skin and soft tissue. Bone subjacent to the Buruli ulcer lesion may become devitalized and necrotic, with the development of sequestra. Metastatic osteomyelitis most likely results from lymphohematogenous spread of *M ulcerans* from a cutaneous lesion. The overlying skin ordinarily is intact, but swelling and inflammation develop over the site of bone involvement.

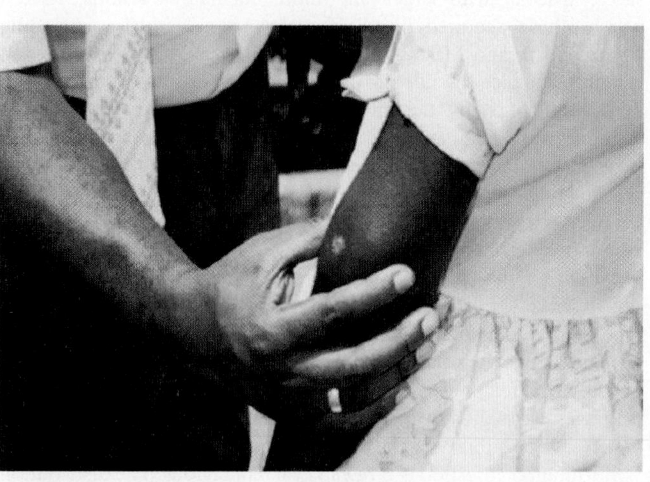

**FIGURE 267-2** Nodular lesion of Buruli ulcer in a Ghanaian child. Note incipient ulceration.

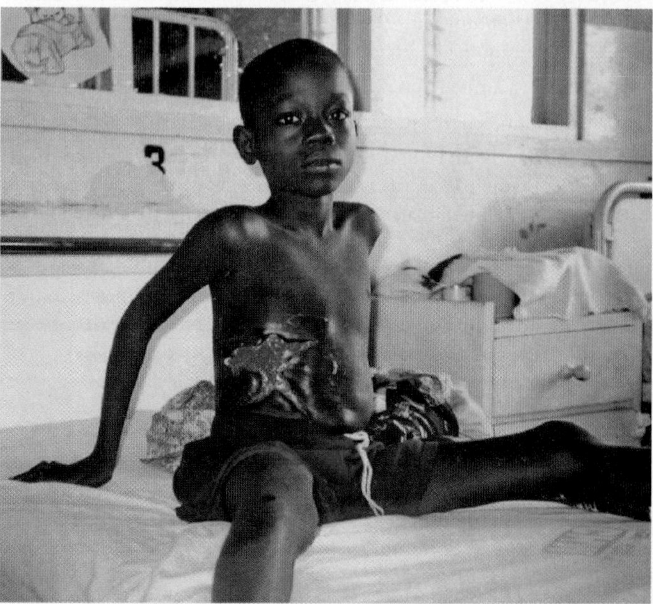

**FIGURE 267-3** Ghanaian boy with a well-developed plaque of Buruli ulcer on his right flank and abdomen. The ulceration in the plaque is stellate.

Bone scans are helpful in diagnosis. If the condition goes untreated, a draining fistula may develop. Both contiguous and metastatic osteomyelitis often result in deformity and amputation.

Other diagnoses that can be mistaken for Buruli ulcers include papules from insect bites, verruca vulgaris, pityriasis, or granuloma annulare; nodules from lipomas, sebaceous cysts, onchocerciasis, or furuncles; plaques from leprosy, mycosis, necrobiosis, psoriasis, or Mkar disease (granuloma multiforme); edema from bacterial cellulitis, necrotizing fasciitis, actinomycosis, elephantiasis, or pyomyositis; and ulcers from cutaneous tuberculosis, tropical phagedenic ulcer, noma, stasis ulcer, leishmaniasis, or injection abscesses.

## DIAGNOSIS

An accurate clinical diagnosis can often be made by an experienced observer. The WHO guidelines classify the lesion(s) clinically into 3 categories based on the type of lesion. Category 1 includes single nodules, papules, plaques, and ulcers less than 5 cm in diameter. Category 2 includes single plaques and ulcers 5 to 15 cm in diameter, as well as edematous lesions. Category 3 includes single plaques and ulcers over 15 cm in diameter, as well as the presence of multiple lesions, joint involvement, or osteomyelitis, or a lesion at critical sites, such as genital organs or the head and neck.

Laboratory confirmation is important, both from the public health perspective and the individual patient, especially when clinical expertise wanes. WHO recommends that national control programs strengthen the laboratory confirmation of cases and ensure that at least 70% of all reported cases are laboratory-confirmed by positive PCR. In the ulcerative forms, a Ziehl-Neelsen stain of exudate from the undermined edge obtained with a cotton swab will reveal clusters of extracellular acid-fast bacilli, although this test is less than 60% sensitive. The same material, obtained by swab after decontamination, may be used for culture. Sensitivity of culture is 20% to 60% on Löwenstein-Jensen or other suitable mycobacterial media. The incubation temperature must be 30°C to 32°C. If culture cannot be performed locally, transport media may be inoculated with material from the cotton swab and maintained at 4°C while in transport to a specialized laboratory. Molecular biologic analysis techniques consisting of quantitative PCR for the identification of *M ulcerans* have the highest sensitivity, estimated at 90%. Tissue for histopathologic analysis should be obtained from the edge of the ulcer or presumed center of edematous or plaque lesions and must include all levels of the integument, including the fascia. Fixation in 10% buffered formalin is adequate.

## TREATMENT

Antibiotic therapy is highly effective for Buruli ulcer, with high treatment success and a low relapse rate with 8 weeks of rifampin and streptomycin. "All oral" regimens are also used, especially in Australia, in which streptomycin is replaced by clarithromycin. In mice, rifampin and clofazimine also cleared *M ulcerans* infection. Streptomycin and, to a lesser extent, rifampin are associated with rare but important side effects, some of which require stopping treatment. For streptomycin, treatment should be stopped if hearing impairment or vertigo with nystagmus develops. For rifampin, treatment should be stopped if hepatitis, jaundice, or acute renal failure develops; these side effects are generally associated with intermittent therapy of doses over 10 mg/kg. Streptomycin is also contraindicated during pregnancy.

Some patients, especially those with large lesions, will in addition require surgical intervention to remove necrotic tissue, cover large skin defects, and correct deformities. Current WHO guidelines moreover recommend wound care and the prevention of disability. Physiotherapeutic evaluation and management are imperative for all Buruli ulcer patients. Bone lesions are difficult to manage and should be referred to specialists to minimize disabilities.

Heat therapy without surgical excision has been successful for appropriate lesions but must be applied assiduously with all necessary controls to prevent iatrogenic burns. In a recent phase II study, 92% of patients achieved cure of their primary lesion at 6 months and 84% remained disease free at 24 months, suggesting that this effective approach can serve as home-based treatment.

Given the high prevalence of HIV in several countries where Buruli ulcer is endemic and an association between HIV and severe forms of Buruli, WHO has issued specific guidelines that recommend that all Buruli patients are offered voluntary counseling and testing for HIV infection and that those with advanced immunosuppression receive antiretroviral therapy after the initiation of Buruli treatment.

Without treatment, Buruli ulcer often leads to deforming depressed scars, contracture deformities, or amputations. A few deaths attributed to severe edematous Buruli ulcer have been observed. The stigma of the deformities and the socioeconomic burden of the disease often are marked. With early appropriate treatment, including antibiotics, the prognosis usually is excellent.

## PREVENTION

In an endemic tropical, rural setting, where children usually are scantily attired, preventing contamination of the skin from environmental sources is virtually impossible. Wearing trousers seems to prevent development of infection. Protected water supplies in villages would reduce exposure somewhat; however, such protective measures usually are futile in rural areas of developing countries and hard to justify when the transmission route is still uncertain. Some other effective preventive measures include frequent use of soap for washing, treating injuries with soap and/or application of antibiotic powder, contact with rapidly flowing water, and use of bed nets and insect repellent.

Vaccination with bacilli Calmette-Guérin (BCG) has a moderate protective effect against *M ulcerans* infections for 6 to 12 months. BCG vaccination has a prophylactic effect against osteomyelitis in Buruli ulcer in children.

## SUGGESTED READINGS

Portaels F, ed. *Laboratory Diagnosis of Buruli Ulcer: A Manual for Health-Care Providers*. Geneva, Switzerland: World Health Organization; 2014.

Vincent QB, Ardant MF, Marsollier L, Chauty A, Alcaïs A, Franco-Beninese Buruli Research Group. HIV infection and Buruli ulcer in Africa. *Lancet Infect Dis*. 2014;14:796-797.

Vogel M, Bayi PF, Ruf MT, et al. Local heat application for the treatment of Buruli ulcer: results of a phase II open label single center non comparative clinical trial. *Clin Infect Dis*. 2016;62:342-350.

Williamson HR, Mosi L, Donnell R, Aqqad M, Merritt RW, Small PL. *Mycobacterium ulcerans* fails to infect through skin abrasions in a guinea pig infection model: implications for transmission. *PLoS Negl Trop Dis*. 2014;8:e2770.

World Health Organization. Treatment of *Mycobacterium ulcerans* disease (Buruli ulcer). Geneva, World Health Organization, 2012 (WHO/HTM/NTD/IDM/2012.1). Available at: http://apps.who.int/iris/bitstream/10665/77771/1/9789241503402_eng.pdf.

# 268 *Mycoplasma* Infections

Gueorgui Dubrocq

## INTRODUCTION

Mycoplasmas are bacteria that make up 1 genus of a special class called Mollicutes. The species are widespread in nature and can affect humans, plants, and animals. They are the smallest self-replicating microorganisms (0.2 μm) and are capable of a cell-free existence. A small genome and limited biosynthetic capabilities are responsible for their biological characteristics and requirements for complex growth media.

Mycoplasmas are unique from other bacteria due to their lack of cell wall around the cell membrane. Lack of rigid cell walls allows them to be presented in pleomorphic shapes not susceptible to antibiotics that inhibit cell wall synthesis like penicillins and other β-lactam antibiotics, and they are unaffected by the Gram staining method. There are over 120 *Mycoplasma* species, of which 14 have been isolated in humans. The most common species causing disease in humans include *Mycoplasma pneumoniae, Mycoplasma hominis*, and *Mycoplasma genitalium*.

The best-characterized human *Mycoplasma* disease is respiratory tract infection due to *M pneumoniae*, a prominent cause of the atypical pneumonia syndrome. *M hominis*, another member of the genus, is associated with a variety of genitourinary and perinatal conditions, including postpartum maternal sepsis, neonatal skin infections, meningitis, and bacteremia. Problems associated with *M genitalium* include pelvic inflammatory disease, salpingitis, and nongonococcal urethritis in sexually active individuals.

## *MYCOPLASMA PNEUMONIAE*

### PATHOGENESIS AND EPIDEMIOLOGY

The most common route of transmission of *M pneumoniae* from person to person is by inhalation of respiratory droplets expelled through coughing. During infection, *M pneumoniae* can be found within the mucosal secretions from the nose, throat, and trachea. Upon reaching the respiratory tract epithelium, it attaches to the host cell using a specialized terminal tip structure. P1 and other supporting proteins (eg, P30, P40, and P90) promote adhesion and binding to host cells via sialic acid receptors. Damage to host cells is related to hydrogen peroxide and superoxide radicals interacting with host cell toxins leading to deterioration of epithelial cells and their associated cilia and, ultimately, cell lysis. A potential candidate protein of *M pneumoniae* that may be involved in causing direct damage to the respiratory tract is a pertussis toxin–like protein termed community-acquired respiratory distress syndrome (CARDS) toxin.

Various reports state that the most distinguishable pathologic feature is an increase of plasma cell–rich lymphocytic infiltration in the peribronchovascular areas with accumulation of macrophages, neutrophils, and lymphocytes in the alveolar spaces. The immunologic response following infection and the immunity of the host generate an inflammatory reaction that plays an important role in the progression of *M pneumoniae* pulmonary and extrapulmonary manifestations.

*M pneumoniae* infection can occur throughout life and mainly infects the upper and lower respiratory tracts of children and adults worldwide. It is most common in school-aged children and young adults. Gender and race do not appear to play a role. *M pneumoniae* causes an estimated 20% to 40% of community-acquired pneumonia cases in the general population and up to 70% of cases in closed-setting populations. An estimated 2 million cases occur each year in the United States, making this organism second only to *Streptococcus pneumoniae* as a cause of pneumonia-related hospitalization in adults. The rate varies annually, but cyclic epidemics have been observed every 3 to 5 years. The infection can occur at any time during the year but is more common in the summer and early fall. Spread of infection is facilitated by prolonged close contact with symptomatic person(s) within closed settings. Outbreaks are most common in crowded settings such as childcare centers, schools, hospitals, college dormitories, nursing homes, and military barracks. The incubation period is usually 1 to 3 weeks and can be as long as 4 weeks. Asymptomatic carriage after infection may persist for several weeks, and immunity is not long lasting.

### CLINICAL MANIFESTATIONS

*M pneumoniae* symptoms are variable and include cough, malaise, fever, and occasional headache. The most frequent recognizable clinical presentation of *M pneumoniae* infection is tracheobronchitis. As most infections are mild and self-limited, it has led to the term "walking pneumonia." In the acute phase of infection, a dry cough develops that may progress to a wet cough in 3 to 4 days. Coughing is often worse at night and may persist for 3 to 4 weeks. Approximately 10% of infected school-aged children will develop pneumonia with cough and widespread rales on physical exam within days after onset of symptoms. Radiographic findings are variable as it can present with bilateral diffuse infiltrates or focal abnormalities such as consolidation, effusion, or hilar adenopathy. Unusual pulmonary manifestations include perfusion defects, noncardiogenic pulmonary edema, massive pleural effusions, and lung abscesses. Other syndromes that may be seen are upper respiratory infections, pharyngitis, and wheezing illness, particularly in children with a history of asthma. Because these clinical findings are nonspecific, *M pneumoniae* disease tends to be underdiagnosed.

The nonspecificity and usually mild symptoms of *M pneumoniae* infection are often coupled with a paucity of physical findings. The patient's complaints often appear greater than is suggested by examination. The pharynx can be erythematous in patients with complaints of sore throat. If lymphadenopathy is present, it typically presents as cervical adenopathy. If severe pneumonia is present, scattered crackles and rhonchi can be heard usually over one of the lower lobes. Children and adults with conditions known to be associated with impaired antibody production (eg, sickle cell disease, Down syndrome, hypogammaglobulinemia syndromes) are known to be susceptible to severe respiratory disease due to *M pneumoniae*.

The signs and symptoms of *M pneumoniae* respiratory disease are similar to those caused by multiple respiratory viruses, including rhinovirus, adenovirus, influenza, parainfluenza, respiratory syncytial virus, human metapneumovirus, and coronaviruses. Infection due to *Chlamydia pneumoniae* and *Bordetella pertussis* may also mimic disease due to *M pneumoniae*. Co-infection with *Streptococcus pneumoniae* typically is associated with a greater degree of pulmonary consolidation and a greater increase in the white blood cell count than is seen with *M pneumoniae* pneumonia.

*M pneumoniae* infection has been known to cause a wide variety of extrapulmonary manifestations (Table 268-1), but the pathogenesis remains largely unknown. Possible explanations include the following: (1) direct type, in which the bacterium is present at the site of inflammation and local cytokines are produced by the bacterium; (2) indirect type, in which the bacterium is not present at the site of inflammation and immune modulations, such as autoimmunity or formation of immune complexes, play a role; and (3) vascular occlusion type, in which obstruction of blood flow is induced either directly or indirectly by the bacterium. Limitations of definitive diagnostic testing (see below) have made it difficult to prove a causal role for many of these conditions.

Central nervous system (CNS) complications compose the bulk of extrapulmonary manifestations. A respiratory illness often precedes 2 to 14 days before CNS findings in most patients. The mechanism behind these manifestations remains unknown but is thought to be a postinfectious phenomenon in most cases. Neurologic complications are most often self-limited, but they may be severe, life-threatening, and associated with long-term sequelae.

Dermatologic manifestations, most commonly a maculopapular rash, may occur in approximately 10% of children with *M pneumoniae* infection. It has been acknowledged that *M pneumoniae* is one of the most frequent agents identified in "typical Stevens-Johnson syndrome (SJS)" presenting with fever, conjunctivitis, stomatitis, and generalized cutaneous lesions. The presence of another distinct form mimicking SJS and without skin lesions is widely noticed and called atypical SJS. Although universal agreement has not been established, it is presently referred to as *M pneumoniae*–associated mucositis or *M pneumoniae*–induced rash and mucositis.

Hematologic, cardiovascular, gastrointestinal, musculoskeletal, respiratory, renal, and other inflammatory manifestations have been reported in rare cases. While Kawasaki disease associated with *M pneumoniae* infection is not unusual in Japan, the disease association is rarely reported outside of Asia. Cases of glomerulonephritis with or without interstitial nephritis have been reported along with multiple skin lesions. This leads to the speculation that circulating immune complexes containing mycoplasmal cell components are

**TABLE 268-1 EXTRAPULMONARY DISEASE REPORTED DUE TO *MYCOPLASMA PNEUMONIAE* INFECTION**

| |
|---|
| **Hematologic** |
| Hemolytic anemia (Coombs positive) |
| Hemophagocytic syndrome |
| Thrombocytopenic purpura |
| Infectious mononucleosis |
| Disseminated intravascular coagulation |
| Splenic infarct |
| **Dermatologic** |
| Erythema nodosum |
| Erythema multiforme |
| Urticaria |
| Mucositis |
| Stevens-Johnson syndrome |
| Subcorneal pustular dermatosis |
| Anaphylactoid purpura |
| Cutaneous leukocytoclastic vasculitis |
| **Neurologic** |
| Meningoencephalitis |
| Acute disseminated encephalomyelitis |
| Stroke |
| Aseptic meningitis |
| Cerebellitis |
| Acute cerebellar ataxia |
| Opsoclonus myoclonus syndrome |
| Myelitis |
| Striatal and thalamic necrosis |
| Psychological disorders |
| Guillain-Barré syndrome |
| Cranial/peripheral neuropathies |
| **Musculoskeletal** |
| Arthritis |
| Rhabdomyolysis |
| **Renal** |
| Glomerulonephritis |
| IgA nephropathy |
| Priapism |
| Renal artery embolism |
| **Cardiac** |
| Pericarditis |
| Myocarditis |
| Kawasaki disease |
| Endocarditis |
| Cardiac or aortic thrombus |
| **Gastrointestinal** |
| Hepatitis |
| Pancreatitis |
| **Respiratory** |
| Pulmonary embolism |
| **Sensory** |
| Otitis media |
| Conjunctivitis |
| Iritis |
| Uveitis |
| Sudden hearing loss |

probably involved in the pathogenesis. A few cases of pulmonary embolism have been reported in association with *M pneumoniae*. Production of antiphospholipid antibodies has been shown to be an underlying mechanism for thrombus formation.

## DIAGNOSIS

Routine laboratory tests are chiefly used to exclude other conditions. Blood leukocyte levels and differential counts are usually within normal limits, but there may be mild leukocytosis. Erythrocyte sedimentation rate may be elevated during the course of the disease.

Chest radiography for *M pneumoniae* shows no characteristic pattern, but some features may be seen more frequently when compared to other types of pneumonia. Bronchopneumonia is the most common presentation, although segmental parenchymal infiltration can also be seen. Involvement of one or both lower lobes is the most common presentation, although either upper lobe can be involved as well. Hilar lymphadenopathy and pleural effusions can occur and are usually unilateral, small, and transient. Empyemas and lung abscesses are rare.

Experts consider the most reliable diagnosis for acute *M pneumoniae* infection is a combination of 2 or more separate laboratory methods, such as serology and polymerase chain reaction (PCR). Serologic diagnosis of *M pneumoniae* infection is a 4-fold increase in antibody titer measured in paired acute and convalescent sera. The sensitivity of serologic tests depends on the time point of the first serum and on the availability of paired sera for seroconversion to immunoglobin (Ig) G and/or rise in antibody titer. Serum IgM emerges within 1 week of initial infection and about 2 weeks before IgG; unfortunately, it may persist for several months, limiting its utility in diagnosis of acute disease. In the past, cold agglutinins and complement fixation tests were widely used. Problems with cold agglutinins included a lack of specificity for *M pneumoniae*, as autoantibodies in the blood can be elevated from other diseases or syndromes. For complement fixation tests, a single 1:64 titer was considered an indication of recent *M pneumoniae* infection, but the test lacks sensitivity and specificity. Newer *M pneumoniae* antibody assays may have similar problems. Cultures, although not available in most diagnostic laboratories, may require 2 to 6 weeks to complete, and results require collection of a convalescent specimen. Thus, both culture and serologic tests may offer only retrospective diagnosis.

PCR tests for *M pneumoniae* are replacing other tests as they are rapid and yield positive results earlier in the course of the disease than serologic tests. The PCR assay detects *M pneumoniae* even when only a small number of organisms are present in respiratory secretions and other body fluids. PCR performed on respiratory tract specimens (nasal wash, nasopharyngeal swab, pharyngeal swab) has a sensitivity and specificity between 80% and 100%. However, because asymptomatic shedding of *M pneumoniae* can persist for several weeks following infection, the significance of a positive PCR (or culture) in the absence of an associated antibody response is not known. From a practical viewpoint, diagnosis most often is based on clinical and epidemiologic features. Severe or unusual presentations may require attempted laboratory diagnosis using combined antibody testing and PCR.

## TREATMENT

Because *Mycoplasma* organisms lack a cell wall, they do not respond to β-lactam agents. Agents that interfere with DNA synthesis and have the best minimum inhibitory concentrations against *M pneumoniae* include quinolones, macrolides, and tetracyclines. Sensitivity to the aminoglycosides and chloramphenicol is variable.

Pneumonia due to *M pneumoniae* can be self-limited, making it difficult to assess antibiotic efficacy. To date, there is insufficient evidence in the literature to support a beneficial effect of macrolides in the treatment of community-acquired lower respiratory tract infection due to *M pneumoniae* in children. If choosing to treat *M pneumoniae* pneumonia, macrolides such as azithromycin should be considered first. Several comparative studies in children with laboratory-documented *M pneumoniae* infection have demonstrated that clarithromycin (15 mg/kg/d divided into twice-daily doses for 10 days) and azithromycin (10 mg/kg—maximum 500 mg—on day 1, followed by 5 mg/kg—maximum 250 mg—on days 2–5) are as effective as erythromycin in achieving clinical cure. Erythromycin is usually administered to preadolescent children at an oral dose of 30 to 40 mg/kg/d divided into 4 evenly spaced administrations for 10 to 14 days and is usually effective and minimizes symptomatic relapses. Doxycycline is an effective alternative therapy for children older than 7 years. Adult doses of erythromycin (1–2 g/d divided into 4 doses) or doxycycline (100 mg twice daily) can be used in adolescents weighing more than 60 kg. Fluoroquinolones such as moxifloxacin, gemifloxacin, ofloxacin, and levofloxacin have been studied in adults with atypical pneumonia and have been beneficial.

Macrolide-resistant strains of *M pneumoniae* are becoming increasingly common. Resistant organisms have been isolated from children with respiratory tract infection in Japan since 2000 and have since been continuously reported in increasing percentages in eastern Asian countries. However, prevalence of macrolide resistance varies among countries. Restriction fragment length polymorphism or gene sequence analysis has demonstrated that a point mutation in domain V of 23S rRNA reduced the affinity of macrolide for the large subunit (50S) of the bacterial ribosome. In the United States, the macrolide-resistant *M pneumoniae* rates from 2012 through 2014 were approximately 13%.

Despite limitations in our understanding of the importance of antimicrobials in treating *M pneumoniae* infections, antibiotic therapy should continue to be used for patients with community-acquired pneumonia when the differential diagnosis includes *M pneumoniae, C pneumoniae*, and *S pneumoniae*. It is impractical to establish a microbial cause for each patient, though reasonable efforts should be made to determine the cause of infection in hospitalized patients so that optimal antibiotic therapy can be provided.

Natural *M pneumoniae* disease appears to confer only limited protective immunity as reinfections have been documented as soon as 13 months after the original infection in young children, and repeated episodes of pneumonia have been seen within 4 to 10 years in older children. Prolonged therapy may be required for immunocompromised children. Because there is some evidence that extrapulmonary complications result from the host inflammatory response, rather than, or in addition to, damage from infection, both corticosteroids and immune globulin have been used in an attempt to ameliorate symptoms in the most severe cases, such as encephalitis or SJS. Moreover, anticoagulation therapy appears promising for vascular occlusion–type manifestations.

### PREVENTION

Outbreaks of infection due to *M pneumoniae* in closed populations have been reported, and there is evidence that prophylactic azithromycin therapy is 60% to 75% effective in preventing transmission of infection in those settings. Vaccine development continues to be an area of interest as it may help reduce morbidity from pneumonia, secondary complications of *M pneumoniae* infection, and the impact of macrolide-resistant strains. Recombinant proteins as vaccine candidates have been studied in animals with mixed results.

## *MYCOPLASMA HOMINIS*

Six *Mycoplasma* species colonize the genitourinary tract in humans, but only 2, *M hominis* and *M genitalium*, have been clearly linked to human disease. Prospective studies have attempted to define a relationship between *M hominis* and low birth weight, miscarriage, and premature delivery without consistent success. However, *M hominis* has been associated with a variety of conditions in premature newborns, which include meningitis, bacteremia, pneumonia, and subcutaneous abscesses. In older children and adults, *M hominis* has been associated with CNS disease, arthritis, wound infections, bacteremia, endocarditis, and respiratory tract infection. Most case reports in the literature involve patients who are immunocompromised or in the postpartum state.

### EPIDEMIOLOGY

*M hominis* can be part of the flora of sexually experienced women and may play a role in premature labor, chorioamnionitis, salpingitis, postpartum endometritis, pyelonephritis, and bacterial vaginosis. Colonization in men is less common. *M hominis* has also been detected on the skin and mucous membranes and in gastric aspirates of newborn infants whose mothers are colonized or infected. Studies have also demonstrated by culture the presence of *M hominis* in the cord blood of infants born prematurely.

### DIAGNOSIS

*M hominis* can be isolated on blood agar and in broth media used for the routine isolation of bacteria from blood. PCR assays for detection of *M hominis* have used 16S rRNA as the gene target. Theoretical advantages of the PCR assay over the culture include that no viable organisms are necessary, its limit of detection is better, and results can be available within 1 day. Serologic tests for *M hominis* using the techniques of microimmunofluorescence, metabolism inhibition, and enzyme immunoassay have been developed and used in research settings, but no assays have been standardized or made commercially available in the United States.

### TREATMENT

*M hominis* infection can be treated with tetracyclines, although resistance has been reported. Clindamycin and fluoroquinolones are alternatives. Unlike the other mycoplasmas that cause infection in humans, *M hominis* is usually resistant to erythromycin and azithromycin.

## *MYCOPLASMA GENITALIUM*

Isolation of *M genitalium* was first reported in 1981, and like *M hominis*, it is found in the genitourinary tract. Understanding of the epidemiology and clarification of the link between *M genitalium* and disease in humans has been made difficult by its fastidious growth requirements, but PCR identification has provided evidence that this organism may play a role in pelvic inflammatory disease, nongonococcal urethritis, endometritis, and cervicitis. There is insufficient evidence to attribute pregnancy outcome or neonatal disease to *M genitalium* infection. *M genitalium* is susceptible to doxycycline, macrolides, and moxifloxacin. Various studies have shown that azithromycin-sensitive strains have at least 100-fold more activity in vitro against *M genitalium* than any of the quinolones or tetracyclines. There are now cases of emerging strains resistant to both azithromycin and moxifloxacin. *M genitalium* is weakly sensitive to the other fluoroquinolones such as ciprofloxacin and ofloxacin.

### SUGGESTED READINGS


American Academy of Pediatrics. *Mycoplasma pneumoniae* and other *Mycoplasma* species infections. In: Kimberlin DW, Brady MT, Jackson MA, Long SS, eds. *Red Book: 2015 Report of the Committee on Infectious Diseases*. 30th ed. Washington, DC: American Academy of Pediatrics; 2015:568-571.

Biondi E, McCulloh R, Alverson B, Klein A, Dixon A, Ralston S. Treatment of mycoplasma pneumonia: a systematic review. *Pediatrics*. 2014;133:1081-1090.

Blanchard A, Bébéar C. The evolution of *Mycoplasma genitalium*. *Ann N Y Acad Sci*. 2011;1230:e61-e64.

Meyer Sauteur PM, Unger WW, Nadal D, Berger C, Vink C, van Rossum AM. Infection with and carriage of *Mycoplasma pneumoniae* in children. *Front Microbiol*. 2016;7:329.

Narita M. Classification of extrapulmonary manifestations due to *Mycoplasma pneumoniae* infection on the basis of possible pathogenesis. *Front Microbiol*. 2016;7:23.

Olson D, Watkins LKF, Demirjian A, et al. Outbreak of *Mycoplasma* pneumonia-associated Stevens-Johnson syndrome. *Pediatrics*. 2015;136:e386-e394.

Parrott GL, Kinjo T, Fujita J. A compendium for *Mycoplasma pneumoniae*. *Front Microbiol*. 2016;7:513.

Winchell JM. *Mycoplasma pneumoniae*—a national public health perspective. *Curr Pediatr Rev*. 2013;9:323-333.

# 269 *Neisseria gonorrhoeae*

Melissa Del Castillo

## INTRODUCTION

A commonly reported infectious disease in the United States, gonorrhea is sexually transmitted and principally affects adolescents and young adults. Infants can be infected by passage through an infected birth canal. Children can acquire the disease through sexual play, molestation, and sexual abuse. The principal manifestation of the uncomplicated infection is a urethral or vaginal discharge; however, localized infections of the fallopian tubes, joints, conjunctiva, pharynx, and anus, as well as disseminated infection, can occur.

## PATHOGENESIS AND EPIDEMIOLOGY

The gonococcus is a gram-negative kidney bean–shaped diplococcus, nonmotile and nonencapsulated, and fastidious in its nutritional requirements. It grows best aerobically in carbon dioxide with increased humidity on a medium of chocolate agar with antibiotics (Thayer-Martin medium) that suppress the growth of other microorganisms. Gonococci grow in small colonies that are easily identified; they elaborate indophenoloxidase—the basis for identification by an oxidase test. However, definitive identification (required in more complicated clinical settings and for medicolegal purposes) requires the use of specific fluorescein-conjugated antibody staining or sugar fermentation.

*Neisseria gonorrhoeae* infects nonciliated columnar and transitional epithelial cells. Attachment to the cells is mediated by pili and the outer-membrane opacity proteins. Within 24 to 48 hours after attachment, the organism synthesizes enzymes to facilitate penetration to submucosal tissues. The host produces a neutrophil response, which results in sloughing of the epithelium, submucosal abscesses, and a purulent exudate. *N gonorrhoeae* is capable of invading the bloodstream and disseminating to other sites, such as the joints and meninges. Bacteremic spread is also more likely to occur in conjunction with menstruation, which facilitates spread to the upper genital tract (salpingitis). Deficiency of one of the terminal components of the complement system (especially factors 5, 6, 7, or 8) places the patient at increased risk of disseminated, chronic, or recurrent gonococcal disease.

Gonococcal infections are limited to humans, and transmission is almost always sexual (genital, anal, or oral). The US rate of reported gonorrhea cases reached a historic low of 98.1 cases per 100,000 people in 2009. However, the rates of gonorrhea infections have been increasing slightly each year since then, to a rate of 110.7 cases per 100,000 people in 2014 (a total of 350,062 cases were reported to the Centers for Disease Control and Prevention [CDC] in 2014). The increase in gonorrhea has been observed primarily among men. Rates increased among individuals age 20 to 24 years and in older age groups, but decreased among younger age groups. Gonorrhea infections have increased in South and West United States but have decreased in the Northeast and Midwest. Sexual transmission and risk factors for gonococcal infection are further discussed in Chapter 228.

## CLINICAL MANIFESTATIONS

The incubation period of gonorrheal infection is 2 to 7 days. Infection may occur in the newborn period, in prepubertal children, and in sexually active adolescents and adults. The majority of infected males present with urethritis, which has been described at all ages, even in the newborn. Most gonococcal infections in the mature female are asymptomatic, but there may be thick purulent cervical or urethral discharge and pain upon manipulation of the cervix, which is indicative of pelvic inflammatory disease (PID). The following types of gonococcal infections are of particular relevance to the pediatrician.

## LOCALIZED INFECTIONS

### Pharyngeal

Pharyngeal infection is increasingly common in adults and adolescents as a result of orogenital sexual practices and has been reported in children who are victims of sexual abuse. The clinical findings, when present, are cryptic tonsillitis, pharyngitis and erythema, and swelling of the soft palate. These infections are typically asymptomatic otherwise. Infection is diagnosed by culture of the organism. Nucleic acid amplification test (NAAT) is not cleared by the US Food and Drug Administration (FDA) for use on oropharyngeal specimens; however, some laboratories have met standardized regulatory requirements and established performance specifications for using NAAT on oropharyngeal and rectal samples.

### Vulvovaginitis

*N gonorrhoeae* is one of the etiologic agents to consider in preadolescent girls with vulvovaginitis. Before puberty, the vaginal mucosa is more susceptible to infection than it is in the mature female. The majority of gonococcal infections in girls younger than 9 years of age result from sexual abuse. Typically, girls with vulvovaginitis present with a voluminous thick green or creamy vaginal discharge. Asymptomatic infections with labial erythema and scanty secretions have been described. Because the endocervical glands in the prepubertal female are not developed, infection rarely spreads to the fallopian tubes and upper genital tract, although tubal infection or peritonitis can rarely occur. Septic complications, such as arthritis, have also been reported.

### Cervicitis

In postpubertal females, the endocervix is the primary site of infection. A mucopurulent discharge from the cervical os is frequently accompanied by severe pelvic pain upon manipulation of the cervix. The infection may ascend from the vagina or cervix to the upper genital tract to cause inflammation of the endometrium (endometritis), fallopian tubes (salpingitis), ovaries (oophoritis), or the pelvic peritoneal cavity (pelvic peritonitis).

### Urethritis

Infection in young men usually presents with a purulent urethral discharge; it is commonly associated with dysuria, frequency of urination, and meatal erythema. Gonococcal urethritis occurs in preadolescent boys, in whom it is usually the result of sexual experimentation or molestation. Urethritis can also occur in women.

### Anorectal Infections

Anorectal gonorrhea occurs in children who have been molested, in sexually active young men and women, and in the neonate. Symptoms include rectal pain, tenesmus, mucopurulent rectal discharge, and rectal bleeding. On inspection, the mucous membrane is friable and erythematous, and a discharge may be present.

### Pelvic Inflammatory Disease (Salpingitis)

Infection rarely spreads to the upper genital tract in prepubertal girls. However, with the onset of menarche and sexual intercourse, some 10% to 20% of young women with gonorrhea will develop tubal infections. Infection can spread along the paracolic gutters to the liver, causing Fitz-Hugh Curtis syndrome (see Chapter 228).

### Gonococcal Ophthalmia

Unilateral or bilateral gonococcal ophthalmia can occur at any age, but it notoriously afflicts the newborn infant, who is infected by contact with gonococci from the birth canal. Instillation of silver nitrate solution into the eyes of all newborns shortly after birth had greatly reduced but not completely eliminated gonococcal ophthalmia neonatorum; the current practice of using erythromycin ointment for prophylaxis is of uncertain efficacy in an era of decreased gonococcal susceptibility to macrolides.

The appearance of a purulent or serosanguinous discharge from the eye 2 to 7 days after delivery should prompt a gram-stained smear and culture for *N gonorrhoeae*. Purulent discharge occurring within 48 hours of birth is most often the result of chemical conjunctivitis; during the second week of life, the likely diagnosis is *C trachomatis*. Edema, congestion of lids and conjunctiva, periorbital swelling, and adherence of eyelashes ("matting") due to purulent exudate are typical of gonococcal ophthalmia. A Gram stain of the exudate shows polymorphonuclear leukocytes, some containing intracellular diplococci. Spontaneous recovery may occur, but permanent damage, such as iridocyclitis and corneal ulceration, occurs in about one-third of untreated individuals. In view of the serious consequences of gonococcal ophthalmitis, with perforation of the globe of the eye and blindness, treatment should be commenced as early as feasible, based on a gram-stained smear, without awaiting cultural confirmation. Infants with suspected gonococcal ophthalmia should have a blood culture and lumbar puncture and should be treated with systemic antibiotics until results of the cultures are known.

## DISSEMINATED INFECTIONS

Disseminated disease constitutes less than 1% of gonococcal infections. Hematogenous spread of gonococci can originate from local infections and can occur at any age; there is a predisposition to dissemination during the neonatal period, during pregnancy, and at the time of menses, as well as in drug users, patients with accompanying liver disease, and individuals with terminal complement deficiencies. Disseminated gonococcemia in the neonatal period may be associated with scalp abscesses secondary to fetal monitoring through scalp electrodes, arthritis, and meningitis.

Arthritis and tenosynovitis are the most common manifestations in adolescents and adults. During the phase of bacteremia, a migratory polyarthritis is typical. All joints may be affected, but knees, ankles, and wrists are most frequently affected. Accompanying skin lesions are common (arthritis-dermatitis syndrome) and consist of clusters of erythematous or hemorrhagic lesions about 2 mm in diameter, whose centers are gray or black because of necrosis, or hemorrhage, or both. Skin lesions are found more frequently on the extremities, clustered around joints. At the time of bacteremia, cultures of joint fluid are rarely positive, but later bacteria may localize to 1 or more joints, at which time there may be purulent effusion containing viable gonococci.

More than 30 instances of gonococcal meningitis have been reported among newborn infants and adults. Infection may present as a typical pyogenic meningitis, but frequently, the simultaneous presence of urethritis, arthritis, or cutaneous lesions affords clues to its cause.

## DIAGNOSIS

In gonococcal ophthalmia, vulvovaginitis, and urethritis, examination of a stained smear of the purulent discharge will usually reveal intracellular gram-negative diplococci. Although this finding is virtually diagnostic, confirmatory cultures are important for precise bacteriologic identification, especially for medicolegal purposes. In females, symptoms are usually insufficient evidence for presumptive diagnosis, and gram-stained smears of secretions from the vagina or endocervix are frequently negative. The presence of nonpathogenic *Neisseria* species (eg, *N sicca, N subflava*) may occasionally result in false-positive smears.

Disseminated disease is difficult to diagnose because cultures of blood, joint fluid, or skin lesions show growth of gonococci in less than one-third of patients; even under optimal circumstances in which all 3 tissues are cultured, fewer than 50% of suspected cases are confirmed bacteriologically.

Specimens should be collected using swabs made of a synthetic fiber and transported in a medium that will keep the organisms alive (eg, Transgrow agar, a modification of Thayer-Martin medium, or other similar medium). Rapid diagnosis using DNA probes, enzyme immunoassays, and DNA amplification techniques (NAAT) in urine and secretions from the vagina, endocervix, or urethra provide increased sensitivity. However, cultures are still the preferred testing method if there are medicolegal concerns such as sexual abuse.

## TREATMENT

The CDC provides guidelines for treatment of sexually transmitted infections including gonococcal infections. Emergence of fluoroquinolone resistance among *N gonorrhoeae* strains prompted the CDC to cease recommending fluoroquinolone use for treatment in 2007. Because the minimum concentrations of cefixime needed to inhibit in vitro growth of *N gonorrhoeae* began to increase in 2006, the CDC now recommends dual therapy with ceftriaxone plus azithromycin. Most states have laws allowing minors to be treated for sexually transmitted infections without parental consent in order to encourage teenagers to seek therapy even though they are unwilling to have their parents know that they are sexually active.

## UNCOMPLICATED INFECTIONS IN ADOLESCENTS

The treatment regimen for uncomplicated infections (eg, vaginal, cervical, urethral, rectal) in adolescents is ceftriaxone 250 mg intramuscularly in a single dose plus azithromycin 1 g orally in a single dose. If ceftriaxone is unavailable, an alternative regimen is cefixime 400 mg orally in a single dose plus azithromycin 1 g orally as a single dose. However, it is important to keep in mind emerging resistance to oral cephalosporins.

## UNCOMPLICATED INFECTIONS IN THE PHARYNX

Pharyngeal infections can be more difficult to eradicate than genital infections. The recommended regimen for treatment of gonococcal oropharyngeal infection is 250 mg ceftriaxone intramuscularly in a single dose plus azithromycin 1 g orally as a single dose.

## CONJUNCTIVITIS IN ADOLESCENTS

The recommended treatment is a single 1-g dose of ceftriaxone plus azithromycin 1 g orally in a single dose. A one-time lavage of the infected eye with saline solution can be considered.

## DISSEMINATED INFECTIONS IN ADOLESCENTS

The treatment of disseminated gonococcal infection is 1 g ceftriaxone intramuscularly or intravenously every 24 hours plus azithromycin 1g orally in a single dose. Alternative treatments include 1 g cefotaxime or ceftizoxime intravenously every 8 hours plus azithromycin 1 g orally as a single dose. Data are limited regarding alternative regimens for persons allergic to β-lactam drugs. However, spectinomycin, 2 g every 12 hours, can be used. Hospitalization and consultation with an infectious disease expert are recommended for initial therapy. The duration of treatment for disseminated gonococcal infection has not been systematically studied and should be determined in consultation with an infectious disease specialist.

Typically, with substantial clinical improvement and guided by antimicrobial susceptibility, most patient with arthritis-dermatitis syndrome can switch to an oral agent in 24 to 48 hours, for a total treatment course of at least 7 days. The recommended therapy for meningitis and endocarditis is 1 to 2 g of ceftriaxone intravenously every 12 hours plus azithromycin 1 g orally once, for a duration of 10 to 14 days for meningitis and at least 4 weeks for endocarditis.

## OPHTHALMIA NEONATORUM

The key to treatment is parenteral administration of an effective antimicrobial agent. Because of the high prevalence of penicillin resistance, ceftriaxone 25 to 50 mg/kg intravenously or intramuscularly should be administered in a single dose. Although 1 dose of ceftriaxone is sufficient therapy for neonatal conjunctivitis, most infants receive antibiotics for 48 to 72 hours until blood and cerebrospinal fluid cultures are found to be negative. No data exist on the use of dual therapy with azithromycin.

## DISSEMINATED INFECTIONS AND SCALP ABSCESSES IN INFANTS

Treatment consists of ceftriaxone 25 to 50 mg/kg/d intravenously or intramuscularly in a single daily dose for 7 days (10–14 days if meningitis is documented). Cefotaxime, 25 mg/kg intravenously or intramuscularly every 12 hours, may be used instead of ceftriaxone.

### ALLERGIC TO OR INTOLERANT OF PENICILLIN OR CEPHALOSPORINS

Treatment with spectinomycin in a single dose of 40 mg/kg (maximum of 2 g) is recommended. There are data in adults with the use of either gemifloxacin 320 mg orally once plus azithromycin 1 g orally once, or gentamicin 240 mg intramuscularly once plus azithromycin 2 g orally once. However, no data for these regimens exist in children.

## PREVENTION

Part of management of gonorrhea is to identify and treat the sexual contacts of the patient; therefore, patients should be instructed to refer sexual partners for evaluation and treatment (see Chapter 228). Persons having sexual contact with the infected patient within the 60 days preceding onset of symptoms or gonorrhea diagnosis should be referred for testing and presumptive treatment. Patients and their partners should abstain from any sexual contact for 7 days after they have completed treatment and after resolution of symptoms.

## SUGGESTED READINGS

Barbee LA, Kerani RP, Dombrowski JC, Soge OO, Golden MR. A retrospective comparative study of 2-drug oral and intramuscular cephalosporin treatment regimens for pharyngeal gonorrhea. *Clin Infect Dis.* 2013;56:1539-1545.

Bissessor M, Whiley DM, Fairley CK, et al. Persistence of *Neisseria gonorrhoeae* DNA following treatment for pharyngeal and rectal gonorrhea is influenced by antibiotic susceptibility and reinfection. *Clin Infect Dis.* 2015;60:557-563.

Darling EK, McDonald H. A meta-analysis of the efficacy of ocular prophylactic agents used for the prevention of gonococcal and chlamydial ophthalmia neonatorum. *J Midwifery Womens Health.* 2010;55:319-327.

Kirkcaldy RD, Weinstock HS, Moore PC, et al. The efficacy and safety of gentamicin plus azithromycin and gemifloxacin plus azithromycin as treatment of uncomplicated gonorrhea. *Clin Infect Dis.* 2014;59:1083-1091.

Patton ME, Kidd S, Llata E, et al. Extragenital gonorrhea and chlamydia testing and infection among men who have sex with men—STD Surveillance Network, United States, 2010–2012. *Clin Infect Dis.* 2014;58;1564-1570.

Rietmeijer CA, Mettenbrink CJ. Recalibrating the gram stain diagnosis of male urethritis in the era of nucleic acid amplification testing. *Sex Trans Dis.* 2012;39:18-20.

Workowski KA, Bolan GA. Sexually transmitted diseases treatment guidelines, 2015. *MMWR Recomm Rep.* 2015;64:1-137.

# 270 *Neisseria meningitidis*

Madan Kumar

## INTRODUCTION

*Neisseria meningitidis* is a common commensal bacterium of the human upper respiratory tract. Colonization infrequently leads to disseminated disease, but the resulting meningitis and sepsis can be fulminant and rapidly fatal in healthy children and adults. Among survivors, 11% to 19% are left with disabilities such as neurologic deficit, hearing loss, or limb amputation. Despite advances in vaccine technology, *N meningitidis* remains a significant worldwide pathogen and the cause of epidemic meningitis. Children and young adults bear most of the burden of disease.

## PATHOGENESIS AND EPIDEMIOLOGY





*N meningitidis* are gram-negative, aerobic diplococci that grow well on enriched medium such as chocolate or Mueller-Hinton agar in an atmosphere of 5% to 10% carbon dioxide. Organisms are divided into 13 serogroups based on the structure of their capsular polysaccharide, but only 6 (A, B, C, Y, W-135, and X) account for most of the disease, with groups A, B, C, and Y predominating. Molecular subtyping methods (eg, multilocus enzyme electrophoresis, pulsed-field gel electrophoresis, or DNA sequence analysis) are useful for the characterization of outbreaks and the identification of disease-causing clones.

Meningococci are transmitted by aerosol or contact with secretions and colonize the respiratory mucosa. Focal spread can lead to respiratory tract infection, including pneumonia. Invasion through epithelial surfaces leads to bloodstream dissemination, allowing the bacteria to seed the meninges, pericardium, or large joints. The loss of protective maternal antibody renders the infant susceptible until endogenous antibody is induced by carriage of *N meningitidis* and *Neisseria lactamica*, a nonpathogenic species, as well as cross-reactive antibody induced by normal enteric organisms.

*N meningitidis* enters the nasopharynx and attaches to nonciliated epithelial cells, probably through the binding of the pili to the CD46 receptor (a membrane cofactor protein) and the subsequent binding of opacity-associated proteins, Opa and Opc, to the CD66e (carcinoembryonic antigen) and heparan sulfate proteoglycan receptors, respectively (Fig. 270-1). The attached organisms are engulfed by the cells, enter phagocytic vacuoles, and may then pass through the cells. IgA1 protease (an outer-membrane protein) cleaves lysosome-associated membrane protein and may promote the survival of *N meningitidis* in epithelial cells. PorB (another outer-membrane protein) crosses the cell membrane and arrests the maturation of the phagosome. In the bloodstream, the organisms release endotoxin in the form of blebs (vesicular outer-membrane structures) that contain 50% lipooligosaccharide and 50% outer-membrane proteins, phospholipids, and capsular polysaccharide. The endotoxin and probably other components stimulate cytokine production and the alternative complement pathway. *N meningitidis* crosses the blood-brain barrier endothelium by entering the subarachnoid space, possibly through the choroid plexus of the lateral ventricles.

Humans are the only reservoir for *N meningitidis.* Approximately 10% of the general population are asymptomatic, nasopharyngeal carriers. Peak colonization rates of 24% to 37% occur in healthy adolescents and young adults. The colonization rate increases even more under conditions of crowding in which people from diverse regions are brought together, such as with military recruits, pilgrims, or prisoners. The majority of these strains are not pathogenic, but carriage often results in protective serum antibodies. Even colonization with a virulent clone infrequently leads to disease, but when dissemination occurs, it is often in the first week after acquisition. Serum bactericidal antibody that activates complement has been shown to be responsible for blocking the dissemination of meningococci from the nasopharynx. Baseline endemic disease can be punctuated with localized outbreaks or epidemics caused by virulent, genetically related (focal complex) strains.

Exposure to tobacco smoke, concurrent viral infection of the upper respiratory tract, household crowding, and chronic underlying illness all increase the risk of developing disseminated disease. Several studies have looked at the risk of meningococcal disease in college students in the United States and the United Kingdom. While the risk was higher for domestic college students residing in dormitories compared to those residing in other types of accommodations, the overall incidence among college students was similar or slightly lower than that seen in the general population of similar age. In the United Kingdom, college students had higher rates of meningococcal disease compared with nonstudents, and risk was associated with residence in dormitories.

Underlying immune defects increase the risk of invasive meningococcal disease but account for only a small percentage of disease. These include functional and anatomic asplenia as well as several genetic defects. X-linked properdin deficiency predisposes to fatal meningococcemia, and defects in the terminal complement components (C5 to C9)

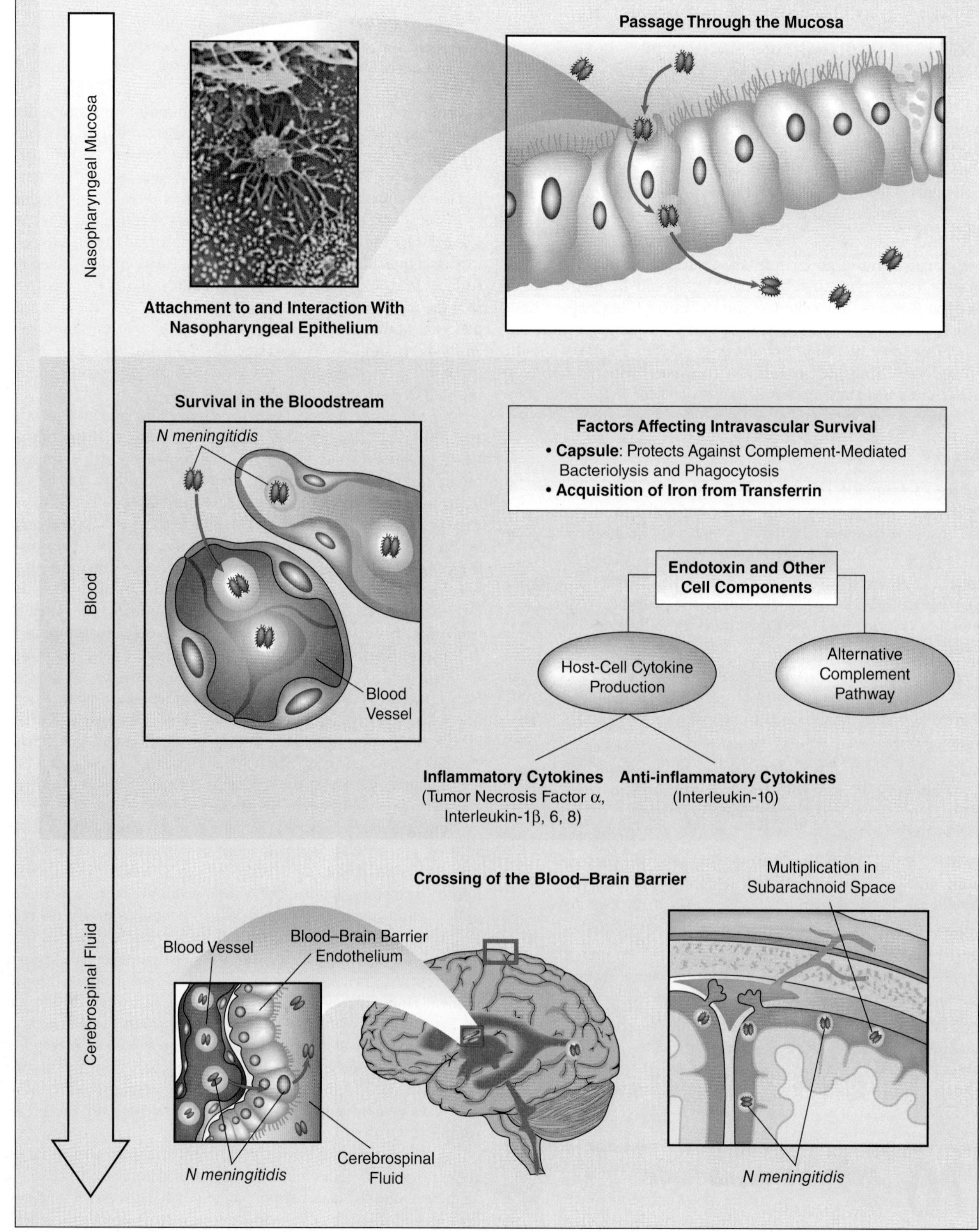


**FIGURE 270-1** Colonization of *Neisseria meningitidis* in the nasopharynx and entry into the bloodstream and cerebrospinal fluid.

increase the risk for recurrent infections. Polymorphisms in genes encoding for mannose-binding lectin, the Fcγ-receptor II (CD32) and III (CD16), plasminogen activator inhibitor (PAI-1), and Toll-like receptor 4 (TLR4) are associated with increased frequency or severity of disease.

Meningococcal disease occurs worldwide. Serogroups B and C cause most of the disease in industrialized nations, including the United States. Recently, group Y has increased in prevalence domestically and now accounts for one-third of cases. Serogroup A and, to a lesser extent, serogroup C predominate in developing countries, with a much higher incidence of 25 cases per 100,000 population. Figure 270-2 shows the global serogroup distribution of invasive meningococcal disease.

Serogroup A causes the highest incidence of disease globally. Sub-Saharan Africa, known as the meningitis belt, experiences yearly outbreaks during the dry season. Epidemics, with rates up to 1000 cases

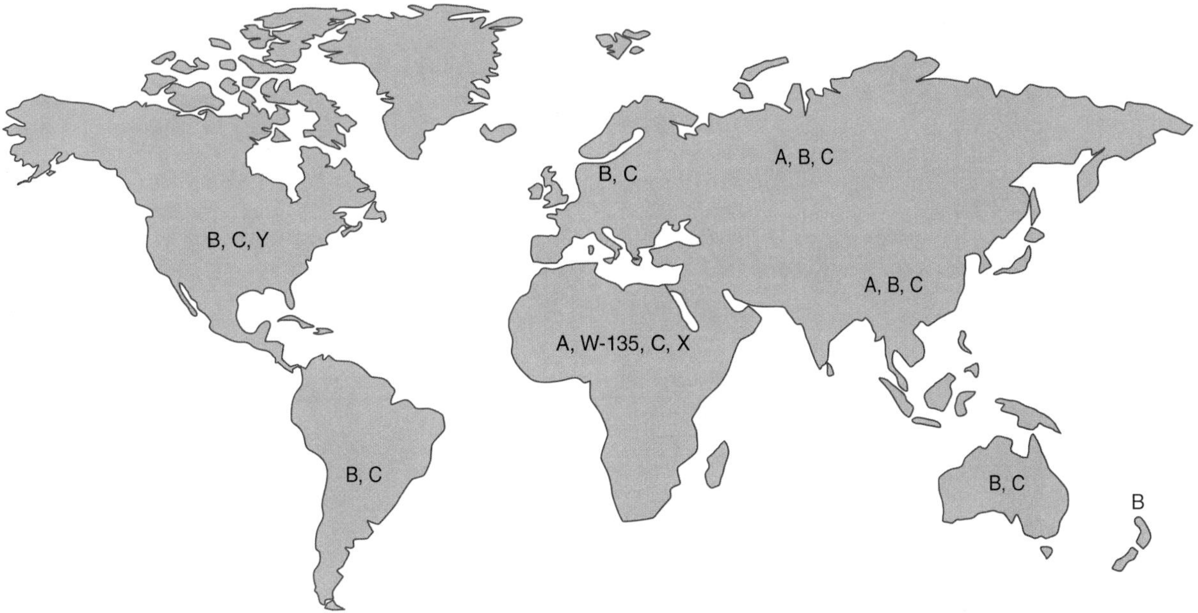


**FIGURE 270-2** Global serogroup distribution of invasive meningococcal disease.

per 100,000 people, have occurred every 5 to 12 years in this region, spreading from east to west. They are responsible for about 3000 to 10,000 deaths annually. Serogroup A epidemics have also occurred in China and Russia. Serogroup B is associated with a lower incidence of disease but has been associated with prolonged outbreaks in Europe, Cuba, South America, and New Zealand. Serogroup C has caused major epidemics in sub-Saharan Africa and Brazil and also focal outbreaks in Canada and Western Europe. Serogroup W has emerged as a cause of outbreaks associated with the Hajj (pilgrimage to Mecca) and in Africa, with a recent epidemic in Burkina Faso. Previously rare, serogroup X has emerged as the cause of a recent epidemic in Niger.

In the United States, the rate of meningococcal disease remained relatively stable at 0.9 to 1.5 cases per year per 100,000 people between 1960 and 1999, or 2500 to 3000 cases per year. The rate of disease then declined yearly until 2004, after which it has remained steady. Since 2005, only an estimated 800 to 1000 cases have been reported annually. Meningococcal disease varies seasonally, with the highest attack rates occurring in the winter and early spring. The prevalence of serum bactericidal antibody is lowest in infants 6 to 24 months of age, and this window of susceptibility correlates with the peak incidence of meningococcal disease. Rates drop during childhood, and then a second, smaller peak occurs during adolescence and early adulthood.

## CLINICAL MANIFESTATIONS

Meningococcal disease can manifest as several different clinical syndromes as summarized in Table 270-1. Meningitis without shock occurs in about 50% of cases (higher in developing countries) and is indistinguishable from other forms of purulent meningitis. Fever, headache, and neck stiffness are sometimes accompanied by photophobia, nausea, and altered mental status. Infants often present with irritability and lethargy and occasionally a bulging anterior fontanel. Bacteria are isolated from the blood in up to 75% of cases. This can present as occult bacteremia in young children being evaluated for fever without a source or as transient bacteremia associated with fever and a nonspecific rash. Meningococcal sepsis occurs in 5% to 10% of patients and is characterized by fever and petechial or purpuric rash. This can progress to fulminant meningococcal septicemia (purpura fulminans) and is associated with rapid growth of meningococci in the bloodstream, resulting in very high concentrations of organisms and endotoxin. Patients present with severe, persistent shock with little or no signs of meningitis. The development of a profound inflammatory response leads to progressive circulatory collapse; severe coagulopathy; and impaired pulmonary, renal, and adrenal function. Disseminated intravascular coagulation results in thrombotic lesions in the skin, limbs, kidneys, adrenals (Waterhouse-Friderichsen syndrome), and choroid plexus and lungs; multiorgan failure ensues. Vascular complications often lead to limb amputation and extensive skin loss (Fig. 270-3)

Pneumonia occurs in 5% to 15% of patients with disseminated meningococcal disease and tends to occur in older children. Other, less common respiratory tract infections include otitis media and epiglottitis. Focal infections occur less frequently and include septic arthritis, purulent pericarditis, conjunctivitis, urethritis, osteomyelitis, primary peritonitis, and endophthalmitis. Chronic meningococcemia is a rare manifestation that can last weeks to months and is characterized by prolonged intermittent fevers, rash, and arthralgias.

## DIAGNOSIS

The culture of *N meningitidis* from a normally sterile site, including blood, cerebrospinal fluid (CSF), and less frequently, synovial, pleural, and pericardial fluid, remains the cornerstone of diagnosis. In the absence of antibiotic treatment, the blood culture is positive in 40% to 75% and the CSF culture in 80% to 90% of cases. Once antibiotics have been initiated, the sensitivity of a culture rapidly decreases. The Gram stain of CSF remains important in the evaluation of a patient with meningitis and can rapidly and accurately determine the diagnosis. Up to 75% of cases of meningitis will have a positive culture result in the absence of antibiotics.

**TABLE 270-1 INFECTIOUS SYNDROMES ASSOCIATED WITH MENINGOCOCCAL DISEASE**

| |
|---|
| Meningitis |
| Bacteremia |
| Meningococcemia (purpura fulminans and the Waterhouse-Friderichsen syndrome) |
| Respiratory tract infection |
| Pneumonia |
| Epiglottitis |
| Otitis media |
| Focal infection |
| Conjunctivitis |
| Septic arthritis |
| Urethritis |
| Purulent pericarditis |
| Chronic meningococcemia |

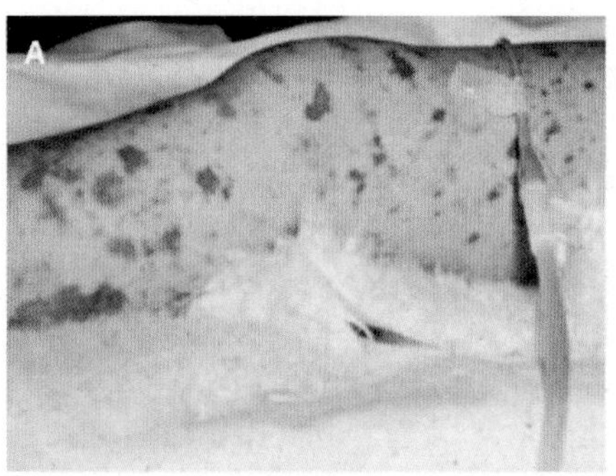

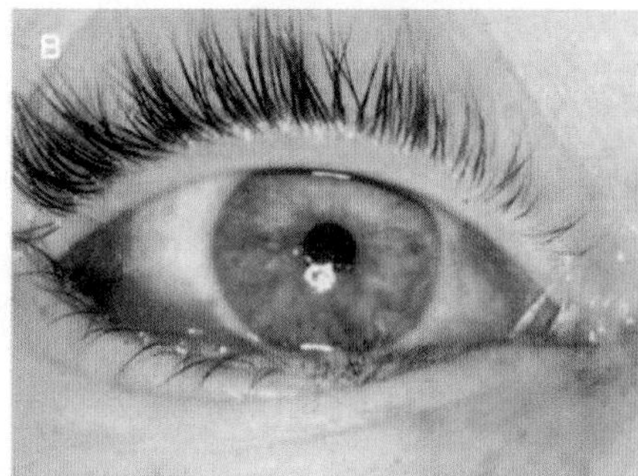

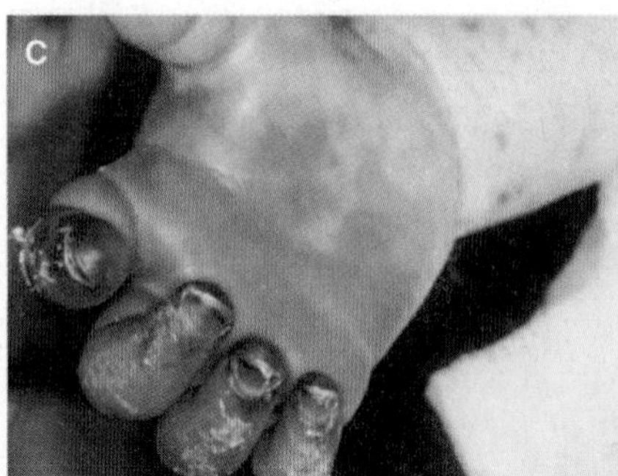

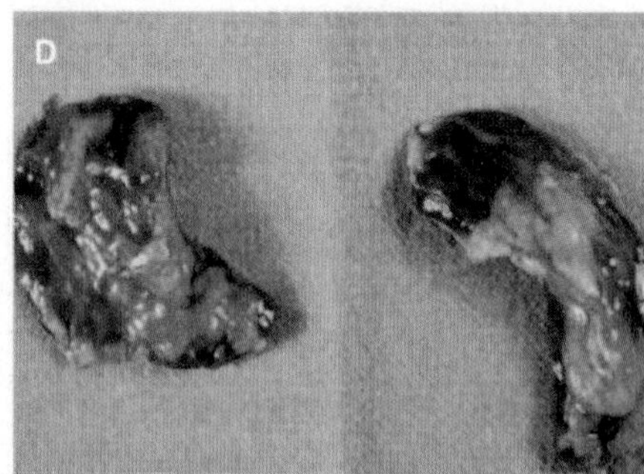

**FIGURE 270-3** Fulminant meningococcal septicemia: **A:** Fulminant meningococcal septicemia with ecchymoses, **B:** eye with intraocular hemorrhage, **C:** thrombosis and gangrene in the fingers of a child, and **D:** hemorrhagic adrenal glands.

Recently, polymerase chain reaction (PCR) has emerged as a very useful tool in the diagnosis of meningococcal disease and has the advantage of being rapid and more sensitive than culture or antigen detection. Since viable bacteria are not necessary, PCR is less affected by pretreatment with antibiotics. A prospective study of children found that real-time PCR of blood and CSF had a sensitivity of 96%, specificity of 100%, positive predictive value of 100%, and negative predicted value of 99%.

## TREATMENT

The antibiotics penicillin, cefotaxime, ceftriaxone, and chloramphenicol are effective in treating meningococcal infections, although decreased susceptibility to penicillin, secondary to alterations in penicillin-binding protein, has been reported worldwide. The clinical significance of this intermediate resistance is uncertain, as both failure and success in treatment have been reported. US surveillance studies reported that 3% to 30% of strains showed intermediate resistance to penicillin. Decreased susceptibility to penicillin has been reported worldwide and varies by country. Some areas of Spain have reported that more than 55% of strains were not fully penicillin susceptible. Most mean inhibitory concentrations (MICs) of penicillin have ranged from 0.06 to 0.8 μg/mL. High-level penicillin resistance (MIC > 1 μg/mL), β-lactamase–producing strains, and chloramphenicol resistance remain rare. Because susceptibility testing of meningococcus is not standardized, most clinical laboratories do not perform such testing.

Rapid initiation of antibiotics is crucial in the treatment of meningococcal disease as CSF is sterilized within 3 to 4 hours after starting intravenous antibiotics and plasma endotoxin levels fall by 50% within 2 hours. Empirical antimicrobial therapy for purulent meningitis is based on age and predisposing factors. For children 1 month of age or older, empiric therapy should include a third-generation cephalosporin (eg, ceftriaxone or cefotaxime). Empiric therapy will often also include an agent such as vancomycin for potential meningitis from gram-positive bacteria such as *Streptococcus pneumoniae*. Once *N meningitidis* is isolated, therapy can be completed with penicillin, ampicillin, or a third-generation cephalosporin. Five to 7 days of intravenous antibiotic are recommended.

With the advent of antibiotics in the 20th century, the mortality rate for meningococcal disease declined dramatically, but has since remained stable at 9% to 12%. The mortality rate for meningococcal sepsis is much higher and reaches 40%. Of survivors, 11% to 19% are left with sequelae including hearing loss, neurologic disability, or need for limb amputation. One multicenter surveillance study of invasive meningococcal disease in children found an overall mortality of 8%, which varied by age. Children who were 11 years of age or older had a higher mortality rate of 21% compared with a rate of 4.8% for children younger than 11 years of age. Hearing loss occurred in 12.5% of children with meningitis. Other less common sequelae included limb amputation, skin necrosis, ataxia, and hemiplegia. Immune-mediated complications such as pericarditis and arthritis can occur several days after the onset of illness when the patient is otherwise improving.

## PREVENTION

The risk of meningococcal disease is increased among close contacts. Hence, chemoprophylaxis is indicated for household members, childcare center contacts, and anyone directly exposed to the patient's oral secretions (Table 270-2) beginning 7 days before onset of illness in the index patient. The risk of secondary disease is highest in the first 7 days of illness in the index patient, and chemoprophylaxis should be given as soon as possible, preferably within 24 hours of diagnosis. Nasopharyngeal cultures are not useful in determining the need for prophylaxis. Rifampin, ciprofloxacin, and ceftriaxone have been shown to be effective. Rifampin 10 mg/kg (maximum 600 mg) orally every 12 hours is given to children 1 month of age or older for 2 days. In infants younger than 1 month of age, each dose is reduced to 5 mg/kg. Rifampin is not recommended for pregnant women. Ceftriaxone is given in a single intramuscular dose of 125 mg for children younger than 15 years of age and 250 mg for individuals 15 years of age or older. For nonpregnant individuals, ciprofloxacin in a single 20-mg/kg oral dose (maximum 500 mg) is also an acceptable alternative. Failure of appropriate prophylaxis has been reported but remains rare.

In the United States, there is 1 vaccine available that uses capsular polysaccharides alone that is targeted against serotypes A, C, Y, and W-135 (MPSV4) and is licensed for individuals older than 2 years of age. There are 3 meningococcal polysaccharide (A/C/Y/W-135) and protein conjugate vaccines (MenACWY) licensed for individuals age 9 months through 55 years (MenACWY-D), 2 months through 55 years (MenACWY-CRM), and 6 weeks through 18 months (HibMenCY-TT). All persons age 11 to 18 years should receive a meningococcal

| TABLE 270-2 DISEASE RISK FOR CONTACTS OF INDIVIDUALS WITH MENINGOCOCCAL DISEASE |
|---|
| **High risk: chemoprophylaxis recommended (close contacts)** |
| • Household contact, especially young children |
| • Childcare or nursery school contact during 7 days before onset of illness |
| • Direct exposure to index patient's secretions through kissing or through sharing toothbrushes or eating utensils, markers of close social contact, during 7 days before onset of illness |
| • Mouth-to-mouth resuscitation, unprotected contact during endotracheal intubation during 7 days before onset of illness |
| • Frequently slept or ate in same dwelling as index patient during 7 days before onset of illness |
| • Passengers seated directly next to the index case during airline flights lasting more than 8 hours |
| **Low risk: chemoprophylaxis not recommended** |
| • Casual contact: no history of direct exposure to index patient's oral secretions (eg, school or work) |
| • Indirect contact: only contact is with a high-risk contact, no direct contact with the index patient |
| • Healthcare professionals without direct exposure to patient's oral secretions |
| **In outbreak or cluster** |
| • Chemoprophylaxis for people other than those at high risk should be administered only after consultation with local health authorities |

conjugate vaccination. People at increased risk of invasive meningococcal disease (eg, persons with terminal complement component deficiencies, persons with anatomic or functional asplenia, travelers to or residents of countries in which *N meningitidis* meningitis is hyperendemic or epidemic) should be immunized with a conjugate vaccine beginning at 2 months of age.

Two vaccines have recently been licensed for use against meningococcal B strains. The Advisory Committee on Immunization Practices (ACIP) of the CDC and the American Academy of Pediatrics (AAP) recommend that patients at high risk of meningococcal disease (ages 10 and older) should receive a serogroup B vaccine series. Meningococcal vaccine recommendations are changing rapidly as new information is gathered. Practitioners should consult current resources (ACIP or AAP) for guidance.

## SUGGESTED READINGS


American Academy of Pediatrics. Meningococcal infections. In: Kimberlin DW, Brady MT, Long SS, Jackson MA, eds. *Red Book: 2015 Report of the Committee on Infectious Diseases*. 30th ed. Elk Grove Village, IL: American Academy of Pediatrics; 2015:547-556.

Centers for Disease Control and Prevention. Prevention and control of meningococcal disease: recommendations of the Advisory Committee on Immunization Practices (ACIP). *Morb Mortal Wkly Rep.* 2013;62:1-22.

MacNeil JR, Bennett N, Farley MM, et al. Epidemiology of infant meningococcal disease in the United States, 2006-2012. *Pediatrics.* 2015;153:e305-e311.

MacNeil JR, Rubin L, Folaranmi T, Ortega-Sanchez IR, Patel M, Martin SW. Use of serogroup B meningococcal vaccines in adolescents and young adults: recommendations of the Advisory Committee on Immunization Practices, 2015. *Morb Mortal Wkly Rep.* 2015;64:1171-1176.

Rouphael NG, Stephens DS. *Neisseria meningitidis*: biology, microbiology, and epidemiology. *Methods Mol Biol.* 2012;799:1-20.

Terranella A, Beekmann SE, Polgreen PM, Cohn A, Wu HM, Clark TA. Practice patterns of infectious disease physicians for management of meningococcal disease. *Pediatr Infect Dis J.* 2012;31:e208-e212.

Zalmanovici Trestioreanu A, Fraser A, Gafter-Gvili A, Paul M, Leibovici L. Antibiotics for preventing meningococcal infections. *Cochrane Database Syst Rev.* 2013;10:CD004785.


# 271 Nocardiosis

Nahed Abdel-Haq



## INTRODUCTION

Nocardiosis is an uncommon gram-positive infection with protean clinical manifestations. It is caused by a soilborne aerobic actinomycete of the family Nocardiaceae and is acquired mostly through the respiratory tract. Members of the family Nocardiaceae reproduce by fragmenting into bacillary and coccoid elements but are distinguished by filamentous growth with true branching. These organisms appear as gram-positive branching filaments and are weakly acid-fast. *Nocardia* species grow readily on simple media as pigmented colonies due to rudimentary aerial mycelia.

## PATHOGENESIS AND EPIDEMIOLOGY

The immune response to *Nocardia* is both humoral and cellular. The neutrophils inhibit the spread of infection; however, the cell-mediated immune response is vital in preventing dissemination. Killing of the organism occurs via cytotoxic T lymphocytes and activated macrophages. *Nocardia* may persist in neutrophils and macrophages by production of enzymes that inactivate the myeloperoxidase system. Nocardiosis produces suppurative necrosis and abscess formation typical of pyogenic infection. In contrast to the pronounced tissue fibrosis seen in actinomycosis, nocardiosis seldom provokes more than a loose wall of granulation tissue. This absence of encapsulation accounts for the tendency of this organism to disseminate from its initial pulmonary focus. Sulfur granules are not formed by this organism except in the skin in the lymphocutaneous or mycetoma syndromes.

The genus *Nocardia* contains at least 80 species that were characterized by molecular methods. Species from the *Nocardia asteroides* complex (*N cyriacigeorgica*, *N farcinica*, *N abscessus*, and *N nova*) are the most common cause of human disease in the United States. Other species that are associated with human disease that belong to the *Nocardia* genus but are not identified as part of the *N asteroides* complex include *N brasiliensis* and *N otitidiscaviarum* complex. *Nocardia* species can be skin contaminants and respiratory tract saprophytes. They are ubiquitous in the environment and can be found worldwide as saprophytes in soil, fresh and salt water, and decaying organic material, including vegetation and animal deposits. Some species may be more prevalent than others in certain geographic areas with specific climates. Infections with *Nocardia* appear to be more prevalent in the southwestern United States. Possible explanations include the facilitation and dispersal of *Nocardia* by the dusty, dry, and windy conditions in these areas. *N brasiliensis* is most frequently found in tropical and subtropical areas. In the United States, *N brasiliensis* is prevalent in the southeastern and southwestern states. Most systemic diseases in humans are caused by *N asteroides. N farcinica* has been reported to cause more severe disease and disseminated infections than other species. *N farcinica* and *N otitidiscaviarum* are increasingly reported in invasive infections and may have clinical implication due to their antibiotic resistance. Human beings acquire pulmonary infections by inhaling contaminated dust particles from environmental sources, whereas traumatic inoculation through the skin is responsible for subcutaneous disease. There is no evidence for airborne, animal-to-person, or person-to-person spread. Nosocomial outbreaks have been linked to environmental sources. Dust contaminating air systems in the operating rooms or the transplant units has been suggested as the source. About 15% of all patients with nocardiosis are children.

## CLINICAL MANIFESTATIONS

*Nocardia* can cause both localized and disseminated infections in humans. Although typically considered as an opportunistic infection, *Nocardia* can cause various clinical syndromes in immunocompetent patients. The most characteristic features of *Nocardia* are its ability to disseminate to any organ and its tendency for relapse despite appropriate antibiotic treatment.

## PULMONARY INFECTION

Pulmonary infection is the most common manifestation of nocardial disease. It occurs mostly in immunocompromised patients with frequent dissemination and death. Hematogenous dissemination particularly involves the nervous system and soft tissues. Predisposing conditions include steroid use, chronic granulomatous disease, hematologic malignancies, bone marrow and solid organ transplantation, human immunodeficiency virus infection, and alveolar proteinosis. In solid organ transplant recipients, high-dose corticosteroids, cytomegalovirus infection in the preceding 6 months, and high median calcineurin inhibitor serum levels in the preceding 30 days were independent risk factors for nocardiosis. Patients with bronchiectasis and cystic fibrosis are predisposed to colonization with *Nocardia*; infection may develop in the setting of steroid therapy. Patients receiving tumor necrosis factor inhibitors, particularly infliximab, may be at increased risk of *Nocardia* infection.

Species from the *N asteroides* complex are the etiologic agents most often isolated from pulmonary lesions. Lung involvement may be acute, subacute, or chronic. Symptoms are nonspecific and may resemble other chronic lung infections. Fever, night sweats, malaise, productive cough, pleuritic pain, anorexia, and weight loss are frequent. In addition to plain radiographs, computed tomography (CT) of the lungs is frequently needed to delineate extent of the disease. Radiologic findings include single or multiple nodules. Cavitation is a common finding. Lesions may appear as a localized infiltrate, a solitary lung abscess, necrotizing pneumonia, or progressive nodular fibrosis. Empyema, which can form sinus tracts to the chest wall resembling actinomycosis, may be seen. Local extension of lung lesions may cause mediastinitis or pericarditis. The differential diagnosis includes tuberculosis; actinomycosis; fungal infections, especially *Aspergillus*; *Rhodococcus equi* (in HIV-infected patients); and tumor. In high-risk patients, the diagnosis should be suspected when soft tissue swellings or abscesses and/or central nervous system (CNS) mass lesions develop in conjunction with a current or chronic pulmonary infection.

## EXTRAPULMONARY INFECTION

Hematogenous dissemination occurs in 30% of patients with pulmonary infection. Metastatic subcutaneous abscesses are common with pulmonary infection, as are hepatic and renal lesions. Although extrapulmonary nocardiosis usually occurs with concomitant lung lesions, some patients may present solely with extrapulmonary disease. CNS involvement occurs in 20% of patients with *Nocardia* infections and 44% of patients with disseminated disease. Affected patients most frequently present with discrete brain lesions or abscesses. Brain lesions may be single or multiple. Less frequently, *Nocardia* meningitis occurs, often with concomitant parenchymal involvement. The cerebrospinal fluid typically shows neutrophilic pleocytosis, hypoglycorrhachia, and elevated protein. Patients with CNS involvement may develop signs of increased intracranial pressure such as headache, confusion, and altered mental status. Seizures are common in patients with brain abscess. Fever and leukocytosis may be absent in patients with nocardial CNS disease mimicking a noninfectious etiology such as malignancy. The clinical progression of CNS disease is rapid in patients with underlying immune disorders. Normal hosts, in contrast, develop a more insidious and indolent disease process. Because *Nocardia* commonly causes metastatic brain lesions, especially in immunocompromised patients, brain imaging using magnetic resonance imaging (MRI) or CT should be done in those who have had *Nocardia* isolated from other sites even in the absence of neurological symptoms. Similarly, nocardiosis should always be suspected in any patient who presents with a brain lesion and has concurrent or recent lung findings. Brain imaging typically reveals single or multiple abscesses or cavitary lesions associated with peripheral and ring enhancement as well as surrounding edema.

Primary cutaneous disease occurs mainly in immunocompetent hosts following local trauma and subsequent environmental, often soil, wound contamination. *N brasiliensis* is responsible for the majority (80%) of these infections. Clinical manifestations include ulcerations, wound infection, pyoderma, superficial cellulites, and subcutaneous abscesses. Lymphocutaneous syndrome that resembles sporotrichosis is another presentation and is characterized by a subcutaneous nodule or abscess with lymphangitis and regional lymphadenopathy. The primary lesion is characterized by ulceration and purulence (pyoderma). It is usually caused by *N brasiliensis* and may be associated with traumatic injury. Skin infections with *Nocardia* may also follow a cat scratch and have been reported in postoperative sternal wound infections. Primary cutaneous infections should be distinguished from hematogenous dissemination in immunocompromised patients.

Mycetoma or Madura foot is a localized and slowly progressive chronic infection of the skin that may extend to involve the subcutaneous tissues and bone, usually involving the foot. It is characterized by a slowly progressive swelling consisting of a granulomatous mass and sinus tracts that drain purulent material that may occasionally contain sulfur granules. Evidence of systemic disease such as fever or malaise is lacking; local pain is rare. Most cases are due to *N brasiliensis*. Walking barefoot predisposes for this condition in endemic areas due to repeated trauma and inoculation of *Nocardia* from contaminated soil. *Nocardia* mycetoma occurs endemically in the tropics.

*Nocardia* bacteremia is mostly associated with central venous catheter–related infections mainly in cancer patients. Primary ocular nocardiosis is uncommon. Keratitis and endophthalmitis have been reported. Infection may develop in healthy people following minor trauma to the eye or may follow eye surgery. Other risk factors include corneal lens implants and topical corticosteroids. Other rare complications of *Nocardia* infection include peritonitis (during peritoneal dialysis), synovitis/arthritis, osteomyelitis, peritonsillar abscess, ventriculitis associated with a ventriculoperitoneal shunt, and cervicofacial infection resembling actinomycosis.

## DIAGNOSIS

Because the clinical and radiologic findings of nocardiosis are nonspecific, the diagnosis depends on the identification of the microorganism in a clinical sample obtained from the site of infection. As pulmonary involvement is reported in the majority of cases, respiratory samples are key to diagnosis. The diagnosis of pulmonary nocardiosis in some cases may be established by sputum analysis and culture. However, because *Nocardia* can be a respiratory saprophyte, bronchoalveolar lavage or lung biopsy is frequently needed to confirm the diagnosis due to the wide differential diagnosis and high frequency of co-infections in immunocompromised patients.

An invasive procedure such as tissue biopsy is often required to establish the diagnosis of nocardiosis. The most important diagnostic finding is appearance of the organisms on the Gram-stained smear of the clinical specimen. This will reveal the typical delicate, weakly gram-positive, irregularly stained, and beaded branching filaments surrounded by acute inflammatory cells. Many *Nocardia* species are acid-fast, in contrast to other branching gram-positive rods. Biopsy material should be stained by the Brow-Brenn (tissue Gram stain) and modified Fite (tissue acid-fast) stains.

The diagnosis is confirmed by culture. If *Nocardia* is suspected in a clinical specimen, the laboratory needs to be notified to optimize recognition and recovery of the organism. Using selective media for culture, blind subculture of negative blood culture bottles and prolonged incubation can increase recovery of *Nocardia* species. Cultures from sterile sites will grow in 2 to 14 days. In mixed cultures from respiratory secretions, rapidly growing bacteria may obscure small *Nocardia* colonies, and colonial characteristics sufficient to arouse suspicion often take 2 to 4 weeks to develop. Susceptibility testing should be conducted on all isolates from immunocompromised patients, patients with life-threatening illness or CNS involvement, and patients who are intolerant or not responding to initial treatment.

Limited *Nocardia* speciation may be done using a battery of biochemical laboratory tests. However, accurate identification of different species is accomplished by molecular methods such as 16s rRNA gene sequencing. Antibiotic susceptibility profiles are predictable for several *Nocardia* species. Because different *Nocardia* species vary in their antibiotic resistance patterns and clinical outcome, it is essential to send these isolates to a reference laboratory for precise molecular speciation and susceptibility testing.

## TREATMENT

A sulfonamide-containing regimen such as trimethoprim-sulfamethoxazole (TMP/SMX) or a sulfonamide alone is considered the treatment of choice. Sulfisoxazole (150 mg/kg every 4–6 hours) has been used. Sulfadiazine is less soluble in urine than other sulfonamides and may cause oliguria, azotemia, and crystalluria and thus should be avoided. TMP/SMX (15 mg/kg trimethoprim and 75 mg/kg sulfamethoxazole) is the most frequently used sulfonamide for nocardiosis, especially when intravenous treatment is desired. Patients unable to tolerate sulfonamides may receive minocycline, ampicillin, or erythromycin. Antibiotic resistance of *Nocardia* species has been increasing over time. Thus all clinically significant *Nocardia* isolates should have susceptibility testing performed. TMP/SMX should be avoided or used with caution in patients who are receiving other nephrotoxic medications such as cyclosporine. Nocardiosis has been reported in immunocompromised patients who are receiving TMP/SMX 3 times weekly for *Pneumocystis jirovecii* prophylaxis.

Due to the rising incidence of sulfonamide resistance in *Nocardia* species and poor clinical response in immunocompromised patients, most clinicians now administer combination drug therapy at least initially. Situations that favor this approach include CNS nocardiosis, overwhelming or disseminated disease, and nocardiosis in immunocompromised or HIV-infected patients. An empirical regimen consisting of TMP/SMX, amikacin, and either ceftriaxone or imipenem has been used in such situations. Treatment is continued with 2 agents to which the organism is susceptible. Duration of therapy depends on clinical response and immune status of the host. Initial treatment should be given intravenously for at least 6 weeks until the patient improves clinically and antibiotic susceptibility testing is available. Patients who respond to the initial treatment and who do not have CNS disease may be switched to an oral antibiotic such as TMP/SMX, minocycline, or amoxicillin-clavulanate. Because of the high mortality and the possibility of CNS disease, a 2- or 3-drug combination is usually required for the first 6 to 12 months. All patients with CNS involvement as well as immunocompromised patients regardless of the site of diseases should be treated for a total duration of at least 1 year and at least 3 months after apparent cure because of the risk of relapse. Patients with acquired immunodeficiency syndrome and persistently low CD4 counts may need lifelong suppressive therapy.

Linezolid, an oxazolidinone antibiotic, has been shown to have excellent in vitro activity against all clinically significant *Nocardia* species. Linezolid may be useful as part of initial combination therapy while awaiting cultures and susceptibility testing. It has been successfully used to treat patients with nocardiosis, including those who failed therapy with other antibiotics. However, linezolid use for more than 4 weeks is associated with hematologic toxicity in addition to reports of peripheral and optic neuropathy with long-term use. Thus, patients should be closely monitored when receiving long-term treatment with linezolid for nocardiosis.

Primary cutaneous *Nocardia* infections following inoculation injury in immunocompetent patients may be treated with a single oral agent. Trimethoprim-sulfamethoxazole and minocycline are the most commonly used antibiotics. Alternatively, amoxicillin-clavulanate, doxycycline, macrolides, fluoroquinolones, and linezolid may be used if susceptible in vitro. Patients with lymphocutaneous disease usually respond to a 6- to 12-week course of treatment. However, patients with mycetoma usually require treatment for 6 to 12 months. Tetracyclines are not used in children age 8 years and younger because of potential dental staining. Fluoroquinolones are not approved for use in children younger than 18 years of age.

Patients who do not show clinical improvement within the first 2 weeks of treatment should be carefully reevaluated. Poor response or progression of the disease indicates treatment failure. This may be due to drug resistance, the presence of an abscess that requires drainage, or poor tissue penetration of the antibiotic. Immunocompromised patients with nocardiosis who have poor response to appropriate therapy should be evaluated for possible concomitant pathogens such as *Aspergillus*, *P jirovecii*, and *Mycobacterium tuberculosis*.

Surgical drainage of empyema and mediastinal fluid collections is essential for good outcome. Localized pleuropulmonary disease usually does not require surgery. Drainage of abscesses is required in patients who fail to respond to antibiotic therapy; however, antimicrobial treatment of brain abscesses without surgery has been successful in some cases. Because immunosuppressive therapy predisposes patients to nocardiosis, lowering the doses of these medications or stopping them, if possible, may be helpful during the course of treatment.

The mortality of nocardiosis is still high (15–26%) despite specific therapy. Mortality is higher (60%) in cancer patients. Factors associated with poor outcome include underlying corticosteroid use, Cushing disease, the presence of dissemination involving 2 or more noncontiguous organs, CNS involvement, and fulminant disease at initial evaluation. Chemotherapy and concomitant cytomegalovirus infection are other risk factors of increased mortality in cancer patients.





## SUGGESTED READINGS

Coussement J, Lebeaux D, van Delden C, et al. Nocardia infection in solid organ transplant recipients: a multicenter European case-control study. *Clin Infect Dis*. 2016;63:338-345.

Hardak E, Yigla M, Berger G, Sprecher H, Oren I. Clinical spectrum and outcome of *Nocardia* infection: experience of 15-year period from a single tertiary medical center. *Am J Med Sci*. 2012;343:286-290.

Lebeaux D, Morelon E, Suarez F, et al. Nocardiosis in transplant recipients. *Eur J Clin Microbiol Infect Dis*. 2014;33:689-702.

Schlaberg R, Fisher MA, Hanson KE. Susceptibility profiles of *Nocardia* isolates based on current taxonomy. *Antimicrob Agents Chemother*. 2014;58:795-800.

Wang HL, Seo YH, LaSala PR, Tarrand JJ, Han XY. Nocardiosis in 132 patients with cancer: microbiological and clinical analyses. *Am J Clin Pathol*. 2014;142:513-523.

Welsh O, Vera-Cabrera L, Salinas-Carmona MC. Current treatment for *Nocardia* infections. *Expert Opin Pharmacother*. 2013;14:2387-2398.

Wilson JW. Nocardiosis: updates and clinical overview. *Mayo Clin Proc*. 2012;87:403-407.

# 272 *Pasteurella multocida*

Morven S. Edwards

## INTRODUCTION

*Pasteurella multocida*, formerly known as *Pasteurella septica*, was renamed *P multocida* or "killer of many" because it affects many different animal species. The first report of human infection caused by *P multocida* was published in 1919. The primary importance of the organism in pediatrics is in animal bites in which *P multocida*, alone or in concert with other organisms, is the most common infecting organism.

## PATHOGENESIS AND EPIDEMIOLOGY

There are several species in the genus *Pasteurella*. The most common human pathogen is *P multocida*, but infection also can be caused by one of the related species such as *P canis* or *P dagmatis*. There are 3 subspecies of *P multocida*: *multocida*, *septica*, and *gallicida*. More than one-half of human infections are caused by *P multocida* subspecies *multocida*. Defining the subspecies aids in epidemiologic investigation but is not necessary in the usual clinical setting.

There are 3 major clinical expressions of disease caused by *P multocida* depending on the portal of entry. Focal infection is initiated by direct inoculation of the organism into the subcutaneous tissue, bone, or joint space after a cat scratch or bite or a dog bite. The organism produces endotoxin, which may promote the inflammatory reaction that is observed, often within hours, after inoculation.

Respiratory tract infection occurs as a consequence of inhalation of *P multocida*. Animal-to-human but not human-to-human spread has been documented. The organism has low pathogenicity in the respiratory tract, and infection has been documented almost exclusively in the setting of altered host resistance.

Invasive infection occurs when hematogenous dissemination complicates primary soft tissue or pulmonary infection. Bacteremic infection is a particular risk for children with hepatic dysfunction and reduced efficiency of reticuloendothelial clearance mechanisms.

The organism is found as a component of the oral flora of 70% to 90% of cats and 25% to 50% of dogs. Other animals, including rabbits, rats, or pigs, also harbor the organism in respiratory tract or oral secretions. Carriage of *P multocida* by humans is uncommon, but commensal carriage can occur as a consequence of frequent animal contact. The usual mode of transmission is direct inoculation from the bite or scratch of a colonized animal. *P multocida* has been implicated as causal in 50% of dog and 80% of cat bite wound infections.

## CLINICAL MANIFESTATIONS

Focal infection, usually manifested as cellulitis, develops rapidly after inoculation of *P multocida*. The average time of onset of erythema, swelling, and pain is within 24 hours after an animal bite or scratch. Infections due to *P multocida* characteristically develop watery gray or serosanguinous drainage. Infection in the subcutaneous space can result in abscess formation and regional lymphadenopathy. Infection also can present as tenosynovitis, septic arthritis, or osteomyelitis. These expressions of infection usually occur after cat bites, which tend to penetrate tissue spaces more deeply than do dog bites. Joint stiffness with cellulitis of the hand is a finding suggestive of tendon sheath involvement.

When *P multocida* infection is not related to an animal bite, the most common focus of infection is the respiratory tract. The clinical manifestations are those expected for children with exacerbations of chronic underlying conditions, such as bronchiectasis or chronic bronchitis. Several cases of pleural empyema and of lung abscess have occurred.

Meningitis, with or without bacteremia, is the most common manifestation of invasive infection caused by *P multocida*. Most children diagnosed as having *Pasteurella* meningitis are younger than 1 year of age, and most have had contact with a pet within the household. These infections usually are associated with animal contact, such as licking, that does not violate cutaneous barriers. The presenting features include lethargy, irritability, and fever, similar to bacterial meningitis caused by other bacterial pathogens.

*P multocida* urinary tract infection can occur in children with obstructive uropathy, and peritonitis can occur in patients with chronic renal disease who are receiving peritoneal dialysis. The organism has been isolated from children with periappendiceal abscess or with peritonitis in association with appendicitis. It is not known whether these infections result from hematogenous spread or from ingestion of the organism. There are reports of unusual manifestations of infection due to *P multocida* such as ocular infections, tonsillitis, endocarditis, hepatic abscess, or infection of a ventriculoperitoneal shunt. Brain abscess has resulted from a dog bite that penetrated a small child's skull.

## DIAGNOSIS

*P multocida* is a small, nonmotile gram-negative rod that grows well on standard media, including blood, chocolate, and Mueller-Hinton agars. Colonies resemble enterococci on blood agar plates. If *P multocida* is suspected, laboratory personnel should be alerted so that appropriate confirmatory biochemical testing can be performed. Laboratory differentiation from morphologically similar organisms, such as *Haemophilus influenzae*, is not difficult.

Isolation of the organism from the drainage of skin lesions caused by bite wounds or from other sites of focal infection, such as joint fluid or aspirate of the subperiosteum, is diagnostic. Pleural fluid or sputum can yield the organism in patients with pulmonary infection. In disseminated infection, *P multocida* can be isolated from cultures of blood or, with meningeal involvement, from cerebrospinal fluid.

## TREATMENT

Penicillin is the drug of choice. Other effective oral agents include ampicillin, amoxicillin, amoxicillin-clavulanate, cefuroxime, cefpodoxime, cefixime, doxycycline, and fluoroquinolones. Susceptibility testing should be performed, but β-lactamase–producing strains have been recovered only rarely. Because polymicrobial infection should be assumed after an animal bite, empiric therapy consisting of oral amoxicillin-clavulanate or intravenous ampicillin-sulbactam should be initiated while culture results are pending. Parenterally administered broad-spectrum cephalosporins such as cefotaxime and ceftriaxone have good activity and have been used successfully to treat invasive *P multocida* infection.

In children who are allergic to β-lactam agents, the optimal treatment for *P multocida* infection is problematic. Doxycycline is effective, but tetracyclines should be administered to children younger than 8 years of age only after assessment of the risk-to-benefit ratio. Azithromycin exhibits good activity against *P multocida*. An oral alternative for empiric treatment of dog or cat bite wounds in penicillin-allergic children is trimethoprim-sulfamethoxazole *plus* clindamycin or, alternatively, an extended-spectrum cephalosporin *plus* clindamycin. Trimethoprim-sulfamethoxazole is effective against *P multocida* as well as *Staphylococcus aureus*. Clindamycin is active against anaerobes, as well as streptococci and most strains of *S aureus*. These combinations or carbapenem monotherapy can be employed parenterally for wounds of severity warranting hospitalization.

The usual duration of therapy is 7 to 10 days for focal soft tissue infections. A longer treatment course is required for septic arthritis and osteomyelitis. For pulmonary or disseminated infection, including meningitis, 10 to 14 days of therapy are usually required. Infected animal bite wounds should be adequately debrided. Infected collections of fluid should be drained, and devitalized tissue removed. Consultation with a specialist in hand surgery is appropriate for tendon sheath involvement. Preventive treatment for rabies should be instituted only if clinical circumstances warrant.

## PREVENTION

Educational interventions regarding appropriate interactions with domestic animals and limiting interactions with wild animals can help to prevent *P multocida* infections.

## SUGGESTED READINGS

American Academy of Pediatrics. Bite wounds. In: Kimberlin DW, Brady MT, Jackson MA, Long SS, eds. *Red Book: 2015 Report of the Committee on Infectious Diseases*. 30th ed. Elk Grove Village, IL: American Academy of Pediatrics; 2015:205-210.

American Academy of Pediatrics. *Pasteurella* infections. In: Kimberlin DW, Brady MT, Jackson MA, Long SS, eds. *Red Book: 2015 Report of the Committee on Infectious Diseases*. 30th ed. Elk Grove Village, IL: American Academy of Pediatrics; 2015:596-597.

Boyce JD, Seemann T, Alder B, Harper M. Pathogenomics of *Pasteurella multocida*. *Curr Top Microbiol Immunol*. 2012;361:23-38.

Goldstein EJC, Citron DM, Merriam CV, Tyrrell KL. Ceftaroline versus isolates from animal bite wounds: comparative in vitro activities against 243 isolates, including 156 *Pasteurella* species isolates. *Antimicrob Agents Chemother*. 2012;56:6319-6323.

Guet-Revillet H, Levy C, Andriantahina I, et al. Paediatric epidemiology of *Pasteurella multocida* meningitis in France and review of the literature. *Eur J Clin Microbiol Infect Dis*. 2013;32:1111-1120.

# 273 Pertussis

Joshua K. Schaffzin and Beverly L. Connelly

## INTRODUCTION

Despite relatively high coverage with an effective vaccine, pertussis continues to cause morbidity and mortality worldwide. The World Health Organization estimated in 2014 that approximately 89,000 children died from pertussis. The United States has seen a steady rise in case incidence to the highest levels in 60 years. The reemergence of pertussis in the United States and elsewhere punctuates the need for pediatricians to be aware of pertussis epidemiology and presentation in all ages. Early recognition of disease allows implementation of effective measures to prevent spread and further harm.

## PATHOGENESIS AND EPIDEMIOLOGY

*Bordetella* are small, fastidious, aerobic, gram-negative coccobacilli that require enriched media for isolation. *B pertussis* is a respiratory pathogen of humans only and is the sole cause of epidemic pertussis. *B parapertussis* is a closely related species that accounts for less than 5% of clinical pertussis. *B bronchiseptica* occasionally causes disease in the immunocompromised host but is better recognized as a veterinary pathogen. Less related genetically, *B holmesii* has been reported to cause respiratory illness and rarely joint infection in normal hosts and invasive infection in asplenic and immunocompromised patients.

*B pertussis* produces numerous virulence factors, including toxins and attachment agents, many of which are antigenic and included in the acellular vaccine. The link of each virulence factor to clinical illness has been difficult to elucidate due to lack of an animal model for experimentation. However, a recently developed model in infant baboons has the potential to address unanswered questions. The bacteria attach to ciliated epithelial cells of the respiratory tract, induce ciliary paralysis and local inflammation, and thicken and decrease clearance of secretions. *B pertussis* is not invasive. Pertussis toxin, necessary but not sufficient to cause clinical pertussis, is secreted by the bacteria and affects G-protein function, which prevents migration of lymphocytes to the area of infection, and inhibits the function of neutrophils, macrophages, monocytes, and lymphocytes. Adenylate cyclase toxin invades phagocytes and induces high levels of cyclic adenosine monophosphate (AMP), which impairs immune cell function and induces apoptosis. Other cell-surface proteins, including filamentous hemagglutinin, pertactin, and fimbrial agglutinogens, are involved in bacterial attachment to ciliated respiratory epithelium. Pertactin-deficient *B pertussis* strains have been described and hypothesized to evade vaccine immunity, although this has not borne out in surveillance studies. The function of additional factors, including tracheal cytotoxin, surface lipooligosaccharide, and cytoplasmic heat-labile toxin, is less well characterized.

Pertussis occurs year-round in the United States, although the disease usually peaks in the summer and fall in most locations and occurs in 3- to 5-year epidemic cycles. Humans are the only reservoir for the causative agent, *B pertussis*, which does not cause prolonged colonization or persist in the environment. Thus, transmission occurs from person to person via respiratory droplets. Higher transmission rates among close household versus community (eg, school) contacts have been reported, with attack rates following household exposure as high as 90% for unimmunized children and at least 30% in adults. Attack rates are lower when household members are vaccinated or cases are treated soon after disease identification. Communicability is highest early in the disease (catarrhal phase), but may persist for weeks in some individuals. Unrecognized disease serves as a reservoir for spread of infection.

Infants younger than 6 months of age have the highest burden of disease, with the highest rates of hospitalizations and mortality among those under 3 months of age. Based on Centers for Disease Control and Prevention (CDC) surveillance data from 2000 to 2003, 86% of hospitalizations for pertussis occur in infants less than 3 months of age. Apnea and respiratory distress were the most frequent complications, followed by pneumonias. The frequency of complications declines with increasing age; however, posttussive emesis, protracted cough (≥ 3 months), sleep disturbances, and weight loss are common in adults with pertussis; subcutaneous emphysema, pulled muscles, and even broken ribs may occur in adults following paroxysmal coughing. The characteristic "whoop" is often absent in older individuals. It is not until the nagging, forceful cough has persisted for 2 or more weeks that adolescents and adults come to medical attention. Even then, diagnosis may be delayed or disease may go unrecognized because of a low index of suspicion.

According to the CDC, the number of reported cases of pertussis in the United States has increased steadily since 1980. Over 48,000 cases were reported in 2012, the most since 1955. Large outbreaks and epidemics have been reported in many areas, including California and Ohio in 2010, Florida in 2013, and California in 2014. In 2014, infants younger than 6 months old had the highest reported rate of pertussis (169.0 per 100,000 population), but adolescents age 11 to 19 years contributed approximately one-third of reported cases. Adult caretakers with undiagnosed pertussis are frequently found to be the source for pertussis in infants. Nosocomial spread by healthcare workers has been well documented.

## CLINICAL MANIFESTATIONS

The incubation period of pertussis is usually 5 to 10 days but may be up to 3 weeks. Clinical pertussis is a protracted illness with 3 identifiable stages: the catarrhal, the paroxysmal, and the convalescent stages. The catarrhal stage is the most contagious phase and is indistinguishable from a common cold. During this stage, organism burden is highest, but fever is minimal or absent; rhinorrhea, sneezing, mild cough, and sometimes mild conjunctival suffusion last from a few days to a couple of weeks. In the young infant, signs and symptoms may be minimal or absent in the catarrhal stage.

Apnea, choking, or gasping may herald the paroxysmal stage in young infants. Observation in a setting in which assisted ventilation is available is prudent in the very young infant who presents with these features. Seemingly insignificant stimuli may provoke frightening episodes of coughing in the young infant, which may be sufficiently protracted to result in hypoxia and cyanosis. Forceful coughing can result in subconjunctival and scleral hemorrhages, upper-body petechiae, umbilical and inguinal hernias, subcutaneous emphysema, rib fractures, and even central nervous system hemorrhages. The characteristic inspiratory "whoop" of pertussis occurs in toddlers and older children at the end of a paroxysm as air is finally sucked in through a partially closed glottis. Posttussive emesis is common at all ages. Feeding becomes a major problem for the young infant and may actually provoke the paroxysm; the immediate postparoxysmal period may provide a refractory period during which feeding is possible. The severity of the child's paroxysms contrasts sharply with the lack of distress seen between coughing spells. Most of the complications from pertussis occur in the paroxysmal stage, which may last from 1 to 6 weeks.

During the convalescent period, coughing in the young infant may actually become louder, although generally less distressing. Overall, the paroxysmal coughing gradually lessens in severity and frequency during convalescence. Paroxysms may disappear, only to reappear in a milder form during a subsequent respiratory illness over the ensuing year. Persons with pertussis are considered infectious from onset of the catarrhal stage through the third week of the paroxysmal stage or until 5 days after starting treatment.

In addition to the immediate complications already mentioned, infectious and noninfectious complications of pertussis are numerous. Uncomplicated pertussis is usually an afebrile disease, so fever should prompt evaluation for a secondary bacterial infection. Otitis media and pneumonia are the most common secondary infections. Other pulmonary complications include atelectasis, emphysema, pneumothorax, and pulmonary hypertension. Coughing and vomiting may result in esophageal tears with hematemesis and melena. Neurologic complications include hypoxic encephalopathy, seizures, and intracranial bleeds. Nutritional compromise and resultant failure to thrive are common in young infants recovering from pertussis. Risk of death in the young infant is between 0.04% and 1%.

Classic pertussis in the nonimmune host is difficult to confuse with other illnesses. In the immunized individual, symptoms are less likely to be characteristic. A coughing illness for more than 2 weeks and/or posttussive emesis should arouse suspicion. In infants presenting with apnea, respiratory syncytial virus or other viral infection and serious bacterial illness need to be excluded.

*B pertussis* is the cause of epidemic pertussis as well as of most sporadic pertussis. *B parapertussis* may cause a similar syndrome that is less severe and of shorter duration. Protracted coughing illness mimicking pertussis may also be seen with adenovirus, *Mycoplasma*, and *Chlamydia*. Ancillary features of the illness such as sore throat, headache, or swollen lymph nodes, as well as knowledge of epidemiologically significant local pathogens, will aid diagnostically.

## DIAGNOSIS

Classical pertussis should be readily diagnosed based on clinical features. The presence of absolute peripheral lymphocytosis (> 10,000 lymphocytes/μL) is supportive evidence for systemically active pertussis toxin. Absolute lymphocyte counts of more than 20,000 cells/μL are not uncommon, and total white blood cell counts more than 100,000 cells/μL have been reported. The chest x-ray in pertussis is often normal, although shagginess along the cardiac border, peribronchial consolidation, and atelectasis may be seen. The presence of a focal infiltrate in a febrile child with pertussis may indicate a secondary bacterial process.

Recovery of *B pertussis* in culture has long been the gold standard for the diagnosis of pertussis. Nasopharyngeal specimens should ideally be obtained within the first 2 to 3 weeks of illness. Because of the fastidious growth requirements for *B pertussis*, cultures are most accurate in a laboratory experienced in *B pertussis* isolation. Nasopharyngeal samples should be obtained at the bedside, placed directly on selective or specific transport media, and incubated for 7 or more days. Asymptomatic carriage of *B pertussis* is extremely rare.

Polymerase chain reaction (PCR) testing on nasopharyngeal swab specimens for pertussis is becoming the most widely used diagnostic procedure, although assays are not standardized across clinical laboratories. PCR has proven to be sensitive and specific for the diagnosis of pertussis and is an accepted alternative to culture for case confirmation of *B pertussis* infection. Nasopharyngeal specimens should ideally be obtained within the first 0 to 3 weeks following cough onset, but may remain positive through 4 weeks. PCR can yield a false-positive result through contamination, and possibly due to the presence of *B holmseii*. To mitigate this, the CDC has provided a best practices statement for healthcare providers using PCR for diagnosing pertussis, which includes considering pretest probability and specimen collection timing with respect to cough onset and methodology.

Following natural infection, antibodies develop to several *B pertussis* antigens. These responses do not confer lifetime immunity but rather wane in 7 to 20 years. Immunization with whole-cell vaccine likewise results in response to multiple antigens, but responses last only 6 to 12 years. The acellular pertussis vaccines are well tolerated, offer very targeted responses, but do not have durability of response. Recent outbreaks and increases in disease incidence suggest the protection afforded by acellular vaccines may be as short as 4 to 5 years.

Serologic diagnosis of pertussis is not generally recommended. Standardized tests for routine serologic diagnosis are not widely available. Currently, the most generally accepted serologic criterion for diagnosis of pertussis is the use of an enzyme-linked immunosorbent assay to demonstrate a significant increase in immunoglobulin (Ig) G serum antibody concentrations against pertussis toxin between acute and convalescent specimens or a single point test collected 2 to 8 weeks following cough onset, available through the CDC. Results may not correlate with clinical disease and can be difficult to interpret in a highly immunized population.

In the past, a direct fluorescent antibody (DFA) test on secretions from a nasopharyngeal swab has been used for rapid presumptive diagnosis. However, inexperience in performing this test results in numerous false-positive and false-negative results, and thus DFA is no longer recommended by the CDC.

## TREATMENT

Treatment for clinical pertussis is primarily supportive. Hospitalization is indicated for all infants with severe paroxysms associated with cyanosis or apnea. Infants with potentially fatal pertussis may appear to be amazingly well between paroxysms. Caution should be exercised when suctioning these young, exhausted infants because it may precipitate a paroxysm. Admission to an intensive care setting is indicated if emergent response to paroxysms cannot be managed on the ward. Supplemental oxygen, intravenous fluids, and nutritional support are frequently required in severe and protracted disease. Some have suggested that early extracorporeal membrane oxygenation with leukodepletion in the most severe cases may decrease mortality. Cough suppressants, expectorants, mucolytic agents, bronchial dilators, anti-inflammatory agents, antihistamines, steroids, antipertussis toxin immunoglobulin, and sedatives are not proven to be beneficial in treating pertussis. Other adjunctive therapies under investigation involve manipulation of airway ion channels and phospholipid signaling. Young infants should remain hospitalized until nutrition is adequate, no supportive intervention is required during paroxysms, disease is unchanged or improved for at least 48 hours, and the infant's care can be safely managed at home.

Antibiotic therapy has no discernible effect on the course of the illness once the paroxysms are well established; however, treatment may ameliorate disease expression for those who are treated in the catarrhal phase. Clinicians should strongly consider treating prior to test results if clinical history is strongly suggestive or patient is at risk for severe or complicated disease (eg, infants). All suspected and confirmed cases of pertussis should be treated in order to minimize secondary spread. CDC recommends treating patients > 1 year of age within 3 weeks of cough onset and those ≤ 1year of age and pregnant women within 6 weeks of cough onset. Treatment and postexposure prophylaxis dosing is based on age and weight (Table 273-1). Macrolides are the drugs of choice for the treatment of pertussis and may improve infant survival. Studies have demonstrated that both azithromycin and clarithromycin are as effective as erythromycin at eliminating *B pertussis* from the nasopharynx, although there are no data in infants younger than 1 month of age. Because of the known association of erythromycin and infantile hypertrophic stenosis, it is not a preferred agent for use in neonates and should be used only if azithromycin is not available. There are data demonstrating that 7 days of erythromycin estolate are as effective as 14 days, which may reflect the improved penetration of this erythromycin formulation over others. Stomach upset is the most commonly reported side effect of erythromycin and frequently is a reason for patient noncompliance. In 2013, the FDA issued a warning that azithromycin may cause prolonged QT interval. Resistance to erythromycin has been reported but is believed to be limited at this time. β-Lactam antibiotics are not effective against *B pertussis*.

## PREVENTION

Local health officials should be notified of all cases in order to assist in outbreak control within the community. Household and daycare contacts of confirmed pertussis patients, as well as persons at high risk or who will have close contact with someone at risk of severe illness, should receive antibiotic prophylaxis within 21 days of onset of cough in the index case. Prophylaxis is indicated regardless of prior immunization status. Macrolides are the drugs of choice at the same dosages used for therapy. Efficacy of trimethoprim-sulfamethoxazole as a chemoprophylactic agent has not been evaluated.

Hospitalized patients should be managed in respiratory isolation (droplet precautions) until 5 days after the initiation of macrolide therapy. A private room is preferred; however, culture-positive cases may be cohorted. Untreated patients should remain in isolation until 3 weeks after the onset of paroxysms.

**TABLE 273-1 RECOMMENDED ANTIMICROBIAL TREATMENT AND POSTEXPOSURE PROPHYLAXIS FOR PERTUSSIS, BY AGE GROUP**

| | Primary Agents | | | Alternate Agent[a] |
|---|---|---|---|---|
| Age Group | Azithromycin | Erythromycin | Clarithromycin | TMP-SMZ |
| < 1 month | Recommended agent. 10 mg/kg daily in a single dose for 5 days (only limited safety data available) | Not preferred. Erythromycin is associated with infantile pyloric stenosis. Use if azithromycin is unavailable; 40–50 mg/kg daily in 4 divided doses for 14 days | Not recommended (safety data unavailable) | Contraindicated for infants age < 2 months (risk for kernicterus) |
| 1–5 months | 10 mg/kg daily in a single dose for 5 days | 40–50 mg/kg daily in 4 divided doses for 14 days | 15 mg/kg daily in 2 divided doses for 7 days | Contraindicated at age < 2 months. For infants ≥ 2 months, TMP 8 mg/kg daily, SMZ 40 mg/kg daily in 2 divided doses for 14 days |
| Infants (age ≥ 6 months) and children | 10 mg/kg in a single dose on day 1, then 5 mg/kg daily (maximum 500 mg) on days 2–5 | 40–50 mg/kg daily (maximum 2 g/d) in 4 divided doses for 14 days | 15 mg/kg daily in 2 divided doses (maximum 1 g/d) for 7 days | TMP 8 mg/kg daily, SMZ 40 mg/kg daily in 2 divided doses for 14 days |
| Adults | 500 mg in a single dose on day 1, then 250 mg daily on days 2–5 | 2 g/d in 4 divided doses for 14 days | 1 g/d in 2 divided doses for 7 days | TMP 320 mg/d, SMZ 1600 mg/d in 2 divided doses for 14 days |

[a]Trimethoprim-sulfamethoxazole (TMP-SMZ) can be used as an alternative agent to macrolides in patients age ≥ 2 months who are allergic to macrolides, who cannot tolerate macrolides, or who are infected with a rare macrolide-resistant strain of *Bordetella pertussis*.

Adapted with permission from Centers for Disease Control and Prevention. Recommended antimicrobial agents for the treatment and postexposure prophylaxis of pertussis: 2005 CDC guidelines. *Morb Mortal Wkly Rep*. 2005;54:RR-14; available at: http://www.cdc.gov/mmwr/preview/mmwrhtml/rr5414a1.htm

Immunization is the principal method of prevention. Current recommendations include vaccination of children beginning in infancy with booster doses for school-age children and preteens. Following introduction of the preteen booster, an initial reduction in cases was observed in the United States, but rates soon began to rise to historic levels. One hypothesis for this shift is the transition from whole-cell to acellular pertussis vaccine, where the birth cohort who did not receive whole-cell vaccine had more rapidly waning immunity following the preteen booster. Two strategies to prevent illness in infants 0 to 6 months of age have been proposed. The preferred strategy is immunizing pregnant women during the third trimester, which has been shown to be safe and effective. A secondary strategy is cocooning, where all individuals having close contact with infants < 6 months old are immunized. Immunizations are discussed further in Chapter 239.

## SUGGESTED READINGS


Burns DL, Meade BD, Messionnier NE. Pertussis resurgence: perspectives from the working group meeting on pertussis on the causes, possible paths forward, and gaps in our knowledge. *J Infect Dis*. 2014;209:S32-35.

Edwards KM, Berbers GA. Immune responses to pertussis vaccines and disease. *J Infect Dis*. 2014;209:S10-15.

Farizo KM, Burns DL, Finn TM, Gruber MF, Pratt RD. Clinical evaluation of pertussis vaccines: US Food and Drug Administration regulatory considerations. *J Infect Dis*. 2014;209:S28-S31.

Kilgore PE, Salim AM, Zervos MJ, Schmitt HJ. Pertussis: microbiology, disease, treatment, and prevention. *Clin Microbiol Rev*. 2016;29:449-486.

Melvin JA, Scheller EV, Miller JF, Cotter PA. *Bordetella pertussis* pathogenesis: current and future challenges. *Nat Rev Microbiol*. 2014;12:274-288.

Skoff TH, Martin SW. Impact of tetanus toxoid, reduced diphtheria toxoid, and acellular pertussis vaccinations on reported pertussis cases among those 11 to 18 years of age in an era of waning pertussis immunity: a follow-up analysis. *JAMA Pediatr*. 2016;170:453-458.

Winter K, Zipprich J, Harriman K, et al. Risk factors associated with infant deaths from pertussis: a case-control study. *Clin Infect Dis*. 2015;61:1099-1106.


# 274 Plague

Nicole Akar-Ghibril and Bernhard L. Wiedermann

## INTRODUCTION

Plague is a zoonotic infection primarily maintained in rodents and fleas. Humans are incidental hosts, and transmission from rodents to humans is most commonly by flea bites. This disease still exists worldwide and likely has been responsible for at least 3 devastating pandemics—the Justinian Plague (Byzantine Empire, 541–542), the Black Death (Europe and Middle East, 1346–1353), and the plague pandemic in the mid-19th century, which started in China.

## PATHOGENESIS AND EPIDEMIOLOGY

Plague is caused by *Yersinia pestis,* a pleomorphic, gram-negative, non–spore-forming coccobacillus that exhibits bipolar staining with Wright-Giemsa or Wayson stains. When cultures are obtained from clinical samples (eg, blood, sputum, lymph node aspirates), the organism can be recovered on blood, chocolate, or MacConkey's agar. Care should be taken if the clinician is suspecting *Y pestis* since many of the automated identification systems may not accurately identify this pathogens, confusing it with similar organisms (eg, *Yersinia enterocolitica*, *Yersinia pseudotuberculosis*).

The clinical presentation of plague is most often dictated by the portal of entry of the organism into the host. When the portal of entry is through the skin (eg, flea bite or contact with infected animals), the organisms most commonly settle out in the lymph nodes and form buboes, but *Y pestis* can just as easily disseminate throughout the bloodstream to distant organs. The severity of disease is determined by the extent of endotoxin production. Organisms that can continue to replicate within the host macrophages without being killed have the ability to produce high levels of endotoxin. When the portal of entry is the lungs, severe pneumonia, endotoxemia, and septicemia are more likely to occur, causing a fatal infection if not appropriately recognized and treated.

The geographic distribution of plague is largely confined to the semiarid areas of most continents, with the exception of Australia. Enzootic foci occur in Africa, Asia, North America, and South America, with the majority of human cases in Africa. Most cases occur in rural areas. North American foci occur primarily in the southwestern United States and the Pacific coastal region. The disease exists almost entirely in the sylvatic form, among a number of wild rodent species. Urban plague, the cause of the epidemics of the European Middle Ages, is dependent on the Norwegian rat and a flea (*Xenopsylla cheopis*) but is now quite rare. The last epidemic of urban US plague occurred in 1924 to 1925 in Los Angeles. Currently, a median of 8 cases of human plague are reported annually in the United States, although preliminary data from 2015 suggested a slight increase.

In the United States and Canada, the epidemiology is complex and involves a number of different rodent hosts and flea vectors, as well as domestic animals. Most commonly, the bubonic or septicemic form of infection is acquired by human exposure to infected tissues or from the bites of fleas of wild rodents such as prairie dogs, ground squirrels, chipmunks, rabbits, and other wild rodent species. Domestic animals, especially cats, may become infected after contact with wildlife and may transmit the infection to humans. Pneumonic plague is transmissible from person to person, bypassing both the rat reservoir and the flea vector. Human cases were linked to an infected domestic dog in Colorado in 2014. In this latter outbreak, human-to-human transmission also may have occurred, the first time this mode of transmission had been seen in the United States since 1924.

## CLINICAL MANIFESTATIONS

In the United States, most human plague cases occur from May to September and usually present as 1 of 3 primary forms: bubonic, septicemic, or pneumonic. Bubonic plague accounts for the vast majority of cases (80–95%), followed by septicemic (10–20%) and then pneumonic.

The incubation period of bubonic and septicemic plague is usually 2 to 6 days. Skin lesions are infrequently present at the site of initial infection (eg, flea bite). The first symptom usually consists of sudden onset of fever (39°C/102.2°F or higher), often accompanied by chills. Within hours to a few days, exquisitely tender, often erythematous or swollen lymph nodes are present; severe pain may occur prior to swelling. Any node may be involved, but the most frequently involved are the inguinal or femoral nodes, followed by axillary and cervical nodes. The nodes enlarge rapidly, forming the characteristic bubo. There may be erythema of the overlying skin. Buboes may vary in diameter from 1 to several centimeters. The buboes increase in size over several days until they become fluctuant and the overlying skin hemorrhagic. With clinical recovery, the lymph node abscess clears slowly, often healing within 2 weeks after onset, although occasionally the process may become chronic, with the formation of ulcers and draining fistulas.

Fever may be accompanied by profound malaise, severe headache, photophobia, abdominal pain, nausea, vomiting, diarrhea, restlessness, delirium, myalgias, and weakness. Fever usually peaks during the first 24 hours and then continues at slightly lower levels for 3 to 4 days, with occasional morning remissions. The temperature may then fall, sometimes achieving nearly normal levels, followed almost immediately by a second steep rise. If no complications or pulmonary disease develop, the fever again gradually declines after days 7 to 10 of illness, often in association with spontaneous rupture of the buboes. Although uncommon, seizures may occur secondary to fever or to the presence of concomitant meningitis.

Bacteremia occurs regularly during the early phase of the disease in both mild and severe forms. In some instances, the reticuloendothelial system clears the bloodstream of organisms. In other individuals, these defenses are overwhelmed, and a septic phase develops, during which the patient may succumb to overwhelming endotoxemia. Frequent signs are marked tachycardia, tachypnea, and hypotension. The bacteria may spread through the blood to the respiratory system, producing secondary pneumonia with pulmonary hemorrhages, edema, abscesses, or bronchitis. In addition, other organs, such as the brain and meninges, may become infected. Hemorrhages often occur in the skin, or more massive subcutaneous bleeding may be found. The affected areas have a distinctive red or black discoloration. A disseminated intravascular coagulation syndrome leading to gangrene of the skin, appendages, and various other organs may occur in patients who survive the initial endotoxemia.

Pneumonic plague can be rapidly fatal. It is acquired by inhaling infected aerosol (primary pneumonic plague) or following hematogenous seeding of the lungs with *Y pestis* (secondary pneumonic plague). The incubation period of primary pneumonic disease is very short, often less than 24 hours. The bacteria multiply rapidly within the alveoli, resulting in the absorption of massive amounts of endotoxin. Symptoms include cough, dyspnea, pleuritic chest pain, and hemoptysis. Hemorrhages occur in the lungs, with epithelial desquamation and bleeding into respiratory tissues. Radiologically, the process may resemble a lobar or bronchial pneumonia or massive pulmonary edema (ie, respiratory distress syndrome). The use of plague as a bioweapon is likely to be disseminated by aerosols, and thus, primary pneumonic plague is likely to be the most common presentation in weaponized plague.

A relatively mild form of plague (*pestis minor*) occurs rarely and may remain unrecognized. These patients demonstrate minimal toxicity, a low-grade fever, and simple lymphadenitis rather than buboes. This clinical picture is the result of infection with a strain of *Y pestis* lacking 1 or more virulence factors.

## DIAGNOSIS

Plague should be suspected in a patient in an endemic area who presents with the symptoms noted earlier. The bubonic form is usually accompanied by significant leukocytosis up to 50,000/μL, whereas in the pneumonic and septicemic forms, leukopenia or leukocytosis may be found with varying proportions of immature polymorphonuclear leukocytes. Classic bubonic plague can be recognized readily on clinical grounds, but the signs and symptoms of the septicemic form are similar to those of other gram-negative septicemias. Tularemia, especially when tick-borne, may greatly resemble plague, but the site of the initial bite is usually more evident with tularemia.

A presumptive diagnosis is established by detecting bipolar ("safety pin") staining, gram-negative organisms in blood cultures, sputum smears, or aspirates of the affected lymph nodes (buboes). A positive fluorescent antibody-staining test (often directed against the F1 capsular protein) permits rapid presumptive and species-specific diagnosis. Serologic tests for antibodies to *Y pestis* are also available (eg, passive hemagglutination of anti-F1 antibodies), but a rise in antibody may not occur until 2 weeks after the initial onset of symptoms. A single titer equal to 1:10 or greater provides a presumptive diagnosis. A 4-fold rise or fall over 3 to 6 weeks or a single titer equal to 1:128 or greater is considered diagnostic. Culture of the organism confirms diagnosis, but *Y pestis* has been misidentified by automated identification systems. Also, because plague is considered a potential bioterrorism agent, its isolation in most clinical laboratories in the United States is restricted to genus and presumptive species based on phenotypic criteria. Final specific identification is performed in appropriate public health laboratories. Polymerase chain reaction assay for *Y pestis pla* gene has been tested but is not routinely used.

## TREATMENT

Intravenous gentamicin or a fluoroquinolone (eg, levofloxacin or ciprofloxacin) is the medication used most commonly in the United States to treat plaque. Other likely effective agents include streptomycin, doxycycline, and chloramphenicol. Treatment is generally continued for 2 days after body temperature returns to normal or for a total of 10 to 14 days. Note that gentamicin is less effective when abscesses are present, such as with bubonic disease, and alternative or dual therapy should be considered. Chloramphenicol, a less desirable choice generally, is preferred only in the treatment of known or suspected plague meningitis or when treatment with tetracycline or aminoglycosides is contraindicated or unavailable. A wild-type *Y pestis* strain resistant to multiple drugs was reported in Madagascar. Another strain resistant to streptomycin also has been reported.

Nonspecific therapy is the same as that employed for patients with other forms of gram-negative sepsis and consists primarily of the treatment of shock, seizures, respiratory problems, and high fevers. With present management, bubonic plague has a mortality of 10% to 20%; the mortality with septicemic forms is slightly higher; mortality from pneumonic disease, previously almost universally fatal, was 36% in a recent US report. Worldwide, untreated bubonic plague is fatal in 50% to 90% of cases.

## PREVENTION

Hospitalized patients with suspected plague should be placed on droplet precautions until 48 hours after starting effective antimicrobial therapy to prevent the potential spread of infection from possible pulmonary involvement. Therapy should be initiated as soon as the diagnosis is suspected and not await definitive diagnosis. Standard isolation precautions should be enacted for non–pneumonic plague patients. Bodily fluids, secretions, and pus should be handled with gloves. Personnel caring for patients who are coughing should wear face masks and goggles. Careful attention must be paid to waste disposal because feces often contain *Y pestis.*

Individuals with unprotected close contact to patients with pneumonic plague should be treated prophylactically with doxycycline (if ≥ 8 years) or ciprofloxacin for 7 days.

Preventive measures against the sporadic form of plague that occurs in the United States are not feasible because *Y pestis* is so widespread. However, in those areas of the world where the disease is transmitted by the rodent-flea-human cycle, continuous flea control, accompanied by rodent controls, is indicated.

Inactivated whole-cell and live-attenuated vaccines have been used for persons at high risk of exposure; however, these vaccines are no longer available in the United States. New vaccines are currently in development.

## SUGGESTED READINGS


American Academy of Pediatrics. Plague. In Kimberlin DW, Brady MT, Jackson MA, Long SS, eds. *Red Book: 2015 Report of the Committee on Infectious Diseases.* 30th ed. Elk Grove Village, IL: American Academy of Pediatrics; 2015:624-626.

Centers for Disease Control and Prevention. Human plague—United States, 2015. *MMWR Morb Mortal Wkly Rep.* 2015;64: 918-919.

Centers for Disease Control and Prevention. Plague. Available at http://www.cdc.gov/plague/index.html. Accessed May 25, 2017.

Kugeler KJ, Staples JE, Hinckley AF, Gage KL, Mead PS. Epidemiology of human plague in the United States, 1900–2012. *Emerg Infect Dis.* 2015; 21:16-22.

Runfola JK, House J, Miller L, et al. Outbreak of human pneumonic plague with dog-to-human and possible human-to-human transmission—Colorado, June–July 2014. *MMWR Morb Mortal Wkly Rep.* 2015;64:429-434.

Tourdjman M, Ibraheem M, Brett M, et al. Misidentification of *Yersinia pestis* by automated systems, resulting in delayed diagnoses of human plague infections—Oregon and New Mexico, 2010–2011. *Clin Infect Dis.* 2012;55:e58-e60.


# 275 Pneumococcal Infections

Sandra R. Arnold

## INTRODUCTION

*Streptococcus pneumoniae, Staphylococcus aureus,* and group A *Streptococcus pyogenes* are the 3 most important bacterial pathogens causing infections in otherwise well children. In 2005, it was estimated that *S pneumoniae* caused 700,000 to 1 million deaths in children younger than 5 years of age. Most of these children lived in developing countries.

There are 90 immunologically and chemically distinct capsular polysaccharides that determine virulence. Based on antigenic similarities, the 90 types have been grouped into 45 serotypes. Relatively few serotypes cause most disease, which has led to development of polyvalent vaccines.

*S pneumoniae* can cause infection in almost any tissue or organ. The vast majority of infections in children occur in the middle ear, sinuses, lungs, meninges, and bloodstream. In 2000, the US Food and Drug Administration (FDA) approved and the Advisory Committee on Immunization Practices recommended the heptavalent pneumococcal conjugate vaccine (PCV7) for routine use in infants and young children. While this vaccine had an impressive effect on the incidence of invasive pneumococcal disease in vaccine recipients and the general population, serotype replacement of vaccine serotypes with other strains able to cause invasive disease limited effectiveness and led to the development and release in 2010 of the 13 valent vaccine (PCV13), which included the serotypes that emerged following release of PCV7. In addition, there is a 10 valent vaccine (PCV10), containing 3 of the additional 6 serotypes in PCV13, which is licensed in some countries. Use of pneumococcal conjugate vaccines has been limited in low-income countries where they are most needed.

## PATHOGENESIS AND EPIDEMIOLOGY

Invasive pneumococcal disease is preceded by colonization of the nasopharynx, the organism having been acquired through respiratory droplet spread from a colonized individual. Colonization of the nasopharynx typically leads to type-specific immunity and clearance. Capsular polysaccharide facilitates nasopharyngeal colonization and also inhibits phagocytosis of the organisms by neutrophils. Antibodies against capsular polysaccharides are protective; however, pneumococci can undergo capsular switching and evade immunity. Other surface components include choline binding proteins, which promote adherence, and pneumococcal surface protein A (PspA), which inhibits complement deposition and, thus, uptake by phagocytes. Cell wall components such as lipoteichoic acid stimulate the inflammatory response with accumulation of fluid, white blood cells, and cytokines, leading to symptomatology. Pneumolysin is a virulence factor released upon autolysis of the bacteria that is capable of lysing a variety of host cells including red and white blood cells and respiratory epithelial cells.

Bacterial adherence in the respiratory tract and subsequent spread to cause upper and lower respiratory tract infection is facilitated by the presence of viral respiratory pathogens resulting in exposure of muscosal receptors. Bacteremia occurs when colonizing bacteria gain access to the bloodstream. Phosphorylcholine in the cell wall binds to the platelet activating factor receptor. This results in the bacterial uptake and transportation across the cell (epithelial or endothelial), leading to bacterial invasion of the bloodstream. Pneumococci can cause infection in a variety of tissues via bacteremic spread. Most commonly and importantly, it leads to meningitis but can also seed other sites and cause localized disease.

Local and circulating antibody and an intact complement pathway are the most important factors mediating the outcome of *S pneumoniae*–invasive pneumococcal disease. Circulating antibody may be acquired as the result of maternal transmission (neonates), nasopharyngeal colonization, immunization, or infection. Individuals who have had no previous contact with a virulent strain and, therefore, have no serotype-specific circulating antibody are at risk for developing infection. Serotype-specific or cross-reactive antibody adheres to the capsule, which results in capsular swelling and "stickiness," enhancing opsonization and phagocytosis by neutrophils. Without antibody attached to the organism, these cells are unable to phagocytose the organisms, which can reproduce unhindered. Infants under 2 years of age are at high risk for invasive pneumococcal disease as they are unable to produce anticapsular antibody after infection or following immunization with purified polysaccharide vaccine.

Children in daycare centers have an increased risk, presumably as a result of the spread of and colonization by virulent serotypes. Children who are not breastfed are also at higher risk. The risk of invasive pneumococcal disease is increased approximately 2-fold to 4-fold for American Indians, Alaskan natives, and African Americans; however, significant narrowing or elimination of these racial/ethnic disparities in invasive pneumococcal disease incidence has been documented with the use of PCV7 and PCV13.

Increased risk for invasive pneumococcal disease also occurs among children with immunodeficiency, including defects in humoral immunity; human immunodeficiency virus infection; asplenia or splenic dysfunction including sickle hemoglobinopathies; and recently described defects of the innate immune system. Other populations at risk include children with cancer, central nervous system disorders or craniofacial anomalies, congenital heart disease, asthma, chronic kidney disease (especially nephrotic syndrome), liver disease, recent trauma, burns, or near drowning. Children who have received cochlear implants, particularly those with a positioner, are at increased risk for pneumococcal meningitis. Children with these conditions continue to be overrepresented among patients with invasive pneumococcal disease (IPD) despite protection with conjugate vaccine and are more likely to suffer from infections due to nonvaccine serotypes than children without comorbidities. Recent nasopharyngeal colonization with a new serotype almost always precedes infection. Colonization rates are highest in infants and preschool children, where they may be as high as 35%. PCV7 included the 7 most common serotypes causing colonization and infection in children (4, 6B, 9V, 14, 18C, 19F, and 23F) in the United States. These serotypes and the cross-reactive serotypes (6A, 9A, 9L, 18B, and 18F) caused the majority of bacteremia, meningitis, and otitis media due to *S pneumoniae* and accounted for more than 80% of penicillin-resistant colonizing serotypes.

Following widespread use of PCV7, the rates of IPD in children due to vaccine serotypes virtually disappeared in the United States and other countries. Overall rates of IPD among vaccinated children under 5 declined the most, but rates also declined among unvaccinated children and adults. Coincident with the reduction in IPD was a reduction in the incidence of disease due to penicillin and multidrug-resistant strains of pneumococcus by 50% across all age groups. This resulted, predominantly, from interruption of transmission of vaccine serotype antibiotic-resistant strains by blocking acquisition and spread of these strains.

The reduction in IPD following introduction of PCV7 was somewhat offset by an increase in disease caused by nonvaccine serotypes. Serotype 19A emerged in the early 2000s causing IPD, complicated otitis media, mastoiditis, and chronic sinusitis, a large proportion of which were due to a multidrug-resistant strain. Although all-cause and pneumococcal pneumonia cases declined with PCV7, pneumonia hospitalizations complicated by empyema in children increased, with non-PCV7 serotypes (1, 3, 19A, and 7F) causing the bulk of disease.

PCV13 was licensed in the United States in February 2010. It covers the additional serotypes 1, 3, 5, 6A, 7F, and 19A. PCV10 (1, 4, 5, 6B, 7F, 9V, 14, 18C, 19F, and 23F) is also licensed and used in many countries. Following replacement of PCV7 by PCV13 in the US immunization schedule, IPD fell by 64% in children under 5 years of age compared to expected rates had PCV7 continued. The incidence of IPD in adults also fell, more modestly, after PCV13 introduction. Although the effect of PCV7 on the incidence of pneumococcal meningitis was significant, PCV13 has had a more modest effect, with the majority of cases caused by nonvaccine serotypes and some persistence of meningitis caused by serotype 19A despite its inclusion in the vaccine. In 2013, the rate of IPD in children under 5 was 8.7 per 100,000, compared to 87.4 cases per 100,000 children under 5 years in 1999 and 19 cases per 100,000 in 2010 (year of introduction of PCV13).

## CLINICAL MANIFESTATIONS

In the pre-PCV7 era, *S pneumoniae* was the predominant organism causing occult bacteremia (92% of cases). In the postvaccine era, this entity has virtually disappeared.

Pneumococcal pneumonia rates have declined in the postvaccine era, but in children beyond the neonatal period, *S pneumoniae* remains the leading cause of typical bacterial pneumonia in the United States. In infants and young children, bronchopneumonia with scattered distribution of parenchymal consolidation is commonly seen on x-rays. In older children and adults, lobar consolidation is more common, although nonconsolidative patterns can be seen. Other radiographic findings can include pleural fluid, lung abscess resulting from necrosis, and, infrequently, pneumatoceles. Symptoms may range from mild fever and nonspecific respiratory symptoms with or without cough to high fever with toxicity and severe respiratory impairment. In infants and toddlers, fever, vomiting, abdominal distension, and pain may suggest appendicitis. The classic clinical presentation in older children and adults, following a viral prodrome, is the abrupt onset of high fever with chills, dyspnea, and cough with rust-colored sputum. Patients with right upper lobe pneumonia can have nuchal rigidity suggestive of meningitis. Pneumococcal pneumonia is often complicated by parapneumonic effusions. Despite declining hospital admissions for pneumonia, rates of pneumonia complicated by parapneumonic effusion or empyema increased before and after PCV7 with non-PCV7 serotypes (1, 3, 7F, and 19A). The effect of PCV13 on empyema incidence remains to be seen.

Local spread from the colonized nasopharynx may result in acute otitis media, sinusitis, conjunctivitis, and periorbital cellulitis. Other important but uncommon infections resulting from metastatic seeding following *S pneumoniae* bacteremia are meningitis, acute bacterial endocarditis, pericarditis, pyogenic arthritis, osteomyelitis, and cellulitis. All of these infections are covered in more detail in other chapters. In children with defective humoral immunity, functional or anatomic asplenia, and/or complement defects, fulminant septicemia occurs with *S pneumoniae*. Pneumococcal peritonitis may be uniquely seen in children with nephrotic syndrome.

Pneumococcal meningitis has a case fatality rate of 5% to 10% in developed countries. Hearing loss is the most common neurologic sequela, occurring in up to 10% of infections; other neurologic sequelae occur with less frequency, ranging from mild to severe. Fulminant pneumococcal sepsis is unusual but can occur, especially among immunocompromised or asplenic individuals. Pneumococcal pneumonia may be complicated by pleural effusion or empyema necessitating a chest tube or surgical procedure to hasten resolution. Mastoiditis is an uncommon complication of otitis media and can be associated with meningitis or brain abscess. Mastoiditis admissions declined after the introduction of PCV7 but rebounded to pre-PCV7 levels with the emergence of serotype 19A. Since introduction of PCV13, the number of pneumococcal isolates from middle ear and mastoid samples has fallen overall, mostly driven by a fall in serotype 19A infections. Invasive pneumococcal infections may rarely be complicated by hemolytic-uremic syndrome.

## DIAGNOSIS

Pneumococcal infections can only be diagnosed with certainty if the organism is isolated from a normally sterile site, such as blood; cerebrospinal fluid; joint, pleural, pericardial, or middle ear fluid; or a bone or abscess aspirate. Every attempt should be made to obtain these cultures before starting antibiotics in order to document the etiology and perform antimicrobial susceptibility testing.

Nasopharyngeal cultures are of no value because almost all young children are colonized with *S pneumoniae* at some time. Lower respiratory tract secretions obtained by tracheal aspirate or bronchoalveolar lavage or needle aspirate of infected lung tissue may be helpful but are rarely justified. Sputum obtained by spontaneous expectoration or induction with hypertonic saline is of uncertain value in children.

Polymerase chain reaction (PCR) has been used to detect *S pneumoniae* in sterile body fluids such as cerebrospinal fluid and pleural fluid and can be a useful adjunct to Gram stain and culture, especially in patients pretreated with antibiotics. PCR of whole blood is not routinely available for clinical use and appears to improve on blood culture detection marginally. Urinary antigen tests for *S pneumoniae* are useful in adults but in children lack specificity because colonizing bacteria are often detected. Latex agglutination, enzyme immunoassay, and immunochromatic assays on body fluids, in general, are as effective as Gram stains. Inflammatory markers such as leukocytes, elevated erythrocyte sedimentation rate, and C-reactive protein are frequently associated with IPD but are not specific for IPD and should never be used to restrict antibiotics to cover *S pneumoniae* alone.

## TREATMENT

Penicillin and all β-lactam drugs act on *S pneumoniae* by inhibiting the activity of transpeptidase enzymes (also called penicillin-binding proteins), which build the peptidoglycan lattice or scaffolding of the cell wall. Through the process of transformation, *S pneumoniae* acquires mutated penicillin-binding proteins from other resistant streptococcal species. Changes have resulted in a slow but steady increase of the minimal inhibitory concentrations for β-lactam antibiotics. Multidrug resistance occurs in penicillin-resistant pneumococci and includes resistance to cefotaxime, macrolides, trimethoprim-sulfamethoxazole, chloramphenicol, tetracycline, and increasingly, clindamycin and the fluoroquinolones. Vancomycin is the only drug to which no strains have yet become resistant. Resistant strains may spread from person to person, throughout communities, and across international borders.

The definition of antimicrobial susceptibility is based on achievable levels of the antibiotic at the site of infection and varies by antibiotic. The breakpoints for susceptibility for penicillin and cefotaxime are provided in Table 275-1.

All patients with suspected bacterial meningitis should be treated initially with vancomycin at 60 mg/kg and ceftriaxone at 100 mg/kg up to 2 g every 12 hours. After susceptibilities are available, antibiotic modifications can be made. For susceptible organisms, aqueous penicillin G 250,000 U/kg per day divided every 4 hours or ampicillin 300 mg/kg per day divided every 6 hours is appropriate. For patients with penicillin- and cephalosporin-resistant *S pneumoniae*, vancomycin and ceftriaxone should be continued and the addition of rifampin considered. Therapy is usually continued for 10 days but may extend for longer periods. The use of dexamethasone as adjunctive therapy for bacterial meningitis remains unresolved. Results from a meta-analysis of clinical trials of steroids in meningitis, including cases of pneumococcal meningitis, suggest a benefit in the prevention of hearing loss if steroids are given before or concomitantly with antibiotics.

For nonmeningeal IPD in the immunocompetent host, empiric use of vancomycin is not generally indicated because treatment failures are rare with penicillin and cephalosporins for bacteremia and pneumonia. Plasma levels of recommended agents, including the β-lactam antibiotics, are well in excess of the minimum inhibitory concentration of even the highly resistant strains isolated thus far. No clear therapeutic failures have yet been reported for nonmeningeal invasive infections when recommended doses of systemic β-lactam agents are used in patients with normal host defenses. Less experience is available for patients with fulminant and potentially life-threatening invasive infections, particularly in immunocompromised hosts. In patients with fulminant and potentially life-threatening invasive infections, particularly in immunocompromised hosts, the addition of vancomycin to the usual regimen for an invasive, nonmeningeal infection may be justified, providing the vancomycin is discontinued after susceptibilities reveal that therapy with β-lactam agents should be successful. Treatment failures with the use of newer macrolides and fluoroquinolones (the latter in adults) to treat bacteremia and pneumonia due to nonsusceptible strains have been reported; thus, empiric monotherapy with these agents for community-acquired pneumonia should take into account the antibiotic-resistance patterns and the severity of illness. Linezolid was licensed for the treatment of gram-positive community-acquired and nosocomial pneumonia in children in 2002 and is a treatment option for suspected or confirmed multidrug-resistant pneumococcal pneumonia; it may be most useful when infection (either primary or coinfection) with methicillin-resistant *S aureus* cannot be excluded.

High doses of amoxicillin (80–90 mg/kg/d) remain the treatment of choice for otitis media caused by *S pneumoniae*. A guideline for the management of community-acquired pneumonia in children was published for the first time in 2011 and recommend amoxicillin as first choice for outpatients and ampicillin for inpatients with nonsevere pneumonia in vaccinated children in areas with less than 10% high-level penicillin resistance.

**TABLE 275-1 BREAKPOINTS FOR *STREPTOCOCCUS PNEUMONIAE* SUSCEPTIBILITY TO PENICILLIN AND THIRD-GENERATION CEPHALOSPORINS (μg/mL)**

| | Susceptible | Intermediate | Resistant |
|---|---|---|---|
| Penicillin | ≤ 2[a] | 4 | ≥ 8 |
| Cefotaxime/ceftriaxone (meningeal) | ≤ 0.5 | 1 | ≥ 2 |
| Cefotaxime/ceftriaxone (nonmeningeal) | ≤ 2 | 2 | ≥ 4 |

[a]The breakpoint for penicillin susceptibility in meningitis remains ≤ 0.06 μg/mL.

## PREVENTION

The 23-valent pneumococcal capsular polysaccharide vaccine (PPSV23) licensed in 1977 covers 90% of the serotypes causing IPD in the United States. This vaccine elicits type-specific antibody responses in children older than 5 years of age and adults, but not for children younger than 2 years of age.

Currently there are 3 PCVs licensed around the world, PCV7 (Prevnar 7), PCV13 (Prevnar 13), and PCV10 (Synflorix). In addition to the PCV7 serotypes (4, 6B, 9V, 14, 18C, 19F, and 23F), PCV10 contains 3 additional serotypes, 1, 5, and 7F. PCV13 contains the serotypes in PCV10 plus 3, 6A, and 19A. PCV13 is currently recommended by the Advisory Committee on Immunization Practices (ACIP) in the United States for routine immunizations of infants as a 4-dose series at 2, 4, 6, and 12 to 15 months of age. If a child received 4 doses of PCV7, a single dose of PCV13 at 14 to 59 months is recommended. Children with underlying medical conditions placing them at risk for IPD should receive a supplemental dose of PCV13 up to 71 months of age. In addition, these children should receive PPSV23 between 2 and 18 years of age more than 8 weeks after completing recommended PCV13 doses.

Novel pneumococcal vaccines are based on pneumococcal proteins that contribute to virulence and are common to all serotypes. Several candidate protein vaccine antigens have been identified and tested, with the most promising being a combination of pneumolysin, pneumococcal surface protein A, and choline-binding protein A.

## SUGGESTED READINGS


Abdelnour A, Arguedas A, Dagan R, et al. Etiology and antimicrobial susceptibility of middle ear fluid pathogens in Costa Rican children with otitis media before and after the introduction of the 7-valent pneumococcal conjugate vaccine in the National Immunization Program: acute otitis media microbiology in Costa Rican children. *Medicine*. 2015;94:e320.

Adegbola RA, DeAntonio R, Hill PC, et al. Carriage of *Streptococcus pneumoniae* and other respiratory bacterial pathogens in low and middle-income countries: a systematic review and meta-analysis. *PLoS One*. 2014;9:e103293.

Ciapponi A, Elorriaga N, Rojas JI, et al. Epidemiology of pediatric pneumococcal meningitis and bacteremia in Latin America and the Caribbean: a systematic review and meta-analysis. *Pediatr Infect Dis J*. 2014;33:971-978.

Maraga NF. Pneumococcal infections. *Pediatr Rev*. 2014;35:299-310.

Ngo CC, Massa HM, Thornton RB, Cripps AW. Predominant bacteria detected from middle ear fluid of children experiencing otitis media: a systematic review. *PLoS One*. 2016;11:e0150949.

Plosker GL. 13-valent pneumococcal conjugate vaccine: a review of its use in infants, children and adolescents. *Paediatr Drug*. 2013;15:403-423.

Wu DB, Chaiyakunapruk N, Chong HY, Beutels P. Choosing between 7-, 10- and 13-valent pneumococcal conjugate vaccine in childhood: a review of economic evaluations (2006-2014). *Vaccine*. 2015;33:1633-1658.

# 276 Rat-Bite Fever

Lorry G. Rubin

## INTRODUCTION

Rat-bite fever is an acute febrile illness with arthritis and rash that occurs as a result of the bite of a rodent, usually a rat. Two distinct microorganisms, *Streptobacillus moniliformis* and *Spirillum minus,* the agent of sodoku in Asia, cause this infection.

## PATHOGENESIS AND EPIDEMIOLOGY

*S moniliformis*, the main etiologic agent of rat-bite fever, is a fastidious, gram-negative, pleomorphic, and often filamentous and beaded facultative anaerobic bacillus. In addition to rat-bite fever, *S moniliformis* causes an overlapping syndrome, Haverhill fever, also known as erythema arthriticum epidemicum. A second *Streptobacillus* species, *S hongkongensis,* has been described to cause a rat-bite fever-like syndrome not associated with rat contact. Sodoku caused by *S minus* is currently rare in the United States.

*S moniliformis* is a normal and asymptomatic inhabitant of the upper respiratory tract of rodents and may be excreted in rat urine. Humans are infected by the bite of a rat (or mouse, squirrel, cat, or weasel) or, less commonly, by a scratch from a rat, by handling a dead animal, or by contact with rat-eating carnivores. Approximately 50% of cases reported are in children, and pet rats are a source of infection. Infection may also be acquired by ingestion of milk or water contaminated with rat excreta, as occurred in epidemic form in 1916 in Haverhill, Massachusetts, resulting in the name "Haverhill fever."

## CLINICAL MANIFESTATIONS

Seven to 10 days (range 2–21 days) after a rat bite, there is an abrupt onset of fever accompanied by chills, headache, vomiting, muscle pain, and sore throat. Fifty percent develop asymmetric polyarthralgia or polyarthritis typically involving the knees and ankles that may reflect either sterile effusions or septic arthritis with *S moniliformis* present in the joint fluid. Several days later, there is a maculopapular and sometimes petechial, pustular, or purpuric rash, which is most prominent on the extremities, including the palms and soles. The bite wound has usually healed, and the site exhibits no or minimal inflammation. Generalized adenopathy commonly occurs. Young children often have diarrhea and weight loss. Many of the clinical features are similar to Rocky Mountain spotted fever and disseminated gonococcal infection. Left untreated, the infection follows a relapsing course lasting a mean of 3 weeks, but may have a fatal outcome or result in arthritis persistent for several months. Other reported manifestations of *S moniliformis* infection include fever without a focus, osteomyelitis, septic arthritis without a rash, amnionitis, brain abscess, disseminated fatal infection in infants, endocarditis, hepatitis, meningitis, spinal epidural abscess, brain abscess, cutaneous abscess, myocarditis, nephritis, and pneumonia. Patients with Haverhill fever exhibit fever followed by rash and polyarthritis/polyarthralgia; vomiting and pharyngitis are more prominent manifestations than in patients with rat-bite fever.

Sodoku disease, due to *S minus,* has an incubation period of 1 to 4 weeks. There is fever that may be relapsing, ulceration at the previously healed bite site, and regional lymphadenopathy, and there may be an associated rash.

## DIAGNOSIS

The diagnosis is established by recovering *S moniliformis* from cultures of blood or joint fluid, but the organism is fastidious and slow growing. Broth enriched with blood, serum, or ascitic fluid, or blood or chocolate agar incubated in a $CO_2$-supplemented environment should be used. Sodium polyanethol sulfonate can inhibit growth of *S moniliformis,* but it has been recovered using Bactec™ (Becton Dickinson and Company, Franklin Lakes, NJ) blood culture media that contains this anticoagulant. Identification of isolates often is established using nucleic acid amplification with specific primers; matrix-assisted laser desorption/ionization time-of-flight mass spectrometry (MALDI-TOF MS) has also been used. Direct detection of organism from clinical specimens can be established by nucleic acid amplification of 16S RNA using broad-range primers followed by sequencing or electrospray ionization followed by mass spectrometry. At least 25% of infected patients have a false-positive nontreponemal serologic test for syphilis.

*S minus* is a spirillum-like organism that cannot be grown in vitro and is identified by dark-field microscopic examination of material from an ulcer or blood smear.

## TREATMENT

Penicillin given for 10 to 14 days is the treatment of choice for rat-bite fever, although penicillin-resistant strains have been reported rarely. The organism is susceptible to many antibiotics in addition to penicillin, including ampicillin, cefuroxime, cefotaxime, tetracycline (doxycycline), vancomycin, and streptomycin. Doxycycline is an acceptable alternative in penicillin/cephalosporin-allergic patients. Isolates are resistant to sulfonamides, trimethoprim-sulfamethoxazole, and colistin. For therapy of endocarditis, the addition of streptomycin to high-dose penicillin should be considered. Disease caused by *S minus* also responds rapidly to therapy with penicillin.

## PREVENTION

Avoidance of contact with rats and their excreta or wearing gloves during such contacts is the best means of prevention. Because the attack rate of rat-bite fever after a rat bite is approximately 10%, individuals sustaining rat bites should be observed closely, and penicillin prophylaxis can be considered, although its efficacy is unknown.

## SUGGESTED READINGS


Adam JK, Varan AK, Pong AL, McDonald EC. Notes from the field: fatal rat-bite fever in a child: San Diego County, California, 2013. Centers for Disease Control and Prevention (CDC). *MMWR Morb Mortal Wkly Rep.* 2014;63:1210-1211.

Edwards R, Finch RG. Characterisation and antibiotic susceptibilities of *Streptobacillus moniliformis. J Med Microbiol.* 1986;21:39-42.

Sato R, Kuriyama A, Nasu M. Rat bite fever complicated by vertebral osteomyelitis. *J Infect Chemother.* 2016;22:574-576.

Zhinden R. *Actinobacillus, Capnocytophaga, Eikenella, Kingella, Pasteurella,* and other fastidious or rarely encountered gram-negative rods. In: Jorgensen JH, Pfaller MA, Carroll KC, et al, eds. *Manual of Clinical Microbiology.* 11th ed. Washington, DC: American Society for Microbiology; 2015:652-666.


# 277 Relapsing Fever

Andrés E. Alarcón and Bernhard L. Wiedermann

## INTRODUCTION

Relapsing fever is a vector-borne, remittent febrile illness, transmitted by lice and ticks, which is caused by several species of spirochetes of the bacterial genus *Borrelia.* Two clinical forms are distinguished by their vectors: louse-borne and tick-borne relapsing fevers.

## PATHOGENESIS AND EPIDEMIOLOGY

*Borrelia* do not infect blood cells directly, but the concentration of the spirochetes in the blood correlates directly with severity. Repeated episodes of spirochetemia, each involving a different predominant antigenic variant, account for the cyclic nature of the disease. IgM antibodies help clear the more common variant each time, but other variants proliferate between episodes. Organisms can be sequestered in the liver, spleen, central nervous system, and/or bone marrow. Periodic relapses continue to occur until the antigenic variations are eliminated or the patient receives effective treatment.

Louse-borne (epidemic) relapsing fever is caused by *Borrelia recurrentis.* The vector is the body louse, *Pediculus humanus,* which becomes infected by ingesting blood from infected humans, and the disease is transmitted when the louse is crushed and the spirochetes (*Borrelia*) penetrate human skin of a new host. Epidemic *Borrelia* infection has disappeared from the United States, along with louse-borne typhus. Louse-borne relapsing fever does occur in other areas of the world, mainly confined to the Horn of Africa (Ethiopia), Sudan, regions of Peru, and Bolivia. In afflicted regions, it is prevalent among the homeless, refugee populations, and confined populations exposed to famine and war.

Tick-borne (endemic) relapsing fever is a zoonosis caused by *Borrelia hermsii,* and less commonly by *Borrelia turicatae, Borrelia parkeri,* and *Borrelia mazzottii.* It is transmitted to humans by soft-bodied ticks of the genus *Ornithodoros* (especially *Ornithodoros hermsii* and *Ornithodoros turicata*) and, less commonly, the genus *Carios.* In contrast to louse-borne relapsing fever, humans are incidental hosts for the *Borrelia*-causing tick-borne relapsing fever. Animal reservoirs include rodents, other mammals, reptiles, and birds. Ticks causing endemic relapsing fever are distributed worldwide with the exception of Antarctica and Australia. *Borrelia* may be transmitted from the *Ornithodoros* tick to the host in a matter of minutes, often with a painless nocturnal bite. Patients frequently are unaware of a tick bite or exposure. As reported by the Centers for Disease Control and Prevention in 2015, most cases of tick-borne relapsing fever in the United States occur in the Rocky Mountain regions of the western states. Three states account for approximately 70% of the 504 reported cases from 1990 to 2011: California, 33%; Washington, 25%; and Colorado, 11%. Exposure to rodent-infested cabins or caves is important to human infection with *Borrelia*-associated tick-borne disease. Most cases of autochthonous transmission in the United States are caused by *B hermsii.* Cases of *B turicatae* infection have been reported mainly in Texas with tick exposures while spelunking in caves infested with rodents; 1 case of infection has been reported with *B parkeri.*

## CLINICAL MANIFESTATIONS

After a variable incubation period (4 to > 18 days, mean of 7 days for tick-borne disease; 4–8 days for louse-borne disease), the illness starts abruptly with fever, chills, headache, myalgia, and arthralgia. Conjunctivitis, petechiae of the mucous membranes and or skin, and hepatosplenomegaly with tenderness may be present. This first phase of illness typically lasts 3 to 6 days and subsides spontaneously. During the next approximately 7 days, the infected patient experiences extreme fatigue and may have a diffuse maculopapular rash but is afebrile or has only a low-grade fever.

Return of fever and chills signals the relapse phase of the disease. Several such relapses can occur (up to 13 in tick-related cases, while they are fewer in number in louse-borne disease), although the duration of relapses typically becomes shorter and the symptoms milder over time. Relapsing fever may resolve even among untreated patients with tick-borne disease. Myocarditis, hepatosplenomegaly, brain edema, and diffuse petechiae are prominent in fatal cases of tick-borne disease. The case fatality rate for untreated tick-borne relapsing fever is between 4% and 10%, mainly occurring in infants, the elderly, and immunocompromised hosts. With appropriate therapy, case fatality rates are less than 5% in tick-borne disease. The case fatality rate can surpass 30% in untreated louse-borne relapsing fever, and this high rate may be attributed to the associated comorbidities of living in famine, crowded conditions, and refugee camps. Louse-borne relapsing fever can be associated with particularly severe Jarisch-Herxheimer reactions on initiation of treatment.

Tick-borne relapsing fever is not typically transmitted from human to human; however, congenital, vertical transmission from an infected mother to infant can occur, resulting in abortion, prematurity, or severe infection of the neonate. Children and pregnant women tend to have a more prolonged disease course.

The infectious differential diagnosis includes malaria, typhoid fever, rat-bite fever, brucellosis, dengue, yellow fever, leptospirosis, meningococcemia, hepatitis, and rickettsial diseases. Other infectious differentials to consider include influenza, enterovirus, Colorado tick fever (*Coltivirus*), Powassan virus, Heartland virus, *Borrelia burgdorferi* (Lyme borreliosis), *Borrelia mayonii,* lymphocytic choriomeningitis virus, *Babesia microti* and *Babesia duncani* (babesiosis), *Anaplasma phagocytophilum* (human granulocytic anaplasmosis), *Ehrlichia chaffeensis* (human monocytic ehrlichiosis) and *Ehrlichia ewingii,* and the potentially emerging tick-borne infection of *Borrelia miyamotoi.* The periodic fever disorders, such as the periodic fever, aphthous stomatitis, pharyngitis, and adenitis (PFAPA) syndrome, may resemble relapsing fever, but PFAPA is milder and the intervals between febrile episodes are longer. Noninfectious differentials to consider include juvenile idiopathic arthritis and occult malignancy.

## DIAGNOSIS

Louse-borne relapsing fever may be suspected, along with typhus, when body lice (not head lice or crab lice) are prevalent, particularly with crowded and unsanitary conditions. With the endemic form, the disease should be suspected in patients with appropriate symptoms who have had exposure to environments where *Ornithodoros* or *Carios* ticks are located. Due to increasing migration patterns and returning travelers from endemic areas, it is important to consider a broad differential of infectious diseases that may show similar clinical finding to those of louse-borne (epidemic) or tick-borne (endemic) relapsing fever.

A definitive diagnosis is made by demonstrating the *Borrelia* spirochete on a blood smear. Spirochetes can be observed by dark-field microscopy and in Wright, Giemsa, or acridine orange–stained preparations of either thick or thin blood smears, with highest sensitivity in blood obtained while the person is febrile. Culture of the spirochetes in a modified Kelly medium or in mouse inoculation has decreased sensitivity but may be used in attempt to confirm the diagnosis. Immunofluorescence testing and polymerase chain reaction primers and probes have been developed but may not be commercially available. Serologic tests are available at certain reference labs, are not well standardized, and require a 4-fold serologic convalescent rise; cross-reactions occur with other spirochetes, including *B burgdorferi* (Lyme disease), *Treponema pallidum* (syphilis), and leptospirosis.

## TREATMENT

Treatment recommendations for tick-borne relapsing fever are based on retrospective studies and case reports. Expert consensus is that treatment with penicillin, tetracyclines (preferably doxycycline), or erythromycin is effective. Erythromycin and penicillin are considered the drugs of choice for children younger than 8 years of age and for pregnant women. Intravenous penicillin is an effective drug for the initial illness, especially when central nervous system involvement is suspected or in patients who cannot tolerate oral medications. Parenteral ceftriaxone or penicillin G for 14 days is recommended for meningitis and encephalitis.

Doxycycline, penicillin, and erythromycin have been used as single-dose treatment for louse-borne disease. In 2011, meta-analysis of 6 randomized controlled trials in Ethiopia showed that there was no significant difference between tetracycline and penicillin in regard to mortality rate; relapse was reduced with tetracycline, but treatment with tetracycline had higher rates of a Jarisch-Herxheimer reaction. Jarisch-Herxheimer reactions in children are generally milder than those in adults. For the febrile louse-borne patient, some experts suggest initiating therapy with a low-dose oral penicillin (7.5 mg/kg of phenoxymethyl penicillin in a single dose) or intravenous aqueous penicillin G (10,000 U/kg by infusion over 30 minutes). Following this first dose, gradual clearing of spirochetes and defervescence should occur; thereafter, therapy with an oral formulation with doxycycline or erythromycin should be continued to complete a 7- to 10-day course to prevent relapse. In patients with tetracycline contraindication, erythromycin may be used as a substitute.

Control and avoidance of the vectors responsible for relapsing fever are the mainstays of prevention for this disease. Rodent control and prevention of infestation of homes and cabins are essential. Environmental use of insecticides on interior walls of primitive buildings and dwellings has reduced the frequency of disease caused by ticks. Good personal hygiene and prompt treatment of louse infestation with effective pediculocides can aid in controlling this vector. Use of insect repellents containing DEET (*N,N*-diethyl-*m*-toluamide) or picaridin on the skin or permethrin on clothing is an important adjunct to prevention of tick-borne disease. Tick-borne disease is reportable to the state health department in most western US states, and louse-borne disease is reportable to the World Health Organization.

## SUGGESTED READINGS


American Academy of Pediatrics. *Borrelia* infections (relapsing fever). In: Kimberlin DW, Brady MT, Jackson, MA, Long SS, eds. *Red Book: 2015 Report of the Committee on Infectious Diseases*. 30th ed. Elk Grove Village, IL: American Academy of Pediatrics; 2015: 265-267.

Centers for Disease Control and Prevention. Louse-borne relapsing fever (LBRF). Available at http://www.cdc.gov/relapsing-fever/resources/louse.html. Accessed October 25, 2016.

Centers for Disease Control and Prevention. Tickborne relapsing fever in a mother and newborn child—Colorado, 2011. *MMWR Morb Mortal Wkly Rep*. 2011;61:174-176.

Centers for Disease Control and Prevention. Tick-borne relapsing fever (TBRF). Available at http://www.cdc.gov/relapsing-fever/clinicians/index.html. Accessed October 25, 2016.

Centers for Disease Control and Prevention. Tickborne relapsing fever-United States, 1990-2011. *MMWR Morb Mort Wkly Rep*. 2015;64:58-60.

Guerrier G, Doherty T. Comparison of antibiotic regimens for treating louse-borne relapsing fever: a meta-analysis. *Trans R Soc Trop Med Hyg*. 2011;105:483-490.

Molloy PJ, Telford SR 3rd, Chowdri HR, et al. *Borrelia miyamotoi* disease in the northeastern united states: a case series. *Ann Intern Med*. 2015;163(2):91-98.


# 278 *Salmonella*, *Shigella*, and *Escherichia coli*

Daniel Leung and Andrew T. Pavia

## INTRODUCTION

The family Enterobacteriaceae is a large, heterogeneous group of gram-negative bacteria. Many are normal inhabitants of the gastrointestinal tract of humans and other animals, but members also frequently cause disease in human beings. Among the Enterobacteriaceae, *Salmonella, Shigella, Yersinia,* and a number of specific phenotypes of *Escherichia coli* are important causes of gastroenteritis. In addition to diarrhea, these organisms cause a variety of extraintestinal infections. Each genera includes a heterogenous group of organisms that vary in their epidemiology and clinical characteristics. Enterobacteriaceae possess 3 major antigenic groups that react with antisera: (1) the O or somatic antigens; (2) the H or flagellar antigens; and (3) the K or capsular antigens. Serotyping has historically been an important means of subtyping these enteric pathogens; this technique is being partially superseded by our increasing ability to identify genotypic and phenotypic markers of virulence.

## *SALMONELLA*

*Salmonella* are gram-negative, aerobic, non–lactose-fermenting, nonsporulating, flagellated bacilli. The genus *Salmonella* consists of only 2 species, *S enterica* and *S bongori*. Further, *Salmonella* are divided into approximately 2500 serotypes based on the somatic antigen (the major determinant) plus one or more less strongly reacting minor somatic antigens. Serotyping is performed by state health department laboratories after initial isolation of the organism. Serotyping is extraordinarily useful for epidemiologic purposes but not necessary for initial clinical management. The majority of human infections are caused by serotypes of *S enterica*, including Typhimurium, Enteritidis, and Typhi. The nomenclature of *Salmonella* has been simplified recently, with serotypes designated after species (eg, *S enterica* serotype Typhimurium is often simplified to *S* Typhimurium). Because several serotypes represent the majority of isolates, additional epidemiologic subtyping can be useful. Plasmid profile analysis, bacteriophage typing, restriction endonuclease analysis, ribotyping, pulsed-field gel electrophoresis, and antimicrobial susceptibility have all been used as epidemiologic tools.

### PATHOGENESIS AND EPIDEMIOLOGY

There are several distinctive steps in the development of a *Salmonella* infection. Upon reaching the small intestine, the bacteria must attach to the epithelium. Chromosomally encoded long, polar fimbriae; thin, aggregative fimbriae; and plasmid-encoded fimbriae are important in this process. *Salmonella* invade M cells (mucosal antigen-presenting immune cells) and nonphagocytic epithelial cells. Within macrophages, they may not only survive but multiply. The ability of strains to survive and reproduce in macrophages is correlated with virulence in animal models. The organism directs its own endocytosis through a complex mechanism encoded in a "pathogenicity island," a large collection of contiguous virulence genes. Interestingly, a key component of invasion is a type 3 secretion system, which is similar to systems mediating the invasiveness of *Yersinia* and enteropathic and enterohemorrhagic *E coli*. Diarrhea is probably induced by local inflammation, by induction of inflammatory mediators, and in some strains, by one or more enterotoxins or cytotoxins. When examined histologically, the organism is prominent in Peyer's patches. In some cases of nontyphoid salmonellosis and in all cases of typhoid, the organisms reach the regional lymphatics. Bacteremia may result.

There are several important barriers that the organism must overcome to cause infection. The organism must survive gastric acid, which can rapidly kill *Salmonella*. Reduced gastric acidity as a result of extremes of age, medications, surgery, *Helicobacter pylori* infection, and foods that buffer gastric acid increases the number of organisms that reach the small intestine. Normal intestinal flora are an important barrier. Prior treatment with antibiotics, particularly those that disrupt the predominant intestinal flora, increases the risk of infection with both antibiotic-resistant and antibiotic-sensitive strains. This has been demonstrated experimentally and in outbreak investigations. The third and most complex barrier is the host immune system. Although cell-mediated immunity appears to be the primary immunologic defense against *Salmonella* infections, the importance of antibody responses for invasive infection has been increasingly recognized. Susceptibility appears to be highest in the first few months of life, reflecting the developing immune system and low gastric acidity. Children with human immunodeficiency virus (HIV) infection, transplant recipients, and others on immunosuppressive agents and children with advanced malignancies are at increased risk. Reticuloendothelial dysfunction is also associated with increased risk of *Salmonella* infection, including sickle cell disease, hemolytic anemias, and malaria.

Bacteremia and mesenteric adenitis are the rule with *S* Typhi but much less common with other nontyphoid *Salmonella*. However, the rate of bacteremia and extraintestinal infection varies by serotype, reflecting distinct but incompletely understood differences in virulence. Reptiles, birds, poultry, cattle, and pigs serve as the major reservoirs for nontyphoidal *Salmonella*. In contrast, human beings are the only reservoir for *S* Typhi and Paratyphi A. The primary animal

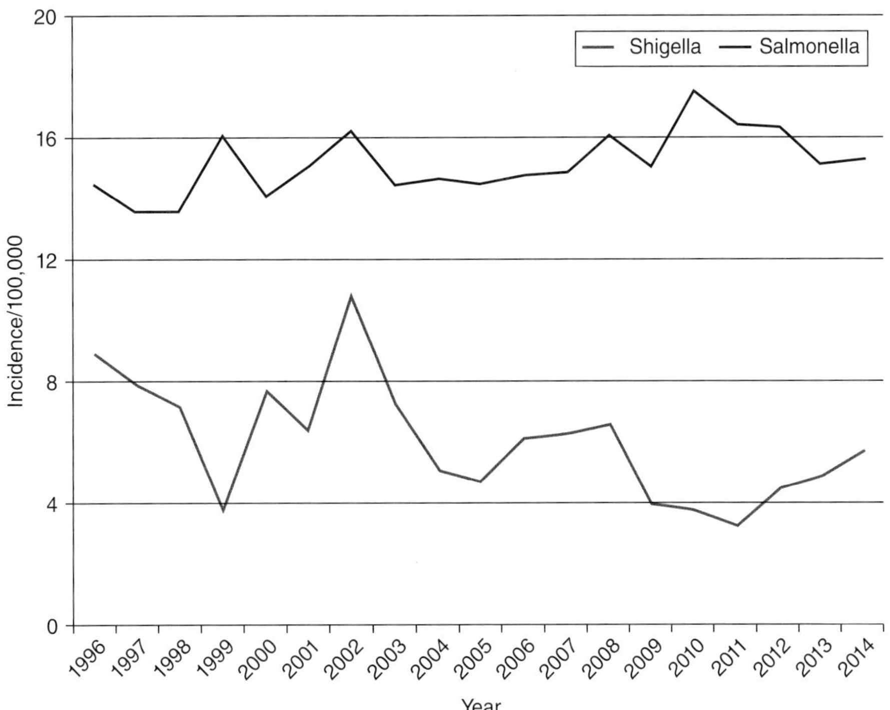


**FIGURE 278-1** Annual incidence of culture-confirmed *Salmonella* and *Shigella* infections based on the Centers for Disease Control and Prevention FoodNet Surveillance System, United States, 1996–2014. (Reproduced with permission from the Centers for Disease Control [CDC] https://www.cdc.gov/foodnet/reports/annual-reports-2014.html.)

reservoir varies by serotype and can serve as a clue to the source of contamination. For example, *S* Hadar and *S* Heidelberg are primarily associated with chickens; *S* Enteritidis with eggs; *S* Choleraesuis with pigs; and *S* Marinum and *S* Urbana with reptiles. Nevertheless, nontyphoidal *Salmonella* is one of the most commonly reported bacterial causes of foodborne outbreaks in the United States (Fig. 278-1).

In the United States, the highest incidence of nontyphoid *Salmonella* infection is in the first year of life, with greater than 110 laboratory-confirmed cases per 100,000 population per year (Fig. 278-2). Thereafter, rates of isolation decline rapidly by age 5 years and remain constant throughout adulthood. *Salmonella* infections show a seasonal pattern, with a consistent peak in the summer and fall. Infection with *S* Typhi and S Paratyphi A, which causes typhoid fever, in the United States is uncommon (approximately 400 reported cases per year) and rarely occurs in children less than 1 year of age. However, typhoid fever remains an important problem in many developing countries.

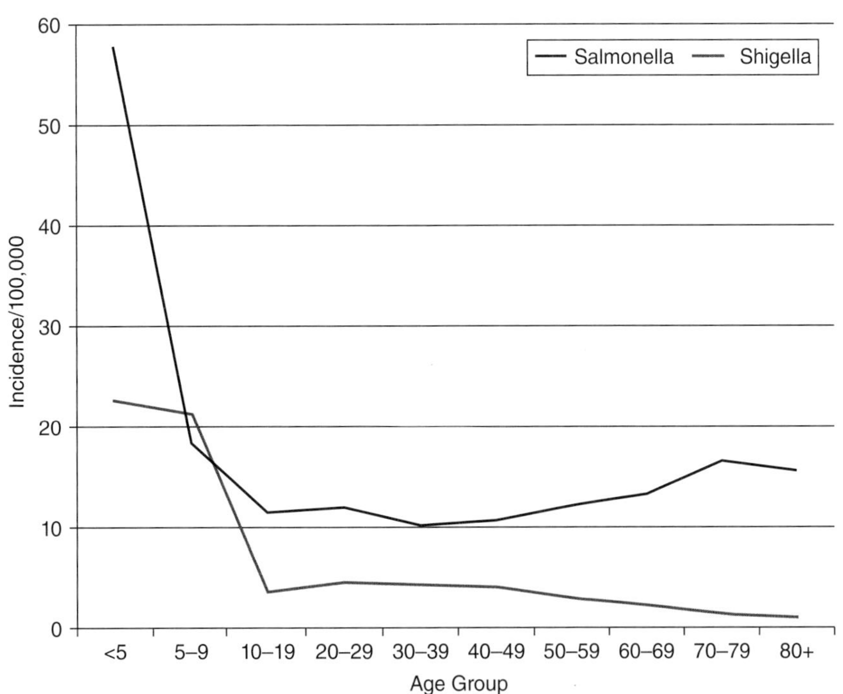


**FIGURE 278-2** Age-specific incidence of culture-confirmed *Salmonella* and *Shigella* infections based on the Centers for Disease Control and Prevention FoodNet Surveillance System, United States, 1996–2014. (Reproduced with permission from the Centers for Disease Control [CDC] https://www.cdc.gov/foodnet/reports/annual-reports-2014.html.)

In the United States, > 85% of S Typhi and Paratyphi A infections are related to foreign travel.

*Salmonella* infections are acquired through ingesting the organism, most often from food, but waterborne, person-to-person, and animal-to-person transmission can occur. The majority of cases are sporadic; recognized outbreaks account for a minority of cases but provide insight into the epidemiology. Important common source outbreaks have occurred as a consequence of contaminated milk, cheese, shell eggs, produce, ice cream, and roast beef.

Since the mid-1980s, low-level contamination of the yolks of intact shell eggs with *S* Enteritidis has been an increasing problem, although rates have recently declined. Prominent outbreaks in the last 2 decades have been traced to contaminated ice cream, tomatoes, cantaloupe, sprouts, dry cereal, dog food, and peanut butter. Iguanas and other pet reptiles and amphibians have emerged as an important source of infection for young children.

Sentinel surveillance demonstrates that *Salmonella* are becoming increasingly resistant to ampicillin, chloramphenicol, streptomycin, tetracycline, kanamycin, cephalosporins, and aminoglycosides. Some of these agents are rarely used in human disease but are routinely added to animal feed as growth promoters.

The dose necessary to cause clinical infection is estimated to be $10^5$ to $10^{10}$ organisms, based on volunteer studies in adults. However, the number of organisms necessary to cause illness is substantially lower in other situations, including more virulent organisms, low gastric acidity, prior use of antibiotics, infants, the elderly, and defective cell-mediated immunity. Because of the relatively large number of organisms necessary to produce disease, water and person-to-person spread are less frequent sources of infection than food, which can support multiplication of the organism. Contaminated water may play a larger role in typhoid fever. Spread of *Salmonella* in childcare centers is unusual.

Following infection, nontyphoid *Salmonella* are excreted in feces for a median of 5 weeks. Excretion is more prolonged in children less than 5 years of age and for people who have had symptomatic infections. In children younger than 5 years of age, 2.6% continue to excrete nontyphoid *Salmonella* beyond 1 year, compared to fewer than 1% of patients age 5 years and older. Two to 4% of adults infected with *S* Typhi become chronic carriers, often excreting the organism for the remainder of their lives. Long-standing infection of the gallbladder plays a role in chronic carriage. Despite the large number of chronic excretors of nontyphoid *Salmonella,* carriers are rarely implicated in outbreaks or sporadic disease. In contrast, chronic carriers play a pivotal role in typhoid fever.

The source of *Salmonella* is not as well understood among infants. Chronic or transient asymptomatic carriage by the mother and cross-contamination during food preparation are probably important. Exposure to reptiles and riding in a shopping cart next to poultry products are associated with infection. Nursery outbreaks of salmonellosis occur. Contaminated medical devices such as rectal thermometers, suction equipment, and baths have led to nosocomial spread of disease. Breastfeeding is protective.

## CLINICAL MANIFESTATIONS

The range of clinical manifestations of *Salmonella* infection includes asymptomatic infection, gastroenteritis, bacteremia, focal infection, urinary tract infection, and enteric fever. These symptom complexes may overlap. The incubation period for gastroenteritis is 6 to 72 hours (mean, 36 hours); for enteric fever, it is 7 to 21 days (usually 7–14 days). The incubation period is affected by the inoculum size.

### Gastroenteritis

Diarrhea is the most common manifestation of salmonellosis. The diarrhea may be profuse and watery, reflecting predominant small-bowel involvement, or may involve smaller volume stools associated with mucous and fecal leukocytes, reflecting colonic involvement. Bloody diarrhea occurs in approximately 25% of cases and is more common in young children. Fever, when present, tends to be highest at the onset. Headache, chills, anorexia, nausea, vomiting, and malaise may be present. Symptoms usually last 2 to 5 days, although diarrhea may be prolonged. The most common complication of *Salmonella* gastroenteritis is dehydration and metabolic acidosis, occasionally progressing to hypovolemic shock. Infected children also may have concurrent bacteremia, may develop prolonged secretory diarrhea, or may manifest failure to thrive after acute infection.

### Bacteremia

Bacteremia may occur during acute *Salmonella* gastroenteritis. Factors that increase the risk include age, underlying systemic illness, hemoglobinopathy, immunosuppression, and serotype of the infecting organism. In children with uncomplicated gastroenteritis, "silent" bacteremia occurs in 5% to 10%. The risk of bacteremia is markedly increased in infants less than 3 months of age, most likely because of the immaturity of their cell-mediated immune response. Other conditions associated with increased risk of bacteremia include malnutrition; hemolytic anemias, especially sickle cell anemia; collagen vascular disease; schistosomiasis; bartonellosis; hematogenous or gastrointestinal tract malignancy; diabetes mellitus; previous therapy with antimicrobial agents; corticosteroids; and HIV infection. *Salmonella* bacteremia is common among adults and children with acquired immunodeficiency syndrome (AIDS). Frequently, *Salmonella* bacteremia in AIDS patients presents with fever and a paucity of gastrointestinal symptoms. The illness is often prolonged, and relapses after therapy are common. After relapse, lifetime secondary prophylaxis may be necessary.

Patients with *Salmonella* bacteremia during acute gastroenteritis cannot be readily recognized by clinical examination. Although fever usually is present and the patient appears acutely toxic, these signs may be indistinguishable from those of acute gastroenteritis without bacteremia.

### Focal Infection

Focal suppurative infections occur in about 10% of patients with bacteremia. *Salmonella* bacteremia can result in suppurative complications of almost any organ or tissue. Infection can result in pneumonia; empyema; pyelonephritis; abscesses of brain, liver, spleen, muscle, or other soft tissue; or endovascular infection. Endocarditis most often involves abnormal or prosthetic valves, but infection of normal valves can occur. Endovascular infections can also involve arteriovenous fistulas, preexisting aneurysms (classically atherosclerotic aneurysms), or endarteritis. *S* Choleraesuis has a propensity for causing endovascular infections. Osteomyelitis caused by *Salmonella* tends to occur in injured or infarcted bone. This probably explains the predisposition of children with hemoglobinopathies, especially sickle cell disease, to develop this complication. Meningitis is rare, occurring most often in neonates or young infants and in AIDS patients. Mortality is high, even since the advent of third-generation cephalosporins.

### Enteric Fever

The prototypic enteric fever is typhoid fever caused by *S* Typhi, accounting for 80% of enteric fever in the United States, although clinically indistinguishable enteric fever is also seen with infections by *S* Paratyphi A (20% of US cases) and, less commonly, by other "nontyphoidal" serotypes such as *S* Choleraesuis. The enteric fever caused by nontyphoidal *Salmonella* generally has less morbidity than typhoid, in that the duration of fever is briefer, patients do not appear to be as ill, and complications and relapses occur less frequently.

Approximately 400 *S* Typhi isolates are reported yearly to the Centers for Disease Control and Prevention. More than 85% of patients report international travel within the 30 days before onset of illness. The onset of enteric fever is insidious, in contrast to bacteremia due to other gram-negative bacteria. The number of bacteria ingested influences attack rate and the length of the incubation period. The initial signs of infection are malaise, anorexia, headache, myalgias, and fever. The fever begins insidiously, is hectic, and gradually rises over the initial week to as high as 40°C (104°F). A relative bradycardia disproportionate to the temperature elevation is characteristic. Although diarrhea may be present during the initial stages, constipation becomes a more prominent symptom as the illness progresses. Hepatomegaly and splenomegaly, often with diffuse abdominal tenderness, are common. The abdomen may be mildly tender, but marked distension, dilated loops, or significant tenderness may indicate ileus. Leukopenia is not uncommon.

Rose spots occur in a small proportion of patients toward the second week. They are discrete (2–4 mm), palpable, erythematous lesions on the trunk. Biopsy of a rose spot reveals nests of mononuclear cells and usually yields *S* Typhi. However, rose spots are often sparse, transient, and difficult to spot on dark-skinned children. The natural course of illness is persistence of fever for 2 to 3 weeks, with slow recovery. Signs and symptoms of a chronic inflammatory process are often apparent by this time.

Complications are common. Most fatalities are the result of intestinal hemorrhage or perforation, resulting from necrosis of infected Peyer's patches. The overall mortality is 3% to 6% with treatment. Predictors of mortality include intestinal perforation, seizures, septic shock, pneumonia, delirium, and coma. Late focal infections, such as meningitis, endocarditis, osteomyelitis, and pneumonia, are rare. Relapse, a recurrence of the manifestations of typhoid fever after initial clinical response, occurred in 8% to 12% of patients who did not receive antimicrobial therapy but may be higher in the antibiotic era.

Children younger than 2 years of age often have mild illness, often resembling a mild, nonspecific febrile illness. Classic typhoid fever can occur in this age group, although it is the exception. In endemic areas such as South Asia, children age 2 to 4 years old have the highest incidence of disease.

## DIAGNOSIS

Identification of *Salmonella* from normally sterile sites such as blood, cerebrospinal fluid (CSF), and joint fluid does not require special media. However, selective media are necessary to identify *Salmonella* in stool because of the vast number of other bacteria. Media range from low to high selectivity. MacConkey, deoxycholate agar, and eosin-methylene blue (EMB) agar are low-selectivity media; *Salmonella-Shigella* (SS), Hektoen enteric (HE), and xylose lysine deoxycholate (XLD) agar are widely used media of medium selectivity; and bismuth sulfite agar is highly selective. Stool specimens that are placed in enrichment broth prior to plating on agar media will have an increase in the yield of organisms.

*Salmonella* should always be considered in a child with gastroenteritis. More severe disease; fever; headache; evidence of dysentery; immune deficiency; recent immigration from endemic areas; exposure to reptiles; undercooked meat or eggs; or an ongoing common source outbreak should increase suspicion.

The diagnosis can be made by stool culture or molecular testing. If fresh stool cannot be obtained, a rectal swab can be used for both culture and molecular tests. For culture, the yield is higher from fresh stool, and the use of enrichment broths in the microbiology lab also improves sensitivity. Blood cultures are negative in the majority of children with *Salmonella* gastroenteritis, and febrile agglutination tests (eg, Widal test) are of no value. Gastroenteritis with fever, especially in a child under 2 years old, is usually an indication for obtaining a blood culture. CSF cultures should be obtained when salmonellosis is suspected in infants less than 3 months of age, even in the absence of elevated temperature, because of the increased risk in this age group.

For suspected enteric fever, serial blood cultures should be obtained. Because the concentration of organisms is low, culturing larger volumes of blood and up to 3 specimens increases the yield. In untreated patients with typhoid fever, 3 blood cultures during the first week have approximately a 90% yield. The yield decreases over time with a concomitant increase in positive stool cultures. Bone marrow culture is the most sensitive procedure for recovery of *S* Typhi. Culture of bile obtained by a swallowed capsule (string test) is also sensitive, but not as sensitive as the combination of blood and bone marrow cultures.

The Widal test is problematic and no longer considered an appropriate diagnostic method. It measures the titer of agglutinating serum antibodies against the O and H antigens of *S* Typhi. In untreated disease, only one-half to two-thirds of patients have a 4-fold or greater increase. Moreover, the Widal test is not specific. In endemic areas, antibody may represent past infection, and there is cross-reactivity with antibody from nontyphoid *Salmonella* infections. In the future, polymerase chain reaction (PCR) or other immunologic tests may increase the sensitivity and turnaround time for detection of bacteremia.

## TREATMENT

The type of illness caused by *Salmonella* directs the selection and duration of antimicrobial therapy. Uncomplicated *Salmonella* gastroenteritis requires no antimicrobial therapy; antibiotics do not shorten the clinical illness, as demonstrated in carefully conducted trials. In addition, antimicrobials may select for resistant strains and prolong *Salmonella* carriage. Antimicrobial therapy should be given to patients with enteric fever, bacteremia from nontyphoid strains, and disseminated infection with localized suppuration. Antimicrobial therapy also should be considered in infants younger than 3 to 6 months and in patients with enterocolitis who have HIV disease or other underlying conditions that impair host resistance.

Ampicillin, chloramphenicol, and trimethoprim-sulfamethoxazole (TMP-SMX) have in vitro activity and historically have been successful in treating patients with nontyphoid *Salmonella* infections (Table 278-1). Resistance to these agents has increased in recent years. Therefore, all isolates should be tested for susceptibility. Cefotaxime and ceftriaxone are useful for ampicillin-resistant strains and are the drugs of choice for *Salmonella* meningitis. Therapy for uncomplicated

**TABLE 278-1 ANTIMICROBIAL THERAPY FOR PATIENTS WITH *SALMONELLA* INFECTIONS**

| Syndrome | Infants | Children | Healthy Adolescents and Adults | Immunocompromised Adults |
|---|---|---|---|---|
| Gastroenteritis | Ampicillin[a] 200 mg/kg/d IV divided q6h or ceftriaxone 100 mg/kg/d IV qd or trimethoprim-sulfamethoxazole 10 mg/kg/d IV or PO divided q12h or cefotaxime 200 mg/kg/d divided q6h | Not recommended | Not recommended | Ampicillin[a] 1 g IV q4h or ceftriaxone 2 g IV qd or trimethoprim-sulfamethoxazole 160 mg IV or PO q12h or fluoroquinolone (eg, ciprofloxacin 500 mg IV or PO q12h, ofloxacin 300 mg PO q12h, or levofloxacin 500 mg PO daily) |
| Extraintestinal infection | Ampicillin[a] or ceftriaxone or cefotaxime | Ampicillin[a] or ceftriaxone or cefotaxime | Ampicillin[a] or ceftriaxone or cefotaxime or fluoroquinolone | Ampicillin[a] or ceftriaxone or cefotaxime or fluoroquinolone |
| Typhoid fever | Ceftriaxone 100 mg/kg/d for 10–14 days or cefotaxime 200 mg/kg/d for 10–14 days | Ceftriaxone 100 mg/kg/d for 10–14 days or cefotaxime 200 mg/kg/d for 10–14 days or cefixime 8 mg/kg/d PO for 5 days or ciprofloxacin 30 mg/kg/d PO divided q12h or azithromycin 10–20 mg/kg/d PO for 7 days | Fluoroquinolone for 7–14 days or ceftriaxone 2 g IV qd for 10–14 days or cefixime 400 mg PO qd for 5 days or azithromycin 10–20 mg/kg/d PO for 7 days | Fluoroquinolone for 7–14 days or ceftriaxone 2 g IV qd for 10–14 days or azithromycin 500 mg PO for 7 days |

[a]Resistance is increasing worldwide. Use only for susceptible isolates.

IV, intravenous; PO, oral; q, every; qd, every day.

bacteremia is usually given for 10 to 14 days; at least 7 days of therapy should be intravenous. Meningitis should be treated for at least 3 weeks. Fluoroquinolones have been very effective in the treatment of adults, although resistance is increasing. The use of fluoroquinolones is no longer contraindicated in children, but the risks and benefits of choosing these agents over other drugs should be weighed carefully.

Ampicillin, amoxicillin, and TMP-SMX are traditional first-line drugs for typhoid fever and effective therapy for susceptible *S* Typhi. Multidrug-resistant *S* Typhi is a rapidly emerging problem worldwide; fluoroquinolones have now become the drug of choice for empiric treatment of typhoid fever in most regions. Short courses of oral cefixime demonstrate acceptable success rates, but the time to clinical improvement is slower than with ceftriaxone or fluoroquinolones. Patients whose isolates have elevated minimum inhibitory concentrations to ciprofloxacin or resistance to nalidixic acid have higher failure rates when treated with fluoroquinolones. Therefore, due to increasing quinolone resistance in South Asia, returning travelers from that region should be treated empirically with azithromycin, ceftriaxone, or cefixime until susceptibility results are available.

Survival of patients with delirium, stupor, or coma associated with typhoid fever is improved by brief, high-dose corticosteroid therapy administered concurrently with antibiotics. Dexamethasone has been used at an initial dose of 3 mg/kg followed by 8 doses of 1 mg/kg every 6 hours. Aggressive surgical intervention, together with broad-spectrum antibiotics (including anti-*Salmonella* therapy), has improved survival in typhoid fever complicated by intestinal perforation with peritonitis.

The chronic asymptomatic carriage of *S* Typhi can be extremely difficult to eradicate, especially if there is obstructive hepatobiliary disease such as gallstones. Success has been achieved with a combination of 6 weeks of ampicillin or amoxicillin with probenecid in patients who have normally functioning gallbladders without evidence of cholelithiasis. In adults, ciprofloxacin has been reasonably successful in eradicating the organism in chronic carriers. Cholecystectomy is recommended for carriers who have relapsed after therapy or who cannot tolerate antimicrobial therapy. Patients who excrete nontyphoid *Salmonella* do not need antimicrobial therapy.

The mortality of *Salmonella* infections ranges from 0.5% to 1.4%. Most deaths are associated with bacteremia, sepsis, or meningitis. Malnutrition, extremes of age, and underlying disease strongly influence mortality. The fatality rate for typhoid fever in hospitalized patients is less than 2% for industrialized nations and variably higher in resource-limited settings. Coma, shock, and abdominal perforation are predictors of mortality.

## PREVENTION

Improvements in sanitation, waste disposal, and safe drinking water have led to a dramatic decrease in *S* Typhi infections but have had little impact on the control of nontyphoid *Salmonella*. Prevention of nontyphoid *Salmonella* involves many fronts. The amount of *Salmonella*, particularly antimicrobial-resistant *Salmonella*, reaching the consumer depends on practices in agriculture, food transportation, and food preparation.

Two vaccines against typhoid fever are available for civilian use in the United States: an orally administered, live-attenuated oral vaccine prepared from the Ty21a strain of *S* Typhi, and an injectable vaccine made from purified Vi polysaccharide. The vaccines are of roughly equal efficacy. The oral Ty21a vaccine is licensed for children age 6 years and older, although it is immunogenic in children age 2 years and older. It requires 4 oral doses and must be repeated every 5 years. The Vi polysaccharide vaccine is licensed for children older than 2 years. It requires a single injection but must be repeated every 2 years. Vaccination against typhoid fever is recommended for persons with intimate exposure with a known carrier, for microbiologists, and for travelers to endemic areas. The risk to travelers is greatest with prolonged stay or with exposure to potentially contaminated food or water. Protein-conjugated Vi polysaccharide vaccines have been shown to very effective in young children and have been licensed in other countries but are not currently licensed in the United States.

# SHIGELLA

*Shigella* are divided into 4 species (serogroups) and over 40 serotypes based on serologic and biochemical reactions: *S dysenteriae* (serogroup A), *S flexneri* (serogroup B), *S boydii* (serogroup C), and *S sonnei* (serogroup D). Groups A, B, and C contain multiple serotypes, but there is only a single serotype of *S sonnei*. *Shigella* are gram-negative, non-lactose-fermenting aerobic, nonmotile bacilli, closely related to *E coli*. They do not survive well in the environment, and delays in plating stool specimens may significantly reduce the recovery rate. Selective media must be used to identify *Shigella* in stool to suppress routine flora and to make *Shigella* distinguishable from other Enterobacteriaceae. Several media are available, including MacConkey bile salt, XLD, and HE. The use of 2 or more media improves the recovery rate, as does broth enrichment. Even optimal handling of stool specimens may not result in isolation of the organism.

## PATHOGENESIS AND EPIDEMIOLOGY

The cardinal features of the pathogenesis of shigellosis are its ability to invade cells and to incite an inflammatory response. In the colon, *Shigella* bind to M cells and translocate across them. The bacteria invade macrophages within Peyer's patches and induce apoptosis with subsequent release of interleukin-1, migration of polymorphonuclear cells, and intense inflammatory response. *Shigella* then invade enterocytes, lyse the cytoplasmic vacuoles, and move to the cytoplasm, where they divide and subsequently invade adjacent cells. The pathologic changes that accompany this include superficial ulcerations of the mucosa, inflammation, hemorrhages, edema, and friability. Involvement is typically worse in the rectosigmoid and distal colon.

*S dysenteriae* type 1 also encodes genes for Shiga toxin, a potent inhibitor of protein synthesis. Shiga toxin is responsible for the increased virulence of this organism and its association with the hemolytic uremic syndrome (HUS). Other species of *Shigella* produce enterotoxins (ShET1 and ShET2) that are distinct from Shiga toxin and are not associated with HUS. The epidemiology of shigellosis differs between developed and less developed countries. *S sonnei* is the most frequently isolated species in the United States and Western Europe, accounting for 60% to 80% of *Shigella* infections; *S flexneri* is second in frequency. In sub-Saharan Africa and the Indian subcontinent, the predominant species is *S flexneri*, accounting for half of infections in children, with *S sonnei* emerging as the second most prevalent (approximately 30%). *S dysenteriae* is rare in high-income countries and is decreasing in prevalence even in low- and middle-income countries, accounting for < 5% of infections in children worldwide.

High attack rates occur among young children, children in childcare centers, men who have sex with men, residents of facilities for the mentally ill, and persons living on Native American reservations. The highest attack rate for shigellosis is in children 1 to 4 years old (see Fig. 278-2). Breastfeeding is clearly protective. Attack rates among children in developing countries are dramatically higher. *Shigella* infections show a distinct seasonal peak during July through October, but infections occur year-round.

*Shigella* infection is acquired through fecal–oral exposure. Unlike *Salmonella* infections, however, person-to-person transmission plays a key role. As few as 10 to 100 organisms can cause disease, based on volunteer studies. Humans are the primary reservoir of *Shigella*; higher primates can become infected but do not play a significant role in the epidemiology. Crowding, poor sanitation, inadequate supplies of water for washing, lack of soap, and the presence of diapered children are risk factors for the spread of *Shigella*. Outbreaks of shigellosis in childcare centers are common. The spread in childcare centers plays a central role in sustaining endemic shigellosis in communities. Outbreaks have also occurred as a consequence of swimming in contaminated lakes and pools. There have been many foodborne outbreaks from an ever-expanding list of vehicles; fresh fruits and vegetables have assumed a prominent role in recent years. In developing countries, waterborne spread and close contact fuel ongoing transmission.

The role of asymptomatic carriers in the epidemiology of shigellosis is not completely understood. In one study, 17% of children excreted *Shigella* for at least 1 month after the acute illness, and 11% excreted *Shigella* for at least 2 months. In highly exposed populations, asymptomatic carriage and/or prolonged excretion may be more common.

## CLINICAL MANIFESTATIONS

The clinical manifestations of shigellosis vary. The incubation period can be as short as 12 hours or as long as 5 days, but most often, it is 24 to 48 hours. Most illness begins with fever, malaise, anorexia, and occasionally vomiting or headache. Diarrhea usually begins as watery diarrhea and may progress within hours or days to dysentery. Typical symptoms of dysentery include frequent small-volume stools containing mucus and blood associated with lower abdominal cramps and tenesmus. However, the diarrhea may remain watery and copious. Asymptomatic infection also occurs.

Physical findings include fever, systemic toxicity, increased bowel sounds, and lower abdominal tenderness. The child may have signs of dehydration. Rectal prolapse may occur in 5% to 8% of patients. In general, *S sonnei* causes milder illness with fewer complications, *S flexneri* tends to be more severe, and *S dysenteriae* tends to cause the most severe dysentery and extraintestinal complications. The white blood cell count is usually elevated. Leukemoid reactions with as many as 50,000 cells/μL occasionally occur.

Shigellosis is less common in neonates and young infants than in children older than 1 year, but infants and neonates are more likely to be severely dehydrated or hypothermic, are twice as likely to die, and are less likely to have classic findings such as high fever, bloody diarrhea, abdominal tenderness, and rectal prolapse. Thus, a high index of suspicion and a low threshold for obtaining stool cultures are appropriate for young infants with diarrhea.

A variety of complications of shigellosis occur. Dehydration, hypoglycemia, hyponatremia, hypernatremia, and hypokalemia can occur; hypoglycemia and hyponatremia are associated with an increased mortality rate. Seizures are a common extraintestinal manifestation and occur exclusively in children. Isolated seizures are usually not associated with any long-term neurologic sequelae. Ekiri syndrome, a severe toxic encephalopathy with seizures, rapid progression, and high mortality, is a rare complication of shigellosis.

Bacteremia is uncommon in healthy children but is more common with HIV infection and severe malnutrition. In about half of bacteremic children, there may be polymicrobial bacteremia caused by other organisms that have traversed the injured gut. Extraintestinal suppurative complications such as osteomyelitis, meningitis, septic arthritis, and splenic abscess are rare. HUS is an important complication of *S dysenteriae* type 1 infection, reported in 1% to 4% of children; it is seen occasionally with *S flexneri*. Reactive arthritis and Reiter syndrome (arthritis, urethritis, and iritis in conjunction with HLA-B27) are unusual postinfectious complications of *Shigella*, usually occurring in adolescents or adults.

## DIAGNOSIS

*Shigella* should be suspected in children with fever and diarrhea, particularly if there are seizures, or in children with small-volume diarrhea with abdominal cramping, blood, white blood cells, or mucus in the stool. Many patients with *S sonnei*, however, do not have bloody diarrhea. The diagnosis hinges on the recovery of *Shigella* from a fresh stool specimen or a rectal swab. By bacterial culture methods, recovery is easier early in the course of the disease. *Shigella* may not survive transportation. If rectal swabs are used, they should be placed in appropriate transport media, such as Cary-Blair media. Specimens should be processed immediately by the clinical microbiology laboratory. Even with optimal handling, false-negative cultures will occur. In volunteer studies, cultures were negative in 20% of volunteers. Presumptive identification of *Shigella* requires at least 48 hours; definitive identification may require 72 hours.

PCR can be used to detect *Shigella* in stool, appears to be very sensitive, and is increasingly available as part of multiplex gastrointestinal pathogen panels. In developed countries, the frequency of *Shigella* and *E coli* O157:H7 infection in children with bloody diarrhea is similar. Making the distinction is critical, because shigellosis responds to antimicrobial therapy but *E coli* O157:H7 infections do not, and some evidence suggests that antimicrobials increase the risk of HUS. Fortunately, currently available PCR and enzyme-based immunoassays for Shiga toxin allow the diagnosis of *E coli* O157:H7 and other enterohemorrhagic *E coli* in about 24 hours.

## TREATMENT

Fluid and electrolyte therapy are key components of management. Although shigellosis is a self-limited disease for most patients, antibiotic treatment during acute dysentery will reduce the duration of fever and diarrhea. Table 278-2 lists antimicrobial therapy for patients with shigellosis. Treatment of milder disease or later in the course has only modest clinical benefit but leads to more rapid cessation of shedding, usually within 1 to 2 days. This reduces the likelihood of secondary spread and is particularly important in settings such as childcare centers and institutions. This public health benefit must be weighed against the public health risk of enhanced selection of antimicrobial-resistant disease from treating mild disease with antibiotics.

Antibiotic-resistant *Shigella* have emerged rapidly throughout the world. Local resistance patterns and travel history must be taken into consideration. Ampicillin was once the drug of choice for *Shigella*, but resistance is now close to universal. TMP-SMX is effective for sensitive strains. However, resistance is increasingly common, and therefore,

**TABLE 278-2 ANTIMICROBIAL THERAPY FOR PATIENTS WITH SHIGELLOSIS**

| Antibiotic | Children | Maximum Dose[a] | Comments |
|---|---|---|---|
| Ampicillin | 100 mg/kg/d divided q6h | 500 mg qid | Resistance is very common; use only if susceptible strain |
| Trimethoprim-sulfamethoxazole | 10 mg/kg/d (trimethoprim) divided q12h | 160 mg bid (1 DS tablet) divided q12h | Resistance is increasingly common, even in United States |
| Nalidixic acid | 55 mg/kg/d divided q6h | 1 g qid | Not licensed in the United States for this indication, but the empiric drug of choice in many regions |
| Cefixime | 8 mg/kg/d divided q12h | 400 mg/d | Not licensed in the United States for this indication; poor efficacy in adults |
| Ceftriaxone | 50 mg/d IV or IM as single dose × 3 days | 1–2 g IV or IM qd | Not licensed in the United States for this indication |
| Azithromycin | 12 mg/kg PO once, then 6 mg/kg daily for 4 days | 500 mg PO once, then 250 mg daily | Emerging resistance worldwide |
| Ciprofloxacin | 20 mg/kg/d divided q12h | 500 mg bid for 5 days | If alternatives are active, they may be preferred for young children; resistance increasing worldwide |
| Other fluoroquinolones | Limited data | Varies | Efficacy and resistance similar to ciprofloxacin |

[a]Maximum adult/adolescent dose.

bid, twice a day; DS, double-strength; IM, intramuscular; IV, intravenous; PO, oral; q, every; qd, every day.

TMP-SMX can no longer be considered a reliable drug for empiric therapy without considering local epidemiology.

Resistant strains of *S sonnei* and *S flexneri* may be susceptible to fluoroquinolones, ceftriaxone, cefixime, and azithromycin. A clinical trial of cefixime in children in Israel suggested good efficacy, but in a trial among adults in Bangladesh, it was not effective. Azithromycin was effective in a single trial, but the widespread use of this drug may lead to more resistance. For severe shigellosis, intravenous or intramuscular ceftriaxone is effective. Although fluoroquinolones are not approved for use in children because of lingering concerns over arthropathy, 2 clinical trials in children with severe shigellosis suggested that ciprofloxacin and norfloxacin are safe and effective. Unfortunately, strains of *Shigella* resistant to fluoroquinolones and cephalosporins are commonly encountered in sub-Saharan Africa and Asia and, more recently, in the United States. Although still uncommon, azithromycin resistance has been increasingly reported, including in the United States.

Antidiarrheal agents that reduce gastrointestinal tract motility should not be used in infants and children with infectious diarrhea. Their use in children with shigellosis is associated with toxic megacolon and with HUS in patients with *E coli* O157:H7.

Shigellosis usually resolves completely in 7 to 10 days if untreated. A postdiarrheal enteropathy may occur, particularly following *S dysenteriae* infection. Growth delay and exacerbation of malnutrition may follow shigellosis, particularly in children with preexisting malnutrition. In developed countries, the mortality is less than 1%. In developing countries, the mortality can range from 10% to 30%. Risk factors for death include infection with *S dysenteriae* type 1, malnutrition, very young age, and bacteremia.

## PREVENTION

Simple measures of hygiene can greatly reduce the incidence of *Shigella* infections in resource-poor settings. These measures include the provision of appropriate sanitation, safe drinking water, and soap and water for hand washing. Provision of narrow-mouthed water containers that cannot be contaminated by dirty hands is a cost-effective prevention tool. Breastfeeding is a practical strategy to prevent disease in infants.

Prevention of shigellosis in developed countries depends on control of person-to-person transmission and identification of foodborne outbreaks. Within childcare centers, control measures include adequate number of sinks, methods to clean diaper-changing surfaces, prohibiting food handlers from diaper changing, cohorting of sick children, and frequent staff education. Control of spread in childcare centers is likely to impact community-wide transmission. In other institutional outbreaks, cohorting and contact isolation are important measures. Antibiotic treatment of infected persons may curtail outbreaks in closed settings. Antibiotic prophylaxis is ineffective and risks the emergence of resistance.

Both killed and live-attenuated oral vaccines have been studied but have provided only partial, transient, serotype-specific immunity. Several candidate vaccines are in development, the most advanced of which include polysaccharide conjugates and oral live-attenuated cells with deletion of enterotoxin genes.

# *ESCHERICHIA COLI*

*E coli* are gram-negative, lactose-fermenting, motile, facultative bacilli belonging to the family Enterobacteriaceae. *E coli* can be grouped by serotype, defined by the 171 somatic (O) and 56 flagellar antigens. Thus, *E coli* O157:H7 is an example of a specific serotype. *E coli* are the most common flora of the gastrointestinal tract and probably serve useful symbiotic functions. Most are nonpathogenic, but some possess specific virulence traits that enable them to cause meningitis, urinary tract infection, or diarrhea. The diarrhea-causing *E coli* fall into 5 distinct phenotypes (also referred to as pathotypes; Table 278-3). Each phenotype possesses unique genes encoding virulence traits, each with their own pathogenesis. There is substantial heterogeneity in the number and type of virulence genes even within phenotypic categories, complicating the interpretation of studies.

**TABLE 278-3 CHARACTERISTICS OF *ESCHERICHIA COLI* ASSOCIATED WITH DIARRHEA**

| Type | Pathogenesis | Epidemiology |
|---|---|---|
| Enteropathogenic (EPEC) | Attaching and effacing lesions | Acute and chronic diarrhea in infants |
| Enterotoxigenic (ETEC) | Enterotoxins (LT and ST) induce accumulation of cAMP and cGMP | Watery diarrhea in infants in developing countries and travelers |
| Enteroinvasive (EIEC) | Direct invasion plus exotoxins, similar to *Shigella* | Diarrhea with fever in all ages |
| Shiga toxin–producing (STEC); also called enterohemorrhagic (EHEC) | Attaching and effacing lesions; Shiga toxin | Hemorrhagic colitis in all ages; hemolytic uremic syndrome, highest rates in children |
| Enteroaggregative (EAEC) | Not fully defined; adhesion molecules, enterotoxin, and cytotoxin identified | Persistent diarrhea in children in developing world and travelers; may be important in developed countries |

cAMP, cyclic adenosine monophosphate; cGMP, cyclic guanosine monophosphate.

Because *E coli* is the most common facultative organism in stool, identifying diarrhea-causing *E coli* in stool specimens is difficult. Colonies of *E coli* must be individually tested for specific virulence traits using bioassays, assays for specific toxins, phenotypic adherence assays, DNA probes for virulence genes, or PCR. Many of these assays are available only in research laboratories.

Shiga toxin–producing *E coli* (STEC), also known as enterohemorrhagic *E coli* (EHEC), are able to cause an attaching and effacing lesion in intestinal mucosa and secrete Shiga toxin (previously called Vero toxin or Shiga-like toxin). Because Shiga toxin is the defining virulence factor, the preferred terminology for this group of organisms is now Shiga toxin–producing *E coli* (STEC). At least 12 serotypes of *E coli* are STEC, but one serotype, *E coli* O157:H7, is the predominant strain in much of the world. Because it is much easier to screen for *E coli* O157:H7, its importance relative to other serotypes of STEC has been overestimated, and non-O157:H7 serotypes may account for more than half of STEC infections in the United States (Fig. 278-3). Unlike most *E coli*, *E coli* O157:H7 ferments sorbitol slowly, which led to the development of a simple microbiologic screen, sorbitol MacConkey (SMAC) agar. With the exception of *E coli* O157:H7, STEC must be identified in the lab by detection of Shiga toxin by immunoassays or the Shiga toxin gene by PCR. Additional serogroup identification may be performed at the public health laboratory based on O and H antigen serology of the colony.

Enterotoxigenic *E coli* (ETEC) belong to many serotypes. They produce one or both of the enterotoxins ST and LT, which cause secretory diarrhea without invading or damaging enterocytes. They can be identified in the laboratory by detection of enterotoxin by immunoassays or detection of the enterotoxin gene by DNA probe or by PCR.

Enteropathogenic *E coli* (EPEC) are an important cause of diarrhea in infants in developing countries and were responsible for numerous nursery outbreaks in industrialized countries during the 1950s and 1960s. In the laboratory, EPEC are usually identified by the presence of the EAF plasmid, which can be detected by colony blot with the *eae* and *bfpA* genes by gene probe or by PCR. Recent studies have also described the emergence of an atypical EPEC, which does not have the EAF plasmid and is *bfpA* negative. By definition, EPEC do not secrete Shiga toxin. Adherence assays can also be used, although they are cumbersome and require considerable expertise.

Enteroinvasive *E coli* (EIEC) are strains of *E coli* that closely resemble *Shigella* in their genetics, biochemical characteristics, and clinical manifestations. Identification of EIEC was traditionally performed by isolating strains of *E coli* with a positive Sereny test (guinea pig keratoconjunctivitis). Gene probes for the invasiveness gene *ipaC* are used to screen colony blots of *E coli* for EIEC, although PCR for the *ipaH* gene is becoming the favored assay for EIEC.

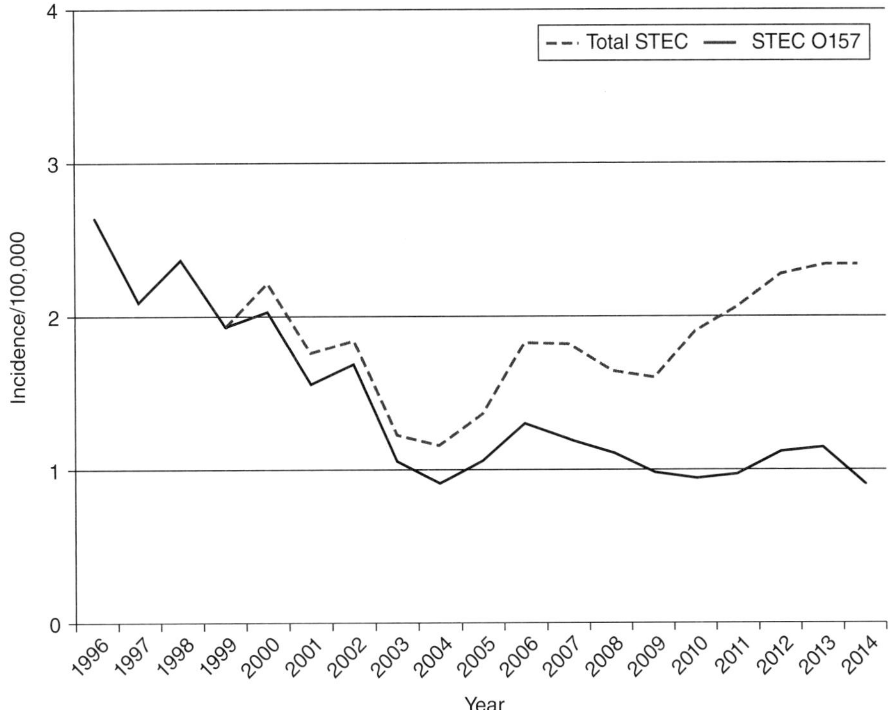


**FIGURE 278-3** Annual incidence of laboratory-confirmed Shiga toxin–producing *E coli* (STEC) O157:H7 and total STEC infections based on the Centers for Disease Control and Prevention FoodNet Surveillance System, United States, 1996–2014. Note that non-O157:H7 STEC infections were not reported before 1999, and the availability of testing for non-O157:H7 STEC has increased over time. (Reproduced with permission from the Centers for Disease Control [CDC] https://www.cdc.gov/foodnet/reports/annual-reports-2014.html.)

Enteroaggregative *E coli* (EAEC) are the most recent phenotype of *E coli* demonstrated to cause diarrhea. They are defined as strains that do not secrete LT or ST and that adhere to Hep-2 cells or a cover slip with a "stacked brick" pattern of adherence. This test is only available in research laboratories and a few reference laboratories, is tedious, and requires care and expertise. Several genetic markers of virulence factors that can be detected by probe or PCR have been found that identify EAEC, including EAST1, CVD432, and several adherence markers. Most recently, studies have used the presence of *aaiC* (chromosomally encoded), *aggR*, and *aatA* (both plasmid encoded) genes to define EAEC, although the optimal use of these markers remains unclear.

An *E coli* O104:H4 strain with the phenotypic characteristics of EAEC that also produces Shiga toxin has caused several outbreaks, including a large outbreak in Germany characterized by high rates of HUS.

## PATHOGENESIS AND EPIDEMIOLOGY

All diarrhea-causing *E coli* are transmitted by fecal-oral contact, but they differ in the infectious dose, the susceptible population, the geographic patterns, and the relative importance of food, water, and person-to-person transmission.

The incubation period for STEC is usually 3 to 4 days, although it ranges from 1 to 9 days. *E coli* O157:H7 are quite acid tolerant and probably are less affected by the gastric acid barrier than other enteric pathogens. On reaching the intestine, STEC adhere to enterocytes, primarily in the colon. A characteristic attaching and effacing lesion occurs, similar to what occurs with EPEC. Histology shows edema and submucosal hemorrhage. The defining virulence factor for STEC is the ability to produce Shiga toxin (Stx), one of the most potent protein inhibitors of protein synthesis known. There are 2 major subtypes of Stx: Stx1 and Stx2, with numerous minor variants of Stx2. Other putative virulence factors include a hemolysin, lipopolysaccharide (LPS), iron utilization genes, and EAST. The attaching and effacing lesion is mediated by genes encoded in the locus of enterocyte effacement (LEE), a 35-kb pathogenicity island that is identical to the island found in EPEC.

The pathogenesis of HUS is not fully understood, but available evidence supports the following sequence: (1) binding of STEC to enterocytes promotes production of tumor necrosis factor and interleukin-1, which may upregulate endothelial expression of toxin receptors; (2) Stx and LPS probably reach the systemic circulation; (3) LPS sensitizes endothelial cells to cell damage due to Stx; (4) endothelial cell damage leads to platelet aggregation, white cell activation and adherence, and microvascular damage; and (5) fibrin thrombi occur in the kidneys and potentially in many other sites, including brain, spinal cord, heart, lung, pancreas, and colon. HUS is discussed further in Chapter 468.

The pathogenesis of ETEC is fairly similar to *Vibrio cholerae*. Symptoms follow an incubation period of 14 to 48 hours. ETEC colonize the surface of the small-bowel epithelium but do not invade. Binding is mediated by surface fimbriae (or pili), referred to as colonization fimbriae (CFAs). Diarrhea is caused by 1 of 2 toxins: heat-labile toxin (LT) or heat-stable toxin (ST). Strains may produce 1 or both toxins. LT is 80% homologous to cholera toxin at the protein sequence level and has a similar structure and a similar function. LT induces adenylate cyclase, leading to increased levels of cyclic adenosine monophosphate. This activation of chloride channels results in increased chloride secretion, leading to passive efflux of water and watery diarrhea. ST binds to guanylate cyclase, a membrane-spanning enzyme, and stimulates the production of cyclic guanosine monophosphate.

The incubation period for EPEC is 6 to 48 hours. EPEC adhere to the epithelial cell through a process thought to be mediated by the bundle-forming pilus, encoded in the EAF plasmid. Genes within the LEE are activated, leading to secretion of a molecule called intimin and activation of a type III secretion system. The microvillus structure is dissolved. Intimate adherence supervenes, with activation of the cell's cytoskeleton, leading to production of a pedestal lesion. The mechanisms by which this cascade causes diarrhea are not fully understood.

The pathophysiology of EIEC is virtually identical to *Shigella*. It invades and divides within enterocytes, causing intense inflammation.

Much less is understood about the pathogenesis of diarrhea caused by EAEC. Not all strains cause diarrhea in laboratory animals or in human volunteers. EAEC adhere to intestinal epithelium through the actions of fimbriae and form biofilm, which allows for local immune evasion. EAST1, an enterotoxin associated with secretion, is present in most strains associated with diarrhea, and a number of cytotoxins have been identified. EAEC causes an inflammatory response, characterized by induction of interleukin-8 release from epithelial cells. Increased mucus production is seen in patients, animals, and volunteers, but the mechanism is not known. *E coli* O157:H7 and other STECs have emerged as some of the most important enteric pathogens in developed countries. They are a relatively common cause of nonbloody and bloody diarrhea in developed countries of North and South America, Europe, and Japan. STECs are responsible for upward of 90% of postdiarrheal HUS and an unknown proportion of cases of thrombotic thrombocytopenic purpura (TTP). *E coli* O157:H7 currently accounts for less than half of STEC infections in the United States, and the incidence of non-O157 infections is increasing (see Fig. 278-3); however, the true incidence is not known, because many laboratories do not use techniques to identify STEC. The Centers for Disease Control and Prevention estimates the disease burden using the FoodNet active surveillance system. The incidence is highest among children younger than 5 years (4.4/100,000 person-years), but infection occurs in all age groups. STEC infections show a clear seasonal pattern, with peak incidence in the summer and fall in the Northern Hemisphere.

The natural reservoir of STEC is dairy cattle; however, other animals that can carry the organism include goats, sheep, pigs, deer, and elk. Outbreaks are most often the result of consumption of hamburger meat or raw milk. Several outbreaks have followed swimming in contaminated water in lakes, ponds, and swimming pools. Other outbreaks have been the result of visits to petting zoos and consumption of roast beef, apple cider, unpasteurized apple juice, salami, municipal water, and produce, including leaf lettuce, spinach, and alfalfa and radish sprouts. Most cases are sporadic, and consumption of undercooked hamburger and farm visits are risk factors for sporadic cases. The infectious dose for *E coli* O157:H7 is low, estimated from one outbreak to be less than 700 organisms. Person-to-person transmission has been documented in institutions, childcare centers, homes with young children, and, rarely, hospitals.

ETEC is an important cause of diarrhea in 2 groups: young children in developing countries and travelers to developing countries. In recent large multinational studies, ETEC was the top bacterial pathogen associated with diarrhea in infants. The incidence of symptomatic ETEC disease drops sharply with age in endemic countries. However, travelers from developed countries lack immunity. Twenty to 40% of traveler's diarrhea is due to ETEC. Transmission generally results from contamination of water and food in conditions of poor sanitation and requires a relatively high inoculum. Several outbreaks of ETEC have been identified in the United States, and sporadic cases are increasingly recognized with use of multiplex PCR platforms. EPEC is most commonly associated with diarrhea in infants and is a large contributor to both morbidity and mortality due to diarrhea in infants in developing countries. Diarrhea due to typical EPEC rarely occurs in adults. The epidemiology of atypical EPEC is emerging, with some studies demonstrating incidence exceeding that of typical EPEC, although its association with diarrhea continues to be questioned.

EAEC was initially identified as a pathogen in developing countries and later associated with persistent diarrhea among persons with HIV infection. There is also increasing recognition that it is responsible for a large proportion of cases of traveler's diarrhea. Recent studies showing that these organisms were an important cause of diarrhea in children in Baltimore and New Haven have challenged the assumption that EAEC disease is limited to developing countries. Little is known about modes of transmission or infectious dose of EAEC, though it is thought to be transmitted by fecal-oral route with a human reservoir.

## CLINICAL MANIFESTATIONS

STEC most often cause hemorrhagic colitis, characterized by vomiting, bloody diarrhea, and severe abdominal cramps. Fecal leukocytes may be present but are not prominent. Asymptomatic carriage and nonbloody diarrhea also occur. HUS—the triad of thrombocytopenia, hemolytic anemia, and renal failure—occurs in 5% to 10% of children infected with *E coli* O157:H7, although there has been wide variability. The rate may be lower for non-O157 strains. Leukocytosis during the diarrheal illness has been consistently reported to be a predictor of HUS. Risk factors for HUS include young age, use of antimotility agents, and, possibly, use of antimicrobial agents. The data implicating antimicrobial agents are based on in vitro studies that demonstrate that antimicrobial agents upregulate toxin production and epidemiologic data. A limited number of retrospective epidemiologic studies and a single prospective study demonstrated an association between antibiotic use and HUS or death, as did a recent meta-analysis. Given the lack of evidence of benefit and the potential for harm, antibiotics should be avoided during STEC infection. In adults, STEC infection may lead to TTP.

ETEC causes large-volume watery diarrhea. Fever and vomiting may occur but are uncommon. The diarrhea may be mild and self-limited, or it may lead to massive fluid loss and dehydration. Blood, mucus, and fecal white cells are very uncommon. Duration is typically less than 1 week.

EPEC diarrhea typically occurs in children less than 2 years old. Diarrhea is usually watery and profuse. Vomiting and low-grade fever are common. While most cases are associated with acute disease, persistent diarrhea may occur.

EIEC causes abdominal cramps, tenesmus, fever, and small-volume stools. Blood and mucus may be present but may be less common than with some of the more virulent strains of *Shigella*.

EAEC most often occurs as a watery diarrhea without vomiting and with low-grade fever. Mucoid diarrhea is common, and in some series, bloody diarrhea occurred in up to one-third of patients. Of particular importance is the association of EAEC with persistent diarrhea. In malnourished children, persistent diarrhea is associated with malnutrition and contributes to increased mortality.

Currently, STECs are associated with the greatest morbidity in developed countries. Five to 10% of infected patients develop HUS; the mortality from HUS is 2% to 5%. The major complications of ETEC infection are related to dehydration and electrolyte disturbances. Severe complications of ETEC infection should be uncommon in a setting with good rehydration facilities. However, ETEC contributes a substantial proportion of the approximately 3 million deaths that occur as a consequence of diarrhea among infants and young children in developing countries. Although several nursery epidemics caused by EPEC in the 1940s and 1950s reported mortality rates approaching 50%, the current mortality is less than 1% in developed countries. The persistent diarrhea associated with EAEC is associated with growth failure and increased mortality. As rehydration services improve in developing countries, persistent diarrhea accounts for an increasing proportion of diarrheal mortality.

## DIAGNOSIS

Diagnosis of infection by diarrhea-causing *E coli* is difficult. Techniques for the diagnosis of STEC are widely available in clinical laboratories, although many do not test routinely. Techniques for diagnosing the other 4 phenotypes are largely limited to research and public health laboratories, although this may change with the increasing availability of multiplex PCR assays. Etiologic diagnosis may be advantageous in outbreaks and in the evaluation of patients with severe or persistent diarrhea, especially in the setting of foreign travel and the immunocompromised.

Screening with SMAC agar, an inexpensive technique that should be available in all clinical microbiology laboratories, can identify *E coli* O157:H7. To detect other serotypes of STEC, methods that detect Stx are necessary. Commercial enzyme immunoassays are available, although there is increasing use of molecular assays. When used on supernatants of 24-hour broth cultures, enzyme immunoassay is highly sensitive and specific. Some laboratories may routinely screen all stools for STEC, whereas others screen only bloody stools or only when specific testing is requested.

ETEC cannot be identified by biochemical characteristics or serotype. Definitive diagnosis is based on detection of toxin in *E coli* colonies by bioassay in the suckling mouse assay, the Y1 adrenal cell assay, enzyme immunoassay, DNA probes, or PCR primers directed against the genes encoding LT and ST.

Serotyping was once the gold standard for identifying EPEC strains; it is no longer considered the primary method. According to a consensus definition, EPEC strains are those that can cause an attaching and effacing lesion in the Hep-2 adherence assay and that lack Stx. Genotypic diagnosis relies on DNA probes and PCR primers for the *eae* gene, the *bfp* gene, and the EAF plasmid.

EIEC can be diagnosed by demonstrating that an isolate with the biochemical characteristics of *E coli* contains *Shigella* invasiveness genes. An enzyme immunoassay to detect the *ipaC* gene has been developed, although PCR for the *ipaH* gene is now widely used for both research and in the clinic.

The gold standard for diagnosing EAEC is the Hep-2 adherence assay, in which tested *E coli* isolates demonstrate the stacked brick configuration. PCR for the *aaiC, aggR,* or *aatA* genes is commonly used to identify EAEC in research studies, although more studies are needed to determine optimal targets for this pathogen.

## TREATMENT

As for all diarrheal illness in children, the cornerstone of therapy is careful replacement of fluids and electrolytes. The treatment of STEC is supportive. As noted earlier, the use of antimicrobial agents in STEC may be associated with an increased risk of HUS. Although this remains controversial, there are no data supporting any clinical benefit, so it is prudent to avoid all antimicrobials.

Antimicrobial therapy is clearly useful in shortening the course of ETEC infections in travelers, as demonstrated in numerous studies in many settings. TMP-SMX, doxycycline, bacampicillin, furazolidone, rifaximin, and fluoroquinolones have demonstrated efficacy. However, resistance to TMP-SMX is common in some regions. Treatment of EPEC with TMP-SMX, oral gentamicin, and oral colistin is effective, although symptomatic therapy may suffice. Antibiotics used to treat *Shigella* can be used in EIEC, although clear data are lacking. The optimal treatment of EAEC infection is unknown, but small studies have reported clinical response to ciprofloxacin among HIV-infected patients and travelers with EAEC infection. Rifaximin was more effective than placebo among travelers in a small study.

Antimotility agents should be avoided in persons with inflammatory or bloody diarrhea and in infants and children with diarrhea. Antimotility agents in low dose and for a brief period are safe for treating secretory diarrhea in adults. Bismuth subsalicylate reduces the severity of diarrhea in patients with ETEC infections, although salicylate absorption occurs. The general rule is that the amount of salicylate absorbed from 30 mL of Pepto-Bismol is similar to that of one 325-mg aspirin tablet.

## PREVENTION

The most important measures for prevention of ETEC, EPEC, EAEC, and EIEC are improvements in sanitation, including proper disposal of human waste, access to water and soap for hand washing, and clean sources of food for weaning. Breastfeeding is protective and should be encouraged. Nosocomial transmission of diarrhea causing *E coli* occurs; therefore, careful enteric precautions should be followed.

To prevent STEC, hamburger and other beef products should be cooked thoroughly and protected from contamination from raw meat. Unpasteurized milk and apple juice should be avoided. Because several outbreaks of *E coli* O157:H7 were caused by diapered children in swimming pools and ponds, this is a potential area for intervention.

To prevent ETEC infection, travelers to developing countries should avoid ice, salads, and those raw fruits and vegetables without peels. They should drink only boiled or carbonated water or beverages or bottled water from a reliable source. Infant formula should be prepared from boiled water. Routine use of prophylactic antibiotics is not recommended, particularly for children. Bismuth subsalicylate can be used for prophylaxis in adolescents and adults, but the aspirin exposure represents a relative contraindication for young children.

Because preliminary studies with inactivated ETEC vaccines prove that protective vaccines are feasible, several approaches are under active investigation.

## SUGGESTED READINGS

Crim SM, Griffin PM, Tauxe R, et al. Preliminary incidence and trends of infection with pathogens transmitted commonly through food: Foodborne Diseases Active Surveillance Network, 10 U.S. sites, 2006-2014. *MMWR Morb Mortal Wkly Rep*. 2015;64:495-499.

Croxen MA, Law RJ, Scholz R, Keeney KM, Wlodarska M, Finlay BB. Recent advances in understanding enteric pathogenic *Escherichia coli*. *Clin Microbiol Rev*. 2013;26:822-880.

Crump JA, Sjölund-Karlsson M, Gordon MA, Parry CM. Epidemiology, clinical presentation, laboratory diagnosis, antimicrobial resistance, and antimicrobial management of invasive *Salmonella* infections. *Clin Microbiol Rev*. 2015;28:901-937.

Date KA, Newton AE, Medalla F, et al. Changing patterns in enteric fever incidence and increasing antibiotic resistance of enteric fever isolates in the United States, 2008-2012. *Clin Infect Dis*. 2016;63:322-329.

Denno DM, Shaikh N, Stapp JR, et al. Diarrhea etiology in a pediatric emergency department: a case control study. *Clin Infect Dis*. 2012;55:897-904.

Freedman SB, Xie J, Neufeld MS, et al. Shiga toxin-producing *Escherichia coli* infection, antibiotics, and risk of developing hemolytic uremic syndrome: a meta-analysis. *Clin Infect Dis*. 2016;62:1251-1258.

Kotloff KL, Nataro JP, Blackwelder WC, et al. Burden and aetiology of diarrhoeal disease in infants and young children in developing countries (the Global Enteric Multicenter Study, GEMS): a prospective, case-control study. *Lancet*. 2013;382:209-222.

Platts-Mills JA, Babji S, Bodhidatta L, et al. Pathogen-specific burdens of community diarrhoea in developing countries: a multisite birth cohort study (MAL-ED). *Lancet Glob Health*. 2015;3:e564-e575.

Scallan E, Mahon BE, Hoekstra RM, Griffin PM. Estimates of illnesses, hospitalizations and deaths caused by major bacterial enteric pathogens in young children in the United States. *Pediatr Infect Dis J*. 2013;32:217-221.

Stockmann C, Pavia AT, Graham B, et al. Detection of 23 gastrointestinal pathogens among children who present with diarrhea. *J Pediatr Infect Dis Soc*. doi:10.1093/jpids/piw020 [Epub ahead of print on May 4, 2016].

# 279 Staphylococcal Infections

Matthew C. Washam and Beverly L. Connelly

## INTRODUCTION

Staphylococci are ubiquitous inhabitants of the skin and mucous membranes of humans and other mammals. They exist in a commensal relationship until a breach in a cutaneous or mucosal barrier permits staphylococci access to deeper tissues and the bloodstream or until a foreign body or medical device provides a foothold. The production of coagulase, an enzyme that clots plasma, distinguishes *Staphylococcus aureus* from other medically important staphylococci. Those that do not produce coagulase are grouped collectively as coagulase-negative staphylococci (CoNS) and represent the most common resident bacteria of humans. All staphylococci are nonmotile, non–spore-forming, facultative anaerobic bacteria. In gram-stained specimens, they appear as gram-positive cocci in clusters, as well as in pairs and tetrads. Peptidoglycans and lipoteichoic acids form the basic cell wall structures of staphylococci, and most exhibit microcapsule formation. Colony morphology followed by selected biochemical reactions allows identification of pathogenic staphylococci. Typical 24-hour *S aureus* colonies are larger, yellow pigmented, and surrounded by a small zone of hemolysis. Colonies of *Staphylococcus epidermidis* are typically small, white or beige, and approximately 1 to 2 mm in diameter after overnight incubation. Small-colony variants of *S aureus,* important in some persistent infections, may be missed initially because of their pinpoint size. Staphylococcal colonies in general will be catalase-positive, distinguishing them from streptococci.

## COAGULASE-NEGATIVE *STAPHYLOCOCCUS*

### PATHOGENESIS AND EPIDEMIOLOGY

Most infections attributed to CoNS are facilitated by the formation of biofilm on host tissue or medical device surfaces. CoNS can attach directly to foreign bodies via hydrophobic interactions mediated by cell wall–anchored proteins, the surface charge of teichoic acids, and van der Waals forces. Host extracellular matrix and plasma proteins including fibrinogen, fibronectin, and collagen can cover foreign bodies and serve as additional attachment sites for CoNS via covalent binding with staphylococcal cell wall–anchored adhesins. Following attachment, the bacteria multiply to form multilayered cell aggregates mediated by polysaccharide intercellular adhesin and proteinaceous adhesins resulting in biofilm formation. Biofilms are key to the pathogenesis of foreign body–associated infections, providing CoNS with a physical barrier to evade both host immune responses and systemic antimicrobial therapy. *Staphylococcus saprophyticus* is uniquely outfitted as a genitourinary pathogen because of a novel cell wall–anchored protein involved in adherence to uroepithelial cells, redundant urine adaptive transporter systems, and urease. The virulence factors for *Staphylococcus lugdunensis* are unclear but likely involve its production of extracellular glycocalyx, which assists immune evasion, and enzymes such as esterase, protease, and lipases, which facilitate tissue invasion.

CoNS colonize virtually all normal skin with a predilection for areas of higher humidity, such as the anterior nares, axillae, inguinal and gluteal regions, umbilicus, the antecubital and popliteal spaces, as well as conjunctiva. Because of the commensal nature of the CoNS, they are often recovered in specimens from superficial sites and may be recovered from body fluids and deep sites when inadequate or improper collection techniques have been employed. Recovery of CoNS from a normally sterile body site must be interpreted in light of the clinical circumstances of the patient. Of the more than 40 species, at least 19 are indigenous to humans, with *S epidermidis* being the most common of the resident CoNS. Certain species display select colonizing ecological niches: *Staphylococcus haemolyticus* and *Staphylococcus hominis* (axillae and pubic areas high in apocrine glands), *Staphylococcus capitis* (sebaceous glands of the forehead and scalp), *Staphylococcus auricularis* (ear), and *S saprophyticus* (genitourinary tract). Other medically relevant CoNS species include *S lugdunensis*, *Staphylococcus cohnii*, *Staphylococcus pettenkoferi*, and *Staphylococcus warneri*.

*S lugdunensis* has been recognized for its propensity to cause severe infections of skin and soft tissue in the absence of underlying risk factors, particularly in the perineal and gluteal areas. *S lugdunensis* endocarditis has a predilection for native valves and may result in a fulminant course similar to that of *S aureus*. Identification in the laboratory may be difficult because *S lugdunensis* may produce clumping factor, a heat-stable DNAse easily misidentified as coagulase on initial slide screening tests for *S aureus*.

### CLINICAL MANIFESTATIONS

#### Device-Related Infections

CoNS are the leading causes of medical device–related infections due to their ability to colonize foreign bodies and form biofilms. *S epidermidis* has been associated with approximately 34% of catheter-associated bloodstream infections and approximately 40% of the cases of bacterial peritonitis in patients undergoing continuous ambulatory peritoneal dialysis. Hemodialysis catheters and ventriculoperitoneal shunt catheters frequently fall victim to CoNS and to *S epidermidis* in particular. *S lugdunensis* may be an emerging cause of a variety of these infections. Contamination of the device with resident commensal organisms at the time of insertion may play a principal role in risk for subsequent infection. Breaks in sterile technique while manipulating the device may serve to introduce colonizing organisms at a time remote from insertion. The biologic characteristics of these organisms and their ability to escape immune surveillance facilitate prolonged smoldering shunt infections that may manifest only as intermittent device malfunctions. A high index of suspicion is required to make the appropriate diagnosis, as up to half of patients with CoNS shunt infections do not display overt signs of central nervous system inflammation.

#### Bacteremia

Determining whether a positive blood culture for CoNS in the presence of a catheter equates with disease can be problematic when only a single blood culture is obtained. Obtaining multiple blood cultures from different sites, including a percutaneous blood culture, can be useful in differentiating true infection from either contamination or catheter colonization without concomitant bloodstream infection. CoNS are a major cause of bacteremia in children receiving chemotherapy for malignancies as well as infants in the neonatal intensive care unit, especially very-low-birth-weight infants. CoNS are more recently recognized as causes of native-valve endocarditis in normal as well as compromised hosts. Risks for infection due to CoNS include the presence of intravascular devices, loss of integrity of skin or mucosal barriers, parenteral nutrition (specifically intravenous lipid), and use of immunosuppressive drugs. These trends may change as quality improvement initiatives focus efforts on preventing infections related to central venous line insertion and line care. To the extent that skin and mucosal colonization serves as the portal of entry for bacteremia, however, CoNS infections will continue to plague intravascular catheter use.

#### Urinary Tract Infections

*S saprophyticus* is the second most common cause of uncomplicated urinary tract infections (UTIs) in adolescent females and young women, although it is the cause in only 0.3% to 3% of UTIs in all ages. *S saprophyticus* is most often detected in the presence of a symptomatic UTI; however, asymptomatic carriage may occur in a small number of healthy women. Urethral trauma associated with intercourse is speculated to be a significant risk factor preceding infection in some cases. Diagnosis requires recognition that colony counts may be falsely low ($< 10^5$ colony-forming units (cfu)/mL) because of the bacteria's clumping factor. Other CoNS may be implicated in catheter-associated UTIs and should prompt catheter removal.

### TREATMENT

Virtually all *S epidermidis* produce β-lactamase, and more than 80% of *S epidermidis* isolates are methicillin-resistant. Until speciation and formal susceptibility testing are available, vancomycin is the drug of choice for invasive CoNS infections. Central nervous system/shunt infections require higher dosing of vancomycin to achieve adequate concentrations in the cerebrospinal fluid. The addition of gentamicin or rifampin to vancomycin should be considered for severe infections. Nearly all CoNS will be susceptible to linezolid, and about half will be susceptible to clindamycin, trimethoprim/sulfamethoxazole, and gentamicin; fewer will be susceptible to macrolides. Unlike other CoNS, *S lugdunensis* is generally susceptible to penicillins and cephalosporins with only about 20% producing β-lactamase. Since β-lactams generally exhibit superior efficacy when compared to vancomycin, use of a penicillin or a cephalosporin would be preferred to treat *S lugdunensis* if it is β-lactamase–negative. *S saprophyticus* is generally susceptible to ampicillin, cephalosporins, trimethoprim/sulfamethoxazole, and ciprofloxacin, among others drugs commonly used to treat UTIs.

## STAPHYLOCOCCUS AUREUS

### PATHOGENESIS AND EPIDEMIOLOGY

*S aureus* colonization and infections begin with bacterial adherence to host tissues. Surface-expressed proteins, such as clumping factor B and wall-associated teichoic acid, are mediators of adhesion and attachment to nasal epithelial cells. After establishing colonization, evidence suggests that virulence genes are downregulated until exposure of the bacteria to host tissues beyond the mucosal surface or skin occurs. The triggers activating virulence genes to initiate infection, however, remain unknown.

Once beyond the mucosal and skin barrier, surface and secreted molecules aid in the ability of *S aureus* to evade innate immune defenses to survive in the extracellular space. These molecules are present in varying combinations among *S aureus* populations. The secreted hemolysins (α, β, δ, γ) as well as phospholipase C and hyaluronidase enhance spreading and tissue invasion by *S aureus*. Protein A on the surface of *S aureus* binds to the Fc portion of IgG in a nonphysiologic manner inhibiting phagocytosis. The polysaccharide capsule along with expression of clumping factor A and complement inhibitors further help *S aureus* avoid opsonophagocytosis. *S aureus* secretes a chemotaxis inhibitor protein that functions in concert with the extracellular adherence protein to inhibit neutrophil recruitment to the site of infection. Reactive oxygen and nitrogen species produced by neutrophils are inactivated by the antioxidant enzymes catalase and superoxide dismutase. Extracellular serine proteases cleave and inactivate IgG and neutrophil defensins. Panton-Valentine leukocidin (PVL), a pore-forming toxin expressed in less than 5% of *S aureus* isolates, acts mainly on neutrophils and is associated with skin and soft tissue infections as well as necrotizing disease.

The mechanisms by which *S aureus* evades adaptive immune defense and infects the human host repeatedly throughout life are not as well understood. Protein A has been shown to deplete B-cell precursors. Toxic shock syndrome toxin-1 (TSST-1) and enterotoxins A, B, C1-3, D, E, G, and H act as superantigens to suppress B cells and induce both T-cell proliferation as well as cytokine and tumor necrosis factor release. These exotoxins may also alter T-cell function by targeting the T-cell receptor activation pathway.

The severity and extent of invasion by *S aureus* are dependent on the complex interplay between host defenses and virulence factors of the bacteria. Infections may be mild and self-limited or severe and life-threatening, especially in individuals with underlying risk factors. Carriage is an important risk factor for the development of infection in patients undergoing selected surgeries, hemodialysis, or peritoneal dialysis, as well as those with indwelling catheters, underlying conditions such as diabetes, immune deficiencies, or intravenous drug use. *S aureus* is also responsible for an array of toxin-mediated diseases that may be either mild or potentially life-threatening, as in toxic shock syndrome in otherwise healthy individuals.

Like CoNS, the pathogenesis of *S aureus* is aided by the ability to form biofilms through the covalent binding of staphylococcal cell wall–anchored adhesins to human matrix proteins coating medical device surfaces. Several of the staphylococcal adhesins have disease-specific associations: fibronectin-binding protein A participates in endothelial invasion, clumping factors A and B are important in endocarditis, and sialoprotein-binding protein is associated with bone and joint infections. Unlike CoNS, biofilm-associated infections due to *S aureus* have the propensity to disseminate widely and require device removal for optimal management. Failure to remove a device may result in recrudescent disease once treatment with antibiotics stops.

Initially susceptible to penicillin following its discovery in 1928, *S aureus* quickly developed resistance due to acquisition of β-lactamase–producing genes. Methicillin, the first semisynthetic antistaphylococcal penicillin, was first used clinically in 1959 with methicillin resistance noted by 1961. Resistance to methicillin is conveyed by an altered penicillin-binding protein 2a encoded by a chromosomal *mecA* gene. This gene also confers cross-resistance to other β-lactam antibiotics, including most currently available cephalosporins. The *mecA* gene is carried within the mobile staphylococcal cassette chromosome *mecA* (SCC*mecA*). Identification of resistance in clinical laboratories today currently uses oxacillin instead of methicillin; however, the older name, methicillin-resistant *S aureus* (MRSA), has continued in common usage.

Prior to the 1990s, most MRSA were associated with healthcare exposure. These strains carried SCC*mec* types I to III that also conferred resistance to multiple other classes of antibiotics. Beginning in the 1990s, however, MRSA infections began emerging in individuals without previous healthcare exposure via strains carrying a novel SCC*mec* type IV. This SCC*mec* element is smaller than the previous healthcare-associated elements and carries fewer resistance genes but is more likely to encode for PVL. The predominant community-associated MRSA strain identified by pulse-field gel electrophoresis currently circulating in the United States, USA300, nearly always carries genes for PVL. USA300 has emerged in otherwise healthy individuals as a cause of recurrent skin and soft tissue infections as well as severe invasive diseases such as necrotizing pneumonia, necrotizing fasciitis, and osteoarticular disease associated with deep vein thromboses.

Initially susceptible to most antibiotics except β-lactams, increasing resistance to tetracyclines, fluoroquinolones, and clindamycin has emerged as the USA300 epidemic has progressed. Vancomycin has been the mainstay of treatment for severe MRSA infections in pediatrics, but resistance to this agent has emerged as well. Mutations involving the *vraSR* and *graSR* genes have been associated with conversion to vancomycin intermediate-resistant *S aureus* (VISA). First identified in 2002, strains of vancomycin-resistant *S aureus* (VRSA) have been found to carry the *vanA* gene acquired from vancomycin-resistant *Enterococcus*. The principal site for *S aureus* colonization is the nares, although the pharynx, axillae, vagina, and damaged skin are also important reservoirs. Nasal carriage may be persistent (~20%), intermittent (~60%), or absent (~20%) with prevalence as high as 85% in high-risk populations. Individuals who are intermittently colonized may be recolonized with the same strain or different strains.

MRSA emerged as a cause of serious healthcare-associated infections in the 1970s and now accounts for greater than 50% of the *S aureus* isolates in US hospitals. In the late 1990s, community-associated MRSA emerged as a cause of severe infections in individuals without underlying risk factors. The clinical and microbiologic characteristics of the initial community-associated strains demonstrated distinct differences from healthcare-acquired MRSA strains. As the reservoirs merge over time, however, the differences between community and healthcare association are fading. Prevalence of MRSA colonization is 1.5% to 3%, much less than that of methicillin-susceptible *S aureus* (MSSA); however, individuals colonized with MRSA are up to 10 times more likely to experience an infection than those colonized with MSSA.

### CLINICAL MANIFESTATIONS

#### Skin and Soft Tissue Infection

Staphylococcal impetigo may appear as erythematous-crusted papules and pustules, often at the site of minor trauma such as an insect bite, and may be indistinguishable from infection caused by pyogenic streptococci. Bullous impetigo is more classically staphylococcal in origin and appears as flaccid coalescent pustules and bullae on previously undamaged skin. Cleavage of the skin in bullous impetigo occurs at a very superficial layer mediated by the local production of enterotoxins A and B and does not result in scarring, unlike infections involving deeper skin layers. Furuncles occur when focal infection involves the hair follicle and surrounding tissues; carbuncles occur when multiple furuncles coalesce. Recurrent infections and soft tissue abscesses are commonly associated with MRSA and result in frequent emergency room visits. The increasing prevalence of MRSA has been associated with an increase in deep soft tissue infections such as myositis, pyomyositis, necrotizing fasciitis, and thrombophlebitis.

Recurrent *S aureus* skin and soft tissue infections are a common clinical syndrome. While the majority are not associated with primary immune deficiencies, recurrent staphylococcal infections in early childhood may be the presenting feature for patients with neutrophil dysfunction such as chronic granulomatous disease. Other rare primary immune deficiencies associated with recurrent superficial *S aureus* infections include hyper-IgE syndrome, leukocyte adhesion molecule deficiency, Wiskott-Aldrich syndrome, and severe congenital neutropenia.

#### Bacteremia

*S aureus* bacteremia may occur as a primary event in a normal host or may be in association with an underlying medical condition such as an immune deficiency, indwelling medical device, wound infection, diabetes, or intravenous drug use. Bacteremia without a source should raise suspicion for an undiagnosed occult deep site infection, including osteoarticular or endovascular infection. *S aureus* is responsible for 20% of neonatal intensive care unit bacteremias, which are usually catheter-associated and can be frequently complicated by metastatic foci. Up to 40% of catheter-related *S aureus* bacteremias in cancer patients are associated with systemic or metastatic complications. Septic shock, disseminated intravascular coagulation, septic thromboses, osteoarticular infections, endocarditis, meningitis, acute respiratory distress syndrome, and death may complicate *S aureus* bacteremia even in previously healthy hosts. In bacteremia where an intravascular catheter is implicated, it is important to remove the device. Failure to remove a catheter that is associated with *S aureus* bacteremia increases the risk of metastatic complications. Rapidly positive blood cultures for *S aureus* likely reflect increased bacterial loads that are associated with prolonged bacteremia, an endovascular source, increased risk for distant complications (metastatic infections), and increased mortality. *S aureus* bacteremia occurring on multiple successive days is associated with poor outcomes. Metastatic seeding of secondary sites may occur in as many as half of all patients, and recognition of the distant site may be delayed.

#### Bone and Joint Infections

*S aureus* is the most common cause of osteomyelitis in children. Hematogenous seeding of the metaphysis of long bones, often with a history of antecedent minor trauma, is typical. Bacteremia may present in up to 50% of cases. MRSA strains appear to be associated with the development of deep venous thrombosis in association with osteomyelitis, from which septic emboli may rapidly develop. Radiographic evidence of periosteal reaction or bone lucencies may not be apparent until well into the second week of infection. Magnetic resonance imaging of focal physical findings may facilitate early aspirate and biopsy for culture confirmation in nonbacteremic patients.

*S aureus* is also the most common cause of pyogenic arthritis in children and the most common cause of nongonococcal arthritis in adolescents and adults. Staphylococcal arthritis may occur as an extension of intracapsular metaphyseal bone infection (eg, at the elbow, shoulder, or hip) or may occur as an independent complication of staphylococcal bacteremia. Risk factors also include penetrating and nonpenetrating trauma, rheumatoid arthritis, diabetes, and other chronic debilitating diseases, and immunosuppression. Presentation is usually acute. Adequate drainage of the joint, either open or closed, is essential to minimize joint destruction. Removal of any prosthetic material is usually required.

#### Lower Respiratory Tract Infections

*S aureus* can cause rapidly progressive necrotizing pneumonia. Enhanced inflammatory responses and extensive tissue destruction have been associated with PVL-expressing strains of *S aureus,* dominated by the USA300 strain. The presence of pneumatoceles on a chest radiograph is strongly suggestive of staphylococcal disease. Pleural effusions and empyema accompany most cases and should be promptly drained.

#### Endocarditis

*S aureus* is a leading cause of infective endocarditis (IE). The prevalence of IE among pediatric patients with *S aureus* bacteremia may be as high as 12% in at-risk populations. The risk of acquiring IE is highest among patients with valvular heart disease (eg, rheumatic valves, bicuspid aortic valves), congenital heart disease (eg, coarctation, patent ductus arteriosus, ventricular septal defect), and prosthetic cardiac valves and among intravenous drug abusers. Infective endocarditis that develops in association with a chronic catheter is associated with greater long-term mortality. Bacteremia in association with *S aureus* IE may be sustained (≥ 7 days) even with appropriate antibiotics. Septic emboli are common and may be peripheral or central. Neurologic sequelae are common with mitral and prosthetic valve involvement. Cardiac complications are especially common with aortic valvular involvement and include valvular destruction, myocardial abscess and fistula formation, and development of conduction abnormalities. Hematogenous dissemination to any tissue may occur.

#### Central Nervous System Infections

*S aureus* central nervous system infections are associated with neurosurgical procedures, penetrating trauma, foreign bodies, direct extension from a contiguous site, and hematogenous dissemination from a distant site. Shunt infections, meningitis, brain abscesses, subdural empyema, and epidural abscesses may occur. Primary staphylococcal infection of the central nervous system is rare. Cyanotic congenital heart disease with right-to-left shunting poses a significant risk for brain abscess due to staphylococci as well as other organisms. Because the earliest symptoms in young children are nonspecific, the diagnosis of epidural abscess is often delayed until signs of cord compression are present.

#### Surgical Wound and Foreign Body Infections

The risk of *S aureus* wound infection following surgery increases in the presence of underlying chronic disease, immunodeficiency, and the presence of a foreign body. Local and systemic complications include wound dehiscence, tissue abscesses, septic thrombophlebitis, bacteremia, sepsis, and metastatic infections. Primary treatment of surgical wounds is debridement. Foreign bodies involved with staphylococcal infections generally must be removed; antibiotics are adjunctive.

*S aureus* is a major cause of morbidity and mortality in hemodialysis patients. Local infection at the access site may progress to abscess formation and be complicated by bacteremic disease. *S aureus* is a leading cause of exit- and tunnel-site infections in patients on chronic peritoneal dialysis as well. Nasal carriage of *S aureus* appears to be a major risk factor for subsequent infections in each of these patient groups. *S aureus* is second to CoNS as a causative agent in intravascular device–related infections in other settings.

#### Toxin-Mediated Syndromes

The most common clinical syndromes associated with extracellular toxins produced by *S aureus* are toxic shock syndrome (TSS), staphylococcal scalded skin syndrome, and staphylococcal foodborne disease.

TSS results from infection or colonization with a strain of *S aureus* that produces TSST-1, which acts as a superantigen to activate T cells at orders of magnitude above antigen-specific activation and results in massive cytokine release. Enterotoxins B and C are structurally very similar to TSST-1 and may be responsible for TSS in the absence of TSST-1. Although first described in young women in association with tampon use (menstrual TSS), TSS of nonmenstrual origin now accounts for more than half of all cases. Unlike streptococcal TSS, staphylococcal TSS is not commonly associated with bacteremia. Any infection with a toxin-producing strain may pose a risk. Symptoms of TSS include fever, headache, chills, vomiting, diarrhea, sore throat, and myalgias. Hypotension, capillary leak syndrome, and respiratory distress may ensue. Diffuse erythroderma resembling sunburn is often described during the course of illness, and desquamation may be a late finding. TSS must be differentiated from septic shock, streptococcal toxic shock, scarlet fever, meningococcemia, Rocky Mountain spotted fever, Kawasaki syndrome, severe drug reactions, leptospirosis, and measles. Early intensive supportive care is essential in the care of TSS. Although mucosal colonization alone can serve as the nidus for toxin production, any identified focus of infection should be drained and treated. Clindamycin is often recommended because of its ability to inhibit protein synthesis, but should not be used alone to treat infections in critically ill patients unless susceptibility data are known.

Staphylococcal scalded skin syndrome, often referred to as Ritter syndrome in young infants, is a blistering dermatitis mediated by exfoliative toxins enterotoxin A and B. Widespread hematogenous dissemination of the toxin produces fever and tender erythema that may rapidly progress to bullae formation. Minimal friction applied to the skin results in sloughing of the superficial layers of skin (Nikolsky sign). Bacteremia may or may not be present. Protection may be afforded to older children by naturally occurring antitoxin antibodies present in up to 50% of 10-year-olds. Thus, a less-severe syndrome resembling streptococcal "scarlet fever" may be seen in older children where sloughing is generally absent, but superficial desquamation is often seen in the convalescent phase.

Staphylococcal foodborne disease is the most common cause of food poisoning in the United States. Foods are contaminated by toxin-producing strains of *S aureus* during preparation and then maintained at a temperature suitable for toxin elaboration prior to ingestion by unsuspecting individuals. The incubation period for staphylococcal foodborne disease is short, usually less than 4 hours; nausea, vomiting, and abdominal cramps follow. Fever and headache may occasionally be present. In most individuals, staphylococcal foodborne disease is self-limited, although severe dehydration and prostration and even death may be seen in a few individuals. Specific antistaphylococcal treatment is not indicated.

## TREATMENT

The emerging problem of antibiotic resistance has complicated the treatment of *S aureus* infections. Clinicians should be familiar with local antibiograms and take into consideration the prevalence of MRSA within the community as well as the potential consequences of treatment failure when planning therapy for suspected *S aureus* infections. Cultures should be obtained whenever possible to guide therapy. When faced with a severely ill patient in whom *S aureus* infection is suspected, treatment to cover methicillin-resistant strains should be initiated until culture results and susceptibility data are available.

Local skin care and cleansing may no longer be sufficient therapy for minor superficial infections. Topical mupirocin is a useful adjunctive antibacterial therapy for well-circumscribed impetigo, although mupirocin resistance is increasing. Evaluation for potential bacteremia and treatment with systemic antistaphylococcal therapy should be considered for the neonate with bullous impetigo, especially when the prevalence of MRSA is high or when nursery outbreaks have been reported.

Cellulitis without abscess may be due to either streptococci or staphylococci; therefore, empirical antibiotic therapy for cellulitis should be effective against both. In areas of low MRSA prevalence, antibiotics such as cephalexin, amoxicillin plus clavulanate, or dicloxacillin may be effective. Soft tissue abscesses have emerged as a common presentation for MRSA. Lesions should be incised and the drainage sent for culture. In many circumstances, drainage and wound care will be sufficient for these lesions. However, antibiotics should be considered for more severe local disease or when disease has progressed in spite of incision and drainage.

Clindamycin, doxycycline or minocycline (if over 8 years of age), and trimethoprim-sulfamethoxazole (TMP/SMX) provide coverage for many MRSA cases. Because of widespread resistance, the macrolides may not provide optimal management for MSSA or MRSA infections. *S aureus* isolates that appear erythromycin-resistant and clindamycin-susceptible by routine in vitro susceptibility testing may exhibit resistance to clindamycin during therapy ("inducible resistance"), resulting in therapeutic failures. The D-test is used in clinical laboratories to detect this phenomenon; D-test–positive strains are considered clindamycin-resistant. Linezolid, an oxazolidinone class antibiotic that is bacteriostatic for *S aureus*, has been useful for the management of skin and soft tissue infections resulting from MRSA. Linezolid is virtually 100% bioavailable following oral administration. Fluoroquinolones are not optimal for *S aureus* because resistance develops rapidly. Vancomycin is the drug of choice for the treatment of severe or limb-threatening infections in pediatrics when MRSA is a possibility. However, because β-lactam agents exhibit superior antistaphylococcal activity over vancomycin, they should be used in susceptible organisms. MRSA strains with a vancomycin minimal inhibitory concentration (MIC) of 2 μg/mL or greater may exhibit prolonged bacteremia in spite of high serum vancomycin concentrations.

Newly developed antibiotics against resistant gram-positive organisms offer expanded treatment options for invasive MRSA infections for patients who cannot tolerate or clinically fail vancomycin therapy; however, experience in pediatrics is limited and these drugs are not US Food and Drug Administration-approved for use in children < 18 years of age. Daptomycin, a novel bactericidal lipopeptide, has been approved in adults to treat complicated skin and soft tissue infections and bloodstream infections. Available in a once-daily intravenous formulation, the rapid bactericidal activity of daptomycin makes it attractive for treatment of MRSA endocarditis or endovascular disease. Daptomycin is inhibited by pulmonary surfactant and thus is not indicated for treatment of pneumonia. Ceftaroline, a new broad-spectrum cephalosporin, is approved for use in adults for complicated skin and soft tissue infections and community-acquired pneumonia. Other recently approved antibiotics in adults include oritavancin, dalbavancin, and tedizolid (approved for bacterial skin and soft tissue infections). Ceftobiprole, a broad-spectrum cephalosporin with MRSA activity, is approved in Europe for treatment of pneumonia and bacterial skin and soft tissue infections.

Duration of therapy is dependent on the nature of the infection. For limited skin and soft tissue infections, oral therapy for 5 to 7 days is usually sufficient. Initial treatment with a parenteral agent should be considered in patients suspected of having a more serious disease. For moderate to severe soft tissue infections such as pyomyositis, 10 to 14 days of antibiotics are recommended with evidence of appropriate clinical response. Treatment of catheter-associated bacteremia should last at least 14 days. Septic arthritis should be treated for at least 3 weeks and acute osteomyelitis should be treated for 4 to 6 weeks based on resolution of inflammation. In general, staphylococcal endocarditis should be treated for at least 6 weeks with a bactericidal agent. Combination therapy with an aminoglycoside (gentamicin) is sometimes advocated for severe endovascular infections; data supporting the addition of gentamicin for more than 3 to 5 days are lacking. Combination therapy with rifampin is sometimes advocated for treatment of device-related infections due to its ability to penetrate biofilms. Adjunctive therapy with rifampin has been associated with poor outcomes for staphylococcal bacteremia and IE and thus is not recommended unless complicated by involvement of bone, joint, or cerebrospinal fluid where enhanced penetration may be beneficial. Involvement of an infectious disease specialist is recommended.

## PREVENTION

There are limited data to support the routine attempt to eradicate staphylococcal colonization. However, eradication of the carrier state may be desirable in certain patients at high risk (such as patients in the pediatric or neonatal intensive care unit), in patients with a history of repeated staphylococcal infections, or in order to terminate outbreaks in a healthcare setting. Regimens are not standardized. Decolonization strategies have been employed including topical 2% mupirocin applied to the nasal vestibules alone or in combination with antiseptic baths, hand sanitizing, hot-water laundering, and the daily sanitizing of razors and other personal items. Dialysis patients may receive some benefit, although mupirocin resistance emerges with prolonged use. A 5- to 7-day regimen of nasal mupirocin in combination with daily bathing using a 2% chlorhexidine gluconate solution has been advocated as a preoperative regimen to reduce postoperative infections. A similar strategy combined with either oral rifampin or doxycycline has been used to reduce transmission and to decrease infections in a hospital outbreak setting. Repeated or prolonged use of either mupirocin or systemic antibiotics is discouraged because of the likely emergence of resistance. In general, prevention strategies that focus on good personal hygiene should be advocated first.

Becker K, Heilmann C, Peters G. Coagulase-negative staphylococci. *Clin Microbiol Rev*. 2014;27:870-926.

Gostelow M, Gonzalez D, Smith PB, Cohen-Wolkowiez M. Pharmacokinetics and safety of recently approved drugs used to treat methicillin-resistant *Staphylococcus aureus* infections in infants, children, and adults. *Expert Rev Clin Pharmacol*. 2014;7:327-340.

Liu C, Bayer A, Cosgrove S, et al. Clinical practice guidelines by the Infectious Diseases Society of America for the treatment of methicillin-resistant *Staphylococcus aureus* infections in adults and children. *Clin Infect Dis*. 2011;52:1-38.

Moellering RC. MRSA: the first half century. *J Antimicrob Chemother*. 2012;67:4-11.

Rodvold KA, McConeghy KW. Methicillin-resistant *Staphylococcus aureus* therapy: past, present, and future. *Clin Infect Dis*. 2014;58:S20-S27.

Septimus EJ, Schweizer ML. Decolonization in prevention of health care-associated infections. *Clin Microbiol Rev*. 2016;29:201-222.

Shallcross LJ, Fragaszy E, Johnson AM, Hayward AC. The role of the Panton-Valentine leucocidin toxin in staphylococcal disease: a systematic review and meta-analysis. *Lancet Infect Dis*. 2013;13:43-54.

# 280 Streptococcus Group A Infections

Mark R. Schleiss

## INTRODUCTION

Descriptions of what were likely *Streptococcus pyogenes* infections are found in the earliest written records of human history. *S pyogenes* was likely responsible for the apparent scarlet fever epidemic described by Hippocrates in the 5th century BC. The first modern description of streptococcal infection was the demonstration of the organism in patients with erysipelas and wound infection in 1874. The organism was designated *Streptococcus pyogenes* by Rosenbach in the late 19th century. In the early 1930s, Rebecca Lancefield's classification of the β-hemolytic strains into characteristic distinct serogroups led to the recognition that serogroup A isolates (*S pyogenes*) were the strains most commonly responsible for pharyngitis and impetigo/pyoderma. *S pyogenes* is one of the most important infectious agents encountered in clinical practice causing infections of the upper respiratory tract and skin. *S pyogenes* also causes a variety of severe systemic infections, including toxic shock syndrome and life-threatening skin and soft tissue infections. Infection with this pathogen is also causally linked to 2 serious nonsuppurative complications, acute rheumatic fever and acute glomerulonephritis.

## PATHOGENESIS AND EPIDEMIOLOGY

Streptococci are gram-positive cocci that tend to grow as pairs and chains. When cultured on sheep or horse blood agar plates, a characteristic zone of complete hemolysis (β-hemolysis) is observed. *S pyogenes* (group A streptococci) may be identified either by serologic means or latex agglutination techniques. Additional typing of group A streptococci for epidemiologic purposes is based on variation in the M and T proteins and *emm* genes (see below). The somatic cellular constituents as well as the extracellular enzymes and toxins responsible of *S pyogenes* are responsible for many of pathogenic effects observed in vivo. These also are summarized in Table 280-1. The major virulence factor of the organism is the M protein. This protein is anchored to the cell membrane and transverses and penetrates the cell wall. Functionally, the M proteins inhibit phagocytosis, which is a primary virulence mechanism for survival in tissues. Immunity to M protein appears to be a key determinant in protection against infection. In the nonimmune host, M protein mediates its antiphagocytic effect by inhibiting activation of the alternate complement pathway. Genes related to the M protein gene (*emm*) are called the M gene superfamily and include immunoglobulin-binding proteins. Other streptococcal cell wall antigens are important in the pathogenesis and epidemiologic typing of *S pyogenes*. Most strains are enveloped in a hyaluronic acid capsule that serves as an accessory virulence factor by inhibiting phagocytosis. Lipoteichoic acid and protein F are cell wall constituents that play roles in the adherence of *S pyogenes* to fibronectin on the surface of human epithelial cells, an important event in the initiation of the infectious process. Serum opacity factor (OF) is a lipoproteinase associated with M protein that is useful in classifying strains that are not identifiable by M typing.

**TABLE 280-1 SUMMARY OF THE MOLECULAR DETERMINANTS RESPONSIBLE FOR *STREPTOCOCCUS PYOGENES* PATHOGENICITY**

| |
|---|
| **Intrinsic (Somatic) Constituents** |
| M protein |
| Hyaluronic acid |
| Lipoteichoic acid |
| Protein F |
| Serum opacity factor |
| T protein |
| Envelope protease (SpyCEP) |
| **Extracellular Proteins** |
| Pyogenic exotoxins (SPEs) |
| Streptolysin O |
| Streptolysin S |
| Extracellular DNAases |
| Hyaluronidase |
| Streptokinase |
| NADase |

Group A streptococci also produce a large variety of extracellular enzymes and toxins. The family of streptococcal pyogenic exotoxins (SPE) includes SPEs A, B, C, and F. These toxins are responsible for the rash of scarlet fever. They also produce other pathogenic effects, including pyrogenicity, cytotoxicity, and enhancement of susceptibility to endotoxin. Streptococcal pyogenic exotoxin B is a precursor for a cysteine protease that functions as a virulence factor. Isolates associated with streptococcal toxic shock syndrome encode certain SPEs (A, C, and F) functioning as superantigens. These antigens induce a marked febrile response, induce proliferation of T lymphocytes, and induce synthesis and release of multiple cytokines, including tumor necrosis factor, interleukin-1β, and interleukin-6. *S pyogenes* elaborates 2 extracellular hemolysins, streptolysin O and streptolysin S. Streptolysin O is toxic to eukaryotic cells, including myocytes. Streptolysin S is capable of damaging polymorphonuclear leukocytes and subcellular organelles. *S pyogenes* cell envelope serine protease (SpyCEP) functions to degrade and inactivate the chemoattractant interleukin-8 (IL-8), impairing host neutrophil recruitment. Other extracellular products elaborated by *S pyogenes* include deoxyribonucleases (DNAses A–D), hyaluronidase, and streptokinase.

*S pyogenes* is highly communicable. Respiratory droplet spread is the major route for transmission of strains associated with upper respiratory tract infection, although skin-to-skin spread is known to occur with strains associated with pyoderma. Foodborne outbreaks are not rare and often are associated with egg-containing foods. Although uncommon, nursery outbreaks of group A streptococcal infections have been reported. The incidence of pharyngeal infection with group A streptococci is highest in children age 5 to 15 years. Indeed, group A streptococcal pharyngitis has been described as an "occupational disease" of school-aged children. *S pyogenes* also has the potential to produce outbreaks of disease in younger children in group daycare. In temperate zones, pharyngeal infection is most common during late autumn, winter, and early spring. Group A streptococcal skin infections occur most frequently during the summer in temperate climates but can occur year-round in warmer climates.

## CLINICAL MANIFESTATIONS

### Streptococcal Pharyngitis

Acute pharyngitis represents one of the most common reasons children are seen by primary care physicians. Yet, despite the common nature of the infection, the optimal diagnostic and therapeutic approaches to the child with pharyngitis or tonsillitis remain sources of uncertainty. In general, decisions about laboratory testing and antibiotic therapy should be made only after careful consideration of clinical findings and epidemiologic considerations. The most important historical information in the evaluation of the complaint of sore throat is that of the presence or absence of other symptoms of upper respiratory infection. Children with bona fide streptococcal pharyngitis rarely, if ever, have cough, rhinorrhea, or symptoms of a viral upper respiratory infection (URI), and the diagnosis of streptococcal pharyngitis can almost always be excluded with the clinical findings of coryza, hoarseness, cough, or conjunctivitis. Identification of a positive throat swab in a child with a viral URI may reflect the asymptomatic carrier state, and antibiotics to eliminate carriage are not generally warranted. Although the findings of cough and coryza are important exclusionary criteria, the pediatrician must be aware that the signs and symptoms of streptococcal pharyngitis may also be nonspecific and vary greatly depending on the age of the patient, the severity of the infection, or the seasonal timing of the illness. Young infants may not present with classic signs and symptoms of pharyngitis. Streptococcal upper respiratory tract infections in infants and toddlers may instead be characterized by low-grade fever, anorexia, and a serous nasal discharge (so-called streptococcosis). Conversely, some patients with acute streptococcal pharyngitis may present with a toxic appearance, manifesting high fever, malaise, headache, and severe pain on swallowing. Vomiting and abdominal pain may be prominent early symptoms, simulating gastroenteritis or even acute appendicitis.

On physical examination, children with group A streptococcal pharyngitis classically demonstrate tonsillopharyngeal erythema, a red edematous uvula, palatal petechiae, and tender anterior cervical adenitis. Typically, tonsils are enlarged and erythematous with patchy exudate on the surface. The papillae of the tongue may be red and swollen (so-called strawberry tongue). Cutaneous petechiae have even been noted, and a scarlatiniform rash may be present. When the characteristic rash of scarlet fever is present, a clinical diagnosis can be made with increased confidence. However, it is difficult to consistently make the diagnosis of streptococcal pharyngitis on clinical grounds alone. Therefore, even the most experienced clinician should consider bacteriologic confirmation of the diagnosis whenever possible. Obtaining appropriate diagnostic testing for group A streptococcal pharyngitis before therapy is instituted may prevent unnecessary antibiotic prescriptions for viral pharyngitis.

If performed correctly, a throat swab cultured on a blood agar plate has a sensitivity of 90% to 95% in detecting the presence of *S pyogenes* in the pharynx. The specimen should be obtained from the surface of both tonsils/tonsillar fossae and from the posterior pharyngeal wall. Concern has been expressed regarding the delay of 24 to 48 hours required for bacteriologic culture, and clinicians often feel pressure to initiate therapy immediately, prior to obtaining culture results. Since treatment of streptococcal sore throat as long as 9 days after onset of symptoms is still effective in preventing rheumatic fever, initiation of antibiotics is rarely of urgent importance. Early antibiotic therapy may have beneficial effects in relieving symptoms and allowing an earlier return to school or daycare, but may have disadvantages. Some studies suggest that children receiving immediate antibiotic therapy are more likely to have symptomatic recurrences in the months following treatment than are children who delay the initiation of therapy by 48 hours. Delaying antibiotics may allow for an immune response to occur that protects the child against reinfection. These questions continue to be sources of uncertainty in the management of streptococcal pharyngitis.

When the diagnosis of streptococcal pharyngitis seems particularly likely based on clinical findings or when an immediate decision about antibiotic therapy is required, the use of rapid antigen detection tests can be of value in confirming the diagnosis. Current guidelines recommend confirmation of group A streptococcal pharyngitis in children with a rapid antigen detection test (RADT), with follow-up cultures in RADT-negative cases. A throat culture should be performed for children with negative RADT results, and treatment is indicated when the results of either test are positive. Most rapid antigen detection kits use antibody for detection of the group A carbohydrate antigen in the cell wall. The specificity of these antibody tests is superior to their sensitivity. Currently available rapid streptococcal tests have a sensitivity of 70% to 90% compared with standard throat cultures. The sensitivity may depend on the inoculum obtained in the clinical sample. The sensitivity may be no greater than 75% for colonization (or light growth on culture) to approximately 95% in symptomatic pharyngitis (where culture usually reveals a heavy growth). The recent development of molecular methods may offer alternatives to improve speed and accuracy in the diagnosis of streptococcal pharyngitis. These tests have been shown to have superior sensitivity and specificity to RADT and culture and are being adopted by many clinical laboratories, although a positive result must still be interpreted within the context of a patient's signs and symptoms. When identified by culture, group A *Streptococcus* does not require antibiotic susceptibility testing, since antibiotic resistance to cell wall–active agents has not been described.

### Scarlet Fever

When a fine, diffuse erythematous rash (Fig. 280-1) is present in the setting of acute streptococcal pharyngitis, the illness is known as *scarlet fever*. The modes of streptococcal transmission, age distribution, and other epidemiologic features are identical to those for streptococcal pharyngitis. The rash is induced by the pyrogenic exotoxins SPE A, B, C, and F. It often is noticed initially on the neck and upper chest. It is a diffuse, finely papular, erythematous eruption producing a bright red discoloration of the skin, which blanches on pressure. The texture is that of fine sandpaper. The flexor skin creases, particularly in the antecubital fossae, and the groin area may be unusually prominent (Pastia lines). The circumoral skin is pale, giving the appearance of pallor. Small vesicular lesions (miliary sudamina) may appear on the abdomen, hands, and feet. Toward the end of the first week of illness, the rash fades, followed by desquamation over the trunk that progresses to the hands and feet. Scarlet fever may be confused with roseola, Kawasaki disease, drug eruptions, and toxin-mediated *Staphylococcus aureus* infections.

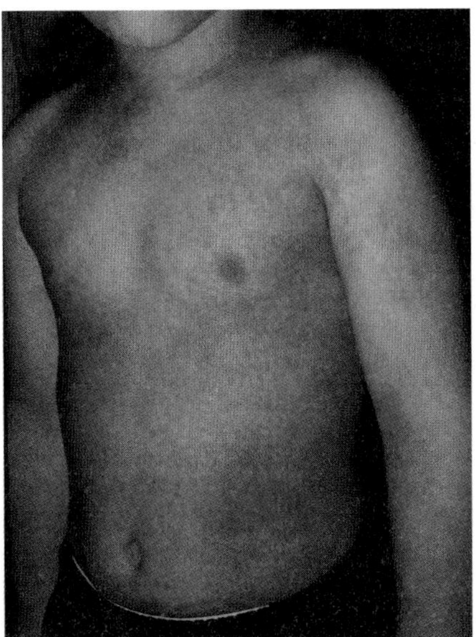

**FIGURE 280-1** Erythematous scarlatiniform rash of scarlet fever. (Reproduced with permission from Knoop KJ, Stack LB, Storrow AB, et al: The Atlas of Emergency Medicine, 3rd ed. New York: McGraw-Hill, 2010. Photo contributor: Lawrence B. Stack, MD.)

### Streptococcal Skin Infections

The most common form of skin infection due to group A *Streptococcus* is superficial pyoderma. Also referred to as streptococcal impetigo (or impetigo contagiosa), it occurs commonly in tropical climates, but can be highly prevalent in temperate climates as well, particularly during the summer months. Major risk factors that predispose to this infection include local injury to skin caused by insect bites, scabies, atopic dermatitis, and minor trauma. This form of streptococcal infection is usually painless, and the patient is usually afebrile. Streptococcal impetigo usually has the highest incidence in young children (ages 2–5 years). Streptococcal impetigo usually appears first as a discrete papulovesicular lesion surrounded by a localized area of redness. The vesicles rapidly become purulent and then crusted, in contrast to the classic bullous appearance of impetigo resulting from *S aureus*. Lesions are most commonly encountered on the face and extremities. If untreated, streptococcal impetigo is usually a mild but chronic illness, often spreading to other parts of the body. Regional lymphadenitis may be observed. Pyoderma-associated group A strains such as M/*emm* 49, M/*emm* 55, and M/*emm* 57 are associated with poststreptococcal glomerulonephritis. The M/*emm* types that give rise to streptococcal tonsillitis (eg, types 1, 3, 4, 5, 6, 12) uncommonly cause streptococcal impetigo.

Deeper soft tissue infections may occur as the result of *S pyogenes*. A deeply ulcerated form of streptococcal impetigo, ecthyma, may complicate streptococcal impetigo. This form of infection tends to involve deeper layers of the skin and is encountered mainly in the tropics. Streptococcal cellulitis is an acute, rapidly spreading infection of skin and subcutaneous tissue that can follow burns, wounds, surgical incisions, varicella infection, and mild trauma. In contrast to impetigo, pain, tenderness, swelling and erythema, and systemic toxicity are common, and patients may have associated bacteremia. Prompt antibiotic therapy and careful serial examination are crucial, as cellulitis may progress to necrotizing fasciitis. Perianal cellulitis and vaginitis should be considered in children who complain of perineal discomfort or vaginal discharge. Erysipelas is now a relatively rare acute streptococcal infection involving the deeper layers of the skin and the underlying connective tissue. The face is a commonly involved site, especially in adults. The skin over the affected area is swollen, red, and very tender, and superficial blebs may be present. The most characteristic finding in erysipelas is the sharply defined, slightly elevated border, in contrast to the indistinct border of streptococcal cellulitis. Cultures obtained by leading edge needle aspiration of inflamed areas will often result in a positive culture.

### Necrotizing Fasciitis

Necrotizing fasciitis resulting from *S pyogenes* (so-called streptococcal gangrene) is an acute, rapidly progressive, severe deep infection of the fascia and subcutaneous tissues and is associated with extensive destruction of superficial and deep fascia. Recent varicella infection has proven to be an important risk factor for necrotizing fasciitis, although routine childhood immunization against chickenpox has substantially reduced this complication. The onset is heralded by diffuse erythematous swelling, followed by development of necrosis. With decreased perfusion and minimal inflammation in the setting of necrotic changes, the patient will exhibit exquisite pain at the affected site that seems incompatible with the degree of swelling noted. This dissociation between the lack of inflammation and the magnitude of pain is an important diagnostic clue. As the lesion progresses, often quite rapidly, the skin becomes bluish gray. It is not uncommon for large hemorrhagic bullae to appear over the area. The area of involvement under the skin is usually much larger than seems evident from the superficial examination of skin. Compartment syndromes often occur. Repeated surgical debridement of necrotic tissue is crucial. Differentiating streptococcal cellulitis from necrotizing fasciitis can be difficult; therefore, careful frequent serial physical examinations are crucial. Surgical consultation early in the course of infection is essential, since debridement of devitalized tissue is required.

### Streptococcal Toxic Shock Syndrome

Streptococcal toxic shock syndrome (TSS) is characterized by hypotension and multiple organ failure. Criteria currently endorsed by the Red Book committee of the American Academy of Pediatrics are outlined in Table 280-2. There is considerable overlap with streptococcal necrotizing fasciitis; most cases occur in association with soft tissue infections. However, streptococcal TSS may occur in association with other focal streptococcal infections, including pharyngeal infection. Renal impairment occurs in approximately 80% of patients, and hepatic dysfunction occurs in 65%. Acute respiratory distress syndrome is often present in severe cases and should be looked for. The pathogenesis of streptococcal toxic shock syndrome appears to be related in part to the ability of certain SPEs (A, C, and F). Most commonly, SPE A is implicated. These toxins function as superantigens capable of stimulating production of inflammatory cytokines, in particular tumor necrosis factor. These inflammatory mediators trigger capillary leak, hypotension, and end-organ damage

**TABLE 280-2 CLINICAL CASE DEFINITION FOR STREPTOCOCCAL TOXIC SHOCK**

I. Isolation of group A *Streptococcus*
- From a sterile site (blood, cerebrospinal fluid, tissue biopsy, peritoneal fluid)
- From a nonsterile body site (throat, sputum, perineum, superficial skin lesion)

II. Clinical signs of severe illness
- Hypotension (systolic blood pressure < 90 mm Hg in adults or < fifth percentile for age in children)

**AND**

Two or more of the following signs:
- Renal impairment (creatinine concentration of 2 mg/dL or 2× upper limit of normal for age)
- Coagulopathy (platelet count ≤ 100,000/μL or presence of disseminated intravascular coagulation)
- Hepatic involvement (elevated alanine aminotransferase, SST, or bilirubin concentration ≥ 2× upper limit for age
- Acute respiratory distress syndrome
- Generalized rash (erythematous, macular; may demonstrate desquamation)
- Soft tissue necrosis (necrotizing fasciitis, myositis, gangrene)

Data from Red Book 2015: 2015 Report of the Committee on Infectious Diseases, 30th ed. Chicago: American Academy of Pediatrics; 2015.

### Other Suppurative Complications

Suppurative complications resulting from the spread of streptococci to adjacent structures are occasionally observed. Cervical adenitis, peritonsillar abscess, retropharyngeal abscess, otitis media, mastoiditis, and sinusitis occur in children in whom the primary illness has gone unnoticed or in whom treatment of the pharyngitis has been incomplete. *S pyogenes* may cause pneumonia, parapneumonic effusion, and epiglottitis. Group A *Streptococcus* is a common etiology of acute hematogenous osteomyelitis. Isolated bacteremia, meningitis, and endocarditis have been described, but these are relatively rare manifestations of group A streptococcal infection.

### Postinfectious Complications Of A Group A Streptococcal Infection

Acute rheumatic fever (ARF) is discussed in detail in Chapter 230. Only 25% to 40% of ARF patients have a positive throat culture at the time of presentation. The most reliable evidence of an antecedent group A streptococcal infection is often identification of a serologic response to the organism.

Glomerulonephritis can follow group A streptococcal infections of either the pharynx or the skin. Its occurrence requires the presence of so-called nephritogenic strains of group A streptococci in the community. Type 12 is one of the most common M/*emm* serotypes causing poststreptococcal glomerulonephritis after pharyngitis, and M/*emm* type 49 is a type commonly related to pyoderma-associated nephritis. The latent period between the group A streptococcal infection and the onset of glomerulonephritis varies from 1 to 2 weeks after streptococcal pharyngitis, but is approximately 21 days after pyoderma. Like ARF, the pathogenesis of poststreptococcal glomerulonephritis appears to be immunologically mediated (see Chapter 468).

Sydenham chorea is the most common cause of acquired chorea in children and occurs most commonly between ages 5 and 15 years. It is a cardinal feature of rheumatic fever and is sufficient alone to make a diagnosis. Sydenham chorea usually occurs several weeks to months after untreated *S pyogenes* infection (see Chapter 558). In 1998, a syndrome known as pediatric autoimmune neuropsychiatric disease associated with streptococci (PANDAS) was described. Patients are usually prepubertal children who develop multiple neuropsychiatric symptoms (tics and obsessive-compulsive behavior), and it was suggested that this was temporally related to group A streptococcal infection. Whether or not this syndrome is related to streptococcal infection remains unconfirmed. There is no evidence from controlled studies to support the efficacy of continuous or suppressive antimicrobial therapy for these children (see Chapter 558).

## TREATMENT

Treatment approaches for group A streptococcal infections vary depending on the clinical syndrome. Worldwide, penicillin remains the most widely used therapy. Remarkably, no penicillin-resistant clinical isolates of *S pyogenes* have ever been encountered. Penicillin therefore remains a drug of choice (except in penicillin-allergic individuals) for pharyngeal infections as well as for complicated or invasive infections. For streptococcal pharyngitis, the oral penicillin of choice is penicillin V. In many clinical trials, a dose of 40 mg/kg/d has been used. In general, 250 mg 2 or 3 times daily is recommended for most children. In young children, amoxicillin has been used because of its better taste (50 mg/kg once daily [maximum = 1000 mg] for 10 days; alternate: 25 mg/kg [maximum = 500 mg] twice daily for 10 days). The most common reason for penicillin failure is noncompliance. When oral treatment is prescribed, the necessity of completing a full course of therapy must be emphasized. Parenteral therapy with benzathine penicillin G is another option. In children weighing more than 27 kg, a dose of 1,200,000 units has been the recommended dose, and in children weighing less than 27 kg, 600,000 units are recommended. Injections with preparations that contain procaine penicillin are less painful. The total dose of penicillin is calculated based on the amount of benzathine penicillin G, as procaine penicillin is rapidly excreted.

Even in compliant patients, recent reports have suggested that penicillin fails to eradicate *S pyogenes* from up to 30% of treated patients. Many theories have been proposed to explain these apparent penicillin failures. The presence of β-lactamase–producing normal flora (particularly mouth anaerobes) has been proposed as a potential mechanism by which penicillin could become inactivated, rendering it ineffective. However, the validity of this theory has never been conclusively demonstrated. It is more likely that many of the "failures" of penicillin therapy occur in patients in whom streptococcal pharyngitis has not been defined rigorously enough. As noted earlier, some of these patients are streptococcal carriers with intercurrent viral pharyngitis.

For penicillin-allergic patients, several alternative treatment options are available. Oral cephalosporins are effective in the treatment of streptococcal pharyngitis and generally are safe to use in the penicillin-allergic patient. First-generation cephalosporins are adequate and are often the least expensive option. Cefdinir has been approved by the US Food and Drug Administration for use in a 5-day treatment course for streptococcal pharyngitis. Erythromycin estolate and erythromycin ethylsuccinate are both effective, although caution must be taken to note local antibiotic resistant rates, as > 5% of isolates of *S pyogenes* may be erythromycin resistant in some regions of the United States, and up to 30% in some European countries. Newer macrolides and azalides such as clarithromycin and azithromycin have similar susceptibility profiles to that of erythromycin. Azithromycin is approved for treatment of streptococcal pharyngitis (pediatric dose of 12 mg/kg on the first day [maximum of 500 mg], followed by 6 mg/kg [maximum of 50 mg] on days 2–5) and may be used in penicillin-allergic patients. Shorter-course regimens of azithromycin have been described but appear to be associated with increased risks of treatment failure. Oral clindamycin (7 mg/kg/dose 3 times daily [maximum = 300 mg/dose] for 10 days) is also an acceptable alternative for treatment of penicillin-allergic patients.

Treatment of the child with recurrent culture-positive pharyngitis can be a difficult clinical management problem. It may be difficult to differentiate a streptococcal carrier from the child with recurrent bona fide streptococcal pharyngitis. Although most streptococcal carriers do not require intervention, there are situations in which eradication of the carrier state is desirable. These include families in which there is inordinate anxiety about streptococci, families in which "ping pong" spread has been occurring, or when tonsillectomy is being considered only because of chronic carriage. A course of clindamycin (20 mg/kg/d in 3 divided doses for 10 days) has been shown to be effective in eradicating the carrier state. Other options for the carrier state include penicillin plus rifampin, amoxicillin/clavulanate, and benzathine penicillin plus oral rifampin.

Antibiotic therapy for a patient with streptococcal impetigo can prevent local extension of the lesions, spread to distant infectious foci, and transmission of the infection, although the ability of antibiotics to prevent poststreptococcal glomerulonephritis has not been clearly demonstrated. Patients with superficial, isolated lesions and no systemic signs can be treated with topical mupirocin. However, if there are widespread lesions or systemic signs, oral therapy with a β-lactamase–stable agent should be used, since mixed infections with *S pyogenes* and *S aureus* are common.

Patients with invasive group A streptococcal infections (eg, necrotizing fasciitis, TSS, sepsis) should typically be treated with intravenous penicillin in combination with clindamycin. The use of an inhibitor of protein synthesis (such as clindamycin) is useful, since in vivo evidence of the lack of efficacy of penicillin in deep tissue infections has been observed in animal models. This effect, first described by Eagle in 1952, appears to be the result of reduced expression of penicillin-binding proteins, the molecular targets of penicillin, in the setting of the high inoculum of organisms encountered in overwhelming infections. Supportive care, including fluids, pressors, and often mechanical ventilation, is also a critical aspect of management of invasive streptococcal skin and soft tissue infections. Prompt and repeated surgical drainage, debridement, or fasciotomy is often indicated. For infections such as osteomyelitis, penicillin is generally the treatment of choice, although clindamycin is an acceptable alternative, particularly for penicillin-allergic patients.

## PREVENTION

Long-term antibiotic prophylaxis to prevent streptococcal infections is recommended for patients with a history of acute rheumatic fever or rheumatic heart disease. The recommended regimen is 3 to 4 weekly injections of 1.2 million IU of intramuscular benzathine penicillin G, 250 mg of oral penicillin V twice a day, or 0.5 to 1 g of sulfadiazine daily. Although no controlled studies have been carried out, 250 mg of erythromycin twice daily has been used in some patients in this category. For patients without carditis, prophylaxis is recommended to age 18 years and at least 5 years after the last attack. For documented carditis, prophylaxis is continued to at least 25 years and often longer. For patients with persistent valvular disease, prophylaxis for 10 years after the last episode of acute rheumatic fever or until 40 years of age (whichever is longer) is recommended.

The role of prophylaxis for household contacts of patients with either acute streptococcal infection or nonsuppurative complications is also controversial. Some authorities recommend that all contacts should be cultured if there is a family history of rheumatic fever or when a patient with acute glomerulonephritis is identified. An alternative approach is to treat all household contacts in the setting of acute poststreptococcal glomerulonephritis (PSGN), in an effort to reduce household transmission of nephritogenic strains. For invasive group A streptococcal infections (necrotizing fasciitis, TSS), there are no convincing data on which to predict risk to household contacts. However, given the devastating nature of these infections, empiric antibiotic therapy of household contacts should sometimes be considered.

The role of antibiotic prophylaxis for household contacts of patients with acute streptococcal pharyngitis is generally limited to contacts of patients who have had rheumatic fever. Some experts believe that members of the family should have throat cultures, and those family members who prove to be positive should be treated. In instances in which PSGN is present in the family, it has been shown that many members of the family may have subclinical infection and therefore should be cultured and treated, as indicated. Apart from rheumatic fever prophylaxis and the prevention of intrafamilial spread, there are few strategies available to prevent streptococcal infection. Vaccines containing multiple M-protein peptide epitopes have been engineered and show efficacy in animal models and in some preliminary studies with human subjects. Until a vaccine is available, clinicians must remain attentive to the diverse range of diseases caused by this important pediatric pathogen.

## SUGGESTED READINGS

Andreoni F, Zürcher C, Tarnutzer A, et al. Clindamycin affects group A streptococcus virulence factors and improves clinical outcome. *J Infect Dis.* 2017;215:269-277.

Carapetis JR, Beaton A, Cunningham MW, et al. Acute rheumatic fever and rheumatic heart disease. *Nat Rev Dis Primers.* 2016;2:15084.

de Almeida Torres RS, dos Santos TZ, Torres RA, et al. Management of contacts of patients with severe invasive group A streptococcal infection. *J Pediatric Infect Dis Soc.* 2016;5:47-52.

DeMuri GP, Wald ER. The Group A streptococcal carrier state reviewed: still an enigma. *J Pediatric Infect Dis Soc.* 2014;3:336-342.

Felsenstein S, Faddoul D, Sposto R, Batoon K, Polanco CM, Dien Bard J. Molecular and clinical diagnosis of group A streptococcal pharyngitis in children. *J Clin Microbiol.* 2014;52:3884-3889.

Lean WL, Arnup S, Danchin M, Steer AC. Rapid diagnostic tests for group A streptococcal pharyngitis: a meta-analysis. *Pediatrics.* 2014;134:771-781.

Nelson GE, Pondo T, Toews KA, et al. Epidemiology of invasive group A streptococcal infections in the United States, 2005-2012. *Clin Infect Dis.* 2016;63:478-486.

Shulman ST, Bisno AL, Clegg HW, et al. Clinical practice guideline for the diagnosis and management of group A streptococcal pharyngitis: 2012 update by the Infectious Diseases Society of America. *Clin Infect Dis.* 2012;55:1279-1282.

Walker MJ, Barnett TC, McArthur JD, et al. Disease manifestations and pathogenic mechanisms of Group A *Streptococcus*. *Clin Microbiol Rev.* 2014;27:264-301.

Wong CJ, Stevens DL. Serious group A streptococcal infections. *Med Clin North Am.* 2013;97:721-736.

# 281 Group B *Streptococcus*

Morven S. Edwards

## INTRODUCTION

Group B *Streptococcus* has been a common cause of invasive infection in neonates and young infants for several decades. Group B *Streptococcus* also is an important cause of maternal obstetrical morbidity and fetal loss. The incidence of early-onset group B streptococcal neonatal infections has declined 85% in the United States in association with universal culture-based screening of pregnant women and administration of intrapartum antibiotic prophylaxis to women colonized with group B *Streptococcus*.

## PATHOGENESIS AND EPIDEMIOLOGY

Group B streptococci are gram-positive cocci that grow readily as white to gray-white colony-forming units with a narrow zone of β-hemolysis when inoculated on blood agar. Group B streptococci have been classified, based on capsular polysaccharide antigens, into 10 types. Contemporary data indicate that types Ia, III, and V predominate in early-onset disease, accounting for more than three-fourths of isolates from infants with invasive infection. Together with types Ib and II, these 5 types account for approximately 98% of isolates from infant invasive early-onset disease. Among late-onset cases of group B streptococcal infection, type III strains predominate, accounting for more than one-half of infections. Serotype IV, formerly uncommon, appears to be emerging as a cause of invasive disease in neonates.

Rates of maternal rectal and vaginal colonization with group B streptococci during pregnancy range from 20% to 30%. Without interruption of transmission, approximately 50% of infants delivered of a colonized mother acquire mucous membrane colonization. The risk for invasive disease among colonized infants is approximately 1%. This risk is increased when there is premature onset of labor, maternal chorioamnionitis, a prolonged interval between rupture of membranes and delivery, twin pregnancy, or maternal postpartum bacteremia, among other factors. Heavy maternal colonization also increases the risk for neonatal infection. Fetal aspiration of infected amniotic fluid can result in the development of congenital pneumonia with symptoms at or shortly after birth.

## CLINICAL MANIFESTATIONS

The clinical features of early-onset and later-onset group B streptococcal infections are shown in Table 281-1. Risk for early-onset infection is increased in the setting of maternal obstetric complications, but term infants usually present with no risk factors other than maternal colonization. The 3 common presentations for early-onset disease are septicemia without a focus, pneumonia, and meningitis. Most infants (~75%) present with respiratory signs, including tachypnea, grunting, or cyanosis. Radiographic findings can be suggestive of surfactant deficiency, transient tachypnea, or congenital pneumonia. Other signs of early-onset infection include temperature or vascular instability, poor feeding, and lethargy. Clinical signs suggesting meningeal involvement can be unapparent at the initial presentation, but seizures develop within 24 hours of presentation in 50% of infants with meningitis.

The common presentations for late-onset infection are bacteremia without a focus of infection and meningitis. The presentation for bacteremia without a focus can be insidious, with detection of infection when a sepsis evaluation is undertaken for an otherwise well-appearing febrile infant. Approximately one-third of infants have a history of upper respiratory tract infection that precedes the development of bacteremia. For infants with meningitis, the initial signs of infection include fever, lethargy, irritability, poor feeding, and tachypnea. Some infants with late-onset meningitis have a fulminant presentation with seizures, poor perfusion, and septic shock developing over several hours. These infants have large numbers of bacteria visible in the cerebrospinal fluid Gram stain. They usually respond poorly to supportive care and tend to have a rapidly fatal outcome or, if they survive, to have major neurologic sequelae.

Less common presentations for late-onset disease include focal soft tissue infection or osteomyelitis. Group B streptococcal osteomyelitis can have an indolent or an acute presentation and is characterized by single-bone involvement, often the proximal humerus. The signs of infection include swelling, erythema, and pain overlying the involved bone. Inflammatory signs tend to be less prominent than those of staphylococcal osteomyelitis, and group B streptococcal osteomyelitis can be misdiagnosed as Erb palsy. The hip, knee, and ankle joints are usual sites of involvement for septic arthritis. Monoarticular involvement is the rule. Adenitis or cellulitis caused by group B streptococci usually is unilateral and can involve facial or submandibular sites or the genital or inguinal region. Infants with cellulitis or adenitis often have bacteremia, but collections of purulence also yield the organism.

The designation *late, late-onset infection* is appropriate for infants older than 3 months of age who develop group B streptococcal sepsis. Late, late-onset infection can account for 20% of all late-onset disease. These infants usually have a history of prematurity and prolonged hospitalization. Bacteremia without a focus is a common presentation.

## DIAGNOSIS

Isolation of group B streptococci from a normally sterile body site such as the blood or cerebrospinal fluid or from the site of focal infection such as bone, joint, or abscess fluid is diagnostic. Abnormalities

**TABLE 281-1 DIFFERENTIAL CHARACTERISTICS OF EARLY- VERSUS LATE-ONSET GROUP B STREPTOCOCCAL INFECTIONS IN EARLY INFANCY**

| Characteristics | Early Onset | Late Onset | Late, Late Onset |
|---|---|---|---|
| Age on onset | < 7 days (median 1 hour) | 7 days–3 months (median 27 days) | > 3 months |
| Obstetric complications | Common | Uncommon | Varies |
| Prematurity | Common | Uncommon | Common |
| Clinical presentations | Septicemia (25–40%) | Bacteremia without focus (40–50%) | Bacteremia without focus (common) |
| | Pneumonia (35–55%) | Meningitis (30–40%) | Bacteremia with a focus |
| | Meningitis (5–10%) | Osteoarthritis, cellulitis, or adenitis (5–10%) | |
| Infecting capsular types | Ia, Ib, II, III, V | III (75–80%) | Unknown |
| Case fatality rate | 5–10% | 2–6% | Low |

of the white blood cell count, such as neutropenia or elevation of the ratio of immature to total neutrophils, can be found in association with group B streptococcal infection, as well as in neonatal sepsis caused by other bacterial pathogens.

## TREATMENT

Penicillin G is the drug of choice. Initial therapy for suspected infection should consist of ampicillin and an aminoglycoside. This combination is synergistic in vitro and in vivo for killing group B streptococci and provides broad-spectrum coverage for other potential pathogens in the newborn. When the diagnosis is confirmed, penicillin G alone should be continued to complete a 10-day parenteral course of therapy for sepsis or pneumonia and a 14-day minimum course of therapy for meningitis. Treatment should be continued for 2 to 3 weeks for treatment of group B streptococcal septic arthritis and 3 to 4 weeks for treatment of osteomyelitis. The dose of penicillin for the treatment of group B streptococcal sepsis (200,000 U/kg/d) is lower than that recommended for the treatment of meningitis (400,000–500,000 U/kg/d). This higher dose is given for meningitis because the inoculum of bacteria in the cerebrospinal fluid can be as high as 10 million to 100 million colony-forming units per milliliter, and the goal of therapy is to exceed the minimal inhibitory concentration of the infecting isolate by a substantial margin.

A blood culture should be performed to document that antimicrobial therapy has achieved bloodstream sterility for infants with sepsis. For those with meningitis, a repeat lumbar puncture should be performed after 24 to 48 hours of therapy and before discontinuing therapy. The cerebrospinal fluid findings after 14 days of therapy can suggest inadequate resolution of the inflammatory response as indicated by a proportion of neutrophils exceeding 25% to 30% of the total or a protein concentration in excess of 200 mg/dL. In this circumstance, it is advisable to continue antimicrobial therapy for an additional week and to repeat a lumbar puncture. It is rarely necessary to continue antibiotic treatment for longer than 3 weeks.

For infants with meningitis, cranial magnetic resonance imaging should be obtained before discontinuing antibiotic therapy. Cranial imaging gives information regarding the adequacy of resolution of cerebritis or ventriculitis. On occasion, cerebral imaging can reveal a previously unsuspected abscess or infarct that will influence the duration of therapy or prognosis.

Supportive care for infants with group B streptococcal infection includes attention to the details of fluid management, ventilation, and support of vascular volume. Seizures should be anticipated in infants with meningitis and controlled to limit brain edema and hypoxia. For infants with bone or joint infection, open or closed aspiration can be required to establish the diagnosis and to drain purulent material. A drainage procedure is required to preserve vascular supply of the hip or shoulder joints.

The mortality rate from group B streptococcal disease has declined markedly and now stands at 5% to 10% for early-onset disease. The mortality rate for late-onset disease ranges from 2% to 6%. Term infants surviving sepsis usually have no sequelae of infection. Premature infants with septic shock and periventricular leukomalacia can have residual neurologic impairment. Approximately one-half of infants surviving group B streptococcal meningitis have severe (~20%) or mild to moderate (25%) long-term neurologic sequelae. Features at discharge associated with death in infancy or severe impairment include failed hearing screen, abnormal neurologic examination at the time of discharge, and abnormal end-of-therapy cranial imaging. Infections, including those caused by group B streptococci, in extremely low-birth-weight infants are associated with poor neurodevelopmental outcomes in early childhood. Infants usually recover fully from bone or joint infection, but impairment of joint function or bone growth has occurred.

## PREVENTION

Recognition that intrapartum antibiotic administration could prevent early-onset neonatal group B streptococcal infection dates to the 1980s. National standards for intrapartum antibiotic prophylaxis were first implemented in 1996. Current guidelines from the Centers for Disease Control and Prevention, last updated in 2010, recommend universal culture-based screening of all pregnant women at 35 to 37 weeks of gestation to determine maternal group B streptococcal colonization status and administration of intrapartum antibiotic prophylaxis to all carriers. Swabbing both the lower vagina and rectum optimizes the culture yield. The average early-onset disease incidence in the era of universal culture-based screening is 0.2 to 0.3 cases per 1000 live births.

A risk-based method is recommended for women in whom group B streptococcal colonization status is not known at the onset of labor or rupture of membranes. Factors known to increase risk for early-onset infection, including onset of labor or delivery before 37 weeks of gestation, rupture of membranes 18 hours or more before delivery, or intrapartum fever, warrant use of intrapartum antibiotic prophylaxis. The strategy also targets women with group B streptococcal bacteriuria during pregnancy, as well as women who have had a previous infant with invasive group B streptococcal infection. Intrapartum antibiotic prophylaxis should be administered for women with an intrapartum nucleic acid amplification test positive for group B *Streptococcus*.

Penicillin G is the antimicrobial of choice and ampicillin an alternative for intrapartum chemoprophylaxis. Cefazolin is recommended for women who are allergic to penicillin but at low risk for anaphylaxis. Vancomycin use is reserved for penicillin-allergic women with a high risk for anaphylaxis for whom the susceptibility pattern of the group B streptococcal isolate does not permit use of clindamycin. Overall, an 85% decline in the incidence of early-onset disease has been documented since guidelines for intrapartum chemoprophylaxis became available.

Management of a neonate whose mother received intrapartum antibiotic prophylaxis is dependent on the infant's clinical status, the gestational age of the infant, and the duration of prophylaxis before delivery. Symptomatic infants and those born to mothers with chorioamnionitis should undergo full diagnostic evaluation or limited evaluation, respectively, and should receive empiric antibiotic therapy. A limited evaluation consists of a blood culture at birth and complete blood count with differential and platelet count at birth or at 6 to 12 hours of life. For well-appearing infants of 37 weeks of gestation or more born to mothers who had an indication for prophylaxis but received no or inadequate prophylaxis and for whom the duration of membrane rupture before delivery was less than 18 hours, the infant should be observed for at least 48 hours and no diagnostic testing is indicated. If the infant is well appearing and either less than 37 weeks of gestation or the duration of membrane rupture before delivery was 18 hours or longer, the infant should undergo a limited evaluation and observation for at least 48 hours.

Intrapartum antibiotic prophylaxis is considered an interim intervention, and its use has not reduced the incidence of late-onset group B streptococcal infection, which remains constant at 0.2 to 0.3 cases per 1000 live births. A comprehensive program for prevention of group B streptococcal infection awaits the licensure of protein polysaccharide conjugate vaccines now under development.

## SUGGESTED READINGS


American Academy of Pediatrics. Group B streptococcal infections. In: Kimberlin DW, Brady MT, Jackson MA, Long SS, eds. *Red Book: 2015 Report of the Committee on Infectious Diseases*. 30th ed. Elk Grove Village, IL: American Academy of Pediatrics; 2015:745-750.

Baker CJ, Carey VJ, Rench MA, et al. Maternal antibody at delivery protects neonates from early onset group B streptococcal disease. *J Infect Dis*. 2014;209:781-788.

Centers for Disease Control and Prevention. Prevention of perinatal group B streptococcal disease. Revised guidelines from CDC, 2010. *MMWR Morbid Mortal Wkly Rep*. 2010;59(No. RR-10):1-32.

Edwards MS, Nizet V, Baker CJ. Group B streptococcal infections. In: Wilson CB, Nizet V, Maldonado YA, Remington JS, Klein JO, eds. *Remington and Klein's Infectious Diseases of the Fetus and Newborn Infant*. 8th ed. Philadelphia, PA: Elsevier Saunders; 2016:411-456.

Edwards MS, Rench MA, Baker CJ. Relevance of age at diagnosis to prevention of late-onset group B streptococcal disease by maternal immunization. *Pediatr Infect Dis J*. 2015;34:538-539.

Ferrieri P, Lynfield R, Creti R, Flores AE. Serotype IV and invasive group B streptococcal disease in neonates, Minnesota, USA, 2000-2010. *Emerg Infect Dis*. 2013;19:551-558.

Levent F, Baker CJ, Rench MA, Edwards MS. Early outcomes of group B streptococcal meningitis in the 21st century. *Pediatr Infect Dis J*. 2010;29:1109-1112.

Libster R, Edwards KM, Levent F, et al. Long-term outcomes of group B streptococcal meningitis. *Pediatrics*. 2012;130:e8-e15.


# 282 Nongroup A or B *Streptococcus*

Cicely W. Fadel and Bernhard L. Wiedermann

## INTRODUCTION

Nongroup A or B streptococci are a diverse group of gram-positive microorganisms that may be commensal or may be associated with severe, even life-threatening, infections.

## PATHOGENESIS AND EPIDEMIOLOGY

Nongroup A or B streptococci that are pathogenic for humans fall into 3 categories: viridans streptococci, β-hemolytic streptococci groups C and G (*Streptococcus dysgalactiae*), and nonenterococcal group D *Streptococcus*. These organisms are normal commensal flora of the upper airway and asymptomatic colonizers of the skin (groups C and G), gastrointestinal tract, or female genital tract. Viridans streptococci, so named because of the Latin *viridis*, or green, comprise a group of at least 30 species, subdivided into several groups including *anginosis* (previously *milleri*), *mitis, salivarius,* and *mutans.* Growth on blood agar may elicit α, γ, or occasionally β-hemolysis. β-Hemolytic groups C and G each comprise 2 strains, which are identifiable by colony size. Colonies greater than 0.5 mm are considered to be pathogenic, whereas colonies less than 0.5 mm are nonpathogens. *Streptococcus bovis* (also called *S gallolyticus*) is the only nonhemolytic group D species; it must be differentiated from enterococci, which also carry group D antigens.

Viridans streptococci do not share any of the pathogenic features of pyogenic streptococci. Their propensity to cause disease is primarily related to a high frequency of transient bacteremia following dental procedures or loss of integrity of mucosal membranes. Some strains of viridans streptococci, particularly *S mutans, S sanguis,* and *S mitis,* appear to have enhanced ability to adhere to damaged heart valves and vegetations. Members of the *S anginosus* group (SAG; includes *S intermedius, S constellatus,* and *S anginosus*) have a propensity for abscess formation. Large-colony groups C and G streptococci possess virulence factors in common with group A streptococci such as hemolysins, extracellular proteins, and M proteins.

## CLINICAL MANIFESTATIONS

Viridans streptococci are recognized as a major organism causing bacterial endocarditis. The majority of children with bacterial endocarditis (see Chapter 230) have underlying congenital heart defects and usually have undergone cardiac surgery; rheumatic heart disease also is a risk factor. Endocarditis due to viridans streptococci is typically subacute in presentation, with fever and fatigue in the background of a changing cardiac murmur. An elevated erythrocyte sedimentation rate and anemia are the most common laboratory findings. When compared to acute endocarditis, viridans streptococcal endocarditis tends to respond to therapy more quickly with more rapid defervescence and clearing of the bacteremia. Complications and the need for heart surgery are significantly less frequent with viridans streptococcal infections.

Viridans streptococci are also important pathogens in immunocompromised hosts. In cancer patients and children receiving hematopoietic stem cell transplants, viridans streptococci are a major cause of bacteremia, mainly associated with indwelling vascular catheters, mucositis, gastrointestinal toxicity, and neutropenia. Pneumonia and septic shock are common complications. Rare cases of early-onset sepsis have also been described in neonates.

SAG streptococci are increasingly reported causing complicated abscesses associated with sinusitis and with central nervous system, pulmonary, and intra-abdominal infections. These abscesses often are polymicrobial.

Group C and group G streptococci have been implicated as a cause of epidemic pharyngitis from foodborne infections in children and adults, but controversy remains as to whether these organisms are causes of pediatric pharyngitis. Infrequently, group C and group G streptococci can cause a variety of pyogenic infections including pneumonia, epiglottitis, osteomyelitis, septic arthritis, pyomyositis, brain abscess, meningitis, cellulitis, endocarditis, sinusitis, urinary tract infections, bacteremia, and toxic shock syndrome. These organisms are not known to cause acute rheumatic fever.

Group D streptococci (*S bovis*) rarely cause disease in children. There are a few reports of endocarditis (seen mainly in adults), meningitis, and bacteremia, particularly in newborns.

## DIAGNOSIS

Streptococci are readily recovered from standard blood culture media. Complex media containing 5% sheep's blood are usually recommended for subculture of blood isolates and for the culture of streptococci from throat swabs. Colony size and hemolytic pattern determine the initial classification. There is no consensus on whether a predominance of large-colony group C or G streptococci from throat cultures should be reported. Viridans streptococci are usually differentiated from *S pneumoniae* by a lack of optochin disk susceptibility or bile solubility, from *S bovis* by a lack of bile esculin reaction, and from enterococci by negative PYR (L-pyrrolidonyl-β-naphthylamide) hydrolysis. Speciation of viridans streptococci may be accomplished through biochemical reactions available in several commercial kits. There are limited data to support the clinical relevance of speciation at this point. It is important, however, to realize that because viridans streptococci are not common skin flora, their recovery from blood culture should be carefully scrutinized before discounting them as contaminants.

## TREATMENT

Group C and G streptococci remain susceptible to penicillin; third-generation cephalosporins are also suitable treatment alternatives. The addition of gentamicin for endocarditis and other serious infections may be useful if high-level gentamicin resistance is not present. Despite the resistance of some isolates to clindamycin, it can be used to enhance bacterial killing and inhibit toxin production in the setting of necrotizing fasciitis or toxic shock syndrome. Clindamycin should not be used alone for treatment unless susceptibility has been shown.

Resistance of group D streptococci to non–β-lactam antibiotics is common, and an increasing incidence of penicillin resistance is emerging among viridans streptococci and group D streptococci. This is particularly true in the setting of neutropenic hosts. Therapy must be guided by susceptibility testing, which is best performed with the E test or agar dilution. Treatment of pharyngitis associated with group C and G streptococci is controversial, but treatment of endocarditis resulting from viridans streptococci or *S bovis* is complex and determined by antibiotic susceptibility. High-quality guidelines from the American Heart Association/Infectious Diseases Society of America are available to assist in diagnosis and treatment decisions.

## SUGGESTED READINGS


American Academy of Pediatrics. Non-group A or B streptococcal and enterococcal infections. In: Kimberlin DW, Brady MT, Jackson MA, Long SS, eds. *Red Book*. 29th ed. Elk Grove Village, IL: American Academy of Pediatrics; 2015:750-753.

DeSimone DC, Tleyjeh IM, de Sa DD, et al. Incidence of infective endocarditis caused by viridans group streptococci before and after publication of the 2007 American Heart Association's endocarditis prevention guidelines. *Circulation*. 2012;126:60-64.

Doern CD, Burnham CA. It's not easy being green: the viridans group streptococci, with a focus on pediatric clinical manifestations. *J Clin Microbiol*. 2010;48(11):3829-3835.

Krzyściak W, Pluskwa KK, Jurczak A, Kościelniak D. The pathogenicity of the *Streptococcus* genus. *Eur J Clin Microbiol*. 2013;32:1361-1376.

Miah MS, Nix P, Koukkoullis A, Sandoe J. Microbial causes of complicated acute bacterial rhinosinusitis and implications for empirical antimicrobial therapy. *J Laryngol Otol*. 2016;130:169-175.


# 283 Syphilis

Amol Purandare

## INTRODUCTION

Syphilis is a sexually transmitted infection caused by *Treponema pallidum*. The organism is a motile, thin spirochete 6 to 20 μm long that has the appearance of a helical coil on dark-field microscopy or immunofluorescence. It is a fastidious organism, with a short life span out of host, and is unable to grow on culture media.

## PATHOGENESIS AND EPIDEMIOLOGY

Human beings are the only host. Sexual contact is the predominant form of transmission, although it may also occur via very close physical contact with infected mucosal surfaces. Congenital syphilis may occur transplacentally or by passage through an infected birth canal. Transmission by transfusion has also been documented.

After invasion into the patient, the organism rapidly multiplies and disseminates through the perivascular lymphatics and the systemic circulation. Within 3 to 4 weeks, an inflammatory response occurs at the site of initial inoculation, resulting in the characteristic lesion, the chancre (not present in congenital syphilis). If treatment is not received, secondary syphilis develops with clinical manifestations in the skin, mucous membranes, and central nervous system as part of an inflammatory response. Tertiary syphilis may follow with involvement of any organ system. The host immune response is responsible for many of the clinical findings associated with this infection. Long clinically latent periods are common between stages; the infection may persist through the patient's lifetime with a variety of clinical manifestations. Syphilis causes significant complications if untreated and facilitates the transmission of human immunodeficiency virus (HIV).

Syphilis rates in the United States had declined steadily from 1990 to an all-time low of 2.1 cases per 100,000 population in 2001, but since then have risen almost annually in all disease forms and in all age, sex, racial, and ethnic groups. In 2015, 23,872 cases of primary and secondary syphilis were reported, a rate of 7.5 per 100,000 population, which is the highest in the United States since 1994. The increase in rates is largely attributed to increased syphilis cases in men having sex with men, but budget cuts in public health services funding and an increase in HIV infection also played important roles.

Congenital syphilis rates in the United States declined from 2008 to 2012 from 10.5 to 8.4 cases per 100,000 live births. However, the number of new congenital syphilis cases increased to 12.4 cases per 100,000 (a total of 487 cases) by 2015.

## POSTNATALLY ACQUIRED SYPHILIS

### CLINICAL MANIFESTATIONS

Children and adolescents who acquire syphilis follow a clinical course similar to adults. In infected children, sexual abuse must be presumed and laws require that a report be made and an investigation take place.

The incubation period is approximately 3 weeks (10–90 days) followed by the appearance of the primary stage, which is characterized by a painless, indurated chancre that appears at the site of contact—the glans penis, the labia, or within the vagina. Primary lesions may also appear on the lips or tongue, within the anus, or on the cervix (Fig. 283-1A). Regional lymph nodes are usually very enlarged, hard, and painless. The chancre is usually positive for spirochetes when examined by either dark-field microscopy or immunofluorescence—the best ways to make the diagnosis. The serologic tests for syphilis may not yet be positive during the primary stage. The chancre usually disappears in 3 to 5 weeks without treatment, to be followed by the secondary stage. Secondary syphilis usually appears 6 to 10 weeks after the infection and is characterized by malaise, fever, adenopathy, and a generalized cutaneous rash that may be macular, papular, papulosquamous, or bullous (Fig. 283-1B). Mucous patches are also common. Alopecia and condylomas may occur later. The patient is very infectious at this stage: the lesions are often positive for treponemes by either dark-field microscopy or immunofluorescence. Serologic tests for syphilis are positive at this stage. As the secondary stage subsides, the patient enters the latent phase. The patient continues to be seropositive without clinical manifestations. Late manifestations of syphilis (tertiary stage) are gummatous lesions, which are probably the result of hypersensitivity, as well as cardiovascular disease and neurosyphilis, both the result of longstanding vascular capillary disease and endarteritis. Tertiary syphilis is not a disease of children and thus is beyond the scope of this text. An unusual form of syphilis, ocular syphilis, usually presents as posterior or panuveitis, may be increasing in the United States, and may occur at any stage of syphilis.

### DIAGNOSIS

The diagnosis of syphilis depends on correlating clinical findings with those of the serologic tests, smears of fluid from lesions, and results of examination of the spinal fluid. There are 2 general categories of serologic tests for syphilis: nontreponemal antigen tests and treponemal antigen tests. Nontreponemal antigen tests use a component of normal tissue (eg, beef-heart cardiolipin) as an antigen to measure reagin, a nonspecific antibody formed by syphilitic patients. The most common

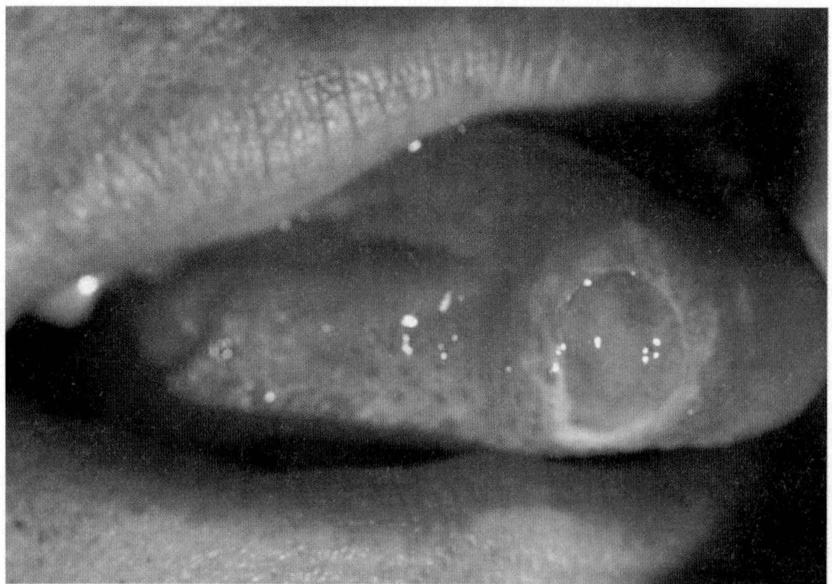

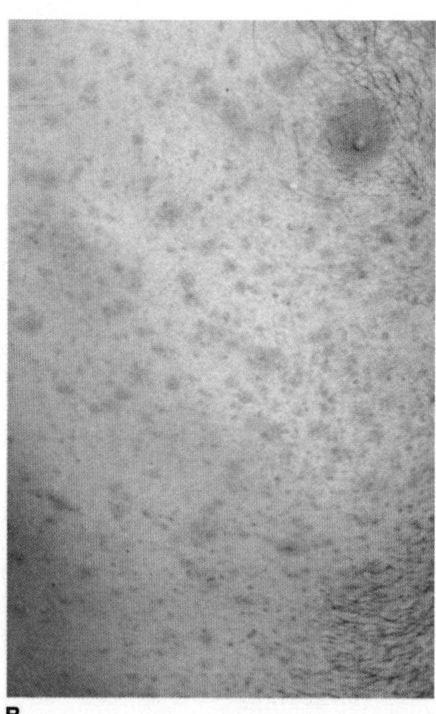

**FIGURE 283-1** Primary and secondary syphilis. A 24-year-old male with painful lesion on the tongue and disseminated rash. **A:** Extragenital primary ulceration on the tip of the tongue. **B:** A disseminated papulosquamous eruption, ie, secondary syphilis, was present at the time of the examination. (Reproduced with permission from Wolff K, Johnson RA: *Fitzpatrick's Color Atlas & Synopsis of Clinical Dermatology*, 6th ed. New York: McGraw-Hill; 2009.)

nontreponemal tests are the Venereal Disease Research Laboratory (VDRL) and the rapid plasma reagin (RPR) flocculation tests. Older tests that use complement fixation (Kolmer and Wassermann) are less commonly used. The VDRL test usually becomes positive 4 to 6 weeks after the infection (several weeks after the primary lesion appears) and is almost always positive at a high titer (> 1:32) during the secondary stage. The titer often falls during the latent phase, as it does following therapy. False-positive reactions are encountered in nonvenereal treponemal infections and, more importantly, in a wide variety of disease states, including infectious mononucleosis, collagen vascular diseases, malaria, drug addiction, many febrile diseases, and, occasionally, pregnancy. The RPR test is a simpler test than the traditional VDRL, capable of automation, and in all other respects comparable to VDRL.

Of the treponemal antigen tests, the most widely used are the *Treponema pallidum* particle agglutination (TPPA) and fluorescent treponemal antibody absorption test (FTA-ABS) assays. These tests are both sensitive and specific for treponemal antibody and are used extensively to determine whether positive nontreponemal antigen tests are true positives or false positives. These tests are positive in most patients with primary syphilis and in virtually all patients with secondary disease; they usually remain permanently positive despite successful treatment. False-positive tests occur rarely in mixed connective tissue and autoimmune diseases and other spirochetal diseases including Lyme disease. A microhemagglutination assay for antibody to *T pallidum* (MHA-TP) is comparable to the FTA-ABS and TPPA tests; however, it is no longer widely available. Other treponemal tests, typically using enzyme immunoassay or chemiluminescence, are sometimes used as preliminary screening tests, but this approach is not the preferred screening approach of the Centers for Disease Control and Prevention (CDC). Each of the treponemal assays measure IgG and therefore do not distinguish true infection in an infant from maternally derived antibody.

Examination of dried smears of fluid or smears taken from syphilitic lesions can be performed by either dark-field microscopy or immunofluorescence to provide an early and specific diagnosis. In selected patients, the spinal fluid should be examined for neurosyphilis. Positive findings for neurosyphilis include an elevated white blood cell count, an increase in the total protein and gamma globulin, and a positive reagin (VDRL) test. The VDRL is the preferred test to examine the spinal fluid; the FTA-ABS is highly sensitive but less specific (more false positives).

## TREATMENT

Early syphilis (primary, secondary, or latent of less than 1 year in duration) should be treated with a single injection of 2.4 million units of benzathine penicillin given intramuscularly for people older than 1 month of age. Syphilis of more than 1 year in duration should be treated with benzathine penicillin 2.4 million units intramuscularly once a week for 3 consecutive weeks. In penicillin-allergic individuals, tetracycline or doxycycline given orally for 2 weeks for early syphilis or 4 weeks for late syphilis provides an alternative. Macrolide use may be effective in some populations, but is not recommended for first-line use and is associated with treatment failures. Likewise, there have been clinical studies that indicate 2 weeks of ceftriaxone therapy are effective, but optimal use has not been established. The treatment of neurosyphilis and that of pregnant women require a different therapeutic approach. Penicillin is the best therapeutic agent and the only one shown to protect the fetus. There are no effective alternatives to penicillin in pregnancy, and the current recommendation is that pregnant women with penicillin allergy be desensitized first and then treated with penicillin.

Penicillin treatment may be complicated by a Jarisch-Herxheimer reaction manifested by fever, headache, myalgia, and an aggravated clinical picture lasting less than 24 hours ascribed to sudden massive destruction of spirochetes and release of their toxic products. Treatment with antipyretics is useful for management; in rare severe cases, corticosteroids have been initiated.

In addition to treating the patient, sexual partners should be treated. Syphilis is a reportable disease in the United States, and when diagnosed, the patient should be examined for other sexually transmitted diseases, including HIV.

## PREVENTION

Education about sexually transmitted diseases and how to prevent them (eg, condom use) is important. The early identification and appropriate treatment of patients with syphilis may prevent spread to others. Follow-up evaluation and appropriate treatment of sexual contacts of patients with syphilis are also important.

## CONGENITAL SYPHILIS

Congenital syphilis results from the transplacental infection of the developing fetus. An infected pregnant woman has a high probability of transmitting the infection to the fetus. Treponemal organisms can cross the placenta at any stage of pregnancy, but appear to elicit little tissue response before the 15th week of gestation. The rate of vertical transmission is 70% to 100% for primary syphilis, 40% for early-latent syphilis, and 10% for latent disease. Adequate treatment of the mother with penicillin protects the fetus, but the mother may become re-infected. Fetal mortality is high—17% to 25% of infected infants die in utero; another 23% die perinatally. The signs and symptoms are varied and may appear at any time between birth and 3 months of life, with 5 weeks as the median time of onset for those infants appearing normal at birth.

### CLINICAL MANIFESTATIONS

#### Early Congenital (Prenatal) Syphilis

Untreated syphilis in the pregnant woman can result in stillbirth, spontaneous abortion, nonimmune hydrops, premature delivery, perinatal death, and early or late congenital syphilis. Women with primary or secondary syphilis are more likely to have infants with adverse outcomes compared to women with early- or late-latent syphilis. Most live-born syphilitic infants have no visible lesions at birth. When lesions are present, they are most commonly on the skin and in the bones. In the first week of life, syphilis may produce bullous lesions of the skin on the palms and soles (Fig. 283-2). No other syphilitic skin lesion at any age forms bullae or vesicles. The more usual pattern of skin involvement is a diffuse, symmetric, copper-colored maculopapular rash that is most intense on the face, palms, and soles. It is an infiltrative lesion that when gently scraped with a scalpel yields serum teeming with treponemes. Thus, either dark-field microscopy or direct fluorescent antibody examination may result in a rapid and definitive diagnosis. If left untreated, most syphilitic infants will eventually have some kind of skin lesion. Many varieties of papular skin rashes may occur and recur over the next months, with a high predilection for oral or anal mucocutaneous sites. Perioral lesions may result in scarring, with fissures that persist. The recurrences become progressively less symmetric with time. The perianal condylomatous lesion (condyloma latum), seen in adults, is also seen in infancy.

A characteristic mucous membrane lesion of infants that has no counterpart in the adult is snuffles, a rhinitis producing a serous discharge that frequently becomes secondarily infected. Postinflammatory scarring beneath the nose is called rhagades. The lesion may extend to the nasal cartilage and cause sufficient damage to result in saddle-nose deformity.

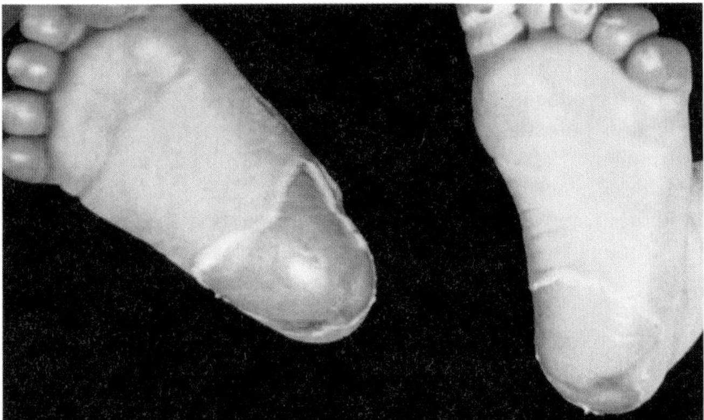

**FIGURE 283-2** Bullous eruptions on the soles of a newborn with early prenatal syphilis. Bullae have ruptured and now present as erosions ("syphilitic pemphigus"). (Reproduced with permission from Wolff K, Goldsmith LA, Katz SI, et al: *Fitzpatrick's Dermatology in General Medicine*, 7th ed. New York: McGraw-Hill; 2008.)

Congenital syphilis produces widespread lesions in the skeleton, resulting in osteochondritis at metaphyseal plates, a generalized symmetric periosteal elevation, and symmetrically occurring osteomyelitic lesions on radiographs. The humerus is the most commonly involved bone, with the tibia next, which often has a highly characteristic pattern with a bilateral moth-eaten appearance; indeed, if other bones are involved, these 2 bones are almost sure to be involved as well. A bilateral moth-eaten appearance of the medial aspects of the proximal tibia that is highly characteristic of congenital syphilis has been described. More than 90% of infants with congenital syphilis manifest skeletal lesions that begin between 1 and 3 months of age; the process is usually self-limited, with healing occurring spontaneously over the next few months, regardless of treatment. Radiographic findings usually disappear by age 5 months. The bone lesions are often asymptomatic. Occasionally, there is pain, often manifested by a pseudoparalysis that may be unilateral, involving either an arm or a leg (parrot paralysis). Later in infancy, there may be recurring isolated bone lesions; dactylitis, frequently asymmetric, is a typical example.

Central nervous system involvement with abnormal cerebrospinal fluid (CSF) findings is present in 40% to 60% of infants with syphilis. Jaundice as a manifestation of syphilitic hepatitis sometimes appears early in congenital syphilis and is resolved with treatment. Syphilitic pneumonitis, or pneumonia alba, is uncommon and usually is only present in fatal cases. Other viscera are involved less commonly. Splenomegaly and generalized lymphadenopathy are frequent manifestations of the early systemic illness. The epitrochlear nodes commonly enlarge. Involvement of the kidney, when present, takes the form of a glomerulonephritis that presents as nephrotic syndrome. Syphilis is responsible for almost half of all nephrotic syndromes in patients less than 6 months of age.

#### Late Congenital Syphilis

Late congenital syphilis may be suspected from the stigmata, from the presence of continued active disease, or from persistently positive tests in an otherwise asymptomatic child. Hutchinson triad, described in the 19th century, includes Hutchinson teeth, interstitial keratitis, and eighth nerve deafness. The most common stigmata are Hutchinson teeth, a screwdriver or peg-shaped deformity of the upper central incisors of the second dentition. Molars may have extra cusps and are referred to as "Mulberry" molars. They are poorly formed and crumble under normal use. All syphilitic teeth demonstrate deficient enamel and decay more readily than normal teeth. Hutchinson incisors are visible by radiography in its pre-eruptive site from about age 1 year.

Interstitial keratitis begins between ages 5 and 16 years. The keratitis is an intense inflammatory vascular infiltration of the cornea that may be accompanied by an iritis, which may be followed by a dense cicatricial scar that produces blindness. Although usually bilateral, it may appear in one eye before it appears in the other eye. The lesion is not prevented by treatment given after the first year of disease. Early stages are characterized by marked photophobia, lacrimation, and a hazy appearance of the cornea. Later, scarring occurs.

Other active forms of late disease are gummas and osteitis, which are among the late benign syphilitic lesions. The palate and nasal septum are predilectional sites for destructive gummas, with saddle nose and perforated palatal deformities possible end results. Persistent periostitis gives rise to thickened clavicles and to a usually asymmetric saber shin. Clutton joints are symmetric synovial effusions, usually of the knees, that are sometimes painless, but which are more often warm and painful.

An important form of active late congenital syphilis involves the central nervous system, most commonly meningovascular. Paresis, a potentially more dangerous form of central nervous system syphilis, occurs in juveniles, and may be detected in a preparetic state by examination of CSF. The examination shows complement-fixing antibody, pleocytosis, and elevation of protein concentration. If untreated, parenchymal involvement may be severe and eventually irreversible. Juvenile tabes dorsalis rarely occurs.

Any form of late congenital syphilis may have become spontaneously seronegative by the time the disease is recognized. Paradoxically, some patients become serofast, signifying an indefinitely high serologic titer unresponsive to treatment, even though therapy is otherwise successful.

## DIAGNOSIS

An accurate diagnosis is difficult, particularly in the first few days or weeks of life, unless the newborn has classic signs and symptoms. Serologic tests on the infant may only reflect maternally derived IgG antibody and thus may not confirm infection of the newborn. If the infant is not infected, the maternal antibodies eventually disappear but sometimes require as long as 15 months. In an infected untreated infant, a rising RPR titer can be anticipated. Antitreponemal IgM antibody testing has been the focus of active research, but these tests are not yet available.

In clinical situations where the diagnosis is in doubt, one must consider the status of the maternal infection, whether the mother has been treated, the serologic tests in the infant, the clinical findings in the infant, and the results of bone radiographs and examination of CSF. Usually one can conclude that infection in the infant is possible, probable, or unlikely. The American Academy of Pediatrics (AAP) Committee on Infectious Diseases provides detailed guidelines for evaluation, treatment, and follow-up.

## TREATMENT

Because the probability of neurosyphilis cannot be definitively ruled out in most neonates, benzathine penicillin should not be used because it does not provide a treponemicidal level in CSF. The regimens of choice in proven or highly probable congenital syphilis in infants 4 weeks or younger are as follows:

- Aqueous crystalline penicillin G 100,000 to 150,000 U/kg/d (administered as 50,000 U/kg intravenously every 12 hours during the first 7 days of life and every 8 hours thereafter) for a total of 10 days; or
- Procaine penicillin G 50,000 U/kg intramuscularly daily in a single dose for 10 days; adequate CSF concentrations may not be achieved with this regimen.

The penicillin G treatment regimen for children > 4 weeks of age is 200,000 to 300,000 U/kg/d administered as 50,000 U/kg intravenously every 4 to 6 hours for 10 days. If 1 or more days of therapy are missed, the entire course needs to be restarted. Follow-up is particularly important for these infants. They should be seen frequently with a careful developmental evaluation, including vision and hearing testing. Nontreponemal tests should be repeated 3, 6, and 12 months after therapy. Titers are expected to decline and become nonreactive or stabilize at very low levels. In infants with congenital neurosyphilis or in those children not evaluated for neurosyphilis, the CSF should also be examined toward the end of therapy. Repeat treatment should be considered if the titer increases or fails to decrease 4-fold within 1 year.

## PREVENTION

Serologic tests for syphilis should be performed in all pregnant women prior to delivery and are required by law in many states. No infant should leave the hospital without the serologic status of the infant's mother having been documented at least once during pregnancy. Serologic testing also should be performed at delivery in communities and populations at risk for congenital syphilis. Serologic tests can be nonreactive among infants infected late during their mother's pregnancy. Penicillin is the only drug that, when given during pregnancy, reliably protects the fetus. If other drugs such as erythromycin are used, the infant should be treated again after birth. The infected pregnant woman's sexual partners must also be treated because the mother could become reinfected and could also reinfect her infant after penicillin therapy. Because most open lesions and possibly blood are contagious, standard precautions are recommended for all patients with suspected or proven syphilis until therapy has been administered for at least 24 hours.

## SUGGESTED READINGS


American Academy of Pediatrics. Syphilis. In: Kimberlin DW, ed. *Red Book: 2015 Report of the Committee on Infectious Diseases*. 30th ed. Elk Grove Village, IL: American Academy of Pediatrics; 2015:755-768.

Bowen V, Su J, Torrone E, Kidd S, Weinstock H. Increase in incidence of congenital syphilis — United States, 2012–2014. *MMWR Morb Mortal Wkly Rep*. 2015;64:1241-1245.

Centers for Disease Control and Prevention. Sexually transmitted diseases treatment guidelines, 2015. *MMWR Recomm Rep*. 2015;64:34-51.

Cohen SE, Klausner JD, Engelman J, Phillip S. Syphilis in the modern era: an update for physicians. *Infect Dis Clin North Am*. 2013;27:705-722.

US Preventive Services Task Force (USPSTF), Bibbins-Domingo K, Gorssman DC, et al. Screening for syphilis infection in nonpregnant adults and adolescents: US Preventive Services Task Force recommendation statement. *JAMA*. 2016;315:2321-2327.

Woolston S, Cohen SE, Fanfair RN, Lewis SC, Marra CM, Golden MR. Notes from the field: a cluster of ocular syphilis cases—Seattle, Washington, and San Francisco, California, 2014–2015. *MMWR Morb Mortal Wkly Rep*. 2015;64:1150-1151.


# 284 Tetanus

Amol Purandare

## INTRODUCTION

Tetanus is an acute illness caused by an exotoxin produced by the vegetative form of *Clostridium tetani*. The tetanus bacillus is a gram-positive, spore-forming obligate anaerobe. It is widely distributed in the soil in most parts of the world. *Clostridium tetani* is normally present in the intestines of horses, cattle, and other herbivora and is found in 2% to 30% of normal human fecal flora. The highest number of colonized persons occurs in agricultural communities. The tetanus organism is a wound contaminant and does not cause tissue destruction or inflammation.

## PATHOGENESIS AND EPIDEMIOLOGY

Contamination of wounds by spores of the tetanus bacillus occurs without clinical signs of infection. Anaerobic conditions in the wound allow conversion of spores to the vegetative form and the subsequent production of a plasmid-encoded exotoxin, tetanospasmin, which acts at the myoneural junction of skeletal muscles and on neuronal membranes in the spinal cord to block inhibitory pulses to motor neurons, producing spasms of muscles. This requires a low oxidation-reduction potential, which is achieved in deep puncture wounds, crushing injuries, and burns. Contamination with dirt, soil, or manure provides a heavy inoculum of organisms; however, *C tetani* spores are ubiquitous, and any wound has the potential to become contaminated.

Although some toxin diffuses into the surrounding muscles, most toxin is distributed hematogenously to neural tissues. Some evidence suggests that tetanus toxin also travels along axis cylinders to reach the spinal cord and medulla. The exotoxin tetanospasmin consists of binding and toxin components. Tetanospasmin binding occurs to gangliosides at the myoneural junction, and toxin interferes with neuromuscular transmission by inhibition of acetylcholine release. The toxin's action in the central nervous system lowers the threshold of reflexes in which the lower motor neurons are involved and induces susceptibility to reflex spasms and convulsions. The toxin combines with high affinity to neural tissue, and binding is essentially irreversible by antitoxin. Thus, only toxin circulating in the blood can be neutralized by antitoxin. Tetanospasmin also affects the sympathetic nervous system, resulting in labile hypertension, tachycardia, profuse sweating, and increased urinary excretion of catecholamines.

Tetanus is rare in the United States, with an average of 29 cases annually. Mortality in the United States is approximately 13%, but of course, it is much higher in resource-poor countries. Globally, in 2013, approximately 49,000 infants died from neonatal tetanus, in large part because of the practice of applying animal excreta to the umbilical stump for hemostasis. The increasing use of prophylaxis in the care of wounds of all kinds and the widespread use of active immunization have greatly reduced the incidence in older children.

## CLINICAL MANIFESTATIONS

Two overlapping clinical forms of tetanus are observed: generalized and localized. The generalized form is the result of widespread distribution of toxin; the localized form is caused by distribution of toxin in the vicinity of the portal of entry. A subset of the local form is cephalic tetanus, occurring with injuries to the head and neck and presenting initially with cranial nerve dysfunction. Localized tetanus can progress to become generalized. In children, local tetanus is rare, presenting with stiffness in a single group of muscles, such as those of the jaw, the muscles of deglutition, or muscles in other parts of the body. The generalized form is more common, especially in the developing world.

Mean incubation period is 5 to 12 days after inoculation. Shorter incubation periods are associated with higher mortality rates. The local wound is often unremarkable and appears to be trivial, likely because more severe injuries are more likely to result in medical attention, where appropriate tetanus prophylactic measures can be administered. The onset is insidious, with gradually increasing stiffness of muscles, particularly those of the neck and jaw and the large muscles of the back and lower extremities. Within 24 hours of the onset of first symptoms, the disease is generally fully evident with marked stiffness or spasms of the jaw and neck (trismus). Swallowing may be difficult, and other parts of the body musculature progressively become involved. Cutaneous, auditory, or visual stimulation and attempts at voluntary motion initiate paroxysmal contraction of the muscles of the body as a whole that lasts for 5 or 10 seconds. During the spasm, the entire body becomes rigid; the head is retracted, the back is arched in opisthotonos, the legs and feet are extended, and the arms are outstretched, with fists clenched and thumbs adducted. The jaws are immobile, and the face assumes a tonic expression known as *risus sardonicus* consisting of raised eyebrows, narrowing of the palpebral fissures, downward and outward stretching of the angles of the mouth, and the upper lip pressed firmly against the teeth. Consciousness is not lost, and the patient is usually very apprehensive.

At first, spasms are infrequent, with complete relaxation between episodes and only mild discomfort. With progression, spasms become more numerous, more prolonged, and painful. Relaxation between the seizures is then only partial, and a considerable degree of rigidity persists. The paroxysms may affect the respiratory muscles or those of the larynx, with fatal results. Partial or complete relaxation occurs during sleep or with anesthesia, and sedatives may afford some relief. Spasm of the sphincters with retention of urine is common. Sweating is sometimes marked, but fever is usually absent. Aspiration may occur during spasms or seizures. The duration of tetanus in fatal infections is seldom more than 3 or 4 days and may be less than 24 hours. Death usually results from respiratory failure, and body temperature sometimes shows an abrupt terminal rise. Patients who recover seldom have much fever; after several days, the paroxysms gradually decrease in frequency and the muscular rigidity diminishes, although several weeks may elapse before they disappear entirely. Trismus is often the last symptom to disappear. Unless the patient suffers anoxic brain injury, most survivors have no sequelae.

Tetanus neonatorum usually follows introduction of *C tetani* into the umbilical cord stump. The illness usually starts between the third and tenth day of life and is manifested by excessive crying and unwillingness or inability to suck. These symptoms are rapidly followed by trismus, sustained tonic contractions, spasms, and convulsions. Anoxia, exhaustion, and caloric deprivation result in death.

## DIAGNOSIS

Tetanus must be diagnosed clinically. The causative organism, *C tetani,* may not be demonstrable, but finding the organisms alone cannot confirm the diagnosis. Fortunately, there are few diseases with which tetanus is apt to be confused. The history of a wound, the onset with trismus, the facial expression, and the spasm accentuated by external stimuli are quite characteristic. Meningitis may be difficult to rule out without lumbar puncture. The differentiation from rabies is discussed in Chapter 316. Muscle spasms resulting from a dystonic reaction are easily confused with tetanus, but its causes are likely to be elicited in the medical history.

Local tetanus should be considered when stiffness of muscles and irritability to local mechanical stimuli develop in the neighborhood of a wound, particularly a compound fracture.

Laboratory studies are rarely specific. Cerebrospinal fluid findings are normal; peripheral leukocytosis may be present. Wounds should be débrided and can be cultured for *C tetani*, although as stated above, a positive culture alone is not sufficient for diagnosis, and recovery of the organism from wounds is uncommon.

## TREATMENT

The management of tetanus includes careful supportive measures, control of spasms and seizures, prevention of complications, and administration of antitoxin to prevent the binding of additional toxin. Noise and unnecessary disturbance should be minimized to decrease the frequency of spasms. Maintenance of oxygenation is of prime importance. Some experts recommend routine intubation or tracheotomy and the use of assisted ventilation to reduce the risk of respiratory arrest, anoxia, and aspiration. Management of the airway includes suctioning of secretions accumulating in the pharynx and the tracheobronchial tree. Support of fluid, electrolyte, and caloric balance may be accomplished through an indwelling nasogastric tube or total parenteral nutrition.

Several classes of drugs have been used in the symptomatic management of this disease to control pain and to treat severe anxiety, seizures, spasms, and secretions. Diazepam, barbiturates, and meprobamate, in high doses given by continuous or intermittent intravenous (IV) administration, are useful. Most centers now manage tetanus with continuously administered neurologic blocking agents or general anesthesia with complete support of ventilation, fluids, and nutrition.

Tetanus antitoxin in sufficient quantity may prevent unbound toxin from reaching the central nervous system but does not displace bound toxin. The dose of antitoxin should be gauged by the severity of the disease, not by the size of the patient. Human tetanus immune globulin (TIG) in doses of 3000 to 6000 U, given intramuscularly, is recommended. IV immunoglobulin is an alternative if TIG is not available. Equine antitoxin is used in some countries but is not available in the United States.

It is essential that injuries receive proper surgical care, but extensive operative intervention is neither necessary nor indicated. Metronidazole 30 mg/kg/d for 7 to 10 days can decrease the number of toxin-producing organisms and is the drug of choice; penicillin G is an alternative.

## PREVENTION

All age groups are susceptible to tetanus. Protection is afforded only by active or passive immunization; even development of clinical tetanus does not confer immunity. Recommendations for active immunization are summarized in Chapter 239. Following immunization, an antitoxin level of 0.01 IU/mL is considered protective. If an individual has completed a primary series of tetanus immunization, a booster using tetanus/diphtheria (Td) or tetanus/diphtheria toxoids/acellular pertussis (Tdap) vaccine will only be needed at the time of injury for clean, minor wounds if it has been more than 10 years since the last booster. For wounds that are dirty or neglected or where the blood supply is severely compromised, a booster of Td or Tdap will be needed at the time of injury if it has been more than 5 years since the last booster.

**TABLE 284-1 SUMMARY GUIDE TO TETANUS PROPHYLAXIS IN ROUTINE WOUND MANAGEMENT**

| History of Adsorbed Tetanus Toxoid | Clean Minor Wounds | | All Other Wounds[a] | |
|---|---|---|---|---|
| | DTaP, Tdap, or Td[b] | TIGc | DTaP, Tdap, or Td[b] | TIG[c] |
| Unknown or < 3 doses | Yes | No | Yes | Yes |
| ≥ 3 doses | No if < 10 y since last tetanus-containing vaccine | No | No[d] if < 5 y since last tetanus-containing vaccine | No |
| | Yes if ≥ 10 y since last tetanus-containing vaccine | | Yes if ≥ 5 y since last tetanus-containing vaccine | |

[a]Such as, but not limited to, wounds contaminated with dirt, feces, soil, and saliva; puncture wounds; avulsions; and wounds resulting from missiles, crushing, burns, and frostbite.

[b]DTaP is used for children younger than 7 years. Tdap is preferred over Td for underimmunized children age 7 years and older who have not received Tdap previously.

[c]Intravenous immune globulin should be used when TIG is not available.

[d]More frequent boosters are not needed and can accentuate adverse effects.

DTaP, diphtheria, tetanus, and pertussis; Td, tetanus toxoid with diphtheria toxoid adsorbed; Tdap, booster tetanus, reduced diphtheria toxin, and acellular pertussis; TIG, human tetanus immune globulin.

Modified with permission from Kimberlin DW: *Red Book: 2015 Report of the Committee on Infectious Diseases*, 30th ed. Elk Grove Village, IL: American Academy of Pediatrics; 2015.

Passive immunization is needed in addition to toxoid only if the primary series was never completed or if more than 10 years have elapsed since the previous booster. If passive immunization is needed, the product of choice is human TIG 250 U intramuscularly. The human preparation provides longer protection and causes fewer adverse reactions than antitoxin of animal origin. The latter should be used only if TIG is not available and only after suitable sensitivity testing. The dose of TIG is 3000 to 5000 U intramuscularly. Td or Tdap should always be given as a booster when TIG is given to a child older than age 7 years, whereas infant diphtheria and tetanus toxoids and acellular pertussis vaccine (DTaP) or infant diphtheria and tetanus toxoids (DT) should be given at the beginning of a series to unimmunized children younger than age 7 years. If Td and TIG are given concurrently, separate syringes and sites should be used, and only adsorbed toxoid is recommended in this situation.

Wound cleansing and debridement is an additional essential step in preventing tetanus. Recommendations for tetanus prophylaxis in routine wound management are shown in Table 284-1.

## SUGGESTED READINGS


American Academy of Pediatrics. Tetanus. In: Kimberlin DW, Brady MT, Jackson MA, Long SS, eds. *Red Book: 2015 Report of the Committee on Infectious Diseases*. 30th ed. Elk Grove Village, IL: American Academy of Pediatrics; 2015:773-778.

Centers for Disease Control and Prevention. Tetanus. http://www.cdc.gov/tetanus/index.html. Accessed October 27, 2016.

Centers for Disease Control and Prevention. Tetanus. In: Hamborsky J, Kroger A, Wolfe S, eds. *Epidemiology and Prevention of Vaccine-Preventable Diseases*. 13th ed. Washington, DC: Public Health Foundation; 2015. http://www.cdc.gov/vaccines/pubs/pinkbook/tetanus.html. Accessed October 27, 2016.

Centers for Disease Control and Prevention. Tetanus surveillance: United States, 2001-2008. *MMWR Morb Mortal Wkly Rep*. 2011;60:365-369.

Ergonul O, Egeli D, Kahyaoglu B, Bahar M, Etienne M, Bleck T. An unexpected tetanus case. *Lancet*. 2016;16:746-752.


# 285 Q Fever

Gordon E. Schutze

## INTRODUCTION

*Coxiella burnetii* is an obligate intracellular pleomorphic gram-negative coccobacillus that was originally named *Rickettsia burnetii*. Extensive changes in the taxonomy of rickettsiae based on the sequencing of the 16S rRNA have resulted in the removal of *C burnetii* from the order Rickettsiales.

## PATHOGENESIS AND EPIDEMIOLOGY

Cattle, sheep, and goats are the primary reservoirs for infections resulting from *C burnetii*, although an increasing number of cases have been reported following occasional contact with cats, rabbits, and dogs in an urban setting. Infection in humans most often occurs after inhalation of aerosolized organisms or with ingestion of raw milk or fresh goat cheese. Reactivation of infection can occur in female mammals during pregnancy where high concentrations of *C burnetii* can be found in the placenta, resulting in animal-to-human transmission during parturition of such animals by direct aerosol transmission. Tick vectors may be important in maintaining animal reservoirs but are usually not responsible for human disease. Infection can also occur due to contact with contaminated wool, straw, bedding material, or laundry. Q fever is endemic in virtually every country in the world, especially those areas where cattle are raised and sheep and goats are herded. Little is known about the pathologic process associated with infection because most patients recover from their illness. Evidence for human intrauterine infection has also been reported.

## CLINICAL MANIFESTATIONS

The incubation period for Q fever is usually between 14 and 22 days (range 2–6 weeks). The severity of illness in children is varied and difficult to document because published data on infections in children are limited. Acute illness in older patients is usually manifested by an abrupt onset of fever, chills, weakness, headache, and anorexia. Cough and chest pain should alert the clinician to the possibility of pneumonia, which occurs in approximately 50% of patients. Symptoms are exacerbated during temperature spikes, whereas patients frequently feel well during afebrile intervals. In patients younger than age 3 years, the presentation is usually one of persistent fever without respiratory manifestations. Although pneumonitis is a hallmark of this illness, Q fever is a systemic illness. Hepatosplenomegaly and gastrointestinal manifestations (eg, vomiting, abdominal pain) are frequently noted (50–80%); rash is unusual in adults but may be more likely to develop in children. Most patients with Q fever improve with or without specific antimicrobial therapy, although a relapsing illness has been described.

A small number of patients (< 1% of adults) do not clear the organism and develop a chronic illness. The risk for developing chronic infection, however, is correlated with advancing age. Therefore, children are infrequently diagnosed with chronic illness. Endocarditis is the major form of chronic Q fever, but chronic relapsing or multifocal osteomyelitis and chronic hepatitis have been described. Endocarditis occurs almost exclusively in patients who have had previous valvular heart disease or immunosuppression. Bone involvement can be demonstrated in patients with chronic Q fever and is more prevalent among children than it is among adults. Chronic Q fever is difficult to treat and often ends in death.

## DIAGNOSIS

Q fever should be suspected in febrile patients who live in high-prevalence areas and who are in contact with domestic farm animals. In the United States, animal handlers and laboratory workers make up a significant portion of reported infection. Chest roentgenographic findings for Q fever pneumonia are nonspecific and are similar to those associated with pneumonia caused by viruses, *Mycoplasma pneumoniae*, or *Chlamydophila pneumoniae*. Multiple round opacities are commonly seen even in patients who are clinically asymptomatic. Q fever endocarditis is rare, vegetations are rarely detected, and blood cultures are usually negative. The diagnostic clue in this situation is valvular heart disease, in association with an unexplained infectious or inflammatory syndrome. Q fever should also be considered in patients with purpuric eruptions, renal insufficiency, stroke, and unexplained hepatosplenomegaly. A normal white blood cell count with thrombocytopenia and elevated liver function tests are associated with Q fever.

The approach to the diagnosis of Q fever is serologic. Specific phase I and II immunofluorescent, enzyme immunoassay, complement fixation, and immune adherence hemagglutination antibody tests using paired (acute and convalescent) serum specimens make up the diagnostic method of choice. In acute Q fever, antibody titers to phase II antigens are higher than antibody titers to phase I antigens, whereas in chronic forms, elevated phase I titers are more commonly found. Because patients with previous infection remain seropositive for prolonged periods, single positive titers cannot be used to establish a diagnosis. The use of DNA detection for *C burnetii* by polymerase chain reaction may be a useful tool during the first 2 weeks of illness and prior to antibiotic administration. Because *C burnetii* has been transmitted with minimal exposures in laboratory settings, routine isolation by clinical laboratories for diagnostic purposes is not recommended.

## TREATMENT

Acute Q fever can be a self-limited disease, and many patients recover without the use of antimicrobial therapy. If antimicrobial agents are used, doxycycline is the drug of choice, as treatment can hasten the recovery by several days. It should be noted, however, that the initiation of therapy late in the course of illness has little effect on the course of the acute infection, and in order to prevent complications, antimicrobial therapy needs to be started within 3 days of the onset of symptoms. As with the rickettsial diseases, many experts consider that the benefits of using doxycycline in treating Q fever exceed any potential risk of teeth staining and would use it at any age. Trimethoprim-sulfamethoxazole can be used as an alternative to doxycycline in the younger patient. Treatment of chronic Q fever is prolonged, lasting a minimum of 18 months and, in certain instances, as long as 3 years. For Q fever endocarditis, the combination of doxycycline and hydroxychloroquine is the treatment of choice.

## PREVENTION

Adherence to proper hygiene when handling infected parturient animals or their excrement and consuming pasteurized milk and milk products can decrease the risk of infection.

## SUGGESTED READINGS


American Academy of Pediatrics. Q fever (*Coxiella burnetii* infection). In: Kimberlin DW, Brady MT, Jackson MA, Long SS, eds. *Red Book: 2015 Report of the Committee on Infectious Diseases*. 30th ed. Elk Grove Village, IL: American Academy of Pediatrics; 2015:656-658.

Bart IY, Schabos Y, van Hout RWNM, Leenders ACAP, de Vries E. Pediatric acute Q fever mimics other common childhood illness. *PLoS One*. 2014;9:e88677.

Dahlgren FS, Haberling DL, McQuiston JH. Q fever is underestimated in the United States: a comparison of fatal Q fever cases from two national reporting systems. *Am J Trop Med Hyg*. 2015;92:244-246.

Dahlgren FS, McQuiston JH, Massung RF, Anderson AD. Q fever in the United States: summary of case reports from two national surveillance systems, 2000-2012. *Am J Trop Med Hyg*. 2015;92:247-255.

Gunn TM, Raz GM, Turek JW, Farivar RS. Cardiac manifestations of Q fever infection: case series and a review of the literature. *J Card Surg*. 2013;28:233-237.

Million M, Roblot F, Carles D, et al. Reevaluation of the risk of fetal death and malformation after Q fever. *Clin Infect Dis*. 2014;59:256-260.

Million M, Thuny F, Richet H, Raoult D. Long-term outcome of Q fever endocarditis: a 26-year personal survey. *Lancet Infect Dis*. 2010;10:527-535.




# 286 Tularemia

Jessica Snowden, Gwenn Skar, and Stephanie H. Stovall

## INTRODUCTION

Tularemia is a highly infectious zoonotic disease caused by several subspecies of the gram-negative bacterium *Francisella tularensis* (Table 286-1). *Francisella tularensis* is a small, aerobic, nonmotile gram-negative bacterium first identified in 1911 by Dr. Edward Francis, after an outbreak of plague-like disease in rodents in Tulare County, California. Infection has been reported in humans since 1914. In the United States, nearly all human cases of tularemia are caused by the *F tularensis* subspecies *tularensis* (type A, 66%) or *F tularensis* subspecies *holarctica* (type B, 34%).

## PATHOGENESIS AND EPIDEMIOLOGY

Mammals provide the primary reservoir for *F tularensis*, including ground squirrels, rabbits, hares, voles, muskrats, water rats, and other rodents. Human infection typically occurs after handling infected animals or after a bite from an arthropod vector. In the United States, biting flies and ticks are the primary arthropod vectors. In Europe and the former Soviet Union, ticks and mosquitoes have been reported to transmit infection. Infection can also occur after ingestion of contaminated food or water or after inhalation of the organism from decaying animal carcasses, contaminated straw, or other sources. There have been several large waterborne outbreaks of tularemia in Europe and the former Soviet Union. The largest airborne outbreak of tularemia was reported among farmers in Sweden in the 1960s, attributed to the aerosolization of organisms from rodent-infested hay. There has been no documented person-to-person transmission of tularemia.

Once the organism gains access into the body, it begins to multiply and then spreads to the local lymph nodes. Once in the lymph nodes or tissues (eg, skin, liver, spleen, lungs) necrosis begins (eg, ulceration of the skin at the tick bite site) and true granulomas develop, often leading to microabscess or abscess formation. The caseating granulomas that form can be indistinguishable from those caused by infections with *Mycobacterium tuberculosis*. The severity of illness is determined by the virulence of the organism, the inoculum size, the portal of entry of the organism, and the immune system of the host.

Infections with *F tularensis* are found only in the Northern Hemisphere. In the United States, cases are reported from the eastern seaboard, Arkansas, Missouri, Oklahoma, and the central mountain regions. Other endemic areas include Eurasia, particularly the former

**TABLE 286-1** ***FRANCISELLA TULARENSIS* SUBSPECIES**

| Subspecies | Geographic Distribution | Clinical Characteristics |
|---|---|---|
| *tularensis* (type A) | North America (70%) | More virulent; lagomorph exposure |
| *holarctica* (type B) | North America (30%), Europe, Siberia, Japan | Less virulent; rodent exposure |
| *mediasiatica* | Central Asia, some parts of former Soviet Union | Little data are known about this subspecies |
| *novicida* | North America | Not recognized by all antibody-based testing |

Soviet Union, Japan, and the Scandinavian countries. Tularemia is not a World Health Organization (WHO) reportable disease. The incidence of disease is believed to have decreased significantly around the world in the past 50 years, largely attributed to the decrease in wild rabbits sold in markets and the introduction of clean water supplies.

In the United States, 1939 marked the peak incidence of tularemia, with 2300 cases reported that year. In contrast, a mean of 126 cases per year was reported in the United States in the period from 2001 to 2010. Cases have been reported in all states except Hawaii, with over 40% of all cases originating from Arkansas, Missouri, and Oklahoma.

There have been 2 reported outbreaks of pneumonic tularemia in the United States, both occurring in Martha's Vineyard (1978 and 2000). The first outbreak was attributed to dogs shaking and aerosolizing *F tularensis* after rolling in infected animal carcasses. The second was likely caused by brush cutting over infected animal carcasses, effectively aerosolizing the bacteria.

The groups at highest risk include those who live in rural areas, farmers, hunters, forestry workers, and laboratory workers. Over 70% of those infected are male, reflecting their greater participation in these higher risk activities. Human outbreaks tend to parallel outbreaks among wildlife reservoirs or surges in the wildlife populations. Most infections occur between May and September, corresponding to times of higher tick and other arthropod vector activity. Cases reported in the winter months usually occur in hunters and trappers who handle infected carcasses.

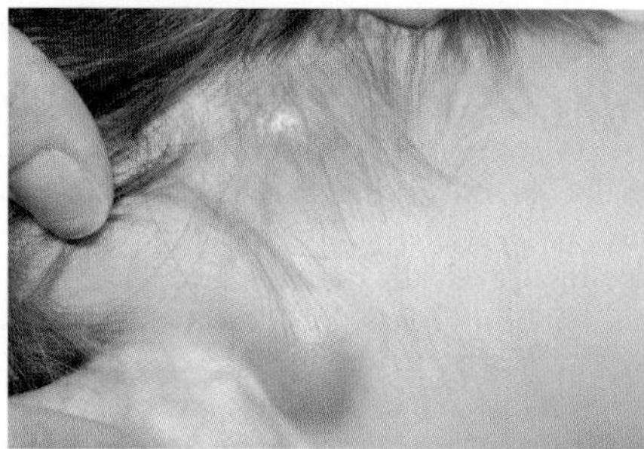

A

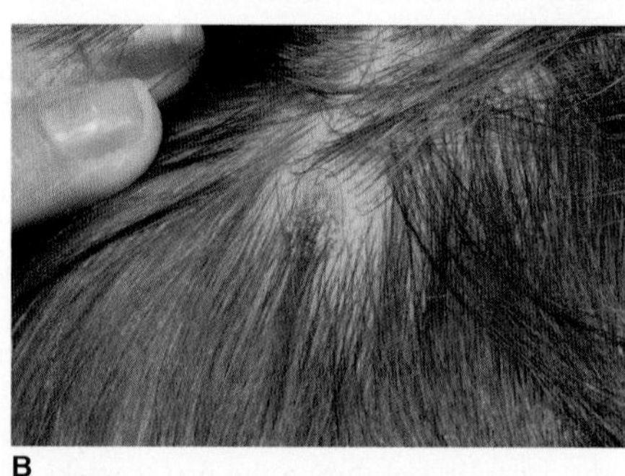

B

**FIGURE 286-1** Toddler with regional lymphadenopathy (**A**) and scalp ulcer (**B**) caused by ulceroglandular tularemia.

## CLINICAL MANIFESTATIONS

The clinical syndromes associated with *F tularensis* infection vary according to the site of entry. The incubation period, from exposure to initial disease manifestations, is typically 3 to 6 days but can range from 1 to 14 days depending on the size of the inoculum. Most patients report a prodromal period with the sudden onset of chills, fever (38–40°C), headache, and generalized aches.

Ulceroglandular and glandular tularemia represent 65% of reported cases of tularemia, occurring more commonly in younger patients (median age, 37 years and 11 years, respectively). The patient with ulceroglandular tularemia typically has an ulcer at the site of bacterial entry and regional lymphadenopathy. Usually, patients are infected via the bite of an arthropod vector or cuts or abrasions on their hands when directly handling infected animal carcasses. A papule develops at the site of bacterial entry that becomes pustular and eventually ulcerates. These ulcers are tender and can persist for months without proper treatment. Regional lymph nodes begin to enlarge within several days after the ulcer develops (Fig. 286-1A). Glandular tularemia occurs via the same disease process as ulceroglandular tularemia, but there is no ulcer noted. Glandular tularemia is reported more commonly in children, who often present with tender lymphadenopathy and no history of ulceration or other skin lesion. In some cases, the ulcer is not recognized before it heals spontaneously and patients present with lymphadenopathy alone. The regional lymphadenopathy in both ulceroglandular and glandular tularemia is very tender, with erythema of the overlying skin and eventual suppuration in some cases (Fig. 286-1B). Young children commonly have involvement of the lymph nodes in the neck, while adults more commonly have inguinal nodes involved. This simply reflects the location of the tick bites (eg, head in children, legs in adults).

Pneumonic tularemia is caused by the inhalation of as few as 10 *F tularensis* organisms. Patients most commonly present with a dry or slightly productive cough, retrosternal chest pain, and constitutional symptoms consistent with the tularemia prodrome described above. Patients may also have purulent sputum, hemoptysis, dyspnea, tachypnea, or pleuritic chest pain. Most commonly, there will be ill-defined infiltrates on chest radiographs, although hilar adenopathy and pleural effusions have also been reported. The difference in virulence between type A and type B tularemia is most pronounced in pneumonic tularemia. Type A infection leads to fulminant disease, whereas type B is much milder and frequently presents with only hilar adenopathy. Pneumonic disease is the most likely manifestation expected if tularemia were used as a biologic weapon and should be suspected in any outbreak of rapidly progressive respiratory disease that fails to respond to traditional therapy.

The other clinical syndromes seen after tularemia infection are relatively rare. Typhoidal tularemia is tularemia sepsis without any localizing symptoms, most likely acquired through inhalation. Patients present with a flu-like prodrome, progressing to mental status changes and shock. They may have prominent gastrointestinal symptoms such as abdominal pain and diarrhea or pulse-temperature dissociation. If untreated, typhoidal tularemia is fatal in 30% to 60% of cases.

Oculoglandular tularemia occurs when the conjunctiva are the initial site of infection, usually following the transfer of bacteria on a patient's fingertips from infected tissue to the eye. Patients present with ulcers and nodules on the conjunctiva, with associated photophobia, chemosis, and vasculitis. Without treatment, infection spreads to the preauricular lymph nodes. Oropharyngeal tularemia occurs following ingestion of infected food or water and is also very rare. Patients present with a sore throat, tonsillar enlargement, and a yellow-white pseudomembrane on physical examination. They may also have associated lymphadenopathy, which is typically unilateral. After ingestion of infected food or water, patients may also present with stomatitis alone. The differential diagnosis of tularemia is presented in Table 286-2.

## DIAGNOSIS

Routine laboratory evaluations are of limited usefulness in the diagnosis of tularemia. A complete blood count can be completely normal or may have a slightly increased white blood cell count with increased mononuclear cells. Liver function tests and inflammatory markers such as erythrocyte sedimentation rate and C-reactive protein are only slightly elevated.

Definitive diagnosis of tularemia is complicated by its poor growth with routine laboratory culture and the exposure risk it presents to microbiology staff. The organism can be cultured from lymph node tissues, sputum samples, blood samples, pharyngeal washings, and fasting gastric aspirates (if inhalational), but the laboratory should be notified that tularemia is suspected so that workers may optimize recovery of this technically difficult organism and protect themselves from accidental inhalation. Cultures should be held for a minimum of 10 days to allow adequate time for colonies to appear on routine microbiology agars. Most labs will not attempt to grow tularemia due to the hazards it imposes on the laboratory workers, and attempts are

**TABLE 286-2 DIFFERENTIAL DIAGNOSIS OF TULAREMIA BY CLINICAL PRESENTATION**

| Clinical Disease | Differential Diagnosis |
|---|---|
| Ulceroglandular | Staphylococcal or streptococcal skin infection |
| | Cutaneous anthrax |
| | Pasteurellosis |
| | Sporotrichosis |
| | Blastomycosis |
| | *Treponema pallidum* |
| | Lymphogranuloma venereum |
| | Viral infection: HSV, VZV |
| Glandular | Viral infection: CMV, HIV, EBV |
| | Atypical mycobacteria |
| | Tuberculosis |
| | Lymphoma |
| | Bacterial lymphadenitis (staphylococci, streptococci) |
| | *Bartonella henselae* |
| | *Toxoplasma gondii* |
| | Plague (*Yersinia pestis*) |
| Pneumonic | Inhalational plague |
| | Inhalational anthrax |
| | Atypical pneumonia: *Mycoplasma, Chlamydia trachomatis, Chlamydia psittaci*, legionellosis |
| | Q fever |
| | Hantavirus pulmonary syndrome |
| | Brucellosis |
| | Toxoplasmosis |
| | Leptospirosis |
| | SARS |
| Typhoidal | Typhoid fever (*Salmonella*) |
| | Brucellosis |
| | Q fever |
| | Rickettsioses |
| | Disseminated bacterial, fungal or mycobacterial infections |

CMV, cytomegalovirus; EBV, Epstein-Barr virus; HIV, human immunodeficiency virus; HSV, herpes simplex virus; SARS, severe acute respiratory syndrome; VZV, varicella-zoster virus.

usually coordinated with public health laboratories. In addition, if tularemia is recovered, it must be reported to the local health authorities because of the potential use of this organism in biologic warfare. Several specific assays are in development, including pulse field gel electrophoresis for differentiating strains, proteome microarray, polymerase chain reaction–based assays, immunohistochemical staining, and direct fluorescent antibody staining, but are available only in select reference and research laboratories at this time.

Diagnosis is usually made by documenting an antibody response to tularemia infection, which appears 10 to 14 days after the onset of symptoms. The most commonly employed agglutination tests will detect combined immunoglobulin M and immunoglobulin G. Tube agglutination testing for tularemia is considered positive with a single titer greater than 1:160 or with a 4-fold increase in titers over the course of the illness. Microagglutination can also be used and is considered positive with a single titer greater than 1:128. Antibody titers can remain elevated for years following infection, although the degree of protection from reinfection this provides is unclear. It is important to note that antibody-based testing would not be useful during an outbreak of tularemia, given the delay in antibody production after onset of disease.

## TREATMENT

Gentamicin and streptomycin remain the drugs of choice for tularemia treatment. Both are bactericidal against *F tularensis* and have been used successfully for decades. Gentamicin is currently more widely available in the United States and is the most commonly used therapy for tularemia. Patients are most often treated with intravenous (IV)/intramuscular (IM) gentamicin for 7 to 10 days with a relatively low rate of relapse if treatment is initiated in the first week of symptoms. Studies are under way to evaluate once-daily gentamicin regimens for tularemia, but there are currently no dosing guidelines for once-daily treatment. Gentamicin is also safe to use during pregnancy for the treatment of tularemia.

Tetracyclines and chloramphenicol are bacteriostatic against *F tularensis* and have been used in the past for treatment, given the ease of oral dosing. These drugs have been associated with a high rate of treatment failure and relapse and are not recommended as first-line therapy for tularemia. Tetracyclines are sometimes used to complete therapy, after a short course of gentamicin, but are rarely used alone. If used, tetracyclines should be given for at least 14 to 21 days, as the relapse rate may be lower with prolonged treatment.

Fluoroquinolones have been shown to have good in vitro activity against *F tularensis*, but their effectiveness against type A tularemia, which is seen more commonly in the United States, is unclear. Although they are not considered first-line therapy, they could be considered for patients who cannot tolerate gentamicin or tetracyclines. Most published studies report the successful use of ciprofloxacin in animal models and outbreak settings, with very little data available on the other fluoroquinolones. In an outbreak in Spain (type B), ciprofloxacin had a lower failure rate and fewer side effects than oral doxycycline. There have also been small reports published in the United States describing the successful use of oral ciprofloxacin in children. *F tularensis* is resistant to β-lactam antibiotics, as well as most macrolides.

Postexposure antibiotics are recommended for high-risk laboratory exposures or biologic attacks but are not recommended for contacts of those infected with tularemia or those with lower risk exposures (eg, tick bites, animal exposure). For laboratory exposures or in a mass casualty situation, the current prophylactic and treatment regimen recommended by the Centers for Disease Control and Prevention (CDC) is oral doxycycline or ciprofloxacin.

Ulceroglandular and glandular tularemia are rarely fatal, even without treatment. Early treatment, within 7 days of onset, is associated with a lower risk of complications and faster healing. If symptoms have been present for greater than 2 weeks before treatment is initiated, the risk of lymph node suppuration is much greater (30–40%). With delayed or no treatment, healing of the ulcer can be prolonged. Pneumonic tularemia has a mortality rate of 30% to 60% if untreated.

## PREVENTION

Patients hospitalized with tularemia require no isolation beyond standard precautions as person-to-person transmission has not been reported with tularemia. Laboratory personnel should be notified before any potential tularemia specimen is submitted for processing. There are currently no widely available vaccines against tularemia in the United States. However, several vaccine approaches are under investigation, including the use of attenuated and killed vaccines, as well as efforts to identify immunogenic subunits for protein or DNA vaccines. Water chlorination has virtually eliminated waterborne epidemics of tularemia in the United States. In endemic areas, the CDC recommends that people wear gloves or other protective equipment when handling dead animals and that insect bites be minimized. Landscapers and other such workers should also check the area thoroughly for any animal carcasses, as brush cutting can aerosolize the organism from decaying animal tissue. Tularemia has been studied for use as a biologic or bioterrorist weapon, so in an outbreak of pulmonary tularemia, appropriate agencies should be notified.

## SUGGESTED READINGS

Boisset S, Caspar Y, Sutera V, Maurin M. New therapeutic approaches for treatment of tularemia: a review. *Front Cell Infect Microbiol.* 2014;4:40-47.

Centers for Disease Control and Prevention (CDC). Tularemia – United States, 2001-2010. *MMWR Morb Mortal Wkly Rep.* 2013;62:963-966.

Chaignat V, Djordjevic-Spasic M, Ruettger A, et al. Performance of seven serological assays for diagnosing tularemia. *BMC Infect Dis.* 2014;14:234-239.

Snowden J, Stovall S. Tularemia: retrospective review of 10 years' experience in Arkansas. *Clin Pediatr (Phila).* 2011;50:64-68.

Sunagar R, Kumar S, Franz BJ, Gosselin EJ. Tularemia vaccine development: paralysis or progress? *Vaccine (Auckl).* 2016;6:9-23.

Tezer H, Ozkaya-Parlakay A, Aykan H, et al. Tularemia in children, Turkey, September 2009-November 2012. *Emerg Infect Dis.* 2015;21:1-7.

Weber IB, Turabelidza G, Patrick S, Griffith KS, Kugeler KJ, Mead PS. Clinical recognition and management of tularemia in Missouri: a retrospective records review of 121 cases. *Clin Infect Dis.* 2012;55:1282-1290.



# 287 *Ureaplasma urealyticum* Infections

Tara M. Randis and Adam J. Ratner

## INTRODUCTION

Shepard first described *Ureaplasma urealyticum* in 1954 after recovery of these organisms from male patients with nongonococcal urethritis. Initially referred to as T-strain ("tiny strain") mycoplasma, these pleomorphic organisms measure less than 500 nm in diameter, lack a cell wall, and are classified as members of the family Mycoplasmataceae. *Ureaplasma* differ from other Mycoplasmataceae in that they produce urease and therefore are capable of generating adenosine triphosphate from hydrolysis of urea. This activity serves as the primary energy source for *Ureaplasma. U urealyticum* has historically been subtyped into 14 serovars. However, recent molecular characterization of these serovars has resulted in a reclassification of *U urealyticum* into 2 distinct species: *U parvum* (serovars 1, 3, 6, and 14) and *U urealyticum* (serovars 2, 4, 5, and 7–13).

## PATHOGENESIS AND EPIDEMIOLOGY

*Ureaplasma* species produce a number of virulence factors including immunoglobulin A protease, phospholipases A and C, hydrogen peroxide, $NH_3$, and the more recently recognized hemolysins. Phospholipases may be of particular importance as they are hypothesized to play a role in the development of preterm labor in colonized, pregnant women by liberating arachidonic acid and increasing prostaglandin synthesis. The multiple-banded antigen (MBA) is a surface lipoprotein and predominant pathogen-associated molecular pattern (PAMP) detected by host immune cells. Reported variations in MBA protein size in vivo are a potential mechanism by which *Ureaplasma* may evade host defenses.

*Ureaplasma* are found on the cervical or vaginal mucosal surfaces of the majority of asymptomatic women and may therefore be considered commensal organisms of the adult female genital tract. Colonization of the male urethra has also been described, although it appears to occur less frequently. Although they may colonize in the absence of symptoms or pathology, there is ample evidence implicating *Ureaplasma* as the primary etiologic agent in a variety of urogenital diseases in both men and women.

Mucosal colonization with *Ureaplasma* occurs less commonly in adolescents and young children than in adults and increases in frequency with the onset of sexual activity. Vertical transmission of *Ureaplasma* with resulting mucosal colonization of the neonate occurs commonly (> 10% of births to colonized mothers) and is increased in frequency in the setting of prolonged rupture of membranes and low birth weight and may persist for several months postnatally.

## CLINICAL MANIFESTATIONS FOR GENITOURINARY INFECTION

*Ureaplasma* species may cause urethritis in both men and women. *U urealyticum* in particular is frequently isolated from male adolescent and adult patients with nongonococcal urethritis. Epididymitis and prostatitis secondary to *U urealyticum* have also been described. The presence of *Ureaplasma* in the urinary tract has been linked to local formation of stones, possibly mediated by urease activity. Colonization and/or infection of the female genital tract are associated with numerous obstetrical complications including infertility, spontaneous abortion, chorioamnionitis, preterm labor, and postpartum endometritis. It is important to note that *Ureaplasma* are capable of invading the intrauterine space, including the maternal-fetal membranes, and are the most common organisms isolated from amniotic fluid and placentas of women delivering preterm.

## ACUTE NEONATAL INFECTION

*Ureaplasma* are now recognized to play an etiologic role in neonatal respiratory disease. These organisms have been isolated from the lungs of stillborn infants with pneumonitis, and subsequent data have supported an etiologic role of *Ureaplasma* in congenital pneumonia. These included isolation of the organism from amniotic fluid as well as the lungs of affected neonates less than 24 hours after birth, the presence of histologic pneumonia, and a concomitant increase in fetal *Ureaplasma*-specific immunoglobulin (Ig) M antibodies. Clinically, the manifestations of congenital *Ureaplasma* pneumonia may be difficult to distinguish from those of respiratory distress syndrome commonly seen in such infants.

*Ureaplasma* infection in the newborn is not limited to the respiratory tract, as these organisms have been isolated from both the blood and cerebrospinal fluid (CSF), particularly in preterm infants. Studies demonstrate that *Ureaplasma* can be isolated from the cord blood of approximately 17% of very low birth weight (VLBW) infants using culture-based techniques. Culture-positive infants have increased rates of systemic inflammatory response syndrome and bronchopulmonary dysplasia (BPD) compared to culture-negative infants. *Ureaplasma* can cause neonatal meningitis and associated complications, including hydrocephalus. A recent study demonstrated the presence of *Ureaplasma* by polymerase chain reaction (PCR) in the blood and/or CSF in 23% of very low birth weight infants. However, the clinical relevance and long-term implications of these findings remain unclear, as most PCR-positive infants were asymptomatic.

The contribution of *Ureaplasma* respiratory tract colonization, occurring in 20% to 45% of low birth weight infants, to the subsequent development of BPD has been widely debated. Two large meta-analyses (performed in 1995 and 2005) demonstrate an increased risk for the development of BPD in infants colonized with *Ureaplasma* compared to noncolonized counterparts. However, individual studies examining this association are plagued with conflicting data. This heterogeneity may be secondary to inconsistencies in defining outcome measures, disparate culture techniques, and variable sample sizes. Furthermore, the multifactorial nature of BPD pathogenesis complicates attempts to directly link exposure and outcome. It is likely that an initial infectious exposure, such as *Ureaplasma* colonization, modulates the newborn's immune responses to subsequent lung injury (eg, mechanical ventilation or oxygen toxicity).

Perinatally acquired *Ureaplasma* has also been associated with an increased risk for the development of other neonatal morbidities including necrotizing enterocolitis, retinopathy of prematurity, and intraventricular hemorrhage.

## OTHER INFECTIONS

Although *Ureaplasma* pneumonia is exceedingly uncommon in older children and adolescents, it may be problematic for the immunocompromised host. Infectious arthritis secondary to *Ureaplasma* has been described, particularly in patients with hypogammaglobulinemia. Case reports implicating *Ureaplasma* species as causative agents in abscesses associated with fetal monitoring, nonimmune fetal hydrops, and surgical wound infections may be found in the literature.

## DIAGNOSIS

Routine culture of the vagina and cervix is not indicated, due to the large number of asymptomatically colonized adults. Similarly, a high rate of perinatal colonization argues against routine screening of asymptomatic newborns. However, evidence of respiratory compromise, pneumonia, sepsis, and/or meningitis in the absence of positive cultures for typical neonatal pathogens warrants consideration of *Ureaplasma* infection. *Ureaplasma* may be difficult to culture, and therefore, careful attention must be given to specimen collection. For maximum yield, specimens must be inoculated into appropriate growth medium at the bedside and processed immediately.

Detection of *Ureaplasma* by PCR-based techniques may exhibit sensitivity superior to traditional culture techniques and has been described in the literature, although its clinical availability remains limited. Efforts to develop serologic assays for the detection of the host immune response to *Ureaplasma* infection are ongoing. However, antibody titers remain difficult to interpret in the setting of chronic colonization.

## TREATMENT

Macrolides are the most widely used antimicrobial agents in treatment of *Ureaplasma* infections. Although newer agents such as azithromycin are most frequently used in older children and adults, erythromycin is the treatment of choice for neonatal infections that do not involve the central nervous system. *Ureaplasma* species are generally susceptible to tetracyclines, although resistance has been reported to occur in as many as 10% of clinical isolates. The ability of tetracycline agents to penetrate the blood-brain barrier makes them a treatment option for infants with meningitis. However, tetracycline use in children under age 8 years is reserved for settings in which the benefits clearly outweigh the risks, as these agents may cause abnormal bone and tooth development in children. Newer-generation fluoroquinolones such as ofloxacin are often active against *Ureaplasma*, although naturally occurring resistance has been documented in adult patients. Notably, *Ureaplasma* are universally resistant to β-lactam antibiotics because they lack a cell wall.

Despite the clear association of *Ureaplasma* colonization with spontaneous abortion, chorioamnionitis, and the onset of preterm labor, the efficacy of antimicrobial treatment both before and during pregnancy in preventing these outcomes remains unclear. Recently published data suggests that early screening and treatment of vaginal infections in pregnant women may reduce the incidence of preterm birth. The ORACLE trial evaluated the use of broad-spectrum, antepartum antibiotics in the setting of premature rupture of fetal membranes and reported some benefits for infants whose mothers received erythromycin. These included a decreased need for oxygen during hospitalization and a trend toward a reduction in the composite primary outcome of neonatal death, chronic lung disease, or major cerebral abnormality before discharge. Although both of these studies suggest that antimicrobial therapy during pregnancy may improve obstetric and neonatal outcomes, their inclusion criteria were not specific for women with *Ureaplasma* infections. A single, recently published case report revealed that maternal azithromycin administration effectively eradicated a culture-confirmed intra-amniotic *Ureaplasma* infection in the setting of threatened preterm delivery. Data suggests that treatment of couples colonized with *Ureaplasma* may reduce the incidence of spontaneous pregnancy loss. At this time, the most recent Cochrane Review concludes there is insufficient evidence to determine whether giving antibiotics to women with vaginal *Ureaplasma* colonization would prevent these adverse outcomes.

The association of *Ureaplasma* with the subsequent development of BPD raises the possibility that early treatment and eradication of this organism in at-risk infants may be beneficial. To date, 2 small, randomized, prospective, and controlled studies have not shown a benefit for infants receiving erythromycin therapy with respect to rates or severity of BPD. It is possible that postnatal antimicrobial therapy for *Ureaplasma*-associated BPD may not be effective because the responsible inflammatory processes may be initiated in utero. A recent study evaluating azithromycin therapy in preterm infants colonized with *Ureaplasma* demonstrated efficacy in eradication of the organism. Whether this translates to a reduction in the development of BPD for these infants has yet to be determined.

## PREVENTION

The recognition and early treatment of nongonococcal urethritis and/or other female genital tract infections due to *Ureaplasma* can prevent adverse pregnancy outcomes and infections in the neonate.

## SUGGESTED READINGS


Murtha AP, Edwards JM. The role of *Mycoplasma* and *Ureaplasma* in adverse pregnancy outcomes. *Obstet Gynecol Clin North Am.* 2014;41:615-627.

O'Connor O, Ibrahim H, Neal T, Corless CE. Incidence of invasive CNS disease with *Ureaplasma*: where are we now? *Arch Dis Child Fetal Neonatal Ed.* 2014;99:F439-F439.

Paralanov V, Lu J, Duffy LB, et al. Comparative genome analysis of 19 *Ureaplasma urealyticum* and *Ureaplasma parvum* strains. *BMC Microbiol.* 2012;12:88.

Raynes Greenow CH, Roberts CL, Bell JC, Peat B, Gilbert GL, Parker S. Antibiotics for *Ureaplasma* in the vagina in pregnancy. *Cochrane Database Syst Rev.* 2011;9:CD003767.

Sweeney EL, Kallapur SG, Gisslen T, et al. Placental infection with *Ureaplasma* species is associated with histologic chorioamnionitis and adverse outcomes in moderately preterm and late-preterm infants. *J Infect Dis.* 2016;213:1340-1347.

Viscardi RM. *Ureaplasma* species: role in neonatal morbidities and outcomes. *Arch Dis Child Fetal Neonatal Ed.* 2013;99:F87-F92.


# 288 *Yersinia enterocolitica* Infections

Basim I. Asmar

## INTRODUCTION

The genus *Yersinia* is a member of the Enterobacteriaceae family that includes 11 species and is an important cause of foodborne illness. *Yersinia enterocolitica* is a small pleomorphic gram-negative, non-spore-forming coccobacillus that has been classified into 6 biotypes and more than 60 serotypes. The serotypes most often associated with human disease are 0:3, 0:5, 0:8, 0:9, 0:13, and 0:27. Human illness can occur after consumption of *Y enterocolitica*–contaminated food, animal waste, and unchlorinated water. This organism may survive and grow during refrigerated storage. Human illness ranges from self-limited enteritis to potentially life-threatening systemic infection.

## PATHOGENESIS AND EPIDEMIOLOGY

*Yersinia enterocolitica* is an invasive organism and causes disease by tissue destruction. Pathogenic properties include chromosomally mediated effects such as invasion attachment to host cells, iron complexing and uptake, and enterotoxin production. Plasmid-mediated mechanisms include production of outer membrane antigens, calcium dependency for growth, and autoagglutination. Invasion and penetration of the mucosa occur in the ileum, followed by multiplication in Peyer's patches.

Drainage into the mesenteric lymph nodes can lead to systemic infection or mesenteric adenitis. The enterotoxin produced by *Y enterocolitica* appears to play a minor role in causing disease because diarrheal illness can occur in the absence of enterotoxin production. In addition, the toxin appears to be produced only at temperatures lower than 30°C. The plasmid-mediated outer membrane antigens are associated with bacterial resistance to opsonization and neutrophil phagocytosis.

One unique property of *Y enterocolitica* is its inability to chelate iron. Iron is an essential factor for growth of most bacteria. Bacteria produce and release iron-binding chelators known as siderophores that extract iron from transferrin. *Y enterocolitica* does not produce siderophores but has receptors for them and can use siderophores produced by other bacteria including the gastrointestinal flora (eg, deferoxamine produced by *Streptomyces pilosus*). Iron overload substantially increases the pathogenicity of the organism, perhaps through attenuation of the bactericidal activity of the serum. However, to establish extraintestinal infection, an exogenous siderophore (eg, a chelating agent such as deferoxamine) or excess iron is required. It is for this reason that *Y enterocolitica* bacteremia and other systemic infections are more often seen in patients with iron overload and those receiving chelation therapy including patients with thalassemia major with hemosiderosis and some patients with sickle cell disease.

*Yersinia enterocolitica* has been isolated from humans worldwide, but most commonly in cooler climates. The organism has a large animal reservoir, including cattle, sheep, swine, dogs, cats, horses, rodents, and lagomorphs. Streams, lakes, and drinking water have all been contaminated. The most common mode of transmission is ingestion of contaminated food, milk, or water. Person-to-person transmission has not been conclusively proven but probably occurs. Seasonal isolation rates of *Yersinia* indicate that it is more prevalent as a cause of enteritis in winter months in the United States. Because pigs are often infected, persons who eat or handle pork are at risk of getting infected. Diarrheal illness in infants caused by *Y enterocolitica* 0:3 in the United States is associated with household preparation of raw pork intestines (chitterlings). Rarely, severe infections have been transmitted from blood transfusions. Some blood donors may occasionally have transient occult *Y enterocolitica* bacteremia at the time of donation, and the organism can multiply to high concentrations in refrigerated blood.

## CLINICAL MANIFESTATIONS

*Yersinia enterocolitica* may cause illness that ranges from self-limited enteritis to potentially life-threatening infection. The most common clinical syndrome is acute enteritis illness resulting in diarrhea (98%), fever (88%), abdominal pain (65%), and vomiting (38%). The mean duration of diarrhea is 2 weeks (range, 1–28 days). Blood and mucus are found in the stool in 25% to 50% of the children. This clinical presentation is seen most frequently in children younger than age 5 years. Most enteric infections are benign and self-limited; however, intra-abdominal complications occur in a small percentage of patients and include diffuse ulceration, intestinal perforation, peritonitis, intussusception, toxic megacolon, and mesenteric vein thrombosis. In older children and adolescents, *Y enterocolitica* infection is more likely to present with pseudoappendicitis syndrome (mesenteric adenitis). Guarding and rebound tenderness are common; leukocytosis is frequently present. Appendectomy is often performed on these patients; however, at laparotomy, the appendix is normal or slightly inflamed with mesenteric adenitis and terminal ileitis. The organism can be cultured from the ileum as well as the mesenteric nodes.

Septicemia with *Y enterocolitica* is the major complication of enteric infection in the very young and in those with iron overload syndromes. One report indicated that 28% of children younger than age 3 months with *Y enterocolitica* enteritis developed sepsis.

Conditions that seem to predispose to septicemia with this organism include liver disease; hemochromatosis; diabetes mellitus; malnutrition; immunosuppressive therapy; iron overdose; iron overload states such as transfusion-dependent blood dyscrasias (eg, sickle cell diseases, β-thalassemia, aplastic anemia); and chelation therapy. Septicemia can lead to metastatic sites of infection including hepatic and/or splenic abscesses.

Adults with *Yersinia* infection are more susceptible to 2 manifestations that are presumed to be immunologically mediated: arthritis and erythema nodosum. In Scandinavia, reactive arthritis following *Y enterocolitica* infection in adults occurs in about 10% of patients. The initial symptoms may include an acute diarrheal illness with fever and abdominal pain followed in 1 to 2 weeks by an aseptic arthritis. This most commonly involves the knees or ankles, but the small joints of the hands and feet can be affected. Reiter syndrome with reactive arthritis, urethritis, and conjunctivitis/uveitis is seen in 10% of these patients. The synovial fluid may contain a few hundred to > 60,000 white cells per cubic millimeter with predominance of polymorphonuclear leukocytes. Cultures of the joint fluid are sterile, but *Y enterocolitica* antigen has been detected in immune complexes within the affected joints. Reactive arthritis is more common in individuals who are HLA-B27 positive. The illness lasts 1 to 4 months, but can persist for more than a year. Erythema nodosum is seen as a postinfectious syndrome primarily in middle-aged women. In Scandinavia, it occurs in 15% to 20% of patients with *Yersinia* infection. The lesions, usually located on the lower extremities, appear within a few days to several weeks after the intestinal infection and disappear within a month. Erythema nodosum may be associated with fatigue and fever.

Other occasional manifestations of infection with *Y enterocolitica* include exudative pharyngitis (with or without gastrointestinal manifestations), pneumonia, lung abscess, endocarditis, urinary tract infection, cutaneous abscess, and conjunctivitis. The atypical presentations are associated with serotypes other than 0:3, 0:8, and 0:9.

## DIAGNOSIS

Diagnosis of *Y enterocolitica* infection should be made by isolating the organism from appropriate clinical specimens such as stools and sometimes from mesenteric lymph nodes or peritoneal fluid specimens. When infection with *Y enterocolitica* is suspected, the laboratory should be instructed to culture specifically for this organism. Although *Y enterocolitica* can grow on commonly used enteric media, growth is slow and can be overlooked by concomitant growth of multiple isolates of normal flora. The use of selective media such as agar containing cefsulodin, irgasan, and novobiocin (CIN) is more effective than routine enteric media for recovery of the organism from stools.

When the organism cannot be cultured but *Yersinia* is suspected, serologic testing may be of benefit. Tube agglutination test is the standard assay; however, enzyme-linked immunoassays (ELISA) and radioimmunoassays have also been developed. Titer determinations are available through commercial laboratories for the most common serotypes. Agglutinin titers rise 1 week after onset of symptoms and reach a peak in the second week of illness. The usefulness of serologic testing, however, is limited by cross-reactions between *Y enterocolitica* and *Brucella abortus*, *Rickettsia*, *Salmonella* species, and *Morganella morganii*. Children younger than age 1 year are also less likely to develop serologic response than are older children. In addition, some populations may have a high seroprevalence in healthy individuals, which can limit the usefulness of serodiagnosis. An agglutinin titer greater than 1:128, in the appropriate clinical setting, is considered presumptive evidence of infection.

## TREATMENT

In vitro testing indicates that *Y enterocolitica* is susceptible to trimethoprim-sulfamethoxazole, aminoglycosides, chloramphenicol, tetracycline, third-generation cephalosporins, and the quinolones. Strains are often resistant to penicillins, ampicillin, first-generation cephalosporins, and most second-generation cephalosporins. Despite the in vitro testing, the effectiveness of antibiotics in the treatment of uncomplicated gastroenteritis or mesenteric adenitis (ie, pseudoappendicitis syndrome) has not been established. Uncontrolled data suggest some benefit of therapy in patients with prolonged symptoms.

Immunocompromised patients with enterocolitis, patients with septicemia, and those with focal extraintestinal infections should be treated with antimicrobial therapy. Although there are no controlled clinical comparisons of antimicrobials in the treatment of severe *Y enterocolitica* infections in human beings, doxycycline and gentamicin were promising in a mouse model. Trimethoprim-sulfamethoxazole (or doxycycline in older patients) can be used for focal disease. Third-generation cephalosporins, often in combination with an aminoglycoside, were shown to have a successful outcome in the treatment of patients with extraintestinal infection such as septicemia. Selection of appropriate antimicrobial treatment should ultimately be guided by the clinical response of the patient and antimicrobial susceptibility results. Treatment of septicemia in patients with iron overload should include temporary discontinuation of deferoxamine chelation therapy. Recent data indicate that the third-generation cephalosporin cefotaxime is effective in the treatment of *Y enterocolitica* bacteremia in children. Antibiotic treatment has no effect in patients with postinfectious syndromes.

## PREVENTION

Attention to appropriate handling and cooking of pig products, especially intestines, should decrease the risk of infection associated with these food items. Consumption of uncooked meat should be avoided. Refrigeration of cooked meat for prolonged periods of time before consumption should be avoided because *Y enterocolitica* grows at refrigerator temperature. Patients and at-risk individuals should be instructed about appropriate hygiene methods and signs and symptoms of infection.

Outbreaks of illness owing to *Y enterocolitica* are often foodborne and should receive prompt and thorough investigation. Careful handwashing and enteric precautions are required for a prolonged period following infection. In one Canadian report, the duration of excretion of *Y enterocolitica* in the stool ranged from 14 to 97 days (mean 42 days). Spread of the organism occurred in 27 of 57 families studied. Prevention of occupational exposure among butchers and workers engaged in swine slaughter and prevention of cross-contamination of food products not normally harboring *Y enterocolitica* are paramount objectives.

## SUGGESTED READINGS

El Qouqa IA, El Jarou MA, Samaha AS, Al Afifi AS, Al Jarousha AM. *Yersinia enterocolitica* infection among children aged less than 12 years: a case-control study. *Int J Infect Dis.* 2011;15:e48-e53.

Longenberger AH, Gronostaj MP, Yee GY, et al. *Yersinia enterocolitica* infections associated with improperly pasteurized milk products: Southwest Pennsylvania, March-August 2011. *Epidemiol Infect.* 2014;142:1640-1650.

May AN, Piper SM, Boutlis CS. *Yersinia* intussusception: case report and review. *J Paediatr Child Health.* 2014;50:91-95.

Ong KL, Gould LH, Chen DL, et al. Changing epidemiology of *Yersinia enterocolitica* infections: markedly decreased rates in young black children, Foodborne Diseases Active Surveillance Network (FoodNet), 1996-2009. *Clin Infect Dis.* 2012;54:S385-S390.

Rosner BM, Stark K, Höhle M, Werber D. Risk factors for sporadic *Yersinia enterocolitica* infections, Germany 2009-2010. *Epidemiol Infect.* 2012;140:1738-1747.

Rosner BM, Werber D, Höhle M, Stark K. Clinical aspects and self-reported symptoms of sequelae of *Yersinia enterocolitica* infections in a population-based study, Germany 2009-2010. *BMC Infect Dis.* 2013;13:236.

# 289 Rickettsial Infections

Gordon E. Schutze

## INTRODUCTION

Rickettsial infections are caused by pleomorphic gram-negative organisms that contain both DNA and RNA. They are obligate intracellular parasites, have typical bacterial cell walls and cytoplasmic membranes, and divide by binary fission. The order Rickettsiales includes only 2 families, the Anaplasmataceae and the Rickettsiaceae. *Ehrlichia* and *Anaplasma* species are from the family Anaplasmataceae, whereas spotted fever and the typhus group, as well as the causative agent of scrub typhus (*Orientia tsutsugamushi*), are from the family Rickettsiaceae. All of these diseases are commonly referred to as rickettsial diseases.

## PATHOGENESIS

Rickettsial infections have many features in common, including multiplication of the organism in an arthropod host; geographic and seasonal occurrences that are related to the arthropod life cycle, activity, and distribution; zoonotic illnesses with humans as incidental hosts (except for louse-borne typhus); and fever, rash (except some cases of ehrlichiosis and anaplasmosis), headache, myalgias, and respiratory tract symptoms. Ticks become infected by feeding on the blood of infected animals, through fertilization, or by transovarial passage. Once attached, the infected tick is able to transmit the disease to humans during feeding. After attachment to humans has occurred (6–24 hours), rickettsiae are released from the salivary glands and multiply in the endothelial cells lining the small blood vessels, resulting in cell damage. These organisms produce a vasculitis following replication within the endothelial lining and smooth muscle cells of blood vessels, leading to generalized capillary and small-vessel endothelial damage, increased vascular permeability, thrombus formations, and tissue necrosis. This process consumes platelets and results in the characteristic thrombocytopenia. Many of the other initial symptoms and signs are referable to this pathogenesis, which can affect any organ system. Although the thrombus-mediated vascular occlusion that occurs may play a role in severe rickettsial infections, disseminated intravascular coagulation (DIC) occurs rarely. Hyponatremia, which is another laboratory hallmark of many rickettsial infections, is the result of initial active secretion of salt into renal tubules. Subsequently, the syndrome of inappropriate production of antidiuretic hormone (SIADH) can further aggravate the hyponatremic state. Organisms from the typhus (except scrub typhus) and spotted fever groups contain endotoxins, and most will survive only briefly outside of a host (reservoir or vector).

The epidemiology, clinical manifestations, and outcomes of each rickettsial disease are discussed below. Because diagnostic methods and treatment are similar for most rickettsial disorders, these are discussed at the end of the chapter.

## ROCKY MOUNTAIN SPOTTED FEVER

### EPIDEMIOLOGY

According to the Centers for Disease Control and Prevention, from 2006 to 2013, the median number of cases per year for spotted fever rickettsiosis (formerly reported as Rocky Mountain spotted fever [RMSF] until 2010) in the United States was 2426 (range 1815–4470). Of these cases, approximately 76% occurred between April and October, and 8.5% of the cases were in children less than 15 years of age. Although the disease is rare in infants, RMSF has been described to occur in more than 1 family member at the same time. The geographic connotation of its name notwithstanding, RMSF is endemic to much of the Western Hemisphere, including Mexico, Costa Rica, Argentina, Panama, Colombia, and the continental United States. In the United States, RMSF is most common in the south Atlantic states (eg, North Carolina, South Carolina, Georgia, Virginia, and Maryland), the east south central states (eg, Alabama, Mississippi, Tennessee), and the west south central states (eg, Arkansas, Oklahoma). Since 2002, RMSF has become problematic on the tribal lands in Arizona as well. Ticks that transmit the disease vary by region. In the western United States, wood ticks (*Dermacentor andersoni*) are primary carriers and vectors of infection, but the recognition of an unexpected tick vector, the brown dog tick (*Rhipicephalus sanguineus*), has been responsible for outbreaks in Arizona. The dog tick (*Dermacentor variabilis*) in the eastern United States and the Lone Star tick (*Amblyomma americanum*) in the south-central region represent the most common arthropod hosts. Even in areas where most human cases are reported, only approximately 1% to 3% of the tick population will carry the causative agent, *Rickettsia rickettsii*, and very few humans actually become infected despite suffering a tick bite. For all age groups, reported risk factors include exposure to dogs, residence in a wooded area, and male gender.



## CLINICAL MANIFESTATIONS

The incubation period for RMSF is usually 7 days, but ranges from 1 to 14 days, depending on the size of the rickettsial inoculum. The illness is usually characterized by a short prodromal period with headache, malaise, and myalgias. The classic triad of fever, headache, and a centrifugal petechial rash, plus a history of exposure to ticks, is present in only 3% to 18% of patients at their initial evaluation. The onset of fever is usually abrupt and high grade (40–40.5°C [104–104.9°F]). The skin rash, however, begins to appear on average 2 to 3 days after the onset of illness as blanching, 1- to 4-mm macules that later become petechial (Fig. 289-1). The skin rash begins peripherally (eg, wrists, ankles) and spreads centrally; it is common to have involvement of the palms and soles. It is important to note, however, that only 50% of patients have a rash during the first 3 days of illness, and as many as 20% of adults and 5% of children may never develop a rash. Care should also be taken when dealing with patients with darkly pigmented skin because the rash may not be appreciated. The absence of a rash should never delay the institution of appropriate antimicrobial therapy if the historical, clinical, and laboratory findings are compatible with the diagnosis of RMSF. Although physicians rely greatly on a history of tick exposure, in reported series, such information was confirmed in only one-half to two-thirds of documented infections.

Other clinical manifestations include headache, mental confusion, and myalgia. The headache is described by adults and older children as being the most severe headache they have ever experienced, persisting throughout the day and unresponsive to any pain medications. Most of the major complications of this illness occur as a result of a vasculitic mechanism of injury. Complications of severe illness include encephalitis, meningitis, pulmonary edema, respiratory distress syndrome, cardiac arrhythmias, coagulopathy, gastrointestinal bleeding, hepatitis, and skin necrosis.

Long-term sequelae that have been described include paraparesis; hearing loss; peripheral neuropathy; cerebellar, vestibular, and motor dysfunction; language disorders; behavioral disturbances; learning disabilities; bladder and bowel incontinence; and limb amputation. The mortality rate associated with RMSF is 20% to 25% if untreated and 5% with appropriate antimicrobial therapy. Risk factors for an adverse outcome include nonwhite race, male gender, absence of headache, no history of tick attachment, delay in initiating therapy, gastrointestinal symptoms, and no treatment by the fifth day of illness.

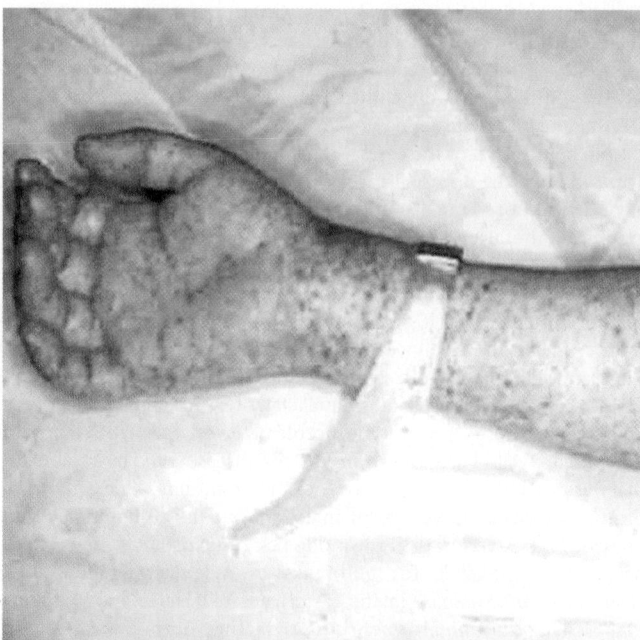

**FIGURE 289-1** Late petechial rash on palm and forearm of a patient with Rocky Mountain spotted fever. (Reproduced with permission from the Centers for Disease Control and Prevention.)

## DIAGNOSIS

The diagnosis of RMSF must be based only on the history and physical examination findings, because specific laboratory tests may not become positive until the second week of infection. Although laboratory abnormalities such as thrombocytopenia, hyponatremia, leukopenia, and elevated liver-associated enzymes may be present in patients with RMSF, none are specific for this illness, and therefore, they cannot be used to confirm a diagnosis. Specific serologic testing should be performed to confirm a diagnosis of RMSF, but most patients will have negative antibody testing at the time of clinical presentation. Thus, diagnosis usually is made later in the course by demonstrating a 4-fold increase in antibody titer between acute and convalescent sera using 1 or more of the specific serologic tests as determined by a number of methods, including complement fixation, immunofluorescent assays, latex agglutination, indirect hemagglutination, or microagglutination tests. Testing is available in most state and local laboratories in highly endemic regions, as well as at the Centers for Disease Control and Prevention (CDC) in Atlanta. A single titer greater than 1:128 can also be used to confirm the diagnosis. *R rickettsii* have been identified by immunofluorescent staining of skin biopsy specimens obtained at the site of the rash with 70% sensitivity and 100% specificity. A polymerase chain reaction assay has been developed to detect *R rickettsii* in blood and biopsy specimens during the acute phase of illness but is not currently widely available.

## OTHER SPOTTED FEVERS

Many new data on *Rickettsia* from the spotted fever group have accumulated over recent years. Prior to 1984, Mediterranean spotted fever (*Rickettsia conorii* subspecies *conorii*), Siberian tick typhus or North Asian tick typhus (*Rickettsia sibirica* subspecies *sibirica*), and Queensland tick typhus (*Rickettsia australis*) were the only other spotted fevers described. Since 1984, new infections have been recognized and described, such as Japanese or Oriental spotted fever (*Rickettsia japonica*), African tick bite fever (*Rickettsia africae*), Flinders Island spotted fever (*Rickettsia honei*), as well as others. More recently, *Rickettsia phillipi* and *Rickettsia parkeri* have been described in the United States and will require a better understanding of their role in human disease. As our knowledge of rickettsiae increases, other new organisms and illnesses will be recognized.

In general, most of the spotted fever rickettsiosis syndromes have similar clinical courses as well as treatments. Those with distinctive clinical features include infections caused by *Rickettsia slovaca* and *R africae*. Tick-borne lymphadenopathy and *Dermacentor*-borne necrosis-eschar-lymphadenopathy (DEBONEL) are descriptive names applied to infections by *R slovaca*. Ticks frequently attach to the scalp, where an eschar appears 7 to 9 days later associated with painful cervical adenopathy. Alopecia at the eschar site may occur, and persistent asthenia of the area may even be present after proper treatment. Fever and rash are seldom present in this disease. African tick fever differs from most other rickettsioses because it is of mild to moderate severity, and it produces painful regional lymphadenopathy, has multiple eschars (Fig. 289-2), and occasionally, has a sparse and sometimes vesicular rash.

# EHRLICHIOSIS

## EPIDEMIOLOGY

In the United States, 4 members of the Anaplasmataceae family are recognized to infect humans: *Anaplasma phagocytophilum*, *Ehrlichia chaffeensis*, *Ehrlichia ewingii*, and an *Ehrlichia muris*–like agent. In other parts of the world, *E muris* (Russia and Japan), *Neorickettsia sennetsu* (Asia) and *Neorickettsia mikurensis* (Europe and Asia) are the more common causes of human disease. Circulating white blood cells are the target of these organisms, and the diseases they cause

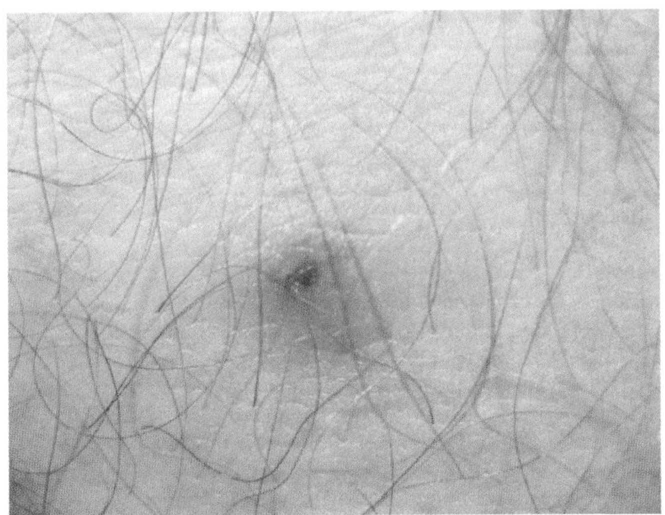

**FIGURE 289-2** Eschar produced from infection with *Rickettsia africae* (African tick fever). (Used with permission from Ryan B. Phelps, MD.)

are often named after the infected white blood cell (eg, *E chaffeensis* infects monocytes and is called human monocytic ehrlichiosis). *E ewingii*, although serologically similar to *E chaffeensis*, actually affects the neutrophils much like *A phagocytophilum* and is usually referred to as human ewingii ehrlichiosis. Human ewingii ehrlichiosis occurs infrequently and is clinically indistinguishable from infections caused by *E chaffeensis* or *A phagocytophilum*.

Human monocytic ehrlichiosis (HME) in humans is caused by *E chaffeensis*. The exact incidence of HME is unknown but has been described to be as high as 330 to 414 per 100,000 population in tick-endemic regions of the United States. The geographic distribution of illness overlaps that of RMSF, as the tick vectors are identical (*A americanum*). According to the CDC, the median number of cases reported over a 6-year period (2008–2013) was 951 per year. The majority of reported cases for *E chaffeensis* and *E ewingii* were from the south central and southeastern parts of the United States (eg, Oklahoma, Arkansas, Missouri, and Virginia). Approximately 78% of reported cases occurred during the 6-month period of April through October with children < 15 years of age comprising approximately 7% of reported cases. The interval from tick exposure to the development of the illness is from 2 days to 3 weeks. White-tailed deer and dogs have been proposed as potential reservoirs of infection from which the tick feeds. Current evidence suggests that *E chaffeensis* is introduced into the dermis of the host by the bite of an infected tick with subsequent hematogenous spread of the organism.

Human granulocytic anaplasmosis (HGA) is caused by *A phagocytophilum* and is transmitted by the blacklegged tick (*Ixodes scapularis*). This tick is also responsible for the transmission of *E muris*–like agent and the causative agents of Lyme disease (*Borrelia burgdorferi*) and babesiosis (*Babesia microti*). Although the majority of illness has been recognized in the United States, HGA has been described in several European countries as well. The prevalence of HGA is not well documented, but rates as high as 52 to 58 cases per 100,000 population have been described in highly endemic regions of Connecticut and Wisconsin in the United States. According to the CDC, the median number of cases reported over a 6-year period (2008–2013) was 2075 per year. The majority of reported cases of *A phagocytophilum* were from the Midwest and northeast parts of the United States (eg, New York, Minnesota, Wisconsin, Connecticut), whereas cases of the *E muris*–like agent have only been reported in Minnesota and Wisconsin. Approximately 80% of reported HGA cases occurred during the 6-month period of April through October with children < 15 years of age comprising approximately 5% of reported cases. Tick and human studies suggest a potential coinfection with comorbidity for HGA and Lyme borreliosis or babesiosis. Human granulocytic anaplasmosis has also been demonstrated to be transmitted perinatally as well as by blood transfusion.

## CLINICAL MANIFESTATIONS

Fever, rash, headache, myalgia, and hepatosplenomegaly are common abnormalities encountered on physical examination in children with HME. The rash associated with HME is more commonly encountered in children than in adults. The rash is generally distributed over the trunk or extremities and may be macular, maculopapular, petechial, or a combination of all 3 types. Life-threatening illness has been reported in children, with up to 25% of all patients with HME requiring intensive care therapy. Long-term sequelae reported to date include foot drop, speech impediment, decreased school performance, renal failure, and hypertension.

Symptoms similar to HME are found in patients with HGA, but the rash is usually absent. The most important feature of HGA is a lack of abnormal findings on physical examination. Peripheral neuropathies (eg, brachial plexus, demyelinating polyneuropathy, isolated facial palsy) can occur in human anaplasmosis and may persist for weeks or months.

## DIAGNOSIS

The recognition of ehrlichiosis can be difficult. Patients who are evaluated during the summer with a history of tick attachment should be considered to be at risk. Elevated liver function tests, thrombocytopenia, and leukopenia (with lymphopenia [HME] or neutropenia [HGA]) are the most common laboratory abnormalities noted. Patients may also have hyponatremia, anemia, and cerebrospinal fluid abnormalities (eg, pleocytosis with a predominance of lymphocytes and an elevated total protein concentration), but none of these laboratory tests are specific for the diagnosis. Although examination of the peripheral smear with a Wright stain looking for intracytoplasmic inclusions (morulae) in the monocytes (HME) or neutrophils (HGA) has been described, it is a very insensitive method for establishing the diagnosis. In addition, doxycycline treatment will adversely affect the ability to detect these inclusions. Detection of specific DNA by polymerase chain reaction is increasingly available at many commercial and state public health laboratories and is currently the best method to confirm infections with *E ewingii* and *E muris*–like agent. In addition to the use of the DNA detection methods, use of serologic testing for confirmation of HME or HGA in patients with compatible history and clinical findings is also available. A 4-fold increase in immunoglobulin (Ig)G–specific antibody titer by indirect immunofluorescence antibody (IFA) assay between acute and convalescent sera is commonly used to establish the diagnosis of HME and HGA.

If a rash is present, ehrlichiosis may be indistinguishable from RMSF. The differential diagnosis in such a patient should also include tularemia, babesiosis, Lyme disease, murine typhus, and Colorado tick fever. Bacterial cultures can help exclude meningococcemia, other bacterial organisms causing sepsis, or endocarditis, whereas viral etiologies such as enterovirus, adenovirus, and Epstein-Barr virus can also be considered. Patients with Kawasaki syndrome are more likely to have conjunctivitis, mucous membrane involvement, and extremity changes as compared to children with RMSF or ehrlichiosis.

# TYPHUS

The incidence of murine typhus (also called endemic typhus or flea-borne typhus) in the United States is unknown since it is not a nationally reportable disease, although it is reportable in some states (eg, California, Texas, Hawaii). Murine typhus is transmitted to human beings by infected feces from the rat flea or the cat flea. Flea bite or the introduction of flea feces into the skin by scratching or through broken skin inoculates *Rickettsia typhi* or *Rickettsia felis* into human tissue. The incubation for murine typhus is 1 to 2 weeks, and the illness usually begins with the abrupt onset of fever. Other important signs and symptoms of infection include headache, chills, rash, nausea, myalgias, arthralgia, and vomiting. Compared with adult populations, children complain less frequently of headaches. The rash begins 6 to 7 days after onset of fever and is usually macular, maculopapular, or papular in appearance. Although a hallmark of rickettsial disease, the presence of rash in endemic typhus is variable and can be found in 20% to 80% of patients.

Historically, epidemic (louse-borne or Sylvatic) typhus (*Rickettsia prowazekii*) has been a significant pathogen, causing massive epidemics of disease during periods of war and famine, accounting for thousands of deaths in prison camps during and after World War II. There have been recent outbreaks in Africa and Central and South America, but not in the United States.

Epidemic typhus has an acute onset beginning 7 to 14 days after exposure to an infected louse. High fever (39–40°C [102.2–104°F]) and headache precede by 3 to 7 days a rash, which has a central distribution, spreading to the extremities but usually sparing the palms and soles. This rash progresses from blanching macules to papules, petechiae, and occasionally ecchymoses. Patients who have recovered from epidemic typhus may retain the organism for an extended period of time, relapsing years later with Brill-Zinsser disease, a milder illness.

Scrub typhus (*O tsutsugamushi*) is a disease transmitted by chiggers and is endemic in Southeast Asia and the southwestern Pacific. The chigger bite results in a papule, enlarging to a bulla that rapidly sloughs, leaving a shallow ulcer. A black crust surrounded by a 1- to 2-cm erythematous, raised circle then forms. At this time, other systemic symptoms begin, at first insidiously with a low-grade fever, headache, chills, and anorexia. Within 5 days, an unremitting fever to 40°C (104°F) and a severe headache are seen in virtually all patients. Generalized lymphadenopathy is the most consistent physical finding, occurring in 80% to 90% of patients. The characteristic rash of scrub typhus is maculopapular and generalized but most apparent on nonexposed skin surfaces.

## RICKETTSIALPOX

Rickettsialpox, a mild infection produced by *Rickettsia akari*, has been reported primarily in New York City, but has been observed in a number of other large cities, especially during periods when large mice populations were being exterminated. Infected mite vectors of *R akari* then attach to human beings, the most available alternative host, and produce disease. Because the skin rash resembles chickenpox, this infectious process was named rickettsialpox. Incubation is estimated at 9 to 14 days as determined by the time period following documented attachment of arthropod vectors. Initially, a red papule appears at the site of the mite bite. This lesion enlarges to form a black eschar, at which time fever is first observed. The rash begins as diffuse nonpruritic macules, progressing to maculopapules and to papulovesicles resembling chickenpox. The palms, soles, and mucous membranes are occasionally involved, but distribution of lesions is quite variable. Fever, chills, and headache persist for about 5 days, but rarely more than 10 days. Upper respiratory and gastrointestinal symptoms are common. Untreated, recovery is still universal, but appropriate antibiotics may shorten duration of symptoms in more severe illness.

## TREATMENT AND PREVENTION OF RICKETTSIAL DISEASE

### TREATMENT

The most important issue when treating rickettsial infections is to avoid delays in treatment. One should not wait for a rash to develop to suspect the diagnosis, nor should one exclude the diagnosis because there is no history of tick bite or based solely on geographic or seasonal reasons. Therapy should be administered when one is clinically suspicious of the infection.

Doxycycline and tetracycline are the antimicrobial agents of choice for most rickettsial infections, and their use should not be delayed in suspected cases regardless of age (Table 289-1). Despite years of intensive education, clinicians in tick-endemic regions still delay in starting empiric antirickettsial therapy. In the past, chloramphenicol was used for children younger than age 9 years because of the side effects (eg, teeth staining) attributed to the use of tetracycline agents. Data now demonstrate that in patients with RMSF, the mortality is higher for those treated with chloramphenicol as compared to those treated with doxycycline. In addition there are data questioning the efficacy of chloramphenicol in the treatment of ehrlichiosis. Regardless of age, children with life-threatening rickettsial illnesses should be treated with doxycycline. The family should be informed of the risks of permanent teeth staining, which appear to be less with doxycycline than tetracycline. The optimal duration of antimicrobial therapy has not been well established for any of the rickettsial diseases because very few comparative clinical trials have examined short-course versus conventional antibiotic management. Patients should, therefore, be managed individually, reserving a briefer course for those with mild illness or for those with a rapid response to therapy. But, as a general approach for more difficult patients, therapy should be continued until patients have been afebrile for 48 to 72 hours and clinically improved.

**TABLE 289-1 AVOIDING DELAY IN TREATING RICKETTSIAL DISEASES**

| |
|---|
| DON'T wait for a rash to develop to suspect the diagnosis. |
| DON'T exclude the diagnosis because there is no history of a tick bite. |
| DON'T exclude the diagnosis solely on geographic or seasonal reasons. |
| DON'T withhold therapy if you are clinically suspicious. |
| DON'T be afraid to use doxycycline at any age for a rickettsial disease. |

Meningococcemia is an important consideration for any toxic patient with a petechial or ecchymotic skin rash. For this reason, empiric therapy often includes coverage for *Neisseria meningitidis* as well as for rickettsial disease. Other pathogens that can produce high fever and petechial rash are enteroviruses, Epstein-Barr virus, group A streptococci, measles virus, and other rickettsiae.

### PREVENTION

Avoidance or control of arthropod vectors remains the first line of defense against rickettsial disease. If high-risk areas cannot be avoided, protective clothing that covers the arms and legs provides an excellent physical barrier to these biting arthropods. Insect repellents for use on the skin such as *N,N*-diethyl-*m*-toluamide (DEET) or picaridin or those used on clothing such as permethrin become important defense mechanisms against ticks. Avoidance of high-risk areas is still the most prudent approach for infants younger than age 1 year because of the potential for systemic reactions with repeated applications of DEET-containing compounds. In general, the higher the DEET concentration in the repellent formulation, the longer the duration of protection; however, this reaches a plateau at about 30% to 35%. DEET and sunscreen combinations are also not recommended because DEET decreases the efficacy of sunscreen, and the recommendations for the use of sunscreen (eg, liberally and often) differ from those of DEET (eg, sparingly and only as required), especially among young children. Although natural-based products such as oil of citronella may have some effects against mosquitoes, the data supporting their use against ticks are lacking.

Ticks must be attached to the human host for at least 6 hours before transmitting the rickettsial organism. Rapid removal of ticks and disinfecting bedding for lice also lessen the possibility of disease transmission. The best method of removing all species of ticks is gentle traction of the attached arthropod using tweezers or similar blunt devices. After removal, the site of attachment should be cleaned with alcohol. Because the risk of transmission of a rickettsial organism following a tick bite is so low, prophylactic antimicrobial agents are not indicated for asymptomatic individuals after a tick bite.

### SUGGESTED READINGS

American Academy of Pediatrics. Rickettsial diseases. In: Kimberlin DW, Brady MT, Jackson MA, Long SS, eds. *Red Book: 2015 Report of the Committee on Infectious Diseases*. 30th ed. Elk Grove Village, IL: American Academy of Pediatrics; 2015:677-680.

Bakken JS, Dumler JS. Human granulocytic anaplasmosis. *Infect Dis North Am*. 2015;29:341-355.

Dahlgren FS, Holman RC, Paddock CD, Callinan LS, McQuiston JH. Fatal Rocky Mountain spotted fever in the United States, 1999-2007. *Am J Trop Med Hyg*. 2012;86:713-719.

Heitman KN, Dahlgren FS, Drexler NA, Massung RF, Behravesh CB. Increasing incidence of ehrlichiosis in the United States: a summary of national surveillance of *Ehrlichia chaffeensis* and *Ehrlichia ewingii* infections in the United States, 2008-2012. *Am J Trop Med Hyg*. 2016;94:52-60.

Folkema AM, Holman RC, McQuiston JH, Cheek JE. Trends in clinical diagnosis of Rocky Mountain spotted fever among American Indians, 2001-2008. *Am J Trop Med Hyg*. 2012;86:152-158.

Green JS, Singh J, Cheung M, Adler-Shohet FC, Ashouri N. A cluster of pediatric endemic typhus cases in Orange County, California. *Pediatr Infect Dis J*. 2011;30:163-165.

Todd SR, Dahlgren FS, Traeger MS, et al. No visible dental staining in children treated with doxycycline for suspected Rocky Mountain spotted fever. *J Pediatr*. 2015;166:1246-1251.

Woods CR. Rocky Mountain spotted fever in children. *Pediatr Clin North Am*. 2013;60:455-470.

Zientek J, Dahlgren FS, McQuiston JH, Regan J. Self-reported treatment practices by healthcare providers could lead to death from Rocky Mountain spotted fever. *J Pediatr*. 2014;164:416-418.



# PART 6 FUNGAL INFECTIONS

## 290 Aspergillosis

Leidy Tovar Padua and Deborah Lehman

### INTRODUCTION

Aspergillosis, caused by any of several species of *Aspergillus*, usually manifests in immunocompromised or debilitated hosts as necrotizing cavitary pulmonary lesions or as hematogenously disseminated foci in multiple organs. *Aspergillus* can also cause a hypersensitivity or allergic pneumonitis in immunocompetent hosts and in patients with chronic pulmonary diseases. This is referred to as allergic bronchopulmonary aspergillosis (ABPA).

### PATHOGENESIS AND EPIDEMIOLOGY

Ubiquitous in nature, *Aspergillus* species are commonly found in soil, in water, and on decaying vegetation. Human exposure to the spores of potentially pathogenic species, particularly *Aspergillus fumigatus*, is unavoidable, yet fungal disease is rare, occurring primarily in immunocompromised hosts. *A fumigatus* has been implicated in most of the disseminated and pulmonary infections, and less common species include *Aspergillus terreus, Aspergillus nidulans, Aspergillus niger*, and *Aspergillus versicolor*. Other pathogenic species have been described recently, such as *Aspergillus lentulus, Neosartorya udagawa*, and *Neosartorya pseudofischeri*. Transmission occurs by inhalation of airborne spores that regularly contaminate the environment; human-to-human transmission or zoonotic transmission has not been documented. Hospital-acquired infections have been described and epidemiologically linked to building demolition and construction, which release fungal spores into the environment. Outbreaks of cutaneous infection have been traced to biomedical devices, such as armboards, contaminated with fungal spores. The primary immune host defense against invasive aspergillosis is the phagocytic function of neutrophils and mononuclear cells. High-risk populations include patients with prolonged neutropenia, those receiving high-dose steroids and/or immunosuppressive agents, stem cell or solid organ transplant recipients, particularly those with graft-versus-host disease, and patients with primary immunodeficiencies and advanced acquired immunodeficiency syndrome (AIDS). There has been a significant increase in the incidence of invasive aspergillosis over the past few decades due to increasing numbers of patients undergoing transplantation, specifically for hematologic malignancies, as well as an increase in the intensity of treatment regimens. Invasive aspergillosis in a patient without underlying disease is infrequent, and an intensive investigation for a predisposing disorder, such as chronic granulomatous disease, should be undertaken.

### CLINICAL MANIFESTATIONS

Infection with *Aspergillus* manifests as 3 distinct syndromes related to host immunocompetence. Two forms of noninvasive aspergillosis are seen in patients with normal or mildly impaired immune systems: pulmonary aspergilloma and ABPA. In contrast, invasive aspergillosis, either local or disseminated disease, affects severely immunosuppressed hosts.

#### Pulmonary Aspergilloma

Pulmonary aspergilloma is the most common form of aspergillosis and occurs when the fungus grows as a dense mass of hyphae and tissue debris within a preexistent cavity caused by a concomitant pulmonary disease such as tuberculosis, lung abscess, or bronchiectasis. A patient with an aspergilloma may be asymptomatic and the lesion noted on incidental radiographic examination; however, an aspergilloma may also lead to life-threatening hemoptysis as a result of invasion of local bronchial blood vessels lining the cavity.

#### Allergic Bronchopulmonary Aspergillosis

ABPA is a hypersensitivity reaction to *A fumigatus* antigens colonizing the respiratory tract of patients with chronic pulmonary disease such as asthma or cystic fibrosis. Recent studies suggest that ABPA occurs in up to 9% of patients with cystic fibrosis and in 7% to 14% of patients with corticosteroid-dependent asthma. Inhalation of fungal spores results in hyphal colonization of the bronchopulmonary tree, leading to mucus plugging, dyspnea, wheezing, and cough. ABPA may eventually lead to large areas of bronchiectasis and systemic inflammation. The pathogenesis of ABPA is not fully understood but most likely results from *Aspergillus*-specific IgE-mediated type I hypersensitivity and an intense Th2 immune response. The sputum of patients with ABPA commonly reveals *Aspergillus* species and eosinophils; pathologic specimens reveal mucoid plugs and granulomatous inflammation, without evidence of tissue invasion.

#### Invasive Aspergillosis

Invasive *Aspergillus* infection can range from locally invasive disease to a disseminated form of disease that occurs in severely immunocompromised patients and is almost always fatal. Pediatric invasive aspergillosis most commonly affects the lungs (59%), followed by the skin and sinuses (10%).

**Invasive Pulmonary Aspergillosis** The most commonly recognized risk factor for invasive pulmonary aspergillosis is prolonged neutropenia. Immunodeficiency such as chronic granulomatous diseases and advanced AIDS are also risk factors for disease. Invasive aspergillosis typically presents as a necrotizing bronchopneumonia with invasion of the pulmonary vessels often accompanied by thrombosis. Widespread embolization to the heart, gastrointestinal tract, skin, kidneys, and

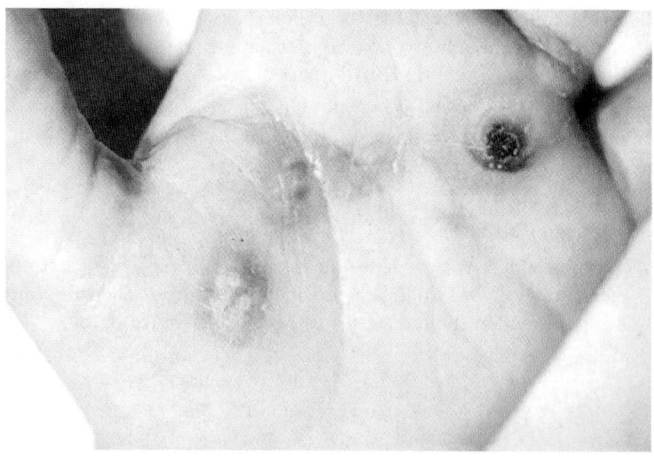

**FIGURE 290-1** Primary cutaneous inoculation with *Aspergillus* from contaminated armboard. (Reproduced with permission from Lichtman MA, Beutler E, Kipps TJ, et al: *Williams Hematology*, 8th ed. New York: McGraw-Hill Education; 2010.)

liver occurs in about one-third of patients. The clinical presentation of invasive aspergillosis is variable, but patients may have prolonged fever and respiratory symptoms, including hemoptysis. Invasion of the central nervous system with occlusion of cerebral vessels may lead to cerebral infarction causing seizures or stupor. The mortality of invasive aspergillosis in children approaches 50% and 90% in those with central nervous system disease or disseminated infection.

**Invasive Fungal Sinusitis** The paranasal sinuses, especially the maxillary sinuses, as well as the external auditory meatus can become colonized by various species of *Aspergillus*. Clinical findings include nasal congestion, fever, facial pain, epistaxis, and ischemia of the palate. If orbital involvement has occurred, facial swelling, proptosis, and cranial nerve abnormalities are suggestive signs. If the individual is immunocompetent, drainage or curettage to define clear margins is usually sufficient treatment. In immunocompromised individuals, the fungus may become invasive, eroding bone and extending into adjacent structures such as the orbit or brain. This complication of *Aspergillus* sinusitis is most commonly seen in patients experiencing a relapse of acute leukemia or in the setting of hematopoietic stem cell transplantation and is much more challenging to control.

**Cutaneous Aspergillosis** Skin and soft tissue infection may result from hematogenous seeding in a highly immunocompromised patient or may be caused by direct invasion of *Aspergillus* spores in contaminated occlusive dressings such as those associated with central venous catheter sites (Fig. 290-1). This direct route of skin infection has been seen in immunocompetent hosts such as burn and trauma patients. It may initially manifest as erythematous macules that develop progressive necrosis or as a cluster of hemorrhagic bullae at sites of intravenous access.

## DIAGNOSIS

### Pulmonary Aspergilloma

Radiologic evidence of a stable single fungal ball in a pulmonary cavity and microbiologic or serologic evidence of *Aspergillus* species in a nonimmunocompromised patient with minimal or no symptoms are considered the diagnostic criteria of pulmonary aspergilloma. Serologic diagnosis of aspergillosis by immunodiffusion and complement fixation tests can be helpful in immunocompetent patients. Precipitins, specific immunoglobulin (Ig) E and IgG antibodies to *Aspergillus* on immunoassay, are reported in more than 90% of aspergillomas and in approximately 70% of ABPA.

### Allergic Bronchopulmonary Aspergillosis

Criteria have been developed to diagnose and classify ABPA. These include a predisposing condition (asthma or cystic fibrosis), elevated serum IgE (typically > 1000 IU/mL), and at least 2 of the following: specific antibodies to *A fumigatus*, radiographic findings consistent with ABPA, and peripheral eosinophilia.

### Invasive Aspergillosis

Sputum can be directly examined for hyphal elements; however, a positive examination must be viewed with caution and interpreted in the context of clinical presentation, as *Aspergillus* can be present in the absence of invasive disease. The diagnosis of invasive aspergillosis in immunocompromised patients is difficult, as the hallmark of disease is tissue invasion, and thus a biopsy is required for definitive diagnosis. A high index of suspicion in severely immunocompromised patients is critical to making a timely diagnosis. Even repeated positive sputum cultures may reflect colonization. Bronchoalveolar lavage (BAL) cultures have approximately 50% sensitivity for focal disease, but are highly predictive of invasive disease when *Aspergillus* is isolated in an immunocompromised patient. In the areas of necrotizing pneumonia, hyphae often can be identified by hematoxylin-eosin stain, but Gomori methenamine silver stain may be necessary to identify typical mycelial structures. The hyphae of *Aspergillus* are 3 to 4 μm in diameter, are septated, and reveal asymmetric dichotomous branching at a 45-degree angle. *Aspergillus* hyphae may be morphologically indistinguishable from other fungi such as *Pseudallescheria boydii* or *Alternaria* species. Sputum and bronchial aspirates should be cultured on Sabouraud dextrose agar.

Chest computed tomography may show surrounding ground-glass infiltrates (halo sign) or a haziness around an area of infiltrate or nodule (air crescent). This represents areas of hemorrhagic infarction as the infection progresses to invade small vessels and is most frequently present early in the course of disease. These signs may be absent in nonneutropenic hosts, and studies have shown that these classic signs of invasive pulmonary aspergillosis are less frequently present in children. More extensive disease may appear as a cavitary lesion or as an area of pulmonary hemorrhage. A large pediatric study found that the most common radiographic presentation of invasive pulmonary aspergillosis was nodules (35%). Only 14.4% of children developed cavitary disease, 6% had a halo sign, and 2% an air crescent sign. Radiographic evidence along with evidence from direct sputum or BAL examination may provide stronger support for the diagnosis, but histopathologic demonstration of invasive hyphae or a positive culture from lung tissue remains the diagnostic gold standard for invasive pulmonary aspergillosis. Because invasive aspergillosis is often rapidly fatal, the finding of hyphal elements or positive cultures from superficial sites such as nasal mucous membranes should prompt a more aggressive search for deep-seated infection (eg, transtracheal aspiration, bronchopulmonary washings, bronchial brush biopsy, and lung biopsy).

Because the patients most at risk for invasive aspergillosis are the ones in whom invasive procedures are most frequently contraindicated, the detection of *Aspergillus* antigens [galactomannan and (1→3)-β-d-glucan] can be useful diagnostic modalities. Galactomannan is a cell wall polysaccharide that is released by the mold during hyphal growth. The assay has proven to be helpful because it can be detected in patients with invasive pulmonary aspergillosis prior to radiographic changes. Galactomannan antigen can be measured in plasma, serum, bronchial fluid, or cerebrospinal fluid. There are several commercial methodologies for detection of galactomannan, but the most sensitive test is an enzyme-linked immunosorbent assay (ELISA)-based method, with sensitivity and specificity of 80.7% and 89.2%, respectively. Lower sensitivity and specificity have been noted in pediatric populations, and sensitivity of this test is lower or almost null in nonneutropenic patients. False-positive results have been seen in patients receiving piperacillin-tazobactam, immunoglobulins, and total parenteral nutrition. False-negative results have been noted in patients receiving antifungal therapy. Cross-reactivity with other fungi (eg, *Penicillium marneffei, Histoplasma capsulatum, Cryptococcus neoformans, Geotrichum* species, *Fusarium* species) has been described. In some specific patient populations, such as high-risk hematopoietic stem cell recipients, biweekly screening for galactomannan by ELISA has been shown to be useful for early diagnosis of invasive disease. β-d-Glucan is a component of the cell wall of most fungi, except for zygomycetes and *Cryptococcus*. This test is also used as a diagnostic tool for invasive fungal infection, although it has variable sensitivities of 55% to 100% and specificities of 71% to 93%, and pediatric data are limited.

Direct detection of *Aspergillus* DNA by polymerase chain reaction (PCR) can be used for early diagnosis of invasive aspergillosis in immunocompromised patients. A multicenter study concluded that sensitivity and specificity of *Aspergillus* PCR were 80% and 81%, respectively. Molecular testing will enable accurate and early diagnosis of invasive aspergillosis in critical patient populations.

## TREATMENT

Patients with aspergillosis require further evaluation and consultation with an infectious diseases specialist. Detailed clinical guidelines on evaluation and management of aspergillosis are available on the Infectious Diseases Society of America Web site (https://www.idsociety.org/Organism/#Aspergillus).

### Pulmonary Aspergilloma

Surgical excision is usually necessary for definitive treatment of an aspergilloma, but often, the risks of surgical intervention outweigh the clinical benefit. A combination of surgical excision and antifungal therapy has been used to manage life-threatening hemoptysis in patients with aspergilloma. Intracavitary instillation of antifungal agents has also been used successfully.

### Allergic Bronchopulmonary Aspergillosis

ABPA involves treating the immunologic response to the *Aspergillus* antigens. Corticosteroids have been the mainstay of treatment, but steroids in combination with antifungal therapy have been demonstrated to improve outcomes. Prednisone is usually initiated at a dose of 0.5 mg/kg/d for 1 to 2 weeks and then given on alternate days for the next 8 weeks. The steroids can then be tapered as symptoms and IgE levels are monitored. A regimen of itraconazole for 16 weeks is commonly used; newer azole agents (voriconazole and posaconazole) have also been used successfully, and antifungal treatment is recommended to reduce the exposure to corticosteroids. Symptomatic improvement followed by recurrence is not uncommon. Small studies have shown that omalizumab, a monoclonal antibody directed against IgE, may benefit patients with poorly controlled asthma or cystic fibrosis and ABPA.

### Invasive Aspergillosis

The mainstay of therapy is early initiation of antifungals upon suspicion for invasive fungal disease. Voriconazole, a triazole, interferes with fungal cell wall formation and is considered first-line therapy for invasive aspergillosis based on adult data, but pharmacokinetics are challenging for pediatric patients younger than 12 years of age where pharmacokinetics are linear rather than nonlinear as is seen in adults. Therapeutic monitoring of levels is critical, and in children < 50 kg, higher voriconazole loading and maintenance dosing are needed. Voriconazole dosing is not defined for children less than 2 years of age; therefore, liposomal amphotericin B is the only agent approved as first-line treatment in this population. Parenteral amphotericin B deoxycholate in high doses of 1.0 to 1.5 mg/kg/d was the standard of care until studies demonstrated that voriconazole was more effective and improved survival in adults with invasive aspergillosis. For fungal rhinosinusitis, amphotericin remains the empiric treatment of choice since voriconazole does not have activity against zygomycete species. Lipid formulations of amphotericin B are less nephrotoxic and are better tolerated at higher doses than amphotericin B deoxycholate. Echinocandin derivatives such as caspofungin, micafungin, and anidulafungin also have anti-*Aspergillus* efficacy but are considered second-line therapeutic agents. Echinocandins act as a noncompetitive inhibitor of an enzyme required for fungal cell wall assembly. This unique mechanism of action makes this new class attractive for synergistic use. Combination antifungal therapy has been suggested for treatment of refractory invasive pulmonary aspergillosis, and combinations of liposomal amphotericin with either voriconazole or an echinocandin have been explored in limited case series and anecdotal clinical reports. Duration of therapy and total optimal dose are not clear, but practice guidelines recommend a period of initial induction therapy during disease stabilization, followed by a period of maintenance therapy until resolution of radiographic changes and completion of immune reconstitution. Surgical resection, in combination with antifungal therapy, is usually necessary in patients with localized aspergillomas, skin and soft tissue infections, sinus infections, and osteomyelitis. Discontinuation or reduction of immunosuppressive therapy is also recommended if possible. Adjunctive therapies such as granulocyte colony-stimulating factor or granulocyte-macrophage colony-stimulating factor are recommended for persistently neutropenic patients; granulocyte transfusions and use of recombinant interferon-γ may be considered for refractory or disseminated disease.

## PREVENTION

Given the high morbidity associated with invasive aspergillosis, an effective prophylactic strategy would be desirable. Randomized trials in adults have demonstrated effectiveness and survival advantage of posaconazole when used for primary chemoprophylaxis; however, pediatric studies are lacking. Multiple regimens have been used in high-risk patients with anecdotal success reported. Secondary prophylaxis is imperative in patients with invasive aspergillosis undergoing further chemotherapy or stem cell transplantation given the high risk of recurrence. The key components to successful identification and treatment of patients with invasive *Aspergillus* infection are a high index of suspicion for infection and empiric antifungal therapy in high-risk patients. Furthermore, highly immunocompromised patients should avoid areas of construction, and the use of high-efficiency air (HEPA) filters has been instituted in many transplantation units. The protective role of surgical masks and N95 respirator masks against mold infections is unknown.

## SUGGESTED READINGS


Elphick HE, Southern KW. Antifungal therapies for allergic bronchopulmonary aspergillosis in people with cystic fibrosis. *Cochrane Database Syst Rev*. 2014;11:CD002204.

Frange P, Bougnoux M-E, Lanternier F, et al. An update on pediatric invasive aspergillosis. *Médecine Mal Infect*. 2015;45:189-198.

Hatipoglu N, Hatipoglu H. Combination antifungal therapy for invasive fungal infections in children and adults. *Expert Rev Anti Infect Ther*. 2013;11:523-535.

Maturu VN, Agarwal R. Prevalence of *Aspergillus* sensitization and allergic bronchopulmonary aspergillosis in cystic fibrosis: systematic review and meta-analysis. *Clin Exp Allergy*. 2015;45:1765-1778.

Molina JR, Serrano J, Sánchez-García J, et al. Voriconazole as primary antifungal prophylaxis in children undergoing allo-SCT. *Bone Marrow Transplant*. 2012;47:562-567.

Patterson TF, Thompson GR 3rd, Denning DW, et al. Practice guidelines for the diagnosis and management of aspergillosis: 2016 update by the Infectious Diseases Society of America. *Clin Infect Dis*. 2016;63:e1-e60.

Reinwald M, Spiess B, Heinz WJ, et al. Aspergillus PCR-based investigation of fresh tissue and effusion samples in patients with suspected invasive aspergillosis enhances diagnostic capabilities. *J Clin Microbiol*. 2013;51:4178-4185.

Tragiannidis A, Roilides E, Walsh TJ, Groll AH. Invasive aspergillosis in children with acquired immunodeficiencies. *Clin Infect Dis*. 2012;54:258-267.

Wattier RL, Dvorak CC, Hoffman JA, et al. A prospective, international cohort study of invasive mold infections in children. *J Pediatr Infect Dis Soc*. 2014;4:1-10.

# 291 Blastomycosis

Nada Harik

## INTRODUCTION

Blastomycosis is a granulomatous fungal infection most commonly caused by *Blastomyces dermatitidis*. A second species, *Blastomyces gilchristii*, has been recently identified from regions in Ontario, Wisconsin, and Minnesota known to be hyperendemic for blastomycosis. Blastomycosis is rare in children, and the infection is often difficult to detect unless considered in the differential diagnosis.

## PATHOGENESIS AND EPIDEMIOLOGY

*Blastomyces* species are thermally dimorphic fungi that exist as a mold in nature and are generally acquired through the inhalation of spores that transform to yeast in the warmer environment of the lungs. Soil exposure is likely necessary to develop blastomycosis. The broad-based budding yeast are typically 8 to 20 μm in diameter. The mycelial phase is characterized by branching septate hyphae that grow as white colonies that eventually turn light brown. Although isolation from natural sources has been very difficult, growth appears to occur in acidic soil in which there is decaying organic matter and high humidity, often in close proximity to rivers and lakes.

The lungs are the usual portal of entry for *B dermatitidis* conidia. Inhaled conidia elicit an inflammatory response characterized by polymorphonuclear leukocytes (PMNs). The few conidia that survive the initial PMN phagocytosis transform to yeast, which are more resistant to phagocytosis by PMNs and alveolar macrophages. Response to the replicating yeast cells results in a mononuclear infiltrate with a granulomatous component. Hematogenous spread of yeast from the lungs may seed any body organ. Development of cell-mediated immunity is believed to be the primary mechanism in prevention of progressive blastomycosis, and lymphocyte reactivity is a marker of specific cellular immunity to *B dermatitidis*.

There is no seasonality to *B dermatitidis* infections, and infections have been reported in all age groups, including newborns. In large surveillance studies of confirmed cases of blastomycosis, pediatric patients compose 3% to 11% of all identified cases. The incubation period from exposure to primary disease is 14 to 106 days (median, 45 days). However, latency with eventual reactivation disease is probable with the finding of newly recognized infection in individuals with no exposure to endemic areas for 3 or more years. Human-to-human transmission is rare.

Cases of blastomycosis are reported from various regions (particularly central Africa), but the vast majority of cases occur in North America. Blastomycosis is most common in the southeastern and south central United States flanking the Ohio and Mississippi River basins, the midwestern United States, the Canadian provinces surrounding the Great Lakes, and areas in Canada and the United States neighboring the Saint Lawrence Seaway. The highest incidence of cases appears to occur in Wisconsin, Minnesota, Mississippi, Kentucky, Tennessee, and Arkansas. In endemic areas, the annual incidence of symptomatic infection is about 1 to 2 per 100,000 population. There are pockets of hyperendemicity, such as northern Wisconsin, where the annual incidence of symptomatic infection may approach 40 per 100,000 population.

Although it is clear that asymptomatic blastomycosis occurs, the distribution and extent have not been determined, because reliable skin tests or seroepidemiologic methods are not available. When careful immunologic studies are performed in outbreaks of blastomycosis, as many as 50% of infected individuals are asymptomatic. Most cases of symptomatic blastomycosis occur sporadically, but there are occasional reports of small outbreaks in communities in which as many as 15 individuals may become infected over a short period of time. The largest reported outbreak involved 55 individuals in Marathon County, Wisconsin, of whom 45% were Hmong. This outbreak suggested that there might be a genetic predisposition to the development of symptomatic blastomycosis.

## CLINICAL MANIFESTATIONS

Pulmonary disease is the most common manifestation of symptomatic blastomycosis. In two 10-year epidemiologic studies of confirmed cases of blastomycosis in Wisconsin and Mississippi (670 and 326 cases, respectively), 75% of the cases involved isolated pulmonary disease. Pulmonary plus extrapulmonary disease occurred in 6% to 16%, whereas isolated extrapulmonary infection occurred in 9% to 18% of cases. In recent studies assessing blastomycosis in children in Manitoba and Wisconsin, pulmonary disease was noted in 79% of children in both studies.

In clinically apparent primary disease with acute pneumonia, onset is typically abrupt, resembling a mild respiratory infection accompanied by low-grade fever, chest pain, and nonproductive cough. These patients are usually detected only in an outbreak situation. As the symptoms increase in severity, spiking fevers, productive cough, and pleuritic chest pain develop. Spontaneous resolution of acute pulmonary blastomycosis is described. Subacute or chronic pneumonia may occur with low-grade fever, productive cough, hemoptysis, weakness, anorexia, and weight loss resembling adult reactivation tuberculosis. Rarely, the illness may be fulminant and resemble acute respiratory distress syndrome. Mortality in such cases may be greater than 50%.

Disseminated blastomycosis is caused by hematogenous spread of the infection from the lungs to other areas of the body. Extrapulmonary disease is often seen in addition to pulmonary infection. Most frequently, extrapulmonary disease involves cutaneous and subcutaneous tissues as well as bone, the central nervous system, and the urogenital tract (only in adults). Cutaneous lesions, the most common extrapulmonary manifestation, initially appear as benign, papulopustular verrucous nodules with a raised irregular border often with crusting and some drainage from an underlying abscess. Lesions may also become ulcerative. The borders are usually sharp and heaped up, and the base commonly contains exudate. As the lesion extends peripherally, the central area heals, leaving a soft, atrophic scar. Osteomyelitis, with lytic bone lesions, is the second most common extrapulmonary infection. The vertebrae, pelvis, sacrum, skull, ribs, and long bones have been reported most frequently, but essentially, any bone may be involved. Granulomatous lesions of the liver and spleen are found in more than 40% of patients with disseminated disease, and the kidneys, prostate, epididymis, bladder, and testes may be involved, causing dysuria, pyuria, and hematuria. Central nervous system (CNS) involvement is rare, especially in immunocompetent individuals. Infection of the CNS may manifest as meningitis, but more commonly, it presents as an epidural or intracranial abscess. Blastomycosis may affect nearly every organ system, and infection has been reported in lymph nodes, eyes, and retropharyngeal soft tissue.

Mortality from blastomycosis is dependent upon age, immune state of the host, and the type of presenting illness. Adults older than age 65 years have a mortality rate from blastomycosis 10 times or greater than that of children. Although a rare infection in immunocompromised hosts when compared to histoplasmosis, cryptococcosis, and coccidioidomycosis, blastomycosis has been documented to cause severe and often fatal infections in patients with many forms of immune deficiency, including those with acquired immunodeficiency syndrome (AIDS), transplantation patients, or patients receiving therapy with corticosteroids and/or tumor necrosis factor-α inhibitors. Regardless of the underlying disorder, blastomycosis in immunocompromised hosts is usually an aggressive disease, often presenting with disseminated, multiple-organ involvement and high, early mortality.

## DIAGNOSIS

Although patients may present to a physician early in the course of infection, diagnosis is often delayed more than 30 days. Typically, patients receive 1 or more courses of antibiotics for bacterial pneumonia before blastomycosis is considered. Clinical diagnosis must be confirmed by laboratory studies, which include microscopic examination of smears, scrapings, aspirates, sputum, and bronchoscopic washings for the characteristic yeast, along with fungal culture. A presumptive diagnosis of blastomycosis can be made by visualization of the classic yeast form of *Blastomyces* in clinical specimens. Calcofluor white or 10% potassium hydroxide (KOH) is used for direct microscopic examination of a multitude of clinical specimens including sputum, skin scrapings, and cerebrospinal fluid (CSF). In biopsy specimens, caseous necrosis usually is absent. Cutaneous lesions typically reveal pseudoepitheliomatous hyperplasia and budding yeasts in pyogranulomas that are characteristic and pathognomonic. In hematoxylin-eosin tissue sections, one may find the characteristic yeast cells with a thick, double-refractive cell wall, but they may be difficult to see. Therefore, routine use should be made of special stains for fungi such as the periodic acid-Schiff and Gomori methenamine silver stain. Characteristics such as yeast size and single broad-based buds help to differentiate *Blastomyces* from *Histoplasma* and *Cryptococcus*.

Definitive diagnosis is made by culture. Cultures of sputum as well as bronchoscopic washings have a high yield in adults. The infected material should be spread on the surface of Sabouraud dextrose agar slants and incubated at room temperature or 30°C (86°F). The yeast phase may be obtained in culture by inoculating glucose blood agar medium and incubating at 37°C (98.6°F). Growth occurs in 1 to 4 weeks. A commercially available molecular DNA probe may be used to confirm the identity of mold growing in culture as *B dermatitidis*. Of note, the DNA probe cannot differentiate between *B dermatitidis* and *B gilchristii*. Polymerase chain reaction followed by sequence analysis is used to differentiate these species.

Given their poor sensitivity and specificity, serologic methods such as complement fixation, immunodiffusion, and enzyme-linked immunosorbent assay (EIA) tests usually are not helpful for diagnosing blastomycosis. The detection of a *B dermatitidis* antigen by EIA on urine, serum, bronchoscopic washings, and CSF is commercially available and has a high overall sensitivity (93%). However, the specificity of the antigen test is poor (79%) due to cross-reactivity with antigens of other fungi, particularly *Histoplasma*. Antigen levels decline with treatment of blastomycosis and may be used to monitor response to therapy.

Radiographic studies of the chest vary widely; there is no characteristic feature of blastomycosis that allows easy differentiation from other pulmonary infections. In acute cases, parenchymal infiltrates, lobar or segmental consolidation, and interstitial infiltrates have all been described. Small pleural effusions occur commonly. In the more chronic form of disease, air-space and interstitial infiltrates are seen, but mass-like infiltrates, pulmonary nodules, and cavitation are more common. Hilar lymphadenitis occurs in ≤ 10% of cases.

## TREATMENT

The prognosis for pulmonary or disseminated blastomycosis is generally good with appropriate therapy. Untreated, widely disseminated disease always has a poor prognosis. A clinical practice guideline for the management of blastomycosis is available from the Infectious Diseases Society of America. The initial treatment of choice for life-threatening or severe blastomycosis is a lipid formulation of amphotericin B. After an induction phase of treatment and noticeable improvement, therapy can be transitioned to itraconazole. A lipid formulation of amphotericin B is also the initial treatment choice for CNS blastomycosis. The preferred step-down therapy for CNS blastomycosis is voriconazole. Itraconazole is the treatment of choice for mild to moderate blastomycosis. Itraconazole serum levels should be checked after 2 weeks of itraconazole therapy. The overall treatment course for blastomycosis is generally 6 to 12 months depending on the severity of infection and the site of infection. Treatment of CNS blastomycosis and blastomycosis in immunocompromised individuals may require life-long suppressive therapy.

## SUGGESTED READINGS


Anderson EJ, Ahn PB, Yogev R, Jaggi P, Shippee DB, Shulman ST. Blastomycosis in children: a study of 14 cases. *J Pediatr Infect Dis Soc*. 2013;2:386-390.

Brown EM, McTaggart LR, Zhang SX, Low DE, Stevens DA, Richardson SE. Phylogenetic analysis reveals a cryptic species *Blastomyces gilchristii*, sp. nov. within the human pathogenic fungus *Blastomyces dermatitidis*. *PLoS One*. 2013;8:e59237.

Castillo CG, Kauffman CA, Miceli MH. Blastomycosis. *Infect Dis Clin North Am*. 2016;30:247-264.

Chapman SW, Dismukes WE, Proia LA, et al. Clinical practice guidelines for the management of blastomycosis: 2008 update by the Infectious Diseases Society of America. *Clin Infect Dis*. 2008;46:1801-1812.

Fanella S, Skinner S, Trepman E, Embil JM. Blastomycosis in children and adolescents: a 30-year experience from Manitoba. *Med Mycol*. 2011;49:627-632.

Frost HM, Anderson J, Ivacic L, Meece J. Blastomycosis in children: an analysis of clinical, epidemiologic, and genetic features. *J Pediatr Infect Dis Soc*. 2017;6(1):49-56.

Smith JA, Gauthier G. New developments in blastomycosis. *Semin Respir Crit Care Med*. 2015;36:715-728.


# 292 *Candida*

Katherine M. Knapp

## INTRODUCTION

*Candida* species are yeast forms that are ubiquitous in nature and frequent colonizers of human skin and mucous membranes of the gastrointestinal, respiratory, and female genital tracts. *Candida* species are the most common cause of human fungal infections, although they rarely cause invasive disease in the absence of mucosal barrier disruption or compromised immune systems. Only a small number of the more than 150 species of *Candida* that have been described are considered to be pathogenic. There are at least 15 *Candida* species associated with human disease, but most invasive infections are due to 5 pathogens: *C albicans*, *C glabrata*, *C tropicalis*, *C parapsilosis*, and *C krusei*. Historically, *C albicans* has accounted for the majority of invasive infections, but in more recent reports, non-*albicans* species have been isolated in half or more of the cases. In addition, the incidence of infections due to *C albicans* isolates that are resistant to azole antifungals is increasing. This changing epidemiology has implications for appropriate treatment of antifungal-resistant *Candida* infections.

## PATHOGENESIS AND EPIDEMIOLOGY

*Candida* species are part of the normal human flora of the skin and mucous membranes. The incidence of colonization with *Candida* species depends on host characteristics such as age and overall health. Neonates are frequently colonized with *Candida* species, and localized oropharyngeal candidiasis (thrush) is not uncommon in this population. Hospitalized and ill children are more frequently colonized than are healthy children. *Candida* species have relatively low virulence factors compared to other organisms and, therefore, rarely cause disease in the normal host. For candidiasis to occur, the host must have impaired resistance to disease, the number of yeast organisms must be high, or both.

Neonates and pregnant women have impaired host resistance to *Candida* species, as do patients with immunodeficiencies (congenital or acquired), induced immunosuppression (due to chemotherapy or corticosteroids), or debilitation (secondary to trauma or surgery). Advances in health care that have decreased mortality for preterm newborns and oncology patients have been associated also with changes in host defense and normal flora, which have in turn led to a larger population at risk for invasive *Candida* infection. These at-risk populations frequently receive multiple and long-term courses of medications, particularly antimicrobials (altering the normal flora), and have defects in mucosal or skin barriers (such as chemotherapy-induced mucositis or the presence of indwelling intravascular catheters), which puts them at high risk for development of candidiasis.

Invasive candidiasis includes candidemia and deep-seated infection. Deep-seated infection usually results from candidemia but may occur through direct inoculation (eg, leaky surgical anastomosis leading to peritonitis). Candidemia is frequently due to translocation of *Candida* species in the gut into the bloodstream. In patients with indwelling central venous catheters, *Candida* species introduced to the bloodstream from the gut or skin colonize the catheter and form a biofilm, which will then persistently release *Candida* into the bloodstream. Candidemia may lead to secondary infections throughout the body, which may in turn cause secondary candidemias.

*Candida* species are the third or fourth most common cause of healthcare-associated bloodstream infections in children in the United States. In recent pediatric studies, *C albicans* accounted for approximately 45% of cases. *C parapsilosis* is the second most common pathogen in pediatrics, accounting for 20% to 25% of bloodstream infections, in both neonates and older children.

## CLINICAL MANIFESTATIONS

Candidiasis may be broadly divided into 2 categories: mucocutaneous infections and invasive disease. Mucocutaneous infection includes involvement of the oropharynx, gastrointestinal tract, female genital tract, skin, and nails. Invasive disease includes candidemia and deep-seated infection due to hematogenous spread or direct inoculation.

### Oropharyngeal and Gastrointestinal Tract Candidiasis

Thrush, almost exclusively the result of *C albicans*, is the most common type of candidiasis in infants and children and is not uncommon in infants up to age 5 months. Thrush may be seen in older infants or children who are receiving antibiotic therapy but are otherwise healthy. Recurrent or recalcitrant thrush in children not receiving antibiotic therapy should prompt an evaluation of the immune system.

The lesions of thrush appear most commonly as pearly white patches on the dorsal and lateral aspects of the tongue, pharynx, gingivae, and buccal mucosa. These patches coalesce into plaques that cause punctate bleeding when removed from the mucosal surface. Removal of the patches by scraping with a tongue depressor reveals an erythematous, eroded base.

Other oropharyngeal infections include acute atrophic candidiasis (glossitis) and angular cheilitis (perlèche). Glossitis usually occurs following the use of broad-spectrum antibiotics that alter the oral bacterial flora. Papillae on the dorsum of the tongue are eroded, which results in a smooth and erythematous tongue that is often painful. This condition typically resolves with discontinuation of the antibiotics. Angular cheilitis (perlèche) is characterized by painful fissuring and erythema at the corners of the mouth, due to habitual licking, although it may also be seen in individuals with iron deficiency or vitamin $B_{12}$ or folate deficiency or in children with poor oral secretion control. Treatment with topical antifungals and/or steroids is useful in persistent cases.

Esophageal candidiasis typically presents with dysphagia. Children may also have nausea or vomiting, and esophagitis may be manifested in infants by decreased oral intake. Esophagitis may occur without oropharyngeal candidiasis.

Although diarrhea and abdominal pain have been reported in patients with *Candida* species recovered from their stool, it is not clear whether symptoms are the result of *Candida* infection or other cause, such as effects of chemotherapy. *Candida* infection may play a role in typhlitis. Gastrointestinal *Candida* lesions are common in immunocompromised pediatric patients and are frequently found at autopsy.

### Vulvovaginitis

Vaginitis caused by *C albicans* occurs commonly and is not necessarily indicative of immunosuppression. Vaginal candidiasis is more frequent in women who are pregnant or taking oral contraceptives. *Candida* vaginitis is characterized by pruritus and a white or watery discharge. The vaginal mucosa is erythematous with white lesions like those seen in thrush. Candidiasis also may also cause papular or ulcerative lesions of the perineum. Penile lesions due to *Candida* species are uncommon, even in sexual partners of women with vaginal candidiasis.

### Cutaneous Candidiasis

Cutaneous candidiasis involves moist areas, such as the perineum and intertriginous areas (eg, gluteal folds, neck, axillae). Infants who suck their fingers may develop sucking blisters, and infection of the nails (onychia) or around the nails (paronychia) may also occur. Paronychia resulting from *Candida* species also may follow other trauma to the nail or surrounding tissue. *Candida* is associated with chronic paronychia, characterized by swollen, erythematous, and tender nail folds, which may occur episodically. Chronic infection may lead to thickening and discoloration of the nail beds.

### Candidemia and Disseminated Infection

Candidemia may represent evidence of disseminated or deep-seated infection, result from hematogenous seeding from the gastrointestinal or urinary tract, or be a transient finding associated with an intravascular catheter. The source of the infection may be difficult to determine, and therefore, candidemia should be treated aggressively with systemic antifungal therapy. Most immunocompromised patients with candidemia will have disseminated disease.

Candidemia that is intravascular and catheter-related may be distinguished from other etiologies by comparison of simultaneous blood cultures drawn from all lumens of the catheter and from a peripheral stick. Candidemia may be said to be catheter-related if the colony count from a culture drawn through a catheter lumen is 10 times that of a culture drawn peripherally. Catheter-related infections resulting from *Candida* species are associated with biofilm formation, which makes treatment very difficult without removing the catheter. It is recommended that intravascular catheters be removed immediately if feasible in all cases of catheter-related candidemia.

In most cases of disseminated candidiasis, the infection is concentrated in 2 or 3 areas, with the lungs, kidneys, liver, spleen, and brain being the organs most commonly affected. Clinical manifestations will depend on the sites and extent of *Candida* infection.

A maculopapular rash in an immunocompromised patient with *Candida* infection is often associated with disseminated disease. The skin lesions that have been described in patients with hematologic malignancies are typically discrete erythematous papules measuring 0.5 to 1.0 cm in diameter, which may have a nodular center. Biopsy of the skin lesions may be necessary for definitive diagnosis in order to exclude other infectious etiologies in an immunocompromised host. Cutaneous lesions also are frequent findings in neonates with disseminated disease: up to half of all neonates have diffuse erythroderma or vesiculopustules.

All neonates with candidemia should be evaluated for disseminated disease. Central nervous system disease may occur in up to one-third of neonates with candidemia. Evaluation of infected neonates should include examination and culture of cerebrospinal fluid (CSF), head ultrasound, ophthalmologic evaluation, and echocardiogram.

### Hepatosplenic Candidiasis

Hepatosplenic candidiasis is seen in patients with hematologic malignancies. Patients may have fever, abdominal pain, and elevation of liver function tests following recovery of neutropenia. Contrast-enhanced computed tomography (CT) is the usual diagnostic imaging modality and is recommended for follow-up evaluations. Biopsy of lesions is frequently nondiagnostic.

### Central Nervous System Candidiasis

Central nervous system (CNS) candidiasis is usually seen with other findings of disseminated candidiasis and frequently occurs along with cardiac candidiasis. *Candida* species may cause a wide variety of CNS findings, including meningitis, vasculitis, thrombosis, mycotic aneurysm, demyelination, abscesses, nodules, and noncaseating granulomas. Patients with CNS candidiasis may not have neurologic findings. *Candida* meningitis is more frequent in preterm newborns and may present as respiratory decompensation. Blood cultures are likely to be sterile, and many patients will not have CSF findings indicative of CNS involvement. All neonates with disseminated disease should have CSF examination and head ultrasound.

In one series of pediatric oncology patients, 11 of 12 cases of *Candida* meningitis were the result of *C tropicalis*, all of which were fatal. In that report, duration of profound neutropenia with fever, antibiotic therapy, and administration of total parenteral nutrition (TPN) were significantly associated with *Candida* meningitis.

#### Ophthalmic Candidiasis

Careful routine ophthalmic examination should be performed in all patients with candidemia or other evidence of disseminated candidiasis. Retinitis is a frequent finding in low-birth-weight neonates with disseminated candidiasis. The typical findings are fluffy white chorioretinal lesions that may extend to the vitreous. Patients may complain of eye pain, blurred vision, or photophobia. Severely neutropenic patients with retinal involvement may not show evidence of retinal lesions; therefore, it is vital to perform ophthalmic examination in these patients following resolution of neutropenia. All neonates with disseminated disease should have an ophthalmologic examination.

#### Cardiac Candidiasis

*Candida* species may cause disease in any part of the heart. Two-thirds of cases of fungal endocarditis are the result of *Candida* species. *Candida* endocarditis is associated with signs and symptoms similar to those seen with subacute bacterial endocarditis, and blood cultures are usually sterile. Vegetations and emboli resulting from *Candida* infection are usually large and may occlude vessels. *Candida* endocarditis is usually associated with systemic candidiasis and indwelling central venous catheters. Valvular involvement usually affects the aortic and mitral valves and may be difficult to visualize by 2-dimensional echocardiography. *Candida* infection of the myocardium may manifest as nonspecific electrocardiographic findings, including QRS changes and marked T-wave changes.

Cardiac candidiasis frequently occurs with CNS involvement; therefore, examination of CSF and performance of CT or magnetic resonance imaging (MRI) of the brain are indicated in all cases of cardiac candidiasis. All neonates with disseminated disease should have an echocardiogram performed.

#### Respiratory Tract Candidiasis

Because *Candida* species are known colonizers of respiratory tract mucosa, their presence in respiratory specimen cultures does not necessarily indicate infection. Candidiasis may affect any site within the respiratory tract and may be associated with oropharyngeal candidiasis.

Laryngeal candidiasis has been reported in HIV-infected children and children receiving immunosuppressive chemotherapy who had oropharyngeal candidiasis and hoarseness. It has also been reported in children receiving inhaled corticosteroids. Laryngeal candidiasis should be considered in any immunosuppressed child with a hoarse cry or voice. Laryngoscopy will reveal the typical white plaques on the vocal cords of these patients.

Bronchial candidiasis occurs rarely and is typically associated with pulmonary parenchymal and systemic disease. Pulmonary candidiasis may manifest as localized pneumonia, diffuse infiltrates, nodular lesions, abscesses, or empyema. The clinical presentation of pulmonary disease is nonspecific, usually characterized by fever and tachypnea. Because recovery of *Candida* species from sputum or bronchial washings may signify only colonization, definitive diagnosis of pulmonary disease requires an invasive procedure such as lung biopsy to demonstrate organisms in tissue specimens.

In addition to causing invasive disease, *Candida* species within the respiratory tract may elicit an allergic response. Polysaccharide and protein extracts of *C albicans* have been shown to trigger exacerbations in asthmatic patients.

#### Musculoskeletal Candidiasis

*Candida* arthritis is usually diagnosed in association with systemic candidiasis and most commonly involves the knee. Joint infection is due to direct inoculation or hematogenous spread and may be associated with a contiguous osteomyelitis. Arthritis in the absence of systemic infection has been reported following prosthetic arthroplasty.

Reported anatomic sites of *Candida* osteomyelitis include the spine, upper and lower extremities, ribs and costochondral junctions, mandible, and sternum. Many *Candida* osteomyelitis cases that have been reported were in neonates or infants younger than age 14 weeks, in whom the lower extremities are the most frequent site of involvement. The axial skeleton is more frequently involved in adults. Multifocal involvement is common, so imaging should be performed to assess for other sites of infection.

#### Peritoneal Candidiasis

*Candida* peritonitis may result from peritoneal dialysis, intestinal surgery, or bowel perforation. As with other causes of peritonitis, abdominal distention, fever, and vomiting may occur. Because the clinical features cannot distinguish fungal from bacterial peritonitis, diagnosis must be made by microbiological examination and culture of peritoneal fluid. Compared to adults, pediatric dialysis patients who develop *Candida* peritonitis usually have more favorable outcomes. Prior antibiotic use, preceding bacterial peritonitis, and infection due to gram-negative organisms are risk factors for development of fungal peritonitis.

#### Candidiasis of the Urinary Tract

The presence of *Candida* in voided urine specimens, even at high colony counts, is not always indicative of urinary tract infection. However, candiduria is frequently seen in patients with urinary tract candidiasis. Candiduria in neonates or neutropenic patients warrants further evaluation for systemic or upper urinary tract disease. Candiduria may be a manifestation of obstructive uropathy ("fungus balls" in the calyces), which may be seen by renal ultrasound or computed tomography. Obstructive uropathy owing to *Candida* species may be seen in patients with indwelling urinary catheters or who have received prolonged antibiotic therapy. *Candida* species may also cause renal microabscesses and papillary necrosis.

Candiduria is often asymptomatic, but *Candida* cystitis may present with dysuria or urethritis, similar to manifestations of bacterial urinary tract infection. White plaques may be seen at the urethral meatus or by cystoscopy on the bladder mucosa. Diabetics and patients with indwelling urinary catheters or receiving prolonged antimicrobial therapy are at risk for development of *Candida* cystitis.

## DIAGNOSIS

Definitive diagnosis of invasive candidiasis entails isolation of *Candida* from a normally sterile body site or a positive tissue biopsy. Negative blood cultures do not exclude invasive disease in immunocompromised patients. The sensitivity of blood culture is about 50%. Direct microscopic examination of specimens mounted in 10% to 20% potassium hydroxide (KOH) or prepared with calcofluor white, Gram, or fluorescent antibody stains will reveal budding yeast cells and/or pseudohyphae. On solid media such as Sabouraud dextrose agar, *Candida* species appear as moist, white, or cream-colored colonies with well-demarcated borders. *C albicans* will produce germ tubes when suspended in serum for a period of 1 to 4 hours, which allows for rapid presumptive identification of this *Candida* species. *Candida* species are definitively identified by biochemical tests of fermentation and assimilation.

There are many new molecular diagnostic tests for candidiasis. The most widely used of these is the β-D-glucan assay, which tests for a component of the fungal cell wall that is not present in mammalian cells. This assay does not distinguish *Candida* species from other fungi and is limited by the false-positive rate among patients most at risk. False-positive β-D-glucan assays may result from hemodialysis, bacterial infections, human blood products, or certain antibiotics (amoxicillin-clavulanate or piperacillin-tazobactam), among many other causes. *Candida* mannan combined antigen-antibody testing has been used in Europe in the diagnosis of culture-negative hepatosplenic and other invasive candidiasis. Many institutions have developed in-house polymerase chain reaction (PCR) testing for *Candida*. PCR studies are limited by the lack of standardized methodologies. Recently, the US Food and Drug Administration approved the T2 Candida Panel (T2 Biosystems, Lexington, MA), which detects *Candida* DNA by PCR and T2 magnetic resonance, which appears promising in early studies. PCR testing offers advantages over other molecular diagnostics by allowing for the potential of species identification and identification of drug resistance.

## TREATMENT

Most mucocutaneous *Candida* infections may be treated topically, with nystatin or azoles. Esophagitis and urinary tract infection may be treated with oral azoles. There are several intravenous antifungals available for treatment of candidemia and deep-seated candidiasis.

Initial therapy for invasive disease prior to identification/susceptibility testing of the organism should be with an echinocandin (eg, caspofungin, micafungin, anidulafungin) or an amphotericin B product (standard amphotericin B deoxycholate or lipid formulations). Echinocandins and amphotericin B are effective against most species of *Candida*. Fluconazole is not appropriate empiric therapy because *C krusei* isolates are resistant to fluconazole, and *C glabrata* isolates are frequently resistant. Other azoles may be considered but often are ineffective for *C glabrata* as well. Some isolates of *C parapsilosis* have decreased susceptibility to echinocandins, but this is of uncertain significance, as *C parapsilosis* infections have been treated effectively with echinocandins despite in vitro resistance. *C lusitaniae* is resistant to amphotericin B, as are some isolates of *C glabrata* and *C krusei*. Amphotericin B products and echinocandins are fungicidal, whereas fluconazole is fungistatic.

### Neonates

Because neonates are more likely to have meningitis as a manifestation of candidiasis, even though up to 50% will have negative blood cultures, amphotericin B deoxycholate is the treatment of choice for any neonate with disseminated disease. Flucytosine is not recommended routinely in addition to amphotericin B deoxycholate in neonates due to toxicity risks and difficulty attaining therapeutic levels, but may be considered as adjunctive therapy in recalcitrant cases. Lipid formulations of amphotericin B have been associated with poorer outcomes in neonates.

### Oropharyngeal and Gastrointestinal Tract Candidiasis

Thrush usually can be treated topically with nystatin or clotrimazole. Systemic therapy may be indicated for immunocompromised patients or in cases refractory to topical therapy. Fluconazole is usually effective therapy in this case, but there is an increasing incidence of non-*albicans* species and azole-resistant *C albicans* isolates that may require alternate therapies.

It is important to address sites that may be colonized with *Candida* to effectively treat thrush in infants. Nystatin may be applied to skin that has sustained contact with the infant's mouth, such as the mother's nipple for breastfed infants or the fingers of infants who habitually suck them. Bottle nipples, pacifiers, or other objects with sustained contact with the infant's mouth should be boiled after each use.

*Candida* esophagitis is treated with oral fluconazole in those who can tolerate oral therapy. Other oral azoles (eg, itraconazole, voriconazole, posaconazole) may be options for fluconazole-resistant *Candida*. Treatment should be for a minimum of 14 to 21 days. Suppressive therapy with fluconazole is recommended for patients with recurrent esophagitis.

### Vulvovaginitis

Vaginal candidiasis may be effectively treated topically. Topical azoles (eg, miconazole, clotrimazole) are often more effective than nystatin. A single 150-mg dose of oral fluconazole has been shown to be an effective option in adolescents and adults. Oral azoles also are options for patients with recurrent or refractory vulvovaginitis.

### Cutaneous Candidiasis

Skin infections may usually be treated effectively with nystatin. Miconazole and clotrimazole are other commonly used options. There are many other topical antifungals available, many of which are significantly more expensive than nystatin.

### Candidemia and Disseminated Infection

Treatment for uncomplicated candidemia should be for 2 weeks from the first negative blood culture, assuming resolution of clinical manifestations. Persistent candidemia occurs frequently in neonates: blood cultures may remain positive for several days after beginning antifungal therapy, and up to 10% may have fungemia for 14 or more days.

Intravascular catheters should be removed as soon as feasible in neonates and nonneutropenic children with candidemia. Delaying removal of catheters more than 1 day after initiating antifungal therapy is associated with increased neurodevelopmental impairment and mortality in neonates. Prompt removal of intravascular catheters should be considered in neutropenic children. The recommendation for removal is not as strong for neutropenic patients, because candidemia is frequently due to gastrointestinal translocation and it may be difficult to adequately assess whether the infection is catheter related, and lack of intravenous access may significantly complicate primary disease therapy in these patients. It is not recommended to immediately replace a catheter over a wire at the same site. Shorter courses of antifungal treatment may be considered in patients with clearance of candidemia following catheter removal if the patient is not immunosuppressed and there is no concern about disseminated disease.

### Hepatosplenic Candidiasis

Treatment should continue until radiographic resolution of lesions. Chemotherapy and/or hematopoietic stem cell transplant does not have to be delayed due to hepatosplenic candidiasis, but antifungal treatment should continue through the periods of neutropenia, in order to prevent relapse. There is some evidence that hepatosplenic candidiasis represents an immune reconstitution syndrome, and therefore, steroids or other anti-inflammatory drugs may be appropriate in some patients, although this has not been well studied.

### Central Nervous System Candidiasis

The combination of an amphotericin B product and flucytosine is the recommended treatment for CNS candidiasis, except for neonates, who should be treated with amphotericin B deoxycholate alone. The addition of flucytosine is recommended beyond the neonatal period because it penetrates the CSF readily, whereas amphotericin B does not. Flucytosine should never be used as monotherapy. Intraventricular administration of amphotericin B is severely toxic and should be an option of last resort. Fluconazole and other azoles have excellent penetration into the CSF, but experience with these agents is limited for *Candida* meningitis.

### Peritoneal Candidiasis

Fluconazole is the recommended agent for first-line therapy in pediatric patients with *Candida* peritonitis related to dialysis. The dialysis catheter should be removed, but there is disagreement about the timing of removal. Data support an option of removing the catheter early, but not immediately, in order to provide peritoneal lavage with fluconazole to help prevent peritoneal adhesions.

### Candidiasis of the Urinary Tract

Isolated candiduria can be treated with a 7-day course of oral fluconazole. Bladder irrigations with amphotericin B (50 μg/mL sterile water) have been used, but as this is not systemic treatment, it is not a recommended therapy. Recurrence is common, and serial urine cultures should be performed to document clearance. Urinary catheters should be removed or replaced as soon as possible in patients diagnosed with candidiasis. For patients with evidence of renal or other systemic *Candida* infection, prolonged intravenous therapy is indicated. Lipid formulations of amphotericin B are not recommended for urinary tract infections because of their decreased renal excretion.

## PREVENTION

Prophylactic antifungal therapy has been shown to reduce the incidence of *Candida* infections in very-low-birth-weight infants (< 1500 g), who are at particular risk. Fluconazole prophylaxis (3–6 mg/kg/dose orally or intravenously twice weekly for 6 weeks) is recommended for extremely low-birth-weight infants (< 1000 g) in nurseries with high rates (> 10%) of invasive candidiasis. Empiric antifungal therapy may be considered when sepsis is suspected in neonates who are extremely premature, who have indwelling catheters, or who have been receiving broad-spectrum antibiotics. Prophylactic antifungal therapy is routinely used in children undergoing hematopoietic stem cell transplantation or myelosuppressive chemotherapy.

## SUGGESTED READINGS


American Academy of Pediatrics. Candidiasis. In: Kimberlin DW, Brady MT, Jackson MA, Long SS, eds. *Red Book: 2015 Report of the Committee on Infectious Diseases*. 30th ed. Elk Grove Village, IL: American Academy of Pediatrics; 2015:275-280.

Castanheira M, Messer SA, Rhomberg PR, Pfaller MA. Antifungal susceptibility patterns of a global collection of fungal isolates: results of the SENTRY Antifungal Surveillance Program (2013). *Diagn Microbiol Infect Dis*. 2016;85:200-204.

Cleveland AA, Harrison LH, Farley MM, et al. Declining incidence of candidemia and the shifting epidemiology of *Candida* resistance in two US metropolitan areas, 2008-2013: results from population-based surveillance. *PLoS One*. 2015;10:e0120452.

Dutta A, Palazzi DL. *Candida* non-*albicans* versus *Candida albicans* fungemia in the non-neonatal pediatric population. *Pediatr Infect Dis J*. 2011;30:664-668.

Ericson JE, Kaufman DA, Kicklighter SD, et al. Fluconazole prophylaxis for the prevention of candidiasis in premature infants: a meta-analysis using patient-level data. *Clin Infect Dis*. 2016;63:604-610.

Fisher BT, Vendetti N, Bryan M, et al. Central venous catheter retention and mortality in children with candidemia: a retrospective cohort analysis. *J Pediatric Infect Dis Soc*. 2015;pii:piv048.

Kullberg BJ, Arendrup MC. Invasive candidiasis. *N Engl J Med*. 2015; 373:1445-1456.

Pappas PG, Kauffman CA, Andes DR, et al. Clinical practice guideline for the management of candidiasis: 2016 update by the Infectious Diseases Society of America. *Clin Infect Dis*. 2016;62:e1-e50.

Steinbach WJ, Roilides E, Berman D, et al. Results from a prospective, international, epidemiologic study of invasive candidiasis in children and neonates. *Pediatr Infect Dis J*. 2012;31:1252-1257.

Tragiannidis A, Tsoulas C, Groll AH. Invasive candidiasis and candidaemia in neonates and children: update on current guidelines. *Mycoses*. 2015;58:10-21.


# 293 Coccidioidomycosis

Ketzela J. Marsh and Mark R. Schleiss

## INTRODUCTION

Coccidioidomycosis is the infection caused by the dimorphic fungi *Coccidioides immitis* or *Coccidioides posadasii*. Although it was initially believed that coccidioidomycosis was an invariably lethal infection, by the mid-1930s, it was recognized that the organism was in fact responsible for a very common, acute, and generally self-limited disease that was known as the San Joaquin Valley fever. In regions where coccidioidomycosis is endemic, Valley fever continues to be an important public health problem. In addition, coccidioidomycosis has emerged in recent years as an important cause of disease in immunocompromised patients, particularly those with human immunodeficiency virus (HIV) infection.

## PATHOGENESIS AND EPIDEMIOLOGY

The life cycle of *Coccidioides* species is complex and demonstrates 2 distinct phases: a saprophytic (vegetative) phase and a parasitic phase. In soil, the organism grows as a mycelium, with branching septated hyphae. As they mature, the mycelia develop rectangular spores (arthroconidia); at this stage, the hyphae become very fragile, and arthroconidia easily become airborne. When inhaled into the lungs (it appears that a single spore can cause disease), the arthroconidia begin the parasitic phase, and spherules form. Spherules are round, double-walled structures that reproduce by formation of spherical internal spores, termed endospores. A single spherule may produce thousands of endospores, and as the spherule ruptures, each endospore may in turn develop into a new spherule, perpetuating the parasitic phase in the tissues. An intense inflammatory response ensues, and the infection stays limited to the lungs and hilar nodes in the majority of patients. Extrapulmonary dissemination can occur, and cutaneous disease has been described after puncture of the skin with a contaminated object.

In general, *Coccidioides* species appear to be confined to the Western Hemisphere. The endemic areas lie in the southwestern United States, encompassing west Texas, New Mexico, Arizona, and California. The organisms can also be found in northwestern Mexico and a few small areas of Central and South America. These endemic areas have arid climates, hot summers, few winter freezes, low altitude, and alkaline soil—ecologic conditions that favor human infection with *Coccidioides.* The organisms are drought resistant, and periodic increases in cases are observed when prolonged drought is followed by periods of heavy rain. Arthroconidia may become airborne after windstorms or disruption of soil by farming or construction work. Since infection requires that arthroconidia be inhaled, person-to-person transmission does not play a role in acquisition of coccidioidomycosis. Hospitalizations for coccidioidomycosis are common, particularly in endemic areas. County of residence, older age, black race, male sex, intercurrent HIV infection, and pregnancy are all risk factors strongly associated with an increased risk for hospitalization.

## CLINICAL MANIFESTATIONS

### Pulmonary

The primary portal of entry in most patients is the lung. Accordingly, signs and symptoms of respiratory tract infection represent the major clinical manifestations of acute coccidioidomycosis in most patients. Pulmonary coccidioidomycosis occurs in 95% of all cases. The majority of individuals with acute coccidioidomycosis will have either asymptomatic infection or mild upper respiratory tract symptoms. Approximately 40% of patients with primary infection will develop a more severe systemic illness 1 to 3 weeks after exposure, characterized by cough, malaise, fever, chills, night sweats, anorexia, and weakness. Lower respiratory tract illness may include pneumonia and parapneumonic effusion. Chest pain may be quite severe in some patients, and hemoptysis is commonly encountered in adult patients, although it is rare in children. The radiographic appearance of acute coccidioidomycosis is nonspecific. Bronchopneumonic infiltrate associated with hilar adenopathy is the most common presentation, although an interstitial pattern may be encountered. Widespread intrathoracic disease ("miliary pattern") may be encountered with disseminated infection.

Pulmonary infections can be divided into 3 main categories: *primary, complicated,* and *residual* pulmonary coccidioidomycosis. Primary infection occurs with inhalation of airborne arthroconidia; remarkably, as few as 10 arthroconidia are capable of producing an infection. Symptomatic disease manifests with predominantly an influenza-like syndrome, with accompanying pneumonia and the presence of a pleural effusion noted on imaging studies. Complicated pulmonary coccidioidomycosis includes both severe and persistent pneumonia, progressive primary coccidioidomycosis, fibrocavitary coccidioidomycosis, coccidioidomycotic empyema, and, rarely, acute respiratory distress syndrome (ARDS). Residual disease comprises 2 entities: pulmonary nodules and fibrosis.

### Cutaneous

An important diagnostic clue in patients with primary coccidioidomycosis is the presence of cutaneous manifestations. The most common skin manifestation of acute coccidioidomycosis is erythema nodosum. The appearance of these lesions, known in California and other endemic regions as the "valley bumps," correlates with the development of cell-mediated immunity and is associated with a lower risk of dissemination. These painful, tender lesions are distributed on the anterior tibial surface. Although not specific for coccidioidomycosis, the finding of erythema nodosum in a child residing in an endemic area strongly suggests recent acute coccidioidomycosis. Less commonly, erythema multiforme may be present, and like erythema nodosum, this rash is also assumed to be immunologically mediated. Interstitial granulomatous dermatitis and Sweet syndrome have recently been recognized as additional reactive signs of the infection. Primary cutaneous infection with *Coccidioides* is rare, with most cases being attributed to laboratory accidents. The skin may also be a target organ in the setting of disseminated infection.

#### Immunocompromised Patients

In recent years, *Coccidioides* species have emerged as major pathogens in immunocompromised patients, particularly those with HIV infection. *Coccidioides* also have an enhanced pathogenic potential in other immunosuppressed patients, such as in transplant recipients, children with congenital immunodeficiencies, and patients on immunosuppressive therapies, including tumor necrosis factor antagonists such as infliximab. Coccidioidomycosis in immunocompromised patients may represent a mix of new and reactivated infections. Diffuse pulmonary disease is common, and lung biopsy is often required to make the diagnosis. Extrapulmonary disease may be difficult to eradicate, necessitating chronic suppressive therapy. Even a remote history of residence or travel to an endemic area should be sought, since the major problem in making the diagnosis is a lack of suspicion of the possibility of coccidioidomycosis.

#### Other

Approximately 0.5% of patients with acute coccidioidomycosis will develop disseminated infection. Dissemination is more common in men, pregnant women, and perhaps individuals from certain ethnic groups (eg, African, Mexican, or Filipino ancestry). Major disseminated disease sites include bones, joints, visceral organs, soft tissue, and the central nervous system (CNS). Paratracheal, hilar, or mediastinal lymphadenopathy can be a common finding in children.

Local pain is the usual hallmark of musculoskeletal coccidioidomycosis, with warmth and swelling accompanying the systemic symptoms of infection. Over one-third of cases of disseminated coccidioidomycosis are complicated by osteomyelitis, which is unifocal in most cases. Any bone can become infected, but the most commonly involved sites are skull, metacarpals, metatarsals, spine, and tibia. Bone scans are more sensitive than plain radiographs in making the diagnosis. When present, vertebral lesions tend to be multiple and pose a high risk for CNS spread. Tendinitis, synovitis, or frank arthritis may result from bloodstream dissemination. Swelling and tenderness are present, most commonly involving the ankle and knee joints. The fungus can usually be cultured from the affected synovial fluid, and synovial biopsy is also recommended in suspect cases.

Coccidioidomycosis meningitis is an important and serious complication of disseminated infection. It typically presents within the first 6 months following primary infection. Importantly, the signs of meningeal irritation common in bacterial meningitis are generally absent. Headache is the most common symptom. Fever, weakness, vomiting, focal neurologic deficits, and meningismus may occur, but many patients are asymptomatic. This makes the decision about whether or not to perform lumbar puncture in all cases of coccidioidomycosis challenging. Current guidelines recommend considering lumbar puncture only when symptoms of CNS involvement are present. If the presence of headache is the primary concern, it is typically persistent and progressive. Cerebrospinal fluid analysis most commonly demonstrates a mononuclear pleocytosis, with decreased glucose and elevated protein levels. *Coccidioides* species are rarely recovered from cerebrospinal fluid, but complement-fixing antibodies for coccidioidin are present in almost all cases. Recent studies of coccidioidal antigen in cerebrospinal fluid suggest that it may be a very sensitive biomarker. Meningitis may be associated with parenchymal involvement evident on magnetic resonance imaging. In children, hydrocephalus complicating basilar inflammation can be found in most patients with *Coccidioides* meningitis.

Other manifestations of disseminated coccidioidomycosis may include seeding of visceral organs, genitourinary tract infection, ophthalmic complications (chorioretinitis), and cutaneous infection. Muscle involvement may occur in disseminated cases, with occasional development of abscesses or draining sinus tracts. Of particular interest to pediatricians is the issue of coccidioidomycosis in pregnancy. Pregnant women are at high risk of dissemination of coccidioidomycosis, presumably due to the physiologic reduction in type 1 T-helper-cell cytokine responses that occurs during pregnancy. Historically, untreated disseminated coccidioidomycosis during pregnancy was thought to be associated with extensive maternal and fetal mortality and was a leading cause of maternal death in endemic areas, demonstrating a dramatically increased risk of dissemination in African American women. As recently as 1995, therapeutic abortions and early deliveries were advocated in certain contexts, although more recent reports suggest that the risk of transplacental infection and fetal complications may have been overstated. Infection in the newborn may also be acquired via the birth canal. The mortality of disseminated disease is higher in neonates than in older children or adults.

## DIAGNOSIS

In addition to conventional roentgenography, computed tomography of the chest may be useful in defining the extent of adenopathy in cases of coccidioidomycosis. Demonstration of the organism by examination and culture of clinical specimens, with confirmation of positive cultures using nucleic acid hybridization methods, remain the definitive diagnostic approaches to establishing the diagnosis of coccidioidomycosis. Sputum, joint fluid, bronchoalveolar lavage fluid, soft tissue aspirates, and deep tissue surgical specimens offer the best yield by culture. Spinal fluid culture is positive by culture only about one-third of the time, and when the diagnosis of meningitis is being considered, multiple lumbar punctures may increase the diagnostic yield. It is important to remember that cultures of *Coccidioides* represent a potentially severe biologic hazard, and laboratory personnel should be alerted to the possibility of the diagnosis prior to processing of specimens. Microscopic examination of clinical specimens may be useful to search for the presence of endospore-containing spherules. Fine-needle aspiration of suspect lesions in soft tissue or bone, synovial biopsies, and skin biopsies all provide suitable specimens for histopathologic evaluation.

Nonculture techniques, such as fungal DNA detection by polymerase chain reaction, colorimetric and antibody-based assays to detect cell wall or capsular polysaccharides, and serology, are also helpful in making the diagnosis of coccidioidomycosis. The mycelial phase antigen, coccidioidin, is the most important target of antibody response. Serum IgM antibodies, called precipitins, can be detected 1 to 3 weeks after onset of symptoms in most cases and are readily identifiable by a variety of immunodiffusion, latex agglutination, or enzyme immunoassay methods. Complement-fixing serum IgG antibodies (CFA) appear later in the course of infection and usually decline 6 to 8 months following primary infection, although antibody may continue to be detectable for years. The CFA titer is a useful marker of disease activity. Sera should be run in paired fashion (acute and convalescent) for titer comparison. Rising titers are a bad prognostic sign, whereas falling titers suggest improvement. In the majority of patients with meningitis, CFA is present in cerebrospinal fluid, and titers parallel the course of meningeal disease. An enzyme immunoassay has been developed that detects and quantifies coccidioidal-specific galactomannan concentrations in urine samples. This test is especially useful in immunocompromised patients in whom antibodies may not be detectable.

Diagnostic skin tests are no longer used, as the interpretation of these tests was problematic. Patients with erythema nodosum may have a severe response to skin tests because of their particularly intense delayed-type hypersensitivity response to coccidioidin antigen. Cutaneous anergy is common in individuals with disseminated coccidioidomycosis, and a negative skin test in such patients does not exclude the diagnosis. However, a newer skin test known as Spherusol (Nielsen BioSciences) is prepared and extracted from laboratory cultures of *C immitis* spherules and appears to be useful in diagnosis. It is specifically approved by the US Food and Drug Administration for the detection and monitoring of the cell-mediated immune response to *Coccidioides* in patients 18 to 64 years of age with an established history of pulmonary coccidioidomycosis.

## TREATMENT

The decision to initiate antifungal therapy in the setting of coccidioidomycosis depends on the extent of disease and the risk factors a patient may have for complicated or disseminated disease. Although most patients with symptomatic primary infection recover spontaneously, treatment is mandated in several clinical settings. Once disease has spread outside the lung (eg, bone, joint, and soft tissue infections, genitourinary tract infections, and CNS involvement), antifungal therapy is almost always warranted. In certain circumstances, individuals with symptomatic primary infection should also be treated, even if disease appears to be limited to the lungs, since the risk of dissemination is high. These patients include pregnant women, young infants, the immunocompromised, and individuals with chronic or debilitating illnesses. The magnitude of the CFA titer at time of diagnosis may also aid decision making regarding therapy. Some studies have reported an association with dissemination and a CFA titer of 1:32 or greater, but this may not be observed in all patients with disseminated disease. An association between CFA titer and the risk of disseminated disease has been confirmed in children, and further investigation of this possibility should be investigated in pediatric patients with titers ≥ 1:32.

Historically, amphotericin B or its lipid congeners have been regarded as the gold standards of therapy for severe pulmonary and disseminated coccidioidomycosis. However, oral fluconazole and itraconazole have replaced amphotericin B as initial therapy for most chronic pulmonary or disseminated infections, including CNS disease. Azoles are avoided in the first trimester of pregnancy but are resumed thereafter. Data remain limited about the use of extended-spectrum azoles such as posaconazole and voriconazole. These agents are typically reserved for use after failure of fluconazole or itraconazole. Itraconazole appears to have efficacy equal to that of fluconazole in the treatment of nonmeningeal infection and has the same relapse rate after therapy is discontinued. However, itraconazole appears to perform better in skeletal lesions, whereas fluconazole performs better in pulmonary and soft tissue infection. Consideration should be given to obtaining serum levels of itraconazole at the onset of long-term treatment, since absorption is unpredictable. The recommended dose of fluconazole is 400 mg daily, although some experts advocate using up to 800 mg daily. The recommended adult dose of itraconazole is 200 mg twice daily. Duration of therapy is individualized depending on the extent of disease and the clinical and radiographic response, but, at minimum, at least 6 months of treatment are required in most patients.

Oral fluconazole is the mainstay of therapy for *Coccidioides* meningitis. Intrathecal amphotericin B is considered only after escalating doses of fluconazole have failed. Because of the extremely high risk of relapse, therapy is typically continued for the life of the patient.

## PREVENTION

Measures to control dust exposure in endemic areas are important especially for immunocompromised patients. Using antifungal prophylaxis or barrier methods (eg, masks) is not practical in most situations.

## SUGGESTED READINGS

Dimitrova D, Ross L. Coccidioidomycosis: experience from a children's hospital in an area of endemicity. *J Pediatr Infect Dis Soc.* 2016;5:89-92.

Galgiani JN, Ampel NM, Blair JE, et al. 2016 Infectious Diseases Society of America (IDSA) clinical practice guideline for the treatment of coccidioidomycosis. *Clin Infect Dis.* 2016;63:e112-e146.

Kassis C, Zaidi S, Kuberski T, et al. Role of *Coccidioides* antigen testing in the cerebrospinal fluid for the diagnosis of coccidioidal meningitis. *Clin Infect Dis.* 2015;61:1521-1526.

McCarty JM, Demetral LC, Dabrowski L, Kahal AK, Bowser AM, Hahn JE. Pediatric coccidioidomycosis in central California: a retrospective case series. *Clin Infect Dis.* 2013;56:1579-1585.

# 294 Cryptococcosis

Leidy Tovar Padua and Deborah Lehman

## INTRODUCTION

Cryptococcosis is a sporadic mycotic disease caused by the yeast-like fungi *Cryptococcus neoformans* and *Cryptococcus gattii*. The incidence of disease with these organisms has increased in the past few decades due to the increased number of individuals living with immunosuppressed conditions.

## PATHOGENESIS AND EPIDEMIOLOGY

*Cryptococcus* species reproduce by budding and vary from 4 to 20 μm in diameter. The fungus is surrounded by a mucopolysaccharide capsule, which aids in its identification in body fluids and tissues. Cryptococcal basidiospores can be found in soil and in avian excrement. The organism can withstand prolonged drying and can persist in the soil for long periods of time. Pigeons are a frequent source of *C neoformans*, but cases have been linked to other birds, including starlings. The birds themselves are likely not infected, but their excreta serve as excellent culture medium for the organism. *C gattii* is commonly associated with eucalyptus tree species and less commonly with several other trees native of tropical, subtropical, and temperate climates. Human disease is initiated by inhalation of cryptococcal cells, although infection via the gastrointestinal tract and direct inoculation into tissues can also be mechanisms of infection. After cryptococcal cells are inhaled, they localize in the pulmonary parenchyma and may cause an isolated pneumonitis or disseminate hematogenously to any organ of the body.

Of the more than 30 species in the genus *Cryptococcus, C neoformans* and *C gattii* are commonly known to be pathogenic to humans. Recently, *Cryptococcus laurentii* has been associated with cases of keratitis, endophthalmitis, cutaneous infection, lung abscess, peritonitis, meningitis, and fungemia. *C neoformans* is responsible for approximately 95% of cryptococcal infections, affecting mostly immunocompromised individuals, and occurs worldwide. *C gattii* more commonly infects immunocompetent hosts and was originally thought to be limited to tropical and subtropical regions. However, since the outbreak of *C gattii* in Vancouver, British Columbia, in 1999, the Pacific Northwest region of the United States has been increasingly affected by *C gattii*, and sporadic cases have been reported in other regions of the country. Interestingly, serologic studies from urban areas in the United States have shown that healthy asymptomatic children have high titers to cryptococcal polysaccharide.

Cryptococcosis is an opportunistic infection and occurs primarily in patients with impaired cell-mediated immunity. Susceptibility to the disease is markedly increased in those with T-cell immune dysfunction. Cryptococcosis has been described in children with acquired immunodeficiency syndrome (AIDS), acute lymphoblastic leukemia, hyper-IgM and -IgE syndromes, and X-linked agammaglobulinemia, as well as in children receiving prolonged corticosteroid therapy. Before the use of highly active antiretroviral therapy (HAART), cryptococcal infection was a major cause of morbidity and mortality in adult patients with advanced human immunodeficiency virus (HIV), infecting up to 10% of individuals with AIDS. In contrast, children infrequently develop cryptococcal disease, and prevalence rates in children with AIDS are reported to be around 1%. Over the past 2 decades, the incidence of cryptococcosis in patients with HIV/AIDS has decreased significantly due to the aggressive use of antiretroviral therapy. However, due to increasing numbers of solid organ transplants and the use of immunosuppressive agents, the number of cases of cryptococcosis in immunocompromised, non–HIV-infected patients continues to be high; it is currently the third most common invasive fungal infection behind infections due to *Candida* and *Aspergillus* in solid organ transplant recipients. The initial host response is thought to be mediated through cell-mediated immunity and is similar to infection with *Mycobacterium tuberculosis*. The organism may stay dormant for long periods of time, only becoming active when there is a decline in the host's immune system.

## CLINICAL MANIFESTATIONS

In immunocompromised hosts, the central nervous system (CNS) is the most common extrapulmonary site of infection, and *Cryptococcus* is the most frequent cause of fungal meningitis. Cryptococcal infection of the CNS is frequently indolent, presenting with nonspecific symptoms such as fever and headache. Focal neurologic deficits and altered mental status are less common and are more typical of advanced disease. Cryptococcal meningitis and meningoencephalitis share many clinical and laboratory features with meningitis caused by *M tuberculosis* and *Coccidioides immitis*. The cerebrospinal fluid (CSF) typically reveals lymphocytosis, elevated protein, and mildly reduced glucose levels. However, CSF parameters may be unremarkable in patients with AIDS due to a lack of inflammatory host response. Slowly progressing symptoms in both immunocompetent and immunocompromised patients may lead to a delay in diagnosis. Untreated cryptococcal meningoencephalitis is generally fatal over weeks to months. CNS infection due to *C gattii* is more commonly associated with elevated intracranial pressure and large mass lesions (cryptococcomas) than *C neoformans*.

Isolated pulmonary infection is most commonly seen in immunocompetent patients and can be asymptomatic, discovered incidentally as a solitary nodule during radiography. When clinically apparent, disease may be associated with cough productive of mucoid sputum, chest pain, fever, weight loss, night sweats, and, occasionally, hemoptysis and respiratory failure. Chest radiographs may show interstitial or focal infiltrates, lymphadenopathy, or, rarely, pleural effusions. In immunocompromised patients, pulmonary disease is most frequently in association with disseminated disease.

*C gattii* infection in immunocompetent individuals may cause an exuberant inflammatory response. Large pulmonary and CNS cryptococcomas are common. Other sites of infection, such as skin, bone, joints, lymph nodes, eye, and placenta, have been reported. Patients with cryptococcal infection isolated from the lungs and other organs should have a lumbar puncture to rule out CNS involvement. Elevated intracranial pressure is a poor prognostic factor in cryptococcal meningitis.

## DIAGNOSIS

The most rapid and reliable way to diagnose cryptococcal infection is to demonstrate cryptococcal capsular polysaccharide antigen in either serum or CSF. Commercially available latex agglutination tests on both CSF and serum have high sensitivities and specificities ranging from 93% to 100%. In severely immunocompromised patients, the only manifestation of cryptococcosis can be a positive cryptococcal antigen in serum or CSF. The polysaccharide antigen test is also useful for follow-up and for predicting prognosis in patients with cryptococcal meningitis. False-positive results have been reported to occur in serum specimens with positive rheumatoid factor or other cross-reacting antigens. False-negative results can sometimes occur with high fungal load, the prozone effect, which can be overcome by diluting out the initial specimen and retesting. Polysaccharide antigen testing on other body fluids, such as bronchoalveolar lavage fluid, has been performed but has not been as well studied. The lateral flow assay is a recently developed rapid screening test for detection of cryptococcal antigen; studies performed in patients with HIV showed a sensitivity and specificity greater than 90% for serum and CSF and a sensitivity in urine of more than 70%. This rapid test has several advantages including rapid results and low cost; it is also easily performed and does not require electricity. Serologic testing for cryptococcal antibodies has poor sensitivity and specificity and has especially unreliable results in patients most at risk for cryptococcosis—severely immunocompromised patients.

*Cryptococcus* can be grown on routine fungal culture media, but cultures are less sensitive than antigen detection when fungal burden is small. Visualization of budding organisms on an India ink wet preparation of the CSF establishes the diagnosis; presence of budding is essential to avoid mistaking leukocytes for yeast. The India ink preparation has an increased sensitivity in patients with AIDS due to the higher number of organisms seen in these patients. In the absence of AIDS, the sensitivity of India ink is less than 50% and requires at least $10^3$ and $10^4$ colony-forming units of yeast to be positive.

## TREATMENT

Detailed clinical guidelines on the management of cryptococcal disease are available on the Infectious Diseases Society of America Web site (https://www.idsociety.org/Organism/#CryptococcalDisease). Immunocompetent hosts with pulmonary disease may experience disease resolution in the absence of any antifungal therapy. However, most infectious diseases experts recommend treatment of patients with isolated pulmonary cryptococcosis with oral azole agents for 6 to 12 months.

Cryptococcal pneumonia associated with CNS involvement, disseminated infection, or severe pneumonia (acute respiratory distress syndrome) should be treated aggressively like CNS disease. High-dose amphotericin B deoxycholate (0.7–1.0 mg/kg/d) in combination with 5-flucytosine (100 mg/kg/d) is recommended. Liposomal preparations of amphotericin are alternative treatments for patients unable to tolerate amphotericin B deoxycholate. Cryptococcal CNS disease requires 3 stages of treatment: induction with high-dose amphotericin and 5-flucytosine for 2 weeks, followed by an 8- to 10-week course of an oral azole agent, and then long-term suppressive therapy of fluconazole at a lower dose. Initial combination therapy has been demonstrated to result in higher rates of CSF sterilization and lower mortality. Because the cure rate in CNS cryptococcosis does not exceed 75% and because relapses are common, patients require lengthy and sometimes lifelong suppressive therapy with an azole agent. Aggressive management of elevated intracranial pressure with repeated lumbar punctures or placement of an intracranial drain is recommended; adjuvant glucocorticoids should be avoided unless in the context of immune reconstitution inflammatory syndrome (IRIS). The newer-generation azoles, such as voriconazole and posaconazole, are also effective in treating cryptococcal infection. The echinocandin agents have no activity against *Cryptococcus*.

## PREVENTION

Cryptoccoccal disease is best prevented by correcting situations that produce immunosuppression in patients. In patients infected with HIV, this would be the early initiation of combination antiretroviral therapy.

## SUGGESTED READINGS


Beardsley J, Wolbers M, Kibengo FM, et al. Adjunctive dexamethasone in HIV-associated cryptococcal meningitis. *N Engl J Med*. 2016;374:542-554.

Harris JR, Lockhart SR, Debess E, et al. *Cryptococcus gattii* in the United States: clinical aspects of infection with an emerging pathogen. *Clin Infect Dis*. 2011;53:1188-1195.

Kabanda T, Siedner MJ, Klausner JD, Muzoora C, Boulware DR. Point-of-care diagnosis and prognostication of cryptococcal meningitis with the cryptococcal antigen lateral flow assay on cerebrospinal fluid. *Clin Infect Dis*. 2014;58:113-116.

Maziarz EK, Perfect JR. Cryptococcosis. *Infect Dis Clin North Am*. 2016;30:179-206.

McKenney J, Bauman S, Neary B, et al. Prevalence, correlates, and outcomes of cryptococcal antigen positivity among patients with AIDS, United States, 1986-2012. *Clin Infect Dis*. 2015;60:959-965.

Perfect JR, Dismukes WE, Dromer F, et al. Clinical practice guidelines for the management of cryptococcal disease: 2010 update by the Infectious Diseases Society of America. *Clin Infect Dis*. 2010;50:291-322.

Williams DA, Kiiza T, Kwizera R, et al. Evaluation of finger stick cryptococcal antigen lateral flow assay in HIV-infected persons: a diagnostic accuracy study. *Clin Infect Dis*. 2015;61:464-467.

Yuanjie Z, Jianghan C, Nan X, et al. Cryptococcal meningitis in immunocompetent children. *Mycoses*. 2012;55:168-171.

# 295 Histoplasmosis

Charles R. Woods

## INTRODUCTION

Histoplasmosis, the most common endemic fungal infection in the United States, is caused by a thermal dimorphic fungus, *Histoplasma capsulatum*. The extent and degree of environmental contamination with the mold are augmented by bird and bat droppings; the latter may contain fungal spores as well as provide factors that stimulate mold growth.

## PATHOGENESIS AND EPIDEMIOLOGY

Infection begins following inhalation of conidia (spores). These convert in the alveoli to the yeast-like invasive forms of the fungus, which are 2 to 4 μm in diameter and ovoid with narrow-based budding. This results in a focus of acute pneumonitis and regional hilar adenitis. In addition to this primary focus, yeast forms also disseminate lymphohematogenously to the reticuloendothelial organs. The host immune response aborts further progression in the vast majority of cases. Inhalation of a large inoculum can lead to acute diffuse lung infection that is severe and sometimes fatal.

Neutrophils arrive early in response but are unable to kill *H capsulatum* cells. Macrophages are able to control infection after stimulation by tumor necrosis factor-α and interferon-γ produced by responding CD4+ Th1 lymphocytes once these arrive. Dendritic cells also may play a fungicidal role via lysosomal hydrolases. Antibodies are produced against multiple *H capsulatum* antigens but do not play a significant role in controlling or preventing infection. The inflammatory infiltrate changes become granulomatous with typical Langhans-type giant cells; caseating necrosis, fibrosis, and calcification may ultimately ensue. Calcification may be evident within a few months after initial infection in children.

The spore-bearing mold form grows in the environment at temperatures less than 35°C, occurs worldwide, and is most commonly found in the United States in the Mississippi River and Ohio River basins (Fig. 295-1). Epidemiologic surveys using histoplasmin skin test reactivity in endemic areas show progressive increases with age. Infections occur as sporadic cases in communitywide outbreaks when dry, windy conditions facilitate aerosolization of spores and as localized clusters caused by disturbance of heavily contaminated microenvironments. Such hyperendemic foci include soil in sites of bird roosts, including stream banks; bat-infested caves; rotting logs; and the attics, wall insulation, and fireplaces of old structures (Table 295-1). The rate of hospitalization among children due to histoplasmosis has historically been approximately 2.5 per million population in the Midwest and South regions of the United States.

## CLINICAL MANIFESTATIONS

The type and severity of symptoms reflect both the intensity of exposure and the adequacy of the host cellular immune response. Primary infection is asymptomatic in 99% of normal hosts who are lightly exposed. Most of the remainder develop nonspecific, transient, flulike respiratory symptoms. Infection is symptomatic in about half of otherwise normal patients who are more heavily exposed. In these patients, fever, cough, and chest pain are common symptoms; chest radiographs often show focal pneumonitis and/or hilar adenopathy. Symptoms are almost always self-limited in otherwise healthy patients and resolve within 2 weeks without treatment. Pulmonary nodules (histoplasmomas) from such infections may persist indefinitely and develop radiographically visible calcifications over months to years. Infrequently, the fever, weight loss, and fatigue persist unabated for more than 4 weeks, and antifungal therapy then may be required. Intense exposure of immunocompetent hosts can cause severe, life-threatening illness characterized by persistent fever, respiratory distress, diffuse reticulonodular chest infiltrates, and sometimes progressive fungal dissemination.

Abnormalities of cellular immune function, whether primary, acquired, or resulting from the relative immaturity of infancy, are risk factors for progressive disseminated histoplasmosis. Patients receiving tumor necrosis factor-α inhibitors are at high risk for disseminated infections. Patients with advanced human immunodeficiency virus (HIV) infection are also at high risk. Severe and disseminating infection can follow primary exposure or result from reactivation of a previously quiescent focus. An immune reconstitution syndrome, in which symptoms of infection follow the administration of effective highly active antiretroviral therapy, has also been recognized. Illness usually begins with isolated fever and weight loss; if untreated, skin lesions, diffuse pulmonary infiltrates, mucosal ulcerations, pancytopenia, and coagulopathy may ensue.

Histoplasmosis in immunosuppressed patients (eg, chemotherapy or other immunosuppressive medications, HIV) may present

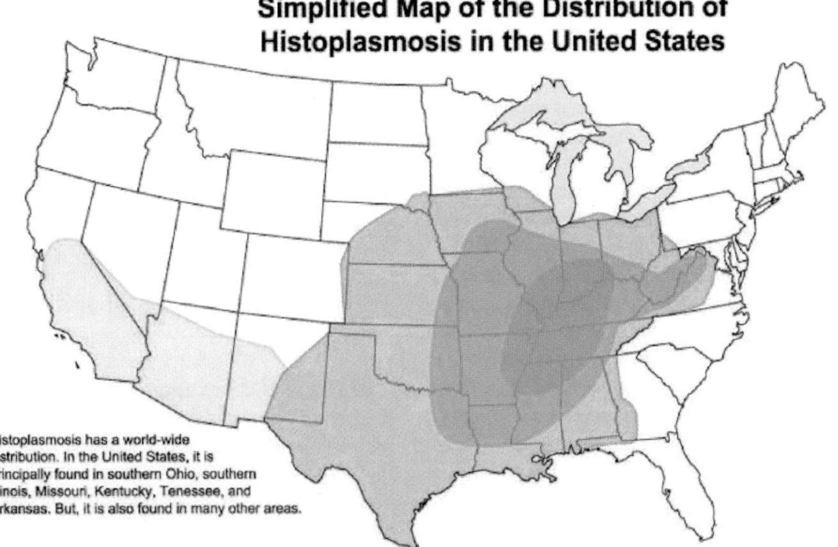


**FIGURE 295-1** Geographic variation in the frequency of reactors to histoplasmin. Darker color indicates higher frequency. (Reproduced with permission from Edwards LB, Acquaviva FA, Livesay VT, et al. An atlas of sensitivity to tuberculin, PPD-B, and histoplasmin in the United States, *Am Rev Respir Dis*. 1969 Apr;99(4):Suppl:1-132.)

**TABLE 295-1 POINT SOURCES/ACTIVITIES ASSOCIATED WITH SPORADIC CHILDHOOD HISTOPLASMOSIS**

| |
|---|
| Cleaning/renovating basements, attics, wall insulation of older homes |
| Cutting firewood or tree stumps, playing in hollow trees |
| Cleaning abandoned building |
| Playing or digging in sites of former bird roosts |
| Gardening |
| Playing in a barn |
| Exploring caves |
| Being downwind of excavation/demolition of contaminated sites |

with fever, diffuse interstitial pulmonary infiltrates, and progressive hypoxia. In these children, symptoms can mimic those caused by cytomegalovirus, numerous respiratory viruses, *Pneumocystis jirovecii*, or many other infectious or noninfectious etiologies. Histoplasmosis also may develop in children after solid organ transplants. About half of such cases occur during the first 2 years after transplant.

The relative immaturity of cellular immunity in otherwise normal infants may predispose them to disseminated histoplasmosis of infancy, a rare but life-threatening infection of children younger than 2 years of age. In some infants, despite what may be relatively minimal exposure to *Histoplasma* spores (ie, low inoculum), progressive dissemination with extensive spread of infection throughout the reticuloendothelial system may occur. The onset of symptoms is usually insidious with initial failure to thrive, variable fever, absent toxicity, and progressive hepatosplenomegaly. After about 4 to 6 weeks, pancytopenia and coagulopathy occur. Mucosal and gastrointestinal ulcerations and hemorrhage often accompany late symptoms; meningitis is common. Chest radiographic abnormalities may remain absent. Disseminated histoplasmosis of infancy is fatal if untreated.

The initial hilar adenopathy of pulmonary histoplasmosis may progress into a mediastinal mass that can mimic malignancy. This manifestation can lead to superior vena cava syndrome or dysphagia. The presence of anterior mediastinal involvement, enlarged cervical lymph nodes, or peripheral blood lymphopenia has high positive predictive value for malignancy. In highly endemic areas, positive serologic evidence for *H capsulatum* infection may not obviate the need for histopathologic confirmation of the diagnosis.

Additional manifestations of histoplasmosis are shown in Table 295-2.

## DIAGNOSIS

The majority of infections are subclinical or self-limited and do not require laboratory confirmation. The recognition of chest radiographic findings of typical granulomas in otherwise well children who reside in endemic areas infrequently requires laboratory confirmation. Laboratory diagnosis is needed to evaluate patients with symptoms that may mimic those caused by other pathogens, especially *Mycobacterium tuberculosis, Blastomyces dermatitidis*, or other causes of granulomatous inflammation. Laboratory diagnosis is also used to differentiate histoplasmosis from neoplasm in patients residing in endemic areas who present with hilar or mediastinal adenopathy. Confirmation of the diagnosis is indicated for patients in whom antifungal therapy is indicated.

Laboratory tests used to diagnose histoplasmosis include culture, histopathologic examination of biopsy specimens, serologic testing, and histoplasmin (antigen) detection and quantification. Direct observation of typical yeast forms in tissue or body fluids and/or isolation of the fungus in culture are diagnostic. Histopathology may show granulomas with or without detectable organisms. The blood, bone marrow, and urine are potential sites from which the organism can be isolated, but cultures are usually negative in mild or moderately severe infections. Disadvantages of these methods are low sensitivities, a delay of 2 weeks required to isolate the fungus in culture, and the need for an invasive procedure to obtain tissue.

The sensitivity and specificity of antibody and antigen assays are variable, with little data for pediatric populations. Serologic tests are used most frequently for diagnosis in children. A single complement-fixation (CF) titer of 1:32 or greater to either the yeast or mycelial phase antigen, or the detection of H or M bands by the immunodiffusion (ID) method, strongly suggests acute or recent infection. About one-third of patients with proven infection (largely adult data) have initial CF titers of 1:8 or 1:16. Host immune response produces M band reactions in most patients; H bands are seen in less than 20%, and most often in more severe or chronic infections. Newer enzyme immunoassay (EIA)-based serologic tests that report IgM and IgG titers may supplant CF

**TABLE 295-2 CLINICAL MANIFESTATIONS OF HISTOPLASMOSIS AND RISK FACTORS FOR DISEASE**

| Presentation | Risk Factors, Manifestations, and Other Comments |
|---|---|
| Asymptomatic infection | Vast majority of cases |
| Subacute pulmonary infection[a] | Most common symptomatic disease; low inhalational inoculum<br>Fever, cough, chest pain, other symptoms with onset 2–4 weeks after exposure; usually self-limited over several weeks<br>May have hilar adenopathy; may lead to mediastinitis |
| Acute pulmonary infection[a] | Follows large inhalational inoculum (often occupational or recreational); young age may predispose; onset within 2 weeks of exposure<br>Diffuse pulmonary infiltrates with respiratory symptoms and signs; may recover without treatment but generally treated; can be fatal |
| Chronic pulmonary infection[a] | Usually seen in adults with underlying lung disease<br>Fever, sweats, chest pain, fatigue; fibrotic cavitary lesions similar to reactivated tuberculosis |
| Progressive disseminated infection | More common at extremes of age and in persons with cellular immunodeficiency conditions (eg, congenital, chemotherapy, advanced HIV, immunosuppression after solid organ or bone marrow transplant) or those receiving TNF-α inhibitors<br>Adenopathy, hepatosplenomegaly, diffuse (can appear miliary) or focal pneumonitis in 70%; enhancing brain lesions in some; skin lesions and lesions in the upper and lower GI tract visible on endoscopy in some; laboratory findings may include anemia, evidence of coagulopathy, and elevated serum concentrations of aminotransferases and ferritin |
| Granulomatous mediastinitis | Caseation of hilar lymph nodes, sometimes with calcification; may impinge upon the esophagus, pulmonary vessels, or trachea |
| Fibrosing mediastinitis | Excessive mediastinal fibrotic, scarring response with significant entrapment of mediastinal structures; very rare under age 20 years; host predisposition likely; superior vena cava syndrome is most common sign |
| Broncholithiasis | Erosion of calcified lymph node into adjacent airway; may cause cough, hemoptysis; lithoptysis may occur |
| Meningitis | Lymphocytic CSF pleocytosis, elevated CSF protein, hypoglycorrhachia with meningitis; usually develops as part of disseminated infection, but can be isolated; may be seen with ventricular shunt infection |
| Primary cutaneous infection | Rare in children; typically fixed ulcerating lesions; skin foci of infection can be seen in disseminated disease |
| Pericarditis | May occur in 5–10% of symptomatic cases; represents inflammatory response from adjacent mediastinal lymph node infection; responds to nonsteroidal anti-inflammatory therapy |
| Erythema nodosum, erythema multiforme or arthritis | Uncommon inflammatory reactions; may occur with mild or severe infection |
| Ocular histoplasmosis syndrome | Peripapillary choroidal neovascularization associated with retinal lesions (which typically are asymptomatic); can occur in children |

[a]Pulmonary histoplasmosis sometimes may closely resemble clinical presentations of sarcoidosis, tuberculosis, and malignancy.

CSF, cerebrospinal fluid; GI, gastrointestinal; TNF, tumor necrosis factor.

and ID over time. Disadvantages of serologic tests are that these may be undetectable early in infection, may cross-react with other fungal antibodies, may remain elevated for 18 months to years following infection, or may be falsely negative in immunocompromised patients.

A quantitative EIA that measures histoplasmin concentration in urine, serum, bronchoalveolar lavage specimens, and cerebrospinal fluid is an important rapid diagnostic test, although most data are from adult populations. Antigen can be detected in urine or serum early on in mild to moderate infections likely to be self-limited, but results are often negative in these patients. Detectable antigenuria occurs in greater than 90% and greater than 80% of patients with disseminated and acute pulmonary infections, respectively. Detectable antigenemia approaches 100% in disseminated infection. Specificity is 99% for patients without fungal disease. Although the EIA cross-reacts with several fungal antigens, especially other dimorphic fungi, clinical findings and exposure risk assessment usually allow accurate interpretation. Antigen testing may also be used to monitor treatment response and to identify early relapse in high-risk patients, since increasing urine *Histoplasma* concentrations precede clinical symptoms. Polymerase chain reaction tests have been developed, but clinical utility is uncertain.

Children with disseminated histoplasmosis should be screened for HIV infection. They may have low CD4 cell counts during the acute phase of disseminated infection during infancy. Evaluation of cellular immunity later in the course may be required to exclude the presence of primary immunodeficiency as a predisposing condition.

## TREATMENT

Most patients with histoplasmosis improve without antifungal therapy, and the strength of the evidence supporting the use of these agents is strongest for only the most serious manifestations (Table 295-3). Antifungal treatment is required for severe and/or progressively disseminating infections and for patients with primary or acquired cellular immune dysfunction. It is also considered for patients with prolonged mild to moderate symptoms (usually exceeding 2–4 weeks); however, evidence for this indication is uncertain. Rheumatologic or hypersensitivity symptoms, such as arthritis, pericarditis, or erythema nodosum, usually improve with supportive treatment. Pericarditis usually responds promptly to indomethacin.

Evidence-based treatment guidelines are summarized in Table 295-4. Amphotericin B is recommended as the initial agent used for treating

**TABLE 295-3 INDICATIONS FOR ANTIFUNGAL THERAPY IN PATIENTS WITH HISTOPLASMOSIS**

| Indication |
|---|
| **Definite Indication, Proven or Probable Efficacy** |
| Acute diffuse pulmonary infection, moderately severe symptoms, or severe symptoms |
| Chronic cavitary pulmonary infection |
| Progressive disseminated infection |
| Central nervous system infection |
| Immunocompromised patients |
| **Uncertain Indication, Unknown Efficacy** |
| Acute focal pulmonary infection, asymptomatic case, or mild symptoms that persist for < 1 month |
| Mediastinal lymphadenitis |
| Mediastinal granuloma |
| Inflammatory syndromes, treated with corticosteroids |
| **Not Recommended, Unknown Efficacy or Ineffective** |
| Mediastinal fibrosis |
| Pulmonary nodule |
| Broncholithiasis[a] |
| Presumed ocular histoplasmosis syndrome[b] |

[a]May require surgical excision.

[b]Surgical excision or intravitreal administration of bevacizumab may be effective.

Reproduced with permission from Wheat LJ, Freifeld AG, Kleiman MB, et al. Management of patients with histoplasmosis: clinical practice guidelines by the Infectious Disease Society of America, *Clin Infect Dis*. 2007 Oct 1;45(7):807-825.

**TABLE 295-4 TREATMENT RECOMMENDATIONS FOR CHILDREN WITH HISTOPLASMOSIS**

| Manifestation | Treatment Recommendations |
|---|---|
| Severe acute pulmonary histoplasmosis | Amphotericin B (AmB)[a] for 1–2 weeks, then itraconazole (Itr) to complete 12 total weeks of therapy |
| Mild to moderate acute or subacute pulmonary histoplasmosis | Symptoms < 4 weeks: none<br>Persistent symptoms[b] for > 4 weeks: Itr for 6–12 weeks |
| Progressive disseminated histoplasmosis in otherwise normal hosts | AmB[a] for 4–6 weeks[c] or<br>AmB for 2–4 weeks followed by Itr to complete 3 total months of therapy[c,d,e,f] |
| Progressive disseminated histoplasmosis in children with underlying immunosuppression that cannot be reversed[g] | Same primary course as for normal hosts[c], followed by potentially lifelong suppressive therapy with Itr (also recommended for children who relapse despite receipt of an appropriate regimen) |
| Mediastinal lymphadenitis | Treatment is usually unnecessary<br>If there are symptoms from compression of airways or the esophagus, prednisone in a tapering regimen over 1–2 weeks plus Itr for 6–12 weeks to reduce risk of progressive disseminated disease |
| Granulomatous mediastinitis[h] | Treatment is usually unnecessary<br>Itr for 6–12 weeks in symptomatic cases<br>Surgical excision may be required for relief of superior vena cava syndrome |
| Meningitis | AmB[a] for 4–6 weeks[i] |
| Pericarditis | NSAID therapy only in mild cases for 2 or more weeks (response usually seen within a few days)<br>Pericardial drainage for hemodynamic compromise<br>Prednisone in a tapering regimen over 1–2 weeks if no response to NSAIDs after several days or for hemodynamic compromise, plus Itr for 6–12 weeks if steroids are administered |
| Rheumatologic (erythema nodosum, arthritis, arthralgia) | NSAID therapy as for pericarditis, followed by prednisone plus Itr as for pericarditis if no response after several days |

[a]Lipid preparations are not preferred over amphotericin B deoxycholate since the latter is usually well tolerated in children.

[b]Persistence of symptoms without improvement.

[c]Longer courses of amphotericin B may be needed for severe cases in (1) infants with prolonged failure to thrive, pancytopenia, coagulopathy, or severe central nervous system infection; (2) patients with large fungal burdens; (3) children receiving tumor necrosis factor-α inhibitors; and (4) children with immunodeficiency conditions that cannot be reversed.

[d]Itraconazole as sole treatment may be considered in progressive disseminated infection when (1) symptoms are only mild to moderate, plus (2) the clinical course and laboratory findings can be closely monitored, plus (3) adherence is expected and absorption of the drug, based on serum levels, is assured.

[e]Itraconazole levels should be obtained during the first month of therapy.

[f]Antigen levels should be monitored during therapy and for 12 months after completion to monitor for relapse. Serum antigen levels should fall within 2 weeks. Urine antigen levels may persist in low concentrations for months and should not be a reason to prolong therapy in the absence of evidence of active infection.

[g]Based on limited data from adults with human immunodeficiency virus (HIV) infection, HIV patients with good immunologic responses (or who have never reached advanced stage) may have itraconazole secondary prophylaxis discontinued after receipt of at least 1 year of therapy plus negative blood cultures and serum and urine antigen levels < 2 ng/mL plus good adherence to antiretroviral therapy that is not failing.

[h]There is no evidence that untreated granulomatous mediastinitis progresses to fibrosing mediastinitis. Neither itraconazole nor surgical resection is indicated solely in effort to prevent the latter.

[i]Meningitis or brain infection occurring as part of progressive disseminated histoplasmosis does not require alteration of the regimen duration unless the manifestations are severe. Longer courses are recommended for adults with meningitis (ie, 4–6 weeks of high-dose liposomal amphotericin B followed by at least 1 year of intraconazole).

NSAID, nonsteroidal anti-inflammatory drug.

Adapted with permission from Wheat LJ, Freifeld AG, Kleiman MB, et al. Management of patients with histoplasmosis: clinical practice guidelines by the Infectious Disease Society of America, *Clin Infect Dis*. 2007 Oct 1;45(7):807-825.

severe manifestations of histoplasmosis. Itraconazole is recommended as initial therapy for mild-to-moderate histoplasmosis and is preferred over other azole antifungal agents. Itraconazole also is used for completion of therapy in most severe cases treated initially with amphotericin B, and serum concentrations should be monitored during the first month in children with disseminated or other severe forms of infection. As with other azoles, potential drug interactions with other concomitant therapies should be addressed. Lifelong suppression (secondary prophylaxis) with itraconazole may be required in patients for whom immunosuppression is not reversible or who relapse despite receiving appropriate therapy.

A brief course of steroids is often a useful adjunctive treatment for patients in whom acutely inflamed lymph nodes impinge on or obstruct adjacent structures. Effective antifungal agents should always be used concomitantly and the patient carefully monitored for signs of progressive dissemination while receiving steroids. Mediastinal fibrosis without evidence of active infection does not benefit from steroids or antifungal agents.

Prevention of infection requires avoidance of high-risk exposure (see Table 295-1) and/or using high-efficiency respiratory protective devices.

## SUGGESTED READINGS


American Academy of Pediatrics Committee on Infectious Diseases. Histoplasmosis. In: *Red Book: 2015 Report of the Committee on Infectious Diseases.* 30th ed. Elk Grove Village, IL: American Academy of Pediatrics; 2015:445-448.

Bahr NC, Antinori S, Wheat JL, Sarosi GA. Histoplasmosis infections worldwide: thinking outside of the Ohio River Valley. *Curr Trop Med Rep.* 2015;2:70-80.

Benedict K, Mody RK. Epidemiology of histoplasmosis outbreaks, United States, 1938-2013. *Emerg Infect Dis.* 2016;22:370-378.

Horwath MC, Fecher RA, Deepe GS Jr. *Histoplasma capsulatum*, lung infection and immunity. *Fut Microbiol.* 2015;10:967-975.

Naeem F, Metzger ML, Arnold SR, Adderson EE. Distinguishing benign mediastinal masses from malignancy in a histoplasmosis-endemic region. *J Pediatr.* 2015;167:409-415.

Richer SM, Smedema ML, Durkin MM, et al. Improved diagnosis of acute pulmonary histoplasmosis by combining antigen and antibody detection. *Clin Infect Dis.* 2016;62:896-902.

Vergidis P, Avery RK, Wheat JL, et al. Histoplasmosis complicating tumor necrosis factor-α blocker therapy: a retrospective analysis of 98 cases. *Clin Infect Dis.* 2015;61:409-417.


# 296 *Malassezia*

Nada Harik

## INTRODUCTION

The genus *Malassezia* (formerly known as *Pityrosporum*) includes 14 species, of which 11 are associated with significant human disease (Table 296-1). Skin diseases are the most common manifestation of *Malassezia* infection. *Malassezia* species, however, can cause invasive infections, especially in neonates and immunocompromised individuals. Confirmed dermatoses caused by *Malassezia* species include tinea versicolor, seborrheic dermatitis, and folliculitis.

| TABLE 296-1 *MALASSEZIA* SPECIES ASSOCIATED WITH HUMAN DISEASE |
|---|
| *M dermatis* |
| *M furfur* |
| *M globosa* |
| *M japonica* |
| *M nana* |
| *M obtusa* |
| *M pachydermatis* |
| *M restricta* |
| *M slooffiae* |
| *M sympodialis* |
| *M yamotoensis* |

## EPIDEMIOLOGY

*Malassezia* species are common inhabitants of human skin, usually found in sebum-rich areas such as the trunk, face, and scalp. Studies on skin colonization have shown that the skin of healthy newborn infants becomes colonized with *Malassezia* species within the first several months of life. Over 50% of prematurely born infants requiring prolonged hospitalization become colonized with *Malassezia* species within 2 weeks of life. Ninety to 100% of adolescents and adults have saprophytic skin colonization with *Malassezia* species. Hospital outbreaks of *Malassezia* infection have been reported.

## CLINICAL MANIFESTATIONS

Tinea versicolor is the prototypic skin disease associated with *Malassezia.* Tinea versicolor lesions are most commonly seen on the chest, back, and upper arms and occur most often in adolescents and young adults. In those who develop tinea versicolor, *Malassezia* transforms from the yeast phase to the mycelial phase. This results in the characteristic "spaghetti and meatballs" appearance of skin scrapings. Heat, moisture, and skin occlusion favor this transformation. *M globosa, M restricta, M sympodialis,* and *M furfur* are the most common causes of tinea versicolor.

Seborrheic dermatitis due to *Malassezia* occurs in 2% to 5% of normal hosts. Seborrheic dermatitis is more common among human immunodeficiency virus (HIV)-infected persons, and its prevalence increases to 70% to 80% in individuals with acquired immunodeficiency syndrome (AIDS). This condition varies from thick greasy scales covering the scalp of infants in the first 3 months of life (cradle cap) to an itchy, papular, erythematous, greasy, scaling rash most commonly found in the nasolabial folds, postauricular scalp, eyebrows, or chest. Dandruff, a mildly pruritic scaling of the scalp without associated inflammation, is felt to represent a milder variant of seborrheic dermatitis.

Folliculitis resulting from *Malassezia* causes acneiform, pruritic lesions most commonly seen over the shoulders, back, and chest. Lesions present as follicle-limited inflammatory papules or papulopustules that may resemble the lesions of disseminated candidiasis. *Malassezia* folliculitis is more common in immunocompromised individuals or those receiving broad-spectrum antibiotics or steroids. Discontinuation of steroids or antibiotics is helpful to aid treatment. *M furfur* is reported to cause eosinophilic pustular folliculitis with pruritus in patients with AIDS, and in its papular form, this lesion is pathologically a vasculitis of the dermis.

*Malassezia* species have been described as a cause of neonatal cephalic pustulosis, characterized by scattered erythematous papules and pustules on the face, scalp, and neck of infants in the first few weeks of life.

Systemic *Malassezia* infections most commonly present as central line–associated fungemia in patients receiving intravenous lipid feedings or total parenteral nutrition. *Malassezia* central line–associated infections are more common in neonates than adults. *M furfur* is the *Malassezia* species most likely to cause central line–associated bloodstream infection. A characteristic syndrome is noted, most often in premature neonates, of fever, bilateral interstitial pulmonary infiltrates, leukocytosis, and thrombocytopenia. This syndrome also has been reported in immunocompromised adults and children with central venous catheters who were not receiving concurrent intravenous lipids. Complications from central line–associated *Malassezia* infections are uncommon but have included meningitis, peritonitis, endocarditis, septic arthritis, and peripheral thromboembolism. *M pachydermatis* is also associated with systemic sepsis in infants. At least 2 nursery outbreaks have been reported; in one, colonization of healthcare workers with *M pachydermatis* by their pet dogs was believed to be a possible source of infection.

## DIAGNOSIS

*Malassezia* species are dimorphic with both yeast and mycelial growth. With the exception of *M pachydermatis,* all other *Malassezia* species are obligatory lipophilic organisms and require lipid supplementation for growth. *Malassezia* species grow within 5 to 14 days on Sabouraud dextrose agar overlaid with sterile olive oil. Isolation on Sabouraud dextrose agar causes colonies to coalesce, making species identification difficult. However, species identification is rarely important in clinical practice. Commercially available media for *Malassezia* isolation include Dixon agar (containing Tween 40 and glycerol monooleate) and Leeming and Notman agar (containing Tween 60, glycerol, and full-fat cow milk). Diagnosis of *Malassezia* central line-associated infection is generally made when blood from culture-negative cases of apparent catheter-associated sepsis is cultured on lipid-enriched media. The use of polymerase chain reaction (PCR) and matrix-assisted laser desorption ionization-time of flight mass spectrometry (MALDI-TOF MS) for rapid identification of *Malassezia* species is promising. Tinea versicolor is diagnosed by the characteristic "spaghetti and meatballs" appearance of skin scrapings when examined under the microscope with 10% potassium hydroxide (KOH). The diagnoses of seborrheic dermatitis and dandruff are usually made on a clinical basis. Culture for *Malassezia* does not confirm the diagnosis because *Malassezia* can be cultured from healthy skin. The diagnosis of *Malassezia* folliculitis can be made by the presence of budding yeast on a skin punch biopsy. Diagnosis of *Malassezia* neonatal cephalic pustulosis can be confirmed by culture of purulent material or by the presence of budding yeast on skin biopsy.

## TREATMENT

*Malassezia* species are generally susceptible to a wide range of topical and systemic antifungal treatments. Tinea versicolor and seborrheic dermatitis can be managed with topical 2.5% selenium sulfide, zinc pyrithione, or azole creams (eg, ketoconazole, itraconazole, fluconazole). Susceptibility to terbinafine varies. Topical terbinafine has been successfully used for treatment of tinea versicolor. However, oral terbinafine is not effective for the treatment of *Malassezia.* Topical corticosteroids are often used for the treatment of seborrheic dermatitis. Oral itraconazole and fluconazole have been shown to be effective for treatment of tinea versicolor and seborrheic dermatitis. Oral therapy is usually reserved for individuals with extensive disease or those who fail a treatment course with topical therapy. Given that cradle cap has a self-limited course, it is typically treated conservatively with topical emollients (vegetable oil, petroleum jelly, mineral oil) and mechanical scale removal (brushing with a soft brush).

*Malassezia* folliculitis may recur after topical antifungal therapy. Systemic therapy with itraconazole or fluconazole may be more effective.

For treatment of central line–associated *Malassezia* infection, therapy includes removal of the catheter and interruption of lipid feedings. A course of intravenous therapy, with conventional or liposomal amphotericin B, is typically used for treatment. An alternative treatment choice is antifungal therapy with an azole (eg, fluconazole, itraconazole). *Malassezia* species are resistant to flucytosine and appear to be resistant to echinocandins. There are reports of successful treatment of central line–associated *Malassezia* infection with catheter removal and no systemic antifungal therapy.

## SUGGESTED READINGS


Gaitanis G, Magiatis P, Hantschke M, Bassukas ID, Velegrakid A. The *Malassezia* genus in skin and systemic diseases. *Clin Microbiol Rev.* 2012;25:106-141.

Gupta AK, Lyons DC. Pityriasis versicolor: an update on pharmacological treatment options. *Expert Opin Pharmacother.* 2014;15:1707-1713.

Hald M, Arendrup MC, Svejgaard EL, et al. Evidence-based Danish guidelines for the treatment of *Malassezia*-related skin diseases. *Acta Derm Venereol.* 2015;95:12-19.

Pedrosa AF, Lisboa C, Gonçalves Rodrigues A. *Malassezia* infections: a medical conundrum. *J Am Acad Dermatol.* 2014;71:170-176.


# 297 Microsporidiosis

James J. Dunn

## INTRODUCTION

Microsporidia is a nontaxonomic term referring to an extensive group of unicellular, spore-forming eukaryotic organisms now reclassified in the kingdom Fungi. Microsporidia lack mitochondria, are obligate intracellular parasites, and have no metabolically active stages outside the host cell. The phylum Microsporidia encompasses more than 160 genera and 1300 species that are pathogenic in nearly all animal phyla and even some protists. To date, at least 16 species of microsporidia have been implicated in human infections (Table 297-1). Mature microsporidial spores possess a characteristic coiled extrusion apparatus consisting of a polar tubule anchored to an anterior disk within the spore. The polar tubule is capable of penetrating the host cell membrane, after which the infective spore contents (sporoplasm) can be injected into the cytoplasm and the reproductive life cycle begins (Fig. 297-1).

**TABLE 297-1 MICROSPORIDIAL SPECIES CAPABLE OF INFECTING HUMANS**

| Microsporidial Species | Site of Infection |
|---|---|
| *Anncaliia algerae* | Eye, muscle, skin |
| *Anncaliia connori* | Disseminated |
| *Anncaliia vesicularum* | Muscle |
| *Encephalitozoon cuniculi* | Disseminated, eye, respiratory tract, urinary tract, liver, peritoneum, intestine, brain |
| *Encephalitozoon hellem* | Disseminated, eye, respiratory tract, urinary tract |
| *Encephalitozoon intestinalis* | Intestine, biliary tract, respiratory tract, urinary tract, bone, skin |
| *Endoreticulatus* species | Muscle, disseminated |
| *Enterocytozoon bieneusi* | Intestine, biliary tract, respiratory tract |
| *Microsporidium africanum* | Eye |
| *Microsporidium ceylonensis* | Eye |
| *Nosema ocularum* | Eye |
| *Pleistophora* species | Muscle |
| *Trachipleistophora anthropophthera* | Disseminated, eye |
| *Trachipleistophora hominis* | Muscle, eye, respiratory tract |
| *Tubulinosema acridophagus* | Disseminated, muscle, liver, respiratory tract, peritoneum, skin |
| *Vittaforma corneae* | Disseminated, urinary tract, eye |

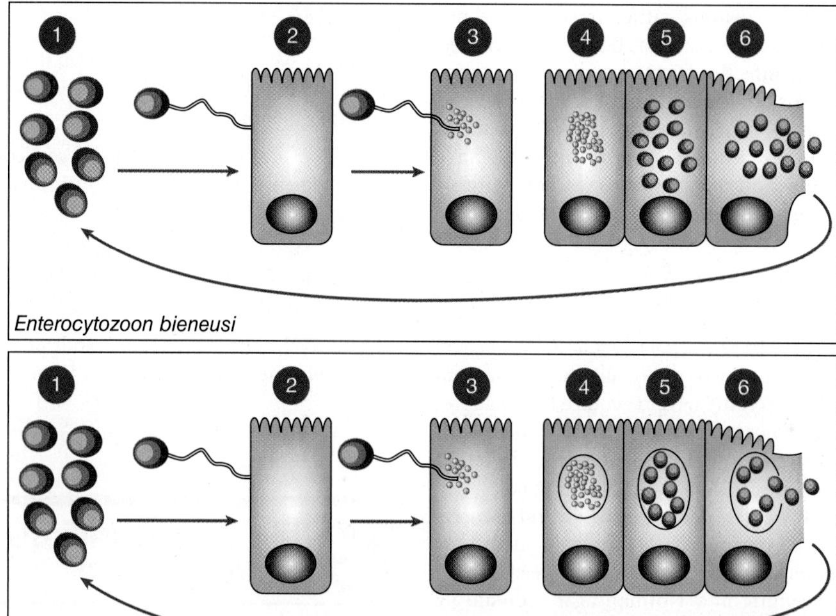


**FIGURE 297-1** Microsporidian life cycle. The intracellular development of *Enterocytozoon bieneusi* and *Encephalitozoon intestinalis* are shown in sequence. (1) The infective spore stage is ingested by a susceptible host. (2, 3) Extrusion of the polar tubule permits injection of the infectious material (sporoplasm) directly into the host cell cytoplasm. (4) The microsporidia develop by sporogony either in the host cell cytoplasm (*E bieneusi*) or inside a parasitophorous vacuole (*E intestinalis*). (5) After undergoing multiple divisions, meronts undergo a sporogenic phase, which, after several more divisions, results in infectious spores that are resistant to adverse environmental conditions. (6) The host cell membrane is disrupted and ruptured as the spores increase in number, releasing spores into the lumen or microenvironment. (Reproduced with permission from Centers for Disease Control and Prevention. Life cycle of microsporidia. http://www.cdc.gov/dpdx/microsporidiosis. Accessed August 30, 2017.)

## PATHOGENESIS AND EPIDEMIOLOGY

Microsporidia are ubiquitous in the environment with an extremely broad host range. Human infections have been documented worldwide. Serosurveys in humans have demonstrated a high prevalence of antibodies to various microsporidia, suggesting that asymptomatic infection may be common. The incidence, reservoirs, and sources of human infection are not well defined, but ingestion of the environmentally highly resistant spores is probably the most important mode of transmission, particularly for *Enterocytozoon bieneusi*, which is almost exclusively found in the gastrointestinal tract. *E bieneusi* infects the enterocytes of the small intestine, producing a limited inflammatory reaction with abnormalities of the villi but rarely invades the lamina propria. Dissemination of *E bieneusi* outside of the gastrointestinal tract is rare, although infection of epithelial cells of the biliary tree and respiratory tract have been noted. *Encephalitozoon* species infect epithelial and endothelial cells, fibroblasts, macrophages, and possibly other cell types. *Encephalitozoon intestinalis* infects primarily enterocytes, but the organism is also found in intestinal lamina propria, and dissemination to the kidneys, airways, and biliary tract appears to occur via infected macrophages. *Encephalitozoon cuniculi* and *Encephalitozoon hellem* also have the capacity to disseminate widely in their hosts.

Microsporidia that infect humans have been found in a variety of animal species, making direct zoonotic transmission a possibility, although very few cases exist. Two genotypes of *E cuniculi* detected in natural infections in rabbits, dogs, and tamarins have been isolated from human immunodeficiency virus (HIV)-infected patients. Originally discovered in humans, *E bieneusi* is increasingly being recognized in various animals. *Encephalitozoon* species have been detected in several avian species, domestic animals in Mexico, and gorillas in Uganda. Transmission is also thought to occur by dust or aerosol based on findings of respiratory and ocular infections. Spores may also be found in environmental water sources, suggesting that waterborne transmission likely plays a role in disease. Contamination of the environment by spores passed in urine and stool is believed to be the mechanism of transmission of these organisms between successive hosts. Although spores may persist in the environment and remain infectious for long periods of time, they can be inactivated through chlorination; ozonation; exposure for 30 minutes to 70% ethanol, 1% formaldehyde, or 2% Lysol; or by autoclaving at 120°C for 10 minutes. Foodborne outbreaks associated with microsporidia have been reported, and microsporidia pathogenic in humans have been detected in fresh produce and milk specimens. Although no congenitally acquired human infections have been reported, studies with mammals suggest that *Encephalitozoon* species can be transmitted transplacentally from mother to offspring.

## CLINICAL MANIFESTATIONS

The propensity of microsporidia to cause disease in humans likely involves the interplay between the immune status of the host and the species of microsporidia involved. Immunocompetent hosts may be asymptomatic or develop transient diarrhea, whereas severely immunocompromised hosts may develop a wide range of clinical manifestations and remain persistently infected. Patients with severe cellular immunodeficiency appear to be at the highest risk for developing microsporidial disease, and microsporidia have long been recognized as opportunistic pathogens causing chronic diarrhea and wasting syndrome in acquired immunodeficiency syndrome (AIDS) patients. The spectrum of diseases associated with microsporidia has now expanded to include infections of practically every organ system including the hepatobiliary system, eyes, sinuses, lung, muscles, urinary tract, and central nervous system (see Table 297-1).

Most cases of microsporidiosis in immunocompetent hosts manifest as self-limiting diarrhea lasting up to 2 to 3 weeks. *E bieneusi* and *E intestinalis* have been reported to cause such cases in travelers to and residents of tropical countries. Clinical manifestations have included watery, nonbloody diarrhea, nausea, diffuse abdominal pain, and fever. Ocular infection with microsporidia, particularly *Vittaforma corneae*, may present as keratoconjunctivitis in immunocompetent hosts. Cases of superficial epithelial keratitis caused by *Encephalitozoon* species have occurred in contact lens wearers. *Encephalitozoon* species have been found as a rare cause of cerebral infection in immunocompetent hosts.

Microsporidiosis is usually seen in individuals with a profound defect in cell-mediated immunity (CD4 cell count < 100/μL). Up to 50% of chronic diarrhea cases of undetermined etiology in HIV-infected patients are caused by microsporidia, in particular *E bieneusi* and *E intestinalis*, although prevalence data vary considerably depending on the population and region studied. Infection has occurred in young adults with advanced AIDS (CD4 count < 50/μL) and severely immunocompromised children. The disease typically presents with afebrile, nonbloody, watery diarrhea with up to 20 bowel movements per day. The diarrhea can be exacerbated by food intake and is associated with progressive weight loss, anorexia, and malabsorption. Children may present with failure to thrive, intermittent abdominal pain, and chronic diarrhea. *E bieneusi* and *E intestinalis* infections of the biliary tract can result in sclerosing cholangitis in AIDS patients. Reports of encephalitis in AIDS patients infected with *E cuniculi* or *Trachipleistophora anthropophthera* indicate that it often mimics that of *Toxoplasma* species central nervous system infection clinically and radiographically.

In immunocompromised patients other than those with HIV, microsporidial infections have been described in organ transplant recipients, patients with hematologic malignancies, patients with rheumatic disease undergoing anti–tumor necrosis factor (TNF)-α therapy, the elderly, and malnourished children. Ocular infection with *E cuniculi*, *E hellem*, *E intestinalis*, or *Trachipleistophora hominis* can result in punctate keratopathy and conjunctivitis characterized by multiple punctate corneal ulcers, photophobia, blurred vision, foreign body sensation, and decreased visual acuity. Ocular involvement may result from disseminated infection with organisms also present in the urine, sputum, and nasal mucosa, but it may also be confined to the eye as a result of direct inoculation. Keratitis and corneal ulcerations have been reported with *Nosema ocularum* and *V corneae*. Interstitial nephritis has been seen in AIDS patients as well as those with renal transplants complicated by microsporidiosis. Microsporidia have been reported to cause necrotizing urethritis and cystitis. Respiratory tract involvement is often seen with disseminated infections in immunocompromised patients and may manifest with myriad symptoms. *E cuniculi*, *E hellem*, and *E intestinalis* infections may present as sinusitis with mucopurulent nasal discharge or lower respiratory tract involvement, which may be asymptomatic or cause bronchiolitis with or without pneumonia. Disseminated infection and myositis have been linked to infection with various microsporidia in immunocompromised hosts, including *Pleistophora* species, *T hominis*, *Anncaliia vesicularum*, *Anncaliia algerae*, *Anncaliia connori*, and *Tubulinosema acridophagus* (see Table 297-1).

## DIAGNOSIS

A definitive diagnosis of microsporidiosis is made by detection of spores in stool, body fluids (duodenal aspirates, urine, bile, sputum, bronchoalveolar lavage fluid, nasal secretions, cerebrospinal fluid, and conjunctival smears), corneal scrapings, or tissue sections. Organisms can be visualized by light microscopy using a variety of specialized stains. Spores of microsporidia vary in size and shape depending on the species, but those that infect humans have spores in the range of 1 to 3 μm × 1.5 to 4 μm in size and are usually ovoid. Although not routinely performed, definitive species identification of microsporidia can be made by ultrastructural analysis using electron microscopy or by molecular typing methods such as species-specific polymerase chain reaction at designated reference laboratories (eg, Centers for Disease Control and Prevention). Some microsporidia have been propagated in cell culture systems, but the isolation of organism has no relevance for diagnostic purposes. Serologic tests for microsporidia have been developed but are used primarily for epidemiologic purposes.

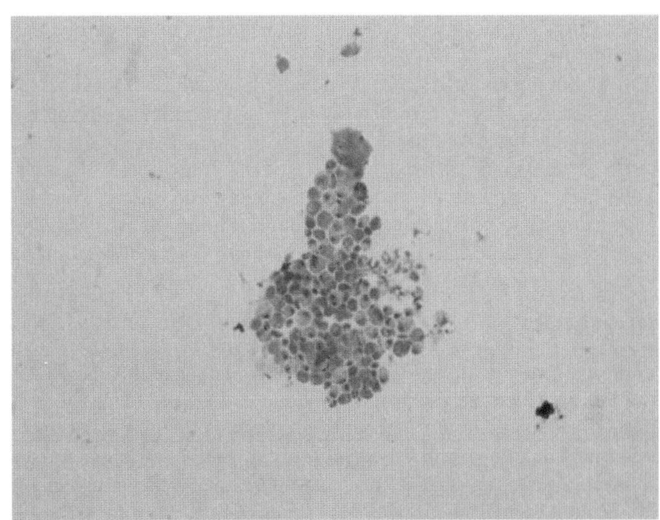

**FIGURE 297-2** Giemsa-stained cerebrospinal fluid cytology specimen with microsporidial spores observed by light microscopy (×1000 magnification).

Organisms in stool can be visualized by light microscopy in thin smears of unconcentrated stool stained most commonly with chromotrope-based (modified trichrome) stains and by fluorescent microscopy using chemifluorescent optical brightening agents such as calcofluor white and Uvitex 2B. These brightening agents stain chitin in the spore wall and will also stain fungi and other fecal elements. However, microsporidial spores can be distinguished from yeast by their uniform oval shape and lack of budding. Spores can be detected in sediments of body fluids obtained by centrifugation using a variety of stains including chemifluorescent optical brightening agents, modified trichrome, Giemsa, Gram, modified acid-fast, and Warthin-Starry silver stains (Fig. 297-2). Paraffin-embedded tissue samples may be examined using routine histologic stains such as hematoxylin-eosin, periodic acid-Schiff, Giemsa, and Steiner silver stains. Since renal involvement with shedding of spores is common in microsporidial species known to cause disseminated human infection, urine sediment should be examined whenever the diagnosis of microsporidiosis is considered. This can have therapeutic implications since microsporidial species that disseminate (eg, *Encephalitozoon* species) can usually be treated with albendazole, whereas those that do not disseminate (eg, *E bieneusi*) would be treated with fumagillin.

## TREATMENT

Since the introduction of combination antiretroviral therapy (cART) in HIV-infected patients, the prevalence of microsporidial infection among AIDS patients has decreased. Improved immune function can result in clinical response of patients with gastrointestinal microsporidiosis, with elimination of the organism and normalization of the intestinal architecture. Likewise, in other non-HIV severely immunocompromised individuals, restoration of immune function is essential.

Among the compounds tested in vitro and in vivo for treatment of microsporidiosis, albendazole and fumagillin have demonstrated the most consistent activity and have been shown to have clinical efficacy in human infections with various microsporidia. Albendazole binds to β-tubulin and is active against *Encephalitozoon* species but has only limited efficacy against *E bieneusi*. Fumagillin and its semisynthetic analogue TNP-470 have been found to have activity in vitro and in vivo against microsporidia including *E cuniculi*, *E hellem*, *E intestinalis*, *V corneae*, and *E bieneusi*. Treatment studies with humans are limited, but AIDS patients and renal transplant recipients treated with fumagillin for 14 days exhibited transient clearing of spores from their stool. The primary side effect of treatment was thrombocytopenia, which was reversible upon stopping fumagillin treatment. Trimethoprim-sulfamethoxazole prophylaxis is not effective for preventing microsporidiosis, and limited and variable success has been reported for other drugs such as metronidazole, furazolidone, nitazoxanide, and atovaquone.

Ocular microsporidiosis has been treated successfully with fumagillin in solution. However, recurrence may occur upon discontinuation of eye drops since the organism is still often present systemically and can be demonstrated in urine or nasal smears. In such cases, the addition of albendazole as a systemic agent should be considered. Keratoplasty appears to provide temporary improvement in some cases, and debulking by corneal scraping may be useful in cases not responding to medical treatment.

## PREVENTION

There are limited data on effective preventive strategies for microsporidiosis, and currently, no prophylactic agents have been identified for these organisms. The most effective prophylaxis is the restoration of immune function in immunocompromised hosts. Although microsporidial spores can survive and remain infective in the environment for prolonged periods, in the hospital environment, spores can be rendered noninfectious by a 30-minute exposure to most of the commonly used disinfectants. Spores are also killed by the methods commonly used for sterilization.

## SUGGESTED READINGS

Champion L, Durrbach A, Lang P, et al. Fumagillin for treatment of intestinal microsporidiosis in renal transplant recipients. *Am J Transplant.* 2010;10:1925-1930.

Decraene V, Lebbad M, Botero-Kleiven S, et al. First reported foodborne outbreak associated with microsporidia, Sweden, October 2009. *Epidemiol Infect.* 2012;140:519-527.

Didier ES, Weiss LM. Microsporidiosis: not just in AIDS patients. *Curr Opin Infect Dis.* 2011;24:490-495.

Galvan AL, Sanchez AM, Valentin MA, et al. First cases of microsporidiosis in transplant recipients in Spain and review of the literature. *J Clin Microbiol.* 2011;49:1301-1306.

Lobo ML, Xiao L, Antunes F, et al. Microsporidia as emerging pathogens and the implication for public health: a 10-year study on HIV-positive and -negative patients. *Int J Parasitol.* 2012;42:197-205.

Matos O, Lobo ML, Xiao L. Epidemiology of *Enterocytozoon bieneusi* infection in humans. *J Parasitol Res.* 2012;2012:981424.

Ramanan P, Pritt BS. Extraintestinal microsporidiosis. *J Clin Microbiol.* 2014;52:3839-3844.

Tham AC, Sanjay S. Clinical spectrum of microsporidial keratoconjunctivitis. *Clin Exp Ophthalmol.* 2012;40:512-518.

Weber R, Deplazes P, Mathis A. Microsporidia. In: Jorgensen JH, Pfaller MA, Carroll KC, et al, eds. *Manual of Clinical Microbiology.* 11th ed. Washington, DC: ASM Press; 2015:2209-2219.

# 298 Sporotrichosis

Charles R. Woods

## INTRODUCTION

Sporotrichosis is an uncommon, chronic mycosis caused by *Sporothrix schenckii*. This ubiquitous plant saprophyte is a dimorphic fungus that grows as a mold at room temperature and as a yeast-like form in tissue. It is distributed worldwide and found most commonly both in warm, highly humid regions and in temperate climates.

## PATHOGENESIS AND EPIDEMIOLOGY

Infection is characterized by isolated cutaneous or subcutaneous necrotizing nodules associated with the indolent development of suppurating nodules along the course of the proximal lymphatics. Extracutaneous and pulmonary forms of the disease occur infrequently. The histopathologic findings of primary cutaneous disease combine features of both granulomatous and pyogenic inflammation. Granulomatous lesions consist of aggregations of epithelioid histiocytes with central areas of necrosis and neutrophils or zones of Langhans giant cells associated with fibroblasts and lymphocytes. Occasionally, areas of microabscesses unassociated with granulomatous reaction may be seen. In chronic disease, pseudoepitheliomatous hyperplasia may be extensive and mimic neoplasm. A common histopathologic feature is the asteroid body, a round basophilic, yeast-like structure surrounded by rays of eosinophilic material thought to represent antigen-antibody complexes. The asteroid body may also be seen in other mycoses.

In 95% of cases, the organism is percutaneously inoculated by contaminated thorns, tree bark, splinters, or animal bites or scratches, especially from cats. Handling of contaminated plant material such as hay or moss also can lead to infection. Rare cases of human-to-human transmission have been reported. Sporotrichosis has been reported in many areas of the United States but is most common along the Mississippi River Valley and in the Plains states. Most cases are sporadic, but single-source outbreaks occur. Infection occurs in all age groups; about 10% to 25% of cases occur in children.

## CLINICAL MANIFESTATIONS

The spectrum of clinical findings in sporotrichosis can be divided into lymphocutaneous, fixed cutaneous, mucosal, extracutaneous (localized or multifocal), and pulmonary. Lymphocutaneous sporotrichosis accounts for 75% of infections. Following inoculation, the average incubation period is 3 weeks but ranges from 5 days to 6 months. Lesions usually involve the upper extremities but may occur on the face and trunk. The primary lesion is a firm, mobile, nontender subcutaneous nodule that enlarges and becomes discolored (Fig. 298-1). After 2 weeks, it undergoes necrosis, leaving a painless ulcer. During the next several weeks, additional lesions develop along the proximal lymphatics; intervening lymphatic channels become thickened, with overlying cutaneous erythema (Fig. 298-2). Lesions can persist for

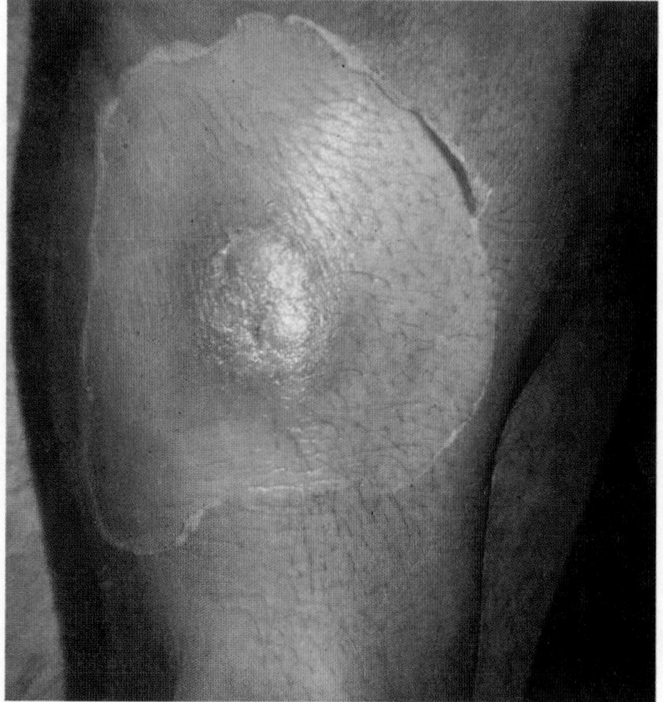

**FIGURE 298-1** The ulcer and surrounding erythema of fixed cutaneous sporotrichosis could be confused with a brown recluse spider bite. (Reproduced with permission from Knoop KJ, Stack LB, Storrow AB, et al: *The Atlas of Emergency Medicine*, 3rd ed. New York: McGraw-Hill; 2010. Photo contributor: Edward J. Otten, MD.)

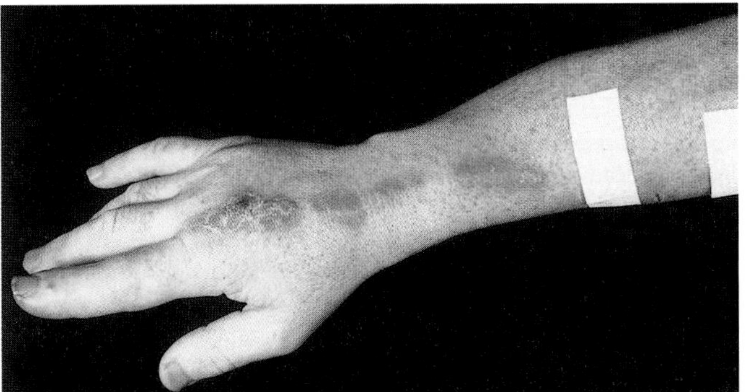

**FIGURE 298-2** Chronic lymphangitic type. An erythematous papule at the site of inoculation on the index finger with a linear arrangement of erythematous dermal and subcutaneous nodules extending proximally in lymphatic vessels of the dorsum of the hand and arm. (Reproduced with permission from Wolff K, Johnson RA: *Fitzpatrick's Color Atlas and Synopsis of Clinical Dermatology*, 6th ed. New York: McGraw-Hill; 2009.)

months to years. Few heal spontaneously, with scarring of the ulcers. Systemic symptoms are absent or mild.

Fixed cutaneous disease accounts for 20% to 25% of cases and is common in children. Infection is limited to the site of inoculation and consists of ulcerative, plaque-like, or maculopapular lesions. These lesions can resolve spontaneously, persist for years, or resolve and recur. Most cutaneous lesions in children occur on the upper extremities and face. Nasal or conjunctival mucosal infection may occur after self-inoculation or inhalation of spores.

Extracutaneous disease accounts for less than 1% of cases and may occur as localized or multifocal disease. Localized extracutaneous infections may result from hematogenous dissemination, spread from contiguous skin lesions, or direct inoculation. Osteoarticular manifestations are a common manifestation of these cases and include destructive arthritis, tenosynovitis, chronic osteomyelitis, and periostitis. The tibiae and the bones of the hands are most often affected. Arthritis is slowly progressive, and symptoms include pain, swelling, and impaired function. Osteoarticular disease usually remains localized but can spread to contiguous structures; dissemination is rare.

Multifocal extracutaneous disease results from hematogenous spread, occurs primarily in immunocompromised hosts, and is rare in children. In adults, predisposing conditions include acquired immunodeficiency syndrome, malignancy, diabetes, sarcoidosis, alcoholism, and long-term corticosteroid therapy. Sporotrichal meningitis is a rare but severe manifestation of disseminated disease primarily seen in immunocompromised patients and has a very poor prognosis. Primary pulmonary sporotrichosis may also occur but is seen mainly in adults and follows inhalation of conidia. It may affect the lung parenchyma or remain localized to the hilar nodes, usually without extracutaneous sites of infection. Apical portions of the lung are involved, and chronic cavitary lesions may result. Lesions can be progressive and fatal. Hilar lymph node enlargement can be the only clinically evident manifestation and may mimic tuberculosis and histoplasmosis.

Painless papulovesicular, ulcerative, or nodular lesions that fail to respond to antibiotics should prompt consideration of sporotrichosis. The differential diagnosis includes infection with *Nocardia* species, *Francisella tularensis*, nontuberculous mycobacteria, *Treponema pallidum*, and *Leishmania*. Nodular lymphangitis can also be seen with infections caused by some pyogenic bacteria such as *Pseudomonas* species, *Bacillus anthracis*, and other mycoses, including blastomycosis, chromoblastomycosis, coccidioidomycosis, cryptococcosis, and histoplasmosis. Nodular lymphangitis can be seen with mycetoma, which may be caused by bacteria or fungi. A careful travel and exposure history may help differentiate these entities.

## DIAGNOSIS

The laboratory diagnosis of sporotrichosis is problematic because histopathologic findings of pyogranulomatous inflammation are not diagnostic, few organisms are found in tissue, and their morphology may not be typical. Fungal culture remains the primary means to determine the diagnosis. *S schenckii* can be isolated from exudate or biopsied tissue, and conversion of the mold to yeast forms is confirmatory. Growth in culture occurs within 8 days in about 90% of cases but may take up to 4 weeks. The organism is more readily recovered from synovial fluid than from cutaneous lesions. In cases of meningitis, the cerebrospinal fluid typically shows a mild pleocytosis with a majority of lymphocytes, elevated protein, and hypoglycorrhachia.

Serologic tests have been developed for *S schenckii* but are of limited utility. Polymerase chain reaction tests for detection of *S schenckii* in clinical specimens have been described.

## TREATMENT

Guidelines for the treatment of sporotrichosis have been published. Itraconazole is currently the recommended treatment for cutaneous and localized lymphocutaneous sporotrichosis for children and adults. Response rates are excellent, and side effects are few. Care must be taken to avoid drug interactions. Serum concentrations should be documented after 2 weeks of therapy to confirm adequate drug exposure. Lesions usually resolve within 1 month of beginning treatment; treatment should be continued for 2 to 4 weeks after all lesions have resolved, which may require a total course of 3 to 6 months of therapy.

Saturated solution of potassium iodide (SSKI) also is an effective treatment of cutaneous disease. This is often used as a therapeutic agent in developing countries because it is inexpensive and available. The mechanism by which iodide therapy works is unknown. (Dosing starts at 1 drop 3 times a day, with dosage increased as tolerated to 1 drop/kg of body weight 3 times a day, up to a maximum of 40–50 drops/kg/dose 3 times a day.) Treatment continues for 6 to 8 weeks after the resolution of lesions. Side effects include anorexia, nausea, a metallic taste, rash, fever, and swelling of the salivary glands. The extended length and inconvenience of treatment with iodide often lead to poor compliance. Iodide therapy cannot be used in pregnancy.

For children with disseminated or visceral sporotrichosis, including meningitis, amphotericin B is recommended as initial therapy. Deoxycholate or lipid preparations may be used. After clinical response is evident, children can be switched to itraconazole to complete a course of therapy of at least 12 months. Pulmonary and disseminated infections do not respond as well as cutaneous infection. In addition to antifungal therapy, excision of localized pulmonary lesions is recommended in adults and may be appropriate in children. Lifelong itraconazole therapy may be required in children with persisting immunodeficiency, including advanced HIV infection without sufficient immunologic reconstitution on antiretroviral therapy.

Itraconazole or initial amphotericin B followed by itraconazole may be used for treatment of isolated osteoarticular disease. Therapy should continue for at least 12 months. Itraconazole may be used for treating less severe or chronic pulmonary disease. Fluconazole may have some effectiveness but should be used only for children who are unable to tolerate amphotericin B or itraconazole.

Amphotericin B is preferred during pregnancy because the azoles have teratogenic potential and SSKI can be toxic to the fetal thyroid.

Local hyperthermia can be effective in treating fixed cutaneous lesions in some patients because *S schenckii* growth is impaired at temperatures exceeding 42°C. This modality may be considered for patients who cannot safely take (eg, pregnant or nursing women) or tolerate the recommended drugs. Local hyperthermia may not be readily tolerated by children.

## PREVENTION

Disease can be prevented by the use of gloves or other clothing that covers exposed skin and protects it from contact with the contaminated thorns, tree bark, splinters, or animal bites or scratches that are responsible for injecting the organism into the skin.

American Academy of Pediatrics. Sporotrichosis. In: Kimberlin DW, Brady MT, Jackson MA, Long SS, eds. *Red Book: 2015 Report of the Committee on Infectious Diseases*. 30th ed. Elk Grove Village, IL: American Academy of Pediatrics; 2015:712-714.

Dhingra D, Durrheim D, Porigneaux P. Sporotrichosis outbreak and mouldy hay in NSW. *Aust Fam Physician*. 2015;44:217-222.

Liu X, Zhang Z, Hou B, et al. Rapid identification of *Sporothrix schenckii* in biopsy tissue by PCR. *J Eur Acad Dermatol Venereol*. 2013;27:1491-1497.

Trotter JR, Sriaroon P, Berman D, Petrovic A, Leiding JW. *Sporothrix schenckii* lymphadenitis in a male with X-linked chronic granulomatous disease. *J Clin Immunol*. 2014;34:49-52.

# 299 Zygomycosis (Mucormycosis)

Rebecca C. Brady

## INTRODUCTION

Zygomycosis is an umbrella term for all diseases caused by fungi of the class Zygomycetes. The more common term *mucormycosis* refers to a group of invasive mycoses caused by members of the order Mucorales, within the class Zygomycetes. *Rhizopus* species are the most commonly isolated agents of mucormycosis.

## PATHOGENESIS AND EPIDEMIOLOGY

The Mucorales are distributed worldwide and commonly grow in decaying organic matter. Although exposure to the airborne spores of these thermotolerant, rapidly growing fungi is universal, human disease is infrequent and is indicative of a serious underlying predisposing condition. Diabetes mellitus, particularly diabetic ketoacidosis, is the most common predisposing condition in patients with mucormycosis. Underlying disease accompanied by acidosis such as uremia, malnutrition, and congenital metabolic aciduria may also predispose to mucormycosis. Additional risk factors include neutropenia, hematologic malignancies, burns, prematurity, corticosteroid therapy, solid organ transplantation, bone marrow transplantation, and deferoxamine therapy for management of iron overload states.

Infection in humans most commonly occurs following inhalation of the spores of Mucorales into the respiratory tract. Spores may also be ingested or introduced directly into abraded skin. Germination of spores occurs with hyphal proliferation and invasion of tissue. Infection may spread by direct extension and hematogenous dissemination. Regardless of the tissue involved, the pathologic hallmark of mucormycosis is hyphal invasion of blood vessels with resultant hemorrhage, thrombosis, infarction, and production of black, necrotic debris. The reasons these fungi target the vasculature are not well understood.

Neutrophils and macrophages are important components of the host response to Mucorales. Thus, defects in their function likely contribute to the pathogenesis of mucormycosis. Iron is an important growth factor for these fungi; hence, interactions between iron molecules and transferrin have been postulated to play a role in predisposing deferoxamine-treated patients to the development of mucormycosis. Because these fungi metabolize ketones and grow optimally at an acid pH, the metabolic conditions encountered in ketoacidotic hosts may enhance their growth.

## CLINICAL MANIFESTATIONS

The clinical manifestations of mucormycosis are classified by site of involvement into rhinocerebral, pulmonary, cutaneous, gastrointestinal, disseminated, and miscellaneous infections. Rhinocerebral infection occurs most frequently and typically presents as facial pain, nasal congestion, and headache in a poorly controlled diabetic patient. From the nasal mucosa and paranasal sinuses, infection may spread to the orbit, resulting in orbital cellulitis, paresis of extraocular muscles, and proptosis. Further extension into the cerebral vasculature and brain can lead to cavernous sinus thrombosis, brain infarcts, and focal neurologic deficits.

Most cases of pulmonary mucormycosis have occurred in neutropenic hosts, especially those receiving chemotherapy for leukemia and lymphoma. Clinically, these patients present with unremitting fever and dyspnea. The chest roentgenogram may show patchy consolidation and cavity formation. Infection progresses rapidly, and hemoptysis may be a fatal complication.

Cutaneous mucormycosis usually occurs at sites of burns, trauma, and invasive procedures in immunosuppressed hosts, including premature infants. The skin lesion may begin as an area of erythema and induration that subsequently develops central necrosis. Skin lesions may also be a manifestation of disseminated infection.

Risk factors for gastrointestinal mucormycosis include malnutrition, prematurity, and underlying gastrointestinal disease. The stomach, ileum, and colon are involved most frequently. Presenting findings may include nonspecific abdominal pain, hematochezia, or melena. Premature infants may experience necrotizing enterocolitis.

Disseminated infection most often follows pulmonary invasion and may spread to the brain, liver, spleen, and other tissues. Clinically, these patients have rapidly progressive multiple organ failure with a high mortality rate. Miscellaneous forms of mucormycosis include endocarditis, osteomyelitis, and pyelonephritis.

## DIAGNOSIS

Mucormycosis must be differentiated from other opportunistic infections in immunosuppressed hosts. Cutaneous mucormycosis may mimic ecthyma gangrenosum, which is commonly due to *Pseudomonas aeruginosa*. Invasion of blood vessels is a major pathologic finding with *Aspergillus* infection. Not surprisingly, the pulmonary, cerebral, and cutaneous manifestations of aspergillosis are clinically indistinguishable from those of mucormycosis. The definitive diagnosis of mucormycosis requires demonstration of hyphal elements invading tissue in a biopsy specimen. Because the Mucorales may colonize body surfaces, swabs of drainage or abnormal tissue are inappropriate. Tissue biopsies, especially of black necrotic lesions, should be sent for histologic examination and for culture. Grinding of tissue should be avoided, because it may disrupt the hyphal elements. Demonstration of irregularly shaped, broad, nonseptate hyphae with right-angle branching by either hematoxylin and eosin or Grocott-Gomori methenamine-silver nitrate staining is the gold standard for diagnosis of mucormycosis. The agents of mucormycosis may be difficult to isolate in culture from infected tissues. Cultures of blood, urine, and cerebrospinal fluid are rarely positive.

## TREATMENT

Successful treatment of mucormycosis requires a coordinated medical and surgical approach. If possible, the underlying predisposing condition should be reversed. Metabolic acidosis should be corrected, and the doses of corticosteroids and other immunosuppressive drugs should be lowered if at all possible. All devitalized tissue should be surgically removed. Often, debridement must be repeated daily for several days. Lipid formulations of amphotericin B are the standard therapy. Some patients can later be transitioned to oral posaconazole. Duration of therapy for antifungals is often hard to define and should be individualized for the specific location of infection in a particular patient.

## PREVENTION

Primary prophylaxis is not recommended. Posaconazole is often prescribed for secondary prophylaxis in immunocompromised patients while they remain at high risk for relapsing mucormycosis.

## SUGGESTED READINGS

Cornely OA, Arikan-Akdagli S, Dannaoui E, et al. ESCMID and ECMM joint clinical guidelines for the diagnosis and management of mucormycosis 2013. *Clin Microbiol Infect.* 2014;20(suppl 3):S5-S26.

Kontoyiannis DP, Lewis RE. Agents of mucormycosis and entomophthoramycosis. In: Bennett JE, Dolin R, Blaser MJ, eds. *Mandell, Douglas, and Bennett's Principles and Practice of Infectious Diseases.* 8th ed. Philadelphia, PA: Elsevier Saunders; 2015:2909-2919.

Lanternier F, Sun HY, Ribaud P, Singh N, Kontoyiannis DP, Lortholary O. Mucormycosis in organ and stem cell transplant recipients. *Clin Infect Dis.* 2012;54:1629-1636.

Petrikkos G, Skiada A, Lortholary O, Roilides E, Walsh TJ, Kontoyiannis DP. Epidemiology and clinical manifestations of mucormycosis. *Clin Infect Dis.* 2012;54(suppl 1):S23-S34.

Walsh TJ, Gamaletsou MN, McGinnis MR, Hayden RT, Kontoyiannis DP. Early clinical and laboratory diagnosis of invasive pulmonary, extrapulmonary, and disseminated mucormycosis (zygomycosis). *Clin Infect Dis.* 2012;54(suppl 1):S55-S60.

Wattier RL, Dvorak CC, Hoffman JA, et al. A prospective, international cohort study of invasive mold infections in children. *J Pediatr Infect Dis Soc.* 2015;4:313-322.

# PART 7 VIRAL INFECTIONS

## 300 Arboviruses

Jason Brophy and Manisha Kulkarni

### INTRODUCTION

Arboviruses (or arthropod-borne viruses) are a heterogeneous group of viruses that share the same usual route of entry into humans: via the bite of an infected mosquito, tick, sandfly, or other arthropod. The life cycle of most arboviruses is characterized by the ability of the virus to replicate in both an arthropod vector and a vertebrate "natural" host (usually birds or small mammals) and by transmission between these 2 organisms at the time of the arthropod's bite (Fig. 300-1). This cycle leads to establishment or maintenance of the virus in a given ecosystem. Humans or domestic animals are only "incidental" hosts for many species of arboviruses, as infection in such hosts (although capable of causing disease) is often a dead end for the virus due to viremia being too low or too transient to contribute to maintenance of the cycle of transmission. Some viruses are specific to a single genus or species of insect, while others are transmissible by multiple vectors. In addition, some arthropods are capable of transovarial transmission, wherein their eggs (which sometimes overwinter and hatch in spring) are infected with the virus, allowing viral maintenance in areas of colder climate.

Ecosystem changes, both natural and anthropogenic, can affect the complex ecology of arboviruses, alter transmission patterns, and drive the emergence and resurgence of diseases in new regions. A global resurgence of several arboviruses has occurred in the last 40 years, most notably of West Nile virus (WNV), dengue viruses (DENV), chikungunya virus (CHIKV), and Zika virus (ZIKV). Their geographic expansion has been associated with a number of factors such as climate

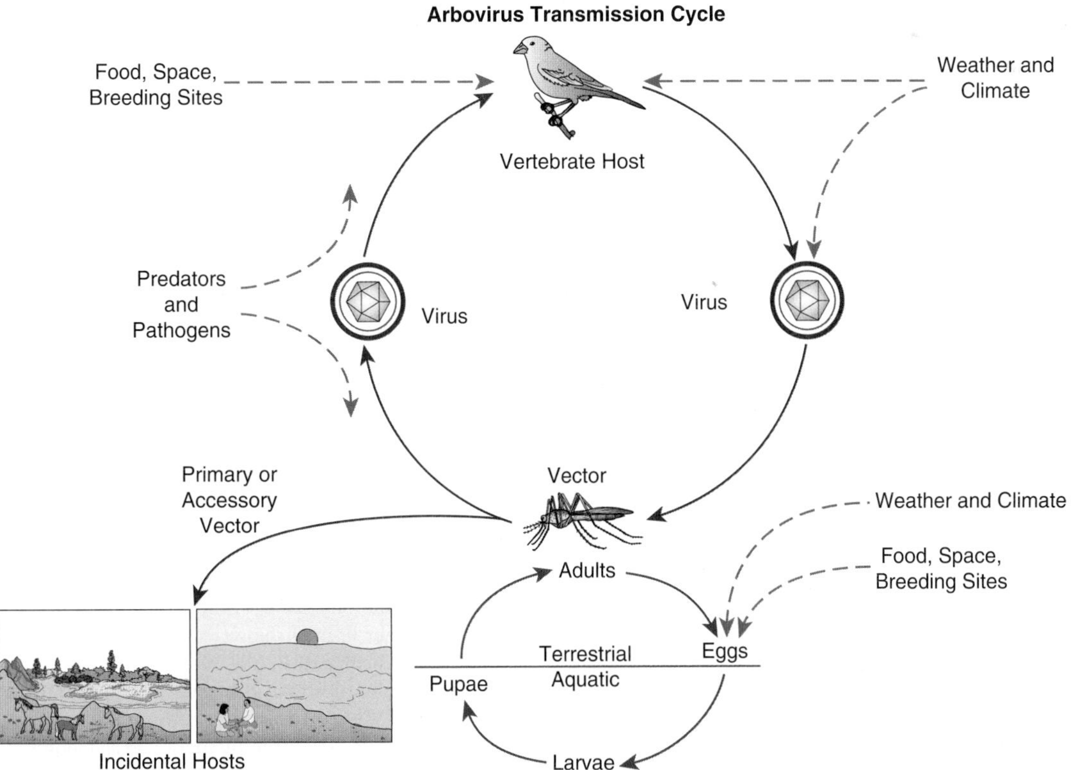


**FIGURE 300-1** Arbovirus transmission cycle. (Reproduced with permission from Centers for Disease Control and Prevention. Division of Vector Borne Infectious Diseases. http://www.cdc.gov/ncidod/dvbid/arbor/schemat.pdf. Accessed November 21, 2017.)

change, expansion of mosquito vector distributions, human population growth and urbanization, and increasing international travel. In particular, the invasion of *Aedes albopictus* mosquitoes into the Americas, Europe, and Africa has driven large-scale epidemics of DENV and CHIKV in these regions. ZIKV has followed the path of DENV and CHIKV emergence in the Americas, spreading to countries with competent vector species including *Aedes aegypti*. Ongoing global change is anticipated to drive further arbovirus emergence, underscoring the current and future importance of this group of viruses.

Arboviruses generally produce 1 of 4 clinical syndromes: (1) central nervous system (CNS) disease, (2) febrile illness with rash, (3) febrile illness with arthropathy, or (4) hemorrhagic fever syndrome. In North America, encephalitis is the most important manifestation of arboviral infection, with several viruses producing sporadic disease as well as outbreaks of infection each year. Table 300-1 provides a list of arboviruses presenting with different symptom complexes and details the vector, reservoir, distribution, incubation period, and population most affected.

## CLASSIFICATION OF ARBOVIRUSES

The term *arbovirus* refers only to viruses in which the mode of infection is by the bite of an infected arthropod. This artificial grouping includes dozens of viruses from a number of different families and genera, including mainly the *Flavivirus* genus, the *Alphavirus* genus, the Bunyaviridae family, and the Reoviridae family (*Coltivirus* genus). These viruses differ phylogenetically and structurally but nonetheless produce similar types of illness.

### Flaviviruses

Flaviviruses are a large group of viruses with worldwide distribution, over 30 of which cause disease in humans. The prototype of the genus is yellow fever virus, from which the genus name is derived (*flavus* being Latin for "yellow"). Eight antigenic groupings have been found, the most important of which are the Japanese encephalitis complex (which includes Japanese encephalitis, St. Louis encephalitis, West Nile, and Murray Valley fever viruses); the dengue complex (DENV 1–4); the tick-borne virus complex (Central European encephalitis [renamed tick-borne encephalitis], Russian spring-summer encephalitis, louping-ill, Powassan, Kyasanur Forest disease, and Omsk hemorrhagic fever viruses); ZIKV; and yellow fever virus.

### Alphaviruses

Alphaviruses are a genus within the Togaviridae family and include a number of medically important arboviruses. These can be roughly divided into New World alphaviruses, which cause CNS disease and include eastern equine, western equine, and Venezuelan equine encephalitis viruses, and Old World alphaviruses, which are more likely to cause syndromes of fever, rash, and arthropathy (chikungunya, O'nyong-nyong, Mayaro, Ross River, Sindbis, and Barmah Forest viruses). This group has been subdivided into antigenic complex groupings including eastern equine encephalitis, western equine encephalitis, Venezuelan equine encephalitis, and Semliki Forest (which includes chikungunya, O'nyong-nyong, and Ross River viruses) and Barmah Forest complexes.

### *Bunyaviridae* Viruses

The Bunyaviridae family includes multiple arthropod-borne viruses as well as viruses transmitted by other modes. The main arboviral genera in this family include the *Bunyavirus* genus (including the California encephalitis group: La Crosse, California, snowshoe hare, and Jamestown Canyon viruses); the *Phlebovirus* genus (which includes Rift Valley fever virus and Toscana virus [TOSV]); and the *Nairovirus* genus (which includes Crimean-Congo hemorrhagic fever virus). The *Hantavirus* genus is also in this family; however, these viruses (which cause pulmonary syndromes as well as hemorrhagic fever with renal syndrome) are transmitted via direct inhalation of rodent excreta or urine rather than by arthropod bite.

### Coltiviruses

*Coltivirus* is a genus within the Reoviridae family, which also includes the well-known rotavirus member. The species included in this genus are Colorado tick fever virus (CTFV) as well as a number of other rare members (Salmon River virus, Eyach virus, and Asian members of the *Seadornavirus* genus, such as Banna and Beijing viruses).

## SYNDROMES CAUSED BY ARBOVIRUSES

### Central Nervous System Arboviral Infections

Arboviral infections can lead to CNS disease of various forms, most commonly including encephalitis, meningitis, and flaccid paralysis. CNS manifestations are usually a rare outcome of infection, with the majority of people developing these infections being asymptomatic or having mild, nonspecific symptoms. This section focuses on those infections that most commonly lead to CNS disease in North America (of which WNV and La Crosse encephalitis virus are the most important) and touches on those that are most important globally (tick-borne encephalitis and Japanese encephalitis viruses [JEV]).

### West Nile Virus

WNV was originally discovered in 1937 in Uganda and is maintained in an enzootic life cycle in birds of the Corvidae family (crows, magpies, jays) via mosquito transmission. A variety of mosquito species have been implicated, but *Culex* species have been the more common vector involved in spread of WNV, particularly in North America. Sporadic epidemics and epizootics (spread within animal populations) were previously observed in Israel (1950s), South Africa (1970s), Algeria, Morocco, Romania, Tunisia, Czech Republic, Congo, Italy, Israel, Russia, and France (1990s), but not in North America until 1999. That year, an outbreak of WNV encephalitis cases was reported in New York City with a strain of virus that was genetically indistinct from epidemic strains in Mediterranean countries, suggesting introduction from that area of the world. A simultaneous epizootic was noted in horses and birds at that time. Since 1999, WNV has spread throughout North America and in 2007 was reported in all continental US states (Fig. 300-2) and in central and western Canada (Ontario, Manitoba, Saskatchewan, and Alberta) with further spread to British Colombia as of 2009. WNV is currently the most commonly diagnosed arboviral infection acquired within North America, accounting for > 90% of domestically acquired neuroinvasive arboviral disease in US national arboviral surveillance. Adults account for the vast majority of cases, with children < 18 years contributing only 4% of cases overall.

While WNV infection occurs predominantly via arthropod transmission to humans, there have also been rare reports of transmission via blood transfusion, organ donation, and congenital, peripartum, or breastfeeding transmission from an acutely infected mother. Screening of blood and organ donors for WNV infection has been initiated in response to these nosocomial transmissions. A seasonal pattern of transmission from July to December has been noted yearly, with the bulk of transmissions taking place during August and September.

After the host is bitten by an infected mosquito, the virus replicates locally in tissue and lymph nodes before resulting in viremia and sometimes crossing the blood-brain barrier to lead to neurologic disease. The incubation period to development of symptoms is 2 to 14 days but can be as long as 21 days in immunocompromised patients. Only about 20% to 25% of individuals will develop symptoms of infection; most of these will develop West Nile fever, while less than 1% will develop CNS manifestations. West Nile fever is characterized by abrupt onset of fever, headache, myalgia, weakness, gastrointestinal symptoms (abdominal pain, nausea/vomiting, diarrhea), and sometimes a transient maculopapular rash. Symptoms often last several days and can be followed by a more prolonged period of fatigue and weakness. Other nonneurologic manifestations that have rarely been observed include hepatitis, pancreatitis, myocarditis, rhabdomyolysis, orchitis, bladder dysfunction, and ocular manifestations such as chorioretinitis, optic neuritis, and retinal hemorrhages.

CNS disease most commonly manifests as meningitis, encephalitis, or flaccid paralysis. WNV meningitis produces the usual symptoms of aseptic or viral meningitis, with fever, headache, and neck stiffness, along with the previously mentioned West Nile fever symptoms;

**TABLE 300-1 ARBOVIRUSES OF IMPORTANCE IN NORTH AMERICA AND GLOBALLY**

| Virus | Vector | Reservoir | Distribution | Incubation Period | Population Most Affected | Salient Clinical Features |
|---|---|---|---|---|---|---|
| **Central Nervous System Syndromes** | | | | | | |
| ***Flaviviruses*** | | | | | | |
| West Nile virus | *Culex pipiens, Aedes albopictus* | Birds | Europe, Africa, Israel, continental United States, central/western Canada | 2–14 days (up to 21 days in immunocompromised) | Young children and elderly | Aseptic meningitis, encephalitis, or flaccid paralysis |
| St. Louis encephalitis virus | *Culex* species | Birds | Continental United States, Canada | 4–21 days | Adults and elderly | Febrile headache, aseptic meningitis, encephalitis with tremor |
| Powassan virus | *Ixodes, Dermacentor* tick species | Small mammals | Northern United States, southern Canada | 1–5 weeks | Children | Encephalitis |
| Tick-borne encephalitis virus | *Ixodes* tick species (*I ricinus* and *I persulcatus*) | Birds, mammals | Eastern Europe, Asia | 4–28 days | Adults | Meningitis or meningoencephalitis |
| Japanese encephalitis virus | *Culex tritaeniorhynchus* and other species | Pigs, birds | Southeast Asia, China, Asian subcontinent, Australia | 5–15 days | Young children | Severe encephalitis |
| Murray Valley encephalitis and Kunjin virus | *Culex annulirostris* | Birds; possibly feral pigs | Australia | 7–28 days | Adults | Encephalitis |
| ***Alphaviruses*** | | | | | | |
| Eastern equine encephalitis virus | *Aedes, Culex, Coquillettidia* species (*Culiseta melanura* is the avian vector) | Birds | United States (mostly eastern seaboard and Gulf states), Canada, South and Central America | 3–10 days | Children and elderly | Fulminant encephalitis |
| Western equine encephalitis virus | *Culex tarsalis, Aedes* species | Birds | Central and western United States, Canada, South America | 2–10 days | Young children | Encephalitis leading to neurologic sequelae |
| Venezuelan equine encephalitis virus | *Culex, Aedes, Mansonia, Psorophora, Deinocerites* species | Small mammals | Southern United States, South and Central America | 1–6 days | Children | Encephalitis |
| ***Bunyaviridae*** | | | | | | |
| La Crosse encephalitis virus | *Aedes triseriatus*; possibly *Aedes albopictus* | Small mammals (chipmunks) | Eastern United States | 5–15 days | Children | Encephalitis |
| Jamestown Canyon virus | *Culex inorata, Aedes* species | Deer | North America | 3–7 days | Adults | Encephalitis |
| California and snowshoe hare viruses | *Aedes, Culex, Anopheles* species | Small mammals | North America | 5–15 days | Adults | Encephalitis |
| Toscanavirus | *Phlebotomus perniciosus, P perfiliewi* | Possibly *Phlebotomus perniciosus, P perfiliewi* | Mediterranean basin (Italy, Spain, France) | Few days to 2 weeks | Children and adults | Aseptic meningitis (one of the most common causes in Italy) |
| ***Coltiviruses*** | | | | | | |
| Colorado tick fever virus | *Dermacentor andersoni* ticks | Small mammals | Western United States, southwestern Canada | 1–14 days | Children and adults | Encephalitis |
| **Rash/Arthralgia Syndromes** | | | | | | |
| ***Flaviviruses*** | | | | | | |
| Zika virus | *Aedes* species | Primates, humans during epidemics | Africa, Asia, South America, Caribbean | 3–12 days | Children and adults | Fever, arthralgia/arthritis, rash; risk of CNS abnormalities in congenital infection, post-infectious Guillain-Barré syndrome |
| ***Alphaviruses*** | | | | | | |
| Chikungunya virus | *Aedes* species | Primates, small mammals, birds (humans during epidemics) | Africa, South/Southeast Asia, South/Central America, Caribbean | 1–12 days | Children and adults | Fever, arthralgia/arthritis, rash |
| Ross River virus | *Aedes, Culex* species | Marsupials, small mammals (humans and horses during epidemics) | Australia, Papua New Guinea, South Pacific islands | 3–21 days | Children and adults | Fever, arthralgia/arthritis, rash |
| Barmah Forest virus | *Aedes* species | Mammals, possibly birds | Australia | 3–21 days | Adults | Fever, arthritis, vesicular rash |

(*Continued*)

**TABLE 300-1 ARBOVIRUSES OF IMPORTANCE IN NORTH AMERICA AND GLOBALLY (CONTINUED)**

| Virus | Vector | Reservoir | Distribution | Incubation Period | Population Most Affected | Salient Clinical Features |
|---|---|---|---|---|---|---|
| O'nyong-nyong virus | *Anopheles funestus, A gambiae* | Unknown | Central and East Africa | > 8 days | Children and adults | Fever, rash, arthralgia, cervical lymphadenopathy |
| Mayaro virus | *Haemagogus* species | Primates, small mammals | South America | Up to 1 week | Adults | Fever, rash, arthritis |
| Sindbis virus | *Culex, Aedes, Culiseta* species | Birds | Africa, Asia, Australia | 8–9 days | Adults | Fever, pruritic rash, arthralgia |
| ***Bunyaviridae*** | | | | | | |
| Oropouche virus | *Culicoides paraensis* (midge) | Unknown | South America | 4–8 days | Children | Fever, arthralgia |
| **Hemorrhagic Fever Viruses (see Table 302-1)** | | | | | | |

CNS, central nervous system.

cerebrospinal fluid analysis often reveals a mild to moderate lymphocytic pleocytosis, elevated protein, and normal glucose. WNV encephalitis can be characterized by the additional findings of altered sensorium, seizures, parkinsonian features (bradykinesia, cogwheel rigidity, postural instability, and masked facies), and other movement disorders such as myoclonus, intentional tremor, and bruxism. Viral infection of the anterior horn cells can produce a poliomyelitis-like presentation with an acute, symmetric, flaccid paralysis. WNV infection has rarely been associated with Guillain-Barré syndrome. Most patients with West Nile fever or aseptic meningitis recover completely, but patients with encephalitis or flaccid paralysis can be left with residual deficits. The case fatality rate of neurologic disease in adults is 5% to 9% but is less than 1% in children. Rare cases of congenital infection have been described, with associated ophthalmologic and CNS malformations; the Centers for Disease Control and Prevention (CDC) has issued recommendations for evaluation of infants born to mothers with WNV infection in pregnancy (http://www.cdc.gov/mmwr/preview/mmwrhtml/mm5307a4.htm).

### St. Louis Encephalitis Virus

St. Louis encephalitis virus (SLEV) is found exclusively in the Western Hemisphere and was the leading cause of epidemic flaviviral

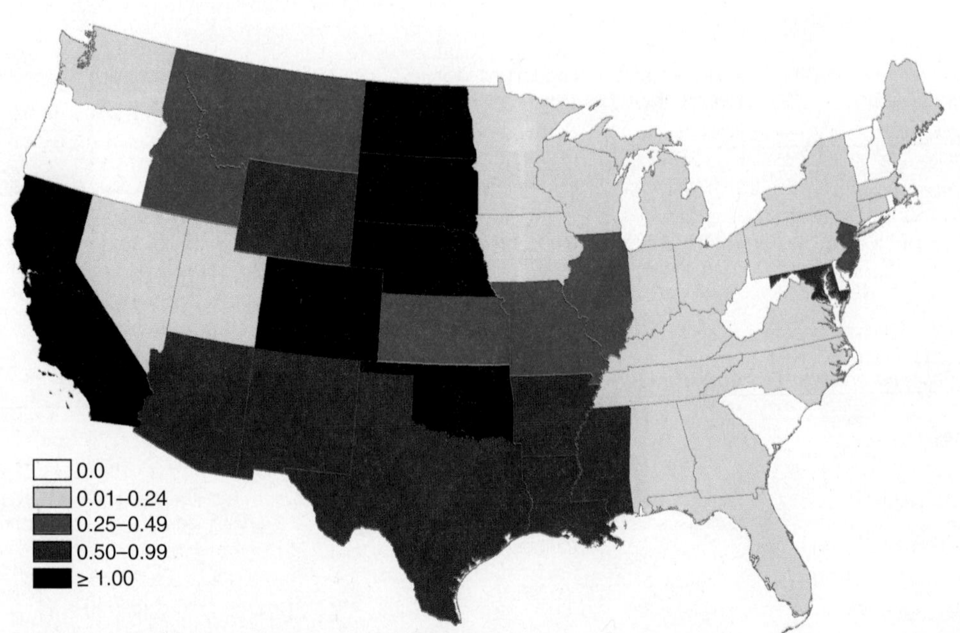


West Nile virus neuroinvasive disease incidence maps present data reported by state and local health departments to CDC's ArboNET surveillance system. This map shows the incidence of human neuroinvasive disease (e.g., meningitis, encephalitis, or acute flaccid paralysis) by state for 2015 with shading ranging from 0.01–0.24, 0.25–0.49, 0.50–0.99, and greater than 1.00 per 100,000 population.

Neuroinvasive disease cases have been reported to ArboNET from the following states for 2015: Alabama, Arizona, Arkansas, California, Colorado, Connecticut, District of Columbia, Florida, Georgia, Idaho, Illinois, Indiana, Iowa, Kansas, Kentucky, Louisiana, Maine, Maryland, Massachusetts, Michigan, Minnesota, Mississippi, Missouri, Montana, Nebraska, Nevada, New Jersey, New Mexico, New York, North Carolina, North Dakota, Ohio, Oklahoma, Pennsylvania, South Dakota, Tennessee, Texas, Utah, Virginia, Washington, Wisconsin, and Wyoming.

**FIGURE 300-2** West Nile virus neuroinvasive disease cases by state, 2015. (Reproduced with permission from Centers for Disease Control and Prevention. Division of Vector Borne Infectious Diseases. http://www.cdc.gov/westnile/resources/pdfs/data/wnv-neuro-incidence-by-state-map_2015_07072016.pdf. Accessed November 21, 2017.)

encephalitis in the United States until the arrival of WNV. It is found throughout the continental United States and historically occurred in parts of Canada. SLEV was first recognized in 1933 in St. Louis, Missouri, and both sporadic cases and focal outbreaks have been observed throughout North America since that time. Similar to WNV, SLEV is maintained in a zoonotic life cycle, with birds as the definitive host, and is transmitted to humans by the bite of *Culex* species of mosquitoes in the late summer and early fall.

Less than 1% of SLEV infections are clinically apparent, and 3 main clinical syndromes are observed: simple febrile headache, meningitis, and encephalitis, with the risk of more severe and neuroinvasive disease increasing with age. After an incubation period of 4 to 21 days, onset of symptoms begins with a flulike prodrome of fever, headache, myalgia, fatigue, and sometimes respiratory or gastrointestinal symptoms. Urologic symptoms, including dysuria, urgency, and incontinence, can also be seen in up to 25% of patients. Those who develop meningitis usually present with typical features of aseptic meningitis. Encephalitis is most commonly associated with altered consciousness and confusion. Other reported features have included generalized weakness without focal findings, tremulousness, cerebellar signs, cranial nerve deficits, abnormal movements (myoclonus, nystagmus), and, less commonly, epileptiform activity.

Laboratory findings with SLEV infection can include a moderate cerebrospinal fluid mononuclear pleocytosis with elevated protein and increased opening pressure, and hyponatremia can be seen as part of the syndrome of inappropriate secretion of antidiuretic hormone. Magnetic resonance imaging can show high signal intensity in the substantia nigra. An extended convalescence can be observed in up to half of patients, characterized by asthenia, irritability, tremulousness, sleep disturbance, depressive symptoms, memory loss, and headache. Overall mortality is reported as 8%, with much higher mortality in the elderly (20%) and much lower mortality in the pediatric population (2%).

### Powassan Virus

Powassan virus encephalitis occurs rarely. Since its discovery in 1958 when it was isolated from the brain of a 5-year-old child from Powassan, Ontario, who died of encephalitis, it has been found to be a rare cause of encephalitis in North America. It is the only tick-borne flavivirus in the Americas and is related to tick-borne encephalitis virus (TBEV) from East Asia. The virus has 2 lineages: the prototype lineage (POWV) is principally transmitted by *Ixodes cookei* ticks, while the deer tick virus (DTV) lineage is transmitted by *Ixodes scapularis* ticks and found in regions with endemic Lyme disease transmission.

While cases of Powassan virus encephalitis have been reported throughout North America and East Asia, overt human disease is felt to be restricted to southern Canada and the northern tier of US states including Wisconsin, Michigan, New York, and Maine. Since the mid-2000s, an increase in incidence has been noted in the north-central United States associated with the DTV lineage. Persons with a history of outdoor activity are most commonly affected by this virus, but in the initial descriptions of POWV, children were disproportionately represented, with one report noting 85% of infections occurring in persons under 20 years of age. More recent case series demonstrated a predominance of older adults.

The clinical presentation of Powassan virus disease is not well characterized because of the low number of cases reported. The incubation period is at least 1 week from exposure with reports of symptoms beginning up to 5 weeks afterward. Prodromal symptoms include sudden onset of illness with sore throat, fatigue, headache, and high fever. Encephalitis cases may be characterized by vomiting, prolonged fever, respiratory distress, lethargy, meningeal irritation, and focal neurologic lesions. One reported case had temporal lobe involvement typical of herpes simplex encephalitis. Laboratory findings include cerebrospinal fluid pleocytosis, initially polymorphonuclear then lymphocytic, as well as normal glucose and elevated protein. The fatality rate is at least 10%, and at least 50% of survivors are left with sequelae, including neurologic abnormalities such as hemiplegia, hypotonia, and spasticity.

### Tick-Borne Encephalitis Virus

TBEV is not found in North America but is the most important tick-borne arbovirus in Europe. It is found predominantly in Eastern Europe and Asia. A dramatic increase in the number of cases has been seen in the last 3 decades, with current estimates of 10,000 to 15,000 clinical cases per year globally. Closely related to Powassan virus, 3 main subtypes of TBEV have been identified: Far Eastern (previously Russian spring-summer encephalitis), Siberian (previously West Siberian encephalitis), and European (previously Central European encephalitis). Some countries have successfully instituted vaccination campaigns to reduce incidence of this infection in at-risk populations, and the need for pretravel vaccination is being increasingly recognized. TBEV is transmitted by ticks that parasitize a variety of bird and mammal species; cases of transmission via ingestion of unpasteurized milk from infected goats, sheep, or cattle have also been reported. Adult males are most commonly affected, but children with outdoor exposures are also at risk.

Few people infected with TBEV develop symptoms. Symptomatic patients most often present in the summer months and report onset of illness approximately 4 to 28 days after exposure (median 8 days). Illness is biphasic, with the initial phase consisting of a nonspecific, flulike illness with fever, malaise, headache, nausea, vomiting, and myalgias lasting less than 1 week. Following resolution of these symptoms, many patients enter a second phase of illness after 4 to 16 days (median 10 days) characterized by fever, vomiting, headache, and meningeal signs. Four TBEV syndromes can occur during the second phase: meningitis, meningoencephalitis, meningoencephalomyelitis, and meningoradiculoneuritis; the former 2 entities are the most common forms in children (approximately two-thirds and one-third of cases, respectively), while the latter 2 are rarely encountered. The most frequent signs noted with encephalitis include tremor (particularly of the tongue and face), somnolence, and ataxia. Laboratory findings typically include leukocytosis, elevated erythrocyte sedimentation rate, and lymphocytic cerebrospinal fluid pleocytosis. While up to 30% of adults may be left with residual neurologic sequelae and up to 2% may die, children commonly fare better, with residual deficits seen in 0% to 4% and few reported deaths. Children who have suffered from TBEV infection are more likely to suffer from impaired attention and psychomotor speed.

### Japanese Encephalitis Virus

JEV is the most important cause of epidemic viral encephalitis worldwide, with current estimates of nearly 68,000 cases annually and approximately 13,000 to 20,000 deaths. This flavivirus is endemic and causes periodic epidemics throughout Southeast Asia, China, and the Asian subcontinent, and has recently spread to parts of Australia (Fig. 300-3). Effective vaccines against JEV have been available for decades and have been incorporated into the childhood vaccination schedules of many Asian countries, leading to dramatic reductions in encephalitis cases in those countries. Meanwhile, the impoverished areas of Southeast Asia still bear the burden of this disease.

JEV is transmitted via mosquitoes that are common in rice fields, and the virus is maintained and amplified in pigs and aquatic bird populations. Due to the association with rice fields and pig farming, rural areas are most heavily affected, although cities with peripheral agricultural development have also seen isolated cases or outbreaks. Most cases (99%) are subclinical, leading to immunity in adolescents and adults, and thus young, nonimmune children suffer the most symptomatic disease.

The incubation period of JEV disease ranges from 5 to 15 days, often followed by a prodromal period of up to a week with nonspecific symptoms including fever, nausea, vomiting, coryza, diarrhea, and rigors. This is followed by the acute phase of disease. While a minority of patients present with aseptic meningitis or acute flaccid paralysis, the majority of those diagnosed with JEV infection have encephalitis. Fever, headache, and altered sensorium (ranging from disorientation to coma) are common and may be accompanied by or may lead to seizures. Other common features include weakness, masklike facies, tremor, generalized hypertonia, cogwheel rigidity, and cranial nerve abnormalities. Neuropsychiatric symptoms, such

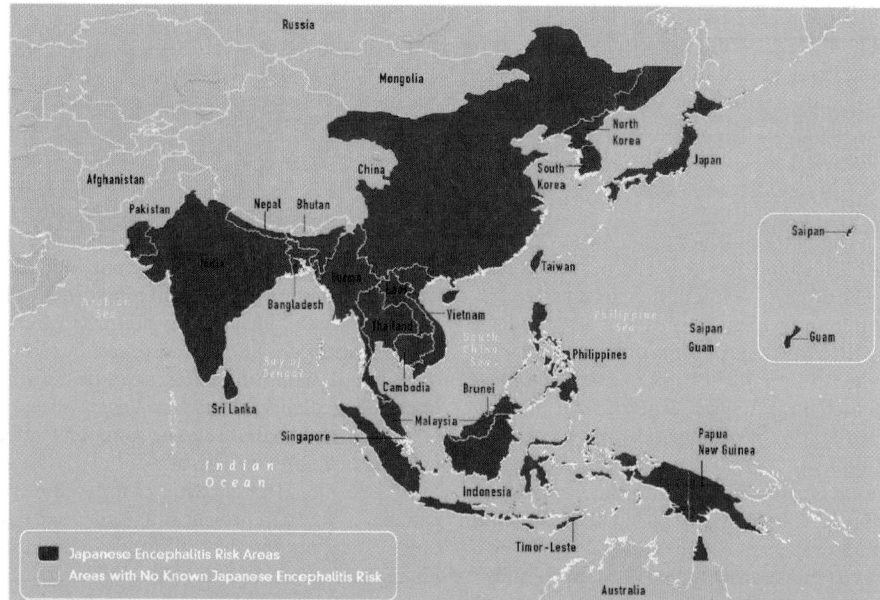


| Data Table: Countries in which Japanese encephalitis virus has been identified | | | |
|---|---|---|---|
| Australia | India | Pakistan | Sri Lanka |
| Bangladesh | Indonesia | Papua New Guinea | Taiwan |
| Brunei* | Japan | Philippines | Thailand |
| Burma | Laos | Russia | Timor-Leste |
| Cambodia | Malaysia | Saipan | Vietnam |
| China | Nepal | Singapore | |
| Guam | North Korea | South Korea | |

*No data but presumed to be endemic.

**FIGURE 300-3** Geographic distribution of Japanese encephalitis virus. (Reproduced with permission from Centers for Disease Control and Prevention. Division of Vector Borne Infectious Diseases. http://www.cdc.gov/japaneseencephalitis/resources/je_map.pdf. Accessed November 21, 2017.)

as mutism in children or abnormal behaviors in older children or adults, may be present. The subacute and convalescent stages manifest a varying degree of neurologic involvement, including focal seizures or asymmetric paralysis, extrapyramidal signs, and rapidly changing CNS signs. Approximately 25% of cases are fatal because of neurologic morbidity of acute infection or complications arising over the course of the illness. Young children are more likely to succumb to JEV infection, and survivors have neurologic sequelae in one-third of cases. These can include impaired cognition, behavioral disturbances, seizure disorders, gait or coordination abnormalities, and psychological deficits. Treatment is supportive.

#### Eastern Equine Encephalitis Virus

Eastern equine encephalitis virus (EEEV) is an alphavirus that was first described in the 1930s following outbreaks in the northeastern United States of encephalitis in horses and then in children and adults. In the United States, its geographic distribution includes the eastern seaboard and Gulf states as well as some inland foci of disease (New York, Georgia, Michigan, and Indiana); Canada and Central and South America have also reported cases. During the last decade, EEEV activity has increased alongside northward expansion of its geographic range. EEEV is maintained in its natural life cycle by transmission between mosquitoes and native bird species and has been most associated with swampy areas. The virus affects humans and horses only via bridging species of mosquitoes, which bite both birds and humans. When humans are infected, those over age 50 and younger than 15 years are at greatest risk of developing severe EEEV disease.

EEEV is distinct from other arboviruses in its propensity to result in fulminant neurologic illness or death, particularly in infants and young children. The incubation period from mosquito bite to development of disease is 3 to 10 days. Prodromal symptoms of fever, headache, confusion, lethargy, myalgias, and gastrointestinal symptoms precede the onset of neurologic symptoms by 5 to 10 days. This is followed by neurologic symptoms such as seizures, nuchal rigidity, altered mental status, muscle twitching or fibrillation, tremors, spasticity, paralysis, and cranial nerve palsies. Rapid progression to coma is possible. Features that may be noted specifically in infants and young children include a short or absent prodrome, fever, altered mental status, seizures, vomiting, cyanosis, and periorbital and upper extremity edema. Cerebrospinal fluid lymphocytic pleocytosis, elevated protein, and increased opening pressure are characteristic, and hyponatremia due to secretion of antidiuretic hormone can be seen. Electroencephalogram demonstrates diffuse slowing consistent with generalized encephalitis, and magnetic resonance imaging can delineate focal lesions in the basal ganglia, thalami, and brainstem. In those who do develop encephalitis, it is typically a fulminant illness leading to coma or death in 30% to 70% of individuals, with the highest mortality rates seen in infants and young children. One-third to one-half of survivors are left with severe neurologic sequelae such as mental retardation, behavioral changes, convulsive disorders, and paralysis; rapid progression to coma, hyponatremia, and high cerebrospinal fluid white blood cell count (> 500 cells/μL) are poor prognostic factors.

#### Western Equine Encephalitis Virus

Western equine encephalitis virus was first described as a cause of viral encephalitis in horses and subsequently in humans in the 1930s. Its distribution has been described in US states and Canadian provinces west of the Mississippi River as well as in countries in South America. Cases typically present in summer in irrigated areas of agriculture. Like other arboviruses, it is maintained in passerine bird populations in which infection is often inapparent. Most human infections are asymptomatic or nonspecific febrile illnesses that do not result in seeking medical attention; the ratio of infection to symptomatic illness is low, reported as less than 1000:1. The exception is in infants, where the ratio is much higher, reported as being nearly 1:1. Most cases are reported in the summer months, with risk factors for infection being male sex, rural residence, and outdoor employment in farming.

Transplacental transmission has been reported when the mother's infection has occurred within days of delivery.

Western equine encephalitis virus disease is characterized by an incubation period of 2 to 10 days and subsequent onset of a short prodrome of 1 to 4 days. Symptoms during the prodrome are similar to those of EEEV, including fever, intense headache, nausea, vomiting, and, occasionally, respiratory symptoms. CNS infection is characterized by lethargy, depressed level of consciousness, nuchal rigidity, photophobia, and vertigo. Infants with Western equine encephalitis virus typically have irritability, seizures, tense fontanel, rigidity, upper motor neuron deficits, and tremors. Children and adolescents may display muscular rigidity/spasticity, tremors, involuntary movements, hyporeflexia, and paralysis. Investigations reveal findings similar to those of EEEV but often milder. Cerebrospinal fluid pressure and protein may be slightly elevated, with a lymphocytic pleocytosis in older children and adolescents or polymorphonuclear pleocytosis in infants. Neurologic sequelae are seen in 30% or more of infants and young children, while the rate in adults is much lower; sequelae can include fatigue, irritability, headache, tremors, and motor and intellectual deficits. The overall case fatality rate is approximately 3%.

### Venezuelan Equine Encephalitis Virus

Venezuelan equine encephalitis virus was first described in the 1930s and has since been described largely as a cause of epizootics of encephalitis in horses in South and Central America, sometimes with coincident human coepidemics. The largest of these began in 1969 in El Salvador and Guatemala and spread throughout Mexico and into Texas by 1971. Since then, Venezuelan equine encephalitis virus has rarely been reported as a cause of encephalitis in southern US states despite the persistence of an endemic focus of infection within the Florida Everglades. Unlike the other equine encephalitis viruses, horses and humans develop significant viremia during infection, which could make them more than simply "dead-end" hosts due to the possibility of a mosquito acquiring the infection from a horse or human and then transmitting it to a new host. Transmitted by multiple mosquito species (*Culex, Aedes, Mansonia, Psorophora*, and *Deinocerites* species), the virus is maintained in small mammal populations.

Human disease with Venezuelan equine encephalitis virus is most often asymptomatic or mildly symptomatic with a nonspecific viral illness, though the risk of significant infection is highest in children. Symptoms begin after an incubation period of 1 to 6 days and include fever, malaise, chills, myalgia, headache, photophonophobia, hyperesthesia, and vomiting. Approximately 4% of children and fewer than 1% of adults progress to severe encephalitis within 7 days of onset of prodrome, and common features include nuchal rigidity, ataxia, seizures, coma, and paralysis. Cytopenias (lymphopenia, neutropenia, and thrombocytopenia) and liver enzyme abnormalities, as well as lymphocytic cerebrospinal fluid pleocytosis, may be observed.

### California Encephalitis Virus

California encephalitis is a CNS disease caused by one of a group of related viruses in the *Bunyavirus* genus. The most common of these is La Crosse encephalitis virus (LACV), while other less common members include California virus (found in California), Jamestown Canyon virus (found throughout the US mainland, Canada, and Alaska), and snowshoe hare virus (found in parts of both the United States and Canada). LACV was first isolated in 1965 from brain tissue from a 4-year-old child in La Crosse, Wisconsin. Its geographic distribution has since been recognized to include predominantly the upper midwestern states of Ohio, Indiana, Illinois, Iowa, Wisconsin, and Minnesota, and less predominantly, the mid-Atlantic and southeastern areas of the United States (Fig. 300-4). The recent introduction to North America of *Aedes albopictus* (another mosquito capable of transmitting LACV) may further extend the geographic range of this disease beyond the eastern United States. The natural hosts for this virus are small mammals, including squirrels and chipmunks. Cases typically occur in summer and autumn months. In national US surveillance of neuroinvasive arboviral disease from 2003 to 2012, LACV was the most common etiology in children; only 12% of cases were in adults > 18 years, suggesting it is a disease of childhood. The Appalachian and midwestern regions have had the highest incidence rates of LACV neuroinvasive disease, with West Virginia, Tennessee, North Carolina, and Ohio reporting 81% of all cases.

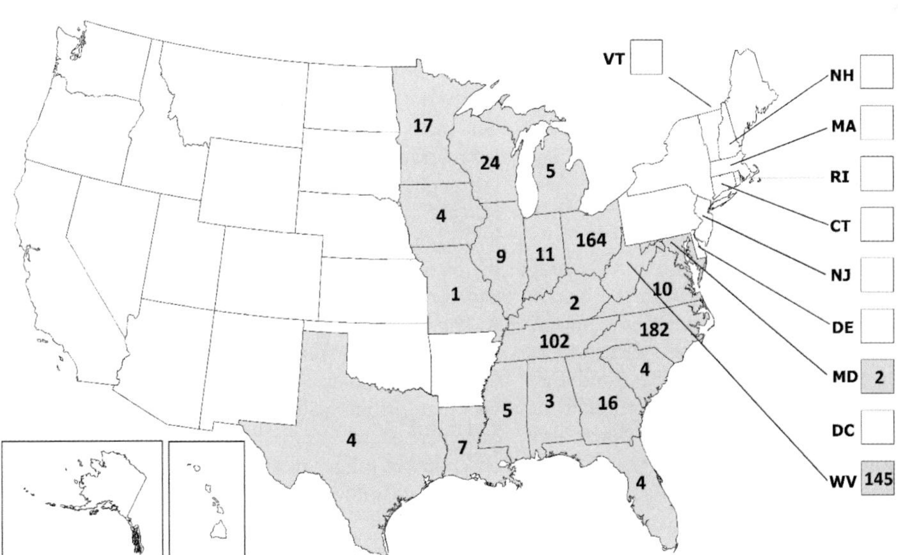


Data table: From 2004 through 2013, La Crosse virus neuroinvasive disease cases have been reported in Alabama (3), Florida (4), Georgia (16), Indiana (11), Illinois (9), Iowa (4), Kentucky (2), Louisiana (7), Maryland (2), Michigan (5), Minnesota (17), Mississippi (5), Missouri (1), North Carolina (182), Ohio (164), South Carolina (4), Tennessee (102), Texas (4), Virginia (10), West Virginia (145) and Wisconsin (24).

**FIGURE 300-4** La Crosse virus neuroinvasive disease cases by state, 2004 to 2013. (Reproduced with permission from Centers for Disease Control and Prevention. Division of Vector Borne Infectious Diseases. http://www.cdc.gov/lac/resources/LACbystate_2004-2013.pdf. Accessed November 21, 2017.)

Symptomatic infection is very uncommon in LACV, but those who develop symptoms are almost all in the pediatric age group, particularly school-aged children. A male predisposition has been found, and proximity to forested areas or artificial mosquito habitats (discarded tires or containers) is a risk factor. The incubation period is 5 to 15 days. Symptomatic infection is usually an encephalitis syndrome, while meningitis and meningoencephalitis are less common presentations. Symptoms include fever, headache, vomiting, meningism, seizures, and disorientation; focal neurologic symptoms are seen in up to 25%. A lymphocytic pleocytosis of 200 cells/mL or less is most often observed with normal glucose and infrequently elevated protein. Hyponatremia can be present due to secretion of antidiuretic hormone. Neurologic sequelae such as seizure disorders, cranial nerve palsies, or hemiparesis may be present in up to 12% of children, while more subtle problems such as cognitive dysfunction and neurobehavioral abnormalities may be more common. Death occurs in less than 1% of those diagnosed with LACV disease.

#### Toscana Virus

TOSV is a sandfly fever virus species of the *Phlebovirus* genus in the Bunyaviridae family. Phleboviruses are transmitted by sandflies (mainly *Phlebotomus* species but other species as well). Naples and Sicilian are the main serocomplexes of sandfly viruses, and TOSV is a serotype of the Naples serocomplex. Although the remaining sandfly viruses typically cause only febrile illnesses, TOSV is distinct in causing neurologic disease as well. TOSV was first isolated from 2 species of sandfly, *Phlebotomus perniciosus* and *Phlebotomus perfiliewi*, in 1971 and was first reported as a cause of neuroinvasive infection in 1985. The distribution of TOSV mirrors that of its vectors, which are found in countries throughout the Mediterranean basin (Italy, France, Spain, Portugal, Slovenia, Croatia, Greece, Turkey, and Cyprus). TOSV is now recognized as one of the most common causes of viral meningitis in summer (July to October, peak in August) in several European countries. The age distribution in most case series demonstrates this to mainly be a disease of young and middle-aged adults, although some children are affected.

While the proportion of asymptomatic cases are unknown, seroprevalence studies in many countries suggest it is a common infection, and thus like other arboviruses, it is suspected that asymptomatic or mild disease is common. For symptomatic cases, illness usually arises 3 to 7 days after sandfly exposure. Cases of febrile illness without neurologic involvement have been described, usually lasting for a few days only. TOSV meningitis symptoms are similar to other forms of aseptic meningitis, including fever, headache, photophobia, nausea and vomiting, and myalgia. Lymphocytic pleocytosis with normal cerebrospinal fluid protein and glucose is typical. Most cases recover without sequelae. Severe meningoencephalitis has also rarely been reported.

#### Colorado Tick Fever Virus

CTFV is a member of the *Coltivirus* genus and is found in the western United States and southwestern Canada, particularly in the Rocky Mountain region. The greatest numbers of cases have been reported in Colorado, Utah, Wyoming, and Montana. Disease distribution corresponds to that of the major vector of CTFV, the wood tick (*Dermacentor andersoni*), which prefers mountainous terrain from 4000- to 10,000-foot elevations. Other species of ticks have also been implicated. The virus is known to be transmitted transtadially (between life stages) in the tick, becoming infected in its larval stage but only capable of transmitting to humans in the adult stage. Unlike some other arboviruses, CTFV is not transmitted transovarially (from adult female to egg). Multiple natural CTFV-amplifying hosts are known to exist, including ground squirrels, chipmunks, marmots, and other mammals. Outdoor exposure is an obvious human risk factor for disease, and a male predominance has been noted. Vertical transmission from mother to fetus has been reported.

The mean incubation period from exposure to infection is 3 to 4 days, with a range from less than 1 day to 14 days. An abrupt onset of illness with symptoms of fever, chills, malaise, myalgia, headache, hyperesthesia, and retro-orbital pain lasting up to 1 week is common, followed by remission of symptoms. Less common findings include conjunctivitis, pharyngitis, lymphadenopathy, splenomegaly, and a papular or petechial rash. Recurrence of symptoms 2 to 3 days later is seen in up to half of cases, giving rise to a diphasic or "saddleback" fever curve. CTFV disease is complicated by CNS manifestations in 5% to 10% of cases, predominantly aseptic meningitis and rarely encephalitis; neurologic manifestations and other severe forms of CTFV disease are more common in younger age groups. Other rare complications of CTFV infection can include pericarditis, myocarditis, orchitis, pneumonia, and hepatitis.

Laboratory findings commonly include leukopenia and thrombocytopenia (which can sometimes be severe). CTFV infects erythroblasts, and the persistence of viremia for up to weeks or months after onset of illness parallels the survival time of red blood cells sheltering the virus. Viral culture methods and molecular diagnostics can thus be used to diagnose disease in addition to the usual serologic methods of diagnosing arboviral infection.

### RASH/ARTHRALGIA ARBOVIRAL INFECTION SYNDROMES

A number of arboviral infections can lead to syndromes that present with prominent symptoms of rash and/or arthralgia. None of these are endemic to North America, although imported cases are becoming more common. ZIKV, a flavivirus that leads to rash/arthralgia symptoms, has garnered major attention due to recent invasion of the Americas. That said, alphaviruses are the most common group of arboviruses causing rheumatologic complaints, but pediatric infection less commonly leads to arthralgia or arthritis than does adult infection. These viruses are listed in Table 300-1.

#### Zika Virus

ZIKV is a flavivirus originally discovered in Uganda in 1947 and previously known to be endemic but with low burden of disease in tropical Africa and Asia. Beginning in 2007, ZIKV epidemics were reported in multiple Pacific Island nations including Yap Island, French Polynesia, New Caledonia, Cook Islands, and Easter Island. In 2015, epidemic spread throughout South America and the Caribbean was documented (Fig. 300-5), affecting large portions of the population in some countries. Imported cases in North America have been widely reported, as well as sexual transmission from imported cases to their nontraveling partners. In 2016, local autochthonous ZIKV transmission via mosquitos was reported in Florida, highlighting once again the risk of introduction of new arboviruses to North America. Spread in the Americas has been attributed to expansion of *Aedes albopictus* and *Aedes aegypti*, mosquito populations that are competent vectors for transmission. While primates have been shown to be the reservoir for ZIKV in Africa, the current epidemic in the Americas is thought to be due to sustained transmission between mosquitos and humans only. ZIKV has come to global attention not due to the severity of clinical illness in the majority of those affected but related to the recognition of 2 major complications of infection: postinfectious Guillain-Barré syndrome and congenital infection.

The incubation period for ZIKV is estimated to be between 3 and 12 days. While 80% of those infected will manifest no clinical symptoms, those who do will commonly present with fever; maculopapular rash that includes palms and soles; arthritis, arthralgias, myalgias, and extremity edema; and conjunctivitis. Symptoms are less abrupt in onset and of milder intensity compared to DENV or CHIKV (which co-circulate with ZIKV in most endemic areas and produce a similar array of manifestations) and tend to last 4 to 7 days in total.

Increased rates of Guillain-Barré syndrome (particularly the acute motor axonal neuropathy type) were noted during the French Polynesian ZIKV epidemic in 2013 and, subsequently, in multiple countries in the Americas. A majority of these patients with Guillain-Barré syndrome recalled an illness with symptoms compatible with ZIKV in the weeks before presentation. Other neurologic manifestations such as myelitis and meningoencephalitis have also been described in association with ZIKV infection.

Of perhaps most concern is the recognition of a congenital ZIKV infection syndrome. This was described initially in Brazil, where a

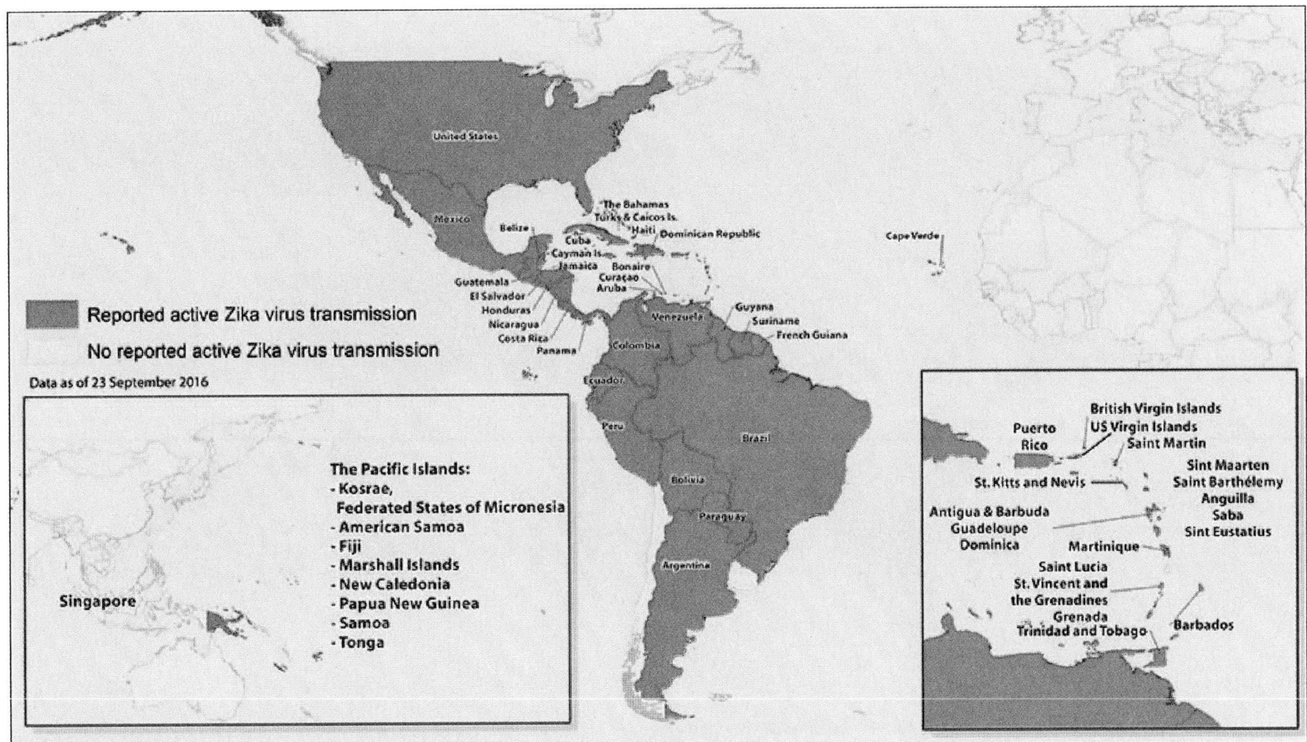


**FIGURE 300-5** Countries and territories with active Zika virus transmission, as of August 31, 2016. (Reproduced with permission from Centers for Disease Control and Prevention. Division of Vector Borne Infectious Diseases. http://www.cdc.gov/zika/geo/active-countries.html. Accessed November 21, 2017.)

dramatic increase in the rate of infants born with microcephaly was noted in northeastern states coincident with ZIKV circulation in 2015. Since then, an array of clinical symptoms resembling other congenital infection syndromes have been noted in infants born to mothers with ZIKV infection in pregnancy. These symptoms include microcephaly, intracranial calcifications, ventriculomegaly and reduced brain volume, polymicrogyria, or other brain malformation; sensorineural hearing loss; chorioretinitis, optic nerve hypoplasia, macular atrophy, or other eye abnormalities; clubfoot; and arthrogryposis. A clear understanding of overall rates of ZIKV transmission, transmission risk by trimester of maternal infection, or symptomatic congenital infection by trimester has not yet been elucidated, but first-trimester exposure seems to carry greater risk for severe fetal effects, and infants born with CNS symptoms have a poor neurodevelopmental prognosis. Any woman with known or suspected ZIKV infection in pregnancy should be assessed by maternal-fetal medicine and infectious diseases specialists and have appropriate monitoring in pregnancy. Guidance on assessment of infants with known ZIKV exposure in utero or suspected congenital ZIKV infection has been issued by multiple expert bodies, including the CDC, with regular updates based on available diagnostic testing modalities. Perinatal infection from mothers with symptoms around the time of delivery has also been reported, with asymptomatic or mild disease described in these infants.

### Chikungunya Virus

CHIKV is an alphavirus that was originally described as part of an outbreak in Tanzania in 1952. The name is derived from the local Makonde language, meaning "that which bends up," which refers to the severe arthralgias common to the disease. CHIKV was previously known to cause infection in various tropical locales, including South and Southeast Asia, islands of the Indian Ocean, and throughout Africa. Recent spread of the virus to the Americas and parts of Europe is attributed to expansion of *Aedes albopictus* and introduction to new regions by viremic travelers (Fig. 300-6). While it is not endemic in the United States, 37 imported cases were reported in 2006 relating to outbreaks in India and islands in the Indian Ocean with an average of 28 imported cases per year since. The first case of locally acquired CHIKV infection in the United States was reported in 2014, highlighting the potential for introduction to North America. It is transmitted by numerous species of *Aedes* mosquitoes, which can inhabit both rural and urban environments. Primates, rodents, and birds are the main reservoirs, although humans can also serve as reservoirs during epidemic periods.

The incubation period for CHIKV is usually 2 to 4 days (though it can range from 1 to 12 days). In children, approximately 35% to 40% of cases are asymptomatic, but in symptomatic cases, typical illness is characterized by abrupt onset of high fever, headache, back pain, myalgia, and arthralgia, with symptom duration of approximately 7 to 10 days. Disease in children has been recognized as somewhat different from that in adults, and severity tends to follow a U-shaped curve, with infants and young children and the elderly being at highest risk. A majority of adults have musculoskeletal symptoms such as arthralgia, which can be severe and mainly affect small joints of the extremities (wrists, ankles, phalanges), whereas only 30% to 50% of children have these symptoms. Extremity edema and joint swelling may also be noted, and in adults, articular symptoms can last from 1 week up to months or years, whereas children rarely have severe or relapsing symptoms. Rash, noted in up to half of cases, is characterized typically as a maculopapular eruption of the trunk and limbs in adults, but as pigmentary changes of the centrofacial area in children and as a bullous rash with sloughing or intertriginous aphthous ulceration in infants < 6 months old; hemorrhagic manifestations with petechiae, purpura, and gingival or mucosal bleeding are noted in approximately 10% of children. Lab findings may include lymphopenia, thrombocytopenia, coagulopathy, or liver transaminase elevation.

More recently, neurologic symptoms have been noted as more common in children with CHIKV infection (up to 25% in one outbreak description in La Reunion), particularly infants < 1 year of age. Neurologic manifestations include encephalopathy (prostration or altered mental status), meningitis, febrile seizures (simple or complex), status epilepticus, and encephalitis; these symptoms occur almost exclusively during the initial presentation with CHIKV symptoms, rather than later during the course of infection. Cerebrospinal fluid pleocytosis appears to be rare, despite the presence of CHIKV by polymerase chain reaction in cerebrospinal fluid being common.

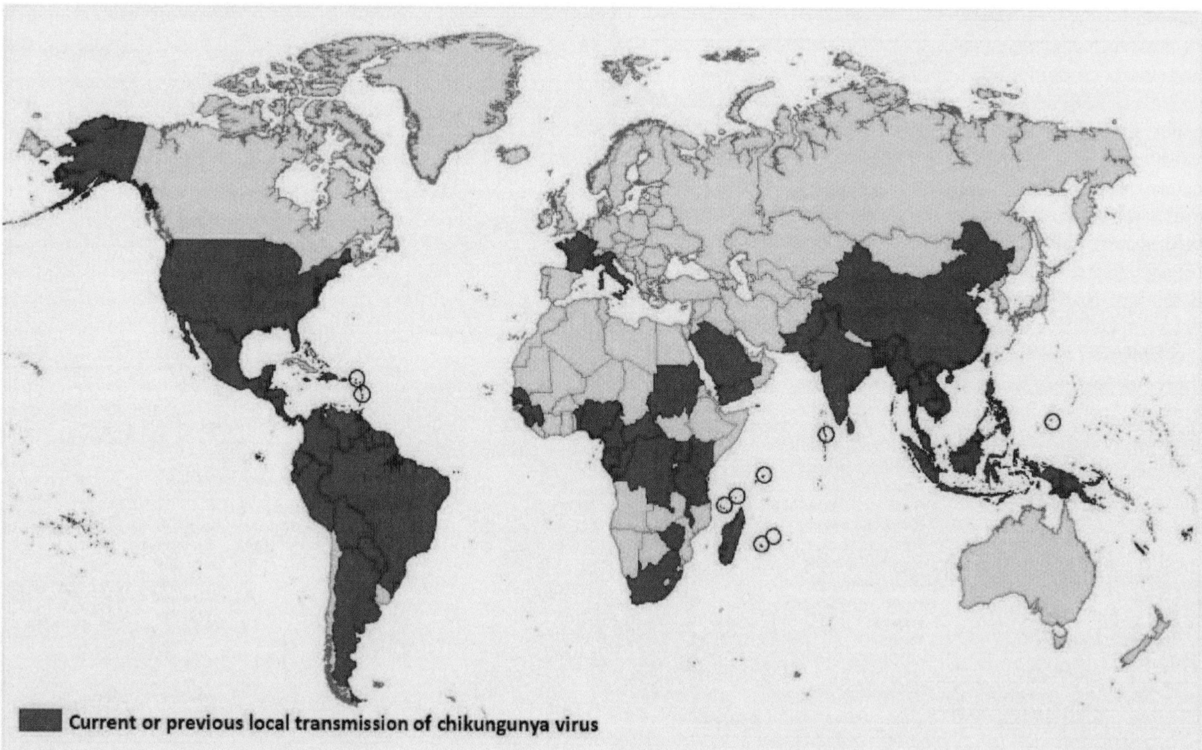


Does not include countries or territories where only imported cases have been documented. This map is updated weekly if there are new countries or territories that report local chikungunya virus transmission.

**Data table: Countries and territories where chikungunya cases have been reported**

**AFRICA**
Benin
Burundi
Cameroon
Central African Republic
Comoros
Dem. Republic of the Congo
Equatorial Guinea
Gabon
Guinea
Kenya
Madagascar
Malawi
Mauritius
Mayotte
Nigeria
Republic of Congo
Reunion
Senegal
Seychelles
Sierra Leone
South Africa
Sudan
Tanzania
Uganda
Zimbabwe

**ASIA**
Bangladesh
Bhutan
Cambodia
China
India
Indonesia
Laos
Malaysia
Maldives
Myanmar (Burma)
Pakistan
Philippines
Saudi Arabia
Singapore
Sri Lanka
Taiwan
Thailand
Timor
Vietnam
Yemen

**EUROPE**
France
Italy

**AMERICAS**
Anguilla
Antigua and Barbuda
Argentina
Aruba
Bahamas
Barbados
Belize
Bolivia
Brazil
British Virgin Islands
Cayman Islands
Colombia
Costa Rica
Curacao
Dominica
Dominican Republic
Ecuador
El Salvador
French Guiana
Grenada
Guadeloupe
Guatemala
Guyana
Haiti
Honduras
Jamaica
Martinique
Mexico
Montserrat
Nicaragua
Panama
Paraguay
Peru
Puerto Rico
Saint Barthelemy
Saint Kitts and Nevis
Saint Lucia
Saint Martin
Saint Vincent & the Grenadines
Sint Maarten
Suriname
Trinidad and Tobago
Turks and Caicos Islands
United States
US Virgin Islands
Venezuela

**OCEANIA/PACIFIC ISLANDS**
American Samoa
Cook Islands
Federal States of Micronesia
French Polynesia
Kiribati
New Caledonia
Papua New Guinea
Samoa
Tokelau
Tonga

**FIGURE 300-6** Countries and territories where chikungunya cases have been reported, as of April 22, 2016. (Reproduced with permission from Centers for Disease Control and Prevention. Division of Vector Borne Infectious Diseases. http://www.cdc.gov/chikungunya/pdfs/chik_world_map_04-22-16.pdf. Accessed November 21, 2017.)

Typical neuroimaging findings include brain edema and white matter changes particularly of the corpus callosum, centrum semiovale, and the periventricular region. The case fatality rate for CHIKV encephalitis has been reported to be as high as 16%, with neurologic sequelae (cerebral palsy, blindness, neurodevelopmental delays) being common among survivors.

Perinatal CHIKV infection has also increasingly been recognized as a significant pediatric disease entity. When the mother is symptomatic in the peripartum period (4 days before to 1 day after delivery), the risk of vertical transmission is approximately 50%. Infants usually develop symptoms 4 to 5 days (range 3–9 days) after birth, including fever, pain, edema of distal extremities, poor feeding, prostration, and rash. A typical evolution of dermatologic involvement was described among perinatally infected infants in La Reunion, with initial erythroderma of the extremities followed by desquamation and eventually brown skin discoloration of limbs and face. Cardiac assessment can reveal coronary artery thickening without aneurysm. Neurologic involvement, including hypotonia, seizures, coma, and intracerebral hemorrhage, has been well described, with similar cerebrospinal fluid and imaging findings as described earlier with the addition of lenticulothalamostriate vasculitis on ultrasound or magnetic resonance imaging. Longitudinal follow-up of perinatally infected children has found that approximately 50% suffer neurodevelopmental delays, and those with more severe neurologic disease (seizures, coma, brain edema) are more likely to be delayed and to develop microcephaly and cerebral palsy. Congenital CHIKV infection has not been described, and adverse infant outcomes do not appear to be increased among mothers with antepartum CHIKV infection, although rare cases of antepartum fetal death with proven fetal infection have been noted.

#### Ross River Virus

Ross River virus (RRV) is another alphavirus responsible for epidemic polyarthritis in Australia, Papua New Guinea, and islands of the South Pacific. Although recognized as an arbovirus similar to CHIKV and others, RRV was only isolated in 1972 from the serum of a 7-year-old aboriginal boy. Thousands of cases of epidemic polyarthritis caused by RRV and the closely related Barmah Forest virus are reported in Australia each year. RRV is transmitted by the bite of species of *Aedes* and *Culex* mosquitoes, and marsupials (kangaroos and wallabies) and small mammals are the natural hosts. Humans and horses are also thought to play a role in epidemic spread and maintenance of RRV.

The incubation period for this illness is 7 to 9 days but can range from 3 to 21 days. Constitutional symptoms of fever, myalgia, sore throat, lymphadenopathy, and coryza may be observed. Rash is present in half of patients, usually maculopapular but sometimes vesicular or purpuric; the extremities, including palms, soles, digits, and face, are affected. Acute onset of joint symptoms, including arthralgias, joint tenderness, warmth, redness, swelling, and restriction of movement, is prominent with RRV, with symmetric involvement of peripheral joints being most common (especially ankles, knees, wrists, hands, and fingers). Symptoms may be intense and prolonged, sometimes extending beyond the acute infection period. Rare cases of meningitis, encephalitis, and glomerulonephritis have been reported. In general, symptoms of infection are less common and less severe in children than in adults, and deaths are extremely rare.

## ARBOVIRAL HEMORRHAGIC FEVER SYNDROMES

Viral hemorrhagic fever infections are caused by a large group of viruses discussed in Chapter 302. Arboviral causes include members of the flavivirus (yellow fever, DENV, Omsk hemorrhagic fever, and Kyasanur Forest disease viruses) and bunyavirus (Congo-Crimean hemorrhagic fever and Rift Valley fever viruses) groups.

## DIAGNOSIS

For most of the arboviruses discussed, diagnosis relies on detection of immunoglobulin (Ig) M and IgG antibodies by enzyme-linked immunosorbent assay (ELISA) in serum and/or cerebrospinal fluid. Serologic cross-reactivity among members of the different families (particularly the flaviviruses) has been noted, sometimes making diagnosis difficult in children coming from areas endemic for other members of the same group. Discrimination between cross-reacting antibodies can be achieved by measuring virus-specific neutralizing antibodies by plaque reduction neutralization testing (PRNT). Viral isolation has been used more commonly in the past but molecular methods such as polymerase chain reaction have been developed for many viruses and likely represent the most reliable and timely modes of diagnosis. While these techniques are not always readily available at the local level, regional or national reference labs usually provide these services. Decisions regarding the best diagnostic assay for testing of specific arboviruses should be made in discussion with institutional microbiologists.

## PREVENTION

Vaccines for yellow fever virus, JEV, and TBEV have been in usage for a number of years, but human vaccines for other arboviruses are not yet available. One DENV vaccine has recently been licensed for use, while other DENV candidate vaccines remain under study. Research is ongoing to develop viable vaccines for CHIKV and ZIKV. Vaccines against the equine encephalitis viruses are available for horses, which may prevent local transmission to humans by reducing virus carriage in the mosquito population.

In the past, vector control programs have been highly successful in controlling arboviruses such as yellow fever virus; however, the resurgence of a number of arboviruses worldwide has not been met with renewed efforts at vector control. During local outbreaks of arboviruses, there may be a role for pesticide use or other attempts to reduce vector populations such as removal of reproductive habitats. Novel methods such as genetically modified mosquitoes and biological control are currently being evaluated. Personal protective measures to avoid exposure should be encouraged to avoid arthropod bites/exposures, such as application of insect repellant, wearing of light-colored clothing with long sleeves and pants, use of screens to keep insects out of dwellings, and prompt removal of ticks when found on children playing outdoors.

## SUGGESTED READINGS


Barzon L, Pacenti M, Sinigaglia A, Berto A, Trevisan M, Palù Gl. West Nile virus infection in children. *Exp Rev Anti-Infect Ther.* 2015;13:1373-1386.

Besnard M, Lastère S, Teissier A, Cao-Lormeau V, Musso D. Evidence of perinatal transmission of Zika virus, French Polynesia, December 2013 and February 2014. *Euro Surveill.* 2014;19:20751.

Charrel R, Bichaud L, de Lamballerie X. Emergence of Toscana virus in the Mediterranean area. *World J Virol.* 2012;1:135-141.

El Khoury M, Camargo J, Wormser G. Changing epidemiology of Powassan encephalitis in North America suggests the emergence of the deer tick virus subtype. *Exp Rev Anti-Infect Ther.* 2013;11:983-985.

Gaensbauer J, Lindsey N, Messacar K, Staples JE, Fischer M. Neuroinvasive arboviral disease in the United States: 2003 to 2012. *Pediatrics.* 2014;134:e642-e650.

Lindsey NP, Lehman JA, Staples JE, Fisher M. West Nile virus and other arboviral diseases - United States, 2014. *Morb Mortal Wkly Rep.* 2015;64:929-934.

Musso D, Gubler DJ. Zika virus. *Clin Microbiol Rev.* 2016;29: 487-524.

Ritz N, Hufnagel M, Gerardin P. Chikungunya in children. *Pediatr Infect Dis J.* 2015;34:789-791.

Russell K, Oliver SE, Lewis L, et al. Update: Interim guidance for the evaluation and management of infants with possible congenital Zika virus infection: United States, August 2016. *Morb Mortal Wkly Rep.* 2016;65:870-878.

Weaver S, Lecuit M. Chikungunya virus and the global spread of a mosquito-borne disease. *N Engl J Med.* 2015;372:1231-1239.

# 301 *Enterovirus* and *Parechovirus* Infections

José R. Romero

## INTRODUCTION

The enteroviruses constitute a genus within the *Picornaviridae* family of viruses. As their family name implies, these viral agents are small (ie, "pico"), ribonucleic acid (RNA) genome (ie, "rna") viruses (ie, "viridae"). Traditionally, the genus *Enterovirus* was speciated into 5 groups: polioviruses, group A coxsackieviruses, group B coxsackieviruses, echoviruses, and numbered enteroviruses (Table 301-1).

The current taxonomic classification of the enteroviruses (EVs) is based on genomic, molecular, and biologic characteristics of the viral isolates and divides the enteroviruses into 13 species. The original enterovirus serotypes have been assigned to the species EVs A to D (see Table 301-1). Together with recently identified types, EVs encompass > 100 types. Additionally, the rhinoviruses, previous assigned to a genus unto themselves, are now considered a species (rhinovirus A–C) within the genus. Lastly, using the revised classification schema, 2 EV serotypes, 22 and 23, have been reassigned to a new genus designated *Parechovirus* (PeV). There are 4 species of PeV (A–D), with those designated as PeV A (19 types) being responsible for disease in humans.

## PATHOGENESIS AND EPIDEMIOLOGY

Morphologically, the EVs and PeVs are small, icosahedral-shaped virions that lack an envelope. The enteroviral capsid is composed of 60 units each of 4 viral capsid proteins: VP1, VP2, VP3, and VP4. The capsid of the PeVs is comprised of 60 units each of 3 viral capsid proteins: VP0, VP3, and VP4. The EVs and PeVs are acid, ether, and chloroform stable and insensitive to nonionic detergents. They are inactivated by heat (> 56°C), ultraviolet light, chlorination, and formaldehyde. These characteristics confer environmental stability to the viruses, permitting them to survive for days to weeks in water and sewage.

The RNA genome of the EVs and PeVs is approximately 7.4 kb in length and serves as a template for viral protein translation and RNA replication (Fig. 301-1). It is organized into a long (~740 nucleotides) 5-nontranslated region (5′NTR), which precedes the single open reading frame. The open reading frame is followed by a short 3′NTR and a terminal polyadenylated tail. The EV 5′NTRs and 3′NTRs play critical roles in the life cycle of the virus. A domain located at the extreme 5′-terminus of the 5′NTR is essential for replication of viral RNA. The 3′NTR has been demonstrated to also play a role in viral RNA replication. Translation of the viral genome is regulated by the internal ribosome entry site within the 5′NTR. For the PVs, the 5′NTR has been documented to be a major determinant of virulence phenotype (ie, the ability to cause paralysis).

Neurovirulence-determining genomic regions have yet to be identified for the nonpolio EVs or PeVs. In animal models of nonpolio EV disease, determinants of virulence for myocarditis and pancreatitis have been variably localized to the 5′NTR and the viral capsid. The 5′NTR of the EVs and PeVs possesses regions of high nucleotide identity in which nucleotide sequences with absolute (or near-absolute) conservation exist for serotypes within each of the genera. These regions have been exploited for the design of primers and probes used for the detection of the EVs and PeVs through nucleic acid amplification techniques (eg, reverse transcription polymerase chain reaction [RT-PCR] and nucleic acid sequence–based amplification [NASBA]).

The EV and PeV open reading frame is subdivided into 3 regions designated P1, P2, and P3. The P1 region codes for structural proteins that form the viral capsid. The capsid protein-coding regions are contiguous to one another, without intervening stop codons. The largest of the capsid proteins is VP1 and contains type-specific epitopes correlating with type. The VP1 coding sequences serve as the target for molecular typing of the EVs and PeVs. The P2 and P3 regions code for 7 nonstructural proteins and their intermediates that are essential for the viral life cycle. Viral cell entry and uncoating are receptor mediated. Viral replication takes place in the cytoplasm of the cell and results in a lytic infection that kills the infected cell.

After oral or respiratory routes of infection, the EVs infect cells in the upper respiratory and, predominantly, the lower gastrointestinal (GI) tracts. While the exact cells responsible for infection in the upper respiratory tract are unknown, it is believed that polioviruses (PVs) infect M cells within Peyer patches or enterocytes in the lower GI tract. EV replication in the GI and upper respiratory tracts results in a primary or minor viremia that leads to seeding of organs (liver, lung, heart, and central nervous system [CNS]) distant from the sites of primary infection. A second, major viremia ensues following replication at these sites. Replication in organs seeded during the minor viremia results in the clinical manifestations of EV infection. Vertical transmission to the fetus is possible during the viremic stages of maternal infection. If the CNS was spared during the minor viremia, it may become infected as a result of the major viremia. This may explain the biphasic nature of illness associated with polio and nonpolio enteroviral infections of the CNS. The mechanism(s) by which the EVs gain entry to the CNS is not yet clearly determined. Viremia has been shown to be essential to development of poliomyelitis in chimpanzees. Free and cell-associated EV can be detected in blood of patients with EV infections, supporting a role for hematogenous entry into the CNS. Pharmacokinetic analysis of intravenously injected PV in a transgenic mouse model suggests that PV can enter the CNS via the vascular system. Primate and transgenic mouse models, supplemented by anecdotal evidence in humans, indicate that PV can also enter the CNS via a neural route using retrograde axonal transport. Thus, it is

**TABLE 301-1 THE ENTEROVIRUSES**

| | | | | | |
|---|---|---|---|---|---|
| **Traditional Classification** | | | | | |
| Species | Poliovirus | Coxsackievirus group A | Coxsackievirus group B | Echovirus | Numbered enteroviruses |
| Strains | Poliovirus 1–3 | Coxsackievirus A1–22, 24[a] | Coxsackievirus B1–6 | Echovirus 1–7, 9, 11–21, 24–27, 29–33[a] | 68–71[a] |
| **Current Classification** | | | | | |
| Species | | Enterovirus A | Enterovirus B | Enterovirus C | Enterovirus D |
| Strains | | Coxsackievirus A2–A8, A10, A12, A14, A16<br>Enterovirus A71, A76, A89–A92, A114, A119, A120, A121 | Coxsackievirus A9<br>Coxsackievirus B1–B6<br>Echovirus 1–7, 9, 11–21, 24–27, 29–33<br>Enterovirus B69, B73–B75, B77–B88, B93, B97, B98, B100, B101, B106, B107, B110–B113 | Poliovirus 1–3<br>Coxsackievirus A1, A11, A13, A17, A19–A22, A24<br>Enterovirus C95, C96, C99, C102, C104, C105, C109, C113, C116–C118 | Enterovirus D68, D70, D94, D111, D120 |

[a]Coxsackievirus A23; echoviruses 8, 10, 22, 23, 28; and enterovirus 72 have been reclassified.

Data from The Pirbright Institute, UK. The Picornaviridae. http://www.picornaviridae.com. Accessed September 25, 2017.

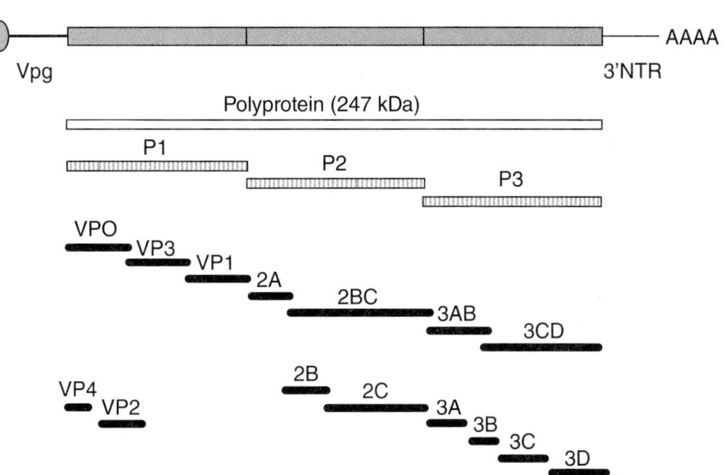


**FIGURE 301-1** Enteroviral genome organization.

probable that the EVs employ multiple means to gain access to the CNS. Viremia and viral replication in the CNS cease once the host produces a type-specific antibody response. Individuals with altered humoral immunity are at risk for severe and chronic EV infections.

The EVs and PeVs are ubiquitous agents with a worldwide distribution. EV and PeV infections exhibit a strong seasonal epidemiology. In regions with temperate climates, the majority of infections occur during the summer and early fall. In the United States, the vast majority of reported infections due to these agents occur from June to October. Infections continue to occur during the winter but with significantly less frequency than during the warmer months of the year. In the world's tropical regions, EV infections occur year-round or with increased incidence during the rainy season.

In the United States and the Americas, as a result of effective vaccination programs against the PVs, these members of the genus no longer circulate endogenously and therefore no longer contribute to annual enteroviral disease burden. With the exception of Pakistan, Nigeria, and Afghanistan, the wild-type PVs have been eradicated from the endemic circulating pool of EVs throughout the world. Although wild-type PV infections no longer occur in North America and the Americas, occasional outbreaks or introductions of vaccine-derived polioviruses (VDPVs) have occurred.

As a result of the use of live attenuated vaccines for the control of the PVs, VDPVs have arisen. VDPVs are derived from the 3 vaccine (Sabin) strains of PV. They are classified into 3 categories: (1) circulating VDPVs (cVDPVs) when there is evidence of person-to-person transmission and that, with rare exception, arise from recombination with naturally circulating types within the EV C species (see Table 301-1); (2) VDPVs that are isolated from individuals with primary immunodeficiencies (iVDPV); and (3) clinical isolates from individuals without immunodeficiency. VDPV-related paralytic disease or isolates have been reported from around the world.

The dominant circulating nonpolio EV types vary by geographic region and by year, and in any given year, multiple EV types may circulate within a community or geographic region. The patterns of circulation vary depending on type. However, the majority of the commonly encountered EVs exhibit an epidemic pattern of circulation. Because widely available tests for the identification of the PeVs have only recently become available, their patterns of circulation have yet to be clearly defined. However, for 1 type, PeV3, the pattern appears to be that of biannually occurring epidemics.

The highest incidence of EV infections is observed in infants under 1 year of age and in toddlers 1 to 4 years of age. Indeed, nearly 45% of cases reported to the Centers for Disease Control and Prevention from 1970 to 2005 occurred in infants under 1 year. The lack of adequate personal hygiene exhibited by children may help to explain the high rates of infection among this population and their caregivers and families. Clinical or serologic evidence of secondary EV infections is observed to occur in more than 50% of susceptible members of households with an infected child. In addition to well-recognized community or nationwide EV outbreaks, outbreaks have been reported to occur in neonatal units and nurseries, schools, childcare centers, camps, and pools, as well as among football teams. Unlike EV, almost all symptomatic PeV infections occur in infants less than 6 months of age and, in particular, those in the first month of life.

It is estimated that a billion or more individuals worldwide are infected with nonpolio EVs annually. In the United States, they are estimated to cause 30 to 50 million infections each year that result in 10 to 15 million symptomatic infections annually. The EVs result in an estimated 30,000 to 50,000 hospitalizations annually for meningitis. Owing to underreporting, this figure may underestimate the actual number of cases.

Humans are the only hosts for the EVs and PeVs, although some EVs have been isolated from nonhuman primates. Most of what is known regarding the pathogenesis of human EV infections has been derived from the study of the PVs in animal models and supplemented by observations in humans. It is believed that the PeVs have a similar pathogenesis but have not been studied. While several modes for transmission of the EVs exist (fecal-oral, respiratory, transplacental, perinatal, self-inoculation), the major route is fecal-oral. For some types (eg, coxsackievirus [CV] A21 and EVs D68, D70, A71), respiratory transmission and self-inoculation are important routes of transmission. Once infected, individuals may shed EVs and PeVs from the respiratory tract for 1 to 2 weeks and from the GI tract for 6 to 8 weeks or longer.

## CLINICAL MANIFESTATIONS

It is important to keep in mind that the vast majority of EV and PeV infections result in a subclinical infection. However, given the large number of EV and PeV infections that occur, it is easy to understand why these viral agents are the preeminent cause of summer and autumnal viral disease each year.

### Undifferentiated Febrile Illness

The EVs and PeVs are common causes of febrile illness without an apparent focus, particularly in infants and toddlers under 2 years of age. This is especially true for the PeVs, for which nearly all infections occur in infants < 6 months of age. This syndrome may result in hospitalization of significant numbers of young infants and children for evaluation of possible bacterial infections. The onset of the illness is typically abrupt with fever (≥ 38°C) in combination with 1 or multiple signs and symptoms: poor feeding, lethargy, irritability, emesis, diarrhea, and upper respiratory tract symptoms. In approximately one-quarter of patients, an exanthem may be present. In EV, fever may be biphasic in nature with an intervening period of euthermia. Older children may complain of abdominal pain. On physical examination, findings are absent or minimal and may consist of mild pharyngeal and conjunctival injection, lymphadenopathy, and exanthems. The duration of illness is generally < 5 days.

Some infants with PeV infection may present with tachycardia, hypotension, and respiratory distress mimicking bacterial sepsis. In

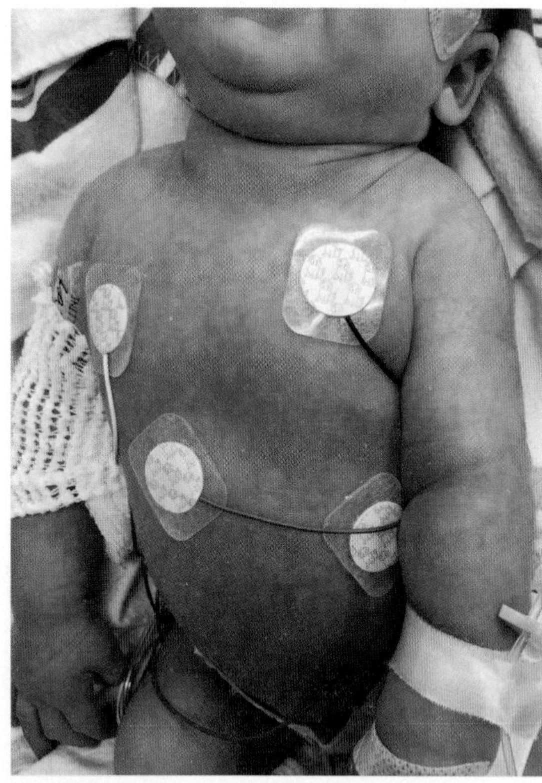

**FIGURE 301-2** Parechovirus erythroderma.

addition to the signs and symptoms listed previously, PeV can result in erythroderma or maculopapular rash involving the palms and soles, extremities, or trunk, in any combination (Fig. 301-2).

#### Central Nervous System Syndromes

The nonpolio EVs are the predominant cause of viral meningitis in children and adolescents, accounting for the overwhelming majority of cases of viral meningitis where an etiology can be determined. Recent evidence suggests that PeVs may also contribute significantly to the burden of meningitis. Members of the EV B species are the principle causes of EV meningitis. Among the PeV types, PeV3 is the principle cause of meningitis.

The clinical presentation of EV and PeV meningitis varies with age. In neonates and young infants, the dominant symptoms consist of fever (≥ 38.0°C) and irritability. In addition to the signs and symptoms discussed earlier in undifferentiated febrile illness, signs of CNS involvement are present. The fontanelle may be full or bulging. Meningoencephalitis in neonates may be manifested by fever, profound lethargy, seizures, full fontanelle, focal neurologic abnormalities, and, much less commonly, nuchal rigidity. Evidence of involvement of other organs (eg, hepatitis, myocarditis, pneumonitis) may be present in severe cases of neonatal meningitis or meningoencephalitis.

In older infants and in children, the onset of EV meningitis is generally abrupt, with fever (38–40°C) being the most common presenting sign. The fever lasts from 1 to 5 days. In some, the pattern of the fever may be biphasic: present for a day, then absent for 2 to 3 days, then reappearing. Young children and infants may be irritable or lethargic and exhibit other nonspecific signs such as poor feeding, emesis, diarrhea, and rash. In infants, the fontanelle may be full. The presence of signs of meningeal irritation (eg, nuchal rigidity, Brudzinski and Kernig signs) increases with advancing age after 3 months and is present in the majority of children older than 1 year. Less than 10% of infants under 3 months of age with EV meningitis have signs of meningeal irritation. Headache, most likely as a result of increased intracranial pressure, is present in nearly all who can report it. The headache may be ameliorated by the performance of a lumbar puncture. Photophobia is a common clinical component of the disease. Seizures occur in < 5% of cases. Nonspecific findings, singly or in combinations, such as rash, malaise, sore throat, abdominal pain, nausea, vomiting, and myalgia, are common. Other nonneurologic EV-associated syndromes, such as herpangina, pleurodynia, and myocarditis, may occur concurrently with the meningitis. In some patients, the entire illness may exhibit a biphasic course consisting of an initial period of nonspecific signs and symptoms (eg, fever, headache, GI symptoms, myalgia) that resolve and subsequently recrudesce, accompanied by evidence of frank neurologic involvement. The duration of EV and PeV meningitis in infants and children is generally < 1 week.

Potential complications of meningitis include coma, increased intracranial pressure, and inappropriate secretion of antidiuretic hormone, but these occur uncommonly.

The presentation of EV meningitis in adolescents and adults is less well characterized than in children and infants. Headache is nearly universally present. In 1 report, 80% of adolescents and adults required narcotic analgesics to control the pain. Photophobia, fever (≥ 37.5°C), signs of meningeal irritation, nausea, emesis, and neck stiffness are reported in greater than two-thirds of patients. Myalgia has been reported in approximately 20% to 90% of patients. Less frequent findings include rash and abdominal pain. The time to full recovery in adults may take up to 2.5 weeks.

Reports of EV encephalitis predominate in children. EV infections may result in generalized or focal encephalitis. Fever, headache, malaise, myalgia and upper respiratory symptoms, nausea, emesis, or diarrhea may precede the onset of the neurologic findings of EV encephalitis. Viral exanthems have occasionally been reported. CNS signs and symptoms may consist of confusion, irritability, weakness, lethargy, and somnolence. The patient may progress to a state of coma. Generalized or focal seizures may occur. Reported focal neurologic findings may include hemiplegia, hemichorea, and paresthesia. The focal nature of the neurologic findings can mimic those seen with herpes simplex encephalitis. Fatal outcomes have been reported.

Encephalitis due to EV A71 deserves special mention. A severe brain stem encephalitis (ie, rhombencephalitis) has been reported primarily in children as a result of EV A71 infection. The illness may have a biphasic presentation with either hand-foot-and-mouth disease (HFMD) or herpangina preceding the onset of myoclonus, the principle neurologic manifestation. The severity of the rhombencephalitis varies. In grade I rhombencephalitis, myoclonic jerks are associated with tremor and/or ataxia. Grade II myoclonus is associated with cranial nerve involvement. In its most severe presentation, grade III, myoclonus is transient and followed by the rapid onset of respiratory distress secondary to neurogenic pulmonary edema, cyanosis, poor perfusion shock, coma, and apnea. Mortality with grade III disease may approach 70%. Reported neurologic sequelae include myoclonus, abducent-nerve palsy, facial diplegia, ataxia, dysarthria, internuclear ophthalmoplegia, and central apnea.

Although acute flaccid paralysis (AFP) has been traditionally linked to the PVs, the cVDPVs, several nonpolio EVs, and some PeVs can also cause this syndrome. In regions of the world where the PVs have been eradicated, the nonpolio EVs and cVDPVs are now the principal causes of EV-associated AFP. Reported nonpolio EV types known to cause AFP include CV A4, A7, A21, A24 B2, B3, and B5; echoviruses 3, 7, 9, 18, 19, and 33; and EV D68, A71, and C105. AFP due to nonpolio EV types tends to be milder than that observed with PV infection. It lacks fever at the time of onset of paralysis, affects the upper extremities and face more frequently, is associated with a more rapid recovery, and is less likely to be associated with atrophy. Interestingly, AFP due to the nonpolio EVs tends to be more severe in infants.

Although not yet conclusively proven, EV D68 may be associated with AFP. During a recent nationwide outbreak of EV D68, > 100 cases of AFP occurred in children with proven EV D68 respiratory tract infection or a syndrome compatible with the same. Upper extremity involvement was seen in 90% of patients and cranial nerve palsies in > 80%. Ninety-two percent of patients had neurologic sequelae.

#### Exanthems and Enanthems

EV infections can result in a plethora of exanthematous syndromes, with any particular type capable of causing several different types of rash. The exanthems of EV infection are more commonly associated with infection of individuals age 15 years or younger. With the exception of CV A16, no single EV type is associated with a unique exanthem. The characteristics of the rashes include maculopapular, macular, papular, morbilliform, rubelliform, vesicular, urticarial, papulopustular, and scarlatiniform. In some cases, a petechial rash reminiscent of that seen with meningococcemia may occur. The rash associated with PeV has been described previously (see above).

One syndrome, HFMD, has been typically associated with CV A16. However, other CVAs and EV A71 may also cause this syndrome. The illness is heralded by low-grade fever, malaise, anorexia, and oral soreness. One to 2 days later, an oral enanthem appears, characterized by macules that rapidly vesiculate and ultimately ulcerate. The evolution of the enanthem may be so rapid that only the ulcerative lesions are seen. The lesions resemble those of aphthous stomatitis and are typically distributed on the buccal mucosa and tongue. They may also occur on the palate, uvula, anterior pillars, and gums. The exanthem occurs in approximately two-thirds of cases and consists of 3- to 7-mm vesicles on slightly erythematous bases. The hands are most commonly involved, followed by the feet and buttocks. Lesions at the latter site tend not to be vesicular. The vesicles predominantly involve the dorsal surfaces of the hands and feet, but the palms and soles are also involved (Fig. 301-3). The illness usually lasts less than a week.

Of note, CV A6 has been associated with more severe HFMD with higher fever and vesiculobullae, bullae, ulcerations, or eschar formation involving the extremities, face, lips and perioral area, buttocks, groin, and perineum. Concentration of lesions in areas of active or dormant eczema (eczema coxsackium) may be seen. Beau lines of the nails or complete shedding of nail (onychomadesis) in the months following the infection can occur.

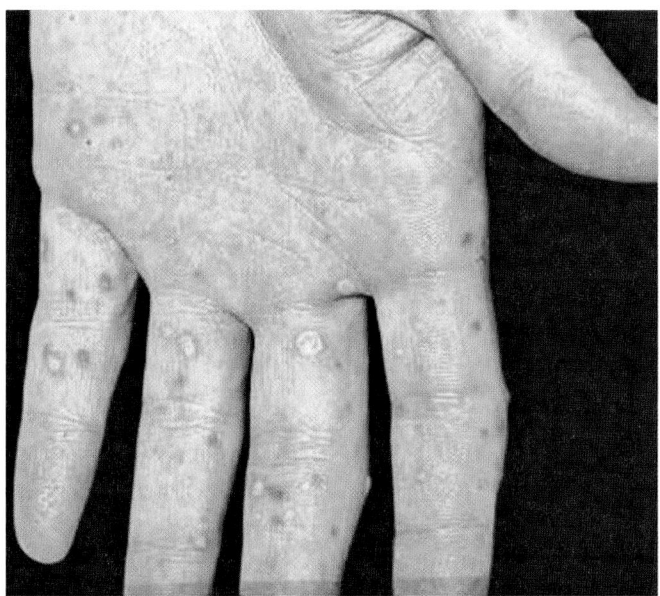

A

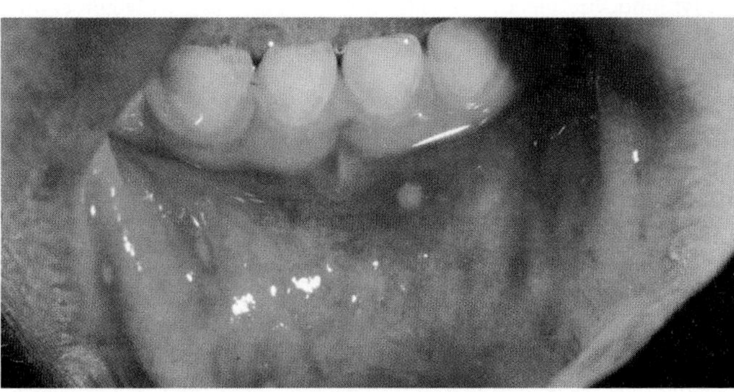

B

**FIGURE 301-3** Hand-foot-and-mouth disease. **A:** Multiple, discrete, small, vesicular lesions on the fingers and palms. **B:** Multiple, superficial erosions and small vesicular lesions surrounded by an erythematous halo on the lower labial mucosa. (Reproduced with permission from Wolff K, Johnson RA: *Fitzpatrick's Color Atlas & Synopsis of Clinical Dermatology*, 6th ed. New York: McGraw-Hill; 2009.)

Herpangina is most commonly caused by the CVAs but has also been associated with CVBs, echoviruses, and numbered EVs. The onset of syndrome is marked by fever to as high as 41°C, with the higher temperatures more commonly seen in younger patients. The enanthem is principally located to the anterior pillars of the tonsillar fauces. It may also be present on the soft palate, uvula, and tonsils. Rarely, involvement of the posterior buccal surfaces and dorsal tip of the tongue may occur. The enanthem consists of papulovesicular, grayish-white lesions, 1 to 2 mm in diameter, with an areola of erythema. Over 2 to 3 days, the lesions progress from papular to vesicular, increase in size (3–4 mm), and ultimately ulcerate (see Fig. 301-3). On average, 5 lesions are present. Associated findings and symptoms include sore throat, mild cervical lymphadenopathy, sialorrhea, anorexia, dysphagia, abdominal pain, and emesis. The illness generally lasts 10 days.

### Respiratory Tract Syndromes

Upper respiratory tract signs and symptoms may accompany EV-associated fevers as well as many of the system- or organ-specific EV syndromes. They may result in both upper and lower respiratory tract syndromes: herpangina, summer cold, pharyngitis, tonsillitis, laryngotracheobronchitis, and pneumonia. The EVs are responsible for up to 15% of etiologically linked upper respiratory tract syndromes. Recently, the use of nucleic acid detection methodologies has demonstrated that 18% of children hospitalized with lower respiratory tract infections and 25% hospitalized with acute wheezing had evidence of EV infection.

The typical EV summer cold consists of nasal congestion, rhinorrhea, and sneezing. Malaise and cough may sometimes be present. Fever and sore throat are minimal or typically absent. The illness lasts less than a week.

Pharyngitis and tonsillitis, alone or in combination (pharyngotonsillitis), has an abrupt onset with fever (38–40°C) in association with sore throat and typically lasts 6 days or less. Examination of the throat reveals erythema and inflammation of the nasopharynx, tonsils, uvula, and soft palate. Petechiae may be present. Cervical lymphadenitis is common.

Pneumonias due to the EVs are clinically indistinguishable from those due to other viral agents. The onset of the illness is gradual, helping to differentiate it from that of bacterial causes, consisting of coryza, anorexia, and low-grade fever. This is followed by a nonproductive cough, tachypnea, retractions, nasal flaring, and, in severe cases, cyanosis. Wheezing may be present if there is concomitant bronchiolitis or bronchospasm. Radiographic findings consist of perihilar infiltrates, patchy consolidation, air trapping, and atelectasis.

Respiratory disease due to EV D68 may be severe. Infants and children with a history of wheezing or asthma are at particular risk for severe disease. Fever is absent in a large proportion of cases. Cough, tachypnea, wheezing, or other abnormalities are present on physical examination in over two-thirds of the cases. Hypoxia is observed in the majority of hospitalized children.

### Muscular Syndromes

Pleurodynia was fully characterized during an outbreak of the syndrome in Bornholm, Denmark, thereby providing its common geographically linked name: Bornholm disease. It is known by other descriptive designations, such as epidemic myalgia and devil's grip. The CVBs are the usual causes of sporadic and epidemic pleurodynia (Bornholm disease), but pleurodynia may also be caused by other EV types.

Pleurodynia is a misnomer for this clinical condition, which is muscular disease with clinical manifestations suggestive of a pleuritic origin. The onset of fever and pain is abrupt in the majority of patients. However, a prodrome of up to 10 days consisting of headache, malaise, anorexia, and vague myalgia may occur. The fever may be biphasic. Referred pain to the lower ribs or the sternum can be paroxysmal and severe. It may radiate to the shoulders, neck, or scapula. During the paroxysms of pain, patients tend to be tachypneic, breath shallowly, and exhibit grunting respirations. The pain may be so severe as to be associated with diaphoresis and pallor. Deep breathing, coughing, sneezing, or other movement accentuates the pain. Abdominal pain may also be present or occur alone and is more commonly seen in children. If the pain is localized to the abdomen, it may be confused with conditions associated with an acute abdomen. Other symptoms include headache, cough, anorexia, nausea, vomiting, and diarrhea. There may be splinting of the chest. Tenderness of the involved muscles and, on abdominal examination, especially in the upper quadrants and periumbilical area may be present but is not pronounced. A pleural friction rub may be heard in a quarter of the patients. The mean duration of the illness is generally less than a week. Enteroviral-related myositis has been observed in patients with agammaglobulinemia and chronic CNS infection. In these patients, cultivable virus is recovered from muscle tissue.

#### Neonatal Infections

The vast majority of EV and PeV infections in neonates are asymptomatic or result in a benign febrile illness. However, infants under 2 weeks of age may be at greater risk for development of severe neonatal EV infections. The greatest risk for increased mortality and severe morbidity is seen when signs and symptoms of infection develop in the first days after delivery. Multiple lines of evidence support in utero acquisition of EV infections and, possibly, PeV infection. Maternal EV illness is manifested as fever, abdominal pain, respiratory symptoms, pleurodynia, or meningitis and has been reported in up to two-thirds of mothers of infected neonates.

As stated previously, the majority of EV- and PeV-infected neonates exhibit a benign and self-limited febrile illness in which the fever resolves in an average of 3 days and other signs and symptoms in about a week. For the EV, a biphasic presentation has been reported in which a mild nonspecific febrile illness precedes the onset of severe disease. Severe neonatal EV disease is a multisystem organ syndrome consisting of combinations of hepatitis, meningoencephalitis, myocarditis, coagulopathy, sepsis, and pneumonia. EV types within the EV B species, in particular echovirus 11, 9, and 6 and the CVBs, are the principal causes of severe disease in the neonate. Two major clinical presentations are encountered: encephalomyocarditis syndrome (severe myocarditis in association with heart failure and meningoencephalitis) and hepatitis-hemorrhage syndrome (severe hepatitis with hepatic failure and disseminated intravascular coagulopathy). The former is predominantly associated with CVB infections; the latter is often associated with echovirus 11 infection. Nonspecific symptoms include fever, temperature instability, irritability, lethargy, hypotonia, poor feeding, emesis, abdominal distension, apnea, retractions, grunting, and rashes. Neurologic involvement may or may not be associated with nuchal rigidity and a bulging anterior fontanelle. CNS involvement may progress to an encephalitic picture: lethargy, seizures, and focal neurologic findings. The latter may be suggestive of herpes simplex virus infections. Myocarditis may be manifested by cardiomegaly, hepatomegaly, poor perfusion, cyanosis, congestive heart failure, metabolic acidosis, and arrhythmias. Clinical findings of severe hepatitis include hepatomegaly, jaundice, increased transaminases, and hyperbilirubinemia. The combination of disseminated intravascular coagulation with other findings of "sepsis" is indistinguishable from that seen in overwhelming bacterial infection. Patients with pneumonia may require mechanical ventilation. Renal failure, intracranial hemorrhage, adrenal hemorrhage, necrotizing enterocolitis, and inappropriate secretion of antidiuretic hormone have been reported.

The risk of death associated with EV infections in neonates is greater than that in older infants and children, reported to be 3.3% in a Centers for Disease Control and Prevention review of cases reported over 20 years.

Severe neonatal PeV infection has also been reported. In addition to the cardiac and hepatic involvement, as described earlier, PeV can cause encephalitis characterized by seizures. Fever, irritability, apnea, and hypotension are common accompaniments. An exanthem (described earlier) is seen in two-thirds of cases. HPeV3 is commonly associated with this syndrome.

#### Cardiac Syndromes

Isolated myocarditis or pericarditis in older children and adults may result from CVB or echovirus infections. The spectrum of illness ranges from benign, self-limited pericarditis to severe, chronic, or fatal myocardial disease. Virus has been isolated from pericardial fluid and heart tissue, particularly in samples obtained within the first 7 to 10 days of disease. Patients present with fever and upper respiratory symptoms followed by the onset of chest pain and shortness of breath. On physical examination, a gallop rhythm might be present as well as a friction rub when auscultating the heart. Echocardiographic findings may demonstrate a decreased ejection fraction or ventricular dilatation. Electrocardiographic findings vary and include low-voltage QRS complexes, ST-segment depressions, and T-wave inversions. Cardiac enzymes are commonly elevated.

#### Nonpolio Enteroviral Infections in Immunocompromised Hosts

Individuals with congenital or acquired B-cell immunodeficiencies are at risk for chronic nonpolio EV and PV infections. Due to a lack or impairment of antibody production, EV cannot be cleared by the host, resulting in chronic infection. Chronic EV infection has been reported in children with X-linked agammaglobulinemia, hyper-IgM syndrome, severe combined immunodeficiency syndrome, and common variable immunodeficiency. Disseminated or prolonged EV infection has been described in patients receiving immunomodulatory therapy, in particular rituximab and obinutuzumab, or chemotherapy, or undergoing bone marrow and solid organ transplantation. Meningoencephalitis, pulmonary infections, and severe gastroenteritis have been reported. These infections can be severe and may result in poor outcomes.

Chronic non-PV meningoencephalitis in patients with X-linked agammaglobulinemia has a subtle presentation. Patients initially complain of persistent headaches and lethargy. As the syndrome progresses, a constellation of neurologic symptoms develops and includes ataxia, loss of cognitive skills and memory, dementia, emotional lability, paresthesias, weakness, dysarthria, and seizures. Nonneurologic manifestations include a dermatomyositis-like syndrome, edema, exanthems, and hepatitis. The cerebrospinal fluid (CSF) demonstrates a persistently elevated protein concentration and pleocytosis. Viral culture and RT-PCR from the CSF are repeatedly positive for EV. Children with humoral immunodeficiency should receive lifelong intravenous immunoglobulin (IVIG) replacement therapy in an attempt to prevent chronic infection. Reports exist of immunodeficient patients developing chronic EV meningoencephalitis despite immunoglobulin therapy.

## DIAGNOSIS

In the case of EV CNS infections, the definitive diagnostic procedure is the lumbar puncture. Cytochemical analysis of the CSF in cases of meningitis or meningoencephalitis typically reveals a mild to moderate lymphocytic pleocytosis. Much less commonly, white cell counts up to or greater than 2000 cells/μL can be encountered. CNS infections with the PeVs can be an exception to this rule as the majority of patients do not demonstrate an increase of white blood cells in the CSF. If the lumbar puncture is performed early in the course of the EV meningitis, a predominantly polymorphonuclear pleocytosis may be present. Reexamination of the CSF several hours later will document a typical lymphocytic pleocytosis. Reports of eosinophilic pleocytosis in association with EV meningitis exist. The CSF protein concentration is mildly to moderately increased. In cases of encephalitis, the sole abnormality may be an elevated protein concentration. Glucose concentration in the CSF is generally normal. However, hypoglycorrhachia may occur and befuddles the assessment, suggesting a bacterial etiology.

In infants, children, and adolescents suspected of having an EV and PeV CNS infection, CSF should be submitted for detection of viral genome by a nucleic acid amplification test (NAAT). Because of the lack of sensitivity of viral culture for detection of the EVs and PeVs in CSF, it should be reserved for instances when NAAT is not available. For neonates with possible EV infections, attempts to detect EV in CSF as well as blood should be made using NAAT, particularly for those with severe EV disease. Additionally, in infants, throat swabs, stool, or rectal swabs should also be submitted for viral culture. The use of samples for viral culture from these sites in older patients to establish the diagnosis of EV and PeV infections should be tempered by the understanding that both may be shed from these sites for weeks to months after infection. Thus, the isolation of an EV or PeV from 1 of these sites may represent residual shedding and not be linked causally to the illness under investigation.

The traditional approach of cell culture for the diagnosis of EV or PeV infections suffers from multiple limitations that lead to a significant lack of sensitivity. No single cell line will support the growth of all members of the EV genus. Additionally, some EV and many PeV types grow poorly or not at all in cell culture. To optimize the isolation of the EV using cell culture, multiple cell lines must be used either individually or as "mixtures." Even using such an approach, some members of the EV genus (eg, CVAs) can only be detected using suckling mouse inoculation, a technique rarely available today in the clinical diagnostic laboratory. Cell culture detection also suffers from a lack of sensitivity for the detection of EV. As many as 25% to 40% of CSF specimens from patients with clinical syndromes consistent with EV CNS disease fail to yield cytopathic effect in cell culture. The time required for isolation and identification of the EVs from CSF is too long to be of clinical utility.

NAATs are rapidly becoming the standard for the detection of the EV and PeV from clinical specimens such as CSF. Regions of conserved nucleotide sequence within the EV and PeV 5′NTR have been used to design primers and probes used in commercial and in-house–developed assays that permit near universal detection of the EV and PeV. When compared to cell culture as the criterion standard, RT-PCR has a sensitivity and specificity that ranges from 86% to 100% and 92% to 100%, respectively. NAATs for detection of the EVs and PeVs from CSF are significantly more sensitive than cell culture. Another significant advantage of NAAT techniques is that the assays can be completed in a matter of hours rather than days, making them clinically useful tools. Multiple reports have documented that RT-PCR–based detection of EV infections of the CNS can shorten hospitalization and reduce cost.

Serologic confirmation of EV infection is generally impractical and not useful in acute management of the patient. While homotypic assays for the detection EV serotype-specific IgM (ie, the CVB-specific IgM and EV A71–specific IgM) and heterotypic assays for the detection of the EV have been reported, they have important limitations. Homotypic assays are useful only if there is suspicion for a specific EV serotype. The IgM response to EV may be nonspecific, resulting in false-positive results. The development of heterotypic assays for the detection of EV is limited by the lack of a common antigen among all serotypes.

Neuroimaging of the CNS using magnetic resonance imaging in patients with EV A71 AFP shows brain stem lesions, most commonly involving the pontine tegmentum; spinal cord lesions, involving the entire central gray matter (acutely) and the anterior horn cells (subacutely); and enhancement of the ventral nerve roots of cervical and cauda equine regions.

## TREATMENT

There is currently no specific treatment for any of the EV infections. Supportive measures include bed rest, antipyretics, and analgesics, as indicated. Immune globulin has been used both in newborn infants and in immunocompromised individuals, such as children with agammaglobulinemia, but its efficacy is not established. Intravenous and intrathecal administration may be necessary to ameliorate or prevent CNS infection in immunocompromised patients.

## PREVENTION AND PROGNOSIS

The overall prognosis for EV infections not involving the CNS outside of the early neonatal period is excellent with respect to mortality and morbidity. The short-term and long-term neurocognitive prognosis following EV meningitis in children appears to be favorable. A controlled study failed to identify differences between patients and controls. In contrast, EV encephalitis can result in more profound long-term sequelae, particularly in the case of EV A71. In these children, CNS and brain stem involvement were associated with neurologic sequelae, delayed neurodevelopment, and reduced cognitive functioning.

EVs are spread primarily by the lack of good hygiene. Handwashing, in particular, prevents this spread since EVs are transmitted via the fecal-oral route and, in rare cases, respiratory droplets. During nursery outbreaks of EV infections, cohorting infected neonates is effective in limiting outbreaks. For patients hospitalized with EV-related syndromes, infection control measures using standard precautions are sufficient.

Use of oral and inactivated PV vaccines has resulted in the near elimination of these viruses worldwide. Vaccines for the prevention of EV A71 disease have recently become available in China, where annual epidemics of EV A71 are common.

Women at the end of their pregnancy should avoid interactions with individuals who potentially have an EV infection. If a pregnant woman has an illness consistent with an EV-related disease and the fetus is doing well, attempts should be made to not deliver the baby. Waiting allows the baby time to acquire protective maternal antibodies.

## SUGGESTED READINGS

Centers for Disease Control and Prevention. Notes from the field: severe hand, foot, and mouth disease associated with coxsackievirus A6—Alabama, Connecticut, California, and Nevada, November 2011-February 2012. *MMWR Morb Mortal Wkly Rep*. 2012;61:213-214.

Khan F. Enterovirus D68: acute respiratory illness and the 2014 outbreak. *Emerg Med Clin North Am*. 2015;33:e19-e32.

Khatami A, McMullan BJ, Webber M, et al. Sepsis-like disease in infants due to human parechovirus type 3 during an outbreak in Australia. *Clin Infect Dis*. 2015;60:228-236.

Maloney JA, Mirsky DM, Messacar K, Dominguez SR, Schreiner T, Stence NV. MRI findings in children with acute flaccid paralysis and cranial nerve dysfunction occurring during the 2014 enterovirus D68 outbreak. *AJNR Am J Neuroradiol*. 2015;36:245-250.

Mathes EF, Oza V, Frieden IJ, et al. "Eczema coxsackium" and unusual cutaneous findings in an enterovirus outbreak. *Pediatrics*. 2013;132:e149-e157.

Messacar K, Schreiner TL, Maloney JA, et al. A cluster of acute flaccid paralysis and cranial nerve dysfunction temporally associated with an outbreak of enterovirus D68 in children in Colorado, USA. *Lancet*. 2015;385:1662-1671.

Romero JR, Selvarangan R. The human Parechoviruses: an overview. *Adv Pediatr*. 2011;58:65-85.

Shoji K, Komuro H, Miyata I, Miyairi I, Saitoh A. Dermatologic manifestations of human parechovirus type 3 infection in neonates and infants. *Pediatr Infect Dis J*. 2013;32:233-236.

Ventarola D, Bordone L, Silverberg N. Update on hand-foot-and-mouth disease. *Clin Dermatol*. 2015;33:340-346.

# 302 Viral Hemorrhagic Fevers

Amy S. Arrington

## INTRODUCTION

Viral hemorrhagic fevers (VHFs) are a diverse group of diseases and include dozens of viruses (Table 302-1). The diseases they cause are either endemic or episodic, with both annual cycles and longer secular trends. Some are associated with high lethality and potential for person-to-person transmission. The challenges for clinicians evaluating suspect cases are to exclude more likely conditions that are potentially

**TABLE 302-1 FEATURES OF VIRAL HEMORRHAGIC FEVERS**

| Family | Virus | Disease | Geographic Region | Epidemiologic Distribution | Incubation Period (days) | Reservoir/Vector |
|---|---|---|---|---|---|---|
| Arenaviridae | Junin[a] | Argentine hemorrhagic fever | Argentina Pampas | Rural | 7–16 | Rodent: *Calomys callosus* |
| | Machupo[a] | Bolivian hemorrhagic fever | Beni Department, Bolivia | Rural | 7–16 | Rodent: *Calomys musculinus* |
| | Guanarito | Venezuelan hemorrhagic fever | Guanarito municipality of Portuguesa State and adjacent regions of Barinas State, Venezuela | Rural | 7–14 | Rodent: *Zygodontomys brevicauda* |
| | Sabía | Sabía-associated hemorrhagic fever | Sao Paulo State, Brazil | Unknown; presumed rural | 8 | |
| | Lassa[a] | Lassa fever | Nigeria, Sierra Leone, Liberia, Guinea | Rural | 2–21 | Rodent: *Matomys* species |
| | Lymphocytic choriomeningitis virus | Lymphocytic choriomeningitis (LCM) | Widespread (domestic, abroad) | Rural | 8–13 | Rodent: *Mus domesticus* |
| Bunyaviridae | Hantaan and related viruses | Hemorrhagic fever with renal syndrome | Asia Europe (rare in Africa and the Americas) | Rural, urban *Rattus*-associated disease, and laboratory-acquired | 4–42 | Rodents: arvicoline and murine genus |
| | Sin Nombre and related viruses (Andes[a]) | Hantavirus pulmonary syndrome | Americas | Rural | 4–35 | Rodents: *Sigmodontine* genus |
| | Crimean-Congo hemorrhagic fever[a] | Crimean-Congo hemorrhagic fever | Africa, Asia, southern Europe | Rural; contacts with ticks, domestic animals | 2–7 | Ticks: *Hyalomma* species |
| | Rift Valley fever | Rift Valley fever | Africa | Rural; contact with mosquitoes, domestic animals | 2–7 | Mosquito: *Aedes* species |
| Filoviridae | Marburg[a] | Marburg hemorrhagic fever | Sub-Saharan Africa | Rural | 3–16 | Cave-dwelling bats (probable) |
| | Ebola[a] | Ebola hemorrhagic fever | Tropical forests, Africa (all strains except Ebola-Reston from Philippines) | Rural | 3–21 | Forest-dwelling bats (probable) |
| | *Cuevavirus* | | | | | |
| Flaviviridae | Dengue | Dengue fever, dengue hemorrhagic fever, dengue shock syndrome | Africa, Americas (excluding the northern and southern extremes) | Urban | 4–7 | Mosquito: *Aedes aegypti, Aedes albopictus* |
| | Yellow fever | Yellow fever | Africa, South America | Rural, urban | 3–6 | Mosquito: *Aedes aegypti*, other *Aedes* species |
| | Omsk hemorrhagic fever | Omsk hemorrhagic fever | Western Siberia | Rural agriculture, winter (muskrat and other rodent transmission) | 2–4 | Tick: *Dermacentor* species |
| | Kyasanur Forest disease | Kyasanur Forest disease | Karnataka State, India | Rural; forests | 2–7 | Tick: *Haemaphysalis* species |

[a]Documented nosocomial transmission.

life-threatening and treatable (especially malaria and typhoid fever); narrow the differential diagnosis based on the travel history; institute appropriate precautions for the diseases in the narrowed differential that are associated with person-to-person transmission; and seek expert guidance for diagnostic confirmation and treatment guidelines.

## PATHOGENESIS AND EPIDEMIOLOGY

The etiologic agents of this syndrome are lipid-enveloped ribonucleic acid (RNA) viruses and include dozens of members from 4 families of viruses: arenaviruses, filoviruses, bunyaviruses, and flaviviruses. All are zoonotic infections and reside in animal reservoirs or insect vectors as opposed to humans, although in many cases, these viruses can be transmitted to humans when the activities of humans and animals overlap. The unprecedented Ebola virus outbreak in 2014 to 2015 perhaps best demonstrates the potential impact of these emerging diseases on the human population worldwide. These agents are localized geographically and are associated with specific vector hosts or reservoirs, although imported cases and infections caused by travel, laboratory accidents, and nosocomial transmission can occur outside their respective ranges.

Most arboviruses (arthropod-borne viruses) are maintained in natural cycles of infection between mosquitoes or ticks and vertebrate hosts. Seasonality of hemorrhagic fever among humans is influenced for the most part by the dynamics of infected arthropod or vertebrate hosts. The viruses may be carried through the winter or dry months by persistence in dormant vectors, by vertical transovarial transmission in mosquitoes, by transstadial transmission in ticks, or in persistently infected vertebrates. In tropical locations, enzootic transmission can occur throughout the year. Human infections occur through accidental exposure to the enzootic cycle or during epizootics. Large urban epidemics occur as a result of vector-borne interhuman transmission of arboviruses like yellow fever and dengue, which produce sufficient viremia in humans to infect mosquitoes. Some arboviruses are primarily transmitted to humans as zoonoses. Zoonotic transmission to humans also occurs with arenaviruses, which cause Lassa and lymphocytic choriomeningitis, and with the hantaviruses, which cause hantavirus pulmonary syndrome. These viruses are spread from the excretions of various persistently or transiently infected rodents to humans through inhalation, ingestion, or direct contact. Filoviruses may be transmitted to humans by bats or other infected mammals. Person-to-person spread of Crimean-Congo hemorrhagic fever, Ebola, and Marburg viruses has led to sizable outbreaks, often with substantial nosocomial transmission. Occasional person-to-person transmission has also been documented for the New World arenaviruses (Junin and Machupo) and Andes virus–related hantavirus pulmonary syndrome.

The largest VHF outbreak in children was the Marburg outbreak in northern Angola in 2004 to 2005, during which approximately 75% of cases occurred in children under the age of 5 years, possibly due to nosocomial transmission in a pediatric ward and from contaminated medical supplies. During periods of hyperendemic or epidemic yellow fever or dengue transmission, adults may have preexisting immunity, so the highest proportion of cases occurs in children and adolescents. Pediatric cases of Lassa fever and town-based Bolivian hemorrhagic fever occur because of peridomestic contact with the vector/reservoir. In contrast, children are rarely affected by sylvatic yellow fever or infection with the New World arenaviruses that are predominantly acquired in forests or fields by hunters and farmers.

## CLINICAL MANIFESTATIONS

Infection in children is determined by a combination of their susceptibility to infection and contact with the reservoir/vector. Compared to adult data, few pediatric cases have been described during outbreaks of Ebola hemorrhagic fever in otherwise susceptible populations, most likely because this disease is primarily spread through direct contact with patients, during funeral practices, or inadvertent exposures in the healthcare setting. Data from the 2014 to 2015 Ebola outbreak described a shorter mean incubation period in children, ranging from 6.9 to 9.8 days, as well as shorter times from symptom onset to hospitalization and from symptom onset to death. Additionally, a study describing the clinical characteristics of children less than 5 years of age diagnosed with Ebola virus disease in the 2014 to 2015 outbreak in Sierra Leone showed that 25% of these patients had no fever either reported in their history before admission or a measured temperature < 38°C on the day of admission.

VHFs typically present with nonspecific signs and symptoms including fever, myalgia, headache, and sometimes gastrointestinal symptoms. Thus, differentiating VHF from other common febrile illnesses can be challenging during the initial stages. The subsequent development of hypotension, a flushed appearance suggesting early vascular injury, petechiae, and hemorrhage should trigger further diagnostic studies. Rash is seen only in Ebola, Marburg, dengue, and Lassa fevers.

The VHFs typically manifest as acute febrile syndromes, although in some cases, these illnesses may evolve into a severe multisystem syndrome characterized by diffuse vascular damage, multiorgan failure, and death. In even the worst cases, hemorrhage occurs in only 50% of patients. High mortality rates in these illnesses typically result from multiorgan failure, severe electrolyte disturbances and hypovolemic shock as opposed to acute hemorrhage. Disease manifestations of VHF in children resemble those in adults, with notable exceptions. Dengue hemorrhagic fever and dengue shock syndrome in infants are thought to be precipitated by decreasing levels of maternal antibody, which is cross-reactive but nonprotective at lower levels. The swollen baby syndrome of Lassa fever is another uniquely pediatric disease.

## DIAGNOSIS

Since each of these diseases occurs in a specific geographic and ecologic pattern, diagnosis requires consideration of the possibility of exposure and an estimation of the incubation period. The suspicion of VHF should immediately trigger safe isolation practices and testing for a specific etiology. The major pitfall in diagnosis among travelers is entertaining the possibility of hemorrhagic fever at the expense of performing a thorough evaluation of more common and treatable conditions, such as malaria or typhoid fever.

Thrombocytopenia is the only universal clinical laboratory feature of VHF, although it may be rare in Lassa fever. Except for hantaviruses, these viruses can be readily isolated from acute-phase samples in specialized laboratories using appropriate biocontainment conditions. Enzyme-linked immunosorbent assays for antigen, immunoglobulin (Ig) M, and IgG antibodies are rapid, sensitive, and specific. The older indirect immunofluorescent antibody, complement fixation, and hemagglutination inhibition assays are less sensitive and specific than enzyme-linked immunosorbent assays. The plaque-reduction neutralization test can be used to detect neutralizing antibodies to some viruses. Nucleic acid tests like polymerase chain reaction and nucleic acid sequence–based assays provide direct and rapid detection of viral RNA in blood and tissue. Immunohistochemical techniques using virus-specific antibodies have improved postmortem tissue diagnosis. The Centers for Disease Control and Prevention's Special Pathogens Branch (phone: 404-639-1115) can provide immediate assistance with appropriate diagnosis and response.

## SPECIFIC INFECTIONS

### Filoviral Hemorrhagic Fevers

The filovirus family consists of 3 viruses, *Ebolavirus*, *Marburgvirus*, and *Cuevavirus*. While members of this family are highly lethal VHFs, Ebola virus has proven to be a pathogen capable of large-scale human morbidity and mortality, with mortality rates ranging from 30% up to 90%. The most recent Ebola virus epidemic in 2014 to 2015 affecting West Africa and beyond demonstrated the ability of these viruses to cause devastating effects, reminded us of the virulence of these agents, and provided new knowledge regarding the pathogenesis and potential treatments for this biologic threat.

The hemorrhagic fevers caused by Marburg and Ebola viruses are among the most lethal: case fatality rates range from approximately 25% to 90% among those with Marburg hemorrhagic fever and 30% to 90% in outbreaks of Ebola hemorrhagic fever. Growing evidence points to cave-dwelling bats as the natural reservoir for Marburg virus, and forest-dwelling bats may be the natural reservoir for Ebola virus. There are 5 known subtypes of Ebola virus (Reston, Sudan, Zaire, Cote d'Ivoire, and Bundibugyo, a newly identified subtype from Uganda) that differ in virulence. Lloviu virus, obtained from bats in Spain (2002), is the only known virus in the *Cuevavirus* family, and the potential to cause human infections remains undetermined because no virus has yet been isolated.

Of the filoviruses that have caused large epidemics in humans, the Zaire subtype of Ebola has caused the highest case fatality rate and was responsible for the largest outbreak to date in 2014 to 2015. Human-to-human spread occurs through direct contact with symptomatic individuals, resulting in chains of transmission that are often amplified in the nosocomial setting. Illness begins with an abrupt onset of fever, prostration, headache, and myalgia. Patients frequently appear restless and anxious, and they later become apathetic and exhibit other encephalopathic signs. After 3 to 8 days, a morbilliform, usually confluent, nonpruritic rash starts on the upper trunk and spreads centrifugally to involve the entire body except the face and neck, and conjunctival injection and edema can be seen. Profuse vomiting and watery diarrhea commence, accompanied by intense abdominal pain. Chest pain is a variable feature that was often noted in the Ebola-Sudan outbreak in 1976 but not in other Marburg and Ebola-Zaire outbreaks. Bleeding occurs in about 50% of patients, primarily from the gastrointestinal tract in the form of melena and hematemesis, but also from the vagina, gums, and nares. Multisystem organ failure from pneumonitis, hepatitis, pancreatitis, and tubulointerstitial nephritis combined with intractable hypotension usually leads to death. Recovery can occur within 7 to 10 days, but convalescence can take weeks to months, and recent data suggest the virus can remain in the bodily fluids of survivors for up to 18 months.

### Arenaviruses

Arenaviruses are classified into 2 distinct groups: Old World (OW) and New World (NW), based primarily on antigenic, phylogenetic, and geographic properties. These viruses cause chronic infections in their hosts, primarily rodents indigenous to Africa, Europe, and the Americas, and enter the human population when humans come into contact with infected animals.

**New World Arenaviruses** The NW group consists of many different arenaviruses, including 4 known to cause human disease—Junin, Machupo, Guanarito, and Sabiá viruses—and are the etiologic agents of Argentine, Bolivian, Venezuelan, and Sabiá hemorrhagic fevers, respectively. These viruses are primarily maintained by rodents indigenous to their respective geographical areas. Argentine hemorrhagic fever is almost exclusively an occupational disease of agricultural workers, although the proportion of pediatric cases is increasing, to approximately 10% of all cases, as increasing numbers of adults in high-risk areas have been vaccinated. Prepartum maternal infection can result in spontaneous abortion, congenital malformations, and neonatal death, as well as maternal death; the virus has also been isolated from breast milk. Bolivian hemorrhagic fever and Venezuelan hemorrhagic fever are acquired in a peridomestic setting, and cases occur in all age groups. All 4 diseases present with a similar nonspecific history of fever, headache, myalgia, weakness, and gastrointestinal symptoms. Photophobia and epigastric abdominal pain may occur, but respiratory signs and symptoms are uncommon. Patients become increasingly toxic and develop a flushed appearance, conjunctival injection, and fine petechial eruptions on the oral pharynx, upper trunk, and axillae. Most enter a convalescent phase after the first week of illness, but more than one-third develop neurologic complications (altered mental status, ataxia, or tremors) or a hypotensive-hemorrhagic phase associated with a capillary leak syndrome. NW arenaviruses have an overall case fatality rate of 10% to 30%.

**Old World Arenaviruses** The OW group consists of a single lineage made up of 5 species, with Lassa virus and lymphocytic choriomeningitis virus (LCMV) being the most well-known. Lassa fever is a common cause of febrile illness in West Africa, particularly Guinea, Liberia, Nigeria, and Sierra Leone, typically from December to March, with as many as 300,000 cases and 5000 deaths annually. The disease is characterized by insidious onset of fever, weakness, myalgia, and generalized malaise followed by lower backache, substernal or epigastric pain, dizziness, cough, and gastrointestinal symptoms. Purulent pharyngitis, conjunctivitis, edema (particularly of the head and neck), and mucosal bleeding are highly specific signs of Lassa fever. Fulminant disease is marked by hypovolemic shock; facial and neck edema; encephalopathy; and respiratory distress due to laryngeal edema, pneumonitis, pulmonary edema, and pleural effusion. Permanent sensorineural hearing loss can occur as a late sequela. Maternal infection can result in maternal and fetal death, especially near term, as well as congenital Lassa fever in neonates. Children younger than 2 years of age with Lassa fever can develop swollen baby syndrome, characterized by widespread edema, abdominal distention, and bleeding. The mortality rate associated with Lassa fever is estimated to be about 15% of those who develop severe cases, and Lassa fever may account for as much as 10% of febrile children admitted to hospitals in endemic areas of West Africa. However, a Lassa fever outbreak in Nigeria between August 2015 and May 2016 resulted in 149 deaths, with a 54% case fatality rate (http://www.who.int/csr/don/27-may-2016-lassa-fever-nigeria/en/).

In contrast, LCMV infections in humans are rarely fatal and have been detected in the human population in Europe, the Americas, Australia, and Japan. Several serologic studies have shown that the prevalence of LCMV antibodies in human populations ranges from 2% to 5%, and human infections with this virus are likely underrecognized and, therefore, underreported. LCMV is most associated with an acute febrile illness and may cause neurologic infections including aseptic meningitis and encephalitis. Although associated with low mortality rates (1%), this disease may cause significant morbidity in certain populations, including the potential for causing congenital hydrocephalus and chorioretinitis in the fetuses of women infected while pregnant.

### Hemorrhagic Fever with Renal Syndrome

Hemorrhagic fever with renal syndrome is caused by 4 murine and arvicoline rodent-borne OW hantaviruses—Hantaan, Dobrova-Belgrade, Seoul, and Puumala—which occur primarily in Asia and Europe. Men, particularly agricultural and forestry workers, are at greatest risk for infection in sylvatic locations. There is an unexplained paucity of cases among children, and it is possible that symptomatic disease may be milder in children. The most severe form of hemorrhagic fever with renal syndrome is caused by Hantaan virus and is classically associated with 5 consecutive phases with characteristic physiologic derangement: febrile, hypotensive, oliguric, diuretic, and convalescence. Hemorrhage is generally noted during the oliguric phase. However, there is considerable variation in the incidence of various manifestations and the severity of individual phases that may overlap.

### Hantavirus Pulmonary Syndrome

Hantavirus pulmonary syndrome is caused by a number of NW sigmodontine rodent-borne hantaviruses indigenous to rural areas of the Americas and is a consequence of sylvatic or peridomestic transmission. As with their OW cousins, there is a relative paucity of pediatric cases. A brief, nondescript febrile prodrome with chills, myalgia, malaise, diarrhea, and headache is generally followed by the precipitous onset of the cardiopulmonary phase with hypotension and increased vascular permeability, resulting in pulmonary edema and hypoxia. Death can occur within 2 days of admission from respiratory failure and cardiogenic shock. In South America, Andes virus infection may be associated with facial flushing, petechiae, and occasionally frank hemorrhage, and it can be transmitted person to person. Overt hemorrhage occurs rarely in severe cases in North America. Bilateral interstitial pulmonary infiltrates in conjunction with shock are a hallmark of severe disease, as is the triad of thrombocytopenia, immature neutrophils, and circulating immunoblasts. Atypical presentations with prominent renal insufficiency and myositis have been reported, as have asymptomatic and mild infections without pulmonary involvement.

### Crimean-Congo Hemorrhagic Fever

Crimean-Congo hemorrhagic fever virus (CCHFV) is also a member of the Bunyaviridae family. It has a wide geographic distribution throughout parts of Africa, the Middle East, Asia, and Eastern Europe, which mirrors the distribution of its vector, the *Hyalomma* genus of ticks. Many types of mammals and perhaps birds serve as reservoirs for the virus as transmitted by ticks, but humans seem to be the only species that develops disease with the infection. In addition to tick bites, contact with human or animal blood (particularly inoculation) also serves as an important route of infection, with numerous nosocomial outbreaks of CCHFV reported. Risk factors for acquisition in endemic areas include outdoor recreational activity, farming, and blood contact through abattoir, veterinary, or healthcare work. Clinical disease with CCHFV usually follows a 3- to 9-day incubation period. Symptom onset is usually abrupt with severe headache, high fever, myalgia, weakness, anorexia, back and abdominal pain, and nausea often accompanied by vomiting. Hyperemia commonly occurs, most notably on the face, mucous membranes, and upper part of the body. Early nonspecific symptoms are followed by more severe manifestations after the sixth day of illness, including hemorrhage from the nose, mouth, and gastrointestinal tract and large ecchymotic areas on the limbs caused by disseminated intravascular coagulation. During this stage, most patients become obtunded with halting speech; dizziness and mild meningeal signs are common. Elevated bilirubin and liver enzyme levels are usually present. Patients may become delirious or comatose; death occurs in approximately 30% of cases.

### Rift Valley Fever

Rift Valley fever virus (RVFV) is a member of the Bunyaviridae family. Rift Valley fever is a primarily mosquito-borne veterinary disease occurring in sub-Saharan Africa and Madagascar, where intermittent epizootics are associated with heavy rainfall and flooding, leading to increased numbers of *Aedes* mosquitos. Livestock epizootics can result in serious losses of domestic livestock from abortions and death. RVFV was first discovered in 1930 after an outbreak in sheep in Kenya and has caused major outbreaks in several countries including Kenya, Tanzania, Somalia, South Africa, Madagascar, Egypt,

Sudan, Mauritania, Senegal, Saudi Arabia, and Yemen. Humans are infected by direct or aerosol exposure to blood from infected animals, from ingestion of raw milk, and through bites of infected mosquitos. Usually it manifests as a self-limited but severe illness characterized by fever, headache, chills, anorexia, myalgia, and prostration, with impaired hepatic and renal function. The illness typically resolves after 2 to 5 days, but a small portion of individuals develop more severe disease: approximately 1% of infected patients develop hemorrhagic fever (although up to 75% were reported to have developed fever in a 2006–2007 outbreak); less than 1%, encephalitis; and 15%, retinitis. The hemorrhagic fever usually involves severe necrotizing hepatitis. Encephalitis, associated with confusion, meningismus, paresis, hallucinations, convulsions, and recrudescence of fever, can occur 1 to 4 weeks after the initial febrile illness, as can retinitis, which can cause permanent vision loss. It remains difficult to estimate morbidity and mortality in humans, but overall mortality with RVFV infection is estimated to be 1% or less, although mortality with severe disease in recent series has been reported to be as high as 29% to 33%, and in the 2006 to 2007 outbreak, up to 76% of infected individuals reported hemorrhage associated with the disease.

#### Dengue Fever

Dengue fever is the most common arboviral infection worldwide. Dengue hemorrhagic fever causes hundreds of thousands of life-threatening infections annually in the tropics, mostly in children. The geographic range of dengue has been expanding dramatically over the past 40 years; it is now hyperendemic in the tropics. Dengue virus is a *Flavivirus* with 4 serotypes, transmitted by *Aedes* species mosquitoes, predominantly *Aedes aegypti*, which are present in most tropical urban areas of the world. *Aedes albopictus* have also been implicated in fairly substantial outbreaks, especially as they have been introduced into new areas, sometimes outcompeting *A aegypti*. In the United States, these mosquitoes can be found in Hawaii year-round and in the southeastern states in the summer months, contributing to an epidemic in Hawaii in 2001 to 2002 and regular autochthonous transmission in southern Texas. Epidemics arise in susceptible populations after the virus is introduced by viremic persons into areas with competent vectors. In areas where transmission is endemic, dengue is principally a disease of childhood. Infections occur in almost 100% of children before 8 years of age. Infections can occur in all age groups when the people exposed are immunologically naïve, such as when a new strain is introduced in a population or when travelers from non-endemic areas travel to dengue-endemic regions.

Asymptomatic dengue virus infection is common. The incubation period for disease in symptomatic individuals is typically 4 to 7 days. Dengue fever can be mild in young children, but in older children and adults, it is associated with significant fever, chills, headache, retro-orbital pain, myalgia, arthralgia, and low back pain accompanied by anorexia, nausea, and vomiting. Facial flushing is common, and in fair-skinned persons, a centrifugally spreading morbilliform rash may be detected late in the illness in more than half of patients. Illness is self-limited and sometimes is complicated by minor hemorrhagic phenomena, such as epistaxis and minor gum, gastrointestinal, and vaginal mucosal bleeding. The tourniquet test (20 or more petechiae appearing below a blood pressure cuff inflated for 5 minutes to halfway between systolic and diastolic pressures) may be positive in one-third of patients. Lowered platelet, total leukocyte, and absolute monocyte and neutrophil counts reflect bone marrow suppression and peripheral destruction of platelets.

The self-limited hemorrhagic phenomena should be differentiated from dengue hemorrhagic fever, characterized by thrombocytopenia, generalized bleeding, and evidence of increased vascular permeability (eg, hemoconcentration, pleural effusions, ascites, or hypoalbuminemia). Advanced cases are called dengue shock syndrome, which is dengue hemorrhagic fever with hypotension and a narrow pulse pressure and causes a case fatality rate as high as 44%. Cross-protective immunity among dengue serotypes is limited, and sequential infection, particularly when dengue 2 virus causes the second infection, increases the risk for dengue hemorrhagic fever and dengue shock syndrome. The onset of hypotension may be precipitous and typically occurs with defervescence. This interval of vascular instability may be as brief as 24 to 48 hours and reverses spontaneously. Hemodynamic monitoring and supportive fluid, cardiovascular support, and avoidance of aspirin reduce dengue hemorrhagic fever mortality from 25% to less than 5%.

#### Yellow Fever

Yellow fever is transmitted between nonhuman primates in the tropical rainforest by *Aedes* species mosquitoes in Africa and *Haemagogus* species mosquitoes in South America. A sylvatic cycle occurs in the moist savanna regions of Africa in which forest *Aedes* species mosquitoes transmit yellow fever between primates and humans. Large epidemics of urban yellow fever can occur in cities in endemic areas of Africa and South America infested by peridomestic *A aegypti* that transmit the disease in a human-mosquito-human cycle, as with dengue. Despite the development of an effective vaccine in the 1940s, outbreaks continue to occur, such as the 2016 outbreak in Angola. Vaccine shortages and poor healthcare structures in endemic countries result in continued outbreaks. Yellow fever epidemics mostly affect children and young adults who have not acquired immunity to yellow fever or to heterologous flaviviruses that may offer some cross-protective immunity and who tend to develop more severe disease with high case fatality rates.

The disease classically has been divided into 3 stages: infection, remission, and intoxication. The period of infection is characterized by sudden onset of fever, headache, malaise, musculoskeletal pain, low back pain, and nausea. Physical signs include conjunctival suffusion, flushing of the skin, and relative bradycardia despite fever, known as Faget sign. In about 15% to 25% of cases, the remission phase is temporary, lasting only 2 to 24 hours, and the illness resumes in a more severe form. Patients in the period of intoxication develop fever, vomiting, abdominal pain, jaundice, hematemesis, and other forms of hemorrhage. Patients are typically dehydrated with hypotension, reduced urinary output, and, frequently, proteinuria. Myocarditis, azotemia, encephalopathy, progressive liver damage, bleeding, and shock can occur; mortality rates in patients who progress to the period of intoxication range from 20% to 50%.

#### Tick-Borne Hemorrhagic Fevers

Kyasanur Forest disease and Omsk hemorrhagic fever are tick-borne flavivirus infections that are seasonally transmitted in the areas of southern and central India and southwestern Siberia, respectively. Kyasanur Forest disease, also called "monkey fever," was first identified after an outbreak of severe disease in people living near the Kyasanur Forest in Karnataka State, India, in the spring of 1957. It is maintained in a forest cycle involving *Haemaphysalis* ticks, birds, and small mammals. It is transmitted by tick bite to nonhuman primates and humans, mainly villagers and lumbermen. Omsk hemorrhagic fever is primarily transmitted directly from infected muskrats to humans during hunting through direct contact with blood, urine, or feces; by tick bite; or through ingestion of unpasteurized milk from infected sheep and goats. Kyasanur Forest disease and Omsk hemorrhagic fever are self-limited illnesses characterized by acute fever, chills, myalgia, headache, vomiting, and diarrhea lasting 4 to 10 days in half of all cases, and hypotension, which can persist for several days. Hemorrhagic manifestations tend to be minor in Omsk hemorrhagic fever. Hepatitis and acute renal failure can occur in both illnesses, and bronchitis, pneumonia, alveolar hemorrhage, and pulmonary edema develop in 40% of cases. Signs of encephalitis appear late in the course of illness in 50% of Kyasanur Forest disease cases but are less prominent in Omsk hemorrhagic fever. The case fatality rate for both illnesses is less than 5%.

### TREATMENT

Treatment for VHFs is limited, and supportive care is essential. Acute infections may range from being asymptomatic or clinically apparent, with progression to critical illness and fatality, to resolution with no serious sequela. Supportive therapy for shock, hemorrhage, and secondary infection is critical for the management of cases of more severe VHFs. Ribavirin is a broad-spectrum antiviral that acts as a purine nucleoside analog with activity against several hemorrhagic viral infections including RVFV and Lassa virus. Anecdotal experience suggests that the use of ribavirin in RVFV may exacerbate or cause encephalitis, and further evidence is necessary to recommend its use. However, in controlled trials of adults, ribavirin reduced mortality and morbidity in Lassa fever and hemorrhagic fever with renal syndrome. Retrospective studies have indicated that ribavirin may decrease mortality among patients with CCHFV and anecdotal experience suggests its efficacy in treating NW arenaviral hemorrhagic fevers. Immunoglobulin has been used with some success in a few cases of CCHFV. Early transfusion of immune plasma is potentially an effective therapy for some hemorrhagic fevers, including Argentine hemorrhagic fever, CCHFV, and Ebola virus, but data are limited, and further studies are needed to confirm the efficacy of this therapy. In the 2014 to 2015 Ebola virus outbreak, convalescent plasma from survivors was utilized, but early studies indicate that this therapy was not associated with a significant improvement in survival.

## PREVENTION

Perhaps the greatest weapon against these viruses remains prevention and control. Vector-borne infections can be prevented by avoiding at-risk locations during the seasons and/or times of day when risk is greatest. Simple measures include covering exposed areas of the body with clothing, avoiding outdoor activities at dusk and dawn when certain vectors are most active, limiting free-standing water to reduce breeding sites, and using insecticide-treated bed nets. Protective clothing and repellents can reduce arthropod exposure and bites. Repellents containing *N,N*-diethyl-meta-toluamide (DEET) or picaridin are the most effective formulations; however, no definitive studies have determined what concentrations of DEET are safe to use in children. The American Academy of Pediatrics has stated that DEET is not harmful to children in concentrations of up to 30% when used appropriately but does not recommended its use in infants under 2 months old. Oil of lemon eucalyptus has also been approved by the US Food and Drug Administration for use as an insect repellent but needs to be applied more frequently and should not be used on children under 3 years of age according to the product label. Permethrin effectively repels and kills mosquitoes and ticks when sprayed on clothing and bed nets and remains effective after several washings.

Practicing good hygiene, including handwashing and avoidance of bodily fluids and blood, is essential to limiting transmission of these viruses. Minimizing human-rodent interactions is the cornerstone of preventing infections with hantaviruses and arenaviruses. Eliminating rodent shelter, excluding rodents, and controlling rodent populations are readily accomplished in urban settings but are more difficult in the rural occupational or recreational setting.

In the case of filoviruses, strict limitations are necessary to prevent infections leading to outbreaks of both Lassa and Ebola viruses. All healthcare workers caring for infected patients should wear appropriate personal protective equipment and avoid exposure to any bodily fluids. All suspected patients should be immediately isolated. To avoid spread of these infections, all individuals in endemic areas should avoid contact with ill or dead bats and nonhuman primates, including exposure to blood, fluids, and raw meat prepared from these animals. People should avoid funeral or burial rituals that require handling the body of someone who has died from these infections and refrain from handling personal effects of patients that may have come into contact with bodily fluids. Prevention of nosocomial transmission, through contact and droplet precautions and decontamination of clinical specimens, is the most critical aspect of the strategy to minimize the risk for the arenaviral and filoviral infections.

Live attenuated vaccines are available for both yellow fever and Argentine hemorrhagic fever, and a formalin-inactivated vaccine for Kyasanur Forest disease virus has been used in India. Inactivated tick-borne encephalitis vaccines may provide some cross-protection against Omsk hemorrhagic fever virus. Yellow fever vaccine is contraindicated in children under 6 months old and not recommended until 9 months of age because of the risk of vaccine-associated encephalitis. Yellow fever immunization is also contraindicated during pregnancy because of a theoretical risk to the fetus. Yellow fever vaccine has been associated with rare neurotropic and viscerotropic severe adverse events that are more common among the elderly. It is safe and effective overall and is required by some countries for entry.

## SUGGESTED READINGS


Anthony SM, Bradfute SB. Filoviruses: one of these things is (not) like the other. *Viruses*. 2015;7:5172-5190.

Burk R, Bollinger L, Johnson JC, et al. Neglected filoviruses. *FEMS Microbiol Rev*. 2016;40:494-519.

Lani R. Tick-borne viruses: a review from the perspective of therapeutic approaches. *Ticks Tick Borne Dis*. 2014;5:457-465.

Linthicum KJ, Britch SC, Anyamba A. Rift Valley fever: an emerging mosquito-borne disease. *Annu Rev Entomol*. 2016;61:395-415.

Mertens M, Schuster I, Sas MA, et al. Crimean-Congo hemorrhagic fever virus in Bulgaria and Turkey. *Vector Borne Zoonotic Dis*. 2016;16:619-623.

Shah T, Greig J, van der Plas LM, et al. Inpatient signs and symptoms and factors associated with death in children aged 5 years and younger admitted to two Ebola management centres in Sierra Leone, 2014: a retrospective cohort study. *Lancet Glob Health*. 2016;4:e495-e501.

Uyeki TM, Mehta AK, Davey RT Jr, et al. Clinical management of Ebola virus disease in the United States and Europe. *N Engl J Med*. 2016;374:636-646.

WHO Ebola Response Team, Agua-Agum J, Ariyarajah A, et al. Ebola virus disease among children in West Africa. *N Engl J Med*. 2015;372:1274-1277.

World Health Organization. Epidemic focus: Lassa fever. *Wkly Epidemiol Rec*. 2016;91:265-266.

Yacoub S, Mongkolsapaya J, Screaton G. The pathogenesis of dengue. *Curr Opin Infect Dis*. 2013;26:284-289.


# 303 Viral Hepatitis

Henry Pollack and William Borkowsky

## INTRODUCTION

Many viruses can infect the liver (Table 303-1). Often, infection occurs as part of a disseminated viremia. In this chapter, we focus mainly on the 5 viruses whose primary target is the liver: the hepatitis viruses A through E (HAV, HBV, HCV, HDV, and HEV).

Hepatitis is both a clinical and a laboratory diagnosis. Inflammation of the liver can result from a variety of causes. The most specific measure of liver injury is the enzyme alanine aminotransferase (ALT), which is primarily released by hepatocytes during injury or death. In the evaluation of a patient with hepatitis, it is also necessary to consider nonviral diseases of the liver (such as autoimmune, drug, congenital, bacterial, rickettsial, or fungal etiologies) that can cause similar symptoms. Because of the large number of potential viral causes of hepatitis, the evaluation of a patient can be confusing and complicated. The clinical context in which disease presents is the key to directing the workup (Table 303-1). If only the transaminases are mildly elevated, then waiting and repeating these tests might avoid an extensive and costly evaluation. Identifying the causative agent may not be critical for an asymptomatic transient elevation of transaminases. In symptomatic disease, it is impossible to establish the causative agent from symptoms alone.

**TABLE 303-1 VIRAL CAUSES OF HEPATITIS BASED ON EPIDEMIOLOGY AND CLINICAL PRESENTATION**

*Epidemic:* Generally HAV or HEV

*Classical clinical features:* HAV, HBV, HCV

*Sporadic:* HBV, HCV

*Clustering within a family:* HBV, HCV, inherited

*Birth, travel, or blood exposure in country where infection is endemic:* East/Southeast Asia (HBV); Africa (HBV); Caribbean and South America, especially Amazon region (HBV); eastern Europe (HBV, HCV); South Asia (HBV [Pakistan HCV > HBV]); foreign travel (HAV > HBV > HEV); injection use (HCV > HBV); transfusion (HCV > HBV)

*Fulminant:* HAV > HBV

*Age:* Newborn and infant (CMV > HSV, HHV-6, enterovirus, LCM, rubella), child or adolescent (EBV, CMV)

*Transient:* Enteroviruses, influenza, viremias (HSV, varicella, HHV-6, HHV-7), parvovirus, adenoviruses, rubella, rubeola, dengue, and yellow fever

*Persistent:* EBV, CMV, HIV, congenital (rubella, CMV, HSV), LCM

*Chronic:* HBV, HCV, HDV

CMV, cytomegalovirus; EBV, Epstein-Barr virus; HAV, hepatitis A virus; HBV, hepatitis B virus; HCV, hepatitis C virus; HDV, hepatitis D virus; HEV, hepatitis E virus; HHV, human herpesvirus; HIV, human immunodeficiency virus; HSV, herpes simplex virus; LCM, lymphocytic choriomeningitis virus.

## HEPATITIS A

HAV is a single-stranded ribonucleic acid (RNA) virus that is classified as a picornavirus. First identified in the 1970s, it is the major cause of infectious hepatitis worldwide. There are several genotypes but only 1 known serotype. HAV causes acute hepatitis and asymptomatic infection but never chronic infection.

### EPIDEMIOLOGY

HAV is the most frequent cause of epidemic hepatitis in the United States, with rates highest in the western United States. According to the most recent data, approximately 1500 to 2000 cases are reported each year. This number represents perhaps half of the estimated new cases. When comparing the 2013 hepatitis A rates of all age groups, persons age 30 to 39 years had the highest rate (0.74 cases per 100,000 population) and persons age 0 to 9 years had the lowest rate (0.14 cases per 100,000 population). The rates of HAV infection have declined by more than 95% in children with the introduction of the HAV vaccine in 1995, especially after the vaccine became part of routine childhood vaccinations in 2006.

Infection occurs primarily via the fecal-oral route because the virus is relatively resistant to gastric acidity, making it an extremely efficient gastrointestinal pathogen. Infection can also occur by percutaneous exposure to blood (intravenous drug use) or exceptionally by transfusion. In 50% of cases, no source is identified. HAV is highly contagious within families and close contacts (sexual partners). Men who have sex with men (MSM) are also at high risk of infection. Epidemics are generally caused by person-to-person transmission or by contaminated food or water products. Daycare outbreaks and communitywide outbreaks were common before the introduction of the vaccine. Travel to countries where HAV is endemic is also a frequent cause of sporadic infection. In countries where it is endemic, infection is usually acquired in childhood and is most of the time asymptomatic.

### PATHOPHYSIOLOGY

HAV replicates in the liver and is excreted in the bile and shed in the stool. The incubation period is between 2 and 6 weeks (average 4 weeks). A period of viremia precedes the presence of virus in stool and continues through the period of elevated liver enzymes. Clinical disease occurs after shedding in stool has begun (Fig. 303-1). The period of peak infectivity is during the 2 weeks prior to jaundice or elevated ALT and alkaline phosphatase, when the viral titer in the stool can be as high as $10^8$ infectious particles per milliliter. Titers in the blood are several orders of magnitude lower, while levels in saliva may attain a few hundred copies and are not associated with transmission of infection. Shedding of virus can persist for several months in young children, presumably due to physiologic immunodeficiency.

### CLINICAL MANIFESTATIONS

The frequency of clinical symptomatology is a function of age, ranging from less than 10% in young children to approximately 50% in older children and more than 80% in adults. Symptomatic acute infection usually begins abruptly with fever, nausea, abdominal pain, malaise, fatigue, anorexia, jaundice, and dark urine. Symptoms generally subside by 2 months. The severity of disease increases with age. Fulminant infection occurs in 1% to 2% of cases. In developing countries, fulminant HAV accounts for almost half of cases of acute liver failure in children.

### DIAGNOSIS

The diagnosis is made serologically by the detection of HAV immunoglobulin (Ig) M during the acute phase of infection. The virus can also be recovered by polymerase chain reaction in the blood or stool. HAV IgG is detected during recovery.

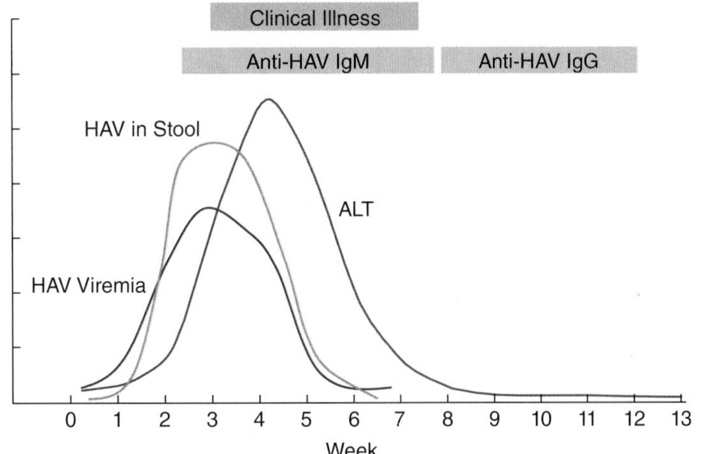


**FIGURE 303-1** Time course of virologic, serologic, and clinical events during acute hepatitis A infection. ALT, alanine aminotransferase; IgG, immunoglobulin G; IgM, immunoglobulin M.

## TREATMENT

In the absence of specific treatment of acute HAV, supportive care remains the mainstay of treatment. Symptoms generally subside after a few weeks. In most cases, the prognosis is excellent. Complications include severe hepatitis and prolonged cholestatic hepatitis and are more common in adolescents, adults, and persons with chronic liver diseases.

In the case of fulminant hepatitis, early referral for liver transplantation is critical, but is still associated with a mortality as high as 50%. Occasionally, relapsing hepatitis lasting up to 6 months may occur after acute HAV. Recovery provides lifelong protection from reinfection.

## PREVENTION

Improved sanitation, purified water, and better hygiene are key strategies in reducing environmental exposure to HAV and preventing large-scale epidemics. An individual can be protected from acquiring disease after exposure to HAV by the use of either γ-globulin injections (0.2 mL/kg intramuscularly) or the HAV vaccine (within 2 weeks of exposure to virus). Immunization against HAV is now recommended starting at age 12 months. Protection is 90% after 1 dose and > 95% after 2 doses (given 6 months apart).

# HEPATITIS B

HBV is the smallest (3.2 kb) and one of the most successful human viruses, having been present among humans for at least 3000 and possibly 30,000 years. It is a circular DNA virus with overlapping open reading frames that encode 5 main proteins: the envelope or surface antigen (HBsAg), the nuclear capsid or core antigen (HBcAg), the e antigen (HBeAg) consisting of the core plus precore, the X protein, and the viral polymerase. The e antigen is not essential for virus replication. HBV replicates using its complex RNA-polymerase cycle. The HBV RNA polymerase explains the virus's high mutation rate and its sensitivity to nucleosides and nucleotides that act on retroviral reverse transcriptases. There are currently 10 known genotypes (A–J) and more subtypes of HBV. Genotypes are geographically distributed and influence outcome and response to certain treatments. The most common genotype among non-Asians in the United States is genotype A, whereas it is genotype B and C among Asians/Pacific Islanders. Genotype E is common in immigrants from West Africa, and D is common in immigrants from the Mediterranean, Middle East, and Pakistan.

## EPIDEMIOLOGY

HBV infects more than 1 billion people and chronically infects 300 million persons, making it one of the most common viral infections worldwide. It is the fifth leading cause of death by an infectious agent and is responsible for 80% of the cases of primary liver cancer worldwide that claim an estimated 500,000 lives each year. It is the number 2 cause of liver transplantation in the United States. Transmission occurs percutaneously, sexually, via mucous membranes, and vertically from mother to infant. Infection acquired in infancy, when chronic infection is most likely to occur, accounts for the largest portion of chronic HBV worldwide. Areas of high prevalence (> 2%) include Asia, Africa, eastern Europe, the Middle East, South Asia, and South America. The seroprevalence in the United States is low, and new cases of acute HBV have declined by more than 90% since the introduction of the hepatitis B vaccine. By contrast, the number of cases of chronic infection has increased to 1.4 million to as high as 2 million with the influx of immigrants from countries of high prevalence. Asians/Pacific Islanders account for approximately 60% of the cases of chronic HBV in the United States, and overall, they are 30 times more likely to be infected with HBV than whites. Other groups with high prevalence are immigrants from African, eastern Europe, Bangladesh, the Caribbean, and the Amazon Basin in South America. Immigrants also account for most of the cases of chronic HBV in children seen in the United States, although there are extremely limited data on the number of actual HBV-infected children. In addition, there are an estimated 20,000 chronically infected pregnant women who deliver each year, but very few of their children (1.5–2%) develop chronic HBV since the implementation of universal perinatal HBV prophylaxis (hepatitis B immune globulin [HBIG] and 3 doses of vaccine starting at birth) in the United States in 1991. The children who become infected despite receiving adequate perinatal prophylaxis are almost always born to mothers who are HBeAg positive (approximately 25–35% of HBV-infected pregnant women), which is generally associated with a viral load of > $10^6$ copies/mL. The overall perinatal prophylaxis failure rate for children born to HBeAg-positive women is around 6% and can be > 25% when the maternal viral load is > $10^9$ copies/mL. Other groups of children who have higher rates of chronic HBV are adolescent males who have sex with males and intravenous drug users.

## PATHOPHYSIOLOGY

The risk of infection is related to the amount of virus inoculum at the time of exposure. HBV can be found in amounts exceeding 1 billion copies/mL in blood in some HBV-infected individuals. The risk of infection from a percutaneous needle stick in an unprotected recipient is around 30%, much higher than that for HCV or human immunodeficiency virus (HIV; 10 and 100 times, respectively). In the case of a neonate born to an HBeAg-positive mother, the risk of infection without perinatal prophylaxis exceeds 90% but drops to less than 30% if the mother is HBeAg negative. HBV is found in lower amounts in saliva, urine, and semen, but these low levels of virus may still play a role in horizontal and sexual transmission.

After exposure, there is local replication, uptake by dendritic cells, then viremia and infection of almost all hepatocytes. Infection occurs through binding of the large surface protein to the newly discovered, species-specific HBV receptor, sodium taurocholate cotransporting polypeptide (NTCP), on hepatocytes. Following entry into the cell, the virus incorporates into the nucleus where it persists in an episomal form consisting of covalently closed circular DNA (cccDNA) that serves as the template for very high viral replication that is extremely difficult to eradicate. HBV can also insert into the host DNA, an event that may cause or contribute to the development of hepatocellular carcinoma.

The incubation period for HBV is usually between 6 and 16 weeks. Whether a person develops chronic infection depends mostly on the age at the time of exposure (> 90% at birth, 40% up to age 5, < 2% in adolescence and young adults), genetic factors (human leukocyte antigen [HLA] class II genes and tumor necrosis factor polymorphisms), the competence of the immune system, and the size of the inoculum. Resolution of acute infection involves T-cell–mediated immunity, either cytokine-mediated or via cytolytic mechanism. HBV by itself is nonnecrotizing and does not cause obvious hepatotoxicity or transaminase release. The stronger the cytolytic response, the greater will be the severity of clinical manifestations. Consequently, the clinical course can range from asymptomatic infection to fulminant infection wherein most of the host's hepatocytes are destroyed by the person's own cytotoxic T cells. If infection persists for longer than 6 months, the patient is considered to have chronic infection. Chronic infection often is accompanied by repeated episodes of T-cell–mediated immunity against infected hepatocytes that leads to flares of ALT and, over time, fibrosis, scarring, and cirrhosis. ALT rises are surrogate markers of the patient's immune response to the virus. Resolution of infection is usually marked by the disappearance of HBsAg and the appearance of HBsAb (Fig. 303-2A). Even after apparent resolution of infection, HBV DNA can be found in the liver and, like varicella, can recrudesce during periods of immune suppression in the nucleus of infected hepatocytes. This is related to the persistence of HBV cccDNA that serves as the transcriptional template of the virus.

The most important determinant of long-term outcome of chronic HBV is the duration of high HBV viral load. The risk of both hepatocellular carcinoma (HCC) and cirrhosis increases markedly with viral loads greater than $10^4$ copies/mL. Other factors include HBV genotype (C and D have higher risk), duration of infection, alcohol exposure, aflatoxin (plant fungus) exposure, co-infection with HIV, HCV, or HDV, and host factors. Integration of HBV genome in host

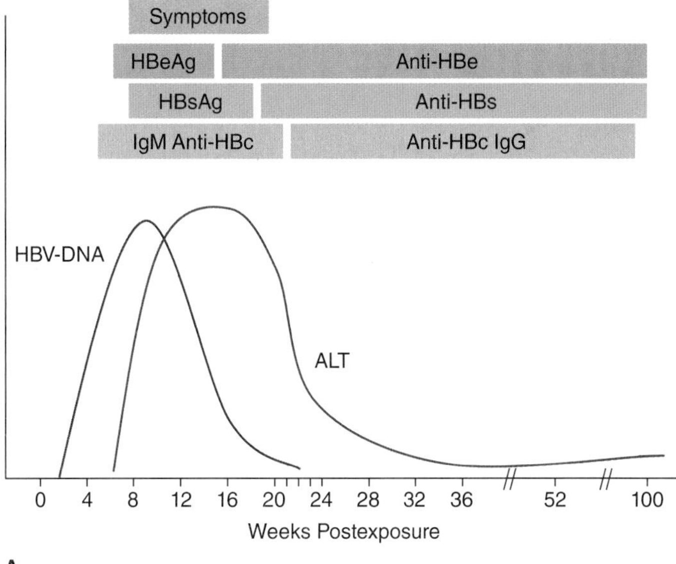


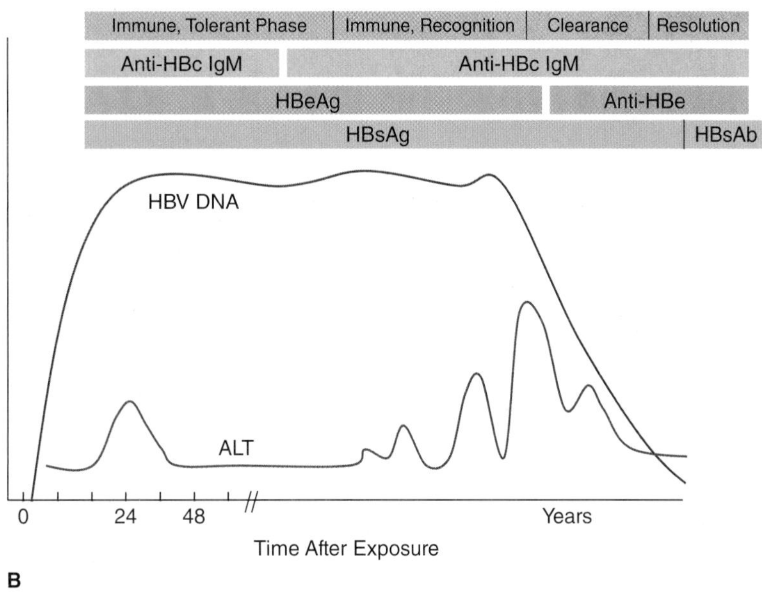


**FIGURE 303-2 A:** Time course of virologic, serologic, and clinical events during the course of acute hepatitis B infection. **B:** Time course of virologic, serologic, and clinical events during the course of chronic hepatitis B infection. Conceptual stages of infection are included in pink. HBc, hepatitis B core antigen; HBe, hepatitis B e antigen; HBs, hepatitis B surface antigen.

DNA is responsible in part for the risk of HCC. In chronic HBV infection, HCC can occur without cirrhosis, distinct from HCC resulting from chronic HCV. This has implications for the different monitoring strategies for HCC in these 2 infections.

## CLINICAL MANIFESTATIONS AND NATURAL HISTORY

The symptoms of acute HBV and chronic HBV infection can sometimes be difficult to distinguish. Acute infection can be asymptomatic or clinically apparent. Severe, acute, and fulminant hepatitis leading to rapid liver failure (bleeding, encephalopathy, low glucose) occurs in about less than 1% of clinically apparent infections. The severity of severe disease is related to both viral and host factors. Although rare in incidence, the most common cause of fulminant HBV in neonates and infants is due to infection with HBeAg-negative virus.

There are usually at least 4 phases of chronic HBV infection (Fig. 303-2B). Initially, the patient goes through an immunotolerant phase characterized by high viral load and normal ALT. At this stage, the infection is usually completely asymptomatic. This phase can last several decades, especially if infection occurred vertically or during early childhood. Viral loads are generally in the $10^8$ to $10^{10}$ copies/mL range. The beginning of an immune response is heralded by a rise in ALT. This begins the phase of immune recognition or activation. If the immune response is effective, the viral load will begin to decline and HBeAg clearance may occur during the phase of immune clearance. During this phase, flares in ALT more than 10 times the upper limit of normal may occur, and occasionally they will be accompanied by jaundice and other symptoms of acute HBV infection. These flares are self-limited, but if they occur often enough, they may lead to marked fibrosis and cirrhosis. In children, these 2 phases occur most frequently during adolescence, often after puberty when the rates of HBeAg clearance can be as high as 15% per year. By the end of adolescence, almost half of children will have spontaneously cleared HBeAg and seroconverted to HBeAb positive. Despite HBeAg clearance, the

HBV viral load can remain at levels that continue to place individuals at risk (although considerably lower than for those who remain HBeAg positive) for cirrhosis and HCC. They will continue to need close monitoring and possible treatment. Some children may clear HBsAg, signaling that the infection has resolved, but this is much less likely to occur (only about 1% per year).

Because of the time it takes to develop cirrhosis, it is much less common in children (< 5%), as is end-stage liver disease and HCC. Most commonly, they occur after 4 to 6 decades, especially in men age 40 to 55 years.

Extrahepatic manifestations of HBV may occur in children but are uncommon. Glomerulonephritis (membranous) occurs in about 1% of children with chronic HBV infection. Other extrahepatic manifestations include arthritis, rashes, periarteritis nodosa, and Giannoti Crosti acrodermatitis.

## DIAGNOSIS AND INITIAL EVALUATION

The diagnosis of acute HBV infection is usually based on serologic evidence of HBsAg and IgM antibody to the HBV core protein (HBcIgMAb) in someone who is acutely ill or recently exposed to the virus. Sometimes the diagnosis is not so straightforward. Generally, HBsAg and DNA can be detected within the first 2 weeks of infection. In acute resolving infection, HBsAg levels will then drop and become negative as it binds to HBsAb. In this "window" period of infection, HBsAg and HBsAb may be undetectable, but HBcIgMAb will remain positive. Eventually, with further resolution of acute infection, HBsAb will become positive and remain positive, as will IgG antibody to HBcAg, while HBcIgM will disappear (see Fig. 303-2A). The presence of antibody to HBV core is also used to distinguish infection versus vaccination when HBsAb is measured.

When HBV infection does not resolve and HBsAg remains positive for more than 6 months, the patient is considered to have chronic HBV infection. Sometimes HBcIgM will also be detected, but in lower titers, and, occasionally, HBsAb may also be present. Usually, the individual is asymptomatic for many years, which is why chronic HBV is often called a "silent infection."

The initial evaluation of a child with chronic HBV should at a minimum include liver enzymes, HBV viral load (quantitative HBV DNA), HBeAg, and HBeAb. Although HBeAg usually correlates with a high viral load, mutations can abolish HBeAg production without affecting viral replication (HBeAg-negative chronic HBV), rendering it unreliable as a surrogate measure of viral load. These tests will provide information that is essential for the proper staging and management of the patient (see next section).

The patient should also be tested for HCV antibody and either vaccinated against HAV or tested for HAV antibody if from a resource-poor country where HAV is usually acquired during childhood. HIV testing should be obtained, especially when there are specific risk factors, as it will affect prognosis and treatment. A baseline liver ultrasound is obtained to eliminate other liver pathology and HCC, but there is no consensus in children how often ultrasounds should be repeated. α-Fetoprotein, a marker for HCC, should be obtained periodically. Genotyping can be done for prognostic purposes and deciding on a specific treatment. Liver biopsy will usually show little, if any, fibrosis and is generally unnecessary because of the availability of other surrogate markers of fibrosis such as the aspartate aminotransferase (AST)-to-platelet ratio index (APRI), Fibrosure test, and liver elasticity (Fibroscan). Hepatic complications are cirrhosis, end-stage liver disease manifestations, and HCC.

## TREATMENT

There are currently 7 approved treatments for chronic HBV in children: α-interferon, which needs to be given parenterally, and 5 oral drugs including 2 nucleoside analogues (lamivudine and entecavir) approved for children 2 years of age and older, 1 nucleoside analogue (telbivudine) approved for children over 16 years, and 2 nucleotide analogues, adefovir and tenofovir, both approved for children over 12 years of age. Because of their high barrier to the development of resistance, entecavir and tenofovir are considered the only oral drugs that should be used as first-line treatment of HBV. Interferon therapy is also considered a first-line treatment. It is approved for chronic HBV as subcutaneous injections 3 times a week. It is often accompanied by flulike symptoms, weight loss, neutropenia, behavioral and mood changes, depression, and decreased growth velocity that is not always transitory. Pegylated interferon, which provides for prolonged blood levels with once-weekly injection, is approved for HBV-infected adults, in whom it has been shown to be much more effective, and in children with chronic HCV, and is often used in HBV-infected children despite the absence of clinical trial data for this indication. Oral drugs act equally on all HBV genotypes, whereas interferon is more effective for genotypes A and B.

### Acute Hepatitis B Infection

The treatment of acute HBV is supportive. The role of antivirals in treating acute uncomplicated HBV is controversial. In fulminant HBV, treatment with oral HBV antiviral medication has been shown to decrease mortality and reduce the need for liver transplant.

### Chronic Hepatitis B Infection

The treatment of chronic HBV in children is complex and evolving. There have been relatively few clinical trials and, therefore, guidelines for treatment of children are more limited compared to adults. Unlike chronic HCV, cure is infrequently achieved. The current goal of HBV treatment is to obtain a durable viral suppression in order to decrease the chance of long-term complications. This is possible with HBsAg loss and HBsAb seroconversion. Unfortunately, HBsAg loss seldom occurs with current treatment (< 10% after treatment with 1 year of interferon or several years of oral treatment). In children who are HBeAg+, HBeAg loss and HBeAb seroconversion are intermediate targets associated with a relatively durable lower viral replication that are achievable in approximately 30% with interferon and 20% with oral therapy after 1 year of treatment. Treatment response is dependent on ALT level and viral load at the time of treatment. When the ALT is more than 5-fold above the upper limit of normal, the chance of HBeAg clearance may be as high as 50%. In children in the immunotolerant phase of HBV, HBeAg clearance is seldom achieved. For children with HBeAg-negative HBV, the only endpoint for stopping treatment is HBsAg loss. Treatment must be balanced against the high cost and potential for adverse effects of long-term medications, the development of antiviral resistance, and the possibility that the patient may spontaneously suppress HBV over time (approximately 50% of children will clear HBeAg before adulthood). The timing of treatment is, therefore, complicated. In general, there is little need to rush into treatment unless early or confirmed cirrhosis is diagnosed. It is customary to monitor liver enzymes, viral load, and the presence of HBeAg for several months before considering treatment. Absolute indications for beginning treatment are evidence of early or established cirrhosis; relative indications are evidence of the immune active phase of hepatitis with ALTs > 2 × ULN and a viral load > 20,000 IU/mL if HBeAg+, or > 2,000 IU/mL if HBeAg negative. Interferon can be given for a relatively short course (24–48 weeks), but it has many side effects and it is proscribed if there is cirrhosis, whereas tenofovir or entecavir can be given for many years with few side effects and little resistance. Some experts recommend interferon initially followed by oral antivirals should significant viremia persist. Others recommend treatment directly with oral antivirals. Patients and their families usually prefer the latter. Oral antivirals should be continued for at least 52 weeks of consolidation treatment after HBeAb seroconversion, should the latter occur. However, as the goals and end points of treatment keep evolving from HBeAg clearance to HBeAb seroconversion with complete HBV DNA suppression to HBsAg loss and HBsAb conversion ("functional cure") and now to even cccDNA elimination ("cure"), the duration of therapy is increasing. As more studies show the importance of maintaining complete viral suppression in order to prevent disease complications, long-term oral antiviral use is becoming more common and is mandatory when there is cirrhosis. Therefore, the decision to begin treatment will very likely commit the patient to long-term antiviral treatment until other more potent treatments are available.

## PREVENTION

HBV infection can be prevented by proper hygiene, proper sterilization of medical equipment, use of barrier methods during sexual intercourse, and use of single-use syringes. Human hepatitis B–specific immunoglobulin (HBIG) has also been used to prevent HBV infection, either before or after exposure. By far, the most effective way to prevent infection is through vaccination, which has been the key to successfully decreasing the incidence of acute and chronic HBV in children in the United States. A number of different vaccines are available. It is estimated that perhaps as many as 5% of vaccines will not respond to vaccine as a function of their HLA genes. Universal vaccination of newborns was first recommended in 1991. This was followed by recommendations for catch-up vaccinations in older children and adolescents (see Chapter 239). Currently, there is a large emphasis on making sure that a birth dose is given to prevent potential instances of mother-to-child transmission when the mother's HBV status is unknown. The durability of the protective effect of the HBV vaccine has been shown to be greater than 20 years. Currently, there is no recommendation for a booster dose after the 3-dose vaccine regimen has been completed.

### Prevention of Mother-to-Child Transmission

Perinatal prophylaxis that combines HBV vaccine and HBIG is extremely effective. The failure rate is less than 2% overall, but 6% in HBeAg-positive women. Mutations in the surface antigen can also lead to failure of binding of antibody. The role of cesarean section is controversial as a method of prophylaxis and is not recommended. Treatment of pregnant women with high levels of viremia (HBeAg+ with HBV DNA > 200,000 IU/mL ($10^6$ copies/mL) with tenofovir or telbivudine is now recommended beginning at 28 to 32 weeks of gestation in order to further reduce the transmission of perinatal HBV. Treatment of pregnant women with lower levels of viremia is not necessary and is discouraged.

### Prevention of Relapse in Immunocompromised Patients

Immunosuppression can result in relapse of viremia. Tenofovir or entecavir is used during cancer chemotherapy and other inducers of immunosuppression to prevent relapse. Similarly, oral HBV antiviral medication is used to prevent and treat acute reactivation of HBV after liver transplantation.

# HEPATITIS C

HCV, originally labeled as non-A, non-B hepatitis, is a 9.5-kb single-stranded RNA. The virus is transcribed as a single polypeptide that is subsequently cleaved into viral proteins, including the envelope, core, polymerase, serine protease, and helicase proteins. These last 3 proteins are important targets for antivirals. There are 6 main genotypes of HCV with additional subtypes. Genotype distribution varies by geographic area. Genotypes 1a and 1b account for approximately 70% of cases of HCV in the United States. Their importance is due to the differences in their response to treatment. Unlike HBV infection, HCV does not incorporate into the nucleus or genome. This distinction makes a huge difference in the duration and outcome of treatment.

## EPIDEMIOLOGY

HCV is transmitted primarily through injection drug use, blood transfusions, or percutaneously from reused, unsterilized instruments or needles used in medical procedures, shaving, or tattooing. Sexual transmission is inefficient (< 5%) but can be enhanced if the host is immunocompromised or among MSM relationships. Mother-to-child vertical transmission occurs in approximately 5% of infants but may be increased 3- to 4-fold if the mother is HIV infected, particularly when the child also is HIV infected. There are an estimated 200 million cases of chronic HCV worldwide and almost 4 million cases in the United States. It is the most important cause of cirrhosis and HCC in the United States, with rates and enormous costs that are steadily increasing. In the United States, the bulk of the infection is in persons born in the decade(s) following 1945 ("baby boomers"). Estimates of the number of children infected are imprecise. The seroprevalence in children under 12 years of age was estimated to be 0.2% and 0.4% for adolescents, based on the 1994 National Health and Nutritional Examination Survey data, or potentially 60,000 to 100,000 children. The rate of new infections in children (perhaps now 1000–2000 per year) has been declining in the United States as a result of testing of blood for HCV since 1990, increased awareness of how the disease is transmitted, and use of needle-exchange programs among injection users. New infections have declined but continue to occur in drug users, the homeless, and incarcerated persons. For adolescents and young adults, transmission by injection or tattooing or sexually in MSM is the main source of infection. It is particularly a problem in adolescents and young adults in correctional facilities, where many become infected. In 2011, a new increase in HCV infections was seen in young, white, nonurban, drug-using and opioid-abusing youth. The major route of new infection in young children in the United States today continues to be via perinatal infection. The mother's HCV viral load is an imprecise predictor of transmission, occurring at higher frequency when the viral load is greater than 106 copies/mL. The benefit of cesarean section in preventing vertical transmission has been controversial, but most studies show no benefit. While HCV can be detected in breast milk at low titer, it is generally felt that transmission does not occur through this route, and present recommendations are not to stop breastfeeding. Reversing a decade-long decline of HCV infection in women of childbearing age to below 1%, there has been a recent sharp increase in HCV infection in rural, white pregnant women in many states, particularly those in the Appalachian region. This has been accompanied by an increase in the number of perinatally infected infants in these areas. In resource-poor countries, transfusion and re-use of unsterilized needles and instruments remain important continued sources of infection for children; therefore, children immigrating from areas with high rates of HCV such as Egypt, Pakistan, eastern Europe, and parts of Africa and Asia should be screened for HCV.

## PATHOGENESIS

During acute HCV infection, transaminases rise during the peak of initial viremia. In about 50% of cases, viremia resolves within 6 months as a result of cell-mediated immune responses (mediated by CD4, CD8, natural killer T cells, and interleukin [IL]-28 status) that control acute infection (Fig. 303-3A). Broad multi-epitope responses, in particular, are associated with resolution of infection. When viremia is not controlled during this phase, chronic infection results (Fig. 303-3B). The outcome of infection, including the long-term complications, is mediated by specific host and viral determinants. Restricted or deficient host response may be a result of direct suppression of dendritic cells and downregulation of cell-mediated immunity by HCV. Almost 50% of infants infected with HCV will spontaneously resolve infection. When this occurs, it is usually within the first months or years of infection.

## CLINICAL MANIFESTATIONS

Acute HCV infection can either be asymptomatic (80%) or present with the classical symptoms of hepatitis, including fever, nausea, vomiting, abdominal pain, diarrhea, and jaundice. These cannot be distinguished from HBV or other viruses. Symptomatic infection is more likely to be seen in adolescents, often after percutaneous exposure from intravenous drug use or tattooing, and is more likely to lead to resolution of infection.

Chronic HCV infection during childhood is usually clinically silent. Fatigue may accompany chronic infection. Extrahepatic symptoms include arthralgias, arthritis, and thrombocytopenia and are uncommon. Cryoglobulinemia, a complication seen in adults, is unusual in children. The most common finding is elevated ALT, which is present in about half of the cases. The disease course is milder than in adults, and cirrhosis or severe fibrosis is uncommon. HCV generally takes decades to become symptomatic. Long-term complications include cirrhosis (< 5% will develop cirrhosis before adulthood), end-stage liver disease, and HCC. The cirrhosis risk for infants who acquired

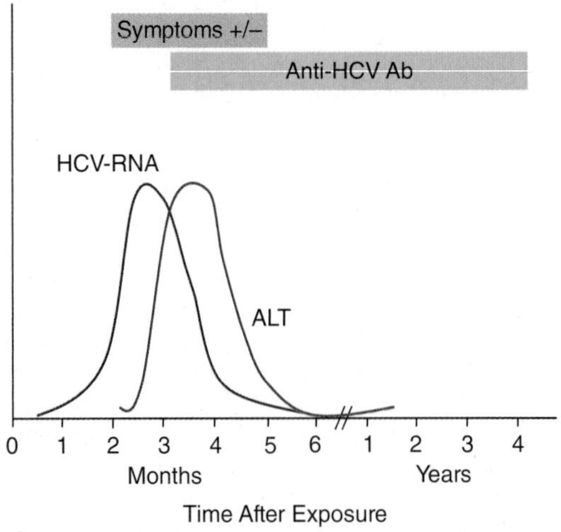


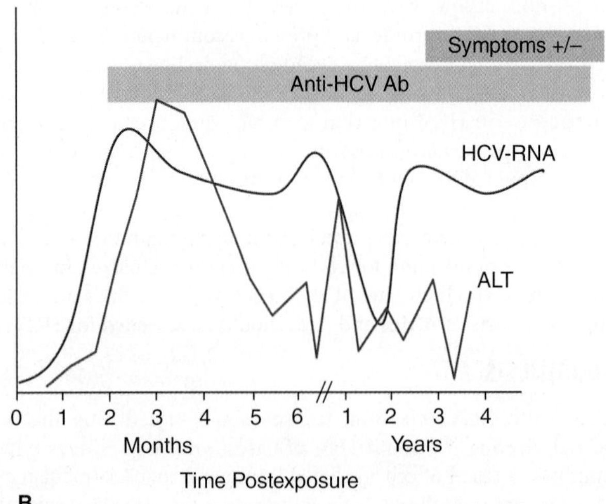


**FIGURE 303-3 A:** Time course of virologic, serologic, and clinical events during a typical course of acute hepatitis C infection. **B:** Time course of virologic, serologic, and clinical events during chronic hepatitis C infection, showing fluctuations in viremia and transaminases.

infection by transfusion is generally less than 5% by age 20, but may be higher for vertically infected and HIV-coinfected children. HCC always occurs as a result of cirrhosis and is very rare in children.

## DIAGNOSIS AND INITIAL EVALUATION

### Who and When to Test

Testing for HCV should be undertaken in persons with unexplained clinical symptoms of hepatitis, persistently elevated liver enzyme tests of unknown etiology, and asymptomatic children and adolescents who are at greater risk of being exposed and infected with HCV. The latter include infants and children born to known HCV-infected women (or drug-using or HIV-infected women who have not been tested for HCV), drug-using or incarcerated youths, and adoptees, refugees, or immigrants from countries with high rates of HCV in Africa (Egypt, Somalia), the Middle East (Yemen, Syria), eastern Europe, Pakistan, and Asia (Cambodia). Repeated or annual testing for those who engage in ongoing risky behavior is recommended.

### Diagnostic Tests

Testing for HCV IgG antibody is usually the first test that is performed (antibody to HCV appears when the person is infected and not when the person is immune, as is the case with HBV infection). The newest third-generation enzyme-linked immunosorbent assays (ELISAs) are very sensitive. To determine whether infection is still ongoing or active and not resolved, an HCV RNA test should be performed. Often this is done reflexively when the HCV antibody is positive. A quantitative HCV RNA test is usually performed as it is almost as sensitive as the qualitative test and provides additional valuable clinical information. Because of fluctuations in levels of viremia, a single negative RNA test is generally not sufficient to exclude ongoing infection. In certain situations, HCV ELISA may not be positive despite infection and HCV RNA tests should be obtained despite negative HCV antibody tests results. This is the case in the early phase (first 2 weeks) of acute infection (see Fig. 303-3A) and, sometimes, in HIV coinfection. In the case of an infant born to a mother who is HCV infected, passively acquired maternal antibody may persist for up to 18 months. To diagnose infant infection earlier, HCV RNA testing is necessary but may be negative in the first few months of life and, in most cases, should be delayed until 3 months of life.

### Initial Evaluation

The initial evaluation of a child with chronic HCV should include liver enzymes and HCV viral load (quantitative RNA). The patient should also be tested for HBV antibody and either vaccinated against HAV or tested for HAV antibody if from a resource-poor country where HAV is usually acquired during childhood. HIV testing should be obtained, especially when there are specific risk factors, as it will affect prognosis and treatment. A baseline liver ultrasound is obtained to eliminate other liver pathology. Genotyping should be done for prognostic purposes and deciding on a specific treatment. Liver biopsy will usually show little if any fibrosis and is generally unnecessary because of the availability of other surrogate markers of fibrosis such as the APRI, Fibrosure test, and liver elasticity (Fibroscan). Hepatic complications such as cirrhosis and end-stage liver disease manifestations are uncommon in childhood, whereas HCC occurs only after cirrhosis is present.

## TREATMENT

In chronic HCV infection, the desired end point of treatment is to achieve complete viral suppression, which will halt and even reverse clinical progression. By convention, if the viral load remains undetectable for 6 months after treatment is discontinued, referred to as a sustained viral response (SVR), the patient is considered "cured." Until recently, the chance of such a response was limited to a relatively small percentage of patients and required taking interferon injections for a year with all of the attendant side effects. Over the past few years, there has been a revolution in the treatment of HCV with the development of potent, safe, well-tolerated oral medications that directly target HCV viral proteins. There are currently at least 11 directly acting antiviral (DAA) drugs that act against the protease (NS2 and NS3 proteins), polymerase (NS5B inhibitors), or NS5A proteins. Within the NS5B inhibitors are nucleoside (NI) and non-nucleoside (NNI) drugs. Different combinations of drugs have been shown to be extremely effective against all genotypes, including the most common and previously hard-to-treat genotype 1 viruses, with SVR rates between 90% and 98%. Although these drugs are very expensive, they are cost-effective. The duration of therapy varies between 8 and 24 weeks depending on genotype and drug combination. For now, only 2 of these drugs, sofosbuvir (Solvadi) and sofosbuvir with ledipasvir (Harvoni) are approved for children, but with several drugs currently in trials in children, this should soon change. These drugs have rendered the use of interferon in the treatment of HCV virtually obsolete. DAAs are so far only approved for children > 12 years of age and while α-interferon and pegylated α-interferon with ribavirin are approved for children 3 years of age and older, current guidelines are to defer treatment of HCV in younger children until the DAAs are approved. This is usually not a problem as HCV is in most cases very mild in the first decade of life. Should one need to treat earlier, in the infrequent situation where the patient has severe fibrosis (stage 3) or cirrhosis (rare in children) and DAAs are not available, pegylated interferon with ribavirin, the other approved drugs for chronic HCV in children, could be used. α-Interferon or pegylated α-interferon with ribavirin are approved for children 3 years of age and older. Treatment regimens and outcomes are dependent on the viral genotype, the magnitude of viremia, and the duration of infection. Combination pegylated interferon plus ribavirin is much more potent, with an SVR rate for genotype 1 infections of approximately 40%. For genotypes 2 and 3, sustained viral response is as high as 80% to 90%. Side effects of interferon include flulike symptoms, neutropenia, hair loss, hypothyroidism, behavioral problems, depression, and decreased growth velocity, which is not always temporary. The major side effect of ribavirin is hemolytic anemia. Indications for treating HCV-infected children used to be relatively complicated because of the duration of therapy, the intensity of side effects, and relatively low response rates to interferon. It took into consideration the patient's symptomatology, degree of hepatic fibrosis, genotype, viral load, age, HIV coinfection, personal and family convenience, risks from side effects, and social conditions including educational status. With the new DAAs with few side effects, a short duration of treatment, and very high cure rates, there is little reason to defer treatment. This is particularly true with adolescents and young adults who use injection drugs or are MSM where the risk of transmitting the virus to others may be very high. Treatment of these high-risk populations should always be accompanied by training in risk-reduction strategies. HIV-coinfected adolescents should be treated with DAAs as soon as feasible because of the higher risk of disease progression in this population. Cure rates are similar to uniquely HCV-infected adolescents. Because of the complicated drug-drug interactions, coinfected children should be treated in specialized centers.

## PREVENTION

There is no anti-HCV vaccine currently available. Development of a vaccine that induces neutralizing antibodies has been hampered by the extraordinary ability of the virus to mutate its envelope. The use of intravenous γ-globulin has not been found to be effective in preventing vertical transmission or infection after percutaneous exposure. While interferon may prevent infection if administered after exposure, the cost and side effects of its use are not warranted, especially given the general low probability of infection occurring and becoming chronic. Counseling on the avoidance of drugs and other risky behavior is currently the only effective way of preventing infection. The screen, diagnose, and treat strategy used in HIV may also decrease risk of transmission to others.

There are currently no means of preventing vertical transmission. Interferon is proscribed during pregnancy and may have serious side effects when given to young infants; newer DAA antivirals may one day find a role (some are pregnancy class B drugs), but the prospect of their use in pregnant women or infants over the next few years is remote.

# HEPATITIS D (DELTA VIRUS)

HDV is a defective RNA virus that is dependent on concurrent infection with HBV to replicate. It uses the same receptor, NTCP, as HBV to infect hepatocytes.

## EPIDEMIOLOGY

HDV is found in approximately 5% of chronic HBV-infected individuals, predominantly in Mediterranean countries, the Middle East, South America, Russia, and South Asia, resulting in 15 to 20 million infections worldwide. It is very uncommon in North America, northern Europe, and East and Southeast Asia and in children. It can be transmitted percutaneously, sexually, and by close family contact either together with HBV (coinfection) or to a person already infected with HBV (superinfection). Vertical transmission is rare if it occurs at all. The pathophysiology of delta virus infection remains obscure. Infection usually results in the downregulation of HBV replication but increases the risk of cirrhosis and HCC through a direct pathogenic effect on hepatocytes, in contradistinction to HBV.

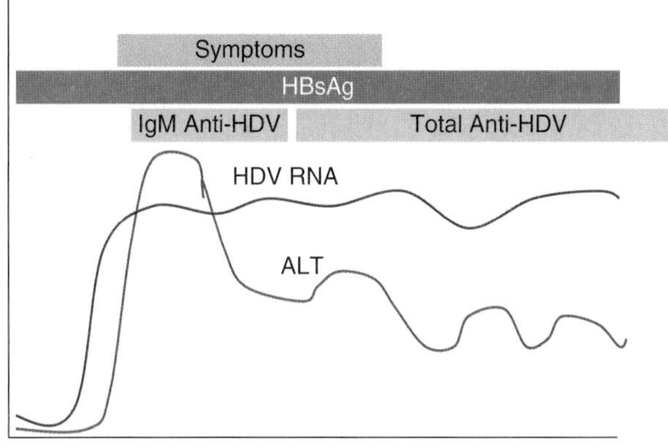


**FIGURE 303-4** Time course of virologic, serologic, and clinical events occurring after superinfection with hepatitis D in a patient with existing chronic hepatitis B infection.

## CLINICAL MANIFESTATIONS

HDV infection can present as an acute fulminant hepatitis if infection of HDV takes place at the same time as infection with HBV. More commonly, it presents as an exacerbation of hepatitis in a person already infected with HBV (Fig. 303-4). HDV infection is associated with a greater chance of developing cirrhosis or HCC. Infection can resolve spontaneously, especially if there is resolution of chronic HBV, with conversion to hepatitis B surface antigen–negative status.

## DIAGNOSIS

Diagnosis is made by serology, either anti-HDV antibody (IgM or IgG) or HDV antigen. Active infection is diagnosed by detecting HDV RNA in the blood.

## TREATMENT

HDV is not sensitive to current anti-HBV nucleosides but has shown some responsiveness to interferon, especially pegylated interferon (up to 40% may resolve) when treatment is given for at least a year. Effective treatment requires resolution of HBV.

## PREVENTION

There is no vaccine for HDV. Prevention of HBV infection through vaccination and the treatment of chronic HBV are currently the best ways to prevent HDV infection.

# HEPATITIS E

HEV is caused by a single-stranded positive-stranded RNA virus that has been recently reclassified as a hepevirus, closely related to the togavirus and calicivirus. There are 7 genotypes. Genotype 1 is the major cause of enterically transmitted acute non-A, non-B hepatitis, whereas genotype 3 is responsible for sporadic cases of chronic HEV.

## EPIDEMIOLOGY

There are around 3 million cases of acute HEV reported worldwide. It is transmitted through the fecal-oral route from contaminated water or food caused mainly by human genotype 1 infection. Large outbreaks of acute HEV occur in South Asia, the Middle East, East Africa, and Central America. Sporadic outbreaks have occurred in the United States, usually from genotype 3 HEV, a zoonotic infection of mainly pigs transmitted primarily by eating undercooked meat. HEV may also be infrequently transmitted from blood donors who are viremic. Chronic infection can occur in persons who are

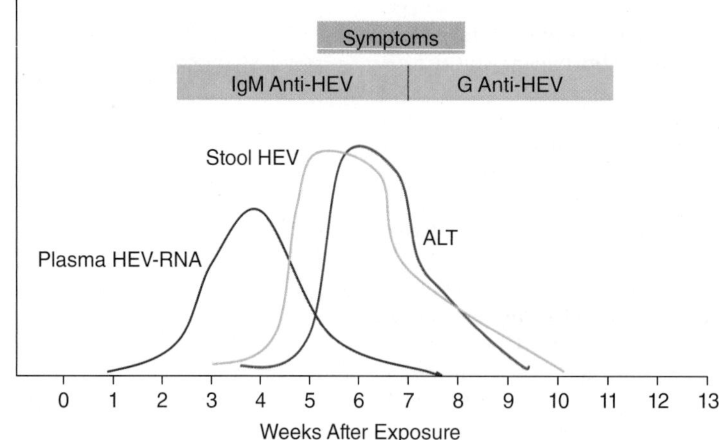


**FIGURE 303-5** Time course of virologic, serologic, and clinical events occurring during infection with hepatitis E virus.

immunocompromised (transplant, chemotherapy, HIV infection) or on hemodialysis. Chronic infections are caused by gentoype 3 virus.

## CLINICAL MANIFESTATIONS

The incubation period of HEV infection is between 15 and 60 days. In hyperendemic regions, acute HEV is usually asymptomatic or associated with only mild symptoms. It is usually a self-limited infection, lasting a few weeks, followed by complete recovery (Fig. 303-5). Extrahepatic manifestations such as pancreatitis, Henoch-Schönlein purpura, thrombocytopenia, hemolytic or aplastic anemia, and diverse neurologic syndromes may occur, but are more common in chronic HEV. Chronic infection often leads to cirrhosis. The major importance of HEV is the mortality it causes in 20% to 60% of women infected during pregnancy from fulminant hepatic failure (encephalopathy, hemorrhage with disseminated intravascular coagulation, or renal failure). Fetal death or premature delivery are common. Vertical infection has been reported in 50% to 100% of infants. Little is known about specific factors affecting transmission. HEV-infected neonates are often symptomatic with hepatitis but usually recover and clear virus. As many as 20% of perinatally HEV-infected infants may succumb to fulminant infection. Chronic infection from perinatal infection has not been reported. Studies of long-term complications and outcome are limited.

## DIAGNOSIS

Diagnosis is made by serology (anti-HEV IgM antibody) or polymerase chain reaction (in research labs).

## TREATMENT

Treatment of acute infection is generally supportive. In the case of chronic infection in immunocompromised individuals, reduction of immune suppression may allow for viral clearance. Ribavirin has been used with success in acute fulminant infection and chronic infection, as has pegylated interferon (in chronic). Both drugs are contraindicated in pregnant women.

## PREVENTION

Several vaccines have been approved outside the United States (China, Nepal) against genotype 1 infections that appear to be effective but are unavailable in the United States. A study of a truncated orf2 protein resulted in over 95% protection when administered in a placebo-controlled phase II trial of young soldiers. A separate vaccine (Hecolin), also based on a truncated orf2 protein, has also been studied in over 100,000 healthy Chinese adults and resulted in similar efficacy while proving safe for pregnant women.

## SUGGESTED READINGS

Goel A, Aggarwal R. Advances in hepatitis E-II: epidemiology, clinical manifestations, treatment and prevention. *Exp Rev Gastroenterol Hepatol.* 2016;20:1-10.

Gonzalez SA, Perrillo RP. Hepatitis B virus reactivation in the setting of cancer chemotherapy and other immunosuppressive drug therapy. *Clin Infect Dis.* 2016;62(suppl 4):S306-S313.

Gotte M, Feld JJ. Direct-acting antiviral agents for hepatitis C: structural and mechanistic insights. *Nature.* 2016;13:338-351.

Infectious Diseases Society of America. HCV guidance: recommendations for testing, managing, and treating hepatitis C. http://hcvguidelines.org. Accessed July 12, 2016.

Jonas MM, Lok ASF, McMahon BJ, et al. Antiviral therapy in management of chronic hepatitis B viral infection in children: a systematic review and meta-analysis. *Hepatology.* 2016;63:307-318.

Lee CK, Jonas MM. Treating HCV infection in children. *Clin Liver Dis.* 2015;5:14-16.

Pan CQ, Duan Z, Dai E, et al. Tenofovir to prevent hepatitis B transmission in mothers with high viral load. *N Engl J Med.* 2016; 374:2324-2334.

Rizzetto M. Hepatitis D virus: introduction and epidemiology. *Cold Spring Harb Perspect Med.* 2015;5:a021576.

Terrault NA, Bzowej NH, Chang K-M, et al. American Association for the Study of Liver Disease. AASLD guidelines for treatment of chronic hepatitis B. *Hepatology.* 2016;63:261-283.

Tran TT. Hepatitis B in pregnancy. *Clin Infect Dis.* 2016;62(suppl 4): S314-S317.

# 304 Herpes Simplex Virus Infections

Claudette L. Poole and David W. Kimberlin

## INTRODUCTION

Herpes simplex virus types 1 (HSV-1) and 2 (HSV-2) are 2 of the 8 members of the human herpesvirus family. Along with varicella-zoster virus (VZV), HSV-1 and HSV-2 belong to the alpha-herpesvirus subfamily and share the characteristic neurotropism and establishment of latency in sensory ganglia, with lifelong infection, periodic reactivation, and reappearance of infectious virus at mucocutaneous sites. Clinical manifestations when present can range from minor

**TABLE 304-1 INFECTIONS CAUSED BY HUMAN HERPESVIRUSES**

| Herpesvirus | Synonym | Approximate Seroprevalence Among Young US Adults (%) | Manifestations | Mode of Transmission |
|---|---|---|---|---|
| HHV-1 | HSV-1 | 50 | Oral mucocutaneous lesions; genital herpes; encephalitis; keratitis; whitlow | Contact with secretions, especially oral |
| HHV-2 | HSV-2 | 25 | Genital mucocutaneous infection; neonatal infection; aseptic meningitis | Contact with secretions, especially genital |
| HHV-3 | VZV | 100 (mostly from vaccination) | Chickenpox; shingles | Contact with infected skin lesions; respiratory secretions for chickenpox |
| HHV-4 | EBV | 75 | Infectious mononucleosis; Burkitt and B-cell lymphoma; immunodeficiency or lymphoproliferation in compromised hosts | Contact with oral secretions, blood, or transplanted organs |
| HHV-5 | CMV | 50 | Infectious mononucleosis; congenital infection; colitis, pneumonitis, retinitis, and hepatitis in compromised host | Contact with oral or genital secretions, urine, breast milk, blood, or transplanted organs |
| HHV-6 | Exanthema subitum | 100 | Roseola, febrile illnesses, and seizure | Contact with oral secretions |
| HHV-7 | | 100 | Roseola, febrile illness | Contact with oral secretions or breast milk |
| HHV-8 | KSHV | < 10 | Kaposi sarcoma | Contact with bodily secretions |

CMV, cytomegalovirus; EBV, Epstein-Barr virus; HHV, human herpesvirus; HSV, herpes simplex virus; KSHV, Kaposi sarcoma herpesvirus; VZV, varicella-zoster virus.

mucocutaneous vesicles to hemorrhagic encephalitis or disseminated disease, but most persons infected with either HSV-1 or HSV-2 are asymptomatic (Table 304-1).

## PATHOGENESIS AND EPIDEMIOLOGY

Herpes simplex viruses are 150 to 200 nm in diameter and consist of a core of linear double-stranded DNA surrounded by an icosahedral capsid, a fibrillous tegument, and a lipid envelope containing viral glycoprotein spikes that mediate attachment and entry into host cells and are responsible for evoking the host response.

There is extensive homology between HSV-1 and HSV-2, rendering serologic distinction difficult. There are at least 60 proteins specified by the virus. Mucocutaneous epithelial cells provide the presumed initial target for viral infection, whereas neural cells in trigeminal and sacral root ganglia constitute the site of latent infection.

Infection of the susceptible host results when herpes simplex virus penetrates through abraded skin or mucosal surfaces. After minimal local replication at the site of inoculation, virus migrates along innervating axons to the sensory ganglia where infectious virus is synthesized. Visible lesions result after the virus returns to the inoculation site via peripheral sensory nerves. Vesicular lesions appear between epidermal and dermal layers and contain large amounts of virus, cell debris, and inflammatory cells. When the host is unable to limit viral replication, such as in newborns and the immunocompromised, viremia may result in multiorgan involvement.

Establishment of latency (eg, HSV-1 in the trigeminal ganglion and HSV-2 in the sacral ganglion) punctuated by episodes of recrudescence characterizes infections caused by HSV. During latency, the HSV genome is maintained in a repressed, noninfectious, "static" state. Periodic reactivation of HSV and spread down the neuraxis is associated with the development of recurrent lesions or asymptomatic viral excretion. A number of stimuli, including direct trauma to ganglia, exposure to ultraviolet lights, stress, hormonal changes, administration of immunosuppressive agents, and serious infection, may precipitate recurrent infections.

The specific immunologic factors that influence the clinical course of HSV infections are not completely understood. Humoral, cell-mediated, and innate immune responses are important in influencing the acquisition of disease, severity of infection, and frequency of recurrences. The important role of antibody in HSV infections is evident by investigations of neonates exposed to HSV at the time of delivery; those exposed to virus in the presence of transplacental acquired neutralizing antibodies are significantly less likely to contract infection. Humoral immunity also influences the course of HSV infections beyond the neonatal period. For example, antibodies against HSV-1 reduce the risk of contracting HSV-2 infection by about 50%, and a first episode of genital infection caused by HSV-2 is less severe in patients with preexisting HSV-1 antibodies than in patients without antibodies.

Cellular immunity is also critical for the control of HSV infections. Clinically severe HSV infections are more common among patients with compromised cellular immunity than among normal hosts, especially in those with impairment of CD4 T cells.

Patients with genetic defects in specific components of their innate immune system, namely, Toll-like receptor 3 and UNC93-B, have been found to be susceptible to herpes encephalitis. The recognition of these patients underscores the importance of these immune mechanisms in controlling herpesvirus. Humans are the only natural reservoirs of HSV. Infections caused by HSV have no seasonal predilection; however, geographic location, socioeconomic status, age, and race influence the prevalence of infection. Children of lower socioeconomic classes and those from developing countries contract HSV-1 earlier in life than children of more affluent socioeconomic classes and children from developed countries. Increased direct person-to-person contact occurring in crowded living conditions probably accounts for these differences.

Primary infection with HSV-1 usually occurs in infancy or childhood, whereas primary infection with HSV-2 occurs after the onset of sexual activity. Acquisition of infection follows intimate mucocutaneous contact (eg, kissing, sexual intercourse) between a susceptible host and one shedding virus. The incubation period for most HSV infections ranges from 2 to 7 days. Twenty-six percent of US children have serologic evidence of HSV-1 infection by 7 years of age. Recent seroepidemiologic studies reveal that the prevalence of HSV-2 is declining somewhat, to approximately 15.5%.

The most devastating form of HSV infection in pediatric patients is neonatal herpes, occurring at an estimated rate of 1 in 3500 to 10,500 deliveries. Genital HSV infection in pregnant women is the major source of virus for the newborn. Approximately 85% of neonatal HSV is acquired at the time of delivery by passage through an infected birth canal, while approximately 10% of cases are acquired postnatally from caregivers shedding virus in oral secretions, on fingers (herpetic whitlow), or from breast lesions.

## CLINICAL MANIFESTATIONS

Most HSV infections in normal children are asymptomatic or of mild to moderate severity. When associated with symptoms, primary infections tend to be more severe than recurrent infections. In contrast, HSV infections in immunocompromised children, even if recurrent, may result in extensive local disease with substantial attendant morbidity.

### Oral Infection (Herpes Labialis/Gingivostomatitis)

Herpes labialis, also known as herpes gingivostomatitis, is the most common HSV infection of childhood, with peak incidence at 1 to 5 years of age. Oral herpes infections are usually caused by HSV-1; however, oral-genital sexual practices may result in HSV-2 infection in the oral cavity. Most primary oral infections are subclinical, although careful examination may detect a few oral ulcers (Fig. 304-1). When symptomatic, the severity and sites of lesions vary: buccal mucosa, tongue, palate, and face may be affected; the gums may also be inflamed and bleed readily. Spread of infection from the oral mucosa to the lips, skin around the mouth, and eyes may occur. Children who frequently suck their fingers may develop concomitant infections of their digits (herpetic whitlow). Submandibular adenopathy, high fever, and irritability often accompany symptomatic oral infection. The most common reason for hospital admission is dehydration resulting from reduced eating and drinking.

The lips, especially at the vermillion border, are the most common site of oral HSV-1 recurrences. Factors associated with recurrent bouts of herpes labialis (cold sores or fever blisters) include intense exposure to sun and/or wind (eg, skiing) and stressful life events. Labial herpes is commonly heralded by a burning sensation or itching 1 to 2 days before lesions develop. In the compromised host, the lips and adjacent facial areas may be involved for prolonged periods. The usual differential diagnosis of herpes labialis includes aphthous stomatitis, herpangina, infectious mononucleosis, and impetigo. Pharyngitis, which cannot be distinguished clinically from other viral and bacterial causes of infection, is a common manifestation of primary HSV infection in older children.

### Cutaneous Infection

Primary and recurrent HSV infections may cause skin vesicles and ulcers on almost any part of the body. Primary skin infections may be accompanied by deep burning pain, edema, lymphadenopathy, and fever. Vesicles may appear singly or in clusters; they tend to become pustular, crust over, and heal within a week, usually leaving no scars. Herpetic whitlow is an eruption that typically occurs on the fingers (Fig. 304-2). It is often painful, and it is easily confused with bacterial infection. Herpes gladiatorum develops in skin area abraded during the course of wrestling after contact with someone who has oral HSV infection. Skin infections also have resulted from other contact sports such as rugby.

HSV cutaneous infection can be particularly severe among patients with burns, diaper rash, or underlying eczema (eczema herpeticum). Erythema multiforme may be associated with either primary or recurrent HSV. The lesions of erythema multiforme can recur with each recrudescence of herpetic infection.

HSV infections of the skin are sometimes difficult to diagnose, particularly when the patient is not seen until the lesions are crusted or pustular, or when the affected skin area is denuded. When HSV skin lesions assume a dermatomal distribution, they may be mistaken for herpes zoster.

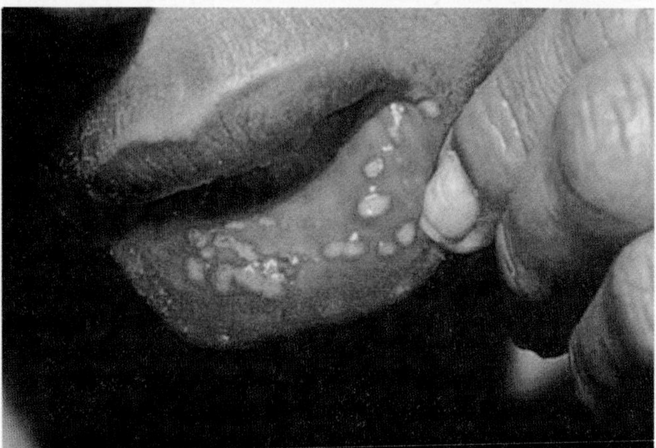

**FIGURE 304-1** Herpes simplex with multiple oral ulcers. (Reproduced with permission from Bondi EE, Jegasothy BV, Lazarus GS: *Dermatology: Diagnosis & Treatment*. Philadelphia: The McGraw-Hill Companies, Inc; 1991.)

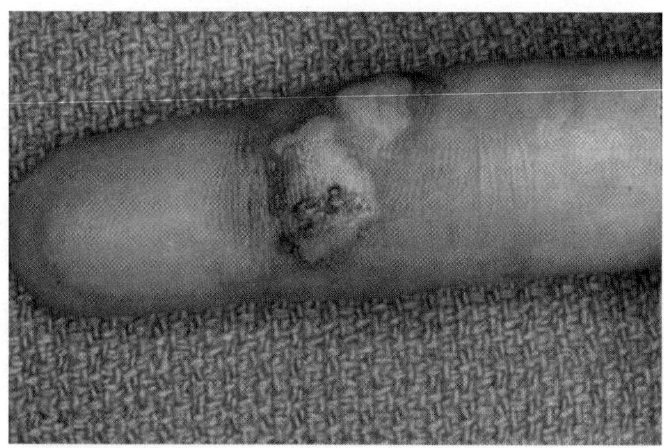

**FIGURE 304-2** Herpetic whitlow with pustules superimposed on erythema and edema of the finger. (Reproduced with permission from McPhee SJ, Papadakis MA: *Current Medical Diagnosis & Treatment 2010*, 49th ed. Philadelphia: The McGraw-Hill Companies, Inc; 2010.)

### Ocular Infection

Herpetic involvement of the eye is of particular concern because it can cause loss of vision. Primary infections may be accompanied by conjunctivitis and tender preauricular nodes, with or without associated keratitis. Conjunctivitis sometimes occurs with recurrent infection, but the most common recurrent form is herpetic keratitis. This entity is readily diagnosed clinically because of the characteristic dendritic, branched, fluorescent-staining corneal ulcers. Deeper ocular involvement, including stromal keratitis and iridocyclitis, occurs occasionally. Corticosteroids, in the absence of antiviral drugs, are contraindicated because they may contribute to deeper ocular involvement. Recurrent ocular infections, in contrast to other sites, tend to get worse with each recurrent episode and can lead to severe corneal scarring and blindness.

### Urogenital Infection

As with other manifestations of HSV infection, genital herpes is a chronic, life-long viral infection. Both HSV-1 and HSV-2 can cause genital herpes. The epidemiology of urogenital HSV infection is changing, with HSV-1 now more common than HSV-2 as a cause of genital mucosal infection in young women in the United States. Most persons infected with either HSV-1 or HSV-2 have mild or unrecognized infections and yet shed the virus intermittently in the anogenital area. As a result, most genital herpes infections are transmitted by persons who are unaware that they have the infection.

Most persons with a symptomatic first-episode genital HSV-2 infection subsequently experience recurrent episodes of genital lesions; recurrences are less frequent after initial genital HSV-1 infection. Genital lesions associated with symptomatic primary infection evolve from vesicles and pustules to ulcers over the first week and a half and then crust and heal during the subsequent 10 days. Lesions are distributed over the labia majora, labia minora, mons pubis, vaginal mucosa, and cervix in women. In men, lesions are typically found on the penile shaft. Individuals who practice anal receptive sex can develop painful proctitis with lesions around the anus and extending onto the buttocks. Local symptoms of itching and pain may precede visible lesions by 1 to 2 days. Tender inguinal adenopathy typically appears during the second or third week of illness and tends to be the last sign to resolve. Constitutional symptoms, including headache, fever, myalgias, and backache, often accompany symptomatic primary genital herpes infection. Extragenital complications of primary HSV infections include aseptic meningitis, mucocutaneous lesions beyond the genital area, pharyngitis, and visceral dissemination.

Approximately 50% of individuals with symptomatic recurrences have local prodromal complaints for several hours to 3 days before the appearance of visible lesions. Sparse genital lesions typically increase in size over the first 3 days, reach a plateau at 6 days, and resolve rapidly. Factors implicated in precipitating recurrences include emotional stress, menses, and sexual intercourse. Of note, about 1% of individuals previously infected with HSV-2 have active viral shedding without symptoms on any given day.

Seroepidemiologic studies show that 17% of adults in the United States are seropositive for HSV-2; however, only 10% to 25% of people with HSV-2 antibodies have a history of genital herpes, illustrating how most genital herpes infections are asymptomatic. When associated with symptoms, primary infections are usually more severe than recurrent infections.

#### Neurologic Infection

HSV is the most common identifiable cause of serious life-threatening sporadic encephalitis. Outside of the neonatal age range, HSV encephalitis is caused by HSV-1, while HSV-2 can cause meningitis, usually as a complication of primary genital infection. Recovery from HSV-2 meningitis is usually complete even without specific therapy, whereas HSV-1 encephalitis has a case fatality rate of 70% if untreated. In addition, HSV can cause both radiculitis and myelitis.

#### Infections in Patients with Compromised Immunity

HSV is a significant pathogen in patients with compromised immune systems. Infection with HSV-2 significantly increases the risk of human immunodeficiency virus (HIV) acquisition. Chronic extensive mucocutaneous ulceration can occur in patients with acquired immunodeficiency syndrome (AIDS). Patients undergoing immunosuppressive therapy for malignancy or transplantation are at risk of developing extensive mucocutaneous disease, most typically from reactivation of latent HSV virus with contiguous spread resulting in either esophagitis or pneumonitis. Acquiring a primary infection with either HSV type 1 or 2 while profoundly immunosuppressed can result in widespread dissemination involving distant areas of skin, lungs, liver, adrenal glands, and central nervous system (CNS). This devastating outcome has been described in severely malnourished children with concomitant measles infection as well. The basic defect common to these conditions has not been ascertained, although a common denominator may be a defect in cellular immunity.

#### Infections in the Neonate

Herpes infections in the neonate may be localized or disseminated. At onset, about 45% of infections are localized to the skin, eyes, and mucosa (SEM), 30% are localized to the CNS, and 25% are disseminated.

Neonatal SEM infection typically presents during the first 1 to 2 weeks of life. Skin lesions characteristically evolve rapidly from macules to vesicles on a red base, but rapid ulceration and skin denudation may confuse the diagnosis. Skin lesions tend to appear at sites of trauma such as the site of attachment of fetal scalp electrodes, the margin of the eyes, or over the presenting body part. HSV infection should be considered whenever any vesicle appears on a neonate. Involvement of the eye may be unilateral or bilateral. Conjunctivitis, keratitis, or chorioretinitis may occur. Outcome of SEM disease is excellent if diagnosis is made promptly and antiviral therapy is administered. However, if untreated, SEM infection can progress to encephalitis or disseminated disease. In the absence of suppressive oral antiviral therapy following treatment of initial disease, recurrent skin lesions commonly occur periodically throughout the first 1 to 2 years of life.

Patients with HSV encephalitis often present with fever, lethargy, irritability, and seizures. Untreated, CNS disease has a mortality of 50%. The use of high-dose parenteral acyclovir therapy during treatment of the acute illness followed by oral suppressive therapy has resulted in a marked decrease in morbidity following neonatal HSV CNS disease.

Disseminated HSV infection is associated with sepsis and coagulopathy. It is often indistinguishable from neonatal bacterial sepsis. In addition to hypoxemia, coagulopathy, and hepatitis, significant respiratory compromise can occur. Chest radiographs are characterized by a diffuse, interstitial pattern that can progress to hemorrhagic pneumonitis. Despite high-dose parenteral acyclovir therapy, mortality is still approximately 30%.

### DIAGNOSIS

The definitive diagnosis of HSV is made by viral culture. HSV can be readily isolated in a number of tissue-culture systems, and cytopathic effects can be detected within 1 to 2 days. Typing of the cultured virus as either type 1 or 2 then can be accomplished by immunofluorescent antibody stains. An optimal sample is obtained by unroofing a vesicle and swabbing the base of a cutaneous lesion or swabbing mucosa or conjunctivae.

Polymerase chain reaction (PCR) is a very sensitive technique for amplifying HSV DNA from cerebrospinal fluid (CSF), blood, and genital mucosa. Its performance from conjunctivae, skin lesions, or mucosal surfaces in neonates, though, has not been established. Results can be reported the same day, and quantitative PCR can report viral loads. PCR has become the gold standard for diagnosing herpes CNS infections, as HSV is very rarely cultured from CSF. If CSF is obtained very early in the course of CNS disease, the HSV PCR may initially be negative, and a repeat lumbar puncture would need to be performed if there remains a high index of suspicion to confirm the diagnosis. In HSV encephalitis, the CSF PCR may remain negative in the first several days of the infection, necessitating either repeat lumbar puncture for PCR or even brain biopsy for both herpes culture and PCR.

Glycoprotein G–based type-specific assays reliably distinguish HSV-1 and HSV-2 antibodies. Since HSV IgG remains positive indefinitely following initial infection, confirming the diagnosis of primary infection necessitates paired sera in which no HSV antibodies are detected in the acute serum and a detectable HSV titer in the convalescent serum is obtained after at least 1 week. Time to seroconversion can be as long as 12 weeks. IgM or IgA antibodies cannot be used to diagnose primary HSV infection because such antibodies also can be found with recurrent infections.

The diagnosis of neonatal HSV requires that conjunctivae, oral, and anal swabs ("surface specimens") be sent for HSV culture, along with an additional swab of any cutaneous lesion. CSF and whole blood should be sent for HSV PCR as well. In addition, surface swabs may be sent for HSV PCR. The diagnosis of SEM disease is determined by the recovery of HSV from the surface swabs with or without positive blood PCR, normal CSF indices, negative CSF HSV PCR, and no evidence of disseminated disease (eg, no thrombocytopenia, elevated alanine aminotransferase, coagulopathy, or pneumonitis).

### TREATMENT

Treatment with antiviral agents for HSV infections depends on the severity of infection and underlying host factors. In general, primary HSV infections are more serious and may require more aggressive treatment. Recurrences are usually self-limited, although treatment can reduce duration of symptoms and viral shedding. Mild gingivostomatitis requires no therapy other than maintenance of proper oral hygiene and perhaps the application of a topical anesthetic. If these infections are severe, antiviral therapy with acyclovir may be indicated. Orally administered acyclovir, valacyclovir, or famciclovir is effective in the treatment of genital HSV infections. In addition, these agents can be used for suppression of recurrent genital lesions as well. Consultation with an ophthalmologist is required for patients with ocular herpes, and treatment for keratoconjunctivitis would include topical trifluridine or ganciclovir.

The early initiation of high-dose intravenous (IV) acyclovir has reduced the mortality and morbidity of neonatal herpes and should be initiated empirically for an infant suspected of HSV infection pending results of the workup. The dosage of acyclovir is 60 mg/kg/day in 3 divided doses (20 mg/kg/dose given every 8 hours) given intravenously. The duration of IV acyclovir is 14 days for neonatal SEM disease and 21 days for CNS or disseminated disease. Infants with ocular involvement, in addition to the parenteral acyclovir therapy, should receive a topical ophthalmic drug (1% trifluridine or 0.15% ganciclovir) in consultation with an ophthalmologist. When there is CNS involvement, a repeat lumbar puncture is required near the completion of the 21-day treatment course to document a negative CSF HSV PCR, with parenteral treatment then being extended in the highly unlikely event that the PCR remains positive. Following completion of the parenteral course of treatment, all infants with neonatal HSV infection should be treated for 6 months with oral suppressive therapy with acyclovir dosed at 300 mg/m$^2$/dose given 3 times per day, with the dose adjusted monthly to account for growth.

Similarly, HSV infections in immunocompromised hosts should be treated with IV acyclovir, with patients frequently being maintained on suppressive therapy for the duration of their immunosuppression. HSV encephalitis in children and adults should be treated with IV acyclovir (30–45 mg/kg/d in 3 divided daily doses) for 14 to 21 days. IV foscarnet should be used for the treatment of severe infections with acyclovir-resistant HSV.

## PREVENTION

Certain preventive measures can be used to reduce the likelihood of contracting HSV infection. For example, exposure of neonates to active maternal genital HSV infection may be reduced by cesarean delivery, especially if performed before or soon after rupture of membranes. Precautions should also be taken to prevent postnatal contact between a neonate and caregivers with nongenital herpetic lesions. Infants with suspected neonatal herpes should be isolated.

## SUGGESTED READINGS

American Academy of Pediatrics. Herpes simplex. In: Kimberlin DW, Brady MT, Jackson MA, Long SS, eds. *Red Book: 2015 Report of the Committee on Infectious Diseases*. 30th ed. Elk Grove, IL: American Academy of Pediatrics; 2015:432-445.

Bernstein DI, Bellamy AR, Hook EW 3rd, et al. Epidemiology, clinical presentation, and antibody response to primary infection with herpes simplex virus type 1 and type 2 in young women. *Clin Infect Dis*. 2013;56:344-351.

Bradley H, Markowitz LE, Gibson T, et al. Seroprevalence of herpes simplex virus type 1 and 2—United States, 1999-2010. *J Infect Dis*. 2014;209:325-333.

Flagg EW, Weinstock H. Incidence of neonatal herpes simplex virus infections in the United States, 2006. *Pediatrics*. 2011;172:e1-e8.

Jones CA, Raynes-Greenow C, Isaacs D. Population-based surveillance of neonatal HSV infection in Australia (1997-2011). *Clin Infect Dis*. 2014;59:525-531.

Kimberlin DW, Whitley RJ, Wan W, et al. Oral acyclovir suppression and neurodevelopment after neonatal herpes. *N Engl J Med*. 2011;365:1284-1292.

Pinninti SG, Angara R, Feja KN, et al. Neonatal herpes disease following maternal antenatal antiviral suppressive therapy: a multicenter case series. *J Pediatr*. 2012;161:134-138.

Workowski KA, Bolan GA, Centers for Disease Control and Prevention. Sexually transmitted diseases treatment guidelines, 2015. *MMWR Recomm Rep*. 2015;64(RR-03):1-137.

# 305 Cytomegalovirus

Mark R. Schleiss

## INTRODUCTION

Cytomegalovirus (CMV) is one of the members of the 8 human herpesviruses and is designated as human herpesvirus type 5 (HHV-5). The clinical manifestations of disease due to CMV vary by age and immune status of the host with asymptomatic infection being the most common in children. CMV is a cause of serious disease in newborn infants, immunocompromised solid organ transplant (SOT) and hematopoietic stem cell transplant (HSCT) patients, and HIV-infected individuals. The virus also is a cause of infectious mononucleosis. Hence, CMV is a pathogen of great importance in all aspects of pediatric medicine.

## PATHOGENESIS AND EPIDEMIOLOGY

Taxonomically, CMV is referred to as a betaherpesvirus, based on its propensity to infect mononuclear cells and lymphocytes and on its molecular phylogenetic relationship to human herpesvirus type 6 (HHV-6) and human herpesvirus type 7 (HHV-7). The virus consists of a double-stranded DNA genome of approximately 235 kbp. As with the other herpesviruses, the structure of the viral particle is that of an icosahedral DNA-containing capsid, surrounded by a lipid bilayer outer envelope that contains the virally encoded glycoproteins, which are the major targets of host neutralizing antibody responses. The proteinaceous layer between the envelope and the inner capsid, the viral tegument, contains proteins that are targets of host cell–mediated immune responses.

Little is known about the molecular mechanisms responsible for the pathogenesis of tissue damage caused by CMV, particularly for congenital CMV infection. Because CMV can infect endothelial cells, it has been postulated that a viral angiitis may be responsible for perfusion failure of developing brain with resultant maldevelopment. Others have postulated a direct teratogenic effect of CMV on the developing fetus. Observation of CMV-induced alternations in the cell cycle and damage to chromosomes supports this speculation, although this hypothesis has been difficult to experimentally verify. Infection of the fetal brain, particularly during the first trimester, induces several perturbations in neural development, including neuronal migration defects. This can lead to the characteristic brain pathologies associated with severe fetal infection.

Immunity to CMV is complex and involves both humoral and cell-mediated responses. Envelope glycoproteins and tegument phosphoproteins are important in humoral and cellular immunity, respectively. More recent investigations into the molecular biology of CMV have revealed the presence of many genes that modulate the host immune responses. These include genes that inhibit major histocompatibility complex (MHC) class I antigen presentation, homologs of cellular G-protein–coupled receptors, a homolog of the cellular major histocompatibility class I gene, homologs of chemokines, and a homolog of the tumor necrosis factor receptor superfamily. These genes may contribute to the ability of CMV to escape immune clearance, which in turn allows for reinfection of seropositive individuals with new CMV strains with different antigenic specificities. CMV immune evasion is an important factor in congenital infection (because of reinfection in seropositive women followed by vertical transmission during pregnancy) and complicates the development of vaccines.

Although most people eventually become infected with CMV, the epidemiology of this infection is complex, and the age at which an individual acquires CMV depends greatly on geographic location, socioeconomic status, cultural factors, and child-rearing practices. In developing countries, most children acquire CMV infection early in life, whereas in developed countries, the seroprevalence of CMV may be well below 50% in young adults of middle-upper socioeconomic status. Congenital CMV disproportionally impacts African American infants and, as such, is an important disease of health disparities.

Transmission of CMV infection may occur throughout life, chiefly via contact with infected secretions. CMV infections in newborns are common, and most are subclinical. Approximately 1% (range, 0.5–2.5%) of all newborns are congenitally infected with CMV. Most infections occur in infants born to mothers with preexisting immunity, and although clinically silent at birth, such infections can lead to long-term sequelae, most notably sensorineural hearing loss. The route of acquisition of congenital CMV infection is believed to be transplacental. CMV may also be transmitted perinatally, both by aspiration of cervicovaginal secretions in the birth canal and by breastfeeding. Toddlers are at high risk to acquire infection in daycare centers and may in turn transmit infection to their parents, usually by contact with body fluids (saliva, urine). In adolescents, sexual activity is a common mode of transmission. So-called "heterophile-negative" mononucleosis can be a presentation of primary infection in adulthood, as described later in this chapter. Blood transfusion–associated CMV was once an important cause of morbidity and mortality, notably in premature infants, but the routine use of leukofiltration in blood banks has largely eliminated the problem of posttransfusion infection.

## CLINICAL MANIFESTATIONS

### Congenital Cytomegalovirus Infection

Current estimates suggest that 30,000 to 40,000 infants in the United States are born annually with congenital CMV infection. Approximately 10% of infants have clinical evidence of disease at birth (Fig. 305-1). The most severe form of congenital CMV infection is referred to as cytomegalic inclusion disease (CID), characterized by intrauterine growth retardation, hepatosplenomegaly, hematologic abnormalities (particularly thrombocytopenia), and cutaneous manifestations such as petechiae and purpura (so-called "blueberry muffin" rash). The most disabling manifestations of CID involve the central nervous system (CNS). Microcephaly, ventriculomegaly, periventricular calcifications, cerebral atrophy, polymicrogyria, cortical dysplasia, chorioretinitis, and sensorineural hearing loss are among the neurologic consequences (Fig. 305-2).

The majority of infants with congenital CMV infection are born to women who have preexisting immunity to CMV. These infants generally are clinically normal at birth but are at risk for neurodevelopmental sequelae, particularly sensorineural hearing loss. Routine newborn hearing screening will miss infants destined to have CMV-associated hearing loss, since hearing loss may not be clinically evident until months or even years after birth. This observation has engendered interest in development of universal newborn screening for congenital CMV infection, since even clinically "silent" cases can lead to long-term consequences that would be amenable to anticipatory monitoring and timely intervention.

### Acquired Cytomegalovirus Infection

**Perinatal Infection** Perinatal acquisition of CMV usually occurs secondary to exposure to infected secretions in the birth canal or via breastfeeding. Most infections are asymptomatic. Indeed, breast milk–acquired CMV infection in term babies has been referred to in some reviews as a form of "natural immunization." However, premature infants who acquire CMV infection perinatally via breast milk may have signs and symptoms of disease, including lymphadenopathy, hepatitis, and pneumonitis, which may, on occasion, be severe. There is no evidence that these infections in premature infants carry any risk of long-term neurologic or neurodevelopmental sequelae, although an association between breast milk–acquired CMV infection and bronchopulmonary dysplasia has been described.

**Cytomegalovirus Mononucleosis** CMV mononucleosis is a disease of young adults. Although it may be acquired by blood transfusion or organ transplantation, it is most commonly acquired via person-to-person transmission. The hallmark symptoms of CMV mononucleosis are fever and severe malaise. An atypical lymphocytosis is present, as is mild elevation of liver enzymes. It may be difficult to clinically differentiate CMV mononucleosis from Epstein-Barr virus (EBV)–induced mononucleosis. As with EBV mononucleosis, the use of β-lactam antibiotics in association with CMV mononucleosis may precipitate a generalized morbilliform rash.

**Transfusion-Acquired Cytomegalovirus Infection** Posttransfusion CMV infection has a presentation similar to that of CMV mononucleosis. Incubation periods range from 20 to 60 days. The use of leukocyte-depleted blood has virtually eliminated the risk of transmission via this mechanism.

**Cytomegalovirus in Immunocompromised Patients** CMV causes a variety of clinical syndromes in immunocompromised patients. CMV disease is observed in the setting of human immunodeficiency virus (HIV) infection, congenital immunodeficiency, malignancy, and SOT/HSCT patients. CMV is a major cause of pneumonitis in the posttransplant setting. The illness usually begins 1 to 3 months following transplantation, and begins with signs and symptoms such as fever and dry, nonproductive cough. The illness progresses quickly, with retractions, dyspnea, and hypoxia becoming prominent. The use of prophylactic antiviral therapy has greatly reduced the risk of this complication. Gastrointestinal tract disease due to CMV can include esophagitis, gastritis, gastroenteritis, pyloric obstruction, hepatitis, pancreatitis, colitis, and cholecystitis. Characteristic signs and symptoms can include nausea, vomiting, dysphagia, epigastric pain, icterus, and watery diarrhea.

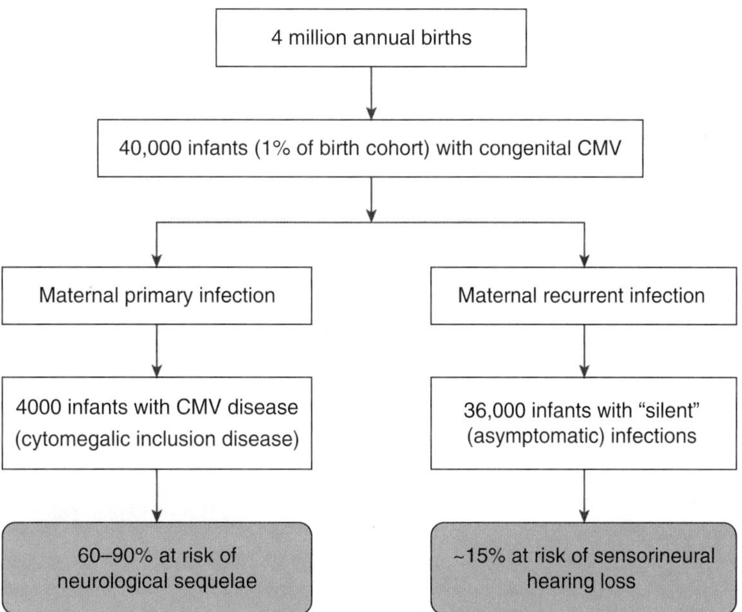


**FIGURE 305-1** Disease outcome profile of congenital cytomegalovirus (CMV) infection. Approximately 10% of cases of congenital CMV infections occur in women with primary infection during pregnancy, and 60% to 90% of these infants have neurologic sequelae. Most infections occur in women with preconception immunity (due to recurrent infection), and although this immunity generally protects against severe disease in the newborn, approximately 15% of these infants still have sequelae, chiefly sensorineural hearing loss.

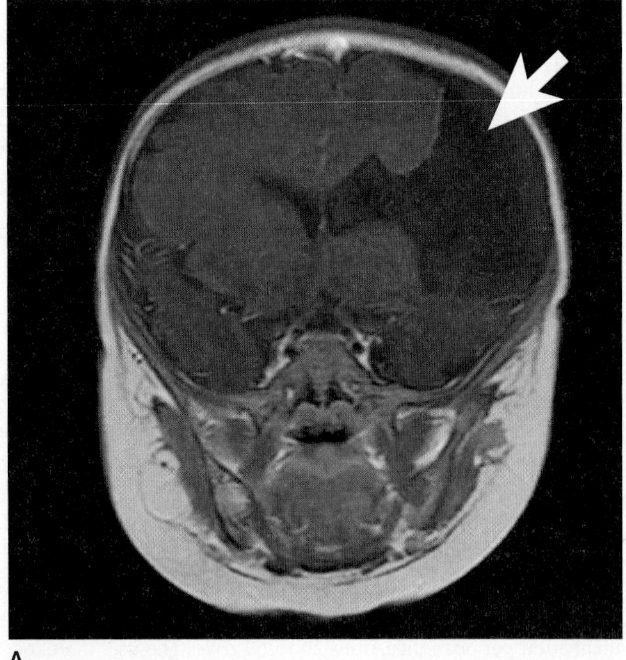

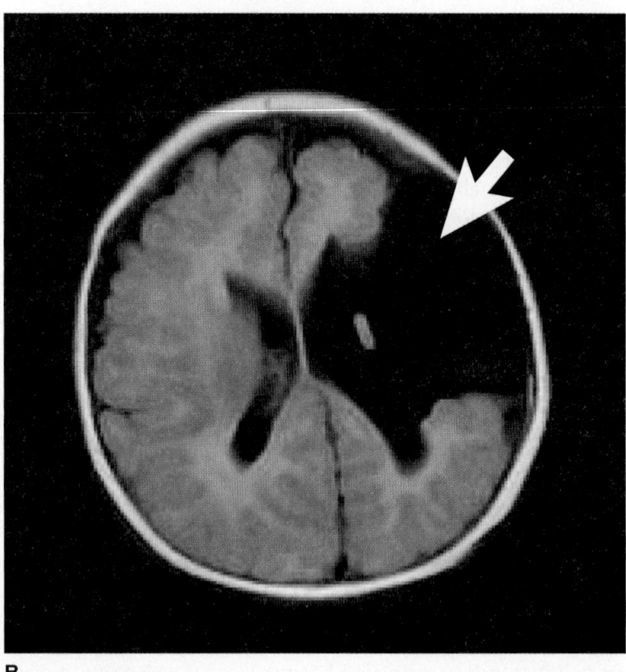

**FIGURE 305-2** Neurodiagnostic imaging abnormalities in infants with symptomatic congenital cytomegalovirus (CMV) infection. In infants with symptomatic congenital CMV infection, a wide range of central nervous system abnormalities are described. Shown are coronal (**A**) and transverse (**B**) T1-weighted MRI images of an infant with congenital CMV infection and profound cortical dysplasia (*arrow*). This infant also had other stigmata of congenital CMV, including sensorineural hearing loss, visceral organomegaly, and thrombocytopenia.

Endoscopy and biopsy are warranted. CMV retinitis was a common disease, particularly in HIV-infected individuals, prior to the advent of combined antiretroviral therapy (cART), with an overall lifetime prevalence of > 90%. CMV produces a necrotic, rapidly progressing retinitis, with characteristic white perivascular infiltrate with hemorrhage ("brushfire retinitis"). Untreated, the disease can progress to total blindness and retinal detachment. Strabismus or failure to fix and follow objects may be important clues to the diagnosis in children.

**Other Cytomegalovirus Syndromes** A variety of other syndromes have been attributed to CMV infection, although cause-and-effect relationships are often difficult to establish. Ménétrier disease is a rare disorder characterized by hyperplasia and hypertrophy of the gastric mucous glands that results in massive enlargement of the gastric folds (Chapter 404). The majority of cases appear to be CMV associated, although the pathogenesis is unknown. Evidence is accumulating that suggests that CMV infection may be a cofactor in the pathogenesis of atherosclerosis, posttransplant vascular sclerosis, postangioplasty restenosis, and malignancies, particularly glioblastoma multiforme. Immunologic control of CMV over a lifetime consumes a substantial portion of an individual's T-cell repertoire. Accordingly, CMV infection may be associated with immunosenescence in elderly individuals.

## DIAGNOSIS

Historically, an important diagnostic study in the evaluation of suspected CMV disease was the viral culture. Blood, urine, saliva, cervicovaginal secretions, cerebrospinal fluid, bronchoalveolar lavage fluid, and tissues from biopsy specimens are all appropriate specimens for culture. The specimen is inoculated onto human cells (usually human foreskin fibroblasts), and the cell culture is monitored for the development of the characteristic CMV-associated cytopathic effect. CMV grows slowly in culture, however, requiring up to 6 weeks of incubation. Due to these limitations, culture-based methodologies have largely been replaced by polymerase chain reaction (PCR) techniques, which appear to have excellent sensitivity. For congenital CMV, PCR should be performed on urine or saliva samples, since some infants with symptomatic congenital infection may not have viremia and PCR of blood samples will accordingly yield false-negative results.

In clinical specimens, one of the classic hallmarks of CMV infection is the cytomegalic inclusion cell. These massively enlarged cells (the characteristic "cytomegaly" from which CMV acquires its name) contain intranuclear inclusions that histopathologically have the appearance of "owl's eyes" (Fig. 305-3). The presence of these cells indicates productive infection in vivo, chiefly in epithelial cells.

Particular care must be taken in the proper approach to diagnosis of congenital CMV in the infant. Emphasis should be placed on diagnostic virology and not serology. Antibody titers in the infant (so-called "TORCH" titers) are seldom of value in establishing the diagnosis of congenital CMV and can often be misleading. The timing of acquisition of diagnostic samples is also of critical importance. Specimens obtained from an infant beyond 3 weeks of age may represent perinatal CMV acquisition (typically by breastfeeding) rather than congenital CMV infection. Outside of the neonatal period, it must be recognized that CMV can be shed from urine for years after infection,

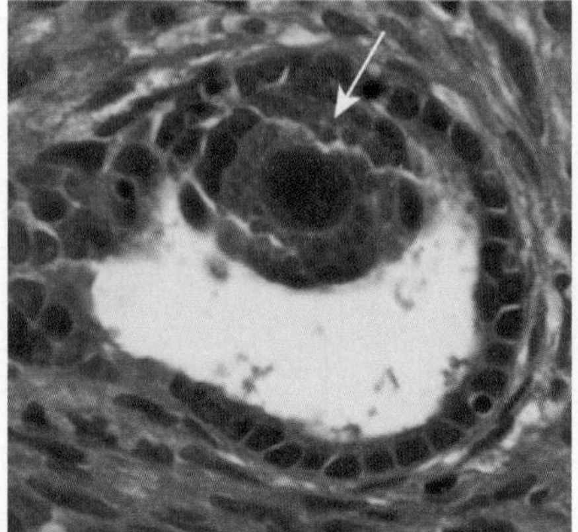

**FIGURE 305-3** Characteristic cytomegalovirus (CMV) inclusion body in biopsy from congenitally infected infant. Classic "owl's eyes" CMV-associated inclusion body noted in renal biopsy of infant with congenital CMV infection and (unrelated) renal disease. Viral inclusion found within renal tubule (*arrow*) in infant with high-grade DNAemia, viruria, and sensorineural hearing loss. This infant had no other stigmata of congenital CMV infection.

so differentiation of CMV infection and CMV disease requires clinical judgment. Lung biopsy or bronchoalveolar lavage may be required for definitive diagnosis of CMV pneumonia and liver biopsy for diagnosis of CMV hepatitis.

The differential diagnosis of congenital CMV infection includes congenital infection with toxoplasmosis; rubella; lymphocytic choriomeningitis virus; and Zika virus. Some aspects of the pathology of congenital CMV mimic those observed with syphilis, neonatal enteroviral disease, and herpes simplex virus. In adolescents with infectious mononucleosis, the major causative pathogen is EBV, although, as noted, CMV produces a clinically indistinguishable syndrome.

## TREATMENT

Nucleoside analogs and other types of viral polymerase inhibitors are available for the treatment of CMV infection. Currently, 5 antiviral therapies are approved by the US Food and Drug Administration for the prophylaxis and/or therapy of systemic CMV infection (see Chapter 240). Experience with these agents is limited in pediatrics, however, and anti-CMV therapy in general should be administered only after consultation with an expert familiar with dosage and side effects.

Ganciclovir was the first compound licensed for treatment of CMV infections. Its use is indicated in immunocompromised children (HIV infection, transplant recipients, other immunocompromised states) when there is clinical and virologic evidence of specific end-organ disease (eg, pneumonitis, enteritis). Ganciclovir is myelosuppressive, which is often a dose-limiting toxicity in immunocompromised patients. Ganciclovir is also commonly used as preemptive or prophylactic therapy in transplant patients at high risk of developing disease (eg, a CMV-seronegative recipient of an organ from a CMV-seropositive donor).

Encouraging data are emerging about the use of ganciclovir in the setting of congenital CMV infection. A trial sponsored by the Collaborative Antiviral Study Group (CASG) demonstrated that a 6-week course of ganciclovir therapy begun in the neonatal period in symptomatically infected infants with congenital CMV infection involving the CNS prevented hearing deterioration at 6 months and that the benefits appeared to persist at or beyond 1 year of age. A subsequent study that examined a 6-month course of antiviral therapy in infants with any symptomatic congenital infection confirmed benefits not only for hearing, but also for neurologic development. Based on these studies, ganciclovir (or the oral prodrug formulation, valganciclovir) should be offered to any infant with symptomatic congenital CMV infection. Infants treated with a 6-month course of valganciclovir require careful clinical and laboratory monitoring, particularly for neutropenia.

FDA-approved alternatives to ganciclovir include foscarnet, cidofovir, and letermovir. Pediatric experience with these agents is limited. Although these drugs are potentially useful in the setting of ganciclovir resistance, the toxicities of these antivirals are significant, and these agents should be used only in exceptional circumstances.

Immunoglobulins have limited value in control of CMV disease. A CMV hyperimmunoglobulin has been shown to decrease the incidence of CMV disease when administered after transplantation to high-risk transplant recipients.

## PREVENTION

Ultimately, control of CMV infection, particularly the devastating sequelae of CID, could be achieved by the development of an effective vaccine. The major target population for a CMV vaccine would likely be adolescents, with the goal of conferring protective immunity, particularly for young women, prior to their entry into their child-bearing years. Although immunization would be unlikely to prevent all congenital infection, there is hope that it would have a significant and major impact on the incidence of CID. Education of young women of childbearing age about the risks of CMV and how to avoid disease transmission is also an important control strategy. Care should be taken to avoid high-risk exposures, including exposure to potentially infectious body fluids such as saliva and urine. Seronegative women who regularly come in close contact with large numbers of young children, particularly in daycare center environments, may be at particularly high risk. Behaviors known to be associated with transmission of infection, such as kissing and sharing eating utensils, can be avoided, and careful handwashing after diaper changes should be stressed. Healthcare workers are not at increased risk for acquiring CMV infection compared to the general population. Screening women for CMV serostatus prior to and during pregnancy may provide valuable information and increase overall knowledge and awareness. CMV causes more disability in newborns than Down syndrome and fetal alcohol syndrome combined, and increased public awareness is required to address this common cause of pediatric disability.





## SUGGESTED READINGS

Boppana SB, Britt WJ. Recent approaches and strategies in the generation of antihuman cytomegalovirus vaccines. *Methods Mol Biol.* 2014;1119:311-348.

Griffiths PD, Mahungu T. Why CMV is a candidate for elimination and then eradication. *J Virus Erad.* 2016;2:131-135.

Kelly MS, Benjamin DK, Puopolo KM, et al. Postnatal cytomegalovirus infection and the risk for bronchopulmonary dysplasia. *JAMA Pediatr.* 2015;169:e153785.

Kimberlin DW, Jester PM, Sánchez PJ, et al. Valganciclovir for symptomatic congenital cytomegalovirus disease. *N Engl J Med.* 2015;372:933-943.

Ljungman P, Boeckh M, Hirsch HH, et al. Definitions of CMV infection and disease in transplant patients for use in clinical trials. *Clin Infect Dis.* 2017;64:87-91.

Pinninti SG, Ross SA, Shimamura M, et al. Comparison of saliva PCR assay versus rapid culture for detection of congenital cytomegalovirus infection. *Pediatr Infect Dis J.* 2015;34:536-537.

Rawlinson WD, Hamilton ST, van Zuylen WJ. Update on treatment of cytomegalovirus infection in pregnancy and of the newborn with congenital cytomegalovirus. *Curr Opin Infect Dis.* 2016;29:615-624.

Swanson EC, Schleiss MR. Congenital cytomegalovirus infection: new prospects for prevention and therapy. *Pediatr Clin North Am.* 2013;60:335-349.

# 306 Epstein-Barr Virus Mononucleosis

W. Garrett Hunt and Guliz Erdem

## INTRODUCTION

Epstein-Barr virus (EBV) is recognized as the major cause of infectious mononucleosis (IM). Most EBV infections are thought to be spread through saliva. Manifestations of EBV infection are varied and range from asymptomatic infection to fulminant lymphoproliferative disease. EBV is also associated with a number of malignancies, including endemic Burkitt lymphoma, nasopharyngeal carcinoma, Hodgkin disease, and a spectrum of posttransplant lymphoproliferative disease.

## PATHOGENESIS AND EPIDEMIOLOGY

EBV is a member of the family Herpesviridae (gamma herpesvirus), which contains linear double-stranded DNA surrounded by a protein capsid with 162 capsomers in an icosahedral arrangement. The nucleocapsid is covered by a lipid-containing envelope derived from the nuclear membrane of the host cell. EBV causes lytic infection of human oropharyngeal and salivary cells and latent infection of human and primate B lymphocytes as well as epithelium of the nasopharynx. It has long been recognized to be lymphotropic for B lymphocytes and to infect both oropharyngeal epithelial cells and myocytes, but it is also true that it infects T lymphocytes and natural killer (NK) cells.

Infection of lymphocytes with linear EBV DNA can transform them into continuously growing lymphoblastoid cell lines containing a circular DNA episome. Once infected, transformed lymphoblastoid cells rarely continue to produce infectious virus in vitro, although EBV antigens can be detected in the cells. The appearance of new antigens on the cell surface of EBV-infected cells is believed to be responsible for the cellular immune response to the virus and for pathogenesis of the resulting disease. The EBV receptor on epithelial cells and B lymphocytes is the CD21 molecule (formerly CR2), which is also the receptor for the C3d fragment of the third component of complement. The virus elicits both humoral and cellular immune responses.

EBV acquired by ingestion appears to first infect either oropharyngeal resting B cells or epithelial cells and then B cells. Subsequently, the virus infects other susceptible B lymphocytes within the lymphoid tissue of the pharynx. During a 30- to 50-day incubation period, virus actively replicates and disseminates throughout the entire lymphoreticular system.

Cell-mediated immune function is essential in the control of and recovery from EBV infection. In EBV IM, the initial infection of B lymphocytes is followed by an extensive proliferation of CD8+ suppressor/cytotoxic T lymphocytes. Subpopulations of these T cells are cytotoxic against EBV-infected lymphoid cells or prevent their proliferation or possibly both. Associated with the increase in these cytotoxic and suppressor cytotoxic T cells is a concomitant decrease in the number of T-helper/inducer cells (CD4+ T lymphocytes), resulting in an inversion of the CD4:CD8 ratio. During lytic infection, several latent viral proteins are also expressed that are kept in check by NK cells and cytotoxic T cells. After convalescence, EBV can be present in memory B cells that express latent membrane protein 2 and EBV nuclear antigen. The virus can undergo reactivation, and some other B cells can undergo lytic replication in the oropharynx, resulting in shedding of virus into saliva or infection of epithelial cells with release of virus. Fatal IM and lymphoproliferative disorders (LPDs), in which B-cell lymphomas develop, have been identified in adults and children with cell-mediated immune defects, particularly in defects with NK cell activity. LPDs have been identified in kidney, heart, and bone marrow transplant recipients and individuals with X-linked lymphoproliferative syndrome, severe combined immunodeficiency syndrome, acquired immunodeficiency syndrome (AIDS), ataxia-telangiectasia, and certain autoimmune diseases.

More recently, EBV has been demonstrated to infect T cells or NK cells, resulting in unique systemic lymphoproliferative diseases such as EBV-associated hemophagocytic lymphohistiocytosis (EBV-HLH) and chronic active EBV (CAEBV) infection, clinical features of which are distinct from the tumor-forming diseases outlined previously. Systemic EBV-related lymphoproliferative disease (EBV-LPD) is now classified into B-cell LPD and T/NK-cell LPD. The former is associated with fulminant IM, whereas the latter is associated with EBV-HLH and CAEBV. EBV-induced posttransplantation lymphoproliferative disorder (EBV-PTLD) is a potentially life-threatening complication after allogeneic hematopoietic cell transplantation that is associated with prolonged impairment of T-cell immune reconstitution. Patients receiving antibodies against T cells, high-dose steroids, or both are also at risk to develop severe EBV infection such as EBV-LPD.

EBV is excreted in oropharyngeal secretions and is transmitted by contact with saliva via kissing or other mucosal contact with contaminated objects. Healthy seropositive individuals intermittently shed EBV in their oropharynx. Mucosal contact with the saliva of these individuals is the likely mechanism of infection in preadolescent and adolescent individuals. Blood products or transplanted tissues can transmit EBV and are particularly problematic for seronegative immunocompromised transplant recipients. There is no evidence of urinary or fecal excretion. Transplacental transmission appears to be rare. Shedding of virus is more frequent in immunosuppressed individuals, 60% of whom may excrete EBV at any one time. Because virus shedding is of a low copy number even in immunocompromised patients, universal isolation precautions are adequate for patients with acute or past EBV infections.

It is important to recognize that acute primary EBV infection is not synonymous with IM. Most EBV infections acquired at any age are asymptomatic. Seroepidemiologic studies demonstrate that from 20% to 100% of children worldwide have antibodies to EBV by 6 years of age. In contrast, in the United States, only 40% to 50% of adolescents are seropositive, with higher socioeconomic groups being less likely to have evidence of prior infection. Seropositivity increases with age in all populations, so that almost all adults have serologic evidence of past EBV infection. Seroconversion is particularly high in college, where 10% to 15% of susceptible persons become infected each year. This group of EBV-naive adolescents in industrialized countries is susceptible to develop EBV-associated IM (EBV-IM), which is much more common in the United States and Western Europe than in unindustrialized countries. Furthermore, the age of EBV acquisition has been increasing in industrialized countries.

The epidemiology of IM is closely related to the age at primary EBV infection. In the United States, the incidence of IM is approximately 50 per 100,000 persons per year, but in individuals 15 to 25 years old, the incidence doubles. Those areas where children are infected at an early age have the lowest incidence of disease. Among susceptible adolescents and young adults, studies measuring both apparent and unapparent EBV infections indicate a clinical-to-subclinical ratio of 1:2 to 1:3. Although the ratio of clinical-to-subclinical infections in young children is not well defined, the incidence of typical IM syndrome is low.

## CLINICAL MANIFESTATIONS

### Infectious Mononucleosis

The incubation period of EBV-IM is 30 to 50 days. The clinical syndrome of EBV-IM is usually preceded by a 3- to 5-day prodrome of malaise, fatigue, headache, nausea, abdominal pain, or some combination of these symptoms. Over the next 7 to 20 days, sore throat and fever gradually increase. The triad of fever, sore throat, and posterior cervical adenopathy occurs in more than 80% of symptomatic patients. Sore throat is often accompanied by evidence of moderate-to-severe pharyngitis, with marked tonsillar enlargement that may be covered with shaggy gray or white exudate. On rare occasions, the tonsillar and peritonsillar swelling can result in airway obstruction. Fine petechiae may cover the uvula and soft palate during the initial week of illness. Throat cultures are positive for group A β-hemolytic streptococci in about 30% of patients, which may represent accompanying disease or pharyngeal colonization in patients with EBV-IM. Fever is present in 85% to 95% of patients, from 39°C (102°F) up to 40.5°C (105°F), and on average lasts 10 days but may persist for weeks. Fatigue and lymphadenopathy may persist longer. Adenopathy most often involves only the bilateral posterior cervical nodes but may involve any node, including anterior cervical, epitrochlear, or even generalized lymph nodes. Nodes may be affected singly or in groups (not necessarily symmetrical) and may be very large or small (the size of grapes); they are most often firm, discrete, and moderately tender to palpation. Splenomegaly, defined as the largest dimension greater than the 95th percentile per age, often results in a spleen that is palpable 2 to 3 cm below the costal margin, and this occurs in about 50% of EBV-IM. Massive splenomegaly may occur, usually defined operationally as a spleen extending well into the left lower quadrant or pelvis or that has crossed the midline of the abdomen and that weighs at least 500 to 1000 g. Rupture is rare but can be a potentially fatal complication. Hepatomegaly occurs in 10% to 30% of patients, but less than 5% of patients develop jaundice. Serum aspartate aminotransferase (AST) and serum lactate dehydrogenase (LDH) are mildly elevated in the majority of patients and may persist for weeks to months. Chronic liver disease, however, does not typically result.

Other clinical findings include bilateral supraorbital edema and rashes. A blanching, erythematous, maculopapular exanthema occurs in about 5% to 15% of patients, but as many as 80% develop this rash if treated with ampicillin or other β-lactam antibiotics (Fig. 306-1). The same rash may occur with cytomegalovirus (CMV)-associated mononucleosis and so does not differentiate CMV- from EBV-associated mononucleosis. Urticarial, bullous, hemorrhagic, and scarlatiniform rashes, as well as the Gianotti-Crosti syndrome, are also associated with IM.

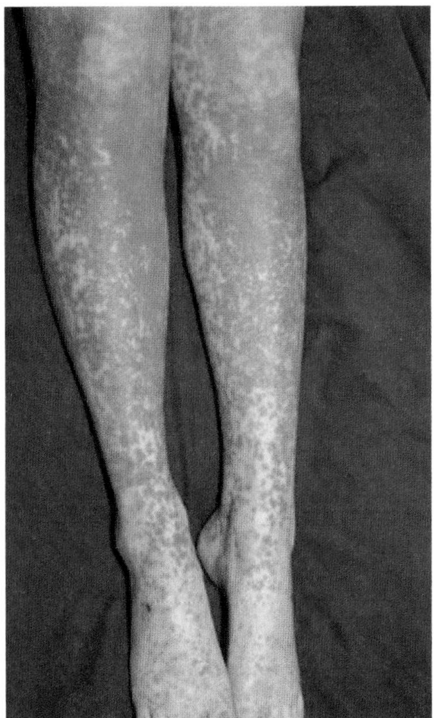

**FIGURE 306-1** Morbilliform rash on the lower extremities in a patient with infectious mononucleosis following treatment with a penicillin derivative. (Reproduced from Wolff K, Goldsmith LA, Katz SI, et al: *Fitzpatrick's Dermatology in General Medicine*, 7th ed. New York: The McGraw-Hill Companies; 2006.)

Neurologic complications include aseptic meningitis, encephalitis, optic neuritis, Guillain-Barré syndrome, transverse myelitis, Bell palsy, and, in numerous more recent epidemiologic studies, multiple sclerosis following EBV-IM. An autoimmune hemolytic anemia occurs in 0.5% to 3% of IM patients and is usually mediated by antibodies against the "i" antigen on the red blood cell. A mild thrombocytopenia below 140,000 platelets/μL, but with absence of profound thrombocytopenia or bleeding, occurs in approximately 50% of patients. Granulocytopenia or thrombocytopenia may occur during the acute illness or in the immediate recovery period. Associated respiratory disease consists of interstitial pneumonia, laryngeal obstruction, pharyngeal edema, and cardiac complications including myocarditis and pericarditis.

#### EBV Infection in Young Children

In children younger than 4 years of age, EBV infection does not usually cause the same symptoms and signs of typical IM as previously described for adolescents in developed countries. When symptomatic, younger children are more likely to exhibit rashes and hepatosplenomegaly. Failure to thrive, otitis media, abdominal pain, and recurrent pharyngitis are also more common in young children. Involvement of the hematopoietic system or the central nervous system or the occurrence of prolonged fever may be the primary or only manifestation of acute EBV infection in this population. In children and adults, EBV infection may be followed by persistent pharyngitis, lymphadenopathy, fever, headaches, arthralgia, fatigue, or psychoneurosis.

#### Other EBV-Related Disorders

Oral hairy leukoplakia of the tongue is a benign EBV-associated lesion commonly noted by human immunodeficiency virus (HIV)-infected persons or on physical exam of these patients by medical care personnel; it is associated with few or no symptoms. Oral hairy leukoplakia is the only lesion presently known to arise as a direct consequence of replication of the linear genome of EBV. X-linked lymphoproliferative disease manifests as fatal EBV-associated disease in males in particular families or sporadically in girls and boys with no family history. In these individuals, EBV infection is usually fatal and is associated with either a lymphoproliferative response, such as fatal mononucleosis, lymphoma, hemophagocytic syndrome, or B-cell immunoblastic sarcoma (seen in 75% of cases), or with an aproliferative response such as agammaglobulinemia, aplastic anemia, agranulocytosis, or late malignancies (seen in 25% of cases). The gene on the X chromosome that is mutated in this disease has been identified as *SAP* (signaling lymphocyte activation molecule [SLAM]–associated protein). The absence of a functional SAP in patients with X-linked lymphoproliferative disease is thought to impair the normal interaction of T and B cells, resulting in unregulated growth of EBV-infected B cells.

Alternatively, although an immunocompromised status is suspected in the development of EBV-HLH, the exact characteristics of host vulnerability are largely unknown. The majority of EBV-HLH cases occur in apparently immunocompetent children. Based on the current diagnostic guidelines from the Histiocyte Society, patients diagnosed with EBV-HLH should fulfill at least 5 of the following 8 criteria: fever, splenomegaly, cytopenia of at least 2 cell lines, hypertriglyceridemia/hypofibrinogenemia, hemophagocytosis, low/absent NK-cell activity, hyperferritinemia, and high soluble interleukin-2 receptor. EBV is also associated with a number of malignant disorders, including nasopharyngeal carcinoma, Burkitt lymphoma, and, to a lesser extent, Hodgkin lymphoma (40–60% of Hodgkin disease in the developed world). EBV is associated with nearly 200,000 new malignancies worldwide each year. EBV DNA or proteins have also been detected in nasal T-cell/NK-cell lymphomas, lymphomatoid granulomatosis, angioimmunoblastic lymphadenopathy, gastric carcinomas, central nervous system lymphomas in nonimmunocompromised patients, and smooth muscle tumors in immunocompromised patients and transplant recipients. Coincident infections with HIV and malaria may increase the risk of EBV-positive malignancies. EBV has also been associated with multiple sclerosis. Genetic variances may exist, such as certain human leukocyte antigen loci, regarding the susceptibility of certain races/ethnicities to EBV infection.

## DIAGNOSIS

The diagnosis of EBV-IM in an immunocompetent child or adolescent is based on clinical manifestations, characteristic blood abnormalities, and positive heterophile or EBV antibodies. By the second week of infection, the relative and absolute numbers of lymphocytes increase, with at least 10% to 20% atypical cells. Early in the disease, the atypical cells, or Downey cells, are both B and T lymphocytes (Fig. 306-2). The atypical lymphocyte has a higher cytoplasm-to-nucleus ratio than a normal lymphocyte. The nucleus has coarse chromatin, and nucleoli are occasionally seen. The cytoplasm is more basophilic and vacuolated than normal. By early convalescence, the majority of

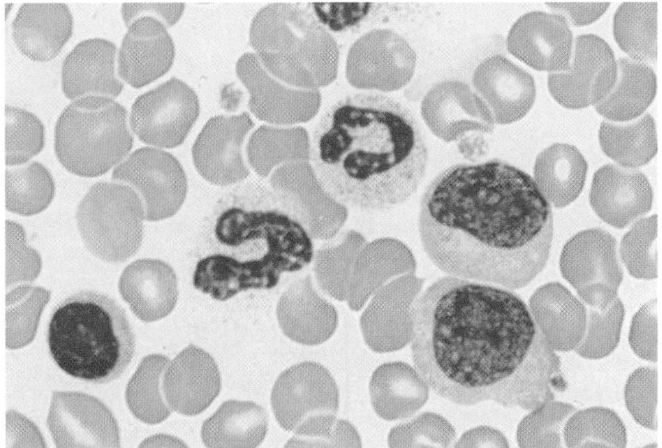

**FIGURE 306-2** Buffy coat from a patient with infectious mononucleosis. Two large reactive lymphocytes. (Reproduced from Lichtman MA, Beutler E, Kipps TJ, et al: *Williams Hematology*, 7th ed. New York: The McGraw-Hill Companies; 2006.)

the atypical lymphocytes are CD8+ suppressor/cytotoxic T cells. The total leukocyte count is usually 10,000 to 20,000 cells/μL but may be as high as 50,000 cells/μL. Leukocyte abnormalities may persist for 4 to 8 weeks.

The heterophile test detects the presence of antibodies induced by the virus that are directed against EBV-specific antigens as well as to nonspecific heterophile antigens, defined as those belonging to nonhuman species. These nonspecific heterophile antibodies cross react with antigens on sheep and horse red blood cells but not those on guinea pig red blood cells. Heterophile antibodies are present in as many as 90% of children older than 4 years of age with EBV-IM. The titer reported is the highest serum dilution at which sheep or horse erythrocytes still agglutinate after serum absorption with guinea pig kidney cells. Such absorption decreases interference (false positives) caused by Forssmann antibodies, directed against antigens on sheep, horse erythrocytes, and guinea pig red blood cells, and by antibodies that are associated with serum sickness. The Paul Bunnell test detected antibodies that agglutinated to equine and ovine erythrocytes but not directed to any known EBV antigens. Therefore, this test was less specific than the heterophile antibody test, which has replaced the Paul Bunnell test. IgM antibodies usually appear during the first or, more commonly, the second or third week of illness and become undetectable by 1 year in about 25% of individuals when using the horse red-cell agglutination test or in 70% when using sheep red-cell agglutinins. A number of rapid spot kits for detecting heterophile antibodies (using equine or ovine erythrocytes) are now available commercially. The correlation between results obtained by the spot and slide tests and the classic tube heterophile test is usually excellent. False-positive monospot tests have occasionally been reported in patients with lymphoma, pancreatitis, mumps, or hepatitis. False-negative tests occur most frequently in children younger than 4 years of age or in older children tested in the first 2 weeks of illness. Following infection with EBV, only 5% to 10% of children younger than 2 years of age have positive heterophile antibodies, in contrast to as many as 50% of children between 2 and 4 years of age.

In older children, the most common cause of heterophile-negative IM is still EBV infection. CMV is the second most common cause of heterophile-negative mononucleosis (see Chapter 305). *Streptococcus pyogenes* pharyngitis, hepatitis A and B, acute toxoplasmosis, rubella, and enteroviral infection may each result in fever, lymphadenopathy, malaise, atypical lymphocytosis, and rash. Throat cultures are positive for group A β-hemolytic streptococci in about 30% of patients, which may confuse the correct diagnosis of EBV. Lymphoma or acute lymphocytic leukemia may similarly present with lymphadenopathy or splenomegaly or both. The heterophile test may be helpful in differentiation. Bone marrow should be examined in any individual who has lymphoproliferative disease without evidence of IM.

**TABLE 306-1 ANTIBODY PATTERNS ASSOCIATED WITH EBV INFECTION STATUS**

| EBV Infection Status | IgM-VCA | IgG-VCA | EBNA | Anti-EA |
|---|---|---|---|---|
| No current or prior EBV infection | – | – | – | – |
| Acute primary EBV infection | ++ | ++++ | – | ++ |
| Recent past EBV infection (< 6 mo) | + | +++ | – | ++ |
| Convalescent/post-EBV infection | – | +++ | + | ± |
| Chronic or reactivation infection | ± | ++++ | ± | +++ |
| EBV-associated malignancies | – | ++++ | ± | +++ |

EA, early antigen; EBNA, Epstein-Barr nuclear antigen; EBV, Epstein-Barr virus; VCA, viral capsid antigen.

The availability of sensitive and specific EBV antibody tests has enabled more accurate diagnosis of EBV infection and disease. Antibodies detected by indirect immunofluorescence include IgG and IgM antibody to viral capsid antigen (IgG-VCA and IgM-VCA); antibodies to early antigens (EAs), which consist of either a diffuse pattern, anti-D (antigen present diffusely in cytoplasm and membrane), or a restricted pattern, anti-R (antigen restricted to cytoplasm only); and IgG antibody to EBV nuclear antigen (EBNA). IgG antibodies to VCA are present in almost 100% of patients during the acute phase of IM. Similarly, more than 95% of patients with IM will have demonstrable IgM-VCA on presentation, and all will have detectable antibody if tested at the appropriate time. Because IgM antibody usually lasts only 2 to 3 months, occasionally the antibody response may not be detected in view of a 30- to 50-day incubation period. Following clinical recovery, IgG-VCA antibody remains detectable throughout life. Antibodies to EAs are present in 70% to 80% of patients with acute IM. Because these antibodies have a relatively similar time course to that of IgM-VCA, they may not often add to the clinical interpretation of acute, subacute, or past EBV infection. That being said, EA may sometimes be useful because these antibodies may persist for 3 to 6 months after IM (as opposed to 2–3 months for IgM-VCA) and may be very elevated in patients with Burkitt lymphoma or CAEBV. IgG antibodies to EBNA appear late in the course of IM and remain detectable for life. Therefore, when antibody to EBNA is absent in the presence of other EBV-specific antibodies, recent infection is likely. Table 306-1 and Figure 306-3 summarize these patterns.

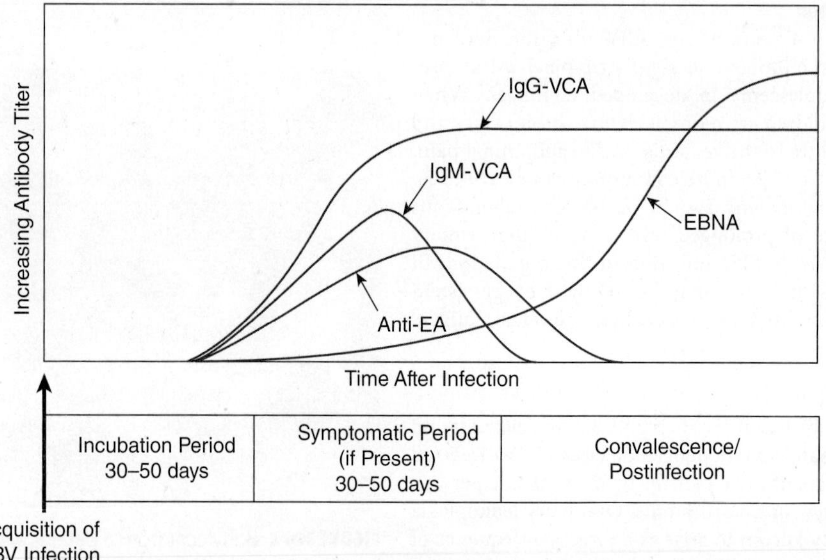


**FIGURE 306-3** Typical course of serum antibody titers in infectious mononucleosis. EA, early antigen (diffuse pattern); EBNA, Epstein-Barr virus nuclear antigen; EBV, Epstein-Barr virus; VCA, viral capsid antigen.

Qualitative and quantitative EBV polymerase chain reaction testing of whole blood or plasma may be used to aid in the diagnosis of EBV infection and disease in patients with primary or acquired immune deficiency or in patients with systemic, severe EBV-associated diseases such as overwhelming IM, hemophagocytic syndrome, or chronic active EBV infection. DNA-DNA hybridization and testing for EBV RNA (electron beam electroreflectance [EBER]) can aid in detection of EBV in histopathologic samples (not to be confused with EBV-encoded small RNAs [EBERs]).

## TREATMENT

Currently, there is no specific antiviral therapy for EBV infections, although symptomatic treatment with antipyretics may be helpful. Forced rest is neither helpful nor indicated, but strenuous activities should be avoided for a minimum of 3 weeks, and contact sports or other activities that may result in abdominal trauma should be avoided for a minimum of 4 weeks and while the spleen is still enlarged (usually 1–3 months). In some instances, vigorous examination of the abdomen can result in splenic rupture, so caution should be used when examining the abdomen of a child with suspected EBV-associated IM. Corticosteroids are not indicated for most patients but may be used for potentially life-threatening complications, including airway obstruction, neurologic complications, fulminant hepatitis, myocarditis, pericarditis, thrombocytopenic purpura, or hemolytic anemia. A short course of prednisone, 1 to 2 mg/kg/d given the first day in divided doses and rapidly tapered over 7 to 10 days, is usually sufficient, although longer courses may be necessary to treat hemolytic anemia and certain neurologic complications.

Specific antiviral therapy has generally not been beneficial in treating EBV infections, although treatment of a suspected acute *S pyogenes* infection with a non–β-lactam antibiotic such as clindamycin is reasonable. Regarding EBV, several nucleotide analogs have in vitro activity but have little clinical effect. Acyclovir treatment of patients with IM results in interruption of viral shedding in the throat, but clinical progression remains unaffected. However, valacyclovir has been shown to decrease the severity and number of symptoms in several studies. Prophylactic interferon-α decreases the incidence of EBV shedding by kidney transplant recipients but is not widely used for prophylaxis or treatment.

Lesions of oral hairy leukoplakia respond to oral or intravenous acyclovir, but they frequently recur in patients with HIV infection after treatment is discontinued. Aggressive, successful antiretroviral therapy frequently results in remission of lesions of oral hairy leukoplakia without specific treatment of EBV. Occasional remissions of polyclonal and monoclonal tumors have been described in persons with LPDs treated with interferon-α and intravenous gamma globulin.

Regarding LPD, acyclovir is generally not considered to be helpful because it is active only during the lytic phase of EBV and not in the latent phase of EBV occurring in lymphoproliferative conditions. Except for the rare occurrence of splenic rupture, severe central nervous system complications, severe hematologic problems, untreated respiratory compromise, and specific immunologic defects, the prognosis for the patient infected with EBV is excellent. Complete clinical recovery, particularly for immunocompetent patients, is to be expected. During convalescence, some patients experience marked fatigue, which occasionally persists for months after the acute infection. Supportive care, including adequate nutrition and hydration as well as over-the-counter pain relievers as needed, is the mainstay of therapy. Treatment of LPD is evolving. In addition to withdrawal/reduction of immune suppression, treatment with anti-CD20 (rituximab) or alternative treatments such as adoptive transfer of EBV-specific T cells have been used.

## PREVENTION

Ganciclovir and valganciclovir have been used to prevent posttransplant EBV disease. Two prophylactic EBV vaccines, gp350 subunit vaccine and CD8 T-cell peptide epitope vaccine, have been evaluated in clinical trials.

## SUGGESTED READINGS


Abdelwahid SA, Mubarak AS, Ahmed AH, Jones IM. Epstein-Barr virus: clinical and epidemiological revisits and genetic basis of oncogenesis. *Open Virol J*. 2015;9:7-28.

American Academy of Pediatrics. Epstein-Barr virus infections. In: Kimberlin DW, Brady MT, Jackson MA, Long SS, eds. *Red Book: 2015 Report of the Committee on Infectious Diseases*. 30th ed. Elk Grove Village, IL: American Academy of Pediatrics; 2015:336-340.

Cohen J. Epstein-Barr virus infection. *N Engl J Med*. 2000;343:481-492.

Dunmire SK, Hogquist KA, Balfour HH. Infectious mononucleosis. *Curr Top Microbiol Immunol*. 2015;390:211-240.

Odumade OA, Hogquist KA, Balfour HH Jr. Progress and problems in understanding and managing primary Epstein-Barr virus infections. *Clin Microbiol Rev*. 2011;24:193-209.

Rasche L, Kapp M, Einsele H, Mielke S. EBV-induced post-transplant lymphoproliferative disorders: a persisting challenge in allogeneic hematopoietic SCT. *Bone Marrow Transplant*. 2014;49:163-167.

Rezk E, Nofal YH, Hamzeh A, Aboujaib MF, AlKheder MA, Al Hammad MF. Steroids for symptom control in infectious mononucleosis. *Cochrane Database Syst Rev*. 2015;11:CD004402.

Rickinson AB. Co-infections, inflammation and oncogenesis: future directions for EBV research. *Semin Cancer Biol*. 2014;26:99-115.


# 307 Human Herpesviruses 6 and 7

Mark R. Schleiss

## HUMAN HERPESVIRUS TYPE 6

### INTRODUCTION

Human herpesvirus-6 (HHV-6) was isolated in tissue culture in 1986 from peripheral blood leukocytes of patients with both lymphoproliferative disorders and human immunodeficiency virus (HIV) infection. It is the major etiologic agent of exanthem subitum (roseola) and has also been implicated in other clinical syndromes. HHV-6 is a prototypical member of the betaherpesvirus family of herpesviruses, which also includes human herpesvirus-7 (HHV-7) and human cytomegalovirus (HCMV). The virus has a double-stranded DNA genome contained within an icosahedral capsid, surrounded by an outer envelope. HHV-6 is subclassified as either variant A or B, based on differences in nucleotide sequence, restriction enzyme profile, and reactivity with monoclonal antibodies. Some experts have suggested that HHV-6A and -6B are sufficiently different from one another that they should be considered distinct, unique herpesviruses. HHV-6B is the subtype associated with exanthem subitum.

### PATHOGENESIS AND EPIDEMIOLOGY

HHV-6 has a tropism for T cells and neuronal cells (particularly oligodendrocytes and microglia). Recent evidence suggests that HHV-6 can be maintained in the host cell in a chromosomally integrated form. The site of integration of the viral genome is the telomere. Approximately 1% of individuals have inherited integrated viral sequences in their genomes, transmitted vertically through the germline, and these individuals characteristically have very high "viral loads" (representing germline inheritance, and not active viral replication) in blood and other sample types when interrogated by PCR. It is unclear whether HHV-6A and HHV-6B chromosomal integration produces any disease phenotype or long-term adverse health consequences, although the integrated viral genome appears capable of becoming excised from the telomeric integration site under some circumstances, potentially allowing for the initiation of viral replication. The clinical consequences of inherited chromosomally integrated HHV-6 have yet to be fully elucidated.

Infection with HHV-6 is ubiquitous, and virtually all children are infected by 2 to 3 years of age. Infection is seldom seen before 6 months of age, presumably due to the protective effect of transplacental antibody. The incidence of infection peaks between 6 and 12 months of age. A recent study in Ugandan infants demonstrated that over 75% of infants acquire HHV-6 infection in the first year of life. HHV-6 can be found in the salivary gland and is shed in saliva of seropositive individuals, suggesting that saliva is the source of virus that leads to person-to-person transmission. Primary infection in children most likely occurs via contact with HHV-6 shed in the secretions of older children or caregivers.

## CLINICAL MANIFESTATIONS

The spectrum of disease associated with primary HHV-6 infection is broad, ranging from asymptomatic infection to (rarely) fatal disseminated disease. Most commonly, primary infection occurs early in life and is manifested as either exanthem subitum or an undifferentiated febrile illness. Reports of HHV-6 infection linked to other clinical syndromes must be interpreted cautiously. Because infection is ubiquitous and persistent in nature, the finding of HHV-6 antibody, or even isolation of the virus, cannot with certainty always prove that HHV-6 is the cause of any given clinical syndrome in older patients.

### Exanthem Subitum

Exanthem subitum (also known commonly as roseola infantum) is a common acute febrile illness of infants and young children characterized by 3 to 5 days of fever followed by rapid defervescence and the appearance of an erythematous macular or maculopapular rash (Fig. 307-1). This entity was first described in 1910, and it was at one time classified as the "sixth disease" among the exanthematous illnesses of childhood. The infection is characterized by onset of viremia preceding development of the rash. The magnitude of the fever can be quite striking. Prior to development of the characteristic rash, there are few other clinical clues to reliably indicate that the febrile ailment is due to HHV-6, although the finding of posterior auricular and occipital adenopathy can be an important clue on physical examination. Because of the high fever and lack of differentiating clinical findings, many young infants will be subjected to extensive laboratory evaluation and empiric antibiotic therapy prior to the onset of the pathognomonic exanthem. In children treated empirically with antimicrobials, the onset of the rash may often be misinterpreted as an antibiotic "allergy." The rash is papular, macular, or maculopapular and appears mainly on the trunk. The pathogenesis of the rash is unknown but is presumed to be immune mediated. The rash usually fades within 3 to 4 days following onset.

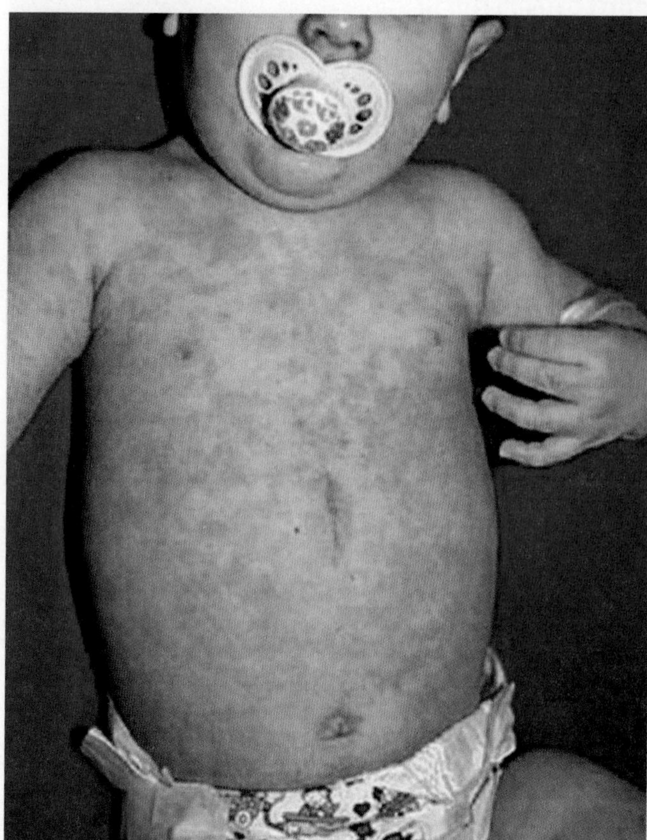

**FIGURE 307-1** Exanthem subitum in an infant showing truncal pink macules and some papules that appeared 1 day after defervescence. (Reproduced with permission from Wolff K, Goldsmith LA, Katz SI, et al: *Fitzpatrick's Dermatology in General Medicine*, 7th ed. New York: McGraw-Hill; 2008.)

### Undifferentiated Febrile Illness

HHV-6 infection can also be a common cause of undifferentiated febrile illness without rash in infants. In 1 study, evidence for acute HHV-6 infection was identified in approximately 10% of children presenting to an emergency department for evaluation of high fever. A peak fever higher than 40°C was found in 65% of the acutely HHV-6–infected children in this study. Inflammation of tympanic membranes and a modest depression in total leukocyte count were the only other features that differentiated these children from those without HHV-6 infection. Because very young infants with high fever due to HHV-6 infection are difficult to discriminate from those with occult bacteremia, many young infants with acute HHV-6 infection are treated empirically with antibiotic therapy, pending the results of blood cultures.

### Central Nervous System Complications

HHV-6 infection can also be associated with central nervous system (CNS) complications in children both with and without rash. Febrile convulsions are the most common complication of HHV-6 infection. In a large study of emergency room visits, HHV-6 accounted for one-third of all febrile seizures in children younger than 2 years. In some children, seizures may be prolonged or recurrent. However, in another prospective, population-based study of 81 children with a well-defined time of acquisition of HHV-6, although 93% had symptoms, none had seizures. The role of primary HHV-6 infection as a cause of neurologic disease in children requires further study. Other neurologic complications reported in acute HHV-6 infection have included encephalitis, meningoencephalitis, and aseptic meningitis. Provocative reports have hypothesized that latent CNS infection with HHV-6 may play a causative role in temporal lobe epilepsy, and controversial reports in adult patients have proposed a link to chronic HHV-6 infection in the CNS and multiple sclerosis (MS). These associations remain unproven (discussed in more detail below).

### Immunocompromised Patients

Immunocompromised patients are at increased risk for disease from HHV-6. Presumably, the majority of such syndromes reflect reactivation of latent infection due to immunosuppression. Reactivation of HHV-6 has been linked to allograft rejection. HHV-6 reactivation may also contribute to an immunomodulatory and immunosuppressive milieu in the transplant patient, which may, in turn, facilitate infection with other opportunistic pathogens, such as cytomegalovirus and fungi, contributing to an increased overall mortality. In hematopoietic stem cell transplant patients, HHV-6 has been implicated as a cause of encephalitis and graft failure.

### Other Human Herpesvirus Type 6 Syndromes

Some less common syndromes are postulated to be causally related to HHV-6 infection. There is evidence to suggest a role for HHV-6 in the pathogenesis of MS. These patients have a higher level of HHV-6 antibody compared to controls, and HHV-6 DNA has been detected by polymerase chain reaction (PCR) assay in brain and/or cerebrospinal fluid from MS patients but not age-matched controls. HHV-6 has been implicated as causing some cases of heterophile-negative mononucleosis. Hepatitis, liver dysfunction, thrombocytopenia, thrombocytopenic purpura, hemophagocytic syndrome, chronic fatigue syndrome, thyroiditis, myocarditis, and prolonged lymphadenopathy have also been described. HHV-6 has also been implicated as a potential cofactor in the pathogenesis of acquired immunodeficiency syndrome (AIDS). An etiological role for HHV-6 (and HHV-7) has been suggested for the rash pityriasis rosea. Both HIV and HHV-6 share a tropism for CD4+ cells, and there is evidence that dual infection may stimulate the replication of HIV. Progression of HIV disease appears to be more rapid in children vertically infected with HIV who are also infected with HHV-6. Congenital infections have been described with HHV-6, as well as HHV-7 (described below), but the clinical significance of these infections is unclear.

## DIAGNOSIS

The diagnosis of primary HHV-6 infection can generally be made clinically in children with exanthem subitum. Primary HHV-6 infection may also be suspected in an irritable infant with high, unexplained fever and no other clinical or laboratory findings suggesting serious bacterial infection. Leukopenia may suggest the diagnosis, of primary HHV-6 infection in a febrile infant but this laboratory abnormality is nonspecific. The differential diagnosis of exanthem subitum includes measles and rubella, but these are currently rare diseases in the United States. A history of recent measles immunization should be sought in the child presenting with fever and rash, recognizing that exanthem due to the vaccine strain is well-recognized in immunized toddlers. The clinician should remember that enteroviral rashes may be indistinguishable from exanthem subitum and can be associated with a prodrome of fever; these are most likely to be encountered in the late summer or early fall. Erythema infectiosum (fifth disease) is usually seen in somewhat older children. Fever is usually not as high as in roseola, and the rash is most prominent on the cheeks (so-called "slapped cheek" appearance). Epstein-Barr virus– and cytomegalovirus-associated infectious mononucleosis can also be associated with an exanthem that can be confused with exanthem subitum, particularly in children who receive β-lactam antibiotics.

In circumstances when specific etiologic diagnosis is necessary, the diagnosis of primary HHV-6 infection may be made by identification of viral genome in blood by use of PCR. Care should be taken to consider the possibility that a positive PCR assay (particularly one demonstrating a very high level of viral DNA) of blood may simply reflect the germline integration of viral genome in that individual (recognizing that this occurs in ~1% of all people). Documenting a 4-fold or greater rise in immunoglobulin (Ig) G titer may be valuable in some clinical circumstances. The virus can be cultured, but culture requires special techniques not available to most diagnostic virology laboratories. The demonstration of HHV-6 DNA in the cerebrospinal fluid may be helpful in the diagnostic evaluation of a child with protracted seizures and may confirm the diagnosis of HHV-6 encephalitis.

## TREATMENT

Treatment of HHV-6 infection is essentially supportive because virtually all infections are self-limited. Some use of empiric antimicrobials in highly febrile children with acute HHV-6 infection is probably unavoidable (before the true diagnosis is known), but care should be taken to not confuse the classic rash of exanthem subitum, which occurs at the time of defervescence, with a drug allergy. For children with HHV-6–related seizures, anticonvulsants may be warranted. In immunocompromised patients with HHV-6 viremia or other disease syndromes, antiviral agents active against cytomegalovirus, in particular ganciclovir and foscarnet, are occasionally employed, but evidence of efficacy from controlled studies is lacking. Antivirals are not recommended for the immunocompetent child with acute HHV-6 infection.

## PREVENTION

Currently, no vaccines or preventative strategies are available for HHV-6. Given the ubiquitous nature of the infection, it is unclear whether prevention strategies are feasible. Strategies for identification and prevention of HHV-6 disease in immunocompromised transplant patients are under investigation.

## HUMAN HERPESVIRUS TYPE 7

HHV-7 is a betaherpesvirus highly related to HHV-6A and HHV-6B and is similarly responsible for the common childhood illness exanthem subitum (roseola infantum). This virus was first isolated from CD4+ T cells of a healthy individual. The high degree of homology with HHV-6 creates difficulty in interpretation of serologic assays (which are largely investigational in nature and not generally useful for clinical practice) because there is considerable cross-reactivity of antibodies between HHV-6 and HHV-7 proteins. As with HHV-6, infection with HHV-7 appears to be ubiquitous, although infection appears to be acquired somewhat later in life than is HHV-6. By 2 years of age, approximately 40% to 45% of children have antibodies to HHV-7, and by 6 years of age, 70% of children are seropositive. Like other betaherpesviruses, HHV-7 can be found in the saliva, suggesting that this is the route that mediates person-to-person transmission.

Primary infection with HHV-7 is clearly associated with exanthem subitum, and the rash is clinically indistinguishable from that caused by HHV-6. It has been estimated that HHV-7 may be responsible for up to 10% of episodes of exanthem subitum. Other manifestations of primary HHV-7 infection include fever of unknown origin, simple febrile seizures, lymphadenopathy, hepatitis, and heterophile-negative mononucleosis. Viremia can occur either as a consequence of primary infection or from reactivation of latent infection. HHV-7 infections play an important, albeit incompletely defined, clinical role in solid organ and hematopoietic stem cell transplant patients.

## SUGGESTED READINGS


Agut H, Bonnafous P, Gautheret-Dejean A. Update on infections with human herpesviruses 6A, 6B, and 7. *Med Mal Infect.* 2017;47: 83-91.

Caserta MT, Hall CB, Schnabel K, et al. Diagnostic assays for active infection with human herpesvirus 6 (HHV-6). *J Clin Virol.* 2010;48:55-57.

Clark DA. Clinical and laboratory features of human herpesvirus 6 chromosomal integration. *Clin Microbiol Infect.* 2016;22:333-339.

Kaufer BB, Flamand L. Chromosomally integrated HHV-6: impact on virus, cell and organismal biology. *Curr Opin Virol.* 2014;9:111-118.

Pantry SN, Medvecsky PG. Latency, integration and reactivation of human herpesvirus-6. *Viruses.* 2017;9(7):194.


# 308 Human Herpesvirus 8 (Kaposi Sarcoma Herpesvirus)

Mark R. Schleiss

## INTRODUCTION

The history of the identification of human herpesvirus-8 (HHV-8; also known as Kaposi sarcoma herpesvirus [KSHV] or Kaposi sarcoma [KS] virus) is unique insofar as the virus was initially "discovered" purely with the use of molecular detection techniques and not traditional viral cell culture. On sequence analysis of tissues amplified from KS patients, the deduced amino acid sequences were found to have strong homology to proteins from the gamma-herpesvirus subfamily, the subfamily of the Herpesviridae that includes Epstein-Barr virus (EBV). This observation was striking in view of the known ability of EBV to persist in lymphocytes, immortalize cells, and produce human malignancies (eg, Burkitt lymphoma and nasopharyngeal carcinoma). Hence, the novel gamma-herpesvirus, HHV-8, appeared to be a new herpesvirus associated with human malignancy—KS.

Structurally, HHV-8 consists of a prototypical enveloped particle, morphologically similar to other herpesviruses. The virus presumably establishes latent infection following primary infection, although the site(s) of latency are unknown. Evolutionarily, HHV-8 appears to have undergone considerable recombination with host genes, and the viral genome contains a variety of transduced cellular oncogenes and chemokine homologs that are probably important in the pathogenesis of KS. It is estimated that 10% of the genes encoded by HHV-8 promote KS development due to mitogenic, antiapoptotic, chemoattractive, angiogenic, or transforming activities.

The epidemiology of primary HHV-8 infection appears to vary considerably worldwide. The routes of acquisition of infection and mechanisms responsible for person-to-person transmission remain uncertain, although a role for salivary transmission in infants has been described. A cross-sectional study of the seroprevalence of HHV-8 in children and adolescents in the United States indicated an overall prevalence of approximately 1%, although considerable regional variation was observed. In sub-Saharan Africa, prevalence in children is much higher, approaching 60% in some studies. In addition to person-to-person routes of infection, HHV-8 can also be transmitted by blood transfusion.

## CLINICAL MANIFESTATIONS

Most primary infections with HHV-8 are probably asymptomatic, although the clinical course of primary symptomatic HHV-8 infections in a case series in immunocompetent children, some of whom had fever and rash, has been described. In this case series, the rash was first noted to appear on the face and it gradually spread to the trunk, arms, and legs. It initially consisted of discrete red macules that blanched with pressure and eventually became papular. The median duration of the rash was 6 days; fever persisted for a median of 10 days, and some children had high fever (temperature 39°C). An upper respiratory tract infection occurred in most of these children, and a lower respiratory tract infection appeared in one-third, although major respiratory complications did not occur during the course of primary HHV-8 infection.

Prior HHV-8 infection appears to be generally necessary, but not sufficient, for the development of KS, which is a multifocal vascular neoplasm involving skin, visceral organs, and lymph nodes. Lesions histopathologically contain distinctive proliferating cells, so-called "spindle" cells, as well as activated endothelial cells, fibroblasts, smooth muscle cells, and infiltrating inflammatory cells. Three variants of KS are described: "classical" KS, which is chiefly an indolent, slowly progressive form of KS seen in elderly, human immunodeficiency virus (HIV)-negative Mediterranean men; "endemic" KS, a variant seen in Africa (including a "lymphadenopathic" form seen predominantly in young children); and "epidemic" KS, seen in HIV-infected patients. All variants are associated with HHV-8. The factors responsible for malignant transformation of HHV-8–infected endothelial cells into tumor are unknown.

Other malignant diseases have been associated with HHV-8, including multicentric Castleman disease (MCD), a lymphoproliferative syndrome associated with HIV infection; and another acquired immunodeficiency syndrome (AIDS)-associated malignancy, primary effusion lymphoma (PEL; Table 308-1). HHV-8 is causally related to these tumors in HIV-negative patients as well. Other malignancies, including skin cancer and multiple myeloma, have been associated with HHV-8 in the literature, but these reports are controversial, and the causal link remains unproven (see Table 308-1). Links between HHV-8 and pemphigus, sarcoidosis, and Kikuchi disease have been postulated, and more recently, there have been associations reported between HHV-8 and hemophagocytic syndromes. Recently, Kaposi sarcoma inflammatory cytokine syndrome (KICS) has been described in both HIV-positive patients and recipients of solid organ transplantation. KICS appears to be driven by lytic reactivation of virus with an associated hyperinflammatory cytokine response.

**TABLE 308-1 DISEASES ASSOCIATED WITH HUMAN HERPESVIRUS 8**

| Definitive Evidence for Causal Relationship |
|---|
| Classical (Mediterranean) Kaposi sarcoma |
| Endemic (African) Kaposi sarcoma |
| Epidemic (AIDS-associated) Kaposi sarcoma |
| Primary effusion lymphoma |
| Castleman disease |
| KICS (Kaposi sarcoma inflammatory cytokine syndrome) |
| **Hypothesized But Unproven Causal Relationship** |
| Multiple myeloma |
| Hemophagocytic syndrome |
| Kikuchi disease |
| Sarcoidosis |
| Pemphigus |
| Bullous pemphigoid |
| Bowen disease |
| Angiosarcoma |
| Salivary gland tumor |

## DIAGNOSIS

In the absence of standardized serologic assays, serodiagnosis of HHV-8 infection is problematic. Tissue from any case of KS, MCD, or PEL that is encountered in a child should be investigated for the presence of HHV-8 DNA sequences, in collaboration with a reference laboratory. HIV serology should also be performed in such patients. AIDS-associated KS has been reported to regress following administration of combined antiretroviral therapy (cART), suggesting that reversal of immunosuppression may promote resolution of the tumor. No controlled trials of specific antiviral therapy have been conducted for KS, although treatment with either oral or intravenous ganciclovir (GCV) was associated with a strongly reduced risk of KS in AIDS patients prior to the advent of cART, suggesting an antiviral effect of GCV against HHV-8. In a cell culture system, the use of the β-adrenergic antagonist propranolol reversed some HHV-8–associated pathologies, suggesting a potential future role for clinical investigation of the utility of this inexpensive and widely available agent in the management of KS in the developing world. Although these are intriguing data, chemotherapy and radiotherapy remain the mainstays of therapy for most cases of KS, as well as other HHV-8–associated tumors.

## SUGGESTED READINGS


De Paoli P, Carbone A. Kaposi's sarcoma herpesvirus: twenty years after its discovery. *Eur Rev Med Pharmacol Sci*. 2016;20:1288-1294.

Dittmer DP, Damania B. Kaposi sarcoma-associated herpesvirus: immunobiology, oncogenesis, and therapy. *J Clin Invest*. 2016;126: 3165-3175.

Dow DE, Cunningham CK, Buchanan AM. A review of human herpesvirus 8, the Kaposi's sarcoma-associated herpesvirus, in the pediatric population. *J Pediatr Infect Dis Soc*. 2014;3:66-76.

Gantt S, Orem J, Krantz EM, et al. Prospective characterization of the risk factors for transmission and symptoms of primary human herpesvirus infections among Ugandan infants. *J Infect Dis*. 2016;214:36-44.

Minhas V, Wood C. Epidemiology and transmission of Kaposi's sarcoma-associated herpesvirus. *Viruses*. 2014;6:4178-4194.

Mularoni A, Gallo A, Riva G, et al. Successful treatment of Kaposi sarcoma-associated herpesvirus inflammatory cytokine syndrome after kidney-liver transplant: correlations with the human herpesvirus 8 miRNome and specific T cell response. *Am J Transplant*. 2017 May 10. doi: 10.1111/ajt.14346.

Olp LN, Minhas V, Gondwe C, et al. Longitudinal analysis of the humoral response to Kaposi's sarcoma-associated herpesvirus after primary infection in children. *J Med Virol*. 2016;88:173-178.

# 309 Varicella-Zoster Virus Infections

Claudette L. Poole and David W. Kimberlin

## INTRODUCTION

Varicella-zoster virus (VZV) is 1 of the 9 human herpesviruses, which include herpes simplex virus (HSV) types 1 and 2, cytomegalovirus, Epstein-Barr virus, and human herpesviruses 6A, 6B, 7, and 8. As with HSV-1 and HSV-2, VZV establishes latency in sensory or autonomic ganglia following primary infection, with the ability for subsequent reactivation. The primary acquisition of VZV results in the clinical disease varicella (chickenpox) with reactivation from latency resulting in zoster (shingles). Live-attenuated varicella vaccine was licensed in the United States in 1995 and, over the past 20 years, has substantially altered the epidemiology of the disease in this country, with rates of varicella and its complications plummeting.

## PATHOGENESIS AND EPIDEMIOLOGY

Humans are the only source of infection of VZV. Transmission occurs when aerosolized virus from skin lesions comes into contact with the mucosa of the upper respiratory tract or conjunctivae of susceptible persons. Although it was long thought that the source of infection was the respiratory tract of infected individuals, very limited virus has been recovered from an infected person's airways and probably represents a much more limited source of infection than aerosolization from skin lesions.

The infectious period extends from up to 48 hours before the appearance of rash until all skin lesions are crusted over, usually about 5 days in normal hosts. Following infectious contact, the incubation period for varicella is 10 to 21 days and up to 28 days following a dose of varicella-zoster immunoglobin (VariZIG).

Infection of cells within the respiratory tract or conjunctivae by inhaled virions is followed by cell-associated spread to local lymph nodes, viremia, and then the development of the vesicular rash approximately 5 days later. Virus can be detected in circulating lymphocytes and monocytes. Cell-to-cell spread of virus within the skin creates infected syncytia with a striking disruption of normal cellular architecture, and VZV-infected keratinocytes appear to elicit a vigorous type I interferon response in neighboring, uninfected cells that restrains horizontal spread of virus and thus may contribute to the topology of the rash.

In the immunocompetent host, VZV viremia and the appearance of new skin lesions are curtailed within a few days by a vigorous cellular immune response comprising both natural killer (NK) and antigen-specific (T-cell) components. Conversely, the failure to mount antigen-specific cellular responses is associated with progressive viral replication and dissemination and a potentially fatal outcome.

Individuals with disorders purely of humoral immunity do not suffer unusually severe or repeated episodes of varicella, indicating that cellular immunity affords sufficient protection against primary infection. However, a host humoral response is detectable within 4 days of the onset of the rash and can confer passive immunity; thus, pooled immunoglobulin derived from VZV-immune donors, known as VariZIG, can be used to protect VZV-exposed subjects at high risk of severe varicella. The presence of VZV-specific antibodies is also the best available correlate of protection against primary infection but is irrelevant to the risk of secondary (reactivation) disease.

Along with measles, varicella is one of the most highly communicable infections in humans, with household attack rates approaching 90%. In the absence of widespread vaccination, outbreaks of varicella occur readily within groups of susceptible children. In unvaccinated populations in temperate climates, seasonal peaks of varicella occur in the spring. These epidemics occur on a background of endemic disease, and 84% of children acquire infection by age 15 years. In contrast, the incidence of varicella in the tropics does not vary by season and tends to be delayed until adolescence or adult life.

Aside from adult age, the greatest risks for severe/fatal varicella are cellular immunocompromise (congenital or acquired), infancy (particularly the neonatal period), and pregnancy (Table 309-1). In the pre-vaccine era, varicella was associated with approximately 11,000 hospitalizations and more than 100 deaths annually in the United States. Much of this burden was borne by previously healthy children. The epidemiology of VZV has been transformed since the introduction of universal varicella vaccination in the mid-1990s, initially as a single dose in 1996 and then as a 2-dose schedule beginning in 2007. The incidence of varicella has been strikingly reduced across all age groups, with concomitant reductions in office visits, hospitalizations, and deaths from varicella. When varicella does occur in a previously immunized child, it produces a much milder form of varicella and is only one-third as transmissible.

## CLINICAL MANIFESTATIONS

### Uncomplicated Varicella

Prodromal symptoms of low-grade fever, headache, and malaise usually precede the characteristic vesicular exanthem by 24 to 48 hours. The rash typically begins as "dew drops on rose petals," appearing on the face, trunk, or scalp and eventually spreading to involve the entire body (Fig. 309-1). The total number of lesions may vary from 50 to 500. The vesicles appear in crops for the first 3 to 5 days of the illness and may be exaggerated in areas of minor trauma or dermatitis, such as sunburn or eczema. The initial tiny vesicles evolve to larger vesicles, filled with clear fluid that becomes cloudy with cellular debris, and finally involute with crust formation. All 3 stages of lesion progression are present at the same time in varicella. The cutaneous lesions of varicella are usually intensely pruritic but not painful; lesions on mucous membranes become shallow ulcers, which may be painful. In the absence of secondary bacterial infection, healing occurs over 7 to 10 days without scar formation, although discrete hypo- or hyperpigmented lesions may persist for several months.

Immunity following varicella usually is lifelong; however, primary infection in circumstances in which immune responses are incomplete may predispose to a second episode of varicella. "Breakthrough" varicella is the term applied to wild-type disease in an individual who has previously received the live-attenuated varicella vaccine. This is generally a highly modified illness in which skin lesions are few (< 10), systemic features such as fever are absent, and transmissibility is reduced by approximately two-thirds compared with unmodified varicella. Not surprisingly, this may pose diagnostic difficulties.

In considering the differential diagnosis of a vesicular rash in children, rarer conditions such as disseminated herpes zoster or herpes simplex should be borne in mind, along with eczema herpeticum, insect bites, scabies, Stevens-Johnson syndrome, and bullous impetigo. Smallpox also is in the differential but is distinguishable from varicella by distinctive centrifugal distribution of pox (more numerous on the extremities than the trunk) and the fact that the skin lesions of smallpox mature simultaneously and hence are all in the same stage of development at any given time in a particular area of the body. Occasionally, drug eruptions may be mistaken for varicella. In the neonate, vesicular eruptions may accompany congenital syphilis, congenital candidiasis, neonatal herpes, pustular melanosis, and histiocytosis. Apparent second episodes of varicella may occur as a consequence of misdiagnosis of the first episode.

Varicella in the normal host is generally a benign self-limited disease. The occurrence of significant fever beyond the first 48 hours of exanthema, as well as the progression of erythema or tenderness around crusting lesions, should raise suspicion for secondary bacterial infection. Likewise, hemorrhagic lesions, significant abdominal pain or vomiting, or altered mental status should alert clinicians to possible complications that require prompt intervention.

### Varicella and Immune Deficiency

Individuals with congenital or acquired immune deficiencies that affect their ability to mount a cellular immune response to VZV are at risk for progressive disseminated varicella, whereas individuals with isolated humoral immune deficiency are not (see Table 309-1). Children being treated for lymphoid malignancy are at particular risk of fatal varicella. Progressive disseminated varicella involves multiple

**TABLE 309-1 PATIENTS AT HIGH RISK OF DEVELOPING SEVERE VARICELLA-ZOSTER VIRUS INFECTIONS AND GUIDANCE TO THERAPY**

| | Varicella | | | Zoster | | |
|---|---|---|---|---|---|---|
| Patient Group | Risk | Treatment | Prevention Strategy[a] | Risk | Treatment | Prevention Strategy[b] |
| Stem cell transplant recipients or | High risk of severe varicella | Yes (IV) | Immunize susceptible family members[c] and | Incidence increased | Yes (IV) | Antiviral prophylaxis |
| Primary combined immunodeficiency (eg, SCID, Wiskott-Aldrich syndrome) | | | VariZIG postexposure prophylaxis | High risk of dissemination | | |
| Children receiving systemic corticosteroids, other immunosuppressive medication[d] | Severe varicella | Yes (IV) | Immunize susceptible family members and VariZIG postexposure prophylaxis | Incidence increased Possibility of dissemination | Yes (IV) | |
| Neonates | Severe varicella, with high mortality rates if acquired peripartum | Yes (IV) | VariZIG postexposure prophylaxis | Increased incidence following varicella in infancy | Consider | |
| HIV positive | Prolonged varicella; rarely severe disease | Yes (consider IV) | Active immunization of child (unless CD4 < 15%) and susceptible family members; if immunosuppressed, avoid exposure and give PEP (VariZIG) | High incidence; recurrences of zoster common | Yes | Antiretroviral therapy (ie, prevention of immunosuppression) |
| Pregnant women | Moderately high risk of severe varicella; risks to unborn child: fetal varicella syndrome, neonatal varicella | Yes (consider IV) | VariZIG PEP | Low | Yes (PO) | |
| Adolescents, adults | Moderate risk of severe varicella | Yes (PO unless ill) | Active immunization—primary or as PEP | Increases with age | Yes (PO) | Zoster vaccine (older than 60 years) |
| Normal children | Low | No | Universal vaccination; vaccine as PEP | Low | Yes (PO) | |

[a]Universal vaccination and infection control strategies reduce exposure across all groups.
[b]Vaccine strain virus appears to reactivate less readily than wild-type VZV; therefore, prior varicella vaccination may be relatively protective against zoster.
[c]Many such patients will receive immunoglobulin replacement and continuous acyclovir prophylaxis, which offer protection against varicella (and, in the case of acyclovir, zoster).
[d]Children being treated for lymphoid malignancy are at particularly high risk.
IV, intravenously; PEP, postexposure prophylaxis; PO, orally; SCID, severe combined immunodeficiency disease; VariZIG, varicella-zoster immunoglobulin.

organ systems. Its onset may be heralded by severe abdominal pain or back pain before the appearance of a rash. Fever reaching to 40°C to 41°C (104°F–105.8°F) may persist for several days. Severe hepatitis, pneumonitis, thrombocytopenia, coagulopathy, encephalitis, and other organ dysfunction may ensue. Mortality is significant, even with treatment and supportive care. Because their ability to terminate viral replication is diminished, immunocompromised individuals with varicella are contagious for an extended period. Individuals with acquired immunodeficiency due to infection with human immunodeficiency virus (HIV) do not appear to be at the same degree of risk for progressive disseminated varicella. Rather, varicella may persist for several weeks to months. The incidence of zoster is extremely high, and recurrent disease is common. Otherwise healthy children receiving courses of high-dose systemic corticosteroids (> 2 mg/kg/d of prednisone or equivalent for 14 days or longer) for asthma or other illness are at risk of developing severe and even fatal varicella.

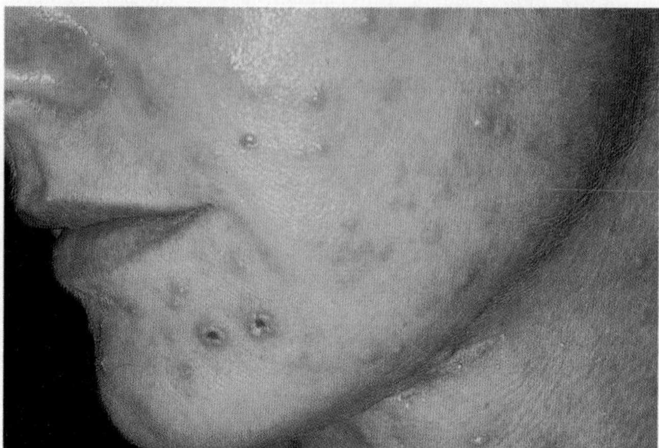

**FIGURE 309-1** Typical varicella lesions. Multiple, very pruritic, erythematous papules, vesicles ("dewdrops on a rose petal"), and crusted papules on erythematous, edematous bases on the face and neck. (Reproduced with permission from Wolff K, Johnson RA: *Fitzpatrick's Color Atlas & Synopsis of Clinical Dermatology*, 6th ed. New York: McGraw-Hill; 2009.)

### Congenital and Neonatal Varicella

When a woman acquires a primary varicella infection during the first 20 weeks of pregnancy, fetal infection can occur, resulting in either miscarriage or infants being born with congenital varicella syndrome (1–2%). The features of congenital varicella syndrome include cutaneous defects, classic cicatricial skin scarring and limb atrophy, microcephaly, cortical atrophy, seizures, chorioretinitis, microphthalmia, and significant neurologic deficits. Autonomic nervous system involvement may manifest as difficulty with sphincter control, intestinal obstruction, Horner syndrome, or other cranial nerve neuropathies (Moebius syndrome). Infants born to mothers who develop varicella less than 5 days before delivery or within 2 days following delivery are at risk of severe or lethal neonatal varicella; mortality approaches 30% when the infection is acquired by the neonate during this critical perinatal window.

## DIAGNOSIS

The diagnosis of VZV infection is usually made clinically. However, with the marked reduction in disease due to the highly successful vaccination program in the United States, the need for laboratory diagnosis has increased both because of lack of familiarity with varicella among parents and younger physicians and due to atypical, mild presentations when breakthrough disease occurs in immunized individuals.

VZV is difficult to culture and requires fluid to be obtained from vesicles in the first few days of eruption. When successful, cytopathic effects in cell culture take many days. Detection of VZV DNA using a polymerase chain reaction (PCR) test currently is the diagnostic method of choice. This testing may be used to distinguish between wild-type and vaccine-strain VZV using genotyping as well as to predict susceptibility to antiviral drugs. During the acute phase of illness, the highest diagnostic yield is to test skin lesions by vesicular fluid aspiration or by swabbing or scraping the scab from crusted skin lesions. Early in the infection, VZV may be detected by PCR testing of saliva or buccal mucosal swabs. Tissue biopsy samples, blood, and cerebrospinal fluid also can be tested by PCR to confirm the diagnosis. Direct fluorescent antibody (DFA) assay can detect VZV using scrapings of a vesicle base in the first 3 to 4 days of the eruption and can provide a result quickly; however, the test is not as sensitive as PCR.

A number of sensitive serologic tests are available to measure antibodies to VZV. These include the fluorescent antibody to membrane antigen (FAMA) method, latex agglutination, and enzyme-linked immunosorbent assay. Antibody to VZV develops within a few days after onset of varicella, persists for many years, and is present before the onset of zoster. VZV infections may be documented by a ≥ 4-fold rise in VZV antibody titer in acute- and convalescent-phase serum specimens. The presence of specific IgM in 1 serum specimen suggests, but does not necessarily prove, recent VZV infection, either varicella or zoster. Persistence of VZV antibody in infants beyond 8 months of age is highly suggestive of intrauterine varicella. Immunity to varicella is highly likely to be present if a positive titer of antibody (measured by a reliable assay) to VZV is demonstrated with a single serum sample from a child or an adult with no history of disease. Serologic methods, however, particularly commercial enzyme-linked immunosorbent assays, may fail to identify many individuals who have been immunized with live-attenuated varicella vaccine due to lack of sensitivity.

## TREATMENT

Treatment with antiviral therapy is dependent on host factors. Antiviral therapy is not recommended for otherwise healthy children with varicella if they are less than 12 years of age, although some would recommend the use of oral acyclovir or valacyclovir for the treatment of secondary household cases as they tend to experience more severe disease. In these children, benefit is only derived if therapy is started promptly as viral replication only occurs in the first 72 hours of illness. Oral acyclovir or valacyclovir should be considered for persons considered at increased risk for severe varicella such as unvaccinated persons older than 12 years, people with chronic cutaneous or pulmonary disorders, people receiving long-term salicylate therapy, and people receiving short, intermittent, or inhaled courses of corticosteroids. Oral acyclovir or valacyclovir should be considered for pregnant women with varicella, with intravenous (IV) acyclovir being administered for more severe disease.

IV acyclovir therapy is recommended for all immunocompromised patients, including patients receiving high-dose corticosteroids for 14 days or more. Therapy should be initiated as soon as possible and should continue until no new lesions develop and all lesions have crusted over. Valacyclovir, which has improved oral bioavailability over oral acyclovir and has been shown to achieve serum levels comparable to IV acyclovir, can be considered in select circumstances. IV acyclovir also is indicated for both term and preterm neonates who develop varicella from their mothers and should be considered for neonates who develop varicella following household exposure. Oral acyclovir is generally not indicated for treatment of young infants because of limited bioavailability and unreliable absorption in infants.

## COMPLICATIONS

The rate of severe or complicated varicella is low among immunocompetent children, but such cases are numerically common in unvaccinated populations. The most frequent complication in the young is secondary bacterial infection of the skin. Many of the other complications of varicella reflect overwhelming viral infection and are more likely to occur in the context of defective cell-mediated immunity.

### Secondary Bacterial Infections

Scratching of the intensely itchy skin lesions of varicella often leads to the introduction of bacteria, typically *Staphylococcus aureus* or *Streptococcus pyogenes*. Local skin infection in a well child can be treated with an oral antibiotic, with close clinical follow-up. Progression of erythema around lesions, formation of bullae, or development of regional lymphadenitis should prompt consideration of intravenous antibiotic therapy. Recent varicella confers a significantly increased risk of invasive bacterial disease, particularly group A streptococcal (GAS) infections; these include necrotizing fasciitis, bacteremia, pneumonia, empyema, and toxic shock syndrome. It has been estimated that varicella directly precedes approximately 15% of invasive GAS infections. Pain in a muscle group, together with circumferential swelling of an extremity, may reflect necrotizing fasciitis despite the lack of significant overlying erythema. Urgent magnetic resonance imaging or ultrasonography can be useful in defining soft tissue involvement. As a result of these severe infectious complications, if a child with varicella appears excessively ill, especially with a recurrence of fever, urgent hospital evaluation is required.

### Varicella Pneumonia

Asymptomatic radiographic changes are common in immunocompetent adults with varicella, but true varicella pneumonia affects only about 1 in 400 adults. Although rates are lower among immunocompetent children, pneumonia commonly accompanies varicella in immunocompromised hosts. Respiratory symptoms (eg, dyspnea, tachypnea, chest tightness, cough) develop in the context of acute varicella, usually 1 to 6 days after the onset of the rash, and may progress rapidly to respiratory failure. The severity of clinical signs is a poor guide to prognosis; therefore, the patient with new respiratory symptoms in the context of varicella should be urgently evaluated. IV antiviral therapy and improved intensive care have markedly improved survival of these patients over recent years, but deaths continue to occur.

### Neurologic Complications

Varicella is classically associated with 3 neurologic pictures: (1) cerebellar ataxia, (2) encephalitis, and (3) Reye syndrome. Rarely, it has been associated with Guillain-Barré syndrome, stroke, transverse myelitis, and aseptic meningitis. Cerebellar ataxia complicates approximately 1 in 4000 cases of varicella and usually follows the onset of rash, making the diagnosis clear. Vomiting and headache often accompany the ataxia, whereas only one-fourth of patients experience neck stiffness or nystagmus. It is not known whether this syndrome results from VZV replication within the central nervous system (CNS) or instead reflects a parainfectious autoimmune process, but the typical timing of onset in the second week following the onset of illness suggests the latter. Cerebrospinal fluid indices may be abnormal, and PCR can be positive for VZV DNA. The role of antiviral therapy is unclear because complete resolution of symptoms is the rule, but antiviral therapy has been proposed for patients with PCR evidence of VZV within the cerebrospinal fluid.

More recent series of suspected viral encephalitis have suggested that VZV may play a major role, especially in patients without evidence of the skin rash associated with varicella. Encephalitis has been reported to complicate 1 to 2 per 100,000 cases of varicella and is marked by fever, altered level of consciousness, headache, photophobia, and seizures. Such patients require urgent diagnostic evaluation and therapy, including antiviral and supportive care. Varicella encephalitis is associated with a low but significant mortality rate; rarely, survivors suffer long-term sequelae.

Reye syndrome, once linked to varicella and influenza in children, has become exceedingly rare since the recognition of an epidemiologic link to the use of aspirin. The syndrome consists of a progressive encephalopathy accompanied by hepatotoxicity and a 30% risk of death.

## PREVENTION

### Active Immunization

Varicella vaccine consists of a live-attenuated virus that is serially propagated and attenuated. It was developed in the early 1970s by Professor Michiaki Takahashi from a boy whose last name was Oka and hence is known as the Oka strain. All unimmunized immunocompetent people greater than 12 months of age should receive 2 doses of the vaccine separated by at least 3 months. Seroprotection rates following the second dose approach 100%, as compared with 76% to 85% following a single dose. In immunocompetent people, varicella vaccine is safe, with reactions being mild. Approximately 25% of people will experience a minor site reaction, and 3% to 5% of children will develop a mild generalized varicella-like rash or a localized rash. These rashes typically consist of 2 to 5 lesions, are maculopapular rather than vesicular, and can appear from 5 to 26 days after immunization. Transmission of vaccine strain virus is exceedingly rare. Vaccination is contraindicated in immunocompromised individuals due to the risk of dissemination and development of severe disease with vaccine strain virus. Protection of these individuals who are unable to receive the vaccine and are most at risk of developing severe disease is afforded by herd immunity by maintaining high population vaccination rates. Healthy persons older than 12 months who are unvaccinated and have been exposed to varicella can have amelioration of clinically apparent disease if vaccine is administered within 5 days of exposure.

### Postexposure Prophylaxis

All high-risk susceptible patients need to be identified and promptly evaluated if an exposure has occurred to a patient with an active case of varicella or to the open skin lesions of zoster. Postexposure prophylaxis primarily is accomplished using VariZIG, although regular IV immunoglobulin or oral antiviral chemoprophylaxis can be considered in certain circumstances (Fig. 309-2).

### Zoster (Shingles)

The establishment of latency in sensory (dorsal root or cranial nerve) and autonomic (including enteric) ganglia provides the opportunity for the subsequent development of zoster, or shingles, should the VZV reactivate subsequently. Latency can occur as a result of primary infection with wild-type VZV in an unvaccinated individual, infection with wild-type VZV in a previously vaccinated individual, or after vaccination with vaccine strain Oka virus. The incidence of zoster increases with increasing age, believed to be in response to declining immunity to VZV. Racial background plays a role; the lifetime incidence of zoster in African Americans is approximately half that reported for whites. Children with malignant disorders, particularly those with lymphomas, acute lymphocytic leukemia, or acquired immunodeficiency syndrome (AIDS), are at increased risk of developing zoster. Immunologically normal children also can develop zoster, especially if varicella was acquired during the first year of life. The risk of developing zoster is reduced in individuals who have been vaccinated.

It was originally proposed that VZV reaches the sensory ganglia via the skin, traveling along sensory nerve axons, yet this process has still not been visualized directly. The establishment of latency may require that neurons are infected by infectious virions, which are produced within the VZV-infected epidermis in close proximity to sensory nerve endings. Latency is characterized by the presence of viral DNA, as well as a limited repertoire of RNA transcripts and viral proteins. Studies of postmortem material have confirmed that around 2% of neurons within dorsal root ganglia support latent infection by VZV. Reactivation of this virus within 1 or more adjacent ganglia produces zoster, with evidence of viral replication in both innervating neurons and satellite cells, as well as expression of the full complement of viral genes. Presumably, nascent viral particles reach the skin by retrograde axonal transport, as has been described for related neurotropic viruses such as HSV. The switch from latent to lytic infection on reactivation is poorly understood in pathophysiologic terms, and indeed, the frequency of asymptomatic reactivation is unknown. Clearly, however, immunosuppression and natural senescence of T-lymphocyte surveillance mechanisms pose a risk for recurrent disease manifested as zoster.

Zoster classically appears as a unilateral process involving a single or possibly 2 adjacent dermatomes. Thoracic dermatomes are most often involved, followed by cranial nerve and lumbosacral regions. The lesions often appear first as patches of erythema, which then develop groups of vesicles. A few scattered lesions, remote from the dermatomes, may appear. The lesions progress over 3 to 5 days and usually dry and crust within 2 weeks. Pain or paresthesia within the involved dermatome may precede the vesicular eruption; pre-eruptive thoracic pain has been mistaken for angina. Persistent pain, known as postherpetic neuralgia (PHN), is relatively uncommon in children, but occurs in 50% of individuals with zoster who are older than 60 years and may be severe and protracted. Zosteriform eruptions in the maxillary division of the fifth cranial nerve may occasionally be due to HSV rather than VZV, and hence, laboratory diagnostic evaluation is advised.

VZV reactivation less frequently may occur in the absence of skin rash (zoster sine herpete); these patients may present with aseptic meningitis or encephalitis as well as with gastrointestinal tract involvement. Visceral zoster can arise from reactivation of latent VZV in the enteric nervous system.

Generalized or disseminated zoster may occur in immunocompromised hosts. The greater the extent of immunosuppression, the higher is the risk of dissemination to noncontiguous dermatomes or to viscera. Multiorgan involvement may precede or follow rash in the untreated immunocompromised host, as has been described for varicella in this high-risk population. Immunosuppressed patients are also at relatively higher risk for PHN.

Zoster should in general prompt specific treatment because antiviral agents given within 72 hours of onset reduce the severity and duration of symptoms and PHN. Oral therapy is usually suitable for immunocompetent persons, but IV acyclovir should be considered in those at risk of severe disease. Pain relief and other supportive measures may be required. In addition, individuals with ophthalmic involvement require specific evaluation and management. Disseminated zoster is a severe systemic illness that may require intensive care, as for severe varicella.

The Oka vaccine strain has been developed into a shingles vaccine, with much higher concentrations of virus compared with those in the varicella monovalent and quadrivalent vaccine products. In addition, a new adjuvanted inactivated vaccine is in development and has demonstrated very encouraging efficacy rates for prevention of both zoster and PHN in adults.

## SUGGESTED READINGS


American Academy of Pediatrics Committee on Infectious Diseases. Varicella-zoster infections. In: *Red Book: 2015 Report of the Committee on Infectious Diseases*. 30th ed. Elk Grove Village, IL: American Academy of Pediatrics; 2015:846-860.

Bialek SR, Perella D, Zhang J, et al. Impact of a routine two-dose varicella vaccination program on varicella epidemiology. *Pediatrics*. 2013;132:e1134-e1140.

Chen J, Gershon AA, Li Z, Cowles RA, Gershon MD. Varicella zoster virus (VZV) infects and establishes latency in enteric neurons. *J Neurovirol*. 2011;17:578-589.

Lal H, Cunningham AL, Godeaux O, et al. Efficacy of an adjuvanted herpes zoster subunit vaccine in older adults. *N Engl J Med*. 2015;372:2087-2096.

Leung J, Harpaz R. Impact of the maturing varicella vaccination program on varicella and related outcomes in the United States: 1994–2012. *J Pediatr Infect Dis Soc*. 2016;5(4):395-402.

Marin M, Marti M, Kambhampati A, Jeram SM, Seward JF. Global varicella vaccine effectiveness: a meta-analysis. *Pediatrics*. 2016;137:e20153741.

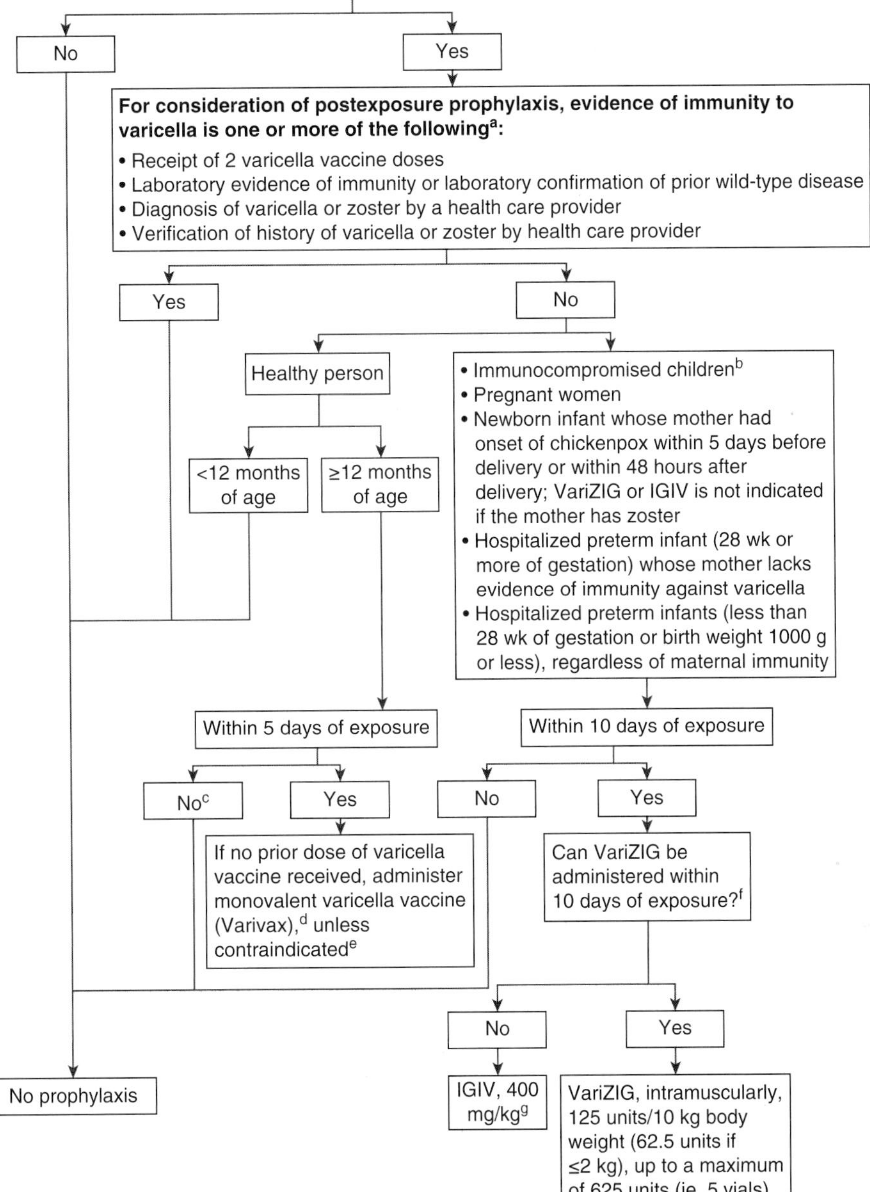


a. People who receive hematopoietic stem cell transplants should be considered nonimmune regardless of previous history of varicella disease or varicella vaccination in themselves or in their donors.

b. Immunocompromised children include those with congenital or acquired T-lymphocyte immunodeficiency, including leukemia, lymphoma, and other malignant neoplasms affecting the bone marrow or lymphatic system; children receiving immunosuppressive therapy, including ≥2 mg/kg/day of systemic prednisone (or its equivalent) for ≥14 days; all children with human immunodeficiency virus (HIV) infection regardless of CD4+ T-lymphocyte percentage; and all hematopoietic stem cell transplant patients regardless of pretransplant immunity status.

c. No postexposure prophylaxis, but age-appropriate vaccination still recommended for protection against subsequent exposures. If the exposure occurred during an outbreak, 2-dose vaccination is recommended for preschool-aged children younger than 4 years for outbreak control.

d. If 1 prior dose of varicella vaccine has been received, a second dose should be administered at ≥4 years of age. If the exposure occurred during an outbreak, a second dose is recommended for preschool-aged children younger than 4 years for outbreak control.

e. Contraindications include patients who are allergic to a vaccine component, or who are immunocompromised (see above footnote), or pregnant. Caution should be used in patients receiving salicylates. Vaccine may not be as effective if patient has recently received Immune Globulin Intravenous, whole blood, or plasma transfusions, and for this reason, it is recommended that varicella vaccine be withheld for 3 to 11 months, depending on the dose, after administration of these products.

f. Varicella Zoster Immune Globulin (VariZIG) was approved by the US Food and Drug Administration in December 2012. The product is manufactured by Cangene Corporation (Winnipeg, Canada) and distributed in the United States by FFF Enterprises (Temecula, California; 800-843-7477; **www.fffenterprises.com**) and ASD Healthcare (Frisco, TX) (telephone, 800-746-6273; online at **www.asdhealthcare.com**).

g. If VariZIG and IGIV are not available, some experts recommend prophylaxis with oral acyclovir (20 mg/kg per dose administered 4 times per day, with a maximum daily dose of 3200 mg) or oral valacyclovir (if >3 months of age; 20 mg/kg per dose administered 3 times per day, with a maximum daily dose of 3000 mg) beginning 7 to 10 days after exposure and continuing for 7 days.

**FIGURE 309-2** Management of exposures to varicella-zoster virus. IVIG, intravenous immunoglobulin; VariZIG, varicella-zoster immunoglobin. (Reproduced with permission from Kimberlin DW, Brady MT, Jackson MA, et al: *Red Book: 2015 Report of the Committee on Infectious Diseases*, 30th ed. Elk Grove Village, IL: American Academy of Pediatrics; 2015.)

Science M, MacGregor D, Richardson SE, Mahant S, Tran D, Bitnun A. Central nervous system complications of varicella-zoster virus. *J Pediatr*. 2014;165:779-785.

Thomas CA, Shwe T, Bixler D, et al. Two-dose varicella vaccine effectiveness and rash severity in outbreaks of varicella among public school students. *Pediatr Infect Dis J*. 2014;33:1164-1168.

van de Wetering MD, Vossen MT, Jansen MH, Caron HN, Kuijpers TW. Varicella vaccination in pediatric oncology patients without interruption of chemotherapy. *J Clin Virol*. 2016;75:47-52.

# 310 Human Immunodeficiency Virus Type 1 Infection

Jonathan Honegger and Joshua R. Watson

## INTRODUCTION

Approximately 2.1 million children younger than age 15 years were living with human immunodeficiency virus type 1 (HIV-1) infection in 2016, including 160,000 newly infected children. In the same year, nearly 120,000 children died from acquired immunodeficiency syndrome (AIDS)-related illnesses, and hundreds of thousands more children lost one or both parents to HIV. HIV clearly continues to exert a devastating effect on global child health. Nevertheless, expanded access to antiretroviral therapy (ART) is turning the tide of this epidemic. The numbers of children newly infected with HIV-1 and children dying of AIDS-related illness in 2016 were approximately half what they were in 2010. For many children with access to ART, HIV-1 has become a manageable, chronic disease rather a certain cause of early death.

## PATHOGENESIS AND EPIDEMIOLOGY

HIV-1 is a retrovirus that preferentially infects activated CD4+ T lymphocytes expressing the cytokine receptors CCR5 or CXCR4, which act as viral co-receptors. Acute HIV infection is marked by high-level viral replication and cytolytic destruction of CD4+ T lymphocytes, particularly the abundant gut-associated CD4+CCR5+ T lymphocytes. This is followed by gradual attrition of circulating CD4+ T-lymphocyte populations as disease progresses. The mechanisms by which HIV-1 infection causes this CD4+ cell decline is not completely established, although possibilities include ongoing lytic infection, destruction of infected cells by host antiviral immune mechanisms, and death or dysfunction of lymphocyte precursors or accessory cells in the thymus and lymph nodes.

Once established, HIV-1 infection invariably persists. In the absence of ART, HIV continuously replicates and infects newly activated CD4+ T lymphocytes. Ongoing generation of viral variants bearing escape mutations in immune epitopes contributes to evasion of host-neutralizing antibodies and cytotoxic T cells. Additionally, HIV-1 genomes integrate into the host chromosomal DNA to establish latent infection. Resting memory CD4+ T lymphocytes appear to be the most important reservoir of latent HIV-1 infection. These cells stably harbor HIV-1 genomes even after years of viral suppression with ART, allowing viral rebound when ART is stopped. Early initiation of combination antiretroviral therapy (cART) may limit the extent of the latent viral reservoir. In addition to CD4+ T lymphocytes, other cells types such as tissue-resident macrophages can also be infected by HIV-1. These cells may also function as long-term viral reservoirs and contribute to organ-specific pathology, although some controversy remains. Even in individuals well controlled on cART, HIV-1 DNA may be recovered from brain, lung, liver, kidney, testes, and other tissues. HIV-1 -related pathology involves many organs, although it is often difficult to know whether injury is primarily a consequence of local virus infection, immune-mediated cytotoxic effects, or associated infectious complications.

The primary modes of HIV-1 transmission include sexual contact, percutaneous exposure, and mother-to-child transmission. The vast majority of pediatric infections have been acquired by mother-to-child transmission, which can occur in utero, at the time of delivery, or postnatally via breast milk. In the absence of ART and other protective measures, the risk of transmission by these routes is 5% to 10%, 10% to 20%, and 5% to 15%, respectively. Transmission during the peripartum period may occur through transplacental passage of virus (in late pregnancy or at the time of labor) or by mucosal exposure to infectious secretions or blood during birth. Many maternal and obstetric factors contribute to the risk of perinatal transmission, including high maternal viral load, advanced maternal disease, prolonged rupture of membranes, and prematurity. However, neither these factors nor other clinical or immunologic data are completely predictive of transmission. Of all identified risk factors, reducing the mother's viral load with ART offers the greatest opportunity to intervene to lower the risk of perinatal transmission.

Rates of mother-to-child transmission of HIV-1 have fallen sharply in countries with widespread access to ART. Other routes of infection in young children, such as child sexual abuse and transfusion of contaminated blood products, result in a very small number of HIV infections in developed nations. In the United States, the number of new HIV-1 diagnoses among children younger than 15 years fell from a high of 2500 per year in the early 1990s to 145 in 2015. New infections among adolescents, mostly acquired by sexual exposure or injection drug use, have not declined as quickly. Over 1600 adolescents aged 15 to 19 years were newly diagnosed with HIV-1 in the United States in 2015.

## CLINICAL MANIFESTATIONS

### Staging

The current Centers for Disease Control and Prevention case definition system for classifying adult and pediatric HIV-1 infections highlights the importance of CD4+ T-cell depletion in the pathogenesis of HIV-1. HIV-1 infection stage is determined by age-based CD4+ T-cell count criteria (Table 310-1). CD4+ T-cell percentage is used for staging when absolute CD4+ T-cell counts are not available. Patients with specific acquired immunodeficiency syndrome (AIDS)-defining clinical illnesses indicative of severe immunosuppression (Table 310-2) are classified as stage 3 regardless of CD4+ T-cell count.

### Infant Infection

Perinatal HIV-1 infection is most often clinically silent at birth. In some instances, adenopathy may be detected in the first month of life. The "incubation period," or interval before symptoms of HIV-1 infection become manifest, is generally shorter following perinatal infection than in adult HIV-1 infection. Viral load (determined by HIV-1 RNA polymerase chain reaction [PCR] quantification) in infants is typically high (> $10^5$ copies/mL) and often does not decline

**TABLE 310-1 HIV INFECTION STAGE[a] BASED ON AGE-SPECIFIC CD4+ T-LYMPHOCYTE COUNT (/μL) OR CD4+ T-LYMPHOCYTE PERCENTAGE OF TOTAL LYMPHOCYTES**

| | Age | | |
|---|---|---|---|
| Immunologic Classification | < 1 Year | 1–5 Years | ≥ 6 Years |
| Stage 1 | ≥ 1500 | ≥ 1000 | ≥ 500 |
| | ≥ 34% | ≥ 30% | ≥ 26% |
| Stage 2: Evidence of moderate immune suppression | 750–1499 | 500–999 | 200–499 |
| | 26–33% | 22–29% | 14–25% |
| Stage 3: Severe immune suppression | < 750 | < 500 | < 200 |
| | < 26% | < 22% | < 14% |

[a]Stage is based on CD4+ T-lymphocyte count. The CD4+ T-lymphocyte percentage is used for staging when the CD4+ T-lymphocyte count is not available. If a stage 3 opportunistic infection (Table 310-2) has been identified, the individual is classified as stage 3 regardless of CD4+ T-lymphocyte test results.

Reproduced with permission from Centers for Disease Control and Prevention (CDC): Revised surveillance case definition for HIV infection—United States, 2014, *MMWR Recomm Rep*. 2014 Apr 11;63(RR-03):1-10.

**TABLE 310-2 STAGE 3-DEFINING OPPORTUNISTIC ILLNESSES IN HIV INFECTION**

| |
|---|
| Bacterial infections, multiple or recurrent[a] |
| Candidiasis of bronchi, trachea, or lungs |
| Candidiasis of esophagus |
| Cervical cancer, invasive[b] |
| Coccidioidomycosis, disseminated or extrapulmonary |
| Cryptococcosis, extrapulmonary |
| Cryptosporidiosis, chronic intestinal (> 1 month in duration) |
| Cytomegalovirus disease (other than liver, spleen, or nodes), onset at age > 1 month |
| Cytomegalovirus retinitis (with loss of vision) |
| Encephalopathy attributed to HIV |
| Herpes simplex: chronic ulcers (> 1 month in duration) or bronchitis, pneumonitis, or esophagitis (onset at age > 1 month) |
| Histoplasmosis, disseminated or extrapulmonary |
| Isosporiasis, chronic intestinal (> 1 month in duration) |
| Kaposi sarcoma |
| Lymphoma, Burkitt (or equivalent term) |
| Lymphoma, immunoblastic (or equivalent term) |
| Lymphoma, primary, of brain |
| *Mycobacterium avium* complex or *Mycobacterium kansasii*, disseminated or extrapulmonary |
| *Mycobacterium tuberculosis* of any site, pulmonary[b], disseminated, or extrapulmonary |
| *Mycobacterium*, other species or unidentified species, disseminated or extrapulmonary |
| *Pneumocystis jirovecii* (previously known as *Pneumocystis carinii*) pneumonia |
| Pneumonia, recurrent[b] |
| Progressive multifocal leukoencephalopathy |
| *Salmonella* septicemia, recurrent |
| Toxoplasmosis of brain, onset at age > 1 month |
| Wasting syndrome attributed to HIV |

[a]Only among children age < 6 years.

[b]Only among adults, adolescents, and children age ≥ 6 years.

Reproduced with permission from Centers for Disease Control and Prevention (CDC): Revised surveillance case definition for HIV infection—United States, 2014, *MMWR Recomm Rep.* 2014 Apr 11;63(RR-03):1-10.

to a stable set point for several years. This protracted high-level viremia is likely due to immune immaturity, but it may also reflect the high thymic output of CD4+ T lymphocytes in early childhood that essentially provides "fuel" for viral replication.

Clinically silent abnormalities of immune function often precede HIV-1–related symptoms. Hypergammaglobulinemia with production of nonfunctional antibodies (polyclonal B-cell stimulation) is more common among HIV-1–infected infants than among adults, typically noted as early as 3 to 6 months of age. Despite the abundance of immunoglobulins, there is an inability to respond to new antigens with appropriate specific immunoglobulin production. This critically affects infants without prior antigen exposure, contributing to the greater frequency and severity of invasive bacterial infections seen in pediatric HIV-1 infection. Frequencies of circulating CD4+ T lymphocytes often drop by 1 to 2 months of age in vertically infected children, but CD4+ depletion may not be readily apparent because of the higher baseline percentage and absolute numbers of lymphocytes in infants and young children than adults. The absolute CD4+ count is not as predictive of the risk for opportunistic infections in infants as it is for older children and adults.

The earliest and most common HIV-1–associated symptoms in infancy are nonspecific and rarely diagnostic. The first abnormalities detected include fever, failure to thrive, hepatosplenomegaly, generalized lymphadenopathy, parotitis, and diarrhea. Prior to the early use of cART, approximately 90% of perinatally HIV-1–infected infants would manifest 1 or more of these symptoms in the first year of life. In 1 study, the conditions that best discriminated between untreated HIV-1–infected and uninfected infants were chronic candidiasis, parotitis, persistent lymphadenopathy, and hepatosplenomegaly.

Approximately 20% of untreated HIV-1–infected infants present with rapidly progressive immune compromise and/or an AIDS-defining condition, such as *Pneumocystis jirovecii* pneumonia (PCP), or serious bacterial or fungal infections within the first 3 to 6 months of life. These infants have a high rate of mortality in the first year of life.

Beyond infancy, common symptoms of untreated HIV-1 infection in childhood include persistent adenopathy, hepatosplenomegaly, recurrent or chronic infections, growth failure, and developmental delay. With the exception of linear growth abnormalities, most of these symptoms are significantly less common and/or less severe with aggressive cART. With successful ART (good adherence and undetectable viral load), opportunistic infections are extremely rare. The development or worsening of HIV-1–related symptoms while receiving effective ART suggests clinical failure and possible resistance to 1 or more of the medications in the treatment regimen.

### Childhood and Adult Infection

Hallmark stages of HIV-1 infection acquired in childhood or adulthood include an acute infection phase (seroconversion syndrome), often with flu-like symptoms and high-grade viremia; followed by a period of immune containment of viral replication, during which the individual is usually free of symptoms; and a final period of progressive symptomatic immune compromise, with increasing viral replication. During the asymptomatic phase, gradual and progressive abnormalities of immune function appear on testing. Viral load is usually lower than during the acute infection phase and may remain relatively stable at a "set point" for months to years. The rapidity with which an infected adult or child progresses through the asymptomatic phase can be predicted to some degree by determining the individual's CD4+ cell count and viral load. Lower CD4+ cell counts and higher viral loads are each independent predictors of more rapid disease progression. The final phase, with symptomatic immune compromise, end-organ dysfunction, and HIV-1–associated malignancies, is correlated with increasing viral replication and often a change in viral tropism from use of cytokine receptor CCR5 to CXCR4, profound attrition of CD4+ T lymphocytes, severe immune dysregulation (not just immune deficiency), and opportunistic infections.

### Associated Clinical Disease

***Pneumocystis jirovecii* Pneumonia** PCP is one of the common AIDS indicator diseases in children and adults, and it previously affected approximately one-third of HIV-1–infected infants and children. The median age for presentation following perinatal HIV-1 infection is approximately 9 months, although there is a peak at 3 to 6 months of age among rapidly progressing and previously unidentified HIV-1–infected infants. Unlike reactivation PCP in adults, this infection is usually a primary infection in HIV-1–infected children, presenting subacutely or abruptly with fever, cough, tachypnea, rales, and often hypoxia. PCP may be difficult to distinguish clinically and radiologically from other pulmonary infections at this age. Extrapulmonary *Pneumocystis* involvement is rarely identified. Because early administration of intravenous trimethoprim-sulfamethoxazole (TMP-SMX) and corticosteroids (for infants with significant oxygen requirement) may lead to marked improvement, diagnostic bronchoalveolar lavage should be considered early in the course of illness in the infant with a consistent clinical presentation and risk factors for HIV-1 infection. In very young infants, PCP may still be associated with a high mortality rate. Milder disease may occur in both young infants and older children.

**Lymphoid Interstitial Pneumonitis** This chronic interstitial infiltration of the lungs by polyclonal B cells and T cells has been described in a small number of HIV-1–infected adults but is seen in 20% to 25% of children with untreated perinatally acquired HIV-1. There may be an association with Epstein-Barr virus infection. The condition is characterized by insidious onset of chronic cough and tachypnea with intermittent exacerbations (often during intercurrent respiratory infections). Chronic chest infiltrates seen on radiograph often suggest the diagnosis. Open-lung biopsy can provide a definitive diagnosis but may be unnecessary in an HIV-1–infected child with consistent clinical findings. Hypoxia is seldom severe until the condition has been present for many years. Improvement with corticosteroid use has been reported. As a presenting symptom of HIV-1 infection, lymphoid interstitial pneumonitis (LIP) is associated with a better prognosis than AIDS indicator diseases and is often seen in a symptom cluster with marked hypergammaglobulinemia, parotitis, hepatosplenomegaly, and massive adenopathy. Initiation of ART has been associated with clinical improvement.

**Recurrent Bacterial Infections** These are defined as 2 or more episodes of sepsis, meningitis, pneumonia, internal abscesses, or bone and joint infection. Prior to aggressive ART, PCP prophylaxis with TMP-SMX, and pneumococcal conjugate vaccine, recurrent bacterial infections were seen in approximately 15% of children with pediatric AIDS. The frequency of bacterial infections is far less in children receiving these protective measures. Less invasive bacterial infections, such as chronic or recurrent sinus infections, otitis media, and pyodermas, are somewhat more common in HIV-1–infected children. *Streptococcus pneumoniae* is the most frequent blood isolate in HIV-1–infected children, although gram-negative enteric (including *Salmonella*), staphylococcal, and even pseudomonal bacteremia are also seen more commonly in HIV-1–infected children.

**Other Opportunistic Infections** More than a dozen specific opportunistic infections meet the AIDS definition (see Table 310-2). After PCP and recurrent bacterial infections, the most common opportunistic infection in pediatric AIDS patients are *Candida* esophagitis and *Mycobacterium avium* complex infection. The most common AIDS-defining viral illnesses include recurrent, prolonged, or disseminated infections with cytomegalovirus (CMV), particularly of the gastrointestinal tract (CMV retinitis occurs in children but is less common than in adults), and recurrent, extensive, and atypical infections with herpes simplex and varicella-zoster. Despite the long list of pathogens causing unusually severe or protracted illness in HIV-1–infected children, common respiratory viruses, including respiratory syncytial virus, seldom cause complicated illness.

**Progressive Neurologic Disease** Central and peripheral nervous system disease occurs more commonly and at an earlier point in HIV-1 disease in children than it does in adults. Prior to availability of ART, as many as 25% of HIV-infected infants had central nervous system (CNS) involvement manifested as a static encephalopathy, usually presenting as developmental delay in the first year of life. Neuroimaging may reveal cerebral atrophy, white matter abnormalities, and/or basal ganglion calcifications, although the severity of imaging abnormalities often does not correlate with clinical findings. Because this progressive syndrome is identified less commonly in the era of cART, it would appear that successful control of viral replication can either prohibit ongoing CNS damage from virus already present in the CNS or reduce new virus entry into the CNS. Capacity of antiretroviral agents to penetrate the CNS is an important consideration in the selection of HIV-1 treatment regimens for infants. Prevention of HIV encephalopathy is one rationale for early initiation of cART in all HIV-1–infected infants.

**Failure to Thrive** Failure to thrive is seen in many infants and children with advanced HIV-1 infection. It is nearly always multifactorial. Metabolic needs are increased by HIV-1 and associated opportunistic infections. Feeding can be hindered by neurologic deficits; generalized malaise; or oral pain from thrush (*Candida albicans* and other yeasts), herpes simplex, and aphthous ulcers. Chronic diarrhea may contribute to malabsorption. Initiation of cART often results in at least partial catch-up growth in weight and height.

**Other Organ Involvement** Hepatic involvement in pediatric HIV-1 infection often takes the form of hepatomegaly with mild-to-moderate, fluctuating transaminitis. Less common is a severe cholestatic hepatitis seen in infected infants in the first year of life, with a poor prognosis. Liver abnormalities may be a result of HIV-1 infection, concomitant infection with the common viruses causing hepatitis (eg, CMV; hepatitis A, B, and C; Epstein-Barr virus), or toxicity from many of the medications used to treat HIV-1. Increased translocation of intestinal bacterial products may contribute to hepatic inflammation in HIV. Renal disease is not uncommon, with proteinuria the most likely finding. Focal glomerulosclerosis and mesangial changes have been identified in children with advanced HIV-1 infection. Without ART, abnormalities may be demonstrable in as many as 50% of children at all stages of HIV-1 disease, although the incidence of symptomatic cardiomyopathy is only 12% to 20%, and it occurs late in advanced disease; ventricular dysfunction and pericardial effusion are the most commonly encountered echocardiographic abnormalities. Despite the frequency of chronic pulmonary disease in HIV-1–infected children, left ventricular involvement is several times more common than is right ventricular involvement. Direct HIV-1 infection, immune-mediated damage, malnutrition, and concomitant infection with myotropic viruses have all been suggested as etiologies for cardiomyopathy. Autoimmune phenomena include Coombs-positive hemolytic anemia, thrombocytopenia, and aphthous ulcers. Kaposi sarcoma and other secondary cancers occur but are uncommon in HIV-1–infected children.

## DIAGNOSIS

Early diagnosis of the infected infant is critically important, but early (prenatal) identification of the infant at risk for HIV-1 infection is equally vital. Only when HIV-1 infection in the pregnant woman is recognized is there an opportunity to implement strategies to prevent transmission and to screen exposed infants. HIV-1 screening and counseling should be a routine part of pregnancy care. Initial testing of the mother should be performed in the first trimester (or first visit if later than first trimester) using current HIV-1/2 combination antibody/antigen assays. Repeat HIV testing in the third trimester (prior to 36 weeks of gestation) is recommended for pregnant women at increased risk for infection. Rapid HIV-1 antibody testing is advised for women who present to labor and delivery with unknown HIV status or ongoing high risk of infection.

The persistence of transplacentally acquired maternal antibody to HIV-1 in the infant complicates the use of conventional IgG antibody tests in diagnosing HIV-1 infection in infancy. Because such HIV-1 antibodies may remain in uninfected infants' blood for up to 24 months, diagnosis of HIV-1 infection in the infant at risk requires the demonstration of HIV-1 nucleic acid in the peripheral blood by nucleic acid tests (NAT), namely HIV-1 DNA PCR or HIV-1 RNA PCR. Although the HIV-1 RNA PCR could be rendered falsely negative in an infected infant who is on antiretroviral prophylaxis, in practice, the current highly sensitive HIV-1 RNA PCR assays function as well as HIV-1 DNA PCR for screening vertically exposed infants. Serial virologic testing with either HIV-1 DNA PCR or HIV-1 RNA PCR can be expected to establish or exclude the diagnosis of HIV infection in an infant by 4 months of age with greater than 99% confidence. Performed appropriately, these tests have an acceptably low rate of false positivity and can be relied on to confirm infection at any age. The sensitivity of each is somewhat lower in the immediate perinatal period (prior to 4 weeks of age), making serial testing necessary. HIV-1 culture and p24 antigen assays are not advised for screening vertically exposed infants. Culture is not widely available and has a slow turnaround time, while p24 antigen assays have lower sensitivity than the HIV-1 NAT assays.

The optimal schedule for testing HIV-exposed infant includes HIV-1 NAT testing at 14 to 21 days, 4 to 6 weeks, and 4 to 6 months of age. Some experts also advise a test in the first 2 to 3 days after birth to identify infants who are viremic at birth from infection presumably acquired in utero. Because zidovudine monotherapy is used commonly in HIV-1–exposed newborns, this early test can help avoid prolonged monotherapy, which could foster development of resistance. *Presumptive* noninfection with HIV-1 can be determined with negative tests at ≥ 2 and ≥ 4 weeks of age (or 1 negative test at ≥ 8 weeks of age).

Definitive exclusion of infection with HIV-1 requires 2 negative virologic tests, with 1 at ≥ 4 weeks of age and 1 at ≥ 4 months of age. Most experts still recommend HIV-1 antibody testing at 24 months of age to ensure noninfection of the child. Before parents are told that a child is infected, confirmation and review of all laboratory tests are imperative.

When infants or children without recognized risk factors for HIV-1 infection present with findings or signs compatible with immunodeficiency, the diagnosis of HIV-1 should be entertained along with other causes of immunodeficiency. That HIV-1 infection is currently the leading cause of immunodeficiency in young children may prove helpful when counseling parents concerning the need to include HIV-1 testing in any comprehensive evaluation of immunodeficiency in children. Although age-based CD4+ lymphocyte parameters are important for staging HIV-1 immunosuppression for surveillance purposes (see Table 310-1), as many as 15% of patients with pediatric AIDS may have a normal absolute number of CD4+ lymphocytes. Neither absolute numbers nor percentage of CD4+ lymphocytes can be relied upon entirely to identify HIV-1–infected infants with immune dysfunction and risk for opportunistic infections. Thus, HIV-1–specific testing should be performed when the possibility of HIV-1 infection needs to be ruled out.

In vertically exposed children over age 24 months or children of any age with nonvertical exposure to HIV, the preferred HIV testing algorithm begins with a fourth-generation HIV-1/2 combination antibody/antigen assay. Inclusion of the p24 antigen test in this combination assay permits potential detection of acute HIV infection prior to seroconversion. A positive antibody/antigen assay should be followed by an HIV-1/HIV-2 antibody differentiating immunoassay to confirm the diagnosis and to distinguish HIV-1 infection from the much rarer HIV-2 infection, which requires distinct testing and management. A negative or indeterminate HIV-1/2 differentiating antibody test could indicate acute infection and should be followed by an HIV-1 RNA PCR. For the child presenting with potential recent exposure and concern for possible acute HIV, HIV-1 RNA PCR should be incorporated in the initial screening testing.

Alternative testing algorithms include enzyme-linked immunosorbent assay–based antibody screening followed by confirmatory Western blot testing. This approach is more likely to miss acute HIV infection and to misclassify HIV-2 infections as HIV-1. Other rare diagnostic pitfalls encountered when using serology alone include HIV-1–infected infants who produce no HIV-1–specific antibody (generally infants with marked immunodeficiency and associated clinical symptoms) and the extremely rare instance of infected infants who become seronegative when transplacental antibody disappears and before endogenous antibody is produced.

## TREATMENT

Care of children with or at risk of HIV-1 infection requires a skilled team approach that includes medical specialists, primary care physicians, nurses, social workers, dietitians, pharmacists, and developmental experts. Extensive psychosocial support is often necessary for families. Early coordination of patient management with a team skilled in the care of children with HIV-1 infection will facilitate later care.

Medical care of infants at risk of HIV-1 infection whose infection status remains uncertain requires careful prospective evaluation for early signs and symptoms of HIV-1 infection. Initial and subsequent visits of the perinatally exposed infant should include a thorough history and physical examination, with particular evaluation for failure to thrive, unexplained fevers, persistent or recurrent oral or diaper candidiasis, parotitis, pulmonary symptoms and findings, generalized lymphadenopathy, hepatomegaly, splenomegaly, neurologic abnormalities, and developmental delay. Because serious bacterial infections or opportunistic infections such as PCP may be the first clinical presentation associated with HIV-1 infection, febrile episodes and respiratory illnesses should be aggressively managed in at-risk infants. Assessment of the infant with HIV-1 nucleic acid and antibody tests should be performed as described in the earlier section on HIV-1 diagnosis. In addition, testing may be required for siblings, parents, and the parents' sexual partners.

Assessment of the HIV-1–infected child should include a thorough physical examination and laboratory evaluation. To test for HIV-associated conditions (eg, cytopenias, kidney disease, hepatitis) and to set the baseline for monitoring of antiretroviral toxicity, complete blood count with differential, comprehensive metabolic panel, urinalysis, and serum lipids should be measured in newly diagnosed children prior to initiation of ART. Immunologic testing (CD4+ cell count and quantitative immunoglobulins) will aid in decisions regarding PCP prophylaxis, intravenous immunoglobulin (IVIG) therapy, and initiation of ART. Quantitative HIV-1 RNA PCR (viral load) and antiretroviral drug-resistance testing should also be obtained at the time of diagnosis. Viral load and CD4+ cell counts are independent predictors for risk of disease progression and should be monitored every 3 to 4 months whether or not the child is started on ART. Clinical well-being in HIV-1–infected children can be estimated by assessment of growth rate (weight, length, and head circumference), developmental achievement, and experience with bacterial and viral infections. Following these clinical and laboratory parameters should assist in decisions concerning initiation and switching ART, prophylaxis for opportunistic infections, nutritional interventions, and psychosocial support efforts.

### Antiretroviral Therapy

Updated information on the most current recommendations for treating HIV-1–infected children can be obtained by accessing the Web site of the HIV/AIDS Treatment Information Service (www.aidsinfo.nih.gov). Because treatment recommendations change frequently, consultation with an expert in pediatric HIV-1 infection is recommended.

ART for HIV-1–infected children has undergone a dramatic evolution over the past 2 decades. What began as serial monotherapy with agents used as soon as they became available has become a more sophisticated use of combination therapies guided by careful monitoring of viral load and clinical and immunologic responses. The currently available antiretroviral agents can be divided into 5 distinct categories: (1) nucleoside/nucleotide reverse transcriptase inhibitors (NRTIs), (2) nonnucleoside reverse transcriptase inhibitors (NNRTIs), (3) protease inhibitors (PIs), (4) integrase strand transfer inhibitors (INSTIs), and (5) entry and fusion inhibitors (Table 310-3). For treatment-naïve children, cART should usually be initiated with a combination of 3 drugs. The most effective regimens have included 2 NRTIs (the so-called "backbone" of cART) in combination with either an NNRTI, protease inhibitor, or INSTI. Considerations when choosing a regimen include patient age, results of antiretroviral resistance testing, barriers to adherence, drug toxicities, and differing drug formulations, among others.

Based on pediatric and adult studies of immediate versus deferred therapy, cART is recommended for all HIV-1–infected children regardless of clinical symptoms, immune status, or viral load, although the urgency and strength of the recommendation vary by age and level

**TABLE 310-3 ANTIRETROVIRAL AGENTS**

| Reverse Transcriptase Inhibitors | | | | |
|---|---|---|---|---|
| Nucleoside/ Nucleotide | Nonnucleoside | Protease Inhibitors | Entry and Fusion Inhibitors | Integrase Inhibitors |
| Abacavir | Delavirdine | Atazanavir | Enfuvirtide | Dolutegravir |
| Didanosine | Efavirenz | Darunavir | Maraviroc | Elvitegravir |
| Emtricitabine | Etravirine | Fosamprenavir | | Raltegravir |
| Lamivudine | Nevirapine | Indinavir | | |
| Stavudine | Rilpivirine | Lopinavir | | |
| Tenofovir | | Ritonavir | | |
| Zidovudine | | Nelfinavir | | |
| | | Saquinavir | | |
| | | Tipranavir | | |

of immune suppression. Because approximately one-sixth of HIV-1–infected children experience rapid progression beginning in the first year of life, initiation of cART is urgent in every child younger than 1 year as soon as the diagnosis is established. Therapy is also considered urgent for children > 1 year of age with an opportunistic illness (infection, HIV-associated malignancy, encephalopathy, or progressive multifocal leukoencephalopathy), as well as for children 1 to 5 years of age with CD4+ cell count < 500 cells/μL and children ≥ 6 years of age with CD4+ cell count < 200 cells/μL.

Once a decision is made to treat, it should be expected that ART will continue for the remainder of the child's life. Factors to be considered in decisions about initiation of therapy include the risk of disease progression as determined by CD4+ cell count and viral load, the potential benefits and risks of therapy, and the ability of the child and caregiver to adhere to administration of the therapeutic regimen. Issues associated with adherence should be fully assessed, discussed, and addressed with the child, if age-appropriate, and caregiver before the decision to initiate therapy is made. Complicating factors include lack of a liquid preparation for some of the medications, tablets in dose forms appropriate for adults only, poor palatability, and the effect of food on absorption. Regimens that do not optimally suppress viral replication are associated with poorer clinical outcomes and a higher likelihood for the development of resistance to the medications being administered.

Innovative measures can assist families in administering these medications to children. Children as young as 3 years can be taught how to take pills. Mixing medications with certain strong-tasting foods or liquids, or coating the mouth with peanut butter, can help with acceptance of medications that are poor tasting. A gastrostomy tube is an effective way to avoid many of the problems associated with the chronic administration of ART. However, tremendous psychosocial support of the child and caregiver, understanding of the difficulty with administering medications, and careful coaching in how best to administer medications may prove to be the most helpful in enhancing adherence to cumbersome combination regimens.

Clinical and laboratory parameters need to be monitored carefully to detect any evidence of medication toxicity or treatment failure. ART adverse events vary by medication, but some of the more common include neuropsychiatric symptoms (eg, abnormal dreams, depression), gastrointestinal symptoms (eg, nausea/vomiting, diarrhea), rash (rarely severe), lipodystrophy, low bone mineral density, dyslipidemia, hyperglycemia, hematologic abnormalities (eg, anemia, neutropenia), lactic acidosis, nephrotoxicity, and hepatotoxicity. To monitor for treatment failure, CD4+ cell count and viral load should be monitored routinely every 3 to 4 months for at least the first 2 years of therapy. In children who are adherent to therapy, have CD4+ cell counts well above the threshold for opportunistic infection risk, and have stable clinical status and viral suppression for more than 2 years, less frequent CD4+ cell count monitoring (every 6–12 months) may be considered. Effective cART should result in maximal viral load reduction by 12 to 16 weeks after initiation of therapy. Virologic failure, defined as a repeated viral load > 200 copies/mL after 6 months of therapy, suggests either a lack of adherence to the prescribed regimen or the presence or development of resistant virus.

Decisions concerning change in ART should be guided primarily by the child's prior medication history and antiretroviral resistance testing, including both past and current resistance test results. The initial antiretroviral regimen that a child receives is the one most likely to achieve a sustained antiviral effect. In cases of virologic failure due to resistance, subsequent regimens are likely to be less effective because of the impact of cross-resistance to prior medications. When resistance is suspected, the optimal approach to changing therapy is to make a complete shift in prescribed medications, with the hope that the new regimen includes at least 2 medications to which the child's virus is susceptible and, optimally, to which the child has not been previously exposed. For example, if the child has already received a PI, it may be appropriate to replace the PI with an NNRTI or INSTI, or vice versa. Alternate categories of ART are now available (eg, entry and fusion inhibitors) and may be sufficiently different from those previously administered to make cross-resistance less likely.

Clinical status at the time of initial presentation appears to correlate with prognosis in perinatally infected children. Perinatally HIV-1–infected infants appear to follow 2 basic patterns of disease progression. Approximately 20% of perinatally infected infants progress rapidly and develop severe immune suppression and stage 3 disease in the first year of life if not treated appropriately. The majority of infants, however, have slower disease progression. Approximately 75% develop severe immune suppression by 6 to 10 years of age.

Since the availability of NNRTIs, PIs, and optimal opportunistic infection prophylaxis, most pediatric HIV-1 treatment centers have documented marked reductions in both new opportunistic infections and mortality in HIV-1–infected children, who now experience immunologic improvement or stabilization with cART. In a multicenter study of > 3500 HIV-1–infected children, most of whom were perinatally infected, mortality decreased from 7.2 deaths per 100 person-years in 1994 to 0.8 deaths per 100 person-years in 2000. Lower CD4+ cell count and presence of an AIDS-defining illness at the time of study entry were associated with increased risk for death. Reductions in mortality over time paralleled increased use of cART. Even though mortality rates in HIV-1–infected children are still 30 times higher than similarly aged children in the United States, with appropriate antiretroviral regimens and strict adherence to administering the prescribed medications, survival well into adulthood should be expected for the majority of HIV-1–infected children.

Persons infected with HIV-1 during adolescence are often not diagnosed until early adulthood. Many at-risk adolescents fail to access systems likely to provide health care, counseling, or testing. Natural history studies in adolescents are incomplete, although HIV-1 infection in adolescents appears to resemble the disease time course, complications, and prognosis in adults.

## PREVENTION

Prevention of HIV-1 infection in children entails the prevention of mother-to-child transmission and prevention of transmission in adolescents who participate in adult risk behaviors. A solution to the worldwide HIV-1 pandemic would be the development of a safe and effective vaccine. Although not currently available, finding an HIV-1 vaccine is a priority of the National Institute of Allergy and Infectious Diseases and is supported by the White House's National HIV/AIDS Strategy for the United States.

### Mother-to-Child Transmission

**Screening and Antiretrovirals During Pregnancy** In the United States, there has been a marked reduction in perinatal HIV-1 transmission. This reduction has been accomplished primarily by first-trimester screening of pregnant women and the successful administration of ART to pregnant HIV-1–infected women. HIV-negative women who are at high risk for acquiring HIV-1 infection (eg, injection drug users, partners are HIV-1 infected or injection drug users, women who exchange sex for money or drugs, women who have had a new sex partner or more than 1 sex partner during this pregnancy, women with signs consistent with the acute retroviral syndrome, women who receive health care in jurisdictions with elevated incidence of HIV-1 or AIDS among women 14–24 years of age) should have repeat testing in the third trimester, preferably prior to 36 weeks of gestation. Zidovudine given to HIV-1–infected pregnant women starting at 14 to 32 weeks of gestation reduced perinatal transmission from 25% to 8%. Further reductions in mother-to-child transmission to < 1% in resource-rich countries have been achieved with the early initiation of cART and monitoring of viral loads during pregnancy. Thus, when HIV-1 infection is diagnosed during pregnancy, initiation of cART as soon as possible is desirable to decrease the risk for perinatal transmission, but maternal status (CD4+ cell count, viral load, pregnancy-related conditions) and the potential fetal effects of drug exposure must also be considered. Further, HIV-1–infected women contemplating pregnancy should be receiving cART and have an undetectable

HIV viral load prior to conception, with the goal to maintain the viral load below the limit of detection throughout pregnancy.

Administration of antiretroviral agents with minimal safety data for use during pregnancy has been fairly liberal because of the obvious benefits associated with appropriate treatment of the mother's HIV-1 infection and the reduction in perinatal transmission. It will be important to monitor both short- and long-term outcomes of infants exposed perinatally to these therapies in order to determine the impact of ART during gestation. Accordingly, healthcare providers caring for HIV-infected pregnant women are strongly encouraged to report prenatal antiretroviral drug exposure to the Antiretroviral Pregnancy Registry (http://www.apregistry.com). Efavirenz has been associated with CNS complications in primate offspring, but human studies linking first-trimester efavirenz exposure to CNS defects and other congenital anomalies are inconclusive. Thus, alternate cART regimens should be considered in women who are planning to become pregnant or are sexually active and not using effective contraception. However, because the risks are primarily limited to the first 5 to 6 weeks of pregnancy, HIV-1–infected women with viral suppression on an efavirenz-based regimen who present for prenatal care in the first trimester can continue the efavirenz-based regimen. Ongoing investigations will help establish whether any of the other currently available antiretroviral agents should be withheld during pregnancy.

**Mode of Delivery** Numerous studies have investigated the impact of the mode of delivery on the rate of perinatal transmission. Cesarean delivery does appear to provide some additional protection to the infant born to the HIV-1–infected woman. However, in the era of cART and the ability to monitor viral load closely, both the risks and the benefits of cesarean delivery must be clearly discussed with prospective parents before any change in the mode of delivery is considered. For pregnant women receiving cART and with a viral load consistently ≤ 1000 copies/mL, the additional benefit of cesarean delivery is minimal and is not routinely recommended. However, cesarean delivery at 38 weeks of gestation is recommended for women with a viral load > 1000 copies/mL or an unknown viral load near the time of delivery, in order to reduce the risk for perinatal transmission.

**Intrapartum Interventions** HIV-1–infected pregnant women should continue their cART regimen as much as possible during labor and prior to scheduled cesarean delivery. Intravenous intrapartum zidovudine decreases the risk for perinatal transmission and should be administered during labor or beginning 3 hours prior to scheduled cesarean delivery to women with an HIV-1 viral load > 1000 copies/mL or an unknown viral load near the time of delivery. Cleansing the birth canal with microbicidal agents has been postulated as another means of reducing transmission at the time of delivery. One study that evaluated chlorhexidine rinses found that they failed to show a benefit. However, stronger concentrations of chlorhexidine, use of other agents, or more frequent application of the rinses may yet provide some benefit. This approach may be particularly valuable in resource-poor countries that cannot pay for expensive ART.

**Infant Prophylaxis** If an infant is born to a mother who is at risk for HIV-1 infection but was not tested in the third trimester, the infant should be tested for HIV-1 antibody using a rapid test as soon as possible after birth. For HIV-1–exposed infants, oral zidovudine (4 mg/kg/dose twice daily in infants with gestational age ≥ 35 weeks) should be initiated as soon as possible after birth and typically continued for a 6-week course. A shorter 4-week course of zidovudine may be considered for the infant if the mother received cART during pregnancy with no concerns for adherence and with consistent viral suppression. For infants born to HIV-1–infected mothers who did not receive antepartum (prior to the onset of labor) antiretrovirals, 3 doses of nevirapine in the first week of life (first dose at birth; second dose 48 hours after the first dose; third dose 96 hours after the second dose) are recommended in addition to the 6-week course of zidovudine. This 2-drug regimen should also be considered when the mother received antepartum ART but had a viral load > 1000 copies/mL near the time of delivery, although available evidence does not clearly indicate whether the addition of nevirapine provides additional protection in this scenario. The most current recommendations for infant antiretroviral prophylaxis based on updated information can be obtained by accessing the Web site of the HIV/AIDS Treatment Information Service (www.aidsinfo.nih.gov).

**Breastfeeding and Premastication** Breastfeeding is associated with HIV-1 transmission, and the duration of breastfeeding appears to have implications for increasing the rate of HIV-1 transmission. For that reason, in areas where safe alternatives to human milk are available, breastfeeding should be avoided. Unfortunately, in many areas of the world where HIV-1 is particularly prevalent (eg, sub-Saharan Africa), safe alternatives to breastfeeding are not readily available. In these areas, the World Health Organization recommends breastfeeding for at least 12 months and up to 24 months or beyond, in conjunction with health services support for maternal cART adherence. When breastfeeding does occur, it should be the only source of milk for the infant. Infants receiving both human milk and infant milk formula have a higher rate of HIV-1 infection than infants who are receiving human milk only. In addition, premastication of infant food by HIV-1–infected caregivers may be associated with HIV-1 transmission and should be discouraged.

***Pneumocystis jirovecii* Pneumonia Prophylaxis** To reduce the risk of PCP, HIV-1–exposed infants should begin PCP prophylaxis with TMP-SMX at 4 to 6 weeks of age unless they have been determined to be presumptively uninfected with HIV-1. They should continue PCP prophylaxis until infection status is established. In uninfected infants, PCP prophylaxis can be discontinued. If HIV-1 infection is proven, PCP prophylaxis is indicated for infants < 1 year of age regardless of CD4+ cell count and for children 1 year of age and older with evidence of severe immune suppression (see Tables 310-1 and 310-2). TMP-SMX is the drug of choice for prophylaxis of PCP and may also provide some protection from serious bacterial infections. TMP-SMX may be given daily, or on 3 consecutive days of the week, or every other day (eg, Monday, Wednesday, Friday). Alternatives to TMP-SMX for patients who cannot tolerate this combination include dapsone, atovaquone, and aerosolized pentamidine.

**Immunizations** Immunization schedules for HIV-1–infected and HIV-1–exposed children should include all vaccines given routinely to children of similar age with some additions (eg, adolescent meningococcal vaccine 2-dose primary series; *Haemophilus influenzae* type b vaccine in previously unvaccinated children age 5–18 years) and some exceptions for live virus vaccines. The most current immunization recommendations may be found on the Centers for Disease Control and Prevention Web site (http://www.cdc.gov/vaccines/schedules/hcp/child-adolescent.html). Varicella and measles-mumps-rubella (MMR) vaccines can be given to asymptomatic HIV-1–infected children without evidence of severe immune suppression (see Tables 310-1 and 310-2) for at least 6 months. However, the quadrivalent measles-mumps-rubella-varicella (MMRV) vaccine should not be administered due to a lack of safety data in HIV-1–infected children. Rotavirus vaccine may be given to HIV-1–exposed infants and HIV-1–infected infants. Inactivated influenza vaccine should be given annually. In addition to routine immunizations, children 2 years of age and older should receive 23-valent pneumococcal polysaccharide vaccine (PPSV23) at least 8 weeks after their last pneumococcal conjugate vaccine dose; a second dose of PPSV23 should be given 5 years after the first.

Adolescent females with HIV-1 infection should have routine cervical cancer screening. A Pap smear is recommended at 6-month intervals for the first year after HIV-1 diagnosis and, if normal, then annually thereafter. For females diagnosed with HIV-1 prior to adolescence, cervical cancer screening is recommended within 1 year of the onset of sexual activity. Some experts also recommend screening for anal cancer by cytology or high-resolution anoscopy for sexually active males and females with HIV-1 infection. Tests for syphilis, gonorrhea, and chlamydia are recommended at least annually for all sexually active HIV-1–infected individuals, as well as trichomonas for sexually active HIV-1–infected females. Hepatitis B virus and hepatitis C virus testing should be performed for children with a history of vertical exposure to these viruses and for all children who acquire HIV-1 by nonvertical routes. Repeat annual testing for hepatitis C virus is advised for adolescents with ongoing risk factors for hepatitis C virus exposure, including injection drug use and sexual activity. Finally, annual testing for latent tuberculosis infection is recommended beginning at 3 to 12 months of age.

#### Sexual and Other Nonoccupational HIV Exposure

Adolescents who participate in behaviors identified with transmission in adults (eg, sexual promiscuity, needle sharing for the injection of illicit drugs or anabolic steroids) represent a growing population of HIV-1–infected children. Abstinence from sexual activity is the only certain way to avoid exposure to HIV-1. In sexually active adolescents, condom use with all types of sexual encounters reduces the risk for HIV-1 transmission and should be strongly encouraged. Altering behavior is difficult in the adolescent population. Outreach education, particularly through the use of peer counselors, has been somewhat successful in taking the message to at-risk youth.

**Postexposure and Preexposure Prophylaxis** Decisions regarding HIV postexposure prophylaxis (PEP) involve a balance of the risk of HIV-1 exposure, the time elapsed from the exposure, the potential side effects of medications, and the likelihood of adherence. Only exposures involving substantial risk for HIV acquisition warrant PEP, and only if PEP can be initiated within 72 hours of the exposure. In many scenarios, the decision for PEP must be made on a case-by-case basis, and consultation with a pediatric HIV healthcare professional is essential. Preferred PEP regimens vary by patient age but generally include 2 NRTIs (eg, tenofovir, emtricitabine, zidovudine, or lamivudine) plus an INSTI (eg, raltegravir or dolutegravir) or PI (lopinavir/ritonavir oral solution) for a 28-day course. Many patients fail to complete the 28-day course due to adverse effects of the medication, interference with their routine, and other reasons. Finally, preexposure prophylaxis (PrEP) is now recommended for certain adults at high risk of HIV infection, but the data on efficacy and safety in adolescents are currently insufficient.

### SUGGESTED READINGS


Brady MT, Oleske JM, Williams PL, et al. Declines in mortality rates and changes in causes of death in HIV-1-infected children during the HAART era. *J Acquir Immune Defic Synd*. 2010;53:86-94.

Luzuriaga K, Mofenson LM. Challenges in the elimination of pediatric HIV-1 infection. *N Engl J Med*. 2016;374:761-770.

National Institutes of Health. Panel on Antiretroviral Therapy and Medical Management of HIV-Infected Children. Guidelines for the use of antiretroviral agents in pediatric HIV infection. http://aidsinfo.nih.gov/contentfiles/lvguidelines/pediatricguidelines.pdf. Accessed September 26, 2016.

National Institutes of Health. Panel on Opportunistic Infections in HIV-Exposed and HIV-Infected Children. Guidelines for the prevention and treatment of opportunistic infections in HIV-exposed and HIV-infected children. Department of Health and Human Services. http://aidsinfo.nih.gov/contentfiles/lvguidelines/oi_guidelines_pediatrics.pdf. Accessed September 26, 2016.

National Institutes of Health. Panel on Treatment of HIV-Infected Pregnant Women and Prevention of Perinatal Transmission. Recommendations for use of antiretroviral drugs in pregnant HIV-1-infected women for maternal health and interventions to reduce perinatal HIV transmission in the United States. http://aidsinfo.nih.gov/contentfiles/lvguidelines/PerinatalGL.pdf. Accessed September 26, 2016.

Puthanakit T, Saphonn V, Ananworanich J, et al. Early versus deferred antiretroviral therapy for children older than 1 year infected with HIV (PREDICT): a multicentre, randomised, open-label trial. *Lancet Infect Dis*. 2012;12:933-941.

The INSIGHT START Study Group. Initiation of antiretroviral therapy in early asymptomatic HIV infection. *N Engl J Med*. 2015;373:795-807.

Tobin NH, Aldrovandi GM. Immunology of pediatric HIV infection. *Immunol Rev*. 2013;254:143-169.

Townsend CL, Byrne L, Cortina-Borja M, et al. Earlier initiation of ART and further decline in mother-to-child HIV transmission rates, 2000-2011. *AIDS*. 2014;28:1049-1057.

Whitmore SK, Taylor AW, Espinoza L, Shouse RL, Lampe MA, Nesheim S. Correlates of mother-to-child transmission of HIV in the United States and Puerto Rico. *Pediatrics*. 2012;129:e74-e81.


# 311 Measles

Roshni Mathew and Yvonne A. Maldonado

## INTRODUCTION

Measles virus infection is one of the most important infectious diseases of humans and has caused millions of deaths since its emergence as a zoonosis thousands of years ago. Prior to the development and widespread use of measles vaccines, measles was estimated to cause between 5 and 8 million deaths worldwide each year. Remarkable progress in reducing measles incidence and mortality has been made through increased measles vaccine coverage. As an example, in the period between 2000 and 2008, there was substantial decrease in measles cases and measles-associated deaths in sub-Saharan Africa due to intensive efforts at increasing measles vaccination coverage through routine vaccination and provision of a second opportunity for measles vaccination through mass measles vaccination campaigns (called supplementary immunization activities [SIAs]). However starting in 2009, there were large outbreaks in these areas and the cause of this resurgence was attributed to suboptimal vaccine coverage due to complacency with the vaccination efforts, which increased the at-risk susceptible population. In the Americas, intensive immunization and surveillance efforts had stopped endemic transmission of measles virus, in part based on the successful Pan American Health Organization strategy of nationwide measles vaccination campaigns and high routine measles vaccine coverage. However, endemic transmission due to a large sustained outbreak of measles in Brazil in 2014 demonstrates that regional measles elimination can be fragile and dependent on global elimination efforts. In the United States, high coverage with 2 doses of measles vaccine has eliminated endemic measles virus transmission. These achievements attest to the enormous public health significance of measles vaccination.

As measles control efforts are increasingly successful, public perceptions of the risk of measles diminish and are replaced by concerns of possible adverse events associated with measles vaccine. As a consequence, numerous limited measles outbreaks have occurred in communities opposed to vaccination on religious or philosophical grounds or because of unfounded fears of serious adverse events. In 2014, the United States experienced a record number of measles cases, with 667 cases from 27 states reported to the Centers for Disease Control and Prevention (CDC), the greatest number of cases since measles elimination was documented in the United States in 2000. Most of these cases occurred in unvaccinated persons. The source of the 2014 outbreaks was primarily importations from endemic areas of the world, and a significant proportion were importations from travelers returning from the Philippines where a large outbreak had been occurring. In 2015, the United States experienced a large, multistate measles outbreak that originated in amusement parks in Orange County, California. Although the source of this outbreak was not identified, it was likely from a person infected overseas. Once again, the majority of patients with measles in this outbreak were either unvaccinated or had unknown vaccination status (total cases in 2015 were 188).

## EPIDEMIOLOGY AND PATHOGENESIS

Measles virus is one of the most contagious human pathogens, and outbreaks can occur in populations in which less than 10% of persons are susceptible. Chains of transmission commonly occur among household contacts, school-age children, and healthcare workers. There are no latent or persistent measles virus infections that result in prolonged contagiousness and no animal reservoirs. Thus, measles virus can only be maintained in human populations by an unbroken chain of acute infections, requiring a continuous supply of susceptible individuals. Newborns become susceptible to measles when passively acquired maternal antibody is lost and are the main source of new susceptible individuals. Unvaccinated children and the small proportion of vaccine nonresponders also contribute to the pool of susceptibles and to the spread of vaccine-preventable infectious diseases.

When endemic, measles has a typical temporal pattern characterized by yearly seasonal epidemics superimposed on longer epidemic cycles of 2 to 5 years or more. In temperate climates, annual measles outbreaks generally occur in the late winter and early spring. These annual outbreaks are likely the result of social networks facilitating transmission (eg, congregation of children at school) and environmental factors favoring the viability and transmission of measles virus. Measles cases continue to occur during the interepidemic period in large populations but at low incidence. The longer cycles occurring every several years result from the accumulation of susceptible persons over successive birth cohorts and the subsequent decline in the number of susceptibles following an outbreak. Secondary attack rates in susceptible household and institutional contacts generally exceed 90%. The average age at which people contract measles depends on the rate of decline of protective maternal antibodies, the amount of contact with infected people, and the vaccine coverage rate. In densely populated urban settings with low vaccination coverage, measles mainly affects infants and young children. As measles vaccine coverage increases or population density decreases, the age distribution shifts toward older children. As vaccination coverage, and thus population immunity, increases further, the age distribution of cases might shift into adolescence and adulthood.

Persons with measles are infectious for several days before and after the onset of rash, when levels of measles virus in blood and body fluids are highest and when the symptoms of cough, coryza, and sneezing are most severe. These symptoms facilitate virus spread. The fact that measles virus is contagious prior to the onset of recognizable disease hinders the effectiveness of quarantine measures. Measles virus can be isolated from urine as late as 1 week after rash onset, and viral shedding may be prolonged in children with impaired cell-mediated immunity.

Medical settings are well-recognized sites of measles virus transmission. Children may present to healthcare facilities during the prodrome when the diagnosis is not obvious, although the child is infectious and likely to infect susceptible contacts. Healthcare workers can acquire measles from infected children and transmit measles virus to others.

Measles virus is a spherical, nonsegmented, single-stranded, negative-sense RNA virus and a member of the *Morbillivirus* genus in the family of Paramyxoviridae. Measles was originally a zoonotic infection, arising from cross-species transmission from animals to humans by an ancestral morbillivirus. Although RNA viruses typically have high mutation rates, measles virus is considered to be an antigenically monotypic virus, meaning that the surface proteins responsible for inducing protective immunity have retained their antigenic structure across time and space. The public health significance is that measles vaccines developed decades ago from a single measles virus strain remain protective worldwide. Measles virus is killed by ultraviolet light and heat. Attenuated measles vaccine viruses retain these characteristics, necessitating a cold chain for transporting and storing measles vaccines.

Measles virus is transmitted primarily by respiratory droplets over short distances and, less commonly, by small-particle aerosols that remain suspended in the air for long periods of time. Airborne transmission appears to be important in certain settings, including schools, pediatricians' offices, hospitals, and enclosed public places, and infectious droplets may persist for several hours after an infected child has left a pediatrician's office. Direct contact with infected secretions can transmit measles virus, but the virus does not survive long on fomites.

Infection is initiated when measles virus reaches epithelial cells in the respiratory tract, oropharynx, or conjunctivae. Wild-type measles virus strains preferentially bind to SLAM (CD150), expressed on activated T cells, B cells, and antigen-presenting cells, whereas laboratory-adapted strains can also bind CD46, which is expressed on all nucleated cells. Measles virus thus infects lymphocytes and dendritic cells, as well as respiratory epithelial cells, which contributes to systemic spread. During the first 2 to 4 days after infection, measles virus proliferates locally in the respiratory mucosa and spreads to draining lymph nodes where further replication occurs. Virus then enters the bloodstream in infected leukocytes, primarily monocytes, producing the primary viremia that disseminates infection throughout the reticuloendothelial system. Further replication results in a secondary viremia that begins 5 to 7 days after infection and disseminates measles virus to tissues throughout the body. Replication of measles virus in these target organs, together with the host immune response, is responsible for the signs and symptoms that occur 8 to 12 days after infection and mark the end of the incubation period.

The incubation period for measles, the time from infection to clinical disease, is approximately 10 days to the onset of fever and 14 days to the onset of rash. The incubation period may be shorter in infants or following a large inoculum of virus and may be longer (up to 3 weeks) in adults.

## CLINICAL MANIFESTATIONS

In most children, the signs and symptoms of measles are highly characteristic. Approximately 10 days after exposure, fever and malaise signal the onset of illness (Fig. 311-1). Cough, coryza, and conjunctivitis follow promptly. A gradual worsening of symptoms accompanies a steady rise in fever over the next 4 days. Two days prior to the appearance of the exanthem, Koplik spots develop. With the onset of rash 14 days after infection, the clinical picture attains maximal severity. Constitutional symptoms throughout this 10-day period vary, but headache, abdominal pain, vomiting, diarrhea, and myalgia are frequent complaints. Fever reaching 40°C (104°F) to 41°C (105.8°F), often accompanied by chills, is not unusual when the rash is most florid. Febrile seizures may occur in children predisposed to them.

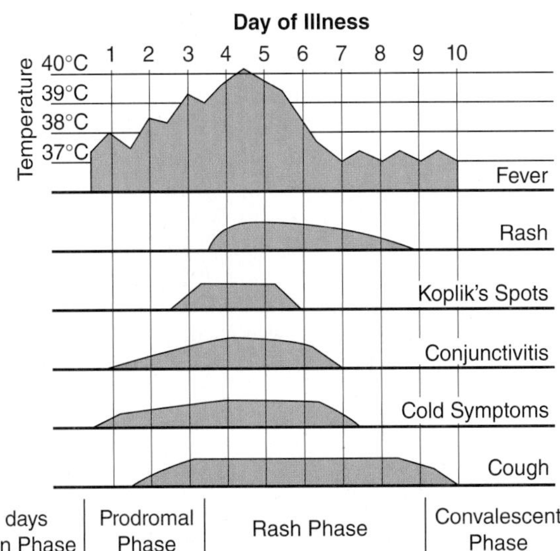


**FIGURE 311-1** Clinical features of measles. (Reproduced with permission from Expanded Programme on Immunization Team. *Manual for the Laboratory Diagnosis of Measles and Rubella Virus Infection*, 2nd ed. Geneva, Switzerland: World Health Organization; 2007.)

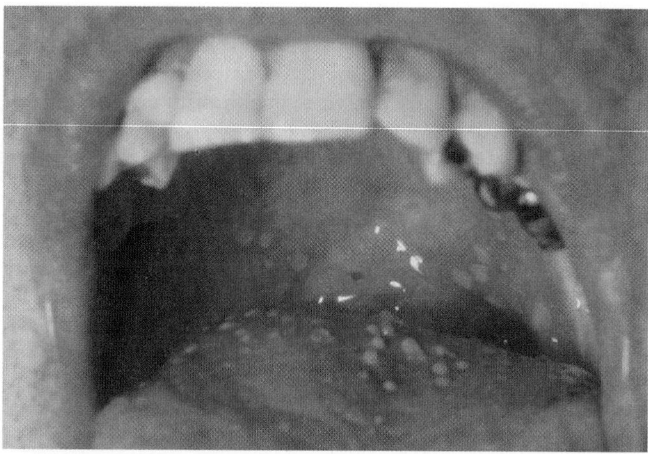

**FIGURE 311-2** Koplik spots.

The conjunctivitis causes edema of the lids, increased lacrimation, and, frequently, photophobia. Sharply demarcated transverse linear injection of the lower lid margins, called a Stimson line, is present before the more generalized conjunctival inflammation obscures it. Among infants with nutritional deficiencies, especially of vitamin A, more severe ocular involvement with corneal ulcers may lead to permanent scarring and loss of vision. A hacking cough progressively increases in frequency and severity. With the abrupt fall in temperature, after rash has covered the entire body, the catarrhal symptoms subside dramatically, but the cough persists for another 7 to 10 days.

Koplik spots, pathognomonic of measles, appear 24 to 48 hours before the exanthem. They consist of bluish white dots about 1 mm in diameter surrounded by a rose-red areola (Fig. 311-2). They tend to appear first on the buccal mucosa opposite the lower molars. Best seen in bright daylight, they are discrete and few in number initially, but within 1 day, they increase rapidly and may spread to cover the entire buccal mucosa. With the onset of rash, they fade, and frequently by the second day of the eruption, they have disappeared.

The rash commences as discrete, irregular, erythematous macules behind the ears, on the neck, and along the hairline. As the rash progresses caudad over the ensuing 24 hours to involve the face, trunk, and arms, careful palpation will reveal a papular component (Fig. 311-3). Involvement of the legs and feet by the end of the second day or early in the third day finds the lesions on the cheeks already coalescent; in severe infections, confluent areas of rash also appear on the trunk and extremities. Although the exanthem ordinarily blanches with pressure, a fine petechial component is often present. The exanthem fades slowly, in the same order of progression as its initial appearance, a process that usually begins by the third or fourth day after onset. Subsidence of the florid eruption is followed by a fine desquamation. In children with protein or cellular immune deficiencies, the desquamation is far more extensive and may be complicated by multiple pyogenic skin abscesses.

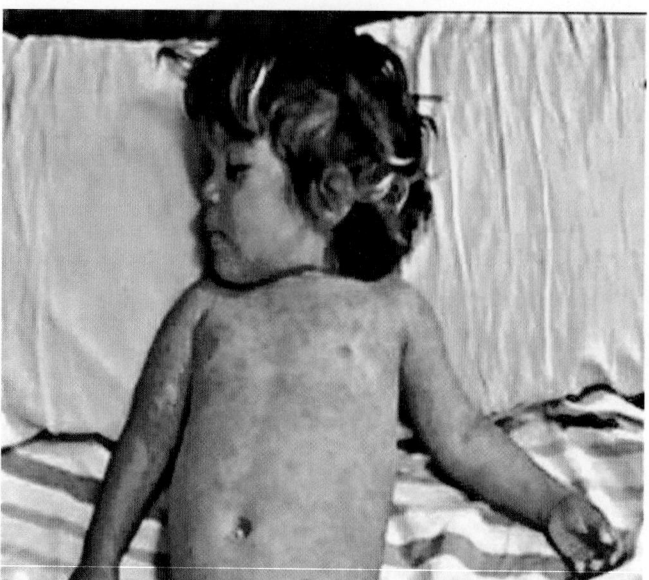

**FIGURE 311-3** Measles rash. (Reproduced with permission from Moss WJ, Griffin DE: Global measles elimination, *Nat Rev Microbiol.* 2006 Dec;4(12):900-908.)

The marked generalized lymphadenopathy and splenomegaly that arise early in the course of the acute illness may persist for several weeks. High fever at the peak of illness may be accompanied by marked irritability, somnolence, or a state of delirium, but these are transient and resolve with the disappearance of pyrexia. They do not correlate with the occurrence of subsequent central nervous system complications. Black measles, a severe form of the disease with a generalized hemorrhagic rash; bleeding from the nose, mouth, and gastrointestinal tract; and marked systemic toxicity, is rare. This form of measles was reported more frequently in the past and probably represented a form of disseminated intravascular coagulation.

The differential diagnosis of measles includes other causes of fever, rash, and conjunctivitis, such as rubella, Kawasaki disease, infectious mononucleosis, roseola, scarlet fever, typhus, Rocky Mountain spotted fever, enterovirus or adenovirus exanthems, and rashes due to drug sensitivity (especially barbiturates, hydantoins, penicillins, and sulfonamides). Rubella is a milder illness, without cough and with distinctive lymphadenopathy usually restricted to the posterior cervical, suboccipital, and postauricular nodes. Roseola (exanthema subitum) has a different sequence of clinical manifestations, with the rash first appearing after the fever subsides. The peripheral blood count and atypical lymphocytes in infectious mononucleosis contrast with the leukopenia of measles.

## DIAGNOSIS

Measles is readily diagnosed on clinical grounds by clinicians familiar with the disease. Koplik spots are especially helpful because they appear early and are pathognomonic of measles. Clinical diagnosis is more difficult during the prodrome and when the rash is attenuated by passively acquired antibodies or prior immunization, or when the rash is absent in immunocompromised or severely malnourished children with impaired cellular immunity. Clinical diagnosis is also more difficult in regions where the incidence of measles is low because other pathogens are responsible for the majority of measles-like illnesses (fever and rash). The CDC case definition for measles requires (1) a generalized maculopapular rash of at least 3 days in duration; (2) fever of at least 38.3°C (101°F); and (3) cough, coryza, or conjunctivitis.

Serology is the most common method of laboratory diagnosis. A positive immunoglobulin (Ig) M on a single serum specimen or a significant increase in serum IgG antibody concentration in paired acute and convalescent serum specimens (collected at least 10 days apart) on a patient with clinical manifestations consistent with measles is considered diagnostic of acute infection. Measles virus–specific IgM antibodies may not be detectable until 4 to 5 days or more after rash onset and usually fall to undetectable levels within 4 to 8 weeks of rash onset.

A number of methods are available for measuring antibodies to measles virus. Neutralization tests are sensitive and specific, the results are highly correlated with immunity to infection, and they provide the most clinically relevant measure of response to immunization. However, they require propagation of measles virus in cell culture and are thus expensive and laborious. Commercially available enzyme immunoassays (EIAs) can detect either IgM or IgG antibodies to measles virus and are the most frequently used diagnostic methods.

Measles can also be diagnosed by isolation of measles virus or identification of measles RNA by reverse transcriptase polymerase chain reaction (RT-PCR) amplification of RNA extracted from clinical specimens, such as urine, blood, or throat or nasopharyngeal secretions. Diagnostic testing for measles should include both serologic and virologic testing. All cases of suspected measles should be reported immediately to the local or state health department without waiting for results of the diagnostic tests.

## TREATMENT

Except for general supportive measures, such as hydration and antipyretics, there is no specific antiviral therapy for persons with uncomplicated measles. Secondary bacterial infections are a major cause of morbidity and mortality following measles, and effective case management involves prompt treatment with antibiotics. Antibiotics are indicated for children with measles who have clinical evidence of bacterial infection, including pneumonia and otitis media. *Streptococcus pneumoniae* and *Haemophilus influenzae* type B were the most common causes of bacterial pneumonia following measles, and vaccines against these pathogens have lowered the incidence of secondary bacterial infections following measles.

Vitamin A treatment results in marked reductions in morbidity and mortality. Although vitamin A deficiency is not a recognized problem in the United States, many American children with measles have low serum vitamin A levels, and these children have increased morbidity following measles. The World Health Organization currently recommends vitamin A for *all* children with acute measles, regardless of their country of residence. Vitamin A for treatment of measles is administered once daily for 2 days, at the following doses: 200,000 IU for children 12 months or older; 100,000 IU for infants 6 through 11 months of age; and 50,000 IU for infants younger than 6 months. An additional (ie, a third) age-specific dose should be given 2 to 4 weeks later to children with clinical signs and symptoms of vitamin A deficiency.

Most children with measles recover and develop long-term protective immunity to reinfection. Measles case fatality rates vary, depending on the average age of infection, nutritional and immunologic status of the population, measles vaccine coverage, and access to health care. Vaccinated children, should they develop disease after exposure, have less severe disease and significantly lower mortality rates. In developed countries, less than 1 in 1000 children with measles dies. In endemic areas in sub-Saharan Africa and Southeast Asia, the measles case fatality rate may be 5% to 10% or higher. Measles is a major cause of child deaths in refugee camps and in internally displaced populations, where measles case fatality rates have been as high as 20% to 30%.

## COMPLICATIONS

A wide variety of complications may be observed during the acute stage of measles or shortly thereafter. The respiratory tract is involved most often, but severe gastroenteritis also occurs. Acute laryngotracheobronchitis (croup) may cause sufficient airway obstruction to require tracheostomy, especially in children younger than 3 years. A rare but almost uniformly fatal interstitial pneumonia (giant cell pneumonia) has been noted in immunocompromised children, including those with human immunodeficiency virus (HIV)-1 infection, who develop a progressive persistent measles virus infection without the typical exanthem and with a unique failure to form measles virus–specific antibodies. The radiographic picture reveals a marked interstitial pattern emanating from both hilar regions.

A benign asymptomatic keratoconjunctivitis that accompanies measles may persist for as long as 4 months. More severe corneal lesions occur in malnourished children. Transient electrocardiographic abnormalities are common, but true myocarditis is rare. The diffuse lymphadenopathy that accompanies measles involves the mesenteric nodes and is believed to cause the abdominal pain that commonly occurs. Symptoms and signs identical to those of acute appendicitis may result in surgical intervention during the prodromal period.

Complications of bacterial origin result principally from invasion of the respiratory tract by pyogenic organisms. Otitis media and bronchopneumonia are most common. Peribronchitis and interstitial pneumonitis are seen in nearly all children with measles and resolve rapidly after the development of rash and the subsidence of fever. A second fever spike, or failure of the initial spike to drop after the eruption has reached its peak, suggests a secondary bacterial infection. The appearance of peripheral leukocytosis with a shift to the left is highly suggestive. A chest radiograph may disclose bronchopneumonia or a pattern of segmental or lobar involvement.

During the early viremic phase of measles, there is a thrombocytopenia of insufficient magnitude to cause spontaneous bleeding. Another rare and unexplained postinfectious complication, thrombocytopenic purpura, appears 4 to 14 days after the rash and may produce marked skin purpura, genitourinary and gastrointestinal bleeding, and epistaxis.

Of those syndromes that can follow measles, the most dreaded are the various central nervous system complications. Uncomplicated measles is frequently accompanied by cerebrospinal fluid pleocytosis and electroencephalographic abnormalities, but there is no evidence that the brain is infected by measles virus. Acute postinfectious measles encephalomyelitis is the most common neurologic complication of measles. It is rare in children younger than 2 years, but occurs in about 1 in 1000 cases of measles in older children and somewhat more frequently in adults. The onset is usually during the first week after the start of the rash and is typically abrupt, with irritability, headache, vomiting, and confusion, and progressing rapidly to obtundation and coma. These manifestations are frequently accompanied by seizures and recurrence or accentuation of fever. A second form of measles encephalitis, subacute sclerosing panencephalitis (SSPE), is a rare delayed complication of measles that occurs in approximately 4 to 11 per 100,000 cases. Typically, SSPE presents in children 7 to 10 years after measles that occurred in early childhood, generally prior to 2 years of age. The onset is insidious, with symptoms of progressive loss of cortical function developing over months. Patients subsequently develop ataxia, progressive mental deterioration, and extrapyramidal dyskinesias, including choreoathetosis and dystonic posturing. The third form of measles encephalitis, measles inclusion body encephalitis (MIBE), is a progressive, generally fatal, measles virus infection of the brain that occurs in immunocompromised patients. Widespread use of measles vaccine has resulted in near disappearance of SSPE in the United States, once again underscoring the importance of routine administration of 2 doses of measles-containing vaccine to all eligible children.

## PREVENTION

Active immunization for measles is discussed in Chapter 239. The proportions of children who develop protective levels of antibody after measles vaccination are approximately 85% at 9 months of age and 95% at 12 months of age.

Human immunoglobulin (Ig) can be given either intramuscularly (IgIM) or intravenously (IgIV) to prevent or modify measles in nonimmune persons if given within 6 days of exposure. Prophylaxis with Ig is recommended for susceptible household and nosocomial contacts who would be at increased risk of complications of measles disease such as infants less than 12 months of age, pregnant women, and severely immunocompromised persons such as patients with severe primary immunodeficiency, patients who have received a bone marrow transplant until at least 12 months after finishing all immunosuppressive treatment or longer in patients who have developed graft-versus-host disease, patients on treatment for acute lymphoblastic leukemia within and until at least 6 months after completion of immunosuppressive chemotherapy, and patients with a diagnosis of acquired immunodeficiency syndrome (AIDS) or HIV-infected persons with severe immunosuppression defined as CD4 percentage < 15% (all ages) or CD4 count < 200 lymphocytes/μL (age > 5 years) and those who have not received the measles, mumps, and rubella (MMR) vaccine since receiving effective antiretroviral therapy. The recommended dose of IgIM is 0.50 mL/kg given intramuscularly (the maximum dose by volume is 15 mL). IgIV at a dose of 400 mg/kg is the recommended Ig preparation for pregnant women without evidence of measles immunity and severely immunocompromised patients.

American Academy of Pediatrics. Measles. In: Kimberlin DW, Brady MT, Jackson MA, Long SS, eds. *Red Book: 2015 Report of the Committee on Infectious Diseases*. 30th ed. Elk Grove Village, IL: American Academy of Pediatrics; 2015:535-547.

Clemmons NS, Gastanaduy PA, Fiebelkorn AP, et al. Measles–United States, January 4–April 2, 2015. *MMWR Morb Mortal Wkly Rep*. 2015;64:373-376.

Fiebelkorn AP, Redd SB, Gastañaduy PA, et al. A comparison of post-elimination measles epidemiology in the United States, 2009-2014 versus 2001-2008. *J Pediatr Infect Dis Soc*. 2017;6(1):40-48.

Gastañaduy PA, Redd SB, Fiebelkorn AP, et al. Measles–United States, January 1-May 23, 2014. *MMWR Morb Mortal Wkly Rep*. 2014;63:496-499.

Liko J, Guzman-Cottrill JA, Cieslak PR. Notes from the field: subacute sclerosing panencephalitis death–Oregon, 2015. *MMWR Morb Mortal Wkly Rep*. 2016;65:10-11.

Moss WJ, Griffin DE. Measles. *Lancet*. 2012;379:153-164.

Phadke VK, Bednarczyk RA, Salmon DA, et al. Association between vaccine refusal and vaccine-preventable diseases in the United States: a review of measles and pertussis. *JAMA*. 2016;315:1149-1158.

Shibeshi ME, Masresha BG, Smit SB, et al. Measles resurgence in southern Africa: challenges to measles elimination. *Vaccine*. 2014;32:1798-1807.

# 312 Molluscum Contagiosum

Jeremy Udkoff and Lawrence F. Eichenfield

## INTRODUCTION

Molluscum contagiosum is a common cutaneous viral infection caused by the poxvirus *Molluscipoxvirus*. Structurally, the virus is brick-shaped, contains double-stranded DNA, and is one of the largest viruses known.

## PATHOGENESIS AND EPIDEMIOLOGY

Molluscum contagiosum can only replicate in the human epidermis and is spread by skin-to-skin contact, autoinoculation, sexual transmission, and contaminated fomites. Once the infection is localized to the epidermis, it replicates and induces the formation of proliferative skin lesions.

Molluscum can present at any age, but the peak incidence is in children between 0 and 4 years, and the majority of cases are found in those younger than 8 years. Most children presenting with molluscum contagiosum are healthy; however, patients with atopic dermatitis or immunosuppressed individuals tend to have larger, more widespread eruptions. While molluscum can be a sexually transmitted disease, this is more common in adults. Outbreaks have been noted among wrestlers, and there is evidence to support that molluscum is more common in swimmers and children with atopic dermatitis. Molluscum contagiosum infection is usually benign and self-limited, with the disease duration lasting several months to several years.

## CLINICAL MANIFESTATIONS

Molluscum lesions typically begin as 3 to 5 mm or larger in diameter, flat-topped, discrete, dome-shaped, flesh-colored to translucent papules, with a central white core, and they umbilicate as they age (Fig. 312-1). Molluscum lesions commonly occur on the trunk, extremities, and face, but may be generalized as well. Groups of lesions often occur in the body folds and intertriginous areas, secondary to skin-to-skin autoinoculation (see Fig. 312-1). Molluscum contagiosum is usually asymptomatic, although an eczematous, red, scaling patch is commonly observed surrounding the lesions and is termed *molluscum dermatitis*. Scratching of the dermatitis may spread the virus. Infrequently, molluscum contagiosum may trigger a papular, eczematous, "id reaction," or a Gianotti-Crosti like reaction, characterized by numerous erythematous and edematous lesions separate from the molluscum lesions.

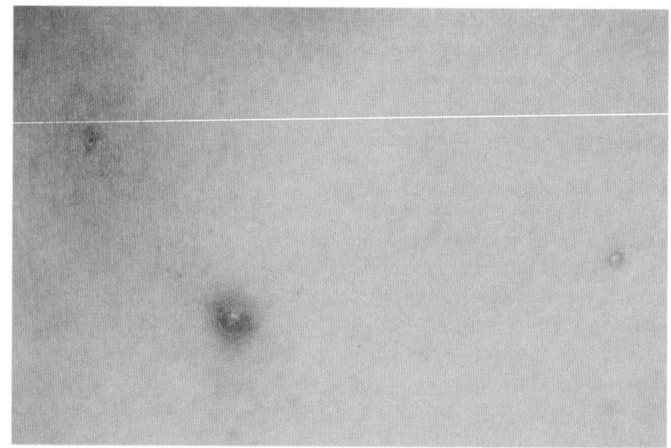

**FIGURE 312-1** View of molluscum lesions. A translucent papule with central white area (*right side of image*), an active inflammatory lesion (*bottom left of image*), and remnant superficial crusting (*upper left corner of image*) are visualized.

## DIAGNOSIS

Molluscum contagiosum is usually diagnosed clinically, based on morphology and distribution. A dermatoscope may assist in visualizing the morphology of the lesions. One may confirm the diagnosis by examining the central core of a molluscum lesion. After appropriate staining, eosinophilic, ovoid, intracytoplasmic inclusions termed *molluscum bodies* may be observed under the microscope. Small, atypical, and giant lesions may be mistaken for bacterial pustules, verrucae, keratosis pilaris, milia, varicella-zoster, or juvenile xanthogranuloma. These conditions should be considered as a part of the differential diagnosis.

## TREATMENT

Reassurance that the condition is self-limited and that the lesions may regress spontaneously, as well as controlling the spread of infection, is a reasonable treatment approach. However, treatment may be indicated for large lesional numbers, to reduce autoinoculation and spread to other individuals, to minimize pruritus or dermatitis, or for cosmetic purposes. Chemical or physical destruction is commonly used to treat molluscum, although there are limited prospective studies to support the various treatment modalities. Chemical treatments include locally destructive chemicals such as cantharidin (0.7% in collodion), which is the most commonly used agent, lactic acid, salicylic acid, trichloroacetic acid, and potassium hydroxide. Other chemical treatments include retinoids, such as tretinoin, and intralesional immunotherapy using *Candida* antigen. Methods of physical destruction include cryotherapy, curettage of the lesions, needle extraction, or pulsed dye laser. These methods usually result in resolution of the molluscum lesion without recurrence (Table 312-1). Tape stripping, topical cidofovir, and oral cimetidine have been reported as therapies for molluscum with minimal evidence basis. Imiquimod cream was not found to be superior to vehicle cream in 2 well-designed clinical studies. Although molluscum contagiosum infections usually resolve completely without sequela, small pitted scars or hypopigmentation may occur spontaneously or secondary to treatment.

## PREVENTION

Children with lesions covered by clothing have a very low risk of spreading disease to others. Because the infection may spread in water,

**TABLE 312-1 COMMON TREATMENT MODALITIES FOR MOLLUSCUM CONTAGIOSUM**

| Treatment | Method | Comments |
|---|---|---|
| Watchful waiting | | Appropriate in uncomplicated cases |
| Cantharidin (in office) (0.7% in flexible collodion) | Apply sparingly with wooden applicator stick | Rinse in 4–6 hours; do not occlude; blistering common; avoid near eyes, anogenital area. May require multiple treatments |
| Cryotherapy (liquid nitrogen) | Two 10–30 seconds cycles | Blistering and pain common; difficult in younger patients |
| Intralesional *Candida* antigen | 1 or more lesions injected monthly | Painful, traumatic, especially in young children |
| Potassium hydroxide (5% solution) | Apply to lesions twice a day for 1 week or until inflammatory response develops | Burning, discomfort, postinflammatory hyper- or hypopigmentation possible |
| Pulse dye laser | Thermal destruction | Painful without proper anesthesia. Useful in recalcitrant lesions |
| Salicylic acid | Apply 12–15% collodion 2–3 times per week | Burning or discomfort possible |
| Surgical removal | Debridement with curette or needle extraction of the central core | Painful, traumatic, especially in young children. Removal of the central core may be more tolerable |
| Tretinoin cream (off-label use; 0.05% cream) | Apply sparingly daily for 6 weeks | Useful for facial lesions; irritation common |

families may be advised to not share towels, sponges, or baths if an affected child has active lesions. In outbreaks (eg, among wrestlers), spread may be decreased by reducing interpersonal body contact and by restricting the sharing of potentially contaminated fomites such as towels.

## SUGGESTED READINGS


Berger EM, Orlow SJ, Patel RR, Schaffer JV. Experience with molluscum contagiosum and associated inflammatory reactions in a pediatric dermatology practice: the bump that rashes. *Arch Dermatol.* 2012;148:1257-1264.

Chen X, Anstey AV, Bugert JJ. Molluscum contagiosum virus infection. *Lancet Infect Dis.* 2013;13:877-888.

Katz KA. Dermatologists, imiquimod, and treatment of molluscum contagiosum in children: righting wrongs. *J Am Med Assoc Dermatol.* 2015;151:125-126.

Olsen JR, Gallacher J, Piguet V, Francis NA. Epidemiology of molluscum contagiosum in children: a systematic review. *Fam Pract.* 2014;31:130-136.

Sterling J. Treatment of warts and molluscum: what does the evidence show? *Curr Opin Pediatr.* 2016;28:490-499.


# 313 Mumps

Dennis L. Murray

## INTRODUCTION

Mumps is a communicable, systemic viral illness most often characterized by parotitis. With widespread use of mumps vaccine in over 114 countries worldwide currently, the disease has become less common. However, due to waning vaccine immunity over time, some disease continues to occur in sporadic outbreaks. A significant number of mumps infections are asymptomatic.

## EPIDEMIOLOGY AND PATHOGENESIS

Humans are the only known natural host of mumps virus, a paramyxovirus closely related to parainfluenza viruses. Mumps is spread by respiratory droplet or through direct contact with saliva. The virus can be isolated from saliva up to 7 days before and through 8 days after parotid swelling. Mumps virus is less contagious than either measles or varicella virus; typically, the incubation period is 16 to 18 days (range, 12–25 days).

A live attenuated mumps virus vaccine was first licensed in the United States in 1967. In the prevaccine era, the incidence of mumps was 50 to 251 cases per 100,000. Following implementation of a single-dose vaccine recommendation, the incidence markedly declined to 2 per 100,000 by 1988. After implementation of a 2-dose recommendation for measles-mumps-rubella vaccine in 1989, mumps incidence declined further to 0.1 case per 100,000 by 1999. By 2005, mumps disease rates had declined 99% compared to the prevaccine era. However, over the past decade, periodic outbreaks of mumps disease have continued to occur, especially in adolescents and young adults, many of whom have received either 1 or 2 doses of vaccine as young children. It is estimated that 1 dose of mumps vaccine is 78% (range, 49–92%) effective and 2 doses of vaccine are 88% (range, 66–95%) effective in preventing mumps disease.

In susceptible, unimmunized populations, 60% to 70% of cases of mumps are associated with parotitis. However, up to 33% of mumps infections may go unrecognized, especially in adults, because the cases do not have parotitis. Given the number of subclinical cases, information regarding a patient's history of mumps infection is notoriously inaccurate.

Following transmission of mumps virus to a susceptible host, the primary site of viral replication is the epithelium of the upper respiratory or gastrointestinal tract or the eye. The virus then quickly spreads to the local lymphoid tissue, and a primary viremia ensues. The parotid gland, central nervous system (CNS), testis or epididymis, pancreas, and/or ovary may be involved. Inflammation in these infected tissues then leads to characteristic symptoms such parotitis, aseptic meningitis, and/or abdominal pain. A secondary viremia occurs a few days after symptoms of illness begin, indicating viral replication within target organs. Virus can be identified in urine for up to 2 weeks following onset of clinical illness.

Lifelong immunity develops in virtually all patients after natural infection, although a second infection has been reported to occur very rarely.

## CLINICAL MANIFESTATIONS

A patient with mumps rarely has severe systemic manifestations. Body temperature is typically only moderately elevated for 3 to 4 days. Symptoms such as abdominal discomfort, anorexia, and headache may precede parotid gland involvement by 1 to 2 days. Parotid swelling, however, may be the first sign of illness; swelling may last 7 to 10 days and be observed on 1 or both sides of the face (Fig. 313-1). Two or 3 days after swelling appears on 1 side of the face, the opposite side may become involved. The submandibular glands may also swell either in addition to the parotid or sometimes in the absence of parotid involvement. Presternal edema is sometimes present.

Typically, the entire parotid gland is involved, including the uncinate lobe, which extends under the back of the ear lobe. The borders of the parotid gland are not discrete, and pressure on the parotid may cause both pain and trismus (spasm of the masticator muscle). The gland swelling also produces discomfort, which can be exacerbated by eating or drinking acidic foods, such as orange juice. The orifice of the Stenson duct may show signs of inflammation.

Mumps virus is neurotropic, and more than 50% of patients with mumps disease have cerebrospinal fluid (CSF) pleocytosis. However, less than 10% have findings typical of aseptic meningitis. Mumps meningitis can occur in the absence of parotid involvement. In the prevaccine era, mumps accounted for roughly 10% of all viral meningitis reported in the United States. CSF findings show predominantly

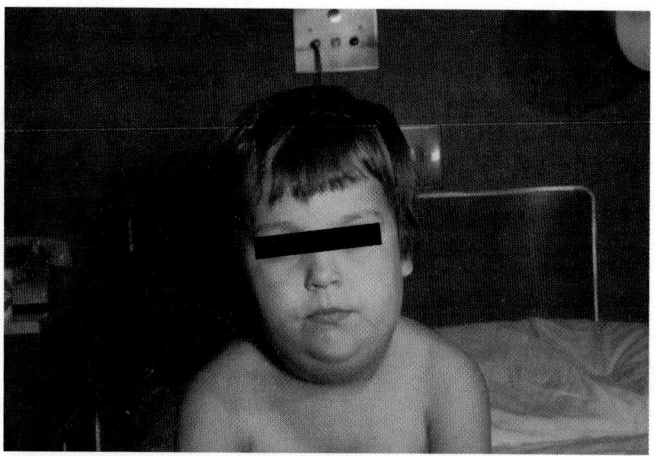

**FIGURE 313-1** Diffuse lymphedema of the neck due to mumps virus infection of the parotid and other salivary glands. (Reproduced with permission from Public Image Library, Centers for Disease Control and Prevention.)

lymphocytic cells, with counts usually < 500 cells/μL; CSF glucose is typically normal to slightly low, with CSF protein normal to slightly high. Evidence of encephalitis occurs rarely in mumps disease.

Some patients with mumps complain of abdominal pain, which could represent involvement of the pancreas or, in the female, the ovaries. Serum amylase is usually elevated during mumps infection, and vomiting can occur.

Complications from mumps disease are more common among adults than children. The most feared complication of mumps in males is orchitis. Although orchitis has been reported to occur in persons as young as 3 years of age, it is seen most frequently in postpubertal males, with the highest incidence in those 15 to 29 years of age. Orchitis is estimated to occur in 14% to 35% of males with mumps disease. The onset of orchitis is usually heralded by fever toward the first week of illness. Severe pain, swelling, and tenderness, which may persist for weeks, are common. Involvement is most often unilateral, but bilateral involvement has been reported. Testicular atrophy may occur after mumps orchitis; unilateral atrophy does not result in sterility, but sterility may occur if the patient has bilateral orchitis. The development of malignancy in mumps-affected testes has been reported.

Other glands may also be occasionally involved with mumps disease. Mastitis is estimated to occur in 31% of females older than 15 who are infected with mumps virus. Findings of oophoritis include emesis, fever, and lower abdominal pain. Involvement of the thyroid gland and the development of diabetes mellitus have both been reported to occur after the onset of mumps. Pancreatic damage has not been documented in cases of diabetes mellitus occurring after either mumps disease or mumps vaccination. Mumps virus involvement of joints, especially knees, can occur but is very rare in children. While complete recovery is usual, symptoms may be protracted. Mumps virus can also involve the heart (myocarditis), kidney (glomerulonephritis), and bone marrow (thrombocytopenia).

An association has been reported between mumps virus infection in the first trimester of pregnancy and an increased rate of fetal demise/spontaneous abortion. There is no convincing evidence, however, that mumps virus, which can cross the placenta, produces congenital malformations. Mumps virus has been isolated from breast milk. Deafness is a known complication associated with mumps disease, occurring in 1 in 20,000 reported cases. Permanent hearing impairment is most often unilateral, with higher tone frequency loss the most severe. Onset of hearing loss is typically sudden and is not related to CNS involvement.

## DIAGNOSIS

Thanks to an effective vaccine, mumps infection in the United States is relatively uncommon now; subsequently, despite periodic mumps outbreaks, many healthcare providers may have not seen cases of mumps and are less likely to suspect mumps in patients presenting with parotitis.

When confronted with a patient with either bilateral or unilateral parotid swelling, a differential diagnosis should include, in addition to mumps, drug effects, metabolic diseases, autoimmune disease such as systemic lupus erythematosus, parotid duct obstruction, and illness caused by other infectious agents including bacteria (both gram-positive and gram-negative organisms as well as acid-fast nontuberculous *Mycobacteria*) and viruses (influenza, parainfluenza, cytomegalovirus, Epstein-Barr virus, enterovirus, lymphocytic choriomeningitis virus, and human immunodeficiency virus [HIV]). Bacterial infection of the parotid gland may be accompanied by purulent drainage from the Stenson duct. In situations where multiple cases of parotid swelling/parotitis are being seen in a relatively short period of time, it is important to remember that mumps virus is the only known cause of epidemic parotitis.

Confirmation of the diagnosis of mumps infection is accomplished by: (1) isolation of the virus in culture; (2) detection of mumps virus nucleic acid by reverse transcriptase polymerase chain reaction (RT-PCR) from either saliva or CSF; (3) detection of mumps-specific immunoglobulin (Ig) M antibody; or (4) demonstration of a significant mumps serum IgG antibody titer rise, quantitatively or semiquantitatively, between acute and convalescent (2 or more weeks apart) serologic assays. RT-PCR is becoming increasingly more available, and consequently, culture is now performed less frequently. A negative IgM test in a previously immunized individual does not eliminate the diagnosis of mumps, because an IgM response may be absent. In addition, again in a previously immunized patient, an IgG titer rise may be blunted by the presence of preexisting antibody. Viral excretion in saliva from a previously immunized person with possible mumps may also be shortened in duration.

Historically, a skin test with mumps antigen was available; however, the test was inaccurate and should not have been used to test for immunity to mumps.

## TREATMENT

Currently, there is no antiviral therapy specific for mumps; supportive therapy includes bed rest, fluids, and fever reduction. Adequate attention to hydration and alimentation is important. Because patients with mumps may have difficulties with acidic foods, the diet should be light with a generous offering of fluids. Analgesics may be needed for headache as well as for discomfort caused by parotitis and/or orchitis.

## PREVENTION

A live attenuated mumps virus vaccine is used in the immunization of children, adolescents, and young adults. The only available mumps vaccines today are as part of combination vaccines with measles and rubella vaccines (MMR) or with measles, rubella, and varicella vaccines (MMRV). While both MMR and MMRV are licensed for use in all children 12 to 15 months of age who are without a true contraindication to the vaccines, MMRV is associated with a higher risk of fever and a slightly increased risk of febrile seizure when compared to giving MMR and a separate varicella vaccine. Either MMR or MMRV can be used for the second dose of vaccine in otherwise healthy children, typically given at 4 to 6 years of age. The second dose of a mumps-containing vaccine may be administered before 4 years of age provided it is given 28 days or more after the initial dose of vaccine (if using MMRV for both doses, the recommended interval is 3 months between doses for those up to 12 years of age). The second dose of mumps-containing vaccine is important because mumps disease continues to occur in highly immunized populations. Because of concern regarding waning immunity to mumps virus during outbreaks, in some populations, the Centers for Disease Control and Prevention (CDC) has issued guidance concerning the use of a third dose of mumps-containing vaccine. In addition, the CDC has proposed criteria for local and state health departments to consider to aid their decision making in case of a mumps outbreak. However, routine use of a third dose of mumps-containing vaccine (given as MMR) is not currently recommended.

Current CDC recommendations indicate that immunity to mumps is established by any of the following: (1) documentation of age-appropriate immunization with live attenuated mumps-containing vaccine—one dose on or after the first birthday for preschool children and adults not at high risk; 2 doses for school-age children, young adults attending post–high school educational institutions, and adults, born after 1957, who work in healthcare facilities or travel internationally; (2) laboratory evidence of immunity; or (3) laboratory evidence of disease.

Mumps vaccine has not been demonstrated to be effective in preventing mumps infection in susceptible individuals after exposure to natural disease. However, mumps-containing vaccine can be given after disease exposure to someone ≥ 12 months of age because immunization will provide protection against subsequent exposures if the patient does not become infected. No increase in reactions or complications from mumps disease is known to occur with immunization during the mumps incubation period. Use of intramuscular serum immunoglobulin or intravenous immunoglobulin (IVIG), unlike use with some other viral diseases, is not effective in preventing mumps infection after exposure and is not recommended.

While the effect of administered γ-globulin (IgG) on the immune response to mumps vaccine is uncertain, mumps-containing vaccine (MMR) should be given 2 weeks before any planned administration of IgG, blood transfusion, or other blood products. Furthermore, to prevent any possible neutralization of the live attenuated virus, MMR and MMRV administration needs to be delayed for 3 to 11 months following receipt of these products.

Adverse reactions to the mumps component of MMR or MMRV are uncommon. Orchitis and parotitis have been rarely reported after receiving mumps-containing vaccine. Causality for temporally related reactions such as febrile seizure, aseptic meningitis, and thrombocytopenia, which may rarely follow mumps-containing vaccine, has yet to be established. Conception should be avoided for a minimum of 28 days after receiving mumps-containing vaccine. Persons receiving high-dose corticosteroids (2 mg/kg/d or > 20 mg/d of prednisone or equivalent) for 14 days or more and who are not otherwise immunocompromised can be immunized with MMR 1 month after the corticosteroids have been discontinued. Persons with immunodeficiency, those with underlying medical conditions causing severe immunocompromise, and those taking medications that are immunosuppressive or who are expected to receive such agents within 4 weeks should not receive either MMR or MMRV. One exception is the patient with HIV infection who is not severely immunocompromised (CD4+ T-lymphocyte percentage ≥ 15%). These patients can receive MMR (not MMRV as it has not been thoroughly studied). Immunocompromised individuals benefit from having all of their close contacts fully immunized. Mumps virus is not transmitted from immunized persons.

Most hypersensitivity reactions following use of mumps-containing vaccines (MMR and MMRV) are related to trace amounts of gelatin, neomycin, or some other component of the vaccine. Mumps-containing vaccines are produced in chick embryo cell culture and do not contain significant amounts of ovalbumin (egg white protein). Children with egg allergy may receive mumps-containing vaccine as MMR without prior testing or the use of special precautions. Persons who have experienced anaphylactic reactions to either gelatin or neomycin should receive mumps-containing vaccine as MMR only in those settings where severe reactions can be properly managed and only after consultation with an allergist or immunologist. Contact dermatitis from neomycin is not a contraindication to receiving a mumps-containing vaccine.

Finally, patients with mumps disease who require hospitalization should be placed into isolation with droplet precautions. Historically, isolation was recommended to continue up until 9 days after the onset of parotitis; however, upon re-evaluation, CDC changed this recommendation to maintaining droplet isolation for 5 days after parotid swelling.

## SUGGESTED READINGS


American Academy of Pediatrics. In: Kimberlin DW, ed. *Red Book 2015 Report of the Committee on Infectious Diseases*. 30th ed. Elk Grove Village, IL: American Academy of Pediatrics; 2015:74-88, 564-568, 856-857.

Centers for Disease Control and Prevention. Mumps. www.cdc.gov/mumps/lab/qa-lab-test-infect.html. Accessed June 11, 2016.

Centers for Disease Control and Prevention. Mumps vaccination. www.cdc.gov/mumps/vaccination.html. Accessed May 6, 2016.

Centers for Disease Control and Prevention. Prevention of measles, rubella, congenital rubella syndrome, and mumps, 2013: summary of recommendations from the Advisory Committee on Immunization Practices (ACIP). *MMWR Rec Rep*. 2013;62(RR04):1-34.

Communication and Education Branch, Centers for Disease Control and Prevention. Chapter 15, Mumps. In: Hamborsky J, Kroger A, Wolfe C, eds. *Epidemiology and Prevention of Vaccine-Preventable Diseases*. 13th ed. Washington, DC: Public Health Foundation; 2015:243-256.

Immunization Action Coalition. www.immunize.org/catg.d/p4211.pdf. Mumps: questions and answers. Item #P4211. Accessed June 1, 2016.

Kutty PK, Kyaw MH, Dayan GH, et al. Guidance for isolation precautions for mumps in the United States: a review of the scientific basis for policy change. *Clin Infect Dis*. 2010;50:1619-1628.

Livingston KA, Rosen JB, Zucker JR, et al. Mumps vaccine effectiveness and risk factors for disease in households during an outbreak in New York City. *Vaccine*. 2014;32:369-374.

Ogbuana IU, Kutty PK, Hudson JM, et al. Impact of a third dose of measles-mumps-rubella vaccine on a mumps outbreak. *Pediatrics*. 2012;130:e1567-e1574.


# 314 Human Parvovirus

Vini Vijayan

## INTRODUCTION

Human parvovirus (HPV) B19 was first discovered in 1975 by Cossart and colleagues while screening healthy blood bank donors' sera. HPV B19 is a small (20–25 nm), single-stranded, nonenveloped DNA virus of the family Parvoviridae, genus *Erythrovirus*. It is the infectious agent of a number of clinical syndromes (eg, erythema infectiosum) and can cause intrauterine infection of the fetus as well.

## PATHOGENESIS AND EPIDEMIOLOGY

Parvovirus infections occur worldwide as sporadic cases or within clustered outbreaks. In temperate climates, cases occur generally in late winter or spring. Parvovirus infections are most commonly recognized during childhood, and approximately 70% occur in children between 5 and 15 years of age. Infection continues at a lower rate throughout adult life, and antibody seroprevalence rates in young adults and elderly are estimated to be 50% and 90%, respectively. Women of child-bearing age in the United States have seroconversion rates of approximately 1.5%.

Parvovirus B19 is readily transmitted from person to person via respiratory droplets, fomites, and close person-to-person contact. Secondary attack rates are approximately 50% within households and variable in school outbreaks. The virus is also transmitted vertically, from mother to child, and hematogenously by blood and blood products, including albumin and plasma. Rarely, nosocomial transmission has been described.

The incubation period from acquisition of the virus to onset of initial symptom is between 4 and 14 days but can be as long as 3 weeks.

Patients are most contagious in the few days preceding the rash, but those with aplastic anemia are considered contagious before the onset of symptoms and for at least 1 week after symptoms.

Viral replication occurs in human erythroid progenitor cells of the bone marrow and blood, leading to cytotoxicity and inhibition of erythropoiesis. Erythroid specificity is due to the virus's cellular receptor, globoside, or blood group P antigen. The antigen is also present on fetal myocardial cells, which may explain the direct myocardial effects seen in fetal infection. Individuals who genetically lack the P antigen are resistant to parvovirus B19 infection.

## CLINICAL MANIFESTATIONS

### Erythema Infectiosum

Parvovirus B19 classically causes erythema infectiosum (EI), or fifth disease, a common childhood exanthem. EI begins as a mild nonspecific prodromal illness that includes fever, malaise, headache, myalgia, nausea, and rhinorrhea typically beginning 5 to 7 days after initial infection and coinciding with the onset of viremia. This is followed by the classic "slapped cheek" or erythematous macular exanthem on the cheeks, which may be accompanied by circumoral pallor or fine desquamation (Fig. 314-1A). One to 4 days following the facial rash, a lacy or reticulated exanthem often develops on the trunk and extremities (Fig. 314-1B). The rash is pruritic in approximately 50% of patients. Classic EI is more common in children than adults. EI is believed to be immunologically mediated, and the rash corresponds to the appearance of immunoglobulin M (IgM) in the serum and clearance of viremia. Recrudescence of the rash can occur after a variety of nonspecific stimuli, such as change in temperature, exposure to sunlight, exercise, or emotional stress.

Rarely, parvovirus B19 can cause papular-purpuric "gloves-and-socks" syndrome (PPGSS), a rash characterized by painful and pruritic papules, petechia, and purpura of hands and feet with a distinct margin at the wrist and ankle joints. The skin changes may progress to petechiae, purpura, and bulla with skin sloughing. PPGSS usually resolves in 1 to 3 weeks without scarring. Other dermatologic manifestations of parvovirus B19 include erythema multiforme, purpuric rash, and pruritus of the soles of the feet.

### Arthropathy

Arthritis and arthralgia occur in < 10% of children but commonly occur in adults, particularly women. The knees are most frequently affected in children, but symmetric polyarthropathy involving the small joints of the hands, wrists, fingers, and feet is typical in adults. Joint pain and swelling can develop after the rash but may be the sole manifestation of infection as well. Arthropathy lasts from 1 to 3 weeks but can persist for months or years. Parvovirus B19 infection has been associated with rheumatoid factor production, and patients may mistakenly be thought to have rheumatoid arthritis. Although parvovirus B19 does not cause erosive arthritis, it has been postulated that the virus may be a trigger for or associated with juvenile rheumatic diseases.

### Transient Aplastic Crisis

Parvovirus B19 can cause transient aplastic crises (TAC) secondary to abrupt cessation of red cell production, which exacerbates or, in compensated states, provokes severe anemia. TAC generally occurs in patients with underlying hemolytic disorders including sickle cell disease, hereditary spherocytosis, thalassemia, pyruvate kinase deficiency, and autoimmune hemolytic anemia. It can also occur with decreased red blood cell production such as with hemorrhage, iron deficiency anemia, or kidney or bone marrow transplantation. Susceptible individuals are unable to compensate for the erythrocyte destruction and have an abrupt decrease in hematocrit and reticulocytopenia. White cell and platelet counts may also decline during TAC, especially in patients with functioning spleens. TAC tends to resolve in 1 to 2 weeks with fall in viremia and as red cell production returns to baseline.

Clinical manifestations include pallor, weakness, and lethargy secondary to severe anemia. Infection is usually self-limited, but severe complications such as congestive heart failure, cerebrovascular accidents, and acute splenic sequestration can develop and may be fatal.

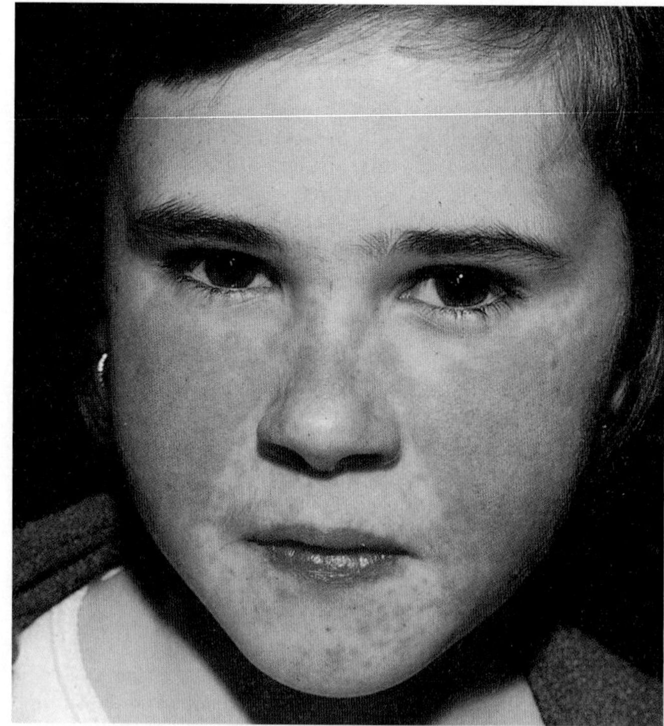

A

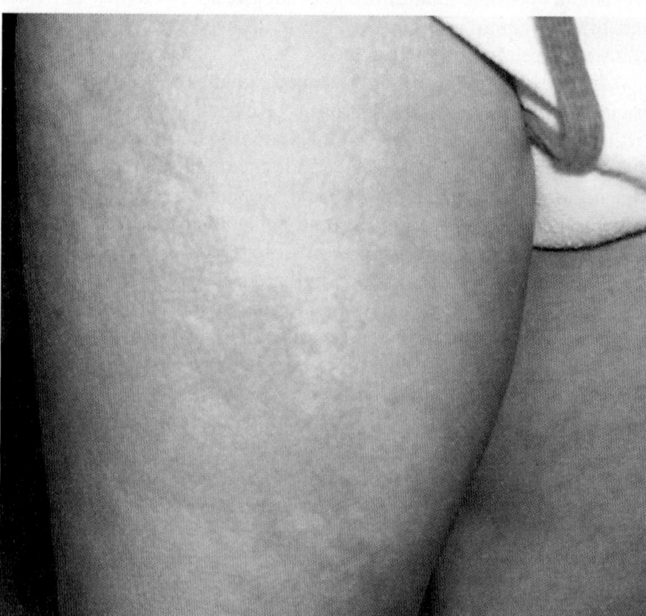

B

**FIGURE 314-1 A:** The classic feature of the rash is a "slapped cheek" appearance on the face, which may be accompanied by circumoral pallor or fine desquamation. (Reproduced with permission from Wolff K, Johnson RA: *Fitzpatrick's Color Atlas & Synopsis of Clinical Dermatology*, 6th ed. New York: McGraw-Hill; 2009.) **B:** The rash then spreads to the trunk and the extremities. It is described as erythematous and macular, often with confluent areas, giving it a reticular or lattice-like appearance.

### Pure Red Cell Aplasia

Immunocompromised hosts, such as those with congenital immunodeficiencies, cancer, organ transplantation, or human immunodeficiency virus (HIV) infection, can develop chronic parvovirus infection characterized by severe anemia. These patients lack protective antibodies and are unable to adequately clear the virus, leading to ongoing bone marrow suppression and high levels of viremia. They do not generally develop the characteristic rash or joint symptoms as antigen–antibody complexes are not formed. Bone marrow examination reveals the presence of scattered giant pronormoblasts, and reticulocytes are absent from the blood.

#### Unusual Manifestations

Rare presentations of parvovirus B19 infection include hemophagocytic syndrome, glomerulonephritis, neurologic complications such as encephalitis and aseptic meningitis, and fulminant hepatitis. Parvovirus B19 infection has also been associated with myocarditis and dilated cardiomyopathy.

#### Infection in Pregnancy

Most intrauterine parvovirus infections do not have adverse outcomes, but rarely, infection in a pregnant woman can lead to fetal loss, stillbirths, or hydrops fetalis. The virus has been found in abortus tissue, and IgM antibodies to the virus have been detected in cord blood. Severe anemia and myocarditis lead to high-output congestive heart failure and may contribute to the hydrops and fetal death in some cases.

The risk of adverse outcomes appears to be limited to infection during the first 20 weeks of gestation. Although previous reports indicated that risk of fetal loss following parvovirus B19 infection during pregnancy was greater than 30%, larger prospective trials have reported lower rates of fetal loss. A large prospective study of 1018 pregnant German women with acute parvovirus B19 infection indicated the overall fetal death rate during pregnancy was 6.3%. The rates of fetal loss in pregnancies infected before and after 20 weeks of gestation were determined to be 11% and < 1%, respectively. Hydrops occurred in 3.9% of pregnancies (40 of 1018 pregnancies) and was more common when infection was diagnosed at ≤ 32 weeks of gestation.

Women diagnosed with acute parvovirus infection during the first half of pregnancy should be counseled that there is no proven risk of parvovirus-induced congenital anomalies, but there is a risk for fetal loss. Pregnant women who are diagnosed with acute infection beyond 20 weeks of gestation should receive weekly ultrasounds to evaluate for fetal hydrops. When severe anemia is suspected on ultrasound findings, the fetus requires close monitoring and assessment of fetal hematocrit by percutaneous umbilical vein sampling. Intrauterine transfusion of red blood cells may be indicated to prevent fetal death from anemia.

### DIAGNOSIS

Parvovirus B19 infection is a clinical diagnosis, and laboratory studies are not usually necessary. Unfortunately, HPV B19 cannot be grown by using routine virologic tissue culture techniques, and definitive diagnosis is made by serologic testing for parvovirus B19–specific IgM and IgG antibodies or detection of parvovirus B19 DNA through nucleic acid amplification testing (NAAT). Parvovirus B19 IgM can be found within 7 to 10 days of exposure and is indicative of acute infection. It persists for 2 to 3 months and sometimes longer. IgG antibodies are detectable by day 7 of illness and persist for life. In immunocompromised patients with TAC or pure red cell aplasia, negative serology does not rule out infection, and parvovirus B19 DNA NAAT may be more useful.

During pregnancy, the laboratory diagnosis of maternal parvovirus B19 infection relies primarily on serology. Congenital infection of the neonate may be diagnosed by parvovirus B19 NAAT on amniotic fluid. This test is also useful in monitoring the quantitative viral load, thereby directing need for transfusions in affected infants.

The differential diagnosis for parvovirus B19 infection depends on the clinical presentation. In some patients, EI may be confused with roseola, rubella, measles, enteroviral infections, infectious mononucleosis, group A streptococcal infection, or acute HIV. The acute polyarthritis syndrome associated with parvovirus B19 infection often mimics rheumatic processes such as juvenile idiopathic arthritis or systemic lupus erythematosus. Transient arthropathy can also be seen in other viral infections such as hepatitis B and C viruses, arboviruses, alphaviruses, and herpesviruses.

### TREATMENT

There is currently no specific antiviral therapy for treating HPV B19. Management varies based on the clinical syndrome. Supportive care with antipyretics, rest, and hydration is effective in treating EI. For patients with arthritis, nonsteroidal anti-inflammatory drugs may provide symptomatic relief. Blood transfusions are often life-saving for patients with TAC. In immunocompromised patients with chronic infection and anemia secondary to parvovirus B19, cessation or reduction of immunosuppression may be sufficient to allow the immune system to mount a response and overcome infection. For those who do not respond to reduction in immunosuppression or if cessation of immunosuppression is not feasible, intravenous immunoglobulin (IVIG) at 400 mg/kg for 5 days or 1000 mg/kg for 3 days has been reported to be beneficial. These patients should be monitored closely for relapse following treatment.

### PREVENTION

The only currently available methods to prevent transmission are good infection control practices, such as hand hygiene. In the hospital setting, those with TAC should be placed in droplet isolation precautions for 7 days. Immunocompromised patients with chronic infection should be placed on droplet precautions for the duration of their hospitalization. Pregnant women at high risk of acquiring parvovirus (teachers, childcare workers, women with young school-age children) might consider serologic testing for IgG to determine their susceptibility. Currently, there is no vaccine available to prevent infection with parvovirus B19, but efforts are under way.

### SUGGESTED READINGS


Adler SP, Koch WC. Human parvovirus infections. In: Remington JS, Klein JO, Wilson CB, Baker CJ, eds. *Remington and Klein's Infectious Diseases of the Fetus and Newborn Infant*. 7th ed. Philadelphia, PA: Saunders Elsevier; 2011:835-855.

Brown KE. Parvovirus B19. In: Mandell GL, Bennett JE, Dolin R, eds. *Mandell, Douglas and Bennett's Principles and Practice of Infectious Diseases*. 7th ed. Philadelphia, PA: Churchill Livingstone Elsevier; 2010;2:2087-2096.

Crabol Y, Terrier B, Rozenberg F, et al. Intravenous immunoglobulin therapy for pure red cell aplasia related to human parvovirus b19 infection: a retrospective study of 10 patients and review of the literature. *Clin Infect Dis*. 2013;56:968-977.

de Haan TR, Beersma MF, Oepkes D, et al. Parvovirus B19 infection in pregnancy: maternal and fetal viral load measurements related to clinical parameters. *Prenat Diagn*. 2007;27:46-50.

de Jong EP, Walther FJ, Kroes AC, Oepkes D. Parvovirus B19 infection in pregnancy: new insights and management. *Prenat Diagn*. 2011;31(5):419-425.

Kimberlin DW, Brady MT, Jackson MA, Long SS, eds. American Academy of Pediatrics Committee on Infectious Diseases. Parvovirus B19. In: *2015 Red Book: Report of the Committee on Infectious Diseases*. 30th ed. Elk Grove Village, IL: American Academy of Pediatrics; 2015:593-596.

Manaresi E, Gallinella G, Venturoli S, et al. Detection of parvovirus B19 IgG: choice of antigens and serological tests. *J Clin Virol*. 2004;29:51-53.


# 315 Rubella

Maria Jevitz Patterson

### INTRODUCTION

Rubella (German measles) is no longer endemic in the United States. Because of its worldwide distribution, imported cases continue to occur, although these sporadic cases do not result in sustained transmission. Rubella is usually a minor illness in adults. Of major significance, however, is the high incidence of a constellation of congenital defects in children whose mothers are infected during early pregnancy. Typical anomalies caused by this congenital infection, known collectively as the congenital rubella syndrome (CRS), include hearing impairment, cardiac defects, cataracts, and developmental delay.

## PATHOGENESIS AND EPIDEMIOLOGY

Rubella is a member of the Togaviridae family (a single serotype and the only member of the genus *Rubivirus*) with an approximately 10-kb (9762 nucleotides) single-stranded, positive-sense polyadenylated RNA genome and a lipid envelope (thus the Latin name of *toga* or *cloak*). The virus was first isolated in 1962 by Weller from the urine of his son. Current proposed nomenclature for wild-type and vaccine rubella viruses employs clades, genotypes, and a more precise sequence database. Rubella shares physicochemical properties with group A arboviruses. The virion is roughly spherical, 60 to 70 nm in diameter, with an icosahedral nucleocapsid composed of multiple copies of a single virus-specified structural capsid protein (C) that is covered by a lipid envelope in which 2 virus-specified structural glycoproteins (E1 and E2) are embedded. E1 appears to function in attachment, fusion, hemagglutination, and neutralization. In addition, there are 2 virus-specified nonstructural proteins (p90 and p150). The virus is thermolabile; inactivation is rapid at 37°C (98.6°F) and at room temperature.

Humans are the only natural host. Direct person-to-person airborne spread by infected nasopharyngeal secretion droplets appears to be the usual mode of transmission. The patient with subclinical infection is also a source of rubella virus. Patients are most contagious for a few days before and after the onset of rash, although virus may be present in pharyngeal secretions for as long as 1 week before and 2 weeks after the onset of rash. Infection acquired postnatally does not produce a chronic carrier state. Prolonged shedding occurs only in patients with CRS, which is characterized by chronic infection; infants may remain contagious for months after birth.

Although rubella occurs in all areas of the world, epidemiologic patterns vary from country to country. Mathematic modeling predicts that elimination of transmission requires approximately 90% immunity among children. Prior to widespread use of rubella vaccines in the United States, when 85% of the population was immune, rubella occurred primarily in children during the elementary school years. A small minority did not become infected until early adulthood. After vaccine introduction, there was a marked shift in epidemiology and a shift in age at which those who are susceptible became infected.

When rubella was endemic in the United States, its seasonal peak occurred in late winter and spring. Its greatest impact resulted from epidemics that occurred at 4- to 7-year intervals in industrialized countries. The last US epidemic (1964–1965) resulted in 12.5 million cases of rubella, 13,350 spontaneous or therapeutic abortions or neonatal deaths, and 20,000 infants born with CRS. Following licensure of the first vaccine in 1969, until 1989, the reported incidence of rubella declined more than 99% in the United States (Fig. 315-1). This was followed by a resurgence in 1989 to 1991, but the reported incidence from 1992 to 1996 was the lowest ever recorded, with an all-time low of 128 cases reported in 1995. In addition, the seasonal peak disappeared, leaving no temporal or geographic clustering. In 2004, endemic rubella transmission elimination was declared achieved in the United States. In 2011, maintenance of elimination was confirmed. Beginning with the 2005–2006 school year, all 50 states required and enforced the second dose of measles-mumps-rubella (MMR) vaccine for school entry. Only 62 cases of rubella (between 2005 and 2011) and 6 cases of CRS (between 2004 and 2013) were reported (Fig. 315-2).

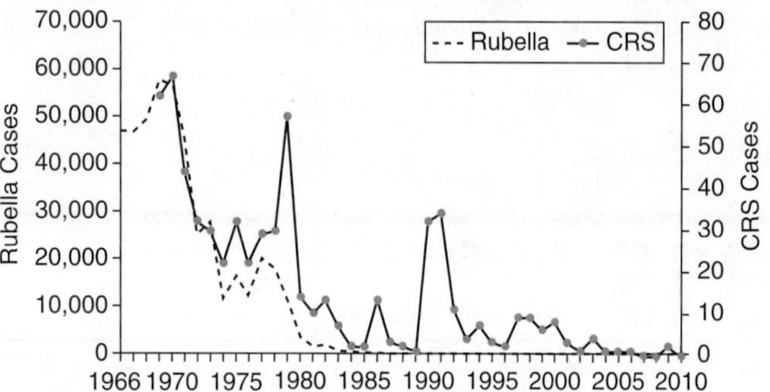


**FIGURE 315-1** Rubella and congenital rubella syndrome: United States 1966–2011. CRS, congenital rubella syndrome. (Data from Centers for Disease Control and Prevention [CDC]: Three cases of congenital rubella syndrome in the postelimination era—Maryland, Alabama, and Illinois, 2012, *MMWR Morb Mortal Wkly Rep*. 2013 Mar 29;62(12):226-229.)

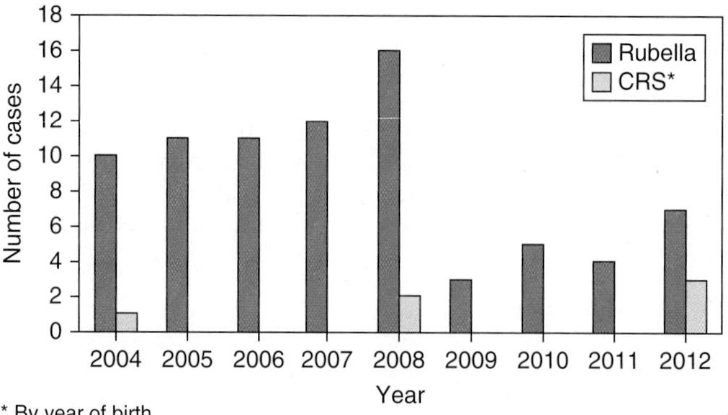


**FIGURE 315-2** Rubella and congenital rubella syndrome: United States 2004–2012. CRS, congenital rubella syndrome. (Reproduced with permission from Hamborsky J, Kroger A, Wolfe S: *Epidemiology and Prevention of Vaccine-Preventable Diseases*, 13th ed. Washington DC: Public Health Foundation. Centers for Disease Control and Prevention; 2015.)

Outbreaks during the years of changing epidemiology in the United States were confined essentially to unimmunized populations, religious communities that traditionally decline vaccination, settings in which young adults congregate, and among persons from countries where rubella vaccine is not routinely used. Many countries have yet to achieve good rubella vaccination rates, which underscores the importance of documenting patient country of origin. A 1995 World Health Organization (WHO) global survey showed that only 78 of 214 countries had national policies for rubella vaccination. In 2011, WHO issued updated guidelines for the introduction of rubella-containing vaccine globally. The following year, the number of reported cases of rubella dropped 86%. By 2014, 46% of children globally had received rubella vaccine. Molecular techniques allowing sequence identification of wild-type and vaccine rubella assist global surveillance, tracking of transmission, investigation of postvaccine cases, confirmation of importations, and documentation of elimination. Although challenges remain (civil unrest, poor healthcare delivery, vaccine hesitancy), the global measles eradication effort should enhance rubella and ultimately CRS elimination.

# POSTNATAL RUBELLA

## CLINICAL MANIFESTATIONS

The clinical manifestations of postnatal rubella range from inapparent infection to a characteristic pattern of adenopathy, rash, and low-grade fever. The incubation period is from 14 to 21 days. Primary replication occurs in the nasopharynx, followed by viremia at approximately days 5 to 7 and rash at days 14 to 17 (Fig. 315-3). A typical clinical course begins with adenopathy involving primarily the postauricular, occipital, and posterior cervical nodes, which may be slightly painful and tender. Although symptoms usually clear promptly as the rash fades, nodes may remain palpable for several weeks. Adolescents and adults may complain of malaise, headache, a low-grade fever, sore throat, and mild coryza during a 1- to 5-day prodromal period that frequently accompanies the onset of adenopathy. In young children, the mild prodrome is usually overlooked.

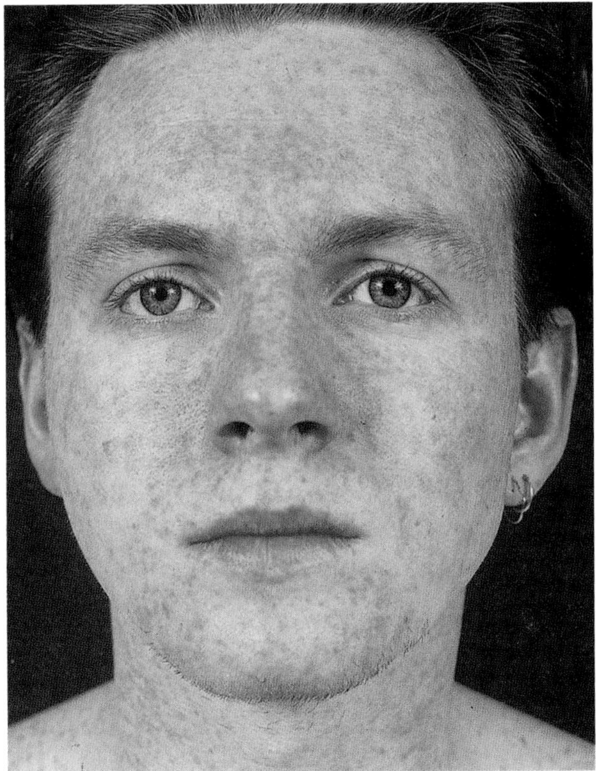

**FIGURE 315-3** Rubella. The rash consists of erythematous macules and papules that appear initially on the face and spread inferiorly to the trunk and extremities, usually within the first 24 hours. (Reproduced with permission from Wolff K, Johnson RA. *Fitzpatrick's Color Atlas & Synopsis of Clinical Dermatology*, 6th ed. New York: McGraw-Hill; 2009.)

The rubella rash is variable but usually brief. It may be no more than a transient blush, but classically it persists for 2 to 3 days in a changing appearance. Initially, small, irregular pink macules begin on the face and spread rapidly (usually within 24 hours) to the neck, trunk, arms, and ultimately legs. By the next day, these lesions may have coalesced, developed a maculopapular component, and become scarlatiniform. The face is frequently clearing by the time a full-blown rash is seen on the lower legs, where coalescence is uncommon. Desquamation is rare.

An exanthem consisting of punctate or slightly larger red spots on the soft palate may be present during the late prodrome and early rash phase. These lesions are not pathognomonic of rubella. Scarlet fever, infectious mononucleosis, measles, and other viral exanthems may be accompanied by similar palatal lesions.

Fever is uncommonly as high as 39°C (102.2°F) to 39.5°C (103.1°F), but may be absent in children. Polyarthralgia and polyarthritis are common manifestations of rubella among women, less common in men, and uncommon in children. Symptoms typically appear with the rash or within several days after its onset, but rarely may precede onset of rash by several days. Joint involvement, frequently symmetric, may range from subjective morning stiffness to full-blown arthritis characterized by swelling, redness, tenderness, and effusion. Objective signs and symptoms usually clear within several days to 2 weeks, but rarely may persist for several months. The proximal interphalangeal joints are affected most frequently, but other joints may be involved. Paresthesia, most typically numbness and tingling, often accompanies, and may outlast, joint symptoms. Joint manifestations in rubella produce no deformity. Joint symptoms are also associated with rubella vaccine, particularly in postpubertal females of HLA-DR2 and HLA-DR5 type. However, no causal relationship between vaccine and persistent joint symptoms has been validated.

Postinfectious encephalitis, clinically indistinguishable from that following measles or varicella, is a rare complication of rubella that occurs less frequently than postmeasles encephalitis. Symptoms and signs of central nervous system involvement usually develop 2 to 4 days after onset of rash.

Many patients have a slight decrease in platelet count during the course of uncomplicated rubella. This thrombocytopenia usually occurs within 1 week after onset of rash. Presenting complaints usually include purpura, epistaxis, bleeding from the gums, hematuria, and gastrointestinal bleeding. Abnormal capillary fragility also contributes to the problem of hemostasis. Prognosis is generally excellent, but fatalities due to uncontrolled central nervous system hemorrhage do occur rarely. Although thrombocytopenia may sometimes be prolonged, most patients become symptom free within 2 weeks. The incidence of thrombocytopenia following vaccine is significantly less than after natural infection.

## DIAGNOSIS

As rubella prevalence has continued to fall, medical professionals have become less experienced in recognizing clinical disease. Diagnosis of rubelliform rashes in acutely ill, febrile children and in young adults requires accurate historical information from parents: vaccine history, source of exposure, prodrome, and progression of rash. Other childhood exanthems (eg, measles, human herpesvirus 6 and 7, adenovirus, enterovirus, parvovirus B19, and various arboviruses), as well as the possibility of primary vaccine failure, should be considered. The predictive value of clinical diagnosis is low. Laboratory testing is required. Rubella can be diagnosed by isolating the virus, detecting viral nucleic acid by polymerase chain reaction (PCR), or demonstrating rising titers of rubella antibody in serum (Fig. 315-4). Virus isolation is less

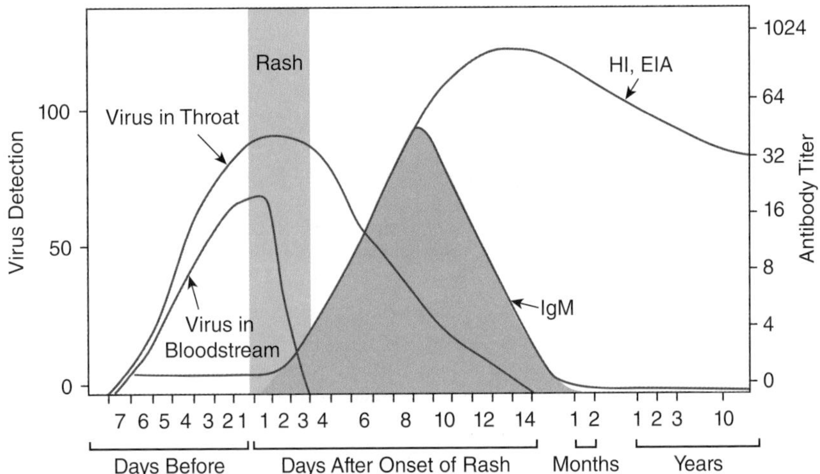


**FIGURE 315-4** Schematic illustration of the natural history of rubella. Virus detection via isolation, polymerase chain reaction, or host immunologic response; see text. EIA, enzyme immunoassay; HI, hemagglutination inhibition; IgM, immunoglobulin M. (Data from Cooper LZ, Krugman S: Clinical manifestations of postnatal and congenital rubella, *Arch Ophthalmol*. 1967 Apr;77(4):434-439.)

practical because of relative lability of rubella virus and the complexity of the assay, and isolation is being replaced by PCR.

Rubella virus may be cultured from the pharynx and serum as early as 1 week before the onset of rash. Virus is promptly cleared from the serum after the rash appears, but persists in pharyngeal secretions, usually for several days after the rash and, uncommonly, for as long as 2 weeks (see Fig. 315-3). Urine, blood, and cerebrospinal fluid (CSF) are also appropriate clinical specimens. Molecular characterization by PCR and sequence analyses provides important epidemiologic information (country of origin or wild-type vs vaccine virus strain).

Rubella serum antibody is measured most commonly now by enzyme immunoassay (EIA), but a variety of test systems based on neutralization, hemagglutination inhibition (the previous serologic standard), latex agglutination, radial hemolysis, and immunoblot have been used. Rapid, sensitive, economical, and reliable diagnosis is critical. A positive immunoglobulin (Ig) M imposes a dilemma in acute rubella diagnosis, especially in pregnant women. The positive predictive value of these assays is lessened in the setting of low incidence where a high proportion of IgM-positive tests may be false positive due to rheumatoid factor, cross-reacting antibody, or other viral infection. IgG avidity testing (measuring strength of antigen/antibody binding) helps confirm or exclude primary infection and clarify diagnostic uncertainty. Interpretation of antibody testing must always be guided by clinical, epidemiologic, and immunization status data.

EIA detects antibody to viral proteins E1, E2, and C. Rubella-specific IgM antibodies are detectable within 24 to 48 hours after onset of the rash, and peak titers are reached within 6 to 12 days. In subclinical rubella (primary rubella without rash), rubella-specific IgM antibodies usually reach detectable levels 14 to 21 days after exposure, a time that corresponds to the onset of rash in clinical disease.

The presence of serum IgG at exposure confirms past rubella infection (or rubella vaccination), indicates protection from another episode of the disease, and in the pregnant woman obviates rubella-induced congenital malformation. Although no antibody titer is absolutely correlated with protection, absence of rubella hemagglutination inhibition or EIA antibodies (< 10 IU) at the time of exposure indicates susceptibility to rubella. The National Health and Nutrition Examination Survey (NHANES III 1988–1994) documented substantial immunity (EIA > 10 IU: 92%, 6–11 year olds; 83%, 12–19 year olds; 85%, 20–29 year olds; 89%, 30–39 year olds; and 93%, > 40 years olds). Subsequent national seropositive rates (1999–2004) showed immunity sufficient to interrupt transmission (children, 96.2%; adolescents, 93.7%; adult women, 91.5%; adult men, 88%). However, with lack of natural boosting from circulating wild-type virus, nearly 10% of women lacked protective antibody to prevent CRS.

### TREATMENT

Rubella is a reportable disease in the United States, and notification should not be delayed awaiting laboratory confirmation. Persons with suspected rubella should be isolated for 7 days after rash onset. Persons who have been exempted from vaccination should be excluded from school as soon as 1 case is confirmed in a community.

### PREVENTION

Widespread use of live attenuated rubella vaccine, first licensed in 1969, has prevented epidemics and even endemicity and protected vaccine recipients from disease, with the ultimate goal of preventing fetal infection and the serious consequences of CRS. The vaccine used exclusively in the United States and most other countries is the subcutaneously administered RA27/3 strain. An aerosolized measles/rubella vaccine is under study. Preterm infants receive vaccine at the same chronologic age as term infants. Recommendations for rubella vaccination are provided in Chapter 239.

Although vaccine immunity is generally less robust than that acquired from wild-type infection, the vaccine stimulates both persistent and long-term humoral and cell-mediated immunity. Primary vaccine failure in up to 5% of those receiving vaccine occurs following the first dose. Determination of immune status requires documentation of 2 doses of MMR or laboratory confirmation.

Rubella was formerly a childhood disease with circulating wild-type virus boosting immunity. Now people rely solely on vaccine-induced immunity. This shifting epidemiology leaves susceptible people in older age groups, further complicated by a shift in first pregnancy to an older age. Continued strong disease surveillance; rapid response to outbreaks; and efforts to identify and vaccinate children, nonimmune adolescents, and women of child-bearing age, using effective strategies to avoid missed opportunities, are critical to continued US efforts to eliminate rubella.

## CONGENITAL RUBELLA

Congenital infection produces a spectrum of illness known as the congenital rubella syndrome (CRS), a result of multiorgan, noninflammatory vasculitis triggered by persistent viral infection. The first link between rubella virus and fetal damage was made by Gregg, an Australian ophthalmologist, in 1941, paving the way for recognition of teratogenesis by subsequent viruses (eg, cytomegalovirus [Chapter 305], zikavirus [Chapter 300]).

### PATHOGENESIS AND EPIDEMIOLOGY

The pathophysiologic basis of rubella's teratogenicity is still not fully elucidated. Rubella demonstrates a vascular endothelial cell tropism, directed in large blood vessels at the inner layer of the vascular wall. At the cellular level, damage is linked to impaired replication, perturbation of cell growth, apoptosis, and postulated interaction between the viral nonstructural protein p90 and host cell regulatory proteins. Timing of infection is of great importance. Prospective studies after laboratory-confirmed rubella in pregnancy have documented that the rate of fetal infection is 90% after symptomatic maternal rubella during the first 12 gestational weeks; it drops to 25% to 30% during the second trimester and rises to 60% to 100% during the last weeks of gestation. During the second trimester, the fetus develops increasing immunologic competence and no longer seems susceptible to the chronic infection characteristic of intrauterine rubella during the early weeks.

In general, earlier infection produces more extensive damage. Cardiac defects, cataracts, and glaucoma occur predominantly after maternal rubella during the first 2 months of pregnancy. Hearing loss and neurologic manifestations may occur any time during the first and, less commonly, into the second trimester. Late in pregnancy, infection does not appear to be teratogenic. Risk after reinfection, although much less than after primary rubella, has been documented.

Maternal infection with rubella during the first trimester of pregnancy frequently results in fetal infection following placental infection during maternal viremia. Potential cases would be born to mothers who are recent immigrants to the United States or who have not received immunization with a rubella-containing vaccine.

### CLINICAL MANIFESTATIONS

The consequences of rubella in utero are varied and unpredictable. Spontaneous abortion, stillbirth, live birth with anomalies (single or multiple), and normal infants are represented in this spectrum. Virtually every organ may be involved, transiently or permanently, some with delayed onset.

During the newborn period, congenital rubella may be manifested by a number of acute conditions that are self-limiting in infants who survive. Neonatal thrombocytopenic purpura, characterized by a variable number of red purple macular "blueberry muffin" lesions, is the most common and striking of these manifestations (Fig. 315-5). It is usually associated with a high incidence of other transient lesions, such as radiolucencies in the metaphyseal portions of the long bones, hepatosplenomegaly, hepatitis, hemolytic anemia, and bulging anterior fontanelle with or without CSF pleocytosis. This clinical picture represents the most severe evidence of congenital infection. Low birth weight, cardiac defects, cataracts, deafness, and developmental delay with or without microcephaly frequently accompany these transient lesions.

Patent ductus arteriosus, with or without stenosis of the pulmonary artery or its branches, and atrial and ventricular septal defects are the most common cardiac lesions encountered. The most characteristic

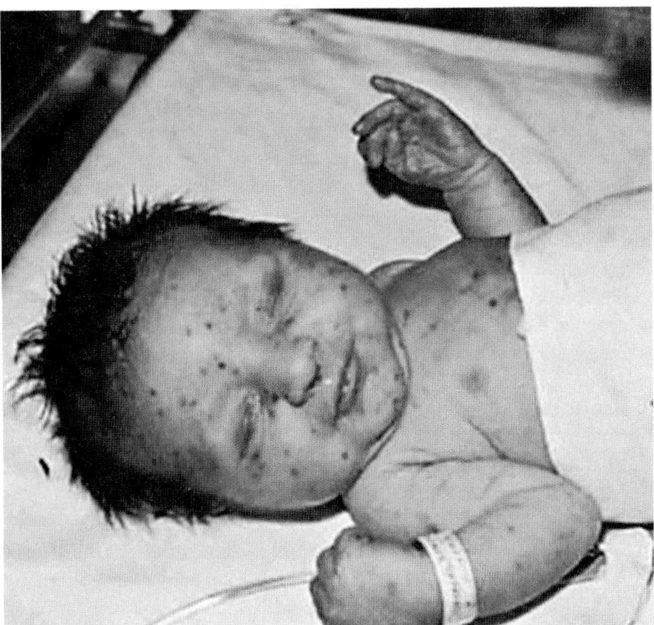

**FIGURE 315-5** Infant with congenital rubella. Note "blueberry muffin" appearance with multiple petechiae. (Used with permission from Louis Z. Cooper.)

ocular anomaly is a pearly nuclear cataract, unilateral or bilateral, frequently associated with microphthalmia. The lesion may be absent at birth or so small that it may not be detected without careful ophthalmoscopic examination. Congenital glaucoma, which might be present at birth or which might develop during infancy, is clinically indistinguishable from hereditary infantile glaucoma. The cornea is enlarged and hazy, the anterior chamber is deep, and ocular tension is increased. Retinopathy, characterized by discrete, patchy black pigmentation, quite variable in size and location, is probably the most common ocular manifestation of congenital rubella. There is no evidence that this anomaly of the pigment epithelium of the retina interferes with vision. However, recognition of this lesion is a valuable aid in the diagnosis of congenital rubella.

Permanent sensorineural deafness caused by damage to the organ of Corti may be severe or mild and bilateral or unilateral. Defects in the middle ear structures have been reported. Deafness and communication disorders may be the only overt manifestations of congenital rubella, especially if maternal infection occurs after the first 8 weeks of pregnancy.

Delayed psychomotor development during infancy is a hallmark of congenital rubella, with the most common consequence of the permanent brain damage being mental retardation, ranging from mild to profound. Behavior disturbances and manifestations of minimal cerebral dysfunction are also common. Less common are severe spastic diplegia and autism.

Progressive rubella panencephalitis, a severe progressive neurologic deterioration beginning during the second decade of life, is a rare complication of congenital rubella. Intellectual deterioration, myoclonus, ataxia, and seizures have progressed to death over the course of several years. High rubella antibody titers in serum and CSF, elevated spinal fluid protein and γ-globulin levels, histopathologic changes of progressive panencephalitis, and isolation of rubella virus from the brain biopsy specimen add to the obvious parallel between this condition and the subacute sclerosing panencephalitis that is a rare and late sequela of measles.

CRS also poses a risk of type 1 diabetes mellitus. By age 10 years, the risk is at least 4 times greater in children with CRS than among healthy children, and by adult life, the risk is 10- to 20-fold greater. In 1 group of adult survivors, 40% had type 1 diabetes. The high prevalence of pancreatic islet cell cytotoxic or surface antibodies in congenital rubella patients with and without type 1 diabetes may reflect the in utero infection of pancreatic cells and play a role in the pathogenesis of type 1 diabetes in genetically susceptible individuals. Thyroiditis also has been described. A comprehensive summary of the early and delayed manifestations of CRS is published elsewhere.

Mortality in a group with various abnormalities due to congenital rubella was approximately 10% and greatest during the first 6 months of life. In a group of 58 infants with neonatal thrombocytopenic purpura, mortality exceeded 35% after the first year of follow-up; this was not usually a consequence of bleeding but of sepsis, congestive heart failure, and general debility.

A number of children with multisystem involvement make excellent adjustments over the years. Among a group of approximately 300 survivors of the 1963 to 1964 US rubella epidemic followed to young adulthood, approximately one-third were leading relatively normal lives; one-third lived with their parents and might have "noncompetitive employment"; and one-third required care in facilities with support personnel present 24 hours a day.

## DIAGNOSIS

Despite the critical clinical management and attendant important implications about termination of pregnancy, prenatal diagnosis suffers from inaccuracy and is not without risk. Maternal serum IgM testing is not recommended unless there is a history of rubella or contact with a person with rubella-like illness. If positive, a second confirmatory and independent assay is required (IgM capture, IgG avidity, or PCR). Women who acquire rubella while pregnant should be monitored for birth outcome. Intrauterine diagnosis can be attempted by reverse transcriptase PCR in chorionic villous samples at 10 weeks of gestation (which does not always prove vertical transmission) or in amniotic fluid at 15 weeks of gestation and 8 or more weeks after maternal infection (sensitivity 87–100%), or by detection of fetal IgM at 22 weeks of gestation in fetal blood from ultrasound-guided cordocentesis. None of these methods predicts fetal infection with complete accuracy. Abnormal test results should be confirmed prior to any intervention. Relying on good clinical and epidemiologic data and conventional serologic assays remains the standard.

The infant with suspected congenital rubella should be evaluated with specimens for viral detection and for rubella-specific IgM. These infants may remain chronically infected for many months after birth and thus are a source of infection for susceptible contacts for a year or more. Virus has been detected in pharyngeal secretions, blood spots, urine, CSF, cataract tissue, and virtually every organ. Reverse transcriptase PCR using dried blood spots, lens aspirates, and oral fluids offers additional evidence for diagnosis in early infancy.

Newborn infants with congenital rubella have serum rubella antibody titers comparable to those of their mothers. Much of this antibody is transplacentally acquired IgG, but the presence of rubella-specific IgM reflects in utero antibody production by the fetus and, when present, is diagnostic of congenital rubella. In all but rare infants, by the end of 1 year, IgG is usually the dominant rubella antibody. Detectable levels of antibody persist for years in most children. A minority, despite congenital infection, have declining titers of antibody beginning during the second year of life. By age 5 years, approximately 20% of children have undetectable levels of antibody. Immunologic tolerance has been proposed as a mechanism for this finding. Loss of antibody cannot be correlated with severity of clinical disease. Rubella antibody that persists in infancy beyond age 6 months without evidence of postnatal infection essentially confirms the diagnosis of congenital rubella.

## TREATMENT

Infants with CRS are contagious as long as they are shedding virus in their pharyngeal secretions. In general, infants who carry rubella for long periods are more severely damaged and delayed in growth and development. There is no specific therapy for congenital rubella. Early detection of auditory and visual impairment and incorporation of adequate educational therapy, including parent education and counseling, are important.

## PREVENTION

CRS is a preventable disease. Despite its low prevalence in the United States, clinicians should remain vigilant. The optimal management of the pregnant woman exposed to rubella is unclear, but practical suggestions have been provided. Documentation of rubella immune status before pregnancy is a pivotal public health strategy, avoiding later diagnostic confusion, preventing misinterpretation of laboratory data, and allowing revaccination if the titer is low. Sadly, lack of implementation of this critical public health strategy in the United States is highlighted by documentation that in late 1998 only 6 states required rubella susceptibility premarital screening and no state required subsequent vaccination. Preconception screening and postpartum immunization remain fundamental to US strategy.

Ideally, postpubertal females should know their immune status before conception and be vaccinated only after assurance that they are not pregnant and can avoid pregnancy for at least 1 month after vaccination. Pregnant women should not be immunized but should be tested for rubella susceptibility. The immediate postpartum period is an excellent time to vaccinate susceptible women, although barriers to postpartum or postabortal vaccination remain challenging. Vaccine virus has been isolated in human breast milk but poses no hazard to the infant. The use of γ-globulin (commercially available human immunoglobulin) in prophylaxis of rubella during pregnancy does not prevent rubella or congenital rubella in a predictable or reliable fashion.

## SUGGESTED READINGS


Centers for Disease Control and Prevention. Rubella and congenital rubella syndrome control and elimination—global progress, 2000-2012. *Morb Mortal Wkly Rep*. 2013;62:983-986.

Centers for Disease Control and Prevention. Three cases of congenital rubella syndrome in the postelimination era—Maryland, Alabama, and Illinois, 2012. *Morb Mortal Wkly Rep*. 2013;62:226-229.

Forrest JM, Turnbull FM, Sholler GF, et al. Gregg's congenital rubella patients 60 years later. *Med J Aust*. 2002;177:664-667.

Gao Z, Wood JG, Burgess MA, Menzies RI, McIntyre PB, MacIntyre CR. Models of strategies for control of rubella and congenital rubella syndrome—a 40 year experience from Australia. *Vaccine*. 2013;31:691-697.

Reef SE, Redd SB, Abernathy E, Kutty P, Icenogle JP. Evidence used to support the achievement and maintenance of elimination of rubella and congenital rubella syndrome in the United States. *J Infect Dis*. 2011;204:S593-S597.

Reef SE, Strebel P, Dabbagh A, Gacic-Dobo M, Cochi S. Progress toward control of rubella and prevention of congenital rubella syndrome worldwide, 2009. *J Infect Dis*. 2011;204:S24-S27.

Sever JL, Nelson KB, Gilkeson MR. Rubella epidemic, 1964: effect on 6,000 pregnancies. *Am J Dis Child*. 1965;110:395-407.

World Health Organization. Rubella virus nomenclature update: 2013. *Wkly Epidemiol Rec*. 2013;88:337-348.


# 316 Rabies

Jin-Young Han

## INTRODUCTION

Rabies typically presents as an acute encephalomyelitis with an extremely high fatality rate. It is primarily a zoonotic infection in humans, and the disease is almost entirely preventable with timely postexposure prophylaxis.

## EPIDEMIOLOGY AND PATHOGENESIS

Rabies is caused by highly neurotropic negative-stranded RNA lyssavirus variants in the family Rhabdoviridae. Infection spreads from terrestrial mammals to humans by introduction of infectious saliva by bites or scratches, through mucous membrane exposures, and rarely, by aerosol inhalations. It is not known to cross intact skin. Rare human-to-human transmissions are reported after organ transplantation.

Transmission by rabid dogs poses the greatest hazard worldwide. A 2015 study estimates that canine rabies causes approximately 59,000 human deaths annually worldwide. The majority of cases occur in Asia and Africa, with India accounting for over 35% of global rabies burden.

With mass vaccination of dogs, canine rabies has been eliminated in the United States. However, unvaccinated dogs and cats can become infected from rabid wildlife. Bats are the source of most human rabies in the United States. In many cases, bat-associated rabies occurs without a recognized bite. Rabies exposure can also occur through contact with skunks, raccoons, coyotes, foxes, and many other species. Rabies is not endemic in rodents or lagomorphs.

Rabies may occur in any climate or season, and susceptibility does not seem to vary with age, sex, or race. The incidence of rabies infection is highest in children, probably because they are more likely to be bitten by dogs and more likely to have multiple bites in high-risk sites. In the United States, an average of 3 human cases occur per year. Some of these cases are due to imported rabies in travelers to canine rabies–endemic areas. The attack rate in persons bitten by rabid animals is difficult to estimate, and it depends on the location of the wound, the depth of the bite, the presence of saliva infected with virus, and the protection afforded by clothing. Following inoculation, rabies virus enters the nerves either directly or after local replication. The nicotinic acetylcholine receptors are believed to be important for viral entry. In vitro studies have identified 2 more putative receptors—neural cell adhesion molecule and p75 neutrophin receptor—with probable role in infection and viral spread. Rabies virus reaches the central nervous system without a viremic phase via axonal transport in a retrograde fashion. Rabies virus localizes to areas of rich cholinergic innervation including amygdala, hippocampus, thalamus, hypothalamus, and basal ganglia. The pathologic changes are minimal, and the infected neurons do not show morphologic signs of degeneration. Perivascular infiltration with lymphocytes, polymorphonuclear leukocytes, and plasma cells is seen histologically. Rabies infection frequently causes cytoplasmic eosinophilic inclusion bodies (Negri bodies) found most commonly in the hippocampus and Purkinje cells of the cerebellum. After infection of the brain, the virus travels via the sensory and autonomic nervous system to the eyes, salivary glands, skin, and viscera.

## CLINICAL MANIFESTATIONS

The average incubation period is 18 to 60 days; the interval, however, can be extremely variable, as short as 5 days and as long as 6 years. It is shorter when the bite is on a well-innervated site such as the head, perineum, or fingertips. The illness begins with a prodrome characterized by general weakness or discomfort, fever, or headache. There may be pain or an itching sensation at the site of the bite. Local motor and sensory symptoms appear to be more common in patients with bat-associated rabies. The prodromal phase lasts 2 to 7 days and is usually followed by the onset of neurologic symptoms.

The rabies infection produces 2 distinct neurologic syndromes: furious and paralytic rabies. Furious rabies is characterized by agitation and confusion with intermittent periods of relative calm, during which the patient is often quite lucid. Twitching, delirium, meningismus, and mild convulsive movements are seen. When the patient attempts to swallow food or liquid, painful, violent spasms of the larynx and pharynx may occur, resulting in hydrophobia. Later, just the sound, smell, or sight of liquid may precipitate these spasms. During these periods, cyanosis may be present, and choking and aspiration are quite common. The temperature is elevated (39.5°C/103.1°F to 40.5°C/104.9°F), and generalized convulsions may occur. Maniacal behavior, such as tearing of clothes and bedding, often occurs. Paralytic rabies is characterized by progressive paralysis, weakness, and paresthesia. This form of rabies may closely resemble Guillain-Barré syndrome early in the course of disease. Ascending paralysis, respiratory depression, hypoventilation, arrhythmias, and hypotension can occur, leading to coma and death.

## DIAGNOSIS

When classic symptoms are present and there is a history of an animal bite, the differential diagnosis is not difficult. It is important to consider the diagnosis even without an obvious exposure, because many patients have had no known contact with rabid animals. Other viral etiologies of encephalitis should be entertained.

The gold standard for diagnosis is the demonstration of virus antigen in brain tissue by direct fluorescence assay. Histologic staining for Negri bodies is neither as sensitive nor specific as other tests, and the presence of Negri bodies is not considered diagnostic. Before death, tests are performed on saliva, serum, spinal fluid, and skin biopsies of hair follicles at the nape of the neck. Virus can be detected from saliva by isolation in cell culture or reverse transcription followed by polymerase chain reaction (RT-PCR). Specimens for biopsy may be obtained from the skin at the back of the neck, which has a heavy concentration of nerve fibers, where it is particularly accessible and useful for immunofluorescence. Negative results should not exclude the diagnosis. RT-PCR of biologic samples such as spinal fluids and tissues may be used for diagnosis where available.

Presence of high titer antibody to rabies virus in the serum is diagnostic if no vaccine or rabies immunoglobulin has been given. Antibody to rabies virus in the cerebrospinal fluid (CSF), regardless of the immunization history, is diagnostic. Viral antibodies usually appear after 7 days of illness in serum. Antibodies appear in the CSF later in the disease course.

## TREATMENT

Currently, there is no effective treatment once symptoms develop. Treatment consists of intensive supportive care, concentrating particularly on support of ventilation and circulation. After a survival of an adolescent in 2004, an aggressive approach to therapy with a Milwaukee protocol is often attempted. However, many experts have argued that the use of this protocol should be discontinued as it has not been proven to be beneficial in research models and in subsequent patients. There is no known role for rabies immune globulin once symptoms have developed in rabies, nor is there any established antiviral therapy.

Until recently, the disease was reported to be uniformly fatal except in rare cases of individuals who contracted the disease despite postexposure prophylaxis. However, a few survivors have been documented, possibly due to a brisk host immune response. Previous preexposure or postexposure prophylaxis had been done in most patients who survived.

## PREVENTION

Vaccinating domesticated pets is the most effective strategy for preventing rabies in humans in the United States. Prevention of human infection includes general public health measures such as mandatory vaccination of and quarantine for traveling pets. Preexposure immunization is also recommended for people in high-risk occupations. Healthcare providers will be protected by following current infection control practices for contact with secretions. Postexposure prophylaxis is often recommended for persons who report a possibly infectious exposure (bite, scratch, or an open wound or mucous membrane contaminated with saliva or other infectious material) from a human with rabies, although human-to-human transmission has not been documented in this manner. Human-to-human transmission has occurred with transplantation of infected organs (eg, cornea, liver) from individuals who died of undiagnosed rabies. Casual contact with an infected person alone does not constitute an exposure and is not an indication for prophylaxis.

Following a possible exposure to a rabid animal, immediate and thorough local treatment of all bite wounds and scratches is a most important means of preventing rabies. At present, thorough washing with soap and water and irrigation of the wound are recommended.

When the decision is made to initiate postexposure prophylaxis, the current recommendations of the Centers for Disease Control and Prevention are that both passive and active immunization be used except in people who have been previously vaccinated. Passive immunization with rabies immune globulin is prepared from the blood of patients with high levels of antibody to rabies. The recommended dose of rabies immune globulin is 20 IU/kg. If possible, the full dose of rabies immune globulin should be infiltrated around the wound; any remaining rabies immune globulin should be given intramuscularly. Outside of the United States, equine antirabies serum is often used. The dose of this material is 40 IU/kg, and it is also given partially around the wound, with the balance given intramuscularly.

Two rabies vaccines are currently available in the United States: human diploid cell vaccine and purified chick embryo cell vaccine. Both are safe and efficacious and can be administered intramuscularly. Four doses are recommended, as soon as possible after exposure and again on days 3, 7, and 14 after the first vaccination. For an immunocompromised individual, postexposure prophylaxis includes a 5-dose regimen (0, 3, 7, 14, and 28 days after exposure). Reactions following vaccine are generally mild, with location reactions being the most common. Persons who need to be vaccinated in other countries may find a nerve tissue vaccine in use, which may induce more severe adverse reactions.

The most common issue involving rabies confronting the physician is whether prophylaxis should be recommended after potential exposure. Many factors influence that decision; these include the species and vaccination status of the biting animal, the nature of the exposure, and the local epidemiology. An unprovoked attack is more likely to occur with a rabid animal, as contrasted to the provoked attack that may ensue when children tease or bother pets while they are feeding. The decision regarding prophylaxis is aided by knowing whether rabies exists in the region and in what animal species. This information can usually be provided by local public health officials. In the United States, it is estimated that approximately 40,000 to 50,000 individuals receive postexposure prophylaxis per year.

Animals whose owners can produce vaccination certificates are considered safe. If vaccination status is unknown, the animal should be considered potentially infectious. Postexposure prophylaxis is assessed depending on the type of animal; recommendations are summarized in Table 316-1. Healthy-appearing domestic dogs and

**TABLE 316-1 RABIES POSTEXPOSURE PROPHYLAXIS**

| Animal Type | Evaluation and Disposition of Animal | Postexposure Prophylaxis Recommendations |
|---|---|---|
| Dogs, cats, and ferrets | Healthy and available for 10 days of observation | Persons should not begin prophylaxis unless animal develops clinical signs of rabies[a] |
| | Rabid or suspected rabid | Immediately vaccinate |
| | Unknown (eg, escaped) | Consult public health officials |
| Skunks, raccoons, foxes, and most other carnivores; bats[b] | Regarded as rabid unless animal proven negative by laboratory tests[c] | Immediate vaccination |
| Livestock, horses, rodents, lagomorphs (rabbits and hares), and other mammals | Consider individually | Consult public health officials. Bites of squirrels, hamsters, guinea pigs, gerbils, chipmunks, rats, mice, other small rodents, rabbits, and hares almost never require rabies postexposure prophylaxis |

[a]During the 10-day observation period, begin postexposure prophylaxis at the first sign of rabies in a dog, cat, or ferret that has bitten someone. If the animal exhibits clinical signs of rabies, the animal should be euthanized immediately and tested.

[b]Bat exposure includes bites, but also any nonverbal person (unable to speak, altered mental status, sleeping) found in a room with a bat could be considered to be exposed.

[c]The animal should be euthanized and tested as soon as possible. Holding for observation is not recommended. Discontinue vaccine if immunofluorescence test results of the animal are negative.

Modified with permission from Human rabies prevention—United States, 1999. Recommendations of the Advisory Committee on Immunization Practices (ACIP), *MMWR Recomm Rep*. 1999 Jan 8;48(RR-1):1-21.

cats that bite human beings should be confined and observed by a veterinarian for 10 days. Illness in the biting animal should be reported to the local health officials and the patient's physician immediately. If an animal must be killed to be captured, it should be done in such a way as not to traumatize the head. Likewise, if the animal dies, the head should be shipped under refrigeration to a competent laboratory for diagnosis. For bites by stray dogs and cats who have disappeared, consultation with the local health officials can also help determine the risk based on local survey data. For wildlife under suspicion, the animal should be killed and its head submitted for laboratory examination. The public health laboratory will perform an examination of the brain using the fluorescent antibody technique. If that examination is negative, one can assume that no rabies was present in the animal's saliva.

Carnivorous animals, such as bats, skunks, foxes, coyotes, wolves, raccoons, and ferrets, should be considered to be infected and receive postexposure prophylaxis. Because of the recent increase in cases without a known bite from a bat, infants, those sleeping, or individuals with altered mental status in the same room with a bat should receive prophylaxis. Farm animals, squirrels, opossums, weasels, muskrats, woodchucks, and mongooses may occasionally be infected and should receive individual consideration. Bites of rodents, lagomorphs, birds, and reptiles seldom require treatment.

## SUGGESTED READINGS


Dupuis M, Brunt S, Appler K, et al. Comparison of automated quantitative reverse transcription-PCR and direct fluorescent-antibody detection for routine rabies diagnosis in the United States. *J Clin Microbiol.* 2015;53:2983-2989.

Feder HM Jr, Petersen BW, Robertson KL, Rupprecht CE. Rabies: still a uniformly fatal disease? Historical occurrence, epidemiological trends, and paradigm shifts. *Curr Infect Dis Rep.* 2012;14:408-422.

Hampson K, Coudeville L, Lembo T, et al. Estimating the global burden of endemic canine rabies. *PLoS Negl Trop Dis.* 2015;9:e0003709.

Jackson AC. Current and future approaches to the therapy of human rabies. *Antiviral Res.* 2013;9:61-67.

Mahadevan A, Suja MS, Mani RS, et al. Perspectives in diagnosis and treatment of rabies viral encephalitis: insights from pathogenesis. *Neurotherapeutics.* 2016;13(3):477-492.

Mani RS, Madhusudana SN. Laboratory diagnosis of human rabies: recent advances. *ScientificWorldJournal.* 2013;2013:569712.

Udow SJ, Marrie RA, Jackson AC. Clinical features of dog- and bat-acquired rabies in humans. *Clin Infect Dis.* 2013;57:689-696.

Wilde H, Hemachudha T. The "Milwaukee protocol" for treatment of human rabies is no longer valid. *Pediatr Infect Dis J.* 2015;34:678-679.

World Health Organization. WHO Expert Consultation on Rabies. Second report. *World Health Organ Tech Rep Ser.* 2013;982:1-139.


# 317 Smallpox

Amy S. Arrington

## INTRODUCTION

Smallpox is a highly infectious disease caused by the variola virus. Two distinct variola viruses (major and minor) exist, and each manifests different clinical characteristics and host mortality. The most common form of smallpox described in the literature was due to variola major, which resulted in severe, disfiguring disease and carried a 30% mortality rate. The mildest form of smallpox was due to variola minor (also known as alastrim), which presented similarly to variola major but with less toxicity and had more superficial lesions that resulted in a faster healing time and lower mortality (1%). The diagnosis of variola minor was based on the assessment of an outbreak and its severity. If there were few deaths (1%), then the disease was determined to be variola minor.

The variola virus, an *Orthopoxvirus* from the family Poxviridae, is a large and complex DNA virus. Variola is genetically homologous to other similar viruses such as vaccinia or those that cause monkeypox, camelpox, and cowpox. For those that receive smallpox vaccine, the high degree of genetic similarity results in protection not only against smallpox, but also monkeypox, camelpox, and cowpox.

## PATHOGENESIS AND EPIDEMIOLOGY

Smallpox is spread by droplet, aerosol, direct person-to-person contact, or direct contact with contaminated fomites. It had a seasonal distribution, with the highest rates occurring in the late winter and early spring. Variola virus enters through the respiratory tract, seeds the mucous membranes, and is transported to the regional lymph nodes where it replicates and enters the lymphatics and blood. The virus is very stable and can survive for long periods (years) in scabs.

Smallpox is one of the oldest recorded infections, with its earliest descriptions dating back to 10,000 BC in Asia and India and the earliest credible evidence being found in Egyptian mummies from over 3000 years ago. The global elimination of smallpox by vaccination remains a major historical and medical milestone, and the last recorded case of smallpox in the world occurred in 1978. Several important factors were crucial in the success of this eradication program: there is no latent or persistent human infection; it is an easily recognizable and diagnosable disease; and vaccination is cost-effective, stable, and easily administered, as well as highly effective against all strains of the virus.

## CLINICAL MANIFESTATIONS

The symptoms of smallpox include high fever, malaise, pain (typically in the back, abdomen, and head), and prostration. Approximately 24 hours before onset of rash, an enanthem occurs on the oral mucosa. In contrast to the similar-appearing varicella (chickenpox), the rash begins on the face, is centrifugal in distribution, and is often present on the palms and soles. Rash progresses from macules to papules and pustules, some of which may become umbilicated. Rash lesions are all in the same stage of development, in contrast to varicella in which macules, papules, and pustules coexist in one area of skin. Smallpox is highly contagious while the rash is evolving, and its evolution may take several weeks. Untreated, unvaccinated patients who develop smallpox have fatality rates as high as 30%, with highest mortality rates seen in infants and adults.

## DIAGNOSIS

Diagnosis of the disease can be made rapidly by viewing vesicular lesions with electron microscopy. Patients in whom the diagnosis of smallpox is seriously being considered should be reported to the Centers for Disease Control and Prevention and local infection control/health department personnel immediately.

## TREATMENT

There is no proven treatment for smallpox. Cidofovir has demonstrated antiviral activity against certain orthopoxviruses in vitro, but its effectiveness against variola is unknown. Newer agents (eg, brincidofovir) are being evaluated in animals. Vaccinia immune globulin (VIG) is reserved for certain complications of immunization with vaccinia virus and has no role in the treatment of smallpox. Special isolation including standard, contact, and airborne precautions must be enforced for hospitalized patients. A negative-pressure ventilated room with high-efficiency particulate air filtration is essential to containment, and the number of staff should be limited and include only those individuals trained in the use of personal protective gear, including an N95 or higher-quality respirator, gloves, and gown, despite immunization status.

## PREVENTION

Originally, cowpox was used to vaccinate against smallpox. Over time, vaccinia virus replaced the cowpox virus in smallpox vaccine preparations and remains that way today. Since the vaccine is not routinely available, it can only be administered by specially trained providers. It is important to note that the vaccinia virus can be transmitted from a vaccine recipient to other persons through direct (skin-to-skin) contact via material from the unhealed vaccination site or through indirect contact by means of fomites. This can result in eczema vaccinatum, a life-threatening complication of vaccinia virus infection no longer seen since use of the vaccine was discontinued.

Routine vaccination against smallpox was discontinued in the United States in 1972 and is not currently available to the general public. However, there is enough smallpox vaccine stockpiled to vaccinate every person in the United States in the event of a smallpox emergency. There was a brief resurrection of use of vaccine in the United States during the early 2000s when there was fear that the virus might be used as an agent of bioterrorism.

## SUGGESTED READINGS


American Academy of Pediatrics Committee on Infectious Diseases. Smallpox (variola). In: *Red Book: 2015 Report of the Committee on Infectious Diseases*. 30th ed. Elk Grove Village, IL: American Academy of Pediatrics; 2015:709-712.

Centers for Disease Control and Prevention. Smallpox fact sheet. Smallpox disease overview. http://emergency.cdc.gov/agent/smallpox/overview/disease-facts.asp. Accessed September 9, 2016.

Henderson DA. The eradication of smallpox: an overview of the past, present and future. *Vaccine*. 2011;29:D7-D9.

Thèves C, Biagini P, Crubézy E. The rediscovery of smallpox. *Clin Microbiol Infect*. 2014;20:210-218.

World Health Organization. Smallpox in the post eradication era. *Wkly Epidemiol Rec*. 2016;91:257-264.




# PART 8 PARASITIC INFECTIONS—NEMATODES

# 318 Antiparasitic Therapy

Fernando J. Bula-Rudas

## INTRODUCTION

Parasitic infections are an important cause of morbidity and mortality worldwide. Parasitic infections occur primarily in the tropical and subtropical areas; nevertheless, due to international travel and immigration, they are becoming important for healthcare practitioners all over the globe. The world of antiparasitic medications can be confusing. Some of the antiparasitic agents are not approved by the US Food and Drug Administration (FDA), and others are approved only for specific indications in children. A few antiparasitic drugs are only available through the Centers for Diseases Control and Prevention (CDC). Several new antiparasitic drugs have become available, and their effectiveness has been determined by their use in countries with endemic infections. Cooperation among governmental and private institutions has made a big impact in helping eradicate or diminish the incidence of parasitic infections in areas with extremely limited resources. Antiparasitic therapy for specific pathogens still could be challenging due to the lack of strong evidence supporting the use for a certain indication. The most recent recommendations for the management of parasitic infections are provided in Tables 318-1 to 318-5, including recommended drugs and dosages for specific parasitic infections. Therapy for malaria is discussed in Chapter 347. The CDC also provides a consultation service for healthcare professionals to assist with the management of parasitic infections by phone, Monday through Friday, 7:30 AM to 4:00 PM EST (1-404-718-4745; after-hours emergencies 1-770-488-7100; email: parasites@cdc.gov).

## TREATMENT OF HELMINTH INFECTIONS

### Nematodes

Benzimidazoles are the most common agents used for the treatment of helminthic infections worldwide. Benzimidazoles can be used for the treatment of hookworms, ascariasis, trichuriasis, pinworms, intestinal and hepatic capillariasis, and trichinellosis. Benzimidazoles along with steroids are recommended in trichinellosis with cardiac or central nervous system (CNS) involvement or in severe cases. Mebendazole is a benzimidazole with broad-spectrum activity against helminths. It acts by inhibiting the formation of the worms' microtubules, thus causing death of the parasite by glucose depletion. Mebendazole is metabolized by the liver, and it is mainly excreted in the feces. It may cause elevation of liver function tests, and hepatitis has been reported when the drug is taken for prolonged courses. Mebendazole can cause transient symptoms of abdominal pain and diarrhea in cases of massive parasitic infection and expulsion of worms. Approximately only 2% of the administered drug is excreted in the urine. Albendazole is recommended for treating toxocariasis (visceral and cutaneous larva migrans) and the filariasis caused by *Mansonella perstans*. Albendazole is better absorbed when ingested with fatty meals, and it has a high volume of distribution in tissues. For this reason, it is the preferred agent for treatment of visceral larva migrans. Its metabolism is hepatic, and adverse effects include increase of liver enzymes. It can also cause bone marrow toxicity. However, in general, systemic side effects are very rare with the dosages used for helminthic infections. Common side effects include transient abdominal pain, diarrhea, nausea, dizziness, and headache. It is labeled as category C in pregnancy; therefore, it should be used only if the potential benefit justifies the potential risk to the fetus. Although albendazole is not excreted in human milk, caution is recommended when given to nursing mothers because it is known to be excreted in animal milk.

The embryotoxic and teratogenic effects of benzimidazoles in animal models have raised concern for their use in children younger than 12 months of age. Albendazole and mebendazole have been used worldwide for routine deworming in young children in developing countries. The evidence is scarce for the safe use of benzimidazoles in children younger than 6 years of age; however, experience suggests that they are safe in this age group. Regular deworming of soil-transmitted helminthic infections (eg, ascariasis, trichuriasis, hookworm) in developing countries improves physical growth and cognitive performance of school-aged children. For this reason, the use of the benzimidazoles for regular deworming is supported in children starting at 12 months of age in areas where local circumstances show that reducing the burden of soil-transmitted helminthic infections is beneficial. Monitoring of drug resistance is recommended, especially in areas where regular deworming is common, since the use of anthelminthic drugs may be higher due to treatment of other infections.

Ivermectin is a semisynthetic, broad-spectrum antiparasitic agent derived from the class of avermectins. It is isolated from the fermentation products of *Streptomyces avermitilis*. It also has activity against

**TABLE 318-1 THERAPY FOR NEMATODE INFECTIONS**

| Infection Site/Microorganism | Drugs of Choice and Dosages | Comments |
|---|---|---|
| **Intestinal Nematodes** | | |
| Hookworms | | |
| *Necator americanus*<br>*Ancylostoma duodenale* | Albendazole[a,b] 400 mg PO once;<br>OR mebendazole 100 mg PO for 3 days or 500 mg PO once;<br>OR pyrantel pamoate[a,c] 11 mg/kg PO QD for 3 days (max 1 g/d) | A repeat dose of albendazole may be necessary. |
| *Ancylostoma caninum* | Albendazole[a,b] 400 mg PO once | May be a cause of eosinophilic colitis. |
| Ascariasis<br>*Ascaris lumbricoides* | First line: albendazole[a,b] 400 mg PO once;<br>OR mebendazole 500 mg PO once or 100 mg TID for 3 days<br>Pregnant women: pyrantel pamoate[a,c] 11 mg/kg PO once (max 1 g/d)<br>Alternatives: ivermectin[a,d] 150–200 µg/kg PO once; nitazoxanide[a] 7.5 mg/kg PO once | Test of cure after therapy is not necessary. |
| Baylisascariasis<br>*Baylisascaris procyonis* | Albendazole[b] 50 mg/kg/d PO divided BID for 20 days AND high-dose corticosteroid therapy for CNS infection | Albendazole 25 mg/kg/d PO daily for 20 days can be considered for prevention in children with known exposure (ingestion of raccoon stool or contaminated soil).<br>Ivermectin may be used in the interim if albendazole is not readily available. |
| Whipworm (trichuriasis)<br>*Trichuris trichiura* | Mebendazole 100 mg PO BID for 3 days or 500 mg once;<br>OR albendazole[a,b] 400 mg PO for 3 days;<br>OR ivermectin[a,c] 200 µg/kg/d PO daily for 3 days;<br>OR mebendazole 100 mg PO BID for 3 days | Treatment can be given for 5–7 days in case of heavy infestation.<br>Ivermectin alone seems to be less effective than albendazole or mebendazole.<br>Mebendazole is no longer available in the United States. |
| Pinworm<br>*Enterobius vermicularis* | Albendazole[a,b]:<br>• < 20 kg: 200 mg PO once<br>• ≥ 20 kg: 400 mg PO once<br>• Repeat in 2 weeks<br>OR pyrantel pamoate[c] 11 mg/kg (max 1 g) PO once, repeat in 2 weeks | Consider treatment of entire household and close contacts in child care or school.<br>To prevent reinfection, retreatment of contacts may be needed. |
| Strongyloidiasis<br>*Strongyloides stercoralis* | Ivermectin[d] 200 µg/kg PO QD for 1–2 days; OR albendazole[a,b] 400 mg PO BID for 7 days | Ivermectin activity is limited to intestinal stages.<br>Albendazole may be used for disseminated disease and longer courses for more severe cases.<br>In immunocompromised patients, especially those with hyperinfection syndrome, parenteral veterinary formulations may be lifesaving. |
| Intestinal capillariasis<br>*Capillaria philippinensis* | Albendazole[a,b] 400 mg PO QD for 10 days; OR<br>Mebendazole 200 mg PO BID for 20 days | |
| Trichinellosis<br>*Trichinella spiralis* | Albendazole[a,b] 20 mg/kg/d (max 400 mg/dose) PO BID for 8–14 days; OR<br>Mebendazole 200–400 mg PO TID for 3 days then 400–500 mg PO TID for 10 days | Treatment not effective for larvae in muscles.<br>Steroids may be used for severe symptoms or cardiac or CNS involvement. |
| **Blood and Tissue Nematodes** | | |
| **Filariasis** | | |
| River blindness<br>*Onchocerca volvulus* | Ivermectin[d] 150 µg PO once;<br>OR doxycycline 200 mg daily for 4–6 weeks followed by Ivermectin[d] given in a single dose | Repeat ivermectin dose every 6–12 months until asymptomatic and no longer exposed.<br>Avoid diethylcarbamazine in *Onchocerca* and *Loa loa* coinfection.<br>Doxycycline may be used to kill adult forms. |
| *Wuchereria bancrofti*<br>*Brugia malayi*<br>*Brugia timori*<br>*Mansonella streptocerca* | Diethylcarbamazine (DEC)[a,e] 6 mg/kg/d PO divided TID for 12 days OR 6 mg/kg/d PO as a single dose<br>For tropical pulmonary eosinophilia: DEC[a,e] 6 mg/kg/d PO divided TID for 12–21 days | In tropical pulmonary eosinophilia, use antihistamines or steroids for allergic reactions followed by doxycycline 200 mg PO daily for 4–6 weeks. |
| *Mansonella ozzardi* | Ivermectin[a,d] 200 µg/kg PO once may be effective | DEC not effective. |
| *Mansonella perstans* | Albendazole[a,d] 400 mg PO BID for 10 days; OR<br>Mebendazole 100 mg PO BID for 30 days | DEC and ivermectin not effective.<br>Doxycycline 200 mg PO daily for 6 weeks (infections acquired in West Africa). |

(Continued)

**TABLE 318-1 THERAPY FOR NEMATODE INFECTIONS (CONTINUED)**

| Infection Site/Microorganism | Drugs of Choice and Dosages | Comments |
|---|---|---|
| *Loa loa* | Diethylcarbamazine[a,e]:<br>Symptomatic with microfilaremia < 8000 MF/mL 8–10 mg/kg/d PO divided TID for 21 days<br>Albendazole[a,b] 200 mg PO BID for 21 days<br>Symptomatic microfliaremia < 8000 MF/mL and failed 2 rounds of DEC<br>Symptomatic with microfliraemia ≥ 8000 MF/mL to reduce level to < 8000 MF/mL prior to treatment with diethylcarbamazine | There is risk of fatal encephalopathy with diethylcarbamazine treatment with microfilaremia loads ≥ 8000 MF/mL. The use of corticosteroids has not been shown to eliminate the risk of encephalopathy.<br>Apheresis followed by diethylcarbamazine should be performed at institutions experienced in apheresis.<br>Doxycycline is not an effective treatment. |
| Hepatic capillariasis<br>*Capillaria hepatica* | Mebendazole 200 mg PO BID for 20 days; OR<br>Albendazole[a,b] 400 mg PO QD for 10 days | |
| **Cutaneous Larva Migrans or Creeping Eruption** | | |
| Dog and cat hookworm<br>*Ancylostoma caninum*<br>*Ancylostoma braziliense*<br>*Uncinaria stenocephala* | Albendazole[a,b] 15 mg/kg/d (max 400 mg) PO qd for 3 days; OR<br>Ivermectin[a,d] 200 µg/kg PO QD for 1–2 days | |
| **Toxocariasis (Visceral and Cutaneous Larva Migrans)** | | |
| Dog and cat roundworms<br>*Toxocara canis*<br>*Toxocara catis* | Visceral larva migrans:<br>• Albendazole[a,b] 400 mg PO BID for 5 days<br>Ocular larva migrans:<br>• Albendazole[a,b] 400 mg PO daily for 2–4 weeks PLUS<br>• Prednisone 0.5–1 mg/kg/d with slow taper | Some experts would treat visceral larva migrans for 20 days.<br>For severe symptoms and ocular larva migrans, topical steroids may be used.<br>Mebendazole 100–200 mg/d PO BID for 5 days and DEC are alternatives. |
| Dracunculiasis (Guinea worm)<br>*Dracunculus medinensis* | No antihelminthic treatment is available<br>Treatment of bacterial superinfection<br>Manual extraction of worm | Global eradication nearly achieved.<br>Restricted to rural, isolated areas of a narrow belt of nations in Africa. |

[a]Not approved by the US Food and Drug Administration for this indication at the time of writing.

[b]Albendazole should be taken with fatty meals to increase oral bioavailability.

[c]Pyrantel pamoate is available without a prescription. The suspension can be mixed with milk or fruit juice.

[d]Safety of ivermectin in children weighting < 15 kg and pregnant women has not been established.

[e]Diethylcarbamazine is available from Centers for Disease Control and Prevention.

BID, twice a day; CNS, central nervous system; PO, orally; QD, once a day; TID, 3 times a day.

Data from Drugs for parasitic infections. *The Medical Letter.* 11(Suppl):2013; and Bradley JS, Nelson JD, eds. *2016 Nelson's Pediatric Antimicrobial Therapy.* 22nd Ed. Washington, DC: American Academy of Pediatrics; 2016.

**TABLE 318-2 THERAPY FOR CESTODE INFECTIONS**

| Infection Site/Microorganism | Drugs of Choice and Dosages | Comments |
|---|---|---|
| **Intestinal (Adult) Tapeworms** | | |
| *Taenia saginata*<br>*Taenia solium*<br>*Hymenolepis nana*<br>*Diphyllobothrium latum*<br>*Dipylidium caninum* | Praziquantel[a] 5–10 mg/kg PO once (25 mg/kg once for *H nana*), then repeat 10 days later; OR<br>Niclosamide[b] 50 mg/kg (max 2 g) PO once (for all except *H nana*) | Nitazoxanide may be effective for treatment of *H nana*, but clinical data are limited. |
| **Tissue (Larval) Tapeworms** | | |
| **Echinococcosis** | | |
| *Echinococcus granulosus* | Albendazole[c] 15 mg/kg/d (max 800 mg/d) PO divided BID for 1–6 months alone or as an adjunctive therapy with surgery or percutaneous treatment | Surgery is the treatment of choice for complicated cysts.<br>Start therapy 4–30 days before and at least 1 month after the surgery.<br>Praziquantel may be used in combination therapy with albendazole. |
| *Echinococcus multilocularis* | Surgical excision is generally the treatment of choice<br>Albendazole[c] 15 mg/kg/d (max 800 mg/d) PO divided BID postoperative should be administered for at least 2 years with monitoring for relapse | Benefit of preoperative albendazole is unknown. |

(Continued)

**TABLE 318-2 THERAPY FOR CESTODE INFECTIONS (CONTINUED)**

| Infection Site/Microorganism | Drugs of Choice and Dosages | Comments |
|---|---|---|
| Cysticercosis<br>*Taenia solium*<br>(*Cysticercus cellulosae*) | Cysticercosis: albendazole[c] 15 mg/kg/d (max 800 mg/d) PO divided BID<br>Neurocysticercosis:<br>• Management of neurologic signs and symptoms when present<br>• Albendazole[c] dose same for cysticercosis PLUS dexamethasone 0.1 mg/kg/d or prednisone 1 mg/kg/d followed by rapid taper; OR<br>• Praziquantel[a] 50 mg/kg/d divided TID for 15 days | Duration of therapy depends on the extent of the infection. Single enhancing lesions: 3–7 days; multiple parenchymal lesions: 10–days; subarachnoid disease: ≥ 28 days.<br>Steroids may not be needed for treatment of single lesions. Therapy can be repeated as necessary.<br>Albendazole is likely to be more effective than praziquantel against extraparenchymal forms of the disease. Combination therapy with albendazole and praziquantal may be more effective than albendazole alone. |

[a]Not approved by US Food and Drug Administration for this indication at the time of writing.

[b]Niclosamide is not available in pharmacies in the United States.

[c]Albendazole should be taken with fatty meals to increase oral bioavailability.

BID, twice a day; PO, oral.

Data from Drugs for parasitic infections. *The Medical Letter.* 11(Suppl):2013; and Bradley JS, Nelson JD, eds. *2016 Nelson's Pediatric Antimicrobial Therapy.* 22nd Ed. Washington, DC: American Academy of Pediatrics; 2016.

some ectoparasites. The systemic form is metabolized in the liver, and its metabolites are excreted in the feces; less than 1% of metabolites are excreted in urine. Ivermectin binds to glutamate-gated chloride channels in nerve and muscle cells of invertebrates, causing paralysis and death of the parasite. It is the drug of choice for strongyloidiasis and onchocerciasis; however, it is not active against all nematodes. It is active against the tissue microfilariae of *Onchocerca volvulus* but not against the adult form.

Ivermectin has shown teratogenic effects in animal models, so it is labeled as category C for its use during pregnancy. The safety and effectiveness of ivermectin have not been established for children weighing less than 15 kg. Since low levels of the drug have been found

**TABLE 318-3 THERAPY FOR TREMATODE INFECTIONS**

| Infection Site/Microorganism | Drugs of Choice and Dosages | Comments |
|---|---|---|
| **Schistosomiasis** | | |
| *Schistosoma haematobium*<br>*Schistosoma japonicum*<br>*Schistosoma mansoni*<br>*Schistosoma mekongi*<br>*Schistosoma intercalatum* | *S haematobium*, *S mansoni*, and *S intercalatum*<br>• Praziquantel[a] 40 mg/kg/d PO divided BID for 1 day<br>*S japonicum* and *S mekongi*<br>• Praziquantel[a] 60 mg/kg/d PO divided TID for 1 day | Oxamniquine is an alternative drug not available in the United States. It is available in Africa and Brazil. |
| **Flukes** | | |
| Liver flukes<br>*Clonorchis sinensis* (Chinese liver fluke)<br>*Opisthorchis viverrini* (Southeast Asian liver fluke)<br>*Metorchi conjunctus* (North American liver fluke)<br>*Opisthorchis felineus* (Cat liver fluke) | Praziquantel[b] 75 mg/kg PO divided TID for 2 days; OR<br>Albendazole[c,d] 10 mg/kg/d PO for 7 days; OR<br>Mebendazole 30 mg/kg/d for 20–30 days | Pediatric and adult doses are the same. |
| Lung flukes<br>*Paragonimus westermani*<br>Other *Paragonimus* species | Praziquantel[c] 75 mg/kg/d PO divided TID for 3 days; OR<br>Triclabendazole[c,e] 10 mg/kg PO once or twice | For CNS involvement, a short course of steroids may be beneficial in addition to praziquantel. |
| Fasciolasis (sheep liver fluke)<br>*Fasciola hepatica* | Triclabendazole[c,e] 10 mg/kg PO once (may receive a second dose in more severe cases); OR<br>Nitazoxanide[c]:<br>• Age 1–3 years: 100 mg PO BID for 7 days<br>• Age 4–11 years: 200 mg PO BID for 7 days<br>• Age ≥ 12 years: 500 mg PO BID for 7 days | *Fasciola hepatica* infections may not respond to praziquantel.<br>Nitazoxanide may be an alternative, but there are limited data about its efficacy. |
| Intestinal flukes<br>*Fasciolopsis buski*<br>*Heterophyes heterophyes*<br>*Metagonimus yokogawi*<br>*Nanophyetus salmincola* | Praziquantel[c] 75 mg/kg divided TID for 1 day | |

[a]Retreatment in 2–6 weeks increases cure.

[b]Praziquantel is US Food and Drug Administration (FDA) approved for treatment of *C sinensis* and *O viverrini*. Not FDA approved for the other flukes.

[c]Not FDA-approved for this indication at the time of writing.

[d]Albendazole should be taken with fatty meals to increase oral bioavailability.

[e]Triclabendazole is not commercially available in the United States. It is available through the Centers for Disease Control and Prevention under an investigational protocol.

BID, twice a day; CNS, central nervous system; PO, oral; TID, 3 times a day.

Data from Drugs for parasitic infections. *The Medical Letter.* 11(Suppl):2013; and Bradley JS, Nelson JD, eds. *2016 Nelson's Pediatric Antimicrobial Therapy.* 22nd Ed. Washington, DC: American Academy of Pediatrics; 2016.

**TABLE 318-4 THERAPY FOR PROTOZOAN INFECTIONS**

| Infection Site/Microorganism | Drugs of Choice and Dosages | Comments |
|---|---|---|
| **Intestinal Protozoa** | | |
| *Entamoeba histolytica* (amebiasis) | | |
| Asymptomatic (colonization) | Paromomycin[a] 25–35 mg/kg/d PO divided TID for 7 days; OR<br>Iodoquinol[b] 30–40 mg/kg/d PO divided TID (max 650 mg/dose) for 20 days; OR<br>Diloxanide furoate[c] 20 mg/kg/d PO divided TID (max 500 mg/dose) for 10 days | Follow-up stool examination is needed to ensure eradication.<br>Screen close contacts. |
| Colitis | Metronidazole[d] 35–50 mg/kg/d PO divided TID for 10 days; OR<br>Tinidazole[d,e] (age > 3 years) 50 mg/kg/d PO (max 2 g) QD for 3 days<br>EITHER followed by paromomycin[a] OR iodoquinol[b] as above to eliminate cysts | Use of steroids and antimotility drugs is not recommended.<br>Nitazoxanide is effective against mild to moderate amebiasis but perhaps less so than metronidazole. |
| Liver abscess or extraintestinal disease | Metronidazole[d] 35–50 mg/kg/d IV (or PO) q8h for 10 days; OR<br>Tinidazole[d,e] (age ≥ 3 years) 50 mg/kg/d PO (max 2 g) QD for 5 days<br>EITHER followed by paromomycin[a] or iodoquinol[b] as above to eliminate cysts<br>Nitazoxanide[f] (age ≥ 12 years) 500 mg BID for 10 days | Serologic assays > 95% positive in extraintestinal amebiasis.<br>Metronidazole can be switched to PO when tolerated.<br>Surgical drainage of abscess may be indicated. |
| Balantidiasis<br>*Balantidium coli* | Tetracycline[g,h] 40 mg/kg/d (max 2 g/d) PO divided QID for 10 days; OR<br>Metronidazole[d] 35–50 mg/kg/d PO divided TID for 5 days | Rare in the United States.<br>Repeat stool examination if symptoms persist after therapy.<br>Nitazoxanide[f] may be effective. |
| Cryptosporidiosis<br>*Cryptosporidium parvum* | Nitazoxanide[f]:<br>• Age 12–47 months: 100 mg PO BID for 3 days<br>• Age 4–11 years: 200 mg PO BID for 3 days<br>• Age ≥ 12 years: 500 mg PO BID for 3 days<br>Paromomycin 30 mg/kg/d divided BID–QID; OR<br>Azithromycin 10 mg/kg/d for 5 days | Treatment in immunocompromised host depends mainly in the recovery of the immune status.<br>Limited efficacy in HIV-infected patients not receiving antiretroviral therapy.<br>Treatment is not always indicated in immunocompetent individuals. |
| Cyclosporiasis<br>*Cyclospora cayetanensis* | Trimethoprim (TMP)-sulfamethoxazole (SMX)[g]; TMP 10 mg/kg/d, SMX 50 mg/kg/d PO divided BID for 7–10 days;<br>OR Nitazoxanide[f] 500 mg PO BID for 7 days | HIV-infected patients may require higher doses or longer therapy. |
| Cystoisosporiasis (formerly isosporiasis)<br>*Cystoisospora belli* | TMP-SMX[g] 8–10 mg TMP/kg/d (max 160 mg TMP/800 mg SMX BID) PO (or IV) divided BID for 7–10 days; OR<br>Ciprofloxacin 500 mg PO BID for 7 days | Usually a self-limited illness in immunocompetent hosts. |
| Dientamoebiasis<br>*Dientamoeba fragilis* | Metronidazole[d] 35–50 mg/kg/d PO divided TID for 10 days (max 500–750 mg/dose); OR<br>Paromomycin[a,g] 25–35 mg/kg/d PO divided TID for 7 days; OR<br>Iodoquinol[b,g] 30–40 mg/kg/d (max 650 mg/dose) PO divided TID for 20 days | Treatment is indicated when no other cause is found for abdominal pain or diarrhea lasting more than a week except *Dientamoeba*.<br>Nitazoxanide[f] may be effective.<br>Albendazole has no activity against *Dientamoeba*. |
| Giardiasis<br>*Giardia intestinalis* | Metronidazole[d,g] 15–30 mg/kg/d (max 250 mg/dose) PO divided TID for 5–7 days; OR<br>Nitazoxanide[f]:<br>• Age 1–3 years: 100 mg/dose PO BID for 3 days<br>• Age 4–11 years: 200 mg/dose BID for 3 days<br>• Age ≥ 12 years: 500 mg/dose BID for 3 days;<br>OR<br>Albendazole 10–15 mg/kg/d (max 400 mg) PO for 5 days<br>Mebendazole 200 mg PO TID for 5 days<br>Tinidazole[d,e] 50 mg/kg/d (max 2 g) for 1 day<br>Alternatives:<br>• Paromomycin[a,g,i] 30 mg/kg/d divided TID for 5–10 days<br>• Furazolidone[c] 6 mg/kg/d in 4 doses for 7–10 days | Higher doses or longer courses may be necessary.<br>Prolonged courses may be considered in immunocompromised.<br>Public health authorities may require treatment of asymptomatic carriers. |
| **Amebic Meningoencephalitis** | | |
| Primary amebic meningoencephalitis (PAM)<br>*Naegleria fowleri* | An effective regimen has not been established<br>Amphotericin B[j] 1.5 mg/kg/d IV QD for 9–30 days ± amphotericin B intrathecally PLUS<br>Rifampin 10 mg/kg/d IV or PO QD or TID PLUS<br>Fluconazole 10 mg/kg/d IV or PO QD; OR<br>Miconazole 350 mg/m²/d IV divided TID PLUS<br>Miltefosine[k]:<br>• ≥ 45 kg: 50 mg PO BID<br>• ≥ 45 kg: 50 mg PO TID PLUS<br>Azithromycin 500 mg IV or PO | Most cases have been fatal in the United States (122/123).<br>Two documented cases of survival in North America (1 in Mexico and 1 in the United States).<br>Survivors received dexamethasone to treat cerebral edema. |

(Continued)

**TABLE 318-4 THERAPY FOR PROTOZOAN INFECTIONS (CONTINUED)**

| Infection Site/Microorganism | Drugs of Choice and Dosages | Comments |
|---|---|---|
| **Granulomatous Amebic Encephalitis (GAE)** | | |
| *Acanthamoeba* species | Treatment uncertain | |
| *Balamuthia mandrillaris* | Miltefosine[k] in combination with fluconazole and pentamidine favored by some experts<br>Other drugs that have been used alone or in combination: rifampin, azoles, pentamidine, sulfadiazine, flucytosine, erythromycin, azithromycin, and caspofungin | |
| Keratitis<br>*Acanthamoeba* species | Biguanide chlorhexidine or polyhexamethylene biguanide (0.02%) combined with propamidine isethionate (0.1%) or hexamidine (0.1%) | Consultation with ophthalmologist as soon as possible.<br>Associated with contact lens use.<br>Topical therapies not approved in the United States but available at compounding pharmacies.<br>Skin and eye infections that have not spread to the central nervous system can be successfully treated with topical therapies alone. |
| **Other Blood and Tissue Protozoa** | | |
| Babesiosis<br>*Babesia microti*<br>*Babesia divergens*<br>*Babesia duncani*<br>*Babesia MO-1* | Clindamycin[g] 30 mg/kg/d IV or PO divided TID (max 600 mg/dose) PLUS<br>Quinine[g,l] 25 mg/kg/d PO (max 650 mg/dose) divided TID for 7–10 days;<br>OR<br>Atovaquone[g,m] 40 mg/kg/d (max 750 mg/dose) divided BID PLUS<br>Azithromycin[g] 12 mg/kg/d (max 500 mg/dose) for 7–10 days | Consultation for management is recommended through CDC.<br>Clindamycin plus quinine is the standard regimen for severely ill patients.<br>Daily monitoring of hematocrit and percentage of parasitized red blood cells (until < 5%) should be done.<br>Higher doses and prolonged treatment may be necessary for asplenic or immunocompromised patients. |
| Toxoplasmosis<br>*Toxoplasma gondii* | Pyrimethamine 2 mg/kg/d PO divided BID for 2 days (max 100 mg) then 1 mg/kg/d (max 25 mg/d) PO daily AND<br>Sulfadiazine[n] 100–200 mg/kg/d (max 6 g/d) PO divided QID; take with supplemental folinic acid (leucovorin) 10–25 mg with each dose of pyrimethamine for 3–6 weeks.<br>In pregnancy: spiramycin[o] 50–100 mg/kg/d PO divided QID<br>Congenital infection: sulfadiazine[n] 100 mg/kg/d PO divided q12h AND pyrimethamine 2 mg/kg PO daily for 2 days (loading dose), then 1 mg/kg PO QD for 2–6 months, then 3 times weekly (Monday-Wednesday-Friday) up to 1 year; with supplemental folinic acid (leucovorin) 10 mg 3 times weekly | Continue treatment for 2 weeks after resolution of illness.<br>Steroids given for ocular or CNS infection.<br>Prolonged therapy recommended if HIV positive. Consult ID specialist.<br>Atovaquone[g] or clindamycin[g] PLUS pyrimethamine may be effective for patients allergic to sulfa drugs.<br>Consult ID specialist for management during pregnancy and congenital infection.<br>Start sulfa after neonatal jaundice has resolved. |
| Trichomoniasis<br>*Trichomonas vaginalis* | Tinidazole 50 mg/kg (max 2 g) PO for 1 dose; OR<br>Metronidazole 500 mg PO TID for 7 days | Treat sexual partners simultaneously.<br>Tinidazole is FDA approved for use in adults and adolescents for this indication.<br>Metronidazole has been associated with higher rates of clinical failure compared to tinidazole. |
| **Trypanosomiasis** | | |
| American trypanosomiasis or Chagas disease<br>*Trypanosoma cruzi* | Benznidazole[p]:<br>• < 12 years: 5–7.5 mg/kg/d PO divided BID for 60 days<br>• ≥ 12 years: 5–7 mg/kg/d PO divided BID for 60 days;<br>OR<br>Nifurtimox[p]:<br>• 1–10 years: 15–20 mg/kg/d divided TID or QID for 90 days<br>• 11–16 years: 12.5–15 mg/kg/d divided TID or QID for 90 days<br>• ≥ 17 years: 8–10 mg/kg/d divided TID or QID for 90–120 days | Side effects from both drugs are common and are more frequent and more severe with increased age. |
| African trypanosomiasis (sleeping sickness)<br>*Trypanosoma brucei gambiense* (West Africa)<br>*Trypanosoma brucei rhodesiense* (East Africa) | | |
| Acute hemolymphatic stage | *Tb gambiense:* pentamidine[g] isethionate 4 mg/kg/d (max 300 mg) IM or IV for 7–10 days<br>*Tb rhodesiense:* suramin[q] 20 mg/kg (max 1 g) IV on days 1, 3, 5, 14, and 21 | Consult tropical medicine specialist. |
| CNS involvement | *Tb gambiense:*<br>• Eflornithine[q] 400 mg/kg/d IV divided BID for 7 days PLUS nifurtimox 5 mg/kg PO TID for 10 days; OR<br>• Eflornithine[q] 400 mg/kg/d IV divided QID for 14 days; OR<br>• Melarsoprol[q] 2.2 mg/d (max 180 mg) IV for 10 days | Consult tropical medicine specialist.<br>Combination of eflornithine and nifurtimox used in rural Africa because difficulty of administering 4 infusions daily.<br>Corticosteroids have been used with melarsoprol to prevent encephalopathy. |

(Continued)

**TABLE 318-4 THERAPY FOR PROTOZOAN INFECTIONS (CONTINUED)**

| Infection Site/Microorganism | Drugs of Choice and Dosages | Comments |
|---|---|---|
| | *Tb rhodesiense:* Melarsoprolol[q] 2–3.6 mg/kg/d (max 200 mg) IV for 3 days; after 7 days, 3.6 mg/kg/d for 3 days; after 7 days, give a 3rd series of 3.6 mg/kg/d for 3 days | |
| **Leishmaniasis** | | |
| *Leishmania donovani* complex (*L donovani, L infantum, L chagasi*) | | |
| *Leishmania mexicana* complex (*L mexicana, L amazonensis, L venezuelensis*) | | |
| *Leishmania major* | | |
| *Leishmania tropica* | | |
| *Leishmania aethiopica* | | |
| *Leishmania viannia* [*L (V) braziliensis, L (V) guyanensis, L (V) paranensis, L (V) peruviansis*] | | |
| Uncomplicated cutaneous | Combination of topical measures: debridement of eschars, cryotherapy, thermotherapy, intralesional pentavalent antimony, and topical paromomycin | Consultation with a specialist is recommended.<br>Topical paromomycin not available in the United States. |
| Complicated cutaneous | Sodium stibogluconate[r] 20 mg/kg/d IV or PO for 10–20 days; OR<br>Miltefosine[s] 2.5 mg/kg/d PO (max 150 mg/d) for 28 days; OR<br>Pentamidine isethionate[g] 2–4 mg/kg/d IV or IM daily or every other day for 4–7 doses or until healed; OR<br>Amphotericin B[g] 0.5–1 mg/kg every other day for 20–30 days | Consultation with a specialist is recommended.<br>There is limited efficacy with azoles, and treatment failure is common. |
| Mucosal | Sodium stibogluconate[r] 20 mg/kg/d IM or IV for 28 days; OR<br>Amphotericin B[g] 0.5–1 mg/kg/d IV daily for 15–20 days or every other day for 4–8 weeks; OR<br>Miltefosine[s] 2.5 mg/kg/d PO (max 150 mg/d) for 28 days | Consultation with a specialist is recommended. |
| Visceral (kala-azar) | Liposomal amphotericin B[t] 3 mg/kg/d on days 1–5, day 14, and day 21; OR<br>Sodium stibogluconate[r] 20 mg/kg/d IM or IV for 28 days or longer; OR<br>Miltefosine[s] 2.5 mg/kg/d PO (max 150 mg/d) for 28 days; OR<br>Amphotericin B[g] 1 mg/kg/d IV daily for 15–20 days or every other day for 4–8 weeks | For immunocompromised patients, the dose of liposomal amphotericin B is 4 mg/kg on days 1–5, 10, 17, 24, 31, and 38. Prolonged therapy indicated on an individual basis.<br>For HIV-coinfected patients, antiretroviral therapy should be started or optimized. |

[a]Paromomycin should be taken with meals.

[b]Iodoquinol should be taken after meals.

[c]Not commercially available in pharmacies in the United States.

[d]Avoid alcohol ingestion during metronidazole and tinidazole therapy and 3 days afterward.

[e]Tinidazole tablets can be crushed and mixed with syrup by pharmacists. It should be taken with food.

[f]Nitazoxanide may be effective against a variety of protozoan and helminth infections. Preliminary data support use of nitazoxanide in children less than 1 year of age. It is FDA approved only for the treatment of giardiasis or cryptosporidiosis.

[g]Not FDA approved for this indication at the time of writing.

[h]Use of tetracyclines is contraindicated in pregnancy and in children < 8 years old. It should be taken 1 hour before or 2 hours after meals and/or dairy products.

[i]Paromomycin is recommended for treatment of symptomatic infection in pregnant women in the second and third trimester.

[j]Although liposomal amphotericin B crosses the blood-brain barrier better than conventional amphotericin, it has shown to be less effective against PAM caused by *Naegleria fowleri* in mice. Aggressive treatment, including the use of intrathecal amphotericin B, should be considered because of the poor prognosis.

[k]Miltefosine is not approved in the United States for treatment of infection with free-living ameba. It is available from the CDC Emergency Operations Center. The drug is contraindicated in breastfeeding and pregnant women.

[l]Quinine should be taken with or after a meal to decrease gastrointestinal adverse effects.

[m]Atovaquone should be taken with meals to increase absorption. It has been used safely in children ≥ 5 kg.

[n]Sulfadiazine should be taken on an empty stomach with adequate water.

[o]Pregnant women who develop toxoplasmosis during the first trimester should be treated with spiramycin. If there is no documented transmission to the fetus after the first trimester, then spiramycin can be continued until term. It is available as an investigational drug through the FDA (301-796-0563).

[p]Benznidazole and nifurtimox are not FDA approved. Both drugs are available from the CDC division of Parasitic Diseases and Malaria (404-718-4745, email: chagas@cdc.gov). Both drugs are contraindicated in pregnancy.

[q]Suramin, eflornithine, and melarsoprolol are not FDA approved. These drugs are available from the CDC division of Parasitic Diseases and Malaria (404-718-4745, email: parasites@cdc.gov).

[r]Sodium stibogluconate available from CDC Drug Service (404-639-3670) under an investigational new drug protocol.

[s]Miltefosine was approved by the FDA in 2014 for this indication in adolescents and nonpregnant women.

[t]Liposomal amphotericin B is the only formulation of amphotericin B FDA approved for treatment of visceral leishmaniasis. Relapse rate in immunocompromised patients is high.

BID, twice a day; CDC, Centers for Disease Control and Prevention; CNS, central nervous system; FDA, US Food and Drug Administration; HIV, human immunodeficiency virus; ID, infectious disease; IM, intramuscular; IV, intravenous; PO, oral; QD, once a day; QID, 4 times a day; TID, 3 times a day.

Data from Drugs for parasitic infections. *The Medical Letter.* 11(Suppl):2013; and Bradley JS, Nelson JD, eds. *2016 Nelson's Pediatric Antimicrobial Therapy.* 22nd Ed. Washington, DC: American Academy of Pediatrics; 2016.

in human milk, some experts recommend delaying maternal treatment until the infant is 7 days old whenever possible. The side effects of ivermectin are mainly seen in patients treated for onchocerciasis with co-infection with *Loa loa*. Patients with high levels of microfilaremia may develop the Mazzotti reaction, which is characterized by severe systemic signs of inflammatory reaction. These patients are also at risk for fatal encephalopathy.

Pyrantel pamoate is an anthelminthic drug that causes neuromuscular blockade in parasites. It has demonstrated effectiveness for *Ascaris lumbricoides*, *Necator americanus* (hookworm), and *Enterobius*

**TABLE 318-5 THERAPY FOR ECTOPARASITE INFESTATIONS**

| Infection Site/ Microorganism | Drugs of Choice and Dosages | Comments |
|---|---|---|
| Lice<br>*Pediculus capitis*<br>*Pediculus humanus*<br>*Phthirus pubis* | Permethrin[a] topical 1% twice, at least 7 days apart; OR<br>Pyrethrin with piperonyl butoxide[a] twice, at least 7 days apart; OR<br>Ivermectin[b] 0.5% topical lotion once<br>Spinosad[c] 0.9% topical suspension twice, at least 7 days apart; OR<br>Benzyl alcohol lotion[a] 5% twice, at least 7 days apart; OR<br>Malathion[d] 0.5% topical twice, at least 7 days apart; OR<br>Ivermectin[e] PO 200 or 400 μg/kg once<br>Eyelash infestation: petrolatum ointment 2–4 times/d for 8–10 days | Some experts recommend manual removal of nits with special combs.<br>Launder bedding and clothing with water temperature > 53.5°C (128.3°F).<br>Permethrin and pyrethrin preferred for children ≥ 2 years of age.<br>Benzyl alcohol lotion and ivermectin lotion for use in children ≥ 6 months of age, spinosad for children age ≥ 4 years, and malathion for children age ≥ 6 years.<br>Skin burning sensation is a common side effect with these topical agents. |
| Scabies<br>*Sarcoptes scabiei* | Permethrin cream 5% applied to entire body (include scalp in infants), leave it on for 8–14 h, then bathe, repeat in 1 week; OR<br>Ivermectin[e,f] 200 μg/kg PO once weekly for 2 doses; OR<br>Crotamiton 10% topical applied overnight on days 1, 2, 3, and 8; bathe in the morning | Medications are only available in the United States with prescription.<br>Launder bedding and clothing with water temperature > 53.5°C (128.3°F).<br>Permethrin is FDA approved for persons at least 2 months of age. |

[a]Retreatment of head lice is usually recommended in 7 to 10 days because pediculocides are not completely ovicidal.

[b]Not ovicidal. Lice from treated eggs die within 48 hours after hatching. Safe for use in children ≥ 6 months of age.

[c]Not ovicidal. Spinosad causes paralysis and death of the parasite. The formulation also includes benzyl alcohol.

[d]Malathion is both ovicidal and pediculocidal.

[e]Not FDA approved for this indication at the time of writing. Ivermectin is not ovicidal. More than 1 dose is usually necessary for eradication. Number of doses and interval have not been established. Safety of ivermectin in children weighting < 15 kg and pregnant women has not been established.

[f]A second dose of ivermectin taken 2 weeks after the first dose increased the cure rate to 95% (comparable with permethrin). Ivermectin alone or with a topical scabicide is the treatment of choice for immunocompromised patients with crusted scabies

FDA, US Food and Drug Administration; PO, oral.

Data from Drugs for parasitic infections. *The Medical Letter.* 11(Suppl):2013; and Bradley JS, Nelson JD, eds. *2016 Nelson's Pediatric Antimicrobial Therapy.* 22nd Ed. Washington, DC: American Academy of Pediatrics; 2016.

*vermicularis* (pinworm). Pyrantel pamoate is available over the counter in the United States. The World Health Organization (WHO) classifies pyrantel pamoate as compatible with breastfeeding. The safety in children has not been established; however, according to WHO, it may be used in children age 1 year and older for mass deworming programs.

Diethylcarbamazine citrate (DEC) is a derivative of the anthelminthic piperazine. It is active against lymphatic filariasis, both microfilaricidal and the adult worm. It is no longer approved by the FDA because these infections are rare in the United States. DEC can be obtained from the CDC after confirmed positive lab results. DEC is the drug of choice for the treatment of lymphatic filariasis. In combination with albendazole, it has shown good results in suppressing microfilaremia and is part of the Global Program for Elimination of Lymphatic Filariasis. DEC is contraindicated in patients with onchocerciasis because of the risk of Mazzotti reaction. In patients with filariasis and co-infection with *L loa,* DEC can cause fatal encephalopathy when there is heavy infestation. Common side effects of DEC include dizziness, gastrointestinal symptoms, fever, headache, and myalgia.

Doxycycline is an antibiotic that has shown positive results for the treatment of onchocerciasis when used in combination with ivermectin. Doxycycline kills *Wolbachia,* which is an endosymbiotic rickettsia-like bacterium that seems to be required for the survival of the *O volvulus* microfilariae. It does not kill the microfilariae, so it should not be used alone. Limited data suggest that treatment of onchocerciasis in patients co-infected with *L loa* is safe when the microfilarial load is less than 8000 microfilariae/mL.

### Cestode and Trematode Infections

Albendazole and praziquantel are the drugs of choice for most of the infections caused by flatworms. The only exception is triclabendazole, which is the drug of choice for treatment of *Fasciola hepatica* (sheep liver fluke). Triclabendazole is a benzimidazole only available through CDC under an investigational protocol. It is not yet approved by the FDA for use in humans, but it is the drug recommended by the WHO to treat fascioliasis. Albendazole decreases the number of microtubules of the intestinal cells in the parasites, thus decreasing their absorptive function. It also depletes the glycogen storages of the parasite, and with subsequent insufficient adenosine triphosphate (ATP) production, it leads to death. It is an effective agent for the treatment of echinococcosis and cysticercosis. See earlier discussion of albendazole in nematode infections for other details.

Praziquantel is active against most trematodes but typically not against *Fasciola* parasites. Praziquantel is a heterocyclic prazino-isoquinolin that causes rapid paralysis of intestinal cestodes and damages the tegument of trematodes. It is the drug of choice for the treatment of schistosomiasis and *Fasciolopsis buski.* The safety of praziquantel has not been established in children less than 4 years of age and pregnant women; however, mass deworming programs and schistosomiasis studies have not reported serious adverse events in these specific groups. Praziquantel is considered category B for its use in pregnancy. The WHO has reports of growing evidence that praziquantel is safe for treating infected children as young as 1 year of age. Praziquantel is metabolized in the liver and is contraindicated for concomitant use with potent cytochrome P450 inducers such as rifampin. It is also contraindicated for the treatment of ocular cysticercosis since parasite destruction may cause irreversible damage. It should not be administered in patients with epilepsy and other CNS involvement such as subcutaneous nodules suggestive of cysticercosis. Its use in patients with schistosomiasis may result in severe systemic inflammatory responses most likely caused by the release of parasitic antigens.

## TREATMENT OF PROTOZOAN INFECTIONS

### Intestinal Protozoa

Metronidazole is a synthetic antiprotozoal and antibacterial agent. It is a nitroimidazole used for anaerobic bacterial infections but is also effective against parasites that use anaerobic metabolism. Most of the parasites that are susceptible to metronidazole are intestinal protozoa such as *Entamoeba histolytica, Entamoeba polecki, Giardia intestinalis, Balantidium coli,* and *Dientamoeba fragilis.* Metronidazole is also the drug of choice for treatment of trichomoniasis, but drug resistance has been reported. Metronidazole is not active against the cysts of *E histolytica;* therefore, a luminal amebicide such as iodoquinol or paromomycin should be used following therapy with metronidazole or tinidazole. Common side effects of metronidazole include unpleasant metallic taste, nausea, vomiting, abdominal discomfort, and diarrhea. It should be used with caution in patients with decreased liver function because plasma clearance of the drug is decreased. Seizures, encephalopathy, aseptic meningitis, and optic and peripheral neuropathy are serious adverse reactions reported mainly with the use of the injectable form. In patients with prolonged use of oral metronidazole, persistent peripheral neuropathy has been reported. Metronidazole causes a disulfiram-like reaction when used concomitantly with alcohol ingestion. Safety for its use in pediatrics has not been established, but its use is supported by the WHO. Teratogenic activity and carcinogenic activity have been documented in oral chronic administration in rodent models; therefore, evaluation of the risks and benefits should be made when given to pregnant women and to nursing mothers.

Tinidazole is an antibacterial agent with antiprotozoal activity that can be used as an alternative drug for the treatment of amebiasis, trichomoniasis, and giardiasis. The mechanism by which this drug is effective against protozoa is unknown. Tinidazole is safe to use in children older than 3 years of age for the treatment of giardiasis and amebiasis. Safety has not been established in younger children. It is available in the United States only in tablets, but they may be crushed and mixed with syrup for those unable to swallow pills.

Paromomycin and iodoquinol are the drugs of choice for the treatment of asymptomatic colonization with *E histolytica*. Both are luminal agents that should follow the treatment of symptomatic intestinal or extraintestinal amebic infections. Paromomycin is an aminoglycoside very similar to neomycin. It has practically no absorption after oral administration, and almost 100% of the drug may be recovered in stool. It is an alternative for the treatment of cryptosporidiosis. Paromomycin is contraindicated in patients with intestinal obstruction. Iodoquinol is an oxyquinoline with poor oral absorption and has activity against the luminal stages of *E histolytica* and *D fragilis*. The mechanism of action is unknown.

Nitazoxanide is a synthetic antiprotozoal agent approved for the treatment of giardiasis and cryptosporidiosis in persons 1 year of age and older. Oral tablets are approved for use in those 12 years of age and older. Nitazoxanide has shown in vitro activity against sporozoites and oocysts of *Cryptosporidium parvum* and trophozoites of *Giardia lamblia*, but studies have not shown it to be superior to placebo for the treatment of cryptosporidiosis in HIV-infected or immunocompromised patients. The mechanism of action is thought to be interference with the electron transfer reactions essential to the anaerobic energy metabolism of the parasite. It should be administered with caution in patients with hepatic and renal disease.

Tetracyclines can be used as an alternative for treatment of *B coli* infection. They are not recommended in children less than 8 years of age and pregnant women.

#### Other Blood and Tissue Protozoa

Treatment regimens are not well established for primary amebic meningoencephalitis (PAM) caused by *Naegleria fowleri* or for granulomatous amebic encephalitis and keratitis caused by *Acanthamoeba* species and *Balamuthia mandrillaris*. In the United States, 122 of the 123 reported cases of PAM have been fatal. The survivor case was reported in California, and the treatment regimen received included amphotericin B, rifampicin, miconazole, dexamethasone, and phenytoin for seizure management. Sulfisoxazole was started but then discontinued after diagnosis of *Naegleria* was made. The other survivor case in North America was reported in Mexico and received a regimen with amphotericin B, rifampicin, fluconazole, ceftriaxone, and dexamethasone.

Miltefosine is an investigational drug that has shown in vitro activity against free-living ameba including *N fowleri*. It has also been successful in patients with disseminated *Acanthamoeba* infection and *Balamuthia*. In the United States, it is available from the CDC Emergency Operations Center.

Skin and eye infections caused by *Acanthamoeba* or *Balamuthia* that have not spread to the CNS can be successfully treated with topical agents. Consultation with an ophthalmologist as soon as the infection is suspected offers better chances of cure. Topical agents used for this purpose are not approved in the United States, but they may be available at compounding pharmacies. These agents include biguanide chlorhexidine or polyhexamethylene biguanide (0.02%) combined with propamidine isethionate (0.1%) or hexamidine (0.1%).

Pyrimethamine in combination with sulfadiazine is the regimen of choice for toxoplasmosis. The safety of pyrimethamine has not been established in children; however, the WHO allows its use in combination with sulfadiazine in children during the first year of life. The doses of pyrimethamine used in toxoplasmosis may produce hematologic adverse reactions such as megaloblastic anemia, leukopenia, thrombocytopenia, and pancytopenia. To prevent the latter, the use of supplemental folinic acid (leucovorin) is recommended in combination with pyrimethamine during the whole duration of the treatment. Clindamycin can be used instead of sulfadiazine in patients allergic to sulfa drugs. Spiramycin is the recommended agent in pregnancy. It is not approved by the FDA but it is available in the United States as investigational therapy.

For the management of babesiosis, consultation through CDC is recommended since most asymptomatic persons do not require medical treatment. Clindamycin plus quinine is the standard regimen for severely ill patients. The combination of atovaquone plus azithromycin has comparable efficacy in adults and is associated with fewer side effects. Atovaquone has been used safely in children who weigh ≥ 5 kg.

Benznidazole and nifurtimox are used for the treatment of *Trypanosoma cruzi* (American trypanosomiasis) in children up to 18 years of age. Neither of the 2 drugs is approved by the FDA, and they are only available in the United States from the CDC. Both drugs are contraindicated in pregnancy and in those with severe hepatic and/or renal disease. Withholding therapy while nursing is recommended as well. Side effects are common and are more frequent and more severe with increased age.

The drugs for treatment of African trypanosomiasis are only available from CDC with the exception of pentamidine, which is approved in the United States. Consultation with a tropical medicine specialist is always recommended. The mechanism of action of pentamidine is not fully understood. In vitro, it seems to interfere with the nuclear metabolism of the protozoan. Pentamidine can be used for the treatment of the acute hemolymphatic stage of *Trypanosoma brucei gambiense* infection. It is given by intravenous infusion or by intramuscular injection.

Suramin, eflornithine, and melarsoprol are only available from the CDC. Suramin is the recommended agent for the first stage of *Trypanosoma brucei rhodesiense* and is also active against *Tb gambiense*, but severe reactions occur in those co-infected with *O volvulus*. The mechanism of action of suramin is not fully understood. It is thought to inhibit DNA metabolism and protein synthesis of the protozoan, and it has limited efficacy in patients with CNS disease. Eflornithine and melarsoprol are indicated in the CNS stage of infection with *Tb gambiense* or *Tb rhodesiense*. Eflornithine inhibits parasite growth. Melarsoprol seems to act by preventing trophozoite multiplication. Nifurtimox can be used in combination with eflornithine or melarsoprol for treatment of the CNS stage of *Tb gambiense* infection. The combination of eflornithine and nifurtimox is preferred in rural Africa because of the difficulty administering 4 intravenous daily infusions with eflornithine alone.

For treatment of leishmaniasis, sodium stibogluconate is available from CDC under an investigational new drug protocol approved by the FDA. It is the only antileishmanial medication available through the CDC. The mechanism of action is unknown. It has been reported as highly effective in most regions with the exception of parts of South Asia. Miltefosine is an oral agent for leishmaniasis. It was approved by the FDA in 2014 for treatment of visceral leishmaniasis caused by *Leishmania donovani* and cutaneous and mucosal leishmaniasis caused by *Leishmania braziliensis, Leishmania guyanensis*, and *Leishmania panamensis* in adults and adolescents. It is contraindicated in pregnancy and women who are breastfeeding. It is not FDA approved for use in children less than 12 years of age. Miltefosine safety in patients less than 12 years old has not been established, but in animal models with juvenile rats, it showed increased sensitivity to drug-induced effects than in adult rats. Amphotericin B and liposomal amphotericin B have been used as rescue therapy for cutaneous and visceral leishmaniasis. Their use is anecdotal, and standard regimens have not been determined. Pentamidine is another alternative; however, it is rarely used in the United States. Pentamidine has the potential for irreversible toxicity, and its effectiveness is variable. There is conflicting data regarding efficacy of oral "-azole" agents.

## TREATMENT OF ECTOPARASITE INFESTATIONS

### Lice

Infestations with lice are treated mainly with topical pediculocide drugs that are available without a prescription in the United States. Permethrin and pyrethrin are the preferred agents for treatment of lice in children 2 years of age and older. Pyrethroids disrupt the sodium channel current in the nerve cell membrane of the parasite. Permethrin (1%) is available in lotion or shampoo and can be used in children 2 months of age and older. Pyrethrins are often combined with piperonyl butoxide, which is an agent that inhibits pyrethrin catabolism in the parasite, hence improving efficacy. Retreatment is usually recommended because these drugs are not completely ovicidal. Recent reports suggest increasing resistance of lice to pyrethrins; however, treatment failures are still attributed to not following appropriately the directions for use.

Topical ivermectin has both pediculocide and ovicidal activity; therefore, retreatment is usually not necessary. Pharmacokinetics of topical ivermectin were observed in a clinical study in children age 6 months to 3 years, and it was determined that the systemic levels were lower than those achieved from oral administration. Safety in patients under 6 months of age has not been established, so its use is not recommended. Oral ivermectin showed no superiority in a study when compared to malathion; therefore, it should be reserved for cases of refractory infestations. Oral ivermectin is not FDA approved for this indication.

Spinosad is a suspension for topical administration only. It interferes with the nicotinic acetylcholine receptor, causing paralysis of the lice. Safety for use in children below the age of 6 months has not been established. The topical suspension that is available in the United States contains benzyl alcohol, which has been associated with death and serious adverse reactions in neonates and low-birth-weight infants; therefore, it should not be used in children below 6 months of age. Benzyl alcohol acts by causing asphyxiation of the lice. Malathion is an organophosphate cholinesterase inhibitor with pediculicidal and ovicidal activity. It requires a longer time of application; thus, there is concern about absorption and toxicity. The safety and effectiveness of malathion in children under 6 years of age have not been well established. None of these drugs for treatment of lice should be applied near the eyes; therefore, petrolatum should be used for eyelash infestation.

### Scabies

Permethrin cream 5% is the drug of choice for the treatment of scabies in the United States. Permethrin kills the *Sarcoptes scabiei* mite and eggs. It is approved by the FDA for use in patients 2 months of age and older and is available only by prescription in the United States. In pregnancy, it should be administered only if absolutely necessary. Transient burning and stinging sensations following application with permethrin cream 10% were the most common adverse reactions in clinical trials and were associated with severity of infestation. Oral ivermectin can also be used for treatment of scabies but is not FDA approved for this indication. It has been reported as a safe and effective treatment for crusted scabies in other countries, and its use in the United States should be considered in patients who have failed treatment with or who cannot tolerate other medications that are FDA approved. The safety of oral ivermectin has not been established in children who weigh less than 15 kg or in pregnant women. Crotamiton lotion and 10% cream are active against *S scabiei* and also act as antipruritic agents. Crotamiton is FDA approved for use only in adults. Its safety and effectiveness for use in pediatric patients have not been determined.

## SUGGESTED READINGS


American Academy of Pediatrics. Drugs for parasitic infections. In: Kimberlin DW, Brady MT, Jackson MA, Long SS, eds. *Red Book: 2015 Report of the Committee on Infectious Diseases.* 30th ed. Elk Grove Village, IL: American Academy of Pediatrics; 2015:927-956.

American Academy of Pediatrics. Preferred therapy for specific parasitic pathogens. In: Bradley JS, Nelson JD, Barnett ED, et al, eds. *2017 Nelson's Pediatric Antimicrobial Therapy.* 23rd ed. Elk Grove Village, IL: American Academy of Pediatrics; 2017:171-187.

Bern C, Montgomery SP, Herwaldt BL, et al. Evaluation and treatment of Chagas disease in the United States. A systematic review. *JAMA.* 2007;298:2171-2181.

Centers for Disease Control and Prevention. Laboratory identification of parasitic diseases of public health concern. Available at http://www.cdc.gov/dpdx/az.html. Accessed May 22, 2017.

Keiser J, Ulteinger J. Efficacy of current drugs against soil-transmitted helminth infections: systematic review and meta-analysis. *JAMA.* 2008;299:1937-1948.

Mackey-Lawrence NM, Petri WA Jr. Amoebic dysentery. *Br Med J Clin Evid.* 2011;2011:0918.

National Institutes of Health. U.S. National Library of Medicine. DailyMed. Available at https://dailymed.nlm.nih.gov/dailymed/index.cfm. Accessed May 22, 2017.

US Food and Drug Administration. FDA approved drug products. Available at http://www.accessdata.fda.gov/scripts/cder/drugsatfda/index.cfm. Accessed May 22, 2017.

World Health Organization. WHO model lists of essential medicines (children). April 2015. 5th ed. Available at http://www.who.int/medicines/publications/essentialmedicines/en/. Accessed May 22, 2017.


# 319 Ascariasis

Ritu Banerjee

## INTRODUCTION

*Ascaris lumbricoides*, an intestinal roundworm, is a soil-transmitted helminth and one of the most common parasites in the world. It causes a variety of clinical manifestations known as ascariasis. Although *A lumbricoides* infects nearly 1 billion people worldwide and causes significant morbidity, it remains a neglected tropical disease.

## PATHOGENESIS AND EPIDEMIOLOGY

*Ascaris* is the largest intestinal roundworm that commonly infects humans: the female measures 20 to 40 cm long, and the male measures 15 to 30 cm long (Fig. 319-1). The female lays approximately 200,000 eggs daily; eggs are broadly ovoid and 45 to 75 μm by 35 to 50 μm. Fertilized eggs have a 3-layer coat with a bile-stained, mamillated outer shell. Unfertilized eggs are broader and longer (ie, approximately 90 μm by 45 μm) and usually lack the mamillated outer coat (Fig. 319-2).

Transmission of *A lumbricoides* is through the fecal-oral route. There is no human-to-human transmission. Infected individuals excrete eggs in their stool. Infection occurs through ingestion of *A lumbricoides* eggs through contaminated food or soil. When eggs are ingested and stimulated by enzymes in the duodenum, the larvae emerge, traverse the intestinal mucosa, and enter the mesenteric lymphatics and venules (Fig. 319-3). They then enter the portal circulation and reach the pulmonary vascular bed, perforate the alveolar wall, ascend the tracheobronchial tree to the epiglottis, and are swallowed. The vast majority of ascarids finally settle in the jejunum, where mature worms mate and females begin laying eggs in 2 to 2.5 months.

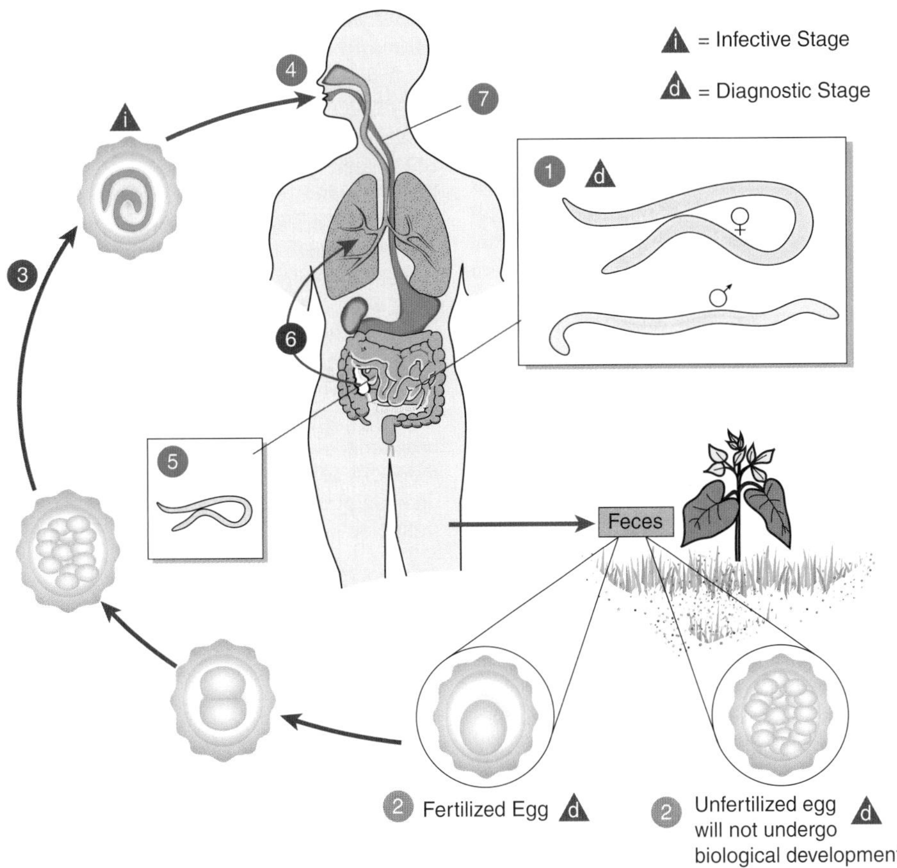


**FIGURE 319-1** Life cycle of *Ascaris lumbricoides*.

After a life span of 10 months to 2 years, they are passed in the stool. A video showing a live worm observed during colonoscopy is available at http://www.youtube.com/watch?v=HOaZCkA8Zvk (accessed July 1, 2016).

The World Health Organization estimates that over 1 billion people worldwide are infected with *A lumbricoides*, predominantly in South and East Asia. Tropical areas with warm, wet climates have year-round transmission of *A lumbricoides* and a high prevalence (approaching 95% in some regions). In the United States, the highest infection rates are among immigrants from developing countries (20–60% infected in some surveys). Young children are infected most frequently, with peak prevalence in school-age children living in the tropics. Intensity of infection, or worm burden, typically decreases significantly after the age of 15 years. *Ascaris* infections tend to cluster in families. Individuals may be asymptomatic and shed eggs for years, thus enhancing transmission. Behavioral and environmental factors are associated with intensity of infection, which is greatest in regions with poverty, malnutrition, and poor sanitation.

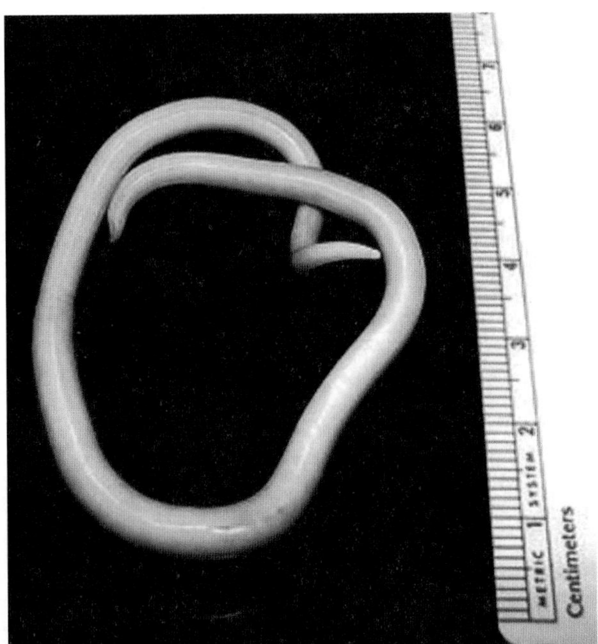


**FIGURE 319-2** *Ascaris lumbricoides* worm.

## CLINCIAL MANIFESTATIONS

The majority of individuals with *Ascaris* have low worm burden and are asymptomatic. In contrast, individuals with heavy worm burden can have a variety of symptoms that correlate with the stage and chronicity of infection.

During the period of larval invasion and migration to the respiratory tract, cough, dyspnea, fever, rales, and dullness to percussion of

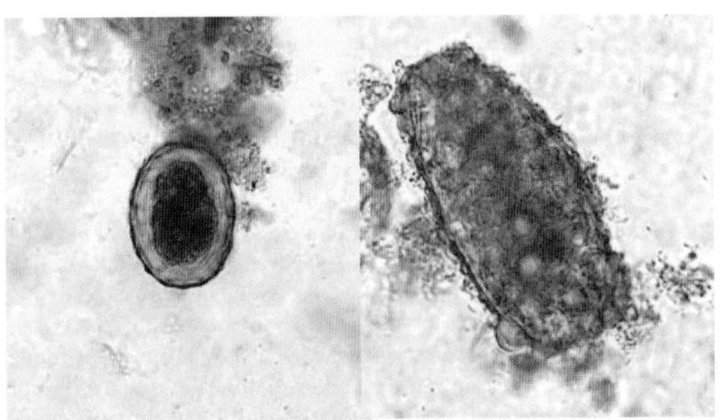

**FIGURE 319-3** *Ascaris lumbricoides* eggs.

the chest may be evident. Invasion of the respiratory system by migrating larvae results in alveolar hemorrhages, and pulmonary damage may be extensive, especially with large numbers of larvae. Hemoptysis may occur, and larvae may be found in the sputum. Shifting, pulmonary infiltrates, and widening of the hilum may be seen, along with eosinophilia (Löffler syndrome). During this phase, other manifestations of hypersensitivity such as urticaria and wheezing may occur with repeated infections. Larvae occasionally may traverse the pulmonary circulation and produce serious lesions in the eye, central nervous system, and kidney, resembling visceral larva migrans caused by *Toxocara* larvae.

Adult worms in the small intestine generally cause few symptoms. In children, the most frequently noted symptoms are vague epigastric pains, nausea, vomiting, and anorexia. Severe, intermittent, colicky abdominal pain may result from partial intestinal obstruction, which is more common in children than in adults, because children have smaller intestinal lumens. The more serious problems encountered with *Ascaris* infection result from migration of adult worms into the bile and pancreatic ducts, where they may cause biliary stone formation, pancreatitis, cholangitis, small bowel perforation, and complete intestinal obstruction, volvulus, or intussusception. Worms occasionally may migrate upward and emerge through the mouth or nose or migrate downward and pass through the rectum. Heavy infections may also lead to malabsorption, malnutrition, poor growth, and cognitive impairment.

*A lumbricoides* causes a Th2 response with increased production of interleukin (IL)-4 and other cytokines. This, in turn, leads to eosinophil, mast cell, and immunoglobulin (Ig) E production associated with atopy and many of the acute clinical manifestations described earlier.

## DIAGNOSIS

The diagnosis of ascariasis is made using a combination of clinical, epidemiologic, and microbiologic information. In a region where *A lumbricoides* is endemic, the differential diagnosis of a child presenting with fever, respiratory symptoms, and pulmonary infiltrates should include bacterial or viral pneumonia, tuberculosis, and *Ascaris*, especially if associated with eosinophilia. *Ascaris* should also be considered in children from endemic regions presenting with acute abdominal pain, signs of bowel obstruction, nonspecific abdominal symptoms, poor growth, asthma, or eosinophilia.

The diagnosis of *Ascaris* is generally confirmed by identifying typical eggs in the feces through light microscopy. Ascaris eggs are usually abundant, and stool concentration is rarely needed to see them. Examining stools from consecutive days increases sensitivity of microscopy. Adult worms can also be passed from the rectum or nose. If a patient brings a spontaneously passed worm to the clinic, a stool should be examined to ascertain whether any other worms remain. Abdominal computed tomographic scans or ultrasonography may be useful to visualize adult worms in the abdomen or biliary tract.

Serologic or antigen tests are performed at specialty laboratories and are not routinely available, but they have been useful diagnostic tests in some unusual cases. Newer polymerase chain reaction methods are more sensitive than direct microscopy for detection of *A lumbricoides* but are costly and not routinely available.

## TREATMENT

Antihelminthic medications are effective and well tolerated. However, reinfection after treatment is common. First-line therapy for *Ascaris* is albendazole or mebendazole. Although not approved by US Food and Drug Administration for this indication, albendazole is widely given as a single dose of 400 mg to adults and to children over 24 months or 200 mg for children 12 to 24 months of age. Second-line treatments for *Ascaris* include ivermectin, pyrantel pamoate, and nitazoxanide. Ivermectin and nitazoxanide are not approved for this indication. The safety of ivermectin has not been established in children < 15 kg.

Intestinal obstruction caused by *Ascaris* often responds to conservative management including nasogastric suction, intravenous fluids, and electrolyte correction. Mineral oil or diatrizoate sodium solution (Gastrografin) can be given to relax the worms. Instillation of piperazine (which is not available in the United States), a drug that paralyzes worms, into a duodenal tube may help. If this fails, the obstructing worms must be removed surgically.

## PREVENTION

Strategies to prevent and control *A lumbricoides* infection consist of (1) improving sanitation and access to clean drinking water, (2) improving health education about the risks of outdoor defecation and importance of hand washing and hygiene, and (3) preventive chemotherapy through mass drug administration. Mass drug administration (usually annually) of a single dose of albendazole to school-age children, without screening stool specimens, has become routine practice in many low- and middle-income countries. Mass treatment of refugees before departure to the United States has also been done to reduce the burden of infection among refugees arriving in the United States. There are international efforts to expand mass drug administration programs, which are considered cost-effective strategies to reduce the morbidity of helminth infections. However, mass drug administration does not prevent reinfection, so additional measures such as improved sanitation and health education are required for sustained control.

## SUGGESTED READINGS


Bieri FA, Gray DJ, Williams GM, et al. Health-education package to prevent worm infections in Chinese schoolchildren. *N Engl J Med.* 2013;368:1603-1612.

Centers for Disease Control and Prevention. Parasites: ascariasis. Available at http://www.cdc.gov/parasites/ascariasis/. Accessed July 2, 2016.

Jia TW, Melville S Utzinger J, King CH, Zhou XN. Soil-transmitted helminth reinfection after drug treatment: a systematic review and meta-analysis. *PLoS Negl Trop Dis.* 2012;6:e1621.

Kappagoda S, Singh U, Blackburn BG. Antiparasitic therapy. *Mayo Clin Proc.* 2011;86:561-583.

Lamberton PHL, Jourdan PM. Human ascariasis: diagnostics update. *Curr Trop Med Rep.* 2015;2:189-200.

Speich B, Moser W, Ali SM, et al. Efficacy and reinfection with soil-transmitted helminths 18-weeks post-treatment with albendazole-ivermectin, albendazole-mebendazole, albendazole-oxantel pamoate and mebendazole. *Parasit Vectors.* 2016;9:123.

Swanson SJ, Phares CR, Mamo B, et al. Albendazole therapy and enteric parasites in the United States-bound refugees. *N Engl J Med.* 2012;366:1498-1507.

Weatherhead JE, Hotez PJ. Worm infections in children. *Pediatr Rev.* 2015;36:341-354.

World Health Organization. Neglected tropical diseases: PCT databank: soil-transmitted helminthiases. Available at http://www.who.int/neglected_diseases/preventive_chemotherapy/sth/en/. Accessed July 2, 2016.


# 320 Baylisascariasis

Tibisay Villalobos-Fry

## INTRODUCTION

Baylisascariasis is an important zoonotic disease caused by the raccoon roundworm *Baylisascaris procyonis*. Baylisascariasis is a potentially severe form of larva migrans in humans that can produce fatal or severe central nervous system disease.

## PATHOGENESIS AND EPIDEMIOLOGY

Humans are a paratenic (intermediate) host, meaning that infection by larval stages of the parasite can occur but the parasite does not complete its lifecycle in the host. Raccoons infected with the roundworms

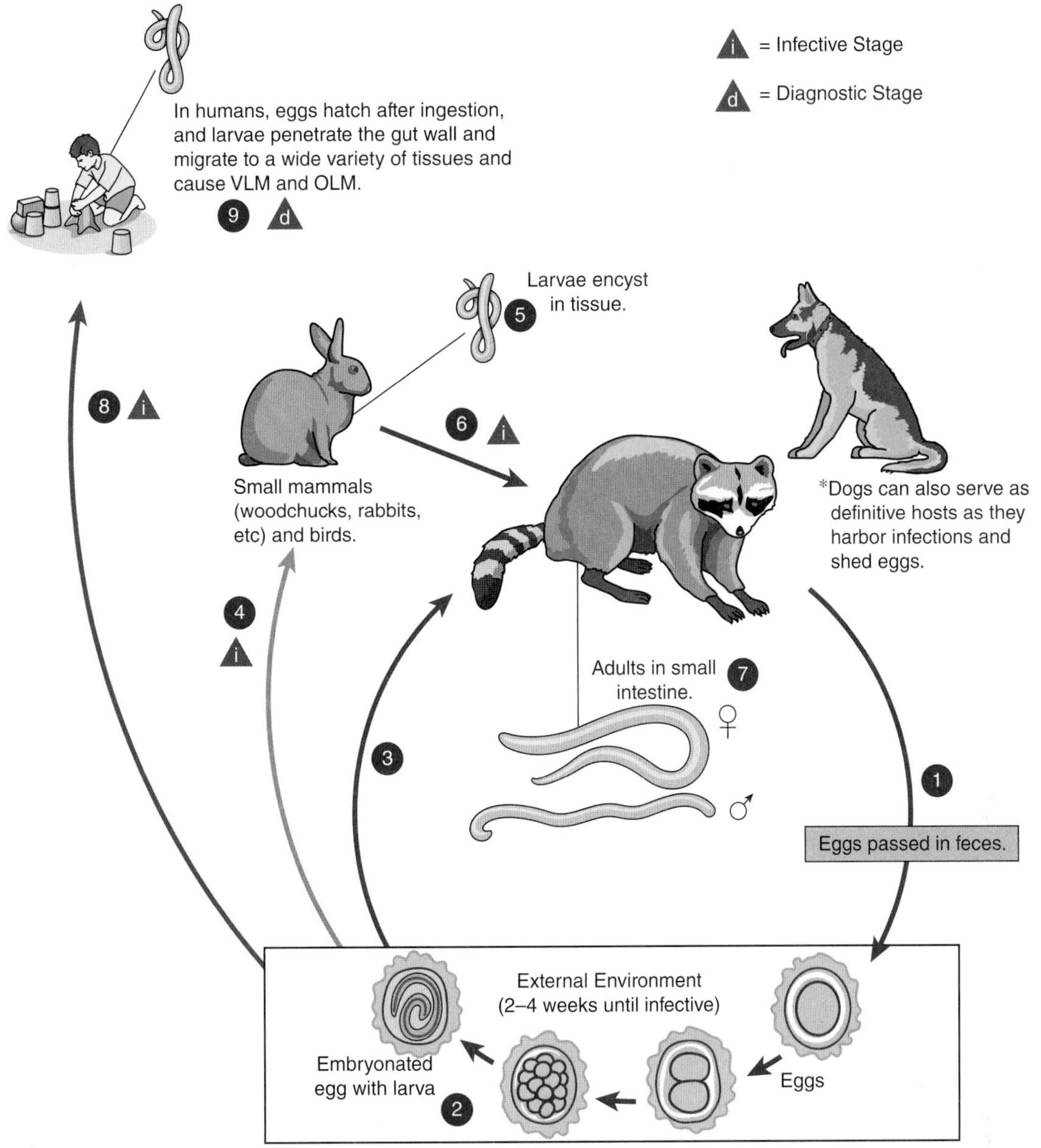

**FIGURE 320-1** Life cycle of *Baylisascaris procyonis*. OLM, ocular larva migrans; VLM, visceral larva migrans. (Reproduced with permission from Centers for Disease Control [CDC].)

shed the eggs in their feces. Adult *Baylisascaris* organisms reside in the raccoon small intestine, and adult *Baylisascaris* females produce a huge number of eggs with estimates as high as greater than 100,000 eggs per worm per day. Adult raccoons may shed millions of eggs per day, which leads to heavy environmental contamination. Humans can become infected when they accidentally ingest infected eggs from objects contaminated with the feces of wild or pet raccoons. People at risk of baylisascariasis infection include young children and developmentally disabled persons who are more likely to place objects with contaminated dirt or animal waste in their mouth. In addition, hunters, taxidermists, and wildlife conservationists who come in contact with animals and their habitats are also at risk (Fig. 320-1).

Infected eggs can be found in tree stumps, decaying trees, or rock piles. In more urban areas, they are often found in attics, chimneys and flat roofs, or patios. The eggs in the soil remain infectious for years. Once ingested, the larvae emerge and migrate to different parts of the body including lung, skeletal muscle, eye, and brain. Approximately 5% to 7% of ingested larvae may enter the brain, where they produce extensive damage before they are enclosed within cystic lesions. The migrating larvae may also cause mechanical damage while they travel throughout the tissue and trigger intense host inflammatory reaction producing eosinophilic granulomas in many organs. The infecting dose of larvae may be related to the disease presentation; when large numbers of embryonated eggs are ingested, larvae may be more likely to penetrate the central nervous system, causing neural larva migrans (NLM) (Fig. 320-2). Death or permanent disability is a common outcome of NLM due to *Baylisascaris*.

Raccoons are the predominant host. *B procyonis* is found in about 50% to 80% of raccoons in North America, but the parasite can also infect other animals, including dogs. It is a well-known cause of larva migrans in animals including mammals and birds. Other *Baylisascaris* species including *Baylisascaris melis* of badgers and *Baylisascaris columnaris* of skunks are also potential causes of human disease. Infected raccoons are found throughout the United States, with higher prevalence in the Midwest, Northeast, and West Coast. Cases of human baylisascariasis have been reported from California, Illinois, Louisiana, Massachusetts, Michigan, Minnesota, Missouri, New York, Oregon, and Pennsylvania.

## CLINICAL MANIFESTATIONS

Symptoms may appear as soon as 1 week after exposure and may include nausea, lethargy, and loss of coordination. The clinical presentation of baylisascariasis depends on the number and the location of larvae in the body.

*B procyonis* can produce visceral larva migrans (VLM), ocular larva migrans (OLM), and NLM with eosinophilic meningoencephalitis:

- VLM often presents with rash, abdominal pain, hepatomegaly, and pneumonitis. Peripheral eosinophilia is common.
- OLM may present as diffuse unilateral subacute neuroretinitis. It is usually seen in older individuals and presents as unilateral loss of vision. Ocular examinations may reveal a migrating larva, larval tracks, or lesions consistent with presence of a nematode larva in the eye. The *Baylisascaris* larvae are 3 to 5 times larger than *Toxocara* and measure 1.5 to 2.0 mm long. Granulomas can be present, and co-infection has been reported.
- NLM may present with mild to severe central nervous system involvement. Signs and symptoms may develop within 2 to 4 weeks after ingestion of large numbers of infective eggs and include weakness, incoordination, ataxia, irritability, weakness, seizures, altered mental status, stupor, and/or coma. Once symptoms and signs of neurologic disease are detected, significant pathology generally is already present, and it may quickly progress to coma and death. Although the disease is rare, fatal or severe baylisascariasis NLM has been reported primarily in children. To date, there have been at least 16 well-documented cases of *Baylisascaris* encephalitis reported.

A number of other parasitic nematode infections may cause similar signs and symptoms, such as infection with larvae of *Toxocara* and *Angiostrongylus* species. The pathogenesis of this disease is similar to that of *Toxocara* infection. However, the clinical course often is more severe because, unlike *Toxocara*, *Baylisascaris* larvae are larger and continue to molt and increase in size, resulting in extensive reaction and damage in the central nervous system, heart, and other internal organs.

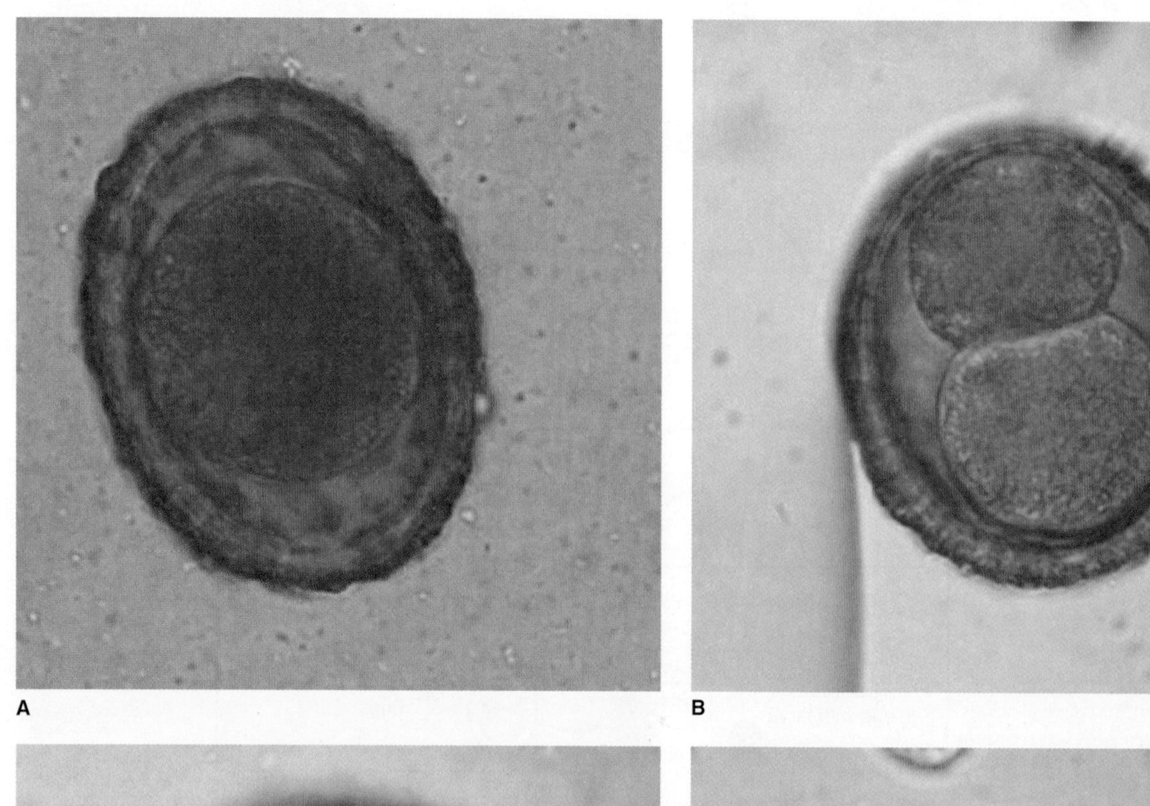


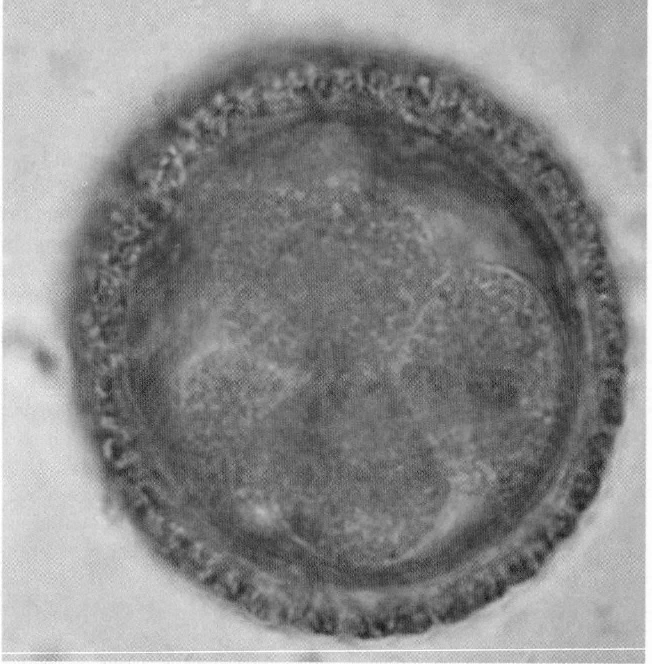


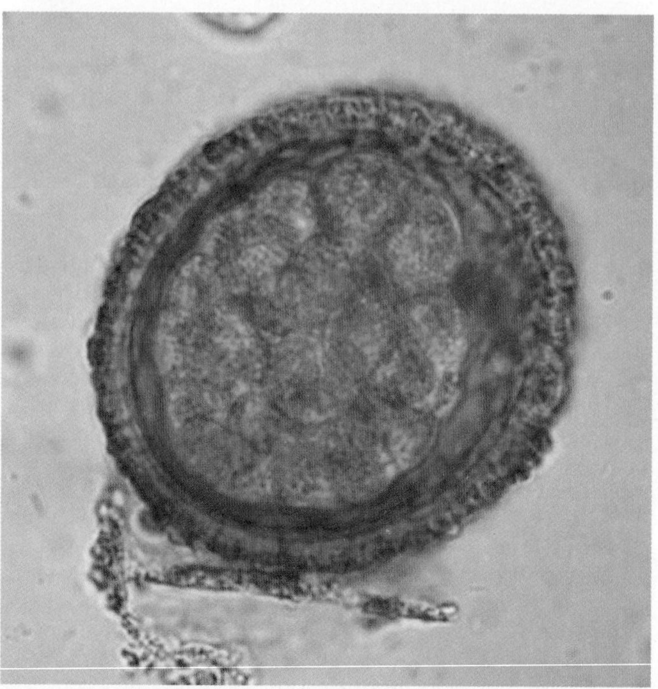


**FIGURE 320-2** Embryonated eggs of *B procyonis*, showing the developing larva inside. (Reproduced with permission from Centers for Disease Control [CDC]. Photo contributor: Dr. Cheryl Davis, Western Kentucky University, KY.)

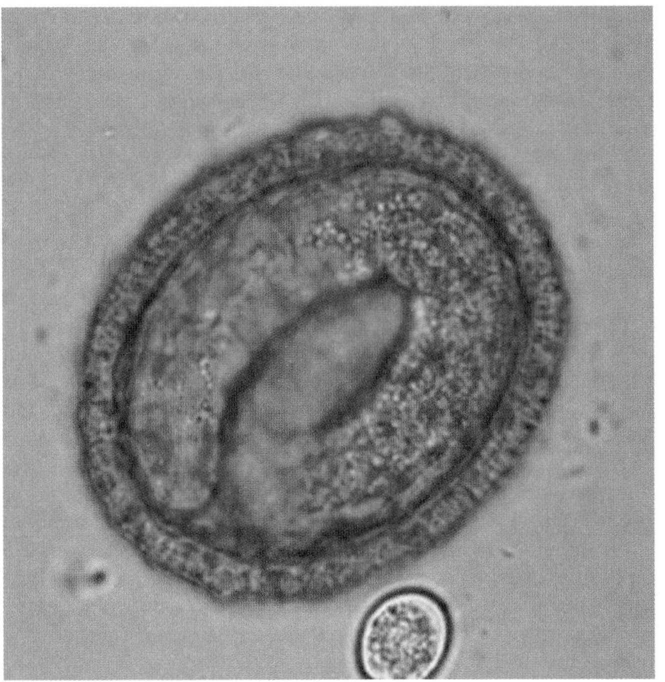

E

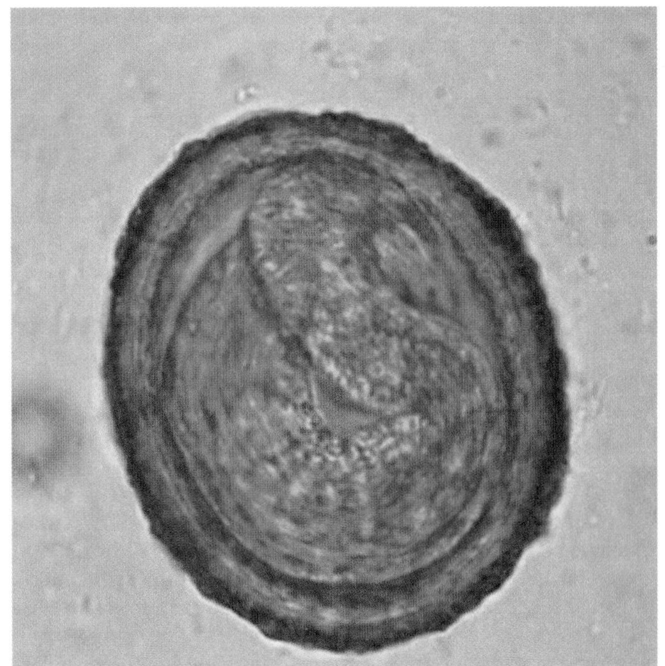

F

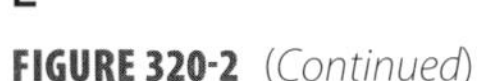

**FIGURE 320-2** *(Continued)*

## DIAGNOSIS

Diagnosis of baylisascariasis can be difficult. Diagnostic findings include eosinophilic pleocytosis in the cerebrospinal fluid (CSF), peripheral eosinophilia, deep white matter abnormalities on brain magnetic resonance imaging, and positive *B procyonis*–specific antibodies in serum and CSF. Patients with OLM are weakly seropositive or frequently seronegative. The recent development of recombinant antigen-based serodiagnostic assays with higher sensitivity and specificity as well as low degree of cross-reactivity when compared to the earlier serologic assays has aided greatly in the early diagnosis of this infection. Examination of tissue biopsies can be extremely helpful if a section of larva is contained, but removing an appropriate piece of tissue where the larva is actually present can be problematic.

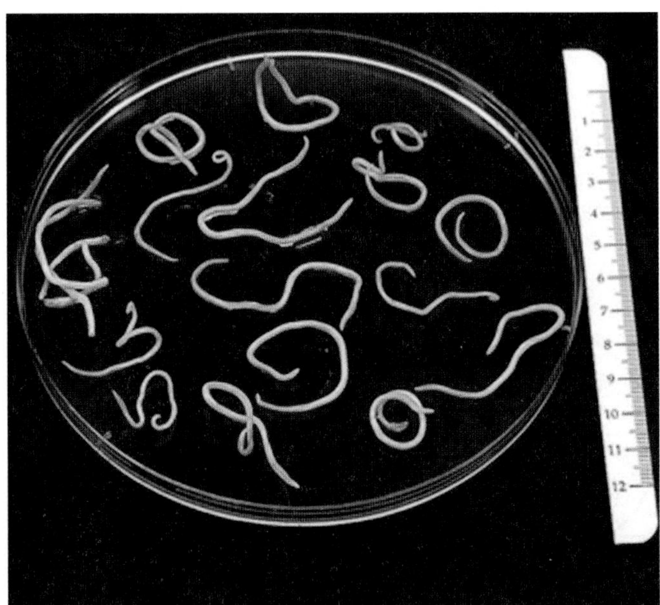

**FIGURE 320-3** *Baylisascaris procyonis* adult worm. (Reproduced with permission from Centers for Disease Control [CDC].)

## TREATMENT

Treatment is most successful when administered within 3 days of exposure. The treatment of choice is albendazole 50 mg/kg/d for 20 days. It should be administered immediately if there is a high index of suspicion. If albendazole is not immediately available, mebendazole or ivermectin may be used. The use of corticosteroids is also indicated. Despite adequate antiparasitic treatment, the outcomes are compromised in NLM because the diagnosis is usually made too late into the disease. Ocular baylisascariasis can be successfully treated with laser photocoagulation therapy.

## PREVENTION

Because of the severity of the disease, prevention is of utmost importance. The best way to prevent baylisascariasis is to avoid contact with raccoons and their feces. Do not feed or adopt wild animals. Discourage raccoons from living near your home. Avoid contact with raccoon feces and use appropriate protection when working in contaminated areas. Greater public and media awareness is critical for the prevention and early treatment of this zoonotic infection (Fig. 320-3).

## SUGGESTED READINGS

Dangoudoubiyam S, Vemulapalli R, Ndao M, Kazacos KR. Recombinant antigen-based enzyme-linked immunosorbent assay for diagnosis of *Baylisascaris procyonis* larva migrans. *Clin Vaccine Immunol.* 2011;18:1650-1655.

Graeff-Teixeira C, Morassutti AL, Kazacos KR. Update on baylisascariasis, a highly pathogenic zoonotic infection. *Clin Microbiol Rev.* 2016;29:375-399.

Liu G, Fennelly G, Kazacos KR, et al. *Baylisascaris procyonis* and herpes simplex virus 2 coinfection presenting as ocular larva migrans with granuloma formation in a child. *Am J Trop Med Hyg.* 2015;93:612-614.

Peters JM, Madhavan VL, Kazacos KR, et al. Good outcome with early empiric treatment of neural larva migrans due to *Baylisascaris procyonis*. *Pediatrics.* 2012;129:e806-e811.

Shafir SC, Sorvillo FJ, Sorvillo T, Eberhard ML. Viability of *Baylisascaris procyonis* eggs. *Emerg Infect Dis.* 2011;17:1293-1295.

# 321 Dracunculiasis

Tibisay Villalobos-Fry

## INTRODUCTION

Dracunculiasis (Guinea worm disease) is caused by *Dracunculus medinensis*, a parasitic worm that infects the subcutaneous and connective tissues and is acquired from drinking contaminated water.

## PATHOGENESIS AND EPIDEMIOLOGY

Humans are the only known reservoir of *D medinensis*. They become infected by drinking unfiltered water containing copepods (plankton) that are infected with larva of *D medinensis*. Once ingested, the copepods die, and the infected larva are set free, penetrating the host's stomach and intestinal wall and entering the abdominal cavity and retroperitoneal space. Maturation into adults takes 60 to 90 days, when copulation occurs, after which male worms die. It takes 8 to 12 months for the female worms to mature and migrate from the deep connective tissue to the subcutaneous tissue and then to the skin surface. The average size of the female worm is 1 m in length by 1 to 2 mm in diameter. More than 90% of the worms emerge from the lower extremities, usually below the knees. There, the female worm induces a painful blister on the skin, generally on the distal lower extremity, which ruptures and ulcerates. When this lesion comes into contact with water, which occurs frequently because infected patients immerse the limb seeking to relieve the local discomfort, the female worm emerges and releases motile larvae into the water. The larvae then might be ingested by a copepod, and if the stagnant water is used for drinking, the cycle begins again (Fig. 321-1).

Approximately 1 year after a person acquires infection from drinking contaminated water, the worm emerges through the skin, usually on the lower extremities. The worldwide campaign to eradicate dracunculiasis began in 1980 at the Centers for Disease Control and Prevention (CDC). In 1986, the World Health Assembly called for dracunculiasis elimination, and the global Guinea Worm Eradication Program (GWEP)—led by the Carter Center and supported by the World Health Organization, United Nations Children's Fund (UNICEF), CDC, and other international organizations—began assisting the ministries of health in countries where dracunculiasis was endemic. In 1986, an estimated 3.5 million cases occurred mostly in Africa and Asia. Although the disease has not been completely eradicated, considerable progress has been made, and the annual numbers of reported cases in 2015 had decreased by 99%. Also in 2015, only 22 cases were reported worldwide—an 83% reduction in cases from the previous year. The disease is now limited to 4 African countries (South Sudan, Mali, Chad, and Ethiopia).

Guinea worm disease (GWD) has a seasonal pattern, with most infections occurring during the dry season when water becomes scarce and surface water dries up and becomes stagnant. GWD occurs in all age groups but is more common in individuals 15 to 45 years old because of the type of outside work they perform; older children who carry water for the household also become infected more often. Many people in affected villages become reinfected often throughout life because immunity does not develop against the parasite.

Almost all cases of the disease occur in isolated rural areas, and the economic impact of the infection is significant because the infection causes temporary or permanent disability in adults and school disruption in children.

A distinctive pattern of the disease has been reported in recent years from Chad, which had eradicated the disease for 10 years but started reporting cases again in 2010, and reemergence has been paralleled by an increased infection among dogs. It has been speculated that the dogs may be eating aquatic animals that are infected with Guinea worm. Studies are currently under way.

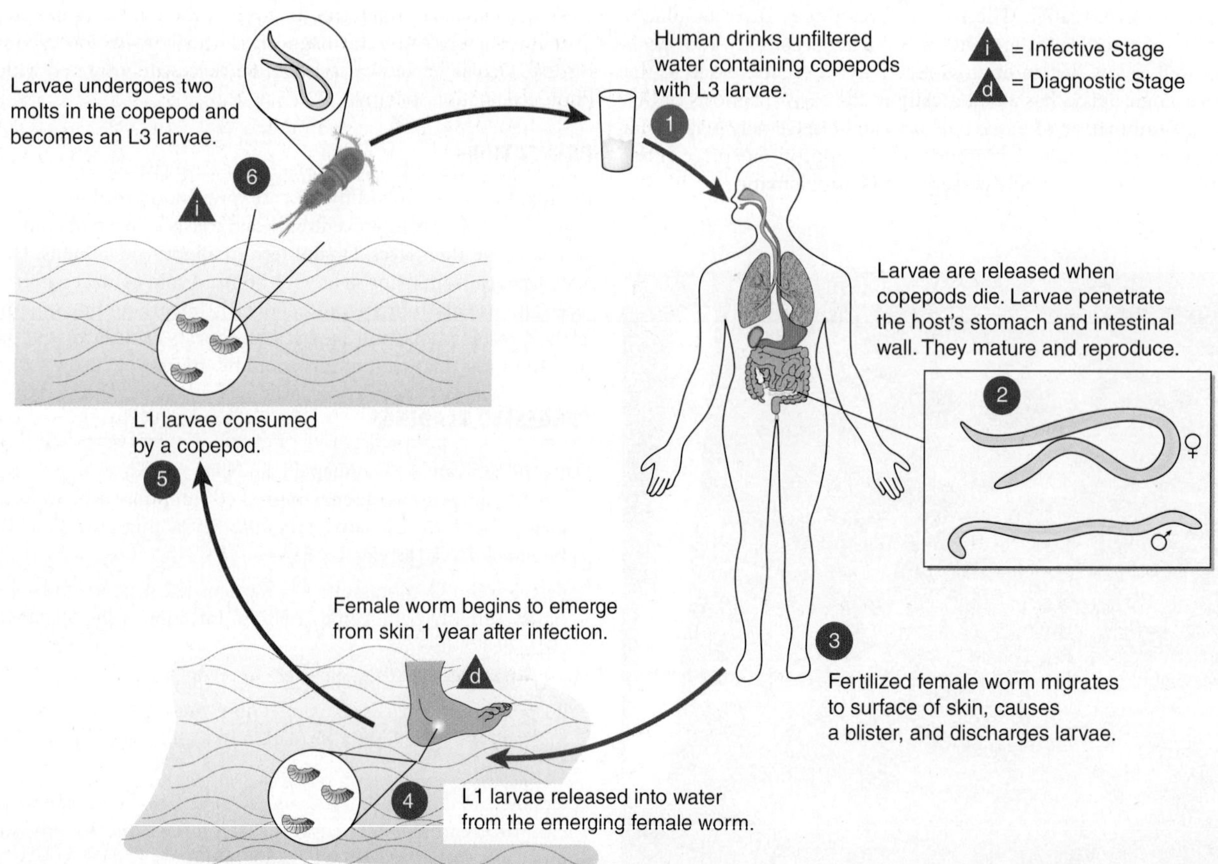


**FIGURE 321-1** Life cycle of *Dracunculus medinensis*. (Used with permission from the Centers for Disease Control and Prevention (CDC) https://www.cdc.gov/parasites/guineaworm/biology.html. Accessed June 30, 2017.)

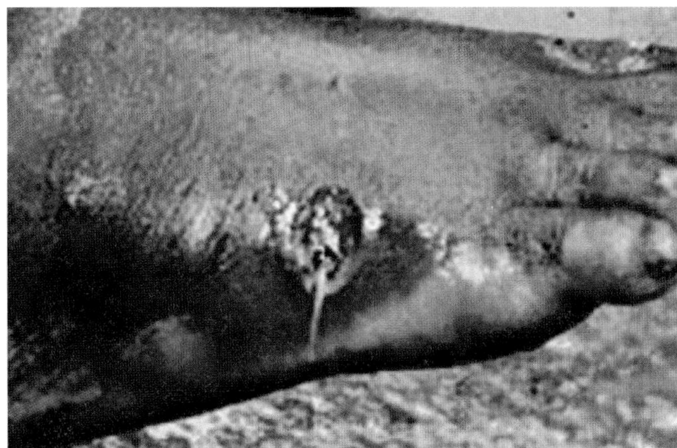

**FIGURE 321-2** Adult female Guinea worm emerging from foot ulcer. (Used with permission from The Carter Center, http://www.cartercenter.org. Accessed June 1, 2016.)

## CLINICAL MANIFESTATIONS

People infected with GWD have no symptoms for approximately 1 year after becoming infected. During the incubation period, there are usually no symptoms since the parasite does not cause symptoms in the deep tissues. However, while migrating to the skin, it may cause hypersensitivity reactions with low-grade fever, itching, rash, nausea, vomiting, and dizziness. On occasion, more severe systemic symptoms with dyspnea and hypotension can occur. A blister will be visible most often (80–90% of cases) on the lower extremities, commonly on the ankle or between the metatarsal bones, but they can occur anywhere (Fig. 321-2). The blister grows larger over several days, causing burning pain. In addition to the pain of the blister, removal of the worm is also very painful. Bacterial superinfection is common if proper care of the wound is not undertaken. Abscesses are also common, as well as septic arthritis. Tetanus can occur in an inadequately immunized person.

## DIAGNOSIS

Dracunculiasis is a clinical diagnosis that can only be made once the skin ulcer appears or the outline of the worm can be seen beneath the skin. Serologic tests are not reliable.

## TREATMENT

The treatment of GWD requires removal of the entire worm and caring for the wound. There is no specific drug to treat GWD.

Wound care involves the following steps:

- Each day, the affected body part is submerged in cool water to encourage the worm to come out.
- The wound is then cleaned.
- Gentle traction is applied until resistance is met to avoid breaking the worm.
- The worm is wrapped around a rolled piece of gauze or stick to maintain some tension of the worm and encourage more of the worm to emerge. This also prevents the worm from slipping back inside.
- Topical antibiotics are applied to the wound to prevent secondary bacterial infections.
- The affected body part is bandaged with fresh gauze to protect the site.
- These steps are repeated daily until the entire worm is removed. The worm can be as long as 1 m in length, so full extraction can take several days to weeks.

## PREVENTION

Providing safe drinking water is the main way to prevent GWD. The GWEP provides guidelines for interventions that focus on stopping the spread of GWD:

- Surveillance and case containment
- Provision of safe drinking water
- Vector control using a chemical larvicide such as temephos (Abate), which is safe for consumption at the concentrations used to treat the water
- Health education and community mobilization

## SUGGESTED READINGS


Al-Awadi AR, Al-Kuhlani A, Breman JG, et al. Guinea worm (dracunculiasis) eradication: update on progress and endgame challenges. *Trans R Soc Trop Med Hyg*. 2014;108:249-251.

Cavendish J. The last bastions of guinea-worm disease. *Bull World Health Organ*. 2014;92:854-855.

Dracunculiasis eradication: global surveillance summary, 2015. *Wkly Epidemiol Rec*. 2016;91:219-236.

Eberhard ML, Ruiz-Tiben E, Hopkins DR, et al. The peculiar epidemiology of dracunculiasis in Chad. *Am J Trop Med Hyg*. 2014;90:61-70.

Hopkins DR, Ruiz-Tiben E, Eberhard ML, Roy SL. Progress toward global eradication of dracunculiasis—January 2013-June 2014. Centers for Disease Control and Prevention (CDC). *Morb Mortal Wkly Rep*. 2014;63:1050-1054.

Lupi O, Downing C, Lee M, et al. Mucocutaneous manifestations of helminth infections: nematodes. *J Am Acad Dermatol*. 2015;73:929-44.


# 322 Enterobiasis (Pinworm)

Jose J. Zayas

## INTRODUCTION

Enterobiasis is caused by the pinworm *Enterobius vermicularis*, a strictly human parasite infecting the gastrointestinal tract.

## PATHOGENESIS AND EPIDEMIOLOGY

Infection occurs by ingestion of embryonated eggs by hand-to-mouth transmission or by oral contact with infected fomites, such as toys, bedding, or clothing. The incubation period from ingestion of an egg until an adult gravid female migrates to the perianal region is 1 to 2 months or longer. Ingested eggs hatch in the duodenum, and the larvae develop into adults in the cecum, where they mate. The yellow-white gravid female pinworms measuring 8 to 13 mm detach from the cecal mucosa and migrate out of the anus onto the perianal and perineal skin, leaving a trail of eggs on the surface of the skin. They do not lay eggs in the colon. Female pinworms usually die after depositing up to 10,000 fertilized eggs within 24 hours on the perianal skin. Eggs average 55 μm by 35 μm and appear flattened on one side and convex on the other. They are fully mature and infective 3 to 8 hours after being deposited, but at normal room temperature, less than 10% of eggs live for 48 hours. Eggs remain infective in an indoor environment usually for 2 to 3 weeks.

Since the female pinworm dies after ovipositing is completed, repeated infections are the result of reinfection from other environmental sources and not from retrograde infection.

Infection occurs worldwide, and clustering of cases in families is common. Prevalence estimates suggest there are 40 million infected persons in the United States, and infection rates in school-aged children vary from 10% to 45%. Infection is unrelated to poor sanitary facilities or tropical climates. Young girls have pinworms more frequently than boys of the same age, and whites are more often infected than African Americans. Infection is most common between early fall and late spring, perhaps related to transmission in schools. For unknown reasons, some individuals seem to be predisposed or vulnerable to reinfection. Unlike soil-transmitted helminths such as *Ascaris*, enterobiasis is more common in urban settings.

## CLINICAL MANIFESTATIONS

Pinworms rarely produce serious pathology, and many infections are asymptomatic. The most common presentation is perianal and perineal pruritus, typically felt at night. Although pruritus probably results from crawling worms, some patients with heavy pinworm infections and many worms in the rectum have little or no itching. Pruritus may provoke such severe scratching that local bleeding, secondary pyogenic infection, and lichenification can occur. Abdominal pain, nausea, and vomiting have been described with heavy worm burden. Adult pinworms may be found in normal and inflamed appendices following surgical removal, but whether or not they cause appendicitis is debated. Eosinophilic enterocolitis has been noted in the presence of pinworms usually without peripheral eosinophilia being observed. Vaginitis and discharge have been observed in young girls. Rarely, pinworms have been found in fallopian tubes, resulting in intra-abdominal ectopic migration and symptomatic granulomatous inflammation in the peritoneal cavity. *Enterobius* infestation of the nasal mucosa has also been observed. Many other clinical entities, such as enuresis, teeth-grinding at night, and weight loss, have been attributed to pinworm infections, but no relationship has been established.

## DIAGNOSIS

Nocturnal perianal pruritus strongly suggests pinworm infection, especially in children. Thin, creamy-white worms are often found if the perianal region is examined when the child is awakened by itching (Fig. 322-1). Since no egg shedding occurs inside the intestinal lumen, ova are not often seen in stools, so examination of stool specimens for ova and parasites is not recommended. The cellophane tape swab technique is the diagnostic method of choice (Fig. 322-2). A 6-cm piece of transparent (not translucent) cellophane tape is folded with its sticky side out over the end of a wooden tongue blade and then firmly applied against either side of the perianal region. Next, the tape is placed sticky side down onto a microscope slide. The swabs should be taken 2 to 3 hours after going to bed or in the morning immediately before the patient gets out of bed. It is recommended that this be done on 3 consecutive days. Slides from specimens may be sealed and stored in the refrigerator until delivered. Serologic tests are not useful for diagnosis, and eosinophilia does not correlate with infection.

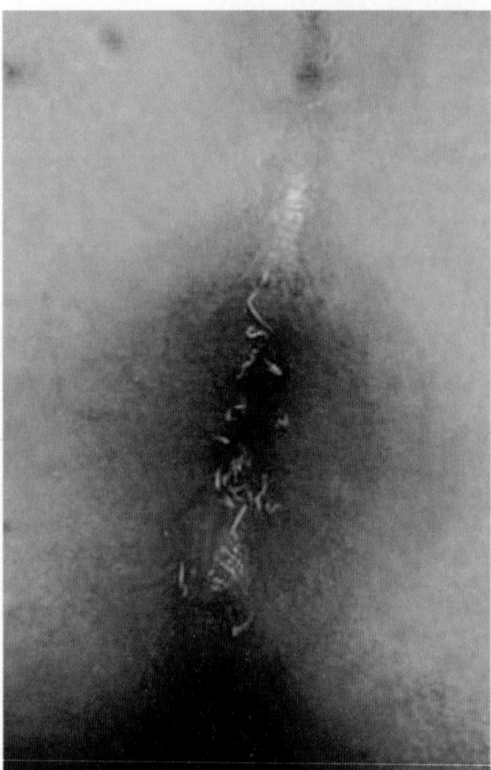

**FIGURE 322-1** Pinworms. Multiple tiny pearly white worms are seen at the anus. (Reproduced with permission from the Centers for Disease Control and Prevention Public Health Image Library.)

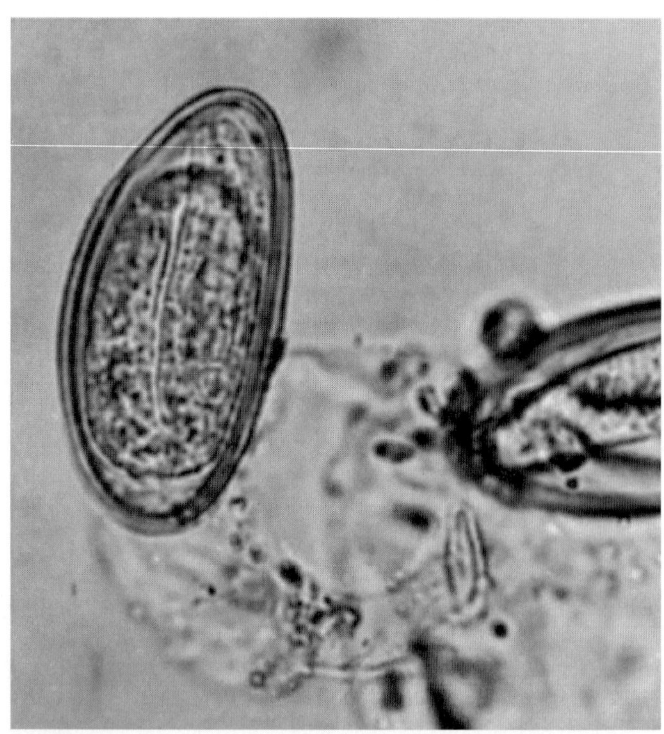

**FIGURE 322-2** *Enterobius vermicularis* ova from the stool of an infected child (cellophane tape technique, 448×).

## TREATMENT

Albendazole (weight < 20 kg: 200 mg, and ≥ 20 kg: 400 mg PO once; repeat in 2 weeks), as a single dose given initially and again 2 weeks later, is the treatment of choice. Mebendazole (100 mg) is as effective but is available in the United States only through compounding pharmacies. Pyrantel pamoate (11 mg/kg; maximum 1 g) is the most frequently used medication in the United States as it is inexpensive and available without a prescription. However, it has greater toxicity, with side effects including anorexia, nausea, vomiting, abdominal cramps, diarrhea, neurotoxic effects, and transient increases in hepatic enzymes. None of the mentioned medications kill *Enterobius* eggs. Therefore, the second dose is given to reduce the risk of autoinoculation. Most studies implementing this strategy result in a nearly 100% cure rate with either mentioned medication. Since infection is often present in several household members, consider treating the entire family excluding anyone who might be pregnant. Repeated infections are common and should be treated in the same fashion as initial infections. Vaginitis is self-limited and does not require separate treatment. Experience with these anthelmintics in children younger than 2 years of age is limited. Treatment of this group should be done with caution, and albendazole is recommended given its safer toxicity profile. Piperazine is no longer used because of lower efficacy and increased toxicity compared with the benzimidazoles.

## PREVENTION

Parents and patients should be reassured that a pinworm infection is not a reflection of poor hygiene or the result of an unclean home. Good hand washing is the most effective means of prevention. Bedclothes, linens, and underclothes of infected children should be handled carefully and not shaken to avoid dispersing ova into the air, and they should be promptly placed into a washer and laundered in hot water followed by a hot dryer to kill any eggs that may be there especially after anthelmintic treatment. Infected persons should bathe well in the morning following treatment, as this frequently removes a large number of infective eggs. Showering is a better method than taking a bath, because showering avoids potentially contaminating the bath water with pinworm eggs. Infected people should not cobathe with others during their time of infection. They should also cut fingernails regularly and avoid biting the nails and scratching around the anus. Control of infection in childcare centers and schools may be difficult because of high rates of reinfection, and in some cases, massive and simultaneous treatment of children and adults in institutions may be necessary.

## SUGGESTED READINGS


American Academy of Pediatrics Committee on Infectious Diseases. Pinworm infection. In: *Red Book: 2015 Report of the Committee on Infectious Diseases*. 30th ed. Elk Grove Village, IL: American Academy of Pediatrics; 2015:520-522.

Centers for Disease Control and Prevention. Enterobiasis (*Enterobius vermicularis*). www.dpd.cdc.gov/DPDx/HTML/Enterobiasis.htm. Accessed on March 3, 2016.

Cranston I, Potgieter N, Mathebula S, Ensink JH. Transmission of *Enterobius vermicularis* eggs through hands of school children in rural South Africa. *Acata Trop*. 2015;150:94-96.

Fleming CA, Kearney DE, Moriarity P, Redmond HP, Andrews EJ. An evaluation of the relationship between *Enterobius vermicularis* infestation and acute appendicitis in a paediatric population—a retrospective cohort study. *Int J Surg*. 2015;18:154-158.

Li HM, Zhou CH, Li ZS, et al. Risk factors for *Enterobius vermicularis* infection in children in Gaozhou, Guangdong, China. *Infect Dis Poverty*. 2015;4:28.


# 323 Lymphatic Filariasis and Onchocerciasis

Daniel E. Dulek

## INTRODUCTION

Filarial worms are parasitic nematodes that dwell within the lymphatics and the subcutaneous tissues. Eight filarial species are associated with human disease, though only 4 cause significant morbidity in children (Table 323-1). These species include the causative agents of lymphatic filariasis—*Wuchereria bancrofti, Brugia malayi*, and *Brugia timori*—and *Onchocerca volvulus*, the causative agent of onchocerciasis. The filarial parasites can be distinguished by their geographic distribution, vector, anatomic location of adult worms, and anatomic location and periodicity of microfilaria detection. Of the human filarial parasites, *W bancrofti* is, by far, the most important in terms of both morbidity and numbers of people infected. *O volvulus* remains an important cause of worldwide morbidity, especially in Africa. With elimination of *O volvulus* from selected transmission zones in the Americas, there is hope of eventual elimination from Africa.

Each filarial parasite is transmitted by biting arthropods, either mosquitoes or flies, and all go through complex life cycles that include a slow maturation (often 3–24 months) from the infective larval stages carried by the insects to the adult worms that live within the lymphatics and lymph nodes (*W bancrofti* and *Brugia* species) or in the subcutaneous tissues (*O volvulus, Loa loa, Mansonella streptocerca*). Infection occurs when male and female adult worms mate and females produce microfilariae offspring, 200 to 400 mm in length, that either circulate in the blood or migrate to the skin while awaiting ingestion by insect vectors. Productive infection is usually not established unless exposure to infective larvae is intense or prolonged. Maturation of microfilariae into macrofilariae requires a transition stage in the vector, and therefore, completion of the filarial life cycle does not occur within the human host. Therefore, while acquisition of and infection with these parasites occurs throughout childhood in endemic regions, most of the pathology associated with these infections is found primarily in older children and adults.

## PATHOGENESIS AND EPIDEMIOLOGY

### Lymphatic Filariasis

Lymphatic filariasis affects approximately 120 million people in Africa, Asia, India, Indonesia, the Philippines, Papua New Guinea, and focal areas of Latin America and the Caribbean. More than 90% of these infections are caused by *W bancrofti* and occur in sub-Saharan Africa, Southeast Asia, and the Western Pacific. Infection with *B malayi* is limited to 10 to 20 million persons in South and Southeast Asia, Indonesia, and the Philippines. *B timori* infection exists only among the islands of southeastern Indonesia and Timor-Leste. Coinfection with *W bancrofti* and *Brugia* species can occur in some regions endemic for both species. In contrast to other vector-borne parasitic diseases such as malaria, several different genera of mosquitoes may transmit lymphatic filariae. These include *Anopheles* species in rural Africa and the Pacific, *Culex* species in urban areas of the world, *Aedes aegypti* in some Pacific islands, and *Mansonia*, which is capable of transmitting only *B malayi*, in South Asia.

The prevalence of microfilaria-producing infection in endemic areas increases with age, apparently correlating with the cumulative exposure. Infection with adult worms in the absence of microfilaremia can occur in 25% or more of children between the ages of 1 and 5 years, depending on the level of filarial endemicity in the community. Productive infection is rare in travelers to or temporary residents of filaria-endemic regions, but can certainly occur with prolonged stays. Overall, microfilarial carrier rates vary significantly among endemic regions, from approximately 10% in the Nile Delta, to 20% to 40% in parts of East Africa, and often greater than 60% in Papua New Guinea.

Disease pathogenesis in lymphatic filariasis most likely is a result of the host inflammatory response to the adult worms causing lymphatic damage rather than a direct result of parasite-mediated tissue destruction. Complex interactions among immune response mediators are thought to explain why certain individuals remain asymptomatic (or subclinical) despite microfilaremia, whereas others develop debilitating lymphedema in the absence of detectable microfilariae. Current research efforts also seek to address the potential influence of filaria-driven immune modulation on coinfections with other pathogens such as malaria, tuberculosis, and intestinal helminths.

### Onchocerciasis

Onchocerciasis affects approximately 18 million people, the overwhelming majority of whom live in sub-Saharan Africa; the rest live in small endemic foci in Latin America and the Arabian Peninsula. Approximately 600,000 of those infected are severely visually impaired as a consequence of onchocercal eye disease (river blindness), the second leading cause of infectious blindness worldwide. Disease transmission is most intense near free-flowing rivers and streams where the blackfly (*Simulium* species) vector breeds. Recently, several foci of endemicity in Latin America have been declared to have eliminated onchocerciasis. In contrast to the situation with lymphatic filariasis, inflammatory responses directed toward onchocercal microfilariae likely account for the major clinical manifestations of dermatitis and ocular inflammation. The precise details of these host-parasite interactions remain largely undeciphered.

## CLINICAL MANIFESTATIONS

### Lymphatic Filariasis

Bancroftian and brugian filariases have very similar clinical presentations. The 3 most common manifestations of the lymphatic filariases are asymptomatic (or subclinical) microfilaremia, acute filarial adenolymphangitis, and lymphatic obstruction. Patients with asymptomatic microfilaremia may have thousands of circulating parasites per milliliter of blood but rarely come to medical attention except through

**TABLE 323-1 EPIDEMIOLOGIC AND BIOLOGIC FEATURES OF THE FILARIAE**

| Species | Endemic Areas | Vector | Microfilariae | Adult Worm Location | Primary Pathology |
|---|---|---|---|---|---|
| *Brugia malayi* | China, India, Malaysia, and some Pacific Island groups | Mosquitoes, including *Anopheles*, *Aedes*, and *Mansonia* species | Bloodborne, sheathed, nocturnally periodic or subperiodic | Lymphatics | Lymphedema, adenolymphangitis |
| *Brugia timori* | Southeastern Indonesia | *Anopheles barbirostris* | Bloodborne, sheathed, nocturnally periodic | Lymphatics | Lymphedema, adenolymphangitis |
| *Loa loa* | Western and central Africa | *Chrysops* species | Bloodborne, sheathed, diurnally periodic | Subcutaneous tissues, including subconjunctiva | Migratory angioedema, conjunctivitis |
| *Mansonella ozzardi* | Central and South America, Caribbean | *Culicoides* species and *Simulium amazonicum* | Skin and blood-borne, unsheathed, nonperiodic | Thoracic and peritoneal cavities, lymphatics | Unknown/poorly defined |
| *Mansonella perstans* | Sub-Saharan Africa, northern coast of South America, Tunisia, and Algeria | *Culicoides* species | Bloodborne, unsheathed, nonperiodic | Serous cavities, mesentery, perirenal and retroperitoneal tissues | Unknown/poorly defined |
| *Mansonella streptocerca* | Western and central Africa | *Culicoides grahamii* | Skin, unsheathed, nonperiodic | Dermis | Pruritus, rash, hypopigmented macules, adenopathy |
| *Onchocerca volvulus* | Sub-Saharan Africa, Latin America, and the Arabian peninsula | *Simulium* species | Skin, unsheathed, nonperiodic | Subcutaneous nodules | Subcutaneous nodules, pruritic dermatitis, lymphadenopathy, keratitis, uveitis, chorioretinitis |
| *Wuchereria bancrofti* | Sub-Saharan Africa, Southeast Asia, western Pacific, Caribbean, and northern coast of South America | Mosquitoes, including *Anopheles*, *Aedes*, and *Culex* species | Bloodborne, sheathed, nocturnally periodic or subperiodic | Lymphatics, lymph nodes | Lymphedema, adenolymphangitis, hydrocele |

the incidental finding of microfilariae in peripheral blood. Many individuals with microfilaremia, however, have some degree of subclinical disease that includes microscopic hematuria and/or proteinuria or dilated and tortuous lymphatics. Such early lymph vessel disease appears to be irreversible, even with antifilarial therapy. With the recent availability of more sensitive imaging techniques in endemic areas, isolated lymph node enlargement without pain or inflammation has become an increasingly recognized manifestation of bancroftian filariasis in children.

The most common symptomatic presentation of lymphatic filariasis in children is acute filarial adenolymphangitis, characterized by high fever, lymphatic inflammation (lymphangitis and lymphadenitis), and transient local edema. Most episodes last between 3 and 7 days and may recur. The lymphangitis is retrograde, extending peripherally from the lymph node draining the area where the adult parasites reside, a finding that helps to distinguish filarial from bacterial lymphangitis. The upper and lower extremities are most commonly involved with both bancroftian and brugian filariasis. Regional lymph nodes are often enlarged, and the entire lymphatic channel can become indurated and inflamed. In brugian filariasis, a single local abscess may form along the involved lymphatic tract and subsequently rupture to the surface.

Persistent infection and recurrent inflammation lead to dilatation and obstruction of lymphatics, resulting in lymphedema or, in the worst cases, elephantiasis (Fig. 323-1). Bacterial and/or fungal superinfection of these poorly vascularized tissues eventually becomes a significant problem. Hydroceles and chyluria result from obstruction of genital lymphatics exclusively with bancroftian filariasis. Chyluria, when it occurs, is characteristically intermittent. Adenolymphangitis with eosinophilia can occur in travelers to endemic regions early in infection. This presumed inflammatory response to developing filarial larvae can resolve with departure from the endemic area; long-term sequelae in travelers are rare.

Tropical pulmonary eosinophilia occurs in an extremely small percentage of individuals infected with filarial parasites. The syndrome consists of cough and wheezing, diffuse lung infiltrates on chest radiograph, and restrictive (with or without obstructive) defects on pulmonary function testing. Extremely high levels of blood eosinophils (> 3000/μL), serum immunoglobulin (Ig) E, and antifilarial IgG are thought to reflect an immunologic hyperresponsiveness to the parasite. Circulating microfilariae are almost never detected in these individuals. Repeated episodes of tropical pulmonary eosinophilia or inadequate treatment can result in chronic interstitial (and irreversible) lung disease.

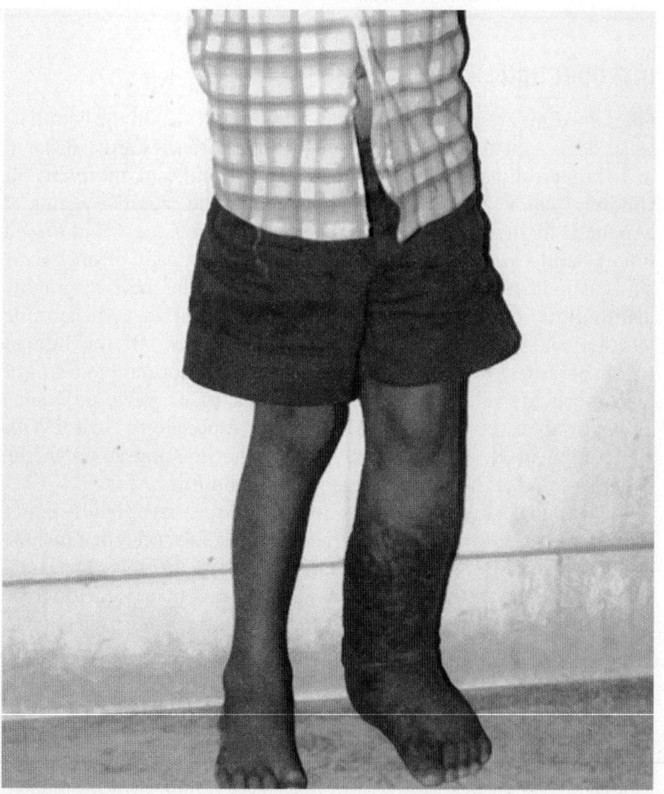

**FIGURE 323-1** Lymphedema and early elephantiasis in a preadolescent.

**FIGURE 323-2** Papular eruption as a consequence of onchocerciasis. (Reproduced with permission from Fauci AS, Braunwald E, Kasper DL, et al: *Harrison's Principles of Internal Medicine*, 17th ed. New York: McGraw-Hill; 2008.)

**Onchocerciasis**

Skin and eye disease are the most common manifestations of onchocerciasis; both may occur in childhood in areas of high transmission. Adult worms in subcutaneous fibrous capsules can be palpated as nodules (onchocercomas), particularly over bony prominences. Microfilariae in the skin induce inflammation that manifests as intense pruritus and papular dermatitis (Fig. 323-2). With long-standing cutaneous inflammation, lichenification, depigmentation ("leopard skin"), and eventual skin atrophy with loss of elastic fibers can occur (Fig. 323-3). Ocular pathology, the most serious consequence of infection, is related to intensity of infection. Lesions may develop in all parts of the eye. The most common early finding is conjunctivitis with photophobia. In the cornea, punctate keratitis—consisting of acute inflammatory reactions surrounding dying microfilariae manifested as "snowflake" opacities—is frequent in younger patients and resolves without apparent complications. Sclerosing keratitis is the leading cause of onchocercal blindness. Anterior uveitis and iridocyclitis occur in up to 5% of infected patients. Complications of the anterior uveal tract (pupillary deformity) may cause secondary glaucoma. Although much rarer than anterior chamber disease, posterior eye disease, including chorioretinitis, chorioretinal atrophy, and optic nerve involvement can lead to constriction of the visual field and eventual blindness.

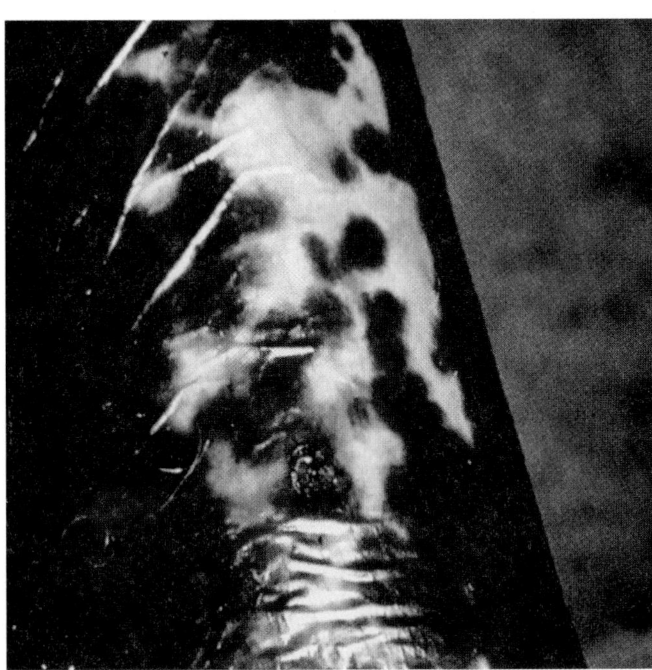

**FIGURE 323-3** Onchocerciasis. Leopard-skin appearance from long-standing infection. (Reproduced with permission from Wolff K, Goldsmith LA, Katz SI, et al: *Fitzpatrick's Dermatology in General Medicine*, 7th ed. New York: McGraw-Hill; 2008.)

## DIAGNOSIS

**Lymphatic Filariasis**

Definitive diagnosis depends on direct identification of parasites. Adult worms can be identified on biopsy or by high-frequency Doppler ultrasound, where the "filarial dance sign" provides sonographic evidence of live adult worms in the inguinal lymph nodes, scrotum, or breast (bancroftian filariasis), or in superficial lymphatic vessels of axilla and proximal extremities (brugian filariasis). Microfilariae are found in the blood almost exclusively between 10:00 PM and 4:00 AM, times that coincide with the nocturnal biting habits of the arthropod vector, except in some areas of the South Pacific where subperiodic forms are common (Fig. 323-4). Filaria-specific antibody testing is highly sensitive but has suffered from cross-reactivity among the filarial species. More recently, 96% to 100% sensitivity and specificity has been demonstrated with a *B malayi* recombinant antigen that detects species-specific IgG4 in an enzyme-linked immunosorbent assay (ELISA)-based assay. For bancroftian filariasis, detection of circulating parasite antigen (ELISA or rapid immunochromatographic testing) is highly sensitive (> 98%) and specific (> 99%), and antigen detection has largely supplanted microscopy because the antigen can be detected in whole blood or serum drawn at any time of the day. Polymerase chain reaction (PCR) detection of filarial DNA in whole blood remains largely a research technique. In children with suspected or proven filariasis, $^{99}$Tc-lymphoscintigraphy is useful in defining the nature and extent of lymphatic damage or dysfunction and in distinguishing lymphedema from other causes of swelling.

Elevated total serum IgE, absolute eosinophil counts, and antifilarial antibodies provide strong supportive evidence for the diagnosis of lymphatic filariasis, but they are commonly elevated in many parasitic infections and therefore must be considered in conjunction with more specific tests. With the extreme IgE elevations seen in tropical

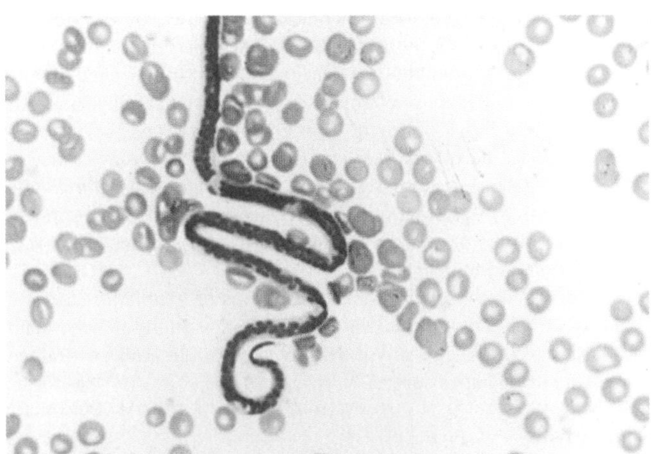

**FIGURE 323-4** Filariasis. Blood film. *Wuchereria bancrofti*. Microfilariae enter the blood about 6 months after infection. (Reproduced with permission from Lichtman MA, Schafer JA, Felgar RE, et al: *Lichtman's Atlas of Hematology*. New York: McGraw-Hill; 2007.)

pulmonary eosinophilia, not only should a chest radiograph and pulmonary function testing results be obtained for help in diagnosis, but also other causes of elevated IgE and eosinophils in children (eg, visceral larva migrans, strongyloidiasis, allergic bronchopulmonary aspergillosis) must be excluded.

### Onchocerciasis

Microfilariae can be recovered from skin snips of the epidermis obtained as superficial (1-mm) skin slices using a scalpel or a corneoscleral punch biopsy. Six skin snips (typically bilaterally from the iliac crests, scapulae, and lower extremities) are recommended for maximal diagnostic yield. When incubated in saline or culture medium, microfilariae may be seen emerging from these snips under low-power microscopy. Microfilariae may also be identified in the anterior chamber of the eye on slit-lamp examination. Adult worms can be identified in excised nodules. Highly sensitive and specific assays to detect *Onchocerca*-specific antibodies in serum and *O volvulus* DNA in skin snips are only available from specialized laboratories.

## TREATMENT

### Lymphatic Filariasis

Diethylcarbamazine (DEC, available from the Centers for Disease Control and Prevention) has both macrofilaricidal and microfilaricidal properties and remains the treatment of choice for the individual with active lymphatic filariasis (microfilaremia, antigen positivity, or adult worms on ultrasound). DEC can be given orally at a dose of 6 mg/kg/d in 3 divided doses for 12 days or 6 mg/kg/d as a single dose. Adverse reactions, typically lasting 24 to 48 hours, may be seen after treatment and consist of fever, chills, myalgia, arthralgia, headache, nausea, and vomiting. These reactions likely reflect immune response to antigens released by dead or dying parasites, and their intensity is directly related to the number of microfilariae circulating in the bloodstream. Treatment of lymphatic filariasis in areas co-endemic for onchocerciasis is complicated by the development of the "Mazzotti" reaction, which can occur within 7 days of initiation of therapy with DEC. This hypersensitivity response to onchocercal antigens following DEC exposure can produce symptoms including fever, tachycardia, hypotension, urticaria, swollen and tender lymph nodes, edema, and abdominal pain. There may also be worsening of ocular inflammation and potentially even death.

As an alternative to DEC, albendazole (400 mg twice a day for 10–21 days) has macrofilaricidal efficacy but no microfilaricidal activity and therefore does not immediately lower blood microfilarial counts. Conversely, the microfilaricidal agent ivermectin (given in a single annual dose of 200–400 μg/kg) achieves sustained suppression of microfilaremia but has no activity against adult worms and is not recommended as monotherapy. Regimens that emphasize combinations of single doses of albendazole and DEC or albendazole and ivermectin have demonstrated sustained microfilaricidal effects. Whether these combinations offer increased efficacy over single-agent therapies in children remains unclear. Interestingly, 6 weeks of daily doxycycline (200 mg/d)—a regimen that targets an intracellular, rickettsiae-like *Wolbachia* endosymbiont—or a 7-day course of DEC/albendazole has both significant macrofilaricidal activity and sustained microfilaricidal activity. Utilization of this regimen in children is limited due to the potential toxicity of prolonged doxycycline administration.

In individuals with chronic manifestations of lymphatic filariasis, treatment regimens emphasize hygiene, prevention of secondary bacterial infections, and physiotherapy. Hydroceles can be drained repeatedly or managed surgically.

### Onchocerciasis

The main goals of therapy are to prevent irreversible lesions (particularly blindness) and to alleviate symptoms. Ivermectin (150 μg/kg given once) is microfilaricidal and is first-line therapy for treatment of onchocerciasis. Ivermectin is given either annually or more often up to 4 times a year, depending on clinical response. Treatment is complicated by pruritus, cutaneous edema, and/or maculopapular rash in 1% to 10% of cases. In areas co-endemic for *O volvulus* and *L loa*, fatal encephalopathy has occurred rarely in individuals with high levels of *L loa* microfilaremia, although few of these reports have involved children. A 6-week course of doxycycline has been demonstrated to be macrofilaristatic (rendering the female adult worms sterile) by targeting the rickettsia-like *Wolbachia* endosymbiont of the filarial parasite. The use of this regimen in children, however, is limited by potential for toxicity as noted earlier.

## PREVENTION

Vaccine development for lymphatic filariasis is still in its infancy. Single-dose combinations of albendazole with either DEC or ivermectin are now being used by filariasis control programs in many countries for annual communitywide treatment with the goal of interrupting transmission of infective larvae. Communitywide treatment strategies are complicated by risk of the Mazzotti reaction (described earlier) in areas co-endemic for lymphatic filariasis and onchocerciasis. Preventive measures also focus on avoidance of exposure to arthropod vectors through combinations of protective clothing and shelter, chemically impregnated bed nets, activity modification, and vector control strategies.

Community-based administration of ivermectin every 6 to 12 months is now being used to interrupt *O volvulus* transmission in endemic areas. This strategy is complicated in *L loa*–endemic areas due to the development of encephalopathy following treatment with ivermectin in persons with high-level *L loa* microfilaremia. Ivermectin administration, in conjunction with vector control, has helped to reduce the prevalence of disease in endemic foci in Africa. In Latin America, this strategy has led to elimination of disease transmission from several endemic foci.

## SUGGESTED READINGS


American Academy of Pediatrics Committee on Infectious Diseases. Lymphatic filariasis. In: *Red Book: 2015 Report of the Committee on Infectious Diseases*. 30th ed. Elk Grove Village, IL: American Academy of Pediatrics; 2015:525-527.

American Academy of Pediatrics Committee on Infectious Diseases. Onchocerciasis. In: *Red Book: 2015 Report of the Committee on Infectious Diseases*. 30th ed. Elk Grove Village, IL: American Academy of Pediatrics; 2015:575-576.

Diaz JH. Ocular filariasis in US residents, returning travelers, and expatriates. *J La State Med Soc*. 2015;167:172-176.

Gayen P, Nayak A, Saini P, et al. A double-blind controlled field trial of doxycycline and albendazole in combination for the treatment of bancroftian filariasis in India. *Acta Trop*. 2013;125:150-156.

Haldaar D, Ghosh D, Mandal D, et al. Is the coverage of mass-drug administration adequate for elimination of Bancroftian filariasis? An experience from West Bengal, India. *Trop Parasitol*. 2015;5:42-49.

Kazura JW. More progress in eliminating transmission of *Onchocerca volvulus* and *Wuchereria bancrofti* in the Americas: a portent of global eradication. *Am J Trop Med Hyg*. 2015;93:1128-1129.

Moya L, Herrador Z, Ta-Tang TH, et al. Evidence for suppression of onchocerciasis transmission in Bioko island, Equatorial Guinea. *PLoS Negl Trop Dis*. 2016;10:e0004829.

Richards F Jr, Rizzo N, Espinoza C, et al. One hundred years after its discovery in Guatemala by Rodolfo Robles, *Onchocerca volvulus* transmission has been eliminated from the central endemic zone. *Am J Trop Med Hyg*. 2015;93:1295-1304.

Walker M, Specht S, Churcher TS, et al. Therapeutic efficacy and macrofilaricidal activity of doxycycline for the treatment of river blindness. *Clin Infect Dis*. 2015;60:1199-1207.

Weil WJ, Curtis KC, Fakoli L, et al. Laboratory and field evaluation of a new rapid test for detecting *Wuchereria bancrofti* antigen in human blood. *Am J Trop Med Hyg*. 2013;89:11-15.

# 324 Hookworm

Christopher Prestel and Rana Chakraborty

## INTRODUCTION

Hookworms are one of the most important neglected tropical diseases globally due to the high human disease burden and the fact that this pathogen is the leading cause of anemia in Africa and Oceania.

## PATHOGENESIS AND EPIDEMIOLOGY

The hookworm life cycle begins with the excretion of fertilized eggs within the feces of an infected individual. The eggs hatch to release first-stage (L1) larvae, which undergo 2 subsequent molts to the infective third stage (L3). These L3 hookworm larvae migrate along moisture and temperature gradients within the soil until they encounter a permissive host. When larvae contact the skin, they quickly penetrate the epidermis and dermis, ultimately invading small blood vessels and entering the venous circulation. They are then carried passively to the heart and lungs, where they lodge in the pulmonary capillaries and break through to the alveolar space. Larvae then migrate up the respiratory tree, are swallowed, and undergo their final developmental molts to the adult stage when they reach the small intestine. Once in the proximal small bowel, the adult worms attach to the mucosal surface and begin to feed (Figs. 324-1 and 324-2). Adult hookworms secrete anticoagulants, platelet inhibitors, and hemoglobin-degrading proteases that facilitate blood feeding and digestion of red blood cells. When the plug of intestinal mucosa at the site of attachment has been digested, the worm releases and reattaches at a new site. Male and female worms mate, and the female releases 10,000 to 30,000 eggs per day into the intestinal lumen. It takes approximately 6 weeks for eggs to appear in the feces of an infected individual.

Two important features of the life cycle distinguish *Ancylostoma* hookworms from *Necator*. First, *Ancylostoma duodenale* can cause infection when ingested, whereas *Necator americanus* can only complete its life cycle in humans following skin penetration. Second, there is epidemiologic evidence to suggest that third-stage larvae of *A duodenale* may arrest within various tissues of their host, ultimately resuming development and completing their life cycle months to years later. Reports of severe disease manifestations in young infants raise the possibility that *A duodenale* may also be transmissible through breast milk.

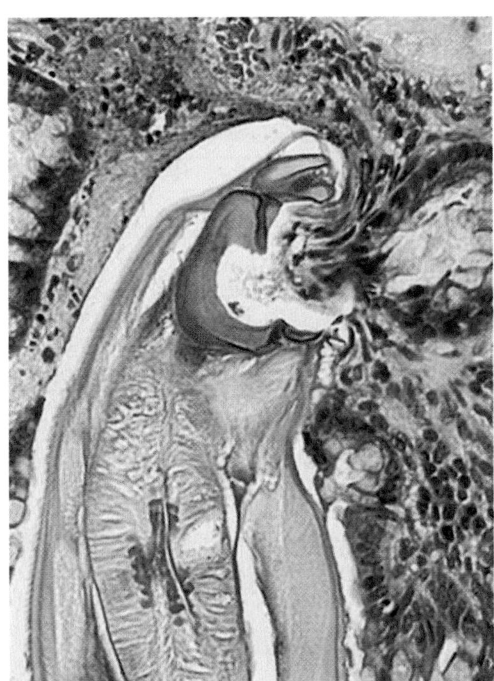

**FIGURE 324-1** Photomicrograph of an adult hookworm attached to the intestine. Note area of hemorrhage adjacent to site of attachment. (Used with permission from R. Bungiro.)

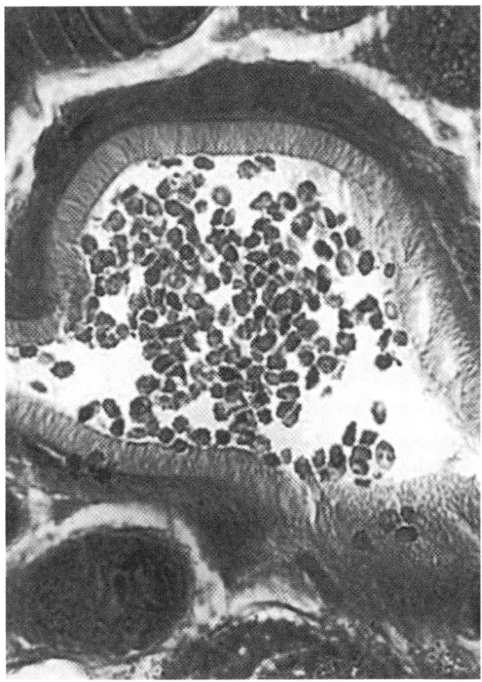

**FIGURE 324-2** Cross-section of adult hookworm showing host red blood cells in the intestine. (Used with permission from R. Bungiro.)

Hookworm infection remains a major health burden in developing countries. In 2010, it was estimated that 438.9 million people globally were infected with hookworms, leading to 3,230,800 years lived with disability. Infections with *A duodenale* occur in focal regions of Africa, Asia, and South America, whereas *N americanus* is the predominant hookworm worldwide, with the greatest number of infections in North and South America, equatorial Africa, much of Southeast Asia, and some Pacific islands. There is significant overlap in the geographic pattern of infection, and mixed infections occur frequently. Although common in southern states in the early part of the 20th century, today there is little evidence of hookworm transmission in the United States. Other species that occasionally cause intestinal disease in humans include *Ancylostoma ceylanicum*, found in India and Southeast Asia, and the dog hookworm *Ancylostoma caninum*, which has been associated with eosinophilic enteritis in Australia. Zoonotic infection with *Ancylostoma braziliense* causes cutaneous larva migrans.

Populations at highest risk for significant disease sequelae include preschool and school-age children, adolescents, and women of childbearing age. Adults who work in agricultural occupations are also at risk for high-intensity infection. Vulnerable populations such as young children and pregnant or lactating women are at greater risk of anemia due to relatively high iron requirements. Unlike *Ascaris lumbricoides* and *Trichuris trichiura*, the intensity of hookworm infection appears to increase with age, defining the elderly as another high-risk group for severe disease.

## CLINICAL MANIFESTATIONS

As third-stage larvae penetrate the skin, a local urticarial eruption, known as ground itch, may occur. Although hookworms frequently penetrate the soles of the feet, it is important to recognize that the parasite can invade any exposed skin surface. The pulmonary migration of hookworms is rarely associated with significant clinical symptoms, although cough and wheezing may develop following infection with a large inoculum. Of note, the pulmonary phase is associated with the development of peripheral eosinophilia and precedes the appearance of eggs in the feces.

The clinically significant manifestations of hookworm infection are primarily attributable to loss of blood and serum proteins that are a consequence of feeding by the adult worm. In light infections, subclinical iron deficiency can also develop if daily iron intake cannot compensate for iron lost through intestinal bleeding. In chronic infections, significant iron deficiency leads to a microcytic, hypochromic anemia. Particularly heavy infections may also manifest as severe protein malnutrition, as the worm drains serum proteins in addition to red blood cells as it feeds. Rarely, high-output heart failure develops as a consequence of chronic, severe hookworm anemia. Importantly, even children with mild infections may suffer impairment of physical and intellectual development, particularly when they also harbor other intestinal nematodes.

Intestinal infection with the dog hookworm *A caninum* is associated with eosinophilic enteritis, an unusual syndrome characterized by abdominal pain, tenderness, and gastrointestinal bleeding. Results of biopsies of the small bowel routinely show massive eosinophilic infiltrates, and occasionally, a single adult canine hookworm has been identified attached to the mucosa. However, there is frequently no direct evidence of hookworm infection in patients with eosinophilic enteritis.

## DIAGNOSIS

The definitive diagnosis of hookworm infection is made by finding characteristic ova in the feces. These thin-shelled, ovoid eggs with granular-appearing contents measure 40 by 60 μm and are generally in the 2- to 4-cell stage when passed in feces. It is important to recognize that many children from the developing world who are infected with hookworm frequently harbor other intestinal nematodes as well, including *A lumbricoides* and *T trichiura*, which are also associated with anemia and malnutrition. Because hookworm egg excretion can be intermittent, multiple stool examinations may be required to confirm the diagnosis. Routine microscopy cannot differentiate between the eggs of *A duodenale* and *N americanus*, although polymerase chain reaction methods have been developed for research purposes. The differentiation between species is not necessary with regard to treatment options. In addition, there are no routinely used serum antibodies or fecal antigen tests for diagnosing hookworm infection. Evaluation for possible hookworm infection is warranted in any traveler, immigrant, or refugee from an endemic area who presents with iron deficiency anemia and/or peripheral blood eosinophilia. It is important to note that the degree of eosinophilia may vary and in light infections is often mild.

## TREATMENT

The treatment of choice for the eradication of intestinal hookworms is a single oral dose of 1 of the benzimidazole anthelmintics, albendazole (400 mg) or mebendazole (500 mg). Mebendazole may also be used as a 100-mg dose orally twice a day for 3 days. Pyrantel pamoate (11 mg/kg/d, maximum of 1 g, for 3 days) is an effective alternative. Nitazoxanide, which has activity against hookworm, is approved for use in children, but not specifically for this indication, and should not be considered a first-line treatment. Additionally, iron supplementation can be considered if anemia is present. Children treated for hookworm frequently experience significant short-term catch-up growth, and studies show short-term improvement in a number of developmental parameters following therapy. Unfortunately, in endemic areas, reinfection with hookworms occurs rapidly, and the benefits of intermittent chemotherapy may be short-lived.

## PREVENTION

Prevention of hookworm infection can be obtained by sanitary disposal of feces and health education. Proper footwear has also helped prevent soil-transmitted helminth infections. Improvements in economic development and reduction of poverty are the most substantial influences on the decreases in helminth infections. School-based deworming programs have offered many benefits to high-risk populations including improved school attendance, school results, and productivity. However, the prevalence and intensity of hookworm infection can return to pretreatment levels in as little as 1 to 2 years. In 2012, the World Health Organization (WHO) urged countries to control schistosomiasis and soil-transmitted helminthiases—including ascariasis, trichuriasis, and hookworm infection. The goal for 2020 is to provide regular treatment to 75% of at-risk preschool and school-aged children in all countries where the WHO operates.

Decreasing efficacy of benzimidazoles in some highly endemic areas has raised concerns about the emergence of hookworm resistance to benzimidazole anthelmintics. Infection with a given hookworm does not confer immunity and allows for repeat infection. For this reason, there has been renewed interest in the development of vaccines and novel chemotherapeutic agents to control hookworm worldwide. Including anthelmintics as part of integrated control programs targeting multiple tropical diseases may confer benefit at both the individual and population levels, including those with coinfections such as human immunodeficiency virus, malaria, and tuberculosis. Clinical trials of recombinant vaccines designed to prevent or ameliorate the clinical sequelae of hookworm infection are currently in progress.

## SUGGESTED READINGS


American Academy of Pediatrics Committee on Infectious Diseases. Hookworm infections. In: *Red Book: 2015 Report of the Committee on Infectious Diseases*. 30th ed. Elk Grove Village, IL: American Academy of Pediatrics; 2015:448-449.

Hotez PJ, Beaumier CM, Gillespie PM, Hayward T, Bottazzi ME. Advancing a vaccine to prevent hookworm disease and anemia. *Vaccine*. 2016;34:3001-3005.

Pullan RL, Smith JL, Jasrasaria R, Brooker SJ. Global numbers of infection and disease burden of soil transmitted helminth infections in 2010. *Parasit Vectors*. 2014;7:37.

Savioli L, Daumerie D, World Health Organization, Department of Control of Neglected Tropical Diseases. 2012 Accelerating work to overcome the global impact of neglected tropical diseases: a roadmap for implementation. www.who.int/neglected_diseases/resources/WHO_HTM_NTD_2012.1/en/. Accessed August 8, 2016.

Smith JL, Brooker S. Impact of hookworm infection and deworming on anaemia in non-pregnant populations: a systematic review. *Trop Med Int Health*. 2010;15:776-795.

Weatherhead JE, Hotez PJ. Worm infections in children. *Pediatr Rev*. 2015;36:341-352.


# 325 Strongyloidiasis

Michael J. Muszynski

## INTRODUCTION

In 1876, a nematode was observed during microscopic examination of stool from a number of French soldiers suffering from severe diarrhea while stationed in French colonial Vietnam. The condition was known as Cochin-China diarrhea, named after the southern region of today's Vietnam. Within 12 years, the etiologic agent and its complex life cycle were defined. The diagnosis of strongyloidiasis can be challenging, and it is frequently overlooked. Adding to the challenging diagnosis is the fact that a large proportion of cases are asymptomatic. The scenario of missed infection leading to chronicity is common in immunocompetent children, and devastating, life-threatening infection can occur in the immunocompromised host. The World Health Organization has recognized the importance of strongyloidiasis by placing it on its official list of neglected diseases.

## PATHOGENESIS AND EPIDEMIOLOGY

Strongyloidiasis is a generally chronic infectious disease caused by the intestinal nematode, *Strongyloides stercoralis*. The phases of development of *Strongyloides* are distinctive and complex. Beginning at the point of human infection, filariform larvae penetrate exposed skin

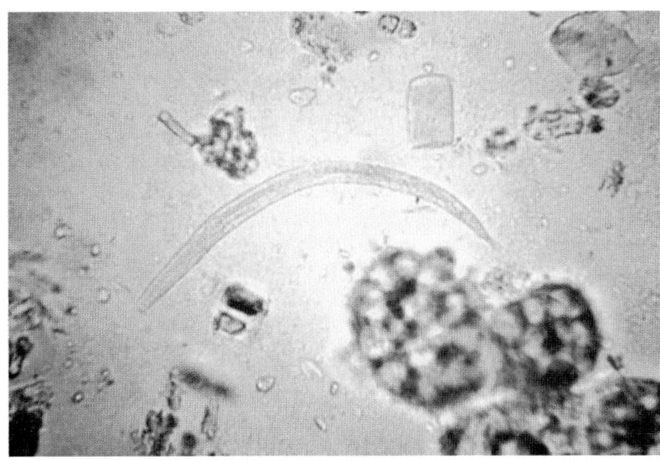

**FIGURE 325-1** Micrograph showing noninfective rhabditiform larva of *Strongyloides stercoralis* in stool specimen with characteristic primordial genital oral, short buccal cavity, and blunter tail. (Reproduced with permission from Centers for Disease Control Public Health Image Library [PHIL].)

using a lytic protease mechanism. They subsequently gain access to the bloodstream by way of lymphatics and venules at their point of entry. Next the larvae are transported by the intravascular circulation to the lungs and break through alveolar walls in order to travel up the trachea to the pharynx where they are swallowed to enter the small bowel. There the larvae mature into adult worms. After successfully mating, the adult female deposits eggs into the intestinal mucosa. In this way, *Strongyloides* is unique among helminths because its eggs are not meant to be secreted in stool. During confinement in the mucosa, eggs develop into noninfective rhabditiform larvae (Fig. 325-1). These larvae then take 2 possible paths. They are either excreted from the body in the stool, or they transform into filariform larvae in the intestine (Fig. 325-2). In this way, any larvae becoming filariform within the gut are infectious to the host and can penetrate the intestine, reenter the blood circulation, and go to the lungs just like the initial infecting larvae. This is called the autoinfection portion of the cycle. Such multiplication in the host is also exclusive among nematodes to *Strongyloides*. The cycle external to the host begins with the rhabditiform larvae that were excreted in the stool into moist soil. From there, this external cycle splits into 2 directions: transformation of rhabditiform larvae into the infective filariform larvae to infect the next human, as described earlier, or maturation of the filariform larvae into free-living adult male and

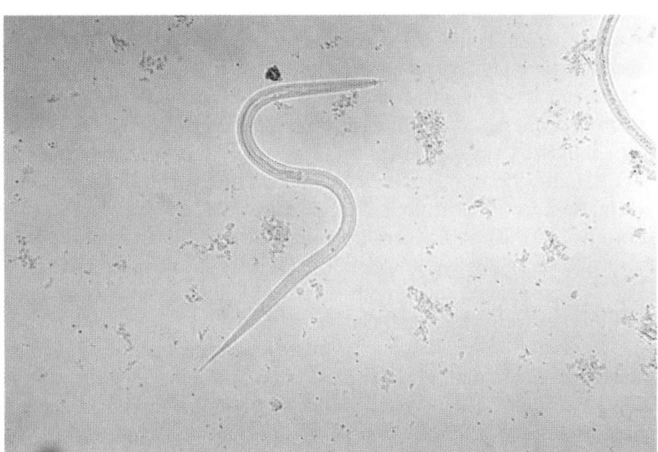

**FIGURE 325-2** Micrograph of infective filariform larva of *Strongyloides stercoralis* in stool specimen demonstrating a longer buccal cavity and total length than rhabditiform larva and a pointed tail. (Reproduced with permission from Centers for Disease Control Public Health Image Library [PHIL]. Photo contributor: Mae Melvin.)

female worms in the soil that mate. Fertilized eggs are laid in the soil, where they eventually hatch as new rhabditiform larvae that, in turn, mature into infective filariform larvae that will await the next human skin contact, and on it goes (Fig. 325-3). The 2 life cycles of *Strongyloides* within the host then predict the potential clinical presentations.

Understanding the life cycles of *S stercoralis* leads to the appreciation of where and how it is acquired and of the conditions it causes. The most common and epidemiologically important point of human contact begins with infectious *S stercoralis* filariform larvae living in warm, moist soil contaminated by human waste. The coexistence of human waste and moist soil in temperate locales explains much of the organism's epidemiology. *Strongyloides* has highest prevalence in the tropics and subtropics, especially in Southeast Asia. Although this organism has a worldwide distribution, it is endemic and on the rise in many parts of the globe, including the Caribbean, Latin America, South America (Columbia, Brazil, and Peruvian Amazon), sub-Saharan Africa, the South Pacific, tropical locales in Australia, and temperate areas of eastern and central Europe and even parts of Spain. The organism is also found in warm regions of many other countries, including the United States, particularly in Appalachia. However, infection acquired within the United States is relatively rare. Imported disease is generally the rule for cases diagnosed in North America. Upwards of 100 to 200 million or more people are infected in 70 countries, and its prevalence is highly underestimated.

*Strongyloides* infection prevalence in refugee populations in the United States is said to be 1% to 4.3% overall, but much higher percentages are seen in groups of immigrants from highly endemic areas such as Vietnam (11.8%), Cambodia (76%), the Sudan (46%), and Somalia (23%). In a 2005 longitudinal analysis, 38% of Southeast Asian immigrants residing in Washington, DC, harbored *Strongyloides*. The infection rate among North Americans traveling abroad is extremely low, even if that travel is to high-prevalence areas, unless there is a history of intimate skin contact with soil.

*Strongyloides* is found particularly in the midst of poverty, in rural and agricultural settings, and even in coal mining. Walking with bare feet on moist soil or any skin contact with soil is central to the organism's life cycle. It should not be surprising that taken worldwide, children compose the largest age group for initial infection. Outdoor play and daily activities of these children commonly done on bare feet are surely pivotal factors. An oral route of infection has also been described in institutionalized individuals, and larvae can enter the body through ingestion of food tainted with infected human feces or contaminated soil in nonhygienic farming practices. A direct fecal-oral route is suspected in some epidemiologic studies, but evidence supporting transmission in household settings is lacking.

## CLINICAL MANIFESTATIONS

Many cases of strongyloidiasis are asymptomatic or have nonspecific findings. Conversely, most infections acquired in the United States are symptomatic and relapsing in nature. In some individuals, infection can be chronic and last for years, giving much explanation as to why the condition is greatly underreported and the prevalence is uncertain. The fact that infection can last for decades was demonstrated in World War II American soldiers who were held as prisoners of war by Japan. Many had documented infection over 3 decades or more after imprisonment. The longest described asymptomatic infection was over 65 years.

As noted, one can predict the symptoms of strongyloidiasis with a good understanding of its life cycles in the host. Thus, dermatologic, pulmonary, and gastrointestinal findings would be expected. The initial presentation of symptomatic patients with normal immune systems often includes vague gastrointestinal symptoms, including nonspecific abdominal pain, cramping, anorexia, indigestion, bloating, diarrhea, nausea, vomiting, and weight loss. Presentations of watery, mucoid diarrhea interchanging with constipation have also been described. Any given patient may have any combination of these symptoms that may then be followed by nonproductive cough with or without wheezing, which occurs in 10% of cases. A pneumonitis much like Löffler syndrome may cause the patient to seek medical attention.

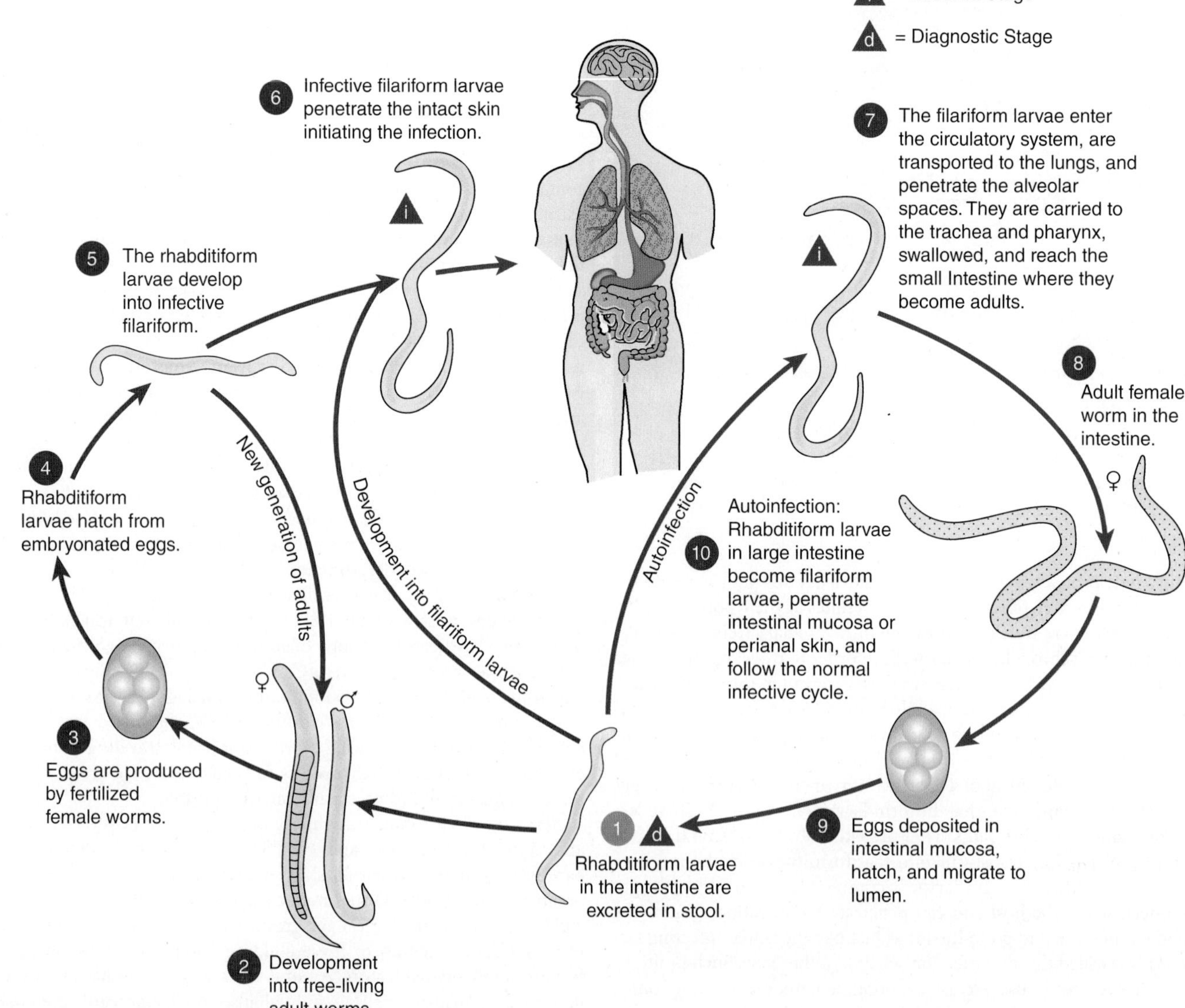


**FIGURE 325-3** Description of the unique and complex life cycles of *Strongyloides stercoralis*. (Reproduced with permission from Centers for Disease Control Public Health Image Library [PHIL].)

Since the organism has reached the gastrointestinal tract, and infectious filariform larvae develop in the bowel, pruritus ani is common. In turn, a larva currens rash can be perianal, on the buttocks, and on the thighs. Larva currens is the only pathognomonic finding for strongyloidiasis, being initially found on the areas that contacted infected soil, especially the feet. Larva currens is an irritatingly pruritic, urticarial rash that occurs in bands that stealthily move in rapid fashion up the body. Its movements have been clocked at 5 to 15 cm/h, hence the name larva currens, which means "racing larva." This rash and its symptoms may also be the only findings in normal hosts suffering from long-term autoinfection.

The autoinfection cycle of *Strongyloides* can result in a dramatic burden of worms in any host. This can be devastating in the immunocompromised patient, resulting in severe hyperinfection syndrome, which involves the same systems as described in normal hosts but with more severe and dramatic presentations. The huge burden of larvae results in penetration into major organs, including lungs, bowel, liver, kidneys, heart, and central nervous system, with the lungs and bowel being the most common sites for severe, high larvae burden disease. The mortality rate for severe disease is 60% to 85%. Basically, any condition with impaired cellular immunity puts an individual with *Strongyloides* infection at risk for this syndrome. A terribly important risk factor is corticosteroid therapy prescribed for any indication. Steroid immune inhibition leads to a prodigious increase in parasite load with impressively vast dissemination to organs. Immunomodulating therapies, including steroid therapy, that lower T-cell immunity are described as the most important risk factors for severe disease. These include chemotherapy, tumor necrosis factor inhibitors, and tacrolimus. Thus, transplant patients are also at increased risk for hyperinfection and severe disease.

*Strongyloides* has an interesting association with human T-cell leukemia virus type 1 (HTLV-1) often with serious consequences. HTLV-1 infection greatly increases the chance of *Strongyloides* dissemination. In turn, the preleukemic phase of HTLV-1 is significantly shortened by the parasite. *Strongyloides* antigen has been hypothesized to set off an aggressive polyclonal T-cell response and activation of HTLV-1 expression and progression to T-cell leukemia. Thus, each condition exacerbates the other.

Other conditions predisposing to severe hyperinfection syndrome include hypogammaglobulinemia, human immunodeficiency virus (HIV) infection, malignancies (particularly lymphoma and leukemia), autoimmune diseases, malabsorption and malnutrition, diabetes mellitus, chronic renal disease, and end-stage renal disease states.

## DIAGNOSIS

It cannot be overemphasized that one must have a heightened index of suspicion to diagnose *Strongyloides* infection. At issue is the frequent nonspecific nature of symptoms and findings and the significant

**TABLE 325-1 THE MANY CLINICAL PRESENTATIONS IN WHICH STRONGYLOIDIASIS SHOULD BE CONSIDERED**

| Patient with Normal Immune System | Immunocompromised Patient |
|---|---|
| Gastrointestinal: | Gastrointestinal: |
| • Nonspecific abdominal pain | • Severe abdominal pain |
| • Epigastric cramping, bloating | • Nausea/vomiting |
| • Chronic diarrhea (watery with mucus) | • Bloody stools |
| • Nausea/vomiting | • Bloody diarrhea |
| • Alternating diarrhea and constipation | • Serious GI bleeding, including massive bleeds |
| • Failure to thrive, unexplained ongoing weight loss | • Ileus |
| • Unexplained GI malabsorption | • GI obstruction |
| • Celiac disease presentation | |
| Pulmonary: | Pulmonary: |
| • Unexplained mild cough | • Severe respiratory distress, dyspnea, |
| • Wheezing mimicking asthma | • Moderate to severe cough |
| • Any unexplained pneumonia | • Wheezing mimicking acute asthma |
| • Transient, migratory pulmonary infiltrates | • Hemoptysis |
| • Eosinophilic pneumonia (Löffler syndrome) | • Acute respiratory distress syndrome (ARDS) |
| Dermatologic: | Dermatologic: |
| • Pruritus ani | • Petechial and purpuric rashes |
| • Pruritic papulovesicular eruptions (especially on feet) | • Jaundice |
| • Creeping eruptions | |
| • Larva currens (pathognomonic) | |
| Systemic: | Systemic: |
| • Eosinophilia | • Gram-negative enteric bacterial sepsis |
| • Unexplained gram-negative enteric bacteremia | • Polymicrobial sepsis |
| • Systemic lupus erythematosus | • Septic shock |
| | Neurologic: |
| | • Meningitis |
| | • Encephalopathy |
| | • New-onset seizures |
| | • Coma |

number of asymptomatic cases. The only physical finding specific to the disease is larva currens. Consideration of *Strongyloides* is important in a fairly broad number of common clinical presentations in normal patients and in important situations involving compromised hosts (Table 325-1). Thus, *Strongyloides* infection can reasonably be added to the differential diagnosis of a host of chief complaints.

Consideration of strongyloidiasis is most important in patients with a suggestive geographic origin or travel history or a history of walking barefoot in soil or of skin contact with soil in endemic settings. It should be considered in any immigrant, refugee, or adoptee from an area of high prevalence, especially if the presentation includes eosinophilia. Unfortunately, eosinophilia occurs in only 25% of refugees with proven asymptomatic infection, so it is an insensitive screening tool for those individuals. Nonetheless, complete blood count testing with white cell differential is recommended in these groups to look for eosinophilia, since its presence very strongly supports the diagnosis.

Eosinophilia is quite common in symptomatic patients from endemic regions of the globe, occurring in 88% of cases, which increases the test's diagnostic sensitivity in this population. Eosinophilia is relatively mild, with numbers between 500 and 1500 eosinophils/μL of blood, corresponding to about 6% to 15% of the total white cell count. The Committee on Infectious Diseases of the American Academy of Pediatrics recommends that adoptee, immigrant, and refugee children with an absolute eosinophil count > 450 cells/μL be automatically tested for *Strongyloides*, since it is the most common cause of chronic eosinophilia due to infection. Eosinophilia is fairly uncommon in disseminated disease and the severe hyperinfection presentations, appearing in less than 16% of such patients.

Any patients with unexplained eosinophilia and/or an epidemiologic history or symptoms suggestive of *Strongyloides* should be tested for the infection, especially if steroid therapy, immunosuppressive therapies, chemotherapies, or transplantation is under consideration. Infected patients must be successfully treated with "proof of cure" before continuing with immunocompromising treatments. Stool studies, serial serology, and resolution of eosinophilia are suggested markers for cure. Multiple case examples are in the literature describing clinical catastrophe or death from severe *Strongyloides* hyperinfection when untreated patients received steroid therapy for wheezing or presumed asthma or other indications.

In general, simple confirmation of *Strongyloides* infection is most problematic in immunocompetent patients due to low numbers of parasites and variable shedding of larvae in the feces. Less than 25 larvae are present per gram of stool in over two-thirds of cases in individuals with normal immunity. Submitting just 1 stool specimen for analysis will miss 70% of infections. A minimum of 3 separately collected, serial stool specimens are recommended for laboratory testing, employing parasite-concentrating techniques and special staining methods. A study reported in 1987 showed that 7 serial stool specimens improved diagnostic sensitivity to nearly 100%, which unfortunately is impracticable in most cases. The laboratory used should be specifically notified that the stool specimen being sent is for *Strongyloides* testing.

Culture plate methods are also available and are more sensitive than direct stool studies. The stool sample is placed on nutrient agar plates and then incubated for 48 hours. Any motile *S stercoralis* larvae will produce visible tracks on the plate as they carry bacteria in their wakes. Duodenal material can also be obtained for testing using a string test (Entero-Test) or by endoscopy for direct examination and culture.

Reliable serologic tests are available from reference laboratories. Sensitive and specific nested polymerase chain reaction methods are in development. Serologic testing for *Strongyloides* is always recommended in the investigation of chronic eosinophilia, in the evaluation of even mild eosinophilia in refugees, immigrants, and international adoptees from endemic areas, and in any individual with suggestive symptoms. Serologic tests can be negative in immunocompromised patients presenting with severe hyperinfection.

In severe hyperinfection cases, the diagnosis is approached in the same fashion as that described for immunocompetent children, but more invasive diagnostic methods are often required. Sputum, induced sputum, and/or specimens obtained endoscopically by bronchoalveolar lavage are useful in worrisome pulmonary presentations in severe disease. Microscopic examination of endoscopic duodenal fluid specimens is highly sensitive in hyperinfection due to the large parasite load. Biopsy of bowel mucosa can be diagnostic (Fig. 325-4).

Blood cultures should be obtained in all patients with severe disseminated infection because of the high rate of associated bacterial sepsis. The most common organisms isolated are *Escherichia coli*, *Klebsiella* species, and bowel streptococci. The massive larval invasion into the gut and migration into the bloodstream form a perfect portal of entry for enteric bacteria to disseminate. Bacterial culture of pulmonary specimens is also important since pulmonary superinfection by enteric organisms is common in severe *Strongyloides* infection. Cerebrospinal fluid studies are often indicated, since gram-negative enteric meningitis is a classic finding in disseminated disease and has a very high mortality without early diagnosis and treatment.

## TREATMENT

All cases of *Strongyloides* infection warrant treatment. Ivermectin is clearly the first drug of choice for all forms of strongyloidiasis (asymptomatic infection, symptomatic infection in normal hosts, disseminated disease, severe disease, and disease in immunocompromised hosts). The dosage is 200 μg/kg, orally, given daily for 1 or 2 days for asymptomatic patients and symptomatic immunologically normal

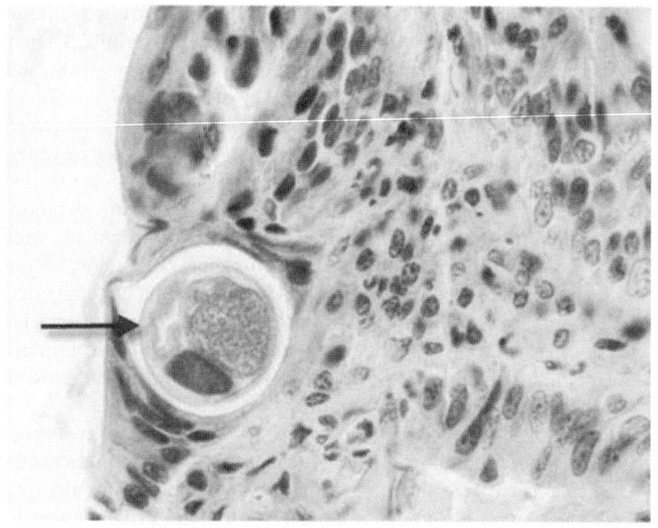

**FIGURE 325-4** Parasitic female *Strongyloides stercoralis* (*red arrow*) on intestinal mucosa biopsy. (Used with permission from Colin Rudolph.)

hosts. Albendazole is an alternative agent given as 400 mg, orally, divided into 2 doses each day for 7 days. Results with albendazole have been variable, and its safety in children less than 6 years of age has not been well established. Limited data suggest it is safe down to 1 year of age.

Severe strongyloidiasis and hyperinfection conditions require longer treatment with ivermectin, usually for 7 to 14 days. Repeat courses of therapy are necessary in cases where the organism has not been completely cleared. Although comparative or definitive efficacy studies are lacking, combination therapy with albendazole and ivermectin has been used in some of the most severe presentations of hyperinfection. In HTLV-1–infected patients, ivermectin therapy has been shown to reverse the progression to the preleukemic and leukemic phases that was induced or amplified by *Strongyloides*.

Patients unable to take oral medication can be treated with intravenous ivermectin, which is available only as a veterinary preparation. Its use must be approved under a single-patient, investigational drug application request to the US Food and Drug Administration.

Expert infectious diseases and tropical medicine specialty consultation is prudent for all patients with severe or complex disease.

## PREVENTION

Prevention measures for strongyloidiasis include avoidance of skin contact with soil in endemic areas, especially bare foot contact. Wearing appropriate footwear greatly decreases infection risk in endemic areas. Appropriate sanitation measures for human waste are the most effective intervention to disrupt the organism's life cycle and thus reduce prevalence. Such methods will additionally prevent a good number of other parasitic, bacterial, and viral diseases related to improper disposing of human waste. Standard precautions—hand hygiene, gowns, gloves, and proper handling of soiled equipment—are recommended for those providing care for infected patients and healthcare providers potentially in contact with patient secretions and bodily fluids.

## SUGGESTED READINGS

Henriquez-Camacho C, Gotuzzo E, Echevarria J, et al. Ivermectin versus albendazole or thiabendazole for *Strongyloides stercoralis* infection. *Cochrane Database Syst Rev*. 2016;1:CD007745.

Luvira V, Watthanakulpanich D, Pittisuttithum P. Management of *Strongyloides stercoralis*: a puzzling parasite. *Int Health*. 2014;6:273-281.

Norsarwany M, Abdelrahman Z, Rahmah N, et al. Symptomatic chronic strongyloidiasis in children following treatment for solid organ malignancies: case reports and literature review. *Trop Biomed*. 2012;3:479-488.

Ostera G, Blum J. Stongyloidiasis: risk and healthcare access for Latin American immigrants living in the United States. *Curr Trop Med Rep*. 2016;3:1-3.

Puthiyakunnon S, Boddu S, Li Y, et al. Strongyloidiasis—an insight into its global prevalence and management. *PLoS Negl Trop Dis*. 2014;8:e3018.

Salvador F, Sulleiro E, Sánchez-Montalvá A, et al. Usefulness of *Strongyloides stercoralis* serology in the management of patients with eosinophilia. *Am J Trop Med Hyg*. 2014;90:830-834.

Takaoka K, Gourtsoyannis Y, Hart JD, et al. Incidence rate and risk factors for giardiasis and strongyloidiasis in returning UK travelers. *J Travel Med*. 2016;5:pii:taw050.

Toledo R, Muñoz-Antoli C, Esteban JG. Strongyloidiasis with emphasis on human infections and its different clinical forms. *Adv Parasitol*. 2015;88:165-241.

# 326 Toxocariasis (Visceral and Ocular Larva Migrans)

Peter J. Hotez

## INTRODUCTION

Toxocariasis is caused by helminth larvae of dogs and cats that ordinarily cannot complete their life cycle in humans (Fig. 326-1). Migrating larvae of zoonotic ascarids may be associated with significant pathology by wandering through extraintestinal viscera, causing tissue necrosis and provoking eosinophilic granulomatous inflammation. The clinical syndromes of visceral larva migrans (VLM), ocular larva migrans (OLM), or covert toxocariasis are most commonly caused by larvae of the dog ascarid *Toxocara canis* and, less frequently, the cat ascarid *Toxocara cati*. Covert toxocariasis refers to infection with either *T canis* or *T cati* that results in either asymptomatic infection or infection associated only with asthma, wheezing, or other pulmonary dysfunctions due to larval lung migrations, or possibly developmental delays due to larval migrations through the brain.

## PATHOGENESIS AND EPIDEMIOLOGY

Adult *Toxocara* live in the dog's small intestine and are 8 to 12 cm long. The ova are deposited with the dog's feces and become infective in approximately 2 weeks. If swallowed by young dogs, second-stage larvae hatch in the small intestine, penetrate the intestinal wall, and migrate through canine tissues where they can undergo arrested development. Some larvae return to the small intestine, where they mature, mate, and oviposit. Arrested larval development more often occurs in female dogs than males, and the dormant larvae in tissues can migrate transplacentally (or possibly enter the mammary tissues) and thereby serve as a source of perinatal and postnatal infection in puppies. In the United States, large numbers of newborn puppies are infected and pose a health risk to those who handle them.

In humans, most VLM cases have been reported in young children 1 to 4 years of age with a history of pica, especially geophagy (defined as the eating of earthy substances). However, OLM is more frequently seen in older children. After a human ingests the embryonated egg, a second-stage larva emerges in the small intestine, penetrates the intestinal wall, and initiates somatic migration that may last for many weeks or months.

The liver and lungs are most often involved with *Toxocara*, the former probably because of the mesenteric venous portal drainage. Tissue granulomas consist of many eosinophils and histiocytes, with an occasional multinucleated foreign body giant cell in an area of necrosis. A portion of a second-stage larva also may be evident. Granulomas can also be found in lung, kidney, lymph node, eyes, brain, heart, and skeletal muscle. OLM results from granulomas in the eye, typically

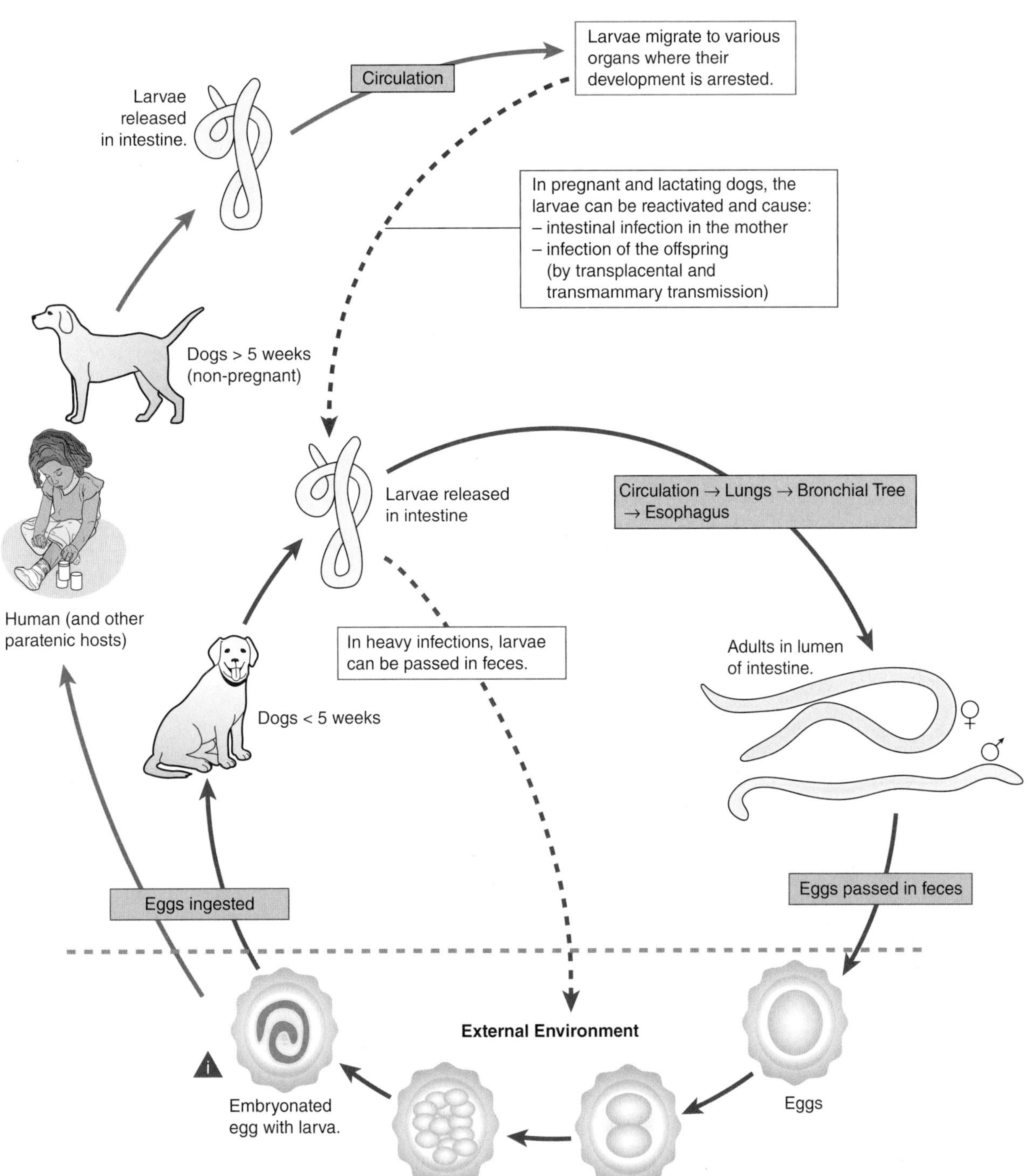


**FIGURE 326-1** The life cycle of *Toxocara canis*.

without evidence of additional visceral involvement. The prevalence of OLM has been estimated to be approximately 1 case per 1000 persons or approximately 1% of people with vision loss.

Toxocariasis is one of the most common human helminth infections in North America and Europe, with the highest occurrence among disadvantaged minority populations. Based on large-scale surveys, the seroprevalence of toxocariasis antibody may exceed 20% among African American and other underrepresented minority children living in poverty in the United States. For that reason, toxocariasis may represent one of the most common parasitic helminth infections in North America. Infection is common in both urban and rural areas, and some studies have linked environmental exposure to *Toxocara* larvae as a contributor to pediatric asthma or developmental delays.

## CLINICAL MANIFESTATIONS

In VLM and covert toxocariasis, clinical presentations vary from eosinophilia discovered by chance in an asymptomatic patient to fever, hepatomegaly, hyperglobulinemia, and marked eosinophilia. Many infections are subclinical. Some children have pulmonary symptoms (notably wheezing and rhonchi), signs of myocarditis, cutaneous nodules, or urticaria. Some children exhibit central nervous system disease, manifested as either cerebritis or epilepsy, a result of larvae migrating through the brain. The acute phase may last 2 to 3 weeks, and in some cases, the resolution of eosinophilia and clinical symptoms may take as long as 18 months. OLM is more common among older children (school-aged and adolescents). The most dramatic symptoms are due to retinal pathology and include visual changes, strabismus, and retinal detachment. Covert toxocariasis may present in children as wheezing or asthma, often with eosinophilia, or developmental delays, without evidence of additional visceral involvement. The burden of disease from asthma or developmental delays in the United States or globally that might be attributed to toxocariasis is unknown, although it is potentially an important avenue for future study.



## DIAGNOSIS

Because *Toxocara* larvae cannot complete their life cycle in order to become adult intestinal worms that release eggs, a stool examination will not reveal human infections with *T canis* or *T cati*. Instead, diagnosis usually is made based on a combination of clinical features and serologic tests. Close association with a dog or cat frequently is disclosed by history, and a history of pica is commonly elicited with VLM, but not OLM. A persistently elevated eosinophil count, a moderate to high increase in γ-globulin, and elevated erythrocyte sedimentation rate all support the diagnosis. If the patient is not blood type AB, one of the antihemagglutinins (anti-A or anti-B) usually is increased, because *Toxocara* larvae contain surface antigens that stimulate isohemagglutinin production. An enzyme immunoassay (EIA) for *Toxocara* antibodies in serum is available through the Centers for Disease Control and Prevention (CDC) and through some private laboratories. The EIA detects antibodies against larval secreted antigens, and when performed by the CDC, the assay has a sensitivity of 78% and a specificity of > 90% at a titer of ≥ 1:32 for patients with VLM. For patients with OLM, the sensitivity is lower at 73%. Therefore, OLM is often diagnosed on the basis of characteristic lesions seen on fundoscopy. There is controversy as to whether elevated anti-*Toxocara* antibodies reflect only previous human exposure or whether it could also represent ongoing larval migrations and infections. This situation is especially relevant to patients with covert toxocariasis who may present with asthma and wheezing or developmental delays. The development of new-generation assays using genetically engineered recombinant parasite antigens might help in addressing some of these issues as well as improving EIA sensitivity and specificity.

Larvae may be detected in biopsy specimens, although most patients do not require surgical procedures for diagnosis. Occasionally, migrating larvae may also be seen in the retina.

## TREATMENT

Albendazole is the treatment of choice for VLM. Typically a 5-day treatment course is used, but longer treatment courses of 20 days have been used in severe cases. The drug should be used with caution because of potential toxicity from allergic responses to dying parasites, while liver and blood functions should be monitored for prolonged courses of albendazole. Although mebendazole is commonly used to treat a number of human helminth infections, the drug is poorly absorbed from the gastrointestinal tract, and therapeutic levels of the drug are often inadequate to treat the tissue-dwelling larvae that cause toxocariasis. The benefit of albendazole in the treatment of covert toxocariasis has not been established. The management and treatment of OLM should be done in consultation with an ophthalmologist and will often require local use of steroids or surgical modalities. The benefit of specific anthelmintic therapy with albendazole for treating OLM has not been established, particularly given the exacerbation of host inflammation that could result.

## PREVENTION

Sandboxes and other play areas where dogs and cats could defecate should be covered, while dogs and cats should be dewormed periodically. Puppies and kittens should be dewormed at 2, 4, 6, and 8 weeks of age, because they usually are heavily infected. Because all forms of toxocariasis are more commonly found in economically disadvantaged areas where stray dogs and cats are found frequently, local animal control initiatives could have an important role in prevention.

## SUGGESTED READINGS


Ahn SJ, Ryoo NK, Woo SJ. Ocular toxocariasis: clinical features, diagnosis, treatment and prevention. *Asia Pac Allergy*. 2014;4:134-141.

Hotez PJ. Neglected infections of poverty in the United States and their effects on the brain. *J Am Med Assoc Psych*. 2014;71:1099-1100.

Lee RM, Moore LB, Bottazzi ME, Hotez PJ. Toxocariasis in North America: a systematic review. *PLoS Negl Trop Dis*. 2014;8:e3116.

Macpherson CN. The epidemiology and public health importance of toxocariasis: a zoonosis of global importance. *Int J Parasitol*. 2013;43:999-1008.

Moreira GM, Telmo Pde L, Mendonca M, et al. Human toxocariasis: current advances in diagnostics, treatment and interventions. *Trends Parasitol*. 2014;30:456-464.

Walsh MG, Haseeb MA. Reduced cognitive function in children with toxocariasis in a nationally representative sample of the United States. *Int J Parasitol*. 2012;42:1159-1163.

Weatherhead JE, Hotez PJ. Worm infections in children. *Pediatr Rev*. 2015;36:341-352.

Woodhall DM, Eberhard ML, Parise ME. Neglected parasitic infections in the United States: toxocariasis. *Am J Trop Med Hyg*. 2014;90:810-813.

Woodhall DM, Flore AE. Toxocariasis: a review for pediatricians. *J Pediatr Infect Dis Soc*. 2014;3:154-159.


# 327 Trichinosis

Haidee Custodio

## INTRODUCTION

*Trichinella* species are nematodes infecting the striated muscle of warm-blooded animals. Human infection with *Trichinella* (called trichinosis, trichinellosis, or trichiniasis) occurs by consumption of raw or insufficiently cooked infected meat. *Trichinella spiralis* is the first of at least 9 *Trichinella* species identified as responsible for disease and is the species most associated with domestic and wild swine. Most human infections are associated with undercooked pork, although horsemeat and wild carnivorous game, such as bear and walrus meat, may also be sources of infection.

## PATHOGENESIS AND EPIDEMIOLOGY

When undercooked meat infected with *Trichinella* cysts is eaten, larvae excyst in the duodenum, invade the mucosa of the small intestine, and develop into tiny adults in 5 to 7 days (Fig. 327-1). Adult nematodes mate in the intestine, fertilized eggs hatch in utero, and larvae are discharged into the gut throughout the 1 to 4 months of the adult female's life. By the second week, larvae are migrating throughout the body, and by the third week, encystment in striated muscle occurs. Here, the larvae may remain viable for years, but they usually die within 6 to 9 months and slowly calcify.

Mucosal petechiae and gastrointestinal bleeding are possible during the intestinal stage of the disease. The primary lesions are in striated muscle, where there is fiber hypertrophy, edema, and degeneration with an acute interstitial inflammatory exudate. The diaphragm is the most commonly involved muscle; infection is also common in the tongue, masseter, intercostal, extraocular, and laryngeal muscles. Eventually, larvae become trapped in an ovoid cyst. Although larvae do not encyst in the heart, their presence there during migration often causes acute myocarditis. Pathology in the central nervous system includes nonsuppurative meningitis or granulomatous inflammatory changes in the basal ganglia, medulla, and cerebellum. In the lungs, larval migration may produce a transient Löffler pneumonitis or

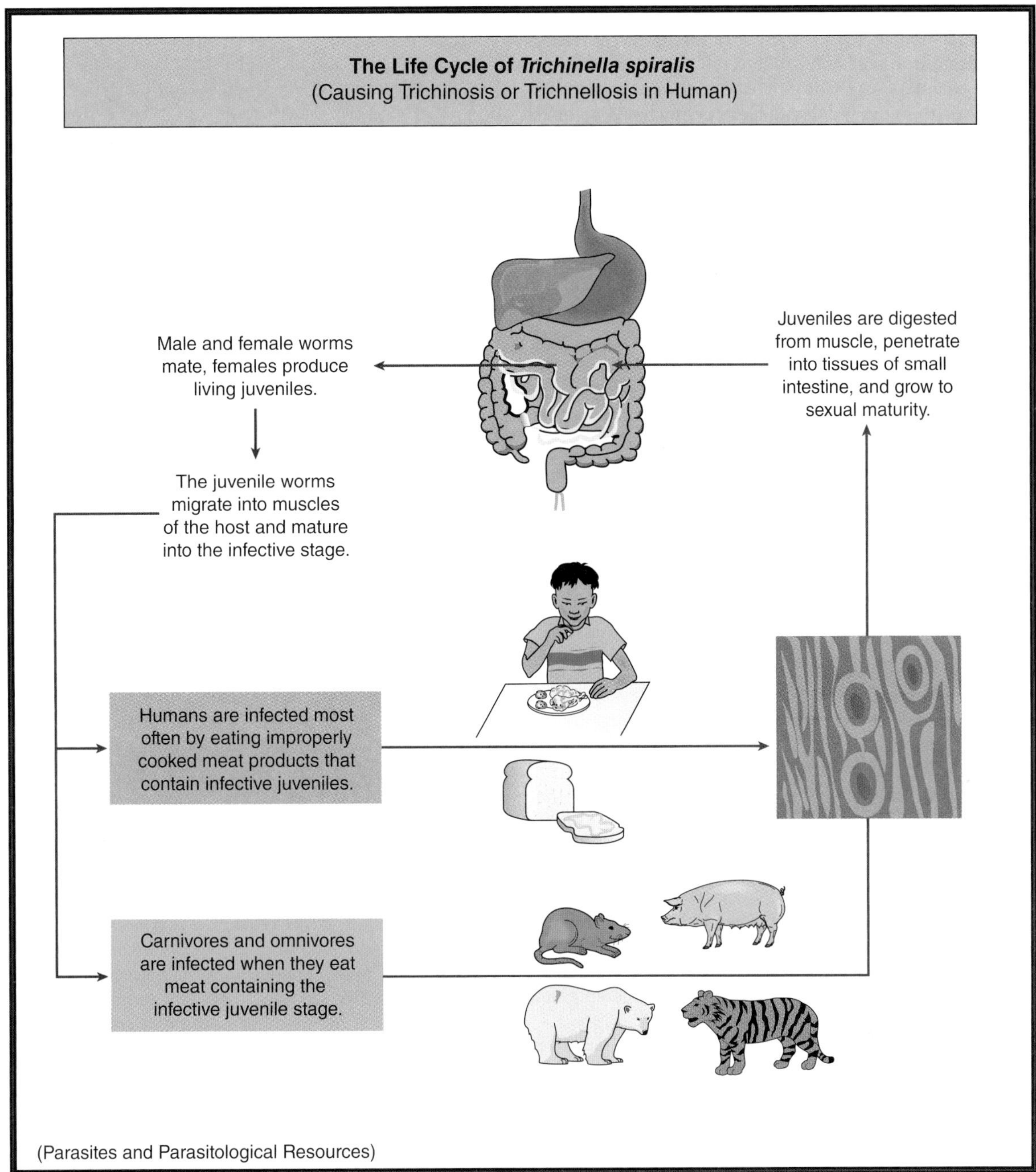


**FIGURE 327-1** *Trichinella spiralis* life cycle. (Reproduced with permission from Stanford University. http://www.stanford.edu/class/humbio103/ParaSites2001/trichinosis/index.html.)

pulmonary edema. Eosinophilia may reach 90% during the height of larval invasion. The host's immunity is directed against both the adult and migrating larvae.

The disease occurs worldwide in both high- and low-income regions, with outbreaks reported in the United States, Mexico, Southeast Asia, and Europe. Because of the mode of transmission, disease is relatively uncommon in predominantly Muslim and Hindu countries where pork is rarely eaten. Most cases are linked to common source outbreaks from contaminated meat. Pork or pork products account for 75% to 80% of infections. While the worldwide prevalence of trichinosis appeared to decline in the 1970s and 1980s, from 1990 on, there has been a resurgence of this disease in both resourced and under-resourced countries. This increase has been attributed both to the mass marketing of meat products, increasing the population at risk from single-source outbreaks, and to the growing proportion of outbreaks attributed to sylvatic (wild animal–associated) *Trichinella* species, either through consumption of wild game or spillover to domestic animals. The disease is naturally perpetuated by cannibalistic rats consumed by higher carnivores, and the practice of feeding pigs garbage containing infected meat maintains the infection in pigs. In the United States, legislative changes in pork production and consumer education on proper cooking of meat led to decline in the number of cases. Recent outbreaks involving consumption of undercooked bear meat emphasize the role of nonpork meat in transmission of infection. In fact, beginning in 1997, US cases associated with nonpork products exceeded those of pork.

## CLINICAL MANIFESTATIONS

Clinical symptoms primarily depend on the number of worms ingested, number of larvae produced, and sites of invasion. Children tend to have typical symptoms but with milder disease than adults, and they rarely present with severe complications. During the intestinal phase of infection, invading larvae and adult worms often cause acute gastrointestinal symptoms such as nausea, vomiting, and diarrhea, as well as fever, diaphoresis, and urticaria. These symptoms may begin within 24 hours of infection and may last up to 7 days. When larvae enter the general circulation, new symptoms may occur, including edema of the eyelids and face, conjunctivitis, splinter hemorrhages of the nailbeds, fever, and both cardiac and respiratory symptoms. Severe muscle tenderness, pain, and spasm occur during muscle invasion.

Primarily during the fourth to eighth weeks of infection, myocarditis may present (approximately 20% of patients), leading to acute congestive heart failure and death in some cases. Arrhythmias are not common, but sudden death occurring in the second to fifth weeks of infection is attributed to arrhythmias. The electrocardiogram may show ST changes and T-wave inversion. Central nervous system symptoms include headache, stiff neck, and psychoses. More severe neurologic complications, such as paresis and paralysis, have been described as rare complications in patients with severe infections, usually occurring in the third week of infection and associated with larval migration to the central nervous system. Ocular involvement, particularly periorbital edema and chemosis, is typical and suggests the diagnosis. Nephropathy may manifest as proteinuria, hematuria, and renal failure. With uncomplicated disease, muscle tenderness is the only persistent symptom, and it gradually diminishes in 12 to 18 months.

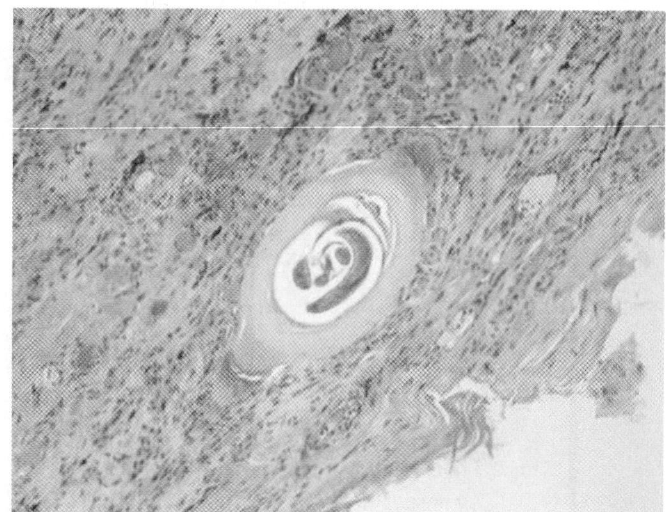

**FIGURE 327-2** *Trichinella* larva encysted in a characteristic hyalinized capsule in striated muscle tissue. (Reproduced with permission from Centers for Disease Control and Prevention (CDC): Trichinellosis associated with bear meat–New York and Tennessee, 2003, *MMWR Morb Mortal Wkly Rep*. 2004 Jul 16;53(27):606-610. Photo contributor: Photo/Wadsworth Center, New York State Department of Health.)

## DIAGNOSIS

Early diagnosis can be difficult given the lack of specific signs and symptoms. Even in late cases where there is multisystem involvement, misdiagnosis can occur, especially in areas where infection is not endemic and clinicians are not familiar with the symptomatology. Eosinophilia in the presence of other characteristic features, such as periorbital edema, fever, and myalgia, should suggest the diagnosis, especially if a history of recent raw meat consumption is elicited.

A rising eosinophilia beginning after 7 to 10 days and peaking at 20 to 21 days is a hallmark of this infection, with differentials that reach 20% to 60% or even higher eosinophils. Leukocytosis is common. Creatinine kinase, lactic acid dehydrogenase, and serum transaminase levels are elevated in more than 50% of patients. Hypoalbuminemia and hypergammaglobulinemia are common, and serum IgE concentration is markedly elevated.

Serologic testing using an enzyme-linked immunoassay, indirect immunofluorescence test, or Western blot is available. Many serologic tests are not reliably positive until after the third week of infection, so testing of acute and convalescent sera may be useful. The enzyme-linked immunoassay is the most specific and most widely used of currently available immunoassays, and a combined diagnostic approach using this assay and indirect immunofluorescence has been suggested to increase sensitivity of case detection. Other tools available in some research and reference laboratories include polymerase chain reaction and tests to detect circulating *Trichinella* larval antigens with monoclonal antibodies, although experience with these tests is limited.

Muscle biopsy may be necessary in some cases to confirm trichinosis. If needed, it should be performed after the second week of infection and taken from a tender muscle mass (Fig. 327-2). Muscle biopsy is necessary only when other diagnostic modalities are unable to confirm the diagnosis.

## TREATMENT

Most patients, including those with severe disease, recover completely as trichinosis is rarely fatal. The benzimidazole drugs, such as mebendazole (where available) and albendazole, are the mainstays of therapy. Steroids generally should be avoided in uncomplicated disease, because animal studies indicate that they may increase the numbers of circulating larvae and prolong the infection. However, steroids should be added in addition to the antiparasitic therapy for central nervous system disease and myocarditis in order to reduce symptoms from inflammation.

## PREVENTION

Because infection primarily results from eating raw or partially cooked meat, proper education in preparing meat and meat products is necessary. The disease can be prevented by cooking pork and wild game meat thoroughly, until it is no longer pink and an internal temperature of 160°F is reached. *Trichinella* larvae may also be killed by freezing. Specific temperature and number of days for freezing depend on the thickness of the meat. In addition, certain species of *Trichinella* such as *Trichinella native* are freeze-resistant and may not be effectively eliminated. Curing and smoking meat do not reliably eliminate *Trichinella* and, hence, are not recommended. In an outbreak of trichinellosis in Germany, postexposure prophylaxis with mebendazole given within 6 days of exposure appeared effective in preventing development of infection.

## SUGGESTED READINGS

Faber M, Schink S, Mayer-Scholl A, et al. Outbreak of trichinellosis due to wild boar meat and evaluation of the effectiveness of post exposure prophylaxis, Germany, 2013. *Clin Infect Dis*. 2015;60:e98-e104.

Murrell KD, Pozio E. Worldwide occurrence and impact of human trichinellosis, 1986–2009. *Emerg Infect Dis*. 2011;17:2194-2202.

Neghina R, Neghina AM, Marincu I, et al. Reviews on trichinellosis (II): neurological involvement. *Foodborne Pathog Dis*. 2011;8:579-585.

Neghina R, Neghina AM, Marincu I. Reviews on trichinellosis (III): cardiovascular involvement. *Foodborne Pathog Dis*. 2011;8:853-860.

Pozio E, Zarlenga DS. New pieces of the *Trichinella* puzzle. *Int J Parasitol*. 2013;43:983-997.

Shimoni Z, Froom P. Uncertainties in diagnosis, treatment and prevention of trichinellosis. *Expert Rev Anti Infect Ther*. 2015;13:1279-1288.

Wilson NO, Hall RL, Montgomery SP, Jones JL. Trichinellosis surveillance–United States, 2008-2012. *Morbid Mortal Wkly Rep Surveill Summ*. 2015;64:1-8.

# 328 Trichuriasis

Amina Ahmed

## INTRODUCTION

Trichuriasis is caused by the intestinal nematode, *Trichuris trichiura*, commonly known as the whipworm. Humans are the principal hosts for this parasite. *T trichiura* is found in coexistence with other soil-transmitted helminths, most commonly *Ascaris lumbricoides* and hookworms (*Ancylostoma duodenale* and *Necator americanus*).

## PATHOGENESIS AND EPIDEMIOLOGY

The life cycle of trichuriasis begins with the passage of eggs in the stool (Fig. 328-1). In optimal soil and temperature conditions, the eggs embryonate in 2 to 4 weeks. After ingestion of eggs via contaminated hands or food, larvae are released into the small intestine and travel to the cecum and colon. In 2 to 3 months, the larvae mature into adult worms that measure approximately 3 to 5 cm in length (Fig. 328-2). The distinctive whiplike anterior portion burrows into the mucosa, while the broader posterior end remains free in the intestinal lumen. Although adult whipworms live preferentially in the cecum and ascending colon, in heavy infections, they can be found throughout the colon and rectum. In those with large worm burdens, the colonic mucosa becomes inflamed, edematous, and friable. One to 2 months after infection, adult females begin to produce 5000 to 20,000 eggs per day. The total life span of the adult is 1 to 3 years.

*T trichiura* is one of the most prevalent human helminthiases, with an estimated 1 billion people infected worldwide. Trichuriasis is found in humid tropical environments and in temperate zones during warm and humid months, with the highest prevalence in Southeast Asia and Africa. It is especially common in poor rural communities with inadequate sanitary conditions and soil contamination with human feces. Transmission of infection occurs by ingestion of the eggs, which contaminate hands, food (raw fruit and vegetables fertilized by human feces), or drink. Children are especially vulnerable to this helminth infection, with the highest rate of infection occurring among those 5 to 15 years of age, presumably because of their high exposure risk and incomplete protective immunity. In endemic communities, people with heavy worm burdens typically represent less than 10% of the population and are the ones who develop overt disease.

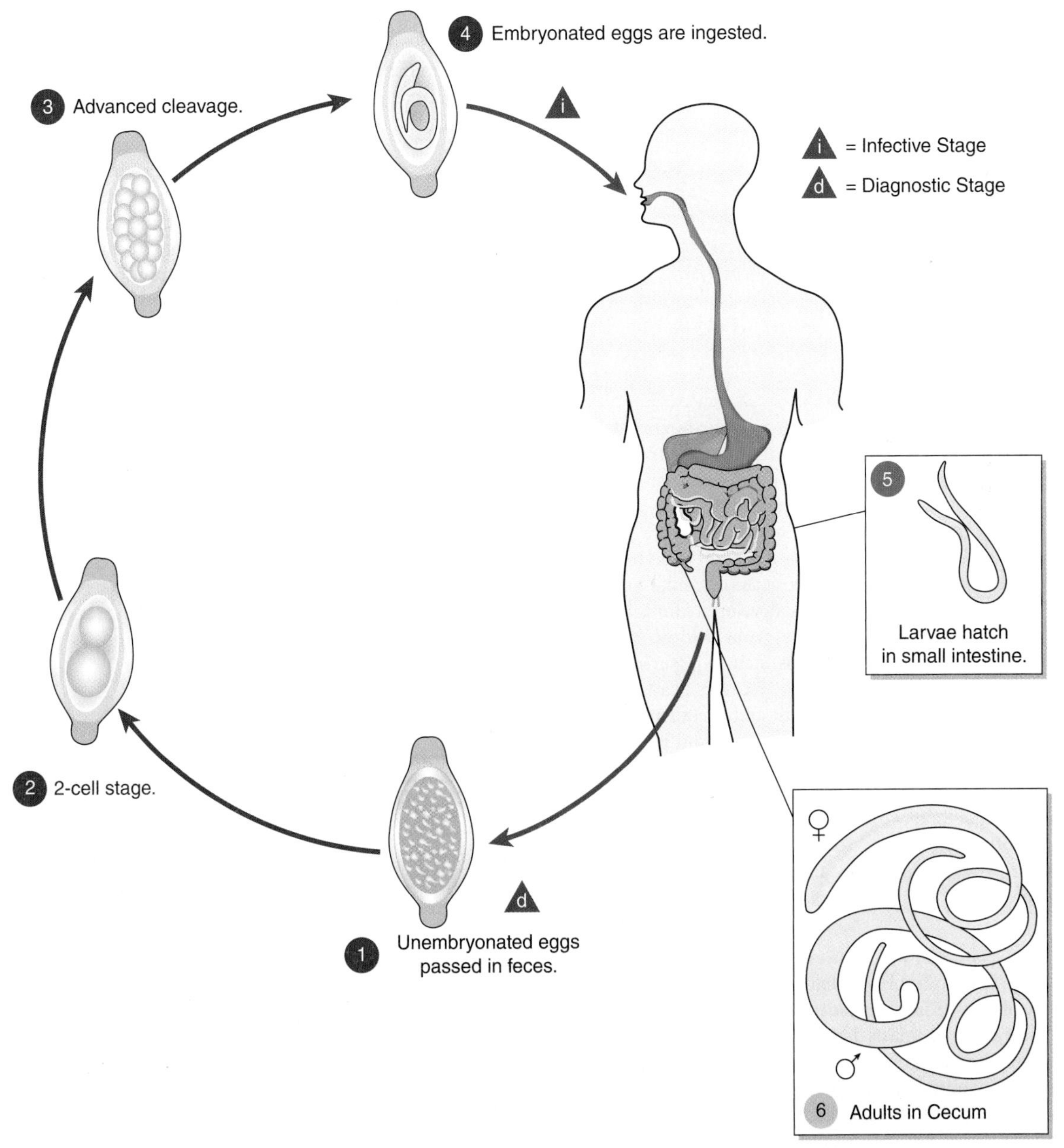


**FIGURE 328-1** Life cycle of *Trichuris trichiura*, the human whipworm.

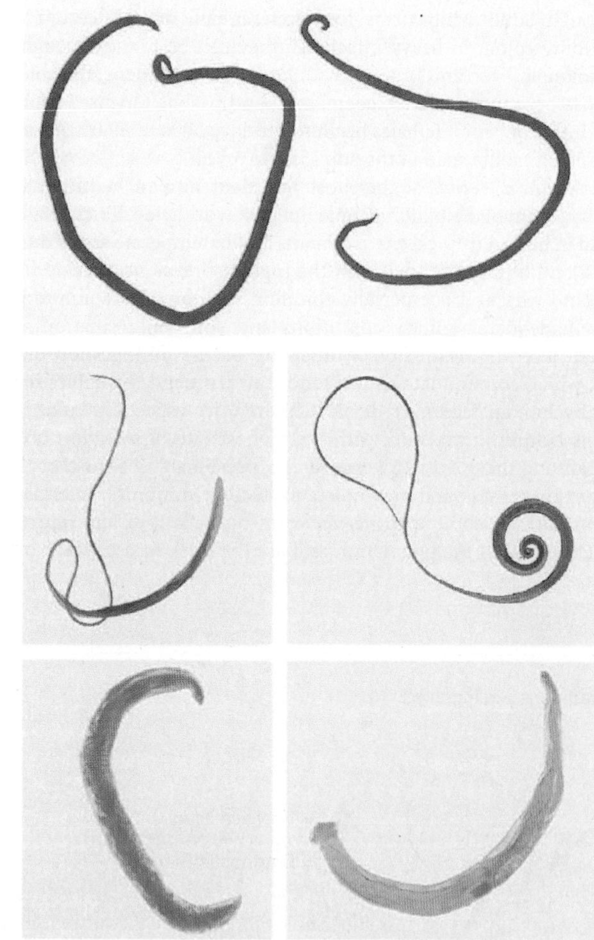

**FIGURE 328-2** Adult female and male *Trichuris trichiura*. (Courtesy Parasites Without Borders [*Parasitic Diseases* 6th ed].)

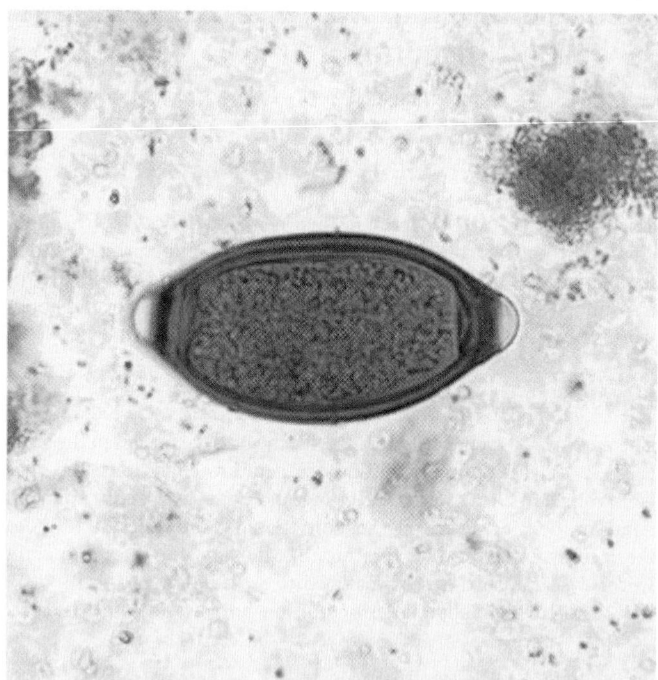

**FIGURE 328-3** Egg of *T trichiura* in an iodine-stained wet mount. (Reproduced with permission from Centers for Disease Control Public Health Image Library [PHIL].)

## CLINICAL MANIFESTATIONS

Although trichuriasis is not highly pathogenic, the amount of disease caused by *T trichiura* is proportional to the intensity of infection. Most infected people harbor fewer than 20 worms, but a small proportion, usually children, may harbor more than 200 worms. Those with low worm burdens are asymptomatic or may only have a peripheral eosinophilia. Inflammation at the site of attachment from large numbers of worms results in a colitis with loose stools containing mucus and blood. Children with chronic colitis develop a clinical disorder resembling inflammatory bowel disease with chronic abdominal pain and diarrhea. Clinical manifestations include anemia, impaired growth, and finger clubbing. Trichuriasis dysentery is a more severe manifestation characterized by tenesmus and frequent and often nocturnal diarrhea with large amounts of mucus and blood. Recurrent rectal prolapse is common, with adult worms visible in prolapsed mucosa. *T trichiura* infection can cause iron deficiency anemia, especially with coexistent hookworm infection. Chronic infection with *T trichiura* and other soil-transmitted helminths is an important cause of malnutrition, growth retardation, and impaired cognitive function in children worldwide.

## DIAGNOSIS

With most *T trichiura* infections being asymptomatic, some index of suspicion is needed to prompt consideration of the diagnosis. The differential diagnosis of trichuriasis depends on the presenting symptom. Eosinophilia may be caused by other intestinal nematodes such as *A lumbricoides*, hookworms, or *Strongyloides stercoralis*. Noninfectious etiologies of eosinophilia include allergy or atopy, drug sensitivity, and malignancy. In children from underdeveloped areas, colitis may be caused by intestinal parasites or protozoal infections such as amebiasis, but can also commonly be caused by bacteria such as *Salmonella*, *Shigella*, and enterohemorrhagic *Escherichia coli*. Inflammatory bowel disease should be considered a potential etiology of chronic colitis in a child. Impaired growth in a child from an underresourced part of the world is often multifactorial and caused by chronic infections due to intestinal parasites, human immunodeficiency virus, or tuberculosis, with malnutrition contributing significantly.

The diagnosis of trichuriasis is confirmed by microscopic examination of a fecal smear for eggs. The eggs are 50 by 20 μm and have a characteristic barrel shape with a hyaline plug at each end (Fig. 328-3). Concentration techniques may increase the yield in light infections. The Kato-Katz fecal thick smear can be used to measure the intensity of infection by estimating the number of egg counts per gram of feces, typically in clinical trial settings to assess the efficacy of treatment.

## TREATMENT

The most widely used drugs for the treatment of trichuriasis are mebendazole and albendazole. These benzimadazoles have a good safety profile and provide broad antihelminthic activity, but single-dose therapy with either agent is associated with suboptimal efficacy against trichuriasis, especially in high infection intensity settings. In a systematic review of 20 randomized controlled trials, some of which included children, cure rates of infection with *T trichiura* following treatment with single-dose albendazole and mebendazole were 28% and 39%, respectively. Cure rates with 3 days of treatment (albendazole 400 mg once daily or mebendazole 100 mg twice daily) are estimated at 70% to 90%. The effectiveness of treatment appears to decrease with greater intensities of infection. For heavy infections, longer courses of therapy of 5 to 7 days are more effective. In endemic settings, treatment success is limited by reinfection and resumption of eggs produced by live worms that survive treatment.

Oxantel pamoate administered as a single dose may offer an alternative option for treatment. Among children in Tanzania, cure rates of 50% to 60% were achieved with a dose range of 15 to 30 mg/kg. Ivermectin has some activity against trichuriasis, although data are limited, and it is not as effective as mebendazole when used as monotherapy. Combination regimens such as albendazole and ivermectin, albendazole and oxantel pamoate, and albendazole and mebendazole have been studied in an effort to increase and broaden the effect of benzimadazoles against *T trichiura* and concurrent helminthic infections. In a recent randomized controlled trial done in children age 6 to 14 years, treatment with albendazole (400-mg single dose) plus oxantel pamoate (20-mg/kg single dose) as well as albendazole plus ivermectin (200 μg/kg) resulted in significantly higher cure rates than mebendazole alone.

In addition to treatment of symptomatic disease, large-scale use of antihelminthic drugs for school-aged children is recommended by the World Health Organization to reduce childhood morbidity associated with trichuriasis and other helminthic infections. Regular deworming of children with benzimadazoles can result in improved iron stores, growth, and cognitive performance. The goal is to keep worm burdens below the level associated with symptoms and pathology, with reduction in transmission as the burden of infective larvae diminishes. Although evidence for a sustained decline in prevalence of infection is limited, regular treatment provided consistently may prevent some of the sequelae associated with chronic infection.

## PREVENTION

Disease prevention can be achieved by improved personal hygiene such as handwashing to prevent ingestion of soil that may be contaminated with human feces. All raw vegetables and fruits should be washed, peeled, or cooked. Transmission of infection may be prevented by improved sanitary conditions and the elimination of use of human feces as fertilizer.

## SUGGESTED READINGS

Geary TG. Are new anthelmintics needed to eliminate human helminthiases? *Curr Opin Infect Dis.* 2012;25:709-717.

Keiser J, Utzinger J. Efficacy of current drugs against soil-transmitted helminth infections. Systematic review and meta-analysis. *J Am Med Assoc.* 2008;299:1937-1948.

Knopp S, Mohammed KA, Speich B, et al. Albendazole and mebendazole administered alone or in combination with ivermectin against *Trichuris trichiura*: a randomized controlled trial. *Clin Infect Dis.* 2010;51:1420-1428.

Moser W, Ali SM, Ame SM, et al. Efficacy and safety of oxantel pamoate in school-aged children infected with *Trichuris trichiura* on Pemba Island, Tanzania: a parallel, randomized, controlled, dose-ranging study. *Lancet Infect Dis.* 2016;16:53-60.

Speich B, Ali SM, Ame SM, et al. Efficacy and safety of albendazole plus ivermectin, albendazole plus mebendazole, albendazole plus oxantel pamoate, and mebendazole alone against *Trichuris trichiura* and concomitant soil-transmitted helminth infections: a four-arm, randomized controlled trial. *Lancet Infect Dis.* 2015;15:277-284.

Speich B, Ame SM, Ali SM, et al. Oxantel pamoate-albendazole for *Trichuris trichiura* infection. *N Engl J Med.* 2014;370:610-620.

# 329 Anisakiasis and Angiostrongyliasis

Lee E. Morris

## ANISAKIASIS

### INTRODUCTION

Anisakiasis is a zoonotic nematode infection that can cause gastric, intestinal, and rarely, ectopic infections in humans. The third-stage larvae of *Anisakis simplex* and *Pseudoterranova decipiens* are the most common parasites to cause this infection after ingestion of raw or insufficiently cooked marine fish, as in sushi, sashimi, ceviche, and salted or smoked fish.

### PATHOGENESIS AND EPIDEMIOLOGY

Adult nematodes are found in the gastrointestinal tract of cetaceans (dolphins, porpoises, and whales), and nematode eggs shed in the feces of these definitive hosts are ingested by small crustaceans, where they develop into third-stage larvae. Crustaceans infected by larval forms are eaten by the fish and cephalopod mollusks, and once infected, the larvae invade the tissues of the fish. Definitive hosts and humans become infected by eating fish containing these larval stages. Most cases are associated with mackerel, squid, yellow tail, cod, haddock, herring, blue fin tuna, and salmon, but other fish may be infected. Once ingested, the larvae usually penetrate the gastric wall, leading to rapid onset of acute abdominal pain, nausea, and vomiting.

There has been a dramatic increase in the incidence of anisakiasis since 1980. This is in part due to (1) improvement in endoscopic procedures needed to make the definitive diagnosis; (2) increasing global demand for seafood and a growing preference for raw or lightly cooked food, especially in Western countries; and (3) the impact of regulatory controls on harvesting of marine mammals, leading to increased populations of potential definitive hosts. Human infection is most common in Japan, where consumption of raw fish is common and approximately 2000 anisakiasis cases are reported annually (accounting for 90% of reported cases worldwide). Incidence is also high in other countries in Asia and is increasing in the United States (approximately 50 annual cases) and Europe (approximately 500 annual cases).

### CLINICAL MANIFESTATIONS

There are 4 major clinical syndromes in humans: gastric (most common), intestinal, ectopic, and allergic disease. Clinical manifestations vary depending on where the worm localizes. In the gastric type, acute gastritis with abrupt onset of severe epigastric pain, nausea, and vomiting may occur, often within the first 12 hours of ingestion. Acute symptoms resolve within a few days, but some may report vague abdominal pain, nausea, and vomiting for weeks to months afterward. More severe symptoms with fever, chills, and urticaria may develop with repeated exposure because of Arthus-type allergic reactions. The relationship between anisakiasis and strong allergic reactions, ranging from urticaria to isolated angioedema and life-threatening anaphylaxis within hours of exposure, has become clearer in recent years. Most cases of allergic manifestations reported have demonstrated elevated immunoglobulin (Ig) E responses against *A simplex*. There is also speculation that initial sensitization may occur from exposure to both dead and live parasitic larvae.

Intestinal anisakiasis may not become symptomatic for up to a week after initial infection. Patients present with severe abdominal pain, nausea, vomiting, and commonly an ileus. Usually, the episode terminates once the worms are regurgitated or expelled by coughing or defecating. Invasion of the gastric or intestinal wall may be associated with a severe eosinophilic granulomatous reaction that may become chronic, causing gastric or right lower quadrant pain and eosinophilia. Occasionally, complications develop such as an intestinal bleed, peritonitis, or perforation by the invading worm causing an acute surgical abdomen. Gastric anisakiasis is often misdiagnosed as peptic ulcer disease or gastritis. Intestinal infection may mimic appendicitis, peritonitis, or other causes of an acute abdomen.

### DIAGNOSIS

Endoscopic gastric examination is diagnostic of infection by direct visual identification, and removal of the parasite endoscopically provides definitive treatment. In cases of intestinal infection, diagnosis can be difficult, but a history of raw seafood consumption and suspicious findings on imaging such as radiographs, ultrasound, or abdominal computed tomography (CT) scans can be useful. Anti–*A simplex* IgG, IgA, and IgE can be helpful, with high sensitivity (range 70–100%) but low specificity (approximately 50%) because there can be a cross-reaction with other parasites including *Ascaris* species and *Toxocara canis*. These serologies also take time to come back and are less helpful in the acute setting because they can be negative early in infection.

## TREATMENT

Although albendazole 400 mg orally twice daily for 6 to 21 days has been successful in some reports, no chemotherapeutic agent has been identified that can treat anisakiasis successfully. Surgical or endoscopic removal of the larvae are the standard methods of treatment for gastric disease, whereas conservative management (eg, intestinal decompression with a nasogastric tube and supportive care) is successful in the majority of intestinal cases, reserving surgical intervention for any complications that may develop. Larvae typically only survive in the human intestine for a few days, with symptoms secondary to inflammation often resolving within 2 to 3 weeks.

## PREVENTION

Prevention, including educating the public on the risks of consuming raw or undercooked fish, remains the best strategy. Proper cooking of fish to at least 60°C (140°F) or freezing to −20°C (−4°F) for 7 days or freezing at −35°C (−31°F) for ≥ 15 hours will kill the larvae.

# ANGIOSTRONGYLIASIS

## INTRODUCTION

*Angiostrongylus cantonensis*, a nematode of rodents that occasionally infects humans, is the cause of angiostrongyliasis. This parasite, also known as the rat lungworm, is the principal cause of eosinophilic meningitis. The organism is widely distributed and found most commonly in the Pacific islands and Southeast Asia; however, it is observed with increasing frequency in North, Central, and South America.

## PATHOGENESIS AND EPIDEMIOLOGY

Larvae are excreted in the feces of infected rats, the definitive host, which are then ingested by snails or slugs where they develop into third-stage larvae. The larvae remain at that stage until the snail is eaten or dies. Once the snail or slug is ingested by a definitive host, the larvae mature into adult worms in the central nervous system (CNS) and then migrate to and reside in the pulmonary arteries and right ventricle where they copulate and lay eggs. The eggs migrate to the lungs and, once developed, move up the trachea to be swallowed and excreted in the definitive host feces. Humans are infected after eating raw snails, slugs, and crustaceans that serve as intermediate hosts for the infective larvae. Other animals can become infected such as freshwater shrimp, land crabs, and frogs, which act as transport hosts that are not required for reproduction of the parasite but may transmit the infection to humans if eaten raw or undercooked. In addition, outbreaks have been associated with eating salads and raw vegetables, presumably due to contamination with mollusk slime. Larvae can be ingested from contaminated hands after handling or playing with mollusks, which is the likely mode of transmission among young children. Once ingested, the larvae enter the circulation and migrate to the meningeal vessels, from which they can migrate into the brain tissue to cause, most commonly, an eosinophilic meningitis, but also meningoencephalitis and ocular disease. These larvae usually do not develop further once they reach the brain and eventually die.

## CLINICAL MANIFESTATIONS

Patients often present after an incubation of 2 weeks with acute severe headache resulting from elevated intracranial pressure (ICP) produced by a widespread inflammatory reaction in the meninges. Associated symptoms can include neck stiffness, nausea, vomiting, and fever. Patients can develop focal neurologic manifestations including cranial nerve deficits, paresthesias, and ataxia. Ocular complications, such as visual disturbances or diplopia associated with headaches, ocular migration, and neurologic sequelae, are reported. Infected children often present with a higher incidence of nausea, vomiting, fever, neck stiffness, cranial nerve palsies, and weakness of the extremities than in adults. Symptoms usually spontaneously resolve within a few weeks, with a mean duration of 20 days. Although long-term sequelae and death are uncommon, severe illness and mortality are seen more often in children and the elderly. Overall, the prognosis for eosinophilic meningitis is good, whereas for encephalitis, prognosis is poor.

## DIAGNOSIS

Diagnosis is difficult and is often made presumptively based on history of ingestion of intermediate hosts, symptoms, and laboratory findings in blood and cerebrospinal fluid (CSF). Although recovery of the nematode from CSF confirms the diagnosis, this is a very infrequent finding. The CSF leukocyte count is often between 150 and 2000 cells/μL, and eosinophilic pleocytosis exceeds 10% in more than 95% of patients. CSF protein may be elevated, and glucose measurements are typically within normal range. Unlike other helminthic infections of the CNS, CT or magnetic resonance imaging of the brain does not demonstrate focal lesions. Various antibody assays to detect the 31-kd and 29-kd antigen of *A cantonensis* in serum are relatively specific; however, immunoassays are not widely available, can cross-react with other parasites, are often only detectable during the convalescent phase of disease, and have not been fully validated. More recently, rapid specific anti–*A cantonensis* IgG serum detection tests and a specific antigen polymerase chain reaction assay have been developed. However, these tests need further evaluation. Other causes of eosinophilic meningitis include gnathostomiasis, neurocysticercosis, cerebral paragonimiasis, *Toxocara canis*, *Baylisascaris*, tuberculous meningitis, and cryptococcal meningitis.

## TREATMENT

Angiostrongyliasis is generally a self-limited disease, but infrequently, deaths do occur. Treatment largely relies on symptomatic relief, such as repeated spinal taps to relieve elevated ICP and anti-inflammatory therapy with corticosteroids. Anthelmintic therapy, such as albendazole (either alone or in combination with corticosteroids), has been attempted, but the benefit of treatment is unclear, and some reports suggest treatment with anthelmintics alone can be detrimental, possibly due to inflammatory reactions to dead worms. Several small trials compared the use of steroids alone to steroids combined with albendazole. Overall results indicated corticosteroid treatment was beneficial for patients, although the role for albendazole remains inconclusive. Albendazole monotherapy is not recommended for treatment of angiostrongyliasis. Most patients do not receive specific therapy and recover spontaneously in 3 to 6 weeks.

*Angiostrongylus costaricensis* is a related parasite with a similar life cycle; it is found in South and Central America as well as in the southern United States. It does not produce eosinophilic meningitis, but results primarily in gastrointestinal pathology. Patients typically present with nausea, vomiting, fever, and abdominal pain. The larvae inhabit the mesenteric arteries, leading to eosinophilic infiltrates with deep ulcerations and fistulae at the site of larval penetration. Infection may present with a palpable mass in the right lower quadrant, and symptoms often are misdiagnosed as acute appendicitis. Peripheral eosinophilia can exceed 60%. Young children are infected more often than adults. Most infections resolve spontaneously; however, treatment with albendazole has been recommended by some, but experience is limited.

## PREVENTION

Preventive measures include educating at-risk populations of the infection, eating adequately cooked intermediate hosts (snails, slugs), and avoiding consumption of unwashed vegetables that may be contaminated.

## SUGGESTED READINGS

Evans-Gilbert T, Lindo JF, Henry S, Brown P, Christie CD. Severe eosinophilic meningitis owing to *Angiostrongylus cantonensis* in young Jamaican children: case report and literature review. *Paediatr Int Child Health*. 2014;34:148-152.

Juric I, Pogorelic Z, Despot R, Mrklic I. Unusual cause of small intestine obstruction in a child: small intestine anisakiasis: report of a case. *Scott Med J*. 2013;58:e32-e36.

Kim T, Song H, Jeong S, et al. Comparison of the clinical characteristics of patients with small bowel and gastric anisakiasis in Jeju Island. *Gut Liver*. 2013;7:23-29.

Martins Y, Tanowitz H, Kazacos K. Central nervous system manifestations of *Angiostrongylus cantonensis* infection. *Acta Trop*. 2015;141:46-53.

Sawanyawisuth K, Chindaprasirt J, Senthong V, et al. Clinical manifestations of eosinophilic meningitis due to infection with *Angiostrongylus cantonensis* in children. *Korean J Parasitol*. 2013;51:735-738.

Senthong V, Chindaprasirt J, Sawanyawisuth K. Differential diagnosis of CNS angiostrongyliasis: a short review. *Hawaii J Med Pub Health*. 2013;72:52-54.

Sohn W, Na B, Kim T, Park T. Anisakiasis: report of 15 gastric cases caused by *Anisakis* type 1 larvae and a brief review of Korean anisakiasis cases. *Korean J Parasitol*. 2015;53:465-470.

Yasunaga H, Horiguchi H, Kuwabara K, Hashimoto H, Matsuda S. Short report: clinical features of bowel anisakiasis in Japan. *Am J Trop Med Hyg*. 2010;83:104-105.

# 330 Schistosomiasis and Foodborne Trematodiasis

Martha Isabel Alvarez-Olmos

## INTRODUCTION

Trematodes, also known as flukes, are a group of flatworms that can cause human disease worldwide affecting millions of people from tropical areas. They have complex life cycles that involve snails as intermediate hosts. They can be divided, depending on their mode of transmission, as bloodborne flukes (*Schistosoma* species); foodborne flukes, which include liver or hepatobiliary flukes (*Clonorchis sinensis, Opisthorchis felineus, Opisthorchis viverrini, Fasciola hepatica*, and *Fasciola gigantica*); lung flukes (*Paragonimus* species); and intestinal flukes (several species). The life cycles are specific for each type of bloodborne and foodborne fluke. The clinical manifestations depend on the fluke's systemic, visceral, or local tropism (Table 330-1).

## SCHISTOSOMIASIS

Schistosomiasis, the most prevalent trematode infection globally (known as bilharziasis in some endemic regions), is a snail-transmitted parasitic condition caused by blood flukes of the genus *Schistosoma*. Among the 25 known species of schistosomas, only 5 cause human disease. There are 2 major forms of schistosomiasis, intestinal and urogenital. The global distribution is shown in Figure 330-1.

### PATHOGENESIS AND EPIDEMIOLOGY

All human schistosomes undergo a similar life cycle, which is complex and requires both intermediate and definitive hosts. The snails are the intermediate hosts where the asexual cycle occurs, and humans are the definitive hosts where the sexual cycle occurs. Schistosomes are cylindrical Platyhelminthes that range from 1 to 2 cm in length. The adult parasites are elongated, cylindrical, and curved. The adult females are larger and thinner and reside in the gynecophoric canal of the adult male.

Individuals can become infected when skin comes in contact with contaminated water and is penetrated by cercariae. Their life cycle begins with seeding of eggs into fresh water through feces (*Schistosoma mansoni* and *Schistosoma japonicum*) or urine (*Schistosoma haematobium*) from infected humans or animal reservoirs. The eggs hatch and release miracidia, which are viable for up to 7 days until they penetrate snails, which serve as intermediate hosts. The stages in the snail include 2 generations of sporocysts followed by production of cercariae, which are released from the snail into the water after 4 to 6 weeks. Cercariae can survive up to 2 days in water but are most infectious to humans during the first few hours after release from the snail. Once the cercariae penetrate human skin, they shed their tails and become schistosomulae, which migrate through the circulation until they reach the liver, where they mature into adult forms over a 2- to 4-week period. The adult worms migrate against portal blood flow to the mesenteric venules of the small and large intestine (*S japonicum* and *Schistosoma mekongi*), the mesenteric venules of the colon (*S mansoni, Schistosoma intercalatum*), or the vesical venous plexus (*S haematobium*). The male schistosome forms a groove on its ventral side in which the female resides. After 3 months, the female worms deposit eggs in the small venules of the mesenteric or perivesical system. The eggs move toward the lumen of the intestine (*S mansoni* and *S japonicum*) or bladder and ureters (*S haematobium*) and are eliminated in feces and urine, respectively. The adult worms usually survive for 5 to 7 years but may persist for up to 30 years.

Most infected individuals do not develop symptomatic illness. The natural course depends on the age of initial exposure, the intensity of ongoing exposure, development of immunity against repeat infection, and genetic susceptibility. Clinical disease is the result of the host immune response to the migrating eggs. Migration of eggs through tissues is associated with inflammation and subsequent fibrosis. Eggs are carried via the splanchnic venous system and may embolize to the liver, lungs, spleen, brain, or spinal cord; less common sites of embolization include skin and peritoneal surfaces. The acute schistosomiasis syndrome, also known as Katayama fever, is a systemic hypersensitivity reaction to schistosome antigens and circulating immune complexes that occurs 3 to 8 weeks after infection, most frequently among nonimmune hosts.

The second phase of infection results from the presence of eggs in capillaries and target organs, resulting in disease. The presence of eggs in the organ leads to inflammation and granuloma formation due to the immune response to antigens. Finally, fibrosis may occur around the eggs. The systemic reaction to eggs can be an early or a delayed hypersensitivity response. The immune response can occur not only to eggs but also to dead adult parasites in venules. When the parasites die, they may cause embolism and/or thrombosis, also resulting in disease.

Schistosomiasis is prevalent in tropical and subtropical areas, especially in poor communities without access to safe drinking water or adequate sanitation. It affects more than 200 million people, resulting in the loss of 1.53 million disability-adjusted life-years (DALYs) and causing up to 200,000 deaths annually. Currently this infection is present in at least 74 countries and continues to spread into additional geographical areas despite new treatment and control measures. The World Health Organization (WHO) estimates that at least 258 million people required frequent preventive treatment in 2014; 90% of these individuals were living in Africa. The infection usually occurs in rural areas where fresh water sources are located, especially below an altitude of 6000 ft (1800 m).

### CLINICAL MANIFESTATIONS

Manifestations of acute schistosomiasis syndrome (Katayama fever) are observed among individuals not living in endemic areas. Because visitors to endemic areas have not developed immunity associated with early exposure, they are at risk for Katayama fever. In contrast, individuals living in endemic areas generally develop chronic infection. The various types of infections that can occur in schistosomiasis are described below.

#### Acute Infection

The onset of clinical manifestations coincides with the beginning of egg production and a period of rapid increase in antigenic burden.

**TABLE 330-1 SCHISTOSOMIASIS AND FOODBORNE TREMATODES**

| Disease | Agent | Endemic Areas | Source of Infections | Age- and Sex-Related Infection Patterns | Main Clinical Aspects |
|---|---|---|---|---|---|
| **Bloodborne flukes** Schistosomiasis | *Schistosoma mansoni* | Sub-Saharan Africa, parts of South America (eg, Brazil), some Caribbean islands | Freshwater, penetration of skin by cercariae from infected snails | School-age children are usually at highest risk of infection<br>Occupation (eg, fishermen) is a risk factor of infection | **Acute form** Fever, urticaria, angioedema, chills, myalgias, arthralgias, diarrhea, cough, abdominal pain, and headache<br>**Chronic form** Intestinal, hepatosplenic, pulmonary, neurologic manifestations; severe malnutrition |
| | *Schistosoma japonicum* | China, Indonesia, the Philippines | | | Idem |
| | *Schistosoma intercalatum* | Parts of Central and West Africa | | | Idem |
| | *Schistosoma mekongi* | Cambodia, Lao People's Democratic Republic (PDR) | | | Idem |
| | *Schistosoma haematobium* | Sub-Saharan Africa, Middle East, some islands in the Indian Ocean | | | **Genitourinary form:** Microscopic or frank hematuria, painful dysuria, hydronephrosis, bladder polyps and tumors; female and male external genital involvement |
| **Foodborne flukes** Lung flukes | Paragonimiasis *Paragonimus westermani* | Cameroon, China, Costa Rica, Ecuador, Equatorial Guinea, Gabon, Guatemala, India, Japan, Lao PDR | Freshwater crustaceans such as crabs or crayfish | School-age children and young adults | Cough, fever, bloody sputum, chest pain, headache, anorexia, night sweats, weight loss<br>Ectopic sites: skin, liver, kidney, peritoneum, epididymis, spinal cord, and brain |
| **Foodborne flukes** Liver flukes | *Opisthorchis viverrini* | Cambodia, Lao PDR, Thailand, Vietnam | Freshwater fish | Low prevalence in young children<br>Highest prevalence and intensities observed in young adults and adults | Asymptomatic<br>**Acute form:** Asthenia, nausea, abdominal discomfort, diarrhea, jaundice, hepatomegaly<br>**Chronic form:** Cholelithiasis, cholangitis, and cholecystitis; liver abscesses and pancreatitis<br>Malnutrition, anemia, developmental retardation<br>Cholangiocarcinoma |
| | *Opisthorchis felineus* | Siberia, Kazakhstan, Russian Federation, Ukraine | Freshwater fish | | |
| | *Clonorchis sinensis* | China, Republic of Korea, Taiwan, Vietnam | Freshwater fish | | |
| | *Fasciola hepatica*<br>*Fasciola gigantica* | Bolivia, Ecuador, Peru, Chile, Egypt, Iran, Cuba, Portugal, France, Spain | Raw vegetables, especially watercress<br>Raw liver of infected animals | | **Acute form**: Fever, anorexia, right upper quadrant pain, ascites, hepatomegaly, jaundice, urticarial rash, respiratory symptoms<br>**Chronic form:** Biliary colic, intermittent jaundice, fatty food intolerance, cholangitis, pancreatitis, cholecystitis, sclerosing cholangitis, biliary cirrhosis<br>**Pharyngeal form:** edema, erythema, and suffocation |
| **Foodborne flukes** Intestinal flukes | *Fasciolopsis buski* | Bangladesh, China, India, Indonesia, Malaysia, Taiwan, Thailand, Vietnam, Lao PDR, Cambodia, Philippines, Liberia, Mexico, Nepal, Pakistan, Panama, Nigeria, Peru, Republic of Korea, Siberia, Sri Lanka | Freshwater plants | School-age children mostly affected | Abdominal pain, diarrhea, constipation, dizziness, headache<br>Severe abdominal pain, fever, and allergic reaction in the moderate to heavy infections |

Data from Steinmann P, Keiser J, Bos R, Tanner M, Utzinger J. Schistosomiasis and water resources development: systematic review, meta-analysis, and estimates of people at risk. Lancet Infect Dis. 2006;6(7):411-425; Utzinger J, Keiser J. Schistosomiasis and soil-transmitted helminthiasis: common drugs for treatment and control. Expert Opin Pharmacother. 2004;5(2):263-285; Keiser J, Utzinger J. Emerging foodborne trematodiasis. Emerg Infect Dis. 2005;11(10):1507-1514; Fang YY. Epidemiologic characteristics of Clonorchiasis sinensis in Guandong province, China. Southeast Asian J Trop Med Public Health. 1994; 25(2):291-295; Sithiathaworn P, Yongvanit P, Tesana S, Pairojkul C. Liver flukes. In: Murrell KD, Fried B, eds. Food-borne Parasitic Zoonoses. New York: Springer; 2007:3-52; Mas-Coma S, Bargues MD, Valero MA. Plant-borne trematode zoonoses: fascioliasis and fasciolopsiasis. In: Murrell KD, Fried B, eds. Food-borne Parasitic Zoonoses. New York: Springer; 2007:293-334; Blair D, Agatsuma T, Wang W. Paragonimasis. In: Murrell KD, Fried B, eds. Food-borne Parasitic Zoonoses. New York: Springer; 2007:117-150.

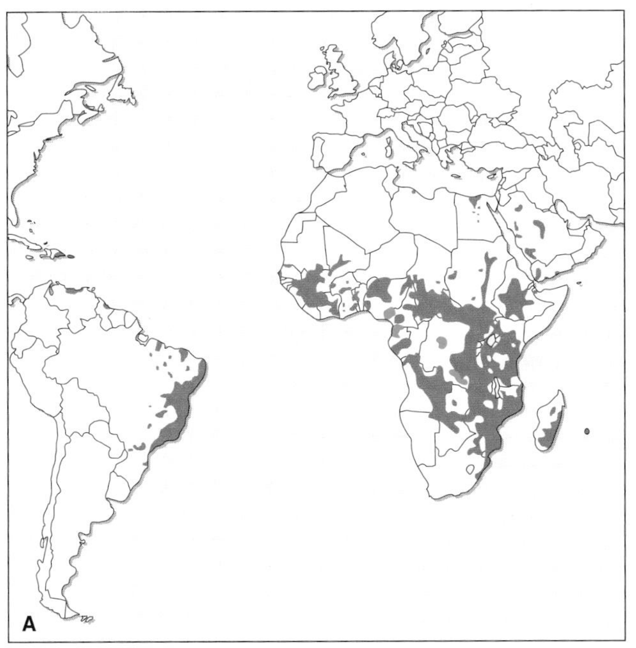


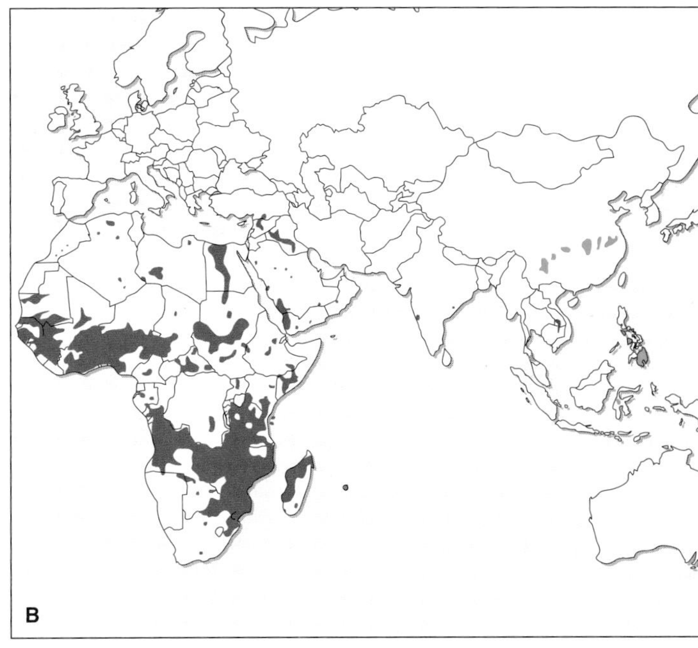


**FIGURE 330-1** Global distribution of schistosomiasis. **A:** *S mansoni* infection (*dark blue*) is endemic in Africa, the Middle East, South America, and a few Caribbean countries. *S intercalatum* infection (*green*) is endemic in sporadic foci in West and Central Africa. **B:** *S haematobium* infection (*purple*) is endemic in Africa and the Middle East. The major endemic countries for *S japonicum* infection (*green*) are China, the Philippines, and Indonesia. *S mekongi* infection (*red*) is endemic in sporadic foci in Southeast Asia. (Reproduced with permission from Kasper D, Fauci AS, Hauser S et al: *Harrison's Principles of Internal Medicine*. 19th ed. New York, NY: McGraw-Hill; 2015.)

Clinical manifestations include sudden onset of fever, urticaria, angioedema, chills, myalgias, arthralgias, diarrhea, cough, abdominal pain, and headache. Katayama fever is caused by a serum sickness–like syndrome. The symptoms are usually mild, with spontaneous resolution in a few days or weeks. In rare cases, neurologic symptoms suggestive of encephalitis can occur. Eosinophilia is present within a few days after onset of symptoms.

Some individuals develop a dermatitis in the form of a pruritic papular or urticarial rash at the site of larval entry after swimming in fresh water. Rash typically appears on the feet or lower legs, commonly known as "swimmer's itch." This reaction to the larvae may sometimes last for days as a maculopapular skin reaction. Bronchial hypersensitivity occurs when the schistosomulae migrate through pulmonary capillaries, and bronchopneumonic infiltrates may be seen on a chest radiograph.

#### Chronic Infection

This is more common among individuals living in endemic areas with ongoing exposure, but it also can occur in individuals with brief exposure. The severity of disease is related to the number of eggs trapped in tissue, their anatomic distribution, the duration and intensity of infection, and the host immune response.

**Intestinal Schistosomiasis** Intestinal infection may be asymptomatic or present with nonspecific manifestations. The most common symptoms include chronic or intermittent abdominal pain, poor appetite, and diarrhea. Ulceration with intestinal bleeding can occur, and there can also be a granulomatous inflammation in the bowel wall with resulting intestinal polyps. In rare cases, an inflammatory mass can lead to obstruction.

**Hepatosplenic Schistosomiasis** Hepatosplenic infection consists of 2 phases depending on the age of the individual and the duration of infection. It leads to a nonfibrotic granulomatous inflammation around trapped eggs in the presinusoidal periportal spaces of the liver. At this stage of the disease, changes are reversible with treatment. Later in the infection, collagen deposition occurs in the periportal spaces and results in periportal fibrosis. This leads to occlusion of the portal veins, portal hypertension with splenomegaly, portocaval shunting, and gastrointestinal varices. Imaging studies at this stage will show the chronic hepatic changes. Ultrasonography (US), computed tomography (CT) scan, and magnetic resonance imaging (MRI) may demonstrate fibrosis around portal vein tributaries, with splenomegaly and presence of collateral vessels. At this stage of disease, the changes are not reversible with treatment.

**Pulmonary Schistosomiasis** Pulmonary disease occurs most frequently among patients with hepatosplenic disease. Eggs embolize in the pulmonary circulation, leading to a granulomatous pulmonary endarteritis, with subsequent pulmonary hypertension and *cor pulmonale*. Dyspnea is the primary clinical manifestation. Chest radiography demonstrates fine miliary nodules.

**Genitourinary Schistosomiasis** When *S haematobium* infects the lower urinary tract, the lower ureters, urinary bladder, seminal vesicles, and occasionally *vas deferens*, prostate and female genital organs may all be involved. The infection provokes granulomatous inflammation resulting in the formation of nodules, tubercles, and micro- or macro-polyps or masses, which often undergo ulceration, fibrosis, and calcification. These patients typically present with microscopic or frank hematuria and frequent, painful micturition. Initially, eggs are excreted in the urine along with microscopic or macroscopic hematuria or pyuria. In chronic infection, eggs produce granulomatous inflammation, ulcerations, and development of pseudopolyps in the vesical and ureteral walls. Dysuria and increased urinary frequency are the common symptoms. Ultrasonography often demonstrates bladder wall irregularities due to granulomas; however, hydronephrosis, bladder polyps, and tumors may also be present. Female genital manifestations include hypertrophic and ulcerative lesions of the vulva, vagina, or cervix. In males, disease manifestations include involvement of epididymis, testicles, spermatic cord, and prostate. The lesions may cause female infertility or may facilitate the transmission of sexually transmitted infections. Schistosomiasis also leads to immune complex glomerulopathy, sometimes leading to nephrotic syndrome.

**Neuroschistosomiasis** Neuroschistosomiasis is a result of embolization of adult worms to the spinal cord or cerebral microcirculation, with subsequent release of eggs leading to an intense inflammatory reaction with local tissue destruction and scarring. It may cause serious neurologic complications involving the spinal cord, including myelopathy, which is more common than cerebral disease. Patients may present with lower limb pain, lower motor dysfunction, bladder paralysis, and bowel dysfunction. A variety of neurologic symptoms, including seizures, motor or sensory impairment, and cerebellar syndrome, may be present.

**Other Manifestations** Some of the other manifestations associated with infections include bacteremia or bacteriuria, which occurs as a result of tissue inflammation due to the migration and presence of eggs. Infection may also result in anemia, malnutrition, and growth retardation. Schistosomiasis may interfere with the host immune response with an increased susceptibility to human immunodeficiency virus (HIV) infection.

## DIAGNOSIS

Direct microscopy of stool and urine can be a very useful tool to confirm the diagnosis of schistosomiasis. More objective laboratory tests include the identification of antigen in the blood, urine, or stool. Serologic assay to detect the presence of antibody in blood can also be helpful in making a diagnosis. Molecular diagnostic tests that detect schistosome DNA are also being used more frequently. However, speciating the organism still depends on egg identification. The available laboratory tests can be divided into screening, diagnostic, and supplementary tests.

Screening tests include serology, urinalysis, and microscopy of urine and/or stool. Serology is a useful screening test to determine if an individual has had an infection in the past since it may take as long as 6 to 12 weeks to become positive. It may be useful in diagnosing acute infection in travelers returning from endemic areas. Serology is more sensitive than microscopic egg detection for demonstration of past infection, especially in those who may have migrated from an endemic area. The available serologic assays include the enzyme-linked immunosorbent assay (ELISA), radioimmunoassay, indirect hemagglutination, or Western blot and complement fixation. The sensitivity and specificity of the serologic technique depend on the antigen used and the stage and intensity of infection. Antibody titer does not correlate with parasite burden, and none of the serologic tests can distinguish between prior infection and active disease. Antibodies persist for many months to years even after successful treatment, so they are not reliable for follow-up.

The gold standard is the detection and demonstration of eggs in stool or urine by microscopy. The tissue biopsy specimens of bladder and rectal mucosa may be used only when eggs are not detected in the stool or urine. A variety of other tests are supportive but not diagnostic of schistosomiasis. These include eosinophilia, anemia, thrombocytopenia, hematuria or pyuria, and elevated liver function tests.

Studies such as US, CT, and MRI also have a role in diagnosing and assessing the severity of target organ pathology and detecting serious complications. US is a useful imaging tool not only for diagnosis of schistosomiasis but also for follow-up. The pattern and regression after treatment can be followed by US, making it a valuable imaging modality. Periportal fibrosis on cross-sectional view appears as "bull's eye" lesion. CT scan provides diagnosis of ectopic schistosomiasis lesions in the central nervous system and lungs. MRI scan can demonstrate spinal and cerebral schistosomiasis, hepatosplenic alterations, and periportal fibrosis and thickening that may not visualized by abdominal US.

Several conditions should be considered in the differential diagnosis of schistosomiasis. If acute febrile illness is the clinical presentation, with or without gastrointestinal manifestations, conditions such as malaria, typhoid fever or other *Salmonella* infections, brucellosis, leptospirosis, acute gastroenteritis, and appendicitis should be considered. If eosinophilia with meningeal signs and fever is present suggesting neuroschistosomiasis, tropical conditions including eosinophilic meningitis, coccidioidomycosis, and neurocysticercosis should be ruled out. In the hepatosplenic presentation, conditions including tropical splenomegaly due to malaria, visceral leishmaniasis, and lymphoproliferative disorders are important considerations. The pruritic rash may mimic cutaneous larva migrans, contact dermatitis, and hot tub folliculitis. In addition, rheumatologic conditions such as systemic lupus erythematosus, as well as allergic and hematologic disorders, should be included in the differential diagnosis of schistosomiasis.

## TREATMENT

All individuals diagnosed with schistosomiasis should be treated. Praziquantel is the drug of choice in adults and children older than 2 years of age. It has the advantage of high efficacy, excellent safety profile, and low cost. However, it is not useful in the very early stages of the disease because it does not act against immature parasites and eggs. Praziquantel does not prevent reinfections. The recommended dose for *S mansoni* and *S haematobium* is 40 mg/kg divided in 2 doses in a single day, whereas the dose for *S japonicum* is 60 mg/kg divided in 3 doses in a single day. Corticosteroids are sometimes used to control inflammatory response along with additional general systemic support for hypersensitivity syndromes such as Katayama fever or transverse myelitis. Prednisolone 0.5 to 1 mg/kg daily up to 20 to 40 mg orally for 5 days is usually recommended.

For chronic infection, praziquantel doses should be given for at least 4 to 6 weeks. With this treatment plan, a cure rate of more than 85% or decrease in the parasite burden by 90% can be achieved. Even though reinfection may occur after treatment, the risk of developing severe disease is diminished and even reversed when treatment is initiated and repeated as necessary. Clinical, laboratory, and radiologic follow-up is important to assess response to treatment and the need for re-treatment with praziquantel. This follow-up in affected individuals is necessary for patients from endemic areas, as well in cases detected in nonendemic areas.

## PREVENTION

Control of schistosomiasis is currently dependent primarily on large-scale treatment of at-risk populations, access to safe water sources, improved sanitation, hygiene education, and snail control.

The control strategy used by the WHO includes large-scale mass drug administration (MDA) of praziquantel, repeated periodically in the at-risk and affected populations. High-risk groups include school-age children and adults, especially those with occupations involving contact with infested water. The frequency of treatment is determined by the prevalence of infection in school-age children. In high-transmission areas, treatment may be repeated every year for a number of years. Recently, prophylactic use of artemether and praziquantel given together every 3 weeks in 5 cycles in school children showed promise.

Although these preventive strategies and health education are key to achieving long-lasting, optimal schistosomiasis control, a vaccine is what is needed to control schistosomiasis. Several candidate vaccines for human schistosomiasis are in development, but none are expected to be released in the near future.

# FOODBORNE TREMATODES: LIVER, LUNG, AND INTESTINAL FLUKES

## PATHOGENESIS AND EPIDEMIOLOGY

Human disease occurs from consumption of contaminated freshwater fish, frogs, shellfish, snails, tadpoles, snakes, and water plants, eaten raw or not well cooked. Parasite eggs are excreted from humans and domestic animals. Once eggs reach a body of freshwater, they develop and release a tiny larva or miracidium, which seeks small aquatic snail species, the first intermediate host. After larval development and asexual multiplication are completed within the snail, cercariae are released. In the foodborne flukes, the cercariae encyst in the flesh of the second intermediate host such as fish (*C sinensis, Opisthorchis* species) or shellfish (*Paragonimus* species) or encyst on aquatic plants (*Fasciola* species, *Fasciolopsis buski*).

Humans become infected after eating raw or uncooked aquatic products harboring metacercariae. The acid pH of the stomach of humans facilitates the excystment, and in the duodenum, the worm burrows into the peritoneal cavity through the intestinal lining. From there, the mature worms reach the lungs (*Paragonimus* species) or bile ducts (*C sinensis, Fasciola* species, and *Opisthorchis* species) through the liver, where the liver flukes reside and excrete eggs. *F buski* is located in the duodenum, and their eggs are excreted in stool. In *Paragonimus* species, eggs are excreted in the sputum or are swallowed and excreted in feces.

The global burden of these foodborne infections is enormous, although exact figures not fully known. In the mid-1990s, it was estimated that over 10% of the global population, or approximately 750 million people, were at risk of foodborne infections caused by trematodes. More recently, it has been estimated that over a billion people globally are at risk, including 601 million for clonorchiasis, 293 million for paragonimiasis, 91 million for fascioliasis, and greater than 60 million for opisthorchiasis.

The most affected regions are located in Southeast Asia and the Western Pacific. Some areas of Central and South America, Europe, and Asia are affected with fascioliasis, with the highest prevalence reported in Bolivia, Peru, Cuba, China, Spain, and the Nile Delta in Egypt. The origin of *F hepatica* is European, and it was spread to their colonies over 5 centuries. Although age distribution of food trematodiasis is not uniform, school-age children and young adults show the highest rates of fascioliasis and paragonimiasis. In contrast, the prevalence of clonorchiasis and opisthorchiasis is low in children and increases with age. Higher prevalence of fascioliasis is seen among women, whereas males are more commonly affected by other foodborne trematodes. These infections have been reported from everywhere in the world except Antarctica, suggesting the role of international travel.

One of the characteristics of these foodborne helminthic conditions is that most individuals harbor just a few worms, while a smaller number of individuals have the highest worm burden. This latter group has the highest risk for disease and environmental contamination. Reinfection after therapy is frequent among heavily infected individuals and communities.

## CLINICAL MANIFESTATIONS

A wide range of clinical manifestations is described with the foodborne trematodes. Light infections tend to be asymptomatic, while large parasite loads, prolonged duration of infection, concomitant parasitic infections, and hypersensitivity are associated with higher morbidity and mortality.

### Liver Flukes

*C sinensis* and *Opisthorchis* species may cause similar clinical features with a benign course, and most infected individuals are asymptomatic if parasitic burden is low. Individuals with higher parasitic burden may present with systemic symptoms and signs including asthenia, nausea, abdominal discomfort or pain, and diarrhea. Jaundice, hepatomegaly, and liver tenderness are frequently observed. Chronic infections with *C sinensis* can be associated with liver and biliary system complications including cholelithiasis, cholangitis, and cholecystitis. Liver abscesses and pancreatitis have also been described. Children with high parasitic burden can develop severe malnutrition, diarrhea, anemia, hepatomegaly, and developmental disability. The risk of cholangiocarcinoma is 5- to 15-fold higher with liver flukes. The carcinogenesis of liver flukes is not completely understood.

With *F hepatica* and *F gigantica* infections, the clinical spectrum in humans is wide and includes acute, chronic, ectopic, and pharyngeal infections. The acute stage is characterized by dyspepsia, fever, anorexia, right upper quadrant pain, hepatomegaly, ascites, urticarial rash, jaundice, and respiratory symptoms. The urticaria is the most common cutaneous presentation during the acute form associated with eosinophilia, jaundice, and gastrointestinal symptoms. The chronic presentation is associated with biliary colic, intermittent jaundice, fatty food intolerance, cholangitis, pancreatitis, and cholecystitis; sclerosing cholangitis and biliary cirrhosis are associated with prolonged or heavy infections. Ectopic forms in the skin can be identified as subcutaneous nodules when the larva migrates under the skin. Sometimes the disease can manifest on the skin as small red vesicles that can progress to painful and serpiginous lesions which can sometimes be vesicular. Other ectopic forms can be found in lung, heart, brain, muscles, genitourinary tract, and eyes. Finally, "halzoun," the pharyngeal form, is described in the Middle East. Halzoun occurs by consumption of raw liver of an infected animal. It is an allergic manifestation characterized by edema and congestion of the pharynx with risk of suffocation. There is no association of fascioliasis with cholangiocarcinoma.

### Lung Flukes

The clinical spectrum caused by *Paragonimus westermani* and related species varies depending on the infection stage, parasite burden, species involved, and individual susceptibility. Cough, fever, bloody sputum, chest pain, headache, and anorexia are the initial symptoms of pulmonary compromise. In the chronic phase, productive cough with brownish sputum and chest pain associated with night sweats are frequently described simulating pulmonary tuberculosis. The symptoms frequently evolve over several months to several years after acquiring the infection. Extrapulmonary manifestations may be present in 30% of patients due to ectopic migration of encysted larvae to skin, liver, kidney, peritoneum, epididymis, spinal cord, and brain, producing localized manifestations. Eosinophilic meningitis is seen with neurologic involvement.

### Intestinal Flukes

The clinical manifestations associated with intestinal fluke infections depend on the level of the parasite burden and the type of parasite. Mild symptoms such as abdominal pain, diarrhea, constipation, dizziness, and headache are described with a lower parasite burden of *F buski*. Severe abdominal pain with gastrointestinal symptoms, fever, and generalized edematous allergic reaction can be seen with moderate to heavy infections and can be fatal in some cases. *Echinostoma* infections may produce transient and mild symptoms including abdominal pain, fatigue, and diarrhea.

## DIAGNOSIS

Eggs of lung flukes, liver flukes, and intestinal flukes can be detected in the feces. In addition, eggs of lung flukes can also be detected in the sputum. Other organic fluids such as bile, gastric washing, or duodenal content may show eggs of liver flukes. There are several coprologic techniques used including direct fecal smears, sedimentation techniques, Kato-Katz thick smear, or formalin-ethyl-acetate technique; the last 2 techniques are the most widely used and have the highest sensitivity for moderate to heavy parasite load. Repeat testing and using different diagnostic techniques result in better detection of foodborne trematodes. Species-specific diagnosis is based on morphology of the eggs and is a challenge due to similarities in features of eggs of various species. Understanding of the geographical distribution and morphology of the adult flukes of the different species is helpful in speciating the eggs. Adult worms can be detected and differentiated in specimens from liver or lung biopsy.

Serologic diagnosis detects antibodies by using various available techniques including indirect hemagglutination assays, indirect fluorescent assays, and ELISA. These tests use different extracts from the various stages of the life cycle of parasites. These tests do have limitations due to cross-reactivity. Several new ELISAs have improved sensitivity and specificity for lung, liver, and intestinal trematode infections. Antibodies to *F hepatica* by ELISA can be detected during the acute phase of the infection. Intradermal tests are also available in which small amounts of diluted antigen are injected into the skin with a local reaction visible after 24 hours. The use of intradermal tests is limited due to their low specificity. These tests are not currently recommended for *C sinensis*.

Polymerase chain reaction (PCR) tests for diagnosis of *O viverrini, C sinensis, Paragonimus* species, and *F hepatica* infections have been recently developed and show high sensitivity and specificity. Cost is a significant limiting factor to the use of PCR in resource-poor countries where these infections are more common.

US, CT, and MRI are useful tests for diagnosis of liver or lung flukes. Cholangiography and endoscopic retrograde cholangiopancreatography (ERCP) can also detect adult liver flukes.

## TREATMENT

Praziquantel is the treatment of choice for all foodborne flukes for children 2 years of age and older. The recommended dose is 75 mg/kg/d divided in 3 doses for 1 day for intestinal flukes and for 2 days for liver flukes, except for *Fasciola*. Praziquantel is not recommended for fascioliasis. For lung flukes, the dose is the same; however, the drug is given for 3 days. Nausea is frequently described during the treatment, and urticaria may be present during the first week after praziquantel use. Biliary obstruction is a side effect that may require surgical removal for liver flukes.

For fascioliasis, triclabendazole, an imidazole derivative, is recommended and is highly effective against all stages of fascioliasis at a dose of 10 mg/kg once (twice in severe cases). It is usually well tolerated, and resistance is very unusual. Nitazoxanide is considered an alternative option and can be used in children but has lower cure rates. Albendazole and mebendazole are not effective. However, albendazole at 10 mg/kg/d for 7 days is an alternative drug for the other liver flukes *C sinensis* and *O viverrini*.

## PREVENTION

Preventive chemotherapy, including regular administration of praziquantel to at-risk populations without prior diagnosis, is promoted by WHO and other international organizations to limit the morbidity of blood- and foodborne trematodes. However, this strategy alone falls short of addressing the root behavioral and environmental causes of these neglected tropical diseases. Education and communication strategies to change human behavior are important. Proper cooking of fish and other aquatic products, including plants, in an endemic area is critical. In addition, water should be boiled before consumption. Food safety measures and improved sanitary conditions are key factors to achieve long-lasting effects on the control or even local elimination of foodborne trematodiasis. Elimination of snails has also been attempted but is not practical. A multipronged approach similar to that for schistosomiasis elimination is recommended to ensure long-term parasite control in areas where foodborne trematodiasis is still rampant.

## SUGGESTED READINGS

Elmorshedy H, Tanner M, Bergquist RN, Sharaf S, Barakat R. Prophylactic effect of artemether on human schistosomiasis mansoni among Egyptian children: a randomized controlled trial. *Acta Trop.* 2016;158:52-58.

Fürst T, Duthaler U, Sripa B, Ultzinger J, Kaiser J. Trematode infections: liver and lung flukes. *Infect Dis Clin North Am.* 2012;26: 399-419.

Knoop S, Becker SL, Ingram KJ, Keiser J, Utzinger J. Diagnosis and treatment of schistosomiasis in children in the era of intensified control. *Expert Rev Anti Infect Ther.* 2013;11:1237-1258.

Lupi O, Downing C, Lee M, et al. Mucocutaneous manifestations of helminth infections: treamatodes and cestodes. *J Am Acad Dermatol.* 2015;73:947-957.

Nyindo M, Lukambagire AH. Fascioliasis: an ongoing zoonotic trematode infection. *BioMed Res Int.* 2015;2015:786195.

Qian MB, Utzinger J, Keiser J, Zhou X-N. Clonorchiasis. *Lancet.* 2016;387:800-810.

Soentjens P, Clerinx J, Aerssens A, Cnops L, Van Esbroeck M, Bottieau E. Diagnosing acute schistosomiasis [letter]. *Clin Infect Dis.* 2014;58:304-305.

Utzinger J, Becker SL, van Lieshout L, van Dam GJ, Knopp S. New diagnostic tools in schistosomiasis. *Clin Microbiol Infect.* 2015;21:529-542.

# 331 Diphyllobothriasis

Miguel M. Cabada, Katherine A. Sota, and Héctor H. García

## INTRODUCTION

Diphyllobothriasis is caused by fish tapeworms of the genus *Diphyllobothrium*. Humans become infected mainly by eating freshwater (perch, pike, and salmonids), but also marine, fish that are raw, partially cooked, or smoked.

## PATHOGENESIS AND EPIDEMIOLOGY

The *Diphyllobothrium* tapeworm lives in the small intestine, where it may reach a length greater than 10 m. The gravid proglottids are wider than they are long, hence the name *broad fish tapeworm*. More than 1 million eggs may be passed in the feces every day with some *Diphyllobothrium* species. The eggs are operculated and measure approximately 60 μm by 40 μm. When the eggs reach water, a ciliated embryo or coracidia develops and is released through the operculum in about 2 weeks. The coracidia is ingested by copepod species (water fleas), and within this first intermediate host, it turns into a procercoid larva in 2 or 3 weeks. When a fish eats the infected copepod (second intermediate host), the procercoid penetrates the fish's intestinal wall and migrates to the muscles, where it grows into a ribbon-like plerocercoid larva (also called a sparganum) in approximately 1 month. Predatory fish such as salmon, pike, perch, and trout may eat the infected fish, and the plerocercoid will again invade the muscle of the new host. When a suitable definitive host eats the infected fish, the plerocercoid larva attaches to the wall of the small intestine and matures into a tapeworm after approximately 5 weeks (Fig. 331-1). Specific characteristics of the life cycle may vary depending on the *Diphyllobothrium* species. While *Diphyllobothrium latum* requires freshwater in ponds or lakes and infects freshwater fish, *Diphyllobothrium pacificum* requires sea water and fish to complete its life cycle. As a consequence, their definitive hosts may vary considerably, including humans, foxes, dogs, bears, seals, and sea lions.

The prevalence of infection is higher in people 20 to 59 years of age and in men. Eighteen species of *Diphyllobothrium* have been reported to infect humans; however, *D latum* causes the biggest burden of infection. *D latum* has a wide geographic distribution including regions of North America, especially Alaska and northern Canada, South America, Northern Europe, Japan, and Russia including Siberia. *Diphyllobothrium nihonkaiense* is an emerging species distributed in the Northern Pacific including China, Japan, Korea, and Eastern Russia. *D pacificum*, probably a phylogenetically distinct clade, is an emerging species causing most infections on the Pacific coast of Peru, Chile, and Ecuador, but with a wider distribution in nature and maybe in humans. Other *Diphyllobothrium* species may infect humans and have regional relevance, such as *Diphyllobothrium dendriticum* in Siberia. The *Diphyllobothrium* life cycle is maintained in nature by other definitive hosts, such as bears, dogs, cats, and sea mammals; humans are usually incidentally involved. Of note, the increasing popularity of sushi, sashimi, ceviche, and other exotic dishes with raw or pickled imported fish may cause *Diphyllobothrium* infections in nonendemic areas or with nonendemic species.

## CLINICAL MANIFESTATIONS

Most patients with diphyllobothriasis are asymptomatic and only notice the infection when they pass a chain of proglottids in the stool. Gastrointestinal complaints are uncommon, but some patients may complain of abdominal pain and diarrhea. Intestinal obstruction associated with vomiting segments of the tapeworm is rarely reported. Megaloblastic anemia has been reported in northern Europe and Chile in association with *D latum* infection. In early reports, clinical manifestations of megaloblastic anemia were found in 2% to 3% of patients with *D latum*, and > 75% of carriers had a low serum level of vitamin $B_{12}$. However, infection with *D latum* alone does not seem to

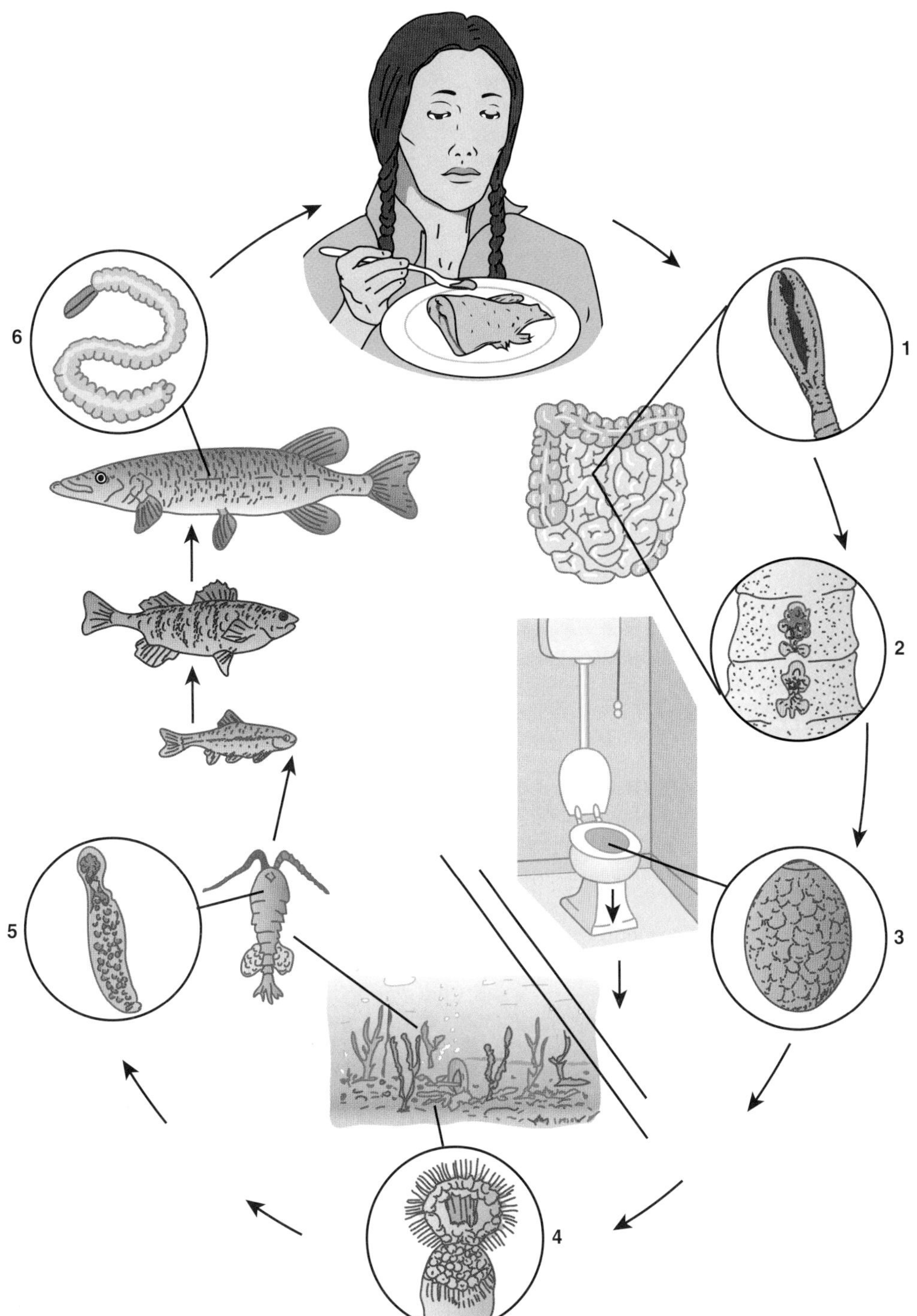


**FIGURE 331-1** 1-6: The scolex (1) of an adult worm attaches by bothria (sucking grooves) to the wall of the small intestine. Mature segments (2) deposit eggs in the gut lumen that are passed in stool (3). Eggs that reach a freshwater pond hatch after a period of development, releasing the ciliated coracidium (4), which develops in the first intermediate (copepod) host into the procercoid (5). Fish—often minnows—feed on the copepods and digest the procercoids free. The procercoids penetrate the gut, pass to the fish musculature, and mature into a nonencysted plerocercoid (6) capable of passing from the gut of one transport fish host to the flesh of a larger piscivorous host. The final transfer occurs when a human or other piscivorous mammal feeds on the infected fish and digests the plerocercoid free. The young worm attaches by its scolex and grows into an adult tapeworm, often 8 m or more in length and up to 2 cm in breadth. (Reproduced with permission from Goldsmith R, Heyneman D: *Tropical Medicine and Parasitology*. New York: The McGraw-Hill Companies, Inc; 1989.)

be a sufficient factor to cause anemia. This condition is the result of several factors, including the location of the tapeworm in the jejunum, the affinity of the geographic strain of *D latum* for vitamin $B_{12}$, and reduced levels of intrinsic factor (eg, atrophic gastritis) or decreased ability to absorb vitamin $B_{12}$. The megaloblastic anemia associated with diphyllobothriasis usually affects individuals over the age of 50. Patients infected with other *Diphyllobothrium* species are not at risk for megaloblastic anemia.

## DIAGNOSIS

Fecal examination allows the identification of *Diphyllobothrium* species eggs. If flatworm segments are available, the central uterine rosette (observed in fresh or stained specimens) and the dimensions of the proglottids are diagnostic. Nonetheless, differentiation to the species level is not always feasible by morphology alone. Sequencing of mitochondrial DNA (eg, cytochrome c oxidase 1 and NADH dehydrogenase subunit 3 genes) and the intertranscribed spacers of the 18S rRNA gene allows the accurate identification of the parasite species and has shed light on the distribution of diphyllobothriasis. Mitochondrial DNA polymerase chain reaction testing in frozen or ethanol-preserved specimens could be a useful tool for the diagnosis of infection in the definitive and intermediate hosts.

## TREATMENT

A single dose of oral praziquantel at 5 to 10 mg/kg is highly effective. However, praziquantel treatment damages the parasite structure and may cause the separation of the scolex from the proximal segments, which may hinder the assessment of treatment response. If the scolex remains attached to the intestine, the flatworm may regrow. Niclosamide is equally effective but is no longer available in the United States. If present, megaloblastic anemia or vitamin $B_{12}$ deficiency should be treated with oral or parenteral vitamin $B_{12}$ after antiparasitic treatment. To recover and identify the flatworm in children, the concomitant administration of praziquantel and a laxative are recommended because young patients may be constipated or cannot evacuate feces intentionally.

## PREVENTION

Diphyllobothriasis is prevented by freezing fish at –20°C for at least 24 hours or –35°C for 15 hours; cooking fish at 55°C or more for at least 5 minutes is sufficient to kill plerocercoid larvae and prevent transmission.

## SUGGESTED READINGS


Arizono N, Yamada M, Nakamura-Uchiyama F, Ohnishi K. Diphyllobothriasis associated with eating raw Pacific salmon. *Emerg Infect Dis.* 2009;15:866-870.

Go YB, Lee Eh, Cho J, Choi S, Chai JY. *Diphyllobothrium nihonkaiense* infections in a family. *Korean J Parasitol.* 2015;53:109-112.

Kuchta R, Brabec J, Kubáčková P, Scholz T. Tapeworm *Diphyllobothrium dendriticum* (Cestoda)—neglected or emerging human parasite? *PLoS Negl Trop Dis.* 2013;7:e2535.

Kuchta R, Serrano-Martinez ME, Scholz T. Pacific broad tapeworm *Adenocephalus pacificus* as a causative agent of globally reemerging diphyllobothriosis. *Emerg Infect Dis.* 2015;21:1697-1703.

Lee SH, Park H, Yu ST. *Diphyllobothrium latum* infection in a child with recurrent abdominal pain. *Korean J Pediatr.* 2015;58:451-453.

Pastor-Valle J, Gonzalez LM, Martin-Clemente JP, Merino FJ, Gottstein B, Garate T. Molecular diagnosis of diphyllobothriasis in Spain, most presumably acquired via imported fish, or sojourn abroad. *New Microbes New Infect.* 2014;2:1-6.

Zhang W, Che F, Tian S, Shu J, Zhang X. Molecular identification of *Diphyllobothrium nihonkaiense* from 3 human cases in Heilongjiang Province with a brief literature review in China. *Korean J Parasitol.* 2015;53:683-688.


# 332 Dipylidiasis

Miguel M. Cabada, Katherine A. Sota, and Héctor H. García

## INTRODUCTION

Dipylidiasis is caused by *Dipylidium caninum*, which is a relatively common tapeworm of dogs and cats worldwide. The infection of humans is a rare occurrence and most often affects infants and children.

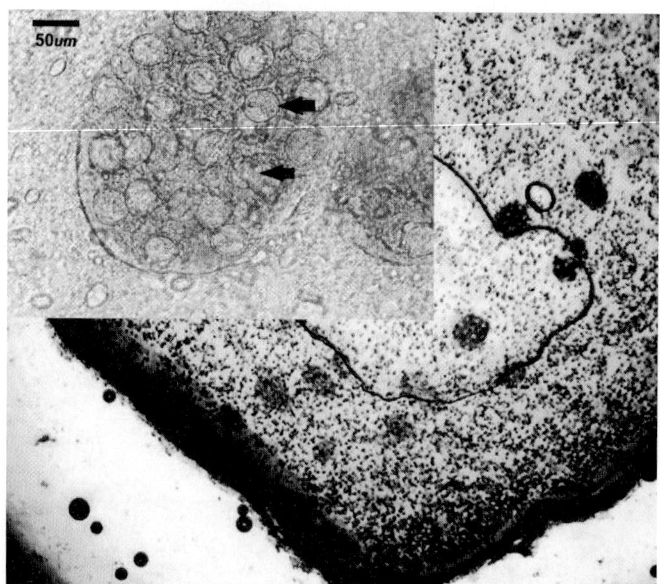


**FIGURE 332-1** *Dipylidium caninum* proglottid. The inset shows an egg sac containing eggs with hooks (*arrows*). (Used with permission from Dr. Miguel M. Cabada, University of Texas Medical Branch and Tropical Medicine Institute–Cusco Branch, Universidad Peruana Cayetano Heredia, Cusco, Peru.)

## PATHOGENESIS AND EPIDEMIOLOGY

Gravid motile proglottids from *D caninum* may actively migrate through the host's anus or be passed with fecal material disintegrating in the environment and dispersing egg-containing sacs (Fig. 332-1). Dog, cat, and human flea larvae and larvae of the dog louse ingest the eggs (35–40 μm) and serve as the intermediate host. In the larvae intestine, oncospheres are released and develop into cysticercoids within the intestinal wall. When a dog, cat, or rarely human ingests an infected adult flea, the cysticercoid larvae are released, and the adult tapeworm measuring between 10 and 70 cm develops in the small intestine of the definitive host in about 3 to 4 weeks after infection. A single flea may contain multiple *Dipylidium* larvae, and infection with more than 1 tapeworm is possible in the definitive host.

This is the most common and widespread adult tapeworm of dogs and cats and can be found worldwide, although not commonly in the United States. Humans acquire the infection by accidental ingestion of infected flea. Dipylidiasis in humans is almost exclusively reported in young children and infants as they are prone to accidentally ingest fleas or have contact with saliva of pets that may contain cysticercoids. In children, gravid proglottids passed in the stool may be confused with other parasites like *Enterobius* or fly larvae, delaying the diagnosis.

## CLINICAL MANIFESTATIONS

The infection by *D caninum* is often asymptomatic, but some patients may show decreased appetite, dyspepsia, abdominal pain, diarrhea, anal pruritus, poor weight gain, and irritability. Clinically, the parents' description of small worms or "maggots" found on diapers or underwear should raise suspicion for dipylidiasis. Eosinophilia and urticaria have been described but are not consistent findings.

## DIAGNOSIS

Microscopic inspection of the sacs of eggs or excreted proglottids passed by the host gives the diagnosis. Isolated eggs are not commonly found in stools because the gravid proglottids do not release eggs within the intestine. Fecal examinations may be falsely negative, because proglottids migrate to the surface of the stool sample and may be mistaken as fly larvae, "maggots," or vegetable matter. The first sign of infection is often the appearance of the proglottids in the stool or in the infant's diaper. The parent should be asked to collect the proglottids in saline solution and bring them to the laboratory.

Specimens could also be preserved in 70% alcohol or 10% neutral buffered formalin if evaluation is expected to be delayed. Compression of the proglottid between glass microscope slides will reveal the bilateral genital pores and egg sacs.

## TREATMENT

Human infection is self-limited unless there are repeated exposures. Praziquantel is effective when administered as a single dose of 5 to 10 mg/kg. Niclosamide can also be used but has only limited availability in the United States.

## PREVENTION

Dipylidiasis may be prevented by deworming cats and dogs and keeping them free of fleas.

## SUGGESTED READINGS


Mani I, Maguire JH. Small animal zoonoses and immuncompromised pet owners. *Top Companion Anim Med.* 2009;24:164-174.

Narasimham MV, Panda P, Mohanty I, Sahu S, Padhi S, Dash M. *Dipylidium caninum* infection in a child: a rare case report. *Indian J Med Microbiol.* 2013;31:82-84.

Taylor T, Zitzmann MB. *Dipylidium caninum* in a 4-month old male. *Clin Lab Sci.* 2011;24:212-214.


# 333 Echinococcosis

Héctor H. García

## INTRODUCTION

Nine species of *Echinococcus* have been recognized to date: *Echinococcus granulosus sensu stricto* (G1 to G3), *Echinococcus equinus* (G4), *Echinococcus ortleppi* (G5), *Echinococcus canadensis* (G6 to G10), *Echinococcus multilocularis, Echinococcus vogeli, Echinococcus oligarthrus, Echinococcus felidis*, and *Echinococcus shiquicus*. All but *E felidis* and *E shiquicus* are able to infect humans with their larval stages. The definitive hosts are canids (eg, dogs, coyotes, wolves, dingoes, jackals), except for *E oligarthrus*, which has been isolated only in wild cats. Humans become accidental intermediate hosts when the eggs from the feces of dogs, wolves, or other canids are ingested.

## PATHOGENESIS AND EPIDEMIOLOGY

Human cystic echinococcosis caused by the larval stage of *E granulosus sensu stricto* (G1 to G3), *E equinus* (G4), *E ortleppi* (G5), and *E canadensis* (G6 to G10) is the most frequent form of disease. The adult worm of *E granulosus* is found in the intestine of dogs, wolves, and other canids. The worm measures only about 0.5 cm in length. It has a scolex with hooks; a neck region; and 1 immature, 1 mature, and 1 gravid proglottid. The dog usually harbors hundreds or thousands of adult tapeworms. The eggs, which are morphologically similar to those of *Taenia* species, are excreted in the feces. When an intermediate host, such as sheep, ingests the eggs, the embryo hatches from the egg, penetrates the intestinal mucosa, and enters lymphatics or blood vessels. The host defense mechanisms destroy many embryos, but those surviving develop into expanding cystic structures called hydatid cysts (Fig. 333-1). The rapidity of cyst growth is quite variable and partially dependent on the tissue localization, but an increase in diameter of 1 cm or more per year is not uncommon, with faster growth in children. Spherical brood capsules arise from the inner germinal membrane of the cyst wall. Protoscolices, the precursors to the scolices of the adult worms, develop from germinal membrane and the inner surface of the brood capsules and accumulate within the cyst as "hydatid sand" (Fig. 333-2). If the cyst, or a portion of it, is eaten by a suitable definitive host, adult tapeworms develop in the small intestine. Hydatid cysts

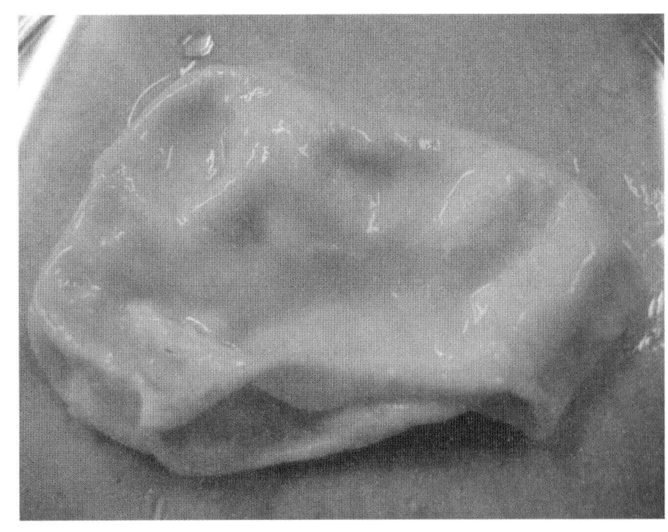

**FIGURE 333-1** A hydatid cyst capsule removed surgically from the lung. (Used with permission from S. Santivañez, 2016.)

are capable of developing in nearly any tissue, including the central nervous system and bone; however, 90% of them develop in either the liver or the lung, most frequently in the liver.

Human infection with hydatid cysts is most common in sheep- and cattle-raising areas such as the countries bordering the Mediterranean, Australia, New Zealand, and the Andean region in South America, particularly Peru and Argentina. In the United States, most infections are found among immigrants from endemic areas. However, there have been foci of infection among Basque shepherds in California, Mormon ranchers in Utah, and Native Americans in Arizona and New Mexico. In Africa, sub-Saharan countries have been demonstrated to be endemic, including reports of very high prevalence rates of human infection in Sudan, Ethiopia, Uganda, and Kenya.

Adult worms of *E multilocularis* are smaller but morphologically similar to *E granulosus*. The larval stage of *E multilocularis* in the intermediate host grows by external budding, resembling a malignant tumor, and does not produce large cystic structures (alveolar hydatid disease). Liver tissue is progressively destroyed, contiguous structures are invaded, and more rarely, metastatic lesions may develop in distant sites. Foxes are usually the definitive hosts, and rodents are intermediate hosts. Hunters and fur traders exposed to foxes and fox fur are at risk. This infection occurs only in the Northern Hemisphere. It has a wide distribution in the northern midwestern states of the

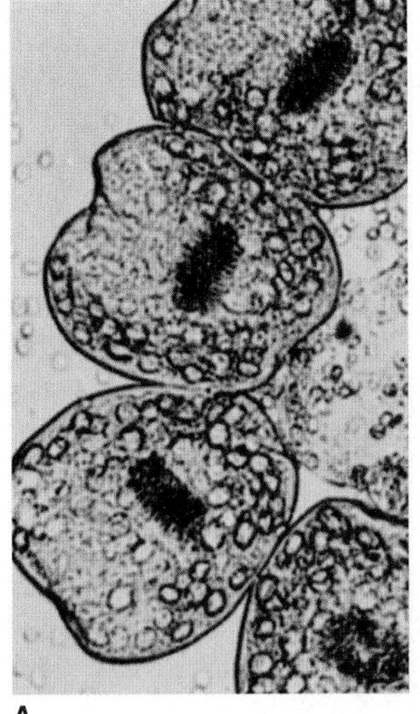



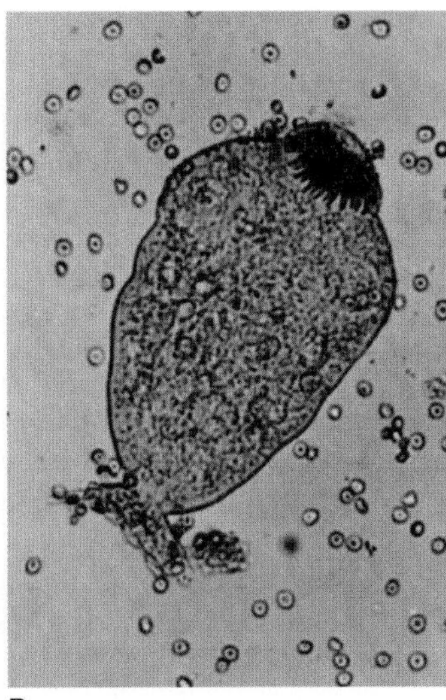



**FIGURE 333-2** Hydatid sand. **A:** Scolices invaginated into cyst membrane (140×). **B:** Evaginated scolex with hooklets; stalk is present, by which the scolex is continuous with the germinal epithelium (140×).

United States, Canada, the former Soviet Union, Switzerland and adjacent countries, and northern Japan. Sled dogs in Arctic villages may be sources of human infection.

Human neotropical echinococcosis, caused by *E vogeli* (polycystic) or *E oligarthrus* (unicystic), occurs much less frequently, and is found in Central and South America. Polycystic disease consists of multiple fluid-filled cysts, up to 3 cm in diameter, often interconnected and multichambered, whereas human infections with unicystic lesions of 1 to 2 cm containing brood capsules of *E oligarthrus* have been reported in the orbit and in the myocardium.

## CLINICAL MANIFESTATIONS

The majority (70%) of subjects with cystic echinococcosis have a single cyst. When multiple cysts are present, they are most commonly in the same organ, but they can develop in multiple sites. In adults, most infections occur in the liver, and the second most frequent site is the lung. Some investigators feel that pulmonary echinococcosis is more common in children and requires special attention and unique surgical approaches. About 20% of children with pulmonary hydatid cysts will also have hepatic cysts. In children, both hepatic and pulmonary cysts are frequently asymptomatic and could remain asymptomatic for a long period of time. Furthermore, because of the higher elasticity of lung parenchyma that allows the rapid growth of the cyst, lung cysts may attain considerable dimensions and lead to parenchymal damage, or conversely, some may resolve by natural evolution. It is not uncommon to find asymptomatic calcified cysts in the liver or spleen of infected adults as an incidental finding on radiologic studies or at autopsy. It takes many years for cysts to die and calcify; therefore, calcifications are rarely seen in children.

Large hepatic cysts may cause pain and tenderness in the right upper quadrant. In some instances, a mass may be palpable. Biliary tract obstruction may develop, depending on the size and location of the hepatic cyst. Between 5% and 15% of hepatic cysts rupture into the biliary tract, causing fever, pain, and jaundice. The release of antigenic cyst fluid may cause severe allergic reactions including anaphylaxis. Patients who survive intraperitoneal cyst rupture are in danger of multiple secondary cysts developing as a secondary infection within the abdomen.

Although pulmonary cysts often are asymptomatic, about one-third of them rupture into a bronchus or into the pleural space. Secondarily infected lung cysts appear as lung abscesses. Cysts that rupture into a bronchus may be coughed up. The patient may describe the membranes in the sputum. Complete evacuation of a pulmonary cyst results in a cure. Partial evacuation of the cyst sets the scene for bacterial growth and the production of a lung abscess.

Bone involvement may present as a bone deformity or as a pathologic fracture. The hydatid cyst begins growth within the marrow cavity. The typical laminated membrane does not develop. Bone destruction by the parasite resembles that caused by tumor or infection. Involvement of the vertebral body causes pain and tenderness to palpation and may produce spinal cord or nerve root compression with neurologic signs and symptoms. Intracranial hydatid cysts are rare and occur most frequently in children. The symptoms are those of an expanding mass, usually causing intracranial hypertension with headache, nausea, and vomiting. Seizures may also develop.

Although alveolar hydatid disease caused by *E multilocularis* has been described in a child as young as 5 years old, it is usually a disease of adults. The progressive destruction of the liver takes many years. Tender hepatomegaly, abdominal masses arising from the liver, and jaundice are common presenting findings. Extension of the parasite into large vessels may result in metastatic lesions in the lungs or brain.

## DIAGNOSIS

A history of exposure to dogs or other canids in an area endemic for echinococcosis is very helpful. For liver echinococcal cyst(s), imaging techniques such as ultrasound are effective in delineating the contents of cystic structures. The presence of daughter cysts can be diagnostic. The World Health Organization (WHO) classification provides a very useful tool for ultrasound staging and follow-up of liver cysts. Features noted from computed tomography (CT) scanning or magnetic resonance imaging (MRI) may be highly characteristic septate densities; furthermore, in terms of staging, MRI reproduces the ultrasound-defined features of echinococcal cyst(s) better than CT. Intact pulmonary cysts appear as sharply demarcated smooth, spherical, or ovoid radiopaque "cannonball" lesions in chest radiograph images. If the cyst has ruptured, an air-fluid level may be present. A collapsed membrane on the surface of the fluid may produce the classic "water lily" sign. CT images provide better definition.

Serologic testing using enzyme-linked immunosorbent assays (ELISAs), immunoblots, or indirect hemagglutination tests is available through a few reference laboratories and the Centers for Disease Control and Prevention. False-negative serologic tests have been problematic, particularly in lung cysts and other sites outside of the liver. Cross-reactivity has been noted with cysticercosis, hymenolepiasis, and other cestode infections. In the past few years, several recombinant antigens from antigen b and antigen 5 (the 2 major antigens from hydatid fluid) as well as specific immunoglobulin (Ig) Gs have been evaluated as tools for diagnosis and patient follow-up.

Examination of the cyst and its contents at surgery proves the diagnosis by the presence of protoscolices and hooklets (hydatid sand). Percutaneous needle aspiration for diagnostic purposes is usually not needed and should be done only after other techniques have failed.

Alveolar hydatid disease is usually suspected when plain films of the liver show amorphous calcification surrounding 2- to 4-mm radiolucent areas. The recent development of a highly sensitive and specific ELISA using an epitope, Em 18, which is not shared with *E granulosus*, appears very promising for diagnosis and for following the response to treatment.

## TREATMENT

The advent of therapy with benzimidazole compounds (initially mebendazole and later albendazole) and the success of percutaneous aspiration and injection techniques make it necessary to carefully reassess the dominant role of surgery in the treatment of cystic hydatid disease caused by *E granulosus*. Antihelminthic therapy alone may be effective. Albendazole has replaced mebendazole as the drug of choice. Recent studies show that a combination of albendazole and praziquantel is more successful than albendazole alone for the treatment of this disease. Smaller, uncomplicated cysts appear to respond to albendazole more readily than do larger cysts. There are reports of central nervous system, muscle, and vertebral and other bone lesions resolving completely with medical therapy. Because of the evolving therapy of cystic echinococcosis, consultation with the Centers for Disease Control and Prevention is advised to obtain current information (contact number: 770-488-7775).

Surgery is still considered appropriate therapy for large liver cysts with multiple daughter cysts, superficial cysts that are subject to spontaneous or traumatic rupture, cysts communicating with the biliary tract, and infected cysts. Surgery should be preceded by antiparasitic treatment to decrease the risk of cyst rupture at surgery, by decreasing pressure inside the cyst and the viability of the protoscolices if rupture occurs. Some authors suggest continuing antiparasitic therapy for 1 month or more following surgery to prevent recurrence and/or the development of secondary cysts. The combination of albendazole plus praziquantel seems more effective than albendazole alone for prevention of secondary infection. It is a common practice to cover the surgical field with pads soaked in hypertonic saline and to introduce a scolicidal substance such as hypertonic saline, alcohol, or cetrimide into the cyst during the surgical procedure. All of the commonly used scolicides have the potential to cause sclerosing cholangitis if there is communication between the cyst contents and the biliary tract.

Percutaneous aspiration, injection of a protoscolicidal agent, and reaspiration (the PAIR technique) have replaced surgery in select cases of liver cystic hydatid disease. The types of cyst that would mostly benefit from PAIR are those in stages I and III of the WHO ultrasound classification of liver cystic hydatid lesions. When feasible, PAIR eliminates the need for open surgery, decreases the hospital stay, and significantly reduces costs.

Alveolar hydatid disease is treated with aggressive surgery, including partial hepatectomy or lobectomy. Unfortunately, less than 30%

of patients have resectable lesions at the time of diagnosis. Long-term albendazole therapy may benefit a significant number of patients with inoperable lesions. Liver transplantation has been used in select patients. However, there is the risk of regrowth and metastatic spread associated with the immunosuppression that is necessary to preserve the transplant. Albendazole also appears to be beneficial in the treatment of polycystic hydatid disease caused by *E vogeli*.

## PREVENTION

Hydatid disease occurs in communities where the dog-livestock cycle is maintained, and usually dogs are given infested offal following unsupervised slaughter. The disease has been eliminated in several countries after very long periods of sustained control, including dog treatment and purge and health education. New tools, including an effective livestock and/or dog vaccine for the larval and tapeworm stage, respectively, may reduce the time required for successful disease control to be achieved.

## SUGGESTED READINGS

Brunetti E, Garcia HH, Junghanss T. Cystic echinococcosis: chronic, complex, and still neglected. *PLoS Negl Trop Dis*. 2011;5:e1146.

Budke CM, Carabin H, Ndimubanzi PC, et al. A systematic review of the literature on cystic echinococcosis frequency worldwide and its associated clinical manifestations. *Am J Trop Med Hyg*. 2013;88:1011-1027.

Giorgio A, Calisti G, de Stefano G, et al. Percutaneous treatment of hydatid liver cysts: an update. *Recent Pat Antiinfect Drug Discov*. 2012;7:231-236.

Manzano-Roman R, Sánchez-Ovejero C, Hernández-González A, et al. Serological diagnosis and follow-up of human cystic echinococcosis: a new hope for the future? *Biomed Res Int*. 2015;2015:428205.

McManus DP. Current status of the genetics and molecular taxonomy of *Echinococcus* species. *Parasitology*. 2013;140:1617-1623.

Nabarro LE, Amin Z, Chiodini PL. Current management of cystic echinococcosis: a survey of specialist practice. *Clin Infect Dis*. 2015;60:721-728.

Sarkar M, Pathania R, Jhobta A, Thakur BR, Chopra R. Cystic pulmonary hydatidosis. *Lung India*. 2016;33:179-191.

Tuxun T, Zhang JH, Zhao JM, et al. World review of laparoscopic treatment of liver cystic echinococcosis—914 patients. *Int J Infect Dis*. 2014;24:43-50.

# 334 Hymenolepiasis

Miguel M. Cabada and Héctor H. García

## INTRODUCTION

Hymenolepiasis, caused by the dwarf tapeworm *Hymenolepis nana*, is the smallest of the adult human tapeworms, can complete its entire life cycle within humans, and is the most common cestode infection in the world.

## PATHOGENESIS AND EPIDEMIOLOGY

The life cycle of *H nana* may vary according to the epidemiologic situation. In endemic areas and among institutionalized individuals, transmission occurs mainly via fecal-oral route. The parasites' eggs are immediately infectious after passed in the stool; thus, autoinfection and person-to-person transmission are possible. Once the eggs are ingested, they hatch in the intestine, and the released oncospheres penetrate the mucosa and form a cysticercoid larva within the villi. In a few days, the cysticercoid matures, leaves the villi, and evaginates in the intestine forming a new tapeworm. In the human host, *H nana* can complete its life cycle without reaching the environment, causing prolonged infections. In this case, eggs hatch in the intestine of the same host and invade the intestinal villi, forming the cysticercoids and then the tapeworms. A third cycle involves rodents as definitive hosts and beetles as intermediate hosts, but it is debatable if humans intervene in this cycle.

The adult tapeworm measures 2 to 4 cm in length. It attaches to the mucosa of the small intestine by a scolex that has 4 circular suckers and a retractable structure called a rostellum. A single host may harbor hundreds or thousands of tapeworms. Conflicting reports associate a high burden of infection with symptoms and complications, particularly in children. There is a strong immune reaction to *H nana* infection, which probably accounts for some of the complications and decreasing prevalence with age.

*H nana* was found in 1.5% of fecal specimens from subjects with gastrointestinal symptoms in the Rocky Mountain region of the United States. Infections occur more frequently in regions with temperate and tropical weather, especially where water and sanitation standards are suboptimal. *H nana* is especially prevalent in the southern part of the former Soviet Union, the Mediterranean, the Indian subcontinent, Africa, and South America. Children are more commonly infected than adults, with prevalence rates reaching 25%. High prevalence rates have been reported in institutionalized children because of fecal-oral transmission.

## CLINICAL MANIFESTATIONS

Data on the clinical manifestations of *H nana* are scarce, and most infections are thought to be asymptomatic or subclinical. However, several studies suggest that children with hymenolepiasis may be more likely to have diarrhea than uninfected children. Other symptoms reported are anorexia, abdominal pain, nausea, vomiting, dizziness, headache, and anal pruritus. Mild eosinophilia may be found with *H nana* infection but is uncommon. *Hymenolepis diminuta* infections are much less common than *H nana* infections, and the clinical differences between these parasites are not known.

## DIAGNOSIS

Routine fecal examinations using concentration techniques for ova and parasites should reveal eggs of *H nana* (Fig. 334-1) or, more rarely, *H diminuta* (Fig. 334-2). However, a single examination may not be

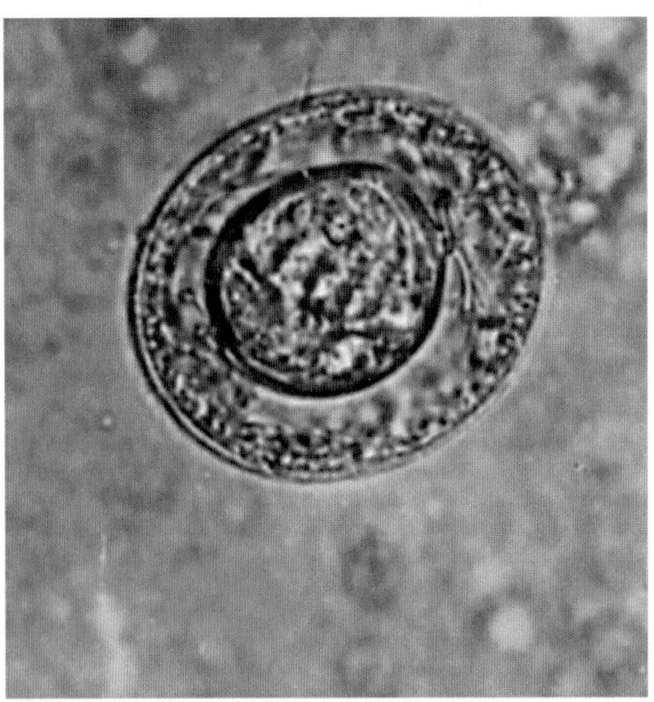

**FIGURE 334-1** *Hymenolepis nana egg recovered from feces. Note polar filaments (448×).*

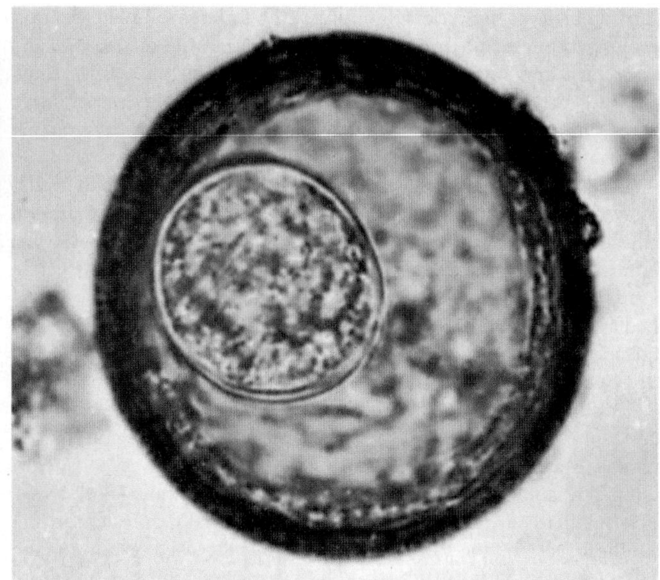

**FIGURE 334-2** *Hymenolepis diminuta* ovum is larger than *Hymenolepis nana*, and polar filaments are absent (448×).

adequate to rule out infection. Tapeworm segments (proglottids) are rarely found in stools since they disintegrate after breaking off from the tapeworm.

## TREATMENT

Praziquantel is the best drug for the treatment of hymenolepiasis. A single oral dose of 25 mg/kg is 100% effective. However, a second dose 10 to 15 days later seems to prevent relapses of hymenolepiasis. Nitazoxanide can be used as an alternative with slightly lower efficacy. Animal studies suggest that 3 doses of ivermectin are highly efficacious to treat *H nana* infection. Since it is common for several individuals within a household to be infected, fecal examinations should be performed on all household members before initiating treatment. Posttreatment fecal examinations should be done at least 1 month after treatment.

## SUGGESTED READINGS


Abdel Hamid MM, Eljack IA, Osman MK, Elaagip AH, Muneer MS. The prevalence of *Hymenolepis nana* among preschool children of displacement communities in Khartoum state, Sudan: a cross-sectional study. *Trav Med Infect Dis.* 2015;13:172-177.

Abrar Ul Haq K, Gul NA, Hammad HM, Bibi Y, Bibi A, Mohsan J. Prevalence of *Giardia intestinalis* and *Hymenolepis nana* in Afghan refugee population of Mianwali district, Pakistan. *Afr Health Sci.* 2015;15:394-400.

Church C, Neill A, Schotthoefer AM. Intestinal infections in humans in the Rocky Mountain region, United States. *J Parasitol.* 2010;96:194-196.

Foletto VR, Vanz F, Gazarini L, Stern CA, Tonussi CR. Efficacy and security of ivermectin given orally to rats naturally infected with *Syphacia* spp., *Giardia* spp. and *Hymenolepis nana*. *Lab Anim.* 2015;49:196-200.

Rohela M, Ngui R, Lim YA, Kalaichelvan B, Wan Hafiz WI, Mohd Redzuan AN. A case report of *Hymenolepis diminuta* infection in a Malaysian child. *Trop Biomed.* 2012;29:224-230.

Thompson RC. Neglected zoonotic helminths: *Hymenolepis nana*, *Echinococcus canadensis* and *Ancylostoma ceylanicum*. *Clin Microbiol Infect.* 2015;21:426-432.

Willcocks B, McAuliffe GN, Baird RW. Dwarf tapeworm (*Hymenolepis nana*): characteristics in the Northern Territory 2002-2013. *J Paediatr Child Health.* 2015;51:982-987.


# 335 Taeniasis and Cysticercosis

Walter Dehority and Gary D. Overturf

## INTRODUCTION

The pork tapeworm *Taenia solium* and the beef tapeworm *Taenia saginata* are the most common tapeworms of humans. The diseases associated with infection by these organisms have been known since ancient times, being found wherever insufficiently cooked pork or beef is eaten. Human infection with the larval stage of *T solium* (*Cysticercus cellulosae*), or cysticercosis, is found in places where adult *T solium* infection is common. *T saginata* infection occurs among those who eat raw or insufficiently cooked beef. As opposed to *T solium*, human infection with larval *T saginata* (*Cysticercus bovis*) almost never occurs. Both parasites are responsible for a tremendous burden of disease globally, with neurocysticercosis due to *T solium* being one of the most important causes of seizures worldwide.

## PATHOGENESIS AND EPIDEMIOLOGY

Humans are the mandatory definitive hosts who disseminate the organism to porcine or bovine intermediate hosts. Transmission to swine usually occurs through contaminated soil, where gravid proglottids are deposited with human feces. Eggs can survive for weeks in moist soil. In cattle, grazing lands, water, or cattle feed that is contaminated with infected human feces are sources of infection. Intrauterine infection of calves has been reported.

Adult worms live in the upper small intestine, with *T solium* measuring 2 to 8 m and *T saginata* measuring 3 to 10 m. The scolex of the pork tapeworm is distinguished by a crown or rostellum with a double row of hooklets. The scolex of *T saginata* is without hooks. The gravid uterus holds thousands of eggs, each with a mature 6-hooked (hexacanth) embryo. Eggs are 30 to 40 µm in diameter and similar in both human *Taenia* species. If the eggs are ingested by a suitable intermediate host such as swine (*T solium*) or cattle (*T saginata*), the embryo is liberated, penetrating the intestinal wall and disseminating via the bloodstream. The embryo of *T solium* may invade all tissues of the body and develop into a cysticercus or bladder worm. Cysticerci are ellipsoidal, white, translucent cysts into which the scolex is inverted. When infected meat is eaten, the cysticercus is activated by gastric juices and bile, which stimulate evagination of the scolex. The scolex attaches to the jejunal wall, and the embryo becomes a mature tapeworm in 10 to 12 weeks for *T saginata* and 5 to 12 weeks for *T solium*. In humans, eggs produced by this mature tapeworm are passed in feces and may be ingested by intermediate hosts (beginning the cycle anew) or ingested by other humans. Human disease is not always contracted through consumption of contaminated meat; transmission from close contacts who are tapeworm carriers that harbor eggs on their hands and fingernails may actually be a more common route. If ingested by humans, the larvae (termed *oncospheres*) escape from the egg and penetrate the duodenum, enter the lymphatic and vascular systems, and are widely disseminated throughout the body causing human *cysticercosis*, which is a serious and sometimes fatal disease. The larval stage may develop in every tissue of the body, a condition known as cysticercosis cellulosae. In tissue, the larvae cause an inflammatory infiltrate of eosinophils, plasma cells, neutrophils, and lymphocytes, with eventual necrosis, fibrosis, and subsequent calcification of the parasite.

Human infection with the pork tapeworm is uncommon in the United States and Canada, although larval infection (ie, cysticercosis) of swine may still occur. In many areas of the world, especially Mexico and parts of South and Central America, Africa, southeastern Europe, India, and China, infection with *T solium* is relatively common. In Mexico City, it accounts for as much as 10% of neurologic admissions and more than 25% of craniotomies; the prevalence in Mexico in the general population is approximately 4%. Cysticercosis is often observed in the United States, particularly in urban centers with large Latin American immigrant populations.

Autochthonous cases of neurocysticercosis have been reported in the United States.

However, because infections with *Taenia* species are not notifiable conditions in most states, the epidemiology of taeniasis in the United States is difficult to assess. Nonetheless, a recent analysis of national hospital discharge data from 2003 to 2012 identified 23,266 hospitalizations in the United States for neurocysticercosis. This was more than the 20,029 hospitalizations for 13 other neglected tropical diseases over the same time period combined. A total of 1493 neurocysticercosis admissions (8.0%) occurred in patients under the age of 20 years, with 74.0% of patients being Hispanic, 9.4% white, 5.5% African American, and 2.3% of Asian-Pacific Islander heritage. Neurocysticercosis in young children is less well described in the literature, with a 2013 review identifying only 27 reports in children under the age of 3 years.

## CLINICAL MANIFESTATIONS

Infection with the adult *T solium* or *T saginata* is either asymptomatic or associated with only mild or moderate complaints including spontaneous discharge of proglottids from the rectum (98%), abdominal pain (36%) or nausea (34%), weakness (25%), loss of appetite (21%) or increased appetite (17%), headache (15%), constipation (9%), dizziness (8%), diarrhea (6%), or pruritus ani (4%). Rarely, infection can cause serious, life-threatening disease by intestinal or appendiceal obstruction or by regurgitation and aspiration of a proglottid. Abdominal pain and nausea are most common in the morning and characteristically relieved by food. Children are more frequently symptomatic than adults. Eosinophilia occurs in 5% to 15% of cases.

Cysticerci have been found in almost every tissue and organ of the body. Small numbers of cysts in muscle or subcutaneous tissue may be of little consequence, but invasion of the eye, brain, or heart may be serious. Cysts are most common (in order of frequency) in subcutaneous tissues, eyes, and brain. Except in the eye, cysts usually provoke development of a fibrous capsule.

A 2013 systematic review of 21 articles encompassing 2312 patients with neurocysticercosis described seizures affecting 78.8% of all patients (78.9% of children) and headache present in 37.9% (27.7% of children). Less common clinical findings in children included cranial nerve palsies (6.0%), altered mental status (4.0%), visual changes (3.5%), and gait abnormalities/ataxia (2.4%). Sensory changes and fever are never present.

Neurocysticercosis may present as a leptomeningitis, resembling tuberculous meningitis, and may cause communicating hydrocephalus. Cysticerci may be present in the ventricles (most commonly the fourth ventricle) causing obstructive hydrocephalus. Cysts that are localized at various sites in brain parenchyma can remain silent for years, only to become evident when the cysts die, provoking an inflammatory response and edema. Cysts often calcify and may be found serendipitously. Spinal cord cysts present as transverse myelitis or arachnoiditis.

Cysts may be found asymptomatically in the vitreous, but if they occur in the retina, there may be visual impairment, scotoma, or retinal detachment. Cysticerci in the myocardium may cause arrhythmias and cardiac failure.

## DIAGNOSIS

Observation of gravid proglottids is required for a specific diagnosis; the presence of *Taenia* eggs in the stool is insufficient. Before initiating therapy, the species of *Taenia* must be identified because disseminated cysticercosis theoretically can be caused iatrogenically in individuals with *T solium* infection if, during therapy, they should regurgitate gravid proglottids into the upper gastrointestinal tract where gastric and duodenal fluids activate the ova.

The species of the proglottid can be identified by pressing the segment between 2 glass microscope slides and counting the main lateral branches of the uterus. *T solium* usually has 7 to 13 branches on each side; *T saginata* usually has 15 to 20 lateral branches on each side (Fig. 335-1). Fecal examination, especially with *T saginata* infection, often is unrewarding because intact gravid proglottids tend to be

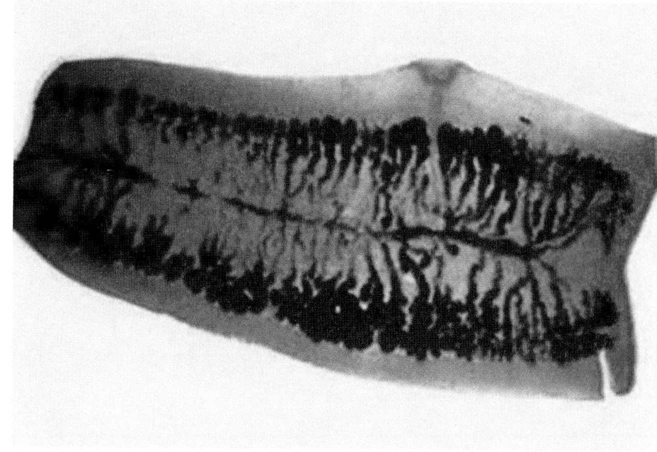

A

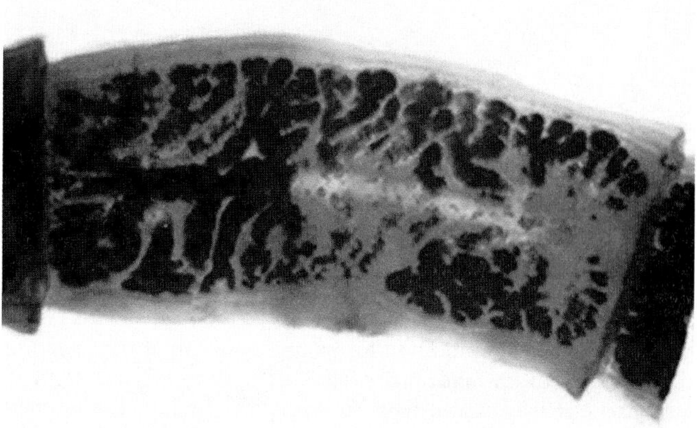

B

**FIGURE 335-1 A:** Mature proglottid of *T saginata*, stained with carmine. Note the number of primary uterine branches (> 12). **B:** Mature proglottid of *T solium*, stained with carmine. Note the number of primary uterine branches (< 13). (Reproduced with permission from Centers for Disease Control and Prevention.)

eliminated or crawl out onto the perianal area before they disintegrate and release their eggs. Thus, the perianal cellophane-tape method, similar to that used to diagnose pinworms, may be more effective for recovering *Taenia* ova.

Approximately 10% of patients with neurocysticercosis have eosinophilia. The findings on lumbar puncture are rarely helpful, and findings range from normal to isolated high protein levels with or without an inflammatory pleocytosis. Eosinophilia may be present occasionally in the cerebrospinal fluid (CSF). A lumbar puncture should not be done in the presence of suspected increased intracranial pressure.

Radiographic findings are often useful. Soft tissue radiographic studies may reveal characteristic numerous, tiny, curvilinear calcifications in the muscle. Magnetic resonance imaging (MRI) or computed tomography (CT) will demonstrate cysts in all stages in the meninges and parenchyma (Fig. 335-2). Contrast enhancement studies with metrizamide often are necessary to demonstrate isodense cysts in the ventricles.

In the past, enzyme-linked immunosorbent assay (ELISA) has been the most frequently used diagnostic method to detect cysticercus antibodies in both serum and CSF. This test can be highly sensitive but may cross-react with other helminth antibodies, especially *Echinococcus*. The enzyme-linked immunoelectrotransfer blot (EITB) is highly specific and sensitive, although sensitivity is low when fewer than 2 parenchymal cysts are present. In a series of children presenting with neurocysticercosis in the United States, fewer than 30% had positive EITB. Examination of the serum is more sensitive than the CSF. In patients with clinical and radiologic features of cysticercosis, negative

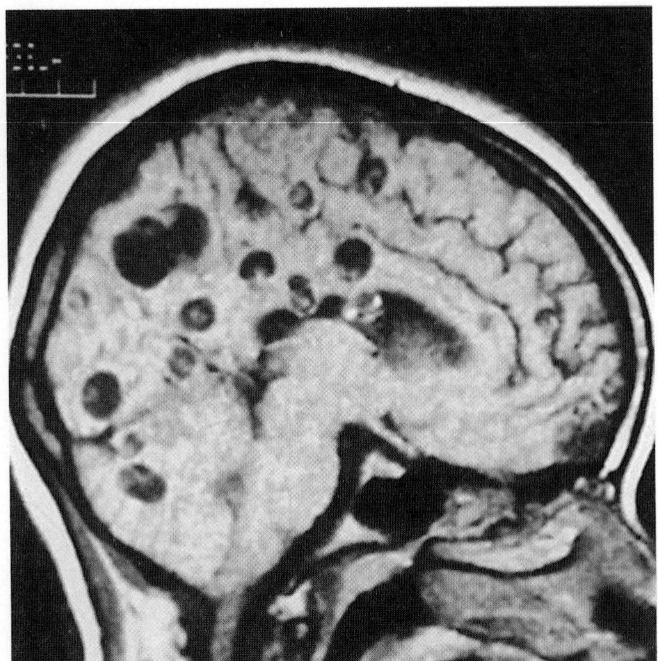

**FIGURE 335-2** Neurocysticercosis. Magnetic resonance image of several cysts, some showing a punctate, dense image corresponding to the scolex. (Used with permission from David Botero and JPS Nobrega, University of Sao Paulo, Brazil.)

serology may be an indication for biopsy, especially if the patient is from an area of low endemicity. Elevated titers in CSF are particularly useful if they exceed those in the serum. Highly positive titers are more often seen in individuals with hydrocephalus or meningeal involvement.

Symptomatology from intestinal infection with the adult tapeworm may be indistinguishable from other common gastrointestinal parasitic infections. Most commonly, the radiographic appearance of neurocysticercosis may mimic *Mycobacterium tuberculosis* infection of the central nervous system.

## TREATMENT

Adult tapeworm infections are treated successfully if the scolex is eliminated. An effective agent with few untoward effects is niclosamide, but this agent is not available in the United States and is approved only for treatment of *T saginata* infections. For *Taenia* infections, the single dose for adults is 2 g chewed thoroughly after a light meal. The WHO recommends a single 1-g oral dose of niclosamide for children > 6 years of age, and for children < 2 years of age 500 mg. For patients with *T solium* infection, therapy probably should be administered in the physician's office. An antiemetic may be administered 30 minutes before the antihelminthic. If the patient does not have a bowel movement within 2 hours, a mild saline purge should be provided. Alternatively, praziquantel is highly active against most tapeworm infections. It can be given in a single dose of 5 to 10 mg/kg in taeniasis.

Until recently, surgical intervention was the only definitive therapeutic option for the treatment of neurocysticercosis. Medical therapy remains controversial, as data from large, well-designed trials are lacking, particularly for the effect of different combinations of antihelminthics, steroids, and antiepileptic drugs at different stages of cyst development (eg, viable, degenerating, calcified). Currently, albendazole is the drug of choice; for children < 60 kg, the daily dose is 15 mg/kg in 2 divided doses for 7 to 28 days, while for children > 60 kg, the dose is 400 mg twice daily. In some studies, shorter courses have been as successful as longer courses of therapy. Corticosteroids (dexamethasone or prednisolone) may be given before and during therapy to ameliorate or attenuate symptoms associated with cyst death, ensuing inflammation, and possible cerebral edema. A 2013 meta-analysis of 5 randomized controlled trials demonstrated that, compared with placebo or no therapy, the use of corticosteroids in neurocysticercosis reduced the risk of seizure recurrence and persistent lesions 6 to 12 months after treatment. However, the quality of trials was poor, and trials evaluating antihelminthic therapy with or without steroids were not found. A 2010 Cochrane review of antihelminthics for neurocysticercosis analyzed data from 9 randomized controlled trials conducted in children (> 700 subjects total) with nonviable (dying) lesions and concluded that seizure recurrence was less common in children treated with albendazole when compared with children receiving no treatment (relative risk, 0.49; 95% confidence interval, 0.32–0.75). Currently, therapy is recommended for children with "active" cysts, indicated on CT as ring-enhancing lesions. Some physicians prefer to treat all children rather than waiting for the natural resolution of the cyst. Others recommend that children be treated only if they are symptomatic. It is uncertain whether children with few cysts, with or without seizures as the predominant symptom, will benefit from treatment. However, a 2013 meta-analysis of 10 randomized controlled trials (765 adults and children) demonstrated a significantly lower risk of seizures and a higher rate of lesion resolution 6 months after therapy with albendazole compared with no antihelminthic treatment in patients with solitary lesions. Controlled studies in children show approximately 50% reduction of cyst size at 3 months after treatment and a 3-fold reduction of seizures in albendazole-treated versus placebo-treated children. The 2013 American Academy of Neurology evidence-based guidelines for the treatment of intraparenchymal neurocysticercosis currently recommend consideration of treatment of intraparenchymal lesions in symptomatic children with albendazole and either dexamethasone or prednisolone. Hydrocephalus, which is a common complication of neurocysticercosis, can only be alleviated by the placement of a ventricular-peritoneal shunt. Intraventricular cysts will not respond to albendazole or praziquantel.

Seizures are not always relieved by treatment of the cysticercosis. Therefore, if a patient with cysticercosis is receiving anticonvulsive therapy, it should be continued and may be required indefinitely. A 2015 Cochrane Review (4 studies, 466 subjects) found no difference in the risk of recurrent seizures between subjects receiving antiepileptic drugs for 6, 12, or 24 months.

## PREVENTION

Given the status of humans as the definitive host for *T solium*, the presence of a domesticated animal as an indeterminate host (the pig, whose exposure to the parasite could theoretically be controlled), and the existence of effective therapies and diagnostic tests, *T solium* transmission could in theory be eradicated or at least controlled in many regions of the world. Avoiding consumption of raw or undercooked pork and beef, prompt diagnosis and treatment of infected individuals, and proper disposal of human waste, particularly near agricultural centers, are all important components of disease prevention.

## SUGGESTED READINGS

Abba K, Ramaratnam S, Ranganathan LN. Anthelmintics for people with neurocysticercosis. *Cochrane Database Syst Rev*. 2010;3:CD000215.

Baird RA, Wiebe S, Zunt JR, Halperin JJ, Gronseth G, Roos KL. Evidence-based guideline: treatment of parenchymal neurocysticercosis. *Neurology*. 2013;80:1424-1429.

Cuello-García CA, Roldán-Benítez YM, Pérez-Gaxiola G, Villarreal-Careaga J. Corticosteroids for neuorcysticercosis: a systematic review and meta-analysis of randomized controlled trials. *Int J Infect Dis*. 2013;17:e583-e592.

Del Brutto OH. Neurocysticercosis in infants and toddlers: report of seven cases and review of published patients. *Pediatr Neurol*. 2013;48:432-435.

Garcia HH, Gonzales I, Lescano AG, et al. Efficacy of combined antiparasitic therapy with praziquantel and albendazole for neurocysticercosis: a double-blind, randomized controlled trial. *Lancet Infect Dis*. 2014;14:687-695.

Garcia HH, Nash TE, Del Brutto OH. Clinical symptoms, diagnosis, and treatment of neurocysticercosis. *Lancet Neurol.* 2014;13:1202-1215.

Gulati S, Jain P, Sachan D, et al. Seizure and radiological outcomes in children with solitary cysticercosis granulomas with and without albendazole therapy: a retrospective case record analysis. *Epilepsy Res.* 2014;108:1212-1220.

O'Neal SE, Flecker RH. Hospitalization frequency and charges for neurocysticercosis, United States, 2003-2012. *Emerg Infect Dis.* 2015;21:969-977.

Otte WM, Singla M, Sander JW, Singh G. Drug therapy for solitary cysticercus granuloma: a systematic review and meta-analysis. *Neurology.* 2013;80:152-162.

Sharma M, Singh T, Mathew A. Antiepileptic drugs for seizure control in people with neurocysticercosis (review). *Cochrane Database Syst Rev.* 2015;10:CD009027.

# 336 Amebiasis

Haidee Custodio

## INTRODUCTION

Amebiasis denotes the disease caused solely by *Entamoeba histolytica*, although there are 2 other morphologically identical *Entamoeba* species that can also infect humans—*Entamoeba dispar* and *Entamoeba moshkovskii*. *E dispar* is about 10 times more prevalent than *E histolytica* in most endemic areas for amebiasis. Recent reports suggest that infection of *E moshkovskii*, which was once considered a free-living amoeba, is also common in some parts of the world such as Bangladesh, India, and Australia. Most cases of *E moshkovskii* infection occur concomitantly with *E dispar* or *E histolytica* infections. Free-living amoebic infections are discussed in Chapter 343.

## PATHOGENESIS AND EPIDEMIOLOGY

*E histolytica* is a protozoan with an invasive, motile trophozoite and infectious cyst stages that is responsible for person-to-person transmission of infection. The trophozoite varies in diameter from approximately 10 to 60 μm, has a clear ectoplasm, and a single nucleus. The cyst averages 12 mm in diameter and has 1 to 4 nuclei (Figs. 336-1 and 336-2). Humans are the only reservoir for *E histolytica*. Cysts that are passed in the feces of infected individuals survive in a moist environment for months. Following their ingestion in contaminated food or water, the cysts travel to the small intestine, the multinucleated metacystic amoeba is activated and emerges through a hole in the cyst wall, and immediately after excysting, it undergoes division into 8 uninucleate trophozoites. These organisms do not colonize the small intestine but are usually carried to the cecum where they become established. In 90% of patients, the trophozoites re-encyst and produce asymptomatic infection, which usually spontaneously resolves within 12 months. In 10% of patients, the parasite causes symptoms. Invasion of trophozoites then occurs, causing intestinal and hepatic abscesses.

Human and parasite genetic differences are likely to play important roles in determining the pathogenicity of infection. Certain human leukocyte antigen (HLA) class II alleles appear to provide independent leptin receptor polymorphisms and appear to provide protection against *E histolytica* infection. On the other hand, *E histolytica* genotypes have been shown to differ among those infected and presenting with no symptoms, diarrhea/dysentery, or liver abscess. A cell-mediated immune response is likely to be important in clearing established infection by generating interferon-γ and tumor necrosis factor-α to activate macrophages and neutrophils to kill the trophozoite. Hepatic lesions illustrate lytic destruction of the hepatic parenchyma with abscess formation. The smallest lesions can measure a few millimeters in diameter, whereas others can extend to destroy most of the liver.

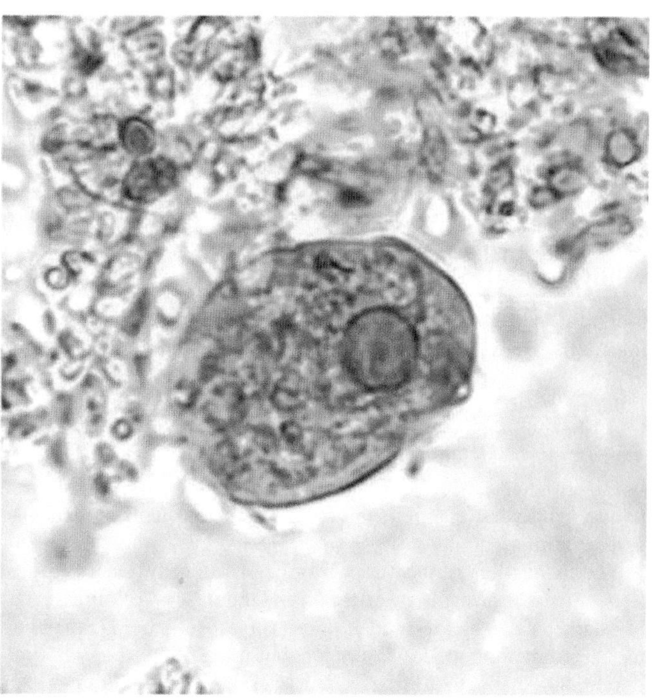

**FIGURE 336-1** Trophozoite of *Entamoeba histolytica/Entamoeba dispar* in direct wet mount stained with iodine. (Reproduced with permission from Centers for Disease Control and Prevention.)

Amebiasis occurs worldwide but is much more common in developing nations. This is a result of contaminated water or food, leading to fecal-oral spread of the cyst. The World Health Organization estimates that *E histolytica* is second only to malaria as a protozoan cause of death. The 1988 Mexican national serosurvey demonstrated serologic evidence of *E histolytica* infection in 8.4% of the population. Nearly half of the children surveyed in a refugee camp in Dhaka, Bangladesh, had evidence of infection by age 5. Amebic dysentery is most common in grade-school children. Amebic liver abscess is 10 times more common in men than in women, being most common in men between the ages of 20 and 50 years. This male sex predominance is not observed in

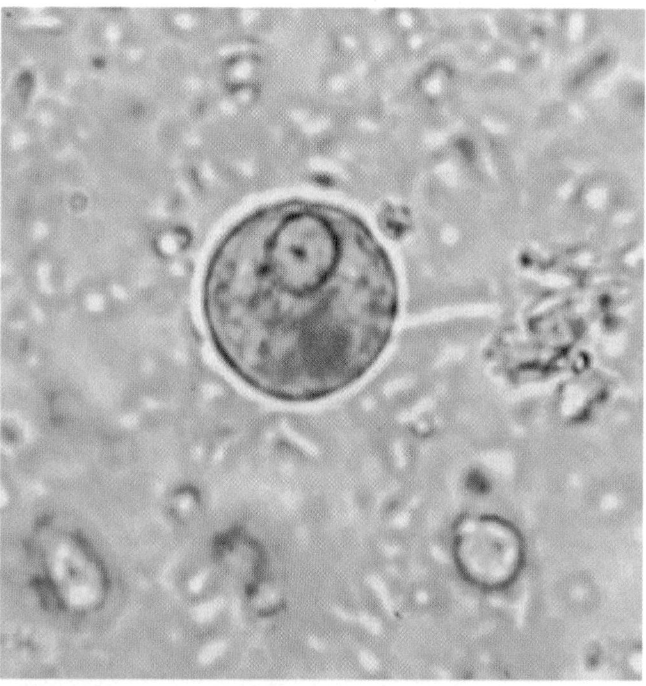

**FIGURE 336-2** Cyst of *Entamoeba histolytica/Entamoeba dispar* in a wet mount stained with iodine. (Reproduced with permission from Centers for Disease Control and Prevention.)

children. Steroid treatment and pregnancy appear to increase susceptibility to life-threatening infection.

In the United States, most infections occur in immigrants or in those who travel to developing countries. Amebic liver abscess may present clinically with symptoms more than 6 months after travel to an endemic area. Residents of institutions for the mentally challenged and human immunodeficiency virus (HIV)-infected individuals are also at greater risk of *E histolytica* infection.

## CLINICAL MANIFESTATIONS

Many infections with *E histolytica* and all *E dispar* or *E moshkovskii* infections are without symptoms. Asymptomatic individuals are referred to as carriers, or cyst passers. It is not unusual for a carrier of *E histolytica* to develop invasive amebiasis months later. Illness that is attributable to amebiasis can have an acute or gradual onset with mild to severe symptoms. Amebiasis occasionally can have a rapid, fulminant course. More often, there is a chronic course of a cyclical nature, consisting of mild symptoms, alternating with moderate to severe manifestations.

The incubation period varies from approximately 4 days to possibly years but is usually a week to several months. Severe disease may be characterized by the sudden onset of frequent, copious diarrhea, usually containing mucus and blood; but more often, the symptoms develop gradually, with irregular bouts of diarrhea, abdominal pain, nausea, and loss of appetite. Weight loss is seen in half of the patients. Erythrophagous trophozoites can be observed in the stool in as many as one-third of cases of amebic colitis. Low-grade fever and leukocytosis are present in less than one-half of patients. If the febrile reaction is marked or if there is considerable polymorphonucleocytosis, an amebic liver abscess should be considered. In severe intestinal disease, palpation of the abdominal wall will reveal exquisite tenderness along the portion of the involved large bowel. Colonoscopy often reveals discrete ulcers that vary in size from a pinhead to large, coalesced lesions with overhanging necrotic edges, but it is not unusual to see a diffusely inflamed mucosa resembling that of a nonspecific ulcerative colitis. Occasionally, the pathologic process extends through the serosa and leads to perforation. Disease may be limited to the cecum. Barium enema examination may be normal.

Amebomas most frequently occur in the cecum, although they have been reported in all parts of the colon. The basic lesion consists of a granulomatous thickening of the colon that results from lytic necrosis followed by secondary pyogenic inflammation, leading to fibrosis, proliferative granulation tissue, and focal abscesses. The lesion may be well localized and can be mistaken for a tumor, or the colonic wall may be extensively involved.

### Liver Abscess

Liver abscess is the most frequent complication of amebiasis. About one-third to almost one-half of patients have no history of diarrhea. Abscesses usually are found in the right lobe of the liver, although this location is not helpful for distinguishing amebic from pyogenic (bacterial) abscesses. Clinically, examination reveals an enlarged liver and tenderness in the right upper quadrant. Polymorphonuclear leukocytosis is usually greater than 12,000/μL, and there is moderate anemia. The erythrocyte sedimentation rate is elevated, and chills with daily remitting fever of 39°C (102.2°F) to 40°C (104°F) are frequent. Abnormalities on routine chest radiography have been reported in 25% to 90% of patients with amebic abscesses of the liver. Frequently, the right hemidiaphragm is elevated, which is of great diagnostic significance when present in the absence of a palpable hepatic mass. Furthermore, there may be consolidation at the base of the right lung or a right pleural effusion. At times, pain is referred to the right shoulder or the right lower quadrant of the abdomen.

Abscesses of the liver's left lobe may present as an epigastric mass that frequently is mistaken for a neoplasm. These may rupture intra-abdominally or into the pericardial sac with dire consequences. A hepatic abscess in the right lobe may extend through the diaphragm into the right chest cavity or the pulmonary parenchyma, subsequently rupturing and draining through a bronchus. Jaundice is seen in approximately 10% of amebic abscesses and usually is mild, but it can be severe with large abscesses. The serum alkaline phosphatase is moderately elevated in about two-thirds of abscesses in adults. Such elevations in children may be difficult to interpret.

### Primary Amebic Abscesses of the Lung and Brain

Primary amebic abscesses of the lung are rare. Lung involvement usually is secondary to hepatic abscess. Similarly, amebic brain abscesses are unusual and secondary to extraintestinal disease, especially hepatic, although several examples of direct hematogenous dissemination from the colon have been reported.

### Amebiasis of the skin

Amebiasis of the skin is usually secondary to perforation of the abdominal wall after an anterior amebic abscess ruptures. It also may occur when the rectum is perforated by a fistula or sinus tract that extends to the perineal skin, or it may occur as perianal extension of amebic colitis. These lesions may be extremely painful and are likely to become secondarily infected.

## DIAGNOSIS

Evaluation for amebic colitis should be considered in all patients with colitis in regions where amebiasis is common. Even in those patients with typical ulcers seen by colonoscopy, parasites may be found either in stool or upon biopsy of lesions.

Identifying *E histolytica* in stool requires a specific antigen detection or polymerase chain reaction (PCR) technique. Microscopy is an obsolete method that is unable to distinguish the more frequent nonpathogenic *E dispar* or *E moshkovskii* from *E histolytica*. In addition, microscopy misses up to two-thirds of the infections detected by antigen tests or PCR. A stool antigen detection test from TechLab (Blacksburg, VA) is the sole antigen detection test commercially available for the specific diagnosis of *E histolytica*. It has comparable sensitivity and specificity to PCR but is much less cumbersome to perform. The antigen detection test takes 2 hours to perform in an enzyme immunoassay (EIA) format and requires fresh (not formalin- or polyvinyl alcohol-fixed) stool samples. Real-time PCR also has a high sensitivity and specificity for diagnosis of *E histolytica, E dispar*, and *E moshkovskii*; however, it requires sophisticated equipment and experienced technicians to perform, which are often absent in many under resourced countries where these parasites are endemic.

Serologic tests are an important adjunct to antigen detection, especially in the case of amebic liver abscess when most such patients do not have detectable parasites in stool. Tests for antiamebic antibodies are approximately 90% sensitive for amebic liver abscess and 70% sensitive for amebic colitis. The serologic tests remain positive for years after an episode of amebiasis. As a result, a substantial number (between 10% and 35%) of residents of countries where amebiasis is endemic have antiamebic antibodies detected by current serologic tests.

Colonoscopy is preferable to sigmoidoscopy for the diagnosis of amebic colitis, because disease may be localized to the cecum or to the ascending colon. Wet preps of material scraped or aspirated from the base of ulcers should be examined for motile trophozoites. Biopsy specimens should be taken from the edge of the ulcers. Periodic acid-Schiff stains the parasites a magenta color and improves detection in biopsies.

Liver abscess usually is diagnosed by serologic tests in combination with a radiologic study (ultrasound, computed tomography [CT], or magnetic resonance imaging) that demonstrates a defect in the liver (Fig. 336-3). Amebic liver abscesses on CT scans are usually round, well-defined, and low-attenuation lesions. The wall commonly enhances with contrast. None of these characteristics is sufficiently specific to differentiate a pyogenic from an amebic liver abscess. Magnetic resonance imaging is not more helpful than CT scans in making the diagnosis of amebic liver abscess. Until more specific diagnostic techniques are developed, the diagnosis of amebic liver abscess relies on detecting the risk factors for *E histolytica* infection, a lesion in the liver, and a positive serologic test. Presence of *E histolytica* lectin antigen in sera and aspirates of liver abscess have been reported in patients with amebic liver abscess. However, prior antiamebic treatment with metronidazole significantly reduces the sensitivity of

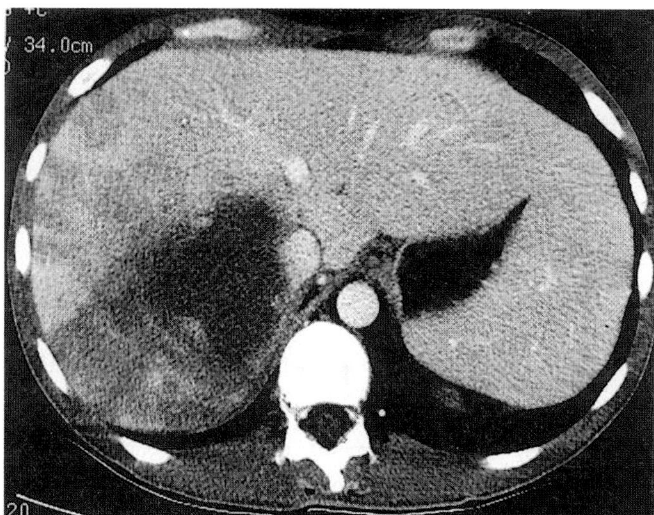


**FIGURE 336-3** Abdominal computed tomography of a large amebic abscess of the right lobe of the liver. (Used with permission from the Department of Radiology, University of California, San Diego.)

amebic antigen detection. Diagnostic aspiration under CT or ultrasonographic guidance may yield typical red-brown "anchovy paste" material, although the aspirate is more often yellow or gray-green. Typically, the aspirate is sterile (ie, no bacteria and no odor). This finding strongly suggests an amebic etiology for the abscess. Amoebae are infrequently seen by direct examination, but they often can be identified in the fluid by antigen detection or PCR.

## TREATMENT

Asymptomatic infection with *E histolytica* should be treated with a luminal agent alone; *E dispar* infection does not require treatment. Oral agents effective against luminal infection include diloxanide furoate (available only through the Centers for Disease Control and Prevention), paromomycin, and iodoquinol (see Table 318-4). Invasive amebiasis (eg, colitis, liver abscess) and moderate or severe intestinal disease should be treated with metronidazole or tinidazole for 10 days followed by a luminal agent; otherwise, patients are at risk of relapsing from residual infection in the intestine.

Paromomycin and diloxanide furoate are associated with primarily gastrointestinal side effects, including diarrhea, nausea, vomiting, and flatulence. Diloxanide furoate is also associated with urticaria and pruritus. Metronidazole and tinidazole have gastrointestinal side effects, including anorexia, nausea, vomiting, diarrhea, and abdominal discomfort. They also have an unpleasant taste and trigger a disulfiram-like intolerance reaction to alcohol.

Fever remits after 3 to 4 days of treatment with metronidazole in the majority of patients with amebic liver abscess. For the rare patient who does not respond to metronidazole alone, the addition of chloroquine and/or percutaneous drainage of the liver abscess are useful.

Antimotility drugs and corticosteroids should not be used as they can worsen the disease.

## PREVENTION

No vaccine is available, but prototype subunit vaccines are under study. Travelers to endemic areas should exercise caution by boiling drinking water, and foods that cannot be cooked should be peeled and washed. Household contacts of cases should be tested and treated if infected, even if they are asymptomatic.

## SUGGESTED READINGS

Ali IK. Intestinal amebae. *Clin Lab Med*. 2015;35:393-422.

American Academy of Pediatrics Committee on Infectious Diseases. Amebiasis. In: *Red Book: 2015 Report of the Committee on Infectious Diseases*. 30th ed. Elk Grove Village, IL: American Academy of Pediatrics; 2015:228-231.

Begum S, Quach J, Chadee K. Immune evasion mechanisms of *Entamoeba histolytica*: progression to disease. *Front Microbiol*. 2015;6:1394.

Gunther J, Shafir S, Bristow B, et al. Short report: amebiasis-related mortality among United States residents, 1990-2007. *Am J Trop Med Hyg*. 2011;85:1038-1040.

Hamzah Z, Petmitr S, Mungthin M, et al. Development of multiplex real-time polymerase chain reaction for detection of *Entamoeba histolytica*, *Entamoeba dispar*, and *Entamoeba moshkovskii* in clinical specimens. *Am J Trop Med Hyg*. 2010;83:909-913.

Kunwar R, Acharya L, Karki S. Trends in prevalence of soil-transmitted helminth and major intestinal protozoan infections among school-aged children in Nepal. *Trop Med Int Health*. 2016;21:703-719.

Mackey-Lawrence NM, Petri WA Jr. Amoebic dysentery. *BMJ Clin Evid*. 2013;2013:0918.

Nair GV, Variyam EP. Noninvasive intestinal amebiasis: *Entamoeba histolytica* colonization without invasion. *Curr Opin Infect Dis*. 2014;27:465-469.

Skappak C, Akierman S, Belga S, et al. Invasive amoebiasis: a review of *Entamoeba* infections highlighted with case reports. *Can J Gastroenterol Hepatol*. 2014;28:355-359.

# 337 Babesiosis

Peter J. Krause

## INTRODUCTION

Babesiosis is a malaria-like illness caused by intraerythrocytic protozoa that are transmitted by the bite of the same hard-bodied ticks (ixodid) that transmit Lyme disease and human granulocytic anaplasmosis. The disease is named after a European microbiologist, Victor Babes, who discovered the causative microorganism. *Babesia* species are parasites of mammals and birds that are currently classified in the subphylum Apicomplexa, together with those organisms that cause malaria (*Plasmodium* species) and toxoplasmosis (*Toxoplasma gondii*) (Fig. 337-1). Only a few of the more than 90 species of *Babesia* that have been described cause disease in humans, including *Babesia microti* from the United States, Asia, and Europe, *Babesia duncani* (WA1) from California and Washington state, MO1 from Missouri, *Babesia divergens* and *Babesia venatorum* from Asia and Europe, and KO1 from Korea.

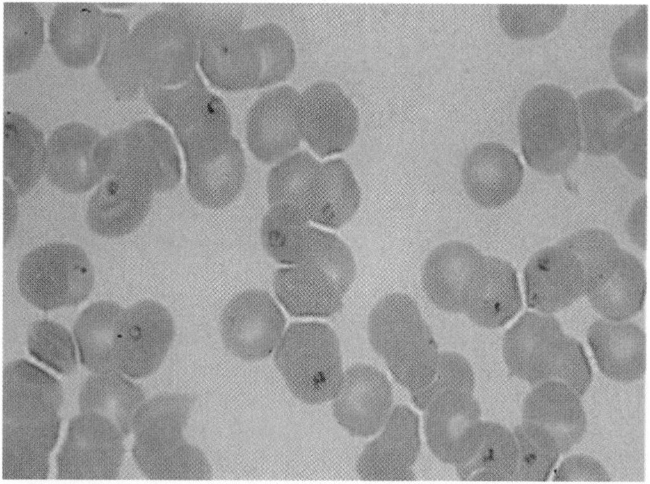

**FIGURE 337-1** Human erythrocytes infected by *Babesia microti* on a thin blood film (1000×).

## PATHOGENESIS AND EPIDEMIOLOGY

The pathogenesis of babesiosis in humans is not well understood. Similar to the *Plasmodium* species, *Babesia* species gain entry into the red blood cell, the organism multiplies into 4 daughter cells (merozoites), and these are released in an asynchronous fashion infecting new red blood cells. Red blood cell lysis is associated with many of the clinical manifestations associated with this disease. *Babesia* are usually found inside the red blood cells but can be demonstrated outside of the red blood cells in heavily parasitized patients. Disease probably results from excessive release of proinflammatory cytokines (eg, tumor necrosis factor) similar to patients with malaria. The spleen plays an important role in protection against *Babesia* species as it has long been recognized that patients without spleens have more severe disease. Most disease occurs in adults, although children seem to be equally susceptible. Almost all cases of disease in children have been reported in neonates, probably as a result of transplacental transmission of the organism or via blood transfusion.

Babesiosis has long been recognized as an economically important disease in livestock, but the first human case was not described until 1957. Over the past 60 years, the epidemiology of the disease has changed from a few isolated cases to the establishment of endemic areas in the northeastern and upper midwestern United States (Fig. 337-2) and in northeastern China, as well as reports from a wide geographic range in America, Africa, Asia, Australia, and Europe. The incidence of babesial infection is similar in children and adults. Human babesiosis is transmitted in the northeastern United States by deer ticks (*Ixodes scapularis*) that feed from infected animal reservoirs (primarily the white-footed mouse, *Peromyscus leucopus*). Nymphal ticks feed in the late spring and summer, and those that are infected transmit *B microti* to rodents or man. Consequently, most human cases of babesiosis occur in the summer. The white-tailed deer is an important host of the deer tick. The recent increase in the deer population is thought to be a major cause of the increased incidence of human babesiosis, anaplasmosis, and Lyme borreliosis. Babesiosis also may be acquired through blood transfusion or, rarely, through transplacental-perinatal transmission. *B microti* is the most common pathogen transmitted through the blood supply in the United States and is associated with a 20% mortality.

## CLINICAL MANIFESTATIONS

The clinical manifestations of babesiosis range from subclinical illness to fulminating disease resulting in death or prolonged convalescence. Symptoms begin after an incubation period of 1 to 6 weeks from the beginning of tick feeding. The unengorged *I scapularis* nymph is about 2 mm in length, and affected persons usually have no recollection of a tick bite. Typical symptoms include intermittent temperature to as high as 40°C (104°F) and 1 or more of the following: chills, sweats, myalgia, arthralgia, nausea, and vomiting. Other less common clinical manifestations are emotional lability and depression, hyperesthesia, headache, sore throat, abdominal pain, conjunctival injection, photophobia, weight loss, and nonproductive cough. While the number of symptoms appears to be similar in children and adults, the duration of symptoms and frequency of hospitalization are greater in adults over 50 years of age. Adults and children who are immunocompromised, especially those who lack a spleen or who have human immunodeficiency virus (HIV) or malignancy, are at increased risk of life-threatening disease. The babesiosis mortality rate in immunocompromised hosts may be as high as 20%. *B microti* may be co-transmitted with the agents causing Lyme disease and anaplasmosis, and this generally results in an increase in the number of symptoms and a longer duration of illness. Asymptomatic babesial infection may persist for months or even years and may result in disease recrudescence or transmission of babesiosis through blood donation.

## DIAGNOSIS

The diagnosis of babesiosis should be considered in any person experiencing fever who has been in an endemic area or who has received a blood transfusion. Specific diagnosis is best made by detecting the organism in red blood cells using Giemsa-stained thin blood

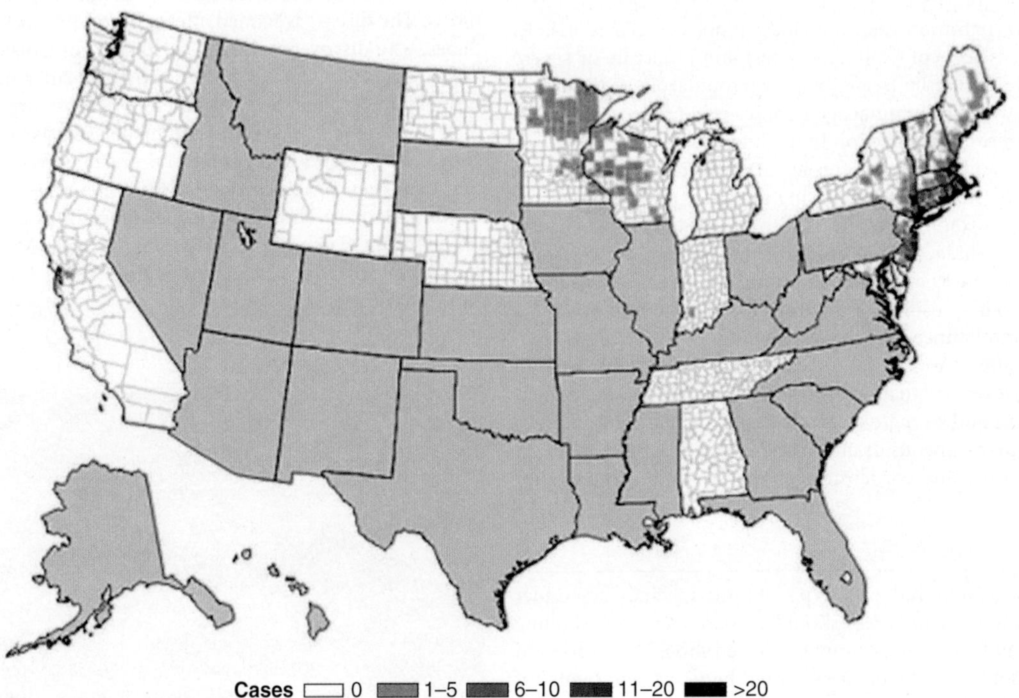


**FIGURE 337-2** Geographic distribution of human cases of babesiosis in the United States. Babesiosis became a nationally notifiable condition in January 2011. As of 2012, babesiosis is reportable in 22 states and the District of Columbia. The figure shows the incidence of babesiosis (number of cases per 100,000 persons) by county of residence in 2012. Human babesiosis caused by *Babesia microti* has long been reported from the Northeast, particularly from Massachusetts to New Jersey, and recently became endemic in northern New England (Maine and New Hampshire) and in the northern mid-Atlantic states (from Pennsylvania to Maryland). *B microti* also causes disease in the upper Midwest, particularly in Wisconsin and Minnesota. *Babesia duncani* has been the etiologic agent along the northwest Pacific Coast. Cases of *Babesia divergens*–like infection have been reported from Washington state, Kentucky, and Missouri. (Adapted with permission from the Centers for Disease Control and Prevention [CDC].)

smears. Severe cases usually are associated with intense parasitemia (10–50%), but parasitemia may be sparse (< 1%), especially early in the course of illness. Other means of detection include amplifying parasite DNA using polymerase chain reaction (PCR) and serology. PCR is highly sensitive and specific and can be rapidly performed; however, scrupulous technique must be maintained to prevent false-positive results. Serology also may help confirm a diagnosis of babesiosis when parasites are scarce or not detectable. A patient's serum often reacts at high titer during the acute illness. An indirect fluorescent antibody (IFA) titer of at least 1:64 generally is considered to be diagnostic. *B microti* antibody often is undetectable within a year or 2 after acute infection.

## TREATMENT

The combination of atovaquone (40 mg/kg/d divided every 12 hours orally [PO]) and azithromycin (12 mg/kg/d given every 24 hours PO) or clindamycin (20–40 mg/kg/d divided every 8 hours PO) and quinine (25 mg/kg/d divided every 8 hours PO) administered for 7 to 10 days should be used to treat babesiosis. Atovaquone and azithromycin are as effective as clindamycin and quinine for mild to moderate disease but are associated with a much lower rate of untoward reactions. Clindamycin and quinine remain the treatment of choice for severe disease. Treatment failures have been reported for both drug combinations in immunocompromised patients, and prolonged therapy in such cases may be necessary. Exchange blood transfusion should be used in the most severe infections, such as those with a high parasitemia (10% or higher), coma, hypotension, congestive heart failure, pulmonary edema, or renal failure. Partial or whole exchange transfusion can rapidly decrease the degree of parasitemia and remove toxic by-products of babesial infection.

## PREVENTION

Prevention of babesiosis can be accomplished by avoiding ticks and tick-infested areas during the transmission season. High-risk groups should be especially careful to avoid areas where deer ticks are found in abundance. When exposure is unavoidable in endemic areas, clothing that covers the lower part of the body should be worn. Tick repellants may be used on skin (DEET [*N,N*-diethyl-meta-toluamide]) or on clothing (eg, permethrine) as directed by the manufacturer. DEET should be used sparingly because of rare reports of serious neurologic complications resulting from excessive application, especially to the face, hands, or abraded skin. Removal of ticks from people and pets should be carried out using tweezers and gently retracting the tick. No data exist to recommend administration of prophylactic antibiotics after a tick bite to prevent babesiosis.

## SUGGESTED READINGS


Centers for Disease Control and Prevention. Babesiosis surveillance – 18 states, 2011. *Morb Mortal Wkly Rep*. 2012;61:505-509.

Diuk-Wasser M, Vannier E, Krause PJ. Coinfection by *Ixodes* tick-borne pathogens: ecological, epidemiological, and clinical consequences. *Trends Parasitol*. 2016;32:30-42.

Herwaldt BL, Linden JV, Bosserman E, Young C, Olkowska D, Wilson M. Transfusion-associated babesiosis in the United States: a description of cases. *Ann Intern Med*. 2011;155:509-519.

Joseph JT, Purtill K, Wong SJ, et al. Vertical transmission of *Babesia microti*, United States. *Emerg Infect Dis*. 2012;18:1318-1321.

Kumar P, Marshall BC, deBlois G, Koch WC. A cluster of transfusion-associated babesiosis in extremely low birthweight premature infants. *J Perinatol*. 2012;32:731-733.

Sanchez E, Vannier E, Wormser GP, Hu LT. Diagnosis, treatment, and prevention of Lyme disease, human granulocytic anaplasmosis, and babesiosis: a review. *J Am Med Assoc*. 2016;315:1767-1777.

Vannier EG, Diuk-Wasser MA, Ben Mamoun C, Krause PJ. Babesiosis. *Infect Dis Clin North Am*. 2015;29:357-370.

Wormser GP, Villfuerte P, Nolan SM, et al. Neutropenia in congenital and adult babesiosis. *Am J Clin Pathol*. 2015;144:94-96.




# 338 Balantidiasis

Camille Sabella

## INTRODUCTION

*Balantidium coli* is the largest protozoan parasite to cause infection in humans. Balantidiasis is a zoonotic infection found in pigs, rodents, cattle, reptiles, birds, fish, annelids, arthropods, and many simian hosts. Domestic pigs are the most important reservoir host and typically the source of human infection. Malnourished individuals and those suffering from concurrent infection are at greater risk of developing balantidiasis.

## PATHOGENESIS AND EPIDEMIOLOGY

The parasite has 2 stages in its life cycle: the trophozoite and the cyst. The cyst is the resting, resistant stage and is the infectious ingested form. The trophozoite form causes manifestations of infection. The cysts are spherical or ovoid with a diameter of 40 to 60 μm and remain viable at room temperature for at least 2 weeks, particularly if kept moist and away from direct sunlight. The motile trophozoite is the form for division. Its shape and size vary with the amount of ingested food, from 30 to 300 μm in length and 30 to 100 μm in width.

Transmission of the parasite occurs by ingestion of cysts. Following ingestion, excystation occurs in the small intestine with the resultant trophozoites colonizing the large intestine. The trophozoites replicate by binary fission and produce infectious cysts, which pass in the stool. Trophozoites may invade the wall of the large intestine or remain in the lumen and disintegrate. In most instances, they fail to cause any signs or symptoms. The parasite feeds upon bacteria and debris in the gut, but also releases enzymes (hyaluronidase) that attack the mucosal surface.

Balantidiasis occurs worldwide but is most prevalent in tropical and subtropical regions and in resource-poor countries, which is a reflection of poor sanitation and inadequate protection of the water supply from sewage contamination. Domestic and wild swine represent a reservoir for human infections. Infection occurs when fecal material from swine contaminates drinking water or food. A relatively high prevalence has been found in New Guinea, southern Iran, South and Central America, central Asia, the Philippines, and some Pacific Islands.

Several cofactors are involved in the pathogenesis of this disease, including the intrinsic virulence of the strain and the host's susceptibility. Symptomatic infection may be observed in cases of malnutrition, alcoholism, hypochlorhydria, and immunodeficiency.

## CLINICAL MANIFESTATIONS

Asymptomatic cyst excretion is the most common outcome of infection. In some patients, the trophozoites invade the mucosa and cause acute colitis, which results from the presence of large ulcerative lesions similar to those produced by *Entamoeba histolytica*. As the trophozoites multiply by binary fission in the mucosa and submucosa, adjacent lesions may anastomose with one another, and the ulcers often extend deeply into the muscularis. Fortunately, perforation or extraintestinal invasion rarely ensues.

Acute colitis may manifest as mild to severe diarrhea that contains mucus and blood, abdominal pain, nausea, vomiting, and often tenesmus. Secondary infection of the colonic lesions by bacteria can worsen the clinical picture. The disease most commonly is self-limiting, with spontaneous eradication and healing. Rarely, chronic infection can ensue and manifests as constipation alternating with bloody diarrhea. Rare complications include typhlitis and perforation of the large intestine. The infection may rarely involve the small intestine, appendix, vagina, uterus, and bladder and, on very rare occasions, may disseminate to the liver and lungs.

## DIAGNOSIS

The diagnosis of balantidiasis rests on finding the characteristic cysts or trophozoites on stool examinations. Trophozoites are short-lived; they will disintegrate unless stool specimens are examined promptly.

Diagnosis is also made by visualizing the organisms in scrapings taken from the periphery of ulcers; by irrigating over an ulcer at colonoscopy and examining aspirated irrigate; or by endoscopic biopsy of an ulcer. The organism is relatively easy to recognize in clinical specimens due to their large size, an outer membrane covered by short cilia, and a single, large kidney bean–shaped nucleus. A history of contact with pigs (eg, farmers, veterinarians, slaughterhouse personnel) is helpful in making the diagnosis.

The differential diagnosis of balantidiasis includes amebic colitis, bacterial causes of colitis, giardiasis, cryptosporidiosis, and inflammatory bowel disease. The appearance and size of the *B coli* trophozoites can help distinguish them from amebic colitis. Appropriate stool culture and antigen detection techniques can help exclude bacterial and other protozoal causes of gastroenteritis.

## TREATMENT

Treatment with a tetracycline product is effective therapy for symptomatic patients. Children less than 8 years of age can be treated with metronidazole, which has been used successfully in children and adults (35–50 mg/kg/d in 3 doses for 5 days; maximum dose 750 mg 3 times a day). Alternatively, iodoquinol may be used (650 mg 3 times a day for 20 days in adults and 40 mg/kg/d in 3 divided doses for 20 days [maximum 2 g/d] in children).

## PREVENTION

Reducing contamination of food and water supplies and human contact with pig feces is the most effective method of prevention.

## SUGGESTED READINGS


American Academy of Pediatrics Committee on Infectious Diseases. *Balantidium coli* infections (balantidiasis). In: *Red Book: 2015 Report of the Committee on Infectious Diseases*. 30th ed. Elk Grove Village, IL: American Academy of Pediatrics; 2015:260.

Bellanger AP, Scherer E, Cazorla A, Grenouillet F. Dysenteric syndrome due to *Balantidium coli*: a case report. *New Microbiol.* 2013;36:203-205.

Hechenbleikner EM, McQuade JA. Parasitic colitis. *Clin Colon Rectal Surg.* 2015;28:79-86.

Sandoval NR, Rios N, Mena A, et al. A survey of intestinal parasites including associated risk factors in humans in Panama. *Acta Trop.* 2015;147:54-63.

Schuster FL, Ramirez-Avila L. Current world status of *Balantidium coli*. *Clin Microbiol Rev.* 2008;21:626-638.


# 339 *Blastocystis hominis*

Vidit Bhargava and Lemuel O. Aigbivbalu

## INTRODUCTION

*Blastocystis hominis* continues to be a subject of controversy. It is the most common single-celled organism detected in human stool samples worldwide. Long considered a protozoan of worldwide distribution, this strict anaerobe has been classified by small subunit rRNA gene analysis into the heterogeneous group of protists, the Stramenopiles, which also includes diatoms and brown algae (kelp). It is most likely an amoeba.

## PATHOGENESIS AND EPIDEMIOLOGY

To date, as many as 17 subtypes of *Blastocystis* species have been isolated. Prevalence greater than 5% in better-resourced countries and as high as 76% in under-resourced countries has been reported. The life cycle of *B hominis* has not been elucidated clearly. Infectivity studies in mice have shown that transmission occurs via the fecal-oral route by a cyst form. These cysts multiply in the epithelial cells of the digestive tract to form vacuolar and amoeboid forms. The vacuolar forms multiply by binary fission and other modes such as budding and ultimately undergo encystment to form the infective cysts, which are shed in the feces of the host. *Blastocystis* may exert its pathologic effects via increasing intestinal permeability, epithelial barrier degradation, and cytokine release from colonic cells, although controversy still exists regarding its exact mechanism. Asymptomatic infection is common; however, some *B hominis* subtypes cause disease rather than colonization when present in large numbers in the absence of other stool pathogens. Others consider *B hominis* an enteric commensal and ascribe response to treatment as elimination of other undetected stool pathogens or resolution of noninfectious etiology. Others suggest it is an opportunistic pathogen.

## CLINICAL MANIFESTATIONS

The most commonly reported symptoms are nonspecific: nausea, mild diarrhea, vomiting, flatulence, and abdominal cramping. Fever, weight loss, and stools with blood, mucus, or leukocytes are uncommon. The ability to cause invasive disease is controversial. Controlled studies fail to confirm a true pathogenic role, although this confusion may be attributed to pathogenic and nonpathogenic ribodeme types, similar to *Entamoeba histolytica* and *Entamoeba dispar*. However, it is also difficult to generate valid control groups, because most stools submitted are obtained from symptomatic patients.

## DIAGNOSIS

Diagnosis can be made by visualization of cysts by direct microscopy and with special stains such as Lugol's iodine and trichome staining of stool specimens (Fig. 339-1). Identification by trichome staining is limited by the organism's great morphologic diversity and the time-consuming nature of the staining procedure. Other diagnostic approaches used to detect the organism in human stool include in vitro culture, indirect fluorescent antibody, host serologic response (enzyme-linked immunosorbent assay), and more recently, polymerase chain reaction (PCR). In vitro culture is considered to be the gold standard for diagnosis of *B hominis*. However, direct fluorescent antibody testing is reported to be rapid, practical, and equally sensitive to culture methods. PCR can detect subtypes of isolate; however, it is extremely costly and nonstandardized.

## TREATMENT

In most patients, adult or pediatric, immunocompetent or immunosuppressed, symptoms resolve spontaneously. Treatment is usually recommended for symptomatic patients in whom other stool pathogens (parasites, bacteria, viruses) and noninfectious etiologies have been ruled out and if the symptoms are protracted with *B hominis* being found in multiple stool specimens. Successful treatment is defined as the complete resolution of symptoms reported by the patient and disappearance of *Blastocystis* in the stool. The drugs of choice for eradication of *Blastocystis* are metronidazole and trimethoprim-sulfamethoxazole. Other drugs that may be used include nitazoxanide, tinidazole, iodoquinol, and paromomycin at antiprotozoan doses.

## PREVENTION

Interventions focused on providing clean water and sanitation along with good hygiene are important in limiting protozoan spread.

## SUGGESTED READINGS


Clark CG, van der Giezen M, Alfellani MA, Stensvold CR. Recent developments in *Blastocystis* research. *Adv Parasitol.* 2013;82:1-32.

Elghareeb AS, Younis MS, El Fakahany AF, Nagaty IM, Nagib MM. Laboratory diagnosis of *Blastocystis* spp. in diarrheic patients. *Trop Parasitol.* 2015;5:36-41.

Kurt Ö, Doğruman Al F, Tanyüksel M. Eradication of *Blastocystis* in humans: really necessary for all? *Parasitol Int.* 2016;65(6 pt B):797-801.

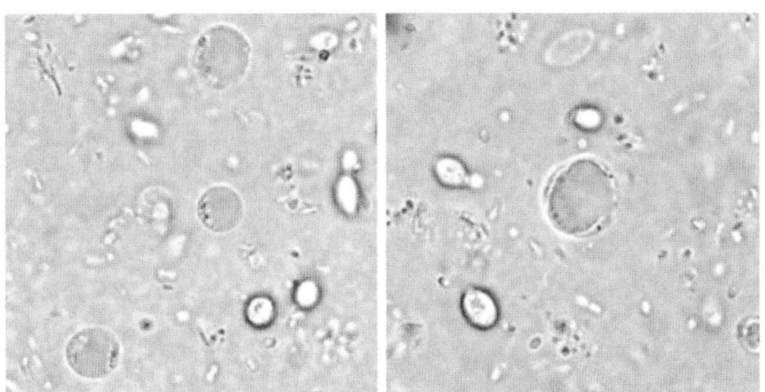
A

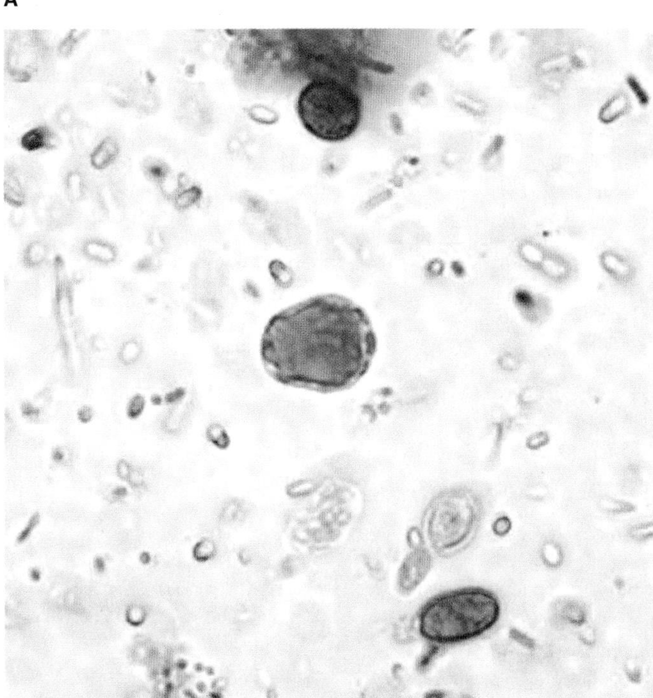
B

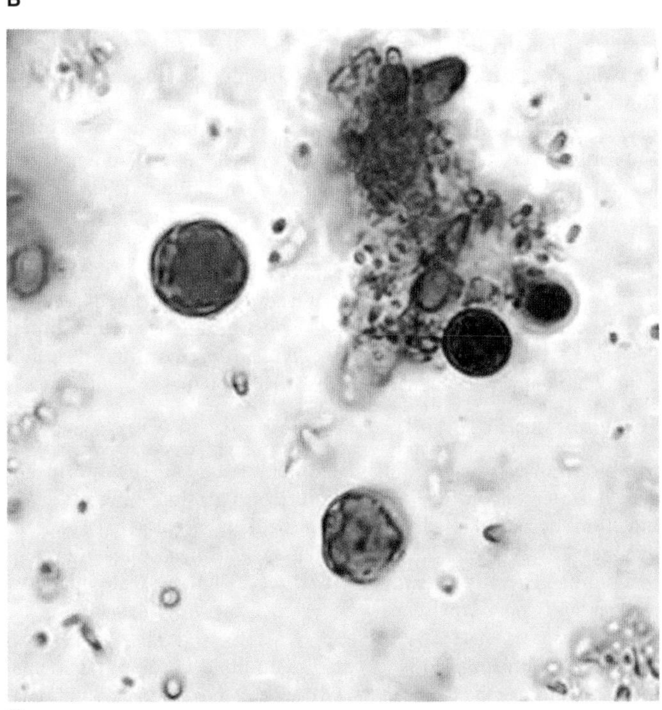
C

**FIGURE 339-1** **A:** *Blastocystis hominis* cyst-like form in a wet mount, unstained. **B:** *B hominis* cyst-like form in a wet mount, stained in iodine. **C:** *B hominis* cyst-like forms undergoing binary fission, stained in iodine. (Reproduced with permission from Centers for Disease Control and Prevention [CDC].)


Parija SC, Jeremiah S. *Blastocystis*: taxonomy, biology and virulence. *Trop Parasitol.* 2013;3:17-25.

Roberts T, Stark D, Harkness J, Ellis J. Update on the pathogenic potential and treatment options for *Blastocystis* sp. *Gut Pathog.* 2014; 6:17.

Speich B, Croll D, Furst T, Utzinger J, Keiser J. Effect of sanitation and water treatment on intestinal protozoa infection: a systematic review and meta-analysis. *Lancet Infect Dis.* 2016;16:87-99.




# 340 Cryptosporidiosis

Haidee Custodio

## INTRODUCTION

*Cryptosporidium* species are tiny (2–6 μm), obligate intracellular parasites related to other coccidian protozoan, including *Toxoplasma, Cyclospora, Isospora, Plasmodium, Eimeria*, and *Sarcocystis. Cryptosporidium* species primarily infect the gastrointestinal tract of a variety of vertebrate hosts, including humans. Host range is largely a function of species, as a given species of parasite most efficiently maintains infection within a few species of hosts.

## PATHOGENESIS AND EPIDEMIOLOGY

*Cryptosporidium* completes its life cycle within a single host (Fig. 340-1). Infection occurs after ingesting the sporulated, thick-walled oocysts. Excystation occurs in the small intestine after exposure to bile salts and pancreatic enzymes, releasing 4 sporozoites. These sporozoites penetrate a surface epithelial cell in the intestinal mucosa and form an intracellular parasitophorous vacuole. They then differentiate into uninuclear trophozoites, which undergo asexual replication (merogony) to form type I meronts. The type I meront can then autoinfect other surface epithelial cells or differentiate into a type II meront. The type II meront then undergoes gametogomy, producing both microgametocytes and macrogametocytes. These gametocytes fertilize to produce oocysts. The life cycle is complete when the oocysts undergo sporogomy, resulting in infectious sporozoites within the oocysts. Approximately 80% of the oocysts produced in this fashion are environmentally resistant, thick-walled cysts that are excreted in the feces. The remaining 20% are thin-walled cysts that undergo another autoinfective stage. The autoinfectious stages are important features in the parasite's life cycle and account for persistent and occasionally severe disease, even when a low inoculum of cysts is ingested.

The principal mode of transmission is fecal-oral, through either a waterborne or person-to-person route. The median infectious dose has been estimated at 132 oocysts, although disease can occur with ingestion of as few as 10 oocysts. Infectious dose tends to be lower with *Cryptosporidium hominis*. Infected individuals may shed oocysts for up to 5 weeks after an acute diarrheal episode.

In the immunocompetent host, *Cryptosporidium* primarily infects the proximal small bowel. The exact mechanism whereby *Cryptosporidium* causes diarrhea is unknown. The organism disrupts epithelial tight junctions in several in vitro epithelial cell models, resulting in a loss of barrier function. Pathologic findings include loss of intestinal epithelium, villous atrophy with loss of epithelial architecture and surface area, and infiltration of the lamina propria with mononuclear and polymorphonuclear cells. Various stages of the parasite can be seen immediately below the brush border of epithelial cells in biopsy samples.

The mechanisms of recovery and immunity to cryptosporidiosis has not been fully elucidated. An intact cell-mediated immune system with CD4 lymphocytes and interferon is crucial for recovery from disease. Animal models support a pivotal role of interferon (IFN)-γ, with IFN-γ knockout models developing severe infections that proceed to chronic forms. Humoral immunity is not completely protective but

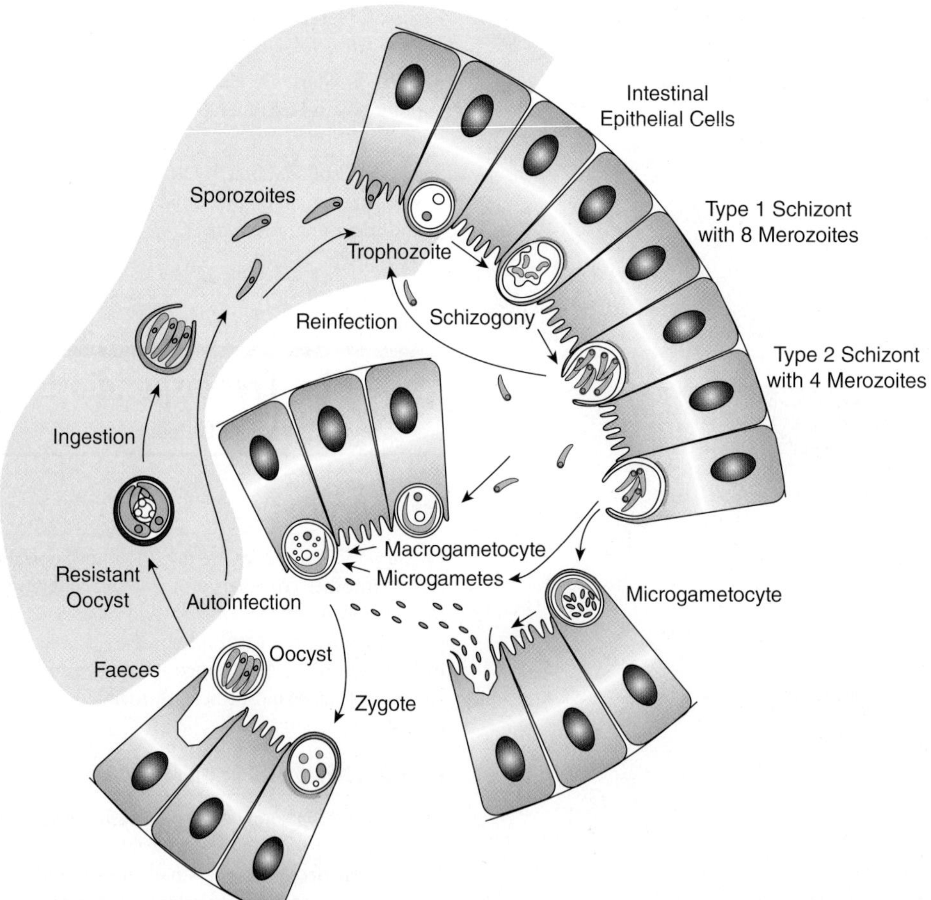


**FIGURE 340-1** *Cryptosporidium* life cycle. (Reproduced with permission from Smith HV, Nichols RA, Grimason AM: Cryptosporidium excystation and invasion: getting to the guts of the matter, *Trends Parasitol.* 2005 Mar;21(3):133-142.)

does decrease the severity of illness and shedding of oocysts. Secretory antibodies are beneficial, as is hyperimmune colostrum.

Over 20 species of *Cryptosporidium* have been described. Two species, *C hominis* and *Cryptosporidium parvum*, account for nearly all of the diseases caused by *Cryptosporidium* species in humans and are the species of public health significance. Humans are the only known reservoir of *C hominis*, whereas *C parvum* affects other vertebrate animals as well as humans.

Cryptosporidia are ubiquitous in the environment and are found in several sources of untreated surface water. The prevalence of disease is higher in developing countries due to less sanitary conditions that promote fecal-oral transmission and the lack of safe water sources. The seroprevalence in developing countries is as high as 75% by age 4, in contrast to the United States, where seroprevalence is approximately 15%. *Cryptosporidium* is 1 of the 4 major pathogens causing moderate to severe diarrhea in children in Africa and Asia irrespective of human immunodeficiency virus (HIV) prevalence. Afflicted infants are at highest risk for death.

Cryptosporidiosis is more common in children than adults. Daycare attendance is a risk factor, and outbreaks have been reported in childcare settings, likely through secondary person-to-person transmission. Travelers to developing countries are at particular risk.

During the acquired immunodeficiency syndrome (AIDS) epidemic, cryptosporidia were recognized as a significant enteric pathogen, causing severe disease in patients with advanced AIDS. Studies show that the incidence of AIDS-associated cryptosporidiosis has declined with the advent of highly active antiretroviral therapy (HAART) in resourced countries.

The oocyst is particularly resistant to disinfectants, including chlorine, bleach, ethanol, and many other hospital, industrial, and household chemicals. However, 6% hydrogen peroxide is an effective cysticide. The resistance to disinfectants coupled with the low infectious dose makes the organism a public health threat and a potential bioterrorism agent; furthermore, it allows for effective waterborne transmission. *Cryptosporidium* is resistant to standard chlorine concentrations in public water systems, and it often escapes filtration systems. The largest waterborne outbreak occurred in 1993 in Milwaukee, Wisconsin, with approximately 400,000 people infected and 69 deaths. As is the case with most diarrheal illnesses, morbidity and productivity loss substantially outpaced mortality.

Airborne transmission has been suggested but not definitively demonstrated. Isolated pulmonary cryptosporidiosis has been described in a case report, although it nearly always occurs in severely immunosuppressed patients with concomitant gastrointestinal disease. Occupational exposure to *C parvum* occurs in farmers and animal handlers, particularly those exposed to cattle.

## CLINICAL MANIFESTATIONS

Symptoms of cryptosporidiosis begin between 2 and 10 days (mean, 7 days) after becoming infected with the parasite. Asymptomatic infection occurs. However, affected patients usually have watery diarrhea. In other cases, vomiting, nausea, and malaise may develop. Symptoms generally persist for 1 to 2 weeks. Occasionally, patients recover and then experience a recurrence of symptoms before the illness ends.

Severe cryptosporidiosis occurs in immunosuppressed patients, including those with advanced AIDS, cancer, hypogammaglobulinemia, severe combined immunodeficiency, and bone marrow and solid organ transplants. Such patients may have severe, life-threatening illness with intractable diarrhea and severe volume loss. Symptoms often last for months to years; wasting, hypovolemia, and weight loss are common. In general, the severity of the diarrheal illness correlates with the severity of immunosuppression.

Children with underlying malnutrition tend to have prolonged episodes of disease with growth shortfalls. Multiple diarrheal episodes in early childhood have been associated with decreased height-for-age scores and decreased cognition and language skills, particularly semantic fluency.

In immunocompromised patients, fluid loss can be massive and can exceed 10 to 20 L/d. Parenteral hydration is usually required to maintain euvolemia in the immunosuppressed host. Other clinical findings include fever, nausea, vomiting, and crampy abdominal pain. Myalgia, malaise, headache, and other flulike symptoms have also been reported.

Extraintestinal infection with *Cryptosporidium* is rare and usually occurs only in severely immunocompromised hosts. In particular, advanced AIDS is associated with biliary cryptosporidiosis, which results in AIDS cholangiopathy. This is due to the synergistic interaction of HIV and *Cryptosporidium* infection, whereby the HIV Tat-1 protein enhances *Cryptosporidium*-induced apoptosis in cholangiocytes. Biliary cryptosporidiosis manifests as acalculous cholecystitis, sclerosing cholangitis, and hepatitis. The clinical presentation includes fever, upper right quadrant pain, jaundice, nausea, vomiting, diarrhea, hyperbilirubinemia, and elevated liver enzymes. Radiographically, the disease resembles sclerosing cholangitis. Pancreatic cryptosporidiosis may also occur.

Respiratory cryptosporidiosis is a rare event and nearly always requires concomitant intestinal disease. It manifests as cough, shortness of breath, wheezing, croup, and hoarseness. Diagnosis is made through isolation of oocysts from sputum or tracheal aspirates.

## DIAGNOSIS

Newer techniques using antigen detection, such as direct fluorescent antibody (DFA) assay and enzyme immunoassays (EIA), and polymerase chain reaction (PCR)-based molecular testing enhance the sensitivity to more than 90% in detecting *Cryptosporidium* in the stool compared with microscopy. Specificity is also high. Rapid tests using immunochromotography lateral flow assays maintain high sensitivity and specificity, are easy to perform, have rapid turnaround time, and require less technical skills compared to microscopy. These tests are becoming widely popular and preferable.

Microscopic examination to identify the characteristic oocysts in the stool may be performed using a modified acid-fast stain or trichrome stain. Sensitivity is low and can miss half of cases. The diagnosis is almost never made on routine ova and parasite stool examination. Concentration techniques with Sheather's sugar solution or zinc sulfate improve the recovery of the parasite.

Extraintestinal cryptosporidiosis remains an elusive diagnosis and requires demonstration of the parasite from an extraintestinal source. This is usually accomplished via biopsy, with the parasite appearing on light microscopy with hematoxylin-eosin stains or electron microscopy. Pulmonary cryptosporidiosis may be diagnosed by finding oocysts in tracheal secretions; however, in the absence of pulmonary biopsy, contamination from swallowed gastrointestinal secretions remains a possibility. However, extraintestinal disease is unlikely in the absence of more easily documented intestinal infection.

## TREATMENT

Placebo-controlled studies have demonstrated that nitazoxanide (> 12 years of age, 500 mg; 4–11 years of age, 200 mg; 1–3 years of age, 100 mg, all twice daily for 3 days) leads to more rapid cessation of diarrhea and more frequent eradication of the organism compared to placebo in HIV-negative adults and children. In severely malnourished children with chronic cryptosporidiosis, cure rates were lower but many cases resolved with retreatment.

In patients with HIV, higher doses or more prolonged therapy (2 weeks) were superior to placebo among those with CD4+ T-cell counts greater than 50/μL but were not better than placebo in those with lower CD4+ counts.

Paromomycin and azithromycin also have in vitro activity against the parasite. Paromomycin in combination with azithromycin has been shown to be effective in case series that largely originate from the pre-HAART AIDS era. Hyperimmune bovine colostrum reduces clinical symptoms and shedding of oocysts, but this is considered experimental therapy.

The cornerstone of therapy in immunosuppressed hosts is restoring immune function. In patients with AIDS, this is accomplished via combined antiretroviral therapy (cART), which serves 2 roles: (1) the restoration of CD4 count allows the host to respond to and eliminate infection, and (2) some cART drugs, particularly protease inhibitors, may have some in vitro activity against the parasite. The clinical relevance of the in vitro activity of protease inhibitors against *Cryptosporidium* is unknown. In bone marrow and solid organ transplant patients, decreasing immune suppression, if possible, greatly enhances cure rates.

Rehydration is also crucial, as large volume of fluid loss is a frequent complication of disease. This often requires parenteral fluid supplementation. Peptidomimetic agents (octreotide and vapreotide) and antimotility agents (loperamide, opiates, and atropine) may help control diarrheal symptoms.

In cases of biliary cryptosporidiosis in severely immunocompromised individuals, drug therapy has been effective. Endoscopic decompression of the biliary system and stenting are helpful in cases of sclerosing cholangitis.

## PREVENTION

Decreasing exposure to oocysts is crucial for immunosuppressed populations and is sensible for immunocompetent populations. Exposure largely occurs through a waterborne source, so all potentially contaminated water must be treated before consumption. Unfortunately, standard chlorination has no effect on oocysts, and even iodine-based water-purification tablets are modestly effective at best. The most reliable way to purify surface water sources involves boiling it for at least 1 minute, which thoroughly inactivates most pathogens, including *Cryptosporidium*. Boiling, however, is labor intensive and time consuming and not often done. Filters with resolutions of less than 1 μm are theoretically effective but are easily clogged and may be bypassed if damaged. In general, immunosuppressed persons should be advised to avoid all untreated surface water sources and potentially risky activities such as camping. Bottled water from a reliable source offers a safe alternative, although its transport may be cumbersome.

Recreational water has been linked to public outbreaks. Since standard chlorination is ineffective, public pools may become potentially contaminated through 1 infected person, particularly a child with diarrhea. For this reason, the Centers for Disease Control and Prevention recommends advising all patrons to avoid swimming during a symptomatic diarrheal illness and for 2 weeks afterward due to shedding of oocysts. While ozonation and ultraviolet treatment are effective cysticidal agents, these methods are highly dependent on water circulation rates; thus, a contaminated pool would remain potentially contaminated for up to 24 hours.

Vaccine development is hampered by the lack of an obvious antigenic target. The parasite has an abbreviated genome, often relying on host enzymes to survive, complicating vaccine development and drug targeting. Furthermore, antigens that result in high antibody titers are not necessarily protective in animal models. The successful vaccine will likely require both the proper mix of antigens and adjuvants and delivery to result in the proper combination of cell-mediated and humoral immunity to the appropriate antigens.

## SUGGESTED READINGS


Barry MA, Weatherhead JE, Hotez PJ, Woc-Colburn L. Childhood parasitic infections endemic to the United States. *Pediatr Clin North Am.* 2013;60:471-485.

Kotloff KL, Nataro JP, Blackwelder WC, et al. Burden and aetiology of diarrhoeal disease in infants and young children in developing countries (the Global Enteric Multicenter Study, GEMS): a prospective, case-control study. *Lancet.* 2013;382:209-222.

McHardy IH, Wu M, Shimizu-Cohen R, et al. Detection of intestinal protozoa in the clinical laboratory. *J Clin Microbiol.* 2014;52:712-720.

O'Connor RM, Shaffie R, Kang G, et al. Cryptosporidiosis in patients with HIV/AIDS. *AIDS*. 2011;25:549.

Shirley DA, Moonah SN, Kotloff KL. Burden of disease from cryptosporidiosis. *Curr Opin Infect Dis*. 2012;25:555-563.

Striepen B. Parasitic infections: time to tackle cryptosporidiosis. *Nature*. 2013;503:189-191.

Yoder JS, Wallace RM, Collier SA, Beach MJ, Hlavsa MC, Centers for Disease Control and Prevention (CDC). Cryptosporidiosis surveillance—United States, 2009-2010. *MMWR Surveill Summ*. 2012;61:1-12.



# 341 Cyclosporiasis

Nizar F. Maraqa

## INTRODUCTION

*Cyclospora cayetanensis* is a coccidian parasite that causes acute or chronic, food- and waterborne diarrhea in both immunocompetent and immunocompromised hosts. *Cyclospora* is a distinct protozoan genus phylogenetically related to other coccidian parasites, including *Cryptosporidium, Cystoisospora, Toxoplasma*, and *Sarcocystis*. Initially described in 1979 as cyanobacteria-like (blue-green algae) bodies in the stools of patients in Papua New Guinea with prolonged diarrhea, anorexia, and fatigue, *Cyclospora* species are now known to be ubiquitous, infecting a variety of animals, birds, reptiles, insectivores, and rodents. However, *C cayetanensis* is the only species that is known to infect humans, and the role of animals as a natural reservoir is uncertain.

## PATHOGENESIS AND EPIDEMIOLOGY

*Cyclospora* are obligate intracellular parasites able to complete all their life cycle within the human host. The species has an anterior polar complex that allows penetration into host cells, but the exact mechanism by which it interacts with human host target cells to cause disease is poorly understood. The oocysts of *C cayetanensis* are spherical to ovoid, about 8 to 10 μm in size, and surrounded by a thick wall. They are smaller than *Cystoisospora belli* and twice the size of *Cryptosporidium parvum*. Infection occurs after the ingestion of sporulated oocysts. During excystation, sporozoites are released and undergo asexual reproduction (merogony and schizogony) and sexual maturation (gametogony) within the host's gastrointestinal epithelium. The gross appearance of the small intestines of symptomatic patients may reveal moderate to severe erythema. Histopathologically, acute and chronic inflammation is seen with intraepithelial lymphocytic infiltrates. Varying degrees of villous atrophy, crypt hyperplasia, parasitophorous vacuoles, reactive hyperemia, and vascular dilatation are observed. All stages of the *C cayetanensis* life cycle have been observed in the enterocytes. As opposed to cryptosporidiosis, when *Cyclospora* oocysts are passed in stools, they are unsporulated and noninfectious, making direct, person-to-person transmission unlikely. Oocysts sporulate in the environment in conditions of high temperature (22–32°C) and humidity in about 1 to 2 weeks producing 2 sporocysts per oocyst. The oocysts can persist in the soil, on food, and in water (where they can survive for 2 months at 4°C and for 7 days at 37°C). The oocysts can be resistant to most disinfectants used in food and water processing (eg, iodine or chlorine). Washing of fruits and vegetables, therefore, may not be sufficient to eliminate the risk of transmission. The high attack rates after foodborne infection suggest a low infective dose of about 10 to 100 organisms, but this has not been precisely quantified.

Although *C cayetanensis* has a broad worldwide geographic distribution, infection is most frequently reported from tropical and subtropical countries, especially Latin America (eg, Peru, Guatemala, Mexico), the Indian subcontinent, Southeast Asia, and Caribbean Islands. In these endemic areas, cyclosporiasis prevalence ranges from 2% to 18%, and infection is associated with poor sanitation and contamination of water, food, and soil, with 70% of infections occurring in people younger than 20 years of age, and the majority (70–90%) being asymptomatic. In some regions, a strong seasonal predominance during the rainy spring and early summer months has been described. Cyclosporiasis prevalence in industrialized countries is estimated at 0.1% to 0.5%, and infection is associated with international travel or the ingestion of contaminated, imported fresh foods. In the United States, where cyclosporiasis infection is nationally notifiable and the disease is reportable in many states, a review of cases reveals that a third of cases are due to travel to endemic areas, while another third are attributed to contaminated food. Among international travelers with gastrointestinal disease, cyclosporiasis was diagnosed in 1% of cases. According to surveillance data from the Centers for Disease Control and Prevention (CDC), there are an estimated 16,264 annual cases of foodborne illness caused by *Cyclospora* (out of an overall 76 million annual cases). Outbreaks of cyclosporiasis in the United States have been attributed to imported fresh produce (eg, raspberries, basil, baby lettuce, snow peas). The use of untreated or poorly treated water for irrigating crops, applying fertilizers, and washing and processing foods has been implicated as a source of contamination for fruits and vegetables. No commercially frozen or canned produce has been implicated. Outbreaks of cyclosporiasis from exposure to recreational water sources and chlorinated swimming pools have also been reported.

## CLINICAL MANIFESTATIONS

*C cayetanensis* infects both immunocompetent and immunocompromised hosts. The incubation period is estimated to be 1 to 14 days, with a median of 7 days. Infection with *Cyclospora* may be asymptomatic (usually in endemic settings), may manifest as mild to moderate self-limiting diarrhea (usually in the healthy host), or may be protracted and severe (usually in the immunocompromised and at the extremes of age). The onset of illness may be abrupt in 30% of cases and usually lasts 7 to 9 weeks in endemic infections and international travelers. In the immunocompetent host in outbreak settings, the mean duration of diarrheal symptoms ranges from 10 to 25 days. However, in the immunocompromised host (particularly in patients with human immunodeficiency virus [HIV]/acquired immunodeficiency syndrome [AIDS]), the illness is usually prolonged with periods of remission and relapse. Diarrhea is characteristically profuse, malodorous, and watery but may contain mucus and/or blood. Nausea, anorexia, abdominal cramps, flatulence, bloating, profound fatigue, and weight loss have been reported. Low-grade fever occurs in half of the patients, and diarrhea may be preceded by a flu-like prodrome.

In the HIV-infected patient, *Cyclospora* causes an insidious chronic diarrheal illness that is indistinguishable from that of other coccidia, (eg, *Cryptosporidium* or *Cystoisospora*). Extraintestinal manifestations of cyclosporiasis are unusual and typically limited to biliary disease in immunocompromised hosts. Weight loss and malabsorption secondary to chronic diarrhea are rare and limited to persons with underlying immunosuppression. Acalculous cholecystitis has been described in AIDS patients infected with *Cyclospora* and is reported to resolve after antiparasitic therapy. Rare cases of Guillain-Barré syndrome or Reiter syndrome following *Cyclospora* infection have been reported. Death due to cyclosporiasis is exceptionally rare.

## DIAGNOSIS

Testing for *Cyclospora* is not routinely done in most laboratories, even when stool is tested for parasites. *Cyclospora* oocysts are visualized in wet mounts of stool as unsporulated, refractile spheres measuring 8 to 10 μm by differential interference microscopy. The oocyst wall exhibits bright blue autofluorescence when viewed by ultraviolet epifluorescence microscopy. Combining these 2 methods provides an efficient and reliable approach to the diagnosis. Concentration of stool by formalin-ethyl acetate sedimentation or other techniques can be employed to maximize oocysts recovery. Symptomatic infected individuals continuously excrete *Cyclospora* oocysts. Nevertheless, examination of multiple stool specimens (eg, 3 specimens collected on alternate days) may increase the yield as the number of excreted oocysts can vary considerably.

Modified safranin staining (with heat) enhances the outline of the oocyst membrane and stains it reddish-orange. The oocyst is variably acid-fast by modified Kinyoun stain, where it can appear light pink to deep purple or remain pale (unstained, ghost cells) on a blue background. However, in areas of limited resources, using lactol-phenol cotton blue (LPCB) staining is a suitable, predictable, simpler, and cheaper alternative to acid-fast stains. *Cyclospora* is not visualized by Gram, Giemsa, or hematoxylin-eosin staining. A sporulation assay may be conducted on a freshly passed oocyst when it is necessary to confirm that the parasite is *Cyclospora*.

In addition to stool, duodenal aspirate or intestinal biopsy may also contain the parasite. In complicated unusual cases, *Cyclospora* has also been identified from bile and pulmonary samples. No serologic assays are available for *Cyclospora*. A number of polymerase chain reaction (PCR) assays have been developed for reliable detection of *C cayetanensis* from clinical and environmental specimens. The combination of epidemiologic history, clinical manifestations, and demonstration of oocysts in the stool is used to confirm the diagnosis.

## TREATMENT

In the immunocompetent patient, the illness is self-limiting. Therapy with trimethoprim-sulfamethoxazole (TMP-SMX) results in eradication of the organism (within 3 days) and clinical improvement without relapse. A 7- to 10-day course of oral TMP-SMX (160 mg TMP plus 800 mg SMX for adults and 5 mg/kg TMP plus 25 mg/kg SMX for children) given twice daily is usually sufficient. In the HIV-infected patient, longer courses may be needed, and recurrent episodes are prevented using secondary prophylaxis with TMP-SMX administered orally, 3 times per week. Efficacy of either ciprofloxacin or nitazoxanide as alternative therapy for cyclosporiasis in patients who cannot tolerate TMP-SMX has been poor. Agents effective against other enteric pathogens (eg, albendazole, azithromycin, norfloxacin, metronidazole, tinidazole, quinacrine, nalidixic acid, tetracycline, doxycycline, and diloxanide furoate) have been reported to be ineffective against *Cyclospora* oocysts.

## PREVENTION

Avoiding food or water that may be contaminated with feces and washing fresh produce before it is consumed are the best ways to prevent infection.

## SUGGESTED READINGS


American Academy of Pediatrics Committee on Infectious Diseases. Cyclosporidiosis. In: *Red Book: 2015 Report of the Committee on Infectious Diseases*. 30th ed. Elk Grove Village, IL: American Academy of Pediatrics; 2015:316-317.

Cachín-Bonilla L. Epidemiology of *Cyclospora cayetanensis*: a review focusing in endemic areas. *Acta Trop*. 2010;115:181-193.

Centers for Disease Control and Prevention (CDC). Parasites: cyclosporiasis (*Cyclospora* infection): resources for health professionals. http://www.cdc.gov/parasites/cyclosporiasis/health_professionals/index.html. Accessed June 14, 2016.

Legua P, Seas C. *Cystoisospora* and *Cyclospora*. *Curr Opin Infect Dis*. 2013;26:479-483.

McHardy IH, Wu M, Shimizu-Cohen R, Couturier MR, Humphries RM. Detection of intestinal protozoa in the clinical laboratory. *J Clin Microbiol*. 2014;52:712-720.

Ortega YR, Sanchez R. Update on *Cyclospora cayetanensis*, a food-borne and waterborne parasite. *Clin Microbiol Rev*. 2010;23:218-234.


# 342 Dientamoebiasis

Dennis L. Murray



## INTRODUCTION

*Dientamoeba fragilis* is a nonflagellate trichomonad parasite that inhabits the human colon and has been associated with both acute and chronic gastrointestinal symptoms. Discovered in 1918, the organism was initially classified as an amoeba, but findings from molecular studies and other methods showed the organism is closely related to trichomonads.

## PATHOGENESIS AND EPIDEMIOLOGY

*D fragilis* infects the mucosal crypts of the large intestine from the cecum to the rectum, with the cecum and proximal colon usually the most affected areas. *D fragilis* is not invasive and does not cause cellular damage. Gastrointestinal symptoms are caused mainly by superficial colonic mucosa irritation. Like *Cryptosporidium parvum*, *D fragilis* can cause disease regardless of the patient's immune status. The exact mechanisms of pathogenicity for this organism are yet to be fully determined.

While animals such as mice can be experimentally infected, humans are likely the natural host for *D fragilis*. The life cycle and mode of transmission of this organism remain poorly defined. Because studies have shown that household contacts may have higher rates of infection, a fecal-oral mode of transmission is most likely.

Worldwide prevalence varies from 0.5% to 16%, and in contrast to many pathogenic protozoa, greater rates of *D fragilis* infection have been reported from countries with higher levels of health standards with increased prevalence of disease in persons residing in crowded living conditions. Serologic surveys suggest that infection occurs mostly during childhood. When adequate laboratory methods are used, *D fragilis* has been described to be more commonly identified than *Giardia* and *Cryptosporidium*.

## CLINICAL MANIFESTATIONS

Both acute and chronic illnesses have been associated with infection due to *D fragilis*. Infected adults and children may present with acute watery diarrhea accompanied by abdominal pain; nausea and vomiting can occur, as can bloating and flatulence. Hematochezia is unusual with these infections. Nongastrointestinal complaints such as fatigue, fever, headache, irritability, malaise, urticaria, and weakness are less common but may occur. *D fragilis* may be associated with chronic abdominal pain lasting months to years as well as bouts of alternating diarrhea and constipation, fatigue, and flatulence. In a study of infected patients, a small percentage (~11%) had no symptoms of infection. On physical examination, usually no specific findings are evident; however, some children have exhibited generalized abdominal tenderness without rebound. No specific mortality is associated with *D fragilis* infection.

## DIAGNOSIS

*D fragilis* should be suspected in patients who have abdominal pain and/or diarrhea for an extended period of time as well as symptomatic household contacts of those patients diagnosed as having an infection with *D fragilis*. Suspicion of infection should be particularly high for persons residing in institutions as well as those who recently traveled outside the United States.

To increase diagnostic yield, stools from symptomatic patients should be collected, on alternate days, for a total of 3 specimens. Collecting a total of 6 specimens increases the diagnostic yield to close to 95%. Stool specimens should be placed into a stool preservative/fixative such as polyvinyl alcohol, sodium acetate–acetic acid–formalin, or Schaudinn's solution to help identify *D fragilis* trophozoites. Because the trophozoites are known to round-up and become granular within 15 minutes at room temperature, immediate placement of the stool into the appropriate fixative is important. Preserved stool should then be stained with iron-hematoxylin, trichrome, or Celestin B stain.

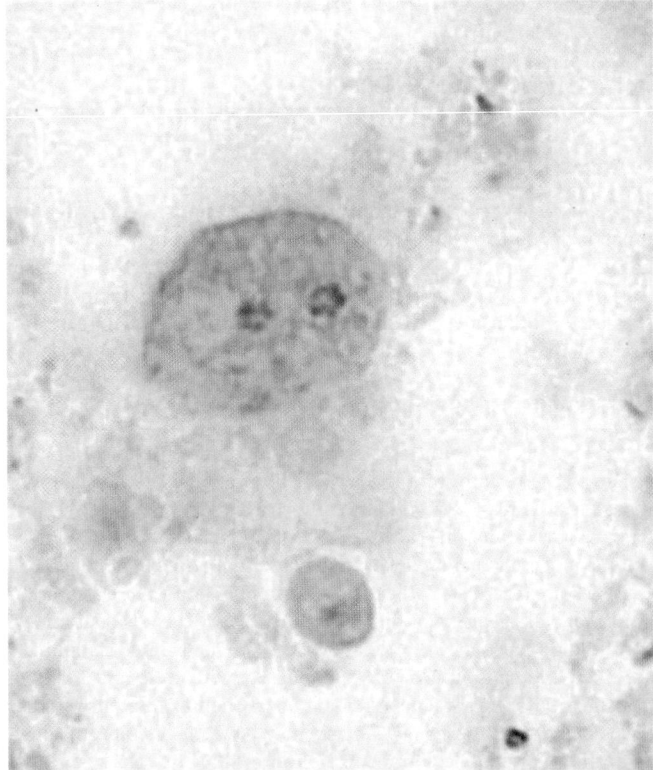

**FIGURE 342-1** *Dientamoeba fragilis*: Note the 2 nuclei in the trophozoite stained with trichrome. (Reproduced with permission from Centers for Disease Control and Prevention. Available at https://www.cdc.gov/dpdx/dientamoeba/index.html. Accessed October 27, 2017.)

Detection of *D fragilis* is apparently not compromised by mercury-free preservative and stain (Ecofix and Ecostain). In infected patients, pleomorphic trophozoites 5 to 15 mm in diameter and containing 1 to 4 nuclei (Fig. 342-1) are seen. The nuclei are distinctive containing 4 to 8 chromatin granules. Interference with the detection of the trophozoites may occur with barium, and this effect on detection of *D fragilis* could last for weeks. Co-infection with other parasites can occur.

Xenic culture methods can be used for diagnosis, as can conventional and real-time polymerase chain reaction (PCR) tests. Real-time PCR may be the most sensitive testing method and, in the future, may become the diagnostic method of choice.

More than 50% of children with *D fragilis* infection may have eosinophilia, whereas only 10% of adults with infection have this finding. Radiology studies, if performed, are usually normal in cases of *D fragilis* infection.

In terms of differential diagnosis for *D fragilis* infection, other parasites such as *Cyclospora*, *Giardia*, and *Entamoeba* need consideration as do both bacterial (eg, *Campylobacter, Escherichia coli, Salmonella*) and viral gastrointestinal pathogens. Other noninfectious etiologies such as inflammatory bowel disease, lactose or protein intolerance, pain somatropin disorder, pediatric malabsorption syndrome, and irritable bowel syndrome with diarrhea, especially for patients with chronic abdominal pain and/or diarrhea, deserve consideration.

## TREATMENT

Most treatment data for *D fragilis* are based on a small number of clinical cases. Few large-scale, double-blind, randomized, placebo-controlled trials testing antimicrobial drug efficacy against *D fragilis* have been undertaken to date. In addition, very little in vitro susceptibility data for medications to treat *D fragilis* infection have been published.

The goal of therapy for *D fragilis* is eradication of the parasite. Due to the lack of sizable clinical trials, all drugs used in the routine therapy of *D fragilis* are considered investigational by the US Food and Drug Administration. The Centers for Disease Control and Prevention has published a list of recommended drugs for *D fragilis* (Resources for Health Professionals: www.cdc.gov/parasites/dientamoeba/health_professionals/).

Treatment is recommended for patients with symptomatic *D fragilis* infection only. The current drug of choice is iodoquinol. Adults should receive 650 mg orally 3 times per day for 20 days. Children require 30-40 mg/kg/d (up to a maximum of 2 g/d) divided into 3 doses for 20 days. Iodoquinol should be taken with food. Alternatively, paromomycin, an aminoglycoside antibiotic poorly absorbed from the gastrointestinal tract, can be used. The paromomycin dosage is 500 mg orally 3 times per day for 7 days in adults and 25 to 35 mg/kg/d (not to exceed the adult maximum) divided into 3 doses for 7 days for children. A syrup formulation of paromomycin is no longer available in the United States.

Tetracycline preparations can be used but have a limited role in the treatment of children due to their side effect profile. Metronidazole and 2 related medications, secnidazole and ornidazole (neither of which are available in the United States), may be effective in treating *D fragilis* infection. Metronidazole, however, has shown a high rate of treatment failure/clinical disease relapse (20%) 2 to 4 weeks after completing therapy. A small number of investigators support the use of a combination of medications to treat cases of persistent diarrhea possibly caused by *D fragilis*. Currently, data are lacking to support such a recommendation in children.

## PREVENTION

Hand washing and the disinfection of surfaces (eg, diapering change tables) contaminated with stool appear to be important in the prevention of disease transmission. In childcare centers the diapering areas should be separate from food preparation areas to prevent food contamination and transmission of gastrointestinal organisms including *D fragilis*.

## SUGGESTED READINGS

American Academy of Pediatrics. Drugs for parasitic infections. In: Kimberlin DW, ed. *Red Book: 2015 Report of the Committee on Infectious Diseases*. 30th ed. Elk Grove Village, IL: American Academy of Pediatrics; 2015:927-956.

Nagata N, Marriott D, Harkness J, et al. Current treatment options for *Dientamoeba fragilis* infections. *Int J Parasitol Drugs Drug Resist*. 2012;2:204-215.

Röser D, Simonsen J, Stensvold CR, et al. Metronidazole therapy for treating dientamoebiasis in children is not associated with better outcomes: a randomized, double blinded and placebo-controlled clinical trial. *Clin Infect Dis*. 2014;58:1692-1699.

Stark D, Barratt J, Chan D, Ellis JT. *Dientamoeba fragilis*, the neglected trichomonad of the human bowel. *Clin Microbiol Rev*. 2016;29:553-560.

Stark D, Garcia LS, Barratt JLM, et al. Description of *Dientamoeba fragilis* cyst and precyst forms from human studies. *J Clin Microbiol*. 2014;52:2680-2683.

Stark D, Roberts T, Marriott D, et al. Detection and transmission of *Dientamoeba fragilis* from environmental and household samples. *Am J Trop Med Hyg*. 2012;86:233-236.

# 343 Free-Living Amebic Infections

Ayesha Mirza

## INTRODUCTION

Organisms of the genera *Naegleria, Acanthamoeba*, and *Balamuthia*, also known as "free-living" amebae, are known to cause meningoencephalitis in humans. Another free-living ameba genus, *Sappinia*, has been isolated from animals but is rarely isolated from humans. *Naegleria fowleri* typically causes primary amebic meningoencephalitis

(PAM), which is usually fulminant in nature, whereas infections caused by *Acanthamoeba* and *Balamuthia mandrillaris* tend to be more indolent. Like *Naegleria*, they primarily affect the central nervous system (CNS) causing granulomatous amebic encephalitis (GAE). Several species of *Acanthamoeba* abound and, besides GAE, are also known to cause amebic keratitis.

## PRIMARY AMEBIC MENINGOENCEPHALITIS

### PATHOGENESIS AND EPIDEMIOLOGY

*N fowleri* exists in 3 forms: trophozoite (infectious form), flagellate, and cysts. Once inhaled into the nasal cavity, this organism makes its way through the nasal mucosa and the cribriform plate and into the CNS via the olfactory nerves. Certain water-related recreational activities such as swimming, diving, and water skiing have been particularly associated with this infection. It is believed that the rapid and sometimes forceful propulsion of water into the nasal cavity propels the organisms through the nose and into the brain. Several factors contribute to the pathogenicity of the organism. These include an intense immune response as well as the release of several cytolytic molecules such as phospholipases, acid hydrolases, and neuraminidases. These induce rapid and fulminant brain swelling, hemorrhage, and necrosis that predominantly affect the frontal lobes leading to necrosis of brain tissue and most often death (Fig. 343-1). Thus far, there have only been 4 reported cases in the literature of individuals who have survived the infection.

Infections have been reported worldwide, predominantly in warmer climates. In the United States, most infections have been reported from the southern states, predominantly Florida and Texas, although in recent years, there have been cases reported from Minnesota, Indiana, and Kansas, suggesting perhaps a change in epidemiology (Fig. 343-2). *N fowleri* are ubiquitous, thermophilic amebae typically found in moist soil as well as warm, freshwater lakes, rivers, streams, swimming pools, tap water, and heating and air conditioning units. Hot tubs, thermal swimming pools, spas, rinsing of nostrils with tap water including irrigation of nostrils as part of management of sinus infections, and the Muslim ritual of ablution have all been associated with infections in different parts of the world. A recent case report linked *N fowleri* infection to swimming pool water supplied from an overland pipe. Most infections have been reported in children and young adults, and there does seem to be a male predominance.

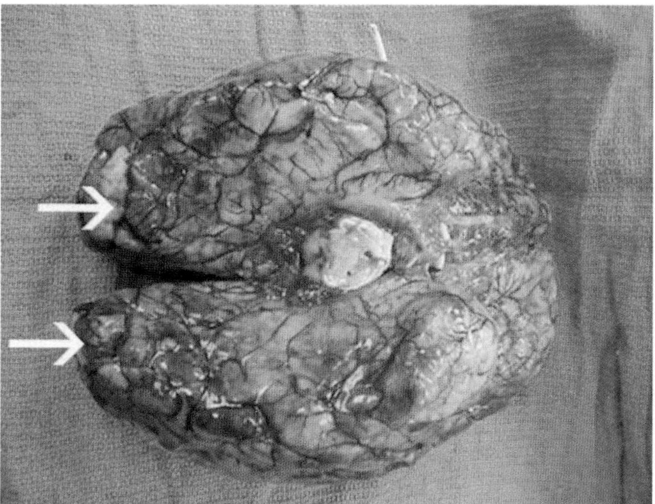

**FIGURE 343-1** Extensive hemorrhage and necrosis is present in the brain in primary amebic meningoencephalitis, mainly in the frontal cortex. (Reproduced with permission from the Centers for Disease Control and Prevention [CDC].)

### CLINICAL MANIFESTATIONS

The usual incubation period is between 2 and 8 days. Initial symptoms are very nonspecific and include headache (often frontal), fever, chills, fatigue, myalgias, and earache. As the illness progresses, patients may complain of drowsiness, irritation, photophobia, disorientation, hallucinations including disturbances of taste and smell, cranial nerve abnormalities, worsening headache, nuchal rigidity, and ultimately seizures, coma, and death. The course is often fulminant, and patients may deteriorate rapidly, making early recognition critical. Death is usually the result of rapid brain edema and herniation.

### DIAGNOSIS

Complete blood counts may reveal leukocytosis with a predominant neutrophilia. Examination of cerebrospinal fluid (CSF) is usually abnormal with increased pleocytosis, abnormal numbers of white and red blood cells, elevated protein (range 24–1210 mg/dL), low glucose (range 1–92 mg/dL), and markedly elevated opening CSF pressures (range 230–560 mm $H_2O$). Motile trophozoites may be seen on CSF wet mount preparations as well as Giemsa/trichrome or Wright staining, which allows detection of typical morphology (Figs. 343-3 and 343-4). Polymerase chain reaction (PCR) tests are available through the Centers for Disease Control and Prevention (CDC). Postmortem brain biopsy specimens have shown collections of trophozoites around blood vessels. (Fig. 343-5)

Radiologic findings either on computed tomography (CT) or magnetic resonance imaging (MRI) may reveal diffuse cerebral edema with effacement of cortical sulci and basilar cisterns as well as meningeal enhancement and areas of hemorrhage and necrosis with or without herniation.

### TREATMENT

Given the fulminant and rapidly progressive nature of *N fowleri* infection, early diagnosis is critical for the institution of appropriate therapy and management of complications. Although there are no clinical trials evaluating the efficacy of 1 treatment regimen over another, intravenous (IV)/intrathecal (IT) amphotericin B (AmB) has long been considered a treatment of choice, based on data available from case reports as well as in vitro studies. Other antimicrobials used for adjunctive therapy include IV/IT azoles (fluconazole, miconazole), azithromycin, rifampin, and most recently, miltefosine. Other macrolides such as clarithromycin, erythromycin, and roxithromycin have been studied in both in vitro and in vivo studies.

To date, there have been 3 survivors in the United States out of a total of 138 reported cases in the literature, and a fourth survivor from Mexico. Early institution of therapy and aggressive management of cerebral edema have been attributed to the good outcome of the second US survivor, a 12-year-old girl with PAM, whereas the third child, an 8-year-old male, survived but has neurologic deficits. As opposed to the previous patient, his treatment was instituted later in the course of his illness, and his cerebral edema was not managed with therapeutic hypothermia.

The CDC recommends the use of conventional deoxycholate AmB for the treatment of PAM. This is due to the lower minimum inhibitory concentration of this agent compared to liposomal AmB preparations, although treatment should not be delayed if deoxycholate AmB is not available. Treatment is generally for 14 days. The anticancer and antileishmaniasis drug miltefosine is also now available through the CDC under an investigational new drug protocol since its use in 2 survivors in 2013 showed some benefit. It has shown efficacy against *N fowleri* as well as the other free-living amebae *Acanthamoeba* and *Balamuthia* in in vitro studies.

In addition to AmB and miltefosine, the CDC also recommends use of azithromycin as part of combination therapy for patients with PAM. Not only has azithromycin shown efficacy against *N fowleri* in in vitro studies, but also azithromycin and AmB have a synergistic effect when used together. Adjunctive therapies such as the use of steroids and therapeutic hypothermia are also equally important in the management of these patients. Specific doses and duration for each of

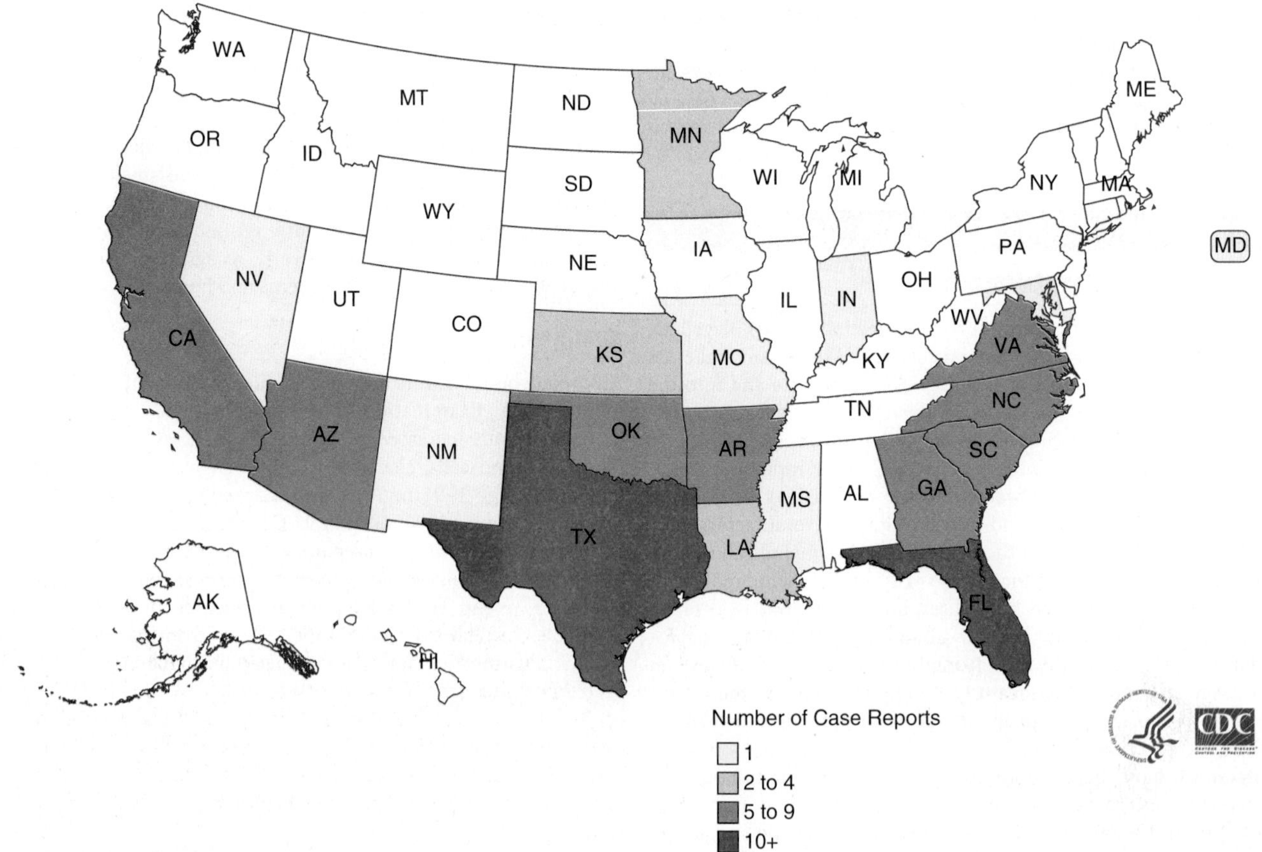


**FIGURE 343-2** Number of case reports of primary amebic meningoencephalitis caused by *Naegleria fowleri* by state of exposure: United States, 1962–2016. (Reproduced with permission from the Centers for Disease Control and Prevention [CDC].)

the medications for PAM can be found at the following CDC Web site: http://www.cdc.gov/parasites/naegleria/treatment-hcp.html.

Given that early signs and symptoms are nonspecific and often suggestive of a viral illness, clinicians should have a high index of suspicion, particularly during the summer months when most infections have been reported. Patients who have a history of participating in water-related recreational activities should be assessed carefully and monitored frequently. Given the rapid progression and overall poor prognosis of this infection, physicians suspecting PAM are strongly encouraged to contact the CDC Emergency Operations Center at 770-488-7100 for assistance with diagnosis and management of cases as soon as one is suspected.

## GRANULOMATOUS AMEBIC ENCEPHALITIS

Like *N fowleri*, the other free-living amebae *Acanthamoeba* species and *B mandrillaris* are found in soil and water sources such as hot springs, thermal swimming pools, spas, showering units, and well water. Both

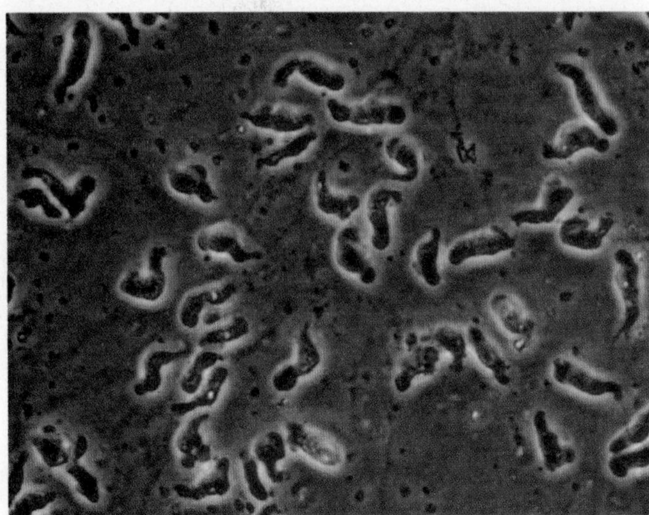

**FIGURE 343-3** A wet mount of *Naegleria fowleri* trophozoites cultured from the CSF of a patient with primary amebic meningoencephalitis (PAM) viewed using phase contrast microscopy. Magnification: 600x. (Reproduced with permission from the Centers for Disease Control and Prevention [CDC].)

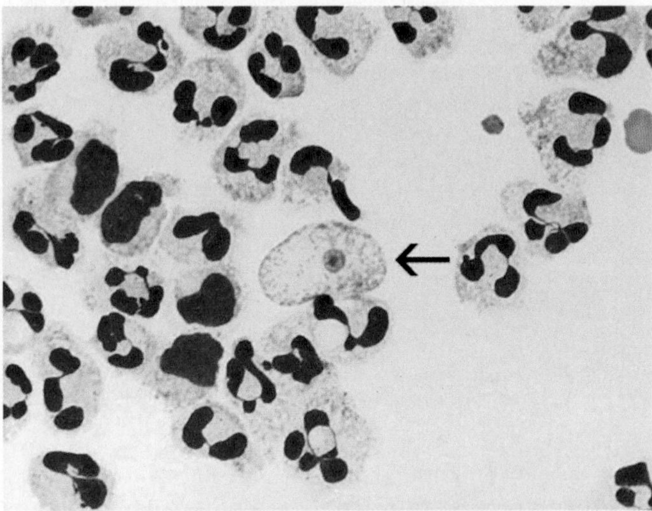

**FIGURE 343-4** A cytospin of fixed cerebrospinal fluid showing a *Naegleria fowleri* trophozoite (*arrow*) stained with Giemsa-Wright amid polymorphonuclear leukocytes and a few lymphocytes. Within the trophozoite, the nucleus and nucleolus can be seen. Magnification: 1000×. (Reproduced with permission from the Centers for Disease Control and Prevention [CDC].)

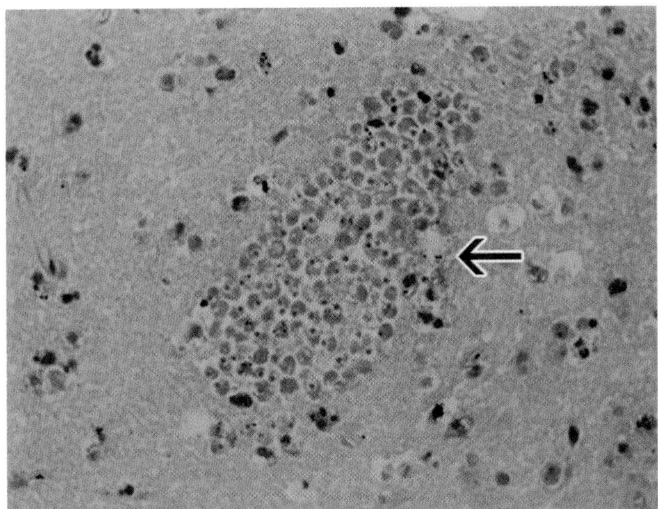

**FIGURE 343-5** A section of the brain from a patient with primary amebic meningoencephalitis stained with hematoxylin and eosin showing a large cluster of *Naegleria fowleri* trophozoites surrounding capillaries. Magnification: 400×. (Reproduced with permission from the Centers for Disease Control and Prevention [CDC].)

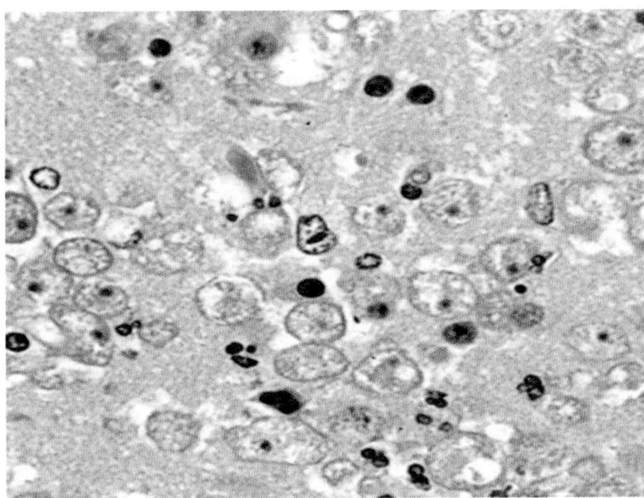

**FIGURE 343-6** Several trophozoites of *Balamuthia mandrillaris* in brain tissue, stained with hematoxylin and eosin. (Reproduced with permission from the Centers for Disease Control and Prevention [CDC].)

exist as trophozoites (infectious stage) and cyst forms; for both, the infectious periods have not been well characterized. *B mandrillaris* has also been isolated from the contact lens storage solution of a case in Germany. Both *Acanthamoeba* and *Balamuthia* can cause GAE and skin and disseminated infections, whereas *Acanthamoeba* species also affect the eyes, causing keratitis. Infections have been reported from immunocompromised patients such as those on systemic steroids and those with diabetes mellitus, cancer, transplantation, and human immunodeficiency virus infection. Keratitis caused by *Acanthamoeba* usually occurs in normal healthy individuals and has been associated with proper and improper contact lens use.

## CLINICAL MANIFESTATIONS

*Balamuthia* and *Acanthamoeba* infections are thought to occur when soil containing the organism comes in contact with human skin damaged by cuts or wounds. Infection may also be acquired when dust containing the ameba is inhaled. Signs and symptoms caused by both infections are similar to those of *N fowleri* infection, with the difference being that the course is usually more indolent and disease may progress over the course of a few weeks to months. Eye infections caused by *Acanthamoeba* may present with eye pain (often out of proportion compared to clinical symptoms), redness, irritation, sensitivity to light, tearing, and the sensation of a foreign body in the eye, whereas skin infections may present as reddish nodules, ulcers, and abscesses. CSF findings in GAE include a predominant lymphocytosis with increased protein concentration and normal or low glucose. Routine Gram staining generally shows no organisms. Imaging studies (CT or MRI) may show multiple ring-enhancing lesions resembling brain abscesses or tumors. Images of *Acanthamoeba*-associated keratitis can be found at the following Web site: http://www.cdc.gov/parasites/acanthamoeba/health_professionals/acanthamoeba_keratitis_images.html.

## DIAGNOSIS

Specific diagnostic tests for *Balamuthia* and *Acanthamoeba* are available through the CDC. These include indirect immunofluorescence, immunohistochemistry, and PCR tests (Figs. 343-6 and 343-7), These are available on blood, CSF, and tissue samples. *Acanthamoeba* eye infections are most commonly diagnosed by an ophthalmologist.

## TREATMENT

Drugs used to treat both infections include miltefosine, azoles such as fluconazole, pentamidine, flucytosine, and sulfadiazine, all usually given as part of combination therapy. *Acanthamoeba* eye infections are amenable to treatment, although early recognition is important for treatment to be successful. Topical eye solutions along with oral antimicrobial therapy have been used for the treatment of keratitis. The prognosis for *Balamuthia* and *Acanthamoeba* CNS infections is very poor. Thus far, more than 200 *Balamuthia* cases have been reported with very few survivors. As with *N fowleri* infections, physicians are urged to contact the CDC Emergency Operations Center for guidance regarding appropriate diagnosis and management of any suspected free-living amebic infections.

## PREVENTION

Strategies to prevent infections from free-living amebae include swimming or playing in pools or hot tubs that are adequately chlorinated. Care should be taken when swimming in areas of fresh water that are stagnant and/or low while the temperature of the water is high.

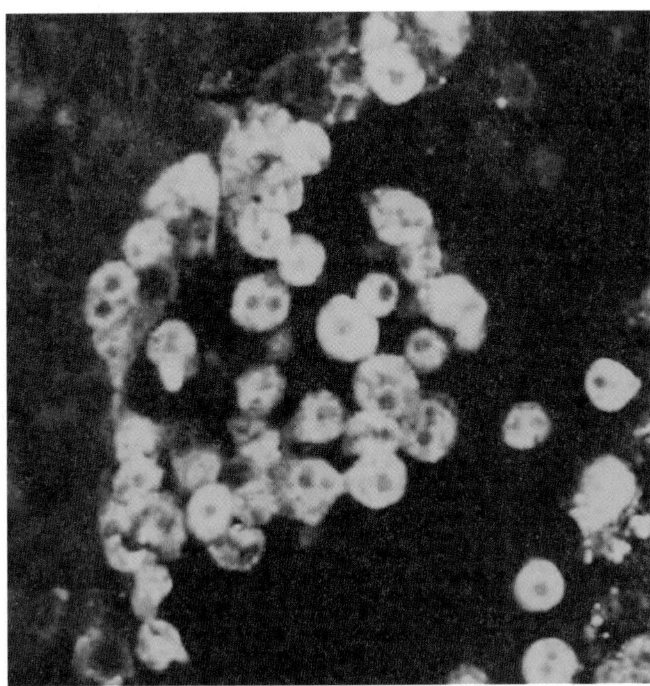

**FIGURE 343-7** Indirect immunofluorescence assay of *Acanthamoeba* species viewed under ultraviolet microscopy. This image was taken at 400× magnification. (Reproduced with permission from the Centers for Disease Control and Prevention [CDC].)

In situations such as these, activities that may lead to water being forcefully sent up the nasal passages (eg, diving) should be avoided. In addition, if using fluids for nasal irrigation, care should be taken to use only bottled or filtered water. Contact lens wearers should clean their lenses as described by the manufacturer. The use of homemade cleaning solutions for contacts and wearing contact lenses while swimming are both strongly contraindicated.

## SUGGESTED READINGS


American Academy of Pediatrics. Amebic meningoencephalitis and keratitis. In: Kimberlin DW, Brady MT, Jackson MA, Long SS, eds. *Red Book: 2015 Report of the Committee on Infectious Diseases.* 30th ed. Elk Grove Village, IL: American Academy of Pediatrics; 2015:231-234.

Centers for Disease Control and Prevention. Acanthamoeba—granulomatous amebic encephalitis (GAE); keratitis. http://www.cdc.gov/parasites/acanthamoeba/. Accessed August 12, 2016.

Centers for Disease Control and Prevention. *Naegleria fowleri* — primary amebic meningoencephalitis (PAM) — amebic encephalitis. http://www.cdc.gov/parasites/naegleria/. Accessed August 12, 2016.

Cope JR, Conrad DA, Cohen N, et al. Use of the novel therapeutic agent miltefosine for the treatment of primary amebic meningoencephalitis: report of 1 fatal and 1 surviving case. *Clin Infect Dis.* 2016;62:774-776.

Cope JR, Eddy BA, Roy SL, et al. Diagnosis, clinical course, and treatment of primary amoebic meningoencephalitis in the United States, 1937-2013. *J Pediatr Infect Dis Soc.* 2015;4:e68-e75.

Kulsoom H, Baig AM, Siddiqui R, et al. Combined drug therapy in the management of granulomatous amoebic encephalitis due to *Acanthamoeba* spp., and *Balamuthia mandrillaris. Exp Parasitol.* 2014;145:S115-S120.

Lopez C, Budge P, Chen J, et al. Primary amebic meningoencephalitis: a case report and literature review. *Pediatr Emerg Care.* 2012;28:272-276.

Visvesvara GS. Amebic meningoencephalitides and keratitis: challenges in diagnosis and treatment. *Curr Opin Infect Dis.* 2010;23:590-594.

Visvesvara GS. Infections with free-living amebae. *Handb Clin Neurol.* 2013;114:153-168.


# 344 Giardiasis

Haidee Custodio

## INTRODUCTION

*Giardia intestinalis* (former names: *Giardia lamblia* or *Giardia duodenalis*) is a protozoan flagellate that is among the most common disease-causing parasites in both developed and developing countries. It is one of the most frequently identified agents of waterborne diarrhea. Cases are especially common in areas with inadequate water and sanitation facilities. Humans are the major reservoir of infection, although other mammals, such as dogs, cats, and beavers, may be colonized and excrete cysts. Massive epidemics have occurred after the contamination of reservoirs, lakes, and streams, especially when community water supplies are not adequately filtered.

## PATHOGENESIS AND EPIDEMIOLOGY

*Giardia* cysts, present in the stool of infected persons, are the infective form. After ingestion, they excyst in the small intestine, yielding trophozoites that subsequently multiply. The trophozoites remain limited to the mucosa, mucus, or lumen of the intestine and are rarely, if ever, invasive (Fig. 344-1). Encystation normally occurs prior to expulsion in the feces. Contamination of oneself and the environment with cysts is common. The number of cysts excreted varies, but it may reach as many as 10 million per gram of stool. Infections are relatively frequent because as few as 10 cysts can infect 30% of inoculated humans.

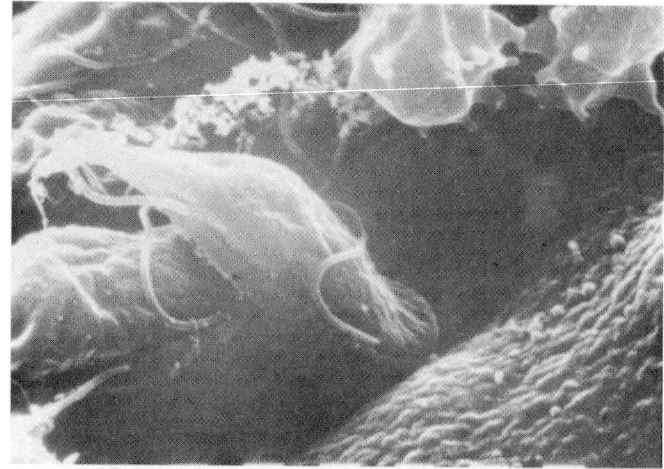

**FIGURE 344-1** *Giardia intestinalis* trophozoite seen by scanning electron microscopy.

The exact pathophysiology of the diarrhea is not known. The most severe cases are characterized by malabsorption and lactose intolerance, with varying degrees of inflammation and villous blunting. Host factors are also determinants of disease outcome; only 40% of humans infected with the same inoculum develop diarrhea. Patients with hypogammaglobulinemia frequently suffer from particularly severe cases of giardiasis. The observation that asymptomatic infections are more common in persons previously infected with *Giardia* also suggests partial immunity.

Although giardiasis affects persons of all age groups, children 0 to 5 years of age are at highest risk. In developing countries, *Giardia* infection has been reported in almost 100% of children who were followed prospectively from birth until age 2 years. In the United States and other developed countries, *Giardia* is prevalent in childcare centers and custodial institutions, among backpackers and others spending time in wooded areas, and among travelers to disease-endemic areas. Among children in childcare centers, *Giardia* cyst carriage has been documented to be as high as 50%, and many of these are asymptomatic carriers who can spread infection to household contacts. Acquisition of infection may occur via the fecal-oral route due to poor hygiene and sexual activity or via waterborne or foodborne transmission.

## CLINICAL MANIFESTATIONS

Clinical manifestations and duration of symptoms vary. Disease ranges from asymptomatic cases to severe, life-threatening diarrhea accompanied by malabsorption and dehydration. Symptoms usually appear approximately 12 to 14 days after presumed exposure. Passage of cysts usually begins 7 to 10 days after inoculation (range, 5–21 days). Symptoms include watery, foul-smelling diarrhea that can be sudden in onset and accompanied by abdominal distension, epigastric cramping, flatus, nausea, vomiting, anorexia, and fatigue. Systemic symptoms such as fever and chills are uncommon. Blood and mucus in the stools do not occur in giardiasis. Most infections resolve after a week; however, some affected patients may continue to have bouts of diarrhea lasting for several months.

In its most florid manifestations, giardiasis results in symptoms and signs associated with severe small intestinal malabsorption and weight loss. Although some patients have severe symptoms at the onset of illness and seek medical care shortly after becoming ill, the majority who seek medical attention complain of remitting abdominal pain, nausea, or weight loss lasting weeks to months.

Urticaria, arthritis, and other extraintestinal manifestations have been associated with giardiasis; however, the mechanisms behind these manifestations remain unclear.

## DIAGNOSIS

Giardiasis is confirmed by detecting the parasite or its antigens in the stool or intestinal lining. Cysts are oval, 8 to 10 µm long by 7 to 10 µm wide, and contain 4 nuclei. When viewed dorsally, the trophozoite has a characteristic pear shape and contains 2 similar nuclei. Trophozoites vary in size from 9 to 21 µm in length and 5 to 15 µm in width. Other features include 4 paired flagella and a ventral sucking disc with which the trophozoite attaches to the intestinal mucosa.

Cysts are the most commonly detected form present in the feces, and trophozoites are almost entirely limited to liquid stools. Merthiolate-iodine-formalin (MIF) concentration improves the detection of cysts. The number of cysts excreted varies, and they may not be detected on any single examination. If initial stool examination is negative, 3 stool examinations spaced 2 days apart are recommended. Careful fecal examination detects over 90% of infected individuals but requires an experienced microscopist.

Commercially available assays for detecting *Giardia* antigen in the stool are more sensitive than stool examination and have similar specificity and the added benefit of being much less time consuming than microscopy. *Giardia* antigens may be detected by immunofluorescent enzyme-linked immunosorbent assays (ELISAs), nonenzymatic immunoassays (some of which combine detection of *Giardia* and *Cryptosporidium* in a single kit), and direct fluorescent antibody tests. These commercial detection tests are similar in cost to microscopy but with better reproducibility and more rapid return of results. Overall, antigen detection tests have a sensitivity of 85% to 98% and a specificity of 90% to 100%. These are becoming more widely used and the preferred tests over microscopy.

Occasionally, cysts are not detected in the feces, and sampling small intestinal fluid by intubation or by the "string test" is useful. For the string test, a capsule attached to an absorbent string is swallowed, and trophozoites attach as the capsule proceeds through the jejunum. After 4 hours, the string is withdrawn and duodenal fluid on the string is examined for trophozoites. Esophagogastroduodenoscopy with biopsy may be diagnostic.

Antibody detection assays are rarely clinically useful, as the relationship between serum antibody and clinical disease is unclear.

## TREATMENT

Because many people are asymptomatically infected, the decision to treat should be based on presence of symptoms such as diarrhea, malabsorption, and failure to thrive. Asymptomatic cyst excreters are generally not treated except in unusual circumstances—for example, when attempting to prevent or control infections in a family with high-risk individuals such as pregnant women or patients with hypogammaglobulinemia or cystic fibrosis.

Metronidazole is frequently prescribed for giardiasis and is a highly effective drug for this indication (80–95% efficacy after 7 days of treatment), but it remains unlicensed in the United States for this purpose. Metronidazole is administered 3 times a day for 5 to 7 days. Tinidazole is approved by the US Food and Drug Administration (FDA) for giardiasis and is considered by some to be first-line therapy because it is highly effective against *Giardia* with single-dose treatment. Treatment failures with metronidazole or tinidazole can be treated with another drug, with longer durations of therapy, and with increased amounts of drug when metronidazole is used. Treatment failures with metronidazole are seen more commonly in immunodeficient patients, including those with acquired immunodeficiency syndrome (AIDS).

Nitazoxanide is a broad-spectrum antiparasitic drug active against a wide range of protozoa and intestinal helminths, as well as some bacteria and viruses. It is also FDA approved for treating giardiasis in children, and a liquid formulation for pediatric patients is available. The drug interferes with anaerobic energy metabolism by inhibiting some enzyme-dependent electron transfer reactions. Clinical trials in children showed efficacy rates of 70% to 85%, similar to those seen with metronidazole therapy. Nitazoxanide is usually administered for 3-day treatment courses, making it an attractive alternative to other treatments that require longer courses of therapy.

Antihelminthic benzimidazole drugs such as albendazole and mebendazole have been shown to have efficacy against *Giardia* similar to that of metronidazole but with fewer adverse effects. Albendazole was given for 5 days or longer in clinical trials for this indication, so the efficacy of single-dose albendazole (as it is frequently given for helminth infections) for giardiasis is not known. Paromomycin, a nonabsorbable aminoglycoside, has limited efficacy (50–70%) but is recommended for treating symptomatic giardiasis in pregnant women because of its lack of systemic absorption.

## PREVENTION

Food or drinks that are likely contaminated should be avoided. Hand washing and attention to personal hygiene including sexual practices are important preventative measures. Potentially contaminated water should be boiled or filtered, because chlorination, freezing, and disinfection by ultraviolet light are not effective against *Giardia*. Affected children are refrained from swimming in bodies of water for at least a week after resolution of symptoms and can return to childcare center once asymptomatic.

## SUGGESTED READINGS


Barry MA, Weatherhead JE, Hotez PJ, Woc-Colburn L. Childhood parasitic infections endemic to the United States. *Pediatr Clin North Am.* 2013;60:471-485.

Einarsson E, Ma'ayeh S, Svärd SG. An up-date on *Giardia* and giardiasis. *Curr Opin Microbiol.* 2016;34:47-52.

Escobedo AA, Hanevik K, Almirall P, et al. Management of chronic *Giardia* infection. *Expert Rev Anti Infect Ther.* 2014;12:1143-1157.

Escobedo AA, Lalle M, Hrastnik NI, et al. Combination therapy in the management of giardiasis: what laboratory and clinical studies tell us, so far. *Acta Trop.* 2016;162:196-205.

Granados CE, Reveiz L, Uribe LG, Criollo CP. Drugs for treating giardiasis. *Cochrane Database Syst Rev.* 2012;12:CD007787.

Halliez MC, Buret AG. Extra-intestinal and long term consequences of *Giardia duodenalis* infections. *World J Gastroenterol.* 2013;19:8974-8985.

McHardy IH, Wu M, Shimizu-Cohen R, et al. Detection of intestinal protozoa in the clinical laboratory. *J Clin Microbiol.* 2014;52:712-720.

Yoder JS, Gargano JW, Wallace RM, Beach MJ. Giardiasis surveillance—United States, 2011-2012. *Morb Mort Wkly Rep Surveill Summ.* 2015; 64:15-25.


# 345 Cystoisosporiasis

Nizar F. Maraqa

## INTRODUCTION

*Cystoisospora belli*, formerly known as *Isospora belli*, is a coccidian unicellular protozoan parasite of the phylum Apicomplexa that primarily infects the human intestinal epithelium and has no known animal reservoir. The parasite is an uncommon cause of diarrhea in immunocompetent hosts and an opportunistic cause of watery diarrhea and weight loss in immunocompromised children and adults.

## PATHOGENESIS AND EPIDEMIOLOGY

Transmission occurs primarily by the fecal-oral route through the ingestion of food or water contaminated with human feces. After the host ingests the mature sporulated oocyst, excystation releases sporozoites in the proximal small bowel, possibly in response to exposure to bile. Occasionally, sporozoites leave the intestinal tract to infect extraintestinal sites, primarily in patients with human immunodeficiency virus (HIV)/acquired immunodeficiency syndrome (AIDS).

However, the sporozoites typically invade the enterocytes of the duodenum and jejunum and mature into trophozoites. The trophozoites then mature into merozoites by asexual replication and invade new enterocytes or replicate sexually to produce immature unsporulated oocysts that are excreted in the stool. While outside the host, the oocysts ripen in 48 to 72 hours into mature sporulated oocysts (the infectious form). This maturation that occurs outside the host may explain why person-to-person transmission is uncommon. The infectious oocysts can remain viable in a cool, moist environment for months.

First described by Virchow in 1860, *C belli* is found worldwide but is more common in tropical and subtropical regions, especially Latin America and the Caribbean Islands (eg, Haiti, Mexico, El Salvador, and Brazil), tropical Africa, the Middle East, Southeast Asia, and Australia. *Cystoisospora* infection is not as common as infections from the closely related genera of *Cryptosporidium*, *Toxoplasma*, or *Cyclospora*. In the United States, sporadic outbreaks (mostly waterborne) of cystoisosporiasis have been reported among institutionalized individuals and attendees of childcare centers. It has been recognized as a cause of diarrhea among travelers to and immigrants from endemic regions and in persons with cell-mediated immunocompromising conditions such as a hematologic malignancy, Hodgkin disease, non-Hodgkin lymphoma, use of steroids or tumor necrosis factor-α antagonists, or HIV/AIDS. In persons with HIV/AIDS, low CD4 cell count (especially < 50 cells/μL), multiple infections, and poor sanitation have been noted as risk factors for cystoisosporiasis. It has been noted that the HIV/AIDS patients receiving trimethoprim-sulfamethoxazole as prophylaxis against pneumocystis pneumonia have a reduced risk of acquiring the disease. It is estimated that between 8% and 40% of HIV/AIDS patients in developing countries are infected with *C belli*. In Africa, cystoisosporiasis is the initial AIDS-defining illness in 2% to 3% of patients. The estimated prevalence of cystoisosporiasis among AIDS patients with chronic diarrhea varies geographically from about 7% to 10% in South America to up to 20% in Africa. Person-to-person transmission seems to be uncommon. In fact, immunocompetent spouses and children cohabitating with HIV/AIDS patients with cystoisosporiasis infection had no evidence of transmission of the infection. However, there have been reports of sexual transmission of cystoisosporiasis among men who have sex with men.

## CLINICAL MANIFESTATIONS

The clinical presentation of cystoisosporiasis is indistinguishable from other coccidian infections such as cryptosporidiosis and cyclosporiasis. The incubation period ranges from 3 to 14 days and is usually followed by a self-limiting diarrhea in the immunocompetent host, the duration of which may be shortened from 2 to 3 weeks to 5 to 7 days with the use of antiparasitic treatment. In contrast, the immunocompromised adult or child usually develops a more protracted and severe diarrhea, which may be acute, chronic, or frequently relapsing without long-term suppressive therapy. In addition to watery nonbloody stools, characteristic symptoms of cystoisosporiasis include crampy abdominal pain and weight loss. Rarely, patients may have fever, headache, anorexia, nausea, vomiting, and myalgia. Fecal blood and leukocytes are absent. However, Charcot-Leyden crystals and, occasionally, mucus may be present in the stool. Unlike other protozoan infections, peripheral eosinophilia may be demonstrated in about half of the patients. Severe volume loss, electrolyte disturbances, and renal insufficiency may develop acutely. Wasting, malabsorption, lactose intolerance, and steatorrhea have also been reported, particularly in the immunosuppressed patient. Extraintestinal presentations such as acalculous cholecystitis, reactive arthritis, and involvement of the lymph nodes, liver, or spleen are rare but have been reported in severely immunosuppressed HIV-infected individuals.

## DIAGNOSIS

The clinical diagnosis of cystoisosporiasis infection is similar to other infectious and noninfectious causes of diarrhea. A combination of epidemiologic, clinical, and laboratory evidence is used to arrive at a definitive diagnosis. Laboratory diagnosis of *C belli* infection is established by identifying the oocyst in feces or by visualizing the intracellular stages of the parasite in biopsy specimens of the intestinal tissue or extraintestinal sites (eg, lymph nodes, liver, spleen, or biliary tract). *Cystoisospora* may not be visualized in the stool by direct fecal smears except in cases of heavy infection, but stool concentration techniques such as flotation or sedimentation methods enhance detection. Modified Kinyoun acid-fast or auramine-rhodamine fluorescent stains are commonly used to identify the translucent oocysts of *Cystoisospora* and other coccidian parasites found in feces. Freshly shed oocysts are thin-walled, ellipsoid, and large (12–20 μm × 20–36 μm in size) and contain 2 sporocysts. Similar to *Cyclospora* species, *C belli* oocysts also exhibit autofluorescence under ultraviolet epifluorescence illumination. A real-time polymerase chain reaction (PCR) for detecting DNA in feces has been developed and seems promising but is not yet readily available for use in clinical practice. Because oocysts may be passed in small amounts and intermittently, multiple stool examinations may be required to detect the organism. Finding the parasite in a duodenal aspirate or intestinal biopsy may occasionally be useful to make a definitive diagnosis. Infection with *C belli* usually remains confined to the small intestine, particularly in the villi. The histopathologic findings of the intestinal mucosa include mild to moderate villous atrophy and crypt hyperplasia. The lamina propria is infiltrated with inflammatory cells, especially eosinophils, plasma cells, and lymphocytes. Routine histologic staining (hematoxylin-eosin) of the intestinal tissue demonstrates the organism in parasitophorous vacuoles. *C belli* appear rounded, elongated, or banana-shaped, and appear pale when stained; the parasite is usually located in the subnuclear region of the mucosal lining. Histologic findings seem to correlate with the severity of the symptoms observed. Differentiation of cystoisosporiasis from cryptosporidiosis may prove challenging, but the smaller (4 × 6 μm) oocysts and presence of 4 sporozoites of *Cryptosporidium* help distinguish it from the much larger *Cystoisospora* oocysts.

## TREATMENT

The anti-infective of choice for *Cystoisospora* infection is trimethoprim (TMP)-sulfamethoxazole (SMX). The typical treatment regimen for adults is TMP 160 mg and SMX 800 mg (1 double-strength tablet) given orally twice daily for 7 to 10 days, whereas children may receive 8 to 12 mg/kg/d of TMP, orally, in 2 divided doses. Patients with HIV/AIDS may need to be treated longer and with higher daily doses (eg, 1 double-strength tablet, orally, 4 times daily for 2–4 weeks). Secondary prophylaxis with TMP-SMX (at 160 mg TMP/800 mg SMX) given orally, 3 times a week, has been proven to decrease the recurrence of symptomatic infection in HIV/AIDS patients. The patient's symptoms generally improve within 72 hours of initiating therapy. Pyrimethamine (50–75 mg, orally, once daily) along with folinic acid may be used in patients who are intolerant of sulfa drugs for treatment of acute infection and for prophylaxis. Ciprofloxacin (500 mg, orally, twice daily in adults) is a second-line medication against *Cystoisospora*. These alternatives may be less effective than TMP-SMX. Secondary prophylaxis with ciprofloxacin (500 mg, orally, once daily) or pyrimethamine (25 mg, orally, once daily) can follow the primary treatment. There are currently insufficient data on the efficacy of nitazoxanide, doxycycline, or roxithromycin to recommend their routine use for cystoisosporiasis.

## SUGGESTED READINGS

Centers for Disease Control and Prevention (CDC). Parasites: cystoisosporiasis (formerly known as isosporiasis). http://www.cdc.gov/parasites/cystoisospora/index.html. Accessed August 12, 2016.

Legua P, Seas C. *Cystoisospora* and *Cyclospora*. *Curr Opin Infect Dis*. 2013;26:479-483.

McHardy IH, Wu M, Shimizu-Cohen R, Couturier MR, Humphries RM. Detection of intestinal protozoa in the clinical laboratory. *J Clin Microbiol*. 2014;52(3):712-720.

# 346 Leishmaniasis

Martha Isabel Alvarez-Olmos

## INTRODUCTION

Leishmaniasis is a group of clinical syndromes caused by the protozoan belonging to the genera *Leishmania*. The clinical spectrum of disease depends on the species causing the infection and includes subclinical infection, self-limited cutaneous and debilitating mucocutaneous disease, severe disseminated disease, and fatal visceral disease. Each condition has a relatively specific geographic distribution, biology, ecology, and natural mammalian reservoir, and its own vector. In nature, *Leishmania* can cause infection in a wide range of vertebrate hosts and is particularly common in canids, rodents, and primates, including humans.

## PATHOGENESIS AND EPIDEMIOLOGY

The genus *Leishmania* belongs to the order Kinetoplastida and to the family Trypanosomatidae. More than 20 species of *Leishmania* affecting humans have been identified and are grouped according to their biochemical and genetic characteristics. They have been classified based on biological, clinical, and epidemiological features as belonging to three major clinical disease groups: (1) cutaneous leishmaniasis (CL), (2) mucocutaneous leishmaniasis (MCL), and (3) visceral leishmaniasis (VL) (Table 346-1).

These single-celled parasites have a complex digenetic life cycle requiring a susceptible vertebrate host and a permissive vector to allow their transmission. They live within the phagocytes of the reticulo-endothelial system of mammals and in the intestinal tract of phlebotomine sandflies. Mammalian *Leishmania* species are present worldwide and are distributed mainly in tropical and subtropical areas of the Old (Europe, Africa, Asia) and the New Worlds (the Americas). In the Old World, the transmission is mainly peridomestic in the semiarid regions. In contrast, in the New World, it is more sylvatic with some species also exhibiting peridomestic transmission. *Leishmania* are obligate intracellular parasites in the vertebrate hosts that live only in the amastigote stage. Morphologically, the species that infect humans are indistinguishable by light microscopy and at the ultrastructural levels. Molecular typing is being recognized as a useful tool for clinical diagnosis, especially in areas where different species coexist. The Old World species of *Leishmania* are found to induce self-limiting disease while the New World species that may affect mucosal surfaces require more aggressive therapy. The main reservoirs of this protozoan are canids (eg, domestic dogs, foxes, jackals, wolves) and rodents.

The female sandfly is the only vector that is known to transmit leishmaniasis. In the Old World the genus *Phlebotomus* is responsible, while in the New World it is the genus *Ludzomyia*. The hematophagous sandfly is a noiseless, white or black 2- to 3-mm arthropod. They are very active and bite outdoors from dusk until dawn, with some exceptions. The sandflies infected with *Leishmania* parasites may bite the same host several times, thereby increasing the transmission risk. The sandfly has limited ability to hop vertically, usually no more than one meter. As a result, it is less likely to bite people living on higher floors of dwellings. These vectors prefer woodlands, and they can be found resting in the tree hollows, rock cracks, and caves. They can also be found in African Savannahs, deserts, and sometimes in mountain areas.

**TABLE 346-1 *LEISHMANIA* SPECIES ASSOCIATED WITH DIFFERENT DISEASE PATTERNS**

| Clinical Syndromes | Type of Infection | *Leishmania* Species |
|---|---|---|
| Cutaneous leishmaniasis (CL) | Old World | *LL mexicana, LL amazonensis, LL venezuelensis, LV braziliensis, LV peruviana, LV panamensis, LV guayanensis* |
| | New World | *L tropica, L aethiopica, L major* |
| Mucocutaneous leishmaniasis (MCL) | Old World | *L aethiopica* |
| | New World | *LV braziliensis, LV panamensis, LV guayanensis* |
| Visceral leishmaniasis (VL) | Old World | *L donovani, L infantum* |
| | New World | *LL chagasi, LL amazonensis* |

Zoonotic and anthroponotic transmission between the sandfly vector and a mammalian reservoir have been identified. Humans with kala-azar, post–kala-azar dermal leishmaniasis (PKDL), and asymptomatic infections are the main reservoirs for anthroponotic cycles. In the zoonotic cycle, dogs are the main domestic reservoirs; however, wild animals in the rain forests of the Americas and the deserts of Central Asia can also act as reservoirs. Humans are incidental or dead-end hosts for *Leishmania*.

The life cycle begins when the promastigote form of the *Leishmania* reaches the blood and is ingested by macrophages, dendritic cells, and neutrophils (Fig. 346-1). Then, the promastigote acquires the aflagellate form and multiplies by binary fission, infecting other cells. The sandfly again takes a blood meal that now has the amastigotes and *Leishmania* completes the cycle within the gut of the sandfly, where they are transformed again into promastigote form. The promastigote form migrates to the proboscis of the sandfly, ready to start the cycle again with a new bite. This is the main form of *Leishmania* transmission. The female sandfly is smaller than a mosquito and produces a painless bite in exposed uncovered areas of the skin. Other means of transmission include contaminated blood transfusions, needle sharing, or transplacental infection of neonates from infected mothers. CL has also been described after accidental occupational exposure in the laboratory.

The immune system plays an important role in the pathogenesis of leishmaniasis. Th1 and Th2 immune responses are induced by the promastigotes within the dendritic cells and presented to the naive T cells. The Th1-CD4 cells are activated and produce interleukin-2 (IL-2), interferon-γ (IFN-γ), and tumor necrosis factor (TNF). The protozoa are killed inside the macrophages activated by IFN-γ while the Treg cells control the damage modulating the antimicrobial response. If the Th2 response predominates, the infections may persist due to inhibition of the Th1 response, such as in the case of disseminated cutaneous leishmaniasis (DCL). The new 17 CD4+ cells produced by naïve T cells are very important for protection against the infections caused by *Leishmania donovani* that progress to disseminated visceral disease, as well as for other types of inflammatory or autoimmune responses. The parasite seems to manipulate cell death and immune response in order to survive, by modifying the maturation process of the fagolysosome, modulating cytokine and chemokine production by host cells, and impairing cell function to enter and infect host cells. The clinical manifestations depend on the type of infecting species and the host's immune response. The variability may result from genomic differences acquired during evolution of *Leishmania*, driving their tropism to skin or to visceral organs depending on the preferential affinity of the parasite to macrophage cell surface receptors. TNF, a cytokine essential for granuloma formation and parasite control, also plays a critical role both in parasite clearance by the liver and in tissue damage of the spleen. Excess TNF in the spleen may cause damage and immunological dysfunction with parasite persistence. In immunosuppressive conditions such as human immunodeficiency virus (HIV), there is an increased risk of VL even with species known to usually cause CL.

The true incidence of leishmaniasis is not accurately determined because of the obvious underreporting of subclinical disease. About 350 million people are at risk for leishmaniasis worldwide, and 10 to 12 million are affected, with 1.3 to 2 million new cases identified annually. *Leishmania* is endemic in more than 90 countries in the tropical and subtropical areas around the world, including the regions of Southern Europe, North Africa, the Middle East, South America, and South Asia. The disease is associated with 3.3 million disability-adjusted life years (DALYs) lost according to the last Global Burden of Disease (GBD) study done in 2013. Global warming and human factors have resulted in a dramatic rise in prevalence of leishmaniasis primarily due to the

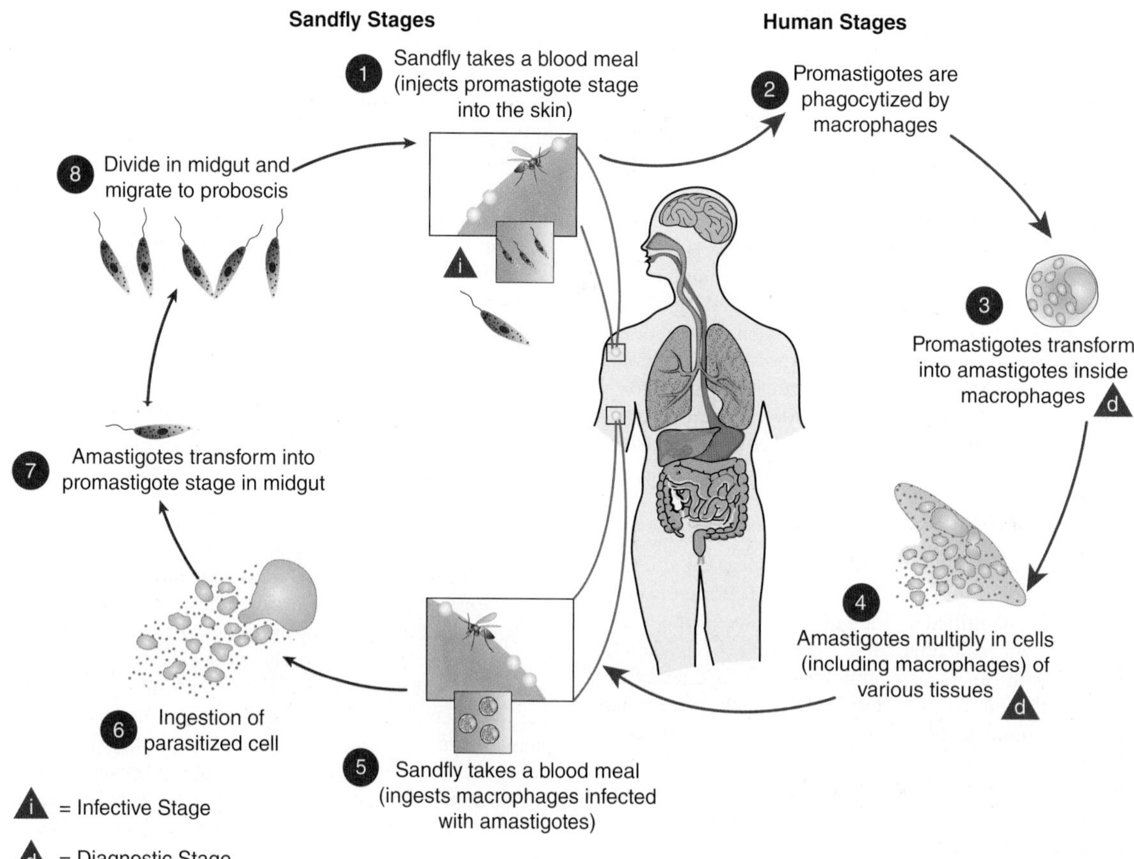


**FIGURE 346-1** Life cycle of *Leishmania* parasite. (Reproduced with permission from the Center for Disease Control and Prevention [CDC]. Public Health Image Library [PHIL].)

increase of vector range and propagation. It is considered the second leading cause of parasite-related death after malaria.

VL, or kala-azar, is a fatal condition if not treated, causing about half a million cases and 20,000 to 30,000 deaths every year. It is more frequent in rural than in urban areas, but it is found in some periurban areas in northeastern Brazil. The Indian subcontinent, East Africa, and Brazil represent 90% of the all human cases with a wide variation among areas, even within the same country. Anthroponotic transmission (human–vector–human) of *L donovani* is prevalent in East Africa and India, causing cycles of recurring outbreaks while zoonotic transmission (vector–human) of *L infantum* causes sporadic cases in the Mediterranean basin, the Middle East, central China, and South America. The coinfection with HIV has increased over time and, especially, in the last two decades. Intravenous drug users (IVDU) are the most affected group in more than 35 countries. Rarely, vertical transmission from mother to infant has been identified with *L infantum*. The transmission risk is higher among mothers with high parasite load, those coinfected with other pathogens, or those receiving immunosuppressive therapy.

CL occurs mainly in the Mediterranean, the Americas, and western Asia with an estimated 0.7 to 1.2 million cases total, about a third in each of the regions. Imported cases of CL into non-endemic developed countries increased during the 1990s and 2000s. The travel clinics report CL among the 10 top dermatologic conditions affecting travelers from Central and South America. Outbreaks of Old World cutaneous leishmaniasis (OWCL) have been identified in military personnel in Iraq and Afghanistan. The mass displacement of people from Syria has led to an epidemic of CL and outbreaks among refugees. Thirteen locally acquired cases of CL in the United States were reported between 2000 and 2007 in Texas and Oklahoma. Use of anti-tumor necrosis factor alpha (anti-TNFα) agents, such as adalimumab for treatment of rheumatologic conditions, has been associated with atypical presentations of visceral, cutaneous, and MCL.

Annually, approximately 35,000 cases of mucosal leishmaniasis occur in Brazil, Peru, and Bolivia. About 2% to 5% of patients infected with *Leishmania braziliensis* and the related species *Leishmania panamensis*, *Leishmania guayanensis*, and *Leishmania amazonensis*. Mucosal involvement of the nose, mouth, pharynx, or larynx may appear from one month to 20 years after primary skin lesions have resolved.

## CLINICAL MANIFESTATIONS

As noted earlier, leishmaniasis has a very wide clinical spectrum. Any *Leishmania* species may produce more than one clinical syndrome and each syndrome may be caused by more than one species. The clinical spectrum ranges from asymptomatic to clinically overt disease, which may be localized to the skin or disseminate to the oral or respiratory mucous membranes or to the reticuloendothelial system.

### Asymptomatic Infection

It is estimated that asymptomatic infection is 5 to 10 times more prevalent than symptomatic VL in immunocompetent hosts. It can be detected by serological evidence of anti-leishmania antibodies or by detection of parasite DNA in blood samples or positive skin reaction to *Leishmania* skin testing (LST). Detection of parasite DNA from blood samples among asymptomatic individuals may reflect recent infection. The role of transmission from asymptomatic carriers cannot be ruled out. Detection of *L donovani* amastigotes by microscopic examination of the blood smears suggests a high level of parasitemia, which could be infectious for the sandfly vector since humans are the only proven reservoir of these anthroponotic species. In endemic areas, individuals with poorly controlled HIV infection have a higher parasitemia, which increases the risk to disease progression by 100 to 2300 times.

### Visceral Leishmaniasis or Kala-Azar

The incubation period for VL usually ranges from 6 weeks to 6 months but can be as short as 10 to 14 days and as long as several years. Children between 1 and 4 years of age are the ones usually affected in Southern Europe, North and West Africa, and Central Asia. In East Africa and India, young adults are the ones frequently affected. The onset of illness can be abrupt or gradual, with systemic manifestations including fever, malaise, weight loss, and progressive splenomegaly with or without hepatomegaly. Abdominal discomfort can be present with firm spleen, which is usually minimally tender. As the disease progresses, anemia and splenic sequestration, hypoalbuminemia, edema, and cachexia may be evident. Hemorrhagic manifestations especially in oral mucosa are explained by thrombocytopenia and liver dysfunction. Darkening of the skin is classically described in South Asia, hence the name of kala-azar or "black fever." Bacterial sepsis is a common complication among Brazilian children, causing pneumonia, otitis media, skin infections, gastroenteritis, and sepsis. Less severe but insidious presentation with low-grade fever, diarrhea, poor growth, hepatomegaly, and splenomegaly has been described in Brazil due to *L infantum* (called *chagasi*). Without treatment, within 2 to 3 years the disease progresses to multiorgan involvement, severe malnutrition, hemorrhages, and sepsis, and is usually fatal. In older age groups, the clinical course is more chronic, with marked emaciation, brittle hair, massive splenomegaly, and lymphadenopathy. Fatality rates are high even with treatment.

Presumed congenital versus peripartum infections have been reported among children born to infected mothers; some of these infants had evidence of placental compromise caused by the parasites. Nephritis and glomerulonephritis have been described in association with immune-complex compromise or cellular inflammatory response, especially among younger children. Hemophagocytic lymphohistiocytosis (HLH) is rare and can be a fatal complication of VL in children. Children with HLH are mostly male, with a mean age of 2 years. It is characterized by prolonged fever, hepatosplenomegaly, pancytopenia, elevated triglyceride levels, low plasma fibrinogen levels, and elevated ferritinemia. No more than 50 children with HLH and VL have been reported, in whom mortality was attributed to bacterial sepsis and hemorrhagic complications.

Coinfection with HIV and tuberculosis increases the mortality rates. When coinfected with HIV, there is a risk of progression of both leishmaniasis and HIV. Parasite infiltration of atypical sites is seen among severely immunosuppressed patients with CD4 of < 50 copies/mL, including gastrointestinal tract, lung, pleural and peritoneal spaces, and skin. Nonulcerative mucocutaneous lesions can also be seen. The main difference in HIV coinfected and immunocompetent individuals is the lower rate of response to treatment and the high risk of disease relapse without antiretroviral therapy in the HIV infected individuals. Relapses may decrease with the use of combination antiretroviral therapy. However, a low level of *Leishmania* DNA can be found in peripheral blood samples of HIV-infected individuals, even with adequate clinical response.

VL has been described among transplant recipients. This condition may be due to new infection from the bite of an infected sandfly, reactivation of latent or asymptomatic infection with the use of immunosuppressive therapy, or acquisition through infected organ transplantation. The clinical presentation could be early, in the first 3 weeks or up to 18 months post-transplantation. The clinical scenario is similar to that described above, with some cases of atypical mucosal involvement. High risk of relapses is possible due to immunosuppression. Early diagnosis and treatment are crucial to control the disease progression and avoid graft dysfunction and loss. Screening for *Leishmania* infection should always be considered in some specific high-risk patients.

#### Post–Kala-Azar Dermal Leishmaniasis

PKDL is a dermatosis observed after treatment for VL caused by *L donovani* in India, Nepal, and Bangladesh in Asia, and in the Sudan and Ethiopia in East Africa. Children are commonly affected in the Sudan, while young adults are commonly affected in India. Skin rash can be present on the face, trunk, and limbs. Rash can be macular, papular, and nodular plaques, which can be of varying degrees of severity, sometimes resembling leprosy without sensorineural compromise. Most cases from the Sudan occur within 6 months of treatment, and they are frequently mild and often resolve without therapy. In contrast, cases from Asia are not self-limited and should always be treated. PKDL is the result of an immunological reaction to *Leishmania* parasites that persist within the skin, providing a reservoir for transmission. The lesions are considered to represent a modified form of *L donovani* infection localized in the skin without visceral involvement.

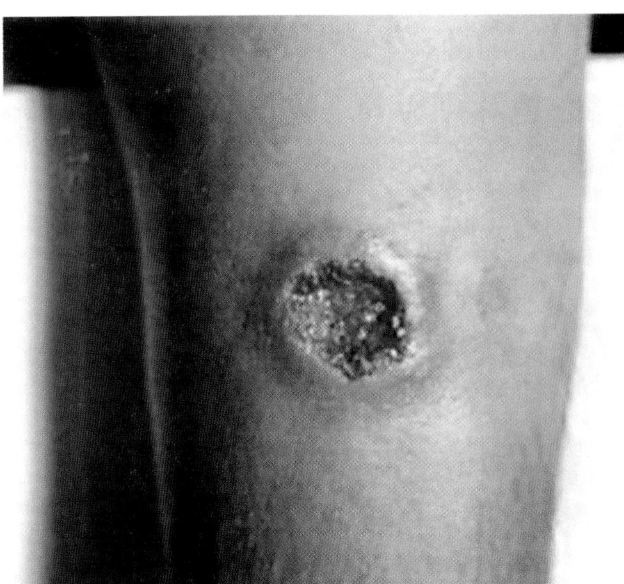

**FIGURE 346-2** Image of a child with cutaneous leishmaniasis. (Reproduced with permission from WHO/TDR/Crump.)

#### Cutaneous Leishmaniasis

CL is the most frequent form of leishmaniasis and is characterized by one or more skin lesions that appear on exposed areas such as the face, neck, and limbs (Fig. 346-2) weeks to months after a bite. The incubation period is from 3 weeks to 6 months. It is widely distributed in tropical and subtropical areas of the world. Although CL affects children of all ages and both genders, it is most commonly diagnosed between 2 and 3 years of age. Adult males are more frequently affected than females due to occupational exposure.

#### Old World Cutaneous Leishmaniasis

OWCL, also known as Oriental sore, Rose of Jericho, Aleppo boil, and Delhi boil, is caused by four species of *Leishmania*: *L major*, *L tropica*, *L aethiopica*, and *L infantum*. A painless papule located at the site of the sandfly bite progresses to ulcers over weeks to months with indurated borders and central erosion. It can be painful if superinfected or located on a joint area. *L infantum* tends to present with a single nodule that may ulcerate and resolves spontaneously within 1 year leaving an atrophic area; *L aethiopica* debuts with localized nodules but is associated with oral and nasal lesions causing local anatomical distortion, and heals over a 2- to 5-year period. Disseminated cutaneous involvement of limbs and face can occur. *L tropica* is characterized by multiple painless dry ulcers healing with disfiguring scars over a period of 1 year or more. *L major* may present with multiple severely inflamed and coalescent ulcers with an exudative base that heals very slowly leaving a disfiguring scar. Regional lymphadenopathy may be present depending on the severity, extension, or associated bacterial infection. DCL may occur in 20% of patients with *L aethiopica* infections.

#### New World Cutaneous Leishmaniasis

New World cutaneous leishmaniasis (NWCL) is known by several other names: American cutaneous leishmaniasis, Chiclero's ulcer, espundia, bush yaws, and uta. There are three main types of clinical presentations of NWCL that are attributed to the differences in parasite virulence and host response: (1) localized CL (LCL), (2) MCL, and (3) DCL. Each of these clinical presentations is associated with a specific *Leishmania* species.

In LCL, the initial papule is similar to that of OWCL, with a few differences. The lesions tend to be larger, with ulcers that are moist, usually associated with regional lymphadenopathy and slow healing. Subcutaneous nodules with sporotrichoid distribution are described. Chiclero's ulcer is the cutaneous presentation caused by *L mexicana*, mainly in the Yucatan, Belize, and Guatemala. The lesions are usually chronic and solitary with rare mucosal involvement, and located on the ear with frequent cartilage and ear destruction.

MCL is a mutilating disease that can be fatal if not treated. Espundia is the most severe form of mucocutaneous disease that is caused by *Viannia* species including *LV braziliensis*, *LV guayanensis*, *LV panamensis*, and *LV amazonensis*. The cutaneous lesions tend to disseminate along lymphatics, similar to sporotrichosis with 5% to 10% mucosal compromise, usually after months and years of initial skin lesions. Nasal obstruction, mucosal bleeding, and increased secretion with sloughing of the dead tissue are frequently described. Nasal mucosa presents with local signs of inflammation and ulceration that progresses and invades the palate, pharynx, and larynx. Nasal cartilage is destroyed with collapse of the nasal bridge with the subsequent typical appearance called "tapir nose."

DCL occurs occasionally and is very similar to OWCL. Clinical and parasitological differences have been proposed recently, classifying them as (1) DL and (2) proper diffuse CL. However, some experts consider them as the clinical spectrum of the same disease.

A wide set of tropical diseases should be included in the differential diagnosis of leishmaniasis. When VL is suspected, lymphoproliferative oncologic conditions should be included in the differential diagnosis as well as infectious tropical conditions such as histoplasmosis, tuberculosis, hepatosplenic schistosomiasis, malaria, and amebic liver abscess, among others. When CL is suspected, conditions such as histoplasmosis, coccidioidomycosis, sporotrichosis, leprosy, cutaneous mycobacterial infections, and skin neoplasia should be considered. MCL should be differentiated from rhinoscleroma, syphilis, tertiary yaws, sarcoidosis, midline granuloma, and neoplasm.

## DIAGNOSIS

Diagnosis is based on the clinical presentation, history of residence and exposure or travel to endemic areas, exclusion of other clinical diagnoses, and confirmation by diagnostic tools. Several diagnostic modalities are currently in use, depending on the convenience and availability. In the United States, the Centers for Disease Control and Prevention (CDC) offer support for diagnosis.

### Histopathology

Skin scraping or biopsy of the most active and youngest lesions should be considered. A dense dermal infiltrate of parasitized histiocytes, lymphocytes, plasma cells, and neutrophils are seen in acute lesions. Small tuberculoid granulomas may replace parasitized histiocytes. Ulceration may be found in the epidermis, with acanthosis, neutrophil microabscesses, or atrophy. The mucosal lesions are characterized by nonspecific chronic inflammation and few parasitized histiocytes with peripheral pseudoepitheliomatous hyperplasia.

In PKDL, the epidermis is atrophic and nonulcerated, with follicular plugging in the facial lesions. These lesions have variable numbers of organisms and histiocytic infiltrates with a large amount of the microorganisms. Necrosis and granulomatous formation with a small amount of organisms are identified in self-limited CL. The amastigotes multiply inside the histiocytes of the human host that can be identified in impression smears or touch preparations.

Aspirate of tissue specimens from the spleen, bone marrow, lymph nodes, liver, and buffy coat of peripheral blood are required. The Leishman-Donovan bodies represent amastigotes with prominent nucleus and eccentric rod-shaped kinetoplast. Promastigotes are not seen in the human host. The main pathologic finding in VL is reticuloendothelial hyperplasia in the spleen and liver with subsequent involvement of the bone marrow, lymph nodes, and other organs.

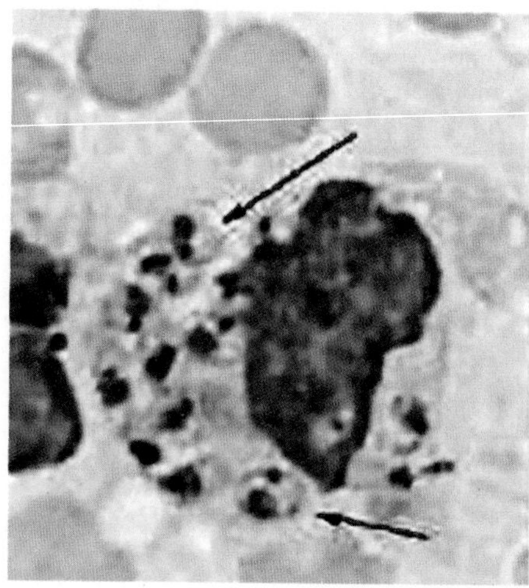

**FIGURE 346-3** Image of amastigotes from a skin biopsy. (Reproduced with permission from the Center for Disease Control and Prevention [CDC]. Public Health Image Library [PHIL].)

Erythrophagocytosis and splenic infarcts can occur with risk of spleen capsule rupture.

### Microscopy

Giemsa stain helps in the identification of amastigotes and hematoxylin-eosin–stained tissue sections may demonstrate amastigotes as basophilic dotlike structures within cytoplasm of histiocytes. For imprint cytology preparation of flat tissue, the slides should be fixed with alcohol and stained with Giemsa (Fig. 346-3) or standard hematoxylin-eosin staining. DNA–DNA hybridization or highly sensitive dot blot test can be used in biopsy specimens. Nuclei and rod-shaped kinetoplasts of amastigotes can also be identified with differential staining of DNA and RNA with acridine orange, and with immunohistochemical staining. Sensitivity in bone marrow specimens is about 60% to 85%, and from spleen aspirates is more than 95%. These are usually the initial screening tests in many laboratories. The usefulness of this test depends in large part on the experience of the microscopist.

### Serology

Serology is available for diagnosis of VL. There are several different methods that are used, including gel diffusion, complement fixation, hemagglutination, immunofluorescence, and countercurrent immunoelectrophoresis. The indirect fluorescent antibody test is useful in immunocompetent patients, especially in children. However, its sensitivity varies in immunocompromised patients with a low of 48% in HIV-infected patients versus 93% in transplant patients. The most commonly used tests in resource-limited settings are the direct agglutination test and the rK39 rapid diagnostic test. The former has demonstrated a sensitivity of > 80% in East Africa. Rapid antigen tests for early diagnosis and treatment are preferred in resource-limited settings. Serology is of limited value in HIV-coinfected individuals. In Europe, more than 40% of VL–HIV-coinfected individuals have a negative serology.

### Molecular Techniques

Several molecular techniques for diagnosis are currently available in some reference laboratories. These tests include nucleic acid amplification techniques (NAAT) with DNA hybridization, qualitative or quantitative real-time PCR (RT-PCR), high-resolution melt analysis, restriction fragment length polymorphism (RFLP), and sequencing and DNA microarrays. Other techniques, such as molecular in situ hybridization using kinetoplast DNA probes, are useful to identify *Leishmania* in tissue slides. Some molecular tests allow better discrimination between species, such as multilocus enzyme typing (MLET), multilocus sequence typing (MLST), and multilocus microsatellite typing (MLMT), which are replacing time-consuming in situ hybridization typing.

The PCR-based methods are now considered the tests of choice because they can differentiate between Old and New World leishmaniasis. PCR is rapid and very sensitive (89–100%) for routine use even with low quality or small amounts of DNA from dermal scrapings of cutaneous lesions. PCR also can be used in bone marrow aspirates, splenic aspirates, and peripheral blood samples with high sensitivity (98%) for VL.

#### *Leishmania* Skin Test

The *Leishmania* skin test (called the Montenegro test) is useful in the diagnosis of acute or recent infection in individuals with CL or MCL infected within 3 months of onset of the signs and symptoms. In the DCL and the localized CL forms, skin testing is useful only in the first month of infection. It is performed using a subcutaneous injection of killed promastigotes that should be read after 48 hours of application. A reaction of ≥ 15 mm is considered positive.

#### Culture

There is a limited role for culture in most diagnostic protocols. Culture is useful for species identification and susceptibility testing. Isolation can take several weeks, thereby limiting its use in clinical practice for rapid diagnosis.

#### Other Laboratory Findings

Laboratory findings in all forms of VL include leukopenia with neutropenia, relative lymphocytosis, and absence of eosinophilia on a peripheral smear. Thrombocytopenia, Coombs-positive hemolytic anemia, hypoalbuminemia lower than 3 g/dL, and hyperglobulinemia greater than 5 g/dL are commonly detected. Several endocrine disturbances have been described among affected patients, including primary adrenal insufficiency, low aldosterone/renin plasma ratio, low daily urinary aldosterone excretion, low transtubular potassium gradient with normal plasma antidiuretic hormone (ADH) concentrations, low plasma parathyroid hormone with hyponatremia and high urinary osmolality, and hypomagnesemia with increased magnesium excretion.

### TREATMENT

There is no ideal therapy for leishmaniasis because of the toxicity profile of the drugs used to treat it. The high cost of drugs limits access in some regions, and lack of efficacy due to emergence of resistance makes treatment of leishmaniasis challenging. Commercial interest in developing new pharmaceutical compounds is very limited due to low return on investment and lack of research into discovery of new chemotherapeutic options. A few alternative drugs have emerged recently, including multiple crude plant extracts from Asia. These new drugs also face challenges similar to older drugs, including difficulties with adherence resulting in treatment failures. Systemic therapy is recommended for VL as well as for all forms of NWCL and PKDL, which are unlikely to heal spontaneously. OWCL can be followed without intervention except in cases with multiple, large, or potentially disfiguring lesions.

There are five drugs that are primarily used for treatment of leishmaniasis. These drugs have specific dose, schedule, indications, toxicity profile, advantages, and disadvantages (Table 346-2). The classic therapy for all types of leishmaniasis has been pentavalent antimonials administrated intravenously or intramuscularly. Intravenous amphotericin B deoxycholate or liposomal and intramuscular paromomycin are additional treatment options. The only oral agent with recognized efficacy for VL is miltefosine. It also has some activity against complicated CL and OWMCL. Oral azoles have also been used in some cases of CL with inconsistent results with ketoconazole while fluconazole has been used and well tolerated with cure rates from 44% to 88%. Azithromycin has limited activity and is only recommended for patients with contraindications to use of other current

**TABLE 346-2 DRUGS FOR THE TREATMENT OF LEISHMANIASIS**

| Drug | Dose and Route | Indication | Advantages | Disadvantages | Toxicity and Side Effects |
|---|---|---|---|---|---|
| Sodium stibogluconate | 20 mg/kg/day IV, IM 28–30 days<br>20 mg/kg/day IV, IM × 10–20 doses IL | VL<br>CL | • Low cost<br>• Availability | • Length of therapy<br>• Resistance (India)<br>• Adverse events | • Cardiac arrhythmia<br>• Liver toxicity<br>• Pancreatitis<br>• Renal toxicity<br>• Fatigue |
| Amphotericin B Deoxycholate | 0.75–1 mg/kg/every other day IV for 28 days | VL<br>CL<br>MCL<br>PKDL | • > 90% response | • Renal toxicity<br>• IV route | • Hypokalemia<br>• Renal dysfunction<br>• Fever, chills<br>• Bone pain |
| Amphotericin B Liposomal | 3–5 mg/kg/day IV<br>3 mg/kg/day × 5 days; additional dose at day 10 15–30 doses every other day | VL<br>MCL<br>CL<br>PKDL | • Less toxicity than amphotericin B deoxycholate<br>• > 95% response<br>• First-line treatment for CL and MCL in nonendemic areas | • High cost<br>• IV route<br>• Limited data in CL | • Hypokalemia |
| Miltefosine | 2.5 mg/kg/day for 28 days (oral) in children aged 2–11 years<br>50 mg/day in children aged ≥ 12 years with weight ≤ 25 kg<br>100 mg/day in children aged ≥ 12 years with weight ≥ 25 kg<br>150 mg/day in ages ≥ 12 years with weight ≥ 50 kg<br>100–150 mg/day for 60–90 days<br>2.5–3.3 mg/kg/day for 28–42 days | VL<br>CL<br>PKDL caused by *L donovani* MCL | • > 95% response (VL)<br>• Oral route | • 60–80% response (CL)<br>• Breastfeeding and pregnancy contraindicated | • Nausea, vomiting, diarrhea<br>• Headache<br>• Motion sickness<br>• Renal dysfunction |
| Paromomycin | 11 mg/kg/day IM for 21 days<br>15% paromomycin/12% methylbenzethonium topical in white soft paraffin twice daily for 3–6 weeks | VL<br>CL | • 95% response<br>• Low cost<br>• Cure rates 17–86% | • IM duration | • Liver toxicity<br>• Rash<br>• Local irritation |

CL, cutaneous leishmaniasis; IM, intramuscular; IL, intralesional; IV, intravenous; MCL, mucocutaneous leishmaniasis; PKDL, post kala-azar dermal leishmaniasis; VL, visceral leishmaniasis.

options. Other alternative therapeutic options for localized use with variable effectiveness include thermotherapy, cryotherapy, surgical excision, laser, intralesional injections of antimonials, or topical application of paromomycin. These localized therapeutic modalities should be used cautiously and only by experienced professionals and at centers that specialize in performing them.

## PREVENTION

The preventive measures are primarily directed toward vector control by eradication or decrease of vector reservoir and prevention of sandfly bites. There is no available vaccine, although some are in development. Measures to control sandfly bites include (1) sleeping under insecticide-treated bed nets with appropriate sized holes to prevent sandflies from passing through them, (2) indoor insecticide spraying to control the vector, (3) use of approved insect repellents on the exposed skin when there is a risk for sandfly bites, (4) use of pretreated clothing to repel insects, (5) sleeping in air conditioning to prevent vector access, and (6) sleeping on higher floors if possible because sandflies cannot fly very high.

Control of the dog (especially stray dog) and rodent populations, which act as reservoirs, can be useful in preventing canine zoonotic transmission. However, the lack of policies to euthanize infected pet dogs limits the elimination of these *Leishmania* reservoirs in some poor-resource settings. Many experts recommend the use of insecticide-impregnated dog collars to prevent acquisition of infection for pet dogs. A canine *Leishmania* vaccine became available in 2011 in the European Union to protect dogs against *L infantum*. However, this vaccine requires booster doses and can decrease but not eliminate the risk of acquiring leishmaniasis.

There is no available vaccine for human use at this time. A safe, effective, and affordable vaccine is essential for controlling leishmaniasis, especially in the under-resourced regions of the world. There are promising candidate vaccines, including those that use antigens, single or multiple chimeric recombinant proteins, plasmid DNA, and viral particles, as well as adjuvants that should be tested and considered for prophylactic vaccination in humans and dogs.

## SUGGESTED READINGS


de Menezes JP, Guedes CE, Petersen AL, et al. Advances in development of new treatment for leishmaniasis. *BioMed Res Int.* 2015;2015:815023. doi: 10.1155/2015/815023.

Garcia LS. Leishmaniasis. In: Cherry JD, Harrison GJ, Kaplan SL, Steinbach WJ, Hotez PJ, eds. *Feigin and Cherry's Textbook of Pediatric Infectious Diseases.* 7th ed. Philadelphia, PA: Saunders; 2014:2947-2958.

Keviric I, Cappel MA, Keeling JH. New World and Old World *Leishmania* infections: A practical review. *Dermatol Clin.* 2015;33:579-593.

Magill AJ. *Leishmania* species: visceral (kala-azar), cutaneous, and mucosal leishmaniasis. In: Bennett JE, Dolin R, Blaser J, eds. *Mandell, Douglas, and Bennett's Principles and Practices of Infectious Diseases.* 8th ed. Philadelphia, PA: Saunders; 2015:3091-3107.

Mongue-Maillo B, López-Vélez R. Miltefosine for visceral and cutaneous leishmaniasis: drug characteristics and evidence-based treatment recommendations. *Clin Infect Dis.* 2015;60:1398-1404.

No JH. Visceral leishmaniasis: revisiting current treatments and approaches for future discoveries. *Acta Tropica.* 2016;155:113-123.

Pace D. Leishmaniasis. *J Infect.* 2014;69:S10-S18.

Sakkas H, Gartzonika C, Levidiotou S. Laboratory diagnosis of human visceral leishmaniasis. *J Vector Borne Dis.* 2016;53:8-16.

Saporto L, Giammanco GM, De Grazia S, Colomba C. Visceral leishmaniasis: host-parasite interactions and clinical presentation in the immunocompetent and in the immunocompromised host. *Inter J Infect Dis.* 2013;17:e572-e576.

Singh S, Sundar S. Developments in diagnosis of visceral leishmaniasis in the elimination era. *J Parasitol Res.* 2015;2015:239469. doi: 10.1155/2015/239469.


# 347 Malaria

Chandy C. John

## INTRODUCTION

Malaria is among the leading infectious causes of morbidity and mortality in children worldwide. Each year, there are more than 200 million clinical cases, causing an estimated 438,000 deaths in 2015, most in sub-Saharan African children under the age of 5 years. Increasing drug resistance, climatic changes, population shifts, economic changes, abandonment of malaria control programs, and insecticide resistance all contributed to a resurgence of malaria in the developing world from the 1970s to the 2000s. Recent World Health Organization (WHO), governmental, and nonprofit foundation support for effective preventative measures—such as insecticide-treated bednets, indoor residual spraying, and the implementation of artemisinin combination therapy as first-line treatment for malaria in many sub-Saharan African countries—has significantly reduced malaria incidence and deaths in many countries.

Diagnostic and treatment approaches differ significantly in malaria-endemic countries as compared to countries like the United States, where almost all malaria is imported. Occasional cases of local transmission have been reported in the United States since elimination of malaria in the United States in 1951, and transfusion-associated malaria also occurs rarely.

Malaria can be a life-threatening illness. Delay in seeking treatment, misdiagnosis, or both are often seen in individuals who die from malaria in the United States. Any febrile child who has been in a malaria-endemic area in the preceding year should be assessed for malaria, and it is critical to obtain an appropriate travel history in children with unexplained febrile illness.

## ORGANISMS AND LIFE CYCLE

*Plasmodium* species can infect many different animals, but most are host-specific. *Plasmodium falciparum* infects all ages of red blood cells, so it generally causes a much higher level of parasitemia than the other *Plasmodium* species. *Plasmodium vivax* and *Plasmodium ovale* preferentially infect reticulocytes and tend to cause a lower level of parasitemia than does *P falciparum*. *Plasmodium malariae* preferentially infects senescent red cells and causes the lowest level parasitemia of the human *Plasmodium* species, but this low-level parasitemia can occasionally persist for decades. It is not clear at this point if *Plasmodium knowlesi* preferentially infects a subset of red cells, but it multiplies rapidly and can cause very high levels of parasitemia. Morphologically, it can be confused with *P malariae* on microscopic examination.

Understanding the malaria parasite life cycle is crucial to understanding malarial infection and disease. The malaria life cycle is summarized in Figure 347-1. Sporozoites are inoculated into the bloodstream by the *Anopheles* mosquito and migrate within minutes to the liver, where they invade hepatic parenchymal cells. Here, the sporozoites undergo asexual multiplication (hepatic schizogony), forming schizonts that rupture the hepatic cells and release merozoites into the bloodstream. Very few hepatic cells are invaded by sporozoites, but multiplication within the hepatic cell produces thousands of merozoites from each sporozoite-infected hepatic cell. The process of liver schizogony lasts from 7 to 10 days for *P falciparum, P ovale*, and *P vivax* and 10 to 14 days for *P malariae. P vivax* and *P ovale* can also produce dormant liver stages (hypnozoites) that can reactivate weeks or months after the initial infection and can cause clinical relapse.

Merozoites released by ruptured hepatic cells invade red blood cells, where they may asexually multiply or undergo sexual differentiation into male and female gametocytes. Parasites established in the red blood cell (trophozoites) that asexually multiply form red blood cell schizonts. These schizonts eventually rupture the red cells containing them and release more merozoites, which continue the cycle of red cell invasion and multiplication.

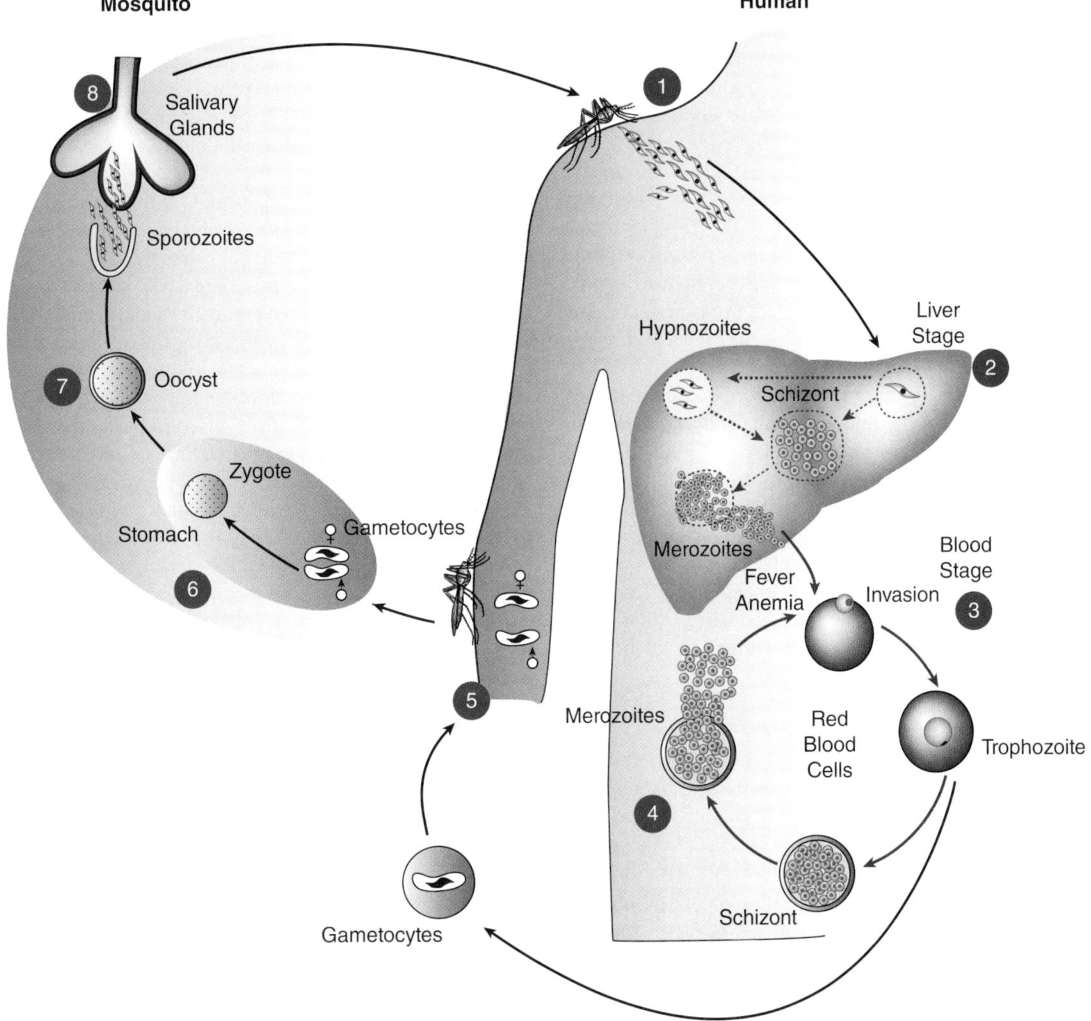


**FIGURE 347-1** Life cycle of the malaria parasite in humans and in the *Anopheles* mosquitoes.

Male and female gametocytes are ingested by mosquitoes with their human blood meal. In the mosquito, the male gametocyte exflagellates, releasing a microgamete that fertilizes the female macrogamete, producing a zygote. The elongated zygote, or ookinete, penetrates the mosquito's stomach wall and forms an oocyst behind it. The oocyst grows and eventually ruptures to release numerous sporozoites, which migrate throughout the mosquito. Those that enter the salivary glands can then infect humans the mosquito bites, thus renewing the cycle of infection.

Malaria can also be acquired by direct blood exposure through blood transfusions. With current blood-screening procedures, such cases are rare in the United States. Congenital malaria, with passage of infection from mother to newborn, can also occur, although it is relatively infrequent in endemic areas. It is seen more frequently in nonimmune women and in women who have an overt attack of clinical malaria during pregnancy. In areas where malaria is endemic, infection during pregnancy, even among semi-immune women, can lead to low birth weight and an increased risk of perinatal mortality.

## PATHOGENESIS AND EPIDEMIOLOGY

Disease from malaria is caused by the blood stages of the parasite. Rupture of red cells and release of merozoites into the blood lead to the fever, chills, and malaise seen in all forms of malaria. *Plasmodium*-infected erythrocytes, opsonized with antibodies or complement, are less deformable than uninfected erythrocytes and are consequently trapped in the spleen, leading to splenomegaly. Anemia and thrombocytopenia are due primarily to splenic consumption of erythrocytes and platelets, but autoimmune hemolysis plays a role in the continued destruction of erythrocytes that can occur for weeks after appropriate treatment. In addition, bone marrow suppression occurs in severe malarial anemia, so the anemia seen is due to both erythrocyte destruction (by autoimmune hemolysis and spleen removal of infected erythrocytes) and impaired erythropoiesis.

The pathogenesis of organ dysfunction in *P falciparum* malaria is complex, and precise mechanisms are still being investigated, but it is clear that organ dysfunction originates in the interactions between infected red blood cells (iRBCs) and the endothelial cells lining vascular organ beds. Cytoadherence of iRBCs in capillaries leads to sequestration of red cells and parasites in microvascular beds, and the resultant local tissue ischemia and hypoxia likely contribute to the renal, gastrointestinal, pulmonary, and central nervous system (CNS) complications seen in *falciparum* malaria. Cytoadherence of iRBCs to endothelial cells is influenced strongly by *P falciparum* export membrane protein-1 (PfEMP-1) *var* antigens, a group of more than 60 antigens that can be turned on and off with successive parasite broods within a single episode of clinical malaria. Specific PfEMP-1 antigens are associated with severe malaria, and these PfEMP-1 antigens bind to specific endothelial cell receptors, among which endothelial protein C receptor (EPCR) appears to be particularly important. Binding of PfEMP to EPCR may block binding of activated protein C to EPCR and induce a loss of EPCR functions, including the barrier-protective effects of activated protein C on endothelial cells. Thus specific PfEMP-1 variants likely play an important role in severe malaria pathogenesis.

A number of additional factors likely contribute to pathogenesis of *P falciparum* complications, often interrelated to PfEMP-1–endothelial cell interactions. Dysregulation of endothelial function, with reduced angiopoietin-1 levels and increased angiopoietin-2 levels, is associated with severe malaria and death in severe malaria. Endothelial cell damage from activation by iRBCs may also cause impairment of the blood–brain barrier (in cerebral malaria) or vascular damage in other organs and may lead to local release of cytokines and other inflammatory factors. In support of this hypothesis, several cytokines, notably tumor necrosis factor (TNF)-α, are present in higher amounts in the cerebrospinal fluid of children with cerebral malaria than in control children. Animal models also strongly support the role of proinflammatory cytokines, particularly TNF-α and interferon (IFN)-γ, in the pathogenesis of severe malaria. Regulatory polymorphisms of cytokine genes also appear to play a role in the development of disease. In contrast, nitric oxide may have a cytoprotective effect in malaria, and low levels of nitric oxide may contribute to development of severe disease.

The hypoglycemia seen in acute *P falciparum* infection is due to both a depletion of glycogen reserves and an increased demand for glucose because of increased anaerobic glycolysis in host tissues and in parasitized erythrocytes. Numerous factors contribute to lactic acidosis, including increased lactate production in parasitized erythrocytes, anaerobic glycolysis induced by seizures, increased metabolic rates caused by fever and anemia, and the decreased oxygen-carrying capacity of the blood in anemia. Lactic acidosis caused by systemic factors such as anemia does not have the prognostic significance of lactic acidosis caused by increased sequestered parasite biomass, and therefore, assessment of lactic acidosis in a patient with severe malaria must take into context the cause of lactic acidosis.

More than 40% of the world's population, or 2.5 billion people, are at risk for malaria in 90 countries in Africa, Asia, South and Central America, and Oceania (Fig. 347-2). For many years, it was thought that malaria in humans was caused by 4 species of *Plasmodium*: *P falciparum, P vivax, P ovale*, and *P malariae*. It is now clear that *P knowlesi*, a *Plasmodium* species that usually infects monkeys, has crossed over to cause malaria in humans in Southeast Asia, notably in Malaysia; it is now considered a fifth human malaria species. *P falciparum* is found mainly in tropical areas, where warm weather ensures the relatively constant presence of the *Anopheles* vector. *P vivax* has the widest geographic distribution of the 4 species and is found in both tropical and temperate areas. *P ovale* is found primarily in sub-Saharan West Africa, where it has largely replaced *P vivax*. *P malariae* can be seen in both tropical and temperate zones but is the least common of the malaria species.

#### Host Genetic Factors

Numerous host genetic factors can affect susceptibility to malarial infection and disease. Protective factors against disease with *P falciparum* include hemoglobinopathies (hemoglobin S [sickle cell trait], hemoglobin C and E, α and β thalassemia, blood group O, and glucose-6-phosphate dehydrogenase [G6PD] deficiency), and specific human leukocyte antigen (HLA) class I and class II alleles; Duffy blood group antigens and hereditary ovalocytosis have been associated with protection against *P vivax*. The best described protective factors are the hemoglobinopathies. Heterozygous carriers of hemoglobin S (sickle cell trait) have an 80% to 95% protection from severe malarial disease, and the high prevalence of hemoglobin S in malaria-endemic areas of sub-Saharan Africa reflect this historic protection. Other hemoglobinopathies, including hemoglobin C and E and α and β thalassemias, have also been associated with some degree of protection from severe malarial disease. Blood group O is also associated with strong protection against severe *P falciparum* malaria. Alterations in erythrocyte structure or function can be protective against malarial infection and disease. The Duffy blood group antigens are critical for invasion of *P vivax* into erythrocytes, and the low frequency of these antigens in West African individuals convincingly correlates with their innate resistance to *P vivax* infection, in contrast to their susceptibility to the other 3 species of human malaria. However, recent studies have demonstrated that some Duffy-null individuals can be infected with *P vivax*, and study into why this occurs is ongoing. Some protective effect has also been seen in individuals who carry the genes for hereditary ovalocytosis and G6PD deficiency. Finally, specific HLAs of the major histocompatibility complex (MHC) may also affect susceptibility to malarial disease, but most associations with protection to date have been of weak strength, and many associations documented in one malaria endemic area have not been confirmed in a different malaria endemic area.

#### Development of Clinical Immunity

Individuals living in malaria-endemic areas never develop complete immunity to clinical disease. However, with repeated exposure to a variety of different malaria strains over several years, they become relatively tolerant to infection. These "semi-immune" individuals often have asymptomatic parasitemia, and when malarial disease does occur, it is generally milder than that seen in nonimmune persons.

The major factors in acquiring immunity to malarial disease are repeated and frequent exposure to *P falciparum*, exposure to multiple strains of *P falciparum*, and age. Acquiring immunity to malarial disease occurs during childhood in malaria-endemic areas, but the pattern of acquisition differs in areas of differing endemicity. In areas of low- and mid-level endemicity, children acquire immunity more slowly than in areas of high-level endemicity. The primary manifestations of disease also tend to differ in areas of varying endemicity. In areas with high endemicity, children develop severe anemia, which is seen most commonly in those age 6 months to 3 years. In areas with low- or mid-level endemicity, cerebral malaria is more common and occurs in a broader age range (6 months to 6 years). In malaria-endemic areas, children less than 6 months old, and especially those

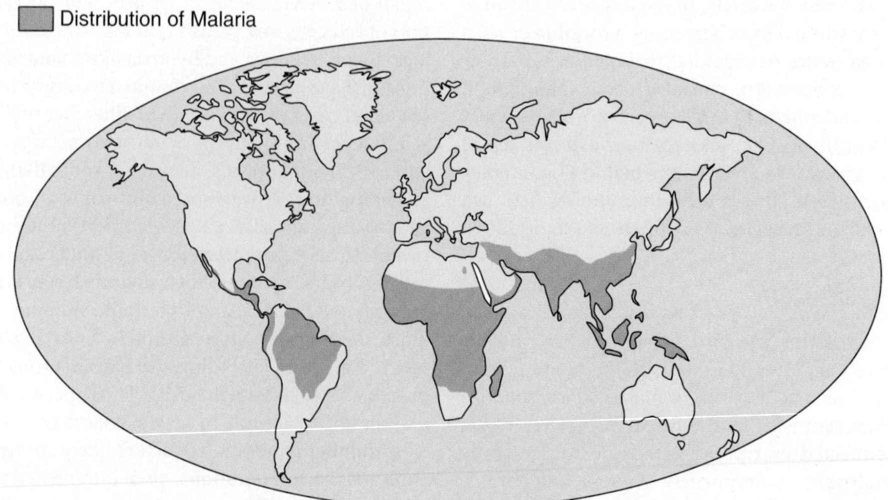


**FIGURE 347-2** Worldwide distribution of malaria. (Reproduced with permission from the Centers for Disease Control and Prevention [CDC]).

less than 3 months old, are protected from malarial infection and disease, thought to be mediated by fetal hemoglobin and passively transferred maternal antibodies.

## CLINICAL MANIFESTATIONS

The clinical presentation of malaria depends on the infected individual's age and level of immunity and on the *Plasmodium* species causing the illness. In the United States, most children who present with malaria are nonimmune. More than 90% of those with *P falciparum* infection (the most common *Plasmodium* species in imported malaria) present within 3 months of travel to or immigration from a malaria-endemic area, while less than 50% of those with *P vivax* or *P ovale* infection present within 3 months; rarely, *P vivax* and *P ovale* may present more than a year after exposure.

Nonimmune individuals, whether children or adults, tend to present with more severe signs and symptoms than semi-immune individuals and may develop severe disease with relatively low-level parasitemia. Prodromal, flulike symptoms occur during the early cycles of erythrocytic infection and may include fever (with no specific pattern), headache, malaise, myalgias, arthralgias, abdominal pain, and diarrhea. Children, especially infants, may not exhibit the classic "febrile paroxysm" seen in adults. In infants, more nonspecific symptoms such as fever, lethargy, decreased appetite, and listlessness may continue to predominate. Vomiting, loose stools, and abdominal pain are very common complaints in both infants and children. Many infants and older children will also have intermittent fevers without a clear pattern, rather than the 48-hour (*P vivax, P ovale, P falciparum*) or 72-hour (*P malariae*) fever patterns classically described with these infections. Children with *P falciparum* in particular may exhibit very irregular fever patterns. Fever is present at some point in the illness in almost all nonimmune children with malaria. Seizures are common in severe malaria. Nonimmune adults frequently exhibit the classic febrile paroxysm, which consists of 3 phases: a brief "cold" phase, with chills and sometimes rigors; a hot phase, with high fever, dry, flushed skin, tachypnea, and thirst; and a sweating stage, with defervescence accompanied by diaphoresis and a feeling of great relief but also great weakness. The paroxysms coincide with the rupture of infected erythrocytes and the release of merozoites, pigment, and cell debris into the circulation.

The physical signs most frequently seen in malaria are hepatomegaly and splenomegaly, which occur in about half of all children with acute malarial disease. In areas where malaria is highly endemic, a large percentage of children develop palpable splenomegaly over time, and the prevalence of splenomegaly in children age 2 to 9 years has been used to define an area's malaria-endemicity pattern. In areas of unstable transmission and in nonimmune individuals, it is less common. Although malaria often leads to some degree of anemia, particularly when not treated immediately, pallor is seen in only 25% of children with malaria in endemic areas and jaundice in only 10% to 15% of children. Scleral icterus may be seen in children. Jaundice is more common in nonimmune adults. Other physical exam findings relate to complications of malaria, such as coma or posturing in children with cerebral malaria or chest indrawing and respiratory distress in children with metabolic acidosis.

Nonimmune children with *P falciparum* malaria often develop complications from the disease. The WHO in the 2015 Guidelines for Treatment of Malaria lists 10 defining criteria for severe malaria, as listed in Table 347-1. The most common of these complications in children are severe malarial anemia, respiratory distress, and impaired consciousness. Each of these complications can contribute to and exacerbate the others, and mortality increases as the number of malarial complications increases.

**TABLE 347-1 WORLD HEALTH ORGANIZATION 2015 CRITERIA FOR SEVERE FALCIPARUM MALARIA**

| |
|---|
| Impaired consciousness (Blantyre coma score < 3 or Glasgow coma score < 11) |
| Prostration (unable to sit, stand, or walk without assistance) |
| Severe malarial anemia (hemoglobin ≤ 5 g/dL), with parasite count > 10,000/µL |
| Multiple seizures (> 2 episodes within 24 hours) |
| Acidosis (base deficit of > 8 mEq/mol or plasma bicarbonate < 15 mol/L or plasma lactate ≥ 5 mmol/L), manifests clinically as respiratory distress |
| Hypoglycemia (glucose < 2.2 mmol/L [40 mg/dL]) |
| Jaundice (plasma bilirubin > 50 µmol/L [3 mg/dL] with a parasite count > 10,000/µL) |
| Significant bleeding |
| Renal impairment (plasma creatinine > 265 µmol/L [3 mg/dL] or blood urea > 20 mmol/L) |
| Shock (compensated, capillary refill ≥ 3 seconds or temperature gradient mid to proximal leg, without hypotension; decompensated, systolic blood pressure < 70 mm Hg, with evidence of impaired perfusion) |
| Pulmonary edema |
| Hyperparasitemia (*Plasmodium falciparum* parasitemia > 10%) |

### Cerebral Malaria

By the WHO definition, cerebral malaria is present in a patient who (1) cannot localize a painful stimulus, (2) has peripheral asexual *P falciparum* parasitemia, and (3) has no other causes of an encephalopathy. The pathophysiology of impaired consciousness in a child with severe malaria is likely the same as that of coma. Recurrent convulsions are a frequent antecedent to subsequent impaired consciousness and coma; according to strict WHO criteria, 50% to 80% of African children with cerebral malaria have a prior history of convulsions.

Cerebral malaria often develops rapidly. Parents typically give a history of 2 to 3 days of fever, followed by abrupt onset of convulsions or severely impaired consciousness. Children with cerebral malaria may progress from a normal sensorium to coma within hours. Focal seizures are occasionally seen, but focal neurologic deficits are rare. Meningeal signs are usually absent. Abnormal posturing, pupillary changes, absent corneal reflexes, Cheyne-Stokes or Kussmaul respirations, and gaze abnormalities may be seen. "Malaria retinopathy" consists of 4 main components: retinal whitening, vessel changes, retinal hemorrhages, and papilledema. Retinal whitening and the vessel color changes are specific to malaria and are not seen in other ocular or systemic conditions. Papilledema is an independent indicator of poor outcome. Malaria retinopathy appears to distinguish children with cerebral malaria from those with coma due to other causes but is impractical as a standard diagnostic tool because it must be assessed with indirect ophthalmoscopy. In addition, children who meet WHO criteria for cerebral malaria but do not have retinopathy may still have *P falciparum* as the primary cause of coma. For this reasons, retinopathy is not a requirement for diagnosis of cerebral malaria. Increased intracranial pressure (ICP), generally not seen in adults with cerebral malaria, is a feature of cerebral malaria in children, and a landmark study from Malawi showed that brain swelling in children with cerebral malaria is a major predictor of death. Studies of interventions that decrease ICP in children with cerebral malaria, including steroids and mannitol, have not shown improved outcomes to date, so understanding and addressing the root cause of increased brain swelling in children with cerebral malaria are key to better outcomes in these children.

The mortality rate for strictly defined cerebral malaria in African children is 16% to 20%. Concurrent respiratory distress, lactic acidosis, or severe malarial anemia increases the mortality rate. Given the severity of cerebral malaria, it is remarkable that only approximately 4% to 6% of children who survive cerebral malaria have long-term neurologic deficits, but studies have demonstrated long-term cognitive impairment in up to 25% of children with cerebral malaria, and recent studies demonstrate behavioral disorders in these children as well.

Nonimmune adults can develop neurologic sequelae after severe malaria, even without cerebral malaria. Neurologic sequelae seen in nonimmune adults may also be seen in nonimmune older children and may include cranial nerve defects, mononeuritis multiplex, polyneuropathy, and cerebellar dysfunction.

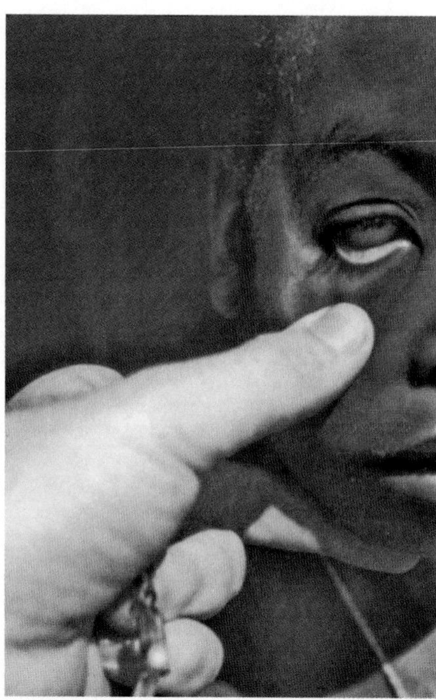

**FIGURE 347-3** Child with conjunctival pallor from severe malarial anemia. (Reproduced with permission from the Centers for Disease Control and Prevention [CDC]. Photo contributor Dr. Lyle Conrad.)

#### Severe Malarial Anemia

Malaria is the leading cause of anemia requiring hospital admission in the African child (Fig. 347-3). Severe anemia is seen most often in children less than 4 years old and is more frequent in areas of very high *P falciparum* transmission. Many children with malaria in endemic areas are already anemic from iron deficiency and hookworm infection, and the sudden worsening of anemia caused by *P falciparum* can lead to congestive heart failure, with subsequent respiratory distress and lactic acidosis. Recent studies documented that children with severe malarial anemia also have long-term cognitive impairment and behavioral disorders, a finding that suggests long-term morbidity from this common problem is even greater than originally thought.

#### Metabolic Dysfunction

Hypoglycemia (a blood glucose level of < 2.2 mmol/L) and lactic acidosis (a plasma lactate of > 5 mmol/L) are seen frequently in children with *P falciparum* malaria, often together, and are independent predictors of mortality. Children are more likely to be hypoglycemic at the time of presentation with *P falciparum* malaria than are adults. Quinine induces hyperinsulinemia in patients with acute malaria, but peripheral insulin resistance increases in acute infection and counters the hypoglycemic effects of elevated insulin levels. Late-onset hypoglycemia may be seen when acute infection has resolved but quinine treatment continues. The signs of hypoglycemia (depressed consciousness, dilated pupils, seizures) may also be seen in cerebral malaria, so checking the blood glucose level is imperative in any severely ill child with malaria. Prolonged lactic acidosis is a strong predictor of mortality. Respiratory distress, another frequent complication of *P falciparum* malaria in children, is most often attributable to underlying metabolic acidosis rather than a primary pulmonary or cardiac process. The pulmonary edema seen in adults is rarely seen in children, and pneumonia is also uncommon in children with severe malaria.

#### Other Complications

Prostration (conscious but unable to sit, drink, or eat) is a common complication of malaria. The exact pathophysiology of this clinical phenomenon is not clear, but it can be associated with mortality as high as 8% even in the absence of other complications. Acute kidney injury in children with severe malaria appears to be more common than previously recognized and may reflect prerenal azotemia, but renal failure requiring dialysis is extremely rare. Similarly, renal failure from glomerulonephritis or massive intravascular hemolysis (blackwater fever) is rarely seen in children in endemic areas, but it appears to be more common in adults. It may occasionally be seen in nonimmune children. Circulatory collapse may be due to concurrent bacterial meningitis or sepsis, which should be ruled out in children with severe malaria. Abnormal bleeding is also an infrequent clinical problem in children with severe malaria. Thrombocytopenia is frequently seen in children with *P falciparum* malaria, but bleeding problems are rare. Mild hyponatremia and hypokalemia are common in *P falciparum* malaria, but adverse outcomes due to either abnormality are rare.

Tropical splenomegaly syndrome is a chronic complication of *P falciparum* malaria in which splenomegaly persists after the acute infection is treated. Massive splenomegaly, hepatomegaly, anemia, and an elevated IgM level are the classic features of this disorder, which is thought to be due to an impaired immune response to *P falciparum* antigens. The only effective therapy for this disorder is lifelong antimalarial prophylaxis, typically with chloroquine. With this treatment, spleen size gradually regresses but increases again if prophylaxis is stopped.

#### Complications from Non-*falciparum* Malaria

In malaria due to *P vivax* and *P ovale*, complications other than anemia (which is seldom as severe as that caused by *P falciparum*) are infrequent. Nonetheless, nonimmune children with *P vivax* and *P ovale* malaria may be acutely ill and profoundly fatigued during recovery from their illness. Death can occur from *P vivax* or *P ovale* infection. Rarely, splenic rupture may occur after trauma. Children and adults with chronic *P malariae* infection may develop nephrotic syndrome, caused by immune complex deposition on glomerular walls. The nephrotic syndrome caused by *P malariae* is poorly responsive to steroids. Because of its rapid life cycle, *P knowlesi* malaria can cause high-level parasitemia and severe seizures and can rapidly lead to death. Since *P knowlesi* can be mistaken for *P malariae* on microscopy, it should be considered in any severely ill patient who acquires malaria in Southeast Asia, particularly in patients who are thought to have *P malariae* infection on microscopy but have high-level parasitemia, as high-level parasitemia with *P malariae* infection is unusual.

## DIAGNOSIS

Malaria is often misdiagnosed in the United States, and many of the deaths caused by malaria in this country are due to a delay in diagnosis. Every febrile child who has been in a malaria-endemic area within the year before presentation should be evaluated for malaria.

Examination of Giemsa-stained thick and thin blood smears remains the primary method for diagnosis of malaria. Thick smears are more sensitive in detecting parasites, but thin smears are necessary for identifying *Plasmodium* species and allow estimation of the degree of peripheral blood parasitemia. It is most important to distinguish *P falciparum* from the other 4 human malaria species. *P falciparum* malaria is suggested by parasitemia that exceeds 2% of red cells, red cells that contain multiple parasites, the almost exclusive presence of ring forms of the parasite, ring forms with a double chromatin dot, and the presence of parasites in all ages of red cells (Fig. 347-4A). The banana-shaped gametocyte is pathognomonic for *P falciparum* malaria (Fig. 347-4B). *P malariae* is characterized by low-level parasitemia and a characteristic band trophozoite (Fig. 347-4C). *P knowlesi* cannot be distinguished on blood slide from *P malariae*, but high parasite density is present in a patient with parasites of the morphology of *P malariae*, especially in a person from an endemic area (Malaysia, Southeast Asia). Schuffner's stippling is characteristic of *P vivax* (Fig. 347-4D) and *P ovale*, although it may be more subtle in *P ovale* infections. *P ovale*–infected cells often have an oval shape in addition to the stippling (Fig. 347-4E).

Asymptomatic parasitemia is common in highly endemic areas, so in these areas, a positive blood smear for malaria does not necessarily implicate malaria as the cause of the patient's illness. In endemic areas,

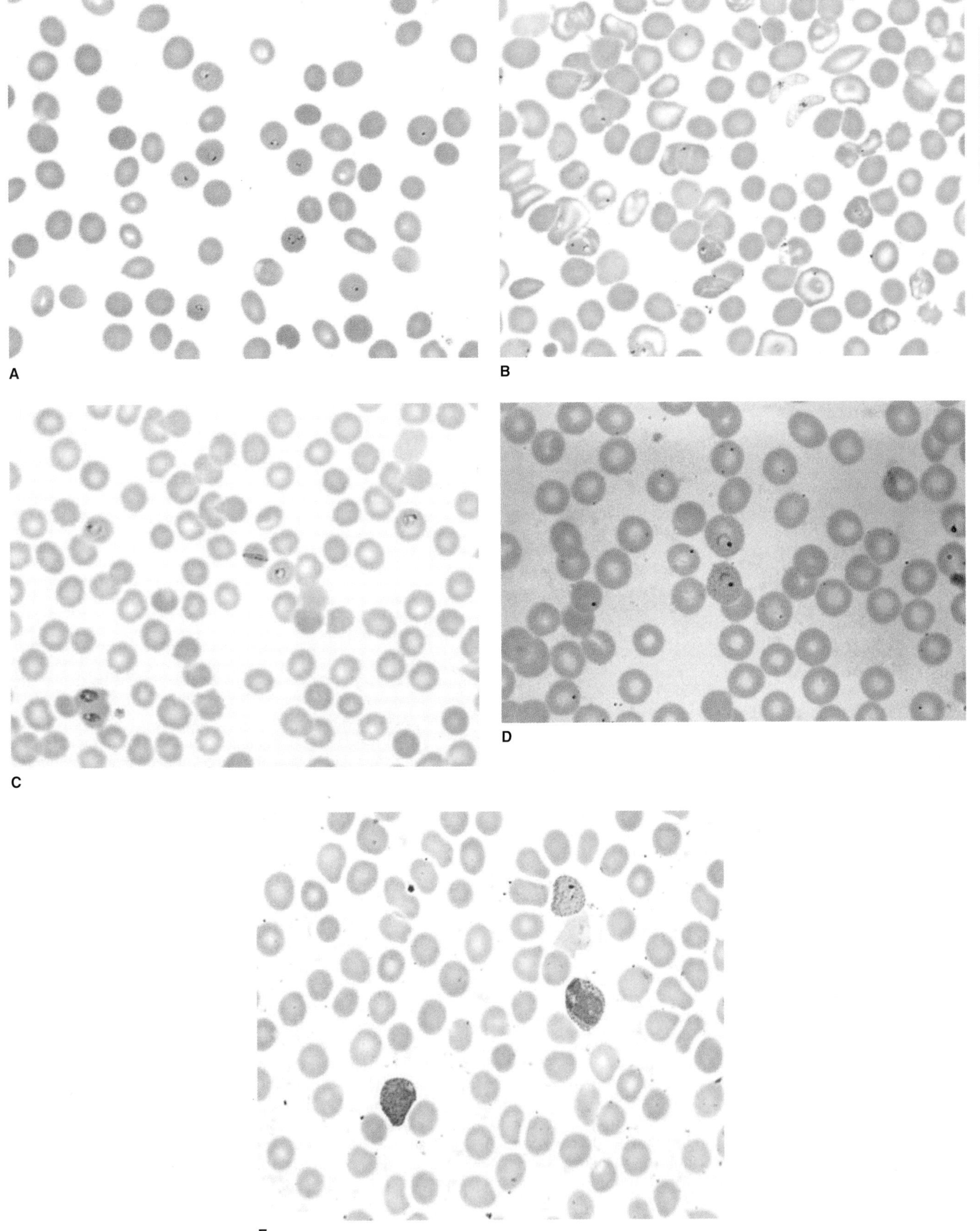


**FIGURE 347-4** *Plasmodium* species appearance on microscopic examination with Giemsa stain. **A:** *Plasmodium falciparum* trophozoite ring forms. **B:** *P falciparum* banana-shaped gametocyte. **C:** *Plasmodium malariae*, with band-shaped trophozoite (center of slide). **D:** *Plasmodium vivax*, showing Schuffner's stippling. **E:** *Plasmodium ovale*. (**C,** Reproduced with permission from the Centers for Disease Control and Prevention [CDC]. Photo contributor Dr. Earl Long; **D,** Reproduced with permission from the Centers for Disease Control and Prevention [CDC]. Photo contributor Steven Glenn; **E,** Reproduced with permission from the Centers for Disease Control and Prevention [CDC]. Photo contributor Dr. Earl Long.)

it can be difficult to distinguish acute malarial disease from other infectious diseases that cause similar symptoms.

In semi-immune individuals living in an area endemic for *P falciparum* malaria, the level of parasitemia may not correlate with severity of disease, although there is a general correlation on a population level. In nonimmune individuals, the level of parasitemia typically does correlate with severity of disease, and high-level parasitemia (> 5%) in a nonimmune individual is frequently accompanied by complications of malaria. However, in nonimmune patients, even low-level parasitemia may be accompanied by severe illness. This may be in part because peripheral blood parasitemia is an imperfect indicator of sequestered parasite load, and persons with a high level of sequestered parasites in end-organ microvasculature may have low-level peripheral blood parasitemia. In a severely ill nonimmune child, malaria blood smears should be repeated every 8 to 12 hours, and at least 3 smears over a 48- to 72-hour period should be obtained before malaria is excluded as a diagnosis. Children have sometimes received treatment with antimalarial medication prior to seeing a physician, and this may lead to a negative blood smear for malaria parasites. If the clinical picture in these individuals is consistent with malaria, and no alternative diagnosis can be made, empirical treatment for malaria may be necessary. Testing with a rapid diagnostic test such as the Binax NOW (see below) is indicated in these children, because the test may remain positive up to 48 hours after treatment begins.

The Binax test is approved by the US Food and Drug Administration (FDA) for rapid diagnosis of malaria. This immunochromatographic test for *P falciparum* histidine-rich protein (HRP2) and aldolase is approved for testing for *P falciparum* and *P vivax* and should also be able to detect *P ovale* and *P malariae*, although sensitivity and specificity for these organisms has not been assessed. Aldolase is present in all 4 of these species, and although the test would be read as positive for *P vivax*, the infection could be due to *P ovale, P knowlesi*, or *P malariae*. The test is simple to perform and can be done in the field or lab in 10 minutes. Other rapid tests for *P falciparum* also show high sensitivity and specificity but are not currently approved by the FDA. Quantitative readings of HRP2 may provide insight into sequestered parasite load, but they are currently done only in research studies. Parasite mRNA or DNA polymerase chain reaction (PCR) testing is more sensitive than the traditional blood smear and allows parasite species and strain identification and can be obtained from reference labs. Because of the time required to obtain results, it is typically used clinically only for confirmation of diagnosis or diagnosis in asymptomatic individuals. PCR testing at a reference lab is currently the only way to identify *P knowlesi* infection.

No other laboratory tests are diagnostic for malaria. Laboratory findings that support the diagnosis include a normocytic, normochromic anemia and thrombocytopenia. In children with concurrent hookworm infection or iron deficiency, microcytosis and hypochromia may be seen. Hypoglycemia, metabolic acidosis, and increased indirect bilirubin are complications in severe malaria. The cerebrospinal fluid (CSF) in children with cerebral malaria is generally unremarkable, with less than 5 white blood cells per milliliter, no red blood cells, a normal protein level, and a normal glucose level relative to serum glucose. Elevated CSF lactate levels are an independent predictor of mortality.

In the nonimmune child returning from a malaria-endemic area, malaria is most likely to be confused with typhoid—which may also present with fever, abdominal pain, vomiting, diarrhea, and malaise—or dengue. The fevers of typhoid are unremitting and generally unaccompanied by chills, rigors, or diaphoresis, and the splenomegaly of typhoid is typically less marked than that of malaria. The classic typhoid "rose spot" exanthem is not seen in malaria, but it is often missing in cases of typhoid as well. In its prodromal phase, malaria can also be confused with viral or bacterial gastroenteritis, including hepatitis A, influenza, enteroviral infection, and other viral illnesses such as influenza. Cerebral malaria may be confused with bacterial or viral meningitis or encephalitis. Babesiosis can cause cyclical fevers and may be mistaken for malaria on blood smear. If blood smears are repeatedly negative for malaria parasites and if antimalarial treatment does not improve symptoms, the differential diagnosis in the traveler returning from a malaria-endemic area should include rickettsial disease, tuberculosis, endocarditis, brucellosis, leptospirosis, trypanosomiasis, kala-azar, histoplasmosis, and noninfectious diseases such as rheumatologic or neoplastic disease.

## TREATMENT

Treatment of malaria can be complex. Physicians without experience in malaria treatment may call the Centers for Disease Control and Prevention (CDC) malaria hotline for expert advice (770-488-7788 Monday–Friday 8–4:30 Eastern US time; or 777-488-7100 at all other times). Four questions must be urgently answered in the evaluation of a child with malaria or suspected malaria: (1) Is the child semi-immune or nonimmune? (2) Does the child have *P falciparum* malaria? (3) Was the child exposed to malaria in an area with chloroquine-resistant or chloroquine-susceptible malaria parasites? (4) Does the child have any evidence of complications from malarial disease by history, examination, or laboratory findings?

All ill-appearing children should be considered nonimmune. Children less than 5 years old, children traveling to or from malaria-endemic areas but originally from a nonendemic area, and children who have been away from an endemic area for more than 6 months should be considered nonimmune. In many malaria-endemic countries, there are large cities where little or no malaria transmission occurs, and individuals from these cities are essentially nonimmune. A well-appearing child over 5 years of age who has arrived within 6 months from a malaria-endemic area but who has *Plasmodium* species infection on blood smear may be considered semi-immune. If there are no physical examination or laboratory findings of concern, and compliance with treatment and good follow-up are certain, such children may be considered for outpatient therapy.

*P falciparum* malaria can be a life-threatening emergency, especially in the nonimmune individual. Any child from a malaria-endemic area with signs and symptoms of severe malaria should be treated for *P falciparum* malaria while awaiting blood smear confirmation. Nonimmune children with documented *P falciparum* malaria should be hospitalized, because clinical decompensation can occur rapidly, even in children with a relatively benign initial presentation. Nonimmune children with *P vivax, P ovale*, or *P malariae* infection can appear quite ill with the initial paroxysm and also typically require hospitalization.

Decisions about antimalarial therapy are based on the chloroquine resistance pattern in the area malaria was acquired. The physician should search carefully for evidence of complications from malarial infection (as outlined in the "Diagnosis" section), because early treatment of these complications may ameliorate the disease process. In children, evidence of hypoglycemia, lactic acidosis, and severe anemia must be sought so that, if present, they can be corrected appropriately.

### Severe *P falciparum* Malaria

In the United States, intravenous quinidine remains the drug of choice for all children with *P falciparum* malaria who require hospitalization, although it has become less available in US hospitals with the advent of newer antiarrythmic drugs. Artesunate is recommended by the World Health Organization (WHO) in preference to quinidine for the treatment of severe malaria based on studies showing a lower mortality in children with severe malaria treated with artensunate. Artesunate has been used worldwide for many years, and it can be obtained on a protocol through the CDC (Table 347-2). Treating *P falciparum* infection with quinine, quinidine, artesunate, or artemether alone has been associated with significant recrudescence rates, which are decreased with the addition of doxycycline, tetracycline, or clindamycin (Table 347-2). High-level quinine resistance, although reported, remains uncommon.

The potential cardiac toxicity of quinidine necessitates that patients receive it as an intravenous infusion, never as a bolus, while on continuous electrocardiographic monitoring. Infusion rates should be reduced if the QT interval is prolonged by more than 25% of the baseline value. Both quinine and quinidine can induce hyperinsulinemic hypoglycemia, which may cause lethargy or unresponsiveness that is

**TABLE 347-2 DRUG TREATMENT OF SEVERE *PLASMODIUM FALCIPARUM* MALARIA IN CHILDREN IN THE UNITED STATES**

| Drug | Dosage and Route of Administration |
|---|---|
| Quinidine gluconate[a] | 10 mg/kg salt (1.0 mg salt = 0.625 mg base) loading dose (max 600 mg) in normal saline over 1–2 h, IV, followed by continuous infusion at 0.02 mg/kg/min, IV, with ECG monitoring, until able to take oral medication or for 7 days |
| **PLUS one of the following:** | |
| Doxycycline | 2.2 mg/kg/day IV every 12 h and then switch to oral doxycycline as soon as the patient can take oral medications. Total therapy is 7 days. For children ≥ 45 kg, use adult dosing (100 mg every 12 h) |
| OR | |
| Clindamycin | 20 mg/kg/day divided 3 times a day for 7 days. If the patient is not able to take oral medications, give 10 mg base/kg loading dose IV followed by 5 mg base/kg IV every 8 h. Switch to oral medications as soon as the patient can tolerate. |

[a]Quinidine gluconate has become less available in United States hospitals with the advent of newer antiarrythmic drugs. If treatment questions arise, please contact the CDC Malaria Hotline: 770-488-7788 (Monday–Friday, 9 am–5 pm, Eastern Time); after hours and holidays, call 770-488-7100 and request to speak with a CDC Malaria Branch clinician.

IV, intravenous; IM, intramuscular; max, maximum.

confused with cerebral malaria; therefore, glucose levels should be followed in severely ill patients who are on these medications. Long-term side effects from either medication are uncommon, and the cinchonism (nausea, dysphoria, tinnitus, and high-tone deafness) seen with quinine resolves with cessation of quinine therapy. When children are ready for oral therapy, CDC guidelines suggest completion of the course with oral quinine plus doxycycline, tetracycline, or clindamycin (see Table 347-2). However, many children do not tolerate oral quinine well, and in practice, a full course of artemether-lumefantrine, now available in the United States, is often given instead of quinine.

Adjunctive treatment for severe malaria includes blood transfusion for children with severe malarial anemia, seizure medication for children with repeated seizures, and intravenous antibiotics in children with hypotension or other signs of sepsis. Exchange transfusion for hyperparasitemia is controversial. Some guidelines still recommend exchange transfusion for parasitemia > 10%, but a recent CDC review concluded that there was little evidence to suggest benefit to patients from exchange transfusion. Similarly, treatment of metabolic acidosis should be aimed at rapid treatment of the underlying cause of the acidosis (malaria), as correction of acidosis itself does not appear to benefit children. Finally, trials for reduction of intracranial pressure in individuals with cerebral malaria using mannitol or steroids have shown either no benefit or harm, and they are not currently recommended in severe malaria treatment.

### Uncomplicated *P falciparum* Malaria

**Chloroquine-Resistant** In the United States, more than 90% of cases of clinical malaria reported to the CDC were acquired in Africa, Asia, or South America, all of which have high-level *P falciparum* chloroquine resistance.

In the United States, artemether-lumefantrine (marketed under the trade name Coartem) and atovaquone-proguanil (marketed under the trade name Malarone) are the preferred alternatives to quinine treatment for uncomplicated chloroquine-resistant *P falciparum* malaria (Table 347-3). Coartem has few side effects, and the side

**TABLE 347-3 DRUG TREATMENT OF UNCOMPLICATED MALARIA IN CHILDREN IN THE UNITED STATES**

| Malaria Species | Drug | Dosage (Oral) |
|---|---|---|
| Chloroquine-resistant *Plasmodium falciparum* | Atovaquone-proguanil (Malarone™) | 5–8 kg: 2 *pediatric* tabs daily for 3 days |
| | | 9–10 kg: 3 *pediatric* tabs daily for 3 days |
| | | 11–20 kg: 1 *adult* tab once daily for 3 days |
| | | 21–30 kg: 2 *adult* tabs once daily for 3 days |
| | | 31–40 kg: 3 *adult* tabs once daily for 3 days |
| | | > 40 kg: 4 *adult* tabs once daily for 3 days |
| | | (Adult tabs: 250 mg atovaquone/100 mg proguanil; pediatric tabs: 62.5 mg atovaquone/25 mg proguanil) |
| | Artemether-lumefantrine[a] (Coartem™) | 5–14 kg: 1 tab q8h × 2 doses, then q12h × 4 doses |
| | | 15–24 kg: 2 tabs q8h × 2 doses, then q12h × 4 doses |
| | | 25–34 kg: 3 tabs q8h × 2 doses, then q12h × 4 doses |
| | | > 35 kg: 4 tabs q8h × 2 doses, then q12h × 4 doses |
| | | (1 tab = 120 mg lumefantrine/20 mg artemether) |
| | Quinine sulfate | 25 mg/kg/d (max 2000 mg) in 3 doses for 3–7 days |
| | **PLUS one of the following:** | |
| | Doxycycline | See Table 347-2 |
| | OR | |
| | Clindamycin | |
| | Mefloquine (Lariam™ or generics)[b] | 13.7 mg base/kg (= 15 mg salt/kg) po as initial dose followed by 9.1 mg base/kg (= 10 mg salt/kg) po given 6–12 h after initial dose; total dose = 25 mg salt/kg |
| Uncomplicated chloroquine-sensitive malaria | Chloroquine phosphate[c] | 10 mg base/kg (max 600 mg base) × 1; 5 mg base/kg 6 h later, then 5 mg base/kg per day for 2 days |
| *Plasmodium vivax* and *Plasmodium ovale* (prevention of relapse) | Primaquine phosphate[d] | 0.6 mg base/kg per day (max 30 mg) for 14 days |

[a]Take with food or whole milk. If patient vomits within 30 minutes of taking a dose, patient should repeat the dose.

[b]Treatment with mefloquine is not recommended in persons who have acquired infections from Southeast Asia due to drug resistance.

[c]Cholorquine and hydroxychloroquine are recommended options. Regimens to treat chloroquine-resistant infections may also be used.

[d]Screen for glucose-6-phosphate dehydrogenase deficiency prior to giving primaquine (see text). Primaquine is used for eradicating liver-stage parasites and should be given at the end of chloroquine treatment.

max, maximum; q, every.

effects of atovaquone-proguanil (abdominal pain, vomiting, nausea, and headache) are usually mild and self-limited. In some studies, an elevation of transaminases was seen with atovaquone-proguanil treatment, but transaminase elevations have not been associated with untoward clinical events. Atovaquone-proguanil should be taken with food or a milky drink. If vomiting occurs within 1 hour of dosing of artemether-lumefantrine, a repeat dose should be given. Because atovaquone-proguanil is also used for prophylaxis, it is typically more easily available than artemether-lumefantrine. Children who took atovaquone-proguanil for malaria prophylaxis should not receive it for treatment of malaria. Instead, artemether-lumefantrine, or, if artemether-lumefantrine is not immediately available, quinine or mefloquine, should be used in children who have received atovaquone-proguanil prophylaxis.

Oral quinine plus doxycycline, tetracycline, or clindamycin (see Table 347-3) can also be used for treatment of uncomplicated chloroquine-resistant *P falciparum* infection but has significantly more side effects than artemether-lumefantrine or atovaquone-proguanil. Children who acquire *P falciparum* infection in border areas of Thailand (where low-level quinine resistance is endemic), who have persistent parasitemia greater than 1%, or who receive clindamycin as their adjunctive therapy should receive a full 7-day course of quinine treatment.

Children frequently vomit after receiving quinine, especially if they are febrile when receiving the drug. Acetaminophen and sponge bathing prior to administration of oral quinine may decrease the likelihood of vomiting. If vomiting occurs within an hour, the full dose of quinine should be repeated. If vomiting occurs after 1 hour, no repeat quinine dosing is necessary. Other side effects of quinine are as noted above. In situations where urgent treatment is required and intravenous medications cannot be given, intrarectal or intramuscular quinine has been used successfully.

Mefloquine can be used to treat chloroquine-resistant malaria, but increasing mefloquine resistance (particularly in Southeast Asia) and significant CNS side effects with treatment dosages make it an inferior choice, to be used only when artemether-lumefantrine, atovaquone-proguanil, or quinine treatment is not an option. Mefloquine should not be used if the child took mefloquine as prophylaxis, and it should not be used in conjunction with quinine or quinidine, as it may potentiate the cardiac side effects of these medications.

**Chloroquine-Sensitive** At the time of publication, chloroquine-sensitive *P falciparum* still exists in the Middle East, Eastern Europe, Central America north of the Panama Canal, Haiti, and the Dominican Republic, but this may change. The CDC Web site (www.cdc.gov) and the malaria hotline (770-488-7788) have up-to-date information on malaria drug resistance in every country. Chloroquine remains the drug of choice for chloroquine-susceptible *P falciparum* malaria (see Table 347-3). It is inexpensive, generally well tolerated, and easy to administer. Side effects include pruritus in dark-skinned patients (which is fairly common) and, in treatment doses, nausea, dysphoria, and rarely a transient neuropsychiatric syndrome or cerebellar dysfunction. Hydroxychloroquine may be used if chloroquine is not available. If there is any doubt as to whether chloroquine resistance is present in the area malaria was acquired, quinine should be used. Quinidine is the preferred drug in the United States for parenteral treatment of chloroquine-sensitive malaria.

#### Malaria Due to *P vivax, P ovale, P malariae,* and *P knowlesi*

Complications due to *P vivax, P ovale,* or *P malariae* are less common than with *P falciparum*, and severe disease is consequently less common as well, but all malaria species can cause significant illness in a nonimmune child, and in some areas, *P vivax* is a more common cause of severe illness than *P falciparum*. Coinfection with *P falciparum* may be missed on blood smear if the slide reader is inexperienced or if the infection inoculum is low. Children hospitalized with non-*falciparum* malaria should be given the same drug treatment regimen as children hospitalized for *falciparum* malaria (see Table 347-2).

CDC guidelines recommend chloroquine or hydroxychloroquine treatment for malaria due to *P vivax, P ovale, P knowlesi*, and *P malariae* (see Table 347-3). High-grade *P vivax* resistance to chloroquine has been reported in Papua New Guinea and Indonesia and, less commonly, in a few other areas of Asia. For *P vivax* acquired in Papua New Guinea or Indonesia, quinine (with doxycycline or tetracycline) or mefloquine is recommended.

Treatment with medications other than chloroquine should be done in consultation with the CDC or a clinician experienced in treating malaria. Patients with *P vivax* and *P ovale* malaria should also receive a 2-week course of primaquine to eradicate dormant liver stages of these parasites. Prior to treatment with primaquine, all patients should be screened for G6PD deficiency. Individuals with the severe form of G6PD deficiency may experience an oxidant hemolysis and methemoglobinemia with primaquine administration and should not receive primaquine. There are currently no effective alternatives to primaquine for liver-stage parasite eradication. Although scattered reports of *P ovale* and *P malariae* chloroquine resistance exist, resistance is not widespread and chloroquine remains first-line therapy for these parasites.

## PREVENTION

For those traveling to endemic areas, avoiding mosquitoes and using barrier protection from mosquitoes are important ways to prevent malaria. The *Anopheles* mosquito feeds from dusk to dawn. During these hours, travelers should remain in well-screened areas, wear clothing that covers most of the body, stay in air-conditioned areas where possible, sleep under a bednet (ideally one impregnated with permethrin), and use insect repellants with *N-N*-diethyl-m-toluamide (DEET) or picaridin. Repellants with low DEET concentrations (< 20%) are effective for only a short period of time. Concentrations of 25% to 35% DEET, to be applied every 6 to 8 hours as needed, are recommended for children. American Academy of Pediatrics recommends using no more than 30% DEET concentration. Picaridin (10–20%) is odorless and does not leave a sticky residue like DEET and can last from 5 to 8 hours. Spraying clothing with permethrin, a synthetic pyrethroid, is a safe and effective method of reducing insect bites in children. Permethrin-sprayed clothes remain effective for at least 2 weeks, even with laundering.

Chemoprophylaxis is the cornerstone of malaria prevention for nonimmune children and adults who travel to malaria-endemic areas (Table 347-4). Weekly mefloquine is the drug of choice for malaria chemoprophylaxis in children and adults traveling to areas with chloroquine-resistant *P falciparum* for more than 4 weeks. The FDA has not approved mefloquine for children who weigh less than 15 kg, but since the risks of acquiring severe malaria outweigh the risks of potential mefloquine toxicity in these children, the CDC recommends that mefloquine prophylaxis be used for all children. The lack of a liquid or suspension formulation sometimes makes mefloquine administration difficult, and potential side effects include nausea and vomiting. Mefloquine is better tolerated by children if it is disguised in other foods. Adults have 10% to 25% incidence of sleep disturbances and dysphoria with mefloquine, but these side effects appear to be less common in children.

Atovaquone-proguanil can also be used for prolonged travel, but must be taken daily and so is better for trips under 4 weeks. It has less side effects than quinine, so it may be preferred to mefloquine for shorter trips to malaria-endemic areas. The side effect of abdominal pain, which is not uncommon, can be decreased by ensuring that the medication is taken with food.

Doxycycline is another alternative for prophylaxis, but it is not recommended for children less than 8 years old, and it must be taken every day. Photosensitivity is a common side effect, and vaginal candidiasis may occur in women on doxycycline prophylaxis. Chloroquine, chloroquine-proguanil, and azithromycin do not provide adequate protection for children traveling to a chloroquine-resistant malaria-endemic area. Daily primaquine has been used successfully as malaria prophylaxis in adults and children in areas endemic for

**TABLE 347-4 RECOMMENDED MALARIA DRUG PROPHYLAXIS IN CHILDREN**

| Area | Drug | Dosage (Oral) |
|---|---|---|
| Chloroquine-resistant area | Mefloquine[a] | ≤ 9 kg 4.6 mg/kg base (5 mg/kg salt) orally, once/week |
| | | > 9–19 kg: 1/4 tab |
| | | > 19–30 kg: 1/2 tab |
| | | > 30–45 kg: 3/4 tab |
| | | > 45 kg 1 tab |
| | OR | |
| | Doxycycline[b] | 2.2 mg/kg daily (max 100 mg) |
| | OR | |
| | Atovaquone/proguanil[c] | Pediatric tabs: 62.5 mg atovaquone/25 mg proguanil |
| | | Adult tabs: 250 mg atovaquone/100 mg proguanil |
| | | 5–8 kg: 1/2 pediatric tab once daily |
| | | > 8–10 kg: 3/4 pediatric tab once daily |
| | | > 10–20 kg: 1 pediatric tab once daily |
| | | > 20–30 kg: 2 pediatric tabs once daily |
| | | > 30–40 kg: 3 pediatric tabs once daily |
| | | > 40 kg: 1 adult tab once daily |
| Chloroquine-sensitive area | Chloroquine phosphate | 5 mg base/kg per week (max 300 mg base) |
| | | < 1 yr: 1/4 tablet |
| | | 1–3 yr: 1/2 tablet |
| | | 4–8 yr: 1 tablet |
| | | 9–14 yr: 2 tablets |
| | | > 14 yr: 3 tablets |

[a]Chloroquine and mefloquine should be started more than 2 weeks prior to departure and continued 4 weeks after last exposure. Mefloquine is contraindicated with a recent history of depression, generalized anxiety disorder, psychosis, or other major psychiatric disorders, seizures, or in persons with cardiac conduction abnormalities.

[b]Doxycycline should be started 1 day prior to departure and continued for 4 weeks after last exposure.

[c]Atovaquone/proguanil (Malarone) should be started 1 to 2 days prior to departure and continued for 7 days after return.

chloroquine-resistant *P falciparum*; however, it has not yet been studied extensively enough in nonimmune children to be recommended as routine chemoprophylaxis for these areas.

In locations where malaria remains chloroquine susceptible, chloroquine is the drug of choice for prophylaxis. The CDC Web site (www.cdc.gov) and hotline number (770-488-7788) are useful resources for determining the current malaria prophylaxis guidelines for specific countries. No prophylaxis is completely effective, and travelers may develop malaria despite taking the recommended malaria chemoprophylaxis.

On leaving an area endemic for *P vivax* or *P ovale* after a prolonged visit (> 3 months), children may require "terminal prophylaxis" with primaquine (0.6 mg/kg base or 1.0 mg/kg salt daily, up to a maximum dose of 30 mg base or 52.6 mg salt, for 14 days) to eliminate extraerythrocytic forms of *P vivax* and *P ovale* and to prevent relapses. Primaquine can cause severe hemolysis in G6PD-deficient individuals, so it is mandatory to rule out G6PD deficiency by laboratory testing before primaquine is prescribed.

Small amounts of antimalarial drugs are secreted into the breast milk of lactating women. The amounts of transferred drug are not considered harmful and do not provide adequate prophylaxis against malaria. Breastfeeding children should take standard doses of malaria chemoprophylaxis. Lactating women should avoid using doxycycline, as prolonged infant exposure to doxycycline via breast milk could be harmful.

In malaria-endemic areas of Africa, studies have demonstrated that insecticide-treated bednets (ITNs) can reduce all-cause mortality in children by 20% in malaria-endemic areas, and large-scale distribution of long-lasting ITNs have significantly reduced mortality from malaria in these areas. Indoor residual spraying with long-lasting pyrethroid insecticides has also significantly decreased malaria transmission in areas, but requires repeated annual or semi-annual application to remain effective in areas of mid- to high-level transmission.

The formulation of a malaria vaccine has been a complex problem because of the many antigens present in both pre-erythrocytic and erythrocytic phases of the parasite, polymorphisms in the parasite, polymorphisms in the human host, and the lack of sustained immunity from natural infection. Numerous malaria vaccine trials are in progress, using components of pre-erythrocytic and erythrocytic malarial antigens. The RTS,S vaccine, a vaccine based on the pre-erythrocytic antigen circumsporozoite protein (CSP), was the first vaccine to show significant efficacy in African children with a protective efficacy of 35% against clinical malaria in children ages 1 to 4 years, but follow-up studies showed much lower long-term efficacy, particularly in children more frequently exposed to malaria. Thus it is unclear whether this vaccine will actually be used in malaria-endemic countries.

Finally, artemisinin combination therapies as first-line treatment for malaria in areas of increasing drug resistance may also help limit transmission by reducing gametocytes, as gametocytes are the form of parasite required for transmission to and development in the *Anopheles* mosquito. A multistrategy approach using some combination of insecticide-treated bednets or indoor residual spraying, artemisinin combination therapy, and a partially effective vaccine may be the most effective way to reduce malaria transmission. Malaria eradication, first proposed in the 1950s but unsuccessful at that time, is now being proposed again. The likelihood of success in malaria eradication will depend on many factors, including the long-term commitment by funding agencies and national governments to this goal; the extent to which effective interventions can be successfully implemented, particularly in difficult-to-reach or politically troubled areas; the development of drug and insecticide resistance; and the continuation of careful malaria surveillance and follow-up after case numbers decrease.

## SUGGESTED READINGS


Bangirana P, Opoka RO, Boivin MJ, et al. Severe malarial anemia is associated with long-term neurocognitive impairment. *Clin Infect Dis*. 2014;59:336-344.

Cullen KA, Mace KE, Arguin PM, Centers for Disease Control and Prevention. Malaria Surveillance–United States, 2013. *Morb Mortal Wkly Rep Surveill Summ*. 2016;65:1-22.

Dondorp AM, Fanello CI, Hendriksen IC, et al. Artesunate versus quinine in the treatment of severe falciparum malaria in African children (AQUAMAT): an open-label, randomised trial. *Lancet*. 2010;376:1647-1657.

Feachem RG, Phillips AA, Hwang J, et al. Shrinking the malaria map: progress and prospects. *Lancet*. 2010;376:1566-1578.

John CC, Kutamba E, Mugarura K, Opoka RO. Adjunctive therapy for cerebral malaria and other severe forms of *Plasmodium falciparum* malaria. *Expert Rev Anti Infect Ther*. 2010;8:997-1008.

Olotu A, Fegan G, Wambua J, et al. Seven-year efficacy of RTS,S/AS01 malaria vaccine among young African children. *N Engl J Med*. 2016;374:2519-2529.

Seydel KB, Kampondeni SD, Valim C, et al. Brain swelling and death in children with cerebral malaria. *N Engl J Med*. 2015;372:1126-1137.

Tan KR, Wiegand RE, Arguin PM. Exchange transfusion for severe malaria: evidence base and literature review. *Clin Infect Dis*. 2013;57:923-928.

Turner L, Lavstsen T, Berger SS, et al. Severe malaria is associated with parasite binding to endothelial protein C receptor. *Nature*. 2013;498:502-505.

World Health Organization. *Guidelines for the Treatment of Malaria*. 3rd ed. Geneva, Switzerland: World Health Organization; 2015:1-313.

# 348 *Pneumocystis* Pneumonia

Francis Gigliotti and Walter T. Hughes

## INTRODUCTION

*Pneumocystis* pneumonia (PCP) occurs almost exclusively in the severely immunocompromised host, especially patients with congenital immunodeficiency diseases, acquired immunodeficiency syndrome (AIDS), and cancer, and those who have had organ transplantation. The increasing use of biologics, such as anti–tumor necrosis factor (TNF), is now putting a new group of patients at risk for developing PCP. Once pneumonia is apparent, the fatality rate is near 100% if untreated. Effective therapeutic and prophylactic drugs are available. The causative agent is an atypical fungus known for the past decade as *Pneumocystis jirovecii.*

## PATHOGENESIS AND EPIDEMIOLOGY

The portal of entry for *Pneumocystis* is believed to be the respiratory tract via the airborne route. In the infected lung, the organism is found in both cystic and extracystic forms. The description of *Pneumocystis* morphology is a carryover from when the organism was felt to be a protozoan. The cyst is a round, oval, or cup-shaped structure approximately 4 to 6 μm in diameter (Fig. 348-1). Within the mature cyst are as many as 8 daughter cells, referred to as sporozoites (or intracystic bodies) that are pleomorphic and often crescent shaped. These cells eventually excyst through breaks in the cyst wall. Outside the cyst, the daughter cell, now termed a trophozoite (or trophic form) varies from 2 to 5 μm in diameter. These thin-walled trophozoites tend to cluster in masses.

In the normal, healthy individual, *Pneumocystis* may lie dormant in the alveoli, eliciting no tissue response and leaving the host asymptomatic. In the severely immunocompromised host, organisms replicate to large numbers, and an extensive diffuse alveolar disease and interstitial infiltration may progress to death.

*Pneumocystis* attaches to the alveolar epithelial cells, and alveolar macrophages ingest and degrade the organisms; this provokes neutrophil, lymphocyte, and monocyte infiltration and cytokine release. Alveolar disruption impedes gas exchange and leads to respiratory failure. The CD4+ T lymphocyte serves to recruit and activate other immune effector cells. There is an increase in CD8+ lymphocytes in the lungs. Surfactant phospholipids are reduced in PCP, further impairing pulmonary function. In untreated patients, this leads to respiratory failure and death.

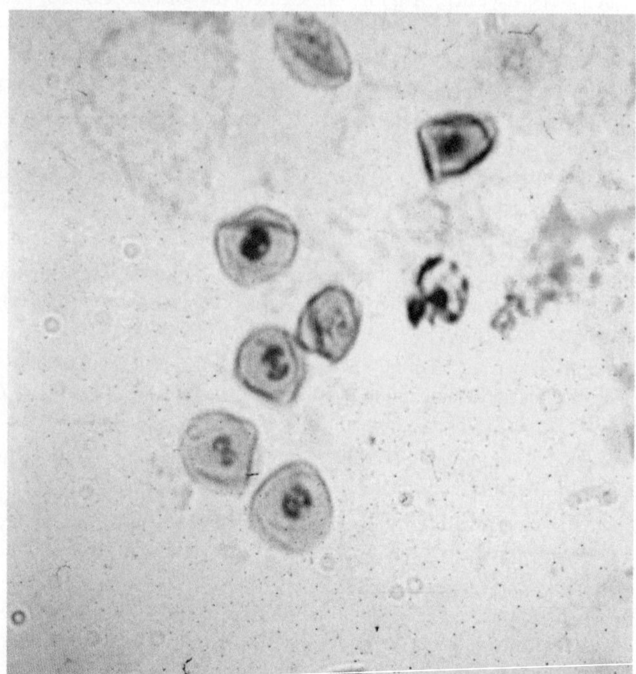

**FIGURE 348-1** Cyst forms of *Pneumocystis* as seen in a bronchoalveolar lavage specimen stained with Gomori methenamine silver nitrate method.

*Pneumocystis* infection is recognized among humans and lower animals worldwide. The natural habitat and mode of transmission in man are unknown, but animal studies suggest animal-to-animal transmission occurs by the airborne route. Animal-to-human transmission has not been reported, and available evidence suggests that human-to-human transmission is possible. Symptomatic infection occurs sporadically in nonimmunocompromised individuals.

PCP was first recognized in humans by Van der Meer and Brug in 1942. During this time, epidemics of interstitial plasma cell pneumonitis were occurring in European infants. In the 1950s, several reports confirmed that *Pneumocystis* was the etiology of epidemics of interstitial plasma cell pneumonitis in these infants. The predisposing risk factor among these children was likely immunodeficiency secondary to malnutrition.

With the advent of immunosuppressive therapy for cancer and methods for diagnosing congenital immunodeficiency disorders, PCP became recognized as an increasingly common and potentially fatal infection in such individuals.

Intrauterine transmission of *Pneumocystis* has also been reported. Of 8 pregnant women with AIDS and PCP, 1 infant had *Pneumocystis* infection. Considerable data show that at least 75% of normal children reaching 4 years of age have acquired antibody to *Pneumocystis* and that more than 90% of normal adults have detectable antibody. Furthermore, a prospective study of otherwise normal infants, age 2 to 12 weeks, with pneumonia showed that 10 of 69 babies had detectable antibody to *Pneumocystis* and that 1 of the 10 infants had PCP. In serial observations of 107 normal infants, *Pneumocystis* DNA was detected in nasopharyngeal aspirates in 74 of the infants tested. In addition, *Pneumocystis* has been associated with sudden infant death syndrome (SIDS), but no cause and effect has been proven. The natural course of PCP can be delineated from studies done before the advent of chemoprophylaxis in 1977 in individuals at high risk for PCP. Data collected at the Centers for Disease Control and Prevention (CDC) revealed 194 documented cases of PCP encountered in the United States during the 3-year period from 1967 to 1970. Twenty-five (12.9%) of these cases had primary immunodeficiency disorders; 91 (47%) had leukemia; 41 (21%) had other malignancies; 22 (11%) were organ transplant recipients, and 15 (8%) had other immunocompromising conditions. From 1962 to 1971, the incidence of PCP was determined in 1251 children with malignancies and 379 patients with nonmalignant neoplasms or immunodeficiency diseases at St. Jude Children's Research Hospital; PCP was found in 4.1%, 0%, and 0% of patients, respectively. The incidence of PCP in cancer patients is influenced more by the extent of immunocompromise from treatment than the primary disease. In a controlled study of 160 children with acute lymphocytic leukemia without PCP prophylaxis and on intensive antileukemia therapy, 20% were found to have developed PCP. Other at-risk populations include those immunosuppressed for solid organ transplantation, rheumatoid arthritis, lupus erythematosus, inflammatory bowel disease, and other connective tissue diseases in adults with CD4+ T-lymphocyte counts less than 250/μL.

A 1999 review of 4581 solid organ transplant recipients who were not receiving prophylaxis found that 4.9% had PCP. A 2006 report showed PCP is emerging as a complication of immunosuppressive therapy for patients with rheumatoid arthritis, lupus erythematosus, and other connective tissue diseases in adults with CD4+ T-lymphocyte counts less than 250/μL.

Patients with HIV are ideal targets for PCP because of a profound defect in their cell-mediated immune responses. Early in the AIDS epidemic, when no antiviral therapy was available and chemoprophylaxis for PCP was not applied, some 75% of adults and 39% of infants with AIDS acquired PCP. In infants and children with human immunodeficiency virus (HIV) infection, PCP occurs most often in infants between 3 and 6 months of age. The use of PCP prophylaxis and combined antiretroviral therapy (cART) has profoundly reduced PCP in patients with AIDS. Before cART (from 1981 to 1988), the incidence of PCP in 3331 HIV-infected children was 1.3 cases per 100 person-years; after the introduction of cART (2001–2004), the incidence of PCP in 2767 HIV-infected patients decreased to less than 0.5 per 100 person-years. The Perinatal AIDS Collaborative Transmission Study showed a 95% decrease in PCP (cases per 100 patient-years), from 5.8 in the pre-HAART era to 0.3 in the HAART era.

While the incidence of PCP has declined in children with AIDS in the United States, the incidence has increased in Africa. From 1992 to 1993, 16% of children dying with AIDS had PCP; 29% of those dying from 1997 to 2000 and 44% of those dying between 2000 and 2001 had PCP.

As with other immunosuppressed states, a highly significant risk factor for PCP in HIV-infected patients is a marked reduction in the CD4+ T-lymphocyte count.

## CLINICAL MANIFESTATIONS

The clinical manifestations of PCP may present abruptly as an acute febrile episode with respiratory symptoms or a more subtle subacute illness with little or no fever. In all cases, tachypnea, cough, dyspnea, and oxygen desaturation occur. Typically, the chest radiograph shows bilateral, diffuse alveolar disease with symmetric reticular (interstitial) or granular opacities (Fig. 348-2). However, by the time pneumonitis is discernible by radiograph, tachypnea, flaring of nasal alae, intercostal retractions, and even cyanosis may be evident on examination. Even with diffuse pneumonitis, rales may not be heard. Once pneumonitis is evident, the infection progresses to a fatal outcome in nearly 100% of cases if untreated.

Atypically, lobar, nodular, or miliary lesions are found. The type of clinical presentation is generally related to the patient's age and the underlying primary disease and its treatment. Presenting features and disease progression are a function of the host's ability to mount an inflammatory response. Infants tend to have the slower subacute course, and older children have the acute onset. Studies have found that HIV-infected patients present with a higher arterial oxygen tension and a lower alveolar-arterial oxygen gradient than other immunocompromised hosts.

In children with severe protein-calorie malnutrition, the onset is often subtle, with chronic diarrhea and weight loss preceding the onset of cough, tachypnea, and dyspnea. Fever is often absent, and symptoms may persist for several days before evidence of pneumonitis is seen on the chest radiograph. By the time pneumonitis is discernible by radiograph, tachypnea, flaring of nasal alae, intercostal retractions, and even cyanosis may be evident on examination. Even with diffuse pneumonitis, rales may not be heard.

It is important to note that both the acute and subacute presentation for PCP may occur in any immunosuppressive disease and in any age group. Hypoxia, as revealed by decreased arterial oxygen tension, is found in essentially all cases of PCP.

A recent study of HIV-infected children with pneumonia showed 4 clinical factors were independently associated with PCP: respiratory rate greater than 59 respirations per minute, arterial hemoglobin saturation ($SaO_2$) less than or equal to 92%, age less than 6 months of age, and the absence of vomiting.

With rare exception, in patients with PCP, the disease and the organisms remain localized to the lungs, even in fatal cases. Although rare, *Pneumocystis* has been found in extrapulmonary sites, including meninges, spleen, liver, pancreas, thyroid, brain, kidneys, bone marrow, heart, lymph nodes, ears, eyes, stomach, intestinal tract, ureter, muscles, adrenal glands, and peritoneum. Usually no clinical manifestations are associated with these infected sites.

## DIAGNOSIS

A definitive diagnosis requires the demonstration of *Pneumocystis* in infected lung tissue or in material from the lung that is obtained by bronchoalveolar lavage (BAL); induced sputum; or open lung, transbronchial, percutaneous, or endobronchial brush biopsies. BAL is usually the preferred procedure for children, although the lung biopsy remains the "gold standard" because it provides histology of the disease. The specimen is stained with Gomori, toluidine blue O, calcofluor white, or Giemsa stains (Figs. 348-1 and 348-3 to 348-6). A fluorescence-conjugated monoclonal antibody (Meriflour; Meridian Bioscience, Cincinnati, OH) is highly sensitive and specific (Fig. 348-7). Serum antibody titers to *Pneumocystis* are of no diagnostic value.

*Pneumocystis* DNA/RNA has been detected in lung tissue, in sputum, and in oral and nasal secretions by polymerase chain reaction (PCR), but standardized assay systems are not generally available, which limits its use in the clinical microbiology laboratory. While lung biopsy is the most sensitive and specific procedure and provides histopathology on the extent of disease process, BAL is usually the procedure initially used because of the possible complications from general anesthesia, pneumothorax, hemorrhage, and pneumomediastinum with biopsy. The reported diagnostic sensitivity of BAL ranges from 89% to greater than 98%.

Due to the dearth of data on induced sputum in infants and children, the sensitivity of the procedure for diagnosis is not known.

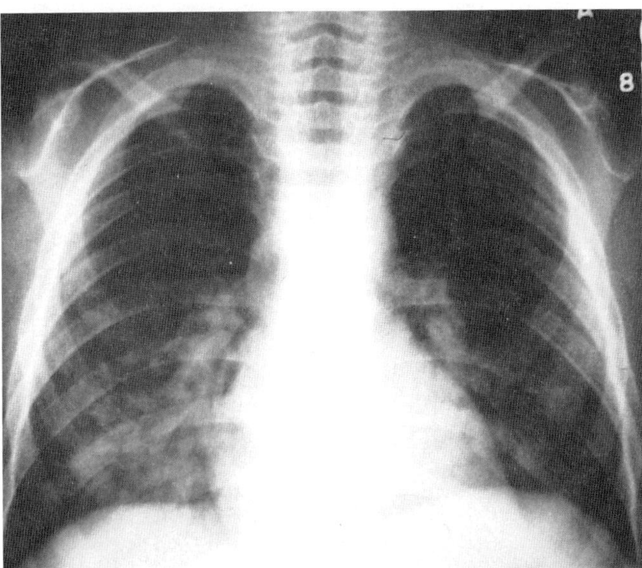

**FIGURE 348-2** Chest radiograph of *Pneumocystis* pneumonia showing bilateral diffuse alveolar disease.

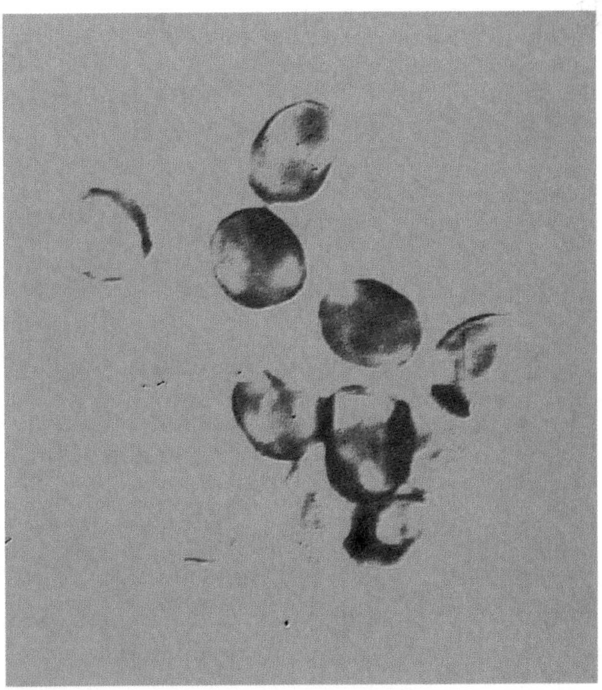

**FIGURE 348-3** Cyst forms of *Pneumocystis* as seen in bronchoalveolar lavage specimen stained with toluidine blue O method.

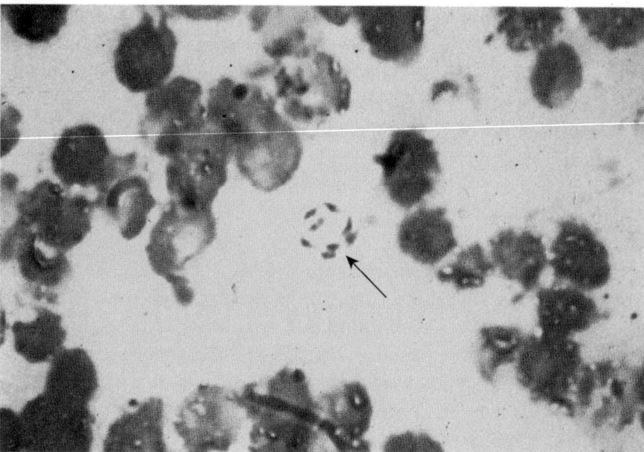

**FIGURE 348-4** *Pneumocystis* sporozoites as seen in bronchoalveolar lavage specimen stained with Giemsa method. Eight crescent-shaped sporozoites (*arrow*) are clustered within the confines of a cyst wall. Giemsa does not stain the cyst wall. Compare organism with background red blood cells for estimation of size.

However, if microscopic methods find *Pneumocystis* in the sputum of a patient of any age who has clinical evidence of pneumonitis, it can be dependably accepted as diagnostic of PCP. If the first induced sputum sample is negative, a BAL is warranted.

Because *Pneumocystis* is highly resistant to acid and because PCP is associated with a massive number of organisms in the lungs, gastric lavage might provide a means to obtain diagnostic specimens (as with acid-fast mycobacteria). Early studies found *Pneumocystis* in gastric aspirates of 23% of children with PCP, and no gastric aspirates in uninfected controls yielded the organism. Other studies yielded a diagnosis of PCP in about half of patients with PCP.

## TREATMENT

Trimethoprim-sulfamethoxazole (TMP-SMX) is the preferred drug for treating *Pneumocystis* pneumonia (Table 348-1). The dosage is based on 20 mg of TMP and 100 mg SMX per kilogram per day orally or three-fourths of this dose given intravenously (IV) in 3 or 4 doses. A 2-week course is usually adequate for patients without AIDS, but at least 3 weeks of treatment is needed for patients with AIDS.

TMP-SMX is usually administered IV at first. When there is evidence of clinical improvement and the patient can take and tolerate oral therapy, the drug combination can be given orally, using either tablets or suspension. The recommended doses provide an effective therapeutic serum concentration of 5 to 10 μg/mL of TMP.

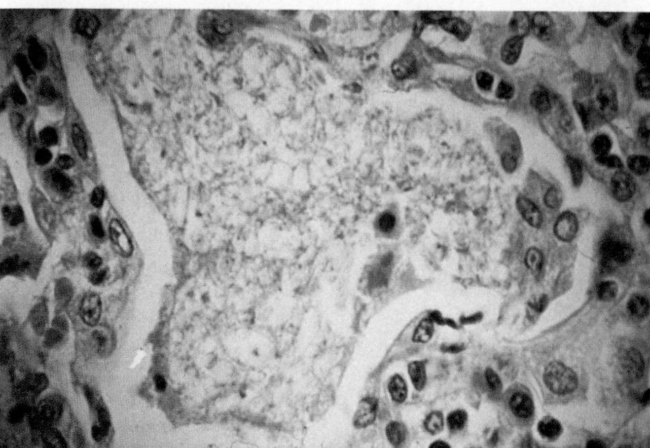

**FIGURE 348-5** Lung biopsy specimen stained with hematoxylin and eosin. This shows alveoli filled with the typical "frothy proteinaceous" material and reactive alveolar macrophages. *Pneumocystis* does not stain with hematoxylin and eosin.

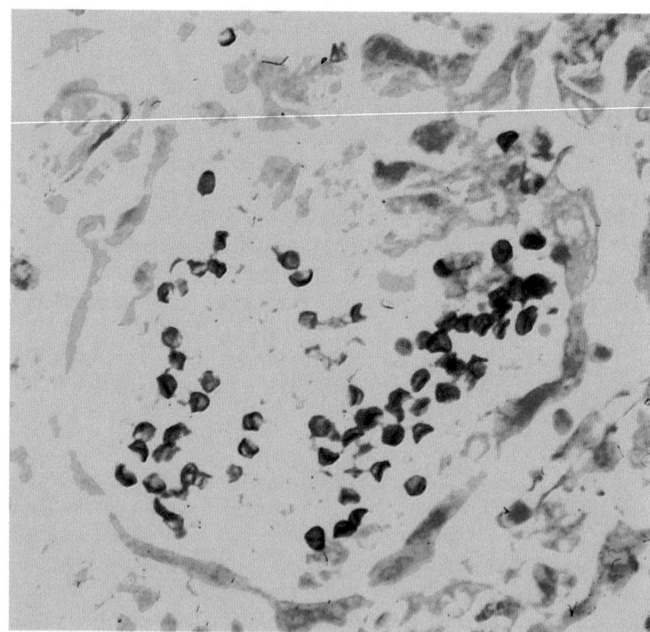

**FIGURE 348-6** Lung biopsy specimen stained with Gomori methenamine silver nitrate method. This shows the dark-staining cyst forms of *Pneumocystis* filling the alveoli.

Because patients who have 1 episode of PCP and recover are at high risk for a recurrent episode, such individuals should be maintained on TMP-SMX as long as their CD4+ totals remain depressed. TMP-SMX is generally well tolerated, but HIV-infected patients have an exceptionally high rate of adverse reactions. These include rash, fever, anorexia, nausea, vomiting, diarrhea, leukopenia, thrombocytopenia, anemia, renal toxicity, and exfoliative skin disorders (Stevens-Johnson syndrome). Unless the reaction is mild and insignificant, TMP-SMX should be discontinued and therapy continued with another drug, usually pentamidine. About 15% of HIV-infected children have substantial adverse reactions to TMP-SMX.

Pentamidine is recommended for patients who cannot tolerate or who do not respond to TMP-SMX. The drug must be administered

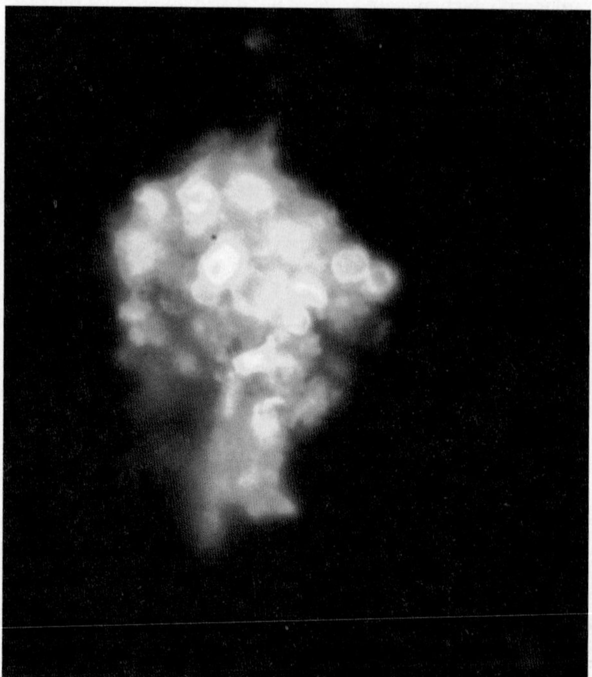

**FIGURE 348-7** *Pneumocystis* cysts and trophozoites in a cluster stained with fluorescein-labeled antibody.

**TABLE 348-1 DRUGS FOR THE TREATMENT OF *PNEUMOCYSTIS* PNEUMONIA (PCP)**

| Drug | Administration | Notations |
|---|---|---|
| Trimethoprim (TMP)-sulfamethoxazole (SMX) | 15–20 mg TMP + 75–100 mg SMX kg/d IV, in 3–4 divided doses. May change to PO as pneumonitis subsides. | Drug of first choice |
| | | Total daily dose not to exceed 960 mg TMP/4800 mg SMX |
| Pentamidine isethionate | 4 mg/kg IV once daily | Drug of second choice |
| | | Total daily dose not to exceed 300 mg |
| | | High toxicity |
| | | Infuse over 1–1.5 h period |
| Atovaquone | Age < 3 mo and > 24 mo = 30–40 mg/kg/d in 2 divided doses PO | Food increases absorption 2–3 times |
| | Age 3 mo to 24 mo = 45 mg/kg/d in 2 divided doses | Few adverse effects |
| | | Approved for mild and moderate PCP |
| Dapsone-trimethoprim | Dapsone 2 mg/kg once daily PO | Do not use dapsone or TMP alone for treatment |
| | AND TMP 15 mg/kg/d PO in 3 divided doses | Total dose of dapsone not to exceed 100 mg/d |
| | | Studied in mild and moderate cases of PCP |
| Clindamycin-primaquine | Clindamycin 40 mg/kg/d IV in 4 divided doses | Not studied in children with PCP |
| | AND primaquine 0.3 mg/kg/d PO | Doses estimated from use in other infections in children |
| | | Exclude G6PD-deficient patients |
| Prednisone | Days 1–5 = 1.0 mg/kg twice daily | Consider use in patients with $PaO_2$ < 70 mm Hg or with alveolar-arterial gradient of > 35 mm Hg |
| | Days 6–10 = 0.5 mg/kg twice daily | |
| | Days 11–21 = 0.5 mg/kg once daily | |

G6PD, glucose-6-phosphate dehydrogenase; IV, intravenous; PO, oral.

parenterally and is frequently associated with nephrotoxicity, hypoglycemia, and other adverse effects. Pentamidine is given as a single IV dose at 4 mg/kg. Pentamidine isethionate is available only by the IV, intramuscular, and aerosol routes. Aerosolized pentamidine is only minimally effective for therapy and should not be used. The IV route is preferred to avoid the severe cutaneous reactions encountered from intramuscular administration. Pentamidine is highly toxic, causing nephrotoxicity, hypokalemia, hypo- and hyperglycemia, pancreatitis, leukopenia, cardiac arrhythmias, and cutaneous sterile abscess and necrosis. Adverse reactions occur in up to 80% of patients receiving pentamidine, and the drug must be discontinued in half the cases.

Other drugs with demonstrated efficacy for treating PCP are atovaquone, dapsone plus trimethoprim, sulfadoxine/pyrimethamine (Fansidar), and clindamycin plus primaquine (see Table 348-1). Atovaquone offers a safe alternative to TMP-SMX and is available only as an oral suspension (750 mg per 5 mL). It has been evaluated for treatment of PCP in adults with AIDS and was found to have therapeutic efficacy related directly to the plasma concentration of the drug. At a mean steady-state concentration of at least 15 μg/mL, therapeutic success was achieved in more than 95% of cases; at levels of 5 to 10 μg/mL, only 69% had successful outcome. Thus, it is essential to emphasize the administration of this medication with food (preferably fatty meals), which will provide a 2- to 3-fold greater plasma concentration than when administered in a fasting state. Adverse events with atovaquone therapy include nausea, vomiting, diarrhea, and rash. No fatal adverse reactions have been reported.

The combination of dapsone and trimethoprim has proven effective in treating PCP in adults with AIDS. Trimethoprim alone has little, if any, effect on PCP but is synergistic to enhance therapeutic efficacy of dapsone. Dapsone alone is effective in only about 61% of cases, while dapsone plus trimethoprim is effective in 100% of cases. Reversible neutropenia is a common adverse effect of dapsone. Other side effects to dapsone are rash, methemoglobinemia, anemia, thrombocytopenia, and elevated transaminases.

Lack of data on the use of clindamycin plus primaquine to treat PCP in children relegates this regimen to cases where the aforementioned regimens cannot be used.

Supportive measures are important in managing PCP. Administering oxygen and using assisted mechanical ventilation are indicated with severe hypoxia. Evidence suggests that using a corticosteroid may enhance survival in patients with moderate and severe PCP. With partial pressure of oxygen ($PaO_2$) values less than 70 mm Hg or an alveolar-arterial gradient of greater than 35 mm Hg, the administration of a corticosteroid such as prednisone is recommended (see Table 348-1).

Once pneumonitis is evident on chest radiograph, PCP is fatal in approximately 100% of cases if untreated. When defervescence reveals signs of clinical improvement from treatment, a decrease in respiratory rate and an increase in $PaO_2$ may be seen at a mean of 4.5 ± 2.5 days and improvement in chest radiograph may be seen at 7.7 ± 4.5 days after treatment begins.

## PREVENTION

*Pneumocystis* pneumonitis can be prevented by the prophylactic use of TMP-SMX in a dosage of 5 mg of TMP and 25 mg of SMX per kilogram per day orally (daily or 3 days a week) in equally divided doses. For patients who cannot tolerate TMP-SMX, atovaquone, dapsone, and aerosolized pentamidine are effective alternatives (Table 348-2). The host is protected for only as long as the drug is administered. Updated CDC and National Institutes of Health (NIH) guidelines established for prophylaxis in infants and children with HIV infection recommend the following individuals receive PCP prophylaxis: all HIV-infected and indeterminate infants age 1 to 12 months; children age 1 through 5 years with CD4+ T-lymphocyte counts of less than 500/μL (or < 15%); and children age 6 years and older with CD4+ T-lymphocyte counts of less than 200/μL (or < 15%). Other patients at high risk for PCP and who warrant prophylaxis are those who have received organ transplants, those who have certain malignancies and congenital immunodeficiency syndromes, and those who require prolonged immunosuppressive therapy.

When deciding which patients should receive chemoprophylaxis, the following high-risk factors should be considered: all HIV-infected patients as defined above; lymphoproliferative malignancies; prolonged corticosteroid therapy; extensive impairment of cell-mediated immunity (eg, severe combined immunodeficiency syndrome, S-linked CD40 ligand deficiency); CD4+ T lymphocyte counts less than 200/μL (15%); severe malnutrition; bone marrow transplant recipients; certain solid organ transplant recipients; previous episode of PCP; brain tumor; and Wegener granulomatosis.

TMP-SMX has been the preferred drug for PCP prophylaxis for 3 decades and has been thoroughly evaluated in children with AIDS and in those with non-AIDS immunosuppressive diseases.

**TABLE 348-2 *PNEUMOCYSTIS* PNEUMONIA PROPHYLAXIS REGIMENS**

| Drug | Administration | Notations |
|---|---|---|
| Trimethoprim (TMP)-sulfamethoxazole (SMX) | 5 mg TMP + 25 mg SMX kg/d or 3 times per week on consecutive days | Drug of choice |
| | | If adverse events, stop drug and consider restarting at desensitizing doses |
| | | Total dose not to exceed 320 mg TMP/1600 mg SMX daily |
| | | Also has broad-spectrum antibiotic activity |
| Atovaquone | Age < 3 mo and > 24 mo = 30 mg/kg once daily | Drug of second choice |
| | Age 4 to 24 mo = 45 mg/kg once daily | Administer with meal (high fat preferred) |
| | | Strong safety record |
| | | No antibacterial effect |
| | | Total daily dose not to exceed 1500 mg/d |
| Dapsone | Age ≥ 1 mo = 2 mg/kg per day PO or 4 mg/kg per week | Drug of second choice |
| | | Monitor for anemia and methemoglobinemia |
| | | Marketed in tablet form only, but syrup may be obtained through compassionate IND |
| | | Total daily dose not to exceed 100 mg daily or 200 mg weekly doses |
| Aerosolized pentamidine | Ages ≥ 5 y = 300 mg once per month | Drug of third choice |
| | | Administer with Respirgard II nebulizer (Marquest, Englewood, CO) |
| | | Watch for cough, sneezing, and bronchospasm |
| | | Good safety record |

IND, investigational new drug.

Generally what is observed with PCP in AIDS patients is somewhat similar to what occurs in non-AIDS patients, except adverse reactions to TMP-SMX are more frequent in HIV-infected patients than in those without HIV. When non–life-threatening adverse effects occur, TMP-SMX can be discontinued; when the reaction has resolved, the drug combination can be restarted with a desensitizing scheme. If the initial adverse reaction is life-threatening, stop TMP-SMX and use an alternative drug. Usually atovaquone or dapsone is the drug of second choice.

Atovaquone is effective and safe for PCP prophylaxis. A major disadvantage of atovaquone is its cost. A month of prophylaxis with atovaquone costs about 40 times that of TMP-SMX. Unlike TMP-SMX, atovaquone has no antibacterial activity but is effective against *Toxoplasma gondii, Babesia* species, and malaria. A prospective controlled study compared atovaquone plus azithromycin with TMP-SMX in 366 HIV-infected children at high risk for PCP. Results showed the regimens were equally effective in preventing PCP and bacterial infections. In a recent study, 86 children with leukemia who were intolerant to TMP-SMX received atovaquone prophylaxis over a period of 172 patient-years. No cases of PCP occurred, and no significant adverse effects were found. Daily atovaquone prophylaxis has been shown to be as effective as aerosolized pentamidine. Dapsone is as effective as atovaquone or aerosolized pentamidine for prophylaxis but is possibly less effective than TMP-SMX. Similarly, no cases of PCP were encountered in peripheral blood stem cell transplant recipients receiving either TMP-SMX or atovaquone, while treatment-limiting adverse reactions occurred in 40% of those on TMP-SMX and none of those given atovaquone.

Dapsone is a sulfone with several known adverse effects; however, it has been proven relatively safe for PCP prophylaxis. The long plasma half-life of dapsone allows its use as a once-a-day or once-a-week dosage administration. This drug is as effective as atovaquone or aerosolized pentamidine for prophylaxis but is possibly less effective than TMP-SMX.

The pediatric dosage for aerosolized pentamidine is 300 mg once a month; the same dose is recommended for adults. This drug is somewhat more cumbersome to administer than dapsone or atovaquone but has the advantage of compliance through direct observational therapy once a month. During and following administration with the Respirgard II nebulizer, patients should be observed for cough and bronchospasm.

Once PCP prophylaxis has been started, it should be continued as long as the susceptible immunocompromised state exists. Usually within 3 to 6 months after completion of chemotherapy, the prophylaxis can be stopped. Recent studies in both adults and children with AIDS show that those on combination antiretroviral therapy who achieve immune reconstitution of CD4+ T lymphocyte to greater than 15% may have PCP prophylaxis discontinued if monitoring with CD4+ T-lymphocyte count is continued.

## SUGGESTED READINGS


Centers for Disease Control and Prevention, National Institutes of Health, and Infectious Diseases Society of America. Guidelines for the prevention and treatment of opportunistic infections among HIV-exposed and HIV-infected children. *Morb Mortal Wkly Rep.* 2009;58(RR-11):1-166.

Centers for Disease Control and Prevention, National Institutes of Health, and Infectious Diseases Society of America. Guidelines for the prevention and treatment of opportunistic infections among HIV-infected adults and adolescents. *Morb Mortal Wkly Rep.* 2009;58(RR-4):1-198.

DeMasi JM, Cox JA, Leonard D, Koh AY, Aquino VM. Intravenous pentamidine is safe and effective as primary *Pneumocystis* pneumonia prophylaxis in children and adolescents undergoing hematopoietic stem cell transplantation. *Pediatr Infect Dis J.* 2013;32:933-936.

Ewald H, Raatz H, Boscacci R, Furrer H, Bucher HC, Briel M. Adjunctive corticosteroids for *Pneumocystis jiroveci* pneumonia in patients with HIV infection. *Cochrane Database Syst Rev.* 2015;4:CD006150.

Morrow BM, Samuel CM, Zampoli M, Whitelaw A, Zar HJ. *Pneumocystis* pneumonia in South African children diagnosed by molecular methods. *BMC Res Notes.* 2014;7:26.

Stern A, Green H, Paul M, Vidal L, Leibovici L. Prophylaxis for Pneumocystis pneumonia (PCP) in non-HIV immunocompromised patients. *Cochrane Database Syst Rev.* 2014;10:CD005590.

# 349 Toxoplasmosis

Despina Contopoulos-Ioannidis and Yvonne A. Maldonado

## INTRODUCTION

*Toxoplasma gondii* is a coccidian parasite that is among the most common parasites that infect humans worldwide. Members of the feline species, domestic or wild cats, are the definitive hosts.

## PATHOGENESIS AND EPIDEMIOLOGY

Cats ingest *Toxoplasma* in the form of tissue cysts (eg, eating infected rodents or oocysts) and excrete oocysts in their feces. The oocysts can remain viable in the soil in a warm and moist environment for as long as 18 months. Oocysts can sporulate within 1 to 5 days and become infectious by releasing sporozoites, becoming an ongoing source of infection for other mammals. Oocysts can also remain viable in salt and fresh water. *T gondii* can be found in nature in 3 forms: (1) oocysts excreted in cat's feces; (2) bradyzoites in tissue cysts; and (3) tachyzoites, the active proliferative form that can infect several different types of cells, seen during acute infections or reactivation of chronic infections.

Humans can become infected by the following routes: (1) ingestion of viable tissue cysts in undercooked *T gondii*–infected meat; (2) ingestion of contaminated food from contact with contaminated surfaces/utensils; (3) ingestion of food contaminated with soil such as unwashed fruits or vegetables; (4) accidental ingestion of soil contaminated with *T gondii* (eg, while cleaning a cat's litter box or during gardening); (5) congenital infection via mother-to-child transmission; (6) drinking contaminated water; (7) via organ transplantation with a *T gondii*–infected organ carrying tissue cysts; (8) rarely from blood transfusion as the duration of parasitemia after acute infection is usually short; and (9) after a laboratory accident with *Toxoplasma*-contaminated material. Additional risk factors recently associated with risk of *T gondii* infections include eating infected raw oysters, clams, or mussels and drinking unpasteurized goat's milk. *Toxoplasma* tissue cysts in meat can be inactivated with cooking at high temperatures (eg, up to 74°C [165°F] for poultry meat) or freezing for at least 48 hours at −20°C (−4°F); processed infected meat that is smoked or dried can still be infectious. Drinking contaminated water has been the source for large community outbreaks. Commonly used water treatments do not efficiently inactivate oocysts. The *T gondii* seroprevalence rates vary in different parts of the world and can range from less than 10% in some northern European countries to 60% to 80% in South America and Africa. In the United States, the overall age-adjusted seroprevalence according to the National Health and Nutrition Examination Survey (NHANES) 2009–2010 survey was 12.4%. However, the seroprevalence in certain socioeconomic and racial subgroups can be as high as 20% to 25%. The age-adjusted seroprevalence of *T gondii* among women of childbearing age in the United States in 2009 to 2010 was 9%. The incidence of acute toxoplasmosis during gestation in the United States has been estimated to range between 0.2 and 1.1 acute infections per 1000 pregnant women, which translates to approximately 800 to 4400 pregnant women being acutely infected during gestation annually. However, the higher rates are derived from an epidemiologic prenatal surveillance study conducted in the United States more than 40 years ago.

The global burden of congenital toxoplasmosis (CT) is high, and it has been estimated that there are approximately 190,000 cases of CT globally per year. In the United States, only 2 states, Massachusetts and New Hampshire, routinely screen newborns for toxoplasmosis. The incidence of CT, according to the most recent data from the New England Newborn Screening Program over the past 9 years (2006–2014), has been reported to be approximately 0.23 cases/10,000 live births. However, the true incidence could be 25% to 50% higher as the sensitivity of the newborn screening blotspot immunoglobulin (Ig) M is only 50% to 75% and fetal losses attributable to severe CT are not captured. In other areas such as Africa and South America, the incidence rate of CT is much higher (20–24 CT cases/10,000 live births and 18–34 CT cases/10,000 live births, respectively). Circulation of more virulent *T gondii* strains that may also cause infections with higher parasite load and absence of routine prenatal screening and treatment may be possible reasons for these differences.

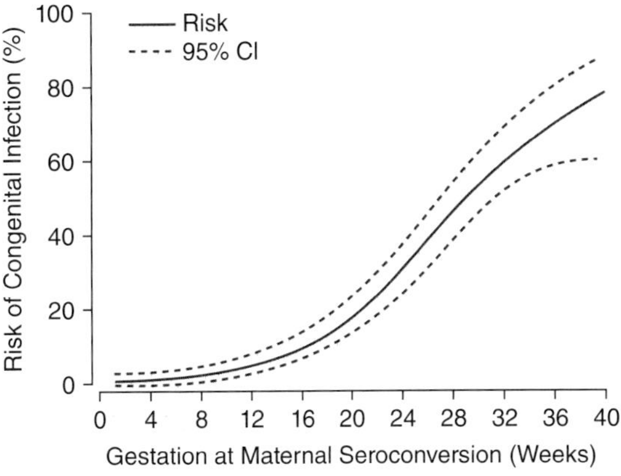


**FIGURE 349-1** Risk of congenital infection by duration of gestation at the time of maternal infection. (Reproduced with permission from Dunn D, Wallon M, Peyron F, et al. Mother-to-child transmission of toxoplasmosis: risk estimates for clinical counselling, *Lancet.* 1999 May 29;353(9167):1829-1833.)

Mother-to-child transmission (MTCT) of *Toxoplasma* can occur in the following ways: (1) transmission of *T gondii* to the fetus from a previously seronegative mother who acquired an acute *Toxoplasma* infection during gestation or within 3 months before conception, which is the most common scenario; (2) occasionally from reactivation of a chronic *Toxoplasma* infection in a previously seropositive pregnant woman who is or becomes severely immunosuppressed or immunocompromised during gestation, particularly in the absence of anti-*Toxoplasma* prophylaxis (eg, in a human immunodeficiency virus [HIV]–infected woman or a woman on immunosuppressive medications or certain monoclonal antibodies); or (3) rare reinfection of a previously seropositive pregnant woman with a new, more virulent *T gondii* strain. The risk of MTCT increases with advanced gestational age at maternal seroconversion (Fig. 349-1). The overall rate of MTCT risk in European cohorts, where acutely infected pregnant women are promptly diagnosed and treated, has been reported to be approximately 25% (6% at 13 weeks; 40% at 26 weeks; 72% at 36 weeks), while the overall rate prior to the introduction of spiramycin was 50% to 60%. The risk of MTCT also increases with absence of prenatal treatment, infections with more virulent strains such as non–type II or atypical strains and/or infections associated with high parasite load. Recently accumulated evidence over the past 10 years from several large European observational cohort studies provides supporting evidence for the effectiveness of prenatal treatment in the decrease of MTCT risk and the amelioration of clinical manifestations of severe CT. Early initiation of prenatal treatment within less than 3 to 4 weeks from the acute maternal primary infection has been shown to be critical. Currently in the United States, universal prenatal screening for CT is not recommended for immunocompetent women, based on the low seroprevalence of infection. However, recently accumulated evidence outside the United States on the effectiveness of prenatal treatment and availability of commercially available screening tests with good diagnostic performance may lead to further evaluation.

## CLINICAL MANIFESTATIONS

Children with toxoplasma infections can present with one of the following clinical scenarios: (1) postnatally acquired acute *Toxoplasma* infection; (2) chronic latent *Toxoplasma* infection; (3) reactivation of chronic latent *Toxoplasma* infection in immunocompromised children, particularly in the absence of appropriate anti-*Toxoplasma* prophylaxis; (4) ocular toxoplasmosis in an infant with CT, from reactivation of eye disease later in life in congenitally infected infants or during a postnatally acquired acute infection; and (5) CT in newborns or young infants.

### Postnatally Acquired Acute *Toxoplasma* Infection

Postnatally acquired acute toxoplasma infection in most immunocompetent individuals may be asymptomatic or may present as a flu-like illness or mononucleosis-like illness, cervical lymphadenopathy that is usually painless, involvement of other lymph node groups, fever, malaise, myalgias, arthralgias, headache, or sore throat. Only 10% to 20% of acute infections in immunocompetent children in the United States and Europe are symptomatic. A small number of atypical lymphocytes may be seen. Occasionally a macular rash, hepatosplenomegaly, and hepatic dysfunction can develop. Approximately 1% of all mononucleosis-like illnesses are caused by *T gondii* infections. The differential diagnosis of toxoplasmic lymphadenopathy includes mononucleosis syndromes from Epstein-Barr virus or cytomegalovirus, human herpesvirus-6 infection, cat scratch disease, tuberculosis, tularemia, lymphoma, or leukemia. The course of acute toxoplasma infection and acute toxoplasmic lymphadenopathy is usually benign and self-limited. Lymphadenopathy usually lasts for approximately 8 weeks, but can occasionally wax and wane for several months. Treatment for acute toxoplasmosis occasionally can be indicated even in immunocompetent individuals if associated with severe or persistent symptoms. Treatment is also indicated for active toxoplasmic chorioretinitis. In certain tropical regions, atypical pneumonitis, disseminated disease with multiorgan failure, and even fatal outcomes have been reported in immunocompetent individuals with acute toxoplasmosis. Aggressive clinical syndromes from toxoplasmosis have also been seen in the United States in immunocompetent individuals likely from acute infections associated with high parasite load (eg, after eating undercooked *T gondii*–infected wild-game meat with high parasite load). Toxoplasmosis should be in the differential diagnosis of individuals with compatible clinical syndromes independent of known risk factors as more than half of acutely infected individuals may not report risk factors.

### Chronic *T gondii* Infection

The immune response to *T gondii* infection transforms the tachyzoites into bradyzoites, which reside in tissue cysts, mainly in the brain and in skeletal and heart muscle, where the parasite survives in a latent form. In immunocompetent individuals, this chronic form generally has no adverse consequences and is usually a latent asymptomatic infection. However, if subsequent immunosuppression occurs, especially impairment of cell-mediated immunity, bradyzoites can be released from cysts and can transform back into tachyzoites, causing recrudescence of active infection.

### Toxoplasmosis in Immunocompromised Host

A wide range of clinical manifestations have been reported to occur during reactivation of a chronic latent infection in immunocompromised individuals (eg, in individuals with transplants or malignancies, or those receiving certain monoclonal antibodies such as adalimumab, alemtuzumab, or infliximab). Reactivation in transplant patients can occur either in a *T gondii*–seropositive recipient or from a *T gondii*–infected donor organ. Approximately 25% of donor *T gondii*–positive/recipient *T gondii*–negative heart transplant recipients develop toxoplasmosis in the absence of anti-*Toxoplasma* prophylaxis. Toxoplasmosis in HIV-infected individuals almost always occurs as a result of reactivation of chronic latent infection.

Toxoplasmosis in immunocompromised individuals can manifest as persistent fever of unknown origin, pneumonitis, hepatitis, myocarditis, brain lesions, meningoencephalitis/myelitis, encephalitis with or without brain abscess, seizures, chorioretinitis, lymphadenopathy, or myositis. Disseminated disease with sepsis-like illness and multiorgan involvement and fatal outcome can also occur if not promptly diagnosed and treated. Toxoplasmosis should be considered in the differential diagnosis in immunocompromised individuals with compatible clinical syndromes (eg, persistent fever, pneumonitis, hepatitis, encephalopathy) and promptly diagnosed and treated.

### Ocular Toxoplasmosis

CT is associated with a higher risk of ocular involvement than postnatally acquired infections. Tissue destruction is probably caused by *T gondii* proliferation and the host's inflammatory response. Toxoplasmic chorioretinitis can occur in newborns or young infants with CT, later in life from reactivation of eye lesions of CT or from postnatally acquired acute infections. It was previously assumed that toxoplasmic chorioretinitis occurs mainly from reactivation of a latent chorioretinal tissue cyst in a chronically infected individual. However, it has been recently shown that patients may also develop ocular disease after an acute *T gondii* infection, and 11.7% of individuals with ocular toxoplasmosis had recently acquired *Toxoplasma* infections. It is estimated that among the 1 million people in the United States estimated to be infected each year with *Toxoplasma*, 2% (approximately 21,000 people) will develop eye disease per year. Eye disease has also been reported to occur during community outbreaks of acute *T gondii* infections (eg, through contamination of municipal water) in up to 20% of documented acute infections. The initial chorioretinal infection may be subclinical, and active lesions may develop months to years later. Recurrences can occur after a congenitally acquired infection or a postnatally acquired infection.

The classic ophthalmologic finding considered diagnostic for ocular toxoplasmosis is a satellite lesion adjacent to an old chorioretinal scar. After resolution of active inflammatory disease, hyperpigmented scars develop and recurrences develop as satellite lesions in the borders of old chorioretinal scars. Ocular disease can have multiple recurrences. Typical ophthalmologic findings include white focal lesions with vitreous inflammatory reaction, focal necrotizing retinitis in the posterior pole, initially a yellowish-white, elevated cotton-like patch, lesions in small clusters, and lesions in varied stages. It is believed that typical and atypical chorioretinal lesions fall within the spectrum of disease that differs only in severity. Acute toxoplasmic chorioretinitis can cause vision impairment, blurred vision, or scotomas. In immunocompetent patients, there is usually only 1 active lesion at a time, while in immunocompromised patients, multiple active lesions can be seen. Although macular lesions have been traditionally described in cases of congenital toxoplasmosis, they have also been seen in postnatally acquired infections. *T gondii* strain virulence and/or parasite load have been associated with the severity of ocular disease in animals. The major factors associated with severity of disease are the duration of active retinal lesions and the intensity of associated inflammatory response. Most uveitis experts agree that treatment of toxoplasmic chorioretinitis is indicated, and the most commonly used treatment regimen includes pyrimethamine plus sulfadiazine (plus prednisone for severe chorioretinitis threatening vision) (Table 349-1). However, there are continuing reservations about its efficacy and absence of consensus on the best treatment.

### Congenital Toxoplasmosis

CT in the fetus can be subclinical or can manifest as intracranial calcifications, hydrocephalus, intrahepatic calcifications, echogenic bowel, hydrops fetalis, pericardial or pleural effusions, ascites, hepatosplenomegaly, intrauterine growth retardation, premature birth, or fetal death. CT in newborns and young infants can cause a wide spectrum of clinical manifestations, ranging from asymptomatic to severely symptomatic disease and neonatal deaths. Visual impairment, learning disabilities, mental retardation, motor abnormalities, and hearing impairment can become apparent several months to years later. The classic triad of chorioretinitis, intracranial calcifications, and obstructive hydrocephalus is most commonly seen in cohorts of children with CT who have not been prenatally diagnosed and treated and/or in countries where more virulent *T gondii* strains are circulating. Chorioretinitis in CT can be unilateral or bilateral, can be associated with vision impairment, and can recur. Based on the 22-year experience from the Lyon cohort, among 142 chorioretinitis cases and 477 CT cases, the initial eye lesion was detected during the

**TABLE 349-1 TREATMENT FOR CHILDREN WITH ACTIVE TOXOPLASMIC CHORIORETINITIS[a,b,c,d]**

| | |
|---|---|
| Pyrimethamine plus sulfadiazine plus folinic acid[e] | **Pyrimethamine (orally [PO]):**<br>1 mg/kg once every 12 hours orally (maximum 50 mg/d) for 2 days, followed by 1 mg/kg once per day orally (maximum 25–50 mg/d)<br>plus<br>**Sulfadiazine (PO):**<br>75 mg/kg (first dose), followed by 50 mg/kg every 12 hours orally (maximum 4 g/d)<br>plus<br>**Folinic acid (leucovorin) (PO):**<br>10–20 mg daily orally<br>Duration: for 1–2 weeks after resolution of clinical manifestations and for ~4–6 weeks total<br>**Prednisone (PO)** (for severe chorioretinitis):<br>0.5 mg/kg every 12 hours (maximum 40 mg/d); short duration |

[a]Data from Long SS, Pickering LK, Prober CG: *Principles and Practice of Pediatric Infectious Diseases*, 4th ed. Philadelphia: Churchill Livingstone Elsevier; 2012.

[b]For older children and adolescents with eye disease in a non–sight-threatening area, experts in the United States have tried alternative regimens (pyrimethamine plus clindamycin or azithromycin followed by clindamycin or azithromycin alone) (limited data).

[c]Treatment is indicated for active toxoplasmic chorioretinitis (due to reactivation of a congenitally acquired or postnatally acquired chronic latent infection or during eye disease associated with acute toxoplasmosis). Preventing reactivation in persons who have had relapse of ocular lesions should be considered in patients with frequent or recurrent chorioretinitis. Two randomized trials (mainly in adults) in Brazil showed that trimethoprim/sulfamethoxazole (TMP/SMX) prophylaxis in patients with recurrent toxoplasmic chorioretinitis for 12 to 20 months decreased significantly the risk of eye recurrences.

[d]Oral prednisone has been used when there is an active ocular inflammatory process (eg, macular lesion, severe vitritis, optic nerve involvement) threatening the vision.

[e]Folinic acid (leucovorin) should be continued for 1 week after the end of therapy (folinic acid should not be substituted with folic acid).

first 2 weeks of life in only 5.6% of children. The remaining children had their first eye lesion detected at a median of 4.2 years; in 75% of cases, the first eye lesion was diagnosed after 7 months of age; and in 50% of cases, after 3 years of age. Additional ocular manifestations in CT include cataract, chorioretinal edema/scars, choroidal neovascular membranes, necrotizing retinitis, central macular or peripheral retinal lesions, single or multiple retinal lesions, vitritis, retinal detachment, microphthalmia-microcornea, optic nerve atrophy, nystagmus, strabismus, amblyopia, and visual impairment. Additional neurologic manifestations in CT include cerebrospinal fluid (CSF) abnormalities including pleocytosis, eosinophilia, and mild lymphocytosis; elevated CSF protein (from slightly above normal up to approximately 1000 mg/dL); ventriculomegaly; obstructive hydrocephalus; and single or multiple intracranial calcifications. Microcephaly and hypoglycorrhachia are uncommon. The clinical spectrum of neurologic manifestations in CT is very broad and can range from subtle neurologic signs to severe encephalopathy. Seizures, hypotonia, or other motor abnormalities, lethargy, cranial nerve palsies, sensorineural hearing loss, and psychomotor retardation can be seen. Additional manifestations of CT include hepatosplenomegaly, skin rashes (maculopapular rash, petechiae, purpura, blueberry muffin rash), myocarditis, pneumonitis, thrombocytopenia, anemia, hepatitis, and/or cholestasis. Rarely, CT can present as a sepsis-like illness with disseminated fulminant neonatal disease with multiorgan failure.

Significant differences exist in the prevalence of severe clinical manifestations from CT between the United States and western European countries (eg, French, Austrian, or German cohorts). US physicians should cautiously extrapolate evidence from such European literature to counsel parents. Also when evaluating infants and children with CT from international settings, they should also be aware that in certain parts of the world severe clinical manifestations of CT are seen more frequently. In the United States, cumulative data from the National Collaborative Chicago-Based Congenital Toxoplasmosis Study showed that among 153 CT cases who were not prenatally treated and referred through 2010, 77% of children had severe disease, 11% had mild disease, and only 12% were asymptomatic. The experience with CT in France is very different. Among 388 prenatally treated CT cases in the Lyon cohort over the past 20 years, 88% of children were asymptomatic, whereas mild disease with intracranial calcifications and extramacular chorioretinitis was seen in 9% of children, and severe disease with hydrocephalus and macular chorioretinitis was seen in 3% of children. Moreover, fetal losses and pregnancy terminations were also rare in the French cohort, occurring in 0.9% and 1% of infected mothers, respectively.

Long-term outcome data for children with CT in the United States are limited. Among children with severe disease at birth, 20% had abnormal motor neurologic outcomes; 27% had an IQ < 70; 16% had decreasing IQ of > 15 point differences between consecutive assessments; 100% had normal audiologic evaluations; 85% had visual impairment; and 36% had recurrences of eye disease. Among children with CT who were asymptomatic at birth or only had mild disease, most had normal neurodevelopmental outcomes except for 8% of children with decreasing IQs between 2 evaluations; 15% had vision impairment, and 9% had recurrences of eye disease. A systematic review reported that sensorineural hearing loss from CT occurs in 0% to 26% of CT cases, and the rate varies according to the presence or absence of postnatal treatment.

The risk of eye disease recurrence was 34% based on 12 years of follow-up from the Lyon cohort. This risk increased to almost 50% when the follow-up was extended to 18 years of age; however, lesions were mainly unilateral in 69% of cases and did not cause visual loss in 81% of cases. Cautious extrapolation of these data is needed for counseling for children with CT in the United States and other countries where different *T gondii* strains are implicated and where children are not prenatally treated. In Brazil, children with ocular toxoplasmosis more frequently have multiple eye lesions, larger lesions, and lesions causing visual impairment and threatening vision. Visual impairment occurred in 87% of cases in Brazil versus 29% in European cohorts.

## DIAGNOSIS

The following tests are available for the laboratory diagnosis of toxoplasmosis: (1) serologic assays, including *Toxoplasma* IgG, IgM, IgA, IgE, IgG avidity, and AC/HS differential agglutination test (acetone [AC]-fixed vs formalin [HS]-fixed tachyzoites); (2) *T gondii* polymerase chain reaction (PCR) in amniotic fluid, blood, CSF, urine, and body fluids such as bronchoalveolar lavage (BAL), pleural fluid, aqueous humor, vitreous fluid, and tissue biopsies; (3) histopathologic and cytologic examination of tissue and body fluids for the identification of tachyzoites or tissue cysts; and (4) isolation of the parasite by mouse subinoculation, now rarely performed even in reference laboratories. For toxoplasmic lymphadenopathy, the classic triad of histopathologic changes includes reactive follicular hyperplasia, irregular clusters of epithelioid histiocytes encroaching on and blurring the margins of germinal centers, and distension of sinuses with monocytoid cells. With lymphadenopathy alone, *T gondii* PCR is rarely positive possibly because lymphadenopathy is mainly a manifestation of the host response to the parasite.

Commercial laboratories in the United States routinely offer only *T gondii* IgG and IgM enzyme-linked immunosorbent assay (ELISA); few also offer IgG avidity, recently approved by the US Food and Drug Administration (FDA), or IgA ELISA. In reference laboratories, an additional panel of tests is offered that can better assist in the estimation of the most likely time of *Toxoplasma* infection. Such tests are the IgG-Dye test, a neutralization assay using live tachyzoites, considered to be the gold-standard IgG test; IgG-avidity interpreted as low, equivocal, or high, with high IgG avidity indicating infection acquired ≥ 4 months before the time of testing and low avidity often seen with recently acquired infections but that can occasionally persist in chronically infected patients; IgM ELISA and IgM immunosorbent agglutination assay (ISAGA); IgA ELISA; IgE ELISA; and the AC/HS differential agglutination test interpreted as an acute, equivocal, or nonacute pattern. This test helps differentiate acute from chronic infection when used with an additional panel of tests. Nonacute patterns indicate infections acquired at least 12 months prior to testing.

*Toxoplasma* IgG antibodies appear within 1 to 2 weeks after acute infection, peak within 1 to 2 months, and usually remain for life at low titers. A negative IgG test excludes *Toxoplasma* infection, with the exception of very early infections within 1 to 2 weeks from sample testing, or in severely immunocompromised patients or those who are unable to produce IgG antibodies. IgG avidity has not been validated for use in newborns with suspected CT, in immunocompromised patients, in cases of reinfection with a different *T gondii* strain, in cases of reactivation of a chronic *T gondii* infection, and for screening of blood and organ donors. IgM antibodies can be used to diagnose acute infections, but a positive IgM needs cautious interpretation and confirmatory testing is required at a reference lab with an additional panel of tests because false-positive IgM results can occur. Moreover, IgM can persist for months after an acute infection.

#### Diagnosis of Congenital Toxoplasmosis

The recommended diagnosis of CT in the fetus can be made by amniotic fluid (AF) PCR in a pregnant woman with evidence of acute primary *T gondii* infection during gestation. Monthly fetal ultrasound monitoring can also detect clinical manifestations in the fetus suggestive of CT.

For the diagnostic workup of newborns or infants with suspected CT, the following serologic and molecular tests should be used: IgG (ELISA or Dye test); IgM ISAGA; IgA ELISA or ISAGA; and PCR from blood, urine, and CSF. Infants with suspected CT should also have CSF cell count, differential, protein, and glucose; complete blood count; and liver function tests. Newborns or infants with suspected CT should be evaluated by testing performed at reference laboratories with the use of a gold-standard panel of tests with higher sensitivity, including tests not offered in commercial nonreference laboratories (eg, IgM ISAGA). An infant's serology should always be tested in parallel with maternal serology.

The diagnosis of CT can be established by 1 of the following 3 findings. First is positive *Toxoplasma* IgG and IgM ISAGA and/or IgA ELISA or ISAGA (or IgE ELISA) in the newborn infant. Serologic testing in the newborn should be obtained as soon as possible after birth, and positive IgM or IgA should be repeated to exclude possible false-positive results from contamination with maternal blood during delivery. Persistence of IgM at or after 5 days of life or persistence of IgA at or after 10 days of life is considered diagnostic of CT. False-positive IgM, usually at low titers, can also be seen in infants who have received transfusion of blood products. False-negative IgM and IgA results in newborns with CT in European cohorts where infants with CT were most likely prenatally treated range between approximately 20% and 50%; in US cohorts, where infants with CT were not prenatally treated, the false-negative rate for IgM ISAGA was 13%; for IgA ELISA, it was 23%; and for the combination of IgM and IgA, the false-negative rate was 7%. False-negative IgM and IgA can also occur if maternal infection was acquired very late in gestation; in such cases, the infant's testing should be repeated 2 to 4 weeks after birth and every 4 weeks until 3 months of age to capture possible late production of these antibodies. The diagnostic performance of *Toxoplasma* IgE is inferior to that of IgM ISAGA and/or IgA and is not included in the routine neonatal panel of tests at the Palo Alto Medical Foundation Toxoplasma Serology Laboratory, the national reference laboratory for toxoplasmosis. The second diagnostic finding is positive *T gondii* PCR in neonatal blood, CSF, and/or urine; a positive anti–*T gondii* IgM in CSF is diagnostic of congenital disease, but testing of the CSF by *T gondii* PCR rather than for IgM is strongly recommended because of the higher sensitivity of CSF PCR testing. The third diagnostic finding is persistence of *T gondii* IgG antibodies beyond 12 months of age and is considered the gold standard for the diagnosis because maternal transplacentally transferred IgG antibodies generally disappear by 6 to 12 months of age. Prenatal treatment can affect the IgG kinetics in the newborn. Disappearance of IgG in the newborn during postnatal treatment does not exclude the diagnosis of CT. Only disappearance of IgG antibodies before 12 months of age in an infant who has not received any postnatal treatment and who is able to produce IgG antibodies can safely exclude the diagnosis of CT.

Newborns and infants with suspected CT should also have a detailed physical examination; evaluation by a pediatric neurologist at birth and every 2 to 3 months afterward during the first year of life and every 4 to 6 months after the first year of life; evaluation by a pediatric ophthalmologist, preferably a pediatric retinal specialist, at birth, every 3 to 4 months during the first year of life, every 4 to 6 months during the second year of life; and every 6 months during the third year and afterward; and a hearing test by auditory brainstem responses at birth and yearly afterward. They should also have the following imaging evaluations: brain imaging for the detection of intracranial calcifications, ventriculomegaly, or hydrocephalus and abdominal ultrasonography for the detection of intrahepatic calcifications and/or hepatosplenomegaly. Head ultrasound, head computed tomography (Fig. 349-2), or head magnetic resonance imaging (MRI) could be considered for brain imaging. Although the role of brain MRI in the workup of newborns and infants with suspected CT has not been systematically evaluated, given the radiation risk from head computed tomography and the successful experience with brain MRI in other congenital infections in detecting intracranial calcifications (eg, in children with congenital cytomegalovirus or congenital Zika virus syndrome), its use may be considered. Head ultrasound has been used mainly in Europe where the rate of symptomatic CT with central nervous system manifestations is low, whereas in the United States, where more severe cases of CT are often seen, computed tomography has been traditionally used as more sensitive for the detection of brain calcifications.

#### Laboratory Diagnosis of Postnatally Acquired Acute Toxoplasmosis

For children older than 6 months of age with suspected postnatally acquired toxoplasmosis, the initial screening could be performed at commercial nonreference laboratories with the following tests: IgG (ELISA), IgG avidity, IgM ELISA, IgA ELISA, IgE ELISA, and differential agglutination test (at reference lab only).

#### Laboratory Diagnosis of Ocular Toxoplasmosis

In patients with eye disease from reactivation of CT, *T gondii* IgG antibodies may be present at low titers and IgM are not present, whereas patients with eye disease during a postnatally acquired acute infection will have a serologic profile of acute infection (positive IgG and IgM and/or IgA and/or IgE). If the response to anti-*Toxoplasma* therapy is not optimal, *T gondii* PCR from vitreous or aqueous humor fluid and/or the Goldman-Witmer coefficient (the ratio of *T gondii* IgG to total IgG antibodies in aqueous fluid divided by the ratio of *T gondii* IgG to total IgG antibodies in serum, with ratios > 2 considered positive) can also assist in the differential diagnosis.

#### Laboratory Diagnosis in Immunocompromised Children with Suspected Toxoplasmosis

Individuals who are anticipated to become immunocompromised should be tested with *T gondii* IgG and IgM antibodies if possible before development of immunosuppression. Serologies after transplantation in previously seropositive individuals are not reliable because they can be negative, unchanged, or even increased without clinical relevance. In immunosuppressed patients with suspected toxoplasmosis, PCR testing of body fluids or tissues (eg, blood, CSF, urine, or other body fluids such as pleural fluid or BAL) may be useful for establishing the diagnosis of active *Toxoplasma* infection via the detection of tachyzoites. *T gondii* PCR screening of blood, although not 100% sensitive because it may be negative in cases of localized reactivation, can be useful for prompt initiation of anti-*Toxoplasma* treatment.

### TREATMENT

Usually immunocompetent children with acute primary toxoplasmosis do not require treatment. However, treatment may be indicated for severe acute toxoplasmosis even in immunocompetent patients when symptoms are severe and persisting (Table 349-2).

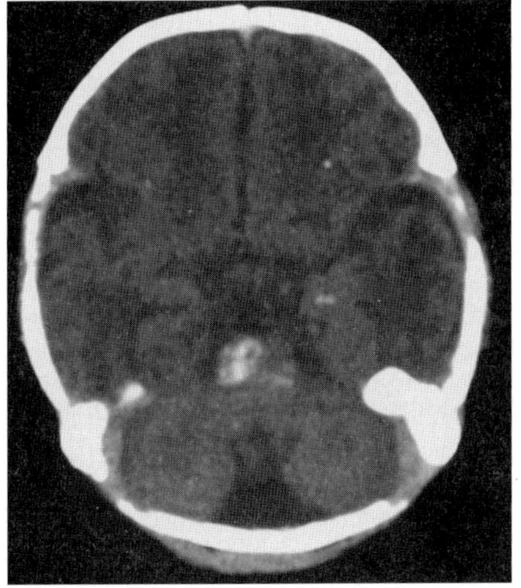
A

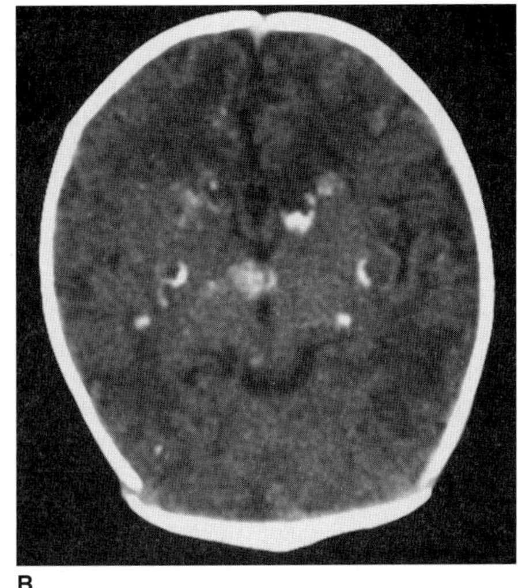
B

**FIGURE 349-2 A and B:** Plain axial computed tomography scan of the brain at age 13 days showing multiple intraparenchymal calcifications, including in the brain stem and basal ganglia.

**TABLE 349-2 TREATMENT FOR IMMUNOCOMPROMISED CHILDREN WITH ACTIVE TOXOPLASMOSIS (FROM REACTIVATION OF A CHRONIC LATENT INFECTION OR FROM AN ACUTE PRIMARY *TOXOPLASMA GONDII* INFECTION) OR IMMUNOCOMPETENT CHILDREN WITH SEVERE/PERSISTING ACUTE TOXOPLASMOSIS[a,b,c,d,e]**

| | |
|---|---|
| **Recommended** | |
| Pyrimethamine (oral [PO]) | 1 mg/kg every 12 hours (maximum 100 mg/d) for 2 days, followed by 1 mg/kg once a day (maximum 25 mg/d; up to 50 mg/d [if < 60 kg] or up to 75 mg/d [if ≥ 60 kg] in older children with severe disease) |
| plus | |
| Folinic acid[f] (PO) | 10–20 mg daily (up to 50 mg/d) |
| plus | |
| Sulfadiazine (PO) | 100–200 mg/kg/d divided every 6 hours (maximum 4–6 g/d for severe disease) |
| **Alternative Preferred Regimen** | |
| Trimethoprim-sulfamethoxazole[g] (intravenous [IV] or PO) | |
| **Alternative Regimens** | |
| Pyrimethamine (plus folinic acid[f]) | |
| plus | |
| Clindamycin[g] (PO or IV) | |
| or | |
| Atovaquone[g] (PO) | |
| **Alternative Regimens with Limited Data** | |
| Pyrimethamine (plus folinic acid) | |
| plus | |
| Clarithromycin[g] (PO) | |
| or | |
| Dapsone[g] (PO) | |
| or | |
| Azithromycin[g] (PO) | |
| Sulfadiazine[g] (PO) | |
| plus | |
| Atovaquone[g] (PO) | |

[a]The Palo Alto Medical Foundation Toxoplasma Serology Laboratory (PAMF-TSL; www.pamf.org/serology; phone: 650-853-4828; fax: 650-614-3292; e-mail: toxolab@pamf.org) and the Toxoplasmosis Center at the University of Chicago (Center of the National Collaborative Chicago-Based Congenital Toxoplasmosis Study, Prof. Rima McLeod; phone: 773-834-4130) can be contacted for assistance with the management of infants with congenital toxoplasmosis.

[b]Preferred regimen: Pyrimethamine (plus folinic acid) plus sulfadiazine.

[c]According to the "Guidelines for the Prevention and Treatment of Opportunistic Infections Among HIV-Exposed and HIV-Infected Children" (AIDSinfo, https://aidsinfo.nih.gov/contentfiles/lvguidelines/PedOIDosingTables.pdf; Updated as of October 29, 2015; accessed June 9, 2016), for treatment of postnatally acquired acute toxoplasmosis in human immunodeficiency virus–infected children, acute induction therapy should include pyrimethamine (plus folinic acid) plus sulfadiazine, followed by chronic suppressive therapy. Duration of treatment: ≥ 6 weeks (longer duration if response at 6 weeks is incomplete or for extensive disease). Alternative regimens for acquired toxoplasmosis for sulfonamide-intolerant patients include pyrimethamine (plus folinic acid) plus clindamycin 5–7.5 mg/kg body weight (maximum, 600 mg/dose) PO or IV given 4 times a day. Other alternative regimens include the following:

TMP/SMX: TMP 5 mg/kg body weight plus SMX 25 mg/kg body weight per dose IV or PO given twice daily has been used as an alternative to pyrimethamine-sulfadiazine in adults but has not been studied in children.

Atovaquone (for adults, 1.5 g by mouth twice daily) in regimens combined with pyrimethamine/leucovorin, with sulfadiazine alone, or as a single agent in patients intolerant to both pyrimethamine and sulfadiazine; these regimens have not been studied in children.

Azithromycin (for adults, 900–1200 mg/d, corresponding to 20 mg/kg/d in children) has also been used in adults combined with pyrimethamine/sulfadiazine, but has not been studied in children.

Corticosteroids (eg, prednisone, dexamethasone) have been used in children with central nervous system disease when cerebrospinal fluid protein is very elevated (> 1000 mg/dL) or if there are focal lesions with significant mass effects, with discontinuation as soon as clinically feasible.

[d]Usually, immunocompetent children with acute primary toxoplasmosis do not require treatment. However, treatment may be indicated for severe acute toxoplasmosis when symptoms are severe and persisting (eg, disease associated with persisting fevers, pneumonitis, myocarditis, hepatitis, myositis, encephalopathy, brain lesions, lymphadenopathy [with severe or persisting symptoms]).

[e]Data from Long SS, Pickering LK, Prober CG: *Principles and Practice of Pediatric Infectious Diseases*, 4th ed. Philadelphia: Churchill Livingstone Elsevier; 2012.

[f]Folinic acid (leucovorin) should be continued for 1 week after the end of therapy (folinic acid should not be substituted with folic acid).

[g]Pediatric doses for these drugs have not been studied in the context of toxoplasmosis. Highest possible doses probably are needed in disseminated or severe cases.

Active chorioretinitis should also be treated (see Table 349-1). Oral prednisone has been used when there is an active inflammatory process that threatens vision through involvement of the macula or optic nerve and active vitritis. Based on adult experience, active eye disease resolves usually within 10 to 14 days after initiation of anti-*Toxoplasma* treatment; treatment should be continued for 1 to 2 weeks after resolution of clinical signs and symptoms of active eye disease and for approximately 4 to 6 weeks total. Close ophthalmologic monitoring is required to determine the optimal duration of therapy. Preventing reactivation in persons who have had relapse of ocular lesions should be considered in patients with frequent or recurrent chorioretinitis; however, there are no pediatric clinical trial data to support this recommendation.

In immunocompromised hosts, reactivation of a chronic infection or acute primary *T gondii* infection is more likely to be life- or sight-threatening and therefore requires therapy. Primary therapy followed by suppressive therapy (secondary prophylaxis) to prevent relapse is recommended unless the immunodeficient state resolves. Recommended treatment regimen for primary therapy includes pyrimethamine plus folinic acid plus sulfadiazine. Alternative regimens are listed in Table 349-2. HIV patients with toxoplasmic encephalitis should be treated for ≥ 6 weeks, followed by suppressive therapy (Table 349-3). Difficulties with long-term therapy include development of hypersensitivity and toxicities from the medication.

Pyrimethamine and sulfadiazine are synergistic against *T gondii*. Both drugs in combination are used to treat infection. Pyrimethamine has a long half-life, about 60 hours, and inhibits dihydrofolate reductase. It can produce reversible bone marrow toxicity, resulting in neutropenia, anemia, and thrombocytopenia. To counter this effect, pyrimethamine is given with folinic acid (leucovorin), and weekly or twice-weekly monitoring of blood counts is recommended, particularly during the daily treatment.

Treatment of infants with suspected or confirmed CT should include pyrimethamine plus folinic acid plus sulfadiazine and should be continued for 12 months (Table 349-4).

**TABLE 349-3 ANTI-*TOXOPLASMA* PROPHYLAXIS (PRIMARY AND SECONDARY)[a]**

| Primary prophylaxis: | Indication: | Recommended: | Alternative regimens: |
|---|---|---|---|
| Prevention of first episode of toxoplasmosis[a,b] | Severe immunosuppression in *T gondii*–seropositive individuals | Trimethoprim (TMP)/ sulfamethoxazole (SMX) (150/750 mg/m²/d) orally once daily | Pyrimethamine 1 mg/kg orally once daily (maximum 25 mg); plus leucovorin 5 mg orally every 3 days<br>plus<br>Dapsone (children 1 month of age or older) 2 mg/kg or 15 mg/m² (maximum 25 mg) orally once daily<br>Atovaquone in children age 1–3 months or > 24 months: 30 mg/kg orally once daily<br>Atovaquone in children age 4–24 months: 45 mg/kg orally once daily, with or without pyrimethamine 1 mg/kg or 15 mg/m² body surface area (maximum 25 mg) orally once daily (plus leucovorin 5 mg orally every 3 days)<br>Acceptable alternative dosage schedules for TMP/SMX:<br>TMP/SMX 150/750 mg/m² body surface area per dose once daily by mouth 3 times weekly on 3 consecutive days per week<br>TMP/SMX 75/375 mg/m² body surface area per dose twice daily by mouth every day<br>TMP/SMX 75/375 mg/m² body surface area per dose twice daily by mouth 3 times weekly on alternate days |
| **Secondary prophylaxis:** | **Indication:** | **Recommended:** | **Alternative regimens:** |
| Suppressive therapy (prevention of recurrence of toxoplasmosis)[a-d] | Prior toxoplasmic encephalitis | Pyrimethamine 1 mg/kg or 15 mg/m² (maximum 25 mg) orally once daily (plus leucovorin 5 mg orally every 3 days) plus sulfadiazine 85–120 mg/kg/d (maximum 2–4 g/d) in 2–4 divided doses, orally, every day | Pyrimethamine 1 mg/kg or 15 mg/m² body surface area, orally, once daily (maximum 25 mg) (plus leucovorin 5 mg orally every 3 days)<br>plus<br>Clindamycin 20–30 mg/kg/d in 3 divided doses orally every day<br>Atovaquone in children age 1–3 months or > 24 months: 30 mg/kg orally once daily<br>Atovaquone in children age 4–24 months: 45 mg/kg orally once daily with or without pyrimethamine 1 mg/kg body weight or 15 mg/m² body surface area (maximum 25 mg) by mouth once daily (plus leucovorin 5 mg by mouth every 3 days)<br>Children age 1–3 months and > 24 months[d]: TMP/SMX 150/750 mg/m² body surface area once daily by mouth<br>Children age 4–24 months[d]: TMP/SMX 150/750 mg/m² body surface area once daily by mouth |

[a]National Institutes of Health. Guidelines for the Prevention and Treatment of Opportunistic Infections Among HIV-Exposed and HIV-Infected Children (October 29, 2015): Primary Prophylaxis of Opportunistic Infections in HIV-Exposed and HIV-infected Children-Summary of Recommendations. AIDSinfo. http://aidsinfo.nih.gov/guidelines. Accessed July 9, 2017.

[b]TMP/SMX and atovaquone are active also against pneumocystis; pyrimethamine-clindamycin does not have activity against *Pneumocystis*; aerosolized pentamidine does not protect against toxoplasmic encephalitis and is not recommended. (National Institutes of Health. Guidelines for the Prevention and Treatment of Opportunistic Infections Among HIV-Exposed and HIV-Infected Children. AIDSinfo. http://aidsinfo.nih.gov/guideline. Accessed July 9, 2017.)

[c]Discontinuation of secondary prophylaxis may be considered if all the following criteria are fulfilled: completed ≥ 6 months of combination antiretroviral therapy; completed initial therapy for toxoplasmic encephalitis; asymptomatic for toxoplasmic encephalitis and, if age 1–6 years, CD4% ≥ 15% for > 6 consecutive months or, if age ≥ 6 years, CD4 > 200 cells/μL for > 6 consecutive months.

[d]Alternative regimens for secondary prophylaxis with very limited data in children. TMP/SMX should only be used if patient is intolerant to other regimens.

**TABLE 349-4 TREATMENT FOR INFANTS WITH CONGENITAL TOXOPLASMOSIS (CT)[a,b,c,d]**

| | |
|---|---|
| Pyrimethamine plus sulfadiazine plus folinic acid[e] | **Pyrimethamine (orally [PO]):**<br>1 mg/kg every 12 hours for 2 days; followed by 1 mg/kg once per day for 2 or 6 months (6 months may be considered for symptomatic cases of CT); followed by 1 mg/kg once a day every Monday, Wednesday, and Friday for a total course of 12 months<br>plus<br>**Sulfadiazine (PO):**<br>50 mg/kg every 12 hours for 12 months<br>plus<br>**Folinic acid (leucovorin) (PO):**<br>10 mg 3 times a week<br>Duration: 12 months<br>**Prednisone (PO)** (for cerebrospinal fluid [CSF] protein ≥ 1 g/dL or severe chorioretinitis):<br>0.5 mg/kg every 12 hours (for short duration, until CSF protein < 1 g/dL or resolution of severe chorioretinitis[f]) |

[a]Data are very sparse for the use of other medications (eg, trimethoprim/sulfamethoxazole or pyrimethamine plus clindamycin) for the treatment of infants with CT and should be avoided. Some centers in Europe are also using as alternative regimen pyrimethamine/sulfadoxine (Fansidar) for subclinical/mild forms of CT; usually after completing the first 2 months of daily therapy with pyrimethamine/sulfadiazine; it can be administered every 10 days (due to the long half-life). Pyrimethamine 1.25 mg/kg every 10 days and sulfadoxine 25 mg/kg every 10 days; and leucovorin 10 mg × 3 per week or 25 mg × 2 per week.

[b]Monitoring for side effects: Complete blood count should be monitored closely (weekly or twice weekly while on daily therapy and monthly afterward); therapy should be discontinued (but not folinic acid) if severe neutropenia develops; there also should be monthly monitoring for proteinuria (while on pyrimethamine/sulfadiazine); gastrointestinal side effects are common at the beginning of therapy; pyrimethamine overdose can also cause seizures.

[c]The Palo Alto Medical Foundation Toxoplasma Serology Laboratory (PAMF-TSL; www.pamf.org/serology; phone: 650-853-4828; fax: 650-614-3292; e-mail: toxolab@pamf.org) and the Toxoplasmosis Center at the University of Chicago (Center of the National Collaborative Chicago-Based Congenital Toxoplasmosis Study, Prof. Rima McLeod; phone: 773-834-4130) can be contacted for assistance with the management of infants with CT.

[d]Data from Long SS, Pickering LK, Prober CG: *Principles and Practice of Pediatric Infectious Diseases*, 4th ed. Philadelphia: Churchill Livingstone Elsevier; 2012.

[e]Folinic acid (leucovorin) should be continued for 1 week after the end of therapy (folinic acid should not be substituted with folic acid).

[f]If steroids are to be used, they should be initiated after the loading dose of anti-*Toxoplasma* medications.

## PREVENTION

Measures for primary prevention are listed in Table 349-5. Pregnant women and immunocompromised individuals, in particular, should be educated about preventive measures, and physicians should reinforce their implementation. Pregnant women and women planning to become pregnant should avoid risks of acquiring acute *T gondii* infections throughout gestation and close to conception. Universal prenatal screening for toxoplasma infections is not currently recommended in the United States, while such screening is routinely implemented in some European countries. Some obstetricians use selective screening of pregnant woman based on risk factors; however, this strategy has been shown to miss approximately 50% of acutely infected pregnant woman who will be asymptomatic and will not report any of the known risk factors. The majority of the women in the United States who were prenatally diagnosed with acute toxoplasmosis either had a mononucleosis-like illness or a fetal ultrasound abnormality suggestive of a congenital infection that led to their subsequent serologic testing for toxoplasmosis. Neonatal screening for toxoplasma infections in the United States is not routinely implemented, except in Massachusetts and New Hampshire as part of the New England Newborn Screening Program. Screening organ donors and transplant recipients prior to transplantation should be routinely implemented as it leads to prompt initiation of anti-*Toxoplasma* prophylaxis and/or treatment, should clinical syndromes compatible with toxoplasmosis develop. Table 349-3 lists the indicated first-line and alternative options for anti-*Toxoplasma* primary and secondary prophylaxis for HIV infected children.

**TABLE 349-5 PREVENTIVE MEASURES FOR PRIMARY PREVENTION**

- Avoiding ingestion of undercooked meat, raw shellfish, unpasteurized goat milk or drinking untreated water.
- All meat should be cooked up to a temperature of 74°C (165°F), eg, for poultry meat. Microwave cooking may not kill tissue cysts. Particular attention should be made when preparing wild-game meat.
- Avoiding eating cured/smoked meat because infected meat that is smoked or dried can still be infectious.
- Freezing of meat for at least 48 hours at −20°C (−4°F) prior to consumption can inactivate tissue cysts, whereas home freezer temperatures do not kill tissue cysts.
- Washing hands after contact with raw meat and after contact with soil.
- Washing fruits and vegetables well before eating, washing surfaces used to prepare raw meat, and avoid drinking untreated water.
- Changing cat litter box daily preferably by a nonimmunocompromised or pregnant individual and avoiding contact with cat feces.
- Avoiding handling or adopting stray cats and trying to keep household cats indoor and avoiding feeding cats uncooked meats.

## SUGGESTED READINGS

American Academy of Pediatrics Committee on Infectious Diseases. *Toxoplasma gondii* infections. In: *Red Book: 2015 Report of the Committee on Infectious Diseases*. 30th ed. Elk Grove Village, IL: American Academy of Pediatrics; 2015:787-796.

Cortina-Borja M, Tan HQ, Wallon M, et al. Prenatal treatment for serious neurological sequelae of congenital toxoplasmosis: an observational prospective cohort study. *PLoS Med.* 2010;7:pii:e1000351.

Gajurel K, Dhakai R, Montoya JG. *Toxoplasma* prophylaxis in haematopoietic cell transplant recipients: a review of the literature and recommendations. *Curr Opin Infect Dis.* 2015;28:283-292.

Hotop AH, Hlobil H, Gross U. Efficacy of rapid treatment initiation following primary Toxoplasma gondii infection during pregnancy. *Clin Infect Dis.* 2012;54:1545-1552.

Montoya JG, Boothroyd BJ, Kovacs JA. *Toxoplasma gondii.* In: Bennett JE, Dolin R, Blaser MJ, eds. *Mandell, Douglas, and Bennett's Principles and Practice of Infectious Diseases.* 8th ed. Philadelphia, PA: Churchill Livingstone Elsevier; 2015:3122-3153.

Olariu TR, Remington JS, McLeod R, Alam A, Montoya JG. Severe congenital toxoplasmosis in the United States: clinical and serologic findings in untreated infants. *Pediatr Infect Dis J.* 2011;30:1056-1061.

Prusa AR, Kasper DC, Pollak A, Gleiss A, Waldhoer T, Hayde M. The Austrian toxoplasmosis register, 1992-2008. *Clin Infect Dis.* 2015;60:e4-e10.

Wallon M, Peyron F, Cornu C, et al. Congenital toxoplasma infection: monthly prenatal screening decreases transmission rate and improves clinical outcome at age 3 years. *Clin Infect Dis.* 2013;56:1223-1231.

# 350 Trypanosomiases

Camille Sabella

## AFRICAN TRYPANOSOMIASIS

### INTRODUCTION

African trypanosomiasis (sleeping sickness) is a parasitic disease transmitted by the tsetse fly of the genus *Glossina* and caused by a group of parasites called trypanosomes. Two forms of human African trypanosomiasis are prevalent, specific to the parasite causing illness: *Trypanosoma brucei gambiense* (Gambian form) is found in West and Central Africa and accounts for 98% of reported cases; and *Trypanosoma brucei rhodesiense* (Rhodesian form) is found in southern and East Africa. Both forms of the illness are present only in Uganda, but in separate zones.

### PATHOGENESIS AND EPIDEMIOLOGY

African trypanosomiasis has a focal distribution but expands outward during epidemics. About 65 million people live in risk areas, and in 1998, the World Health Organization estimated a continent-wide prevalence of both forms of African trypanosomiasis of 300,000 cases. In 2009, the number of cases reported fell below 10,000 for the first time in 50 years and has continued to decrease since that time, with less than 4000 cases reported in 2014. Thirty-six sub-Saharan countries are considered endemic for 1 or the other form of the disease. The Gambian form continues to be a major public health problem over vast areas of Africa, from Sudan in the north to northwest Uganda to the Democratic Republic of the Congo to Angola in the south. The Rhodesian form continues to present a serious health risk in the Lake Victoria Basin, particularly in eastern Uganda, and there are small pockets of disease endemic in other countries of East and Central Africa. A line drawn from north to south through sub-Saharan Africa, roughly following the Rift Valley, differentiates the distribution of the 2 diseases with the Gambian form to the west and the Rhodesian form to the east of this notional line. *T brucei rhodesiense* is a zoonotic parasite, and wild and domestic animals serve as reservoirs. A number of domestic animals species, including pigs, dogs, goats, sheep, and cattle, may carry human-infective trypanosome species. For *T brucei gambiense*, the nature of animal reservoirs and their role in disease transmission are somewhat less certain.

Infection occurs equally among males and females. Although children are infected less frequently because of a decreased risk of exposure. Early central nervous system (CNS) involvement and a fulminant course are more common in children.

All members of the *T brucei* complex share a common morphology, biochemistry, and life cycle (Fig. 350-1). Infective metacyclic trypomastigotes are inoculated into subcutaneous tissue of a human or another mammalian host by a bite from the tsetse fly. They are converted to the pleomorphic blood forms, which can take long, slender forms, or stumpy forms. Within the human host, trypomastigotes multiply in blood, lymph, and extracellular spaces. The CNS eventually is invaded, where multiplication continues unabated. The tsetse fly is infected with ingestion of a blood meal. Trypomastigotes differentiate into procyclic forms in the midgut, where they multiply by binary fission and remain for the next 2 to 3 weeks. Finally, they enter the salivary glands and transform into infective metacyclic trypomastigote forms. When the fly bites another mammal, the parasites are injected into the blood, completing the cycle of infection.

The inoculated metacyclic trypomastigotes transform and multiply locally in the subcutaneous tissue, giving origin to a characteristic

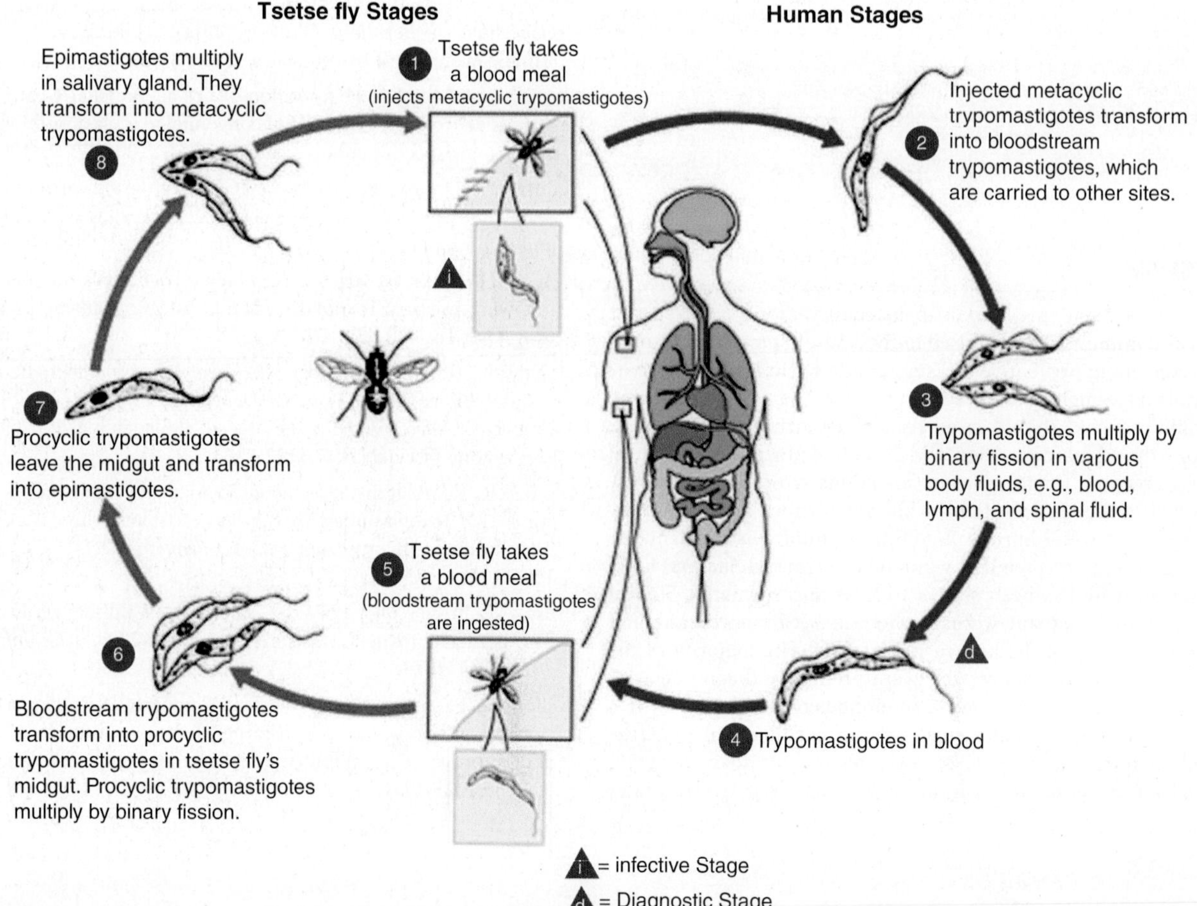


**FIGURE 350-1** Life cycle for organisms causing African trypanosomiasis. (Reproduced with permission from the Centers for Disease Control and Prevention [CDC].)

hard and sometimes painful chancre. By about the 10th day, slender forms reach the bloodstream and lymphatics, and for the next several days, their numbers increase logarithmically, spreading to several tissues. Soon thereafter, the organisms nearly disappear from the bloodstream, only to reappear later. After a variable length of time, trypomastigotes pass through the blood-brain barrier and induce an intense vasculitis, resulting in cerebral edema, demyelination, neuronal damage, and chronic meningoencephalitis.

The parasite survives in the mammalian host by periodically altering its surface antigenic coat, evading the developing immune response of the host. Each successive parasitemic wave represents a new antigenic variant that has emerged to elude the host's antibody response to the previous antigen. The parasite is covered with a variable surface glycoprotein (VSG). Each peak of parasitemia contains a predominant variable antigen type (VAT). The specific antibody response to this coat leads to the destruction of the predominant VAT or homotype. However, within each population of parasites are a number of heterotypes, one of which then becomes the next homotype that is not recognized by the host's immune response. The parasite in each successive wave of parasitemia bears a different VAT. A single trypomastigote may contain as many as 1000 genes, each encoding for a specific VSG.

A marked specific humoral antibody response (predominantly immunoglobulin M [IgM]) follows infection. As a result of polyclonal B-cell activation, there also are many antibodies produced to a wide variety of antigens, including red blood cells, brain, and heart. Circulating immune complexes have been reported regularly, and these may be responsible for the glomerulonephritis often accompanying acute and chronic disease.

## CLINICAL MANIFESTATIONS

Clinical manifestations of infection with *T brucei gambiense* and *T brucei rhodesiense* are similar except that Rhodesian infection presents with a more acute and severe disease, with fewer CNS symptoms, and if untreated, death occurs within weeks to months. Gambian infection has a milder, chronic course, with involvement of lymph nodes, CNS, and a fatal outcome after several years.

In both forms, a trypanosomal chancre may be evident 2 to 3 days after the bite of the fly (Figs. 350-2 and 350-3). Within 1 week, the lesion becomes a large, red, warm, and painful nodule that usually resolves within 3 weeks, leaving residual scarring and depigmentation. In Rhodesian trypanosomiasis, the incubation period typically is 2 to 3 weeks, whereas with Gambian infection, the onset of symptoms may be delayed for several weeks or years. The first stage of the illness is the hemolymphatic stage, characterized by intermittent fevers, chills, headache, and generalized lymphadenopathy. The nodes are discrete, soft, nontender, and contain abundant parasites. In Gambian disease, nodes in the posterior cervical triangle may become enlarged (ie, Winterbottom sign) and, when present, strongly suggest the diagnosis. The spleen and liver may be mildly enlarged. Intermittent fevers may last for months to years with Gambian infection. Arthralgia, weakness, and deep hyperesthesia can be present, often leading to wasting and malnutrition. An irregular, circinate, evanescent rash on the trunk, shoulders, and thighs that is more evident in white persons may appear. Common laboratory abnormalities include a markedly elevated sedimentation rate, hemolytic anemia, elevated hepatic enzymes and abnormal coagulation profiles, hypoalbuminemia, elevated serum immunoglobulin levels (IgM), and thrombocytopenia.

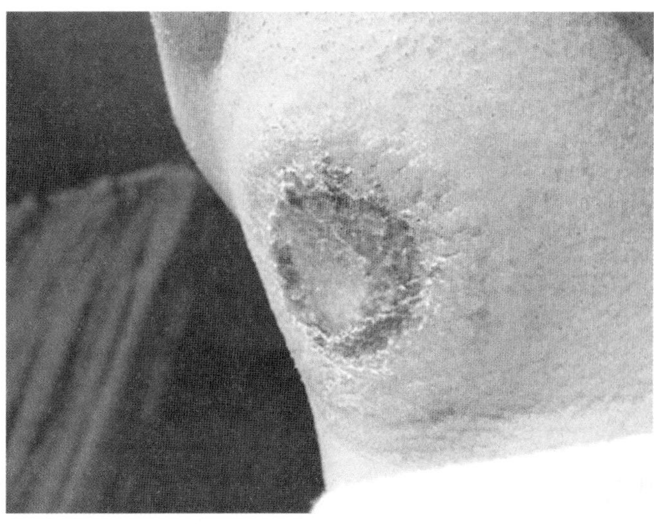

**FIGURE 350-3** Trypanosomal chancre on throat of a patient. (Reproduced with permission from the Centers for Disease Control and Prevention [CDC].)

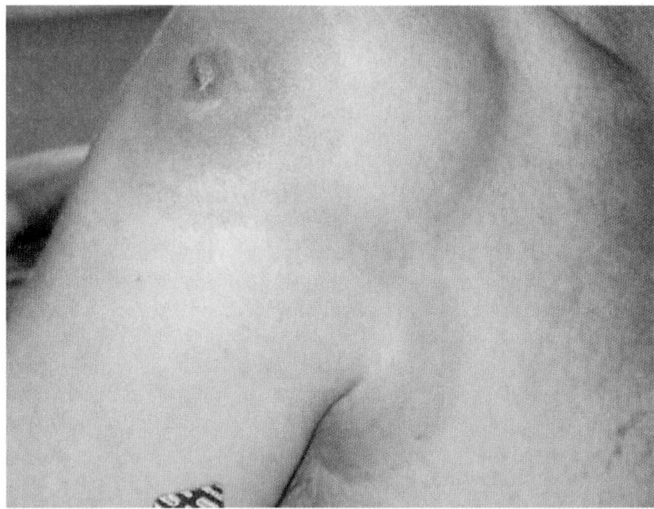

**FIGURE 350-2** Trypanosomal chancre on shoulder with lymphangitis toward axilla. (Reproduced with permission from the Centers for Disease Control and Prevention [CDC].)

Untreated patients with Gambian disease often develop the second stage of illness, the meningoencephalitis stage, characterized by signs of CNS invasion. Severe headaches, disordered sleep, personality and behavior changes, and gradual loss of cognitive function are typical. Tremors, especially of the tongue, hands, and feet, and generalized or focal convulsions may occur. Myocarditis is particularly common and may lead to early death in the Rhodesian form of the disease. Untreated, progressive somnolence and convulsions develop, leading to coma and death in both forms of infection.

## DIAGNOSIS

The diagnosis of human African trypanosomiasis is cumbersome and follows a 3-step approach: screening, parasitologic confirmation (microscopic examination of lymph node and blood specimens), and staging (examination for trypanosomes and for increased white blood cell counts in the cerebrospinal fluid [CSF]). Screening relies on the presence of specific antibodies, which can be detected after the second week of infection. The card agglutination test, a simple, practical, and direct agglutination test for stained trypanosomes, is available for the diagnosis of *T brucei gambiense* and has a specificity of 90% to 95% and a sensitivity of 92% to 100%. Another serologic test for *T brucei gambiense* infection is the latex/*T brucei gambiense*, which is a variant of the card agglutination test but is directed against 3 VATs and has a specificity of up to 99% and a sensitivity between 84% and 100%. Indirect immunofluorescent and enzyme immunoassays are alternative serologic tests that can be used but cannot be readily performed in the field. A monoclonal antibody–based enzyme immunoassay for detection of trypanosome antigens in serum and CSF has a high specificity (99.9%) and sensitivity (94.8% for *T brucei gambiense* and 91.5% for *T brucei rhodesiense*). None of the screening tests can distinguish between current and past infection. Definitive diagnosis depends on demonstration of the parasite from the chancre, in blood, lymph node aspirates, bone marrow, or CSF. Parasitemia is more common during

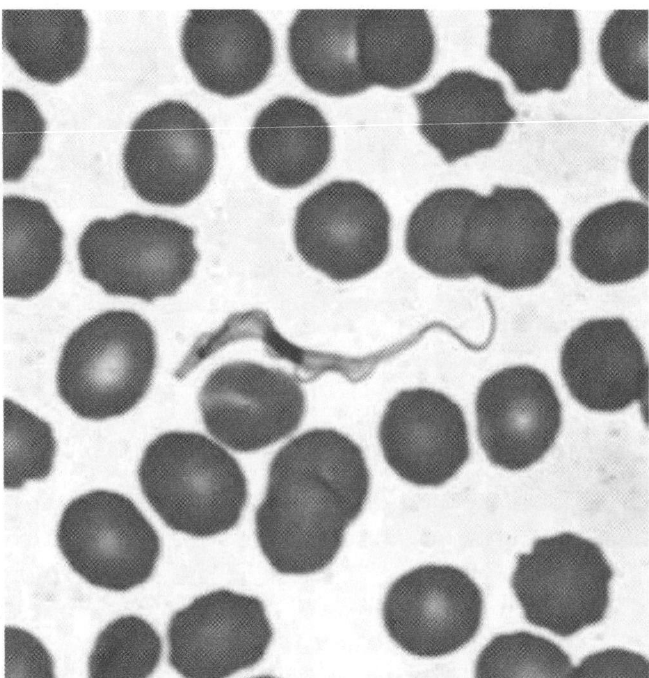

**FIGURE 350-4** *Trypanosoma brucei* in thin blood smear stained with Wright-Giemsa. (Reproduced with permission from the Centers for Disease Control and Prevention [CDC].)

febrile episodes. It is essential to use both thick and thin Giemsa-stained blood smears (Fig. 350-4) as well as to examine the buffy coat from 10 to 20 mL of citrated whole blood or the sediment from 5 mL of centrifuged CSF. Concentration techniques such as the mini-hematocrit centrifugation technique or the miniature anion exchange centrifugation (m-AECT) improve detection levels to 500 and 100 parasites per milliliter by microscopy, respectively. Because of the periodicity of the parasitemia, daily examination of blood films for 10 consecutive days is recommended. *T brucei rhodesiense* is found more frequently in peripheral blood and can be shown in a single microscopic examination in 87% of cases. Examination of wet preparations of cervical lymph node aspirates helps to confirm the diagnosis when trypanosomes are undetected in blood. Intraperitoneal inoculation of 0.5 mL of heparinized blood or CSF into 2 mice is positive in 89% of *T brucei rhodesiense* cases within 2 weeks of inoculation. Highly sensitive and specific conventional and real-time polymerase chain reaction tests have been developed for rapid diagnosis of trypanosomiasis from blood CSF samples.

Staging is performed after diagnosis to determine the presence of CNS involvement. In advanced CNS disease, the CSF shows increased protein concentration; elevated cell counts, predominantly mononuclear; small number of eosinophils; and, frequently, trypomastigotes. The presence of IgM in the CSF is a specific marker for CNS infection. After successful treatment, the IgM level declines gradually, disappearing after approximately 1 year.

The differential diagnosis of the first stage includes any febrile illness common in the geographical area and includes malaria, enteric fever, viral hepatitis, syphilis, brucellosis, visceral leishmaniasis, relapsing fever, and tuberculosis. The second stage of illness needs to be distinguished from other causes of chronic meningoencephalitis, such as tuberculosis, syphilis, and cryptococcal infection. The differential diagnosis of the chancre of African trypanosomiasis includes cutaneous anthrax, syphilis, and African tick bite fever.

## TREATMENT

The choice of treatment depends on the parasite species involved and on the stage of the disease. Hospitalization is required during administration of all the drugs currently used, particularly for the late stage. Early treatment is essential, when the parasite is restricted to the hematolymphatic system, because the prognosis is poor once CNS involvement has occurred.

Suramin and pentamidine do not penetrate the CNS adequately and are useful only in early infection. Pentamidine, as the isethionate salt, is used only against *T brucei gambiense*, as primary resistance of *T brucei rhodesiense* has been observed. Pentamidine is administered intramuscularly at 4 mg/kg/d for 7 to 10 doses, given daily or every second day. Both the liver and kidneys store the drug for months. Common adverse events include hypoglycemia and hypotension. Other serious side effects include nephrotoxicity, hepatotoxicity, and pancreatic toxicity. Suramin, a polysulfonated naphthylamide, inhibits glycolytic enzymes of trypanosomes, and a full course cures early cases of *T brucei gambiense* and *T brucei rhodesiense*. Because suramin is poorly absorbed from the gastrointestinal tract and causes local irritation if given intramuscularly, slow intravenous injection is the best mode of administration. A test dose of 5 mg/kg is given and is followed by a dose of 20 mg/kg intravenously (maximum dose 1 g) on days 1, 3, 7, 14, and 21. Common reactions include joint pain, fever, and paresthesia. Neuropathy, rash, fatigue, anemia, hyperglycemia, hypocalcemia, coagulopathies, neutropenia, renal insufficiency, and transaminase elevation are common. Nephrotoxicity is the most important toxic effect; urinalysis should be done prior to administration of each dose, and the presence of casts or red blood cells in the sediment are indications for alternative therapy.

During the second stage of the disease, drugs that can penetrate into the CSF must be used. Melarsoprol, a derivative of arsenic acid, has the ability to cross the blood-brain barrier and kill both *T brucei gambiense* and *T brucei rhodesiense* parasites residing in the CSF. This agent is considered the first-line treatment for the Rhodesian form of the infection and as second-line therapy for the Gambian form. Various empirically designed, complicated treatment schedules are used. A standardized 10-day course with melarsoprol at 2.2 mg/kg given once a day is as effective as older protocols and has been adopted as the recommended course for *T brucei gambiense* by the World Health Organization. Treatment failures with melarsoprol have been reported in some regions to reach 30%. The most serious side effect is a reactive encephalopathy (arsenic encephalopathy), which can occur in 1% to 10% of treated patients, with mortality in 1% to 5%. Other adverse events are common. These include cutaneous reactions, polyneuropathy, fever, headache, pruritus, hepatotoxicity, cardiac arrhythmias, and thrombocytopenia.

Eflornithine is a selective and irreversible inhibitor of ornithine carboxylase, the first enzyme in polyamine synthesis of trypanosomes. This drug penetrates the CSF and is used for the treatment of the late stage of *T brucei gambiense* infection. The recommended dosage is 400 mg/kg/day intravenously in 4 divided doses for 14 days, although a higher dose is suggested for children and teenagers. Adverse effects appear to be fewer than with melarsoprol and include fever, headache, hypertension, macular rash, peripheral neuropathy, tremor, and gastrointestinal problems including diarrhea. Administration of this compound is cumbersome because of its large volume and frequent dosing regimen. Nifurtimox, a 5-nitrofuran derivative, is active in both stages of *T brucei gambiense* infection and has been studied in combination with eflornithine for the late stage of *T brucei gambiense* infection. This combination produced similar cure rates, shorter duration of therapy, and less adverse effects (likely due to lower cumulative dose of eflornithine) than eflornithine monotherapy. Thus, nifurtimox and eflornithine combination therapy is considered first-line treatment for late-stage *T brucei gambiense* infection. Adverse effects of eflornithine include vomiting, abdominal pain, arthralgias, hearing loss, rash, and bone marrow toxicity. Adverse effects of nifurtimox include gastrointestinal upset, cognitive disturbance, seizures, and allergic reactions. Control programs recommend a follow-up of patients with human African trypanosomiasis for 2 years after treatment, with examinations every 6 months for the presence of trypanosomes and assessment of the white blood cell (WBC) count in CSF. A patient is declared to be cured if no trypanosomes are detected and the WBC count has returned to normal. A recent study reported that patients with CSF WBC of < 5 cells/μL are at low risk for relapse.

After 12 months, the combination of CSF WBC count > 8 cells/μL and latex/IgM end titer > 1:4 predicted treatment failure with 97% specificity and 79% sensitivity. This same combination was 100% specific for treatment failure after 18 and 24 months.

## PREVENTION

The control of trypanosomiasis relies on vector control, surveillance, and early treatment of identified cases. Vector control can curb transmission and has been successfully employed in recent years to eradicate trypanosomiasis using extensive trapping, followed by the sterile insect technique. Tsetse flies can be controlled by using insecticides, such as chlorinated hydrocarbons and synthetic pyrethroids directed at known fly resting sites. Fly traps or screens impregnated with insecticides may be more economical and effective.

Surveillance aims to reduce the human reservoir of infection by detecting and treating early cases of infection. This is important for controlling human disease and reducing the Gambian form of infection. Reducing the size of the human reservoir will reduce the chances of further generations of tsetse becoming infected and passing on the infection, so that transmission will eventually be interrupted. Surveillance is not practical for the Rhodesian form of the infection because asymptomatic human infection is rare. Rather, livestock and other animal hosts of this zoonotic subspecies need to be the focus of control activities. Although chemoprophylaxis with suramin has been shown to be highly effective, this practice is no longer recommended because of the poor risk-benefit associated with the adverse effects of the drug.

# AMERICAN TRYPANOSOMIASIS

## INTRODUCTION

American trypanosomiasis (ie, Chagas disease) is caused by the obligate intracellular protozoan parasite *Trypanosoma cruzi* and threatens more than 120 million (ie, 25%) of the population of Latin America. Transmission usually occurs by vector transfer, transfusion, organ transplant, or congenital transmission.

## PATHOGENESIS AND EPIDEMIOLOGY

Human Chagas disease extends from the southern United States to Chile and Argentina. The Caribbean, Belize, Suriname, and Guyana are reported to be free of this infection. Substantial progress has been made toward the control of Chagas disease in Latin America, from an approximate prevalence of 16 million to 18 million in 1991, to 5.7 million in 2010. The prevalence of infection is greatest in Brazil, Argentina, Bolivia, and Venezuela. There may be up to 300,000 immigrants from endemic countries with latent *T cruzi* infections living in the United States and representing a reservoir for potential transmission of *T cruzi* by blood transfusion or organ donation. The distribution of Chagas disease in the United States includes approximately the southern half of the country; the disease exists almost exclusively as a zoonosis, and only 5 autochthonous cases of Chagas disease have been documented. Despite this apparent low incidence, there is evidence of a relatively high rate of infection among recognized indigenous triatomid bugs in southern states; it has been suggested that Chagas disease is endemic to Texas and that unrecognized cases exist throughout the state. On the other hand, several cases acquired through laboratory accidents, organ transplants, imported infection, and blood transfusion have been reported in the United States and Canada.

*T cruzi* infection can be readily transmitted by blood transfusion (20% infectivity risk). The migration of people infected by *T cruzi* poses a threat to those countries where this insect-transmitted disease does not occur. From 2001 to 2002, the prevalence rate of serologic markers in blood donors ranged from 99 per 1000 in Bolivia to 1.5 per 1000 in Ecuador. Estimates of *T cruzi* seroprevalence in US blood donors range from 0.01% to 0.20% and are higher in geographic regions with higher rates of Hispanic donors. A large multiyear seroprevalence study of *T cruzi* in US blood donors reported an overall seropositive rate for all donations in Los Angeles and Miami to be 1 in 7500 and 1 in 9000 donations, respectively.

Congenital transmission occurs in Latin American countries where Chagas disease is prevalent in women of reproductive age who have chronic *T cruzi* infection. Congenital transmission ranges from 1% or less in Brazil to 7% or more in some regions of Bolivia, Chile, and Paraguay. Finally, in endemic areas, transmission has been associated with the ingestion of contaminated food or drink.

The disease is transmitted by bloodsucking insects that become infected by ingesting trypomastigotes present in the bloodstream of infected mammals. The organisms reach the insect midgut, transform into the multiplying epimastigote stage, and change progressively to infective metacyclic trypomastigotes until they are excreted with feces and urine during feeding. These enter the human body through an abrasion on the skin, intact mucous membrane, or the bite wound.

The vectors of *T cruzi* are insects belonging to the order Hemiptera, family Reduviidae, and subfamily Triatominae. Currently, over 130 species are known, belonging to 5 tribes and 16 genera. However, only a few species of 3 genera—*Triatoma, Rhodnius*, and *Panstrongylus*—are important vectors of *T cruzi* between domestic animals and humans in endemic areas. All 3 genera are widely distributed in the Americas, from Mexico to Argentina and Chile. Twelve species of triatomines are known to occur in the United States, the most important being *Triatoma sanguisuga* in the eastern United States, *Triatoma gerstaeckeri* in the region of Texas and New Mexico, and *Triatoma rubida* and *Triatoma protracta* in Arizona and California. Human Chagas disease develops when humans come into contact with the natural foci of infection and disturb the environment, with the result that infected triatomines move into and colonize human dwellings.

In the mammalian host, the life cycle of *T cruzi* includes 2 developmental stages. The trypomastigote is found in the tissue and bloodstream of infected mammals and is responsible for the intercellular spreading of the infection. The trypomastigote is spindle shaped, measures about 20 μm, and has a kinetoplast located posterior to the nucleus and a flagellum that extends along the outer edge and reaches the anterior end of the body. In stained blood smears, trypomastigotes assume a characteristic C or S shape, with the nucleus just anterior to the middle of the cell (Fig. 350-5). The amastigote is the dividing intracellular form found in the tissues of the mammalian host. Once the cell fills with amastigotes, the amastigotes differentiate into mobile trypomastigotes that burst out, reach the bloodstream, and infect other cells of the body. Every cell in the human body with the exception of neurons and red blood cells could be affected, after which *T cruzi* infection persists in the human body for life. *T cruzi* isolates are grouped in lineages I and II, with type II divided into 5 subtypes, IIa through IIe. In South America, type II is predominantly distributed in Argentina, Chile, Paraguay, and Uruguay, whereas type I is associated with human disease north of the Amazon basin. In Mexico and the United States, most human cases are linked to type I. Lineage I is closely linked to the sylvatic cycle and apparently results in milder infections and morbidity in humans. Type II is closely related to the domestic cycle and produces major infections and morbidity in humans.

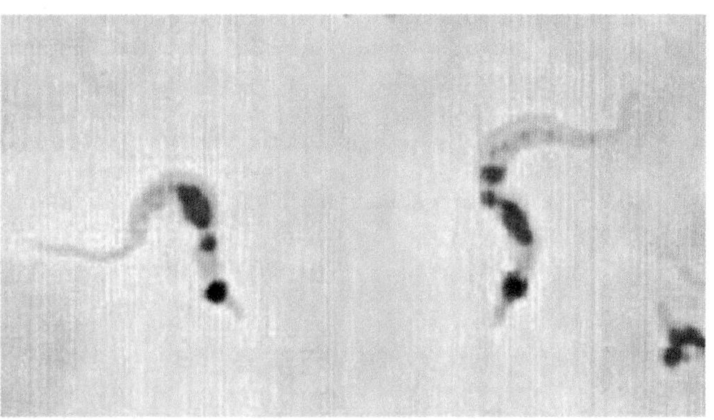

**FIGURE 350-5** *Trypanosoma cruzi* in peripheral blood smear.

Natural infection occurs in a wide variety of peridomestic and sylvatic animals, including birds, guinea pigs, monkeys, opossums, foxes, ferrets, squirrels, armadillos, anteaters, porcupines, rats, and mice. Domestic dogs and cats are believed to be major reservoirs for human infection. However, within the domicile, transmission from human to human through the vector is probably the most common cycle of infection.

## CLINICAL MANIFESTATIONS

The incubation period after transmission is 1 to 2 weeks. Chagas disease is divided into 3 distinct phases: acute, latent, and chronic. In 95% of patients, clinical symptoms during the acute phase are either mild or absent. Shortly after infection, parasites elicit a local inflammatory reaction at the site of entry that gives origin to the chagoma (nodular skin reaction) or the Romaña sign (unilateral periorbital edema, conjunctivitis, and preauricular lymphadenitis). Acute manifestations are usually seen in young children, and severe disease is more common in young infants and immunocompromised hosts. Illness begins with fever, headache, anorexia, and lassitude. Cervical, axillary, and iliac lymphadenopathy; hepatosplenomegaly; vomiting; and rash are common, and occasionally, meningoencephalitis occurs.

The most common and severe manifestations of acute infection (30% of cases) are cardiovascular disturbances from myocarditis, which include cardiomegaly, functional murmurs, and conduction blocks. Examining the blood during the acute phase reveals trypomastigotes, anemia, leukocytosis with a lymphocytosis, elevated erythrocyte sedimentation rate, and increases in serum bilirubin and cardiac enzymes. Five to 10% of patients die of severe myocarditis during the acute phase, but in young infants with meningoencephalitis, mortality can be as high as 50%.

The acute phase subsides after 2 to 3 months, when the disease enters a latent phase for 10 to 40 years or more, during which the patient may be free of clinical symptoms and appear to be in good health. Fewer organisms are found in the peripheral blood during this stage. With increasing age, there is a progressive increase in the number of individuals presenting with electrocardiographic abnormalities.

Chronic cardiomyopathy, which occurs in 30% to 40% of patients, is the most frequent manifestation of chronic Chagas disease; digestive tract disorders are much less frequent (8–10%). The signs and symptoms of chronic cardiomyopathy are secondary to heart failure, arrhythmia, endomyocardial disorders, and embolic complications. Chronic cardiomyopathy may be present by the second and third decades of life; it has even been reported in teenagers and young adults. Megaesophagus and megacolon are caused by destruction of the ganglion cells of the myenteric plexus. Dysphagia, regurgitation with retrosternal burning, and paroxysmal night coughs, which presumably result from aspiration during sleep, are associated with megaesophagus. Chronic constipation, long-term fecal retention, impaction, and volvulus are seen with megacolon.

Congenital transmission occurs in only 0.7% to 2.0% of the cases in which the mother is infected, but the prognosis is poor unless antepartum therapy was initiated. Congenital infection often results in spontaneous abortion, stillbirth, and premature delivery. Newborns who are infected congenitally may have hepatosplenomegaly with jaundice, anemia, petechiae, edema, convulsions secondary to meningoencephalitis, pulmonary edema, and cardiovascular alterations. Many infants die during the first week of life, and those who survive may develop severe neurologic sequelae with mental deficiency and learning disabilities. Congenitally infected children rarely survive until the age of puberty. The heart is enlarged, and thinning of the ventricular wall becomes the starting point for the formation of aneurysms. Mural thrombi may embolize systemically. The myocardium reveals focal myonecrosis, contraction band necrosis, interstitial fibrosis, and lymphocytic infiltration. In addition, the esophagus and colon are frequently affected, with dysfunction and dilatation directly related to peristaltic abnormalities or to aperistalsis caused by destruction of the ganglion cells of the muscle.

Prognosis depends on clinical stage and its complications. The acute phase is most serious in children younger than 2 years of age and is fatal if meningoencephalitis and heart failure develop. Individuals who have severe cardiomyopathy have a poor prognosis, and death usually occurs within a few years from heart failure or cardiac arrhythmia. Chagas disease and human immunodeficiency virus (HIV) mutually affect each other. HIV infection may lead to reactivation of *T cruzi* infection. The disease in some *T cruzi*/HIV–infected patients may have a long, silent clinical course, whereas in others, it may present with meningoencephalitis or myocarditis.

## DIAGNOSIS

Acute Chagas disease should be considered in any infant or child who has been in an endemic area and who develops an acute febrile illness with lymphadenopathy and myocarditis. The laboratory diagnosis of acute Chagas disease can be made by the demonstration of the motile trypomastigotes by direct microscopic examination of fresh anticoagulated blood or buffy coat (see Fig. 350-5). Blood culture employing Novy-MacNeal-Nicolle (NNN), LIT, or other culture media, as well as inoculation of the patient's blood into laboratory animals, may aid in diagnosis at this time as well. Polymerase chain reaction is a sensitive tool used for the diagnosis of acute infection and appears to be the best test for detecting the organism in the recipient of an organ from an infected donor.

During chronic disease, serologic tests are the method of choice in establishing the diagnosis. Antibodies appear in the blood 2 to 3 weeks after infection and persist for years. Antibodies of the IgM isotype predominate during the acute phase, with IgG appearing as the disease progresses. Indirect fluorescence and enzyme-linked immunosorbent assay tests are useful in detecting IgM or IgG antibodies, with a sensitivity and specificity of greater than 95%. Several agglutination tests have been developed that detect the presence of antibodies, including indirect hemagglutination, direct agglutination, latex agglutination, and a flocculation test.

Diagnosis of congenital infection relies on serologic diagnosis of infected mothers, followed by microscopic and polymerase chain reaction–based examination of cord blood and peripheral blood specimens from their infants during the first 1 to 2 months of life. If results of parasitologic testing are negative, the infant should be tested by enzyme-linked immunosorbent assay and immunofluorescent antibody test at 9 to 12 months of age, after the level of transferred maternal antibody has decreased.

False-positive serologic testing can occur with leishmaniasis, malaria, toxoplasmosis, and collagen vascular diseases. Because of the lack of sensitivity and specificity of serologic testing, at least 2 immunologic tests are required to confirm a diagnosis of Chagas disease. When results are discordant, a third assay may be used to confirm or refute the diagnosis, or repeat sampling may be required.

A Chagas disease screening assay for donated blood has been approved by the US Food and Drug Administration.

Differential diagnosis during the acute phase includes visceral leishmaniasis, malaria, brucellosis, schistosomiasis, and infectious mononucleosis. The chronic disease must be distinguished from endomyocardial fibrosis, viral myocarditis, rheumatic heart disease, and achalasia of the esophagus.

## TREATMENT

Treatment is recommended for all cases of acute and congenital Chagas disease, reactivated infection, and chronic infection in individuals age 18 years or younger. In adults age 19 to 50 years without advanced heart disease, treatment may slow development and progression of cardiomyopathy and should generally be offered; treatment is considered optional for those older than 50 years. Nitrofuran and nitroimidazole derivatives are 80% to 90% effective in reducing the parasitemia and in shortening the length and severity of illness, as well as clinical symptoms, in the acute phase of the disease. Because benznidazole is better tolerated, this drug is viewed by most experts as the first-line treatment. Benznidazole (5–7.5 mg/kg/d in 2 divided doses for 60 days) is thought to act by the covalent binding of nitroreduction intermediates to macromolecules. Adverse effects include rash, peripheral neuritis, and granulocytopenia. The recommended dosage of nifurtimox for children ≤ 10 years of age is 15 to 20 mg/kg/d in 3 or 4 divided doses for 90 days; for children 11 to 16 years of age, 12.5 to 15.0 mg/kg/d in 3 or 4 divided doses; and for those ≥ 17 years of age, 8 to 10 mg/kg/d in 3 or 4 divided doses for 90 to 120 days. Many patients develop adverse effects, including weakness, anorexia, nausea, and vomiting. Long-term use is associated with toxic hepatitis, loss of memory, tremor, polyneuritis, and paresthesias.

Negative seroconversion (conversion from positive to negative serologic results) by conventional assays occurs after successful treatment but takes years to decades. Polymerase chain reaction–based techniques are useful in monitoring for treatment failure in persons with acute *T cruzi* infection. Benznidazole and nifurtimox are contraindicated in pregnancy and in patients with severe renal or hepatic dysfunction. Neither drug is approved by the US Food and Drug Administration; both can be obtained from the Centers for Disease Control and Prevention (CDC) and used under investigational protocols (CDC Division of Parasitic Diseases Public Inquiries line: 440-718-4745 or parasites@cdc.gov; the CDC Drug Service: 404-639-3670; or the CDC Emergency Operations Center: 770-488-7100).

## PREVENTION

In endemic countries, transmission of *T cruzi* predominantly occurs via triatomine insect vectors. Accordingly, systematic control strategies include interruption of transmission by the vector and blood-bank screening. A series of multinational programs focusing on the elimination of the domestic insect population through insecticide use, improved screening of blood donors, and improved detection and treatment of congenital cases has led to significant reduction of acute cases and new infections in younger age groups as well as progressive reductions of mortality and morbidity rates. The operational cost to sustain a long-term insecticide spray program and surveillance is the major obstacle in successful vector control. Another concern is the potential development of drug resistance by the vector and/or reinfestation by nondomiciliary triatomines.

Vaccines may be the most practical tool for prevention and control of any form of *T cruzi* infection and transmission. None of the defined vaccine candidates have been shown to provide a sustainable immunologic response or prevent mortality after infection in animal models.

## SUGGESTED READINGS


Bern C. Chagas' disease. *N Engl J Med.* 2015;373:456-466.

Bern C. Chagas disease in the immunosuppressed host. *Curr Opin Infect Dis.* 2012;25:450-457.

Brun R, Blum J, Chappuis F, et al. Human African trypanosomiasis. *Lancet.* 2010;375:148-159.

Centers for Disease Control and Prevention (CDC). Congenital transmission of Chagas disease—Virginia, 2010. *MMWR Morb Mortal Wkly Rep.* 2012;61:477-479.

Eperon G, Balasegaram M, Potet J, et al. Treatment options for second-stage gambiense human African trypanosomiasis. *Expert Rev Anti Infect Ther.* 2014;12:1407-1417.

Kaplinski M, Jois M, Galdos-Cardenas G, et al. Sustained domestic vector exposure is associated with increased Chagas cardiomyopathy risk but decreased parasitemia and congenital transmission risk among young women in Bolivia. *Clin Infect Dis.* 2015;61:918-926.

Lutje V, Seixas J, Kennedy A. Chemotherapy for second-stage human African trypanosomiasis. *Cochrane Database Syst Rev.* 2013;6:CD006201.

Simarro PP, Franco J, Diarra A, Postigo JA, Jannin J. Update on field use of the available drugs for the chemotherapy of human African trypanosomiasis. *Parasitology.* 2012;139:842-846.

Note: Page numbers followed by *f* indicate figures; page numbers followed by *t* indicate tables.

INDEX

**B**

INDEX

INDEX

D

INDEX

**F**

INDEX

INDEX

INDEX

INDEX

INDEX

## O

INDEX

INDEX

INDEX

INDEX

INDEX

X



Y



Z